BRAUNWALD'S

HEART DISEASE

A TEXTBOOK OF CARDIOVASCULAR MEDICINE

Edited by

Douglas P. Zipes, MD, MACC

Distinguished Professor of Medicine, Pharmacology, and Toxicology
Director, Division of Cardiology and the Krannert Institute of Cardiology
Indiana University School of Medicine
Indianapolis, Indiana

Peter Libby, MD

Mallinckrodt Professor of Medicine
Harvard Medical School
Chief, Cardiovascular Division
Brigham and Women's Hospital
Boston, Massachusetts

Robert O. Bonow, MD

Goldberg Distinguished Professor of Cardiology
Northwestern University Feinberg School of Medicine
Chief, Division of Cardiology
Northwestern Memorial Hospital
Chicago, Illinois

Eugene Braunwald, MD, MD (Hon), ScD (Hon), FRCP

Distinguished Hersey Professor of Medicine
Harvard Medical School
Chairman, TIMI Study Group
Brigham and Women's Hospital
Boston, Massachusetts

BRAUNWALD'S

HEART DISEASE

A TEXTBOOK OF CARDIOVASCULAR MEDICINE

7th Edition

ELSEVIER
SAUNDERS

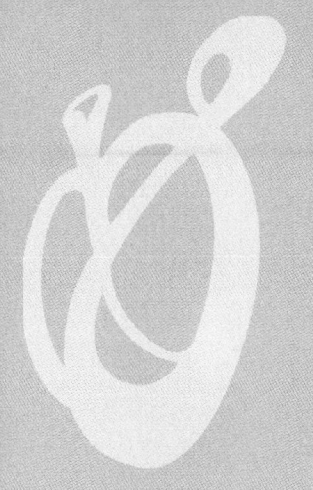

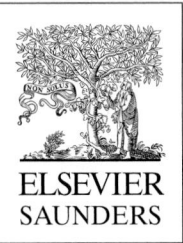

ELSEVIER
SAUNDERS

The Curtis Center
170 S Independence Mall W 300E
Philadelphia, Pennsylvania 19106

BRAUNWALD'S HEART DISEASE: A Textbook of Cardiovascular Medicine, Seventh Edition

Two-volume set	0-7216-0509-5
Single volume	0-7216-0479-X
Two-volume e-dition	1-4160-00038-0
Single volume e-dition	1-4160-00014-3
International edition	0-8089-2305-6
Indian edition	0-8089-2334-X

NOTICE

Medicine is an ever-changing field. Standard safety precautions must be followed, but as new research and clinical experience broaden our knowledge, changes in treatment and drug therapy may become necessary or appropriate. Readers are advised to check the most current product information provided by the manufacturer of each drug to be administered to verify the recommended dose, the method and duration of administration, and contraindications. It is the responsibility of the licensed prescriber, relying on experience and knowledge of the patient, to determine dosages and the best treatment for each individual patient. Neither the publisher nor the authors assume any liability for any injury and/or damage to persons or property arising from this publication.

Library of Congress Cataloging-in-Publication Data

Braunwald's heart disease : a textbook of cardiovascular medicine / [edited by] Douglas P. Zipes . . . [et al.].—7th ed.
p. ; cm.
Rev. ed. of: Heart disease / edited by Eugene Braunwald, Douglas P. Zipes, Peter Libby. 6th ed. 2001.
Includes bibliographical references and index.
ISBN 0-7216-0509-5 (2 vol. set)—ISBN 0-7216-0479-X (Single vol.)—ISBN 0-8089-2305-6 (International ed.)
1. Heart—Diseases. 2. Cardiology. I. Title: Heart disease. II. Zipes, Douglas P. III. Braunwald, Eugene—Heart disease.
[DNLM: 1. Heart Diseases. 2. Cardiovascular Diseases. WG 210 B825 2005]
RC681.H36 2005
616.1′2—dc22 2004050808

Publishing Director: Anne Lenehan
Managing Editor, Developmental Editorial: Deborah Thorp
Publishing Services Manager: Frank Polizzano
Senior Project Manager: Robin E. Davis
Design Manager: Steven Stave

Printed in the United States of America.

Last digit is the print number: 9 8 7 6 5 4 3 2 1

To:

Joan, Debra, Jeffrey, and David

Beryl, Oliver, and Brigitte

Pat, Rob, and Sam

Elaine, Karen, Allison, and Jill

CONTRIBUTORS

Stephan Achenbach, MD
Assistant Professor of Medicine and Cardiology, Friedrich-Alexander University School of Medicine; Staff Cardiologist, Division of Cardiology, Department of Medicine, University Hospital Erlangen, Erlangen, Germany
Computed Tomography of the Heart

David H. Adams, MD
Marie-Josée and Henry R. Kravis Professor and Chair, Department of Cardiothoracic Surgery, Mount Sinai Medical Center, New York, New York
Medical Management of the Patient Undergoing Cardiac Surgery

Elliott M. Antman, MD
Professor of Medicine, Harvard Medical School; Director, Samuel A. Levine Cardiac Unit, Brigham and Women's Hospital, Boston, Massachusetts
ST-Elevation Myocardial Infarction: Pathology, Pathophysiology, and Clinical Features; ST-Elevation Myocardial Infarction: Management; Medical Management of the Patient Undergoing Cardiac Surgery

Karen Antman, MD
Deputy Director for Translational and Clinical Sciences, National Cancer Institute, National Institutes of Health, Bethesda, Maryland
The Patient with Cardiovascular Disease and Cancer

Piero Anversa, MD
Professor, Department of Medicine, Cardiovascular Research Institute, New York Medical College, Valhalla, New York
Myocardial Regeneration

William F. Armstrong, MD
Professor of Medicine, University of Michigan; Associate Clinical Chief, Division of Cardiology, Associate Chair, Department of Internal Medicine, University of Michigan Health System, Ann Arbor, Michigan
Echocardiography

Donald S. Baim, MD
Professor of Medicine, Harvard Medical School; Director, Center for Integration of Medicine and Innovative Technology, Partners Healthcare System and Brigham and Women's Hospital, Boston, Massachusetts
Percutaneous Coronary and Valvular Intervention

Leora B. Balsam, MD
Resident in Surgery, Department of Surgery, Stanford University School of Medicine, Stanford, California
Heart Transplantation

Arthur J. Barsky, MD
Professor of Psychiatry, Harvard Medical School; Director, Psychiatric Research, Brigham and Women's Hospital, Boston, Massachusetts
Psychiatric and Behavioral Aspects of Cardiovascular Disease

Kenneth Lee Baughman, MD
Professor of Medicine, Harvard Medical School; Director, Advanced Heart Disease Section, Brigham and Women's Hospital, Boston, Massachusetts
Myocarditis

Joshua A. Beckman, MS, MD
Assistant Professor of Medicine, Harvard Medical School; Associate Physician, Cardiovascular Division, Brigham and Women's Hospital, Boston, Massachusetts
Diabetes Mellitus, the Metabolic Syndrome, and Atherosclerotic Vascular Disease

George A. Beller, MD
Ruth C. Heede Professor of Cardiology and Professor of Medicine, University of Virginia School of Medicine; Department of Internal Medicine, Cardiovascular Division, University of Virginia Health System, Charlottesville, Virginia
Relative Merits of Cardiac Diagnostic Techniques

Michael A. Bettman, MD
Professor of Radiology, Dartmouth Medical School, Hanover, New Hampshire
The Chest Radiograph in Cardiovascular Disease

Robert O. Bonow, MD
Goldberg Distinguished Professor of Cardiology, Northwestern University Feinberg School of Medicine; Chief, Division of Cardiology, Northwestern Memorial Hospital, Chicago, Illinois
Care of Patients with End-Stage Heart Disease; Nuclear Cardiology; Cardiac Catheterization; Valvular Heart Disease

Eugene Braunwald, MD, MD (Hon), ScD (Hon), FRCP
Distinguished Hersey Professor of Medicine, Harvard Medical School; Chairman, TIMI Study Group, Brigham and Women's Hospital, Boston, Massachusetts
The History; Physical Examination of the Heart and Circulation; Pathophysiology of Heart Failure; Clinical Aspects of Heart Failure; Pulmonary Edema, High-Output Failure; ST-Elevation Myocardial Infarction: Pathology, Pathophysiology, and Clinical Features; Unstable Angina and Non–ST Elevation Myocardial Infarction; Chronic Coronary Artery Disease; Valvular Heart Disease; The Cardiomyopathies

Michael R. Bristow, MD, PhD
Professor of Medicine and Head, Division of Cardiology, University of Colorado Health Sciences Center, Denver, Colorado
Drugs in the Treatment of Heart Failure; Management of Heart Failure

Hugh Calkins, MD, FACC, FAHA
Professor of Medicine, Johns Hopkins University School of Medicine; Director, Arrhythmia Service and Clinical Electrophysiology Laboratory, Johns Hopkins Hospital, Baltimore, Maryland
Hypotension and Syncope

Christopher P. Cannon, MD
Associate Professor of Medicine, Harvard Medical School; Senior Investigator, TIMI Study Group, Cardiovascular Division, Brigham and Women's Hospital, Boston, Massachusetts
Approach to the Patient with Chest Pain; Unstable Angina and Non–ST Elevation Myocardial Infarction

John D. Carroll, MD
Professor of Medicine, Division of Cardiology, University of Colorado Health Sciences Center; Director, Cardiac and Vascular Center and Director, Interventional Cardiology, University of Colorado Hospital, Denver, Colorado
Assessment of Normal and Abnormal Cardiac Function

Agustin Castellanos, MD
Professor of Medicine, University of Miami School of Medicine; Director, Clinical Electrophysiology, University of Miami/Jackson Memorial Medical Center, Miami, Florida
Cardiac Arrest and Sudden Cardiac Death

Bernard R. Chaitman, MD
Professor of Medicine and Director, Cardiovascular Research, St. Louis University School of Medicine, St. Louis, Missouri
Exercise Stress Testing

Jonathan M. Chen, MD
Assistant Professor of Surgery, Columbia University College of Physicians and Surgeons; Attending Surgeon, New York Presbyterian Hospital, New York, New York
Assisted Circulation in the Treatment of Heart Failure

Wilson S. Colucci, MD, FACC
Thomas J. Ryan Professor of Medicine; Professor of Physiology; Director, Myocardial Biology Unit, Boston University School of Medicine; Chief, Cardiovascular Medicine, Boston Medical Center, Boston, Massachusetts
Pathophysiology of Heart Failure; Clinical Aspects of Heart Failure; Pulmonary Edema, High-Output Failure; Primary Tumors of the Heart

Mark A. Creager, MD
Professor of Medicine, Harvard Medical School; Director, Vascular Center; Simon C. Fireman Scholar in Cardiovascular Medicine, Brigham and Women's Hospital, Boston, Massachusetts
Diabetes Mellitus, the Metabolic Syndrome, and Atherosclerotic Vascular Disease; Peripheral Arterial Diseases

Adnan S. Dajani, MD
Professor Emeritus of Pediatrics, Wayne State University School of Medicine; Director Emeritus, Division of Infectious Diseases, Children's Hospital of Michigan, Detroit, Michigan
Rheumatic Fever

Werner G. Daniel, MD
Professor of Medicine and Cardiology, Friedrich-Alexander School of Medicine; Division of Cardiology, Department of Medicine, University Hospital Erlangen, Erlangen, Germany
Computed Tomography of the Heart

Charles J. Davidson, MD
Professor of Medicine, Northwestern University Feinberg School of Medicine; Chief, Cardiac Catheterization Laboratories, Northwestern Memorial Hospital, Chicago, Illinois
Cardiac Catheterization

Vasken Dilsizian, MD
Professor of Medicine and Radiology, University of Maryland School of Medicine; Director of Cardiovascular Nuclear Medicine and Cardiac Positron Emission Tomography, University of Maryland Medical Center, Baltimore, Maryland
Nuclear Cardiology

Pamela S. Douglas, MD
Ursula Geller Professor of Medicine, Chief, Cardiovascular Medicine, Duke University Medical Center, Durham, North Carolina
Cardiovascular Disease in Women

Kim A. Eagle, MD
Albion Walter Hewlett Professor of Internal Medicine; Chief, Clinical Cardiology; Clinical Director, Cardiovascular Center, University of Michigan Health System, Ann Arbor, Michigan
Anesthesia and Noncardiac Surgery in Patients with Heart Disease

Andrew C. Eisenhauer, MD
Assistant Professor of Medicine and Radiology, Harvard Medical School; Director, Interventional Cardiovascular Medicine Service, Brigham and Women's Hospital, Boston, Massachusetts
Endovascular Treatment of Noncoronary Obstructive Vascular Disease

Uri Elkayam, MD
Professor of Medicine, University of Southern California Keck School of Medicine, Los Angeles, California
Pregnancy and Cardiovascular Disease

Linda L. Emanuel, MD, PhD
Buehler Professor of Geriatric Medicine and Director, Buehler Center of Aging, Northwestern University Feinberg School of Medicine, Chicago, Illinois
Care of Patients with End-Stage Heart Disease

Anthony L. Estrera, MD
Assistant Professor of Cardiothoracic and Vascular Surgery, University of Texas Health Science Center, Houston, Texas
Traumatic Heart Disease

Farzan Filsoufi, MD
Assistant Professor of Cardiothoracic Surgery, Mount Sinai School of Medicine, New York, New York
Medical Management of the Patient Undergoing Cardiac Surgery

Stacy D. Fisher, MD
Department of Cardiology, Sinai Hospital of Baltimore, Johns Hopkins University; Mid-Atlantic Cardiovascular Associates, Baltimore, Maryland
Cardiovascular Abnormalities in HIV-Infected Individuals

Lee A. Fleisher, MD, FACC
Professor of Anesthesia and Medicine, University of Pennsylvania School of Medicine; Chair, Department of Anesthesia, University of Pennsylvania Health System, Philadelphia, Pennsylvania
Anesthesia and Noncardiac Surgery in Patients with Heart Disease

J. Michael Gaziano, MD, MPH
Associate Professor of Medicine, Harvard Medical School; Chief, Division of Aging, Brigham and Women's Hospital; Director, Massachusetts Veterans Epidemiology and Research Information Center (MAVERIC), Boston VA Healthcare Systems, Boston, Massachusetts
Global Burden of Cardiovascular Disease; Primary and Secondary Prevention of Coronary Heart Disease

Jacques Genest, MD
Professor of Medicine, McGill University; Chief, Cardiology, McGill University Medical Center, Montréal, Québec, Canada
Lipoprotein Disorders and Cardiovascular Disease

Bernard J. Gersh, MD, DPhil, FRCP
Professor of Medicine, Mayo College of Medicine; Consultant, Division of Cardiovascular Diseases, Mayo Clinic, Rochester, Minnesota
Chronic Coronary Artery Disease

Michael M. Givertz, MD
Assistant Professor of Medicine, Harvard Medical School; Co-Director, Cardiomyopathy and Heart Failure Program, Brigham and Women's Hospital, Boston, Massachusetts
Clinical Aspects of Heart Failure; Pulmonary Edema, High-Output Failure

Ary L. Goldberger, MD
Associate Professor of Medicine, Harvard Medical School; Director, Margret and H. A. Rey Laboratory for Nonlinear Dynamics in Physiology and Medicine, Beth Israel Deaconess Medical Center, Boston, Massachusetts
Electrocardiography

Samuel Z. Goldhaber, MD
Associate Professor of Medicine, Harvard Medical School; Staff Cardiologist and Director, Venous Thromboembolism Research Group; Director, Anticoagulation Service, Brigham and Women's Hospital, Boston, Massachusetts
Pulmonary Embolism

Antonio M. Gotto, Jr., MD, DPhil
Stephen and Suzanne Weiss Dean, Provost for Medical Affairs, Professor of Medicine, Weill Medical College of Cornell University, New York, New York
Lipoprotein Disorders and Cardiovascular Disease

William J. Groh, MD, MPH
Associate Professor of Medicine, Indiana University School of Medicine, Indianapolis, Indiana
Neurological Disorders and Cardiovascular Disease

David L. Hayes, MD
Professor of Medicine, Mayo Medical School, Mayo Clinic College of Medicine; Chair, Division of Cardiovascular Diseases and Internal Medicine, Mayo Clinic, Rochester, Minnesota
Cardiac Pacemakers and Cardioverter-Defibrillators

Otto M. Hess, MD
Professor of Cardiology, Swiss Cardiovascular Center, University Hospital, Bern, Switzerland
Assessment of Normal and Abnormal Cardiac Function

L. David Hillis, MD
Professor and Vice Chair, Department of Medicine; James M. Wooten Chair in Cardiology, University of Texas Southwestern Medical Center, Dallas, Texas
Toxins and the Heart

Mark A. Hlatky, MD
Professor of Health Research and Policy and Professor of Cardiovascular Medicine, Stanford University School of Medicine; Attending Physician, Stanford University Medical Center, Stanford, California
Economics and Cardiovascular Disease

Gary S. Hoffman, MS, MD
Professor of Medicine, Cleveland Clinic Lerner College of Medicine of Case Western Reserve University; Professor of Medicine and Harold C. Schott Chair of Rheumatic and Immunologic Diseases; Director, Center for Vasculitis Care and Research, Cleveland Clinic, Cleveland, Ohio
Rheumatic Diseases and the Cardiovascular System

David R. Holmes, Jr., MD
Professor of Medicine, Mayo Clinic College of Medicine; Consultant, Mayo Clinic Saint Marys Hospital, Rochester, Minnesota
Primary Percutaneous Coronary Intervention in the Management of Acute Myocardial Infarction

Sharon A. Hunt, MD
Professor of Cardiovascular Medicine, Stanford University Medical Center, Stanford, California
Heart Transplantation

Eric M. Isselbacher, MD
Assistant Professor of Medicine, Harvard Medical School; Co-Director, Thoracic Aortic Center, Director, Cardiac Unit Associates, Massachusetts General Hospital, Boston, Massachusetts
Diseases of the Aorta

Samer Kabbani, MD
Assistant Professor of Medicine, University of Vermont College of Medicine; Attending Cardiologist, Fletcher Allen Health Care, Burlington, Vermont
Pericardial Diseases

Norman M. Kaplan, MD
Clinical Professor of Internal Medicine, University of Texas Southwestern Medical Center, Dallas, Texas
Systemic Hypertension: Mechanisms and Diagnosis; Systemic Hypertension: Therapy

Adolf W. Karchmer, MD
Professor of Medicine, Harvard Medical School; Chief, Division of Infectious Diseases, Beth Israel Deaconess Medical Center, Boston, Massachusetts
Infective Endocarditis

Morton J. Kern, MD
Professor of Medicine, Saint Louis University School of Medicine; Director, Cardiac Catheterization Laboratory, Saint Louis University Hospital, St. Louis, Missouri
Coronary Blood Flow and Myocardial Ischemia

Irwin Klein, MD
Professor of Medicine, New York University School of Medicine, New York, New York; Chief, Division of Endocrinology, North Shore University Hospital, Mannasset, New York
Endocrine Disorders and Cardiovascular Disease

Barbara A. Konkle, MD
Associate Professor of Medicine and of Pathology and Laboratory Medicine; Director, Penn Comprehensive Hemophilia and Thrombosis Program, University of Pennsylvania School of Medicine and Health System, Philadelphia, Pennsylvania
Hemostasis, Thrombosis, Fibrinolysis, and Cardiovascular Disease

Peter C. Kouretas, MD, PhD
Cardiothoracic Transplantation Fellow, Department of Cardiothoracic Surgery, Stanford University School of Medicine; Staff Physician and Clinical Instructor, Stanford University Hospital, Stanford, California
Heart Transplantation

Ronald M. Krauss, MD
Adjunct Professor, Department of Nutritional Sciences, University of California, Berkeley, Berkeley, California; Senior Scientist and Director, Atherosclerosis Research, Children's Hospital Oakland Research Institute, Oakland, California
Nutrition and Cardiovascular Disease

Meir H. Kryger, MD, FRCPC
Professor of Medicine, University of Manitoba Department of Medicine; Director, Sleep Disorders Centre, St. Boniface Hospital Research Centre, Winnipeg, Manitoba, Canada
Sleep Disorders and Cardiovascular Disease

Richard E. Kuntz, MD
Associate Professor of Medicine and Chief, Division of Clinical Biometrics, Harvard Medical School, Boston, Massachusetts
Percutaneous Coronary and Valvular Intervention

Gary E. Lane, MD
Assistant Professor, Mayo Medical School; Director, Cardiac Catheterization Laboratory, Mayo Clinic St. Luke's Hospital, Jacksonville, Florida
Primary Percutaneous Coronary Intervention in the Management of Acute Myocardial Infarction

Richard A. Lange, MD
Professor of Medicine and E. Cowles Andrus Professor of Cardiology, Johns Hopkins University School of Medicine, Baltimore, Maryland
Toxins and the Heart

Thomas H. Lee, MSc, MD
Professor of Medicine, Harvard Medical School; Network President, Partners Healthcare System, Boston, Massachusetts
Measurement and Improvement of Quality of Cardiovascular Care; Guidelines: Electrocardiography; Guidelines: Exercise Stress Testing; Guidelines: Use of Echocardiography; Guidelines: Nuclear Cardiology; Guidelines: Management of Heart Failure; Guidelines: Ambulatory Electrocardiography and Electrophysiological Testing; Guidelines: Cardiac Pacemakers and Cardioverter-Defibrillators; Guidelines: Treatment of Hypertension; Approach to the Patient with Chest Pain; Guidelines: Primary Percutaneous Coronary Intervention in Acute Myocardial Infarction; Guidelines: Unstable Angina; Guidelines: Chronic Stable Angina; Guidelines: Percutaneous Coronary and Valvular Intervention; Guidelines: Management of Valvular Heart Disease; Guidelines: Infective Endocarditis; Guidelines: Pregnancy; Guidelines: Reducing Cardiac Risk with Noncardiac Surgery

Annarosa Leri, MD
Associate Professor, Department of Medicine, Cardiovascular Research Institute, New York Medical College, Valhalla, New York
Myocardial Regeneration

Martin M. LeWinter, MD
Professor of Medicine and of Molecular Physiology and Biophysics, University of Vermont College of Medicine; Director, Heart Failure Program, Fletcher Allen Health Care, Burlington, Vermont
Pericardial Diseases

Peter Libby, MD
Mallinckrodt Professor of Medicine, Harvard Medical School; Chief, Cardiovascular Division, Brigham and Women's Hospital, Boston, Massachusetts
The Vascular Biology of Atherosclerosis; Risk Factors for Atherothrombotic Disease; Lipoprotein Disorders and Cardiovascular Disease; Diabetes Mellitus, the Metabolic Syndrome, and Atherosclerotic Vascular Disease; Peripheral Arterial Diseases

Stuart Linas, MD
Professor of Medicine, University of Colorado Health Sciences Center; Chief, Nephrology, Denver Health, Denver, Colorado
Drugs in the Treatment of Heart Failure

Steven E. Lipshultz, MD
Professor and Chair, Department of Pediatrics; Professor of Medicine and of Epidemiology and Public Health, University of Miami School of Medicine; Chief of Staff, Holtz Children's Hospital of the University of Miami–Jackson Memorial Medical Center, Miami, Florida
Cardiovascular Abnormalities in HIV-Infected Individuals

Brian D. Lowes, MD
Associate Professor of Medicine, University of Colorado Health Sciences Center; Director, Heart Failure Program, University Hospital, Denver, Colorado
Management of Heart Failure

Brian F. Mandell, MD, PhD
Professor of Medicine, Cleveland Clinic Lerner College of Medicine of Case Western Reserve University; Vice Chair of Medicine for Education, Cleveland Clinic, Cleveland, Ohio
Rheumatic Diseases and the Cardiovascular System

JoAnn E. Manson, MD, DrPH
Professor of Medicine and Elizabeth F. Brigham Professor of Women's Health, Harvard Medical School; Chief, Division of Preventive Medicine, Co-Director, Connors Center for Women's Health and Gender Biology, Brigham and Women's Hospital, Boston, Massachusetts
Primary and Secondary Prevention of Coronary Heart Disease

Daniel B. Mark, MD, MPH
Professor of Medicine, Duke University Medical Center; Director, Outcomes Research, Duke Clinical Research Institute, Durham, North Carolina
Economics and Cardiovascular Disease

Andrew R. Marks, MD
Professor and Chair, Department of Physiology and Cellular Biophysics; Professor of Medicine; Clyde and Helen Wu Professor of Molecular Cardiology, Columbia University College of Physicians and Surgeons
The Patient with Cardiovascular Disease and Cancer

Barry J. Maron, MD
Director, Hypertrophic Cardiomyopathy Center, Minneapolis Heart Institute Foundation, Minneapolis, Minnesota; Adjunct Professor of Medicine, Tufts University School of Medicine, Boston, Massachusetts
Cardiovascular Disease in Athletes

Kenneth L. Mattox, MD
Professor and Vice Chair, Michael E. DeBakey Department of Surgery, Baylor College of Medicine; Chief of Surgery Service and Chief of Staff, Ben Taub General Hospital, Houston, Texas
Traumatic Heart Disease

Peter A. McCullough, MD, MPH
Consultant Cardiologist and Chief, Division of Nutrition and Preventive Medicine, William Beaumont Hospital, Royal Oak, Michigan
Interface Between Renal Disease and Cardiovascular Illness

Vallerie V. McLaughlin, MD
Associate Professor of Medicine and Director, Pulmonary Hypertension Program, University of Michigan Health System, Ann Arbor, Michigan
Pulmonary Hypertension

John M. Miller, MD
Professor of Medicine, Indiana University School of Medicine; Director, Clinical Cardiac Electrophysiology, Clarian Health System, Indianapolis, Indiana
Diagnosis of Cardiac Arrhythmias; Therapy for Cardiac Arrhythmias

David M. Mirvis, MD
Professor and Director, Center for Health Services Research, University of Tennessee, Memphis, Tennessee
Electrocardiography

David A. Morrow, MD, MPH
Assistant Professor of Medicine, Harvard Medical School; Associate Physician, Brigham and Women's Hospital, Boston, Massachusetts
Chronic Coronary Artery Disease

Robert J. Myerburg, MD
Professor of Medicine and Physiology, University of Miami School of Medicine; Director, Division of Cardiology, University of Miami–Jackson Memorial Hospital, Miami, Florida
Cardiac Arrest and Sudden Cardiac Death

Elizabeth G. Nabel, MD
Scientific Director, National Heart, Lung, and Blood Institute, National Institutes of Health, Bethesda, Maryland
Principles of Cardiovascular Molecular Biology and Genetics

Yoshifumi Naka, MD, PhD
Herbert Irving Assistant Professor of Surgery, Division of Cardiothoracic Surgery, Columbia University College of Physicians and Surgeons; Adjunct Assistant Professor of Cardiothoracic Surgery, Cornell University Weill Medical College; Director, Cardiac Transplantation and Mechanical Circulatory Support Program, Division of Cardiothoracic Surgery, New York Presbyterian Hospital, New York, New York
Assisted Circulation in the Treatment of Heart Failure

Carlo Napolitano, MD, PhD
Senior Scientist, Molecular Cardiology Laboratories, IRCCS Fondazione S. Maugeri, Pavia, Italy
Genetics of Cardiac Arrhythmias

Richard W. Nesto, MD
Associate Professor of Medicine, Harvard Medical School, Boston; Chair, Department of Cardiovascular Medicine, Lahey Clinic Medical Center, Burlington, Massachusetts
Diabetes and Heart Disease

Jeffrey E. Olgin, MD
Associate Professor in Residence and Chief, Cardiac Electrophysiology, University of California, San Francisco, School of Medicine, San Francisco, California
Specific Arrhythmias: Diagnosis and Treatment

Lionel H. Opie, MD, DPhil, DSc, MD (Hon)
Director, Hatter Institute and Cape Heart Center, Faculty of Health Sciences, University of Cape Town; Senior Physician, Department of Medicine, Groote Schuur Hospital, Cape Town, South Africa
Mechanisms of Cardiac Contraction and Relaxation

Richard C. Pasternak, MD
Associate Professor of Medicine, Harvard Medical School; Director, Preventive Cardiology and Cardiac Rehabilitation, Massachusetts General Hospital, Boston, Massachusetts
Comprehensive Rehabilitation of Patients with Cardiovascular Disease

Dudley Pennell, MD, FRCP, FACC, FESC
Professor of Cardiology, Imperial College; Director, Cardiovascular Magnetic Resonance Unit, Royal Brompton Hospital, London, United Kingdom
Cardiovascular Magnetic Resonance

Joseph K. Perloff, MD
Streisand/American Heart Association Professor of Medicine and Pediatrics, Emeritus, Founding Director, Ahmanson/UCLA Adult Congenital Heart Disease Center, David Geffen School of Medicine at UCLA; Los Angeles, California
Physical Examination of the Heart and Circulation

Jeffrey J. Popma, MD
Associate Professor of Medicine, Harvard Medical School; Director, Interventional Cardiology, Brigham and Women's Hospital, Boston, Massachusetts
Coronary Angiography and Intravascular Ultrasound Imaging; Percutaneous Coronary and Valvular Intervention

J. David Port, PhD
Associate Professor of Medicine and Pharmacology, University of Colorado Health Sciences Center, Denver, Colorado
Drugs in the Treatment of Heart Failure

Silvia G. Priori, MD, PhD
Associate Professor, University of Pavia School of Cardiology; Director of Molecular Cardiology, IRCCS Fondazione S. Maugeri, Pavia, Italy
Genetics of Cardiac Arrhythmias

Reed E. Pyeritz, MD, PhD
Professor of Medicine and Genetics, Chief, Division of Medical Genetics, University of Pennsylvania School of Medicine, Philadelphia, Pennsylvania
Genetics and Cardiovascular Disease

Andrew N. Redington, MD, MBBS, MRCP(UK), FRCP(UK), FRCPC
University of Toronto; Head, Division of Cardiology, Hospital for Sick Children, Toronto, Ontario, Canada
Congenital Heart Disease

Stuart Rich, MD
Professor of Medicine and Director, Center for Pulmonary Heart Disease, Rush Medical College, Chicago, Illinois
Pulmonary Hypertension

Paul M. Ridker, MD, MPH
Eugene Braunwald Professor of Medicine, Harvard Medical School; Director, Center for Cardiovascular Disease Prevention, Brigham and Women's Hospital, Boston, Massachusetts
Risk Factors for Atherothrombotic Disease; Primary and Secondary Prevention of Coronary Heart Disease

Robert C. Robbins, MD
Associate Professor, Department of Cardiothoracic Surgery, Stanford University School of Medicine and Stanford Hospital, Stanford, California
Heart Transplantation

David Robertson, MD
Elton Yates Professor of Medicine, Pharmacology, and Neurology; Director, General Clinical Research Center, Vanderbilt University School of Medicine, Nashville, Tennessee
Cardiovascular Manifestations of Autonomic Disorders

Rose Marie Robertson, MD
Professor of Medicine, Vanderbilt University School of Medicine; Chief Science Officer, American Heart Association, Nashville, Tennessee
Cardiovascular Manifestations of Autonomic Disorders

Dan M. Roden, MD
Professor of Medicine and Pharmacology and Director, Division of Clinical Pharmacology, Vanderbilt University School of Medicine, Nashville, Tennessee
The Principles of Drug Therapy

Eric A. Rose, MD
Morris and Rose Milstein/Johnson & Johnson Professor and Chair, Department of Surgery; Surgeon-in-Chief, Columbia University College of Physicians and Surgeons; Director, Surgical Service, New York Presbyterian Hospital, New York, New York
Assisted Circulation in the Treatment of Heart Failure

Kenneth Rosenfield, MD
Lecturer on Medicine, Harvard Medical School; Director, Cardiac and Vascular Invasive Services, Massachusetts General Hospital, Boston, Massachusetts
Endovascular Treatment of Noncoronary Obstructive Vascular Disease

Michael Rubart, MD
Assistant Scientist, Indiana University School of Medicine, Indianapolis, Indiana
Genesis of Cardiac Arrhythmias: Electrophysiological Considerations

Marc S. Sabatine, MD, MPH
Instructor in Medicine, Harvard Medical School; Associate Physician, Cardiovascular Division, Brigham and Women's Hospital, Boston, Massachusetts
Primary Tumors of the Heart

Andrew I. Schafer, MD
Frank Wister Thomas Professor and Chair, Department of Medicine, University of Pennsylvania School of Medicine and Health System, Philadelphia, Pennsylvania
Hemostasis, Thrombosis, Fibrinolysis, and Cardiovascular Disease

Frederick J. Schoen, MD, PhD
Professor of Pathology and Health Sciences and Technology, Harvard Medical School; Executive Vice Chair, Department of Pathology, Brigham and Women's Hospital, Boston Massachusetts
Primary Tumors of the Heart

J. Sanford Schwartz, MD
Professor of Medicine and Health Management and Economics, University of Pennsylvania School of Medicine and The Wharton School, Philadelphia, Pennsylvania
Clinical Decision-Making in Cardiology

Janice B. Schwartz, MD
Clinical Professor of Medicine, Divisions of Cardiology and Clinical Pharmacology, University of California, San Francisco, School of Medicine; Director, Research, Jewish Home of San Francisco, San Francisco, California
Cardiovascular Disease in the Elderly

Peter J. Schwartz, MD
Professor of Cardiology, University of Pavia, Pavia, Italy
Genetics of Cardiac Arrhythmias

Jeffrey F. Smallhorn, MBBS, FRACP, FRCPC
University of Toronto; Hospital for Sick Children, Toronto, Ontario, Canada
Congenital Heart Disease

Nancy K. Sweitzer, MD, PhD
Assistant Professor of Medicine, University of Wisconsin Medical School; Director, Heart Failure Program, University of Wisconsin Hospital and Clinics, Madison, Wisconsin
Cardiovascular Disease in Women

Judith Therrien, MD, FRCPC
McGill University, Department of Medicine; Sir Mortimer B. Davis Jewish General Hospital, Montréal, Québec, Canada
Congenital Heart Disease

James E. Udelson, MD
Associate Professor of Medicine and Radiology, Tufts University School of Medicine; Associate Chief, Division of Cardiology; Director, Nuclear Cardiology; Co-Director, Heart Failure Center, Tufts–New England Medical Center, Boston, Massachusetts
Nuclear Cardiology

Matthew J. Wall, Jr., MD
Professor, Michael E. DeBakey Department of Surgery, Baylor College of Medicine; Deputy Chief of Surgery, Chief of Cardiothoracic Surgery, Ben Taub General Hospital, Houston, Texas
Traumatic Heart Disease

Gary D. Webb, MD, FRCPC
Bitove Family Professor of Adult Congenital Heart Disease and Professor of Medicine, University of Toronto; Director, Toronto Congenital Cardiac Centre for Adults, Toronto General Hospital, Toronto, Ontario, Canada
Congenital Heart Disease

Joshua Wynne, MD, MBA, MPH
Professor of Medicine, Wayne State University; Attending Physician, Detroit Medical Center, Detroit, Michigan
The Cardiomyopathies; Myocarditis

Clyde W. Yancy, MD
Professor of Medicine (Cardiology) and Medical Director, Heart Failure and Heart Transplantation, University of Texas Southwestern Medical Center; Associate Dean of Clinical Affairs, St. Paul University Hospital, Dallas, Texas
Heart Disease in Varied Populations

Douglas P. Zipes, MD, MACC
Distinguished Professor of Medicine, Pharmacology, and Toxicology, Director, Division of Cardiology and the Krannert Institute of Cardiology, Indiana University School of Medicine, Indianapolis, Indiana
Genesis of Cardiac Arrhythmias: Electrophysiological Considerations; Diagnosis of Cardiac Arrhythmias; Therapy for Cardiac Arrhythmias; Cardiac Pacemakers and Cardioverter-Defibrillators; Specific Arrhythmias: Diagnosis and Treatment; Hypotension and Syncope; Cardiovascular Disease in the Elderly; Neurological Disorders and Cardiovascular Disease

PREFACE

The preface to the previous (sixth) edition of *Heart Disease* began, "The accelerating advances in cardiology since the publication of the fifth edition of *Heart Disease* have required the most extensive changes yet made in any revision." That statement applies with even greater emphasis to this edition. The exponential growth curve of new knowledge has never been steeper, and the seventh edition of *Braunwald's Heart Disease* has been created to meet that challenge.

The appearance of the book has been changed radically: the cover shows a holographic MRI of a heart, alternating between systole and diastole, and the pages within are in full color, both to enhance reader appeal and to make figures and images more realistic and understandable. We now have an e-dition that provides electronic access to the entire book and enables the reader to download any figures or tables to his or her own computer and to use them in a PowerPoint format for lectures. The book contains 569 tables and 1503 figures, and the accompanying CD contains additional images and video clips. Finding a particular fact can be done with a flip of a finger in the e-dition, as a reader can electronically scan pages, facts, figures, and references. We recognize that books published on a four-year cycle cannot hope to keep current with the incredible pace of new observations. Therefore, by scanning and summarizing the important articles in the literature, and posting those commentaries on the e-dition site, we will update the e-dition *weekly*. Updates will be keyed to related book content. Finally, having recognized the important issues of professionalism and ethics, for the first time we have included an index listing of potential conflict of interest associations for all contributors.

The contents of this edition have also been comprehensively upgraded. As expected, all of the 51 chapters in the sixth edition that have been retained for the current edition have been thoroughly revised and updated. In addition, 36 new chapters have been included, whose topics range from clinical decision-making to cardiovascular manifestations of autonomic disorders. Fifty-seven new authors have made contributions. Thus, the state-of-the-art information serving as the foundation of the text's intellectual vitality has been retained and strengthened in this edition. Bibliographic citations have been generally limited to sources published in 1998 or later, to avoid the accretion of references that can consume valuable pages without offering the utility of fresh content. Earlier references can be obtained from the reviews cited and from previous editions. We continue to present an understanding of basic mechanisms underlying disease states, but we also emphasize the practical evaluation and treatment of patients with these problems, as well as provide a compendium of current guidelines for the reader's convenience.

Part I includes the general considerations of cardiovascular disease, with chapters on the global burden, economics, *clinical decision making,** *assessment of quality of cardiac care, principles of drug therapy,* and *care of patients with end-stage heart disease.*

Part II continues the tradition of the previous edition, emphasizing history and physical examination, electrocardiography, exercise stress testing, and echocardiography. However, recognizing the increasing importance of new imaging techniques, we include new chapters on *radiology of the heart and great vessels, nuclear cardiology, magnetic resonance imaging, computed tomography,* cardiac catheterization, and coronary angiography and intravascular ultrasonography, as well as a chapter that places the various imaging modalities into perspective.

Heart failure has emerged as one of the most important problems in cardiology, as is reflected in **Part III**. It comprises a chapter on understanding mechanisms of cardiac contraction, *assessment of cardiac function,* pathophysiology of heart failure and its clinical aspects, two chapters on pharmacological treatment, and chapters on *assisted circulation* and *transplantation.*

Almost a quarter of all deaths in the U.S. are due to sudden death, most commonly from a rhythm disturbance, and **Part IV** deals with that issue, beginning with the genesis of arrhythmias. We have a new chapter addressing the growing importance of *genetics and arrhythmias,* and then continue with diagnosis, treatment, pacemakers and defibrillators, specific arrhythmias, cardiac arrest, and syncope.

Preventive cardiology is a mainstay of the cardiologist's role, and we devote multiple chapters to this important initiative in **Part V**, including the biology of atherogenesis, risk factors, hypertension (two chapters), lipoprotein disorders, *diabetes, nutrition,* prevention of coronary heart disease, and *rehabilitation.* In view of the growing importance of diabetes in the practice of cardiology, the current edition now includes a new chapter devoted to the vascular complications of this common condition.

Part VI includes the section on coronary disease, which accounts for the vast majority of heart disease in developed countries. The chapters include *understanding coronary blood flow and ischemia, approach to the patient with chest pain,* pathophysiology, clinical features, and management of ST-segment elevation myocardial infarction (MI), *percutaneous coronary intervention in MI,* unstable angina and non–ST-elevation MI, *chronic coronary artery disease, diabetes and heart disease,* percutaneous coronary and valvular intervention, aortic diseases, peripheral vascular diseases, and *endovascular treatment of noncoronary obstructive vascular disease.*

The rest of the book addresses somewhat less common, but still very important, problems. **Part VII** includes chapters on *congenital heart disease,* valvular heart disease, infective endocarditis, cardiomyopathies, *myocarditis,* HIV and the heart, *toxins,* primary cardiac tumors, *pericardial diseases,* traumatic heart disease, pulmonary embolism and pulmonary hypertension, and *sleep disorders.* **Part VIII** focuses on aspects of molecular biology and genetics. The chapters include *general principles of molecular biology needed by physicians,* genetics, and *myocardial regeneration.*

Part IX focuses on special populations of patients with cardiovascular disease, including *elderly patients, women,* pregnant patients, athletes, patients undergoing cardiac and *noncardiac surgery,* and patients belonging to *varied populations.* **Part X** fills remaining gaps by including cardiovascular disease and disorders of other organs, such as *endocrine disorders,* hematologic issues, rheumatic fever and rheumatic diseases, *oncologic disorders,* behavioral issues, neurological disorders, *renal disorders,* and *autonomic dysfunction.*

Companion volumes continue to supplement the information in *Braunwald's Heart Disease,* and they now include

*New chapters indicated in italics.

Heart Disease Review and Assessment, sixth edition (Lilly), Cardiovascular Therapeutics, second edition (Antman), Molecular Basis of Cardiovascular Disease, second edition (Chien), Clinical Trials in Heart Disease, second edition (Manson), Heart Failure (Mann), Marcus' Cardiac Imaging, second edition (Skorton), Acute Coronary Syndromes (Theroux), and Clinical Cardiovascular Imaging (St. John Sutton and Rutherford). Companion volumes in other areas of cardiology are planned for the near future. The seventh edition of *Braunwald's Heart Disease* continues to serve as the anchor for this collection of books, all of which help the busy scientist and clinician keep up with contemporary issues in cardiovascular diseases.

As always, the goal of this textbook is to educate, stimulate, and serve as a resource for all professionals caring for patients with cardiovascular disease. We are certain that the e-dition will add significant value to accomplishing that end. We could not have accomplished this goal without the help of our editorial associates, Janet Hutcheson, Karen Williams, Cynthia Escobedo, and Kathryn Saxon. The staff at Elsevier has been extremely supportive, and has tolerated our frequent requests for changes to make the book even better. To our editor, Anne Lenehan, developmental editor, Deborah Thorp, and project manager, Robin Davis, we give our thanks.

On the cover is a holographic magnetic resonance image of a cross section of the heart of Dr. Saptarsi Haldar in end-systole and end-diastole courtesy of Dr. Raymond Kwong, both of Brigham and Women's Hospital, reproduced with both of their permissions.

Finally, we thank you, the reader, from medical student to skilled clinician, for showing support for this textbook over the years. You, and our patients, are the driving forces to make this the kind of effort that contributes meaningfully to the education of cardiovascular specialists.

Douglas P. Zipes

Peter Libby

Robert O. Bonow

Eugene Braunwald

2004

PREFACE *Adapted from the First Edition*

Cardiovascular disease is the greatest scourge affecting the industrialized nations. As with previous scourges—bubonic plague, yellow fever, and smallpox—cardiovascular disease not only strikes down a significant fraction of the population without warning but also causes prolonged suffering and disability in an even larger number. In the United States alone, despite recent encouraging declines, cardiovascular disease is still responsible for almost 1 million fatalities each year and more than half of all deaths; almost 5 million persons afflicted with cardiovascular disease are hospitalized each year. The cost of these diseases in terms of human suffering and of material resources is almost incalculable. Fortunately, research focusing on the causes, diagnosis, treatment, and prevention of heart disease is moving ahead rapidly.

In order to provide a comprehensive, authoritative text in a field that has become as broad and deep as cardiovascular medicine, I chose to enlist the aid of a number of able colleagues. However, I hoped that my personal involvement in the writing of about half of the book would make it possible to minimize the fragmentation, gaps, inconsistencies, organizational difficulties, and impersonal tone that sometimes plague multiauthored texts.

Since the early part of the 20th century, clinical cardiology has had a particularly strong foundation in the basic sciences of physiology and pharmacology. More recently, the disciplines of molecular biology, genetics, developmental biology, biophysics, biochemistry, experimental pathology, and bioengineering have also begun to provide critically important information about cardiac function and malfunction. Although *Heart Disease: A Textbook of Cardiovascular Medicine* is primarily a clinical treatise and not a textbook of fundamental cardiovascular science, an effort has been made to explain, in some detail, the scientific bases of cardiovascular diseases.

Eugene Braunwald, 1980

CONTENTS

PART III ■ Heart Failure 457

PART IV ■ Arrhythmias, Sudden Death, and Syncope 653

PART V ■ Preventive Cardiology 921

Look for these other titles in the Braunwald's HEART DISEASE family!

Antman: *Cardiovascular Therapeutics, 2nd Edition: A Companion to Braunwald's Heart Disease*

Chien: *Molecular Basis of Cardiovascular Disease, 2nd Edition: A Companion to Braunwald's Heart Disease*

Lilly: *Heart Disease Review and Assessment to Accompany Heart Disease, Sixth Edition*

Mann: *Heart Failure: A Companion to Braunwald's Heart Disease*

Manson, Buring, Ridker and Gaziano: *Clinical Trials in Heart Disease, 2nd Edition: A Companion to Braunwald's Heart Disease*

St. John Sutton and Rutherford: *Clinical Cardiovascular Imaging: A Companion to Braunwald's Heart Disease*

Theroux: *Acute Coronary Syndromes: A Companion to Braunwald's Heart Disease*

PART I

General Considerations of Cardiovascular Disease

CHAPTER 1

Global Burden of Cardiovascular Disease

J. Michael Gaziano

Over the past two centuries, the Industrial and Technological Revolutions and their associated economic and social transformations have resulted in dramatic shifts in the diseases responsible for illness and death. Cardiovascular disease (CVD) has emerged as the dominant chronic disease in many parts of the world, and early in the 21st century it is predicted to become the main cause of disability and death worldwide. In this chapter, trends in global patterns of disease and the increasing burden of CVD are summarized. The chapter begins with an explanation of the concept of the epidemiological transition, followed by a synopsis of this transition in the United States. This is followed by reviews of the current burden of cardiovascular and other chronic diseases in various regions of the world and global trends in the rates of CVD as well as rates of risk behaviors and factors. The chapter ends with a discussion of the diverse challenges that the increasing burden of CVD poses for the various regions of the world and potential solutions to this global problem.

The Epidemiological Transitions

At the beginning of the 20th century, CVD accounted for less than 10 percent of all deaths worldwide. At the beginning of the 21st century, CVD accounts for nearly half of all deaths in the developed world and 25 percent in the developing world.[1,2] By 2020, it is predicted that CVD will claim 25 million lives annually and that coronary heart disease (CHD) will surpass infectious disease as the world's number one cause of death and disability.

This global rise in CVD is the result of a dramatic shift in the health status of individuals around the world during the course of the 20th century. Equally important, there has been an unprecedented transformation in the dominant disease profile, or the distribution of diseases responsible for the majority of cases of death and debility. Before 1900, infectious diseases and malnutrition were the most common causes of death. These have been gradually supplanted in some (mostly developed) countries by chronic diseases such as CVD and cancer, thanks largely to improved nutrition and public health measures. As this trend spreads to and continues in developing countries, CVD will dominate as the major cause of death by 2020, accounting for at least one in every three deaths (Fig. 1–1).[2]

This shift in the diseases that account for the lion's share of mortality and morbidity is known as the *epidemiological transition*.[3,4] Never occurring in isolation, the epidemiological transition is tightly intertwined with changes in personal and collective wealth (economic transition), social structure (social transition), and demographics (demographic transition). Because the epidemiological transition is linked to the evolution of social and economic forces, it takes place at different rates around the world.

At the beginning of the third millennium, national health and disease profiles

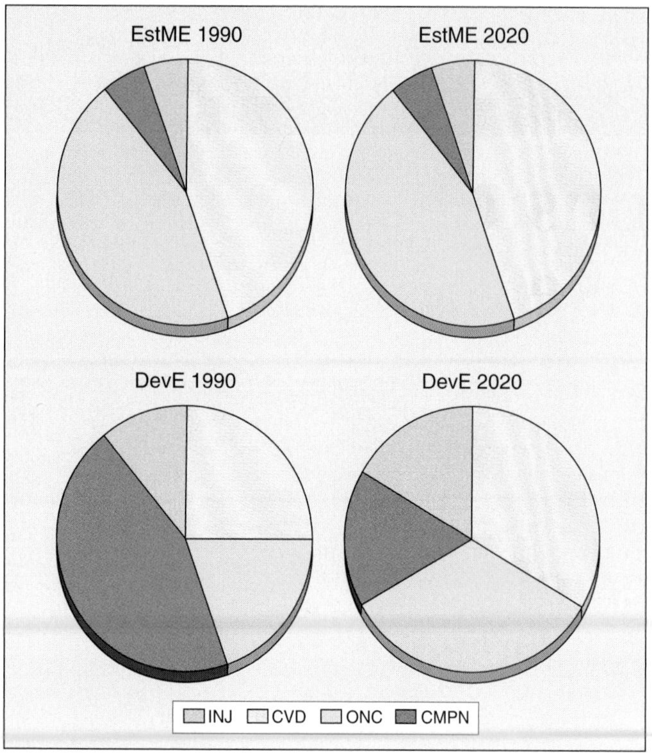

FIGURE 1–1 Changing pattern of mortality, 1990 to 2020. EstMe, Established market economies; DevE, developing economies; INJ, injury; CVD, cardiovascular disease; ONC, other noncommunicable diseases; CMPN, communicable, maternal, perinatal, and nutritional diseases. (From Murray CJL, Lopez AD: The Global Burden of Disease. Cambridge, MA, Harvard School of Public Health, 1996.)

vary widely by country and by region. For example, life expectancy in Japan (81.4 years) is more than twice that in Sierra Leone (34.2 years).[1] In a similar vein, communicable, infectious, maternal, perinatal, and nutritional diseases—the group I diseases defined by Murray and Lopez in their comprehensive analysis of the global burden of disease[2]—account for just 6 percent of deaths in so-called developed countries, compared with 33 percent in India.[2] The vast differences in burden of disease are readily apparent across three broad economic and geographical sectors of the world (Table 1–1). These include the established market economies (EstME) of Western Europe, North America, Australia, New Zealand, and Japan; the emerging market economies (EmgME) of the former socialist states of Eastern Europe; and the developing economies (DevE), which can further be subdivided into six geographical regions: China, India, other Asian countries and islands, sub-Saharan Africa, the Middle Eastern Crescent, and Latin America and the Caribbean. Currently, CVD is responsible for 45 percent of all deaths in EstME, 55 percent of all deaths in EmgME, and only 23 percent of the deaths in DevE.

An excellent model of the epidemiological transition has been developed by Omran.[3] He divides the transition into three basic ages: pestilence and famine, receding pandemics, and degenerative and man-made diseases (Table 1–2). Olshansky and Ault added a fourth stage, delayed degenerative diseases.[4] It is possible that a fifth stage (discussed later) may be emerging in some countries. Although any specific country or region enters these ages at different times, the progression from one to another tends to proceed in a predictable manner.

The Age of Pestilence and Famine

From the epidemiological standpoint, humans evolved under conditions of pestilence and famine and have lived with them for most of recorded history. This age is characterized by the predominance of malnutrition and infectious disease and by the infrequency of CVD as a cause of death. High fertility rates are offset by high infant and child mortality, resulting in a mean life expectancy on the order of approximately 30 years. In the countries that eventually became today's established market economies, the transition through the age of pestilence and famine was relatively slow, beginning in the late 1700s and developing throughout the 1800s. Competing influences prolonged the transition—improvements in the food supply early in the Industrial Revolution that by themselves would have reduced mortality were offset by concentration of the population in urban centers, which led to increases in mortality due to communicable diseases such as tuberculosis, cholera, dysentery, and influenza.

Although the transition through the age of pestilence and famine occurred much later in the emerging market economies and the developing economies, it has also taken place more rapidly, driven largely by the transfer of low-cost agricultural products and technologies and well-established, lower-cost public health technologies. Much of the developing world has emerged from the age of pestilence and famine. In sub-Saharan Africa and parts of India, however, malnutrition and infectious disease remain leading causes of death.

The Age of Receding Pandemics

Rising wealth and the resultant increase in the availability of food help usher in the second phase of the epidemiological transition. Improved nutrition decreases early deaths due to

TABLE 1–1 Burden of Disease for the Three Economic Regions of the World

Sector	Population (Millions) (Percentage of Total World Population)		Cardiovascular Disease (%)		Other Noncommunicable Diseases* (%)		Communicable, Maternal, Perinatal, and Nutritional Conditions (%)		Injuries (%)	
	1990	*2010*	*1990*	*2010*	*1990*	*2010*	*1990*	*2010*	*1990*	*2010*
EstME†	798 (15.2)	874 (12.4)	44.6	43.1	42.8	45.1	6.4	6.2	6.2	5.5
EmgME‡	346 (6.6)	363 (5.2)	54.6	55.0	29.5	32.2	5.6	3.5	10.3	8.8
DevE§	4124 (78.3)	5764 (82.3)	23.0	31.0	17.0	31.2	41.9	24.7	10.7	12.0

*Includes cancer, diabetes, neuropsychiatric conditions, congenital anomalies, and respiratory, digestive, genitourinary, and musculoskeletal diseases.
†EstME = established market economies: United States, Canada, Western Europe, Japan, Australia, and New Zealand.
‡EmgME = emerging market economies: former socialist states of Russian Federation.
§DevE = developing market economies: China, India, other Asian countries and islands, sub-Saharan Africa, Middle Eastern Crescent, and Latin America and the Caribbean.
Adapted from Murray CJL, Lopez AD: The Global Burden of Disease. Cambridge, MA, Harvard School of Public Health, 1996.

TABLE 1–2 Four Typical Stages of the Epidemiological Transition

Stage	Description	Typical Proportion of Deaths due to Cardiovascular Disease (%)	Predominant Types of Cardiovascular Disease
Pestilence and famine	Predominance of malnutrition and infectious diseases as causes of death; high rates of infant and child mortality; low mean life expectancy	<10	Rheumatic heart disease, cardiomyopathies due to infection and malnutrition
Receding pandemics	Improvements in nutrition and public health lead to decrease in rates of deaths due to malnutrition and infection; precipitous decline in infant and child mortality rates	10-35	Rheumatic valvular disease, hypertension, CHD, stroke
Degenerative and man-made diseases	Increased fat and caloric intake and decreased physical activity lead to emergence of hypertension and atherosclerosis; with increased life expectancy, mortality from chronic, noncommunicable diseases exceeds mortality from malnutrition and infectious diseases	35-65	CHD, stroke
Delayed degenerative diseases	Cardiovascular diseases and cancer are the major causes of morbidity and mortality; better treatment and prevention efforts help avoid deaths among those with disease and delay primary events. Age-adjusted CVD mortality declines; CVD affecting older and older individuals	40-50	CHD, stroke, congestive heart failure

CHD = coronary heart disease; CVD = cardiovascular disease.
Adapted from Omran AR: The epidemiologic transition: A theory of the epidemiology of population change. Milbank Mem Fund Q 49:509, 1971; and Olshansky SJ, Ault AB: The fourth stage of the epidemiologic transition: The age of delayed degenerative diseases. Milbank Q 64:355, 1986.

malnutrition and may also reduce susceptibility to infectious diseases. Increased personal and public wealth is associated with public health measures that contribute still further to declines in infectious diseases. These advances, in turn, increase the productivity of the average worker, further improving the economic situation. The change most characteristic of this phase is a precipitous decline in infant and child mortality accompanied by a substantial increase in life expectancy. Examples of countries in this phase of the epidemiological transition are the United States early in the 20th century and China today, where approximately 29 percent of deaths are due to CVD and only 16 percent are due to communicable disease.[2] Changes in nutrition and other aspects of life style that cause lower rates of communicable, maternal, perinatal, and nutritional diseases eventually lead to a greater incidence of CVD.

The Age of Degenerative and Man-Made Diseases

Continued improvements in economic circumstances, combined with urbanization and radical changes in the nature of work-related activities, lead to dramatic life-style changes in diet, activity levels, and behaviors such as smoking. During the age of pestilence and famine, most of the population is deficient in total caloric intake relative to daily caloric expenditure. Easier access to less expensive foods and increased fat content increase total caloric intake, whereas mechanization results in lower daily caloric expenditure. This disparity leads to a higher mean body mass index, blood pressure, and levels of plasma lipids and blood sugar. These changes set the stage for the emergence of hypertensive diseases and atherosclerosis. Cancer rates also rise rapidly during the age of degenerative and man-made diseases. As the average life expectancy increases beyond 50 years, mortality from largely chronic noncommunicable diseases—dominated by CVD—exceeds mortality from malnutrition and infectious diseases.[5,6] Countries currently in this phase of the epidemiological transition are the emerging market economies of the former Soviet socialist states.

The Age of Delayed Degenerative Diseases

In the fourth phase of the epidemiological transition, CVD and cancer remain the major causes of morbidity and mortality. In the industrialized nations, however, major technological advances such as coronary care units, bypass surgery, percutaneous coronary interventions, and thrombolytic therapy are available to manage the acute manifestations of CVD, and preventive strategies such as smoking cessation and blood pressure management are widely implemented. As a result of better treatment and widespread primary and secondary prevention efforts, deaths are prevented among people with disease and primary events are delayed. Life expectancy continues to creep upward as age-adjusted CVD mortality tends to decline, with the average age of people affected by CVD getting increasingly older.

Is There a Fifth Phase of the Epidemiological Transition?

Troubling trends in certain risk behaviors and risk factors may be foreshadowing a new phase of the epidemiological transition. In many parts of the industrialized world, physical activity continues to decline while total caloric intake increases at alarming rates, with the combination resulting in an epidemic of obesity. As a result, rates of type 2 diabetes, hypertension, and lipid abnormalities associated with obesity are increasing. These trends are particularly evident in children. These changes are occurring at a time when measurable improvements in other risk behaviors and risk factors such as smoking have slowed. If these risk factor trends continue, age-adjusted CVD mortality rates, which have declined over the past several decades in developed countries, could increase in the coming years. Evidence that we are approaching an inflection point in the CVD mortality curves is provided by the slowing of the rate of decline in the past few years. This is especially true for age-adjusted stroke death rates.

Changes in Cardiovascular Disease through the Epidemiological Transitions

During the transition from the age of pestilence and famine to the age of delayed degenerative diseases, changes occur in both the character of CVD and total rates of CVD.[6] During the age of pestilence and famine, CVD accounts for only 5 to 10 percent of mortality, with the major forms of CVD related to infection and malnutrition, largely rheumatic heart disease and the infectious and nutritional cardiomyopathies. Given the potentially long latent period of these diseases, they are apparent well into the age of receding pandemics, when they persist as major causes of death along with emerging hypertensive heart disease and stroke. During the age of receding pandemics, CVD accounts for 10 to 35 percent of deaths. CHD rates tend to be low relative to stroke rates. In addition, risk behaviors and risk factors that will foreshadow the next phase become more widespread. During the age of degenerative and man-made diseases, increased caloric intake (particularly from saturated animal fats and processed vegetable fats), reduced daily activity, increased smoking rates, and related changes in the prevalence of hypertension, diabetes, and hyperlipidemia result in further increases in hypertensive diseases and rapid increases in CHD and peripheral vascular disease. During this phase, 35 to 65 percent of all deaths are due to CVD. Typically, the rate of CHD deaths greatly exceeds that of stroke by a ratio of 2:1 to 3:1.

In the fourth phase of the epidemiological transition, the age of delayed degenerative diseases, age-adjusted death rates from CVD begin to fall, leveling off somewhere below 50 percent of total mortality. The decline in stroke rates tends to precede the decline for CHD; thus, the ratio of CHD to stroke deaths increases, typically to between 2:1 and 5:1 (Fig. 1–2).

The decline in CVD rates is the result of two factors: better access to health technology and adoption of healthier life styles. Improvements in health technology and better access to it decrease the likelihood of death among patients presenting with acute manifestations of atherosclerotic disease, although better survival means more and more individuals living longer with conditions such as angina pectoris, congestive heart failure, and cardiac arrhythmias.

Reductions in risk behaviors and factors may make even greater contributions to the decline in age-adjusted rates of death. In many cases, these are the result of concerted efforts by public health and health care communities. In other cases, secular trends also play a role. For example, the widespread availability of fresh fruits and vegetables all year long in developed countries, and thus increased consumption, may have contributed to declining mean cholesterol levels before effective drug therapy was widely available. In general, however, even though age-adjusted rates of CVD continue to decline during the final phase of the epidemiological transition, the prevalence of CVD increases as the population ages.

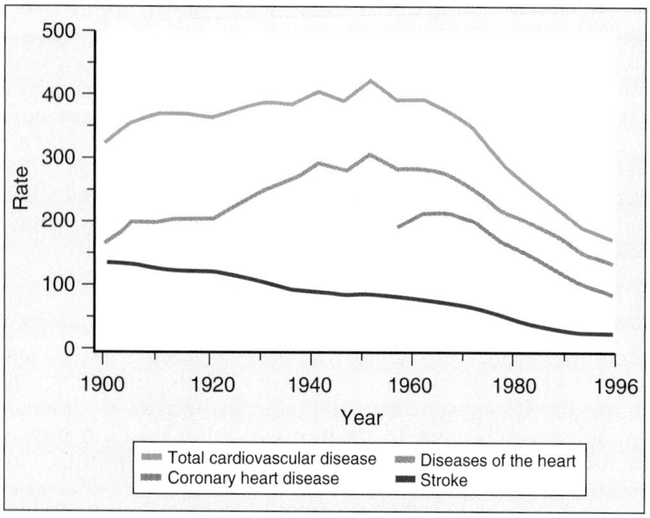

FIGURE 1–2 Increase and decline in heart disease rates through the epidemiological transition in the United States, 1900 to 1996. Rate is per 100,000 population, standardized to the 1940 U.S. population. Diseases are classified according to International Classification of Diseases (ICD) codes in use when the deaths were reported. ICD classification revisions occurred in 1910, 1921, 1930, 1939, 1949, 1958, 1968, and 1979. Death rates before 1933 do not include all states. Comparability ratios were applied to rates for 1970 and 1975. (From Achievements in public health, 1900-1999: Decline in deaths from heart disease and stroke—United States, 1900-1999. MMWR Morbid Mortal Wkly Rep 48:649, 1999.)

ECONOMIC, SOCIAL, AND DEMOGRAPHIC TRANSITIONS

As mentioned earlier, several parallel transformations accompany the epidemiological transition. These include economic, demographic, and social transitions that pave the way for major shifts in a population's health and the nature of the diseases that account for most of the mortality and morbidity.

ECONOMIC TRANSITION. The economic transition is characterized by rising levels of personal wealth. This is usually reflected in increasing per capita income, per capita gross domestic product (GDP), or gross national product (GNP).

SOCIAL TRANSITION. The social transition is driven by industrialization and the changes that accompany it, including urbanization, the development of a public health infrastructure, wider access to health care, and increasing application of health technologies. Industrialization tends to spark a large number of social changes. It is typically accompanied by urbanization, a major social force that has a significant impact on the epidemiological transition. Urbanization affects living standards and life style and affords the opportunity to develop organized health care systems.

In virtually every region of the world, there has been a shift from rural to urban life. For example, in the United States, 60 percent of the population lived in rural settings at the beginning of the 20th century compared with only 20 percent at the beginning of the 21st century. In Asia, Africa, and Latin America, a similar shift has occurred over the second half of the 20th century (Fig. 1-3).

DEMOGRAPHIC TRANSITION. *Demographic transition* refers to shifts in the age structure of a population due to declining fertility and increased survival. During the age of pestilence and famine, individuals 20 years of age and younger may account for 40 to 50 percent of the

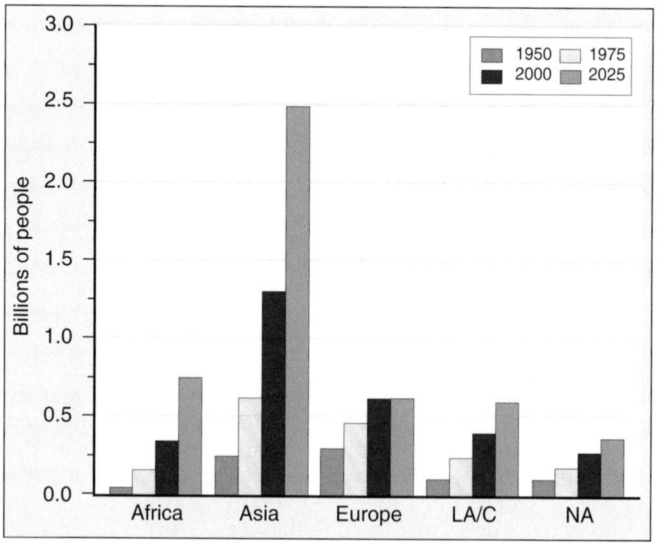

FIGURE 1–3 Number of people living in urban areas, 1950, 1975, 2000, and 2025. LA/C, Latin America and Caribbean; NA, North America. (From Population Division, Department of Economic and Social Affairs: World Urbanization Prospects: The 2001 Revision. New York, United Nations Secretariat, 2002. Number ESA/P/WP.173.)

population. As child and infant mortality rates are reduced in the age of receding pandemics, rapid gains are seen in life expectancy, and the proportion of individuals 20 years of age and younger decreases. Declines in mortality rates are generally followed by declining fertility rates, further flattening the shape of the population distribution curve. As population growth rates fall, the mean age of the population continues to rise slowly as individuals live longer.

The life-style changes associated with the economic and social transitions cause shifts in the profile of risk behaviors and risk factors for disease. These include decreased physical activity, increased smoking, and dramatic changes in diet.

RATE OF CHANGE OF THE EPIDEMIOLOGICAL TRANSITION

Several factors influence how early or how quickly the epidemiological transition occurs in a given country or region. (1) The rate of economic growth relative to population growth affects the rate of adoption of life styles characteristic of established market economies. (2) Regional economic influences can cause great disparities in the rates of transition within a region. (3) The development of low-cost public health technologies, as well as falling costs of unhealthy aspects of the Western life style such as cigarette smoking and consumption of highly processed food, permits currently developing countries to make transitions more rapidly.

SOCIOECONOMIC CLASS. Even within a given country, segments of the population may undergo the transition at varying rates. These factors are related to economic, social, or cultural factors. In fact, epidemiological transitions occur at different rates across economic groups, generally beginning among those with higher socioeconomic status and eventually spreading to those with lower socioeconomic status. The decline in rates of malnutrition and communicable diseases as well as the rise in coronary risk factors and behaviors occur first in the privileged classes; increases in rates of stroke and CHD soon follow. Later, as the middle class grows, the epidemiological transition spreads to a broad enough sector of the population to have a measurable impact on population rates. As more and more of the burgeoning middle class passes through the second and third phases of the transition, CVD and cancer rates become the population's dominant causes of death and disability. People in the lower socioeconomic strata tend to acquire the risk factors and behaviors last, in part because of their economic situation and in part because they tend to engage in more physical activity at work. Compared with people in the upper and middle socioeconomic strata, those in the lowest stratum are less likely to have access to advanced treatments and to acquire and apply information on modification of risk factors and behaviors. Thus, CVD mortality rates decline later among those with lower socioeconomic status. In a developed country such as Canada, for example, CVD mortality rates are highest among the poorest individuals (Fig. 1-4).[7]

The Epidemiological Transition in the United States

Like other established market economies, the United States has proceeded through four stages of the epidemiological transition. Recent trends, however, suggest that the rates of decline of some chronic and degenerative diseases have slowed, suggesting the possibility that the United States is entering a fifth phase characterized by the epidemic of obesity. Given the large amount of economic, social, demographic, and health data available (Table 1–3), the United States is used as a reference point for later comparisons.

THE AGE OF PESTILENCE AND FAMINE

The United States, like virtually all other countries and regions, was born into pestilence and famine. Infectious diseases killed many of the earliest immigrants to the New World. About half of the Pilgrims arriving in the New World in November of 1620 died of infection and malnutrition by the following spring. In addition, the infectious diseases the immigrants brought with them from Europe had a devastating impact on Native American populations.

At the end of the 1800s, the U.S. economy was still largely agrarian, with more than 60 percent of the population living in rural settings. However, industrialization and urbanization were well under way. Per capita income was increasing, and the food supply was improving. Modest gains in life expectancy were apparent throughout the 19th century. By 1900, life expectancy had increased to 47.8 years for men and 50.7 years for women.[8] Infectious diseases—largely tuberculosis, pneumonia, and diarrheal diseases—accounted for more deaths than any other cause.[9] CVD accounted for less than 10 percent of all deaths. Tobacco products were out of the economic reach of a large segment of the population.

THE AGE OF RECEDING PANDEMICS

Early in the 20th century, the pace of industrialization accelerated. The shift from a rural, agriculture-based economy to an urban, industry-based economy had a number of consequences on cardiovascular risk behaviors and factors. Food supplies had become abundant, but urbanization required a dramatic shift in dietary staples. The railway network in place at the turn of the century was capable of moving foodstuffs from the farm to the city. But because the trains were not refrigerated, perishable foodstuffs such as fresh fruits and vegetables could not readily be transported, whereas cereal grains and livestock could. Large slaughter houses and meat-packing plants were established in or near urban areas. As a result, consumption of fresh fruits and vegetables declined and consumption of meat and grains increased, resulting in diets that were higher in fat and processed carbohydrates.[10] In addition, the manufacture of factory-rolled cigarettes made them more portable and more affordable for the mass population.[11]

RAPID SOCIAL CHANGES. The population of urban areas outnumbered that of rural areas for the first time by 1920. By 1930, 56 percent of the population was living in or near urban centers. Infectious disease mortality rates had fallen dramatically, from a crude death rate of approximately 800 per 100,000 population in 1900 to approximately 340 per 100,000 people.[9] Largely as a result of rapidly declining infant, childhood, and adolescent mortality from malnutrition and infectious diseases, life expectancy increased by 10 years between 1900 and 1930, to 57.8 years for men and 61.1 years for women. At the same time, cigarette smoking was on the rise. Age-adjusted CVD mortality rates, at approximately 390 per 100,000 people, were in the midst of their steady climb up from slightly more than 300 per 100,000 people in 1900. This increase was largely driven by rapidly rising CHD rates.

EMERGENCE OF A PUBLIC HEALTH INFRASTRUCTURE. By 1900, a public health infrastructure had emerged: 40 states had health departments and many larger towns had major public works efforts to improve water supply and sewage systems.[9] Municipal use of chlorine to disinfect water was becoming widespread, and improvements in food handling such as pasteurization were introduced.[12] The health care system was growing but still largely comprised general practitioners providing care in the office or home; hospitals were largely for the indigent. The Flexner Report of 1910, which took a careful look at the quality of medical education in the United States and Canada,[13] was the first step toward organized quality improvement in health care personnel that, along with other public health changes, was responsible for dramatic declines in infectious disease mortality rates throughout the century (Fig. 1-5).

THE AGE OF DEGENERATIVE AND MAN-MADE DISEASES

By the middle of the 20th century, the United States was predominantly an urban, industrial economy, with 64 percent of the population living

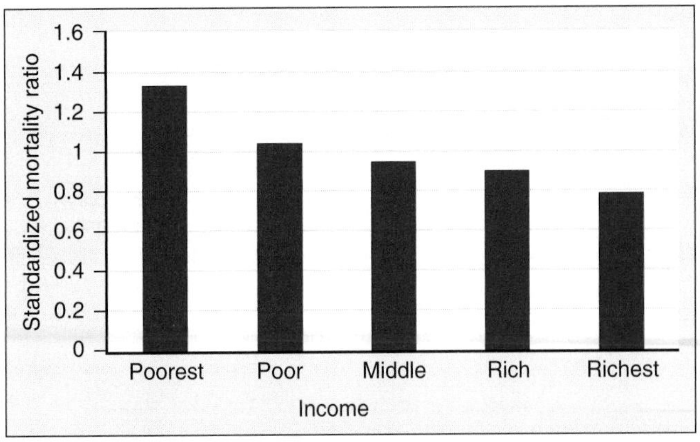

FIGURE 1–4 Cardiovascular disease standardized mortality ratios by neighborhood income for Canadians of European ancestry, ages 35 to 74, in 1986 and 1991. (From Sheth T, Nair C, Nargundjar M, et al: Cardiovascular and cancer mortality among Canadians of European, south Asian, and Chinese origin from 1979 to 1993: An analysis of 1.2 million deaths. Can Med Assoc J 161:132, 1999.)

TABLE 1–3 Trends in the United States During the 20th Century

	1900	1930	1970	2000
Population (millions)	76	123	203	281
Median income (real dollars)	NA	$15,050 (1947)	$26,333	$29,058
Age-adjusted cardiovascular disease mortality (n/100,000)	325	390	699	341
Age-adjusted coronary heart disease mortality (n/100,000)	NA	NA	448	186
Age-adjusted stroke mortality (n/100,000)	140	100	148	57
Urbanization (%)	39	56	74	76
Life expectancy (yr)	49.2	59.3	70.8	76.9
Smoking				
Cigarettes per capita (n)	54	1185	3969	1977
Smokers (%)	NA	NA	37.4	23.3
Total caloric intake (kcal)	3500	3300	3200	3800
Fat intake (% of total calories)	31.6	37.3	41.2	33
Cholesterol level (mg/dl)	NA	NA	216	204
Overweight or obese (%)	NA	NA	47.7	64.5

NA = not available.

Sources: *Population*: US Census Bureau. *Per capita income*: U.S. Bureau of the Census: Current Population Reports, P60-203, Measuring 50 Years of Economic Change Using the March Current Population Survey. Washington, DC, U.S. Government Printing Office, 1998; and U.S. Bureau of the Census: Money Income in the United States, 2000, P60-213. Washington, DC, U.S. Government Printing Office, 2001. *Cardiovascular disease, coronary heart disease, stroke mortality*: Morbidity & Mortality: 2002 Chart Book on Cardiovascular, Lung, and Blood Diseases. Betuesda, MD, National Heart, Lung, and Blood Institute, 2002. *Urbanization*: Measuring America: The Decennial Censuses, 1790 to 2000: U.S. Bureau of the Census, 2002. *Life expectancy*: Arias E: United States life tables, 2000. *In* National Vital Statistics Report vol 51, no 3. Atlanta, GA, National Center for Health Statistics, Centers for Disease Control and Prevention, 2002. *Smoking*: Federal Trade Commission: Cigarette report for 2001. (http://www.ftc.gov/os/2003/06/2001cigreport.pdf) Accessed on 1 July 2003. *Total caloric intake and fat intake*: Nutrient content of the US food supply, 1909-1994: a summary. Washington, DC, US Department of Agriculture, 1998; and Kennedy ET, Bowman SA, Powell R: Dietary-fat intake in the US population. J Am Coll Nutr 18:207, 1999. *Cholesterol level and obesity*: National Center for Health Statistics: Health, United States, 2002. (http://www.cdc.gov/nchs/data/hus/hus02.pdf) Accessed on 15 July 2003.

in urban and suburban settings. With continued mechanization and urbanization, activity levels declined considerably. The rise of suburbs meant that more and more people were driving to work or to shopping rather than walking or bicycling. Prevalence of smoking, one of the major contributors to premature mortality and chronic disease, hit its zenith among adult men at 57 percent in 1955 and among women 10 years later at 34 percent.[14] Annual per capita consumption of cigarettes peaked in 1963 at 4345, or more than half a pack per day for every American.[11]

By 1965, per capita income had risen to approximately $10,000 (in 1997 adjusted dollars).[15] Deaths from infectious diseases had fallen to fewer than 50 per 100,000 population per year, and life expectancy was up to almost 70 years. However, almost 52 percent of men and 34 percent of women were smokers, and fat consumption represented 41 percent of total calories. Age-adjusted CHD mortality rates were at their peak, at approximately 225 per 100,000 people. Stroke rates were also high, at 75 per 100,000.

GROWTH OF THE HEALTH CARE INDUSTRY

One of the most remarkable changes in the years after World War II was the growth of the health care industry. Only some of this growth was stimulated by rises in per capita GDP. In the private sector, the growth of labor unions propelled a major expansion in private health care insurance. In fact, by the late 1950s, more than two thirds of the working U.S. population had some form of private insurance.[16] The federal government also played an important role. Increases in federal funding (the Hill Burton Act of 1948) led to the construction of more hospitals to deal with the acute manifestations of chronic illnesses. These new hospitals drew on the great successes of the military hospitals.[17] In 1966, two key federal insurance programs, Medicare and Medicaid, provided access to medical care for the medically indigent and the elderly. The Health Professions Education Assistance Act of 1966, which provided capitation grants to medical schools, doubled medical school enrollment over the next two decades through expanded class size and estab-

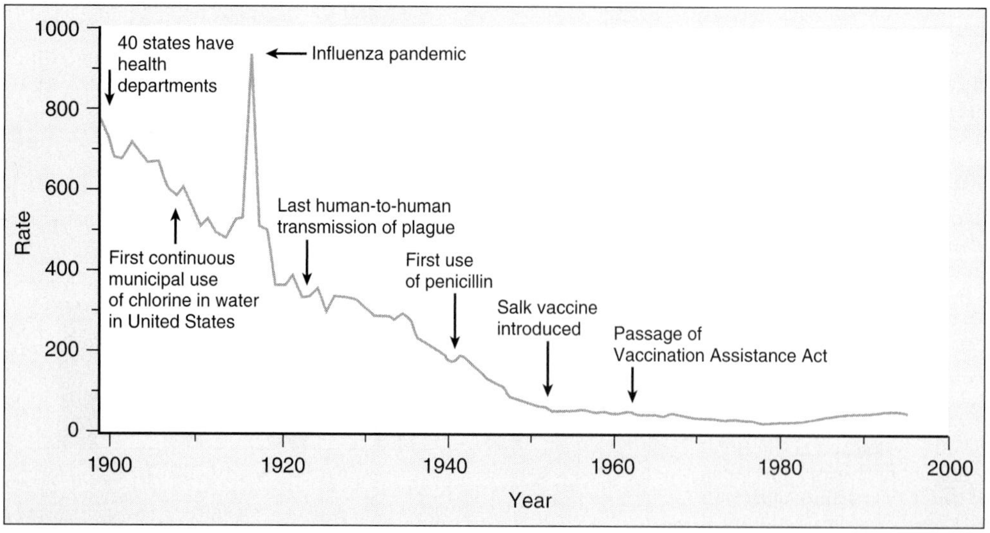

FIGURE 1–5 Decline in mortality due to infectious diseases in the United States, 1900 to 1996. Rate is per 100,000 population per year. (Data on chlorine use from American Water Works Association: Water chlorination principles and practices: AWWA manual M20. Denver, American Water Works Association, 1973. From Achievements in public health 1900-1999: Control of infectious diseases. MMWR Morbid Mortal Wkly Rep 48:621, 1999. Adapted from Armstrong GL, Conn LA, Pinner RW: Trends in infectious disease mortality in the United States during the 20th century. JAMA 281:61, 1999.)

TABLE 1–4 Cardiovascular Disease, United States, 2000

Type	Prevalence* (Millions)	Crude Mortality (Thousands)†	Percentage of Total Deaths†	Rate per 100,000 Population†
Cardiovascular disease	61.8	936.9	38.9	340.4
Hypertension	50	44.6	1.8	16.2
Ischemic heart disease	12.9	515.2	21.4	187.2
Stroke	4.7	167.6	7.0	60.9
Arrhythmia	3.9	37.6	1.6	13.6
Congestive heart failure	4.9	51.5	2.1	18.7
Rheumatic heart disease	NA	3.5	0.2	1.3
Valvular disease (nonrheumatic)	NA	19.7	0.8	7.2

Type	Annual Events* (Thousands)
Myocardial infarction	1100
New	650
Recurrent	450
Stroke	700
New	500
Recurrent	200
CABG	519
PTCA	561
Valve surgery	87
Total costs	$351.8 billion
Direct	$204.3 billion
Indirect	$142.5 billion

*Data from American Heart Association: 2003 Heart and Stroke Statistical Update. Dallas, TX, American Heart Association, 2003.
†From Miniño AM, Arias E, Kochanek KD, et al: Deaths: Final Data for 2000. National Vital statistics reports, vol 50, no 15. Hyattsville, MD, 2002, National Center for Health Statistics.
CABG = coronary artery bypass grafting; CDC, Centers for Disease Control and Prevention; NA = not available; PTCA = percutaneous transluminal coronary angioplasty.

lishment of new medical schools. The establishment of the National Institutes of Health, spurred largely by scientific achievements in medicine made during World War II, not only promoted health-related research but also transformed medical education by providing financial support for the establishment of full-time medical school faculty.

The Age of Declining Degenerative Diseases

A decline in age-adjusted CVD mortality rates began in the mid-1960s, and there have been substantial reductions in rates of mortality from both stroke and CHD since then.[18] These reductions have occurred among both whites and blacks, among men and women, and in all age groups. Age-adjusted CHD mortality rates have fallen approximately 2 percent per year, and stroke rates have fallen 3 percent per year (see Fig. 1–2). Table 1–4 gives a snapshot of CVD in 2000, the last year for which complete statistics are available.

DECLINE IN CARDIOVASCULAR DISEASE MORTALITY. Two main factors have been attributed to the decline in CVD mortality rates: therapeutic advances and prevention measures targeted at people with CVD and those potentially at risk for it.[19-21] Treatments once considered advanced, including the establishment of emergency medical systems, coronary care units, and the widespread use of new diagnostic and therapeutic technologies such as echocardiography, cardiac catheterization, angioplasty, bypass surgery, and implantation of pacemakers and defibrillators are now considered the standard of care. Advances in the pharmaceutical industry have also had a major impact on both primary and secondary prevention. Efforts to improve the acute management of myocardial infarction led to the development of life-saving drugs such as beta blockers, percutaneous coronary intervention thrombolytics, angiotensin-converting enzyme inhibitors, and others (see Chaps. 46 and 47).[22] The widespread use of an "old" drug, aspirin, has also reduced the risk of dying of acute or secondary coronary events. Low-cost pharmacological treatment for hypertension (see Chap. 38) and the development of highly effective cholesterol-lowering drugs such as statins have also made major contributions to reducing deaths from CVD in both primary and secondary prevention (see Chaps. 39 and 42). Such shifts are reflected in the burgeoning cost of medical care. In 1965, Americans spent approximately 5.9 percent of the GDP ($42 billion in unadjusted dollars) on health care.[23] In 2001, the last year for which complete statistics are available, we spent 14.1 percent of the GDP ($1.4 trillion in unadjusted dollars), or $5035 per capita.[24]

In concert with these advances, public health campaigns have also hammered home the message that certain behaviors increase the risk of CVD and that life-style modifications are particularly effective ways to reduce risk. One such success is with smoking cessation. In 1955, 57 percent of men smoked cigarettes,[14] whereas today 26 percent of men smoke. Among women, the prevalence of smoking has fallen from a high of 34 percent in 1965 to 21 percent today. Campaigns beginning in the 1970s resulted in dramatic improvements in the detection and treatment of hypertension.[18] This likely had a profound and immediate effect on stroke rates and a more subtle effect on CHD rates. Similar public health messages concerning saturated fat and cholesterol are largely responsible for the decline in overall fat consumption as a percentage of total calories from approximately 45 percent in 1965 to 34 percent in 1995[25] and the decline in population mean cholesterol levels from 220 mg/dl in the early 1960s to 203 mg/dl in the early 1990s.[18]

A main characteristic of the age of declining degenerative diseases is the steadily rising age at which a first CVD event occurs or at which people die of CVD (Fig. 1–6). Despite declines in age-adjusted mortality, the aging of the population will cause CVD to remain the predominant cause of morbidity and mortality. This, in turn, leads to ever-increasing numbers of individuals with CVD as well as ever-increasing health expenditures related to its treatment. In 2000, for example, CVD was the first-listed diagnosis for 6.3 million inpatients.[26] Hospital discharges included 781,000 for acute myocardial infarction; 716,000 for cardiac dysrhythmias; 999,000 for congestive heart failure; 1,221,000 for cardiac catheterizations; 519,000 for bypass surgery; 1,025,000 for percutaneous coronary interventions; and 327,000 for insertions or revision of a pacemaker or defibrillator. In addition, there were 981,000 hospital discharges for stroke.[27]

At the beginning of the 21st century, the nation is fully industrialized, with only 2 percent of the population involved in farming and a per capita GDP of approximately $36,300. Life expectancy at birth is 74.1 years for men and 79.5 years for women, and at age 65 is 16.3 years for men and 19.2 for women.[28] CVD continues to be the predominant cause of morbidity and mortality, but it afflicts an older

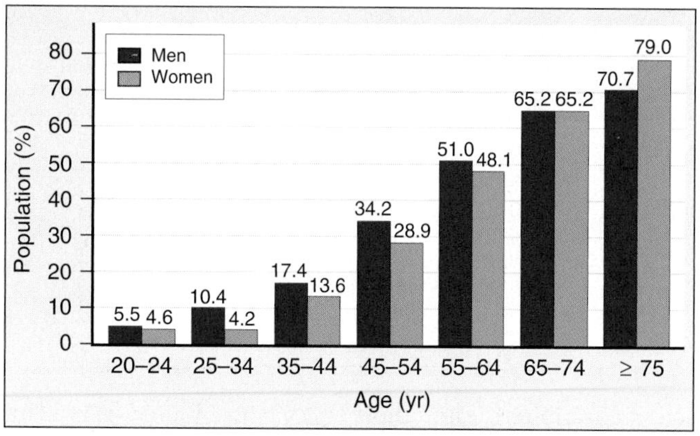

FIGURE 1–6 Estimated prevalence of cardiovascular disease in Americans 20 years of age and older. (From American Heart Association: 2003 Heart and Stroke Statistical Update. Dallas, American Heart Association, 2003.)

population than it did in the middle of the century. Although age-adjusted CVD rates continue to fall, the rate of decline began slowing in the 1990s, with virtually no change in stroke rates for the last 5-year period for which data are available. CHD rates may also be leveling off, owing in part to a slowing in the rate of decline in risk factors such as smoking and increases in other risk factors such as obesity and physical inactivity.

Is the United States Entering a New Phase of the Epidemiological Transition?

Although rates of CHD and stroke death fell 2 to 3 percent per year through the 1970s and 1980s, the rate of decline has slowed.[21] Overweight and obesity are increasing at an alarming pace, and only a minority of the population meets minimal physical activity recommendations. This has resulted in increases in diabetes and hypertension. Rates of detection and treatment of hypertension are stagnant.[29] The decline in smoking rates has leveled off, with approximately 26 percent of men and 21 percent of women classified as current smokers.[14] Even more troubling are increases in childhood obesity and physical inactivity, leading to large increases in diabetes and hypertension among younger individuals.[30,31] These troubling changes in CVD risk behaviors and factors may slow the rate of decline and could even contribute to increases in age-adjusted rates of CVD in the coming years.

Current Worldwide Variations in the Global Burden of Cardiovascular Disease

An epidemiological transition much like the one that occurred in the United States is occurring throughout the world. As in the United States, worldwide CVD rates have risen steadily throughout the 1900s. At the close of the 20th century, 28 percent of all deaths worldwide were due to CVD, whereas communicable diseases accounted for 34 percent of the total.[2] With the ongoing global transition, dominated by the transition in the developing world, CVD is predicted to be the number one cause of death by 2020, accounting for 36 percent of all deaths, whereas communicable diseases will account for barely half that, at 15 percent.[2]

Looking behind the global transition reveals vast discrepancies in regional rates of change. These wide variations began to appear early in the 20th century. Although most of the world remained in the phase of pestilence and famine, economic circumstances in several relatively confined regions changed rapidly, accelerating the pace of their epidemiological transitions. Thus, the global burden of CVD is best understood by examining the differential rates of change in each economic region. In addition to variability in the rate of the transition, there are unique regional features that have modified aspects of the U.S.-style transition in various parts of the world.

In terms of economic development, the world can be divided into two broad sectors, as described in Table 1–1: (1) the developed world, which can be further subdivided into the established market economies (EstME) and the emerging market economies (EmgME); and (2) the developing economies (DevE). Given the diversity within the DevE, it is useful to further subdivide it into six distinct economic/geographic regions: China, India, other Asian countries and Pacific islands, sub-Saharan Africa, the Middle Eastern Crescent, and Latin America and the Caribbean. Currently, four of every five people live in countries with developing economies, and it is these countries that are driving the rates of change in the global burden of CVD.

Like the United States, the rest of the EstME are largely in the fourth phase of the epidemiological transition, with CVD accounting for 45 percent of all deaths in 1990 and communicable diseases accounting for well under 10 percent (see Table 1–1). The EmgME are generally in the third phase of the transition, with CVD accounting for 54 percent of deaths. In the DevE overall, 23 percent of deaths are due to CVD, whereas communicable diseases account for 42 percent of deaths. Across the six subgroups of the DevE, however, there remains a high degree of heterogeneity with respect to the phase of the epidemiological transition, as illustrated by the dominant disease rates in each region (Table 1–5). In sub-Saharan Africa, communicable disease rates still far exceed those of chronic diseases, placing it in the first phase (pestilence and famine). Within regions, there is a great deal of heterogeneity. Some regions of India, for example, appear to be in the first phase, characterized by high rates of infectious and communicable disease, whereas others are in the second or even the third phase. The Middle East appears to be in the third phase of the epidemiological transition. This section briefly describes the difficulties in assessing and comparing disease rates around the world and discusses the regional rates, as well as highlights within-region variations.

Established Market Economies

At the beginning of the 21st century, approximately 840 million people (13.6 percent of the world's population) live in the established market economies of the United States, Canada, Australia, New Zealand, Western Europe, and Japan. In these countries, CHD rates tend to be twofold to fivefold higher than stroke rates. Table 1–6 demonstrates this tendency in selected European countries. There are two notable exceptions. In Portugal, stroke rates for both men and women are higher than CHD rates. The same is true for Japan, where stroke is responsible for far more fatalities than CHD.

Rapid declines in CHD and stroke rates since the early 1970s signal that the EstME countries are in the fourth phase of the epidemiological transition, the age of delayed degenerative diseases. In general, stroke rates have fallen faster than CHD rates, increasing the CHD-to-stroke ratio. In the United States, for example, stroke rates over the past three decades have fallen an average of 3 percent per year, whereas CHD rates have fallen approximately 2 percent per year.

The rates of CVD in Western Europe tend to be similar to those in the United States. However, the absolute rates vary threefold among the countries of Western Europe with a clear north/south gradient, with higher CHD and stroke rates in the

TABLE 1–5 Mortality and Disability-Adjusted Life Years Lost by Disease Category in the Developing World

	Region						
	China	*India*	*Other Asia*	*SSA*	*MEC*	*LatAm*	*Total*
Deaths (%)							
CMPN	15.8	51.0	39.6	64.8	42.7	31.3	41.9
Injury	11.5	8.6	10.1	12.5	9.9	12.9	10.7
Non-CVD, non-CMPN	43.8	16.1	25.9	12.8	19.0	29.5	24.3
All CVD	28.9	24.2	24.4	9.9	28.4	26.2	23.0
Ischemic heart disease	8.6	12.5	8.3	2.5	13.4	11.6	9.0
Stroke	14.3	4.8	7.0	4.7	4.7	8.3	7.5
Rheumatic heart disease	1.8	0.7	0.2	0.2	0.5	0.3	0.7
Other CVD	3.4	5.2	7.3	1.7	8.3	5.3	4.7
Disability-adjusted life-years (%)							
CMPN	24.2	56.4	44.7	65.9	47.7	35.3	48.7
Injury	17.6	14.6	14.4	15.4	11.1	16.4	15.2
Non-CVD, non-CMPN	47.2	20.9	30.8	14.9	28.2	40.3	27.9
All CVD	11.0	8.1	10.1	3.9	11.1	7.9	8.2
Ischemic heart disease	2.9	3.5	2.2	0.8	3.5	3.0	2.5
Stroke	5.2	1.5	2.5	1.6	1.6	2.5	2.4
Rheumatic heart disease	1.1	0.5	0.1	0.2	0.5	0.2	0.5

CMPN = communicable, maternal, perinatal, and nutritional diseases; CVD = cardiovascular disease; LatAm = Latin America; MEC = Middle Eastern Crescent; SSA = sub-Saharan Africa.
Adapted from Murray CJL, Lopez AD: The Global Burden of Disease. Cambridge, MA, Harvard School of Public Health, 1996.

TABLE 1–6 Age-Adjusted, All-Cause and Cardiovascular Mortality in European Countries, 1990-1992*

Country	All Causes	CVD	CHD	Stroke
Established market economies				
Spain				
Men	1323	399	181	93
Women	578	180	52	57
France				
Men	1361	330	142	67
Women	552	122	36	35
Portugal				
Men	1673	593	207	267
Women	805	305	73	158
Finland				
Men	1691	834	631	110
Women	1718	837	587	132
Scotland				
Men	1846	886	655	139
Women	1103	441	273	107
Economies in transition				
Russian Federation				
Men	2881	1343	767	409
Women	1223	657	288	178
Ukraine				
Men	2940	1490	749	606
Women	1379	830	342	408

CHD = coronary heart disease; CVD = cardiovascular disease.
*Per 100,000 men and women aged 45-75 years. From World Heart Federation: Impending Global Pandemic of Cardiovascular Diseases. Barcelona, Prous Science, 1999.

north. The highest CVD rates in the European established market economies (two to three times higher than the median rates) are in Finland, Northern Ireland, and Scotland, where CVD-related mortality exceeds 800 deaths per 100,000 for men and 500 deaths per 100,000 for women.[32] The lowest CVD rates are in the Mediterranean countries of Spain and France, where annual CVD rates are less than 400 and 200 per 100,000 for men and women, respectively. Although both stroke and CHD rates are higher in northern Europe, the disparity in CHD rates is much greater. For example, male CHD rates are 362 percent higher in Finland than in Spain, whereas stroke rates are only 49 percent higher.[32] CVD rates in Canada, New Zealand, and Australia are similar to rates in the United States.

JAPAN. This country is unique among the EstME. As its rates of communicable disease fell in the early part of the 20th century, stroke rates increased dramatically; and by the middle of the century they were the highest in the world. CHD rates, however, did not rise as sharply as they did in other industrialized nations and have remained lower than in any other industrialized country. Overall CVD rates have fallen 60 percent since the 1960s, largely due to a decrease in age-adjusted stroke rates. Japanese men and women currently have the highest life expectancies in the world: 84.7 years for women and 77.9 years for men.[1] The difference between Japan and other industrialized countries may stem in part from genetic factors, but it is more likely that the average plant-based, low-fat diet and resultant low cholesterol levels have played a more important role. As is true for so many countries, Japanese dietary habits are undergoing substantial changes. In the last half of the 20th century, there was an estimated 9.3-fold increase in annual per capita consumption of meat, a 5.2-fold increase in egg consumption, a 7.4-fold increase in milk and dairy consumption, and a 5.3-fold increase in consumption of fats and oils.[33] These changes may explain possible recent increases in CHD.

Emerging Market Economies

As a group, the EmgME countries have the highest rates of CVD mortality in the world. However, there is substantial variability, with some countries experiencing increasing CVD mortality and others experiencing a decline. Overall rates are similar to those seen in the United States in the 1960s, when CVD was at its peak. Although CHD is generally more common than stroke, the CHD-to-stroke ratio is relatively low, approximating 1 : 1 in several countries. This suggests that the EmgME are largely in the third phase of the epidemiological transition.

Within the EmgME, CVD mortality rates vary widely. The highest CVD mortality rates are in Ukraine (1490 for men and 830 for women per 100,000 population) and Russia (1343 and 657 per 100,000), and the lowest rates are in Slovenia (692 and 313 per 100,000).[32] CVD rates for women are particularly high compared with rates in EstME countries. In the former Soviet and Eastern Bloc countries, CVD predominates as the leading cause of death, accounting for approximately 54 percent of deaths, whereas communicable diseases account for only 6 percent. As expected in this phase of the transition, the average age of people who develop and die of CVD is lower than that in the established market economies.

One major difference between the EstME and the EmgME countries is that CVD mortality rates are not falling in many of the latter countries. On the contrary, since the dissolution of the Soviet Union, there has been a surprising increase in CVD rates in some of these countries. In the former socialist countries of the Russian Federation, Belarus, Ukraine, Estonia, Latvia, and Lithuania, there has been a remarkable increase in CVD rates since 1990. In Russia, life expectancy for men has dropped precipitously since 1986, from 71.6 to 59 years today, but has declined only slightly for women, standing now at 72.2 years. The causes of this decline in life expectancy are not entirely clear. Rapid increases in per capita alcohol consumption may represent one possible cause for the increasing CVD rates that underlie this decline. Inadequate health care infrastructure and lack of institution of preventive public health measures also may contribute to worsening CVD mortality rates.

CVD rates have been stable in Bulgaria, Romania, Hungary, and Poland. The only two emerging market economies in which age-adjusted CVD rates have been declining are the Czech Republic and Slovenia. Even so, CVD rates remain generally higher than in Western European countries (Fig. 1–7).

Developing Economies

Approximately 80 percent of the world's inhabitants live in developing economies (DevE). In general, communicable diseases are nearly twice as likely to cause death than CVD in the DevE. Overall, CVD mortality rates are approximately 23 percent, although this represents only 8.2 percent of total lost disability-adjusted life years (DALYs) because cardiovascular diseases tend to affect an older segment of the population than communicable diseases. An infant death due to malnutrition, for example, results in more lost DALYs than a CHD death in the sixth decade of life. There are vast differences within and between the regions and countries that make up the DevE—some are still in the age of pestilence and famine, whereas others are in the second or even third phase of the epidemiological transition (see Table 1–5).

The character of CVD varies greatly by region. Reporting of CVD event rates is often based on sampling rather than on true national data collection efforts. In China, stroke rates far exceed CHD rates, whereas in India the reverse is true. Rheumatic heart disease remains a major problem in India, China, and sub-Saharan Africa but is less of a problem in other Asian countries and Latin America (Table 1–7).

Many factors contribute to the heterogeneity between and within regions of the DevE. First, the distinct regions are at various stages of the economic and social transitions. Second, vast differences in life style and behavioral risk factors exist. For example, per capita consumption of dairy products (and thus consumption of saturated fat) is much higher in India than it is in China. Third, racial and ethnic differences may lead to altered susceptibilities to various forms of CVD. Finally, social, cultural, political, and economic considerations result in vast disparities in the health care structure in each region.

CHINA. The People's Republic of China accounts for one fifth of the world's population; 69 percent of its inhabitants live outside urban centers. Since the 1950s, life expectancy in China has doubled from 35 years to 70 years. Over the same period, the rate of mortality from CVD increased threefold as a percentage of total deaths, from 12 to 36 percent.[34] As in Japan, stroke is by far the leading cause of cardiovascular death. Hemorrhagic stroke predominates over ischemic stroke, and stroke rates are higher among women than men. These lower rates of CHD and high rates of stroke may be due to genetic factors; however, it has also been hypothesized that overall low serum cholesterol levels may contribute to high rates of hemorrhagic stroke.[35]

There appears to be a north/south gradient, with higher CVD rates in northern China than in southern

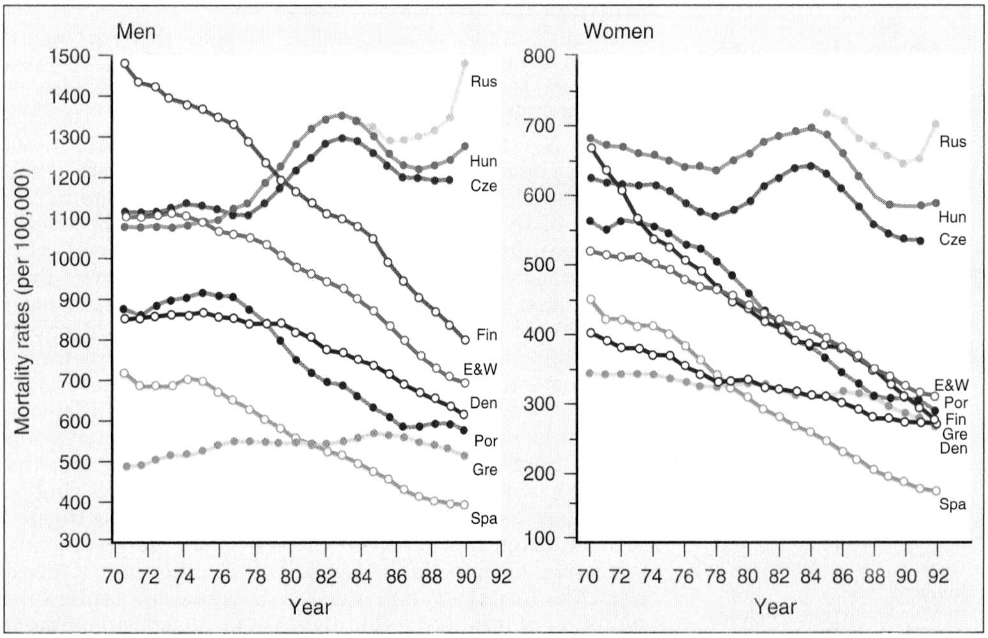

FIGURE 1–7 Time trends in mortality from cardiovascular disease in selected European countries, 1970 to 1992, among men and women aged 45 to 74. Fin = Finland; Hun = Hungary; Rus = Russia; Cze = Czechoslovakia; Por = Portugal; Spa = Spain; Gre = Greece; Den = Denmark; E&W = England and Wales. (From Sans S, Kesteloot H, Kromhout D: The burden of cardiovascular diseases mortality in Europe: Time trends in mortality from CVD in selected European countries. Eur Heart J 18:1231, 1997.)

TABLE 1–7 Rheumatic Heart Disease, Mortality Estimates for 2000

Sector	Number of Deaths (Thousands)	CVD Mortality (%)	DALYs (Thousands)	CVD DALYs (%)
EstME	21	0.6	15	0.8
EmgME	26	1.0	38	2.3
DevE	338	2.8	5697	4.8
India	80,000	2.7	1569	5.5
China	192,000	5.8	2384	8.7
Other Asia	13,000	0.7	159	0.8
Sub-Saharan Africa	19,000	1.8	62	4.7
Middle Eastern Crescent	25,000	1.4	76	3.8
Latin America, Caribbean	9,000	0.8	18	1.9

CVD = cardiovascular disease; DALYs = disability-adjusted life-years; DevE = developing economies; EmgME = emerging market economies; EstME = established market economies.
Adapted from Murray CJL, Lopez AD: The Global Burden of Disease. Cambridge, MA, Harvard School of Public Health, 1996.

China. As is the case in most DevE, there is also an urban/rural gradient for CHD, stroke, and hypertension, with higher rates in urban centers. Regional differences exist in CVD rates, although they are not as great as those seen in India and sub-Saharan Africa. This is likely due to the system of resource distribution that results in less regional difference in the standard of living compared with Africa or India. In general, China appears to be in the third stage of a Japanese-style epidemiological transition, with CVD rates higher than 35 percent, although dominated by stroke and not CHD as they are in the EstME and EmgME. Major features of the transition in China are the rapidly rising rates of cigarette smoking and hypertension, much of which remains untreated.

INDIA. One sixth of the world's population lives in India; approximately three quarters of the more than 1 billion people reside in rural settings. Accurate country-wide data on cause-specific mortality are not available, as death certificate completion is not uniform and the country does not have a centralized registry for CVD deaths. CVD accounts for 24 percent of total deaths.[2] As expected, CVD mortality rates tend to be higher in urban than in rural areas, and CVD is much more prevalent among the upper and middle classes.[36,37]

In contrast to China and much of the rest of Asia, CHD appears to be the dominant form of CVD in India. In 1960, CHD represented 4 percent of all CVD deaths, whereas in 1990 the proportion was greater than 50 percent.[38] CHD death rates are currently about three times higher than stroke rates. This statistic is somewhat unexpected, because stroke tends to be a more dominant factor early in the epidemiological transition. This finding may reflect inaccuracies in cause-specific mortality estimates. However, it may suggest metabolic differences in response to the Western life style of higher-fat diets and lower levels of activity. Based on migration studies, it has been suggested that Indians have an exaggerated insulin insensitivity in response to this life-style pattern that may differentially increase rates of CHD and stroke. Furthermore, the proportion of calories derived from fat, much of which comes from dairy products, is significantly higher in India than in other parts of the developing world.

Although rates of communicable disease remain high, accounting for 51 percent of all deaths and 56 percent of all lost DALYs,[2] the rates are falling rapidly. Thus, India appears to be early in the second phase of the transition, with the urban upper classes in the third phase. As in China, rheumatic heart disease continues to be a major cause of morbidity and mortality (see Table 1-7). Certain remote areas, however, are still in the age of pestilence and famine, with CVD accounting for less than 10 percent of total deaths.[39]

SOUTHEAST ASIA. The diversity of economic circumstances in the countries of Southeast Asia is reflected in the status and character of the epidemiological transition across the region. In South Korea, for example, 57 percent of the population resides in urban centers and the mean annual per capita GNP is $9700, whereas in Cambodia only 19 percent of the population lives in urban centers and the per capita GNP is $240. Average life expectancy in South Korea is 72 years, compared with 53 years in Cambodia.

The rapid economic expansion occurring in several Southeast Asian countries has been accompanied by the expected shift to urbanization and associated life-style changes. In the most industrialized countries, such as Singapore, CVD rates mirror those in the EstME and EmgME, with CVD predominating as a major cause of death and CHD mortality rates twice as high as stroke mortality rates. In other less developed parts of Asia, such as Indonesia and Sri Lanka, the character of disease is similar to that of China. In still others, such as Vietnam and Cambodia, pestilence and famine still predominate.

SUB-SAHARAN AFRICA. In spite of large regional variations, sub-Saharan Africa remains largely in the first phase of the epidemiological transition, with more than 40 percent of all deaths due to infectious and parasitic diseases (see Table 1–5). Life expectancies, as a result, are the lowest in the world.[1] As is the case in India, accurate country-wide data are not generally available, and most data come from urban centers and sampling in rural areas. Overall, CVD is responsible for approximately 10 percent of all deaths in sub-Saharan Africa, with stroke representing the dominant form, in keeping with patterns characteristic of the earlier phases of the epidemiological transition. Even in urban centers, CHD was rare in the middle part of the 20th century.[40] With increasing urbanization, average daily physical activity among urban dwellers is falling and smoking rates are increasing. Hypertension has emerged as a major public health concern, and hypertensive heart disease accounts for the dominance of stroke.[39] Rheumatic heart disease and cardiomyopathies, the latter due mostly to malnutrition, various viral illnesses, and parasitic organisms, are also important causes of CVD mortality and morbidity.

Almost 75 percent of the 40 million adults and children living with HIV/AIDS reside in sub-Saharan Africa.[41] This devastating epidemic is having significant effects on virtually all aspects of health and health care in the region and will definitely influence the natural history of cardiovascular disease. Cardiac involvement is a common sequela of infection with human immunodeficiency virus (HIV) (see Chap. 61). In an autopsy study of adults who died of acquired immunodeficiency syndrome (AIDS), 19 percent had cardiac abnormalities related to HIV infection.[42] Cardiac manifestations can become apparent even earlier in the course of HIV infection. In a prospective study of 952 asymptomatic HIV-infected adults, 8 percent had significant left ventricular dysfunction over 60 months of follow-up.[43] Other cardiovascular-related manifestations of HIV/AIDS include pericardial effusion, infective endocarditis, malignancies such as myocardial Kaposi sarcoma, and myocardial B-cell immunoblastic lymphoma, arrhythmias, and right ventricular and pulmonary disease.[44]

Children with HIV/AIDS are also prone to infection-related cardiovascular disease. These include fetal and congenital cardiovascular malformations, left ventricular dysfunction, myocarditis, vascular disease, dysrhythmias, pericardial disease, cardiovascular tumors, and pulmonary hypertension.[45] In a retrospective study of 68 children with AIDS, predictors of serious cardiac events included recurrent bacterial infections, AIDS-related wasting, encephalopathy, and male gender.[46]

Although much of this research has been conducted in developed countries, reports from Africa describe similar cardiac manifestations of HIV infection.[47,48] At present, few countries in sub-Saharan Africa have the resources to cope adequately with the AIDS epidemic, and few patients receive medications proven to slow the progression of the disease. Thus, opportunistic infections will continue to overshadow cardiac manifestations of AIDS. With the development of public health infrastructures capable of dealing with this disease, cardiac abnormalities should be expected with greater frequency in clinical practice. Use of highly active antiretroviral therapy may further increase the cardiovascular complications of HIV infection.[49,50]

LATIN AMERICA AND THE CARIBBEAN. As a whole, Latin America appears to be in the third phase of the epidemiological transition, although there are vast regional differences. Today, approximately 31 percent of all deaths are attributable to CVD, a figure that is expected to increase to 38 percent by 2020.[2] Although CHD rates are higher than stroke rates (although not to the degree seen in EstME), the combination of these two accounts for more than 75 percent of CVD in this region. CVD rates are beginning to decline in some countries in Latin America and the Caribbean. However, those countries with the lowest CVD rates are facing the steepest increases in CVD mortality rates.[51] Rheumatic heart disease appears to be declining in most countries in this region. Chagas disease remains a major problem in Argentina, Bolivia, Brazil, Chile, Colombia, Costa Rica, Ecuador, El Salvador, Guatemala, Honduras, Mexico, Nicaragua, Paraguay, Peru, Uruguay, and Venezuela, where as much as 30 percent of the population may be infected with the parasite responsible for this disease.

MIDDLE EASTERN CRESCENT. In this region, increasing economic wealth has been characteristically accompanied by urbanization but uncharacteristically accompanied by increasing fertility rates as infant and childhood mortality rates declined. This has resulted in rapid population growth and a young mean age of the population (i.e., 44 percent younger than 15 years of age). The rate of mortality from CVD is increasing rapidly, and CVD is now the leading cause of death, accounting for 25 to 45 percent of total deaths. The adoption of a Western diet has occurred at a rapid rate. As in the established market economies, CHD is the predominant cause of CVD, with about three CHD deaths for every stroke death. Rheumatic heart disease remains a major cause of morbidity and mortality, but the number of hospitalizations for rheumatic heart disease is rapidly declining. This region is entering the third phase of the transition.

Global Trends in Cardiovascular Disease

Estimating global trends in the burden of disease, particularly CVD, is aided by examining regional trends. Because 80 percent or more of the world's population lives in the DevE, global rates of CVD are largely driven by rates in these countries. The acceleration of worldwide CVD rates, for example, is occurring as most DevE countries are entering the second and third phases of the epidemic transition. This section summarizes global and regional estimates for 1990 and 2020 provided by Murray and Lopez.[2]

In 1990, the world population stood at 5.3 billion. CVD accounted for more than 14.3 million deaths, or 28.4 percent of the world's 50 million deaths (Table 1–8). Of these, 6.3 million deaths were due to CHD (44 percent of CVD deaths) and 4.4 million were due to stroke (31 percent of CVD deaths). An estimated 133 million lost DALYs, or 9.7 percent of the total DALYs, were due to CVD.

Expectations for 2020

THE ESTABLISHED MARKET ECONOMIES. By 2020, it is estimated that the world's population will reach 7.8 billion, with much of the growth occurring in the DevE countries (see Table 1–8). In the EstME, population growth (up 13 percent from 1990 to 905 million people) will be fueled by emigration from the DevE. Even this substantial growth, however, represents a gradually shrinking proportion of the world's population, from 15.1 percent in 1990 to 11.5 percent in 2020. In the EmgME, growth will be more modest (up only 5 percent to 365 million people) and also represents a falling world share, from 6.5 percent in 1990 to 4.6 percent in 2020.

TABLE 1–8 Contribution of Various Categories of Disease to Global Mortality

			Total Deaths (%)							
	Population (Millions)	Total Deaths (Millions)	*CMPN*	*Injury*	*Non-CMPN, Non-CVD*	*All CVD*	*IHD*	*Stroke*	*RHD*	*Other CVD*
1990										
World	5267	50.4	34.2	10.1	27.4	28.4	12.4	8.7	0.7	6.7
EstME	798	7.12	6.4	6.2	42.8	44.6	23.4	11.1	0.3	12.0
EmgME	346	3.8	5.6	10.3	29.5	54.6	27.1	16.9	0.7	10.0
DevE	4124	39.5	41.9	10.7	24.3	23.0	9.0	7.5	0.7	5.7
2020										
World	7844	68.3	15.1	12.3	36.4	36.3	16.3	11.3	0.7	8.1
EstME	905	8.6	6.2	5.2	46.3	42.3	22.5	10.6	0.2	9.1
EmgME	365	4.8	2.9	8.6	34.8	53.7	27.0	16.3	0.5	9.9
DevE	6573	54.8	17.6	13.7	34.9	33.8	14.3	10.9	0.8	12.1

CMPN = communicable, maternal, perinatal, and nutritional diseases; CVD = cardiovascular disease; DevE = developing economies; EmgME = emerging market economies; EstME = established market economies; IHD = ischemic heart disease; RHD = rheumatic heart disease.
Adapted from Murray CJL, Lopez AD: The Global Burden of Disease. Cambridge, MA, Harvard School of Public Health, 1996.

Continued rapid growth in the DevE will increase their population by more than 60 percent, from 4.1 billion people in 1990 to 6.6 billion in 2020, or 84 percent of the world's people. By 2020, CVD will be responsible for an estimated 25 million deaths annually (36.3 percent of all deaths), more than twice the number of deaths caused by the combination of communicable, maternal, perinatal, and nutritional conditions. As deaths from these conditions fall from 34.2 percent of the total to 15.1 percent, CVD takes on greater significance. In terms of lost DALYs, those due to CVD are expected to double between 1990 and 2020, from less than 10 percent to greater than 20 percent.

In the EstME, the modest decline in CVD death rates begun in the latter third of the 20th century will continue, with the proportion of total deaths falling from 44.6 to 42.3 percent. The rate of decline, however, appears to be slowing. The absolute number of deaths as well as the prevalence of CVD will continue to increase as the population continues to age. In terms of lost DALYs, the proportion due to CVD will remain stable at about 19 percent.

THE EMERGING MARKET ECONOMIES. In the EmgME, there will be little change in the overall proportion of deaths due to CVD (54.6 percent in 1990 and 53.7 percent in 2020). As a reflection of the anticipated decreases in DALYs lost due to communicable, maternal, perinatal, and nutritional diseases, lost DALYs due to CVD will increase as a proportion of the total (23.2 percent in 1990 to 26 percent in 2020). The average age of those persons afflicted with CVD will increase.

THE DEVELOPING MARKET ECONOMIES. In the DevE, an estimated 9 million persons died of CVD in 1990. By 2020, that figure will more than double to more than 18 million persons annually, accounting for approximately three fourths of all CVD deaths worldwide. What will drive this overall rapid rise in CVD mortality rates in the DevE? One major factor is the projected 60 percent increase in population between 1990 and 2020. Another is that most of the countries that make up the DevE will have entered the third phase of the epidemiological transition by 2020. Substantial declines in communicable disease rates, from 41.2 percent in 1990 to 17.6 percent in 2020, will increase the proportion of DALYs lost due to CVD by more than 50 percent (8.2 percent in 1990 to 13.8 percent in 2020). Because CVD will afflict a younger population in the DevE than in the more developed economies, more than 100 of the 133 million DALYs lost to CVD (75 percent) will occur in this region.

Only in China and sub-Saharan Africa will stroke rates far exceed CHD rates and remain the predominant form of CVD, accounting for about half of all CVD deaths. In the other Asian countries and Latin America, CHD rates will be only slightly greater than stroke rates, whereas the CHD-to-stroke ratio will exceed 2 in India and the Middle Eastern Crescent.

Regional Trends in Risk Factors

As indicated earlier, the global variation in CVD rates is related to temporal and regional variations in known risk behaviors and factors. Discussions of the strength of the associations of the various factors with CVD are found elsewhere in this text (see Chap. 36). Ecological analyses of major CVD risk factors and mortality demonstrate high correlations between expected and observed mortality rates for the three main risk factors—smoking, serum cholesterol, and hypertension[52,53]—and suggest that many of the regional variations are based on differences in conventional risk factors. This section focuses on regional differences in these risk factors that help explain regional variations in the rate and character of the epidemiological transition. Today, the adoption of risky behaviors such as smoking and eating a Western-type diet has preceded the development of advanced health care delivery systems due to economic realities in the DevE.

Tobacco

Smoking represents an important and rapidly growing avoidable global cause of CVD and total death. Worldwide, more than 1.3 billion people smoke cigarettes or other tobacco products.[54] Tobacco currently causes an estimated 4.9 million deaths annually (8.8 percent of all deaths). This represents 1 million more tobacco-related deaths than in 1990, with the increase being most marked in developing countries.[1] If current smoking patterns continue, by 2020 the global burden of disease attributable to tobacco will reach 9 million deaths annually, with 7 million of these in developing countries.[55]

Regionally, the highest per capita cigarette consumption rates are in Europe at 2080 per year, followed closely by the countries of the Western Pacific with 1945 per day and the Americas with 1530; they are the lowest in Africa, where annual per capita consumption is 480 cigarettes (Fig. 1–8).[56]

In the market economies, smoking rates are declining, with the most substantial changes in the EstME. In the United States, for example, 42 percent of adults smoked in 1965, whereas only 23 percent currently smoke.[14] Over the same period, per capita consumption declined from 4200 cigarettes per year to well under 2000.[57] Among young men and women, smoking rates increased through the 1990s but now appear to be declining.[58,59] In the EmgME countries, smoking rates are extremely high—59 percent of men and 26 percent of women smoked in 1995—but are stable or falling.[60]

In the DevE, tobacco represents an important cash crop and source of employment, two things that are often in short supply. On average, about 48 percent of adult men smoke, and smoking rates are increasing about 3.4 percent per year.[56] In some countries included in the DevE, smoking rates among men are staggeringly high, reaching 73 percent in Vietnam[61] and even higher in parts of Nepal.[62] Throughout the developing world, women have traditionally represented only a small proportion of the number of smokers. That is certain to change. In terms of sheer numbers, the number of women living in the DevE will rise from 2.6 billion in 1990 to 3.9 billion by 2020. As women's spending power increases, tobacco companies are targeting them as customers even as woman-specific health education and quitting programs are rare.[63]

A unique feature of the DevE is easy access to smoking during the early stages of the epidemiological transition due

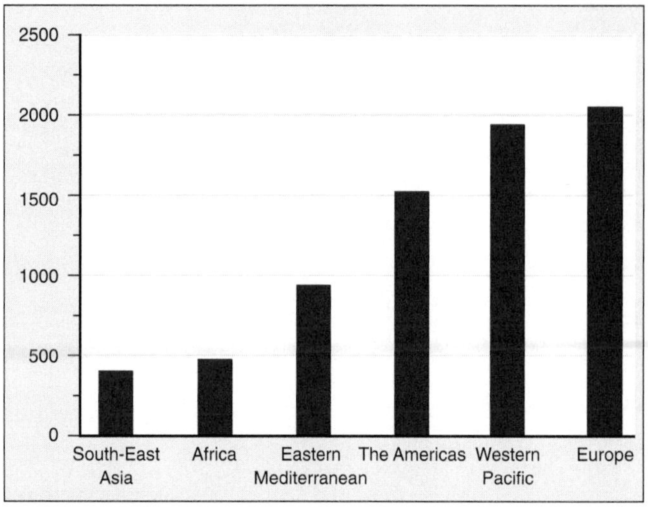

FIGURE 1–8 Annual per capita cigarette consumption in major regions of the world, 2000 estimates. (From World Health Report 1999: Making a Difference. Geneva, World Health Organization, 1999.)

to the availability of relatively inexpensive tobacco products. In the established market economies, cigarette smoking peaked late in the third phase of the transition. In many DevE that are in the first or second stages, however, male smoking rates already exceed the peak rates of the EstME, and rates are expected to continue rising among both men and women. The impact of more widespread smoking earlier in the epidemiological transition means a more rapid increase in CVD rates as the DevE enter the third phase of the transition. In China, which is in the early stages of the epidemiological transition, the 1996 National Prevalence Survey determined that 63 percent of men (but only 3.8 percent of women) were current smokers.[64] A massive retrospective study of 1 million deaths estimated that tobacco was responsible for 13 percent (600,000 deaths) of total mortality in China in 1990 and will account for 3 million deaths a year by 2025.[65]

Diet (see Chap. 41)

With regard to cardiovascular disease, a key element of dietary change is an increase in intake of saturated animal fats and hydrogenated vegetable fats, which contain atherogenic trans fatty acids, along with a decrease in intake of plant-based foods. Although dietary habits clearly vary from country to country, intake of dietary fat tends to be low in many DevE and high in many EstME and generally increases with annual per capita income (Fig. 1–9). Fat contributes less than 20 percent of calories in rural China and India,[66] less than 30 percent in Japan,[67] and well above 30 percent in the United States. Caloric contributions from fat appear to be falling in the EstME. In the United States, for example, the percent of calories from fat has steadily declined over the past 30 years, from 45 percent of calories in 1965 to 34 percent in 1994, although the total amount of fat in the diet has increased slightly since 1989.[68]

Even in the DevE, which are broadly characterized by low fat intake, fat intake varies greatly and tends to increase with industrialization and urbanization. For example, although dietary fat accounts for less than 20 percent of total calories in rural China, in urban areas it contributes more than 30 percent of calories.[69]

Physical Inactivity

One byproduct of the increased mechanization that accompanies the economic transition is decreased physical activity. In the market economies, the widespread prevalence of physical inactivity produces a high population-attributable risk of cardiovascular consequences. In the United States, approximately 25 percent of the population does not participate in any leisure-time physical activity and only 22 percent report engaging in sustained physical activity for at least 30 minutes on 5 or more days a week (the current recommendation).[70,71] The shift from physically demanding, agriculture-based work to largely sedentary industry- and office-based work is occurring throughout the developing world. This is also accompanied by a switch from physically demanding transportation to mechanized transportation.

Obesity (see Chap. 41)

Obesity is clearly associated with increased risk of CHD. However, much of this risk may be mediated by other CVD risk factors, including hypertension, diabetes mellitus, and lipid profile imbalances. Whereas rates of smoking and hypertension tend to increase early in the epidemiological transition, obesity tends to increase later. Worldwide, obesity accounts for approximately 58 percent of diabetes cases, 21 percent of ischemic heart disease cases, 8 to 42 percent of certain cancers, and more than 10 percent of deaths.[1]

In the mid-1980s, the World Health Organization's MONICA Project sampled 48 populations for cardiovascular risk factors. In all but one male population (China), and in most of the female populations, between 50 percent and 75 percent of adults aged 35 to 64 years were overweight or obese.[72] A later follow-up study showed that the prevalence of obesity has continued to increase.[73]

In many EstME, mean body mass index is rising at an alarming rate even as mean plasma cholesterol levels are falling and age-adjusted hypertension levels remain fairly stable during the fourth phase (the age of delayed degenerative diseases).[74] In the United States, this is occurring among all sectors of the population; however, rates are increasing faster among minorities and women.[75] Overweight and obesity are not limited to market economies. In many of the DevE countries, obesity appears to coexist with undernutrition and malnutrition. Although the prevalence of obesity in DevE countries is certainly less than among the market economies, it is on the rise there as well.[74] A study in Mauritius, for example, documented rapid increases in obesity between 1987 and 1992,[76] whereas another study estimated that 44 percent of African women living in the Cape Peninsula were obese.[77]

Excess weight early in life not only increases the likelihood of adult obesity, but it also increases the prevalence of weight-related disorders, including CVD. Further increases in the prevalence of overweight and obesity are to

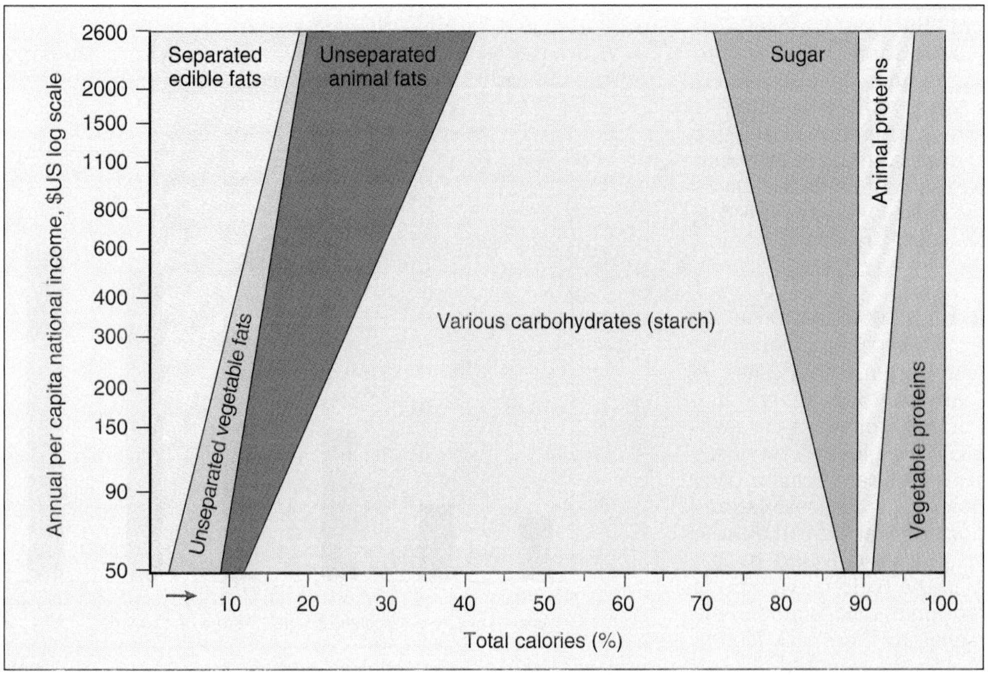

FIGURE 1–9 Association between income and dietary intake, based on country-level sources of energy. (From Drwenowski A, Popkin BM: The nutrition transition: New trends in the global diet. Nutr Rev 55:31, 1997.)

be expected if data on childhood and adolescent obesity are any indication. In Great Britain, for example, waist size and body mass index among youths aged 11 to 16 years increased significantly between 1977 and 1997.[78]

Lipid Levels

The causal association between plasma cholesterol levels and risk of CVD is indisputable. Low levels of high-density lipoproteins and elevated triglycerides are also clearly associated with excess risk of CVD, and this association holds across racial and ethnic divisions. The lipid profile appears to have a greater impact on CHD than on stroke. Worldwide, high cholesterol levels are estimated to cause 56 percent of global ischemic heart disease and 18 percent of strokes, amounting to 4.4 millions deaths annually.[1]

As countries move through the epidemiological transition, mean population plasma cholesterol levels tend to rise. Social and individual changes that accompany urbanization clearly play a role, because plasma cholesterol levels tend be higher among urban residents than among rural residents. This shift is largely driven by greater consumption of dietary fats—primarily from animal products and processed vegetable oils—and decreased physical activity. Cross-cultural differences in mean cholesterol levels reflect this pattern. In rural Nigeria, which is early in the epidemiological transition, mean cholesterol levels are 120 mg/dl (3.1 mmol/l),[79] whereas in the heavily industrialized United States and northern Europe, which are in the fourth phase, mean cholesterol levels are 200 mg/dl (5.2 mmol/l) and 240 mg/dl (6.2 mmol/l),[80] respectively. In the established market economies, mean population cholesterol levels are generally falling. Japan is something of an exception to this pattern, with only relatively recent increases in average serum cholesterol levels.[81,82] This may help explain why CHD rates did not increase in the third phase of Japan's epidemiological transition. If plasma cholesterol levels continue to rise, however, CHD rates may follow in the coming years. In the emerging market economies, mean population cholesterol levels also tend to be high, but levels are stable or rising.

In the DevE, there is wide variation in mean population cholesterol levels. In Asia, cholesterol levels rose steadily in the last decades of the 20th century, generally faster in urban areas than in rural areas.[83] Once as low as 115 mg/dl (3 mmol/l), mean total cholesterol levels now tend to be at or above 190 mg/dl (5 mmol/l). In Singapore, mean population levels reached 250 mg/dl (6.5 mmol/l) in the mid-1980s, but have since fallen. In many countries in Latin America and the Caribbean, cholesterol levels approach those of northern Europe. A population survey in Bogotá, Colombia, for example, found that 46 percent of men had serum cholesterol levels greater than 250 mg/dl (6.5 mmol/l).[84] In sub-Saharan Africa, mean cholesterol levels in rural areas are similar to the low levels seen in China, whereas levels are considerably higher in urban centers.[85] Given the high level of global capacity to produce Western-style food products at low cost, developing countries can now afford to adopt a Western dietary life style earlier in the economic transition than was possible in the past.

As is true for hypertension, rates of hypercholesterolemia are increasing far faster than the resources needed for widespread detection and treatment. Thus, the impact of both of these on atherosclerosis may be far greater than they have been in developed economies.

Hypertension

Hypertension is clearly a risk factor for CHD and stroke (see Chaps. 36 and 37). Elevated blood pressure is an early hallmark of the epidemiological transition. Rising mean population blood pressure is apparent as countries industrialize; emigration from less developed to more developed countries, as well as emigration from rural to urban settings, results in increasing blood pressure levels among emigrants. Among urban-dwelling men and women in India, for example, the prevalence of hypertension is 25.5 percent and 29.0 percent, respectively, whereas it is just 14.0 percent and 10.8 percent, respectively, among those living in rural communities.[86] Although the relative increase in mortality associated with a given increase in blood pressure is similar in various regions of the world, the absolute risk at the same blood pressure level varies greatly.[87] In addition, the overall impact of hypertension may vary depending on the proportion of individuals in a country who have untreated hypertension.

Worldwide, approximately 62 percent of strokes and 49 percent of cases of ischemic heart disease are attributable to suboptimal (<115 mm Hg systolic) blood pressure, and it is thought to account for more than 7 millions deaths annually.[1]

In the EstME, hypertension remains a major cause of CVD morbidity and mortality despite high rates of detection and treatment. Given the relationship of increasing blood pressure with advancing age, the prevalence of hypertension is increasing in most (aging) established market economies. In most of the EstME, the proportion of the population with untreated hypertension is declining, although in the United States there has been a slight reversal of this trend.[29] In the EmgME, the prevalence of hypertension is at least as high as it is in the EstME, whereas rates of treatment are much lower. This may explain, at least in part, the higher stroke rates in these countries in relation to CHD rates.

Across the DevE countries, hypertension rates are quite variable. One major concern in these countries is the high rate of undetected, and therefore untreated, hypertension. In northern Asian countries such as China and South Korea, hypertension is rapidly increasing,[88] with higher rates in urban areas than rural areas. The high rates of hypertension, especially undiagnosed hypertension, throughout Asia likely contribute to the high prevalence of hemorrhagic stroke. An analysis of several large cohort studies from mainland China, Hong Kong, Japan, Singapore, South Korea, Taiwan, Australia, and New Zealand with more than 3 million person-years of follow-up demonstrated continuous log-linear associations between systolic blood pressure and risks of stroke, ischemic heart disease, and total cardiovascular death down to at least 115 mm Hg.[89]

In contrast, rates of hypertension remain relatively low in sub-Saharan Africa. However, the attributable risk of hypertension in urban centers is exceedingly high in most countries of this region owing to lack of available treatment. Data on mean blood pressure levels in the population are limited. High rates of hypertension are apparent only in urban centers, where there are a significant number of hospitalizations for hypertension, largely owing to the very low rates of detection and treatment.[39,90]

In Latin America and the Caribbean, as well as in the Middle Eastern Crescent, hypertension rates are also quite variable. A review of Latin American hypertension studies published between 1995 and 2000, for example, showed overall prevalence of hypertension ranging from 11.1 percent in Chile to 43.0 percent in Cuba, and hypertension control ranging from 22 percent in Chile to 58 percent in Mexico.[91] In these regions, as in others, hypertension rates tend to be highest in more affluent countries and urban centers. However, even in rural areas hypertension can be prevalent. In a screening program in a rural district of Ecuador, 36 percent of the 4284 individuals screened had hypertension; only 4 of these cases were well controlled by treatment.[92] During 2.5 years of follow-up, hypertension-related cardiovascular disease was the main cause of death.

Diabetes Mellitus (see Chap. 40)

Diabetes and impaired glucose tolerance represent strong risk factors for vascular disease, including CHD, cerebrovascular disorders, and peripheral vascular disease. As a consequence of, or in addition to, increasing body mass index and decreasing levels of physical activity, worldwide rates of diabetes—predominantly type 2 diabetes, or non-insulin-dependent diabetes mellitus—are on the rise. According to World Health Organization models, the number of persons with diabetes will swell from 135 million people in 1995 to 300 million in 2025, a 35 percent increase in worldwide prevalence (from 4.0 to 5.4 percent).[93] The largest increases in prevalence of diabetes will be in China (up 68 percent between 1995 and 2025) and India (up 59 percent), followed by Latin America and the Caribbean (41 percent), other Asian countries and the Pacific Islands (41 percent), and the Middle Eastern Crescent (30 percent). The market economies will experience increases between 26 percent and 28 percent.

The prevalence of diabetes varies greatly by geographic region, race, and ethnic composition. There appear to be clear genetic susceptibilities of various racial and ethnic groups. For example, Pima Indians living in the southwestern United States are eight times more likely to develop diabetes than the general U.S. population.[94] Hispanic Americans also tend to have higher rates than white Americans.[95] Migration studies suggest that South Asians and Indians also tend to be at higher risk than those of European extraction.

Diabetes mellitus is associated with a number of other CVD risk factors, including high triglyceride levels, low high-density lipoprotein levels, central obesity, and hypertension. In relative terms, the attributable risk of diabetes is higher in women than in men.

Future Challenges

Although the concept of the epidemiological transition offers tremendous insight into how and why CVD is emerging as the predominant global cause of morbidity and mortality, it does not mandate that this must be so. As has been seen from the experience of established market economies, CVD rates rise in a predictable fashion with increasing rates of risk factors and behaviors. It is equally true that population-based and individual interventions can have an impact on both the rates and the consequences of CVD. This raises the possibility of altering the epidemiological transition to blunt the increase in regional CVD rates or to hasten their decline. The transfer of lower-cost health and food technologies from the EstME to the DevE has produced great gains in the fight against communicable diseases and clearly helped hasten the transition out of the age of pestilence and famine. It is possible that similar interventions could alter the course of later stages.

Given the multifactorial nature of CVD, no single solution will be generally applicable to all geographic and economic regions of the world. In this section are outlined the major challenges facing each economic region, and the various strategies to address these problems are discussed. Appropriate regional strategies depend on a number of factors, including a country or region's stage in the epidemiological transition, the rate of change of the epidemiological transition, individual and collective resources, and cultural and political factors.

Three complementary strategies can be used to reduce morbidity and mortality from CVD (Table 1–9). First, the overall burden of CVD risk factors in the entire population can be lowered through population-wide public health measures. These include detection and surveillance strategies,

TABLE 1–9 Complementary Strategies to Reduce Morbidity and Mortality due to Cardiovascular Disease

Lower overall burden of risk factors in the entire population through population-wide public health measures such as detection and surveillance strategies, public education campaigns, and the institution of low-cost, population-wide preventive interventions.
Identify and target higher-risk subgroups of the population who stand to benefit the most from moderate, cost-effective prevention interventions through screening and targeting preventive interventions such as treatment of hypertension and cholesterol.
Allocate resources to acute and chronic higher-cost treatments and secondary prevention interventions for those with clinically manifest disease.

public education campaigns, and the institution of low-cost, population-wide preventive interventions. National campaigns against cigarette smoking are an example of the public health approach. The second approach involves identifying and targeting higher risk subgroups of the population who stand to benefit the most from moderate, cost-effective prevention interventions. This involves screening and targeting preventive interventions such as treatment of hypertension and cholesterol. Third, resources can be allocated to acute and chronic higher-cost treatments as well as secondary prevention interventions for those with clinically manifest disease. Typically, resources are allocated simultaneously to all three strategies; however, this three-pronged approach has been implemented mostly in EstME with abundant financial resources for health care. In the following sections are outlined the major challenges and possible solutions for each region.

Established Market Economies

Although CVD mortality rates have fallen in most EstME, several important challenges remain. First, socioeconomic and racial disparities in CVD rates continue to linger. In the United States, for example, although rates of CVD mortality have fallen across the population, there are still wide disparities between racial and ethnic groups. Thus, a major goal will be to accelerate the widespread application of preventive and therapeutic technologies to all racial, ethnic, and socioeconomic groups.

Second, the rate of declining CVD mortality appears to be stagnating. Over the past 5 years in the United States, age-adjusted stroke mortality rates have not changed and the decline in CHD rates has slowed. These may be the result of troubling trends in a number of coronary risk factors: although older men and women continue to stop smoking, young adults and teenagers, particularly young women, are smoking at increasing rates; the rates of those appropriately treated for hypertension has decreased slightly in the past 5 years; obesity and diabetes rates are accelerating rapidly. Perhaps most troubling are observations of increasing rates of obesity and decreasing rates of physical activity in children. Taken together, these trends may explain the flattening of mortality curves and may also explain why mortality rates have fallen faster than CVD incidence rates.

In the absence of efforts to reverse these trends in risk factors, we may once again see increasing rates of CVD. More public health dollars need to be directed at anti-smoking efforts that target high-risk groups such as teenage girls and at broader application of guidelines for detecting and managing hypertension and hyperlipidemia. Effective strategies to increase activity and reverse trends in obesity and diabetes must be developed and implemented.

Third, the prevalence of CVD will continue to increase with the increasing mean age of a population even if that population's age-adjusted mortality rates continue to decline. In addition, incremental advances in therapeutic health technology and secondary prevention have led to increasing numbers of people surviving with CVD, which consumes increasing amounts of resources. With the institution of many life-saving strategies among those who present with acute manifestations of atherosclerotic disease, more and more individuals are surviving acute events such as myocardial infarction. For example, approximately one third of those who presented to hospitals with acute myocardial infarction in the 1950s died. Today, in-hospital mortality is less than half that, despite the fact that sicker and older patients are presenting to the hospital. Furthermore, CHD is being diagnosed in increasing numbers of individuals before cardiovascular events. Thousands of pacemakers and defibrillators are implanted each year. As more and more individuals survive longer with CVD, the prevalence of congestive heart failure increases, even as mortality from congestive heart failure is declining.[96,97] Thus, the management of congestive heart failure will consume more and more health care resources.[98] A major challenge for most established market economies will be the increasing financial burden of the management of CVD. More efficient and cost-effective strategies for treating CVD will have to be developed.

Emerging Market Economies

The EmgME region is largely in the third phase of the epidemiological transition. However, the resources available are considerably less than those available in the EstME. Annual per capita GNP in the EmgME ranges from about $1000 to $5000, less than the United States spends per capita on health care alone. This mandates making careful choices in terms of allocating health care dollars to each of the three strategies outlined earlier (see Table 1–9).

In the EmgME, the two overarching goals are to manage the increasing number of people with CVD and to hasten the transition from the third to the fourth phase of the epidemiological transition. This will likely enhance overall productivity in the region, because during the third phase of the epidemiological transition, CVD, and particularly CHD, often afflicts individuals at the age of highest productivity. In terms of challenges facing the former socialist countries, the region can be divided into two categories: those countries with stable or declining rates and those countries with increasing CVD rates. For countries with stable or declining rates, the three-pronged approach used in the EstME should serve as a model. For those countries experiencing rapid rises in CVD rates, an important first step will be implementing more centralized efforts at compiling data on rates of disease and risk factors and then determining the major country-specific contributors to the rise. All countries in this economic sector need more careful tracking and assessment of risk factors in terms of population-attributable risk. Better tracking of CVD rates and risk factors will allow for more careful allocation of scarce preventive resources.

National guidelines that have been developed in the EstME need to be adapted for the EmgME. However, Western guidelines should be modified, taking into account public health and healthcare infrastructure and economic realities. Governments should initiate major public health initiatives aimed at life-style factors, including lowering rates of smoking and drinking, modifying diet, and increasing physical activity. Major public health priorities should include smoking cessation and the detection and control of hypertension, both of which are highly cost effective. The targeting of higher-risk individuals for higher-cost preventive strategies such as pharmacological lowering of cholesterol and blood pressure will initially need to be confined to areas such as urban centers, where the burden is high and the necessary laboratory-based health care infrastructure is available.

Throughout this economic sector, improvements in health care delivery systems will be needed to manage the already high rates of CVD prevalent in these countries. Careful attention must be paid to the transfer of lower-cost health technology, keeping in mind the considerably lower annual health care expenditures in the EmgME countries compared with those in the EstME. An intervention such as the more widespread and appropriate use of aspirin and beta blockers during acute myocardial infarction is an example of an extremely cost-effective life-saving therapy that should be implemented universally before extensive resources are directed at higher-cost interventions such as angioplasty. Personnel issues must also be addressed, given the general shortage of health care professionals in the EmgME.

Developing Economies

The problems facing the DevE may be the most challenging. These countries have rapidly increasing burdens of CVD early in their economic transitions. They often do not have the per capita resources needed to create the three-pronged type of public health and health care infrastructure currently available in the EstME. In many DevE, per capita health care expenditures are less than $50 per year. In addition, there are a number of competing national priorities, including the stimulation of economic growth, social and political change, and the devastation wrought by communicable diseases.

Rising CVD rates will eventually exert a drag on economic growth. Early in the epidemiological transition, CVD deaths occur among younger individuals as opposed to later in the transition. Thus, the economic impact on both the family and national productivity is greater in developing economies than in established market economies. The loss of the head of a household from CVD (or any other disease) has a devastating impact on the health and well-being of the entire family. In Bangladesh, for example, when there is an adult death, a child who depends on that adult has a 12-fold higher probability of death.[99] At present, the data on the economic consequences of CVD in the DevE are limited. Much more work is needed to refine estimates that would permit more thoughtful allocation of health care resources.

As mentioned earlier, the epidemiological transition has been accelerated at least in part by an efficient translation of risk behaviors and the rise in risk factors from the EstME to the DevE early in the economic transition. The rapid spread of cigarette smoking is a prime example of this. A major challenge for developing countries is to attempt to change the natural history of the epidemiological transition. That such alterations are possible is evident from the experience of Japan, in which CHD rates were kept relatively low during a fairly rapid economic transition to an industrial-based economy. Although imbedded cultural practice such as diet likely played a large role, the Japanese experience illustrates that the nature of the transition is variable.

As is true for the EmgME, a critical first step in developing a comprehensive plan for many of the DevE is better assessment of cause-specific mortality and morbidity as well as the prevalence of the major preventable risk factors for CVD. In many areas of the DevE, reliable estimates of the prevalence and incidence of CVD as well as risk behaviors and factors are not available. Improved estimates would enable better allocation of resources based on country-wide burdens of disease. Beginning first in the urban centers and then moving out to rural areas, government agencies will need to make careful assessments of, and create longitudinal surveillance of, rates of disease and risk factors for which low-cost strategies are available. High priorities include smoking and hypertension, for which the population-attributable risks are likely to be high and the cost efficacy favorable. The strategy for the detection and management of high cholesterol must be carefully tailored for each region due to higher costs. Public health approaches aimed at educating the general population about diet and exercise may be useful, but precise estimates of cost efficacy are not available on these even for EstME countries. Drug therapy for cholesterol lowering is likely less cost effective than short-term smoking cessation programs or managing hypertension with low-cost medications.

Once these initial assessments have been made, resources should be carefully allocated to each prong of the overall strategy (see Table 1–9), with most resources dedicated to the first two—national programs for population-wide prevention and guidelines for screening and targeted interventions. Such programs must be based on the population-attributable risk and the available resources. These guidelines must be implemented with low-cost campaigns. Such prevention-directed efforts could blunt the rise in disease rates already apparent in many developed countries. Given the extreme limitations in per capita health care resources in many DevE, the allocation of resources to higher-cost strategies for treating CVD may divert resources from the potentially more effective population-wide efforts. Thus, efforts targeted at interventions and high-technology therapeutics may have to be parsimoniously implemented only in those urban areas where risk is highest. Assistance in the transfer of health care and preventive technologies from countries with developed economies will greatly enhance regional efforts in countries with developing economies.

Summary and Conclusions

We are now halfway through a two-century transition in which CVD will dominate as the major cause of death and disease. Although CVD rates are declining in the EstME, they are increasing in virtually every other region of the world. From a worldwide perspective, the rate of change in the global burden of CVD is accelerating, reflecting the change in the developing economies, which represent more than 80 percent of the world's population, as they move rapidly through the second and third phases of the epidemiological transition. The consequences of this epidemic will be substantial on many levels—individual mortality and morbidity, family suffering, and staggering economic costs, both the direct costs of diagnosis and treatment and the indirect costs of lost productivity.

Each region of the world faces major challenges presented by the epidemic of CVD. There is no single global solution to the rising burden of CVD, given the vast differences in social, cultural, and economic circumstances. The EstME must minimize disparities to reverse unfavorable trends in CVD risk factors and behaviors and deal with the increasing prevalence of CVD in an aging population. To hasten the transition from the third to the fourth phase of the epidemiological transition, the EmgME must find ways to efficiently care for increasing numbers of individuals with CVD as well as to deploy lower-cost prevention strategies. The most complex challenges are those facing the DevE. They must dedicate often minuscule resources to better assessment of rates of death, disease, and CVD risk factors. The allocation of resources to lower-cost preventive strategies will likely be more cost effective than dedicating resources to high-cost management of CVD.

The EstME must continue to bear the burden of research and development into every aspect of prevention and treatment. Through further expansion of the knowledge base, particularly regarding the economic consequences of various treatment and prevention strategies, it is possible that the efficient transfer of low-cost preventive and therapeutic strategies may alter the natural course of the epidemiological transition in every part of the world and thus reduce the excess global burden of preventable CVD.

REFERENCES

Epidemiological Transitions

1. World Health Report 2002: Reducing risks, promoting healthy life. Geneva, World Health Organization, 2002.
2. Murray CJL, Lopez AD: The Global Burden of Disease. Cambridge, MA, Harvard School of Public Health, 1996.
3. Omran AR: The epidemiologic transition: A theory of the epidemiology of population change. Milbank Mem Fund Q 49:509, 1971.
4. Olshansky SJ, Ault AB: The fourth stage of the epidemiologic transition: The age of delayed degenerative diseases. Milbank Q 64:355, 1986.
5. Pearson TA, Jamison DT, Trijo-Gutierrez H: Cardiovascular disease. *In* Jamison DT (ed): Disease Control Priorities in Developing Countries. New York, Oxford University Press, 1993, pp 577-599.
6. Pearson TA: Global perspectives on cardiovascular disease. Evidence Based Cardiovasc Med 1:4, 1997.
7. Sheth T, Nair C, Nargundkar M, et al: Cardiovascular and cancer mortality among Canadians of European, south Asian and Chinese origin from 1979 to 1993: An analysis of 1.2 million deaths. CMAJ 161:132, 1999.
8. National Center for Health Statistics: US Decennial Life Tables for 1989-91, Some Trends and Comparisons of United States Life Table Data, 1900-91. Hyattsville, MD, 1999. DHHS-99-1150-3.
9. Control of infectious diseases. MMWR Morb Mortal Wkly Rep 48:621, 1999.
10. Center for Nutrition Policy: Nutrient content of the US food supply, 1909-1994: A summary. Washington, DC, U.S. Department of Agriculture, 1998.
11. Office on Smoking and Health: Reducing the health consequences of smoking: 25 years of progress. A report of the Surgeon General. Rockville, Maryland, US Department of Health and Human Services, Public Health Service, Centers for Disease Control, 1989. DHHS Publication No. (CDC) 89-8411.
12. Safer and healthier foods. MMWR Morb Mortal Wkly Rep 48:905, 1999.
13. Flexner A: Medical education in the United States and Canada: A report to the Carnegie Foundation for the Advancement of Teaching. Boston, Merrymount Press, 1910.
14. Office on Smoking and Health: Smoking prevalence among U.S. adults. Centers for Disease Control and Prevention, 2002. (*http://www.cdc.gov/tobacco/research_data/adults_prev/prevali.htm*)
15. U.S. Bureau of the Census: Measuring 50 years of economic change using the March Current Population Survey. Washington, DC, U.S. Government Printing Office, 1998, pp P60-203.
16. Starr P: The social transformation of American medicine. New York, Basic Books, 1982.
17. Feldstein PJ: Health care economics. Albany, NY, Delmar Publishers, 1998.
18. Decline in deaths from heart disease and stroke—United States, 1900-1999. MMWR Morb Mortal Wkly Rep 48:649, 1999.
19. Goldman L, Cook EF: The decline in ischemic heart disease mortality rates: An analysis of the comparative effects of medical interventions and changes in lifestyle. Ann Intern Med 101:825, 1984.
20. Hunink MG, Goldman L, Tosteson AN, et al: The recent decline in mortality from coronary heart disease, 1980-1990. The effect of secular trends in risk factors and treatment. JAMA 277:535, 1997.
21. Cooper R, Cutler J, Desvigne-Nickens P, et al: Trends and disparities in coronary heart disease, stroke, and other cardiovascular diseases in the United States: Findings of the national conference on cardiovascular disease prevention. Circulation 102:3137, 2000.
22. Hennekens CH, Albert CM, Godfried SL, et al: Adjunctive drug therapy of acute myocardial infarction—evidence from clinical trials. N Engl J Med 335:1660, 1996.
23. Levit KR, Cowan CA, Lazenby HC, et al: National health spending trends, 1960-1993. Health Aff (Millwood) 13:14, 1994.
24. Levit K, Smith C, Cowan C, et al: Trends in U.S. health care spending, 2001. Health Aff (Millwood) 22:154, 2003.
25. Anand RS, Basiotis PP: Is total fat consumption really decreasing? Washington, DC, US Department of Agriculture, Center for Nutrition Policy and Promotion, 1998. *http://www.usda.gov/agency/cnpp/insght5a.PDF.*
26. American Heart Association: 2003 Heart and Stroke Statistical Update. Dallas, American Heart Association, 2003.
27. Kozak LJ, Hall MJ, Owings MF: National Hospital Discharge Survey: 2000. Hyattsville, MD, National Center for Health Statistics, Centers for Disease Control and Prevention, 2002. Vital Health Statistics, Series 13, No. 153.
28. Arias E: United States life tables, 2000. Hyattsville, MD, National Center for Health Statistics, Centers for Disease Control and Prevention, 2002. National Vital Statistics Report vol 51, no 3.
29. Chobanian AV, Bakris GL, Black HR, et al: The Seventh Report of the Joint National Committee on Prevention, Detection, Evaluation, and Treatment of High Blood Pressure: The JNC 7 Report. JAMA 289:2560, 2003.
30. Fagot-Campagna A, Pettitt DJ, Engelgau MM, et al: Type 2 diabetes among North American children and adolescents: An epidemiologic review and a public health perspective. J Pediatr 136:664, 2000.
31. American Diabetes Association: Type 2 diabetes in children and adolescents. Diabetes Care 23:381, 2000.

Worldwide Variations

32. Sans S, Kesteloot H, Kromhout D: The burden of cardiovascular diseases mortality in Europe. Task Force of the European Society of Cardiology on Cardiovascular Mortality and Morbidity Statistics in Europe. Eur Heart J 18:1231, 1997.

33. Drewnowski A, Popkin BM: The nutrition transition: New trends in the global diet. Nutr Rev 55:31, 1997.
34. Yao C, Wu Z, Wu Y: The changing pattern of cardiovascular diseases in China. World Health Stat Q 46:113, 1993.
35. Okumura K, Iseki K, Wakugami K, et al: Low serum cholesterol as a risk factor for hemorrhagic stroke in men: A community-based mass screening in Okinawa, Japan. Jpn Circ J 63:53, 1999.
36. Singh RB, Niaz MA, Thakur AS, et al: Social class and coronary artery disease in a urban population of North India in the Indian Lifestyle and Heart Study. Int J Cardiol 64:195, 1998.
37. Singh RB, Sharma JP, Rastogi V, et al: Social class and coronary disease in rural population of north India. The Indian Social Class and Heart Survey. Eur Heart J 18:588, 1997.
38. Reddy KS: Cardiovascular diseases in India. World Health Stat Q 46:101, 1993.
39. Bertrand E: Cardiovascular disease in developing countries. *In* Dalla Volta S (ed): Cardiology. New York, McGraw-Hill, 1999, pp 825-834.
40. Muna WF: Cardiovascular disorders in Africa. World Health Stat Q 46:125, 1993.
41. Report on the global HIV/AIDS epidemic. Geneva, United Nations Programme on HIV/AIDS, 2002.
42. Barbaro G, Di Lorenzo G, Grisorio B, Barbarini G: Cardiac involvement in the acquired immunodeficiency syndrome: A multicenter clinical-pathological study. Gruppo Italiano per lo Studio Cardiologico dei Pazienti Affetti da AIDS. AIDS Res Hum Retroviruses 14:1071, 1998.
43. Barbaro G, Di Lorenzo G, Grisorio B, Barbarini G: Incidence of dilated cardiomyopathy and detection of HIV in myocardial cells of HIV-positive patients. Gruppo Italiano per lo Studio Cardiologico dei Pazienti Affetti da AIDS. N Engl J Med 339:1093, 1998.
44. Fisher SD, Lipshultz SE: Epidemiology of cardiovascular involvement in HIV disease and AIDS. Ann N Y Acad Sci 946:13, 2001.
45. Starc TJ, Lipshultz SE, Easley KA, et al: Incidence of cardiac abnormalities in children with human immunodeficiency virus infection: The prospective P2C2 HIV study. J Pediatr 141:327, 2002.
46. Al-Attar I, Orav EJ, Exil V, et al: Predictors of cardiac morbidity and related mortality in children with acquired immunodeficiency syndrome. J Am Coll Cardiol 41:1598, 2003.
47. Danbauchi SS, Okpapi JU: Cardiovascular involvement in HIV/AIDS: Report of 3 cases. West Afr J Med 20:261, 2001.
48. Nzuobontane D, Blackett KN, Kuaban C: Cardiac involvement in HIV infected people in Yaounde, Cameroon. Postgrad Med J 78:678, 2002.
49. Barbaro G: Cardiovascular manifestations of HIV infection. Circulation 106:1420, 2002.
50. Currier JS: Cardiovascular risk associated with HIV therapy. J Acquir Immune Defic Syndr 31 Suppl 1:S16; discussion S24, 2002.
51. Nicholls ES, Peruga A, Restrepo HE: Cardiovascular disease mortality in the Americas. World Health Stat Q 46:134, 1993.

Regional Trends in Risk Factors

52. Kuulasmaa K, Tunstall-Pedoe H, Dobson A, et al: Estimation of contribution of changes in classic risk factors to trends in coronary-event rates across the WHO MONICA Project populations. Lancet 355:675, 2000.
53. The World Health Organization MONICA Project: Ecological analysis of the association between mortality and major risk factors of cardiovascular disease. Int J Epidemiol 23:505, 1994.
54. Shafey O, Dolwick S, Guindon EG: Tobacco Control: Country Profiles. 2nd ed. Atlanta, American Cancer Society, World Health Organization, and International Union Against Cancer, 2003.
55. Peto R, Lopez A: Future worldwide health effects of current smoking patterns. *In* Koop CE, Pearson CE, Schwarz MR (eds): Critical Issues in Global Health. San Francisco, Jossey-Bass, 2001.
56. World Health Report 1999: Making a Difference. Geneva, World Health Organization, 1999.
57. Cigarette report for 2001. Federal Trade Commission, 2003. (*http://www.ftc.gov/os/2003/06/2001cigreport.pdf*)
58. Trends in cigarette smoking among high school students—United States, 1991-2001. MMWR Morb Mortal Wkly Rep 51:409, 2002.
59. Wechsler H, Rigotti NA, Gledhill-Hoyt J, Lee H: Increased levels of cigarette use among college students: A cause for national concern. JAMA 280:1673, 1998.
60. Jha P, Chaloupka FJ: Curbing the epidemic: Governments and the economics of tobacco control. Washington, DC, The World Bank, 1999.
61. Jenkins CN, Dai PX, Ngoc DH, et al: Tobacco use in Vietnam: Prevalence, predictors, and the role of the transnational tobacco corporations. JAMA 277:1726, 1997.
62. Pandey MR, Neupane RP, Gautam A: Epidemiological study of tobacco smoking behaviour among adults in a rural community of the hill region of Nepal with special reference to attitude and beliefs. Int J Epidemiol 17:535, 1988.
63. Mackay J: Women and tobacco: International issues. J Am Med Womens Assoc 51:48, 1996.
64. Yang G, Fan L, Tan J, et al: Smoking in China: Findings of the 1996 National Prevalence Survey. JAMA 282:1247, 1999.
65. Liu BQ, Peto R, Chen ZM, et al: Emerging tobacco hazards in China: 1. Retrospective proportional mortality study of one million deaths. BMJ 317:1411, 1998.
66. Janus ED, Postiglione A, Singh RB, Lewis B: The modernization of Asia: Implications for coronary heart disease. Council on Arteriosclerosis of the International Society and Federation of Cardiology. Circulation 94:2671, 1996.
67. Research Committee on Serum Lipid Level Survey 1990 in Japan: Current state of and recent trends in serum lipid levels in the general Japanese population. J Atheroscler Thromb 2:122, 1996.
68. Kennedy ET, Bowman SA, Powell R: Dietary fat intake in the US population. J Am Coll Nutr 18:207, 1999.
69. Du S, Lu B, Zhai F, Popkin BM: A new stage of the nutrition transition in China. Public Health Nutr 5:169, 2002.
70. U.S. Department of Health and Human Services: Healthy People 2010: Understanding and Improving Health. Washington, DC, U.S. Government Printing Office, 2000.
71. Physical activity trends—United States, 1990-1998. MMWR Morb Mortal Wkly Rep 50:166, 2001.
72. Keil U, Kuulasmaa K: WHO MONICA Project: Risk factors. Int J Epidemiol 18:S46, 1989.
73. Dobson AJ, Evans A, Ferrario M, et al: Changes in estimated coronary risk in the 1980s: Data from 38 populations in the WHO MONICA Project. World Health Organization. Monitoring trends and determinants in cardiovascular diseases. Ann Med 30:199, 1998.
74. Obesity: Preventing and managing the global epidemic. Geneva,World Health Organization, 2000. Technical Report Series, No 894.
75. Mokdad AH, Ford ES, Bowman BA, et al: Prevalence of obesity, diabetes, and obesity-related health risk factors, 2001. JAMA 289:76, 2003.
76. Hodge AM, Dowse GK, Gareeboo H, et al: Incidence, increasing prevalence, and predictors of change in obesity and fat distribution over 5 years in the rapidly developing population of Mauritius. Int J Obes Relat Metab Disord 20:137, 1996.
77. Steyn K, Jooste PL, Bourne L, et al: Risk factors for coronary heart disease in the black population of the Cape Peninsula. The BRISK study. S Afr Med J 79:480, 1991.
78. McCarthy HD, Ellis SM, Cole TJ: Central overweight and obesity in British youth aged 11-16 years: Cross sectional surveys of waist circumference. BMJ 326:624, 2003.
79. Erasmus RT, Uyot C, Pakeye T: Plasma cholesterol distribution in a rural Nigerian population—relationship to age, sex and body mass. Cent Afr J Med 40:299, 1994.
80. Verschuren WM, Jacobs DR, Bloemberg BP, et al: Serum total cholesterol and long-term coronary heart disease mortality in different cultures: Twenty-five-year follow-up of the seven countries study. JAMA 274:131, 1995.
81. Kuzuya M, Ando F, Iguchi A, Shimokata H: Changes in serum lipid levels during a 10 year period in a large Japanese population: A cross-sectional and longitudinal study. Atherosclerosis 163:313, 2002.
82. Yamada M, Wong FL, Kodama K, et al: Longitudinal trends in total serum cholesterol levels in a Japanese cohort, 1958-1986. J Clin Epidemiol 50:425, 1997.
83. Khoo KL, Tan H, Liew YM, et al: Lipids and coronary heart disease in Asia. Atherosclerosis 169:1, 2003.
84. INCLEN Multicentre Collaborative Group: Risk factors for cardiovascular disease in the developing world. A multicentre collaborative study in the International Clinical Epidemiology Network (INCLEN). J Clin Epidemiol 45:841, 1992.
85. Walker AR, Sareli P: Coronary heart disease: Outlook for Africa. J R Soc Med 90:23, 1997.
86. Singh RB, Sharma JP, Rastogi V, et al: Prevalence of coronary artery disease and coronary risk factors in rural and urban populations of north India. Eur Heart J 18:1728, 1997.
87. van den Hoogen PC, Feskens EJ, Nagelkerke NJ, et al: The relation between blood pressure and mortality due to coronary heart disease among men in different parts of the world. Seven Countries Study Research Group. N Engl J Med 342:1, 2000.
88. Gu D, Reynolds K, Wu X, et al: Prevalence, awareness, treatment, and control of hypertension in China. Hypertension 40:920, 2002.
89. Lawes CM, Rodgers A, Bennett DA, et al: Blood pressure and cardiovascular disease in the Asia Pacific region. J Hypertens 21:707, 2003.
90. Seedat YK: Hypertension in developing nations in sub-Saharan Africa. J Hum Hypertens 14:739, 2000.
91. Ordunez P, Silva LC, Rodriguez MP, Robles S: Prevalence estimates for hypertension in Latin America and the Caribbean: Are they useful for surveillance? Rev Panam Salud Publica 10:226, 2001.
92. Anselmi M, Avanzini F, Moreira JM, et al: Treatment and control of arterial hypertension in a rural community in Ecuador. Lancet 361:1186, 2003.
93. King H, Aubert RE, Herman WH: Global burden of diabetes, 1995-2025: Prevalence, numerical estimates, and projections. Diabetes Care 21:1414, 1998.
94. Knowler WC, Pettitt DJ, Saad MF, Bennett PH: Diabetes mellitus in the Pima Indians: Incidence, risk factors and pathogenesis. Diabetes Metab Rev 6:1, 1990.
95. Harris MI, Flegal KM, Cowie CC, et al: Prevalence of diabetes, impaired fasting glucose, and impaired glucose tolerance in U.S. adults. The Third National Health and Nutrition Examination Survey, 1988-1994. Diabetes Care 21:518, 1998.

Future Challenges

96. Haldeman GA, Croft JB, Giles WH, Rashidee A: Hospitalization of patients with heart failure: National Hospital Discharge Survey, 1985 to 1995. Am Heart J 137:352, 1999.
97. Changes in mortality from heart failure—United States, 1980-1995. MMWR Morb Mortal Wkly Rep 47:633, 1998.
98. Malek M: Health economics of heart failure. Heart 82 Suppl 4:IV11, 1999.
99. Howson CP, Reddy KS, Ryan TJ, Bale JR (eds): Control of cardiovascular disease in developing countries. Washington, DC, National Academy Press, 1998.

CHAPTER 2

Economics and Cardiovascular Disease

Mark A. Hlatky • Daniel B. Mark

The United States leads the world in spending on health care, whether measured as a percentage of gross domestic product or as dollars per capita. The decisions made by physicians control the bulk of these expenditures, and society has increasingly called for greater stewardship of the vast resources that doctors command. This chapter discusses some of the key economic principles that underlie clinical and health policy decision-making and reviews important economic studies evaluating management of cardiovascular disorders.

Key Economic Principles

Alternative Uses

A key principle of economics is that all resources have alternative uses, so devoting resources to any particular activity makes them unavailable for different, and perhaps better, uses. Society's application of resources to medical care diminishes the resources available for alternative programs, such as public safety, assistance to the elderly or the poor, or environmental protection. This same principle applies to the resources earmarked to health care: the resources devoted to implantable defibrillators within a health care system might be used to meet alternative health needs, such as treatment of heart failure, prenatal care programs, or provision of vaccinations. Thus, the goal of health economics is to define the most efficient use of the resources available to provide health care to a population of patients.

Societal Perspective

Economic analyses most often employ the societal perspective: how will society as a whole benefit from the new clinical program and what will society have to pay for it? In contrast, clinicians are focused on individual patients. Their traditional role is to be the patient's advocate, to do what is possible for the patient before them, regardless of the value provided to society. Thus, economic analysis is a policy tool for informing spending about populations, not a tool for assisting with bedside decision-making.

Law of Diminishing Returns

An economic principle of special relevance to medicine is the so-called "law of diminishing returns," indicated schematically in Figure 2–1. As resources are initially applied to a particular end, the returns are large, but as further resources are applied, the returns become progressively smaller to the point that there is no further gain, and perhaps even a loss, with application of additional resources. This type of response is familiar to clinicians caring for patients; in the case of acute myocardial infarction (MI), for example, access to defibrillation and hospital monitoring provides great benefits, and the addition of reperfusion therapy further improves patient outcomes. The provision of yet more care may improve outcomes a bit further, but eventually maximum benefit is obtained—this point has been termed the "flat of the curve." A key economic insight is that it is not optimal for society to have medical care operate on the flat of the curve, but rather have it operate on the upsloping portion of the curve (see Fig. 2–1) because the resources that would be spent in moving along the flat of the curve have better alternative uses. A major goal of economic analysis of cardiovascular care is to find the optimal level of resources for a given clinical problem.

As exemplified in Figure 2-1, a key economic measure of value is the cost of adding another unit of medical benefit, or the slope of the curve.[1-3] In economic analysis, the costs and effects of an intervention are always compared with an explicitly defined alternative. Thus, cost-effectiveness analysis assesses the marginal (or incremental) costs required to improve outcomes by one unit. The cost-effectiveness ratio is defined as follows:

$$\frac{\text{Cost}_{\text{new}} - \text{Cost}_{\text{old}}}{\text{Effect}_{\text{new}} - \text{Effect}_{\text{old}}}$$

where $Cost_{new}$ is the total cost of the new program, $Cost_{old}$ is the total cost of the old program, and $Effect_{new}$ and $Effect_{old}$ indicate the medical effectiveness of the new and old programs, respectively. The cost of a program should include all relevant costs: the intervention itself (e.g., streptokinase for an acute MI); the cost of complications induced (e.g., bleeding, stroke) and averted (e.g., heart failure) by therapy; and the costs of concomitant treatments (e.g., mechanical coronary revascularization). The effectiveness of a medical intervention should be assessed using outcomes directly relevant to patients, such as survival and quality of life. Economic analysis commonly measures effectiveness in "quality-adjusted life-years" (QALYs) to assess on a common scale both of these dimensions of improved clinical outcome. Laboratory-based outcome measures (e.g., ejection fraction, serum cholesterol level) are intermediate, surrogate markers of ultimate patient benefit and therefore are not used in economic analysis.

Economies of Scale

A final economic principle of relevance to medical care is that the production of goods and services is often more efficient in larger quantities due to "economies of scale." Costs per patient are lower when the high fixed costs of specialized equipment (e.g., an angiography suite) are spread over more

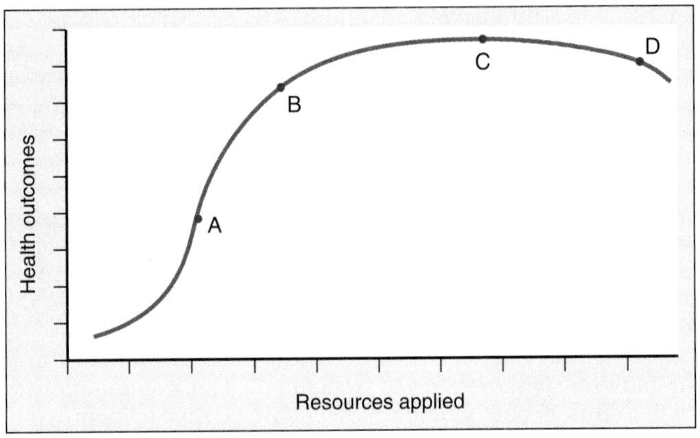

FIGURE 2–1 General relationship between application of health care resources (horizontal axis) and health outcomes (vertical axis). At Point A, outcomes are improving rapidly with increased resources, and treatment is cost-effective. At Point B, outcomes are still improving with increased resources, but at a rate that is less cost-effective. At Point C, increased resources are no longer improving outcome (i.e., "flat at the curve"), and at Point D increased resources actually lead to worse outcomes, through iatrogenic complications and overtreatment.

patients. Also, large-volume facilities can negotiate price discounts from suppliers and achieve more flexible use of personnel with their larger staff. In medical care, there is also evidence that higher patient volumes are associated with greater technical proficiency and better clinical outcomes.[4,5] Of course, beyond a certain scale, the clinical and cost advantages of higher patient volumes will be diminished and the disadvantages may increase (e.g., poorer communication, an impersonal approach to patient care). Nevertheless, there is strong empirical evidence of the value of maintaining a minimum level of clinical volume in procedures such as coronary angioplasty and coronary bypass surgery and in the care of critically ill patients such as those with acute MI.

Medical Costs

Provision of medical care requires resources: the time and energy of physicians, nurses, and other health care professionals; specialized facilities such as intensive care units, angiography suites, and operating rooms; and costly drugs and supplies. Use of these resources has a cost, even if medical care is provided "for free." In principle, the best measure of this cost is what economists term the *opportunity cost*, or what has been lost by not applying resources to their next best use. As a practical matter, cost is measured by the prices paid in a competitive market. The overall cost of a medical program can then be measured as $\Sigma_i P_i Q_i$, where P_i is the price for resource i, Q_i is the quantity of resource i that is used, and the summation is over all i resources used in care of the patient. Modern hospital cost accounting systems facilitate such "microcosting" of medical care services. When microcosting is not feasible, an alternative measure of hospital cost has been found by multiplying the charge for the service by a correction factor (the ratio of costs to charges) from the hospital's annual financial report to the Centers for Medicare and Medicaid Services.

In medical economic studies, the cost of an intervention includes all relevant costs, regardless of who pays for them. The cost of an angioplasty might be borne in part by the insurance company, in part by the patient (e.g., prescription drugs after discharge), and in part by the hospital (e.g., costs over the contracted insurance payment amount). An expensive new therapy in the angioplasty laboratory may reduce total costs in the year after the procedure and therefore be quite economically attractive. Nevertheless, a hospital may resist using the new therapy because its costs are increased. Even programs that save total medical costs can create economic winners and losers, whose incentives and disincentives can distort optimal resource allocation from a societal perspective.

Medical costs and benefits are typically spread over long time intervals, which leads to two related issues regarding measurement. Inflation changes the units of cost measurement, such that a dollar in the year 2003 does not have the same value as a dollar in 2008: it is therefore necessary to standardize all costs to a single metric, such as 2008 dollars. A separate issue is that even if there were no cost inflation, it is still preferable to be paid today than to be paid in 5 years, and, conversely, it is preferable to repay a debt sometime in the future than to repay it immediately. To adjust for these time preferences, medical economic studies typically discount future costs and medical benefits by 3% per year.[2]

Analysis of Specific Interventions

Economic analysis has been applied to treatment of acute illness (e.g., acute MI), procedures (e.g., coronary bypass surgery), treatment of chronic illness (e.g., heart failure), prevention of disease (e.g., reduction of high cholesterol levels), or the use of diagnostic tests (e.g., coronary angiography). In the remainder of this chapter, we illustrate the principles of economic analysis by discussing cardiovascular management strategies drawn from each of these areas. Detailed review of the economics of all cardiovascular therapies is beyond the scope of this chapter.

Application of economic analysis to medical care can be illustrated by the use of thrombolytic therapy for acute MI. Timely reperfusion of the occluded coronary artery improves survival of the patient with an acute MI, and this survival benefit is maintained over long-term follow-up.[6] The added cost of treating an acute MI patient with reperfusion therapy needs to be weighed against the long-term benefit to assess the value provided by this treatment strategy.

The value of streptokinase administration for acute MI compared with no reperfusion therapy can be analyzed using cost-effectiveness analysis. For the purpose of this example, we assume that streptokinase costs \$270 per treatment, and that costs of medical care are otherwise equal in treated and untreated MI patients. We further assume that hospital survival is improved from 88% to 92% by streptokinase treatment, and that the life-expectancy of MI survivors is 15 years, regardless of whether they were treated with streptokinase. Based on these assumptions, the incremental cost-effectiveness of streptokinase for the treatment of acute MI can be calculated as follows:

$$\frac{\Delta\text{Cost}}{\Delta\text{Life expectancy}} = \frac{\$270 - 0}{(0.92)(15\text{ yr}) - (0.88)(15\text{ yr})} = \frac{\$270}{0.6\text{ yr}} = \$450/\text{life-year added}$$

Thus, the expenditure of \$450 on average adds a year to the life of a patient with an acute MI. To judge whether streptokinase therapy for acute MI represents a good value for the money spent (i.e., is "economically attractive") requires a standard of comparison. Renal dialysis currently costs about \$50,000 per patient per year in the United States. The cost of dialysis is covered by the publicly funded Medicare program and provides a good benchmark of how much society is willing to spend to add a life-year. Programs that cost up to \$50,000 per year of life added are generally considered economically attractive, whereas programs with cost-effectiveness ratios greater than \$100,000 per year of life added are generally considered to be economically unattractive. Based on these benchmarks, streptokinase therapy for acute MI is a very economically attractive intervention.

Acute Coronary Syndromes (see Chap. 49)

Thrombolytic Agents

Treatment of acute coronary syndromes (MI, unstable angina) with reperfusion, antithrombotic, and anticoagulant regimens has been extensively investigated. While clinically diverse, these therapies share common features from the perspective of economic evaluation. The therapies for acute coronary syndromes are typically short-term in duration and expensive, and they provide benefit to patients mainly by reducing the short-term risk of hospital death and/or MI.

Tissue plasminogen activator (t-PA) has been extensively studied for the treatment of acute MI. t-PA is much more expensive than streptokinase, the first thrombolytic agent shown to be effective for MI. The cost-effectiveness of t-PA was assessed in the randomized GUSTO-1 trial.[7] In GUSTO-1, the cost of therapy was assessed by assigning standardized costs to each resource consumed (e.g., hospital days, cardiac angiography) and summing the costs over all resources used. Apart from the cost of the thrombolytic agents themselves, hospital and follow-up costs were quite similar in t-PA-treated and streptokinase-treated patients, and the added cost of t-PA ($2200 vs. $270) was not offset by cost savings in other aspects of the patient's care. The 30-day survival rate of t-PA-treated patients was improved by 1%, and the life expectancy of survivors was projected to be 15.4 years. Using these data, the cost-effectiveness of t-PA relative to streptokinase was $27,100 per year of life saved, which was economically attractive by the previously described benchmarks.[7]

The use of streptokinase and t-PA for acute MI provides a striking example of the economic principle of diminishing returns. The greatest gain in clinical outcome comes from using the cheapest effective thrombolytic agent (streptokinase) for acute MI, which improves survival by 4% or more in absolute terms at a net cost of about $270 per patient. t-PA improves survival by a further 1% in absolute terms, but at an added cost of more than $1900 per patient. Thus, the cost-effectiveness of streptokinase relative to placebo ($450 per life-year added) is more favorable than the cost-effectiveness of t-PA relative to streptokinase ($27,100 per life-year added). Simple and cheap therapies usually provide most of the potential improvement in outcomes for a given clinical condition, with smaller and smaller marginal improvements coming at greater and greater cost. This example also illustrates the comparative nature of economic evaluations—the value of a treatment can be assessed only in light of the therapeutic alternatives.

Angioplasty (see Chap. 52)

Primary angioplasty for acute MI has been compared with thrombolytic therapy in several clinical trials, some of which also included an economic evaluation. A quantitative overview of randomized trials showed the survival of patients with acute MI treated with angioplasty is better than patients treated with thrombolysis.[8] The results of economic analysis have been less consistent, with primary angioplasty being less expensive in some studies but more expensive in others.[9-11] The net economic effect of primary angioplasty depends on the patterns of coronary angiography and revascularization in patients treated with thrombolysis. Primary percutaneous coronary intervention (PCI) strategy is relatively less expensive when angiography is routinely performed after thrombolysis, since many patients would have received PCI in the same admission anyway. The primary PCI strategy is more expensive when angiography is infrequent after thrombolysis, however, since primary PCI leads to expensive revascularization procedures that would not otherwise have been performed. A formal cost-effectiveness analysis of primary PCI relative to thrombolysis showed it to be cost-effective when performed in hospitals with existing cardiac angiography laboratories and minimal delay to therapy.[12] This analysis also suggested that it would not be economically justified to build new catheterization laboratories solely to provide primary PCI.[12]

Newer developments in primary coronary intervention for acute MI include the use of stents and adjunctive glycoprotein IIb/IIIa inhibitor therapy, each of which adds to the cost of the procedure. Formal economic evaluations have not yet been reported.

Anticoagulation and Antiplatelet Regimens (see Chap. 80)

Anticoagulant and antiplatelet regimens in the treatment of patients with unstable angina and acute MI have been investigated intensively in clinical trials. Since the newer agents of these classes tend to be more expensive than the standard alternatives (heparin, aspirin), economic evaluation is important. Economic evaluations are difficult to perform in these settings, however, because some or all of the benefit of these therapies comes from reducing nonfatal MI, not hospital mortality. The economic analysis must therefore assess the long-term value of preventing a nonfatal MI.

In one study, low-molecular-weight heparin (enoxaparin) improved clinical outcomes and lowered overall hospital costs relative to unfractionated heparin, largely because the $75 greater cost of enoxaparin was more than recouped by reducing the need for costly revascularization procedures in patients with recurrent ischemia.[13] The combination of better clinical outcomes and lower cost, termed a "dominant" strategy because no tradeoffs between cost and outcome are involved, is clearly economically attractive. Use of eptifibatide, a glycoprotein IIb/IIIa inhibitor, in patients with acute coronary syndrome improved clinical outcomes, primarily nonfatal MI, at a net cost of $1014 per patient. The cost-effectiveness ratio for this drug appears economically attractive ($16,500 per life-year added) based on the assumption that prevention of a nonfatal MI increases life expectancy by approximately 2 years.[14]

Cardiac Procedures and Devices

CORONARY BYPASS GRAFTING (see Chap. 50). In 2001, there were 305,000 coronary bypass surgeries in the United States, as well as 1,051,000 coronary angioplasty procedures.[15] With a total cost of roughly 20 billion dollars a year, the use of coronary revascularization procedures has spurred extensive economic evaluation.

Coronary artery bypass graft surgery (CABG) is an effective treatment for angina in symptomatic patients and extends life expectancy in patients with extensive coronary disease. An overview of randomized clinical trials of surgery versus medical therapy[16] suggests that patients with left main disease may live more than 0.6 years longer after CABG, patients with three-vessel disease may live more than 0.5 years longer, and patients with one- or two-vessel disease may live more than 0.16 years longer (life extension was estimated only over the first 10 years of follow-up). These data suggest that CABG is more economically attractive in patients with more extensive coronary disease at higher risk of death, since the absolute improvement in survival is greatest in these patients whereas the cost of the surgery is roughly the same. An early classic study[17] found that the cost-effectiveness of CABG versus medical therapy for left main disease was $3800 per year of life added, a highly favorable ratio. More recent analyses[18] confirm that the cost-effectiveness of CABG is most favorable in patients with higher clinical risk (more extensive coronary disease, reduced left ventricular function), and greater degrees of angina.

PERCUTANEOUS CORONARY INTERVENTION (see Chap. 52). Despite the extensive use of coronary angioplasty, few randomized trials have compared it with medical therapy. The RITA-2 trial[19] found better angina relief but more cardiac events in patients with stable angina treated by angioplasty compared with medical therapy. Economic data from RITA-2[20] documented that the higher initial cost among the angioplasty patients (2793 British pounds) was undiminished after 3 years of follow-up. A formal cost-effectiveness evaluation of angioplasty compared with medical therapy has not yet been reported.

Coronary angioplasty and bypass surgery have been directly compared in several randomized trials conducted in patients with multivessel disease. The clinical results of these studies have been quite consistent in showing significantly less angina and slightly lower mortality in surgery patients.[21] Economic analysis in the RITA,[22] EAST,[23] ERACI,[24]

BARI,[25] and ARTS[26] trials all documented significantly lower initial costs with coronary angioplasty, roughly one half to two thirds the cost of bypass surgery. The initial cost advantage of angioplasty was almost completely lost over the subsequent follow-up as a result of the frequent need for repeat coronary revascularization procedures among angioplasty-treated patients. At 5 to 8 years of follow-up, the total medical costs averaged 4% to 6% lower in balloon angioplasty patients than in surgery patients.[27,28] The introduction of coronary stents may alter the relative costs of angioplasty and bypass surgery.[26] While long-term follow-up has not yet been reported in the ARTS and SOS trials, which used stents extensively, 1-year follow-up of ARTS shows a $3000 cost advantage for the stent-assigned patients. Economic analysis suggests that bypass surgery is more cost-effective than angioplasty in patients with more extensive coronary disease (i.e., three-vessel disease), whereas angioplasty has a significant cost advantage in patients with less extensive disease, albeit with somewhat less angina relief.[25]

Coronary stents have now become a standard part of percutaneous revascularization. Stents reduce the need for emergency bypass surgery after initial angioplasty and significantly reduce the likelihood of restenosis and repeat revascularization.[29] Use of stents substantially increases the cost of the revascularization procedure, but the higher cost of the stent is only partially offset by the lower incidence of repeat revascularization.[30,31] Consequently, the total cost of patients treated with coronary stents remains 7% to 12% higher than that of patients treated with balloon angioplasty at 1 year of follow-up, with an equivalent incidence of death and nonfatal MI. Drug-coated stents have further reduced the rate of repeat revascularization procedures,[32] but the economic implications of these devices are uncertain. Preliminary data from the SIRIUS trial suggest that the $2880 higher initial cost of patients assigned to a sirolimus-coated stent was narrowed over 1 year of follow-up to only $309 by reduced costs of repeat revascularization procedures.[33] The clinical and economic effects of drug-coated stents in various patient groups are currently undefined and are the subject of ongoing investigation.

IMPLANTABLE CARDIOVERTER DEFIBRILLATOR (see Chap. 31). The implantable cardioverter defibrillator (ICD) has reduced total mortality by 26% among patients at high risk for sudden cardiac death.[34] Because implantation of a defibrillator costs $30,000 or more, many investigators have questioned whether the ICD is worth its high cost.

Several randomized trials have reported data on economic as well as clinical outcomes, including MADIT-1,[35] AVID,[36] and CIDS.[37] In each study, the early costs among ICD patients were considerably higher than those of conventionally treated patients (Table 2–1). Over the next 3 to 5 years, the ICD patients had lower costs, but these savings were only a fraction of the initial ICD cost. With randomized trials showing that ICD-treated patients have higher costs and reduced mortality, cost-effectiveness was performed based on primary data from the trials. The cost-effectiveness of the ICD was most favorable in MADIT-1 (US$27,000 per life-year added) and least favorable in CIDS (C$214,000 per life-year added), primarily because of the degrees of mortality reduction found in the two trials (54% versus 20%). A limitation of the cost-effectiveness analysis within randomized clinical trials is that some clinical benefits and costs occur only after longer follow-up and are not included in the analysis. Lifetime costs and survival were projected for patients with life-threatening ventricular arrhythmias by Owens and coworkers,[38] who found that a 26% relative risk reduction by the ICD translates to a cost-effectiveness ratio of $40,000 per year of life added, a ratio that is in the range generally acceptable in the United States. A current dilemma in health policy is whether prophylactic ICD placement is justified and is worth the expenditure of more than 1 billion dollars per year.

TABLE 2–1 Costs in Implantable Cardiac Defibrillator (ICD) Treated and Conventionally Treated Patients

	Costs		
Study	***ICD***	***Conventional***	***Difference***
MADIT-1[35] (US$)			
Initial therapy	44,565	18,880	25,685
4-year follow-up	52,995	57,100	−4,105
Total	97,560	75,980	21,580
AVID[36] (US$)			
Initial therapy	66,629	34,059	32,570
Follow-up	9,604	14,594	−4,990
Total	76,233	48,653	27,580
CIDS[37] (C$)			
Initial therapy	48,874	7,927	40,948
Follow-up	38,840	30,673	8,167
Total	87,715	38,600	49,115

These studies illustrate several general points about the economic evaluation of procedures and devices. The initial cost of procedures and devices is often quite high, but long-term follow-up is needed to assess the total net cost of the procedure relative to alternative therapies. An expensive procedure may have some or all of its incremental costs recouped through prevention of costly adverse events, such as in the case of bypass surgery relative to balloon angioplasty. The higher cost may be only partially offset by later savings (e.g, coronary stents) or barely recovered at all (e.g., implantable defibrillators). Nevertheless, high initial costs of procedures and devices may be justified if survival is sufficiently improved or quality of life enhanced. These considerations emphasize the importance of a long-term perspective in the economic evaluation of devices and procedures, so that their full costs and benefits can be assessed.

Chronic Disease: Heart Failure (see Chaps. 23, 24)

Economically efficient management of a chronic disease such as heart failure is very different from that of an acute illness or a surgical procedure. In cases of chronic diseases, the cost of care is spread over many years instead of being concentrated at the outset of treatment. Similarly, the benefits of treatment accrue only over a period of prolonged follow-up. Most medical care for chronic disease is delivered in an ambulatory, outpatient setting, and patient adherence to prescribed regimens has a substantial impact on the efficacy of therapy. Improvements in clinical and economic outcomes may come either from better therapies or from better ways to deliver established therapies, or both.

Angiotensin-converting enzyme inhibitors have significantly improved survival of patients with heart failure in randomized trials.[39] An economic appraisal of enalapril therapy based on the SOLVD trial results[40] suggested that the added cost of enalapril was completely offset by the cost savings from fewer hospitalizations for heart failure. Projections of lifetime costs and life expectancy performed using a model suggested that the net lifetime cost per patient was only $25 and that life expectancy was increased by 0.30 life years,[40] yielding an extremely favorable cost-effectiveness ratio of $83 per life-year added. An economic analysis based on the SAVE trial in patients with an ejection fraction less than 40% after an acute MI suggested that captopril therapy was economically attractive for this indication, with more favorable cost-effectiveness ratios in older patients than in younger patients.[41] An overview of economic analyses of heart failure treatment[42] suggests that the use of angiotensin-converting enzyme inhibitors is generally economically attractive.

An overview of randomized trials shows that beta blockade reduces mortality by 35% among patients with congestive heart failure,[43] with hospital admissions for heart failure reduced by a similar degree. A cost-effectiveness model based on published data from clinical trials found that beta blockers for heart failure have a cost-effectiveness ratio between $2500 and $6700 per life-year added,[44] which is certainly acceptable when judged against common benchmarks.

Most hospital admissions for heart failure result from lack of patient adherence to drug or dietary regimens,[45] suggesting that disease management programs could improve clinical outcomes and economic outcomes. An overview of 11 randomized trials[46] found that hospitalizations were reduced by 13% and overall costs were generally lowered by various disease management programs.

Disease Prevention (see Chap. 42)

Disease prevention is very important from a clinical perspective. Some preventive measures are very effective and inexpensive, as exemplified by vaccination programs for common infectious diseases that cut risk by more than 90% at the cost of only a few dollars. Most preventive measures are less effective in reducing the risk of disease and far more costly to implement. Vaccines are relatively inexpensive because they are given only two or three times, whereas drugs to lower serum cholesterol or high blood pressure are given daily for decades. Thus, the cost-effectiveness of preventive programs varies considerably according to the intervention, its effectiveness, and its cost.[47]

Hypercholesterolemia has long been established as a strong, consistent risk factor for coronary atherosclerosis, and HMG-CoA-reductase inhibitors ("statins") clearly reduce the risk of death and nonfatal cardiovascular events.[48] The cost-effectiveness of this class of drugs has been controversial, largely because of the heterogeneity of patients considered for lipid-lowering therapy. Secondary prevention trials have consistently shown substantial reductions in the absolute rate of cardiac events in patients treated with statins. The efficacy of cholesterol lowering in primary prevention (i.e., subjects at high risk of heart disease but without evidence of clinical disease) has been demonstrated in several large randomized trials.

The cost-effectiveness of HMG-CoA reductase therapy to prevent coronary heart disease varies from extremely favorable values in secondary prevention settings to quite unfavorable in some primary prevention settings.[49] The reason for this wide variation is that higher risk patients have a greater absolute benefit from treatment than lower risk patients. The 4S trial[50] of secondary prevention found that lipid-lowering treatment reduced mortality by 32 deaths per 1000 patients treated (Table 2–2). In contrast, the WOSCOPS study[51] of primary prevention found an absolute mortality difference of 5 per 1000 patients treated. The greater clinical efficacy of secondary prevention over primary prevention implies that lipid-lowering therapy is more economically attractive in the secondary prevention setting. Furthermore, the prevention of nonfatal myocardial infarction and revascularization offsets more of the cost of drug therapy in the secondary prevention setting, enhancing its economic attractiveness. Even within the primary prevention setting, treatment of higher risk patients (i.e., those with multiple risk factors, higher cholesterol levels) provides greater absolute risk reduction and hence is more cost-effective than is the treatment of lower risk patients. Formal cost-effectiveness studies suggest that primary prevention with HMG-CoA reductase therapy in low-risk patients is economically unattractive, whereas treatment of higher risk patients is quite cost-effective.[49,52] Clinical guidelines stress the importance of tailoring therapy to the patient's risk profile[53] to achieve optimal results.

Cigarette smoking clearly increases the risk of coronary heart disease events, with evidence of risk reduction after quitting in numerous nonrandomized studies. Although the effectiveness of a physician's advice to stop smoking is low, it does induce some smokers to quit, and because such advice has such a low cost, it has a favorable cost-effectiveness ratio of less than $1000 per year of life added.[54] Use of nicotine replacement strategies as part of a smoking cessation program adds to the number of patients who quit smoking and has a favorable cost-effectiveness ratio.[55] Hospital-based smoking cessation programs have also been shown to be cost-effective.[56] Smoking cessation is a particularly attractive preventive measure, since the interventions are generally short-term and of relatively low cost, and smoking cessation has highly beneficial effects on both cardiac and noncardiac diseases (e.g., various cancers, emphysema) and thus adds considerably to life expectancy.

Diagnostic Testing

Proper selection of diagnostic tests to evaluate various clinical problems has become more challenging as a result of the collision between the forces of technologic innovation, which develop many new tests to examine different facets of a particular disease, and the forces of economic restraint, which insist on their cost-effective use. Economic evaluation of diagnostic tests starts from the premise that the information provided by a test has value only if physicians use the information to change therapy and the change in therapy then improves clinical outcomes. Thus, the effectiveness of a test is gauged not solely by its information content but by its ultimate, indirect effects on patient outcomes.

Tests that provide clinical value do so by adding to what is already known about the patient. In practical terms, the test needs to add independent information to what is available from the clinical history, physical examination, and simpler, cheaper tests. The information value of myocardial perfusion scans in the diagnosis of coronary artery disease, for example, must be judged by how much unique diagnostic and prognostic information they add to the clinical examination and the simpler stress electrocardiogram. The evaluation of diagnostic tests by measuring the incremental value of information they provide is analogous to the way that therapies are evaluated by documenting what they add compared with the best available alternative (e.g., how much better is t-PA than streptokinase for treatment of acute MI). But the additional requirement placed on diagnostic tests is that they add enough information to modify decision-making. A test that is statistically more accurate does not provide value from an economic perspective unless the additional accuracy leads to improved clinical decisions. Demonstrations of a statistical improvement in diagnostic accuracy with new tests are common, but evaluations of the effects of this extra accuracy on clinical management are rare.

The evaluation of chest pain is a critical diagnostic problem that has been carefully analyzed in many studies. Early studies focused on the incremental information provided by noninvasive testing, most commonly the exercise electrocardiogram. These studies, by application of Bayes' rule, showed that the difference between pretest and posttest probability of disease was greatest among patients with an intermediate pretest probability of disease (i.e., between 15% and 85%). More recent

TABLE 2–2 Clinical and Economic Outcomes of Randomized Trials of Lipid-Lowering

	Reductions Per 1000 Patients (n)			Cost per Patient ($)		
Study	*Deaths*	*Myocardial Infarction*	*Revascularization*	*Drug Treatment*	*Complications Prevented*	*Net*
Primary prevention						
WOSCOPS	5	19	8	3700	100	3600
AFCAPS	4	26	31	4654	524	4130
Secondary prevention						
4S	32	47	59	4650	3900	780
CARE	11	18	47	5550	1660	3890

cost-effectiveness analysis extended the earlier studies by considering the health outcomes resulting from detecting (or failing to detect) underlying coronary disease amenable to coronary revascularization.[57-59] These analyses suggest that immediate coronary angiography is reasonable in patients with a very high pretest likelihood of coronary disease, such as an older man with typical exertional angina. In patients with an intermediate probability of coronary disease, noninvasive testing is generally economically attractive in comparison with no testing (cost-effectiveness ratios roughly $30,000 per QALY added), whereas coronary angiography without prior noninvasive testing is not (cost-effectiveness ratio >$65,000 per QALY added, depending on patient characteristics). Alternative noninvasive tests (exercise electrocardiography, exercise single photon emission computed tomography perfusion imaging, stress echocardiography) are close enough in cost-effectiveness that the determining factors in choosing among them are the likelihood of an indeterminate test result and the degree of local expertise with each alternative. The cost-effectiveness of all diagnostic strategies for chest pain are more favorable when stringent, outcome-based guidelines for coronary revascularization are followed.

The use of routine coronary angiography in survivors of acute MI has been controversial, in large part due to conflicting evidence on the efficacy of routine versus selective angiography practices.[60-63] The VANQWISH trial found that routine angiography initially cost $4500 more than a conservative, ischemia-guided strategy, and that this cost difference narrowed to $2200 after 1 years.[64] TIMI-18 found a similar pattern of costs, with the invasive strategy costing $1667 more initially, narrowing to $670 at 6 months' follow-up.[65] FRISC-II also found the invasive approach to be more costly over 1 year.[66] Thus, these clinical trials consistently found the invasive strategy to be more costly than a conservative ischemia-guided approach. The cost-effectiveness of the invasive strategy depended on the clinical results of the trial more than the economic outcomes. Studies that found better clinical results from the invasive strategy (TIMI-18 and FRISC-II) judged it cost-effective, whereas the trial that found poorer clinical outcomes in the invasive strategy (VANQWISH) judged it to be not economically attractive. A synthesis of the clinical and economic evaluations has not yet been performed, but these disparate findings underscore that economic assessment must be closely tied to clinical evaluation. While costs can be readily measured, determination of value requires weighing the added costs against the improvement in outcomes.

Developments in Economic Analysis

Cost-effectiveness analysis has been applied to clinical medicine for just over 20 years. The initial studies were based largely on decision models and related analytical methods and were of more interest to researchers than to clinicians. After considerable experience, consensus on some aspects of the methodology of economic analysis has been reached, although several areas of controversy remain.[1-3] The most important recent development in cost-effectiveness analysis has been the inclusion of economic endpoints as part of randomized trials, providing rigorous evaluation of the efficacy of therapies. As in all arenas of clinical research, the methods of economic evaluation in clinical trials have become more sophisticated, with application of economic models to extend clinical trial findings.[67] Future developments in cost-effectiveness analysis include wider application of economic evaluations in international settings, improved cost-identification methods, and continued development of statistical methods appropriate to cost and outcome data from clinical trials.[68]

REFERENCES

Law of Diminishing Returns

1. Russell LB, Gold MR, Siegel JE, et al: The role of cost-effectiveness analysis in health and medicine. Panel on Cost-Effectiveness in Health and Medicine. JAMA 276:1172, 1996.
2. Weinstein MC, Siegel JE, Gold MR, et al: Recommendations of the Panel on Cost-Effectiveness in Health and Medicine. JAMA 276:1253, 1996.
3. Siegel JE, Weinstein MC, Russell LB, et al: Recommendations for reporting cost-effectiveness analyses. Panel on Cost-Effectiveness in Health and Medicine. JAMA 276:1339, 1996.

Economies of Scale

4. McGrath PD, Wennberg DE, Dickens JD, et al: Relation between operator and hospital volume and outcomes following percutaneous coronary interventions in the era of the coronary stent. JAMA 284:3139, 2000.
5. Tu JV, Austin PC, Chan BTB: Relationship between annual volume of patients treated by admitting physician and mortality after acute myocardial infarction. JAMA 285:3116, 2001.

Analysis of Specific Interventions

6. Franzosi MG, Santoro E, De Vita C, et al: Ten-year follow-up of the first megatrial testing thrombolytic therapy in patients with acute myocardial infarction. Results of the Gruppo Italiano per lo Studio della Sopravivenza nell'Infarto-1 Study. Circulation 98:2659, 1998.

Acute Coronary Syndromes

7. Mark DB, Hlatky MA, Califf RM, et al: Cost effectiveness of thrombolytic therapy with tissue plasminogen activator as compared with streptokinase for acute myocardial infarction. N Engl J Med 332:1418, 1995.
8. Keeley EC, Boura JA, Grines CL: Primary angioplasty versus intravenous thrombolytic therapy for acute myocardial infarction: A quantitative review of 24 randomised trials. Lancet 361:13, 2003.
9. Gibbons RJ, Holmes DR, Reeder GS, et al: Immediate angioplasty compared with the administration of a thrombolytic agent followed by conservative treatment for myocardial infarction. N Engl J Med 328:685, 1993.
10. Stone GW, Grines CL, Rothbaum D, et al: Analysis of the relative costs and effectiveness of primary angioplasty versus tissue-type plasminogen activator: The primary angioplasty in myocardial infarction (PAMI) trial. J Am Coll Cardiol 29:901, 1997.
11. Every NR, Parsons LS, Hlatky M, et al: A comparison of thrombolytic therapy with primary coronary angioplasty for acute myocardial infarction. Myocardial Infarction Triage and Intervention investigators. N Engl J Med 335:1253, 1996.
12. Lieu TA, Gurley RJ, Lundstrom RJ, et al: Projected cost-effectiveness of primary angioplasty for acute myocardial infarction. J Am Coll Cardiol 30:1741, 1997.
13. Mark DB, Cowper PA, Berkowitz SD, et al: Economic assessment of low-molecular-weight heparin (enoxaparin) versus unfractionated heparin in acute coronary syndrome patients. Results from the ESSENCE randomized trial. Circulation 97:1702, 1998.
14. Mark DB, Harrington RA, Lincoff AM, et al: Cost effectiveness of platelet glycoprotein IIb/IIIa inhibition with eptifibatide in patients with non-ST elevation acute coronary syndromes. Circulation 101:366, 2000.

Coronary Procedures and Devices

15. Hall MJ, DeFrances CJ: 2001 National Hospital Discharge Survey. Advance data from vital and health statistics; no. 332. Hyattsville, MD, National Center for Health Statistics, 2003.
16. Yusuf S, Zucker D, Peduzzi P, et al: Effect of coronary artery bypass graft surgery on survival: Overview of 10-year results from randomised trials by the Coronary Artery Bypass Graft Surgery Trialists Collaboration. Lancet 344:563, 1994.
17. Weinstein MC, Stason WB: Cost-effectiveness of coronary artery bypass surgery. Circulation 66:III-56, 1982.
18. Wong JB, Sonnenberg FA, Salem DN, et al: Myocardial revascularization for chronic stable angina: Analysis of the role of percutaneous transluminal coronary angioplasty based on data available in 1989. Ann Intern Med 113:852, 1990.
19. RITA-2 Trial Participants: Coronary angioplasty versus medical therapy for angina: The second Randomised Intervention Treatment of Angina (RITA-2). Lancet 350:461, 1997.
20. Sculpher M, Smith D, Clayton T, et al: Coronary angioplasty versus medical therapy for angina: Health service costs based on the second Randomized Intervention Treatment of Angina (RITA-2) trial. Eur Heart J 23:1291, 2002.
21. Hoffman SN, TenBrook JA, Wolf MP, et al: A meta-analysis of randomized controlled trials comparing coronary artery bypass graft with percutaneous transluminal coronary angioplasty: One- to eight-year outcomes. J Am Coll Cardiol 41:1293, 2003.
22. Henderson RA, Pocock SJ, Sharp SJ, et al: Long-term results of RITA-1 trial: Clinical and cost comparisons of coronary angioplasty and coronary-artery bypass grafting. Lancet 352:1419, 1998.
23. Weintraub WS, Mauldin PD, Becker E, et al: A comparison of the costs of and quality of life after coronary angioplasty or coronary surgery for multivessel coronary artery disease: Results from the Emory Angioplasty Versus Surgery Trial (EAST). Circulation 92:2831, 1995.
24. Rodriguez A, Mele E, Peyregne E, et al: Three-year follow-up of the Argentine randomized trial of percutaneous transluminal coronary angioplasty versus coronary artery bypass surgery in multivessel disease (ERACI). J Am Coll Cardiol 27:1178, 1996.
25. Hlatky MA, Rogers WJ, Johnstone I, et al: Medical care costs and quality of life after randomization to coronary angioplasty or coronary bypass surgery. N Engl J Med 336:92, 1997.
26. Serruys PW, Unger F, Sousa JE, et al: Comparison of coronary-artery bypass surgery and stenting for the treatment of multivessel disease. N Engl J Med 344:1117, 2001.
27. Weintraub WS, Becker ER, Mauldin PD, et al: Costs of revascularization over eight years in the randomized and eligible patients in the Emory Angioplasty Versus Surgery Trial (EAST). Am J Cardiol 86:747, 2000.
28. Hlatky MA, Boothroyd DB, Johnstone IM: Economic evaluation in long-term clinical trials. Statist Med 21:2879, 2002.
29. Brophy JM, Belisle P, Joseph L: Evidence for use of coronary stents: A hierarchical Bayesian meta-analysis. Ann Intern Med 138:777, 2003.
30. Cohen DJ, Krumholz HM, Sukin CA, et al: In-hospital and one-year economic outcomes after coronary stenting or balloon angioplasty. Circulation 92:2480, 1995.

31. Serruys PW, van Hout B, Bonnier H, et al: Randomised comparison of implantation of heparin-coated stents with balloon angioplasty in selected patients with coronary artery disease (Benestent II). Lancet 352:673, 1998.
32. Morice M, Serruys PW, Sousa JE, et al: A randomized comparison of a sirolimus-eluting stent with a standard stent for coronary revascularization. N Engl J Med 346:1773, 2002.
33. Sorelle R: Cardiovascular news. Circulation 107:9024e, 2003.
34. Ezekowitz JA, Armstrong PW, McAlister FA: Implantable cardioverter defibrillators in primary and secondary prevention: A systematic review of randomized, controlled trials. Ann Intern Med 138:445, 2003.
35. Mushlin AI, Hall WJ, Zwanziger J, et al: The cost-effectiveness of automatic implantable cardiac defibrillators: Results from MADIT. Circulation 97:2129, 1998.
36. Larsen G, Hallstrom A, McAnulty J, et al: Cost-effectiveness of the implantable cardioverter-defibrillator versus antiarrhythmic drugs in survivors of serious ventricular tachyarrhythmias. Results of the Antiarrhythmics Versus Implantable Defibrillators (AVID) Economic Analysis Substudy. Circulation 105:2049, 2002.
37. O'Brien BJ, Connolly SJ, Goeree R, et al: Cost-effectiveness of the implantable cardioverter defibrillator: Results from the Canadian Implantable Defibrillator Study (CIDS). Circulation 103:1416, 2001.
38. Owens DK, Sanders GD, Harris RA, et al: Cost-effectiveness of implantable cardioverter defibrillators relative to amiodarone for prevention of sudden cardiac death. Ann Intern Med 126:1, 1997.

Chronic Disease: Heart Failure

39. Flather MD, Yusuf S, Køber L, et al: Long-term ACE-inhibitor therapy in patients with heart failure or left-ventricular dysfunction: A systematic overview of data from individual patients. Lancet 355:1575, 2000.
40. Glick H, Cook J, Kinosian B, et al: Costs and effects of enalapril therapy in patients with symptomatic heart failure: An economic analysis of the studies of left ventricular dysfunction (SOLVD) treatment trial. J Cardiac Fail 1:371, 1995.
41. Tsevat J, Duke D, Goldman L, et al: Cost-effectiveness of captopril therapy after myocardial infarction. J Am Coll Cardiol 26:914, 1995.
42. Weintraub WS, Cole J, Tooley JF: Cost and cost-effectiveness studies in heart failure research. Am Heart J 143:565, 2002.
43. Brophy JM, Joseph L, Rouleau JL: β-blockers in congestive heart failure: A Bayesian meta-analysis. Ann Intern Med 134:550, 2001.
44. Gregory D, Udelson JE, Konstam MA: Economic impact of beta blockade in heart failure. Am J Med 110:74S, 2001.
45. Chin MH, Goldman L: Factors contributing to the hospitalization of patients with congestive heart failure. Am J Public Health 87:643, 1997.
46. McAlister FA, Lawson FME, Teo KK, et al: A systematic review of randomized trials of disease management programs in heart failure. Am J Med 110:378, 2001.

Disease Prevention

47. Krumholz HM, Weintraub WS, Bradford WD, et al: Task Force #2—The cost of prevention: Can we afford it? Can we afford not to do it? J Am Coll Cardiol 40:603, 2002.
48. Ross SD, Allen IE, Connelly JE, et al: Clinical outcomes in statin treatment trials: A meta-analysis. Arch Intern Med 159:1793, 1999.
49. Prosser LA, Stinnett AA, Goldman PA, et al: Cost-effectiveness of cholesterol-lowering therapies according to selected patient characteristics. Ann Intern Med 132:769, 2000.
50. Scandinavian Simvastatin Survival Study Group: Randomised trial of cholesterol lowering in 4444 patients with coronary heart disease: The Scandinavian Simvastatin Survival Study (4S). Lancet 344:1383, 1994.
51. Shepherd J, Cobbe SM, Ford I, et al: Prevention of coronary heart disease with pravastatin in men with hypercholesterolemia. N Engl J Med 333:1301, 1995.
52. Brown AD, Garber AM: Cost effectiveness of coronary heart disease prevention strategies in adults. Pharmacoeconomics 14:27, 1998.
53. Third Report of the National Cholesterol Education Program (NCEP) Expert Panel on Detection, Evaluation, and Treatment of High Blood Cholesterol in Adults (Adult Treatment Panel III): Final report. Circulation 106:3143, 2002.
54. Cummings SR, Rubin SM, Oster G: The cost-effectiveness of counseling smokers to quit. JAMA 261:75, 1989.
55. Song F, Raftery J, Aveyard P, et al: Cost-effectiveness of pharmacological interventions for smoking cessation: A literature review and a decision analytic analysis. Med Decis Making 22(Suppl):S26-S37, 2002.
56. Meenan RT, Stevens VJ, Hornbrook MC, et al: Cost-effectiveness of a hospital-based smoking cessation intervention. Med Care 36:670, 1998.

Diagnostic Testing

57. Shaw LJ, Hachamovitch R, Berman DS, et al: The economic consequences of available diagnostic and prognostic strategies for the evaluation of stable angina patients: An observational assessment to the value of precatheterization ischemia. J Am Coll Cardiol 33:661, 1999.
58. Kuntz KM, Fleischmann KE, Hunink MG, et al: Cost-effectiveness of diagnostic strategies for patients with chest pain. Ann Intern Med 130:709, 1999.
59. Garber AM, Solomon NA: Cost-effectiveness of alternative test strategies for the diagnosis of coronary artery disease. Ann Intern Med 130:719, 1999.
60. Boden WE, O'Rourke RA, Crawford MH, et al: Outcomes in patients with acute non-Q-wave myocardial infarction randomly assigned to an invasive as compared with a conservative management strategy. N Engl J Med 338:1785, 1998.
61. FRagmin and Fast Revascularisation during InStability in Coronary artery disease (FRISC II) Investigators: Invasive compared with non-invasive treatment in unstable coronary-artery disease: FRISC II prospective randomised multicentre study. Lancet 354:708, 1999.
62. Cannon CP, Weintraub WS, Demopoulos LA, et al: Comparison of early invasive and conservative strategies in patients with unstable coronary syndromes treated with the glycoprotein IIb/IIIa inhibitor tirofiban. N Engl J Med 344:1879, 2001.
63. Fox KAA, Poole-Wilson PA, Henderson RA, et al: Interventional versus conservative treatment for patients with unstable angina or non-ST-elevation myocardial infarction: The British Heart Foundation RITA 3 randomised trial. Lancet 360:743, 2002.
64. Barnett PG, Chen S, Boden WE, et al: Cost-effectiveness of a conservative, ischemia-guided management strategy after non-Q-wave myocardial infarction: Results of a randomized trial. Circulation 105:680, 2002.
65. Mahoney EM, Jurkovitz CT, Chu H, et al: Cost and cost-effectiveness of an early invasive vs conservative strategy for the treatment of unstable angina and non-ST-segment elevation myocardial infarction. JAMA 288:1851, 2002.
66. Janzon M, Levin LA, Swahn E, et al: Cost-effectiveness of an invasive strategy in unstable coronary artery disease: Results from the FRISC II invasive trial. Eur Heart J 23:31, 2002.

Developments in Economic Analysis

67. Hlatky MA: Role of economic models in randomized clinical trials. Am Heart J 137:S41, 1999.
68. Diehr P, Yanez D, Ash A, et al: Methods for analyzing health care utilization and costs. Annu Rev Public Health 20:125, 1999.

CHAPTER 3

Clinical Decision-Making in Cardiology

J. Sanford Schwartz

Despite continuing significant advances in medical knowledge and technology, skilled clinical decision-making remains the cornerstone of medical practice. The goal of medical decision-making is to optimize patients' health and health care. This optimization requires integration and application of cognitive skills, medical knowledge, and judgment with social, cultural, and interpersonal sensitivity. Medical decision-making is a multistep process, involving problem identification, selection and assessment of diagnostic information, and choice of interventions.

Medical decision-making is challenging. Medical decisions involve high stakes and are characterized by imperfect information and complex problems that vary in presentation and response to treatment. Medical information is voluminous, widely dispersed, rapidly changing, often conflicting, and of uncertain validity and reliability. Important information is often not available.

All clinical information has diagnostic value, albeit imperfect and subject to error, with imperfect validity and reliability. Thus, all medical decisions are subject to some degree of uncertainty. Paradoxically, the tremendous progress of medical science, while enhancing our ability to diagnose and manage disease and disability, has made medical decision-making ever more complex and difficult.

Medical decision-making is further complicated by *variation* in disease among biological systems and in preferences and values across individuals; *uncertainty* of medical information; and *scarcity* of resources, with resulting need to allocate resources and address trade-offs among benefits, risks, and costs. The decision-making task is made more complex by social, organizational, economic, and environmental factors, including the need to incorporate the perspectives, preferences, values, and needs of patients, families, and providers; highly fragmented financing and delivery systems; inadequate clinical information systems; and misaligned incentives.

The goal of this chapter is to provide a basic framework for approaching, evaluating, and organizing medical information. The chapter discusses cognitive psychological, behavioral, and environmental aspects of decision-making; assessment and use of diagnostic tests; and evaluation and selection of medical practices and interventions. Decision-making related to resource constraints and cost-effectiveness, an increasingly important component of medical decision-making, is discussed in Chapter 2.

Cognitive, Behavioral, and Environmental Influences on Decision-Making

Decision-Making Models

Medical judgment is an inferential process applied to incomplete and inherently uncertain information, requiring integration of observational and diagnostic data with current understanding of disease processes and responses to interventions. Medical reasoning is complex and incompletely understood, involving a combination of heuristic, probabilistic, causal, and deterministic processes.

The first step in medical decision-making involves problem identification and definition through observation, clinical examination, and diagnostic testing. Generation and evaluation of diagnostic hypotheses provide a framework for collection and interpretation of diagnostic information. Medical reasoning and problem solving are iterative, involving modification, refinement, elimination, and addition of diagnostic alternatives. Hypotheses are verified for coherence, adequacy, and parsimony until a limited set of working hypotheses are produced.

Probabilistic reasoning explicitly considers the relationships and associations between clinical variables and is used to reduce the uncertainty inherent in medical decisions. Probabilistic reasoning consists of (1) estimation of prevalence (prior, preexisting, or pretest probability); (2) assessment of conditional probability (frequency of associations between variables and candidate diagnoses and normal individuals); and (3) mathematical calculation of revised probabilities.

Causal reasoning is fundamental to modern medical practice. Causal thinking provides a coherent conceptual framework for explaining clinical observations and outcomes by simulating the natural history of disease and determining the consistency among findings, scientific knowledge, and models of physiology and pathophysiology. Causal models are commonly used when abnormal findings or events are not congruent or compatible with normal physiology. The validity of causal models is a function of the strength, correlation, congruity, and contiguity in time between findings and events.

Deterministic (categorical) reasoning involves use of unambiguous rules derived from medical knowledge to simplify practice and reduce cognitive burden (e.g., ordered, simple structured algorithms to facilitate performance of specific clinical tasks). Frequently used for common, relatively straightforward problems, deterministic thinking is not well suited to complex problems, high levels of uncertainty, multiple complaints, and situations in which underlying logic cannot be precisely defined. Advances in information technology will enhance the utility and practical application of deterministic reasoning.

Heuristic Reasoning

Heuristics are shortcuts used to help cope with cognitive and psychological limitations and reduce information complexity to a manageable level. As expertise increases, data collection, interpretation, and action become more selective and more automatic. Although generally helpful, they may lead to predictable decision-making errors.

Information is interpreted in light of past experience and the context in which it occurs; perceptions are selective and strongly influenced by beliefs, experiences, and expectations. Knowledge and experience may accentuate the impact of preconceived notions on observations (e.g., the same heart sounds may be interpreted somewhat differently depending on what the physician expects to hear). Problem formulation and interpretation are influenced by how information is *framed* (e.g., information ordering or formatting, use of value-laden phrases, presenting events as gains or losses). For example, framing an alternative as trying to "help the patient" versus "doing nothing" biases the decision in favor of intervention.

Decision-making is influenced by inherent human psychological and cognitive factors and constraints. Short-term memory capacity is limited (the average person can consider only up to seven alternatives simultaneously). Memory is context dependent and fallible. Rather than representing accurate recall of past experiences or events, memories are reconstructed from separately stored pieces of information, with missing details filled in by logical inference, resulting in a new blended memory. Medical decisions can be distorted by "cognitive dissonance," aligning beliefs with behavior (either before or after the fact) to reduce or eliminate psychological inconsistencies and contradictions. Thus, before engaging in important medical decisions, physicians should consider how they are motivated by prior belief or expectation to interpret data and how the same findings might be otherwise interpreted in the absence of such motives and expectations.

Physicians often attempt to classify patients' conditions on the basis of their similarity to other patients' conditions (*representativeness*). Although often useful in formulating diagnoses or estimating response to therapy, the representativeness heuristic may, by inappropriately focusing on misleading or noninformative components of clinical presentation, lead to misestimated probabilities (e.g., the frequent underestimation of the probability of acute ischemia in women presenting with chest discomfort), failure to consider the prevalence of alternative possibilities, insensitivity to sample size (giving equal weight to large and small trials although observations based on larger samples should engender greater confidence than those derived from smaller samples), misconceptions of chance (e.g., assuming that if a rare adverse event occurs it will not occur again in the near future), regression to the mean (e.g., failing to recognize that patients tend to present when symptoms worsen and thus misattributing therapeutic benefit to normal waxing and waning of symptoms), and undercorrection for correlation (e.g., overestimating the value of diagnostic tests that measure highly correlated information).

Similarly, there is a tendency to estimate an event's likelihood by the ease with which its occurrence can be recalled (*availability*), resulting in overestimating the probability of events that are familiar, salient, easily imaginable, or recent (e.g., the tendency to assess the likelihood that a patient will respond to a specific antihypertensive drug on the basis of one's experience the last several times the drug was prescribed rather than data from large, rigorous clinical trials) or attempting to predict events that are inherently not predictable (illusory correlation).

Diagnostic information is obtained in a temporal sequence, with initial probability estimates revised as new information becomes available. However, earlier probability estimates (even when based on incomplete information) are typically insufficiently adjusted for subsequent information (*adjustment and anchoring*). For example, initial information suggesting nonischemic chest pain (premenopausal woman) followed by information more suggestive of coronary artery disease (exertional substernal chest discomfort) may result in a lower estimate of the probability of coronary ischemia than if the order of information presentation was reversed. The tendency to view events that already happened as relatively inevitable and obvious (*hindsight bias*) also distorts probability estimates by assigning a higher pre-event probability after the fact than was estimated before the event.

Reduction of Psychological and Heuristic Errors

Cognitive errors occur in all stages of diagnostic reasoning—hypothesis generation, information gathering and processing, data diagnosis, and treatment. The best way to avoid or minimize such errors is to be aware of their existence and undertake conscious actions to override them. Thus, physicians should address the tendency to develop inappropriately narrow search sets by consciously considering alternative perspectives and expanding consideration of the range of potential diagnostic and therapeutic alternatives; reduce uncertainty of predictions by increasing confidence intervals, maintaining alternative hypotheses longer, replacing rejected hypotheses with new hypotheses (instead of just narrowing options as additional information is collected), and seeking and recognizing correlated information; vigilantly seek evidence that either supports competing diagnoses or does not support the working hypothesis, especially for rare but catastrophic conditions; keep accurate records; and explicitly consider why or how results might have turned out differently. Decision-making errors can also be reduced by recognizing common statistical errors, including the narrower confidence intervals associated with larger studies and greater experience, using regression to the mean, and distinguishing between association and causality and statistical versus clinical significance (as may occur in very large studies, where small differences may be statistically significant but not clinically important).

Behavioral and Environmental Influences

Medical decision-making is often presented as a rational, logical sequence, driven by dispassionate evaluation of scientific knowledge. However, medical decisions are influenced by a variety of behavioral, social, organizational, and environmental factors.

People are inherently social organisms; we take behavioral cues from and are concerned with how we are viewed by others (especially our patients and our colleagues). Increasingly, medical decisions are made in conjunction with other people. However, group judgment and decision-making are prone to biases, including insufficient consideration of challenging or disconfirming information, resulting in overconfidence and self-reinforcing judgments and behavior (group attribution error) and polarization of opinion. *Typically, groups perform better than the average member but not as well as the best member.* Errors attributable to group judgment and decision-making can be reduced by brainstorming independently rather than in a group and, within groups, encouraging dissent and criticism, refraining from stating personal preferences at the outset, and appointing a "devil's advocate." For particularly important decisions, decision-making may be improved by creating independent groups to consider the same question and inviting qualified outside experts and colleagues to challenge the group consensus.

Physicians' characteristics (age, knowledge, training, attitudes, experience, practice setting and organization, geographical location, social integration, personality traits, and general decision style such as attitude toward risk) influence decisions, as does *how information is communicated* (characteristics of the message, messenger, and the medium and setting in which it is communicated). Although medical information is communicated through a variety of channels (journals and textbooks, continuing medical education, professional societies, advertising, public media), opinion leaders are most influential. Characteristics of the information itself (e.g., cost, risk, ability to apply, ease of reversibility) also affect decisions.

Education (including clinical practice guidelines) has a major influence on decision-making. However, acceptance and credibility of education are a function of the sponsor, format and context, and previous education and training. Educational efforts can also be distorted or undermined if they conflict with other incentives, practice style, regulations, or professional and local norms and values.

The environment in which medicine is practiced also strongly influences medical decision-making. Administrative structure, process, and regulation can influence physicians' decision-making through construction or elimination of barriers and timely provision of cues, reminders, feedback, and support. However, unless particularly potent or cumbersome, such factors are often easily bypassed and rapidly extinguished. Feedback of credible, relevant data, especially by respected sources and provided on a timely basis (e.g., expert-generated computer reminders at the time of service), may strongly influence medical decisions. Monetary incentives are powerful influencers of decision-making and practice but are difficult to calibrate and must be aligned and consistent with professional, social, cultural, and organizational knowledge, values, and norms. Thus, a wide range of factors exert powerful influence on medical decisions, especially when aligned in combination with one another and reinforced over time.

Diagnostic Decision-Making

Diagnostic tests are used to define medical problems with sufficient precision to guide management of patients. Diagnostic tests are useful to the degree that they provide new information that beneficially affects subsequent diagnostic work-up, clinical management, and health outcome. New information alone is of little value if it does not alter patients' care or health.

Interpretation and use of a diagnostic test are driven by the clinical objective, the test's ability to discriminate between the presence or absence of disease, and the safety, efficacy, effectiveness, and cost-effectiveness of testing and therapy (Fig. 3–1).

For every clinical condition, there is a probability of disease above which intervention is indicated, the "test-treatment threshold," and a probability below which the disease can be excluded with sufficient confidence and other diagnostic possibilities considered, the "test–no treatment threshold." When the probability of disease is between these

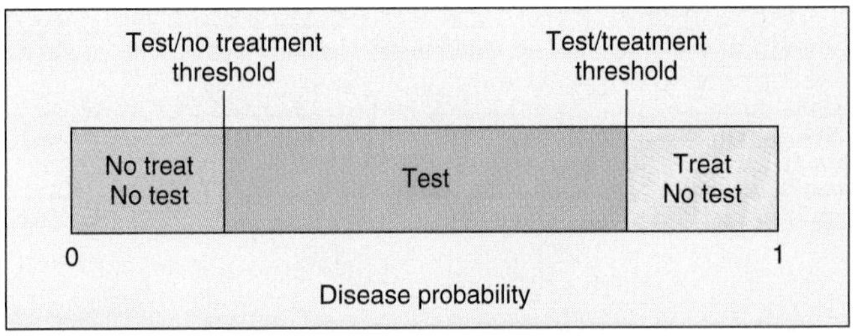

FIGURE 3–1 Schematic diagram of threshold theory of decision-making. (Adapted from Pauker SAG, Kassirer JP: The threshold approach to clinical decision making. N Engl J Med 302:1109, 1980.)

two thresholds, diagnostic tests, singly or in combination, are useful to the degree that they move the probability of disease either above the test-treatment threshold or below the test–no treatment threshold.

Treatment and testing thresholds are determined by diagnostic test performance characteristics (sensitivity and specificity) and the risks, costs, and benefits (mortality, morbidity, and quality of life) of treatment options. Less effective, riskier, or more costly therapy raises both the test-treatment threshold and the test–no treatment threshold (i.e., greater diagnostic certainty is required to institute treatment but less certainty is needed to exclude the disease). Conversely, less diagnostic certainty is required before instituting therapy or testing (lower test-treatment threshold and lower test–no treatment threshold) the more effective, safer, and less costly the treatment. Reduced test risk and cost and improved test performance widen the probability range in which testing is appropriate (higher test-treatment threshold and lower test–no treatment threshold), whereas increased test cost and risk and reduced sensitivity and specificity narrow the range for testing (lower test-treatment threshold and higher test–no treatment threshold). The more serious the disease (i.e., the greater its morbidity and mortality), the lower the test and treatment thresholds.

Diagnostic Test Performance

Although diagnostic tests must be both precise and reliable (yield a consistent result) and valid and accurate (yield a correct result), the primary measure of diagnostic test performance is the ability to distinguish between the presence and absence of a disease. An ideal diagnostic test perfectly discriminates those with disease (true positives [TPs]) and without disease (true negatives [TNs]). However, diagnostic tests detect markers imperfectly correlated with the presence or absence of disease. Thus, in their simplest dichotomous form (interpreted as either positive or negative), two types of misclassification errors occur: people free of a disease incorrectly classified as diseased (false-positives [FPs]) and people with a disease incorrectly classified as nondiseased (false-negatives [FNs]).

Before ordering a diagnostic test, the physician needs to consider the probability of the test's correctly identifying people with and without the disease. *Sensitivity* refers to the proportion of people with disease correctly identified by a diagnostic test, *specificity* the proportion of those without the disease correctly identified by the diagnostic test as nondiseased. When a test has been obtained, however, the physician needs to know the probability that a positive test correctly indicates the presence of disease *(predictive value positive [PV+])* and a negative test correctly identifies those without disease *(predictive value negative [PV−])* (Table 3–1).

For example, exercise stress test performance for detecting coronary ischemia among 1465 men with exercise-induced chest pain, with 1.0 mm of horizontal or downward-sloping

TABLE 3–1 Test Performance Characteristics

	Disease Present	Disease Absent	
Test positive	True-positive (TP)	False-positive (FP)	TP + FP
Test negative	False-negative (FN)	True-negative (TN)	FN + TN
	TP + FN	FP + TN	

Sensitivity = true positives/all patients with disease = TP/TP + FN.
Specificity = true negatives/all patients without disease = TN/TN + FP.
PV+ = true positives/all patients with positve tests = TP/TP + FP.
PV− = true negatives/all patients with negative tests = TN/TN + FN.

TABLE 3–2 Exercise Stress Test Performance Characteristics for Ischemic Congestive Heart Disease in Men Undergoing Cardiac Catheterization

	CHD Present			CHD Absent	
EST positive	815	TP	FP	115	**930**
EST negative	208	FN	TN	327	**535**
	1023			**442**	

Sensitivity = TP/TP + FN = TP/CHD+ = 815/1023 = 0.80.
Specificity = TN/TN + FP = TN/CHD− = 327/442 = 0.74.
PV+ = TP/TP + FP = TP/EST+ = 815/930 = 0.88.
PV− = TN/TN + FN = TN/EST− = 327/442 = 0.61.
CHD = congestive heart disease; EST = exercise stress test; FN = false-negative; FP = false-positive; PV = predictive value; TN = true-negative; TP = true-positive.
Adapted from Weiner DA, Ryan TJ, McCabe CH, et al: Exercise stress testing: Correlation among history of angina, ST-segment response and prevalence of coronary artery disease in the Coronary Artery Surgery Study (CASS). N Engl J Med 301:230, 1979.

ST segment depression, was compared with the resting baseline electrocardiogram (ECG) for at least 0.08 second (considered a positive test) and using the presence of 70 percent narrowing of one or more major coronary arteries on cardiac catheterization as the reference standard against which the exercise stress test was judged (Table 3–2).

Test sensitivity and specificity are not affected by disease prevalence or the pretest probability of disease. In contrast, PV+ increases and PV− decreases as the pretest probability of disease increases. Thus, the higher the prevalence or pretest probability of disease, the more likely a positive test result is to represent a true positive and the less likely a negative test result correctly identifies those without disease. If the pretest probability of disease is very high, even a negative test does not exclude the disease. Conversely, if the pretest probability of disease is very low, a positive test probably represents a false-positive result (Table 3–3).

Biases in Assessing Diagnostic Test Performance

Diagnostic test evaluation is frequently confounded by biases that tend to overstate the diagnostic test performance. The greater the discrepancy between study conditions and the setting in which the test is used, the less applicable the study results are to clinical practice.

REFERENCE ("GOLD") STANDARD PROBLEMS. Test performance should be assessed in relation to an independent reference ("gold") standard that establishes the presence or absence of a disease. However, true disease status is often hard to determine because of safety, cost, ethical, and scientific constraints. Imperfect reference standards result in misclassification errors, distorting estimates of test sensitivity

TABLE 3–3 Relationship Between Predictive Value of Positive Test and Disease Pretest Probability or Prevalence for Hypothetical Tests with Varying Test Sensitivity and Specificity

Pretest Probability	Sensitivity 0.90 Specificity 0.90	Sensitivity 0.95 Specificity 0.95	Sensitivity 0.99 Specificity 0.99
0.001	0.009	0.019	0.09
0.01	0.08	0.16	0.50
0.02	0.15	0.28	0.67
0.05	0.32	0.50	0.84
0.50	0.90	0.95	0.99

From Mulley AG: The selection and interpretation of diagnostic tests. *In* Goroll AH, May L, Mulley AG (eds): Primary Care Medicine. Philadelphia, Lippincott, 1987, p 7.

and specificity. For example, although coronary angiography is an appropriate reference standard for establishing a diagnosis of coronary vessel occlusion, it does not detect patients at increased risk for a cardiac event with nonocclusive coronary lesions (e.g., chemically unstable, thin-walled coronary plaque).

SPECTRUM BIAS. Diagnostic tests should be evaluated on a spectrum of diseased and nondiseased subjects sufficient to estimate test performance in clinically relevant subgroups, including healthy subjects with no disease as well as patients without the disease but with common comorbid conditions, recent onset of asymptomatic disease, established asymptomatic disease, established symptomatic disease, advanced disease, end-stage disease, and other diseases affecting the same anatomical organs. Evaluation of diagnostic tests on an unrepresentative sample results in overestimation of test sensitivity and specificity. For example, exercise stress test sensitivity varies with disease severity (highest in three-vessel disease; intermediate in other multivessel disease; lowest in non–left main single-vessel disease), lesion location (highest for left main lesions and progressively declining for left anterior descending, right coronary, and left circumflex lesions, respectively), and symptom presentation (highest in patients with classical exertional substernal discomfort)[1,2] (see Chap. 10).

REFERRAL, VERIFICATION, AND WORK-UP BIAS. Referral bias occurs when the outcome of the test being evaluated is used to determine which subjects are further evaluated by the reference standard (e.g., the more risky, expensive, or uncomfortable the reference standard, the greater this bias). The specificity of exercise radionuclide angiography was lower in practice than in initial published studies, as physicians used the test to select patients for further, more invasive evaluation by cardiac catheterization.[3] Because people with positive results on the test being evaluated are more likely to receive the reference test, work-up bias often overstates the sensitivity but underestimates the specificity of the test being evaluated.[4]

BLINDED INTERPRETATION. Results of the test being evaluated should be interpreted without knowledge of the reference standard test result or the true diagnosis. When such blinded, independent test interpretation does not occur, test sensitivity and specificity may be overestimated.

UNINTERPRETABLE RESULTS. Uninterpretable or nondiagnostic test results are common. A patient may not be able to exercise to the level of exertion required for a stress test; technicians vary in their ability to obtain high-quality echocardiograms of obese patients or to avoid attenuation of the inferior wall on single-photon emission computed tomography. Such uninterpretable test reports commonly are not included in calculation of diagnostic test performance, resulting in overestimation of test sensitivity, and are especially important when comparing alternative diagnostic tests when the frequency of uninterpretable test results differs among tests.

TEST-INTERPRETER UNIT. A diagnostic test's performance depends on both the test characteristics and the expertise of the person performing the test. This dependence is particularly important for many cardiac tests for which specifics of imaging agents, protocols, and technician and interpreter experience and skill affect test performance. The more important such factors, the more difficult it is to compare or generalize diagnostic performance across tests, interpreters, and sites.

Selection and Use of Diagnostic Tests

True-positive results allow selection of appropriate management, reduce patients' morbidity and mortality, and improve patients' function. True-negative results provide reassurance and avoid unnecessary risk, inconvenience, and cost. In contrast, false-positive results lead to unnecessary testing and treatment and can increase anxiety, and false-negative results lead to delayed or missed diagnosis and treatment, with associated adverse outcomes, unnecessary testing, and increased uncertainty and anxiety.

Tests with high sensitivity are preferred when the costs of missing a diagnosis are high; treatment is effective, safe, and inexpensive; false-positive results do not result in serious harm; and the goal is to minimize false-negative results (as in screening or when attempting to exclude a disease). Tests with high specificity are desired when the goal is to minimize false-positive results: the lower the effectiveness and the greater the risk and expense of therapy (e.g., surgery), the more false-positive results cause serious harm.

Selection of diagnostic tests varies according to the diagnostic process stage (Table 3–4). For example, although a history of chest discomfort has modest sensitivity for clinically significant acute ischemic coronary heart disease, it is not specific (i.e., has a high false-positive rate). Thus, physicians commonly evaluate such patients with an imaging test (e.g., exercise stress test, stress echocardiography, nuclear stress test) that, although more expensive and difficult to perform, has higher sensitivity. However, tests with very high specificity (e.g., coronary angiography) are required before initiating expensive or risky interventions.

The clinician can optimize sensitivity and specificity either by carefully selecting among alternative tests with different test performance characteristics or by altering the cutoff point of a test to emphasize *either* sensitivity *or* specificity (but not both simultaneously).

TABLE 3–4 Test Performance Characteristics Desired at Different Stages of Diagnosis

Objective	Desire	Avoid	Risk	Cost
Screening, case finding	High sensitivity	FN	Minimal	Low
Disease exclusion, R/O disease	High sensitivity	FN	Minimal-moderate	Low-moderate
Disease confirmation, R/in disease	High specificity	FP	Minimal-high	Low-high

FN = false-negative; FP = false-positive; R/in = rule in; R/O = rule out.

Screening

Diagnostic tests are commonly used for screening (detection of disease or elevated risk of disease in apparently well patients prior to the onset of symptoms). Because of the low prevalence of disease among screened populations, tests used for screening purposes always produce a high false-positive rate (low PV+). Unless screening is confined to a population at very high risk (50 percent), even the best screening tests yield more false-positive than true-positive results. Furthermore, the large majority of people being screened do not benefit. Thus, screening is best confined to serious diseases for which safe and effective treatment exists and early detection and treatment significantly improve patients' outcomes. A screening test itself must have high sensitivity (to minimize false-negative results) and specificity and be safe, inexpensive, convenient, and acceptable to the targeted screening population. In addition, because performance of the screening test will result in many false-positive results, appropriate follow-up tests with sufficiently high diagnostic performance and safety and reasonable cost must be available to identify and exclude those without the disease and to confirm the presence of disease in those affected. For this reason, generally even the best screening tests are best confined to populations and patients at increased risk for disease as determined by known risk factors.

The effectiveness and benefits of screening tests and screening testing programs are often overestimated. In deciding whether to screen for a disease, one must determine whether early diagnosis improves outcome. A common pitfall in the evaluation of screening programs is to measure the time between disease detection and death. *Lead time*, the interval between disease detection by screening and the time of usual symptomatic diagnosis, is a function of the rate of biological progression of a disease and screening test sensitivity. Screening effectiveness is often overestimated as a result of artifactual survival prolongation resulting from earlier disease detection in the absence of increased effectiveness of earlier intervention (*lead time bias*); enhanced participation by people more likely to adhere to recommended therapy (*adherence* or *compliance bias*); and unrepresentative impact of detection of prevalent cases in early screening cycles, which have a disproportionate number of slowly progressive cases relative to a larger proportion of more rapidly progressive incident cases in subsequent screening cycles (*prevalence bias*). Therefore, it is essential that promising screening tests and programs be rigorously evaluated by randomized clinical trials over multiple screening cycles before being widely adopted.

Information Content

A diagnostic test's value is a function of the amount of new additional information provided. Even the best diagnostic test does not contribute new diagnostic information when one is certain that the disease either is present or absent. Conversely, diagnostic tests provide the greatest diagnostic information the more uncertain one is prior to testing (intermediate prevalence or pretest probability).

Diagnostic tests are commonly interpreted dichotomously as either positive or negative. The information content of a diagnostic test is greater when one also considers the degree of positivity, as a slightly abnormal test is more likely to be a false-positive result than a markedly abnormal test, which is more likely to be a true-positive. For example, an exercise stress test with 3 mm of ST segment depression at an early stage of exercise is more likely to be a true-positive than an exercise stress test with 1 mm of ST depression at high levels of extended exertion. Similarly, a strongly negative test result is more likely to represent a true-negative than a slightly negative test result, which is more likely to be a false-negative. Borderline test results are commonly of limited diagnostic value. Thus, considering the extent of exercise stress test positivity provides approximately one-third more diagnostic information than interpreting the test as either positive or negative.[5,6]

Use of Likelihood Ratios in Clinical Practice

Sensitivity and specificity are difficult to use clinically because of the computational complexity of revising probabilities. Odds ratios (and likelihood ratios, which express test performance in terms of odds) are interchangeable with probabilities (Table 3–5), can be multiplied by each other, and thus are easier to use to revise disease probability at the bedside.

The likelihood ratio of a positive test (LR+) represents the TP/FP ratio for an interval test result and is obtained by calculating the probability of the positive test result among diseased subjects divided by the probability of the same positive test result among nondiseased subjects.

$$LR+ = \frac{\text{probability (result x)/patients with disease}}{\text{probability (result x)/patients without disease}}$$

TABLE 3–5 Conversion Between Probability and Odds

Odds	Probability
9 : 1	0.90
4 : 1	0.80
3 : 1	0.75
2 : 1	0.67
1 : 1	0.50
1 : 2	0.33
1 : 3	0.25
1 : 4	0.20
1 : 9	0.10

$$\text{Odds} = \frac{\text{probability}}{1 - \text{probability}}$$

Pretest odds × likelihood ratio = posttest odds

where

$$\text{Pretest odds} = \frac{\text{pretest probability disease}}{1 - \text{pretest probability disease}}$$

$$\text{Posttest odds} = \frac{\text{posttest probability disease}}{1 - \text{pretest probability disease}}$$

or

$$LR+ = \frac{\text{sensitivity}}{1 - \text{specificity}} = \frac{\text{probability of T+/patients with disease}}{\text{probability of T+/patients without disease}}$$

An LR+ greater than 1 indicates that the posttest probability of disease is greater than the pretest probability of disease, whereas an LR+ less than 1 indicates that the test result lowered the probability of disease (i.e., the posttest probability of disease is lower than the pretest probability of disease). The higher a test's likelihood ratio, the more likely the test result is to occur in a person with the disease as opposed to a person who is free of the disease, the more likely it is to be a true-positive, and the higher the posttest probability of disease. By providing information for ranges of test results, likelihood ratios maximize the information provided by diagnostic tests. A simple nomogram can be used to convert subjective estimated pretest probability of disease to posttest disease probability for a given LR+, facilitating its clinical use. A literature-based pooled estimate of the diagnostic performance of exercise stress test for congestive heart disease in patients with chest pain syndromes was developed by Diamond and colleagues[7] for various magnitudes of exercise-induced horizontal or downward-sloping ST segment depression, using 50 percent diameter narrowing of at least one coronary artery as the reference standard. Using a dichotomous result criterion of 1.0 ST segment depression as a positive test, exercise stress test sensitivity 0.65 and specificity 0.89. Considering the *degree* of test positivity improves discrimination between those with and without disease (Table 3–6 and Fig. 3–2).

Receiver Operating Characteristic Curves

Diagnostic test sensitivity and specificity depend on the cutoff point chosen between a normal and an abnormal test result. Selection of a cutoff point such that no disease-free people are incorrectly categorized as having disease (specificity = 1.0) results in many false-negative results and low test sensitivity. Conversely, a cutoff point that results in correct identification of all people with disease (sensitivity = 1.0) misclassifies disease-free people as having disease (increased FP), resulting in low test specificity.

A receiver operating characteristic curve is a plot of test sensitivity versus 1 – specificity as the definition of positive test is varied across the full range of clinically relevant values.[8] Table 3–7 illustrates the trade-offs among test sensitivity (true-positive rate), specificity (true-negative rate), and 1 – specificity (false-positive rate) for alternative ST segment positivity criteria for the exercise stress test.

TABLE 3–6 Interval Exercise Stress Test Likelihood Ratios

EST Positivity Criteria (mm ST Segment Depression)	Sensitivity (TP Rate)	1 – Specificity (FP Rate)	Likelihood Ratio (Sensitivity/1 – Specificity)
0.0 ≤ ST < 0.5	0.143	0.625	0.23
0.5 ≤ ST < 1.0	0.208	0.227	0.92
1.0 ≤ ST < 1.5	0.233	0.110	2.12
1.5 ≤ ST < 2.0	0.088	0.021	4.19
2.0 ≤ ST < 2.5	0.133	0.012	11.08
2.5 ≤ ST	0.195	0.005	39.0

EST = exercise stress test; FP = false-positive; TP = true-positive.
Adapted from Diamond GA, Forrester JS: Analysis of probability as an aid in the clinical diagnosis of coronary-artery disease. N Engl J Med 300:1350, 1979.

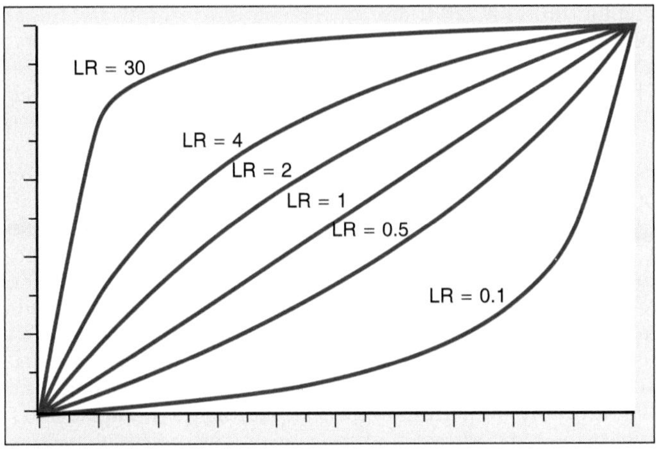

FIGURE 3–2 Relationship of alternative diagnostic test likelihood ratios for a positive test result to pretest and posttest disease probability.

TABLE 3–7 Relationship Between ST Segment Depression Criterion and Exercise Stress Test Sensitivity and Specificity

ST Segment (mm)	Sensitivity	Specificity	1 − Specificity
≥0.5	0.86	0.77	0.23
≥1.0	0.65	0.89	0.11
≥1.5	0.42	0.98	0.02
≥2.0	0.33	0.99	0.01
≥2.5	0.20	0.995	0.005

From Diamond GA, Forrester JS: Analysis of probability as an aid in the clinical diagnosis of coronary artery disease. N Engl J Med 300:1350, 1979.

Given the inherent trade-off between sensitivity and specificity as a test's positivity criterion is varied over a range of cutoff points,[9,10] it is not appropriate or informative to discuss either test sensitivity or specificity without consideration of the other, as test sensitivity can always be increased by adopting a more lenient positivity criterion but only at the expense of decreased specificity and vice versa.

The optimal diagnostic test cutoff point is a function of disease prevalence and estimated pretest probability of disease; test sensitivity and specificity; and the risks, costs, and benefits of correct and incorrect diagnoses (themselves a function of disease severity and the safety, effectiveness, and cost of therapeutic interventions).

$$\frac{\text{sensitivity}}{1-\text{specificity}} = \frac{\text{net cost TN} - \text{net cost FP}}{\text{net cost TN} - \text{net cost FN}} \times \frac{\text{posttest probability no disease}}{\text{posttest probability disease}}$$

Published diagnostic test cutoff points are generally more subjectively determined and thus may not be the most appropriate clinical values to use.

COMPARISON OF PERFORMANCE OF ALTERNATIVE DIAGNOSTIC TEST SYSTEMS. The performance of competing diagnostic tests must be compared over a range of cutoff points, which requires a receiver operating characteristic curve. When using receiver operating characteristic curves to compare the performance of competing diagnostic tests, the superior diagnostic technology is higher and farther to the left in the receiver operating characteristic curve (i.e., sensitivity is greater for any given level of specificity and vice versa), and the greater the area under the receiver operating characteristic curve (or the greater the ROC curve area within a clinically relevant range of test cutoff points), the better the diagnostic test.[7]

TABLE 3–8 Combination Testing: Exercise Stress Test and Radionuclide Angiocardiography

Test Combination Positivity Criterion	Sensitivity	Specificity
EST	0.88	0.46
RNA	0.92	0.34
EST or RNA	0.96	0.29
EST and RNA	0.65	0.68

EST = exercise stress test; RNA = radionuclide angiocardiography.
Campos CT, Chu HW, D'Agostino HJ Jr, Jones RH: Comparison of rest and exercise radionuclide angiocardiography and exercise treadmill testing for diagnosis of anatomically extensive coronary artery disease. Circulation 67:1204, 1983.

Using Tests in Combination

For most problems, multiple diagnostic tests are used in combination to provide the diagnostic information required to guide patients' management. Multiple testing offers the advantages of increased information, improved diagnosis, speed of diagnosis, convenience, and, in some circumstances, reduced cost. However, multiple tests expose patients to increased risks and costs and, at times, diagnostic and therapeutic delay. In addition, as the number of diagnostic tests performed increases, the opportunity for discrepancies among test results increases substantially, increasing the complexity of test interpretation.

When multiple tests are performed, one must adopt criteria for interpreting discrepant test combinations. A test combination may be interpreted as positive if *all* tests are positive (conjunctive positivity criterion). Conversely, a test combination may be interpreted as positive if *any* of the tests performed are positive (disjunctive positivity criteria). Disjunctive criteria for interpreting test combinations increase sensitivity and decrease specificity relative to the individual tests, whereas conjunctive criteria decrease sensitivity but increase specificity relative to the individual tests (Table 3–8).

Thus, conjunctive criteria are preferred when false-positive results are undesirable and specificity is to be maximized. Disjunctive testing is used when false-negative results are undesirable and sensitivity is to be maximized.

TEST CORRELATION AND CONDITIONAL DEPENDENCE. Tests used in combination are often partially correlated with each other. The greater correlation among tests, the less additional information gained from using tests in combination. Tests that measure different aspects of a suspected pathological condition or use different methods of diagnosis (e.g., serological tests and imaging tests) are more likely to provide independent information than test combinations using similar methods.

SEQUENTIAL VERSUS CONCURRENT TESTING. When tests are used in combination, they can be performed either concurrently or sequentially, with performance of subsequent tests based on the results of previous tests. Concurrent test strategies result in faster diagnosis but involve performance of more tests than sequential testing. Thus, sequential testing is generally more appropriate when problem evolution is slow and when costs of slower diagnosis are lower (e.g., outpatients), test risk is high, and the costs of delayed therapy are low. Concurrent testing is preferred when problem evolution is rapid and costs of delay are high (e.g., hospitalized patients), test risk is low, and costs of delayed treatment are high.

Therapeutic Decision-Making

The goal of therapy is to improve the patient's outcome and health. Medical interventions are assessed in terms of *safety* (acceptable side effects), *efficacy* (net benefit under ideal conditions), *effectiveness* (net benefit under routine conditions), and *cost-effectiveness* (incremental benefits relative to incremental costs). Because all interventions in practice have some benefit and risk, the challenge is to determine the trade-offs between benefit and risk in specific patients (i.e., how much net benefit, in which patients, under what conditions).

Therapeutic decision-making requires (1) identifying and defining the potential courses of action, (2) estimating the various potential resulting outcomes and their likelihood of occurrence, (3) assessing the value of each outcome on the basis of the trade-offs between risk and benefit (especially difficult when selecting among alternative competing options), and (4) assessing how patients value alternative outcome states. Although most clinical decisions are made subjectively using a combination of approaches and principles previously discussed, quantitative decision support methods can assist the physician with this complex and challenging task.

Predictive models use various forms of statistical and mathematical regression and related techniques (e.g., neural networks) to identify a parsimonious set of clinical variables that predict a disease state or outcome of therapy. For example, the Jones criteria provide a predictive model for rheumatic fever (see Chap. 82), Framingham risk equations estimate risk of developing congestive heart disease (see Chaps. 21 and 22), and models have been developed to predict the risk of coronary artery bypass graft surgery and coronary angioplasty (see Chap. 52). Predictive models are merely mathematical diagnostic tests, and their interpretation and use are thus subject to the principles described previously for diagnostic tests.

Decision support models are used for a wide range of clinical decisions, ranging from complex problems characterized by high uncertainty, risk, or cost to standardization of management for common, routine problems. Decision models (of which decision analysis is currently the most common and familiar) are prescriptive decision aids (i.e., they seek to improve medical decision-making by proposing how decisions should be made rather than describing how decisions actually are made). In addition to help in guiding clinical decisions, such models are particularly useful for informing clinical decision-making: organizing the salient issues for traditional clinical decision-making, identifying (through single-variable or multivariable sensitivity analysis, where the point estimates of model parameters are varied across a range of plausible values) the critical elements that drive decisions and therefore need to be most precisely defined, and explicitly clarifying trade-offs among safety, effectiveness, and cost.

Decision support models structure clinical decisions, precisely defining the question to be addressed; identifying relevant exhaustive, mutually exclusive alternative actions that may be undertaken and their potential outcomes; and estimating the probability that events will occur and their associated costs and values (i.e., "utilities"). Parameter values are estimated and integrated from the best available experimental (randomized trials), quasiexperimental (observational cohort and case-control studies), and nonexperimental (meta-analysis, models, expert opinion) studies. The expected value of each decision path is calculated and aggregated at each decision node, with the decision providing the highest expected utility the preferred management option. Sensitivity analyses identify the impact of alternative estimates on outcome and decisions and provide an estimate of the robustness of findings.

The primary advantage of decision modeling is its structured, explicit nature, which forces systematic examination of the problem and assignment of explicit values, avoids information processing errors, and focuses attention on parameters that drive clinical decisions. The primary disadvantages are their complexity to develop and explain and the difficulty in maintaining and updating the models. Thus, even when not directly applicable at the point of care of patients, such models are extremely useful for informing general clinical approaches and for guiding development of clinical guidelines.

In theory, in making decisions the physician should act as the patient's agent, choosing the management option the patient would prefer if the patient possessed the same medical information as the physician. For many medical problems there is more than one reasonable management alternative, and the choice is frequently driven by the patient's values and preferences for alternative beneficial outcomes and tolerance for potential adverse events and effects of disease sequelae. Because the physicians' knowledge of the patients' preferences and values is generally incomplete, patients' values and preferences in terms of risk and various potential benefits need to be identified and incorporated into clinical decisions.

Decision support interventions and systems are increasingly attractive methods to supplement physicians' knowledge, providing physicians with reminders and cues by providing timely feedback. However, decision support systems are complex to develop, keep current, and implement, although timely support is facilitated by increasing computerization and especially by the advent of computerized medical record systems.[9-11]

REFERENCES

1. Pauker SG, Kassirer JP: Decision analysis. N Engl J Med 316:250, 1987.
2. Black ER, Panzer RJ, Mayewski RJ, Griner PF: Characteristics of diagnostic tests and principles for their use in quantitative decision making. *In* Black ER, Bordley DR, Tape TG, Panzer RJ (eds): Diagnostic Strategies for Common Medical Conditions. Philadelphia, American College of Physicians, 1999, p 7.
3. Mulley AG: The selection and interpretation of diagnostic tests. *In* Goroll AH, May L, Mulley AG (eds): Primary Care Medicine. Philadelphia, Lippincott, 1987, p 7.
4. Froelicher VF, Myers J: Exercise and the Heart. 3rd ed. Philadelphia, WB Saunders, 1999.
5. Choi BC: Sensitivity and specificity of a single diagnostic test in the presence of work-up bias. J Clin Epidemiol 45:581, 1992.
6. Begg CB, Greenes RA, Iglewicz B: The influence of uninterpretability on the assessment of diagnostic tests. J Chron Dis 39:575, 1986.
7. Diamond GA, Forrester JS: Analysis of probability as an aid in the clinical diagnosis of coronary-artery disease. N Engl J Med 300:1350, 1979.
8. Diamond GA, Hirsch M, Forrester JS, et al: Application of information theory to clinical diagnostic testing. The electrocardiographic stress test. Circulation 63:915, 1981.
9. Hershey JC, Cebul RD, Williams SV: Clinical guidelines for using two dichotomous tests. Med Decis Making 6:68, 1986
10. Schwartz JS, Kinosian B, Pierskalla W, Lee H: Strategies for screening blood for HIV virus antibody: Use of a decision support system. JAMA 264:1704, 1990.
11. Schwartz JS, Dans PE, Kinosian BP: Human immunodeficiency virus test evaluation, performance, and use: Proposals to make good tests better. JAMA 259:2574, 1988.

CHAPTER 4

Measurement and Improvement of Quality of Cardiovascular Care

Thomas H. Lee

Measurement of Quality

In recent years, the measurement and improvement of quality of cardiovascular care have grown in importance due to several factors, including methodological advances in measurement of quality and changes in the health care environment. This trend has been made possible by clinical research that has helped define "evidence-based medicine" for cardiovascular disease—that is, knowledge of which interventions improve patient outcomes. Insight into which interventions should be delivered has naturally led to interest in the reliability with which high-quality care is delivered. At first, health services researchers were the main users of data on quality of cardiovascular care, but today their methods are widely used in quality improvement programs and in publicly available "report cards" for insurance plans, hospitals, and individual physicians.

Interest in such report cards has been intensified by public concerns about quality in the United States and other countries. In 1999, the U.S. Institute of Medicine issued a report that showed serious problems stemming from medical errors leading to harm to patients.[1] In 2001, a follow-up report entitled "Crossing the Quality Chasm" identified major system problems as the source of many errors.[2] During this period, organizations in several countries began disseminating information on quality of care by health care providers to the public to encourage the development of a consumer-based marketplace in which patients use data to improve the quality of their care.[3]

A third report from the Institute of Medicine, released in 2002,[4] recommended that "purchasing strategies should provide rewards to providers who achieve higher levels of quality." Particularly in the United States and England, the health care marketplace began witnessing the introduction of a variety of incentive programs that reward physicians and hospitals whose performance data suggest superior care.

In fact, measurement of quality of cardiovascular care had been building momentum throughout the 1990s, and numerous agencies in the United States are actively involved in the development of measures and dissemination of data (Table 4–1).[5] Statewide report cards on cardiac surgery and percutaneous coronary interventions for hospitals and individual physicians have been introduced in some states.[6-8] The National Committee for Quality Assurance (NCQA) developed measures of quality for managed care organizations known as HEDIS (Healthplan Employers Data and Information Set).[9,10] Most recently, measures for cardiovascular quality of care delivered by hospitals have been introduced by the Joint Commission on Accreditation of Healthcare Organizations (JCAHO),[11] and data on volume of cardiovascular procedures have been disseminated via organizations such as Leapfrog.[12] This phenomenon has not been limited to the United States; detailed data on cardiovascular and other outcomes are available via the Internet for hospitals in the United Kingdom[13] and other countries.

GUIDELINES AND PERFORMANCE MEASURES. Amid calls for caution and expression of concern, health care professionals have responded with a variety of initiatives aimed at improving care. The most prominent of these responses in cardiovascular medicine has been the development of guidelines, particularly those from the American College of Cardiology (ACC) and the American Heart Association (AHA).[14,15] These guidelines often provide the basis for measures of quality (also known as performance measures), but serve a different purpose. Guidelines are written to describe a consensus on the diagnostic or therapeutic interventions appropriate for most patients in most circumstances. Guidelines are written with the expectation that individual physicians will use discretion in the treatment of individual patients, and *not* follow the guidelines in certain cases. Key guidelines are summarized in this text.

In contrast, performance measures build upon the consensus expressed in guidelines to define "rules" or standards of care. As summarized by an AHA/ACC working group, "Performance measures should be explicit actions, performed for carefully specified, easily identified (using clear administrative and/or easily documented clinical criteria) patients for whom adherence should be advocated in all but the most unusual circumstances".[16] When these standards are not met, the implication is that an error has occurred (e.g., failure to recommend aspirin for patients with acute myocardial infarction).

Therefore, performance measures tend to be written to define the minimum standards of adequate care, as opposed to the targets that might define excellent care. For example, NCQA uses a HEDIS measure for cholesterol management in patients who have had acute myocardial infarction, coronary artery bypass graft surgery, or percutaneous coronary interventions. Guidelines from the National Heart, Lung, and Blood Institute encouraged physicians to pursue a target low-density lipoprotein (LDL) cholesterol level below 100 mg/dl for this population,[17] but, as of 2003, the HEDIS measure required managed care organizations to report the percent-age of such patients who achieved an LDL level below 130 mg/dL. The NCQA rationale was that although experts agreed that a level below 100 mg/dl reflects excellent care, the strength of evidence is such that physicians should be faulted only if they allowed patients with coronary disease to have a level above 130 mg/dl.[18]

The practical implication of this relationship between performance measures and guidelines in cardiovascular medicine is that quality measures are usually closely linked to class I indications from the ACC/AHA guidelines—that is, conditions for which there is evidence or general agreement that a given procedure or treatment is useful and effective. Failure to perform

TABLE 4–1 Key Organizations Involved in Measurement of Quality of Cardiovascular Care

Organization	Major Activity	Focus	Web Site
American College of Cardiology (ACC)	Guidelines Applied in Practice (GAP) ACC/AHA Task Force on Performance Measures	Health care providers	www.acc.org
American Heart Association (AHA)	Get with the Guidelines ACC/AHA Task Force on Performance Measures	Health care providers	www.americanheart.org
American Medical Association (AMA)	Physician Consortium for Quality Improvement	Physicians	www.ama-assn.org
Centers for Medicare & Medicaid Services (CMS) (Formerly the Health Care Financing Administration, or HCFA)	National Heart Care Project	Physicians and hospitals	www.cms.gov
Joint Commission on the Accreditation of Healthcare Organizations (JCAHO)	ORYX Initiatives	Accreditation of hospitals	www.jcaho.org
Leapfrog	Publication of volume data for cardiac procedures at hospitals	Hospitals	www.leapfroggroup.org
National Committee for Quality Assurance (NCQA)	Healthplan Employers Data and Information Set (HEDIS) Heart Stroke Provider Recognition Program	Accreditation of health plans; physician provider recognition programs	www.ncqa.org
National Quality Forum	Hospital Performance Measures Project	Hospitals	www.qualityforum.org

Adapted from Sperttus JA, Radford MJ, Every NR, et al: Challenges and opportunities in quantifying the quality of care for acute myocardial infarction: Summary from the Acute Myocardial Infarction Working Group of the American Heart Association/American College of Cardiology First Scientific Forum on Quality of Care and Outcomes Research in Cardiovascular Disease and Stroke. Circulation 107:1681, 2003.

interventions that are less strongly supported by evidence is too often a matter of judgment to use as a quality measure.

METHODOLOGICAL ISSUES. Many of the methodological issues that affect clinical research influence the measurement of cardiovascular quality, with two major additional themes. First, the performance data for individual physicians and hospitals may be made public in some cases; as a general rule, the more widely data are disseminated, the greater the demand for methodological rigor. Second, the collection and analysis of data for quality measurement is rarely funded as well as in clinical trials. Thus, the desire for methodological rigor must be weighed against the cost of collecting and analyzing the data.

Claims Data. The least expensive type of information used for quality measurement is claims data, which are collected for the purposes of mediating payment, not promoting quality of care; thus, there is little or no quality control for claims data regarding issues such as the accuracy of diagnoses. These data have the advantage of being readily available for large populations, but error rates in diagnoses are high, and information that is not required for payment is unavailable (e.g., whether heart failure is due to systolic or diastolic dysfunction, or whether blood pressure levels were controlled).

Retrospective Chart Review. This method can be used to collect more accurate clinical data, but such reviews are expensive and are complicated by the existence of multiple medical records for most patients. Patients generally have separate records at each hospital to which they have been admitted as well as at the office of their primary care physicians and the specialists from whom they have received care; none of these records is complete unless all of these health care providers are part of an integrated delivery system with a single electronic medical record. Even when all records are available for review, data collection from paper records is limited by the completeness, accuracy, and legibility of record-keeping.

Prospective Data Collection. Key data collection for quality measurement is becoming an increasingly common and important tactic for quality improvement. Standard dataforms for patients undergoing cardiac surgery or percutaneous coronary intervention (PCI) are now used at many medical centers. At some institutions, the data collected via these protocols are used for institutional databases or for inter-institutional collaborations, such as the Northern New England Cardiovascular Disease Study Group.[19] Many hospitals now report data on specific cardiovascular patient populations to national databases such as the Society of Thoracic Surgery or the American College of Cardiology's National Catheterization Data Registry. Participation in such databases allows comparison of institutional performance to regional and national benchmarks.

Collection of Patient Outcome Data. Collection of patient outcome data (e.g., 1-year mortality or functional status) is expensive and difficult. Administrative sources such as the National Death Index can provide information on whether individual patients have died within the United States; analogous resources are available in many other countries. However, obtaining information on the cause of death or on the status of patients who have not died requires interviews or surveys. Even when such data are available, the results should be adjusted for clinical and socioeconomic factors that are likely to influence the results. Therefore, many quality measures focus on processes such as the use of medications (e.g., beta blockers after acute myocardial infarction) or tests (e.g., measurement of LDL cholesterol) that are expected to lead to better outcomes.

DEFINITION OF QUALITY. A variety of definitions of quality have been proposed, reflecting the complexity of the health care system and its heterogeneous stakeholders. One of the most widely cited is that of the Institute of Medicine: "The degree to which health services for individual and populations increase the likelihood of desired health outcomes and are consistent with current professional knowledge."[20]

Error Reduction

An increasingly popular operational definition of quality is based on error reduction and the recognition that there are three major types of errors in health care: errors of underuse, overuse, and misuse (Table 4–2).[2,21] *Underuse* is the failure to provide a medical intervention when it is likely to produce a favorable outcome for a patient, such as the failure to prescribe an angiotensin-converting enzyme inhibitor for a patient with left ventricular dysfunction. *Overuse* occurs when an intervention becomes common practice even though its benefits do not justify the potential harm or costs, such as performance of exercise testing in asymptomatic patients with a low risk for cardiovascular disease. *Misuse* occurs when a preventable complication eliminates the benefit of an intervention. An example is continued administration of a statin to a patient with muscle tenderness and weakness, suggesting possible myopathy.

The relationship between guidelines and these three types of errors is close and complex. In ACC/AHA guidelines, class I indications sometimes define "rules" that, if not applied for an appropriate patient, would suggest an error of underuse. Class III indications define potential errors of overuse. The ACC/AHA guidelines tend to focus on two aspects of quality:

- Complying with evidence-based medicine (i.e., doing the right thing for the patient)
- Procedural quality (i.e., performing interventions correctly)

Failure to comply with evidence-based medicine may constitute an error of underuse (e.g., failure to use a beta blocker after acute myocardial infarction) or an error of overuse (e.g., performance of coronary angiography in a patient without clinical evidence of coronary artery disease). Failure to perform an intervention correctly can constitute an error of misuse (e.g., continued administration of a statin in a patient with symptoms of myopathy).

Structure, Process, Outcome. For deeper analysis of quality of health care, Donabedian and others recommend organization of evaluation into three categories—structure, process, and outcome (see Table 4–2).[22] *Structure* describes the components of the local health care system; relevant characteristics include the nurse-to-patient ratios, board certification status of physicians, and availability of computerized physician order entry systems and electronic medical records. *Process* elements of care describe the reliability with which key functions are performed (e.g., smoking cessation counseling for patients with coronary artery disease, administration of angiotensin-converting enzyme inhibitors to patients with left ventricular dysfunction). *Outcome* measures describe clinical outcomes such as mortality and morbidity or efficiency outcomes such as length of stay and overall costs.

A third framework that is increasingly used by organizations to assess their quality of care is that of the Institute of Medicine (see Table 4–2), which describes six dimensions that should serve as aims for improvement. In this structure, measures should be developed to reflect the goal of making health care safe, effective, patient-centered, timely, efficient, and equitable.[2]

- Safe—avoiding injuries to patients from the care that is intended to help them.
- Effective—providing services based on scientific knowledge to all who could benefit and refraining from providing services to those not likely to benefit (avoiding underuse and overuse, respectively).
- Patient-centered—providing care that is respectful of and responsive to individual patient preferences, needs, and values and ensuring that patient values guide all clinical decisions.
- Timely—reducing waits and sometimes harmful delays for both those who receive and those who give care.
- Efficient—avoiding waste, including waste of equipment, supplies, ideas, and energy.
- Equitable—providing care that does not vary in quality because of personal characteristics such as gender, ethnicity, geographic location, and socioeconomic status.

Many organizations are developing an array of measures, with one or two measures in each of these areas.

The ACC and AHA have articulated their own basic principles for selecting performance measures (Table 4–3).[16] Using these principles, AHA/ACC workgroups have reviewed specific domains for measurement of quality for patients with acute myocardial infarction and heart failure (Tables 4–4 and 4–5).[23] Their review notes that no major structural measures of quality fulfill all five of the principles described in Table 4–3. It comments that the evidence and infrastructure to support process measures are more fully developed for acute myocardial infarction than any other medical condition, but these measures are influenced by patient-specific factors such as the long list of relative contraindications to the use of beta blockers. The use of patient outcomes is plagued by expense and the difficulty of performing adequate risk adjustment. The workgroups supported internal use of such performance measures but expressed concern about public dissemination due to methodological limitations.

VOLUME AS A MARKER FOR QUALITY OF CARE. A surrogate marker for quality that is used by the public and by professional organizations is procedure volume. The relationship between volume and patient outcomes has been demonstrated in numerous studies focusing on hospitals and on physicians.[24-31] These relationships are complex; for some procedures, outcomes are associated with the volume for the hospital, whereas for other procedures, outcomes are associated with the volume for the individual physician.[25] The relationship between hospital volume and mortality for major cardiac surgical procedures from one major study is shown in Table 4–6 and Figure 4–1.[26] These findings were based on Medicare claims data from 1994 to 1999, and the study was the largest of its kind to date. Based on such research, organizations in the United States and abroad are publishing volume data for major procedures on their Internet sites to help patients choose their hospital for surgery.[12,13]

The ACC/AHA guidelines acknowledge research on the relationship between volume and outcome in guidelines, such as those for the use of PCI for patients with acute myocardial infarction.[32] These guidelines recommend that PCI should be performed by experienced operators at high-volume facilities (see Table 48G–1).[32] For patients without acute myocardial infarction, these guidelines recommend performance of PCI by higher volume operators

TABLE 4–2 Key Frameworks for Measurement and Improvement of Quality

Framework	Components
Error reduction	Errors of overuse Errors of underuse Errors of misuse
Donabedian[22]	Structure Process Outcome
Institute of Medicine[2]	Safe Effective Patient-centered Timely Efficient Equitable

TABLE 4–3 Basic Principles for Selection of Performance Measures

Principle	Comment
1. The performance measure must be meaningful.	Any potential performance measure must either be a meaningful outcome to patients and society or be closely linked to such an outcome.
2. The measure must be valid and reliable.	To serve as a useful marker of health care quality, it must be possible to measure the structure, process, or outcome of interest.
3. The measure can be adjusted for patient variability.	Interpretation of quality assessments necessitates that the observed outcomes/rates of process adherence be adjusted so that the observed differences between health care systems are due to the performance of those systems and not patient characteristics.
4. The measure can be modified by improvements in the processes of care.	To be a useful measure of quality, there must be an opportunity for motivated providers to improve their performance. This requires that the measures have variability after risk adjustment among providers. In addition, evidence should be available that suggests that alterations in the process of care can favorably influence this measure.
5. It is feasible to measure the performance of health care providers.	Although certain performance measures, such as health status, may fulfill all other criteria, the expense of collecting baseline and follow-up health status may be too great for a health care system to perform on a routine basis. Sensitivity to the fiscal implications of assessing certain performance measures may require limited sampling or avoidance altogether of certain potential measures of health care quality.

Adapted from Quality of Care and Outcomes Research in CVD and Stroke Working Groups: Measuring and improving quality of care: A report from the American Heart Association/American College of Cardiology first scientific forum on the assessment of healthcare quality in cardiovascular disease and stroke. Circulation 101:1483, 2000.

TABLE 4–4 Measures of Quality for Acute Myocardial Infarction

Type	Measures
Structure	Prehospital evaluation, triage, and treatment. Access to invasive and noninvasive cardiac tests and procedures, including transfer protocols to appropriate facilities when the necessary equipment or personnel is not available. Appropriately trained staff with access to cardiovascular specialists for management of patients with complications. Protocols or other management programs that ensure timely delivery of required therapies. Systems to ensure patient education, rehabilitation, and follow-up. Quality-improvement programs that provide for collection and review of data on care that can also be used to identify areas for improvement.
Process	Use of beta blockers at discharge and during admission. Use of aspirin at discharge and during admission. Timely and appropriate acute reperfusion (fibrinolysis or primary angioplasty) The use of angiotensin-converting enzyme inhibitors for patients with depressed left ventricular systolic function. Risk factor assessment and life-style counseling. Cholesterol status assessment and management.
Outcome	Death Readmission Physiological endpoints (e.g., achievement of blood pressure or cholesterol targets) Patient health status Patient satisfaction

TABLE 4–5 Measures of Quality for Heart Failure

Type	Measures
Structure	Availability of clear, evidence-based guidelines. Mechanism to systematically monitor patient care and outcomes. Organizational structure to move patients to appropriate level of care (e.g., access to an advanced heart failure facility). Availability of programs to address end-of-life needs.
Process	Clear documentation of left ventricular function. Use of angiotensin-converting enzyme inhibitors for patients with left ventricular systolic dysfunction. Use of digoxin for patients hospitalized with heart failure and left ventricular systolic dysfunction. Use of beta blockers for patients with NYHA Class II and III heart failure, left ventricular dysfunction, and no contraindication to beta blockers.
Outcome	Mortality Readmission Resource consumption Health status Satisfaction with care

TABLE 4–6 Annual Volume Categories for Hospitals Performing Cardiac Surgery

	Coronary Artery Bypass Graft Surgery (n)	Aortic and Mitral Valve Replacement (n)
Very low	<230	<43
Low	230-348	43-74
Medium	349-549	75-119
High	550-849	120-199
Very high	>849	>199

From Birkmeyer JD, Siewers AE, Finlayon EVA, et al: Hospital volume and surgical mortality in the United States. N Engl J Med 346:1128, 2002.

(>75 cases/year) with advanced technical skills (e.g., subspecialty certification) at high-volume centers (>400 cases/year), associated with on-site cardiovascular surgical programs, except in underserved areas that are geographically far removed from major centers (see Table 52G–1).

Current Quality of Cardiovascular Care

Some of the most comprehensive data on the quality of cardiovascular care have come from the Community Quality Index (CQI) study,[33] which draws upon medical records and self-reported information from random samples of patients from 12 U.S. metropolitan areas (Boston, MA; Cleveland, OH; Greenville, SC; Indianapolis, IN; Lansing, MI; Little Rock, AR; Miami, FL; Newark, NJ; Orange County, CA; Phoenix, AZ; Seattle, WA; and Syracuse, NY). For this study, investigators selected acute and chronic conditions that represented the leading causes of death and disability and developed indicators to assess potential problems with overuse and underuse of key processes. A sampling of the indicators for cardiovascular conditions and the total number of indicators used are summarized in Table 4–7, along with the percentage of recommendations that had been followed for the 6712 study participants. The full list of measures is available at *http://www.rand.org/health/mcglynn_appa.pdf.*

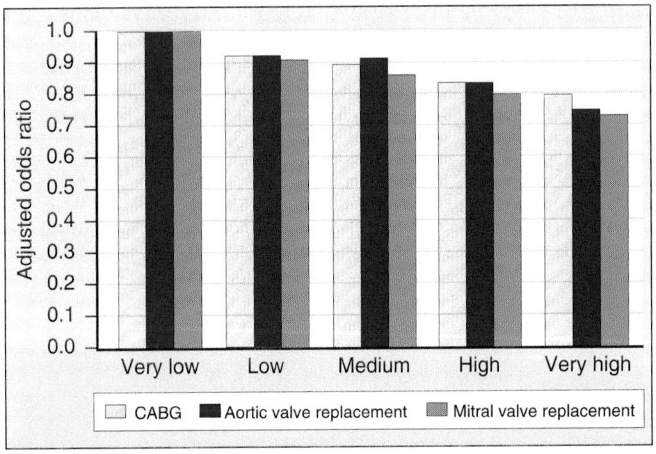

FIGURE 4–1 Relationship of hospital volume and adjusted odds ratio for mortality. Data from reference 26. See Table 4–6 for definition of volume categories. (Data from Birkmeyer JD, Siewers AE, Finlayson EVA, et al: Hospital volume and surgical mortality in the United States. N Engl J Med 346:1128, 2002.)

Rates of compliance with recommendations ranged from 68% for care of coronary disease to 25% for atrial fibrillation. For example, only 45% of patients presenting with a myocardial infarction received beta blockers, and only 61% of participants with a myocardial infarction who were appropriate candidates for aspirin therapy received this drug. It was concluded that patients received about half of the interventions supported by evidence from clinical trials.

HOSPITALS. For hospitals in the United States, measures of cardiovascular care mandated by the JCAHO have recently become important foci for quality improvement. These measures are part of a program called the ORYX Initiative, which integrates outcomes and other performance measurement data into the accreditation process for hospitals. Two of the core foci of the ORYX initiative are acute myocardial infarction and heart failure. It is anticipated that these data will be made public within a few years.

Health services researchers, the JCAHO, and other organizations have converged on several measures of quality of hospital care for acute myocardial infarction and for heart failure (Table 4–8). Review of medical records for Medicare

TABLE 4–7 Selected Cardiovascular Quality of Care Indicators and Classifications Used in the Community Quality Index Study

Condition	Examples of Selected Indicators	Percentage of Recommended Care Received (95% Confidence Interval)
Atrial fibrillation (10 indicators)	Patients with atrial fibrillation >48 hours' duration or of unknown duration who are undergoing elective electrical or chemical cardioversion should receive anticoagulation for at least 3 weeks prior to cardioversion unless they have had a transesophageal echocardiogram within 24 hours of cardioversion that indicates no clot. Patients with atrial fibrillation started on warfarin should have an INR checked within 1 week of the first dose. Patients with atrial fibrillation >48 hours' duration or of unknown duration who do not have contraindications to warfarin should receive warfarin if they are younger than 65 years, with one or more other risk factors for stroke.	25 (18-31)
Congestive heart failure (36 indicators)	Ejection fraction assessed before medical therapy Angiotensin-converting enzyme inhibitors for patients with congestive heart failure and an ejection fraction <40%	64 (55-72)
Coronary artery disease (37 indicators)	Counseling on smoking cessation Avoidance of nifedipine for patients with an acute myocardial infarction	68 (64-72)
Diabetes (13 indicators)	Diet and exercise counseling Angiotensin-converting enzyme inhibitors for patients with proteinuria	45 (43-48)
Hyperlipidemia (7 indicators)	Treatment of high low-density cholesterol levels in patients with coronary artery disease	49 (44-53)
Hypertension (27 indicators)	Life-style modification for patients with mild hypertension Pharmacotherapy for uncontrolled mild hypertension Change in treatment when blood pressure is persistently uncontrolled	65 (53-67)

For full list, see http://www.rand.org/health/mcglynn_appa.pdf.
Data from McGlynn EA, Asch SM, Adams J, et al: The quality of health care delivered to adults in the United States. N Engl J Med 348:2635, 2003.

patients hospitalized from 1998 to 2001 suggests that improvement appears to be taking place for most of these measures.[34] Data for this study were collected by Medicare Quality Improvement Organizations in each state, based on chart reviews of up to 750 inpatients with acute myocardial infarction and up to 800 patients with congestive heart failure per state. However, these data also show marked regional variability. For example, in 2000-2001, use of beta blockers in appropriate patients after acute myocardial infarction varied from 57% in Arkansas to 95% in Rhode Island. Use of an angiotensin-converting enzyme inhibitor for patients with heart failure and an ejection fraction below 0.40 ranged from 43% in Arkansas to 82% in Wyoming and 81% in Vermont.

PHYSICIANS. Cardiovascular surgeons and cardiologists who perform PCI are evaluated on their actual outcomes data via public report cards in some states. In these reports, analyses attempt to adjust for the risk of complications and for emergency procedures, allowing calculation of a risk-adjusted mortality rate for individual physicians and hospitals. Thus far, limited data suggest that the public does not use such data extensively,[35,36] although the public disclosure of performance data is believed to be a powerful driver for individual institutions to improve their care.[8]

Nonprocedural care by physicians is often assessed by HEDIS measures developed by NCQA (Table 4–9).[10] These measures were developed for evaluation of health maintenance organizations, and therefore most rely on analyses of medical and pharmacy claims data. In recent years, however, there has been a shift toward measures that are less focused on measuring processes and are more closely tied to patient outcome. Therefore, measures have been introduced that require review of medical records for some data (e.g., blood pressure and LDL cholesterol levels).

A program called the Heart/Stroke Recognition Program was introduced in 2003 by NCQA in collaboration with the American Heart Association and the American Stroke Association. This program is designed to identify physicians who are providing excellent care to patients who have cardiovascular disease or a history of stroke. It is a voluntary program in which physicians seeking "recognition" must audit a sample of their office records and report on their rates of success in meeting specific performance measures (Table 4–10). A similar physician recognition program for diabetes care has been administered by NCQA for several years, and some employers now pay a bonus to physicians who meet its standards for each of their patients with diabetes. This same

TABLE 4–8 Quality Indicators for Inpatient Care for Medicare Patients

Topic	Indicator	Median State Rates* 1998-1999	Median State Rates* 2000-2001
Acute myocardial infarction	Administration of aspirin within 24 hours of admission	84	85
	Aspirin prescribed at discharge	85	86
	Administration of beta blocker within 24 hours of admission	64	69
	Beta blocker prescribed at discharge	72	79
	Angiotensin-converting enzyme inhibitor prescribed at discharge for patients with left ventricular ejection fraction <0.40	71	74
	Smoking cessation counseling given during hospitalization	40	43
	Time to angioplasty (minutes)	41	45
	Time to thrombolytic therapy (minutes)	120	107
Heart failure	Evaluation of ejection fraction	65	70
	Angiotensin-converting enzyme inhibitor prescribed at discharge for patients with left ventricular ejection fraction <0.40	69	68

*In this study, rates of performance of each measure were calculated from chart reviews in each state. The figures in these columns represent the median performance among the 50 U.S. states.

Data from Jencks SF, Haft ED, Cuerdon T: Change in the quality of care delivered to Medicare beneficiaries, 1998-1999 to 2000-2001. JAMA 289:305, 2003.

TABLE 4–9 Cardiovascular HEDIS Measures

Measure	Description	Mean Performance* (%)
Beta blocker treatment after a heart attack	The percentage of patients ≥35 yrs who were hospitalized and discharged alive during the measurement year with a diagnosis of acute myocardial infarction and who received an ambulatory prescription for beta blockers upon discharge.	92.5
Controlling high blood pressure	The percentage of patients 45-85 yrs who had a diagnosis of hypertension and whose blood pressure was adequately controlled (≤140/90) during the measurement year.	55.4
Cholesterol screening	The percentage of patients 18-75 yrs who had evidence of an acute cardiovascular event (hospitalization for acute myocardial infarction, coronary artery bypass graft, or percutaneous transluminal coronary angioplasty) and whose low-density lipoprotein cholesterol was screened in the year following the event.	77.1
Cholesterol management	The percentage of patients with an acute cardiovascular event whose low-density lipoprotein cholesterol was screened and controlled to less than 130 mg/dl in the year following the event.	59.3

*Data are for commercial population for 2001. Data from http://www.ncqa.org/sohc2002/

TABLE 4–10 Measures of the Heart/Stoke Provider Recognition Program of the National Committee for Quality Assurance

Blood pressure testing
Proportion of patients with blood pressure <130/85 mm Hg
Lipid testing
Proportion of patients with low-density lipoprotein cholesterol <100 mg/dl
Use of aspirin or other antithrombotics
Smoking status and cessation advice

bonus framework may be extended to the Heart/Stroke Recognition Program.

Improvement Strategies

The American College of Cardiology and a wide range of other organizations are attempting to develop and disseminate tools for improvement in the reliability of delivery of evidence-based cardiovascular care. The ACC's Guidelines Applied in Practice Initiative used tactics known as continuous quality improvement (CQI) to help physicians and hospitals improve compliance with guidelines.[37] These CQI tools are based on principles adapted from industrial manufacturers and seek to improve quality and efficiency through repetitive cycles of process and outcomes measurement, design and implementation of interventions to improve the processes of care, followed by remeasurement to assess the impact of interventions.[38]

Research that has evaluated the impact of CQI programs on quality of cardiovascular care have yielded encouraging results. One report demonstrated a positive impact from interventions to improve care for acute myocardial infarction led by local opinion leaders in 37 centers,[39] and collaboratives in which surgeons share data and best practices have been associated with improved outcomes in cardiac surgery.[19] Other studies, however, have been unable to demonstrate significant effects from well-designed CQI programs.[40]

In a large recent study of CQI for improvement of cardiac surgery,[41] the investigators randomly assigned 359 hospitals that performed coronary artery bypass grafting on 267,917 patients between January 2000 and July 2002 and that participated in the Society of Thoracic Surgeons National Cardiac Database. The hospitals were randomly assigned to a control arm or to one of two groups that used CQI interventions aimed at improving preoperative use of beta blockade in all patients and internal mammary artery graft utilization in elderly patients. The intervention groups received measure-specific information, including a call to action to a physician leader, educational products, and periodic longitudinal data with benchmark information. This intervention led to a significant increase in the use of beta blockade at intervention sites (by 7.3% vs 3.6%) and a trend toward an increase in use of internal mammary grafts. Both interventions were associated with statistically significant increases in these practices at lower volume coronary artery bypass grafting sites.

The simplest application of CQI principles is utilization of critical pathways, which are standardized protocols that define the key steps and their timing for procedures or for care of common syndromes such as acute chest pain.[42,43] Whether critical pathways actually improve efficiency and quality is unclear, as some data suggest that improvement associated with them may result simply from focusing physicians' and nurses' attention on the patient population, not from the protocols themselves.[44]

Several studies have demonstrated that outcomes of patients with acute myocardial infarction and other serious cardiovascular conditions are improved if they receive their acute and post-hospitalization care from a cardiologist as opposed to generalist physician.[45-47] Other data demonstrate that team-based care and longitudinal programs known as disease management can improve care for patients with acute myocardial infarction and heart failure.[48,49]

REFERENCES

1. Kohn LT, Corrigan JM, Donaldson MS, et al: To Err is Human: Building a Safer Health System. Washington, DC, National Academy Press, 1999.
2. Committee on Quality of Health Care in America: Crossing the Quality Chasm. Washington, DC, National Academy Press, 2001.
3. Galvin R, Milstein A: Large employers' new strategies in health care. N Engl J Med 347:939, 2002.
4. Leadership by Example, Coordinating Government Roles in Improving Health Care Quality. Washington, DC, National Academy Press, 2002.
5. Bodenheimer T: The American health care system: The movement for improved quality in health care. N Engl J Med 340:488, 1999.
6. Hannan EL, Kilburn H, Racz M, et al: Improving the outcomes of coronary artery bypass surgery in New York State. JAMA 271:761, 1994.
7. Ghali WA, Ash AS, Hall RE, Moskowitz MA: Statewide quality improvement initiatives and mortality after cardiac surgery. JAMA 277:379, 1997.
8. Chassin MR: Achieving and sustaining improved quality: Lessons from New York State and cardiac surgery. Health Aff (Millwood) 21:40, 2002.
9. Iglehart JK: The National Committee for Quality Assurance. N Engl J Med 335:995, 1996.
10. National Committee for Quality Assurance (NCQA): Measuring the Quality of America's Health Care: The Health Plan Employer Data and Information Set (HEDIS). Vol. 2003. Washington, DC; NCQA 2003.
11. Joint Commission on Accreditation of Healthcare Organizations. (http://www.jcaho.org/)
12. Leapfrog Group. (http://www.leapfroggroup.org/)
13. (http://www.drfoster.co.uk/)
14. Gibbons RJ, Smith S, Antman E: American College of Cardiology/American Heart Association clinical practice guidelines: Part I: Where do they come from? Circulation 107:2979, 2003.
15. Gibbons RJ, Smith S, Antman E: American College of Cardiology/American Heart Association clinical practice guidelines: Part II: Evolutionary changes in a continuous quality improvement project. Circulation 107:3101, 2003.
16. Quality of Care and Outcomes Research in CVD and Stroke Working Groups: Measuring and improving quality of care: A report from the American Heart Association/American College of Cardiology first scientific forum on the assessment of healthcare quality in cardiovascular disease and stroke. Circulation 101:1483, 2000.
17. National Cholesterol Education Program: Detection and Treatment of High Blood Cholesterol in Adults (Adult Treatment Panel III) NIH Publication No. 02-5215. 2002.
18. Lee TH, Cleeman JI, Brundy SM, et al: Clinical goals and performance measures for cholesterol management for secondary prevention of coronary heart disease. JAMA 283:94, 2000.
19. O'Connor GT, Plume SK, Olmstead EM, et al, for the Northern New England Cardiovascular Disease Study Group: A regional intervention to improve the hospital mortality associated with coronary artery bypass graft surgery. JAMA 275:841, 1996.
20. Chassin MR, Galvin RW: The urgent need to improve health care quality. JAMA 280:1000, 1998.
21. Lee TH: A broader concept of medical errors. N Engl J Med 347:1965, 2002.
22. Donabedian AL: The quality of care: How can it be assessed? JAMA 260:1743, 1988.
23. Sperttus JA, Radford MJ, Every NR, et al: Challenges and opportunities in quantifying the quality of care for acute myocardial infarction: Summary from the Acute Myocardial Infarction Working Group of the American Heart Association/American College of Cardiology First Scientific Forum on Quality of Care and Outcomes Research in Cardiovascular Disease and Stroke. Circulation 107:1681, 2003.
24. Epstein AE: Volume and outcome—it is time to move ahead. N Engl J Med 346:1161, 2002.
25. Halm EA, Lee C, Chassin MR: Is volume related to quality in health care? A systematic review and methodologic critique of the medical literature. Ann Intern Med 137:511, 2002.
26. Birkmeyer JD, Siewers AE, Finlayson EVA, et al: Hospital volume and surgical mortality in the United States. N Engl J Med 346:1128, 2002.
27. Malenka DJ, McGrath PD, Wennberg DE, et al: The relationship between operator volume and outcomes after percutaneous coronary interventions in high volume hospitals in 1994-1996: The northern New England experience. Northern New England Cardiovascular Disease Study Group. J Am Coll Cardiol 34:1471, 1999.
28. Jollis JG, Peterson ED, DeLong ER, et al: The relation between the volume of coronary angioplasty procedures at hospitals treating Medicare beneficiaries and short-term mortality. N Engl J Med 331:1625, 1994.
29. Magid DJ, Calonge BN, Rumsfeld JS, et al: Relation between hospital primary angioplasty volume and mortality for patients with acute MI treated with primary angioplasty vs thrombolytic therapy. JAMA 284:3131, 2000.
30. Canto JG, Every NR, Magid DJ, et al: The volume of primary angioplasty procedures and survival after acute myocardial infarction: National Registry of Myocardial Infarction 2 Investigators. N Engl J Med 342:1573, 2000.

31. Maynard C, Every NR, Chapko MK, et al: Outcomes of coronary angioplasty procedures performed in rural hospitals. Am J Med 108:710, 2000.
32. Smith SC Jr, Dove JT, Jacobs AK, et al: ACC/AHA guidelines for percutaneous coronary intervention: A report of the American College of Cardiology/American Heart Association Task Force on Practice Guidelines (Committee to Revise the 1993 Guidelines for Percutaneous Transluminal Coronary Angioplasty). J Am Coll Cardiol 37:2239, i-lxvi, 2001.
33. McGlynn EA, Asch SM, Adams J, et al: The quality of health care delivered to adults in the United States. N Engl J Med 348:2635, 2003.
34. Jencks SF, Huff ED, Cuerdon T: Change in the quality of care delivered to Medicare beneficiaries, 1998-1999 to 2000-2001. JAMA 289:305, 2003.
35. Schneider EC, Epstein AM: Use of public performance reports: A survey of patients undergoing cardiac surgery. JAMA 27:1638, 1998.
36. Schneider EC, Epstein AM: Influence of cardiac-surgery performance reports on referral practices and access to care: A survey of cardiovascular specialists. N Engl J Med 335:251, 1996.
37. Mehta RH, Montoye CK, Gallogly M, et al: Improving quality of care for acute myocardial infarction: The Guidelines Applied in Practice (GAP) Initiative. JAMA 287:1269, 2002.
38. Berwick DM: Continuous improvement as an ideal in health care. N Engl J Med 320:53, 1989.
39. Soumerai SB, McLaughlin TJ, Gurwith JH, et al: Effect of local medical opinion leaders on quality of care for acute myocardial infarction. JAMA 279:1358, 1998.
40. Krumholz H, Amatruda J, Smith GL, et al: Randomized trial of an education and support intervention to prevent readmission of patients with heart failure. J Am Coll Cardiol 39:83, 2002.
41. Ferguson TB, Peterson ED, Coombs LP, et al: Use of continuous quality improvement to increase use of process measures in patients undergoing coronary artery bypass graft surgery. A randomized controlled trial. JAMA 290:49, 2003.
42. Pearson SD, Goulart-Fisher D, Lee TH: Critical pathways as a strategy for improving care: problems and potential. Ann Intern Med 123:941, 1995.
43. Nichol G, Walls R, Goldman L, et al: A critical pathway for management of patients with acute chest pain who are at low risk for myocardial ischemia: recommendations and potential impact. Ann Intern Med 127:996, 1997.
44. Pearson SD, Kleefield SF, Roukop JR, et al: Critical pathways intervention to reduce length of hospital stay. Am J Med 110:175, 2001.
45. Jollis JG, DeLong ER, Peterson ED, et al: Outcome of acute myocardial infarction according to the specialty of the admitting physician. N Engl J Med 335:1880, 1996.
46. Ayanian JZ, Hauptman PJ, Guadagnoli E, et al: Knowledge and practices of generalist and specialist physicians regarding drug therapy for acute myocardial infarction. N Engl J Med 331:1136, 1994.
47. Chen J, Radford MJ, Wang Y, et al: Care and outcomes of elderly patients with acute myocardial infarction by physician specialty: The effects of comorbidity and functional limitations. Am J Med 108:460, 2000.
48. DeBusk RF, Miller NH, Superko HR, et al: A case-management system for coronary risk factor modification after acute myocardial infarction. Ann Intern Med 120:721, 1994.
49. Rich MW, Beckham V, Wittenberg C, et al: A multidisciplinary intervention to prevent the readmission of elderly patients with congestive heart failure. N Engl J Med 333:1190, 1995.

CHAPTER 5

The Principles of Drug Therapy

Dan M. Roden

Importance of Correct Drug Use

In 2001, Americans spent $191 billion on pharmaceuticals.[1] Adverse drug reactions are estimated to be the fourth to sixth most common cause of death in the United States, to cost $19 to 27 billion annually, and to account directly for 2% to 3% of all hospital admissions. The prevalence of heart disease and the increasing utilization of not only acute interventional therapies but also long-term preventive therapies translate into a dominant role of cardiovascular drugs in these costs: 19% of all drug costs ($36 billion) in 2001.[1] Moreover, with increasing success not only in heart disease but also in other therapeutic arenas, cardiovascular physicians are increasingly encountering patients receiving multiple medications with which they may not have complete comfort and familiarity. The goal of this chapter is to outline principles of drug action and interaction that allow the safest and most effective therapy in an individual patient.

The Key Decision in Drug Therapy: Risk versus Benefit

The fundamental assumption underlying administration of any drug is that the real or expected benefit exceeds the anticipated risk. The benefits of drug therapy are initially defined in small clinical trials, perhaps involving several thousand patients, prior to a drug's marketing and approval. Ultimately, the efficacy and safety profile of any drug is determined after the compound has been marketed and used widely in hundreds of thousands of patients.

When a drug is administered for the acute correction of a life-threatening condition, the benefits are often self-evident; insulin for diabetic ketoacidosis, nitroprusside for hypertensive encephalopathy, or lidocaine for ventricular tachycardia are examples. Extrapolation of such immediately obvious benefits to other clinical situations may not be warranted, however. The efficacy of lidocaine to terminate ventricular tachycardia led to its widespread use as a prophylactic agent in cases of acute myocardial infarction, until it was recognized that, in this setting, the drug does not alter mortality. The outcome of the Cardiac Arrhythmia Suppression Trial (CAST) highlights the difficulties in extrapolating from an incomplete understanding of physiology to chronic drug therapy. CAST tested the hypothesis that suppression of ventricular ectopic activity (a recognized risk factor for sudden death for myocardial infarction) would reduce mortality; this notion was highly ingrained in cardiovascular practice in the 1970s and 1980s. In CAST, sodium channel-blocking antiarrhythmics did suppress ventricular ectopics, but also unexpectedly increased the rate of mortality threefold. In this instance, the use of arrhythmia suppression as a "surrogate" marker for a desired drug action, reduction in mortality, was inappropriate because the underlying pathophysiology was incompletely understood. Similarly, reduced contractility in cases of heart failure has led to development of a series of drugs with positive inotropic activity, but these also show an increase in mortality, likely due to drug-induced arrhythmias.[2] Nevertheless, clinical trials with these agents do suggest symptom relief. Thus, the prescriber and the patient may elect therapy with positive inotropic drugs, because of this benefit, and recognizing the risk. These examples illustrate the continuing personal relationship between the prescriber and the patient and emphasize the needs for a clear understanding of the expected benefit of therapy, and a clear understanding of disease pathophysiology and its response to drug therapy, in the drug development and prescribing processes.

The risks of drug therapy may be a direct extension of the pharmacological actions for which the drug is actually being prescribed. Excessive hypotension in a patient taking an antihypertensive agent or bleeding in a patient taking a platelet IIb/IIIa receptor antagonist are examples. In other cases, adverse effects develop as a consequence of pharmacological actions that were not appreciated during a drug's initial development and use in patients. Rhabdomyolysis with HMG-CoA reductase inhibitors, angioedema during angiotensin-converting enzyme (ACE) inhibitor therapy, or torsades de pointes during treatment with "noncardiovascular" drugs such as thioridazine or pentamidine are examples. However, these rarer but very serious events may become evident only after a drug has been marketed and extensively used. Even rare adverse effects can alter the overall perception of risk versus benefit and can prompt removal of the drug from the market, particularly if alternate, safer therapies are available; for example, withdrawal of the first insulin-sensitizer, troglitazone, after recognition of hepatotoxicity was further spurred by availability of other new drugs in this class. Further, investigation of the pathophysiology underlying these unusual events has defined new mechanisms underlying variable responses to drug therapy.

Variability in Drug Action

Drugs interact with specific molecular targets to effect changes in whole organ and whole body function. The targets with which drugs interact to produce beneficial effects may or may not be the same as those with which drugs interact to produce adverse effects. Drug targets may be in the circulation, at the cell surface, or within cells. Many newer drugs have been developed to specifically interact with a desired drug target; examples of such targets are HMG-CoA reductase, angiotensin-converting enzyme, G-protein coupled receptors (α, β, AT1, histamine, and many others), and platelet IIb/IIIa receptors. On the other hand, many drugs widely used in cardiovascular therapeutics were developed at a time when the technology to identify specific molecular targets simply was not available; digoxin, amiodarone, and aspirin are examples. In some cases, such agents turn out to have rather specific molecular targets: digoxin's major effect is by inhibition of Na-K-ATPase, whereas aspirin permanently acetylates a specific serine residue on the cyclooxygenase enzyme. However, with the cloning of multiple isoforms of cyclooxygenase has come the recognition that aspirin is in fact targeting multiple molecules; more specific inhibitors have therefore been developed, and their effects are being evaluated in patients with cardiovascular and other types of disease.

MECHANISMS UNDERLYING VARIABILITY IN DRUG ACTION. Two major processes determine how the interaction between a drug and its target molecule can generate variable drug actions in the patient (Fig. 5–1). The first, *pharmacokinetics*, describes drug delivery to and removal from the target molecule and includes the processes of absorption, distribution, metabolism, and excretion. These are collectively termed "drug disposition." Robust techniques—applicable across drugs and drug classes—to analyze drug disposition have been developed and result in a series of principles that can be used to adjust drug dosages to enhance the likelihood of a beneficial effect and to minimize toxicity.

The second process, *pharmacodynamics*, describes how the interaction between a drug and its target generates downstream molecular, cellular, whole organ, and whole body effects. Pharmacodynamic sources of variability in drug action arise from the specifics of the target molecule and the biological context in which the drug-target interaction occurs; thus, methods for analysis of pharmacodynamics tend to be drug class specific. In practice, pharmacodynamic variability often arises as a consequence of disease, especially the disease for which the drug is being prescribed.

One source of pharmacodynamic variability is variability in the target molecule itself; this can arise because of genetic factors, discussed subsequently, or because disease alters the number of target molecules or their state (e.g., changes in extent of phosphorylation). A second source of pharmacodynamic variability arises from our increasing understanding of the molecular pathophysiology of disease: the interaction between drugs and their target molecules occurs in a complex biologic context, so variability in this biology (often a consequence of disease) can affect the extent to which a drug produces desired or undesired effects. Examples include high dietary salt that can inhibit the antihypertensive action of beta blockers, or hypokalemia that increases the risk for drug-induced QT prolongation. The latter clinical observation led to experiments at the basic level to define the underlying mechanism, and these results in turn highlight the value of aggressive potassium supplementation in patients with both congenital and acquired long QT syndromes.

PHARMACOGENETICS AND PHARMACOGENOMICS. This contemporary view of drug actions identifies a series of molecules that mediate drug actions in patients: drug metabolizing enzymes, drug transport molecules, drug targets, and molecules modulating the biology in which the drug-target interaction occurs. The vast majority of these molecules are proteins, so variations in the genes that encode them may therefore contribute to variability in drug actions. Isolated examples of familial aggregation of unusual responses to drug therapy have been recognized for decades and defined the field of *pharmacogenetics*. Such rare aberrant responses recognized in families generally arise as a result of mutations, usually defined as rare DNA variants that are associated with a disease phenotype. With the sequencing of the human genome has come the recognition that DNA variants are extremely common, occurring on average in 1 of 300 base pairs; such variants—termed *polymorphisms*—may or may not alter gene expression or function. The nascent field of *pharmacogenomics* is attempting to define common polymorphisms, or sets of polymorphisms, that underlie variability in drug action.[3] Ultimately, it may be possible to genotype individuals prior to prescribing medications to ensure that benefit is maximized and risk minimized: the concept of "pre-prescription genotyping."

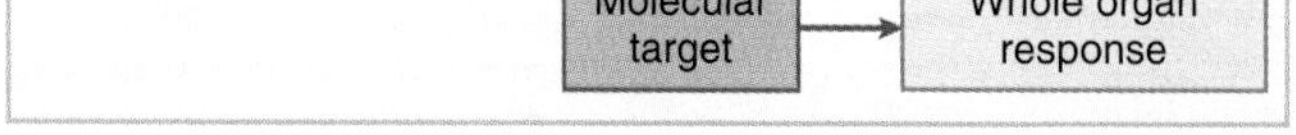

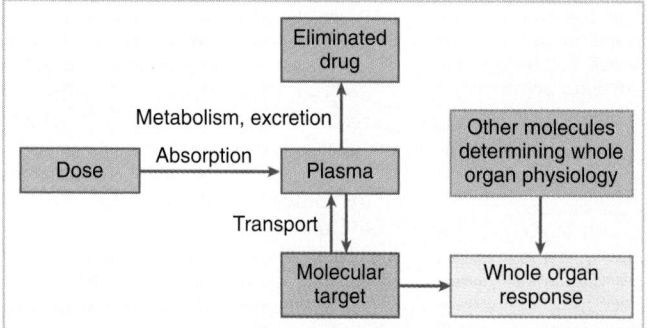

FIGURE 5–1 A model for understanding variability in drug action. When a dose of a drug is administered, the processes of absorption, metabolism, excretion, and transport determine its access to specific molecular targets that mediate beneficial and toxic effects. The interaction between a drug and its molecular target then produces changes in molecular, cellular, whole organ, and ultimately whole patient physiology. This molecular interaction occurs in a complex biologic milieu modulated by multiple factors (some of which are disturbed to cause disease). DNA variants in the genes responsible for the processes of drug disposition (green), the molecular target (blue) or the molecules determining the biological context in which the drug-target interaction occurs (tan) all can contribute to variability in drug action.

Pharmacokinetics

Administration of an intravenous drug bolus results in maximal drug concentrations at the end of the bolus and then a decline in plasma drug concentrations over time (Fig. 5–2A). The simplest case is one in which this decline occurs monoexponentially over time. A useful parameter to describe this decline is the *half-life* (t1/2), the time in which 50% of the drug elimination occurs; after two half-lives, 75% of the drug has been eliminated, after three half-lives 87.5%, and so on.

In some cases, the decline of drug concentrations following administration of an intravenous bolus dose is multiexponential. The most common explanation is that drug is not only eliminated (represented by the terminal portion of the time-concentration plot) but also undergoes more rapid *distribution* to peripheral tissues. Just as elimination may be usefully described by a half-life, distribution half-lives can also be derived from curves such as those shown in Figure 5–2B.

The plasma concentration measured immediately after a bolus dose can be used to derive a volume into which the drug is distributed. When the decline of plasma concentrations is multiexponential, multiple distribution compartments can be defined; these *volumes of distribution* can be useful in considering dose adjustments in cases of disease, but rarely correspond exactly to any physical volume such as plasma or total body water. Indeed, with drugs that are highly tissue bound (such as some antidepressants), volume of distribution can exceed total body volume by orders of magnitude.

Drugs are often administered by nonintravenous routes, such as oral, sublingual, transcutaneous, or intramuscular. With such routes of administration, two differences arise from the intravenous route (see Fig. 5–2A). First, concentrations in plasma demonstrate a distinct rising phase as drug slowly enters plasma. Second, the total amount of drug that actually enters the systemic circulation may be less than that achieved by the intravenous route. The relative amount of drug entering by any route, compared to the same dose administered intravenously, is termed *bioavailability*. Bioavailability may be reduced because drug undergoes metabolism prior to entering the circulation or because drug is simply not absorbed from its site of administration.

Clearance is the most useful way of quantifying drug elimination. Clearance can be viewed as a volume that is "cleared" of drug in any given period of time. Clearance may be organ specific (e.g., renal clearance, hepatic clearance) or whole body clearance.

With repeated doses, drug levels accumulate to a *steady state*, the condition under which the rate of drug administration is equal to the rate of drug elimination in any given period of time. As illustrated in Figure 5–3, the elimination half-life describes not only the disappearance of a drug but also the time course by which a drug accumulates to steady state. It is important to distinguish between steady-state plasma concentrations, achieved in four to five elimination half-lives, and steady-state drug effects, which may take longer to achieve. For some drugs, clinical effects develop immediately upon access to the molecular target: nitrates for angina, nitroprusside to lower blood pressure, and sympathomimetics to treat shock are examples. In other situations, drug effects follow plasma concentrations, but with a lag. An active metabolite may need to be generated to achieve drug effects. Time may be required for translation of the drug effect at the molecular site to a physiologic end point. Inhibition of synthesis of vitamin K-dependent clotting factors by warfarin ultimately leads to a desired elevation of INR, but the development of this desired effect occurs only as levels of clotting factors fall. Penetration of a drug into intracellular or other tissue sites of action may be required prior to development of drug effect; this is widely cited to explain the lag time between administration of amiodarone dosages and development of its effects, although the exact mechanism underlying this phenomenon remains elusive.

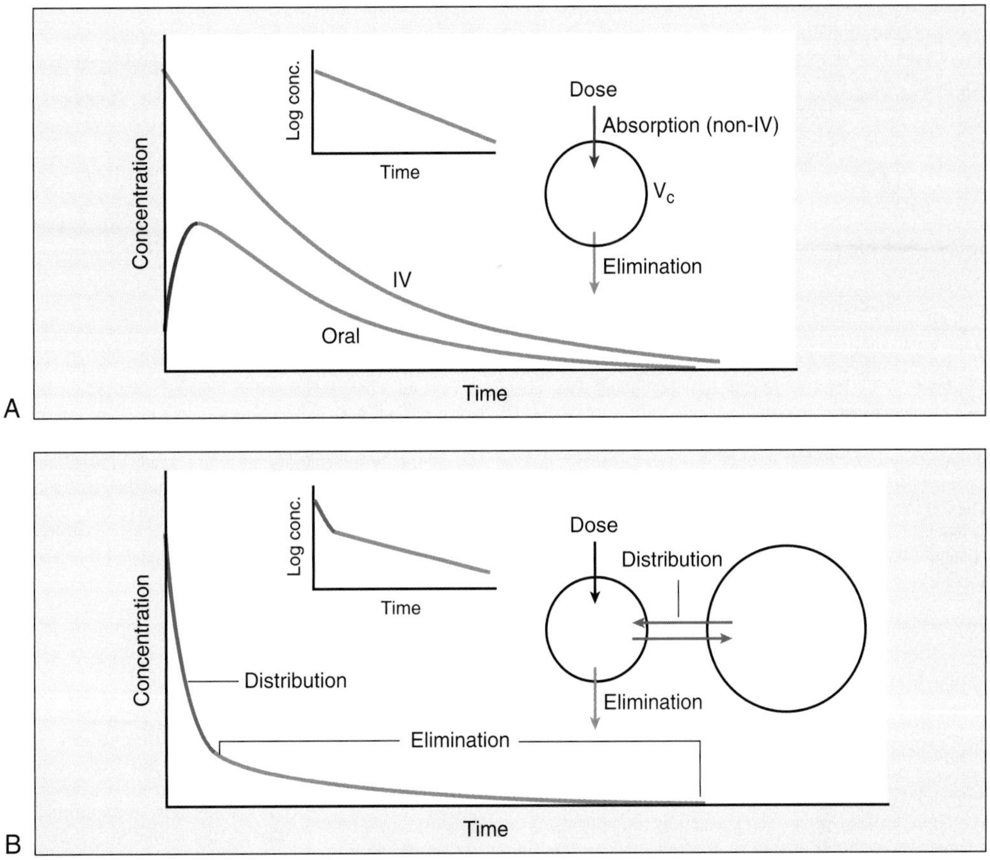

FIGURE 5–2 Models of plasma concentrations as a function of time after a single dose of a drug. **A.** The simplest situation is one in which a drug is administered as a very rapid intravenous bolus into a volume (V_c) into which it is instantaneously and uniformly distributed. Elimination then takes place from this volume. In this case, drug elimination is monoexponential; that is, a plot of the logarithm of concentration versus time is linear, as shown in the inset. When the same dose of drug is administered orally, a distinct absorption phase is required prior to drug entry into V_c. Most absorption (shown here in red) is completed prior to elimination (shown in green), although the processes overlap. In this example, the amount of drug delivered by the oral route is less than that delivered by the intravenous route, assessed by the total areas under the two curves, indicating reduced bioavailability. **B.** In this example, drug is delivered to the central volume, from which it is not only eliminated but also undergoes distribution to the peripheral sites. This distribution process is more rapid than elimination, resulting in a distinct biexponential disappearance curve.

Pharmacokinetic Principles in Managing Drug Therapy

BIOAVAILABILITY AND DOSE ADJUSTMENT. Some drugs undergo such extensive presystemic metabolism that the amount of drug required to achieve a therapeutic effect is much greater (and often much more variable) than that required for the same drug administered intravenously. Thus, small doses of propranolol (5 mg) may achieve heart rate slowing equivalent to that observed with much larger oral doses (80-120 mg). Propranolol is actually well absorbed but undergoes extensive metabolism in the intestine and the liver prior to entering the systemic circulation. Another example is amiodarone, the physicochemical characteristics of which make it only 30% to 50% bioavailable when it is administered orally (the drug is highly lipophilic and thus has limited water solubility). Thus, an intravenous infusion 0.5 mg/min (720 mg/day) is equivalent to 1.5 to 2 gm/day orally.

DISTRIBUTION. Rapid distribution can alter the way in which drug therapy should be initiated. When lidocaine is administered intravenously, it displays a prominent and rapid distribution phase (t1/2 = 8 min) prior to slower elimination (t1/2 = 120 min). As a consequence, an antiarrhythmic effect of lidocaine may be transiently achieved but very rapidly lost following a single bolus, due not to elimination but to rapid distribution. Administration of higher bolus doses to circumvent this problem results in dose-related toxicity, often seizures. Hence, administration of a lidocaine loading dose of 3 to 4 mg/kg should occur over 10 to 20 minutes, as a series of intravenous boluses (e.g., 50-100 mg every 5-10 min) or an intravenous infusion (e.g., 20 mg/min over 10-20 min).

CLEARANCE MECHANISMS. The mechanisms underlying drug elimination from the body are metabolism and excretion. Drug metabolism most often occurs in the liver, although extrahepatic metabolism (in the circulation, the intestine, the lungs, and the kidneys) is increasingly well defined. "Phase I" drug metabolism generally involves oxidation of the drug by specific drug-oxidizing enzymes, a process that renders the drug more water-soluble (and hence more likely to undergo renal excretion). Additionally, drugs or their metabolites often undergo conjugation with specific chemical groups ("phase II") to enhance water solubility; these conjugation reactions are also catalyzed by specific transferases.

The most common enzyme systems mediating drug metabolism are those of the P450 superfamily, termed CYPs. Multiple CYPs are expressed in human liver and other tissues. A major source of variability in drug action is variability in CYP activity, due to variability in CYP expression and/or genetic variants that alter CYP activity. The most abundant CYP in human liver and intestine is CYP3A4 and a closely related isoform, CYP3A5. These CYPs metabolize up to 50% of clinically used drugs. CYP3A activity varies widely among individuals, for reasons that are not entirely clear. One mechanism underlying this variability is the presence of a polymorphism in this CYP3A5 gene that reduces its activity.[4] Table 5–1 lists CYPs and other drug-metabolizing enzymes and emphasizes that genetic variants that alter function are well recognized with some CYPs (2D6, 2C9, 2C19), and a number of phase II enzymes.[5] Table 5–1 also points out that the frequencies of polymorphisms in these genes may vary among ethnic groups and is one explanation for interethnic variability in drug response; another is variability in the frequency of polymorphisms in the genes whose function determines pharmacodynamics, discussed further later.

Reduction in clearance, by disease, drug interactions, or genetic factors, will increase drug concentrations and hence drug effects. An exception is drugs whose effects are mediated by generation of active metabolites. In this case, inhibition of drug metabolism may lead to accumulation of the parent drug but loss of therapeutic efficacy. The anticonvulsant phenytoin is an inhibitor of CYP2C9; when phenytoin is started in a patient receiving the angiotensin receptor blocker losartan, blood pressure control may be lost because of failure of biotransformation of losartan to its active metabolite.[6] This is in contrast to phenytoin effects on CYP3A substrates. In this case, phenytoin acts as a potent inducing agent, increasing gene transcription. Thus, administration of

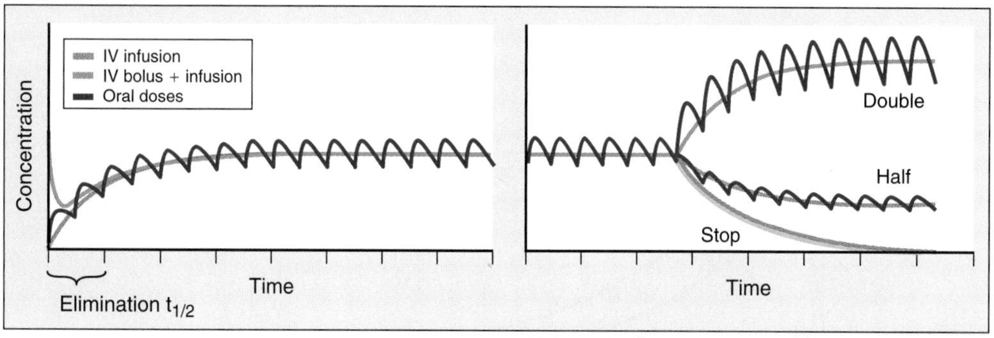

A B

FIGURE 5–3 Time course of drug concentrations when treatment is started or dose is changed. **A.** The hash lines on the abscissa indicate one elimination half-life (t1/2). With a constant rate intravenous infusion (gold), plasma concentrations accumulate to steady state in four to five elimination half-lives. When a loading bolus is administered with the maintenance infusion (blue), plasma concentrations are transiently higher but may dip, as shown here, prior to achieving the same steady state. When the same drug is administered by the oral route, the time course of drug accumulation is identical; in this case, the drug was administered at intervals of 50% of a t1/2 (magenta). Steady-state plasma concentrations during oral therapy fluctuate around the mean determined by intravenous therapy. **B.** This plot shows that dosages are doubled or halved, or the drug is stopped during steady-state administration, and the time required to achieve the new steady state is four or five half-lives and is independent of the route of administration.

phenytoin actually increases CYP3A activity and hence leads to altered effects of CYP3A substrates through this mechanism.

Excretion of drugs, generally into the urine or bile, is accomplished by specific drug-transport molecules, whose level of expression and genetic variation are only now being explored. In fact, drug transporters play a role not only in drug elimination, but also in drug uptake into many cells, including hepatocytes and enterocytes. As with CYPs and other drug-metabolizing enzymes, multiple genes encoding multiple drug uptake and efflux transporters are being identified. The most widely recognized of these is P-glycoprotein, the product of expression of the *MDR1* gene. Originally identified as a factor mediating multiple drug resistance in patients with cancer, *MDR1* expression is now well recognized in normal enterocytes, hepatocytes, renal tubular cells, the endothelium of the capillaries forming the blood-brain barrier, and the testes. In each of these sites, P-glycoprotein expression is restricted to the apical aspect of polarized cells, where it acts to enhance drug efflux. In intestine, P-glycoprotein pumps substrates back into the lumen, thereby limiting bioavailability. In the liver and kidney, it promotes drug excretion into bile or urine. In the central nervous system capillary endothelium, P-glycoprotein-mediated efflux is an important mechanism limiting drug access to the brain.[7]

Clinical Relevance of Polymorphic Drug Metabolism: The Concept of High-Risk Pharmacokinetics

The absence of a specific pathway for drug metabolism, due to genetic factors or to the administration of other drugs, has variable clinical consequences. When a drug uses multiple pathways for its elimination, absence of one of these is unlikely to have major clinical consequences because elimination can be accomplished by alternate pathways. On the other hand, a drug eliminated by only a single pathway carries with it the liability that absence of activity of that pathway will lead to marked accumulation of drug in plasma, failure to form downstream metabolites, and thus a risk of unusual drug responses.

One example was the antihistamine terfenadine, which is eliminated almost exclusively by CYP3A metabolism in the intestine and the liver. Terfenadine itself is a highly potent QT-prolonging agent and is biotransformed to a noncardioactive metabolite (fexofenadine) that mediates the compound's antihistamine actions. Coadministration of terfenadine with CYP3A inhibitors such as ketaconazole or erythromycin led to inhibition of presystemic metabolism, striking elevations of plasma terfenadine concentrations, marked QT prolongation, and torsades de pointes. As a consequence, the drug was withdrawn from the market, and fexofenadine is now marketed as a widely used antihistamine (Allegra).

Similarly, CYP3A inhibition appears to increase the risk of rhabdomyolysis with some but not all HMG-CoA reductase inhibitors, through mechanisms that are not completely understood[8]; fibrates also increase this risk, though the mechanisms are uncertain.

Administration of CYP2D6-metabolized beta blockers to patients with defective enzyme activity (on a genetic basis or due to coadministration of inhibitors) produces exaggerated heart rate slowing. Similarly, the weak beta-blocking actions of the antiarrhythmic propafenone are increased in this setting. The widely used analgesic codeine undergoes CYP2D6-mediated bioactivation to an active metabolite, morphine, and patients with defective CYP2D6 activity display reduced analgesia.[9] A small group of individuals with multiple functional copies of CYP2D6, and hence *increased* enzymatic activity, has been identified; in this group codeine may produce nausea and euphoria, presumably due to rapid morphine generation. Similarly, some antidepressants are CYP2D6 substrates; for these drugs, cardiovascular adverse effects are more common in CYP2D6 poor metabolizers, whereas therapeutic efficacy is more difficult to achieve in ultra-rapid metabolizers.

The concept of high-risk pharmacokinetics extends from drug metabolism to transporter-mediated drug elimination. The most widely recognized example is digoxin, which is eliminated primarily by P-glycoprotein-mediated efflux into bile and urine. Administration of wide range of structurally and mechanistically unrelated drugs has been empirically recognized to increase digoxin concentrations, and the common mechanism appears to be inhibition of P-glycoprotein-mediated elimination (see Table 5–1).[7]

Pharmacodynamics and the Genetics of Drug Responses

Drugs can exert variable effects, even in the absence of pharmacokinetic variability. As indicated in Figure 5–1, this variability can arise as a function of variability in the molecular targets with which drugs interact to achieve their (beneficial and adverse) effects, as well as variability in the broader biologic context within which the drug-target interaction takes place. Simple examples illustrate the point that this is a common mechanism for variability in drug action: the effect of lytic therapy in a patient with no clot is manifestly different from that in a patient with acute coronary thrombosis; the arrhythmogenic effects of digitalis depend on serum potassium; the vasodilating effects of nitrates, beneficial in patients with coronary disease with angina, can be catastrophic in patients with aortic stenosis.

DNA variants in key genes controlling this biological context (as well as genes encoding drug targets themselves) are increasingly recognized as contributors to variability in drug action. Many examples of associations between DNA polymorphisms and disease severity are now reported; there are fewer reports of polymorphisms modulating responses to cardiovascular drugs, and examples are listed in Table 5–2. It is important to recognize that genomic science is in its

TABLE 5–1 Proteins Important in Drug Metabolism and Elimination

Protein	Substrates	Interacting drugs	Genetics
CYP3A4, CYP3A5	Erythromycin, clarithromycin Quinidine, mexiletine Many benzodiazepines Cyclosporine, tacrolimus Many antivirals HMG CoA reductase inhibitors (atorvastatin, simvastatin, lovastatin; not pravastatin) Many calcium channel blockers	*Inhibitors:* Antivirals: ritonavir and others Amiodarone Erythromycin, clarithromycin (not azithromycin) Ketaconazole, itraconazole Many calcium channel blockers *Inducers:* Rifampin Efavirenz, nevirapine St. John's wort Phenytoin Pioglitazone	Highly variable activity in vivo Common coding region polymorphism in CYP3A5 may contribute; more common in blacks than whites No common coding region polymorphisms in CYP3A4
CYP2D6	Some beta-blockers: propranolol, timolol, metoprolol, carvedilol Propafenone Desipramine and other tricyclics Codeine Debrisoquine Dextromethorphan	*Inhibitors:* Amiodarone Fluoxetine Quinidine Paroxetine *Inducers:* Rifampin	Multiple loss of function alleles described. Common (25%) in white and black populations; homozygotes (7%) display the PM phenotype. Reduction of function alleles described in Asian populations but PMs rare. Ultra-rapid metabolizers due to multiple functional copies of CYP2D6 described especially in northern Africa.
CYP2C9	Warfarin Phenytoin Tolbutamide Glyburide Losartan, irbesartan	*Inhibitors:* Amiodarone Zafirlukast *Inducers:* Rifampin Barbiturates	Heterozygotes for common (>50% in some populations) loss of function alleles display reduced enzymatic activity and may have lower warfarin dose requirements. Very low warfarin dose requirements in homozygotes.
CYP2C19	Omeprazole Mephenytoin Nelfinavir		PMs common (~20%) in Asian populations.
P-glycoprotein	Digoxin Fexofenadine Cyclosporine, tacrolimus Many anticancer agents Many antivirals	*Inhibitors:* Amiodarone Quinidine Ketoconazole Erythromycin Itraconazole Verapamil Cyclosporine	DNA polymorphisms common; clinical significance uncertain
N-acetyl transferase	Procainamide Hydralazine Isoniazid		Whites and blacks: 50% fast acetylators, 50% slow acetylators, no non-acetylators Asians: mostly fast acetylators Slow acetylators: increased risk of the lupus syndrome Slow acetylators; increased risk of hepatotoxicity
Thiopurine methyl-transferase	6-mercaptopurine Azathioprine		Homozygotes for loss of function mutations (1/300): increased risk for bone marrow aplasia at usual doses Rapid metabolizers: suboptimal therapeutic response
Pseudo cholinesterase	Succinylcholine		Rare homozygote null individuals: prolonged apnea
UDP-glucuronosyl-transferase	Irinotecan		Polymorphisms cause Gilbert syndrome Enhanced toxicity of some anticancer drugs

More detailed CYP listing available at http://medicine.iupui.edu/flockhart/
PM = Poor metabolizer.

infancy; therefore, reported associations such as these require independent confirmation and assessment of clinical importance and cost-effectiveness before they can or should enter clinical practice.

Polymorphisms in the β_1 and β_2 receptor genes have been associated with variability in heart rate slowing and blood pressure effects with beta blockers and beta agonists.[10-12] An example of tumor genotype determining response to therapy is the anticancer drug herceptin, which is effective only in cancers that do not express the herceptin receptor; since the drug also potentiates anthracycline-related cardiotoxicity, toxic therapy can be avoided in patients who are receptor-negative.[13]

The ACE gene includes a common polymorphism (termed insertion/deletion, or I/D) that determines ACE activity. DD individuals, homozygous for the D allele, have higher plasma ACE activity and thus higher concentrations of the pressor peptide angiotensin than do II individuals. DD patients with heart failure have a worse prognosis than do II or ID subjects and yet have a better response to beta blockers.[14] Almost certainly, this action does not reflect a direct interaction between beta blockers and the ACE protein; rather, the ACE polymorphism likely alters the milieu in which the beta blocker interacts with beta receptors to ameliorate the prognosis in patients with heart failure. Similarly, the effect of hormone replacement therapy on high-density lipoprotein cholesterol has been linked to a polymorphism in the estrogen receptor,[15] and susceptibility to stroke in patients receiving diuretics to a polymorphism in the adducin gene that plays a role in renal tubular sodium transport.[16] Torsades de pointes during QT-prolonging antiarrhythmic therapy has been linked to polymorphisms in ion channel genes; in addition, this adverse effect sometimes arises in patients with clinically latent congenital long QT syndrome, emphasizing the interrelationship among disease, genetic background, and drug therapy.[17,18]

Principles of Dosage Optimization

The goals of drug therapy should be defined prior to initiation of drug treatment. These may include acute correction of serious pathophysiology, acute or chronic symptom relief, or changes in "surrogate" endpoints (such as blood pressure or serum cholesterol or INR) that have been linked to beneficial outcomes in target patient populations. The lessons of CAST and of positive inotropic drugs should make prescribers skeptical about such surrogate-guided therapy in the absence of controlled clinical trials.

When the goal of drug therapy is to acutely correct a disturbance in physiology, the drug should be administered intravenously, in doses designed to rapidly achieve a therapeutic effect. This approach is best justified when benefits clearly outweigh risks. As discussed earlier with lidocaine, large intravenous drug boluses carry with them a risk of enhancing drug-related toxicity, so even with the most urgent of medical indications, this approach is rarely appropriate. An exception is adenosine, which must be administered as a rapid bolus because it undergoes extensive and rapid elimination from plasma by uptake into virtually all cells; as a consequence, a slow bolus or infusion rarely achieves sufficiently high concentrations at the desired site of action (the coronary artery perfusing the atrioventricular node) to terminate arrhythmias.

The time required to achieve steady-state plasma concentrations is determined by elimination half-life, as discussed earlier. The administration of a loading dose may abbreviate this time, but only if the kinetics of distribution and elimination are known *a priori* in an individual subject and the correct loading regimen is chosen; otherwise, overshoot or undershoot during the loading phase may occur. Thus, the initiation of drug therapy by a loading strategy should be used only when the indication is acute.

Two dose-response curves describe the relationship between drug dose and the expected cumulative incidence of a beneficial effect or an adverse effect (Fig. 5–4). The distance along the X axis describing the difference between these

TABLE 5–2 DNA Polymorphisms Implicated in Variable Pharmacodynamics in Cardiovascular Medicine*

Drug	Gene	Reported Association
QT-prolonging drugs	KCNH2/KCNE2 (HERG/MiRP1)†	Increased torsades de pointes risk in patients with KCNE2 T8A[18]
QT-prolonging drugs	KCNQ1 (KvLKQT1)† MinK (KCNE1)† SCN5A†	Increased torsades de pointes risk in patients with KCNE1 D85N, SCN5A S1102Y[22,23]
Beta-blockers	β_1- and β_2-adrenergic receptor	Altered extent of heart rate slowing or blood pressure lowering[10-12]
ACE inhibitors	ACE	Decreased response in DD subjects[24]
β-blockers	ACE	Increased response in DD subjects[19]
Fluvastatin	ABCA1 transporter LDL receptor Paraoxonase	Variable low-density lipoprotein lowering[25-27]
Pravastatin	Cholesteryl ester transfer protein	Variable regression of atherosclerosis[28]
Estrogen	Estrogen receptor	Variable high-density lipoprotein elevation[15]
Lipid-lowering therapy	Hepatic lipase	Variable lipid lowering[29]
Antiplatelet drugs	Platelet glycoprotein IIIa	Variable antiplatelet effects ex vivo[30]
Amiloride	Epithelial sodium channel	Antihypertensive effect in black subjects[31]
Antihypertensive drugs	β_3 G-Protein subunit	Variable blood pressure lowering[32]
Diuretics	α-adducin	Variable myocardial infarction or stroke incidence during antihypertensive therapy[16] Variable blood pressure response (especially with ACE I/D)[33]
ACE inhibitor	Bradykinin B2 receptor	ACE-inhibitor cough[34]

ACE = angiotensin-converting enzyme.
*DNA variants that modulate pharmacokinetics are listed in Table 5–1.
†Mutations in these genes, causing the long QT syndrome, may be clinically silent until challenge with QT prolonging drugs

curves, often termed the *therapeutic ratio* (or index or window), provides an index of the likelihood that a chronic dosing regimen that provides benefits without adverse effects can be identified. Drugs with especially wide therapeutic indices can often be administered at infrequent intervals, even if they are rapidly eliminated (left panels, Fig. 5–4).

When expected adverse effects are serious, the most appropriate treatment strategy is to start at very low doses and re-evaluate the necessity for increasing drug dosages once steady-state drug effects have been achieved. This approach has the advantage of minimizing the risk of dose-related adverse effects but carries with it a need to titrate doses to efficacy. Only when stable drug effects are achieved should increasing drug dosage to achieve the desired therapeutic effect be considered.

The risk of sotalol-related torsades de pointes increases with drug dosage, and so the starting dose should be low. In other cases, anticipated toxicity is relatively mild and manageable. Here, it may be acceptable to start at dosages greater than the minimum required to achieve a therapeutic effect, accepting a greater than minimal risk of adverse effects; some antihypertensives can be administered in this fashion. However, the principle of using the lowest dose possible to minimize toxicity, particularly toxicity that is unpredictable and unrelated to recognized pharmacologic actions, should be the rule.

Occasionally, dose escalation into the high therapeutic range results in no beneficial drug effect and no side effects. In this circumstance, the prescriber should be alert to the possibility of drug interactions, at the pharmacokinetic or pharmacodynamic level. Depending on the nature of the anticipated toxicity, dose escalation beyond the usual therapeutic range may occasionally be acceptable, but only if anticipated toxicity is not serious and is readily manageable.

PLASMA CONCENTRATION MONITORING. For some drugs, curves such as those shown in Figures 5–4A and B relating drug concentration to cumulative incidence of beneficial and adverse effects can be generated. With such drugs, monitoring plasma drug concentrations to ensure that they remain within a desired therapeutic range (i.e., above a minimum required for efficacy and below a maximum likely to produce adverse effects) may be a very useful adjunct to therapy. Monitoring drug concentrations may also be useful to ensure compliance and to detect pharmacokinetically based drug interactions that underlie unanticipated efficacy and/or toxicity at usual dosages. Samples for measurement of plasma concentrations should generally be obtained just prior to the next dose, at steady state. These "trough" concentrations provide an index of the minimum plasma concentration expected during a dosing interval.

On the other hand, patient monitoring, whether by plasma concentration or other physiologic indices, to detect incipient toxicity is best accomplished at the time of anticipated peak drug concentrations. Thus, patient surveillance for QT prolongation during sotalol therapy is best accomplished 1 to 2 hours after administration of a dose of drug at steady state.

There may be a lag between the time courses of drug in plasma and of drug effects, as described earlier. In addition, monitoring plasma drug concentrations relies on the assumption that the concentration measured is in equilibrium with that at the target molecular site. Importantly, it is only the fraction of drug that is not bound to plasma proteins that is available to achieve such equilibration. Variability in the extent of protein binding can therefore affect the free fraction and the anticipated drug effect, even in the face of apparently therapeutic total plasma drug concentrations. Basic drugs such as lidocaine and quinidine not only are bound to albumin but also bind extensively to α_1-acid glycoprotein, an acute phase reactant whose concentrations are increased in a variety of "stress" situations, including acute myocardial infarction. Because of this increased protein binding, drug effects may be blunted despite "therapeutic" drug concentrations in these situations.

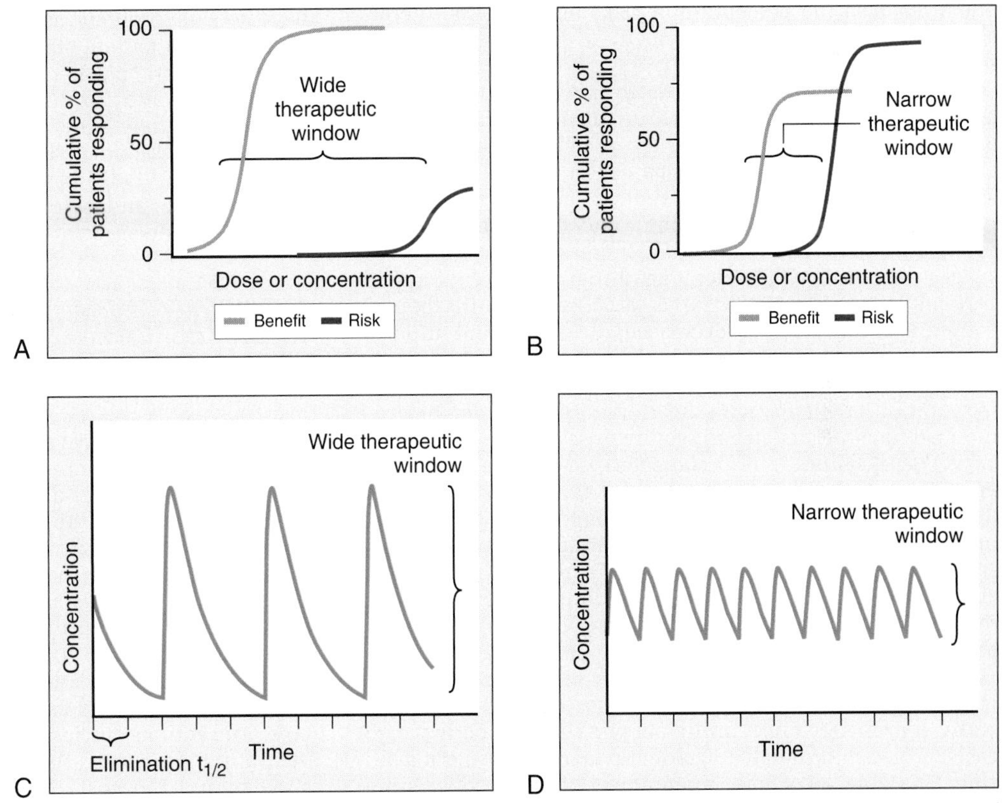

FIGURE 5–4 The concept of a therapeutic ratio. **A** and **B,** Dose- (or concentration) response curves: the solid line in each panel describes the relationship between dose and cumulative incidence of beneficial effects and the dotted line the relationship between dose and dose-related adverse effects (risk). A drug with a wide therapeutic ratio displays separation between the two curves, a high degree of efficacy, and a low degree of dose-related toxicity **(A).** Also, the toxicity would be expected to be mild and readily reversible. Under these conditions, a wide therapeutic ratio can be defined. In part **B,** on the other hand, the curves describing cumulative efficacy and cumulative incidence of adverse effects are positioned near each other, the incidence of adverse effects is higher, and the expected beneficial response is lower; these characteristics define a narrow therapeutic ratio. **C** and **D,** Steady-state plasma concentrations with oral drug administration as a function of time with wide (left) and narrow (right) therapeutic ratios. The hash marks on the abscissae indicate one elimination half-life. When the therapeutic window is wide **(C),** drug administration every three elimination half-lives can produce plasma concentrations that are maintained above the minimum for efficacy and below the maximum beyond which toxicity is anticipated. Panel **D** shows the opposite situation. To maintain plasma concentrations within the narrow therapeutic range, the drug must be administered more frequently.

It is unusual for a healthy patient to receive chronic drug therapy with a single agent. Rather, the rule is polypharmacy in patients with varying degrees of specific organ dysfunction. Although treatment with an individual agent may be justified, the practitioner should also recognize the risk of unanticipated drug effects, particularly drug toxicity, in these settings.

The presence of advanced renal disease mandates that the dosages of drugs eliminated primarily by renal excretion be reduced. Digoxin, dofetilide, and sotalol are examples. A requirement for dose adjustment in cases of less severe renal dysfunction is dictated by available clinical data, and the likelihood of serious toxicity if drug accumulates in plasma due to impaired elimination. Renal failure reduces the protein binding of some drugs (e.g., phenytoin); in this instance, a total drug concentration value in the therapeutic range may actually represent a toxic value of unbound drug.

Very advanced liver disease is characterized by decreased hepatic drug metabolism and portocaval shunts that decrease clearance (and particularly first-pass clearance). Moreover, such patients frequently have other profound disturbances of homeostasis, such as coagulopathy, severe ascites, and altered mental status. These pathophysiologic features of advanced liver disease can profoundly affect not only the dose of a drug required to achieve a potentially therapeutic effect but also the perception of risks and benefits, thereby altering the prescriber's assessment of the actual need for therapy.

Heart disease similarly carries with it a number of disturbances of drug elimination and drug sensitivity that may alter either the therapeutic doses or the practitioner's perception of the desirability of therapy, based on evaluation of risks and benefits. Patients with left ventricular hypertrophy often have baseline QT prolongation, and thus risks of QT-prolonging antiarrhythmias may increase; most guidelines suggest avoiding QT-prolonging antiarrhythmics in such patients (see Table 72–3). In cases of heart failure, hepatic congestion can lead to decreased clearance and thus an increased risk for toxicity with usual doses of certain drugs. Some sedatives, lidocaine, and beta blockers are examples. In addition, patients with heart failure may demonstrate reduced renal perfusion and require dose adjustments on this basis. Heart failure is also characterized by a redistribution of regional blood flow. This can lead to reduced volume of distribution and enhanced risk for drug toxicity. Lidocaine is probably the best-studied example: loading doses of lidocaine should be reduced in patients with heart failure because of altered distribution, whereas maintenance doses should be reduced in cases both of heart failure and of liver disease because of altered clearance.

Age is also a major factor in determining drug doses as well as sensitivity to drug effects. Doses in children are generally administered on a milligram per kilogram body weight basis, although firm data to guide therapy are often not available. Variable postnatal maturation of drug disposition systems may present a special problem in the neonate. Elderly persons often have reduced creatinine clearance, even in the face of a normal serum creatinine level, and dosages of renally excreted drugs should be adjusted accordingly. Systolic dysfunction with hepatic congestion is more common in the elderly. Vascular disease and dementia are common in the elderly and can lead to increased postural hypotension and risk of falling. Thus, therapies such as sedatives, tricyclic antidepressants, or anticoagulants should be initiated only when the practitioner is convinced that the benefits of such therapies outweigh this increased risk.

Drug Interactions

Multiple mechanisms, and examples, of interactions on a pharmacokinetic or pharmacodynamic basis have been presented in this chapter. Table 5–3 summarizes these and other mechanisms that may underlie important drug interactions. Drug interactions may be based on altered pharmacokinetics (absorption, distribution, metabolism, and excretion). In addition, drugs can interact at the pharmacodynamic level. A trivial example is coadministration of two antihypertensive drugs leading to excessive hypotension. Similarly, coadministration of aspirin and warfarin leads to an increased risk for bleeding, although benefits of the combination can also be demonstrated.

The most important principle in approaching a patient receiving polypharmacy is to recognize this potential. A complete medication history should be obtained from each patient at regular intervals; patients will often omit topical medications such as eye drops, "health food" supplements, and medications prescribed by other practitioners unless specifically prompted. Each of these, however, carries a risk of important systemic drug actions and interactions. Beta blocker eye drops can produce systemic beta blockade, particularly with CYP2D6 substrates in patients with defective CYP2D6 activity. St. John's wort induces CYP3A and P-glycoprotein activity and thus can markedly lower plasma concentrations of drugs such as cyclosporine and oral contraceptives.[19,20] As with many other interactions, this may not be a special problem as long as both drugs are continued. However, if a patient stabilized on cyclosporine stops taking St. John's wort, plasma concentrations of the drug can rise dramatically and toxicity ensue. Similarly, initiation of St. John's wort may lead to markedly lowered cyclosporine concentrations and a risk of organ rejection. A number of other "health foods" have been associated with very serious drug toxicity and withdrawal from the market; phenylpropanolamine-associated stroke is one recent example.[21]

Prospects for the Future

The last 20 years have seen dramatic advances in the treatment of heart disease, due in no small part to the development of highly effective and well tolerated drug therapies, such as HMG-CoA reductase inhibitors, ACE inhibitors, and beta blockers. These developments, along with improved nonpharmacological approaches, have led to dramatically enhanced survival of patients with advanced heart disease. Thus, polypharmacy in an aging and chronically ill population is becoming increasing common. In this milieu, drug effects become increasingly variable, reflecting interactions among drugs, underlying disease and disease mechanisms, and genetic backgrounds.

An increasing understanding of the genetic basis of variable drug actions carries with it the promise of reducing such variability. However, the logistics of implementing such a strategy and the costs of individualizing therapy based on genetics are major outstanding issues. An alternate view is that effective therapies are available and have not been adequately delivered to populations that would benefit. The two views are not mutually exclusive. In the face of such increasing complexity, the relationship between the individual prescriber and the individual patient remains the centerpiece of modern therapeutics. Each initiation of drug therapy represents a new clinical experiment, and prescribers must be continually vigilant regarding the possibility of unusual drug effects that may provide initial clues to unanticipated and important mechanisms of beneficial and adverse drug effects.

TABLE 5–3 Drug Interactions: Mechanisms and Examples

Mechanism	Drug	Interacting Drug	Effect
Decreased bioavailability	Digoxin	Antacids	Decreased digoxin effect due to decreased absorption
Increased bioavailability	Digoxin	Antibiotics	By eliminating gut flora that metabolize digoxin, some antibiotics may increase digoxin bioavailability. Note: some antibiotics also interfere with P-glycoprotein (expressed in the intestine and elsewhere), another effect that can elevate digoxin concentration.
Induction of hepatic metabolism	*CYP3A substrates:* Quinidine Mexiletine Verapamil Cyclosporine	Phenytoin Rifampin Barbiturates St. John's wort	Loss of drug effect due to increased metabolism Similar effects with the CYP2C9 substrate warfarin, except with phenytoin
Inhibition of hepatic metabolism	*CYP2C9:* Warfarin Losartan	Amiodarone Phenytoin	Decreased warfarin requirement Diminished conversion of losartan to its active metabolite, with decreased antihypertensive control
	CYP3A substrates: Quinidine Cyclosporine HMG-CoA reductase inhibitors: lovastatin, simvastatin, atorvastatin; not pravastatin Cisapride, terfenadine, astemizole*	Ketoconazole Itraconazole Erythromycin Clarithromycin Some calcium blockers Some HIV protease inhibitors (especially ritanovir)	Increased risk for drug toxicity
	CYP2D6 substrates: Beta blockers (see Table 5–1) Propafenone Desipramine Codeine	Quinidine (even ultra-low dose) Fluoxetine	Increased beta-blockade Increased beta-blockade Increased adverse effects Decreased analgesia (due to failure of biotransformation to the active metabolite morphine)
Inhibition of drug transport	*P-glycoprotein substrates:* Digoxin	Amiodarone Quinidine Verapamil Cyclosporine Itraconazole Erythromycin	Digoxin toxicity
	Renal tubular transport: Dofetilide	Verapamil Cimetidine	Slightly increased plasma concentration and QT effect
	Monoamine transporter substrates: Guandrel	Tricyclic antidepressants	Blunted antihypertensive effects
Pharmacodynamic interactions	Aspirin + warfarin		Increased therapeutic anti-thrombotic effect; increased risk of bleeding
	Nonsteroidal anti-inflammatory drugs	Warfarin	Increased risk of gastrointestinal bleeding
	Antihypertensive drugs	Nonsteroidal anti-inflammatory drugs	Loss of blood pressure lowering
	QT-prolonging antiarrhythmics	Diuretics	Increased torsades de pointes risk due to diuretic-induced hypokalemia
	Supplemental potassium	Angiotensin-converting enzyme inhibitors	Hyperkalemia
	Sildenafil	Nitrates	Increased and persistent vasodilation; risk of myocardial ischemia

*These drugs have been withdrawn or their availability highly restricted because they can produce torsades de pointes, particularly when their metabolism is inhibited.

Importance of Correct Drug Use

1. (http://cms.hhs.gov/statistics/nhe/historical/t2.asp; http://www.americanheart.org/downloadable/heart/10461207852142003HDSStatsBook.pdf)
2. Cohn JN, Goldstein SO, Greenberg BH, et al: A dose-dependent increase in mortality with vesnarinone among patients with severe heart failure. Vesnarinone Trial Investigators. N Engl J Med 339:1810, 1998.

Variability in Drug Action

3. Roden DM, George AL Jr: The genetic basis of variability in drug responses. Nat Rev Drug Discovery 1:37, 2002.
4. Kuehl P, Zhang J, Lin Y, et al: Sequence diversity in CYP3A promoters and characterization of the genetic basis of polymorphic CYP3A5 expression. Nat Genet 27:383, 2001.
5. Meyer UA: Pharmacogenetics and adverse drug reactions. Lancet 356:1667, 2000.
6. Fischer TL, Pieper JA, Graff DW, et al: Evaluation of potential losartan-phenytoin drug interactions in healthy volunteers. Clin Pharmacol Ther 72:238, 2002.
7. Fromm MF, Kim RB, Stein CM, et al: Inhibition of P-glycoprotein-mediated drug transport: A unifying mechanism to explain the interaction between digoxin and quinidine. Circulation 99:552, 1999.

Clinical Relevance of Polymorphic Drug Metabolism

8. Thompson PD, Clarkson P, Karas RH: Statin-associated myopathy. JAMA 289:1681, 2003.
9. Caraco Y, Sheller J, Wood AJ: Impact of ethnic origin and quinidine coadministration on codeine's disposition and pharmacodynamic effects. J Pharmacol Exp Ther 290:413, 1999.

Pharmacodynamics

10. Sofowora GG, Dishy V, Muszkat M, et al: A common beta1-adrenergic receptor polymorphism (Arg389Gly) affects blood pressure response to beta-blockade. Clin Pharmacol Ther 73:366, 2003.
11. Dishy V, Sofowora GG, Xie HG, et al: The effect of common polymorphisms of the beta2-adrenergic receptor on agonist-mediated vascular desensitization. N Engl J Med 345:1030, 2001.
12. Johnson JA, Terra SG: β-Adrenergic receptor polymorphisms: Cardiovascular disease associations and pharmacogenetics. Pharm Res 19:1779, 2002.
13. Chien KR: Myocyte survival pathways and cardiomyopathy: Implications for trastuzumab cardiotoxicity. Semin Oncol 27:9, 2000.
14. McNamara DM, Holubkkov R, Janosko K, et al: Pharmacogenetic interactions between β-blocker therapy and the angiotensin-converting enzyme deletion polymorphism in patients with congestive heart failure. Circulation 103:1644, 2001.
15. Al Khatib SM, Granger CB, Huang Y, et al: Sustained ventricular arrhythmias among patients with acute coronary syndromes with no ST-segment elevation: Incidence, predictors, and outcomes. Circulation 106:309, 2002.
16. Psaty BM, Smith NL, Heckbert SR, et al: Diuretic therapy, the alpha-adducin gene variant, and the risk of myocardial infarction or stroke in persons with treated hypertension. JAMA 287:1680, 2002.
17. Yang P, Kanki H, Drolet B, et al: Allelic variants in long QT disease genes in patients with drug-associated torsades de pointes. Circulation 105:1943, 2002.
18. Sesti F, Abbott GW, Wei J, et al: A common polymorphism associated with antibiotic-induced cardiac arrhythmia. PNAS 97:10613, 2000.

Drug Interactions

19. Dresser GK, Schwarz UI, Wilkinson GR, et al: Coordinate induction of both cytochrome P4503A and MDR1 by St John's wort in healthy subjects. Clin Pharmacol Ther 73:41, 2003.
20. Zhou S, Gao Y, Jiang W, et al: Interactions of herbs with cytochrome P450. Drug Metab Rev 35:35, 2003.
21. Kernan WN, Viscoli CM, Brass LM, et al: Phenylpropanolamine and the risk of hemorrhagic stroke. N Engl J Med 343:1826, 2000.
22. Splawski I, Timothy KW, Tateyama M, et al: Variant of SCN5A sodium channel implicated in risk of cardiac arrhythmia. Science 297:1333, 2002.
23. Wei J, Yang IC, Tapper AR, et al: *KCNE1* polymorphism confers risk of drug-induced long QT syndrome by altering kinetic properties of IKs potassium channels. Circulation 100:I-495, 1999.
24. Kuznetsova T, Staessen JA, Wang JG, et al: Antihypertensive treatment modulates the association between the D/I ACE gene polymorphism and left ventricular hypertrophy: A meta-analysis. J Hum Hypertens 14:447, 2000.
25. Turban S, Fuentes F, Ferlic L, et al: A prospective study of paraoxonase gene Q/R192 polymorphism and severity, progression and regression of coronary atherosclerosis, plasma lipid levels, clinical events and response to fluvastatin. Atherosclerosis 154:633, 2001.
26. Salazar LA, Hirata MH, Quintao EC, et al: Lipid-lowering response of the HMG-CoA reductase inhibitor fluvastatin is influenced by polymorphisms in the low-density lipoprotein receptor gene in Brazilian patients with primary hypercholesterolemia. J Clin Lab Anal 14:125, 2000.
27. Lutucuta S, Ballantyne CM, Elghannam H, et al: Novel polymorphisms in promoter region of ATP binding cassette transporter gene and plasma lipids, severity, progression, and regression of coronary atherosclerosis and response to therapy. Circ Res 88:969, 2001.
28. Kuivenhoven JA, Jukema JW, Zwinderman AH, et al: The role of a common variant of the cholesteryl ester transfer protein gene in the progression of coronary atherosclerosis. The Regression Growth Evaluation Statin Study Group. N Engl J Med 338:86, 1998.
29. Zambon A, Deeb SS, Brown BG, et al: Common hepatic lipase gene promoter variant determines clinical response to intensive lipid-lowering treatment. Circulation 103:792, 2001.
30. Szczeklik A, Sanak M, Undas A, et al: Platelet glycoprotein IIIa P1A polymorphism and effects of aspirin on thrombin generation response. Circulation 103:33e, 2001.
31. Baker EH, Duggal A, Dong Y, et al: Amiloride, a specific drug for hypertension in black people with T594M variant? Hypertension 40:13, 2002.
32. Siffert W: Cardiovascular pharmacogenetics: On the way toward individually tailored drug therapy. Kidney Int Suppl 84:S168, 2003.
33. Sciarrone MT, Stella P, Barlassina C, et al: ACE and alpha-adducin polymorphism as markers of individual response to diuretic therapy. Hypertension 41:398, 2003.
34. Mukae S, Aoki S, Itoh S, et al: Bradykinin B2 receptor gene polymorphism is associated with angiotensin-converting enzyme inhibitor-related cough. Hypertension 36:127, 2000.

CHAPTER 6

Care of Patients with End-Stage Heart Disease

Linda L. Emanuel • Robert O. Bonow

Care for the incurable patient has been a defining part of medicine from its earliest origins, as reflected in the emphasis on comfort in the writings of 5th century BC Greek physician Hippocrates.[1] In recent decades, advances in cardiopulmonary resuscitation, cardiovascular surgery, and implantable devices have stimulated medical ethics discussions of who should receive resuscitation and when life really ends. End-of-life and palliative care more generally remain a defining part of the practice of cardiology. For instance, the primary indication for coronary artery bypass, stents (see Chap. 50), and other procedures is symptom control and quality of life; in this sense, a significant amount of care provided by cardiologists is quality palliative care. At the same time, consideration of the types of care sought by those who are facing death and dying needs more attention.[2-4] For instance, one study found that of the 15 guidelines on congestive heart failure (see Chap. 24), none had significant mention of palliative care and only six had moderate mention.[5] By explicitly integrating palliative care considerations into the new patient assessment, treatment decision-making, continuity of care planning, and systems of care delivery, cardiovascular medicine can further advance the quality of care it provides.[6]

Epidemiology (see Chap. 1)

The characteristic cardiovascular death is sudden (see Chap. 33). However, cardiovascular conditions are also chronic and can afflict children and young adults as well as the elderly. In 2000, about 65 million Americans had chronic cardiovascular conditions, and between 1976 and 1980, approximately 1 million children and young adults were living with congenital heart defects.

The site of death has also evolved. Nearly 60% of Americans died as inpatients in hospitals in 1980; by 2000, about 40% died in the hospital. Although this trend corresponds with patient and family preferences, patients with cardiovascular disease are least represented among those receiving home care and hospice care. In 2000, approximately 20% of all decedents received hospice care, with cancer patients accounting for more than 70% of hospice users. Among patients with nine cancer diagnoses, 15% to 34% of decedents used hospice, whereas among patients with myocardial infarction and congestive heart failure diagnoses, 7% and 8% of decedents, respectively, used hospice.[7] Patients in need of palliative care can be ambulatory, in long-term care, or in the hospital. Consequently, palliative care is needed in a full range of settings.

Palliative Care

Because terminally ill patients have a wide variety of advanced diseases, often with multiple symptoms demanding relief and requiring a noninvasive therapeutic regimen to be delivered in a commodious care setting, their care requires some of the most complex and demanding cognitive skills for assessments and interventions. Fundamental to ensuring quality palliative and end-of-life care is a focus on four broad domains of the illness experience: (1) physical symptoms; (2) mental or psychological symptoms; (3) social needs, including relationships, practical issues, and economic issues; and (4) existential or spiritual needs. Palliative care also includes support for the family, including for their bereavement. Recent empirical studies have confirmed that these domains coincide with the experiences and preferences for care of patients with advanced illness and for their families. A whole-person assessment screens for and evaluates needs in each of these four domains. Goals for care are discerned and decided on in discussion with the patient and/or family based on the assessment in each of these domains. Although physicians are responsible for certain, especially technical, interventions and for coordinating the interventions, they depend on an interdisciplinary team and the family to provide all of them. Importantly, failing to address any one of the domains is likely to preclude a good death, and therefore a well coordinated, effectively communicating interdisciplinary team takes on special importance in end-of-life care.

Assessment, Goals, and Care Planning

WHOLE-PERSON ASSESSMENT. The assessment of physical and mental symptoms should follow a modified version of the traditional history and physical examination that emphasizes symptoms. Questions should discern sources of suffering and how much these symptoms interfere with the patient's life. Standardized assessment questions are available from clinically relevant scales such as the Memorial Symptom Assessment Scale; these have the advantage of ensuring that the assessment is comprehensive. For a patient with late end-stage disease for whom the care goal is quality of being, tests and aspects of the physical examination that are uncomfortable should be carefully evaluated for their benefit-to-burden ratio for the patient. Since a focused physical examination may be all that is reasonable, these skills need to be well developed.

In the area of social needs, health care providers should screen for financial needs, the status of important relationships, care giving needs, and access to medical care. Relevant questions may include the following: *How often is there someone to feel close to? How much help do you need with things like getting meals or getting around? How much trouble do you have getting the medical care you need?* In the area of existential needs, providers should assess distress and the patient's sense of being emotionally and existentially settled and of finding purpose or meaning.[8] Helpful assessment questions can include the following: *How much are you able to find meaning since your illness began?* It is helpful to ask about the patient's perception of his or her care, as follows: *How much do you feel your doctors and nurses respect you? How clear is the information from us about what to expect regarding your illness? How much do you feel that the medical care you are getting fits with your goals?* If concern is detected in any areas, deeper evaluation questions are warranted.[9]

COMMUNICATION. Communication is arguably as powerful an intervention in medicine as any invasive procedure. Poor communication has significant adverse consequences, and quality communication allows for navigating difficult situations in the best available fashion. Communication requires both effective "signal output" and effective reception, so the clinician must assist the patient and family with their ability to receive difficult information as well as offer the information in an accessible way.

A seven-step guide for communicating important information has been developed by Buckman: (1) Prepare, mentally and physically by (2) setting up a quiet environment with room for face-to-face discussion and accommodating items such as a chair, a box of tissues, a pen and paper to write down information, and perhaps a beverage. (3) Begin by asking what the patient and/or family know and/or understand and then (4) ask how they prefer to receive new information and how much they want who to know. (5) Give the new information according to their preferences. (6) Allow for emotional responses and (7) plan for the next steps in care, including identification of the next concrete steps.[10] See Table 6–1 for suggested wording and the rationale behind each step.

PROGNOSIS. Among patients with an equally poor prognosis, 75% of cancer patients reported that they knew they would likely die, whereas only 54% of non-cancer patients, many of whom had cardiac diagnoses, reported the same.[11,12]

TABLE 6–1 Elements of Communicating Bad News: The P-SPIKES Approach

Acronym	Steps	Aim of the Interaction	Preparations, Questions, or Phrases
P	Preparation	Mentally prepare for the interaction with the patient and/or family.	Review what information needs to be communicated. Plan how you will provide emotional support. Rehearse key steps and phrases in the interaction.
S	Setting of the interaction	Ensure the appropriate setting for a serious and emotionally charged discussion.	Ensure that patient, family, and appropriate social supports are present. Devote sufficient time—do not squeeze in a discussion. Ensure privacy and prevent interruptions by people or beeper. Bring a box of tissues.
P	Patient's perception and preparation	Begin the discussion by establishing the baseline and whether the patient and family can grasp the information. Ease tension by having the patient and family contribute.	Start with open-ended questions to encourage participation. Possible phrases to use: *What do you understand about your illness?* *When you first had symptom X, what did you think it might be?* *What did Dr. X tell you when he sent you here?* *What do you think is going to happen?*
I	Invitation and information needs	Discover what information needs the patient and/or family have and what limits they want regarding the bad information.	Possible phrases to use: *If this condition turns out to be something serious, do you want to know?* *Would you like me to tell you the full details of your condition? If not, then who would you like me to talk to?*
K	Knowledge of the condition	Provide the bad news or other information to the patient and/or family sensitively.	Do not just dump the information on the patient and family. Interrupt and check that the patient and family are understanding. Possible phrases to use: *I feel badly to have to tell you this, but. . . .* *Unfortunately, the tests showed. . . .* *I'm afraid the news is not good. . . .*
E	Empathy and exploration	Identify the cause of the emotions—e.g. poor prognosis. Empathize with the patient and/or family's feelings. Explore by asking open-ended questions.	Strong feelings in reaction to bad news are normal. Acknowledge what the patient and family are feeling. Remind them that such feelings are normal even if frightening. Give them time to respond. Remind patient and family you won't abandon them. Possible phrases to use: *I imagine this is very hard for you.* *You must be upset. Tell me how you are feeling.* *I wish the news were different.* *I'll do whatever I can to help you.*
S	Summarizing and strategic planning	Delineate for the patient and the family the next steps, including additional tests or interventions.	It is the unknown and uncertain that increase anxiety. Recommend a schedule with goals and landmarks. Provide your rationale for the patient and/or family to accept or reject. If the patient and/or family are not ready to discuss the next steps, schedule a follow-up visit.

Adapted from Buchman R: How to Break Bad News: A Guide for Health Care Professionals. Baltimore, Johns Hopkins University Press, 1992.

The established gap between prognosis in late-stage cardiovascular conditions and the patients' expectation of death, the continuous stream of life-prolonging cardiovascular therapies and devices, the difficulty in establishing accurate prognoses in individual cases, and the need to sustain hope may be only four of multiple factors that conspire to keep poor prognosis from triggering appropriate forms of palliative care.

Clinicians should provide population-based statistics regarding prognosis to patients and families and allow these statistics rather than individual predictions to trigger the kinds of whole-patient assessments and continuous goal assessment conversations that follow palliative care guidelines. This in turn will allow patients and families not only to follow plans for care that are appropriate but also to achieve the kinds of psychological, social, and existential engagements that people tend to seek when going through the last stages of life.[13-15] Generally, clinicians should share population-based prognosis at the time of diagnosis and then introduce a palliative care framework of whole-patient assessment and continuous goal adjustment from the time when clinical indicators suggest a prognosis of 6 months or less. When sharing prognostic information, use language such as, *"Of all the people with your condition in America, about half will go on to live for more than 3 years and about half will die within 3 years."* Continue by saying something like this: *"We will hope for the best but also plan for the worst so that we are not caught unprepared and you can live your life with a positive attitude."* The conversation can go further if the clinician then says something such as, *"Many people have special things they want to accomplish in this phase of their life, such as a project, a trip, or coming to terms in a personal relationship. I encourage you to think about what that might be for you so that I can do my best to tailor our medical care to your goals."* For patients with cardiovascular illnesses, it is often helpful to point out that, *"The good news is that we can expect you to feel well and function pretty normally. Often people with cardiac disease avoid the long phases of disability and suffering that other illnesses can cause. The counterpart is that people sometimes do not engage in the growth that often comes at the end of life or they become overly fearful of dying suddenly. Preparation of the kind we just mentioned can bring the best of both worlds. So let's keep an open discussion about your goals for care."*

CONTINUOUS GOAL ASSESSMENT. Goals for care are numerous. They range from cure of a specific condition, to delaying the course of an incurable disease, to adapting to progressive disability without disrupting the family, to finding peace of mind or personal meaning, to dying in a manner that leaves loved ones with a positive "departure memory." Discernment of goals for care can be approached through a seven-step protocol: (1) Ensure that information is as complete as is reasonably possible and is understood by all relevant parties (see sections on Whole-Patient Assessment and on Communication). (2) Explore what the patient and family are hoping for. (3) Share all the options with the patient and family. Delineate some relevant goals that are also realistic. (4) Respond empathetically to the patient and family as they adjust to declining realistic expectations. (5) Make a plan, emphasizing what can be done toward the realistic goals. (6) Follow through with the plan. (7) Review and revise this plan periodically, considering at every encounter whether the goals of care should be reviewed with the patient and/or family. If a patient or family member has difficulty letting go of an unrealistic goal, suggest that while hoping for the best, it is still prudent to have a plan for other outcomes as well.

ADVANCE CARE PLANNING. Advance care planning is a process of planning for future medical care in case the patient becomes incapable of making medical decisions. Ideally, it starts before a health care crisis or the terminal phase of an illness. However, although 80% of Americans endorse advance care planning, only 20% have actually made advance care plans. A similarly small proportion of health care providers have completed their own advance care planning. A good first step is for health care providers to start with themselves. Personal planning makes the providers aware of the critical and charged choices in the process and allows them to truthfully tell their patients that they have done this themselves. With experience, advance care planning discussions need not take long.

Steps in effective advance care planning involve the following: (1) introducing the topic, (2) structuring a discussion, (3) reviewing plans that have been discussed by the patient and family, (4) documenting the plans, (5) updating them periodically, and (6) implementing the advance care directive (Table 6–2). Raising the topic can be done efficiently as a routine matter, analogous to insurance or estate planning, and is recommended for all patients. Structuring a focused discussion (step 2) is the central skill. Identify the health care proxy and recommend his or her involvement in the discussion. Select a worksheet, preferably one that has been evaluated and demonstrated to produce reliable and valid expressions of patient preferences, and orient the patient and proxy to it. Discuss with the patient and proxy one scenario as an example to demonstrate how to think about the issues. It is often helpful to begin with a scenario in which the patient is likely to have settled preferences, such as being in a persistent vegetative state. Ask the patient and proxy to discuss and complete the worksheet for the other scenarios. If appropriate, suggest that they involve family members in the discussion. On a return visit, go over the patient's preferences, checking and resolving any medical or logical inconsistencies. After having the patient and proxy sign the document, place it in the medical chart and be sure that copies are provided to relevant family members and care sites. Since patients' preferences can change, review these documents periodically or after an illness episode or personal experience.

Types of Documents. Two broad types of advance care planning documents exist. The first includes living wills or instructional directives; these advisory documents describe the types of decisions that should direct care. Some are specific, delineating scenarios and interventions. Among these, some are for general use and others are for a specific type of disease, such as cancer or human immunodeficiency virus; some are available in multiple languages.[16] Less specific directives can be general statements or can describe the values that should guide decisions. Health care proxy forms appoint an individual to make decisions. A combined directive that both directs care and designates a proxy is generally recommended, and the directive should clearly indicate whether the patient's preferences or the proxy's choice should take precedence if they conflict.

The U.S. Supreme Court has established that patients have a constitutional right to refuse or terminate life-sustaining interventions, and that mentally incompetent patients may do so by having previously provided "clear and convincing evidence" of their advance preferences.[17,18] As of 2003, all states and the District of Columbia also have living will or health care proxy legislation. State variations exist but are less important than they could be, since the Constitution has been interpreted to require states to honor any clear advance care directive. A potentially misleading distinction relates to statutory as opposed to advisory documents. Statutory documents are drafted to fit relevant state statutes. They tend to be written with the goal of protecting clinicians from legal action if they follow the patient's stated wishes. Advisory documents are drafted to reflect the patient's wishes. Both are legal, the first under State and the second under common or

TABLE 6–2 Steps in Advance Care Planning

Step	Goals to be Achieved and Measures to Cover	Useful Phrases or Points to Make
Introducing advance care planning	Ask the patient what he or she knows about advance care planning and if he or she has already completed an advance care directive. Indicate that you as a physician have completed advance care planning. Indicate that you try to perform advance care planning with all patients regardless of prognosis. Explain the goals of the process as empowering the patient and ensuring that you and the proxy understand the patient's preferences. Provide the patient with relevant literature, including the advance care directive that you prefer to use. Recommend that the patient identify a proxy decision-marker who should attend the next meeting.	"I'd like to talk with you about something I try to discuss with all my patients. It's called advance care planning. In fact, I feel that this is such an important topic that I have done this myself. Are you familiar with advance care planning or living wills?" "Have you thought about the type of care you would want if you ever became too sick to speak for yourself? That is the purpose of advance care planning." "There is no change in health that we have not discussed. I am bringing this up now because it is sensible for everyone, no matter how well or ill, old or young." Have many copies of advance care directives available, including in the waiting room, for patients and families.
Structured discussion of scenarios and patient preferences	Affirm that the goal of the process is to follow the patient's wishes if the patient loses decision-making capacity. Elicit the patient's overall goals related to health care. Elicit the patient's preferences for specific interventions in a few salient and common scenarios. Help the patient define the threshold for withdrawing and withholding interventions. Define the patient's preference for the role of the proxy.	Use a structured worksheet with typical scenarios. Begin the discussion with persistent vegetative state and consider other scenarios, such recovery from an acute event with serious disability, asking the patient about his or her preferences regarding specific interventions, such as ventilators, nasogastric feedings, and CPR proceeding to less invasive interventions, such as blood transfusions and antibiotics.
Review the patient's preferences	After the patient has made choices of interventions, review them to ensure that they are consistent and that the proxy is aware of them.	
Document the patient's preferences	Formally complete the advance care directive and have witness sign it. Provide a copy for the patient and the proxy. Insert a copy into the patient's medical record.	
Update the directive	Periodically, and with major changes in health status, review with the patient the existing choice made and make any modifications.	
Apply the directive	The directive goes into effect only when the patient becomes unable to make medical decisions for him- or herself. Re-read the directive to be sure about its content. Discuss your proposed actions based on the directive with the proxy.	

constitutional law. However, it is simpler to honor a statement that complies with all laws, so if a patient is not using a statutory form, then it is appropriate to attach a statutory form to the advance care directive being used.

Interventions

PHYSICAL SYMPTOMS AND THEIR MANAGEMENT. The most common physical and psychological symptoms among all terminally ill patients include pain, fatigue, insomnia, anorexia, dyspnea, depression, anxiety, and nausea and vomiting (Table 6–3). In the last days of life, terminal delirium is also common. Patients with advanced cancer experience an average of 11.5 symptoms. Statistics on symptoms for late-stage cardiovascular patients are not available. However, almost one third of cardiovascular deaths involve additional causes, so the cardiologist managing patients in end-stage disease should be able to manage symptoms from noncardiac conditions as well. Symptom management skills are well described elsewhere.[19]

SOCIAL NEEDS AND THEIR MANAGEMENT.

Financial Burdens. Dying can impose substantial economic strains on patients and families (see Chap. 2). In the United States, about 20% of terminally ill patients and their families have to spend more than 10% of family income on health care costs over and above health insurance premiums. Between 10% and 30% of families have sold assets, used savings, or taken out a mortgage to pay for the patient's health care costs. Nearly 40% of terminally ill patients report that the cost of their illness was a moderate or great economic hardship for their family.

One source of economic burden is related to medical costs. The second, more universal source of economic burden is a decline in the patient's income. In 20% of cases, a family member stopped working to provide care. Economic burden is associated with poor physical functioning and needs for housekeeping, nursing, and personal care. That is, more

TABLE 6–3 Managing Changes in the Patient's Condition during the Final Days and Hours

Change in the Patient's Condition	Potential Complication	Family's Possible Reaction and Concern	Advice and Intervention
Profound fatigue	Bedbound with development of pressure ulcers that are prone to infection, malodor, and pain, as well as joint pain.	Patient is lazy and giving up.	Reassure family and caregivers that terminal fatigue will not respond to interventions and should not be resisted. Use an air mattress if necessary.
Anorexia	None	Patient is giving up. Patient will suffer from hunger and will starve to death.	Reassure family and caregivers that the patient is not eating because he or she is dying; not eating at the end of life does not cause suffering or death. Forced feeding, whether oral, parenteral, or enteral, does not reduce symptoms or prolong life.
Dehydration	Dry mucosal membranes (see below).	Patient will suffer from thirst and die of dehydration.	Reassure family and caregivers that terminal dehydration does not cause suffering because patients lose consciousness before any symptom distress. Intravenous hydration can worsen symptoms of dyspnea by pulmonary or peripheral edema as well as prolong dying process.
Dysphagia	Inability to swallow oral medications needed for palliative care.		Do not force oral intake. Discontinue unnecessary medications that may have been continued including antibiotics, diuretics, antidepressants, and laxatives. If swallowing pills is difficult for patient, convert essential medications (analgesics, antiemetics, anxiolytics, and psychotropics) to oral solutions, buccal, sublingual, or rectal administration.
"Death rattle"—noisy breathing		Patient is choking and suffocating.	Reassure the family and caregivers that this is caused by secretions in the oropharynx and the patient is not choking. Reduce secretions with scopolamine (0.2-0.4 mg Sc every 4 hours or 1-3 patches every 3 days) Reposition patient to permit drainage of secretions. Do not suction. Suction can cause patient and family discomfort and is usually ineffective.
Apnea, Cheyne-Stokes respirations, dyspnea		Patient is suffocating.	Reassure family and caregivers that unconscious patients do not experience suffocation or air hunger. Apneic episodes are frequently a premorbid change. Opioids or anxiolytics may be used for dyspnea. Oxygen is unlikely to relieve dyspneic symptoms and may prolong the dying process.
Urinary or fecal incontinence	Skin breakdown if days until death. Potential transmission of infectious agents to caregivers.	Patient is dirty, malodorous, and physically repellent.	Remind family and caregivers to use universal precautions. Frequent changes of bedclothes and bedding. Use diapers, urinary catheter, or rectal tube if diarrhea or high urine flow occur.
Agitation or delirium	Day/night reversal. Hurt to self or caregivers.	Patient is in horrible pain and going to have a horrible death.	Reassure family and caregivers that agitation and delirium do not necessarily connote physical pain. Depending on the prognosis and goals of treatment, consider evaluating for causes of delirium and modify medications. Manage symptoms with haloperidol, chlorpromazine, diazepam, or midazolam.
Dry mucosal membranes	Cracked lips, mouth sores, and candidiasis can also cause pain. Malodor.	Patient may be malodorous, physically repellent.	Use baking soda mouthwash or saliva preparation every 15-30 minutes. Use topical nystatin for candidiasis. Coat lips and nasal mucosa with petroleum jelly every 60-90 minutes. Use ophthalmic lubricants every 4 hours or artificial tears every 30 minutes.

debilitated and less well-off patients experience greater economic burdens. Economic burdens tend to increase the psychological distress of families and patients. Assistance from a social worker, early on if possible, to ensure access to available benefits may be helpful. Many people are unaware of options, including insurance benefits, the Family Medical Leave Act, and other sources of assistance.

Relationships. Closing the narrative of lived relationships is a nearly universal need. When asked if sudden death or death after an illness is preferable, respondents often initially select the former but soon change to the latter as they reflect on the importance of saying goodbye. Bereaved family members who have not had the chance to say goodbye often have a difficult grief process. Since many of the deaths in cardiology are sudden (see Chaps. 32 and 33), this issue is of particular importance. Patients and their families should be encouraged to settle what they would like to, even though it is more difficult to anticipate the time of death.

Care of seriously ill patients requires efforts to facilitate the types of encounters and time spent with family and friends that are necessary to meet these needs. Family and close friends may need to be accommodated with unrestricted visiting hours for inpatients, including, in some cases, sleeping near the patient even in institutional settings. Assistance for patients and family members who are unsure about how to create or help preserve memories, whether by providing materials such as a scrap book or memory box or by offering suggestions and informational resources, can be deeply appreciated. Taking photographs and creating videos or audiotapes can be especially helpful to patients with life-shortening illness who have younger children.

Family Caregivers. Caring for seriously ill patients places a heavy burden on families. Families are required to provide transportation, homemaking, and other services. Typically, paid professionals, such as home health nurses and hospice, supplement family care giving; only about one quarter of all caregiving is exclusively paid professional assistance. The trend toward more out-of-hospital deaths will increase reliance on families for end-of-life care. About three quarters of the caregivers of terminally ill patients are female—wives, daughters, and even sisters. Consequently, women tend to be able to rely less on family for caregiving assistance and may need more paid assistance. About 20% of terminally ill patients report substantial unmet needs for nursing and personal care.

This makes it imperative to inquire about unmet needs and facilitate family or paid professional services. Assistance from religious or community groups can often be mobilized by phone calls from the medical team to someone the patient or family identifies.

Existential Needs and Their Management. Dying is one of the ultimate existential challenges. Religion and spirituality are important to dying patients. Approximately 70% of patients report becoming more religious or spiritual when they became terminally ill, and many find comfort in practices such as prayer. Some studies suggest that women and older patients are more likely to experience greater interest in religion and spirituality. On the other hand, about 20% of terminally ill patients become less religious, frequently feeling alienated by becoming terminally ill. For other patients, the need is for existential meaning and purpose that is distinct from, and maybe even an antireligious form of, spirituality. Among patients with cardiovascular conditions, clinical experience suggests that fear of sudden death is common. Further, the well-recognized accomplishment of personal growth and relationship resolution characteristic among patients who foresee death in the near future is less apparent among patients with cardiovascular illnesses.[20] This may reflect the rarer recognition of mortality among heart patients as compared with cancer patients.

Health care providers are often hesitant about involving themselves in the religious, spiritual, and existential experiences of their patients, because it may seem private, related to alternative lifestyles, or "soft." But physicians and other members of the interdisciplinary team should be able to at least detect spiritual need. Screening questions have been developed for a physician's spiritual history taking. Spiritual distress can amplify other types of suffering and even masquerade as, for instance, intractable physical pain or anxiety. The screening questions in the whole-person assessment are usually sufficient. Deeper evaluation and intervention is rarely appropriate for the physician unless no other member of the team is available or suitable. Pastors may be helpful, whether from the medical institution or from the patient's community.

Precisely how religious practices, spirituality, and existential explorations can be facilitated and improve end-of-life care is not well established. In at least one study, only 36% of respondents indicated that a clergy member would be comforting. Nevertheless, this increase in religious and spiritual interest among a substantial proportion of dying patients underscores the importance of inquiring how this need can be addressed in individual patients.

Managing the Last Stages of Life

WITHDRAWING AND WITHHOLDING LIFE-SUSTAINING TREATMENT. For centuries, it has been deemed ethical to withhold or withdraw life-sustaining interventions. For patients who are incompetent and terminally ill but have not completed an advance care directive, next-of-kin can exercise this right, although this may be restricted in some states depending on how clear and convincing the evidence is of the patient's preferences. In theory, a patient's right to refuse medical therapy can be limited by four countervailing interests: (1) preservation of life; (2) prevention of suicide; (3) protection of third parties such as children; and (4) preserving the integrity of the medical profession. In practice, these interests almost never override the right of competent patients or incompetent patients who have left explicit advance care directives to decline unwanted intervention.

Physicians' Orders Regarding Cardiopulmonary Resuscitation and Other Life-Sustaining Treatments. Whenever a patient is a suitable candidate for a Do Not Resuscitate (DNR) order, he or she deserves to have had a comprehensive discussion about goals of care, a plan of care, and possibly also advance care planning. Use of predesigned forms such as the Physicians Orders for Life-Sustaining Treatments (POLST) in place of limited DNR orders can encourage these more comprehensive and coherent approaches to creating plans of care. In general, an isolated DNR order with no reference to other life-sustaining treatment preferences can be considered a red flag that should prompt a physician to include or return to a whole-patient assessment and a comprehensive plan for care with goal-tailored treatment choices.

Mechanical Ventilation. Perhaps the most challenging intervention to withdraw is mechanical ventilation. There are two approaches: "terminal extubation," which is the removal of the endotracheal tube, and "terminal wean," which is the gradual reduction of the FIO_2 or ventilator rate. Some physicians recommend the terminal wean because patients do not develop upper airway obstruction and the distress caused by secretions or stridor with this approach; however, it is reported that terminal weaning can prolong the dying process. To ensure comfort for conscious or semiconscious patients, a common practice is to inject a bolus of midazolam (2-4 mg) prior to withdrawal followed by 5 to 10 mg of morphine and a continuous infusion of morphine (50% of the bolus dose per hour). (Higher doses are needed for patients already receiving anxiolytics and opioids.) Remove any neuromuscular blocking agents so that patients can show any discomfort, which in turn can allow medication titration or additional boluses of morphine or midazolam. Families need to be warned that up to 10% of patients unexpectedly survive for 1 day or more after mechanical ventilation is stopped.

FUTILE CARE. Beginning in the late 1980s, some commentators argued that physicians could terminate futile treatments demanded by families of terminally ill patients. There is no objective definition or standard of futility. The term conceals subjective value judgments about when a treatment is not beneficial. A more practical approach acknowledges that in many cases in which futility concerns are raised, there are underlying communication gaps or unresolved personal issues that are best dealt with in team or family meetings. Occasionally, true value differences exist; these may be best handled with assistance from an ethics committee.

EUTHANASIA AND PHYSICIAN-ASSISTED SUICIDE. Terminating life-sustaining intervention and providing opioids to manage symptoms are not to be confused with euthanasia or physician-assisted suicide. Both the former, unlike the latter, have long been considered ethical by the medical profession and legal by courts.

A growing body of data indicates that depression, hopelessness, and worries about loss of dignity or autonomy are the primary factors motivating a desire for euthanasia or physician-assisted suicide. While any of these can occur in patients with cardiovascular conditions, there appear to be fewer requests in this population than among patients with cancer or acquired immunodeficiency syndrome. Perhaps the characteristic sudden death among cardiac patients helps to avoid some of the fears of indignity and dependence associated with a slow, highly symptomatic decline. Nonetheless, multiple symptoms and chronic disability do occur in patients with end-stage heart disease, and requests for physician-assisted suicide or euthanasia also occur. Cardiologists should know how to respond to such requests.

After receiving a request for euthanasia or physician-assisted suicide, the physician should probe with empathetic, open-ended questions to help elucidate the underlying cause for the request such as: *"What makes you want to consider this option?"* Endorsing either moral opposition or moral support for the act tends to be counterproductive, lending an impression either of being judgmental or of endorsing the worthlessness of the patient's life. Health care providers must reassure the patient of continued care and commitment. Simultaneously, the patient should be educated about (1) alternative, less controversial options, such as symptom management and withdrawing any unwanted treatments; (2) the reality of euthanasia and/or physician-assisted suicide, since the patient is likely to have misconceptions about its effectiveness; and (3) the legal implications of the choice. As indicated, depression, hopelessness, and other symptoms of psychological distress, as well as physical suffering and economic burdens, are likely factors motivating the request. Health care providers should identify the factors motivating the request and aggressively treat those factors. After these interventions and clarification of options, most patients proceed with a less controversial approach of declining life-sustaining interventions, possibly including refusal of nutrition and hydration.

CARE DURING THE LAST HOURS. Most lay people have limited experiences with the actual dying process and death. They frequently do not know what to expect of the final hours, and afterwards. There is no rehearsal and no second chance. Therefore, the family must be prepared, especially if the plan is for the patient to die at home.

For patients with heart failure, there may be several last days of life with characteristic pathophysiologic changes such as increased orthopnea and nocturnal dyspnea. Patients experience extreme weakness and fatigue and become bed bound. This can lead to bedsores. If death is imminent and the sores are causing less distress than the dressing changes and frequent turning do, it is reasonable to cease these usual types of care. Dry mucosal membranes should be cared for with frequent oral swabbing, lip lubricants, and artificial tears. These activities can provide the family with a form of care to substitute for those that no longer help, such as feeding. With loss of the gag reflex and dysphagia, patients can also accumulate airway and pharyngeal secretions, producing noises during respiration sometimes called "the death rattle." Scopolamine can reduce this condition. Dying patients also have changes in respiration with periods of apnea or Cheyne-Stokes breathing. Decreased intravascular volume and cardiac output cause tachycardia, hypotension, peripheral coolness, and livedo reticularis (skin mottling). Patients can also have urinary and fecal incontinence at death as the sphincters lose their tone. Most importantly, changes occur in consciousness and neurological function, leading to two very different paths to death (Fig. 6–1). Patients with hallucinations and seizures may need a palliative care specialist's attention.

Each of these terminal changes can cause distress to patients and families. Informing families of what to expect, even by providing an information sheet, can help relieve this distress. For instance, it can be calming to know that patients stop eating because they are dying, not dying because they have stopped eating, or that the "death rattle" is not a sign of suffocation, or that mottling tends to mean that death is near.

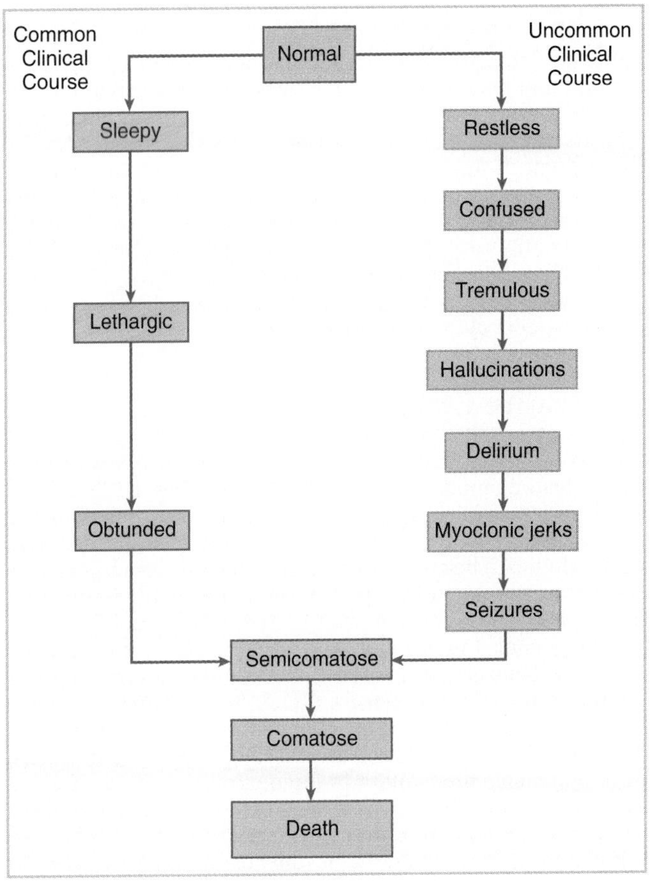

FIGURE 6–1 Common and uncommon clinical courses of the last days of terminally ill patients . (Adapted from Advance Planning. Module 4: Palliative Care. *In* Ferris FD, Flannery JS, McNeal HB, et al (eds): A Comprehensive Guide for the Care of Persons with HIV Disease. Mount Sinai and Casey Hospice, Toronto, Ontario, 1995. Available at http://www.cpsonline.info/content/resources/hivmodule4.html.)

It is claimed that hearing and touch are the last senses to stop functioning. Families should be encouraged to communicate with and touch the patient, even if he or she is unconscious.

When the plan is for the patient to die at home, the family needs to know how to determine when death has occurred, including the cardinal signs of cessation of cardiac function and respiration, fixed pupils, coolness, changes in skin color and texture, and incontinence. Remind the family that the eyes may remain open. It helps to have a plan of who the family and caregivers will contact when the patient is dying or has died. Without a plan, they may panic and call 911, unleashing a cascade of unwanted events from arrival of emergency personnel and resuscitation to hospital admission. Family and caregivers should be instructed to contact hospice, the covering physician, or the on-call member of the palliative care team. There is no reason to contact the coroner, unless the state requires it for all deaths. Similarly, unless foul play is suspected, the health care team need not contact the coroner either.

Just after the patient dies, even the best prepared family may experience shock and bereavement and be distraught. They need time to assimilate the event and be comforted. Health care providers should write a bereavement card or letter to the family. It can be appropriate, although it is not obligatory, to attend the funerals of patients to lend support to the grieving family and to find an opportunity for closure for the physician.

Death is a strong predictor of poor health and even mortality for the surviving spouse. It may be important to alert the spouse's physician about the death so that he or she can be aware of symptoms that might require professional attention.

SUDDEN DEATH. Sudden death may "short-change" patients of the growth that often happens in the last phase of life and that may make it easier for bereaved family members to accommodate to the death. Even adult children of patients who have died suddenly may be excessively influenced by the sudden disappearance of their parent, without a chance to say goodbye, and by the fear of suffering the same fate. Preparedness through discussion, planning, and engaging the benefits of the consciously trodden last paths in life can help, as can extended bereavement counseling. The services of a social worker or other professional with expertise in the area should almost always be considered.

Palliative Care Services

HOW AND WHERE. For nearly two decades, hospice has been a leading model of palliative care services. Patients who use hospice tend to appreciate the care, and their families tend to adjust better than others in similar situations.[21] In 1983, Medicare began paying for hospice services under Part A, the hospital insurance part of reimbursement. To be eligible, a patient must be certified by two physicians as having a prognosis of 6 months or less if the disease runs its usual course. Prognoses are probabilistic by their nature; patients are not required to die within 6 months but rather to have a condition from which half the people with it would be deceased within 6 months. Patients sign a hospice enrollment form that states their intent to forgo curative services related to their terminal illness, but they can still receive medical services for other comorbid conditions. Patients can also disenroll and re-enroll later; that is, the hospice Medicare benefit can be reinvoked later in order to secure traditional Medicare benefits in the interim. Payments to hospice are per diem rather than fee-for-service and are intended to cover comprehensive care, including physician services for the medical direction of the interdisciplinary team, regular home care visits by registered nurses and licensed practical nurses, home health aide and homemaker services, dietary counseling, chaplain services, social work services, and bereavement counseling as well as medical equipment, supplies, and medications. Additional clinical care, including care by the primary physician, is covered by Medicare Part B, even while the hospice Medicare benefit is in place. By 1996, the mean length of enrollment in hospice was 65 days, with the median being less than 24 days. Since then, the length of enrollment has declined. Physicians should initiate earlier referrals to hospice to allow more time for patients to receive palliative care.

Until relatively recently, hospice had been the main way of securing palliative services for terminally ill patients. Efforts are now directed at ensuring continuity of palliative care across settings and through time. Increasingly, these same types of palliative care services are available as consultative services in hospitals, in day care and other outpatient settings, and in nursing homes. For instance, in the United States, although the vast majority of hospice care is provided in residential homes, just over 10% now occurs in nursing homes. In addition, palliative care consultations for non-hospice patients can be billed as for other consultations under Medicare Part B, the physician reimbursement part. Many supporters believe that palliative care should be offered to patients regardless of their prognosis. A patient and his or her family should not have to make an "either curative care or palliative care" choice, in large part because it can be psychologically stressful to embrace mortality. Although provision of palliative care, as needed, from the onset of illness onward is ideal, discontinuities in care can make this challenging. Documentation of goals, orders for life-sustaining treatment that are comprehensive and standardized,[22] advance care planning, and the date of the most recent update can help coordinate care across care sites, among members of the care team, and along the illness trajectory of changing goals for care.

OUTCOME MEASURES. Care near the end of life cannot be measured by most of the traditional validated outcome measures, since palliative care does not consider death a bad outcome. Similarly, family and patients may seek different elements of quality of life that are not included in standard measures when their active engagement is with dying well. Symptom control, enhanced family relationships, and quality of bereavement are difficult to measure and are rarely the primary focus of carefully developed or widely used outcome measures. Nevertheless, outcomes are as important in end-of-life care as in any other field of medical care. Specific end-of-life care instruments are being developed both for assessment and for outcome measures, such as The Brief Hospice Inventory, NEST, and the Palliative Care Outcomes Scale. The field of end-of-life care is ready to enter an era of evidence-based practice and continuous improvement within established institutions.

Acknowledgment

Portions of this chapter are derived from previous writings by Ezekiel and Linda Emanuel.

RESOURCES

The Education in Palliative and End-of-Life Care (EPEC) Project: www.epec.net.
The End of Life/Palliative Education Resource Center (EPERC): www.eperc.mcw.edu.
The National Comprehensive Cancer Network (NCCN) palliative care guidelines, 2002: www.nccn.org.

REFERENCES

1. Asimov I: Asimov's Biographical Encyclopedia of Science and Technology. 2nd ed. Garden City, NY, Doubleday, 1982.

2. Hanratty B, Hibbert D, Mair F, et al: Doctor's perceptions of palliative care for heart failure: Focus group study. Br Med J 325:581, 2002.
3. Easson AM, Crosby JA, Librach SL: Discussion of death and dying in surgical textbooks. Am J Surg 182:34, 2001.
4. Rabow MW, McPhee SJ: Deficiencies in end-of-life care content in medical textbooks. J Am Geriatr Soc 50:397, 2002.
5. Personal communication from R. Arnold.
6. Emanuel L, Alexander C, Arnold R, et al: Palliative care in disease management guidelines. Copies available from American Hospice Foundation, 2004, Washington, DC.
7. Iwashyna T, Zhang JX, Christakis NA: Disease-specific patterns of hospice and related healthcare use in an incidence cohort of seriously ill elderly patients. J Pall Med 5:531, 2002.

Assessment Goals and Care Planning

8. Lo B, et al: Discussing religious and spiritual issues at the end of life: A practical guide for physicians. JAMA 287:749, 2002.
9. Emanuel LL, Alpert H, Emanuel EJ: Concise screening questions for clinical assessments of terminal care: The needs near the end of life care screening tool (NEST). J Palliat Med 4:465, 2001.
10. Buckman R: How to break bad news: A guide for health care professionals. Baltimore, The Johns Hopkins University Press, 1992, pp 65-97.
11. Lamont EB, Christakis NA: Complexities in prognostication in advanced cancer: JAMA 290:98, 2003.
12. Foley K: *In* Seale & Cartwright, 1994.
13. Emanuel EJ, Emanuel LL: The promise of a good death. Lancet 351(Suppl 2):SII21, 1998.
14. Singer PA, et al: Quality end-of-life care: Patients' perspectives. JAMA 281:163, 1999.
15. Webb M: The Good Death: The New American Search to Reshape the End of Life. New York, Bantam Books, 1997.
16. Emanuel LL: The Health Care Directive: Learning how to draft advance care documents. J Am Geriatrics Soc 39:1221, 1991. (www.medicaldirective.org)
17. President's Commission for the Study of Ethical Issues in Medicine and Biomedical and Behavioral Research: Deciding to Forego Life-Sustaining Treatment. Washington, DC, US Government Printing Office, 1983.
18. *Vacco v Quill*, 95-1858; and *State of Washington v Glucksberg*, 96-110.

Interventions

19. An ASCO Curriculum: Optimizing Cancer Care—The importance of symptom management. Vols I & II. Dubuque, IA, Kendal/Hunt Publishing Company, 2001, p 52002.
20. Byock I: Dying Well: The Prospect for Growth at the End of Life, New York, Putnam/Riverhead, 1998.
21. Christakis NA, Iwashyna TJ: The health impact of health care on families: A matched cohort study of hospice use by decedents and mortality outcomes in surviving, widowed spouses. Soc Sci Med 57:465, 2003.
22. Center for Ethics in Health Care: Physician Orders for Life-Sustaining Treatment (POLST) forms. Portland, OR, Oregon Health Sciences University, 1997.

PART II

Examination of the Patient

CHAPTER 7

The History

Eugene Braunwald

Importance of the History

Specialized examinations of the cardiovascular system, presented in Chapters 9 through 18, provide a large portion of the database required to establish a specific anatomical diagnosis of cardiac disease and to determine the extent of functional impairment of the heart. The development and application of these methods are a triumph of modern medicine. However, their appropriate use is to supplement but not to supplant a careful clinical examination. The clinical examination, consisting of the history and physical examination (see Chap. 8), remains the cornerstone of the assessment of the patient with known or suspected cardiovascular disease. For example, the initial clinical evaluation is at least as accurate in predicting coronary anatomy and survival as the exercise stress test.[1] There is a temptation in cardiology, as in many other areas of medicine, to carry out expensive, and occasionally uncomfortable or even hazardous, procedures to establish a diagnosis when a detailed and thoughtful history and a thorough physical examination are sufficient. Obviously, it is undesirable to subject patients to the unnecessary risks, discomfort, and expenses inherent in many specialized tests when a diagnosis can be made on the basis of the clinical examination or when management will not be altered significantly as a result of these tests.

With the increasing emphasis on the cost of medical care, it is likely that there will be a resurgence of interest in the relatively inexpensive clinical examination. On the other hand, it must be appreciated that there may be little correlation between the intensity of symptoms and the severity of heart disease; asymptomatic persons may have a life-threatening condition, whereas persons with many symptoms referable to the cardiovascular system may have no or mild heart disease.

THE ROLE OF THE HISTORY. The overreliance on laboratory tests has increased as physicians attempt to use their time more efficiently by delegating responsibility for taking the history to an assistant or nurse or even by limiting the history to a questionnaire. I consider this to be an undesirable trend for the patient with known or suspected heart disease. First, it must be appreciated that the history remains the richest source of information concerning the patient's illness,[2] and any practice that might diminish the quality or quantity of information provided by the history is likely ultimately to impair the quality of care. Second, the physician's attentive and thoughtful taking of a history establishes a bond with the patient. This bond is frequently valuable in securing the patient's compliance in following a complex treatment plan, undergoing hospitalization for an intensive diagnostic workup or a hazardous operation, and, in some instances, accepting that heart disease is not present at all.

A careful history allows the physician to evaluate the impact of the disease, or the fear of disease, on the various aspects of the patient's life and to assess the patient's personality, affect, and emotional stability; often it provides a glimpse of the patient's responsibilities, fears, aspirations, and threshold for discomfort as well as the likelihood of compliance with one or another therapeutic regimen. Whenever possible, the physician should question not only the patient but also relatives or close friends to obtain a clearer understanding of the extent of the patient's disability and the impact of the disease on both the patient and the family. For example, the patient's spouse is much more likely than the patient to provide a history of Cheyne-Stokes (periodic) respiration.

The combination of the widespread fear of cardiovascular disorders and the deep-seated emotional, symbolic, and sometimes even religious connotations surrounding the heart may, on the one hand, lower the threshold for the development of symptoms that mimic those of organic heart disease in persons with normal cardiovascular systems. On the other hand, they may cause so much dread that serious symptoms are denied by patients with established heart disease. Patients with established heart disease are often frightened, anxious, and/or depressed; these symptoms may be as troubling as those resulting from the pathophysiology of their disorder. These and other psychological symptoms can be identified only by a careful history.[2]

TECHNIQUE. Several approaches can be employed in obtaining the medical history. I believe that patients should first be given the opportunity to relate their experiences and complaints in their own way. Although time consuming and likely to include much seemingly irrelevant information, this technique provides considerable insight into the patient's intelligence, emotional make-up, and attitude toward his or her symptoms and gives the patient the satisfaction that he or she has been "heard" by the physician. After the patient has given an account of the illness, the physician should direct the discussion and obtain information concerning the onset and chronology of symptoms; their location, quality, and intensity; the precipitating, aggravating, and alleviating factors; the setting in which the symptoms occur and any associated symptoms; and the response to therapy.

Of course, a detailed general medical history, including the personal past history, occupational history, nutritional history, and review of systems, must be obtained. Of particular interest is a history of thyroid disease, recent dental extractions or manipulations, or catheterization of the bladder as well as a report of earlier examinations that showed abnormalities of the cardiovascular system as reflected in restriction from physical activity at school and in rejection for life insurance, employment, or military service. Personal habits such as exercise, cigarette smoking, alcohol intake, and parenteral use of drugs—illicit and otherwise—should be ascertained. The medications taken and the reasons given to the patient should be obtained.

Adults should be routinely questioned about the presence of or history of the major risk factors for coronary artery disease (see Chap. 36): cigarette smoking, hypertension, hypercholesterolemia, diabetes mellitus, and a family history of premature coronary artery disease. The exact nature of the patient's work, including physical and emotional stresses, should be assessed. The increasing appreciation of the importance of genetic influences in many forms of heart disease (see Chap. 70) underscores the importance of the family history.

Myocardial and coronary function that may be adequate at rest are often inadequate during exertion; therefore, specific attention should be directed to the influence of activity on the patient's symptoms. Thus, a history of chest discomfort and/or undue shortness of breath that appears only during activity is characteristic of heart disease, whereas the opposite pattern (i.e., the appearance of symptoms at rest and their remission during exertion) is almost never observed in patients with heart disease but is more characteristic of functional disorders.

It is important also to assess the "tempo" of the progression of symptoms. A decline in the threshold for severe anginal discomfort across a 2-week period is much more likely to signify a high risk of an adverse outcome, such as cardiac death or myocardial infarction, than a similar decline occurring over 2 years. Similarly, the history of a "breakthrough" of symptoms despite maintenance of a previously successful regimen should be noted, because it, too, may be a harbinger of a poor outcome and may dictate a change in therapeutic strategy.

As the patient relates the history, important nonverbal clues are often provided. The physician should observe the patient's attitude, reactions, and gestures while being questioned, as well as the choice of words or emphasis. Tumulty has aptly likened obtaining a meaningful clinical history to playing a game of chess[3]: "The patient makes a statement and based upon its content, and mode of expression, the physician asks a counter-question. One answer stimulates yet another question until the clinician is convinced that he understands precisely all of the circumstances of the patient's illness."

Cardinal Symptoms of Heart Disease

Dyspnea (see Chap. 22)

Dyspnea is defined as an abnormally uncomfortable awareness of breathing[4]; it is one of the principal symptoms of cardiac and pulmonary disease and ranges from an increased awareness of breathing to intense respiratory distress.[5,6] Dyspnea occurs after strenuous exertion in normal, healthy, well-conditioned subjects and after only moderate exertion in those who are healthy but unaccustomed to exercise (dyspnea of deconditioning). It should therefore be regarded as abnormal only when it occurs at rest or at a level of physical activity not expected to cause this symptom.

Dyspnea is associated with a wide variety of diseases of the heart and lungs, chest wall, and respiratory muscles as well as with anxiety.[7] Among patients with cardiac dyspnea, this symptom is most commonly associated with and caused by pulmonary congestion, as occurs in cases of left ventricular failure or mitral stenosis. The interstitial and alveolar edema stiffens the lungs and stimulates respiration by activating "J" receptors in the lung. Less frequently, cardiac dyspnea occurs secondary to a reduced cardiac output, without pulmonary engorgement, as in cases of tetralogy of Fallot. Table 7–1 provides a list of the various syndromes that may cause dyspnea and the primary pathophysiological mechanisms that are responsible. Both Borg and Noble[8] and the American Thoracic Society (Table 7–2)[9] have developed scales that are useful in quantitating the severity of dyspnea.

The sudden development of dyspnea suggests pulmonary embolism, pneumothorax, acute pulmonary edema, pneumonia, or airway obstruction. In contrast, in most forms of chronic heart failure, dyspnea progresses slowly over weeks or months. Such a protracted course may also occur in patients with a variety of unrelated conditions, including obesity, pregnancy, and bilateral pleural effusion. Inspiratory dyspnea suggests obstruction of the upper airways, whereas expiratory dyspnea characterizes obstruction of the lower airways. Exertional dyspnea suggests the presence of organic diseases, such as left ventricular failure (see Chap. 22) or chronic obstructive lung disease (see Chap. 67), whereas dyspnea developing at rest may occur in patients with pneumothorax, pulmonary embolism, pulmonary edema, or anxiety neurosis.

Dyspnea that occurs only at rest and is absent on exertion is almost always functional. A functional origin is also suggested when dyspnea, or simply a heightened awareness of breathing, is accompanied by brief stabbing pain in the region of the cardiac apex or by prolonged (more than 2 hours) dull chest pain. It is often associated with difficulty in getting enough air into the lungs, claustrophobia, and sighing respirations that are relieved by exertion, by taking a few deep breaths, or by sedation. Dyspnea in patients with panic attacks is usually accompanied by hyperventilation. A history of relief of dyspnea by bronchodilators suggests asthma as the cause, whereas relief of dyspnea by rest and diuretics suggests left ventricular failure. Dyspnea accompanied by wheezing may be secondary to left ventricular failure (cardiac asthma) or primary bronchial constriction (bronchial asthma).

In patients with chronic heart failure, dyspnea is a clinical expression of pulmonary venous and capillary hypertension (see Chap. 22). It occurs either during exertion or in resting patients in the recumbent position, in whom it is relieved promptly by sitting upright or standing (orthopnea). Patients with left ventricular failure soon learn to sleep on two or more pillows to avoid this symptom. In patients with heart failure, dyspnea is often accompanied by edema of the lower extremities, upper abdominal pain (due to congestive hepatomegaly), and nocturia.

TABLE 7–1 Disorders Causing Dyspnea and Limiting Exercise Performance, Pathophysiology, and Discriminating Measurements

Disorders	Pathophysiology	Measurements that Deviate from Normal
Pulmonary		
Air flow limitation	Mechanical limitation to ventilation, mismatching of $\dot{V}_A/\dot{Q}$, hypoxic stimulation to breathing	$\dot{V}_E$ max/MVV, expiratory flow pattern, V_D, V_T; $\dot{V}O_2$ max, $\dot{V}_E/\dot{V}O_2$, $\dot{V}_E$ response to hyperoxia, $(A-a)\ PO_2$
Restrictive	Mismatching $\dot{V}_A/\dot{Q}$, hypoxic stimulation to breathing	
Chest wall	Mechanical limitation to ventilation	$\dot{V}_E$ max/MVV, $PACO_2$, $\dot{V}O_2$ max
Pulmonary circulation	Rise in physiological dead space as fraction of V_T, exercise hypoxemia	V_D/V_T, work-rate-related hypoxemia, $\dot{V}O_2$ max, $\dot{V}_E/\dot{V}O_2$, $(a-ET)PCO_2$, O_2-pulse
Cardiac		
Coronary	Coronary insufficiency	ECG, $\dot{V}O_2$ max, anaerobic threshold $\dot{V}O_2$, $\dot{V}_E/\dot{V}O_2$, O_2-pulse, BP (systolic, diastolic, pulse)
Valvular	Cardiac output limitation (decreased effective stroke volume)	
Myocardial	Cardiac output limitation (decreased ejection fraction and stroke volume)	
Anemia	Reduced O_2-carrying capacity	O_2-pulse, anaerobic threshold $\dot{V}O_2$, $\dot{V}O_2$ max, $\dot{V}_E/\dot{V}O_2$
Peripheral circulation	Inadequate O_2 flow to metabolically active muscle	Anaerobic threshold $\dot{V}O_2$, $\dot{V}O_2$ max
Obesity	Increased work to move body; if severe, respiratory restriction and pulmonary insufficiency	$\dot{V}O_2$-work-rate relationship, PAO_2, $PACO_2$, $\dot{V}O_2$ max
Psychogenic	Hyperventilation with precisely regular respiratory rate	Breathing pattern, PCO_2
Malingering	Hyperventilation and hypoventilation with irregular respiratory rate	Breathing pattern, PCO_2
Deconditioning	Inactivity or prolonged bed rest; loss of capability for effective redistribution of systemic blood flow	O_2-pulse, anaerobic threshold $\dot{V}O_2$, $\dot{V}O_2$ max

$\dot{V}_A$ = alveolar ventilation; $\dot{Q}$ = pulmonary blood flow; $\dot{V}_E$ = minute ventilation; MVV = maximum voluntary ventilation; V_D/V_T = physiological dead space/tidal volume ratio; O_2 = oxygen; $\dot{V}O_2 = O_2$ consumption; $(A-a)PO_2$ = alveolar-arterial PO_2 difference; $(a-ET)PCO_2$ = arterial-end tidal PCO_2 difference.
Modified from Wasserman D: Dyspnea on exertion: Is it the heart or the lungs? JAMA 248:2042, 1982, Copyright 1982, the American Medical Association.

TABLE 7–2 American Thoracic Society Scale of Dyspnea

Descriptions	Grade	Degree
Not troubled by shortness of breath when hurrying on the level or walking up a slight hill	0	None
Trouble by shortness of breath when hurrying on the level or walking up a slight hill	1	Mild
Walks more slowly than people of the same age on the level because of breathlessness or has to stop for breath when walking at own pace on the level	2	Moderate
Stops for breath after walking about 100 yards or after a few minutes on the level	3	Severe
Too breathless to leave the house; breathless on dressing or undressing	4	Very severe

From Fishman AP: Approach to the patient with respiratory symptoms. *In* Fishman's Pulmonary Diseases and Disorders. 3rd ed. New York, McGraw-Hill, 1998, pp 361-393.

Paroxysmal nocturnal dyspnea is caused by interstitial pulmonary edema and sometimes intraalveolar edema, most commonly as a consequence of left ventricular failure (see Chap. 22). This condition, usually beginning 2 to 4 hours after the onset of sleep and often accompanied by cough, wheezing, and sweating, may be quite frightening. Paroxysmal nocturnal dyspnea is often ameliorated by the patient's sitting on the side of the bed or getting out of bed; relief is not instantaneous but usually requires 15 to 30 minutes. Although paroxysmal nocturnal dyspnea secondary to left ventricular failure is usually accompanied by coughing, a careful history often discloses that the dyspnea precedes the cough, not vice versa. Nocturnal dyspnea associated with pulmonary disease is usually relieved after the patient rids himself or herself of secretions rather than specifically by sitting up.

Patients with pulmonary embolism usually experience sudden dyspnea that may be associated with apprehension, palpitation, hemoptysis, or pleuritic chest pain (see Chap. 66). The development or intensification of dyspnea, sometimes associated with a feeling of faintness, may be the only symptom of the patient with pulmonary emboli. Pneumothorax and mediastinal emphysema also cause acute dyspnea, accompanied by sharp chest pain. Dyspnea is a common "anginal equivalent" (see Chap. 50), that is, a symptom secondary to myocardial ischemia that occurs in place of typical anginal discomfort. This form of dyspnea may or may not be associated with a sensation of tightness in the chest, is present on exertion or emotional stress, is relieved by rest (more often in the sitting than in the recumbent position), is similar to angina in duration (i.e., 2 to 10 minutes), and is usually responsive to or prevented by nitroglycerin.

APPROACH TO THE PATIENT. The approach to the patient is shown in Figure 7–1. Measurement of Brain Natriuretic Peptide (BNP) has been shown to be a valuable laboratory test in the evaluation of dyspnea, especially in patients presenting to the Emergency Department[11] (see Chaps. 21 and 22).

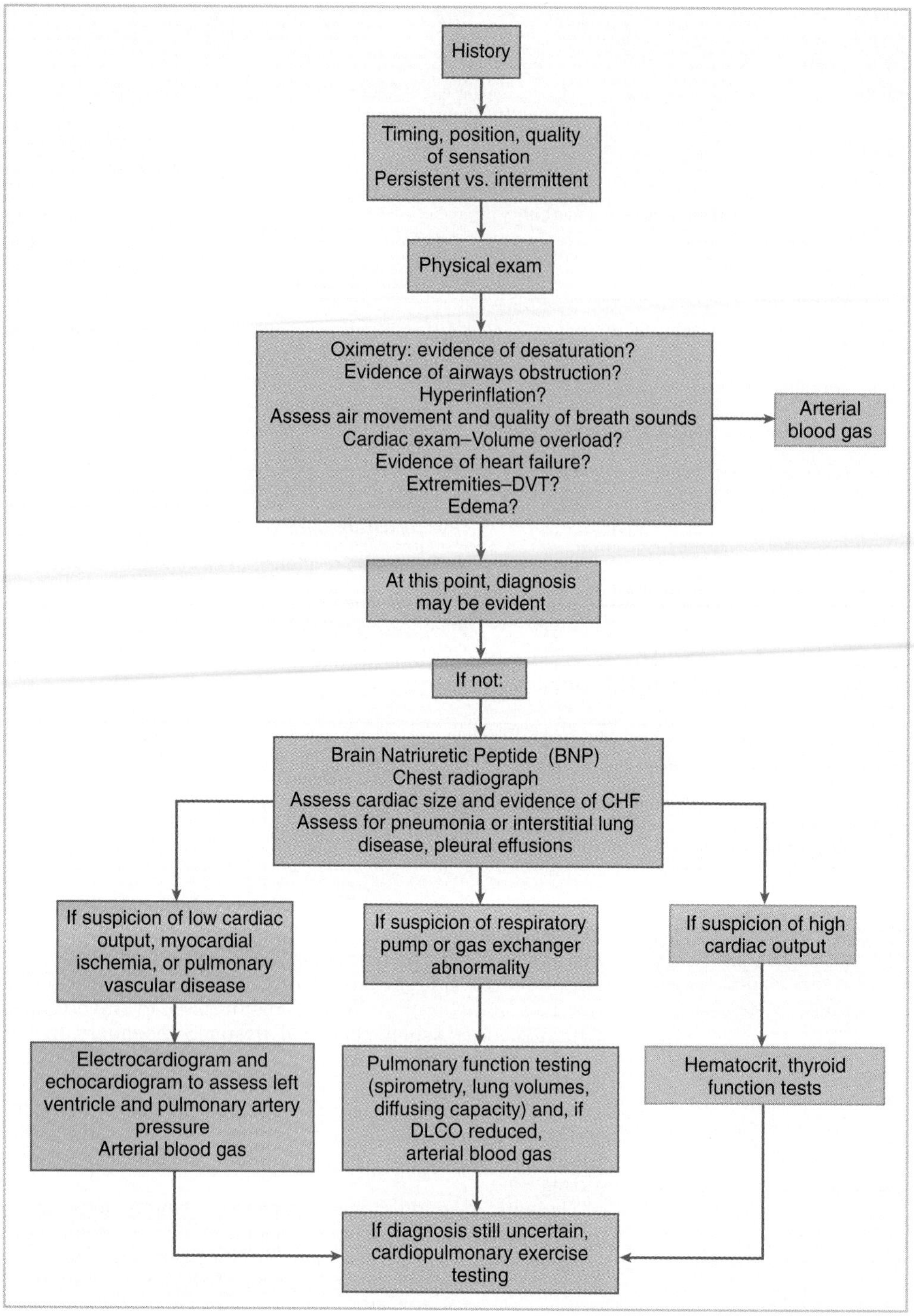
History
Timing, position, quality of sensation
Persistent vs. intermittent
Physical exam
Oximetry: evidence of desaturation?
Evidence of airways obstruction?
Hyperinflation?
Assess air movement and quality of breath sounds
Cardiac exam–Volume overload?
Evidence of heart failure?
Extremities–DVT?
Edema?
Arterial blood gas
At this point, diagnosis may be evident
If not:
Brain Natriuretic Peptide (BNP)
Chest radiograph
Assess cardiac size and evidence of CHF
Assess for pneumonia or interstitial lung disease, pleural effusions
If suspicion of low cardiac output, myocardial ischemia, or pulmonary vascular disease
If suspicion of respiratory pump or gas exchanger abnormality
If suspicion of high cardiac output
Electrocardiogram and echocardiogram to assess left ventricle and pulmonary artery pressure
Arterial blood gas
Pulmonary function testing (spirometry, lung volumes, diffusing capacity) and, if DLCO reduced, arterial blood gas
Hematocrit, thyroid function tests
If diagnosis still uncertain, cardiopulmonary exercise testing

FIGURE 7–1. Algorithm for the evaluation of the patient with dyspnea. The pace and completeness with which one approaches this framework depend on the intensity and acuity of the patient's symptoms. In the patient with severe, acute dyspnea, for example, an arterial blood gas measurement may be one of the first laboratory evaluations, whereas it might not be obtained until much later in the work-up in a patient with chronic breathlessness of unclear cause. A therapeutic trial of a medication, for example, a bronchodilator, may be instituted at any point if one is fairly confident of the diagnosis based on the data available at that time. DVT = deep venous thrombosis; CHF = congestive heart failure; DLCO = diffusing capacity of the lung for carbon monoxide. (From Schwartzstein RM, Feller-Kopman, D.: Approach to the patient with dyspnea. *In* Braunwald E, Goldman L [eds]: Primary Cardiology. 2nd ed. Philadelphia, WB Saunders, 2003, pp 101-116.)

Chest Pain or Discomfort

(see Chaps. 45, 46, and 49)

Although chest pain or discomfort is one of the cardinal manifestations of heart disease, such pain may originate not only in the heart but also (1) in a variety of noncardiac intrathoracic structures, such as the aorta, pulmonary artery, bronchopulmonary tree, pleura, mediastinum, esophagus, and diaphragm; (2) in the tissues of the neck or thoracic wall, including the skin, thoracic muscles, cervicodorsal spine, costochondral junctions, breasts, sensory nerves, and spinal cord; and (3) in subdiaphragmatic organs such as the stomach, duodenum, pancreas, and gallbladder (Table 7–3). Pain of functional origin or factitious pain may also occur in the chest.

In obtaining the history of a patient with chest pain, it is helpful to have a mental checklist and to ask the patient to describe the location, radiation, and character of the discomfort; what causes and relieves it, especially the extent and timing of relief by sublingual nitroglycerin; the duration, frequency, and pattern of recurrence of the discomfort; the setting in which it occurs; and associated symptoms. It is also particularly useful to observe the patient's gestures. The patient's clenching of the fist in front of the sternum while describing the sensation (Levine sign) is a strong indication of an ischemic origin of the pain.

QUALITY OF DISCOMFORT. Angina pectoris may be defined as a discomfort in the chest and/or adjacent area associated with myocardial ischemia but without myocardial necrosis.[12-15] *Angina* means tightening, not pain. Thus, the discomfort of angina often is described not as pain at all but rather as an unpleasant sensation; "pressing," "squeezing," "strangling," "constricting," "bursting," and "burning" are some of the adjectives commonly used to describe this sensation. "A band across the chest," "a weight in the center of the chest," and "a vise tightening around the chest" are other frequent descriptors.

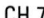

It is characteristic of angina pectoris that the intensity of effort required to incite it may vary from day to day and throughout the day in the same patient, but often a careful history will uncover explanations for this, such as meals ingested, weather, emotions, and the like. The anginal threshold is lower in the morning than at other times of the day. When the threshold for angina is quite variable, defies any pattern, and is prominent at rest, the possibility that myocardial ischemia is caused by coronary

TABLE 7–3 Cardiovascular Causes of Chest Pain

Condition	Location	Quality	Duration	Aggravating or Relieving Factors	Associated Symptoms or Signs
Angina	Retrosternal region: radiates to or occasionally isolated to neck, jaw, epigastrium, shoulder, or arms—left common	Pressure, burning, squeezing, heaviness, indigestion	<2-10 min	Precipitated by exercise, cold weather, or emotional stress; relieved by rest or nitroglycerin; atypical (Prinzmetal) angina may be unrelated to activity, often early morning	S_4, or murmur of papillary muscle dysfunction during pain
Rest or unstable angina	Same as angina	Same as angina but may be more severe	Usually <20 min	Same as angina, with decreasing tolerance for exertion or at rest	Similar to stable angina, but can be pronounced. Transient cardiac failure can occur
Myocardial infarction	Substernal and can radiate like angina	Heaviness, pressure, burning, constriction	Sudden onset, 30 min or longer, but variable	Unrelieved by rest or nitroglycerin	Shortness of breath, sweating, weakness, nausea, vomiting
Pericarditis	Usually begins over sternum or toward cardiac apex and can radiate to neck or left shoulder; often more localized than the pain of myocardial ischemia	Sharp, stabbing, knifelike	Lasts many hours to days; may wax and wane	Aggravated by deep breathing, rotating chest, or supine position; relieved by sitting up and leaning forward	Pericardial friction rub
Aortic dissection	Anterior chest; can radiate to back	Excruciating, tearing, knifelike	Sudden onset, unrelenting	Usually occurs in setting of hypertension or predisposition such as Marfan syndrome	Murmur of aortic insufficiency, pulse or blood pressure asymmetry; neurological deficit
Pulmonary embolism (chest pain often not present)	Substernal or over region of pulmonary infarction	Pleuritic (with pulmonary infarction) or angina-like	Sudden onset; minutes to <1 hr	Can be aggravated by breathing	Dyspnea, tachypnea, tachycardia; hypotension, signs of acute right-sided heart failure, and pulmonary hypertension with large emboli; rales, pleural rub, hemoptysis with pulmonary infarction
Pulmonary hypertension	Substernal	Pressure; oppressive		Aggravated by effort	Pain usually associated with dyspnea; signs of pulmonary hypertension

From Andreoli TE, Bennett JC, Carpenter CCJ, Plum F: Evaluation of the patient with cardiovascular disease. *In* Cecil Essentials of Medicine, 4th ed. Philadelphia, WB Saunders, 1997, p 11.

spasm should be considered.[15] A history of prolonged, severe anginal chest discomfort accompanied by profound fatigue often signifies acute myocardial infarction. Thus, a careful history not only may indicate the cause of the pain (i.e., myocardial ischemia) but also can provide a clue to the mechanism.

When dyspnea is an "anginal equivalent," the patient may describe the mid-chest as the site of the shortness of breath, whereas true dyspnea is usually not well localized. Other anginal equivalents are discomfort limited to areas that are ordinarily sites of secondary radiation, such as the ulnar aspect of the left arm, lower jaw, teeth, neck, or shoulders, and the development of gas and belching, nausea, "indigestion," dizziness, and diaphoresis. When angina radiates to the arms, it is often described as a "painful heaviness." Anginal equivalents above the mandible or below the umbilicus are quite uncommon.

LOCATION. Embryologically, the heart is a midline viscus; thus, cardiac ischemia produces symptoms that are characteristically felt substernally or across both sides of the chest (Fig. 7–2). Some patients complain of discomfort only to the left or less commonly only to the right of the midline. If the pain or discomfort can be localized to the skin or superficial structures and can be reproduced by localized pressure, it usually arises from the chest wall and is not caused by myocardial ischemia. If the patient can point directly to

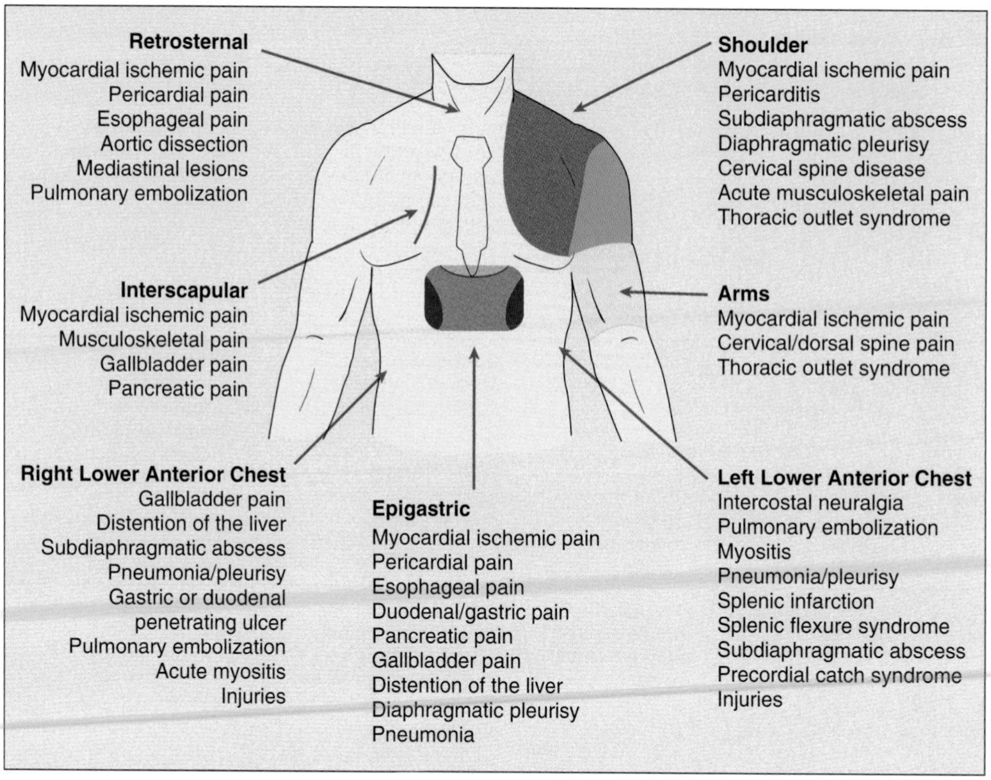

FIGURE 7–2. Differential diagnosis of chest pain according to location where pain starts. Serious intrathoracic or subdiaphragmatic diseases are usually associated with pains that begin in the left anterior chest, left shoulder, or upper arm, the interscapular region, or the epigastrium. The scheme is not all inclusive (e.g., intercostal neuralgia occurs in locations other than the left, lower anterior chest area). (From Miller AJ: Diagnosis of Chest Pain. New York, Raven Press, 1988, p 175.)

the site of discomfort with the tip of a finger, and if that site is quite small (<3 cm in diameter), it is usually not angina pectoris.

Pain that is localized to the region of or under the left nipple or that radiates to the right lower chest is usually noncardiac in origin and may be functional or due to costochondritis, gaseous distention of the stomach, or the splenic flexure syndrome.[16] Like other symptoms arising in deeper structures, angina tends to be diffuse and eludes precise localization. Although pain due to myocardial ischemia often radiates to the arm, especially the ulnar aspect of the left arm, wrist, epigastrium, or left shoulder, such radiation may also occur in patients with pericarditis and disorders of the cervical spine. Radiation of pain from the chest to the neck and jaws is typical of myocardial infarction.

DURATION. The duration of the pain is important in determining its origin. Angina pectoris is relatively brief, usually lasting from 2 to 10 minutes. However, if the pain is very brief (i.e., a momentary, lancinating, sharp pain, or other discomfort that lasts less than 15 seconds), angina can usually be excluded; such a short duration points instead to musculoskeletal pain, pain due to a hiatal hernia, or functional pain. Chest pain that is otherwise typical of angina but that lasts for more than 10 minutes or occurs at rest is typical of unstable angina.[12] Chest pain lasting for hours can be seen with acute myocardial infarction, pericarditis, aortic dissection, musculoskeletal disease, herpes zoster, anxiety, and cocaine abuse.[13]

PRECIPITATING AND AGGRAVATING FACTORS. Angina pectoris occurs characteristically on exertion, particularly when the patient is hurrying or walking up an incline. Thus, the development of chest discomfort or pain during walking, typically in the cold and up an incline or against a wind, especially after a heavy meal, is typical of angina pectoris. Angina may also be precipitated by strong emotion or fright, by a nightmare, by working with the arms over the head, by hurrying, by cold exposure, or by smoking a cigarette. Prinzmetal (variant) angina characteristically occurs at rest and may or may not be affected by exertion[15]; however, classic angina, although most often precipitated by effort, may progress to unstable angina, which is characterized by ischemic discomfort at rest (see Chap. 49).

DIFFERENTIAL DIAGNOSIS. Chest pain that occurs after protracted vomiting can be due to the Mallory-Weiss syndrome (i.e., a tear in the lower portion of the esophagus). Pain that occurs while the patient is bending over is often radicular and can be associated with osteoarthritis of the cervical or upper thoracic spine. Chest pain occurring on moving the neck can be due to a herniated intervertebral disc.

ESOPHAGEAL AND OTHER GASTROINTESTINAL PAIN

Substernal and epigastric discomfort after swallowing can be caused by esophageal spasm or esophagitis, often with acid reflux, with or without a hiatal hernia.[17-19] These conditions can also be associated with substernal or epigastric burning pain that is brought on by eating or by lying down after meals and that can be relieved by antacids. Pain due to esophageal spasm has many of the features of and may be difficult to differentiate from angina pectoris. A history of acid reflux into the mouth (water brash) and/or dysphagia can be a useful diagnostic clue pointing to esophageal disease. The chest discomfort secondary to esophageal reflux is most common after meals, occurs in the supine position or on bending, and can be relieved by nitroglycerin.

The discomfort produced by peptic ulcer disease is characteristically located in the mid-epigastrium. It can also resemble angina pectoris, but its characteristic relationship to food ingestion and its relief by antacids are important differentiating features. The pain of acute pancreatitis, like that of acute myocardial infarction, may be predominantly in the epigastrium. However, unlike the pain of myocardial infarction, pancreatic pain is usually transmitted to the back, is position sensitive, and can be relieved in part by leaning forward.[16]

OTHER CAUSES

The chest discomfort of unstable angina[12] and acute myocardial infarction (see Chaps. 46 and 49) is similar in quality, location, and character to that of chronic stable angina pectoris; however, it usually radiates more widely than does chronic stable angina, is more severe, and therefore is generally referred to by the patient as true pain rather than discomfort. The development of pain in patients with these conditions is usually unrelated to unusual effort or emotional stress, often with the patient at rest or even sleeping. Characteristically, nitroglycerin does not provide complete or lasting relief. The chest discomfort of pulmonary hypertension (see Chap. 67) may be identical to that of typical angina[20]; it is caused by right ventricular ischemia or dilation of the pulmonary arteries.

Acute pericarditis (see Chap. 64) is frequently preceded by a history of a viral upper respiratory infection. The inflammation causes pain that is sharper than anginal discomfort, is more left sided than central, and is often referred to the neck, upper shoulders, and back. The pain of pericarditis lasts for hours and is little affected by effort but is often aggravated by breathing, turning in bed, swallowing, or twisting the body; unlike the discomfort produced by ischemia, the pain of acute pericarditis may lessen when the patient sits up and leans forward.

Aortic dissection (see Chap. 53) is suggested by the sudden development of persistent, very severe pain with radiation to the back and into the lumbar region, often in a patient with a history of hypertension. An expanding thoracic aortic aneurysm may erode the vertebral bodies and cause localized, severe, boring pain that may be worse at night.

Chest-wall pain due to costochondritis or myositis is common in patients who present with fear of heart disease.[21] It is associated with local costochondral and muscle tenderness, which can be aggravated by moving or coughing. Chest-wall pain can also accompany chest injury. In patients with the Tietze syndrome, the discomfort is localized to swollen costochondral and costosternal joints, which are painful on palpation. When herpes zoster affects the left chest, it can mimic myocardial infarction. However, its persistence, its localization to a dermatome, the extreme sensitivity of the skin to touch, and the appearance of the characteristic vesicles allow recognition of this condition. The preeruptive stage of herpes zoster can mimic myocardial ischemia as a tight localized band across the chest.

The pain of pulmonary embolism (see Chap. 66) usually commences suddenly and in patients who are at rest, and it is accompanied by shortness of breath. It is typically described as tightness in the chest and is accompanied or followed by pleuritic chest pain (i.e., sharp pain in the side of the chest that is intensified by respiration or cough). Functional or psychogenic chest pain (see Chap. 84) can be one feature of an anxiety state called *Da Costa syndrome* or *neurocirculatory asthenia*.[22-24] It differs from angina pectoris in that it is usually localized to the cardiac apex and consists of a dull, persistent ache that lasts for hours and is often accentuated by or alternates with attacks of sharp, lancinating stabs of inframammary pain of 1 or 2 seconds' duration. The condition may occur with emotional strain and fatigue, bears little relation to exertion, and may be accompanied by precordial tenderness. Attacks can be associated with palpitation, hyperventilation, numbness and tingling in the extremities, sighing, dizziness, dyspnea, generalized weakness, faintness, severe fatigability, and a history of panic attacks and other signs of emotional instability or depression. The pain may not be completely relieved by any medication other than analgesics, but it is often attenuated by many types of interventions, including rest, exertion, tranquilizers, and placebos. Patients with Da Costa syndrome usually are young (<40 years), are female, and have high scores on depression and anxiety scales.[24]

RELIEF OF PAIN

Rest and sublingual nitroglycerin characteristically relieve the discomfort of chronic stable angina in 1 to 5 minutes. If more than 10 minutes transpire before relief, the diagnosis of chronic stable angina becomes questionable and instead unstable angina, acute myocardial infarction, or pain not caused by myocardial ischemia at all is the cause. Although nitroglycerin commonly relieves the pain of angina pectoris, response to this drug is nonspecific, since the discomfort caused by esophageal spasm and esophagitis can also be relieved. Angina pectoris is alleviated by quiet standing or sitting; sometimes resting in the recumbent position does not relieve angina. Chest pain secondary to acute pericarditis is characteristically relieved by leaning forward, whereas pain that is relieved by food or antacids may be due to peptic ulcer disease or esophagitis. Pain that is alleviated by holding the breath in deep expiration is commonly due to pleuritic inflammation. Some patients with upper gastrointestinal disease or anxiety report relief of symptoms after belching.

CHEST PAIN IN WOMEN (see Chap. 73). Chest discomfort that is atypical for angina pectoris is more common in women than in men, perhaps because of the higher prevalence of vasospastic and of microvascular angina and nonischemic causes of chest pain in women.[25-27] Women with epicardial coronary artery disease more often report chest discomfort at rest, during sleep, or during mental stress than do men.

ACCOMPANYING SYMPTOMS. The physician should always be concerned about the patient with the combination of severe chest discomfort and profuse sweating. This combination frequently signals a serious disorder, such as acute myocardial infarction but also acute pulmonary embolism or aortic dissection. Severe chest pain accompanied by nausea and vomiting is also often due to myocardial infarction. The latter diagnosis, as well as pneumothorax, pulmonary embolism, or mediastinal emphysema, is suggested by pain associated with shortness of breath. Chest pain accompanied by palpitation may be due to the acute myocardial ischemia precipitated by a tachyarrhythmia-induced increase in myocardial oxygen consumption in the presence of coronary artery disease. Chest pain accompanied by hemoptysis suggests pulmonary embolism with infarction or lung tumor, whereas pain accompanied by fever occurs in patients with pneumonia, pleurisy, and pericarditis. Functional pain is commonly accompanied by frequent sighing, anxiety, or depression.

APPROACH TO THE PATIENT (see Chap. 45). This is summarized in the algorithm shown in Figure 7-3 (see also Fig. 45-3). After administration of emergency treatment, if necessary, a focused history and physical examination should allow determination of a cardiac or possible cardiac cause. The 12-lead electrocardiogram and cardiac markers of necrosis (CK-MB and troponin) are then helpful in guiding therapy.[28,29]

Cyanosis

Cyanosis, both a symptom and a physical sign, is a bluish discoloration of the skin and mucous membranes resulting from an increased quantity of reduced hemoglobin or of abnormal hemoglobin pigments in the blood perfusing these areas.[30,31] It may go unnoticed by the patient and is more commonly described by a family member. There are two principal forms of cyanosis: (1) central cyanosis, characterized by decreased arterial oxygen saturation due to right-to-left shunting of blood or impaired pulmonary function, and (2) peripheral cyanosis, most commonly secondary to cutaneous vasoconstriction due to low cardiac output or exposure to cold air or water; if peripheral cyanosis is confined to a single extremity, localized arterial or venous obstruction should be suspected. A history of cyanosis localized to the hands suggests Raynaud's phenomenon. Patients with central cyanosis due to congenital heart disease or pulmonary disease characteristically report that it worsens during exertion, whereas the resting peripheral cyanosis of congestive heart failure may be accentuated only slightly, if at all, during exertion.

Central cyanosis usually becomes apparent at a mean capillary concentration of 4 gm/dl reduced hemoglobin (or 0.5 gm/dl methemoglobin). In general, a history of cyanosis in light-skinned people is rarely elicited unless arterial saturation is 85 percent or less; in people with darker skin, arterial saturation has to drop far lower before cyanosis is perceptible.

Although a history of cyanosis beginning in infancy suggests a congenital cardiac malformation with a right-to-left shunt, hereditary methemoglobinemia is another, albeit rare, cause of congenital cyanosis; the diagnosis of this condition is supported by a family history of cyanosis in the absence of heart disease.

A history of cyanosis limited to the neonatal period suggests the diagnosis of atrial septal defect with transient right-to-left shunting or, more commonly, pulmonary parenchymal disease or central nervous system depression. Cyanosis beginning at the age of 1 to 3 months may be reported when spontaneous closure of a patent ductus arteriosus causes a reduction of pulmonary blood flow in the presence of right-sided obstructive cardiac anomalies, most commonly tetralogy of Fallot. If cyanosis appears at the age of 6 months or later in childhood, it may be due to the development or progression of obstruction to right ventricular outflow in patients with ventricular septal defect. A history of the development of cyanosis in a patient with congenital heart disease between 5 and 20 years of age suggests Eisenmenger syndrome with right-to-left shunting as a consequence of a progressive increase in pulmonary vascular resistance (see Chap. 56). Cyanosis secondary to a pulmonary arteriovenous fistula also usually appears first in childhood.

Syncope (see Chap. 34)

Loss of consciousness results most commonly from reduced perfusion of the brain. The history is extremely valuable in

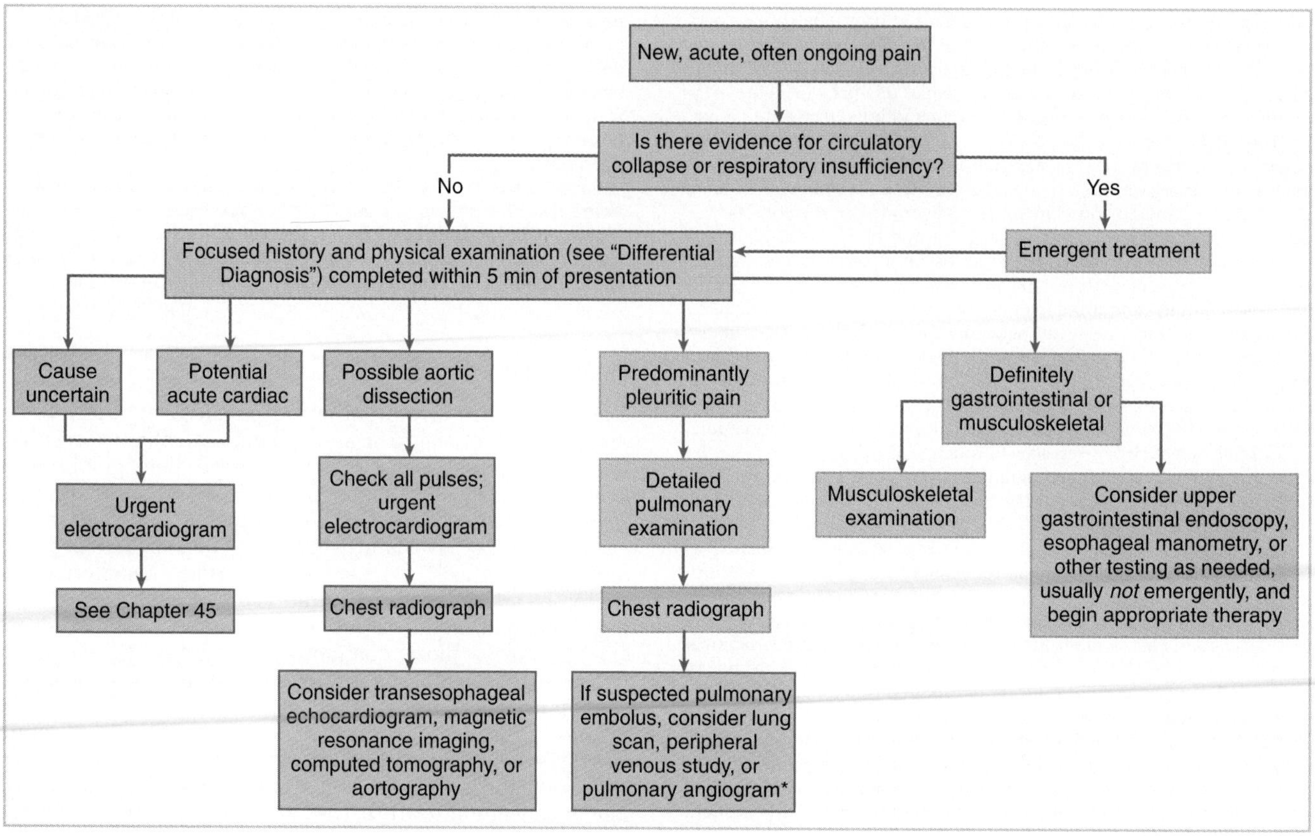
New, acute, often ongoing pain
Is there evidence for circulatory collapse or respiratory insufficiency?
No
Yes
Emergent treatment
Focused history and physical examination (see "Differential Diagnosis") completed within 5 min of presentation
Cause uncertain
Potential acute cardiac
Possible aortic dissection
Predominantly pleuritic pain
Definitely gastrointestinal or musculoskeletal
Urgent electrocardiogram
See Chapter 45
Check all pulses; urgent electrocardiogram
Chest radiograph
Consider transesophageal echocardiogram, magnetic resonance imaging, computed tomography, or aortography
Detailed pulmonary examination
Chest radiograph
If suspected pulmonary embolus, consider lung scan, peripheral venous study, or pulmonary angiogram*
Musculoskeletal examination
Consider upper gastrointestinal endoscopy, esophageal manometry, or other testing as needed, usually *not* emergently, and begin appropriate therapy

FIGURE 7–3. Diagnostic approach to the patient with new, acute, often ongoing chest pain. *Spiral computed tomographic scan should also be considered. (From Goldman L: Approach to the patient with chest pain. *In* Braunwald E, Goldman L [eds]: Primary Cardiology. 2nd ed. Philadelphia, WB Saunders, 2003, pp 83-100, Adapted from Goldman L: Chest discomfort and palpitation. *In* Fauci A, Braunwald E, et al [eds]: Harrison's Principles of Internal Medicine. 14th ed. New York, McGraw-Hill, 1998, p 61.)

the differential diagnosis of syncope. Several daily attacks of loss of consciousness suggest (1) Stokes-Adams attacks (i.e., transient asystole or ventricular fibrillation in the presence of atrioventricular block); (2) other cardiac arrhythmias; or (3) a seizure disorder (i.e., petit mal epilepsy). These diagnoses are suggested when the loss of consciousness is abrupt and occurs over 1 or 2 seconds; a more gradual onset suggests vasodepressor syncope (i.e., the common faint) or syncope due to hyperventilation or, much less commonly, hypoglycemia.

CARDIAC SYNCOPE. This condition is usually of rapid onset without aura and is usually not associated with convulsive movements, urinary incontinence, or a postictal confusional state. Syncope in aortic stenosis[32-34] is usually precipitated by effort. Patients with syncope secondary to a convulsive disorder often have a prodromal aura preceding the seizure. Injury from falling is common, as are urinary incontinence and a postictal confusional state, associated with headache and drowsiness. Unconsciousness developing gradually and lasting for a few seconds suggests vasodepressor (neurocardiogenic) syncope or syncope secondary to postural hypotension[35,36] (see Chap. 87), whereas a longer period of unconsciousness suggests aortic stenosis or hyperventilation. Hysterical fainting is usually not accompanied by any untoward display of anxiety or change in pulse, blood pressure, or skin color, and there may be a question whether any true loss of consciousness occurred. It is often associated with paresthesias of the hands or face, hyperventilation, dyspnea, chest pain, and feelings of acute anxiety.

REGAINING CONSCIOUSNESS. Consciousness is usually regained quite promptly in patients with syncope of cardiovascular origin but more slowly in patients with convulsive disorders. When consciousness is regained after vasodepressor syncope, the patient is often pale and diaphoretic with a slow heart rate, whereas after a Stokes-Adams attack, the patient's face is often flushed and there may be cardiac acceleration.

DIFFERENTIAL DIAGNOSIS. A family history of syncope or near-syncope can often be elicited in patients with hypertrophic cardiomyopathy (see Chap. 59) or ventricular tachyarrhythmias associated with QT prolongation (see Chap. 29). A history of syncope during childhood suggests the possibility of obstruction to left ventricular outflow—valvular, supravalvular, or subvalvular aortic stenosis. In patients with hypertrophic cardiomyopathy, syncope may be posttussive and occurs characteristically in the erect position, when arising suddenly, after standing erect for long periods, and during or immediately after cessation of exertion. Patients with syncope secondary to orthostatic hypotension may have a history of drug therapy for hypertension or of abnormalities of autonomic function, such as impotence, disturbances of sphincter function, peripheral neuropathy, and anhidrosis.[36]

Calkins and coworkers demonstrated the value of the clinical history in differentiating between serious arrhythmias (ventricular tachycardia or atrioventricular block) and neurocardiogenic syncope. Features predictive of the former were male gender, age older than 54 years, two or fewer episodes of syncope, and duration of warning of 5 seconds or less. On the other hand, features of syncope due to neurocardiogenic syncope included palpitations, blurred vision, nausea, diaphoresis, or lightheadedness before syncope, and nausea, warmth, diaphoresis, or fatigue after syncope.[37]

Palpitation (see Chap. 29)

Palpitation is a common symptom defined as an unpleasant awareness of the forceful or rapid beating of the heart. Patients describe it as pounding, jumping, racing, or irregularity of the heart beat, a "flip flopping" or "rapid fluttering" in the chest, or pounding in the neck.[38-40] It can be brought about by a variety of disorders involving changes in cardiac rhythm or rate, including all forms of tachycardia, ectopic beats, compensatory pauses, augmented stroke volume due to valvular regurgitation, hyperkinetic (high cardiac output) states, and the sudden onset of bradycardia. In the case of premature contractions, the patient is more commonly aware of the post-extrasystolic beat than of the premature beat itself.

DIFFERENTIAL DIAGNOSIS. Palpitation characterized by a slow heart rate may be due to atrioventricular block or sinus node disease. When palpitation begins and ends abruptly, it is often due to a paroxysmal arrhythmia such as paroxysmal atrial or junctional tachycardia, atrial flutter, or atrial fibrillation, whereas a gradual onset and cessation of the attack suggest sinus tachycardia and/or an anxiety state. A history of chaotic, rapid heart action suggests the diagnosis of atrial fibrillation; fleeting and repetitive palpitation suggests multiple ectopic beats. A history of dizziness, presyncope, or syncope with palpitations may be due to ventricular tachycardia and may be an ominous prognostic sign.

Some patients have taken their pulse during palpitation or have asked a companion to do so. A regular rate between 100 and 140 beats per minute suggests sinus tachycardia, a regular rate of approximately 150 beats per minute suggests atrial flutter, and a regular rate exceeding 160 beats per minute suggests paroxysmal supraventricular tachycardia.

A history of palpitation during strenuous physical activity is normal, whereas palpitation during mild exertion suggests either that the individual is severely deconditioned or the presence of heart failure, atrial fibrillation, anemia, or thyrotoxicosis. When palpitation can be relieved suddenly by stooping, breath-holding, or induced gagging or vomiting (i.e., by vagal maneuvers), the diagnosis of paroxysmal supraventricular tachycardia is suggested. Palpitation followed by angina suggests that myocardial ischemia has been precipitated by increased oxygen demands induced by the rapid heart rate. Palpitations are frequently accompanied by, and are often caused by, anxiety, panic reactions, or emotionally startling experiences.[40]

A directed history is useful in elucidating the cause of palpitation (Table 7–4). Is there a history of cocaine or amphetamine abuse? Thyrotoxicosis? Anemia? Do the palpitations occur after heavy cigarette smoking or caffeine ingestion? Is there a family history of syncope, arrhythmia, or sudden death?

DIAGNOSTIC APPROACH TO THE PATIENT. The diagnostic approach is shown in Figure 7–4. The key decision points are the determination of whether structural heart disease is present and whether the patient complains of severe symptoms, including syncope and presyncope.

Edema

LOCALIZATION. Localization is helpful in elucidating the cause of edema.[41,42] Unilateral leg edema is most commonly due to deep venous thrombosis or cellulitis. A history of edema of the legs that is most pronounced in the evening is characteristic of heart failure or bilateral chronic venous insufficiency. Inability to fit the feet into shoes is a common early symptom. In most patients, any visible edema of both lower extremities is preceded by a weight gain of at least 3 to 5 kg. Cardiac edema is generally symmetrical. As it progresses, it usually ascends to involve the legs, thighs, genitalia, and abdominal wall. In patients with heart failure who are largely confined to bed, the edematous fluid localizes in the sacral area. Edema may be generalized (anasarca) in patients with the nephrotic syndrome, severe heart failure, and hepatic cirrhosis. These three conditions can be distinguished by consideration of the history, physical examination, and simple laboratory tests (Table 7–5).

A history of edema around the eyes and face is characteristic of the nephrotic syndrome, acute glomerulonephritis, angioneurotic edema, hypoproteinemia, and myxedema. A history of edema limited to the face, neck, and upper arms may be associated with obstruction of the superior vena cava, most commonly by carcinoma of the lung, lymphoma, or aneurysm of the aortic arch. A history of edema restricted to one extremity is usually due to venous thrombosis or lymphatic blockage of that extremity.

ACCOMPANYING SYMPTOMS. A history of dyspnea associated with edema is most frequently due to heart failure, but it may also be observed in patients with large bilateral pleural effusions, elevation of the diaphragm due to ascites, angioneurotic edema with laryngeal involvement, and pulmonary embolism. When dyspnea precedes edema, the underlying disorder is usually left ventricular dysfunction, mitral stenosis, or chronic lung disease with cor pulmonale. A history of jaundice suggests that edema may be of hepatic origin, whereas edema associated with a history of ulceration and pigmentation of the skin of the legs is most commonly due to chronic venous insufficiency or postphlebitic syndrome. When cardiac edema is not associated with

TABLE 7–4 Items to be Covered in History of Patient with Palpitation

Does the Palpitation Occur:	If So, Suspect:
As isolated "jumps" or "skips"?	Extrasystoles
In attacks known to be of abrupt beginning, with a heart rate of 120 beats/min or over, with regular or irregular rhythm?	Paroxysmal rapid heart action
Independent of exercise or excitement adequate to account for the symptom?	Atrial fibrillation, atrial flutter, thyrotoxicosis, anemia, febrile states, hypoglycemia, anxiety state
In attacks developing rapidly though not absolutely abruptly, unrelated to exertion or excitement?	Hemorrhage, hypoglycemia, tumor of the adrenal medulla
In conjunction with the taking of drugs?	Tobacco, coffee, tea, alcohol, epinephrine, ephedrine, aminophylline, atropine, thyroid extract, monoamine oxidase inhibitors
On standing?	Postural hypotension
In middle-aged women, in conjunction with flushes and sweats?	Menopausal syndrome
When the rate is known to be normal and the rhythm regular?	Anxiety state

From Goldman L, Braunwald E: Chest discomfort and palpitation. *In* Isselbacher KJ, Braunwald E, et al (eds). Harrison's Principles of Internal Medicine, 13th ed. New York, McGraw-Hill, 1994.

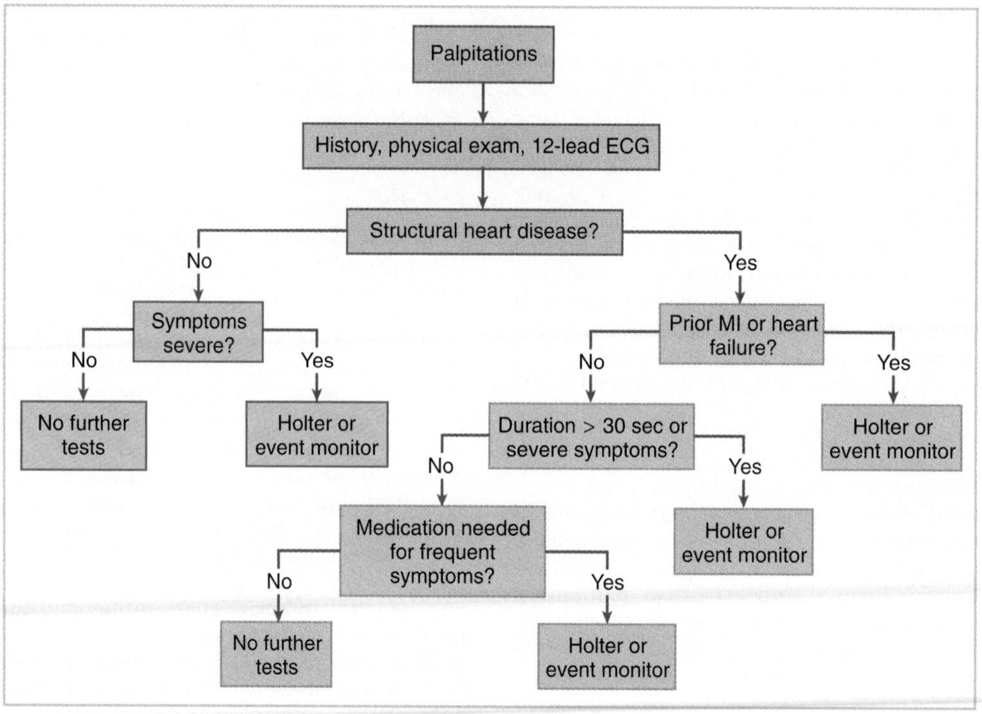

FIGURE 7–4. Diagnostic approach to the patient with palpitations. (From Hlatky MA: Approach to the patient with palpitations. *In* Braunwald E, Goldman L [eds]: Primary Cardiology, 2nd ed. Philadelphia, WB Saunders, 2003, pp 129-136.)

TABLE 7–5 Principal Causes of Generalized Edema: History, Physical Examination, and Laboratory Findings

Organ System	History	Physical Examination	Laboratory Findings
Cardiac	Dyspnea with exertion prominent—often associated with orthopnea—or paroxysmal nocturnal dyspnea	Elevated jugular venous pressure, ventricular (S_3) gallop; occasionally with displaced or dyskinetic apical pulse; peripheral cyanosis, cool extremities, small pulse pressure when severe	Elevated urea nitrogen-to-creatinine ratio common; elevated uric acid; serum sodium often diminished; liver enzymes occasionally elevated with hepatic congestion
Hepatic	Dyspnea infrequent, except if associated with a significant degree of ascites; most often a history of ethanol abuse	Frequently associated with ascites; jugular venous pressure usually normal or low; blood pressure typically lower than in patients with renal or cardiac disease; one or more additional signs of chronic liver disease (jaundice, palmar erythema, Dupuytren contracture, spider angiomas, male gynecomastia or testicular atrophy, caput medusae); asterixis and other signs of encephalopathy may be present	If severe, reductions in serum albumin, cholesterol, other hepatic proteins (transferrin, fibrinogen); liver enzymes may or may not be elevated, depending on the cause and acuity of the liver injury; tendency toward hypokalemia, respiratory alkalosis; magnesium and phosphorus levels often markedly reduced if associated with ongoing ethanol intake; uric acid typically low; macrocytosis from folate deficiency
Renal	Usually chronic; associated with uremic signs and symptoms, including decreased appetite, altered (metallic or fishy) taste, altered sleep pattern, difficulty concentrating, restless legs or myoclonus; dyspnea can be present, but is generally less prominent than in patients with heart failure	Blood pressure often high; hypertensive or diabetic retinopathy in selected cases; nitrogenous fetor; periorbital edema may predominate; pericardial friction rub in advanced cases with uremia	Elevation of serum creatinine and urea nitrogen most prominent; also frequent hyperkalemia, metabolic acidosis, hyperphosphatemia, hypocalcemia, anemia (usually normocytic)

S_3, third heart sound.

From Chertow GM: Approach to the patient with edema. *In* Braunwald E, Goldman L (eds): Primary Cardiology. 2nd ed. Philadelphia, WB Saunders, 2003, pp 117-127.

orthopnea, it may be due to interference with filling of the right side of the heart, such as tricuspid valve disease or constrictive pericarditis. A history of leg edema after prolonged sitting (particularly in the elderly) may be due to simple venous stasis and not be associated with disease at all.

COUGH

Cough, one of the most frequent of all cardiorespiratory symptoms, may be defined as an explosive expiration that provides a means of clearing the tracheobronchial tree of secretions and foreign bodies.[43,44] It can be caused by a variety of infectious, neoplastic, or allergic disorders of the lungs and tracheobronchial tree. Cardiovascular disorders most frequently responsible for cough include those that lead to pulmonary venous hypertension, interstitial and alveolar pulmonary edema, pulmonary infarction, and compression of the tracheobronchial tree (aortic aneurysm).

Cough due to pulmonary venous hypertension secondary to left ventricular failure or mitral stenosis tends to be dry, irritating, spasmodic, and nocturnal. When cough accompanies exertional dyspnea, it suggests either chronic obstructive lung disease or heart failure, whereas in a patient with a history of allergy and/or wheezing, cough is often concomitant with bronchial asthma. A history of a combination of cough with hoarseness without upper respiratory disease may be due to pressure of a greatly enlarged left atrium on an enlarged pulmonary artery compressing the recurrent laryngeal nerve.

The character of the sputum may be helpful in the differential diagnosis. Thus, a cough producing frothy, pink-tinged sputum occurs in cases of pulmonary edema, whereas blood-streaked sputum suggests tuberculosis, bronchiectasis, carcinoma of the lung, or pulmonary infarction.

HEMOPTYSIS

The expectoration of blood or of sputum, either streaked or grossly contaminated with blood, may be due to (1) escape of red blood cells into the alveoli from congested vessels in the lungs (acute pulmonary edema); (2) rupture of dilated endobronchial vessels that form collateral channels between the pulmonary and bronchial venous systems (mitral stenosis); (3) necrosis and hemorrhage into the alveoli (pulmonary infarction); (4) ulceration of the bronchial mucosa or the slough of a caseous lesion (tuberculosis); (5) minor damage to the tracheobronchial mucosa, produced by excessive coughing of any cause, which can result in mild hemoptysis; (6) vascular invasion (carcinoma of the lung); or (6) necrosis of the mucosa with rupture of pulmonary-bronchial venous connections (bronchiectasis).

The history is often decisive in pinpointing the cause of hemoptysis.[43,45] Recurrent episodes of minor bleeding are observed in patients with chronic bronchitis, bronchiectasis, tuberculosis, and mitral stenosis. Rarely, these conditions result in the expectoration of large quantities of blood (i.e., more than one-half cup). Massive hemoptysis can also be due to rupture of a pulmonary arteriovenous fistula; exsanguinating hemoptysis may occur with rupture of an aortic aneurysm into the bronchopulmonary tree.

Hemoptysis associated with shortness of breath suggests mitral stenosis (see Chap. 57); in this condition, the hemoptysis is often precipitated by sudden elevations in left atrial pressure with effort, especially during pregnancy, and is attributable to rupture of small pulmonary or bronchopulmonary anastomosing veins. Blood-tinged sputum in patients with mitral stenosis may also be due to transient pulmonary edema; in these circumstances, it is usually associated with severe dyspnea. A history of hemoptysis associated with acute pleuritic chest pain suggests pulmonary embolism with infarction. Hemoptysis associated with congenital heart disease and cyanosis suggests Eisenmenger syndrome.

FATIGUE

Fatigue is among the most common symptoms in patients with impaired cardiovascular function. However, it is also one of the most nonspecific of all symptoms. In patients with impaired systemic circulation as a consequence of a depressed cardiac output, fatigue may be associated with muscular weakness. In other patients with heart disease, fatigue may be caused by drugs, such as beta-adrenoceptor blocking agents. It may be the result of excessive blood pressure reduction in patients treated too vigorously for hypertension or heart failure. In patients with heart failure, fatigue may also be caused by excessive diuresis and by diuretic-induced hypokalemia. Extreme fatigue sometimes precedes or accompanies acute myocardial infarction.

OTHER SYMPTOMS

Nocturia is a common early complaint in patients with congestive heart failure. Anorexia, abdominal fullness, right upper quadrant discomfort, weight loss, and cachexia are symptoms of advanced heart failure (see Chap. 22). Anorexia, nausea, vomiting, and visual changes are important signs of digitalis intoxication (see Chap. 23). Nausea and vomiting occur frequently in patients with acute myocardial infarction. Hoarseness may be caused by compression of the recurrent laryngeal nerve by an aortic aneurysm, a dilated pulmonary artery, or a greatly enlarged left atrium. A history of fever and chills is common in patients with infective endocarditis (see Chap. 58).

The History in Specific Forms of Heart Disease

Just as the history is of central importance in determining whether a specific symptom is caused by heart disease, it is equally valuable in elucidating its cause. A few examples are given here, whereas considerably greater detail is provided in chapters that deal with each specific disease entity.

HEART DISEASE IN INFANCY AND CHILDHOOD
(see Chap. 56)

The history is particularly helpful in establishing the diagnosis of congenital heart disease. In view of the familial incidence of certain congenital malformations (see Chap. 70), a history of congenital heart disease, cyanosis, or heart murmur in the family should be ascertained. Rubella in the first 2 months of pregnancy is associated with a number of congenital cardiac malformations (patent ductus arteriosus, atrial and ventricular septal defect, tetralogy of Fallot, and supravalvular aortic stenosis). A maternal viral illness in the last trimester of pregnancy may be responsible for neonatal myocarditis. Exertional syncope in a child with congenital heart disease suggests a lesion in which the cardiac output is fixed, such as aortic or pulmonic stenosis. Exertional angina in a child suggests severe aortic stenosis, pulmonary stenosis, primary pulmonary hypertension, or anomalous origin of the left coronary artery. A history of syncope or faintness with straining and associated with cyanosis suggests tetralogy of Fallot.

In infants or children with cardiac murmurs, it is important to ascertain by history as precisely as possible when the murmur was first detected. Murmurs due to either aortic or pulmonic stenosis are usually audible within the first 48 hours of life, whereas those produced by a ventricular septal defect are usually apparent a few days or weeks later. On the other hand, the murmur produced by an atrial septal defect often is not heard until age 2 to 3 months.

Frequent episodes of pneumonia early in infancy suggest a large left-to-right shunt, and a history of excessive diaphoresis occurs in patients with left ventricular failure, most commonly due to ventricular septal defect in this age group. A history of squatting is most frequently associated with tetralogy of Fallot or tricuspid atresia. Dysphagia in early infancy suggests the presence of an aortic arch anomaly such as double aortic arch or an anomalous origin of the right subclavian artery passing behind the esophagus. A history of headaches, weakness of the legs, and intermittent claudication is compatible with the diagnosis of coarctation of the aorta. Weakness or lack of coordination in a child with heart disease suggests cardiomyopathy associated with Friedreich ataxia or muscular dystrophy (see Chap. 85). A cerebrovascular accident in a cyanotic patient may be due to cerebral thrombosis or abscess or paradoxical embolization.

MYOCARDITIS AND CARDIOMYOPATHY. Rheumatic fever (see Chap. 81) is suggested by a history of sore throat followed by rash and chorea (St. Vitus dance). Chorea is characterized by twitching or clumsiness for a few months in childhood, as well as by frequent episodes of epistaxis and growing pains (i.e., nocturnal pains in the legs). A history of dyspnea following an influenza-like illness with myalgia suggests acute myocarditis. Carcinoid heart disease (see Chap. 59) is associated with a history of diarrhea, bronchospasm, and flushing of the upper chest and head. A history of diabetes, particularly if resistant to insulin and associated with bronzing of the skin, suggests hemochromatosis, which can be associated with heart failure due to cardiac infiltration.

Amyloid heart disease (see Chap. 59) is often associated with a history of postural hypotension and peripheral neuropathy. Hypertrophic cardiomyopathy (see Chap. 59) is often associated with a family history of this condition and sometimes with a family history of sudden death. The characteristic symptoms are angina, dyspnea, and syncope, which occur during or immediately after exercise.

HIGH-OUTPUT HEART FAILURE. Patients with symptoms of heart failure (breathlessness and excess fluid accumulation) with warm extremities often have high-output heart failure (see Chap. 22). They should be questioned about a history of anemia and of its common causes and accompaniments, such as menorrhagia, melena, peptic ulcer, hemorrhoids, sickle cell disease, and the neurological manifestations of vitamin B_{12} deficiency. Also, in such patients an attempt should be made to elicit a history of thyrotoxicosis (weight loss, polyphagia, diarrhea, diaphoresis, heat intolerance, nervousness, breathlessness, muscle weakness, and goiter [see Chap. 79]). Patients with beriberi heart disease responsible for high-output heart failure often have a history characteristic of peripheral neuritis, alcoholism, poor eating habits, fad diets, or upper gastrointestinal surgery.

COR PULMONALE. Patients with chronic cor pulmonale (see Chap. 67) frequently present with a history of smoking, chronic cough and sputum production, dyspnea, and wheezing relieved by bronchodilators. Alternatively, they have a history of pulmonary emboli, phlebitis, and the sudden development of dyspnea at rest, with palpitations, pleuritic chest pain, and, in the case of massive infarction, syncope.

PERICARDITIS. In patients in whom pericarditis or cardiac tamponade is suspected (see Chap. 64), an attempt should be made to elicit a history of chest trauma, a recent viral infection, recent cardiac surgery, neoplastic disease of the chest with or without radiation therapy, myxedema, scleroderma, tuberculosis, or contact with tuberculous patients. In patients with chronic constrictive pericarditis, ascites often precedes edema, which in turn usually precedes exertional dyspnea.

INFECTIVE ENDOCARDITIS. The diagnosis of infective endocarditis is suggested by a history of fever, severe night sweats, anorexia, and weight loss and embolic phenomena expressed as hematuria, back pain, petechiae, tender finger pads, and a cerebrovascular accident (see Chap. 58).

Drug-Induced Heart Disease

Because a wide variety of cardiac abnormalities can be induced by drugs, a meticulous history of drug intake is of great importance. Table 7–6 summarizes the major drugs responsible for various cardiovascular manifestations.

TABLE 7–6 Cardiovascular Manifestations of Adverse Reactions to Drugs

Acute Chest Pain (Nonischemic)	**Cardiomyopathy**	**Hypertension**
Bleomycin	Adriamycin	Clonidine withdrawal
	Daunorubicin	Corticotropin
Angina Exacerbation	Emetine	Cyclosporine
Alpha blockers	Lithium	Erythropoietin
Beta-blocker withdrawal	Phenothiazines	Glucocorticoids
Ergotamine	Sulfonamides	Monoamine oxidase inhibitors with sympathomimetics
Excessive thyroxine	Sympathomimetics	Nonsteroidal anti-inflammatory drugs
Hydralazine		Oral contraceptives
Methysergide	**Fluid Retention/Congestive Heart Failure/Edema**	Sympathomimetics
Minoxidil	Beta-blockers	Tricyclic antidepressants with sympathomimetics
Nifedipine	Calcium blockers	
Oxytocin	Carbenoxolone	**Pericardial Effusion**
Vasopressin	Diazoxide	Minoxidil
	Estrogens	Oral contraceptives
Arrhythmias	Mannitol	Thromboembolism
Adenosine	Minoxidil	
Adriamycin	NSAIDs	**Prolonged QT Interval/Torsades de Pointes**
Anticholinesterases	Phenylbutazone	Amiodarone
Atropine	Steroids	Amitriptyline
Beta blockers	Verapamil	Chlorpromazine
Daunorubicin		Diphenylhydramine
Digitalis	**Pericarditis**	Disopyramide
Emetine	Emetine	Haloperidol
Erythromycin	Hydralazine	Ibutilide
Guanethidine	Methysergide	Pentamidine
Lithium	Procainamide	Procainamide
Papaverine		Sotalol
Pentamidine	**Hypotension (see also Arrhythmias)**	Terfenadine
Phenothiazines, particularly thioridazine	Amiodarone	Trimethoprim-sulfamethoxazole
Sympathomimetics	Calcium channel blockers, e.g., nifedipine	
Terfenadine		
Theophylline	**Diuresis**	
Thyroid hormone	Interleukin-2	
Tricyclic antidepressants	Levodopa	
Verapamil	Morphine	
	Nitroglycerin	
Atrioventricular Block	Phenothiazines	
Clonidine	Protamine	
Methyldopa	Quinidine	
Verapamil	Sildenafil	

Modified from Wood AJ: Adverse reactions to drugs. *In* Braunwald E, Fauci A, Kasper D, et al (eds): Harrison's Principles of Internal Medicine. 15th ed. New York, McGraw-Hill, 2001.

Catecholamines, whether administered exogenously or secreted by a pheochromocytoma (see Chap. 79), may produce myocarditis and arrhythmias. Digitalis glycosides can be responsible for a variety of tachyarrhythmias and bradyarrhythmias as well as gastrointestinal, visual, and central nervous system disturbances (see Chap. 23). Paradoxically, the administration of antiarrhythmic drugs is one of the major causes of serious cardiac arrhythmias (see Chap. 29). For example, quinidine may cause QT prolongation, ventricular tachycardia of the torsades de pointes variety, syncope, and sudden death, presumably due to ventricular fibrillation.

Disopyramide, beta-adrenoceptor blockers, and the calcium channel antagonists diltiazem and verapamil may depress ventricular performance, and, in patients with ventricular dysfunction, these drugs may precipitate heart failure. Alcohol is also a potent myocardial depressant and may be responsible for the development of cardiomyopathy (see Chap. 59), arrhythmias, and sudden death. Tricyclic antidepressants may cause orthostatic hypotension and arrhythmias. Lithium, also used in the treatment of psychiatric disorders, can aggravate preexisting cardiac arrhythmias, particularly in patients with heart failure in whom the renal clearance of this ion is impaired. Cocaine can cause coronary spasm with resultant myocardial ischemia, myocardial infarction, and sudden death (see Chap 62).[13,46]

The anthracycline compounds doxorubicin (Adriamycin) and daunorubicin, which are widely used because of their broad spectrum of activity against various tumors, may cause or intensify left ventricular failure, arrhythmias, myocarditis, and pericarditis (see Chap. 83). Cyclophosphamide, an antineoplastic alkylating agent, may also cause left ventricular dysfunction, whereas 5-fluorouracil and its derivatives may be responsible for angina secondary to coronary spasm. Radiation therapy to the chest may cause acute and chronic pericarditis (see Chap. 64), pancarditis, or coronary artery disease; furthermore, it may enhance the aforementioned cardiotoxic effects of the anthracyclines.

Assessing Cardiovascular Disability
(Table 7–7)

One of the greatest values of the history is in categorizing the degree of cardiovascular disability, so that a patient's status can be followed over time, the effects of a therapeutic intervention assessed, and patients compared with one another. The Criteria Committee of the New York Heart Association has provided a widely used classification that relates functional activity to the ability to carry out "ordinary" activity.[47] The term *ordinary* is, of course, subject to widely varying interpretation, as are terms such as *undue fatigue* that are used in this classification, and this has limited its accuracy and reproducibility. More recently, the New York Heart Association changed its evaluation from functional activity to a broader one, called *cardiac status*, which takes account

TABLE 7–7 A Comparison of Three Methods of Assessing Cardiovascular Disability

Class	New York Heart Association Functional Classification	Canadian Cardiovascular Society Functional Classification	Specific Activity Scale
I	Patients with cardiac disease but without resulting limitations of physical activity. Ordinary physical activity does not cause undue fatigure, palpitation, dyspnea, or anginal pain.	Ordinary physical activity, such as walking and climbing stairs, does not cause angina. Angina with strenuous or rapid or prolonged exertion at work or recreation.	Patients can perform to completion any activity requiring ≤7 metabolic equivalents (e.g., can carry 24 lb up eight steps; carry objects that weigh 80 lb; do outdoor work [shovel snow, spade soil]; do recreational activities [skiing, basketball, squash, handball, jog/walk 5 mph])
II	Patients with cardiac disease resulting in slight limitation of physical activity. They are comfortable at rest. Ordinary physical activity results in fatigue, palpitation, dyspnea, or anginal pain.	Slight limitation of ordinary activity. Walking or climbing stairs rapidly, walking uphill, walking or stair climbing after meals, in cold, in wind, or when under emotional stress, or only during the few hours after awakening. Walking more than two blocks on the level and climbing more than one flight of ordinary stairs at a normal pace and in normal conditions.	Patients can perform to completion any activity requiring ≤5 metabokic equivalents (e.g., have sexual intercourse without stopping, garden, rake, weed, roller skate, dance fox trot, walk at 4 mph on level ground) but cannot and do not perform to completion activities requiring ≥7 metabolic equivalents.
III	Patients with cardiac disease resulting in marked limitation of physical activity. They are comfortable at rest. Less than ordinary physical activity causes fatigue, palpitation, dyspnea, or anginal pain.	Marked limitation of ordinary physical activity. Walking one to two blocks on the level and climbing more than one flight in normal conditions.	Patients can perform to completion any activity requiring ≤2 metabolic equivalents (e.g., shower without stopping, strip and make bed, clean windows, walk 2.5 mph, bowl, play golf, dress without stopping) but cannot and do not perform to completion any activities requiring ≥5 metabolic equivalents.
IV	Patient with cardiac disease resulting in inability to carry on any physical activity without discomfort. Symptoms of cardiac insufficiency or of the anginal syndrome may be present even at rest. If any physical activity is undertaken, discomfort is increased.	Inability to carry on any physical activity without discomfort—anginal syndrome *may be* present at rest.	Patients cannot or do not perform to completion activities requiring ≥2 metabolic equivalents. *Cannot* carry out activities listed above (Specific Activity Scale, Class III).

From Goldman L, Hashimoto B, Cook EF, Loscalzo A: Comparative reproducibility and validity of systems for assessing cardiovascular functional class: Advantages of a new specific activity scale. Circulation 64:1227, 1981. Copyright 1981, American Heart Association.

of symptoms and other data gathered from the patient.[47] Cardiac status is classified as (1) uncompromised, (2) slightly compromised, (3) moderately compromised, and (4) severely compromised.

Somewhat more detailed and specific criteria were provided by the Canadian Cardiovascular Society,[48] but this classification is limited to patients with angina pectoris. Goldman and coworkers[49] developed a specific activity scale in which classification is based on the estimated metabolic cost of various activities. This scale appears to be more reproducible and to be a better predictor of exercise tolerance than either the New York Heart Association classification or the Canadian Cardiovascular Society criteria.

A key element of the history is to determine whether the patient's disability is stable or progressive. A useful way to accomplish this is to inquire whether a specific task that now causes symptoms (e.g., dyspnea after climbing two flights of stairs) did so 3, 6, and 12 months previously. Precise questioning on this point is important because a gradual reduction of ordinary activity as heart disease progresses may lead to an underestimation of the apparent degree of disability.[50]

REFERENCES

1. Sandler G: The importance of the history in the medical clinic and the cost of unnecessary tests. Am Heart J 100:928, 1980.
2. Sapira JD: The history. *In* The Art and Science of Bedside Diagnosis. Baltimore, Urban & Schwartzenberg, 1990, pp 9-45.
3. Tumulty PA: Obtaining the history. *In* The Effective Clinician. Philadelphia, WB Saunders, 1973, pp 17-28.
4. Scano G, Ambrosino N: Pathophysiology of dyspnea. Lung 180:131, 2002.
5. Schwartzstein RM, Feller-Kopman D: Approach to the patient with dyspnea. *In* Braunwald E, Goldman L (eds): Primary Cardiology, 2nd ed. Philadelphia, WB Saunders, 2003, pp 101-116.
6. Mahler DA, Fierro-Carrion G, Baird JC: Evaluation of dyspnea in the elderly. Clin Geriatr Med 19:19, 2003.
7. Michaelson E, Hollrah S: Evaluation of the patient with shortness of breath: An evidence based approach. Emerg Med Clin North Am 17:221, 1999.
8. Borg G, Noble B: Perceived exertion. *In* Wilmore JH (ed): Exercise and Sports. Science Reviews. New York, Academic Press, 1974, pp 131-153.
9. American Thoracic Society: Dyspnea: Mechanisms, assessment, and management. A consensus statement. Am J Respir Crit Care Med 159:321, 1999.
10. Logeart D, Saudubray C, Beyne P, et al: Comparative value of Doppler echocardiography and B-type natriuretic peptide assay in the etiologic diagnosis of acute dyspnea. J Am Coll Cardiol 40:1794, 2002.
11. Collins SP, Ronan-Bentle S, Storrow AB: Diagnostic and prognostic usefulness of natriuretic peptides in emergency department patients with dyspnea. Ann Emerg Med 41:532, 2003.
12. Yeghiazarians Y, Braunstein JB, Askari A, et al: Unstable angina pectoris. N Engl J Med 342:101, 2000.
13. Weber JE, Shofer FS, Larkin GL, et al: Validation of a brief observation period for patients with cocaine-associated chest pain. N Engl J Med 348:510, 2003.
14. Crea F, Gaspardone A: Mechanisms and significance of anginal pain. Cardiologia 44:233, 1999.
15. Mayer S, Hillis LD: Prinzmetal's angina. Clin Cardiol 21:243, 1998.
16. Horwitz LD, Groves BM (eds): Signs and Symptoms in Cardiology. Philadelphia, JB Lippincott, 1985.
17. Boivin M, Peterson WG: Management of complicated gastroesophageal reflux disease: Atypical chest pain. Can J Gastroenterol 11:91B, 1997.
18. Lemire S: Assessment of clinical severity and investigation of uncomplicated gastroesophageal reflux disease and noncardiac angina-like chest pain. Can J Gastroenterol 11:37B, 1997.
19. Chauhan A, Mullins PA, Taylor G, et al: Cardioesophageal reflex: A mechanism for "linked angina" in patients with angiographically proven coronary artery disease. J Am Coll Cardiol 27:1621, 1996.
20. Zimmerman D, Parker BM: The pain of pulmonary hypertension: Fact or fancy? JAMA 246:2345, 1981.
21. Spalding L Reay E, Kelly C: Cause and outcome of atypical chest pain in patients admitted to hospital. J R Soc Med 96:122, 2003.
22. Carter CS, Servan-Schreiber D, Perlstein WM: Anxiety disorders and the syndrome of chest pain with normal coronary arteries: Prevalence and pathophysiology. J Clin Psychiatry 58:70, 1997.
23. Mayou R: Chest pain, palpitations, and panic. J Psychosom Res 44:53, 1998.
24. Serlie AW, Erdman RA, Passchier J, et al: Psychological aspects of non-cardiac chest pain. Psychother Psychosom 64:62, 1995.
25. Douglas PS, Ginsberg GS: The evaluation of chest pain in women. N Engl J Med 334:1311, 1996.
26. Marroquin OC, Holubkov R, Edmindowicz D, et al: Heterogeneity of microvascular dysfunction in women with chest pain not attributable to coronary artery disease: Implications for clinical practice. Am Heart J 145:628, 2003
27. D'Antono B, Dupuis G, Fleet R, et al: Sex differences in chest pain and prediction of exercise-induced ischemia. Can J Cardiol 19:515, 2003.
28. Goldman L: Approach to the patient with chest pain. *In* Braunwald E, Goldman L (eds): Primary Cardiology, 2nd ed. Philadelphia, WB Saunders, 2003, pp 83-101.
29. Rao SV, Ohman EM, Granger CB, et al: Prognostic value of isolated troponin elevation across the spectrum of chest pain syndromes. Am J Cardiol 91:936, 2003.
30. Braunwald E: Hypoxia and cyanosis. *In* Kasper DL, et al (eds): Harrison's Principles of Internal Medicine. 16th ed. New York, McGraw-Hill, 2005.
31. Fishman AP: Cyanosis and clubbing. *In* Fishman A, et al (eds): Fishman's Pulmonary Diseases and Disorders. 3rd ed. New York, McGraw-Hill, 1998, pp 382-383.
32. Linzer M, Yang EH, Estes NA III, et al: Diagnosing syncope: I. Value of history, physical examination, and electrocardiography. Clinical Efficacy Assessment Project of the American College of Physicians. Ann Intern Med 126:989, 1997.
33. Linzer M, Yang EH, Estes NA III, et al: Diagnosing syncope: II. Unexplained syncope. Clinical Efficacy Assessment Project of the American College of Physicians. Ann Intern Med 127:76, 1997.
34. Kochar MS: Management of postural hypotension. Curr Hypertens Rep 2:457, 2000.
35. Cadman CS: Medical therapy of neurocardiogenic syncope. Cardiol Clin 19:203, 2001.
36. Mathias CJ, Kimber JR: Postural hypotension: Causes, clinical features, investigation and management. Annu Rev Med 50:317, 1999.
37. Calkins H, Shyr Y, Frumin H, et al: The value of the clinical history in the differentiation of syncope due to ventricular tachycardia, atrioventricular block, and neurocardiogenic syncope. Am J Med 98:365, 1995.
38. Zimetbaum P, Josephson ME: Evaluation of patients with palpitations. N Engl J Med 338:1369, 1998.
39. Hlatky MA: Approach to the patient with palpitations. *In* Braunwald E, Goldman L (eds): Primary Cardiology. 2nd ed. Philadelphia, WB Saunders, 2003, pp 129-136.
40. Barsky AJ: Palpitations, arrhythmias, and awareness of cardiac activity. Ann Intern Med 134:832, 2001.
41. Braunwald E: Edema. *In* Kasper DL, et al (eds): Harrison's Principles of Internal Medicine. 16th ed. New York, McGraw-Hill, 2005.
42. Chertow GM: Approach to the patient with edema. *In* Braunwald E, Goldman L (eds): Primary Cardiology. 2nd ed. Philadelphia, WB Saunders, 2003, pp. 117-128.
43. Weinberger S: Cough and hemoptysis. *In* Kasper DL, et al (eds): Harrison's Principles of Internal Medicine. 16th ed. New York: McGraw-Hill, 2005.
44. Patrick H, Patrick F: Chronic cough. Med Clin North Am 79:361, 1995.
45. Corder R: Hemoptysis. Emerg Med Clin North Am 21:421, 2003.
46. Isner JM, Chokshi SK: Cocaine and vasospasm. N Engl J Med 321:1604, 1989.
47. The Criteria Committee of the New York Heart Association: Nomenclature and Criteria for Diagnosis. 9th ed. Boston, Little, Brown, 1994.
48. Campeau L: Grading of angina pectoris. Circulation 54:522, 1975.
49. Goldman L, Hashimoto B, Cook EF, Loscalzo A: Comparative reproducibility and validity of systems for assessing cardiovascular functional class: Advantages of a new specific activity scale. Circulation 64:1227, 1981.
50. Goldman L, Cook EF, Mitchell N, et al: Pitfalls in the serial assessment of cardiac functional status: How a reduction in "ordinary" activity may reduce the apparent degree of cardiac compromise and give a misleading impression of improvement. J Chronic Dis 35:763, 1982.

CHAPTER 8

Physical Examination of the Heart and Circulation

Eugene Braunwald • Joseph K. Perloff

Importance of the Physical Examination

A common pitfall in cardiovascular medicine is the failure by the cardiologist to recognize that a patient's heart disease is part of a systemic illness. Equally important is the failure by the noncardiologist to recognize the presence of a cardiac disorder that is a component of a systemic illness whose major effect may be on other organ systems. To avoid these two pitfalls, patients known to have or suspected of having heart disease require not only a detailed examination of the cardiovascular system but also a careful general physical examination. For example, the presence of coronary artery disease should prompt a careful search for frequent noncardiac concomitant conditions such as atherosclerosis of the carotid arteries and of the arteries of the lower extremities and aorta. Conversely, the very high incidence (approximately 50 percent) of coronary artery disease in patients with cerebrovascular disorders must be considered in dealing with patients with these conditions.

As stated by Mangione and coworkers,[1] "There are still many reasons to promote the teaching of bedside diagnostic skills such as cardiac auscultation. Among these are cost-effectiveness, the possibility of making inexpensive serial observations, the early detection of critical findings, the intelligent and well-guided selection of costly diagnostic technology, and the therapeutic value of the physical contact between physician and patient."

Shaver and Tavel have pointed out that in this era of cost containment in the practice of medicine, and the great expense of many "high-tech" diagnostic procedures, the physical examination remains a relatively inexpensive, useful "test."[2,3] An additional benefit is that the actual physical contact, that is, the "laying on of hands" by the physician creates a valued closer bond with the patient at a time when the patient's encounter with the medical care system is often so impersonal.

The General Physical Examination

General Appearance

An assessment of the patient's general appearance is usually begun with a detailed inspection at the time that the history is being obtained.[4-7] The general build and appearance of the patient, the skin color, and the presence of pallor or cyanosis should be noted, as well as the presence of shortness of breath, orthopnea, periodic (Cheyne-Stokes) respiration (see Chap. 22), and distention of the neck veins. If the patient is in pain, is he or she sitting quietly (typical of angina pectoris); moving about, trying to find a more comfortable position (characteristic of acute myocardial infarction); or most comfortable sitting upright (heart failure) or leaning forward (pericarditis)? Simple inspection also reveals whether the patient's whole body shakes with each heartbeat and whether Corrigan pulses (bounding arterial pulsations, as occur with the large stroke volume of severe aortic regurgitation, arteriovenous fistula, or complete atrioventricular [AV] block) are present in the head, neck, and upper extremities. Malnutrition and cachexia, which occur in severe chronic heart failure (see Chap. 22), may also be readily evident. The distinctive general appearance of the Marfan syndrome (see Chap. 70) is often apparent: long extremities with an arm span that exceeds the height; a longer lower segment (pubis to foot) than upper segment (head to pubis); and arachnodactyly (spider fingers).

HEAD AND FACE

Examination of the face often aids in the recognition of many disorders that can affect the cardiovascular system. For example, myxedema (see Chap. 79) is characterized by a dull, expressionless face, periorbital puffiness, loss of the lateral eyebrows, a large tongue, and dry, sparse hair. An earlobe crease occurs more frequently in patients with coronary artery disease than in those without this condition.[8] Bobbing of the head coincident with each heartbeat (de Musset sign) is characteristic of severe aortic regurgitation. Facial edema may be present in patients with tricuspid valve disease or constrictive pericarditis.

EYES

External ophthalmoplegia and ptosis due to muscular dystrophy of the extraocular muscles occur in patients with the Kearns-Sayre syndrome, which may be associated with complete heart block. Exophthalmos and stare occur in patients with hyperthyroidism, an important cause of high-output cardiac failure (see Chaps. 22 and 79). Blue sclerae can be seen in patients with osteogenesis imperfecta, a disorder that may be associated with aortic dilatation, regurgitation, and dissection and with prolapse of the mitral valve (see Chap. 70).

FUNDI

Examination of the fundi allows classification of arteriolar disease in patients with hypertension and may also be helpful in the recognition of arteriosclerosis. Beading of the retinal artery may be present in patients with hypercholesterolemia. Hemorrhages near the discs with white spots in the center (Roth spots) occur in patients with infective endocarditis. Embolic retinal occlusions can occur in patients with rheumatic heart disease, left atrial myxoma, and atherosclerosis of the aorta or arch vessels. Papilledema can be present not only in patients with malignant hypertension (see Chap. 37) but also in those with cor pulmonale with severe hypoxia (see Chap. 67).

SKIN AND MUCOUS MEMBRANES

Central cyanosis (due to intracardiac or intrapulmonary right-to-left shunting) involves the entire body, including warm, well-perfused sites such as the conjunctivae and the mucous membranes of the oral cavity. Peripheral cyanosis (due to reduction of peripheral blood flow, such as occurs in patients with heart failure and peripheral vascular disease) is characteristically most prominent in cool, exposed areas that may not be well perfused, such as the extremities, particularly the nail beds and nose. Polycythemia can often be suspected from inspection of the conjunctivae, lips, and tongue, which are darkly congested in cases of polycythemia and pale in cases of anemia.

Bronze pigmentation of the skin and loss of axillary and pubic hair occur in patients with hemochromatosis (which may result in cardiomyopathy owing to iron deposits in the heart). Jaundice may be observed in patients after pulmonary infarction as well as in patients with congestive hepatomegaly or cardiac cirrhosis. Lentigines, which are small brown macular lesions on the neck and trunk that begin at about age 6 and do not increase in number with sunlight, are observed in patients with pulmonic stenosis and hypertrophic cardiomyopathy.[9]

Several types of xanthomas (cholesterol-filled nodules) are found either subcutaneously or over tendons in patients with hyperlipoproteinemia (see Chap. 39). Premature atherosclerosis frequently develops in these individuals. Tuberoeruptive xanthomas, present subcutaneously or on the extensor surfaces of the extremities (Fig. 8–1), and xanthoma striatum palmare, which produce yellowish, orange, or pink discoloration of the palmar and digital creases, occur most commonly in patients with type III hyperlipoproteinemia. Patients with xanthoma tendinosum (i.e., nodular swellings of the tendons, especially of the elbows, extensor surfaces of the hands, and Achilles tendons) usually have type II hyperlipoproteinemia. Eruptive xanthomas are tiny yellowish nodules, 1 to 2 mm in diameter on an erythematous base, that may occur anywhere on the body and are associated with hyperchylomicronemia and are therefore often found in patients with type I and type V hyperlipoproteinemia.

Hereditary telangiectases are multiple capillary hemangiomas occurring in the skin, lips (Fig. 8–2), nasal mucosa, and upper respiratory and gastrointestinal tracts and resemble the spider nevi seen in patients with liver disease. When present in the lung, they are associated with pulmonary arteriovenous fistulas and cause central cyanosis.

EXTREMITIES

A variety of congenital and acquired cardiac malformations are associated with characteristic changes in the extremities. Among the congenital lesions, short stature, cubitus valgus, and medial deviation of the extended forearm are characteristic of Turner syndrome (see Chap. 56). Patients with the Holt-Oram syndrome[10] (atrial septal defect with skeletal deformities) often have a thumb with an extra phalanx, a so-called fingerized thumb, which lies in the same plane as the fingers, making it difficult to appose the thumb and fingers. In addition, they may exhibit deformities of the radius and ulna, causing difficulty in supination and pronation.

Arachnodactyly is characteristic of Marfan syndrome (see Chap. 70). Normally, when a fist is made over a clenched thumb, the thumb does not extend beyond the ulnar side of the hand, but it usually does so in patients with Marfan syndrome.

Systolic flushing of the nail beds, which can be readily detected by pressing a flashlight against the terminal digits (Quincke sign), is a sign of aortic regurgitation and of other conditions characterized by a greatly widened pulse pressure. Differential cyanosis, in which the hands and fingers (especially on the right side) are pink and the feet and toes are cyanotic, is indicative of patent ductus arteriosus with reversed shunt due to pulmonary hypertension (see Chap. 67); this finding can often be brought out by exercise. On the other hand, reversed differential cyanosis, in which cyanosis of the fingers exceeds that of the toes, suggests Taussig-Bing anomaly with pulmonary vascular disease and reversed flow through a patent ductus arteriosus. Alternatively, it may occur with transposition of the great arteries, pulmonary hypertension, preductal narrowing of the aorta, and reversed flow through a patent ductus arteriosus.[11]

CLUBBING OF THE FINGERS AND TOES

Clubbing of the digits is characteristic of central cyanosis (cyanotic congenital heart disease or pulmonary disease with hypoxia) (Fig. 8–3). It may also appear within a few weeks of the development of infective endocarditis. The earliest forms of clubbing are characterized by increased glossiness and cyanosis of the skin at the root of the nail.[12] After obliteration of the normal angle between the base of the nail and the skin, the soft tissue of the pulp becomes hypertrophied, the nail root floats freely, and its loose proximal end can be palpated. In the more severe forms of clubbing, bony changes occur (i.e., hypertrophic

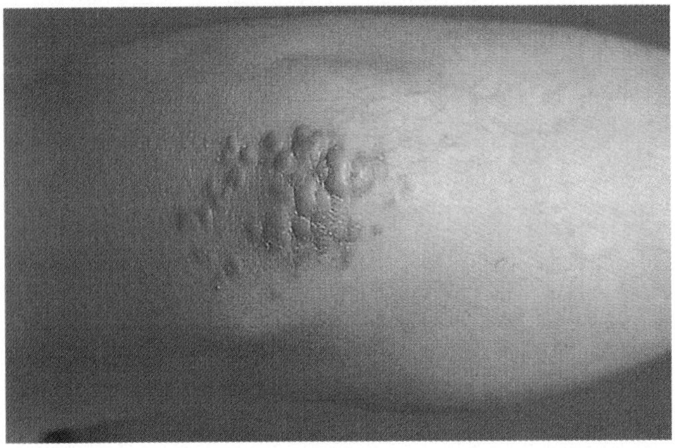

FIGURE 8–1 Eruptive xanthomas on the elbow. Lipid deposition in the skin (xanthoma tuberosum) can be seen in young patients with homozygous familial hypercholesterolemia. It affects the buttocks and palms. There is also joint involvement. (From Zatouroff M: Physical Signs in General Medicine. 2nd ed. London, Mosby-Wolff, 1996, p 99.)

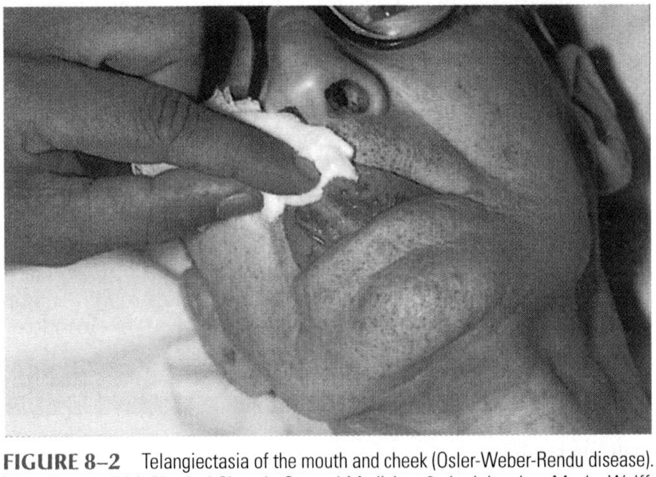

FIGURE 8–2 Telangiectasia of the mouth and cheek (Osler-Weber-Rendu disease). (From Zatouroff M: Physical Signs in General Medicine. 2nd ed. London, Mosby-Wolff, 1996, p 168.)

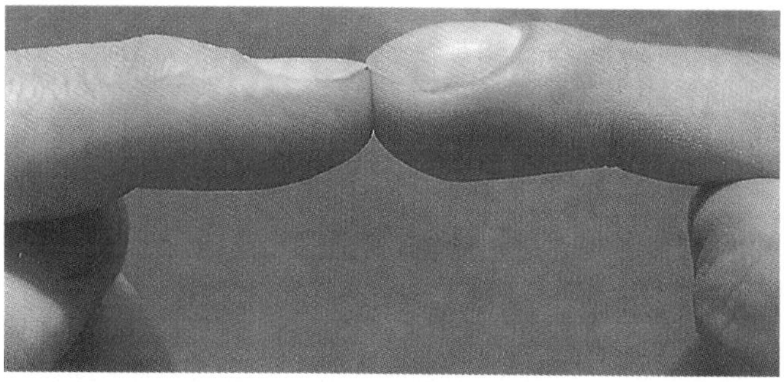

FIGURE 8–3 Nail clubbing (right) and a normal nail (left). (From Zatouroff M: Physical Signs in General Medicine. 2d ed. London, Mosby-Wolff, 1996, p 239.)

osteoarthropathy); these changes involve the terminal digits and in rare instances even the wrists, ankles, elbows, and knees. Unilateral clubbing of the fingers is rare but can occur when an aortic aneurysm interferes with the arterial supply to one arm.

Osler nodes are small, tender, purplish erythematous skin lesions caused by infected microemboli and occurring most frequently in the pads of the fingers or toes and in the palms of the hands or soles of the feet,[13] whereas Janeway lesions are slightly raised, nontender hemorrhagic lesions in the palms of the hands and soles of the feet; both of these lesions as well as petechiae occur in patients with infective endocarditis (see Chap. 58). When petechiae occur under the nail beds, they are termed *splinter hemorrhages.*

EDEMA. The presence of edema of the lower extremities is a common finding in patients with congestive heart failure (see Chap. 22)[14]; however, if it is present in only one leg, it is more likely due to obstructive venous or lymphatic disease than to heart failure. Firm pressure on the pretibial region for 10 to 20 seconds may be necessary for the detection of edema. In patients confined to bed, edema appears first in the sacral region. Edema may involve the face in children with heart failure of any cause and in adults with heart failure associated with marked elevation of systemic venous pressure (e.g., constrictive pericarditis and tricuspid valve disease).

Chest and Abdomen

Examination of the thorax should begin with observations of the rate, effort, and regularity of respiration. The shape of the chest is important as well; thus, a barrel-shaped chest with low diaphragm suggests emphysema, bronchitis, and cor pulmonale. Inspection of the chest is an integral part of the cardiac examination. It may reveal a bulging to the right of the upper sternum caused by an aortic aneurysm. The latter can also produce a venous collateral pattern caused by obstruction of the superior vena cava. *Kyphoscoliosis* of any cause can cause cor pulmonale; this skeletal abnormality, as well as pectus excavatum (funnel chest)[15,16] and pectus carinatum (pigeon breast), is often present in patients with Marfan syndrome.

Left ventricular failure and other causes of elevation of pulmonary venous pressure can cause pulmonary rales; wheezing is sometimes audible in patients with pulmonary edema (cardiac asthma).

Painful enlargement of the liver may be due to venous congestion; the tenderness disappears in cases of long-standing heart failure. Hepatic systolic expansile pulsations occur in patients with severe tricuspid regurgitation, and presystolic pulsations can be felt in patients with tricuspid stenosis and sinus rhythm. Patients with constrictive pericarditis also often have pulsatile hepatomegaly, the contour of the pulsations resembling those of the jugular venous pulse in this condition. When firm pressure over the abdomen causes cervical venous distention (that is, when there is abdominojugular reflux, right-sided heart failure[17]) constrictive pericarditis (see later), or tricuspid valve disease is usually present. Ascites is also characteristic of heart failure, but it is especially characteristic of tricuspid valve disease and chronic constrictive pericarditis.

Splenomegaly can occur in the presence of severe congestive hepatomegaly, most frequently in patients with constrictive pericarditis or tricuspid valve disease. The spleen may be enlarged and painful in patients with infective endocarditis as well as after splenic embolization. Splenic infarction is frequently accompanied by an audible friction rub.

Both kidneys may be palpably enlarged in patients with hypertension secondary to polycystic disease. Auscultation of the abdomen should be carried out in all patients with hypertension; a systolic bruit secondary to renal artery stenosis may be audible near the umbilicus or in the flank.

Atherosclerotic aneurysms of the abdominal aorta are usually readily detected on palpation of the abdomen below the umbilicus (see Chap. 53), except in markedly obese patients. In patients with coarctation of the aorta, no abdominal pulsations are palpable despite the presence of prominent arterial pulses in the neck and upper extremities; arterial pulses in the lower extremities are reduced or absent.

Jugular Venous Pulse

Important information concerning the dynamics of the right side of the heart can be obtained by observation of the jugular venous pulse.[5,18-21] The internal jugular vein is ordinarily examined; the venous pulse can usually be analyzed more readily on the right than on the left side of the neck, because the right innominate and jugular veins extend in an almost straight line cephalad to the superior vena cava, thus favoring transmission of hemodynamic changes from the right atrium, whereas the left innominate vein is not in a straight line and may be kinked or compressed by a variety of normal structures, by a dilated aorta, or by an aneurysm.

During the examination, the patient should be lying comfortably. Although the head should rest on a pillow, it must not be at a sharp angle from the trunk. One can examine the jugular venous pulse effectively by shining a light tangentially across the neck. Most patients with heart disease are examined most effectively in the 45-degree position, but in patients in whom venous pressure is high, a greater inclination (60 or even 90 degrees) is required to obtain visible pulsations, whereas in those in whom jugular venous pressure is low, a lesser incline (30 degrees) is desirable.

The internal jugular vein is located deep within the neck, where it is covered by the sternocleidomastoid muscle and is therefore not usually visible as a discrete structure except in the presence of venous hypertension. However, its pulsations are transmitted to the skin of the neck, where they are usually easily visible. Sometimes examiners experience difficulty in differentiating between the carotid and jugular venous pulses in the neck, particularly when the latter exhibits prominent v waves, as occurs in patients with tricuspid regurgitation, in whom the valves in the internal jugular veins may be incompetent. There are several helpful clues to avoid this difficulty, however:

1. The arterial pulse is a sharply localized rapid movement that may not be readily visible but that strikes the palpating fingers with considerable force; in contrast, the venous pulse, although more readily visible, often disappears when the palpating finger is placed lightly on or below the pulsating area.
2. The arterial pulse usually exhibits a single upstroke, whereas (in patients in sinus rhythm) the venous pulse has two peaks and two troughs per cardiac cycle.
3. The arterial pulsations do not change when the patient is in the upright position or during respiration, whereas venous pulsations usually disappear or diminish greatly in the upright position and during inspiration, unless the venous pressure is greatly elevated.
4. Compression of the root of the neck does not affect the arterial pulse but usually abolishes venous pulsations, except in the presence of extreme venous hypertension.

Two principal observations can usually be made from examination of the neck veins: the level of venous pressure and the type of venous wave pattern. To estimate jugular venous pressure, the height of the oscillating top of the distended proximal portion of the internal jugular vein, which reflects right atrial pressure, should be determined. The upper limit of normal is 4 cm above the sternal angle, which corresponds to a central venous pressure of approximately 9 cm H_2O, since the right atrium is approximately 5 cm below the sternal angle. When the veins in the neck collapse in a subject breathing normally in the horizontal position, it is likely that the central venous pressure is subnormal. When obstruction of veins in the lower extremities is responsible for edema, pressure in the neck veins is not elevated and the abdominal-jugular reflux is negative.

ABDOMINAL-JUGULAR REFLUX. With the patient positioned to make the jugular vein easily visible, steady, firm pressure is supplied to the periumbilical region for 10 to 30 seconds with the patient breathing quietly[17-20]; increased respiratory excursions, straining, and the Valsalva maneuver should be avoided. In normal subjects, jugular venous pressure rises less than 3 cm H_2O and only transiently while abdominal pressure is continued, whereas in patients with right or left ventricular failure and/or tricuspid regurgitation, the jugular venous pressure remains elevated for more than 15 seconds. A positive abdominal-jugular reflux suggests right ventricular systolic and/or diastolic dysfunction, tricuspid valve disease, constrictive pericarditis, or central venous pressure.

PATTERN OF THE VENOUS PULSE. The events of the cardiac cycle, shown in Figure 19–19 provide an explanation for the details of the jugular venous waveform (Fig. 8–4). The A wave in the venous pulse results from venous distention due to right atrial systole, whereas the X descent is due to atrial relaxation and descent of the floor of the right atrium during right ventricular systole. The C wave, which occurs simultaneously with the carotid arterial pulse, is an inconstant wave in the jugular venous pulse and/or interruption of the X descent after the peak of the A wave. The continuation of the X descent after the C wave is referred to as the X′ descent. The V wave results from the rise in right atrial pressure when blood flows into this chamber during ventricular systole when the tricuspid valve is shut, and the Y descent (i.e., the downslope of the V wave) is related to the decline in right atrial pressure when the tricuspid valve reopens. After the bottom of the Y descent (the Y trough) and beginning of the A wave is a period of relatively slow filling of the atrium or ventricle, the diastasis period, a wave termed the H wave.

ALTERATIONS IN DISEASE. Elevation of jugular venous pressure reflects an increase in right atrial pressure and occurs in cases of heart failure, reduced compliance of the right ventricle, pericardial disease, hypervolemia, obstruction of the tricuspid orifice, and obstruction of the superior vena cava. During inspiration, the jugular venous pressure normally declines but the amplitude of the pulsations increases. Kussmaul sign[19,20] is a paradoxical rise in the height of the jugular venous pressure during inspiration, which typically occurs in patients with chronic constrictive pericarditis and sometimes in patients with congestive heart failure and tricuspid stenosis.

The A wave is particularly prominent in patients with conditions in which the resistance to right atrial contraction is increased, such as right ventricular hypertrophy, pulmonary hypertension, and tricuspid stenosis (see Fig. 8–4A). The A wave can also be tall in cases of left ventricular hypertrophy when the thickened ventricular septum interferes with right ventricular filling. Tall A waves are present in patients with sinus rhythm and tricuspid stenosis or atresia, right atrial myxoma, or reduced compliance and/or marked hypertrophy of the right ventricle. Cannon (amplified) A waves are noted in patients with AV dissociation when the right atrium contracts against a closed tricuspid valve. In cases of atrial fibrillation, the A wave and X descent disappear and the V wave and Y descent become more prominent. In cases of right ventricular failure and sinus rhythm, there may be increases in

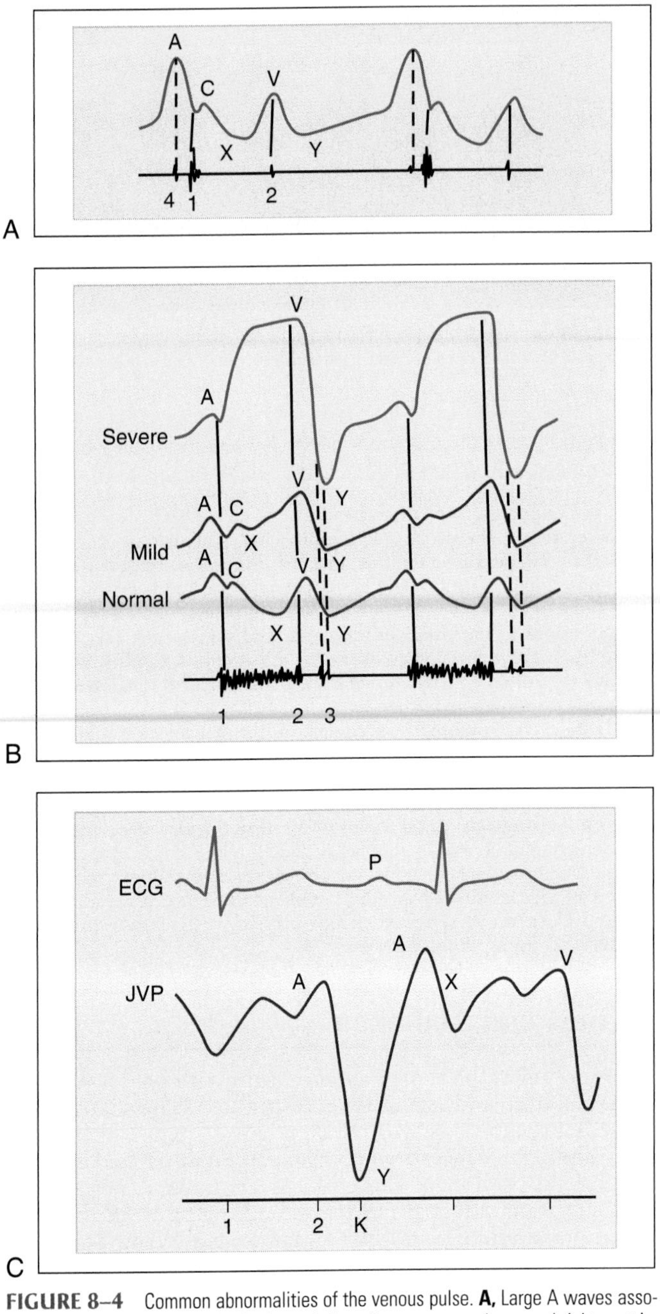

FIGURE 8–4 Common abnormalities of the venous pulse. **A,** Large A waves associated with elevated right ventricular end-diastolic pressure or decreased right ventricular compliance. Increased A wave size or giant A waves are seen when there is severe right ventricular hypertrophy, usually associated with right ventricular systolic hypertension. A right ventricular S4 is often present in such cases. **B,** Augmented V wave in tricuspid regurgitation. As reflux across the tricuspid valve increases in severity, the systolic V valve becomes higher as well as broader. The X descent disappears and the Y descent is progressively accentuated with increasing severity of tricuspid regurgitation. With severe tricuspid regurgitation, the systolic wave may be so dominant as to mimic the carotid arterial pulsations; the entire lower neck will swell with each right ventricular systole. **C,** Constrictive pericarditis. In this condition, right ventricular diastolic pressure is greatly elevated. This elevation results in a prominent Y descent following tricuspid valve opening. The abrupt rise in venous pressure during right ventricular filling is due to the noncompliant right ventricular chamber encased in an unyielding pericardial shell. The venous pulse contour in constrictive pericarditis often takes on an M or W configuration. A pericardial knock (K), a high-frequency early diastolic filling sound, typically is present. (From Abrams J: Synopsis of Cardiac Physical Diagnosis. 2nd ed. Boston, Butterworth Heinemann, 2001, pp 23-35.)

prominence of both A and V waves. A steeply rising H wave is observed (or recorded) in patients with restrictive cardiomyopathy, constrictive pericarditis, and right ventricular infarction. The X descent may be prominent in patients with large A waves, as well as in patients with right ventricular volume overload (atrial septal defect).

Constrictive pericarditis (see Fig. 8–4C) is characterized by a rapid and deep Y descent followed by a rapid rise to a diastolic plateau (H wave) without a prominent A wave; occasionally, the X descent is prominent in patients with this condition as well, causing a W-shaped jugular venous pulse. However, it is in patients with cardiac tamponade that the X descent is most prominent. A prominent V wave or a C-V wave (i.e., fusion of the C and V waves in the absence or attenuation of an X descent) occurs in patients with tricuspid regurgitation, sometimes causing a systolic movement of the earlobe (see Fig. 8–4B, *center*) and a right-to-left head movement with each ventricular systole. Equal A and V waves are seen in patients with atrial septal defect; the Y descent is gradual when right atrial emptying is impeded, as in tricuspid stenosis, and rapid when it is unimpeded, as in tricuspid regurgitation. A steep Y descent is seen in patients with any condition in which there is myocardial dysfunction, ventricular dilatation, and an elevated central venous pressure.

Sphygmomanometric Measurement of Arterial Pressure

One can estimate systolic arterial pressure without a sphygmomanometer by gradually compressing the brachial artery while palpating the radial artery; the force required to obliterate the radial pulse represents the systolic blood pressure, and, with practice, one can often estimate this level within 15 mm Hg. Ordinarily, however, a sphygmomanometer is used to obtain an indirect measurement of arterial pressure. The cuff should fit snugly around the arm, with its lower edge at least 1 inch above the antecubital space, and the diaphragm of the stethoscope should be placed close to or under the edge of the sphygmomanometer cuff. The width of the cuff selected should be at least 40 percent of the circumference of the limb to be used.

The standard size, with a 5-inch-wide cuff, is designed for adults with an arm of average size. When this cuff is applied to a large upper arm or a normal adult thigh, arterial pressure is overestimated, leading to spurious hypertension in the obese patient (arm circumference >35 cm)[22]; when it is applied to a small arm, the pressure is underestimated. The cuff width should be approximately 1.5 inches in infants and small children, 3 inches in young children (2 to 5 years), and 8 inches in obese adults. The rubber bag should be long enough to extend at least halfway around the limb (10 inches in adults). In patients with rigid, sclerotic arteries, the systolic pressure may also be overestimated, by as much as 30 mm Hg. Mercury manometers are, in general, more accurate and reliable than the aneroid type; the latter should be calibrated at least once yearly.

BLOOD PRESSURE IN THE UPPER EXTREMITIES. To measure arterial pressure in an upper extremity,[23,24] the patient should be seated or lying comfortably and relaxed, the arm should be slightly flexed and at heart level, and the arm muscles should be relaxed. The cuff should be inflated rapidly to approximately 30 mm Hg above the anticipated systolic pressure. The cuff is then deflated slowly, no faster than 3 mm Hg/sec; the pressure at which the brachial pulse can be palpated is close to the systolic pressure.

The cuff should be deflated rapidly after the diastolic pressure is noted and a full minute allowed to elapse before pressure is remeasured in the same limb. Although excessive pressure on the stethoscope head does not affect systolic pressure, it does erroneously lower diastolic readings.

BLOOD PRESSURE IN THE LOWER EXTREMITIES. With the patient lying on the abdomen, an 8-inch-wide cuff should be applied with the compression bag over the posterior aspect of the mid-thigh and should be rolled diagonally around the thigh to keep the edges snug against the skin. Auscultation should be carried out in the popliteal fossa. To measure pressure in the lower leg, an arm cuff is placed over the calf and auscultation is carried out over the posterior tibial artery. Regardless of where the cuff is applied, care must be taken to avoid letting the rubber part of the balloon of the cuff extend beyond its covering and to avoid placing the cuff on so loosely that central ballooning occurs.

KOROTKOFF SOUNDS. There are five phases of Korotkoff sounds (i.e., sounds produced by the flow of blood as the constricting blood pressure cuff is gradually released). The first appearance of a clear, tapping sound (phase I) represents the systolic pressure. These sounds are replaced by soft murmurs during phase II and by louder murmurs during phase III, as the volume of blood flowing through the constricted artery increases. The sounds suddenly become muffled in phase IV, when constriction of the brachial artery diminishes as arterial diastolic pressure is approached. Korotkoff sounds disappear in phase V, which is usually within 10 mm Hg of phase IV.

Diastolic pressure measured directly through an intraarterial needle and external manometer corresponds closely to phase V. In cases of severe aortic regurgitation, however, when the disappearance point is extremely low, sometimes 0 mm Hg, the sound of muffling (phase IV) is much closer to the intraarterial diastolic pressure than is the disappearance point (phase V). When the difference between phases IV and V of the Korotkoff sounds exceeds 10 mm Hg, both pressures should be recorded (e.g., 142/54/10 mm Hg).

Korotkoff sounds may be difficult to hear and arterial pressure difficult to measure when arterial pressure rises at a slow rate (as in cases of severe aortic stenosis), when the arteries are markedly constricted (as in cases of shock), and when the stroke volume is reduced (as in cases of severe heart failure). Very soft or inaudible Korotkoff sounds can often be accentuated by having the patient dilate the blood vessels simply by opening and closing the fist repeatedly. Sometimes in states of shock, the indirect method of measuring blood pressure is unreliable and arterial pressure should be measured through an intraarterial needle.

The Auscultatory Gap. The auscultatory gap is a silence that sometimes separates the first appearance of the Korotkoff sounds from their second appearance at a lower pressure. The phenomenon tends to occur when there is venous distention or reduced velocity of arterial flow into the arm. If the first muffling of sounds is considered to be the diastolic pressure, it will be overestimated. If the second appearance is taken as the systolic pressure, it will be underestimated. On the other hand, sounds transmitted through the arterial tree from prosthetic aortic valves may be responsible for falsely high readings.

BLOOD PRESSURE IN THE BASAL CONDITION. To determine arterial pressure in the basal condition, the patient should have rested in a quiet room for 5 to 10 minutes. It is desirable to record the arterial pressure in both arms at the time of the initial examination; differences in systolic pressure between the two arms that exceed 10 mm Hg when measurements are made simultaneously or in rapid sequence[24] suggest obstructive lesions involving the aorta or the origin of the innominate and subclavian arteries or supravalvular aortic stenosis (in which pressure in the right arm exceeds that in the left). In patients with vertebral-basal artery insufficiency, a difference in pressure between the arms may signify that a subclavian "steal" is responsible for the cerebrovascular symptoms.

To be certain from physical examination that the systolic pressure is different in the two arms or in the upper and lower extremities, two examiners should measure the pressures simultaneously and then switch extremities and measure the pressures again.

ORTHOSTATIC HYPOTENSION. To determine whether orthostatic hypotension is present, arterial pressure should be determined with the patient in both the supine and the erect positions. Regardless of the patient's posture, however, the brachial artery should be at the level of the heart to avoid superimposition of the effects of gravity on the recorded pressure.

Normally, the systolic pressure in the legs is up to 20 mm Hg higher than in the arms, but the diastolic pressures are usually virtually identical. The recording of a higher diastolic pressure in the legs than in the arms suggests that the thigh cuff is too small. When systolic pressure in the popliteal artery exceeds that in the brachial artery by more than 20 mm Hg (Hill sign), aortic regurgitation is usually present.[25] Blood pressure should be measured in the lower extremities in patients with hypertension to detect coarctation of the aorta or when obstructive disease of the aorta or its immediate branches is suspected.

Arterial Pulse

The volume and contour of the arterial pulse are determined by a combination of factors, including the left ventricular stroke volume, the ejection velocity, the relative compliance and capacity of the arterial system, and the pressure waves that result from the antegrade flow of blood and reflections of the arterial pressure pulse returning from the peripheral circulation (Table 8–1).[25,26] Bilateral palpation of the carotid, radial, brachial, femoral, popliteal, dorsalis pedis, and posterior tibial pulses should be part of the examination of all cardiac patients (Fig. 8–5). The frequency, regularity, and shape of the pulse wave and the character of the arterial wall should be determined.

The carotid pulse provides the most accurate representation of the central aortic pulse.[26,27] The brachial artery is the vessel ordinarily most suitable for appreciating the rate of rise of the pulse and the contour, volume, and consistency of the peripheral vessels. This artery is located at the medial aspect of the elbow, and it may be helpful to flex the patient's arm to improve palpation; palpation of the artery should be carried out with the thumb exerting pressure on the artery until its maximal movement is detected. A normal rate of rise of the arterial pulse suggests that there is no obstruction to left ventricular outflow, whereas a pulse wave of small amplitude with normal configuration suggests a reduced stroke volume.

THE NORMAL PULSE. The pulse in the ascending aorta normally rises rapidly to a rounded dome (Fig. 8–6); this initial rise reflects the peak velocity of blood ejected from the left ventricle. A slight anacrotic notch or pause is frequently recorded, but only occasionally felt, on the ascending limb of the pulse. The descending limb of the central aortic pulse is less steep than is the ascending limb, and it is interrupted by the incisura, a sharp downward deflection related to closure of the aortic valve. Immediately thereafter, the pulse wave

TABLE 8–1 Classification of Abnormal Pulses

Name	Meaning	Comments
General Abnormalities		
Hypokinetic	Related to a decreased rate of LV pressure development, a decreased LV stroke volume, and/or obstruction of LV outflow	Low amplitude, may or may not have a slow rate of rise
Hyperkinetic	Related to an increased rate of LV pressure development and/or to a large LV stroke volume with decreased peripheral resistance	Prominent fluctuation in the diameter of an artery Pulse pressure can be: Increased (aortic regurgitation, patent ductus arteriosus, arteriovenous fistulas, fever, anemia, exercise) Normal (HOCM, MR)
Specific Abnormalities		
Pulsus parvus et tardus	Pulse with slow rate of pressure increase, small pulse pressure, late	AS
Bisferiens pulse	A pulse with two palpable beats during systole	Occurs in HOCM and in mixed AS/AR. Can also occur in cases of rapid ejection of an increased stroke volume (e.g., exercise, fever, patent ductus arteriosus) Best appreciated in the carotid artery
Dicrotic pulse	A twice-beating or double pulse produced by a combination of the systolic wave followed by an exaggerated dicrotic (diastolic) wave	Low-volume pulse, with shortened ejection period. Observed both in central and peripheral arteries. Observed in cases of cardiac tamponade, hypovolemic shock, severe cardiac failure
Pulsus alternans	Beats occur at constant intervals but with a regular alternation of the peak of the pressure pulse and/or the rate of rise of the ascending limb.	Strong and weak pulses occur in consecutive beats. Pulses alternate in systolic pressure by ≥20 mm Hg Caused by alternating strength of cardiac contraction with consecutive beats, signifies severely depressed cardiac function Best palpated in radial or femoral artery
Bigeminal pulse	Regular coupling of two beats with the interval between a pair of beats greater than between the coupled beats themselves.	Observed with premature ectopic beats coupled to a sinus beat, 3 : 2 Wenckebach atrioventricular block and nonconducted atrial premature systole following every second sinus beat
Pulsus paradoxus	Abnormal exaggeration (>10 mm Hg) of the normal decrease in systolic blood pressure during inspiration	Observed in cases of cardiac tamponade, constrictive pericarditis, restrictive cardiomyopathy, hypotensive shock, severe obstructive pulmonary disease, large pulmonary embolism

AR = aortic regurgitation; AS = aortic stenosis; HOCM = hypertrophic obstructive cardiomyopathy; LV = left ventricular; MR = mitral regurgitation.
Modified from Vlachopoulos C, O'Rourke M: Genesis of the normal and abnormal pulse. Curr Prob Cardiol 25:297, 2000.

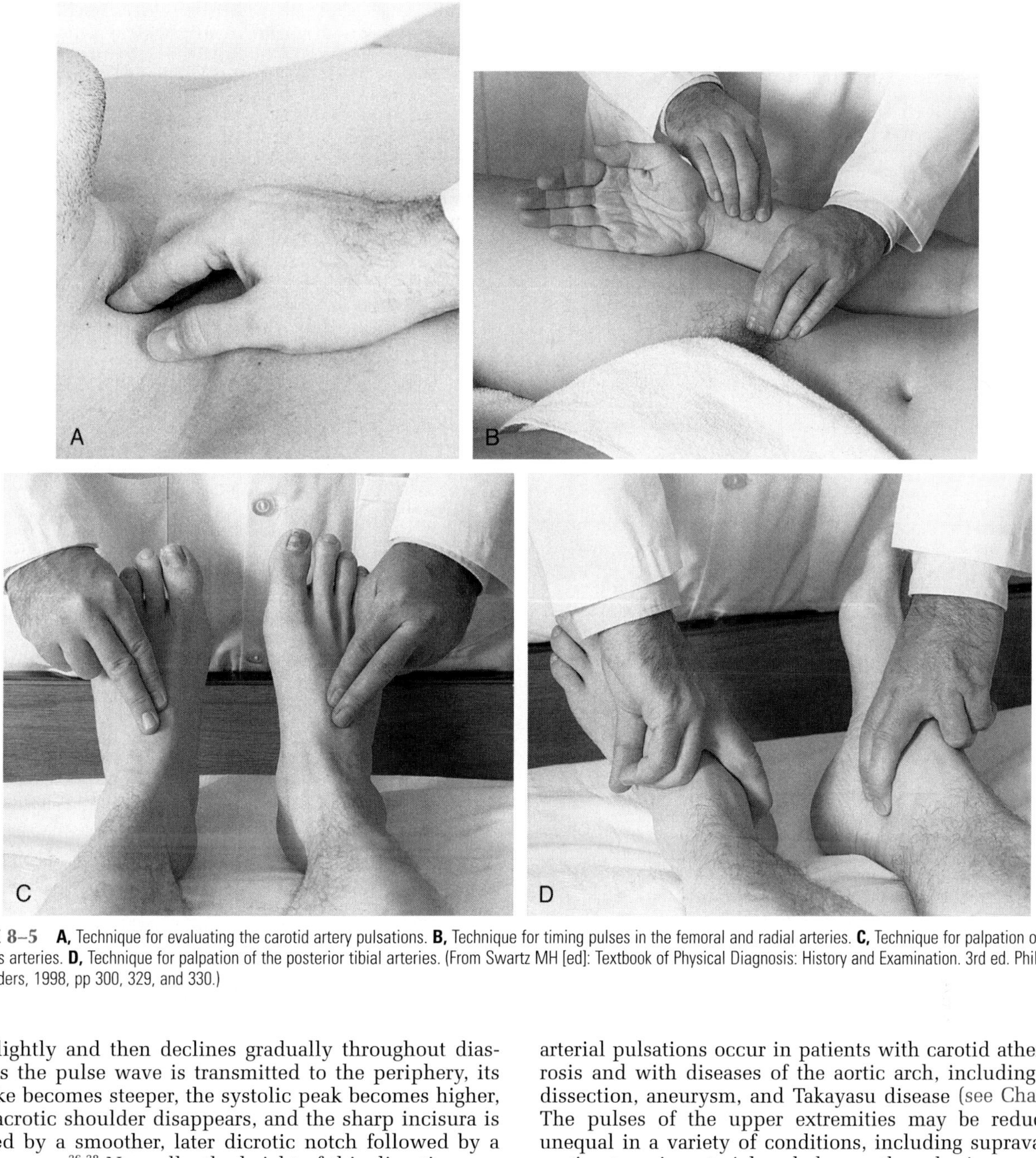

FIGURE 8–5 **A,** Technique for evaluating the carotid artery pulsations. **B,** Technique for timing pulses in the femoral and radial arteries. **C,** Technique for palpation of the dorsalis pedis arteries. **D,** Technique for palpation of the posterior tibial arteries. (From Swartz MH [ed]: Textbook of Physical Diagnosis: History and Examination. 3rd ed. Philadelphia, WB Saunders, 1998, pp 300, 329, and 330.)

rises slightly and then declines gradually throughout diastole. As the pulse wave is transmitted to the periphery, its upstroke becomes steeper, the systolic peak becomes higher, the anacrotic shoulder disappears, and the sharp incisura is replaced by a smoother, later dicrotic notch followed by a dicrotic wave.[26-28] Normally, the height of this dicrotic wave diminishes with age, hypertension, and arteriosclerosis. In the central arterial pulse (central aorta and innominate and carotid arteries), the rapidly transmitted impact of left ventricular ejection results in a peak in early systole, referred to as the *percussion wave;* a second, smaller peak, the *tidal wave,* presumed to represent a reflected wave from the periphery, can often be recorded but is not normally palpable. In older subjects, however, particularly those with increased peripheral resistance, as well as in patients with arteriosclerosis and diabetes, the tidal wave may be somewhat higher than the percussion wave; that is, the pulse reaches a peak in late systole. In peripheral arteries, the pulse wave normally has a single sharp peak.

ABNORMAL PULSES. When peripheral vascular resistance and arterial stiffness are increased, as in patients with hypertension or with the increased arterial stiffness that accompanies normal aging, there is an elevation in pulse wave velocity and the pulse contour has a more rapid upstroke and greater amplitude.[29] Reduced or unequal carotid arterial pulsations occur in patients with carotid atherosclerosis and with diseases of the aortic arch, including aortic dissection, aneurysm, and Takayasu disease (see Chap. 53). The pulses of the upper extremities may be reduced or unequal in a variety of conditions, including supravalvular aortic stenosis, arterial embolus or thrombosis, anomalous origin or aberrant path of the major vessels, and cervical rib or scalenus anticus syndrome. Asymmetry of right and left popliteal pulses is characteristic of iliofemoral obstruction. Weakness or absence of radial, posterior tibial, or dorsalis pedis pulses on one side suggests arterial insufficiency. In cases of coarctation of the aorta, the carotid and brachial pulses are bounding, rise rapidly, and have large volumes, whereas in the lower extremities, the systolic and pulse pressures are reduced, their rate of rise is slow, and there is a late peak. This delay in the femoral arterial pulses can usually be readily detected by simultaneous palpation of the femoral and brachial arterial pulses (see Fig. 8–5B).

In patients with fixed obstruction to left ventricular outflow (valvular aortic stenosis and congenital fibrous subaortic stenosis), the carotid pulse rises slowly (pulsus tardus) (see Fig. 8–6B); the upstroke is frequently characterized by a thrill (the carotid shudder); and the peak is reduced, occurs late in systole, and is sustained. There is a notch on the upstroke of the carotid pulse (anacrotic notch) that is so

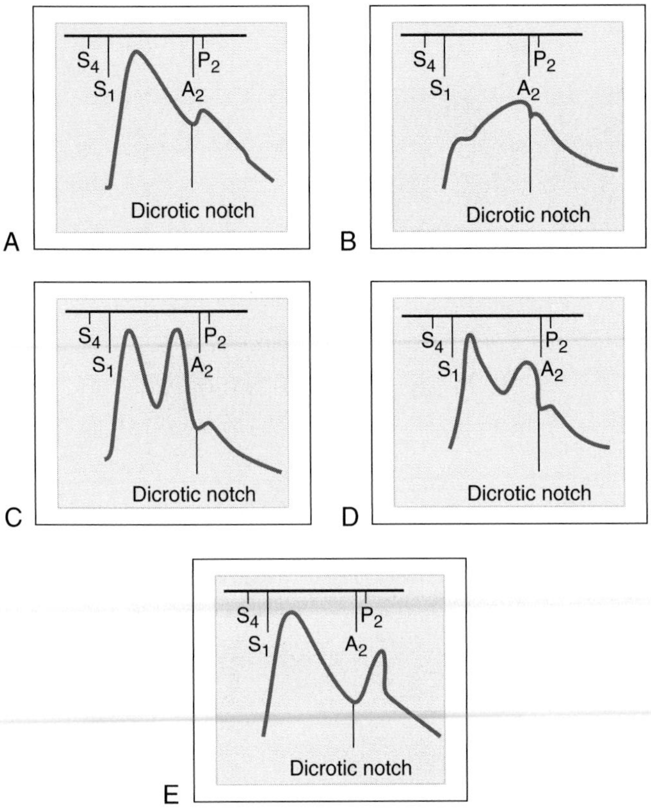

FIGURE 8–6 Schematic diagrams of the configurational changes in carotid pulse and their differential diagnoses. Heart sounds are also illustrated. **A,** Normal. **B,** Anacrotic pulse with a slow initial upstroke. The peak is close to S_2. These features suggest fixed left ventricular outflow obstruction, such as occurs with valvular aortic stenosis. **C,** Pulsus bisferiens with both percussion and tidal waves occurring during systole. This type of carotid pulse contour is most frequently observed in patients with hemodynamically significant aortic regurgitation or combined aortic stenosis and regurgitation with dominant regurgitation. It is rarely observed in patients with mitral valve prolapse or in normal individuals. **D,** Pulsus bisferiens in hypertrophic obstructive cardiomyopathy. It is rarely appreciated at the bedside by palpation. **E,** A dicrotic pulse results from an accentuated dicrotic wave and tends to occur in patients with sepsis, severe heart failure, hypovolemic shock, cardiac tamponade, and aortic valve replacement. A_2 = aortic component of the second heart sound; P_2 = pulmonic component of the second heart sound; S_1 = first heart sound; S_4 = atrial sound. (From Chatterjee K: Bedside evaluation of the heart: The physical examination. *In* Chatterjee K, Parmley W [eds]: Cardiology: An Illustrated Text/Reference. Philadelphia, JB Lippincott, 1991, pp 3.11-3.51; and Braunwald E: The clinical examination. *In* Braunwald E, Goldman L [eds]: Primary Cardiology. 2nd ed. Philadelphia, Elsevier, 2003, pp 36.)

distinct that two separate waves can be palpated in what is termed an *anacrotic pulse. Pulsus parvus* is a pulse of small amplitude, usually because of a reduction of stroke volume. *Pulsus parvus et tardus* refers to a small pulse with a delayed systolic peak, which is characteristic of severe aortic stenosis. This type of pulse is more readily appreciated by palpating the carotid rather than a more peripheral artery. Patients with severe aortic stenosis and heart failure usually exhibit simply a reduced pulse amplitude (i.e., pulsus parvus), and the delay in the upstroke is not readily apparent. However, this delay is readily recorded. In elderly patients with inelastic peripheral arteries, the pulse may rise normally despite the presence of aortic stenosis.

The carotid arterial pulse may be prominent or exaggerated in a patient with any condition in which pulse pressure is increased, including anxiety, the hyperkinetic heart syndrome, anemia, fever, pregnancy, or other high cardiac output states (see Chap. 22), as well as in patients with bradycardia and peripheral arteriosclerosis with reduction in arterial distensibility. In patients with mitral regurgitation or ventricular septal defect, the forward stroke volume (from the left ventricle into the aorta) is usually normal but the fraction ejected during early systole is greater than normal; hence, the arterial pulse is of normal volume (the pulse pressure is normal) but the pulse may rise abnormally rapidly.[30] Exaggerated or bounding arterial pulses may be observed in patients with an elevated stroke volume, with sympathetic hyperactivity, and in patients with a rigid, sclerotic aorta. In patients with aortic regurgitation, there is a very brisk rate of rise with an increased pulse pressure.

AORTIC REGURGITATION. The *Corrigan* or *water-hammer pulse* of aortic regurgitation consists of an abrupt upstroke (percussion wave) followed by rapid collapse later in systole but no dicrotic notch. Corrigan pulse reflects a low resistance in the reservoir into which the left ventricle rapidly discharges an abnormally elevated stroke volume, and it can be exaggerated by raising the patient's arm. In cases of acute aortic regurgitation, the left ventricle may not be significantly dilated, and premature closure of the mitral valve may occur and limit the volume of aortic reflux; therefore, the aortic diastolic pressure may not be very low, the arterial pulse not bounding, and the pulse pressure not widened despite a serious abnormality of valve function (see Chap. 57).

Signs characteristic of severe chronic aortic regurgitation include "pistol shot" sounds heard over the femoral artery when the stethoscope is placed on it (Traube sign); a systolic murmur heard over the femoral artery when the artery is gradually compressed proximally; a diastolic murmur when the artery is compressed distally (Duroziez sign[25]), and Quincke sign (phasic blanching of the nail bed). Of these, Duroziez sign is the most predictive of severe aortic regurgitation. Bounding arterial pulses are also present in patients with patent ductus arteriosus or large arteriovenous fistulas; those in hyperkinetic states such as thyrotoxicosis, pregnancy, fever, and anemia; those in severe bradycardia; and in arteries proximal to coarctation of the aorta. In patients with the Hill sign[25] of aortic regurgitation (or any condition leading to an increased stroke volume or the hyperkinetic circulatory state), the indirectly recorded systolic pressures in the lower extremities exceed that in the arms by more than 20 mm Hg. Other signs of increased pulse pressure include Becker sign (visible pulsations of the retinal arterioles) and Mueller sign (pulsating uvula).

BISFERIENS PULSE. A bisferiens pulse (see Fig. 8–6C) is characterized by two systolic peaks, the percussion and tidal waves, separated by a distinct midsystolic dip; the peaks may be equal, or either one may be larger. This type of pulse is detected most readily by palpation of the carotid and, less commonly, of the brachial arteries. It occurs in conditions in which a large stroke volume is ejected rapidly[31] and is observed most commonly in patients with pure aortic regurgitation or with a combination of aortic regurgitation and stenosis; it may disappear as heart failure supervenes (see Fig 8–6D).[26,31]

A bisferiens pulse also occurs in patients with hypertrophic obstructive cardiomyopathy, but the bifid nature may only be recorded, not palpated; on palpation, there may merely be a rapid upstroke. In these patients, the initial prominent percussion wave is associated with rapid ejection of blood into the aorta during early systole, followed by a rapid decline as obstruction becomes manifest in midsystole and by a tidal (reflected) wave. In some patients with hypertrophic cardiomyopathy with no or little obstruction to left ventricular outflow, the arterial pulse is normal or simply hyperkinetic in the basal state, but obstruction and a bisferiens pulse can be elicited by means of the Valsalva maneuver or inhalation of amyl nitrite. Occasionally, a bisferiens pulse is observed in patients in hyperkinetic circulatory states, and very rarely it occurs in normal individuals.

DICROTIC PULSE. Not to be confused with a bisferiens pulse, in which both peaks occur in systole, is a dicrotic pulse, in which the second peak is in diastole immediately after S_2 (see Fig. 8–6E).[27-29,31-33] The normally small wave that follows aortic valve closure (i.e., the dicrotic notch) is exaggerated and measures more than 50 percent of the pulse pressure on direct pressure recordings and in which the dicrotic notch is low (i.e., near the diastolic pressure). A dicrotic wave may be present in normal hypotensive subjects with reduced peripheral resistance, as occurs in fever, and it may be elicited or exaggerated by inhalation alone or the inhalation of amyl nitrite. Rarely, a dicrotic pulse is noted in healthy adolescents or young adults, but it usually occurs in conditions such as cardiac tamponade,[29] severe heart failure, and hypovolemic shock, in which a low stroke volume is ejected into a soft elastic aorta. In patients with these conditions, the dicrotic pulse is due to a reduction of the systolic wave with preservation of the incisura.

PULSUS ALTERNANS (ALTERNATING STRONG AND WEAK PULSES). Mechanical alternans is a sign of depression of left ventricular function (see Chap. 22).[34,35] Although more readily recognized on sphygmomanometry, when the systolic pressure alternates by more than 20 mm Hg, pulsus alternans can be detected by palpation of a peripheral (femoral or brachial) pulse more frequently than by a more central pulse. Palpation should be carried out with light pressure and with the patient's breath held in mid-expiration to avoid the superimposition of respiratory variation on the amplitude of the pulse. Pulsus alternans is generally accompanied by alternation in the intensity of the Korotkoff sounds and occasionally by alternation in intensity of the heart sounds. Rarely, pulsus alternans is so marked that the weak beat is not perceived at all.[36] Aortic regurgitation, systemic hypertension, and reducing venous return by administration of nitroglycerin or by tilting the patient into the upright position all exaggerate pulsus alternans and assist in its detection. Pulsus alternans, which is frequently precipitated by a premature ventricular contraction, is characterized by a regular rhythm and must be distinguished from pulsus bigeminus, which is usually irregular.

PULSUS BIGEMINUS. A bigeminal rhythm is caused by the occurrence of premature contractions, usually ventricular, after every other beat and results in alternation of the strength of the pulse, which can be confused with pulsus alternans. However, in contrast to the pulsus alternans, in which the rhythm is regular, in pulsus bigeminus the weak beat always follows the shorter interval. In normal persons or in patients with fixed obstruction to left ventricular outflow, the compensatory pause after a premature beat is followed by a stronger-than-normal pulse. In patients with hypertrophic obstructive cardiomyopathy, however, the post-premature ventricular contraction beat is weaker than normal because of increased obstruction to left ventricular outflow (see Chap. 59).[37]

PULSUS PARADOXUS. Pulsus paradoxus is an exaggerated reduction in the strength of the arterial pulse during normal inspiration due to an exaggerated inspiratory fall in systolic pressure (more than 10 mm Hg during quiet breathing) (see Chap. 64). When marked (i.e., an inspiratory reduction of pressure greater than 20 mm Hg), the paradoxical pulse can be detected by simple palpation of the brachial arterial pulse[38]; in severe cases, there is inspiratory disappearance of the pulse. Milder degrees of a paradoxical pulse can be readily detected on sphygmomanometry: the cuff is inflated to suprasystolic levels and is deflated slowly at a rate of about 2 mm Hg per heartbeat; the peak systolic pressure during exhalation is noted.[39,40] The cuff is then deflated even more slowly, and the pressure is again noted when Korotkoff sounds become audible throughout the respiratory cycle. Normally, the difference between the two pressures should not exceed 10 mm Hg during quiet respiration. (Pulsus alternans can also be detected by this maneuver by noting whether peak systolic pressure or the intensity of the Korotkoff sounds alternates when the breath is held.)

Pulsus paradoxus represents an exaggeration of the normal decline in systolic arterial pressure with inspiration. It results from the reduced left ventricular stroke volume and the transmission of negative intrathoracic pressure to the aorta. It is a frequent, indeed characteristic, finding in patients with cardiac tamponade,[41,42] occurs less frequently (in about half) in patients with chronic constrictive pericarditis,[19] and is also observed in patients with emphysema and bronchial asthma (who have wide respiratory swings of intrapleural pressure),[39] as well as in patients with hypovolemic shock, pulmonary embolus, pregnancy, and extreme obesity. Aortic regurgitation tends to prevent the development of pulsus paradoxus despite the presence of cardiac tamponade. Reversed pulsus paradoxus (an inspiratory rise in arterial pressure) may occur in hypertrophic obstructive cardiomyopathy.

THE ARTERIAL PULSE IN VASCULAR DISEASE (see Chap. 54). Examination of the arterial pulses is of critical importance in the diagnosis of extracardiac obstructive arterial disease. Systematic bilateral palpation of the common carotid, brachial, radial, femoral, popliteal, dorsalis pedis,[42] and posterior tibial vessels (see Fig. 8–5C and D), as well as palpation of the abdominal aorta (both above and below the umbilicus), should be part of every examination in patients suspected of having ischemic heart disease.[43] A normal aorta is often palpable above the umbilicus, but a palpable aorta below the umbilicus suggests the presence of an aneurysm of the abdominal aorta. To diminish cold-induced vasoconstriction, peripheral pulses should be palpated after the patient has been in a warm room for at least 20 minutes. Absent or weak peripheral pulses usually signify obstruction. However, the dorsalis pedis and posterior tibial arteries may be absent in approximately 2 percent of normal persons because they pursue an aberrant course.

Arterial bruits should be sought at specific anatomical sites. When the lumen diameter is reduced by approximately 50 percent, a soft short systolic bruit is heard; as the obstruction becomes more severe, the bruit becomes high pitched, louder, and longer. With approximately 80 percent diameter reduction, the murmur spills into early diastole, but it disappears with more severe stenosis or complete occlusion. Arterial bruits are augmented by elevation of the cardiac output (e.g., as occurs in patients with anemia), by poor development of collaterals, and by increased arterial outflow (as occurs with regional exercise).

The Cardiac Examination

Inspection

The cardiac examination proper should commence with inspection of the chest, which can usually best be accomplished with the examiner standing at the side or foot of the bed or examining table.[4] Respirations—their frequency, regularity, and depth—as well as the relative effort required during inspiration and exhalation, should be noted. Simultaneously, one should search for cutaneous abnormalities, such as spider nevi (seen in patients with hepatic cirrhosis and Osler-Weber-Rendu disease). Dilation of veins on the anterior chest wall with caudal flow suggests obstruction of the superior vena cava, whereas cranial flow occurs in patients with obstruction of the inferior vena cava. Precordial prominence is most striking if cardiac enlargement developed before puberty, but it may also be present, although to a lesser extent, in patients in whom cardiomegaly developed in adult life, after the period of thoracic growth.

A heavy muscular thorax, contrasting to less developed lower extremities, can occur in patients with coarctation of the aorta, in which collateral arteries may be visible in the axillae and along the lateral chest wall. The upper portion of the thorax exhibits symmetrical bulging in children with stiff lungs in whom the inspiratory effort is increased. A "shield chest" is a broad chest in which the angle between the manubrium and the body of the sternum is greater than normal, and it is associated with widely separated nipples; shield chest is frequently observed in patients with Turner and Noonan syndromes (see Chap. 56). Careful note should be made of other deformities of the thoracic cage, such as kyphoscoliosis, which may be responsible for cor pulmonale (see Chap. 67); and ankylosing spondylitis, sometimes associated with aortic regurgitation (see Chap. 82).

Pectus excavatum,[15,16] a condition in which the sternum is displaced posteriorly, is commonly observed in patients with Marfan syndrome, homocystinuria, Ehlers-Danlos syndrome, and Hunter-Hurler syndrome and in a small fraction of patients with mitral valve prolapse. This thoracic deformity rarely compresses the heart or elevates the systemic and pulmonary venous pressures, and the signs of heart disease are more often apparent rather than real.[44] Displacement of the heart into the left thorax, prominence of the pulmonary artery, and a parasternal midsystolic murmur, all key features of this deformity, may falsely suggest the presence of organic heart disease. Lack of normal thoracic kyphosis (i.e., the straight back syndrome) is often associated with expiratory splitting of S_2, a parasternal midsystolic murmur, and prominence of the pulmonary artery on radiography.

CARDIOVASCULAR PULSATIONS. Cardiovascular pulsations should be looked for on the entire chest but specifically in the regions of the cardiac apex, the left parasternal region, and the third left and second right intercostal spaces. Prominent pulsations in these areas suggest enlargement of the left ventricle, right ventricle, pulmonary artery, and aorta, respectively. A thrusting apex exceeding 2 cm in diameter suggests left ventricular enlargement; systolic retraction of the apex may be visible in cases of constrictive pericarditis. Normally, cardiac pulsations are not visible lateral to the midclavicular line; when present there, they signify cardiac enlargement unless there is thoracic deformity or congenital absence of the pericardium. Shaking of the entire precordium with each heartbeat can occur in patients with severe valvular regurgitation, large left-to-right shunts, especially patent ductus arteriosus, complete AV block, hypertrophic obstructive cardiomyopathy, and various hyperkinetic states. Aortic aneurysms may produce visible pulsations of one of the sternoclavicular joints of the right anterior thoracic wall.

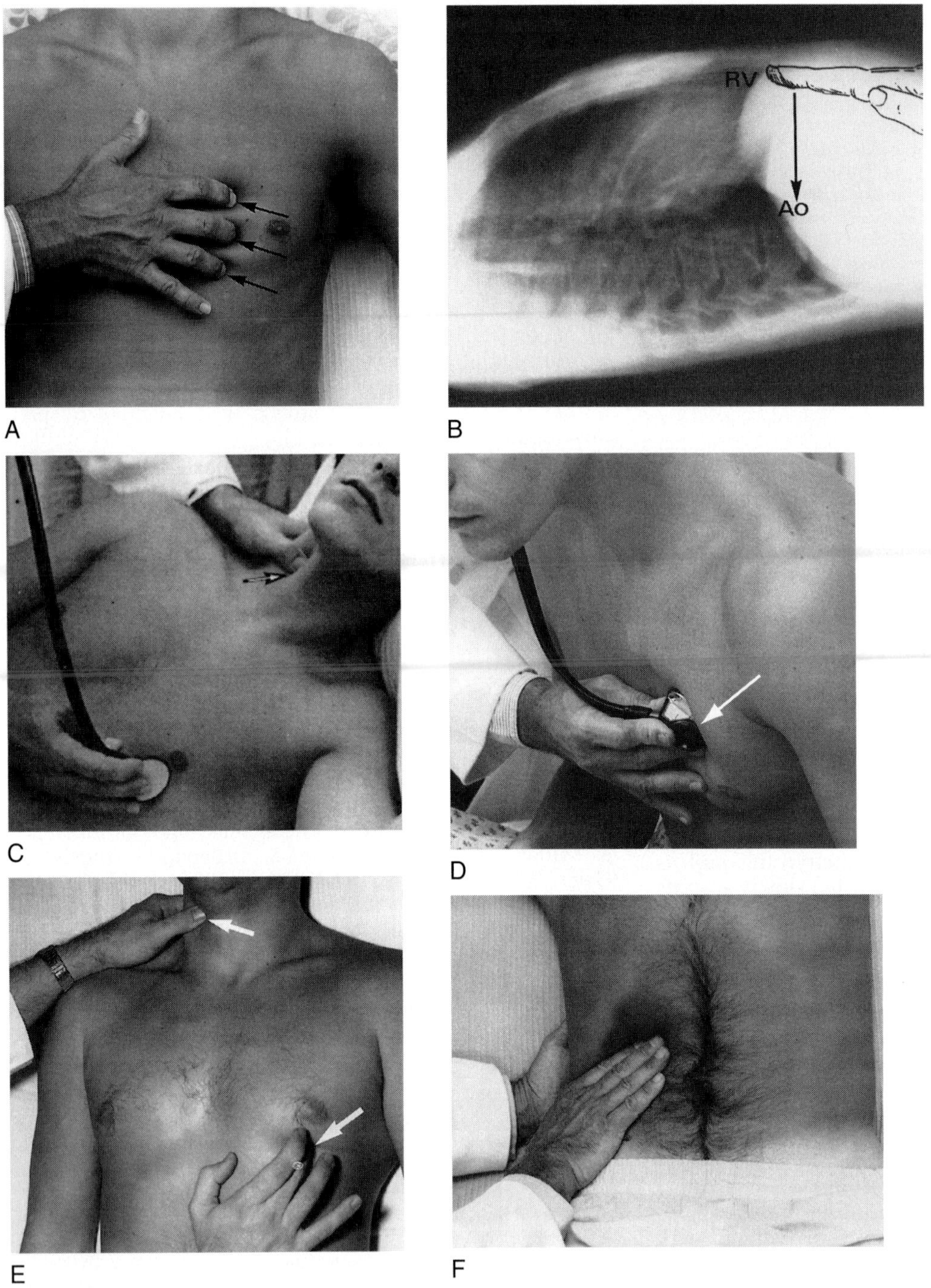

FIGURE 8–7 **A,** Palpation of the anterior wall of the right ventricle by applying the tips of three fingers in the third, fourth, and fifth interspaces, and left sternal edge (arrows), during full held exhalation. Patient is supine with the trunk elevated 30 degrees. **B,** Subxiphoid palpation of the inferior wall of the right ventricle (RV) with the relative position of the abdominal aorta (Ao) shown by the arrow. **C,** The bell of the stethoscope is applied to the cardiac apex while the patient lies in a partial left lateral decubitus position. The thumb of the examiner's free left hand is used to palpate the carotid artery for timing purposes. **D,** The soft, high-frequency early diastolic murmur of aortic regurgitation or pulmonary hypertensive regurgitation is best elicited by applying the stethoscopic diaphragm very firmly to the mid-left sternal edge. The patient leans forward with breath held in full exhalation. **E,** Palpation of the left ventricular impulse with a fingertip (arrow). The patient's trunk is 30 degrees above the horizontal. The examiner's right thumb palpates the carotid pulse for timing purposes. **F,** Palpation of the liver. The patient is supine with knees flexed to relax the abdomen. The flat of the examiner's right hand is placed on the right upper quadrant just below the expected inferior margin of the liver; the left hand is applied diametrically opposite. (From Perloff JK: Physical Examination of the Heart and Circulation. 3rd ed. Philadelphia, WB Saunders, 2000.)

Palpation

Pulsations of the heart and great arteries that are transmitted to the chest wall are best appreciated when the examiner is positioned on the right side of a supine patient. To palpate the movements of the heart and great arteries, the examiner should use the fingertips or the area just proximal thereto. Precordial movements should be timed with the simultaneously palpated carotid pulse or auscultated heart sounds.[45] The examination should be carried out with the chest completely exposed and elevated to 30 degrees, with the patient both supine and in the partial left lateral decubitus positions (Fig. 8–7).[2] Rotating the patient into the left lateral decubitus position with the left arm elevated over the head causes the heart to move laterally and increases the palpability of both normal and pathological thrusts of the left ventricle. The subxiphoid region, which allows palpation of the right ventricle, should be examined with the tip of the index finger during held inspiration. Obese, muscular, emphysematous, and elderly persons may have weak or undetectable cardiac pulsations in the absence of cardiac abnormality, and thoracic deformities (e.g., kyphoscoliosis, pectus excavatum) can alter the pulsations transmitted to the chest wall. In the course of cardiac palpation, precordial tenderness may be detected; this finding can result from costochondritis (Tietze syndrome) and can be an important indication that chest pain is not due to myocardial ischemia.

LEFT VENTRICLE. The left ventricular impulse, also referred to as the cardiac impulse, the apex beat, and the apical thrust, is normally produced by left ventricular contraction and is the lowest and most lateral point on the chest at which the cardiac impulse can be appreciated and is normally above the anatomical apex. Normally, the left ventricular impulse is medial and superior to the intersection of the left midclavicular line and the fifth intercostal space and is palpable as a single, brief outward motion. Although it may not be palpable in the supine position in as many as half of all normal subjects older than 50 years of age, the left ventricular impulse can usually be felt in the left lateral decubitus position. Displacement of the apex beat lateral to the midclavicular line or more than 10 cm lateral to the midsternal line is a sensitive but not specific indicator of left ventricular enlargement. However, when the patient is in the left lateral decubitus position, a palpable apical impulse that has a diameter of more than 3 cm is an accurate sign of left ventricular enlargement.[46] Thoracic deformities—particularly scoliosis, straight back, and pectus excavatum—can result in the lateral displacement of a normal-sized heart.

APEX CARDIOGRAM. This recording reflects the movement of the chest wall and represents the pulsation of the entire left ventricle. Its contour differs from what is perceived on palpation of the apex.

SYSTOLIC MOTION

During isovolumetric contraction, the heart normally rotates counterclockwise (as one faces the patient), and the lower anterior portion of the left ventricle strikes the anterior chest wall, causing a brief outward motion followed by medial retraction of the adjacent chest wall during ejection. The peak outward motion of the left ventricular impulse occurs simultaneously with, or just after, aortic valve opening; then the left ventricular apex moves inward. In asthenic persons, in patients with mild left ventricular enlargement, and in subjects with a normal left ventricle but an augmented stroke volume, as occurs in anxiety and other hyperkinetic states, and in cases of mitral or aortic regurgitation, the cardiac impulse may be overactive but with a normal contour; that is, the outward thrust during systole is exaggerated in amplitude but is not sustained during ejection.

HYPERTROPHY AND DILATATION. With moderate or severe left ventricular concentric hypertrophy, the outward systolic thrust persists throughout ejection, often lasting up to the second heart sound,[47] and this motion is accompanied by retraction of the left parasternal region. The left ventricular heave or lift, which is more prominent in patients with concentric hypertrophy than in those with left ventricular dilatation without volume overload, is characterized by a sustained outward movement of an area that is larger than the normal apex; that is, it is more than 2 to 3 cm in diameter. In patients with left ventricular enlargement, the systolic impulse is displaced laterally and downward into the sixth or seventh interspaces. In patients with volume overload and/or sympathetic stimulation, the left ventricular impulse is hyperkinetic; that is, it is brisker and larger than normal.

OTHER CONDITIONS. Left ventricular aneurysm produces a larger-than-normal area of pulsation of the left ventricular apex. Alternatively, it may produce a sustained systolic bulge several centimeters superior to the left ventricular impulse, sometimes termed an *ectopic impulse*.

A double systolic outward thrust of the left ventricle is characteristic of patients with hypertrophic obstructive cardiomyopathy (see Chap. 54), who may also often exhibit a typical presystolic cardiac expansion, thus resulting in three separate outward movements of the chest wall during each cardiac cycle.[48] Constrictive pericarditis is characterized by systolic retraction of the chest, particularly of the ribs in the left axilla (Broadbent sign).

DIASTOLIC MOTION

The outward motion of the apex characteristic of rapid left ventricular diastolic filling is most readily palpated with the patient in the left lateral decubitus position and in full exhalation. The outward motion is accentuated when the inflow of blood into the left ventricle is accelerated. This occurs in cases of mitral regurgitation, when the volume of the left ventricle is increased or when its function is impaired.[4] This motion is the mechanical equivalent of and occurs simultaneously with a third heart sound (S_3).

PRESYSTOLIC EXPANSION. When the atrial contribution to ventricular filling is augmented, as occurs in patients with reduced left ventricular compliance associated with concentric left ventricular hypertrophy, myocardial ischemia, and myocardial fibrosis, a presystolic pulsation (usually accompanying a fourth heart sound [S_4]) is palpable, resulting in a double outward movement of the left ventricular impulse. This presystolic expansion is most readily discernible during exhalation, when the patient is in the left lateral decubitus position, and it can be confirmed by detecting the motion of the stethoscope placed over the left ventricular impulse or by observing the motion of an X mark over the left ventricular impulse. Presystolic expansion of the left ventricle can be enhanced by sustained handgrip. In patients with ischemic heart disease, presystolic pulsation is usually associated with a reduction in left ventricular compliance.

RIGHT VENTRICLE

Except in the first few months of life, the right ventricle normally is not palpable. A palpable anterior systolic movement (replacing systolic retraction) in the left parasternal region, best felt by the proximal palm or fingertips and with the patient supine, usually represents right ventricular enlargement or hypertrophy.[4] In patients with pulmonary emphysema, even an enlarged right ventricle is not readily palpable at the left sternal edge but is better appreciated in the subxiphoid region. Exaggerated motion of the entire parasternal area (i.e., a hyperdynamic impulse with normal contour) usually reflects increased right ventricular stroke volume, as occurs in patients with atrial septal defect or tricuspid regurgitation.

PULMONARY ARTERY

Pulmonary hypertension and increased pulmonary blood flow frequently produce a prominent systolic pulsation of the pulmonary trunk in the second intercostal space just to the left of the sternum. This pulsation is often associated with a prominent left parasternal impulse, reflecting right ventricular enlargement, or with hypertrophy and a palpable shock synchronous with the second heart sound, reflecting forceful closure of the pulmonic valve.

LEFT ATRIUM

An enlarged left atrium or a large posterior left ventricular aneurysm can make right ventricular pulsations more prominent by displacing the right ventricle anteriorly against the left parasternal area; in patients with severe mitral regurgitation, an expanding left atrium may be responsible for marked left parasternal movement, even in the absence of right ventricular hypertrophy. Movement imparted by the systolic expansion of the left atrium can be appreciated by placing the index finger of one hand at the left ventricular apex and the index finger of the other in the left parasternal region in the third intercostal space.

AORTA. Enlargement or aneurysm of the ascending aorta or aortic arch may cause visible or palpable systolic pulsations of the right or left sternoclavicular joint and may also cause a systolic impulse in the suprasternal notch or the first or second right intercostal space.[4]

THRILLS

The flat of the hand or the fingertips usually best appreciate thrills, which are vibratory sensations that are palpable manifestations of loud, harsh murmurs having low- to medium-frequency components. Because the vibrations must be quite intense before they are felt, far more information can be obtained from the auscultatory than from the palpatory features of heart murmurs. High-pitched murmurs such as those produced by valvular regurgitation, even when loud, are not usually associated with thrills.

PERCUSSION

Palpation is far more helpful than is percussion in determining cardiac size. However, in the absence of an apical beat, as occurs in patients with pericardial effusion or in some patients with dilated cardiomyopathy, heart failure, and marked displacement of a hypokinetic apical beat, the left border of the heart can be approximately outlined by means of percussion. Also, percussion of dullness in the right lower parasternal area may, in some instances, aid in the detection of a greatly enlarged right atrium. Percussion aids materially in determining visceral situs, that is, in ascertaining the side on which the heart, stomach, and liver are located.

Cardiac Auscultation

Principles and Technique

The modern binaural stethoscope is a well-crafted, airtight instrument with earpieces selected for comfort, with metal tubing joined to single flexible 12-inch-long, thick-walled rubber tubing (internal diameter of 1/8 inch), and with dual chest pieces—diaphragm for high frequencies, bell for low or lower frequencies—designed so that the examiner can readily switch from one chest piece to the other.[49,50] When the bell is applied with just enough pressure to form a skin seal, low frequencies are accentuated; when the bell is pressed firmly, the stretched skin becomes a diaphragm, damping low frequencies. Variable pressure with the bell provides a range of frequencies from low to medium.

Cardiac auscultation is best accomplished in a quiet room with the patient comfortable and the chest fully exposed. The topographical areas for auscultation (Fig. 8–8) are best designated by descriptive terms: cardiac apex, left and right sternal borders interspace by interspace, and subxiphoid. Auscultation should begin at the cardiac apex (best identified in the left lateral decubitus) and contiguous lower left sternal edge (inflow), proceeding interspace by interspace up the left sternal border to the left base and then to the right base (outflow). In addition, the stethoscope should be applied regularly to the axillae, the back, the anterior chest on the opposite side, and above the clavicles. In patients with increased anteroposterior chest dimensions (emphysema), auscultation is often best achieved by applying the stethoscope in the epigastrium (subxiphoid).

During auscultation, the examiner is generally on the patient's right; three positions are routinely employed: left lateral decubitus (assuming left thoracic heart), supine, and sitting. One should begin auscultation by applying the stethoscope to the cardiac apex with the patient in the left lateral decubitus position (see Fig. 8-7C). Identification of S_1 can usually be established by simultaneous palpation of the carotid artery with the thumb of the free left hand. Once the S_1 is identified, analysis then proceeds by systematic, methodical, sequential attention to early, middle, and late systole; S_2; then early, middle, and late diastole (presystole); and returning to S_1. When auscultation at the apex has been completed, the patient is turned into the supine position. Each topographical area—lower to upper left sternal edge interspace by interspace and then the right base—is interrogated using the same systematic sequence of analysis (see Fig. 8-7D).

Assessment of pitch or frequency ranging from low to moderately high can be achieved by variable pressure of the stethoscopic bell, whereas for high frequencies the diaphragm should be employed. It is practical to begin by using the stethoscopic bell with varying pressure at the apex and lower left sternal edge, changing to the diaphragm when the base is reached. Low frequencies are best heard by applying the bell just lightly enough to achieve a skin seal. High-frequency events are best elicited with firm pressure of the diaphragm, often with the patient sitting, leaning forward in full, held exhalation.

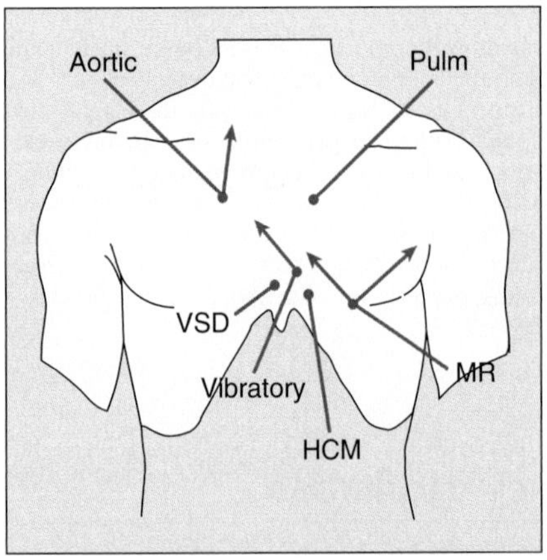

FIGURE 8–8 Maximal intensity and radiation of six isolated systolic murmurs. HCM = hypertrophic cardiomyopathy; MR = mitral regurgitation; Pulm = pulmonary; VSD = ventricular septal defect. (From Barlow JB: Perspectives on the Mitral Valve. Philadelphia, FA Davis, 1987, p 140.)

Heart Sounds

Heart sounds are relatively brief, discrete auditory vibrations that can be characterized by intensity (loudness), frequency (pitch), and quality (timbre). S_1 identifies the onset of ventricular systole, and S_2 identifies the onset of diastole. These two auscultatory events establish a framework within which other heart sounds and murmurs can be placed and timed.[4,48,50]

The basic heart sounds are the S_1, S_2, S_3, and S_4 (Fig. 8–9). Each of these events can be normal or abnormal. Other heart sounds are, with few exceptions, abnormal or iatrogenic (e.g., prosthetic valve sounds, pacemaker sounds). Heart sounds within the framework established by S_1 and S_2 are designated as "early systolic, midsystolic, late systolic," and "early diastolic, mid-diastolic, late diastolic (presystolic)."[2]

For example, an early systolic sound might be an ejection sound (aortic or pulmonary) or an aortic prosthetic sound. Midsystolic and late systolic sounds are typified by the click or clicks of mitral valve prolapse but occasionally are "remnants" of pericardial rubs. Early diastolic sounds are represented by opening snaps (usually mitral), an early S_3 (constrictive pericarditis, less commonly mitral regurgitation), the opening of a mechanical inflow prosthesis, or the abrupt seating of a pedunculated mobile atrial myxoma ("tumor plop"). Mid-diastolic sounds are generally S_3 or summation

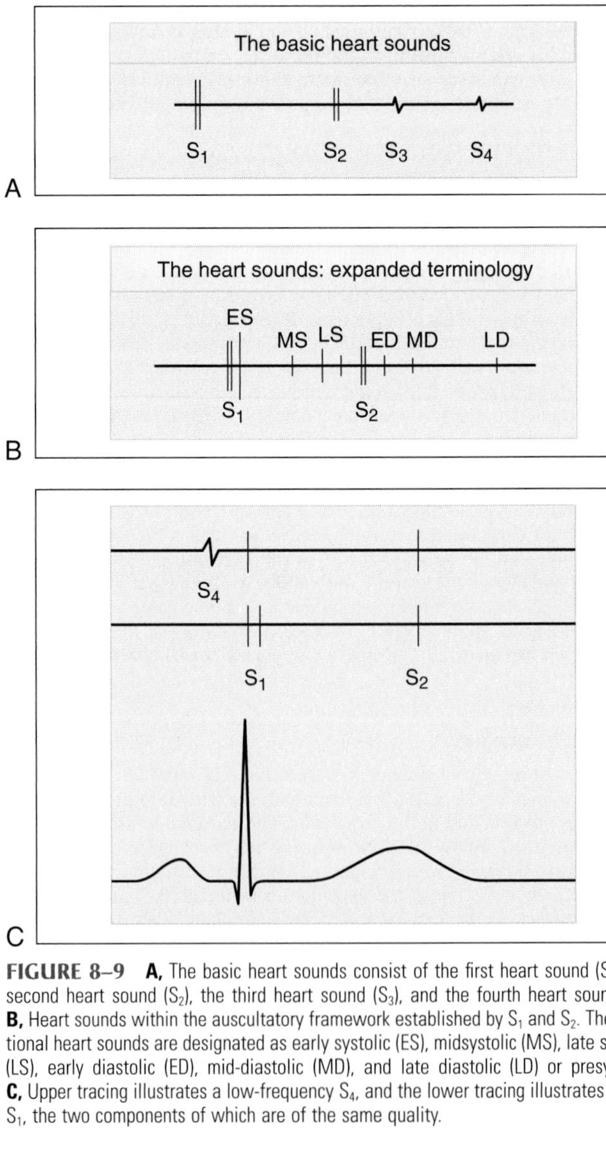

FIGURE 8–9 **A,** The basic heart sounds consist of the first heart sound (S_1), the second heart sound (S_2), the third heart sound (S_3), and the fourth heart sound (S_4). **B,** Heart sounds within the auscultatory framework established by S_1 and S_2. The additional heart sounds are designated as early systolic (ES), midsystolic (MS), late systolic (LS), early diastolic (ED), mid-diastolic (MD), and late diastolic (LD) or presystolic. **C,** Upper tracing illustrates a low-frequency S_4, and the lower tracing illustrates a split S_1, the two components of which are of the same quality.

TABLE 8–2 Factors Affecting the Intensity of S_1

Loud S_1
Short PR interval (<160 msec)
Tachycardia or hyperkinetic states
"Stiff" left ventricle
Mitral stenosis
Left atrial myxoma
Holosystolic mitral valve prolapse
Soft S_1
Long PR interval (>200 msec)
Depressed left ventricular contractility
Premature closure of mitral valve (e.g., acute aortic regurgiation)
Left bundle branch block
Extracardiac factors (e.g., obesity, muscular chest, chronic obstructive pulmonary disease, large breasts)
Flail mitral leaflet

From Abrams J: Synopsis of Cardiac Physical Diagnosis. 2nd ed. Boston, Butterworth Heinemann, 2001, p 60.

sounds (synchronous occurrence of S_3 and S_4). Late diastolic or presystolic sounds are almost always S_4 sounds, rarely pacemaker sounds.

First Heart Sound

S_1 consists of two components (see Fig. 8–9C). The initial component is most prominent at the cardiac apex when the apex is occupied by the left ventricle. The second component, if present, is normally confined to the lower left sternal edge, is less commonly heard at the apex, and is seldom heard at the base. The first major component is associated with closure of the mitral valve and coincides with abrupt arrest of leaflet motion when the cusps, especially the larger and more mobile anterior mitral cusp, reach their fully closed positions. The origin of the second component of S_1 has been debated but is generally assigned to closure of the tricuspid valve based on an analogous line of reasoning.[4,48-51]

Opening of the semilunar valves with ejection of blood into the aortic root or pulmonary trunk usually produces no audible sound in the normal heart. In cases of complete right bundle branch block, S_1 is widely split as a result of delay of the tricuspid component.[52] In cases of complete left bundle branch block, S_1 is single as a result of delay of the mitral component.[53]

When S_1 is split, its first component is normally louder. The softer second component is confined to the lower left sternal edge but may also be heard at the apex. Only the louder first component is heard at the base. The intensity of the S_1, particularly its first major audible component, depends chiefly on the position of the bellies of the mitral leaflets, especially the anterior leaflet, at the time the left ventricle begins to contract. S_1 is therefore loudest when the onset of left ventricular systole finds the mitral leaflets maximally recessed into the left ventricular cavity, as in the presence of a rapid heart rate, a short PR interval (Table 8–2),[54] short cycle lengths in atrial fibrillation, or mitral stenosis with a mobile anterior leaflet. When this mobility is lost, the intensity of S_1 decreases.

Early Systolic Sounds

Aortic or pulmonary ejection sounds are the most common early systolic sounds (Table 8–3).[55] *Ejection sound* is preferred to the term *ejection click*, with the latter designation best reserved for the midsystolic to late systolic clicks of mitral valve prolapse (see Chap. 57). Ejection sounds coincide with the fully opened position of the relevant semilunar valve, as in congenital aortic valve stenosis (Fig. 8–10), bicuspid aortic valve in the left side of the heart, or pulmonary valve stenosis in the right side of the heart.[4,48,50] Ejection sounds are relatively high frequency events and, depending on intensity, have a pitch similar to that of S_1. An ejection sound originating in the aortic valve (congenital aortic stenosis or bicuspid aortic valve) or in the pulmonary valve (congenital pulmonary valve stenosis) indicates that the valve is mobile because the ejection sound is caused by abrupt cephalad doming.[56] Less certain is the origin of an ejection sound within a dilated arterial trunk distal to a normal semilunar valve (Fig. 8–11A). Origin of the sound is assigned either to opening movement of the leaflets that resonate in the arterial trunk or to the wall of the dilated great artery. Aortic ejection sounds do not vary with respiration.

TABLE 8–3 Conditions Associated with Ejection Sound or Click

Aortic
Congenital valvular aortic stenosis
Bicuspid aortic valve
Aortic regurgitation
Aortic aneurysm
Aortic root dilatation
Systemic hypertension
Severe tetralogy of Fallot
Pulmonic
Pulmonary valve stenosis
Idiopathic dilatation of the pulmonary artery
Atrial septal defect
Chronic pulmonary hypertension
Tetralogy of Fallot (with pulmonic valve stenosis)
Pseudo-ejection sound
Prominent splitting of S_1
Increased T_1 (Ebstein's anomaly; atrial septal defect)
Hypertrophic cardiomyopathy
Early nonejection click of holosystolic mitral valve prolapse
High-pitched S_4 (S_1 confused for ejection sound)

From Abrams J: Synopsis of Cardiac Physical Diagnosis. 2nd ed. Boston, Butterworth Heinemann, 2001, p 100.

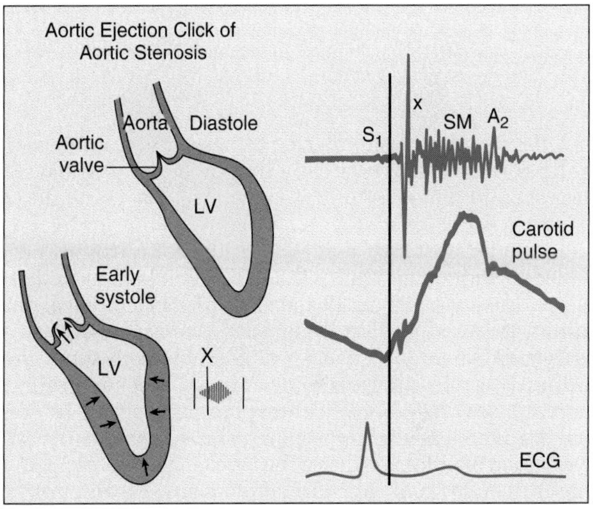

FIGURE 8–10 Ejection click associated with aortic stenosis due to a congenitally bicuspid valve. Note the high-frequency, high-amplitude sound that follows S_1 and is coincident with the onset of ejection into the aorta. The aortic ejection sound is formed by sudden cessation of the opening motion of the abnormal valve leaflets (doming). Note also the delayed carotid upstroke and long systolic murmur. (From Abrams J: Synopsis of Cardiac Physical Diagnosis. 2nd ed. Boston, Butterworth Heinemann, 2001, p 135.)

Midsystolic to Late Systolic Sounds

The most common midsystolic to late systolic sounds are associated with mitral valve prolapse (see Chap. 57).[4,57] The

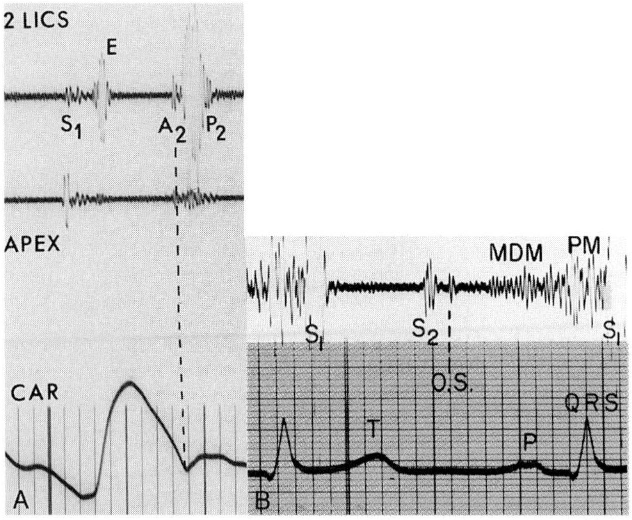

FIGURE 8–11 **A,** Tracings from a 32-year-old woman with an ostium secundum atrial septal defect, pulmonary hypertension, and a small right-to-left shunt. In the second left intercostal space (2 LICS), the first heart sound is followed by a prominent pulmonary ejection sound (E). The second sound remains split. The pulmonic component (P_2) is very loud and is transmitted to the apex. CAR = carotid pulse. **B,** Phonocardiogram recorded in the left lateral decubitus position over the left ventricular impulse in a patient with pure rheumatic mitral stenosis. The first heart sound (S_1) is loud. The second heart sound (S_2) is followed by an opening snap (OS). There is a mid-diastolic murmur (MDM). The prominent presystolic murmur (PM) goes up to the subsequent loud S_1.

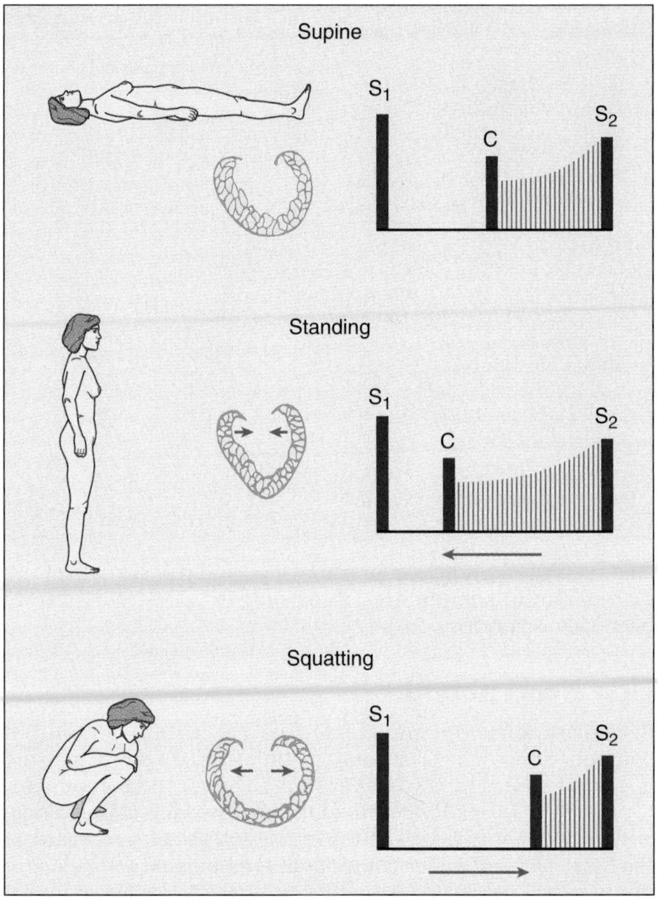

FIGURE 8–12 A midsystolic nonejection sound (C) occurs during mitral valve prolapse and is followed by a late systolic murmur that crescendos to the second heart sound (S_2). Standing decreases venous return; the heart becomes smaller; C moves closer to the first heart sound (S_1) and the mitral regurgitant murmur has an earlier onset. With prompt squatting, venous return increases; the heart becomes larger; C moves toward S_2 and the duration of the murmur shortens. (From Shaver JA, Leonard JJ, Leon DF: Examination of the Heart. Part IV: Auscultation of the Heart. Dallas, American Heart Association, 1990, p 13. Copyright 1990, American Heart Association.)

term *click* is appropriate because these midsystolic to late systolic sounds are of relatively high frequency. Midsystolic to late systolic clicks of mitral valve prolapse coincide with maximal systolic excursion of a prolapsed anterior leaflet (or scallop of the posterior leaflet) into the left atrium and are ascribed to sudden tensing of the redundant leaflets and elongated chordae tendineae. Physical or pharmacological interventions that reduce left ventricular volume, such as the Valsalva maneuver, or a change in position from squatting to standing (Fig. 8–12) causes the clicks to occur earlier in systole.[57] Conversely, physical or pharmacological interventions that increase left ventricular volume, such as squatting or sustained hand grip, delay the clicks. Multiple clicks are thought to arise from asynchronous tensing of different portions of redundant mitral leaflets, especially the triscalloped posterior leaflet.

Second Heart Sound (Table 8–4)

S_2, like S_1, has two components. The first component of the second heart sound is designated "aortic" (A_2) and the second "pulmonic" (P_2) (Fig. 8–13).[58,59] Each component coincides with the incisura of its great arterial pressure pulse. Inspiratory splitting of S_2 is due chiefly to a delay in P_2, less to earlier timing of A_2.[60] During inspiration, the pulmonary arterial incisura moves away from the descending limb of the right ventricular pressure pulse because of an inspiratory increase in capacitance of the pulmonary vascular bed, delaying P_2.[61] Exhalation has the opposite effect. The earlier inspiratory timing of A_2 is attributed to a transient reduction in left ventricular volume coupled with unchanged impedance (capacitance) in the systemic vascular bed. Normal respiratory variations in the timing of S_2 are therefore ascribed principally to the variations in impedance characteristics (capacitance) of the pulmonary vascular bed and secondarily to an inspiratory increase in right ventricular volume as originally proposed. When an increase in capacitance of the pulmonary bed is lost because of a rise in pulmonary vascular resistance, inspiratory splitting of S_2 narrows and, if present at all, reflects an increase in right ventricular ejection time and/or earlier timing of A_2.

The frequency compositions of the aortic and pulmonary components of S_2 are similar, but their normal amplitudes differ appreciably, the aortic component being the louder, reflecting the differences in systemic (aortic) and pulmonary arterial closing pressures. Splitting of S_2 is most readily identified in the second left intercostal space, because the softer P_2 is normally confined to that site, whereas the louder A_2 is heard at the base, sternal edge, and apex.[4,58]

ABNORMAL SPLITTING OF THE SECOND HEART SOUND (Fig. 8–14). Three general categories of abnormal splitting are recognized: (1) persistently single, (2) persistently split (fixed or nonfixed), and (3) paradoxically split (reversed). When S_2 remains single throughout the respiratory cycle, one component is absent or the two components are persistently synchronous. The most common cause of a single S_2 is inaudibility of the P_2 in older adults with increased anteroposterior chest dimensions. In the setting of congenital heart disease, a single S_2 due to absence of the pulmonary component is a feature of pulmonary atresia, severe pulmonary valve stenosis, dysplastic pulmonary valve, or complete transposition of the great arteries. Conversely, a single S_2 due to inaudibility of the A_2 occurs when the aortic

TABLE 8–4 Causes of Splitting of the Second Heart Sound

Normal Splitting	Reversed Splitting
Delayed pulmonic closure	**Delayed aortic closure**
Delayed electrical activation of the right ventricle	Delayed electrical activation of the left ventricle
Complete right bundle branch block (proximal type)	Complete left bundle branch block (proximal type)
Left ventricular paced beats	Right ventricular paced beats
Left ventricular ectopic beats	Right ventricular ectopic beats
Prolonged right ventricular mechanical systole	Prolonged left ventricular mechanical systole
Acute massive pulmonary embolus	Complete left bundle branch block (peripheral type)
Pulmonary hypertension with right-sideed heart failure	Left ventricular outflow tract obstruction
Pulmonic stenosis with intact septum (moderate to severe)	Hypertensive cardiovascular disease
Decreased impedance of the pulmonary vascular bed (increased hangout)	Arteriosclerotic heart disease
Normotensive atrial septal defect	Chronic ischemic heart disease
Idiopathic dilatation of the pulmonary artery	Angina pectoris
Pulmonic stenosis (mild)	Decreased impedance of the systemic vascular bed (increased hangout)
Atrial septal defect, postoperative (70%)	Poststenotic dilatation of the aorta secondary to aortic stenosis or insufficiency
	Patent ductus arteriosus
Early aortic closure	**Early pulmonic closure**
Shortened left ventricular mechanical systole (left ventriculer ejection time)	Early electrical activation of the right ventricle
Mitral regurgitation	Wolff-Parkinson-White syndrome, type B
Ventricular septal defect	

Modified from Shaver JA, O'Toole JD: The second heart sound: Newer concepts. Parts 1 and 2. Mod Concepts Cardiovasc Dis 46:7 and 13, 1977.

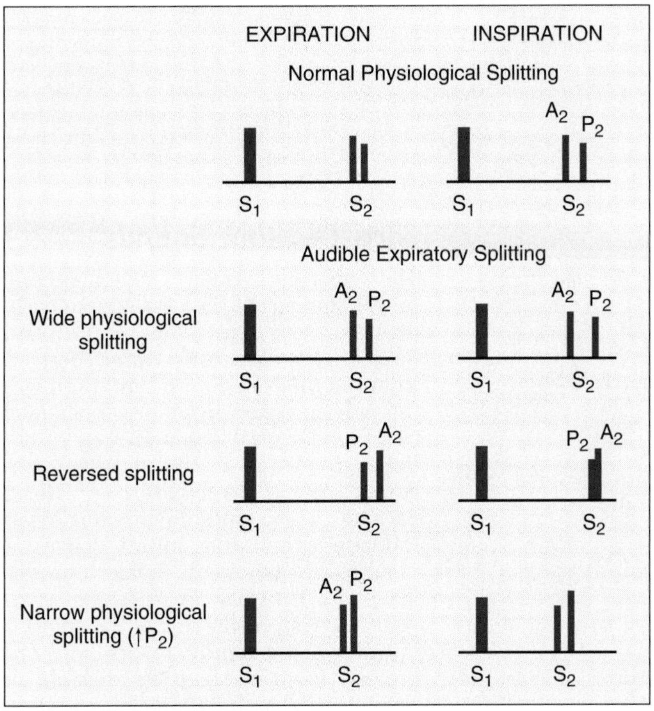

FIGURE 8–13 **Top,** Normal physiological splitting. During expiration (left), the aortic (A_2) and pulmonic (P_2) components of the second heart sound are separated by less than 30 milliseconds and are appreciated as a single sound. During inspiration (right), the splitting interval widens, and A_2 and P_2 are clearly separated into two distinct sounds. **Bottom,** Audible expiratory splitting. In contrast to normal physiological splitting, two distinct sounds are easily heard during expiration. Wide physiological splitting is caused by a delay in P_2. Reversed splitting is caused by a delay in A_2, resulting in paradoxical movement; that is, with inspiration P_2 moves toward A_2, and the splitting interval narrows. Narrow physiological splitting occurs in patients with pulmonary hypertension, and both A_2 and P_2 are heard during expiration at a narrow splitting interval because of the increased intensity and high-frequency composition of P_2. (From Shaver JA, Leonard JJ, Leon DF: Examination of the Heart, Part IV, Auscultation of the Heart. Dallas, American Heart Association, 1990, p 17. Copyright 1990, American Heart Association.)

valve is immobile (severe calcific aortic stenosis) or atretic (aortic atresia).

Persistent Splitting of S_2. This term applies when the two components remain audible (or recordable) during both inspiration and exhalation (see Fig. 8–14). Persistent splitting may be due to a delay in P_2, as in cases of simple complete right bundle branch block,[58] or to early timing of the A_2, as occasionally occurs in cases of mitral regurgitation. Normal directional changes in the interval of the split (greater with inspiration, lesser with exhalation) in the presence of persistent audibility of both components defines the split as *persistent* but not *fixed.*

Fixed Splitting of S_2. This term applies when the interval between the A_2 and P_2 is not only wide and persistent but also remains unchanged during the respiratory cycle.[50] Fixed splitting is an auscultatory hallmark of uncomplicated ostium secundum atrial septal defect (Fig. 8–15; see Chap. 56). A_2 and P_2 are widely separated during exhalation and exhibit little or no change in the degree of splitting during inspiration or with the Valsalva maneuver. The wide splitting is caused by a delay in the P_2 because a marked increase in pulmonary vascular capacitance prolongs the interval between the descending limbs of the pulmonary arterial and right ventricular pressure pulses ("hangout"), and therefore delays the pulmonary incisura and the P_2. The capacitance (impedance) of the pulmonary bed is appreciably increased, and the right ventricular stroke volume is not influenced by respiration, so there is little or no additional increase during inspiration and little or no inspiratory delay in the P_2. Phasic changes in systemic venous return during respiration in patients with atrial septal defect are associated with reciprocal changes in the volume of the left-to-right shunt, minimizing respiratory variations in right ventricular filling. The net effect is the characteristic wide, fixed splitting of the two components of the S_2.[55]

Paradoxical (Reversed) Splitting of S_2. This term refers to a reversed sequence of semilunar valve closure, the P_2 preceding the A_2. Common causes of paradoxical splitting are complete left bundle branch block[62] or a right ventricular pacemaker, both of which are associated with initial activation of the right side of the ventricular septum, and delayed activation of the left ventricle owing to transseptal (right-to-left) depolarization.[63] When the S_2 splits paradoxically, its

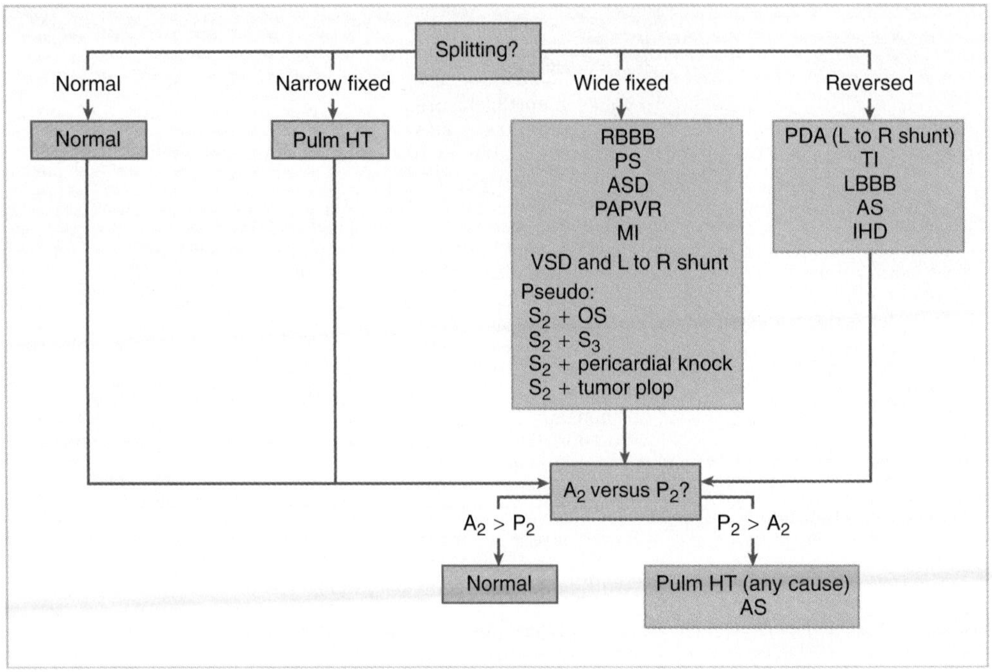

FIGURE 8–14 Decision tree for splitting of the second heart sound (S_2). A_2 = aortic valve closure; AS = aortic stenosis; ASD = atrial septal defect; IHD = ischemic heart disease; L to R shunt = left-to-right shunt; LBBB = left bundle branch block; MI = mitral insufficiency; OS = opening snap; P_2 = pulmonic valve closure; PAPVR = partial anomalous pulmonary venous return; PDA = patent ductus arteriosus; PS = pulmonic stenosis; Pulm HT = pulmonary hypertension; RBBB = right bundle branch block; S_3 = third heart sound; TI = tricuspid insufficiency; VSD = ventricular septal defect. (From Braunwald E: The clinical examination. *In* Braunwald E, Goldman L [eds]: Primary Cardiology. 2nd ed. Philadelphia, Elsevier, 2003; and Sapira JD: The Art and Science of Bedside Diagnosis. Baltimore, Urban and Schwartzenberg, 1990.)

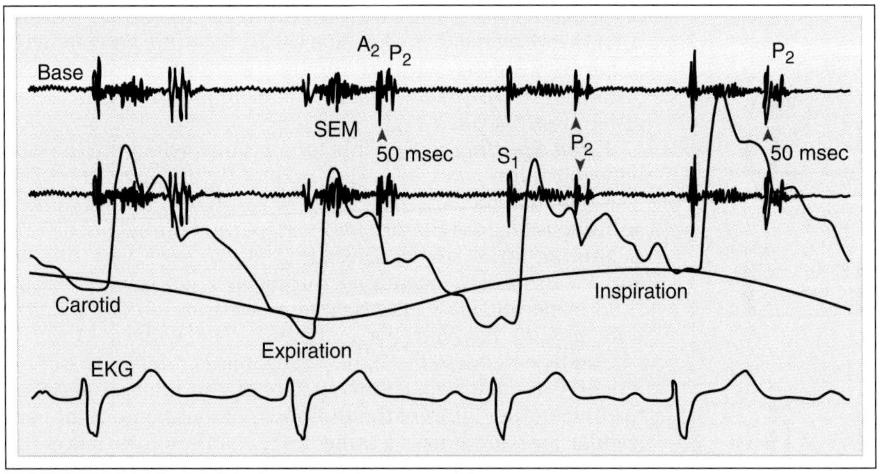

FIGURE 8–15 Simultaneous base and apex phonocardiograms recorded with the carotid pulse during quiet respiration in a young woman with a large atrial septal defect. Wide fixed splitting of the second heart sound (S_2) is present, and the pulmonic component (P_2) is easily recorded at the apex. A prominent systolic ejection murmur (SEM) is recorded at the base and is attributable to the large stroke volume across the right ventricular outflow tract. The tricuspid component of S_1 is prominent at the apex. EKG = electrocardiogram. (From Shaver JA: Innocent murmurs. Hosp Med 14:8, 1978. Copyright 1999, Quadrant Healthcom, Inc.)

two components separate during exhalation and become single (synchronous) during inspiration (see Fig. 8–13). Inspiratory synchrony is achieved as the two components fuse because of a delay in the P_2, less to earlier timing of the aortic component.

ABNORMAL LOUDNESS (INTENSITY) OF THE TWO COMPONENTS OF S_2

Assessment of intensity requires that both components be compared when heard simultaneously at the same site. The relative softness of the normal P_2 is responsible for its localization in the second left intercostal space, whereas the relative loudness of the normal A_2 accounts for its audibility at all precordial sites (see earlier). An increase in intensity of the A_2 occurs with systemic hypertension. The intensity of A_2 also increases when the aorta is closer to the anterior chest wall, owing to root dilatation or transposition of the great arteries or when an anterior pulmonary trunk is small or absent, as in pulmonary atresia.[55]

A loud P_2 is a feature of pulmonary hypertension, and the loudness is enhanced by dilatation of a hypertensive pulmonary trunk. An accentuated P_2 can be transmitted to the middle or lower left sternal edge and, when very loud, throughout the precordium to the apex and right base. A moderate increase in loudness of the P_2 sometimes occurs in the absence of pulmonary hypertension when the pulmonary trunk is dilated, as in cases of ostium secundum atrial septal defect or when there is a decrease in anteroposterior chest dimensions (loss of thoracic kyphosis) that places the pulmonary trunk closer to the chest wall.[64]

Early Diastolic Sounds

The opening "snap" of rheumatic mitral stenosis is the best known early diastolic sound (see Figs. 8–11B and 8–26). The diagnostic value derived from the pitch, loudness, and timing of the opening snap in the assessment of rheumatic mitral stenosis was established by Wood in his classic monograph, *An Appreciation of Mitral Stenosis.*[65] An audible opening snap indicates that the mitral valve is mobile, or at least its longer anterior leaflet is. The snap is generated when superior systolic bowing of the anterior mitral leaflet is rapidly reversed toward the left ventricle in early diastole in response to high left atrial pressure. The mechanism of the opening snap is therefore a corollary to the loud S_1, which is generated by abrupt superior systolic displacement of a mobile anterior mitral leaflet that was recessed into the left ventricle during diastole by high left atrial pressure until the onset of left ventricular isovolumetric contraction (see earlier). The designation "snap" is appropriate because of the relatively high frequency of the sound.

The timing of the opening snap relative to the A_2 has important physiological meaning.[4] A short A_2/opening snap interval generally reflects the high left atrial pressure of severe mitral stenosis. In older subjects with systolic hypertension, however, mitral stenosis of appreciable severity can occur without a short A_2/opening snap interval because the elevated left ventricular systolic pressure takes longer to fall below the left atrial pressure. In the presence of atrial fibrillation, the A_2/opening snap interval varies inversely with cycle length, because (all else being equal) the higher the left atrial pressure (short cycle length), the earlier the stenotic valve opens and vice versa.

Early diastolic sounds are not confined to the opening snap of rheumatic mitral stenosis but include the pericardial "knock" of chronic constrictive pericarditis.[66] The term "knock" has also been applied to an early diastolic sound in patients with pure severe mitral regurgitation with reduced left ventricular compliance. Both the pericardial knock and the knock of mitral regurgitation are rapid filling sounds that are early and loud because a high-pressure atrium rapidly decompresses across an unobstructed mitral valve into a recipient ventricle whose compliance is impaired.

Early diastolic sounds are sometimes caused by atrial myxomas (see Chap. 63).[67] The generation of such a sound, called a tumor "plop," requires a mobile myxoma attached to the atrial septum by a long stalk. The "plop" is believed to result from abrupt diastolic seating of the tumor within the right or left AV orifice.[67]

An early diastolic sound can also be generated by the opening movement of a mechanical prosthesis in the mitral position. This opening sound is especially prominent with a ball-in-cage prosthesis (Starr-Edwards) and less prominent with a tilting disc prosthesis (Bjork-Shiley).

Mid-diastolic and Late Diastolic (Presystolic) Sounds (Fig. 8–16)

Mid-diastolic sounds are, for all practical purposes, either normal or abnormal S_3 sounds, and most, if not all, late diastolic or presystolic sounds are S_4 sounds. Each sound coincides with its relevant diastolic filling phase.[68] In sinus rhythm, the ventricles receive blood during two filling phases. The first phase occurs when ventricular pressure drops sufficiently to allow the AV valve to open; blood then flows from atrium into ventricle. This flow is designated the "rapid filling phase," accounting for about 80 percent of normal ventricular filling. The rapid filling phase is not a passive event in which the recipient ventricle merely expands in response to augmented inflow volume. Rather, ventricular relaxation is an active, complex, energy-dependent process (see Chaps. 19 and 20).

S_3 is generated during the rapid filling phase.[69] The second filling phase—diastasis—is variable in duration, usually accounting for less than 5 percent of ventricular filling. The third phase of diastolic filling is in response to atrial contraction, which accounts for about 15 percent of normal ventricular filling. S_4 is generated during the atrial filling phase. Both S_3 and S_4 occur within the recipient ventricle as that chamber receives blood. The addition of either an S_3 or an S_4 to the cardiac cycle produces a triple rhythm. If both S_3 and S_4 are present, a quadruple rhythm is produced. When diastole is short or the PR interval is long, S_3 and S_4 occur simultaneously to form a summation sound.[4]

Children and young adults often have a normal (physiological) S_3 but do not have a normal S_4. A normal S_3 sometimes persists beyond the age of 40 years, especially in women. After that age, however, especially in men, S_3 is likely to be abnormal. An S_4 is sometimes heard in healthy older adults without clinical evidence of heart disease, particularly after exercise.[4] Such observations have led to the conclusion, still debated, that such an S_4 may be normal in the elderly.

ATRIAL CONTRIBUTION TO FILLING. Because an S_4 requires active atrial contribution to ventricular filling, the sound disappears when coordinated atrial contraction ceases, as in atrial fibrillation. When the atria and ventricles contract independently as in complete heart block, an S_4 or summation sound occurs randomly in diastole because the relationship between the P wave and the QRS of the electrocardiogram is random. S_3 and S_4 are events caused by rapid ventricular filling, so obstruction of an AV valve, by impeding ventricular inflow, removes one of the prime preconditions for the generation of these filling sounds. Accordingly, the presence of an S_3 or S_4 implies an unobstructed (or relatively unobstructed) AV orifice on the side of the heart in which the sound originates. An S_3 or S_4 originating from the right ventricle often responds selectively and distinctively to respiration, becoming more prominent during inspiration.[4] The inspiratory increase in right atrial flow is converted into an inspiratory augmentation of both mid-diastolic and presystolic filling.

S_3 and S_4, either normal or abnormal, are relatively low frequency events that vary considerably in intensity (loudness), that originate in

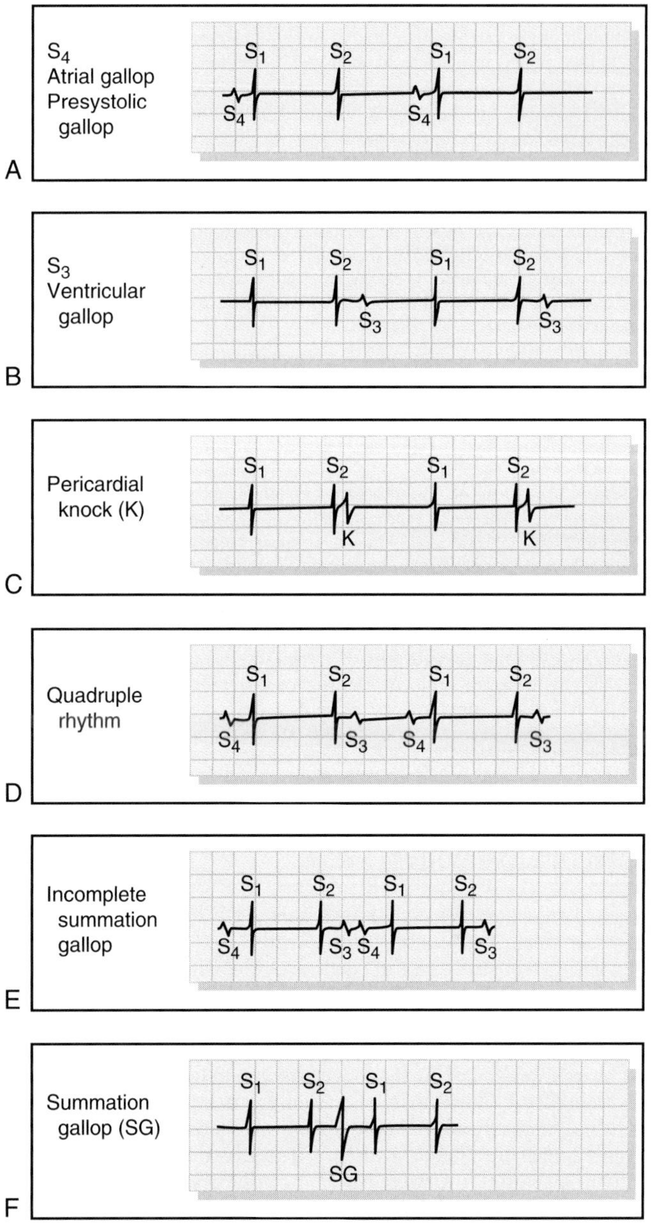

FIGURE 8–16 Diastolic filling sounds. **A,** the fourth heart sound (S_4) occurs in presystole and is frequently called an *atrial* or *presystolic gallop.* **B,** The third heart sound (S_3) occurs during the rapid phase of ventricular filling. It is a normal finding that is commonly heard in children and young adults but disappears with increasing age. When it is heard in a patient with cardiac disease, it is called a pathologic S_3 or ventricular gallop and usually indicates ventricular dysfunction or atrioventricular valvular incompetence. **C,** In constrictive pericarditis, a sound in early diastole, the pericardial knock (K) is heard earlier and is louder and higher pitched than the usual pathologic S_3. **D,** A quadruple rhythm results if both S_4 and S_3 are present. **E,** At faster heart rates, S_3 and S_4 occur in rapid succession and may give the illusion of a mid-diastolic rumble. **F,** When the heart rate is sufficiently rapid, the two rapid phases of ventricular filling reinforce each other, and a loud summation gallop (SG) may appear; this sound may be louder than either S_3 or S_4 alone. S_1 = first heart sound; S_2 = second heart sound. (From Braunwald E: The clinical examination. *In* Braunwald E, Goldman L [eds]: Primary Cardiology. 2nd ed. Philadelphia, Elsevier, 2003, pp 29-46; and Shaver JA: Examination of the Heart. Part 4: Auscultation. Dallas, American Heart Association, 1990.)

either the left or right ventricle, and that are best elicited when the bell of the stethoscope is applied with just enough pressure to provide a skin seal. An S_3 or S_4 originating from the left ventricle should be sought over the left ventricular impulse identified with the patient in the left lateral decubitus position. An S_3 or S_4 originating from the right ventricle should be sought over the right ventricular impulse (lower left sternal edge, occasionally subxiphoid) with the patient supine. An understanding of these simple principles sets the stage for bedside detection. The same principles can be used to advantage to distinguish an S_4 preceding a single S_1 from splitting of the two components of the S_1 (see Fig. 8–9C). The two components of S_1 are similar in frequency (pitch) although not in intensity (loudness) but differ in pitch from a preceding S_4. Selective pressure with the bell of the stethoscope enhances these distinctions.

AUDIBILITY OF S_3. This is improved by isotonic exercise that augments venous return and mid-diastolic AV flow. A few sit-ups usually suffice to produce the desired increase in venous return and acceleration in heart rate that increase the rate and volume of AV flow. Venous return can be increased by simple passive raising of both legs with the patient supine. The heart rate is also transiently increased by vigorous coughing. Left ventricular S_4, especially in patients with ischemic heart disease, can be induced or augmented when resistance to left ventricular discharge is increased by sustained hand-grip (isometric exercise; see later).

In the presence of sinus tachycardia, atrial contraction may coincide with the rapid filling phase, making it impossible to determine whether a given filling sound is an S_3, an S_4, or a summation sound. Carotid sinus massage transiently slows the heart rate, so the diastolic sound or sounds can be assigned their proper timing in the cardiac cycle.[4]

CAUSES OF S_3 AND S_4. The normal S_3 is believed to be caused by sudden limitation of longitudinal expansion of the left ventricular wall during brisk early diastolic filling.[70-73] The majority of abnormal S_3 sounds are generated by altered physical properties of the recipient ventricle and/or an increase in the rate and volume of AV flow during the rapid filling phase of the ventricle. An abnormal S_4 occurs when augmented atrial contraction generates presystolic ventricular distention (an increase in end-diastolic segment length) so that the recipient chamber can contract with greater force.[74-76] Typical substrates are the left ventricular hypertrophy of aortic stenosis or systemic hypertension or the right ventricular hypertrophy of pulmonary stenosis or pulmonary hypertension in the right side of the heart.[74] S_4 sounds are also common in ischemic heart disease and are almost universal during angina pectoris or acute myocardial infarction.

Heart Murmurs

A cardiovascular murmur is a series of auditory vibrations that are more prolonged than a sound and are characterized according to timing in the cardiac cycle, intensity (loudness), frequency (pitch), configuration (shape), quality, duration, and direction of radiation.[4,50,77] When these features are established, the stage is set for diagnostic conclusions.[2,76,78] The principal causes of heart murmurs are listed in Table 8–5.

Intensity or loudness is graded from 1 to 6, based on the original recommendations of Samuel A. Levine in 1933. A grade 1 murmur is so faint that it is heard only with special effort. A grade 2 murmur is soft but readily detected; a grade 3 murmur is prominent but not loud; a grade 4 murmur is loud (and usually accompanied by a thrill); a grade 5 murmur is very loud. A grade 6 murmur is loud enough to be heard with the stethoscope just removed from contact with the chest wall. The factors affecting the loudness of heart murmurs are listed in Table 8–6. Frequency or pitch varies from high to low. The configuration or shape of a murmur is best characterized as crescendo, decrescendo, crescendo-decrescendo (diamond-shaped), plateau (even), or variable (uneven). The duration of a murmur varies from short to long, with all gradations in between. A loud murmur radiates from its site of maximal intensity, and the direction of radiation is sometimes diagnostically useful.

There are three broad categories of murmurs: systolic, diastolic, and continuous. A systolic murmur begins with or after S_1 and ends at or before S_2 on its side of origin. A

TABLE 8–5 Principal Causes of Heart Murmurs

A. Organic Systolic Murmurs
  1. Midsystolic (ejection)
    a. Aortic
      (1) Obstructive
        (a) Supravalvular—supraaortic stenosis, coarction of the aorta
        (b) Valvular—aortic stenosis and sclerosis
        (c) Infravalvular—HOCM
      (2) Increased flow, hyperkinetic states, aortic regurgitation, complete heart block
      (3) Dilatation of ascending aorta, atheroma, aortitis, aneurysm of aorta
    b. Pulmonary
      (1) Obstructive
        (a) Supravalvular—pulmonary arterial stenosis
        (b) Valvular—pulmonic valve stenosis
        (c) Infravalvular—infundibular stenosis
      (2) Increase flow, hyperkinetic states, left-to-right shunt (e.g., ASD, VSD)
      (3) Dilatation of pulmonary artery
  2. Pansystolic (regurgitant)
    a. Atrioventricular valve regurgitation (MR, TR)
    b. Left-to-right shunt to ventricular level

B. Early Diastolic Murmurs
  1. Aortic regurgitation
    a. Valvular: rheumatic deformity; perforation postendocarditis, posttraumatic, postvalvulotomy
    b. Dilatation of valve ring: aorta dissection, annuloectasia, cystic medial necrosis, hypertension
    c. Widening of commissures: syphilis
    d. Congenital: biscuspid valve, with VSD
  2. Pulmonic regurgitation
    a. Valvular: postvalvulotomy, endocarditis, rheumatic fever, carcinoid
    b. Dilatation of valve ring: pulmonary hypertension; Marfan syndrome
    c. Congenital: isolated or associated with tetralogy of Fallot, VSD, pulmonic stenosis

C. Mid-Diastolic Murmurs
  1. Mitral stenosis
  2. Carey-Coombs murmur (mid-diastolic apical murmur in acute rheumatic fever)
  3. Increased flow across nonstenotic mitral valve (e.g., MR, VSD, PDA, high-output states, and complete heart block)
  4. Tricuspid stenosis
  5. Increased flow across nonstenotic tricuspid valve (e.g., TR, ASD, and anomalous pulmonary venous return)
  6. Left and right atrial tumors

D. Continuous Murmurs
  1. PDA
  2. Coronary arteriovenous fistula
  3. Ruptured aneurysm of sinus of Valsalva
  4. Aortic septal defect
  5. Cervical venous hum
  6. Anomalous left coronary artery
  7. Proximal coronary artery stenosis
  8. Mammary souffle
  9. Pulmonary artery branch stenosis
  10. Bronchial collateral circulation
  11. Small (restrictive) ASD with mitral stenosis
  12. Intercostal arteriovenous fistula

A and *C*, Modified from Oram S (ed): Clinical Heart Disease. London, Heinemann, 1981. *D*, Modified from Fowler NO (ed): Cardiac Diagnosis and Treatment. Hagerstown, MD, Harper & Row, 1980.

ASD = atrial septal defect; HOCM = hypertrophic obstructive cardiomyopathy; MR = mitral regurgitation; PDA = patent ductus arteriosus; TR = tricuspid regurgitation; VSD = ventricular septal defect.

From Norton PJ, O'Rourke RA: Approach to the patient with a heart murmur. *In* Braunwald E, Goldman L, (eds): Primary Cardiology. 2nd ed. Philadelphia, Elsevier, 2003, pp 151–168.

TABLE 8–6 Factors Affecting the Loudness of Heart Murmurs
Increased intensity
High cardiac output (hyperdynamic) states
Thin chest wall
Narrow thoracic diameter; for example, "straight back," pectus excavatum
Anemia (decreased blood viscosity)
Tortuous aorta (close to chest wall)
Decreased intensity
Obesity
Muscular or thick chest wall
Obstructive lung disease
Barrel chest (increased anteroposterior diameter)
Pericardial thickening or fluid
Decreased cardiac output (congestive heart failure, low ejection fraction)

From Abrams J: Synopsis of Cardiac Physical Diagnosis. 2nd ed. Boston, Butterworth Heinemann, 2001, p 115.

diastolic murmur begins with or after S_2 and ends before the subsequent S_1. A continuous murmur begins in systole and continues without interruption through the S_2 into all or part of diastole. The following classification of murmurs is based on their timing relative to S_1 and S_2.

Systolic Murmurs

Systolic murmurs are classified according to their time of onset and termination as midsystolic, holosystolic, early systolic, or late systolic (Fig. 8–17).[77,79,80] A midsystolic murmur begins after S_1 and ends perceptibly before S_2. The termination of a systolic murmur must be related to the relevant component of S_2. Accordingly, midsystolic murmurs originating in the left side of the heart end before A_2; midsystolic murmurs originating in the right side of the heart end before P_2. A holosystolic murmur begins with S_1, occupies all of systole, and ends with the S_2 on its side of origin. Holosystolic murmurs originating in the left side of the heart end with A_2, and holosystolic murmurs originating in the right side of the heart end with P_2.

The term *regurgitant systolic murmur*, originally applied to murmurs that occupied all of systole, has fallen out of use because "regurgitation" can be accompanied by holosystolic, midsystolic, early systolic, or late systolic murmurs.[2] Similarly, the term *ejection systolic murmur*, originally applied to midsystolic murmurs, should be discarded, because midsystolic murmurs are not necessarily due to "ejection."[4]

MIDSYSTOLIC MURMURS. Midsystolic murmurs occur in five settings: (1) obstruction to ventricular outflow, (2) dilatation of the aortic root or pulmonary trunk, (3) accelerated systolic flow into the aorta or pulmonary trunk, (4) innocent (normal) midsystolic murmurs,[55] and (5) some forms of mitral regurgitation. The physiological mechanism of outflow midsystolic murmurs reflects the pattern of phasic flow across the left or right ventricular outflow tract as originally described by Leatham (Fig. 8–18).[58] Isovolumetric contraction generates S_1. Ventricular pressure rises, the semilunar valve opens, flow commences, and the murmur begins. As flow proceeds, the murmur increases in crescendo; as flow decreases, the murmur decreases in decrescendo. The murmur ends before ventricular pressure drops below the pressure in the central great artery, at which time the aortic and pulmonary valves close, generating A_2 and P_2.

AORTIC VALVE STENOSIS (see Chap. 57). This is associated with a midsystolic murmur, which may have an early systolic peak and a short duration, a relatively late peak and a prolonged duration, or all gradations in between. Whether long or short, however, the murmur retains a symmetrical diamond shape beginning after S_1 (or with an aortic ejection sound), rising in crescendo to a systolic peak, and declining in decrescendo to end before A_2. The high-velocity jet within the aortic root results in radiation of the murmur upward, to the right (second right intercostal space), and into the neck. An important variation occurs in older adults with previously normal trileaflet aortic valves rendered sclerotic or stenotic by fibrocalcific changes. The accompanying murmur in the second right intercostal space is harsh, noisy, and impure (see Fig.

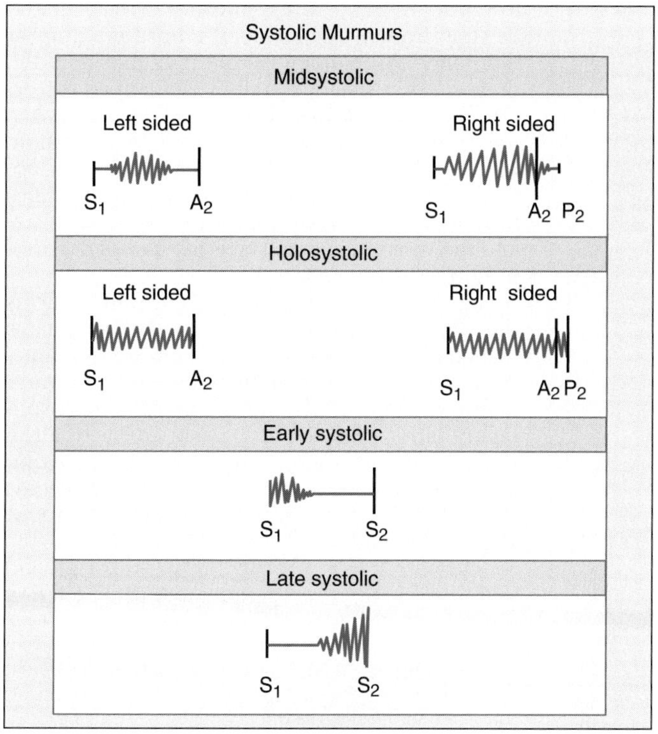

FIGURE 8–17 Systolic murmurs as illustrated here are descriptively classified according to their time of onset and termination as midsystolic, holosystolic, early systolic, and late systolic. The termination of the murmur must be related to the component of the second heart sound on its side of origin, that is, the aortic component (A_2) for systolic murmurs originating in the left side of the heart and the pulmonic component (P_2) for systolic murmurs originating in the right side of the heart.

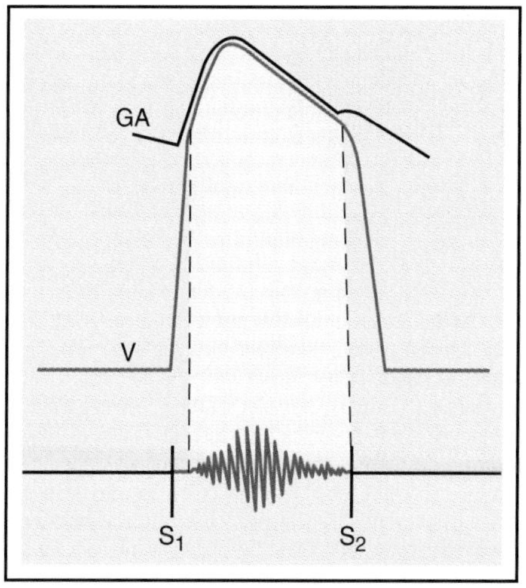

FIGURE 8–18 Illustration of the physiological mechanism of a midsystolic murmur generated by phasic flow into aortic root or pulmonary trunk. Ventricular (V) and great arterial (GA) pressure pulses are shown with phonocardiogram. The midsystolic murmur begins after the first heart sound (S_1), rises in crescendo to a peak as flow proceeds, then declines in decrescendo as flow diminishes, ending just before the second heart sound (S_2) as ventricular pressure falls below the pressure in the great artery.

8–10), whereas the murmur over the left ventricular impulse is pure and often musical.

The high-frequency apical midsystolic murmur of aortic sclerosis or stenosis should be distinguished from the high-frequency apical murmur of mitral regurgitation, a distinction that may be difficult or impossible, especially if A_2 is soft or absent. However, when premature ventricular contractions are followed by pauses longer than the dominant cycle length, the apical midsystolic murmur of aortic stenosis or sclerosis increases in intensity in the beat after the premature contraction, whereas the intensity of the murmur of mitral regurgitation (whether midsystolic or holosystolic) remains relatively unchanged. The same patterns hold after longer cycle lengths in atrial fibrillation.

PULMONARY VALVE STENOSIS (see Chap. 56). This is prototypical of a midsystolic murmur originating in the right side of the heart.[55] The murmur begins after S_1 or with a pulmonary ejection sound, rises in crescendo to a peak, then decreases in a slower decrescendo to end before a delayed or soft P_2. The length and configuration of the murmur are useful signs of the severity of obstruction.[55] When the ventricular septum is intact (Fig. 8–19, *left*), as obstruction becomes more severe, the murmur lengthens and envelops A_2, and P_2 becomes softer. When obstruction to right ventricular outflow is accompanied by a ventricular septal defect (tetralogy of Fallot), the midsystolic murmur becomes shorter with increased severity of obstruction (see Fig. 8–19, *right*).

ACCELERATED FLOW. Short, soft midsystolic murmurs originate within a dilated aortic root or dilated pulmonary trunk. Midsystolic murmurs are also generated by rapid ejection into a normal aortic root or pulmonary trunk, as during pregnancy, fever, thyrotoxicosis, or anemia. The pulmonary midsystolic murmur of ostium secundum atrial septal defect results from rapid ejection into a dilated pulmonary trunk (see Fig. 8–17).

INNOCENT (NORMAL) MURMURS. These are, except for the systolic mammary souffle, all midsystolic.[53] The normal vibratory midsystolic murmur (Still murmur) is short, buzzing, pure, and medium in frequency (Fig. 8–20) and is believed to be generated by low-frequency periodic vibrations of normal pulmonary leaflets at their attachments or periodic vibrations of a left ventricular false tendon.[81,82] A second type of innocent midsystolic murmur occurs in children, adolescents, and young adults and represents an exaggeration of normal ejection vibrations within the pulmonary trunk. This normal pulmonary midsystolic murmur is relatively impure and is best heard in the second left intercostal space, in contrast to the vibratory midsystolic murmur of Still, which is typically heard between the lower left sternal edge and apex. Normal pulmonary midsystolic murmurs are also heard in patients with diminished anteroposterior chest dimensions (e.g., loss of thoracic kyphosis).

The most common form of "innocent" midsystolic murmur in older adults has been designated the "aortic sclerotic" murmur (see earlier). The cause of this functionally benign murmur is fibrous or fibrocalcific thickening of the bases of otherwise normal aortic cusps as they insert into the sinuses of Valsalva.[55] As long as the fibrous or fibrocalcific thickening is confined to the base of the leaflets, the free edges remain mobile. No commissural fusion and no obstruction occur. The Gallavardin dissociation phenomenon associated with such an aortic valve was described earlier.

MIDSYSTOLIC MURMUR OF MITRAL REGURGITATION. The clinical setting is usually ischemic heart disease associated with left ventricular regional wall motion abnormalities. The physiological mechanism responsible for the midsystolic murmur of mitral regurgitation in this setting reflects impaired integrity of the muscular component of the mitral apparatus, with early systolic competence of the valve, and midsystolic incompetence, followed by a late systolic decline in regurgitant flow. These midsystolic murmurs are unrelated to "ejection."

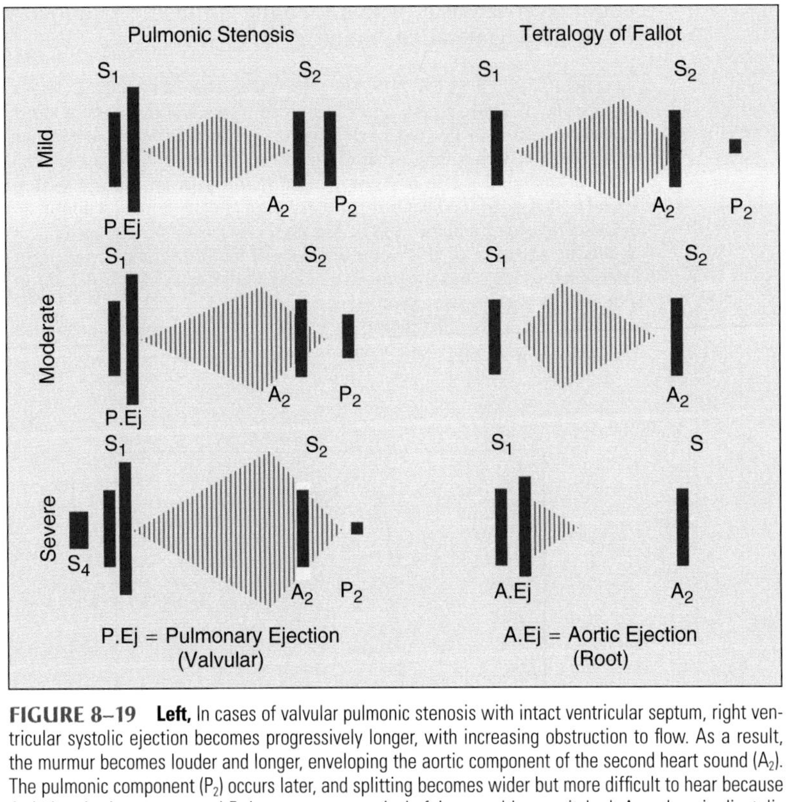

FIGURE 8–19 **Left,** In cases of valvular pulmonic stenosis with intact ventricular septum, right ventricular systolic ejection becomes progressively longer, with increasing obstruction to flow. As a result, the murmur becomes louder and longer, enveloping the aortic component of the second heart sound (A_2). The pulmonic component (P_2) occurs later, and splitting becomes wider but more difficult to hear because A_2 is lost in the murmur and P_2 becomes progressively fainter and lower pitched. As pulmonic diastolic pressure progressively decreases, isometric contraction shortens until the pulmonary valvular ejection sound fuses with the first heart sound (S_1). In cases of severe pulmonic stenosis with concentric hypertrophy and decreasing right ventricular compliance, a fourth heart sound appears. **Right,** In cases of tetralogy of Fallot with increasing obstruction at the pulmonic infundibular area, an increasing amount of right ventricular blood is shunted across the silent ventricular septal defect, and flow across the obstructed outflow tract decreases. Therefore, with increasing obstruction the murmur becomes shorter, earlier, and fainter. P_2 is absent in patients with severe tetralogy of Fallot. A large aortic root receives almost all cardiac output from both ventricular chambers, and the aorta dilates and is accompanied by a root ejection sound that does not vary with respiration. (From Shaver JA, Leonard JJ, Leon DF: Examination of the Heart. Part IV: Auscultation of the Heart. Dallas, American Heart Association, 1990, p 45. Copyright 1990, American Heart Association.)

HOLOSYSTOLIC MURMURS. Just as the term *midsystolic* is preferable to *ejection systolic*, the term *holosystolic* is preferable to *regurgitant* because holosystolic murmurs are not necessarily due to regurgitant flow. A holosystolic murmur begins with S_1 and occupies all of systole up to the S_2 on its side of origin (see Figs. 8–17 and 8–21).[4,50] Such murmurs are generated by flow from a vascular bed whose pressure or resistance throughout systole is higher than the pressure or resistance in the vascular bed receiving the flow. Holosystolic murmurs occur in the left side of the heart with mitral regurgitation, in the right side of the heart with high-pressure tricuspid regurgitation, between the ventricles through a restrictive ventricular septal defect, and between the great arteries through aortopulmonary connections.

The timing of holosystolic murmurs reflects the physiological and anatomical mechanisms responsible for their genesis. Figure 8–21 illustrates the mechanism of the holosystolic murmur of mitral regurgitation or high-pressure tricuspid regurgitation. Ventricular pressure exceeds atrial pressure at the very onset of systole (isovolumetric contraction), so regurgitant flow begins with the S_1. The murmur persists up to or slightly beyond the relevant component of the S_2, provided that ventricular pressure at end systole exceeds atrial pressure and provided that the AV valve remains incompetent.

Direction of radiation of the intraatrial jet of mitral regurgitation determines the chest wall distribution of the murmur.[83] When the direction of the intraatrial jet is forward and medial against the atrial septum near the origin of the aorta, the murmur radiates to the left sternal edge, to the base, and even into the neck. When the flow generating the murmur of mitral regurgitation is directed posterolaterally within the left atrial cavity, the murmur radiates to the axilla, to the angle of the left

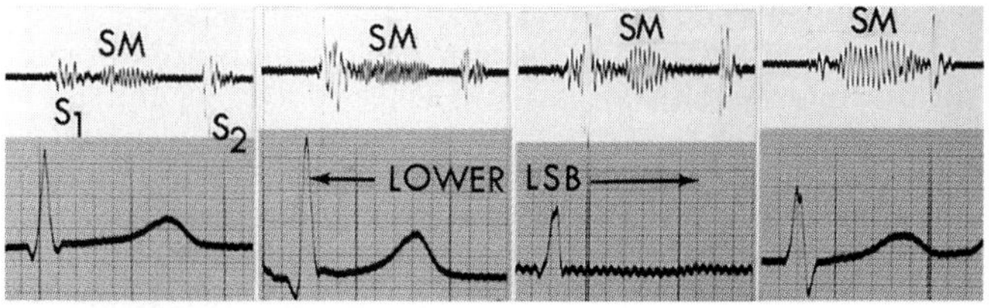

FIGURE 8–20 Four vibratory midsystolic murmurs (SM) from healthy children. These murmurs, designated *Still murmur*, are pure, medium frequency, relatively brief in duration, and maximal along the lower left sternal border (LSB). The last of the four murmurs was from a 5-year-old girl who was febrile. After defervescence, the murmur decreased in loudness and duration.

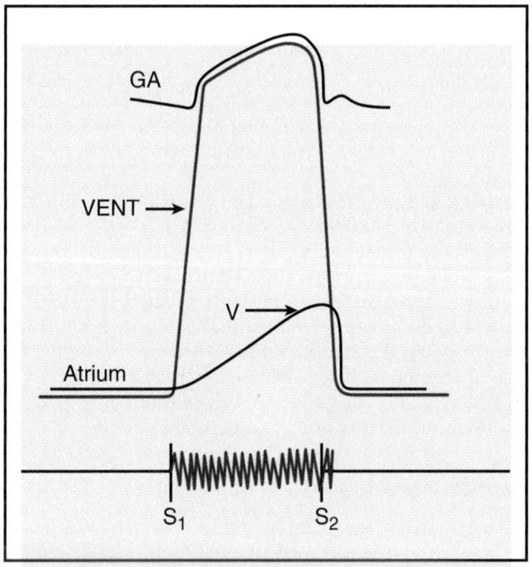

FIGURE 8–21 Illustration of great arterial (GA), ventricular (VENT), and atrial pressure pulses with phonocardiogram showing the physiological mechanism of a holosystolic murmur in some forms of mitral regurgitation and in high-pressure tricuspid regurgitation. Ventricular pressure exceeds atrial pressure at the very onset of systole, so regurgitant flow and murmur commence with the first heart sound (S_1). The murmur persists up to or slightly beyond the second heart sound (S_2) because regurgitation persists to the end of systole (ventricular pressure still exceeds atrial pressure). V = atrial v wave.

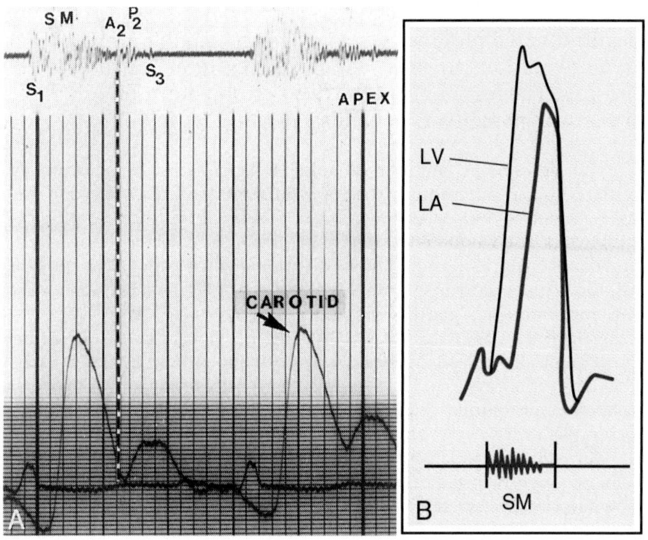

FIGURE 8–22 **A,** Phonocardiogram recorded from the cardiac apex of a patient with acute severe mitral regurgitation due to ruptured chordae tendineae. There is an early systolic decrescendo murmur (SM) diminishing if not ending before the aortic component (A_2) of the second heart sound. **B,** Left ventricular (LV) and left atrial (LA) pressure pulses with schematic illustration of the phonocardiogram showing the relationship between the decrescendo configuration of the early systolic murmur and late systolic approximation of the tall left atrial v wave and left ventricular end-systolic pressure. Regurgitant flow diminishes or ceases. The murmur therefore is early systolic and decrescendo, paralleling the hemodynamic pattern of regurgitation. P_2 = pulmonic component of the second heart sound; S_1 = first heart sound; S_3 = third heart sound.

scapula, and occasionally to the vertebral column, with bone conduction from the cervical to the lumbar spine.

The *murmur of tricuspid regurgitation* is holosystolic when there is a substantial elevation of right ventricular systolic pressure, as schematically illustrated in Figure 8-21. A distinctive and diagnostically important feature of the tricuspid murmur is its selective inspiratory increase in loudness—Carvallo sign. The tricuspid murmur is occasionally audible only during inspiration. The increase in intensity occurs because the inspiratory augmentation in right ventricular volume is converted into an increase in stroke volume and in the velocity of regurgitant flow. When the right ventricle fails, this capacity is lost; thus, Carvallo sign vanishes.

The murmur of an uncomplicated restrictive ventricular septal defect (see Chap. 56) is holosystolic because left ventricular systolic pressure and systemic resistance exceed right ventricular systolic pressure and pulmonary resistance from the onset to the end of systole. Holosystolic murmurs are perceived as such in patients with large aortopulmonary connections (aortopulmonary window, patent ductus arteriosus) when a rise in pulmonary vascular resistance abolishes the diastolic portion of the continuous murmur, leaving a murmur that is holosystolic or nearly so.[55]

EARLY SYSTOLIC MURMURS. Murmurs confined to early systole begin with S_1, diminish in decrescendo, and end well before S_2, generally at or before midsystole (see Fig. 8–17). Certain types of mitral regurgitation, tricuspid regurgitation, or ventricular septal defects are the substrates.

Acute severe mitral regurgitation is accompanied by an early systolic murmur or a holosystolic murmur that is decrescendo, diminishing if not ending before S_2 (Fig. 8–22A).[84] The physiological mechanism responsible for this early systolic decrescendo murmur is acute severe regurgitation into a relatively normal-sized left atrium with limited distensibility. A steep rise in left atrial V wave approaches the left ventricular pressure at end systole; a late systolic decline in left ventricular pressure favors this tendency (see Fig. 8–22B). The stage is set for regurgitant flow that is maximal in early systole and minimal in late systole. The systolic murmur parallels this pattern, declining or vanishing before S_2.

An early systolic murmur is a feature of tricuspid regurgitation with normal right ventricular systolic pressure.[85] An example is tricuspid regurgitation caused by infective endocarditis in drug abusers. The mechanisms responsible for the timing and configuration of the early systolic murmur of low-pressure tricuspid regurgitation are analogous to those just described for mitral regurgitation. The crest of the right atrial V wave reaches the level of normal right ventricular pressure in later systole; the regurgitation and murmur are therefore chiefly, if not exclusively, early systolic. These murmurs are of medium frequency because normal right ventricular systolic pressure generates comparatively low velocity regurgitant flow, in contrast to elevated right ventricular systolic pressure, which generates a high-frequency holosystolic murmur (see earlier).

Early systolic murmurs also occur through ventricular septal defects, but under two widely divergent anatomical and physiological circumstances. A soft, pure, high-frequency, early systolic murmur localized to the middle or lower left sternal edge is typical of a very small ventricular septal defect in which the shunt is confined to early systole.[55] A murmur of similar timing and configuration occurs through a nonrestrictive ventricular septal defect when an elevation in pulmonary vascular resistance decreases or abolishes late systolic shunting.

LATE SYSTOLIC MURMURS. The term *late systolic* applies when a murmur begins in middle to late systole and proceeds up to the S_2 (see Fig. 8–17). The late systolic murmur of mitral valve prolapse is prototypical (see Fig. 8–12).[86] One or more middle to late systolic clicks often introduce the murmur. The responses of the late systolic murmur and clicks to postural maneuvers are illustrated in Figure 8–12.

The late systolic murmur of mitral valve prolapse is occasionally replaced by an intermittent, striking, and sometimes disconcerting systolic "whoop" or "honk," either spontaneously or in response to physical maneuvers. The whoop is of high frequency, musical, widely transmitted, and occasionally loud enough to be disturbing to the patient. The musical whoop is thought to arise from mitral leaflets and chordae tendineae set into high-frequency periodic vibration.

SYSTOLIC ARTERIAL MURMURS. Systolic murmurs can originate in anatomically normal arteries in the presence of normal or increased flow or in abnormal arteries because of tortuosity or luminal narrowing. Detection of systolic arterial murmurs requires auscultation at nonprecordial sites.

The supraclavicular systolic murmur, often heard in children and adolescents, is believed to originate at the aortic origins of normal major brachiocephalic arteries.[55] The configuration of these murmurs is crescendo-decrescendo, the onset is abrupt, the duration is brief, and the intensity at times is surprisingly loud, with radiation below the clavicles. Normal supraclavicular systolic murmurs decrease or vanish in response to hyperextension of the shoulders, which is achieved by bringing the elbows back until the shoulder girdle muscles are drawn taut.

In older adults, the most common cause of a systolic arterial murmur is atherosclerotic narrowing of a carotid, subclavian, or iliofemoral artery. A variation on this theme is the "compression artifact" that can be induced in the femoral artery in the presence of free aortic regurgitation. When the femoral artery is moderately compressed by the examiner's stethoscopic bell, a systolic arterial murmur is generated. Further compression causes the systolic murmur to continue into diastole, a sign described in 1861 by Duroziez.[55] The eponym is still in use.

A systolic "mammary souffle" is sometimes heard over the breasts because of increased flow through normal arteries during late pregnancy or more especially in the postpartum period in lactating women.[55] The murmur begins well after S_1 because of the interval between left ventricular ejection and the arrival of flow at the artery of origin.

A systolic arterial murmur is present in the interscapular region over the site of coarctation of the aortic isthmus.[55] Transient systolic arterial murmurs originating in the pulmonary artery and its branches are occasionally heard in normal neonates because the angulation and disparity in size between the pulmonary trunk and its branches set the stage for turbulent systolic flow. These normal or innocent pulmonary arterial systolic murmurs disappear with maturation of the pulmonary bed, generally within the first few weeks or months of life.[55] Similar if not identical pulmonary arterial systolic murmurs are generated at sites of congenital stenosis of the pulmonary artery and its branches. Rarely, a pulmonary arterial systolic murmur is caused by luminal narrowing after a pulmonary embolus.[74]

Diastolic Murmurs

Diastolic murmurs, like systolic murmurs, are classified according to their time of onset as early diastolic, mid-diastolic, or late diastolic (presystolic) (Fig. 8–23). An early diastolic murmur begins with A_2 or P_2, depending on its side of origin. A mid-diastolic murmur begins at a clear interval after S_2. A late diastolic or presystolic murmur begins immediately before S_1.

Early Diastolic Murmurs

CHRONIC AORTIC REGURGITATION. An early diastolic murmur originating in the left side of the heart occurs in cases of aortic regurgitation (see Chap. 57). This murmur is heard best with the diaphragm of the stethoscope, with the patient leaning forward and during a held, deep exhalation (see Fig. 8–7D). The murmur begins with the aortic component of S_2 (Fig. 8–24A), that is, as soon as left ventricular pressure falls below the aortic incisura. The configuration of the murmur tends to reflect the volume and rate of regurgitant flow. In cases of chronic aortic regurgitation of moderate severity, the aortic diastolic pressure consistently and appreciably exceeds left ventricular diastolic pressure, so the decrescendo is subtle and the murmur is well heard throughout diastole. In cases of chronic severe aortic regurgitation, the decrescendo is more obvious, paralleling the dramatic decline in aortic root diastolic pressure. Selective radiation of the murmur of aortic regurgitation to the right sternal edge implies aortic root dilatation, as in patients with Marfan syndrome. When an inverted cusp is set into high-frequency periodic vibration by aortic regurgitation, the accompanying murmur is musical, early diastolic, and decrescendo (see Fig. 8–24B).

ACUTE AORTIC REGURGITATION. The diastolic murmur of acute severe aortic regurgitation differs importantly from the murmur of chronic severe aortic regurgitation as just described (Fig. 8-25). When regurgitant flow is both sudden *and* severe (as may occur in cases of infective endocarditis or aortic dissection), the diastolic murmur is relatively short because the aortic diastolic pressure rapidly equilibrates with the steeply rising diastolic pressure in the unprepared, nondilated left ventricle; the pitch of the murmur is likely to be medium and it may be quite soft (grade 2). These auscultatory features are in contrast to the long, pure, high-frequency, blowing and often loud (grade 4) early diastolic murmur of chronic severe aortic regurgitation (see Figs. 8-24 and 8-25).

Pulmonary Regurgitation. The Graham Steell murmur of pulmonary hypertensive pulmonary regurgitation begins with a loud P_2 because the elevated pressure exerted on the incompetent pulmonary valve begins at the moment that right ventricular pressure drops below the pulmonary arterial incisura. The high diastolic pressure generates high-velocity regurgitant flow and results in a high-frequency blowing murmur that may last throughout diastole. Because of the persistent and appreciable difference between pulmonary arterial and right ventricular diastolic pressures, the amplitude of the murmur is usually relatively uniform throughout most, if not all, of diastole.

Mid-Diastolic Murmurs

By definition, mid-diastolic murmurs begin at a clear interval after S_2 (Figs. 8–23 and 8–26). The majority of mid-diastolic murmurs originate across mitral or tricuspid valves during the rapid filling phase of the cardiac cycle (AV valve obstruction or abnormal patterns of AV flow) or across an incompetent pulmonary valve in the absence of pulmonary hypertension.

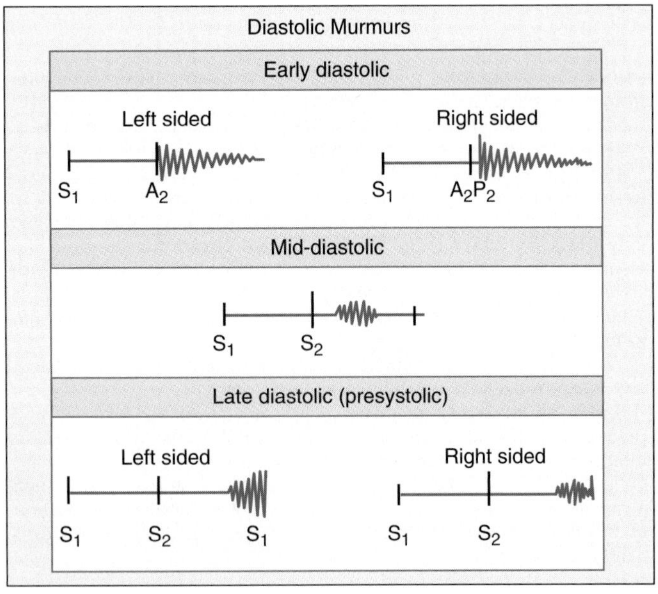

FIGURE 8–23 Diastolic murmurs are descriptively classified according to their time of onset as early diastolic, mid-diastolic, or late diastolic (presystolic). Diastolic murmurs originate in either the left or the right side of the heart.

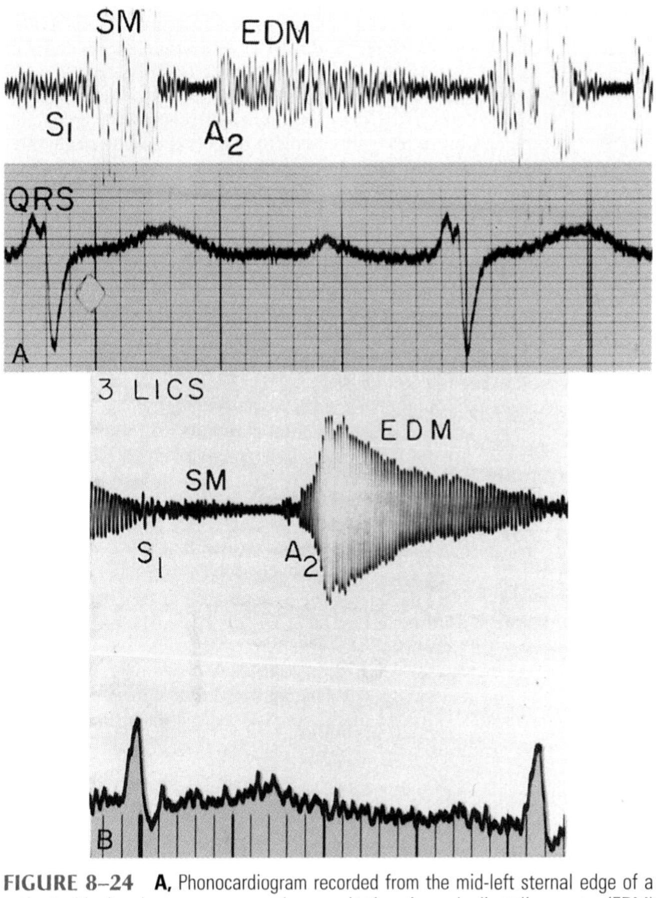

FIGURE 8–24 **A,** Phonocardiogram recorded from the mid-left sternal edge of a patient with chronic pure severe aortic regurgitation. An early diastolic murmur (EDM) proceeds immediately from the aortic component of the second heart sound (A_2). The murmur has an early crescendo followed by a late long decrescendo. There is a prominent midsystolic flow murmur (SM) across an unobstructed aortic valve. **B,** Phonocardiogram in the third left intercostal space (3 LICS) records a high-frequency, musical, early diastolic decrescendo murmur (EDM) caused by eversion of an aortic cusp. S_1 = first heart sound; SM = midsystolic murmur.

The mid-diastolic murmur of rheumatic mitral stenosis is a prime example.[87] The murmur characteristically follows the mitral opening snap (see Fig. 8–11B). Because the murmur originates within the left ventricular cavity, transmission to the chest wall is maximal over the left ventricular impulse. Care must be taken to place the bell of the stethoscope lightly against the skin precisely over the left ventricular impulse with the patient turned into the left lateral decubitus position (see Fig. 8–7C). Soft mid-diastolic murmurs are reinforced when the heart rate and mitral valve flow are transiently increased by vigorous voluntary coughs or a few sit-ups. In patients with atrial fibrillation, the duration of the mid-diastolic murmur is a useful sign of the degree of obstruction at the mitral orifice. A murmur that lasts up to S_1 even after long cycle lengths indicates that the stenosis is severe enough to generate a persistent gradient even at the end of long diastoles.

The mid-diastolic murmur of tricuspid stenosis occurs in the presence of atrial fibrillation. The tricuspid mid-diastolic murmur differs from the mitral mid-diastolic murmur in two important respects: (1) the loudness of the tricuspid murmur increases with inspiration, and (2) the tricuspid murmur is confined to a relatively localized area along the left lower sternal edge. The inspiratory increase in loudness occurs because inspiration is accompanied by an augmentation in right ventricular volume, by a fall in right ventricular diastolic pressure, and by an increase in gradient and flow rate across the stenotic tricuspid valve.[4] The murmur is localized to the lower left sternal edge because it originates within the inflow portion of the right ventricle and is transmitted to the overlying chest wall.

Mid-diastolic murmurs across unobstructed AV valves occur in the presence of augmented volume and velocity of flow. Examples in the left side of the heart are the mid-diastolic flow murmur of pure mitral regurgitation and the mid-diastolic mitral flow murmur that accompanies a large left-to-right shunt through a ventricular septal defect (Fig. 8–27A). Mid-diastolic murmurs due to augmented flow across unobstructed tricuspid valves are generated by severe tricuspid regurgitation or by a large left-to-right shunt through an atrial septal defect (see Fig. 8–27B). These mid-diastolic murmurs indicate appreciable AV valve incompetence or large left-to-right shunts and are often preceded by an S_3, especially in the presence of mitral or tricuspid regurgitation.

Short, mid-diastolic AV flow murmurs occur intermittently in patients with complete heart block when atrial contraction coincides with the phase of rapid diastolic filling. These murmurs are believed to result from antegrade flow across AV valves that are closing rapidly during filling of the recipient ventricle. A similar mechanism is believed to be responsible for the Austin Flint murmur (see Fig. 8–25).[88,89]

A mid-diastolic murmur is a feature of pulmonary valve regurgitation, provided that the pulmonary arterial pressure is not elevated. The diastolic murmur typically begins at a perceptible interval after P_2 is crescendo-decrescendo, and ends well before the subsequent S_1.[55] The diastolic pressure exerted on the incompetent pulmonary valve is negligible at the inception of P_2, so regurgitant flow is minimal. Regurgitation accelerates as right ventricular pressure dips below the diastolic pressure in the pulmonary trunk; at that point, the murmur reaches its maximum intensity. Late diastolic equilibration of pulmonary arterial and right ventricular pressures eliminates regurgitant flow and abolishes the murmur before the next S_1.

Late Diastolic or Presystolic Murmurs

A late diastolic murmur occurs immediately before S_1, that is, in presystole (see Fig. 8–23). With few exceptions, the late

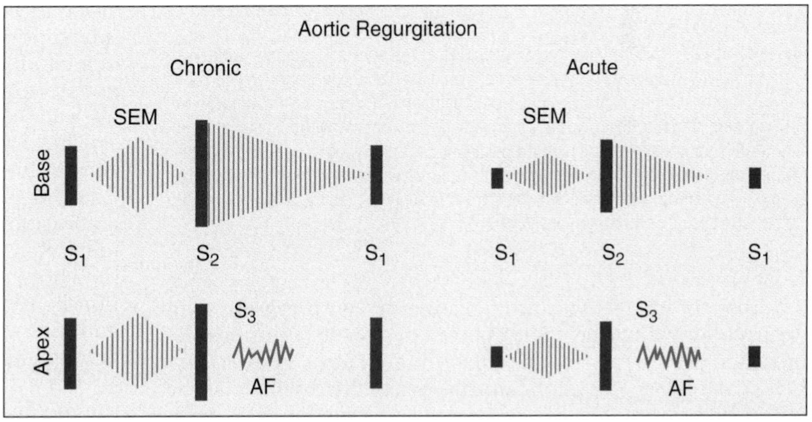

FIGURE 8–25 Contrast between the auscultatory findings in patients with chronic and acute aortic regurgitation. In a patient with chronic aortic regurgitation, a prominent systolic ejection murmur resulting from the large forward stroke volume is heard at the base and the apex and ends well before the second heart sound (S_2). The aortic diastolic regurgitant murmur begins with S_2 and continues in a decrescendo fashion, terminating before the first heart sound (S_1). At the apex, the early diastolic component of Austin Flint murmur (AF) is introduced by a prominent third heart sound (S_3). A presystolic component of the AF is also heard. In cases of acute aortic regurgitation, there is a significant decrease in the intensity of the systolic ejection murmur compared with that of chronic aortic regurgitation because of the decreased forward stroke volume. The S_1 is markedly decreased in intensity because of preclosure of the mitral valve, and at the apex the presystolic component of the AF murmur is absent. The early diastolic murmur at the base ends well before S_1 because of equilibration of the left ventricle and aortic end-diastolic pressures. Significant tachycardia is usually present. (From Shaver JA: Diastolic murmurs. Heart Dis Stroke 2:100, 1994.)

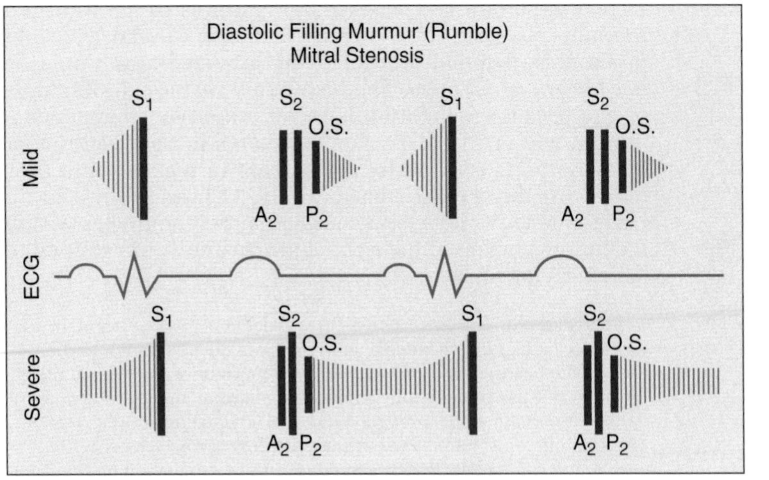

FIGURE 8–26 Diastolic filling murmur (rumble) in mitral stenosis. In cases of mild mitral stenosis, the diastolic gradient across the valve is limited to the two phases of rapid ventricular filling in early diastole and presystole. The rumble may occur during either period or during both periods. As the stenotic process becomes severe, a large pressure gradient exists across the valve during the entire diastolic filling period, and the rumble persists throughout diastole. As the left atrial pressure becomes greater, the interval between aortic component of the second heart sound (A_2) and the opening snap (O.S.) shortens. In cases of severe mitral stenosis, secondary pulmonary hypertension develops and results in a loud pulmonic component of the second heart sound (P_2) and the splitting interval usually narrows. S_1 = first heart sound; S_2 = second heart sound; ECG = electrocardiogram. (From Shaver JA, Leonard JJ, Leon DF: Examination of the Heart. Part IV: Auscultation of the Heart. Dallas, American Heart Association, 1990, p 55. Copyright 1990, American Heart Association.)

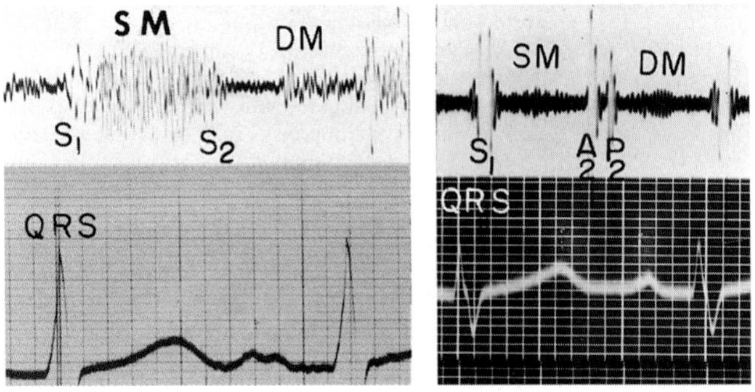

FIGURE 8–27 **A,** Phonocardiogram recorded at the apex of a patient with a moderately restrictive ventricular septal defect and increased pulmonary arterial blood flow. The mid-diastolic murmur (DM) results from augmented flow across the mitral valve. **B,** Phonocardiogram at the lower left sternal edge of a patient with an ostium secundum atrial septal defect and increased pulmonary arterial blood flow. A mid-diastolic murmur resulted from augmented flow across the tricuspid valve. SM = holosystolic murmur; S_1 = first heart sound; S_2 = second heart sound; A_2 and P_2 = aortic and pulmonic components of a conspicuously split S_2.

diastolic timing of the murmur coincides with the phase of ventricular filling that follows atrial systole and implies the presence of sinus rhythm and coordinated atrial contraction. Late diastolic or presystolic murmurs usually originate at the mitral or tricuspid orifice because of obstruction, but occasionally because of abnormal patterns of presystolic AV flow.

The best known presystolic murmur accompanies rheumatic mitral stenosis in sinus rhythm as AV flow is augmented in response to an increase in the force of left atrial contraction (Figs. 8–11B and 8–28A).[65] Presystolic accentuation of a mid-diastolic murmur is occasionally heard in patients with mitral stenosis with atrial fibrillation, especially during short cycle lengths; however, the timing is actually early systolic, and the mechanism differs from the true presystolic murmur as described earlier and as shown in Figure 8–28A.

TRICUSPID STENOSIS. In patients with tricuspic stenosis who are in sinus rhythm, a late diastolic or presystolic murmur typically occurs in the absence of a perceptible mid-diastolic murmur (see Fig. 8–28B). This is so because the timing of tricuspid diastolic murmurs reflects the maximal acceleration of flow and gradient, which is usually negligible until a powerful right atrial contraction occurs.[4] The presystolic murmur of tricuspid stenosis is crescendo-decrescendo and relatively discrete, fading before S_1 (see Fig. 8–28B). This is in contrast to the presystolic murmur of mitral stenosis, which tends to rise in a crescendo up to S_1 (see Fig. 8–28A). The most valuable auscultatory sign of tricuspid stenosis in sinus rhythm is the effect of respiration on the intensity of the presystolic murmur. Inspiration increases right atrial volume, provoking an increase in right atrial contractile force that coincides with a fall in right ventricular end-diastolic pressure. The result is an increase in the tricuspid gradient, in the velocity of tricuspid flow, and in the intensity of the tricuspid stenotic presystolic murmur (Fig. 8–29).

THE AUSTIN FLINT MURMUR (see Fig. 8–25). In 1862, Austin Flint described a presystolic murmur in patients with aortic regurgitation and proposed a mechanism that was astonishingly perceptive[88-91]: "Now in cases of considerable aortic insufficiency, the left ventricle is rapidly filled with blood flowing back from the aorta as well as from the auricle, before the auricular contraction takes place. The distention of the ventricle is such that the mitral curtains are brought into coaptation; and when the auricular contraction takes place, the mitral direct current passing between the curtains throws them into vibration and gives rise to the characteristic blubbering murmur."[88]

Continuous Murmurs

The term *continuous* appropriately applies to murmurs that begin in systole and continue without interruption through S_2 into all or part of diastole (Fig. 8–30). The presence of murmurs throughout both phases of the cardiac cycle (holosystolic followed by holodiastolic) is not the criterion for the designation "continuous." Conversely, a murmur that fades completely before the subsequent S_1 may be continuous, provided that the systolic portion of the murmur proceeds without interruption through S_2.

Continuous murmurs are generated by uninterrupted flow from a vascular bed of higher pressure or resistance into a vascular bed of lower pressure or resistance without phasic interruption between systole and diastole. Such murmurs are due chiefly to (1) aortopulmonary connections, (2) arteriovenous connections, (3) disturbances of flow patterns in arteries, and (4) disturbances of flow patterns in veins (Table 8–7).

The best known continuous murmur is associated with the aortopulmonary connection of patent ductus arteriosus (see Chap 56; Fig. 8–31). The murmur characteristically peaks just before and after S_2, which it envelops, decreases in late diastole (often appreciably), and may be soft or even absent before the subsequent first heart sound.[55] George Gibson's description in 1900 was even more precise.[92] "It persists through S_2 and dies away gradually during the long pause. The murmur is rough and thrilling. It begins softly and increases in intensity so as to reach its acme just about, or immediately after, the incidence of the second sound, and from that point gradually wanes until its termination."

ARTERIOVENOUS CONTINUOUS MURMURS. These can be congenital or acquired and are represented in part by arteriovenous fistulas, coronary arterial fistulas, anomalous origin of the left coronary artery from the pulmonary trunk, and communications between the sinus of Valsalva and the right side of the heart.[55] The configuration, location, and intensity of arteriovenous continuous murmurs vary considerably among these different lesions. Acquired systemic arteriovenous fistulas are created surgically by forearm shunts for hemodialysis. Congenital arteriovenous continuous murmurs occur when a coronary arterial fistula enters the pulmonary trunk, right atrium, or right ventricle. At the right ventricle, the continuous murmur can be either softer or louder in systole, depending on the degree of compression exerted on the fistulous coronary artery by right ventricular contraction.[55] Rupture of a congenital aortic sinus aneurysm into the right side of the heart results in a continuous murmur that tends to be louder in either systole or diastole, sometimes creating a to-and-fro impression.[55]

ARTERIAL CONTINUOUS MURMURS. These originate in either constricted or nonconstricted arteries. A common example of a continuous murmur arising in a constricted artery is carotid or femoral arterial atherosclerotic obstruction. Not surprisingly, these murmurs are characteristically louder in systole and more often than not are purely systolic.

Disturbances of flow patterns in normal, nonconstricted arteries sometimes produce continuous murmurs. The "mammary souffle" described earlier,[4] an innocent murmur heard during late pregnancy and the puerperium, is an arterial murmur that, when continuous, is typically louder in systole and maximal over either lactating breast.

Continuous murmurs in nonconstricted arteries originate in the large systemic-to-pulmonary arterial collaterals in certain types of cyanotic congenital heart disease, typically tetralogy of Fallot with pulmonary atresia. These continuous murmurs are randomly located throughout the thorax because of the random location of the aortopulmonary collaterals.[55] They are also heard in coarctation of the aorta (see Chap. 56).

CONTINUOUS VENOUS MURMURS. These are well represented by the innocent cervical venous "hum" (Fig. 8–32). The hum is by far the most common type of normal continuous murmur, universal in healthy children, and frequently present in healthy young adults, especially during pregnancy. Thyrotoxicosis and anemia, by augmenting cervical venous flow, initiate or reinforce the venous hum. The term *hum* does not necessarily characterize the quality of these cervical venous murmurs, which may be rough and noisy and are occasionally accompanied by a high-pitched whine.[55] The hum is truly continuous, although

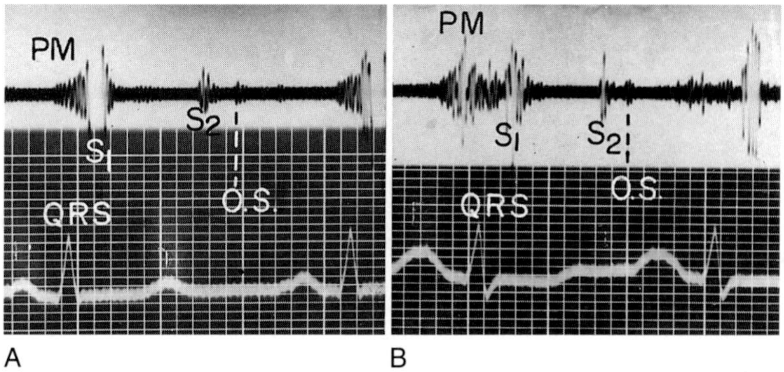

FIGURE 8–28 **A,** Phonocardiogram from the cardiac apex of a patient with pure rheumatic mitral stenosis. A presystolic murmur (PM) rises in a crescendo that is interrupted by a loud first heart sound (S_1). **B,** Phonocardiogram from the lower left sternal edge of a patient with rheumatic tricuspid stenosis. The first cycle is during inspiration and is accompanied by a prominent presystolic murmur (PM) that is crescendo-decrescendo, decreasing before the S_1. During exhalation (second cycle), the presystolic murmur all but vanishes. S_2 = second heart sound; OS = mitral opening snap.

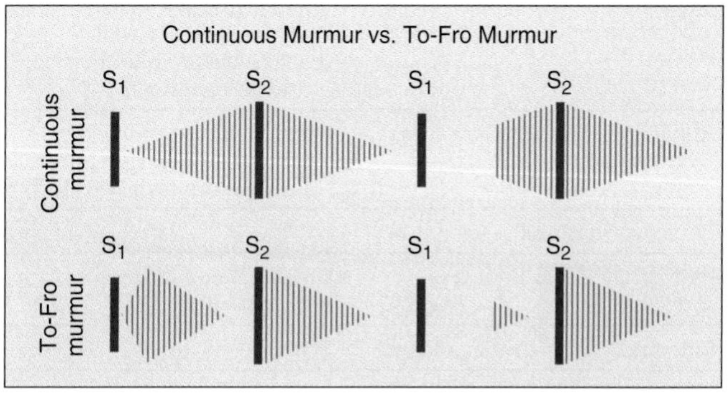

FIGURE 8–30 Comparison of continuous murmurs and to-fro murmurs. During abnormal communication between high-pressure and low-pressure systems, a large pressure gradient exists through the cardiac cycle, producing a continuous murmur. A classic example is patent ductus arteriosus. At times, this type of murmur is confused with a to-fro murmur, which is a combination of systolic ejection murmur and a murmur of semilunar valve incompetence. A classic example of a to-fro murmur is aortic stenosis and regurgitation. A continuous murmur crescendos to around the second heart sound (S_2), whereas a to-fro murmur has two components. The midsystolic ejection component decrescendos and disappears as it approaches S_2. S_1 = first heart sound. (From Shaver JA, Leonard JJ, Leon DF: Examination of the Heart. Part IV: Auscultation of the Heart. Dallas, American Heart Association, 1990, p 55. Copyright 1990, American Heart Association.)

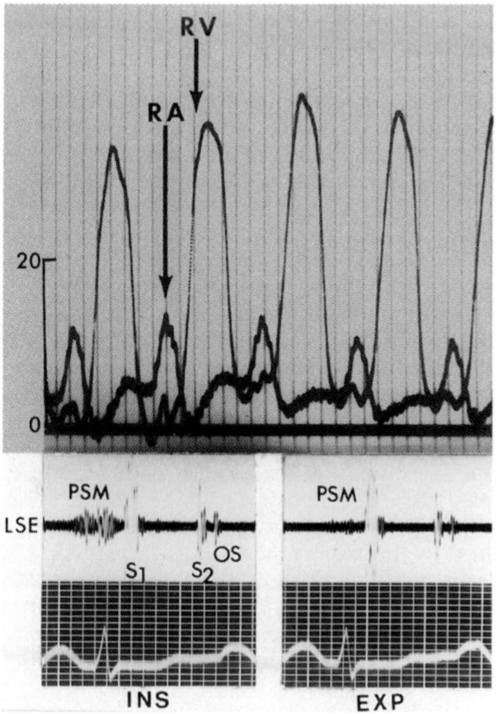

FIGURE 8–29 Pressure pulses and phonocardiogram illustrating the physiological mechanism of the respiratory variation in the presystolic murmur of tricuspid stenosis. During inhalation, a fall in intrathoracic pressure and an increase in systemic venous return result in an increase in the right atrial (RA) A wave and a decline in right ventricular (RV) end-diastolic pressure, so the presystolic murmur (PSM) increases in loudness. During exhalation, the right atrial A wave declines, the RV diastolic pressure increases, the tricuspid gradient is at its minimum, and the PSM all but vanishes. LSE = left sternal edge; S_1 = first heart sound; S_2 = second heart sound; INS = inspiration; EXP = expiration.

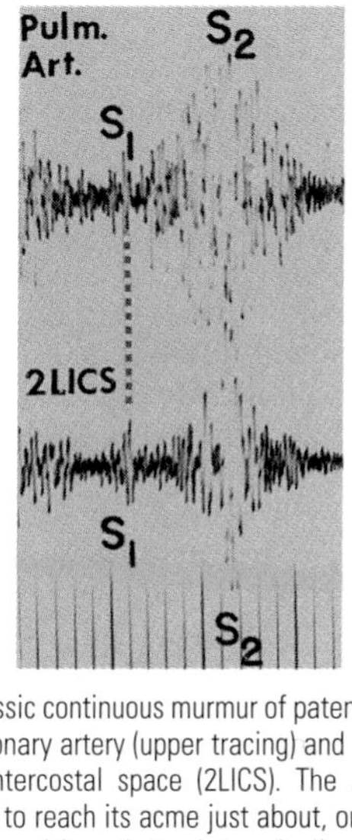

FIGURE 8–31 The classic continuous murmur of patent ductus arteriosus recorded from within the main pulmonary artery (upper tracing) and simultaneously on the chest wall at the second left intercostal space (2LICS). The murmur "begins softly and increases in intensity so as to reach its acme just about, or immediately after, the incidence of the second sound, and from that point gradually wanes until its termination," as originally described by Gibson in 1900.[92] Pulm. Art. = pulmonary artery; S_1 = first heart sound; S_2 = second heart sound.

TABLE 8–7 Differential Diagnosis of Continuous Thoracic Murmurs (in Order of Frequency)

Diagnosis	Key Findings
Cervical venous hum	Disappears on compression of the jugular vein
Hepatic venous hum	Often disappears with epigastric pressure
Mammary souffle	Disappears on pressing hard with stethoscope
Patent ductus arteriosus	Loudest at second left intercostal space
Coronary arteriovenous fistula	Loudest at lower sternal borders
Ruptured aneurysm of sinus of Valsalva	Loudest at upper right sternal border, sudden onset
Bronchial collaterals	Associated signs of congenital heart disease High-grade coarctation Brachial pedal arterial pressure gradient
Anomalous left coronary artery arising from pulmonary artery	Electrocardiographic changes of myocardial infarction
Truncus arteriosus	
Pulmonary artery branch stenosis	Heard outside the area of cardiac dullness
Pulmonary arteriovenous fistula	Same as above
Atrial septal defect with mitral stenosis or atresia	Altered by the Valsalva maneuver
Aortic-atrial fistulas	

Adapted from Sapira JD: The Art and Science of Bedside Diagnosis. Baltimore, Urban & Schwartzenberg, 1990.

typically louder in diastole. The mechanism of the venous hum is unsettled. Silent laminar flow in the internal jugular vein may be disturbed by deformation of the vessel at the level of the transverse process of the atlas during head rotation designed to elicit the hum.[93]

Approach to the Patient with a Heart Murmur

Although a careful physical examination with emphasis on detailed auscultation is useful in establishing a cardiac diagnosis or excluding serious cardiac disease in a patient with a heart murmur, echocardiography is decisive in confirming the diagnosis and determining the severity of the condition (Fig. 8–33). As delineated by O'Rourke,[77] the approach to the patient with a heart murmur depends on its intensity, timing, location, response to maneuvers, and the presence of other cardiac and noncardiac symptoms and signs. Patients with diastolic murmurs, or continuous murmurs that are not cervical venous hums, or mammary souffles of pregnancy, should ordinarily go to two-dimensional and Doppler echocardiography, and subsequent work-up, including cardiac consultation, is guided by the echocardiographic findings. In general, echocardiography is also advised for patients with systolic murmurs having the following characteristics: (1) loud murmur (i.e., grade 3 or higher); (2) holosystolic or late systolic murmur, especially at the left sternal edge or apex; (3) systolic murmurs that become louder or longer during the strain of the Valsalva maneuver (suggesting the diagnosis of hypertrophic obstructive cardiomyopathy or

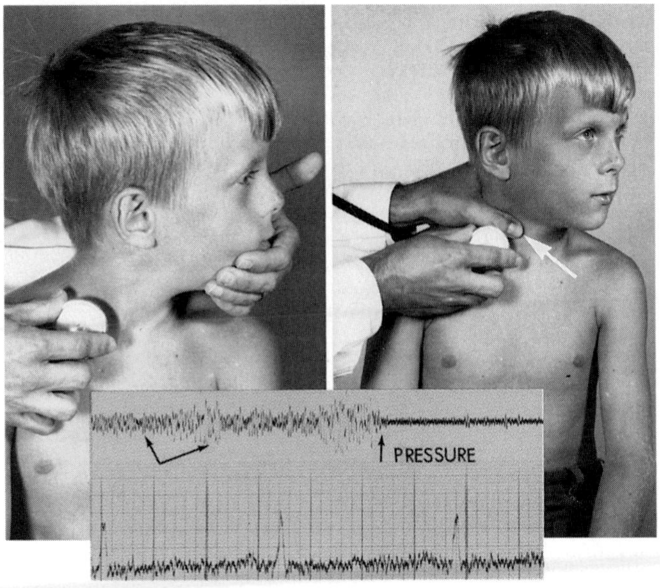

FIGURE 8–32 The phonocardiogram shows the continuous murmur of a normal venous hum. The diastolic component is louder (paired arrows). Digital pressure over the right internal jugular vein (vertical arrow) abolishes the murmur. The photographs show maneuvers used to elicit or abolish the venous hum. **Left,** The bell of the stethoscope is applied to the medial aspect of the right supraclavicular fossa as the examiner's left hand grasps the patient's chin from behind and pulls it tautly to the left and upward, stretching the neck. **Right,** The patient's head has returned to a more neutral position, and digital compression of the right internal jugular vein (arrow) abolishes the hum.

mitral valve prolapse respectively); (4) other systolic murmurs in patients with clinical findings suggesting infective endocarditis (see Chap. 58), thromboembolism, or syncope; (5) a systolic murmur accompanied by an abnormal electrocardiogram.

According to this schema, a large majority of patients with heart murmurs (i.e., patients with grade 1 or grade 2 midsystolic murmurs) without any other clinical manifestations of cardiac disease ordinarily do not require extensive work-up.

Pericardial Rubs (see Chap. 64)

In sinus rhythm, the typical pericardial "rub" is triple phased, that is, midsystolic, mid-diastolic, and presystolic. Recognition is simplest when all three phases are present and when the characteristic superficial scratchy, leathery quality is evident. Pericardial rubs may be more readily detected when the patient is on elbows and knees (Fig. 8–34), a physical maneuver designed to increase the contact of visceral and parietal pericardium (see earlier). The term *rub* is appropriate because the auscultatory sign is generated by abnormal visceral and parietal pericardial surfaces "rubbing" against each other. In the supine position, firm pressure with the stethoscopic diaphragm during full held exhalation reinforces visceral and parietal pericardial contact and accentuates the rub. Apposition of visceral and parietal pericardium can be even better achieved by examination while the patient rests on elbows and knees.

Of the three phases of the pericardial rub, the systolic phase is the most consistent,[94] followed by the presystolic phase. In atrial fibrillation, the presystolic component necessarily disappears. The diagnosis of a pericardial rub is least secure when only one phase remains, which is typically the midsystolic. The most common clinical setting in which pericardial rubs are heard is immediately after open heart surgery. However, auscultation often detects instead a "crunch" synchronous with the heartbeat, especially in the left lateral decubitus position. This is not a pericardial rub but is Hamman sign caused by air in the mediastinum.[95] Pericardial rubs are frequently audible in patients with acute pericarditis. They may become softer or even disappear in the presence of a large pericardial effusion.

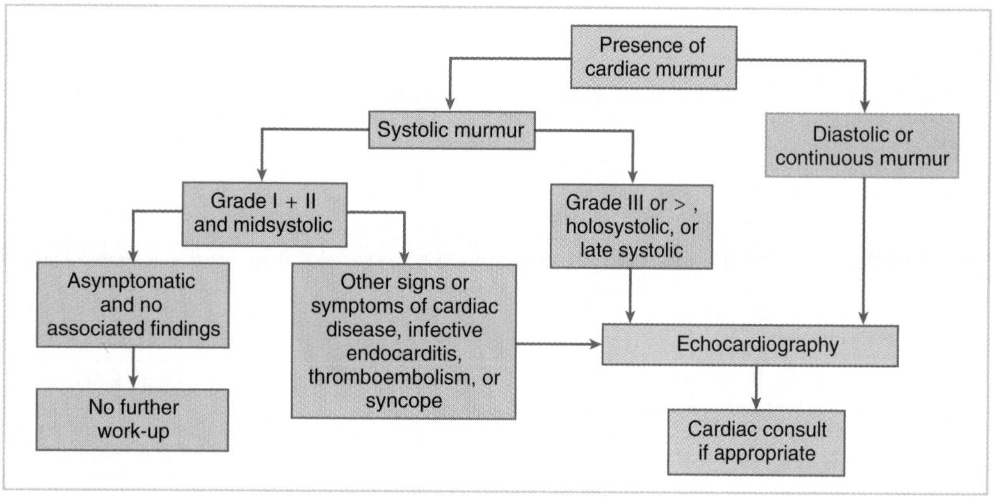

FIGURE 8–33 A schematic approach to the work-up of a patient with a cardiac murmur according to whether the murmur is probably innocent or secondary to cardiac pathology. This algorithm is particularly relevant to children and adults younger than 40 years, and echocardiography is recommended before cardiac consultation. (From Norton PJ, O'Rourke RA: Approach to the patients with a heart murmur. *In* Braunwald E, Goldman L [eds]: Primary Cardiology. 2nd ed. Philadelphia, Elsevier, 2003.)

Dynamic Auscultation

Dynamic auscultation refers to the technique of altering circulatory dynamics by a variety of physiological and pharmacological maneuvers and determining the effects of these maneuvers on heart sounds and murmurs.[96,97] The conditions and interventions most commonly employed in dynamic auscultation include respiration, postural changes, the Valsalva maneuver, premature ventricular contractions, isometric exercise, and one of the vasoactive agents—amyl nitrite, methoxamine, or phenylephrine.

Respiration

SECOND HEART SOUND. The splitting of S_2 is most audible along the left sternal border and can usually be appreciated when A_2 and P_2 are separated by more than 0.02 second. The effects of respiration on the splitting of the second heart sound were discussed earlier (see Second Heart Sound).

DIASTOLIC SOUNDS AND EJECTION SOUNDS. When S_3 and S_4 originate from the right ventricle, they are characteristically augmented during inspiration and diminished during exhalation, whereas they exhibit the opposite response when they originate from the left side of the heart. Like other left-sided events, the opening snap of the mitral valve may become softer during inspiration and louder during exhalation, owing to respiratory alterations in venous return, whereas the opening snap of the tricuspid valve behaves in the opposite fashion. Inspiration also diminishes the intensity of ejection sounds in pulmonary valve stenosis because the elevation of right ventricular diastolic pressure causes partial presystolic opening of the pulmonary valve and therefore less upward motion of the valve during systole. On the other hand, respiration does not affect the intensity of aortic ejection sounds, except in cases of tetralogy of Fallot with pulmonary atresia.

MURMURS. Respiration exerts more pronounced and consistent alterations on murmurs originating from the right than from the left side of the heart. During inspiration, the diastolic murmurs of tricuspid stenosis (see Fig. 8–29) and low-pressure pulmonary regurgitation, the systolic murmurs of tricuspid regurgitation (Carvallo sign),[98] and the presystolic murmur of Ebstein anomaly may all be accentuated. The inspiratory reduction in left ventricular size in patients with mitral valve prolapse increases the redundancy of the mitral valve and therefore the degree of valvular prolapse; consequently, the midsystolic click and the systolic murmurs occur earlier during systole and may become accentuated.[99]

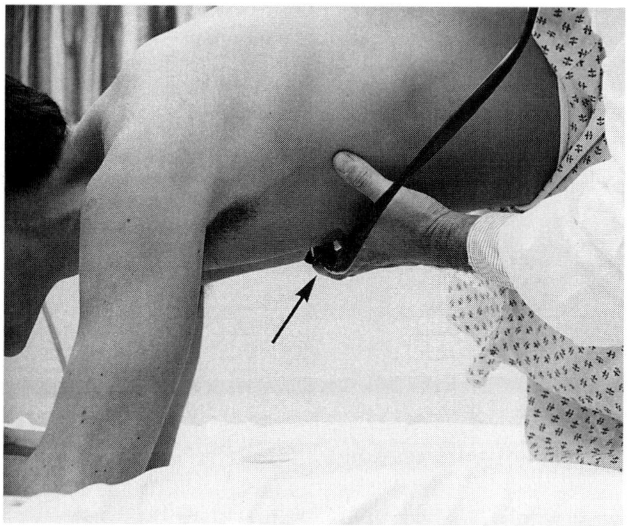

FIGURE 8–34 A technique for eliciting a pericardial rub. The diaphragm of the stethoscope is firmly applied to the precordium (arrow) while the patient rests on elbows and knees.

THE VALSALVA MANEUVER. This maneuver consists of a relatively deep inspiration followed by forced exhalation against a closed glottis for 10 to 20 seconds. The patient should first be instructed on how to perform the maneuver. Simulation by the examiner is a simple means of doing so. The examiner then places the flat of the hand on the abdomen to provide the patient with a force against which to strain and to permit assessment of the degree and duration of the straining effort.[100,101]

The normal response to the Valsalva maneuver consists of four phases. Phase I is associated with a transient rise in systemic arterial pressure as straining commences. Phase II is accompanied by a perceptible decrease in systemic venous return, systolic pressure, and pulse pressure (small pulse) and by reflex tachycardia. Phase III begins promptly with cessation of straining and is associated with an abrupt, transient decrease in arterial pressure. Phase IV is characterized by an overshoot of systemic arterial pressure and reflex bradycardia. During phase II, S_3 and S_4 are attenuated and the A_2-P_2 interval narrows or is abolished. As stroke volume and systemic arterial pressure fall, the systolic murmurs of aortic and pulmonary stenosis and of mitral and tricuspid regurgitation diminish and the diastolic murmurs of aortic and pulmonary regurgitation and of tricuspid and mitral stenosis soften. As left ventricular volume is reduced, the systolic murmur of hypertrophic obstructive cardiomyopathy amplifies and the click and late systolic murmur of mitral valve prolapse begin earlier. In phase III, the sudden increase in systemic venous return is accompanied by wide splitting of the S_2 and by augmentation of murmurs and filling sounds in the right side of the heart. Murmurs and filling sounds in the left side of the heart return to control levels and may transiently increase during the overshoot of phase IV.

In patients with atrial septal defect, mitral stenosis, or heart failure, the Valsalva maneuver provokes a "square wave" response, negating the four phases and their auscultatory equivalents. The Valsalva maneuver should not be performed in patients with ischemic heart disease because of the accompanying fall in coronary blood flow.

THE MULLER MANEUVER. This maneuver is the converse of the Valsalva maneuver but is less frequently employed because it is not as useful. In this maneuver, the patient forcibly inspires while the nose is held closed and the mouth is firmly sealed for about 10 seconds. The Muller maneuver exaggerates the inspiratory effort, widens the split S_2, and augments murmurs and filling sounds originating in the right side of the heart.

POSTURAL CHANGES AND EXERCISE (Fig. 8-35)

Sudden assumption of the lying position from the standing or sitting position or sudden passive elevation of both legs results in an increase in venous return, which augments first right ventricular and, several cardiac cycles later, left ventricular stroke volume. The principal auscultatory changes include widening of the splitting of S_2 in all phases of respiration and augmentations of right-sided S_3 and S_4 and, several cardiac cycles later, left-sided S_3 and S_4. The systolic murmurs of pulmonic valve stenosis and aortic stenosis, the systolic murmurs of mitral and tricuspid regurgitation and ventricular septal defect, and most functional systolic murmurs are augmented. On the other hand, because left ventricular end-diastolic volume is increased, the systolic murmur of hypertrophic obstructive cardiomyopathy is diminished and the midsystolic click and late systolic murmur associated with mitral valve prolapse are delayed and sometimes attenuated (see Fig. 8-12).

Rapid standing or sitting up from a lying position or rapid standing from a squatting posture has the opposite effect; in patients in whom there is relatively wide splitting of S_2 during exhalation—a finding that may be confused with fixed splitting—the width of the splitting is reduced, so that a normal pattern emerges during the respiratory cycle. No change in splitting occurs in patients with true fixed splitting. The decrease in venous return reduces stroke volume and innocent pulmonary flow murmurs as well as the murmurs of semilunar valve stenosis and of AV valve regurgitation. The auscultatory changes in hypertrophic cardiomyopathy and mitral valve prolapse are opposite to those on assumption of the lying posture just described.

SQUATTING. A sudden change from standing to squatting increases venous return and systemic resistance simultaneously. Stroke volume and arterial pressure rise, and the latter may induce a transient reflex bradycardia. The auscultatory features include augmentation of S_3 and S_4 (from both ventricles) and as a consequence of an increase in stroke volume, the systolic murmurs of pulmonary and aortic stenosis and the diastolic murmurs of tricuspid and mitral stenosis become louder, with right-sided events preceding left-sided events. Squatting may make audible a previously inaudible murmur of aortic regurgitation.

The elevation of arterial pressure increases blood flow through the right ventricular outflow tract of patients with tetralogy of Fallot and increases the volume of mitral regurgitation and of the left-to-right shunt through a ventricular septal defect, thereby increasing the intensity of the systolic murmur in these conditions. Also, the diastolic murmur of aortic regurgitation is augmented consequent to an increase in aortic reflux. The combination of elevated arterial pressure and increased venous return increases left ventricular size, which reduces the obstruction to outflow and thus the intensity of the systolic murmur of hypertrophic obstructive cardiomyopathy; the midsystolic click and the late systolic murmur of mitral valve prolapse are delayed.

OTHER POSITIONAL CHANGES. Assumption of the left lateral recumbent position accentuates the intensity of S_1, S_3, and S_4 originating from the left side of the heart; the opening snap and the murmurs associated with mitral stenosis and regurgitation; the midsystolic click and late systolic murmur of mitral valve prolapse; and the Austin Flint murmur associated with aortic regurgitation. Sitting up and leaning forward (see Fig. 8-10D) make the diastolic murmurs of aortic and pulmonary regurgitation more readily audible.

Stretching the neck to elicit a venous hum is illustrated in Figure 8-32. Passive elevation of the legs with the patient supine transiently increases venous return and augments S_3.

ISOMETRIC EXERCISE. This can be carried out simply and reproducibly using a calibrated handgrip device or hand ball. (It is useful to carry out isometric exercise bilaterally simultaneously.) Isometric exercise should be avoided in patients with ventricular arrhythmias and myocardial ischemia, both of which can be intensified by this activity. Handgrip should be sustained for 20 to 30 seconds, but a Valsalva maneuver during the handgrip must be avoided. Isometric exercise results in transient but significant increases in systemic vascular resistance, arterial pressure, heart rate, cardiac output, left ventricular filling pressure, and heart size.

As a consequence, (1) S_3 and S_4 originating from the left side of the heart become accentuated; (2) the systolic murmur of aortic stenosis is diminished as a result of reduction of the pressure gradient across the aortic valve[102]; (3) the diastolic murmur of aortic regurgitation and the systolic murmurs of rheumatic mitral regurgitation and ventricular septal defect increase in intensity; (4) the diastolic murmur of mitral stenosis becomes louder consequent to the increase in cardiac output; and (5) the systolic murmur of hypertrophic obstructive cardiomyopathy diminishes and the systolic click and late systolic murmur of mitral valve prolapse are delayed because of the increased left ventricular volume.

PHARMACOLOGICAL AGENTS (see Fig. 8-35)

AMYL NITRITE. Inhalation of amyl nitrite is carried out by placing an ampule in gauze near the supine patient's nose and then crushing the ampule. The patient is asked to take three or four deep breaths over 10 to 15 seconds, after which the amyl nitrite is removed. The drug produces marked vasodilatation, resulting in the first 30 seconds in a reduction of systemic arterial pressure and 30 to 60 seconds later in a

Diagnosis	Systolic Murmur	Second Sound	Effect of Posture: Erect	Effect of Posture: Squatting	Amyl Nitrite	Phenylephrine
			Changes in intensity of systolic murmur			
1. Hypertrophic obstructive cardiomyopathy		Variable ie - reversed partially reversed narrow or normal	↑	↓	↑	↓
2. Mitral regurgitation a. Pure severe		widely split	↓	↑	↓	↑
b. Papillary muscle dysfunction		normal or partially reversed	↑↓	↑	↓	↑
c. Billowing posterior leaflet		normal	↑↓	↑	↓	↑
d. Rheumatic of moderate degree		slightly wide	↓	↑	↓	↑
3. Valvular aortic stenosis: mild to mod		narrow or partially reversed	↓	↑	↑	—
3. Valvular aortic stenosis: marked		reversed	↓	↑	↑	—
4. Ventricular septal defect		slightly wide	—↓	↑	↓	↑
5. Innocent vibratory systolic murmur		normal	↓	—	↑	↓

— No change from control ↑ ↑ Degree of increase ↓ ↓ Degree of decrease

FIGURE 8–35 Diagrammatic representation of the character of the systolic murmur and of the second heart sound in five conditions. The effects of posture, amyl nitrite inhalation, and phenylephrine injection on the intensity of the murmur are shown. (Modified from Barlow JB: Perspectives on the Mitral Valve. Philadelphia, FA Davis, 1987, p 138.)

reflex tachycardia, followed in turn by a reflex increase in cardiac output, velocity of blood flow, and heart rate.[4,97,101,103] The major auscultatory changes occur in the first 30 seconds after inhalation. S_1 is augmented, and A_2 is diminished. The opening snaps of the mitral and tricuspid valves become louder, and as arterial pressure falls, the A_2/opening snap interval shortens. An S_3 originating in either ventricle is augmented, owing to greater rapidity of ventricular filling; but because mitral regurgitation is reduced, the S_3 associated with this lesion is diminished. The systolic murmurs of aortic valve stenosis, pulmonary stenosis, hypertrophic obstructive cardiomyopathy, tricuspid regurgitation, and functional systolic murmurs are all accentuated.

The response to amyl nitrite is useful in distinguishing (1) the systolic murmur of aortic stenosis (which is augmented) from that of mitral regurgitation (which is diminished)[103]; (2) the systolic murmur of tricuspid regurgitation (augmented) from that of mitral regurgitation (diminished); (3) the systolic murmur of isolated pulmonary stenosis (augmented) from that of tetralogy of Fallot (diminished); (4) the diastolic rumbling murmur of mitral stenosis (augmented) from the Austin Flint murmur of aortic regurgitation (diminished); and (5) the early blowing diastolic murmur of pulmonary regurgitation (augmented) from that of aortic regurgitation (diminished).

In patients with tetralogy of Fallot, the reduction of arterial pressure increases the right-to-left shunt and decreases the blood flow from the right ventricle to the pulmonary artery and diminishes the midsystolic murmur. The increase in cardiac output augments the diastolic murmurs of mitral and tricuspid stenosis and of pulmonary regurgitation and the systolic murmur of tricuspid regurgitation. However, as a result of the fall in systemic arterial pressure, the systolic murmurs of mitral regurgitation and ventricular septal defect, the diastolic murmurs of aortic regurgitation, and the Austin Flint murmur as well as the continuous murmurs of patent ductus arteriosus and of systemic arteriovenous fistula are all diminished. The reduction of cardiac size results in an earlier appearance of the midsystolic click and late systolic murmur of mitral valve prolapse; the intensity of the systolic murmur exhibits a variable response.

METHOXAMINE AND PHENYLEPHRINE. These agents increase systemic arterial pressure and exert an effect opposite to that of amyl nitrite. Phenylephrine is preferred because of its shorter duration of action; when administered intravenously it elevates systolic pressure by approximately 30 mm Hg for only 3 to 5 minutes. Both drugs cause reflex bradycardia and decreased contractility and cardiac output. They should not be used in the presence of congestive heart failure and systemic hypertension.

After administration, the intensity of S_1 is usually reduced, and the A_2/mitral opening snap interval becomes prolonged. The responses of S_3 and S_4 are variable. As a result of the increased arterial pressure, the diastolic murmur of aortic regurgitation, the systolic murmurs of mitral regurgitation, ventricular septal defect, and tetralogy of Fallot, and the continuous murmurs of patent ductus arteriosus and systemic arteriovenous fistula all become louder. On the other hand, as a consequence of the increase in left ventricular size, the systolic murmur of hypertrophic obstructive cardiomyopathy becomes softer and the click and late systolic murmur of mitral valve prolapse are delayed. The reduction in cardiac output diminishes the systolic murmur of aortic valve stenosis, functional systolic murmurs, and the diastolic murmur of mitral stenosis. The rumbling diastolic murmurs of mitral regurgitation and the Austin Flint murmur also diminish.

REFERENCES

The General Physical Examination

1. Mangione S, Nieman LZ, Gracely E, et al: The teaching and practice of cardiac auscultation during internal medicine and cardiology training: A nationwide survey. Ann Intern Med 119:47, 1993.
2. Shaver JA: Cardiac auscultation: A cost-effective diagnostic skill. Curr Probl Cardiol 20:441, 1995.
3. Tavel M: Cardiac auscultation: A glorious past—but does it have a future? Circulation 93:1250, 1996.
4. Perloff JK: Physical Examination of the Heart and Circulation. 3rd ed. Philadelphia, WB Saunders, 2000.
5. Roldan CA, Abrams J (eds): Evaluation of the Patient with Heart Disease: Integrating the Physical Exam and Echocardiography. Philadelphia: Lippincott Williams & Wilkins, 2002, pp 383.
6. Swartz MH (ed): Textbook of Physical Diagnosis: History and Examination. 3rd ed. Philadelphia, WB Saunders, 1998.
7. O'Rourke RA, Braunwald E: Physical Examination of the Cardiovascular System. *In* Kasper DL et al (eds): Harrison's Principles of Internal Medicine. 16th ed. New York: McGraw-Hill, 2005.
8. Kirkham N, Murrels T, Melcher SH, Morrison EA: Diagonal ear lobe creases and fatal cardiovascular disease: A necropsy study. Br Heart J 61:361, 1989.
9. Woywodt A, Welzel J, Haase H, et al: Cardiomyopathic lentiginosis/LEOPARD syndrome presenting as sudden cardiac arrest. Chest 113:1415, 1998.
10. Basson CT, Cowley GS, Solomon SD, et al: The clinical and genetic spectrum of the Holt-Oram syndrome (heart-hand syndrome). N Engl J Med 330:885, 1994.
11. Buckley MJ, Mason DT, Ross J Jr, Braunwald E: Reversed differential cyanosis with equal desaturation of the upper limbs: Syndrome of complete transposition of the great vessels with complete interruption of the aortic arch. Am J Cardiol 15:111, 1965.
12. Fishman AP: Approach to the patient with respiratory symptoms. *In* Fishman AP (ed): Pulmonary Diseases and Disorders. New York, McGraw-Hill, 1998, pp. 361-394.
13. Yee J, McAllister CK: The utility of Osler's nodes in the diagnosis of infective endocarditis. Chest 92:751, 1987.
14. Braunwald E: Edema. *In* Kasper DL, et al (eds): Harrison's Principles of Internal Medicine. 16th ed. New York, McGraw-Hill, 2005.
15. Willekes CL, Backer CL, Mavroudis C: A 26-year review of pectus deformity repairs, including simultaneous intracardiac repair. Ann Thorac Surg 67:511, 1999.
16. Fonkalsrud EW, Bustorff-Silva J: Repair of pectus excavatum and carinatum in adults. Am J Surg 177:121, 1999.
17. Wiese J: The abdominojugular reflux sign. Am J Med 109:59, 2000.
18. Butman SM, Ewy GA, Standen JR, et al: Bedside cardiovascular examination in patients with severe chronic heart failure: Importance of rest or inducible jugular venous distension. J Am Coll Cardiol 22:968, 1993.
19. Perloff JK: The jugular venous pulse and third heart sound in patients with heart failure. N Engl J Med 345:612, 2001.
20. Bilchick KC, Wise RA: Paradoxical physical findings described by Kussmaul: Pulsus paradoxus and Kussmaul's sign. Lancet 359:1940, 2002.
21. Drazner MH, Rame JE, Stevenson LW, Dries DL: Prognostic importance of elevated jugular venous pressure and a third heart sound in patients with heart failure. N Engl J Med 345:574, 2001.
22. Linfors EW, Feussner JR, Blessing CL, et al: Spurious hypertension in the obese patient: Effect of sphygmomanometer cuff size on prevalence of hypertension. Arch Intern Med 144:1482, 1984.
23. Nelson WP, Egbert AM: How to measure blood pressure accurately. Prim Cardiol 10:14, 1984.
24. Gould BA, Hornung RS, Kieso HA, et al: Is the blood pressure the same in both arms? Clin Cardiol 8:423, 1985.
25. Sapira JD: Quincke, de Musset, Duroziez, and Hill: Some aortic regurgitations. South Med J 74:459, 1981.
26. Vlachopoulos C, O'Rourke M: Genesis of the normal and abnormal pulse. Curr Prob Cardiol 25:297, 2000.
27. Perloff JK: The physiologic mechanisms of cardiac and vascular physical signs. J Am Coll Cardiol 1:184, 1983.
28. Brown DV: Dicrotic pulse in pericardial tamponade. J Cardiothorac Vasc Anesth 16:742, 2002.
29. Safar ME, Levy BI, Struijker-Boudier H: Current perspectives on arterial stiffness and pulse pressure in hypertension and cardiovascular diseases. Circulation 107:2864, 2003.
30. Elkins RC, Morrow AG, Vasko JS, Braunwald E: The effects of mitral regurgitation on the pattern of instantaneous aortic blood flow: Clinical and experimental observations. Circulation 36:45, 1967.
31. Talley JD: Recognition, etiology, and clinical implications of pulsus bisferiens. Heart Dis Stroke 3:309, 1994.
32. Smith D, Craige E: Mechanisms of the dicrotic pulse. Br Heart J 56:531, 1986.
33. Talley JD: Dicrotism: Examples and review of the dicrotic pulse. J Ark Med Soc 92:507, 1996.
34. Morpurgo M, Boutarin J: Right-sided pulsus alternans: A neglected phenomenon. Cardiologia 40:803, 1995.
35. Lab MJ, Seed WA: Pulsus alternans. Cardiovasc Res 27:1407, 1993.
36. Rosenthal E: Extreme pulsus alternans presenting as 2:1 electromechanical dissociation. Br Heart J 74:695, 1995.
37. Brockenbrough EC, Braunwald E, Morrow AG: A hemodynamic technic for the detection of hypertrophic subaortic stenosis. Circulation 23:189, 1961.
38. Fowler NO: Pulsus paradoxus. Heart Dis Stroke 3:68, 1994.
39. Pearson MG, Spence DP, Ryland I, Harrison BD: Value of pulsus paradoxus in assessing acute severe asthma. BMJ 307:659, 1993.
40. Jay GD, Onuma K, Davis R, et al: Analysis of physician ability in the measurement of pulsus paradoxus by sphygmomanometry. Chest 118:348, 2000.
41. Swami A, Spodick DH: Pulsus paradoxus in cardiac tamponade: A pathophysiologic continuum. Clin Cardiol 26:215, 2003.
42. Mowlavi A, Whiteman J, Wilhelmi BJ, et al: Dorsalis pedis arterial pulse: Palpation using a bony landmark. Postgrad Med J 78:746, 2002.
43. Hirsch AT: Recognition and management of peripheral arterial disease. *In* Braunwald E, Goldman L (eds): Primary Cardiology. 2nd ed. Philadelphia: Elsevier, 2003.
44. Beiser GD, Epstein SE, Stampfer M, et al: Impairment of cardiac function in patients with pectus excavatum. N Engl J Med 287:267, 1972.

The Cardiac Examination

45. Abrams J: Precordial palpation. *In* Horwitz LD, Groves BM (eds): Signs and Symptoms in Cardiology. Philadelphia, JB Lippincott, 1985, pp. 156-177.
46. Ellen SD, Crawford MH, O'Rourke RA: Accuracy of precordial palpation for detecting increased left ventricular volume. Ann Intern Med 99:628, 1983.
47. Ellen SD, et al: Accuracy of precordial palpation for detecting increased left ventricular volume. Ann Intern Med 99:628, 1983.
48. Ranganathan N, Juma Z, Sivaciyan V: The apical impulse in coronary heart disease. Clin Cardiol 8:20, 1985.

49. Adolph RJ: In defense of the stethoscope. Chest 114:1235, 1998.
50. Abrams J: Synopsis of cardiac physical diagnosis. 2nd ed. Boston: Butterworth Heinemann, 2001.

Heart Sounds

51. O'Toole JD, Reddy PS, Curtiss EL, et al: The contribution of tricuspid valve closure to the first heart sound: An intracardiac micromanometer study. Circulation 53:752, 1976.
52. Brooks N, Leech G, Leatham A: Complete right bundle branch block: Echophonocardiographic study of the first heart sound and right ventricular contraction times. Br Heart J 41:637, 1979.
53. Burggraf GW: The first heart sound in left bundle branch block: An echophonocardiographic study. Circulation 63:429, 1981.
54. Leech G, Brooks N, Green-Wilkinson A, Leatham A: Mechanism of influence of PR interval on loudness of first heart sound. Br Heart J 43:138, 1980.
55. Perloff JK: The Clinical Recognition of Congenital Heart Disease. 5th ed. Philadelphia, WB Saunders, 2003.
56. Mills PG, Brodie B, McLaurin L, et al: Echocardiographic and hemodynamic relationships of ejection sounds. Circulation 56:430, 1977.
57. Lembo NJ, Dell'Italia JL, Crawford MH, O'Rourke RA: Bedside diagnosis of systolic murmurs. N Engl J Med 318:1572, 1988.
58. Leatham A: Splitting of the first and second heart sounds. Lancet 2:607, 1954.
59. Kupari M: Aortic valve closure and cardiac vibrations in the genesis of the second heart sound. Am J Cardiol 52:152, 1983.
60. Curtiss EI, Matthews DG, Shaver JA: Mechanism of normal splitting of the second heart sound. Circulation 51:157, 1975.
61. Shaver JA, Nadolny RA, O'Toole JD, et al: Sound-pressure correlates of the second heart sound. Circulation 49:316, 1974.
62. Xiao HB, Faiek AH, Gibson DG: Re-evaluation of normal splitting of the second heart sound in patients with classical left bundle branch block. Int J Cardiol 45:163, 1994.
63. Hultgren HN, Craige E, Nakamura T, Bilisoly J: Left bundle branch block and mechanical events of the cardiac cycle. Am J Cardiol 52:755, 1985.
64. Tokushima T, Utsunomiya T, Ogawa T, et al: Contrast-enhanced radiographic computed tomographic findings in patients with straight back syndrome. Am J Card Imaging 10:228, 1996.
65. Wood P: An appreciation of mitral stenosis: I. Clinical features. BMJ 1:1051, 1954; II. Investigations and results. BMJ 1:1113, 1954.
66. Tyberg TI, Goodyer AVN, Langou RA: Genesis of the pericardial knock in constrictive pericarditis. Am J Cardiol 46:570, 1980.
67. Bass NM, Sharatt GJP: Left atrial myxoma diagnosed by echocardiography with observations on tumor movement. Br Heart J 35:1332, 1973.
68. Van de Werf F, Minten J, Carmeliet P, et al: Genesis of the third and fourth heart sounds. J Clin Invest 73:1400, 1984.
69. Van de Werf F, Boel A, Geboers J, et al: Diastolic properties of the left ventricle in normal adults and in patients with third heart sounds. Circulation 69:1070, 1984.
70. Drzewiecki GM, Wasicko MJ, Li JK: Diastolic mechanics and the origin of the third heart sound. Ann Biomed Eng 19:651, 1991.
71. Glower DD, Murrah RL, Olsen CO, et al: Mechanical correlates of the third heart sound. J Am Coll Cardiol 19:450, 1992.
72. Downes TR, Dunson W, Stewart K, et al: Mechanism of physiologic and pathologic S_3 gallop sounds. Am Soc Echocardiol 5:211, 1992.
73. Tribouilloy CM, Enriquez-Sarano M, Mohty D, et al: Pathophysiologic determinants of third heart sounds: A prospective clinical and Doppler echocardiographic study. Am J Med 111:96, 2001.
74. Adolph RJ: The fourth heart sound. Chest 115:1480, 1999.
75. Baracca E, Scorzoni D, Brunazzi MC, et al: Genesis and acoustic quality of the physiological fourth heart sound. Acta Cardiol 50:23, 1995.
76. Ishikawa M, Sakata K, Maki A, et al: Prognostic significance of a clearly audible fourth heart sound detected a month after an acute myocardial infarction. Am J Cardiol 80:619, 1997.

Heart Murmurs

77. O'Rourke R: Approach to the patient with a heart murmur. *In* Braunwald E, Goldman L (eds): Primary Cardiology. 2nd ed. Philadelphia: Elsevier, 2003, pp 155-173.
78. Grewe K, et al: Differentiation of cardiac murmurs by auscultation. Curr Probl Cardiol 13:699, 1988.
79. Lembo NJ, et al: Bedside diagnosis of systolic murmurs. N Engl J Med 318:1572, 1988.
80. Ecchells E, et al: Does this patient have an abnormal systolic murmur? JAMA 277:564, 1997.
81. Joffe HS: Genesis of Still's innocent systolic murmur. Br Heart J 67:206, 1992
82. Donnerstein RL, Thomsen VS: Hemodynamic and anatomic factors affecting the frequency content of Still's innocent murmur. Am J Cardiol 74:508, 1994.
83. Perloff JK, Roberts WC: The mitral apparatus: Functional anatomy of mitral regurgitation. Circulation 46:227, 1972.
84. Ronan JA, Steelman RB, DeLeon AC, et al: The clinical diagnosis of acute severe mitral insufficiency. Am J Cardiol 27:284, 1971.
85. Rios JC, Massumi RA, Breesman WT, Sarin RK: Auscultatory features of acute tricuspid regurgitation. Am J Cardiol 23:4, 1969.
86. Fontana ME: Mitral valve prolapse and floppy mitral valve: Physical examination. *In* Mitral Valve: Floppy Mitral Valve, Mitral Valve Prolapse, Mitral Valvular Regurgitation. 2nd ed. Armouk, NY, Futura, 2000, pp 283-304.
87. Fortuin NJ, Craige E: Echocardiographic studies of genesis of mitral diastolic murmurs. Br Heart J 35:75, 1973.
88. Flint A: On cardiac murmurs. Am J Med Sci 44:23, 1862.
89. Landzberg JS, Tflugfelder PW, Cassidy MM, et al: Etiology of the Austin Flint murmur. J Am Coll Cardiol 20:408, 1992.
90. Reddy PS, Curtiss EL, Salerni R: Sound-pressure correlates of the Austin Flint murmur: An intracardiac sound study. Circulation 53:210, 1976.
91. Berman P: Austin Flint—America's Laennec revisited. Arch Intern Med 148:2053, 1988.
92. Gibson GA: Persistence of the arterial duct and its diagnosis. Edinb Med J 8:1, 1900.
93. Cutforth R, Wideman J, Sutherland RD: The genesis of the cervical venous hum. Am Heart J 80:488, 1970.
94. Spodick DH: Auscultatory phenomena in pericardial disease. *In* Spodick DH: The Pericardium: A Comprehensive Textbook. New York, Marcel Dekker, 1997, pp 27-39.
95. Hamman L: Mediastinal emphysema. JAMA 128:1, 1945.

Dynamic Auscultation

96. Grewe K, Crawford MH, O'Rourke RA: Differentiation of cardiac murmurs by dynamic auscultation. Curr Probl Cardiol 13:671, 1988.
97. Lembro NJ, Dell'Italia LJ, Crawford MH, O'Rourke RA: Bedside diagnosis of systolic murmurs. N Engl J Med 318:1572, 1988.
98. Cha SD, Gooch AS: Diagnosis of tricuspid regurgitation. Arch Intern Med 143:1763, 1983.
99. Barlow JB: Perspectives on the Mitral Valve. Philadelphia, FA Davis, 1987.
100. Vrewe K, Crawford MH, O'Rourke RA: Differentiation of cardiac murmurs by dynamic auscultation. Curr Probl Cardiol 13:671, 1988.
101. Nishimura RA, Tajik AJ: The Valsalva maneuver and response revisited. Mayo Clin Proc 61:211, 1986.
102. McCraw DB, Siegel W, Stonecipher HK, et al: Response of the heart murmur intensity to isometric (handgrip) exercise. Br Heart J 34:605, 1972.
103. Barlow J, Shillingford J: The use of amyl nitrite in differentiating mitral and aortic systolic murmurs. Br Heart J 20:162, 1958.

CHAPTER 9

Electrocardiography

David M. Mirvis • Ary L. Goldberger

The electrocardiogram (ECG), as used today, is the product of a series of technological and physiological advances pioneered over the past two centuries.[1] Early demonstrations of the heart's electrical activity reported during the last half of the 19th century, for example, by Marchand and others, were closely followed by direct recordings of cardiac potentials by Waller in 1887. Invention of the string galvanometer by Willem Einthoven in 1901 provided a reliable and direct method for registering electrical activity of the heart. By 1910, use of the string galvanometer had emerged from the research laboratory into the clinic.

Subsequent achievements built on the very solid foundation supplied by the early electrocardiographers. The result has become a widely used and invaluable clinical tool for the detection and diagnosis of a broad range of cardiac conditions, as well as a technique that has contributed to the understanding and treatment of virtually every type of heart disease. Electrocardiography remains the most direct method for assessing abnormalities of cardiac rhythm. Furthermore, the ECG is essential in the management of major metabolic abnormalities such as hyperkalemia and certain other electrolyte disorders, as well as in assessing drug effects and toxicities such as those caused by digitalis, antiarrhythmic agents, and tricyclic antidepressants. More than 7 million ECGs are performed in the United States each year, making ECG the most commonly performed as well as the oldest cardiovascular laboratory procedure.

Fundamental Principles

Use of the ECG for any of these clinically important purposes is the final outcome of a complex series of physiological and technological processes. This sequence is depicted in Figure 9-1. First, an extracellular cardiac electrical field is generated by ion fluxes across cell membranes and between adjacent cells. These ion currents are synchronized by cardiac activation and recovery sequences to generate a cardiac electrical field in and around the heart that varies with time during the cardiac cycle. This electrical field passes through numerous other structures, including the lungs, blood, and skeletal muscle before reaching the body surface. These elements, known as *transmission factors,* differ in their electrical properties and perturb the cardiac electrical field as it passes through them.

The potentials reaching the skin are then detected by electrodes placed in specific locations on the extremities and torso and configured to produce leads. The outputs of these leads are amplified, filtered, and displayed by a variety of electronic devices to construct an ECG recording. Finally, diagnostic criteria are applied to these recordings to produce an interpretation. The criteria have statistical characteristics that determine the clinical utility of the findings. Each of these steps influences the final product—the clinical ECG—and are considered in detail in this chapter to provide a foundation for considering the common abnormalities found in clinical practice and as a basis for further learning.

GENESIS OF THE CARDIAC ELECTRICAL FIELD

CARDIAC ELECTRICAL FIELD GENERATION DURING ACTIVATION. Transmembrane ionic currents are ultimately responsible for the cardiac potentials that are recorded as an ECG. Current may be analyzed as though carried by positively charged or negatively charged ions. Through a purely arbitrary choice, electrophysiological currents are considered to be the movement of positive charge. A positive current moving in one direction is equivalent to a negative current of equal strength moving in the opposite direction.

The process of generating the cardiac electrical field during activation can be illustrated by considering the events in a single cardiac fiber, 20 mm in length, that is activated by a stimulus applied to its left-most margin (Fig. 9-2A). Transmembrane potentials (V_m) are recorded as the difference between intracellular and extracellular potentials (ϕ_e and ϕ_i, respectively). Figure 9-2B plots V_m along the length of the fiber at the instant during the propagation (t_o) at which activation has reached the point designated as X_0. As each site is activated, the polarity of the transmembrane potential is converted from negative to positive. Thus, sites to the left of the point X_0, which have already undergone excitation, have positive transmembrane potentials (that is, the inside of the cell is positive relative to the outside of the cell), whereas those to the right of X_0 (which remain in a resting state) have negative transmembrane potentials. Near the site undergoing activation (site X_0), the potentials reverse polarity over a short distance.

Figure 9-2C displays the direction and magnitude of transmembrane currents (I_m) along the fiber at the instant (t_o) at which excitation has reached site X_0. Current flow is inwardly directed in fiber regions that have undergone activation (that is, to the left of point X_0) and outwardly directed in neighboring zones still at rest (that is, to the right of X_0). Sites of outward current flow are *current sources* and those with inward current flow are *current sinks*. As depicted in the figure, current flow is most intense in each direction near the site of activation X_0. Because the border between inwardly and outwardly directed currents is relatively sharp, we can visualize these currents as though they were limited to the sites of maximal current flow, as depicted in Figure 9-2D, and separated by distance d that is usually 1.0 mm or less. As activation proceeds along the fiber, the source-sink pair moves to the right at the speed of propagation for the particular type of fiber.

Two point sources of equal strength but of opposite polarity located very near each other, such

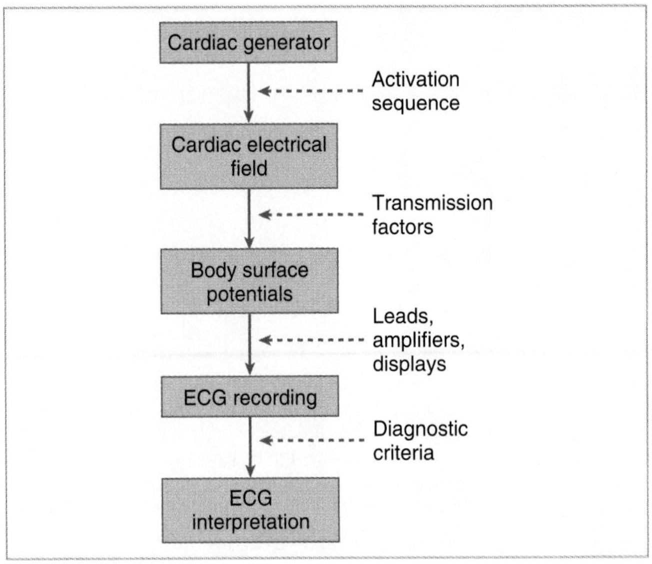

FIGURE 9–1 Schematic representation of the factors resulting in recording the electrocardiogram (ECG). The major paths leading to the ECG are marked by solid arrows and factors influencing or perturbing this path are shown with dashed arrows.

as the current source and the current sink depicted in Figure 9-2D, can be represented as a *current dipole*. Thus, activation of a fiber can be modeled as a current dipole that moves in the direction of propagation of activation. Such a dipole is fully characterized by three parameters: strength or dipole moment, location, and orientation. In this case, the location of the dipole is the site undergoing activation (point X_0), and its orientation is in the direction of activation (that is, from left to right along the fiber). Dipole moment is proportional to the rate of change of intracellular potential with respect to distance along the fiber, that is, action potential shape.

A current dipole produces a characteristic potential field with positive potentials projected ahead of it and negative potentials projected behind it. The actual potential recorded at any site within this field is directly proportional to the dipole moment, inversely proportional to the square of the distance from the dipole to the recording site, and directly proportional to the cosine of the angle between the axis of the dipole and a line drawn from the dipole to the recording site.

This example from one cardiac fiber can be generalized to the more realistic case in which multiple adjacent fibers are activated in synchrony to produce an activation front. Activation of each fiber creates a dipole oriented in the direction of activation. The net effect of all the dipoles in this wave front is a single dipole equal to the (vector) sum of the effects of all the simultaneously active component dipoles. Thus, an activation front propagating through the heart can be represented by a single dipole that projects positive potentials ahead of it and negative potentials behind it.

This relationship between activation direction, orientation of the current dipole, and polarity of potentials is a critical one in electrocardiography. It describes a fundamental relationship between the polarity of potentials sensed by an electrode and the direction of movement of an activation front: an electrode senses positive potentials when an activation front is moving toward it and negative potentials when the activation front is moving away from it.

The dipole model, though useful in describing cardiac fields and understanding clinical electrocardiography, has significant theoretical limitations. These limits derive primarily from the inability of a single dipole to accurately represent more than one wave front that is propagating through the heart at any one instant. As will be discussed, during much of the time of ventricular excitation, more than one wave front is present.

Solid Angle Theorem. One important and commonly used method of estimating the potentials projected to some point away from an activation front is an application of the *solid angle theorem*. A *solid angle* is a geometric measure of the size of a region when viewed from a distant site. It equals the area on the surface of a sphere of unit radius constructed around an electrode that is cut by lines drawn from the recording electrode to all points around the boundary of the region of interest.

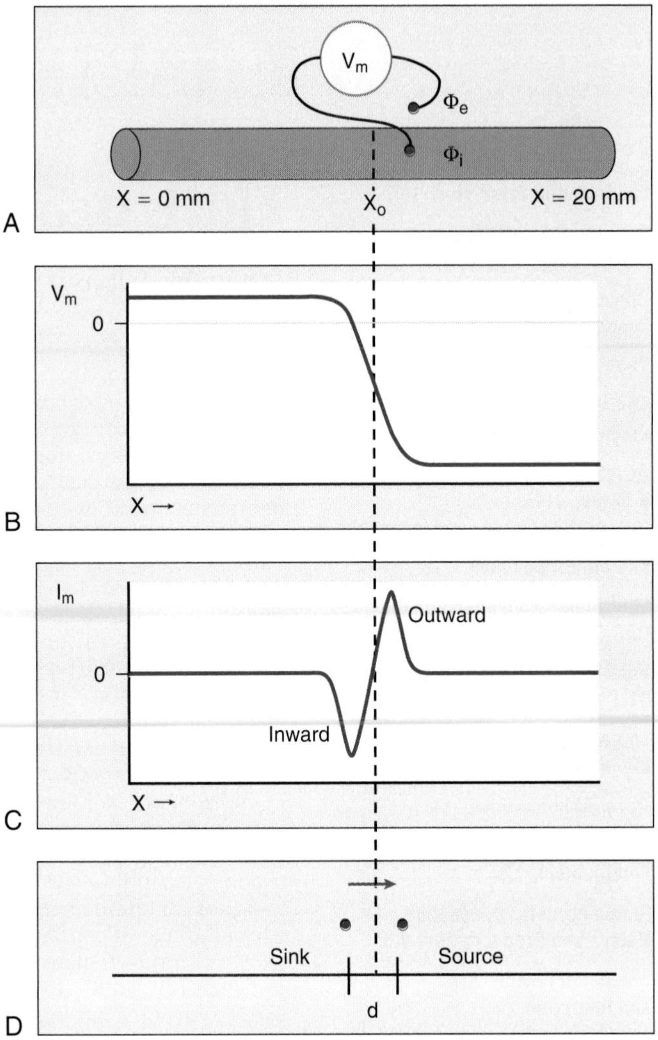

FIGURE 9–2 Example of potentials and currents generated by the activation of a single (e.g., ventricular) cardiac fiber. **A,** Intracellular (ϕ_i) and extracellular (ϕ_e) potentials are recorded with a voltmeter (Vm) from a fiber 20 mm in length. The fiber is stimulated at site X = 0 mm, and propagation proceeds from left to right. **B,** Plot of transmembrane potential (Vm) at the instant in time at which activation reaches point X_0 as a function of the length of the fiber. Positive potentials are recorded from activated tissue to the left of site X_0, and negative ones are registered from not yet excited areas to the right of site X_0. **C,** Membrane current (I_m) flows along the length of the fiber at time t_0. The outward current is the depolarizing current that propagates ahead of activation site X_0, while an inward one flows behind site X_0. **D,** Representation of the sites of peak inward and outward current flow as two point sources, a sink (at the site of peak inward current flow) and a source (at the site of peak outward current flow) separated by distance d. The dipole produced by the source-sink pair is represented by the arrow. (Modified from Barr RC: Genesis of the electrocardiogram. *In* MacFarlane PW, Lawrie TDV [eds]: Comprehensive Electrocardiography. New York, Pergamon, 1989.)

This region may be a wave front, a zone of infarction, or any other region in the heart.

The solid angle theorem states that the potential recorded by a remote electrode (Φ) is defined by the following equation:

$$\Phi = (\Omega/4\pi)(V_{m2} - V_{m1})K$$

where Ω is the solid angle, $V_{m2} - V_{m1}$ is the potential difference across the boundary under study, and K is a constant reflecting differences in intracellular conductivity. This equation indicates that the recorded potential equals the product of two factors. First, the solid angle reflects spatial parameters, such as the size of the boundary of the region under study and the distance from the electrode to that boundary. The potential will rise as the boundary size increases and as the distance to the electrode shrinks. A second set of parameters includes nonspatial factors, such as the potential difference across the surface and intracellular and extracellular conductivity. Nonspatial effects include, as one example, myocardial ischemia, which changes transmembrane action potential shapes and alters conductivity.

CARDIAC ELECTRICAL FIELD GENERATION DURING VENTRICULAR RECOVERY. The cardiac electrical field during recovery (phases 1 through 3 of the action potential) differs in fundamental ways from that described for activation. First, intercellular potential differences and hence the directions of current flow during recovery are the opposite of those described for activation. As a cell undergoes recovery, its intracellular potential becomes progressively more negative. Hence, for two adjacent cells, the intracellular potential of the cell whose recovery has progressed further is more negative than that of an adjacent, less recovered cell. Intracellular currents then flow from the less toward the more recovered cell. An equivalent dipole can then be constructed for recovery, just as for activation. Its orientation, however, points from less to more recovered cells. Thus, the recovery dipole is oriented away from the direction of propagation of the activation front, that is, in the direction opposite that of the activation dipole.

The moment, or strength, of the recovery dipole also differs from that of the activation dipole. As described previously, the strength of the activation dipole is proportional to the rate of change in transmembrane potential. Rates of change in potential during the recovery phases of the action potential are considerably slower than during activation, so that the dipole moment at any one instant during recovery is less than during activation.

A third difference between activation and recovery is the rate of movement of the activation and recovery dipoles. Activation is rapid (as fast as 1 msec in duration) and occurs over only a small distance along the fiber. Recovery, in contrast, lasts 100 msec or longer and occurs simultaneously over extensive portions of the fiber.

These features result in characteristic ECG differences between activation and recovery patterns. All other factors being equal (an assumption that is often not true, as described later), ECG waveforms generated during recovery of a linear fiber with uniform recovery properties may be expected to be of opposite polarity, lower amplitude, and longer duration than those due to activation. As will be described, these features are explicitly demonstrated in the clinical ECG.

THE ROLE OF TRANSMISSION FACTORS. These activation and recovery forces exist within a complex three-dimensional physical environment (the *volume conductor*). The structures within the volume conductor modify the cardiac electrical field in significant ways. They are called *transmission factors* to emphasize their effects on transmission of the cardiac electrical field throughout the body and can be grouped into four broad categories: cellular factors, cardiac factors, extracardiac factors, and physical factors.

Cellular factors determine the intensity of current fluxes that result from local transmembrane potential gradients and include intracellular and extracellular resistance and the concentration of relevant ions, especially the sodium ion. Lower ion concentrations reduce the intensity of current flow and lower extracellular potentials.

Cardiac factors affect the relationship of one cardiac cell to another. Two major factors are (1) *anisotropy*, that is, the property of cardiac tissue that results in greater current flow and more rapid propagation along the length of a fiber than transversely, and (2) the presence of connective tissue between cardiac fibers that disrupts effective electrical coupling between adjacent fibers. These factors alter the paths of extracellular currents and produce changes in the amplitude and configuration of recorded electrograms. Recording electrodes oriented along the long axis of a cardiac fiber register larger potentials than do electrodes oriented perpendicular to the long axis, and waveforms recorded from fibers with little or no intervening connective tissue are narrow in width and smooth in contour, whereas those recorded from tissues with abnormal fibrosis are prolonged and heavily fractionated.

Extracardiac factors encompass all the tissues and structures that lie between the activation region and the body surface, including the ventricular walls, intracardiac and intrathoracic blood volume, the pericardium, and the lungs, as well as skeletal muscle, subcutaneous fat, and skin. These tissues alter the cardiac field because of differences in the electrical resistivity of adjacent tissues, that is, the presence of electrical inhomogeneities within the torso. For example, intracardiac blood has much lower resistivity (162 Ω-cm) than do the lungs (2150 Ω-cm). When the cardiac field encounters the boundary between two tissues with differing resistivity, the field is altered.

Other transmission factors reflect basic laws of physics. First, changes in the distance between the heart and the recording electrode reduce potential magnitudes in accord with the inverse square law; that is, amplitude decreases in proportion to the square of the distance. A related factor is the effect of eccentricity. The heart is located eccentrically within the chest; it lies closer to the anterior than to the posterior of the torso, so that the right ventricle and the anteroseptal aspect of the left ventricle are located closer to the anterior chest wall than are other parts of the left ventricle and the atria. Therefore, ECG potentials will be higher anteriorly than posteriorly, and waveforms projected from the anterior of the left ventricle to the chest wall will be greater than those generated by posterior ventricular regions.

As a result of all of these factors, body surface potentials have an amplitude of only 1 percent of the amplitude of transmembrane potentials and are smoothed in detail so that surface potentials have only a general spatial relationship to the underlying cardiac events. The modifying effect of these physical structures is a biophysical one dependent on the physical properties of the structures and the related laws of physics, in contrast to the biological cardiac generators, whose output is dependent on cellular structure and physiological and biochemical processes. Thus, ECG potentials on the body surface are dependent on both biological and biophysical properties.[2] Although changes in torso inhomogeneities within physiological ranges appear to have little impact on ECG potentials,[3] pathological changes such as those produced by anasarca do have an impact on the ECG recording.[4]

Recording Electrodes and Leads

Potentials generated by the cardiac electrical generator and modified by transmission factors are processed by a series of electrical and electronic devices to yield a clinical ECG (Fig. 9–3). They are first sensed by electrodes placed on the torso that are configured to form various types of leads.

ELECTRODE CHARACTERISTICS. Electrodes used to sense the cardiac electrical field are not passive devices that merely detect the field. Rather, they are intricate systems that are affected by the properties of the dermal and epidermal layers of the skin, the electrolytic paste applied to the skin, the electrode itself, and the mechanical contact between the electrode and skin. The net effect is a complex electrical circuit that includes resistances, capacitances, and voltages produced by these different components and the interfaces between them. Each of these factors modifies the cardiac potentials registered by the electrodes before they are displayed as an ECG.

The ECG leads can be subdivided into two general types, ***bipolar leads*** and ***unipolar leads***. A bipolar lead consists of two electrodes placed at two different sites. These leads register the difference in potential between these two sites. The actual potential at either electrode is not known, and only the difference between them is recorded. One electrode is designated as the positive input; the potential at the other, or negative, electrode is subtracted from the potential at the positive electrode to yield the bipolar potential.

Unipolar leads, in contrast, measure the absolute electrical potential at one site. To do so requires a *reference site*—that is, a site at which the potential is deemed to be zero. The reference site may be a location far away from the active electrode (as in an experimental preparation) or, as in clinical electrocardiography, a specially designed electrode configuration (described later). The unipolar recording is then the potential sensed by a single electrode at one site—the *recording* or *active* or *exploring electrode*—in relation to the designated zero or reference potential.

Clinical Electrocardiographic Lead Systems

The standard clinical ECG includes recordings from 12 leads. These 12 leads include three *bipolar* (leads I, II, and III), six *unipolar precordial leads* (leads V_1 through V_6), and three *modified unipolar limb leads* (the augmented limb leads aV_r, aV_l, and aV_f). Definitions of the positive and negative inputs for each lead are listed in Table 9–1.

BIPOLAR LIMB LEADS. Bipolar limb leads record the potential differences between two limbs, as detailed in Table 9–1 and illustrated in Figure 9–4. As bipolar leads, the output is the potential difference between two limbs. Lead I

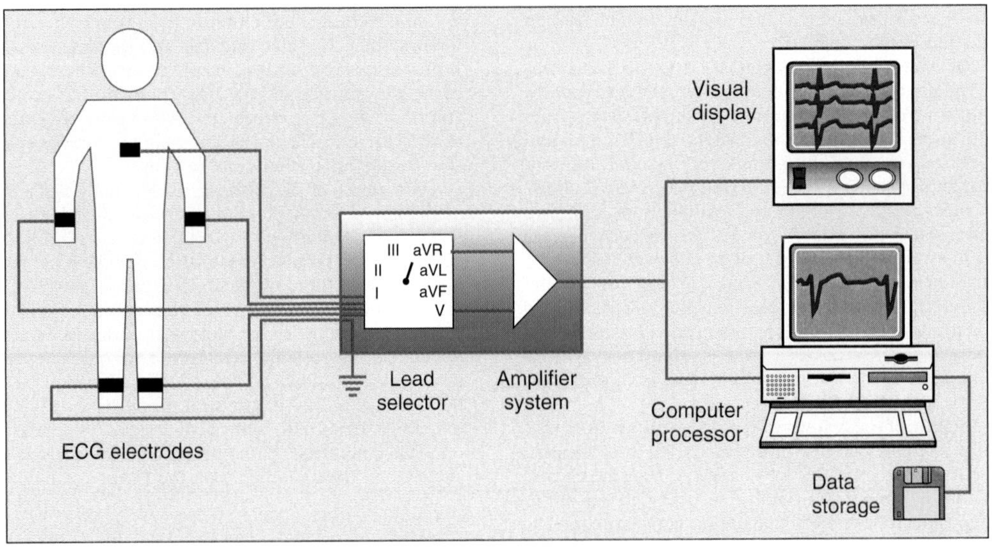

FIGURE 9–3 Components used in the recording and processing of an electrocardiogram. (From Mirvis DM: Electrocardiography: A Physiologic Approach. St Louis, Mosby-Year Book, 1993.)

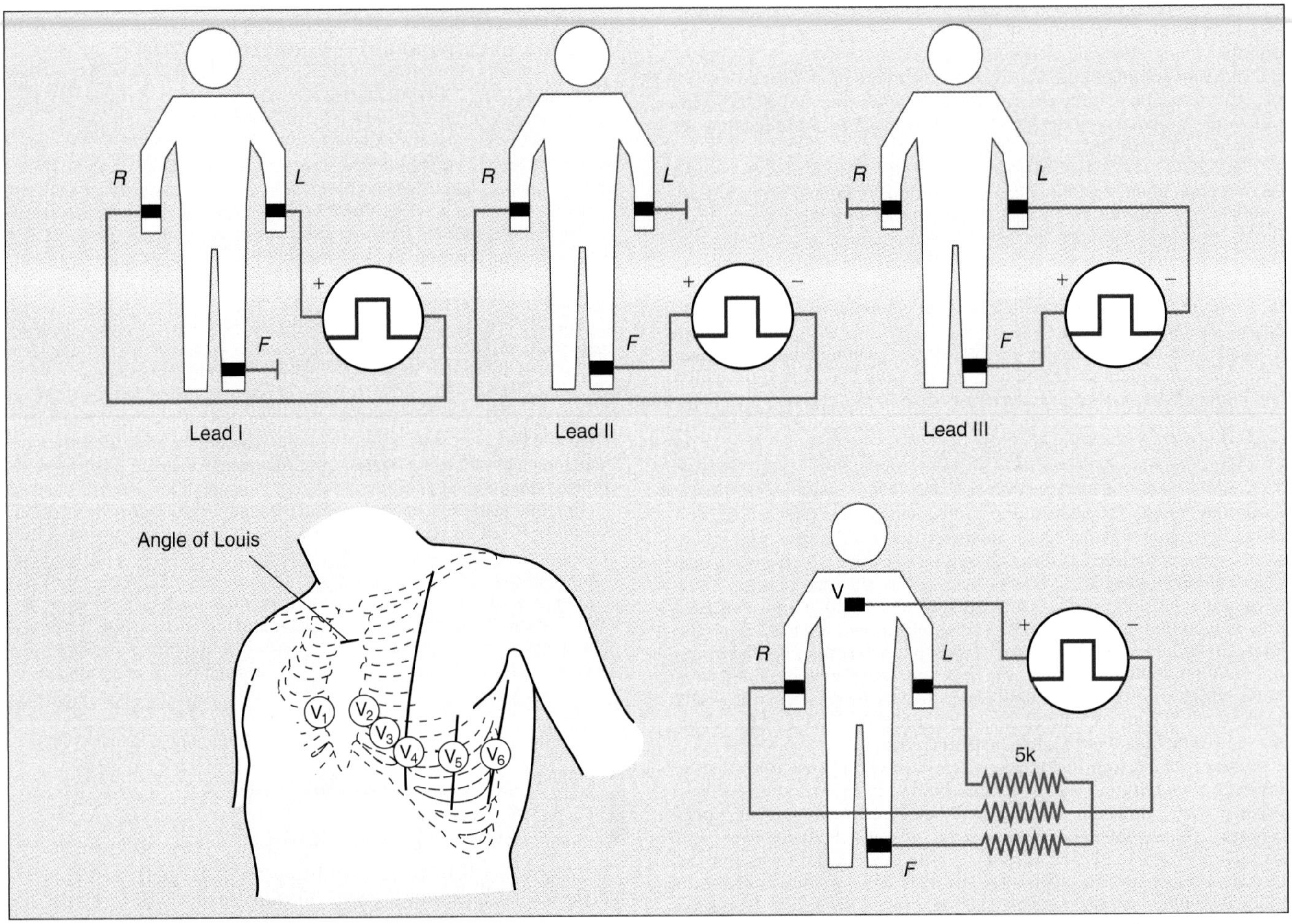

FIGURE 9–4 **Top,** Electrode connections for recording the three bipolar limb leads I, II, and III. R, L, and F indicate locations of electrodes on the right arm, the left arm, and the left foot, respectively. **Bottom,** Electrode locations and electrical connections for recording a unipolar precordial lead. Left, The positions of the exploring electrode (V) for the six precordial leads. Right, Connections to form the Wilson central terminal for recording a precordial (V) lead. (From Goldberger AL: Clinical Electrocardiography: A Simplified Approach. 6th ed. St Louis, CV Mosby, 1999.)

TABLE 9–1 Location of Electrodes and Lead Connections for the Standard 12-Lead Electrocardiogram and Additional Leads		
Lead Type	**Positive Input**	**Negative Input**
Bipolar limb leads		
Lead I	Left arm	Right arm
Lead II	Left leg	Right arm
Lead III	Left leg	Left arm
Augmented Unipolar Limb Leads		
aV_r	Right arm	Left arm plus left leg
aV_l	Left arm	Right arm plus left leg
aV_f	Left leg	Left arm plus left arm
Precordial Leads*		
V_1	Right sternal margin, 4th intercostal space	Wilson central terminal
V_2	Left sternal margin, 4th intercostal space	Wilson central terminal
V_3	Midway between V_2 and V_4	Wilson central terminal
V_4	Left midclavicular line, 5th intercostal space	Wilson central terminal
V_5	Left anterior axillary line†	Wilson central terminal
V_6	Left midaxillary line†	Wilson central terminal
V_7	Posterior axillary line†	Wilson central terminal
V_8	Posterior scapular line†	Wilson central terminal
V_9	Left border of spine†	Wilson central terminal

*The right-sided precordial leads V_3R to V_6R are taken in mirror image positions on the right side of the chest.

†Leads V_5 to V_9 are taken in the same horizontal plane as V_4.

represents the potential difference between the left arm (positive electrode) and the right arm (negative electrode), lead II displays the potential difference between the left foot (positive electrode) and the right arm (negative electrode), and lead III represents the potential difference between the left foot (positive electrode) and the left arm (negative electrode). The electrode on the right foot serves as a ground and is not included in these leads.

The electrical connections for these leads are such that the potential in lead II equals the sum of potentials sensed in leads I and III. That is,

$$I + III = II$$

This relationship is known as *Einthoven's law* or Einthoven's equation.

UNIPOLAR PRECORDIAL LEADS AND THE WILSON CENTRAL TERMINAL. The unipolar precordial leads register the potential at each of the six designated torso sites (see Fig. 9–4, bottom, left panel) in relation to a theoretical zero reference potential. To do so, an exploring electrode is placed on each precordial site and connected to the positive input of the recording system (see Fig. 9–4, bottom, right panel).

The negative, or reference, input is composed of a compound electrode (that is, a configuration of more than one electrode connected electrically) known as the *Wilson central terminal.* This terminal is formed by combining the output of the left arm, right arm, and left leg electrodes through 5000-Ω resistances (see Fig. 9–4, bottom, right panel). The result is that each precordial lead registers the potential at a precordial site with reference to the average potential on three limbs. The potential recorded by the Wilson central terminal remains relatively constant during the cardiac cycle, so the output of a precordial lead is determined predominantly by time-dependent changes in the potential at the precordial site.

AUGMENTED UNIPOLAR LIMB LEADS. The three augmented limb leads aV_r, aV_l, and aV_f are modified or augmented unipolar leads. The exploring electrode (Fig. 9–5) is the right arm electrode for lead aV_r, the left arm electrode for lead aV_l, and the left foot electrode for aV_f. It is the reference electrode that is modified. Instead of consisting of a full Wilson central terminal composed of the output from three limb electrodes, the reference potential for the augmented unipolar limb lead is the mean of the potentials sensed by only two of the three limb electrodes; the electrode used for the exploring electrode is excluded from the reference electrode. For lead aV_l, for example, the exploring electrode is on the left arm and the reference electrode is the mean output of the electrodes on the right arm and the left foot. Similarly, for lead aV_f, the reference potential is the mean of the output of the two arm electrodes.

This modified reference system was designed to increase the amplitude of the output. The output of the limb leads without augmentation tended to be small, in part because the same electrode potential was included in both the exploring

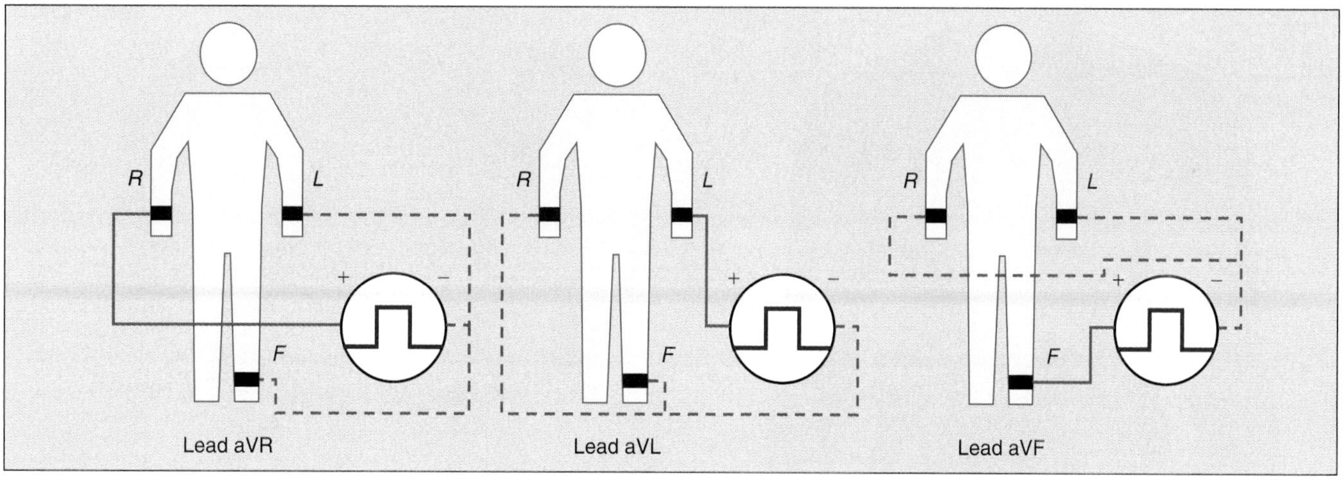

FIGURE 9–5 Electrode locations and electrical connections for recording the three augmented unipolar leads aV_r, aV_l, and aV_f. Dotted lines indicate connections to generate the reference electrode potential.

and the reference potential input. Eliminating this duplication results in a theoretical increase in amplitude of 50 percent.

OTHER LEAD SYSTEMS. Other lead systems can be used for specific purposes. For example, additional unipolar right precordial leads can be used to assess right ventricular lesions, and locations posterior to V_6 can be used to help detect acute posterior-lateral infarctions[5] (see Table 9-1). Such posterior locations include lead V_7 with the exploring electrode at the left posterior axillary line at the vertical level of V_6, lead V_8 with the exploring electrode on the left midscapular line, lead V_4R with the exploring electrode on the right midclavicular line in the 4th intercostal space, and so forth. A vertical parasternal bipolar pair can facilitate detection of P waves for diagnosing arrhythmias.

Precordial and anterior-posterior thoracic electrode arrays of up to 150 (or more) electrodes can be used to display the spatial distribution of body surface potentials as body surface isopotential maps.[6] Other arrays have sought to reduce rather than expand the number of electrodes and reconstruct the full 12-lead ECG from as few as three bipolar leads.[7] Modified lead systems are also used in ambulatory ECG recording and exercise stress testing, as described elsewhere, and for bedside cardiac monitoring.

Other lead systems that have had clinical utility include those designed to record a vectorcardiogram (VCG). The VCG depicts the orientation and strength of a single cardiac dipole or vector at each instant during the cardiac cycle. Lead systems for recording the VCG are referred to as *orthogonal systems* because they record the three orthogonal or mutually perpendicular components of the dipole moment: the horizontal (x axis), frontal (y axis), and sagittal or anteroposterior (z axis) axes. An example of a normal VCG is shown in Figure 9-6. Clinical use of the VCG has waned in recent years, but the VCG can be useful in certain situations, and, as described below, vectorial principles remain essential to understanding the physiology and pathology of ECG waveform genesis.[8]

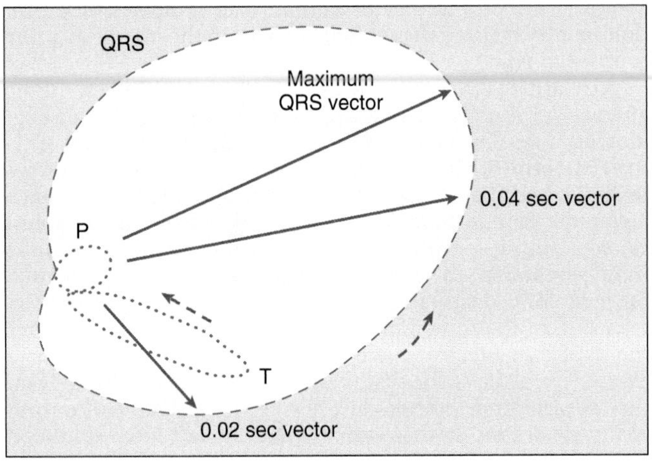

FIGURE 9–6 Example of a frontal plane vectorcardiogram. The three loops (QRS, T, and P) mark the ends of instantaneous vectors during the P wave, the QRS complex, and the T wave. Long arrows correspond to heart vectors 0.02 and 0.04 second into the QRS complex, at the instant of maximal vector strength during the QRS complex. Short arrows identify the direction in which the QRS and T loops are inscribed.

LEAD VECTORS AND HEART VECTORS

A lead can be represented as a vector (the *lead vector*). For simple bipolar leads, such as leads I, II, and III, the lead vectors are directed from the negative electrode toward the positive one (Fig. 9-7). For unipolar leads such as the augmented limb and precordial leads, the origin of the lead vectors lies at the midpoint of the axis connecting the electrodes that make up the compound electrode. That is, for lead aV_L, the vector points from the midpoint of the axis connecting the right arm and left leg electrodes toward the left arm (see Fig. 9-7, left). For the precordial leads, the lead vector points from the center of the torso to the precordial electrode site (see Fig. 9-7, right).

Instantaneous cardiac activity can also be approximated as a single dipole representing the vector sum of the various active wave fronts (the *heart vector*). Its location, orientation, and intensity vary from instant to instant because of the changing pattern of cardiac activation.

The amplitude and polarity of the potentials sensed in a lead equal the length of the projection of the heart vector on the lead vector multiplied by the length of the lead vector:

$$V_L = (H)(\cos\theta)(L)$$

where L and H are the length of the lead and heart vectors, respectively, and θ is the angle between the two vectors, as illustrated in Figure 9-8.

If the projection of the heart vector on the lead vector points toward the positive pole of the lead axis, the lead will record a positive potential. If the projection is directed away from the positive pole of the lead axis, the potential will be negative.

The lead axes of the six frontal plane leads can be overlaid to produce the hexaxial reference system. As depicted in Figure 9-9, the six lead axes divide the frontal plane into 12 segments, each subtending 30 degrees.

The Electrical Axis

The concepts of the heart vector and the lead vector allow calculation of the mean electrical axis of the heart. The mean force during activation is represented by the area under the QRS waveform measured as millivolt-milliseconds. Areas above the baseline are assigned a positive polarity and those

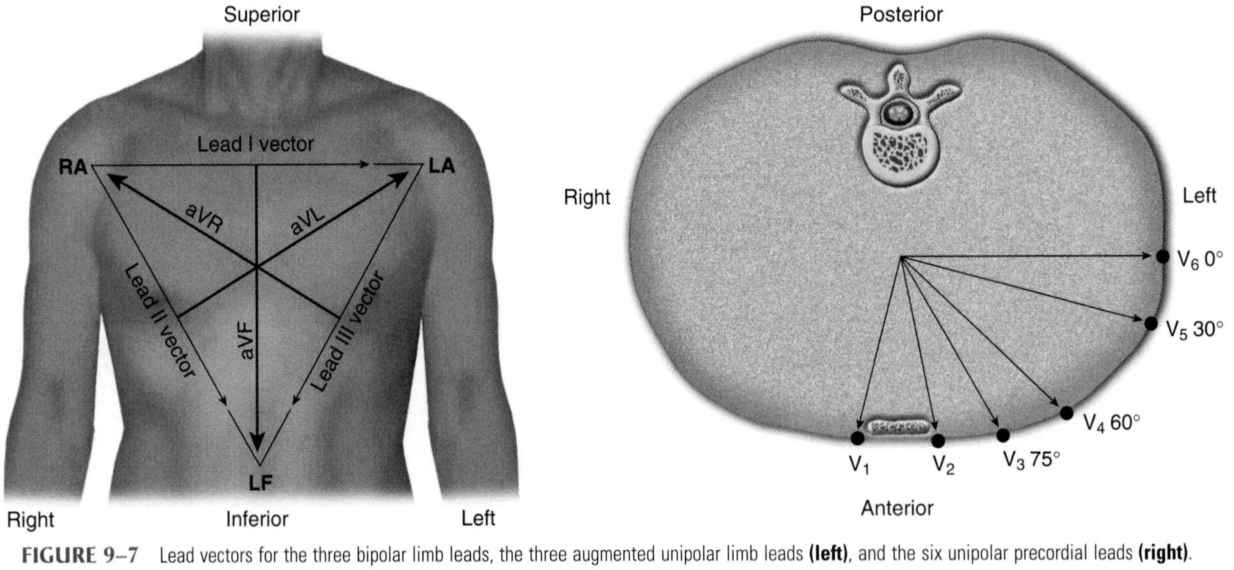

FIGURE 9–7 Lead vectors for the three bipolar limb leads, the three augmented unipolar limb leads **(left)**, and the six unipolar precordial leads **(right)**.

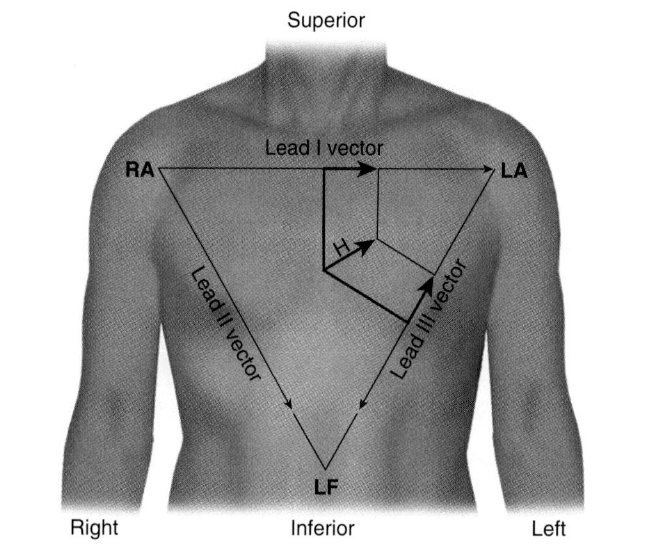

FIGURE 9–8 The heart vector H and its projections on the lead axes of leads I and III. Voltages recorded in lead I will be positive and potentials in lead III will be negative.

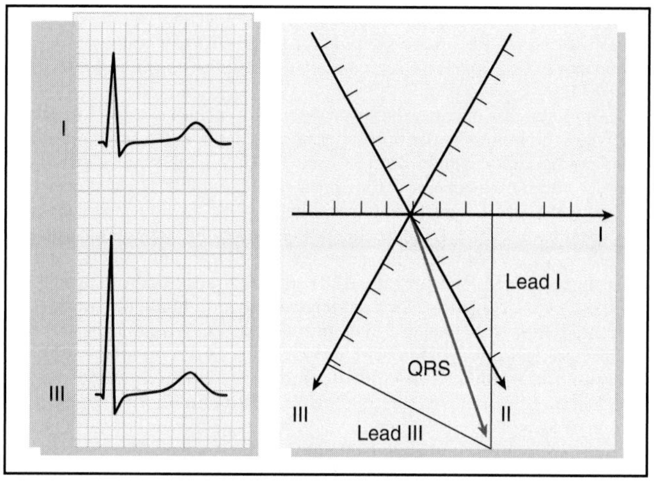

FIGURE 9–10 Calculation of the mean electrical axis during the QRS complex from the areas under the QRS complex in leads I and III. Magnitudes of the areas of the two leads are plotted as vectors on the appropriate lead axes, and the mean QRS axis is the sum of these two vectors. (From Mirvis DM: Electrocardiography: A Physiologic Approach. St Louis, Mosby-Year Book, 1993.)

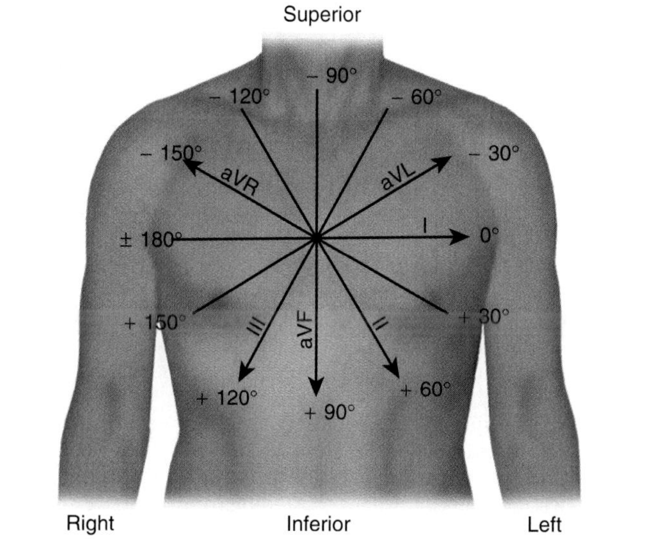

FIGURE 9–9 The hexaxial reference system composed of the lead axes of the six frontal plane leads. The lead axes of the six frontal plane leads have been rearranged so that their centers overlay one another. These axes divide the plane into 12 segments, each subtending 30 degrees. Positive ends of each axis are labeled with the name of the lead.

below the baseline have a negative polarity. The overall area equals the sum of the positive and the negative areas.

The process for computing the axis of the mean force during activation is illustrated in Figure 9–10. It is the reverse of that used to compute potential magnitudes in the leads from the orientation and moment of the heart vector. The area in each lead (typically two are chosen) is represented as a vector oriented along the appropriate lead axis in the hexaxial reference system (see Fig. 9–9), and the mean electrical axis equals the resultant or the sum of the two vectors. An axis directed toward the positive end of the lead axis of lead I, that is, oriented directly away from the right arm and toward the left arm, is designated as an axis of 0 degrees. Axes oriented in a clockwise direction from this zero level are assigned positive values and those oriented in a counterclockwise direction are assigned negative values.

The mean electrical axis in the horizontal plane can be computed in an analogous manner by using the areas and the lead axes of the six precordial leads (see Fig. 9–7, right). A horizontal plane axis located along the lead axis of lead V_6 is assigned a value of 0 degrees, and those directed more anteriorly have positive values.

This process can be applied to compute the mean electrical axis for other phases of cardiac activity. Thus, the mean force during atrial activation will be represented by the areas under the P wave, and the mean force during ventricular recovery will be represented by the areas under the ST-T wave. In addition, the instantaneous electrical axis can be computed at each instant during ventricular activation by using voltages at a specific instant rather than using areas to calculate the axis.

The orientation of the mean electrical axis represents the direction of the activation front in an "average" cardiac fiber. The direction of the front, in turn, is determined by the interaction of three factors: the anatomical position of the heart in the chest, the properties of the cardiac conduction system, and the activation properties of the myocardium. Differences in the anatomical position of the heart within the chest would be expected to change the relationship between cardiac regions and the lead axes and would thus change recorded voltages. Similarly, changes in conduction patterns, even of minor degree, can significantly alter relationships between activation (or recovery) of various cardiac areas and, hence, the direction of instantaneous as well as mean electrical force. In practice, differences in anatomy contribute relatively little to shifts in axis; the major influences on the mean electrical axis are the properties of the conduction system and cardiac muscle.

Electrocardiographic Display Systems

Another group of factors that determines ECG waveforms includes the characteristics of the electronic systems used to amplify, filter, and digitize the sensed signals. ECG amplifiers are differential amplifiers; that is, they amplify the difference between two inputs. For bipolar leads, the differential output is the difference between the two active leads; for unipolar leads, the difference is between the exploring electrode and the reference electrode. This differential configuration significantly reduces the electrical noise that is sensed by both inputs and hence is canceled. The standard amplifier gain for routine electrocardiography is 1000 but can vary from 500 (*half-standard*) to 2000 (*double standard*).

Amplifiers respond differently to the range of signal frequencies included in an electrophysiological signal. The *bandwidth* of an amplifier defines the frequency range over which the amplifier accurately amplifies the input signals. Waveform components with frequencies above or below the bandwidth can be artifactually reduced or increased in amplitude. In addition, recording devices include high- and low-pass filters that intentionally reduce the amplitude of specific frequency ranges of the signal. Such reduction in amplitude may be done, for example, to reduce the effect of body motion or line voltage frequencies, that is, 60 Hz interference. For routine electrocardiography, the standards of the American Heart Association require a bandwidth of 0.05 to 100 Hz.

Amplifiers for routine electrocardiography include a capacitor stage between the input and the output terminals; they are *capacitor coupled*. This configuration blocks direct-current (DC) voltage while permitting flow of alternating-current (AC) signals. Because the ECG waveform can be viewed as an AC signal (which accounts for the waveform shape) that is superimposed on a DC baseline (which determines the actual voltage levels of the recording), this coupling has significant effects on the recording process. First, unwanted DC potentials, such as those produced by the electrode interfaces, are eliminated. Second, elimination of the DC potential from the final product means that ECG potentials are not calibrated against an external reference level. ECG potentials must be measured in relation to an internal standard. Thus, amplitudes of waves are measured in millivolts or microvolts relative to another portion of the waveform. The TP segment, which begins at the end of the T wave of one cardiac cycle and ends with onset of the P wave of the next cycle, is usually the most appropriate internal ECG baseline.

An additional issue is the digitizing or sampling rate for computerized systems. Too low a sampling rate will miss brief signals such as notches in QRS complexes or brief bipolar spikes and reduce the precision and accuracy of waveform morphologies. Too fast a sampling rate may introduce artifacts, including high-frequency noise, and requires excessive digital storage capacity. In general, the sampling rate should be at least twice the frequency of the highest frequencies of interest in the signal being recorded. Standard electrocardiography is most commonly performed with a sampling rate of 500 Hz, with each sample representing a 2 msec period.

Cardiac potentials can be processed for display in numerous formats. The most common of these formats is the classic scalar ECG. Scalar recordings depict the potentials recorded from one lead as a function of time. For standard electrocardiography, amplitude is displayed on a scale of 1 mV to 10 mm vertical displacement and time as 400 msec/cm on the horizontal scale. Other display formats are used for ambulatory electrocardiography and for bedside ECG monitoring.

The Normal Electrocardiogram

The heart is activated with each cardiac cycle in a very characteristic manner determined by the anatomy and physiology of working cardiac muscle and the specialized cardiac conduction systems. The waveforms and intervals that make up the standard ECG are displayed in the diagram in Figure 9–11, and a normal 12-lead ECG is shown in Figure 9–12. The

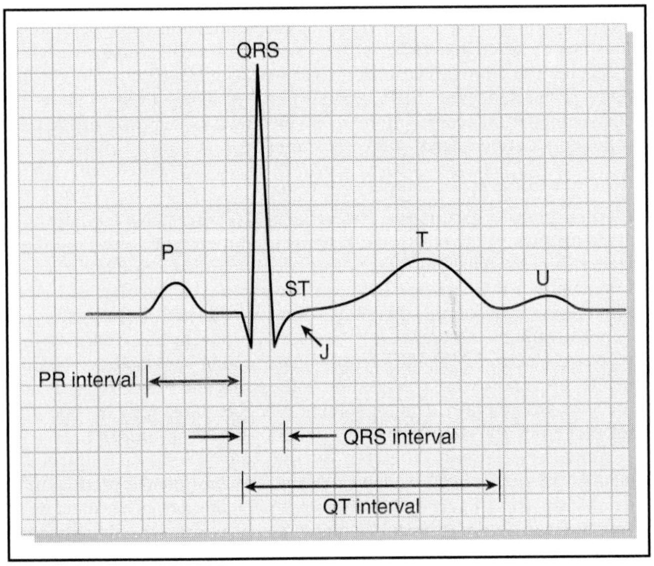

FIGURE 9–11 The waves and intervals of a normal electrocardiogram. (From Goldberger AL: Clinical Electrocardiography: A Simplified Approach. 6th ed. St Louis, CV Mosby, 1999.)

TABLE 9–2 Normal Values for Durations of Electrocardiographic Waves and Intervals in Adults

Wave/Interval	Duration (msec)
P wave duration	<120
PR interval	<120
QRS duration	<110-120*
QT interval (corrected)	≥440-460*

*See text for further discussion.

P wave is generated by activation of the atria, the *PR segment* represents the duration of atrioventricular (AV) conduction, the *QRS complex* is produced by activation of both ventricles, and the *ST-T wave* reflects ventricular recovery. Table 9–2 includes normal values for the various intervals and waveforms of the ECG.

Atrial Activation and the P Wave

Atrial activation[9,10] under normal conditions begins with impulse generation in the atrial pacemaker complex in or near the sinoatrial (SA) node. The rate of discharge of the SA node, and hence the heart rate, is determined by parasympathetic and sympathetic tone, the intrinsic properties of the SA node, extrinsic factors such as mechanical stretch, and various pharmacological effects (see Chap. 27).

HEART RATE VARIABILITY. Increasing attention is being directed to the beat-to-beat changes in heart rate, termed *heart rate variability,* to gain insight into neuroautonomic control mechanisms and their perturbations with aging, disease, and drug effects.[11] For example, high-frequency (0.15-0.5 Hz) fluctuations mediated by the vagus nerve occur phasically, with heart rate increasing during inspiration and decreasing during expiration. Attenuation of this respiratory sinus arrhythmia, and related short-term heart rate variability, is a consistent marker of physiological aging and also occurs with diabetes mellitus, congestive heart failure, and a wide range of other cardiac and noncardiac conditions that alter autonomic tone.[12] Lower frequency (0.05-0.15 Hz) physiological oscillations in heart rate are associated with baroreflex activation and appear to be jointly regulated by sympathetic and parasympathetic interactions. A variety of complementary signal processing techniques are being developed to analyze heart rate variability, including the very low-frequency (<0.05 Hz) components and circadian rhythms. These methods include time-domain statistics, frequency-domain techniques based on spectral (Fourier) methods, and tools derived from nonlinear dynamics. For further discussion, see Chapter 29.

Once the impulse leaves this pacemaker site within the SA node, atrial activation spreads in several directions. First, propagation is rapid along the crista terminalis and moves anteriorly toward the lower portion of the right atrium. It also spreads across the anterior and posterior surfaces of the atria toward the left atrium. The last area to be activated is over the inferolateral aspect of the left atrium, which is activated by convergence of these anterior and posterior wave fronts moving from right to left. Although right atrial activation begins before activation of the left atrium, activation occurs simultaneously in both atria during much of the overall atrial activation time. At the same time, activation spreads through the interatrial septum, beginning high on the right side and moving around the fossa ovalis to reach the top of the interventricular septum. These patterns are largely determined by the complex anatomical and functional properties of the atrial musculature.

The pattern of atrial activation noted above produces the normal P wave. Activation beginning high in the right atrium

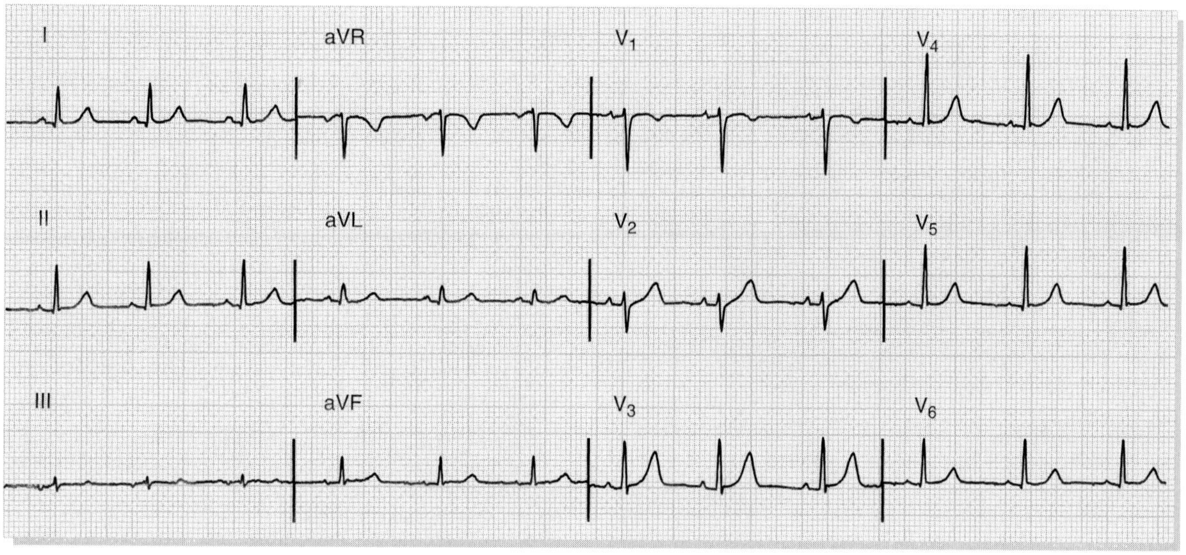

FIGURE 9–12 Normal electrocardiogram recorded from a 48-year-old woman. The vertical lines of the grid represent time, with lines spaced at 40 msec intervals. Horizontal lines represent voltage amplitude, with lines spaced at 0.1 mV intervals. Every fifth line in each direction is typically darkened. The heart rate is approximately 72 beats/min; the PR interval, QRS, and QT_c durations measure about 140, 84, and 400 msec, respectively; and the mean QRS axis is approximately +35 degrees.

and proceeding simultaneously leftward toward the left atrium and inferiorly toward the AV node corresponds to a mean frontal plane P wave axis of approximately 60 degrees. Based on this orientation of the heart vector, normal atrial activation projects positive or upright P waves in leads I, II, aV_l, and aV_f. The pattern in lead III may be either upright or downward, depending on the exact orientation of the mean axis, that is, upright if the mean axis is more positive than +30 degrees and downward otherwise.

P wave patterns in the precordial leads correspond to the direction of atrial activation wavefronts in the horizontal plane. Atrial activation early in the P wave is over the right atrium and is oriented primarily anteriorly; later it shifts posteriorly as activation proceeds over the left atrium. Thus, the P wave in the right precordial leads (V_1 and, occasionally, V_2) is commonly biphasic, with an initial positive deflection followed by a later negative one. In the more lateral leads, the P wave is upright and reflects right-to-left spread of the activation fronts.

P wave duration is normally less than 120 msec and is usually measured in the lead with the widest P wave. The amplitude in the limb leads is normally less than 0.25 mV and the terminal negative deflection in the right precordial leads is normally less than 0.1 mV in depth.

Atrial depolarization is followed by atrial repolarization. The potentials generated by atrial repolarization are not usually seen on the surface ECG because of their low amplitude (usually less than 100 μV) and because they are superimposed on the much higher amplitude QRS complex. They may be observed as a low-amplitude wave with a polarity opposite that of the P wave (the T_a wave) during heart block and may have special significance in influencing ECG patterns during exercise testing. Deviation of the PR segment (corresponding to the atrial ST segment) is, as described later, also an important marker of acute pericarditis and, more rarely, atrial infarction.

Atrioventricular Node Conduction and the PR Segment

The PR segment is the isoelectric region beginning with the end of the P wave and ending with the onset of the QRS complex. It forms part of the PR interval, which extends from the onset of the P wave to the onset of the QRS complex. The PR interval is usually best measured in the leads with the shortest PR intervals (to avoid missing various preexcitation syndromes). The normal PR interval measures 120 to 200 msec in duration.

The PR segment is the temporal bridge between atrial activation and ventricular activation. It is during this period that activation of the AV node, the bundle of His, the bundle branches, and the intraventricular specialized conduction system occurs. As noted earlier, atrial repolarization also occurs during this period. Most of the conduction delay during this segment is due to slow conduction within the AV node.

Upon exiting the AV node, the impulse traverses the bundle of His to enter the bundle branches and then travels through the specialized intraventricular conduction paths to finally activate ventricular myocardium. The PR segment appears isoelectric because the potentials generated by these structures are too small to produce detectable voltages on the body surface at the normal amplifier gains used in clinical electrocardiography. The standard ECG detects only activation and recovery of working myocardium, not the specialized conduction system. Signals from elements of the conduction system have been recorded from the body surface by using very high gains (over 25,000) and signal-averaging techniques or, in clinical settings, from intracardiac recording electrodes placed against the base of the interventricular septum near the bundle of His, as described in Chapter 29.

Ventricular Activation and the QRS Complex

Ventricular excitation is the product of two temporally overlapping functions, endocardial activation and transmural activation. Endocardial activation is guided by the anatomical distribution and physiology of the His-Purkinje system. The broadly dispersed ramifications of this tree-like (fractal) system[13] and the rapid conduction within it result in depolarization of most of the endocardial surfaces of both ventricles within several milliseconds and the simultaneous activation of multiple endocardial sites.

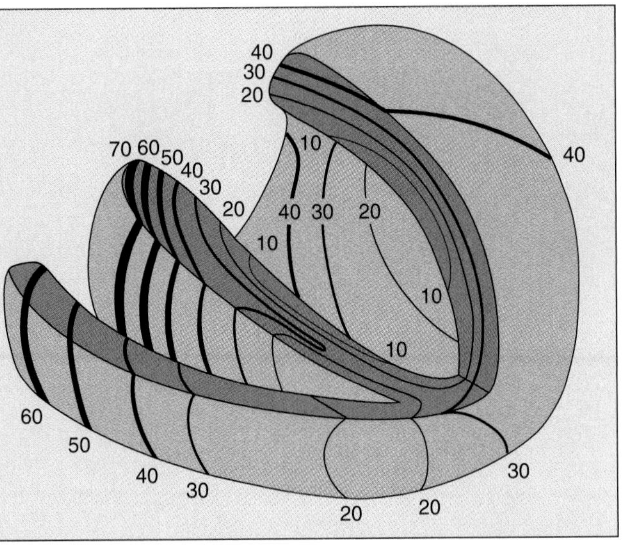

FIGURE 9–13 Activation sequence of the normal right and left ventricles. A portion of the left and right ventricles has been removed so that the endocardial surfaces of the ventricles and the interventricular septum can be seen. Isochrone lines connect sites that are activated at equal instants after the earliest evidence of ventricular activation. (From Durrer D: Electrical aspects of human cardiac activity: A clinical-physiological approach to excitation and stimulation. Cardiovasc Res 2:1, 1968.)

The sequence of ventricular endocardial activation is depicted in Figure 9-13. Earliest activity begins in three sites: (1) the anterior paraseptal wall of the left ventricle, (2) the posterior paraseptal wall of the left ventricle, and (3) the center of the left side of the septum. These loci generally correspond to the sites of insertion of the three branches of the left bundle branch. Wavefronts spread from these sites in anterior and superior directions to activate the anterior and lateral walls of the left ventricle. The posterobasal areas of the left ventricle are the last to be activated. Septal activation begins in the middle third of the left side and spreads across the septum from left to right and from apex to base.

Excitation of the right ventricle begins near the insertion point of the right bundle branch close to the base of the anterior papillary muscle and spreads to the free wall. The final areas to be involved are the pulmonary conus and the posterobasal areas. Thus, in both ventricles, the overall endocardial excitation pattern begins on septal surfaces and sweeps down and around the anterior free walls to the posterior and basal regions in an apex-to-base direction.

The activation fronts then move from endocardium to epicardium. Excitation of the endocardium begins at sites of Purkinje-ventricular muscle junctions and proceeds by muscle cell-to-muscle cell conduction in an oblique direction toward the epicardium.

LIMB LEADS. The sequence of endocardial and transmural activation results in the characteristic waveforms of the QRS complex. QRS patterns are described by the sequence of waves constituting the complex. An initial negative deflection is called the *Q wave*; the first positive wave is the *R wave;* and the first negative wave after a positive wave is the *S wave.* A second upright wave following an S wave is an *R′ wave.* Tall waves are denoted by capital letters and smaller ones by lowercase letters. A monophasic negative complex is referred to as a *QS complex*. Thus, for example, the overall QRS complex may be described as qRS if it consists of an initial small negative wave (the q wave) followed by a tall upright one (the R wave) and a deep negative one (an S wave). In an RSr′ complex, initial R and S waves are followed by a small positive wave (the r′ wave). In each case, the deflection must cross the baseline to be designated a discrete wave.

Septal Q Waves. The complex pattern of activation described can be simplified into two vectors representing septal and left ventricular free wall activation (Fig. 9-14). Initial activation of the interventricular septum corresponds to a vector oriented from left to right in the frontal plane and anteriorly in the horizontal plane, as determined by the anatomical position of the septum within the chest. This arrangement produces an initial positive wave in leads with axes directed to the right (lead aVr) or anteriorly (lead V_1). Leads with axes directed to the left (leads I, aV_l, V_5, and V_6) will register initial negative waves (septal q waves). These initial forces are normally of low amplitude and are brief (less than 30–40 msec).

Absence of these septal q waves is often a normal variant and not associated with any cardiac disease. However, absence or, particularly, loss of septal q waves may be a sign of septal infarction, various forms of conduction defects, or fibrosis, and commonly correlates with other ECG evidence of myocardial infarction and left ventricular mechanical dysfunction.[14-16]

Subsequent parts of the QRS complex reflect activation of the free walls of the left and right ventricles. Because right ventricular muscle mass is considerably smaller than that of the left ventricle, it contributes little to normal QRS complexes recorded in the standard ECG. Thus, the second phase of the normal QRS can be considered to represent only left ventricular activity with relatively little oversimplification.

Axis Positions. The forms of the QRS complex frontal plane leads are variable and reflect differences in the mean QRS electrical axis. The normal mean QRS axis in adults lies between −30 degrees and +90 degrees. Mean QRS axes more positive than +90 degrees represent *right axis deviation,* and those more negative than −30 degrees represent *left axis deviation*. Mean axes lying between −90 and −180 degrees (or equivalently between +180 and +270 degrees) are referred to as *extreme axis deviations*. The designation *indeterminate axis* is applied when all six extremity leads show biphasic (QR or RS) patterns; this finding can occur as a normal variant or may be seen in a variety of pathological conditions.

The wide span of the normal axis results in a range of QRS patterns, especially in the inferior leads. This characteristic can be understood by referring to the hexaxial reference system in Figure 9–9. If the mean axis is near 90 degrees, the QRS complex in leads II, III, and aV_f will be predominantly upright with qR complexes; lead I will record an isoelectric RS pattern because the heart vector lies perpendicular to the lead axis. This configuration is commonly referred to

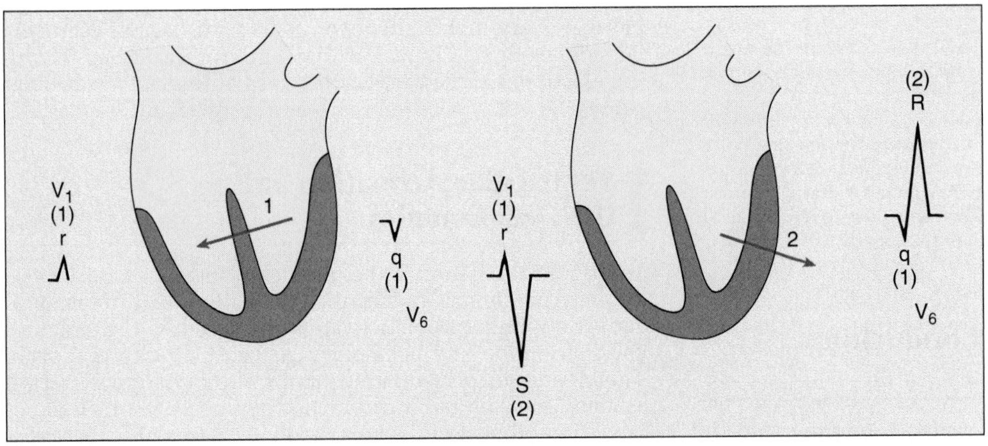

FIGURE 9–14 Schematic representation of ventricular depolarization as two sequential vectors representing septal **(left)** and left ventricular free wall **(right)** activation. QRS waveforms generated by each stage of activation in leads V_1 and V_6 are shown.

as a *vertical heart* position, although it is not necessarily related to the anatomical position of the heart within the chest. If the mean axis is nearer 0 degrees, the patterns will be reversed; lead I (and aV_l) will register a predominantly upright qR pattern, and leads II, III, and aV_f will show rS or RS patterns, a configuration often referred to as a *horizontal heart* pattern.

PRECORDIAL LEADS. In the precordial leads V_1 and V_2, free wall activation generates S waves following the initial r waves generated by septal activation. These S waves are produced by the spread of activation in the free wall to the left and posteriorly, with generation of a heart vector directed away from the axes of these leads. Thus, these leads are characterized by rS patterns.

Patterns in the midprecordial leads V_3 and V_4 are more variable. Potentials sensed in these leads reflect, as in the case of the right precordial leads, the activation front in the ventricular free wall approaching the exploring electrode, followed by its moving leftward and posteriorly to more remote regions of the left ventricle. This front generates an R or r wave and later an S wave to produce rS or RS complexes in these leads. As the exploring electrode moves laterally to the left, however, the R wave becomes more dominant and the S wave becomes smaller because of the greater time period during which the activation front moves toward the positive end of the electrode.

Thus, in the precordial leads, the QRS complex is usually characterized by consistent progression from an rS complex in the right precordial leads to a qR pattern in the left precordial leads. The point during this transition at which the pattern changes from an rS to an Rs configuration, that is, the lead in which an isoelectric RS pattern is present, is known as the *transition zone* and normally occurs in leads V_3 or V_4. An example of a normal precordial QRS pattern is shown in Figure 9–12. Transition zones shifted to the right, to lead V_2, are referred to as *early transitions,* and those shifted leftward to V_5 or V_6 are *delayed transitions.* These variations in the horizontal plane axis are sometimes described as *counterclockwise* and *clockwise rotations*, respectively, of the heart, although these descriptors do not necessarily correlate with cardiac anatomical findings.[17]

QRS DURATION. The upper normal value for QRS duration is traditionally given as less than 120 msec (and often as <110 msec) measured in the lead with the widest QRS duration. In a survey of 1224 healthy men with normal QRS morphology and frontal plane axis, the 98 percent upper boundary of QRS duration measured by a multilead, automated computer algorithm was 116 msec. Women, on average, have somewhat smaller QRS durations than men (by about 5 to 8 msec).

INTRINSICOID DEFLECTION. An additional feature of the QRS complex is the intrinsicoid deflection. An electrode overlying the ventricular free wall will record a rising R wave as transmural activation of the underlying ventricular free wall proceeds. Once the activation front reaches the epicardium, the full thickness of the wall under the electrode will be in an active state, with no propagating electrical activity. At that moment, the electrode will register negative potentials from remote cardiac areas still undergoing activation. The sudden reversal of potential with a sharp downslope is the intrinsicoid deflection and marks the timing of activation of the epicardium under the electrode.

Ventricular Recovery and the ST-T Wave

The normal ST-T wave begins as a low-amplitude, slowly changing wave (the *ST segment*) that gradually leads to a larger wave, the *T wave.* Onset of the ST-T wave is the junction, or *J point*, and is normally at or near the isoelectric baseline of the ECG (see Figs. 9–11 and 9–12).

The polarity of the ST-T wave is generally the same as the net polarity of the preceding QRS complex. Thus, T waves are usually upright in leads I, II, aV_l, aV_f, and the lateral precordial leads. They are negative in lead aVr and variable in leads III and V_1 through V_3.

Recovery, like activation, occurs in a characteristic geometrical pattern. Differences in recovery timing occur both across the ventricular wall and between regions of the left ventricle. Transmural differences in recovery times are the net result of two effects—differences in action potential duration across the ventricular wall and the relatively slow spread of activation across the wall. As activation moves from endocardium to epicardium, sites further away from the endocardium are activated later and later in sequence. However, action potential durations are longest near the endocardium and shortest near the epicardium, which produces a transmural gradient in recovery periods. Differences in action potential duration are greater than differences in activation times, so recovery is completed near the epicardium before it is completed near the endocardium. For example, one endocardial site may be excited 10 msec earlier than the overlying epicardium (that is, transmural activation may require 10 msec), and the action potential duration at the endocardium may be 22 msec longer than on the epicardium. As a result, recovery will be completed 12 msec earlier in the epicardium than in the endocardium.

The resulting recovery dipole will then be directed from sites of less recovery (the endocardium) toward sites of greater recovery (near the epicardium). The orientation of this dipole is in the same direction as transmural activation dipoles. This orientation is opposite to the expected direction as described earlier in this chapter; this difference is due to the presence of nonuniform recovery properties across the wall. If recovery times were uniform across the wall (or if differences in recovery times were less than differences in transmural activation times), the recovery dipole would have been directed toward the endocardium, that is, in the direction opposite the activation dipole. The result, in normal persons, is concordant QRS and ST-T wave patterns.

Regional differences in recovery properties likewise exist. Under normal conditions, it is the transmural gradients that predominantly determine ST patterns. However, as will be described, these regional differences account for the discordant ST-T patterns observed with intraventricular conduction defects.

THE QRST ANGLE. This concordance between orientation of the QRS complex and ST-T wave can also be expressed vectorially. An angle can be visualized between the vector representing the mean QRS force and that representing the mean ST-T force—the *QRST angle*. This angle in the frontal plane is normally less than 60 degrees and usually less than 30 degrees. Abnormalities of the QRST angle reflect abnormal relationships between the properties of activation and recovery.

THE VENTRICULAR GRADIENT. If the two vectors representing mean activation and mean recovery forces are added, a third vector known as the *ventricular gradient* is created. This third vector represents the net area under the QRST complex. The concept of the ventricular gradient was originally developed to assess differences in the properties of ventricular activation and recovery. According to this concept, the more variability that exists in regional repolarization properties, the greater the difference between the QRS and ST-T areas will be. In other words, the ventricular gradient correlates with the magnitude of regional differences in recovery properties. In addition, because changes in activation patterns produced, for example, by bundle branch block cause corresponding changes in recovery patterns (see later), no change in the ventricular gradient typically results. The ventricular gradient should thus allow a measure of regional recovery properties that is independent of the activation pattern. This measurement has possible relevance to the genesis of reentrant arrhythmias that are due, in part, to abnormal regional variations in refractory periods.

THE U WAVE. The T wave may be followed by an additional low-amplitude wave known as the *U wave.* This late repolarization wave, usually less than 0.1 mV in amplitude, normally has the same polarity as the preceding T wave and is largest in the midprecordial leads and at slow heart rates. Its basis in cardiac electrophysiology is uncertain; it may be caused by repolarization of the Purkinje fibers, by the long action potential of midmyocardial cells (M cells), or by delayed repolarization in areas of the ventricle that undergo late mechanical relaxation.[18,19]

THE QT INTERVAL. A final interval of the ECG waveform is the QT interval, which is measured from the beginning of the QRS complex to the end of the T wave in the lead with the longest interval and without prominent U waves.[20] It includes the total duration of ventricular activation and recovery and, in a general sense, corresponds to the duration of the ventricular action potential.

The normal QT interval is defined by its duration, measured in milliseconds. Like the ventricular action potential duration, the duration of the QT interval decreases as heart rate increases. Thus, the normal range for the QT interval is rate dependent. One formula for relating QT interval duration to heart rate was developed by Bazett in 1920. The result is computation of a corrected QT interval, or QT_c, by using the following equation:

$$QT_c = QT/(R - R)^{1/2}$$

where the QT and RR intervals are measured in seconds. The normal QT_c is generally accepted to be less than or equal to 440 msec. Some studies suggest that it may be 20 msec longer,[20a] and it is slightly longer, on average, in women (see Chap. 32). When the T wave overlaps with the beginning of a U wave, the QT interval is sometimes referred to as the *QT(U) interval*; this designation is particularly appropriate when considering the ECG effects of certain metabolic abnormalities that alter the duration of repolarization and the amplitude of the U wave (see later).

The Bazett formula, while widely used to adjust the QT interval duration for the effects of heart rate, has limited accuracy in predicting the effects of heart rate on the QT interval.[20,20b] Many other formulas and methods for correcting the QT interval for the effects of heart rate, including logarithmic, hyperbolic, and exponential functions, have been developed and tested, but they also have limitations. These limitations result from both physiological and computational problems. The substantial variation in the relationship between QT interval duration and heart rate among different patient groups reduces the accuracy of any single correction formula. In addition, these formulas do not account for the effects of autonomic tone on the QT interval independent of the effects on rate. They also do not account for the relatively slow adaptation of repolarization to changes in rate; for example, several minutes may be required for the QT interval to reach a new steady state after an abrupt change in heart rate. The normal corrected QT interval can vary by more than 75 msec during a 24-hour period.[20b]

A second property of the QT interval is that its duration is lead dependent; that is, the duration of the QT interval varies from lead to lead. In normal persons, the QT interval varies between leads by up to 50 msec and is longest in the midprecordial leads V_2 and V_3. This range of intervals, referred to as *QT interval dispersion*, may be related to electrical instability and the risk of ventricular arrhythmogenesis, as described further below.[21]

NORMAL VARIANTS. These descriptions of the waveforms of the normal ECG represent patterns most often observed in normal adults. Understanding the limitations of assigning and interpreting the normal ranges of ECG measurements is important. Values for many of the intervals and amplitudes to be described vary widely within the population as a function of age, race, gender, body habitus, and the geometric position of the heart within the torso. Variation may also occur within an individual over time as a function of autonomic tone and activity level. Thus, what is normal in one condition may be abnormal in another. Some variations have already been described in this chapter, including, for example, variations in rate, QRS axis, and QT intervals.

Common variations occur in patterns of the ST segment and the T wave. These variations are important to recognize because they may be mistaken for significant abnormalities; for example, as many as 40% of Olympic athletes have "abnormal" electrocardiograms, whereas fewer than 5% of these athletes have structural cardiac disease.[22] ST-T patterns are affected by maneuvers that change autonomic tone. For example, changing body position, hyperventilating, drinking cold water, and performing the Valsalva maneuver can produce modest ST segment depression and slight T wave inversion in as many as one third of subjects.

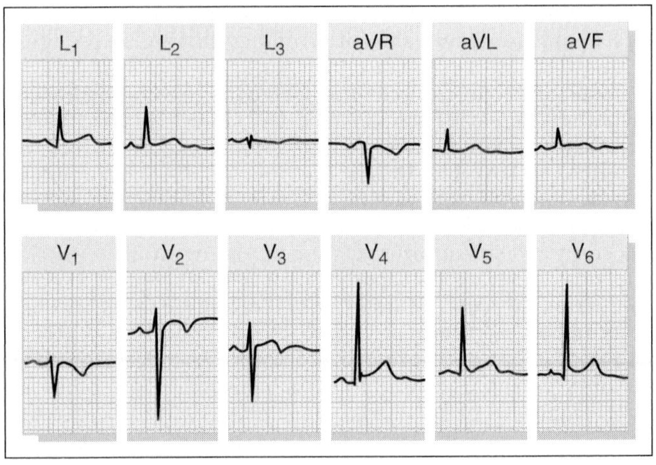

FIGURE 9–15 Normal tracing with a juvenile T wave inversion pattern in leads V_1, V_2, and V_3, as well as early repolarization pattern manifested by ST segment elevation in leads I, II, aV_f, V_4, V_5, and V_6. (Courtesy of C. Fisch, M.D.)

T waves can be inverted in the right precordial leads (Fig. 9–15). In adults, this inversion reflects the uncommon, but not necessarily abnormal, persistence of patterns commonly seen in infants and children. T waves can be inverted in all precordial leads at birth and usually become more limited to the right side of the chest as time passes; by the age of 10 years, T wave inversion is generally limited to leads V_1 and V_2. A persistent juvenile pattern is more common in women than in men and among the black population than among other racial or ethnic groups.

Second, the ST segment can be elevated, especially in the midprecordial leads (Fig. 9–16). The elevation begins from an elevated J point, is usually concave in form, is commonly associated with notching of the downstroke of the QRS complex, and can reach 0.3 mV in amplitude.[23,24] This pattern is more common at slow than at rapid heart rates and is most prevalent in young adults, especially among black men. Although this physiological ST segment elevation pattern is commonly referred to as *early repolarization*, clinical studies have failed to demonstrate an earlier than normal onset of ventricular recovery. This physiologic variant may be related to relative enhancement of vagal tone in healthy subjects and is also prevalent in those with high (T5 or above) spinal cord injuries where sympathetic outflow is interrupted.[25]

The Abnormal Electrocardiogram

Atrial Abnormalities

Various pathological and physiological events alter the normal sequence of atrial activation and produce abnormal P wave patterns in the ECG. Three general categories of P wave changes are described here, including those reflecting abnormal sites or patterns of activation, those caused by left atrial abnormalities, and those resulting from right atrial abnormalities.

Abnormal Sites of Atrial Activation

Shifts in the site of initial activation away from the SA node to other, ectopic sites can lead to major changes in the pattern of atrial activation and, hence, in the morphology of P waves.[26] These shifts can occur either as escape rhythms if the normal SA nodal pacemaker fails or as accelerated ectopic rhythms if the automaticity of an ectopic site is enhanced (see AV dissociation, Chapter 32). The resulting ECG abnormalities most commonly include recording negative P waves in the leads in which P waves are normally upright (leads I, II, aV_f, and V_4 through V_6), with or without shortening of the PR interval.

P wave patterns can suggest the site of impulse formation based on simple vectorial principles. For example, a negative P wave in lead I can predict a left atrial rhythm. Inverted P waves in the inferior leads normally correspond to a posterior atrial site. However, because of the uncertainties with this localization, these ECG patterns can, as a group, be referred to as *ectopic atrial rhythms*. Apparent left atrial rhythms can arise in the pulmonary veins and play a role in precipitating atrial fibrillation (see Chap. 32).

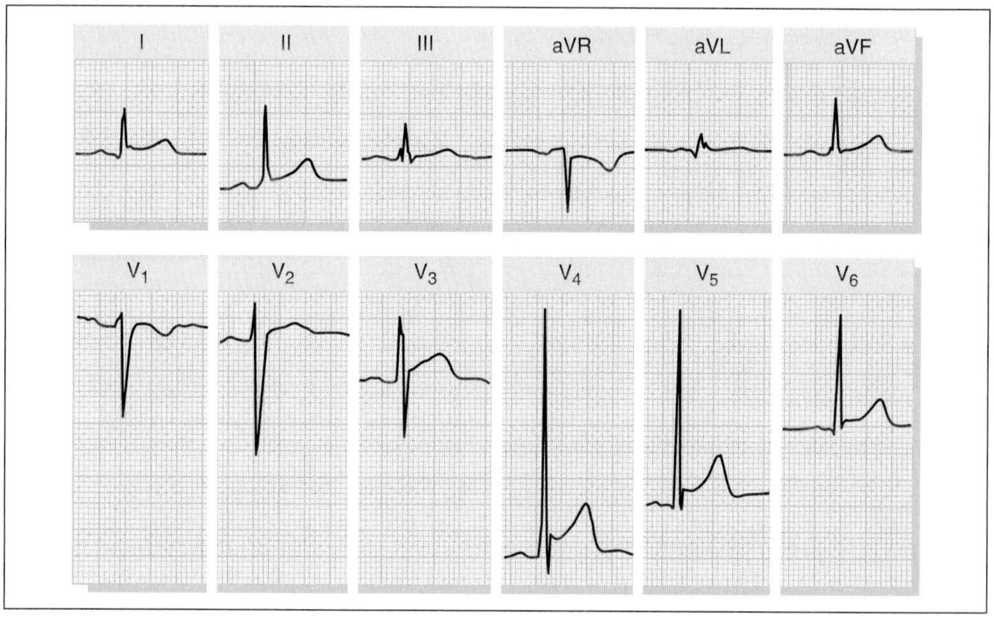

FIGURE 9–16 Normal variant pattern with functional ST elevations ("early repolarization" variant). These benign ST segment elevations are usually most marked in the midprecordial leads (V_4 here). Note the absence of reciprocal ST depression (except in lead aV_r), as well as the absence of PR segment deviation, which may be helpful in the differential diagnosis of ischemia and pericarditis, respectively. Note also that lead II has a baseline recording shift. (From Goldberger AL: Myocardial Infarction: Electrocardiographic Differential Diagnosis. 4th ed. St Louis, Mosby-Year Book, 1991.)

Left Atrial Abnormality

ECG ABNORMALITIES. Anatomical or functional abnormalities of the left atrium alter the morphology, duration, and amplitude of the P waves in the clinical ECG. Specific abnormalities include increases in the amplitude and duration of the P wave in the limb leads, as well as an increase in the amplitude of the terminal negative portion of the P wave in lead V_1. These features are illustrated in Figures 9–17 and 9–18.

DIAGNOSTIC CRITERIA. Commonly used criteria for diagnosing left atrial abnormality are listed in Table 9–3.

MECHANISMS FOR ECG ABNORMALITIES. Abnormal ECG patterns can reflect increases in left atrial mass or chamber size or conduction delays within the atria. Increasing mass causes increased P wave amplitudes. Because the left atrium is activated (in general) late during P wave inscription, the increased electrical force accounts for the prolonged P wave duration and the augmented P terminal force in the right precordial leads.

These patterns also correlate with a delay in interatrial conduction. This delay prolongs P wave duration and shortens the PR segment. It also reduces the overlap between right and left atrial activation, so the ECG patterns generated by each atrium may be separated as two humps in lead II (*P mitrale*).

DIAGNOSTIC ACCURACY. The diagnostic accuracy of these criteria is limited. Comparison of the various ECG abnormalities to echocardiographic criteria for left atrial enlargement demonstrates limited sensitivity but high specificity for standard ECG criteria. For example, recent studies have demonstrated that the presence of classic P mitrale patterns has a sensitivity of only 20 percent but a specificity of 98 percent for detecting echocardiographically enlarged left atria.[27] Other studies have reported better correlations of these ECG abnormalities with ventricular dysfunction (e.g., with reduced ventricular compliance) than with atrial morphology. Because of the correlation of these ECG features with high atrial pressure, intraatrial conduction defects, and ventricular dysfunction, as well as increased atrial size, these ECG abnormalities are preferably referred to as criteria for left atrial abnormality rather than left atrial enlargement.

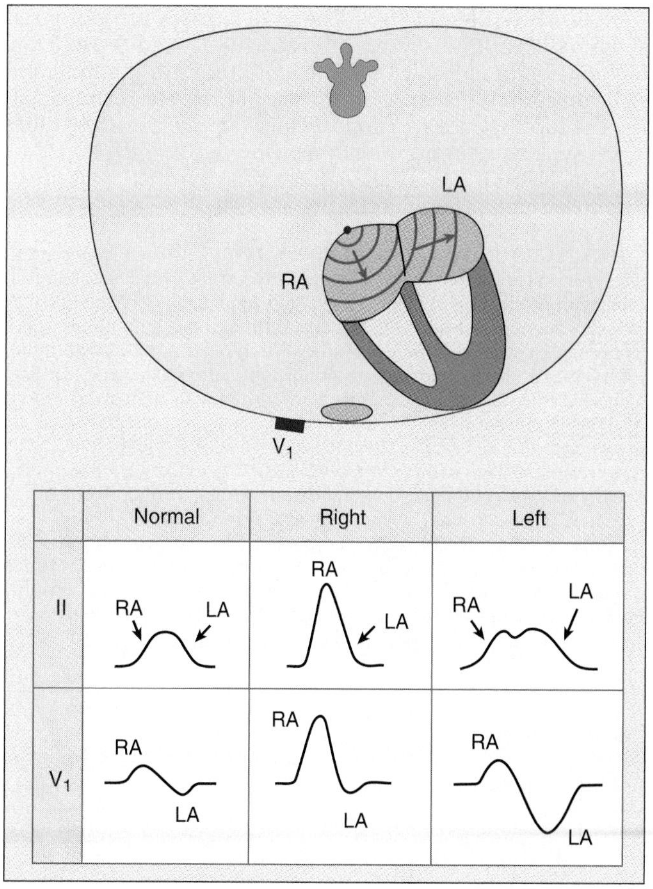

FIGURE 9–17 Schematic representation of atrial depolarization **(diagram)** and P wave patterns associated with normal atrial activation **(left panel)** and with right **(middle panel)** and left **(right panel)** atrial abnormalities. (Modified from Park MK, Guntheroth WG: How to Read Pediatric ECGs. 3rd ed. St Louis, Mosby-Year Book, 1993.)

TABLE 9–3 Common Diagnostic Criteria for Left and Right Atrial Abnormalities*

Left Atrial Abnormality	Right Atrial Abnormality
Prolonged P wave duration of >120 msec in lead II	Peaked P waves with amplitudes greater than 0.25 mV in lead II (P pulmonale)
Prominent notching of the P wave, usually most obvious in lead II, with an interval between the notches of >40 msec (P mitrale)	Rightward shift of the mean P wave axis to above 75 degrees
Ratio between the duration of the P wave in lead II and the duration of the PR segment of >1.6	Increased area under the initial positive portion of the P wave in lead V_1 to >0.06 mm-sec
Increased duration and depth of the terminal negative portion of the P wave in lead V_1 (the P terminal force) so that the area subtended by it exceeds 0.04 mm-sec	
Leftward shift of the mean P wave axis to between −30 and +45 degrees	

*In addition to criteria based on P wave morphologies, right atrial abnormalities are suggested by QRS changes, including (1) Q waves (especially qR patterns) in the right precordial leads without evidence of myocardial infarction and (2) low amplitude (under 600 μV) QRS complexes in lead V_1 with a threefold or greater increase in lead V_2.

CLINICAL SIGNIFICANCE. The ECG findings of left atrial abnormality are associated with more severe left ventricular dysfunction in patients with ischemic heart disease and with more severe valve damage in patients with mitral or aortic valve disease. Patients with left atrial changes also have a higher than normal incidence of paroxysmal atrial tachyarrhythmias.

Right Atrial Abnormality

ECG ABNORMALITIES. The ECG features of right atrial abnormality are illustrated in Figures 9–17 and 9–18. They include abnormally high P wave amplitudes in the limb and right precordial leads. As in the case of left atrial abnormality, the term *right atrial abnormality* is preferred over other terms such as *right atrial enlargement.*

DIAGNOSTIC CRITERIA. Criteria commonly used to diagnose right atrial abnormality are listed in Table 9–3.

MECHANISMS FOR ECG ABNORMALITIES. Greater right atrial mass generates greater electrical force early during overall atrial activation, with production of taller P waves and augmentation of the initial P wave deflection in lead V_1. In patients with chronic lung disease, the abnormal P pattern may reflect a more vertical heart position within the chest caused by pulmonary hyperinflation rather than true cardiac damage. The QRS changes commonly associated with right atrial abnormalities correspond to the underlying pathologic condition that is producing the right atrial hemodynamic changes—right ventricular hypertrophy (RVH), which produces tall R waves in the right precordial leads, and a shift of the position of the heart within the chest by obstructive lung disease, which produces initial Q waves.

DIAGNOSTIC ACCURACY. The finding of right atrial abnormality has limited sensitivity but high specificity. Echocardiographic correlations have shown, for example, that P pulmonale has very low sensitivity but very high specificity for detecting right atrial enlargement.

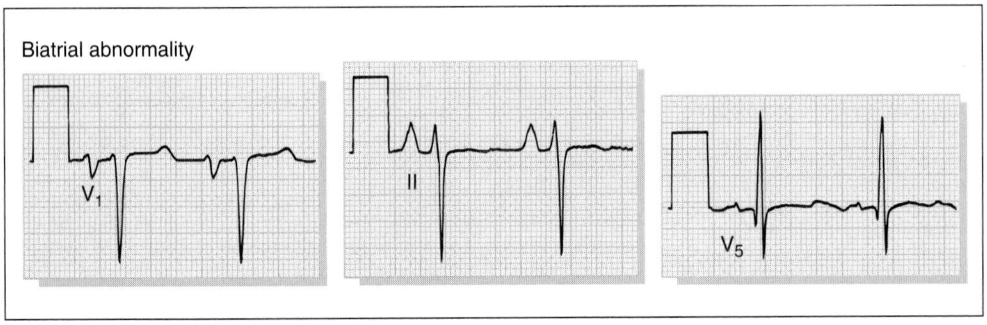

FIGURE 9–18 Biatrial abnormality, with tall P waves in lead II (right atrial abnormality) and an abnormally large terminal negative component of the P wave in lead V_1 (left atrial abnormality). The P wave is also notched in lead V_5.

CLINICAL SIGNIFICANCE. Patients with chronic obstructive pulmonary disease and this ECG pattern have more severe pulmonary dysfunction, as well as significantly reduced survival.[28] However, comparison of ECG and hemodynamic parameters has not demonstrated a close correlation of P wave patterns and right atrial hypertension.

Other Atrial Abnormalities

Patients with abnormalities in both atria—that is, *biatrial abnormality*—can have ECG patterns reflecting each defect. Suggestive findings include large biphasic P waves in lead V_1 and tall and broad P waves in leads II, III, and aV_f (see Fig. 9–18).

P wave and PR segment changes can also be seen in patients with atrial infarction or pericarditis. The changes caused by these conditions are described later in this chapter.

Ventricular Hypertrophy and Enlargement

Left Ventricular Hypertrophy and Enlargement

ECG ABNORMALITIES. Left ventricular hypertrophy (LVH) or enlargement produces changes in the QRS complex, the ST segment, and the T wave. The most characteristic finding is increased amplitude of the QRS complex. R waves in leads facing the left ventricle (that is, leads I, aV_l, V_5, and V_6) are taller than normal, whereas S waves in leads overlying the right ventricle (that is, V_1 and V_2) are deeper than normal. These changes are illustrated schematically in Figure 9–19.

ST-T wave patterns vary widely in patients with left ventricular enlargement and hypertrophy. ST segment and T wave amplitudes can be normal or increased in leads with tall R waves. In many patients, however, the ST segment is depressed and followed by an inverted T wave (Fig. 9–20). Most often, the ST segment slopes downward from a depressed J point and the T wave is asymmetrically inverted. These repolarization changes usually occur in patients with QRS changes but can appear alone. Particularly prominent inverted T waves, or so-called *giant negative T waves*, are characteristic of hypertrophic cardiomyopathy with predominant apical thickening, especially in patients from the Pacific Rim (*Yamaguchi syndrome*) (see Fig. 9–49).

Other ECG changes seen in cases of LVH include widening and notching of the QRS complex. An increase in QRS duration beyond 110 msec and a delay in the intrinsicoid deflection may reflect the longer duration of activation in a thickened ventricular wall or damage to the ventricular conduction system. Notching of the QRS complex may also be observed.

These ECG features are most typical of LVH induced by pressure or "systolic overload" of the left ventricle. Volume overload or "diastolic overload" can produce a somewhat different ECG pattern, including tall, upright T waves and sometimes narrow (less than 25 msec) but deep (0.2 mV or greater) Q waves in leads facing the left side of the septum (Fig. 9–20). The diagnostic value of these changes in predicting the underlying hemodynamics is, however, very limited.

MECHANISMS FOR ECG ABNORMALITIES. High voltages can be produced by any of several mechanisms. They can be due directly to an increase in left ventricular mass. This increase in mass is due to an enlargement in cell size, with an increase in surface area increasing transmembrane current flow and an increase in the number of intercalated disks enhancing intercellular current flow. This effect is augmented by an increase in the size of activation fronts moving across the thickened wall; these larger wavefronts subtend larger solid angles and result in higher body surface voltage.

The high voltage as well as QRS prolongation can also be due to conduction system delays. The delay in intrinsicoid deflection is a result of the prolonged transmural activation time required to activate the thickened wall, as well as delayed endocardial activation. Notching of the QRS complex can be produced by the fractionation of activation wavefronts by intramural scarring associated with wall thickening and damage.

In addition, changes in transmission factors can contribute to ECG abnormalities. Left ventricular enlargement can shift the position of the heart so that the lateral free wall lies closer than normal to the chest wall, which, as described earlier, would increase body surface potentials in accordance with the inverse square law.

Also, ventricular dilatation increases the size of the highly conductive intraventricular blood pool. This enhanced blood volume results in an increase in potentials produced by transmural activation fronts, a phenomenon referred to as the *Brody effect*.

Repolarization abnormalities can reflect a primary disorder of repolarization that accompanies the cellular processes of hypertrophy. Alternatively, they can reflect subendocardial ischemia. Patients with coronary artery disease have a higher prevalence of ST-T abnormalities with LVH than do those without coronary artery disease. Ischemia can be induced in the absence of coronary artery disease by the combination of high oxygen demand caused by high wall tension and limited blood flow to the subendocardium of the thickened wall.

DIAGNOSTIC CRITERIA. Many sets of diagnostic criteria for LVH have been developed on the basis of these ECG abnormalities (Fig. 9–21). Details of widely used criteria are presented in Table 9–4. Most commonly used methods assess the presence or absence of LVH as a binary function based on an empirically determined

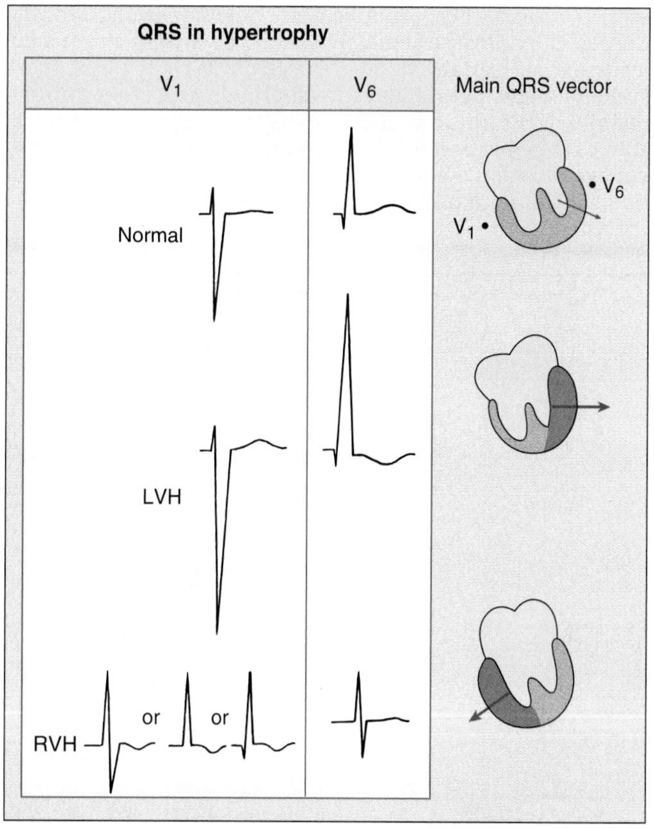

FIGURE 9–19 Left ventricular hypertrophy (LVH) increases the amplitude of electrical forces directed to the left and posteriorly. In addition, repolarization abnormalities can cause ST segment depression and T wave inversion in leads with a prominent R wave (formerly referred to as a "strain" pattern). Right ventricular hypertrophy (RVH) can shift the QRS vector to the right; this effect is usually associated with an R, RS, or qR complex in lead V_1, especially when due to severe pressure overload. T wave inversions may be present in the right precordial leads. (From Goldberger AL: Clinical Electrocardiography: A Simplified Approach. 6th ed. St Louis, CV Mosby, 1999.)

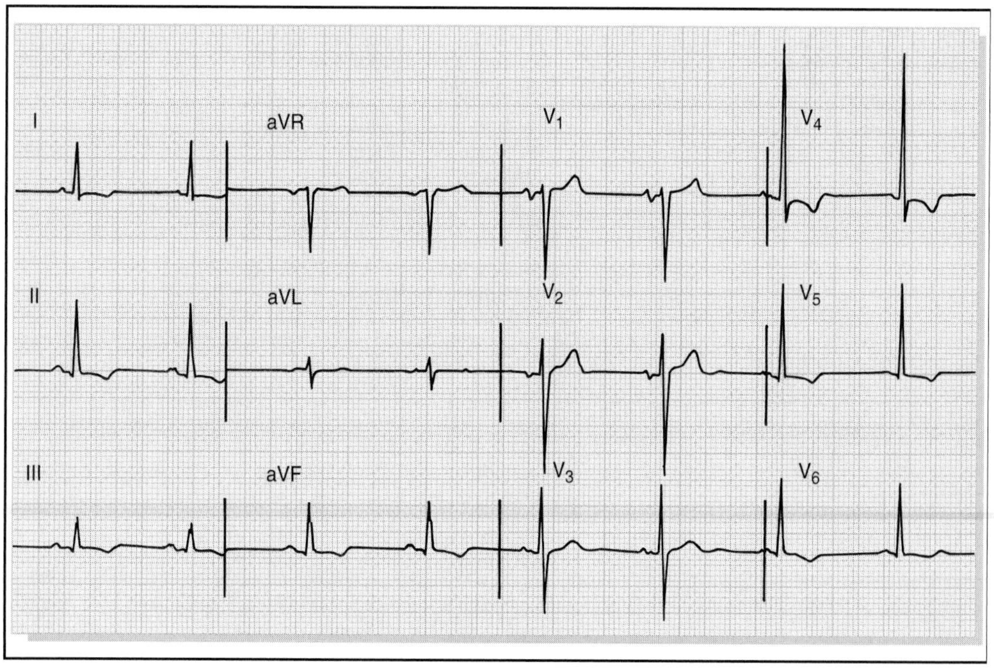

FIGURE 9–20 Marked left ventricular hypertrophy (LVH) pattern with prominent precordial lead QRS voltages. ST depression and T wave inversion can be seen with severe LVH in leads with a predominant R wave (compare with Fig. 9–21). Left atrial abnormality is also present.

set of criteria. For example, the Sokolow-Lyon and the Cornell[29,30] voltage criteria require that voltages in specific leads exceed certain values. The Romhilt-Estes point score system assigns point values to amplitude and other criteria; definite LVH is diagnosed if 5 points are computed, and probable LVH is diagnosed if 4 points are computed. The Cornell voltage-duration method includes measurement of QRS duration as well as amplitudes.

Other methods seek to quantify left ventricular mass as a continuum. Diagnosis of LVH can then be based on a computed mass that exceeds an independently determined threshold. Two recently developed sets of criteria applying this approach are the Cornell regression equation and the Novacode system.

Diagnostic Accuracy. The relative diagnostic accuracy of these methods has been tested by radiographic, echocardiographic, and autopsy measurements of left ventricular size as standards. In general, these studies have reported low sensitivity and high specificity. Sensitivities are lowest (approximately 10 to 30 percent) for the Sokolow-Lyon and Romhilt-Estes criteria and higher for the Cornell voltage and voltage-duration criteria and for the Cornell and Novacode regression methods (35 to 50 percent). In contrast, specificities for all measures vary from 85 percent to 95 percent. Thus, all methods are limited as screening tests in which high sensitivities (few false-negatives) are critical but have good reliability as diagnostic tests when few false-positives are desired.

Repolarization abnormalities associated with ECG findings increase the correlation with anatomical LVH. ST and T wave abnormalities

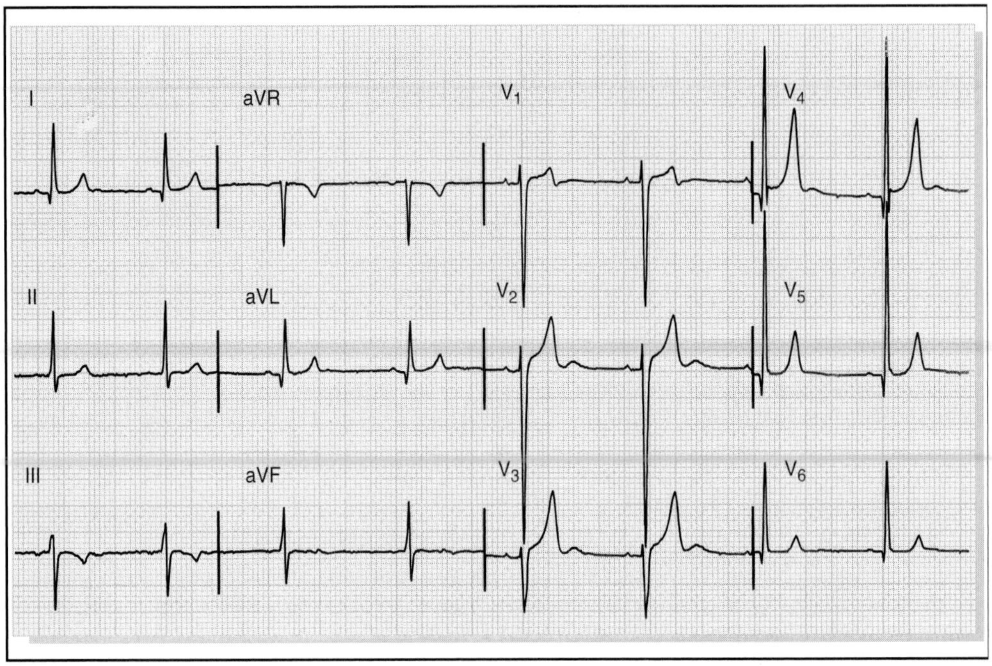

FIGURE 9–21 Left ventricular hypertrophy with prominent positive anterior T waves from a patient with severe aortic regurgitation. This pattern has been described with "diastolic overload" syndrome but has limited sensitivity and specificity. Serum potassium level was normal.

TABLE 9–4 Common Diagnostic Criteria for Left Ventricular Hypertrophy

Measurement	Criteria	
Sokolow-Lyon index	$S_{V1} + (R_{V5}$ or $R_{V6}) > 3.5$ mV	
	$R_{aVl} > 1.1_1$ mV	
Romhilt-Estes point score system*	Any limb lead R wave or S wave ≥2.0 mV	3 points
	or S_{V1} or $S_{V2} \geq 3.0$ mV	3 points
	or R_{V5} to $R_{V6} \geq 3.0$ mV	3 points
	ST-T wave abnormality (no digitalis therapy)	3 points
	ST-T wave abnormality (digitalis therapy)	1 point
	Left atrial abnormality	3 points
	Left axis deviation (≥30 degrees)	2 points
	QRS duration ≥90 msec	1 point
	Intrinsicoid deflection in V_5 or V_6 ≥50 msec	1 point
Cornell voltage criteria	$S_{V3} + S_{aVl} \geq 2.8$ mV (for men)	
	$S_{V3} + S_{aVl} \geq 2.0$ mV (for women)	
Cornell regression equation	Risk of LVH = $1/(1 + e^{-exp})$, where exp = $4.558 - 0.092\ (R_{aVl} + S_{V3}) - 0.306\ T_{V1} - 0.212$ QRS $- 0.278\ PTF_{V1} - 0.859$ (sex), voltages are in mV, QRS is QRS duration in msec, PTF is the area under the P terminal force in lead V_1 (in mm-sec), and sex = 1 for men and 2 for women; LVH is present if exp < −1.55.	
Cornell voltage-duration measurement[55]	QRS duration X Cornell Voltage <2436	
	QRS duration X sum of voltages in all leads >17,472	
Novacode criterion (for men)	LVMI (gm/m²) = $-36.4 + 0.010\ R_{V5} + 0.20\ S_{V1} + 0.28\ S^{\dagger}_{III} + 0.182\ T_{(neg)}V_6 - 0.148\ T_{(pos)}aVr + 1.049\ QRS_{duration}$	
	where neg and pos refer to amplitudes of the negative and positive portions of the T waves, respectively; $S^{\dagger}_{III}$ indicates the amplitude of the S, Q, and QS wave, whichever is larger	

LVH = left ventricular hypertrophy; LVMI = left ventricular mass index.

*Probable left ventricular hypertrophy is diagnosed if 4 points are present and definite left ventricular hypertrophy is diagnosed if 5 or more points are present.

are associated with a three-fold greater prevalence of anatomical LVH in patients without coronary artery disease and a fivefold greater risk among patients with coronary disease.[31] The prevalence of anatomical LVH increases with the magnitude of the ST-segment depression.[32]

Which diagnostic criteria are met may have pathophysiological and clinical implications. Most patients with ECG criteria for LVH meet criteria for one set of criteria but not others.[30] Those meeting Cornell criteria have different patterns of left ventricular geometry than do those meeting Sokolow-Lyon criteria.[33]

Accuracy of the diagnostic criteria vary with demographic and related features of the populations studied. For example, precordial voltages are often higher among African Americans than among white persons, which leads to a higher prevalence of false-positive ECG diagnoses of left ventricular hypertrophy among African Americans with hypertension.[34]

Several reasons can be suggested for the limited accuracy of these criteria. Many of the clinical studies that were used to define the criteria included a disproportionate number of white men, thus limiting applicability of the tests to other populations. In addition, the criteria for dichotomous tests such as the Sokolow-Lyon and Cornell voltage criteria are based on quantitative differences in normally occurring measures, that is, QRS voltage, between normal and abnormal cohorts. These tests by their nature are limited to detecting only the extreme end of the spectrum of LVH, because milder degrees overlap with findings in normal populations. Finally, these voltage measurements are subject to the influence of many noncardiac factors, such as body habitus, which blurs the distinction between normal and abnormal.[35]

CLINICAL SIGNIFICANCE. The presence of ECG criteria for LVH identifies a subset of the general population with a significantly increased risk for cardiovascular morbidity and mortality.[36] This increased risk is particularly apparent in women and in people in whom ST-T wave abnormalities are present; the relative risk of cardiovascular events for patients with LVH voltage criteria alone is approximately 2.8, whereas the relative risk increases to more than 5.0 if ST segment depression is also present.[37] Interestingly, positive diagnoses of LVH by Sokolow-Lyon criteria and by Cornell criteria have independent prognostic value.[38]

In patients with cardiac disease, the ECG finding of LVH correlates with more severe disease, including higher blood pressure in hypertensive patients and greater ventricular dysfunction in patients with hypertension or coronary artery disease. In contrast, effective treatment of hypertension reduces ECG evidence of LVH and decreases the associated risk of cardiovascular mortality (see Chap. 38).

Patients with repolarization abnormalities have, on average, more severe degrees of LVH and more commonly have symptoms of left ventricular dysfunction, in addition to a greater risk of cardiovascular events.

Right Ventricular Hypertrophy and Enlargement

ECG ABNORMALITIES. The right ventricle is considerably smaller than the left ventricle and produces electrical forces that are largely concealed by those generated by the larger left ventricle. Thus, for RVH to be manifested on the ECG, it must be severe enough to overcome the concealing effects of the larger left ventricular forces. In addition, increasing dominance of the right ventricle changes the ECG in fundamental ways, whereas an enlarged left ventricle produces predominantly quantitative changes in underlying normal waveforms.

The ECG changes associated with moderate to severe concentric hypertrophy of the right ventricle include abnormally tall R waves in anteriorly and rightward directed leads (leads aV_r, V_1, and V_2) and deep S waves and abnormally small r waves in leftward directed leads (I, aV_l, and lateral precordial leads) (Fig. 9–22). These changes result in a reversal of normal R wave progression in the precordial leads, a shift in the frontal plane QRS axis to the right, and sometimes the presence of S waves in leads I, II, and III (so-called *$S_1S_2S_3$ pattern*).

Several other ECG patterns of RVH also exist. Less severe hypertrophy, especially when limited to the outflow tract of the right ventricle that is activated late during the QRS complex, produces less marked changes. ECG abnormalities may be limited to an rSr′ pattern in V_1 and persistence of s (or S) waves in the left precordial leads. This pattern is typical of right ventricular volume overload as produced by an atrial septal defect.

Chronic Obstructive Pulmonary Disease. Chronic obstructive pulmonary disease can induce ECG changes by producing RVH, changes in the position of the heart within the chest, and hyperinflation of the lungs (Fig. 9–23). QRS changes caused by the insulating and positional changes produced by hyperinflation of the lungs include reduced amplitude of the QRS complex, right axis deviation in the

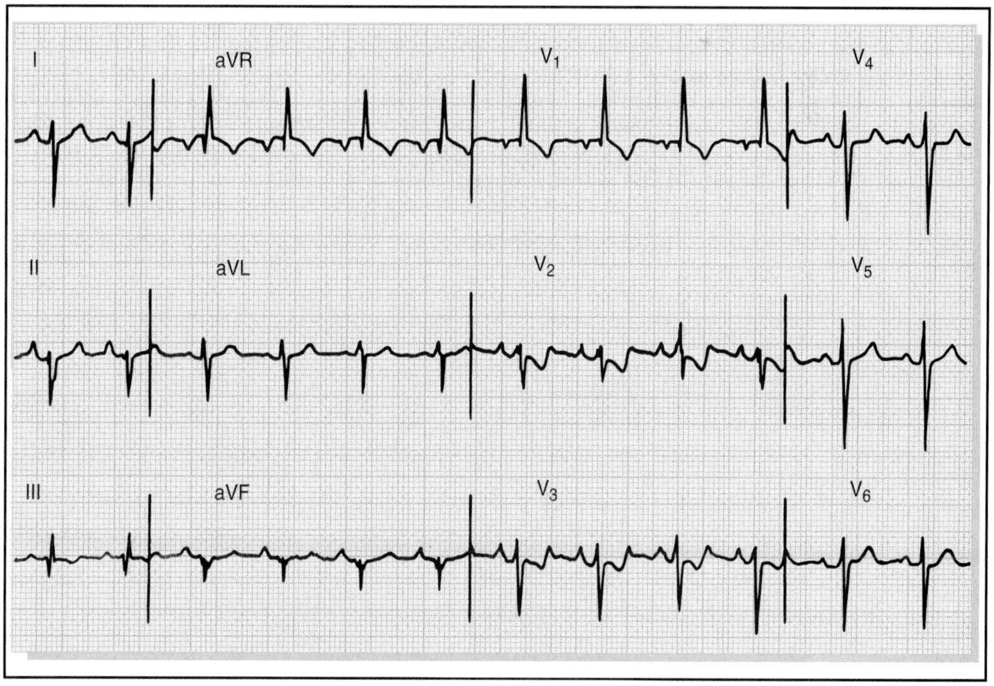

FIGURE 9–22 Right ventricular hypertrophy pattern most consistent with severe pressure overload. Note the combination of findings, including (1) a tall R wave in V_1 (as part of the qR complex), (2) right axis deviation, (3) T wave inversion in V_1 through V_3, (4) delayed precordial transition zone (rS in V_6), and (5) right atrial abnormality. An S_1Q_3 pattern is also present and can occur with acute or chronic right ventricular overload syndromes.

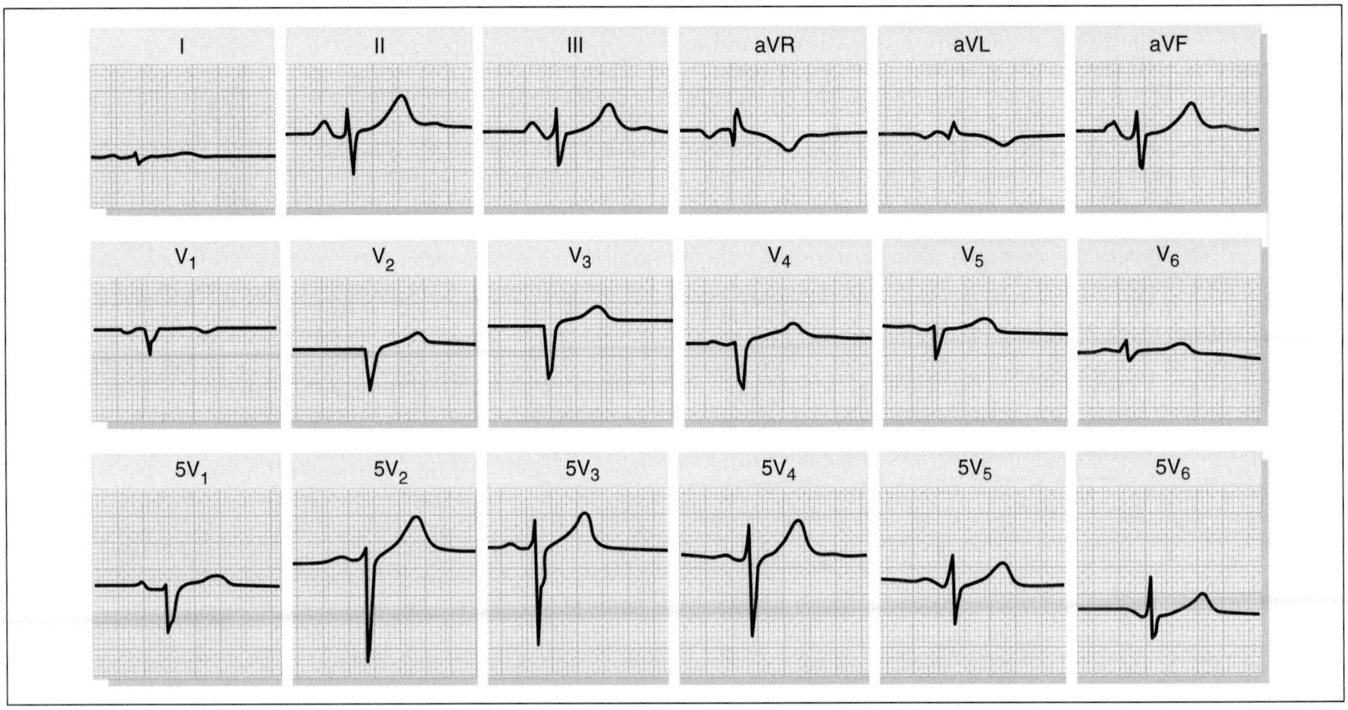

FIGURE 9–23 Pulmonary emphysema simulating anterior infarction in a 58-year-old man with no clinical evidence of coronary disease. Note the relative normalization of R wave progression with placement of the chest leads an interspace below their usual position ($5V_1$, $5V_2$, and so forth). (From Chou TC: Pseudo-infarction (noninfarction Q waves). *In* Fisch C [ed]: Complex Electrocardiography. Vol 1. Philadelphia, FA Davis, 1973.)

frontal plane, and delayed transition in the precordial leads (probably reflecting a vertical and caudal shift in heart position because of hyperinflation and a flattened diaphragm). Evidence of true RVH includes (1) marked right axis deviation (more positive than 110 degrees), (2) deep S waves in the lateral precordial leads, and (3) an $S_1Q_3T_3$ pattern, with an S wave in lead I (as an RS or rS complex), an abnormal Q wave in lead III, and an inverted T wave in the inferior leads.

Pulmonary Embolism. Finally, acute right ventricular pressure overload such as produced by pulmonary embolism can produce a characteristic ECG pattern (Fig. 9–24), including (1) a QR or qR pattern in the right ventricular leads; (2) an $S_1Q_3T_3$ pattern with an S wave in lead I and new or increased Q waves in lead III and sometimes aV_f, with T wave inversions in those leads; (3) ST segment deviation and T wave inversions in leads V_1 to V_3; and (4) incomplete or complete right bundle branch block (RBBB). Sinus tachycardia is usually present. Arrhythmias such as atrial fibrillation can also occur. However, even with major pulmonary artery obstruction, the ECG is notoriously deceptive and may show little more than minor or nonspecific waveform changes, or it may even be normal. The classic $S_1Q_3T_3$ pattern occurs in only about 10 percent of cases of acute pulmonary embolism (see Chaps. 66 and 67). Furthermore, the specificity of this finding is limited, because it can occur acutely with other causes of pulmonary hypertension.

DIAGNOSTIC CRITERIA. These ECG abnormalities form the basis for the diagnostic criteria for RVH. The most commonly relied on criteria for the ECG diagnosis of RVH are listed in Table 9–5.

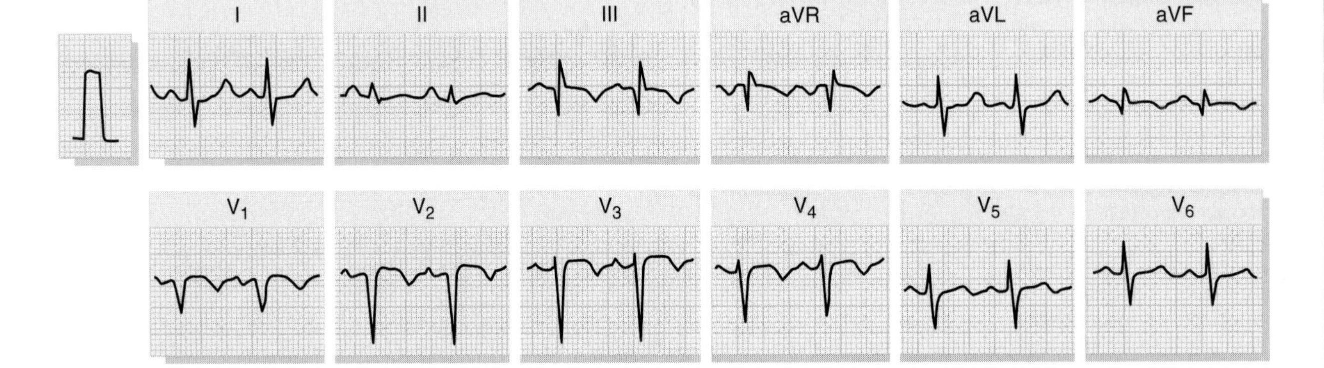

FIGURE 9–24 Acute cor pulmonale secondary to pulmonary embolism simulating inferior and anterior infarction. This tracing exemplifies the classic pseudoinfarct patterns sometimes seen: an $S_1Q_3T_3$, a QR in V_1 with poor R wave progression in the right precordial leads ("clockwise rotation"), and right precordial to midprecordial T wave inversion (V_1 to V_4). Sinus tachycardia is also present. The S_1Q_3 pattern is usually associated with a QR or QS complex, but not an rS, in aV_r. Furthermore, acute cor pulmonale per se does not cause prominent Q waves in II (only in III and aV_f). (From Goldberger AL: Myocardial Infarction: Electrocardiographic Differential Diagnosis. 4th ed. St Louis, Mosby-Year Book, 1991.)

TABLE 9–5 Common Diagnostic Criteria for Right Ventricular Hypertrophy

Criterion	Sensitivity (%)	Specificity (%)
R in $V_1 \geq 0.7$ mV	<10	—
QR in V_1	<10	—
R/S in $V_1 > 1$ with R > 0.5 mV	<25	89
R/S in V_5 or $V_6 < 1$	<10	—
S in V_5 or $V_6 \geq 0.7$ mV	<17	93
R in V_5 or $V_6 \geq 0.4$ mV with S in $V_1 \geq 0.2$ mV	<10	—
Right axis deviation (≥+90 degrees)	<14	99
S_1Q_3 pattern	<11	93
$S_1S_2S_3$ pattern	<10	—
P pulmonale	<11	97

From Murphy ML, Thenabadu PN, de Soyza N, et al: Reevaluation of electrocardiographic criteria for left, right and combined cardiac ventricular hypertrophy. Am J Cardiol 53:1140, 1984

MECHANISMS FOR ECG ABNORMALITIES. These ECG patterns result from three effects of RVH. First, current fluxes between hypertrophied cells are stronger than normal and produce higher than normal voltage on the body surface. Second, activation fronts moving through the enlarged right ventricle are larger than normal and produce higher surface potentials, as predicted by the solid angle theorem. Third, the activation time of the right ventricle is prolonged. This last effect is particularly important in producing ECG changes; right ventricular activation now ends after the completion of left ventricular activation, so its effects are no longer canceled by the more powerful forces of the left ventricle and may merge in the ECG. Because the right ventricle is located anteriorly as well as to the right of the left ventricle, the effects produce increased potentials in leads directed anteriorly and to the right, especially late during the QRS complex. As noted, changes in cardiac position in patients with obstructive lung disease can produce ECG changes without intrinsic cardiac electrophysiological derangements.

Diagnostic Accuracy. The sensitivity and specificity of the individual ECG criteria are also shown in Table 9–5. As in the case of ECG criteria for other abnormalities, the sensitivities of individual criteria are low and specificities are high. If any one feature is present, the sensitivity rises to more than 50 percent with a specificity of more than 90 percent; requiring any two features to make a diagnosis markedly reduces the sensitivity and raises the specificity to very high levels. These low sensitivities may reflect the marked degree of hypertrophy required to produce ECG abnormalities.

CLINICAL SIGNIFICANCE. The ECG evidence of RVH has limited value in assessing the severity of pulmonary hypertension or lung disease. QRS changes do not generally appear until ventilatory function is significantly depressed, with the earliest change commonly being a rightward shift in the mean QRS axis, and correlation with either ventilatory function or hemodynamics is poor. The presence of right atrial abnormality, an $S_1S_2S_3$ pattern, or both is associated with reduced survival, especially if an increased arterial-alveolar oxygen gradient is also present. ECG findings of acute right ventricular overload in patients with pulmonary embolism correspond to obstruction of more than 50 percent of the pulmonary arterial bed and significant pulmonary hypertension.

Biventricular Enlargement

Enlargement or hypertrophy of both ventricles produces complex ECG patterns.[39] In contrast to biatrial enlargement, the result is not the simple sum of the two sets of abnormalities. The effects of enlargement of one chamber may cancel the effects of enlargement of the other; for example, anterior forces produced by RVH may be canceled by enhanced posterior forces generated by LVH. In addition, the greater left ventricular forces generated in LVH increase the degree of RVH needed to overcome the dominance of the left ventricle.

Because of these factors, specific ECG criteria for either RVH or LVH are seldom observed with biventricular enlargement. Rather, ECG patterns are usually a modification of the features of LVH and include (1) tall R waves in both the right and left precordial leads, (2) vertical heart position or right axis deviation in the presence of criteria for LVH, (3) deep S waves in the left precordial leads in the presence of ECG criteria for LVH, or (4) a shift in the precordial transition zone to the left in the presence of LVH. The presence of prominent left atrial abnormality or atrial fibrillation with evidence of right ventricular or biventricular enlargement (especially LVH with a vertical or rightward QRS axis) should suggest chronic rheumatic valvular disease (Fig. 9–25) (see Chap. 57).

Intraventricular Conduction Delays and Preexcitation

The ECG patterns described in this section reflect abnormalities in the conduction system (see Chap. 29).

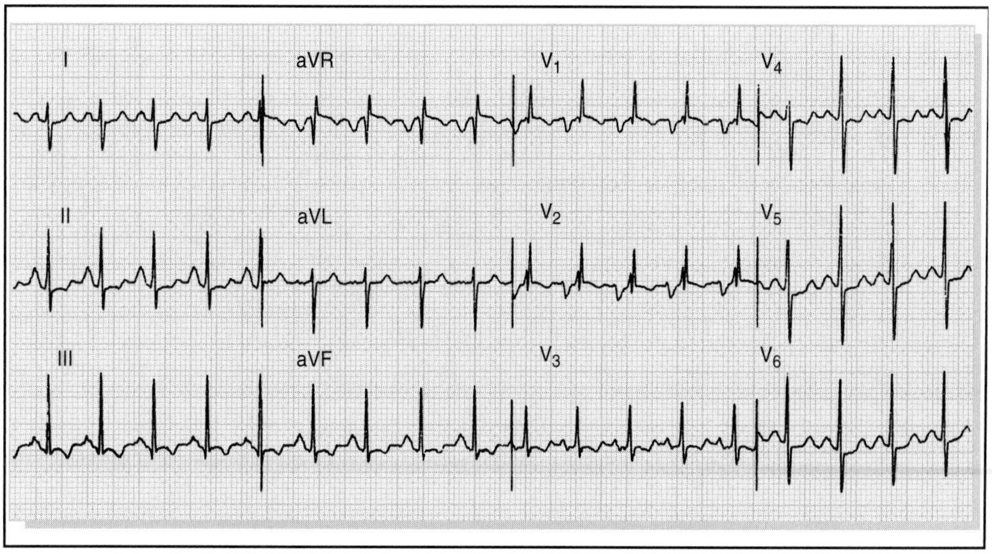

FIGURE 9–25 This electrocardiogram from a 45-year-old woman with severe mitral stenosis shows multiple abnormalities. The rhythm is sinus tachycardia. Right axis deviation and a tall R wave in lead V_1 are consistent with right ventricular hypertrophy. The very prominent biphasic P wave in lead V_1 indicates left atrial abnormality/enlargement. The tall P waves in lead II suggest concomitant right abnormality. Nonspecific ST-T changes and incomplete right bundle branch block are also present. The combination of right ventricular hypertrophy and marked left or biatrial abnormality is highly suggestive of mitral stenosis. (From Goldberger AL: Clinical Electrocardiography: A Simplified Approach. 6th ed. St Louis, CV Mosby, 1999.)

Under normal conditions, activation of the left ventricle begins simultaneously at the insertion sites of the fascicles. Delayed conduction in a fascicle—*fascicular block*—results in activation of these sites sequentially rather than simultaneously. This produces an abnormal sequence of early left ventricular activation that, in turn, leads to characteristic ECG patterns. Even modest delays in conduction through the affected structure may be enough to alter ventricular activation patterns sufficiently to produce characteristic ECG patterns; complete block of conduction is not required.

LEFT ANTERIOR FASCICULAR BLOCK. Damage to the left anterior fascicle is a very common occurrence because of the delicate nature of the structure. The ECG features of left anterior fascicular block (LAFB) are listed in Table 9–6 and illustrated in Figure 9–26. The most characteristic finding is marked left axis deviation. However, LAFB is not synonymous with left axis deviation. Axis shifts to between −30 and −45 degrees commonly reflect other conditions, such as LVH, without conduction system damage and are best referred to as *left axis deviation* rather than LAFB.

TABLE 9–6 Common Diagnostic Criteria for Unifascicular Blocks

Left anterior fascicular block
Frontal plane mean QRS axis of −45 to −90 degrees with rS patterns in leads II, III, and aV_f and a qR pattern in lead aV_l
QRS duration less than 120 msec
Left posterior fascicular block
Frontal plane mean QRS axis of ±120 degrees
RS pattern in leads I and aV_l with qR patterns in inferior leads
QRS duration of less than 120 msec
Exclusion of other factors causing right axis deviation (e.g., right ventricular overload patterns, lateral infarction)

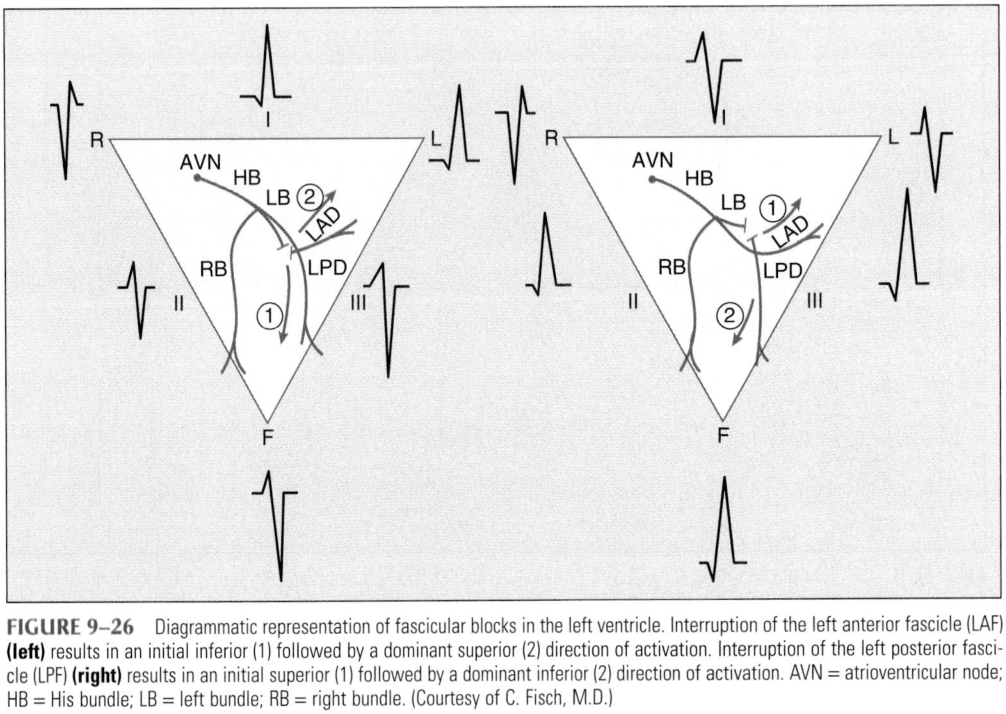

FIGURE 9–26 Diagrammatic representation of fascicular blocks in the left ventricle. Interruption of the left anterior fascicle (LAF) **(left)** results in an initial inferior (1) followed by a dominant superior (2) direction of activation. Interruption of the left posterior fascicle (LPF) **(right)** results in an initial superior (1) followed by a dominant inferior (2) direction of activation. AVN = atrioventricular node; HB = His bundle; LB = left bundle; RB = right bundle. (Courtesy of C. Fisch, M.D.)

Left axis shift is a result of delayed activation of the anterosuperior left ventricular wall. Delayed activation causes unbalanced inferior and posterior forces early during ventricular activation and unopposed anterosuperior forces later during the QRS complex. The abnormal pattern results in initial r waves followed by deep S waves in the inferior leads (left axis deviation with rS patterns) and a qR pattern in left-looking leads (leads aV_l and usually V_5 and V_6). Initial q waves in these leads reflect the normal left-to-right activation of the septum. LAFB can also produce prominent changes in the precordial leads; V_4 through V_6 commonly show deep S waves related to superiorly directed late QRS forces. The overall QRS duration is not prolonged; fascicular block alters only the sequence of left ventricular activation but does not by itself prolong the overall duration of ventricular excitation or the QRS complex.

Left anterior fascicular block is common in persons without overt cardiac disease, as well as in persons with a wide range of diseases. It has minimal or no independent prognostic significance. Commonly associated cardiac and systemic conditions include myocardial infarction, especially occlusion of the left anterior descending coronary artery, LVH, hypertrophic and dilated cardiomyopathy, and degenerative diseases. The development of LAFB with rS complexes in II, III, and aV_f can mask the Q waves of a prior inferior myocardial infarction.

LEFT POSTERIOR FASCICULAR BLOCK. Conduction delay in the left posterior fascicle is considerably less common than delay in the anterior fascicle because of its thicker structure and more protected location near the left ventricular inflow tract. Conduction delay results in sequential activation of the anterosuperior left ventricular free wall, followed by activation of the inferoposterior aspect of the left ventricle, that is, the reverse of the pattern observed with LAFB.

The ECG features of left posterior fascicular block (LPFB), listed in Table 9–6 and illustrated in Figure 9–26, reflect this altered activation pattern. Right axis deviation with rS patterns in leads I and aV_l, as well as qR complexes in the inferior leads, is the result of early unopposed activation forces from the anterosuperior aspect of the left ventricle (producing the initial q and r waves) and late unopposed forces from the inferoposterior free wall (generating the late S and R waves). As in the case of LAFB, the overall activation time of the ventricles is not prolonged and the QRS duration remains normal.

Left posterior fascicular block, like LAFB, can occur in patients with almost any cardiac disease but is unusual in otherwise healthy persons. Other conditions that enhance electrical forces from the right ventricle, such as right ventricular enlargement and extensive lateral infarction, can produce similar ECG patterns and must be excluded before a diagnosis of LPFB is made.

OTHER FORMS OF FASCICULAR BLOCK. The ECG evidence of left septal fascicular block has also been described. These patterns are adduced to reflect conduction delay in the third fascicle of the left bundle branch system—the septal fascicle—that inserts high on the left side of the interventricular septum. Among the ECG changes that are attributed to this form of block is the absence of septal q waves reflecting an abnormal sequence of septal activation.[16]

Left Bundle Branch Block

Left bundle branch block (LBBB) results from conduction delay or block in any of several sites in the intraventricular conduction system, including the main left bundle branch, in each of the two fascicles, or, less commonly, within the fibers of the bundle of His that become the main left bundle branch. The result is extensive reorganization of the activation pattern of the left ventricle.

ECG ABNORMALITIES. LBBB produces a prolonged QRS duration, abnormal QRS complexes, and ST-T wave abnormalities (Fig. 9–27). Commonly accepted diagnostic criteria for LBBB are listed in Table 9–7. Basic requirements include a prolonged QRS duration to 120 msec or beyond; broad, sometimes notched R waves in leads I and aV_l and the left precordial leads; narrow r waves followed by deep S waves in the right precordial leads; and absent septal q waves. R waves are typically tall and S waves are deep. The mean QRS axis with LBBB is highly variable; it can be normal, deviated to the left or, less often, deviated to the right.[40] Left axis deviation is associated with more severe conduction system disease that includes the fascicles as well as the main left bundle,[41] whereas right axis deviation suggests dilated cardiomyopathy with biventricular enlargement.[40] In addition to these features, some electrocardiographers require a delayed intrinsicoid deflection (60 msec or greater) to diagnose LBBB.

ST-T wave changes are also prominent with LBBB. In most cases, the ST wave and the T wave are discordant with the QRS complex; that is, the ST segment is depressed and the T wave is inverted in leads with positive QRS waves (leads I, aV_l, V_5, and V_6), while the ST segment is elevated and the T wave is upright in leads with negative QRS complexes (leads V_1 and V_2).

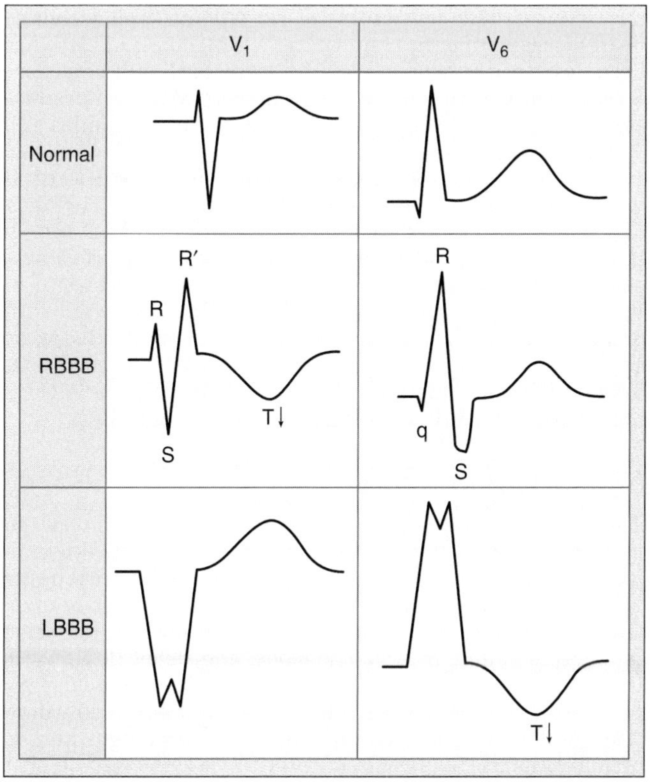

FIGURE 9–27 Comparison of typical QRS-T patterns in right bundle branch block (RBBB) and left bundle branch block (LBBB) with the normal pattern in leads V_1 and V_6. Note the secondary T wave inversions (arrows) in leads with an rSR′ complex with RBBB and in leads with a wide R wave with LBBB. (From Goldberger AL: Clinical Electrocardiography: A Simplified Approach. 6th ed. St Louis, CV Mosby, 1999.)

TABLE 9–7 Common Diagnostic Criteria for Bundle Branch Blocks

Complete left bundle branch block
QRS duration ≥120 msec
Broad, notched R waves in lateral precordial leads (V_5 and V_6) and usually leads I and aV_l
Small or absent initial r waves in right precordial leads (V_1 and V_2) followed by deep S waves
Absent septal q waves in left-sided leads
Prolonged intrinsicoid deflection (>60 msec) in V_5 and V_6*
Complete right bundle branch block
QRS duration ≥120 msec
Broad, notched R waves (rsr′, rsR′, or rSR′ patterns) in right precordial leads (V_1 and V_2)
Wide and deep S waves in left precordial leads (V_5 and V_6)

*Criterion required by some authors.

An incomplete form of LBBB may result from lesser degrees of conduction delay in the left bundle branch system. Left ventricular activation begins, as in complete LBBB, on the right side of the septum, but much of left ventricular activation occurs through the normal specialized conduction system. ECG features include (1) loss of septal q waves (reflecting reversal of the normal pattern of septal activation), (2) slurring and notching of the upstroke of R waves (because of the presence of competing activation fronts), and (3) modest prolongation of the QRS complex (between 100 and 120 msec).

MECHANISMS FOR ECG ABNORMALITIES. The ECG abnormalities of LBBB result from an almost completely reorganized pattern of left ventricular activation. Initial septal activation occurs on the right (rather than on the left) septal surface, resulting in the absence of normal septal q waves in the ECG.

The excitation wave then spreads slowly, by conduction from muscle cell to muscle cell, to the left side of the septum; the earliest left ventricular activation begins as late as 30 to 50 msec into the QRS complex. Endocardial activation of the left ventricle may then require an additional 40 to more than 180 msec, depending largely on the functional status of the distal left bundle and Purkinje systems.[42] Thus, the overall QRS complex is prolonged and can be very wide in patients with, for example, diffuse ventricular scarring from prior myocardial infarction.

Once left ventricular activation begins, it proceeds in a relatively simple and direct manner around the free wall and, finally, to the base of the heart. This is in contrast to the multicentric, overlapping patterns of activation seen under normal conditions. Direct progression of activation across the left ventricle projects continuous positive forces to left-sided leads and continuous negative ones to right-sided leads. Spread predominantly through working muscle fibers rather than the specialized conduction system results in notching and slurring as a consequence of discontinuous anisotropy, as described earlier.

The discordant ST-T wave pattern is a result of the transventricular recovery gradients referred to earlier. With LBBB, the right ventricle is activated and recovers earlier than the left, so recovery vectors or dipoles are directed toward the right and away from the left. Hence, positive ST-T waves will be registered over the right ventricle and negatives ones over the left ventricle. These transventricular gradients play only a minor role in normal conduction because the simultaneous activation of multiple regions cancels the forces that they produce; with bundle branch block, activation is sequential, so cancellation is reduced. Because the ST-T wave changes with LBBB are generated by abnormalities in conduction, they are called *secondary T wave abnormalities*; as will be discussed later, ST-T wave changes produced by direct abnormalities of the recovery process are referred to as *primary T wave abnormalities.*

CLINICAL SIGNIFICANCE. LBBB usually appears in patients with underlying heart disease. It is associated with significantly reduced long-term survival and with 10-year survival rates as low as 50 percent, probably reflecting the severity of the underlying cardiac disease. Among patients with coronary artery disease, the presence of LBBB correlates with more extensive disease, more severe left ventricular dysfunction, and reduced survival rates. The duration of the QRS complex in LBBB correlates inversely with left ventricular ejection fraction.[43] Patients with associated left or right axis deviation have more severe clinical manifestations.

In addition to the hemodynamic abnormalities produced by these underlying conditions, the abnormal ventricular activation pattern of LBBB itself induces hemodynamic perturbations, including abnormal systolic function with dysfunctional contraction patterns, reduced ejection fraction and lower stroke volumes, and abnormal diastolic function; reversed splitting of the second heart sound and functional mitral regurgitation are common. In addition, functional abnormalities in phasic coronary blood flow and reduced coronary flow reserve caused by delayed diastolic relaxation[44] often result in septal or anteroseptal defects on exercise perfusion scintigraphy in the absence of coronary artery disease. Pharmacological vasodilator stress testing with dipyridamole or adenosine, or stress echocardiography (exercise or dobutamine), appear more specific than standard exercise scintigraphy in diagnosing left anterior descending coronary stenosis in the presence of LBBB.[45,46]

A major impact of LBBB lies in obscuring or simulating other ECG patterns. The diagnosis of LVH is complicated by the increased QRS amplitude and axis shifts intrinsic to LBBB; in addition, the very high prevalence of anatomical LVH in combination with LBBB makes defining criteria with high specificity difficult. The diagnosis of infarction may be obscured; as will be described, the emergence of abnormal Q waves with infarction is dependent on a normal initial sequence of ventricular activation, which is absent with LBBB. In addition, ECG patterns of LBBB, including low R wave amplitude in the midprecordial leads and ST-T wave changes, can simulate anterior infarct patterns.

Right Bundle Branch Block

Right bundle branch block is a result of conduction delay in any portion of the right-sided intraventricular conduction system. The delay can occur in the main right bundle branch itself, in the bundle of His, or in the distal right ventricular conduction system. The latter is the common cause of RBBB after right ventriculotomy performed, for example, to correct the tetralogy of Fallot. The high prevalence of RBBB corresponds to the relative fragility of the right bundle branch, as suggested by the development of RBBB after minor trauma produced by right ventricular catheterization.

ECG ABNORMALITIES. Major features of RBBB are illustrated in Figure 9–27, and commonly used diagnostic criteria are listed in Table 9–7. As with LBBB, the QRS complex duration exceeds 120 msec. The right precordial leads show prominent and notched R waves with rsr′, rsR′, or rSR′ patterns, while leads I, aV_L, and the left precordial leads demonstrate wide S waves that are longer in duration than the preceding R wave. Septal q waves are preserved because the initial ventricular activation remains unchanged. The ST-T waves are, as in LBBB, discordant with the QRS complex, so T waves are inverted in the right precordial leads (and other leads with a terminal R′ wave) and upright in the left precordial leads and in leads I and AV_L.

The mean QRS axis is not altered by RBBB. Axis shifts can occur, however, as a result of the simultaneous occurrence of fascicular block along with RBBB. This concurrence of RBBB with either LAFB (producing left axis deviation) or LPFB (producing right axis deviation) is termed *bifascicular block*.

Features indicative of incomplete RBBB, produced by lesser delays in conduction in the right bundle branch system, are commonly seen. This finding is most frequently characterized by an rSr′ pattern in lead V_1 with a QRS duration between 100 and 120 msec.

MECHANISMS FOR ECG ABNORMALITIES. With delay or block in the proximal right bundle branch system, activation of the right side of the septum is initiated after slow transseptal spread of activation from the left septal surface. The right ventricular free wall is then excited slowly, with variable participation of the specialized conduction system. The result is delayed and slowed activation of the right ventricle with much or all of the right ventricle undergoing activation after depolarization of the left ventricle has been completed.

Because left ventricular activation remains relatively intact, the early portions of the QRS complex are normal. Delayed activation of the right ventricle causes prolongation of the QRS duration and a reduction in the cancellation of RV activation forces by the more powerful left ventricular activation forces. The late and unopposed emergence of right ventricular forces produces increased anterior and rightward voltage in the ECG. Discordant ST-T wave patterns are generated by the same mechanisms as for LBBB; with RBBB, recovery forces are directed toward the earlier-activated left ventricle and away from the right. Although these ECG changes of incomplete RBBB are commonly attributed to conduction defects, they can reflect RVH without intrinsic dysfunction of the conduction system.

CLINICAL SIGNIFICANCE. RBBB is a common finding in the general population, and many persons with RBBB have no clinical evidence of structural heart disease. In the group without overt heart disease, the ECG finding has no prognostic significance. However, the new onset of RBBB does predict a higher rate of coronary artery disease, congestive heart failure, and cardiovascular mortality. When cardiac disease is present, the coexistence of RBBB suggests advanced disease with, for example, more extensive multivessel disease and reduced long-term survival in patients with ischemic heart disease. An entity known as the *Brugada syndrome* has been described in which a RBBB-like pattern with persistent ST segment elevation in the right precordial leads is associated with susceptibility to ventricular tachyarrhythmias and sudden cardiac death[47] (see Chap. 32).

Right bundle branch block interferes with other ECG diagnoses, although to a lesser extent than does LBBB. The diagnosis of RVH is more difficult to make with RBBB because of the accentuated positive potentials in lead V_1. RVH is suggested, although with limited accuracy, by the presence of an R wave in lead V_1 that exceeds 1.5 mV and a rightward shift of the mean QRS axis. The usual criteria for LVH can be applied but have lower sensitivities than with normal conduction. The combination of left atrial abnormality or left axis deviation with RBBB also suggests underlying LVH.

Multifascicular Blocks

The term *multifascicular block* refers to conduction delay in more than one of the structural components of the specialized conduction system—that is, the left bundle branch, the left anterior and posterior fascicles of the left bundle branch, and the right bundle branch. Conduction delay in any two fascicles is called *bifascicular block,* and delay in all three fascicles is called *trifascicular block*. The term *bilateral bundle branch block* is sometimes used to refer to concomitant conduction abnormalities in the left and right bundle branch systems.

Bifascicular block can have several forms. These include (1) RBBB with LAFB, which is characterized by the ECG pattern of RBBB plus left axis deviation beyond −45 degrees (Fig. 9–28), (2) RBBB with LPFB, with an ECG pattern of RBBB and a mean QRS axis deviation to the right of +120 degrees (Fig. 9–29), or (3) LBBB that may be caused by delay in both the anterior and posterior fascicles. This form of LBBB represents one of the inadequacies of current ECG terminology and the simplification inherent in the trifascicular schema of the conduction system. The electrophysiological consequences of these abnormalities are discussed in Chapters 29, 30, and 31.

Trifascicular block involves conduction delay in the right bundle branch plus delay in either the main left bundle branch or both the left anterior and the left posterior fascicles. The resulting ECG pattern is dependent on (1) the relative degree of delay in the affected structures, and (2) the shortest conduction time from the atria to the ventricles through any one fascicle. Ventricular activation begins at the site of insertion of the branch with the fastest conduction time and spreads from there to the remainder of the ventricles. For example, if delay in the right bundle branch is less than the delay in the left main bundle branch, activation will begin in the right ventricle and the QRS pattern will resemble that of LBBB. If the delay were greater in the right bundle branch than in the left bundle branch, the ECG pattern would be that of RBBB. The fascicle with the greatest delay can vary with, for example, the heart rate and lead to changing or alternating conduction patterns, as illustrated in Figure 9–30.

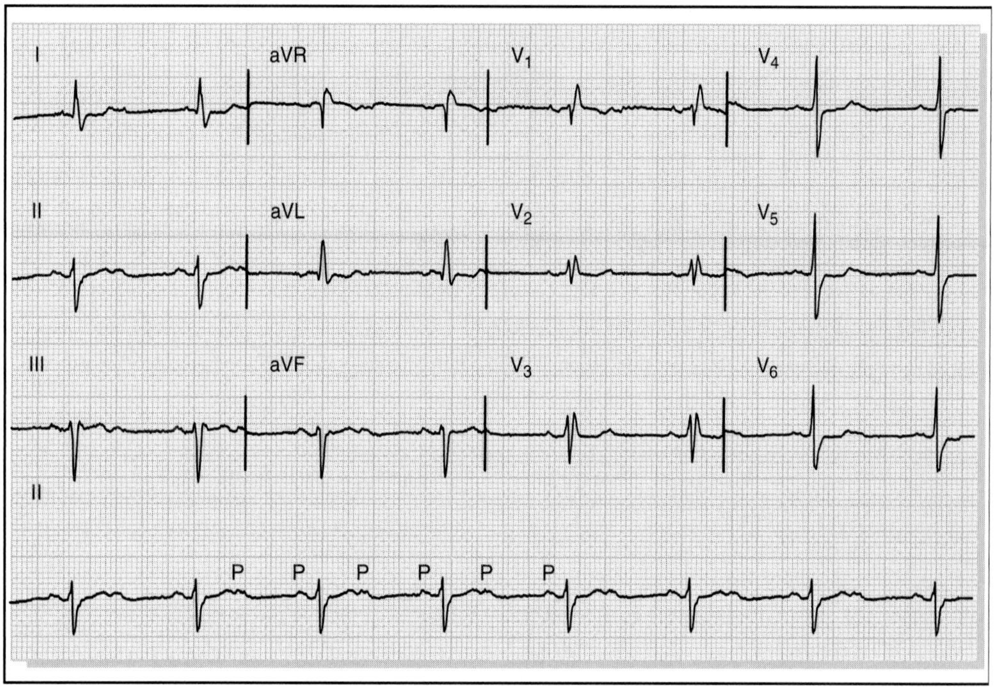

FIGURE 9–28 Sinus rhythm at 95 beats/min with 2 : 1 atrioventricular block. Conducted ventricular beats show a pattern consistent with bifascicular block with delay or block in the right bundle and left anterior fascicle. The patient underwent pacemaker implantation for presumed infra-Hisian block.

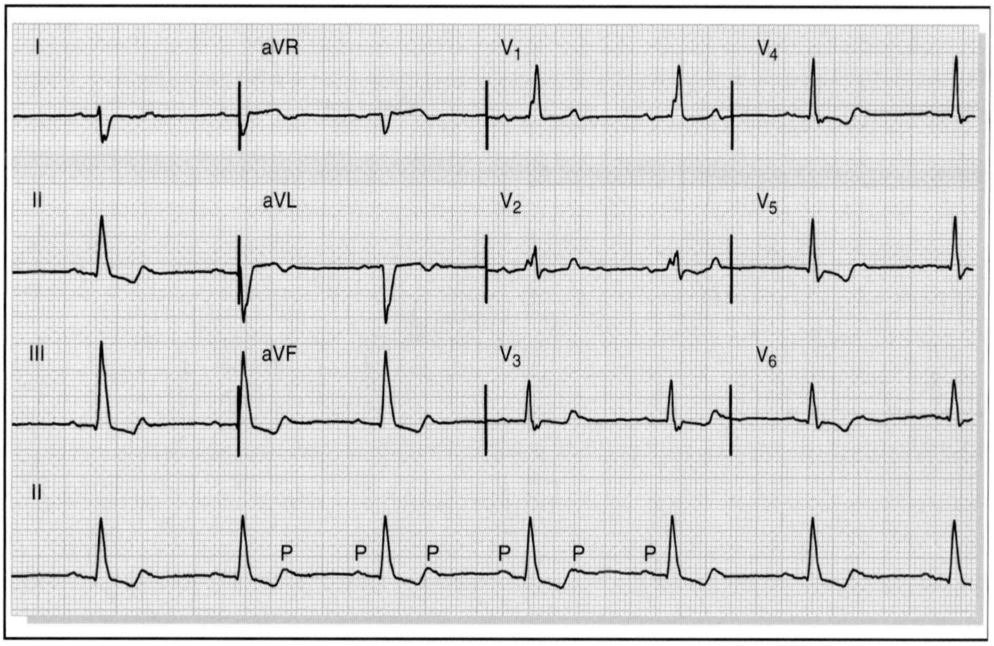

FIGURE 9–29 Sinus rhythm with a 2 : 1 atrioventricular block. QRS morphology in the conducted leads is consistent with bifascicular block with delay or block in the right bundle and left posterior fascicle. Subsequently, complete heart block was also noted. The patient underwent pacemaker implantation for presumed infra-Hisian block.

What distinguishes ECG patterns of trifascicular block from those of bifascicular block is an increased overall AV conduction interval that results specifically from prolongation of the His-ventricular time. In bifascicular block, conduction time through the unaffected fascicle (and hence, overall AV conduction time) is normal. In trifascicular block, however, the delay in conduction through even the least affected fascicle is abnormal and results in relative prolongation of the overall AV conduction interval. (Note that only delay, not block, of conduction is required. If block were present in all fascicles, conduction would fail and complete heart block would result. This situation is perhaps best illustrated by cases of alternating bundle branch block [see Fig. 9-30]; if the block were total in one bundle branch, development of block in the other would produce complete AV block rather than a change in bundle branch block patterns.) Thus, a diagnosis of trifascicular block requires an ECG pattern of bifascicular block *plus* evidence of prolonged AV conduction.

Detecting AV conduction delay is best accomplished by intracardiac recordings as a prolongation of the His-ventricular interval. On the surface ECG, AV conduction delay may be manifested as a prolonged PR interval. However, the PR interval includes conduction time in the AV node as well as in the intraventricular conduction system. Prolonged intraventricular conduction may be insufficient to extend the PR interval beyond normal limits, whereas a prolonged PR interval can reflect delay in the AV node rather than in all three intraventricular fascicles. Thus, the finding of a prolonged PR interval in the presence of an ECG pattern of bifascicular block is not diagnostic of trifascicular block, whereas the presence of a normal PR interval does not exclude this finding (see Chap. 29).

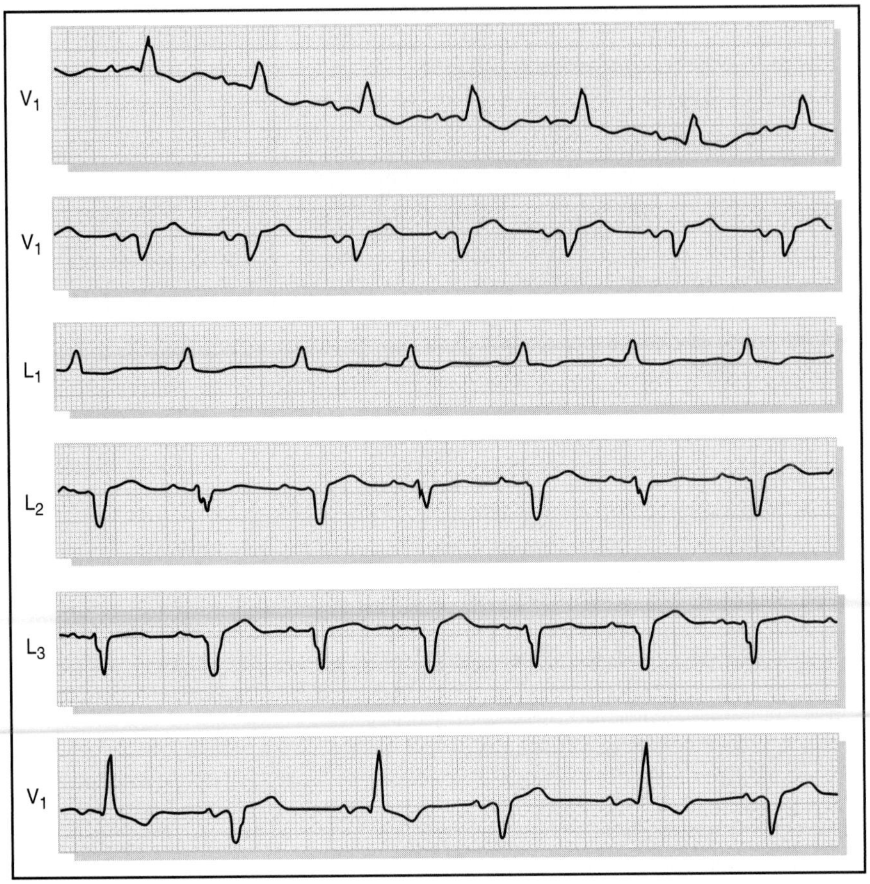

FIGURE 9–30 Multifascicular block manifested by alternating bundle branch blocks and PR intervals. **Top panel,** V_1 right bundle branch block (RBBB) with a PR interval of 280 msec. **Middle panel,** V_1 left bundle branch block (LBBB) with a PR interval of 180 msec. **Lower panel,** RBBB alternating with LBBB, along with alternation of the PR interval. The electrocardiographic records shown in leads I, II, and III (L1 to L3) exhibit left anterior fascicular block. An alternating bundle branch block of this type is consistent with trifascicular conduction delay. (From Fisch C: Electrocardiography of Arrhythmias. Philadelphia, Lea & Febiger, 1990, p 433.)

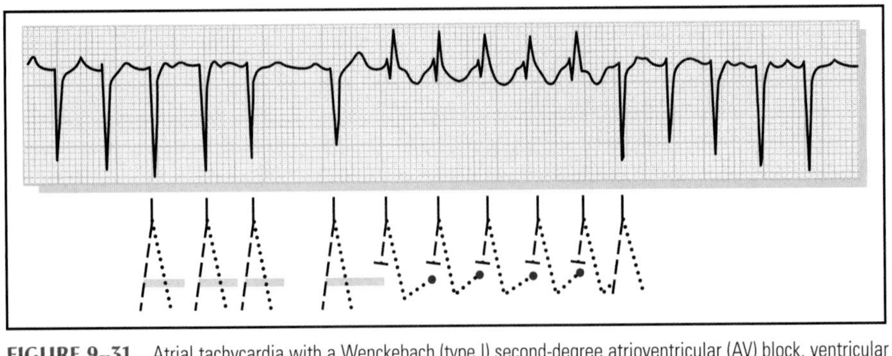

FIGURE 9–31 Atrial tachycardia with a Wenckebach (type I) second-degree atrioventricular (AV) block, ventricular aberration resulting from the Ashman phenomenon, and probably concealed transseptal conduction. The long pause of the atrial tachycardia is followed by five QRS complexes with right bundle branch block (RBBB) morphology. The RBBB of the first QRS reflects the Ashman phenomenon. The aberration is perpetuated by concealed transseptal activation from the left bundle (LB) into the right bundle (RB) with block of anterograde conduction of the subsequent sinus impulse in the RB. Foreshortening of the R-R cycle, a manifestation of the Wenckebach structure, disturbs the relationship between transseptal and anterograde sinus conduction, and RB conduction is normalized. In the ladder diagram below the tracing, the solid lines represent the His bundle, the dashes represent the RB, the dots represent the LB, and the solid horizontal bars denote the refractory period. P waves and the AV node are not identified in the diagram. (Courtesy of C. Fisch, M.D.)

The major clinical implication of a multifascicular block is its relation to advanced conduction system disease. It may be a marker for advanced myocardial disease and may identify patients at risk for heart block (see Figs. 9–28 and 9–29), as discussed in Chapters 30 and 31.

Rate-Dependent Conduction Block (Aberration)

Intraventricular conduction delays can result from the effects of changes in the heart rate, as well as from fixed pathological lesions in the conduction system. Rate-dependent block or aberration can occur at either high or low heart rates. In acceleration (tachycardia)-dependent block, conduction delay occurs when the heart rate exceeds a critical value. At the cellular level, this aberration is the result of encroachment of the impulse on the relative refractory period (usually in phase 3 of the action potential) of the preceding impulse, which results in slower conduction. This form of block is relatively common and can have the ECG pattern of RBBB or LBBB (Figs. 9–31 and 9–32).

In deceleration (bradycardia)-dependent block, conduction delay occurs when the heart rate falls below a critical level. Although the mechanism is not clearly established, it may reflect abnormal phase 4 depolarization of cells so that activation occurs at lower resting potentials. Deceleration-dependent block is less common than acceleration-dependent block and is usually seen only in patients with significant conduction system disease (Fig. 9–33).

Other mechanisms of ventricular aberration include concealed conduction (anterograde or retrograde) in the bundle branches (see Figs. 9-31 and 9-32), premature excitation, depressed myocardial conduction as a result of drug effects or hyperkalemia (see Fig. 9-52, top), and the effect of changing cycle length on refractoriness (the Ashman phenomenon) (see Chaps. 29 and 32). The duration of the refractory period is a function of the immediately preceding cycle length: the longer the preceding cycle, the longer the subsequent refractory period. Therefore, abrupt prolongation of the immediately preceding cycle can result in aberration as part of a long cycle-short cycle sequence. These so-called Ashman beats usually have a RBBB morphology (see Fig. 9-31).

WOLFF-PARKINSON-WHITE PRE-EXCITATION. This abnormality is discussed in Chapter 32.

Myocardial Ischemia and Infarction

The ECG remains a key test in the diagnosis of acute and chronic coronary syndromes.[48] The findings vary considerably, depending importantly on four major factors: (1) the duration of the ischemic process (acute vs. evolving/chronic), (2) its extent (transmural vs. nontransmural), (3) its topography (anterior vs. inferior-posterior and right ventricular), and (4) the presence of other underlying abnormalities (e.g., LBBB, Wolff-Parkinson-White

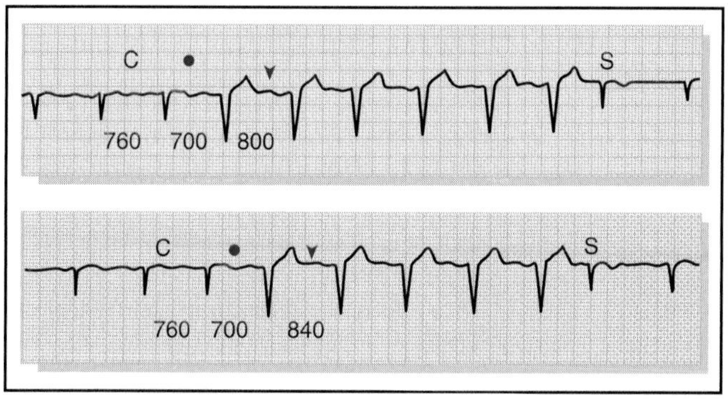

FIGURE 9–32 Acceleration-dependent QRS aberration with the paradox of persistence at a longer cycle and normalization at a shorter cycle than what initiated the aberration. The duration of the basic cycle (C) is 760 msec. Left bundle branch block (LBBB) appears at a cycle length of 700 msec (dot) and is perpetuated at cycle lengths of 800 (arrowhead) and 840 (arrowhead) msec; conduction normalizes after a cycle length of 600 msec. Perpetuation of LBBB at a cycle length of 800 and 840 msec is probably due to transseptal concealment, similar to that described in Figure 9–31. Unexpected normalization of the QRS (S) following the atrial premature contraction is probably due to equalization of conduction in the two bundles; however, supernormal conduction in the left bundle cannot be excluded. (From Fisch C, Zipes DP, McHenry PL: Rate dependent aberrancy. Circulation 48:714, 1973.)

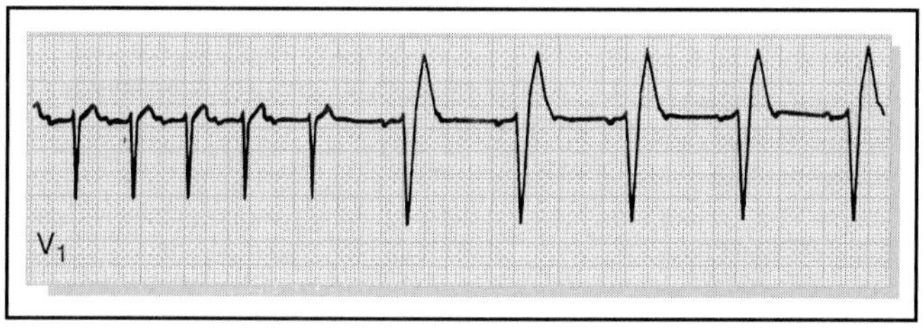

FIGURE 9–33 Deceleration-dependent aberration. The basic rhythm is sinus with a Wenckebach (type I) atrioventricular (AV) block. With 1 : 1 AV conduction, the QRS complexes are normal in duration; with a 2 : 1 AV block or after the longer pause of a Wenckebach sequence, left bundle branch block (LBBB) appears. Slow diastolic depolarization (phase 4) of the transmembrane action potential during the prolonged cycle is implicated as the cause of the LBBB. (Courtesy of C. Fisch, M.D.)

syndrome, or pacemaker patterns) that can mask or alter the classic patterns.

Repolarization (ST-T Wave) Abnormalities

The earliest and most consistent ECG finding during acute ischemia is deviation of the ST segment as a result of a current-of-injury mechanism. Under normal conditions, the ST segment is usually nearly isoelectric because virtually all healthy myocardial cells attain approximately the same potential during early repolarization, that is, during the plateau phase of the ventricular action potential.

Ischemia, however, has complex time-dependent effects on the electrical properties of myocardial cells. Severe, acute ischemia can reduce the resting membrane potential, shorten the duration of the action potential in the ischemic area, and decrease the rate of rise and amplitude of phase 0 (Fig. 9–34). These changes cause a voltage gradient between normal and ischemic zones that leads to current flow between these regions. These currents of injury are represented on the surface ECG by deviation of the ST segment.

Both *diastolic* and *systolic injury currents* have been proposed to explain ischemic ST elevations (Fig. 9-35). According to the diastolic-current-of-injury hypothesis, ischemic ST elevation is attributable to negative (downward) displacement of the electrical "diastolic" baseline (the TQ segment of the ECG). At least partly because of transmembrane

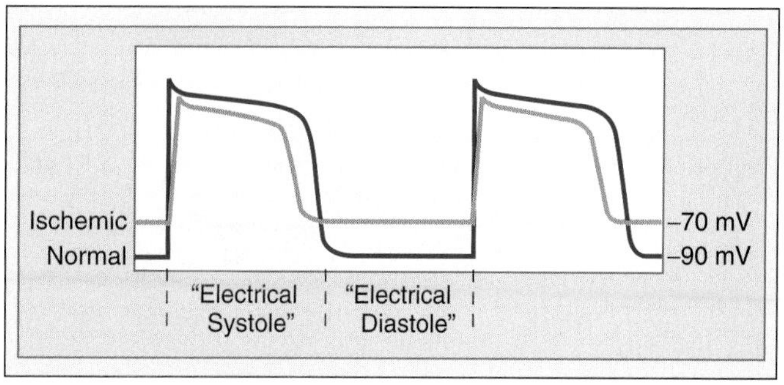

FIGURE 9–34 Acute ischemia may alter ventricular action potentials by inducing lower resting membrane potential, decreased amplitude and velocity of phase 0, and an abbreviated action potential duration (pathological early repolarization). These electrophysiological effects create a voltage gradient between ischemic and normal cells during different phases of the cardiac electrical cycle. The resulting currents of injury are reflected on the surface electrocardiogram by deviation of the ST segment (see Figure 9–35).

leakage of intracellular potassium ions, ischemic cells may remain relatively depolarized during phase 4 of the ventricular action potential (i.e., lower membrane resting potential) (see Fig. 9-34).[49] Depolarized muscle carries a negative extracellular charge relative to repolarized muscle. Therefore, during electrical diastole, current (the diastolic current of injury) will flow between the partly or completely depolarized ischemic myocardium and the neighboring normally repolarized uninjured myocardium. The injury current vector will be directed away from the more negative ischemic zone toward the more positive normal myocardium. As a result, leads overlying the ischemic zone will record a negative deflection during electrical diastole and produce depression of the TQ segment.

TQ segment depression, in turn, appears as ST segment elevation because the ECG recorders in clinical practice use AC-coupled amplifiers that automatically "compensate" for any negative shift in the TQ segment. As a result of this electronic compensation, the ST segment will be proportionately elevated. Therefore, according to the diastolic-current-of-injury theory, ST segment elevation represents an apparent shift. The true shift, observable only with DC-coupled ECG amplifiers, is the negative displacement of the TQ baseline.

Current evidence suggests that ischemic ST elevations (and hyperacute T waves) are also related to systolic injury currents. Three factors may make acutely ischemic myocardial cells relatively positive in comparison to normal cells with respect to their extracellular charge during electrical systole (QT interval). These are (1) pathological early repolarization (shortened action potential duration), (2) decreased action potential upstroke velocity, and (3) decreased action potential amplitude (see Fig. 9-34). The presence of one or more of these effects will establish a voltage gradient between normal and ischemic zones during the QT interval such that the current-of-injury vector will be directed toward the ischemic region. This systolic-current-of-injury mechanism will result in primary ST elevation, sometimes with tall positive (hyperacute) T waves.

When acute ischemia is transmural (whether caused by diastolic or systolic injury currents or both), the overall ST vector is usually shifted in the direction of the outer (epicardial) layers, and ST elevation and sometimes tall positive (hyperacute) T waves are produced over the ischemic zone (Fig. 9–36). Reciprocal ST depressions can appear in leads reflecting the contralateral surface of the heart. Occasionally, the reciprocal changes can be more apparent than the primary ST elevations. When ischemia is confined primarily to the subendocardium, the overall ST vector typically shifts toward the inner ventricular layer and the ventricular cavity such that the overlying (e.g., anterior precordial) leads show ST segment depression with ST elevation in lead aV_r (see Fig. 9–36). This subendocardial ischemic pattern is the typical finding during spontaneous episodes of angina pectoris or during symptomatic or asymptomatic ("silent") ischemia induced by exercise or pharmacological stress tests (see Chaps. 10 and 46).

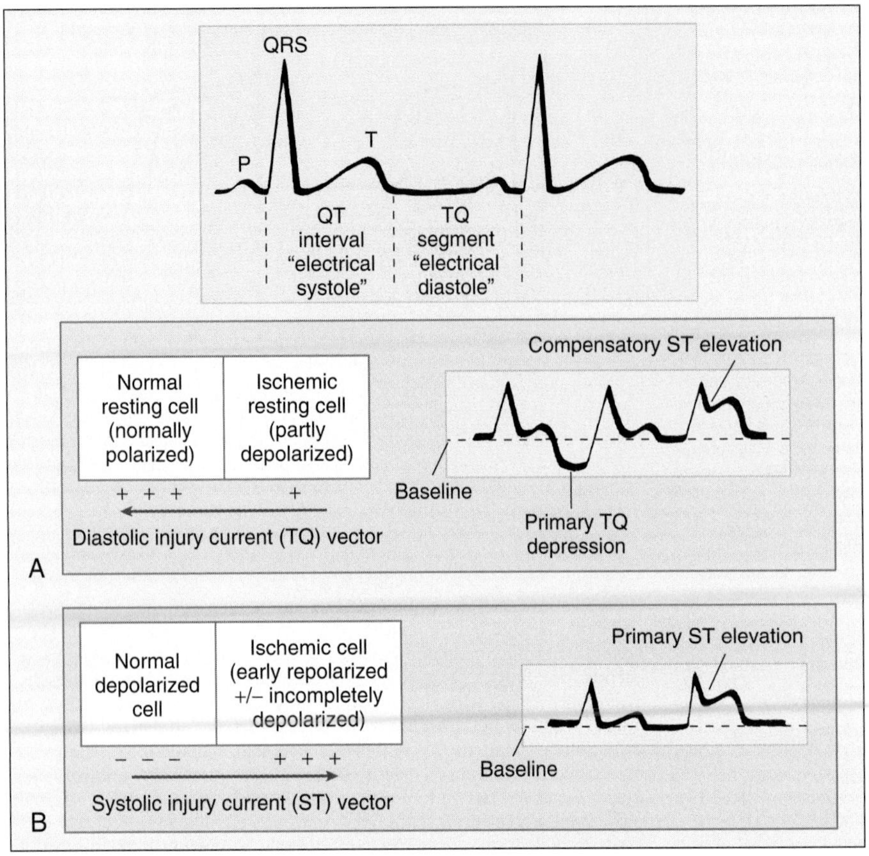

FIGURE 9–35 Pathophysiology of ischemic ST elevation. Two basic mechanisms have been advanced to explain the elevation seen with acute myocardial injury. **A,** Diastolic current of injury. In this case (first QRS-T complex), the ST vector will be directed away from the relatively negative, partly depolarized, ischemic region during electrical diastole (TQ interval), and the result will be primary TQ depression. Conventional alternating-current electrocardiograms compensate for the baseline shift, and an apparent ST elevation (second QRS-T complex) results. **B,** Systolic current of injury. In this case, the ischemic zone will be relatively positive during electrical systole because the cells are repolarized early and the amplitude and upstroke velocity of their action potentials may be decreased. This injury current vector will be oriented toward the electropositive zone, and the result will be primary ST elevation. (Modified from Goldberger AL: Myocardial Infarction: Electrocardiographic Differential Diagnosis. 4th ed. St Louis, Mosby-Year Book, 1991.)

can occur with slight or even absent ST-T changes. Furthermore, a relative increase in T wave amplitude (hyperacute T waves) can accompany or precede the ST elevations as part of the injury current pattern attributable to ischemia with or without infarction (Fig. 9–37).

QRS Changes

With actual infarction, depolarization (QRS) changes often accompany repolarization (ST-T) abnormalities (Fig. 9–38). Necrosis of sufficient myocardial tissue can lead to decreased R wave amplitude or Q waves in the anterior, lateral, or inferior leads as a result of loss of electromotive forces in the infarcted area. Local conduction delays caused by acute ischemia can also contribute to Q wave pathogenesis in selected cases. Abnormal Q waves were once considered markers of transmural myocardial infarction, while subendocardial (nontransmural) infarcts were thought to not produce Q waves. However, careful experimental and clinical ECG-pathological correlative studies have indicated that transmural infarcts can occur without Q waves and that subendocardial infarcts can sometimes be associated with Q waves.[52] Accordingly, infarcts are better classified electrocardiographically as "Q wave" or "non-Q-wave" rather than transmural or nontransmural, based on the ECG. The findings may be somewhat different with posterior or lateral infarction (Fig. 9–39). Loss of depolarization forces in these regions can reciprocally *increase* R wave amplitude in lead V_1 and sometimes V_2, rarely without causing diagnostic Q waves in any of the conventional leads.

The differential diagnosis of prominent right precordial R waves is given in Table 9–8.

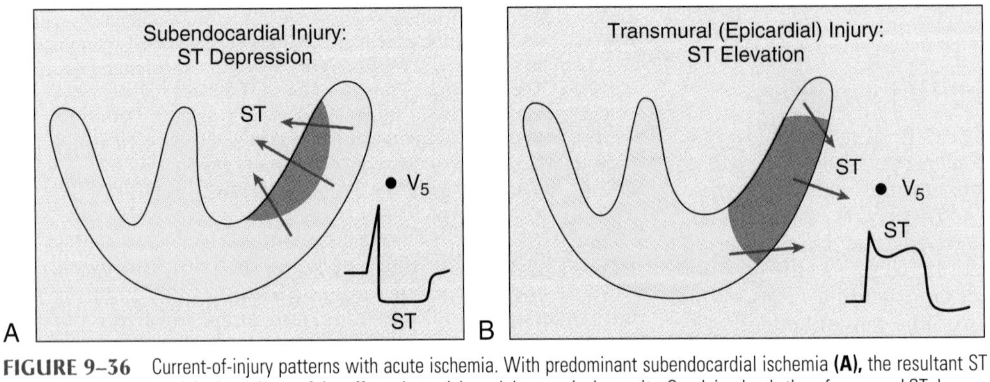

FIGURE 9–36 Current-of-injury patterns with acute ischemia. With predominant subendocardial ischemia **(A)**, the resultant ST vector is directed toward the inner layer of the affected ventricle and the ventricular cavity. Overlying leads therefore record ST depression. With ischemia involving the outer ventricular layer **(B)** (transmural or epicardial injury), the ST vector is directed outward. Overlying leads record ST elevation. Reciprocal ST depression can appear in contralateral leads.

Evolution of Electrocardiographic Changes

Ischemic ST elevation and hyperacute T wave changes occur as the earliest sign of acute infarction and are typically followed within a period ranging from hours to days by evolving T wave inversion and sometimes Q waves in the same lead distribution (see Fig. 9–38). T wave inversion from evolving or chronic ischemia correlates with increased ventricular action potential duration, and these ischemic changes are often associated with QT prolongation. The T wave inversion can resolve after days or weeks or persist indefinitely. The extent of the infarct may be an important determinant of T wave evolution.[53] In one series, T waves that were persistently negative for more than 1 year in leads with Q waves were associated with a

Multiple factors can affect the amplitude of acute ischemic ST deviations. Profound ST elevation or depression in multiple leads usually indicates very severe ischemia. Conversely, prompt resolution of ST elevation following thrombolytic therapy[50] or primary angioplasty[51] is a specific marker of successful reperfusion. These relationships are not universal, however, since severe ischemia or even infarction

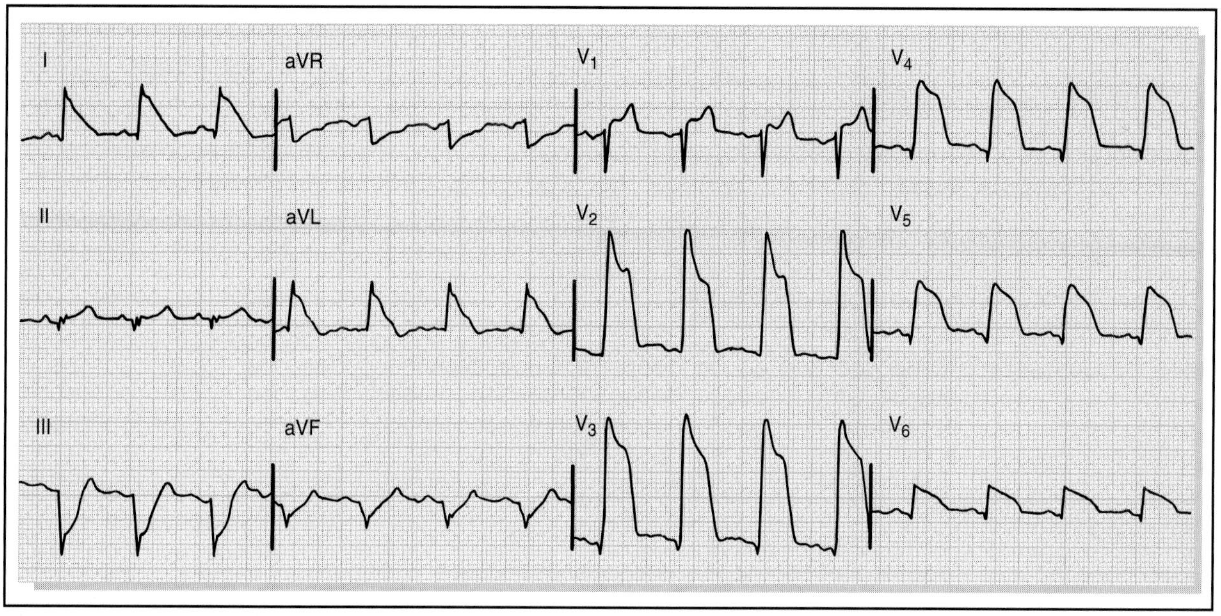

FIGURE 9–37 Hyperacute phase of extensive anterior-lateral myocardial infarction. Marked ST elevation melding with prominent T waves is present across the precordium, as well as in leads I and aV_l. ST depression, consistent with a reciprocal change, is seen in leads III and aV_f. Q waves are present in leads V_3 through V_6. Marked ST elevations with tall T waves caused by severe ischemia are sometimes referred to as a *monophasic current-of-injury* pattern. A paradoxical increase in R wave amplitude (V_2 and V_3) may accompany this pattern. This tracing also shows left axis deviation with small or absent inferior R waves, which raises the possibility of a prior inferior infarct.

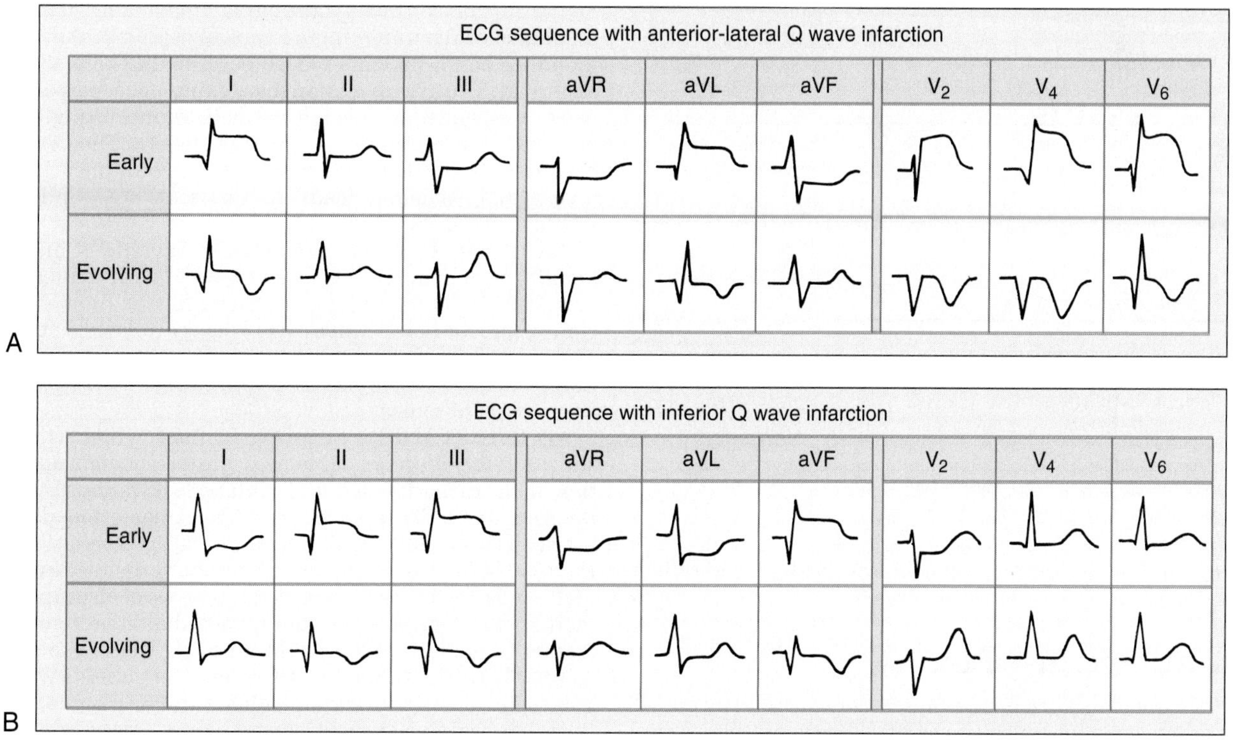

FIGURE 9–38 Sequence of depolarization and repolarization changes with **(A)** acute anterior-lateral and **(B)** acute inferior wall Q wave infarctions. With anterior-lateral infarcts, ST elevation in leads I, aV_l, and the precordial leads can be accompanied by reciprocal ST depression in leads II, III, and aV_f. Conversely, acute inferior (or posterior) infarcts can be associated with reciprocal ST depression in leads V_1 to V_3. (Modified from Goldberger AL: Clinical Electrocardiography: A Simplified Approach. 6th ed. St Louis, CV Mosby, 1999.)

transmural infarction with fibrosis of the entire wall; in contrast, T waves that were positive in leads with Q waves correlated with nontransmural infarction with viable myocardium within the wall.

In the days to weeks or longer following infarction, the QRS changes can persist or begin to resolve. Complete normalization of the ECG following Q wave infarction is uncommon but can occur, particularly with smaller infarcts and when the left ventricular ejection fraction and regional wall motion improve. This is usually associated with spontaneous recanalization or good collateral circulation[54] and is a good prognostic sign. In contrast, persistent Q waves and ST elevation several weeks or more after an infarct correlate strongly with a severe underlying wall motion disorder (akinetic or dyskinetic zone), although not necessarily a frank ventricular aneurysm. The presence of an rSR′ or similar

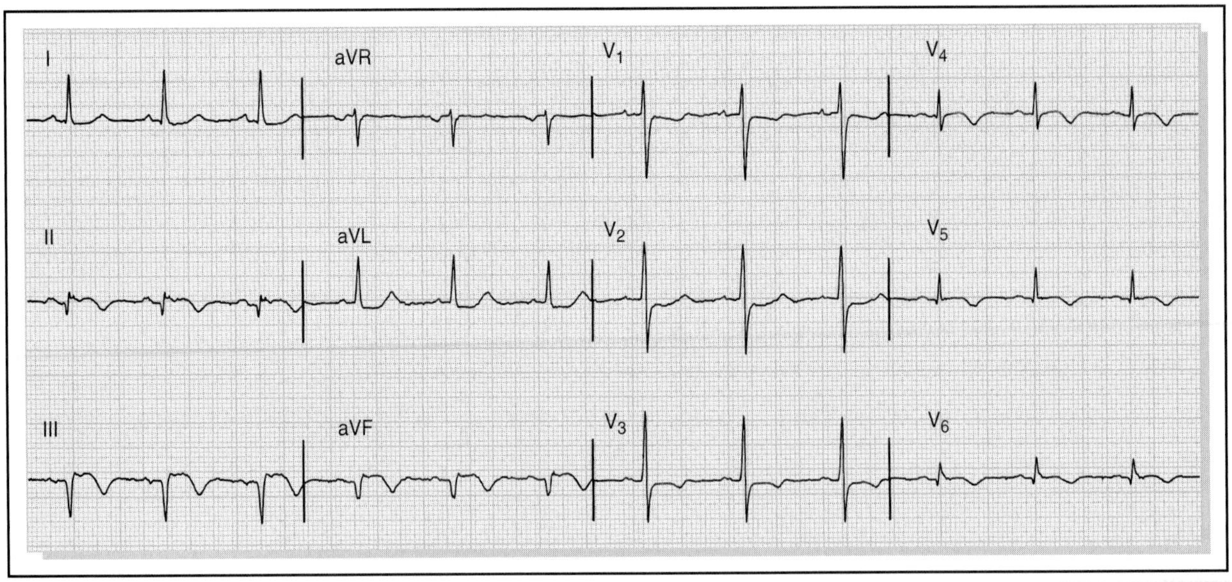

FIGURE 9–39 Evolving inferoposterolateral infarction. Note the prominent Q waves in II, III, and aV_f, along with ST elevation and T wave inversion in these leads, as well as V_3 through V_6. ST depression in I, aV_l, V_1, and V_2 is consistent with a reciprocal change. Relatively tall R waves are also present in V_1 and V_2.

TABLE 9–8 Differential Diagnosis of Tall R Waves in V_1/V_2

Physiological/positional factors
Misplacement of chest leads
Normal variants
Displacement of heart toward right side of chest (dextroversion): congenital or acquired
Myocardial injury
Posterior (and/or lateral) myocardial infarction (see Fig. 9–39)
Duchenne muscular dystrophy (see Chap. 71)
Ventricular enlargement
Right ventricular hypertrophy (usually with right axis deviation)
Hypertrophic cardiomyopathy
Altered ventricular depolarization
Right ventricular conduction abnormalities
Wolff-Parkinson-White patterns (caused by posterior or lateral wall preexcitation)

Modified from Goldberger AL: Clinical Electrocardiography: A Simplified Approach. 6th ed. St Louis, CV Mosby, 1999.

complex in the mid-left chest leads or lead I is another reported marker of ventricular aneurysm.

Other Ischemic ST-T Patterns

Reversible transmural ischemia caused, for example, by coronary vasospasm may cause transient ST segment elevation (Fig. 9–40). This pattern is the ECG marker of Prinzmetal variant angina (see Chap. 49). Depending on the severity and duration of such noninfarction ischemia, the ST elevation can either resolve completely within minutes or be followed by T wave inversion that can persist for hours or even days. Some patients with ischemic chest pain have deep coronary T wave inversion in multiple precordial leads (e.g., V_1 through V_4), with or without cardiac enzyme elevations. This finding is typically caused by severe ischemia associated with a high-grade stenosis in the proximal left anterior descending coronary artery system (LAD-T wave pattern). The T wave inversion can actually be preceded by a transient ST elevation that resolves by the time the patient arrives at the hospital. These T wave inversions, in the setting of unstable angina, can correlate with segmental hypokinesis of the anterior wall and suggest a "myocardial stunning" syndrome. The natural history of this syndrome is unfavorable, with a high incidence of recurrent angina and myocardial infarction. On the other hand, patients whose baseline ECG already shows abnormal T wave inversion can experience paradoxical T wave normalization (pseudonormalization) during episodes of acute transmural ischemia (Fig. 9–41). The four major classes of acute ECG-coronary artery syndromes in which myocardial ischemia leads to different ECG findings are summarized in Figure 9–42.

ISCHEMIC U WAVE CHANGES. Alterations in U wave amplitude or polarity have been reported with acute ischemia or infarction. For example, exercise-induced transient inversion of precordial U waves has been correlated with severe stenosis of the left anterior descending coronary artery.[55] Rarely, U wave inversion can be the earliest ECG sign of acute coronary syndromes.

QT INTERVAL DISPERSION. Increasing interest has been shown in the effects of acute myocardial ischemia and infarction on the disparity among QT intervals in various ECG leads, referred to as *QT dispersion*.[56] The greater the difference between maximum and minimum QT intervals, that is, increased QT dispersion, the greater the variability in myocardial repolarization. An increased index has been proposed as a marker of arrhythmia risk after myocardial infarction and as a marker of acute ischemia with atrial pacing.[56] The practical utility of QT dispersion measurements, in patients with coronary syndromes and certain other cardiac pathologies, is a focus of ongoing investigation and debate[57] (see Chap. 27).

Localization of Ischemia or Infarction

The ECG leads are more helpful in localizing regions of transmural than subendocardial ischemia. As examples, ST elevation and/or hyperacute T waves are seen in (1) one or more of the precordial leads (V_1 through V_6) and in leads I and aV_l with acute transmural anterior or anterolateral wall ischemia; (2) leads V_1 to V_3 with anteroseptal or apical[58] ischemia; (3) leads V_4 to V_6 with apical or lateral ischemia; (4) leads II, III, and aV_f with inferior wall ischemia; and (5) right-sided precordial leads with right ventricular ischemia. Posterior wall infarction, which induces ST elevation in leads placed over

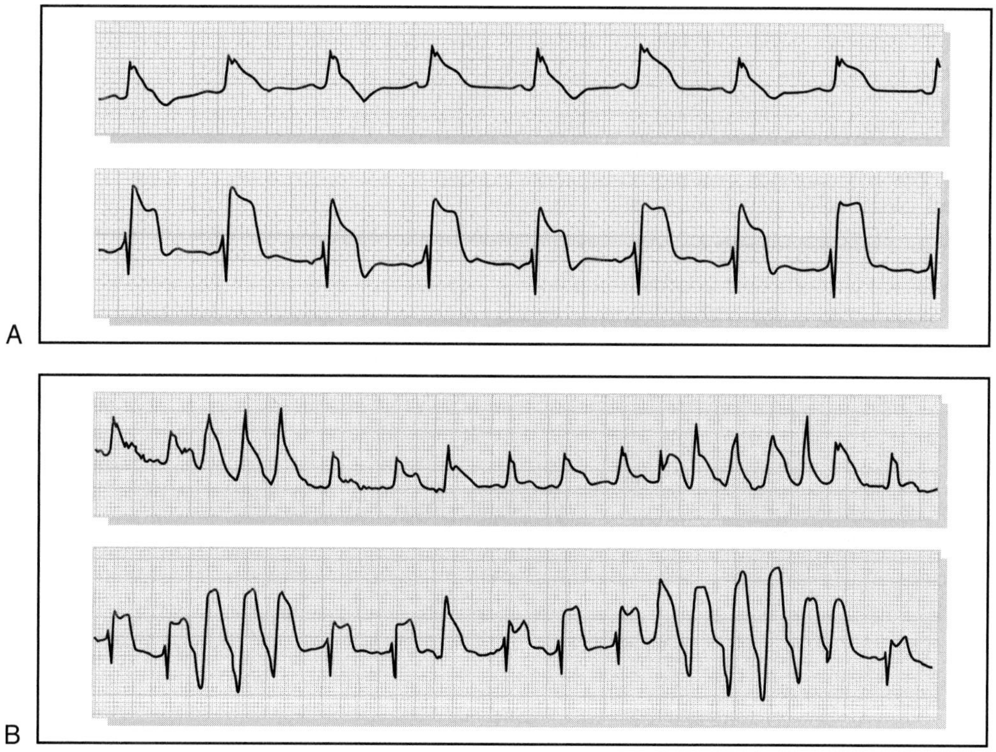

FIGURE 9–40 **A,** Prinzmetal angina with ST segment and T wave alternans. **B,** ST segment and T wave alternans associated with nonsustained ventricular tachycardia. (Courtesy of C. Fisch, M.D.)

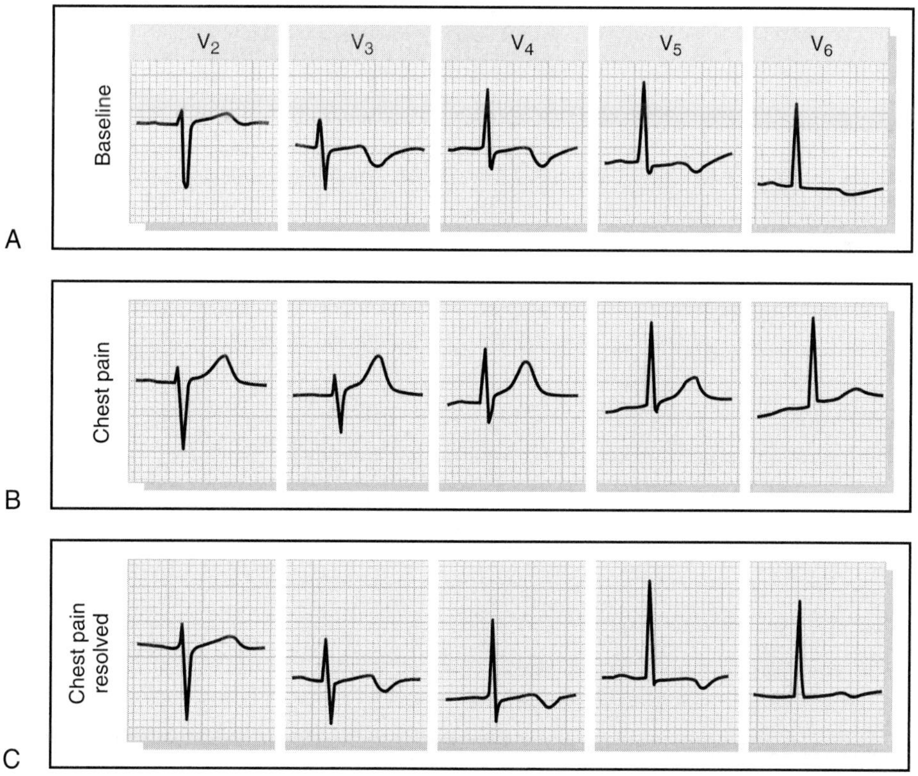

FIGURE 9–41 Pseudo (paradoxical) T wave normalization. **A,** The baseline electrocardiogram of a patient with coronary artery disease shows ischemic T wave inversion. **B,** T wave "normalization" during an episode of ischemic chest pain. **C,** Following resolution of the chest pain, the T waves have reverted to their baseline appearance. (From Goldberger AL: Myocardial Infarction: Electrocardiographic Differential Diagnosis. 4th ed. St Louis, Mosby-Year Book, 1991.)

the back of the heart, such as leads V_7 to V_9,[5,59] can be induced by lesions in the right coronary artery or left circumflex artery. These lesions can produce both inferior and posterior-lateral injury, which may be indirectly recognized by reciprocal ST depression in leads V_1 to V_3.[60] Similar ST changes can also be the primary ECG manifestation of anterior subendocardial ischemia. Posterior inferior wall infarction with reciprocal changes can be differentiated from primary anterior wall ischemia by the presence of ST segment elevations in posterior leads.

The ECG can also provide more specific information about the location of the occlusion within the coronary system *(the culprit lesion)*.[48] In patients with an inferior wall myocardial infarction, the presence of ST segment elevation in lead III exceeding that in lead II, particularly when combined with ST elevation in V_1, is a useful predictor of occlusion in the proximal to midportion of the right coronary artery (Fig. 9–43). In contrast, the presence of ST segment elevation in lead II equal to or exceeding that in lead III, especially in concert with ST depression in leads V_1 to V_3 or ST elevation in leads I and aV_l, strongly suggests occlusion of the left circumflex coronary artery or a distal occlusion of a dominant right coronary artery. Right-sided ST elevation is indicative of acute right ventricular injury[61,62] and usually indicates occlusion of the proximal right coronary artery. Of note is the finding that acute right ventricular infarction can project an injury current pattern in leads V_1 through V_3 or even V_4, thereby simulating anterior infarction. In other cases, simultaneous ST elevation in V_1 (V_2R) and ST depression in V_2 (V_1R) can occur (Fig. 9–43). These and many other criteria proposed for localization of the site of coronary occlusion based on the initial ECG[48,63-67] require additional validation in test populations.

In some cases, ischemia can affect more than one region of the myocardium (e.g., inferolateral) (see Fig. 9–38). Not uncommonly, the ECG will show the characteristic findings of involvement in each region. Sometimes, however, partial normalization can result from cancellation of opposing vectorial forces. Inferior lead ST segment elevation accompanying acute anterior wall infarction suggests either occlusion of a left anterior descending artery that extends onto the inferior wall of the left ventricle

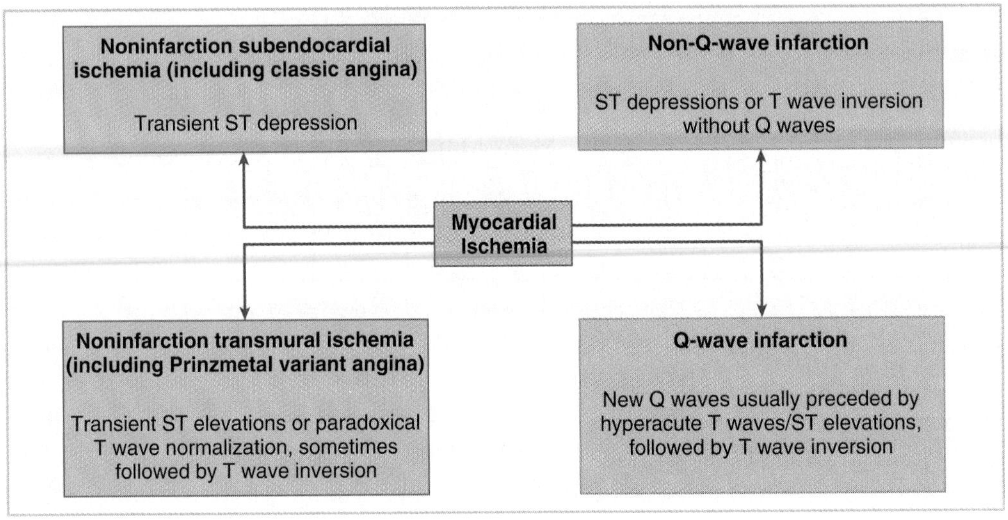

FIGURE 9–42 Variability of electrocardiogram (ECG) patterns with acute myocardial ischemia. The ECG may also be normal or nonspecifically abnormal. Furthermore, these categorizations are not mutually exclusive. For example, a non-Q-wave infarct can evolve into a Q wave infarct, ST elevation can be followed by a non-Q-wave infarct, or ST depression and T wave inversion can be followed by a Q wave infarct. (Modified from Goldberger AL: Myocardial Infarction: Electrocardiographic Differential Diagnosis. 4th ed. St Louis, Mosby-Year Book, 1991.)

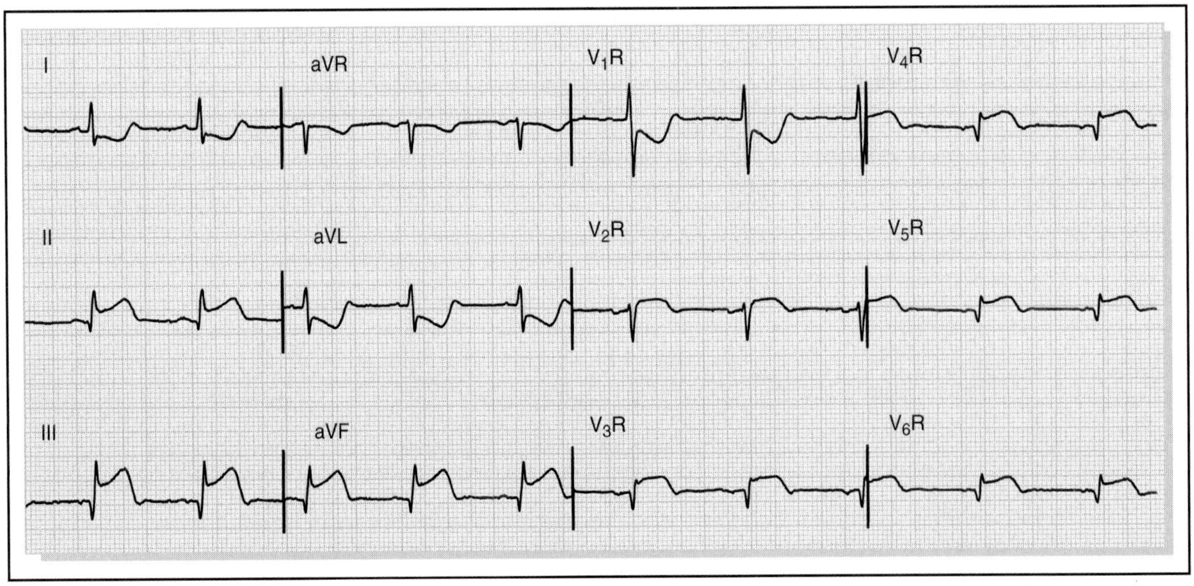

FIGURE 9–43 Acute right ventricular infarction with acute inferior wall infarction. Note the ST elevation in the right precordial leads, as well as in leads II, III, and aV_f, with reciprocal change in I and aV_l. ST elevation in lead III greater than in lead II and right precordial ST elevation are consistent with proximal to middle occlusion of the right coronary artery. The combination of ST elevation in conventional lead V_1 (V_2R here) and ST depression in lead V_2 (lead V_1R here) has also been reported with acute right ventricular ischemia/infarction.

(the "wrap around" vessel) or multivessel disease with jeopardized collaterals.[68]

Electrocardiographic Diagnosis of Bundle Branch Blocks and Myocardial Infarction

The diagnosis of myocardial infarction is often more difficult in cases in which the baseline ECG shows a bundle branch block pattern, or a bundle branch block develops as a complication of the infarct. The diagnosis of Q wave infarction is not usually impeded by the presence of RBBB, which affects primarily the terminal phase of ventricular depolarization. The net effect is that the criteria for the diagnosis of a Q wave infarct in a patient with RBBB are the same as in patients with normal conduction (Fig. 9–44). The diagnosis of infarction in the presence of LBBB is considerably more complicated and confusing, because LBBB alters both the early and the late phases of ventricular depolarization and produces secondary ST-T changes. These changes may both mask and mimic the findings of myocardial infarction. As a result, considerable attention has been directed to the problem of diagnosing acute and chronic myocardial infarction in patients with LBBB[69,70] (Fig. 9–45).

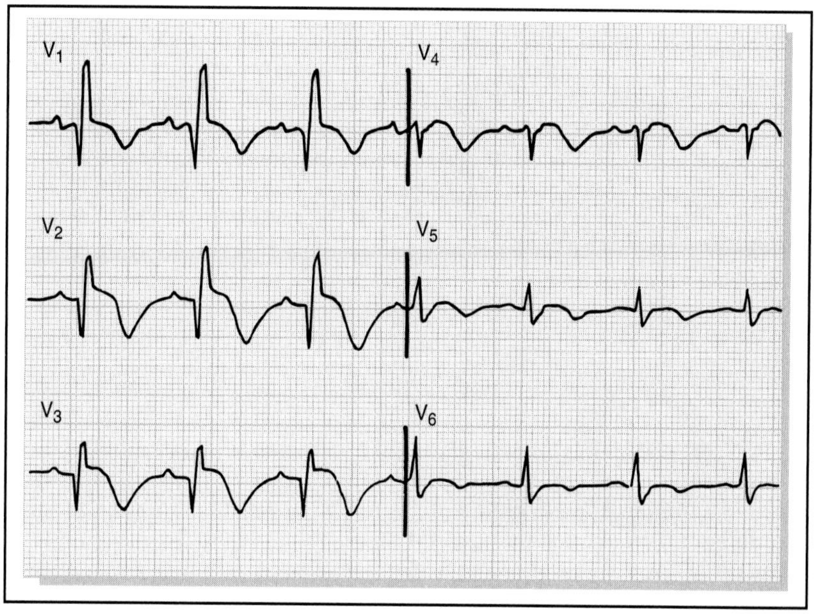

FIGURE 9–44 Right bundle branch block with acute anterior infarction. Loss of anterior depolarization forces results in QR-type complexes in the right precordial to midprecordial leads, with ST elevations and evolving T wave inversions (V_1 through V_6).

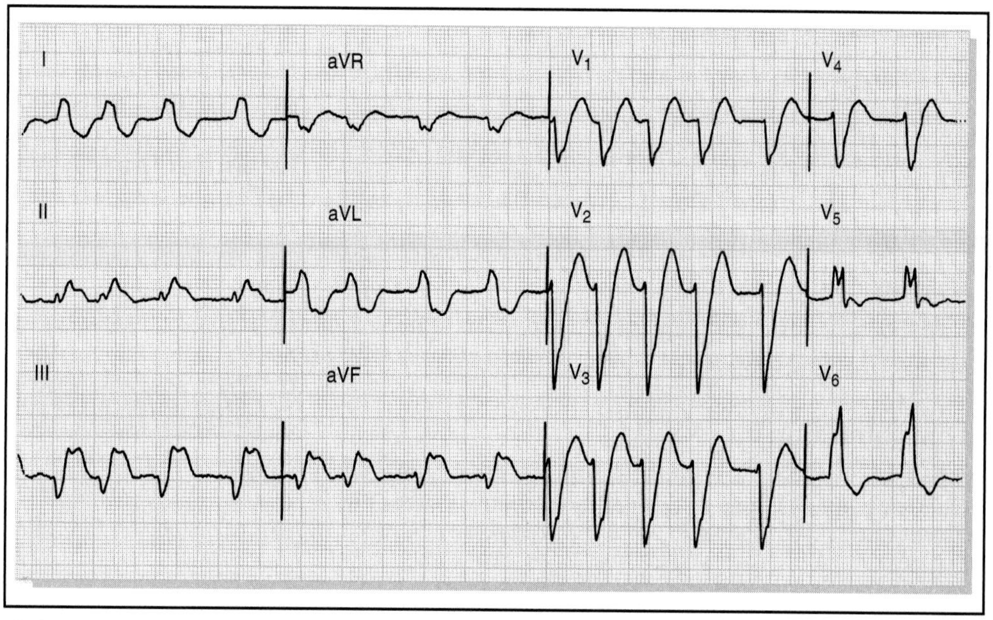

FIGURE 9–45 Complete left bundle branch block with acute inferior myocardial infarction. Note the prominent ST segment elevation in leads II, III, and aV_f, with reciprocal ST segment depression in I and aV_l superimposed on secondary ST-T changes. The underlying rhythm is atrial fibrillation.

Infarction of the left ventricular free (or lateral) wall ordinarily results in abnormal Q waves in the midprecordial to lateral precordial leads (and selected limb leads). However, the initial septal depolarization forces with LBBB are directed from right to left. These leftward forces produce an initial R wave in the midprecordial to lateral precordial leads, usually masking the loss of electrical potential (Q waves) caused by the infarction. Therefore, acute or chronic left ventricular free wall infarction by itself will not usually produce diagnostic Q waves in the presence of LBBB. Acute or chronic infarction involving both the free wall and the septum (or the septum itself) may produce abnormal Q waves (usually as part of QR-type complexes) in leads V_4 to V_6. These initial Q waves probably reflect posterior and superior forces from the spared basal portion of the septum (Fig. 9–46). Thus, a wide Q wave (≥40 msec) in one or more of these leads is a reliable sign of underlying infarction. The sequence of repolarization is also altered in LBBB, with the ST segment and T wave vectors being directed opposite the QRS complex. These changes can mask or simulate the ST segment changes of actual ischemia.

The following points summarize the ECG signs of myocardial infarction in LBBB: (1) ST segment elevation with tall positive T waves are frequently seen in the right precordial leads with uncomplicated LBBB. Secondary T wave inversions are characteristically seen in the lateral precordial leads. However, the appearance of ST elevations in the lateral leads or ST depressions or deep T wave inversions in leads V_1 to V_3 strongly suggests underlying ischemia. More marked ST elevations (≥0.5 mV) in leads with QS or rS waves may also be due to acute ischemia, but false-positive findings occur, especially with large-amplitude negative QRS complexes.[69] (2) The presence of QR complexes in leads I, V_5, or V_6 or in II, III, and aV_f with LBBB strongly suggests underlying infarction. (3) Chronic infarction is also suggested by notching of the ascending part of a wide S wave in the midprecordial leads or the ascending limb of a wide R wave in V_5 or V_6. Similar principles

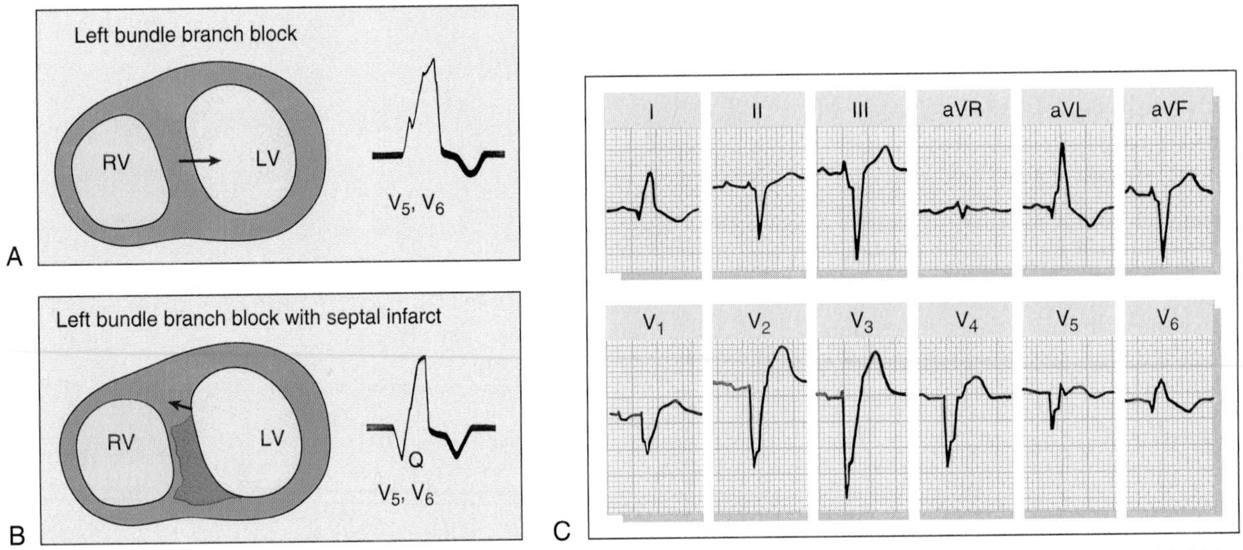

FIGURE 9–46 **A,** With uncomplicated left bundle branch block, early septal forces are directed to the left. Therefore, no Q waves will be seen in V_5 and V_6 **(right panel)**. **B,** With left bundle branch block complicated by anteroseptal infarction, early septal forces can be directed posteriorly and rightward **(left panel)**. Therefore, prominent Q waves may appear in V_5 and V_6 as a paradoxical marker of septal infarction **(right panel)**. **C,** Anterior wall infarction (involving septum) with left bundle branch block. Note the presence of QR complexes in leads I, aV_l, V_5, and V_6. (**A** and **B** adapted from Dunn MI, Lipman BS: Lipman-Massie Clinical Electrocardiography. 8th ed. Chicago, Year Book, 1989.)

can apply to the diagnosis of acute and chronic infarction in the presence of right ventricular pacing.[71] Comparison between an ECG exhibiting the LBBB prior to the infarction and the present ECG is often helpful to show these changes.

The diagnosis of concomitant LAFB and inferior wall infraction can also pose challenges. This combination can result in loss of the small r waves in the inferior leads, so that leads II, III, and aVF show QS, not rS, complexes. LAFB, however, will occasionally hide the diagnosis of inferior wall infarction. The inferior orientation of the initial QRS forces caused by the hemiblock can mask inferior Q waves, with resultant rS complexes in II, III, and aVF. In other cases, the combination of LAFB and inferior wall infarction will produce qrS complexes in the inferior limb leads, with the initial q wave the result of the infarct and the minuscule r wave the result of the hemiblock.

Atrial Infarction

A number of ECG clues to the diagnosis of atrial infarction have been suggested, including localized deviations of the PR segment (e.g., PR elevation in V_5 or V_6), changes in P wave morphology, and atrial arrhythmias. The sensitivity and specificity of these signs are limited, however. Diffuse PR segment changes (PR elevation in aV_r with depression in the inferolateral leads) with acute infarction usually indicate concomitant pericarditis (see later).

Electrocardiographic Differential Diagnosis of Ischemia and Infarction

The ECG has important limitations in both sensitivity and specificity in the diagnosis of coronary syndromes. An initially normal ECG does not exclude ischemia or even acute infarction.[72] However, a normal ECG throughout the course of an alleged acute infarct is distinctly uncommon. As a result, prolonged chest pain without diagnostic ECG changes should always prompt a careful search for noncoronary causes of chest pain (see Chap. 47). Pathological Q waves can be absent even in patients with depressed left ventricular function caused by severe coronary disease and a previous infarct. As noted, the diagnosis of acute or chronic infarction can be completely masked by ventricular conduction disturbances, especially those resulting from LBBB, as well as ventricular pacing and Wolff-Parkinson-White preexcitation. On the other hand, diagnostic confusion can arise because Q waves, ST elevation, ST depression, tall positive T waves, and deep T wave inversion can be seen in a wide variety of noncoronary settings.

Noninfarction Q Waves

Q waves simulating coronary artery disease can be related to one (or a combination) of the following four factors (Table 9–9): (1) physiological or positional variants, (2) altered ventricular conduction, (3) ventricular enlargement, and (4)

TABLE 9–9 Differential Diagnosis of Noninfarction Q Waves (with Selected Examples)

Physiological or positional factors
Normal-variant "septal" Q waves
Normal-variant Q waves in V_1-V_2, III, and aV_f
Left pneumothorax or dextrocardia: loss of lateral R wave progression
Myocardial injury or infiltration
Acute processes: myocardial ischemia without infarction, myocarditis, hyperkalemia (rare cause of transient Q waves)
Chronic myocardial processes: idiopathic cardiomyopathies, myocarditis, amyloid, tumor, sarcoid
Ventricular hypertrophy/enlargement
Left ventricular (poor R wave progression*)
Right ventricular (reversed R wave progression† or poor R wave progression, particularly with chronic obstructive lung disease)
Hypertrophic cardiomyopathy (can simulate anterior, inferior, posterior, or lateral infarcts) (see Fig. 9–47)
Conduction abnormalities
Left bundle branch block (poor R wave progression*)
Wolff-Parkinson-White patterns

Modified from Goldberger AL: Clinical Electrocardiography: A Simplified Approach. 6th ed. St Louis, CV Mosby, 1999.
*Small or absent R waves in the right precordial to midprecordial leads.
†Progressive decrease in R wave amplitude from V_1 to the midlateral precordial leads.

myocardial damage or replacement. Depending on the electrical axis, prominent Q waves (as part of QS- or QR-type complexes) can also appear in the limb leads (aV_l with a vertical axis and III and aV_f with a horizontal axis). A QS complex can appear in lead V_1 as a normal variant and rarely in leads V_1 and V_2. Prominent Q waves can be associated with a variety of other positional factors that alter the orientation of the heart vis-à-vis a given lead axis. Poor R wave progression, sometimes with actual QS waves, can be due solely to improper placement of chest electrodes above their usual position. In cases of dextrocardia, provided that no underlying structural abnormalities are present, normal R wave progression can be restored by recording leads V_2 to V_6 on the right side of the chest. A rightward mediastinal shift in left pneumothorax can contribute to the apparent loss of left precordial R waves. Other positional factors associated with poor R wave progression include pectus excavatum, congenitally corrected transposition of the great vessels, and congenital absence of the left pericardium.

An intrinsic change in the sequence of ventricular depolarization can lead to pathological, noninfarct Q waves. The two most important conduction disturbances associated with pseudoinfarct Q waves are LBBB and the Wolff-Parkinson-White preexcitation patterns. With LBBB, QS complexes can appear in the right precordial to midprecordial leads and occasionally in one or more of leads II, III, and aV_f. Depending on the location of the bypass tract, WPW preexcitation can mimic anteroseptal, lateral, or inferior-posterior infarction. LAFB is often cited as a cause of anteroseptal infarct patterns; however, LAFB has only minor effects on the QRS complex in horizontal plane leads. Probably the most common findings are relatively prominent S waves in leads V_5 and V_6. Poor R wave progression is not a routine feature of LAFB, although some authors have reported minuscule q waves in leads V_1 to V_3 in this setting. These small q waves can become more apparent if the leads are recorded one interspace above their usual position and disappear in leads one interspace below their usual position. As a general clinical rule, however, prominent Q waves (as part of QS or QR complexes) in the right precordial to midprecordial leads should *not* be attributed to LAFB alone.

Poor R Wave Progression. In contrast, poor R wave progression is commonly observed with LVH and with acute or chronic right ventricular overload. Q waves in such settings can reflect a variety of mechanisms, including a change in the balance of early ventricular depolarization forces and altered cardiac geometry and position. A marked loss of R wave voltage, sometimes with frank Q waves from V_1 to the lateral chest leads, can be seen with chronic obstructive pulmonary disease (see Fig. 9-23). The presence of low limb voltage and P pulmonale can serve as additional diagnostic clues. This loss of R wave progression may, in part, reflect right ventricular dilation. Furthermore, downward displacement of the heart in an emphysematous chest can play a major role in the genesis of poor R wave progression in this syndrome. Partial or complete normalization of R wave progression can be achieved in such cases simply by recording the chest leads an interspace lower than usual (see Fig. 9-23).

Other Pseudoinfarct Patterns in Ventricular Overload. A variety of pseudoinfarct patterns can occur with acute cor pulmonale caused by pulmonary embolism. Acute right ventricular overload in this setting can cause poor R wave progression and sometimes right precordial to midprecordial T wave inversion (right ventricular "strain"), mimicking anterior infarction. The classic $S_1Q_3T_3$ pattern can occur but is neither sensitive nor specific. A prominent Q wave (usually as part of a QR complex) can also occur in lead aV_f along with this pattern (see Fig. 9-24). However, acute right overload by itself does not cause a pathological Q wave in lead II. Right heart overload, acute or chronic, may also be associated with a QR complex in lead V_1 and simulate anteroseptal infarction.

Pseudoinfarct patterns are an important finding in patients with hypertrophic cardiomyopathy, and the ECG can simulate anterior, inferior, posterior, or lateral infarction. The pathogenesis of depolarization abnormalities in this cardiomyopathy is not certain. Prominent inferolateral Q waves (II, III, aV_f, and V_4 to V_6) and tall right precordial R waves are probably related to increased depolarization forces generated by the markedly hypertrophied septum (Fig. 9-47). Abnormal septal depolarization can also contribute to the bizarre QRS complexes.

Q Wave Pathogenesis with Myocardial Damage. Loss of electromotive force associated with myocardial necrosis contributes to R wave loss and Q wave formation in cases of myocardial infarction. This mechanism of Q wave pathogenesis, however, is not specific for coronary artery disease with infarction. Any process, acute or chronic, that causes sufficient loss of regional electromotive potential can result in Q waves. For example, replacement of myocardial tissue by electrically inert material such as amyloid or tumor can cause noninfarction Q waves. A variety of dilated cardiomyopathies associated with extensive myocardial fibrosis can be characterized by pseudoinfarct patterns. Ventricular hypertrophy can also contribute to Q wave pathogenesis in this setting. Finally, Q waves caused by myocardial injury, whether ischemic or nonischemic in origin, can appear transiently and do not necessarily signify irreversible heart muscle damage. Severe ischemia can cause regional loss of electromotive potential without actual cell death ("electrical stunning" phenomenon). Transient conduction disturbances can also cause alterations in ventricular activation and result in noninfarctional Q waves. In some cases, transient Q waves may represent unmasking of a prior Q wave infarct. New, but transient, Q waves have been described in patients with severe hypotension from a variety of causes, as well as with tachyarrhythmias, myocarditis, Prinzmetal angina, protracted hypoglycemia, phosphorus poisoning, and hyperkalemia.

ST-T Changes Simulating Ischemia

The differential diagnosis of ST segment elevation includes acute pericarditis (see Chap. 64) (Fig. 9–48), acute myocarditis (see Chap. 60), normal-variant "early repolarization" (see Fig. 9–16), and a number of other conditions[73,74] listed in Table 9–10. Acute pericarditis, in contrast to acute myocardial infarction, typically induces diffuse ST segment elevation, usually in most of the chest leads and also in leads I, aV_l, II, and aV_f. Reciprocal ST depression is seen in lead aV_r.

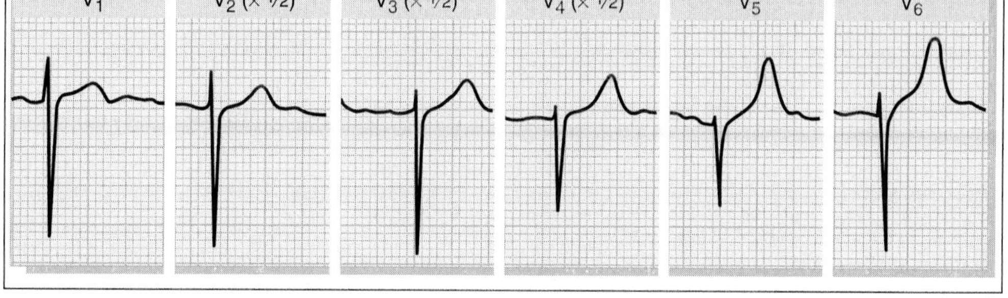

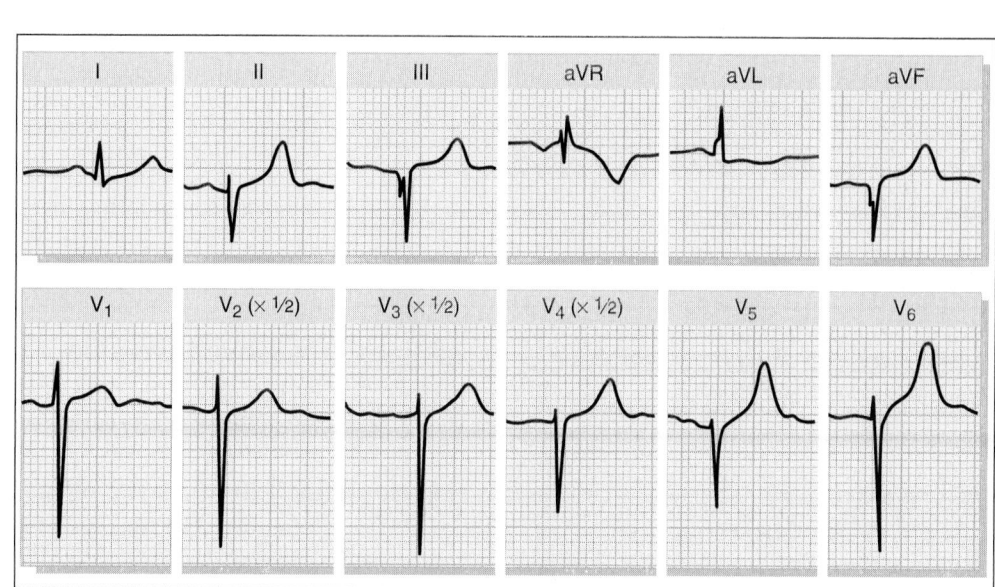

FIGURE 9–47 Hypertrophic cardiomyopathy simulating inferolateral infarction. This 11-year-old girl had a family history of hypertrophic cardiomyopathy. Note the W-shaped QS waves and the qrS complexes in the inferior and lateral precordial leads. (From Goldberger AL: Myocardial Infarction: Electrocardiographic Differential Diagnosis. 4th ed. St Louis, Mosby-Year Book, 1991.)

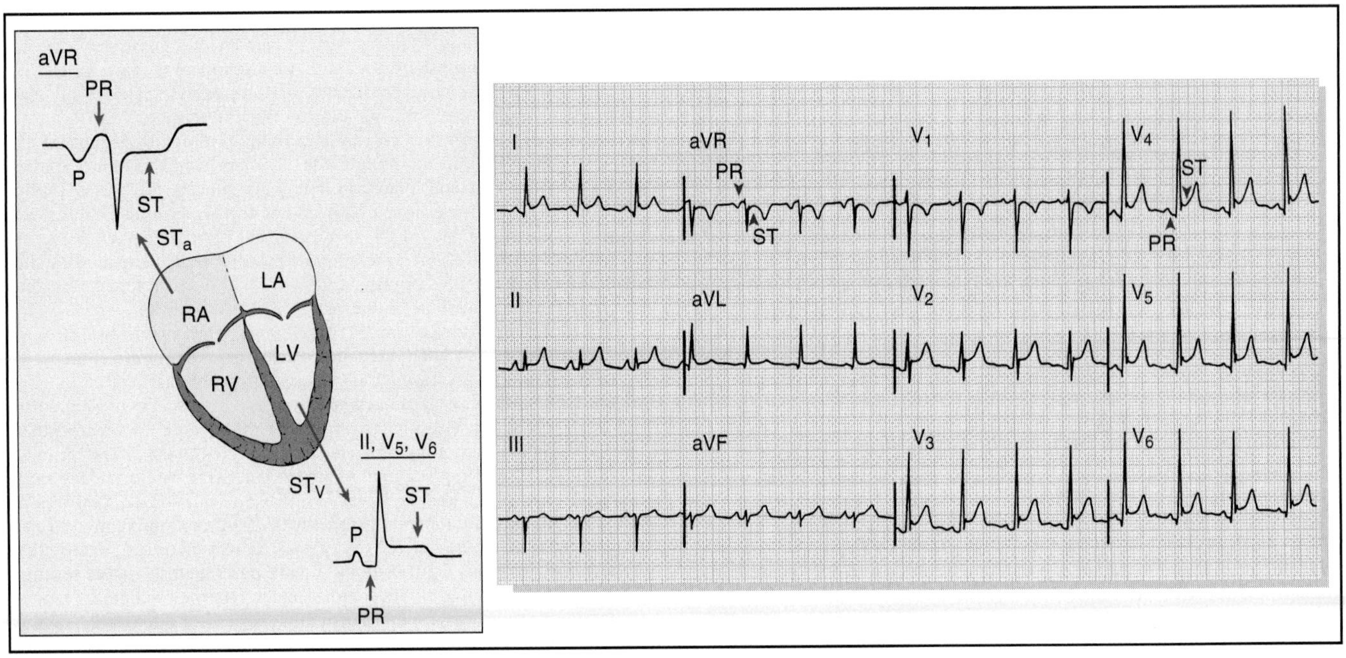

FIGURE 9–48 Acute pericarditis is often characterized by two apparent injury currents: one atrial, the other ventricular. The atrial injury current vector (ST_a) is usually directed upward and to the right and produces PR segment elevation in aV_r with reciprocal PR depression in II, V_5, and V_6. The ventricular injury current (ST_V) is directed downward and to the left, associated with ST elevation in II, V_5, and V_6 with reciprocal ST depression in aV. This characteristic PR-ST segment discordance is illustrated in the bottom-most tracing. Note the diffuse distribution of ST segment elevation in acute pericarditis (e.g., I, II, and V_2 through V_6, with reciprocal changes in aV_r and perhaps minimally in V_1). Note the PR segment elevation in aV. (From Goldberger AL: Myocardial Infarction: Electrocardiographic Differential Diagnosis. 4th ed. St Louis, Mosby-Year Book, 1991.)

TABLE 9–10 Differential Diagnosis of ST Segment Elevation
Myocardial ischemia/infarction Noninfarction, transmural ischemia (Prinzmetal angina pattern) (see Fig. 9–40) Acute myocardial infarction (see Fig. 9–37) Post myocardial infarction (ventricular aneurysm pattern)
Acute pericarditis (see Fig. 9–48)
Normal variant ("early repolarization" pattern) (see Fig. 9–16)
LVH/LBBB (V_1-V_2 or V_3 only)
Other (rarer) Myocardial injury Myocarditis (may look like myocardial infarction or pericarditis) Tumor invading the left ventricle Trauma to the ventricles
Hypothermia (J wave/Osborn wave) (see Fig. 9–53)
After DC-cardioversion
Intracranial hemorrhage
Hyperkalemia*
Brugada pattern (RBBB-like pattern and ST elevations in right precordial leads)*
Type 1C antiarrhythmic drugs*
Hypercalcemia*

LBBB = left bundle branch block; LVH = left ventricular hypertrophy; RBBB = right bundle branch block.

Modified from Goldberger AL: Clinical Electrocardiography: A Simplified Approach. 6th ed. St Louis, CV Mosby, 1999.

*Usually localized to V_1 to V_2.

An important clue to acute pericarditis, in addition to the diffuse nature of the ST elevation, is the frequent presence of PR segment elevation in aVR, with reciprocal PR segment depression in other leads, caused by a concomitant atrial current of injury[75] (see Fig. 9–48). Abnormal Q waves do not occur with acute pericarditis, and the ST elevation may be followed by T wave inversion after a variable period. Myocarditis can, in some patients, exactly simulate the ECG pattern of acute myocardial infarction, including ST elevation and Q waves. These pseudoinfarct findings can be associated with a rapidly progressive course and increased mortality.

A variety of factors such as digitalis, ventricular hypertrophy, hypokalemia, and hyperventilation can cause ST segment depression mimicking subendocardial ischemia. Similarly, tall positive T waves do not invariably represent hyperacute ischemic changes but can reflect normal variants, hyperkalemia, cerebrovascular injury, and left ventricular volume loads resulting from mitral or aortic regurgitation, among other causes. ST elevation and tall positive T waves are also common findings in leads V_1 and V_2 with LBBB or LVH patterns. In addition, tall T waves may be seen occasionally in the left chest leads with LVH, especially with volume (diastolic) overload syndromes (see Fig. 9–21).

T Wave Inversion

When caused by physiological variants, T wave inversion is sometimes mistaken for ischemia. T waves in the right precordial leads can be slightly inverted, particularly in leads V_1 and V_2. Some adults show persistence of the juvenile T wave pattern (see Fig. 9–15), with more prominent T wave inversion in right precordial to midprecordial leads showing an rS or RS morphology. The other normal variant that can be associated with prominent T wave inversion is the early repolarization pattern (see Fig. 9–16). Some subjects with this variant have prominent, biphasic T wave inversion in association with the ST elevation. This pattern, which may simulate the initial stages of an evolving infarct, is most prevalent in young adult black males and among athletes. These functional ST-T changes are probably due to regional disparities in repolarization and can be normalized by exercise.

PRIMARY AND SECONDARY T WAVE INVERSIONS. A variety of pathological factors can alter repolarization and cause prominent T wave inversion (Fig. 9–49). As noted earlier, T wave alterations are usefully classified as primary or secondary. Primary T wave changes are caused by alterations in the duration or morphology of ventricular action potentials in the absence of changes in the activation sequence. Examples include ischemia, drug effects, and metabolic factors. Prominent primary T wave inversion (or in some cases, tall positive T waves) is also a well-described feature of the ECG in cerebrovascular accidents, particularly with subarachnoid hemorrhage. The so-called cerebrovascular accident T wave pattern is characteristically diffuse, with a widely splayed appearance usually associated with marked QT prolongation (Fig. 9–49). Some studies have implicated structural damage (myocytolysis) in the hearts of patients with such T wave changes, probably induced by excessive sympathetic stimulation mediated via the hypothalamus. A role for concomitant vagal activation in the pathogenesis of such T wave changes, which are usually associated with bradycardia, has also been postulated. Similar T wave changes have been reported after truncal vagotomy, radical neck dissection, and bilateral carotid endarterectomy. In addition, the massive diffuse T wave inversion seen in some patients after Stokes-Adams syncope may be related to a similar neurogenic mechanism. Patients with subarachnoid hemorrhage can also show transient ST elevation, as well as arrhythmias, including torsades de pointes. Ventricular dysfunction can even occur.

In contrast to these primary T wave abnormalities, secondary T wave changes are caused by altered ventricular activation, without changes in action potential characteristics. Examples include bundle branch block, Wolff-Parkinson-White preexcitation, and ventricular ectopic or paced beats. In addition, altered ventricular activation (associated with QRS interval prolongation) can induce persistent T wave changes that appear after normal ventricular depolarization has resumed. The term *cardiac memory T wave changes* has been used in this context to describe repolarization changes subsequent to depolarization changes caused by ventricular pacing, intermittent LBBB, intermittent Wolff-Parkinson-White preexcitation, and other alterations of ventricular activation.[76] Finally, the designation *idiopathic global T wave inversion* has been applied in cases in which no identifiable cause for often marked, diffuse repolarization abnormalities can be found. An unexplained female preponderance has been reported. Major causes of prominent T wave inversion are summarized in Table 9–11, with selected examples in Figure 9–49.

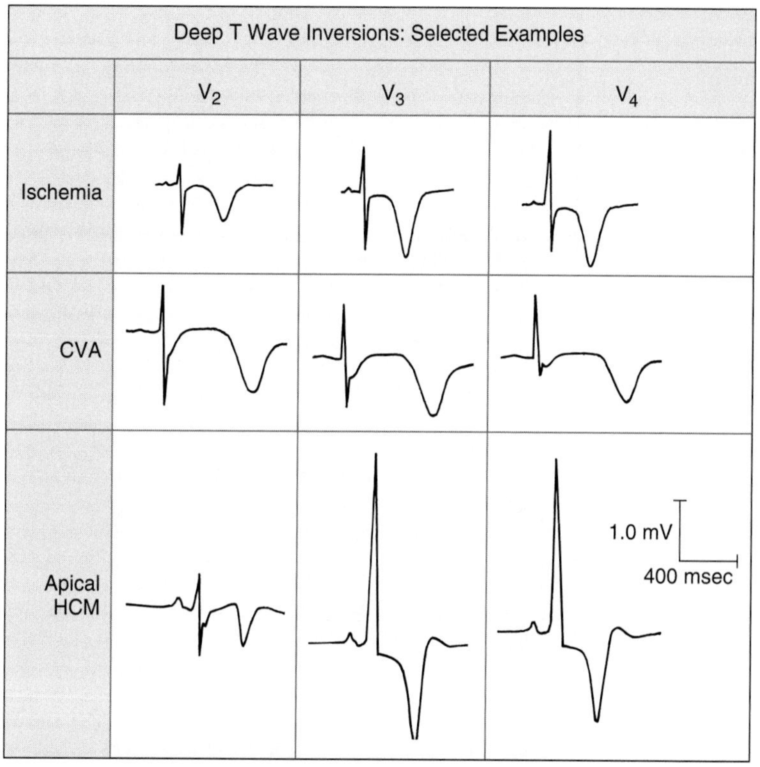

FIGURE 9–49 Deep T wave inversion can be due to a variety of causes (see Table 9–11). Note the marked QT prolongation in conjunction with the cerebrovascular accident (CVA) T wave pattern caused here by subarachnoid hemorrhage. Apical hypertrophic cardiomyopathy (HCM) is another cause of deep T wave inversion that can be mistaken for coronary disease. (From Goldberger AL: Deep T wave inversions. ACC Curr J Rev Nov/Dec:28, 1996.)

TABLE 9–11 Differential Diagnosis of Prominent T Wave Inversion

Normal variants Juvenile T wave pattern (see Fig. 9–15) Early repolarization
Myocardial ischemia/infarction (see Fig. 9–49)
Cerebrovascular accident (especially intracranial bleeding) and related neurogenic patterns (e.g., radical neck dissection, Stokes-Adams syndrome) (see Fig. 9–49)
Left or right ventricular overload Classic "strain" patterns Apical hypertrophic cardiomyopathy (Yamaguchi syndrome) (see Fig. 9–49)
Post-tachycardia T wave pattern
Idiopathic global T wave inversion syndrome
Secondary T wave alterations: bundle branch blocks, Wolff-Parkinson-White patterns
Intermittent left bundle branch block, preexcitation, or ventricular pacing ("memory T waves")

Modified from Goldberger AL: Clinical Electrocardiography: A Simplified Approach. 6th ed. St Louis, CV Mosby, 1999.

Drug Effects

Numerous drugs can affect the ECG, often in association with nonspecific ST-T alterations. More marked changes, as well as AV and intraventricular conduction disturbances, can occur with selected agents. The proarrhythmic effects of "antiarrhythmic" medications are described in Chapter 30.

Digitalis effect refers to the relatively distinctive "scooped" appearance of the ST-T complex and shortening of the QT interval, which correlates with abbreviation of the ventricular action potential duration (Fig. 9–50). Digitalis-related ST-T changes can be accentuated by an increased heart rate during exercise and result in false-positive stress test results[70] (see Chap. 10). Digitalis effect can occur with therapeutic or toxic doses of the drug. The term *digitalis toxicity* refers specifically to systemic effects (nausea and

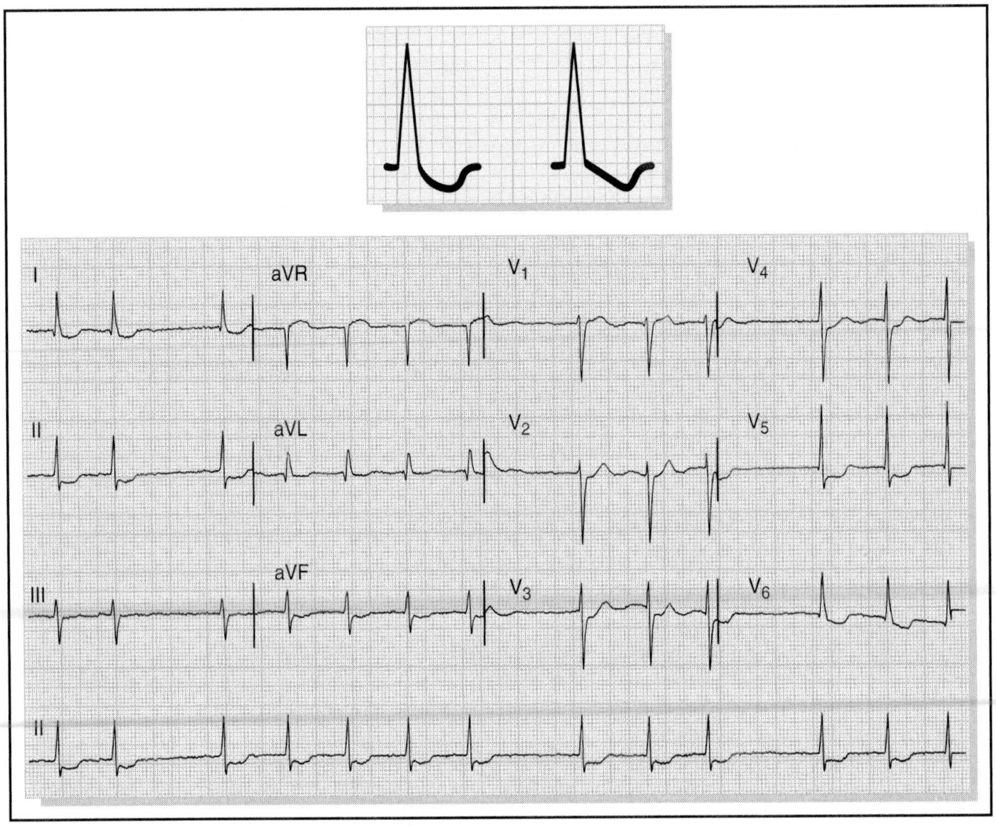

FIGURE 9–50 **Top,** Digitalis effect. Digitalis glycosides characteristically produce shortening of the QT interval with a "scooped" or downsloping ST-T complex. (From Goldberger AL: Clinical Electrocardiography: A Simplified Approach. 6th ed. St Louis, CV Mosby, 1999.) **Bottom,** Digitalis effect in combination with digitalis toxicity. The underlying rhythm is atrial fibrillation. A "group beating" pattern of QRS complexes with shortening of the R-R intervals is consistent with nonparoxysmal junctional tachycardia with exit (atrioventricular Wenckebach) block. ST segment depression and "scooping" (V_6) are consistent with digitalis effect, although ischemia or left ventricular hypertrophy cannot be excluded. Findings are strongly suggestive of digitalis excess; the serum digoxin level was greater than 3 ng/ml. Digitalis effect does not necessarily imply digitalis toxicity, however.

anorexia, among other effects) or conduction disturbances and arrhythmias caused by drug excess or increased sensitivity.

The ECG effects and toxicities of other cardioactive agents can be anticipated, in part, from ion channel effects (see Chap. 27). Inactivation of sodium channels by class 1 agents (e.g., quinidine, procainamide, disopyramide, flecainide) can cause QRS prolongation. Class 1A and class 3 agents (e.g., amiodarone, dofetilide, ibutilide, sotalol) can induce an acquired long QT(U) syndrome (see Chap. 30). Psychotropic drugs (e.g., tricyclic antidepressants and phenothiazines), which have class 1A-like properties, can also lead to QRS and QT(U) prolongation.[78] Toxicity can produce asystole or torsades de pointes. Right axis shift of the terminal 40 msec frontal plane QRS axis was reported to be a helpful marker of tricyclic antidepressant overdose.

Electrolyte and Metabolic Abnormalities

In addition to the structural and functional cardiac conditions already discussed, numerous systemic metabolic aberrations affect the ECG, including electrolyte abnormalities and acid-base disorders, as well as systemic hypothermia.

CALCIUM. Hypercalcemia and hypocalcemia predominantly alter the action potential duration. An increased extracellular calcium concentration shortens the ventricular action potential duration by shortening phase 2 of the action potential. In contrast, hypocalcemia prolongs phase 2 of the action potential. These cellular changes correlate with abbreviation and prolongation of the QT interval (ST segment portion) with hypercalcemia and hypocalcemia, respectively (Fig. 9–51). Severe hypercalcemia (e.g., serum Ca^{2+} >15 mg/dl) can also be associated with decreased T wave amplitude, sometimes with T wave notching or inversion. Hypercalcemia sometimes produces a high takeoff of the ST segment in leads V_1 and V_2 and can thus simulate acute ischemia (see Table 9–10).

POTASSIUM. Hyperkalemia is associated with a distinctive sequence of ECG changes (Fig. 9–52A). The earliest effect is usually narrowing and peaking (tenting) of the T wave. The QT interval is shortened at this stage, associated with decreased action potential duration. Progressive extracellular hyperkalemia reduces atrial and ventricular resting membrane potentials, thereby inactivating sodium channels, which decreases V_{max} and conduction velocity. The QRS begins to widen and P wave amplitude decreases. PR interval prolongation can occur, followed sometimes by second- or third-degree AV block. Complete loss of P waves may be associated with a junctional escape rhythm or so-called sinoventricular rhythm. In the latter instance, sinus rhythm persists with conduction between the SA and AV nodes and occurs without producing an overt P wave. Moderate to severe hyperkalemia occasionally induces ST elevations in the right precordial leads (V_1 and V_2) and simulates an ischemic current-of-injury pattern. However, even severe hyperkalemia can be associated with atypical or nondiagnostic ECG findings.[79] Very marked hyperkalemia leads to eventual asystole, sometimes preceded by a slow undulatory (sine-wave) ventricular flutter-like pattern. The ECG triad of

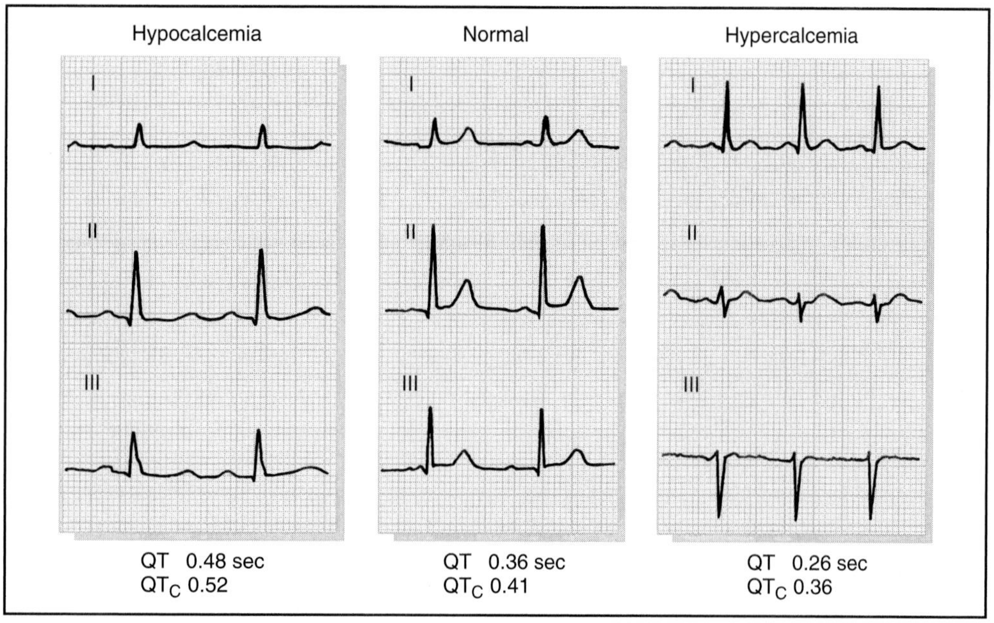

FIGURE 9–51 Prolongation of the QT interval (ST segment portion) is typical of hypocalcemia. Hypercalcemia may cause abbreviation of the ST segment and shortening of the QT interval. (From Goldberger AL: Clinical Electrocardiography: A Simplified Approach. 6th ed. St Louis, CV Mosby, 1999.)

(1) peaked T waves (from hyperkalemia), (2) QT prolongation (from hypocalcemia), and (3) LVH (from hypertension) is strongly suggestive of chronic renal failure.

The electrophysiological changes associated with hypokalemia, in contrast, include hyperpolarization of myocardial cell membranes and increased action potential duration. The major ECG manifestations are ST depression with flattened T waves and increased U wave prominence (Fig. 9–52B). The U waves can exceed the amplitude of T waves. Clinically, distinguishing T waves from U waves can be difficult or impossible from the surface ECG. Indeed, apparent "U" waves in hypokalemia and other pathologic settings may actually be part of T waves whose morphology is altered by the effects of voltage gradients between M, or midmyocardial cells, and adjacent myocardial layers.[80] The prolongation of repolarization with hypokalemia, as part of an acquired long QT(U) syndrome, predisposes to torsades de pointes. Hypokalemia also predisposes to tachyarrhythmias from digitalis.

MAGNESIUM. Specific ECG effects of mild to moderate isolated abnormalities in magnesium ion concentration are not well characterized. Severe hypermagnesemia can cause AV and intraventricular conduction disturbances that may culminate in complete heart block and cardiac arrest (Mg^{2+} >15 mEq/L). Hypomagnesemia is usually associated with hypocalcemia or hypokalemia. Hypomagnesemia can potentiate certain digitalis toxic arrhythmias. The role of magnesium deficiency in the pathogenesis and treatment of the acquired long QT(U) syndrome with torsades de pointes is discussed in Chapters 27 and 30.

OTHER FACTORS. Isolated hypernatremia or hyponatremia does not produce consistent effects on the ECG. Acidemia and alkalemia are often associated with hyperkalemia and hypokalemia, respectively. Systemic hypothermia may be associated with the appearance of a distinctive convex elevation at the junction (J point) of the ST segment and QRS complex (J wave or Osborn wave) (Fig. 9–53). The cellular mechanism of this type of pathological J wave appears to be related to an epicardial-endocardial voltage gradient associated with the localized appearance of a prominent epicardial action potential notch.

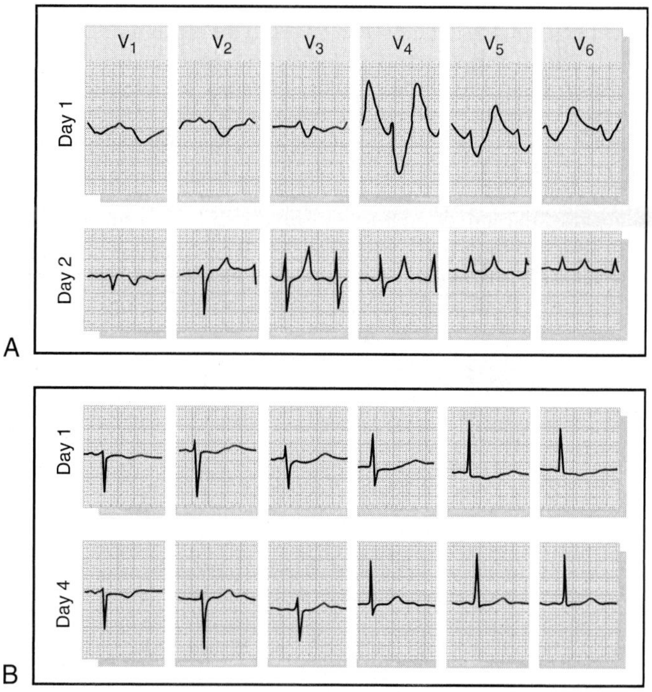

FIGURE 9–52 Electrocardiographic changes in hyperkalemia **(A)** and hypokalemia **(B)**. **A,** On day 1, at a K^+ level of 8.6 mEq/liter, the P wave is no longer recognizable and the QRS complex is diffusely prolonged. Initial and terminal QRS delay is characteristic of K^+-induced intraventricular conduction slowing and is best illustrated in leads V_2 and V_6. On day 2, at a K^+ level of 5.8 mEq/liter, the P wave is recognizable with a PR interval of 0.24 second, the duration of the QRS complex is approximately 0.10 second, and the T waves are characteristically "tented." **B,** On day 1, at a K^+ level of 1.5 mEq/liter, the T and U waves are merged. The U wave is prominent and the QU interval is prolonged. On day 4, at a K^+ level of 3.7 mEq/liter, the tracing is normal. (Courtesy of C. Fisch, M.D.)

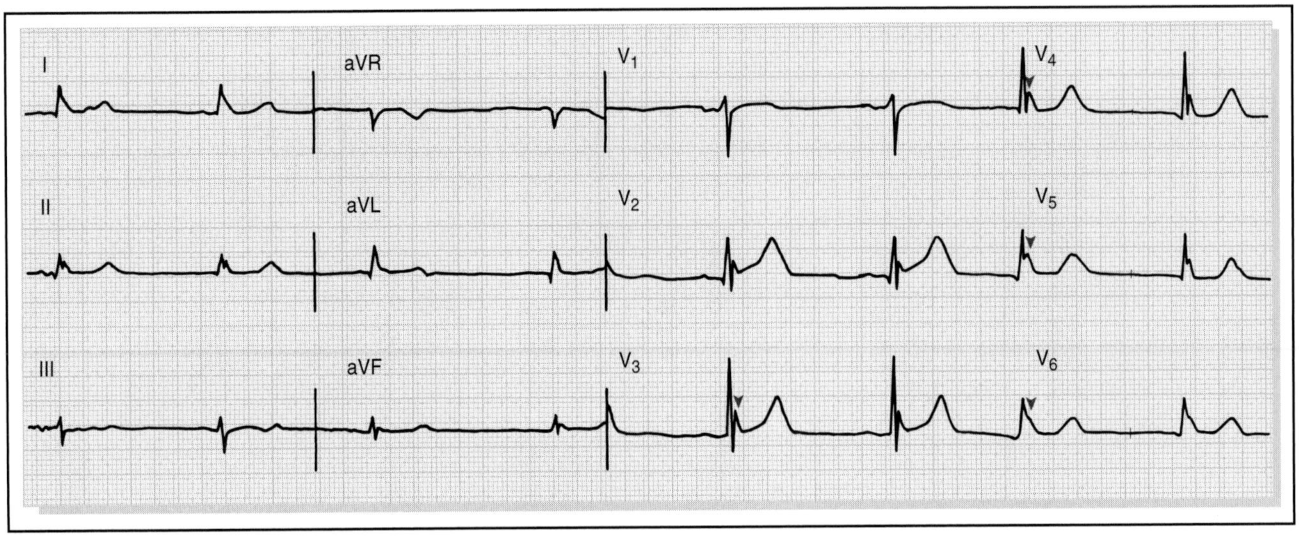

FIGURE 9–53 Systemic hypothermia. The arrows (V_3 through V_6) point to the characteristic convex J waves, termed *Osborn waves*. Prominent sinus bradycardia is also present. (From Goldberger AL: Clinical Electrocardiography: A Simplified Approach. 6th ed. St Louis, CV Mosby, 1999.)

Nonspecific QRS and ST-T Changes

Low QRS voltage is said to be present when the total amplitude of the QRS complexes in each of the six extremity leads is 0.5 mV or less or 1.0 mV or less in leads V_1 through V_6. Low QRS voltage can relate to a variety of mechanisms (Table 9–12), including increased insulation of the heart by air (chronic obstructive pulmonary disease) or adipose tissue (obesity); replacement of myocardium, for example, by fibrous tissue (ischemic or nonischemic cardiomyopathy), amyloid, or tumor; or short-circuiting (shunting) effects due to low resistance of the fluids (especially with pericardial or pleural effusions, or anasarca). The combination of relatively low limb voltage (QRS voltage ≤0.8 mV in each of the limb leads), relatively prominent QRS voltage in the chest leads (SV_1 or SV_2+RV_5 or RV_6 ≥3.5 mV), and poor R wave progression (R wave less than the S wave in V_1 through V_4) has been reported as a relatively specific, but not sensitive sign of dilated-type cardiomyopathies (ECG-congestive heart failure triad).

TABLE 9–12 Causes of Low-Voltage QRS Complexes
Adrenal insufficiency
Anasarca
Artifactual or spurious, e.g., unrecognized standardization of the electrocardiogram at half the usual gain (i.e., 5 mm/mV)
Cardiac infiltration or replacement (e.g., amyloidosis, tumor)
Cardiac transplantation, especially with acute or chronic rejection
Cardiomyopathies, idiopathic or secondary*
Chronic obstructive pulmonary disease constrictive pericarditis
Hypothyroidism (usually with sinus bradycardia)
Left pneumothorax (mid-left chest leads)
Myocardial infarction, extensive
Myocarditis, acute or chronic
Normal variant
Obesity
Pericardial effusion or tamponade (latter usually with sinus tachycardia)
Pleural effusions

*Dilated cardiomyopathies can be associated with a combination of relatively low limb lead voltage and prominent precordial voltage.

Many factors in addition to ischemia (e.g., postural changes, meals, drugs, hypertrophy, electrolyte and metabolic disorders, central nervous system lesions, infections, pulmonary diseases) can affect the ECG. Ventricular repolarization is particularly sensitive to these effects, which can lead to a variety of nonspecific ST-T changes. The term is usually applied to slight ST depression or T wave inversion or to T wave flattening without evident cause. Care must be taken to not overinterpret such changes, especially in subjects with a low prior probability of heart disease. At the same time, subtle repolarization abnormalities can be markers of coronary or hypertensive heart disease or other types of structural heart disease and probably account for the association of relatively minor but persistent nonspecific ST-T changes with increased cardiovascular mortality in middle-aged men and women.[81]

Alternans Patterns

The term *alternans* applies to conditions characterized by the sudden appearance of a periodic beat-to-beat change in some aspect of cardiac electrical or mechanical behavior. These abrupt changes (AAAA → ABAB pattern) are reminiscent of a generic class of subharmonic (period-doubling) bifurcation patterns observed in perturbed nonlinear control systems.[13,82] Many different examples of electrical alternans have been described clinically[83,84] (Table 9–13); a number of others have been reported in the laboratory.[85] Most familiar is total electrical alternans with sinus tachycardia, a specific but not highly sensitive marker of pericardial effusion with tamponade physiology (Fig. 9–54) (see Chap. 64). This finding is associated with an abrupt transition from a 1:1 to a 2:1 pattern in the "to-fro" swinging motion of the heart in the effusion. Other alternans patterns are due to primary electrical rather than mechanical causes. ST-T alternans has long been recognized as a marker of electrical instability in cases of acute ischemia, where it may precede ventricular tachyarrhythmia[86] (see Fig. 9–40). Considerable interest has recently been shown in the detection of microvolt T wave (or ST-T) alternans as a noninvasive marker of the risk of

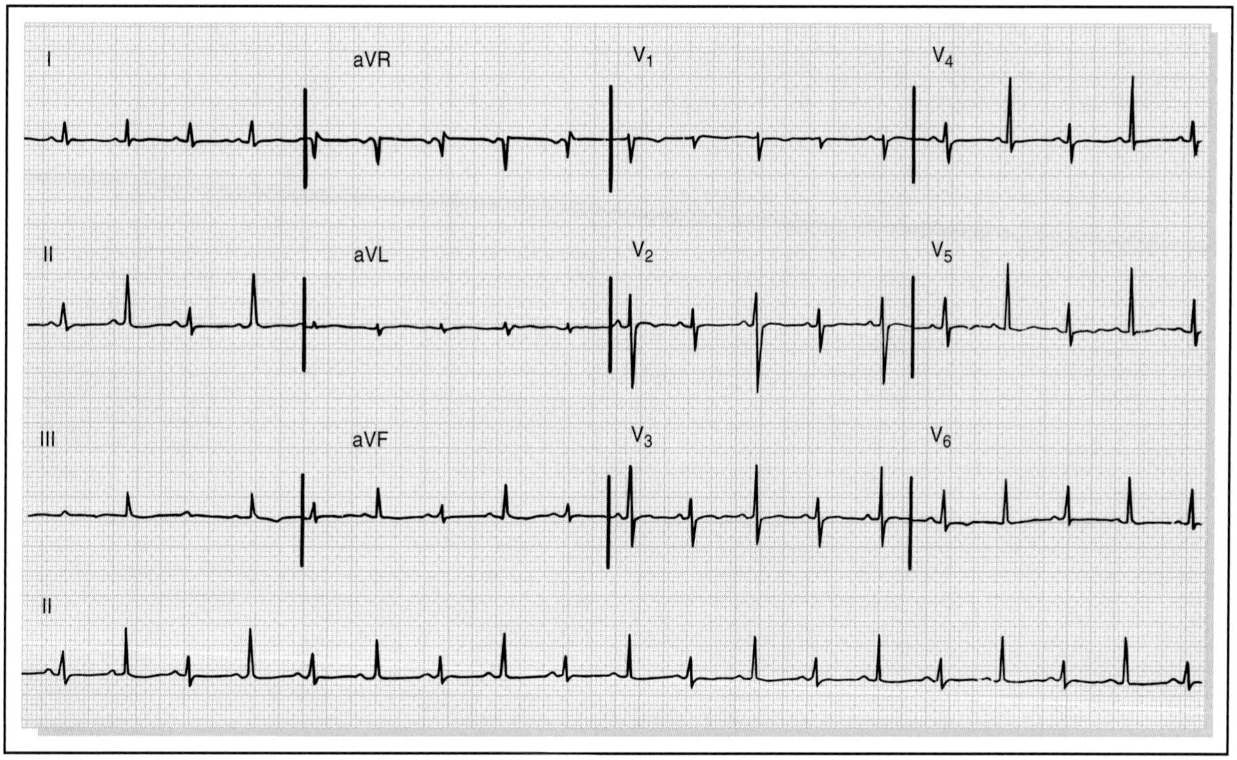

FIGURE 9–54 Total electrical alternans (P-QRS-T) caused by pericardial effusion with tamponade. This finding, particularly in concert with sinus tachycardia and relatively low voltage, is a highly specific, although not sensitive, marker of cardiac tamponade.

TABLE 9–13 Examples of Alternans Patterns in Electrocardiographic Diagnosis

Pattern	Comment
P wave alternans	Rarely reported; e.g., in pulmonary embolism
"Total" electrical alternans (P-QRS-T) with sinus tachycardia	Swinging-heart mechanism in pericardial effusion/tamponade* (see Fig. 9–54)
PR interval alternans	Dual AV nodal pathway physiology; alternating bundle branch block (see Fig. 9–30)
ST segment alternans	Can precede ischemic ventricular tachyarrhythmias (see Fig. 9–40)
T wave (or ST-T) alternans	Can precede nonischemic or ischemvc ventricular tachyarrhythmias
TU wave alternans	Can precede torsades de pointes in long QT(U) syndromes, congenital or acquired (see Fig. 9–55)
QRS alternans in supraventricular or ventricular tachycardias	Most common with AV reentrant tachycardias (concealed bypass tract)
R-R (heart rate) alternans	With sinus rhythm, e.g., in congestive heart failure With non–sinus rhythm tachyarrhythmias, e.g., PSVT
Bidirectional tachycardias	Usually ventricular in origin; may be caused by digitalis excess
Intermittent bundle branch/fascicular blocks or Wolff-Parkinson-White patterns	Rarely occur on beat-to-beat basis (see Fig. 9–31)

*Also case report of QRS-T alternans with sinus tachycardia in acute pulmonary embolism.
AV = atrioventricular; PSVT = paroxysmal supraventricular tachycardia.

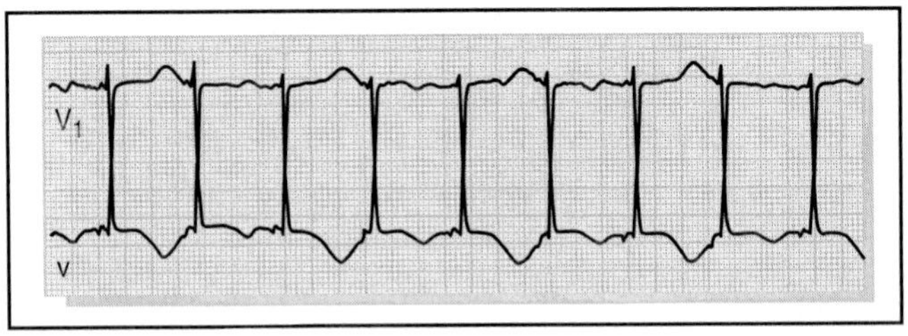

FIGURE 9–55 The QT(U) interval is prolonged (approximately 600 msec) with TU wave alternans. The tracing was recorded in a patient with chronic renal disease shortly following dialysis. This type of repolarization alternans may be a precursor to torsades de pointes. (Courtesy of C. Fisch, M.D.)

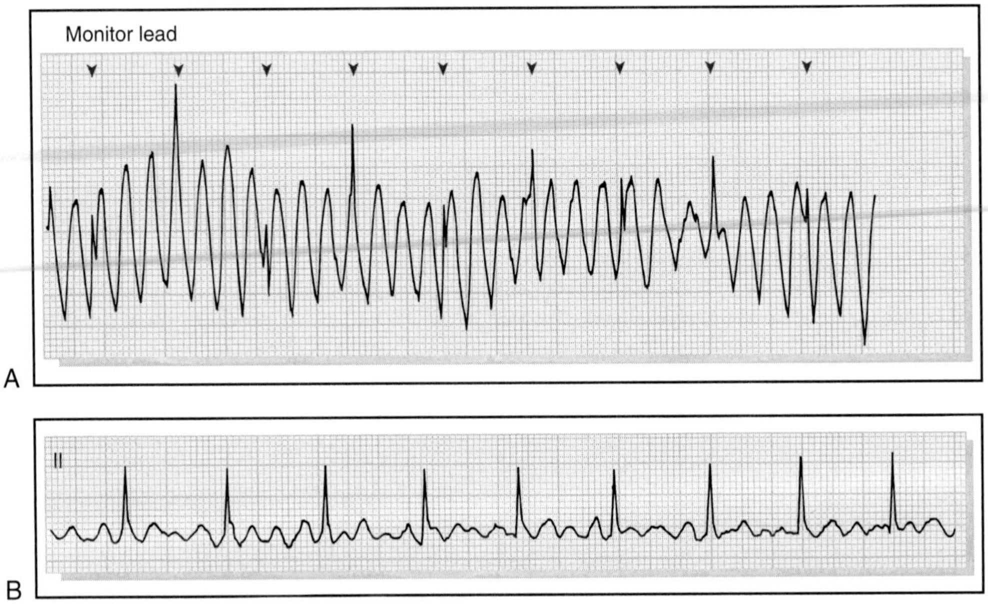

FIGURE 9–56 Artifacts simulating serious arrhythmias. **A,** Motion artifact mimicking ventricular tachyarrhythmia. Partly obscured normal QRS complexes (arrows) can be seen with a heart rate of about 100 beats/min. **B,** Parkinsonian tremor causing baseline oscillations mimicking atrial fibrillation. The regularity of QRS complexes may provide a clue to this artifact.

ventricular tachyarrhythmia in patients with chronic heart disease[87,88] (see Chap. 29). Similarly, TU wave alternans (Fig. 9–55) may be a marker of imminent risk of a ventricular tachyarrhythmia such as torsades de pointes in hereditary or acquired long QT syndromes.[89]

Clinical Issues in Electrocardiographic Interpretation

These principles and diagnostic ECG guidelines are, finally, subject to appropriate use in the clinical setting. Their effectiveness as a diagnostic tool depends on factors such as the indications for the procedure, the clinical context in which the ECG is used, and proper technique and skills of the ECG reader.

INDICATIONS FOR AN ECG. Limited attention has been paid to the indications for an ECG, probably because of its seeming simplicity and low cost. Because specific indications have not been accepted, there is wide variation in the use of the procedure.[90] However, the cumulative expense of low-cost tests performed at high volume is significant, and the risk to the patient of false diagnoses of cardiac disease can be damaging.

In patients with known cardiac disease, ECGs are warranted as part of a baseline examination; after therapy known to produce ECG changes that correlate with therapeutic responses, progression of disease, or adverse effects; and for intermittent follow-up with changes in signs or symptoms or relevant laboratory findings or after significant intervals (usually 1 year or longer), even in the absence of clinical changes. In patients suspected of having cardiac disease or at high risk for cardiac disease, an ECG is appropriate as part of an initial evaluation in the presence of signs or symptoms suggesting cardiac disease; in patients with important risk factors such as cigarette abuse, diabetes mellitus, peripheral vascular disease, or a family history of cardiac disease (including long QT interval syndromes and ventricular preexcitation); during therapy with cardioactive medications; and during follow-up if clinical events develop or at prolonged intervals (usually 1 year or more) if clinically stable. Preoperative tracings are appropriate for patients with known or suspected cardiac disease, although this application too may be questioned, especially if the cardiac condition is hemodynamically insignificant or the procedure is simple.

It has been common practice to include an ECG as part of routine health examinations, before any surgical procedure, and on any admission to a hospital in patients without current evidence of cardiac disease and without major risk factors. These ECGs are assumed to be of value in detecting any unknown abnormalities, serving as a baseline against which to compare later tracings, and assessing future risk of cardiovascular events. There is little evidence to support these practices. The overall sensitivity of the ECG for identifying specific patients who will have future events and the number of therapeutic or diagnostic changes provoked by routine ECG findings are too low to warrant universal screening.[91] The routine recording of the ECG before noncomplex surgery has also been questioned because of its limited value in risk stratification.[92] In these cases, use of the ECG should be based on clinical judgment rather than rigid protocol requirements. Flexible guidelines for ordering ECGs on general hospital admission and preoperatively have been proposed on the basis of age, gender, medical history, and physical examination.

KNOWLEDGE OF THE CLINICAL CONTEXT AND PRIOR ECG FINDINGS. Although most ECGs are read without a priori knowledge of the clinical condition of the patient, the accuracy and the value of the interpretation are enhanced by having clinical information about the patient. Such knowledge can include, for example, information about drug therapy, which can be a cause of observed ECG abnormalities, or prior myocardial infarction, which can produce ECG changes mimicking acute ischemia.[93]

Similarly, the availability of prior ECGs can improve the clinical value of the ECG. For example, knowledge of prior ECG patterns can improve diagnostic accuracy and triage decisions for patients with current ECG and clinical evidence of ischemia or infarction, as well as improve the proper interpretation of, for example, bundle branch block in the setting of acute infarction.[94]

TECHNICAL ERRORS AND ARTIFACTS. Technical errors can lead to significant diagnostic mistakes that can result in false diagnoses that place patients at risk for unneeded and potentially dangerous diagnostic tests and treatments and unnecessarily use limited health care resources.[95] Misplacement of one or more ECG electrodes is a common cause for errors in ECG interpretation. Some misplacements produce ECG patterns that can aid in identification of the error.[96,97] Reversal of the two arm electrodes, for example, results in an inverted P and QRS waveforms in lead I but not in lead V_6, two leads that would normally be expected to have similar polarities. Others are not as obvious. For example, placing the right precordial electrodes too high on the chest can yield patterns that mimic those produced by anterior myocardial infarction (poor R wave progression) or intraventricular conduction delay (rSr′ patterns). Electrical or mechanical artifacts such as produced by poor electrode contacts or tremors can simulate life-threatening arrhythmias[95] (Fig. 9–56), and excessive body motion can cause excessive baseline wander that may simulate an ST segment shift of myocardial ischemia or injury.

READING ERRORS. Errors in interpreting ECGs are common.[98-100] Studies assessing the accuracy of routine interpretations have demonstrated significant numbers of errors that can lead to clinical mismanagement, including failure to appropriately detect and triage patients with acute myocardial ischemia and other life-threatening situations. Organizations such as the American College of Cardiology have proposed minimal training and experience standards for electrocardiographers to help reduce these potentially serious errors.[100]

A final issue concerns overreliance on computerized interpretations. Computer systems have facilitated storage and retrieval of large numbers of ECGs and, as diagnostic algorithms have become more accurate, have provided important adjuncts to the clinical interpretation of ECGs. However, the current systems are not sufficiently accurate,[101] especially in the presence of rhythm disturbances or complex abnormalities, to be relied on in critical clinical environments without expert review. New analysis techniques based on artificial intelligence concepts may lead to future improvements,[102,103] and new hardware technology may result in expanded deployment of systems for prompt expert interpretation.[104]

ECGS FOR SELF-ASSESSMENT. A number of websites feature ECGs for self-assessment and clinical instruction. ECG Wave-Maven (http://ecg.bidmc.harvard.edu), for example, provides free access to more than 200 ECG case studies with answers and multimedia adjuncts.[105]

REFERENCES

Introduction and Fundamental Principles

1. Fisch C: Centennial of the string galvanometer and the electrocardiogram. J Am Coll Cardiol 26:1737, 2000.
2. Mirvis DM: Physiology and biophysics in electrocardiography. J Electrocardiol 29:175, 1996.
3. Ramanathan C, Rudy Y: Electrocardiographic imaging: I. Effect of torso inhomogeneities on body surface electrocardiographic potentials. J Cardiovasc Electrophysiol 12:229, 2001.
4. Madias JE, Bazaz B, Agarwal H, et al: Anasarca-mediated attenuation of the amplitude of electrocardiogram complexes: A description of a heretofore unrecognized phenomenon. J Am Coll Cardiol 38:756, 2001.
5. Novak PG, Davies C, Gin KG: Survey of British Columbia cardiologists' and emergency physicians: Practice of using nonstandard ECG leads (V_4R to V_6R and V_7 to V_9) in the diagnosis and treatment of acute myocardial infarction. Can J Cardiol 15:967, 1999.
6. Taccardi B, Punske BB, Lux RL, et al: Useful lessons from body surface mapping. J Cardiovasc Electrophysiol 9:773, 1998.
7. Horacek BM, Warren JW, Stovicek P, Feldman CL: Diagnostic accuracy of derived versus standard 12-lead electrocardiograms. J Electrocardiol 33(Suppl I):155, 2000.
8. Hurst JW: The use of the Grant method to interpret electrocardiograms. J Am Coll Cardiol 39:1878, 2002.

The Normal Electrocardiogram

9. Debbas NMG, Jackson SHD, de Jonghe D, et al: Human atrial depolarization: Effects of sinus rate, pacing and drugs on the surface electrocardiogram. J Am Coll Cardiol 33:358, 1999.
10. Markides V, Schilling RJ, Ho SY, et al: Characterization of left atrial activation in the intact human heart. Circulation 107:733, 2003.
11. Stovut DP, Wenstrom JC, Moeckel RB, et al: Respiratory sinus dysrhythmia persists in transplanted human hearts following autonomic blockade. Clin Exp Pharmacol Physiol 25:322, 1998.
12. Mietus JE, Peng CK, Henry I, Goldsmith RL, Goldberger AL: The pNNx-fiiles: Re-examining a widely-used heart rate variability measure. Heart 88:378, 2002.
13. Goldberger AL, Amaral LAN, Hausdorff JM, et al: Fractal dynamics in physiology: Alterations with disease and aging. Proc Natl Acad Sci U S A 99(suppl 1):2466, 2002.
14. Mathew TC, Shankariah L, Spodick DH: Electrocardiographic correlates of absent septal q waves. Am J Cardiol 82:809, 1998.
15. Yotsukura M, Toyofuku M, Tajino K, et al: Clinical signifiicance of the disappearanc of septal Q wave after the onset of myocardial infarction: Correlation with location of responsible coronary lesions. J Electrocardiol 32:15, 1999.
16. MacAlpin RN: In search of left septal fascicular block. Am Heart J 144:948, 2002.
17. MacLeod RS, Ni Q, Erschler PR, et al: Effects of heart position on the body surface electrocardiogram. J Electrocardiol 33(Suppl):229, 2000.
18. Surawicz B: U wave: Facts, hypotheses, misconceptions, and misnomers. J Cardiovasc Electrophysiol 9:1117, 1998.
19. Wu J, Wu J, Zipes DP: Early afterdepolarizations, U waves and torsades de pointes. Circulation 105:675, 2002.
20. Bednar MM, Harrigan EP, Anziano RJ, et al: The QT interval. Prog Cardiovasc Dis 43(Suppl I):1-45, 2001.
20a. Molnar J, Zhang F, Weiss J, et al: Diurnal pattern of QTc interval: How long is prolonged? Possible relation to circadian triggers of cardiovascular events. J Am Coll Cardiol 27:76, 1996.
20b. Malik M: Is there a physiologic QT/RR relationship? J Cardiovasc Electrophysiol 13:1211, 2002.
21. Franz MR, Zabel M: Electrophysiological basis of QT dispersion measurements. Prog Cardiovasc Dis 47:311, 2000.
22. Pellicia A, Maron BJ, Culasso F, et al: Clinical signifiicance of abnormal electrocardiographic patterns in trained athletes. Circulation 102:278, 2000.
23. Mehta M, Jain AC, Mehta A: Early repolarization. Clin Cardiol 27:59, 1999.
24. Surawicz B, Parikh SR: Prevalence of male and female patterns of early repolarization in the normal ECG of males and females from childhood to old age. J Am Coll Cardiol 40:1870, 2002.
25. Marcus RR, Kalisetti D, Raxwal V, et al: Early repolarization in patients with spinal cord injury: Prevalence and clinical signifiicance. J Spinal Cord Med 25:33, 2002.

Atrial Abnormalities; Ventricular Hypertrophy and Enlargement

26. Pinter A, Molin F, Savard P, et al: Body surface mapping of retrograde P waves in the intact dog by simulation of accessory pathway re-entry. Can J Cardiol 16:175, 2000.
27. Hazen MS, Marwick TH, Underwood DA: Diagnostic accuracy of the resting electrocardiogram in detection and estimation of left atrial enlargement: An echocardiographic correlation in 551 patients. Am Heart J 79:819, 1997.
28. Incalzi RA, Fuso L, De Rosa M, et al: Electrocardiographic signs of cor pulmonale: A negative prognostic finding in chronic obstructive pulmonary disease. Circulatio 99:1600, 1999.
29. Okin PM, Roman MJ, Devereux RB, et al: Time-voltage QRS area of the 12-lead electrocardiogram: Detection of left ventricular hypertrophy. Hypertension 31:937, 1998.
30. Okin PM, Devereux RB, Jern S, et al: Baseline characteristics in relation to electrocardiographic left ventricular hypertensive patients: The Losartan Intervention for End-point Reduction Study. Hypertension 36:766, 2000.
31. Okin PM, Devereux RB, Nieminen MS, et al: Relationship of the electrocardiographic strain pattern to left ventricular structure and function in hypertensive patients. Losartan Intervention For Endpoint. J Am Coll Cardiol 38:514, 2001.
32. Okin PM, Devereux RB, Fabsitz RR, et al: Quantitative assessment of electrocardiographic strain predicts increased left ventricular mass: The Strong Heart Study. J Am Coll Cardiol 40:1395, 2002.
33. Tomita S, Veno H, Takata M, et al: Relationship between electrocardiographic voltage and geometric patterns of left ventricular hypertrophy in patients with essential hypertension. Hypertens Res 21:259, 1998.
34. Rautaharju PM, Park LP, Gottdiener JS, et al: Race-and-sex-specifiic ECG models for lef ventricular mass in older populations. Factors infliuencing overestimation of left ve-tricular hypertrophy prevalence by ECG criteria in African-Americans. J Electrocardiol 33:205, 2000.
35. Okin PM, Jern S, Devereux RB, et al: Effect of obesity on electrocardiographic left ventricular hypertrophy in hypertensive patients: The losartan intervention for endpoint (LIFE) reduction in hypertension study. Hypertension 35:13, 2000.
36. Mirvis DM: The electrocardiogram as a prognostic tool. ACC Curr Rev J 4:181, 1999.
37. Menotti A, Seccareccia F: Electrocardiographic Minnesota code fiindings predictin short-term mortality in asymptomatic subjects. The Italian RIFLE Pooling Project (Risk Factors and Life Expectancy). G Ital Cardiol 27:40, 1997.
38. Sundstom J, Lind L, Arnlov J, et al: Echocardiographic and electrocardiographic diagnoses of left ventricular hypertrophy predict mortality independently of each other in a population of elderly men. Circulation 103:2346, 2001.

39. Jain A, Chandna H, Silber EN, et al: Electrocardiographic patterns of patients with echocardiographically determined biventricular hypertrophy. J Electrocardiol 32:269, 1999.

Intraventricular Conduction Delays and Preexcitation

40. Childers R, Lupovich S, Sochanski M, Knoarzewska H: Left bundle branch block and right axis deviation: A report of 36 cases. J Electrocardiol 33(Suppl):93, 2000.
41. Ducceschi V, Sarubbi B, D'Andrea A, et al: Electrophysiologic signifiicance of leftwar QRS axis deviation in bifascicular and trifascicular block. Clin Cardiol 21:597, 1998.
42. Mehdirad AA, Nelson SD, Love CJ, et al: QRS duration widening: Reduced synchronization of endocardial activation or transseptal conduction time? Pacing Clin Electrophysiol 21:1589, 1998.
43. Das MK, Cheriparambil K, Bedi A, et al: Prolonged QRS duration (QRS >/=170 ms) and left axis deviation in the presence of left bundle branch block: A marker for poor ventricular function? Am Heart J 142:756, 2001.
44. Skalidis EI, Kochiadakis GE, Koukouraki SI, et al: Phasic coronary flow pattern an flow reserve in patients with left bundle branch block and normal coronary arteries. J Am Coll Cardiol 33:1338, 1999.
45. Wagdy HM, Hodge D, Christian TF, et al: Prognostic value of vasodilator myocardial perfusion imaging in patients with left bundle branch block. Circulation 97:1563, 1998.
46. Peteiro J, Monserrat L, Martinez D, Castro-Beiras A: Accuracy of exercise echocardiography to detect coronary artery disease in left bundle branch block unassociated with either acute or healed myocardial infarction. Am J Cardiol 85:890, 2000.

Myocardial Ischemia and Infarction

47. Antzelevitch C, Brugada P, Brugada J, et al: Brugada syndrome: 1992-2003. A historical perspective. J Am Coll Cardiol 41:1665, 2003.
48. Zimetbaum PJ, Josephson ME: Use of the electrocardiogram in acute myocardial infarction. N Engl J Med 348:933, 2003.
49. Kleber AG: ST-segment elevation in the electrocardiogram: A sign of myocardial ischemia. Cardiovasc Res 45:111, 2000.
50. de Lemos JA, Antman EM, Giugliano RP, et al: ST-segment resolution and infarct-related artery patency and flow after thrombolytic therapy. Am J Cardiol 85:299, 2000.
51. van't Hof AW, Liem A, de Boer MJ, et al: Clinical value of 12-lead electrocardiogram after successful reperfusion therapy for acute myocardial infarction. Zwolle Myocardial Infarction Study Group. Lancet 350:615, 1997.
52. Phibbs B, Marcus F, Marriott HJ, et al: Q-wave versus non-Q-wave myocardial infarction: A meaningless distinction. J Am Coll Cardiol 33:576, 1999.
53. Bosimini E, Giannuzzi P, Temporelli PL, et al: Electrocardiographic evolutionary changes and left ventricular remodeling after acute myocardial infarction: Results of the GISSI-3 Echo substudy. J Am Coll Cardiol 35:127, 2000.
54. Nagase K, Tamura A, Mikuriya Y, et al: Signifiicance of Q-wave regression after anterior wall acute myocardial infarction. Eur Heart J 19:742, 1998.
55. Chikamori T, Kitaoka H, Matsumura Y, et al: Clinical and electrocardiographic profiile producing exercise-induced U-wave inversion in patients with severe narrowing of the left anterior descending coronary artery. Am J Cardiol 80:628, 1997.
56. Hohnloser SH: Effect of coronary ischemia on QT dispersion. Prog Cardiovasc Dis 42:351, 2000.
57. Malik M: QT dispersion: time for an obituary? Eur Heart J 12:955, 2000.
58. Bogaty P, Boyer L, Rousseau L, Arsenault M: Is anteroseptal myocardial infarction an appropriate term? Am J Med 113:37, 2002.
59. Schmitt C, Lehman G, Schmieder S, et al: Diagnosis of acute myocardial infarction in angiographically documented occluded infarct vessel: Limitations of ST-segment elevation in standard and extended ECG leads. Chest 120:1540, 2001.
60. Matetzky S, Freimark D, Chouraqui P, et al: Signifiicance f ST segment elevations in posterior chest leads (V_7 to V_9) in patients with acute inferior myocardial infarction: Application for thrombolytic therapy. J Am Coll Cardiol 31:506, 1998.
61. Menown IBA, Allen J, Anderson JMcC, et al: Early diagnosis of right ventricular or posterior infarction associated with inferior wall left ventricular acute myocardial infarction. Am J Cardiol 85:934, 2000.
62. Porter A, Herz I, Strasberg B: Isolated right ventricular infarction presenting as anterior wall myocardial infarction on electrocardiography. Clin Cardiol 20:971, 1997.
63. Kosuge M, Kimura K, Ishikawa T, et al: New electrocardiographic criteria for predicting the site of coronary artery occlusion in inferior wall acute myocardial infarction. Am J Cardiol 82:1318, 1998.
64. Herz I, Assali AR, Adler Y, et al: New electrocardiographic criteria for predicting either the right or left circumfllex artery as the culprit coronary artery in inferior wall acut myocardial infarction. Am J Cardiol 80:1343, 1997.
65. Assali AR, Sclarovsky S, Herz I, et al: Comparison of patients with inferior wall acute myocardial infarction with versus without ST-segment elevation in leads V_5 and V_6. Am J Cardiol 81:81, 1998.
66. Arbane M, Goy JJ: Prediction of the site of total occlusion in the left anterior descending coronary artery using admission electrocardiogram in anterior wall acute myocardial infarction. Am J Cardiol 85:487, 2000.
67. Yamaji H, Iwasaki K, Kusachi S, et al: Prediction of acute left main coronary artery obstruction by 12-lead electrocardiography. ST segment elevation in lead aVR with less ST segment elevation in lead V1. J Am Coll Cardiol 38:1348, 2001.
68. Yip HK, Chen MC, Wu CJ, et al: Acute myocardial infarction with simultaneous ST-segment elevation in the precordial and inferior leads: Evaluation of anatomic lesions and clinical implications. Chest 123:1170, 2003.
69. Madias JE, Sinha A, Ashitani R, et al: A critique of the new ST-segment criteria for the diagnosis of acute myocardial infarction in patients with left bundle-branch block. Clin Cardiol 10:652, 2001.
70. Laham CL, Hammill SC, Gibbons RJ: New criteria for the diagnosis of healed inferior wall myocardial infarction in patients with left bundle branch block. Am J Cardiol 79:19, 1997.
71. Sgarbossa EB, Pinski SL, Gates KB, et al: Early electrocardiographic diagnosis of acute myocardial infarction in the presence of ventricular paced rhythm. GUSTO-1 investigators. Am J Cardiol 77:423, 1996.
72. Welch RD, Zalenski RJ, Frederick PD, et al: Prognostic value of a normal or nonspecifiic initial electrocardiogram in acute myocardial infarction. JAMA 286:1977, 2001.
73. Kok LC, Mitchell MA, Haines DE, et al: Transient ST elevation after transthoracic cardioversion in patients with hemodynamically unstable ventricular tachyarrhythmia. Am J Cardiol 85:878, 2000.
74. Krishnan SC, Josephson ME: ST segment elevation induced by class IC antiarrhythmic agents: Underlying electrophysiologic mechanisms and insights into drug-induced proarrhythmia. J Cardiovasc Electrophysiol 9:1167, 1998.
75. Baljepally R, Spodick DH: PR-segment deviation as the initial electrocardiographic response in acute pericarditis. Am J Cardiol 81:1505, 1998.

Drug Effects, Electrolyte and Metabolic Abnormalities; Nonspecific QRS and ST-T Abnormalities; Alternans Patterns

76. Shvilkin A, Danilo P, Wang J, et al: Evolution and resolution of long-time cardiac memory. Circulation 97:1810, 1998.
77. Sundqvist K, Jogestrand T, Nowak J: The effect of digoxin on the electrocardiogram of healthy middle-aged and elderly patients at rest and during exercise: A comparison with the ECG reaction induced by myocardial ischemia. J Electrocardiol 35:213, 2002.
78. Reilly JG, Ayis SA, Ferrier IN, et al: QT_c-interval abnormalities and psychotropic drug therapy in psychiatric patients. Lancet 355:1048, 2000.
79. Martinez-Vea A, Bardaji A, Garcia C, et al: Severe hyperkalemia with minimal electrocardiographic manifestations: A report of seven cases. J Electrocardiol 32:45, 1999.
80. Antzelevitch C, Shimizu W, Yan GX, et al: The M cell: Its contribution to the ECG and to normal and abnormal electrical function of the heart. J Cardiovasc Electrophysiol 10:1124, 1999.
81. Greenland P, Xie X, Liu K, et al: Impact of minor electrocardiographic ST-segment and/or T-wave abnormalities on cardiovascular mortality during long-term follow-up. Am J Cardiol 91:1068, 2003.
82. Ho KK, Moody GB, Pang CK, et al: Predicting survival in heart-failure case and control subjects by use of fully automated methods for deriving non-linear and conventional indices of heart rate dynamics. Circulation 96:442, 1997.
83. Fisch C, Mandrola JM, Rardon DP: Electrocardiographic manifestations of dual atrioventricular node conduction during sinus rhythm. J Am Coll Cardiol 29:1015, 1997.
84. Maury P, Racka F, Piot C, Davy JM: QRS and cycle length alternans during paroxysmal supraventricular tachycardia: what is the mechanism? J Cardiovasc Electrophysiol 13:92, 2002.
85. Hall K, Christini DJ, Tremblay M, et al: Dynamic control of cardiac alternans. Phys Rev Lett 78:4518, 1997.
86. Laguna P, Moody GB, Garcia J, et al: Analysis of the ST-T complex of the electrocardiogram using the Karhunen-Loève transform: Adaptive monitoring and alternans detection. Med Biol Eng Comput 37:175, 1999.
87. Pastore JM, Girouard SD, Laurita KR, et al: Mechanism linking T-wave alternans to the genesis of cardiac fiibrillation. Circulation 99:1385, 1999.
88. Gold MR, Bloomfiield DM, Anderson KP, et al: A comparison of T-wave alternans, signa averaged electrocardiography and programmed ventricular stimulation for arrhythmia risk stratifiication. J Am Coll Cardiol 36:2247, 2000.
89. Shimizu W, Antzelevitch C: Cellular and ionic basis for T-wave alternans under long Q-T conditions. Circulation 99:1499, 1999.

Clinical Issues in Electrocardiographic Interpretation

90. Stafford RS, Misra B: Variation in routine electrocardiogram use in academic primary care practice. Arch Intern Med 161:2351, 2001.
91. Ashley EA, Raxwal VK, Froelicher VF: The prevalence and prognostic signifiiance of electrocardiographic abnormalities. Curr Probl Cardiol 25:1, 2000.
92. Murdoch CJ, Murdoch DR, McIntyre P, et al: The preoperative ECG in day surgery: A habit? Anaesthesia 54:907, 1999.
93. Hatala R, Norman GR, Brooks LR: Impact of a clinical scenario on accuracy of electrocardiogram interpretation. J Gen Intern Med 14:126, 1999.
94. Pope JH, Aufderheide TP, Ruthazer R, et al: Missed diagnoses of cardiac ischemia in the emergency department. N Engl J Med 342:1163, 2000.
95. Knight BP, Michaud GF, Strickberger SA, et al: Clinical consequences of electrocardiographic artifact mimicking ventricular tachycardia. N Engl J Med 341:1270, 1999.
96. Ho KK, Ho SK: Use of the sinus P wave in diagnosing electrocardiographic limb lead misplacement not involving the right leg (ground) lead. J Electrocardiol 34:161, 2001.
97. Hurst JW: Electrocardiographic crotchets or common errors made in the interpretation of the electrocardiogram. Clin Cardiol 21:211, 1998.
98. Sur DK, Kaye L, Goad J, Morena A: Accuracy of electrocardiogram reading by family practice residents. Fam Med 32:315, 2000.
99. Goodacre S, Webster A, Morris F: Do computer generated ECG reports improve interpretation by accident and emergency room house offiicers? Postgrad Med J 7:455, 2001.
100. Kadish AH, Buxton AE, Kennedy HL, et al: ACC/AHA clinical competence statement on electrocardiography and ambulatory electrocardiography. Circulation 104:3169, 2001.
101. Spodick D: Computer treason: Intraobserver variability of an electrocardiographic computer system. Am J Cardiol 80:102, 1997.
102. Hedén B, Öhlin H, Rittner R, et al: Acute myocardial infarction detected in the 12-lead ECG by artifiicial neural networks. Circulation 96:1798, 1997.
103. Holst H, Ohlsson M, Peterson C, Edenbrandt L: A confiident decision support syste for interpreting electrocardiograms. Clin Physiol 19:410, 1999.
104. Pettis KS, Savona MR, Leibrandt PN, et al: Evaluation of the efficacy of hand-held co-puter screens for cardiologists' interpretation of 12-lead electrocardiograms. Am Heart J 138:765, 1999.
105. McClennen S, Nathanson LA, Safran C, Goldberger AL: ECG Wave-Maven: An Internet-based electrocardiography self-assessment program for students and clinicians. Med Educ Online 8:2, 2003. (http://www.med-ed-online.org/issue2.htm#v8)

Electrocardiography

Guidelines for the performance of electrocardiograms (ECGs) have evolved little in recent years. The most widely cited guidelines were published by the American College of Cardiology and American Heart Association (ACC/AHA) in 1992.[1] These guidelines make recommendations on the use of ECGs in patients with and without cardiovascular disease. Other guidelines were published by the American Heart Association in 1987,[2] by a task force assembled by the Canadian government in 1991,[3] and by the US Preventive Task Force (USPTF) in 1996.[4] Standards for clinical competence were recommended more recently (in 2001) by an ACC/AHA task force.[5]

Patients with Known Cardiovascular Disease or Dysfunction

The ACC/AHA guidelines[1] endorse the use of ECGs in the baseline evaluation of all patients with known cardiovascular disease and for the evaluation of response to therapies likely to produce ECG changes (Table 9G–1). These guidelines use the older ACC/AHA convention of classifying indications according to one of three classes. Class I indications are conditions for which it is generally agreed that ECGs are useful. Class II indications are conditions for which opinions differ with

TABLE 9G–1 ACC/AHA Guidelines for Electrocardiography in Patients with Known Cardiovascular Disease or Dysfunction

Indication	Class I (appropriate)	Class II (equivocal)	Class III (inappropriate)
Baseline or initial evaluation	All patients	None	None
Response to therapy	Patients in whom prescribed therapy is known to produce ECG changes that correlate with therapeutic responses or progression of disease. Patients in whom prescribed therapy may produce adverse effects that may be predicted from or detected by ECG changes.	None	Patients receiving pharmacological or nonpharmacological therapy not known to produce ECG changes or to affect conditions that may be associated with such changes.
Follow-up	Patients with a change in symptoms, signs, or relevant laboratory findings. Patients with an implanted pacemaker or antitachycardia device. Patients with symptoms such as the following conditions, even in the absence of new symptoms or signs, after an interval of time appropriate for the condition or disease: Syncope and near-syncope Unexplained change in the usual pattern of angina pectoris Chest pain New or worsening dyspnea Extreme and unexplained fatigue, weakness, and prostration Palpitation New signs of congestive heart failure A new organic murmur or pericardial friction rub New findings suggesting pulmonary hypertension Accelerating or poorly controlled systemic arterial hypertension Evidence of a recent cerebrovascular accident Unexplained fever in patients with known valvular disease New onset of cardiac arrhythmia or inappropriate heart rate Chronic known congenital or acquired cardiovascular disease		Adult patients whose cardiovascular condition is usually benign and unlikely to progress (e.g., patients with asymptomatic mild mitral valve prolapse, mild hypertension, or premature contractions in the absence of organic heart disease) Adult patients with chronic stable heart disease seen at frequent intervals (i.e., 4 months) and who have no new or unexplained findings.
Before surgery	All patients with known cardiovascular disease or dysfunction except as noted under Class II.	Patients with hemodynamically insignificant congenital or acquired heart disease, mild systemic hypertension, or infrequent premature complexes in the absence of organic heart disease.	None

TABLE 9G–2 ACC/AHA Guidelines for Electrocardiography in Patients Suspected of Having or Who Are at Increased Risk for Cardiovascular Disease or Dysfunction

Setting	Class I (appropriate)	Class II (equivocal)	Class III (inappropriate)
Baseline or initial evaluation	All patients suspected of having or being at increased risk for cardiovascular disease. Patients who may have used cocaine, amphetamines, or other illicit drugs known to have cardiac effects. Patients who may have received an overdose of a drug known to have cardiac effects.	None	None
Response to therapy	To assess therapy with cardioactive drugs in patients with suspected cardiac disease. To assess the response to the administration of any agent known to result in cardiac abnormalities or ECG abnormalities (e.g., antineoplastic drugs, lithium, and antidepressant agents).	To assess the response to administration of any agent known to alter serum electrolyte concentrations.	To assess the response to administration of agents known not to influence cardiac structure or function.
Follow-up	The presence of any change in clinical status or laboratory findings suggesting interval development of cardiac disease or dysfunction. Periodic follow-up (e.g., every 1 to 5 yr) of patients known to be at increased risk for cardiac disease. Follow-up of patients after resolution of chest pain.	None	Follow-up ECGs more often than once yearly are not indicated in patients who remain clinically stable, who are not at increased risk for the development of cardiac disease, and who have not been demonstrated to have cardiac disease with previous studies.
Before surgery	As part of the preoperative evaluation of any patient with suspected, or at increased risk of developing, cardiac disease or dysfunction.	None	None

TABLE 9G–3 ACC/AHA Guidelines for Electrocardiography in Patients with No Apparent or Suspected Heart Disease or Dysfunction

Setting	Class I (appropriate)	Class II (equivocal)	Class III (inappropriate)
Baseline or initial evaluation	Persons aged 40 or more years undergoing physical examination. Before administration of pharmacological agents known to have a high incidence of cardiovascular effects (e.g., antineoplastic agents). Before exercise stress testing. People of any age who are in special occupations that require very high cardiovascular performance (e.g., fire fighters, police officers) or whose cardiovascular performance is linked to public safety (e.g., pilots, air traffic controllers, critical process operators, bus or truck drivers, and railroad engineers).	To evaluate competitive athletes	Routine screening or baseline ECGS in asymptomatic persons younger than 40 yr with no risk factors.
Response to therapy	To evaluate patients in whom prescribed therapy (e.g., doxorubicin) is known to produce cardiovascular effects.	None	To assess treatment that is known to not produce any cardiovascular effects.
Follow-up	To evaluate asymptomatic persons >40 yr of age.	None	To evaluate asymptomatic adults who have had no interval change in symptoms, signs, or risk factors and who have had a normal ECG within the recent past.
Before surgery	Patients >40 yr of age. Patients being evaluated as a donor for heart transplantation or as a recipient of a noncardiopulmonary transplant.	Patients 30–40 yr of age	Patients younger than 30 yr with no risk factors for coronary artery disease.

respect to the usefulness of ECGs. Class III indications are conditions for which it is generally agreed that ECGs have little or no usefulness.

The ACC/AHA guidelines do not comment on the frequency of follow-up ECGs but do endorse the use of serial ECGs for patients with known cardiovascular disease whenever there are changes in symptoms, signs, or laboratory findings. Even in the absence of such changes, follow-up ECGs are considered appropriate for patients with syndromes such as syncope, chest pain, and extreme fatigue. Follow-up ECGs are not considered appropriate for patients with mild chronic cardiovascular conditions that are not considered likely to progress (e.g., mild mitral valve prolapse). ECGs at each visit are considered inappropriate for patients with stable heart disease who are seen frequently (e.g., within 4 months) and have no evidence of clinical change.

Before surgical procedures, ECGs are considered appropriate for all patients with known cardiovascular disease or dysfunction, except those with insignificant or mild conditions such as mild systemic arterial hypertension.

Patients with Suspected Cardiovascular Disease or at High Risk for Cardiovascular Disease

The ACC/AHA guidelines make similar recommendations for patients with suspected cardiovascular disease and those who are at high risk for such conditions for the use of ECGs at baseline, for evaluation of the response to therapy, and before surgery (Table 9G–2). In the follow-up of patients at increased risk for heart disease, ECGs every 1 to 5 years are considered appropriate, but routine screening ECGs more frequently than yearly are not supported for patients who remain clinically stable, as long as they had not been previously demonstrated to have heart disease.

Patients without Known or Suspected Heart Disease

The various guidelines differ in their recommendations for the use of ECGs to screen for cardiovascular disease in healthy people. In the ACC/AHA guidelines, ECGs are considered appropriate screening tests in patients without apparent or suspected heart disease who are 40 years of age or older (Table 9G–3). Earlier guidelines from the AHA recommended that ECGs be obtained at ages 20, 40, and 60 years.[2] In contrast, the U.S. Preventive Services Task Force and the task force assembled by the Canadian government did not find evidence to support the use of screening ECG.[3,4]

The ACC/AHA guidelines recommend ECGs for patients for whom drugs with a high incidence of cardiovascular effects (e.g., chemotherapy) or exercise testing is planned and for people of any age in occupations with high cardiovascular demands or whose cardiovascular status might affect the safety of many other people (e.g., airline pilots). ECGs are considered appropriate before surgery in patients 40 of age or older and are equivocal in patients between the ages of 30 and 40 years in these guidelines. More recent guidelines from the ACC/AHA for perioperative evaluation[6] found good evidence for ECGs before noncardiac surgery in asymptomatic patients with diabetes (Table 76G–1), but otherwise do not strongly endorse routine preoperative ECG testing in patients without cardiovascular symptoms.

Clinical Competence

The ACC/AHA Clinical Competence Statement on electrocardiography[5] provides an overview for minimal standards for performance and interpretation of ECGs. In addition to making recommendations for the list of diagnoses with which ECG interpreters should be familiar, the Statement asserts that computer interpretations must be reviewed by an experienced electrocardiographer. The Task Force recommended a minimum of 100 ECG interpretations a year to maintain competence.

References

1. Schlant RC, Adolph RJ, DiMarco JP, et al: Guidelines for electrocardiography: A report of the American College of Cardiology/American Heart Association Task Force on Assessment of Diagnostic and Therapeutic Cardiovascular Procedures (Committee on Electrocardiography). J Am Coll Cardiol 19:473, 1992.
2. Grundy SM, Greenland P, Herd A, et al: Cardiovascular and risk factor evaluation of healthy American adults: A statement for physicians by an ad hoc committee appointed by the Steering Committee, American Heart Association. Circulation 75:1340A, 1987.
3. Hayward RSA, Steinberg EP, Ford DE, et al: Preventive care guidelines: 1991. Ann Intern Med 114:758, 1991.
4. US Preventive Task Force: Guide to Clinical Preventive Services. 2nd ed. Baltimore, Williams & Wilkins, 1996.
5. Kadish AH, Buxton AE, Kennedy HL, et al: ACC/AHA clinical competence statement on electrocardiography and ambulatory electrocardiography: A report of the American College of Cardiology/American Heart Association/American College of Physicians-American Society of Internal Medicine Task Force on Clinical Competence (ACC/AHA Committee to Develop a Clinical Competence Statement on Electrocardiography and Ambulatory Electrocardiography); Circulation104:3169, 2001.
6. Eagle KA, Berger PB, Calkins H, et al: ACC/AHA guideline update for perioperative cardiovascular evaluation for noncardiac surgery: A report of the American College of Cardiology/ American Heart Association Task Force on Practice Guidelines (Committee to Update the 1996 Guidelines on Perioperative Cardiovascular Evaluation for Noncardiac Surgery). 2002. American College of Cardiology Web site. (http:/www.acc.org/clinical/guidelines/perio/dirIndex.htm)

CHAPTER 10

Exercise Stress Testing

Bernard R. Chaitman

Exercise is a common physiological stress used to elicit cardiovascular abnormalities not present at rest and to determine the adequacy of cardiac function.[1-11] Exercise electrocardiography (ECG) is one of the most frequent noninvasive modalities used to assess patients with suspected or proven cardiovascular disease. The test is mainly used to estimate prognosis and to determine functional capacity, the likelihood and extent of coronary artery disease (CAD), and the effects of therapy. Hemodynamic and ECG measurements combined with ancillary techniques such as metabolic gas analysis, radionuclide imaging, and echocardiography enhance the information content of exercise testing in selected patients.[5]

Exercise Physiology

Anticipation of dynamic exercise results in an acceleration of ventricular rate due to vagal withdrawal, increase in alveolar ventilation, and increased venous return primarily as a result of sympathetic venoconstriction.[12] In normal persons, the net effect is to increase resting cardiac output before the start of exercise. The magnitude of hemodynamic response during exercise depends on the severity of the exercise and the amount of muscle mass involved. In the early phases of exercise in the upright position, cardiac output is increased by an augmentation in stroke volume mediated through the use of the Frank-Starling mechanism and heart rate; the increase in cardiac output in the latter phases of exercise is primarily due to a sympathetic-mediated increase in ventricular rate. At fixed submaximal workloads below anaerobic threshold, steady-state conditions are usually reached after the second minute of exercise, following which heart rate, cardiac output, blood pressure, and pulmonary ventilation are maintained at reasonably constant levels.[1,8] During strenuous exertion, sympathetic discharge is maximal and parasympathetic stimulation is withdrawn, resulting in vasoconstriction of most circulatory body systems, except for that in exercising muscle and in the cerebral and coronary circulations. Venous and arterial norepinephrine release from sympathetic postganglionic nerve endings, as well as plasma renin levels, are increased; the catecholamine release enhances ventricular contractility. As exercise progresses, skeletal muscle blood flow is increased, oxygen extraction increases by as much as threefold, total calculated peripheral resistance decreases, and systolic blood pressure, mean arterial pressure, and pulse pressure usually increase. Diastolic blood pressure does not change significantly. The pulmonary vascular bed can accommodate as much as a sixfold increase in cardiac output with only modest increases in pulmonary artery pressure, pulmonary capillary wedge pressure, and right atrial pressure; in normal individuals, this is not a limiting determinant of peak exercise capacity.

Cardiac output increases by four- to sixfold above basal levels during strenuous exertion in the upright position, depending on genetic endowment and level of training.[12] The maximum heart rate and cardiac output are decreased in older individuals, partly because of decreased beta-adrenergic responsivity.[13,14] Maximum heart rate can be estimated from the formula 220 − age in years, with a standard deviation of 10 to 12 beats per minute. The age-predicted maximum heart rate is a useful measurement for safety reasons. However, the wide standard deviation in the various regression equations used and the impact of drug therapy limit the usefulness of this parameter in estimating the exact age-predicted maximum for an individual patient.[15]

In the postexercise phase, hemodynamics return to baseline within minutes of termination of exercise. Vagal reactivation is an important cardiac deceleration mechanism after exercise and is accelerated in well-trained athletes but blunted in patients with chronic heart failure (see also section on heart rate). Intense physical work or significant cardiorespiratory impairment may interfere with achievement of a steady state, and an oxygen deficit occurs during exercise. The total oxygen uptake in excess of the resting oxygen uptake during the recovery period is the oxygen debt.

PATIENT'S POSITION

At rest, the cardiac output and stroke volume are higher when the person is in the supine position than when the person is in the upright position. With exercise in normal supine persons, the elevation of cardiac output results almost entirely from an increase in heart rate, with little augmentation of stroke volume. In the upright posture, the increase in cardiac output in normal individuals results from a combination of elevations in stroke volume and heart rate. A change from supine to upright posture causes a decrease in venous return, left ventricular end-diastolic volume and pressure, stroke volume, and cardiac index. Renin and norepinephrine levels are increased. End-systolic volume and ejection fraction are not significantly changed. In normal individuals, end-systolic volume decreases and ejection fraction increases to a similar extent from rest to exercise in the supine and upright positions. The magnitude and direction of change in end-diastolic volume from rest to maximum exercise in both positions are small and may vary according to the patient population studied. The net effect on exercise performance is an approximate 10 percent increase in exercise time, cardiac index, heart rate, and rate pressure product at peak exercise in the upright as compared with the supine position.

Cardiopulmonary Exercise Testing

Cardiopulmonary exercise testing involves measurements of respiratory oxygen uptake ($\dot{V}O_2$), carbon dioxide production ($\dot{V}CO_2$), and ventilatory parameters during a symptom-limited exercise test. During testing, the patient usually wears a nose clip and breathes through a nonrebreathing valve that separates expired air from room air. Important measurements of expired gas are PO_2, PCO_2, and air flow. Ventilatory measurements include respiratory rate, tidal volume, and minute ventilation ($\dot{V}e$). PO_2 and PCO_2 are sampled breath by breath or by use of a mixing chamber. The $\dot{V}O_2$ and $\dot{V}CO_2$ can be computed from ventilatory volumes and differences between inspired and expired gases.[4,5] Under steady-state conditions, $\dot{V}O_2$ and $\dot{V}CO_2$ measured at the mouth are equivalent to total-body oxygen consumption and carbon dioxide production. The relationship between work output, oxygen consumption, heart rate, and cardiac output during exercise is linear (Fig. 10–1). $\dot{V}O_2$max is the product of maximal arterial-venous oxygen difference and cardiac output and represents the largest amount of oxygen a person can use while performing dynamic exercise involving a large part of total muscle mass. The $\dot{V}O_2$max decreases with age, is usually less in women than in men, and can vary among individuals as a result of genetic factors.[4,5] $\dot{V}O_2$max is diminished by degree of cardiovascular impairment and by physical inactivity. In untrained persons, the arterial-mixed venous oxygen difference at peak exercise is relatively constant (14 to 17 volume-percent), and $\dot{V}O_2$max is an approximation of maximum cardiac output. Measured $\dot{V}O_2$max can be compared with predicted values from empirically derived formulas based on age, sex, weight, and height.[3-5] Most clinical studies that use exercise as a stress to assess cardiac reserve report peak $\dot{V}O_2$ that is the highest $\dot{V}O_2$ attained during graded exercise testing rather than $\dot{V}O_2$max. Peak exercise capacity is decreased when the ratio of measured to predicted $\dot{V}O_2$max is less than 85 to 90 percent. Oximetry, performed noninvasively, can be used to monitor arterial oxygen saturation, and the value normally does not decrease by more than 5 percent during exercise.[6] Estimates of oxygen saturation during strenuous exercise using pulse oximetry can be unreliable in some patients.

ANAEROBIC THRESHOLD. Anaerobic threshold is a theoretical point during dynamic exercise when muscle tissue switches over to anaerobic metabolism as an additional energy source. All tissues do not shift simultaneously, and there is a brief interval during which exercise muscle tissue shifts from predominantly aerobic to anaerobic metabolism.[4,5] Lactic acid begins to accumulate when a healthy untrained subject reaches about 50 to 60 percent of the maximal capacity for aerobic metabolism. The increase in lactic acid becomes greater as exercise becomes more intense, resulting in metabolic acidosis. As lactate is formed, it is buffered in the serum by the bicarbonate system, resulting in increased carbon dioxide excretion, which causes reflex hyperventilation. The gas exchange anaerobic threshold is the point at which $\dot{V}e$ increases disproportionately relative to $\dot{V}O_2$ and work; it usually occurs at 40 to 60 percent of $\dot{V}O_2$max in normal, untrained individuals with a wide range of normal values between 35 and 80 percent. Below the anaerobic threshold, carbon dioxide production is proportional to oxygen consumption. Above the anaerobic threshold, carbon dioxide is produced in excess of oxygen consumption. There are several methods to determine anaerobic threshold, which include (1) the V-slope method, the point at which the rate of increase in $\dot{V}CO_2$ relative to $\dot{V}O_2$ increases (see Fig. 10–1); (2) the point at which the $\dot{V}O_2$ and $\dot{V}CO_2$ slopes intersect; and (3) the point at which the ratio of $\dot{V}e/\dot{V}O_2$ and end-tidal oxygen tension begins to increase systematically without an immediate increase in the $\dot{V}e/\dot{V}O_2$ (see Fig. 10–1). The anaerobic threshold is a useful parameter because work below this level encompasses most activities of daily living. Anaerobic threshold is often reduced in patients with significant cardiovascular disease. An increase in anaerobic threshold with training can enhance an individual's capacity to perform sustained submaximal activities, with consequent improvement in quality of life and daily living. Changes in anaerobic

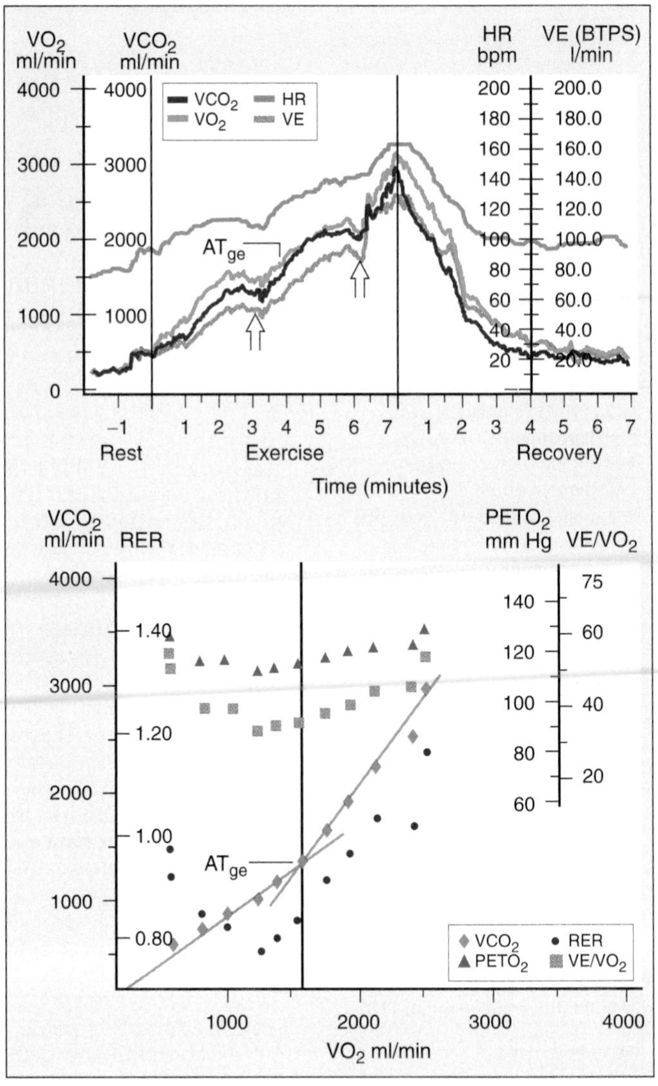

FIGURE 10–1 Cardiopulmonary exercise test in a healthy 53-year-old man using the Bruce protocol. The progressive linear increase in work output, heart rate (HR), and oxygen consumption ($\dot{V}O_2$) is noted, with steady-state conditions reached after 2 minutes in each of the first two stages **(top)**. Open arrows indicate the beginning of each new 3-minute stage. The subject completed 7 minutes and 10 seconds of exercise, and peak $\dot{V}O_2$ was 3.08 liters/min. The anaerobic threshold (AT_{ge}), determined by the V-slope method, is the point at which the slope of the relative rate of increase in $\dot{V}CO_2$ relative to $\dot{V}O_2$ changes; it occurred at a $\dot{V}O_2$ of 1.5 liters/min, or 49 percent of peak $\dot{V}O_2$, within predicted values for a normal sedentary population **(bottom)**. The AT_{ge} determined by the point at which the $\dot{V}O_2$ and $\dot{V}CO_2$ slopes intersect (1.8 liters/min) **(top)** is slightly greater than the AT_{ge} determined by the V-slope method **(bottom)**. The V-slope method usually provides a more reproducible estimate of AT_{ge}. $PETO_2$ = end-tidal pressure of oxygen; RER = respiratory exchange ratio; $\dot{V}e/\dot{V}O_2$ = ratio of ventilation to oxygen uptake.

threshold and peak $\dot{V}O_2$ with repeat testing can be used to assess disease progression, response to medical therapy, and improvement in cardiovascular fitness with training.

VENTILATORY PARAMETERS. In addition to peak $\dot{V}O_2$, minute ventilation and its relation to $\dot{V}CO_2$ and oxygen consumption are useful indices of cardiac and pulmonary function.[4,5,16,17] The respiratory exchange ratio represents the amount of carbon dioxide produced divided by the amount of oxygen consumed. The respiratory exchange ratio ranges from 0.7 to 0.85 at rest and is partly dependent on the predominant fuel used for cellular metabolism (e.g., the respiratory exchange rate for predominant carbohydrate use is 1.0, whereas the respiratory exchange ratio for predominant fatty acid use is 0.7). At high exercise levels, carbon dioxide production exceeds $\dot{V}O_2$, and a respiratory exchange ratio greater than 1.1 often indicates that the subject has performed at maximal effort.

METABOLIC EQUIVALENT. In current use, the term *metabolic equivalent* (MET) refers to a unit of oxygen uptake in a sitting, resting person; 1 MET is equivalent to 3.5 ml O_2/kg/min of body weight. Measured $\dot{V}O_2$ in ml O_2/min/kg divided by 3.5 ml O_2/kg/min determines the number of METs associated with activity. Work activities can be calculated in multiples of METs; this measurement is useful to determine exercise prescriptions, assess disability, and standardize the reporting of submaximal and peak exercise workloads when different protocols are used. An exercise workload of 3 to 5 METs is consistent with activities such as raking leaves, light carpentry, golf, and walking at 3 to 4 mph. Workloads of 5 to 7 METs are consistent with exterior carpentry, singles tennis, and light backpacking. Workloads in excess of 9 METs are compatible with heavy labor, handball, squash, and running at 6 to 7 mph. Estimating $\dot{V}O_2$ from work rate or treadmill time in individual patients may lead to misinterpretation of data if exercise equipment is not correctly calibrated, when the patient holds on to the front handrails, or if the patient fails to achieve steady state, is obese, or has peripheral vascular disease, pulmonary vascular disease, or cardiac impairment. $\dot{V}O_2$ does not increase linearly in some patients with cardiovascular or pulmonary disease as work rate is increased, and $\dot{V}O_2$ can thus be overestimated. The measurements obtained with cardiopulmonary exercise testing are useful in understanding an individual patient's response to exercise and can be useful in the diagnostic evaluation of a patient with dyspnea.[3-5,8]

Exercise Protocols

The main types of exercise are isotonic or dynamic exercise, isometric or static exercise, and resistive (combined isometric and isotonic) exercise. Dynamic protocols most frequently are used to assess cardiovascular reserve, and those suitable for clinical testing should include a low-intensity warm-up phase. In general, 6 to 12 minutes of continuous progressive exercise during which the myocardial oxygen demand is elevated to the patient's maximal level is optimal for diagnostic and prognostic purposes.[8] The protocol should include a suitable recovery or cool-down period. If the protocol is too strenuous for an individual patient, the test must be terminated early, and there is no opportunity to observe clinically important responses. If the exercise protocol is too easy for an individual patient, the prolonged procedure tests endurance and not aerobic capacity. Thus, exercise protocols should be individualized to accommodate a patient's limitations. Protocols may be set up at a fixed duration of exercise for a certain intensity to meet minimal qualifications for certain industrial tasks or sports programs.

STATIC EXERCISE. This form of isometric exercise generates force with little muscle shortening and produces a greater blood pressure response than dynamic exercise.11 Cardiac output does not increase as much as with dynamic exercise, because increased resistance in active muscle groups limits blood flow. In a common form of static exercise, the patient's maximal force on a hand dynamometer is recorded. The patient then sustains 25 to 33 percent of maximal force for 3 to 5 minutes while ECG and blood pressure are recorded. The increase in myocardial $\dot{V}O_2$ is often insufficient to initiate an ischemic response.

ARM ERGOMETRY. Arm crank ergometry protocols involve arm cranking at incremental workloads of 10 to 20 W for 2- or 3-minute stages. The heart rate and blood pressure responses to a given workload of arm exercise usually are greater than those for leg exercise. A bicycle ergometer with the axle placed at the level of the shoulders is used, and the subject sits or stands and cycles the peddles so that the arms are alternately fully extended. The most common frequency is 50 rpm. In normal individuals, maximal $\dot{V}O_2$ and $\dot{V}e$ for arm cycling approximates 50 to 70 percent of the same measures as leg cycling. Peak $\dot{V}O_2$ and peak heart rate are approximately 70 percent of the measures during leg testing. Arm ergometry exercise protocols for risk stratification of patients with suspected or documented CAD before noncardiac surgery can be used as a stressor when leg exercise is not possible or insufficient to test cardiac reserve.

BICYCLE ERGOMETRY. Bicycle protocols involve incremental workloads calibrated in watts or kilopond-meters per minute (kpm). One watt is equivalent to approximately 6 kpm. Because exercise on a cycle ergometer is not weight bearing, kpm or watts can be converted to oxygen uptake in milliliters per minute. In mechanically braked bicycles, work is determined by force and distance and requires a constant pedaling rate of 60 to 80 rpm, according to the patient's preference. Electronically braked bicycles provide a constant workload despite changes in pedaling rate and are less dependent on a patient's cooperation. They are more costly than a mechanically braked bicycle but are preferred for diagnostic and prognostic assessment. Most protocols start with a power output of 10 or 25 W/min (150 kpm), usually followed by increases of 25 W every 2 or 3 minutes until endpoints are reached. Younger subjects can start at 50 W, with increases in 50-W increments every 2 minutes. A ramp protocol differs from the staged protocols in that the patient starts at 3 minutes of unloaded pedaling at a cycle speed of 60 rpm. Work rate is increased by a uniform amount each minute, ranging from 5- to 30-W increments, depending on a patient's expected performance. Exercise is terminated if the patient is unable to maintain a cycling frequency above 40 rpm. In the cardiac catheterization laboratory, hemodynamic measurements can be made during supine bicycle ergometry at rest and at one or two submaximal workloads.

The bicycle ergometer is associated with a lower maximal $\dot{V}O_2$ and anaerobic threshold than the treadmill; maximal heart rate, maximal $\dot{V}e$, and maximal lactate values are often similar. The bicycle ergometer has the advantage of requiring less space than a treadmill; it is quieter and permits sensitive precordial measurements without much motion artifact. However, in North America, treadmill protocols are more widely used in the assessment of patients with coronary disease.

TREADMILL PROTOCOL. The treadmill protocol should be consistent with the patient's physical capacity and the purpose of the test. In healthy individuals, the standard Bruce protocol is popular, and a large diagnostic and prognostic data base has been published using this protocol.[1,2,7,8] The Bruce multistage maximal treadmill protocol has 3-minute periods to allow achievement of a steady state before workload is increased (Figs. 10–1 and 10–2). In older individuals or those whose exercise capacity is limited by cardiac disease, the protocol can be modified by two 3-minute warm-up stages at 1.7 mph and 0 percent grade and 1.7 mph and 5

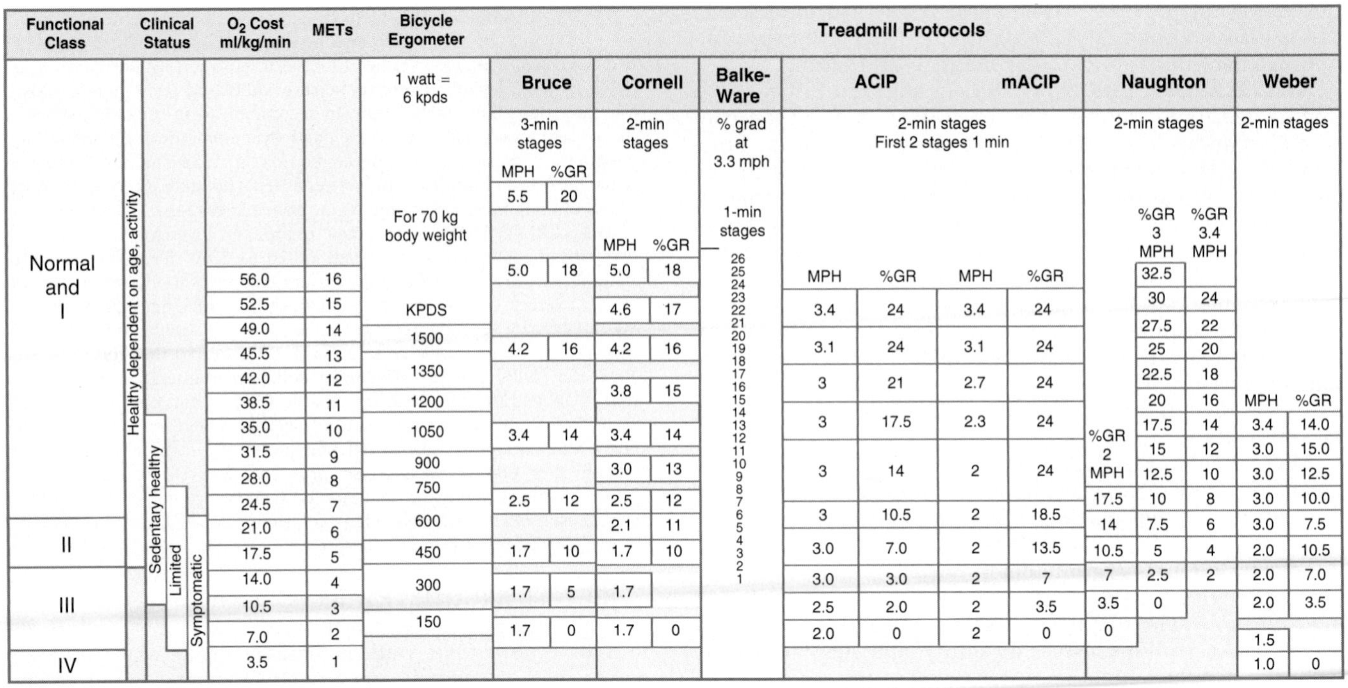
Functional Class
Clinical Status
O_2 Cost ml/kg/min
METs
Bicycle Ergometer
Treadmill Protocols
1 watt = 6 kpds
For 70 kg body weight
KPDS
Bruce
3-min stages
Cornell
2-min stages
Balke-Ware
% grad at 3.3 mph
1-min stages
ACIP
mACIP
2-min stages First 2 stages 1 min
Naughton
2-min stages
Weber
2-min stages
Normal and I
II
III
IV
Healthy dependent on age, activity
Sedentary healthy
Limited
Symptomatic
56.0 16
52.5 15
49.0 14
45.5 13
42.0 12
38.5 11
35.0 10
31.5 9
28.0 8
24.5 7
21.0 6
17.5 5
14.0 4
10.5 3
7.0 2
3.5 1
1500
1350
1200
1050
900
750
600
450
300
150
MPH %GR
5.5 20
5.0 18
4.2 16
3.4 14
2.5 12
1.7 10
1.7 5
1.7 0
MPH %GR
5.0 18
4.6 17
4.2 16
3.8 15
3.4 14
3.0 13
2.5 12
2.1 11
1.7 10
1.7
1.7 0
26 25 24 23 22 21 20 19 18 17 16 15 14 13 12 11 10 9 8 7 6 5 4 3 2 1
MPH %GR MPH %GR
3.4 24 3.4 24
3.1 24 3.1 24
3 21 2.7 24
3 17.5 2.3 24
3 14 2 24
3 10.5 2 18.5
3.0 7.0 2 13.5
3.0 3.0 2 7
2.5 2.0 2 3.5
2.0 0 2 0
%GR 2 MPH
17.5
14
10.5
7
3.5
0
%GR 3 MPH
32.5
30
27.5
25
22.5
20
17.5
15
12.5
10
7.5
5
2.5
0
%GR 3.4 MPH
24
22
20
18
16
14
12
10
8
6
4
2
MPH %GR
3.4 14.0
3.0 15.0
3.0 12.5
3.0 10.0
3.0 7.5
2.0 10.5
2.0 7.0
2.0 3.5
1.5
1.0 0

FIGURE 10–2 Estimated oxygen cost of bicycle ergometer and selected treadmill protocols. The standard Bruce protocol starts at 1.7 mph and 10 percent grade (5 METs), with a larger increment between stages than protocols such as the Naughton, ACIP, and Weber, which start at less than 2 METs at 2 mph and increase by 1- to 1.5-MET increments between stages. The Bruce protocol can be modified by two 3-minute warm-up stages at 1.7 mph and 0 percent grade and 1.7 mph and 5 percent grade. METs = metabolic equivalents. (Adapted from Fletcher GF, Balady G, Amsterdam EA, et al: Exercise Standards for Testing and Training. A statement for healthcare professionals from the American Heart Association. Circulation 104:1694, 2001. Copyright 2001 American Heart Association.)

percent grade. A limitation of the Bruce protocol is the relatively large increase in $\dot{V}O_2$ between stages and the additional energy cost of running as compared with walking at stages in excess of Bruce's stage III. The Naughton and Weber protocols use 1- to 2-minute stages with 1-MET increments between stages; these protocols may be more suitable for patients with limited exercise tolerance, such as patients with compensated congestive heart failure. The Asymptomatic Cardiac Ischemia Pilot (ACIP) trial and modified ACIP (mACIP) protocols use 2-minute stages with 1.5-MET increments between stages after two 1-minute warm-up stages with 1-MET increments. The ACIP protocols were developed to test patients with established CAD and result in a linear increase in heart rate and $\dot{V}O_2$, distributing the time to occurrence of ST segment depression over a wider range of heart rate and exercise time than protocols with more abrupt increments in workload between stages.[2] The mACIP protocol produces a similar aerobic demand as the standard ACIP protocol for each minute of exercise and is well suited for short or elderly individuals who cannot keep up with a walking speed of 3 mph (see Fig. 10–2).

Ramp protocols start the patient at relatively slow treadmill speed, which is gradually increased until the patient has a good stride. The ramp angle of incline is progressively increased at fixed intervals (e.g., 10 to 60 seconds), starting at zero grade with the increase in grade calculated on the basis of the patient's estimated functional capacity such that the protocol will be complete at 6 to 12 minutes.[8] In this type of protocol, the rate of work increase is continuous and steady-state conditions are not reached. A limitation of ramp protocols is the need to estimate functional capacity from an activity scale; underestimation or overestimation of functional capacity occasionally results in an endurance test or premature cessation. One formula for estimating $\dot{V}O_2$ from treadmill speed and grade is as follows:

$$\dot{V}O_2\ (\text{ml } O_2/\text{kg/min}) = (\text{mph} \times 2.68) + (1.8 \times 26.82 \times \text{mph} \times \text{grade} \div 100) + 3.5$$

The peak $\dot{V}O_2$ is usually the same regardless of treadmill protocol used; the difference is the rate of time at which the peak $\dot{V}O_2$ is achieved.

It is important to encourage patients not to grasp the handrails of the treadmill during exercise, particularly the front handrails. Functional capacity can be overestimated by as much as 20 percent in tests in which handrail support is permitted, and $\dot{V}O_2$ is decreased. Because the degree of handrail support is difficult to quantify from one test to another, more consistent results can be obtained during serial testing when handrail support is not permitted.

The 6-Minute Walk Test. The 6-minute walk test can be used for patients who have marked left ventricular dysfunction or peripheral arterial occlusive disease and who cannot perform bicycle or treadmill exercise. Patients are instructed to walk down a 100-foot corridor at their own pace, attempting to cover as much ground as possible in 6 minutes. At the end of the 6-minute interval, the total distance walked is determined and the symptoms experienced by the patient are recorded. The 6-minute walk test as a clinical measure of ambulatory function requires highly skilled personnel following a rigid protocol to elicit reproducible and reliable results. The coefficient of variation for distance walked during two 6-minute walk tests was 10 percent in one series of patients with peripheral arterial occlusive disease.[18]

TECHNIQUES. Patients should be instructed not to eat, drink caffeinated beverages, or smoke for 3 hours before testing and to wear comfortable shoes and loose-fitting clothes. Unusual physical exertion should be avoided before testing. A brief history and physical examination should be performed, and patients should be advised about the risks and benefits of the procedure. A written informed consent form is usually required. The indication for the test should be known. The supervising physician should be made aware of any recent deterioration in the patient's clinical status. The test should not be performed in subjects who are markedly hypertensive (e.g., >220/120 mm Hg) or who have unexplained hypotension (e.g., systolic blood pressure <80 mm Hg) or other contraindications to exercise testing (see section on safety and risks of exercise testing). In many laboratories, the presence or absence of atherosclerotic risk factors is noted and cardioactive medication recorded. A 12-lead ECG should be obtained with the electrodes at the distal extremities. The timing of cardioactive medication ingestion before testing depends on the test indication.

After the standard 12-lead ECG is recorded, torso ECGs should be obtained with the patient in the supine position and in the sitting or standing position. Postural changes can elicit labile ST-T wave abnormalities. Hyperventilation is not recommended before exercise. If a false-positive test result is suspected, hyperventilation should be performed after the test, and the hyperventilation tracing compared with the maximal ST segment abnormalities observed. The ECG and blood pressure should be recorded in both positions, and patients should be instructed on how to perform the test.

Adequate skin preparation is essential for high-quality recordings, and the superficial layer of skin needs to be removed to augment signal-to-noise ratio. The areas of electrode application are rubbed with an alcohol-saturated pad to remove oil and rubbed with free sandpaper or a rough material to reduce skin resistance to 5000 ohms or less. Silver chloride electrodes with a fluid column to avoid direct metal-to-skin contact produce high-quality tracings; these electrodes have the lowest offset voltage. The electrode fluid column can dry out over time and should be verified prior to application. This can be a cause of poor-quality tracings.

Cables connecting the electrodes and recorders should be light, flexible, and properly shielded. In a small minority of patients, a fishnet jersey may be required over the electrodes and cables to reduce motion artifact. The electrode-skin interface can be verified by tapping on the electrode and examining the monitor or by measuring skin impedance. Excessive noise indicates that the electrode needs to be replaced; replacement before the test rather than during exercise can save time. The ECG signal can be digitized systematically at the patient's end of the cable by some systems, reducing power line artifact. Cables, adapters, and the junction box have a finite life span and require periodic replacement to obtain the highest quality tracings. Exercise equipment should be calibrated regularly. Room temperature should be between 64° and 72°F (18° and 22°C) and humidity less than 60 percent.

Treadmill walking should be demonstrated to the patient. The heart rate, blood pressure, and ECG should be recorded at the end of each stage of exercise, immediately before and immediately after stopping exercise, at the onset of an ischemic response, and for each minute for at least 5 to 10 minutes in the recovery phase. A minimum of three leads should be displayed continuously on the monitor during the test. There is some controversy about optimal patient position in the recovery phase. In the sitting position, less space is required for a stretcher, and patients are more comfortable immediately after exertion. The supine position increases end-diastolic volume and has the potential to augment ST segment changes.[19]

Electrocardiographic Measurements

LEAD SYSTEMS. The Mason-Likar modification of the standard 12-lead ECG requires that the extremity electrodes be moved to the torso to reduce motion artifact. The arm electrodes should be located in the most lateral aspects of the infraclavicular fossae, and the leg electrodes should be in a stable position above the anterior iliac crest and below the rib cage. The Mason-Likar modification results in a right-axis shift and increased voltage in the inferior leads and may produce a loss of inferior Q waves and the development of new Q waves in lead aV_L. Thus, the body torso limb lead positions cannot be used to interpret a diagnostic resting 12-lead ECG. The more cephalad the leg electrodes are placed, the greater is the degree of change and the greater is the augmentation of R wave amplitude.

Bipolar lead groups place the negative, or reference, electrode over the manubrium (CM_5), right scapula (CB_5), RV_5 (CC_5), or on the forehead (CH_5), and the active electrode at V_5 or a proximate location to optimize R wave amplitude. In bipolar lead ML, which reflects inferior wall changes, the negative reference is at the manubrium and the active electrode in the left leg position. Bipolar lead groups may provide additional diagnostic information, and in some medical centers, lead CM_5 is substituted for lead aV in the Mason-Likar–modified lead system. Bipolar leads are frequently used when only a limited ECG set is required (e.g., in cardiac rehabilitation programs). The value of adding right precordial leads to improve test sensitivity is controversial.[20,21] The use of more elaborate lead set systems is usually reserved for research purposes.

Types of ST Segment Displacement

In normal persons, the PR, QRS, and QT intervals shorten as heart rate increases. P amplitude increases, and the PR segment becomes progressively more downsloping in the inferior leads. J point, or junctional, depression is a normal finding during exercise (Fig. 10–3). In patients with myocardial ischemia, however, the ST segment usually becomes more horizontal (flattens) as the severity of the ischemic response worsens. With progressive exercise, the depth of ST segment depression may increase, involving more ECG leads, and the patient may develop angina. In the immediate postrecovery phase, the ST segment displacement may persist, with downsloping ST segments and T wave inversion, gradually returning to baseline after 5 to 10 minutes (Figs. 10–4 and 10–5). Ischemic ST segment displacement may be seen only during exercise, emphasizing the importance of adequate skin preparation and electrode placement to capture high-quality recordings during maximum exertion (Fig. 10–6). In about 10 percent of patients, the ischemic response may appear only in the recovery phase. This is a relevant finding, and the prevalence of reversible perfusion defects by single-photon emission computed tomography criteria are comparable to those observed when the ischemic ST segment response occurs both during and after exercise.[22-24] Patients should not leave the exercise laboratory area until the postexercise ECG has returned to baseline. Figure 10–7 illustrates eight different ECG patterns seen during exercise testing.

Measurement of ST Segment Displacement

For purposes of interpretation, the PQ junction is usually chosen as the isoelectric point. The TP segment represents a true isoelectric point but is an impractical choice for most routine clinical measurements. The development of 0.10 mV (1 mm) or greater of J point depression measured from the PQ junction, with a relatively flat ST segment slope (e.g., <0.7 to

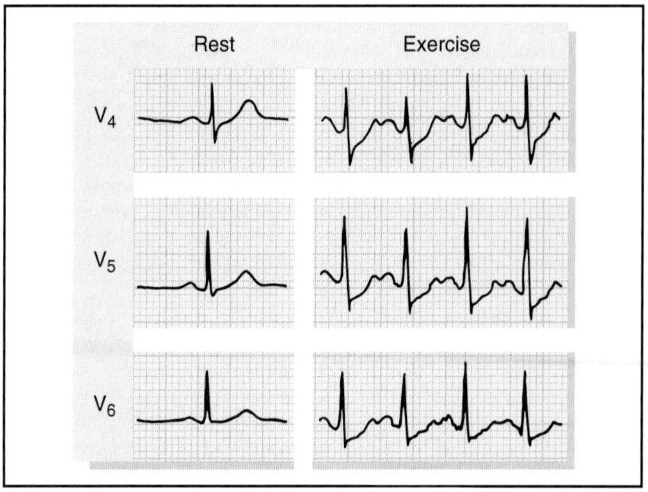

FIGURE 10–3 J point depression of 2 to 3 mm in leads V_4 to V_6 with rapid upsloping ST segments depressed approximately 1 mm 80 msec after the J point. The ST segment slope in leads V_4 and V_5 is 3.0 mV/sec. This response should not be considered abnormal.

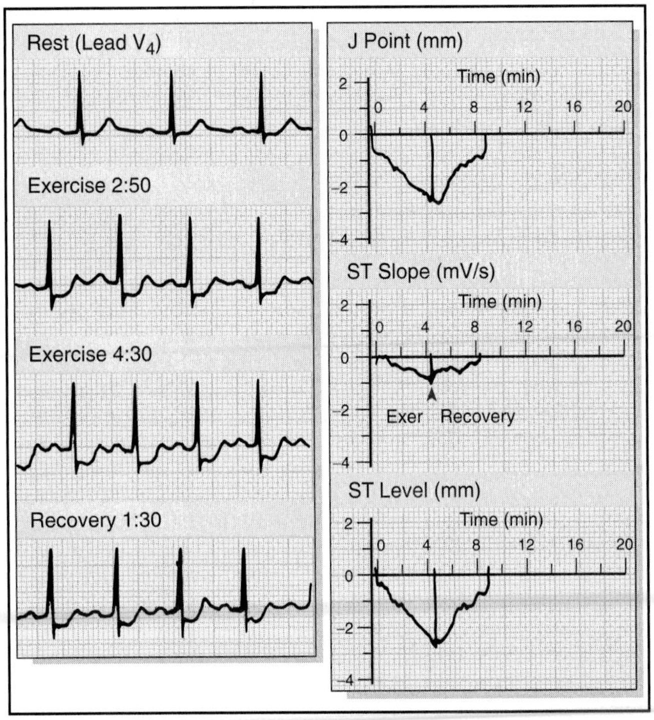

FIGURE 10–4 Bruce protocol. In lead V_4, the exercise electrocardiographic (ECG) result is abnormal early in the test, reaching 0.3 mV (3 mm) of horizontal ST segment depression at the end of exercise. The ischemic changes persist for at least 1 minute and 30 seconds into the recovery phase. The **right** panel provides a continuous plot of the J point, ST slope, and ST segment displacement at 80 msec after the J point (ST level) during exercise and in the recovery phase. Exercise ends at the vertical line at 4.5 minutes (red arrow). The computer trends permit a more precise identification of initial onset and offset of ischemic ST segment depression. This type of ECG pattern, with early onset of ischemic ST segment depression, reaching more than 3 mm of horizontal ST segment displacement and persisting several minutes into the recovery phase, is consistent with a severe ischemic response.

1 mV/sec), depressed 0.10 mV or more 80 msec after the J point (ST 80) in three consecutive beats with a stable baseline is considered to be an abnormal response (Fig. 10–8). When the ST 80 measurement is difficult to determine at rapid heart rates (e.g., >130 beats/min), the ST 60 measurement should be used. The ST segment at rest may occasionally be depressed. When this occurs, the J point and ST 60 or ST 80 measurements should be depressed an additional 0.10 mV or greater to be considered abnormal.

When the degree of resting ST segment depression is 0.1 mV or greater, the exercise ECG becomes less specific, and myocardial imaging modalities should be considered.[1,2,8,25] In patients with early repolarization and resting ST segment elevation, return to the PQ junction is normal. Therefore, the magnitude of exercise-induced ST segment depression in a patient with early repolarization should be determined from the PQ junction and not from the elevated position of the J point before exercise. Exercise-induced ST segment depression does not localize the site of myocardial ischemia, nor does it provide a clue about which coronary artery is involved. For example, it is not unusual for patients with isolated right CAD to exhibit exercise-induced ST segment depression only in leads V_4 to V_6, nor is it unusual for patients with disease of the left anterior descending coronary artery to exhibit exercise-induced ST segment displacements in leads II, III, and aV_f. Exercise-induced ST segment elevation is relatively specific for the territory of myocardial ischemia and the coronary artery involved.

UPSLOPING ST SEGMENTS. Junctional or J point depression is a normal finding during maximal exercise, and

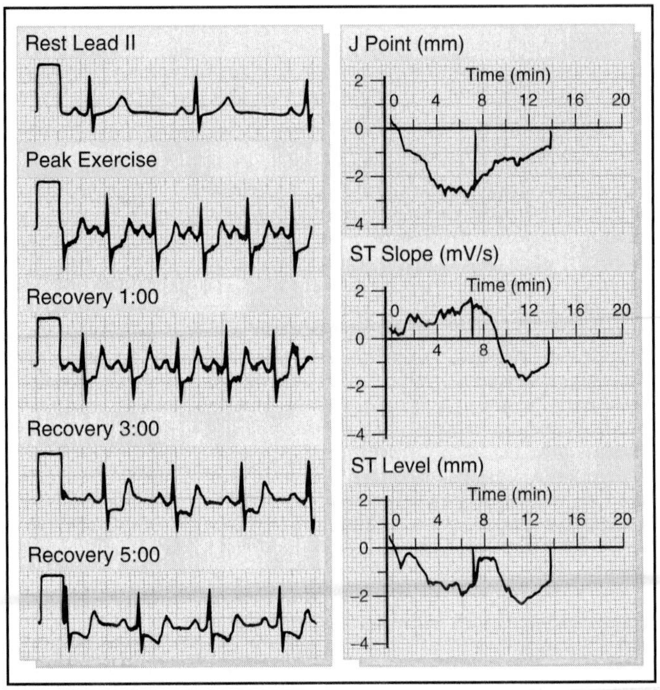

FIGURE 10–5 Bruce protocol. In this type of ischemic pattern, the J point at peak exertion is depressed 2.5 mm, the ST segment slope is 1.5 mV/sec, and the ST segment level at 80 msec after the J point is depressed 1.6 mm. This "slow upsloping" ST segment at peak exercise indicates an ischemic pattern in patients with a high pretest prevalence of coronary disease. A typical ischemic pattern is seen at 3 minutes of the recovery phase when the ST segment is horizontal and 5 minutes after exertion when the ST segment is downsloping. Exercise is discontinued at the vertical line in the **right** panels at 7.5 minutes.

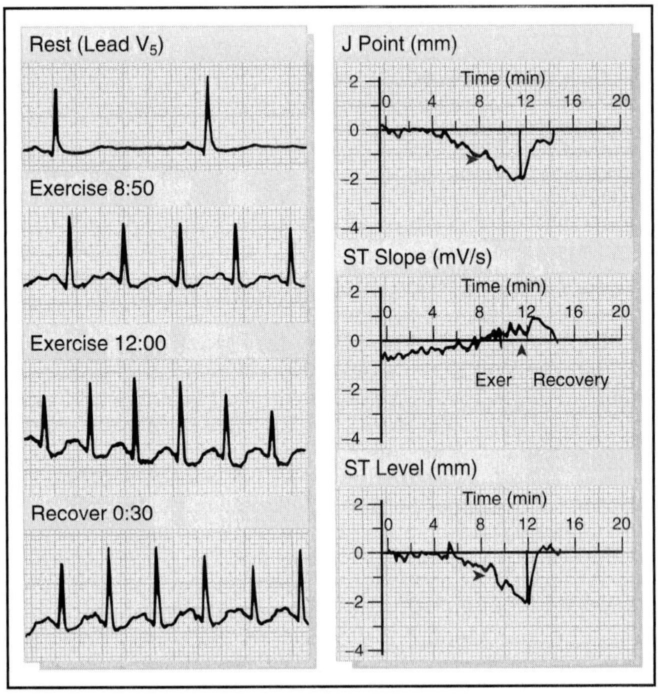

FIGURE 10–6 Bruce protocol. The exercise electrocardiographic (ECG) result is not yet abnormal at 8:50 minutes but becomes abnormal at 9:30 minutes (horizontal arrows, **right**) of a 12-minute exercise test and resolves in the immediate recovery phase. This ECG pattern in which the ST segment becomes abnormal only at high exercise workloads and returns to baseline in the immediate recovery phase may indicate a false-positive result in an asymptomatic individual without atherosclerotic risk factors. Exercise myocardial imaging would provide more diagnostic and prognostic information if this were an older person with several atherosclerotic risk factors. Vertical arrow indicates termination of exercise.

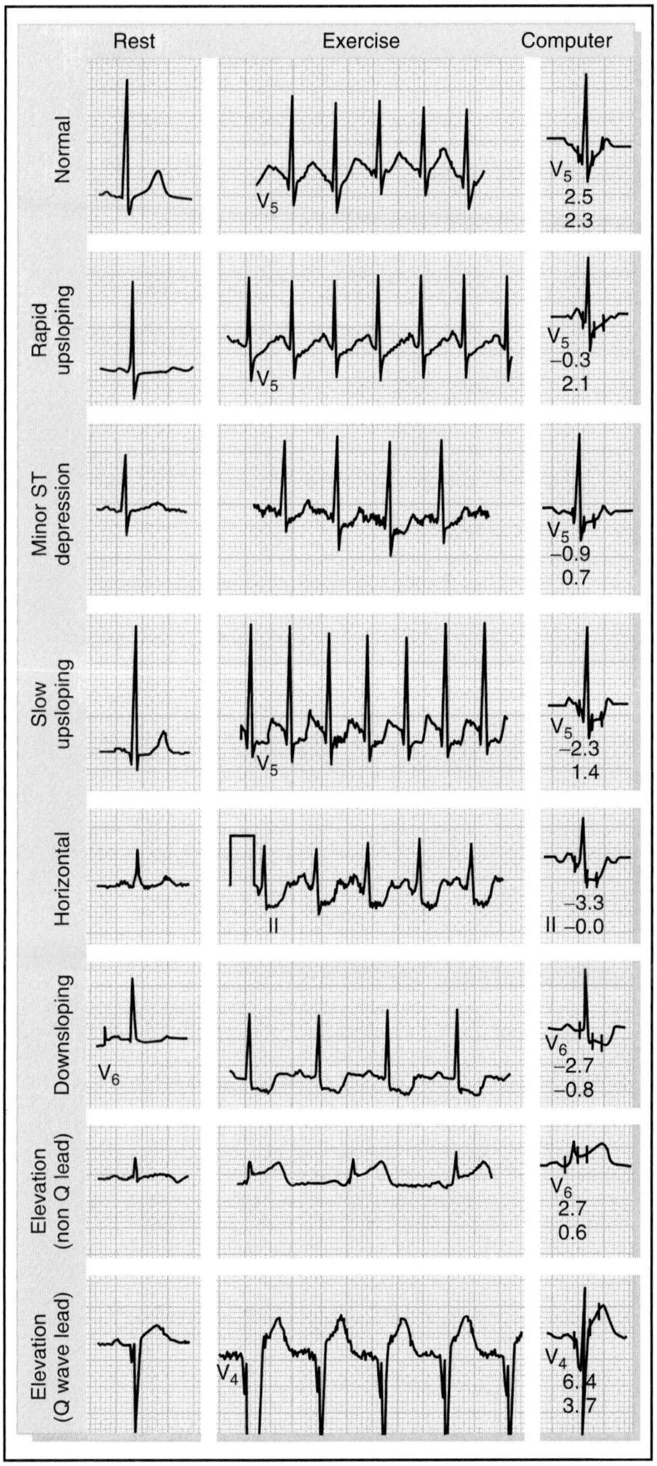

FIGURE 10–7 Illustration of eight typical exercise electrocardiographic (ECG) patterns at rest and at peak exertion. The computer-processed incrementally averaged beat corresponds with the raw data taken at the same time point during exercise and is illustrated in the last column. The patterns represent worsening ECG responses during exercise. In the column of computer-averaged beats, ST 80 displacement (top number) indicates the magnitude of ST segment displacement 80 msec after the J point relative to the PQ junction or E point. ST segment slope measurement (bottom number) indicates the ST segment slope at a fixed time point after the J point to the ST 80 measurement. At least three noncomputer average complexes with a stable baseline should meet criteria for abnormality before the exercise ECG result can be considered abnormal (see Fig. 10–9). The normal and rapid upsloping ST segment responses are normal responses to exercise. J point depression with rapid upsloping ST segments is a common response in an older, apparently healthy population. Minor ST depression can occur occasionally at submaximal workloads in patients with coronary disease; in this illustration, the ST segment is depressed 0.09 mV (0.9 mm) 80 msec after the J point. The slow upsloping ST segment pattern often demonstrates an ischemic response in patients with known coronary disease or those with a high pretest clinical risk of coronary disease. Criteria for slow upsloping ST segment depression include J point and ST 80 depression of 0.15 mV or more and ST segment slope of more than 1.0 mV/sec. Classic criteria for myocardial ischemia include horizontal ST segment depression observed when both the J point and ST 80 depression are 0.1 mV or more and ST segment slope is within the range of 1.0 mV/sec. Downsloping ST segment depression occurs when the J point and ST 80 depression are 0.1 mV and ST segment slope is −1.0 mV/sec. ST segment elevation in a non-Q wave noninfarct lead occurs when the J point and ST 60 are 1.0 mV or greater and represents a severe ischemic response. ST segment elevation in an infarct territory (Q wave lead) indicates a severe wall motion abnormality and in most cases is not considered an ischemic response. (From Chaitman BR: Exercise electrocardiographic stress testing. *In* Beller GA [ed]: Chronic Ischemic Heart Disease. *In* Braunwald E [series ed]: Atlas of Heart Diseases. Vol 5. Chronic Ischemic Heart Disease. Philadelphia, Current Medicine, 1995, pp 2.1-2.30.)

a rapid upsloping ST segment (>1 mV/sec) depressed less than 0.15 mV (1.5 mm) after the J point should be considered to be normal (see Fig. 10–3). Occasionally, however, the ST segment is depressed 0.15 mV (1.5 mm) or greater at 80 msec after the J point. This type of slow upsloping ST segment may be the only ECG finding in patients with well-defined obstructive CAD and may depend on the lead set used (see Figs. 10–5 and 10–7). In patient subsets with a high CAD prevalence, a slow upsloping ST segment depressed 0.15 mV or greater at 80 msec after the J point should be considered abnormal. The importance of this finding in asymptomatic individuals or those with a low CAD prevalence is less certain. Increasing the degree of ST segment depression at 80 msec after the J point to 0.20 mV (2.0 mm) or greater in patients with a slow upsloping ST segment increases specificity but decreases sensitivity.[1,2,7,8]

ST SEGMENT ELEVATION. Exercise-induced ST segment elevation may occur in an infarct territory where Q waves are present or in a noninfarct territory. The development of 0.10 mV (1 mm) or greater of J point elevation, persistently elevated greater than 0.10 mV at 60 msec after the J point in three consecutive beats with a stable baseline, is considered an abnormal response (see Fig. 10–7). This finding occurs in approximately 30 percent of patients with anterior myocardial infarctions and 15 percent of those with inferior ones tested early (within 2 weeks) after the index event and decreases in frequency by 6 weeks. As a group, postinfarct patients with exercise-induced ST segment elevation have a lower ejection fraction than those without, a greater severity of resting wall motion abnormalities, and a worse prognosis. Exercise-induced ST segment elevation in leads with abnormal Q waves is not a marker of more extensive CAD and rarely indicates myocardial ischemia. Exercise-induced ST

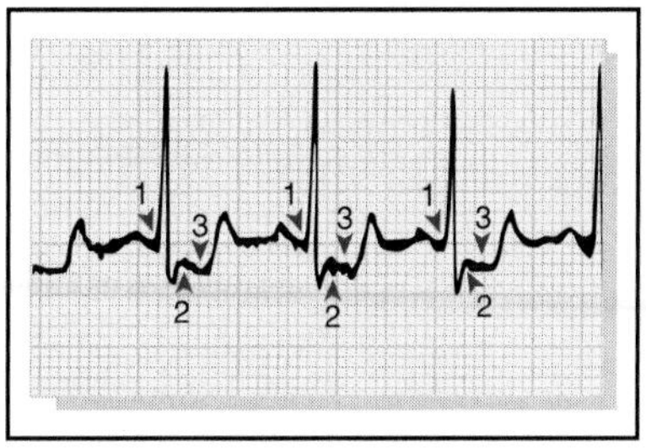

FIGURE 10–8 Magnified ischemic exercise–induced electrocardiographic pattern. Three consecutive complexes with a relatively stable baseline are selected. The PQ junction (1) and J point (2) are determined; the ST 80 (3) is determined at 80 msec after the J point. In this example, average J point displacement is 0.2 mV (2 mm) and ST 80 is 0.24 mV (24 mm). The average slope measurement from the J point to ST 80 is −1.1 mV/sec.

segment elevation may occasionally occur in a patient who has regenerated embryonic R waves after an acute myocardial infarction; the clinical significance of this finding is similar to that observed when Q waves are present.

When ST segment elevation develops during exercise in a non-Q wave lead in a patient without a previous myocardial infarction, the finding should be considered as likely evidence of transmural myocardial ischemia caused by coronary vasospasm or a high-grade coronary narrowing (Fig. 10–9). This finding is relatively uncommon, occurring in approximately 1 percent of patients with obstructive CAD. The ECG site of ST segment elevation is relatively specific for the coronary artery involved, and myocardial perfusion scintigraphy usually reveals a defect in the territory involved.

T WAVE CHANGES. The morphology of the T wave is influenced by body position, respiration, hyperventilation, drug therapy, and myocardial ischemia/necrosis. In patient populations with a low CAD prevalence, pseudonormalization of T waves (inverted at rest and becoming upright with exercise) is a nondiagnostic finding (Fig. 10–10). In rare instances, this finding may be a marker for myocardial ischemia in a patient with documented CAD, although it would need to be substantiated by an ancillary technique, such as the concomitant finding of a reversible myocardial perfusion defect.[26]

OTHER ELECTROCARDIOGRAPHIC MARKERS. Changes in R wave amplitude during exercise are relatively nonspecific and are related to the level of exercise performed. When the R wave amplitude meets voltage criteria for left ventricular hypertrophy, the ST segment response cannot be used reliably to diagnose CAD, even in the absence of a left ventricular strain pattern. Loss of R wave amplitude, commonly seen after myocardial infarction, reduces the sensitivity of the ST segment response in that lead to diagnose obstructive CAD. Adjustment of the extent of ST segment depression by R wave height in individual leads has not been consistently shown to improve the diagnostic value of the exercise ECG for CAD. U wave inversion can occasionally be

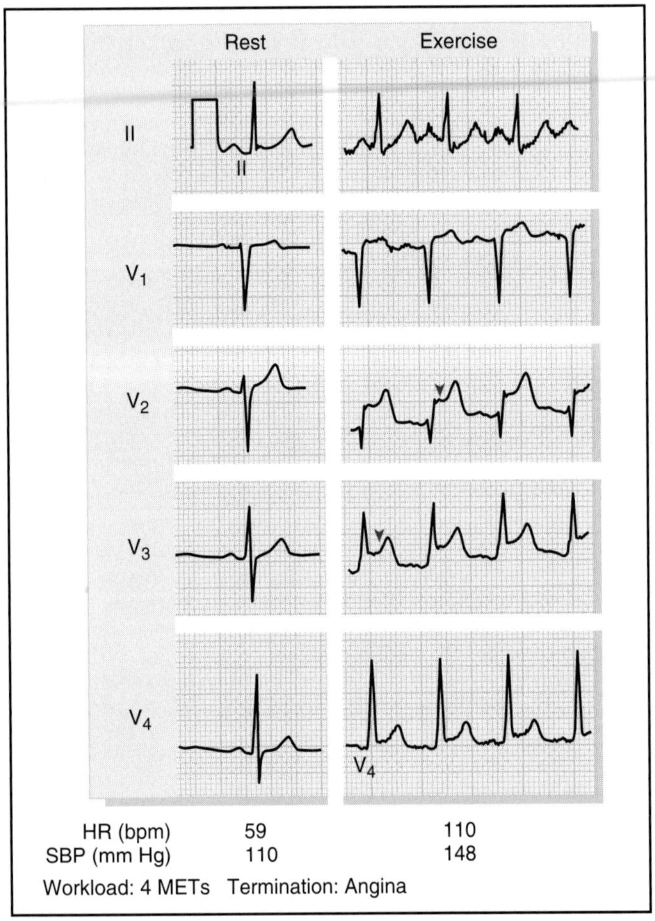

FIGURE 10–9 A 48-year-old man with several atherosclerotic risk factors and a normal resting electrocardiographic (ECG) result developed marked ST segment elevation (4 mm [arrows]) in leads V_2 and V_3 with lesser degrees of ST segment elevation in leads V_1 and V_4 and J point depression with upsloping ST segments in lead II, associated with angina. This type of ECG pattern is usually associated with a full-thickness, reversible myocardial perfusion defect in the corresponding left ventricular myocardial segments and high-grade intraluminal narrowing at coronary angiography. Rarely, coronary vasospasm produces this result in the absence of significant intraluminal atherosclerotic narrowing. HR = heart rate; METs = metabolic equivalents; SBP = systolic blood pressure. (From Chaitman BR: Exercise electrocardiographic stress testing. *In* Beller GA [ed]: Chronic Ischemic Heart Disease. *In* Braunwald E [series ed]: Atlas of Heart Diseases. Vol 5. Chronic Ischemic Heart Disease. Philadelphia, Current Medicine, 1995, pp 2.1-2.30.)

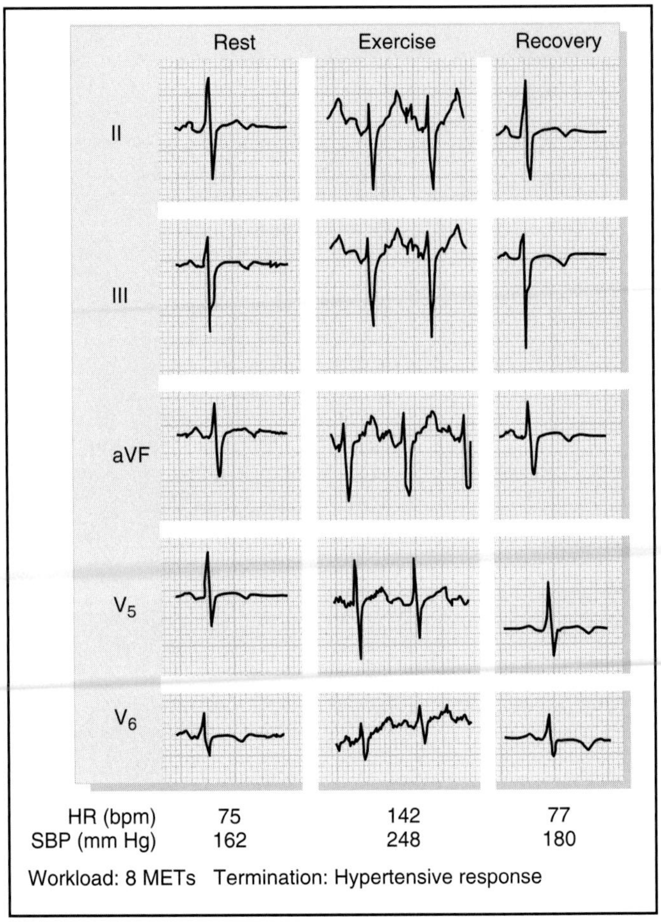

FIGURE 10–10 Pseudonormalization of T waves in a 49-year-old man referred for exercise testing. The patient had previously been seen for typical angina. The resting electrocardiogram in this patient with coronary artery disease shows inferior and anterolateral T wave inversion, an adverse long-term prognosticator. The patient exercised to 8 METs, reaching a peak heart rate of 142 beats/min and a peak systolic blood pressure of 248 mm Hg. At that point, the test was stopped because of hypertension. During exercise, pseudonormalization of T waves occurs, and it returns to baseline (inverted T wave) in the postexercise phase. The patient denied chest discomfort, and no arrhythmia or ST segment displacement was noted. Transient conversion of a negative T wave at rest to a positive T wave during exercise is a nonspecific finding in patients without prior myocardial infarction and does not enhance the diagnostic or prognostic content of the test; however, the ability to exercise to 8 METs without ischemic changes in the ST segment places this patient into a subset of lower risk. HR = heart rate; METs = metabolic equivalents; SBP = systolic blood pressure. (From Chaitman BR: Exercise electrocardiographic stress testing. *In* Beller GA [ed]: Chronic Ischemic Heart Disease. *In* Braunwald E [series ed]: Atlas of Heart Diseases. Vol 5. Chronic Ischemic Heart Disease. Philadelphia, Current Medicine, 1995, pp 2.1-2.30.

seen in the precordial leads at heart rates of 120 beats/min. Although this finding is relatively specific for CAD, it is relatively insensitive.[27]

COMPUTER-ASSISTED ANALYSIS

The use of computers has facilitated the routine analysis and measurements required from exercise ECG and can be performed on-line as well as off-line. When the raw ECG data are of high quality, the computer can filter and average or select median complexes from which the degree of J point displacement, ST segment slope, and ST displacement 60 to 80 msec after the J point (ST 60 to 80) can be measured. The selection of ST 60 or ST 80 depends on the heart rate response. At ventricular rates greater than 130 beats/min, the ST 80 measurement may fall on the upslope of the T wave, and the ST 60 measurement should be used instead. In some computerized systems, the PQ junction or isoelectric interval is detected by scanning before the R wave for the 10-msec interval with the least slope. J point, ST slope, and ST levels are determined (see Figs. 10–4, 10–5, and 10–6); the ST integral can be calculated from the area below the isoelectric line from the J point to ST 60 or ST 80. Computerized treatment of ECG complexes permits reduction of motion and myographic artifacts. However, the averaged or median beats may occasionally be erroneous because of ECG signal distortion caused by noise, baseline wander, or changes in conduction, and identification of the PQ junction and ST segment onset can be imperfect. Therefore, it is crucial to ensure that the computer-determined averages or median complexes reflect the raw ECG data, and physicians should program the computer to print out raw data during exercise and inspect the raw data to be certain that the QRS template is accurately reproduced and the placement of the fiducial points are correctly placed at the PQ junction and J point before accepting the automatic measurements.

ST/HEART RATE SLOPE MEASUREMENTS. Heart rate adjustment of ST segment depression appears to improve the sensitivity of the exercise test, particularly the prediction of multivessel CAD.[28] The ST/heart rate slope depends on the type of exercise performed, number and location of monitoring electrodes, method of measuring ST segment depression, and clinical characteristics of the study population. Calculation of maximal ST/heart rate slope in mV/beats/min is performed by linear regression analysis relating the measured amount of ST segment depression in individual leads to the heart rate at the end of each stage of exercise, starting at the end of exercise. An ST/heart rate slope of 2.4 mV/beats/min is considered abnormal, and values that exceed 6 mV/beats/min are suggestive evidence of three-vessel CAD. The use of this measurement requires modification of the exercise protocol such that increments in heart rate are gradual, as in the Cornell protocol, as opposed to more abrupt increases in heart rate between stages, as in the Bruce or Ellestad protocols, which limit the ability to calculate statistically valid ST segment heart rate slopes. The measurement is not accurate in the early postinfarction phase. A modification of the ST segment/heart rate slope method is the ST segment/heart rate index calculation, which represents the average change of ST segment depression with heart rate throughout the course of the exercise test. The ST/heart rate index measurements are less than the ST/heart rate slope measurements, and a ST/heart rate index of 1.6 is defined as abnormal. A slight increase in the prognostic content of ST segment/heart rate slope measurements as compared with standard criteria was demonstrated in the Multiple Risk Factor Interventional Trial.[1,8]

Mechanism of ST Segment Displacement

PATHOPHYSIOLOGY OF THE MYOCARDIAL ISCHEMIC RESPONSE. Myocardial oxygen consumption ($M\text{O}_2$) is determined by heart rate, systolic blood pressure, left ventricular end-diastolic volume, wall thickness, and contractility (see Chap. 44).[1,2,7,8,12] The rate-pressure or double product (heart rate × systolic blood pressure) increases progressively with increasing work and can be used to estimate the myocardial perfusion requirement in normal persons and in many patients with coronary artery disease. The heart is an aerobic organ with little capacity to generate energy through anaerobic metabolism. Oxygen extraction in the coronary circulation is nearly maximal at rest. The only significant mechanism available to the heart to increase oxygen consumption is to increase perfusion, and there is a direct linear relationship between $M\text{O}_2$ and coronary blood flow in normal individuals. The principal mechanism for increasing coronary blood flow during exercise is to decrease resistance at the coronary arteriolar level. In patients with progressive atherosclerotic narrowing of the epicardial vessels, an ischemic threshold occurs, and exercise beyond this threshold can produce abnormalities in diastolic and systolic ventricular function, ECG changes, and chest pain. The subendocardium is more susceptible to myocardial ischemia than the subepicardium because of increased wall tension, causing a relative increase in myocardial oxygen demand in the subendocardium.

Dynamic changes in coronary artery tone at the site of an atherosclerotic plaque may result in diminished coronary flow during static or dynamic exercise instead of the expected increase that normally occurs from coronary vasodilation in a normal vessel; that is, perfusion pressure distal to the stenotic plaque actually falls as during exercise, resulting in reduced subendocardial blood flow (Fig. 10–11).[29,30] Thus, regional left ventricular myocardial ischemia may result not only from an increase in myocardial oxygen demand during exercise but also from a limitation of coronary flow as a result of coronary vasoconstriction, or inability of vessels to sufficiently vasodilate at or near the site of an atherosclerotic plaque.

Some patients with chronic angina have a warm-up phenomenon that can be demonstrated using sequential exercise testing.[31-33] Under these conditions, the time to angina and ischemic ST segment depression can be prolonged and can occur at a higher rate-pressure product on the second of two exercise tests performed within 10 to 30 minutes of each other. Improvement in performance on the second test is related to the magnitude of myocardial ischemia produced on the first test, and, usually, myocardial ischemia of more than moderate intensity is required to produce the warm-up response.

In normal persons, the action potential duration of the endocardial region is longer than that of the epicardial region,

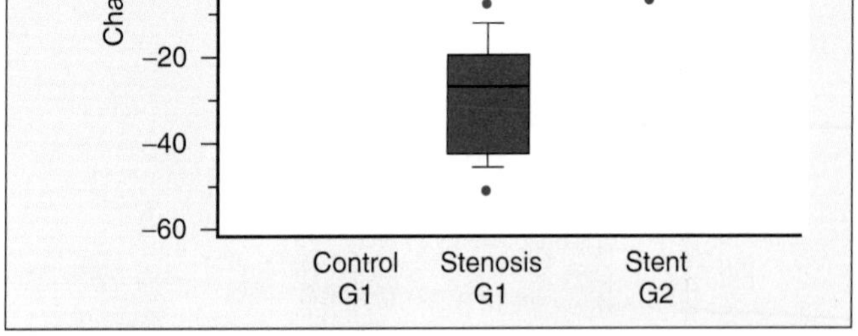

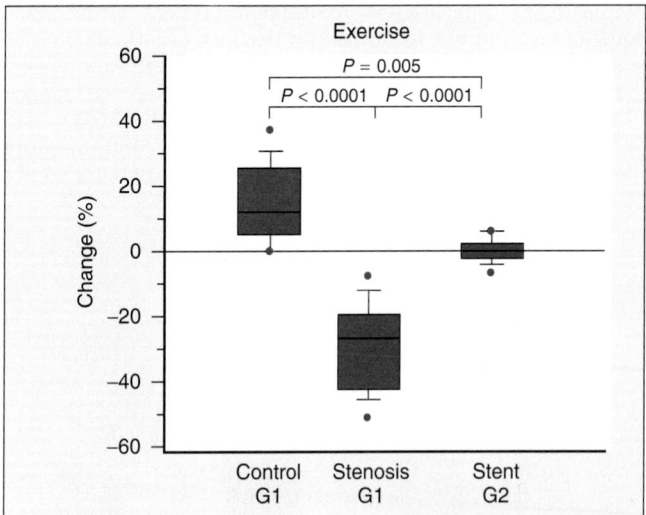

FIGURE 10–11 Box plot of exercise-induced changes of the left coronary artery in a control group of 12 patients with chronic angina and single vessel disease (G1) and results for 14 patients studied 10 months after coronary stenting (G2). In control group G1, the mean percentage diameter stenosis of the stenotic segment was 59 percent; during exercise, the stenotic segment exhibited coronary vasoconstriction (average −29 percent compared with rest) compared with a control segment in the same vessel that showed vasodilation (+15 percent compared with rest). Sublingual nitroglycerin induced maximal vasodilation in the nonstenotic segment (+36 percent) and mild vasodilation (+10 percent) in the stenotic segments (not shown). Exercise does not elicit any vasomotion in stent group G2, and vessel diameter remains unchanged. (From Maier W, Windecker S, Kung A, et al: Exercise-induced coronary artery vasodilation is not impaired by stent placement. Circulation 105:2373, 2002.)

and ventricular repolarization is from epicardium to endocardium. The action potential duration is shortened in the presence of myocardial ischemia, and electrical gradients are created, resulting in ST segment depression or elevation, depending on the surface ECG leads. At the molecular level, activation of sarcolemmal ATP-sensitive potassium (K_{ATP}) channels by ischemic ATP depletion may play a role. Transgenic mice with homozygous knockout of the Kir6-2 channel gene, which encodes the pore-forming subunit of cardiac surface K_{ATP} channels, lack the ability to generate an ST segment elevation response to acute coronary occlusion.[34] Increased myocardial oxygen demand associated with a failure to increase or an actual decrease in regional coronary blood flow usually causes ST segment depression; ST segment elevation may occasionally occur in patients with more severe coronary flow reduction.

Nonelectrocardiographic Observations

The ECG is only one part of the exercise response, and abnormal hemodynamics or functional capacity is just as important as, if not more important than, ST segment displacement.

BLOOD PRESSURE. The normal exercise response is to increase systolic blood pressure progressively with increasing workloads to a peak response ranging from 160 to 200 mm Hg, with the higher range of the scale in older patients with less compliant vascular systems.[1,7,8,35] As a group, black patients tend to have a higher systolic blood pressure response than white patients. At high exercise workloads, it is sometimes difficult to obtain a precise determination of systolic blood pressure by auscultation. In normal persons, the diastolic blood pressure does not usually change significantly. Failure to increase systolic blood pressure beyond 120 mm Hg, a sustained decrease greater than 10 mm Hg repeatable within 15 seconds, or a fall in systolic blood pressure below standing resting values during progressive exercise when the blood pressure has otherwise been increasing appropriately is abnormal and reflects either inadequate elevation of cardiac output because of left ventricular systolic pump dysfunction or an excessive reduction in systemic vascular resistance.[36] Exertional hypotension ranges from 3 to 9 percent and is higher in patients with three-vessel or left main CAD. Conditions other than myocardial ischemia that have been associated with a failure to increase or an actual decrease in systolic blood pressure during progressive exercise are cardiomyopathy, cardiac arrhythmias, vasovagal reactions, left ventricular outflow tract obstruction, ingestion of antihypertensive drugs, hypovolemia, and prolonged vigorous exercise.

It is important to distinguish between a decline in blood pressure in the postexercise phase and a decrease in or failure to increase systolic blood pressure during progressive exercise. The incidence of postexertional hypotension in asymptomatic subjects was 1.9 percent in 781 asymptomatic volunteers in the Baltimore Longitudinal Study on Aging, with a 3.1 percent incidence noted in subjects younger than 55 years and a 0.3 percent incidence in patients older than 55 years.[37] In this series, most hypotensive episodes were symptomatic, and only two patients had hypotension associated with bradycardia and vagal symptoms. Although ST segment abnormalities suggestive of ischemia occurred in one third of the patients with hypotension, none of the patients had a cardiac event during 4 years of follow-up. Rarely, in young patients, vasovagal syncope can occur in the immediate postexercise phase, progressing through sinus bradycardia to several seconds of asystole and hypotension before reverting to sinus rhythm. An abnormal hypertensive blood pressure response in patients with a high prevalence of CAD is associated with more extensive CAD and more extensive myocardial perfusion defects. Occasionally, a marked hypertensive response may cause new exercise-induced wall motion abnormalities in the absence of coronary disease.[38]

MAXIMAL WORK CAPACITY. This variable is one of the most important prognostic measurements obtained from an exercise test (Fig. 10–12).[1,2,7,8,10,39-41] Maximal work capacity in normal individuals is influenced by familiarization with the exercise test equipment, level of training, and environmental conditions at the time of testing. In patients with known or suspected CAD, a limited exercise capacity is associated with an increased risk of cardiac events, and, in general, the more severe the limitation, the worse the CAD extent and prognosis. In estimating functional capacity, the amount of work performed (or exercise stage achieved) expressed in METs, not the number of minutes of exercise, should be the parameter measured. Estimates of peak functional capacity for age and gender have been well established for most of the exercise protocols in common use, subject to the limitations described in the section on cardiopulmonary testing. Comparison of an individual's performance against normal standards provides an estimate of the degree of exercise impairment. There is a rough correlation between observed peak functional capacity during exercise treadmill testing and estimates derived from clinical data and specific activity questionnaires.

Serial comparison of functional capacity in individual patients to assess significant interval change requires a careful examination of the exercise protocol used during both tests, of drug therapy and time of ingestion, of systemic blood pressure, and of other conditions that might influence test performance. All these variables need to be considered before attributing changes in functional capacity to

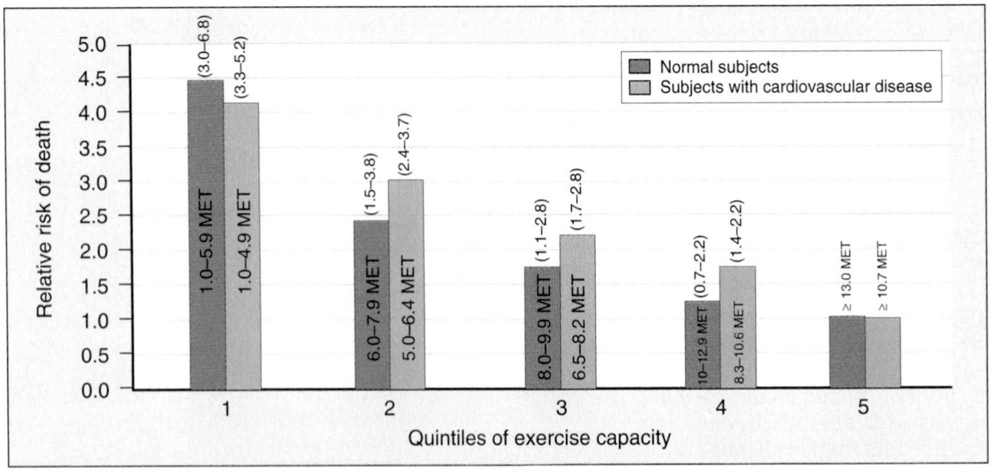

FIGURE 10–12 Age-adjusted relative risks of all-cause mortality by quintile of exercise capacity in 2534 subjects with a normal exercise test result and no history of cardiovascular disease and 3679 subjects with an abnormal exercise test result or history of cardiovascular disease. The mean duration of follow-up was 6.2 ± 3.7 years. Quintile 5 was used as the reference category. For each 1-MET increase in exercise capacity, the survival improved by 12 percent (From Myers J, Prakash M, Froelicher V, et al: Exercise capacity and mortality among men referred for exercise testing. N Engl J Med 346:793, 2002.)

progression of CAD or worsening of left ventricular function. Major reductions in exercise capacity usually indicate significant worsening of cardiovascular status; modest changes may not.[42]

SUBMAXIMAL EXERCISE. The interpretation of exercise test results for diagnostic and prognostic purposes requires consideration of maximal work capacity. When a patient is unable to complete moderate levels of exercise or reach at least 85 to 90 percent of age-predicted maximum, the level of exercise performed may be inadequate to test cardiac reserve. Thus, ischemic ECG, scintigraphic, or ventriculographic abnormalities may not be evoked and the test may be nondiagnostic. Nondiagnostic test results are more common in patients with peripheral vascular disease, orthopedic limitation, or neurological impairment and in patients with poor motivation. Pharmacological stress imaging studies should be considered in this setting.[1,2]

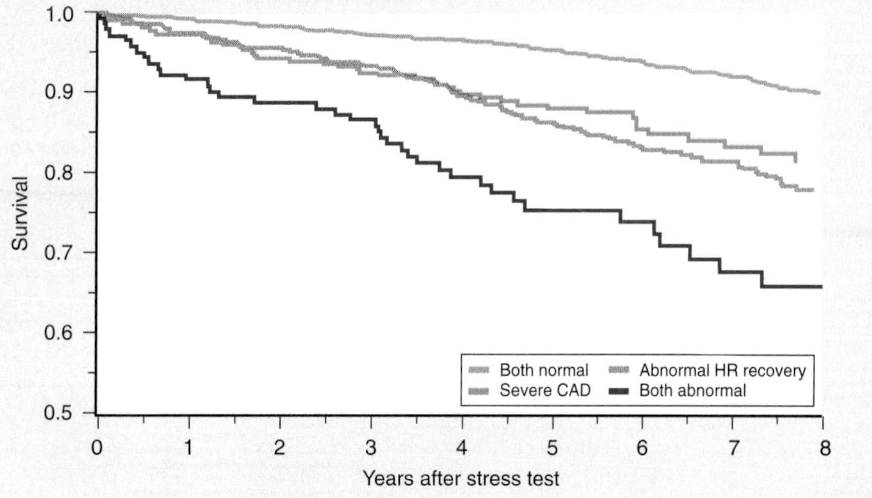

No. at risk									
Both normal	1817	1802	1784	1666	1415	1170	868	706	475
Severe CAD	280	273	264	251	210	161	127	90	79
Abnl HR rec	697	678	665	614	508	395	299	243	143
Both abnormal	141	129	125	117	84	51	49	40	29

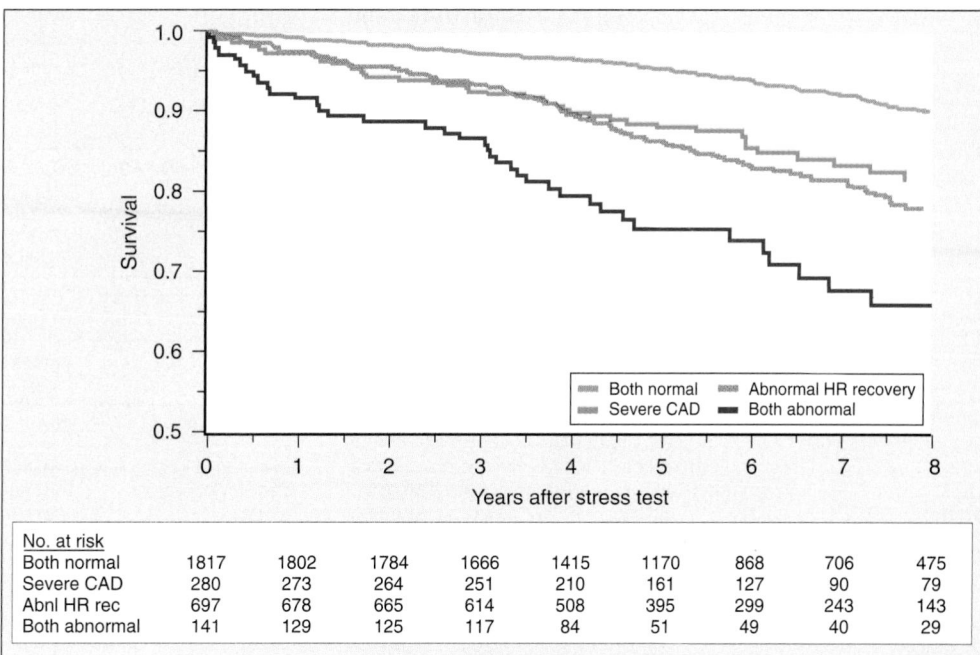

FIGURE 10–13 Six-year follow-up in 2935 patients who underwent an exercise test and coronary angiography. After adjustment for age, gender, standard risk factors, medications, exercise capacity, coronary disease extent, and left ventricular function, abnormal heart rate recovery (Abnl HR rec) was an independent predictor of mortality. The survival plot illustrates a mortality gradient with the worst prognosis in patients with abnormal heart rate recovery and severe coronary artery disease (CAD). (From Vivekananthan DP, Blackstone EH, Poithier CE, et al: Heart rate recovery after exercise is a predictor of mortality, independent of the angiographic severity of coronary disease. J Am Coll Cardiol 42:831, 2003.)

HEART RATE RESPONSE. The sinus rate increases progressively with exercise, mediated in part through sympathetic and parasympathetic innervation of the sinoatrial node and circulating catecholamines. In some patients who may be anxious about the exercise test, there may be an initial overreaction of heart rate and systolic blood pressure at the beginning of exercise, with stabilization after approximately 30 to 60 seconds. An inappropriate increase in heart rate at low exercise workloads may occur in patients who are in atrial fibrillation, physically deconditioned, hypovolemic, or anemic or who have marginal left ventricular function; this increase may persist for several minutes in the recovery phase. In some patients, heart rate (HR) fails to increase appropriately with exercise and is associated with an adverse prognosis.[43-45] Chronotropic incompetence is determined by decreased heart rate sensitivity to the normal increase in sympathetic tone during exercise and is defined as inability to increase heart rate to at least 85 percent of age-predicted maximum or as an abnormal heart rate reserve. Heart rate reserve is calculated as follows:

$$\%HRR_{Used} = (HR_{peak} - HR_{rest})/(220 - \text{age} - HR_{rest})$$

The term *chronotropic index* refers to a heart rate increment per stage of exercise that is below normal or a peak heart rate below predicted at maximal workloads. It reflects an inability to use up all of the heart rate reserve. This finding may indicate autonomic dysfunction, sinus node disease, drug therapy such as beta blockers, or a myocardial ischemic response. When the chronotropic index is 80 percent or less, long-term mortality is increased. Chronotropic incompetence should not be used to estimate prognosis in patients on beta blocker therapy. Abnormal heart rate recovery (HRR) refers to a relatively slow deceleration of heart rate following exercise cessation. This type of response reflects decreased vagal tone and is associated with increased mortality.[46,47]

$$HRR = HR_{peak} - HR_{1\ \text{minute later}}$$

When the postexercise phase includes an upright cool down, a value 12 beats/min or less is abnormal. For patients undergoing stress echocardiography or otherwise assuming a supine position immediately after exercise, a value 18 beats/min or less is abnormal. When HRR is measured 2 minutes into recovery, a value 22 beats/min or less is abnormal. The prognostic value of abnormal HRR is independent of the exercise level attained, beta blocker usage, severity of coronary disease, left ventricular function, chronotropic incompetence, Duke treadmill score, and presence of exercise-induced angina or ischemic ECG abnormalities (Fig. 10–13). A submaximal heart rate response in a patient who is poorly motivated to complete the test or has a physical impairment that limits ability to perform sufficient exercise to test heart rate reserve (resulting in a nondiagnostic test, as described earlier) should be distinguished from a patient with chronotropic incompetence and an adequate test for prognostic estimates.

RATE-PRESSURE PRODUCT. The heart rate–systolic blood pressure product, an indirect measure of myocardial oxygen demand, increases progressively with exercise, and the peak rate-pressure product can be used to characterize cardiovascular performance. Most normal individuals develop a peak rate pressure product of 20 to 35 mm Hg × beats/min × 10^{-3}. In many patients with significant ischemic heart disease, rate-pressure products exceeding 25 mm Hg × beats/min × 10^{-3} are unusual. However, the cutpoint of 25 mm Hg × beats/min × 10^{-3} is not a useful diagnostic parameter; significant overlap exists between patients with disease and those without disease. Furthermore, cardioactive drug therapy significantly influences this measurement.

CHEST DISCOMFORT. Characterization of chest discomfort during exercise can be a useful diagnostic finding, particularly when the symptom complex is compatible with typical angina pectoris. In some patients, the exercise level during the test may exceed that which the patient exhibits in day-to-day activities. Exercise-induced chest discomfort usually occurs after the onset of ischemic ST segment abnormalities and may be associated with diastolic hypertension. In some patients, however, chest discomfort may be the only signal that obstructive CAD is present. In patients with chronic stable angina, exercise-induced chest discomfort occurs less frequently than ischemic ST segment depression. The severity of myocardial ischemia in a patient with exercise-induced angina and a normal ECG can often be assessed using a myocardial imaging technique.[1,2] The new development of an S_3, holosystolic apical murmur, or basilar rates in the early recovery phase of exercise enhances the diagnostic accuracy of the test.

EXERCISE TEST INDICATIONS

The most frequent indications for exercise testing are to aid in establishing the diagnosis of CAD, in determining functional capacity, and in estimating prognosis. The indications continue to evolve, with some that are uniformly accepted and others that are more controversial. The American Heart Association and American College of Cardiology Exercise Task Force determined several categories of test indications drawn from a large body of published literature on exercise testing[1] (see Guidelines section). Exercise testing should not be used to screen very low-risk, asymptomatic individuals because the test has limited diagnostic and prognostic value in this situation, and the resultant undesirable consequences of a false-positive exercise test result may be unnecessary follow-up, additional procedures, anxiety, and exercise restrictions.[7,8] Most asymptomatic subjects who are enrolled in an exercise screening program for CAD and who die suddenly of cardiac causes have had a previous normal exercise test result. In patients with established CAD, low-risk patients with an estimated annual mortality rate of less than 1 percent do not require repeat testing for several years after their initial evaluation. Higher risk patients (estimated annual mortality > 3%) might require more frequent follow-up testing on an annual basis in the absence of a change of symptoms.[48]

TABLE 10–1 Terms Useful in Evaluation of Test Results

Term	Definition
True positive (TP)	Abnormal test result in individual with disease
False positive (FP)	Abnormal test result in individual without disease
True negative (TN)	Normal test result in individual without disease
False negative (FN)	Normal test result in individual with disease
Sensitivity	Percentage of patients with CAD who have an abnormal result = TP/(TP + FN)
Specificity	Percentage of patients without CAD who have a normal result = TN/(TN + FP)
Predictive value	Percentage of patients with an abnormal result who have CAD = TN/(TN + FN)
Test accuracy	Percentage of true test results = (TP + TN)/total number tests performed
Likelihood ratio	Odds of a test result being true abnormal test result: sensitivity/(1 – specificity) normal test result: specificity/(1 – sensitivity)
Relative risk	Disease rate in persons with a positive test result/disease rate in persons with a negative test result

CAD = coronary artery disease.

Diagnostic Use of Exercise Testing

Appreciation of the noninvasive test literature to diagnose CAD requires an understanding of standard terminology such as *sensitivity, specificity*, and *test accuracy* (Table 10–1).[1,2,7,8] In patients selected for coronary angiography, the sensitivity of the exercise ECG in patients with CAD is approximately 68 percent, and specificity is 77 percent. In patients with single-vessel disease, the sensitivity ranges from 25 to 71 percent, with exercise-induced ST displacement most frequent in patients with left anterior descending CAD, followed by those with right CAD and those with isolated left circumflex CAD. In patients with multivessel CAD, sensitivity is approximately 81 percent and specificity is 66 percent. The sensitivity and specificity for left main or three-vessel CAD are approximately 86 percent and 53 percent, respectively. The exercise ECG tends to be less sensitive in patients with extensive anterior wall myocardial infarction and when a limited exercise ECG lead set is used. Approximately 75 to 80 percent of the diagnostic information on exercise-induced ST segment depression in patients with a normal resting ECG is contained in leads V_4 to V_6. Exercise ECG is less specific when patients in whom false-positive results are more common are included, such as those with valvular heart disease, left ventricular hypertrophy, marked resting ST segment depression, or digitalis therapy. Table 10–2 lists the more common causes of noncoronary exercise–induced ST segment depression.

The traditional reference standard against which the exercise ECG has been measured is a qualitative assessment of the coronary angiogram using 50 to 70 percent obstruction of the luminal diameter as the angiographic cutpoint. Limitations are inherent in angiographic classification of patients according to whether they have one-, two-, or three-vessel CAD, and the length of the coronary artery narrowing and the impact of serial lesions are not accounted for in correlative studies comparing diagnostic exercise testing with coronary angiographic findings. Other approaches, including intracoronary Doppler flow studies and quantitative coronary angiography, have been proposed to assess coronary vascular reserve; these may be more accurate than qualitative assessment of the angiogram.[49,50] The magnitude of coronary atherosclerosis in a coronary vessel is often underestimated on a luminal angiogram when intravascular ultrasonographic studies are performed.[51] A normal coronary angiogram does not eliminate the possibility that a patient's symptoms may be ischemic in origin. In a study of 20 patients with ischemic-appearing ST segment depression during exercise and normal findings on coronary angiography (syndrome X), intravenous adenosine infusion produced chest pain and subendocardial hypoperfusion detected with cardiac magnetic resonance

TABLE 10–2 Noncoronary Causes of ST Segment Depression

Severe aortic stenosis	Glucose load
Severe hypertension	Left ventricular hypertrophy
Cardiomyopathy	Hyperventilation
Anemia	Mitral valve prolapse
Hypokalemia	Intraventricular conduction disturbance
Severe hypoxia	Preexcitation syndrome
Digitalis use	Severe volume overload (aortic, mitral regurgitation)
Sudden excessive exercise	Supraventricular tachyarrhythmias

imaging in 95 percent of subjects, as compared with 40 percent in a control group.[52]

Selective referral of patients with a positive test result for further study both decreases the rate of detection of true-negative test results and increases the rate of detection of false-positive results, thus increasing sensitivity and decreasing specificity.[1,2,7,8] Froelicher and colleagues, in a study of 814 consecutive patients who presented with angina pectoris and agreed to undergo both exercise testing and coronary angiography, reported exercise ECG sensitivity of 45 percent and specificity of 85 percent for obstructive CAD using visual analysis in this population with reduced work-up bias.[53] Computerized ST segment measurements were similar to visual ST segment measurements in this study. A false-positive result is more common when only the inferior lead group (leads 2, 3, aV_f) is abnormal at high exercise workloads.

BAYES' THEOREM. The depth of exercise-induced ST-segment depression and the extent of the myocardial ischemic response can be thought of as continuous variables. Cutpoints such as 1 mm of horizontal or downsloping ST segment depression as compared with baseline cannot completely distinguish patients with disease from those without disease, and the requirement of more severe degrees of ST segment depression to improve specificity will decrease sensitivity. Sensitivity and specificity are inversely related, and false-negative and false-positive results are to be expected when ECG or angiographic cutpoints are selected to optimize the diagnostic accuracy of the test.

The use of Bayes' theorem incorporates the pretest risk of disease and the sensitivity and specificity of the test (likelihood ratio) to calculate the posttest probability of coronary disease. The patient's clinical information and exercise test results are used to make a final estimate about the probability of CAD. Atypical or probable angina in a 50-year-old man or a 60-year-old woman is associated with approximately 50 percent probability for CAD before exercise testing is performed. The diagnostic power of the exercise test is maximal when the pretest probability of CAD is intermediate (30 to 70 percent).

MULTIVARIATE ANALYSIS. Multivariate analysis of noninvasive exercise tests to estimate posttest risk also can provide important diagnostic information. Multivariate analysis offers the potential advantage that it does not require that the tests be independent of each other or that sensitivity and specificity remain constant over a wide range of disease prevalence rates (see section on prognosis). However, the multivariate technique depends critically on how patients are selected to establish the reference data base.[54,55] Both bayesian and multivariate approaches are commonly used to provide diagnostic and prognostic estimates of patients with CAD.

SEVERITY OF ELECTROCARDIOGRAPHIC ISCHEMIC RESPONSE. The exercise ECG result is more likely to be abnormal in patients with more severe coronary arterial obstruction, with more extensive CAD, and after more strenuous levels of exercise. Early onset of angina, ischemic ST segment depression, and fall in blood pressure at low exercise workloads are the most important exercise parameters associated with an adverse prognosis and multivessel CAD.[1,2,7,8] Additional adverse markers include profound ST segment displacement, ischemic changes in five or more ECG leads, and persistence of the changes late in the recovery phase of exercise (Table 10-3).

Exercise Testing in Determining Prognosis

Exercise testing provides not only diagnostic information but also, more importantly, prognostic data. The value of exercise testing to estimate prognosis must be considered in light of what is already known about a patient's risk status. Left ventricular dysfunction, CAD extent, electrical instability, and noncoronary comorbid conditions must be taken into consideration when estimating long-term outcome.

ASYMPTOMATIC POPULATION. The prevalence of an abnormal exercise ECG result in middle-aged asymptomatic men ranges from 5 to 12 percent. Rywik and colleagues studied 1083 volunteers from the Baltimore Longitudinal Study of Aging to determine the prognostic value of different types of exercise ECG response for cardiac events defined as onset of angina, myocardial infarction, or cardiac death. After a 7.9-year follow-up, horizontal or downsloping ST segment depression 1 mm or greater or intensification of minor pre-exercise ST segment depression to 1 mm or greater independently predicted cardiac events.[56] In earlier studies from other institutions, the risk of developing a cardiac event such as angina, myocardial infarction, or death in men was approximately nine times greater when the test result was abnormal than when it was normal; however, over 5 years of follow-up, only one in four men suffered a cardiac event, and this was most commonly the development of angina. The data illustrate the difficulty in identifying asymptomatic subjects destined to develop abrupt changes in plaque morphology based on an abnormal exercise electrocardiogram. The future risk of cardiac events is greatest if the test result is strongly positive or if an asymptomatic subject has atherosclerotic risk factors such as diabetes, hypertension, hypercholesterolemia, smoking history, or familial history of premature coronary disease (Fig. 10–14).[56-58] Target extracardiac end-organ damage such as peripheral vascular disease, proteinuria, or stroke further escalates the risk in accordance with bayesian

TABLE 10–3 Exercise Parameters Associated with an Adverse Prognosis and Multivessel Coronary Artery Disease

Duration of symptom-limiting exercise < 5 METs
Failure to increase systolic blood pressure ≥ 120 mm Hg, or a sustained decrease ≥ 10 mm Hg, or below rest levels, during progressive exercise
ST segment depression ≥ 2 mm, downsloping ST segment, starting at <5 METs, involving ≥5 leads, persisting ≥5 min into recovery
Exercise-induced ST segment elevation (aV excluded)
Angina pectoris at low exercise workloads
Reproducible sustained (>30 sec) or symptomatic ventricular tachycardia
Acute systemic illness (pulmonary embolism, aortic dissection)

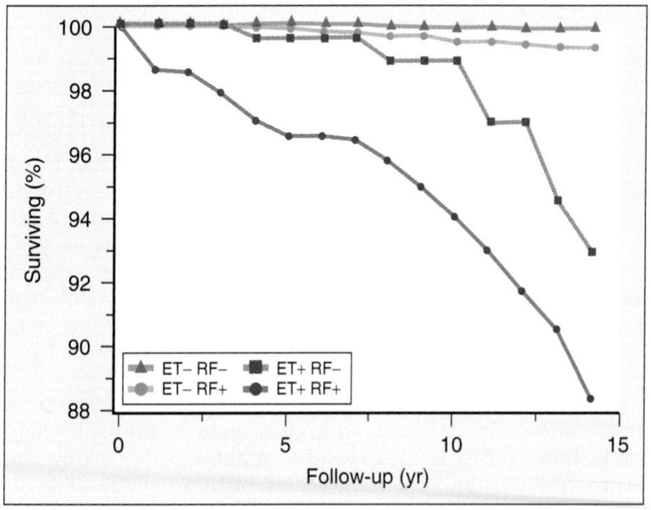

FIGURE 10–14 In 25,927 apparently healthy asymptomatic men 20 to 82 years of age followed for an average 8.4 years, cardiac event-free survival was worse in the patient subset with conventional atherosclerotic risk factors (RF+) and an abnormal exercise test (ET+). The age-adjusted relative risk (not shown) increased with the number of risk factors. In contrast, the event rate in subjects without risk factors (RF–) and an ET+ was not significantly different than in subjects with a normal exercise test (ET–) in the first 5 years of follow-up. (Gibbons LW, Mitchell TL, Wei M, et al: Maximal exercise test as a predictor of risk for mortality from coronary heart disease in asymptomatic men. Am J Cardiol 86:53, 2000.)

principles. Selection of asymptomatic subjects for an exercise test should be based on the atherosclerotic risk profile that can be used to provide a global risk estimate of the likelihood of death, myocardial infarction, or stroke. Appropriate asymptomatic subjects for exercise testing would be those with an estimated annual risk greater than 1 or 2 percent per year.[59] In asymptomatic middle-aged or older men with several atherosclerotic risk factors, a markedly abnormal exercise response is associated with a significantly increased risk of subsequent cardiac events, particularly when there is additional supporting evidence for underlying CAD (e.g., coronary calcification, abnormal results of thallium scan, and the like). Blumenthal and colleagues studied 734 asymptomatic siblings of persons with documented coronary disease and reported abnormal exercise perfusion results in 153 subjects, 95 percent of whom had mild to moderate atherosclerosis at angiography. Luminal narrowings of greater than 50 percent were found in 70 percent of subjects with an abnormal exercise ECG and scan.[58] Serial change of a negative exercise ECG result to a positive one in an asymptomatic person carries the same prognostic importance as an initially abnormal test result. However, when an asymptomatic individual with an initially abnormal test result has significant worsening of the ECG abnormalities at lower exercise workloads, this finding may indicate significant CAD progression and warrants a more aggressive diagnostic work-up. The prevalence of an abnormal exercise ECG result in middle-aged asymptomatic women ranges from 20 to 30 percent.[1,2,7,8] In general, the prognostic value of an ST segment shift in women is less than in men. Although the use of multivariate scores to predict CAD in women has improved diagnostic accuracy, false-positive results continue to be a problem in many patients, and supplemental imaging techniques are often necessary to enhance the diagnostic performance of the test.[1,2]

SYMPTOMATIC PATIENTS. Exercise testing should be routinely performed (unless this is not feasible or unless there are contraindications) before coronary angiography in patients with chronic ischemic heart disease. Patients who have excellent exercise tolerance (e.g., >10 METs) usually have an excellent prognosis regardless of the anatomical extent of CAD.[1,2,39-41] The test provides an estimate of the functional significance of angiographically documented coronary artery stenoses. The impact of exercise testing in patients with proven or suspected CAD was studied by Weiner and colleagues in 4083 medically treated patients in the CASS study.[60] A high-risk patient subset was identified (12 percent of the population), with an annual mortality rate of 5 percent when exercise workload was less than Bruce stage I (<4 METs) and the exercise ECG exhibited 0.1 mV (1 mm) or greater ST segment depression. A low-risk patient subset (34 percent of the population) who were able to exercise into Bruce stage III or higher and who had a normal exercise ECG result had an annual mortality rate of less than 1 percent over 4 years of follow-up. Similar ECG and workload parameters were useful in risk-stratifying patients with three-vessel CAD likely to benefit from coronary bypass grafting.

Mark and colleagues developed a treadmill score based on 2842 consecutive patients with chest pain in the Duke data bank; these patients underwent treadmill testing using the Bruce protocol and cardiac catheterization.[61] Patients with left bundle branch block (LBBB) or those with exercise-induced ST elevation in a Q wave lead were excluded. The treadmill (TM) score is calculated as follows:

$$\text{TM score} = \text{exercise time} - (5 \times \text{ST deviation}) - (4 \times \text{treadmill angina index})$$

Angina index was assigned a value of 0 if angina was absent, 1 if typical angina occurred during exercise, and 2 if angina was the reason the patient stopped exercising. Exercise-induced ST deviation was defined as the largest net ST displacement in any lead. The 13 percent of patients with a treadmill score of −11 or less had a 5-year survival rate of 72 percent, as compared with a 97 percent survival rate among the 34 percent of patients at low risk with a treadmill score of +5 or greater. The score added independent prognostic information to that provided by clinical data, coronary anatomy, and left ventricular ejection fraction. The stratified annual mortality rates predicted from the treadmill score were less in 613 outpatients referred for exercise testing from the same institution (Fig. 10–15).[62] The score worked equally well in men and women, although women had a lower overall risk than men for similar scores. The Duke treadmill score is not as effective in estimating risk in subjects 75 years of age or older (see section on elderly patients).[63] Exercise scoring systems can be used to identify prognostically intermediate- to high-risk patients in whom coronary angiography would be indicated to define coronary anatomy.[54,55,64] However, the decision to perform coronary revascularization should take into consideration the fact that in patients with less extensive CAD (e.g., one to two vessels narrowed and well-preserved left ventricular function), a similar degree of exercise-induced myocardial ischemia does not carry the same significant increased risk of cardiac events as in patients with more extensive disease (e.g., three vessels narrowed or impaired left ventricular function). When estimating prognosis in individual patients from the population-based data collected in the previous two decades, consideration should be given to the fact that actual survival rates in the current era are likely to be greater because of more aggressive treatment of atherosclerotic risk factors and use of noninvasive testing to identify the highest risk subjects that benefit from coronary revascularization.

SILENT MYOCARDIAL ISCHEMIA (see Chap. 50). In patients with documented CAD, the presence of exercise-induced ischemic ST segment depression confers increased risk of subsequent cardiac events regardless of whether angina occurs during the test.[65] The magnitude of the prognostic gradient in patients with an abnormal exercise ECG result with or without angina varies considerably in the published literature, most likely a feature of patient selection. In the CASS data bank, 7-year survival in patients with silent or symptomatic exercise-induced myocardial ischemia was similar in patients stratified by coronary anatomy and left ventricular function, with the worst survival in patients with the most extensive CAD. In the ACIP trial, coronary revascularization was a more effective treatment strategy to reduce exercise-induced myocardial ischemia than was medical therapy.

ACUTE CORONARY SYNDROMES (see Chaps. 47 and 49)

The incidence of exercise-induced angina or ischemic ST segment abnormalities in patients who have an acute coronary syndrome and who undergo a predischarge low-level protocol ranges from 30 to 40 percent. The finding of ischemic ST segment changes or limiting chest pain is associated with a significantly increased risk of subsequent cardiac events in men and postmenopausal women.[66-68] The absence of these findings identifies a low-risk patient subset. The prognostic risk assessment after an acute coronary syndrome should incorporate findings from the history, physical examination, resting 12-lead ECG, and level of serum markers to optimize mortality and morbidity estimates and to categorize patients into low-, intermediate-, and high-risk groups.[67] Exercise testing should be considered in the outpatient evaluation of low-risk patients with unstable angina (biomarker negative) who are free of active ischemic symptoms for a minimum of 8 to 12 hours, and in hospitalized low- to intermediate-risk ambulatory patients who are free of angina or heart failure symptoms for at least 48 hours.[69] In many intermediate- or high-risk patients, coronary angiography will have been performed during the acute phase of the illness; coronary disease extent, left ventricular function, and degree of coronary revascularization, if performed, should then be incorporated with the exercise test data to determine the overall predischarge prognostic risk estimate.

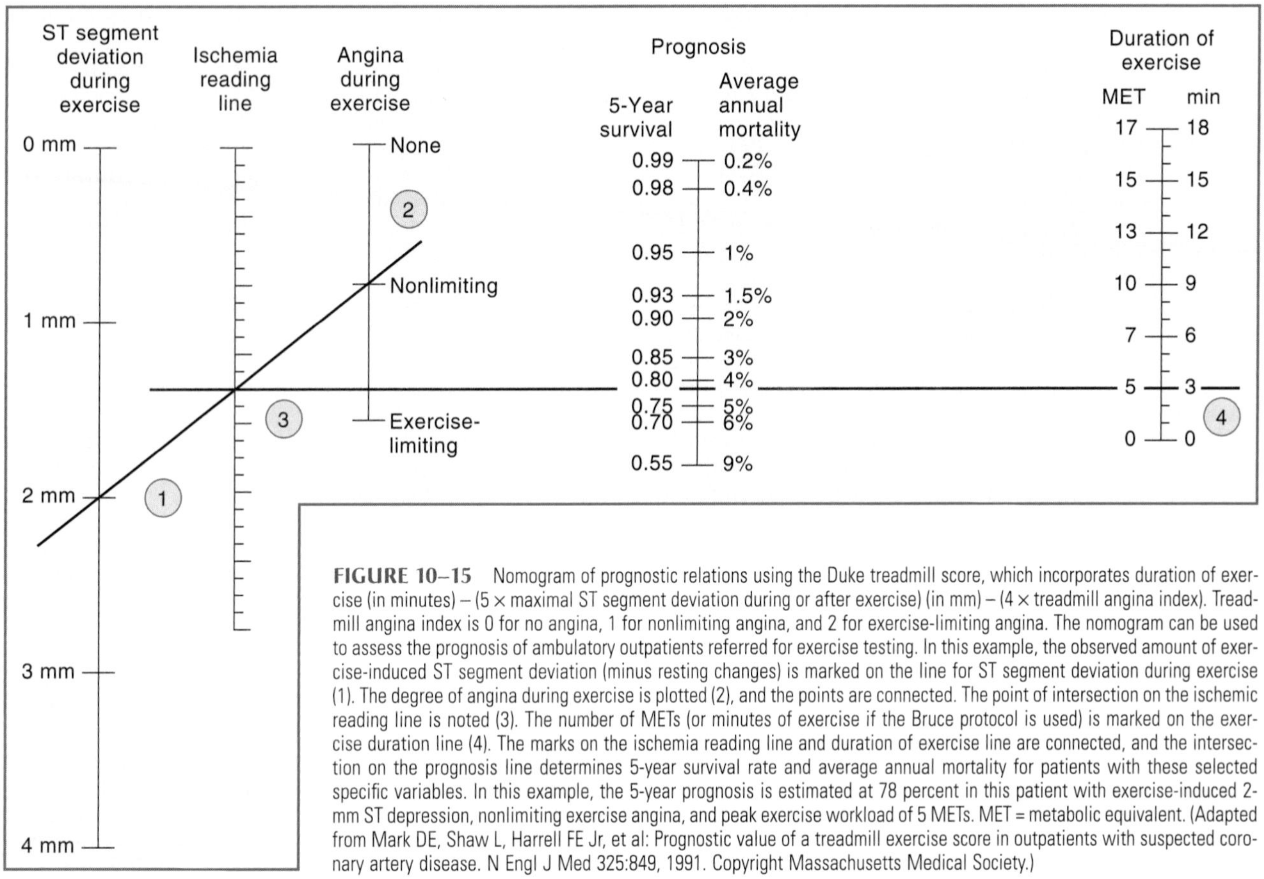

FIGURE 10–15 Nomogram of prognostic relations using the Duke treadmill score, which incorporates duration of exercise (in minutes) – (5 × maximal ST segment deviation during or after exercise) (in mm) – (4 × treadmill angina index). Treadmill angina index is 0 for no angina, 1 for nonlimiting angina, and 2 for exercise-limiting angina. The nomogram can be used to assess the prognosis of ambulatory outpatients referred for exercise testing. In this example, the observed amount of exercise-induced ST segment deviation (minus resting changes) is marked on the line for ST segment deviation during exercise (1). The degree of angina during exercise is plotted (2), and the points are connected. The point of intersection on the ischemic reading line is noted (3). The number of METs (or minutes of exercise if the Bruce protocol is used) is marked on the exercise duration line (4). The marks on the ischemia reading line and duration of exercise line are connected, and the intersection on the prognosis line determines 5-year survival rate and average annual mortality for patients with these selected specific variables. In this example, the 5-year prognosis is estimated at 78 percent in this patient with exercise-induced 2-mm ST depression, nonlimiting exercise angina, and peak exercise workload of 5 METs. MET = metabolic equivalent. (Adapted from Mark DE, Shaw L, Harrell FE Jr, et al: Prognostic value of a treadmill exercise score in outpatients with suspected coronary artery disease. N Engl J Med 325:849, 1991. Copyright Massachusetts Medical Society.)

MYOCARDIAL INFARCTION

Exercise testing after myocardial infarction (both non-ST and ST elevation) is useful to determine (1) risk stratification and assessment of prognosis, (2) functional capacity for activity prescription after hospital discharge, and (3) assessment of adequacy of medical therapy and need to use supplemental diagnostic or treatment options.[1,2,7,8] The incidence of fatal or nonfatal cardiac events associated with exercise testing after myocardial infarction is low. The risk of events is approximately twofold greater for symptom-limited protocols compared with submaximal tests, although the overall fatal event rate is extremely low with both types of exercise protocols. A low-level exercise test (achievement of 5 to 6 METs or 70 to 80 percent of age-predicted maximum) is frequently performed before hospital discharge to establish the hemodynamic response and functional capacity.[1,2,70] The ability to complete 5 to 6 METs of exercise or 70 to 80 percent of age-predicted maximum in the absence of abnormal ECG or blood pressure is associated with a 1-year mortality rate of 1 to 2 percent and may help guide the timing of early hospital discharge.[71] Parameters associated with increased risk include inability to perform or complete the low-level predischarge exercise test, poor exercise capacity, inability to increase or a decrease in exercise systolic blood pressure, and angina or exercise-induced ST segment depression at low workloads. Many postinfarct patients referred for exercise testing have been prescribed beta-adrenergic blocking agents and angiotensin-converting enzyme inhibitors. Although beta-adrenergic blocking drugs may attenuate the ischemic response, they do not interfere with poor functional capacity as a marker of adverse prognosis and should be continued in patients referred for testing. The relative prognostic value of a 3- to 6-week postdischarge exercise test is minimal once clinical variables and the results of the low-level predischarge test are adjusted for. For this reason, the timing of the exercise test after the infarct event favors predischarge exercise testing to allow implementation of a definitive treatment plan in patients in whom coronary anatomy is known as well as risk stratification of patients in whom coronary anatomy has not yet been determined. There is a trend toward early predischarge exercise testing (within 3 to 5 days) in uncomplicated cases after acute myocardial infarction.[71] A 3- to 6-week test is useful in clearing patients to return to work in occupations involving physical labor in which the MET expenditure is likely to be greater than that performed on a predischarge test.

The goals and basic principles of the predischarge evaluation have not been changed by the advent of reperfusion or direct percutaneous transluminal coronary angioplasty therapy for acute infarction. After receiving intravenous thrombolytic therapy or direct coronary angioplasty, patients with uncomplicated myocardial infarction tend to exhibit exercise-induced angina and ST segment depression less frequently than do consecutive postinfarct patients before these treatment strategies were widely applied. The occurrence of reciprocal ST segment depression associated with exercise-induced ST segment elevation in patients who undergo testing approximately 6 to 8 weeks after Q wave infarction with single-vessel disease may indicate residual tissue viability in the infarct-related area.[72] In patients with negative T waves after infarction, stress-induced normalization of the T waves may also indicate higher coronary flow reserve than in patients unable to normalize their T waves.[26]

RISK STRATIFICATION IN THE EMERGENCY DEPARTMENT. Patients who present to the emergency department are a heterogeneous population with a large range of pretest risk for CAD. Clinical algorithms can identify lower risk persons who can safely be further risk-stratified using exercise testing.[69,73,74] In one series of 1000 symptomatic low-risk patients with chest pain possibly of cardiac origin who presented to the emergency department, Amsterdam and colleagues reported a positive, intermediate, and nondiagnostic exercise test result in 13, 64, and 23 percent, respectively.[75] There were no adverse effects of exercise testing. The cost-effectiveness of this approach has been demonstrated in both low- and intermediate-risk patients. The accuracy of exercise testing in the emergency department setting follows bayesian principles, with the greatest diagnostic and prognostic estimates in intermediate-risk clinical patient subsets. Exercise testing in the emergency department should not be performed when (1) new or evolving ECG abnormalities are noted on the rest tracing, (2) the levels of cardiac enzymes are abnormal, (3) the patient cannot adequately perform exercise, (4) the patient reports worsening or persistent chest pain symptoms, or (5) clinical risk profiling indicates that imminent coronary angiography is likely. Several series of clinically low-risk subjects reported 6-month cardiac event rates less than 1 percent with a normal exercise test result.[76]

PREOPERATIVE RISK STRATIFICATION BEFORE NONCARDIAC SURGERY (see Chap. 77). Exercise ECG before elective noncardiac surgery provides an objective measurement of functional capacity and the potential to identify the likelihood of perioperative myocardial ischemia in patients with a low ischemic threshold.[77] In patients with intermittent claudication and no prior history of cardiac disease, approximately 20 to 25 percent will have an abnormal exercise ECG result. In patients with a prior history of myocardial infarction or an abnormal resting ECG, 35 to 50 percent will have an abnormal exercise ECG result. The risk of perioperative cardiac events and adverse long-term outcome is significantly increased in patients with abnormal exercise ECG results at low workloads. Coronary angiography with revascularization, when feasible, should be considered in such patients before noncardiac operative interventions that are considered high risk, such as aortic and other major vascular surgery and anticipated prolonged procedures associated with large fluid shifts or blood loss.[78-80]

CONGESTIVE HEART FAILURE. Cardiac and peripheral compensatory mechanisms are activated in patients with chronic congestive heart failure to partly or fully restore impaired left ventricular performance. Abnormal baroreflex function and increased norepinephrine spillover, sympathetic discharge, downregulation of beta-adrenergic receptors, and depletion of myocardial sympathetic stores characterize the disease process resulting in the hemodynamic response to exercise.[81-84] There is a wide range of exercise capacity in patients who have a markedly reduced ejection fraction, with some patients having near-normal peak exercise capacity. The magnitude of exercise capacity impairment is a function of the relative inability to augment stroke volume and abnormalities in skeletal muscle metabolism, which may be the predominant cause of functional limitation in a significant proportion of patients with heart failure. Fatigue may be related to altered skeletal muscle metabolism secondary to chronic physical deconditioning, impaired perfusion, and chronic anemia.[81,85-87] In a series of 26 heart failure patients with chronic anemia, peak $\dot{V}O_2$ was significantly increased when hemoglobin was increased from 11 to 14 g/dl with erythropoietin, iron, and folate administration.[86] Symptoms in patients with congestive heart failure are related to an excessive increase in blood lactate during low exercise levels, reduction in quantity of oxygen consumed at peak exertion, and disproportionate increase in ventilation at submaximal and peak workloads. The increased ventilatory requirement assessed by the hyperventilatory response to exercise and increase in pulmonary dead space leads to rapid, shallow breathing during exercise. Dyspnea and fatigue are the usual reasons for exercise termination.

Peak $\dot{V}O_2$ measurements in patients with compensated congestive heart failure are useful in risk-stratifying patients with congestive heart failure to determine the subsequent incidence of cardiac events (Fig. 10–16).[81,84,88-90] The ability to achieve a peak $\dot{V}O_2$ of greater than 20 ml O_2/kg/min and anaerobic threshold greater than 14 ml O_2/kg/min is associated with a relatively good long-term prognosis and maximal cardiac output greater than 8 liters/min/m^2. Patients who are unable to achieve a peak $\dot{V}O_2$ of 10 ml O_2/kg/min and anaerobic threshold of 8 ml O_2/kg/min have a poor prognosis, and their maximal exercise cardiac output is usually less than 4 liters/min/m^2. Failure of $\dot{V}O_2$ to decrease within 30 seconds after peak exertion is associated with more severe reductions in left ventricular ejection fraction and moderate to severe impairment of pulmonary gas exchange. Inability to increase oxygen pulse (milliliters of oxygen per beat) is related to a lack of or a minimal increase of stroke volume. A blunted heart rate response caused by postsynaptic desensitization of beta-adrenergic receptors is not uncommon in patients with congestive heart failure. Exercise protocols that limit exercise duration to 5 to 7 minutes are associated with the most reproducible peak $\dot{V}O_2$ measurements in patients with heart

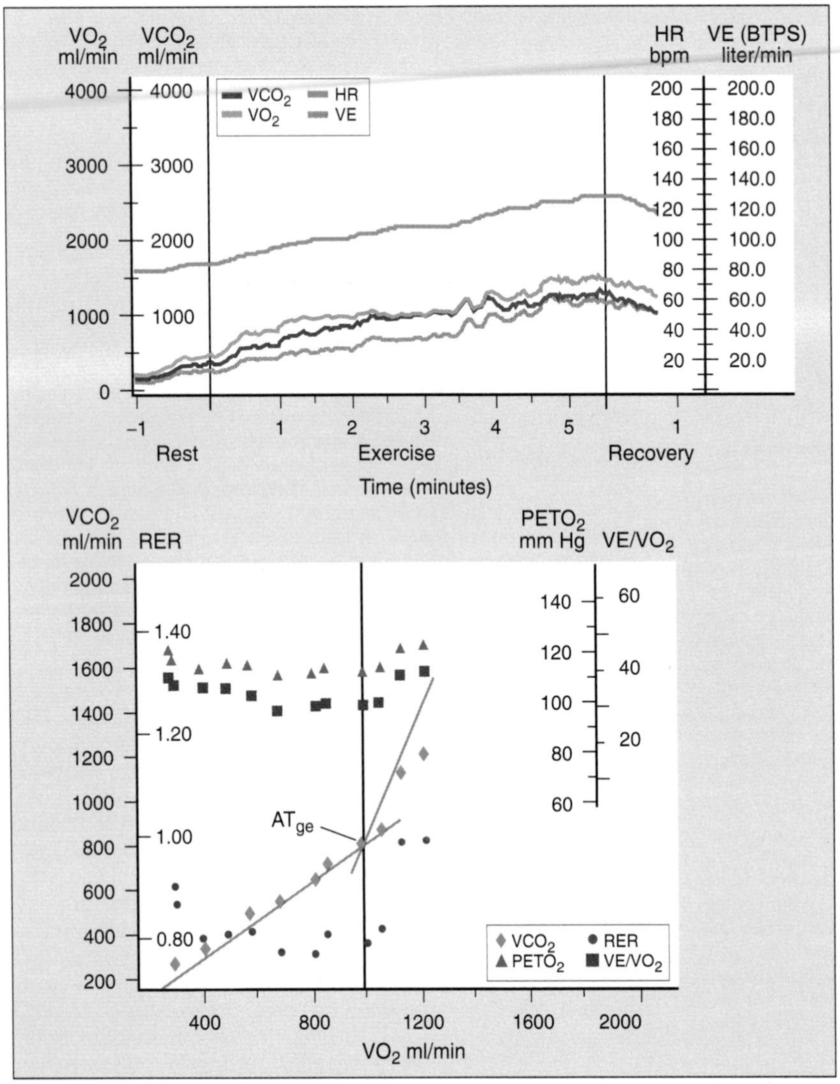

FIGURE 10–16 Cardiopulmonary exercise test in a 51-year-old man with cardiomyopathy in New York Heart Association Class III. A modified Bruce protocol was used. The patient reached a peak $\dot{V}O_2$ of 14 ml O_2/kg/min (4 METs), 44 percent of predicted for age, gender, and weight **(top)**. Anaerobic threshold (AT_{ge}) occurred at a $\dot{V}O_2$ of 977 ml/min **(bottom)**. The blunted cardiopulmonary response is typical for a patient with severe cardiomyopathy and marked impairment of cardiac reserve. This patient was listed for cardiac transplantation. METs = metabolic equivalents; $PETO_2$ = end-tidal pressure of oxygen.

failure. The interpretation of cardiopulmonary exercise test results in patients with heart failure can occasionally be difficult, because some patients hyperventilate during exercise, producing falsely low peak oxygen consumption, and it can be difficult to distinguish patients who are deconditioned from those who have impaired exercise performance and low peak $\dot{V}O_2$ due to cardiac pathology. Randomized controlled trials of long-term moderate exercise training in patients with chronic heart failure report a 15 to 20 percent improvement in peak $\dot{V}O_2$ and prolonged onset of anaerobic metabolism.[89] Thus, clinical decisions such as listing a patient for cardiac transplantation based on peak $\dot{V}O_2$ measurements need to take into consideration interval training effects.[89,90] The 6-minute walk test also can be used to evaluate functional capacity and to estimate prognosis in patients unable to exercise on a bicycle ergometer or treadmill.[91] However, in patients with moderate to severe heart failure, peak $\dot{V}O_2$ measurements are more reliable than the walking test for clinical decisions.[92]

Cardiac Arrhythmias and Conduction Disturbances

The genesis of cardiac arrhythmias includes reentry, triggered activity, and enhanced automaticity (see Chap. 27). Increased catecholamines during exercise accelerate impulse conduction velocity, shorten the myocardial refractory period, increase the amplitude of afterpotentials, and increase the slope of phase 4 spontaneous depolarization of the action potential. Other potentiators of cardiac rhythm disturbance include metabolic acidosis and exercise-induced myocardial ischemia. Ventricular premature complexes occur frequently during exercise testing and increase with age. Repetitive forms occur in 0 to 5 percent of asymptomatic subjects without suspected cardiac disease and are not associated with an increased risk of cardiac death. Exercise-induced ventricular ectopic activity is not a useful diagnostic marker of ischemic heart disease in the absence of ischemic ST segment depression. Suppression of ventricular ectopic activity during exercise is a nonspecific finding and may occur in patients with CAD as well as in normal subjects. The prognostic importance of ventricular arrhythmias in patients with chronic ischemic heart disease after adjustment for baseline, clinical, and left ventricular function characteristics is small. Approximately 20 percent of patients with known heart disease and 50 to 75 percent of sudden cardiac death survivors have repetitive ventricular beats induced by exercise. In patients with a recent myocardial infarction, the presence of exercise-induced repetitive forms is associated with an increased risk of subsequent cardiac events. Beta-adrenergic blocking drugs may suppress exercise-induced ventricular arrhythmias. Exercise-induced ventricular arrhythmias tend to be more frequent in the recovery phase of exercise because peripheral plasma norepinephrine levels continue to increase for several minutes after cessation of exercise, and vagal tone is high in the immediate recovery phase. Five-year all-cause mortality rates are significantly greater in patients who have frequent ventricular ectopy or repetitive ventricular beats in the recovery phase of exercise as compared with those who have ventricular arrhythmias that occur only during exercise.[93] The test is useful in evaluating the effects of antiarrhythmic drugs, detecting supraventricular arrhythmias, treating patients with chronic atrial fibrillation to test for ventricular rate control, and exposing possible drug toxicity in patients placed on antiarrhythmic drugs.

EVALUATION OF VENTRICULAR ARRHYTHMIAS. Exercise testing is useful in the assessment of patients with ventricular arrhythmias and has an important adjunctive role along with ambulatory monitoring and electrophysiological studies.[1,2,7,8,93,94] Exercise testing provokes repetitive ventricular premature beats in most patients with a history of sustained ventricular tachyarrhythmia, and in approximately 10 to 15 percent of such patients, spontaneously occurring arrhythmias are observed only during exercise testing (Fig. 10–17). Frequent ventricular ectopy that occurs in the early postexercise phase is associated with a worse long-term prognosis than ventricular ectopy that occurs only during exercise (Fig. 10–18). In patients with adrenergic-dependent rhythm disturbances (including monomorphic ventricular tachycardia and polymorphic ventricular tachycardia related to long-QT syndromes), ambulatory electrocardiography or event monitoring may fail to capture the arrhythmia, particularly if the patient is relatively sedentary.[95,96] Paradoxical prolongation of the QT_C interval greater than 10 msec with exercise identifies patients likely to develop a proarrhythmic effect on type 1A antiarrhythmic drugs. Exercise-induced widening of the QRS complex in patients using type 1C drugs may favor reentry induction of ventricular tachycardia. Amiodarone therapy increases the QRS duration during exercise by approximately 6 percent in patients with a QRS duration less than 110 msec, as compared with 15 percent in patients with a QRS duration longer than 110 msec.

SUPRAVENTRICULAR ARRHYTHMIAS. Supraventricular premature beats induced by exercise are observed in 4 to 10 percent of normal persons and up to 40 percent of patients with underlying heart disease. Sustained supraventricular tachyarrhythmias occur in only 1 to 2 percent of patients, although the frequency may approach as much as 10 to 15 percent in patients referred for management of episodic supraventricular arrhythmias. The presence of supraventricular arrhythmias is not diagnostic for ischemic heart disease.

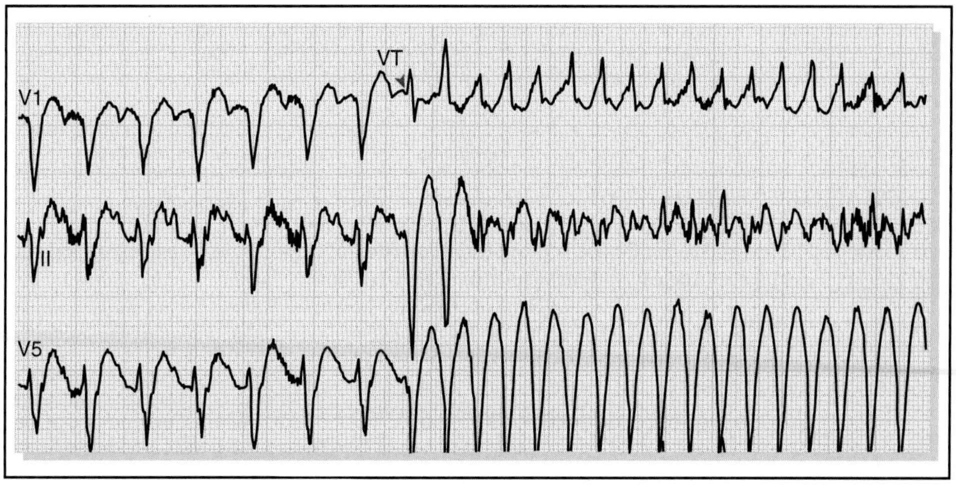

FIGURE 10–17 A 67-year-old man with ischemic cardiomyopathy referred for exercise testing had a left bundle branch block and first-degree atrioventricular (AV) block on the resting ECG. There was no worsening of the AV conduction disturbance immediately before onset of ventricular tachycardia (VT) (arrow). At 4:55 minutes into the test, a 27-beat run of VT was noted, reproducing the patient's symptoms of dizziness and chest pounding. The exercise test proved useful in directing subsequent patient management to treatment of the ventricular arrhythmia.

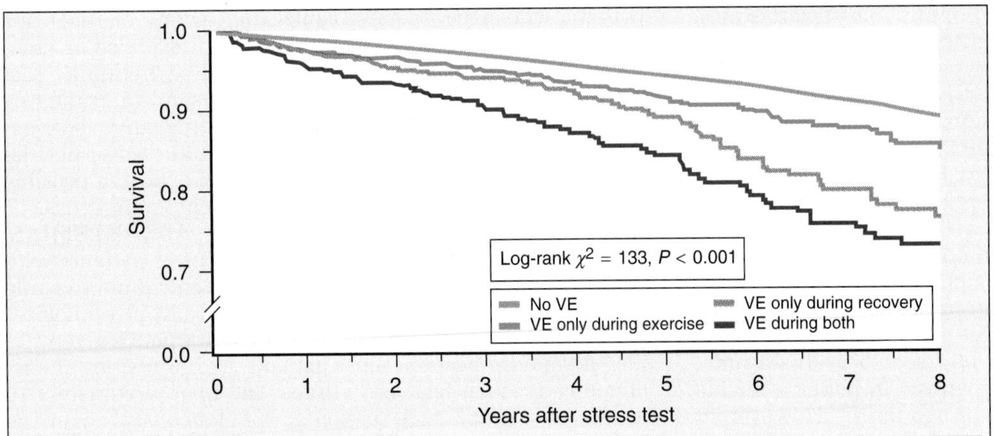

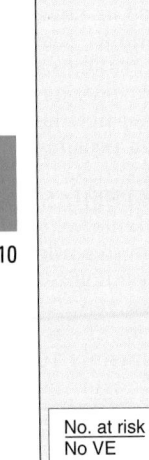

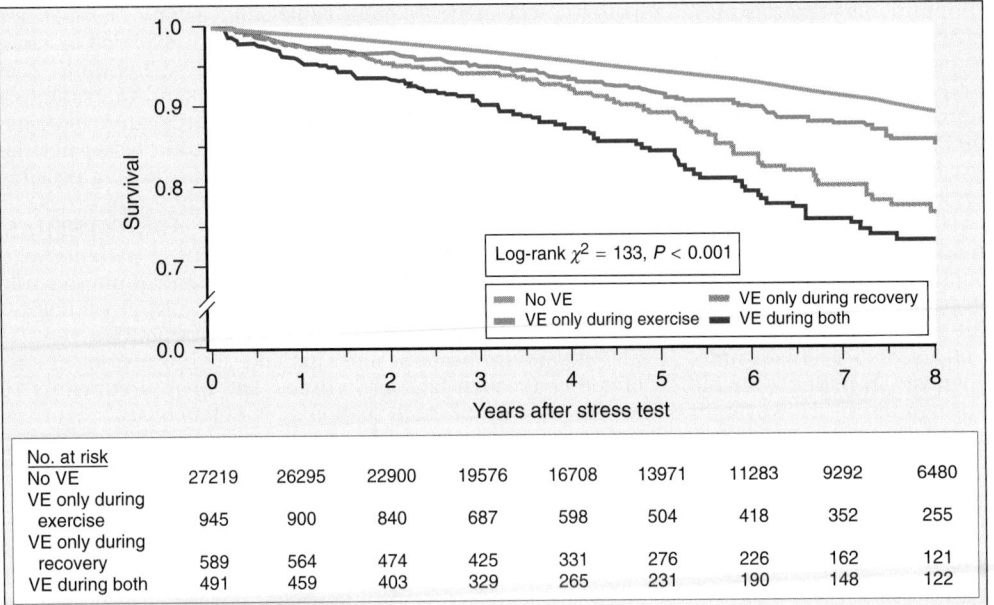

No. at risk									
No VE	27219	26295	22900	19576	16708	13971	11283	9292	6480
VE only during exercise	945	900	840	687	598	504	418	352	255
VE only during recovery	589	564	474	425	331	276	226	162	121
VE during both	491	459	403	329	265	231	190	148	122

FIGURE 10–18 In this series of 29,244 subjects, frequent ventricular ectopy occurred in 3 percent of subjects only during exercise, in 2 percent of subjects only during recovery from exercise, and in 2 percent of subjects during both exercise and recovery. The prognosis of patients who had postexercise-induced frequent ventricular ectopy was worse than the prognosis of subjects who had frequent ventricular ectopy only during exercise. The mean follow-up time was 5.3 years. (From Frolkis JP, Pothier CE, Blackstone EH, et al: Frequent ventricular ectopy after exercise as a predictor of death. N Engl J Med 348:781, 2003.)

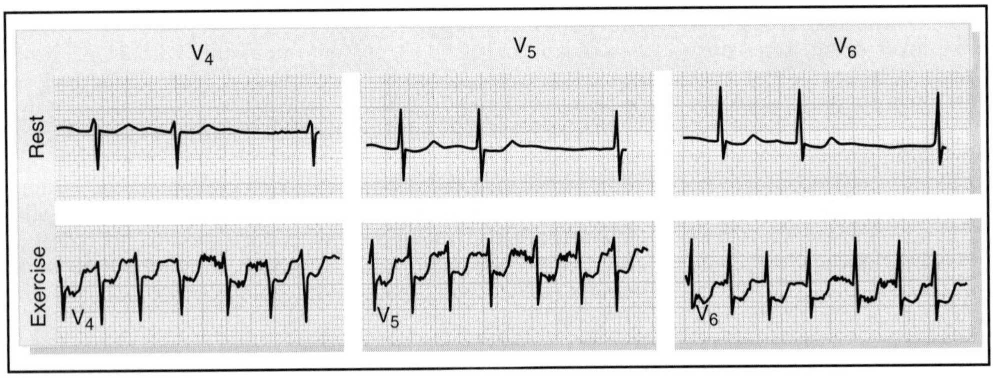

FIGURE 10–19 A 75-year-old woman with chronic atrial fibrillation and a 6-month history of atypical chest pain underwent mitral valve repair 1 year before testing, at which time nonobstructive coronary disease was noted. The patient exercised for 6 minutes, achieving a peak heart rate of 176 beats/min and peak blood pressure of 170/90 mm Hg. The resting electrocardiogram shows atrial fibrillation with a controlled ventricular response and minor ST segment depression. At peak exertion, marked ST segment depression is seen in the anterior leads, consistent with either digitalis effect or myocardial ischemia. In this type of patient, initial exercise testing with myocardial perfusion tracers or echocardiography would provide more useful diagnostic information than exercise testing alone.

ATRIAL FIBRILLATION. Patients with chronic atrial fibrillation tend to have a rapid ventricular response in the initial stages of exercise, and 60 to 70 percent of the total change in heart rate usually occurs within the first few minutes of exercise (Fig. 10–19). The effect of digitalis preparations and beta-adrenergic and selected calcium antagonists such as diltiazem on attenuating this rapid increase in heart rate for individual patients can be measured using exercise testing. Pharmacological control of the ventricular rate does not necessarily result in a significant increase in exercise capacity, which in many patients is related to the underlying cardiac disease process and not to adequacy of control of the ventricular rate.

SINUS NODE DYSFUNCTION. In general, patients with sinus node dysfunction have a lower heart rate at submaximal and maximal workloads compared with control subjects. However, as many as 40 to 50 percent of patients will have a normal exercise heart rate response.

ATRIOVENTRICULAR BLOCK. Exercise testing may help determine the need for atrioventricular (AV) sequential pacing in selected patients. In patients with congenital AV block, exercise-induced heart rates are low and some patients develop symptomatic rapid junctional rhythms that can be suppressed with DDD devices. In patients with acquired conduction disease, exercise can occasionally elicit advanced AV block.

LEFT BUNDLE BRANCH BLOCK. Exercise-induced ST segment depression is found in most patients with left bundle branch block (LBBB) and cannot be used as a diagnostic or prognostic indicator regardless of the degree of ST segment abnormality. In patients who are referred to a tertiary center and in whom exercise testing is carried out, the new development of exercise-induced transient left hemiblock is 0.3 percent and the new development of LBBB is 0.4 percent, with a slightly greater incidence in older patients.[97] The relative risk of death or other major cardiac events in patients with exercise-induced LBBB is increased approximately threefold over the risk in patients without this abnormality. In one series, permanent LBBB was reported in approximately half of patients who developed transient LBBB during exercise and who were monitored for an average of 6.6 years. High-grade AV block did not develop in any of the patients in this 15-patient series. The development of ischemic ST segment depression before the LBBB pattern appears or in the recovery phase after the LBBB has resolved does not attenuate the diagnostic yield of the ST segment shift. The ventricular rate at which the LBBB appears and disappears can be significantly different (Fig. 10-20).

RIGHT BUNDLE BRANCH BLOCK. The resting ECG in patients with right bundle branch block (RBBB) is frequently associated with T wave and ST segment changes in the early anterior precordial leads (V_1 to V_3). Exercise-induced ST depression in leads V_1 to V_4 is a common finding in patients with RBBB and is nondiagnostic (Fig. 10-21). The new development of exercise-induced ST segment depression in leads V_5 and V_6 or leads 2 and aV_f, reduced exercise capacity, and inability to adequately increase systolic blood pressure are useful in detecting patients who have CAD and a high clinical pretest risk of disease. The presence of RBBB decreases the sensitivity of the test. The new development of exercise-induced RBBB is relatively uncommon, occurring in approximately 0.1 percent of tests.

PREEXCITATION SYNDROME. The presence of Wolff-Parkinson-White syndrome invalidates the use of ST segment analysis as a diagnostic method for detecting CAD in preexcited as well as normally conducted beats; false-positive ischemic changes are frequently registered (Fig. 10–22).[98] In patients with persistent preexcitation, exercise may normalize the QRS complex, with disappearance of the delta wave in 20 to 50 percent of cases, depending on the series studied. Abrupt disappearance of the delta wave is presumptive evidence of a longer anterograde effective refractory period of the accessory pathway. Progressive disappearance of the delta wave is less reassuring and occurs when the improvement in AV node conduction is greater than in the accessory pathway; this finding does not preclude a possible significant or even critical shortening of the anterograde effective refractory period in the accessory pathway under the influence of sympathetic stimulation. Exercise-induced disappearance of the delta wave is more frequent with left-sided than right-sided accessory pathway positions. Although tachyarrhythmias appearing during an exercise test in patients with Wolff-Parkinson-White syndrome are rare, when they do occur, they provide an opportunity to evaluate AV conduction velocity. The presence of Wolff-Parkinson-White syndrome does not cause a limitation of physical work capacity.

CARDIAC PACEMAKERS AND IMPLANTABLE CARDIOVERTER-DEFIBRILLATOR DEVICES. The exercise protocol used to assess chronotropic responsiveness in patients before and after cardiac pacemaker insertion should adjust for the fact that many patients with such devices are older individuals and may not tolerate high exercise workloads or abrupt and relatively large increments in work between stages of exercise. An optimal physiological cardiac pacemaker should normalize the heart rate response to exercise in proportion to oxygen uptake and should increase heart rate 2 to 4 beats/min for an increase in $\dot{V}O_2$ of 1 ml O_2/kg/min, with a slightly steeper slope for patients with severe left ventricular function impairment.[99] The exercise test can be particularly useful in evaluating sensor-triggered rate-adaptive pacing, in terms of both maximum heart rate achieved and rate of increase in heart rate during progressive exercise. Exercise testing can also be used to assess performance following cardiac resynchronization therapy in patients with heart failure and ventricular conduction delay.[100]

When testing patients with an implantable cardioverter-defibrillator device, the program detection interval of the device should be known. If the implantable cardioverter-defibrillator device is implanted for ventricular fibrillation or fast ventricular tachycardia, the rate will normally exceed that attainable during sinus tachycardia and the test can be terminated as the heart rate approaches 10 beats/min below the detection interval of the device. In patients with slower programmed detection rates, the implantable cardioverter-defibrillator can be reprogrammed to a faster rate to avoid accidental discharge during exercise testing or can be temporarily deactivated by a magnet. Exercise testing can be used to test the efficacy of tachycardic detection algorithms that apply criteria such as suddenness of onset and R-R variability.

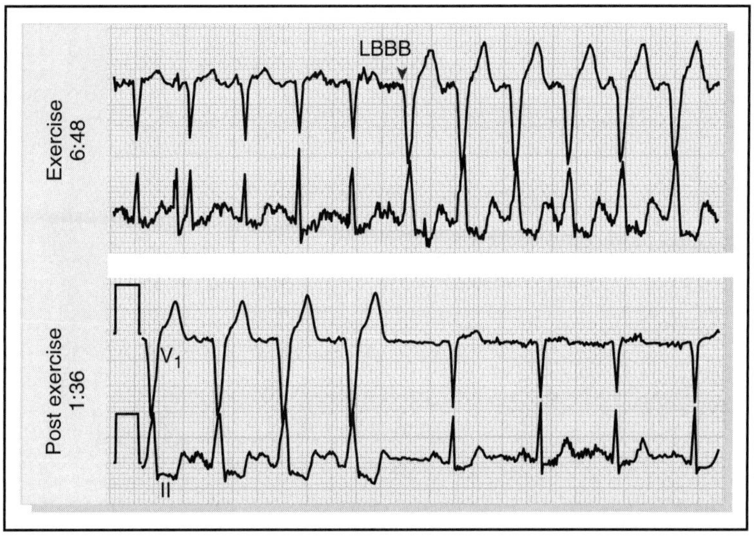

FIGURE 10–20 A 58-year-old hypertensive diabetic man with prior history of cigarette smoking was referred for evaluation of dyspnea and early fatigability during exercise. At 6:48 minutes into the test, the patient developed a rate-related left bundle branch block (LBBB) at a heart rate of 133 beats/min, which persisted during exercise and resolved at 1:36 minutes into the postexercise phase. The abnormal 2.5 to 3 mm downsloping ST segment depression in lead II during the LBBB is nondiagnostic for coronary artery disease because of the conduction disturbance. The test was stopped because of dyspnea at a peak heart rate of 138 beats/min (85 percent of predicted) and estimated workload of 6 METs. Peak blood pressure at the end of exercise was 174/94 mm Hg. Time to onset and offset of LBBB occurred at different ventricular rates related to fatigue in the left bundle, a common finding. METs = metabolic equivalents.

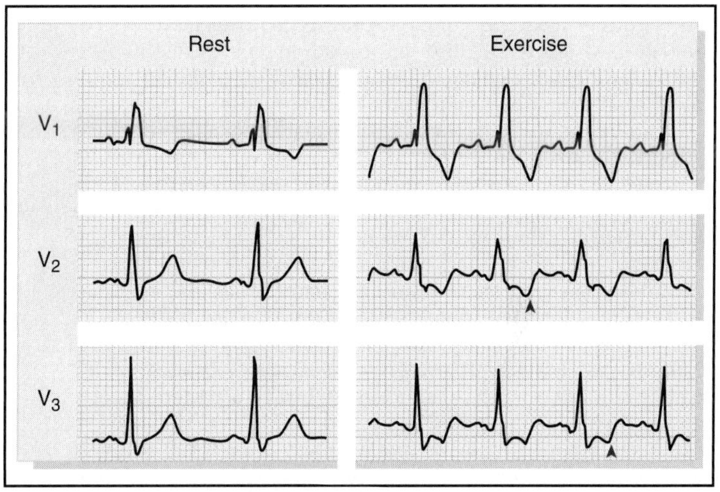

FIGURE 10–21 Exercise-induced ST segment depression is noted in leads V_2 to V_3 (arrows) in this patient with a resting right bundle branch block (RBBB) pattern. Exercise-induced horizontal or downsloping ST segment responses in the early anterior precordial leads (V_1 through V_4) are common in patients with RBBB and are secondary to the conduction disturbance. The presence of this finding in leads V_1 through V_4 is not diagnostic of obstructive coronary disease; however, if ischemic changes are seen in leads II, aV_F, or in leads V_5 or V_6, the specificity for coronary disease is improved.

Specific Clinical Applications

INFLUENCE OF DRUGS AND OTHER FACTORS. Patients with CAD demonstrate individual variability in time to onset of exercise-induced angina, time to onset of exercise-induced ischemic ST segment depression of 0.1 mV or greater, and cardiovascular efficiency during exercise testing.[7,8] The average individual variability in time to onset of exercise-induced myocardial ischemia or peak anaerobic capacity approximates as much as 20 percent in placebo-controlled trials of antianginal drugs. Average increases in exercise duration approach 40 to 60 seconds after 2 to 4 weeks and as much as 90 seconds after 12 weeks of placebo therapy.[101] Variability can be reduced by patients' familiarization with the exercise protocol and equipment, controlling for antianginal drug therapy at the time of testing, and stable test performance conditions. When two or three exercise tests are conducted within weeks of each other, the greatest increase in exercise time usually occurs between the first test and the second test. In one series of 24 subjects with stable

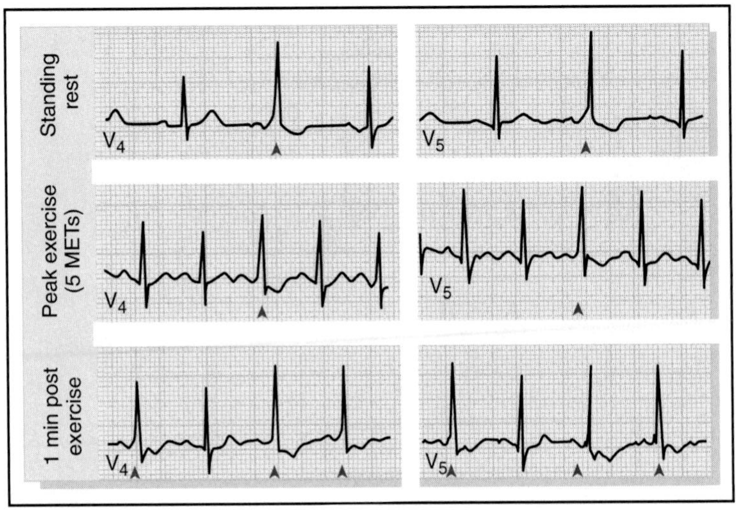

FIGURE 10–22 A 61-year-old man with atypical angina and a hiatal hernia was referred for diagnostic exercise testing. The test was stopped because of dyspnea. The standing resting ECG shows an intermittent Wolff-Parkinson-White pattern (arrows). In the nonpreexcited beats, ST segment depression does not occur either at peak exercise or in the postexercise phase. However, in the preexcited beats (arrows), an additional 1.3 mm of downsloping ST segment depression is noted as compared with baseline during and after exertion. METs = metabolic equivalents.

angina of less than class II, exercise time was increased by approximately 1 minute and time to onset of angina or ischemic ST segment depression by 3 minutes when two exercise tests were performed 15 minutes apart.[102] The mechanisms of the attenuation response with reexercise may be the results of ischemic preconditioning, familiarization with the exercise protocol, and improved musculoskeletal efficiency but do not appear to be dependent on exercise protocol intensity or downregulation of myocardial contractility induced by the initial ischemic stimulus.[31-33] In cold-sensitive individuals, exercise testing in a cooler environment results in onset of ischemic ST segment depression earlier than under normal temperature-controlled conditions. Conditions that increase carbon monoxide levels, such as chronic cigarette smoking, lower the ischemic response threshold.

Digitalis glycosides can produce exertional ST segment depression even if the effect is not evident on the resting ECG and can accentuate ischemic exercise-induced ST segment changes, particularly in older individuals. Absence of ST segment deviation during an exercise test in a patient receiving a cardiac glycoside is considered a valid negative response. Hypokalemia in patients on long-term diuretic therapy can be associated with exercise-induced ST segment depression. Antiischemic drug therapy with nitrates, beta-blocking drugs, or calcium channel blocking drugs prolongs the time to onset of ischemic ST segment depression, increases exercise tolerance, and, in a small minority of patients (10 to 15 percent), may normalize the exercise ECG response in patients with documented CAD.[7,8] The time and dose of drug ingestion may affect exercise performance. In some laboratories, cardioactive drug therapy is withheld for three to five half-lives and digitalis for 1 to 2 weeks before diagnostic testing. This is impractical in many cases, however.

WOMEN. The diagnostic accuracy of exercise-induced ST segment depression for obstructive CAD is less in women than in men. The decreased sensitivity results in part from a lower prevalence and extent of CAD in young and middle-aged women. Women tend to have a greater release of catecholamines during exercise, which could potentiate coronary vasoconstriction and augment the incidence of abnormal exercise ECG results, and false-positive results have been reported to be more common during menses or preovulation, or in postmenopausal women on isolated estrogen replacement therapy.[103,104] In a series of 976 symptomatic women referred for exercise testing and coronary angiography, low-, moderate-, and high-risk Duke treadmill scores were associated with CAD of 75 percent or greater luminal narrowing in 19.1, 34.9, and 89.2 percent of subjects, respectively. The frequency of three-vessel disease (75 percent or greater luminal narrowing) or left main CAD was 3.5, 12.4, and 46 percent, respectively. In a retrospective population-based cohort study of 1452 men and 741 women, exercise-induced angina, ischemic ECG changes, and workload were strongly associated with all-cause mortality and cardiac events in both sexes. The relationship between workload and outcome was linear, with an increment of 1 MET in workload associated with a 20 to 25 percent reduction in risk of death and cardiac events.[105] Alexander and colleagues compared the Duke treadmill score in 976 women and 2249 men; the 2-year mortality rate for women was 1, 2.2, and 3.6 percent for low-, moderate-, and high-risk scores, respectively, as compared with 1.7, 5.8, and 16.6 percent in men. In this report, women had a similar frequency of angina on the treadmill as men, but exertional angina in women was less often correlated with the presence of CAD.[106]

Morise and colleagues reported mortality rates ranging from 0.2 percent for a low-risk score to 7 percent for a high-risk score based on five clinical and three exercise test variables after an average 2.6-year follow-up in 442 symptomatic women referred for their first exercise test (Fig. 10–23).[55] Thus, in women with established CAD, exercise testing provides useful prognostic information for risk stratification and identification of low risk and higher risk patient subsets.

HYPERTENSION. Exercise testing has been used in an attempt to identify patients who have an abnormal blood pressure response and are destined subsequently to develop hypertension. In asymptomatic normotensive individuals, an exaggerated exercise systolic and diastolic blood pressure response during exercise or an exaggerated peak systolic

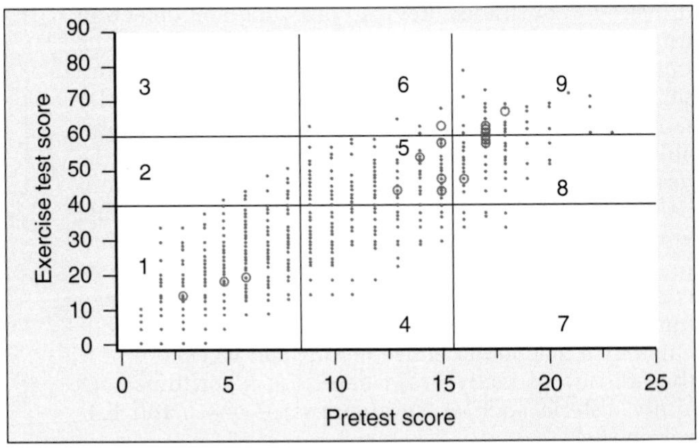

FIGURE 10–23 Scatter plot of exercise score as a function of pretest score for 1678 women referred for exercise testing. Points for those alive (closed circles) and dead (open circles) are shown. Heavy gridlines represent cutpoints for low-intermediate and intermediate-high risk groups for each score. Lowest risk patients (lowest pretest risk and lowest exercise score) are in sector 1 and highest risk patients (highest pretest risk and highest exercise score) in sector 9. Mortality after a mean 2.6-year follow-up was greatest in women with at least an intermediate pretest clinical score and exercise test score. Clinical variables include age, symptoms, diabetes, smoking, and estrogen status. Exercise ECG score variables include ST depression, peak heart rate, and Duke angina index. (From Morise AP, Lauer MS, Froelicher VF: Development and validation of a simple exercise test score for use in women with symptoms of suspected heart disease. Am Heart J 144:818, 2002.)

blood pressure response to 214 mm Hg or greater or an elevated systolic or diastolic blood pressure at the third minute of recovery is associated with significant increased long-term risk of hypertension (Fig. 10–24).[35,107,108] Severe systemic hypertension may interfere with subendocardial perfusion and cause exercise-induced ST segment depression in the absence of atherosclerosis, even when the resting ECG does not show significant ST or T wave changes. Beta- and calcium channel blocking drugs decrease submaximal and peak systolic blood pressure in many hypertensive patients. Exercise tolerance is decreased in patients with poor blood pressure control.

ELDERLY PATIENTS. Maximal aerobic capacity ($\dot{V}O_2max$) declines 8 to 10 percent per decade in sedentary men and women, with an approximately 50 percent reduction in exercise capacity between the ages of 30 and 80 years.[1,2,63] The exercise protocol in elderly patients should be selected according to estimated aerobic capacity. In patients with limited exercise tolerance, the test should be started at the slowest speed with a 0 percent grade and adjusted according to the patient's ability. Older patients may need to grasp the handrails for support. The frequency of abnormal exercise ECG patterns is greater in older than in younger individuals, and the risk of cardiac events is significantly increased because of a concomitant increase in prevalence of more extensive CAD.[1,2,40,109,110] The greater test sensitivity of the exercise ECG in elderly individuals is accompanied by a slight reduction in specificity. Cardiac arrhythmias, chronotropic incompetence, and hypertensive responses are more common in older individuals. The value of exercise testing to estimate prognosis in elderly subjects was evaluated in 3107 patients from Olmstead County, of whom 512 were 65 years of age or older. Workload expressed in METs was the only variable associated with all-cause mortality in subjects 65 years of age or older, whereas workload and exercise-induced angina were predictive of cardiac death or nonfatal myocardial infarction.[110] In elderly subjects 75 years of age or older, the Duke treadmill scoring system is less effective in estimating prognosis.[63] Most elderly patients tend to be categorized as intermediate risk, primarily because they cannot exercise long enough to be classified as low risk.

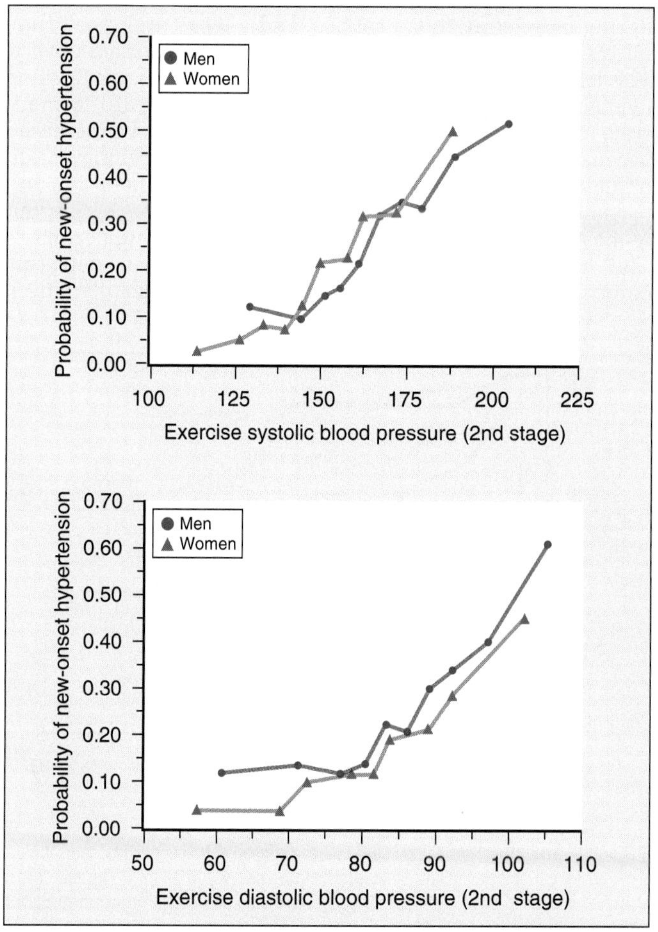

FIGURE 10–24 Probability of developing systemic hypertension within 8 years after exercise testing as a function of exercise-induced systolic **(top)** and diastolic **(bottom)** blood pressure responses in men and women. Crude probabilities of developing hypertension are displayed for mean systolic or diastolic blood pressure value for each exercise response during the second stage of treadmill testing. (From Singh JP, Larson MG, Manolio TA, et al: Blood pressure response during treadmill testing is a risk factor for new onset hypertension. The Framingham Heart Study. Circulation 99:1831, 1999.)

DIABETES MELLITUS. Coronary atherosclerosis and peripheral vascular disease are significantly increased in adult diabetic patients as compared with nondiabetic patients (see Chap. 51); the likelihood of atherosclerosis correlates closely with the duration of diabetes and the presence of microvascular disease, peripheral vascular disease, and autonomic neuropathy.[111] In patients with autonomic dysfunction and sensory neuropathy, anginal threshold may be increased, and abnormal exercise-induced heart rate and blood pressure responses are common. Once CAD is established, the incidence of exercise-induced ECG changes is similar to the incidence in nondiabetic persons.[112] The probability of an adverse cardiac outcome in a diabetic person as compared with a nondiabetic person for a similar abnormal exercise test result is likely to be increased because of the increased risk of dyslipidemia, impaired fibrinolysis, and hypertension associated with the diabetic process. Patients with diabetes who wish to enroll in a moderate- to high-intensity exercise program are considered to have a class IIa indication for exercise testing.[1] Further research is required to determine optimal noninvasive test procedures to diagnose early endothelial dysfunction and the presence and extent of obstructive CAD in patients with diabetes.

VALVULAR HEART DISEASE AND HYPERTROPHIC CARDIOMYOPATHY. The hemodynamics of exercise provide an excellent opportunity to measure gradients across stenotic valves, to assess ventricular function in patients with primary valvular regurgitation or mixed lesions, and to assess pulmonary and systemic vascular resistance (see Chap. 57).[113-115] The use of echocardiographic Doppler techniques (see Chap. 11) is particularly valuable in evaluating patients whose symptoms are out of proportion to the degree of hemodynamic abnormalities observed at rest and in assessing the results of valvulotomy or valve replacement. Clinical and exercise noninvasive assessment of patients with valvular heart disease can provide useful information on the timing of operative intervention and help achieve a more precise estimate of a patient's degree of incapacitation than can assessment of symptoms alone.[114] Studies of adults with moderate to severe aortic stenosis (e.g., valve area 0.5 to 1.5 cm^2 and mean gradients of 18 to 64 mm Hg) show that exercise testing can be safely performed when appropriate exercise protocols and precautions are used. Exercise testing is useful in evaluating aortic valve gradients during low-output flow states and with Doppler echocardiography provides important data on left ventricular functional reserve. Hypotension during exercise in asymptomatic patients with aortic stenosis may be a sufficient reason to consider valve replacement.[113] In patients with mitral stenosis, excessive heart rate response to relatively low levels of exercise, reduction of cardiac output with exercise (manifested by exercise-induced hypotension), and chest pain (ischemia secondary to low output or pulmonary hypertension) are indicators that favor earlier valve repair. In patients with mitral valve prolapse without regurgitation at rest, exercise-induced mitral regurgitation has been associated with the subsequent development of progressive mitral regurgitation, heart failure symptoms, or syncope.

Peak $\dot{V}O_2$ and anaerobic threshold are reduced in symptomatic patients with hypertrophic cardiomyopathy as compared with sedentary subjects (see Chap. 59). In a 50-patient series of hypertrophic cardiomyopathy, 59 percent of symptomatic subjects were unable to achieve a peak $\dot{V}O_2$ of 60 percent of predicted; only two patients achieved a peak $\dot{V}O_2$ greater than 80 percent of predicted.[116] Inability to increase blood pressure by 20 mm Hg during exercise may result from exercise-induced left ventricular systolic dysfunction and is associated with an adverse prognosis.[117] Abnormal blood pressure responses in patients with hypertrophic cardiomyopathy may normalize after transcoronary alcohol septal ablation, associated with only a slight increase in exercise time.[118]

CORONARY REVASCULARIZATION

CORONARY BYPASS GRAFTING (see Chap. 50). The degree of improvement in exercise-induced myocardial ischemia and aerobic capacity after coronary bypass grafting depends in part on the degree of revascularization achieved and on left ventricular function. Exercise-induced ischemic ST segment depression may persist when incomplete revascularization is achieved, albeit at higher exercise workloads. It also may persist in approximately 5 percent of patients in whom complete revascularization has been achieved. It usually takes at least 6 weeks of convalescence before maximum exercise can be performed. The natural history of saphenous vein grafts and internal mammary artery conduits is different, and serial conversion from an initially normal to an abnormal exercise ECG result over time depends in part on the type of conduit used and on CAD progression in nongrafted vessels. Stress imaging studies are likely to provide more useful information regarding the site and extent of myocardial ischemia after coronary revascularization procedures than the exercise electrocardiogram and are the preferred modality when noninvasive testing is performed for management decisions. The diagnostic and prognostic utility of exercise testing late after coronary revascularization (e.g., 5 to 10 years) is much greater than early (<1 year) testing, because a late abnormal exercise response is more likely to indicate graft occlusion, stenosis, or progression of CAD, particularly in the presence of typical angina or conditions of accelerated atherosclerosis such as diabetes mellitus, hemodialysis, or immunosuppressive therapy.[119] In selected patients with severe left ventricular dysfunction and symptomatic heart failure, coronary bypass surgery is associated with a significant increase in exercise capacity when a large amount of dysfunctional but viable myocardium (e.g., >25% of left ventricular mass) is revascularized.[120]

PERCUTANEOUS CORONARY INTERVENTION (see Chap. 52). The risk of restenosis after percutaneous coronary intervention (PCI) is time dependent; stent restenosis usually occurs within the first 12 months after PCI, and it is anticipated that rates of restenosis will be greatly reduced with the use of drug-eluting stents. In the early post-PCI phase (<1 month), an abnormal exercise ECG result may be secondary to a suboptimal result, impaired coronary vascular reserve in a successfully dilated vessel, or incomplete revascularization.[30,121-123] Thus, exercise electrocardiography has a low diagnostic accuracy to detect restenosis or an incomplete dilation in the periprocedural phase. The optimal time to perform an exercise test after PCI depends in part on the success of the procedure and the degree of revascularization obtained. In an otherwise asymptomatic patient, a 6- to 12-month postprocedure test allows sufficient time to document restenosis should it occur and allows the dilated vessel an opportunity to heal. Serial conversion of an initially normal exercise test result after PCI to an abnormal result in the initial 6 months after the procedure, particularly when it occurs at a lower exercise workload, is usually associated with restenosis. The use of exercise myocardial imaging in selected patients enhances the diagnostic content of the test and can help localize the territory of myocardial ischemia and guide indications for repeat coronary angiography in patients who have undergone multivessel/multilesion PCI. In general, routine periodic monitoring of asymptomatic patients after a coronary revascularization procedure (coronary artery bypass grafting or PCI) without a specific indication is not useful.

CARDIAC TRANSPLANTATION (see Chap. 26). Cardiopulmonary exercise testing is useful in selecting patients with end-stage heart failure for cardiac transplantation. A peak $\dot{V}O_2$ of less than 12 to 14 ml O_2/kg/min or 40 to 50 percent of predicted $\dot{V}O_2$ is associated with 2-year survival rates ranging from 30 to 50 percent (Fig. 10–25).[84] The use of percentage of predicted $\dot{V}O_2$, which adjusts an individual patient's peak $\dot{V}O_2$ for age, gender, and weight rather than weight alone, has been shown to further enhance prognostic estimates in patients who have a low peak exercise $\dot{V}O_2$. In patients with initial poor exercise capacity awaiting heart transplantation, the ability to increase peak oxygen uptake with increased peak oxygen pulse identifies a relatively lower risk group in whom cardiac transplantation may be able to be deferred if the patient's clinical status is stable.

Exercise performance in transplant recipients is influenced by the fact that the donor heart is surgically denervated without efferent parasympathetic or sympathetic innervation and by the occurrence of rejection and scar formation, systemic and pulmonary vascular resistance, level of training, and development of coronary atherosclerosis in the graft.[124] Maximal oxygen uptake and work capacity are reduced after cardiac transplantation compared with measures in age-matched control subjects but usually are markedly improved compared with preoperative findings.[125] Abnormalities of the ventricular rate response include a resting tachycardia due to parasympathetic denervation, a slow heart rate response during mild to moderate exercise, a more rapid response during more strenuous exercise, and a more prolonged time for the ventricular rate to return to baseline during recovery. The transplanted heart relies heavily on the Frank-Starling mechanism to increase cardiac output during mild to moderate exercise. Systemic vascular resistance may be increased because of cyclosporine therapy. Sympathetic reinnervation of the sinus node may occur after cardiac transplantation and partially restore a normal heart rate response to exercise, but in most patients will not return exercise capacity to normal.[126] The exercise ECG is relatively insensitive in detecting coronary artery vasculopathy after cardiac transplantation.

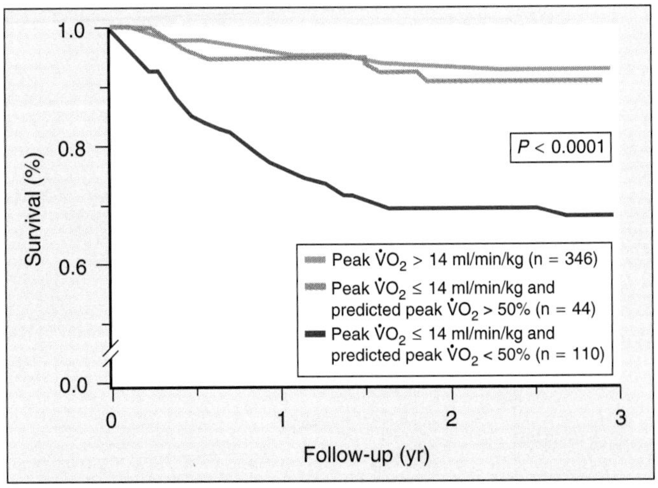

FIGURE 10–25 The 3-year survival of patients with congestive heart failure referred for cardiac transplant evaluation with a peak $\dot{V}O_2$ of 14 ml O_2/kg/min or less stratified according to predicted peak $\dot{V}O_2$ greater than 50 percent or less. The 91 ± 5 percent 3-year survival rate of the 44 patients with a predicted $\dot{V}O_2$ greater than 50 percent was similar to the survival rates of patients with a peak $\dot{V}O_2$ greater than 14 ml O_2/kg/min and significantly greater than the 61 ± 5 percent survival rate of the 110 patients with a peak $\dot{V}O_2$ of 50 percent or less. The data indicate that a low peak $\dot{V}O_2$ and percentage predicted $\dot{V}O_2$ identify high-risk patients with congestive heart failure whose survival may be improved by cardiac transplantation. (From Osada N, Chaitman BR, Miller LW, et al: Cardiopulmonary exercise testing identifies low risk patients with heart failure and severely impaired exercise capacity considered for heart transplantation. J Am Coll Cardiol 31:577, 1998.)

However, the new development of an abnormal exercise ECG result several years after cardiac transplantation may indicate focal intraluminal narrowing.

Safety and Risks of Exercise Testing

Exercise testing has an excellent safety record. The risk is determined by the clinical characteristics of the patient referred for the procedure. In nonselected patient populations, the mortality is less than 0.01 percent and morbidity is less than 0.05 percent.[127] The risk is greater when the test is performed soon after an acute ischemic event. In a survey of 151,941 tests conducted within 4 weeks of an acute myocardial infarction, mortality was 0.03 percent, and 0.09 percent of patients tested either had a nonfatal reinfarction or were resuscitated from cardiac arrest.[128] The relative risk of a major complication is about twice as great when a symptom-limited protocol is used as compared with a low-level protocol. Nevertheless, in the early postinfarction phase, the risk of a fatal complication during symptom-limited testing is only 0.03 percent. The risk is less for low-risk patients who are seen in the emergency department and who undergo exercise testing for risk stratification. Exercise testing can be safely performed in patients with compensated congestive heart failure, with no major complications reported in 1286 tests in which a bicycle ergometer was used.[129] The risk of exercise testing in patients referred for life-threatening ventricular arrhythmias was examined by Young and colleagues[130] in a series of 263 patients who underwent 1377 tests; 2.2 percent developed sustained ventricular tachyarrhythmias that required cardioversion, cardiopulmonary resuscitation, or antiarrhythmic drugs to restore sinus rhythm. The ventricular arrhythmias were more frequent in tests performed on antiarrhythmic drug therapy as compared with the baseline drug-free state. In contrast to the high risk in the aforementioned patient subsets, the risk of complications in asymptomatic subjects is extremely low, with no fatalities reported in several series.[1,7,8]

The risk of incurring a major complication during exercise testing can be reduced by performing a careful history and physical examination before the test and observing patients closely during exercise with monitoring of the ECG, arterial pressure, and symptoms. The standard 12-lead ECG should be verified before the test for any acute or recent changes. The contraindications to exercise testing are well defined (Table 10–4). Patients with critical obstruction to left ventricular outflow are at increased risk of cardiac events during exercise. In selected patients, low-level exercise can be useful in determining the severity of the left ventricular outflow tract obstruction. The cool-down period should be prolonged to at least 2 minutes in patients with left ventricular outflow tract obstruction or stenotic valves to avoid sudden pressure-volume shifts that occur in the immediate postexercise phase.

TABLE 10–4 Absolute Contraindications to Exercise Testing
Acute myocardial infarction (<2 d)
High-risk unstable angina
Decompensated heart failure
Uncontrolled cardiac arrhythmias with symptoms or hemodynamic compromise
Advanced atrioventricular block
Acute myocarditis or pericarditis
Severe symptomatic aortic stenosis
Severe hypertrophic obstructive cardiomyopathy
Uncontrolled hypertension
Acute systemic illness (pulmonary embolism, aortic dissection)

Uncontrolled systemic hypertension is a contraindication to exercise testing. Patients should continue antihypertensive drug therapy on the day of testing. Patients who present with systemic arterial pressure readings of 220/120 mm Hg or greater should rest for 15 to 20 minutes, and their blood pressure should be remeasured. If blood pressure remains at these levels, the test should be postponed until the hypertension is better controlled.

A resuscitator cart and defibrillator should be available in the room where the test procedure is carried out, and appropriate cardioactive medication should be available to treat cardiac arrhythmias, AV block, hypotension, and persistent chest pain. An intravenous line should be started in high-risk patients such as those being tested for adequacy of control of life-threatening ventricular arrhythmias. The equipment and supplies in the cart should be checked on a regular basis. A previously specified routine for cardiac emergencies needs to be determined; this includes patient transfer and admission to a coronary care unit if necessary.

Clinical judgment is required to determine which patients can be safely tested in an office as opposed to a hospital-based setting. The experience is acquired through training programs and maintenance of clinical competency.[131,132] High-risk patients, such as those with major left ventricular dysfunction, recent angina pectoris, cardiac syncope, or important ventricular ectopy on the pretest examination, should be tested in the hospital. Low-risk patients, such as asymptomatic individuals and those with a low pretest risk of disease, can be tested by specially trained nurses or physician assistants who have received advanced cardiac life support certification, with a physician in close proximity.

Termination of Exercise

The use of standard test indications to terminate an exercise test reduces risk (Table 10–5). Termination of exercise should be determined in part by the patient's recent activity level. The rate of perceived patient exertion can be estimated by the Borg scale. The scale is linear, with values of 9 for very light; 11 for fairly light; 13 for somewhat hard; 15 for hard; 17 for very hard; and 19 for very, very hard. Borg readings of 14 to 16 approximate anaerobic threshold, and readings of 18 or greater approximate a patient's maximum exercise capacity. It is helpful to grade exercise-induced chest discomfort on a 1 to 4 scale, with 1 indicating the initial onset of chest discomfort and 4 the most severe chest pain the patient has ever experienced. The exercise technician should note the onset of grade 1 chest discomfort on the work sheet, and the test should be stopped when the patient reports grade 3 chest pain. In the absence of symptoms, it is prudent to stop exercise when a patient demonstrates 0.3 mV (3 mm) or greater of ischemic ST segment depression or 0.1 mV (1 mm) or greater of ST segment elevation in a noninfarct lead without an abnormal Q wave. Significant worsening of ambient ventricular ectopy during exercise or the unsuspected appearance of ventricular tachycardia is an indication to terminate exercise. A progressive, reproducible decrease in systolic blood pressure of 10 mm Hg or more may indicate transient left ventricular dysfunction or an inappropriate decrease in systemic vascular resistance and is an indication to terminate exercise. The test should be stopped if the arterial blood pressure is 250 to 270/120 to 130 mm Hg or higher. Ataxia can indicate cerebral hypoxia.

The exercise test report should contain basic demographic data, the indication for testing, a brief description of the patient's profile, and exercise test results (Table 10–6).

TABLE 10–5 Indications for Terminating Exercise Testing
Absolute indications
Drop in systolic blood pressure of >10 mm Hg from baseline blood pressure despite an increase in workload, when accompanied by other evidence of ischemia
Moderate to severe angina (grade 3/4)
Increasing nervous system symptoms (e.g., ataxia, dizziness, or near-syncope)
Signs of poor perfusion (cyanosis or pallor)
Technical difficulties in monitoring ECG or systolic blood pressure
Subject's desire to stop
Sustained ventricular tachycardia
ST elevation (≥1.0 mm) in noninfarct leads without diagnostic Q waves (other than V_1 or aV)
Relative indications
Drop in systolic blood pressure of ≥10 mm Hg from baseline blood pressure despite an increase in workload, in the absence of other evidence of ischemia
ST or QRS changes such as excessive ST depression (>3 mm of horizontal or downsloping ST segment depression) or marked axis shift
Arrhythmias other than sustained ventricular tachycardia, including multifocal PVCs, triplets of PVCs, supraventricular tachycardia, heart block, or bradyarrhythmias
Fatigue, shortness of breath, wheezing, leg cramps, or claudication
Development of bundle branch block of intraventricular conduction delay that cannot be distinguished from ventricular tachyardia
Increasing chest pain
Hypertensive response

ECG = electrocardiogram; PVCs = premature ventricular contractions.
Modified from Fletcher GF: Exercise standards: A standard for healthcare professionals from the American Heart Association Writing Group. Circulation 91:580, 1995.

TABLE 10–6 Exercise Test Report Information
Demographic data: name, patient identifier, date of birth/age, gender, weight, height, test date
Indication(s) for test
Patient descriptors: atherosclerotic risk profile, drug usage, resting ECG findings
Exercise test results
Protocol used
Reason(s) for stopping exercise
Hemodynamic data: rest and peak heart rate, rest and peak blood pressure, percent maximum achieved heart rate, maximum rate of perceived exertion (Borg scale), peak workload, peak METs, total exercise duration in minutes
Evidence for myocardial ischemia: time to onset and offset of ischemic ST segment deviation or angina, maximum depth of ST segment deviation, number of abnormal exercise ECG leads, abnormal systemic blood pressure responses
General comments

ECG = electrocardiogram; METs = metabolic equivalents.

REFERENCES

1. Gibbons RJ, Balady GJ, Bricker JT, et al: ACC/AHA 2002 guideline update for exercise testing. Summary article: A report of the ACC/AHA Task Force on Practice Guidelines (Committee to Update the 1997 Exercise Testing Guidelines). J Am Coll Cardiol 40:1531, 2002.
2. Fletcher GF, Balady GJ, Amsterdam EA, et al: Exercise standards for testing and training: A statement for healthcare professionals from the American Heart Association. Circulation 104:1694, 2001.
3. Balady GJ, Berra KA, Golding LA, et al: ACSM's Guidelines for Exercise Testing and Prescription. 6th ed. Philadelphia, Lippincott Williams & Wilkins, 2000.
4. Wasserman K, Hansen JE, Sue DY, et al: Principles of Exercise Testing and Interpretation. 3rd ed. Philadelphia, Lippincott Williams & Wilkins, 1999.
5. American Thoracic Society/American College of Chest Physicians: Statement on cardiopulmonary exercise testing. Am J Respir Crit Care Med 167:211, 2003.
6. Hadeli KO, Siegel EM, Sherrill DL, et al: Predictors of oxygen desaturation during submaximal exercise in 8,000 patients. Chest 120:88, 2001.
7. Ellestad MH: Stress Testing: Principles and Practice. 4th ed. Philadelphia, FA Davis, 1996.
8. Froelicher VF, Myers J: Exercise and the Heart. 4th ed. Philadelphia, W.B. Saunders, 2000.
9. Fletcher GF, Flipse TR, Kligfield P, et al: Current status of ECG stress testing. Curr Probl Cardiol 23:353, 1998.
10. Fleg JL, Pina IL, Balady GJ, et al: Assessment of functional capacity in clinical and research applications: An advisory from the Committee on Exercise, Rehabilitation, and Prevention, Council on Clinical Cardiology, American Heart Association. Circulation 102:1591, 2000.
11. Pollock ML, Franklin BA, Balady GJ, et al: AHA Science Advisory. Resistance exercise in individuals with and without cardiovascular disease: Benefits, rationale, safety, and prescription. An advisory from the Committee on Exercise, Rehabilitation, and Prevention, Council on Clinical Cardiology, American Heart Association. Position paper endorsed by the American College of Sports Medicine. Circulation 101:828, 2000.

Exercise Physiology

12. Guyton AC, Hall JE: Textbook of Medical Physiology. 10th ed. Philadelphia, WB Saunders, 2000.
13. Correia LCL, Lakatta EG, O'Connor FC, et al: Attenuated cardiovascular reserve during prolonged submaximal cycle exercise in healthy older subjects. J Am Coll Cardiol 40:1290, 2002.
14. Williams MA, Fleg JL, Ades PA, et al: Secondary prevention of coronary heart disease in the elderly (with emphasis on patients ≥75 years of age): An American Heart Association scientific statement from the Council on Clinical Cardiology Subcommittee on Exercise, Cardiac Rehabilitation, and Prevention. Circulation 105:1735, 2002.
15. Tanaka H, Monahan KD, Seals DR: Age-predicted maximal heart rate revisited. J Am Coll Cardiol 37:153, 2001.
16. Gonzalez-Alonso J, Calbet JA: Reductions in systemic and skeletal muscle blood flow and oxygen delivery limit maximal aerobic capacity in humans. Circulation 107:824, 2003.
17. Hollenberg M, Tager IB: Oxygen uptake efficiency slope: An index of exercise performance and cardiopulmonary reserve requiring only submaximal exercise. J Am Coll Cardiol 36:194, 2000.
18. Montgomery PS, Gardner AW: The clinical utility of a six-minute walk test in peripheral arterial occlusive disease patients. J Am Geriatr Soc 46:706, 1998.
19. Badruddin SM, Ahmad A, Mickelson J, et al: Supine bicycle versus post-treadmill exercise echocardiography in the detection of myocardial ischemia: A randomized single-blind crossover trial. J Am Coll Cardiol 33:1485, 1999.

Electrocardiographic Measures

20. Michaelides AP, Psomadaki ZD, Dilaveris PE, et al: Improved detection of coronary artery disease by exercise electrocardiography with the use of right precordial leads. N Engl J Med 340:340, 1999.
21. Sabapathy R, Bloom HL, Lewis WR, Amsterdam EA: Right precordial and posterior chest leads do not increase detection of positive response in electrocardiogram during exercise treadmill testing. Am J Cardiol 91:75, 2003.
22. Rywik TM, Zink RC, Gittings NS, et al: Independent prognostic significance of ischemic ST segment response limited to recovery from treadmill exercise in asymptomatic subjects. Circulation 97:2117, 1998.
23. Soto JR, Watson DD, Beller GA.: Incidence and significance of ischemic ST-segment depression occurring solely during recovery after exercise testing. Am J Cardiol 88:670, 2001.
24. Akutsu Y, Shinozuka A, Nishimura H, et al: Significance of ST-segment morphology noted on electrocardiography during the recovery phase after exercise in patients with ischemic heart disease as analyzed with simultaneous dual-isotope single photon emission tomography. Am Heart J 144:335, 2002.
25. Fearon WF, Lee DP, Froelicher VF: The effect of resting ST segment depression on the diagnostic characteristics of exercise treadmill testing. J Am Coll Cardiol 35:1206, 2000.
26. Mobilia G, Zanco P, Desideri A, et al: T wave normalization in infarct-related electrocardiographic leads during exercise testing for detection of residual viability: Comparison with positron emission tomography. J Am Coll Cardiol 32:75, 1998.
27. Miwa K, Nakagawa K, Hirai T, Inoue H: Exercise-induced U-wave alterations as a marker of well-developed and well-functioning collateral vessels in patients with effort angina. J Am Coll Cardiol 35:757, 2000.
28. Okin PM, Prineas RJ, Grandits G, et al: Heart rate adjustment of exercise induced ST segment depression identifies men who benefit from a risk factor reduction program. Circulation 96:2899, 1997.

29. Julius BK, Vassalli G, Mandinov L, Hess OM: Alpha-adrenoreceptor blockade prevents exercise-induced vasoconstriction of stenotic coronary arteries. J Am Coll Cardiol 33:1499, 1999.
30. Maier W, Windecker S, Kung A, et al: Exercise-induced coronary artery vasodilation is not impaired by stent placement. Circulation 105:2373, 2002.
31. Kelion AD, Webb TP, Gardner MA, Ormerod OJM, Banning AP: The warm-up effect protects against ischemic left ventricular dysfunction in patients with angina. J Am Coll Cardiol 37:705, 2001.
32. Bogaty P, Poirier P, Boyer L, et al: What induces the warm-up ischemia/angina phenomenon: Exercise or myocardial ischemia? Circulation 107:1858, 2003.
33. Lambiase PD, Edwards RJ, Cusack MR, et al: Exercise-induced ischemia initiates the second window of protection in humans independent of collateral recruitment. J Am Coll Cardiol 41:1174, 2003.
34. Li RA, Leppo M, Miki T, et al: Molecular basis of electrocardiographic ST-segment elevation. Circ Res 87:837, 2000.

Nonelectrocardiographic Measures

35. Miyai N, Arita M, Miyashita K, et al: Blood pressure response to heart rate during exercise test and risk of future hypertension. Hypertension 39:761, 2002.
36. Reman A, Zelos G, Andrews NP, et al: Blood pressure changes during transient myocardial ischemia: Insights into mechanisms. J Am Coll Cardiol 30:1249, 1997.
37. Fleg JL, Lakatta EG: Prevalence and significance of postexercise hypotension in apparently healthy subjects. Am J Cardiol 57:1380, 1986.
38. Ha JW, Juracan EM, Mahoney DW, et al: Hypertensive response to exercise: A potential cause for new wall motion abnormality in the absence of coronary artery disease. J Am Coll Cardiol 39:323, 2002.
39. Myers J, Prakash M, Froelicher V, et al: Exercise capacity and mortality among men referred for exercise testing. N Engl J Med 346:793, 2002.
40. Spin JM, Prakash M, Froelicher VF, et al: The prognostic value of exercise testing in elderly men. Am J Med 112:453, 2002.
41. Florenciano-Sanchez R, Castillo-Moreno JA, Molina-Laborda E, et al: The exercise test that indicates a low risk of events. Differences in prognostic significance between patients with chronic stable angina and patients with unstable angina. J Am Coll Cardiol 38:1974, 2001.
42. Miller TD, Chaliki HP, Christian TF, et al: Usefulness of worsening clinical status or exercise performance in predicting future events in patients with coronary artery disease. Am J Cardiol 88:1294, 2001.
43. Lauer MS, Francis GS, Okin PM, et al: Impaired chronotropic response to exercise stress testing as a predictor of mortality. JAMA 281:524, 1999.
44. Elhendy A, Mahoney DW, Khandheria BK, et al: Prognostic significance of impairment of heart rate response to exercise: Impact of left ventricular function and myocardial ischemia. J Am Coll Cardiol 42:823, 2003.
45. Chaitman BR: Abnormal heart rate responses to exercise predict increased long-term mortality regardless of coronary disease extent. The question is why? J Am Coll Cardiol 42:2049, 2003.
46. Shetler K, Marcus R, Froelicher VF, et al: Heart rate recovery: Validation and methodologic issues. J Am Coll Cardiol 38:1980, 2001.
47. Vivekananthan DP, Blackstone EH, Pothier CE, Lauer MS: Heart rate recovery after exercise is a predictor of mortality, independent of the angiographic severity of coronary disease. J Am Coll Cardiol 42:831, 2003.

Diagnostic Applications

48. Gibbons RJ, Abrams J, Chatterjee K, et al: ACC/AHA 2002 guideline update for the management of patients with chronic stable angina: A report of the American College of Cardiology/American Heart Association Task Force on Practice Guidelines (Committee to update the 1999 Guidelines for the Management of Patients with Chronic Stable Angina). 2002. (http://www.acc.org/clinical/guidelines/stable/stable.pdf)
49. Danzi GB, Pirelli S, Mauri L, et al: Which variable of stenosis severity best describes the significance of an isolated left anterior descending artery lesion? Correlation between quantitative coronary angiography, intracoronary Doppler measurements and high dose dipyridamole echocardiography. J Am Coll Cardiol 31:526, 1998.
50. Schulman SP, Lasorda D, Farah T, et al: Correlations between coronary flow reserve measured with a Doppler guide wire and treadmill exercise testing. Am Heart J 134:99, 1997.
51. Nishioka T, Amanullah AM, Luo H, et al: Clinical validation of intravascular ultrasound imaging for assessment of coronary stenosis severity. J Am Coll Cardiol 33:1870, 1999.
52. Panting JR, Gatehouse PD, Yang GZ, et al: Abnormal subendocardial perfusion in cardiac syndrome X detected by cardiovascular magnetic resonance imaging. N Engl J Med 346:1948, 2002.
53. Froelicher VF, Lehmann KG, Thomas R: Veterans Affairs Cooperative Study in Health Services #016 (QUEXTA) Study Group. The electrocardiographic exercise test in a population with reduced workup bias: Diagnostic performance, computerized interpretation and multivariable prediction. Ann Intern Med 128:965, 1998.
54. Froelicher V, Shetler K, Ashley E: Better decisions through science: Exercise testing scores. Prog Cardiovasc Dis 44:395, 2002.
55. Morise AP, Lauer MS, Froelicher VF: Development and validation of a simple exercise test score for use in women with symptoms of suspected coronary artery disease. Am Heart J 144:818, 2002.

Prognostic Applications

56. Rywik TM, O'Connor FC, Gittings NS, et al: Role of nondiagnostic exercise-induced ST-segment abnormalities in predicting future coronary events in asymptomatic volunteers. Circulation 106:2787, 2002.
57. Laukkanen JA, Kurl S, Lakka TA, et al: Exercise-induced silent myocardial ischemia and coronary morbidity and mortality in middle-aged men. J Am Coll Cardiol 38:72, 2001.
58. Blumenthal RS, Becker DM, Yanek LR, et al: Detecting occult coronary disease in a high-risk asymptomatic population. Circulation 107:702, 2003.
59. Greenland P, Smith SC, Grundy SM: Improving coronary heart disease risk assessment in asymptomatic people: Role of traditional risk factors and noninvasive cardiovascular tests. Circulation 104:1863, 2001.
60. Weiner DH, Ryan T, McCabe CH, et al: Prognostic importance of a clinical profile and exercise test in medically treated patients with coronary artery disease. J Am Coll Cardiol 3:772, 1984.
61. Mark DB, Hlatky MA, Harrell FE, et al: Exercise treadmill score for predicting prognosis in coronary heart disease. Ann Intern Med 106:793, 1987.
62. Mark DB, Shaw L, Harrell FE Jr, et al: Prognostic value of a treadmill exercise score in outpatients with suspected coronary artery disease. N Engl J Med 325:849, 1991.
63. Kwok JMF, Miller TD, Hodge DO, Gibbons RJ: Prognostic value of the Duke treadmill score in the elderly. J Am Coll Cardiol 39:1475, 2002.
64. Morise AP, Haddad WJ, Beckner D: Development and validation of a clinical score to estimate the probability of coronary artery disease in men and women presenting with suspected coronary disease. Am J Cardiol 102:350, 1997.
65. Stone PH, Chaitman BR, Forman S, et al: Prognostic significance of myocardial ischemia detected by ambulatory electrocardiogram, exercise treadmill testing, and resting electrocardiogram to predict cardiac events by 1 year (the Asymptomatic Cardiac Ischemia Pilot [ACIP] Study). Am J Cardiol 80:1395, 1997.
66. Safstrom K, Nielsen NE, Bjorkholm A, et al: Unstable coronary artery disease in postmenopausal women: Identifying patients with significant coronary artery disease by basic clinical parameters and exercise test. Eur Heart J 19:899, 1998.
67. Braunwald E, Antman EM, Beasley JW, et al: ACC/AHA 2002 guideline update for the management of patients with unstable angina and non-ST-segment elevation myocardial infarction: A report of the American College of Cardiology/American Heart Association Task Force on Practice Guidelines (Committee on the Management of Patients With Unstable Angina). 2002. (http://www.acc.org/clnical/guidelines/unstable/unstable.pdf)
68. Goyal A, Samaha FF, Boden WE, et al: Stress test criteria used in the conservative arm of the FRISC-II trial underdetects surgical coronary artery disease when applied to patients in the VANQWISH trial. J Am Coll Cardiol 39:1601, 2002.
69. Stein RA, Chaitman BR, Balady GJ, et al: Safety and utility of exercise testing in emergency room chest pain centers: An advisory from the Committee on Exercise, Rehabilitation and Prevention, Council on Clinical Cardiology, American Heart Association. Circulation 102:1463, 2000.
70. Peterson ED, Shaw L, Califf RM, et al: Risk stratification after myocardial infarction. Ann Intern Med 126:561, 1997.
71. Senaratne MP, Smith G, Gulamhusein SS: Feasibility and safety of early exercise testing using the Bruce protocol after acute myocardial infarction. J Am Coll Cardiol 35:1212, 2000.
72. Nakano A, Lee JD, Shimizu H, et al: Reciprocal ST segment depression associated with exercise induced ST-segment elevation indicates residual viability after myocardial infarction. J Am Coll Cardiol 33:620, 1999.
73. de Filippi CR, Rosanio S, Tocchi M, et al: Randomized comparison of a strategy of predischarge coronary angiography versus exercise testing in low-risk patients in a chest pain unit: In-hospital and long-term outcomes. J Am Coll Cardiol 37:2050, 2001.
74. Diercks DB, Gibler B, Liu T, et al: Identification of patients at risk by graded exercise testing in an emergency department chest pain center. Am J Cardiol 86:289, 2000.
75. Amsterdam EA, Kirk JD, Diercks DB, et al: Immediate exercise testing to evaluate low-risk patients presenting to the emergency department with chest pain. J Am Coll Cardiol 40:251, 2002.
76. Farkouh ME, Smars PA, Reeder GS, et al: A clinical trial comparing a chest pain observation unit with routine admission in patients with unstable angina. N Engl J Med 339:1882, 1999.
77. Eagle KA, Berger PB, Calkins H, et al: ACC/AHA guidelines for perioperative cardiovascular evaluation for noncardiac surgery update: executive summary: A report of the American College of Cardiology/American Heart Association Task Force on Practice Guidelines (Committee to Update the 1996 Guidelines on Perioperative Cardiovascular Evaluation for Noncardiac Surgery). Circulation 105:1257, 2002.
78. Chaitman BR, Miller DD: Perioperative cardiac evaluation for noncardiac surgery noninvasive cardiac testing. Prog Cardiovasc Dis 40:405, 1998.
79. Best PJ, Tajik AJ, Gibbons RJ, et al: The safety of treadmill exercise stress testing in patients with abdominal aortic aneurysms. Ann Intern Med 129:628, 1998.
80. McGlade DP, Poon AB, Davies MJ: The use of a questionnaire and simple exercise test in the preoperative assessment of vascular surgery patients. Anaesth Intensive Care 29:520, 2001.
81. Pina IL, Apstein CS, Balady GJ, et al: Exercise and heart failure: A statement from the American Heart Association Committee on Exercise, Rehabilitation, and Prevention. Circulation 107:1210, 2003.
82. de Jonge N, Kirkels H, Lahpor JR, et al: Exercise performance in patients with end-stage heart failure after implantation of a left ventricular assist device and after heart transplantation: An outlook for permanent assisting? J Am Coll Cardiol 37:1794, 2001.
83. Wasserman K, Zhang YY, Gitt A, et al: Lung function and exercise gas exchange in chronic heart failure. Circulation 96:2221, 1997.
84. Osada N, Chaitman BR, Miller LW, et al: Cardiopulmonary exercise testing identifies low risk patients with heart failure and severely impaired exercise capacity considered for heart transplantation. J Am Coll Cardiol 31:582, 1998.
85. Duscha BD, Annex BH, Keteyian SJ, et al: Differences in skeletal muscle between men and women with chronic heart failure. J Appl Physiol 90:280, 2001.
86. Mancini DM, Katz SD, Lang CC, et al: Effect of erythropoietin on exercise capacity in patients with moderate to severe chronic heart failure. Circulation 107:294, 2003.
87. Duscha BD, Annex BH, Green HJ, Pikppen AM: Deconditioning fails to explain peripheral skeletal muscle alterations in men with chronic heart failure. J Am Coll Cardiol 39:1170, 2002.

88. Myers J, Gullestad L, Vagelos R, et al: Clinical, hemodynamic, and cardiopulmonary exercise test determinants of survival in patients referred for evaluation of heart failure. Ann Intern Med 129:293, 1998.
89. Belardinelli R, Georgiou D, Cianci G, et al: Randomized, controlled trial of long-term moderate exercise training in chronic heart failure. Effects on functional capacity, quality of life, and clinical outcome. Circulation 99:1173, 1999.
90. Metra M, Faggiano P, D'Aloia A, et al: Use of cardiopulmonary exercise testing with hemodynamic monitoring in the prognostic assessment of ambulatory patients with chronic heart failure. J Am Coll Cardiol 33:943, 1999.
91. Shah MR, Hasselblad V, Gheorghiade M, et al: Prognostic usefulness of the six-minute walk in patients with advanced congestive heart failure secondary to ischemic or non-ischemic cardiomyopathy. Am J Cardiol 88:987, 2001.
92. Opasich C, Pinna GD, Mazza A, et al: Six-minute walking performance in patients with moderate-to-severe heart failure. Eur Heart J 22:488, 2001.

Arrhythmias and Conduction Disturbances

93. Frolkis JP, Pothier CE, Blackstone EH, Lauer MS: Frequent ventricular ectopy after exercise as a predictor of death. N Engl J Med 348:781, 2003.
94. Partington S, Myers J, Cho S, et al: Prevalence and prognostic value of exercise-induced ventricular arrhythmias. Am Heart J 145:139, 2003.
95. Takenaka K, Ai T, Shimizu W: Exercise stress test amplifies genotype-phenotype correlation in the LQT1 and LQT2 forms of the long-QT syndrome. Circulation 107:838, 2003.
96. Dillenburg RF, Hamilton RM: Is exercise testing useful in identifying congenital long QT syndrome? Am J Cardiol 89:233, 2002.
97. Grady TA, Chiu AC, Snader CE, et al: Prognostic significance of exercise-induced left bundle branch block. JAMA 279:153, 1998.
98. Shah PP, Nair M, Dhall A, et al: False-positive exercise stress electrocardiogram due to accessory pathway in the absence of manifest preexcitation. Pacing Clin Electrophysiol 23:1051, 2000.
99. Janosik DL: Effect of exercise on pacing hemodynamics. *In* Ellenbogen KA, Neal Kay G, Wilkoff BL (eds): Clinical Cardiac Pacing. 2nd ed. Philadelphia, WB Saunders, 1999.
100. Auricchio A, Kloss M, Trautmann SI, et al: Exercise performance following cardiac resynchronization therapy in patients with heart failure and ventricular conduction delay. Am J Cardiol 89:198, 2002.

Specific Clinical Applications

101. Chaitman BR: Measuring antianginal drug efficacy using exercise testing for chronic angina: Improved exercise performance with ranolazine, a pFOX inhibitor. Curr Probl Cardiol 27:527, 2002.
102. Bogaty P, Kingma JG Jr, Robitaille NM, et al: Attenuation of myocardial ischemia with repeated exercise in subjects with chronic stable angina: Relation to myocardial contractility, intensity of exercise and the adenosine triphosphate-sensitive potassium channel. J Am Coll Cardiol 32:1665, 1998.
103. Bokhari S, Bergmann SR: The effect of estrogen compared to estrogen plus progesterone on the exercise electrocardiogram. J Am Coll Cardiol 40:1092, 2002.
104. Henzlova MJ, Croft LB, Diamond JA: Effect of hormone replacement therapy on the electrocardiographic response to exercise. J Nucl Cardiol 9:385, 2002.
105. Roger VL, Jacobsen SJ, Pellika PA, et al: Gender differences in use of stress testing and coronary heart disease mortality: A population based study in Olmsted County, Minnesota. J Am Coll Cardiol 32:345, 1998.
106. Alexander KP, Shaw LJ, Delong ER, et al: Value of exercise treadmill testing in women. J Am Coll Cardiol 32:1657, 1998.
107. Singh JP, Larson MG, Manolio TA, et al: Blood pressure response during treadmill testing as a risk factor for new-onset hypertension. The Framingham Study. Circulation 99:1831, 1999.
108. Allison TG, Corderio MA, Miller TD, et al: Prognostic significance of exercise-induced systemic hypertension in healthy subjects. Am J Cardiol 83:371, 1999.
109. Era P, Schroll M, Hagerup L, Shult-Larsen Jurgensen K: Changes in bicycle ergometer test performance and survival in men and women from 50 to 60 and from 70 to 80 years of age: Two longitudinal studies in the Glostrup (Denmark) population. Gerontology 47:136, 2001.
110. Goraya TY, Jacobsen SJ, Pellikka PA, et al: Prognostic value of treadmill exercise testing in elderly persons. Ann Intern Med 132:862, 2000.
111. Rutter MK, McComb JM, Brady S, Marshall SM: Silent myocardial ischemia and microalbuminuria in asymptomatic subjects with non-insulin-dependent diabetes mellitus. Am J Cardiol 83:27, 1999.
112. Caracciolo EA, Chaitman BR, Forman SA, et al: Diabetics with coronary disease have a prevalence of asymptomatic ischemia during exercise treadmill testing and ambulatory ischemia monitoring similar to that of nondiabetic patients. An ACIP database study. Circulation 93:2097, 1996.
113. Bonow RO, Carabello B, deLeon AC Jr, et al: ACC/AHA guidelines for the management of patients with valvular heart disease: A report of the American College of Cardiology/American Heart Association Task Force on Practice Guidelines (Committee on Management of Patients with Valvular Heart Disease). J Am Coll Cardiol 32:1486, 1998.
114. Borer JS, Hockreiter C, Herrold EM, et al: Prediction of indications for valve replacement among asymptomatic or minimally symptomatic patients with chronic aortic regurgitation and normal left ventricular performance. Circulation 97:518, 1998.
115. Otto CM, Burwash IG, Legget ME, et al: Prospective study of asymptomatic valvular aortic stenosis: Clinical, echocardiographic, and exercise predictors of outcome. Circulation 95:2262, 1997.
116. Jones S, Elliott PM, McKenna WJ, et al: Cardiopulmonary responses to exercise in patients with hypertrophic cardiomyopathy. Heart 80:60, 1998.
117. Ciampi Q, Betocchi S, Lombardi R, et al: Hemodynamic determinants of exercise-induced abnormal blood pressure response in hypertrophic cardiomyopathy. J Am Coll Cardiol 40:278, 2002.
118. Kim JJ, Lee CW, Park SW, et al: Improvement in exercise capacity and exercise blood pressure response after transcoronary alcohol ablation therapy of septal hypertrophy in hypertrophic cardiomyopathy. Am J Cardiol 83:1220, 1999.
119. Krone RJ, Hardison RM, Chaitman BR, et al: Risk stratification after successful coronary revascularization: The lack of a role for routine exercise testing. J Am Coll Cardiol 38:136, 2001.
120. Marwick TH, Zuchowski C, Lauer MS, et al: Functional status and quality of life in patients with heart failure undergoing coronary bypass surgery after assessment of myocardial viability. J Am Coll Cardiol 33:750, 1999.
121. Ferrari M, Schnell B, Werner GS, et al: Safety of deferring angioplasty in patients with normal coronary flow velocity reserve. J Am Coll Cardiol 33:82, 1999.
122. Dagianti A, Rosanio S, Penco M, et al: Clinical and prognostic usefulness of supine bicycle exercise echocardiography in the functional evaluation of patients undergoing elective percutaneous transluminal coronary angioplasty. Circulation 95:1176, 1997.
123. Garzon P, Sheppard R, Eisenberg MJ, et al: Comparison of event and procedure rates following percutaneous transluminal coronary angioplasty in patients with and without previous coronary artery bypass graft surgery (the Routine versus Selective Exercise Treadmill Testing after Angioplasty [ROSETTA] Registry). Am J Cardiol 89:251, 2002.
124. Kavanagh T, Mertens DJ, Shephard RJ: Long-term cardiorespiratory results of exercise training following cardiac transplantation. Am J Cardiol 91:190, 2003.
125. Osada N, Chaitman BR, Donohue TJ, et al: Long-term cardiopulmonary exercise performance after heart transplantation. Am J Cardiol 79:451, 1997.
126. Wilson RF, Johnson TH, Haidet GC, et al: Sympathetic reinnervation of the sinus node and exercise hemodynamics after cardiac transplantation. Circulation 101:2727, 2000.

Safety and Risks of Exercise Testing

127. Stuart RJ, Ellestad MH: National survey of exercise stress testing facilities. Chest 77:94, 1980.
128. Hamm LF, Crow RS, Stull GA, Hannan P: Safety and characteristics of exercise testing early after acute myocardial infarction. Am J Cardiol 63:1193, 1989.
129. Tristani FE, Hughes CV, Archibald DG, et al: Safety of graded symptom-limited exercise testing in patients with congestive heart failure. Circulation 76:VI-54, 1987.
130. Young DZ, Lampert S, Graboys TB, Lown B: Safety of maximal exercise testing in patients at high risk for ventricular arrhythmia. Circulation 70:184, 1984.
131. Beller GA, Bonow RO, Fuster V, et al: ACC revised recommendations for training in adult cardiovascular medicine core cardiology training II (COCATS 2) (Revision of the 1995 COCATS Training Statement). J Am Coll Cardiol 39:1242, 2002.
132. Rodgers GP, Ayanian JZ, Balady G, et al: American College of Cardiology/American Heart Association clinical competence statement on stress testing. A report of the American College of Cardiology/American Heart Association/American College of Physicians—American Society of Internal Medicine Task Force on Clinical Competence. J Am Coll Cardiol 36:1441, 2000.

GUIDELINES *Thomas H. Lee*

Exercise Stress Testing

Several sets of guidelines for the performance of exercise testing have been published by the American Heart Association and by committees commissioned jointly by the American College of Cardiology and the American Heart Association (ACC/AHA).[1-5] Use of exercise testing is addressed in guidelines for specific clinical syndromes, including acute myocardial infarction,[6] chronic stable angina,[7] valvular heart disease,[8] and congestive heart failure.[9] Recommendations for optimal use of treadmill exercise testing are also closely related to guidelines for use of nuclear cardiology tests for detection of myocardial ischemia.[10]

STANDARDS FOR TESTING AND TRAINING

The AHA published standards for performance of exercise testing in 2001,[1] which define absolute and relative contraindications to exercise testing; these recommendations were slightly modified in ACC/AHA guidelines published in 2002 (Table 10G–1). "Relative" contraindications are those that can be superseded if clinicians believe that the benefits of testing outweigh the risks of exercise. The AHA standards also provide recommendations for specific testing

TABLE 10G–1 ACC/AHA Guidelines: Absolute and Relative Contraindications to Exercise Testing
Absolute
Acute myocardial infarction (within 2 days)
High-risk unstable angina
Uncontrolled cardiac arrhythmias causing symptoms or hemodynamic compromise
Symptomatic severe aortic stenosis
Uncontrolled symptomatic heart failure
Acute pulmonary embolus or pulmonary infarction
Acute myocarditis or pericarditis
Acute aortic dissection
Relative
Left main coronary stenosis
Moderate stenotic valvular heart disease
Electrolyte abnormalities
Severe arterial hypertension (suggested definition: systolic blood pressure > 200 mm Hg and/or diastolic blood pressure > 100 mm Hg)
Tachyarrhythmias or bradyarrhythmias
Hypertrophic cardiomyopathy and other forms of outflow tract obstruction
Mental or physical impairment leading to inability to exercise adequately
High-degree atrioventricular block

From Gibbons RJ, Balady GJ, Bricker JT, et al: ACC/AHA 2002 guideline update for exercise testing: Summary article. A report of the ACC/AHA Task Force on Practice Guidelines (Committee to update the 1997 Exercise Testing Guidelines). Circulation 106:1883, 2002.

procedures, such as patient instructions for preparation for the procedure. This Scientific Statement does not offer explicit recommendations on when and whether beta blockers or other drugs (e.g., vasodilators, digitalis, diuretics) should be discontinued before testing.

Indications for termination of exercise testing from this Scientific Statement were updated in the most recent ACC/AHA guidelines on exercise testing[4] and are summarized in Table 10G–2. Again, relative indications for termination of testing are those that can be superseded when the clinician considers the benefits of continued exercise to exceed the risks.

Exercise testing should be performed under the supervision of a physician, who should be in the vicinity and immediately available during all exercise tests. However, the Scientific Statement indicates that a properly trained nonphysician (i.e., a nurse, physician assistant, or exercise physiologist or specialist) can perform the direct supervision for healthy younger persons and those with stable chest pain syndromes.[1] An ACC/AHA Clinical Competence Statement on exercise testing published in 2000 describes a "majority opinion" of its authors that supervising physicians should participate in at least 50 exercise test procedures during training and perform at least 25 exercise tests per year.[2] This Statement also lists specific skills that are needed for competent test supervision and interpretation, and recommends that medical centers have a program of quality assurance to ensure systematic review and critique of a significant sample of exercise tests. Because computer processing can lead to an overestimation of ST depression, ACC/AHA guidelines recommend that the interpreting physician always be supplied with raw electrocardiographic (ECG) tracings in addition to any computerized summaries.[4]

TABLE 10G–2 ACC/AHA Guidelines: Indications for Terminating Exercise Testing
Absolute
Drop in systolic blood pressure of >10 mm Hg from baseline blood pressure despite an increase in workload, when accompanied by other evidence of ischemia
Moderate to severe angina
Increasing nervous system symptoms (e.g., ataxia, dizziness, or near-syncope)
Signs of poor perfusion (cyanosis or pallor)
Technical difficulties in monitoring electrocardiogram or systolic blood pressure
Subject's desire to stop
Sustained ventricular tachycardia
ST elevation (≥1.0 mm) in leads without diagnostic Q waves (other than V_1 or aV_R)
Relative
Drop in systolic blood pressure of >10 mm Hg from baseline blood pressure despite an increase in workload, in the absence of other evidence of ischemia
ST or QRS changes such as excessive ST depression (>2 mm of horizontal or downsloping ST segment depression) or marked axis shift
Arrhythmias other than sustained ventricular tachycardia, including multifocal PVCs, triplets of PVCs, supraventricular tachycardia, heart block, or bradyarrhythmias
Fatigue, shortness of breath, wheezing, leg cramps, or claudication
Development of bundle-branch block or IVCD that cannot be distinguished from ventricular tachycardia
Increasing chest pain
Hypertensive response (suggested definition: systolic blood pressure > 250 mm Hg and/or a diastolic blood pressure of > 115 mm Hg)

ECG = electrocardiogram; ICD = implantable cardioverter-defibrillator discharge; IVCD = intraventricular conduction delay; PVCs = premature ventricular contractions.

From Gibbons RJ, Balady GJ, Bricker JT, et al: ACC/AHA 2002 guideline update for exercise testing: Summary article. A report of the ACC/AHA Task Force on Practice Guidelines (Committee to Update the 1997 Exercise Testing Guidelines). Circulation 106:1883, 2002.

Clinical Indications for Exercise Testing

Guidelines published by the ACC/AHA in 1997[3] and updated in 2002[4] assess the appropriateness of exercise testing in specific clinical settings. The complete guidelines are available at *www.americanheart.org* or *www.acc.org*. As with other ACC/AHA guidelines, these recommendations classify indications into one of three classes, including two levels of the intermediate group, as follows:

Class I: Conditions for which there is evidence and/or general agreement that exercise testing is useful and effective.

Class II: Conditions for which there is conflicting evidence and/or a divergence of opinion about the usefulness/efficacy of performing exercise testing.

Class IIa: Weight of evidence/opinion is in favor of usefulness/efficacy.

Class IIb: Usefulness/efficacy is less well established by evidence/opinion.

Class III: Conditions for which there is evidence and/or general agreement that exercise testing is not useful/effective and in some cases may be harmful.

Diagnosis of Obstructive Coronary Artery Disease

When the clinical question is whether obstructive coronary disease is present or absent in a patient (i.e., diagnosis), the ACC/AHA guidelines consider exercise testing most appropriate for patients with an "intermediate" pretest probability of coronary artery disease, such as patients with atypical or probable angina or younger patients with typical angina. Definitions of pretest risk status according to age, gender, and symptoms are summarized in Table 10G–3. Patients with high or low pretest probability of coronary disease are less likely to have their management altered by exercise testing; hence, exercise testing is not strongly supported by these guidelines in these populations (Table 10G–4). Exercise electrocardiography is considered appropriate in patients with complete right bundle branch block and less than 1 mm of resting ST depression, but not in patients with electrocardiographic patterns more likely to lead to uninterpretable tracings. The 2002 ACC/AHA guidelines lower the threshold for using an imaging technology in patients with minor ST depression. The prior ACC/AHA guidelines considered exercise electrocardiography "the first test option" in such patients,[3] whereas the 2002 update has changed this phrase to "a reasonable first test option."

Risk Assessment and Prognosis in Patients with Coronary Disease

The ACC/AHA guidelines emphasize that exercise testing should be used to improve risk stratification as part of a process that begins with assessment of routinely available data from the clinical examination and other laboratory tests. The decision of whether to order an exercise test should reflect the chances that test results might alter management, and the interpretation of the results should be considered in the context of the patient's overall clinical status.

The recommendations endorse routine use of exercise testing for risk stratification of patients with suspected or known coronary disease (Table 10G–5), whether stable or after a change in clinical status. The guidelines emphasize the importance of consideration of multiple types of data from the exercise test (e.g., exercise duration) and encourage use of tools such as the Duke Treadmill Score[11] to integrate these data into a risk prediction.

For patients with unstable angina, the guidelines support exercise testing early (8-12 hours) after presentation in patients with a low clinical risk of complications (Table 10G–6) if they have been free of active ischemic or heart failure symptoms. A longer delay (2-3 days) is recommended for patients with an intermediate risk of complications, although the guidelines indicate that there is good supportive evidence for earlier exercise testing as part of chest pain management protocols for stable patients from this population if there is no evidence of active ischemia (Class IIa indication). More detailed recommendations on exercise testing in chest pain centers were provided in a Science Advisory Statement from the American Heart Association in 2000.[5]

The guidelines discourage exercise testing for patients in whom the procedure would be dangerous (e.g., high-risk unstable angina patients); unlikely to add accurate information (e.g., patients with certain resting ECG abnormalities); or unlikely to change management

TABLE 10G–3 Pretest Probability of Coronary Artery Disease by Age, Gender and Symptoms

Age (yr)	Gender	Typical/Definite Angina Pectoris	Atypical/Probable Angina Pectoris	Nonanginal Chest Pain	Asymptomatic
30-39	Men	Intermediate	Intermediate	Low	Very low
	Women	Intermediate	Very low	Very low	Very low
40-49	Men	High	Intermediate	Intermediate	Low
	Women	Intermediate	Low	Very low	Very low
50-59	Men	High	Intermediate	Intermediate	Low
	Women	Intermediate	Intermediate	Low	Very low
60-69	Men	High	Intermediate	Intermediate	Low
	Women	High	Intermediate	Intermediate	Low

From Gibbons RJ, Balady GJ, Bricker JT, et al: ACC/AHA 2002 guideline update for exercise testing: Summary article. A report of the ACC/AHA Task Force on Practice Guidelines (Committee to Update the 1997 Exercise Testing Guidelines). Circulation 106:1883, 2002.

TABLE 10G–4 ACC/AHA Guidelines for Exercise Testing to Diagnose Obstructive Coronary Artery Disease

	Indication
Class I (indicated)	Adult patients (including those with complete right bundle branch block or less than 1 mm of resting ST depression) with an intermediate pretest probability of CAD on the basis of gender, age, and symptoms (specific exceptions are noted under Classes II and III below).
Class IIa (good supportive evidence)	Patients with vasospastic angina.
Class IIb (weak supportive evidence)	1. Patients with a high pretest probability of CAD by age, symptoms, and gender. 2. Patients with a low pretest probability of CAD by age, symptoms, and gender. 3. Patients with less than 1 mm of baseline ST depression and taking digoxin. 4. Patients with electrocardiographic criteria for left ventricular hypertrophy and less than 1 mm of baseline ST depression.
Class III (not indicated)	1. Patients with the following baseline ECG abnormalities: • Preexcitation (Wolff-Parkinson-White) syndrome • Electronically paced ventricular rhythm • Greater than 1 mm of resting ST depression • Complete left bundle branch block 2. Patients with a documented myocardial infarction or prior coronary angiography demonstrating significant disease who have an established diagnosis of CAD; however, ischemia and risk can be determined by testing.

CAD = coronary artery disease.

TABLE 10G–5 ACC/AHA Guidelines: Risk Assessment and Prognosis in Patients with Symptoms or a Prior History of Coronary Artery Disease

	Indication
Class I (indicated)	1. Patients undergoing initial evaluation with suspected or known CAD, including those with complete right bundle branch block or less than 1 mm of resting ST depression. Specific exceptions are noted below in Class IIb. 2. Patients with suspected or known CAD, previously evaluated, now presenting with significant change in clinical status. 3. Low-risk unstable angina patients 8 to 12 hours after presentation who have been free of active ischemic or heart failure symptoms. 4. Intermediate-risk unstable angina patients 2 to 3 days after presentation who have been free of active ischemic or heart failure symptoms.
Class IIa (good supportive evidence)	Intermediate-risk unstable angina patients who have initial cardiac markers that are normal, a repeat ECG without significant change, and cardiac markers 6 to 12 hours after the onset of symptoms that are normal and no other evidence of ischemia during observation.
Class IIb (weak supportive evidence)	1. Patients with the following resting ECG abnormalities: • Preexcitation (Wolff-Parkinson-White) syndrome • Electronically paced ventricular rhythm • 1 mm or more of resting ST depression • Complete left bundle branch block or any interventricular conduction defect with a QRS duration longer than 120 msec. 2. Patients with a stable clinical course who undergo periodic monitoring to guide treatment.
Class III (not indicated)	1. Patients with severe comorbidity likely to limit life expectancy and/or candidacy for revascularization. 2. High-risk unstable angina patients.

CAD = coronary artery disease; ECG = electrocardiogram.

TABLE 10G–6 ACC/AHA Classification System for Risk of Death or Nonfatal Myocardial Infarction in Patients with Unstable Angina

Feature	High Risk (at least one of the following features must be present)	Intermediate Risk (no high-risk feature but must have one of the following features)	Low Risk (no high- or intermediate-risk features, but may have any of the following features)
History		Prior MI, peripheral or cerbrovascular disease, or CABG, prior aspirin use	
Character of pain	Prolonged, ongoing (>20 min) pain at rest	Prolonged (>20 min) resting angina, now resolved, with moderate or high likelihood of CAD Rest angina (<20 min) or relieved with rest or sublingual NTG	New-onset or progressive CCSC III or IV angina in the past 2 weeks with moderate or high likelihood of CAD
Clinical findings	Pulmonary edema, most likely related to ischemia New or worsening MR murmur S3 or new/worsening rales Hypotension, bradycardia, tachycardia Age older than 75 years	Age older than 70 yr	
ECG findings	Angina at rest with transient ST changes ≥ 0.05 mV BBB, new or presumed new/sustained ventricular tachycardia	T-wave inversions greater than 0.2 mV Pathological Q waves	Normal or unchanged ECG during an episode of chest discomfort
Biochemical cardiac markers	Elevated (e.g., troponin T or I greater than 0.1 mg/ml)	Slightly elevated (e.g., troponin T > 0.01 but <0.1 mg/ml)	Normal

BBB = bundle branch block; CABG = coronary artery bypass graft; CAD = coronary artery disease; CCSC = Canadian Cardiovascular Society Classification; ECG = electrocardiogram; MI = myocardial infarction; MR = mitral regurgitation.

From Gibbons RJ, Balady GJ, Bricker JT, et al: ACC/AHA 2002 guideline update for exercise testing: Summary article. A report of the ACC/AHA Task Force on Practice Guidelines (Committee to update the 1997 Exercise Testing Guidelines). Circulation 106:1883, 2002.

(e.g., patients with stable clinical courses or who were poor candidates for revascularization) (see Table 10G–5).

After Acute Myocardial Infarction

Recommendations for the use of exercise testing after acute myocardial infarction (Table 10G–7) reflect an overall strategy for risk stratification and management that is described in ACC/AHA guidelines on acute myocardial infarction.[6] In this approach (Fig. 10G–1), if patients' clinical data suggest a high risk for complications, the patients should undergo invasive evaluation to determine whether they are candidates for coronary revascularization procedures (strategy I). For patients with apparently low risk for complications, two strategies for performing exercise testing are endorsed. One uses a symptom-limited exercise test at 14 to 21 days (strategy II). An alternative strategy for low-risk patients (strategy III) is to perform a submaximal exercise test at 4 to 7 days after myocardial infarction or just before hospital discharge. If the exercise test result is negative, a second

TABLE 10G–7 ACC/AHA Guidelines for Exercise Testing after Acute Myocardial Infarction

	Indication
Class I (indicated)	1. Before discharge for prognostic assessment, activity prescription, evaluation of medical therapy (submaximal at about 4 to 76 days).* 2. Early after discharge for prognostic assessment, activity prescription, evaluation of medical therapy, and cardiac rehabilitation if the predischarge exercise test was not done (symptom-limited; about 14 to 21 days).* 3. Late after discharge for prognostic assessment, activity prescription, evaluation of medical therapy, and cardiac rehabilitation if the early exercise test was submaximal (symptom-limited; about 3 to 6 weeks).*
Class IIa (good supportive evidence)	After discharge for activity counseling and/or exercise training as part of cardiac rehabilitation in patients who have undergone coronary revascularization.
Class IIb (weak supportive evidence)	1. Patients with the following electrocardiographic abnormalities: • Complete left bundle-branch block • Preexcitation syndrome • Left ventricular hypertrophy • Digoxin therapy • Greater than 1 mm of resting ST segment depression • Electronically paced ventricular rhythm 2. Periodic monitoring in patients who continue to participate in exercise training or cardiac rehabilitation.
Class III (not indicated)	1. Severe comorbidity likely to limit life expectancy and/or candidacy for revascularization. 2. At any time to evaluate patients with acute myocardial infarction who have uncompensated congestive heart failure, cardiac arrhythmia, or noncardiac conditions that severely limit their ability to exercise. 3. Before discharge to evaluate patients who have already been selected for, or have undergone, cardiac catheterization. Although a stress test may be useful before or after catheterization to evaluate or identify ischemia in the distribution of a coronary lesion of borderline severity, stress imaging tests are recommended.

*Exceptions are noted under Classes IIb and III.

TABLE 10G–8 ACC/AHA Guidelines for Exercise Testing with Ventilatory Gas Analysis

	Indication
Class I (indicated)	1. Evaluation of exercise capacity and response to therapy in patients with heart failure who are being considered for heart transplantation. 2. Assistance in the differentiation of cardiac versus pulmonary limitations as a cause of exercise-induced dyspnea or impaired exercise capacity when the cause is uncertain.
Class IIa (good supportive evidence)	Evaluation of exercise capacity when indicated for medical reasons in patients in whom the estimates of exercise capacity from exercise test time or work rate are unreliable.
Class IIb (weak supportive evidence)	1. Evaluation of the patient's response to specific therapeutic interventions in which improvement of exercise tolerance is an important goal or endpoint. 2. Determination of the intensity for exercise training as part of comprehensive cardiac rehabilitation.
Class III (not indicated)	Routine use to evaluate exercise capacity.

symptom-limited exercise test can be repeated at 3 to 6 weeks for patients undergoing vigorous activity during leisure time activities, at work, or exercise training as part of cardiac rehabilitation. Exercise imaging tests are reserved for patients with equivocal exercise electrocardiography tests or those with electrocardiography findings that preclude interpretation of ST changes. The extent of ischemia on noninvasive studies helps determine whether patients should undergo cardiac catheterization.

Exercise Testing with Ventilatory Gas Analysis

Although measurement of maximal oxygen uptake is the best index of aerobic capacity, the ACC/AHA guidelines do not support ventilatory gas analysis as part of routine exercise testing or for routine measurement of exercise capacity (Table 10G–8). Ventilatory gas analysis is recommended when it is most likely to change management, such as in patients being considered for transplantation or those in whom clinical differentiation between pulmonary and cardiac causes of exercise limitation is difficult. Some support is provided for ventilatory gas exchange for patients in whom estimates of exercise capacity from other sources (e.g., exercise test time) are unreliable, but the guidelines discourage use of this technology for assessment of response to therapy or as a routine part of cardiac rehabilitation.

Special Populations

Exercise electrocardiography has poorer overall test performance in women compared with men, but the ACC/AHA guidelines recommend that exercise electrocardiography be the first-choice noninvasive test for coronary disease in women.[4] This recommendation reflects the fact that stress imaging technologies also have poorer sensitivity and higher false-positive rates in women, leading to the conclusion that there was insufficient evidence to recommend them as the initial diagnostic test in women.

The ACC/AHA guidelines discourage routine exercise testing for asymptomatic persons without known coronary artery disease (Table 10G–9) and conclude that only weak evidence is available to support its appropriateness for asymptomatic patients with multiple risk factors or patients about to embark on an exercise program. The guidelines are more supportive of exercise testing of patients with diabetes who are about to start vigorous exercise programs, owing to the high risk for atherosclerotic disease in this population.

TABLE 10G–9 ACC/AHA Guidelines for Exercise Testing in Asymptomatic Persons without Known Coronary Artery Disease (CAD)

	Indication
Class I (indicated)	None
Class IIa (good supportive evidence)	Evaluation of asymptomatic persons with diabetes mellitus who plan to start vigorous exercise.
Class IIb (weak supportive evidence)	1. Evaluation of persons with multiple risk factors as a guide to risk reduction therapy.* 2. Evaluation of asymptomatic men older than 45 years and women older than 55 years: • Who plan to start vigorous exercise (especially if sedentary) or • Who are involved in occupations in which impairment might impact public safety or • Who are at high risk for CAD due to other diseases (e.g., peripheral vascular disease and chronic renal failure)
Class III (not indicated)	Routine screening of asymptomatic men or women.

*Multiple risk factors are defined as hypercholesterolemia (>240 mg/dl), hypertension (systolic blood pressure > 140 mm Hg or diastolic blood pressure > 90 mm Hg), smoking, diabetes, and family history of heart attack or sudden cardiac death in a first-degree relative younger than 60 years. An alternative approach might be to select patients with a Framingham risk score consistent with at least a moderate risk of serious cardiac events within 5 years.

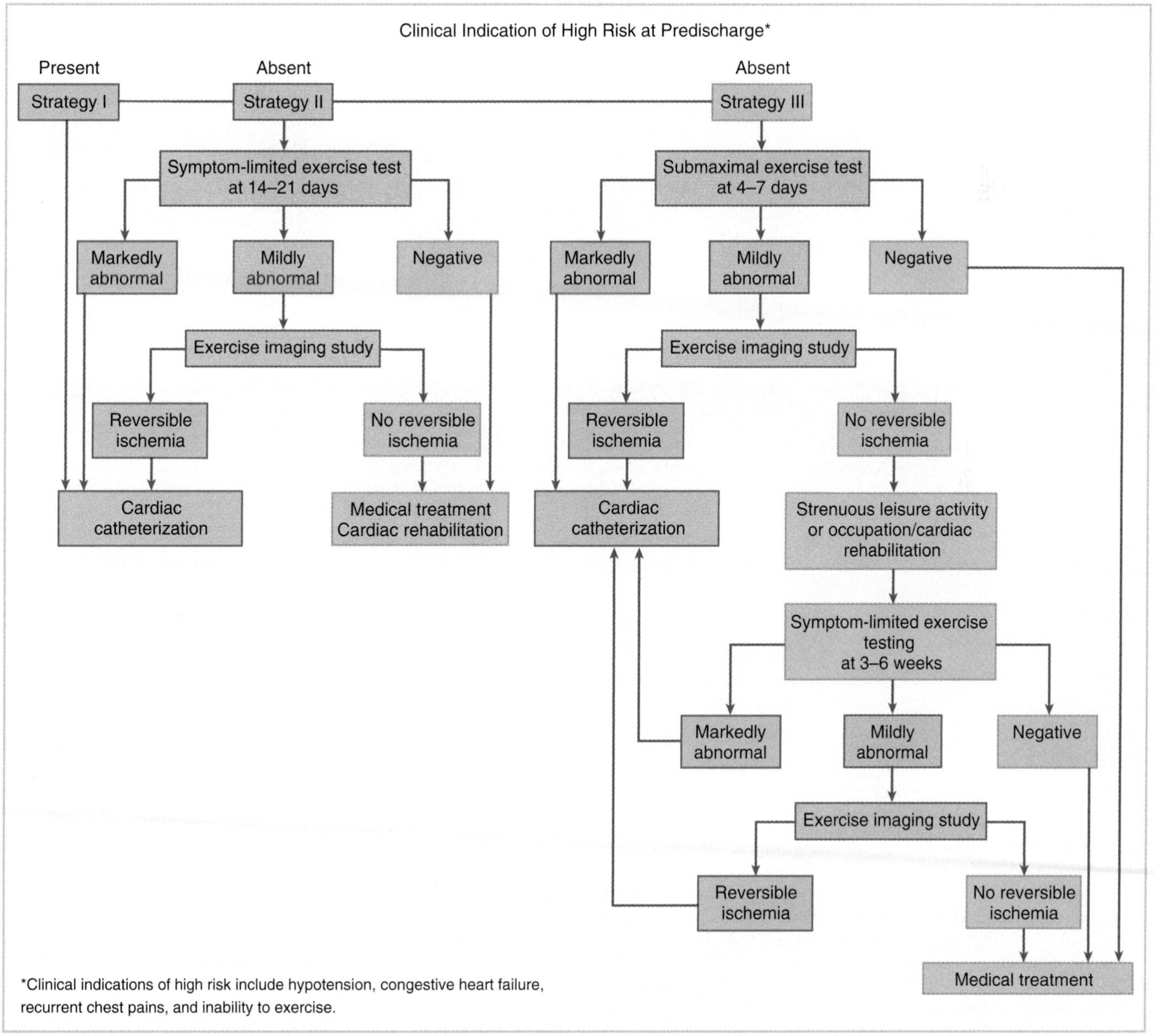

FIGURE 10G–1. Strategies for exercise test evaluation soon after myocardial infarction.

TABLE 10G–10 ACC/AHA Guidelines for Exercise Testing in Patients with Valvular Heart Disease

	Indication
Class I (indicated)	In chronic aortic regurgitation, assessment of functional capacity and symptomatic responses in patients with a history of equivocal symptoms.
Class IIa (good supportive evidence)	1. In chronic aortic regurgitation, evaluation of symptoms and functional capacity before participation in athletic activities. 2. In chronic aortic regurgitation, prognostic assessment before aortic valve replacement in asymptomatic or minimally symptomatic patients with left ventricular dysfunction.
Class IIb (weak supportive evidence)	Evaluation of exercise capacity in patients with valvular heart disease.
Class III (not indicated)	Diagnosis of coronary artery disease in patients with moderate to severe valvular disease or with the following baseline electrocardiographic abnormalities: • Preexcitation • Electronically paced ventricular rhythm • Greater than 1 mm ST depression • Complete left bundle branch block

TABLE 10G–11 ACC/AHA Guidelines for Exercise Testing Before and After Revascularization

	Indication
Class I (indicated)	1. Demonstration of ischemia before revascularization. 2. Evaluation of patients with recurrent symptoms that suggest ischemia after revascularization.
Class IIa (good supportive evidence)	After discharge for activity counseling and/or exercise training as part of cardiac rehabilitation in patients who have undergone coronary revascularization.
Class IIb (weak supportive evidence)	1. Detection of restenosis in selected, high-risk asymptomatic patients within the first 12 months after percutaneous coronary intervention. 2. Periodic monitoring of selected, high-risk asymptomatic patients for restenosis, graft occlusion, incomplete coronary revascularization, or disease progression.
Class III (not indicated)	1. Localization of ischemia for determining the site of intervention. 2. Routine, periodic monitoring of asymptomatic patients after percutaneous coronary intervention or coronary artery bypass grafting without specific indications.

TABLE 10G–12 ACC/AHA Guidelines for Exercise Testing for Investigation of Heart Rhythm Disorders

	Indication
Class I (indicated)	1. Identification of appropriate settings in patients with rate-adaptive pacemakers. 2. Evaluation of congenital complete heart block in patients considering increased physical activity or participation in competitive sports.
Class IIa (good supportive evidence)	1. Evaluation of patients with known or suspected exercise-induced arrhythmias. 2. Evaluation of medical, surgical, or ablative therapy in patients with exercise-induced arrhythmias (including atrial fibrillation).
Class IIb (weak supportive evidence)	1. Investigation of isolated ventricular ectopic beats in middle-aged patients without other evidence of coronary artery disease. 2. Investigation of prolonged first-degree atrioventricular block or type I second-degree Wenckebach block, left bundle branch block, right bundle branch block, or isolated ectopic beats in young patients considering participation in competitive sports.
Class III (not indicated)	Routine investigation of isolated ectopic beats in young patients.

Exercise testing is useful for assessing functional capacity in patients with valvular heart disease, particularly patients with regurgitant lesions (Table 10G–10). The guidelines note that exercise testing is usually not needed for symptomatic patients with stenotic valvular heart disease, and that severe aortic stenosis is classically considered a contraindication to exercise testing. However, the guidelines acknowledge that there are subsets of asymptomatic patients with stenotic valvular lesions in whom exercise testing may help assess functional capacity, for goals such as determination of whether they are truly asymptomatic.

The ACC/AHA guidelines support the use of exercise testing as part of the evaluation of patients before revascularization with coronary artery bypass grafting (CABG) or percutaneous coronary interventions and for evaluation of recurrent symptoms or part of the rehabilitation process. However, the guidelines do not support routine periodic exercise testing of asymptomatic patients after revascularization (Table 10G–11).

The guidelines endorse exercise testing for patients with heart rhythm disorders when the test is intended to diagnose exercise-induced arrhythmias or evaluate therapy (e.g., settings for rate-adaptive pacemakers, or impact of therapy for patients with exercise-induced arrhythmias). However, there is little support for exercise testing for heart rhythm abnormalities that, in isolation, are not associated with a higher risk of cardiovascular complications, such as isolated ventricular or atrial premature beats (Table 10G–12).

References

1. Fletcher GF, Balady GJ, Amsterdam EA, et al: Exercise standards for testing and training: A statement for healthcare professionals from the American Heart Association. Circulation 104:1694, 2001.
2. Rodgers GP, Ayanian JZ, Balady G, et al: American College of Cardiology/American Heart Association clinical competence statement on stress testing. Circulation 102:1726, 2000.
3. Gibbons RJ, Balady GJ, Beasley JW, et al: ACC/AHA guidelines for exercise testing: A report of the American College of Cardiology/American Heart Association Task Force on Practice Guidelines (Committee on Exercise Testing). J Am Coll Cardiol 30:260, 1997.
4. Gibbons RJ, Balady GJ, Bricker JT, et al: ACC/AHA 2002 guideline update for exercise testing: Summary article. A report of the ACC/AHA Task Force on Practice Guidelines (Committee to Update the 1997 Exercise Testing Guidelines). Circulation 106:1883, 2002.
5. Stein RA, Chaitman BR, Balady GJ, et al: Safety and utility of exercise testing in emergency room chest pain centers. An advisory from the Committee on Exercise, Rehabilitation, and Prevention, Council on Clinical Cardiology, American Heart Association. Circulation 102:1463, 2000.
6. Ryan TJ, Antman EM, Brooks NH, et al: ACC/AHA guidelines for the management of patients with acute myocardial infarction: 1999 update. A report of the American College of Cardiology/American Heart Association Task Force on Practice Guidelines (Committee on Management of Acute Myocardial Infarction). (http://www.acc.org)
7. Gibbons RJ, Abrams J, Chatterjee K, et al: ACC/AHA 2002 guideline update for the management of patients with chronic stable angina: Summary article. A report of the American College of Cardiology/American Heart Association Task Force on Practice Guidelines (Committee on the Management of Patents With Chronic Stable Angina). Circulation 107:149, 2003.
8. Bonow RO, Carabello B, de Leon AC Jr, et al: ACC/AHA guidelines for the management of patients with valvular heart disease: Executive summary. A report of the American College of Cardiology/American Heart Association Task Force on Practice Guidelines (Committee on Management of Patients With Valvular Heart Disease). Circulation 98:1949, 1998.
9. Hunt SA, Baker DW, Chin MH, et al: ACC/AHA guidelines for the evaluation and management of chronic heart failure in the adult: A report of the American College of Cardiology/American Heart Association Task Force on Practice Guidelines (Committee to Revise the 1995 Guidelines for the Evaluation and Management of Heart Failure). American College of Cardiology Web site, 2001. (http://www.acc.org/clinical/guidelines/failure/hf_index.htm)
10. Committee on Nuclear Imaging: Guidelines for Clinical Use of Cardiac Radionuclide Imaging. A Report of the American College of Cardiology/American Heart Association Task Force on the Assessment of Cardiovascular Procedures. J Am Coll Cardiol 25:521, 1995.
11. Mark DB, Shaw L, Harrell FE Jr, et al: Prognostic value of a treadmill exercise score in outpatients with suspected coronary artery disease. N Engl J Med 325:849, 1991.

CHAPTER 11

Echocardiography

William F. Armstrong

Principles of Cardiac Ultrasonography

Echocardiography is a group of interrelated applications of ultrasound including two-dimensional imaging, M-mode echocardiography, Doppler techniques, and contrast echocardiography. All of these techniques rely on sound in the frequency range of 2 to 10 MHz. Typically, adult imaging is performed at frequencies ranging from 2 to 5 MHz. For pediatric and specialized adult applications, higher frequencies of 7.5 and 10 MHz can also be used. This chapter deals with the clinical utility of echocardiographic techniques as they relate to the majority of forms of disease encountered in adult patient populations. It is important to have an understanding of the basic physical principles of ultrasound and image generation to understand the limitations and advantages of the technique.

Principles of Ultrasound Physics and Instrumentation

Cardiac ultrasonography relies on sound waves in the frequency of 2 to 10 MHz. Although typically displayed as a sine wave traveling through space, ultrasound actually consists of a pulsatile pressure phenomenon transmitted through a medium as alternating areas of pressure increase and pressure rarification. The periodicity of the pressure waveform, or its cycle, is expressed as frequency. A sound wave has several characteristics (Fig. 11–1), many of which are related. ***Frequency*** is the number of complete cycles occurring per second and is the inverse of ***wavelength*** (λ), which is the length of a single cycle. ***Amplitude*** is the power, or ability of the wave to transfer energy to the conducting medium or other insonated object. As the pressure wave propagates through a medium, the amplitude of the pressure change diminishes due to attenuation. The emitted sound wave is described as having an initial or fundamental frequency. This fundamental frequency is preserved during a propagation through a conducting medium, and a portion of the sound energy is reflected back at the same fundamental frequency.

A recent adaptation of cardiac ultrasonography relies on the generation of harmonic frequencies during transmission of the ultrasound beam. Traditionally, transducers have had narrow bandwidth elements that transmit and receive at narrowly defined frequencies. Modern transducers have a wide bandwidth that allows transmission and receipt of ultrasound over a broad range of frequencies. The traditional view of harmonics is that an insonated object may resonate and hence reflect back ultrasound not only at the fundamental, transmitted frequency but also at harmonics of that frequency. In the traditional view of harmonics, an object can be imaged at 2 MHz but reflect ultrasound back at 2 MHz and at 4 and 8 MHz harmonics (Fig. 11–2). Recently, it has been recognized that the transmission of ultrasound through tissue actually creates harmonic frequencies during propagation. Because the transmitted frequency is not a narrow discrete frequency but rather a broad range of frequencies, the full range of reflected frequencies and the resultant harmonics are likewise substantially broader than originally conceived. This is the premise for what has been termed ***tissue harmonic imaging***. Harmonic frequencies increase in strength with depth of penetration but represent only a small portion of the total reflected ultrasound energy. The advantage of the reflected harmonic frequencies is that they are free of near-field reverberation and shadowing effect. This results in an increased signal-to-noise ratio of the harmonic signal.[1-3] This type of imaging shows tremendous promise for improved visualization of the myocardium but at the cost of a minor reduction in resolution. Additionally, tissue signature is brighter than usual, and there is loss of detail for evaluation of fine valvular structures.

For clinical imaging, the ultrasound energy is both generated and received by a transducer attached to an imaging platform. Ultrasound energy is generated by an electrically stimulated piezoelectric crystal. The ultrasound energy generated is modified by the physical elements of the transducer, which serves to provide damping functions as well as some focusing function. In its simplest application, a piezoelectric crystal emits ultrasound at a single discrete frequency that is not altered by either the transducer or during propagation. In modern scanners, broad-band technology is used such that the emitted ultrasound consists of not just a single frequency but a range of frequencies. For any given transducer, there is not only a center "fundamental" frequency but also a range of frequencies both greater and lesser than the fundamental frequency, each of which has less amplitude than the fundamental frequency. This results in the substantially greater ability to determine tissue signature than is possible with a single discrete fundamental frequency. The imaging beam is emitted as a series of pulses, each of which contains several cycles of ultrasound. The number of pulses emitted per second is the pulse repetition frequency.

The ultrasound beam has several characteristics that are determined by the

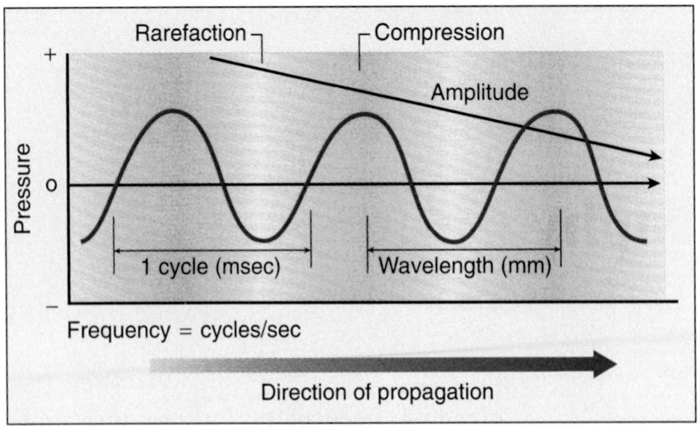

FIGURE 11–1 Schematic representation of a sound wave. The sound wave is typically described as a sine wave but actually represents alternating areas of pressure compression and rarification in a medium. Several characteristics that describe the sound wave, including amplitude, wavelength, and cycle, are schematized. Frequency is the number of cycles per second and, for clinical ultrasonography, ranges between 2.0 and 10 MHz. Amplitude (diagonal line) diminishes with distance from the sound source.

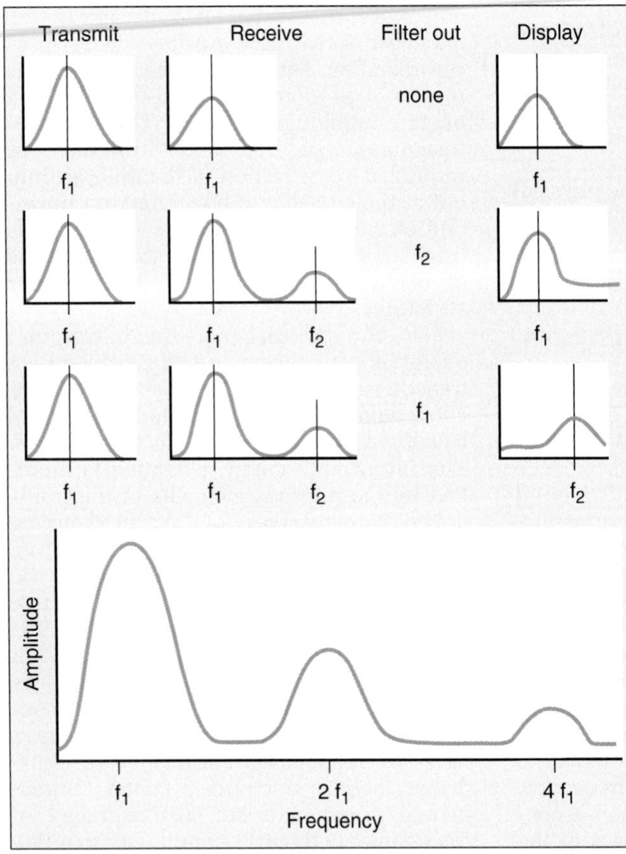

FIGURE 11–2 Schematic of second harmonics. A modern broadband transducer emits and receives ultrasound over a fairly broad range. Its central frequency is noted as the fundamental frequency (f_1). The frequency spectrum can also be described as a series of harmonics or multiples of that frequency, as noted. Harmonics are generated during transmission, with each successive harmonic being twice the preceding in frequency. Each successive harmonic has a substantially reduced amplitude, as noted. For detection of harmonics, selective filtering for receipt of the targeted frequency is employed, as is selective amplification of that frequency to enhance returning signals in the harmonic range. The bottom schematic depicts the phenomenon of multiple harmonics, each twice the frequency of the preceding, but with diminished amplitude. The top three schematics depict receiving and display characteristics of a narrow band (single frequency) transducer at the top and selective filtering to display either the fundamental (f_1) or harmonic (f_2) frequency.

transducer and that impact both its ability to penetrate a medium and its resolution for separating two objects in space. Low-frequency ultrasound provides a greater depth of penetration than does high-frequency ultrasound. Conversely, image resolution is greater with higher frequencies and less with low frequencies. Because ultrasound is propagated through tissue, it attenuates (loses energy) as well as losing the directional integrity of the beam. This results in far field dispersion of the ultrasound beam, so that it effectively images a larger area in the far field, more distant from the transducer face, than in the near field. It is within the near field that resolution is greatest. The distance of the near field from the transducer face can be calculated as outlined in Figure 11–3.

It should be emphasized that there are several forms of resolution, including axial, lateral, contrast, and temporal resolution (Fig. 11–4). *Axial resolution* refers to the ability to separate objects that fall in the direction of ultrasound propagation. *Lateral resolution* applies to the ability to detect objects that lie side by side within the ultrasound beam. *Contrast resolution* refers to the ability to detect objects of differing acoustic reflectivity, and *temporal resolution* refers to the ability to determine separation in time of events by ultrasound.

The amount of ultrasound energy delivered to the field can be controlled by the output of the transducer. For clinical

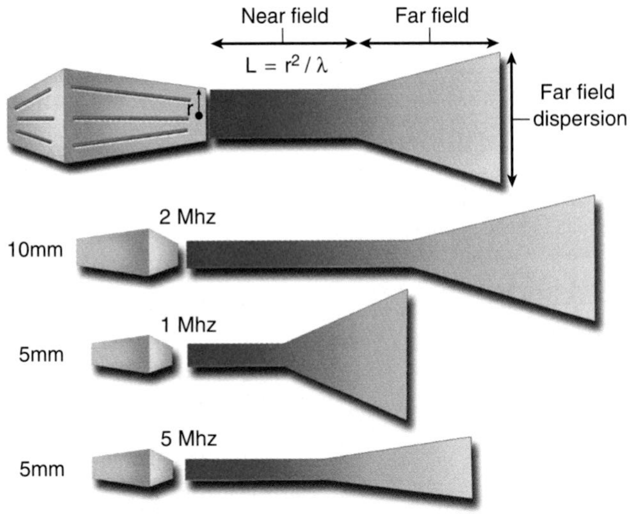

FIGURE 11–3 Schematic of a typical ultrasound transducer. The ultrasound transducer emits ultrasound from a series of piezoelectric crystals. The beam has several components, including a near field (Fresnel zone) with relatively narrow beam width and a far field where there is divergence of the ultrasound beam. Ultrasound intensity decreases with distance from the transducer face. The length of the near field can be calculated as $L = r^2/\lambda$. Changes in the transducer diameter and frequency have predictable effects on the near and far field characteristics, as is noted in the lower two illustrations. Higher frequencies preserve the length of the near field compared to lower frequencies, as do larger transducer diameters.

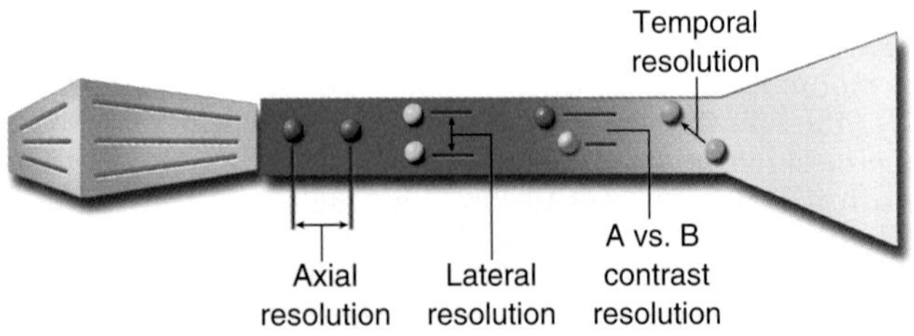

FIGURE 11–4 Schematic representation of different forms of ultrasound resolution. The four types of resolution—axial, lateral, temporal, and contrast—are all illustrated in the schematized ultrasound beam.

purposes, the delivered ultrasound power is typically described as a mechanical index. Mechanical index is defined as the peak negative acoustic pressure divided by the square root of the transmission frequency. For routine clinical imaging, a mechanical index of 1.0 to 1.6 is typically used. As the ultrasound energy delivered increases, it may result in destruction of microbubbles, so for contrast imaging a lower mechanical index is necessary.

THE DOPPLER PRINCIPLE

The Doppler principle states that the frequency of ultrasound reflected from a stationary object is identical to the transmitted frequency. If an object is moving toward the transducer, the reflected frequency will be higher than the transmitted frequency; and conversely, if an object is moving away from the transducer, the reflected frequency will be lower. The difference between the transmitted and received frequencies is the Doppler shift (Fig. 11-5). The magnitude of the Doppler shift is determined by the velocity and direction of the moving object and can be calculated by the Doppler equation. The Doppler equation relates the angle of interrogation, the Doppler shift, or change in frequency between the transmitted and reflected frequency, and a constant that is equal to the speed of sound in water to the velocity and direction of the moving object (Fig. 11-6). A major contributor to this equation is the angle θ, with which the interrogating beam intercepts flow. For maximum accuracy, interrogation should be directly in the line of flow, that is $\theta = 0$ degrees. Because the cosine of 0 degrees equals 1.0, solving the Doppler equation is a fairly straightforward process. With increasing angle of incidence (θ), cosine θ becomes progressively less than 1.0, and when incorporated into the equation results in a systematic and increasingly severe underestimation of the true velocity. For practical purposes, an angle of interrogation θ less than 20 degrees is essential to ensure clinically accurate information. The Doppler shift data that are generated are typically displayed as velocity rather than the actual frequency shift. By convention, motion toward the transducer is displayed above a "zero crossing line" and motion away from the transducer below the line (Fig. 11-7).

Pulsed versus Continuous-Wave Doppler. Doppler ultrasonography is used in two basic methods. The first is pulsed Doppler, which can be considered a "steerable stethoscope," in which a sample volume of variable size can be superimposed on the two-dimensional echocardiographic image. Range gating is used to ensure that only Doppler shifts from one discrete site are interpreted for velocity calculations. Thus, pulsed Doppler allows determination of direction and flow velocity at a precise point within the cardiac system. It is limited, however, in its maximum detectable velocity by the Nyquist limit. The Nyquist limit is defined as one-half of the pulse repetition frequency. For typical imaging systems, the maximum recordable velocity with pulsed Doppler is 1.5 to 2 m/sec. Many stenotic and regurgitant velocities exceed this limit, at which point the spectral display is paradoxically recorded as a velocity in the opposite direction of the moving target. This phenomenon is known as "aliasing" (Fig. 11-8).

Continuous-wave Doppler simultaneously and continuously transmits and interrogates the returning ultrasound beam for Doppler shifts. The line of interrogation is identifiable; however, the precise location of the maximum velocity must be deduced by integrating the interrogation line direction with known cardiac anatomy. Although continuous-wave Doppler imaging provides less precise localization of gradients, it is not constrained by velocity limits and hence can record velocities exceeding those that can be detected with pulsed Doppler.

Multigate Doppler. In an effort to increase the maximum velocity detectable with pulsed Doppler, a technique of multigating can be employed in which multiple pulsed gates are simultaneously employed, thus increasing the effective Nyquist limit. Multigate Doppler allows detection of velocities as high as 3.5 to 5 m/sec with the ability to identify one of the gates as the site of origin. In large part, multigate Doppler has been supplanted by steerable continuous wave Doppler methodology.

Color Flow Doppler. Color flow Doppler imaging represents a variation on multigate pulsed Doppler imaging and thus is subject to its velocity limitations. In color flow Doppler, instead of only a single site being interrogated for a Doppler shift, a variably sized matrix of sampling points can be created and used to simultaneously interrogate velocity over a large area of the heart. Because this represents multiple pulsed sample volumes, each of which must be independently interrogated, frame rates are relatively low for color Doppler flow imaging. Color flow imaging is the display solution for managing the data that are derived from thousands of sample sites simultaneously.[4,5] The typical color flow display algorithm involves displaying velocities toward the transducer in varying shades of red, and those heading away from the transducer in varying shades of blue with either the intensity or hue paralleling the actual velocity. If multiple velocity shifts are present at an interrogation point, this is defined as "variance" and may be colored in a yellow or green "confetti-like" image.

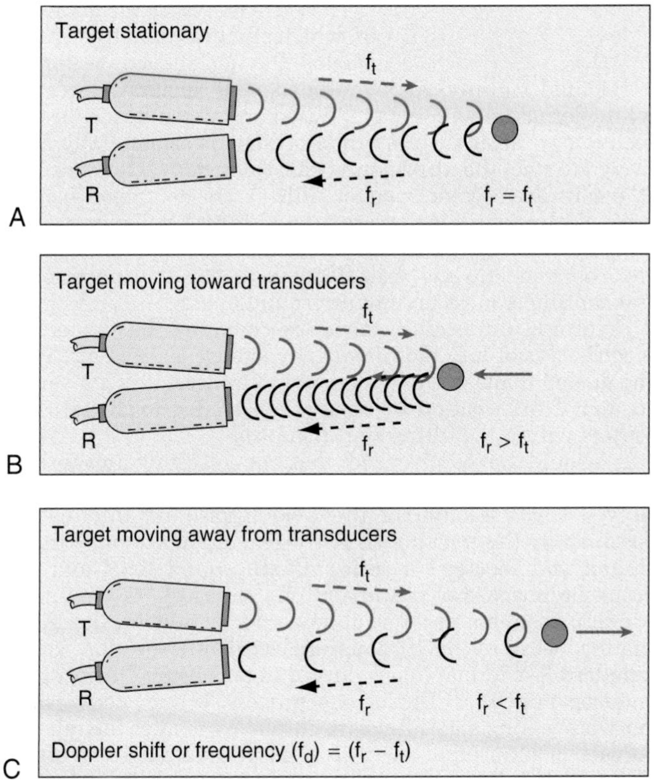

FIGURE 11–5 Demonstration of the Doppler effect. In each instance, the transmitted ultrasound beam is denoted emanating from the upper transducer and the returning beam off the reflecting object (orange circle) coming to the lower transducer. The upper panel depicts a stationary target in which the transmit frequency (f_t) is equal to the returning frequency (f_r) and there is no Doppler shift. The middle panel depicts an object moving toward the transducer in which the returning frequency (f_r) is greater than the transmit frequency (f_t). In the lower schematic, the object is moving away from the transducer, and the returning frequency (f_r) is less than the transmit frequency (f_t). The Doppler shift (f_d) equals the difference between these two frequencies. (From Feigenbaum H: Echocardiography. 4th ed. Malvern, PA, Lea & Febiger, 1986.)

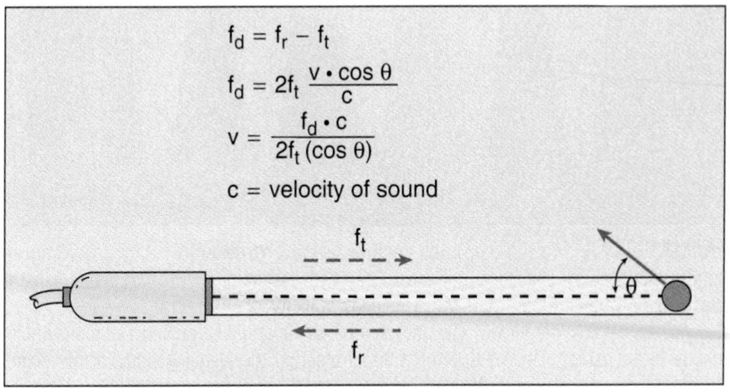

FIGURE 11–6 Demonstration of the Doppler equation for determining the velocity of a moving object. The Doppler shift (f_d) is calculated as the difference between the returning (f_r) and transmit (f_t) frequencies. The Doppler equation relates the Doppler shift (f_d) to the transmit frequency, the angle of interrogation (θ), the velocity of the moving object (V), and the speed of sound (C). The equation can be rearranged to solve for velocity as is noted in the third equation. (From Feigenbaum H: Echocardiography. 4th ed. Malvern, PA, Lea & Febiger, 1986.)

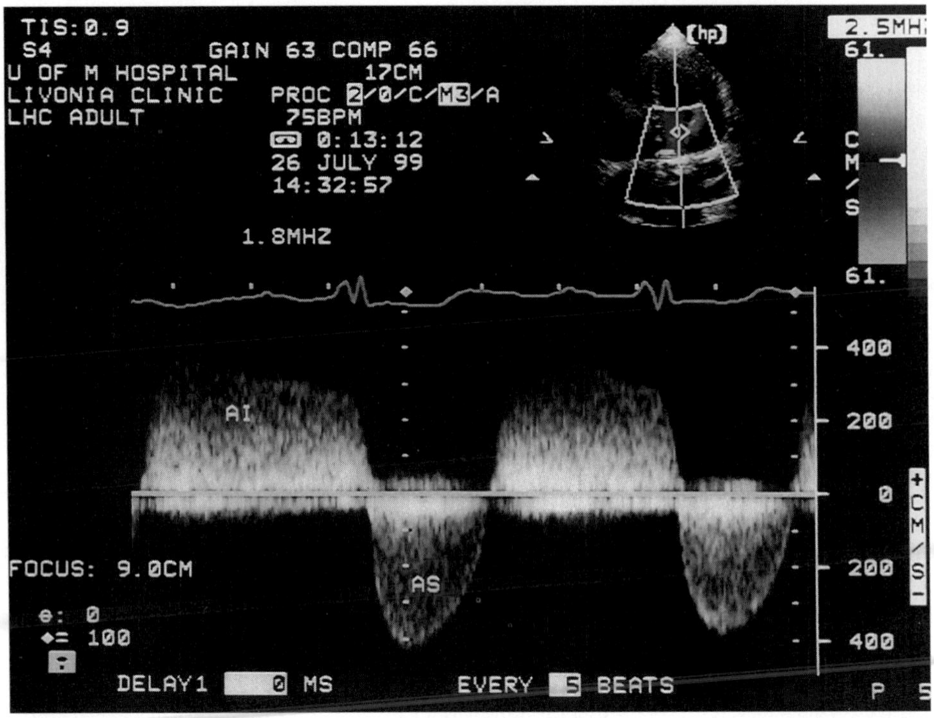

FIGURE 11–7 Combination of aortic stenosis (AS) and aortic insufficiency (AI), demonstrating the directional nature of spectral Doppler. The continuous-wave Doppler is recorded from the apex of the left ventricle along a line oriented through the aortic valve. Aortic stenosis is present with a peak velocity of 4 m/sec (400 cm/sec) that is directed away from the transducer and hence recorded below the zero crossing line. Aortic insufficiency is also present and is noted as a diastolic signal recorded above the zero crossing line.

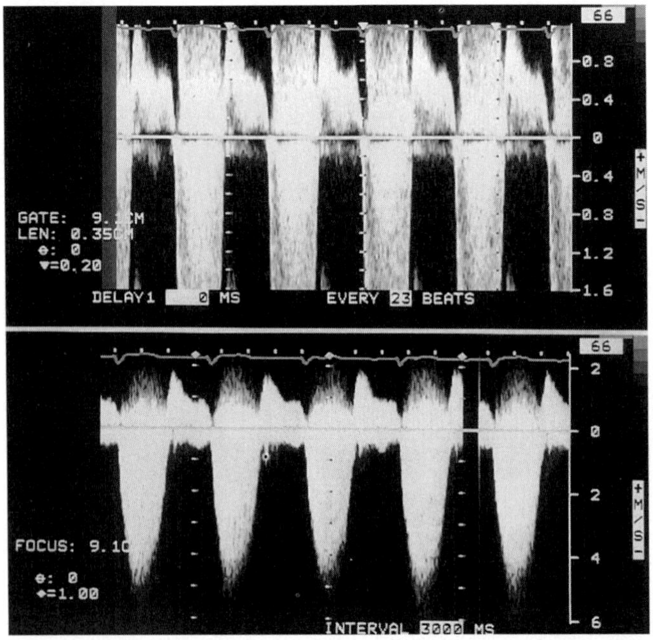

FIGURE 11–8 Pulsed **(top)** and continuous-wave **(bottom)** Doppler recording of mitral regurgitation. The lower panel recorded with continuous wave Doppler is free of the aliasing phenomenon, and the true peak velocity of the mitral regurgitation jet (5.5 m/sec) is fully displayed. The top panel was recorded in pulsed Doppler, which results in "aliasing." Once the velocity has exceeded the Nyquist limit (in this case, 1.6 m/sec) the signal is paradoxically displayed above the zero crossing line.

Image Generation

An ultrasound platform consists of several components. Modern scanners have highly computerized platforms for analog to digital conversion of returning ultrasound signals and then manipulation and display of the signal to provide either anatomical information (two-dimensional echocardiography) or information regarding velocity of motion (Doppler information) or other highly specialized applications such as tissue characterization.

An ultrasound transducer consists of a series of piezoelectric crystals, which when electrically activated, emit ultrasound energy. A transducer will be described by its frequency range as well as the number of crystals or channels incorporated in its face. This typically will range from 128 to 512 channels in modern scanners. Recently, scanners with a rectangular array of piezoelectric crystals (rather than a linear array) have been developed that allow a three-dimensional beam to be propagated in real time. Incorporated into the transducer construction is damping material to allow a crystal to be excited but then rapidly become quiescent, as well as filters to control the range of frequencies received and an effective "lens," which focuses the resulting ultrasound beam.

There are two basic mechanisms by which an ultrasound transducer creates the fan-shaped sector of ultrasound required for two-dimensional imaging. Virtually all modern scanners rely on phased array scan heads. In this technology, firing of individual crystals is sequentially controlled to steer the ultrasound beam through its 90-degree arc. A mechanical sector scanner utilizes one to three discrete piezoelectric crystals that are rotated at high velocity to then create an arc. In either instance, the piezoelectric crystals incorporated into the scan head serve the dual purpose of transmitting and receiving ultrasound energy.

Returning ultrasound energy is converted by the piezoelectric crystal into radiofrequency energy. This energy is in the analog domain. For processing purposes, it is converted to digital information by high-speed analog to digital converters within the ultrasound platform.

It should be emphasized that the resulting image that appears on the screen of the ultrasound platform contains only a small fraction of the total ultrasound information received by the transducer. Early-generation scanners transmitted and received a series of ultrasound lines and the resulting image was comprised of a series of "rastor lines." Modern scanners use a scan converter to convert the information being received along angles of interrogation into a standard X-Y format image devoid of evidence of the original interrogation lines. During the process of scan conversion, post-processing algorithms are employed to alter the relative impact of ultrasound in various amplitude ranges to create the aesthetically pleasing ultrasound image characteristic of current scanners.

Controls available for image manipulation include either enhancing or suppressing the signal from any given receipt depth. As the depth of imaging is directly related to the time of transit, this alteration is known as time-gain compensation. Current-generation scanners display images in 128 to 512 shades of gray, each of which can be assigned using a variety of post-processing algorithms designed for enhancement of myocardial texture, suppression of highly reflective objects or to enhance the ultrasound signature of faint objects. In an effort to enhance visual detection of anatomical boundaries and spectral Doppler signals, the fundamental gray scale image can be colorized. This has shown promise for detection and tracking of endocardial boundaries and for visualization of faint spectral Doppler signals.

When ultrasound interacts with a reflective surface, its interaction can be described as either specular or scattering. Specular reflectors generally reflect ultrasound energy back as a unified predictable beam. If the angle of the reflector is perpendicular to the beam, energy will be reflected back directly. If the reflector is tangential to the beam reflection can also be tangential to the original line of propagation. In any event, a portion of the ultrasound energy is reflected back as a discrete signal. Conversely, scattering reflectors tend to scatter the ultrasound beam and result in substantial lessening of its reflective amplitude. Biological examples of a specular reflector would be a bright pericardial echo or mechanical valve prosthesis. These objects reflect ultrasound back directly. Tissue tends to be a more scattering reflector that scatters the beam, which results in substantial dispersion of ultrasound energy, only a portion of which is reflected directly back to the transducer.

Ultrasound Image Formats

The simplest image to understand is the M-mode echocardiogram. An M-mode echocardiogram is acquired by interrogating returning ultrasound signals along a single line of interrogation. Each returning packet is analyzed for its round trip transit time, which is then converted to a distance from the transducer face. It is then displayed as a discrete point. The intensity of the point is directly related to the amplitude of the returning signal. Ultrasound reflected off of a highly reflective object such as a fibrotic or calcified structure has greater amplitude and hence is displayed as a brighter dot. Ultrasound reflected from a diffuse reflector such as myocardium is displayed as a fainter dot. This process is repeated at a frequency of 1000 to 3000 per second and then recorded. Early M-mode echocardiograms were recorded on a strip chart recorder at speeds of 25 to 100 mm/sec. Modern M-mode echocardiograms are recorded on a scrolling video screen. It is uncommon to use a dedicated M-mode transducer in contemporary practice. Using the electronic steering capability of a modern two-dimensional scanner, the operator can select a single line of interrogation within the 90-degree sector and obtain an M-mode interrogation line along that sector. The M-mode interrogation line can be "swept" over an area of cardiac anatomy and the image then displayed as a series of side-by-side M-mode interrogation lines (Fig. 11–9). M-mode echocardiography was once the mainstay of anatomical diagnosis but has been largely abandoned in favor of modern 90-degree two-dimensional sector scanning. M-mode echocardiography does confer substantially higher temporal resolution than two-dimensional echocardiography and in some instances may provide a higher degree of axial resolution than two-dimensional scanning. In general, however, its clinical role, especially as a stand-alone technique, has been largely supplanted by two-dimensional scanning.

Color M-Mode

Color M-mode echocardiography examines routine M-mode scanning with superimposed color Doppler information. As with M-mode echocardiography, the x axis represents time and the y axis represents distance from the transducer. Along the single line of interrogation, Doppler information is then color-encoded and superimposed on the M-mode display (Fig. 11–10). This technique provides high temporal resolution for timing intracardiac flow and can have particular value in determining the timing of a regurgitant valvular lesion and in determining the rate of inflow into the left ventricle. It is limited in that it provides information regarding velocity of flow in only one dimension.

THE ANATOMICAL ECHOCARDIOGRAPHIC EXAMINATION

The mainstay of the echocardiographic examination is transthoracic two-dimensional echocardiography. The fan-shaped scan plane is directed into the chest to provide tomographic imaging planes of the heart and great vessels (Figs. 11-11 to 11-17). Each returning ultrasound signal is then registered and converted to a two-dimensional image of the interrogated plane. This process is repeated 20 to 120 times per second, resulting in a frame rate of 20 to 120 Hz. The sequence of imaged frames results in a real-time moving image of the heart. The frame rate for two-dimensional imaging is dependent on line density and scanning depth. Smaller areas can be imaged at substantially higher (100-140 Hz) frame rates than larger sectors, which typically are imaged at 40 to 60 Hz.

For the transthoracic examination, patients are typically placed in a left lateral position and scanned from several different left intercostal spaces. The standard transthoracic views (Table 11-1) are recorded from parasternal and apical transducer positions. Subcostal and suprasternal transducer positions can also be used. From any transducer position, the Doppler modalities, including pulsed, continuous-wave, and color flow imaging, can be recorded. Other imaging windows, such as the right sternal border, can be used for specific examinations.

Traditionally, two-dimensional echocardiograms and Doppler echocardiograms have been recorded on videotape for subsequent analysis and activities. With modern ultrasonography equipment, the image is acquired in a digital format and stored as such. Digital images can be displayed side by side or as a quad screen containing multiple views for visualization simultaneously. Digital images can be transmitted to remote sites for review and are free from degradation seen when the source image is transferred to analog videotape.

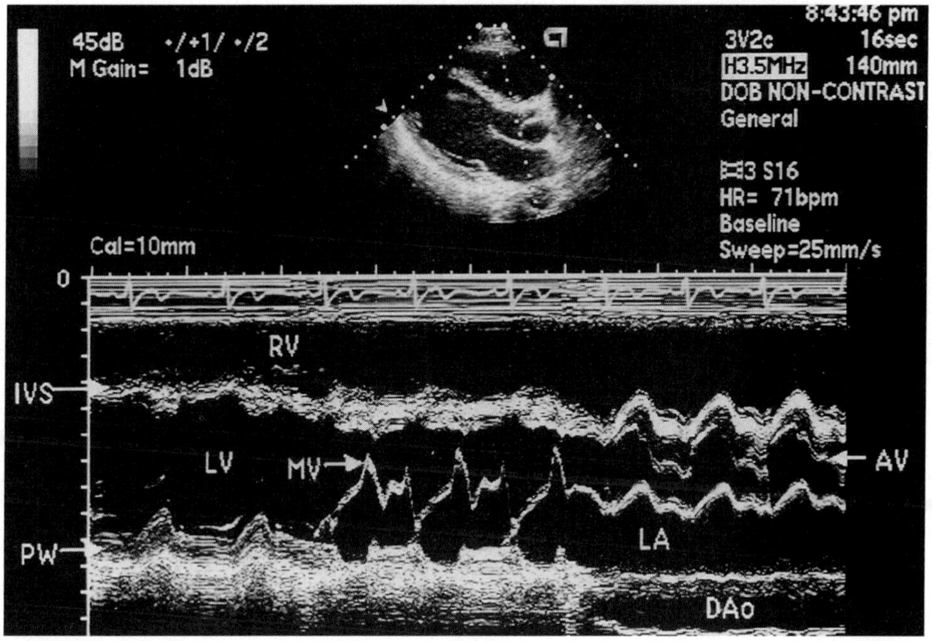

FIGURE 11–9 Normal M-mode echocardiogram in which the M-mode beam is swept from the aortic valve through the mitral valve and to the level of the papillary muscles. Note the normal box-like opening of the aortic valve and the biphasic, "M"-shaped opening pattern of the mitral valve. There is posterior motion of the ventricular septum synchronous with anterior motion of the posterior wall. AV = aortic valve; DAo = descending aorta; LA = left atrium; LV = left ventricle; MV = mitral valve; RV = right ventricle.

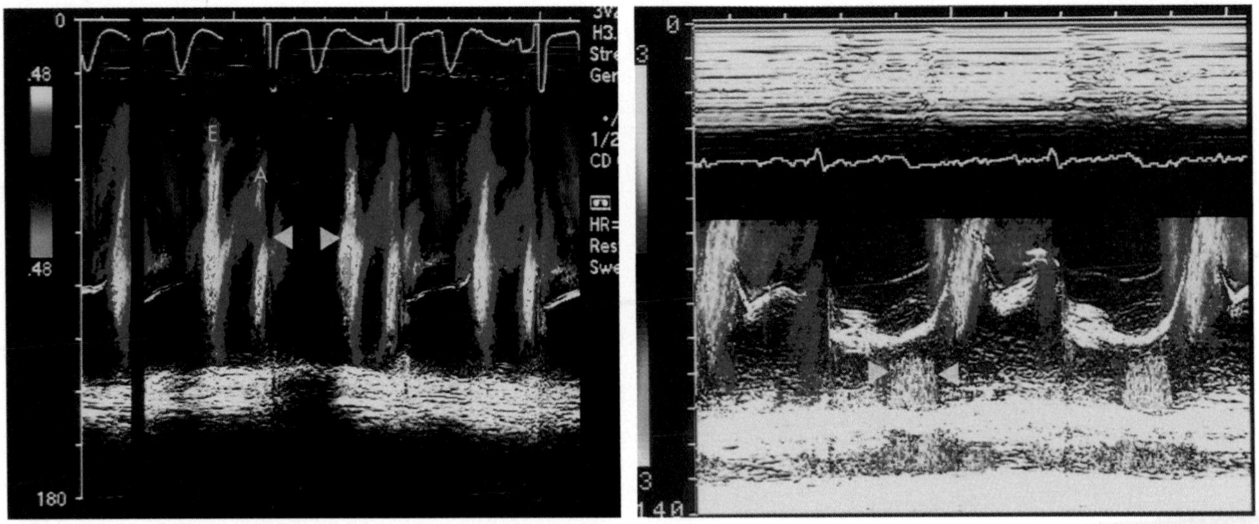

FIGURE 11–10 Color M-mode echocardiography. With this methodology, color flow imaging is superimposed on an M-mode echocardiogram. This provides excellent temporal resolution for timing intracardiac events. The **left panel** was recorded in a normal, disease-free individual from the apex of the left ventricle. Notice that both early and late (E and A) mitral inflow can be detected. The systolic interval (white arrowheads) is devoid of flow. The **right panel** was recorded in a patient with mitral valve prolapse and late systolic mitral regurgitation. Note the prominent early flow velocity through the mitral valve and a late systolic regurgitant flow (white arrowheads).

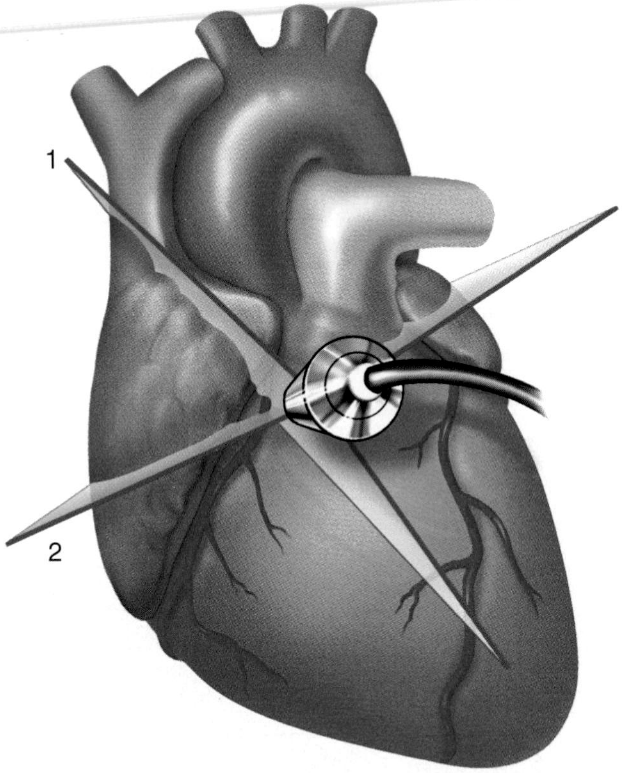

FIGURE 11–11 Schematic of the transducer orientation used for acquiring parasternal views. The scanning plane of the ultrasound beam is superimposed on a schematic of the heart. Plane 1 represents a parasternal long-axis view in which the right ventricular outflow tract, proximal portion of the aorta and aortic valve, anterior ventricular septum, cavity of the left ventricle containing the mitral valve, and inferoposterior wall of the left ventricle can be visualized. Scanning plane 1 results in an ultrasound image, as noted in Figure 11–12. Scanning plane 2 is obtained by rotating the transducer 90 degrees and can be used to obtain a family of short-axis views of the heart (see Fig. 11–14). (From Feigenbaum H: Echocardiography. 4th ed. Malvern, PA, Lea & Febiger, 1986.)

TABLE 11–1 Two-Dimensional Echocardiographic Examination

Parasternal Approach
Long-axis plane
Root of aorta—aortic valve, left atrium, left ventricular outflow tract
Body of left ventricle—mitral valve
Left ventricular apex
Right ventricular inflow tract—tricuspid valve
Short-axis plane
Root of the aorta—aortic valve, pulmonary valve, tricuspid valve, right ventricular outflow tract, left atrium, pulmonary artery, coronary arteries
Left ventricle—mitral valve
Left ventricle—papillary muscles
Left ventricle—apex
Apical Approach
Four-chamber plane
Four chambers
Four chambers with aorta
Long-axis plane
Two chambers—left ventricle, left atrium
Two chambers with aorta
Subcostal Approach
Four-chamber plane—all four chambers and both septa
Short-axis plane
Left ventricle
Right ventricle
Inferior vena cava
Suprasternal Approach
Four-chamber plane
Arch of aorta—descending aorta
Long-axis plane
Arch of aorta—pulmonary artery, left atrium

Examination and Appearance of the Normal Heart

PARASTERNAL LONG-AXIS VIEW. In this view (Fig. 11–12), the inferoposterior wall and interventricular septum are visualized, each of which is mildly concave toward the other. The normal ascending aorta is visualized, including its annulus, the sinuses of Valsalva, and the proximal portion of the ascending aorta. The anterior and posterior leaflets of the mitral valve can be visualized in the parasternal long-axis view, with the anterior leaflet appearing more elongated. Typically, the posterolateral papillary muscle is also visualized from this transducer position. Anterior to the aorta, a portion of the right ventricular outflow tract is visualized. By medially angulating the transducer, the right ventricular inflow tract can be visualized in which the inferior vena cava, right atrium, tricuspid valve, and right ventricle are visualized (Fig. 11–13). From the parasternal transducer position, a series of short-axis views can be obtained by rotating the transducer 90 degrees (Fig. 11–14). At the base of the heart, the circular aorta and the aortic valve with three equally sized leaflets are visualized, as well as the right ventricular outflow tract, which is seen as an inverted "U" overlying the aorta. By angling the transducer toward the apex, a short-axis view of the mitral valve can be visualized from which the actual orifice can be seen and its area measured. With further angulation, the circular cavity of the left ventricle is visualized, including the papillary muscles. The normal left ventricle has circular geometry, whether it is visualized at the level of the mitral valve, papillary muscles, or apex. In the short-axis projections at the level of the mitral valve and below, the right ventricle appears as a more trabeculated crescent-shaped structure.

APICAL VIEWS. From this transducer position, the normal left ventricle has a bullet-shaped geometry. The anterior and posterior mitral valve leaflets can be visualized. The left atrium and pulmonary veins are visualized as well (Fig. 11–15). In the four-chamber view, the right ventricle appears as a triangular structure. The tricuspid valve inserts into the annulus of the right ventricle at a position slightly more apical than the mitral valve. This results in a small portion of the ventricular septum (the atrioventricular septum) falling between the septal leaflets of the tricuspid and mitral valves. By rotating the transducer 90 degrees from the four-chamber view, a two-chamber view of the left ventricle and left atrium can be obtained (see Fig. 11–15).

SUBCOSTAL AND SUPRASTERNAL VIEWS. In addition to parasternal and apical transducer positions, subcostal and suprasternal positions also provide imaging windows in adult patients. The subcostal transducer position can be very effective in patients with chronic lung disease in whom parasternal and apical views are obscured by intervening lung tissue. For subcostal imaging, patients are placed in the supine position with the knees bent and the transducer placed in the subxiphoid position. Imaging during held inspiration often is effective at bringing the heart into optimal position. Views similar to a four-chamber view as well as a series of short-axis views can be obtained from this transducer position. The subcostal views also provide excellent visualization of the atrial septum and the connection between the inferior vena cava (IVC) and right atrium (Fig. 11–16).

SUPRASTERNAL VIEWS. These views are obtained by placing the transducer in the suprasternal notch. This transducer position may be somewhat uncomfortable for many patients. It provides a view of the arch and adjacent ascending and descending aorta. In the majority of patients, the great vessels and portions of the main pulmonary artery are also seen (Fig. 11–17).

Anatomic Variants

Several well-recognized anatomical and developmental variants can be seen with echocardiography. It is important to recognize these as normal variants to avoid confusion with pathological structures.

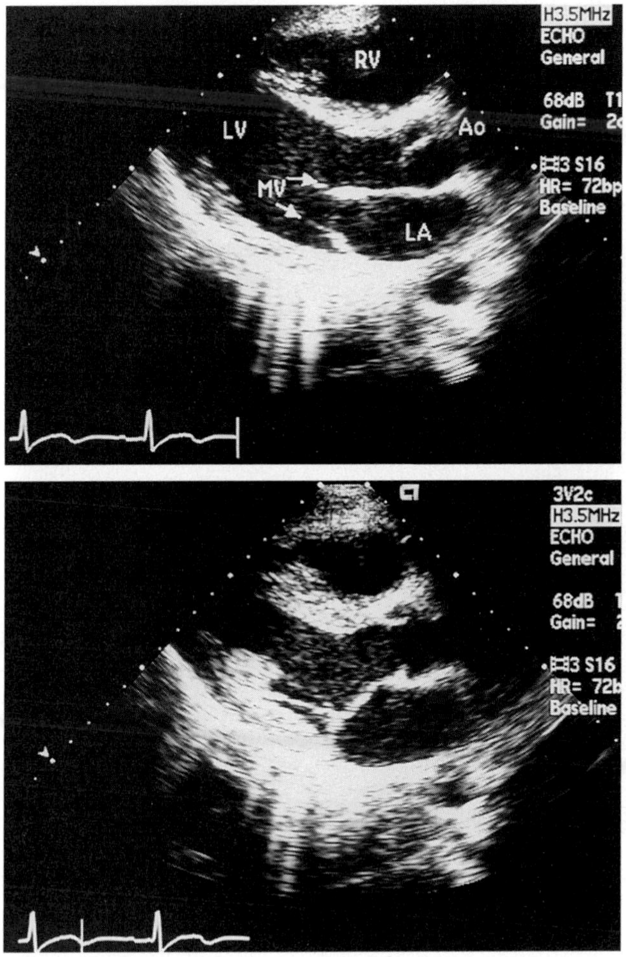

FIGURE 11–12 Parasternal long-axis view of the left ventricle in diastole **(top)** and systole **(bottom)**. Chambers and cardiac structures are as noted. This view corresponds to plane 1 of Figure 11–11. Ao = aorta; LA = left atrium; LV = left ventricle; MV = mitral valve; RV = right ventricular outflow tract.

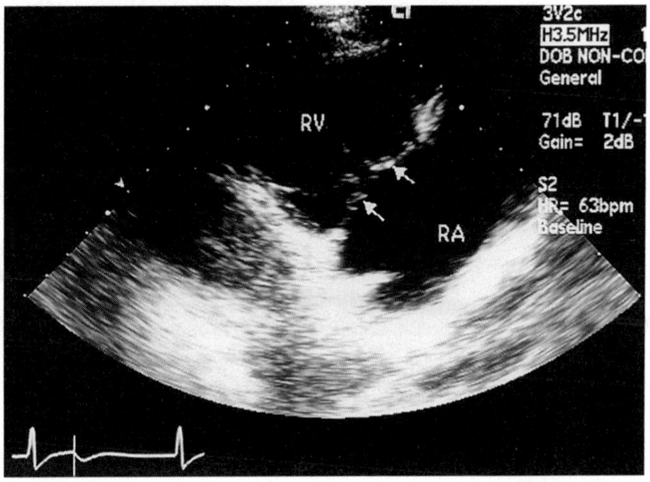

FIGURE 11–13 Two-dimensional echocardiogram of the right ventricular inflow tract, recorded from the parasternal transducer position. RA = right atrium; RV = right ventricle.

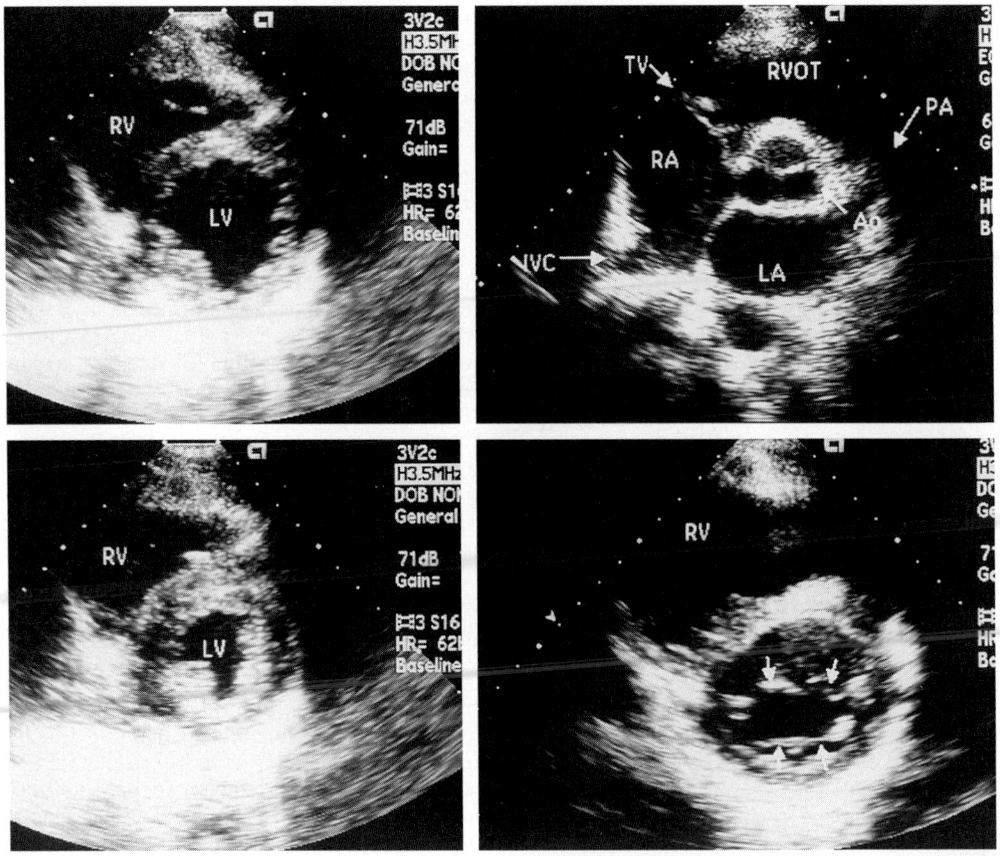

FIGURE 11–14 Short-axis two-dimensional echocardiograms, the two **left panels** are recorded at the level of the papillary muscles in diastole **(top)** and systole **(bottom)**. Note the symmetrical thickening of the myocardium and inward motion of the endocardium representing normal ventricular function in systole. The **top right panel** is recorded at the level of the aortic valve, and the **bottom right panel** is recorded at the level of the mitral valve in diastole. Ao = aorta; IVC = inferior vena cava; LA = left atrium; LV = left ventricle; PA = pulmonary artery; RA = right atrium; RV = right ventricle; RVOT = right ventricular outflow tract; TV = tricuspid valve.

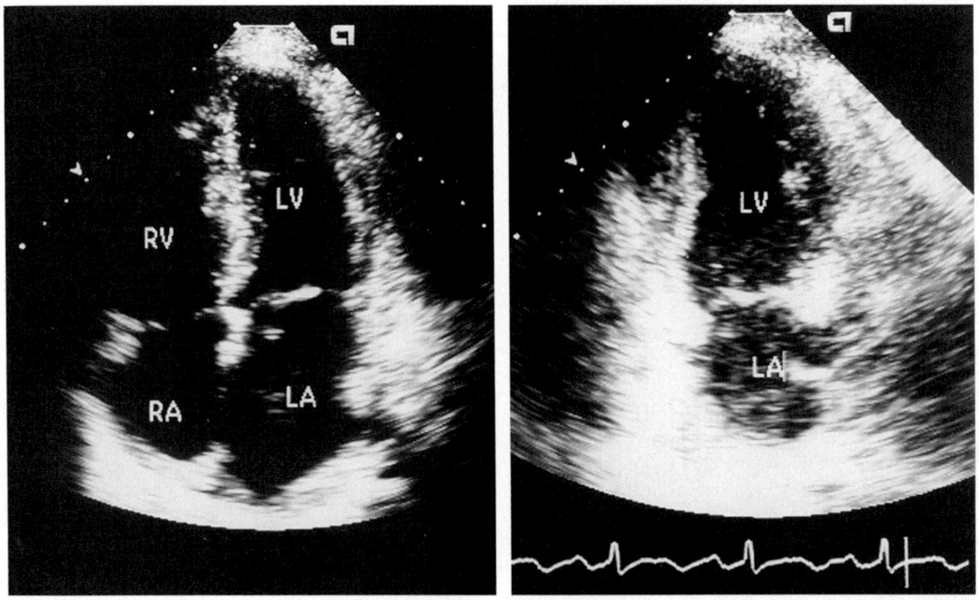

FIGURE 11–15 Apical four- and two-chamber views of the left ventricle. Note the normal "bullet-shaped" geometry of the left ventricle and the more triangular right ventricle. Note also the more apical insertion of the tricuspid valve compared with the mitral valve. LA = left atrium; LV = left ventricle; RA = right atrium; RV = right ventricle.

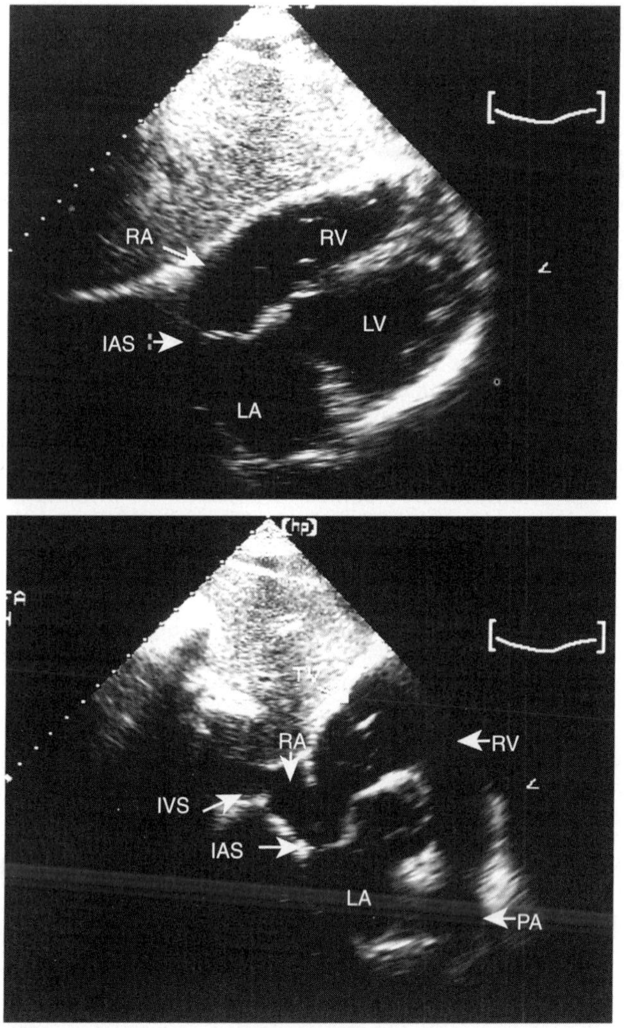

FIGURE 11–16 Two-dimensional echocardiograms recorded from the subcostal transducer position. The **upper panel** is a subcostal four-chamber view in which all four cardiac chambers are visualized as well as the plane of the mitral and tricuspid valves. The atrial septum is visualized in its entire length in this view. The **lower panel** was recorded in a short-axis view at the level of the aortic valve from the subcostal position. The right atrium (RA), tricuspid valve (TV), right ventricle (RV), and pulmonary artery (PA) are visualized as well as the circular aorta. The interatrial septum (IAS) and inferior vena cava (IVC) are both visualized in this view as well. LA = left atrium; LV = left ventricle.

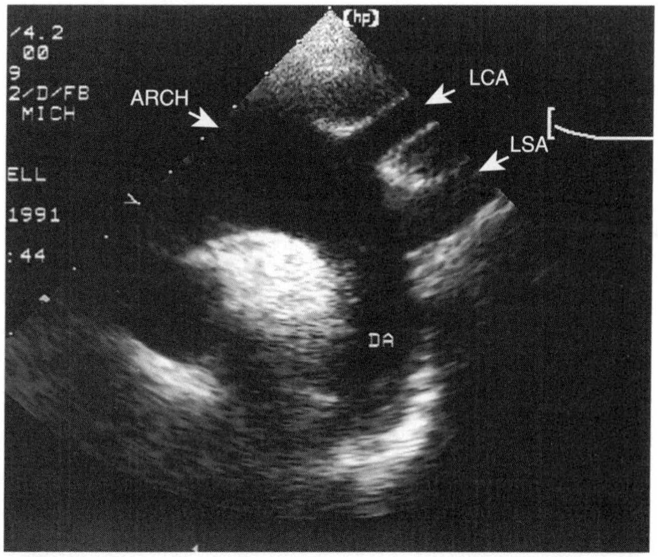

FIGURE 11–17 Two-dimensional echocardiogram recorded from a suprasternal transducer position. The arch of the aorta (ARCH) as well as a portion of the ascending and descending aorta can be visualized. Note also the great vessels arising from the arch (arrows). DA = descending aorta; LCA = left carotid artery; LSA = left subclavian artery.

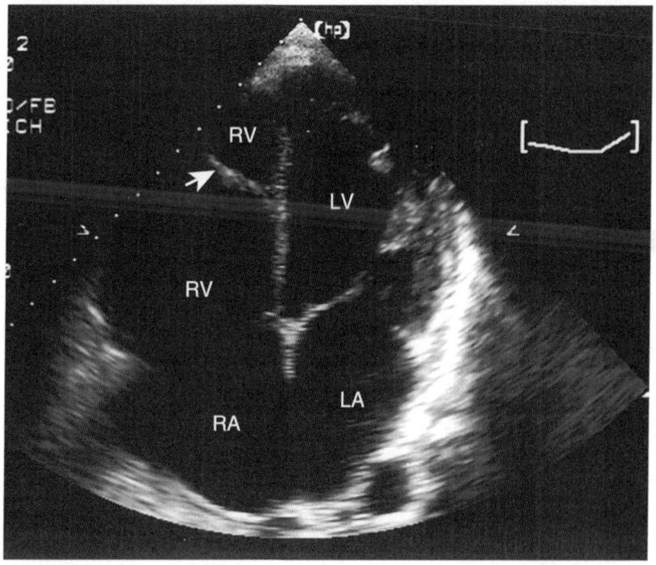

FIGURE 11–18 Apical four-chamber view of the heart revealing a prominent moderator band. The moderator band (arrow) appears as a muscle density structure traversing the apex of the right ventricle. This is a normal anatomical structure that should not be confused with a pathological process. LA = left atrium; LV = left ventricle; RA = right atrium; RV = right ventricle.

MUSCLE TRABECULATIONS. The right ventricle is more heavily trabeculated than the left, and, similarly, the right atrium is more trabeculated than the left atrium. High-resolution scanning virtually always detects multiple muscle trabeculations in the right ventricle, the most prominent of which is the moderator band, which is a muscular structure traversing from the lateral wall to the septum of the right ventricle near the apex (Fig. 11–18). On occasion, secondary muscle bundles are likewise noted. In any situation in which right ventricular hypertrophy occurs, the trabeculations become more prominent. It is important to recognize this phenomenon to avoid confusing a heavily trabeculated right ventricle with tumor, vegetation, thrombus, or other pathological mass.

The left ventricle is typically less trabeculated than the right, and other than the papillary muscles it is not common to note muscular tissue protruding into the left ventricle. Occasionally, a trabeculated left ventricular apex is encountered, the degree of which rarely approaches that seen in the right ventricle. Not infrequently, pseudochordae are seen in the left ventricular apex. Anatomically, these are structures similar to mitral valve chordae but that take an aberrant course, typically across the apex of the left ventricle. They are less often seen in the left ventricular outflow tract. They are more easily visualized in patients with cardiomyopathy and dilated hearts than in normal hearts, where they may lie against the endocardium and therefore not be visible.

RIGHT AND LEFT ATRIAL STRUCTURES. Several developmental remnants can be noted in the right atrium. These include the eustachian valve (Fig. 11–19) and Chiari network. In the embryo, a continuous membrane courses from the IVC to the coronary sinus to direct oxygenated blood from the IVC directly across the foramen ovale. During cardiac development, this membrane regresses. In the majority of patients, a small remnant known as the eustachian

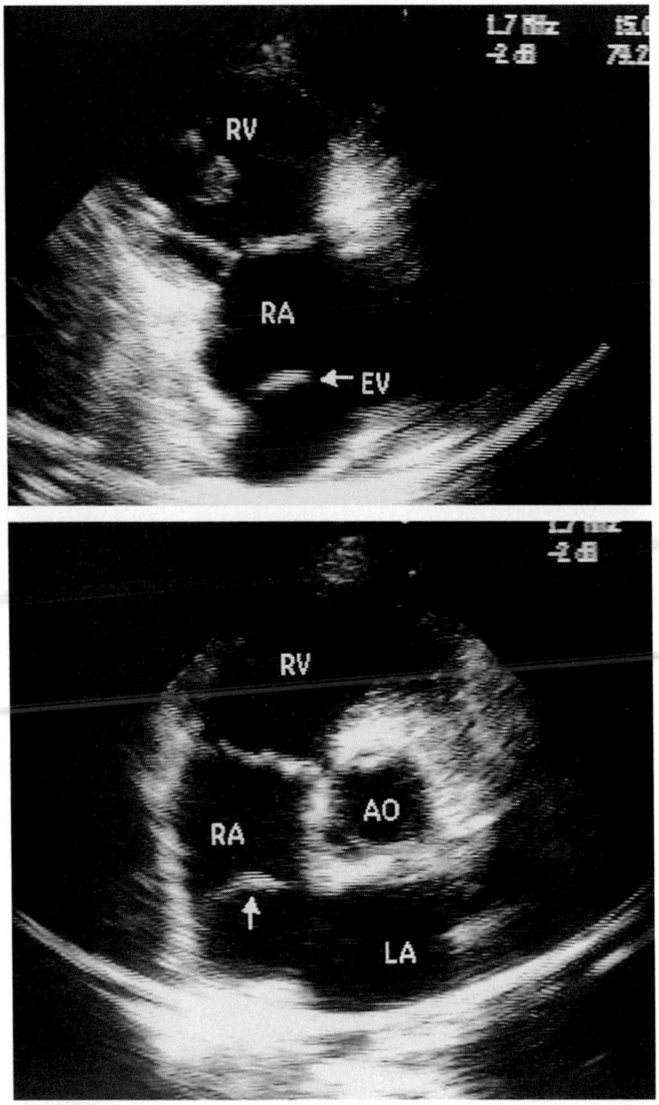

FIGURE 11–19 Transthoracic parasternal echocardiograms recorded in a patient with a prominent eustachian valve (EV). This is a normal anatomical variant that should not be confused for a mass, vegetation, or other pathological structure. The **top panel** is a right ventricular inflow tract view recorded from the left sternal border. Both the right atrium (RA) and right ventricle (RV) can be seen, and the tricuspid valve is closed. Note the linear echo arising from the junction of the right atrium and inferior vena cava coursing into the body of the right atrium. In real time this linear echo has highly mobile motion, mimicking valvular motion. The **bottom panel** is recorded in a parasternal short-axis view at the base of the heart. The same linear echo is noted in the bottom of the right atrium (arrow). AO = aorta.

valve can be seen at the right atrial–IVC junction. A second remnant is occasionally seen attached to the coronary sinus. This is known as a Chiari network and consists of a fine filamentous membrane with multiple perforations. On rare occasions, a "complete eustachian valve" is seen as a linear echo coursing from the IVC to the coronary sinus. In this instance, it has many perforations and rarely, if ever, is truly obstructive. Either the eustachian valve or a Chiari network can result in redirection of blood flow within the atrium and unusual patterns of blood flow noted with contrast echocardiography.

The right atrial appendage is typically visualized only with transesophageal echocardiography (TEE). It is a more trabeculated structure than the left atrial appendage, and, on occasion, trabeculae in the right atrial appendage have been confused for thrombi. Recognizing the full range of appearance of the right atrial appendage is essential to avoid this error.

The left atrium has a smoother wall than the right atrium. Using modern scanners, the left atrial appendage is often partially visualized with transthoracic imaging, either in the apical two-chamber view or in a parasternal short-axis view. It is optimally visualized with TEE, where it has the appearance of a "dog's ear" (Fig. 11–20). A substantial percentage of individuals have a multilobed left atrial appendage, which can result in a confusing appearance because the septation between the two lobes may be confused for thrombus.[6]

ATRIAL SEPTUM. The normal interatrial septum is visualized both in its primum and in its more superior portions, connected by the thin tissue of the foramen ovale. There is substantial variation in the thickness and prominence of the more muscular primum and superior portions of the atrial septum. A commonly encountered anomaly of the atrial septum is lipomatous atrial hypertrophy in which there is benign infiltration by lipomatous tissue of the primum and superior atrial septum (Fig. 11–21). The valve of the foramen ovale is spared, resulting in a "dumbbell" configuration of the atrial septum. The amount of infiltration is highly variable and can range from less than 1.0 cm to 5 cm or more. The tissue is homogeneous and somewhat brighter than the normal atrial septum. Because of its characteristic appearance, it should not be confused with intracardiac tumor or thrombus.

QUANTIFICATION OF VENTRICULAR PERFORMANCE

Echocardiography provides an excellent method for quantification of ventricular function. Linear measurements such as wall thickness, internal chamber dimension, and the derived parameters such as fractional shortening traditionally have been obtained from M-mode echocardiography. Normal values for adults and children are well established (Table 7–2).[7-11] Global ventricular function and cardiac volumes can be measured with a variety of algorithms using two-dimensional echocardiography. The most commonly employed method for quantitation of ventricular volume is Simpson's rule (Fig. 11–22). Once the chamber volumes have been determined, ejection fraction can be calculated. Calculation of ejection fraction represents only a small aspect of quantification of ventricular performance. Determination of left ventricular

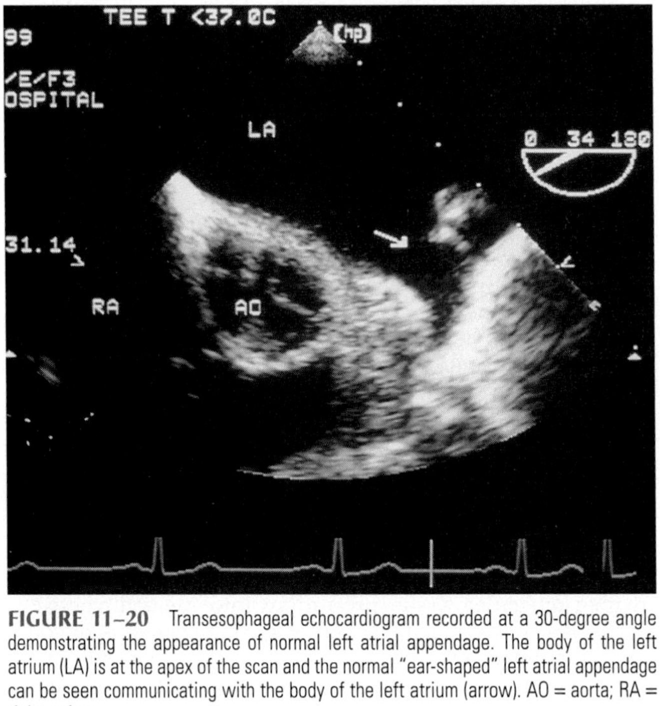

FIGURE 11–20 Transesophageal echocardiogram recorded at a 30-degree angle demonstrating the appearance of normal left atrial appendage. The body of the left atrium (LA) is at the apex of the scan and the normal "ear-shaped" left atrial appendage can be seen communicating with the body of the left atrium (arrow). AO = aorta; RA = right atrium.

TABLE 11–2 Normal Values of M-Mode Echocardiographic Measurements in Adults

	Range	Mean	No. of Subjects
Age (yrs)	13-54	26	134
Body surface area (M^2)	1.45-2.22	1.8	130
RVD—flat (cm)	0.7-2.3	1.5	84
RVD—left lateral (cm)	0.9-2.6	1.7	83
LVID—flat (cm)	3.7-5.6	4.7	82
LVID—left lateral (cm)	3.5-5.7	4.7	81
Posterior LV wall thickness (cm)	0.6-1.1	0.9	137
Posterior LV wall amplitude (cm)	0.9-1.4	1.2	48
IVS wall thickness (cm)	0.6-1.1	0.9	137
Mid IVS amplitude (cm)	0.3-0.8	0.5	10
Apical IVS amplitude (cm)	0.5-1.2	0.7	38
Left atrial dimension (cm)	1.9-4.0	2.9	133
Aortic root dimension (cm)	2.0-3.7	2.7	121
Aortic cusps' separation (cm)	1.5-2.6	2.9	93
Fractional shortening* (%)	34-44	36	20
Rate of circumferential shortening (Vcf)† or normalized shortening velocity (circ/sec)	1.02-1.94	1.3	38

d = end diastole; IVS = interventricular septum; LV = left ventricle; LVID = left ventricular internal dimension; RVD = right ventricular dimension; s = end systole.
*(LVIDd – LVIDs) ÷ LVIDd
†(LVIDd – LVIDs) ÷ (LVIDd × Ejection time)

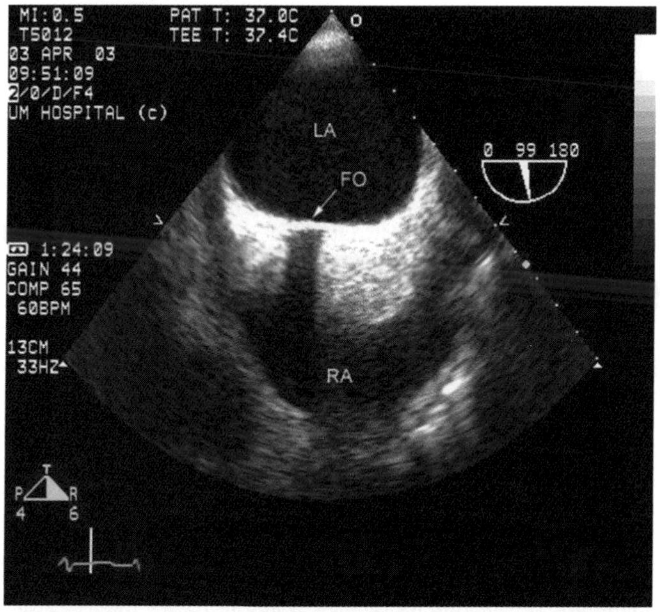

FIGURE 11–21 Transesophageal echocardiogram in a longitudinal view recorded in a patient with marked lipomatous atrial hypertrophy. Note the two large masses bulging off the atrial septum into the cavity of the right atrium, which represent lipomatous deposits. The foramen ovale (FO) is spared in the infiltrative process. LA = left atrium; RA = right atrium.

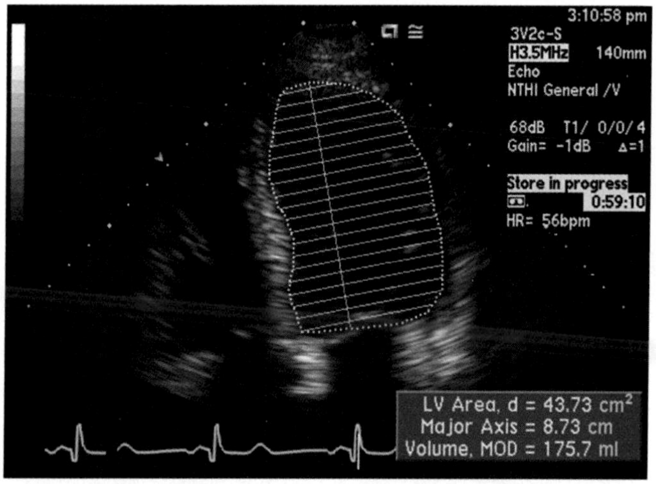

FIGURE 11–22 Apical four-chamber view from which left ventricular volume has been calculated using Simpson's rule. The endocardium has been traced and automatically subdivided into a series of discs. The volume of each of the discs is then calculated as disc area (πr^2) multiplied by the height of each disc. The volume of each separate disc is then summed to provide the volume of the ventricle (175.7 ml in this example).

volume requires manual tracings of the endocardial border in diastole and systole. Instrumentation exists that can automatically determine the endocardial border and calculate volumes and ejection fraction (Fig. 11-23).[12] Application of this technology requires high-quality images with a favorable signal-to-noise ratio. These automatically determined ventricular volumes can be combined with arterial pressure measurements to create pressure-volume loops for more sophisticated evaluation of ventricular performance.[13]

Left ventricular mass can be measured by several different methods.[14,15] One of the earliest was the "cube" method, which used M-mode septal, posterior wall, and left ventricular internal dimensions and assumed normal ventricular geometry. More recently, several two-dimensional methods have been shown to provide enhanced accuracy, especially in abnormally shaped ventricles.[15]

Normal wall motion consists of simultaneous myocardial thickening and inward motion of the endocardium toward the center of the chamber. In adults, the most common cause of a regional wall motion abnormality is myocardial ischemia or infarction. The extent of a wall motion abnormality can be measured in several different ways. Echocardiography is a tomographic technique that visualizes all of the cardiac walls. Traditionally, for quantitative purposes, the left ventricle is divided into 16 segments (Fig. 11-24). More recently, in an effort to provide better concordance with other imaging techniques, a 17-segment model has been proposed in which the true apex is considered the 17th segment.[16] Each segment can be attributed to one of the three major epicardial coronary arteries. There is substantial overlap in the posterior segments and inferior and lateral apical segments. For each of these segments, a wall motion score can be assigned (Fig. 11-25). This is a unitless hierarchical number in which 1 represents normal motion; 2, hypokinesis; 3, akinesis; and 4, dyskinesis. Each wall is then assigned a score, and the average score for the visualized segments is calculated. This number is directly proportional to the extent and severity of wall motion abnormalities.[17] There are several variations on a wall motion score, including addition of scores for aneurysm, mild hypokinesis, and hyperkinesis. The wall motion score can be calculated for all segments of the left ventricle or separately for anterior and posterior segments, representing the left anterior descending, right, and circumflex coronary artery territories. An M-mode interrogation line can be used to quantify endocardial excursion and myocardial thickening in any targeted segment (Fig. 11-26).

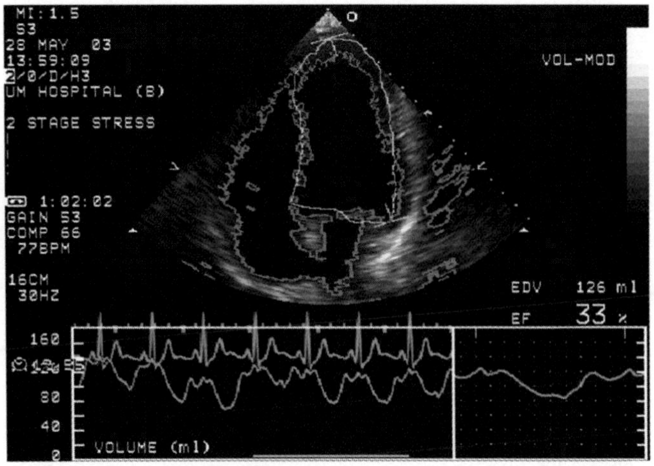

FIGURE 11–23 Apical four-chamber image in which an algorithm for automatic border detection has been used to determine instantaneous left ventricular volume. The white line outlining the endocardial border has been automatically drawn by the ultrasound machine. A graphic output of instantaneous ventricular volume (end diastolic volume = 126 ml) and ejection fraction (33%) is presented below the echocardiographic image.

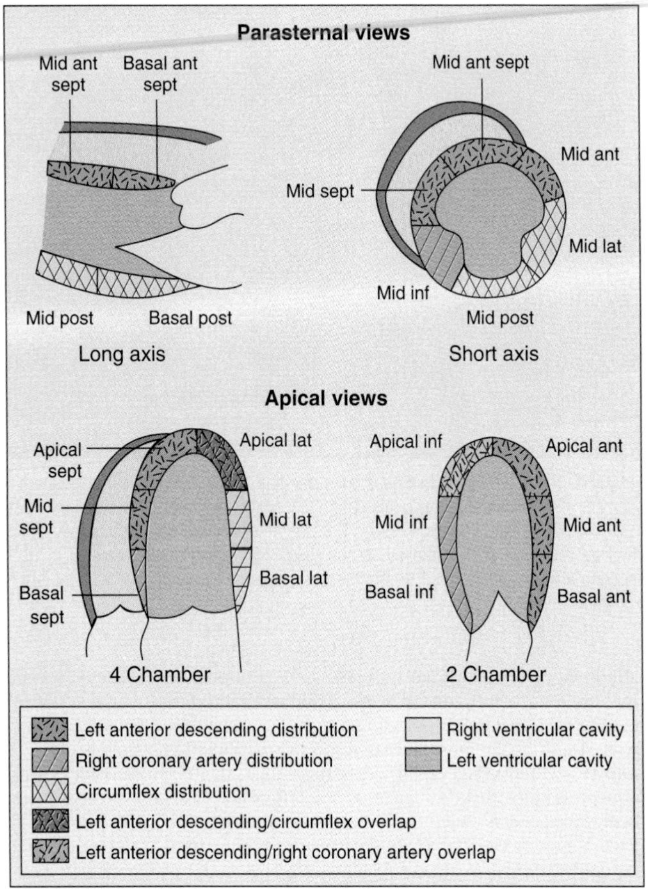

FIGURE 11–24 Schematic representation of a 16-segment model for segmenting the left ventricle. Each segment has been assigned to one of the three major coronary arteries with areas of overlap in the apex and posterior walls noted as well. ant = anterior; inf = inferior; lat = lateral; post = posterior; sept = septum.

There are several more complex methods for quantification of left ventricular function. Most rely on tracing the endocardial border in diastole and systole in either a short-axis or an apical view. Radians are then constructed from the center of mass, and either changes in radian length or changes in area subtended by an arc are then quantified.

Variants of Normal Wall Motion Patterns

ABNORMALITIES OF SEPTAL MOTION. The interventricular septum is a shared wall between the right and left ventricles, and thus its motion can be affected by processes in either ventricle. Myocardial ischemia and infarction cause a fairly characteristic absence of systolic thickening and dyskinesis of the septum. There are multiple nonischemic causes for septal wall motion abnormalities as well.

CONDUCTION DISTURBANCES. Both left bundle branch block and Wolff-Parkinson-White syndrome, with a septal pathway, can result in abnormalities of septal motion. Left bundle branch block characteristically causes an early systolic downward motion followed by relaxation of the ventricular septum and a secondary downward contraction. This is best appreciated with M-mode echocardiography. This phenomenon is most common in the proximal anterior septum and is less prominent in the distal septum. A similar pattern is seen in patients with ventricular pacing; however, the maximum location of abnormal motion is highly variable, depending on the location of the pacemaker lead.

Wolff-Parkinson-White syndrome results in ventricular preexcitation in a localized area of the left or right ventricle. The preexcited area contracts slightly earlier than the remainder of the heart and can be seen in the ventricular septal, posterior or lateral walls. The abnormality associated with Wolff-Parkinson-White syndrome is less dramatic than that seen with left bundle branch block. Although newer two-dimensional scanning instruments have temporal resolution sufficient to detect an abnormality of wall motion due to a conduction disturbance, the high temporal resolution of M-mode echocardiography may be necessary for precise identification of the wall motion abnormalities.

CONSTRICTIVE PERICARDITIS. Constrictive pericarditis interferes with the normal sequence of right and left ventricular filling and results in subtle septal wall motion abnormalities. This typically causes early downward motion of the septum, followed by paradoxical motion. Multiple patterns of septal motion abnormalities have been noted in constrictive pericarditis. As with electrical conduction disturbances, these may be best identified with M-mode echocardiography.

VENTRICULAR OVERLOAD. Either a volume or a pressure overload of the right ventricle results in a ventricular septal motion abnormality. In each instance, the right ventricle is dilated. In a pure volume overload, there is diastolic flattening of the ventricular septum so that the left ventricular geometry in diastole assumes a D shape rather than circular geometry. Because this is a low-pressure phenomenon, the left ventricle becomes circular in early systole before the onset of ventricular ejection (Fig. 11–27). A right ventricular pressure overload results in flattening of the septum not only in diastole but also in systole. The degree of flattening is directly proportional to the elevation in right ventricular systolic pressure. Frank reversal of septal curvature is seen in individuals with systemic level right-sided heart pressures.

A final septal motion abnormality that is commonly encountered is the "postoperative septum." This abnormality is characterized by paradoxical anterior motion of the septum in systole, with preserved myocardial thickening. Often posterior wall excursion appears exaggerated. This phenomenon may be seen in any form of cardiac surgery in which the pericardium has been opened. It often resolves 3 to 5 years after surgery.

Principles of the Doppler Examination

NORMAL FLOW PATTERNS. All four cardiac valves can be interrogated using either pulsed, continuous wave, or

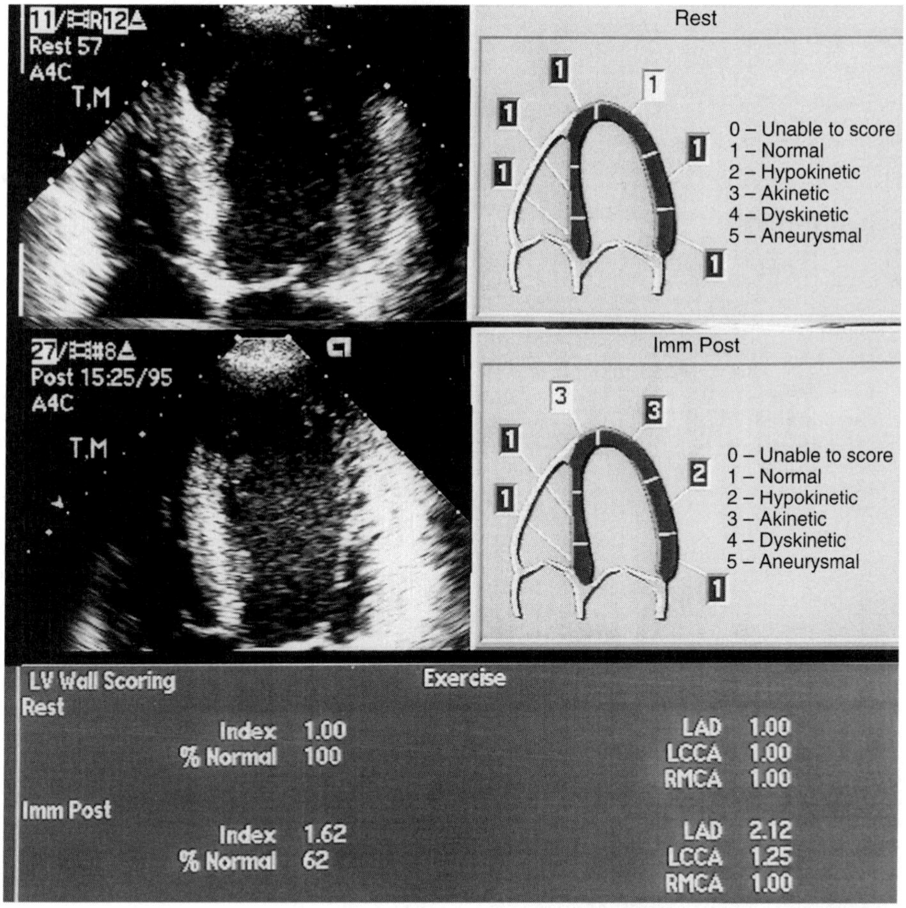

FIGURE 11–25 Wall motion score algorithm. For each of the predefined segments (typically 16), a score of 1 to 4 is assigned, with 1 representing normal motion and 4 representing dyskinetic motion. The wall motion score index equals the sum of these scores divided by the number of scored segments. Because each of the wall segments can be attributed to one of the coronary artery territories (see Fig. 11–24), wall motion scores can be calculated for the left anterior descending (LAD), left circumflex (LCCA), and right (RMCA) coronary arteries. The representative scores are as noted in the right-hand schematics, and both the global and regional wall motion scores at rest and with stress are noted in the bottom graphic.

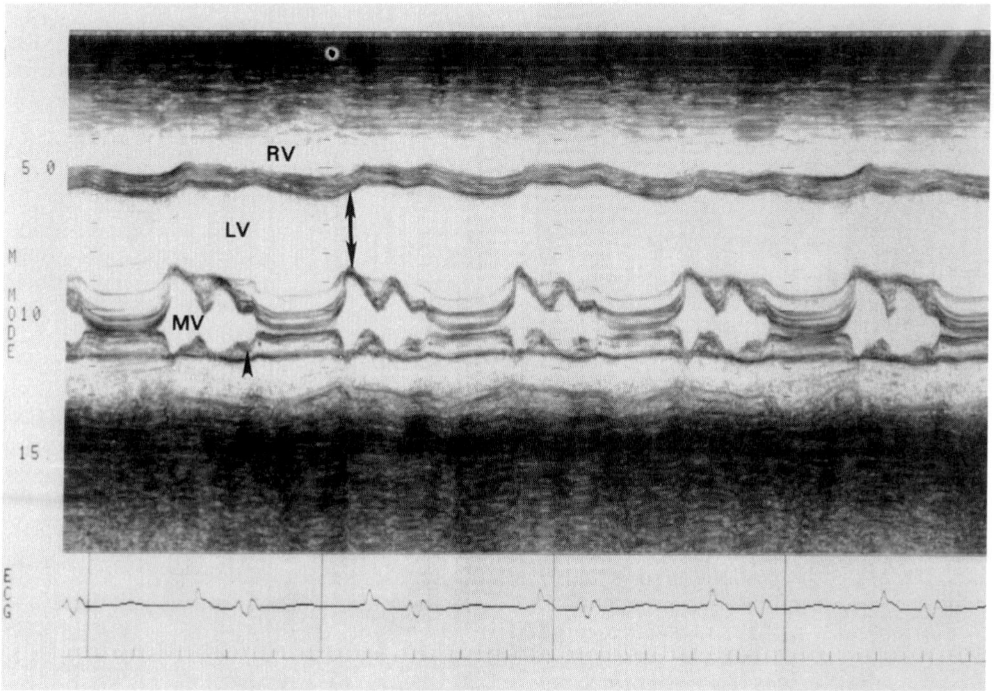

FIGURE 11–26 M-mode echocardiogram recorded in a patient with severe left ventricular systolic dysfunction. Note the dilated left ventricle (LV) and a decreased excursion of the septum and posterior wall compared with the normal example seen in Figure 11–9. There is additional evidence of left ventricular systolic dysfunction in that the mitral valve E point septal separation is increased (double-headed arrow). Evidence of elevated end-diastolic pressure is noted in the "B bump" (arrowhead), which delays final closure of the mitral valve (MV). RV = right ventricle.

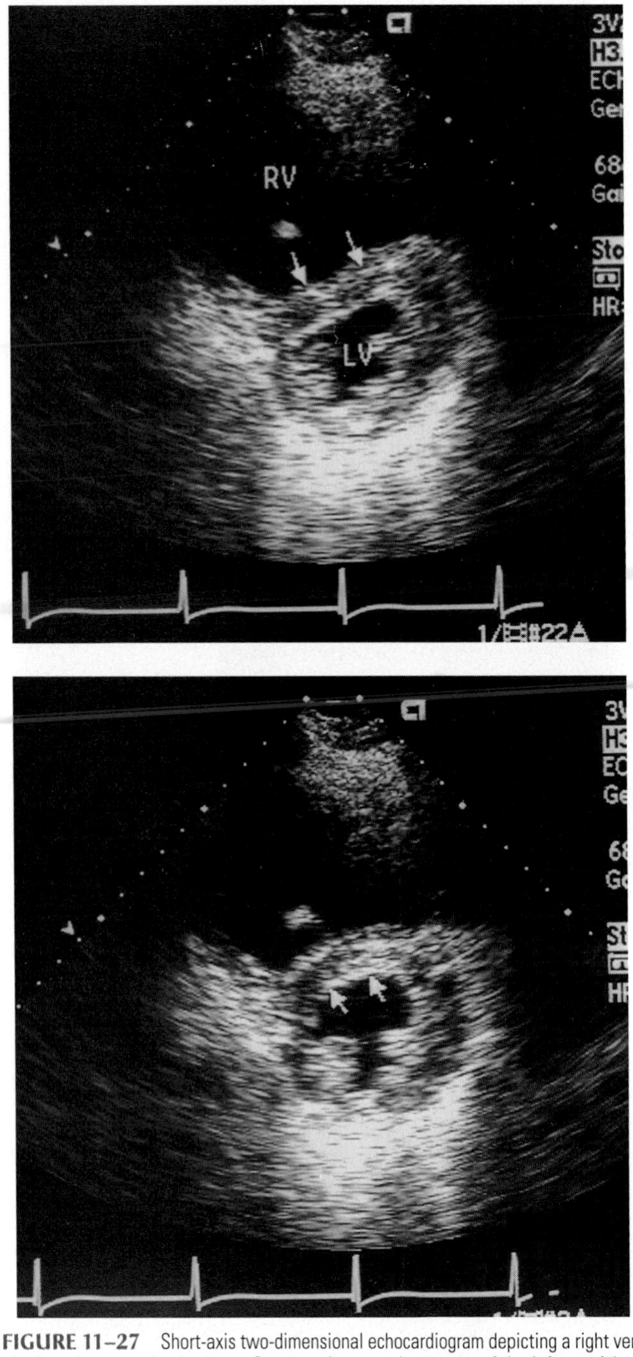

FIGURE 11–27 Short-axis two-dimensional echocardiogram depicting a right ventricular volume overload pattern. Compare the normal geometry of the left ventricle in a short-axis view (see Fig. 11–14) to that noted here. In the right ventricular volume overload pattern, there is dilation of the right ventricle (RV) and flattening of the ventricular septum (downward pointing arrows) so that in diastole the ventricle takes on a D-shaped configuration rather than circular geometry. With systole, there is restitution of normal circular geometry (upward arrows). LV = left ventricle.

color flow Doppler. Substantial physiological data can be derived from the recorded signals. Figure 11–28 is a representation of normal Doppler flow patterns across the four cardiac valves. Highly sensitive Doppler instrumentation frequently picks up mild amounts of physiological regurgitation, which is more common for the tricuspid and pulmonic than for the aortic and mitral valves. In the normal heart under physiological circumstances, the maximum velocity typically encountered is less than 1.5 m/sec. Pulmonary vein and hepatic vein flows can also be recorded in the majority of patients (Fig. 11–29).

Color flow Doppler provides the ability to track mitral and tricuspid inflow patterns and left and right ventricular outflow as well as to detect abnormal flow. Normal mitral inflow appears as a red encoded signal moving from the mitral orifice along the lateral wall to the left ventricular apex, where it reverses course and appears as a blue encoded signal along the septum. The flow profile accelerates with atrial systole. With systole, the organized flow in the left ventricular outflow tract appears as a series of color shifts as the accelerating flow exceeds the relatively low Nyquist limit of color Doppler imaging. Pathological flow will be detected either as turbulence due to a restricted orifice, such as flow through a stenotic valve, or as a regurgitant flow signal in a downstream chamber. The above scheme represents traditional color flow imaging algorithms. Many alternative color schemes and variance maps can be employed as well. It should be emphasized that the visualized jet area is heavily dependent on Doppler gain settings. At higher heart rates, the relatively low frame rate of color flow imaging also compromises accuracy. Substantial experience and attention to technical detail are essential to provide accurate clinical information from color flow Doppler imaging.

CALCULATION OF PRESSURE GRADIENTS. By interrogating the spectral Doppler profile, valuable physiological information can be derived. Once the velocity of the target has been determined, this information can be used to determine pressure gradients across an orifice using the Bernoulli equation. The Bernoulli equation contains many elements, including convective acceleration and viscous friction (Fig. 11–30). Of note, convective acceleration and viscous friction are relatively weak contributors in most biological systems and can be effectively ignored. The Bernoulli equation in its simplest form states that ΔP (the pressure gradient across a restrictive orifice) is $4V^2$, where V is the peak instantaneous velocity of flow through the restrictive orifice. In reality, the equation incorporates not only the peak instantaneous velocity at the restrictive orifice but also the velocity noted in the acceleration zone, V_1. For most clinically relevant conditions such as severe aortic stenosis, V_2 is substantially greater than V_1 and hence V_1 can effectively be ignored. There are several instances in which the V_1 velocity must be included. These include the obvious case of a serial obstruction, as well as situations in which V_1 is relatively large compared with V_2, such as in milder degrees of aortic stenosis and aortic stenosis combined with aortic insufficiency.

DOPPLER CALCULATION OF RIGHT VENTRICULAR SYSTOLIC PRESSURE. Obviously, application of the Bernoulli equation allows calculation of gradients across stenotic valves, but likewise it can be used to calculate a gradient between any high-pressure and low-pressure chambers. A commonly used application of the Bernoulli equation is the determination of the right ventricular systolic pressure.[18-20] Tricuspid regurgitation is very common in many disease states. By determining the peak velocity of a tricuspid regurgitation jet, one can then calculate the right ventricular–to–right atrial pressure gradient (Fig. 11–31). A key component of this is estimation of right atrial pressure. Approaches to this determination include assigning an empirical constant, assigning a floating constant of 5, 10, or 15 mm Hg (depending on the size of the right atrium, severity of regurgitation, and appearance of the inferior vena cava), or assigning a floating constant of 10 percent of the peak gradient. Each of these methods appears to result in satisfactory estimation of intercardiac pressure.

CALCULATION OF FLOW. Because the Doppler spectral profile provides a highly accurate measure of the velocity of the moving blood, this value, when combined with a measured or calculated area, can provide data regarding actual volumetric flow (Figs. 11-32 and 11-33). Multiplying the cross-sectional area of the flow times the velocity time integral

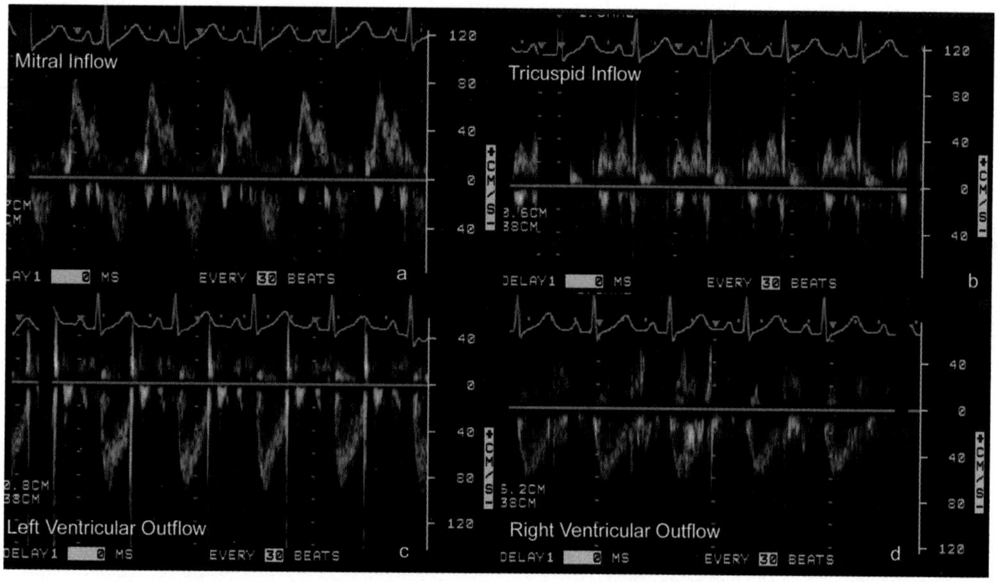

FIGURE 11–28 Composite pulsed Doppler tracings of normal flow in all four cardiac valves. Note the marked similarity between the aortic and pulmonary flow velocities, with a lower velocity in the pulmonary flow due to its larger diameter. Similarly, there is a lower velocity of tricuspid flow, but a similar relationship of early (e-wave) and atrial related (a-wave) flow when compared to mitral inflow.

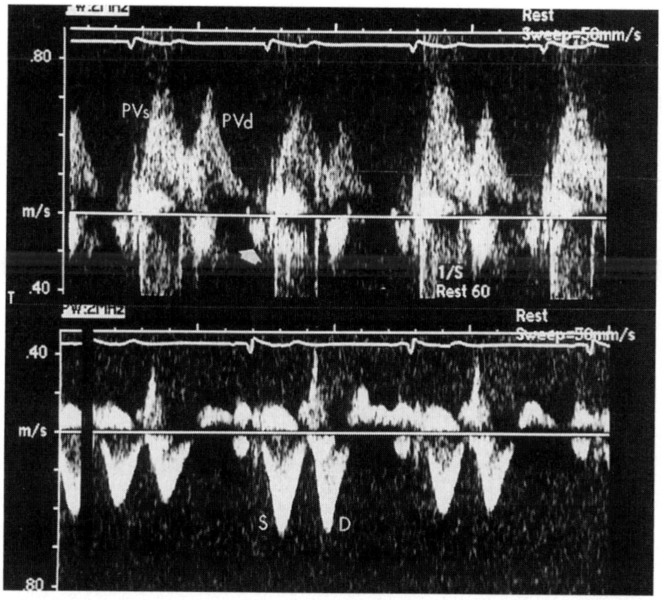

FIGURE 11–29 Normal pulmonary **(upper panel)** and hepatic **(lower panel)** vein flows. Nearly continuous, multiphasic flow is seen in the normal pulmonary and hepatic veins. Note that there is higher velocity of pulmonary vein inflow during ventricular systole then during diastole.

yields the actual volume of flow during that pulse interval. If the left ventricular outflow tract is interrogated, this value then represents the forward stroke volume of the left ventricle. This, in turn, can be used to calculate cardiac output.[21] The greatest source of error in this calculation is often determination of the cross-sectional area of the left ventricular outflow tract, which may not assume circular geometry. Additionally, because of the formula for determining area ($A = \pi r^2$), any error in measuring the diameter of the flow channel is squared. Thus, determination of stroke volume and cardiac output may have greater clinical value in following serial trends than in precise determination of volumetric flow. For clinical purposes, however, this remains a valuable technique. Similar calculations of flow volume can be performed for the pulmonic and mitral valves as well.

An expansion of volume flow calculation involves the "continuity equation" (Fig. 11–34).[22] The underlying principle of the continuity equation is that the volume of flow entering a channel must equal the volume of flow exiting that channel. If the cross-sectional area is equal at the entrance and exit points, then flow velocity will likewise be equal at those two points. If, however, the cross-sectional area decreases at the downstream site, then, of necessity, velocity must increase to maintain the same volumetric flow. The continuity equation can be applied for determination of aortic valve area in aortic stenosis and less often for mitral valve area or other conditions.

Color Doppler flow imaging can be used to determine volumetric flow as well. Flow converging on a relatively restrictive area will accelerate as it nears the downstream exit. Because of the relatively low Nyquist limit of color flow Doppler imaging, this results in a series of aliasing lines where the color flow signal will alternately change from blue to red. By purposely utilizing relatively low Nyquist limits, the echocardiographer can determine the distance from the actual flow exit point to one of the aliasing lines. Because the velocity at which flow aliases is known, the velocity of flow at that point is likewise known. If one assumes that flow converges at equal velocities symmetrically toward an orifice, then by applying the geometric formula for a hemisphere, one can determine the surface area of flow in motion at any of the aliasing points that represents an identifiable velocity (Fig. 11–35). From this, one can then calculate the actual volume of flow from this proximal isovelocity surface area as velocity times surface area.[23,24] In general terms, for any given Nyquist limit, the larger the proximal isovelocity surface area, the greater the amount of flow involved. Therefore, quantitation of proximal isovelocity surface area allows an additional clue as to the volume of regurgitant flow. Proximal isovelocity surface area calculations can be performed for any flow that accelerates toward a relatively restrictive orifice, including mitral regurgitation, aortic insufficiency, and shunt lesions. The major limitation of the use of proximal isovelocity surface area is the assumption that flow moves in a hemispherical manner. This assumption is true only for flow converging on a relatively flat surface. If flow is channeled through a funnel, corrections must be made for a surface area less than a full hemisphere.[25]

Close inspection of a regurgitant jet between either ventricle and its corresponding atrium can also provide clues to ventricular performance. In early systole, ventricular pressure exceeds atrial pressure by a wide margin and thus ejection of blood into the downstream atrium is at low resistance, resulting in a high dP/dt that corresponds to the forcefulness of ventricular contraction.[26] If myocardial failure occurs, the ability of the ventricle to eject forcefully is compromised and dP/dt decreases. This is also noted in spectral Doppler echocardiography of continuous-wave ejection parameters by a decrease in the ejection velocity slope (Fig. 11–36). Actual dP/dt can be calculated by determining the time in milliseconds between a regurgitant velocity of 1 and 3 m/sec. This corresponds to a pressure difference of 32 mm Hg. If the time over which this pressure difference is obtained is measured, a noninvasive dP/dt can be calculated.

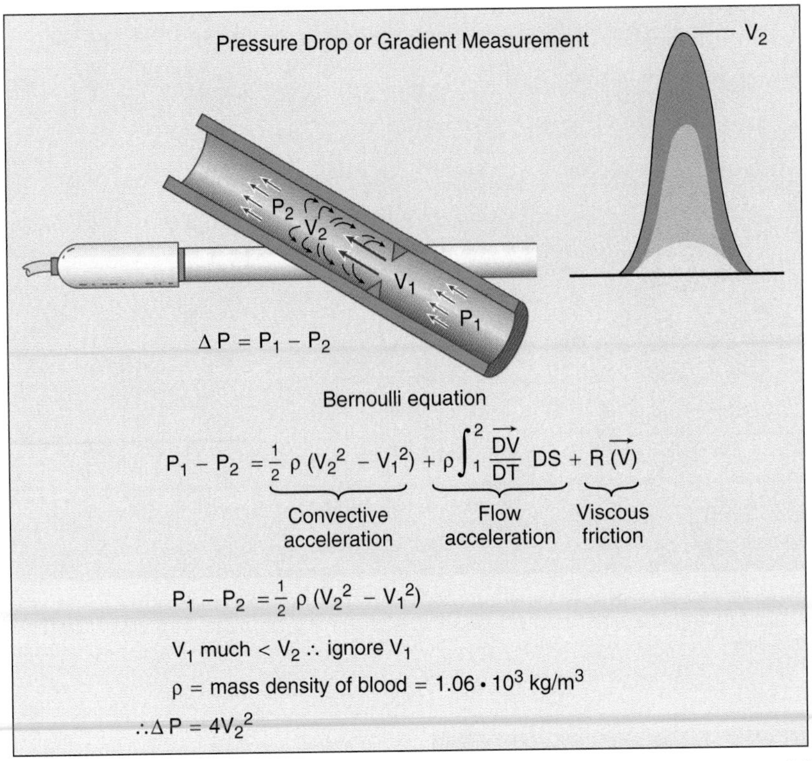

FIGURE 11–30 The Bernoulli equation can be used to calculate a pressure gradient across any restrictive orifice. The components of the Bernoulli equation are convective acceleration, flow acceleration, and viscous friction. The full equation can be modified to $P_1 - P_2 = (V_2^2 - V_1^2) \times 4$ and further simplified in the absence of a significant V_1 velocity to $\Delta P = 4V^2$. P_1 = pressure proximal to an obstruction; P_2 = pressure distal to an obstruction; V_1 = velocity proximal to an obstruction; V_2 = Doppler velocity distal to an obstruction. (From Feigenbaum H: Echocardiography. 4th ed. Malvern, PA, Lea & Febiger, 1986.)

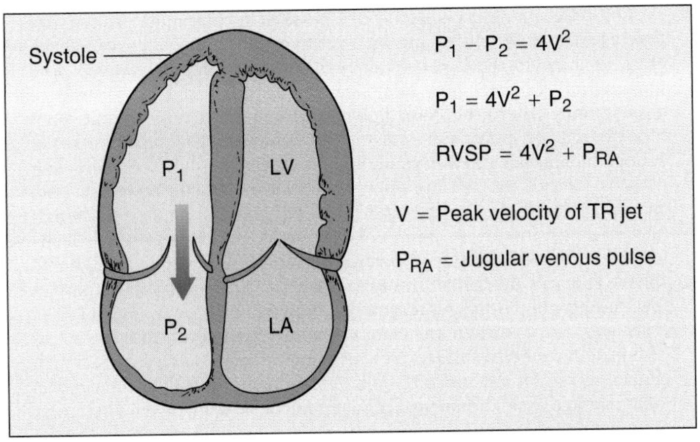

FIGURE 11–31 Measurement of right ventricular systolic pressure (RVSP) using the tricuspid regurgitation jet. The gradient between the right ventricle and right atrium ($P_1 - P_2$) can be calculated from the velocity of the tricuspid regurgitation jet using the modified Bernoulli equation ($\Delta P = 4V^2$). Actual right ventricular systolic pressure is then calculated as the sum of the pressure gradient between the two chambers and an assumed right atrial pressure (P_{RA}). Right atrial pressure can be estimated from examination of the jugular veins, by evaluation of the inferior vena cava for collapse during inspiration, or by using an empirical or floating constant (see text for further details). LA = left atrium; LV = left ventricle. (From Feigenbaum H: Echocardiography. 5th ed. Malvern, PA, Lea & Febiger, 1994.)

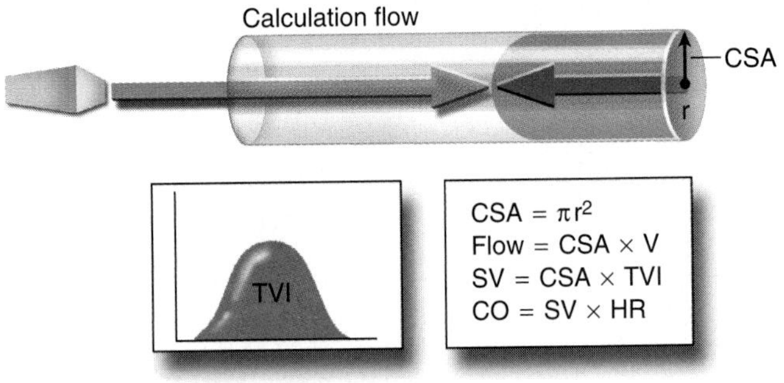

FIGURE 11–32 Schematic demonstration of the method for determining flow using a combination of Doppler and two-dimensional echocardiography. Flow can be calculated as the product of the cross-sectional area of the chamber or vessel through which flow is occurring (CSA) and the velocity of flow. The time-velocity integral (TVI) is used to calculate pulsatile flow. Cross-sectional areas are calculated as noted in the schematic, and cardiac output (CO) can then be calculated as the product of stroke volume (SV) and heart rate (HR).

The continuous-wave spectral profile can also provide clues as to the nature of obstruction in many disease states. The spectral profile provides high temporal resolution for determining the timing of pressure gradients. Thus, the contour of the spectral profile provides clues as to whether an obstruction is fixed or develops over time, in which case the peak gradient will occur late rather than early. The latter is classic for dynamic obstruction in cases of hypertrophic cardiomyopathy. Close examination of a regurgitant profile can also reveal evidence that atrial pressure has become acutely elevated toward the end of ejection when velocities taper off rapidly in the latter half of systole.

Much attention has been paid to mitral valve inflow patterns as they relate to diastolic function of the left ventricle.[27-30] This assessment must be done in patients who are in sinus rhythm, during which there are discrete E and A wave velocities of the mitral valve inflow. In normal individuals, early velocities exceed later velocities and the E to A ratio is typically greater than 1.2. With impaired relaxation of the left ventricle, this ratio declines and the rate of decay of the E wave velocity likewise decreases. Figure 11–37 schematizes several mitral valve Doppler inflow patterns. There are a number of other influences on the E to A ratio, including age and heart rate. With a pathological increase in left ventricular stiffness accompanied by excess volume, there is an augmentation of the normal E to A ratio. This increased E to A ratio is classic for a restrictive cardiomyopathy and constrictive pericarditis but is also typically seen in patients with end-stage heart disease of virtually any type who have markedly elevated diastolic pressures. It is imperative to incorporate the anatomical and other Doppler information into an assessment of mitral valve inflow patterns in an effort to provide clinically relevant information.

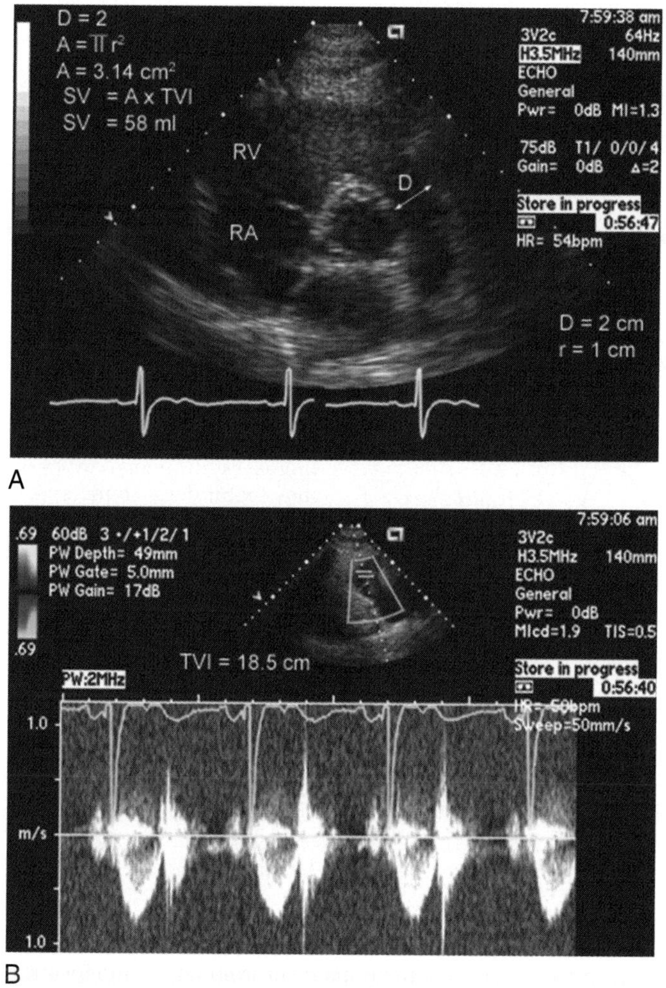

FIGURE 11–33 Demonstration of the calculation of stroke volume from a two-dimensional echocardiogram and pulsed wave Doppler in the right ventricular outflow tract. **A,** Recorded at the level of the aortic valve and right ventricular outflow tract, from which a proximal pulmonary artery diameter (D) of 2 cm can be measured. **B,** Pulsed wave Doppler at the same, from which a time velocity integral (TVI) of 18.5 cm can be determined. The calculations for determination of stroke volume are superimposed on the upper panel and result in a calculated stroke volume of 58 ml. RA = right atrium; RV = right ventricle.

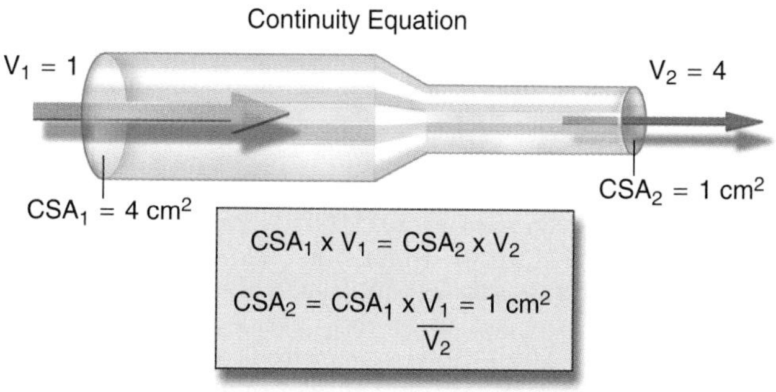

FIGURE 11–34 Schematic demonstration of the continuity equation. The continuity equation states that flow through a structure is equal at both the entrance and exit points. If there is a change in flow area, it must be accompanied by a directionally appropriate and proportionate change in velocity. In the example schematized, flow enters a chamber with a cross-sectional area (CSA_1) of 4 cm^2 and a velocity of 1, giving a flow of 4 ml. Downstream flow must also be 4 ml, but across the exiting cross-sectional area (CSA_2) has been reduced to 1 cm^2. Of necessity, the downstream velocity then must increase to 4. In clinical practice, the entrance cross-sectional area and entrance velocity are typically known, as is the exit velocity and the equation is solved for the exit cross-sectional area, as noted in the schematic.

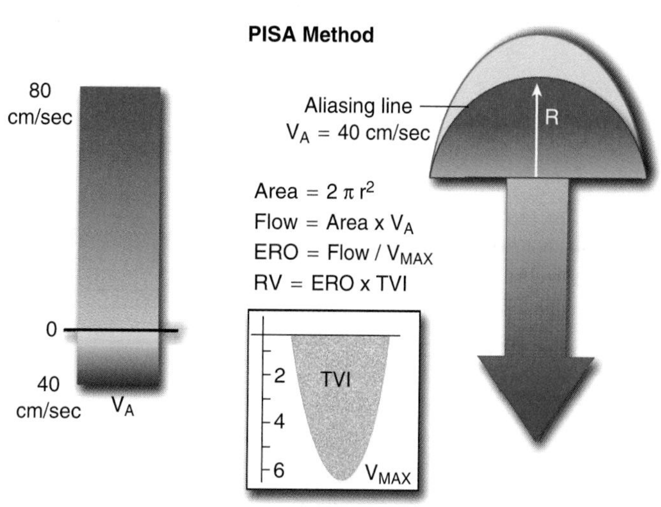

FIGURE 11–35 Demonstration of the proximal isovelocity surface area (PISA) method for determining flow. The figure on the **right** is a schematized color flow image of the acceleration of flow toward a regurgitant orifice in a patient with mitral regurgitation. The boundary between color shifts represents an aliasing line at which velocity has exceeded the Nyquist limit (V_A), which is displayed on the color bar (40 cm/sec). The calculations necessary to determine flow are as noted in the middle panel. For any given aliasing line, a hemisphere of flow is assumed. The surface area of a hemisphere is calculated as $2\pi r^2$. Flow is equal to the product of the surface area times the velocity, which is determined from the Nyquist limit. ERO = effective regurgitant orifice; TVI = time velocity integral.

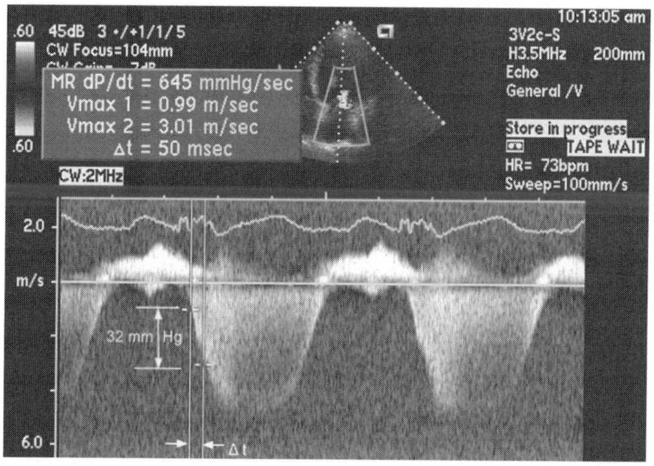

FIGURE 11–36 Use of the mitral regurgitation spectral display to determine positive and negative dP/dt of left ventricular contraction. The spectral mitral regurgitation jet is displayed at high sweep speed to maximize temporal resolution. The time in milliseconds (Δt) required for velocity to increase from 1 to 3 m/sec is then measured. This time is then divided into 32 mm Hg (the pressure difference between 1 and 3 m/sec) to determine dP/dt noninvasively (645 mm Hg/sec in this example).

Doppler can be used to evaluate the inflow patterns of the hepatic and pulmonary veins as well. Both hepatic and pulmonary vein inflow are biphasic with predominant flow in ventricular systole (see Fig. 11-29). Examination of the flow patterns can provide valuable clues in a variety of disease states, including mitral regurgitation, restrictive and constrictive processes, and other diseases that elevate right or left ventricular diastolic pressure.

Additional Imaging Formats and Techniques

Transesophageal Echocardiography

For this technique, the ultrasound transducer has been miniaturized and mounted on the tip of a flexible gastroscope-like instrument. The mechanics of the instrument allow both flexion and lateral motion of the tip to optimize views. Early transesophageal echocardiography (TEE) probes provided

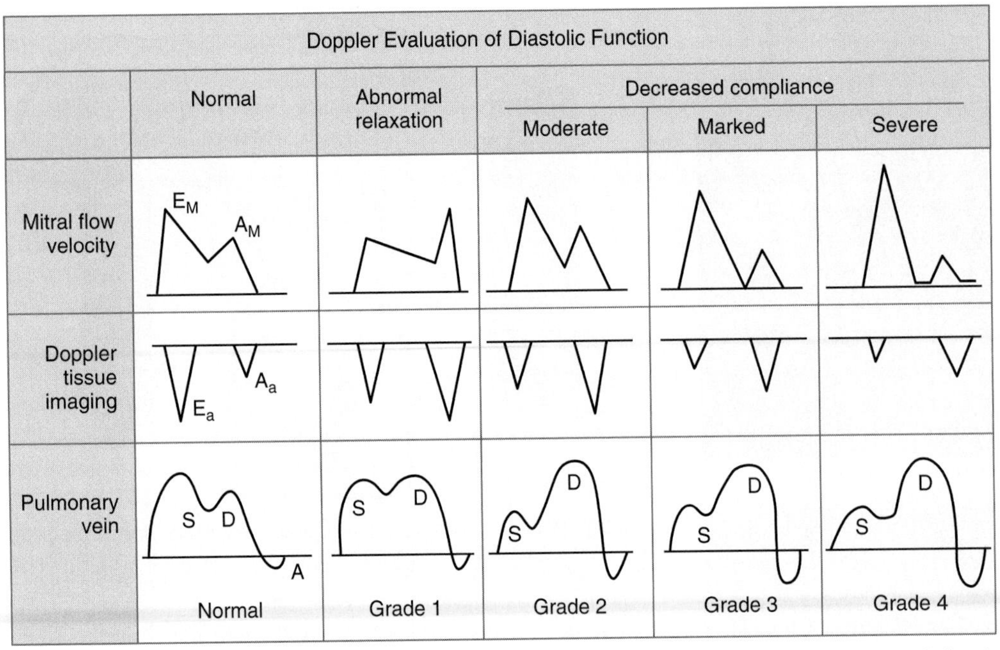

FIGURE 11–37 Schematic representation of mitral inflow, Doppler tissue imaging of the annulus, and pulmonary vein flow in normal and abnormal diastolic states. Normal mitral inflow is biphasic and consists of an early velocity (E_M) and a late flow velocity related to atrial contraction (A_M). Doppler tissue imaging of the annulus results in a similar pattern of early and late (E_A and A_A) annular velocities opposite in direction to the mitral inflow velocity. In patients with normal diastolic function, both E_M and E_A exceed A_M and A_A. In disease-free states, pulmonary vein flow is multiphasic, with roughly equal systolic and diastolic forward flow and a relatively narrow low velocity retrograde pulmonary vein a-wave. With varying degrees of diastolic dysfunction, there are predictable changes in mitral flow velocity, Doppler tissue annular velocities, and pulmonary vein velocities as noted in the schematic.

only a single plane of interrogation, with subsequent probes providing two perpendicularly oriented planes that could be viewed in alternate fashion. Modern TEE probes contain an array of ultrasound crystals at the tip of the probe that allow rotation of the ultrasound scanning plane through 360 degrees.

There are specific indications and contraindications to TEE as well as well-recognized inherent risks. TEE is indicated in patients in whom transthoracic echocardiography (TTE) is either unlikely to provide diagnostic information or has been nondiagnostic. Specific situations in which TEE is of proven incremental yield include detection of aortic dissection, evaluation of the mechanism of mitral regurgitation, evaluation of the left atrial appendage for thrombus prior to cardioversion of atrial fibrillation, and evaluation of patients for source of cardiac emboli. TEE is relatively contraindicated in individuals with significant esophageal pathology.

Transesophageal echocardiography is typically performed under intravenous conscious sedation after application of local anesthesia to the oropharynx. The exact choice of intravenous agents is institutionally dependent but frequently consists of a combination of narcotics and a benzodiazepine agent. Complications associated with TEE include those associated with the agents used for conscious sedation as well as complications related to the mechanical aspects of probe insertion. The latter can involve trauma to any aspect of the teeth, gums, oropharynx, or esophagus. Esophageal complications are most likely to arise in individuals with preexisting esophageal disorders. Trauma to the oropharynx, teeth, and gums is more likely in patients who are uncooperative.

There is a family of standardized views that are obtained during the TEE examination.[31] Most echocardiographers begin by examining the heart from behind the left atrium because this view provides a fairly rapid means for orienting the operator. Figures 11–38 and 11–39 outline views in the horizontal and longitudinal planes that correspond to 0- and 90-degree scanning planes using a multidirectional rotating transducer. Figures 11–40 and 11–41 are transesophageal echocardiograms recorded from several of the transducer positions schematized in Figures 11–38 and 11–39.

Three-Dimensional Echocardiography

Three-dimensional echocardiography remains a technique in evolution for which increases in image processing technology and speed have allowed substantial advancement in the last several years. There are two basic approaches to acquiring a three-dimensional data set. The first involves collection of the entire series of two-dimensional image planes. The location in space of each of these planes is known and registered for subsequent three-dimensional reconstruction. The localization of each plane can be performed by two methods. The first and oldest was by using a transducer positioning device which automatically recorded the precise location and angulation of the transducer from which the location and orientation of each acquired imaging plane could be determined. This resulted in collection of a data set composed of multiple two-dimensional images of known orientation and location that could then be compiled into a three-dimensional data set. Typically, this involved an external device that attached to the transducer for image localization. An advancement on this technique is available using a rotating scan head, as is found in multiplane transesophageal probes. The same technology has been adapted to TTE. With this technique, the imaging plane is rotated through 180 degrees while the transducer is held in a fixed position, thereby providing a 360-degree view around a point of reference. The location and orientation of each imaging plane is automatically known based on the angle of rotation of the transducer. Each individual image is then stored, and the three-dimensional data set can be derived.

The newest method for obtaining a three-dimensional echocardiogram involves transducers with a rectangular, rather than lineal, crystal array.[32-35] This type of transducer intrinsically scans in three dimensions and acquires a three-dimensional volume set, as opposed to creating a three-dimensional volume set from individual two-dimensional imaging planes. Limitations of current technology and processor capacity have limited three-dimensional echocardiography to structural imaging only in most systems. Increasing processor speed and computational capacity as well as transducer capability have allowed three-dimensional color reconstruction as well in select circumstances.

Once the three-dimensional data set is acquired with any of these techniques, there are several ways of displaying the information. These include identifying a desired two-dimensional plane in the three-dimensional data set and displaying it as a two-dimensional echocardiogram. This has

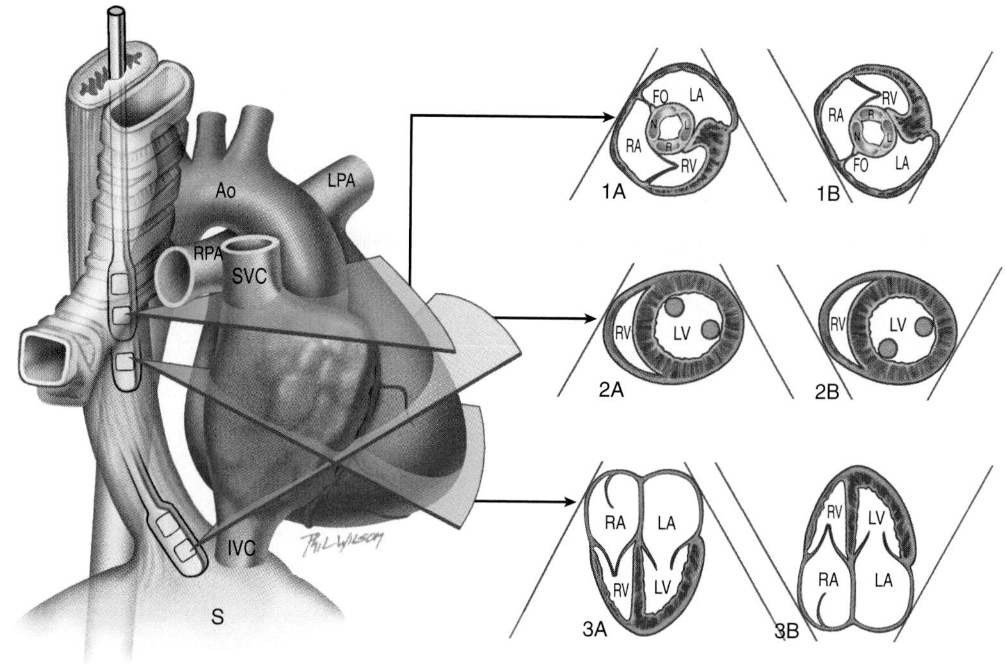

FIGURE 11–38 Schematic demonstrating the transesophageal echocardiographic images that can be obtained in a horizontal plane. Figures **2A** and **2B** are obtained from the transgastric location, **3A** and **3B** from the midesophageal position, and **1A** and **1B** from the upper esophageal position. (Images can be displayed with the apex of the sector either up [A figures] or the apex down [B figures].) Echocardiographic images corresponding to figures 1A, 2A, and 3A are presented in Figure 11–40. Ao = aorta; FO = fossa ovalis; IVC = inferior vena cava; LA = left atrium; LPA = left pulmonary artery; LV = left ventricle; RA; right atrium; RPA = right pulmonary artery; RV = right ventricle; S = stomach; SVC = superior vena cava. (From Feigenbaum H: Echocardiography. 5th ed. Malvern, PA, Lea & Febiger, 1994.)

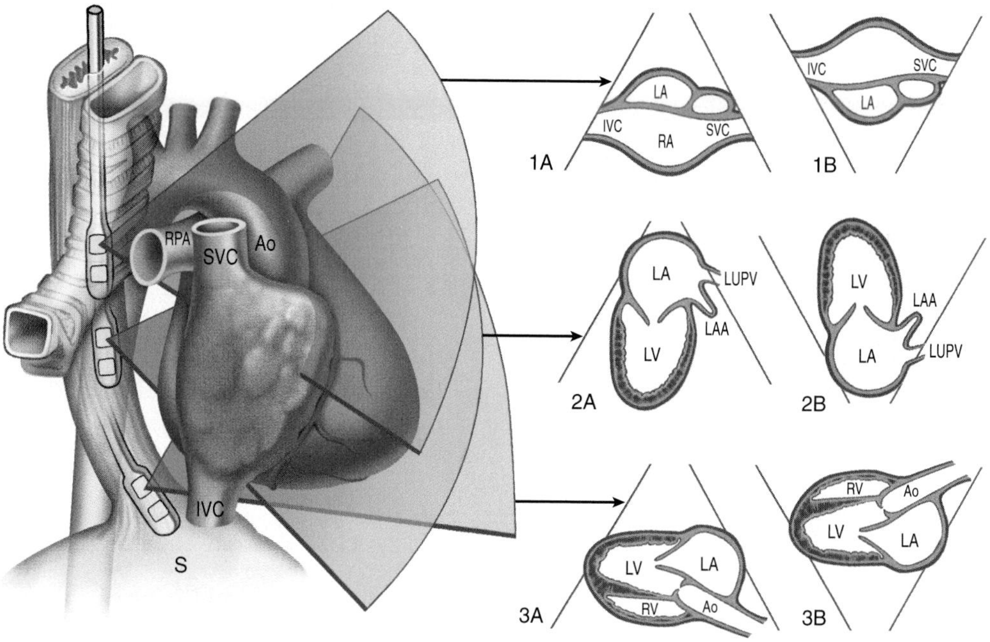

FIGURE 11–39 Transesophageal echocardiographic views obtained in the longitudinal transducer position. The **A** series of figures are recorded with the apex down and the **B** series with the apex up. **3A** and **3B** are recorded in the gastric position, **2A** and **2B** from the midesophagus, and **1A** and **1B** from the upper esophagus. Ao = aorta; IVC = inferior vena cava; LA = left atrium; LAA = left atrial appendage; LUPV = left upper pulmonary vein; LV = left ventricle; RA = right atrium; RPA = right pulmonary artery; RV = right ventricle; S = stomach; SVC = superior vena cava. (From Feigenbaum H: Echocardiography. 5th ed. Malvern, PA, Lea & Febiger, 1994.).

the advantage of allowing the operator to select a nontraditional imaging plane for precise quantitation or for viewing a structure that may lie in an off-axis position (Fig. 11–42). This technique has shown preliminary applicability in stress echocardiography, in which an entire three-dimensional data set can be rapidly acquired and then separate two-dimensional images extracted for subsequent analysis.

The second method for display of a three-dimensional data set is in a "surface-rendered" image in which the multiple two-dimensional planes are blended into a pseudo-three-dimensional image. Obviously, for display either as hard

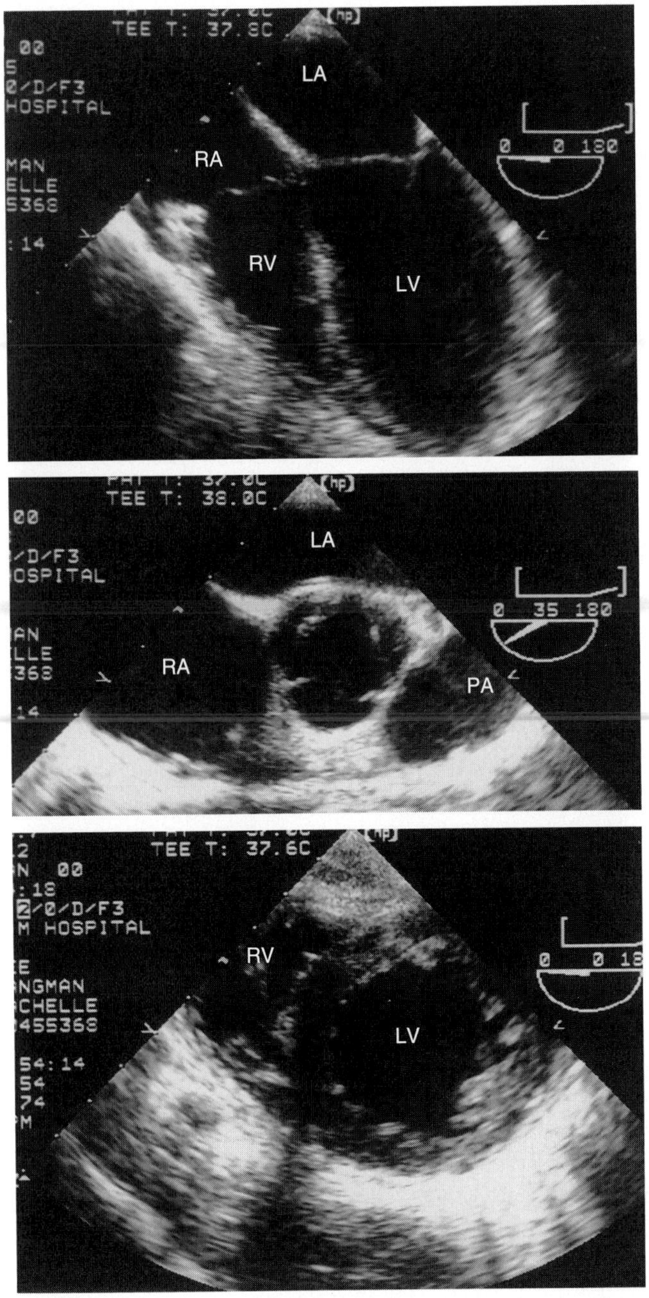

FIGURE 11–40 Transesophageal echocardiograms recorded in a horizontal plane. The **upper** and **lower panels** were recorded in a true 0-degree plane at a high level behind the left atrium and at a midesophageal level, respectively. In the left atrial view, a typical four-chamber view of the heart is obtained in which all four cardiac chambers as well as the mitral and tricuspid valves are clearly visualized. The lower panel was recorded at 0 degrees with the probe inserted deeper in the esophagus. A typical short-axis view of the left ventricle is obtained in which a circular left ventricle and crescent-shaped right ventricle are seen. This view is analogous to a parasternal short-axis view; however, the orientation is inverted such that the inferior wall is at the top of the image and the anterior wall at the bottom. The **middle panel** was recorded at 35 degrees and with pull back of the transducer slightly from the position needed for view in the upper panel. This provides a short-axis view at the base of the heart at which the circular aorta with an open aortic valve is clearly visualized. LA = left atrium, LV = left ventricle; PA = pulmonary artery; RA = right atrium; RV = right ventricle.

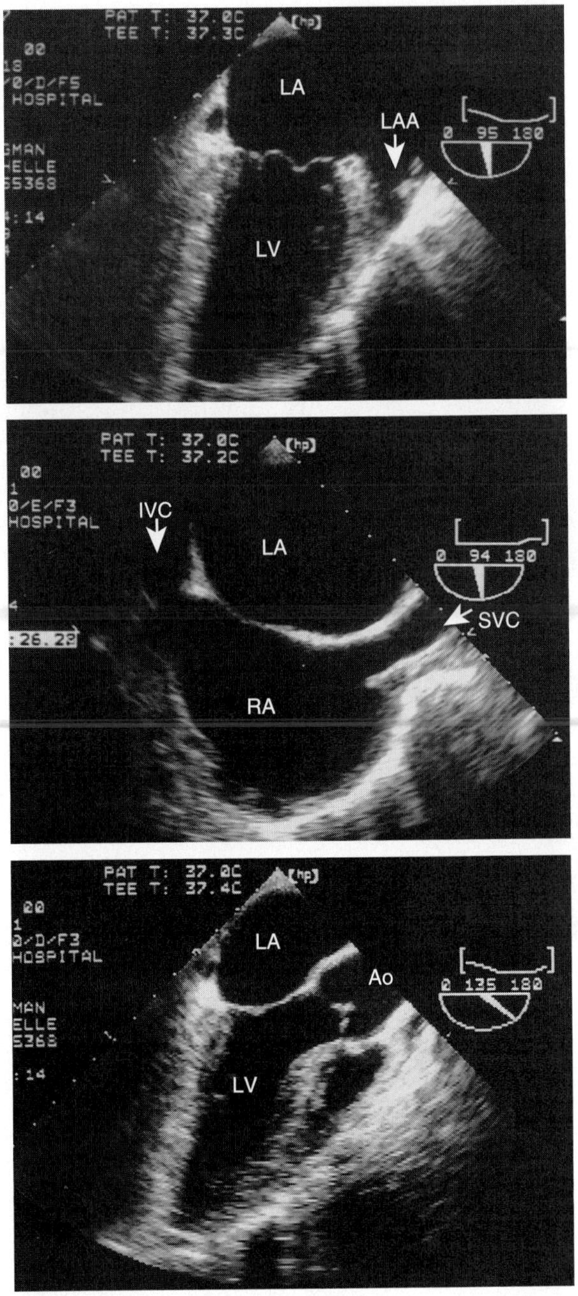

FIGURE 11–41 Transesophageal echocardiographic images recorded in view orthogonal to the horizontal images seen in Figure 11–40. The **top panel** is recorded at the same level in the esophagus as the top panel in Figure 11–40 at a 95-degree angle. In this view, the left atrium (LA) and left ventricle (LV) as well as left atrial appendage (LAA) are clearly visualized. Distinct scallops of the closed mitral valve are also well seen. The **middle panel** is likewise recorded at the same level in the esophagus with rotation of the probe clockwise. In this view, the left atrium and right atrium (RA) as well as inferior vena cava (IVC) and superior vena cava (SVC) are clearly visualized. The **bottom panel** was recorded at 135 degrees. This view provides excellent visualization of the left ventricular outflow tract and proximal aorta (Ao).

copy or on a video screen, no true third dimension is available; however, surface rendering adds depth to the apparent image (Fig. 11–43).

Proven advantages of three-dimensional echocardiography have been its ability to allow precise special characterization of complex lesions such as more complex forms of congenital heart disease,[36] more accurate identification of flail leaflets, and detection of complications of endocarditis. An additional advantage is in the quantitation of ventricular volumes, especially in irregularly shaped ventricles in which the ability to calculate precise volumes clearly exceeds that available from routine two-dimensional scanning.[37]

Intravascular Ultrasonography

Intracardiac ultrasonography is a discipline largely employed by the invasive cardiologist in the catheterization laboratory (see Chap. 18). This ultrasound technique relies on ultraminiaturization of ultrasound transducers that are then incorporated into the tip of intracardiac catheters. The catheters can be as small as 5 French for intracoronary work or as large as 10 or 12 French, which can be used inside cardiac chambers. Typically, either a phased array of crystals is placed circumferentially around the catheter tip or a single crystal, often reflected by a mirror, is mechanically rotated at the tip of a catheter. In either instance, high frequencies of 10 to 40 MHz are used. The smaller catheters can be placed, through a guiding catheter, into epicardial coronary arteries. They provide a high-resolution view of cardiac and intravascular anatomy (Fig. 11–44) and have provided previously unavailable visualization of morphology within the coronary

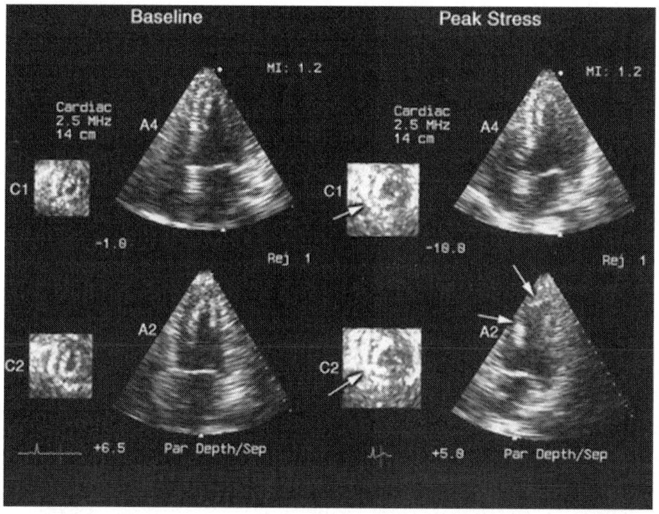

FIGURE 11–42 Apical real-time three-dimensional systolic frames at baseline and at peak stress in a patient with inducible ischemia. Arrows point to the inducible left ventricular wall motion abnormality at peak stress in A2, C1, and C2 images. (From Ahmad et al: Real-time three-dimensional dobutamine stress echocardiography in assessment of ischemia: Comparison with two-dimensional dobutamine stress echocardiography. J Am Coll Cardiol 37:1303, 2001; with permission from the American College of Cardiology Foundation.)

artery and characterization of the intracoronary tissue.[38,39] Calcification and atherosclerosis can be identified and the eccentric or concentric nature of plaque likewise determined. Intracoronary ultrasonography has been instrumental in determining the success of interventions such as stent deployment in coronary artery disease.[40,41] Figure 11–45 depicts intracoronary ultrasound studies demonstrating increasing degrees of severity of atherosclerosis. A closely related technology is the use of miniaturized Doppler wires for monitoring intracoronary flow velocity.[42] Intravascular ultrasonography has also been used in the evaluation of patients with known or suspected aortic dissection, in which case it provides a high-resolution intraluminal view of dissection pathology and yields incremental information with respect to the origin of branch vessels. It has been instrumental in refining the techniques of emergent fenestration in stenting for acute type III dissections.

More recently, a 10 French catheter with a 64-element linear array (oriented along the long access of the catheter) was introduced for intracardiac use (Fig. 11–46).[43-45] This transducer provides steering in both anteroposterior and lateral directions and provides imaging for wide-angle two-dimensional real-time imaging, pulsed and continuous-wave Doppler, and color flow imaging. This device has shown tremendous promise for monitoring of interventional procedures such as atrial septostomy, mitral balloon valve valvotomy, and atrial septal defect closure.

Tissue Characterization

Tissue characterization refers to the detailed evaluation of the entire reflected ultrasound signal in an effort to extract information regarding actual tissue character. Typically, this has relied on evaluation of data in the radiofrequency signal component before processing into a diagnostic, visual image. One of the more promising applications has been in evaluating the cyclic variation in returning ultrasound signal intensity (cyclic variation in backscatter) as a marker of myocardial ischemia.[46,47]

Doppler Tissue Interrogation

The original application of Doppler echocardiography was for determination of the direction and velocity of blood flow.

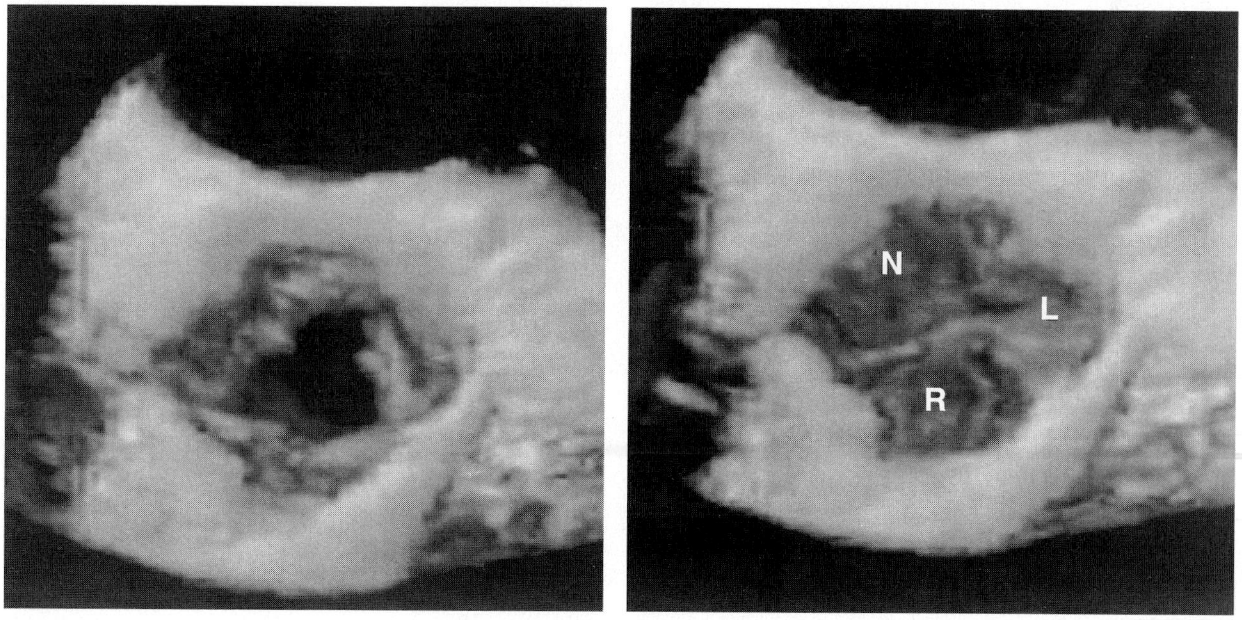

FIGURE 11–43 Surface-rendered three-dimensional echocardiogram showing a normal aortic valve. The panel on the **left** shows the valve in the open position, and a roughly triangular orifice is seen. The image has been captured at mid-opening. At the **right,** the valve is seen in the closed position and the right (R), left (L), and noncoronary (N) cusps are clearly visualized.

As such, original Doppler instrumentation provided filters to exclude highly reflective, slowly moving objects such as myocardium and to exclusively interrogate relatively rapid moving structures with faint reflectivity such as red blood cells. This resulted in the characteristic spectral profiles seen of moving blood in the cardiovascular system. By altering the amplitude and velocity filters, Doppler methodology can be used to determine the direction and velocity of motion of tissue such as left ventricular myocardium. All of the traditional Doppler display methods such as pulsed spectral displays or color encoding can be employed with this technique.

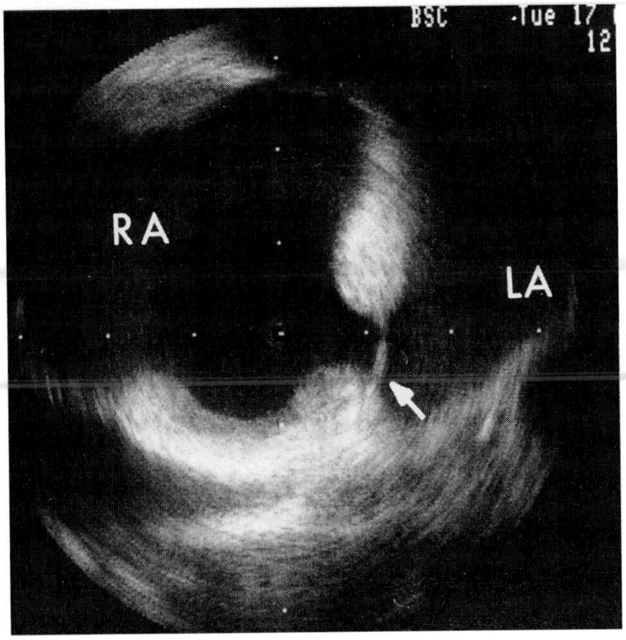

FIGURE 11–44 Intracardiac ultrasonographic image recorded from within the cavity of the right atrium (RA). Note the fairly thick tissue at the primum and more superior aspect of the atrial septum and the very thin valve of the foramen ovale (arrow). LA = left atrium.

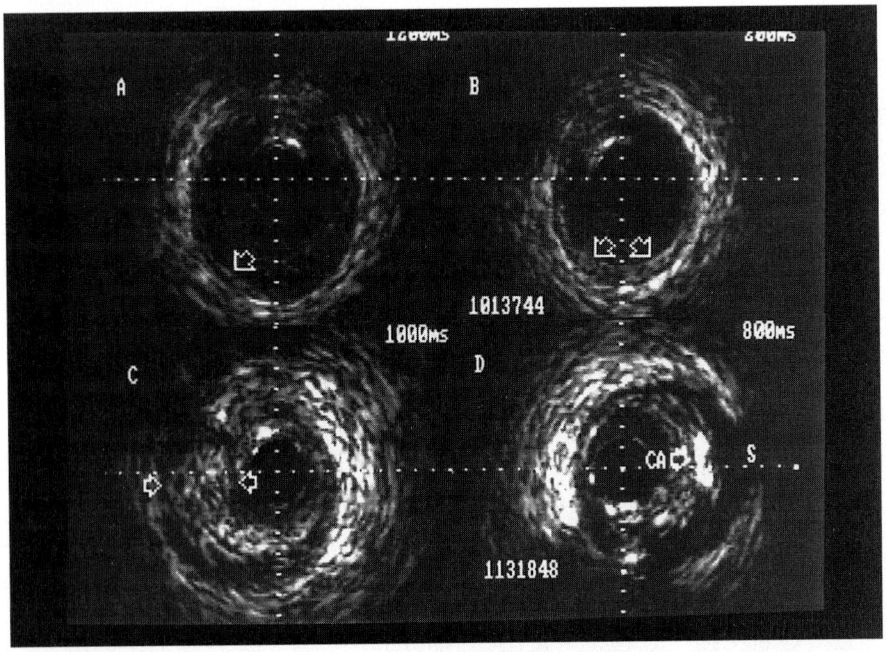

FIGURE 11–45 Intracoronary ultrasonographic images demonstrating the different severity of coronary atherosclerosis. **A,** Small rim of thickened intima (arrow). **B,** Larger amount of eccentric intimal thickening (arrows). **C,** Massive atherosclerotic plaque that is wider (arrows) than the residual lumen. **D,** Calcification in the plaque (CA) produces shadowing (S). (From Feigenbaum H: Echocardiography. 5th ed. Malvern, PA, Lea & Febiger, 1994.)

"Doppler Tissue Imaging" refers to the technique of determining directional velocity of tissue structures rather than the moving blood pool (Figs. 11–37 and 11–47). Doppler evaluation of annular motion has shown tremendous promise for the evaluation of diastolic function. When evaluated from an apical transducer, position annular motion is opposite in direction to the mitral inflow signal. The early annular velocity (Ea) exceeds late annular velocity (Aa) in a manner similar to the mitral valve E/A (see Fig. 11–37). This is a methodology that has shown tremendous promise and clinical applicability for characterizing detailed myocardial motion characteristics.[48-54]

Doppler tissue imaging records the velocity of motion of myocardium and can be targeted to discrete segments with sample volumes similar to that for routine Doppler interrogation. The information thus recorded is converted to velocity of tissue motion (centimeters per second). Several derivative calculations also provide valuable information. If both the velocity of motion and the duration of motion are known, then the absolute magnitude of motion can also be calculated.[54] Doppler tissue imaging can be used to calculate direction and velocity of motion in two adjacent myocardial segments of known distance of separation. From this strain, reflecting the relative velocity of either separation or closure between these two points can be calculated. This can further be developed into "strain rate imaging," which integrates the rate of distance change between two adjacent points over time, which in turn is a parameter that can be color-encoded over a segment of the myocardium. Both experimental animal and clinical data suggest that strain rate imaging can provide an increased level of resolution and accuracy for identification of subtle wall motion abnormalities in patients with ischemic and those with nonischemic heart disease.[55-61]

CONTRAST ECHOCARDIOGRAPHY

Contrast echocardiography is a rapidly evolving field that currently plays a number of routine clinical roles and has shown tremendous investigative promise for assessing myocardial perfusion.[62,63] All forms of contrast echocardiography rely on the fact that microbubbles, when injected into the blood pool, are intense echo reflectors. This pertains to the simplest contrast agent, agitated saline, as well as to the new, commercially available perfluorocarbon agents. Reflectivity of a microbubble is substantially greater than that of tissue, and as such in low concentration they create a highly reflective target. The interaction of the ultrasound beam with contrast is quite complex and occurs on three basic levels.

Depending on the power of the insonating ultrasound beam, the interaction may be simple reflection back at the fundamental frequency,[64,65] generation and reflection back of harmonic frequencies, or "stimulated acoustic omission."[66] The first and simplest interaction is pure reflection. This is characterized by reflection back of an intensive echo target from each individual microbubble. This was the phenomenon capitalized on for routine saline contrast echocardiography, which is used on a routine basis for detection of intracardiac shunts and enhancement of tricuspid regurgitation signals. Modern perfluorocarbon-based agents reflect back not only at the fundamental frequency but also at a harmonic of the insonating frequency. If these agents are insonated at a fundamental frequency and transducer receiving characteristics "tuned" to the harmonic frequency, the relative contribution of reflection from the oscillating microbubble (generating harmonic energy) is relatively greater than that from the sur-

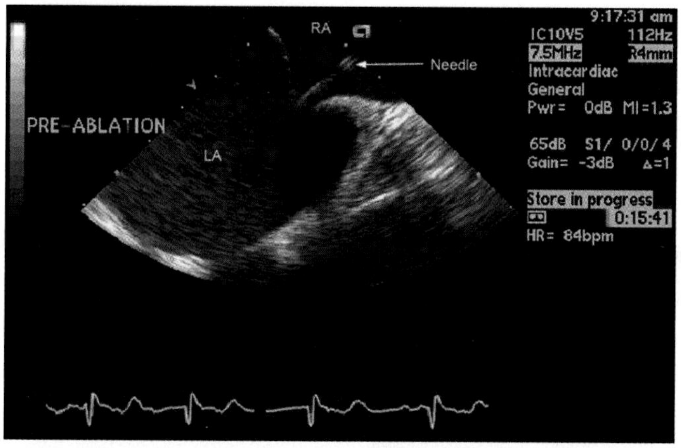

FIGURE 11–46 Image recorded from within the right atrium (RA) in a patient undergoing a transeptal puncture (needle) to gain access to a the left atrium (LA). Note the "tenting" of the atrial septum just prior to actual puncture.

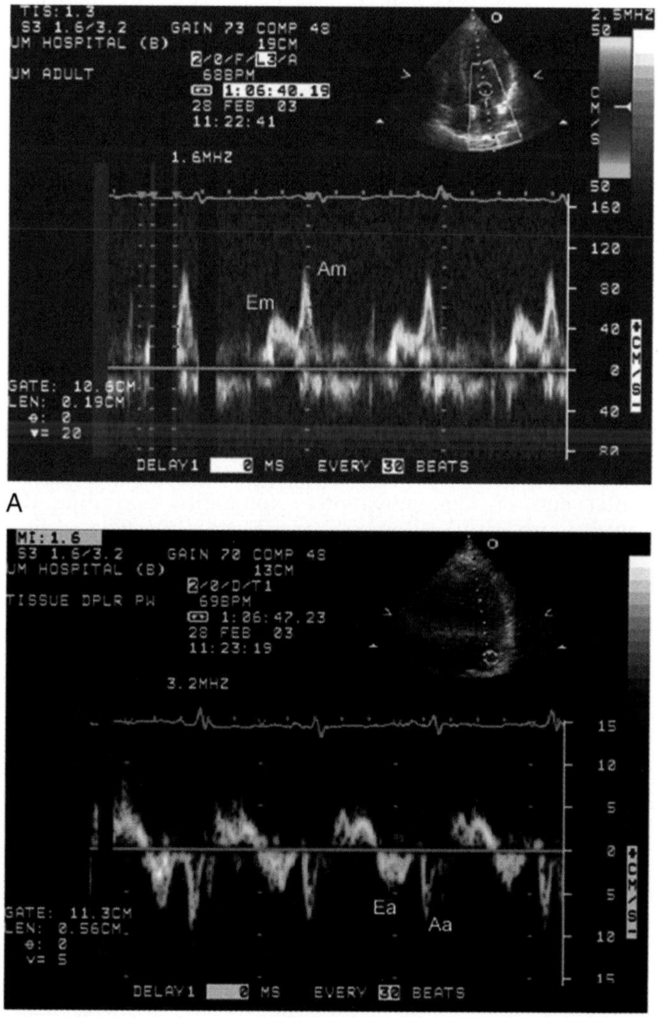

A

B

FIGURE 11–47 Mitral inflow velocity and Doppler tissue annular recording in a patient with diastolic dysfunction and impaired relaxation. Note the reversed E/A ratio, **(A)**, which is paralleled by a reduced annular E_A/A_A ratio.

rounding blood pool or tissue. This provides a *relatively* contrast-specific mode of imaging.

It has recently been recognized that interaction of bubbles with a ultrasound beam of significant amplitude results in actual disruption of the microbubble with subsequent loss of its reflectivity.[67-69] The initial interaction, however, results in an intense ultrasound signal emanating from the disrupted bubbles that contains an entire family of harmonic and subharmonic frequencies. Immediately following disruption of the microbubble in the blood pool, there is absence of any contrast-specific signal.

Microbubbles can be detected in the blood pool or tissue either using direct reflection in the fundamental or harmonic domains or by their creation of Doppler shifts after higher energy insonation. One of the more promising methods for contrast-specific imaging involves transmission of two sequential pulses that are 180 degrees out of phase with each other.[70] If these pulses reflect back in an unaltered manner and then are summed, the result is zero signal, as the sum of two waveforms 180 degrees out of phase results in cancellation of the signal. If, however, the signals interact with a microbubble capable of altering the insonating beam frequency, then each will be reflected back, no longer 180 degrees out of phase with the other, and the sum of the two signals results in the detectable ultrasound signal. Because tissue will not alter the frequency of the insonating beam, this results in a substantial degree of contrast specificity for this imaging modality. This type of phase shift analysis employs analysis in a Doppler domain rather than pure ultrasound reflection. A variation on this methodology is to emit two pulses of different amplitude and on receipt of the signal, amplify the weaker signal to match the transmitted amplitude of the stronger. This also, after subtraction of the two returning signals, results in a more contrast-specific imaging mode.

In clinical practice, contrast echocardiography is used on a daily basis for detection of shunts, typically using agitated saline. This can be accomplished easily in the clinical laboratory by vigorously agitating saline with a small amount of room air (typically 9.5 ml sterile saline plus 0.5 ml air) between two 10 ml syringes connected by a three-way stopcock. Vigorous agitation creates a population of microbubbles, 50 to 300 μm in diameter. These bubbles are relatively unstable and subject to rapid coalescence and should be injected quickly. After intravenous injection, they will appear in the right heart as a dense cloud of echoes, but because of their relatively large size, they are filtered by the pulmonary capillary bed. In the absence of a right-to-left shunt, these bubbles are confined to the right heart and cannot be used for visualization for left heart structures. Their appearance in the left heart is indirect evidence of a pathological right-to-left shunt.

The commercially developed perfluorocarbon agents contain populations of substantially smaller (typically 4-6 μm) microbubbles of near uniform size.[71] Because perfluorocarbons have low diffusibility, these microbubbles have substantial persistence after injection and because of their size can cross the pulmonary capillary bed and thus opacify left heart structures. They are currently approved for enhancing left heart border definition (Fig. 11–48). When used for this purpose, they have been shown to improve the ability to identify the left ventricular endocardial border in routine studies,[62,72,73] in the intensive care unit,[74,75] and during stress echocardiography,[76-78] and to enhance the accuracy of quantification.[79] They can also be used to enhance left-sided Doppler signals[80,81] and to improve detection of left ventricular thrombus.[82] Contrast agents currently in development use microbubbles that can be targeted to thrombus[83] or to endothelium.[84,85] When using these agents, it is important to recognize that they will be disrupted by high-amplitude ultrasound. For this reason, contrast-specific imaging algorithms utilize low mechanical index, typically less than 0.5, to provide smooth homogeneous imaging of the agent within the left ventricular cavity. Use of a higher mechanical index results in bubble destruction.

Because these new perfluorocarbon agents pass the pulmonary cavity bed, they will be present in all distally perfused tissues, including the myocardium, kidney, and liver. Their presence in the myocardium can be used as a marker of intact myocardial perfusion (to be discussed subsequently). Myocardial perfusion contrast echocardiography is a complex field currently in evolution that requires highly specific imaging formats and analysis algorithms.

ADVANTAGES AND LIMITATIONS OF ECHOCARDIOGRAPHY

As with any diagnostic technique, echocardiography has distinct advantages and disadvantages. Cardiac ultrasonography itself carries no risk to the patient, operator, bystanders, pregnant women, or fetus. Specialized examinations such as contrast echocardiography, TEE, and stress echocardiography carry the minimal additional risk associated with the procedural modifications necessary for their undertaking. Modern ultrasound instruments are capable of visualizing all four

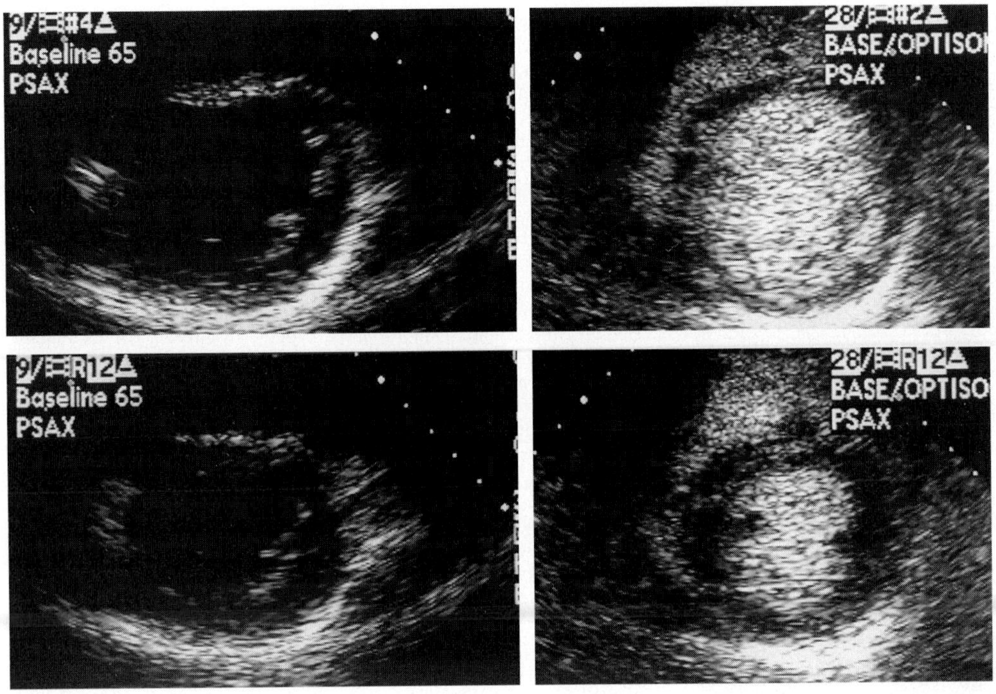

FIGURE 11–48 Demonstration of left ventricular cavity contrast enhancement after intravenous injection of a perfluorocarbon-based agent. The panels on the **left** were recorded before administration of contrast agent, and those on the **right** after opacification of the left ventricular cavity. Note the enhanced ability to identify the left ventricular cavity and distinguish it from the endocardial border after cavity opacification.

cardiac chambers, all four cardiac valves, and the great vessels. They provide high-resolution tomographic views in unlimited planes, which facilitates the ability to diagnose virtually all forms of anatomical cardiovascular disease. The addition of Doppler interrogation allows determination of physiological parameters as they relate to blood flow and myocardial velocities.

Echocardiography does have specific limitations because ultrasound does not transmit well through calcified structures such as bone, and an appropriate acoustic window is necessary for optimal visualization. In neonates and infants, ultrasound can pass through noncalcified cartilage and the windows available exceed those in adults. In the adult population, a noncalcified window must be obtained that typically is in the intercostal spaces or from the subxiphoid positions. In patients with narrow intercostal spaces, imaging can be problematic. A greater limitation is the degree to which the air-filled structures reflect ultrasound. Intervening lung tissue in patients with obstructive lung disease can result in suboptimal or even inadequate imaging.

Another area of concern for echocardiography is its potential for overuse. Because of the absence of risk from routine ultrasonography, overuse by less than adequately trained individuals has become a recent concern. The American College of Cardiology, American Heart Association, and American Society of Echocardiography have outlined recommendations for appropriate training in echocardiography and likewise recommendations on its appropriate clinical use.[86,87]

Clinical Applications of Echocardiography

Acquired Valvular Heart Disease (see Chap. 57)

Mitral Valve Disease

Virtually all types of mitral valve disease can be characterized anatomically using echocardiography. Doppler techniques provide accurate physiological information that complements the anatomical assessment. Figure 11–49 outlines the closure pattern of the normal mitral valve and the valve in multiple disease states, each of which are discussed.

MITRAL STENOSIS. Mitral stenosis was the first valvular lesion to be comprehensively evaluated with echocardiography. Two-dimensional echocardiography and Doppler ultrasonography remain the mainstay of diagnosis and characterization of this lesion. In the vast majority of adult patients, mitral stenosis is the result of rheumatic heart disease, with rarer cases of congenital mitral stenosis being encountered in adult patients. Rarely, heavy calcification of the mitral annulus results in functional restriction of the left ventricular inflow and can result in a left atrial to left ventricular gradient mimicking the physiological effects of valvular mitral stenosis.

The hallmark of mitral stenosis on two-dimensional echocardiography is thickening and restriction of motion of both mitral valve leaflets, with the predominant pathological process being fibrosis and fusion of the leaflet tips and proximal chordae (Fig. 11–50). In more advanced cases, the body of the leaflet itself may become involved and in even more advanced cases substantial calcification occurs within the leaflet and on the subvalvular apparatus, including the chordae and papillary muscle tips (Fig. 11–51). The earliest effect of rheumatic disease on the mitral valve is the result of inflammation and thickening of leaflet tips that restricts the motion of the tips while allowing free motion of the body of the leaflets. This results in a characteristic "doming" motion of the mitral valve in diastole. The appearance of the anterior leaflet in diastole has also been described as having a "hockey stick" configuration. Restriction of the tips results in a funnel-like mitral valve apparatus with the restrictive orifice being at the tips of the leaflets. This appearance is easily recognized from TTE in both the parasternal long-axis and apical four-chamber views. With careful attention to detail, the actual restrictive orifice of the mitral valve can be visualized and planimetered from a parasternal short-axis view (Fig. 11–52). This planimetered area correlates well with the area determined in the hemodynamic laboratory. M-mode echocardiography was the initial diagnostic tool for evaluation of mitral stenosis. By using this technique, the thickened leaflets could be identified as well as the restricted motion. The restricted motion pattern results in a flattening of the E-F slope of the mitral valve (Fig. 11–53). The E-F slope can be quantified and tracked as a measure of stenosis severity but provides no truly quantitative value by today's standards.

Assessment of Severity. In addition to determining the anatomical extent and severity of the stenotic lesion, assessment of physiological significance is made using Doppler echocardiography. Color flow imaging is instrumental in determining the degree of concurrent mitral regurgitation. Both continuous-wave and pulsed Doppler echocardiography can

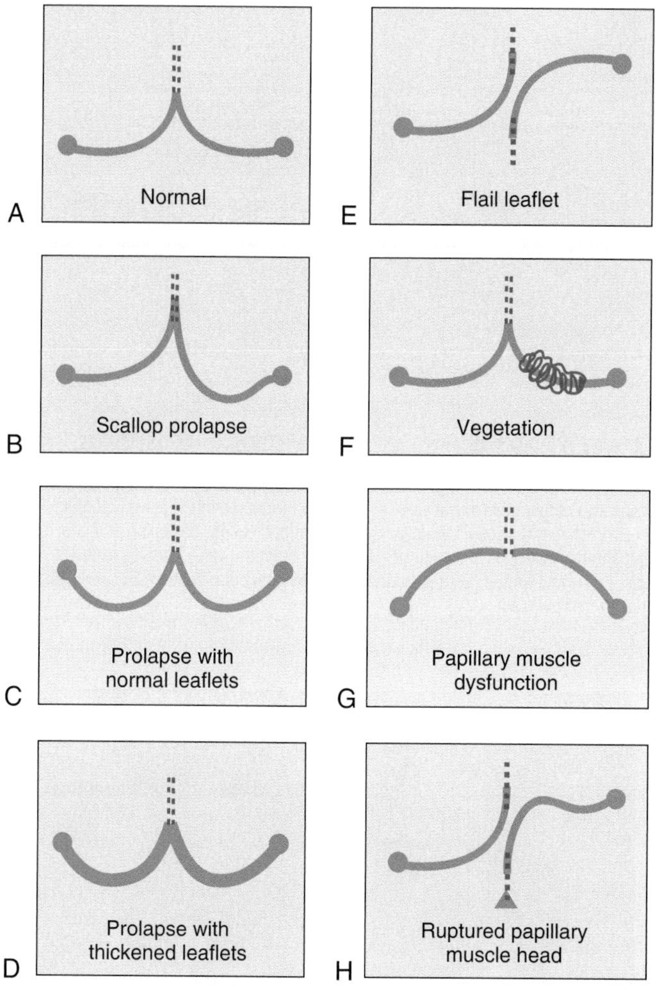

FIGURE 11–49 Schematic outlining both normal and abnormal mitral valve closure patterns in apical 4 chamber view. See text for details.

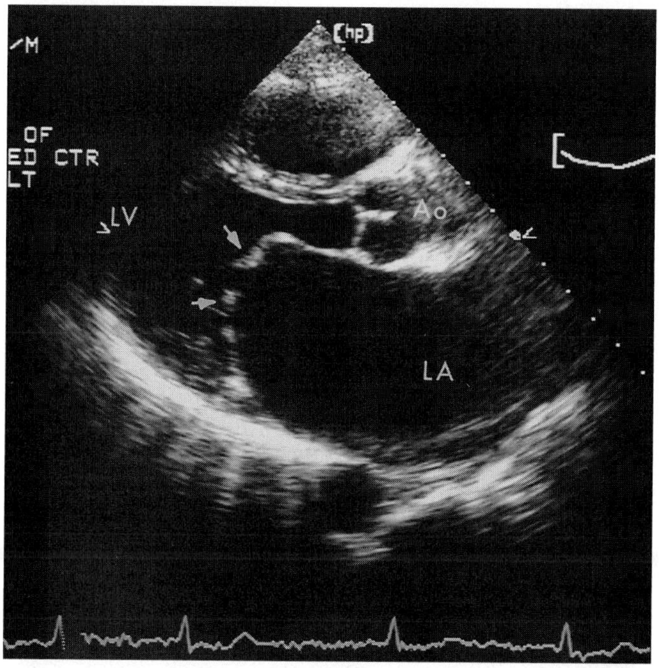

FIGURE 11–50 Parasternal long-axis view of a patient with mitral stenosis and a pliable noncalcified mitral valve leaflet. Note the "doming" motion of the mitral valve leaflets (arrowheads). Valves with these morphological features are excellent candidates for percutaneous balloon valvotomy. Ao = aorta; LA = left atrium; LV = left ventricle.

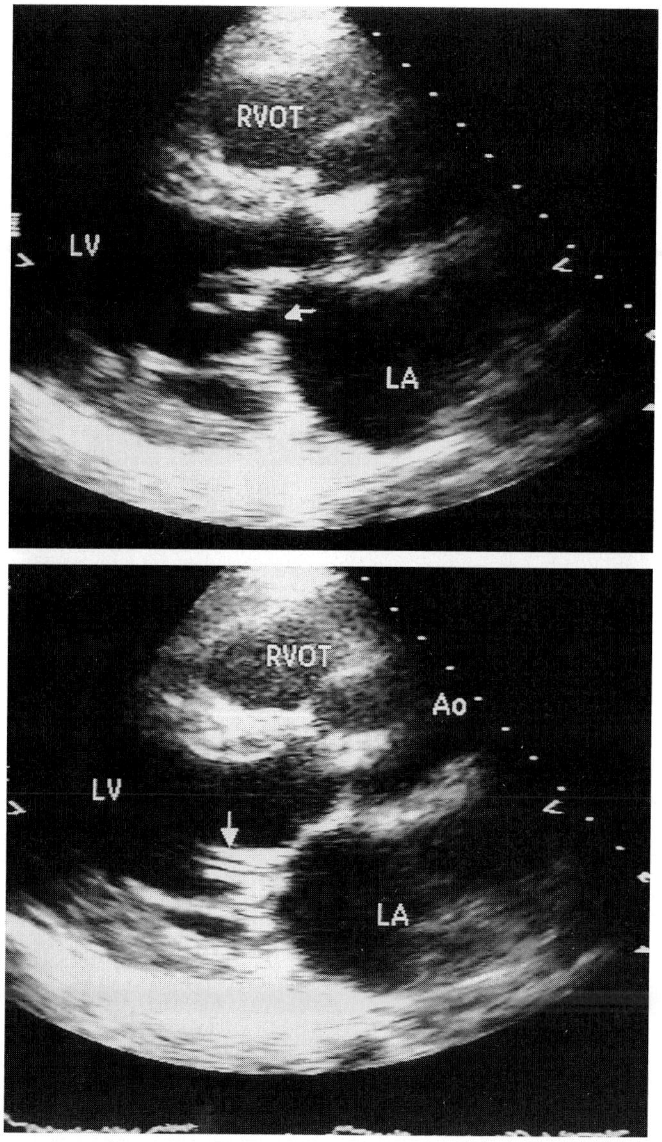

FIGURE 11–51 Parasternal long-axis view in diastole **(top)** and systole **(bottom)** in a patient with rheumatic heart disease and mitral stenosis. In the top panel, note the diffuse thickening of the mitral valve. The reduced orifice can be seen in this end-diastolic frame (arrow). The bottom panel was recorded in systole and provides a view of the chordal apparatus, which can be seen to be diffusely thickened and fibrotic. Valves with this appearance are less ideal candidates for percutaneous intervention than the valve presented in Figure 11–50. Ao = aorta; LA = left atrium; LV = left ventricle; RVOT = right ventricular outflow tract.

be obtained at rest and with exercise and provide accurate quantification of the transvalvular gradient (Fig. 11-54).[88-90] Determination of the transvalvular gradient should be performed in patients both at rest and with modest degrees of exercise. A population of symptomatic patients exists who have relatively unimpressive gradients at rest that increase dramatically with mild exercise.

A second Doppler method for determining the severity of mitral stenosis involves calculating the pressure half-time ($P_{1/2}t$), which is the time in milliseconds required for the peak pressure gradient to decline to one half of its original value.[91,92] The pressure half-time can be related to an anatomical valve area by the following formula:

$$\text{mitral valve area} = P_{1/2}t \div 220 \text{ msec}$$

This relationship is probably valid only for isolated mitral stenosis and is not accurate for quantitation of the mitral valve orifice if concurrent mitral regurgitation or significant aortic insufficiency is present. The relationship also has diminished accuracy in cases in which left ventricular diastolic compliance is markedly abnormal, such as in patients with

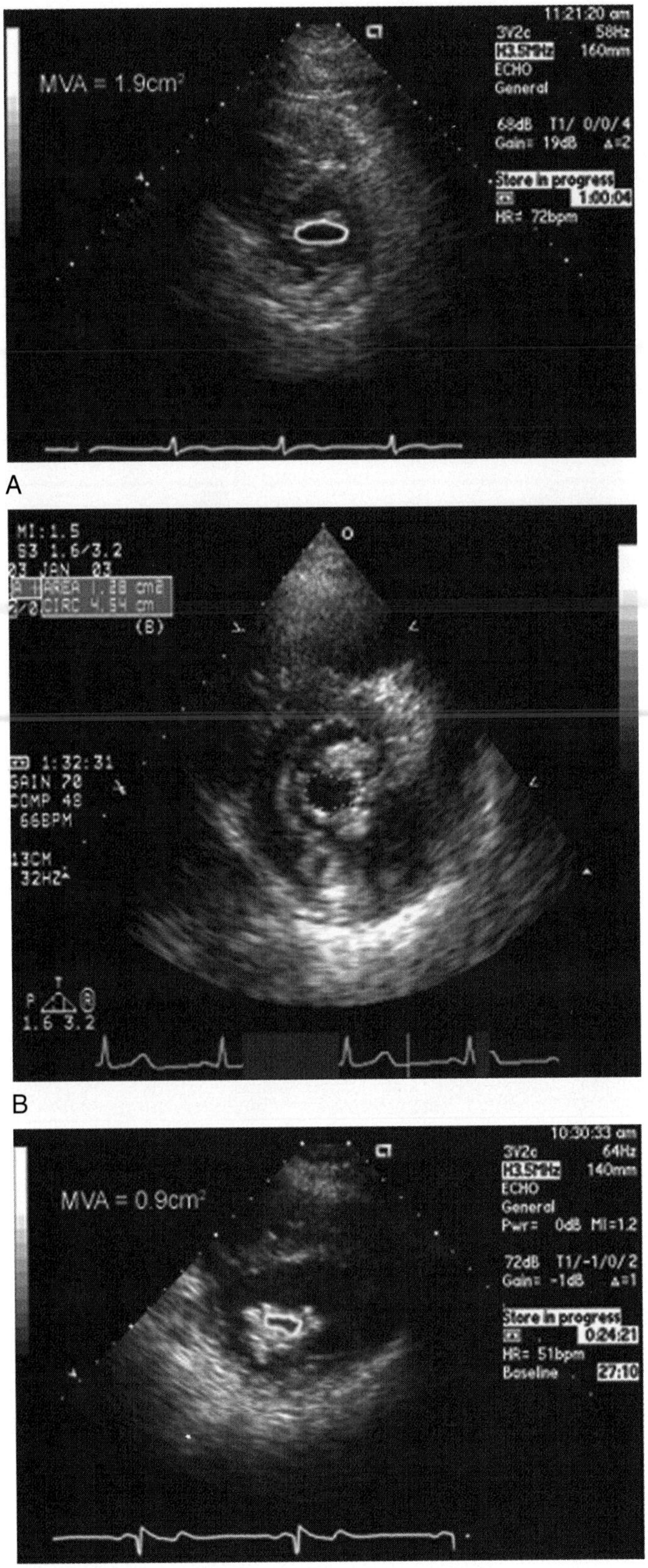

FIGURE 11–52 Mitral valve area. Three examples of planimetry of the stenotic mitral valve orifice. In each instance, a relatively regularly shaped mitral orifice can be planimetered. The planimetered values are superimposed in each figure.

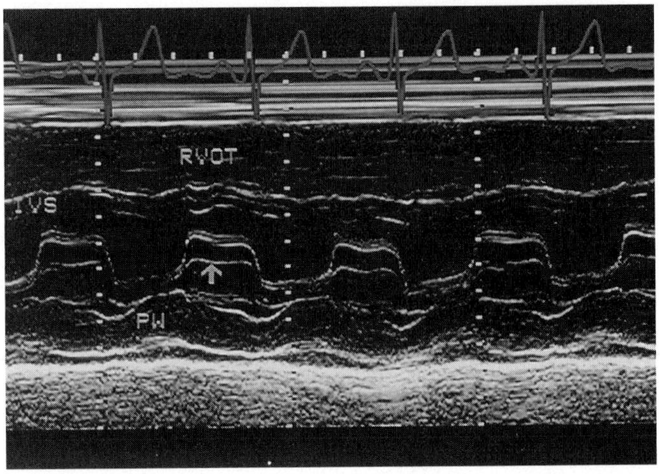

FIGURE 11–53 M-mode echocardiogram recorded in a patient with typical mitral stenosis. Compare this mitral valve opening pattern to the mitral valve motion in Figure 11–9. With mitral stenosis there is thickening of the leaflets, flattening of the E-F slope, and anterior motion of the posterior leaflet during mitral valve opening (arrow) in diastole. FW = left ventricular free wall; IVS = interventricular septum; RVOT = right ventricular outflow tract.

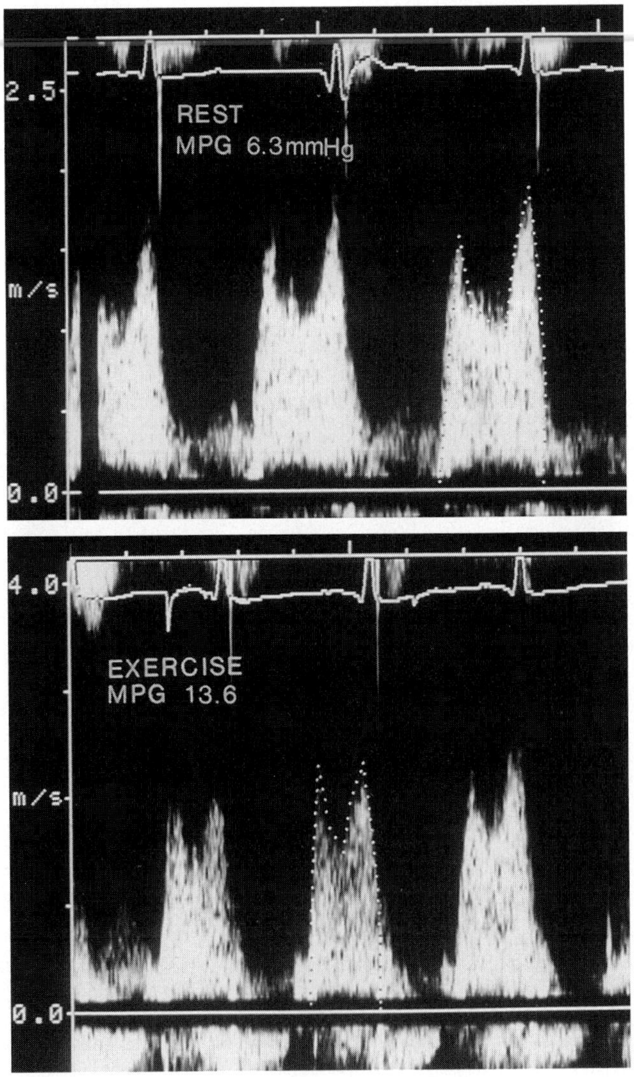

FIGURE 11–54 Transmitral Doppler recordings obtained in a patient with mitral stenosis at rest **(top)** and with exercise **(bottom)**. Heart rate has increased from 85 to 110 beats/min, resulting in an increase in the mean pressure gradient from 6.3 to 13.6 mm Hg.

severe hypertension or aortic stenosis and immediately after mitral balloon valvotomy.[93]

Other more detailed methods for determining the mitral valve area involve determination of quantitative mitral valve flow. This can be performed using the continuity equation in a manner analogous to that for aortic stenosis. Either flow and dimensions at the level of the mitral valve annulus or forward going flow in the left ventricular outflow tract can be used in this equation. Obviously, this approach has limitations in patients with concurrent regurgitation or multivalve disease.

Secondary effects of mitral stenosis include left atrial dilation with subsequent blood stasis and thrombus formation and secondary pulmonary hypertension. Evaluation of the left atrium for blood stasis and thrombus typically requires TEE (Fig. 11-55). The aortic, tricuspid, and pulmonic valves can likewise be directly interrogated for evidence of rheumatic involvement. The most common significant sequelae of mitral stenosis is development of secondary pulmonary hypertension with subsequent right heart dysfunction and tricuspid regurgitation. As with other diseases in which the right side of the heart is evaluated, the tricuspid regurgitation jet can be interrogated for determination of right ventricular systolic and pulmonary artery systolic pressures.

It is important to fully evaluate the anatomical features of mitral stenosis in patients in whom a mitral balloon valvotomy is contemplated. Four features of mitral valve anatomy have been identified that correlate with the success of this procedure. These include valve pliability, thickening, calcification, and subvalvular involvement. Each of these can be quantified on a score of 0 to 4 and a total score tabulated. Scores above 8 represent valves less likely to be successfully treated with a percutaneous approach.[94-96] More recent studies have suggested a disproportionate impact of calcification and subvalvular involvement on the likelihood of successful balloon valvotomy.

MITRAL REGURGITATION. Two-dimensional echocardiography and Doppler techniques can be used to detect the presence and severity of mitral regurgitation, to determine the cause of regurgitation and to look for secondary effects. Mitral regurgitation can be due to a wide variety of cardiac conditions, many of which are presented in schematic form in Figure 11–49. Often, mitral regurgitation will first be documented using Doppler color flow imaging. In the presence of significant mitral regurgitation, volume overload of left ventricle and left atrium occurs, resulting in dilation of these chambers, the degree of which is dependent on both the severity and duration of mitral regurgitation. The cause of mitral regurgitation is determined by assessing the anatomy of the left ventricle and the mitral valve apparatus. Many forms of mitral regurgitation are due to intrinsic disease of the mitral valve, such as mitral regurgitation concurrent with mitral stenosis, myxomatous degeneration with mitral valve prolapse, chordal rupture, endocarditis, and infarct-related papillary muscle rupture. Functional forms of mitral regurgitation also occur in which the mitral valve may be anatomically normal but fails to coapt because of dilation of the left ventricle. This can occur due to either cardiomyopathy or coronary artery disease. In the vast majority of instances, the anatomical and functional abnormality responsible for mitral regurgitation can be documented with TTE. On occasion, TEE is necessary to refine the anatomical assessment and may be particularly helpful in identifying rupture of a papillary muscle head and flail leaflets and in detecting smaller vegetations or perforations.[97,98]

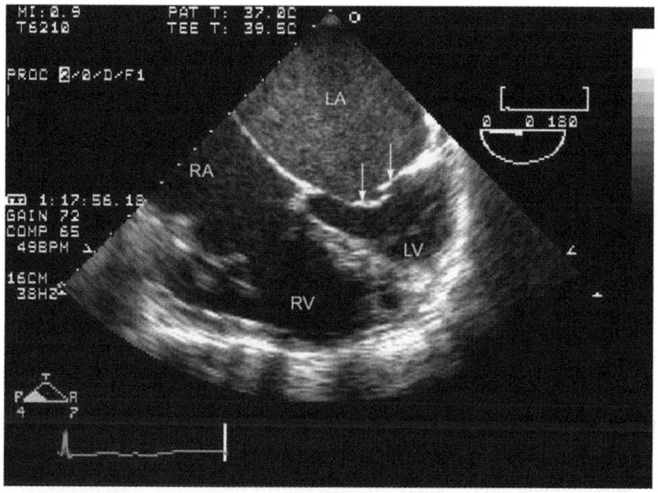

FIGURE 11–55 Transesophageal echocardiogram recorded in a patient with severe rheumatic mitral valvular stenosis and marked biatrial and right ventricular enlargement. This frame was recorded in diastole. Note the thickened immobile mitral leaflets, which have not appropriately separated in diastole. Note also the dense, spontaneous echo contrast in the body of the left atrium, which in real time appears as a mass of swirling echoes. LA = left atrium; LV = left ventricle; RA = right atrium; RV = right ventricle.

Assessment of Severity. Doppler color flow imaging is used to determine the severity of mitral regurgitation. The size of the regurgitant jet within the left atrium is directly proportional to the severity of mitral regurgitation. Multiple studies have confirmed the relationship between the size of the regurgitant jet and the severity of regurgitation determined with angiography or other techniques. Typically, the size of the jet is indexed to the size of the left atrium. Figure 11-56 demonstrates examples of mitral regurgitation. Jets that are peripheral or impinging on a wall, rather than central, cause predictable underestimation of severity. A regurgitant jet impinging on a wall results in a smaller color flow area than an equivalent central regurgitant volume.[99] The underlying mechanism of this phenomenon is that a regurgitant jet "recruits" the adjacent blood flow into motion. As color Doppler flow detects cells in motion, irrespective of their origin, the visualized regurgitant jet is the sum of the regurgitant volume and the recruited blood. A centrally oriented jet recruits in all of its dimensions, whereas a jet adjacent to a wall recruits only on its free surface, hence being relatively smaller than an equal volume of central regurgitation. A jet impinging on a wall underestimates the regurgitant volume by approximately 40 percent. In cases of moderate and severe mitral regurgitation, flow in the pulmonary veins may reverse direction in systole. A variation on this finding is attenuation of normal forward flow in the pulmonary vein during ventricular systole. More recently, three-dimensional reconstruction of mitral regurgitation jets has been shown to be feasible.[100,101] The incremental value of this method has not yet been shown.

Several characteristics of a regurgitant jet can give clues as to its origin. In the presence of normal ventricular function, an anatomically normal mitral valve closes along a 2- to 3-mm-long line of overlap of the leaflets (*zona coapta*). This overlap of leaflet tissue results in more efficient closure of the mitral valve than does tip-to-tip closure. With left ventricular dilatation, the papillary muscles are displaced apically and laterally, pulling the mitral valve leaflet toward the apex.[102,103] This results in a systolic doming of the leaflets and tip-to-tip closure of the mitral valve leaflet rather than overlapping in the *zona coapta* (Fig. 11-57). Tip-to-tip closure is inefficient and results in variable degrees of mitral regurgitation. In extreme examples, the leaflet tips may fail to coapt at all and the actual regurgitant orifice can be directly visualized. These jets are typically central in location. By using either color Doppler M-mode or careful interrogation of the spectral display, the timing of the mitral regurgitation jet can also be determined. Lesions such as mitral prolapse may result in regurgitant confined to midsystole and late systole.

Anatomical disruption of any portion of the mitral valve will result in regurgitation. This can range from a few ruptured chordae with isolated prolapse of a single scallop to disruption of an entire papillary muscle head with flail of an entire leaflet. TEE is often incrementally helpful in determining the precise degree of anatomical disruption of the valve (Fig. 11-58). Irrespective of the cause of a flail leaflet, the resultant jet is often highly eccentric and its flow is directed opposite the leaflet bearing the pathological lesion; that is, a flail posterior mitral valve leaflet results in an anteriorly directed jet. A highly eccentric jet should lead to a higher index of suspicion of a flail leaflet. Three-dimensional echocardiography has shown promise for detailed assessment of mitral valve pathology in mitral regurgitation (Fig. 11-59).

Quantitation of mitral regurgitation is heavily dependent on the color Doppler flow area. Other techniques for quantifying mitral regurgitation rely on determining the width of the jet at its origin (*vena contracta*) and on evaluation of the proximal isovelocity surface area. In general terms, for any given Nyquist limit, the larger the size is of the proximal isovelocity surface area, the greater the degree of regurgitation. Calcula-

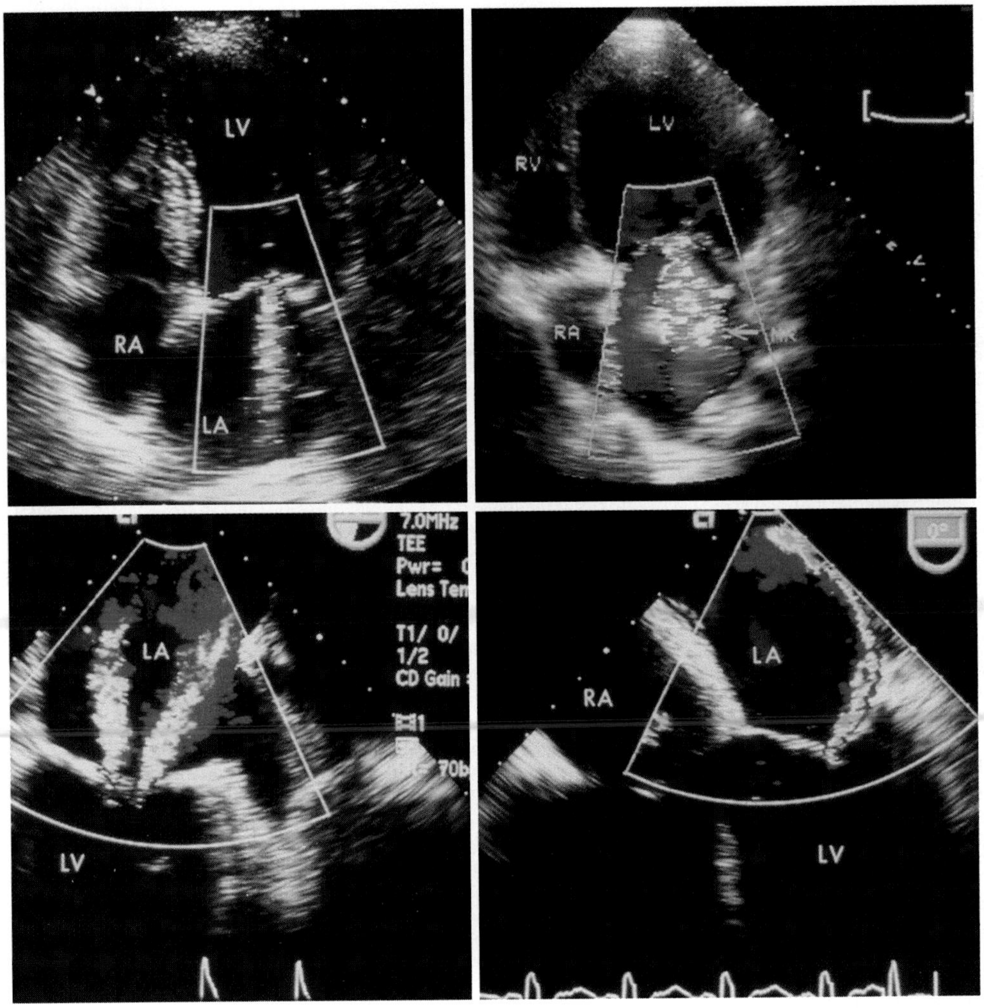

FIGURE 11–56 Four panels depicting varying degrees of mitral regurgitation; the two **top panels** are apical four-chamber transthoracic views showing, on the **left,** mild mitral regurgitation and, on the **right,** moderate to severe mitral regurgitation. On the left, note the relatively narrow jet directed from the tips of the mitral valve toward the posterior left atrial wall. On the right, note the larger jet, filling approximately 40 percent of the left atrial cavity. The two **bottom panels** are transesophageal echocardiograms. On the **left,** note the mitral regurgitation occurring in two discrete jets and, on the **right,** the highly eccentric jet, which courses along the extreme lateral wall of the left atrium. LA = left atrium; LV = left ventricle; RA = right atrium; RV = right ventricle.

tion of flow volume from proximal isovelocity surface area has already been discussed and can be applied to determine regurgitant volume. In addition to calculating flow volume using proximal isovelocity surface area, several derivative measurements can also be made (Fig. 11-60). The surface area of the isovelocity of flow represents the area of flow and, when multiplied by the aliasing velocity, results in regurgitant flow. This volume of regurgitant flow, when divided by the peak velocity, results in calculation of effective regurgitant orifice.[104,105] All of these measurements assume holosystolic mitral regurgitation. It should be emphasized that there are many instances in which mitral regurgitation may be confined to only a portion of systole. A classic example is mitral prolapse with regurgitation confined to the later half or third of systole. While there are no strict guidelines, when mitral regurgitation is identified as being confined to only a portion of systole, the assessment of severity whether based on the size of the regurgitant jet at one point in time or regurgitant flow must be adjusted accordingly for the partial duration of flow. A secondary finding seen in cases of moderate and severe mitral regurgitation is reversal of systolic flow in the pulmonary veins. In practice, combining observations from all these techniques is often beneficial for quantifying mitral regurgitation. Table 11-3 outlines the various criteria for determining severity of mitral regurgitation.

MITRAL VALVE PROLAPSE. The detection and characterization of mitral valve prolapse remains a common use of echocardiography. Early studies suggested a prevalence of prolapse of up to 21 percent in otherwise healthy young females. It should be emphasized that many individuals identified as having mitral prolapse in these earlier studies today are recognized to simply have normal bowing of the mitral valve. The normal mitral valve closure pattern is for the tips of the leaflets to point toward the left ventricular apex and for there to be gentle bowing of the leaflet with a concavity toward the apex of the left ventricle. Based largely on dimensional reconstruction techniques, the mitral valve annulus is known not to be a planar structure but rather to have complex three-dimensional geometry. Depending on the tomographic plane of interrogation, a portion of one or both leaflets may bow behind the imaginary annular line. In the presence of otherwise anatomically normal thin leaflets, this represents a variation of normal and does not represent pathological mitral valve prolapse.

The most extreme forms of mitral valve prolapse involve myxomatous degeneration of the valves with visible leaflet thickening (defined as greater than 3 to 5 mm in thickness) and either marked symmetrical bowing of the valve behind the majority of the annular plane or highly asymmetrical buckling of one or both leaflets into the plane of the left atrium (Figs. 11–61 and 11–62). This will be associated

TABLE 11–3 Mitral Regurgitation Severity*

	I (Mild)	II	III	IV (Severe)
MR = JET (% LA)	<15	15-30	35-50	>50
Spectral Doppler	Faint	—	—	Dense
Vena Contracta	<3 mm	—	—	>6 mm
Pulmonary vein flow	S > D	—	—	Systolic Reversed
RV (ml)	<30	30-44	45-59	≥60
ERO (cm²)	<0.2	0.2-0.29	0.3-0.39	30.40
PISA	Small	—	—	Large

D = antegrade flow in diastole; ERO = effective regurgitant orifice; % LA = percentage of left atrial area encompassed by the MR jet with color flow Doppler; MR = mitral regurgitation; PISA = proximal isovelocity surface area; RV = regurgitant volume; S = antegrade flow in systole.

*For some parameters, the observation is valid at the extremes of MR severity and there may be marked overlap in intermediate (grades II, III) MR. In these instances, no value is presented.

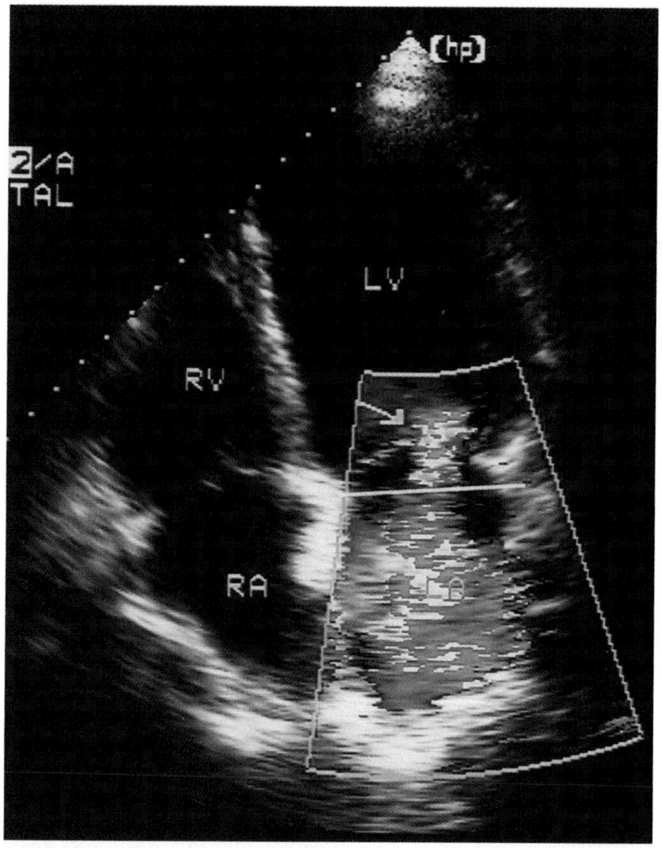

FIGURE 11–57 Apical four-chamber view in a patient with a dilated cardiomyopathy and severe mitral regurgitation due to a dilated annulus and abnormal mitral valve coaptation. The solid horizontal white line represents the plane of the mitral annulus. Note that the mitral valve closes well within the cavity of the left ventricle. The actual origin of the mitral regurgitation jet can be seen as it accelerates toward the regurgitant orifice (arrow) and is likewise displaced into the cavity of the left ventricle. LA = left atrium; LV = left ventricle; RA = right atrium; RV = right ventricle.

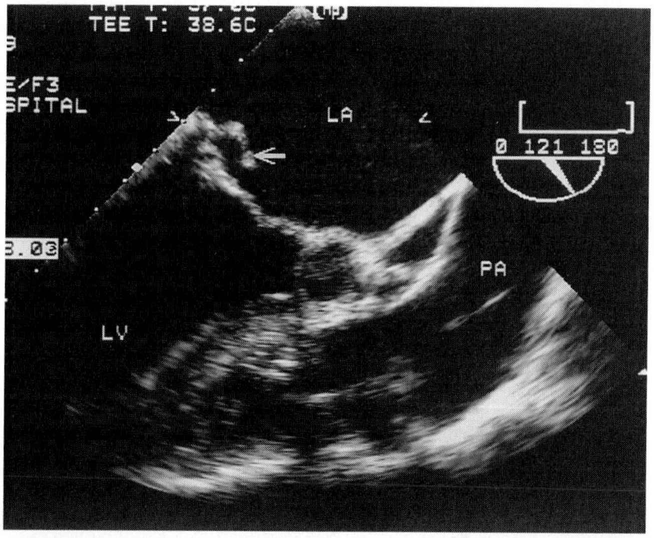

FIGURE 11–58 Transesophageal echocardiogram recorded in a patient with a flail posterior mitral valve leaflet. The echocardiogram is recorded in a longitudinal view in which the left atrium (LA), left ventricle (LV), and pulmonary artery (PA) are visualized. Because flail leaflets occur in atypical locations, it is often necessary to scan in unusual planes to identify the leaflet. In this projection, a substantial portion of the posterior leaflet (arrow) can be seen to protrude into the left atrium, with the tip of the leaflet no longer attached to the chordal apparatus.

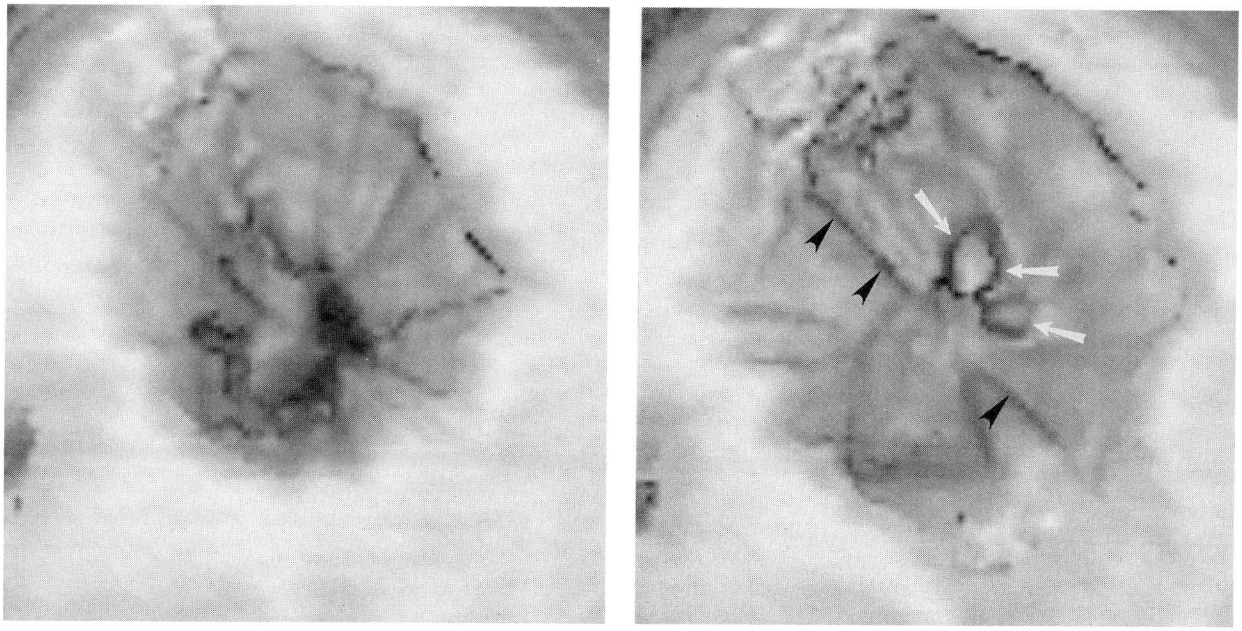

FIGURE 11–59 Three-dimensional echocardiogram recorded in a patient with a partial flail mitral anterior leaflet. For both panels, the orientation is a view of the mitral valve from within the left atrium. The left panel was recorded in diastole, and the unrestricted orifice can be seen. The right panel was recorded in mid-systole. Note the two scallops of the anterior leaflet that protrude into the left atrium (arrows).

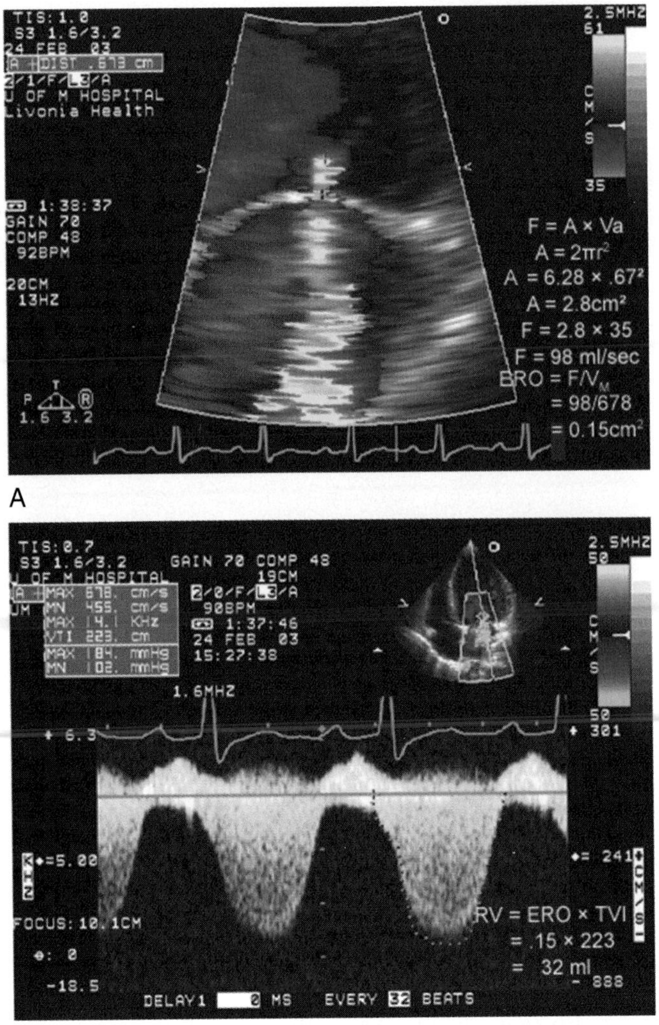

FIGURE 11–60 Example for calculation of regurgitant flow and effective regurgitant orifice (ERO) and regurgitant volume using the PISA technique. See Figure 11–35 for a schematic representation of these calculations as well. **A,** Color Doppler image from which the diameter of the convergence zone can be calculated as 0.67 cm. The aliasing limit is 35 cm^2. **B,** Continuous wave spectral display of the mitral regurgitation jet from which the VTI and V_{MAX} can be determined. From this, the regurgitant volume can be calculated as 32 ml. Using the calculation schematized in Figure 11–35, flow can be calculated as 98 ml/sec, and the effective regurgitant orifice as 0.15 cm^2.

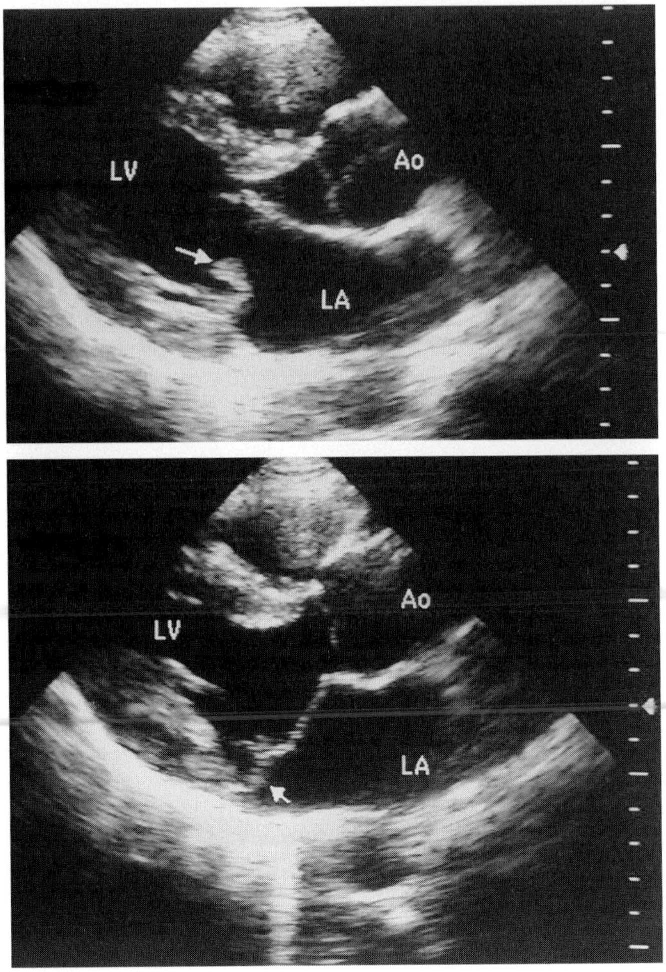

FIGURE 11–61 Parasternal long-axis view in diastole **(top)** and systole **(bottom)** in a patient with mitral valve prolapse and myxomatous changes. In the upper panel, note the open mitral valve and the diffuse thickening of the posterior mitral valve leaflet (arrow). The lower panel was recorded in systole. Note that both leaflets prolapse behind the plane of the mitral valve annulus. The prolapse of the posterior leaflet is somewhat more prominent (arrow). Ao = aorta; LA = left atrium; LV = left ventricle.

with variable degrees of mitral regurgitation, which may be either holosystolic or confined to middle to late systole. Because of the eccentric buckling of the myxomatous valve, the mitral regurgitation jet can be eccentric rather than central. The key aspects to the diagnosis of mitral valve prolapse rely not on the mere detection of a valve that buckles into the plane of the left atrium but on characterization of the valve morphology. As mentioned earlier, normal thin leaflets that bow gently into the left atrial plane probably represent a variation of normal closure patterns. Patients with thickened redundant valves and myxomatous changes of the leaflet have a true form of structural heart disease. It is these individuals who are most at risk for endocarditis, spontaneous rupture of chordae, and progressive mitral regurgitation (see Chap. 57). It also appears that there is a higher than usual incidence of ventricular arrhythmias and neurological events in this subset of patients.

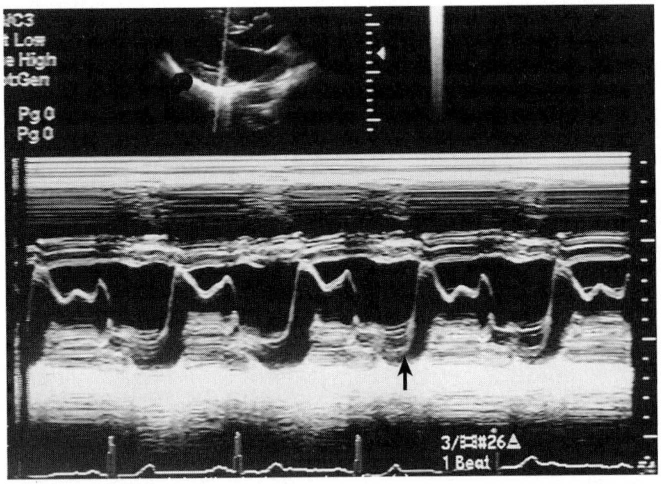

FIGURE 11–62 M-mode echocardiogram of the mitral valve recorded in the same patient noted in Figure 11–61. Note that the posterior leaflet is diffusely thickened and in systole prolapses posteriorly from the normal closure line (arrow).

Aortic Valve Disease

AORTIC STENOSIS. Aortic stenosis is most commonly due to one of three pathological processes: a bicuspid aortic valve, rheumatic heart disease, or degenerative aortic stenosis. On rare occasions, aortic stenosis can be the result of endocarditis or radiation heart disease. Bicuspid aortic valve typically manifests as a hemodynamically significant lesion in the fourth or fifth decade of life and calcific degenerative aortic stenosis in the seventh decade and beyond. Rheumatic aortic valve disease will virtually always be seen in patients who have concurrent rheumatic mitral valve disease.

The bicuspid aortic valve is the single most common congenital cardiac defect and occurs in approximately 2 percent of the population. There is a broad range of anatomical and physiological abnormalities associated with this condition. The bicuspid aortic valve is commonly thought of as a two-leaflet valve with roughly equal leaflet proportions. There is a range of abnormality in the "bicuspid valve" that includes nearly unicuspid valves and distribution of leaflet tissue other than 50/50 percent. Bicuspid aortic valves are commonly described as having either an anteroposterior or a lateral orientation of the leaflets. In reality, virtually any direction of the major coaptation can be seen. TTE is a reliable method for detecting the bicuspid aortic valve. With the use of this technique, the hallmark of the bicuspid valve will be eccentric closure of the leaflets within the aorta. In approximately 80 percent of cases, two rather than three leaflets can be directly visualized (Fig. 11–63). With closer scrutiny by way of TEE, what at first appears to be a true bicuspid valve often is found to represent a three-leaflet valve with unequal leaflet sizes and fusion of one of the three commissures, resulting in a functional bicuspid valve (Fig. 11–64). In this instance, there will be three coronary sinuses and normal orientation of the coronary arteries. In a true two-leaflet bicuspid aortic valve, there will be only two coronary sinuses and variable location of the coronary ostia. It is important to examine the opening pattern of the aortic valve to determine that it is functionally bicuspid. There is a strong association between coarctation of the aorta and bicuspid valve. When either of these conditions is clinically suspected, the other should also be considered.

Degenerative calcific valves appear as three-leaflet structures with marked thickening of the leaflets. Thickening and calcification may be more prominent at the base of the leaflets than at the tips. There is a broad range of immobility and stenosis, depending on the duration and severity of disease. In advanced cases, the degree of calcification may be so extensive that it is not possible to identify discrete valve cusps.

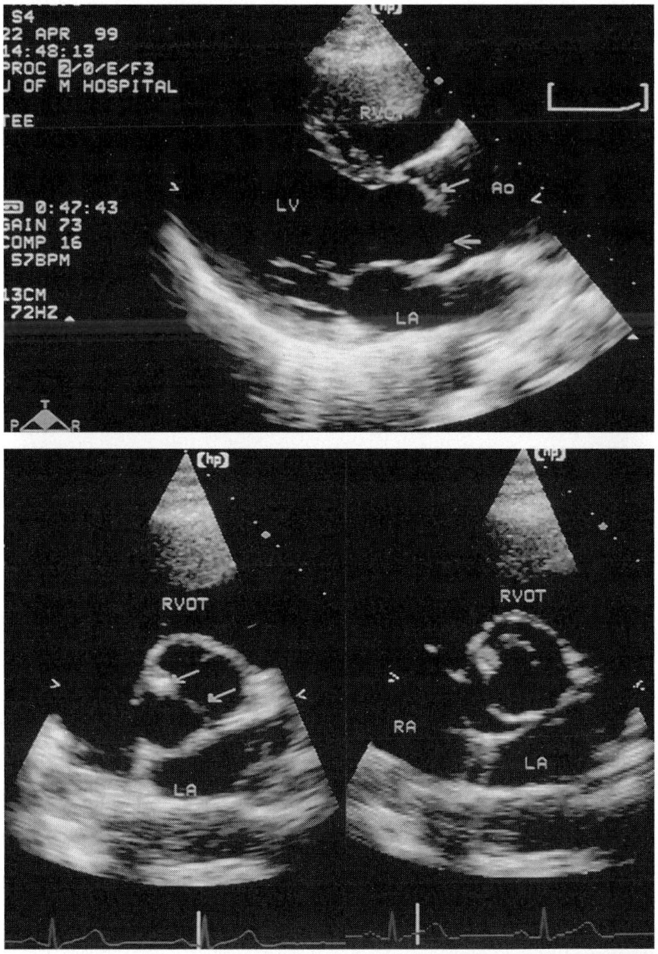

FIGURE 11–63 Transthoracic echocardiogram in a patient with bicuspid aortic valve. In the **upper panel,** note that the leaflets of the aortic valve do not open all the way to the margins of the aorta but are "tethered" in lumen of the proximal aorta. The two bottom panels are recorded in the short-axis view at the base of the heart. The **lower left panel** was recorded in diastole and reveals the closed bicuspid valve with a single commissure oriented from 10 o'clock to 4 o'clock (arrows). The **lower right panel** is recorded in systole, and the oval opening of the bicuspid valve can be appreciated within the circular aorta. Ao = aorta; LA = left atrium; LV = left ventricle; RA = right atrium; RVOT = right ventricular outflow tract.

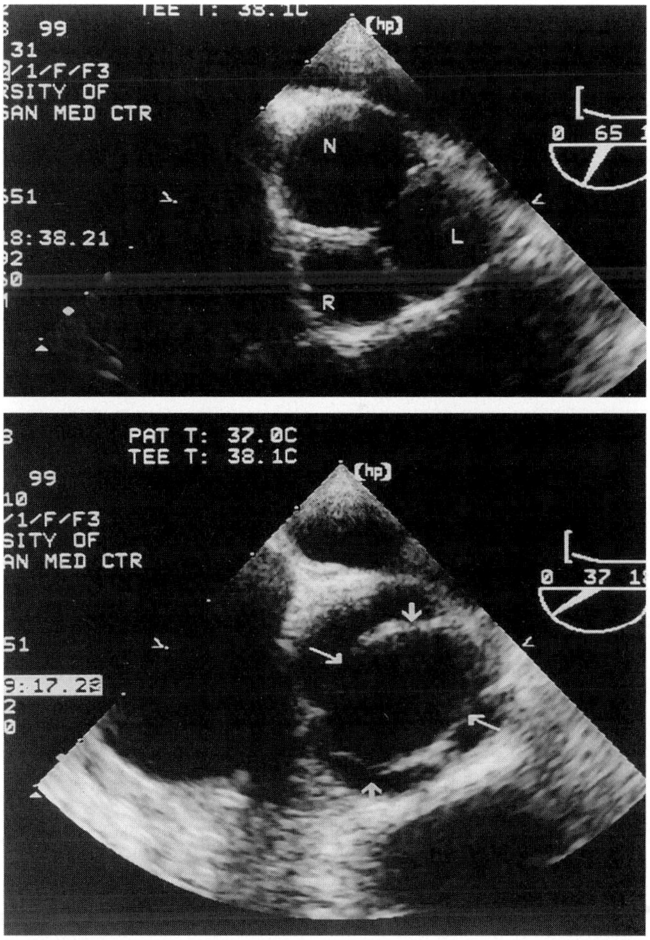

FIGURE 11–64 Transesophageal echocardiogram recorded in a patient with an anatomical three-leaflet valve with a fused commissure resulting in a functional bicuspid aortic valve. In the **top panel,** note the three cusps (N = noncoronary, L = left coronary, R = right coronary). The upper frame was recorded in diastole, and the closure lines would suggest the presence of three leaflets. The **lower panel** is recorded in systole, and instead of opening fully to the margins of the aorta with a circular orifice, the valve opens with an oval, fishmouth-shaped orifice. Note that the commissure between the right and left cusps is fused, resulting in a functionally bicuspid valve.

Rheumatic aortic stenosis typically results in leaflet thickening along the commissural edges. It will be seen almost exclusively in the presence of rheumatic mitral stenosis.

Once aortic stenosis is anatomically defined, secondary effects can also be evaluated. These include poststenotic dilation of the aorta and left ventricular hypertrophy. Assessment of left ventricular systolic function should also be undertaken.

Assessment of Severity. Doppler echocardiography is essential for assessment of the physiological significance of aortic stenosis (Fig. 11-65). In cases of clinically significant aortic stenosis, the gradient is likely to exceed 50 mm Hg. This corresponds to a Doppler velocity of approximately 3.5 m/sec, which is out of the range for accurate quantitation using pulsed-wave Doppler. For this reason, continuous-wave Doppler is essential for quantitation. From continuous-wave Doppler, both instantaneous peak and mean gradients can be determined using the Bernoulli equation. Either on-line or off-line outlining of the spectral display and automatic calculation of these values can be performed. In some instances, determination of the gradient at rest and with exercise may be beneficial. The gradients determined from Doppler echocardiography correlate very well with simultaneously determined invasive measurements. This correlation is maximal during simultaneous measurement and when micromanometer tip catheters are used (Fig. 11-66).[106] The commonly measured "peak to peak" gradient determined in the catheterization laboratory has no basis in physiological reality and will not correspond to either a peak instantaneous or a mean gradient determined by either micromanometer catheters or Doppler interrogation. In most instances, cardiac output and hence stroke volume are augmented in the catheterization laboratory compared with rest. For this reason, Doppler-determined gradients in the echocardiography laboratory may be lower than a catheterization-determined gradient. In asymptomatic patients, it may be beneficial to assess the aortic valve gradient at rest and with exercise.

On occasion, the Doppler gradient significantly underestimates the measured gradient. This is common with nonsimultaneous recordings, as noted earlier, but also occurs when the angle of interrogation (θ) exceeds 20 degrees. Off-angle interrogation is the single most common cause for underestimation of an aortic stenosis gradient. In instances in which there is a serial obstruction consisting of both valvular and subvalvular obstruction, both the V1 and the V2 component of the Bernoulli equation must be incorporated.

The actual valve orifice is usually not visualized to a reliable degree from TTE. TEE can be used to obtain a direct measurement of the aortic valve orifice in many patients with aortic stenosis. In cases of severe aortic stenosis, the orifice may be highly irregular and not all portions of it may lie in the same plane. With scrupulous attention to detail, it is possible in many instances to directly planimeter the area (Fig. 11-67).[107]

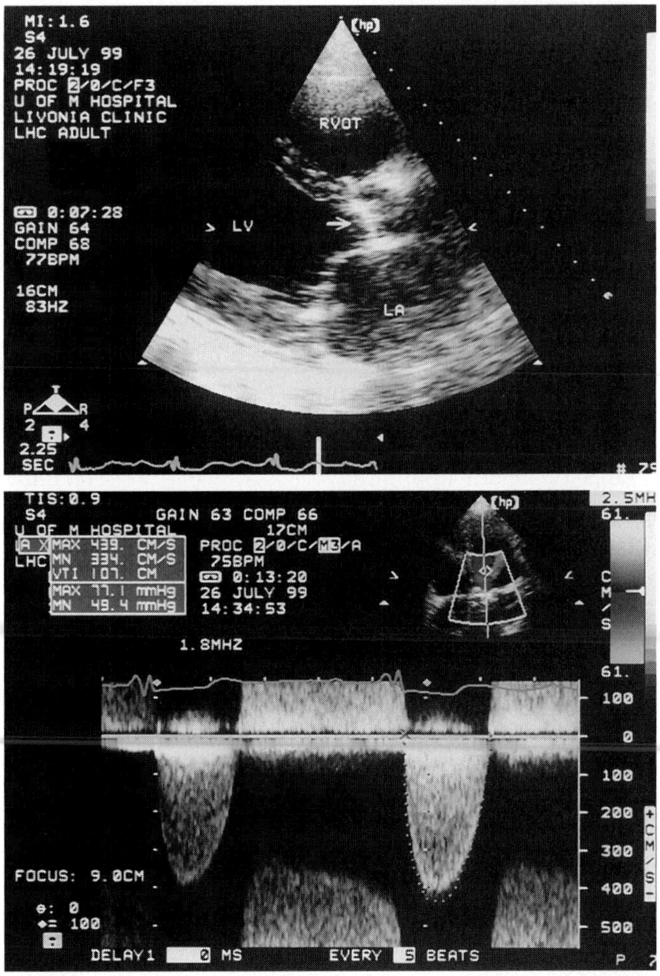

FIGURE 11–65 Echocardiogram recorded in a patient with severe aortic stenosis. The **top panel** is a parasternal long-axis view recorded in systole. Left ventricular function is diminished. The aortic valve is markedly thickened and partially calcified. Its motion is markedly reduced and in systole it appears that the valve occludes the orifice (arrow). The **lower panel** is a continuous-wave Doppler recorded from the apex of the left ventricle along a line aimed through the stenotic aortic valve. Note the aortic stenosis signal below the zero crossing line. The peak velocity is 430 cm/sec, which corresponds to a maximum gradient of 77 mm Hg and a mean gradient of 49.4 mm Hg. LA = left atrium; LV = left ventricle; RVOT = right ventricular outflow tract.

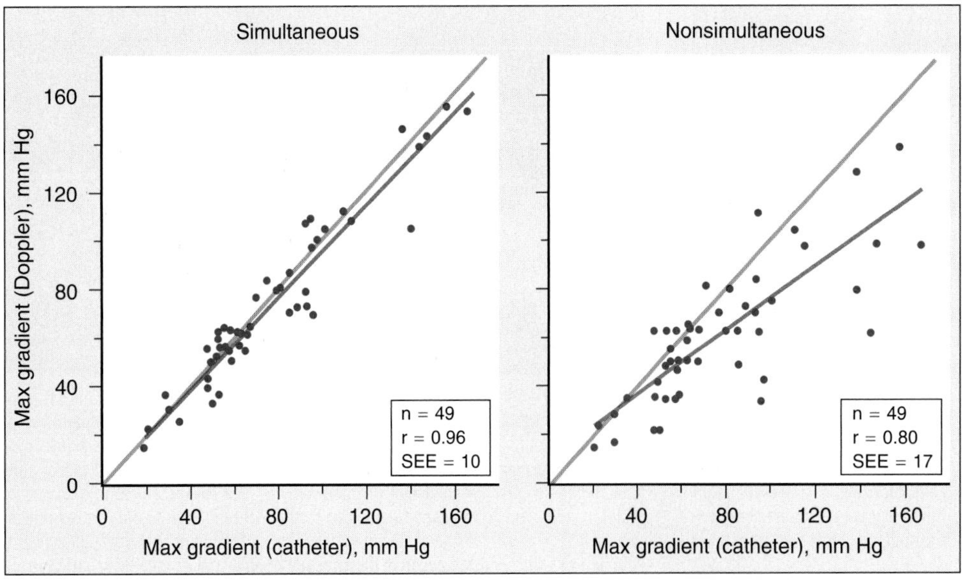

FIGURE 11–66 Graphic comparison of Doppler- and catheterization-determined gradients in patients with aortic stenosis. On the **left** are simultaneously recorded gradients and on the **right** are nonsimultaneous gradients. Note the stronger correlation between Doppler and catheterization when gradients are obtained in a simultaneous manner. (From Currie PJ, Hagler DJ, Seward JB, et al: Instantaneous pressure gradient: A simultaneous Doppler and dual catheter correlative study. J Am Coll Cardiol 7:800, 1986; with permission from the American College of Cardiology Foundation.)

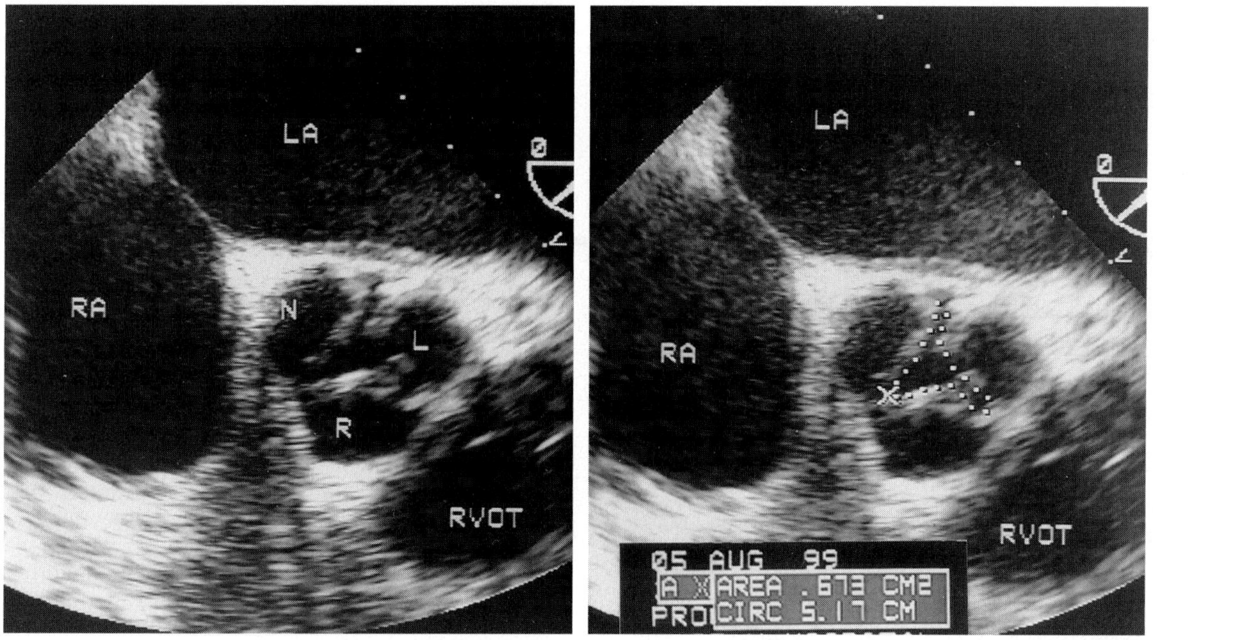

FIGURE 11–67 Transesophageal echocardiogram recorded in a patient with severe aortic stenosis. In the **left panel,** note the three aortic valve cusps (N = noncoronary, L = left coronary, R = right coronary). The leaflets are diffusely thickened and have restricted opening motion. The **right panel** is the same systolic frame in which the stenotic area of the aortic valve has been planimetered. Note that the area of the aortic valve is calculated as 0.67 cm^2, consistent with severe aortic stenosis. LA = left atrium; RA = right atrium; RVOT = right ventricular outflow tract.

An additional method for determining the aortic valve area relies on the continuity equation (Figs. 11-34 and 11-68).[108] Typically, in aortic stenosis, the left ventricular outflow tract area can be determined, assuming circular geometry. Pulsed Doppler is then used to determine the velocity of flow at that site. The product of the two is volumetric flow in the outflow tract. At the stenotic orifice, continuous-wave Doppler is used to determine the velocity integral. The algebraic equation can then be solved for the aortic valve area. A modification of this technique uses mitral valve flow instead of left ventricular outflow. Because the velocity of flow increases at the restrictive orifice, several investigators have suggested using the V1/V2 ratio as a marker of significant aortic stenosis. Other methods for determining the severity of aortic stenosis involve calculation of aortic valve resistance[109] and using echo-Doppler data in variations of the Gorlin formula.

From a practical standpoint, it is often not necessary to determine an aortic valve area. In a patient with thickened restricted leaflets and a mean gradient exceeding 50 mm Hg, the presence of severe aortic stenosis is clinically assured. Likewise, in a patient with normal ventricular function and a low peak gradient (20-25 mm Hg), the likelihood of significant aortic stenosis becomes negligible. Patients with reduced left ventricular function, typically with a left ventricular ejection fraction of 25 to 35 percent, and a modest transvalvular gradient of 25 to 30 mm Hg are problematic. This situation may either represent mild aortic valve disease and unrelated left ventricular dysfunction or, conversely, critical aortic stenosis with secondary left ventricular dysfunction. In the latter situation, patients will benefit from aortic valve replacement, whereas for the former situation, medical management is indicated. Dobutamine infusion, while monitoring left ventricular function and transvalvular gradients, can be a useful means for separating these two entities.[110] If left ventricular function augments with a dobutamine infusion and the gradient increases to clinically pertinent levels, the diagnosis is most likely severe aortic stenosis with secondary left ventricular dysfunction, and these patients will benefit from valve replacement. Conversely, if ventricular function improves without a change in the gradient, it is less likely that the aortic stenosis is the limiting factor.

AORTIC REGURGITATION. Detection and quantitation of aortic regurgitation rely predominantly on Doppler techniques. Using color flow imaging, the regurgitant jet can be visualized in the left ventricular outflow tract from several different planes (Fig. 11–69). In the majority of instances, there is an underlying anatomical abnormality of the aortic valve such as endocarditis, disease of the aortic root, rheumatic valve disease, or a bicuspid valve.

Several features of the regurgitant jet have been investigated as markers of the severity of aortic regurgitation.[111] Unlike mitral regurgitation, in which the overall jet size correlates well with regurgitation severity, neither the overall size nor the depth of penetration of the aortic regurgitation jet correlates strongly with the severity of aortic regurgitation. This is in large part due to the difficulty in separating the regurgitant flow stream from mitral valve inflow. A greater degree of success has been obtained by measuring either the width or the cross-sectional area of the regurgitant jet in the outflow tract and indexing this to the width or cross-sectional area of the outflow tract (Fig. 11–70). These measurements are dependent on imaging the jet in its true minor axis, and an eccentric jet, crossing tangentially across the outflow tract, will result in a disproportionately sized jet compared with its true dimension. TEE often provides more accurate visualization of the true direction and size of the regurgitant jet.

Assessment of Severity. By using continuous-wave Doppler from the apex, one can record the actual flow velocity profile of the regurgitant jet (Fig. 11-71). The velocity of the regurgitant jet is directly related to pressure gradient between the aorta and the left ventricle. If this gradient remains high throughout diastole, the slope of velocity and pressure decay is relatively flat. This implies a relatively mild degree of aortic regurgitation in which there has been little equilibration of aortic and left ventricular diastolic pressures. Conversely, with severe aortic regurgitation (especially if acute), there is a greater degree of equilibration of left ventricular and aortic diastolic pressures and the terminal aortic regurgitation velocities are relatively low, resulting in a fairly steep slope of velocity decay over the diastolic pressure curve. The pressure half-time of the regurgitant jet, defined as the time in milliseconds required for the initial transvalvular diastolic gradient to decline to one half of its peak value, can be calculated and is inversely related to the severity of aortic regurgitation. A pressure half-time less than 400 msec correlates with severe aortic regurgitation. In high-quality studies, the continuity equation can be used to calculate the aortic regurgitant volume. It should be noted that any concurrent disease that also increases left ventricular diastolic pressure will also cause a steeper slope of the aortic regurgitation flow signal. Quantitation of aortic regurgitation has also been performed using the proximal isovelocity surface area method.

Several secondary Doppler and anatomical features should also be noted in cases of aortic regurgitation. The proximal aorta often has progressive dilation with long-standing aortic regurgitation.[112] Left ventricu-

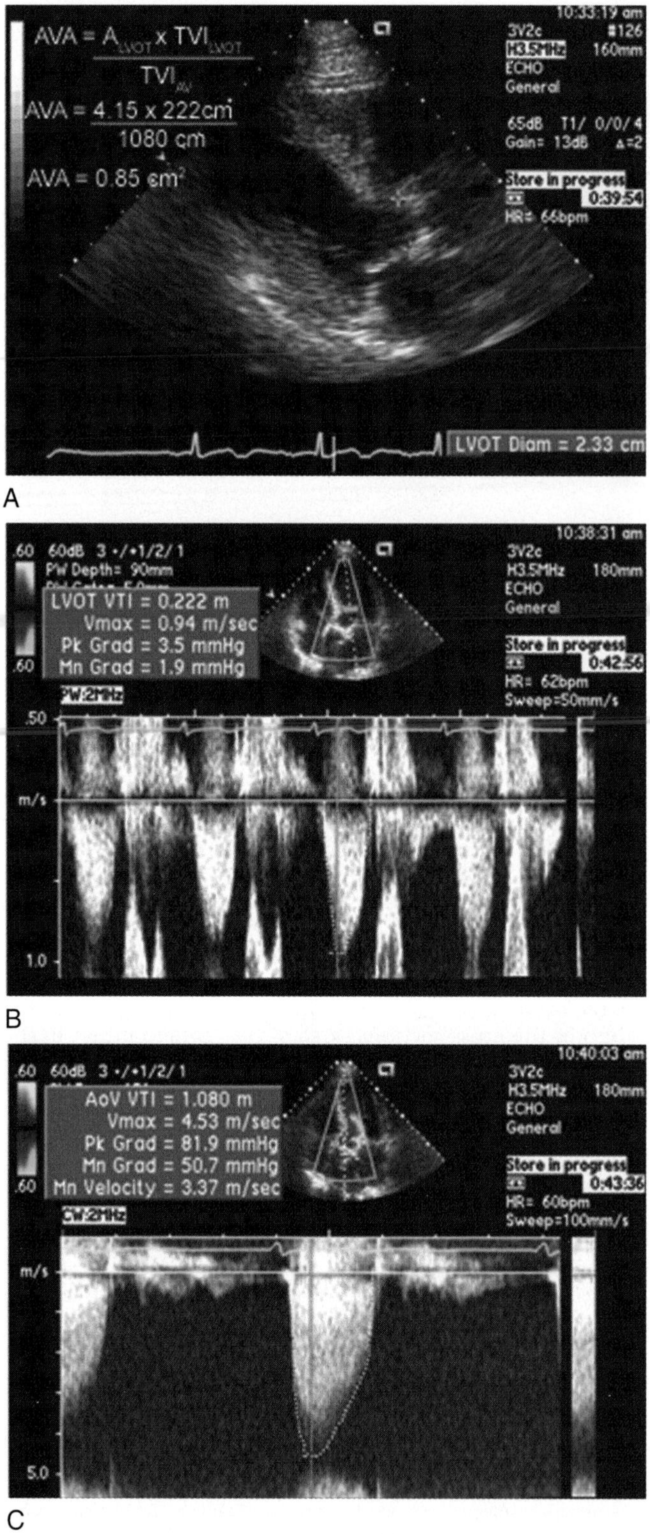

FIGURE 11–68 Transthoracic echocardiogram demonstrating the continuity equation for determining aortic valve area (AVA) in aortic stenosis. **A,** Parasternal long-axis view in which the thickened aortic valve can be appreciated; the left ventricular outflow tract diameter is measured as 2.33 cm. The overall calculations for AVA are presented in the text superimposed in the figure. **B,** Time-velocity integral (TVI) recorded from an apical four-chamber view with a sample volume in the left ventricular outflow tract (LVOT). The TVI is 222 cm. **C,** Spectral continuous wave Doppler of the aortic stenosis jet from which a peak gradient of 81.9 mm Hg and a TVI of 1080 cm are obtained. The calculation of aortic valve area is as noted in the text superimposed on the upper panel. In this instance, the aortic valve area calculates to 0.85 cm^2.

lar dilation is a natural consequence of long-standing hemodynamically significant aortic regurgitation. Left ventricular size can be normal in the acute phase. With moderate and severe aortic regurgitation, diastolic flow reversal in the descending thoracic aorta can frequently be detected from the suprasternal notch. Two-dimensional echocardiography often reveals an indentation of the anterior mitral valve leaflet during diastole. This is due to the impinging regurgitant jet that distorts the symmetrical opening pattern of the mitral leaflet. This is typically seen only in cases of moderate and severe aortic insufficiency. With M-mode echocardiography, fine high-velocity flutter of the anterior mitral leaflet and occasionally the septum can be appreciated (Fig. 11-72). Table 11-4 outlines many of these findings as they relate to the severity of aortic insufficiency.

Timing of Surgery. Aortic valve replacement is the most appropriate therapy in virtually all patients with symptomatic aortic regurgitation. Echocardiography also plays a significant role in the evaluation of these patients and in the timing of surgery in many asymptomatic patients. This decision is based largely on left ventricular size and performance rather than on the Doppler assessment of severity. Traditional echocardiographic findings that represent indications for surgery have included dilation of the left ventricle beyond 75 mm in diastole or beyond 55 mm in systole in association with fractional shortening or ejection fraction below the normal range (see Chap. 57). Additionally, a serial decline in left ventricular ejection fraction or progressive dilation of the left ventricle of 1.0 cm or more over a 12-month duration typically represents an indication for valve replacement.

Tricuspid Valve Disease

TRICUSPID REGURGITATION. Probably due to the complex closure pattern of the tricuspid valve, minimal and mild degrees of tricuspid regurgitation are commonly seen in normal disease-free individuals. The most common form of tricuspid valve disease is annular dilation due to right-sided heart overload, resulting in abnormal leaflet coaptation and tricuspid regurgitation. This is typically secondary to pulmonary hypertension, which most commonly is due to left-sided heart pathology. Tricuspid regurgitation due to annular dilation can be the result of virtually any form of heart disease that results in elevation of right ventricular pressure or volume. In these cases, the tricuspid valve typically appears anatomically normal but is found to be regurgitant. Quantitation of tricuspid regurgitation is done in a manner similar to that for mitral regurgitation and in clinical practice usually is a qualitative assessment (Fig. 11–73).[113] Minimal and mild degrees of tricuspid regurgitation are nearly ubiquitous in adult populations, even in the absence of identifiable structural heart disease. Moderate and severe tricuspid regurgitation and tricuspid regurgitation in association with elevated right ventricular systolic pressure are

TABLE 11–4 Aortic Insufficiency Severity*

	I	II	III	IV
Jet height (%LVOT)	<25	25-46	47-64	>65
Jet area/LVOT (short axis) (%)	<5	5-24	25-59	≥60
Reversal in descending aorta?	No	No	—	Yes
Spectral density	Faint	—	—	Dense
Pressure half-time (msec)	>400	—	—	≤250
Mitral preclosure?	No	—	—	Yes

LVOT = left ventricular outflow tract.

*For some parameters, the observation is valid at the extremes of mitral regurgitation severity and there may be marked overlap in intermediate (grades II, III) mitral regurgitation. In these instances, no value is presented.

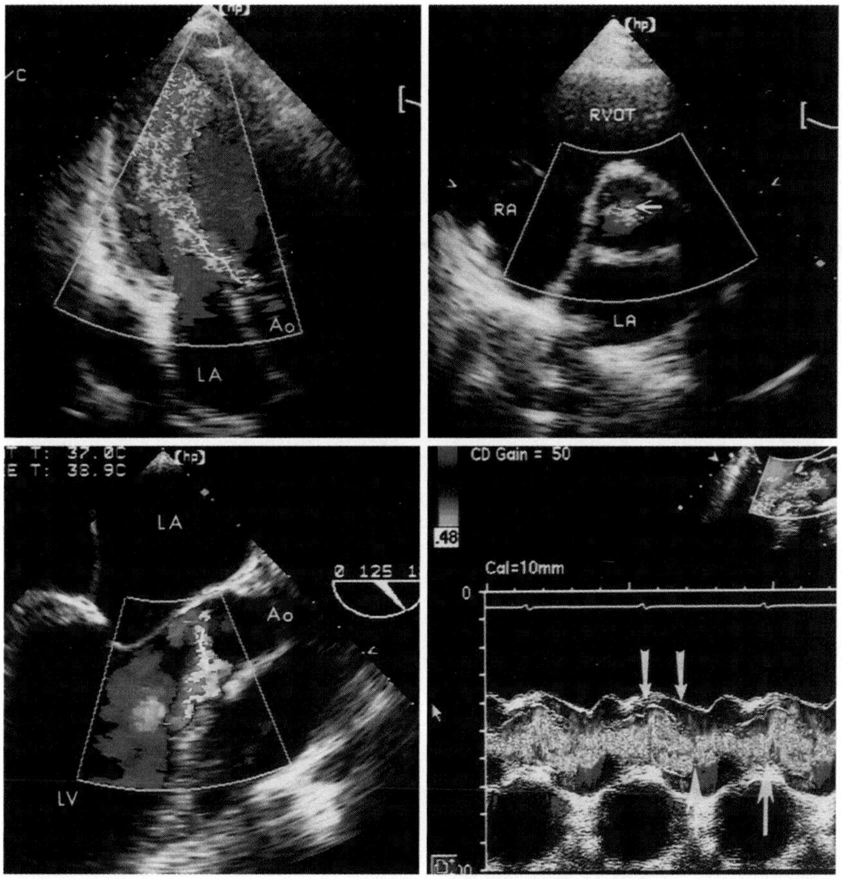

FIGURE 11–69 Composite of echocardiograms recorded in patients with aortic regurgitation. The two **top panels** were recorded in the same patient and show, on the left, an apical long-axis view and, on the right, a parasternal short-axis view. In the apical long-axis view, note the fairly extensive confetti-like aortic regurgitation jet arising from the proximal aorta and traversing to the left ventricular apex. Note also that the aortic regurgitation jet velocities merge with the mitral inflow velocities, rendering quantitation problematic. The **top right panel** is recorded in the same patient and shows a central aortic regurgitation jet. The **bottom left panel** is a transesophageal echocardiogram recorded in a longitudinal view. Note the highly eccentric aortic regurgitation jet that appears to fill the entire width of the left ventricular outflow tract. This apparent filling of the left ventricular outflow tract is due to the posterior to anterior jet direction (white arrow) rather than to a substantial true width of the jet. The **bottom right panel** is a color M-mode echocardiogram recorded in a patient with aortic insufficiency in which the normal systolic flow can be appreciated as well as a continuous diastolic flow in the lumen of the aorta that represents aortic insufficiency. The two downward pointing arrows denote the duration of systole, and the two upward pointing arrows indicate the duration of diastole. Ao = aorta; LA = left atrium; LV = left ventricle; RA = right atrium; RVOT = right ventricular outflow tract.

typically associated with cardiac pathology. Primary tricuspid valve disease can result in tricuspid regurgitation as well. Involvement by rheumatic heart disease, endocarditis, trauma with rupture of a papillary muscle, Ebstein anomaly, radiation heart disease, carcinoid heart disease, and tricuspid valve prolapse all have characteristic anatomical features that result in regurgitation. TEE can be useful in determining the feasibility of tricuspid valve repair. Carcinoid heart disease is a rare abnormality but has classic echocardiographic features (Fig. 11–74). In this syndrome, the leaflets appear stiffened and immobile. The annulus is secondarily dilated and the leaflets may fail to coapt. This lesion is typically associated with severe tricuspid regurgitation without elevation in right ventricular systolic pressure.

Irrespective of the cause of tricuspid regurgitation, one can capitalize on this lesion to calculate right ventricular systolic pressure, as noted in the section on Doppler calculations.[18-20] In the absence of obstruction to right ventricular outflow, this pressure equals pulmonary artery systolic pressure (see Fig. 11–31). Calculation of right ventricular systolic pressure can be measured both at rest and with exercise and is a valuable means of noninvasively determining pulmonary artery systolic pressures.

TRICUSPID STENOSIS. Isolated tricuspid stenosis is a very rare clinical entity. Tricuspid stenosis can be seen in individuals with rheumatic heart disease, in which case concurrent mitral stenosis will invariably be present. The carcinoid syndrome can result in tricuspid stenosis as well. Calculation of transvalvular gradients across the tricuspid valve is done in a manner identical to that for the mitral valve. In the majority of cases, tricuspid valve stenosis is associated with regurgitation.

Pulmonic Valve Disease

Primary disease of the pulmonic valve is uncommon in adult patients. Occasional patients with pulmonic stenosis (Fig. 11–75), either in isolation or in combination with other congenital lesions, may be encountered in the practice of adult cardiology. Congenital pulmonic stenosis results in thickening of the leaflets and restricted motion on two-dimensional echocardiography. Because the orientation of the pulmonary outflow tract is anterior to posterior, Doppler interrogation is quite easily performed within an angle of integration (θ) close to 0 degrees. The degree of stenosis and regurgitation across the pulmonic valve is determined in a manner analogous to that for the aortic valve. In the presence of pulmonic regurgitation, the pressure gradient between the pulmonary artery and right ventricle in diastole can be calculated, and from this an estimate of pulmonary artery diastolic pressure can be obtained.[114] This is done by calcu-

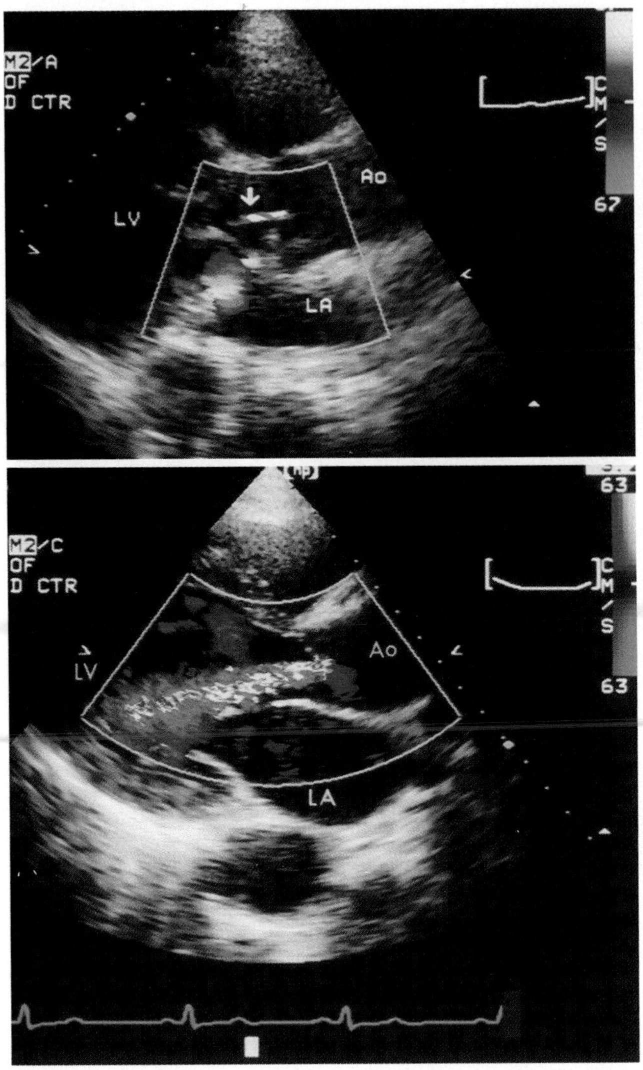

FIGURE 11–70 Parasternal long-axis two-dimensional echocardiograms in a patient with minimal **(top)** and a patient with moderate **(bottom)** aortic regurgitation. In the top panel, note the thin color jet of aortic regurgitation that fills less than 10 percent of the left ventricular outflow tract, compared with the wider aortic insufficiency profile, filling more than one third of the left ventricular outflow tract in the lower panel. Ao = aorta; LA = left atrium; LV = left ventricle.

lating the end-diastolic pulmonary artery–to–right ventricular gradient and adding an assumed right ventricular diastolic pressure.

Several characteristic patterns of pulmonary valve motion should be recognized on M-mode echocardiography. The first is that of pulmonic stenosis in which there is an augmented "a" wave but otherwise normal motion. In the presence of infundibular stenosis, coarse fluttering of the pulmonic valve is seen. In the presence of significant pulmonary hypertension, there is midsystolic notching of the pulmonic valve and loss of the pulmonary valve "a" wave. These findings are qualitative and may be seen only in the more advanced cases. In modern practice, determination of pulmonary artery hemodynamics relies heavily on Doppler interrogation.

Evaluation of the right ventricular outflow tract or pulmonary artery Doppler flow profile can provide valuable clues in patients with known or suspected pulmonary hypertension. Normally, after the onset of ejection, pulmonary artery flow reaches its maximum velocity 120 to 160 msec after the onset of ejection. In cases of pulmonary hypertension, this acceleration time is progressively shortened (Fig. 11–76). There is a linear and inverse correlation between the ejection time, defined as the time from onset of ejection to reaching peak velocity, and pulmonary artery systolic and mean pressures. In general, a pulmonary artery acceleration time less than 70 msec implies presence of a pulmonary artery systolic pressure exceeding 70 mm Hg. Other findings in pulmonary hypertension include notching of the pulmonary artery flow profile on spectral Doppler.

Miscellaneous Valvular Heart Diseases

Several miscellaneous forms of valvular heart disease deserve comment. Recently, attention has been drawn to the association between the use of anorectic drugs, particularly the combination of phentermine and fenfluramine (PhenFen), and development of valvular heart disease.[115,116] The exact incidence of diet drug–related valvular heart disease is unknown. Most studies have suggested that the predominant lesions are similar to that seen in carcinoid or ergot heart disease. The leaflets of the mitral valve and chordae appear thickened and immobile, and mitral regurgitation is present. Aortic insufficiency also has been noted in association with the use of these drugs, and it often appears out of proportion to the anatomical abnormalities noted on the aortic valve. Recent studies have suggested that these lesions may regress after exposure to the drugs has terminated.[117]

Radiation therapy can result in valvular dysfunction, most often thickening and insufficiency. The severity of the valvular insufficiency is dependent on the degree of anatomical damage to the valve, and the precise valves involved are dependent entirely on the radiation portal and dose. Typically, more anterior structures are involved and there may be concurrent myocardial dysfunction due to radiation myocarditis.

EVALUATION OF PROSTHETIC HEART VALVES

Modern echocardiographic techniques play a role in both preoperative and postoperative management of patients with prosthetic heart valves. Two-dimensional echocardiography can be used to determine the appropriate prosthesis size to implant in the aortic position and the need for additional procedures, such as aortic annuloplasty, to enlarge a pathologically small aortic root.[118-120] Evaluation of prosthetic heart valves can be a complex and time-consuming process. Prosthetic heart valves can be divided into three basic groups: mechanical prostheses, such as single or dual disc valves or ball and cage valves; stented bioprostheses, which use either porcine aortic valves or bovine pericardium for valve leaflets; and a newer generation of stentless porcine valves that at this time are approved for use only in the aortic position.[119] Each valve has unique echocardiographic characteristics, and different valves can be evaluated to varying degrees using TTE and TEE. Doppler echocardiography is obviously crucial for determining the presence of regurgitation and the flow characteristics of a valve. It is often not possible to fully evaluate a prosthetic valve with TTE, and TEE is often necessary. This is particularly true for visualization of mitral prostheses. Even with TEE, complete anatomical visualization of an aortic mechanical prosthesis can be problematic. For all but the new stentless aortic prosthesis, the sewing ring is characteristically visualized as an echo-dense circular structure within the appropriate annulus.

The ball and cage valve is typically visualized as an echo-dense sewing ring with three wire struts forming the cage and an echogenic ball moving within the cage. The ball itself may appear either as a spherical structure or as a single echo-dense line in motion. Single-disc mechanical prostheses are visualized as a sewing ring in which the disc can be seen to move. Typically, from the transthoracic route, all one sees is a single, bright echo-dense line with phasic motion during the cardiac cycle above and into the plane of the sewing ring. The discs of a two-disc valve cast a smaller echo signature, and actual disc motion can be difficult to discern from TTE. Using TEE, both leaflets of a two-disc valve are easily visualized in the mitral position and have a characteristic butterfly wing motion (Fig. 11–77). Identifying motion of both leaflets in the aortic position is more problematic. Stented porcine valves are visualized as a sewing ring in which three separate leaflets can be seen. These leaflets have the characteristics of a normal aortic valve. With fibrosis and degeneration or endocarditis, the leaflets may become thickened and brighter than usual (Fig. 11–78). The newer stentless prosthesis and aortic

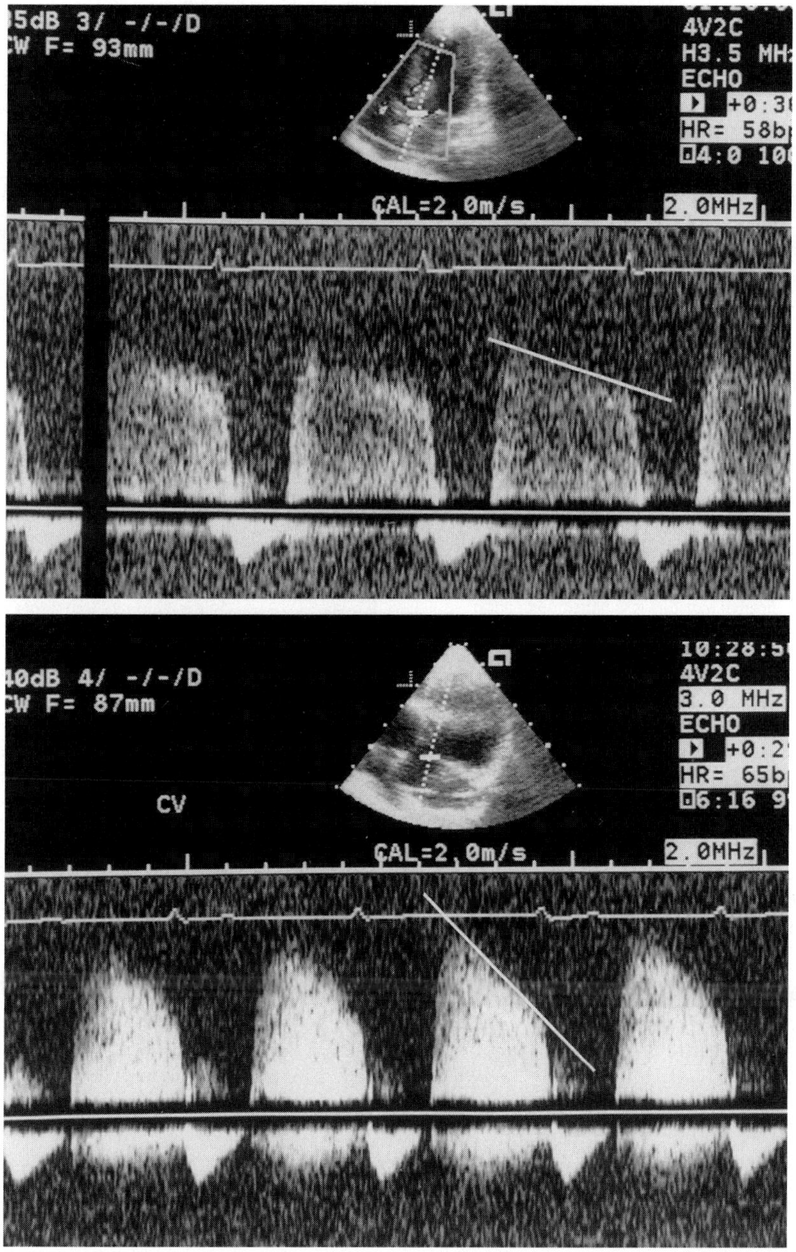

FIGURE 11–71 Continuous-wave spectral recordings of patients with mild **(top)** and severe **(bottom)** aortic insufficiency. Note the relatively flat slope pressure decay and faint spectral signal intensity in the mild insufficiency and a denser spectral signal and steeper slope of pressure decay, denoting near equalization of aortic and left ventricular diastolic pressures, seen in severe aortic insufficiency.

homograft valves can be difficult to distinguish from a native aortic valve. Depending on the implantation technique, there may be few clues as to the presence of a stentless prosthesis other than subtle echodensities at the line of attachment in the annulus or, if implanted within the native aorta, a double-density aortic wall can be seen.

Complete evaluation of prosthetic valves requires detailed Doppler assessment. Color flow imaging is used to determine the presence and severity of regurgitation. The combination of the sewing ring and/or the mechanical valve itself results in substantial reverberation and shadowing and dramatically reduces the ability to interrogate structures posterior to the mechanical prosthesis or sewing ring with Doppler. There is frequently a minimal amount of physiological regurgitation in mechanical prostheses that represents a combination of the closing velocity of the disc or ball and small physiological leaks at the closure lines. It is not uncommon to see minimal degrees of regurgitation in association with a stented or nonstented bioprosthesis. Valvular regurgitation in prosthetic valves can be quite eccentric, and one must use caution in applying rules for determining severity of regurgitation. This is particularly true for paravalvular regurgitation (Fig. 11–79). Three-dimensional echocardiography and Doppler have shown promise for providing incremental information regarding the location and size of a paravalvular leak.

Spectral Doppler is used to determine pressure gradients across prosthetic valves. Stentless bioprostheses behave in a manner nearly identical to native aortic valves and typically have a peak gradient of 10 to 15 mm Hg. Because of narrowing of the outflow tract by a sewing ring, a stented prosthesis often has a higher transvalvular gradient. The magnitude of this gradient is dependent on both flow and the size of the valve. Because of the wide range of anticipated gradients, it is crucial to establish a baseline for prosthetic valves at a time when they are known to be functioning normally. This avoids the problem of subsequent detection of a peak gradient that can be as high as 50 mm Hg. This may be due to the combination of a high flow state and a narrow orifice because of the sewing ring and may not represent valve deterioration. Doppler evaluation for the gradient across a mechanical prosthesis is complicated by several factors, including phenomena of localized gradients and pressure recovery.[121,122] As flow accelerates through the noncircular orifice of a mechanical prosthesis, there are areas of rapid flow acceleration that occur over very short distances. This acceleration results in instantaneous

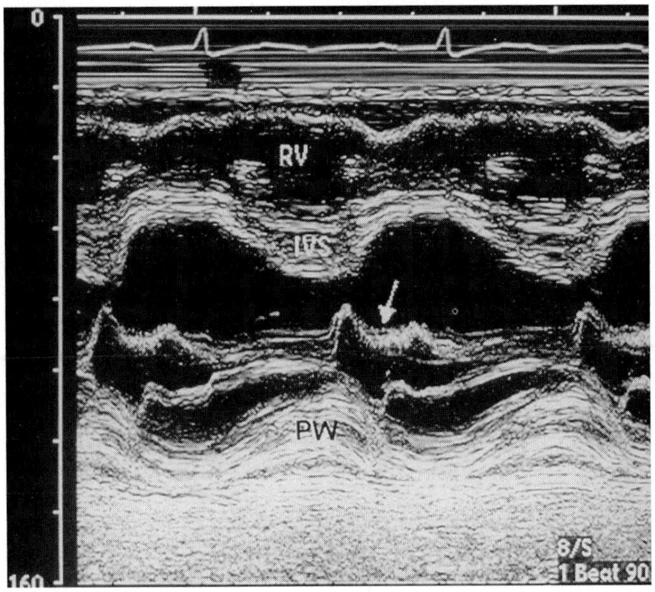

FIGURE 11–72 M-mode echocardiogram recorded in a patient with aortic insufficiency. Note the fine fluttering of the mitral valve leaflet secondary to impingement by the aortic insufficiency jet. IVS = interventricular septum; PW = posterior wall; RV = right ventricle.

peak velocities of 3 to 4 m/sec, corresponding to gradients of 36 to 64 mm Hg. These pressure gradients occur over a very limited distance (1-2 mm) within the sewing ring and do not reflect the true left ventricular-to-proximal aorta pressure difference measured in the hemodynamic laboratory. As with a stented bioprosthesis, it is crucial to obtain an early baseline pressure gradient across a mechanical prosthesis at a time when it is known to function normally for subsequent comparison. This is best done by performing a full echocardiographic and Doppler examination at the time of the first follow-up visit after implantation.

Dysfunction of prosthetic valves occurs due to valvular dehiscence, in which case a paravalvular leak can be seen (see Fig. 11-79), or there may be endocarditis, thrombosis, or pannus interfering with motion of a mechanical valve. Typically, either stenosis or regurgitation can occur. If the mechanical valve becomes obstructed by pannus, vegetation, or thrombus, the transvalvular gradient typically will increase, although in some instances it may remain stable or even decline. Regurgitation is usually seen in conjunction with restriction of the leaflet unless the leaflet has been restricted in a fully closed position. In cases of suspected dysfunction of a prosthesis, TEE adds incremental value and is essential for complete evaluation.

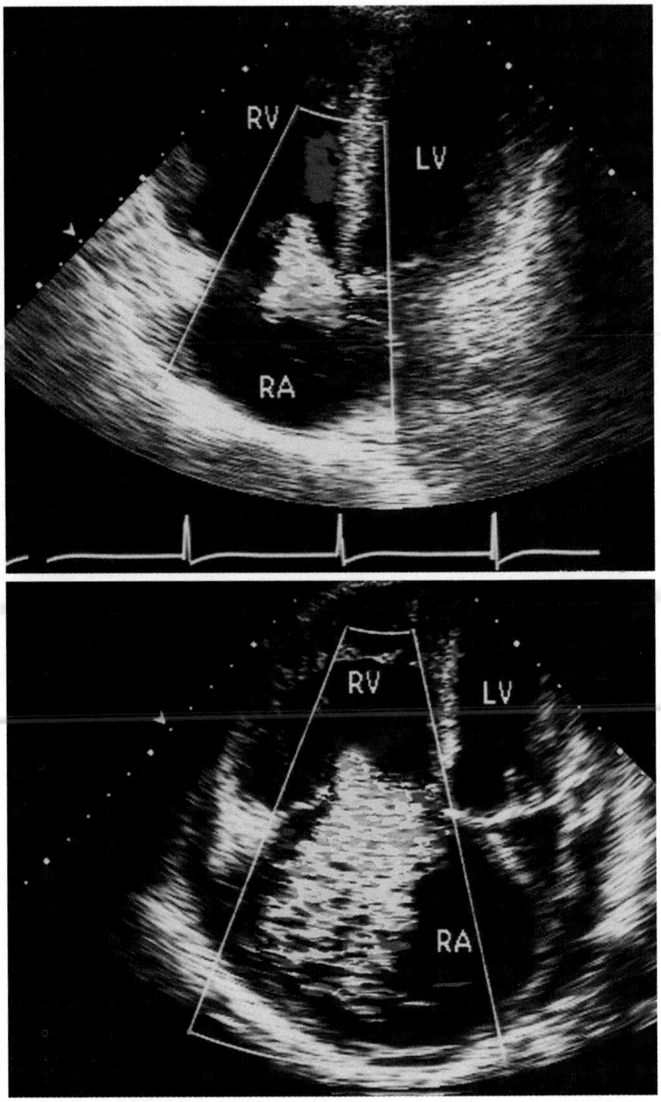

FIGURE 11–73 Two-dimensional echocardiograms with color flow imaging of patients with tricuspid regurgitation. **Top,** Echocardiogram is recorded in a patient with a mild degree of tricuspid insufficiency. **Bottom,** Echocardiogram of a patient with severe tricuspid regurgitation. LV = left ventricle; RA = right atrium; RV = right ventricle.

ASSESSMENT OF MITRAL VALVE REPAIR

Transesophageal echocardiography has been instrumental in determining the success of mitral valve repair. The preoperative echocardiogram is highly reliable as a means for determining which patients are candidates for mitral valve repair, and intraoperative monitoring is an integral part of the surgical routine in determining success of repair. From a surgical perspective, the mitral valve is considered to have two leaflets, each with three scallops. The anterior leaflet scallops are designated A1, A2, A3 and the posterior scallops P1, P2, and P3. Each scallop can be viewed from many transesophageal imaging planes.[123,124] In general, patients with elongated redundant valves, those with pathological lesions of the posterior leaflet, and those with smaller vegetations or perforations are excellent candidates for mitral valve repair. Patients with a rheumatic origin of their condition and those with fibrotic leaflets are less likely to have good long-term results.

The postoperative transesophageal echocardiogram is used to determine transvalvular gradients to exclude iatrogenic mitral stenosis and determine the degree, if any, of residual mitral regurgitation. Other adverse sequelae of mitral valve repair include development of dynamic left ventricular outflow tract obstruction, which likewise can be assessed with TEE before the patient is removed from the operating room. Figures 11–58 and 11–80 are examples from a patient before and after successful mitral valve repair.

Infective Endocarditis (see Chap. 58)

Infective endocarditis represents an invasive infection, usually by a bacterial organism of the endothelial lining of the heart, most commonly on one of the four cardiac valves. Left-sided valves are more commonly involved than right-sided valves. The echocardiographic hallmark of bacterial endocarditis is formation of a vegetation on a valvular surface. Pathologically, a vegetation consists of a combination of thrombus, necrotic valvular debris, inflammatory material, and bacteria. Over time, a vegetation may become sterile, at which point only the residua of the inflammatory response with variable degrees of the thrombotic component persist. By echocardiography, a vegetation has the appearance of an irregularly shaped oscillating mass attached to a valve leaflet (Figs. 11–81 and 11–82). Classically, these are seen on the

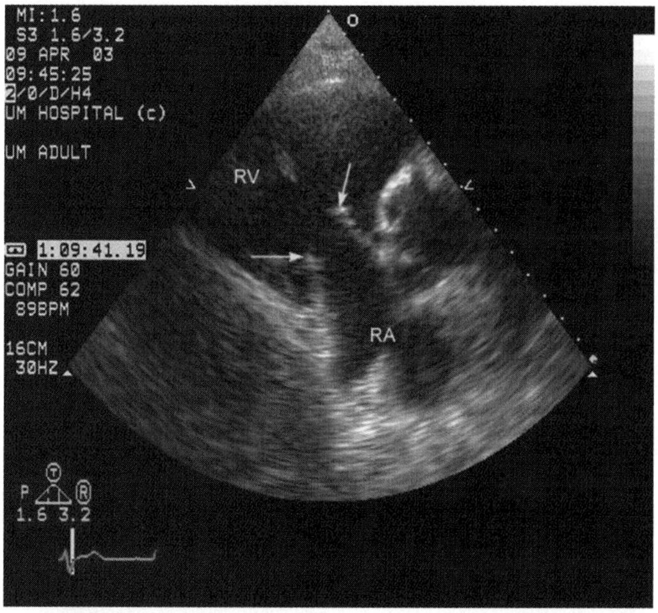

FIGURE 11–74 Right ventricular inflow tract view recorded in a patient with carcinoid disease and tricuspid regurgitation. The right atrium (RA) and right ventricle (RV) are both visualized in this systolic frame. The tricuspid valve leaflets are abnormally dense and immobile. In this systolic frame, the leaflets fail to coapt with the leaflet tip separated by approximately 2 cm. In real time, the leaflets are nearly immobile.

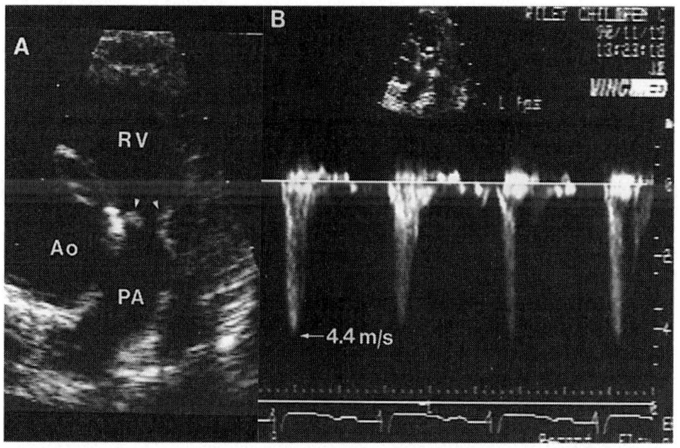

FIGURE 11–75 Two-dimensional **(A)** and continuous-wave Doppler **(B)** recorded in a patient with valvular pulmonic stenosis. The two-dimensional study shows a thickened pulmonic valve with restricted motion (arrowheads). The continuous-wave Doppler shows a peak velocity of 4.4 m/sec, which is consistent with a systolic gradient of approximately 78 mm Hg. Ao = aorta; PA = pulmonary artery; RV = right ventricle. (From Feigenbaum H: Echocardiography. 5th ed. Malvern, PA, Lea & Febiger, 1994.)

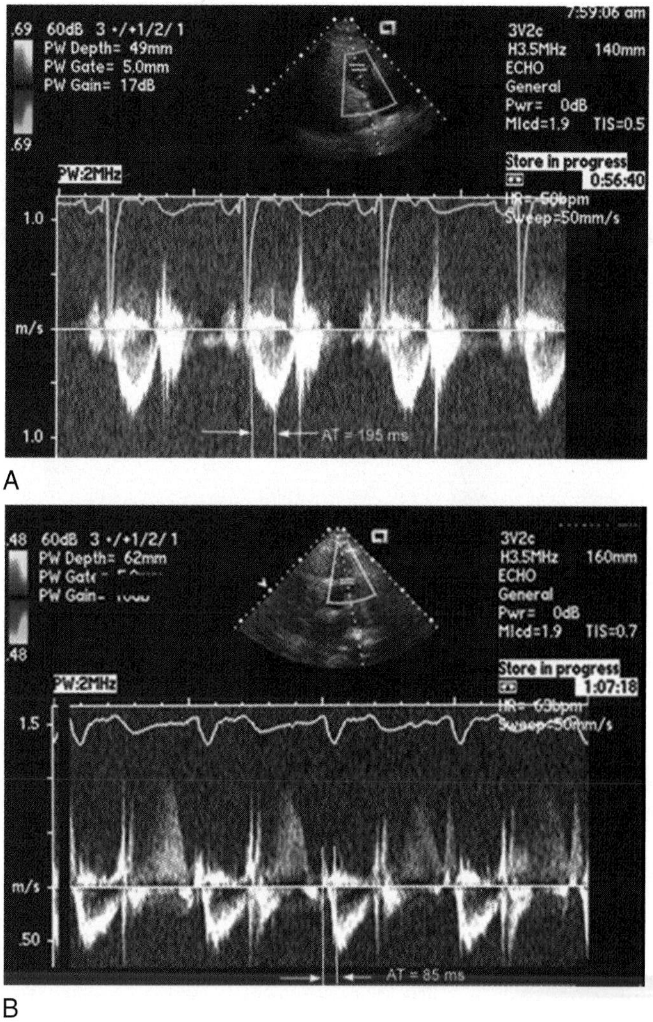

FIGURE 11–76 Pulsed-wave Doppler in the right ventricular outflow tract demonstrating the impact of pulmonary hypertension of the contour of the outflow tract signal. **A,** Signal from a normal individual. Note the normal acceleration time, defined as the time in milliseconds from onset of ejection to reaching peak velocity. In this instance, the acceleration time is approximately 200 msec. **B,** Recorded in a patient with pulmonary hypertension. Note the shortened acceleration time (85 msec).

downstream, low-pressure side of a valve. Therefore, one typically anticipates a vegetation on the left atrial side of the mitral valve and on the left ventricular outflow tract side of the aortic valve. In reality, larger vegetations can exist on both sides of a valve and atypical locations are not uncommon. In screening for vegetations, small unrelated masses or surface irregularities are not infrequently encountered, and thus the specificity for defining a vegetation is not 100 percent. Several large-scale studies have demonstrated that echocardiography may play an incremental role in rapidly establishing the diagnosis of endocarditis, and at least one algorithm for defining endocarditis has used echocardiography as an intrinsic component of the diagnosis.[125,126] Noninfectious vegetation, such as those seen in association with connective tissue disease, are also detected with echocardiographic imaging.

In addition to detection of a vegetation in patients with suspected endocarditis, echocardiography can be used to determine the functional significance and degree of anatomical impairment due to endocarditis and to evaluate complications of endocarditis. Typically, endocarditis results in valvular regurgitation and only rarely in significant valvular stenosis. Because of the variable location of vegetations and the highly variable degree to which the valvular surface may be interrupted, regurgitant lesions in patients with endocarditis are more often eccentric than seen in other forms of valvular heart disease.

Several studies have attempted to use echocardiographic features of vegetations as a marker for the likelihood of requiring surgery or progressing to heart failure. In general, larger and more mobile vegetations are more likely to be associated with embolic events than are smaller sessile vegetations.[127] Vegetations due to *Staphylococcus aureus* are more likely to result in abscess formation and less likely to be sterilized with antibiotics.

Complications of Endocarditis. Complications include progressive valvular regurgitation leading to congestive heart failure, abscess formation, failure to sterilize, and embolic phenomena. Intracardiac abscesses are most commonly

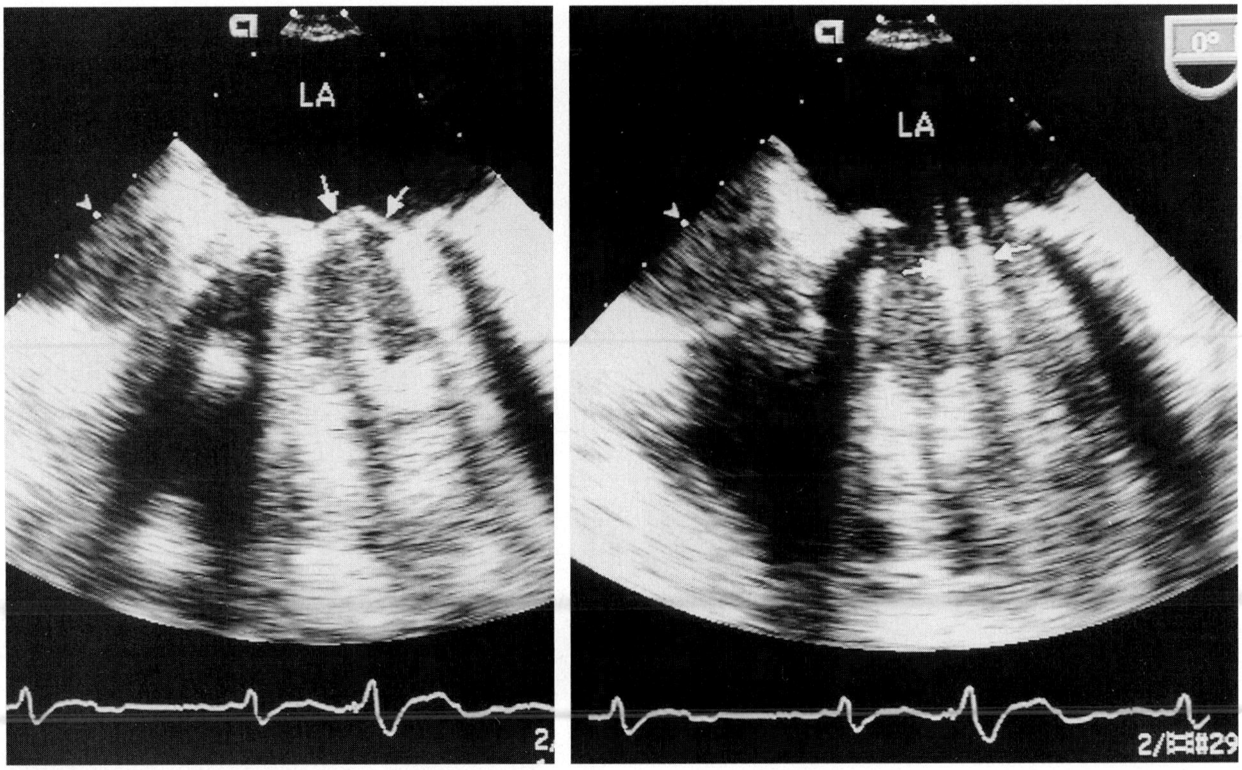

FIGURE 11–77 Transesophageal echocardiogram of a patient with a normally functioning St. Jude mitral valve prosthesis. The scans are recorded at 0 degrees from behind the left atrium. The **left panel** is recorded in systole. Note the two closed leaflets of the prosthetic valve (arrows). The **right panel** is recorded in diastole. Note that the two leaflets now have a parallel position, pointing into the cavity of the left ventricle (arrows). Note the substantial shadowing from the sewing ring and discs, which reduces the ability to visualize the left ventricular cavity. LA = left atrium.

encountered in the relatively avascular areas of the heart. For aortic valve endocarditis, this includes the aorta/mitral valve junction, and for mitral and tricuspid valve disease the annular structures. Less commonly, intramyocardial abscess or abscess within a papillary muscle is encountered.

TRANSESOPHAGEAL ECHOCARDIOGRAPHY. The relative diagnostic value of TTE and TEE has been evaluated in several studies. Because of the higher quality, higher resolution imaging afforded by TEE, virtually all studies have demonstrated an increased sensitivity for detection of vegetations with TEE (see Fig. 11–82). Often the clinical diagnosis of endocarditis has included detection of vegetations, and, thus, many of these studies tend to overstate the sensitivity of TEE. Most studies have also suggested that when a high-quality, entirely normal transthoracic echocardiogram has been obtained in which there is no evidence of valvular mass or thickening and no evidence of pathological regurgitation, the yield in proceeding to TEE is relatively low. Because TEE provides a high-resolution view of the heart, it also detects many limited areas of valvular thickening that are not related to an infectious process. Thus, its specificity for excluding the diagnosis of endocarditis may be less than optimal.

There are several situations in which there is a proven advantage to TEE in patients with endocarditis. Perhaps the most well established is the detection of abscesses, particularly in the aortic root (Fig. 11–83).[128] Data suggest that detection rates from the transthoracic approach are less than 30 percent, whereas sensitivity for detecting an abscess in the aortic root with TEE exceeds 95 percent. Additionally, TEE provides more accurate characterization of the size and mobility of vegetations and detection of multiple vegetations in endocarditis. Finally, TEE is more accurate for determining the cause of valvular regurgitation than is TTE. TEE can identify valvular perforations, ruptured chordae, and flail leaflets with a higher degree of reliability than can TTE.

CALCIFICATION OF THE MITRAL ANNULUS

Fibrosis and calcification of the mitral annulus are common findings with increasing age and can be seen in younger patients with renal disease and other metabolic abnormalities that result in abnormal calcium metabolism (Fig. 11-84). The degree of calcification can range from limited, focal deposits in the annulus to larger deposits resulting in a mass effect. In advanced degrees, the basal aspects of the posterior mitral valve leaflet may be involved. In rare situations, annular calcification can result in functional restriction of the mitral valve orifice and a left atrial-left ventricular pressure gradient. Only in advanced and rare cases does the degree of obstruction result in pressure gradients likely to cause symptoms or result in secondary pulmonary hypertension. More commonly, mitral annular calcification is associated with varying degrees of mitral regurgitation. Heavy annular calcification may result in a lower likelihood of successful valve replacement and is a situation in which paravalvular regurgitation is not uncommon after mitral valve replacement. Statistically, it also has been associated with embolic events and other adverse cardiovascular outcomes.[129]

Congenital Heart Disease (see Chap. 56)

Modern two-dimensional echocardiographic techniques provide a comprehensive means for evaluating virtually all forms of congenital heart disease found in both adults and children. Additionally, echocardiography can be used to evaluate repaired and palliated congenital heart disease. In the modern era, it is unusual for cardiac catheterization or other techniques to be necessary for defining the anatomical anomaly in congenital heart disease. Cardiac magnetic resonance imaging (MRI) may provide incremental information regarding pulmonary artery anatomy and complex venous and great artery connections. Doppler echocardiography often provides the majority of physiological information necessary for the clinical decision-making.

It has become increasingly uncommon to make the diagnosis of congenital heart disease de novo in adult populations. Because of the increased access to well-trained pediatricians, family practitioners, and pediatric cardiologists, the majority of "significant" congenital heart lesions are detected in childhood and adolescence. Thus, the number and nature of lesions "escaping" detection until adulthood has changed over the past several decades. The single most common congenital lesion to be detected in adulthood, other than the bicuspid aortic valve, is the atrial septal defect. There are infrequent cases of ventricular septal defect and other anomalies that escape detection to adulthood. This section deals only with the more common entities likely to be encountered in adult populations and evaluation of the more common repaired and palliated lesions.

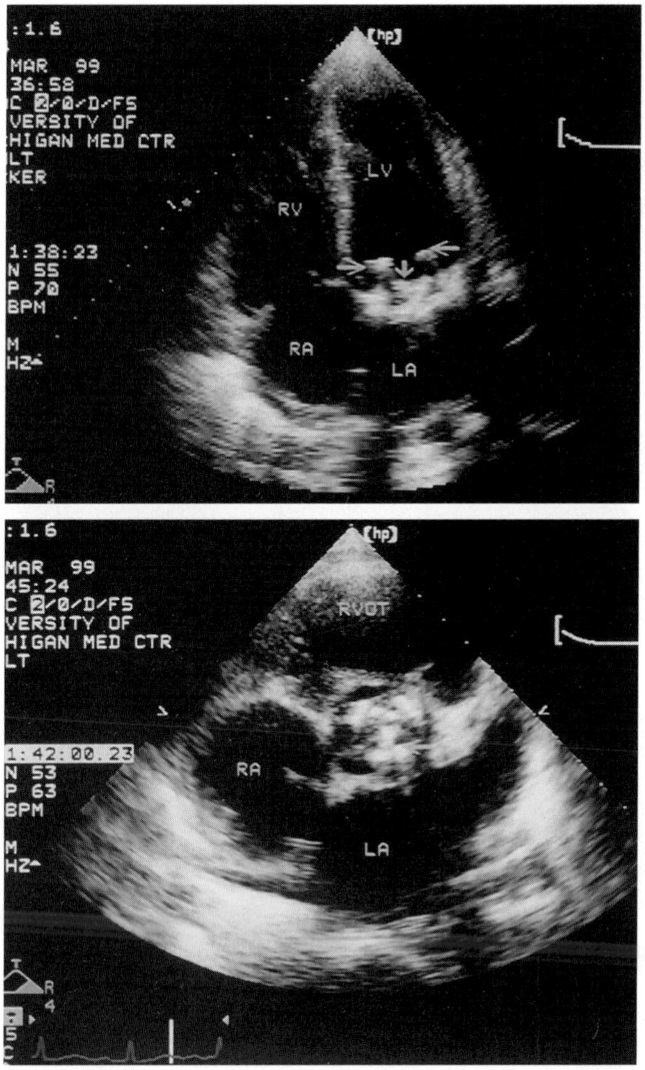

FIGURE 11–78 Apical four-chamber **(top)** and parasternal short-axis views **(bottom)** recorded in a patient with stented porcine bioprostheses in the mitral **(top)** and aortic **(bottom)** positions. In the **top panel,** the horizontally oriented arrows denote the struts of the stented porcine valve that protrude in the cavity of the left ventricle. Within the struts note the echo-dense mass that represents vegetation. In the **lower panel,** the three struts of the porcine bioprosthesis can be visualized at 2, 6, and 10 o'clock positions. Within the sewing ring of the bioprosthesis are noted several echo densities that represent vegetations. LA = left atrium; LV = left ventricle; RA = right atrium; RV = right ventricle; RVOT = right ventricular outflow tract.

Intracardiac Shunts

ATRIAL SEPTAL DEFECT. The most common shunt lesion to be detected de novo in adulthood is the atrial septal defect. Because atrial septal defects result in a relatively innocent murmur, they are often overlooked in childhood and may escape detection until adolescence or adulthood. Atrial septal defects result in a left-to-right shunt at a level of the atrium and, consequently, a diastolic volume overload of the right ventricle. The volume overload pattern of the right ventricle is manifest as dilation of the right ventricle and usually the right atrium. Additionally, the septum is "flattened" and the left ventricle, rather than assuming circular geometry, has a D-shaped geometry (see Fig. 11–27). This septal flattening is present predominantly in diastole, and during systole the septum assumes its normal circular geometry. This right ventricular volume overload pattern, which is typically seen in atrial septal defects, is also seen in any other lesion resulting in right ventricular diastolic volume overload, including significant pulmonary insufficiency, tricuspid regurgitation, and anomalous pulmonary venous return. On M-mode echocardiography, the right ventricular volume overload pattern is characterized as paradoxical septal motion. It is now recognized that this "paradoxical" septal motion actually represents restitution of normal circular geometry with the onset of ventricular systole.

Detection of a right ventricular volume overload pattern may be the first clue to the presence of an atrial septal defect, after which further interrogation of the atrial septum should be undertaken to identify the location of the defect. The three most common locations of an atrial septal defect are secundum, primum, and sinus venosus, representing approximately 70 percent, 15 percent, and 15 percent of atrial septal defects, respectively. Rarer forms of atrial septal defect, including the unroofed coronary sinus, are also encountered.

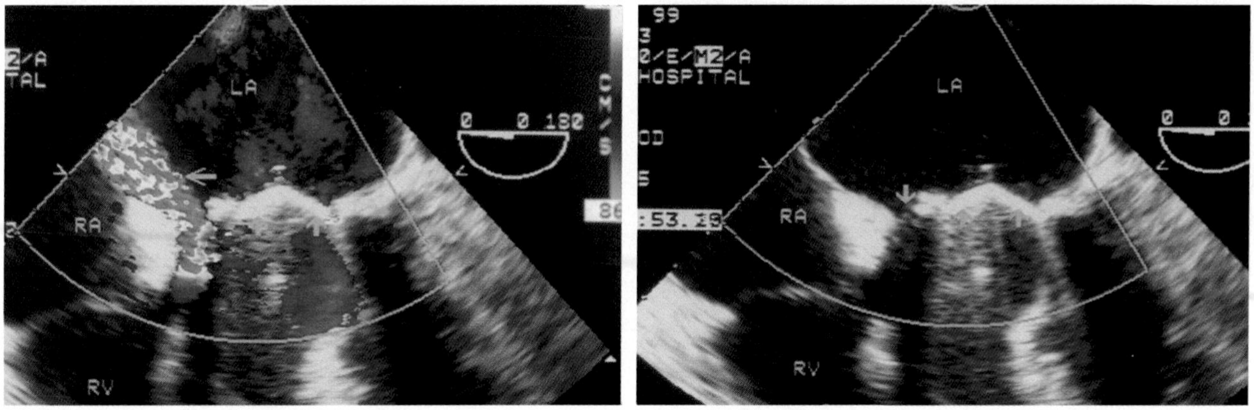

FIGURE 11–79 Transesophageal echocardiogram recorded in a patient with a St. Jude mitral valve replacement and a paravalvular leak, resulting in moderate mitral regurgitation. **Left,** Recorded in systole. Note the two discs of the St. Jude prosthesis in their closed position (up-pointing arrows). Immediately outside the boundary of the sewing ring is a distinct color jet (horizontal arrow) representing an eccentric mitral regurgitation jet arising from outside the border of the sewing ring. **Right,** The same image with color suppressed. Again note the closed leaflets of the St. Jude valve. With the color suppressed, a distinct gap between the sewing ring and tissue (down-pointing arrow) can be seen, representing partial valve dehiscence. LA = left atrium; RA = right atrium; RV = right ventricle.

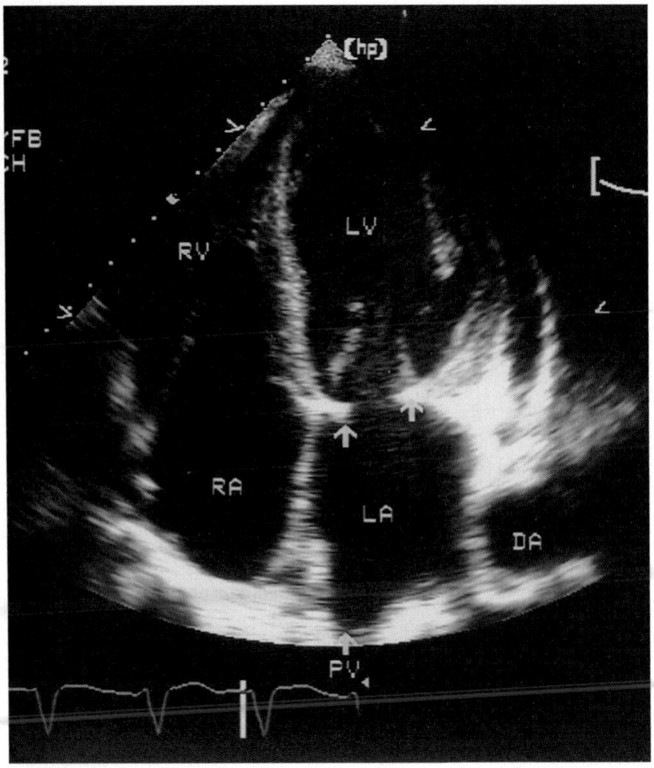

FIGURE 11–80 Two-dimensional echocardiogram recorded in a patient after mitral valve repair and annuloplasty ring. The ring is seen as an echo-dense structure in the annulus (arrows). DA = descending aorta; LA = left atrium; LV = left ventricle; PV = pulmonary vein; RA = right atrium; RV = right ventricle.

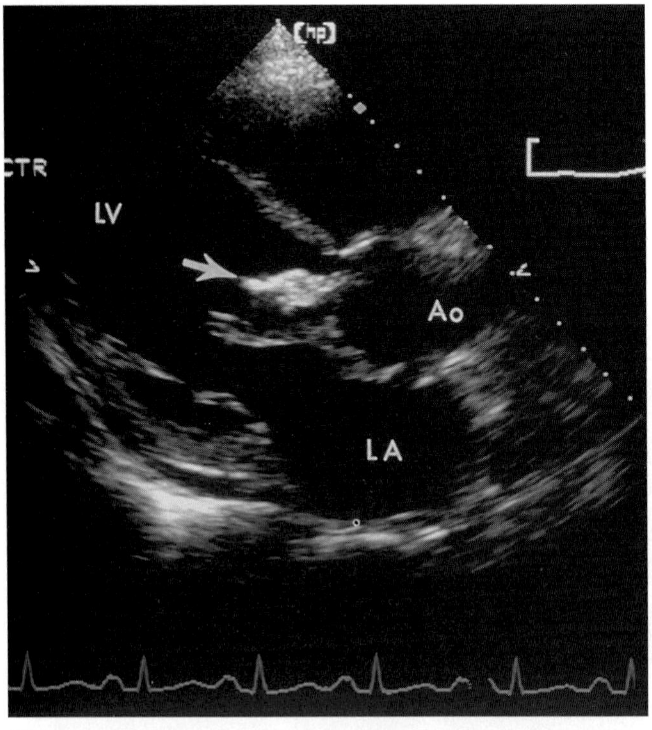

FIGURE 11–81 Parasternal long-axis view of patient with aortic valve vegetation. Note the relatively echo-dense, irregular mass prolapsing into the left ventricular outflow tract in this diastolic frame (arrow). Ao = aorta; LA = left atrium; LV = left ventricle.

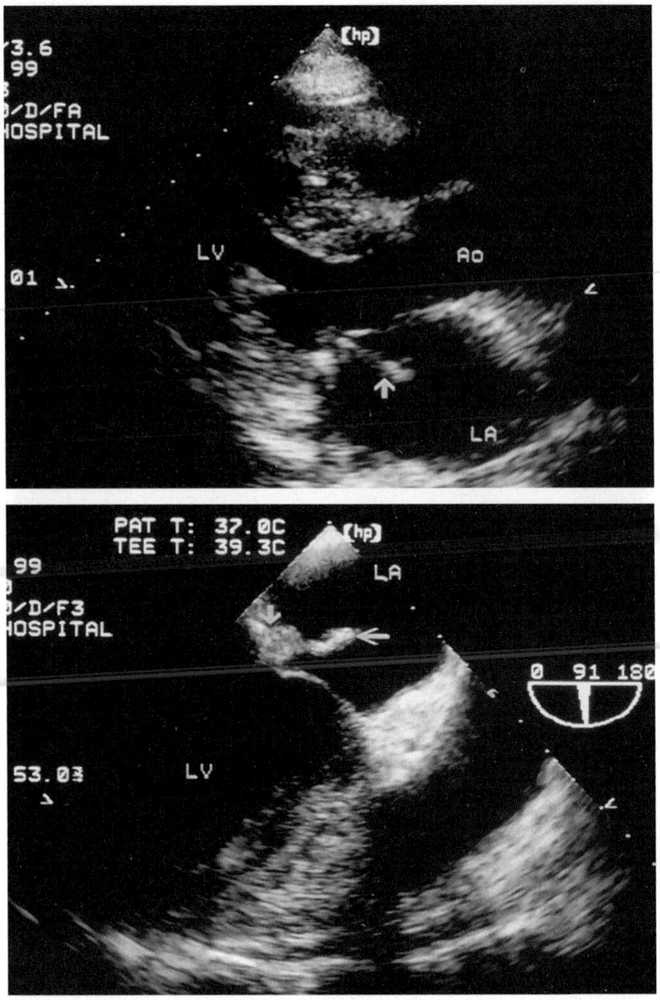

FIGURE 11–82 Transthoracic **(top)** and transesophageal echocardiogram **(bottom)** recorded in a patient with a mitral valve vegetation. In the transthoracic parasternal long-axis view, a highly mobile filamentous echo can be seen prolapsing into the left atrium (LA) during systole. This is consistent with a highly mobile vegetation. A systolic frame from the transesophageal echocardiogram is presented in the bottom panel. Again, the highly filamentous mobile echo is noted (horizontal arrow). In addition, there is a more sessile 8 mm diameter mass attached to the mitral valve (downward pointing arrow). Ao = aorta; LV = left ventricle.

Whereas the secundum atrial septal defect is an isolated entity, there are strong associations between sinus venosus atrial septal defect and malalignment of the pulmonary veins, resulting in functional anomalous pulmonary venous return. A primum atrial septal defect is a variant of endocardial cushion defect in which a small, perimembranous ventricular septal defect and anomalies of the mitral valve may also be encountered. The classic mitral valve abnormality associated with a primum defect is a cleft mitral valve with varying degrees of mitral regurgitation.

On occasion, a right ventricular volume overload pattern is encountered but no anatomical defect can be visualized. In these instances, contrast echocardiography using agitated saline can be a valuable means of detecting the right-to-left component of interatrial shunting. Of the three common types of atrial septal defect, the sinus venosus defect is most likely to escape direct visualization on a transthoracic echocardiogram. TEE is nearly 100 percent specific and sensitive in detection of all types of atrial septal defects, including sinus venosus defects (Fig. 11–85).[130,131] With TEE, the atrial septal defect is visualized as a loss of tissue. The size of the defect can be accurately measured, and color flow

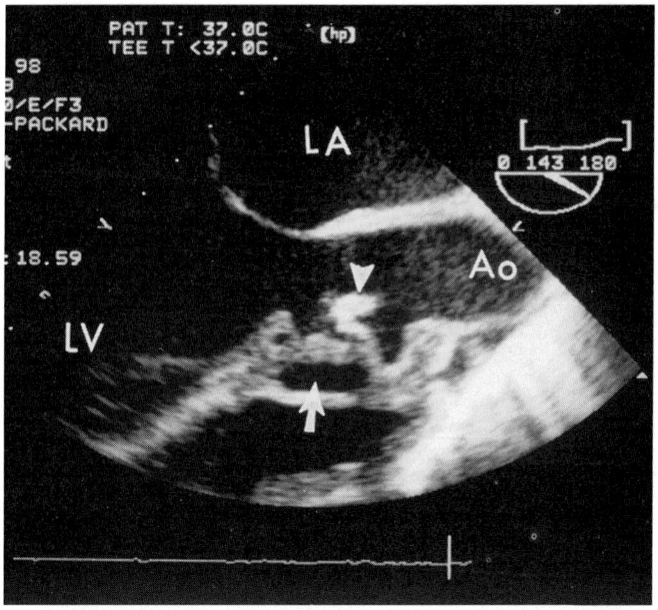

FIGURE 11–83 Transesophageal echocardiogram recorded in a patient with an aortic root abscess, obtained in a longitudinal orientation. Note the thickened aortic valve with superimposed vegetation (arrowhead) and the echo-free space (arrow) between the wall of the aorta and the right ventricular outflow tract, which represents a periaortic abscess. Ao = aorta; LA = left atrium; LV = left ventricle.

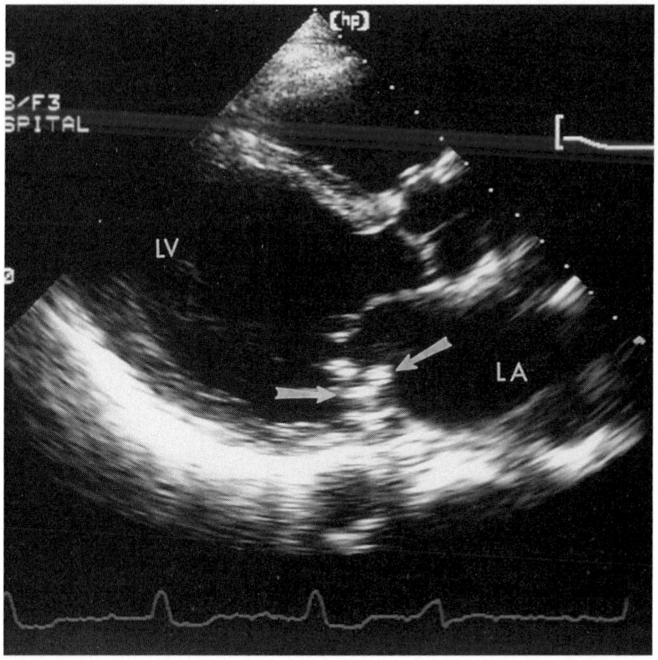

FIGURE 11–84 Two-dimensional echocardiogram recorded in a patient with renal insufficiency and calcification of the mitral annulus. Mitral annular calcium appears as an echo-dense mass in the mitral annulus (arrows). LA = left atrium; LV = left ventricle.

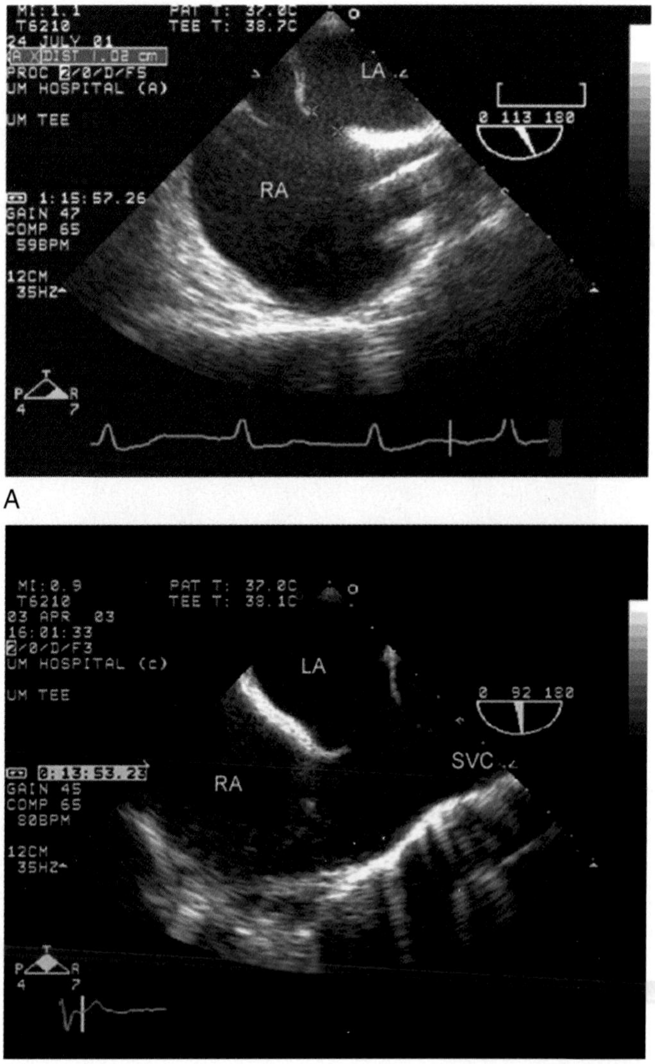

FIGURE 11–85 Transesophageal echocardiograms in a patient with a secundum atrial septal defect **(A)** and a sinus venosus defect **(B)**. The margins of the secundum defect are easily seen and the defect can be measured approximately 1 cm in maximum dimension. In panel B, there is a larger defect at the junction of the atrial septum and superior vena cava (SVC). LA = left atrium; RA = right atrium.

imaging can be used to identify abnormal transatrial flow patterns (Fig. 11–86). Often the diagnosis can be established with a degree of accuracy and confidence so that catheterization is not necessary before surgical repair or percutaneous closure.

Once identified, further characterization of the atrial septal defect can be undertaken using two-dimensional echocardiography and Doppler techniques. Three-dimensional echocardiography can provide valuable clues as to the complex shape of an atrial septal defect.[132] TEE can be an invaluable technique for determining the integrity of the tissues surrounding the atrial septal defect and plays a valuable role in determining the feasibility of percutaneous closure.[133,134] Defects less than 2 cm in diameter and with relatively firm tissue at the margins are more likely to be successfully closed, compared with large defects and those with fairly thin tissue at the margin or multiple perforations.

Numerous attempts have been made to quantify the ratio of pulmonary and systemic flow in intracardiac shunt lesions, including atrial septal defect. The majority of these attempts have been by calculating the instantaneous stroke volume of the pulmonary outflow tract and left ventricular outflow tract (see section on Doppler calculations). This calculation has been fairly reproducible and has correlated with hemodynamic assessment in the animal laboratory and in children. Because of the margin of error for measuring the dimension of the outflow tract, it has seen less use in adult patients. In general, the threshold for recommending closure of an atrial septal defect has diminished to a Qp/Qs (pulmonary/systemic flow ratio) of 1.5 or less. Detection of a right

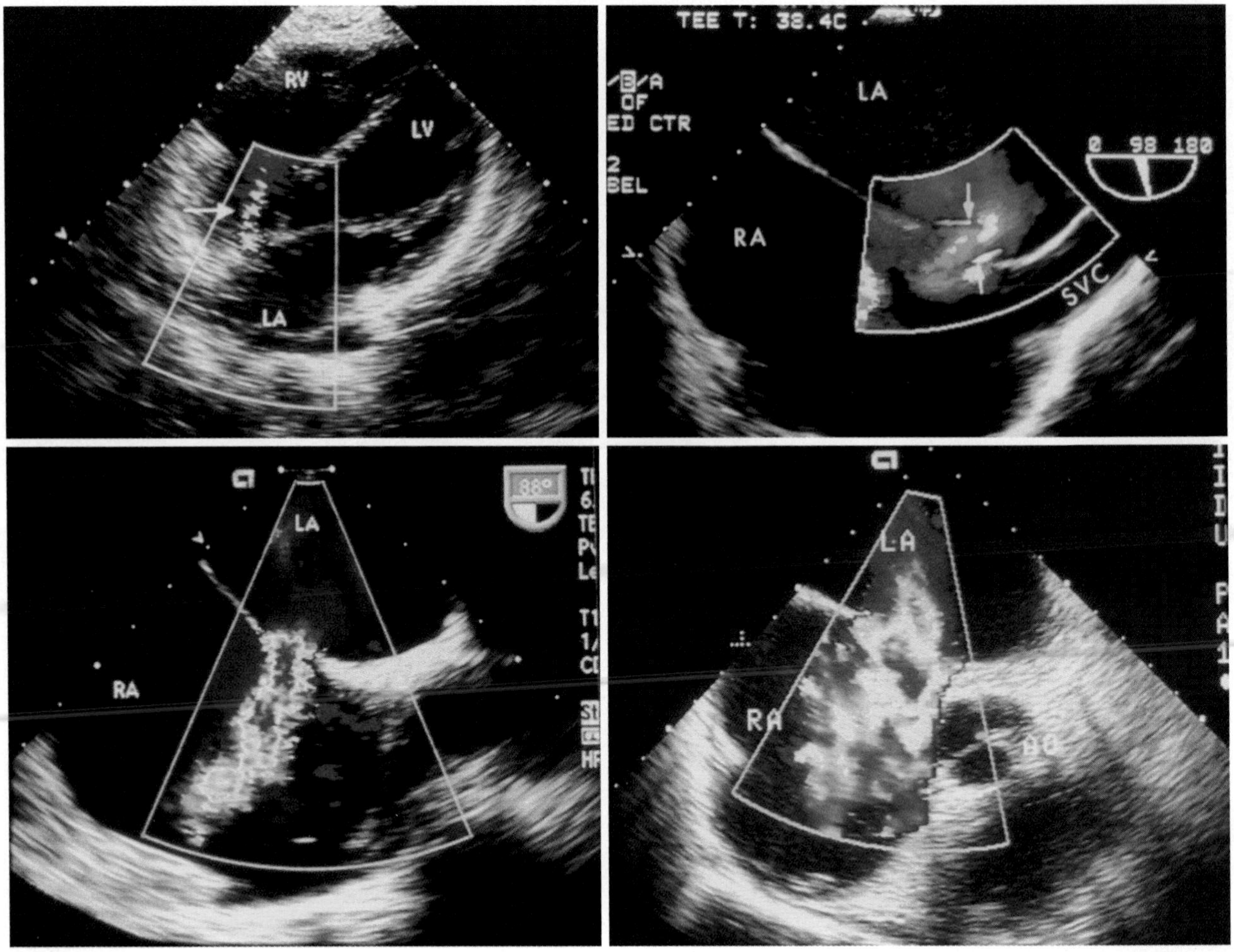

FIGURE 11–86 Four illustrations of patients with atrial septal defects. **Top left,** Recorded from a subcostal transducer position in a patient with a small atrial septal defect (also illustrated in the lower left panel). From the subcostal transducer position, the entire length of the atrial septum can be visualized. There is a defect approximately 7 mm in diameter in the secundum portion of the atrial septum with a color flow signal coursing from the left atrium into the right atrium (arrow), consistent with secundum septal defect. **Bottom left,** Transesophageal echocardiogram from the same patient presented on the top left. The size of the defect can be more accurately appreciated, and again there is a distinct color flow image coursing from the left atrium into the right atrium. **Top right,** Longitudinal view of the atrial septum showing a large patent foramen. Note the margins of the atrial septal tissue (arrows). The atrial septal tissue does not oppose, in this case leaving a 1 cm defect, through which flow shunts from the left atrium to the right atrium. **Bottom right,** Recorded in a patient with a large secundum defect. Note the color flow image denoting a substantial flow from left atrium to right atrium. The defect is approximately 2 cm in diameter. AO = aorta; LA = left atrium; LV = left ventricle; RA = right atrium; RV = right ventricle; SVC = superior vena cava.

ventricular volume overload pattern denotes a shunt of at least this level, and thus the majority of detected atrial septal defects fall into the range that warrant closure.

Repaired Atrial Septal Defect. Depending on the magnitude of the initial shunt and the age at which an atrial septal defect is repaired, the two-dimensional echocardiogram may revert to normal with respect to chamber sizes or show evidence of residual right-sided heart dilation. In instances in which the defect was large and repaired only late, residual right ventricular dysfunction, varying degrees of pulmonary hypertension, and right ventricular hypertrophy may persist throughout adulthood. Depending on the nature of the repair technique, the atrial septum can appear anatomically normal or can reveal areas of echo density consistent with the type of patch material used. In general, the right ventricular volume overload pattern resolves but can be replaced by a postoperative septal motion pattern.

Other Abnormalities of the Atrial Septum. In addition to atrial septal defect, anomalies such as aneurysm of the atrial septum, lipomatous atrial hypertrophy, and patent foramen ovale[135] can be detected. The aneurysmal atrial septum is not infrequently associated with small perforations and minor degrees of either right-to-left or left-to-right atrial shunting (Fig. 11–87). Contrast echocardiography can detect minor degrees of right-to-left shunting in both of these situations.

Anomalous Pulmonary Venous Return. A final congenital lesion that results in a right ventricular volume overload pattern is anomalous pulmonary venous return. A variation on anomalous return is seen in patients with sinus venosus atrial septal defects who have functional anomalous return due to malalignment of the right superior pulmonary vein such that its flow is directed into the superior vena cava and right atrium. True anomalous pulmonary venous return often results in creation of a venous chamber posterior to the left atrium, which then drains to the right atrium.

VENTRICULAR SEPTAL DEFECT. Although the ventricular septal defect represents the most common congenital intracardiac shunt encountered in infants and children, it accounts for a small percentage of defects detected de novo in adults. A substantial number of small ventricular septal defects close spontaneously during childhood and thus are not present in adults, whereas the larger defects result in symptoms and are detected in childhood. Furthermore, the smaller persistent defects are associated with prominent pathological murmurs and unlikely to be confused for a flow murmur, and therefore these individuals come to medical attention promptly. On occasion, patients with small ventricular septal defects escape detection to adulthood, when the defects are found on the basis of a pathological murmur. Ventricular septal defects occur

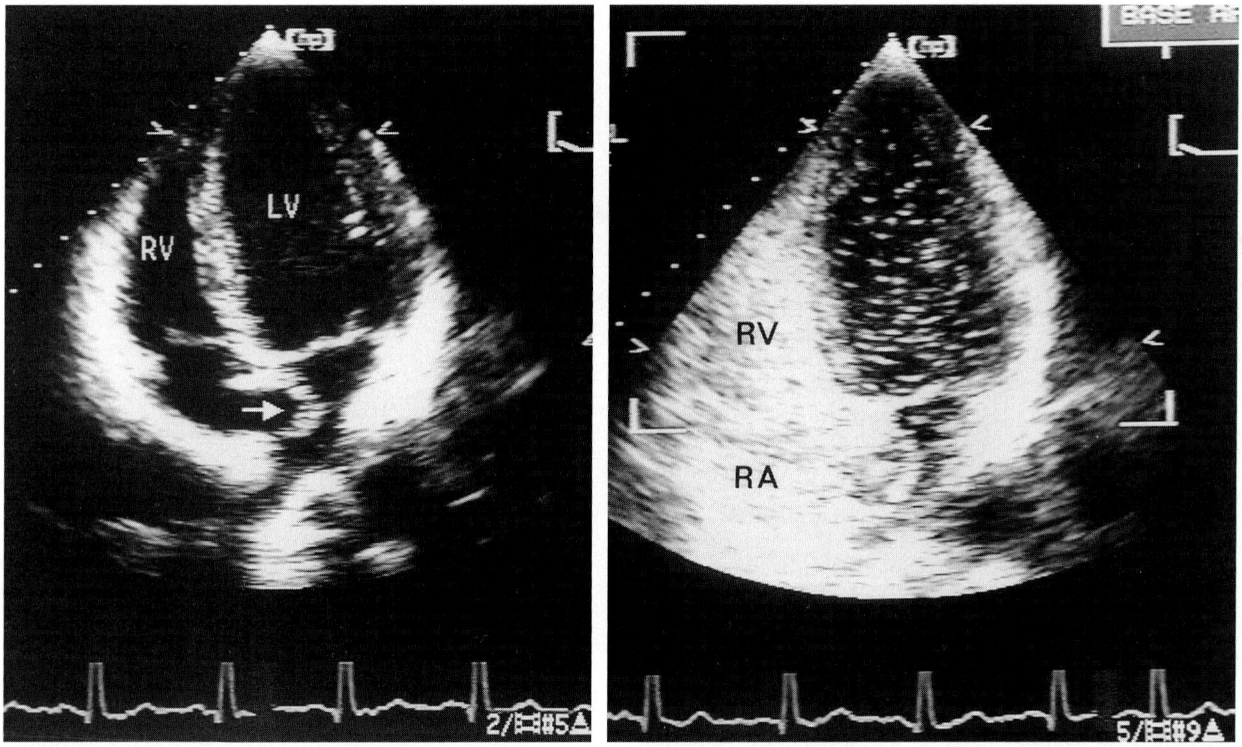

FIGURE 11–87 Apical four-chamber view recorded in a patient with an atrial septal aneurysm. Note the marked bulging of the atrial septum into the cavity of the left atrium **(A)**. **B,** Recorded after injection of saline contrast medium. Note that the contrast medium has filled the right ventricular cavity, and numerous individual microbubbles are seen in the cavity of both the left atrium and left ventricle, consistent with a right-to-left shunt through fenestrations in the atrial septal aneurysm. LV = left ventricle; RA = right atrium; RV = right ventricle.

in several different locations, which are denoted echocardiographically in Figure 11–88. The most common location is a small perimembranous septal defect; however, other locations, including supracristal, are not uncommonly encountered. Muscular defects can occur anywhere within the muscular septum and may take a serpiginous route through the septal myocardium. Small apical defects are frequently multiple.

A ventricular septal defect can be visualized as a dropout of myocardial tissue with communication between the left and right ventricles. The resolution of TTE, using 3- and 5-MHz transducers, is such that most defects below a 3 mm size may not be directly visualized. It is uncommon to directly visualize small muscular defects that may take an angulated or serpiginous course through the ventricular septum. Color Doppler imaging over areas of the septum is a reliable means for detecting the abnormal transseptal flow (Fig. 11–89). It is often necessary to scan in unusual and atypical planes to identify flow through the septum, especially when searching for a muscular defect. For the isolated small perimembranous defect, continuous-wave Doppler can be used to determine the velocity of flow from the left ventricle to the right ventricle and hence the transventricular pressure gradient. This can then be subtracted from arm blood pressure to estimate right ventricular systolic pressure. With the use of this methodology, the small restrictive ventricular septal defect can be characterized as a defect resulting in little or no chamber dilation, having small anatomical extent on two-dimensional scanning, and associated with a high transventricular gradient.

The magnitude of shunting through a ventricular septal defect can be calculated using several Doppler techniques. Larger ventricular septal defects may be associated with substantial left-to-right shunts and development of secondary pulmonary hypertension. In this instance, the right ventricle will be dilated and hypertrophied. By using the tricuspid regurgitation signal, right ventricular systolic pressure can be calculated. In the presence of a ventricular septal defect, it is important to look for associated anomalies of the right ventricular outflow tract and pulmonary valve. Pulmonic stenosis and right ventricular outflow tract obstruction are both protective of the pulmonary circuit and will lead to the scenario of elevated right ventricular systolic pressure with elevation or even normal pulmonary artery pressures. This has obvious clinical implications with respect to surgical intervention.

Closed and Repaired Ventricular Septal Defect. As noted earlier, many small ventricular septal defects close spontaneously in infancy and

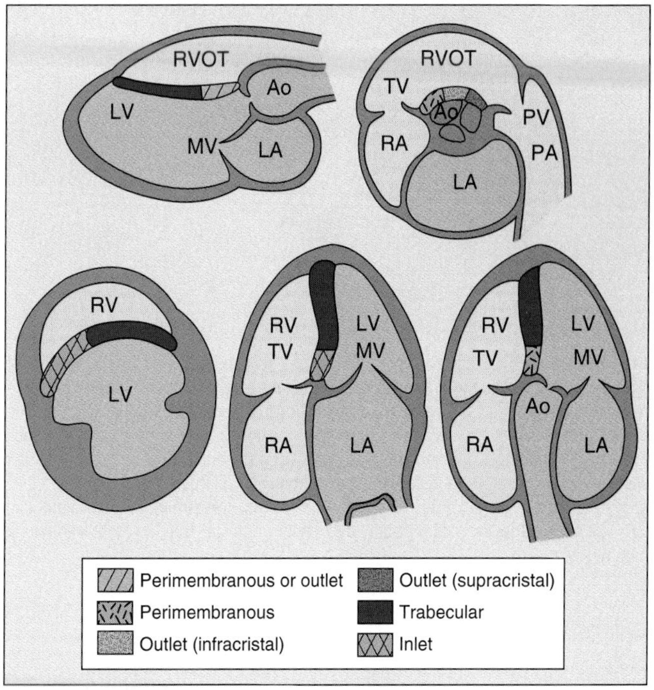

FIGURE 11–88 Schematic depicting the location of different ventricular septal defects compared with the different echocardiographic views. Ao = aorta; LA = left atrium; LV = left ventricle; MV = mitral valve; PV = pulmonary vein; RA = right atrium; RV = right ventricle; RVOT = right ventricular outflow tract; TV = tricuspid valve. (From Feigenbaum H: Echocardiography. 5th ed. Malvern, PA, Lea & Febiger, 1994.)

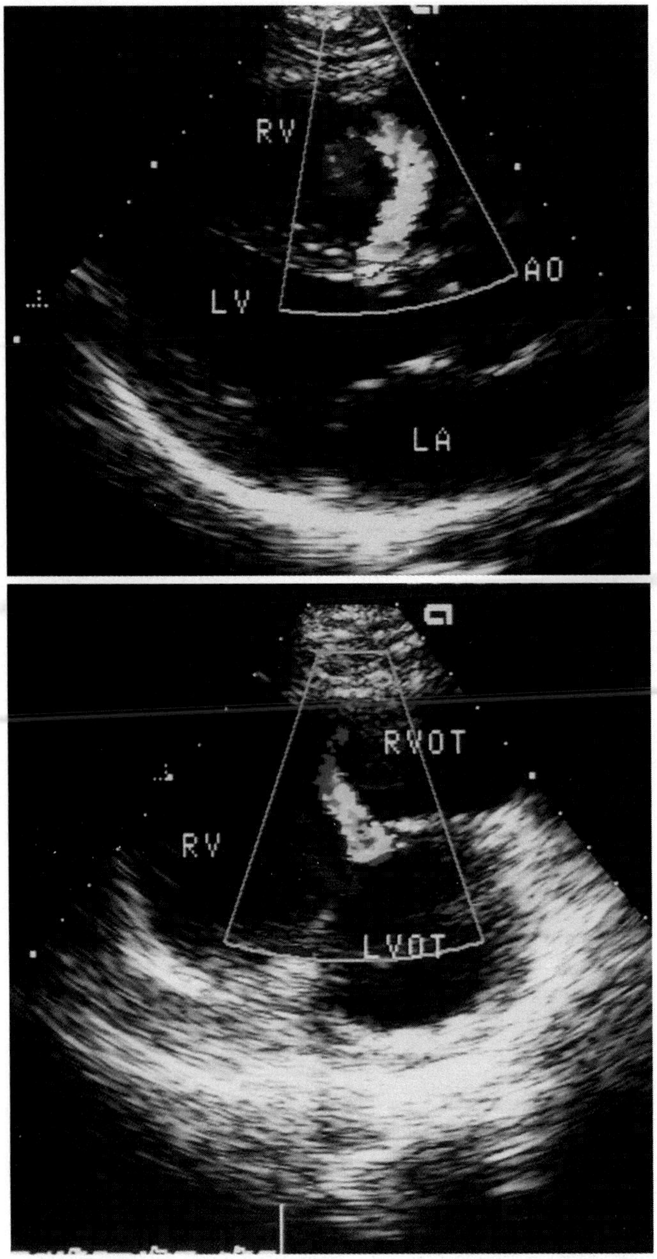

FIGURE 11–89 Parasternal two-dimensional echocardiographic views in a patient with a moderate-sized perimembranous ventricular septal defect. The **upper panel** is recorded in a parasternal long-axis view and shows the proximal anterior septum. The **lower panel** is recorded in a short-axis view at the base of the heart. Note in each instance the distinct color jet arising on the left ventricular side of the ventricular septum and coursing in the right ventricular outflow tract. This is consistent with left-to-right ventricular septal defect flow. AO = aorta; LA = left atrium; LV = left ventricle; LVOT = left ventricular outflow tract; RV = right ventricle; RVOT = right ventricular outflow tract.

childhood. This occurs by way of two basic mechanisms. The first is fusion of a portion of the tricuspid leaflet to the ventricular septal defect. In this case, one may visualize a very thin membrane closing the actual ventricular septal defect. The second mechanism appears to be growth of additional tissue from the margins of the ventricular septal defect. In this instance, there may be irregular tissue closing the ventricular septal defect, the extent of which can be highly variable. In many instances, a thin-walled aneurysm may be noted in the area of the previous ventricular septal defect. The aneurysm typically bows into the right ventricular outflow tract. A small residual left-to-right shunt may be encountered that often is of little hemodynamic significance but that may result in a murmur and pose a risk for endocarditis.

Other Congenital Disorders

TETRALOGY OF FALLOT. Tetralogy of Fallot represents a constellation of lesions, including a ventricular septal defect with overriding aorta, obstruction to right ventricular outflow tract at either the infundibular or valvular level, and right ventricular hypertrophy (Fig. 11–90). The fourth component is a right-sided aortic arch. Before correction, the lesion is characterized by a ventricular septal defect in which the tip of the ventricular septum is directed not at the anterior wall of the aorta but at the aortic lumen. Varying degrees of right ventricular outflow tract obstruction, including true valvular stenosis and infundibular muscular stenosis, can be seen. Tetralogy of Fallot represents the most common cyanotic congenital lesion to be encountered that is likely to result in survival to adulthood and, furthermore, the most common complex lesion to be encountered in the adult population after repair.

Preoperatively, tetralogy of Fallot represents a broad spectrum of ventricular septal defect size and outflow tract obstruction. Postoperatively, varying degrees of residual abnormalities can be encountered, ranging from a nearly normal-appearing heart to one in which there are substantial degrees of right ventricular dysfunction and residual right ventricular outflow tract obstruction. Two-dimensional echocardiography and Doppler techniques can be a definitive means for following these individuals with respect to recovery of right ventricular function and development of complications such as recurrent right ventricular outflow tract obstruction and residual ventricular septal defect.

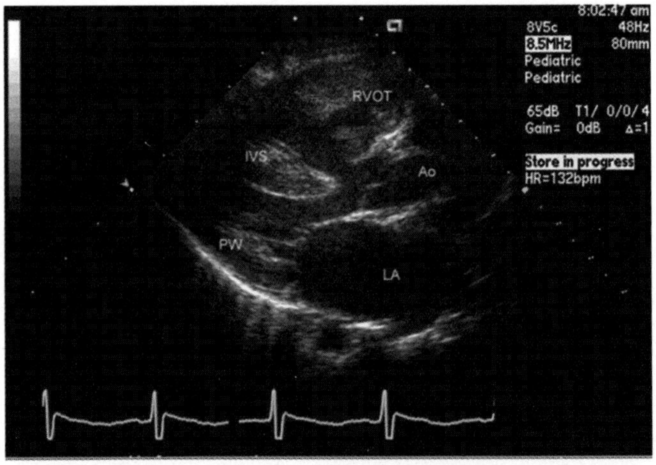

A

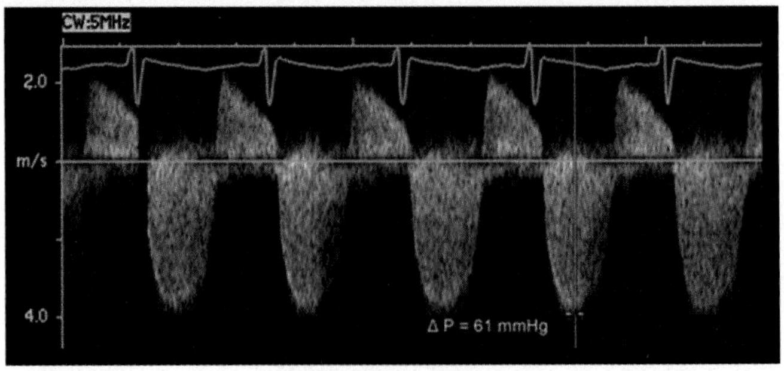

B

FIGURE 11–90 **A,** Two-dimensional echocardiogram recorded in a patient with an unrepaired tetralogy of Fallot. Note the large ventricular septal defect and the overriding aorta. Because of the overriding aorta, both right and left ventricular outflow is directed toward the aorta. **B,** Continuous wave Doppler recorded through the right ventricular outflow tract. Note the peak gradient of 61 mm Hg. Ao = aorta; IVS = interventricular septum; LA = left atrium; PW = posterior wall; RVOT = right ventricular outflow tract.

PULMONIC STENOSIS. Isolated pulmonic stenosis is a relatively common congenital lesion. As with the bicuspid aortic valve, its hemodynamic severity ranges from negligible to severe and life threatening early in infancy. Because of the orientation of the proximal pulmonary artery and pulmonic valve, it is easily interrogated with Doppler. Underestimation of pulmonic valve gradients due to off-angle interrogation is uncommon. Anatomically, the stenotic pulmonary valve appears somewhat thickened and has "doming" motion (see Fig. 11–75). On M-mode echocardiography, there may be an accentuation of the pulmonic valve "a" wave. In adult patients, it is not uncommon for valvular pulmonic stenosis to be associated with secondary infundibular hypertrophy with concurrent right ventricular outflow tract obstruction. Thus, it is important to evaluate both the subvalvular and valvular aspects of the pulmonary valve in adult patients. Less frequently, peripheral pulmonic stenosis will be encountered. Identification and characterization of the peripheral pulmonary arteries in adult populations can be quite problematic and constitute an area in which MRI can play an incremental and valuable role.

ABNORMALITIES OF THE LEFT VENTRICULAR OUTFLOW TRACT. The most common abnormality of left ventricular outflow is the bicuspid aortic valve, which has been discussed previously. Additionally, both tunnel and discrete subaortic stenosis are occasionally encountered in adult patients. Tunnel aortic stenosis is visualized as a diffuse narrowing of the left ventricular outflow tract and more often is identified in children. Discrete, membranous subvalvular stenosis occasionally escapes detection until adulthood and is characterized by the presence of a thin membrane or ridge that encircles the left ventricular outflow tract (Fig. 11–91). Components of the membrane may be attached to the ventricular septum and to the anterior mitral valve leaflet. The membrane itself can be difficult to visualize from TTE positions and may require TEE for complete visualization. The obstructing membrane results in turbulence in the left ventricular outflow tract, which can be detected with color Doppler flow imaging and eventually results in secondary pathology of the aortic valve with subsequent aortic insufficiency. M-mode echocardiography often reveals characteristic coarse systolic fluttering of the aortic valve leaflets. This finding can help distinguish valvular from subvalvular obstruction. This should be contrasted to hypertrophic cardiomyopathy, in which anatomical abnormalities of the aortic valve and aortic insufficiency are uncommon and a single notch representing valve preclosure may be noted.

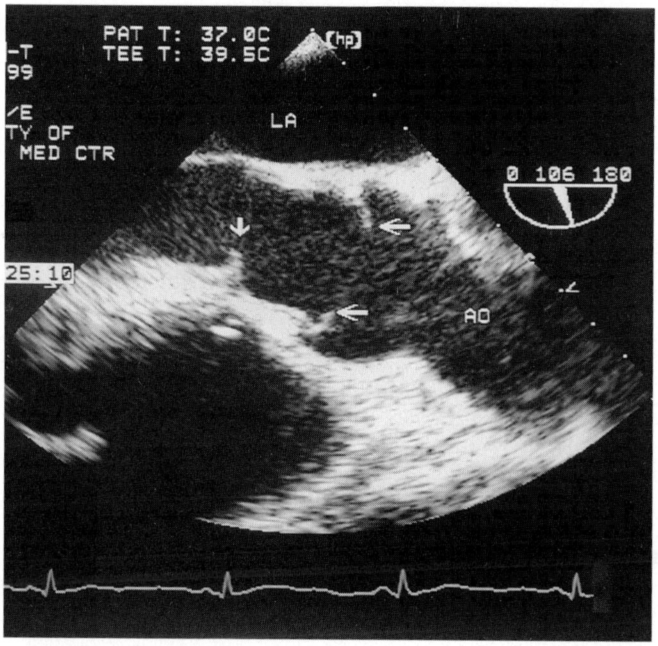

FIGURE 11–91 Transesophageal echocardiogram in a longitudinal plane of the left ventricular outflow tract demonstrating a small, discrete subaortic membrane (downward pointing arrow). The aortic leaflets are mildly thickened (horizontal arrows). This small membrane was not visualized from the transthoracic echocardiogram. AO = aorta; LA = left atrium.

CONGENITAL ABNORMALITIES OF THE MITRAL VALVE. Congenital abnormalities of the mitral valve, likely to be encountered in adult populations, include the previously mentioned cleft mitral valve, seen in association with a primum atrial septal defect as well as congenital mitral stenosis. The latter can occur either in the presence of a single papillary muscle, in which all chordae attach to a central point, rendering an otherwise unremarkable valve functionally stenotic, or in a valve that is intrinsically stenotic but with two papillary muscle attachments. Functionally, these patients present in a manner nearly identical to that of patients with rheumatic mitral stenosis. Awareness of the anatomical features of congenital mitral stenosis is necessary to separate it from rheumatic causes. In many instances, the congenital lesion will be characterized by an obstructive but eccentrically directed mitral valve orifice without the characteristic chordal and leaflet thickening. Transvalvular gradients can be measured across the congenitally stenotic mitral valve but may require unusual transducer angulations and lines of interrogation.

Cor triatriatum represents a membrane within the body of the left atrium that likewise may be obstructive. Transthoracic imaging may suffice for identification of the membrane (Fig. 11-92), but in many instances TEE, which affords a more accurate view of the left atrium, is necessary. A final congenital abnormality of the mitral valve is the submitral ring or web. This represents a membrane attached near the mitral annulus within the left atrium that is variably obstructive to flow.

ANOMALIES OF THE TRICUSPID VALVE. The most common congenital tricuspid valve anomaly to escape detection to adulthood is Ebstein anomaly. In this situation, the lateral leaflet is elongated and tethered to the lateral wall of the right ventricle and the septal leaflet is relatively small and apically displaced. This results in conversion of a portion of the right ventricle to an "atrialized" right ventricle (Figs. 11-93 and 11-94). Tricuspid regurgitation is invariably present and results in dilation of the right side of the heart in general but predominantly of the right atrium and atrialized right ventricle. Atrial septal defect is a common association with Ebstein anomaly and should be considered in all instances. Because the coaptation of the tricuspid valve is displaced toward the apex of the right ventricle, the apical location of the convergence zone of the tricuspid regurgitation jet may be one of the clues to the presence of this anomaly.

Once identified, it is important to characterize several features of Ebstein anomaly that have direct relevance to the feasibility of surgical repair. Surgical repair can be undertaken in individuals with a relatively large functional right ventricle, compared with the atrialized portion, and in whom there is not extensive tethering of the lateral leaflet.

Tricuspid Atresia. Tricuspid atresia is usually detected in infancy and after palliation may allow survival to adulthood. In patients with tricuspid atresia, there is no functional tricuspid valve tissue, although the tricuspid annulus may be closed by a thin membrane with small perforations. Because of the atretic tricuspid valve, right ventricular hypoplasia coexists. Obviously, a complete form of tricuspid atresia is incompatible with life unless a concurrent atrial or ventricular septal defect is present.

PERSISTENT DUCTUS ARTERIOSUS. Persistent ductus arteriosus represents persistence of the normal communication between the descending thoracic aorta and the left pulmonary artery. The size of the communication varies from 1 or 2 mm to a centimeter or more. The magnitude of left-to-right shunting is dependent on the size of the defect. Initially, persistent ductus rsults in a continuous left-to-right shunt at the great artery level that may result in left-sided heart volume overload early in childhood and adolescence. Because of the increased pulmonary flow, pulmonary hypertension may develop, in which case only the systolic component of the shunt persists. Echocardiographic detection of persistent ductus arteriosus is dependent on detection of left-sided heart enlargement and/or an abnormal pulmonary

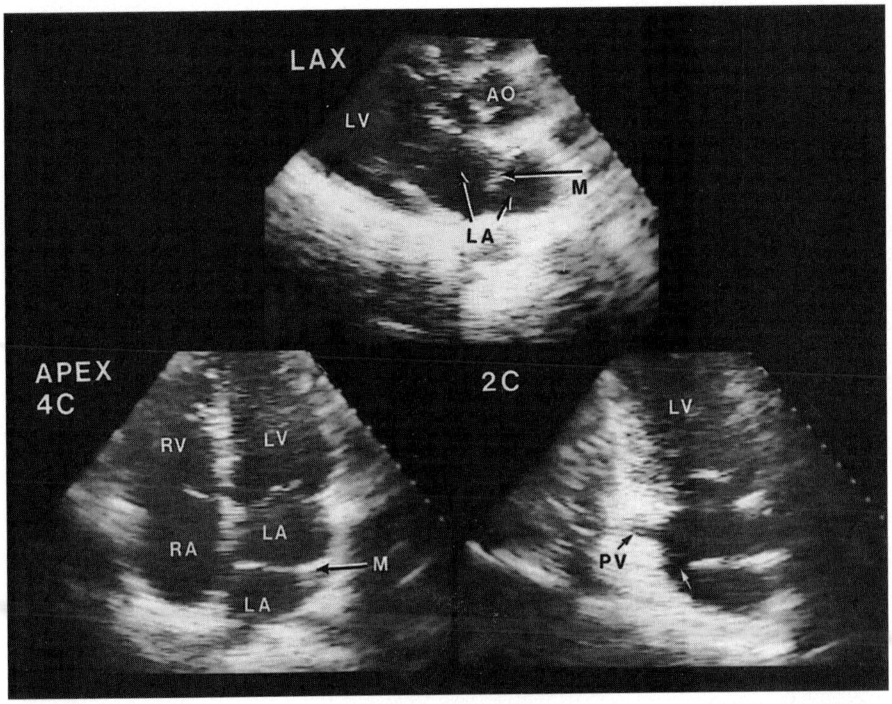

FIGURE 11–92 Transthoracic echocardiogram recorded in a patient with *cor triatriatum* in the parasternal long-axis view **(top)** and apical views **(bottom)**. A linear echo courses posteriorly from the area of the aorta (AO). From the apical views, the membrane (M) can be seen to divide the left atrium (LA) into two chambers. LV = left ventricle; PV = pulmonary vein; RA = right atrium; RV = right ventricle. (From Feigenbaum H: Echocardiography. 5th ed. Malvern, PA, Lea & Febiger, 1994.)

artery flow pattern. With the use of suprasternal notch views, it is occasionally possible to directly visualize the ductus. More commonly, Doppler interrogation of the proximal pulmonary artery is the initial clue to the presence of a persistent ductus. By using either color Doppler flow imaging or pulsed Doppler, one can detect continuous turbulent flow in the proximal pulmonary artery (Fig. 11–95). Further careful interrogation will frequently identify the origin of the abnormal flow from the descending aorta into the left main pulmonary artery.

COARCTATION OF THE AORTA. Narrowing or coarctation of the aorta occurs after the takeoff of the left subclavian artery. It results in reduction of systolic pressure distally and may present in adulthood as a secondary cause of systemic hypertension. The anatomical extent of coarctation may be visualized from the suprasternal notch, and continuous-flow Doppler can be used to determine the coarctation gradient (Fig. 11–96). There is a strong association between coarctation and bicuspid aortic valve; and whenever coarctation is discovered, efforts should be made to define the aortic valve anatomy.

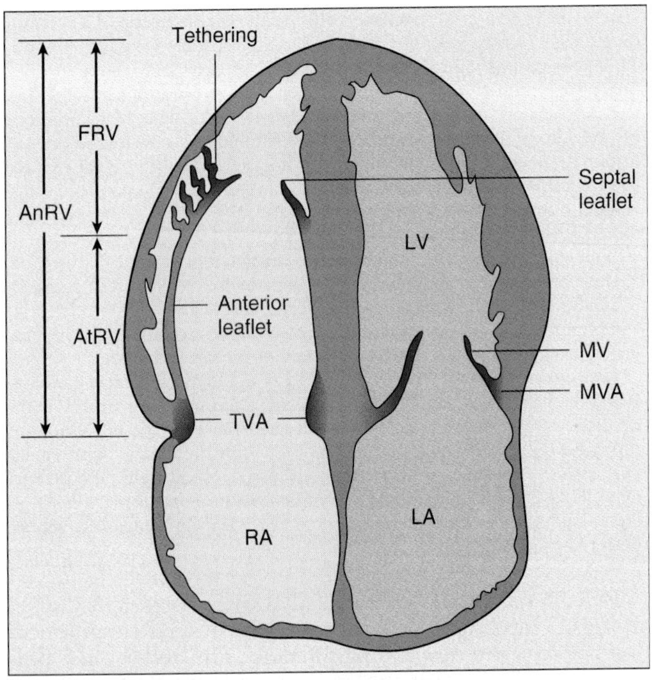

FIGURE 11–93 Schematic of the anatomical and echocardiographic abnormalities seen in Ebstein anomaly, including apical displacement of the septal leaflet and elongation and tethering of the lateral leaflet. Both the functional (FRV) and atrialized right ventricle (AtRV) are noted. AnRV = anatomic right ventricle; LA = left atrium; LV = left ventricle; MV = mitral valve; MVA = mitral valve annulus; RA = right atrium; TVA = tricuspid valve annulus. (From Feigenbaum H: Echocardiography. 5th ed. Malvern, PA, Lea & Febiger, 1994.)

TRANSPOSITION OF THE GREAT ARTERIES. *Transposition* refers to the situation in which there is ventricular-arterial discordance. This is defined as a connection of the left ventricle to the pulmonary artery and the right ventricle to the aorta. Two forms of transposition may be encountered. D-Transposition is an isolated malposition of the great vessels due to failure of the conotruncos to appropriately coil. In this situation, the pulmonary artery is attached to the left ventricle, which receives blood from the left atrium. The aorta is attached to the right ventricle, which receives blood from the right atrium. This results in two parallel circulations and is obviously not compatible with life in the absence of an intracardiac shunt such as a persistent ductus or large ventricular or atrial septal defect. This lesion is invariably detected in infancy and is not encountered in adult patients, other than in surgically corrected or palliated forms. Previously, surgical correction of transposition consisted of creation of an atrial septal defect early and subsequent surgical creation of a baffle that directed right atrial blood into the left ventricle and left atrial blood flow into the right ventricle. Currently, an anatomical switch of the great arteries is the preferred surgical procedure. L-Transposition occurs when there is both inversion of the ventricles and transposition of the great arteries (Fig. 11–97). In this situation, blood flows from the anatomical right atrium through an anatomical mitral valve into the anatomical left ventricle and then into the pulmonary artery. Blood returning to the left atrium flows through an anatomical tricuspid valve into an anatomical right ventricle and then to the aorta. This results in "corrected" transposition, in which physiological blood flow is maintained.

In either type of transposition, the great arteries no longer have the circular and crescent orientation but rather arise from the heart in a parallel fashion. In adult patients, it can be difficult to directly visualize the parallel nature of the great vessels. Clues to the presence of congenitally "corrected" transposition include the presence of a trabeculated ventricle with a more apically placed valve in a left and posterior position. L-Transposition is compatible with survival into the fourth and fifth decade. After this period of time, substantial hypertrophy of the anatomical right ventricle occurs and right ventricular dysfunction is not uncommon. Regurgitation of the anatomical tricuspid valve in the systemic circuit is also quite common in adult patients.

COMPLEX CONGENITAL HEART DISEASE. The echocardiographic and clinical evaluation of complex congenital heart disease is best undertaken by individuals with specific interest and training in the area and is beyond the scope of this chapter. Three-dimensional echocardiography has been a valuable adjunct in evaluating the complex anatomy seen in complex lesions (Fig. 11–98).

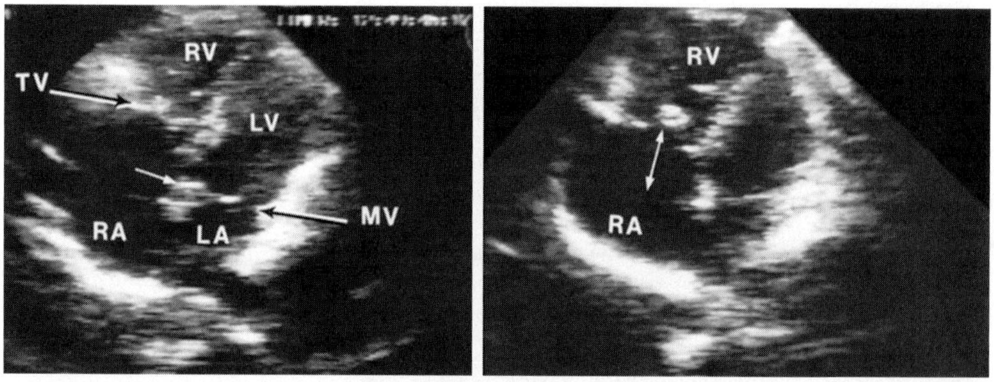

FIGURE 11–94 Two-dimensional echocardiogram recorded in a patient with Ebstein anomaly. Note the small, apically displayed septal leaflet and the elongated lateral leaflet that is tethered to the myocardium of the right ventricular lateral wall. LA = left atrium; LV = left ventricle; MV = mitral valve; RA = right atrium; RV = right ventricle; TV = tricuspid valve. (From Feigenbaum H: Echocardiography. 5th ed. Malvern, PA, Lea & Febiger, 1994.)

Diseases of the Pericardium (see Chap. 64)

Pericardial Effusion

Detection of pericardial effusion was one of the earliest uses of echocardiography, and modern ultrasonographic techniques remain the predominant diagnostic tool for detection, quantitation, and determination of the physiological significance of pericardial effusion. A pericardial effusion is viewed as an echo-free space surrounding the heart, most commonly seen posteriorly (Fig. 11–99). Most clinical laboratories document the presence of pericardial effusion and quantify it as minimal, small, moderate, or large. A minimal effusion represents the 5 to 20 ml of normal pericardial fluid seen in disease-free individuals. This is most frequently noted as an echo-free space, confined to the posterior atrioventricular

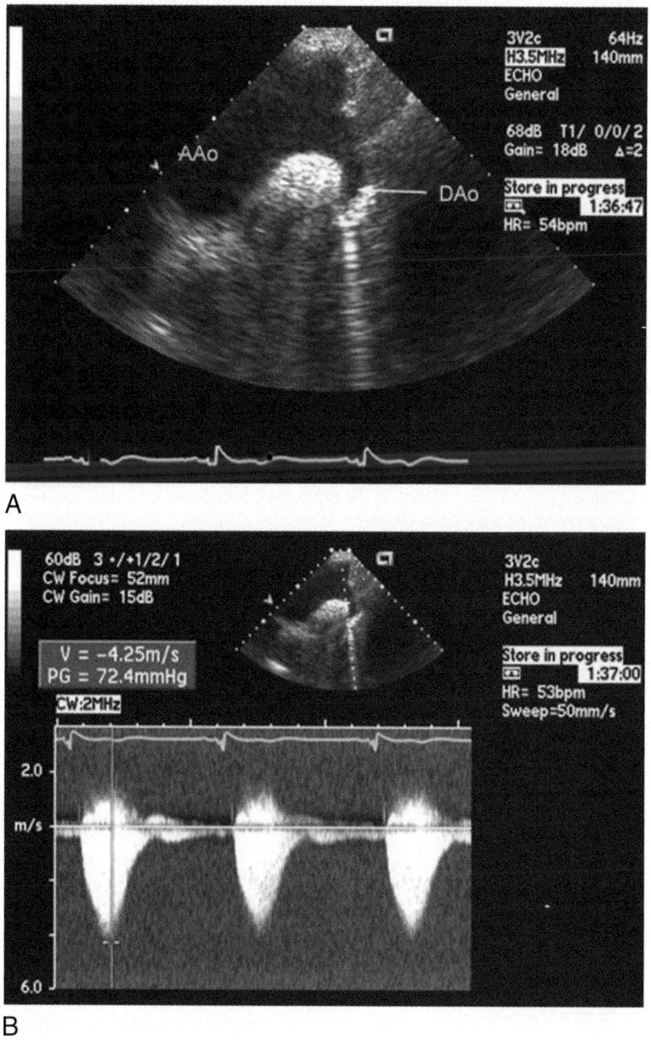

FIGURE 11–96 Coarctation of the aorta. **A,** Suprasternal two-dimensional echocardiogram revealing a dilated ascending aorta (AAo) and a markedly narrowed descending aorta (DAo). The actual tissue of the coarctation is not easily visualized in this image. **B,** Continuous-wave Doppler through the descending thoracic aorta, revealing a peak pressure gradient across the area of narrowing of 72 mm Hg.

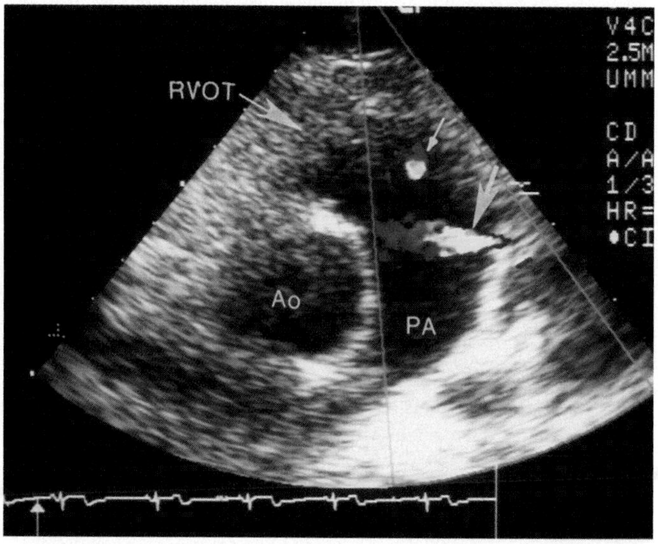

FIGURE 11–95 Parasternal short-axis view at the level of the great vessels recorded in a patient with persistent ductus arteriosus. Note the dilated pulmonary artery (PA) and the abnormal color flow signal (large arrow) that originates from the area of the descending thoracic aorta and flows into the pulmonary artery distal to the pulmonary valve. In this diastolic frame, note the small pulmonic insufficiency jet (small white arrow). Ao = aorta; RVOT = right ventricular outflow tract.

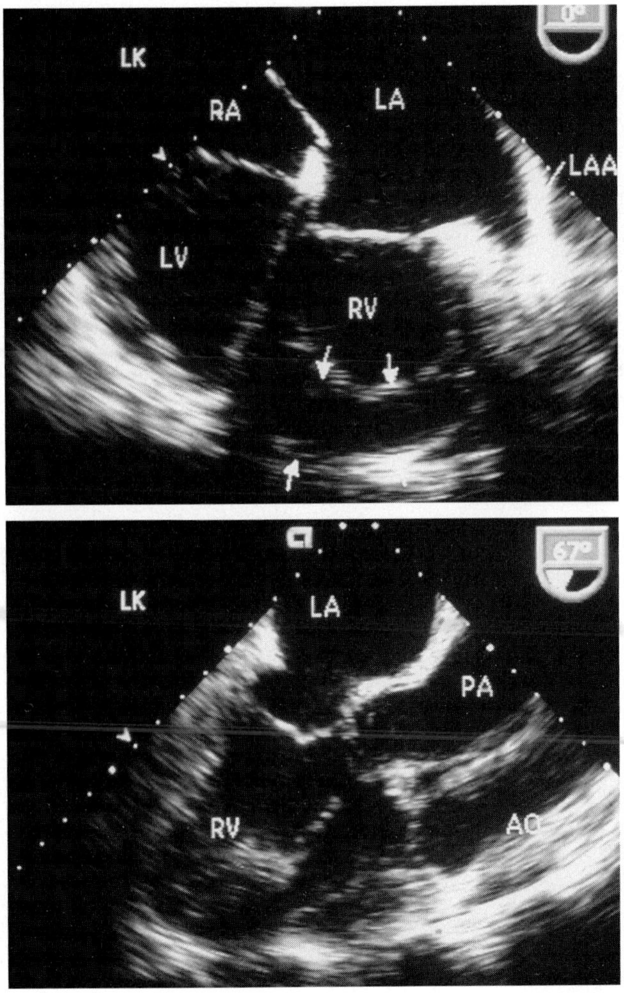

FIGURE 11–97 Transesophageal echocardiogram in an adult patient with L-transposition of the great vessels. In the **top panel,** the connection of the anatomical right atrium to the anatomical left ventricle and the communication of the anatomical left atrium, through an anatomical tricuspid valve, into an anatomical right ventricle can be appreciated. Note the normal-appearing left atrial appendage (LAA). Note also the marked hypertrophy of the right ventricular trabeculations, which nearly obliterate the apex of the anatomical right ventricle (RV) (arrows). There is apical displacement of the atrioventricular valve contained within the anatomical right ventricle, compared with the atrioventricular (mitral) valve connecting the right atrium (RA) to the left ventricle (LV). The **lower panel** depicts the parallel orientation of the pulmonary artery (PA) and aorta (AO). The more anteriorly placed aorta is in communication with the anatomical right ventricle.

groove often only in systole. A small pericardial effusion is defined as less than 5 mm in maximum dimension, which is visualized throughout the cardiac cycle. Moderate pericardial effusions typically are 15 to 20 mm in dimension and tend to be more circumferential. Large effusions are defined as those larger than 20 mm. Because patients are scanned in a supine or left lateral position, the fluid tends to pool and to be mostly visible in the posterior aspects of the imaging planes. Numerous attempts have been made to quantify the amount of pericardial fluid but have not seen uniform acceptance. The majority of laboratories use the semiquantitative scheme noted earlier. Three-dimensional echocardiography has shown some promise for enhanced localization and quantitation of pericardial effusion. The most commonly employed technique for quantifying the volume of effusion is to image the effusion in orthogonal planes and determine the intrapericardial volume using Simpson's rule. The entire cardiac silhouette can then likewise be traced and the total cardiac volume determined. The difference between the pericardial and cardiac volumes represents the volume of pericardial fluid. Although theoretically accurate, there are practical limitations to tracing both the cardiac and pericardial volumes that render this technique less than optimal and of little true clinical utility.

Other aspects of a pericardial effusion also can be noted with echocardiography. Soft tissue density masses, thickening of the visceral pericardium, and presence of fibrinous strands can all be identified. All of these features are more common in patients with marked inflammatory or malignant causes for pericardial effusion. Additionally, the nature of the fluid can be further characterized as clear or "cloudy." The hallmark of the benign, idiopathic effusion is a clear echo-free space, whereas malignancy, bacterial infection, and hemorrhagic effusions are more likely to have solid components or stranding.

Cardiac Tamponade

Several echocardiographic findings are reliable indicators of elevated intrapericardial pressure, which in turn correlate with hemodynamic compromise or clinical tamponade. One of the earliest described was collapse of the right ventricular outflow tract during early diastole. This is best visualized in the parasternal views but can also be appreciated in the four-chamber view. The precise timing and duration of right ventricular collapse can best be determined with M-mode echocardiography. Cardiac tamponade occurs when pericardial effusion of sufficient magnitude has accumulated to result in equilibration of intrapericardial and passively determined intracardiac pressures. Immediately after mechanical systole, the ventricle begins to relax, with a greater degree of active relaxation attributed to the left ventricle compared with the right. This results in disproportionate or favored filling of the left ventricle with a transient elevation in intrapericardial pressure, which results in turn in early diastolic collapse of the highly compliant right ventricular outflow tract (Figs. 11–100 and 11–101). Detection of transient outflow tract collapse is a reliable marker that intrapericardial pressure is elevated and hemodynamic compromise is present. It is correlated with the presence of overt tamponade but also has been seen in patients who subsequently developed tamponade. The atrial corollary of this phenomenon is exaggerated atrial emptying. Because of elevated intrapericardial pressures, filling of the right ventricle is impeded in early diastole (a manifestation of which is early diastolic right ventricular collapse) and occurs to an exaggerated degree with atrial systole. This results in a delayed and exaggerated contraction of the right atrium with actual invagination of the atrial wall in late diastole (Fig. 11–102). This echocardiographic sign of hemodynamic compromise is more sensitive than right ventricular diastolic collapse but less specific, because it occurs earlier in the course of intrapericardial pressure elevation. Right ventricular collapse may be absent even in the presence of elevated pericardial pressures in patients with right ventricular hypertrophy or significant pulmonary hypertension. In the presence of loculated effusion or in complex situations, either right- or left-sided chambers may be differentially compressed.

Doppler echocardiography can also provide valuable clues as to the hemodynamic significance of pericardial effusions. In patients with hemodynamically significant effusions, there is exaggerated interplay between right and left ventricular filling, occurring with phases of the respiratory cycle. Clinically, this is manifest as an exaggerated pulsus paradoxus. Echocardiographically exaggerated respiratory variation can be documented by examining the left ventricular and right ventricular outflow tract flows in systole and noting exaggerated phasic variation in velocities and time velocity integrals (Fig. 11–103). Similarly, in patients with a hemodynamically significant effusion, ventricular filling is impeded. The normal respiratory variation of the tricuspid valve is 25 percent, with a greater velocity in inspiration than expiration, and the normal mitral valve shows the opposite pattern with a variation of approximately 15 percent. In patients with hemodynamically significant effusions, there is a greater than usual variation in this respiratory pattern (Fig. 11–104).

Constrictive Pericarditis

Although chronic constrictive pericarditis remains an elusive diagnosis, echocardiography and Doppler evaluation can provide valuable clues as to its presence. The classic form of constrictive pericarditis is calcific constrictive pericarditis after tuberculosis infection. In contemporary times, constric-

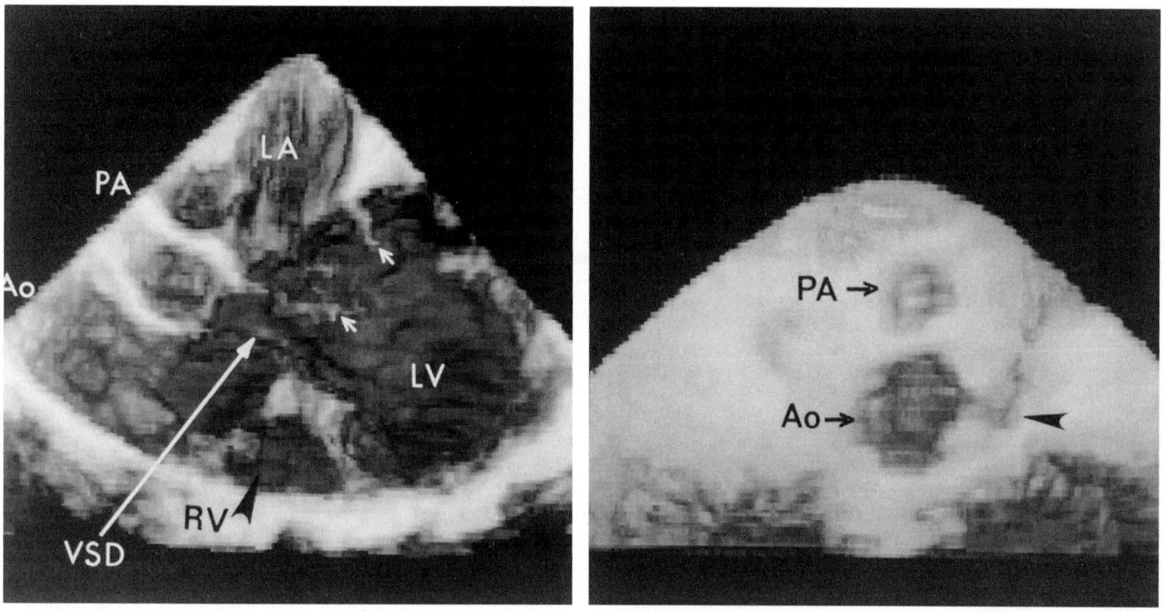

FIGURE 11–98 Three-dimensional echocardiogram of a patient with a ventricular septal defect, transposition, and double outlet right ventricle. Note the small right ventricular cavity and the parallel orientation of the two great vessels. Ao = aorta; LA = left atrium; LV = left ventricle; PA = pulmonary artery; RV = right ventricle; VSD = ventricular septal defect.

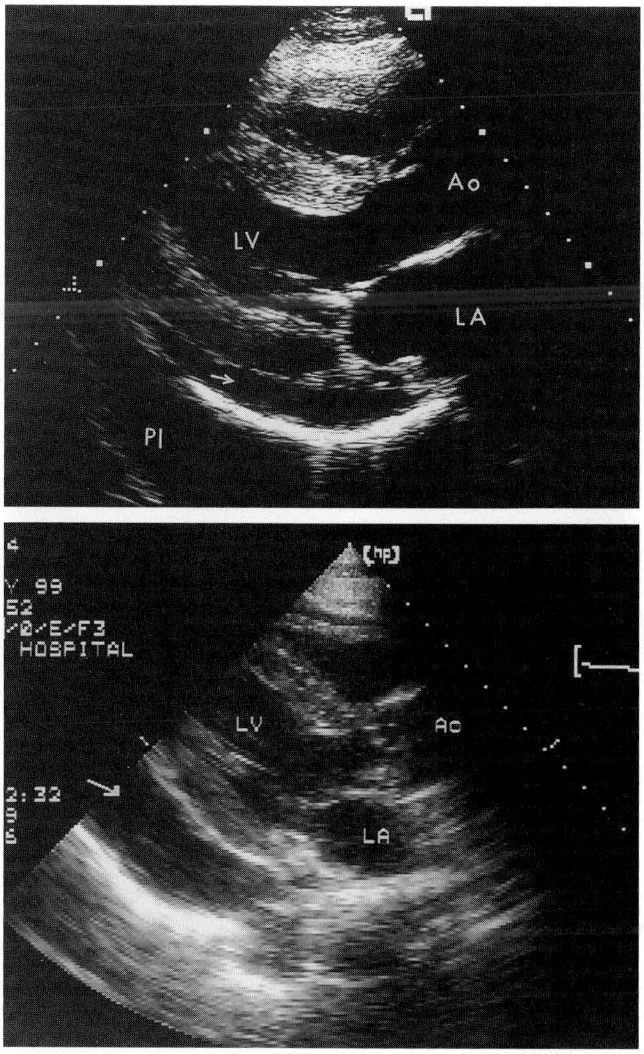

FIGURE 11–99 Transthoracic parasternal long-axis echocardiograms recorded in a patient with a small **(top)** pericardial effusion. Note the echo-free space confined to the area posterior to the heart (arrow). The **bottom panel** reveals a similar pattern but with a larger echo-free space (arrow). Ao = aorta; LA = left atrium; LV = left ventricle; Pl = pleural effusion.

tion is more likely to be related to nontuberculous infections, hemorrhagic effusions, cardiac surgery, or irradiation. The clinical presentation and echocardiographic appearance often vary from those classically described with calcific constriction. Numerous attempts have been made to quantify pericardial thickness using echocardiography. Routine transthoracic imaging has not been an accurate means for detecting pericardial thickening. TEE has shown more promise but has not seen clinical acceptance. Intracardiac ultrasonography does provide a high-resolution view of the pericardium but is an invasive procedure and has been validated in only a small number of patients. Determination of pericardial thickening is probably more accurately done with computed tomography (CT) or MRI.

In the absence of direct ultrasonographic documentation of thickened pericardium, there are indirect signs of pericardial constriction that should be evaluated in suspected cases, including abnormalities of ventricular septal motion. The abnormalities of septal motion that occur are an exaggerated respiratory variation in septal position with marked bowing of the ventricular septum toward the left ventricle during inspiration. Additionally, when viewed from the parasternal long-axis position, an abnormality of septal motion is often detected. This frequently is seen as a downward motion of the ventricular septum in early systole, followed by a brief anterior motion, which can be confused with a conduction disturbance and is best detected with M-mode scanning.

The Doppler hallmarks of cardiac constriction include exaggerated respiratory variation of mitral and tricuspid inflows with a pathologically elevated E/A ratio (Fig. 11–105).[136,137] Additionally, deceleration time is abnormally short and may vary to a disproportionate degree during the respiratory cycle. Examination of the IVC frequently reveals dilation. The normal multiphasic hepatic vein flow is replaced by monophasic flow, occurring predominantly in systole.

The diagnosis of constrictive pericarditis in large part remains one of exclusion. From an echocardiographic standpoint, this diagnosis should be suspected in individuals with symptoms consistent with that diagnosis (i.e., edema, fatigue, and apparent low output state), normal left ventricular systolic function, and no valvular heart disease. Detection of

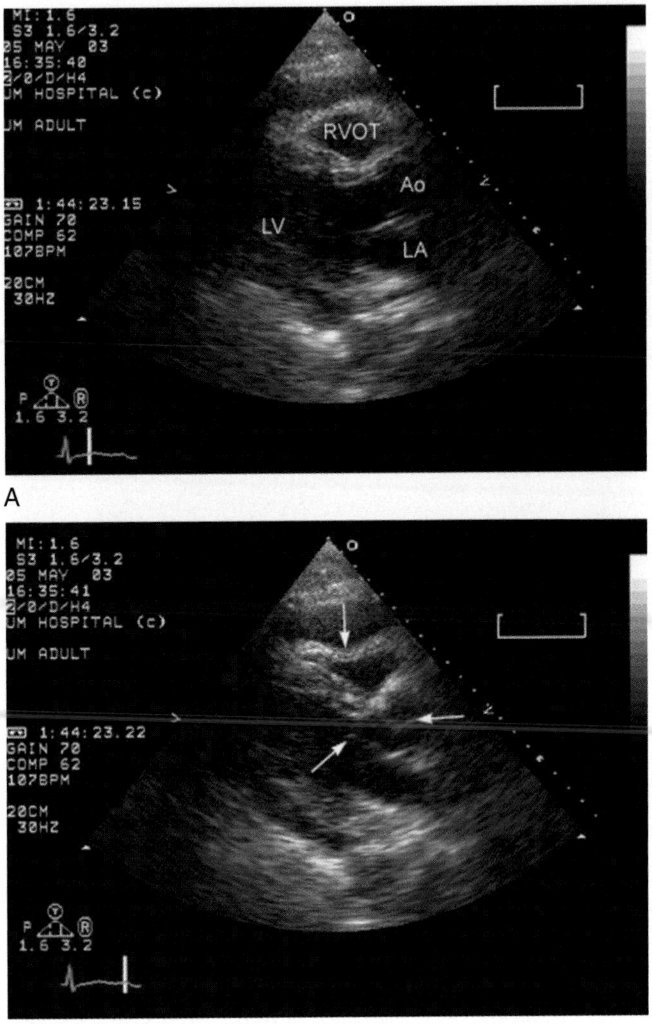

FIGURE 11–100 Parasternal long-axis view of a patient with a moderate pericardial effusion and collapse of the right ventricular outflow tract in early diastole. **A,** Recorded in midsystole to late systole (see electrocardiogram in lower left of figure). The right ventricular outflow tract (RVOT) has a normal configuration. **B,** Recorded in early diastole; note the open mitral valve and closed aortic valve (arrows). There is distinct inward collapse of the RVOT (downward pointing arrow) at this point in the cardiac cycle. Ao = aorta; LA = left atrium; LV = left ventricle.

abnormal septal motion, exaggerated respiratory variation, and an elevated E/A ratio provide the majority of the confirmatory evidence of this diagnosis.

MISCELLANEOUS CONDITIONS OF THE PERICARDIUM. Congenital absence of the pericardium occurs in both partial and complete forms. In the complete form, there is a marked abnormality of septal motion with exaggerated intracardiac motion within the thorax. In the partial form, varying degrees of septal motion abnormality can be detected, depending on the degree to which the pericardium is anatomically deficient. Pericardial cysts are detected as echo-free spaces adjacent to the heart. The diagnosis should probably be confirmed by CT or MRI as well.

Cardiomyopathies (see Chap. 59)

Cardiomyopathies can be divided into three basic types: dilated cardiomyopathy of any cause, hypertrophic cardiomyopathy, and restrictive cardiomyopathy.

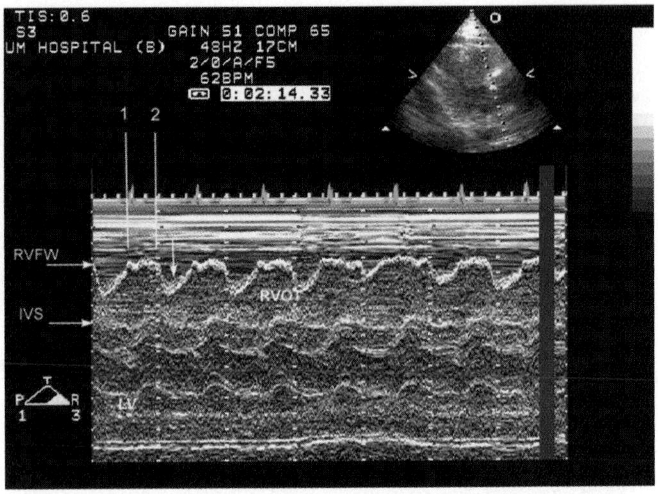

FIGURE 11–101 M-mode echocardiogram recorded in a patient with evidence of hemodynamic compromise. The M-mode beam traverses the right ventricular outflow tract (RVOT), right ventricular free wall (RVFW), and interventricular septum (IVS). Note the distinct diastolic collapse of the right ventricular free wall. Point 1 represents end diastole and the right ventricle is fully expanded. Point 2 represents end systole, at which point the right ventricle has remained expanded. Note that following end systole, there is a dramatic downward motion of the RVFW (arrow), representing collapse of the RVFW, which is indicative of elevated intrapericardial pressure.

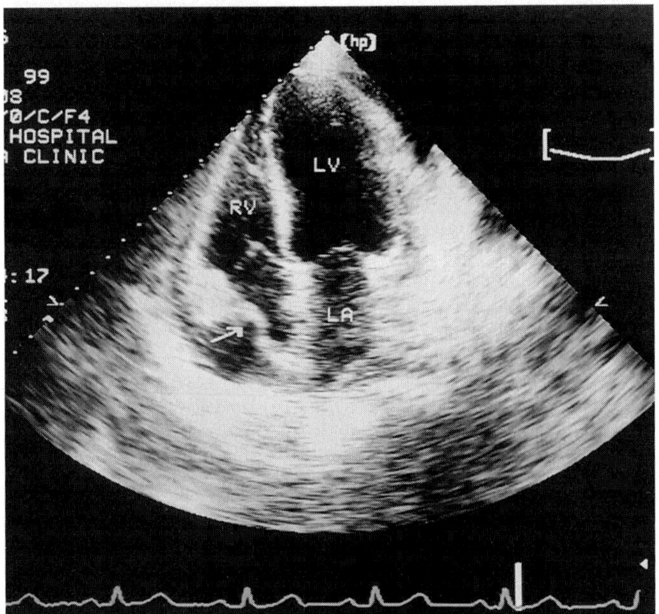

FIGURE 11–102 Apical four-chamber view recorded in a patient with a moderate pericardial effusion and evidence of hemodynamic compromise. The frame is recorded in early ventricular systole, immediately after atrial contraction. Note that the right atrial wall is indented inward and its curvature is frankly reversed (arrow), implying elevated intrapericardial pressure above right atrial pressure. LA = left atrium; LV = left ventricle; RV = right ventricle.

Dilated Cardiomyopathy

Irrespective of the cause of a dilated cardiomyopathy, left ventricular dilation with global systolic dysfunction is noted (Figs. 11–106 and 11–107). Depending on the duration of the disease, left atrial dilation likewise occurs; if significant mitral regurgitation is present, secondary pulmonary hypertension with right-sided heart dilation is common. The range of systolic dysfunction in patients with dilated cardiomyopathy is quite broad, and ejection fraction ranges from less

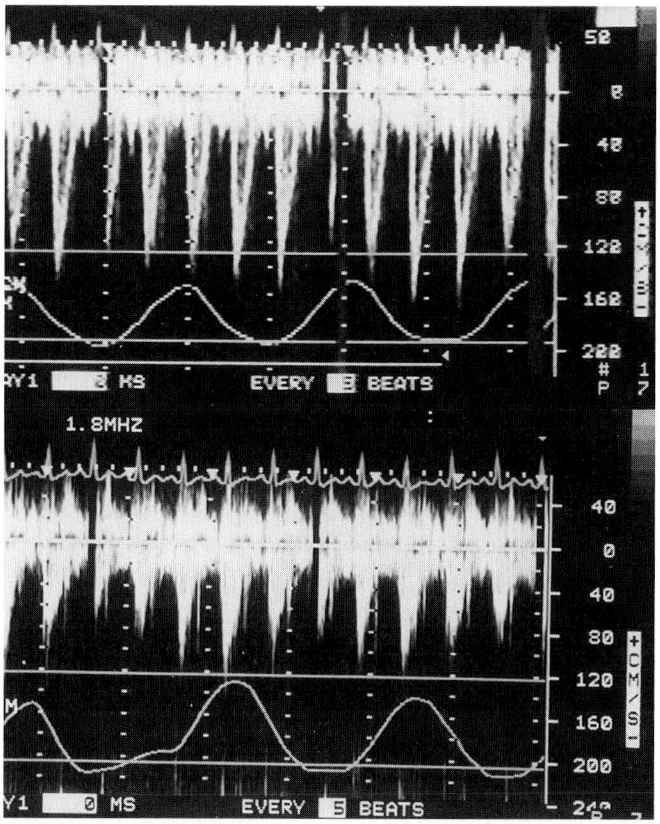

FIGURE 11–103 Pulsed-wave spectral Doppler recorded through the left ventricular outflow tract **(top)** and right ventricular outflow tract **(bottom)** in a patient with hemodynamic compromise due to pericardial effusion. Note the respirometry line on the bottom of each tracing. There is exaggerated respiratory velocity of flow in both the left ventricular and right ventricular outflow tracts. Note the reciprocal nature of the flow variation, with flow increasing during expiration and decreasing in early inspiration for the left ventricular outflow tract and the opposite pattern seen in the right ventricular outflow tract.

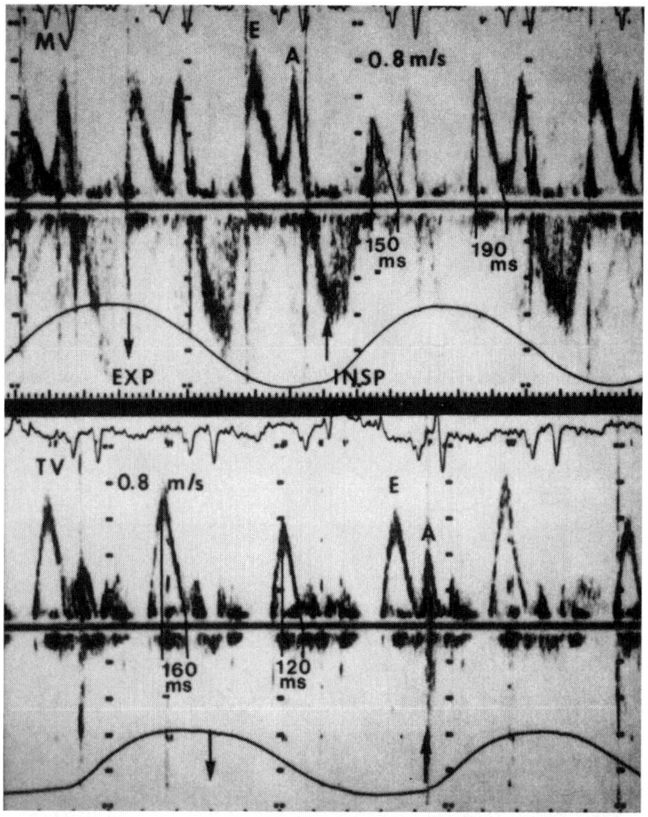

FIGURE 11–105 Pulsed Doppler recording through the mitral valve **(top)** and tricuspid **(bottom)** in a patient with constrictive pericarditis. Note the respirometer tracing for each. There is exaggerated respiratory variation in inflow velocities in both the mitral and tricuspid valves. Note also that the deceleration time is shorter with inspiration (150 msec) than with expiration in the mitral tracing. Reciprocal changes are noted in the tricuspid valve flow patterns. (From Oh JK, Hatle LK, Seward JB, et al: Diagnostic role of Doppler echocardiography in constrictive pericarditis. J Am Coll Cardiol 23:154, 1994; with the permission of the American College of Cardiology Foundation.)

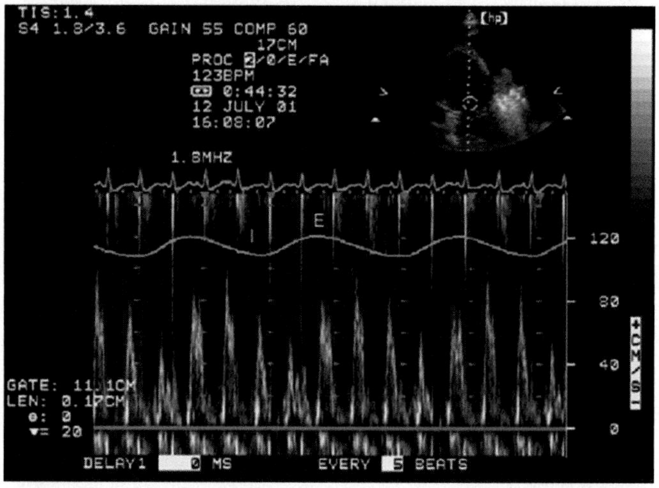

FIGURE 11–104 Pulsed Doppler of the mitral valve inflow in a patient with hemodynamically significant pericardial effusion. Note the exaggerated respiratory variation of inflow with greater than 25 percent variation in e-wave velocity. A respirometer tracing is superimposed on the pulsed Doppler flow velocity. E = expiration; I = inspiration.

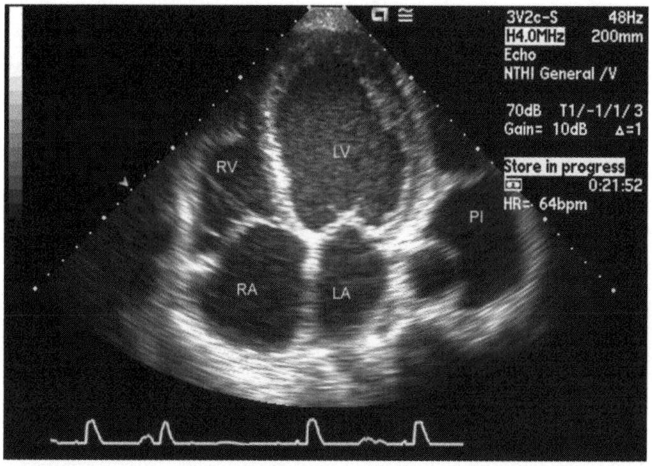

FIGURE 11–106 Apical four-chamber view of a patient with a dilated cardiomyopathy. Note the dilation of all four chambers and the relatively spherical geometry of the left ventricular cavity. Incidental note is made of a pleural effusion (PI). LA = left atrium; LV = left ventricle; RA = right atrium; RV = right ventricle.

than 10 percent to only mildly diminished. Although dilated cardiomyopathy is a global process, because of regional wall stress and loading conditions, regional heterogeneity of function is seen.[138] Typically, the proximal portions of the inferoposterior and posterolateral walls have relatively preserved systolic function, whereas the more distal walls, the ventricular septum, and apex appear more severely compromised. This pattern of wall motion may initially be confused with ischemic heart disease. The absence of frank scar or aneurysm and the absence of any truly normally functioning segments

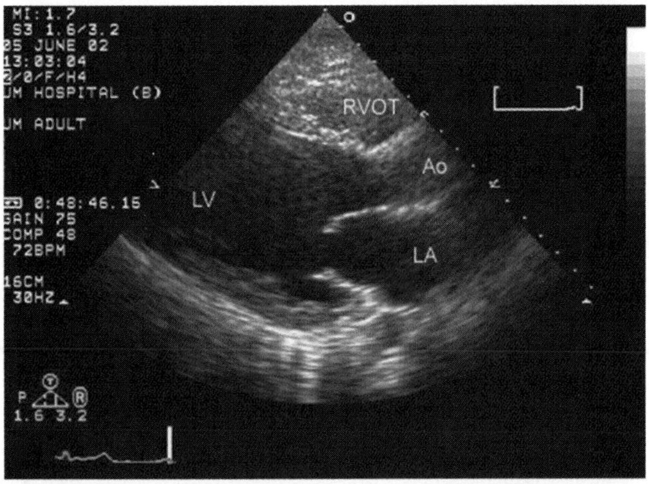

A

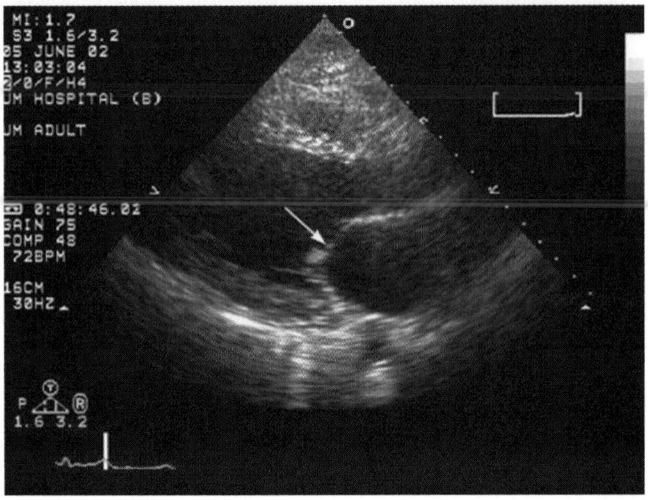

B

FIGURE 11–107 Parasternal long-axis views of a patient with a dilated cardiomyopathy recorded in diastole **(A)** and systole **(B)**. Note in the lower panel, the mitral valve is now closed (arrow), however, there is little visible change in the size of the left ventricular cavity. Ao = aorta; LA = left atrium; LV = left ventricle; RVOT = right ventricular outflow tract.

should lead the observer to appropriately make a diagnosis of nonischemic cardiomyopathy. The echocardiographic appearance of nonischemic cardiomyopathy is not dependent on its cause, and patients with alcoholic, doxorubicin (Adriamycin)–induced, idiopathic, or postviral causes all have a similar echocardiographic appearance.

As a consequence of left ventricular dilation, the bullet-shaped geometry of the left ventricle is often distorted and the left ventricle becomes more spherical. This has the effect of drawing the papillary muscles away from the mitral valve annulus and results in functional mitral regurgitation due to abnormal coaptation of the mitral valve (see Fig. 11–57).[102,103] Mitral regurgitation severity may range from mild to severe, and, as a consequence, left atrial dilation to some degree is invariably present. Because of the diffuse nature of the initial insult, the right ventricle can be primarily affected with dilation and hypokinesis and also secondarily affected due to subsequent pulmonary hypertension. Other complications of dilated cardiomyopathy that should be evaluated include the presence of left ventricular thrombus and, in certain circumstances, development of left atrial thrombi. Detection of the latter requires TEE. The magnitude of secondary tricuspid regurgitation and pulmonary hypertension can be reliably determined from Doppler evaluation of the tricuspid valve. Evaluation of diastolic properties of the left ventricle may provide valuable prognostic information. Generally, mitral valve inflow patterns showing a "restrictive pattern" with a high E/A ratio or pseudonormalization confer a substantially worse prognosis.[139-141] Other echocardiographic features associated with a worse prognosis include increased left atrial size[142] and mitral and tricuspid regurgitation.[143]

HYPERTROPHIC CARDIOMYOPATHY

Hypertrophic cardiomyopathy is a heterogeneous disease in which there is inappropriate, pathological hypertrophy of the left ventricle and, less commonly, the right ventricle. The classic form of hypertrophic cardiomyopathy was previously termed *idiopathic hypertrophic subaortic stenosis*. In this entity, there is characteristic disproportionate hypertrophy of the proximal ventricular septum with dynamic left ventricular outflow tract obstruction (Fig. 11-108). Because hypertrophic cardiomyopathy is a heterogeneous disease, the preferred terminology is *hypertrophic cardiomyopathy*, secondarily described as focal, concentric, apical, and with or without obstruction.

From an echocardiographic perspective, outflow obstructive hypertrophic cardiomyopathy is associated with systolic anterior motion of the mitral valve. This results in development of a dynamic systolic gradient that develops in the left ventricular outflow tract over the course of systole (Fig. 11-109). Thus, the maximum gradient is in late systole as opposed to early or midsystole, which is characteristic of a fixed valvular or other discrete obstruction. Systolic anterior motion of the mitral valve can be detected with two-dimensional echocardiography, typically from the parasternal long-axis view, and also with M-mode echocardiography (Fig. 11-110). Although Doppler echocardiography remains the definitive examination for detection and quantification of outflow tract obstruction, secondary evidence of outflow tract obstruction can be

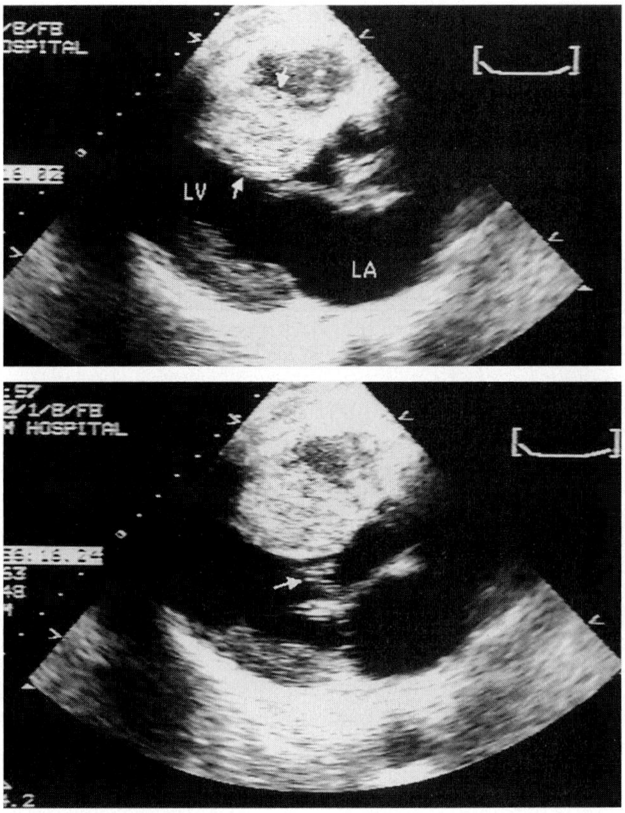

FIGURE 11–108 Parasternal long-axis views recorded in a patient with a hypertrophic cardiomyopathy. The **top panel** is diastole and the **bottom panel** is systole. (Note this image has been recorded in tissue harmonic imaging and therefore myocardial signatures and brightness are increased. No assumptions regarding tissue characterization should be made from a tissue harmonic image.) In the top panel, note the marked thickening of the ventricular septum (white arrows), which measures approximately 3 cm in thickness. The posterior wall was only mildly hypertrophied. The bottom panel was recorded in systole, and systolic anterior motion of the mitral valve (arrow) is clearly seen. LA = left atrium; LV = left ventricle.

obtained from the M-mode echocardiogram. Systolic anterior motion of the mitral valve that remains in contact with the septum for 40 percent of the systolic cycle is more likely to be associated with significant hemodynamic obstruction. Additionally, the outflow tract obstruction results in a characteristic systolic notching pattern on the aortic valve that is best visualized with M-mode echocardiography.

Mitral regurgitation is common in patients with obstructive hypertrophic cardiomyopathy, and the continuous wave of Doppler spectral profile of the mitral regurgitation may occasionally be confused with outflow tract obstruction. It should be kept in mind that the mitral regurgitation velocity will peak relatively early, whereas the outflow tract obstruction has a characteristic late-peaking "dagger-like" appearance.

Other variants of hypertrophic cardiomyopathy include mid-cavity obstruction, in which case the maximum gradient is typically at the papillary muscle level. An additional form of hypertrophy includes concentric left ventricular hypertrophy that may have no associated outflow tract obstruction. In this instance, patients can be highly symptomatic because of a relatively small left ventricular cavity with markedly elevated diastolic pressures. Additionally, the small cavity, even with supernormal systolic functions, results in a low stroke volume and cardiac output. Occasionally, patients are encountered who have isolated hypertrophy of the lateral or inferior walls (Fig. 11–111). A final variant of hypertrophic cardiomyopathy is the apical variant, which is more common in Asian populations. Deep T-wave inversions across the precordium are seen in this variant. By definition, it is not obstructive.

Two-dimensional echocardiography and Doppler imaging can be used to follow the status of outflow tract gradients at rest or exercise and after either pharmacological, surgical, or, more recently, catheter-based septal reduction therapy.[144] A reduction in both the outflow tract gradient and the severity of mitral regurgitation can be documented after successful therapy. On occasion, patients present with what appears to be a "burned-out" hypertrophic cardiomyopathy. In this instance, unexplained pathological hypertrophy is present with a relatively normal-sized left ventricle that is diffusely hypokinetic. Frequently, systolic function has deteriorated to the point that there is no longer an outflow tract gradient. Any of the forms of hypertrophic cardiomyopathy can result in long-standing elevation of diastolic pressure and secondary pulmonary hypertension.

Restrictive and Infiltrative Cardiomyopathy

Restrictive cardiomyopathies are a family of diseases in which systolic function is relatively preserved until very late stages but the ventricular myocardium is pathologically stiff, leading to chronic elevation of diastolic pressure. Symptoms result because of the elevated diastolic pressures. By definition, obstruction is not present, nor is there a primary cause for abnormal myocardial relaxation. The most common form of restrictive cardiomyopathy is the idiopathic restrictive cardiomyopathy most often seen in the elderly. In this disease, both atria are dilated, wall thickness tends to be at the upper normal limit or mildly hypertrophied, systolic function is within normal limits or only mildly depressed, and there is Doppler evidence of abnormal ventricular filling. Typically, this is manifest as an elevated E/A ratio without exaggerated respiratory variation.

Other causes of restrictive physiology include infiltrative cardiomyopathies, the most common of which is cardiac amyloidosis. Other rarer causes include the glycogen storage diseases and association with other systemic diseases.

Cardiac amyloidosis can manifest as either a primary or a secondary entity and is often associated with amyloid deposits in other organs. Amyloid deposition in the myocardium results in hypertrophy in the absence of hypertension and abnormal myocardial texture, which is noted as a bright "speckling" appearance (Fig. 11–112). Caution is advised when using second harmonic imaging, because this type of instrumentation leads to the appearance of an abnormal myocardial signature as well. There is often evidence of diastolic dysfunction. In the early phases, a reduced E/A ratio with a flat deceleration slope is seen. Later, an elevated E/A ratio occurs, associated with a short deceleration time. This pattern has been associated with a worse prognosis.[145] In patients with advanced amyloid, virtually all cardiac structures, including valve leaflets, are involved. In late phases, systolic dysfunction is seen.

DISTINCTION OF RESTRICTIVE AND CONSTRICTIVE PHYSIOLOGY. The distinction between constrictive pericarditis and a restrictive cardiomyopathy is often clinically problematic. Echocardiography can play several valuable roles in this clinical situation. The first is in the exclusion of primary valvular disease, left ventricular dysfunction, and pulmonary hypertension, which may have resulted in the clinical presentation. Typically, patients in whom this dilemma arises have preserved right and left ventricular systolic function with signs and symptoms of heart failure. Signs and symptoms of right-sided failure often predominate. Other than detection of cardiac amyloid or in patients in whom there are classic findings of constriction, the separation of these two entities relies heavily on Doppler echocardiography. In both cases, the E/A ratio is elevated, but in cases of constriction there is a greater than usual respiratory variation

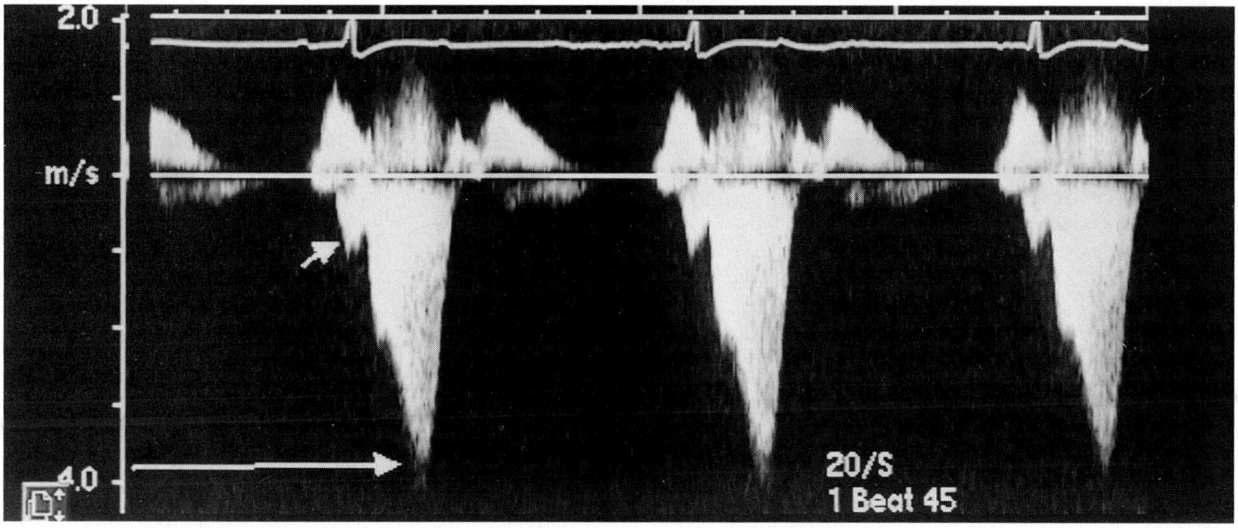

FIGURE 11–109 Continuous-wave Doppler recorded from the apex of the left ventricle with the interrogation being directed through the left ventricular outflow tract in a patient with an obstructive hypertrophic cardiomyopathy. Note the late peaking systolic gradient with a peak velocity of approximately 3.8 m/sec (corresponding to a peak pressure gradient of 58 mm Hg). Additionally (small arrow), there is evidence of presystolic forward flow in the left ventricular outflow tract, following atrial systole. This is consistent with a hypertrophied and noncompliant ventricle in which atrial contraction results in presystolic flow in the outflow tract.

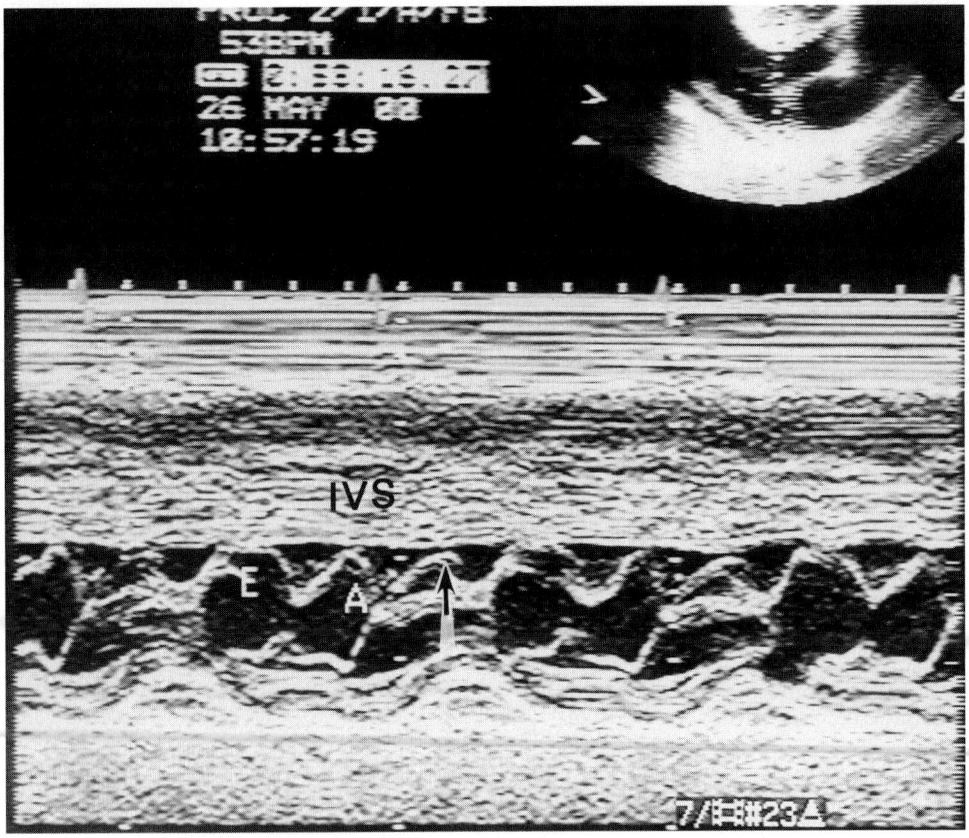

FIGURE 11–110 M-mode echocardiogram recorded in the same patient depicted in Figure 11–108. Note the markedly thickened ventricular septum. The mitral valve as seen directly below the ventricular septum and the E and A waves in diastole are noted. Note in systole there is anterior motion of the mitral valve (black/white arrow).

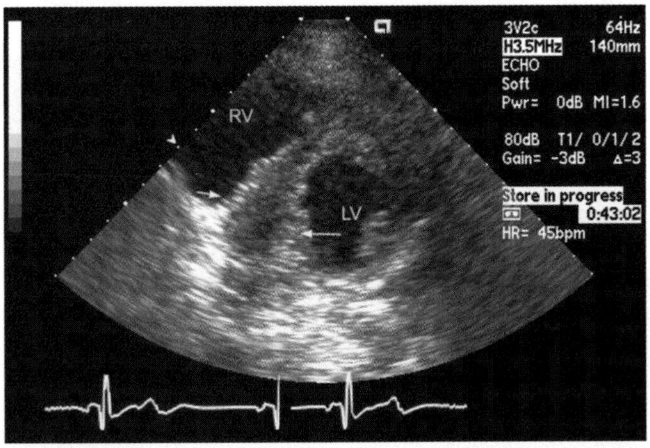

FIGURE 11–111 Transthoracic two-dimensional echocardiogram in a short axis at the midventricular level in a patient with hypertrophic cardiomyopathy. This is a variant of hypertrophic cardiomyopathy in which the predominant hypertrophy is in the true inferior wall and inferior septum. The full thickness of the inferior septum and wall are as noted by the arrows. LV = left ventricle; RV = right ventricle.

in inflow velocities.[146,147] Deceleration time is short in both but varies to a greater degree in restrictive than in constrictive processes. Examination of pulmonary and hepatic vein flow can be helpful as well. In both instances, vein flow is monophasic, but in cases of restriction, there is a greater degree of flow reversal in late diastole coincident with inspiration. Doppler tissue imaging to interrogate the velocity of myocardial relaxation can also play a role. Most patients with restrictive disease have delayed relaxation and delayed motion of the annulus compared with patients with constrictive pericarditis.[148] The diagnosis of constrictive pericarditis and its separation from restrictive diseases remains problematic even in experienced hands, and many atypical cases of each process exist. Both processes can also coexist, and this combination is not uncommon after radiation therapy, in which there may be a constrictive component in the pericardium but a restrictive component to the right ventricle due to radiation injury.

Ischemic Heart Disease

BASIC PRINCIPLES. Myocardial ischemia and infarction result in regional disturbances of ventricular contraction. After acute reduction in coronary flow, both diastolic and systolic dysfunction occur. Normal systolic contraction consists of both myocardial thickening and inward motion of the endocardium (see Figs. 11–12 and 11–14). Immediately after the onset of ischemia, myocardial thickening ceases and, depending on the size of the anatomical area and the severity of ischemia, the wall can become frankly dyskinetic (Figs. 11–113 and 11–114). If blood flow is not restored, myocardial necrosis results and the wall motion abnormality persists. Over a period of approximately 6 weeks, actual tissue loss occurs, and there is replacement by fibrous tissue and a scar forms.

Myocardial Infarction (see Chap. 46)

As noted earlier, myocardial necrosis, once established, results in a permanent wall motion abnormality. The degree of transmural involvement required before wall motion becomes abnormal is approximately 20 percent. The implication of this is that nontransmural myocardial infarction will result in hypokinesis or akinesis of the wall, even though the majority of the myocardial mass may still be perfused and viable. A tethering effect of nontransmural infarction or ischemia results in dysfunction of the entire wall thickness. Because the balance of the myocardium is intrinsically normal, it is capable of overriding this effect during either pharmacological stimulation or stress, therefore resulting in substantial cardiovascular reserve in segments that may be akinetic at rest. The regional wall motion score is directly related to the size of the myocardial infarction; however, because of the tethering phenomenon, wall motion abnormalities overestimate the true anatomical extent.[149]

Tethering occurs in several different forms. The most common occurs in substantial size myocardial infarction where the infarcted area may be frankly dyskinetic. During systole, the dyskinetic segment drags the normal myocardium outward. Thus, this normal myocardium, which intrinsically has the capacity to contract, is tethered to the abnormal myocardium and is functionally abnormal. The opposite phenomenon can occur in patients with relatively small infarctions in whom, during cardiovascular stress, the normal

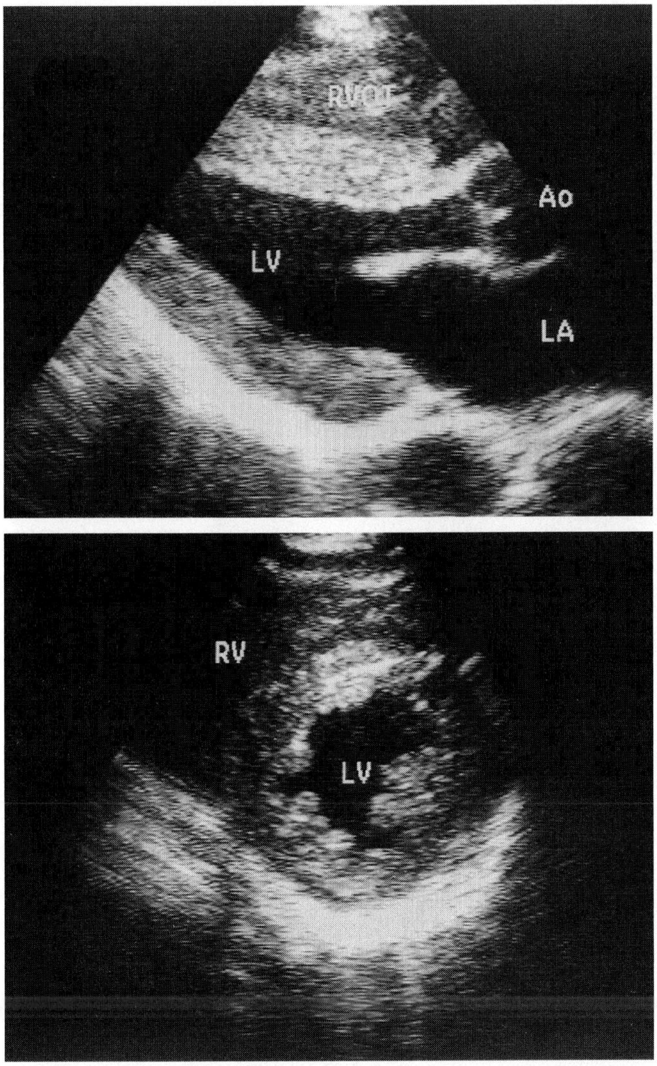

FIGURE 11–112 Two-dimensional echocardiogram recorded in a patient with cardiac amyloid. In both the parasternal long-axis view **(top)** and short-axis view **(bottom)**, note the homogeneous echo intensity of the myocardium. Both the mitral and aortic valves are also thickened. In real time, the myocardium takes on a speckled appearance. Ao = aorta; LA = left atrium; LV = left ventricle; RV = right ventricle.

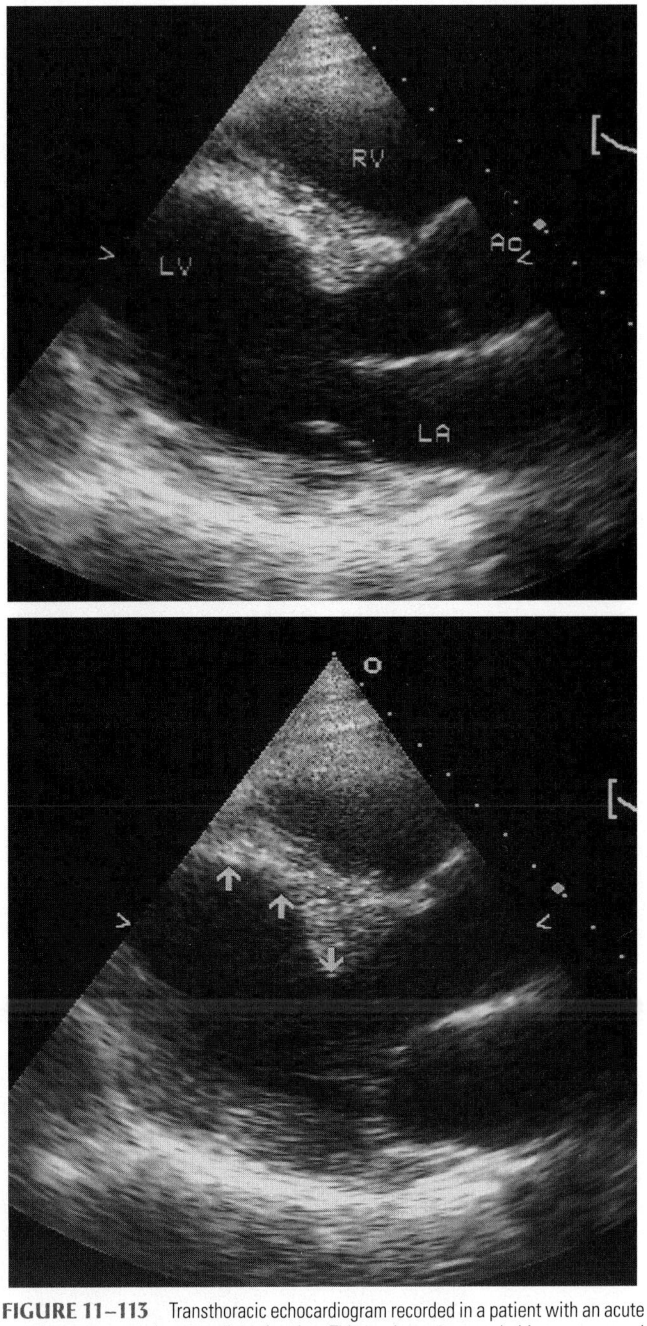

FIGURE 11–113 Transthoracic echocardiogram recorded in a patient with an acute anterior anteroseptal myocardial infarction. This tracing was recorded in a parasternal long-axis view, in diastole **(top)** and in systole **(bottom)**. In the lower panel, note the normal downward motion of the proximal portion of the ventricular septum and the dyskinesis of the more distal portions of the anterior septum (upward arrows). Ao = aorta; LA = left atrium; LV = left ventricle; RV = right ventricle.

healthy adjacent myocardium contracts more vigorously and drags the abnormal segment with it, thus masking the wall motion abnormality. A final form of tethering is "vertical" tethering, in which ischemic or infarcted subendocardial layers exert a disproportionate effect on overall myocardial contractility. Because only 20 percent of the myocardium needs to be involved in the ischemic or infarction process for the entire wall to become dysfunctional, nontransmural (non-Q-wave myocardial infarction) results in a wall motion abnormality that is indistinguishable from that of transmural infarction.

More recently advanced Doppler-based methods have been used to detect and quantify wall motion abnormalities. Both Doppler tissue imaging and strain rate imaging have shown promise as a sensitive means for detecting systolic and diastolic abnormalities during ischemia.[150,151]

Depending on the location and size of the necrotic area, ventricular remodeling will also occur. Remodeling takes several forms and ranges from formation of a frank aneurysm (Figs. 11–115 and 11–116) to progressive left ventricular dilation. Echocardiographically, an aneurysm is defined as a noncontracting area of myocardium with abnormal geometry in both diastole and systole.

In clinical echocardiography, a regional wall motion abnormality, conforming to a known coronary distribution, is the hallmark of acute ischemia or myocardial infarction. Detection of a wall motion abnormality with echocardiography can be a valuable adjunct in the diagnosis of ischemia in patients who are presenting with chest pain.[152-154] After successful reperfusion, wall motion abnormalities typically will resolve. The time course over which they resolve is variable and may range from 12 hours to 2 weeks. Typically, wall motion abnormalities recover within 72 hours if blood flow has been restored in a timely fashion.

At the time of a patient's presentation with acute myocardial infarction, there are several echocardiographic findings that relate to prognosis. As with all imaging techniques, the

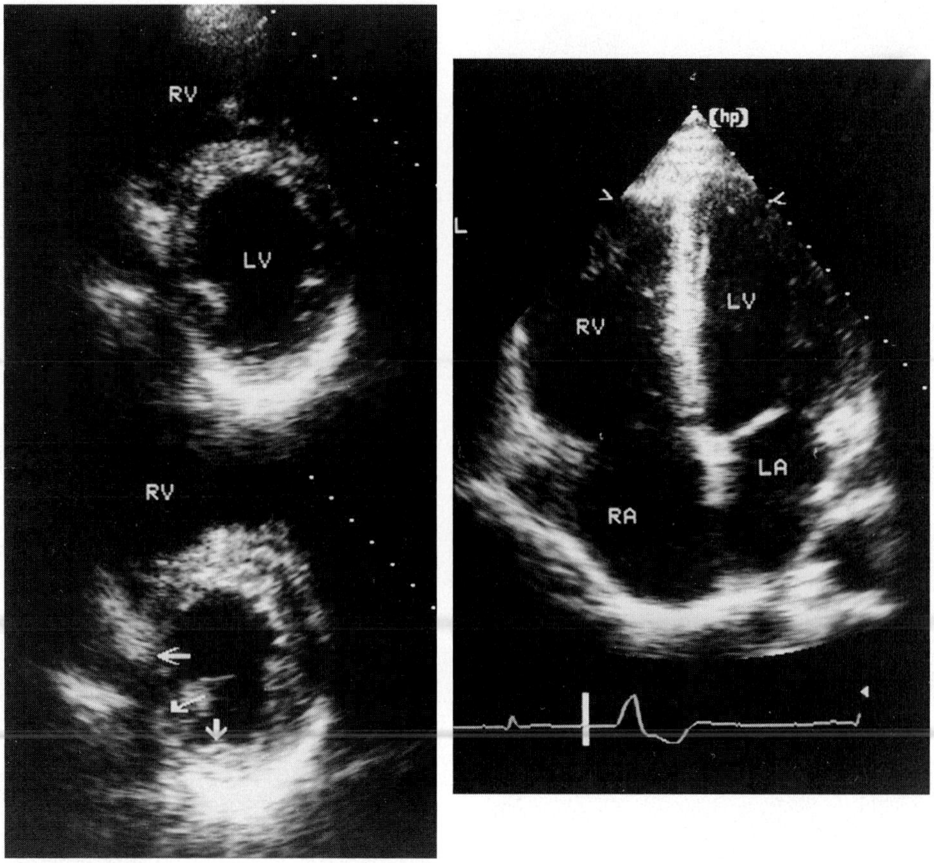

FIGURE 11–114 Two-dimensional echocardiogram recorded in a patient with an inferior myocardial infarction complicated by right ventricular infarction. The **left panel** shows two parasternal short-axis views recorded at the level of the papillary muscles. The **top left** is recorded in diastole. Note the full-thickness myocardium and the circular geometry of the left ventricle (LV). In systole **(bottom left)**, the inferior wall (arrows) becomes frankly dyskinetic and fails to show normal systolic thickening, whereas the remaining walls thickened appropriately and moved inward. The **right panel** is an apical four-chamber view demonstrating a dilated right ventricle (RV) that is globally hypokinetic in real time. This is consistent with right ventricular involvement. LA = left atrium; RA = right atrium.

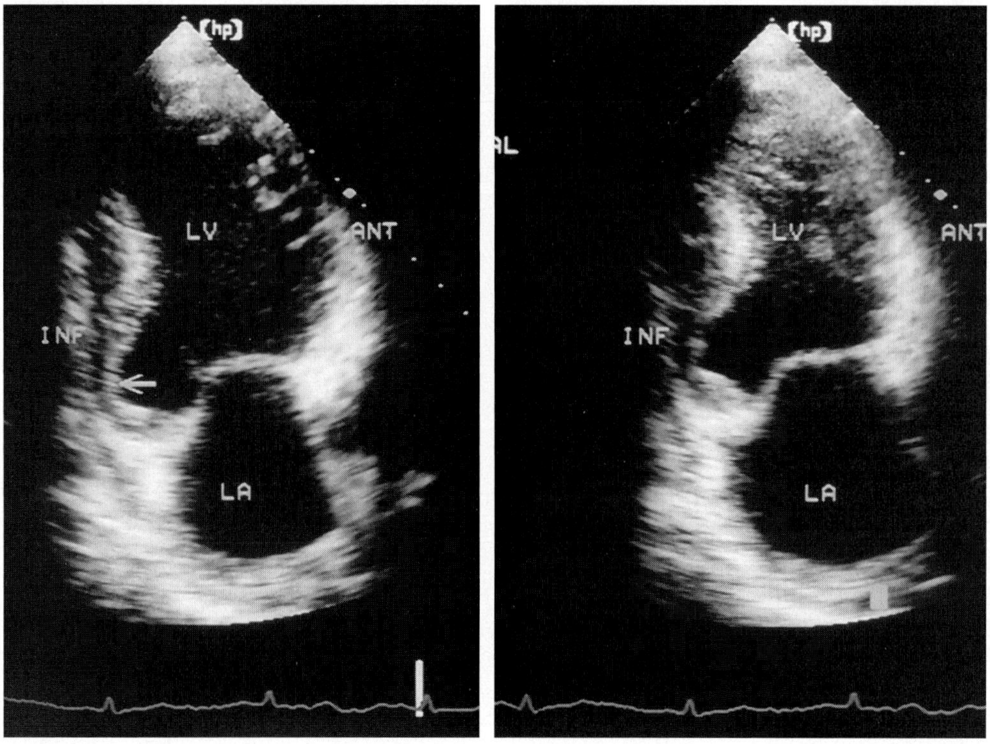

FIGURE 11–115 Apical two-chamber view of a patient with a remote inferior myocardial infarction. The proximal third of the inferior wall (INF) is thin, with distorted geometry consistent with a basilar aneurysm. The **right panel** was recorded in systole, and this area can be seen to bulge further compared with the remaining ventricular walls, which contract normally. ANT = anterior; INF = inferior; LA = left atrium; LV = left ventricle.

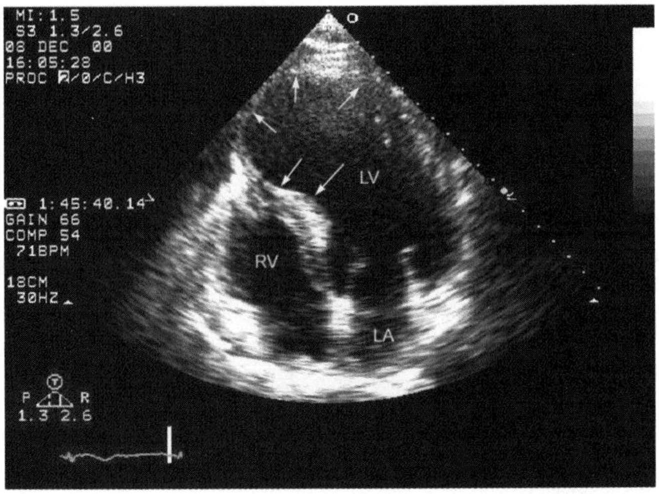

FIGURE 11–116 Apical four-chamber view recorded in a patient with a large anteroapical aneurysm. Note the marked distortion in geometry seen in this diastolic frame with marked aneurysmal bulging of the distal septum and apex (arrows). LA = left atrium; LV = left ventricle; RV = right ventricle.

TABLE 11–5 Complications of Myocardial Infarction Detected by Echocardiography

EARLY
Pericardial effusion
Infarct expansion
Thrombus formation
Myocardial rupture
Free wall
Ventricular septal defect
Papillary muscle
Functional mitral regurgitation
Right ventricular infarction
LATE
Infarct expansion
Left ventricular aneurysm
Left ventricular thrombus
Pericardial effusion
Functional mitral regurgitation

greater the degree of left ventricular dysfunction found, the greater the likelihood is of complications such as the development of heart failure and death.[155] The size of the myocardial infarction can be approximated with echocardiography by calculating a wall motion score or by calculation of an ejection fraction. Both of these values can be tracked over time to determine the recovery of function. Evaluation of the mitral valve inflow with Doppler echocardiography provides valuable prognostic information as well. Because myocardial ischemia causes immediate diastolic abnormalities, mitral valve inflow patterns become abnormal early in the course of myocardial infarction. One can anticipate an abnormal (typically reduced) E/A ratio in patients with myocardial ischemia. With more substantial areas of ischemia and greater degrees of diastolic dysfunction, an increased E/A ratio, suggesting restrictive physiology, can be seen. This is of more ominous prognostic significance.[156,157] Additionally, development of mitral regurgitation in association with myocardial infarction confers a worse prognosis.

COMPLICATIONS OF MYOCARDIAL INFARCTION. Table 11-5 outlines the complications of myocardial infarction that can be reliably detected using two-dimensional echocardiography. Virtually all mechanical complications are accurately identified.

Left ventricular thrombi may form in the first 24 hours after myocardial infarction and are most commonly seen in anterior infarctions with large areas of apical dyskinesis. They are far less common in cases of inferior wall myocardial infarction. Thrombi can present either as laminar, pedunculated, or mobile masses (Fig. 11-117). There is a substantially greater likelihood of subsequent embolization in mobile and pedunculated thrombi than in sessile and laminar thrombi.

Infarct expansion is defined as progressive dilation of the infarct zone without recurrent myocardial necrosis.[158] This can occur either acutely, after myocardial infarction, in which case it can be confused with reinfarction, or more chronically over the first 3 to 6 months. When infarct expansion (remodeling) occurs acutely it is seen in the substrate of necrotic and highly friable myocardium. Acute infarct expansion manifests as an aneurysm appearing in the first 72 hours, is the anatomical precursor of free wall rupture and ventricular septal defect, and carries a grave prognosis. Chronic infarct expansion occurs over several months, and the likelihood of mechanical complications is low. It results in tethering of normal walls and progressive chamber dilation with reduction in overall systolic performance. It has been linked to development of both arrhythmias and progressive congestive heart failure.

Pericardial effusion occurs in approximately 40 percent of patients with transmural myocardial infarction. It is often asymptomatic and detected only with echocardiographic scanning. A pericardial effusion occurring in the presence of acute infarct expansion is far more worrisome and may be one of the earlier signs of partial myocardial rupture.

Myocardial Rupture. The myocardium can rupture in one of three locations. In each case, infarct expansion usually precedes rupture. Free wall rupture complicates approximately 3 percent of unintervened acute myocardial infarction and is usually not a survivable event. Clinically, patients with myocardial rupture present with recurrent pain and rapidly develop pericardial effusion and tamponade, and death results. In rare instances, echocardiography has been used to document the presence of free wall rupture and allow emergency corrective surgery. A pseudoaneurysm forms when a partial rupture spontaneously seals off, resulting in an extra cardiac chamber, the walls of which consist of pericardium and thrombus. It typically connects to the left ventricle with a narrow mouth, distinguishing it from a true aneurysm, which communicates with the left ventricular cavity by way of a wide opening.

Rupture of either a papillary muscle or the ventricular septum results in signs and symptoms of heart failure and a prominent holosystolic murmur, owing to acute mitral regurgitation or ventricular septal defect (Figs. 11-118, 11-119, and 11-120). Two-dimensional echocardiography is a highly accurate technique for separating the two entities. Because of the critically ill nature of these individuals, many of them are intubated and TEE may be necessary to establish the diagnosis. Once the diagnosis is established, the degree of mechanical disruption can be determined. Additionally, echocardiography can be used to assess left and right ventricular function. Both of these are critical components of risk assessment when planning surgical intervention. Ventricular septal defect with concurrent right ventricular dysfunction carries a substantially greater risk of mortality.

RIGHT VENTRICULAR INFARCTION. Some degree of right ventricular dysfunction accompanies a large proportion of patients with inferior infarction due to occlusion of the proximal right coronary artery. Both systolic and diastolic dysfunction occur, and variable degrees of tricuspid regurgitation are common. Depending on which right ventricular branches are involved, the right ventricular wall motion abnormality can be either apical or more laterally located. Frequently, all that is noted is right ventricular dilation with fairly uniform hypokinesis of the right ventricle (see Fig. 11-114).[159] In many instances, right ventricular ischemia is a transient phenomenon and there is fairly rapid recovery of function. An additional complication of right ventricular infarction is the opening of a patent foramen ovale with subsequent right-to-left shunting. Shunts of significant size can result in arterial oxygen desaturation. The presence of a right-to-left shunt can be reliably documented with saline contrast echocardiography.

In patients with severe multivessel disease, an ischemic cardiomyopathy can develop. This term refers to diffuse global left ventricular systolic dysfunction as a consequence of severe, multivessel coronary artery disease. In many cases, there have been multiple, unrecognized acute myocardial infarctions. This type of cardiomyopathy presents as a nearly globally hypokinetic ventricle, often with patchy areas of wall thinning but without distinct aneurysm. Secondary mitral regurgitation is common and is due to papillary muscle dysfunction and dilation of the mitral valve annulus.

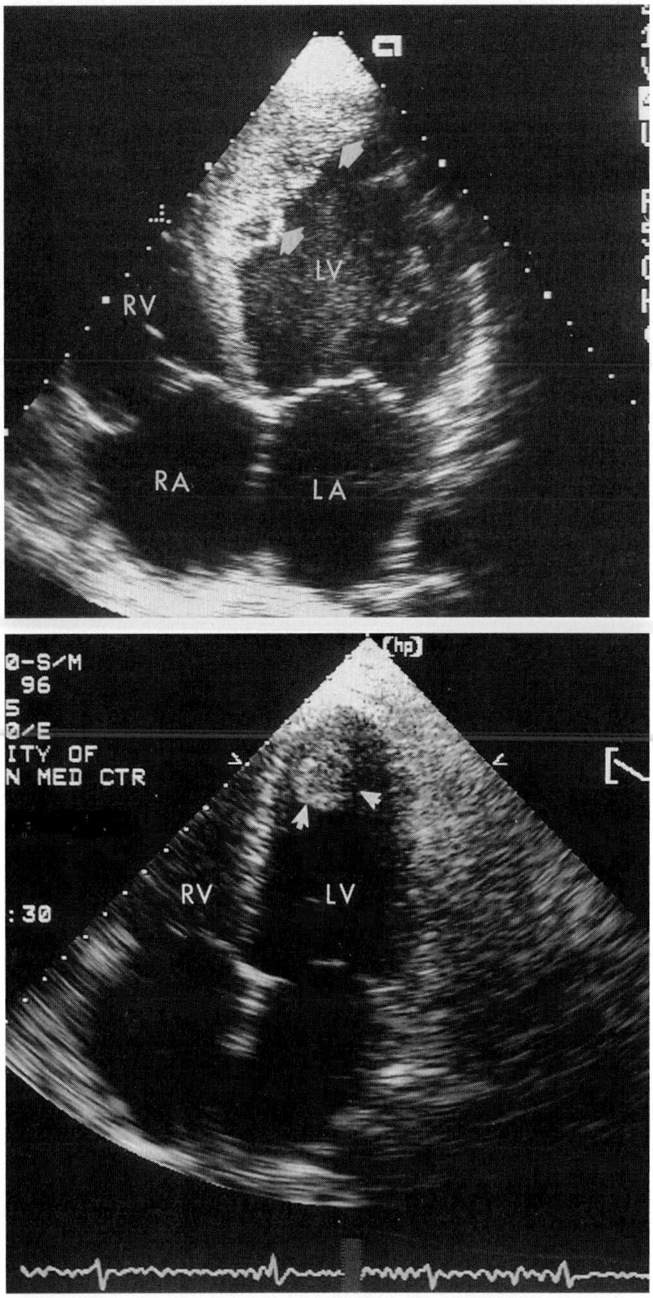

FIGURE 11–117 Apical four-chamber views recorded in two different patients with anterior infarct and left ventricular thrombus. The **top panel** denotes a large laminar thrombus filling a substantial portion of the apex and adherent to the ventricular septum (arrows). The **bottom panel** denotes a smaller, more spherical thrombus in the apex of the patient with a more limited apical myocardial infarction (arrows). LA = left atrium; LV = left ventricle; RA = right atrium; RV = right ventricle.

Myocardial Stunning and Hibernation (see Chap. 44)

There are two phenomena that result in potentially reversible myocardial dysfunction.[160] The first of these is myocardial stunning, which occurs after a severe acute ischemic insult. In this scenario, flow is restored and there is no myocardial necrosis. The exact physiological causes of myocardial stunning are not fully understood, but the syndrome results in spontaneous recovery of myocardial function after restitution of blood flow. Typically, myocardial function recovers in 1 to 7 days. Echocardiography can be used to track recovery of function in patients with this syndrome, and dobutamine stress echocardiography is an excellent means of predicting viability.

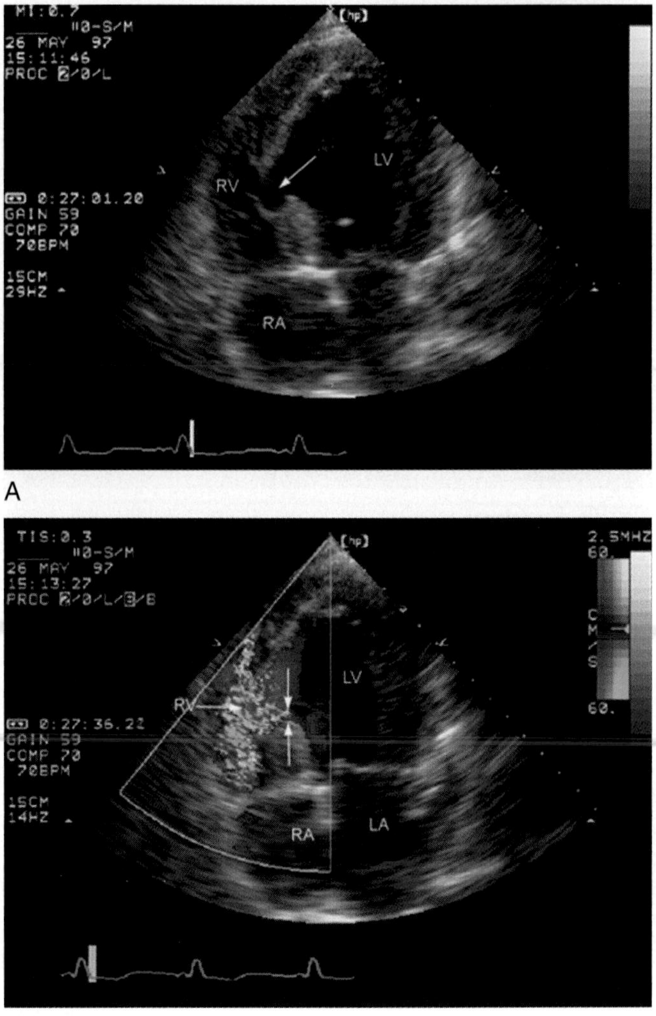

FIGURE 11–118 Apical four-chamber views in a patient with an acute anteroseptal myocardial infarction and a postinfarct ventricular septal defect. **A,** Routine two-dimensional image; **B,** accompanying color Doppler image. In panel **A**, there is a distinct break in the continuity of the ventricular septum (arrow) representing the ventricular septal defect with communication between the left and right ventricle. In panel **B**, color Doppler flow imaging has been used to demonstrate the high-velocity turbulent flow from the left ventricle to the right ventricle. LA = left atrium; LV = left ventricle; RA = right atrium; RV = right ventricle.

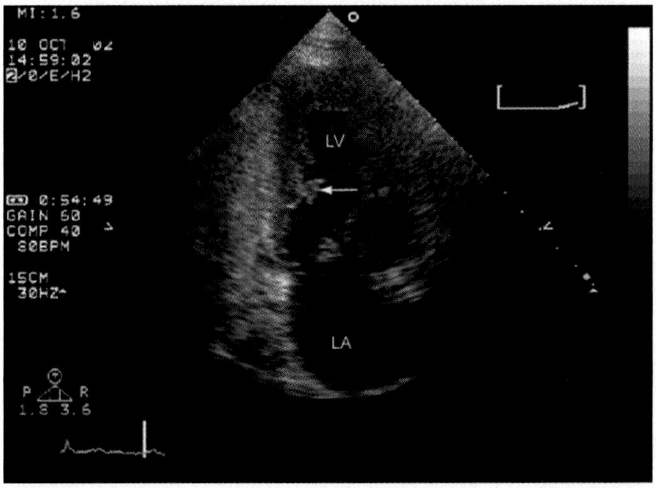

FIGURE 11–119 Transthoracic apical view demonstrating a ruptured papillary muscle in a patient with an acute myocardial infarction. Significant mitral regurgitation was present in this patient, in whom a remnant of the papillary muscle head (arrow) can be seen along the inferior wall. LA = left atrium; LV = left ventricle.

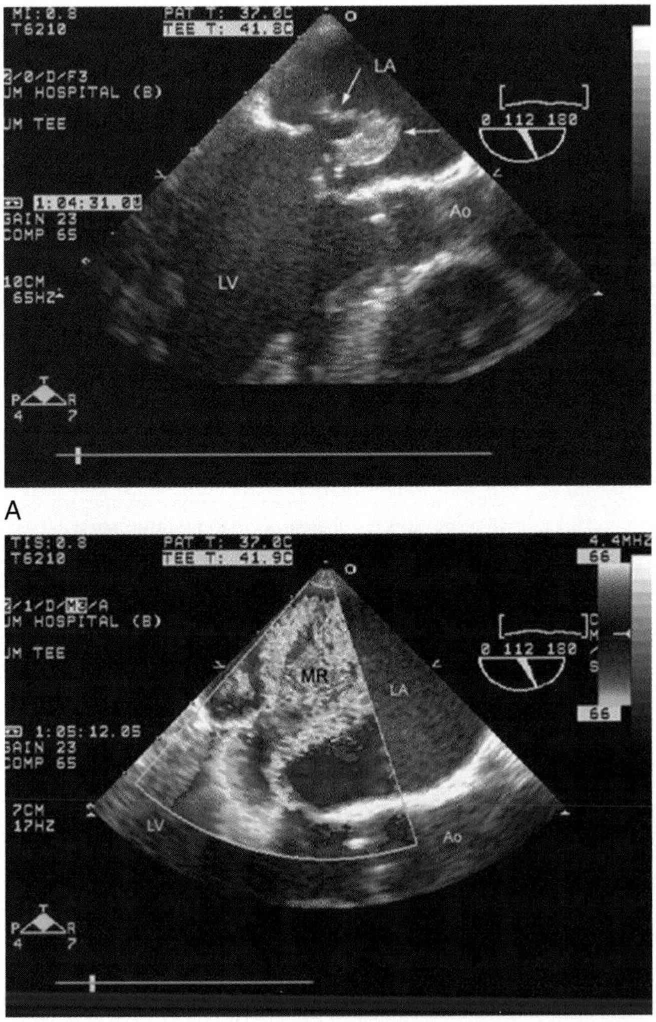

FIGURE 11–120 Transesophageal echocardiogram recorded in a patient with an acute myocardial infarction and complete rupture of a papillary muscle. **A,** Recorded in a longitudinal view in systole; a large, bulky muscular mass can be seen prolapsing into the left atrium (arrows). This represents the body of a papillary muscle. **B,** Recorded in the same view, using color flow imaging; demonstrates the presence of severe mitral regurgitation. Ao = aorta; LA = left atrium; LV = left ventricle.

Myocardial hibernation is a similar phenomenon usually encountered in a chronic case. Conceptually, hibernation represents myocardial dysfunction related to reduced coronary blood flow with no identifiable acute event. In many instances, what has been termed "myocardial hibernation" may represent repetitive stunning. In either scenario, functional recovery of the myocardium occurs after successful revascularization. As in cases of stunning, dobutamine stress echocardiography is an excellent means for detecting hibernation myocardium.[161-164]

Stress Echocardiography

Stress echocardiography is a family of examinations in which two-dimensional echocardiographic monitoring is undertaken before, during, and after cardiovascular stress. It has been shown to be a cost-effective means for evaluating patients presenting with chest pain. The form of cardiovascular stress can include exercise with treadmill or bicycle ergometry. By evaluating wall motion at rest and then comparing myocardial performance at stress, one obtains indicators of inducible ischemia that can be assigned to specific coronary territory (Figs. 11–25 and 11–121). Although treadmill exercise is often more familiar to patients, it is limited by the need to image only at rest and after exercise. It is not possible to successfully image an upright walking individual. Bicycle exercise provides the opportunity to image at each sequential stage of stress, and therefore peak exercise images are available.

For patients incapable of physical exercise, pharmacological stress, most commonly employing a dobutamine infusion, can be used. These protocols typically rely on an incremental infusion protocol of 10, 20, 30, and 40 μg/kg/min, augmented by atropine to obtain an adequate heart rate response when necessary. Images can be obtained at each stage of dobutamine infusion. Patients with significant obstructive coronary disease develop regional wall motion abnormalities identical to those seen during physical stress. The safety record of dobutamine has been excellent, and its accuracy appears equivalent to that of exercise echocardiography. An alternative to dobutamine is dipyridamole infusion, which relies on provocation of ischemia by differential vasodilation in normal and diseased arteries.

All of the different exercise echocardiography modalities have been validated against coronary arteriography as a standard and appear to have accuracy equivalent to the competing radionuclide procedures (Table 11–6; see also Chap. 13).[165-179] In general, the sensitivity of thallium scintigraphy tends to be slightly higher than that of exercise echocardiography, whereas the specificity of exercise echocardiography typically has been higher than that of thallium. As with all other forms of cardiovascular stress, exercise echocardiography has distinct advantages and disadvantages. Even in experienced laboratories, there may be a 5 percent failure rate due to suboptimal imaging. Patients in whom adequate levels of cardiovascular stress have not been obtained will not have positive study findings, even in the presence of coronary disease. The clinical utility and value of stress echocardiography has been specifically evaluated in female populations. In female populations, it appears to be an effective clinical tool for diagnosis and prognosis, but with a slightly lower overall accuracy than seen in male patients. Accuracy also appears to be preserved in the elderly and in hypertensive patients. Accuracy can be reduced in patients with left bundle branch block, who have a septal wall motion abnormality due to the conduction disturbance.

In addition to the diagnosis of coronary disease, stress echocardiography has been used extensively for determining patient prognosis in general populations[180-187] and after myocardial infarction[188,189] as well as in tracking results of percutaneous interventions. It plays a major role in determining myocardial viability in suspected cases of stunning or hibernation.[161-164] Dobutamine stress echocardiography has seen substantial success in determining preoperative risk assessment in patients undergoing noncardiac surgery.[190] Its accuracy for predicting cardiac events of myocardial infarction and death after major vascular surgery is equivalent to or greater than that of competing thallium scintigraphic techniques.

Myocardial Contrast Echocardiography

Myocardial contrast echocardiography is a field in evolution that shows tremendous promise for providing information about myocardial perfusion from contrast enhanced echocardiograms.[191-194] It should be emphasized that its utilization remains investigational, and a substantial amount of technical skill and expertise as well as specialized imaging equipment may be required for its appropriate utilization. As noted in the section on contrast echocardiography, modern perfluorocarbon-based agents are capable of transpulmonary passage, after which they perfuse virtually all organs, including the ventricular myocardium (Fig. 11-122). The appearance of contrast in the myocardium parallels the distribution of myocardial blood flow, and parameters of its appearance in the myocardium parallel actual coronary flow.

In the simplest analysis, the absence of contrast in the ventricular myocardium implies the absence of significant capillary level flow, whereas homogeneous opacification of the myocardium implies normal capillary flow. Intermediate levels of contrast appearance suggest delayed capillary flow and suggest the presence of underlying obstructive coronary artery disease. Animal experimentation has demonstrated that the presence of contrast in the ventricular myocardium is a highly accurate marker of perfused versus nonperfused myocardium and accurately identifies infarct areas following total coronary occlusion. Similarly, total absence of contrast in the myocardium in human clinical studies has been correlated with the presence of myocardium infarction (Fig. 11-123). Preserved capillary flow as demonstrated by myocardial contrast echocardiography is also an accurate predictor of myocardial viability.[195,196]

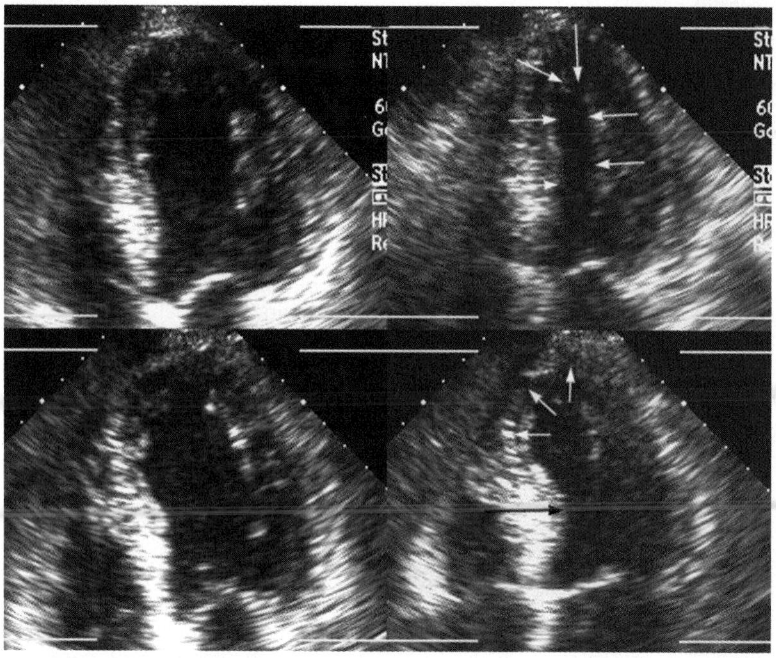

FIGURE 11–121 Stress echocardiogram in a patient with an obstructive lesion of the left anterior descending coronary artery. All four panels are four-chamber views. The **upper panels** were recorded at rest and reveal normal motion of all walls (white arrows); the **lower panels** were recorded immediately following stress. The **right lower panel** is an end-systolic frame immediately following exercise in which normal appropriate motion of the proximal septum (black arrow) is noted. The more distal portions of the septum and apex, however, were frankly dyskinetic (white arrows) indicating ischemia in the left anterior descending artery distribution.

In an effort to refine the technique, it is important to determine the time-of-appearance curve contrast in the myocardium. To create a time-activity curve of contrast in the myocardium requires creation of "a bolus effect" in which contrast flows into a previously unopacified myocardium. The most effective method for creating a bolus effect is to use a myocardial perfusion agent as a continuous infusion in which its presence in the bloodstream can be considered constant and therefore, its presence in the coronary bed stable. To create a bolus effect the mechanical index of the ultrasound beam is transiently increased to acutely destroy all of the contrast in the myocardium, after which the myocardium refills with contrast and its appearance time and intensity can then be tracked.[191] This maneuver can be repeated on multiple occasions to create several different time-activity curves, either under basal conditions or during pharmacological vasodilation. Figure 11-124 is an example of using this technique in which four different bolus effects have been created by transient bubble destruction and then tracking the appearance of contrast. In each example, baseline and vasodilation contrast has been destroyed, leaving a relatively dark appearance to the myocardium. The contrast-enhanced frames for each were recorded five cardiac cycles after bubble destruction. Under basal circumstances, there is definite visible contrast in the myocardium. However, during pharmacological vasodilation, at the same point after destruction, there is a more dramatic contrast effect in the myocardium, implying faster refill time.

Two different characteristics of the appearance curve have relevance for coronary disease. The actual intensity of contrast in the myocardium is directly related to capillary volume (as opposed to being related to actual flow). The plateau level of myocardial intensity is referred to as alpha (α) and the appearance rate or time constant of appearance as beta (β). The product of the two is directly proportional to myocardial blood flow.[191] In the

TABLE 11–6 Accuracy of Stress Echocardiography for Detection of Coronary Artery Disease

			Sensitivity		Specificity	
Study	**Stress**	**No. of Patients**	**%**	***No.***	**%**	***No.***
Armstrong et al.[165]	Treadmill	123	88		86	
Crouse et al.[166]	Treadmill	228	97	170/175	64	34/35
Marwick et al.[167]	Treadmill	150	84	96/114	86	31/36
Roger et al.[168]	Treadmill	150	83	50/60	62	56/90
Beleslin et al.[169]	Treadmill	136	88	105/119	82	14/17
Quinones et al.[170]	Treadmill	112	74	64/86	88	22/26
Ryan et al.[171]	Bike	309	91	193/211	77	76/98
Cohen et al.[172]	Bike	52	78	29/37	87	13/15
Hecht et al.[173]	Bike	180	93	127/137	86	37/43
Luotolahti et al.[174]	Bike	118	93	101/108	70	7/10
Marwick et al.[175]	DSE	217	72	102/142	83	62/75
Ling et al.[176]	DSE	183	93	151/162	62	13/21
Marcovitz and Armstrong[177]	DSE	141	96	105/109	66	21/32
Beleslin et al.[169]	DSE	136	82	98/119	77	13/17
Takeuchi et al.[178]	DSE	120	85	63/74	93	43/46

DSE = dobutamine stress echocardiography.

presence of significant coronary stenosis, the time constant of appearance (β) will be reduced; however, the actual eventual intensity (α) will be equivalent to that in a nondisease state. Creation of time-activity curves such as depicted in Figure 11–124 can provide valuable information regarding the presence of a flow-limiting obstructive coronary lesion. Myocardial contrast echocardiography can be recorded either in real time or using intermittent imaging at variable imaging intervals (1:1, 1:2, 1:4, 1:8, etc.) from which time-intensity curves can be developed.

It should be emphasized that detection of contrast within the myocardium requires highly specialized imaging algorithms, typically relying on analysis of sequential pulses. Much of the contemporary analysis of myocardial contrast cardiograms occurs in a Doppler domain rather than the gray-scale imaging domain. Limitations of the technique include the substantial learning curve, the requirement for highly specialized imaging platforms, and the tendency for more distal structures to be shadowed and thus mimic absence of perfusion. With continued development of agents and imaging platforms as well as experience, myocardial contrast echocardiography has shown tremendous promise as a technique that can give information similar to that provided by competing rate radionuclide perfusion methodologies.

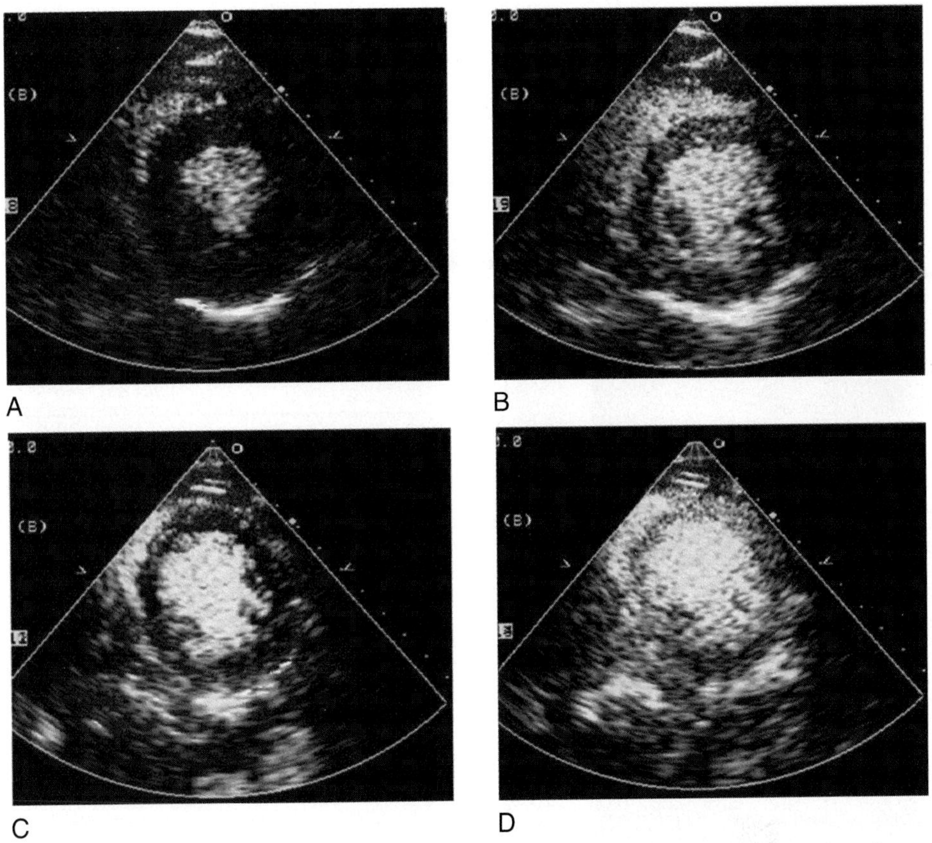

FIGURE 11–122 Myocardial contrast echocardiogram recorded in a patient without obstructive coronary disease. **A** and **B**, Recorded under basal conditions; **C** and **D**, recorded during dipyridamole infusion. Panels **A** and **C** were recorded immediately after a burst of high-intensity ultrasound intended to destroy contrast. Note the relatively dark appearance of the myocardium. Panels **B** and **D** were recorded five cardiac cycles after purposeful microbubble destruction. Under basal conditions **(B)**, note the definite but relatively faint opacification of the myocardium. Panel **D** was recorded five cardiac cycles after purposeful destruction but during infusion of dipyridamole to create a hyperemic response. The intensity of contrast at an equivalent time point after purposeful destruction is substantially greater during dipyridamole infusion than under basal conditions.

DIRECT VISUALIZATION OF CORONARY ARTERIES

Using high-frequency transducers, it is possible to directly visualize the proximal portions of the left main and right coronary arteries (Fig. 11–125). This can be done to identify their takeoff and to exclude anomalous origin of a coronary artery.[197] With scrupulous attention to detail, one can visually characterize the wall of the left main and proximal left interior descending coronary artery and detect areas of atherosclerotic involvement and calcification. Detection of calcification within the proximal left anterior descending coronary artery appears to be a potentially reliable marker that significant obstructive coronary artery disease is present.[198] Proximal coronary artery aneurysms can also be detected in children with Kawasaki disease. Either from the transesophageal or the transthoracic approach, it is also possible to place a Doppler sample volume in the coronary artery lumen and to quantify phasic flow in the coronary artery.[199] It is also possible to use Doppler echocardiography to determine the velocity of flow in the coronary sinus. This can be done both under basal conditions and after vasodilation.

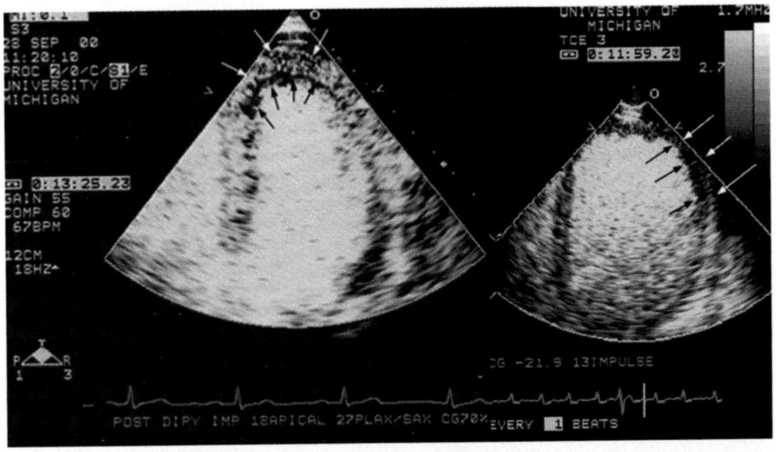

FIGURE 11–123 Myocardial contrast echocardiograms recorded in patients with disease of the mid-left anterior descending coronary artery. Both were recorded using a technique similar to that used for Figure 11–122. **Left,** Selective lack of myocardial contrast in the subendocardium at the apex (black arrows), indicative of absent perfusion in that territory. **Right,** Recorded in a patient with prior lateral wall infarction and reveals transmural loss of contrast effect in the area between the black and white arrows.

Diseases of the Aorta (see Chap. 53)

Transthoracic echocardiography visualizes the proximal 3 to 5 cm of the ascending aorta and portions of the descending thoracic aorta behind the left atrium from parasternal positions. In the majority of patients, a portion of the aortic arch can be visualized from the suprasternal transducer position. The sensitivity for detecting aortic disease is relatively poor from the transthoracic approach. If disease of the aorta is suspected, TEE is usually necessary. TEE provides a high-resolution view of the ascending aorta and descending thoracic aorta as far as the gastroesophageal junction but does not

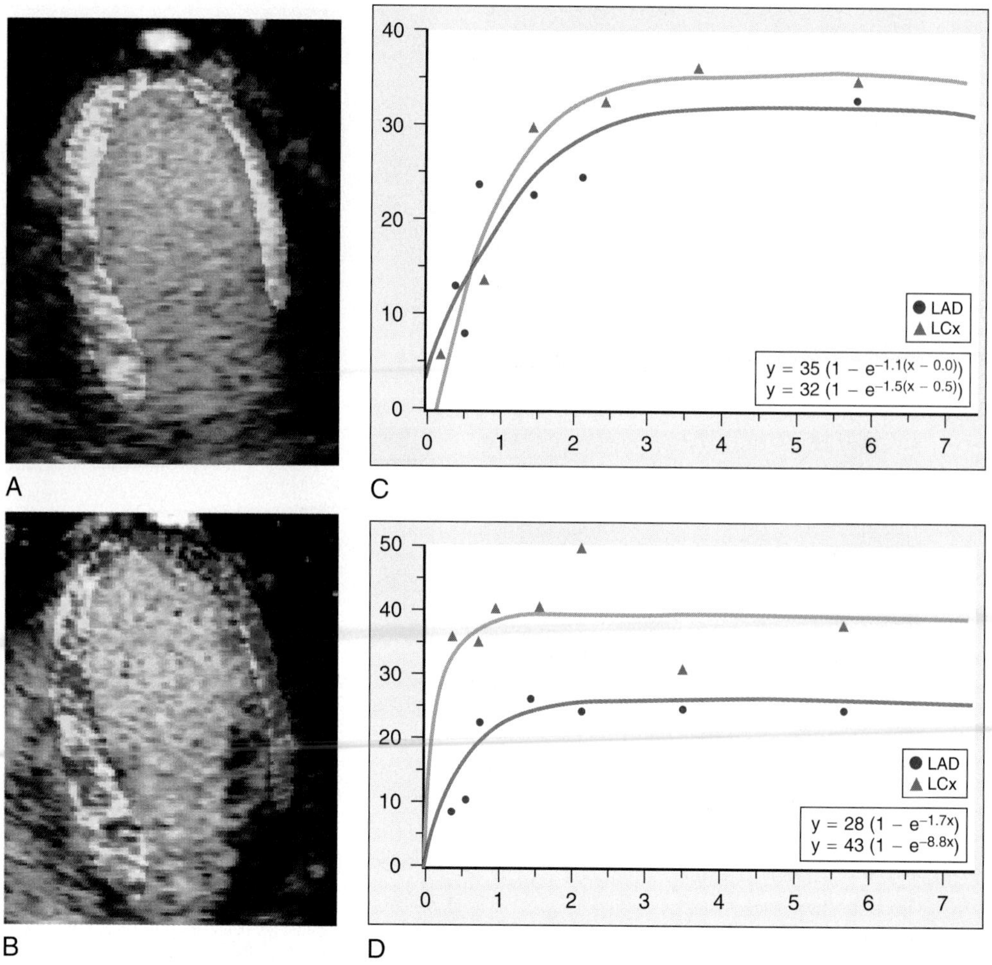

FIGURE 11–124 **A** and **B,** Background subtracted color-coded images from an apical two-chamber view from a patient with a 60 percent left anterior descending artery stenosis. Panel A represents the contrast appearance (contrast minus baseline) at baseline and panel B during hyperemia induced by intravenous adenosine infusion. **C,** Graph representing the time-intensity curve in the left anterior descending (LAD) and left circumflex (LCx) distributions. Note the similar appearance of the curves with respect to their peak video intensity and rate of rise of contrast intensity. **D,** Note the dramatic difference of appearance curves in the LAD and circumflex territories with a substantially reduced video intensity and slower rate of rise to a plateau in a diseased LAD artery, versus the normal circumflex territory. (From Wei K, Ragosta M, Thorpe J, et al: Noninvasive quantification of coronary blood flow reserve in humans using myocardial contrast echocardiography. Circulation. 103:2560, 2001; with permission from the American Heart Association.)

visualize the abdominal aorta. Additionally, there is a very limited area of the aortic arch that may be suboptimally viewed. In many centers, TEE has become the preferred and standard examination for evaluation of patients with suspected aortic disease.

AORTIC DISSECTION. Acute aortic dissection is a life-threatening disease requiring emergency surgical intervention. TTE can be used for early screening and is valuable for detecting aortic dilation, determining whether secondary aortic insufficiency is present, and assessing left ventricular function. Its accuracy for actual detection of the aortic dissection flap and determining its extent is not adequate as a stand-alone technique. TEE has proven to be a highly accurate and reliable technique for diagnosing and excluding aortic dissection, determining its extent, identifying communication points, assessing the severity of aortic insufficiency, and obviously determining complications such as rupture and adventitial hematoma. The accuracy for detection of acute aortic dissection is equivalent to that of CT and MRI (Table 11–7).[200-203]

Aortic dissection is classified by several schemes, all of which are designed to distinguish dissection of the ascending aorta from that confined to the descending thoracic aorta. A dissection flap appears as a thin linear echo within the lumen of the aorta (Fig. 11–126). In patients with connective tissue disease and relatively nonatherosclerotic aortas, the intimal flap is frequently highly mobile. It may take a spiral course as it courses through the descending thoracic aorta. More chronic dissections appear as a linear echo dividing the aorta into two or more lumens. In this instance, the intimal flap may appear thicker and less mobile than in the acute setting. In cases of acute dissection of the ascending aorta, dilation of the ascending aorta is seen in virtually all instances. Other echocardiographic findings of acute aortic dissection include presence of pleural effusion and of adventitial hematoma, which appears as a homogeneous echo-dense mass outside the wall of the aorta tracking along its course.

Specific cardiac features to be noted in aortic dissection include the presence or absence of pericardial effusion and of aortic insufficiency. Aortic insufficiency can be due either to sinotubular dilation with abnormal aortic cusp coaptation, direct extension of the dissection into the annulus, disruption of the support for the aortic valve, or, less commonly, prolapse of a portion of the intimal flap through the aorta, resulting in a conduit for insufficiency.[204]

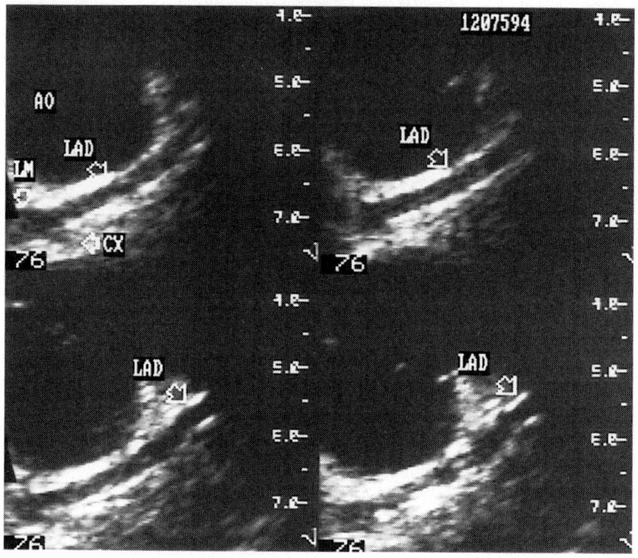

FIGURE 11–125 Transthoracic echocardiogram of the left coronary artery. The left main (LM), left anterior descending (LAD), and a proximal portion of the circumflex (CX) coronary artery are clearly visualized.

TABLE 11–7 Accuracy of Transesophageal Echocardiography for Detection of Aortic Dissection

Study	Year	No. of Patients	No. with Dissection	Sensitivity (n [%])	Specificity (n [%])
Erbel et al.[200]	1989	164	82	81/82 (99)	80/82 (98)
Hashimoto et al.[201]	1989	22	22	22/22 (100)	N/A
Ballal et al.[202]	1991	61	34	33/34 (97)	27/27 (100)
Nienaber et al.[203]	1993	110	44	43/44 (98)	20/26 (77)

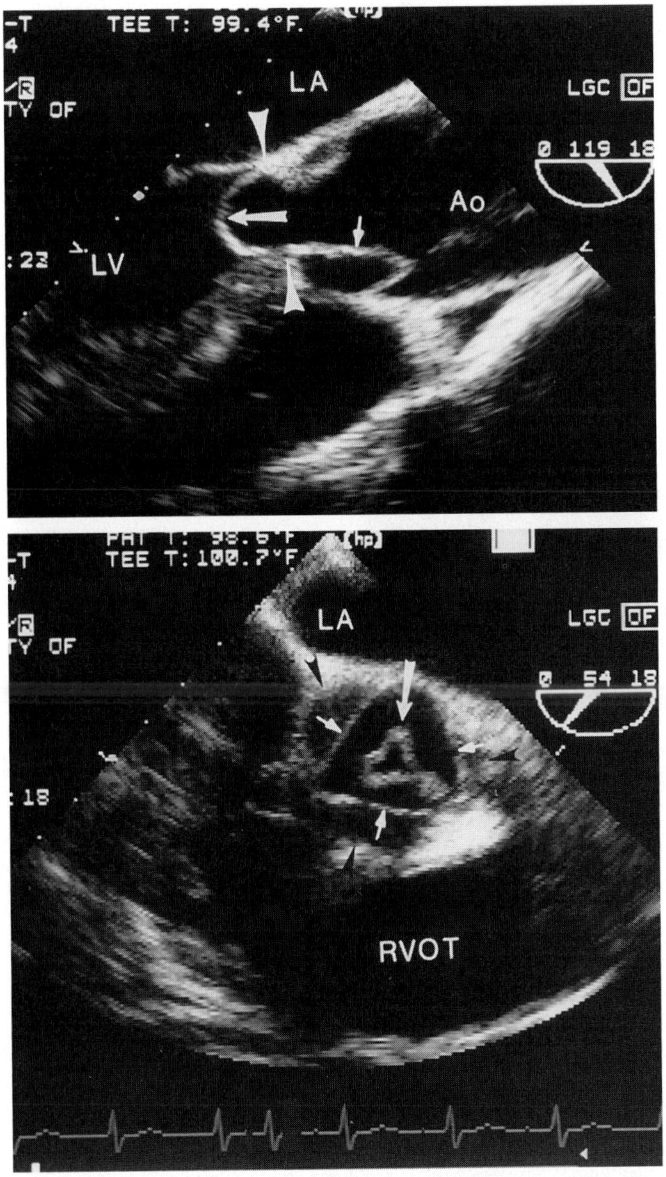

FIGURE 11–126 Transesophageal echocardiogram recorded in a patient with an acute type A dissection of the aorta. The **top panel** is a longitudinal view of the ascending aorta. Note the dilation of the proximal aorta and the thin linear echo present in both in the lumen of the aorta, a portion of which prolapses through the aortic valve into the left ventricular outflow tract (arrows). The white arrowheads denote the actual margins of the aortic annulus. The **bottom panel** is recorded in a view orthogonal to the upper panel and reveals the external diameter of the aorta (black arrowheads) as well as the open three-leaflet aortic valve (small white arrows). Within the actual orifice of the aortic valve is a portion of the dissection tear (large white arrow). Ao = aorta; LA = left atrium; LV = left ventricle; RVOT = right ventricular outflow tract.

The phenomenon of intramural hematoma has recently received much attention. Intramural hematoma often occurs in the setting of underlying atherosclerotic disease and is the result of spontaneous rupture and hemorrhage in the medial layers of the aorta.[205] The syndrome of acute intramural hemorrhage is virtually identical to acute dissection from the standpoint of clinical presentation. Intramural hemorrhage may be a focal process resulting in local breakdown in the medial layers or can result in creation of a dissection plane through the media. By definition, there is no communication between the lumen and the medial space.

AORTIC ANEURYSM. Aneurysm of the ascending aorta, arch, and descending thoracic aorta can be diagnosed and characterized with TEE. Characteristics of the aneurysm as fusiform or discrete and the extent of atherosclerotic involvement and secondary thrombus formation can all be determined. Because thoracic aneurysm without dissection is a chronic process requiring serial evaluation, most centers rely more heavily on CT or MRI for elective follow-up of chronic thoracic aortic aneurysms.

ATHEROSCLEROTIC DISEASE. The transesophageal echocardiogram is an excellent tool for determining the extent and nature of atherosclerotic involvement of the thoracic aorta (Fig. 11–127).[206,207] Atherosclerotic disease can be characterized as focal or diffuse and further characterized as mild, moderate, and severe. Complex and mobile components likewise can be noted and have relevance for embolic phenomena.

MARFAN SYNDROME AND DISEASE OF THE PROXIMAL AORTA. Marfan syndrome is a heritable disorder of connective tissue that results in abnormalities in the proximal aorta. The underlying pathological condition is cystic medial necrosis, which results in characteristic dilation of the proximal aorta, most prominent in the sinuses of Valsalva. There is secondary effacement of the sinotubular junction and dilation of the ascending aorta. Because the predominant area of dilation is in the proximal aorta, TTE often suffices for screening (Fig. 11–128). Complications of the aortic process in patients with Marfan syndrome include progressive dilation with secondary aortic insufficiency and development of aortic dissection. Echocardiography has seen tremendous success in the serial evaluation of these individuals and in the timing of elective surgery.

SINUS OF VALSALVA ANEURYSM. In addition to the characteristic symmetrical dilation seen in patients with Marfan syndrome, aneurysms can arise in the sinus of Valsalva. These range from relatively small and discrete to large "windsock" aneurysms that protrude into the right ventricular outflow tract. On occasion, rupture occurs, leading to a continuous shunt from the aorta into the downstream chamber. The most common site for a sinus of Valsalva aneurysm to rupture is into the right atrium or the right ventricular outflow tract. In this instance, remnants of the aneurysm can be seen prolapsing into the right ventricular outflow tract and high-velocity turbulent flow is noted in the downstream chamber. Because of the rupture, coarse fluttering of the right coronary cusp of the aortic valve may be noted.

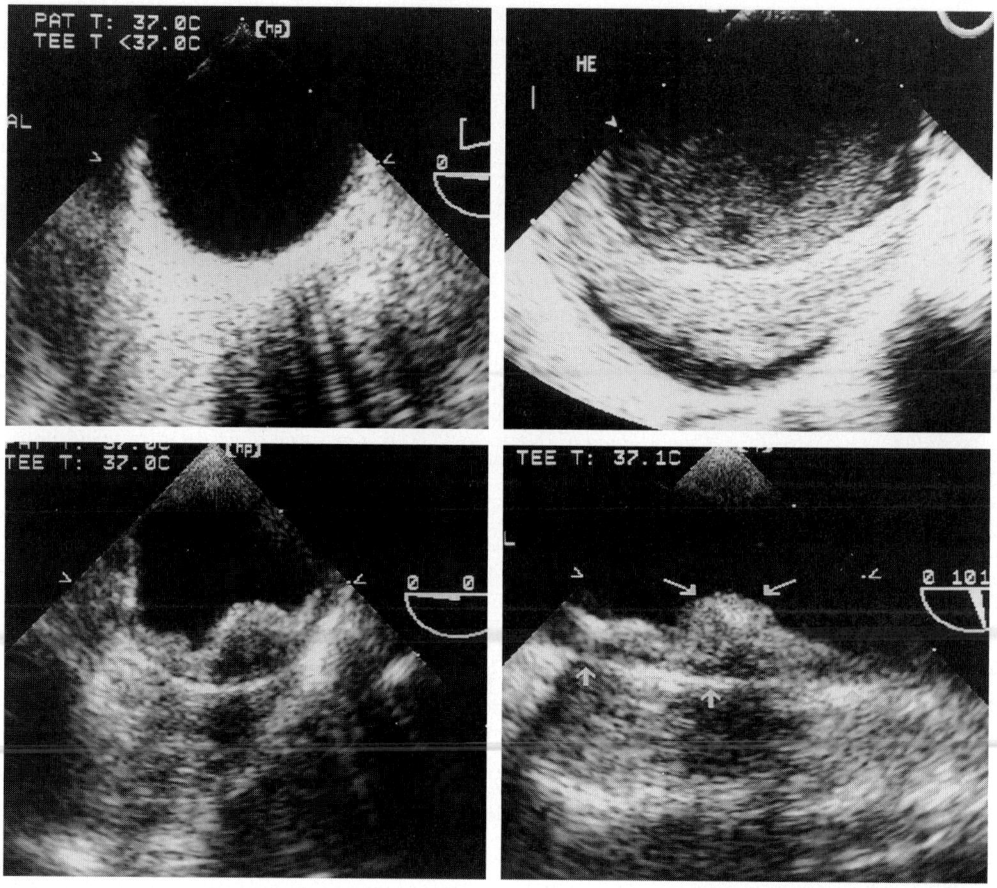

FIGURE 11–127 Transesophageal echocardiograms recorded in three different patients, visualizing the descending thoracic aorta. The **upper left panel** is recorded in a normal, disease-free aorta. Notice the circular geometry and the lack of any thickening or irregularity in the wall of the aorta. The **upper right panel** was recorded in a patient with a large descending thoracic aortic aneurysm measuring approximately 6 cm in its greatest dimension. Note the substantial atherosclerosis present as well as the vague, smoke-like echoes in the lumen of the aorta representing stagnant blood. There is also a lucency posterior to the wall representing spontaneous intramural hemorrhage. The **lower panels** were recorded in a patient with moderately severe atherosclerotic disease of the thoracic aorta. The panel on the **left** was recorded in the transverse view of the aorta. Note the irregular contour of the lumen, which is due to atherosclerotic involvement of the wall. The panel on the **right** was recorded at the same level of the aorta but in a longitudinal projection. The up-pointing arrows denote the outer wall of the aorta. Note the irregularity in the aortic lumen and the protruding atheroma (arrows).

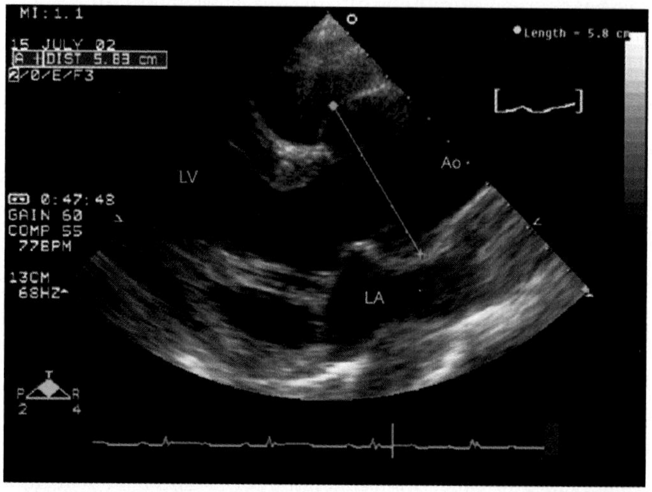

FIGURE 11–128 Transthoracic echocardiogram in a patient with Marfan syndrome. Note the marked dilation of the sinuses of proximal aorta (arrow). Ao = aorta; LA = left atrium; LV = left ventricle.

CARDIAC MASSES AND TUMORS (see Chap. 63)

Echocardiography is the primary screening tool for patients with known or suspected intracardiac tumors. Cardiac tumors can be divided into those that are primary to the heart and those that are secondary or metastatic. They can be further divided into benign and malignant types.

Atrial Myxoma. The most common benign primary tumor of the heart is the atrial myxoma. Approximately 75 percent of atrial myxomas are isolated, pedunculated tumors in the left atrium attached to the area of the foramen ovale by a stalk (Fig. 11–129). Less common locations include the right atrium and either ventricle, pulmonary vein, or vena cava. The classic left atrial myxoma is a smooth, relatively homogeneously echo-dense mass with substantial mobility. It moves into the orifice of the mitral valve in diastole and prolapses back into the left atrium in systole. Depending on its size, it may result in functional obstruction of the mitral valve, thereby mimicking mitral stenosis. Concurrent mitral regurgitation is not uncommon. In the presence of a typical appearance of a myxoma, the diagnosis is virtually certain from an echocardiographic standpoint, and no further evaluation may be necessary. Because of the tendency to cause obstruction of the mitral valve, secondary pulmonary hypertension can occur. Additionally, emboli from the surface of the myxoma are not uncommon.

Other Primary Cardiac Tumors. Cardiac lipomas are benign primary cardiac tumors with a broad range of appearances. They are most common in the body of the left ventricle and occasionally may be present as pedunculated masses. Although unlikely to embolize, they can be associated with superimposed thrombus, which can embolize. Echocardiography is useful for identification of the mass but is unable to precisely identify it as lipomatous tissue. MRI has substantially succeeded in tissue characterization of these masses.

Papilloma. Benign papillomas occasionally occur on valvular structures. These appear as homogeneous, usually spherical masses, typically less than 1 cm in diameter.[208] They may appear on the mitral valve chordae and occasionally on the aortic valve. As with other cardiac tumors, they have been associated with emboli. The main differential diagnosis is between benign papilloma and vegetation.

Cardiac Malignancies. The majority of cardiac malignancies represent metastatic disease, most commonly from esophagus, lung, or breast. Diffuse malignancy, such as lymphoma, can also involve the heart either primarily or secondarily. Metastatic disease of the heart is virtually always associated with pericardial involvement as well. The appearance of metastatic disease in the heart is typically of mobile echo-dense masses attached to the endothelium (Fig. 11–130), although isolated intramural masses and diffuse myocardial invasion have also been noted.

There are several primary malignant tumors of the heart, including angiosarcoma and rhabdomyoma. Rhabdomyoma is more common in children. Cardiac malignancies are relatively rare and can appear in virtually any chamber in adults. There is a greater prevalence of sarcoma and rhabdomyoma in the right atrium (Fig. 11–131) and right ventricle and involving the veins or great vessels than in the actual body of the heart.

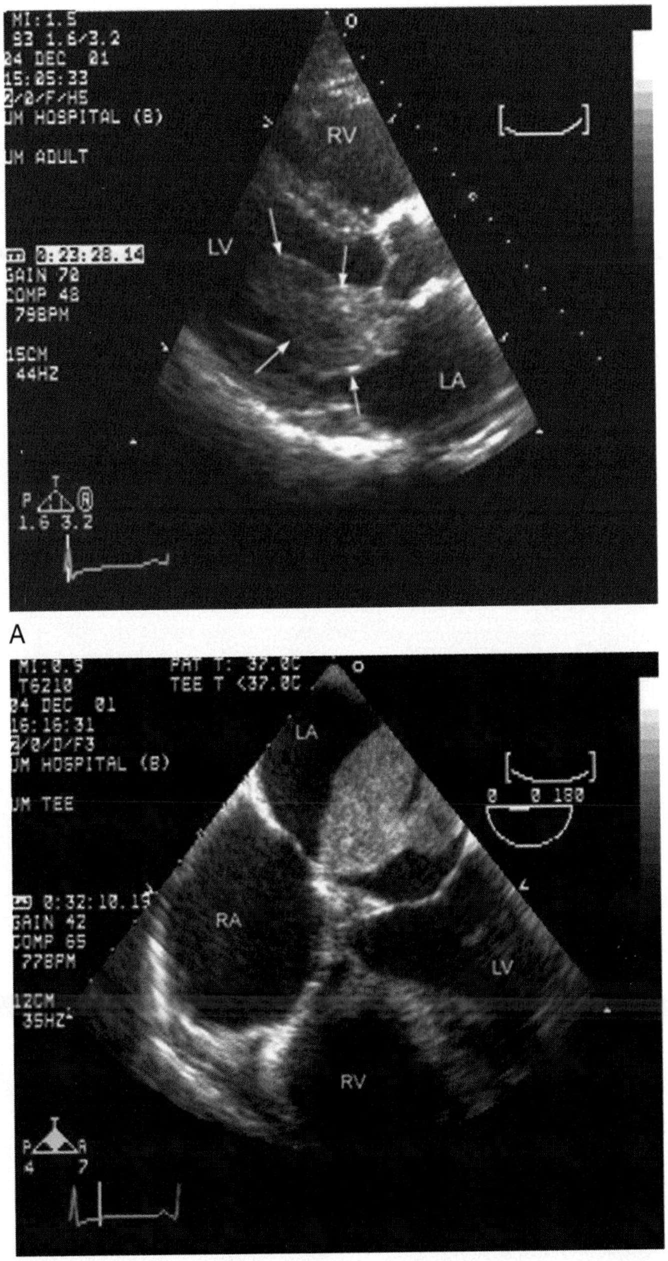

FIGURE 11–129 Transthoracic **(A)** and transesophageal **(B)** echocardiograms recorded in a patient with a large left atrial myxoma. Panel **A** is recorded in diastole. Note the large bulky mass (white arrows) essentially filling the entire mitral orifice. Panel **B** is recorded in the same patient. Note the irregular bilobed appearance of the mass and its attachment to the atrial septum by a relatively narrow stalk. LA = left atrium; LV = left ventricle; RA = right atrium; RV = right ventricle.

Intracardiac Thrombus. Thrombi can occur in any chamber of the heart but are most common in the left ventricular apex (see Fig. 11–117) after myocardial infarction or in the setting of cardiomyopathy, and in the left atrium in the setting of mitral stenosis or atrial fibrillation. Ventricular thrombi have been discussed previously.

Atrial thrombi appear as echo-dense masses within the body of the left atrium but more commonly in the left atrial appendage. The left atrial appendage has a fine muscular ridge-like network (pectinate muscles) that can be confused with small thrombi. Because thrombi occur in the presence of stasis, spontaneous contrast with "smoke-like" echoes is frequently seen in the left atrium and left atrial appendage as well.

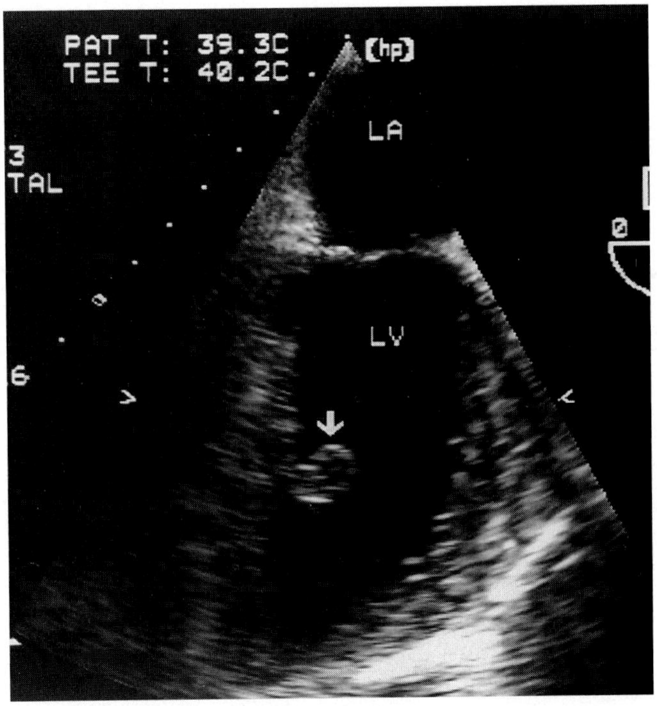

FIGURE 11–130 Transesophageal echocardiogram recorded in a long-axis view of the left atrium (LA) and left ventricle (LV) in a patient with an intracardiac tumor. Note the approximately 1 cm diameter, spherical mass attached to the posterior wall of the left ventricle by a thin stalk (arrow).

Specific Clinical Utilization of Echocardiography

The previous discussion represents an outline of the diagnostic capabilities of echocardiography. There are several specific clinical situations in which echocardiography can be used and that should be understood by the clinician. Table 11–8 outlines the role of different echocardiographic modalities in clinical problem-solving.

EVALUATION OF DYSPNEA AND CONGESTIVE HEART FAILURE. Two-dimensional echocardiography is recommended as an initial part of the evaluation in patients with known or suspected congestive heart failure (see Chap. 24). Evaluation of ventricular function can be undertaken, and determination of both primary and secondary valvular abnormalities can likewise be accurately assessed. Doppler echocardiography can play a valuable role with respect to determining diastolic function and establishing the diagnosis of diastolic heart failure. Heart failure with normal systolic function but abnormal diastolic relaxation accounts for 30 to 40 percent of patients presenting with congestive heart failure. Because the therapy of this condition is distinctly different from that of systolic dysfunction, establishing the appropriate cause and diagnosis is essential. This can be effectively done with the combination of two-dimensional echocardiography and Doppler echocardiography.

CARDIAC SOURCE OF EMBOLUS. It has become increasingly recognized that many neurological events and large artery occlusions are the result of embolization from the heart or other major vascular structures. Identifying patients who are most likely to have a cardiac source of embolus has been problematic, but in general, any patient with abrupt occlusion of a major vessel or younger individual (typically younger than 45 years of age) with a neurological event should be suspected of having a potential cardiac

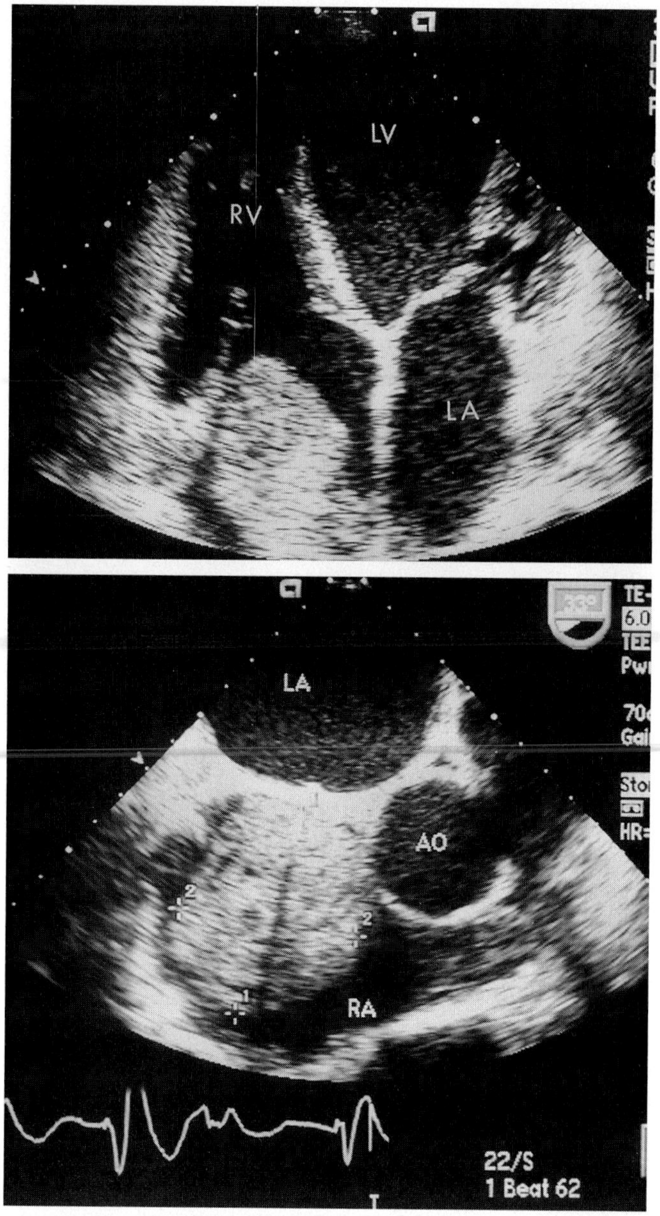

FIGURE 11–131 Apical four-chamber view **(top)** and transesophageal echocardiogram **(bottom)** in a patient with a large right atrial mass. In the top panel, the mass can be seen arising from the area of the inferior vena cava and essentially filling the right atrium (RA). A similar appearance is seen in the transesophageal echocardiogram **(bottom)**, where the mass appears adjacent to the atrial septum. AO = aorta; LA = left atrium; LV = left ventricle; RV = right ventricle.

cause. Additionally, older individuals with neurological events but who do not have identifiable vascular disease require screening for a cardiac cause. Several large-scale surveillance studies have demonstrated prevalence and range of abnormalities associated with neurological and embolic events.[209-211]

One of the more common abnormalities to identify in this situation is a patent foramen ovale with or without a right-to-left shunt identified by contrast echocardiography (see Fig. 11–87).[212,213] TEE is often required for complete evaluation because TTE is not sufficient to exclude left atrial thrombus or evaluate the thoracic aorta for atherosclerotic degree. A potential cardiac source of embolus will be identified in many patients with neurological and other embolic events, but the identification of such a lesion does not necessarily prove cause and effect. The degree to which atherosclerotic disease of the aorta and patent foramen ovale are causative rather than coexistent with other causes often remains unproven. In a substantial number of patients, highly mobile strands and areas of fibrosis may be noted on either the aortic or the mitral valve. The clinical implication of these anomalies is unknown.

ATRIAL FIBRILLATION. Echocardiography plays a crucial role in the evaluation of patients with atrial fibrillation (see Chap. 30). Patients with atrial fibrillation should be characterized as having underlying heart disease or having a structurally normal heart, in which case a diagnosis of lone atrial fibrillation can be made. Determination of the underlying cardiac anatomy is essential for decision-making regarding the likelihood of conversion to and maintenance of

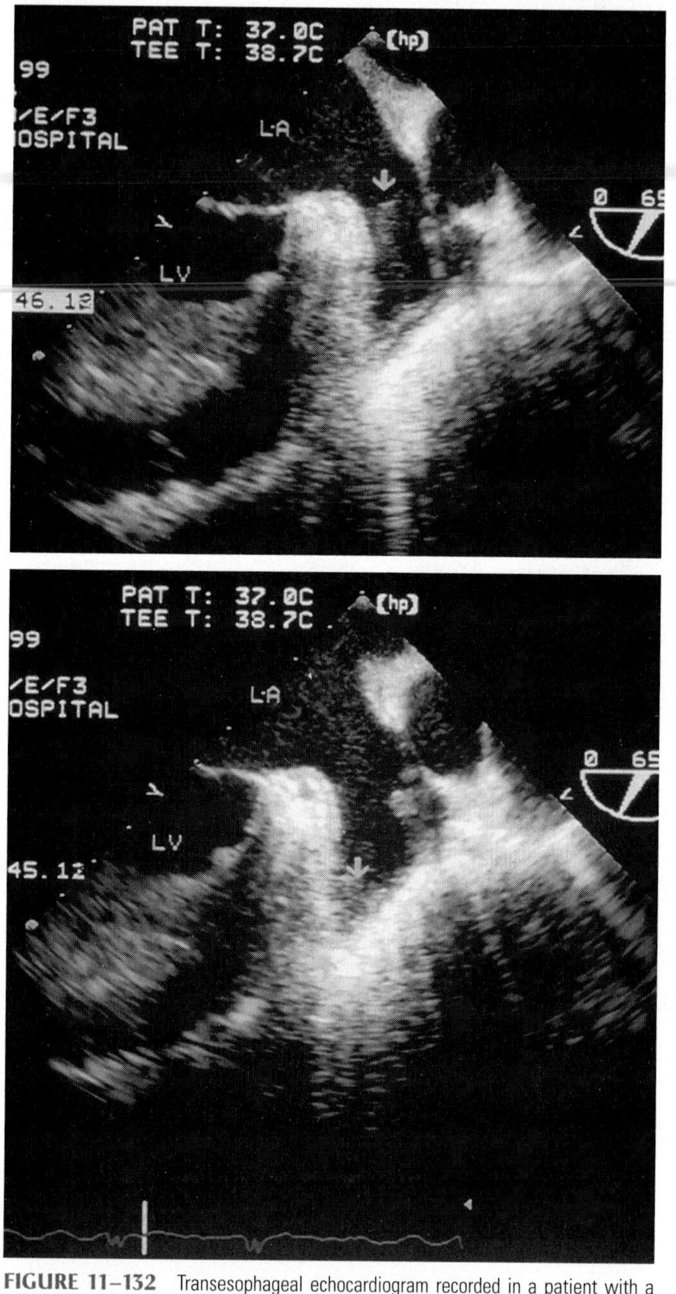

FIGURE 11–132 Transesophageal echocardiogram recorded in a patient with a recent neurological event. There is vague echo mass **(top)**, which in real time has a swirling smoke-like appearance (downward pointing arrow). At a slightly different transducer position, the actual apex of the left atrial appendage can be seen to contain a filling defect consistent with thrombus, noted between the two vertically oriented arrows. LA = left atrium; LV = left ventricle.

TABLE 11–8 Clinical Utility of Echocardiography

Situation	2D	Doppler	CFD	Continuous Wave	TEE	Stress
Pericardial disease	1	2	3	4	4	N/A
Valvular heart disease						
Murmur	1	1	1	3	4	N/A
Mitral stenosis	1	1	1	—	3	3
Mitral regurgitation	1	1	1	—	3	N/A
Aortic stenosis/regurgitation	1	1	1	—	3	3
Prosthetic heart valve dysfunction	1	1	1	—	2	N/A
Coronary artery disease						
Chest pain syndrome	1	3	3	4	4	1
Rule out coronary artery disease	1	3	3	4	4	1
Diagnose acute myocardial infarction	1	3	3	4	4	N/A
Complications of infarction						
Aneurysm	1	3	3	4	4	N/A
Thrombus	1	3	3	4	4	N/A
Ventricular septal defect/papillary muscle rupture	1	1	1	3	2	N/A
Assess left ventricular function	1	1	2	4	4	3
Congenital heart disease	1	1	1	3	3	3
Atrial septal defect	1	1	1	2	2	4
Cardiomyopathy						
Dilated	1	1	1	4	4	3
Hypertrophic	1	1	1	4	4	3
Endocarditis	1	1	1	4	2	N/A
Pulmonary hypertension						
Known	1	1	1	2	3	3
Occult	1	1	1	2	3	2
Congestive heart failure	1	1	1	4	4	3
Stroke/source of embolus	1	2	2	1	2	N/A
Aortic dissection	2	2	1	4	1	N/A
Dyspnea evaluation	1	1	1	1	4	1

1 = Indicated and essential; 2 = often required—may add, informative; 3 = necessary in select instances for specific question; 4 = rarely necessary; 2D = two-dimensional; CFD = color flow Doppler; TEE = transesophageal echocardiography; N/A = not available.
From Armstrong WF: Echocardiography. *In* Kelly's Textbook of Medicine. 4th ed. Philadelphia, Lippincott Williams & Wilkins, 2000.

sinus rhythm and for determining the embolic potential and hence the need for long-term anticoagulation. In general, patients with normal cardiac anatomy are unlikely to sustain an embolic event and highly likely to revert to sinus rhythm and have sinus rhythm maintained. Conversely, patients with cardiomyopathy and severe mitral stenosis are less likely to be maintained in sinus rhythm and have a higher likelihood of embolic events. Thus, these individuals are candidates for long-term anticoagulation. TEE has also been proposed as a management tool in determining the timing for elective cardioversion.[214-216] Immediately after electrical cardioversion, there is an increased likelihood of embolization. Embolization in this setting arises either from a preexisting thrombus or, more likely, from atrial stunning with subsequent thrombus formation (Fig. 11–132). A strategy of TEE to exclude left atrial thrombus, followed immediately by cardioversion, has been demonstrated to be an efficient means of restoring sinus rhythm without requiring long-term pre-cardioversion anticoagulation. After cardioversion, atrial stunning occurs and the likelihood of new thrombus formation is actually transiently enhanced. For this reason, anticoagulation is indicated in virtually all patients after cardioversion for 6 weeks to 6 months. Although TEE-guided cardioversion has been demonstrated to be a safe alternative to the standard approach of 3 weeks of aortic coagulation followed by cardioversion, it has not been shown to result in a higher success rate for either initial conversion to sinus rhythm or maintenance of sinus rhythm at 1 year.

PULMONARY EMBOLUS (see Chap. 66). Patients with pulmonary embolus may present with atypical symptoms. In this instance, TEE and TTE can provide valuable clinical information.[217-219] In a patient presenting with a combination of chest pain and dyspnea, with or without evidence of venous stasis, detection of right heart dilation and dysfunction and/or elevation of pulmonary artery pressures can be valuable clues to the nature of the underlying process. Direct visualization of large pulmonary emboli is occasionally possible with either TTE or TEE, but more usually with TEE. Additionally, by using either technique, embolus in transit can be detected as a highly mobile serpiginous mass, typically entrapped in the tricuspid valve apparatus and less commonly spanning a patent foramen ovale. Detection of a typical serpiginous mass in the right atrium identifies a patient at substantial risk for further embolization and is a clinical situation requiring emergency therapy (Fig. 11–133).

PULMONARY HYPERTENSION (see Chap. 67). Pulmonary hypertension represents an elusive diagnosis. Clinically, pulmonary hypertension can occur either as a primary phenomenon or secondary to a variety of either cardiac or pulmonary processes. The majority of patients with established pulmonary hypertension have identifiable abnormalities on echocardiography, including variable degrees of right ventricular enlargement and hypertrophy (Fig. 11–134).[220,221] As noted earlier, pulmonary artery pressures can be estimated from the velocity of the tricuspid regurgitation jet (see Fig. 11–31). In patients with only mild elevation of pulmonary

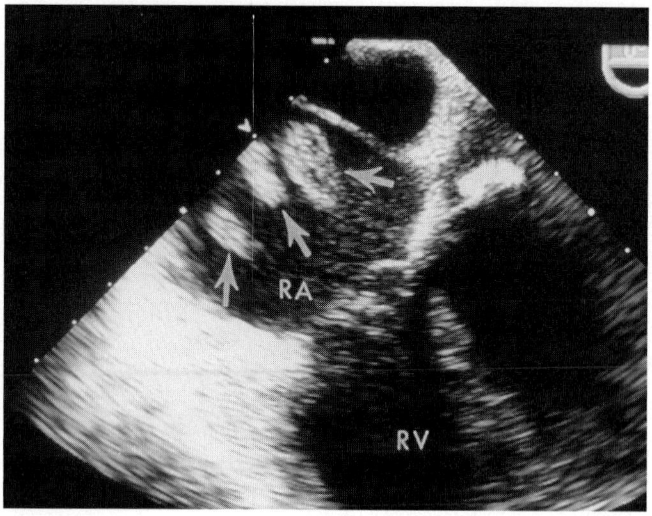

FIGURE 11–133 Transesophageal echocardiogram recorded in a patient with pulmonary embolus, found to have "thromboembolism in transit." Image was recorded at 0 degrees. The dilated right atrium and right ventricle are obvious. Three highly mobile components of a long serpiginous thrombus can be seen in the right atrium (arrows). RA = right atrium; RV = right ventricle.

pressure, exercise echocardiography can be used to track pulmonary artery pressures with stress and provides valuable information regarding the presence of occult, exercise-induced pulmonary hypertension.[222] Doppler echocardiography can also be used to follow pulmonary artery pressures during therapy.

FETAL ECHOCARDIOGRAPHY. Because cardiac ultrasonography carries no risk to the pregnant woman or fetus and is fully noninvasive, it can be used to make the antepartum diagnosis of congenital heart disease. This should be undertaken only by pediatric echocardiographers with appropriate experience in the technique. Many major intracardiac abnormalities can be detected at the end of the first trimester, and the majority of physiologically significant abnormalities can be detected in utero in the second trimester. This technique has seen substantial use in identifying fetuses with congenital heart defects who may warrant urgent transfer to a neonatal intensive care unit or an emergency intervention for life-threatening cardiac problems immediately after birth.

EVALUATION AND MONITORING OF INVASIVE AND INTERVENTIONAL PROCEDURES. Two-dimensional echocardiography, often using TEE, has seen substantial success as a means of monitoring invasive procedures. This includes direct online monitoring of pericardiocentesis and assistance in localization and placement of catheters for electrophysiological ablation as well as online monitoring of endomyocardial biopsy. Additionally, TEE is an instrumental component of transcatheter closure of atrial septal defects in the catheterization laboratory[223,224] and often used in other

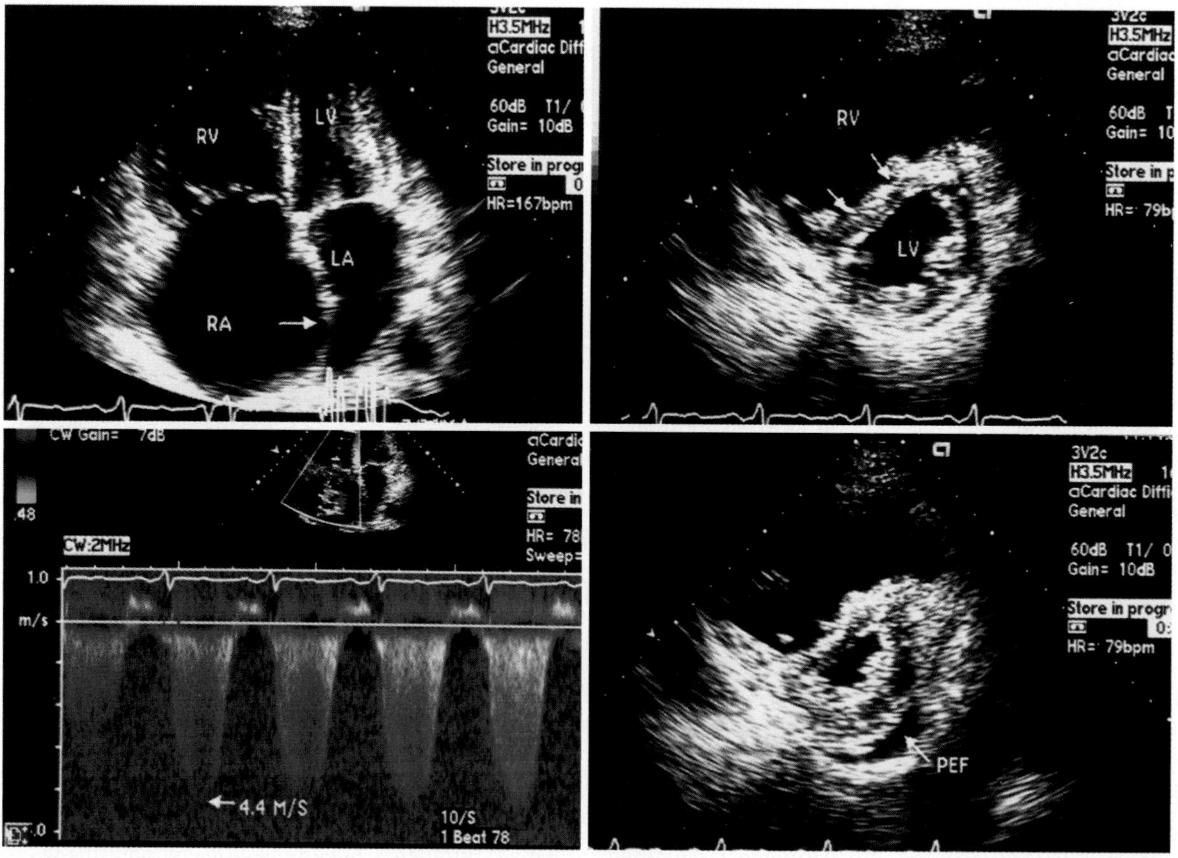

FIGURE 11–134 Composite images recorded in a patient with severe pulmonary hypertension. The **upper left panel** is an apical four-chamber view in which marked dilation of the right ventricle (RV) and right atrium (RA) can be appreciated. Notice the bowing of the atrial septum from right to left, implying that right atrial pressure exceeds left atrial pressure. The two **right panels** are recorded in a parasternal short-axis view and demonstrate a classic right ventricular pressure in volume overload pattern with flattening of the ventricular septum in both diastole and systole. The **lower left panel** is a continuous-wave Doppler recording of the tricuspid regurgitation jet, from which a peak velocity of 4.4 m/sec, corresponding to a right ventricular-right atrial pressure gradient of 77 mm Hg, can be calculated. Addition of right atrial pressure (assumed to be 15 mm Hg) results in an estimated right ventricular systolic pressure of 92 mm Hg in this instance. LA = left atrium; LV = left ventricle; PEF = pericardial effusion.

procedures where a transatrial approach is necessary for therapy, such as mitral balloon valvotomy.

REFERENCES

Principles of Cardiac Ultrasonography

1. Senior R, Soman P, Khattar RS, et al: Improved endocardial visualization with second harmonic imaging compared with fundamental two-dimensional echocardiographic imaging. Am Heart J 138:163, 1999.
2. Skolnick DG, Sawada SG, Feigenbaum H, et al: Enhanced endocardial visualization with noncontrast harmonic imaging during stress echocardiography. J Am Soc Echocardiogr 12:559, 1999.
3. Sozzi FB, Poldermans D, Bax JJ, et al: Second harmonic imaging improves sensitivity of dobutamine stress echocardiography for the diagnosis of coronary artery disease. Am Heart J 142:153, 2001.
4. Stevenson JG: Appearance and recognition of basic Doppler concepts in color flow imaging. Echocardiography 6:451, 1989.
5. Ritter SB: Red, green and blue: The flag of Doppler color flow mapping: Flow mapping. Echocardiography 6:369, 1989.
6. Veinot JP, Harrity PJ, Gentile F, et al: Anatomy of the normal left atrial appendage: A quantitative study of age-related changes in 500 autopsy hearts: Implications for echocardiographic examination. Circulation 96:3112, 1997.

Quantification of Ventricular Function

7. Huwez FU, Houston AB, Watson J, et al: Age and body surface area related normal upper and lower limits of M mode echocardiographic measurements and left ventricular volume and mass from infancy to early adulthood. Br Heart J 72:276, 1994.
8. Chuang ML, Hibberd MG, Salton CJ, et al: Importance of imaging method over imaging modality in noninvasive determination of left ventricular volumes and ejection fraction: Assessment by two- and three-dimensional echocardiography and magnetic resonance imaging. J Am Coll Cardiol 35:477, 2000.
9. Marcus R, Krause L, Weder AB, et al: Sex-specific determinants of increased left ventricular mass in the Tecumseh Blood Pressure Study. Circulation 90:928, 1994.
10. Pearlman JD, Triulzi MO, King ME, et al: Limits of normal left ventricular dimensions in growth and development: Analysis of dimensions and variance in the two-dimensional echocardiograms of 268 normal healthy subjects. J Am Coll Cardiol 12:1432, 1988.
11. Weyman AE: Appendix A: Normal Cross-Sectional Echocardiographic Measurements. *In* Principles and Practice of Echocardiography. Philadelphia, Lea & Febiger, 1994.
12. Yvorchuk KJ, Davies RA, Chan KL: Measurement of left ventricular ejection fraction by acoustic quantification and comparison with radionuclide angiography. Am J Cardiol 74:1052, 1994.
13. Gorcsan J 3rd, Romand JA, Mandarino WA, et al: Assessment of left ventricular performance by on-line pressure-area relations using echocardiographic automated border detection. J Am Coll Cardiol 23:242, 1994.
14. Devereux RB, Alonso DR, Lutas EM, et al: Echocardiographic assessment of left ventricular hypertrophy: Comparison to necropsy findings. Am J Cardiol 57:450, 1986.
15. Byrd BF 3rd, Finkbeiner W, Bouchard A, et al: Accuracy and reproducibility of clinically acquired two-dimensional echocardiographic mass measurements. Am Heart J 118:133, 1989.
16. Cerqueira MD, Weissman NJ, Dilsizian V, et al: Standardized myocardial segmentation and nomenclature for tomographic imaging of the heart: A statement for healthcare professionals from the Cardiac Imaging Committee of the Council on Clinical Cardiology of the American Heart Association. Circulation 105:539, 2002.
17. Bourdillon PD, Broderick TM, Sawada SG, et al: Regional wall motion index for infarct and noninfarct regions after reperfusion in acute myocardial infarction: Comparison with global wall motion index. J Am Soc Echocardiogr 2:398, 1989.

Doppler Examination

18. Chan KL, Currie PJ, Seward JB, et al: Comparison of three Doppler ultrasound methods in the prediction of pulmonary artery pressure. J Am Coll Cardiol 9:549, 1987.
19. McQuillan BM, Picard MH, Leavitt M, et al: Clinical correlates and reference intervals for pulmonary artery systolic pressure among echocardiographically normal subjects. Circulation 104:2797, 2001.
20. Scapellato F, Temporelli PL, Eleuteri E, et al: Accurate noninvasive estimation of pulmonary vascular resistance by Doppler echocardiography in patients with chronic heart failure. J Am Coll Cardiol 37:1813, 2001.
21. Moulinier L, Venet T, Schiller NB, et al: Measurement of aortic blood flow by Doppler echocardiography: Day to day variability in normal subjects and applicability in clinical research. J Am Coll Cardiol 17:1326, 1991.
22. Taylor R: Evolution of the continuity equation in the Doppler echocardiographic assessment of the severity of valvular aortic stenosis. J Am Soc Echocardiogr 3:326, 1990.
23. Recusani F, Bargiggia GS, Yoganathan AP, et al: A new method for quantification of regurgitant flow rate using color Doppler flow imaging of the flow convergence region proximal to a discrete orifice: An in vitro study. Circulation 83:594, 1991.
24. Shiota T, Jones M, Teien DE, et al: Evaluation of mitral regurgitation using a digitally determined color Doppler flow convergence "centerline" acceleration method: Studies in an animal model with quantified mitral regurgitation. Circulation 89:2879, 1994.
25. Pu M, Vandervoort PM, Griffin BP, et al: Quantification of mitral regurgitation by the proximal convergence method using transesophageal echocardiography: Clinical validation of a geometric correction for proximal flow constraint. Circulation 92:2169, 1995.
26. Kolias TJ, Aaronson KD, Armstrong WF: Doppler-derived dP/dt and -dP/dt predict survival in congestive heart failure. J Am Coll Cardiol 36:1594, 2000.
27. Oh JK, Appleton CP, Hatle LK, et al: The noninvasive assessment of left ventricular diastolic function with two-dimensional and Doppler echocardiography. J Am Soc Echocardiogr 10:246, 1997.
28. Nishimura RA, Tajik AJ: Evaluation of diastolic filling of left ventricle in health and disease: Doppler echocardiography is the clinician's Rosetta Stone. J Am Coll Cardiol 30:8, 1997.
29. Wachtell K, Smith G, Gerdts E, et al: Left ventricular filling patterns in patients with systemic hypertension and left ventricular hypertrophy (the LIFE study). Losartan Intervention For Endpoint. Am J Cardiol 85:466, 2000.
30. Firstenberg MS, Levine BD, Garcia MJ, et al: Relationship of echocardiographic indices to pulmonary capillary wedge pressures in healthy volunteers. J Am Coll Cardiol 36:1664, 2000.

Transesophageal and Three-Dimensional Imaging

31. Seward JB, Khandheria BK, Freeman WK, et al: Multiplane transesophageal echocardiography: Image orientation, examination technique, anatomic correlations, and clinical applications. Mayo Clin Proc 68:523, 1993.
32. Takuma S, Zwas DR, Fard A, et al: Real-time, 3-dimensional echocardiography acquires all standard 2-dimensional images from 2 volume sets: A clinical demonstration in 45 patients. J Am Soc Echocardiogr 12:1, 1999.
33. Collins M, Hsieh A, Ohazama CJ, et al: Assessment of regional wall motion abnormalities with real-time 3-dimensional echocardiography. J Am Soc Echocardiogr 12:7, 1999.
34. Balestrini L, Fleishman C, Lanzoni L, et al: Real-time 3-dimensional echocardiography evaluation of congenital heart disease. J Am Soc Echocardiogr 13:171, 2000.
35. Ahmad M, Xie T, McCulloch M, et al: Real-time three-dimensional dobutamine stress echocardiography in assessment stress echocardiography in assessment of ischemia: Comparison with two-dimensional dobutamine stress echocardiography. J Am Coll Cardiol 37:1303, 2001.
36. Salustri A, Spitaels S, McGhie J, et al: Transthoracic three-dimensional echocardiography in adult patients with congenital heart disease. J Am Coll Cardiol 26:759, 1995.
37. Schmidt MA, Ohazama CJ, Agyeman KO, et al: Real-time three-dimensional echocardiography for measurement of left ventricular volumes. Am J Cardiol 84:1434, 1999.

Intravascular Imaging

38. Pinto FJ, Chenzbraun A, Botas J, et al: Feasibility of serial intracoronary ultrasound imaging for assessment of progression of intimal proliferation in cardiac transplant recipients. Circulation 90:2348, 1994.
39. de Feyter PJ, Kay P, Disco C, et al: Reference chart derived from post-stent-implantation intravascular ultrasound predictors of 6-month expected restenosis on quantitative coronary angiography. Circulation 100:1777, 1999.
40. Schiele F, Meneveau N, Gilard M, et al: Intravascular ultrasound-guided balloon angioplasty compared with stent: Immediate and 6-month results of the multicenter, randomized Balloon Equivalent to Stent Study (BEST). Circulation 107:545, 2003.
41. Oemrawsingh PV, Mintz GS, Schalij MJ, et al: Intravascular ultrasound guidance improves angiographic and clinical outcome of stent implantation for long coronary artery stenoses: Final results of a randomized comparison with angiographic guidance (TULIP Study). Circulation 107:62, 2003.
42. Di Mario C, Krams R, Gil R, et al: Slope of the instantaneous hyperemic diastolic coronary flow velocity-pressure relation: A new index for assessment of the physiological significance of coronary stenosis in humans. Circulation 90:1215, 1994.
43. Fu M, Hung JS, Lo PH, et al: Intracardiac echocardiography via the transvenous approach with use of 8F 10-MHz ultrasound catheters. Mayo Clin Proc 74:775, 1999.
44. Bruce CJ, Packer DL, Seward JB: Transvascular imaging: Feasibility study using a vector phased array ultrasound catheter. Echocardiography 16:425, 1999.
45. Packer DL, Stevens CL, Curley MG, et al: Intracardiac phased-array imaging: Methods and initial clinical experience with high resolution, under blood visualization: Initial experience with intracardiac phased-array ultrasound. J Am Coll Cardiol 39:509, 2002.

Tissue Characterization and Doppler Tissue Imaging

46. Milunski MR, Mohr GA, Perez JE, et al: Ultrasonic tissue characterization with integrated backscatter: Acute myocardial ischemia, reperfusion, and stunned myocardium in patients. Circulation 80:491, 1989.
47. Iwakura K, Ito H, Kawano S, et al: Detection of TIMI-3 flow before mechanical reperfusion with ultrasonic tissue characterization in patients with anterior wall acute myocardial infarction. Circulation 107:3159, 2003.
48. Garcia MJ, Rodriguez L, Ares M, et al: Myocardial wall velocity assessment by pulsed Doppler tissue imaging: Characteristic findings in normal subjects. Am Heart J 132:648, 1996.
49. Derumeaux G, Ovize M, Loufoua J, et al: Assessment of nonuniformity of transmural myocardial velocities by color-coded tissue Doppler imaging: Characterization of normal, ischemic, and stunned myocardium. Circulation 101:1390, 2000.
50. Pasquet A, Armstrong G, Beachler L, et al: Use of segmental tissue Doppler velocity to quantitate exercise echocardiography. J Am Soc Echocardiogr 12:901, 1999.
51. Wang M, Yip GW, Wang AY, et al: Peak early diastolic mitral annulus velocity by tissue Doppler imaging adds independent and incremental prognostic value. J Am Coll Cardiol 41:820, 2003.
52. Waggoner AD, Bierig SM: Tissue Doppler imaging: A useful echocardiographic method for the cardiac sonographer to assess systolic and diastolic ventricular function. J Am Soc Echocardiogr 14:1143, 2001.
53. Kukulski T, Jamal F, D'Hooge J, et al: Acute changes in systolic and diastolic events during clinical coronary angioplasty: A comparison of regional velocity, strain rate, and strain measurement. J Am Soc Echocardiogr 15:1, 2002.
54. Cain P, Baglin T, Khoury V, et al: Automated regional myocardial displacement for facilitating the interpretation of dobutamine echocardiography. Am J Cardiol 89:1347, 2002.

55. Stoylen A, Slordahl S, Skjelvan GK, et al: Strain rate imaging in normal and reduced diastolic function: Comparison with pulsed Doppler tissue imaging of the mitral annulus. J Am Soc Echocardiogr 14:264, 2001.
56. D'Hooge J, Heimdal A, Jamal F, et al: Regional strain and strain rate measurements by cardiac ultrasound: Principles, implementation and limitations. Eur J Echocardiogr 1:154, 2000.
57. Edvardsen T, Gerber BL, Garot J, et al: Quantitative assessment of intrinsic regional myocardial deformation by Doppler strain rate echocardiography in humans: Validation against three-dimensional tagged magnetic resonance imaging. Circulation 106:50, 2002.
58. Hoffmann R, Altiok E, Nowak B, et al: Strain rate measurement by Doppler echocardiography allows improved assessment of myocardial viability inpatients with depressed left ventricular function. J Am Coll Cardiol 39:443, 2002.
59. Belohlavek M, Pislaru C, Bae RY, et al: Real-time strain rate echocardiographic imaging: Temporal and spatial analysis of postsystolic compression in acutely ischemic myocardium. J Am Soc Echocardiogr 14:360, 2001.
60. Pislaru C, Belohlavek M, Bae RY, et al: Regional asynchrony during acute myocardial ischemia quantified by ultrasound strain rate imaging. J Am Coll Cardiol 37:1141, 2001.
61. Kukulski T, Jamal F, Herbots L, et al: Identification of acutely ischemic myocardium using ultrasonic strain measurements: A clinical study in patients undergoing coronary angioplasty. J Am Coll Cardiol 41:810, 2003.

Contrast Echocardiography

62. Mulvagh SL, DeMaria AN, Feinstein SB, et al: Contrast echocardiography: Current and future applications. J Am Soc Echocardiogr 13:331, 2000.
63. Kaul S: Myocardial contrast echocardiography: 15 years of research and development. Circulation 96:3745, 1997.
64. Becher H, Tiemann K, Schlief R, et al: Harmonic power Doppler contrast echocardiography: Preliminary clinical results. Echocardiography 14:637, 1997.
65. Senior R, Kaul S, Soman P, et al: Power doppler harmonic imaging: A feasibility study of a new technique for the assessment of myocardial perfusion. Am Heart J 139:245, 2000.
66. Tiemann K, Becher H, Bimmel D, et al: Stimulated acoustic emission nonbackscatter contrast effect of microbubbles seen with harmonic power Doppler imaging. Echocardiography 14:65, 1997.
67. Villarraga HR, Foley DA, Aeschbacher BC, et al: Destruction of contrast microbubbles during ultrasound imaging at conventional power output. J Am Soc Echocardiogr 10:783, 1997.
68. Wei K, Skyba DM, Firschke C, et al: Interactions between microbubbles and ultrasound: In vitro and in vivo observations. J Am Coll Cardiol 29:1081, 1997.
69. Skyba DM, Price RJ, Linka AZ, et al: Direct in vivo visualization of intravascular destruction of microbubbles by ultrasound and its local effects on tissue. Circulation 98:290, 1998.
70. Simpson DH: Pulse inversion Doppler: A new method for detecting nonlinear echoes from microbubble contrast agents. IEEE Trans Ultrasonics Ferroelectrics Frequency Control 20:16, 1998.
71. Goldberg BB, Liu JB, Forsberg F: Ultrasound contrast agents: A review. Ultrasound Med Biol 20:319, 1994.
72. Cohen JL, Cheirif J, Segar DS, et al: Improved left ventricular endocardial border delineation and opacification with OPTISON (FS069), a new echocardiographic contrast agent: Results of a phase III multicenter trial. J Am Coll Cardiol 32:746, 1998.
73. Main ML, Grayburn PA: Clinical applications of transpulmonary contrast echocardiography. Am Heart J 137:144, 1999.
74. Reilly JP, Tunick PA, Timmermans RJ, et al: Contrast echocardiography clarifies uninterpretable wall motion in intensive care unit patients. J Am Coll Cardiol 35:485, 2000.
75. Yong Y, Wu D, Fernandes V, et al: Diagnostic accuracy and cost-effectiveness of contrast echocardiography on evaluation of cardiac function in technically very difficult patients in the intensive care unit. Am J Cardiol 89:711, 2002.
76. Dolan MS, Riad K, El-Shafei A, et al: Effect of intravenous contrast for left ventricular opacification and border definition on sensitivity and specificity of dobutamine stress echocardiography compared with coronary angiography in technically difficult patients. Am Heart J 142:908, 2001.
77. Rainbird AJ, Mulvagh SL, Oh JK, et al: Contrast dobutamine stress echocardiography: Clinical practice assessment in 300 consecutive patients. J Am Soc Echocardiogr 14:378, 2001.
78. Shimoni S, Zoghbi WA, Xie F, et al: Real-time assessment of myocardial perfusion and wall motion during bicycle and treadmill exercise echocardiography: Comparison with single photon emission computed tomography. J Am Coll Cardiol 37:741, 2001.
79. Thomson HL, Basmadjian AJ, Rainbird AJ, et al: Contrast echocardiography improves the accuracy and reproducibility of left ventricular remodeling measurements: A prospective, randomly assigned, blinded study. J Am Coll Cardiol 38:867, 2001.
80. von Bibra H, Becher H, Firschke C, et al: Enhancement of mitral regurgitation and normal left atrial color Doppler flow signals with peripheral venous injection of a saccharide-based contrast agent. J Am Coll Cardiol 22:521, 1993.
81. von Bibra H, Sutherland G, Becher H, et al: Clinical evaluation of left heart Doppler contrast enhancement by a saccharide-based transpulmonary contrast agent. The Levovist Cardiac Working Group. J Am Coll Cardiol 25:500, 1995.
82. Thanigaraj S, Schechtman KB, Perez JE: Improved echocardiographic delineation of left ventricular thrombus with the use of intravenous second-generation contrast image enhancement. J Am Soc Echocardiogr 12:1022, 1999.
83. Takeuchi M, Ogunyankin K, Pandian NG, et al: Enhanced visualization of intravascular and left atrial appendage thrombus with the use of a thrombus-targeting ultrasonographic contrast agent (MRX-408A1): In vivo experimental echocardiographic studies. J Am Soc Echocardiogr 12:1015, 1999.
84. Lindner JR, Dayton PA, Coggins MP, et al: Noninvasive imaging of inflammation by ultrasound detection of phagocytosed microbubbles. Circulation 102:531, 2000.
85. Leong-Poi H, Christiansen J, Klibanov AL, et al: Noninvasive assessment of angiogenesis by ultrasound and microbubbles targeted to alpha(v)-integrins. Circulation 107:455, 2003.
86. Cheitlin MD, Alpert JS, Armstrong WF, et al: ACC/AHA Guidelines for the Clinical Application of Echocardiography. A report of the American College of Cardiology/American Heart Association Task Force on Practice Guidelines (Committee on Clinical Application of Echocardiography). Developed in collaboration with the American Society of Echocardiography. Circulation 95:1686, 1997.
87. Quinones MA, Douglas PS, Foster E, et al: American College of Cardiology/American Heart Association clinical competence statement on echocardiography: A report of the American College of Cardiology/American Heart Association/American College of Physicians—American Society of Internal Medicine Task Force on Clinical Competence. Circulation 107:1068, 2003.

Acquired Valvular Heart Disease

88. Nishimura RA, Rihal CS, Tajik AJ, et al: Accurate measurement of the transmitral gradient in patients with mitral stenosis: A simultaneous catheterization and Doppler echocardiographic study. J Am Coll Cardiol 24:152, 1994.
89. Wang A, Ryan T, Kisslo KB, et al: Assessing the severity of mitral stenosis: Variability between noninvasive and invasive measurements in patients with symptomatic mitral valve stenosis. Am Heart J 138:777, 1999.
90. Leavitt JI, Coats MH, Falk RH: Effects of exercise on transmitral gradient and pulmonary artery pressure in patients with mitral stenosis or a prosthetic mitral valve: A Doppler echocardiographic study. J Am Coll Cardiol 17:1520, 1991.
91. Fredman CS, Pearson AC, Labovitz AJ, et al: Comparison of hemodynamic pressure half-time method and Gorlin formula with Doppler and echocardiographic determinations of mitral valve area in patients with combined mitral stenosis and regurgitation. Am Heart J 119:121, 1990.
92. Loperfido F, Laurenzi F, Gimigliano F, et al: A comparison of the assessment of mitral valve area by continuous wave Doppler and by cross sectional echocardiography. Br Heart J 57:348, 1987.
93. Thomas JD, Wilkins GT, Choong CY, et al: Inaccuracy of mitral pressure half-time immediately after percutaneous mitral valvotomy: Dependence on transmitral gradient and left atrial and ventricular compliance. Circulation 78:980, 1988.
94. Hernandez R, Banuelos C, Alfonso F, et al: Long-term clinical and echocardiographic follow-up after percutaneous mitral valvuloplasty with the Inoue balloon. Circulation 99:1580, 1999.
95. Palacios IF, Sanchez PL, Harrell LC, et al: Which patients benefit from percutaneous mitral balloon valvuloplasty? Prevalvuloplasty and postvalvuloplasty variables that predict long-term outcome. Circulation 105:1465, 2002.
96. Wang A, Krasuski RA, Warner JJ, et al: Serial echocardiographic evaluation of restenosis after successful percutaneous mitral commissurotomy. J Am Coll Cardiol 39:328, 2002.
97. Himelman RB, Kusumoto F, Oken K, et al: The flail mitral valve: Echocardiographic findings by precordial and transesophageal imaging and Doppler color flow mapping. J Am Coll Cardiol 17:272, 1991.
98. Shyu KG, Lei MH, Hwang JJ, et al: Morphologic characterization and quantitative assessment of mitral regurgitation with ruptured chordae tendineae by transesophageal echocardiography. Am J Cardiol 70:1152, 1992.
99. Chao K, Moises VA, Shandas R, et al: Influence of the Coanda effect on color Doppler jet area and color encoding: In vitro studies using color Doppler flow mapping. Circulation 85:333, 1992.
100. De Simone R, Glombitza G, Vahl CF, et al: Three-dimensional color Doppler: A clinical study in patients with mitral regurgitation. J Am Coll Cardiol 33:1646, 1999.
101. Sugeng L, Spencer K, Mor-Avi V, et al: Dynamic three-dimensional color flow Doppler: An improved technique for the assessment of mitral regurgitation. Echocardiography 20:265, 2003.
102. Kwan J, Shiota T, Agler DA, et al: Geometric differences of the mitral apparatus between ischemic and dilated cardiomyopathy with significant mitral regurgitation: Real-time three-dimensional echocardiography study. Circulation 107:1135, 2003.
103. Otsuji Y, Handschumacher MD, Liel-Cohen N, et al: Mechanism of ischemic mitral regurgitation with segmental left ventricular dysfunction: Three-dimensional echocardiographic studies in models of acute and chronic progressive regurgitation. J Am Coll Cardiol 37:641, 2001.
104. Vandervoort PM, Rivera JM, Mele D, et al: Application of color Doppler flow mapping to calculate effective regurgitant orifice area: An in vitro study and initial clinical observations. Circulation 88:1150, 1993.
105. Rodriguez L, Thomas JD, Monterroso V, et al: Validation of the proximal flow convergence method: Calculation of orifice area in patients with mitral stenosis. Circulation 88:1157, 1993.
106. Currie PJ, Hagler DJ, Seward JB, et al: Instantaneous pressure gradient: A simultaneous Doppler and dual catheter correlative study. J Am Coll Cardiol 7:800, 1986.
107. Tribouilloy C, Shen WF, Peltier M, et al: Quantitation of aortic valve area in aortic stenosis with multiplane transesophageal echocardiography: Comparison with monoplane transesophageal approach. Am Heart J 128:526, 1994.
108. Ray R: Evolution of the continuity equation in the Doppler echocardiographic assessment of the severity of valvular aortic stenosis. J Am Soc Echocardiogr 3:326, 1990.
109. Ford LE, Feldman T, Carroll JD: Valve resistance. Circulation 89:893, 1994.
110. Lin SS, Roger VL, Pascoe R, et al: Dobutamine stress Doppler hemodynamics in patients with aortic stenosis: Feasibility, safety, and surgical correlations. Am Heart J 136:1010, 1998.
111. Evangelista A, del Castillo HG, Calvo F, et al: Strategy for optimal aortic regurgitation quantification by Doppler echocardiography: Agreement among different methods. Am Heart J 139:773, 2000.
112. Padial LR, Oliver A, Sagie A, et al: Two-dimensional echocardiographic assessment of the progression of aortic root size in 127 patients with chronic aortic regurgitation: Role of the supraaortic ridge and relation to the progression of the lesion. Am Heart J 134:814, 1997.

113. Mugge A, Daniel WG, Herrmann G, et al: Quantification of tricuspid regurgitation by Doppler color flow mapping after cardiac transplantation. Am J Cardiol 66:884, 1990.
114. Stephen B, Dalal P, Berger M, et al: Noninvasive estimation of pulmonary artery diastolic pressure in patients with tricuspid regurgitation by Doppler echocardiography. Chest 116:73, 1999.
115. Jollis JG, Landolfo CK, Kisslo J, et al: Fenfluramine and phentermine and cardiovascular findings: Effect of treatment duration on prevalence of valve abnormalities. Circulation 101:2071, 2000.
116. Gardin JM, Schumacher D, Constantine G, et al: Valvular abnormalities and cardiovascular status following exposure to dexfenfluramine or phentermine/fenfluramine. JAMA 283:1703, 2000.
117. Gardin JM, Weissman NJ, Leung C, et al: Clinical and echocardiographic follow-up of patients previously treated with dexfenfluramine or phentermine/fenfluramine. JAMA 286:2011, 2001.
118. Abraham TP, Kon ND, Nomeir AM, et al: Accuracy of transesophageal echocardiography in preoperative determination of aortic annulus size during valve replacement. J Am Soc Echocardiogr 10:149, 1997.
119. Bridgman PG, Bloomfield P, Reid JH, et al: Prediction of stentless aortic bioprosthesis size with transesophageal echocardiography and magnetic resonance imaging. J Heart Valve Dis 6:487, 1997.
120. Oh CC, Click RL, Orszulak TA, et al: Role of intraoperative transesophageal echocardiography in determining aortic annulus diameter in homograft insertion. J Am Soc Echocardiogr 11:638, 1998.
121. Vandervoort PM, Greenberg NL, Powell KA, et al: Pressure recovery in bileaflet heart valve prostheses. Localized high velocities and gradients in central and side orifices with implications for Doppler-catheter gradient relation in aortic and mitral position. Circulation 92:3464, 1995.
122. Baumgartner H, Khan S, DeRobertis M, et al: Effect of prosthetic aortic valve design on the doppler-catheter gradient correlation. J Am Coll Cardiol 19:324, 1992.
123. Kodavatiganti R: Intraoperative assessment of the mitral valve by transoesophageal echocardiography: An overview. Ann Cardiac Anaesth 5:127, 2002.
124. Shanewise JS, Cheung AT, Aronson S, et al: ASE/SCA guidelines for performing a comprehensive intraoperative multiplane transesophageal echocardiography examination: Recommendations of the American Society of Echocardiography Council for Intraoperative Echocardiography and the Society of Cardiovascular Anesthesiologists Task Force for Certification in Perioperative Transesophageal Echocardiography. Anesth Analg 89:870, 1999.
125. Yvorchuk KJ, Chan KL: Application of transthoracic and transesophageal echocardiography in the diagnosis and management of infective endocarditis. J Am Soc Echocardiogr 7:294, 1994.
126. Durack DT, Lukes AS, Bright DK: New criteria for diagnosis of infective endocarditis: Utilization of specific echocardiographic findings. Duke Endocarditis Service. Am J Med 96:200, 1994.
127. Heinle S, Wilderman N, Harrison JK, et al: Value of transthoracic echocardiography in predicting embolic events in active infective endocarditis. Duke Endocarditis Service. Am J Cardiol 74:799, 1994.
128. Leung DY, Cranney GB, Hopkins AP, et al: Role of transoesophageal echocardiography in the diagnosis and management of aortic root abscess. Br Heart J 72:175, 1994.
129. Fox CS, Vasan RS, Parise H, et al: Mitral annular calcification predicts cardiovascular morbidity and mortality: The Framingham Heart Study. Circulation 107:1492, 2003.

Congenital Heart Disease

130. Watanabe F, Takenaka K, Suzuki J, et al: Visualization of sinus venosus-type atrial septal defect by biplane transesophageal echocardiography. J Am Soc Echocardiogr 7:179, 1994.
131. Hausmann D, Daniel WG, Mugge A, et al: Value of transesophageal color Doppler echocardiography for detection of different types of atrial septal defect in adults. J Am Soc Echocardiogr 5:481, 1992.
132. Dall'Agata A, McGhie J, Taams MA, et al: Secondum atrial septal defect is a dynamic three-dimensional entity. Am Heart J 137:1075, 1999.
133. Mazic U, Gavora P, Masura J: The role of transesophageal echocardiography in transcatheter closure of secundum atrial septal defects by the Amplatzer septal occluder. Am Heart J 142:482, 2001.
134. Mullen MJ, Dias BF, Walker F, et al: Intracardiac echocardiography guided device closure of atrial septal defects. J Am Coll Cardiol 41:285, 2003.
135. Kerut EK, Norfleet WT, Plotnick GD, et al: Patent foramen ovale: A review of associated conditions and the impact of physiological size. J Am Coll Cardiol 38:613, 2001.

Pericardial and Myocardial Disease

136. Oh JK, Hatle LK, Seward JB, et al: Diagnostic role of Doppler echocardiography in constrictive pericarditis. J Am Coll Cardiol 23:154, 1994.
137. Myers RB, Spodick DH: Constrictive pericarditis: Clinical and pathophysiologic characteristics. Am Heart J 138:219, 1999.
138. Bach DS, Beanlands RS, Schwaiger M, et al: Heterogeneity of ventricular function and myocardial oxidative metabolism in nonischemic dilated cardiomyopathy. J Am Coll Cardiol 25:1258, 1995.
139. Hansen A, Haass M, Zugck C, et al: Prognostic value of Doppler echocardiographic mitral inflow patterns: Implications for risk stratification in patients with chronic congestive heart failure. J Am Coll Cardiol 37:1049, 2001.
140. Yong Y, Nagueh SF, Shimoni S, et al: Deceleration time in ischemic cardiomyopathy: Relation to echocardiographic and scintigraphic indices of myocardial viability and functional recovery after revascularization. Circulation 103:1232, 2001.
141. Whalley GA, Doughty RN, Gamble GD, et al: Pseudonormal mitral filling pattern predicts hospital re-admission in patients with congestive heart failure. J Am Coll Cardiol 39:1787, 2002.
142. Rossi A, Cicoira M, Zanolla L, et al: Determinants and prognostic value of left atrial volume in patients with dilated cardiomyopathy. J Am Coll Cardiol 40:1425, 2002.
143. Koelling TM, Aaronson KD, Cody RJ, et al: Prognostic significance of mitral regurgitation and tricuspid regurgitation in patients with left ventricular systolic dysfunction. Am Heart J 144:524, 2002.
144. Faber L, Seggewiss H, Ziemssen P, et al: Intraprocedural myocardial contrast echocardiography as a routine procedure in percutaneous transluminal septal myocardial ablation: Detection of threatening myocardial necrosis distant from the septal target area. Catheter Cardiovasc Interv 47:462, 1999.
145. Klein AL, Hatle LK, Taliercio CP, et al: Prognostic significance of Doppler measures of diastolic function in cardiac amyloidosis: A Doppler echocardiography study. Circulation 83:808, 1991.
146. Tabata T, Kabbani SS, Murray RD, et al: Difference in the respiratory variation between pulmonary venous and mitral inflow Doppler velocities in patients with constrictive pericarditis with and without atrial fibrillation. J Am Coll Cardiol 37:1936, 2001.
147. Garcia MJ, Rodriguez L, Ares M, et al: Differentiation of constrictive pericarditis from restrictive cardiomyopathy: Assessment of left ventricular diastolic velocities in longitudinal axis by Doppler tissue imaging. J Am Coll Cardiol 27:108, 1996.
148. Palka P, Lange A, Donnelly JE, et al: Differentiation between restrictive cardiomyopathy and constrictive pericarditis by early diastolic doppler myocardial velocity gradient at the posterior wall. Circulation 102:655, 2000.

Acute Myocardial Infarction

149. Force T, Kemper A, Perkins L, et al: Overestimation of infarct size by quantitative two-dimensional echocardiography: The role of tethering and of analytic procedures. Circulation 73:1360, 1986.
150. Derumeaux G, Loufoua J, Pontier G, et al: Tissue Doppler imaging differentiates transmural from nontransmural acute myocardial infarction after reperfusion therapy. Circulation 103:589, 2001.
151. Gotte MJ, van Rossum AC, Twisk JWR, et al: Quantification of regional contractile function after infarction: Strain analysis superior to wall thickening analysis in discriminating infarct from remote myocardium. J Am Coll Cardiol 37:808, 2001.
152. Sabia P, Abbott RD, Afrookteh A, et al: Importance of two-dimensional echocardiographic assessment of left ventricular systolic function in patients presenting to the emergency room with cardiac-related symptoms. Circulation 84:1615, 1991.
153. Elhendy A, van Domburg RT, Bax JJ, et al: Significance of resting wall motion abnormalities in 2-dimensional echocardiography in patients without previous myocardial infarction referred for pharmacologic stress testing. J Am Soc Echocardiogr 13:1, 2000.
154. Kontos MC, Kurdziel K, McQueen R, et al: Comparison of 2-dimensional echocardiography and myocardial perfusion imaging for diagnosing myocardial infarction in emergency department patients. Am Heart J 143:659, 2002.
155. Burns RJ, Gibbons RJ, Yi Q, et al: The relationships of left ventricular ejection fraction, end-systolic volume index and infarct size to six-month mortality after hospital discharge following myocardial infarction treated by thrombolysis. J Am Coll Cardiol 39:30, 2002.
156. Moller JE, Sondergaard E, Poulsen SH, et al: Pseudonormal and restrictive filling patterns predict left ventricular dilation and cardiac death after a first myocardial infarction: A serial color M-mode Doppler echocardiographic study. J Am Coll Cardiol 36:1841, 2000.
157. Moller JE, Egstrup K, Kober L, et al: Prognostic importance of systolic and diastolic function after acute myocardial infarction. Am Heart J 145:147, 2003.
158. Picard MH, Wilkins GT, Gillam LD, et al: Immediate regional endocardial surface expansion following coronary occlusion in the canine left ventricle: Disproportionate effects of anterior versus inferior ischemia. Am Heart J 121:753, 1991.
159. Mehta SR, Eikelboom JW, Natarajan MK, et al: Impact of right ventricular involvement on mortality and morbidity in patients with inferior myocardial infarction. J Am Coll Cardiol 37:37, 2001.

Myocardial Stunning and Hibernation

160. Kloner RA, Bolli R, Marban E, et al: Medical and cellular implications of stunning, hibernation, and preconditioning: An NHLBI workshop. Circulation 97:1848, 1998.
161. Bax JJ, Poldermans D, Elhendy A, et al: Improvement of left ventricular ejection fraction, heart failure symptoms and prognosis after revascularization in patients with chronic coronary artery disease and viable myocardium detected by dobutamine stress echocardiography. J Am Coll Cardiol 34:163, 1999.
162. Bonow RO: Identification of viable myocardium. Circulation 94:2674, 1996.
163. Bolognese L, Buonamici P, Cerisano G, et al: Early dobutamine echocardiography predicts improvement in regional and global left ventricular function after reperfused acute myocardial infarction without residual stenosis of the infarct-related artery. Am Heart J 139:153, 2000.
164. Allman KC, Shaw LJ, Hachamovitch R, et al: Myocardial viability testing and impact of revascularization on prognosis in patients with coronary artery disease and left ventricular dysfunction: A meta-analysis. J Am Coll Cardiol 39:1151, 2002.

Stress Echocardiography

165. Armstrong WF, O'Donnell J, Ryan T, et al: Effect of prior myocardial infarction and extent and location of coronary disease on accuracy of exercise echocardiography. J Am Coll Cardiol 10:531, 1987.
166. Crouse LJ, Harbrecht JJ, Vacek JL, et al: Exercise echocardiography as a screening test for coronary artery disease and correlation with coronary arteriography. Am J Cardiol 67:1213, 1991.
167. Marwick TH, Nemec JJ, Pashkow FJ, et al: Accuracy and limitations of exercise echocardiography in a routine clinical setting. J Am Coll Cardiol 19:74, 1992.
168. Roger VL, Pellikka PA, Oh JK, et al: Identification of multivessel coronary artery disease by exercise echocardiography. J Am Coll Cardiol 24:109, 1994.
169. Beleslin BD, Ostojic M, Stepanovic J, et al: Stress echocardiography in the detection of myocardial ischemia: Head-to-head comparison of exercise, dobutamine, and dipyridamole tests. Circulation 90:1168, 1994.

170. Quinones MA, Verani MS, Haichin RM, et al: Exercise echocardiography versus 201Tl single-photon emission computed tomography in evaluation of coronary artery disease. Analysis of 292 patients. Circulation 85:1026, 1992.
171. Ryan T, Segar DS, Sawada SG, et al: Detection of coronary artery disease with upright bicycle exercise echocardiography. J Am Soc Echocardiogr 6:186, 1993.
172. Cohen JL, Ottenweller JE, George AK, et al: Comparison of dobutamine and exercise echocardiography for detecting coronary artery disease. Am J Cardiol 72:1226, 1993.
173. Hecht HS, DeBord L, Shaw R, et al: Digital supine bicycle stress echocardiography: A new technique for evaluating coronary artery disease. J Am Coll Cardiol 21:950, 1993.
174. Luotolahti M, Saraste M, Hartiala J: Exercise echocardiography in the diagnosis of coronary artery disease. Ann Med 28:73, 1996.
175. Marwick T, D'Hondt AM, Baudhuin T, et al: Optimal use of dobutamine stress for the detection and evaluation of coronary artery disease: Combination with echocardiography or scintigraphy, or both? J Am Coll Cardiol 22:159, 1993.
176. Ling LH, Pelikka PA, Mahoney DW: Atropine augmentation in dobutamine stress echocardiography. J Am Coll Cardiol 28:551, 1996.
177. Marcovitz PA, Armstrong WF: Accuracy of dobutamine stress echocardiography in detecting coronary artery disease. Am J Cardiol 69:1269, 1992.
178. Takeuchi M, Araki M, Nakashima Y, et al: Comparison of dobutamine stress echocardiography and stress thallium-201 single-photon emission computed tomography for detecting coronary artery disease. J Am Soc Echocardiogr 6:593, 1993.
179. Kwok Y, Kim C, Grady D, et al: Meta-analysis of exercise testing to detect coronary artery disease in women. Am J Cardiol 83:660, 1999.
180. Chuah SC, Pellikka PA, Roger VL, et al: Role of dobutamine stress echocardiography in predicting outcome in 860 patients with known or suspected coronary artery disease. Circulation 97:1474, 1998.
181. Poldermans D, Fioretti PM, Boersma E, et al: Long-term prognostic value of dobutamine-atropine stress echocardiography in 1737 patients with known or suspected coronary artery disease: A single-center experience. Circulation 99:757, 1999.
182. Marwick TH, Case C, Sawada S, et al: Prediction of mortality using dobutamine echocardiography. J Am Coll Cardiol 37:754, 2001.
183. Bholasingh R, Cornel JH, Kamp O, et al: Prognostic value of predischarge dobutamine stress echocardiography in chest pain patients with a negative cardiac troponin T. J Am Coll Cardiol 41:596, 2003.
184. Kamalesh M, Matorin R, Sawada S: Prognostic value of a negative stress echocardiographic study in diabetic patients. Am Heart J 143:163, 2002.
185. Elhendy A, Mahoney DW, Khandheria BK, et al: Prognostic significance of the location of wall motion abnormalities during exercise echocardiography. J Am Coll Cardiol 40:1623, 2002.
186. McCully RB, Roger VL, Mahoney DW, et al: Outcome after abnormal exercise echocardiography for patients with good exercise capacity: Prognostic importance of the extent and severity of exercise-related left ventricular dysfunction. J Am Coll Cardiol 39:1345, 2002.
187. Arruda-Olson AM, Juracan EM, Mahoney DW, et al: Prognostic value of exercise echocardiography in 5,798 patients: Is there a gender difference? J Am Coll Cardiol 39:625, 2002.
188. Carlos ME, Smart SC, Wynsen JC, et al: Dobutamine stress echocardiography for risk stratification after myocardial infarction. Circulation 95:1402, 1997.
189. Shaw LJ, Peterson ED, Kesler K, et al: A metaanalysis of predischarge risk stratification after acute myocardial infarction with stress electrocardiographic, myocardial perfusion, and ventricular function imaging. Am J Cardiol 78:1327, 1996.
190. Shaw LJ, Eagle KA, Gersh BJ, et al: Meta-analysis of intravenous dipyridamole-thallium-201 imaging (1985 to 1994) and dobutamine echocardiography (1991 to 1994) for risk stratification before vascular surgery. J Am Coll Cardiol 27:787, 1996.

Myocardial Contrast Echocardiography

191. Wei K, Jayaweera AR, Firoozan S, et al: Quantification of myocardial blood flow with ultrasound-induced destruction of microbubbles administered as a constant venous infusion. Circulation 97:473, 1998.
192. Heinle SK, Noblin J, Goree-Best P, et al: Assessment of myocardial perfusion by harmonic power Doppler imaging at rest and during adenosine stress: Comparison with (99m)Tc-sestamibi SPECT imaging. Circulation 102:55, 2000.
193. Porter TR, Xie F, Silver M, et al: Real-time perfusion imaging with low mechanical index pulse inversion Doppler imaging. J Am Coll Cardiol 37:748, 2001.
194. Masugata H, Peters B, Lafitte S, et al: Quantitative assessment of myocardial perfusion during graded coronary stenosis by real-time myocardial contrast echo refilling curves. J Am Coll Cardiol 37:262, 2001.
195. Balcells E, Powers ER, Lepper W, et al: Detection of myocardial viability by contrast echocardiography in acute infarction predicts recovery of resting function and contractile reserve. J Am Coll Cardiol 41:827, 2003.
196. Shimoni S, Frangogiannis NG, Aggeli CJ, et al: Identification of hibernating myocardium with quantitative intravenous myocardial contrast echocardiography: Comparison with dobutamine echocardiography and thallium-201 scintigraphy. Circulation 107:538, 2003.
197. Angelini P, Velasco JA, Flamm S: Coronary anomalies: Incidence, pathophysiology, and clinical relevance. Circulation 105:2449, 2002.
198. Gradus-Pizlo I, Sawada SG, Wright D, et al: Detection of subclinical coronary atherosclerosis using two-dimensional, high-resolution transthoracic echocardiography. J Am Coll Cardiol 37:1422, 2001.
199. Watanabe N, Akasaka T, Yamaura Y, et al: Noninvasive detection of total occlusion of the left anterior descending coronary artery with transthoracic Doppler echocardiography. J Am Coll Cardiol 38:1328, 2001.

Disease of the Aorta

200. Erbel R, Engberding R, Daniel W, et al: Echocardiography in diagnosis of aortic dissection. Lancet 1:457, 1989.
201. Hashimoto S, Kumada T, Osakada G, et al: Assessment of transesophageal Doppler echography in dissecting aortic aneurysm. J Am Coll Cardiol 14:1253, 1989.
202. Ballal RS, Nanda NC, Gatewood R, et al: Usefulness of transesophageal echocardiography in assessment of aortic dissection. Circulation 84:1903, 1991.
203. Nienaber CA, von Kodolitsch Y, Nicolas V, et al: The diagnosis of thoracic aortic dissection by noninvasive imaging procedures. N Engl J Med 328:1, 1993.
204. Keane MG, Wiegers SE, Yang E, et al: Structural determinants of aortic regurgitation in type A dissection and the role of valvular resuspension as determined by intraoperative transesophageal echocardiography. Am J Cardiol 85:604, 2000.
205. Song JK, Kim HS, Kang DH, et al: Different clinical features of aortic intramural hematoma versus dissection involving the ascending aorta. J Am Coll Cardiol 37:1604, 2001.
206. Di Tullio MR, Sacco RL, Savoia MT, et al: Aortic atheroma morphology and the risk of ischemic stroke in a multiethnic population. Am Heart J 139:329, 2000.
207. Tunick PA, Kronzon I: Atheromas of the thoracic aorta: Clinical and therapeutic update. J Am Coll Cardiol 35:545, 2000.

Specific Clinical Applications

208. Sun JP, Asher CR, Yang XS, et al: Clinical and echocardiographic characteristics of papillary fibroelastomas: A retrospective and prospective study in 162 patients. Circulation 103:2687, 2001.
209. Labovitz AJ: Transesophageal echocardiography and unexplained cerebral ischemia: A multicenter follow-up study. The STEPS Investigators. Significance of Transesophageal Echocardiography in the Prevention of Recurrent Stroke. Am Heart J 137:1082, 1999.
210. McNamara RL, Lima JA, Whelton PK, et al: Echocardiographic identification of cardiovascular sources of emboli to guide clinical management of stroke: A cost-effectiveness analysis. Ann Intern Med 127:775, 1997.
211. Meissner I, Whisnant JP, Khandheria BK, et al: Prevalence of potential risk factors for stroke assessed by transesophageal echocardiography and carotid ultrasonography: The SPARC study. Stroke Prevention: Assessment of Risk in a Community. Mayo Clin Proc 74:862, 1999.
212. Homma S, Di Tullio MR, Sacco RL, et al: Characteristics of patent foramen ovale associated with cryptogenic stroke: A biplane transesophageal echocardiographic study. Stroke 25:582, 1994.
213. Steiner MM, Di Tullio MR, Rundek T, et al: Patent foramen ovale size and embolic brain imaging findings among patients with ischemic stroke. Stroke 29:944, 1998.
214. Klein AL, Grimm RA, Black IW, et al: Cardioversion guided by transesophageal echocardiography: The ACUTE Pilot Study. A randomized, controlled trial. Assessment of Cardioversion Using Transesophageal Echocardiography. Ann Intern Med 126:200, 1997.
215. Silverman DI, Manning WJ: Role of echocardiography in patients undergoing elective cardioversion of atrial fibrillation. Circulation 98:479, 1998.
216. Klein AL, Murray RD, Grimm RA: Role of transesophageal echocardiography-guided cardioversion of patients with atrial fibrillation. J Am Coll Cardiol 37:691, 2001.
217. Grifoni S, Olivotto I, Cecchini P, et al: Short-term clinical outcome of patients with acute pulmonary embolism, normal blood pressure, and echocardiographic right ventricular dysfunction. Circulation 101:2817, 2000.
218. Ribeiro A, Lindmarker P, Johnsson H, et al: Pulmonary embolism: One-year follow-up with echocardiography Doppler and five-year survival analysis. Circulation 99:1325, 1999.
219. Miniati M, Monti S, Pratali L, et al: Value of transthoracic echocardiography in the diagnosis of pulmonary embolism: Results of a prospective study in unselected patients. Am J Med 110:528, 2001.
220. Bossone E, Duong-Wagner TH, Paciocco G, et al: Echocardiographic features of primary pulmonary hypertension. J Am Soc Echocardiogr 12:655, 1999.
221. Raymond RJ, Hinderliter AL, Willis PW, et al: Echocardiographic predictors of adverse outcomes in primary pulmonary hypertension. J Am Coll Cardiol 39:1214, 2002.
222. Bossone E, Rubenfire M, Bach DS, et al: Range of tricuspid regurgitation velocity at rest and during exercise in normal adult men: Implications for the diagnosis of pulmonary hypertension. J Am Coll Cardiol 33:1662, 1999.
223. Ewert P, Berger F, Daehnert I, et al: Diagnostic catheterization and balloon sizing of atrial septal defects by echocardiographic guidance without fluoroscopy. Echocardiography 17:159, 2000.
224. Cooke J, Gelman J, Harper R: Echocardiologists' role in the deployment of the Amplatzer atrial septal occluder device in adults. J Am Soc Echocardiogr 14:588, 2001.

Use of Echocardiography

Jointly, the American College of Cardiology and the American Heart Association (ACC/AHA) published guidelines for the use of echocardiography in 1997,[1] and, in collaboration with several other professional societies, issued recommendations regarding standards of clinical competence in 2003.[2] Recommendations regarding the use of echocardiography are also included in guidelines for specific clinical syndromes, such as management of heart failure (see Chap. 24), valvular heart disease (see Chap. 57), and suspected endocarditis (see Chap. 58). These recommendations are included in appendices for chapters devoted to those syndromes.

The 1997 guidelines provide recommendations for the use of echocardiography in various clinical settings, using the standard three-class system of ACC/AHA guidelines. The guidelines specify situations in which echocardiography is considered likely or unlikely to contribute information that improves the management of patients. They also make recommendations on the frequency with which Doppler echocardiography should be repeated for some clinical issues. In general, the guidelines urge restraint in the use of echocardiography for patients whose initial evaluations indicated minimal or mild abnormalities, unless there is a change in clinical status.

Murmurs and Valvular Heart Disease

The ACC/AHA guidelines for use of echocardiography in patients with known or suspected valvular heart disease reflect the critical role of this test in assessing cardiac structure and function (Table 11G–1). Accordingly, echocardiography is considered appropriate in any patient with cardiorespiratory symptoms and a heart murmur, and any asymptomatic patient with a murmur in whom there is a reasonable probability of structural heart disease. However, the guidelines also emphasize that echocardiography is not a substitute for a careful clinical evaluation. The guidelines repeatedly state that this test is not appropriate in patients with murmurs or other clinical findings that an experienced observer identifies as functional or innocent. Serial or follow-up testing is discouraged in the absence of any change in symptoms or signs.

For patients with known or suspected valvular stenosis, the guidelines support the use of echocardiography for assessing severity of valvular stenosis and ventricular dysfunction. Reevaluation with echocardiography is considered appropriate with changing symptoms or signs, and also for patients with severe valvular stenosis even if asymptomatic. Pregnancy in a patient with valvular stenosis is considered a sufficient change in clinical status to justify echocardiographic evaluation.

Doppler echocardiography is the test of choice to evaluate valvular regurgitation and assess the need for surgical intervention. Because left ventricular dysfunction is such a critical issue in the management of such patients, serial use of echocardiography is appropriate in asymptomatic patients with severe regurgitation or with left ventricular dilatation, as well as in those with changes in symptoms or signs or who have become pregnant. The guidelines were less supportive of routine serial echocardiography for patients with mild to moderate valvular regurgitation without chamber dilatation or clinical symptoms.

The guidelines emphasize that diagnosis of mitral valve prolapse should be made on the basis of the physical examination, in part due to the high rates of false-positive results with echocardiography. Specifically discouraged is the use of echocardiography to exclude mitral valve prolapse in patients with ill-defined symptoms but no other clinical evidence for this condition.

Echocardiography is strongly supported in virtually all patients with known or suspected infective endocarditis. (ACC/AHA guidelines on the use of echocardiography in this setting are discussed in the Guidelines in Chap. 58). Similarly, the guidelines support the use of echocardiography before and after operative interventions for valvular heart disease. The incremental value of transesophageal echocardiography over transthoracic echocardiography is acknowledged for several clinical issues related to patients for whom procedures are contemplated or have been performed. Specific recommendations about the ideal interval for repeat evaluations in patients without changes in symptoms or signs are not made.

Chest Pain and Ischemic Heart Disease

Ischemic heart disease and other cardiac conditions (e.g., pericarditis and acute aortic dissection) are major diagnostic considerations in the evaluation of acute chest pain; accordingly, the ACC/AHA guidelines support the use of echocardiography when routinely available clinical data, including the electrocardiogram, are not diagnostic and in patients with suspected aortic dissection or severe hemodynamic instability (Table 11G–2). This test was not considered necessary for routine use in patients with a high likelihood of myocardial ischemia or infarction.

For patients with suspected acute myocardial ischemic syndromes, echocardiography is considered an appropriate tool for detection of ischemia or injury when other data are not conclusive; for evaluations of left and right ventricular function; and for detection of mechanical complications such as ruptured papillary muscles or a mural thrombus. Once the diagnosis of acute ischemic heart disease is established, the ACC/AHA guidelines support the use of echocardiography to assess the extent of myocardial injury and assess ventricular function, and to help assess prognosis as part of pharmacological or exercise stress testing. The guidelines were less certain but generally supportive of the use of echocardiography for assessment of the location and severity of disease in patients with ongoing ischemia, or for assessment of myocardial viability when patients were candidates for coronary revascularization (Class IIa).

For patients with chronic ischemic heart disease, the guidelines support echocardiography as appropriate for assessment of ventricular function and as a method for assessing myocardial viability and jeopardy through exercise or pharmacological stress testing. However, the guidelines explicitly state that echocardiography should not be routinely substituted "for treadmill exercise testing in patients for whom electrocardiographic (ECG) analysis is expected to suffice" (see Table 11G–2).

Cardiomyopathy and Assessment of Left Ventricular Function

Echocardiography is the ideal first test for assessment of global and regional left ventricular function and is therefore the preferred first-line test for patients with symptoms or signs consistent with left ventricular dysfunction (Table 11G–3). Transesophagealechocardiography (TEE) is recommended when transthoracic echocardiography (TTE) is not diagnostic. Echocardiography is also recommended for assessment of left ventricular hypertrophy, restrictive cardiomyopathy, and heart failure due to diastolic dysfunction. Use of this test is discouraged for routine evaluation of clinically stable patients in whom no change in management is contemplated and in patients with edema but normal venous pressures and no evidence of heart disease.

Pericardial Disease

Echocardiography remains the test of choice for detection of pericardial effusion, and an appropriate test for diagnosis of other pericardial disease (see Table 11G–3). The guidelines discourage the use of

TABLE 11G–1 ACC/AHA Guidelines for Use of Echocardiography in the Evaluation of Patients with Murmurs or Valvular Heart Disease

Indication	Class I (Indicated)	Class IIa (Good Supportive Evidence)	Class IIb (Weak Supportive Evidence)	Class III (Not Indicated)
Evaluation of heart murmurs	1. A murmur in a patient with cardiorespiratory symptoms. 2. A murmur in an asymptomatic patient if the clinical features indicate at least a moderate probability that the murmur is reflective of structural heart disease.	1. A murmur in an asymptomatic patient in whom there is a low probability of heart disease but in whom the diagnosis of heart disease cannot be reasonably excluded by the standard cardiovascular clinical evaluation.		1. In an adult, an asymptomatic heart murmur that has been identified by an experienced observer as functional or innocent.
Valvular stenosis	1. Diagnosis; assessment of hemodynamic severity. 2. Assessment of LV and RV size, function, and/or hemodynamics. 3. Reevaluation of patients with known valvular stenosis with changing symptoms or signs. 4. Assessment of changes in hemodynamic severity and ventricular compensation in patients with known valvular stenosis during pregnancy. 5. Reevaluation of asymptomatic patient with severe stenosis.	1. Assessment of the hemodynamic significance of mild to moderate valvular stenosis by stress Doppler echocardiography. 2. Reevaluation of patients with mild to moderate aortic stenosis with LV dysfunction or hypertrophy even without clinical symptoms.	1. Reevaluation of patients with mild to moderate aortic valvular stenosis with stable signs and symptoms.	1. Routine reevaluation of asymptomatic adult patients with mild aortic stenosis having stable physical signs and normal LV size and function. 2. Routine reevaluation of asymptomatic patients with mild to moderate mitral stenosis and stable physical signs.
Native valvular regurgitation	1. Diagnosis; assessment of hemodynamic severity. 2. Initial assessment and reevaluation (when indicated) of LV and RV size, function, and/or hemodynamics. 3. Reevaluation of patients with mild to moderate valvular regurgitation with changing symptoms. 4. Reevaluation of asymptomatic patient with severe regurgitation. 5. Assessment of changes in hemodynamic severity and ventricular compensation in patients with known valvular regurgitation during pregnancy. 6. Reevaluation of patients with mild to moderate regurgitation with ventricular dilation without clinical symptoms. 7. Assessment of the effects of medical therapy on the severity of regurgitation and ventricular compensation and function.		1. Reevaluation of patients with mild to moderate mitral regurgitation without chamber dilation and without clinical symptoms. 2. Reevaluation of patients with moderate aortic regurgitation without chamber dilation and without clinical symptoms.	1. Routine reevaluation in asymptomatic patients with mild valvular regurgitation having stable physical signs and normal LV size and function.
Mitral valve prolapse (MVP)	1. Diagnosis; assessment of hemodynamic severity, leaflet morphology, and/or ventricular compensation in patients with physical signs of MVP.	1. To exclude MVP in patients who have been diagnosed but without clinical evidence to support the diagnosis. 2. To exclude MVP in patients with first-degree relatives with known myxomatous valve disease. 3. Risk stratification in patients with physical signs of MVP or known MVP.		1. Exclusion of MVP in patients with ill-defined symptoms in the absence of a constellation of clinical symptoms or physical findings suggestive of MVP or a positive family history. 2. Routine repetition of echocardiography in patients with MVP with no or mild regurgitation and no changes in clinical signs or symptoms.

TABLE 11G–1 ACC/AHA Guidelines for Use of Echocardiography in the Evaluation of Patients with Murmurs or Valvular Heart Disease—cont'd

Indication	Class I (Indicated)	Class IIa (Good Supportive Evidence)	Class IIb (Weak Supportive Evidence)	Class III (Not Indicated)
Interventions for valvular heart disease and prosthetic valves	1. Assessment of the timing of valvular intervention based on ventricular compensation, function, and/or severity of primary and secondary lesions. 2. Selection of alternative therapies for mitral valve disease (such as balloon valvuloplasty, operative valve repair, valve replacement).* 3. Use of echocardiography (especially TEE) in performing interventional techniques (eg, balloon valvotomy) for valvular disease. 4. Postintervention baseline studies for valve function (early) and ventricular remodeling (late). 5. Reevaluation of patients with valve replacement with changing clinical signs and symptoms; suspected prosthetic dysfunction (stenosis, regurgitation) or thrombosis.*	1. Routine reevaluation study after baseline studies of patients with valve replacements with mild to moderate ventricular dysfunction without changing clinical signs or symptoms.	1. Routine reevaluation at the time of increased failure rate of a bioprosthesis without clinical evidence of prosthetic dysfunction.	1. Routine reevaluation of patients with valve replacement without suspicion of valvular dysfunction and unchanged clinical signs and symptoms. 2. Patients whose clinical status precludes therapeutic interventions.

*TEE may provide incremental value in addition to information obtained by TTE.
LV = left ventricular; MVP = mitral valve prolapse; RV = right ventricular; TEE = transesophageal echocardiography; TTE = transthoracic echocardiography.

TABLE 11G–2 ACC/AHA Guidelines for Use of Echocardiography in the Evaluation of Patients with Chest Pain and Known or Suspected Ischemic Heart Disease

Indication	Class I (Indicated)	Class IIa (Good Supportive Evidence)	Class IIb (Weak Supportive Evidence)	Class III (Not Indicated)
Patients with chest pain	1. Diagnosis of underlying cardiac disease in patients with chest pain and clinical evidence of valvular, pericardial, or primary myocardial disease. 2. Evaluation of chest pain in patients with suspected acute myocardial ischemia, when baseline ECG is nondiagnostic and when study can be obtained during pain or soon after its abatement. 3. Evaluation of chest pain in patients with suspected aortic dissection. 4. Chest pain in patients with severe hemodynamic instability.			1. Evaluation of chest pain for which a noncardiac cause is apparent. 2. Diagnosis of chest pain in a patient with electrocardiographic changes diagnostic of myocardial ischemia/infarction.
Diagnosis of acute myocardial ischemic syndromes	1. Diagnosis of suspected acute ischemia or infarction not evident by standard means. 2. Measurement of baseline LV function. 3. Patients with inferior myocardial infarction and bedside evidence suggesting possible RV infarction. 4. Assessment of mechanical complications and mural thrombus (TEE is indicated when TTE studies are not diagnostic).	1. Identification of location/severity of disease in patients with ongoing ischemia.		1. Diagnosis of acute myocardial infarction already evident by standard means.

TABLE 11G–2 ACC/AHA Guidelines for Use of Echocardiography in the Evaluation of Patients with Chest Pain and Known or Suspected Ischemic Heart Disease—cont'd

Indication	Class I (Indicated)	Class IIa (Good Supportive Evidence)	Class IIb (Weak Supportive Evidence)	Class III (Not Indicated)
Risk assessment, prognosis, and assessment of therapy in acute myocardial ischemic syndromes	1. Assessment of infarct size and/or extent of jeopardized myocardium 2. In-hospital assessment of ventricular function when the results are used to guide therapy. 3. In-hospital or early postdischarge assessment of the presence/extent of inducible ischemia whenever baseline abnormalities are expected to compromise electrocardiographic interpretation.*	1. In-hospital or early postdischarge assessment of the presence/extent of inducible ischemia in the absence of baseline abnormalities expected to compromise ECG interpretation.* 2. Assessment of myocardial viability when required to define potential efficacy of revascularization (dobutamine stress echocardiography). 3. Reevaluation of ventricular function during recovery when results are used to guide therapy. 4. Assessment of ventricular function after revascularization.	1. Assessment of long-term prognosis (≥2 years after acute myocardial infarction).	1. Routine reevaluation in the absence of any change in clinical status.
Diagnosis and prognosis of chronic ischemic heart disease	1. Diagnosis of myocardial ischemia in symptomatic individuals.* 2. Assessment of global ventricular function at rest. 3. Assessment of myocardial viability (hibernating myocardium) for planning revascularization. (dobutamine stress echocardiography) 4. Assessment of functional significance of coronary lesions (if not already known) in planning percutaneous transluminal coronary angioplasty.*		1. Diagnosis of myocardial ischemia in selected patients with an intermediate or high pretest likelihood of coronary artery disease.* 2. Assessment of an asymptomatic patient with positive results from a screening treadmill test. 3. Assessment of global ventricular function with exercise.*	1. Screening of asymptomatic persons with a low likelihood of coronary artery disease. 2. Routine periodic reassessment of stable patients for whom no change in therapy is contemplated. 3. Routine substitution for treadmill exercise testing in patients for whom ECG analysis is expected to suffice.
Assessment of interventions in chronic ischemic heart disease	1. Assessment of LV function when needed to guide institution and modification of drug therapy in patients with known or suspected LV dysfunction. 2. Assessment for restenosis after revascularization in patients with atypical recurrent symptoms.*	1. Assessment for restenosis after revascularization in patients with typical recurrent symptoms.*		1. Routine assessment of asymptomatic patients after revascularization.

*Exercise or pharmacological stress echocardiogram.
ECG = electrocardiogram; LV = left ventricular; RV = right ventricular; TEE = transesophageal echocardiography; TTE = transthoracic echocardiography.

echocardiography when findings are unlikely to change management and note that pericardial friction rubs are common after acute myocardial infarction and the early postoperative period after cardiac surgery, and echocardiography is not routinely needed in such settings. Echocardiographic assessment of pericardial thickness to assess the diagnosis of constrictive pericarditis is not supported by these guidelines, which note that other technologies (computed tomography or magnetic resonance imaging) provide more accurate data.

Cardiac Masses and Tumors

Echocardiography is also the first-line test for detection of cardiac masses and tumors and is therefore considered appropriate in patients with syndromes suggestive of such abnormalities (e.g., patients with arterial emboli of unknown origin or patients with auscultatory findings suggesting intermittent obstruction of intracardiac flow) (see Table 11G–3). Other candidates include patients with malignancies with a high incidence of cardiovascular involvement, such as hypernephroma, metastatic melanoma, or malignancies of intrathoracic organs.

Diseases of the Great Vessels

Transthoracic echocardiography is often adequate for detection of abnormalities of the aortic root and proximal pulmonary vasculature, but TEE is a far more sensitive tool for evaluation of most conditions affecting the great vessels. Therefore, TEE is the procedure of choice for evaluation of possible aortic dissection or rupture (see Table

TABLE 11G–3 ACC/AHA Guidelines for Use of Echocardiography in the Evaluation of Left Ventricular Function and Other Cardiovascular Anatomy

Indication	Class I (Indicated)	Class IIa (Good Supportive Evidence)	Class IIb (Weak Supportive Evidence)	Class III (Not Indicated)
Patients with dyspnea, edema, or cardiomyopathy	1. Assessment of LV size and function in patients with suspected cardiomyopathy or clinical diagnosis of heart failure.* 2. Edema with clinical signs of elevated central venous pressure when a potential cardiac cause is suspected or when central venous pressure cannot be estimated with confidence and clinical suspicion of heart disease is high.* 3. Dyspnea with clinical signs of heart disease. 4. Patients with unexplained hypotension, especially in the intensive care unit.* 5. Patients exposed to cardiotoxic agents, to determine the advisability of additional or increased dosages. 6. Reevaluation of LV function in patients with established cardiomyopathy when there has been a documented change in clinical status or to guide medical therapy.		1. Reevaluation of patients with established cardiomyopathy when there is no change in clinical status. 2. Reevaluation of patients with edema when a potential cardiac cause has already been demonstrated.	1. Evaluation of LV ejection fraction in patients with recent (contrast or radionuclide) angiographic determination of ejection fraction. 2. Routine reevaluation in clinically stable patients in whom no change in management is contemplated. 3. In patients with edema, normal venous pressure, and no evidence of heart disease.
Pericardial disease	1. Patients with suspected pericardial disease, including effusion, constriction, or effusive-constrictive process. 2. Patients with suspected bleeding in the pericardial space, e.g., trauma, perforation. 3. Follow-up study to evaluate recurrence of effusion or to diagnose early constriction. Repeat studies may be goal directed to answer a specific clinical question. 4. Pericardial friction rub developing in acute myocardial infarction accompanied by symptoms such as persistent pain, hypotension, and nausea.	1. Follow-up studies to detect early signs of tamponade in the presence of large or rapidly accumulating effusions. A goal-directed study may be appropriate. 2. Echocardiographic guidance and monitoring of pericardiocentesis.	1. Postsurgical pericardial disease, including postpericardiotomy syndrome, with potential for hemodynamic impairment. 2. In the presence of a strong clinical suspicion and nondiagnostic TTE, TEE assessment of pericardial thickness to support a diagnosis of constrictive pericarditis.	1. Routine follow-up of small pericardial effusion in clinically stable patients. 2. Follow-up studies in patients with cancer or other terminal illness for whom management would not be influenced by echocardiographic findings. 3. Assessment of pericardial thickness in patients without clinical evidence of constrictive pericarditis. 4. Pericardial friction rub in early uncomplicated myocardial infarction or early postoperative period after cardiac surgery.
Cardiac masses and tumors	1. Evaluation of patients with clinical syndromes and events suggesting an underlying cardiac mass. 2. Evaluation of patients with underlying cardiac disease known to predispose to mass formation for whom a therapeutic decision regarding surgery or anticoagulation will depend on the results of echocardiography. 3. Follow-up or surveillance studies after surgical removal of masses known to have a high likelihood of recurrence (i.e., myxoma). 4. Patients with known primary malignancies when echocardiographic surveillance for cardiac involvement is part of the disease staging process.		1. Screening persons with disease states likely to result in mass formation but for whom no clinical evidence for the mass exists.	1. Patients for whom the results of echocardiography will have no impact on diagnosis or clinical decision-making.

TABLE 11G–3 ACC/AHA Guidelines for Use of Echocardiography in the Evaluation of Left Ventricular Function and Other Cardiovascular Anatomy—cont'd

Indication	Class I (Indicated)	Class IIa (Good Supportive Evidence)	Class IIb (Weak Supportive Evidence)	Class III (Not Indicated)
Suspected thoracic aortic disease	TEE: 1. Aortic dissection. 2. Aortic aneurysm. 3. Aortic rupture. 4. Degenerative or traumatic aortic disease with clinical atheroembolism. 5. Follow-up of aortic dissection, especially after surgical repair when complications or progression is suspected. TTE: 1. Aortic aneurysm (especially for aortic root aneurysm). 2. Aortic root dilation in Marfan or other connective tissue syndromes. 3. Follow-up of aortic dissection, especially after surgical repair without suspicion of complication or progression. 4. First-degree relative of a patient with Marfan syndrome or other connective tissue disorder.			

LV = left ventricular; TEE = transesophageal echocardiography; TTE = transthoracic echocardiography.

11G–3). Because TTE is a less invasive and expensive procedure than TEE, it is recommended for follow-up of patients after repair of aortic dissection who do not have suspicion of complications or progression and of first-degree relatives of patients with Marfan syndrome or other connective tissue disorders.

Pulmonary Disease

Primary pulmonary disease often compromises the quality of TTE, but echocardiography can be an appropriate test for evaluation of the right ventricle and right-sided heart pressures that may be abnormal in patients with conditions such as pulmonary hypertension and pulmonary emboli (Table 11G–4). When other clinical data were not diagnostic, the ACC/AHA guidelines considered echocardiography appropriate for attempts to distinguish cardiac and noncardiac causes of dyspnea. However, echocardiography was not considered necessary for routine evaluation of patients with pulmonary disease or patients with pulmonary disease without changes in clinical status.

Systemic Hypertension

Use of echocardiography in patients with hypertension is supported by the ACC/AHA guidelines when the assessment of left ventricular function or hypertrophy is likely to influence management. An example of such a case would be a patient with mild hypertension in whom the detection of left ventricular hypertrophy would lead to initiation of drug therapy. The guidelines explicitly state that not every patient with hypertension should have a left ventricular function assessment and discourage serial echocardiograms to assess changes in left ventricular mass as patients are treated.

Neurological Disease and Other Cardioembolic Disease

The ACC/AHA guidelines support the use of echocardiography for evaluation of patients with embolic events affecting any major peripheral or visceral artery (see Table 11G–4). Echocardiography was considered clearly appropriate in patients with neurological events without evidence of cerebrovascular disease; its appropriateness in patients with neurological events and known intrinsic cerebrovascular disease was less clear (Class IIb). Echocardiography was discouraged when results would not influence management, such as in patients in whom anticoagulation was absolutely discouraged.

Arrhythmias and Palpitations

Because arrhythmias can be a manifestation of underlying structural heart disease, the ACC/AHA guidelines consider echocardiography appropriate in several subsets of patient with arrhythmias and palpitations (see Table 11G–4). However, echocardiography is discouraged in most patients with palpitations or isolated ventricular premature complexes if they do not have other evidence for structural or arrhythmic cardiac disease. The guidelines support the use of echocardiography as an adjunct to some advanced electrophysiological procedures.

The 1997 ACC/AHA guidelines support the use of TEE to assess risk of thromboembolic events in patients under atrial fibrillation if the need to proceed to cardioversion is urgent and an extended course of anticoagulation is not desirable (see Table 11G–4). There is also limited support for this strategy if the duration of atrial fibrillation is less than 48 hours. However, these guidelines were written before more recent research demonstrating the safety of using TEE to assess risk for thromboembolic events for patients undergoing elective cardioversion of atrial fibrillation of more than 48 hours' duration.[3] Therefore, future revisions of these guidelines can be expected to provide even more support for the use of TEE as an alternative to conventional management with several weeks of anticoagulation.

The ACC/AHA guidelines discourage the routine use of echocardiography for the evaluation of classic neurogenic syncope or for patients in whom there was no suspicion of cardiac disease (see Table 11G–4). Echocardiography is considered appropriate for patients with clinical evidence of cardiac disease or periexertional syncope. The guidelines are somewhat supportive of the use of echocardiography in patients with syncope who are in high-risk professions, such as airline pilots (Class IIa).

Text continued on page 270.

TABLE 11G–4 ACC/AHA Guidelines for Use of Echocardiography in the Evaluation of Other Clinical Syndromes

Indication	Class I (Indicated)	Class IIa (Good Supportive Evidence)	Class IIb (Weak Supportive Evidence)	Class III (Not Indicated)
Pulmonary disease	1. Suspected pulmonary hypertension. 2. Pulmonary emboli and suspected clots in the right atrium or ventricle or main pulmonary artery branches.* 3. For distinguishing cardiac versus noncardiac cause of dyspnea in patients in whom all clinical and laboratory clues are ambiguous.* 4. Follow-up of pulmonary artery pressures in patients with pulmonary hypertension to evaluate response to treatment. 5. Lung disease with clinical suspicion of cardiac involvement (suspected cor pulmonale).	1. Measurement of exercise pulmonary artery pressure. 2. Patients being considered for lung transplantation or other surgical procedure for advanced lung disease.*		1. Lung disease without any clinical suspicion of cardiac involvement. 2. Reevaluation studies of RV function in patients with chronic obstructive lung disease without a change in clinical status.
Hypertension	1. When assessment of resting LV function, hypertrophy, or concentric remodeling is important in clinical decision-making (see LV function). 2. Detection and assessment of functional significance of concomitant coronary artery disease (stress echocardiography). 3. Follow-up assessment of LV size and function in patients with LV dysfunction when there has been a documented change in clinical status or to guide medical therapy.	1. Identification of LV diastolic filling abnormalities with or without systolic abnormalities. 2. Assessment of LV hypertrophy in a patient with borderline hypertension without LV hypertrophy on ECG to guide decision-making regarding initiation of therapy. A limited goal-directed echocardiogram may be indicated for this purpose.	1. Risk stratification for prognosis by determination of LV performance.	1. Reevaluation to guide antihypertensive therapy based on LV mass regression. 2. Reevaluation in asymptomatic patients to assess LV function.
Neurological events or other vascular occlusive events	1. Patients of any age with abrupt occlusion of a major peripheral or visceral artery. 2. Younger patients (typically <45 years) with cerebrovascular events. 3. Older patients (typically >45 years) with neurological events without evidence of cerebrovascular disease or other obvious cause. 4. Patients for whom a clinical therapeutic decision (e.g., anticoagulation) will depend on the results of echocardiography.	1. Patients with suspicion of embolic disease and with cerebrovascular disease of questionable significance.	1. Patients with a neurological event and intrinsic cerebrovascular disease of a nature sufficient to cause the clinical event.	1. Patients for whom the results of echocardiography will not impact a decision to institute anticoagulant therapy or otherwise alter the approach to diagnosis or treatment.
Arrhythmias and palpitations	1. Arrhythmias with clinical suspicion of structural heart disease. 2. Arrhythmia in a patient with a family history of a genetically transmitted cardiac lesion associated with arrhythmia such as tuberous sclerosis, rhabdomyoma, or hypertrophic cardiomyopathy. 3. Evaluation of patients as a component of the work-up before electrophysiological ablative procedures.	1. Arrhythmia requiring treatment. 2. TEE guidance of transseptal catheterization and catheter placement during ablative procedures.	1. Arrhythmias commonly associated with, but without clinical evidence of, heart disease. 2. Evaluation of patients who have undergone radiofrequency ablation in the absence of complications. (In centers with established ablation programs, a postprocedural echocardiogram may not be necessary.)	1. Palpitation without corresponding arrhythmias or other cardiac signs or symptoms. 2. Isolated premature ventricular contractions for which there is no clinical suspicion of heart disease.
Before cardioversion	1. Evaluation of patient for whom a decision concerning cardioversion will be impacted by knowledge of prognostic factors (e.g., LV function, coexistent mitral valve disease).	1. Patients with atrial fibrillation of <48 hours duration and other heart disease (TEE only)	1. Patients with atrial fibrillation of <48 hours duration and no other heart disease (TEE only). 2. Patients with mitral valve disease or hypertrophic	1. Patients requiring emergent cardioversion. 2. Patients who have been on long-term anticoagulation at therapeutic levels and

Continued

TABLE 11G–4 ACC/AHA Guidelines for Use of Echocardiography in the Evaluation of Other Clinical Syndromes–cont'd

Indication	Class I (Indicated)	Class IIa (Good Supportive Evidence)	Class IIb (Weak Supportive Evidence)	Class III (Not Indicated)
	TEE only: 1. Patients requiring urgent (not emergent) cardioversion for whom extended precardioversion anticoagulation is not desirable.* 2. Patients who have had prior cardioembolic events thought to be related to intraatrial thrombus.* 3. Patients for whom anticoagulation is contraindicated and for whom a decision about cardioversion will be influenced by TEE results.* 4. Patients for whom intraatrial thrombus has been demonstrated in previous TEE.*		cardiomyopathy who have been on long-term anticoagulation at therapeutic levels before cardioversion (TEE only). 3. Patients undergoing cardioversion from atrial flutter.	who do not have mitral valve disease or hypertrophic cardiomyopathy before cardioversion. 3. Precardioversion evaluation of patients who have undergone previous TEE and with no clinical suspicion of a significant interval change.
Patients with syncope	1. Syncope in a patient with clinically suspected heart disease. 2. Periexertional syncope.	1. Syncope in a patient in a high-risk occupation (e.g., pilot).	1. Syncope of occult origin with no findings of heart disease on history or physical examination.	1. Recurrent syncope in a patient in whom previous echocardiographic or other testing demonstrated a cause of syncope. 2. Syncope in a patient for whom there is no clinical suspicion of heart disease. 3. Classic neurogenic syncope.
Screening	1. Patients with a family history of genetically transmitted cardiovascular disease. 2. Potential donors for cardiac transplantation. 3. Patients with phenotypic features of Marfan syndrome or related connective tissue diseases. 4. Baseline and reevaluations of patients undergoing chemotherapy with cardiotoxic agents.		1. Patients with systemic disease that may affect the heart.	1. The general population. 2. Competitive athletes without clinical evidence of heart disease.
Critically ill	1. The hemodynamically unstable patient 2. Suspected aortic dissection (TEE)			1. The hemodynamically stable patient not expected to have cardiac disease. 2. Reevaluation follow-up studies on hemodynamically stable patients.
Critically injured	1. Serious blunt or penetrating chest trauma (suspected pericardial effusion or tamponade). 2. Mechanically ventilated multiple-trauma or chest trauma patient. 3. Suspected preexisting valvular or myocardial disease in the trauma patient. 4. The hemodynamically unstable multiple-injury patient without obvious chest trauma but with a mechanism of injury suggesting potential cardiac or aortic injury (deceleration or crush). 5. Widening of the mediastinum, postinjury suspected aortic injury (TEE). 6. Potential catheter, guidewire, pacer electrode, or pericardiocentesis needle injury with or without signs of tamponade.	1. Evaluation of hemodynamics in multiple-trauma or chest trauma patients with pulmonary artery catheter monitoring and data disparate with clinical situation. 2. Follow-up study on victims of serious blunt or penetrating trauma.		1. Suspected myocardial contusion in the hemodynamically stable patient with a normal ECG.

TABLE 11G–4 ACC/AHA Guidelines for Use of Echocardiography in the Evaluation of Other Clinical Syndromes—cont'd

Indication	Class I (Indicated)	Class IIa (Good Supportive Evidence)	Class IIb (Weak Supportive Evidence)	Class III (Not Indicated)
Adult patient with congenital heart disease	1. Patients with clinically suspected congenital heart disease, as evidenced by signs and symptoms such as a murmur, cyanosis, or unexplained arterial desaturation, and an abnormal ECG or x-ray suggesting congenital heart disease. 2. Patients with known congenital heart disease on follow-up when there is a change in clinical findings. 3. Patients with known congenital heart disease for whom there is uncertainty as to the original diagnosis or when the precise nature of the structural abnormalities or hemodynamics is unclear. 4. Periodic echocardiograms in patients with known congenital heart lesions and for whom ventricular function and atrioventricular valve regurgitation must be followed (e.g., patients with a functionally single ventricle after Fontan procedure, transposition of the great vessels after Mustard procedure, L-transposition and ventricular inversion, and palliative shunts). 5. Patients with known congenital heart disease for whom following pulmonary artery pressure is important (e.g., patients with moderate or ventricular septal defects, atrial septal defects, single ventricle, or any of the above with an additional risk factor for pulmonary hypertension). 6. Periodic echocardiography in patients with surgically repaired (or palliated) congenital heart disease with the following: change in clinical condition or clinical suspicion of residual defects, LV or RV function that must be followed, or when there is a possibility of hemodynamic progression or a history of pulmonary hypertension. 7. To direct interventional catheter valvotomy, radiofrequency ablation valvotomy interventions in the presence of complex cardiac anatomy.		1. A follow-up Doppler echocardiographic study, annually or once every 2 years, in patients with known hemodynamically significant congenital heart disease without evident change in clinical condition.	1. Multiple repeat Doppler echocardiography in patients with repaired patent ductus arteriosus, atrial septal defect, ventricular septal defect, coarctation of the aorta, or bicuspid aortic valve without change in clinical condition. 2. Repeat Doppler echocardiography in patients with known hemodynamically insignificant congenital heart lesions (e.g., small atrial septal defect, small ventricular septal defect) without a change in clinical condition.

*TEE is indicated when TTE studies are not diagnostic.

ECG = electrocardiogram; LV = left ventricular; RV = right ventricular; TEE = transesophageal echocardiography; TTE = transthoracic echocardiography.

Screening

The ACC/AHA guidelines do not support using echocardiography to screen for heart disease in the general population or asymptomatic athletes (see Table 11G–4). Examples of settings in which screening echocardiography may be appropriate include those involving patients with a family history of genetically transmitted cardiovascular diseases, those involving potential donors for heart transplantation, and serial evaluation of patients receiving potentially cardiotoxic chemotherapy.

Critically Ill and Injured Patients

Echocardiography is often useful for establishing the diagnosis in hemodynamically unstable, critically ill and injured patients (see Table 11G–4). TEE is particularly useful if injury to the aorta or spontaneous dissection is suspected.

Adult Patients with Congenital Heart Disease

Echocardiography is useful for diagnosis of congenital heart disease in adults, and for follow-up of manifestations of disease such as ventricular function and hemodynamically significant shunts. The guidelines discourage the overuse of serial echocardiography in patients without changes in clinical status, particularly if they are known to have lesions of minor hemodynamic significance, such as small atrial or ventricular septal defects.

Standards for Clinical Competence

A joint statement on standards for Clinical Competency was issued in 2003 by the ACC/AHA and other professional societies. It described three levels of expertise and standards for the duration and depth of training. Level I training (3 months, 75 examinations performed, 150 examinations interpreted) constitutes the minimum amount of training that must be achieved by all trainees in adult cardiovascular medicine. Level II training (6 months, 150 cases performed, 300 cases interpreted) is the minimum training for physicians who perform and interpret echocardiograms independently. Level III training (12 months, 300 cases performed, 750 cases interpreted) is appropriate for physicians who direct echocardiography laboratories and supervise quality control systems for interpretation of tests. Different criteria are recommended for experienced echocardiographers who completed training before these guidelines were established.

For competence in TEE, trainees in cardiovascular medicine should perform at least 25 esophageal intubations with an echocardiographic probe and perform approximately 50 TEEs under the supervision of a level III trained echocardiographer. To maintain competence in TEE, the task force recommends a minimum of 25 to 50 cases per year.

References

1. Cheitlin MD, Alpert JS, Armstrong WF, et al: ACC/AHA guidelines for the clinical application of echocardiography: A report of the American College of Cardiology/American Heart Association Task Force on Practice Guidelines (Committee on Clinical Application of Echocardiography). Circulation 95:1686, 1997.
2. Douglas PS, Foster E, Gorcsan J, et al: ACC/AHA clinical competence statement on echocardiography: A report of the American College of Cardiology/American Heart Association/American College of Physicians-American Society of Internal Medicine Task Force on Clinical Competence (Committee on Echocardiography). J Am Coll Cardiol 41:687, 2003.
3. Klein AL, Grimm RA, Murray RD, et al: Use of transesophageal echocardiography to guide cardioversion in patients with atrial fibrillation. N Engl J Med 344:1411, 2001.

CHAPTER 12

The Chest Radiograph in Cardiovascular Disease

Michael A. Bettmann

The chest radiograph was one of the first types of x-ray films to be used clinically.[1] It remains the most common x-ray examination and one of the most difficult examinations to interpret. It contains a large amount of anatomical and physiological information, but it is difficult and sometimes even impossible to interpret objectively. There are major variations in information as a function of radiographic technique, body habitus, age, underlying physiological status, and training and focus of the interpreter. The aims of this chapter are to review the way chest radiographs are obtained, to present a basic approach to how to interpret them, and to discuss and illustrate common as well as characteristic findings that are relevant to cardiovascular disease.

Technical Considerations

The usual chest radiograph consists of a frontal and a lateral view. The frontal is a posteroanterior (PA) view, with the patient standing with the chest toward the film. The lateral is also taken with the patient standing, with the left side toward the film. For both, the x-ray tube is kept at a distance of 6 feet from the film. The rationale for these conventions is based on simple physics. X-rays are created by first inducing a high current across a diode, thereby generating electrons. These electrons are aimed at a metal target, the rotating anode, which gives off the x-rays. The x-rays are allowed to emerge only through a small opening in the tube, the focal spot. The ability of the x-rays to penetrate structures is determined by the combination of kilovoltage, milliamperage, and time used to produce them. These factors also determine the exposure to the patient.[2,3]

In theory, x-rays emerge from the x-ray tube as a point source, remain parallel, and do not diverge from each other, and there is no geometrical distortion of structures as they pass through the body and are recorded on film. In practice, the x-rays diverge from the focal spot and are not parallel. As a result, when they are captured on film there is geometrical distortion as a function of the distance from the midline of the x-ray beam and the distance of the structures from the film. The farther from the tube an object is, the more parallel are the x-rays that penetrate it. Conversely, the closer to the tube the object and the film are, the more the incident x-rays must diverge to cover the edges of the object. Thus, the farther an object is from the source, the less geometrical distortion is encountered. The greater the distance from the source, however, the more energy must be applied to penetrate the object to be imaged and expose the x-ray film. That is, in simple terms, resolution is improved by increasing the source-image distance (SID) but tube energy and thus exposure to the patient must also be increased with increasing SID. As a result, a standard convention has been developed: standard chest radiographs are obtained with an SID of 6 feet. X-rays are blocked from the film to varying degrees by various structures, leading to shades of gray that allow discrimination between the heart, which is fluid filled and is relatively impervious to x-rays, and the air-filled lung parenchyma, which blocks few x-rays.

Several practical observations result from the physics of chest radiographs. If patients are unable to stand, chest radiographs are not generally obtained with the chest toward the film (PA). With the standard PA view, the heart appears smaller and its size and contour are more accurately depicted than on a portable film, which is usually an anteroposterior (AP) view (i.e., the tube is in front of the patient and the film is behind) with resultant greater divergence of x-rays because the heart lies relatively anteriorly and the SID is short. Similarly, on a standard lateral film, the right ribs appear larger than the left (Fig. 12–1). In both cases, this effect occurs because a structure is further from the film. As a result, there is increased divergence of the x-rays from the midline point source, and relative magnification. The side of an effusion, therefore, can generally be delineated on a lateral radiograph.

There are several inherent practical limitations to portable chest radiographs. Most are obtained with patients positioned either supine or semisupine. The degree of inspiration is therefore likely to be substantially less than with an erect film. Further, portable radiographs are invariably taken as AP views and the SID is less than 6 feet, of necessity, because of the nature of the portable x-ray machine and also because of the usual position of the patient, sitting or lying in a bed. Most portable x-ray units are not able to generate sufficient energy to penetrate a patient adequately and expose the film from 6 feet. Space constraints and the patient's position are additional hurdles. Also, because exposure time must usually be longer than with fixed units, edge definition is compromised. For all these reasons, the inherent resolution is poorer with portable radiographs, and the accuracy is limited. Because of the lower available kilovoltage with portable x-ray units and the longer exposure time that is necessary, radiation exposure to the patient is also greater than with a standard PA film. Portable films are most useful for answering relatively simple questions, such as whether the pacemaker or implantable cardioverter-defibrillator (ICD) is properly positioned, whether the endotracheal tube is in the correct location, and whether the mediastinum is midline (Fig. 12–2).[2,4,5]

Other questions cannot be answered accurately from a portable chest x-ray film. If the film is obtained with the patient in a less than upright position, it is impossible to exclude even a sizable pneumothorax or pleural effusion. Because of the patient's

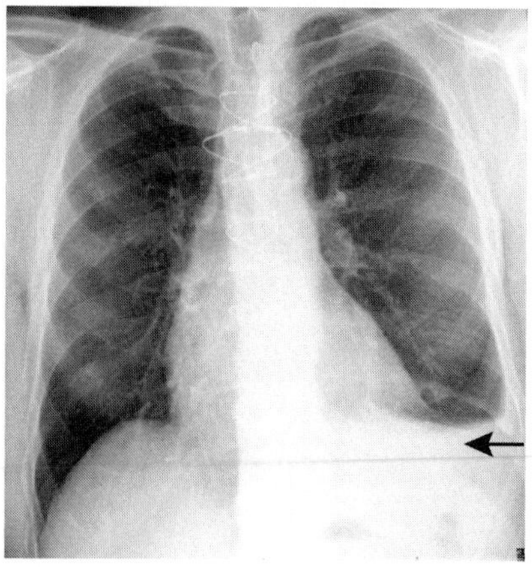

A

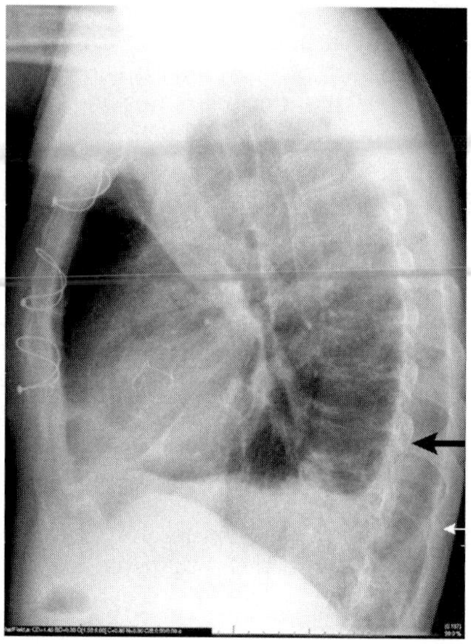

B

FIGURE 12–1 Standard upright chest radiographs of a 74-year-old man who has undergone aortic valve replacement. **A,** Posteroanterior view shows median sternotomy wires, a left pleural effusion (arrow), and normal pulmonary vascular pattern. **B,** Lateral view. Note that the right ribs (small arrow) are magnified compared with the left (large arrow), and the effusion can be localized to the left.

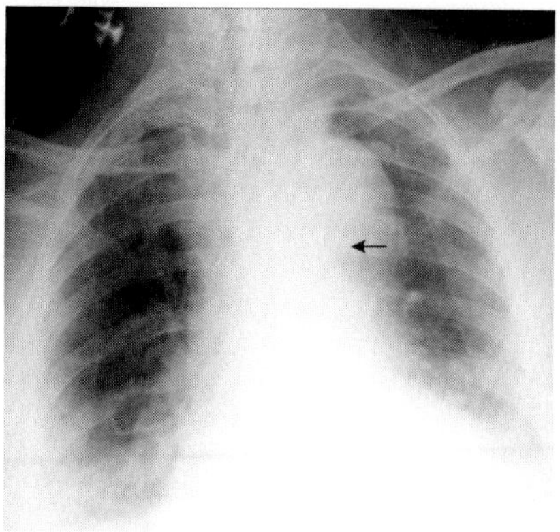

A

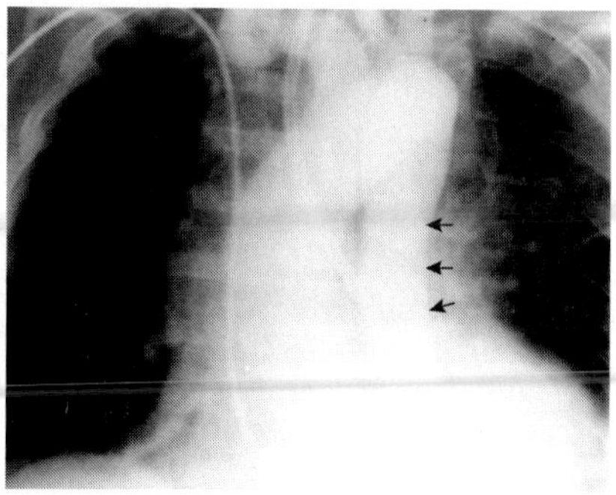

B

FIGURE 12–2 **A,** Portable chest radiograph of a 70-year-old man with spontaneous dissection of the thoracic aorta. Portable frontal view cannot accurately demonstrate heart size or pulmonary vascularity but shows a double density (arrow) at the level of the descending aorta. Note also widened superior mediastinum, with nasogastic tube deviated toward the right. **B,** Levo phase of a right-heart angiogram shows an evident Stanford type B dissection, with a flap (arrows) beginning at the level of the left subclavian artery, and filling of the true (but not the false) lumen of the descending aorta.

position, conventional SID, and the limited tube output, it is impossible to evaluate heart size and contour or status of pulmonary vascularity. It may be possible to say that there is or is not acute pulmonary edema, but it is not possible to judge whether or not there is cardiomegaly, mild to moderate congestive heart failure, or the presence or absence of a small infiltrate.

Digital Imaging

Chest radiographs have generally been recorded on high-resolution x-ray film. With optimal technique and a cooperative patient who can hold a deep inspiration, the result is a study that clearly and accurately depicts very small structures, such as the contour of small pulmonary arteries. With the advent of digital radiography (DR), a filmless form of radiography, chest radiographs are increasingly stored on digital media. There are two principal ways to do this. The first is computed radiography (CR), which is widely available. It is essentially a digital conversion of conventionally obtained chest radiographs. The second method, DR, is the direct recording of images by digital means, without conversion of analog to digital information. There is, then, an inherent difference, with the elimination of added noise and lost information that occurs with this conversion. CR is accomplished with a reusable plate to record the images, which are then converted to a digital format. True DR can be accomplished in many ways. The most promising is "flat plate" technology, for reasons of resolution, utility, and (in the long term) cost. It involves the use of an image-sensing plate that directly converts the incident photons into a digital signal rather than producing a transient conversion as with an image intensifier, producing a reusable CR plate, or altering a silver iodide crystal in a film emulsion, as in standard film radiography. DR is truly "filmless"; CR can be either, and the classic chest radiograph relies on film that is exposed and developed.[6-11]

Resolution with DR may be marginally decreased because the pixel size is larger than that of the silver iodide crystals in the emulsion on x-ray film.[6,9,11] Such a decrease, however, is generally below the ability of the eye to detect. At this time, DR equipment is more costly than either standard radiographic rooms or CR rooms. Both DR and CR have significant advantages for several reasons. First, with the widespread adoption of picture archiving and communication systems (PACSs), films that are obtained digitally or are directly converted to digital format are immediately available for review at any location where there is a PACS-enabled workstation. This system obviates the problem of lost films (all films are digitally archived) and the need to go to a remote location to review a film.[12,13] Also, each film is available for review immediately after it is obtained and stored. In addition, the exposure dose is generally lower, and the need to repeat films because of inadequacy is limited if not eliminated. There is less need to repeat films because of the inherent ability to manipulate the image after it is obtained; the relative density (window and level), magnification, and even area included can be altered without reexposure. Most PACSs now utilize the Internet for gaining access to images, further simplifying availability.

There are several additional basic considerations. The first is radiation exposure. The radiation necessary for PA and lateral chest films is usually minimal in terms of radiation effects, regarding both the dose of a single study and the cumulative dose of repeated chest x-ray studies. Radiation dose is always a consideration in the pediatric age group, however, for obvious reasons.[2] It is also a consideration in patients who undergo interventional cardiology procedures.[3-5] Excluding oncological radiology, the majority of recently reported cases of radiation skin damage have occurred in patients who have undergone repeated prolonged interventional procedures. In this setting, it is important to be alert to any additional radiation exposure. Consequently, each extra chest film should be ordered with care. DR is important in this regard, because it generally provides a lower radiation dose to the patient.

The Normal Chest Radiograph

Reading standard PA and lateral chest radiographs is a daunting task. The amount of information present is huge, and there are countless relevant variables. It is imperative to have a systematic approach, based on an assessment first of anatomy and then of physiology. This approach, of course, is based on an understanding of what is normal.[14,15]

In the standard PA chest study, the overall heart diameter is normally less than half the transverse diameter of the thorax (Fig. 12–3). The heart overlies the thoracic spine, roughly three-fourths to the left of the spine and one-fourth to the right. The mediastinum is narrow superiorly, and normally the descending aorta can be defined from the arch to the dome of the diaphragm, on the left. Below the aortic arch, the pulmonary hila are seen, slightly higher on the left than the right. On the lateral film (Fig. 12–4), the left main pulmonary artery can be seen coursing superiorly and posteriorly compared with the right. On both frontal and lateral views, the ascending aorta (aortic root) is normally obscured by the main pulmonary artery and both atria. The location of the pulmonary outflow tract is usually clear on the lateral film.

Cardiac Chambers and Aorta

On the normal chest film, it is not usually possible to define individual cardiac chambers. It is imperative, however, both to know their normal position and to examine the film to determine whether the size and location of each are within the normal range. On the PA view, the right contour of the mediastinum contains the right atrium but also the ascending aorta and the superior vena cava. The right ventricle, as is clear on echocardiography, is located partially overlying the left ventricle on both frontal and lateral views.[16] The left atrium is located just inferior to the left pulmonary hilum. In normal persons, there is a concavity at this level, the location of the left atrial appendage. The atrium constitutes the upper portion of the posterior contour of the heart on the lateral film but cannot be separated from the left ventricle. The left ventricle constitutes the prominent, rounded apex of the heart on the frontal view as well as the sloping inferior portion of the mediastinum on the lateral (see Fig. 12–4B).

The apex is often not clearly delineated for a reason related to x-ray attenuation. The heart is evident and distinguishable from the lungs because it contains water-density blood rather than air. Because blood attenuates x-rays to a greater extent than air, the heart appears relatively white (less so than bones) and the lungs relatively black (less so than the edges of the film where there is no interposed tissue). A fat pad of varying thickness surrounds the apex of the heart (Fig. 12–5). Fat has a density greater than that of air and marginally less than that of blood. As it covers the ventricular apex, the fat pad is relatively thick and dense. As it thins out toward the left lateral chest wall, it is progressively less dense—hence the hazy, poorly marginated appearance of the apex. Similarly, a fat pad may be seen on the lateral chest film as a wedge-shaped density overlying the anterior aspect of the left ventricle. The pericardial sac cannot normally be defined (Fig. 12–6). The borders of the cardiac silhouette are normally moderately but not completely sharp in contour. Even though the exposure time for a chest x-ray is very short (less than 100 milliseconds), there is usually sufficient cardiac motion to cause minor haziness of the silhouette. If a portion of the heart border does not move, as in the case of a left ventricular aneurysm, the border is unusually sharp (Fig. 12–7). The aortic arch, however, is usually visible, as the aorta courses posteriorly and is surrounded by air. Most of the descending aorta is also visible. The position and the size of each can be easily evaluated (Fig. 12–8) using the frontal and lateral views.

Lungs and Pulmonary Vasculature

Lung size varies as a function of inspiratory effort, age, body habitus, water content, and intrinsic pathological processes. For example, because lung distensibility decreases with age, the lungs appear subtly but progressively smaller with advancing age, even with maximal inspiratory effort. Also, with increasing left ventricular dysfunction, the interstitial fluid in the lungs increases and lung expansion decreases. On the other hand, the lungs appear both larger and blacker in the presence of chronic obstructive lung disease with bulla formation (Fig. 12–9). As lung expansion decreases, the heart appears relatively slightly larger even though it does not

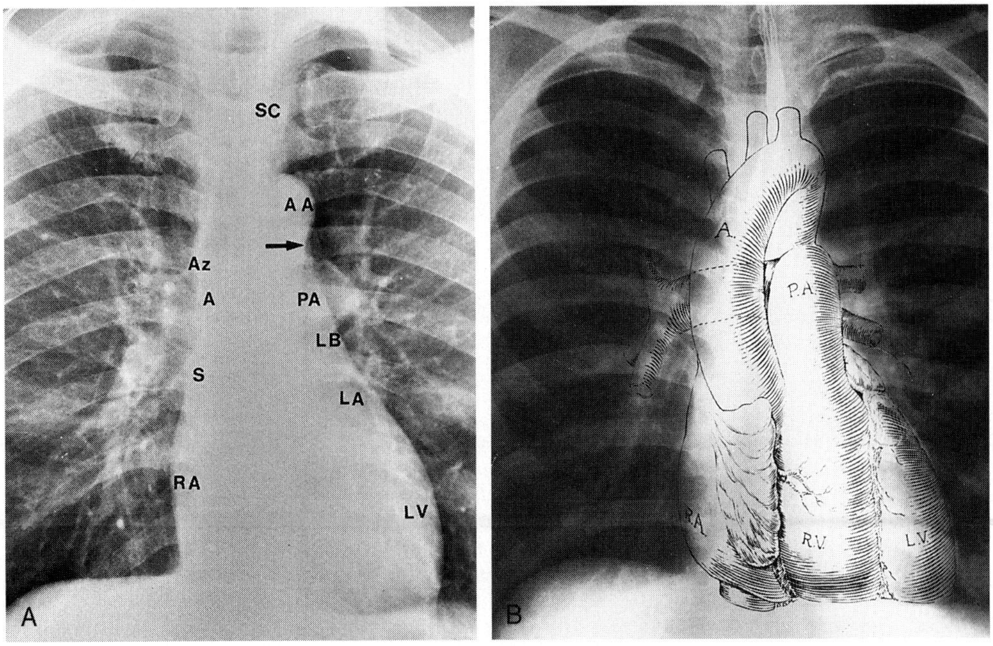

FIGURE 12–3 Frontal projection of the heart and great vessels. **A,** Left and right heart borders in the frontal projection. **B,** A line drawing in the frontal projection demonstrates the relationship of the cardiac valves, rings, and sulci to the mediastinal borders. A = ascending aorta; AA = aortic arch; Az = azygous vein; LA = left atrial appendage; LB = left lower border of pulmonary artery; LV = left ventricle; PA = main pulmonary artery; RA = right atrium; S = superior vena cava; SC = subclavian artery.

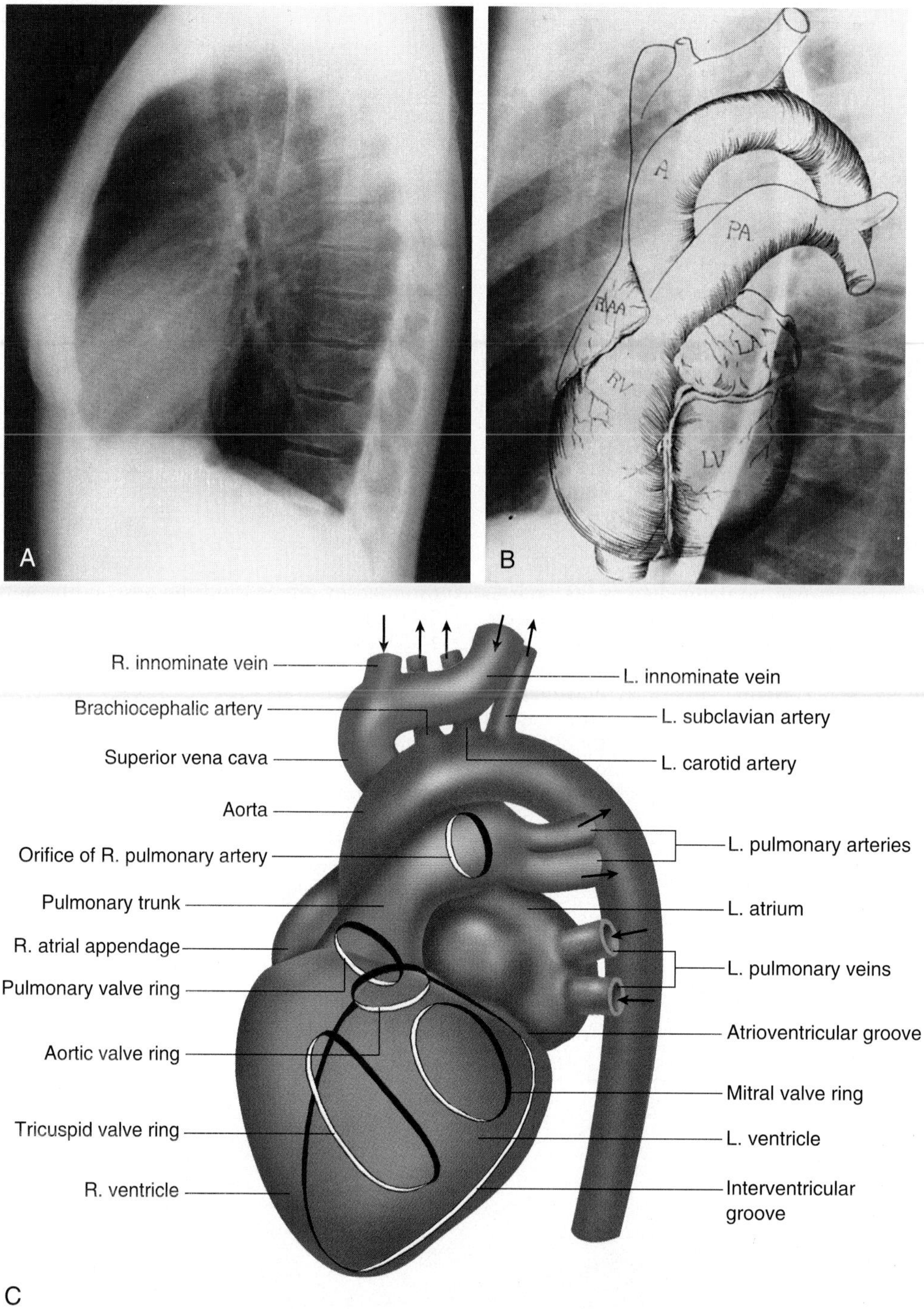

FIGURE 12–4 **A,** Lateral chest radiograph. **B,** Superimposed anatomical drawing of the cardiac chambers and great vessels. **C,** Diagram of the lateral projection of the heart showing the position of the cardiac chambers, valve rings, and sulci. Arrows indicate direction of blood flow.

change in size. However, the heart does not exceed half the transverse diameter of the chest in a good-quality PA film unless there is true cardiomegaly. It is important to keep in mind that evident enlargement may be due to enlargement of the heart overall, to dilation of one or more chambers, or to pericardial fluid (Fig. 12–10). In patients with chronic obstructive pulmonary disease, the heart often appears small or normal in size even in the presence of cardiac dysfunction (see Fig. 12–9).

In normal subjects, pulmonary vascularity has a predictable pattern.[17] Pulmonary arteries are usually easily visible centrally in the hila and progressively less so more peripherally. The central main right and left pulmonary arteries are usually not individually identifiable, as they lie within the mediastinum (see Figs. 12–3 and 12–4). If the lung is thought of in three zones, the major arteries are central, the clearly distinguishable small arteries in the middle zone, and the small arteries and arterioles that are normally below the limit of resolution in the outer zone. The visible small arteries have sharp, easily defined margins. As noted earlier, this is because of the sharp border between water-density and air-density structures. In the standard, standing frontal view, the arteries in the lower zone are larger than those in the upper zone, at an equal distance from the hila. This

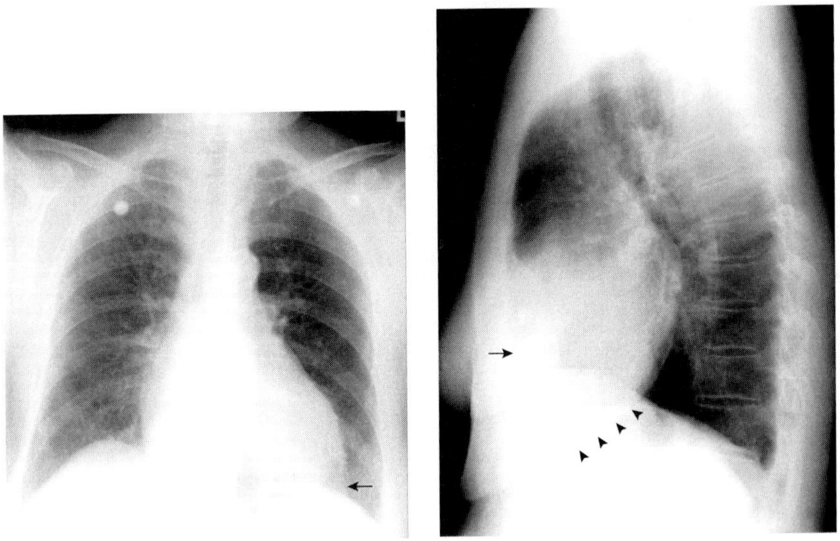

FIGURE 12–5 Chest radiographs of a 70-year-old woman with rheumatic heart disease and combined aortic stenosis and mitral stenosis. Her pulmonary capillary wedge pressure is 30 mm Hg. **A,** Posteroanterior view. There is evidence of chronically elevated pulmonary venous pressures with moderate (not marked) pulmonary vascular redistribution. There is moderate left ventricular enlargement and prominence of the left atrial appendage. **B,** Lateral view. Note enlargement of the left ventricle, extending below the diaphragm and compressing the gastric bubble (arrowheads).

Also note the apical fat pad, seen as the hazy density on the frontal view (**A,** arrow), and the anterior, retrosternal, well-delineated, wedge-shaped density on the lateral view (**B,** arrow).

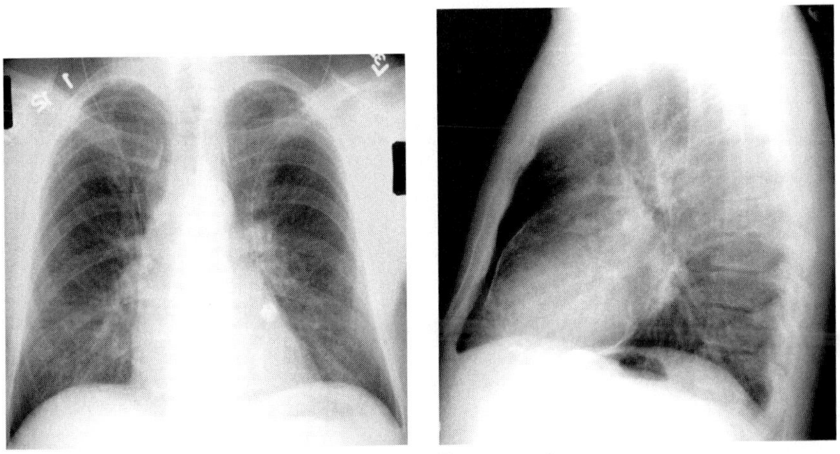

FIGURE 12–6 Chest radiographs of a 45-year-old man with calcific pericarditis. **A,** Posteroanterior view is essentially normal. **B,** Lateral view demonstrates thin, irregular calcification of pericardium around the left ventricular contour.

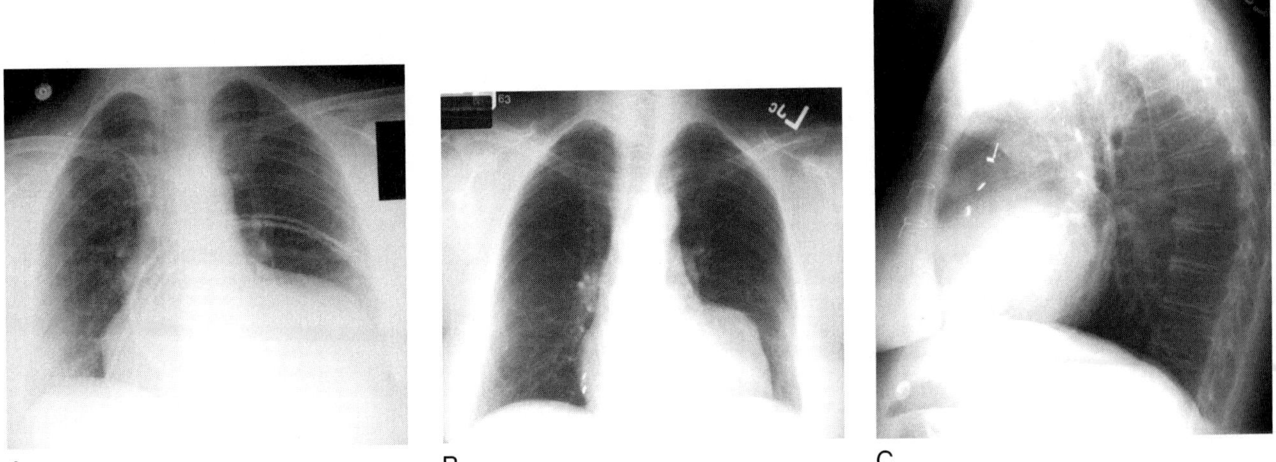

FIGURE 12–7 Chest radiographs of a 53-year-old woman with coronary artery disease and heart failure following a large anterolateral myocardial infarction. **A,** Frontal, portable view suggests cardiomegaly and heart failure. Sharp, horizontal contour of the left ventricle is suggestive of anterior wall aneurysm. **B** and **C,** Posteroanterior and lateral views after revascularization and aneurysmectomy demonstrate persistence of an abnormal contour of the left ventricle, consistent with recurrent aneurysm, and clips on side branches of saphenous vein graft to right coronary artery.

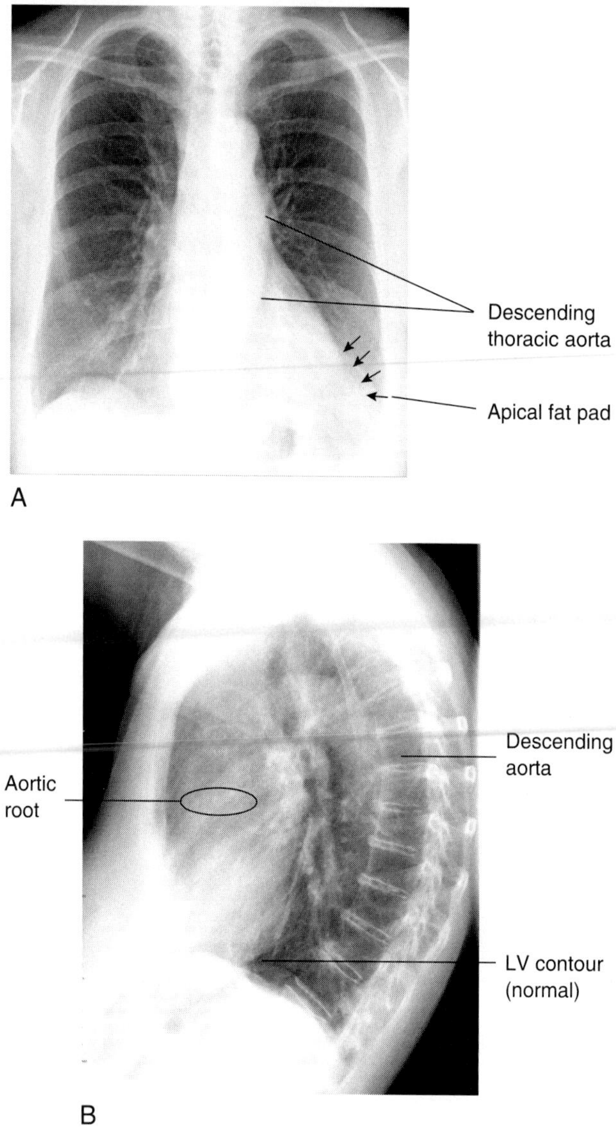

FIGURE 12–8 Chest radiographs of a 67-year-old woman with aortic stenosis. **A,** The posteroanterior view shows a normal cardiac size and pulmonary vascular pattern and enlargement of the aortic root. Note also prominence of the apical fat pad (arrows) on the left and no real cardiomegaly. Note also moderate pectus excavatum (causing blurring of the right heart border). **B,** The lateral view shows normal pulmonary vasculature and enlargement of the aortic root. There is moderate pectus excavatum. There is no visible aortic valve calcification or left ventricular enlargement.

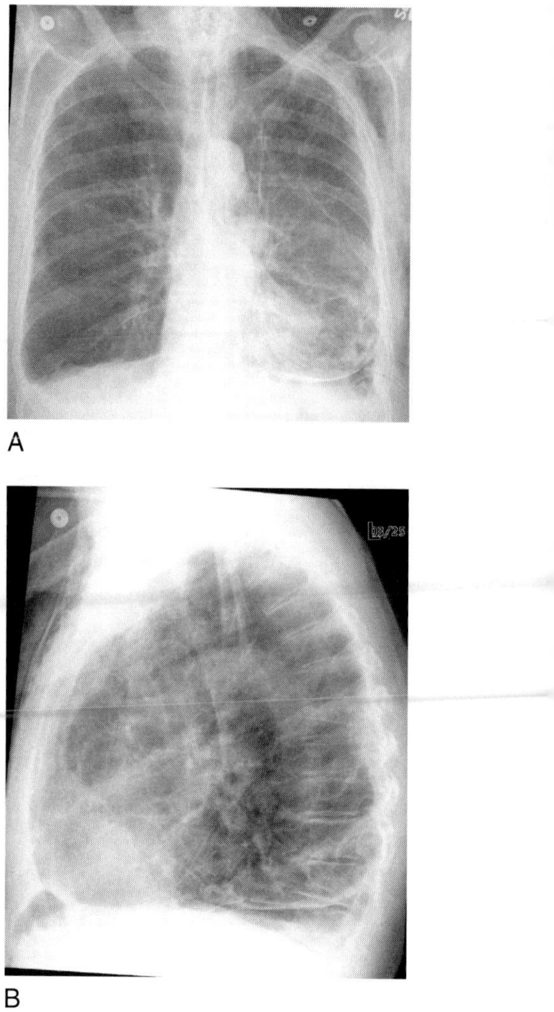

FIGURE 12–9 Patient with severe bullous chronic obstructive lung disease (COPD), spontaneous pneumothorax, and subcutaneous emphysema. Posteroanterior **(A)** and lateral **(B)** views of the chest show loculation of the left-sided pneumothorax to the inferior lateral region because of bullae and fibrosis. Note small cardiac silhouette, secondary to severe COPD.

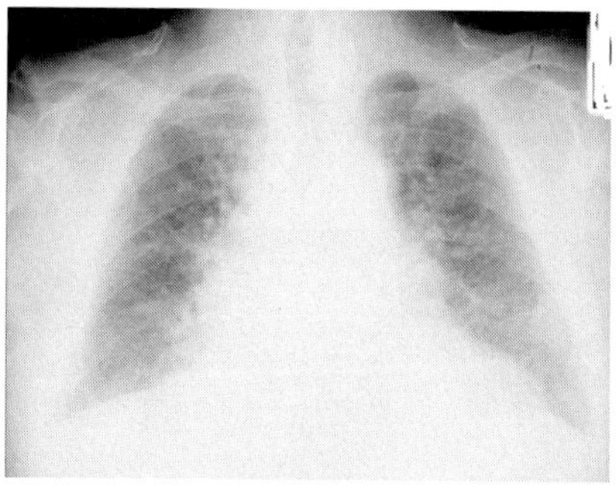

FIGURE 12–10 Chest film of a 63-year-old man with end-stage renal disease. There is marked enlargement of the cardiac silhouette secondary to pericardial effusion associated with renal failure. Note also marked pulmonary vascular redistribution.

appearance is related to the effect of gravity on the normal, low-pressure lung circulation. That is, gravity leads to slightly greater intravascular volume at the lung bases than in the upper zones. This effect is also seen in a normal perfusion lung scan. Because the radionuclide is generally administered with the patient supine, there is a greater concentration posteriorly than anteriorly, as confirmed in the count rates. If the patient is sitting or standing when the radionuclide is injected, the count rate is greater at the lung base than at the apices.

The angles that the lungs make with the diaphragm are normally very sharp and can be delineated bilaterally on both frontal and lateral views. The pleura is usually tightly applied, not separated from the ribs on the PA or lateral view. The contour that the inferior vena cava (IVC) makes with the heart is clearly seen on the lateral film (see Fig. 12–1B). Its relationship to the cardiac contour varies markedly, depending on minor degrees of rotation of the patient. That is, the IVC lies on the right of the mediastinum and posterior to the contour of the heart. This contour is made up of the left atrium and ventricle, which lie toward the left side of the thorax. If the patient is placed laterally with the left side against the film, the right is relatively slightly magnified compared with the left (see Fig. 12–1B). If the patient rotates minimally anterior or posterior to true lateral, the relationship between the IVC and the left-sided contours changes substantially. This change is worth noting, as in the past a formula has been employed (using the "Riegler sign") to determine left ventricular enlargement as a function of its relationship to the IVC.[18] This sign, although sometimes still used, is not accurate and should not be used.[19,20]

Normal Variations

Anatomical variables and aging present challenges in the evaluation of chest radiographs in addition to those posed by decreased lung compliance. The aorta and great vessels normally dilate and become more tortuous and prominent with increasing age, leading to widening of the superior mediastinum. As noted, the heart appears larger because of decreasing lung compliance, although unless there is true cardiac disease it is less than half the transverse diameter of the chest on a PA view. There are additional important anatomical considerations. Patients who are obese are likely to have a degree of inhibition of maximal lung expansion that may make a normal heart appear slightly larger. Patients with pectus excavatum have a narrowed AP diameter of the chest, increasing the transverse diameter (Fig. 12–11; see Fig. 12–8). Consequently, the heart may appear enlarged on the frontal view but the narrow AP diameter seen on the lateral view explains this. There may also be lack of definition of the right heart border on the frontal view because of compression by the sternum. Marked kyphosis or scoliosis can also cause the heart or mediastinum to look abnormal. It is thus important to examine the spine and other bone structures systematically when looking at a chest radiograph. Delineation of all anatomical abnormalities is beyond the scope of this chapter. For an in-depth discussion, *Fraser and Pare's Diagnosis of Diseases of the Chest*[21] is a useful reference.

Evaluating the Chest Radiograph in Heart Disease

Cardiovascular disease states cause various and complex changes in the appearance of the chest radiograph. Overall cardiomegaly can be judged with reasonable accuracy on the frontal view by noting whether or not the diameter of the heart exceeds half the diameter of the thorax. Cardiomegaly is probably most often seen as a result of ischemic cardiomyopathy following one or more myocardial infarctions (Fig. 12–12). Cardiomegaly is a common finding but a nonspecific one (Fig. 12–13; see Fig. 12–10).[22-26] A systematic approach to the evaluation of a chest radiograph is imperative, to distinguish normal from abnormal and to define the underlying pathology and pathophysiology. The first step is to decide what type of film is being evaluated—PA and lateral, PA alone, or AP (either portable or one obtained in the AP view because the patient is unable to stand). The next step is to determine whether prior films are available for comparison.[27] Many abnormalities are put into appropriate perspective by determining whether or not they are new. Common examples are a prominent aortic arch, a visible major fissure related to prior inflammatory process, or a widened superior mediastinum related to substernal thyroid.

There are many ways of proceeding, and it is most appropriate that each person develop his or her own system. Any system should include a routinely utilized, deliberate attempt to look at areas that are easily ignored. These include the thoracic spine, the neck (for masses and tracheal position), the costophrenic angles, the lung apices, the retrocardiac space, and the retrosternal space. Looking at these areas allows definition of mediastinal position and cardiac and aortic situs and the presence of pleural effusions, scarring, or diaphragmatic elevation. Next, the lung fields are evaluated. This evaluation should involve a careful search for infiltrates or masses even when looking at a chest radiograph for cardiovascular abnormalities, keeping in mind that many people with coronary artery disease have a history of tobacco abuse and are, therefore, at increased risk for lung malignancies. The overall size of the cardiac silhouette, its position, and the location of the ascending and descending aorta are then evaluated. Dextrocardia and a right descending aorta are rare, particularly in adults, but are easy to check for. They are important to recognize because of their association with congenital cardiac and abdominal situs abnormalities. It is also important to look at the site and the position of the stomach. This information can be used to differentiate between a high diaphragm and a pleural effusion (see Fig. 12–1). It can also provide information about other pathological processes (see Fig. 12–13).

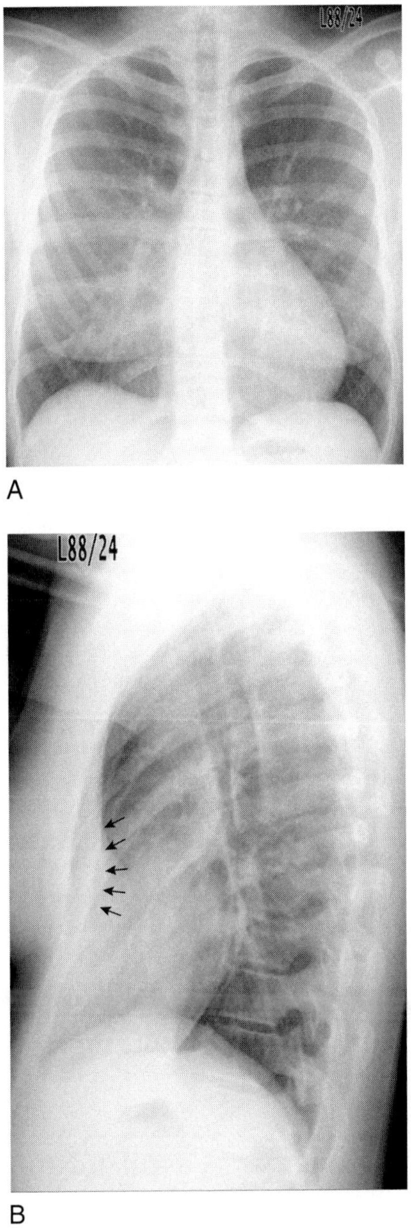

FIGURE 12–11 Chest radiographs of a 12-year-old girl with marked pectus excavatum. **A,** The posteroanterior (PA) view shows suggestion of mild cardiomegaly and haziness of the right heart border. Note sharp contour of cardiac apex related to absence of a fat pad. **B,** Lateral view confirms pectus deformity (arrows) and narrow anteroposterior diameter of the chest, explaining the appearance on the PA film.

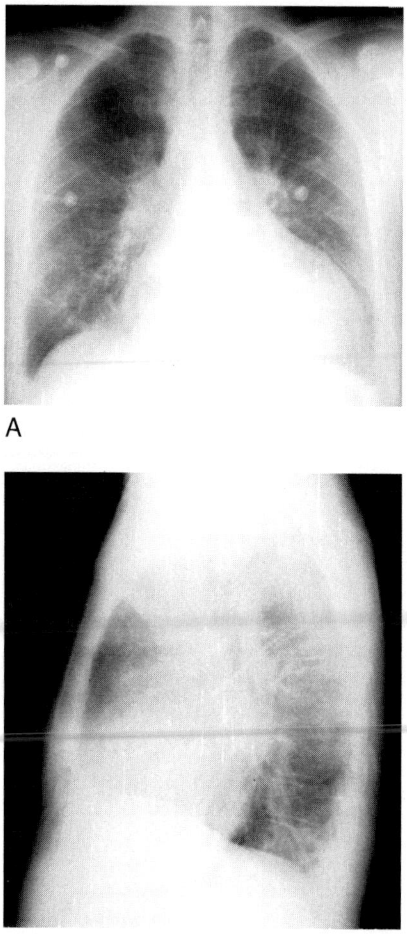

FIGURE 12–12 Chest radiographs of a 53-year-old man with severe ischemic cardiomyopathy and marked cardiomegaly. Frontal **(A)** and lateral **(B)** views show markedly enlarged cardiac silhouette, without clear enlargement of individual chambers, and marked pulmonary vascular redistribution.

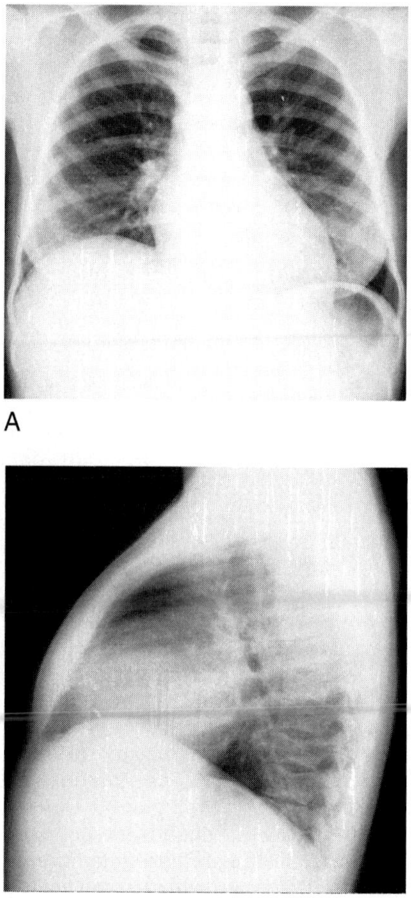

FIGURE 12–13 Chest radiographs of a 22-year-old woman with sickle cell disease. There is mild cardiomegaly and plethoric pulmonary vascularity secondary to anemia with a resultant high-output state. **A,** Gastric bubble is lateral in position related to autosplenectomy. **B,** "Fish mouth" vertebral bodies, characteristic of sickle cell disease.

Lungs and Pulmonary Vasculature

Evaluation of the pulmonary vascular pattern is difficult and imprecise but very important. As noted earlier, it varies with the patient's position (erect versus supine) and is altered substantially by underlying pulmonary disease. It is best to define pulmonary vascularity by looking at the middle zone of the lungs (i.e., the third of the lungs between the hilar region and the peripheral region laterally) and comparing a region in the upper lung field with a region in the lower at equal distances from the hilum.[17] Vessels should be larger in the lower lung but sharply marginated in both upper and lower zones. In normal persons, the vessels taper and bifurcate and are difficult to define in the outer third of the lung. They normally cannot be seen near the pleura (see Fig. 12–8).

Two distinct patterns of abnormality are recognizable. In patients with a high-output state (e.g., pregnancy, severe anemia as in sickle cell disease, hyperthyroidism) or left-to-right shunt, because pulmonary arterial flow is increased, the pulmonary vessels are seen more prominently than usual in the periphery of the lung (Fig. 12–14; see Fig. 12–13). They are uniformly enlarged, but their margins remain clear. In situations with elevated pulmonary artery pressure, the vessel borders become hazy, the lower zone vessels constrict and the upper zone vessels enlarge, and vessels become visible farther toward the pleura, in the outer third of the lungs (see Fig. 12–12). With increasing left ventricular end-diastolic pressure (LVEDP) or left atrial pressure, interstitial edema increases and ultimately pulmonary edema occurs. There is usually a reasonable correlation between the pulmonary vascular pattern and pulmonary capillary wedge pressure (PCWP). At a PCWP of less than 8 mm Hg, the vascular pattern is normal. As the PCWP increases to 10 to 12 mm Hg, the lower zone vessels appear equal in diameter to or smaller than the upper zone vessels. At pressures of 12 to 18 mm Hg, the vessel borders become progressively hazier because of increasing extravasation of fluid into the interstitium. This effect is sometimes evident as *Kerley B lines,* which are horizontal, pleural-based, peripheral linear densities. As PCWP increases above 18 to 20 mm Hg, pulmonary edema occurs, with interstitial fluid present in sufficient amounts to cause a perihilar "bat wing" appearance (Fig. 12–15).

Again, these typical appearances may be altered for various reasons. In patients with extensive pulmonary fibrosis or multiple bullae, the vascular pattern is abnormal at baseline, and as the PCWP increases, it does not change in predictable ways as definable on a chest radiograph. In patients with chronic congestive heart failure, there are chronic changes in the pulmonary vascular pattern that do not correlate with the changes that occur in patients with normal left ventricular pressure at baseline. For example, a patient with a chronic elevation of LVEDP to 25 to 30 mm Hg resulting from ischemic myopathy or other cause may have a normal

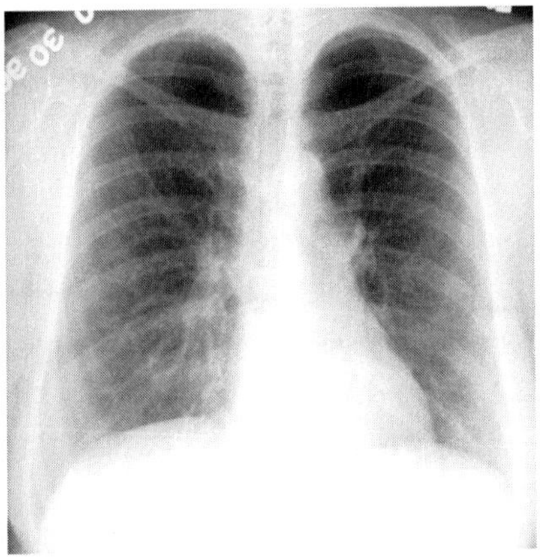

A

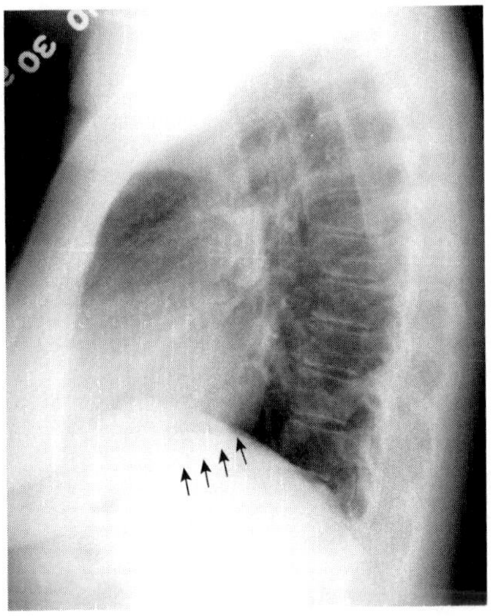

B

FIGURE 12–14 Chest radiographs of a 47-year-old asymptomatic woman with a small atrial septal defect. **A,** The posteroanterior view shows a normal cardiac contour, with mild pulmonary vascular plethora. at the periphery of the lung fields. **B,** Lateral view shows mild prominence of the left ventricle (arrows).

pulmonary vascular pattern or moderate rather than marked redistribution (see Fig. 12–5). Characteristically, heart size increases with increasing pulmonary vascular redistribution. If pulmonary edema is independent of left ventricular dysfunction, however, as may occur at high altitude or following cerebral trauma, the heart size may remain normal. Despite these limitations, it is important to evaluate the pulmonary vascular pattern routinely, as it does provide relevant information.

Cardiac Chambers and Great Vessels

Evaluation of the heart must also be done systematically. After assessing overall size and pulmonary vascular pattern—as a reflection of left-heart physiological status—the individual chambers should be examined. As noted, it is not possible to define clearly individual chambers in a normal chest radiograph (see Figs. 12–3 and 12–4). Furthermore, when the cardiac silhouette is enlarged, it is most often related to biventricular failure, and, again, individual chamber enlargement is not visible (see Fig. 12–12). In acquired valvular disease and in many types of congenital heart disease, however, individual chamber enlargement is present and crucial to plain film (and often clinical) diagnosis.[14,22,28] This

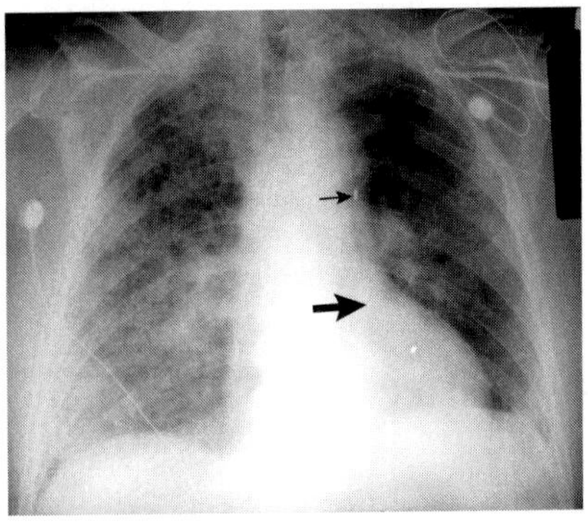

FIGURE 12–15 Patient with acute pulmonary edema. Note engorged hila bilaterally, with typical pattern of pulmonary edema on the right. Also note intraaortic counterpulsation balloon with radiopaque tip at the top of the descending aorta (arrow) and the balloon expanded in the aorta below it (large arrow).

information is now readily available with other, more expensive imaging modalities, namely cardiac echocardiography, magnetic resonance imaging (MRI), and computed tomography (CT) (see also Chaps. 11, 14, and 15).[29] Plain films remain important nonetheless as they allow fairly straightforward and inexpensive assessment of changes over time and are routinely and quickly available.[30-33]

RIGHT ATRIUM. Right atrial enlargement is essentially never isolated except in the presence of congenital tricuspid atresia or Ebstein anomaly, both rarely encountered even in the pediatric age group. The right atrium may dilate in the presence of pulmonary hypertension or tricuspid regurgitation, but right ventricular dilation usually predominates and prevents definition of the atrium. The right atrial contour blends with that of the superior vena cava, right main pulmonary artery, and right ventricle. In adults, therefore, it is virtually impossible to define, and in fact it is pointless to try.

RIGHT VENTRICLE. The classic signs of right ventricular enlargement are a "boot-shaped" heart and filling in of the retrosternal airspace.[16] The former is due to transverse displacement of the apex of the right ventricle as it dilates (Fig. 12–16A). Because in adults it is rare for the right ventricle to dilate without left ventricular dilation, this boot shape is not often obvious. It is most commonly seen in congenital heart disease, classically in tetralogy of Fallot. As the right ventricle dilates, it expands superiorly as well as laterally and posteriorly, filling in the retrosternal airspace (Fig. 12–17; see Fig. 12–16B). The classic teaching is that in a lateral chest radiograph in normal patients the soft tissue density is confined to less than one-third of the distance from the suprasternal notch to the tip of the xyphoid. If the soft tissue fills in more than half of this distance, it is a reliable indication of right ventricular enlargement.

There are other causes of increased soft tissue density in this region, and history and other findings must be considered. Common causes that are generally easy to distinguish from right ventricular enlargement include retrosternal adenopathy, midmediastinal mass (e.g., lymphoma or thymoma), marked dilation of the main pulmonary artery (Fig. 12–18A and B), and marked aortic root dilation (see Fig. 12–8). By far the most common cause of increased retrosternal soft tissue, however, is prior median sternotomy with resultant scarring (see Fig. 12–7C). Right ventricular enlargement is most often seen in mitral valve disease, secondary to pulmonary hypertension (see Fig. 12–17A and B). Less commonly, it is the result of primary pulmonary hypertension.

LEFT ATRIUM. Several classic signs define left atrial enlargement.[14,34] First is dilation of the left atrial appendage,

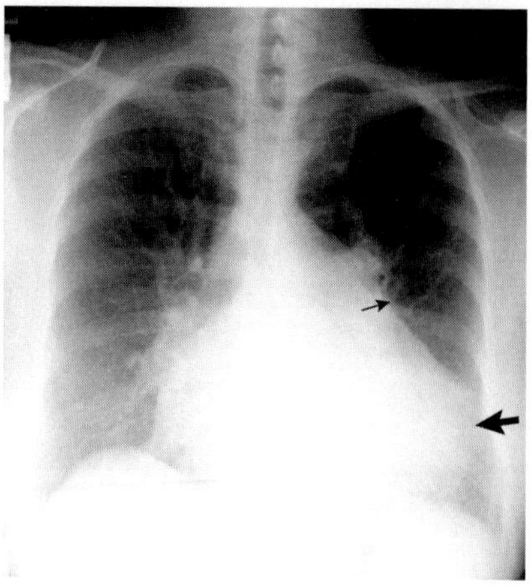

A

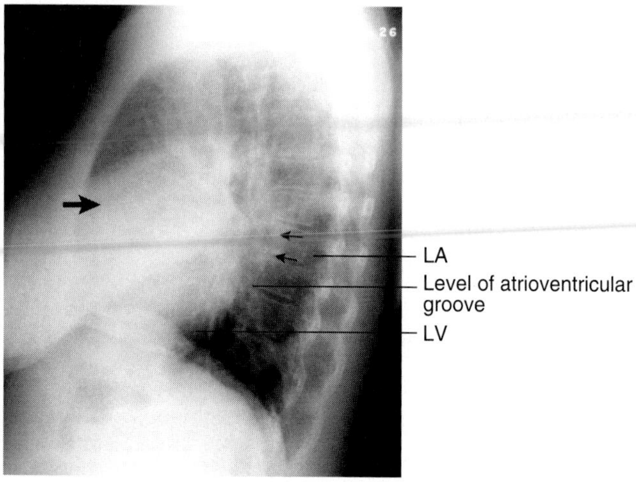

B

FIGURE 12–16 Chest radiographs of a 59-year-old woman with history of rheumatic heart disease and mitral stenosis. **A,** The posteroanterior view demonstrates enlarged cardiac silhouette, with suggestion of a double density seen through the heart (left atrial enlargement), prominent convexity of the left atrial appendage (arrow), and slightly elevated cardiac apex (large arrow), suggestive of right ventricular (rather than left ventricular) enlargement. There is significant elevation of the pulmonary venous pressures. **B,** The lateral view confirms marked right ventricular (arrow) and left atrial (small arrows) enlargement. Note filling in of the retrosternal airspace. LA = left atrium; LV = left ventricle.

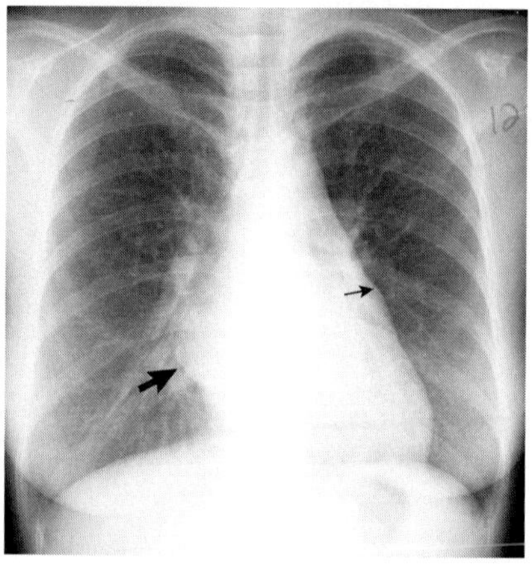

A

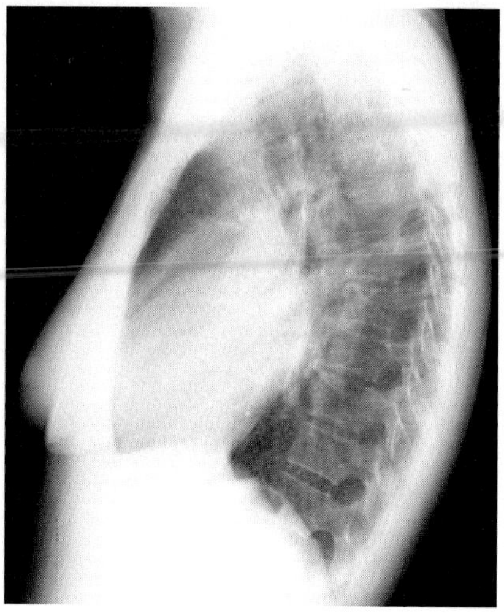

B

FIGURE 12–17 Chest radiographs of a 39-year-old Asian woman with rheumatic mitral stenosis. **A,** Frontal view shows normal heart size, mild vascular redistribution, and marked, focal enlargement of the left atrium (small arrow), which extends to the right of the midline (large arrow). There is elevation of the left main stem bronchus. **B,** Lateral view shows dilated right ventricle, with filling in of the retrosternal airspace. The left ventricle is normal in size and contour.

which is seen as a focal convexity where there is normally a concavity between the left main pulmonary artery and the left border of the left ventricle on the frontal view (Fig.12–19A). Second, because of its location, as the left atrium enlarges, it elevates the left main stem bronchus. In so doing, it widens the angle of the carina (see Fig. 12–19A).[35] Third, as the left atrium enlarges posteriorly, it may cause focal bowing of the middle to low thoracic aorta toward the left. This bowing is distinguishable from the tortuosity seen with progressive atherosclerosis, which involves the descending thoracic aorta either in its upper portion or throughout. Next, with marked left atrial enlargement, a double density can be seen on the frontal view, as the left atrium projects laterally toward the right as well as posteriorly and is surrounded by lung (see Figs.12–17A and 12–19A). Finally, on the lateral film, left atrial enlargement appears as a focal, posteriorly directed bulge (see Fig. 12–19B).

Isolated left atrial enlargement in the adult is most often seen in mitral stenosis, and definable left atrial enlargement is the hallmark of mitral valve disease (see Chap. 57). In mitral stenosis, the left atrium is enlarged, there is progressive evidence of pulmonary vascular redistribution (often with Kerley B lines), and there is ultimately enlargement of the right ventricle. The left ventricle, however, remains normal in size (see Figs. 12–17 and 12–19). In mitral regurgitation, the left atrium and ventricle both enlarge because of increased flow (Fig. 12–20). The pulmonary vascular redistribution is more variable in mitral regurgitation than in mitral stenosis, as is right ventricular dilation. It is also important to note mitral annulus calcification: it is common but does not have a strong association with valvular dysfunction. It does, however, have an association with premature coronary artery disease (Fig. 12–21).[36]

LEFT VENTRICLE. Left ventricular enlargement is characterized by a prominent, downwardly directed contour of the apex, as distinguished from the transverse displacement seen with right ventricular enlargement. The overall cardiac contour is also usually enlarged, although this is nonspecific. It is also important to evaluate the left ventricle on the lateral film. Here, it is seen as a posterior bulge, below the level of the mitral annulus (Fig. 12–22). It may also be seen inferiorly, pushing the gastric bubble (see Fig. 12–14B). Enlargement in this way is an illustration of findings that lie outside the usual confines of the chest. This is another example of the value of looking at the entire chest radiograph. Focal left ventricular enlargement in adults is most commonly seen in the presence of aortic insufficiency (with aortic root dilation; see Fig. 12–22) or mitral regurgitation (with left atrial dilation; see Fig. 12–19). Left ventricular dilation is less common with aortic stenosis, although it can occur, accompanied by congestive heart failure.[18-20,28,37]

PULMONARY ARTERIES. The main pulmonary artery can appear abnormal in many situations. In the presence of pulmonic stenosis, the main pulmonary artery and the left pulmonary artery dilate (see Fig. 12–18A and B). This dilation is thought to be due to the jet effect through the stenotic valve, coupled with the anatomy. That is, the main pulmonary artery continues straight into the left main pulmonary artery, but the right comes off at a fairly sharp angle and is not generally affected by the jet. This enlargement can be seen with a prominent left hilum on the frontal view and a prominent pulmonary outflow tract on the lateral. It is important to remember that the pulmonic valve lies higher than and more peripherally in the outflow tract than the aortic valve (see Fig. 12–4). It is also located anterior to the aortic valve on the lateral view.

AORTA. The aorta dilates in different ways as a function of the underlying pathology. It is often possible to define the pathology not only by the pattern of aortic dilation but also by associated cardiac abnormalities.[38] On the frontal chest radiograph, aortic dilation is seen as a prominence to the right of the middle mediastinum (Fig. 12–23A). There is also a prominence in the anterior mediastinum on the lateral view, behind and superior to the pulmonary outflow tract (see Figs. 12–5, 12–8, and 12–23B). Dilation of the aortic root is probably most commonly seen in the presence of long-term, poorly controlled systemic hypertension. Enlargement of the aortic root is also seen in the presence of aortic valve disease.

In aortic valve stenosis (see Chap. 57), there is usually focal dilation of the aortic root, often subtle, and often without left ventricular enlargement (see Figs. 12–8 and 12–23). It is important to look for this, as there are often no other signs on the chest radiograph, even in the presence of a very small valve area.[37] The left ventricle generally hypertrophies in response to increased resistance to outflow rather than dilating as it does in response to the increased flow volume that occurs with aortic insufficiency. This wall thickening with hypertrophy is seen with echocardiography, CT, or MRI, but the ventricle may appear entirely normal on the chest radiograph despite tight aortic valve stenosis. Aortic valve calcification is pathognomonic of significant aortic valve disease (see Fig. 12–23B), but it is usually difficult to see on a chest radiograph because of the overlying soft tissue densities and the minimal blurring caused by cardiac motion, even with a

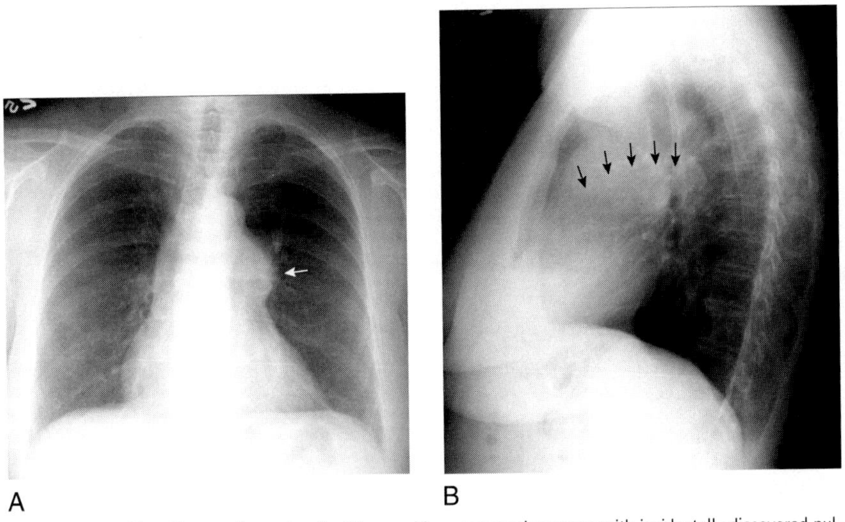

FIGURE 12–18 Chest radiographs of a 56-year-old asymptomatic woman with incidentally discovered pulmonic stenosis. **A,** Posteroanterior view shows marked enlargement of the main pulmonary trunk extending into the left main pulmonary artery (arrow). **B,** Lateral view confirms prominence of the pulmonary outflow tract and main and left pulmonary arteries (arrows).

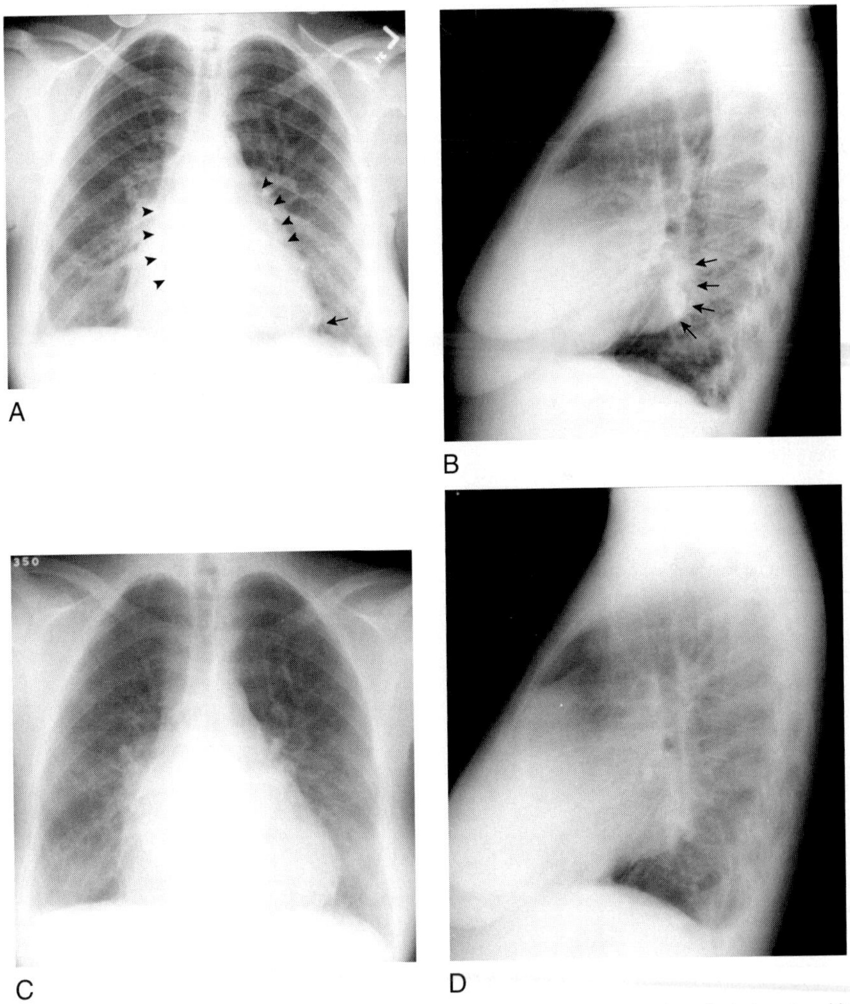

FIGURE 12–19 Chest radiographs of a 60-year-old woman with severe progressive mitral stenosis, with serial films spanning 4 years. **A,** Initial posteroanterior (PA) view shows enlargement of the left atrium (arrowheads), prominence of the hilar vessels, and pulmonary venous redistribution. Transverse angle of the apex suggests right ventricular enlargement (arrow). **B,** Initial lateral view confirms this, with filling in of the retrosternal airspace. Note also severe left atrial enlargement (arrows). **C** and **D,** PA and lateral views 4 years later show progressive left atrial and right ventricular enlargement, with increased double density of the left atrium on the frontal view with prominent focal bulge on the lateral view above the level of the left ventricular contour. There is increased density in the retrosternal airspace.

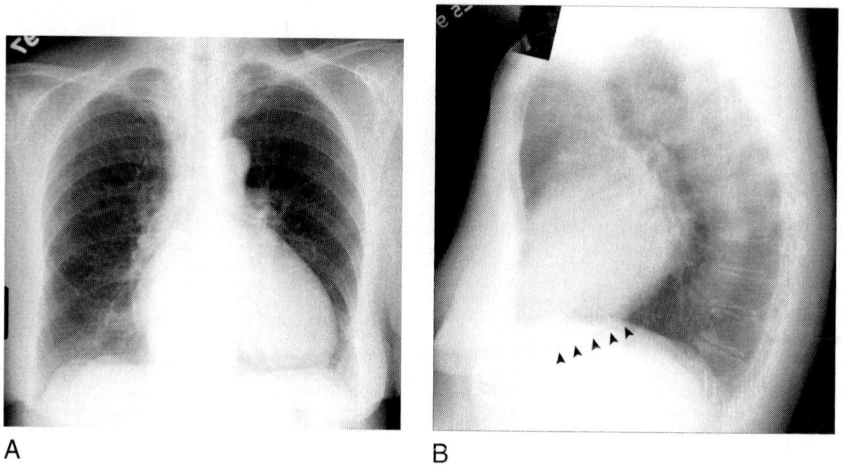

FIGURE 12–20 Chest films of a 78-year-old woman with pure mitral regurgitation and atrial fibrillation. **A,** Posteroanterior view shows enlargement of the left atrium and left ventricle with mild pulmonary vascular redistribution. **B,** Lateral view confirms these findings. Arrowheads indicate prominent left ventricular contour.

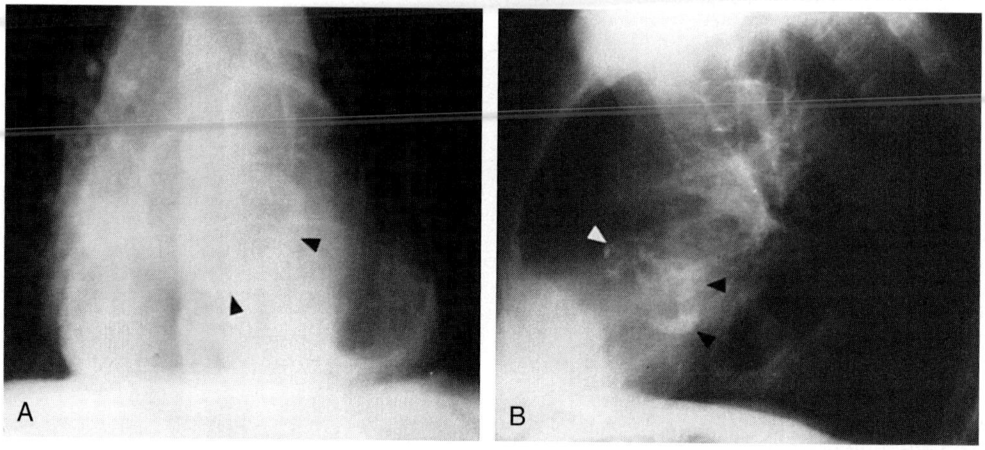

FIGURE 12–21 **A,** Mitral valve calcification in the posteroanterior projection. **B,** Mitral valve calcification in the lateral projection. Valve calcification (black arrows) lies below the line drawn from the left main bronchus to the anterior costophrenic sulcus, which localizes it to the mitral valve. The aortic valve in this projection lies more anteriorly and above the line (white arrows).

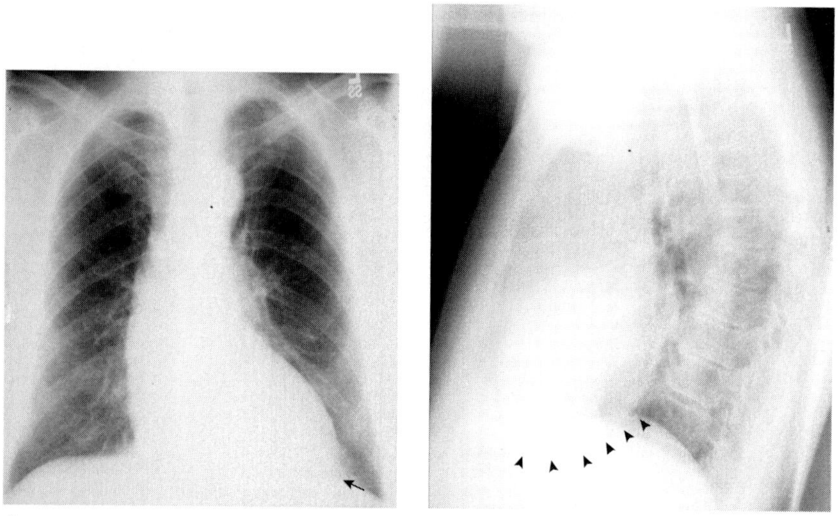

FIGURE 12–22 Chest radiographs of a 63-year-old man with chronic aortic regurgitation. **A,** Posteroanterior view shows downward displacement of the apex (arrow), suggestive of left ventricular enlargement. There is prominence and enlargement of the ascending aorta, creating a convex right border of the mediastinum. **B,** Lateral view shows prominent left ventricular enlargement (arrowheads). The aortic root is markedly enlarged in the retrosternal airspace but is separate from the sternum (in contrast to findings in right ventricular enlargement; see Figs. 12–16B and 12–17B).

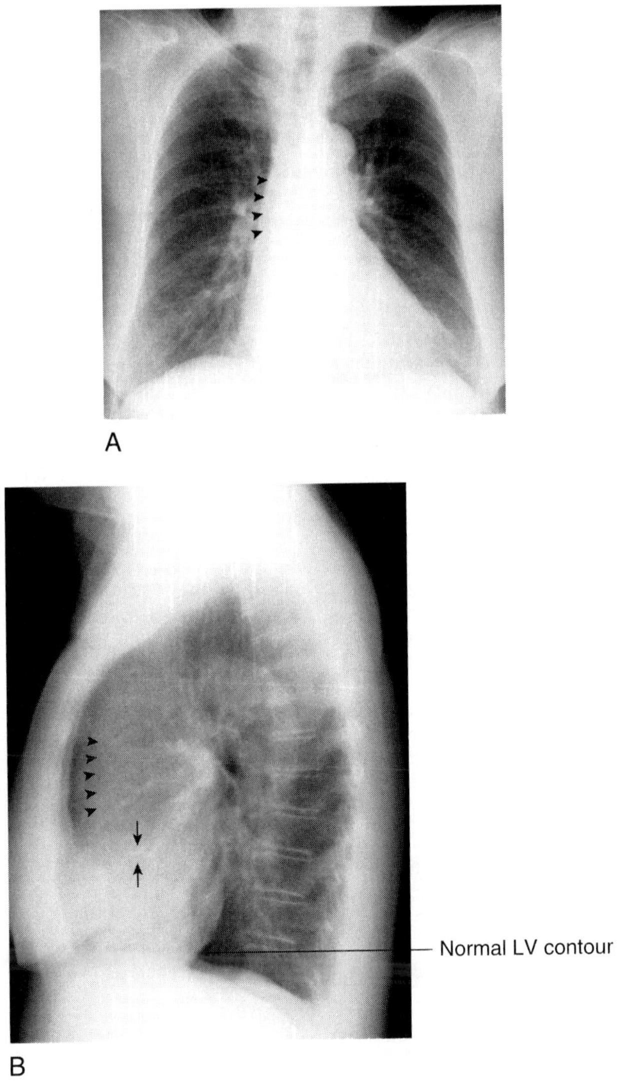

FIGURE 12–23 Chest radiographs of a 65-year-old woman with severe aortic stenosis. **A,** Frontal view shows prominent aortic root, to the right of the midline (arrowheads). Note absence of cardiomegaly and presence of normal pulmonary vascular pattern. **B,** Lateral view demonstrates calcification of the aortic valve leaflets (arrows), suggestive of a bicuspid valve. There is a prominent, mildly dilated aortic root (arrowheads).

very stenotic valve. Calcification, if present, is much more easily seen with fluoroscopy. Despite the decreased resolution of fluoroscopy compared with a standard chest radiograph, real-time visualization facilitates definition of calcification.[39-41]

It is important to remember that there is a subset of patients with aortic stenosis who present with left ventricular decompensation. In these patients, there is left ventricular and aortic root enlargement, and to distinguish this from aortic regurgitation it is important to look carefully for aortic valve calcification. It is not possible on a chest radiograph to establish definitively the etiology of aortic stenosis: rheumatic versus bicuspid valve versus degenerative. It can be helpful, however, to remember that rheumatic disease essentially always involves the mitral valve (see Chap. 57), and the absence of signs of mitral stenosis generally indicates that the etiology is not rheumatic (see Fig. 12–5).

In aortic regurgitation, aortic involvement is usually more diffuse than in aortic stenosis and more easily seen (see Chap. 57). In pure aortic regurgitation, the left atrium is not usually enlarged. Over time, however, dilation of the mitral annulus may occur secondary to the left ventricular dilation with resultant mitral regurgitation and left atrial dilation. Although aortic regurgitation classically occurs secondary to rheumatic fever (with associated mitral valve disease), congenital defects, or degenerative valve disease, it may also be caused by disease of the aortic root, including cystic medial necrosis, with or without Marfan syndrome. In cystic medial necrosis, the involvement is diffuse, and there is generally dilation of the aorta from the level of the valve at least through the arch (see Chap. 53). In tertiary syphilis, now rarely seen, the characteristic finding is marked dilation of the aorta from the root to the arch, with abrupt return to normal diameter at this level. With cystic medial necrosis, the transition of diameter is gradual. Aneurismal dilation of the ascending aorta also occurs in cystic medial necrosis and may be hard to define as distinct from the heart itself. Other aortic abnormalities, such as acute (see Fig. 12–2B) or chronic dissection and traumatic rupture or pseudoaneurysm, are better defined with CT. A chest radiograph may delay appropriate diagnosis and intervention in acute trauma, for example, in the case of suspected aortic rupture. The findings on the chest films are generally nonspecific indirect ones, such as the presence of mediastinal widening, blood at the left apex or a large left effusion (presumably blood), or rib fractures. Spiral or multislice CT can provide a rapid and accurate answer (see Chap. 15).

Pleura and Pericardium

The pleura and pericardium also require systematic evaluation (see Chap. 64). The pericardium is rarely distinctly definable on plain films of the chest (see Fig. 12–10).[42] There are two situations, however, in which it can be seen. In the presence of a large pericardial effusion, the visceral and the parietal pericardium separate. Because there is a fat pad associated with each, it is sometimes possible on the lateral film to make out two parallel lucent lines, usually in the area of the cardiac apex, with density (fluid) between them. Echocardiography, MRI, and CT, however, are all far more reliable for defining a pericardial effusion (see Chaps. 11, 14, and 15). Nonetheless, if the cardiac silhouette is enlarged on the chest radiograph is important to look for specific explanations. Although cardiac dilation and valvular disease are more common causes, the presence of an unsuspected effusion is worth considering. Classically, the cardiac silhouette has a "water bottle" shape in the presence of a pericardial effusion, but such a shape is not in itself diagnostic.

Both pleural and pericardial calcification can occur, but they are often not obvious (see Fig.12–6). Pericardial calcification is associated with a history of pericarditis, most often related to tuberculosis but also with other etiologies, such as a viral process. It is usually thin and linear and follows the contour of the pericardium. Because the calcification is thin, it is often seen only on one view, as in Figure 12–6. Myocardial calcification secondary to a large myocardial infarction with transmural necrosis is rare but can generally be distinguished from pericardial calcification. It tends to appear thicker, more focal, and less in conformance with the outer contour of the heart. Pleural calcification is essentially pathognomonic for asbestos exposure. It is associated with a high risk of malignant mesothelioma but is not diagnostic of such a tumor. It is generally easy to distinguish from pericardial calcification by its location.

Specific Conditions

The multitude of findings associated with cardiac disease are beyond the scope of this chapter, but several entities and situations are worth considering as they are either common or characteristic of certain disease states. As noted, the most common explanation for cardiomegaly and pulmonary vascular redistribution is ischemic heart disease.[20,23,24] In most patients with an acute myocardial infarction, the cardiac silhouette is not enlarged but there is pulmonary vascular redistribution, consistent with an acute increase in LVEDP. This condition is most easily defined when the chest radiograph is compared with a prior or subsequent one. After infarction, a variety of alterations can occur. Left ventricular aneurysms, either true (generally in the distribution of the left anterior descending artery) (see Fig. 12–7A) or false (usually involving the base or the posterior wall) are uncommon.[43,44] Although the location usually differs, the appearance of both is similar; there is focal prominence (of the anterolateral cardiac contour with true aneurysms), there may be linear myocardial calcification, and the margin is unusually sharp because the area of the aneurysm does not have normal cardiac motion. Again, this is best seen in comparison with prior chest radiographs.

It is impossible to define a postinfarction ventricular septal defect on the chest radiograph because the presentation is usually characterized by cardiac dilation and failure. On presentation, there is generally enlargement of the cardiac silhouette and evidence of heart failure, both nonspecific findings. After percutaneous repair, however, the septal repair device can often be identified (Fig. 12–24).[45]

Chest radiographs provide a wealth of physiological and anatomical information. As such, they play a central role in the evaluation and management of patients with a wide variety of cardiovascular and other disorders. Portable chest films should be used as infrequently as possible because the information they provide is limited and may even be misleading (for example, in defining cardiomegaly or in ruling out a pneumothorax or effusion). Standard 6-foot frontal and lateral chest films, on the other hand, are almost always of value. Whether recorded conventionally or digitally, if they are evaluated carefully using a systematic approach and when possible are compared with prior chest radiographs, it is hard to overestimate their importance.

Implantable Devices

A final important and broad area concerns the chest radiograph following surgery or other procedures. In these situations, it is crucial to recognize devices that have been implanted and changes that may occur. Devices include various valve prostheses,[46] pacemakers[47] and ICDs (Fig. 12-25), and intraaortic counterpulsation balloons (see Fig. 12-15). There are also clear changes that occur after surgery, such as the presence of clips on the side branches of saphenous veins used for coronary artery bypass grafting (see Fig. 12-7B and C) and retrosternal blurring (Fig. 12-26) and effusions (see Fig. 12-1).[48] Some such findings may be temporary, such as lines and tubes associated with surgery and effusions. Pacers and ICDs present specific questions. The first is the patency of the leads,[49,50] and the second is the position of the tip. Although course and tip position are generally confirmed fluoroscopically at the time of placement, malposition can occur. The ends of the wires (if there are two

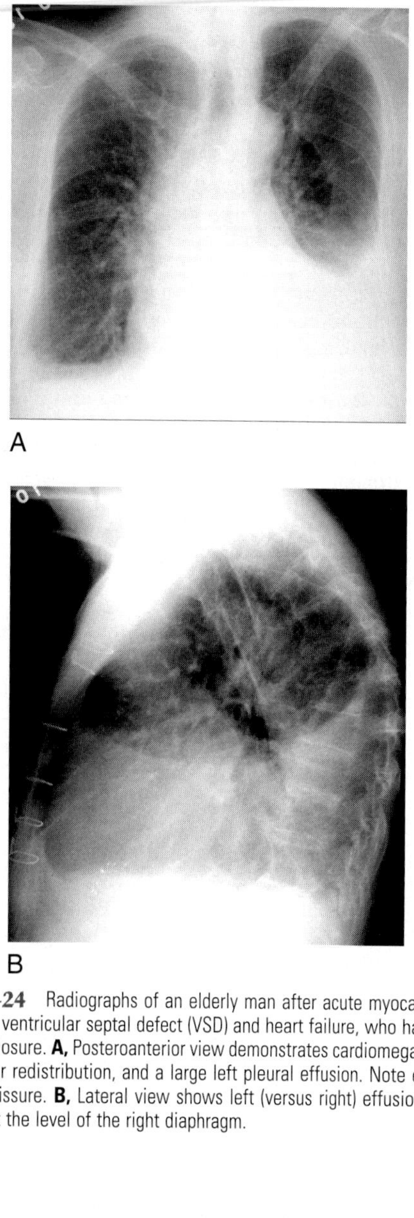

FIGURE 12–24 Radiographs of an elderly man after acute myocardial infarction complicated by ventricular septal defect (VSD) and heart failure, who has undergone a percutaneous closure. **A,** Posteroanterior view demonstrates cardiomegaly, marked pulmonary vascular redistribution, and a large left pleural effusion. Note effusion outlining left major fissure. **B,** Lateral view shows left (versus right) effusion and the VSD repair device at the level of the right diaphragm.

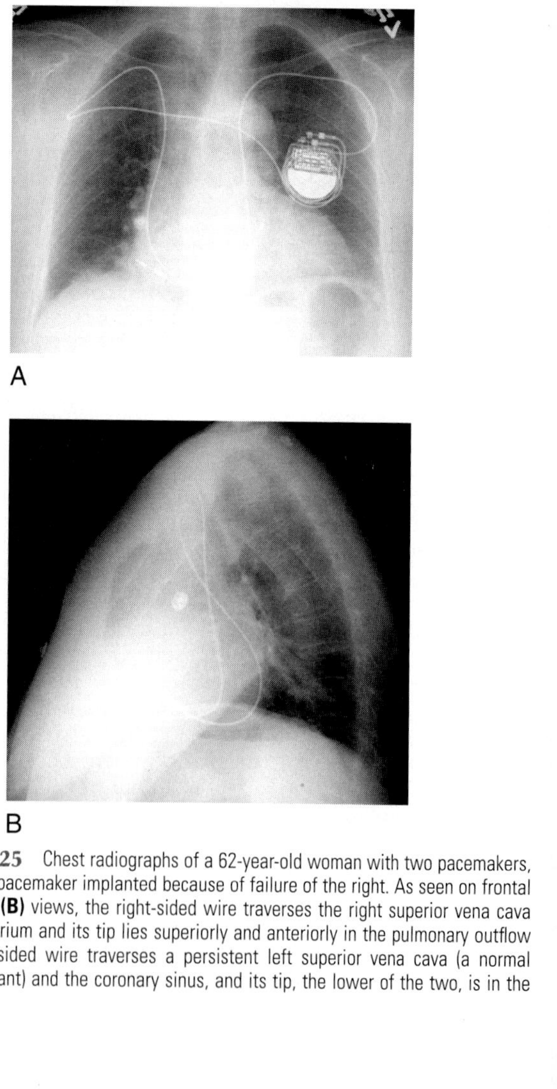

FIGURE 12–25 Chest radiographs of a 62-year-old woman with two pacemakers, with left-sided pacemaker implanted because of failure of the right. As seen on frontal **(A)** and lateral **(B)** views, the right-sided wire traverses the right superior vena cava and the right atrium and its tip lies superiorly and anteriorly in the pulmonary outflow tract. The left-sided wire traverses a persistent left superior vena cava (a normal anatomical variant) and the coronary sinus, and its tip, the lower of the two, is in the right atrium.

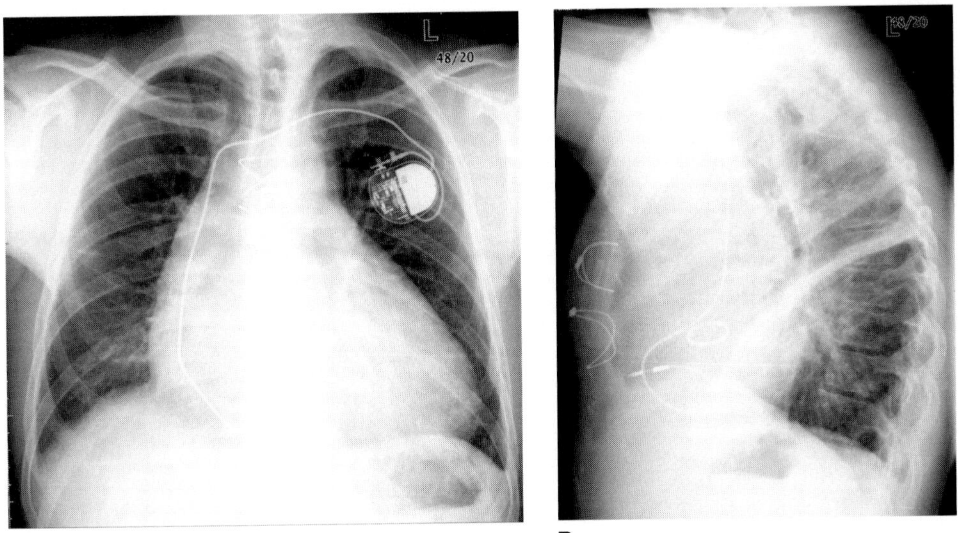

A B

FIGURE 12–26 Chest radiographs of a 28-year-old man who has undergone aortic valve replacement with a porcine bioprosthesis. **A,** Posteroanterior view. There is marked left ventricular (LV) enlargement with downwardly displaced apex. Note pacemaker wire with tip in the right ventricular (RV) apex. **B,** Lateral view confirms primary LV dilation, shows position of the aortic valve, and also shows the tip of the pacing wire in the RV apex. This confirms LV versus RV dilation.

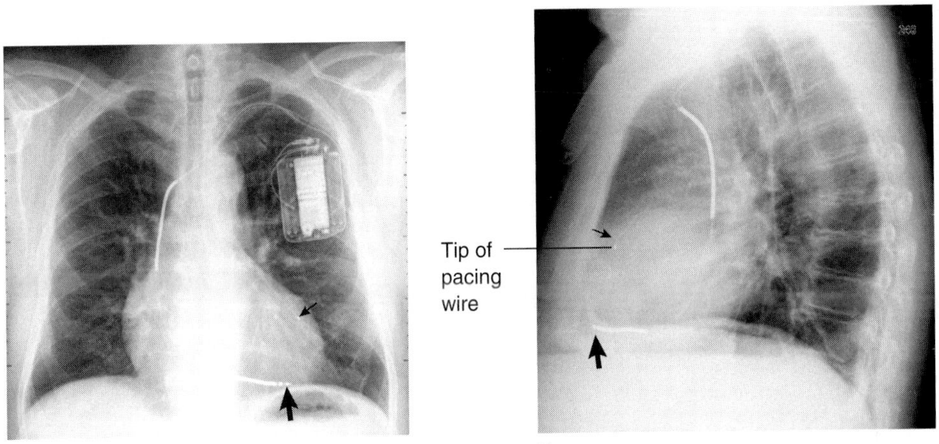

A B

FIGURE 12–27 **A** and **B,** Chest radiographs of a 78-year-old man after aortic valve replacement. Note wire position (arrow), through coronary sinus into great coronary vein (running parallel to the left anterior descending coronary artery), and biventricular enlargement. Also note position of AICD tip in right ventricular apex (large arrow).

leads) should be in the anterolateral wall of the right atrium and the apex of the right ventricle. If the leads are not so positioned, the reasons should be carefully determined (Fig. 12–27). That is, are they positioned because of error or because of anatomical variants, such as a persistent left superior vena cava that empties into the coronary sinus and then the right atrium (see Fig. 12–25)?[51] The position of the wires and of valve prostheses can help in the definition of specific chamber enlargement (see Fig. 12–27).

REFERENCES

1. Williams FH: A method for more fully determining the outline of the heart by means of a fluoroscope together with other uses of the instrument in medicine. Boston Me Surg J 135:335, 1896.

Technical Considerations

2. Hintenlang KM, Williams JL, Hintenlang DE: A survey of radiation dose associated with pediatric plain-fiilm chest X-ray examinations. Pediatr Radiol 32:771, 2002.
3. Wagner LK, Eifel PJ, Geise RA: Potential biological effects following high x-ray dose interventional procedures. J Vasc Intervent Radiol 5:71, 1994.
4. Krivopal M, Shlobin OA, Schwartzstein RM: Utility of daily routine portable chest radiographs in mechanically ventilated patients in the medical ICU. Chest 123:1607, 2003.
5. Shiralkar S, Rennie A, Snow M, et al: Doctors' knowledge of radiation exposure: Questionnaire study. BMJ 327:371, 2003.
6. Rong XJ, Shaw CC, Liu X, et al: Comparison of an amorphous silicon/cesium iodide fllat-panel digital chest radiography system with screen/fiilm and computed radiogrhy systems: A contrast-detail phantom study. Med Phys 28:2328, 2000.
7. Garmer M, Hennigs SP, Jäger HJ, et al: Digital radiography versus conventional radiography in chest imaging: Diagnostic performance of a large area fllat-panel detector in clinical CT-controlled study. AJR 174:75, 2000.
8. Chotas HG, Dobbins JT, Ravin CE: Principles of digital radiography with large-area electronically readable detectors: A review of the basics. Radiology 210:595, 1999.
9. Bacher K, Smeets P, Bonnarens K, et al: Dose reduction in patients undergoing chest imaging: Digital amorphous silicon fllat-panel detector radiography versus conventiona fiilm-screen radiography and phosphor-based computed radiography. AJR 181:923, 2003.
10. Schaefer-Prokop C, Uffmann M, Eisenhuber E, et al: Digital radiography of the chest: Detector techniques and performance parameters. J Thorac Imaging 18:124, 2003.
11. Ganten M, Radeleff B, Kampschulte A, et al: Comparing image quality of fllat-panel ches radiography with storage phosphor radiography and fiilm-screen radiography. AJ 181:171, 2003.
12. Honeyman-Buck J: PACS adoption. Semin Roentgenol 38:256, 2003.
13. Weatherburn GC, Ridout D, Strickland NH, et al: A comparison of conventional fiilm CR hard copy and PACS soft copy images of the chest: Analyses of ROC curves and inter-observer agreement. Eur J Radiol 47:206, 2003.

The Normal Chest Radiograph

14. Baron MG: The cardiac silhouette. J Thorac Imaging 15:230, 2000.
15. Ohye RG, Kulik TA: Images in cardiovascular medicine. Normal chest x-ray. Circulation 105:2455, 2002.
16. Boxt LM: Radiology of the right ventricle. Radiol Clin North Am 37:379, 1999.

17. Sharma S, Bhargave A, Krishnakumar R, et al: Can pulmonary venous hypertension be graded by the chest radiograph? Clin Radiol 53:899, 1998.
18. Hoffman RB, Rigler LG: Evaluation of left ventricular enlargement in the lateral projection of the chest. Radiology 85:93, 1965.
19. Freeman V, Mutatiri C, Pretorius M, et al: Evaluation of left ventricular enlargement in the lateral position of the chest using the Hoffman and Rigler sign. Cardiovasc J S Afr 14:134, 2003.
20. Jung G, Landwehr P, Schanzenbacher G, et al: Value of thoracic radiography in the assessment of cardiac size. A comparison with left ventricular cardiography. Rofo Fortschr Geb Rontgenstr Neuen Bildgeb Verfahr 162:368, 1995.
21. Fraser RS, Muller NL, Colman N, et al (eds): Fraser and Pare's Diagnosis of Diseases of the Chest. 4th ed. Philadelphia, WB Saunders, 1999.

Evaluating the Chest Radiograph in Heart Disease

22. Satou GM, Lacro RV, Chung T, et al: Heart size on chest x-ray as a predictor of cardiac enlargement by echocardiography in children. Pediatr Cardiol 22:218, 2001.
23. Thomas JT, Kelly RF, Thomas SJ, et al: Utility of history, physical examination, electrocardiogram, and chest radiograph for differentiating normal from decreased systolic function in patients with heart failure. Am J Med 112:437, 2002.
24. Ernst ER, Shub C, Bailey KR, et al: Radiographic measurements of cardiac size as predictors of outcome in patients with dilated cardiomyopathy. J Card Fail 7:13, 2001.
25. Petrie MC: It cannot be cardiac failure because the heart is not enlarged on the chest X-ray. Eur J Heart Fail 5:117, 2003.
26. Perez AA, Ribeiro AL, Barros MV, et al: Value of the radiological study of the thorax for diagnosing left ventricular dysfunction in Chagas' disease. Arq Bras Cardiol 80:208, 2003.
27. Berbaum KS, Smith WL: Use of reports of previous radiologic studies. Acad Radiol 5:111, 1998.
28. Murphy ML, Blue LR, Thenabadu PN, et al: The reliability of the routine chest roentgenogram for determination of heart size based on specifiic ventricular chambe evaluation at postmortem. Invest Radiol 20:21, 1985.
29. Schmermund A, Rensing BJ, Sheedy PF, et al: Reproducibility of right and left ventricular volume measurements by electron-beam CT in patients with congestive heart failure. Int J Card Imaging 14:201, 1998.
30. Ferri C, Emdin M, Nielsen H, et al: Assessment of heart involvement. Clin Exp Rheumatol 21:S24, 2003.
31. Rothrock SG, Green SM, Costanzo KA, et al: High yield criteria for obtaining non-trauma chest radiography in the adult emergency department population. J Emerg Med 23:117, 2002.
32. Oeppen RS, Fairhurst JJ, Argent JD: Diagnostic value of the chest radiograph in asymptomatic neonates with a cardiac murmur. Clin Radiol 57:736, 2002.
33. Gardiner S: Are routine chest x ray and ECG examinations helpful in the evaluation of asymptomatic heart murmurs? Arch Dis Child 88:638, 2003.
34. Lipton MJ, Coulden R: Valvular heart disease. Radiol Clin North Am. 37:319, 1999.
35. Murray JG, Brown AL, Anagnostou EA, et al: Widening of the tracheal bifurcation on chest radiographs: Value as a sign of left atrial enlargement. AJR 164:1089, 1995.
36. Atar S, Jeon DS, Luo H, et al: Mitral annular calcifiication: A marker of severe coronar artery disease in patients under 65 years old. Heart 89:161, 2003.
37. Rodan BA, Chen JT, Halber MD, et al: Chest roentgenographic evaluation of the severity of aortic stenosis. Invest Radiol 17:453, 1982.
38. Yamamoto H, Shavelle D, Takasu J, et al: Valvular and thoracic aortic calcium as a marker of the extent and severity of angiographic coronary artery disease. Am Heart J 146:153, 2003.
39. Cook C, Styles C, Hopkins R: Calcifiication on the chest X-ray: A pictorial rview. Hosp Med 62:210, 2001.
40. Li J, Galvin HK, Johnson SC, et al: Aortic calcifiication on plain chest radiograph increases risk for coronary artery disease. Chest 121:1468, 2002.
41. Kiryu S, Raptopoulos V, Baptista J, et al: Increased prevalence of coronary artery calcifiication in patients with suspected pulmonary embolism. Acad Radiol 10:840, 2003.
42. Wang ZJ, Reddy GP, Gotway MB, et al: CT and MR imaging of pericardial disease. Radiographics 23:S167, 2003.
43. Kao CL, Chang JP: Left ventricular pseudoaneurysm secondary to left ventricular apical venting. Tex Heart Inst J 30:162, 2003.
44. Brown SL, Gropler RJ, Harris KM: Distinguishing left ventricular aneurysm from pseudoaneurysm. A review of the literature. Chest 111:1403, 1997.
45. Kim JH, Siegel MJ, Goldstein JA, et al: Radiologic fiindings of 2 commonly used cardia septal occluders with clinical correlation. J Thorac Imaging 18:183, 2003.
46. Bordlee RP: Cardiac valve reconstruction and replacement: A brief review. Radiographics 12:659, 1992.
47. Bejvan SM, Ephron JH, Takasugi JE, et al: Imaging of cardiac pacemakers. AJR 169:1371, 1997.
48. Kurihara Y, Yakushiji YK, Nakajima Y, et al: The vertical displacement sign: A technique for differentiating between left and right ribs on the lateral chest radiograph. Clin Radiol 54:367, 1999.
49. Morishima I, Sone T, Tsuboi H, et al: Follow-up X rays play a key role in detecting implantable cardioverter defiibrillator lead fracture: A case of incessant inappropriat shocks due to lead fracture. Pacing Clin Electrophysiol 26:911, 2003.
50. Drucker EA, Brooks R, Garan H, et al: Malfunction of implantable cardioverter defiibrilators placed by a nonthoracotomy approach: Frequency of malfunction and value of chest radiography in determining cause. AJR 165:275, 1995.
51. Schummer W, Schummer C, Frober R: Persistent left superior vena cava and central venous catheter position: Clinical impact illustrated by four cases. Surg Radiol Anat 25:315, 2003.

CHAPTER 13

Nuclear Cardiology

James E. Udelson • Vasken Dilsizian • Robert O. Bonow

The era of noninvasive radionuclide cardiac imaging in humans began in the early 1970s, with the first reports of noninvasive evaluation of resting myocardial blood flow. Since that time, there have been major advances in the technical ability to image cardiac physiology and pathophysiology, including that of myocardial blood flow, myocardial metabolism, and ventricular function. Just as important has been a major growth in the understanding of how to apply the image information to care of patients and the effect of that information on clinical decision-making. Ultimately, the role of information derived from any imaging procedure is to enhance the clinician's decision-making process to improve symptoms or clinical outcomes, or both.

Technical Aspects of Image Acquisition, Display, and Interpretation

Single-Photon Emission Computed Tomography Imaging of Perfusion and Function

The most commonly performed imaging procedure in nuclear cardiology is single-photon emission computed tomography (SPECT) imaging of myocardial perfusion. Following injection of the chosen radiotracer, the isotope is extracted from the blood by viable myocytes and retained within the myocyte for some period of time. Photons are emitted from the myocardium in proportion to the magnitude of tracer uptake, in turn related to perfusion. The standard camera used in nuclear cardiology studies, a gamma camera, captures the gamma ray photons and converts the information into digital data representing the *magnitude of uptake* and the *location of the emission*. The photoemissions collide along their flight path with a detector crystal. There, the gamma photons are absorbed and converted into visible light events (a "scintillation event"). Emitted gamma rays are selected for capture and quantitation by a *collimator* attached to the face of the camera-detector system. Most often, parallel hole collimators are used so that only photon emissions coursing perpendicular to the camera head and parallel to the collimation holes are accepted (Fig. 13–1). This arrangement allows better appropriate *localization of the source* of the emitted gamma rays. Photomultiplier tubes, the final major component in the gamma camera, sense the light-scintillation events and convert the events into an electrical signal to be further processed (see Fig. 13–1). The final result of SPECT imaging is the creation of multiple tomograms, or slices, of the organ of interest, comprising a digital display representing radiotracer distribution throughout the organ.[1] With SPECT myocardial perfusion imaging (MPI), the display represents the distribution of perfusion throughout the myocardium.

SPECT Image Acquisition

In order to construct the three-dimensional model of the heart from which tomograms are created, the myocardial perfusion data must be sampled from multiple angles over 180 or 360 degrees around the patient (Fig. 13–2A). Multiple images, each comprising 20 to 25 seconds of emission data, are collected. Each one of the separate "projection" images constitutes a two-dimensional snapshot of myocardial perfusion from the angle at which the projection was acquired. Then, the imaging information from each of the angles is *back projected* onto an imaging matrix, creating a reconstruction of the organ of interest (see Fig. 13–2B). The reader is referred to detailed reviews for more extensive information on the technical aspects of SPECT imaging and image reconstruction.[2,3]

SPECT Image Display

From the three-dimensional reconstruction of the heart, computer processing techniques are used to identify the long axis of the left ventricle, and standardized tomographic images in three standard planes are derived. *Short-axis* images, representing "donut-like" slices of the heart cut perpendicular to the long axis of the heart, are displayed beginning toward the apex and moving toward the base. This tomographic orientation is similar to the short-axis view in two-dimensional echocardiography, although shifted counterclockwise (Fig. 13–3A). Tomographic slices cut parallel to the long axis of the heart and also parallel to the long axis of the body are termed *vertical long-axis* tomograms (see Fig. 13–3B), and slices also cut parallel to the long axis of the heart but perpendicular to the vertical long axis slices are known as *horizontal long-axis* tomograms (see Fig. 13–3C). From all of these tomographic planes, the entire three-dimensional myocardium is sampled and displayed, minimizing overlap of structures.

Basics of Quality Control

The quality of SPECT MPI and the "accuracy" of the representation of regional myocardial perfusion are dependent on multiple quality control issues. These issues include the stability of the tracer distribution in the organ of interest during the acquisition interval, the absence of motion of the patient or organ of interest or both during the acquisition, and the absence of overlying structures that would attenuate the photon emissions from one region relative to another region across the different projection images. Those issues are related to the patient and the organ being imaged, and other quality control issues involve the camera and detector system, including the uniformity of photon detection efficiency across the camera face as well as the stability of the camera across the entire orbit of acquisition.[4]

It is important when interpreting SPECT images to be aware of possible sources of image artifacts.[5] Discrete motion of the patient (and thus motion of the heart outside its original field) causes an abnormality in the final images that may be corrected with motion correction software. Imaging artifacts commonly occur because of the effects of overlying structures that attenuate photon emissions. These include breast attenuation in women and attenuation of the inferobasal wall related to the diaphragm, most commonly seen in men. Strategies to overcome quality problems such as attenuation are described subsequently.

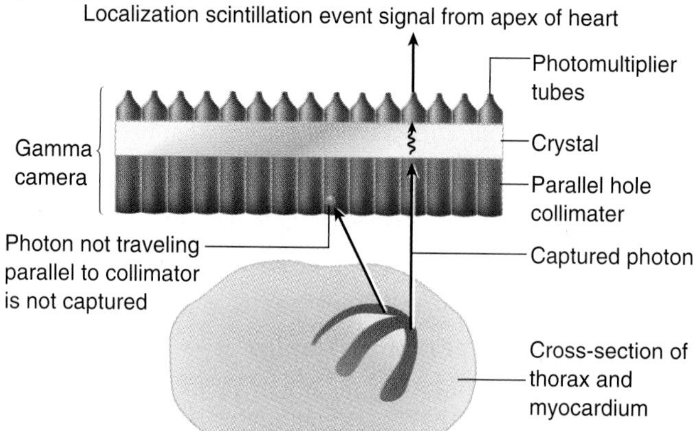

FIGURE 13–1 Capture of emitted photons by a gamma camera. Emissions are captured by a parallel hole collimator, allowing photons to interact with a detector crystal, and are recorded as scintillation events. The event is localized on the basis of where the photon interacts with the crystal.

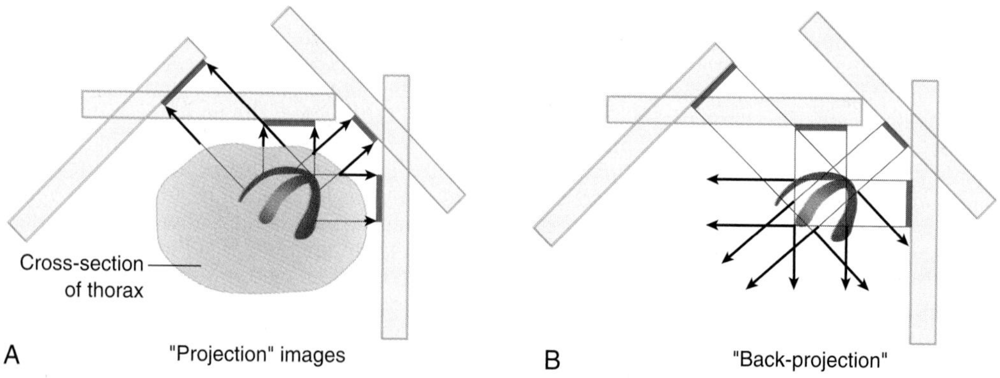

FIGURE 13–2 **A,** Single-photon emission computed tomography imaging technique. The gamma camera collects photon emission information from multiple angles around the body in order to reconstruct a three-dimensional image of the organ of interest. **B,** Back-projection technique during computer processing. Scintillation events as seen by the camera are back projected onto a matrix to reconstruct an image of the organ of interest.

SPECT Perfusion Tracers and Protocols

Thallium-201. Thallium-201 was introduced in the 1970s and propelled the clinical application of MPI as an adjunct to exercise treadmill testing. Thallium-201 is a monovalent cation with biological properties similar to those of potassium. As potassium is the major intracellular cation in muscle and is virtually absent in scar tissue, thallium-201 is a well-suited radionuclide for differentiating normal and ischemic from scarred myocardium.[6] Thallium-201 emits 80 keV of photon energy and has a physical half-life of 73 hours. The initial myocardial uptake early after intravenous injection of thallium is proportional to regional blood flow. First-pass extraction fraction (the proportion of tracer extracted from the blood as it passes through the myocardium) is high, in the range of 85 percent. It is transported across the myocyte cell membrane by the Na^+,K^+-adenosine triphosphatase (ATPase) transport system and by facilitative diffusion. Peak myocardial concentration of thallium occurs within 5 minutes of injection, with rapid clearance from the intravascular compartment. Although the initial uptake and distribution of thallium are primarily a function of blood flow, the subsequent *redistribution* of thallium, which begins within 10 to 15 minutes after injection, is unrelated to flow but is related to the rate of thallium clearance from myocardium, linked to the concentration gradient between myocytes and the blood levels of thallium (Fig. 13–4A). Thallium clearance is more rapid from normal myocardium with high thallium activity compared with myocardium with reduced thallium activity (ischemic myocardium), a process termed "differential washout" (see Fig. 13–4B).

Thallium studies can be divided into protocols in which thallium-201 is administered during stress or at rest.[6] Following stress, the reversal of a thallium defect from the initial peak stress to delayed 3- to 4-hour or 24-hour redistribution images is a marker of reversibly ischemic, viable myocardium. When thallium is injected at *rest*, the extent of thallium defect reversibility from the initial rest images to delayed redistribution images (at 3 to 4 hours) reflects viable myocardium with resting hypoperfusion. When scarred myocardium is present, the initial rest or stress thallium defect persists over time, termed an "irreversible" or "fixed" defect. However, in some patients with coronary artery disease (CAD), the initial uptake of thallium during stress may be severely decreased, and tracer accumulation from the recirculating thallium in the blood during the redistribution phase may be slow or even absent because of rapid decline of thallium levels in the blood. The result is that some severely ischemic but viable regions may show no redistribution on either early (3- to 4-hour) or late (24-hour) imaging, *even if viable myocardium is present*. Viable myocardium in this situation can be revealed by raising blood levels of thallium by reinjecting a small dose (1 mCi) of thallium at rest. Thus, in some patients, thallium reinjection is necessary to identify viable myocardium when there are irreversible defects on stress-redistribution images.

Technetium-99m–Labeled Tracers. Tc 99m–labeled myocardial perfusion tracers were introduced in the clinical arena in the 1990s.[7] Technetium-99m emits 140 keV of photon energy and has a physical half-life of 6 hours. Despite the excellent myocardial extraction and flow kinetics properties of thallium, its energy spectrum of 80 keV is suboptimal for conventional gamma cameras (ideal photopeak in the 140-keV range). In addition, thallium's long physical half-life (73 hours) limits the amount of thallium that may be administered in order to stay within acceptable radiation exposure parameters. Thus, Tc 99m–labeled tracers improve on these two limitations of thallium. Although three Tc 99m–labeled tracers (sestamibi, teboroxime, and tetrofosmin) have received U.S. Food and Drug Administration approval for detection of CAD, only sestamibi and tetrofosmin are available for clinical use at present.

Sestamibi and tetrofosmin are lipid-soluble cationic compounds with first-pass extraction fraction in the range of 60 percent. Myocardial uptake and clearance kinetics of both tracers are similar. They cross the sarcolemmal and mitochondrial membranes of myocytes by passive distribution, driven by the transmembrane electrochemical gradient, and they are retained within the mitochondria.[7] There is minimal redistribution with these

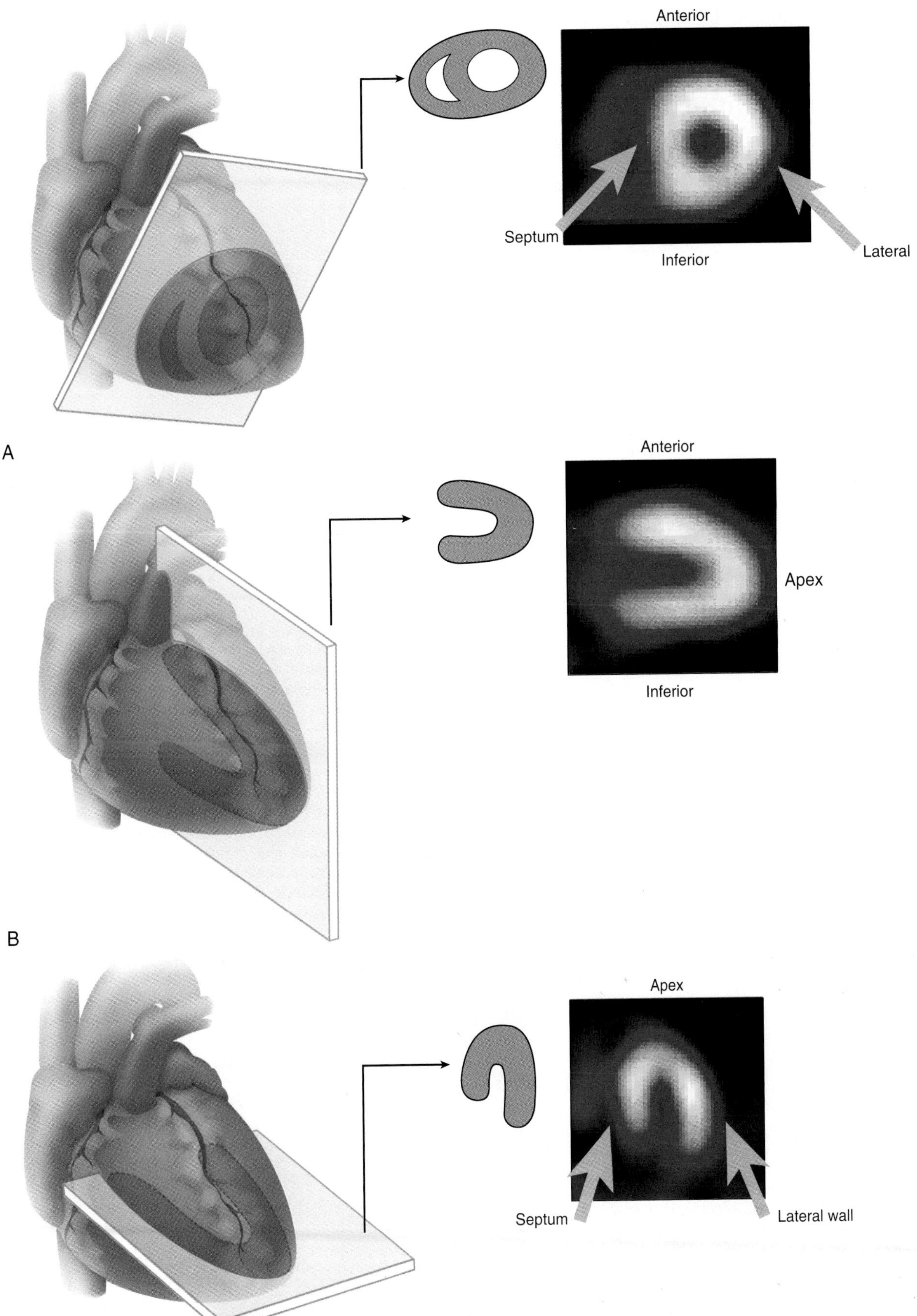

FIGURE 13–3 Standard single-photon emission computed tomography imaging tomographic display. **A,** The short-axis images each represent a portion of the anterior, lateral, inferior, and septal walls. **B,** Vertical long-axis images are displayed from left to right from the septal edge to the lateral wall and represent the anterior wall, apex, and inferior wall. **C,** Horizontal long-axis images are displayed from left to right from inferior to superior, representing the septum, apex, and lateral walls.

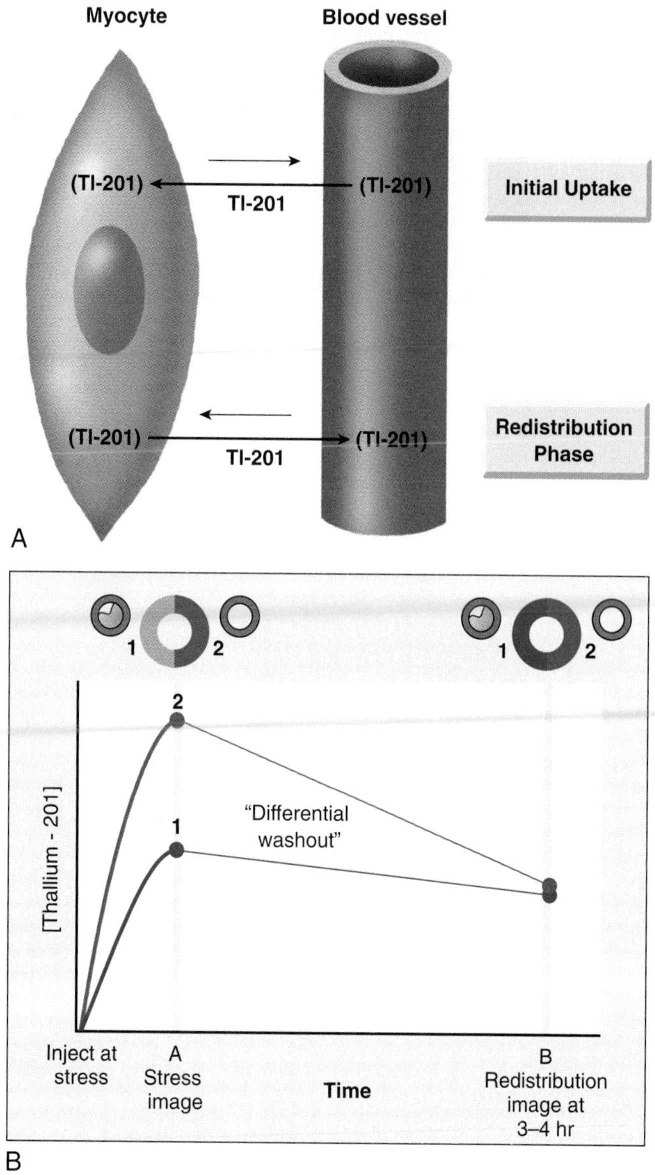

FIGURE 13–4 Thallium-201 redistribution. **A,** After initial uptake into the myocyte, an equilibrium is created between the intracellular and extracellular concentrations of thallium. After blood levels diminish during the redistribution phase, the equilibrium favors egress of thallium out of the myocyte. **B,** On the basis of that equilibrium, thallium concentration diminishes over time in zones of normal uptake, while diminishing more slowly in zones with less initial thallium uptake, i.e., those with diminished flow reserve or ischemia. In this example, segment 1 of the myocardial schematic is supplied by an artery with an 80 percent stenosis and segment 2 is supplied by a normal artery. During peak stress, normal blood flow reserve is present in segment 2; blunted flow reserve, based on the presence of stenosis, is present in segment 1, and there is less initial thallium uptake into segment 1 (time point A). Thallium washout is more rapid from the territory with initially normal uptake and slower from the ischemic zone, creating the phenomenon of differential washout. When redistribution imaging is done 3 to 4 hours later, (time point B), thallium concentrations are equal in segments 1 and 2. Thus, a reversible stress defect is seen in segment 1, based on the redistribution properties and differential washout. (Adapted from Dilsizian V: SPECT and PET techniques. *In* Dilsizian V, Narula J [eds]: Atlas of Nuclear Cardiology. Braunwald E (series ed). Philadelphia. Current Medicine, 2003, pp 19-46.)

tracers compared with thallium. Thus, myocardial perfusion studies with Tc 99m–labeled tracers require *two separate injections, one at peak stress and the second at rest.*

There are three basic protocols[8] with Tc 99m–labeled tracers: (1) a single-day study, in which myocardial blood flow is interrogated at rest and at peak stress, or in the reverse order, as long as the first injected dose is low (8 to 10 mCi) and the second injected dose is high (22 to 30 mCi); (2) a 2-day study, (commonly performed in patients with large body habitus) in which higher doses of the tracer are injected (20 to 30 mCi) both at rest and at peak stress in order to optimize myocardial count rate; and (3) a dual-isotope technique, which combines injection of thallium at rest followed by injection of a Tc 99m tracer at peak stress. The last approach takes advantage of the favorable properties of each of the two tracers, including high-quality gated SPECT images from Tc-99m and the potential of acquiring redistribution images from thallium (either at 4 hours prior to the stress study or at 24 hours after the Tc 99m activity has decayed).

A comparison of the properties of the available isotopes for perfusion imaging is shown in Table 13–1.

SPECT Image Interpretation

SPECT myocardial perfusion images may be evaluated visually, with the interpreter describing the perfusion pattern findings. Because the imaging data are digital, computer-aided quantitative analysis may also be used.[9]

For visual interpretation, the key elements to be reported include the *presence and location of perfusion defects* and whether defects on stress images are *reversible* on the rest images (implying stress-induced ischemia) or whether stress perfusion defects are *irreversible or "fixed"* (often implying myocardial infarction [MI]). Moreover, substantial literature has documented that the *extent* and the *severity* of the perfusion abnormality are independently associated with clinical outcomes.[10] Extent of perfusion abnormality refers to the amount of myocardium or vascular territory that is abnormal, and the severity refers to the magnitude of reduction in tracer uptake in abnormal zone relative to normal. Examples of stress and rest SPECT myocardial perfusion abnormalities of varying extents and severity are shown in Figure 13–5.

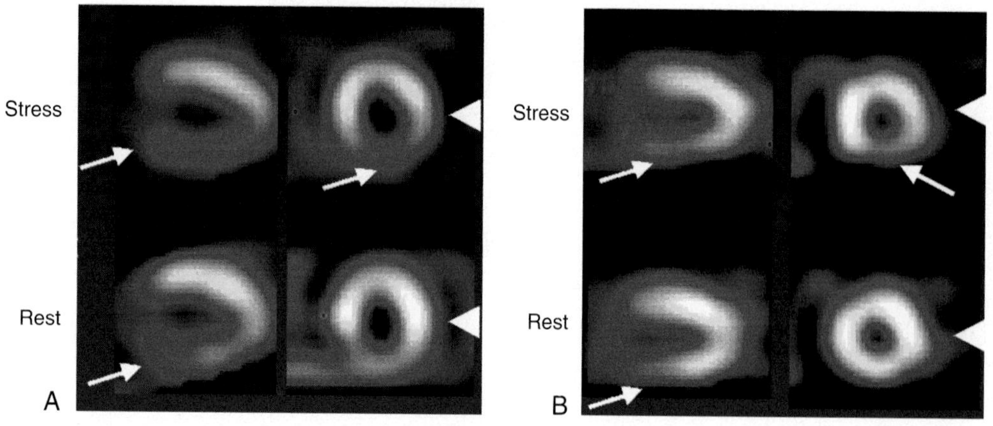

FIGURE 13–5 Abnormal single-photon emission computed tomography images of different extent and severity. **A,** A large, moderately severe, reversible inferior wall defect (arrows) reflecting a severe flow reserve abnormality. **B,** A milder reversible inferior wall defect (arrows) reflecting a less severe stenosis or a more severe stenosis with well-developed collaterals minimizing the defect severity. In both patients, there is also a mild lateral wall reversible defect (arrowheads). Note how the lateral wall brightens relative to the septum on the rest images compared with the stress images.

To minimize subjectivity in image interpretation,

TABLE 13–1 Properties of SPECT Tracers

Tracer	Physical Half-Life (hr)	Uptake	Myocardial Clearance	"Differential Washout"	Maximum Extraction Fraction
Thallium-201	73	Active	~50% at 6 hr	Yes	~0.70
Tc 99m sestamibi	6	Passive	Minimal	Minimal	0.39
Tc 99m tetrafosmin	6	Passive	Minimal	Minimal	0.24
Tc 99m teboroxime	6	Passive	~50% at 10 min	Yes	0.72

SPECT = single-photon emission computed tomography.
From Gerson MC, McGoron A, Roszell N, et al: Myocardial perfusion imaging: Radiopharmaceuticals and tracer kinetics. *In* Gerson MC (ed): Cardiac Nuclear Medicine. New York, McGraw Hill, 1997, pp 3-27.

semiquantitative visual analysis or fully quantitative computer analysis may be applied to MPI data.[11] With semiquantitative visual analysis, a score is assigned to represent perfusion for each of multiple segments of the myocardium. A segmentation model has been standardized for this approach by dividing the myocardium into 17 segments[12] on the basis of three short-axis slices and a representative long-axis slice to depict the apex (Fig. 13–6). Perfusion is graded on a scale of 0 to 4, with 0 representing normal perfusion and 4 representing a very severe perfusion defect. Scores for all 17 segments are added to create the "summed" score. The summed score from the stress images (summed stress score, SSS) represents the extent and severity of stress perfusion abnormality, the magnitude of perfusion defect related to *both ischemia and infarction*. The sum of the 17 segmental scores from the rest image (the summed rest score, SRS) represents the *extent of infarction*. The summed difference score (SDS) is derived by subtracting SRS from the SSS and represents the extent and severity of *stress-induced ischemia*. As discussed subsequently, a substantial literature has validated these scores as predictors of natural history outcomes.

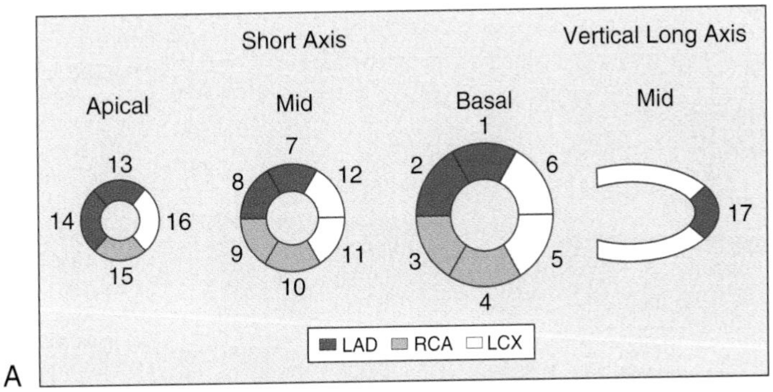

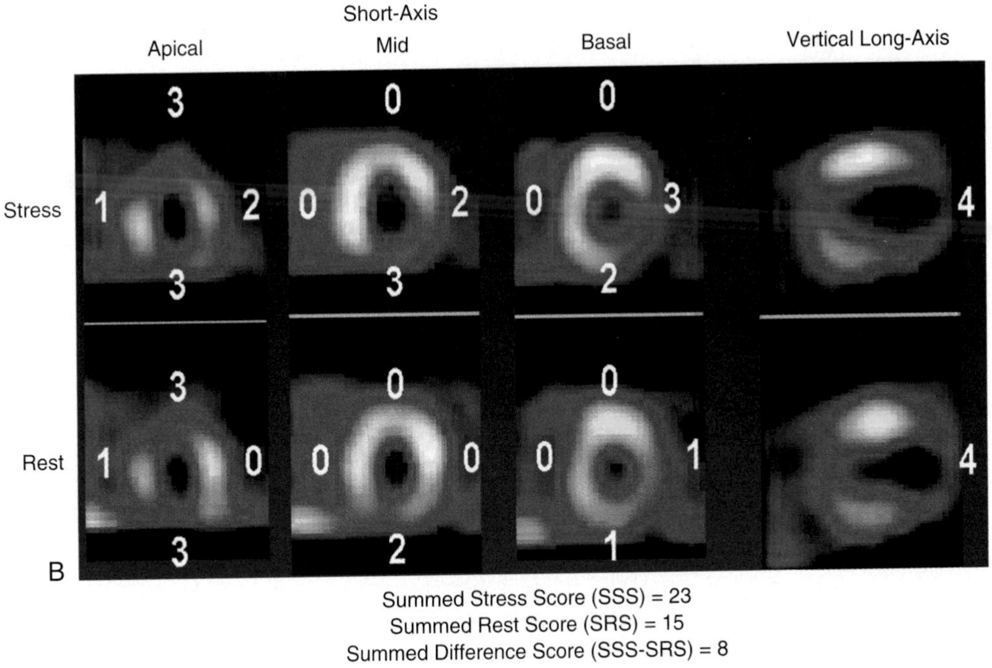

FIGURE 13–6 **A,** Standard segmental myocardial display for semiquantitative visual analysis in a 17-segment model. **B,** Segmental scoring of a patient whose stress and rest single-photon emission computed tomography perfusion images show a severe apical fixed defect (in the vertical long axis), extending into the inferoapical and anteroapical walls (in the apical short axis), with evidence of reversible defects in the inferior and lateral walls (in the middle and short axis). The summed stress score (SSS) represents extensive perfusion abnormality at stress (reflecting ischemia and infarct), the summed rest score (SRS) represents the extent of infarct, and the summed difference score (SDS) represents the extent of ischemia. LAD = left anterior descending (artery); LCX = left circumflex (coronary artery); RCA = right coronary artery.

Because SPECT MPI data are a digital representation of radiotracer distribution, the data can be analyzed quantitatively. The most common technique involves creation of a *circumferential profile* of relative tracer activity around the tomogram of interest, such as a short-axis tomogram.[13] With this technique, the 360 degrees around the tomogram are sampled at every 3 to 6 degrees, along a ray extending from the center of the image. The maximum counts at a picture element ("pixel") along the ray, usually occurring in the midportion of the myocardium, are recorded for each angle. The data may be plotted to create a profile of the perfusion pattern of that tomogram relative to the most "normal" area of uptake, which is assigned a value of 100 percent uptake (Fig. 13–7A). Circumferential profiles for an individual patient can be compared directly with a composite profile representing normal perfusion.[13,14] The

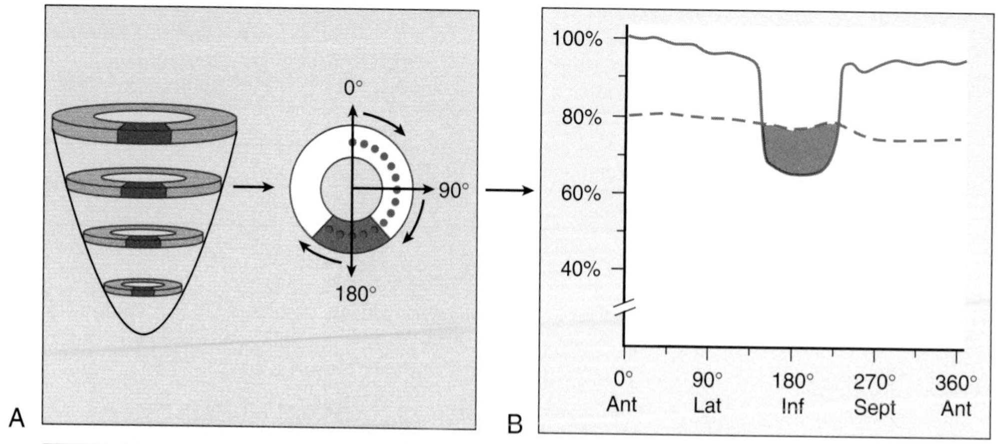

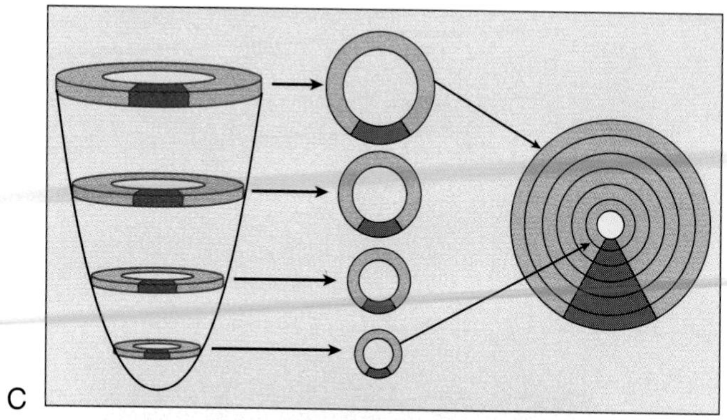

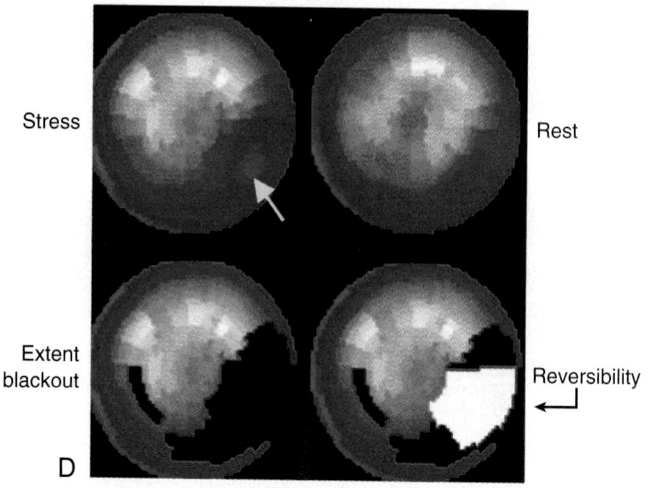

FIGURE 13–7 Quantitative analysis of single-photon emission computed tomography imaging. **A,** Circumferential profile analysis of tracer uptake along rays emanating from the center of the short-axis tomogram. The data are plotted relative to location around the myocardium and "normalized" to the point of peak uptake, which is assigned a value of 100 percent. From this procedure, a circumferential profile of tracer uptake around the myocardium is developed for each short-axis tomogram. In this example, there is a perfusion defect in the inferior wall (purple area). **B,** The patient's data are compared with lower limits of normal (dashed line) derived from a group of subjects without coronary artery disease of the same gender. From this comparison, the quantitative extent and severity of the perfusion abnormality can be derived (orange area). **C,** Data from the individual short-axis tomograms can be combined to create a bull's-eye polar plot, representing a two-dimensional compilation of all of the three-dimensional short-axis perfusion data. The inferior wall perfusion defect (gray area) is seen on the two-dimensional map. **D,** Example of a bull's-eye polar plot for a patient with a reversible defect of the inferolateral wall (yellow arrow on the stress bull's-eye plot, upper left). The "blackout" area (on the extent blackout plot, lower left) represents the myocardium that falls below the lower limits of normal, and in the reversibility plot (lower right) the white area represents the extent of that abnormality that is reversible (ischemic) on rest imaging. (Images courtesy of Ernest Garcia, Ph.D.)

normal perfusion data are often created from studies performed in normal subjects with a very low clinical probability of CAD or in those with known normal coronary arteries (see Fig. 13–7B). A quantitative extent of abnormality can be derived (the total amount of myocardium that falls below the lower limit of normal) as well as a derivation of the severity of the perfusion abnormality (the depth of the patient's perfusion abnormality relative to the lower limit of normal).

Most contemporary computer systems and analysis programs have the ability to create "bull's-eye" or "polar" maps representing perfusion of the entire three-dimensional myocardium in a two-dimensional plot (see Fig. 13–7C). Quantitative data may be derived on the extent of global perfusion abnormality, abnormality within vascular territories, as well as the extent of reversible and fixed defects (see Fig. 13–7D).

ADDITIONAL IMPORTANT SIGNS IN SPECT IMAGING ANALYSIS BEYOND MYOCARDIAL PERFUSION. There are other abnormal findings that provide additional information beyond that provided by the perfusion pattern alone, including lung uptake of tracer (particularly thallium-201) and transient ischemic dilation of the left ventricle.

Lung Uptake. In some patients, substantial tracer uptake is apparent throughout the lung fields following stress that is not present at rest (Fig. 13–8A). Patients with lung uptake often have severe multivessel disease, elevation of pulmonary capillary wedge pressure during exercise, and decreases in ejection fraction (EF) during exercise, all implying extensive myocardial ischemia.[15] It is likely that elevation in left atrial and pulmonary pressures slows pulmonary transit of the tracer, allowing more time for extraction or transudation into the interstitial spaces of the lung, accounting for this imaging sign.

Lung uptake of thallium-201 has been more extensively validated than lung uptake of the technetium-99m tracers sestamibi and tetrofosmin. There is minimal splanchnic or background activity after thallium stress injection, allowing image acquisition earlier after stress. In addition, the redistribution properties of thallium mandate that imaging begin relatively early after stress, and thus lung uptake may be more apparent.

With the technetium-99m perfusion tracers, liver uptake is more prominent than the heart immediately after injection; thus, image acquisition should begin 15 to 30 minutes after exercise stress injection and 30 to 60 minutes after pharmacological stress.[8] Thus, lung uptake, even if it had been present early after stress, may be missed with technetium-99m tracers because of the more delayed onset of imaging compared with thallium.

Transient Ischemic Dilation of the Left Ventricle. Transient ischemic dilation (TID) refers to an imaging pattern in which the left ventricle or left ventricular (LV) cavity appears larger on the stress images than at rest (see Fig. 13–8B).[16] For patients in whom the entire left ventricle appears larger during stress, the pathophysiology is probably related to extensive ischemia and prolonged postischemic systolic dysfunction, resulting in a dilated, dysfunctional left ventricle during the stress acquisition relative to the rest acquisition. In other patients, the epicardial silhouette appears similar at stress and rest, but there is apparent dilation in the LV cavity. This probably represents diffuse subendocardial ischemia (relatively less tracer uptake in the subendocardium creating the appearance of an enlarged cavity) and is also associated with severe and extensive CAD. Contemporary processing systems can automatically quantify TID.[17]

Both lung uptake and TID provide clues to more extensive CAD than may have been suspected from the perfusion pattern alone. Both signs have been associated with angiographically extensive and severe CAD and with unfavorable long-term outcomes and thus are considered "high-risk" findings.

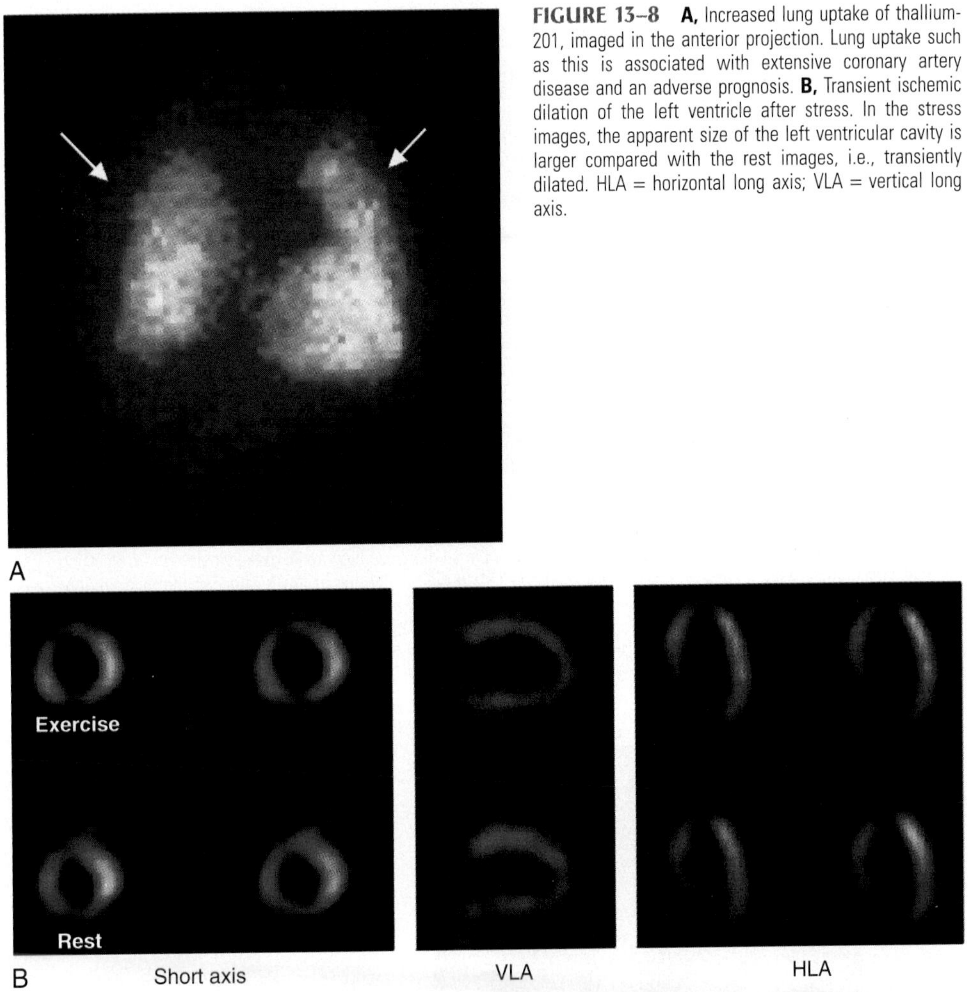

FIGURE 13–8 **A,** Increased lung uptake of thallium-201, imaged in the anterior projection. Lung uptake such as this is associated with extensive coronary artery disease and an adverse prognosis. **B,** Transient ischemic dilation of the left ventricle after stress. In the stress images, the apparent size of the left ventricular cavity is larger compared with the rest images, i.e., transiently dilated. HLA = horizontal long axis; VLA = vertical long axis.

COMMON NORMAL VARIATIONS IN SPECT IMAGING

Normal variations in perfusion images can be falsely interpreted as a defect. These perturbations from a completely homogeneous tracer pattern throughout the myocardium are related to structural variations of the myocardium as well as technical factors associated with image acquisition.

One example is the "dropout" of the upper septum because of the muscular septum merging with the membranous septum (Fig. 13–9A). Apical thinning is another variation of normal that can be mistaken for a perfusion defect (see Fig. 13–9B). The apex is anatomically thinner than other myocardial regions, creating this appearance. In normal SPECT images, the lateral wall may often appear brighter than the contralateral septum (see Fig. 13–9C). This is not due to a difference in lateral versus septal wall myocardial blood flow. Rather, during a SPECT acquisition, the camera is physically closer to the lateral myocardial wall (in close proximity to the lateral chest wall) than to the septum, thus subject to less soft tissue attenuation and associated with more efficient count capture. A careful review of a series of normal volunteers or subjects with a low probability of CAD with one's own equipment is an important step in minimizing the influence of these normal variations on the sensitivity and specificity for detecting CAD.[9]

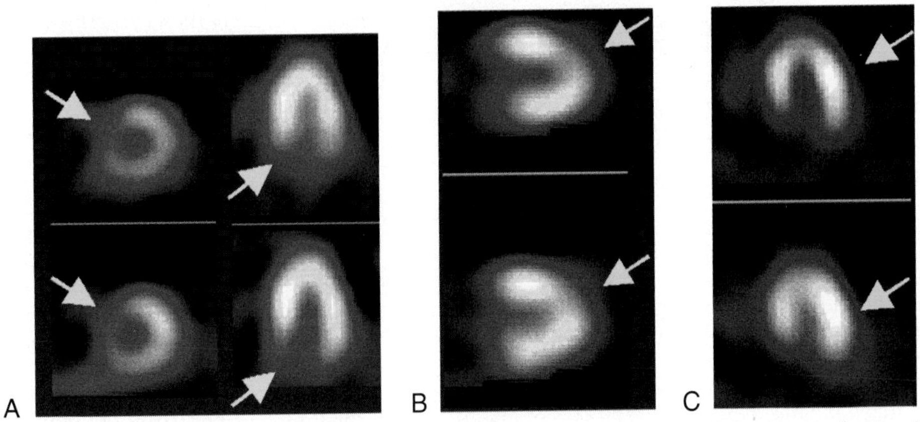

FIGURE 13–9 Normal variations in single-photon emission computed tomography perfusion imaging. **A,** Normal "dropout" of the basal septum. **B,** Normal apical thinning. **C,** The lateral wall is often slightly "hotter" than the septum, another normal variation.

Technical Artifacts Affecting Image Interpretation

Breast Attenuation. In patients with large or dense breasts, significant attenuation may create artifacts varying considerably in their appearance and location (Fig. 13–10A and B). A review of the cine display of the raw projection images may reveal the presence of potential breast attenuation.[5] Gender-matched quantitative data bases have had a favorable although modest impact on this issue, as such data bases generally consist of subjects who are of average body and breast size.

Several approaches toward minimizing the impact of breast tissue have been taken in order to improve specificity (lowering the false-positive rate) in women. Most well documented is the use of technetium-99m–based agents with SPECT imaging with electrocardiographic (ECG) gating. In the setting of a mild to moderately severe fixed defect, most often of the anterior or anterolateral wall, that may represent breast attenuation artifact versus nontransmural MI, the *presence of preserved wall motion suggests the absence of infarct* and supports the interpretation of attenuation artifact (see Fig. 13–10A, bottom). Specificity for ruling out CAD in women has been improved significantly with this technique,[18] as discussed subsequently.

Inferior Wall Attenuation. Inferior wall attenuation artifacts are commonly encountered in SPECT imaging. This

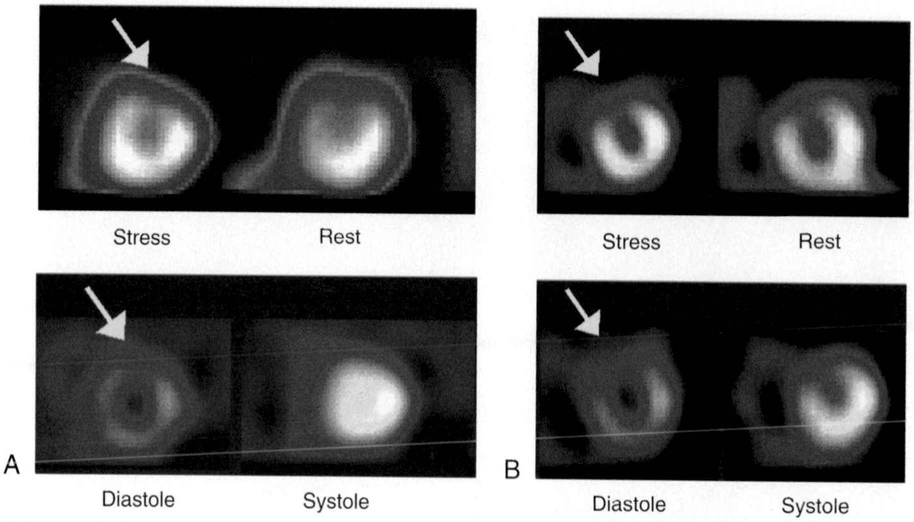

FIGURE 13–10 Breast attenuation artifact. **A,** Top row: a mild fixed anterior defect related to a possible breast attenuation artifact. In the bottom row, diastolic and systolic frames from an electrocardiographic-gated single-photon emission computed tomography (SPECT) acquisition demonstrating preserved wall thickening in the territory of the mild anterior fixed defect. The preserved wall thickening supports the conclusion that the mild defect is an attenuation artifact. **B,** A more severe anterior fixed defect is unlikely to represent an artifact on the basis of the severity and is more likely to represent myocardial infarction. In the bottom row, diastolic and systolic frames from the gated SPECT acquisition demonstrate abnormal thickening, supporting the interpretation of infarct rather than artifact.

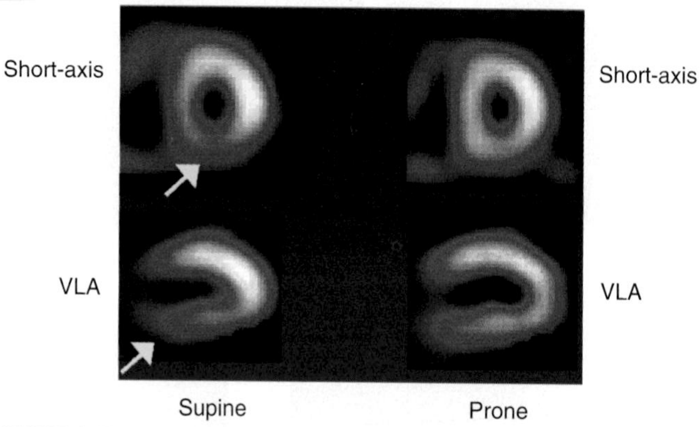

FIGURE 13–11 **Left,** Attenuation of the inferior basal wall (yellow arrows) possibly related to attenuation by overlying left hemidiaphragm. Most commonly, this appears as a tapering of the inferior wall seen best on the vertical long-axis (VLA) image. **Right,** One solution to the problem of inferior wall attenuation is reimaging the patient in the prone position.

artifact may be caused by extracardiac structures such as the diaphragm overlapping the inferior wall (Fig. 13–11). In addition, during a SPECT acquisition, the longer distance from the inferior wall to the camera means that photons must traverse a greater degree of tissue before reaching the detectors, which may increase the degree of scatter and attenuation.

As with breast attenuation artifact detection, the demonstration of preserved wall thickening by gated SPECT imaging may be helpful in distinguishing attenuation artifact from infarct. The patient's positioning may also minimize the degree of attenuation. When patients are imaged in the *prone* position,[19] the inferior wall is brought closer to the detector, although sometimes at the expense of image quality for the anterior wall (see Fig. 13–11).

Artifacts Related to Extracardiac Tracer Uptake. Tracer in extracardiac structures can cause artifacts in SPECT images. When such a structure is near the heart, increased counts may reach the detector. This may falsely elevate the number of counts the system assigns to the nearby cardiac wall, so that the cardiac region is displayed as falsely "hotter." A second possibility occurs when a nearby hot extracardiac structure causes a "ramp filter" or "negative lobe" artifact.[20] This artifact is due to a hot extracardiac structure "stealing" counts from the heart during the calculation of the summed SPECT images. The adjacent myocardium appears falsely "cool." If substantial extracardiac uptake is noted, image acquisition may be repeated after waiting a longer period of time before imaging. Having the patient drink cold water may enhance clearance of tracer from visceral organs, particularly bowel.

Attenuation Correction

Advances in camera hardware and computer software have led to new methods of *correcting for attenuation,* with the goal of reducing false-positive scans stemming from attenuation artifacts. Attenuation correction techniques use an associated transmission scan of an isotope distinct from the perfusion tracer to create a patient-specific "attenuation map." This map is then used to "correct" the patient's emission data (the perfusion images) for tissue attenuation specific to the patient. There are several methodologies for attenuation correction, reviewed in detail elsewhere.[21]

Although attenuation correction is a relatively new technique, there is now substantial validation of its effectiveness in improving the specificity of SPECT imaging for CAD.[22] At this writing, the hardware and software required for attenuation correction are not yet widely available, although its use is likely to grow given the published data. When such attenuation correction algorithms are used, it is important to interpret the original, uncorrected images as well as the corrected images.

Gated SPECT Display, Interpretation, and Quantitation

An important advance in the use and application of SPECT MPI has been the incorporation of ECG-gated SPECT perfusion imaging for *simultaneous assessment of LV function as well as perfusion.* Prior to the use of gated SPECT, comprehensive information on both perfusion and function required separate testing modalities, such as SPECT MPI and a separate radionuclide ventriculogram or echocardiogram

Electrocardiographically Gated Radionuclide Techniques to Assess the Physiology of Ventricular Function

To assess parameters of cardiac function with echocardiography, LV endocardial borders are drawn over several beats to derive parameters such as EF. With contrast left ventriculography, endocardial borders are drawn for either one beat or an average of several beats to calculate EF. In contrast, the commonly used radionuclide techniques to assess ventricular function create *one cardiac cycle for analysis that represents an average of several hundred beats* acquired over a period of 8 to 15 minutes, using a technique known as ECG gating (Fig. 13–12).

During an ECG-gated image acquisition, the patient's ECG is monitored simultaneously with the image.[23] As the peak of an R wave is detected, the "gate" opens and a set number of milliseconds of imaging information is stored in a "frame." For a typical gated SPECT acquisition, each R-R interval is divided into eight frames. For example, if the patient's resting heart rate is 60 beats/min (1000 milliseconds per beat), an eight-

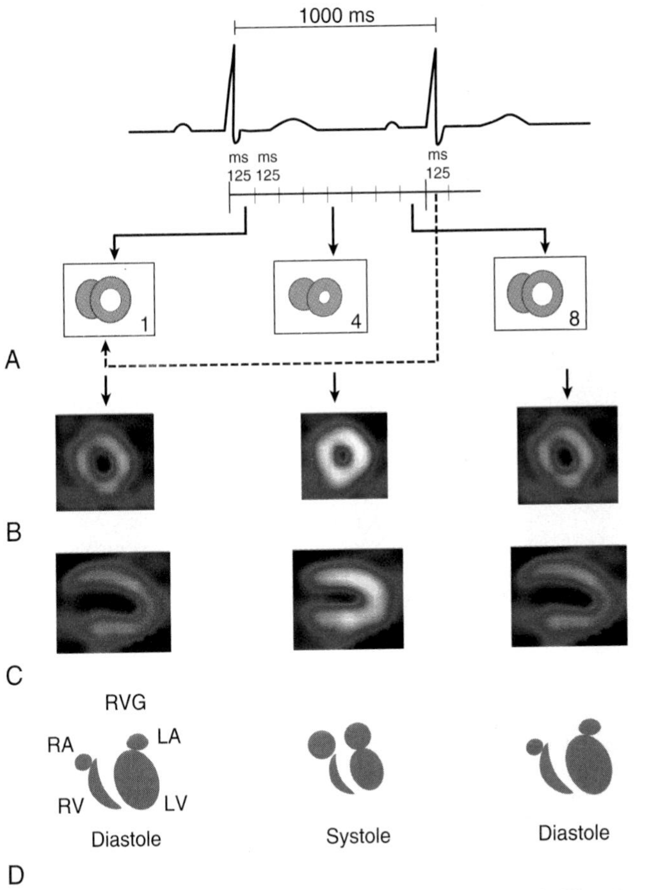

FIGURE 13–12 Basis for the technique of electrocardiographic (ECG) gating. **A,** The scintigraphic acquisition data are collected in conjunction with the electrocardiogram. The R-R interval is divided into a prespecified number of frames (in this example eight frames). At a heart rate of 60 beats/min (1000 msec/beat), each of the eight frames would comprise 125 milliseconds. For the first 125 milliseconds after the peak of the initial R wave, all imaging data are recorded in frame 1; the second 125 milliseconds are recorded in frame 2 and so on until the peak of the next R wave is detected, and this is repeated for each beat in the acquisition. Frame 1 thus represents the end-diastolic events, and one of the frames in the middle of the acquisition (frame 4 in this example) represents end-systolic events. **B,** Examples of gated single-photon emission computed tomography perfusion imaging. Short-axis images are seen at end diastole and at end systole. **C,** Similar timing with images displayed from the vertical long-axis orientation. Visually, wall thickening and brightening are seen across the course of systole. These events represent regional wall thickening and changes in global function across the cardiac cycle. **D,** ECG-gated equilibrium radionuclide ventriculographic (RVG) images are shown at diastole and at end systole. LA = left atrium; LV = left ventricle; RA = right atrium; RV = right ventricle. (Adapted from Germano G, Berman DS: Acquisition and processing for gated SPECT: Technical aspects. *In* Germano G, Berman DS [eds]: Clinical gated cardiac SPECT. Armonk, NY, Futura Publishing, 1999, pp 93-114.)

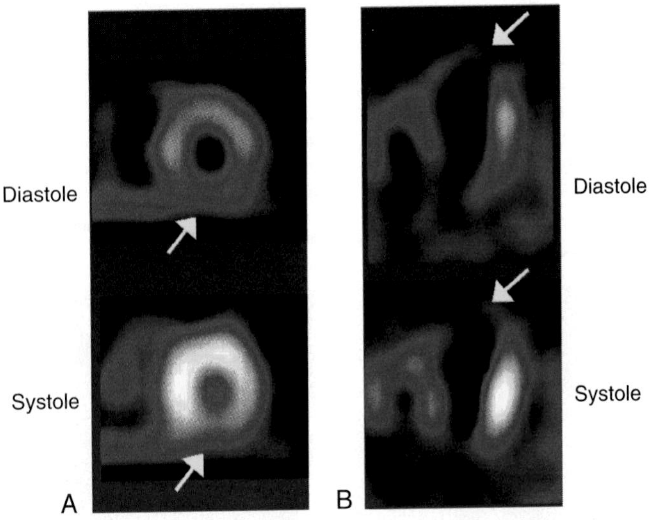

FIGURE 13–13 Examples of regional dysfunction detected by ECG-gated single-photon emission computed tomography perfusion imaging. **A,** The *hypokinetic* inferior region appears to brighten less (arrows) than the other regions from diastole to systole. **B,** The *akinetic* apex in the horizontal long axis (arrows) appears to have no change from diastole to systole, in contrast to the normally thickening (brightening) lateral walls.

frame acquisition across the cardiac cycle comprises 125 milliseconds per frame. After the first 125 milliseconds of imaging data have been recorded in frame 1, the gate closes and then instantly reopens, allowing the second 125 milliseconds of information to be recorded in frame 2 (see Fig. 13–12). This sequence continues through the prespecified number of frames throughout the cardiac cycle. When the R wave of the next beat is detected by the ECG-gated system, the sequence is repeated for each beat that occurs throughout the image acquisition.

The number of counts recorded during any individual cardiac cycle is insufficient to create an interpretable image. When several hundred beats have been recorded, an average cardiac cycle representing all the recorded beats can be reconstructed by redisplaying the frames sequentially in a cine or movie format. The first few frames represent systolic events, and the latter frames represent diastolic events (see Fig. 13–12).

High-quality ECG-gated images require that included cardiac cycles have reasonably homogeneous beat lengths. This is usually accomplished by "beat-length windowing," whereby the computer acquisition system is programmed to accept beats into the acquisition of only certain cycle lengths. Typically, the beat length represented by the average heart rate of the patient (1000 milliseconds in the preceding example) along with beat lengths of ±10 to 15 percent around the average length is allowed into the acquisition. Cardiac cycles with cycle lengths above or below that limit are rejected. For example, the short cardiac cycle from the R wave of a normal beat to the R wave of a premature ventricular contraction (PVC) would not be allowed into the acquisition, nor would the long cycle representing the post-PVC pause. This makes physiological sense; the short pre-PVC beat and the more prolonged post-PVC beat have distinctly different systolic and diastolic characteristics than the beats during normal sinus rhythm.

ECG-Gated SPECT Imaging. The technique most commonly used to assess ventricular function clinically is ECG-gated SPECT imaging.[23] Normal regional systolic function is depicted as brightening of the wall during systole (see Fig. 13–12B). The wall appears to thicken, and there is apparent endocardial excursion. Assessment of regional LV function by gated SPECT imaging is based on an effect known in imaging physics as the *partial volume effect*, sometimes referred to as the *recovery coefficient* effect. When objects being imaged fall below a certain thickness threshold, count (or photon) recovery from the object is related not only to the tracer concentration within that object but also to the thickness of the object.[24] For the myocardium, usually all thicknesses fall below that threshold for SPECT imaging. Although tracer concentration within the myocardium is constant during a gated SPECT image acquisition, the recovery of counts (and thus the brightness of the object being imaged) is related to wall thickness. Hence, during systolic wall thickening, it appears that the LV wall is becoming brighter and thicker, even though the isotope concentration per gram of myocardial tissue is actually unchanged. This principle forms the basis for gated SPECT imaging.

Regional myocardial function is usually assessed visually, in a manner similar to the analysis performed in echocardiography. Regions that brighten normally have normal regional systolic performance, and those with diminished but apparent brightening are labeled hypokinetic. Regions with slight brightening are interpreted as severely hypokinetic and regions with no apparent brightening as akinetic (Fig. 13–13). Regional function can also be analyzed by quantitative techniques and displayed in a polar map format.

Quantitative Analysis of Global Left Ventricular Function by Gated SPECT Imaging

All contemporary camera-computer systems have software capable of quantitative analysis of global LV function. These computer-based methodologies are fully automated and thus extremely reproducible. The most common method involves automated interrogation of the apparent epicardial and endocardial borders of all of the tomograms in all three orthogonal planes (Fig. 13–14A). These multiple two-dimensional contours are then reconstructed to create a surface-rendered three-dimensional display representing global LV function across a typical cardiac cycle (see Fig. 13–14B) that can be viewed from any direction by simple maneuvering of the computer display screen or cursor.[23] The three-dimensional display is accompanied by automated calculation of EF and LV volumes.

EF measurements from automated analysis of ECG-gated SPECT perfusion imaging have been extensively validated against other quantitative techniques assessing LV function, such as equilibrium radionuclide ventriculography (RVG), invasive measures of contrast left ventriculography, and cardiac magnetic resonance imaging.[23] Across a wide range of ventricular function, and even in the setting of severe perfusion defects, ECG-gated SPECT imaging provides robust, highly reproducible estimates of LVEF.

The incorporation of ECG-gated SPECT imaging into a SPECT acquisition is now routine in MPI and is recommended as standard by contemporary guidelines.[25] As discussed subsequently, the addition of LV function data to the perfusion information provides incremental and independent prognostic information as well as being of practical importance in management decisions. Gated SPECT imaging has also been an important advance in helping to differentiate attenuation artifacts from infarct, as regions with persistent low counts that show normal motion and thickening represent soft tissue artifacts rather than scar. Thus, gated SPECT has improved the specificity of perfusion imaging for ruling out CAD, particularly in women.[18]

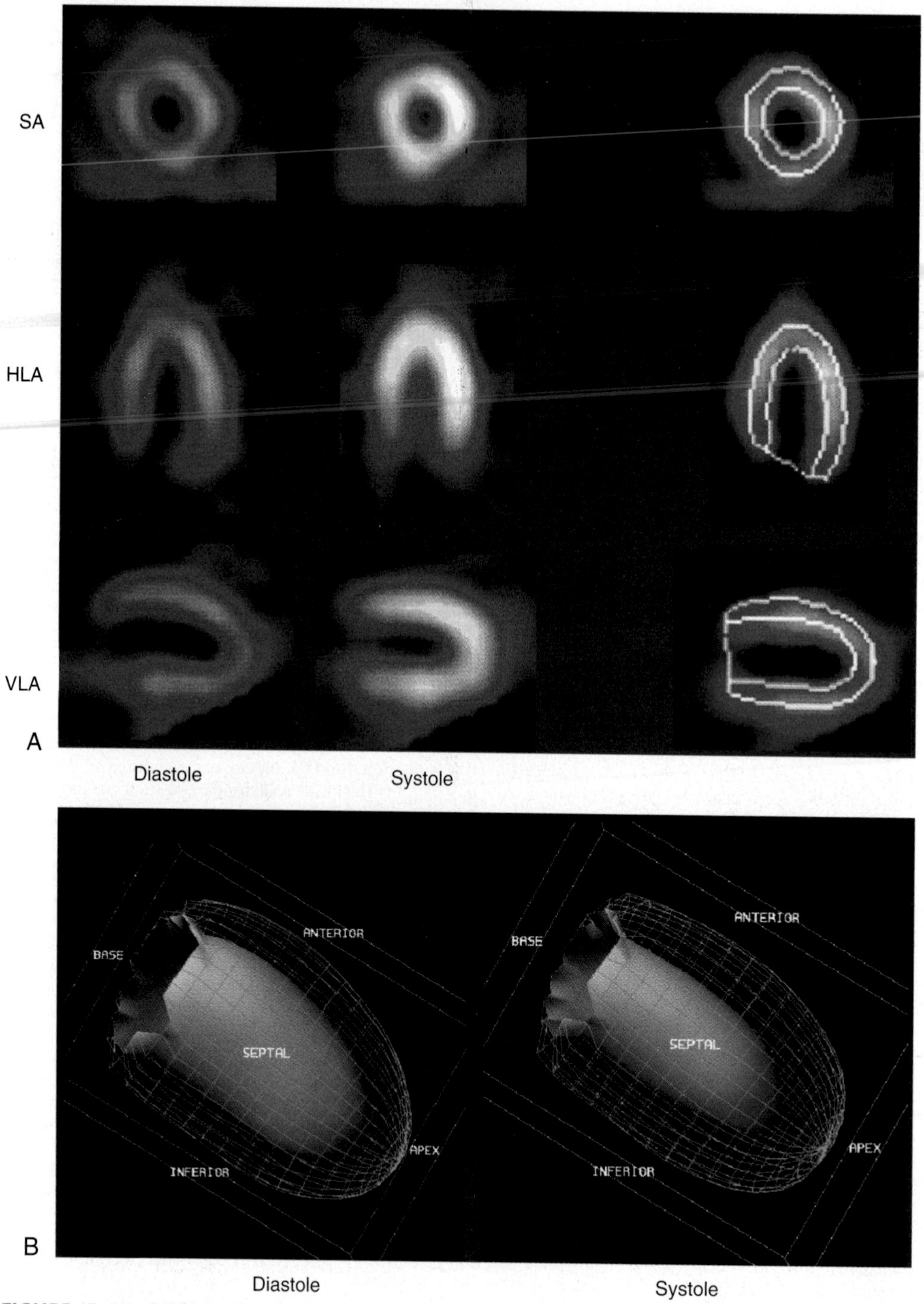

FIGURE 13–14 **A,** ECG-gated single-photon emission computed tomography (SPECT) perfusion images in short axis (SA), vertical long axis (VLA), and horizontal long axis (HLA), shown frozen at diastole (left column) and at end systole (middle column). Endocardial and epicardial borders are shown on the diastolic frames as automatically assigned by the software analysis program (right column). **B,** From the contours that are created from all of the two-dimensional tomograms, a three-dimensionally surface-rendered image of the left ventricle can be created and displayed in multiple orientations here frozen at end diastole (left) and end systole (right). The green "mesh" represents the epicardium, and the gray surface represents the endocardium. Ejection fraction is quantitated from the volume change. During image interpretation, gated SPECT images are displayed in the cine format, as an endless loop movie rather than as the still frames depicted here.

Planar Myocardial Perfusion Imaging

Prior to the widespread application of tomographic (SPECT) perfusion imaging techniques, planar imaging was the standard acquisition and display methodology. In planar imaging, three separate two-dimensional images are obtained with the gamma camera following radiotracer injection and uptake into the myocardium.[26] The three standard views are an anterior, a left anterior oblique, and a more lateral view (Fig. 13–15).

Using planar imaging, the imaging views are standard and the reader must account for the different orientations of the heart in assignng regional abnormalities. In contrast, because the tomographic slices of SPECT imaging are constructed perpendicular and parallel to an assigned long axis, SPECT images are oriented in a uniform manner for display and interpretation without influence by the individual patient's cardiac orientation.

An advantage of planar imaging over SPECT imaging is its simplicity. Each of the three views can be acquired

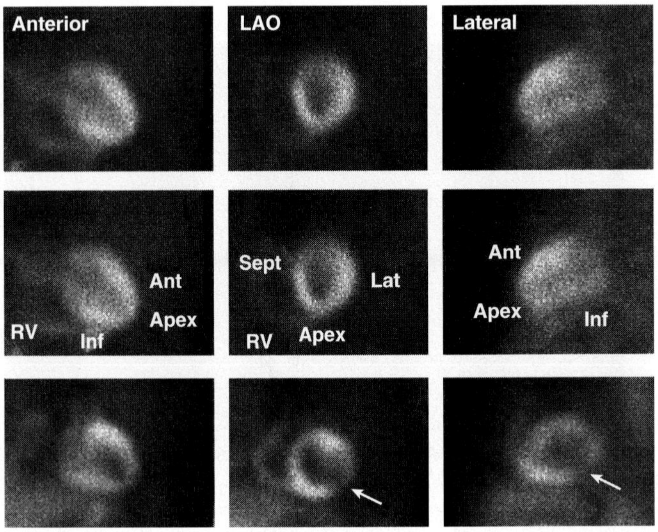

FIGURE 13–15 Examples of planar myocardial perfusion imaging. **Top row:** A normal stress planar perfusion study in the anterior, shallow left anterior oblique (LAO), and more lateral views. Tracer uptake is uniform throughout the myocardial walls. **Middle row:** The same normal planar stress perfusion images are shown, with the myocardial walls that are seen in each view labeled. The anterior wall (ant), apex, and inferior (inf) walls are seen in the anterior view as well as the right ventricle (RV). The septum (sept), apex, and lateral walls (lat) and the RV are seen in the shallow LAO view, and the anterior wall, apex, and inferior walls are seen in the lateral view. **Bottom row:** Example of an abnormal planar study showing a lateral wall stress perfusion defect in the shallow LAO view (arrow), extending into the inferior wall in the lateral view (arrow). Rest images are not shown. (Courtesy of Kim A. Williams, M.D.)

over 5 to 8 minutes with patients lying on a table with their arms by their side. Planar imaging is less affected by patients' motion than is SPECT imaging. With planar imaging, there is no extensive image processing as with SPECT, which creates many more sources of potential error and artifact. However, given the two-dimensional nature of planar imaging, in each of the standard views there is substantial overlap of myocardial regions and less ability to differentiate smaller and particularly milder perfusion abnormalities. The more standard orientation of SPECT imaging lends itself to easier understanding of the localization of perfusion abnormalities.

The original data on the sensitivity and specificity of perfusion imaging for CAD, as well as the prognostic value of perfusion imaging, were developed using planar imaging and later revalidated using SPECT imaging. In contemporary practice, planar imaging may be used for patients who do not tolerate the position that must be maintained during a SPECT acquisition, those who have difficulty coping with the larger SPECT camera being so close to the body, or those with large body habitus that surpasses the weight and size limits of SPECT systems.[10]

Quantitative analytical techniques such as the circumferential profile technique were originally developed using planar perfusion imaging.[2] A substantial literature has documented that when quantitative analysis is applied to planar perfusion imaging, there is an improvement in the sensitivity to detect multivessel CAD.

Radionuclide Angiography or Ventriculography

Radionuclide angiography (RNA), also known as RVG or blood pool imaging, may be performed by *first-pass* or by *equilibrium gated* techniques.[27,28] The equilibrium technique is often referred to as multiple gated acquisition (MUGA) scanning. Although the two techniques use distinct tracers and data recording, they provide similar results for global EF and chamber volumes. Both techniques provide a highly reproducible means to quantify global LV and right ventricular (RV) EF.

Equilibrium Radionuclide Angiography or Ventriculography (Gated Blood Pool Imaging)

In equilibrium RVG studies, data are recorded in a computer system synchronized with the R wave of the patient's ECG, similar to ECG-gated SPECT (see Fig. 13–12). Most commonly, technetium-99m labeling is applied to red blood cells or albumin. Image contrast is usually better with ^{99m}Tc-labeled red blood cells, but ^{99m}Tc-labeled albumin is preferable in patients in whom red blood cell labeling may be difficult. Labeling of red blood cells with ^{99m}Tc pertechnetate requires a reducing agent, stannous pyrophosphate, which is administered 15 to 30 minutes prior to pertechnetate injection. The reader is referred to reviews of red blood cell labeling techniques for additional detail.[29]

Image Acquisition. Although few counts are recorded during a single ECG-gated cardiac cycle, the summation of counts from 800 to 1000 cardiac cycles produces an average cardiac cycle with high resolution. Images of the heart are usually acquired in three standard projections: anterior, left anterior oblique (best separation of the left and right ventricles), and left lateral (or left posterior oblique). The minimum framing rate for a resting RVG study is 16 frames/cycle (about 50 msec/frame).[27] For quantitative assessment of diastolic indices and regional EF, the framing rate should be increased to 32 frames/cycle (about 25 msec/frame). For adequate counting statistics, images are acquired for a preset count of at least 250,000 per frame or count density of 300 counts per pixel, which corresponds to an acquisition time of 5 to 10 minutes per projection. For exercise studies, adequate counts can be obtained in the best septal view with a 2-minute acquisition using a high-sensitivity collimator. Arrhythmias such as multiple PVCs can adversely affect the study if these beats account for more than 10 percent of the total. In patients with atrial fibrillation, there may be considerable beat-to-beat variability, and the mean EF obtained over the period of acquisition may underestimate the actual LVEF.[27]

Image Display and Analysis. Qualitative inspection of equilibrium studies as an endless cinematic loop of the cardiac cycle (see Fig. 13–12D) allows assessment of (1) the size of heart chambers and great vessels; (2) regional wall motion; (3) global function (qualitative assessment) (Fig. 13–16A and B); (4) ventricular wall thickness, pericardial effusion, or paracardiac pericardial fat pad or mass; and (5) extracardiac uptake (such as splenomegaly). Quantification of systolic and diastolic indices and volumes is derived from the ventricular time-activity curve,[30] which is analogous to the angiographic time-volume curve (Fig. 13–17). In addition to the time-activity curve, functional images, such as amplitude and phase images, can be produced that have been useful in characterizing regional asynergy and asynchrony.

First-Pass Radionuclide Angiography or Ventriculography

In first-pass RVG studies, the bolus of radioactivity passes initially through the right chambers of the heart, then through the lungs, and finally through the left-sided chambers of the heart. Radiopharmaceuticals used for this purpose must produce adequate counts in a short period of time at an acceptably low radiation dose to the patient.[28] Although both technetium-99m diethylenetriaminepentaacetic acid (DTPA) and ^{99m}Tc pertechnetate have short intravascular residence time, ^{99m}Tc-DTPA is the recommended radionuclide of choice because the DTPA salt enhances renal excretion.

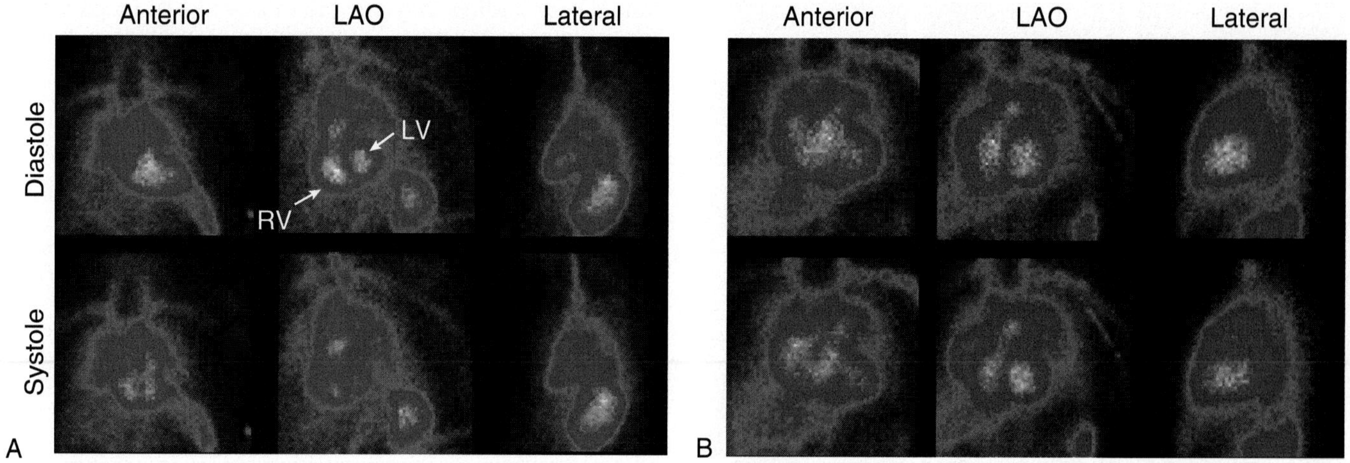

FIGURE 13–16 Equilibrium radionuclide ventriculography (RVG). The isotope (Tc99m) is labeled to red blood cells, and hence the images represent the blood "pools" in the left ventricle (LV), the right ventricle (RV), the other cardiac chambers and the great vessels, as well as the spleen. Typically, three views are obtained, as shown. **A,** Normal left ventricular function, with end-diastolic images in the top row and end-systolic images in the bottom row. LV and RV volumes diminish from diastole to systole. **B,** Images obtained in a patient with LV dysfunction. There is significant LV and RV dilatation at both end diastole (top) and end systole (bottom), and severely dimished LV systolic function (i.e., much less volume change from end diastole to end systole compared to the study in panel A). LAO = left anterior oblique projection.

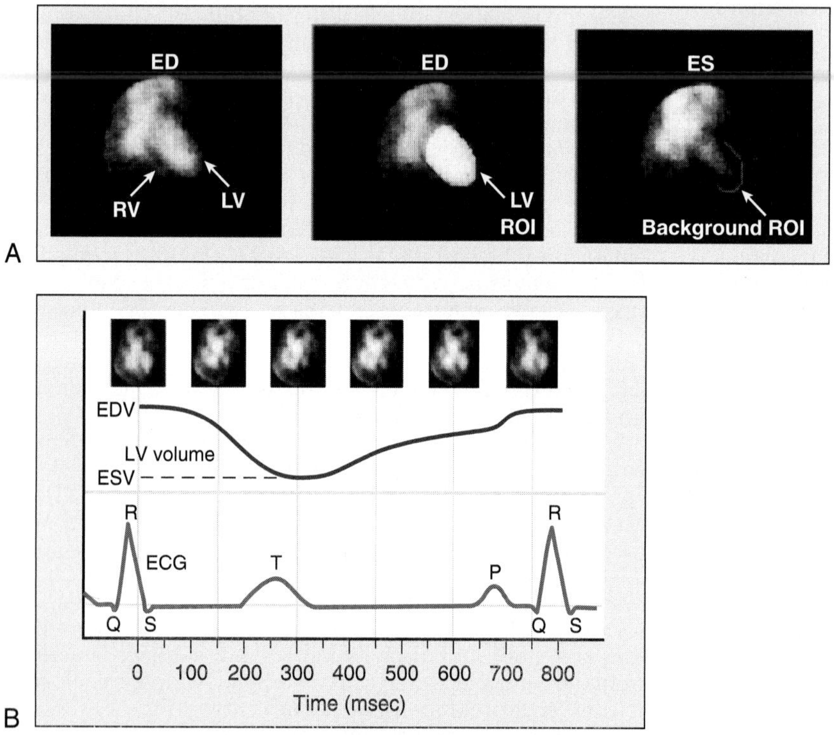

FIGURE 13–17 Quantitative analysis of equilibrium ECG-gated radionuclide ventriculography. **A,** The left anterior oblique view of the left ventricle (LV) and right ventricle (RV) is shown at end diastole (ED) **(left)**, with a region of interest (ROI) identifying the LV contour at end diastole **(middle)** and a "background" ROI drawn at end systole (ES) **(right)**, used to correct for count activity in front of and behind the LV. In **B,** a time-activity curve is demonstrated that illustrates the change in counts within the regions of interest shown in A across a cardiac cycle. Because count activity is related to LV chamber volume, the time-activity curve represents the relative volume change of the LV chamber across a cardiac cycle, from end diastole to end systole and back to end diastole. EDV = end-diastolic volume; ESV = end-systolic volume. (From Green MV, Bacharach SL, Douglas MA, et al: The measurement of left ventricular function and the detection of wall motion abnormalities with high temporal resolution ECG-gated scintigraphic angiocardiography. IEEE Trans Nucl Sci NS-23, 1976.)

Image Acquisition. Images are acquired very rapidly as the tracer passes through the heart chambers. Separation of the right and left ventricles is achieved because of the temporal separation of the bolus. Image quality is related to the injection technique, which should be rapid (over 2 to 3 seconds) in order to achieve an uninterrupted bolus (Fig. 13–18). Images are acquired in the supine position following the rapid injection of 25 mCi of tracer through an 18-gauge or larger intravenous catheter placed in the medial antecubital or external jugular vein. The shallow (20 to 30 degree) right anterior oblique projection is used to optimize separation of the atria and great vessels from the ventricles and to view the ventricles parallel to their long axes. Although the right anterior oblique view maximizes overlap of the right and left ventricles, this is not a problem in most patients because the timing of tracer appearance reliably identifies each chamber sequentially. A 1-mCi tracer dose may be used to ensure proper positioning so that the right and left ventricles are in the field of view.

Image Analysis. To identify the RV and LV phases, regions of interest are drawn around the right and left ventricles at end diastole.[28] Time-activity curves are generated, and cycles around and including the peak time-activity curve are used to calculate EFs. In general, two to five cardiac cycles are summed for the RV phase, and five to seven cycles are summed for the LV phase. From these data, quantitative analysis of LV and RV EF is performed.

COMPARISON OF EQUILIBRIUM AND FIRST-PASS TECHNIQUES

Advantages of the first-pass technique are the high target-to-background ratio, more distinct temporal separation of the cardiac chambers, and rapidity of imaging. RV EF may be more readily assessed using the first-pass technique because of the more distinct separation of this structure from the other chambers with that technique. Advantages of equilibrium technique are the potential for repeated assessment of cardiac function during rapidly varying physiological conditions, high count density, and acquisition of images in multiple projections. In contemporary practice, the equilibrium technique is performed more commonly.[10]

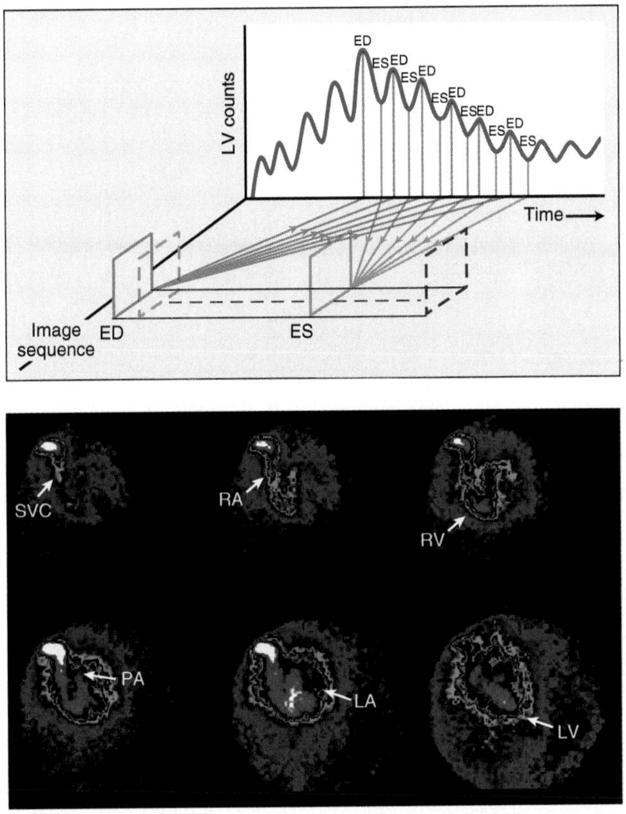

A

B

FIGURE 13–18 First-pass radionuclide ventriculography. **A,** First-pass image acquisition and analysis. ED = end diastole; ES = end systole. (From Bacharach SL, Green MV, Borer JS: Instrumentation and data processing in cardiovascular nuclear medicine: Evaluation of ventricular function. Semin Nucl Med 9:257-274, 1979.) **B,** Individual frames from a first-pass radionuclide ventriculography acquisition, illustrating the path of the bolus isotope through the superior vena cava (SVC), the right atrium (RA), the right ventricle (RV), the pulmonary outflow tract and lungs (pulmonary artery, PA), the left atrium (LA), and the left ventricular (LV) phase, from which the isotope bolus is then distributed systemically.

TABLE 13–2 Properties of Selected Positron-Emission Tomography Tracers

Tracer	Produced	Half-Life	Compound
Perfusion			
Oxygen-15	Cyclotron	2.1 min	H_2O
Nitrogen-13	Cyclotron	10 min	NH_3
Rubidium-82	Generator	76 sec	RbCl
Metabolism			
Carbon-11	Cyclotron	20.4 min	Acetate Palmitate
Fluorine-18	Cyclotron	110 min	Deoxyglucose

Adapted from Bergmann SR: Positron emission tomography of the heart. *In* Gerson MC (ed): Cardiac Nuclear Medicine. New York, McGraw-Hill, 1997, pp 267-300.

POSITRON-EMISSION TOMOGRAPHY

Because of the quantitative capabilities of positron-emission tomography (PET), measurement of myocardial perfusion and metabolism can be obtained with PET in absolute quantitative terms, a potential advantage compared with SPECT imaging. The radiotracers used in PET are labeled with positron-emitting isotopes that have chemical and physical properties identical to those of naturally occurring elements, such as carbon, oxygen, nitrogen, and fluorine. *Incorporating such elements allows interrogation of physiologically relevant processes in normal and diseased states.*[31] Although most positron-emitting radiotracers are cyclotron produced with short half-lives, the development of *generator-produced* positron-emitting isotopes, such as rubidium, makes it feasible for laboratories to perform cardiac PET studies without an on-site cyclotron.

Clinically available cardiac PET radiotracers fall within two broad categories: those that evaluate myocardial perfusion and those that evaluate myocardial metabolism (Table 13–2).[10] The perfusion tracers, rubidium-82 and [^{13}N]ammonia, and the myocardial metabolic tracer ^{18}F-labeled 2-fluoro-2-deoxyglucose (FDG) have received U.S. Food and Drug Administration approval.

Image Acquisition. PET employs camera systems designed to optimize the detection of positron-emitting radioisotopes. The process by which a positron-emitting radionuclide attempts to stabilize over time is termed beta decay, which occurs when the nucleus of an atom emits a positron, a positively charged beta particle. A negatively charged beta particle represents an electron (Fig. 13–19A). After a high-energy positron is emitted from a nucleus, it travels a few millimeters in tissue and collides with an electron. This collision results in complete annihilation of both the positron and the electron, with conversion to energy in the form of electromagnetic radiation composed of two high-energy gamma rays, each with 511-keV energy. The discharged gamma rays travel in perfectly opposite directions (180 degrees from each other). PET detectors can be programmed to register only events with temporal *coincidence* of photons that strike at directly opposing detectors (see Fig. 13–19B). The outcome of such selective *coincidence detection* is an improvement in spatial and temporal resolution of PET compared with SPECT imaging.[32] Unlike the procedure in SPECT, in which an extrinsic collimator is used to limit the direction at which photons enter the detector, the coincidence detection with PET provides intrinsic collimation and improves the sensitivity of the camera. An attenuation scan is acquired (using a rod source or external ring of radioactivity) before emission data collection in order to measure photon attenuation correction factors.

In addition, an important distinction between PET and SPECT is in the ease of labeling primary substrates for energy metabolism and membrane receptor subtypes in the heart, allowing the interrogation of such pathways in vivo. Moreover, dynamic mode with PET scanning allows potential analysis of the *change in tracer content* in a specific region of interest in the heart with time.

Image Analysis. Emission data are displayed as tomograms in the horizontal and vertical long-axis and short-axis views.[32] If the data are acquired in dynamic mode, with appropriate mathematical modeling, myocardial perfusion and metabolic data can be displayed in absolute terms: in milliliters per gram per minute for blood flow and moles per gram per minute for metabolism.

PET Perfusion Tracers. PET perfusion tracers can be divided into two types: (1) freely diffusible tracers, which accumulate and wash out from myocardial tissue as a function of blood flow, and (2) nondiffusible tracers, characterized by retention in myocardial tissue as a function of blood flow.[31] The rapid physiological washout of the freely diffusible tracers, such as ^{15}O-labeled water, makes it possible to repeat studies in rapid sequence. The images of the distribution of such tracers are usually not visually meaningful; mathematical modeling is done to arrive at flow values at each pixel. An advantage of freely diffusible tracers is that they do not depend on a metabolic trapping mechanism that might change as a function of a changing metabolic environment.

The nondiffusible flow tracers are easier to image as the tracer is retained in myocardium for a reasonable length of time. Rubidium-82 and [^{13}N]ammonia fall into this second category of flow tracers—the more microsphere-like flow tracers. Rubidium-82 is a cation, with biological properties similar to those of potassium and thallium. Uptake across the sarcolemmal membrane reflects active transport by the Na^+,K^+-ATPase pump. In experimental studies, its extraction fraction does not change significantly over a wide range of metabolic conditions. However, the very short half-life of 75 seconds for ^{82}Rb means that any trapped ^{82}Rb quickly disappears from the myocardium by physical decay. Despite its short half-life, ^{82}Rb is easily obtained as it is generator produced, and it can be used clinically without the need for an on-site cyclotron.

[^{13}N]Ammonia is an extractable perfusion tracer, with a physical half-life of 10 minutes. Its transport across cell membranes may occur by passive diffusion or by the active Na-K transport mechanism. Retention of [^{13}N]ammonia in the myocyte involves metabolic trapping. As with rubidium-82, myocardial uptake of ammonia reflects absolute blood flows up to 2 to 3 ml/gm/min and plateaus at more hyperemic flows. The use of this tracer to assess myocardial blood flow has been extensively validated in both experimental and clinical studies.[32]

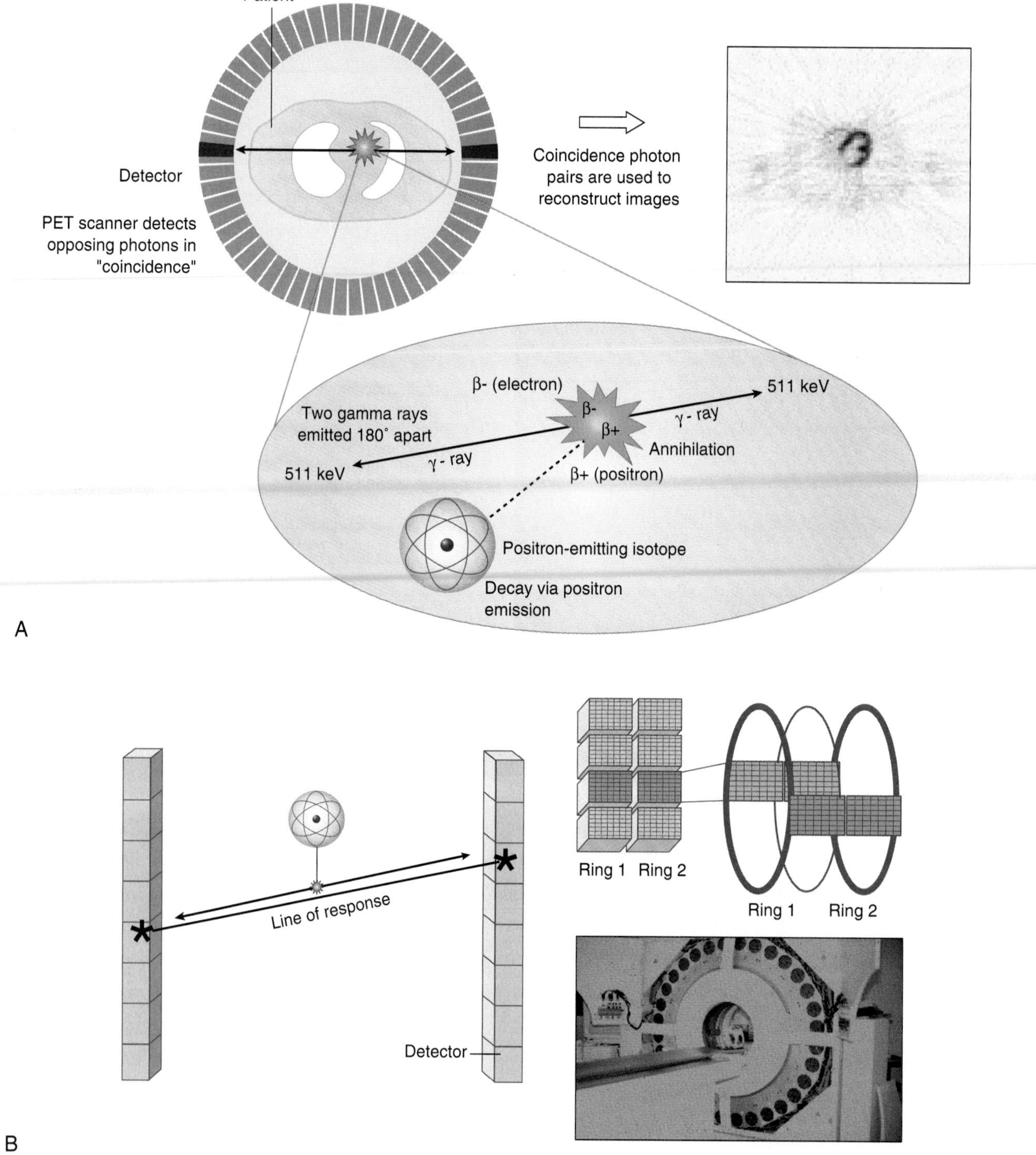

FIGURE 13–19 **A,** Schematic of positron and electron beta particle emission as the basis of positron-emission tomography (PET) imaging. **B,** Schematic of PET camera coincidence detection. (Courtesy of Martin Logde and Bruce Line.)

Assessment of the Physiology and Pathophysiology of Myocardial Blood Flow, Myocardial Metabolism, and Ventricular Function

Assessment of Myocardial Blood Flow by Radionuclide Imaging

Resting Myocardial Blood Flow

Myocardial blood flow at rest is tightly regulated in order to provide nutritive perfusion to viable, contractile myocytes. SPECT tracers to image myocardial blood flow are commonly referred to as "perfusion tracers," that is, *the magnitude of regional tracer uptake is proportional to the magnitude of regional myocardial blood flow*. However, although these tracers are delivered to regions of myocardium by perfusion, they require viable myocyte cell membranes for uptake and retention in order to be visualized.[33] Thus, the uptake and retention of the tracers reflect regional flow differences, with myocyte cell membrane integrity being a prerequisite. Although visualization of myocardial regions suggests the presence of working, viable cell membranes, lack of visualization of myocardium does not necessarily suggest the absence of viable cells. Decreased regional myocardial tracer uptake at rest could reflect either lack of cell membrane integrity in an area of infarcted myocardium or reduced blood flow secondary to hibernating but viable myocardium. A severe reduction in tracer activity usually signifies infarction, and a more moderate reduction in regional activity of a blood flow tracer *alone* cannot always differentiate hibernating from partially scarred myocardium in patients with ischemic LV dysfunction. In that setting, techniques that assess intact cellular metabolic processes, e.g., FDG, or myocardial potassium space, e.g., thallium-201 redistribution, are sometimes used as an adjunct to resting myocardial blood flow.[34]

Imaging Myocardial Infarction. In patients with prior MI, blood flow to the infarcted region is usually diminished, often severely, and there are few viable myocytes within the scarred territory.[10] Thus, severely reduced uptake of a radionuclide perfusion tracer in a resting study is a good marker of presence, location, and extent of MI (Fig. 13–20).

Assessment of Infarct Size. Contemporary studies have used ^{99m}Tc sestamibi to provide an assessment of infarct size.[35] As there is minimal clearance out of the myocardium following initial uptake, images acquired even hours after initial injection represent a "snapshot" of blood flow conditions and tracer uptake at the time of injection.

Infarct size as assessed by quantitative analysis of resting sestamibi uptake has been validated against many other measures of infarct size.[36] Moreover, a significant association between sestamibi infarct size and mortality over long-term follow-up has been demonstrated. Many clinical trials now use final infarct size by sestamibi SPECT imaging as an early post-MI surrogate endpoint to assess new agents to reduce infarct size.

When a tracer such as sestamibi is injected *during acute infarction* in the setting of an occluded infarct-related artery *before reperfusion therapy*, the resulting defect, even when imaged hours later after successful reperfusion, represents the *risk area* of the occluded artery.[35] A second injection of sestamibi at rest with subsequent imaging can be done at a later time during the post-MI course and represents *final infarct size*. The change in defect size between the initial image acquired in the acute stage and the later image represents the *magnitude of salvaged myocardium from reperfusion*. Hence, SPECT imaging at rest in the early postinfarct period can provide important information regarding final infarct size and infarct zone viability.

Assessment of Myocardial Perfusion During Stress

Coronary blood flow must respond rapidly to changing metabolic conditions and oxygen demand in order to meet the nutrient needs of myocytes being called on to contract more quickly and with more force. Oxygen extraction by the myocardium is near maximum at rest; thus, any increase in oxygen demand can be met only through increasing coronary blood flow to deliver more oxygen per unit time. The major determinants of coronary blood flow include the perfusion pressure at the head of the system (principally aortic diastolic pressure) and the downstream resistance, residing predominantly in the coronary *arteriolar* bed. Because aortic diastolic pressure during exercise varies little from the resting value, the major mechanism responsible for increasing coronary blood flow during stress involves a reduction in coronary vascular resistance. During *exercise* stress, coronary blood flow can increase approximately two to three times over resting levels. During *pharmacological* stress to minimize coronary arteriolar resistance, with intravenous coronary arteriolar vasodilator agents such as dipyridamole or adenosine (discussed further later), coronary blood flow can increase up to four to five times over resting levels. The magnitude of blood flow increase secondary to any stress relative to resting flow values is termed *coronary blood flow reserve*.[37]

PERFUSION TRACERS AND CORONARY BLOOD FLOW RESERVE. The ideal perfusion tracer should track myocardial blood flow across the entire physiologically relevant range of blood flow achievable in animal models and in humans (Fig. 13–21). It should be taken up rapidly, as the hemodynamic conditions during peak stress are not maintained for long periods of time. The ideal tracer should be taken up (extracted) as completely as possible out of the bloodstream, and it should be retained in myocardium for a sufficient period to be imaged. Moreover, perturbations in metabolic conditions, such as ischemia, or commonly used cardioactive drugs should neither influence nor interfere with uptake so that the resulting regional tracer concentrations primarily reflect myocardial perfusion.[33]

Despite the excellent first-pass myocardial extraction (85 percent), the energy spectrum of thallium is lower (69 to 80 keV) than optimum for current gamma cameras. The 140-keV energy spectrum of ^{99m}Tc perfusion tracers results in less scatter and soft tissue attenuation, with improved spatial resolution compared with thallium.[8] However, the first-pass myocardial extraction of both sestamibi and tetrofosmin is only in

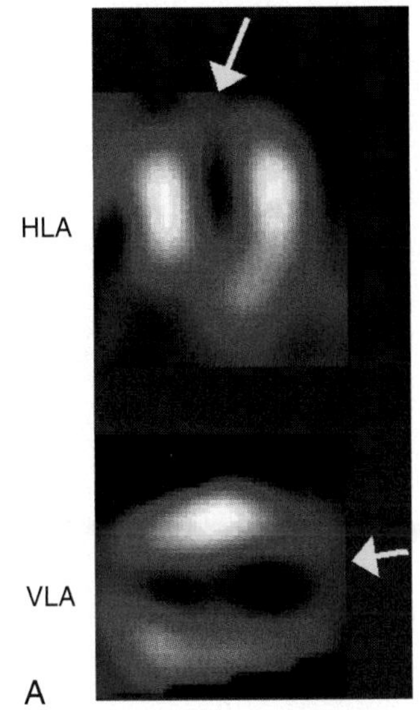

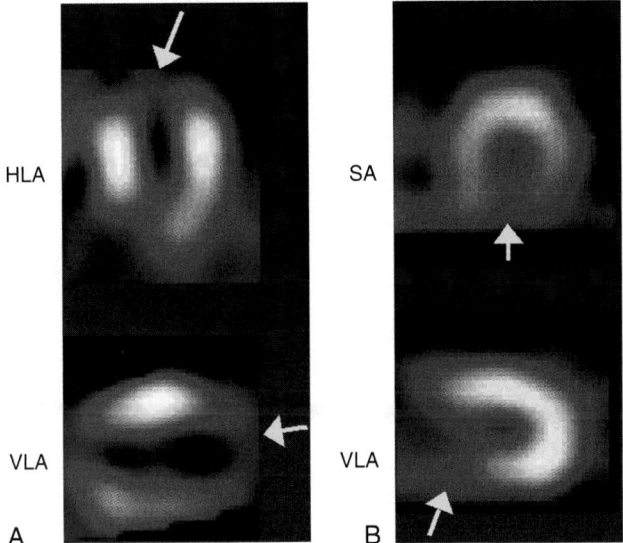

FIGURE 13–20 Single-photon emission computed tomography perfusion images demonstrating myocardial infarction in different locations. **A,** An apical infarction (arrow) in the horizontal long-axis (HLA) and vertical long-axis (VLA) views. **B,** An inferior infarction in the short-axis (SA) and VLA views. In both studies, the *severity* of the defect suggests minimal myocyte viability within those territories.

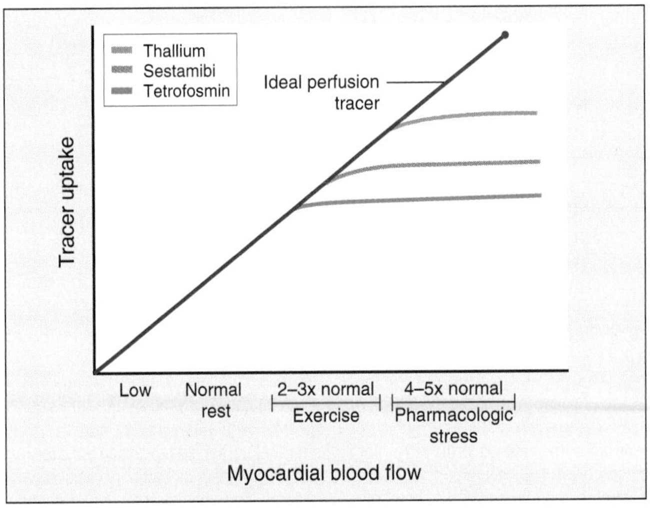

FIGURE 13–21 The relation between myocardial blood flow and perfusion tracer uptake. The ideal perfusion tracer would track myocardial blood flow across the entire range of physiologically relevant flows. However, the available perfusion tracers "roll off" at higher levels of flow. The different tracers begin to reach a plateau at different levels of myocardial blood flow, as demonstrated in this schematic example based on multiple studies in animal models.

the 60 percent range with nonlinear extraction at high flows. Thus, none of the clinically available SPECT perfusion tracers have all of the properties of an ideal perfusion tracer (see Fig. 13–21). Nonetheless, regional differences in myocardial tracer uptake during exercise or pharmacological stress have provided important diagnostic as well as prognostic information.[10]

The PET perfusion tracer [^{13}N]ammonia displays an extraction fraction exceeding 90 percent; rubidium-82 has a lower extraction fraction and reaches a plateau more rapidly at hyperemic range of flow. In the clinical setting, the evaluation of regional myocardial blood flow and flow reserve with [^{13}N]ammonia and rubidium-82 has also been validated for detecting and localizing CAD.[10] Because exercise studies are difficult to perform in the PET scanner and attenuation correction with PET requires close alignment of transmission and emission data, most PET studies evaluating coronary flow reserve use pharmacological rather than exercise stress.

EFFECT OF A CORONARY STENOSIS ON CORONARY BLOOD FLOW RESERVE. In animal models in which discrete coronary stenoses of varying degrees were induced, *resting* coronary blood flow was maintained by autoregulatory dilation of the downstream arteriolar resistance vessels until a stenosis between 80 and 90 percent diameter was reached (Fig. 13–22). As stenosis severity increases further, the arteriolar vasodilatory capacity to maintain resting flow is exhausted, at which point resting coronary blood flow diminishes.[38]

In contrast, *maximum coronary blood flow reserve* begins to decrease when the upstream coronary stenosis reaches 50 percent diameter. There are three levels of resistance that influence coronary blood flow: that provided by the large conductance epicardial vessels (R1), the coronary arteriolar resistance (R2), and the resistance in the subendocardium by wall tension from the ventricular chamber (R3) (see Fig. 13–22). Under normal conditions, most of the resistance at rest is provided by R2, and most of the increase in coronary flow during heightened demand occurs through reduction of resistance at this level, potentially increasing flow as much as four times as demand increases. Normal epicardial vessels dilate slightly (R1 decreases slightly) in response to increased coronary flow as a consequence of normal endothelial cell function. Depending on the type of exercise that is performed, the R3 component may remain unchanged or may increase, with an increase in chamber radius and wall tension. Achieving maximal flow is predominantly dependent on the vasodilatory capacity of the downstream resistance vessels.[37,38] With a coronary stenosis, in which some vasodilatory reserve has been used to maintain resting flow, less vasodilatory reserve is available to minimize resistance during stress. Thus, in a vessel with a moderate stenosis, *coronary blood flow reserve* is blunted and detectable by a perfusion tracer (see Fig. 13–22).

In contrast to animal models, human CAD is more complex. Stenoses may not be discrete, the length and complexity of the stenosis may affect the coronary reserve, and impaired endothelial function plays a role.[39] In subjects with preserved endothelial function, the increased coronary flow during stress leads to coronary arterial and arteriolar vasodilation, contributing to maximal coronary flow reserve. Endothelial function is often abnormal with early atherosclerosis, or risk factors for atherosclerosis, contributing to the blunting of coronary flow reserve.[40] The development of collaterals to the distal perfusion bed of a myocardial territory with a severe upstream coronary stenosis also influences blood flow at rest and during stress.[41]

With SPECT imaging, *relative* regional differences of tracer uptake can be detected and quantified (Fig. 13–23), whereas with PET imaging, *absolute* regional coronary blood flow at rest and during stress (in milliliters per gram per minute) can be quantified.[32]

Detecting Stress-Induced Ischemia Versus Infarct with Myocardial Perfusion Imaging. In standard practice, stress and rest myocardial perfusion images are compared in order to determine the presence, extent, and severity of stress-induced perfusion defects and to determine whether such defects represent regions of myocardial ischemia or infarction.[8,9,10] *Regions with stress-induced perfusion abnormalities, which have normal perfusion at rest, are termed reversible perfusion defects and represent viable regions with blunted coronary blood flow reserve* (Fig. 13–24). Strictly speaking, SPECT MPI is demonstrating stress induced reversible abnormalities in perfusion reserve, although these findings are often referred to as "ischemia." Regional myocardial *tissue ischemia* per se is not being demonstrated, although it is indeed often present, based on a mismatch between oxygen supply and demand. Perfusion abnormalities at stress that are *irreversible*, or *fixed*, as seen on resting images (unchanged from stress to rest) most often represent infarction, particularly if the defect is severe (see Fig. 13–24). When both viable myocardium and scarred myocardium are present, thallium redistribution or technetium 99m tracer reversibility is incomplete, giving the appearance of

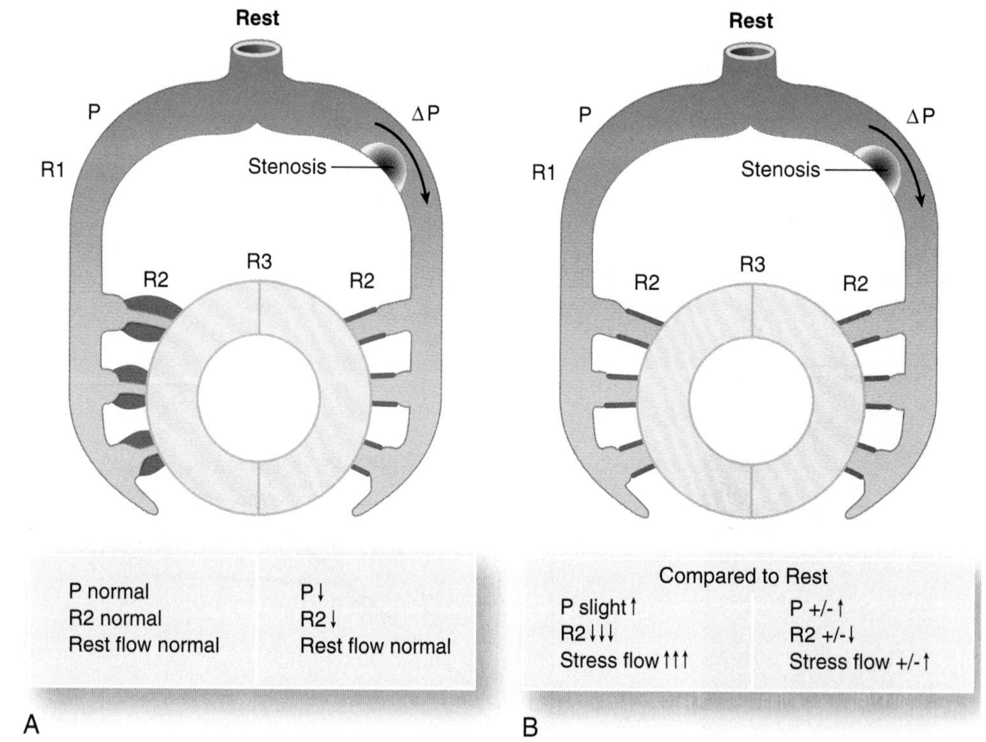

FIGURE 13–22 Effect of coronary resistance on coronary blood flow reserve. **A,** At rest, flow is driven by the pressure head (P) at the proximal end of the system. R1 refers to resistance offered by the large epicardial conductance vessels. R2 represents the coronary arteriolar resistance, which predominantly regulates coronary blood flow. R3 represents the resistance provided by wall tension in the subendocardium. At rest in the normal vessel, some vasoconstrictor resistance is present. In the setting of an epicardial coronary stenosis, blood flow at rest can be maintained, as coronary resistance can be lowered downstream (R2 decreased) by autoregulatory dilation. Thus, with lower resistance, flow may be maintained despite the lower pressure head at the distal end of stenosis. **B,** With a demand stress or with the administration of coronary arteriolar vasodilators, perfusion increases substantially in the area supplied by the normal epicardial artery as R2 decreases. However, there is blunted flow reserve in the area supplied by the stenosis because most vasodilator reserve at the R2 level has been used to maintain resting flow. (Adapted from Follansbee WP: Alternatives to leg exercise in the evaluation of patients with coronary artery disease: Functional and pharmacologic stress modalities. *In* Gerson MC [ed]: Cardiac Nuclear Medicine. New York, McGraw-Hill, 1997, pp 193-236.)

partial reversibility on the delayed thallium or rest technetium 99m images.

Exercise Stress to Induce Coronary Hyperemia

SPECT MPI is commonly performed with exercise stress to induce coronary hyperemia, particularly suitable for patients with exertional symptoms, as this provides the opportunity to link the *symptoms* induced during exercise to the location, extent, and severity of abnormal perfusion patterns.[10] Moreover, performing exercise stress in conjunction with MPI allows the opportunity to incorporate additional information on functional capacity, stress-induced ECG changes or arrhythmias, and utilization of heart rate reserve and heart rate recovery in the assessment of CAD probability or prognosis.[42]

Physiology of Exercise Stress–Induced Coronary Hyperemia. During exercise, systolic pressure rises but diastolic pressure usually changes little. Thus, the driving pressure for coronary perfusion is relatively unchanged, and increases in flow necessary to match increased demand occur predominantly by reducing arteriolar resistance. In the presence of coronary stenosis, if a degree of downstream resistance has been reduced to maintain resting flow, coronary flow reserve during exercise stress is blunted.[37,38]

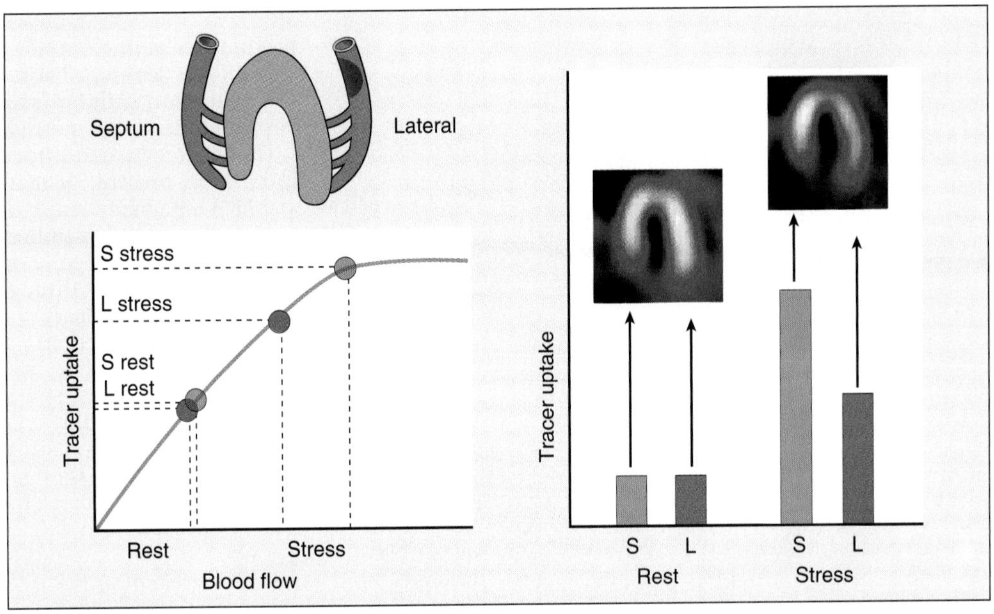

FIGURE 13–23 Illustration of coronary blood flow reserve abnormalities, the concomitant perfusion tracer concentration differences, and the resulting tomographic images. **Left,** The myocardial blood flow profiles at rest and stress of two myocardial regions are shown, with region S (septum) supplied by a normal epicardial artery and region L (lateral wall) supplied by an artery with a significant epicardial coronary stenosis. Blood flow at stress is diminished in region L compared with S. **Right,** The perfusion tracer uptake profile is demonstrated with myocardial blood flow on the y-axis. Tracer uptake is diminished in region L relative to S during stress. In the resulting perfusion images, a relative "defect" of tracer uptake is seen in the lateral wall compared with the septum, whereas at rest both regions demonstrate similar tracer uptake. The lateral wall thus demonstrates a reversible perfusion defect, reflecting the blunted coronary blood flow reserve and indirectly reflecting the presence of the coronary stenosis.

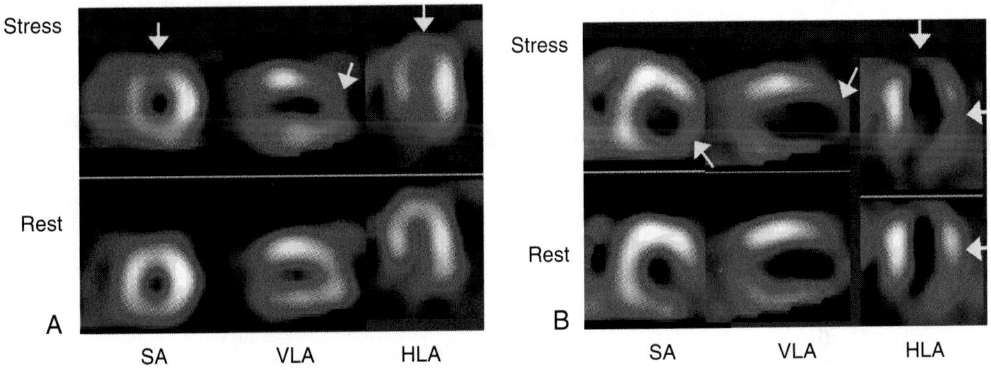

FIGURE 13–24 **A,** Example of single-photon emission computed tomography anterior and apical reversible perfusion defects (arrows), representing inducible regional myocardial ischemia in the short axis (SA), vertical long axis (VLA), and horizontal long axis (HLA). **B,** Example of irreversible or fixed defects of the inferolateral wall in the SA and of the apex in the VLA image (arrows), representing predominant myocardial infarction. There is also evidence of a reversible lateral wall defect (arrowhead) in the HLA image representing lateral wall ischemia.

Pharmacological Stress to Induce Coronary Hyperemia

Exercise stress is the preferred modality for inducing coronary hyperemia as it allows a correlation between exertional symptoms and the perfusion pattern and provides information on exercise duration, workload achieved, and the presence and extent of ischemic ECG changes, all of which provide important diagnostic and prognostic information.[10] However, a substantial proportion of patients are incapable of attaining a sufficient level of exercise. Patients with exertional symptoms may not exercise adequately to reproduce these symptoms, and patients may not achieve more than 85 percent of the maximum predicted heart rate for age (see Chap. 10), considered the optimal level of exertion to achieve coronary hyperemic responses.[10,42] As the population ages and comorbid disease states such as peripheral vascular disease and diabetes increase, the proportion of patients referred for stress testing who are unable to achieve adequate levels of exercise will increase.

In such patients, *pharmacological stress testing* can be used to induce coronary hyperemia. The most widely used agents for pharmacological stress testing can be divided into those that act as coronary arteriolar vasodilators, adenosine and dipyridamole, and adrenergic agents such as dobutamine.[43]

Mechanism of Coronary Arteriolar Vasodilator Pharmacological Stress. Stimulation of adenosine A_{2a} receptors on the smooth muscle cells leads to enhanced production of adenylate cyclase, increased intracellular cyclic adenosine monophosphate, and other effects that produce vasorelaxation. With maximal arteriolar vasodilation (maximal decrease in coronary resistance), coronary blood flow increases to near-maximum levels.

Adenosine is a powerful, endogenous molecule that acts as a regulator of blood flow in many organ beds, including the coronary circulation. It has many other effects mediated by different receptor subtypes (Fig. 13–25). Adenosine A_1 recep-

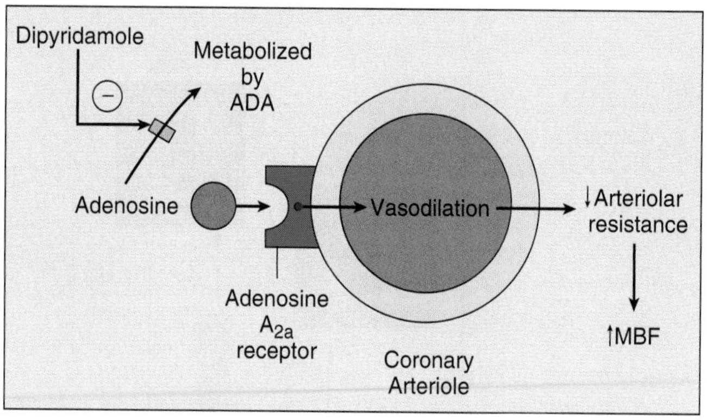

FIGURE 13–25 Schematic of the mechanism of action of dipyridamole and adenosine. Exogenously administered adenosine acts directly on its receptor to result in coronary arteriolar vasodilation and thus an increase in myocardial blood flow (MBF) as resistance is minimized. The adenosine A_{2a} receptor mediates coronary arteriolar vasodilation, which is the basis for pharmacological stress testing. Dipyridamole blocks the intracellular retransport of adenosine and also inhibits adenosine deaminase (ADA), resulting in increased intracellular and interstitial concentrations of adenosine, which then interacts with its receptor. (Adapted from Follansbee WP: Alternatives to leg exercise in the evaluation of patients with coronary artery disease: Functional and pharmacologic stress modalities. *In* Gerson MC [ed]: Cardiac Nuclear Medicine. New York, McGraw-Hill, 1997, pp 193-236.)

tors are present in the sinus node and atrioventricular (AV) node and mediate diminished heart rate and AV nodal conduction. Adenosine A_{2b} receptors are present in bronchioles and the peripheral vasculature, and stimulation may result in bronchial constriction and peripheral vasodilation. Adenosine A_3 receptors are less well characterized but appear to be important in the preconditioning response.

Initial studies of adenosine demonstrated that a dose of 140 μg/kg/min induced maximal coronary hyperemia, with no further increase in maximum coronary blood flow at higher doses.[44] Following the onset of intravenous adenosine infusion, maximum coronary flow occurs at an average of 84 seconds with a range of up to 125 seconds. Dipyridamole blocks the intracellular retransport of adenosine and inhibits adenosine deaminase, responsible for the intracellular breakdown of adenosine.[44] Thus, dipyridamole acts as an indirect coronary arteriolar vasodilator, increasing intracellular and interstitial concentrations of adenosine (see Fig. 13–25).

Heterogeneity of Coronary Hyperemia with Pharmacological Stress. With the administration of dipyridamole or adenosine, the resistance vessels in the area subtended by a normal epicardial vessel dilate, diminishing coronary resistance and resulting in an increment in coronary blood flow four to five times above normal. Coronary resistance in a bed supplied by a stenotic epicardial vessel is diminished at rest (i.e., coronary vasodilator reserve has been utilized), and only minor or no further reductions can take place. Thus, myocardial blood flow in that territory does not change or may even decrease slightly because of the peripheral vasodilation and drop in diastolic blood pressure characteristic of pharmacological stress. The net result of these changes is heterogeneity in myocardial blood flow (increased in the normal territory and relatively unchanged in the territory supplied by the stenotic epicardial vessel). Perfusion tracer administration in this setting demonstrates a defect in the area supplied by the stenotic vessel (see Fig. 13–22).[44,45]

During exercise stress, the increase in myocardial oxygen demand and limitation of oxygen supply create a supply-demand mismatch often resulting in cellular ischemia. With pharmacological stress, the perfusion defect may represent merely the heterogeneity in coronary flow reserve. "Demand" may change little during pharmacological stress; there is often a reduction in blood pressure accompanied by a reflex although modest increase in heart rate, so that double product, reflecting oxygen demand, changes little during the vasodilator "stress." Thus, a supply-demand mismatch may not occur and cellular ischemia may not be present despite vasodilator-induced perfusion defects.[44]

Under certain conditions, true myocardial ischemia may indeed be present, related to development of a *coronary steal*.[38] This phenomenon appears to occur when the myocardial perfusion bed supplied by a severe epicardial stenosis is also dependent on collateral vessels from remote coronary arteries. Blood flow through coronary collaterals is dependent on perfusion pressure, particularly if the collaterals are jeopardized; that is, their parent blood vessel is compromised by a moderate coronary stenosis. In this setting, administration of a vasodilator stress agent diminishes the perfusion pressure supplying the collaterals, and collateral flow diminishes. Flow to the bed supplied by a severe epicardial stenosis may then *decrease* compared with resting flow, and the diminished supply may create supply-demand mismatch and true myocardial ischemia.

Hemodynamic Effects of Vasodilator Pharmacological Stress. Dipyridamole and adenosine both result in adenosine receptor–mediated systemic as well as coronary vasodilation, resulting in an average 8 to 10 mm Hg reduction in systolic and diastolic blood pressure, often accompanied by a reflex increase in heart rate.[44] The magnitude of the heart rate increase is variable, usually between 10 and 20 beats/min. A blunted heart rate response may be observed in patients who are taking beta blockers or in diabetic patients with underlying autonomic insufficiency.

Side Effects and Symptoms Associated with Vasodilator Pharmacological Stress. The symptoms and side effects associated with pharmacological vasodilator stress are the result of stimulation of the adenosine A_1, A_{2b}, and A_3 receptors and are common.[43-46] Following dipyridamole stress, approximately 50 percent of patients experience some side effect. In a large registry study, more than 80 percent of patients undergoing adenosine stress experienced untoward symptoms or side effects, or both, most commonly flushing, chest pain, or shortness of breath.[43-45]

As a result of adenosine's effect on the conduction system, AV block may develop during adenosine administration. Approximately 10 percent of patients manifest first-degree AV block, with 5 percent developing either second- or third-degree AV block. AV block is more common in patients who are studied while taking beta blockers or heart rate–lowering calcium channel blockers. Patients with baseline evidence of second- or third-degree AV block in the absence of a pacemaker should not receive adenosine. However, patients with first-degree AV block or left bundle branch block (LBBB) appear to tolerate adenosine infusion well, without an exacerbation of conduction abnormalities.[8,10]

Ischemic ST depression is observed in 10 to 15 percent of patients undergoing pharmacological vasodilator stress, probably representing the physiological consequence of induction of a coronary steal and regional myocardial ischemia. Such patients often have extensive and severe perfusion defects on imaging and more often have collateralized multivessel disease on angiography.

Chest pain, even typical angina pectoris, develops commonly during pharmacological vasodilator stress testing. Although it may reflect regional myocardial ischemia based on a coronary steal, chest pain may also occur in patients with no ischemic ECG changes and with normal perfusion studies because of involvement of adenosine A_1 receptors in the nociceptive pathway influencing the sensation of chest pain.[43-46] Thus, chest pain by itself is a nonspecific finding during vasodilator pharmacological stress.

In early reports of dipyridamole testing, infrequent but severe episodes of bronchospasm occurred, probably related to a nonspecific adenosine receptor–mediated mechanism. Thus, patients with a significant history of reactive airways disease should not undergo vasodilator stress testing.[8,10] However, patients with obstructive lung disease without a reactive airways component generally tolerate the procedure well.

Reversing the Effects of Vasodilator Pharmacological Stress. Methylxanthine compounds such as theophylline and caffeine act as competitive antagonists of adenosine at the receptor level, and infusion of intravenous aminophylline antagonizes the effects of dipyridamole or adenosine.[8,10] As adenosine has a very short half-life (~20 to 30 seconds), administration of aminophylline is rarely required during adenosine testing, as simply stopping the infusion results in cessation of symptoms within 20 to 30 seconds. Following intravenous dipyridamole, infusion of aminophylline at approximately 1 to 2 mg/kg, given over 30 seconds, reverses side effects (as well as the coronary vasodilator effects), usually within 1 to 2 minutes. As the coronary vasodilator effects are reversed as well, reversal of the dipyridamole effect should be delayed until at least 1 to 2 minutes after radionuclide administration if clinically safe, or the true stress perfusion pattern may not be manifest. Generally, side effects from vasodilator pharmacological stress, although common, may be tolerated for this period of time. However, with more severe side effects such as severe shortness of breath or bronchospasm or with more dramatic ST segment abnormalities, reversal of the dipyridamole effect more quickly is prudent. As caffeine is a methylxanthine compound and antagonizes the effect of adenosine at its receptor, it is critical that patients be instructed to withhold caffeine, ideally for 24 hours prior to vasodilator pharmacological stress testing.

In some patients, myocardial ischemia provoked during vasodilator stress testing triggers a cascade of events that maintains ischemia even after reversal of the vasodilator effect with aminophylline. The sensation of chest pain may drive a heightened sympathetic response, with an elevation of heart rate and blood pressure. In that setting, when aminophylline has been given to reverse the effects of the vasodilator, it is safe to administer sublingual nitroglycerin or other measures to relieve myocardial ischemia. It is *not safe* to give sublingual nitroglycerin *prior to* aminophylline to treat signs of myocardial ischemia. Because systemic vasodilation is present during vasodilator stress testing, administration of nitroglycerin prior to aminophylline may result in substantial systemic hypotension. Thus, aminophylline should always be given first to reverse the effect of the vasodilator, after which it is safe to pursue other anti-ischemic measures.

In contemporary practice, a small number of patients may be encountered who are taking oral dipyridamole preparations for their antiplatelet effects. As dipyridamole is an adenosine deaminase inhibitor and prevents the usual rapid breakdown of adenosine, infusion of intravenous adenosine in patients receiving oral dipyridamole may be accompanied by a far more prolonged adenosine effect than usual. Thus, for adenosine testing, oral dipyridamole compounds must be stopped at an appropriate period of time before testing. Oral dipyridamole as background therapy does not complicate the performance of intravenous dipyridamole testing.

Protocols for Pharmacological Stress Testing. The accepted protocols for performing vasodilator pharmacological stress testing are listed in Table 13–3.[8,10] Since the original descriptions of these protocols, iterations have been studied, with the goal of shortening the test procedure or minimizing side effects, or both,[47,48] by shortening the duration of the adenosine infusion or adding low-level exercise.

Handgrip exercise may be used in order to raise peripheral blood pressure and thus coronary perfusion pressure. Reports are mixed on whether image quality is improved. This approach may be useful in patients with borderline low blood pressure prior to the test to avoid significant hypotension.

Low-level treadmill exercise has been increasingly applied in combination with vasodilator stress testing. Although no clear advantage in diagnostic performance has been demonstrated, a reduction in side effects of pharmacological stress testing has been demonstrated, as well as a reduction in extracardiac tracer uptake that improves image quality.[47,48]

TABLE 13–3 Pharmacological Stress Protocols

	Dose (μg/kg/min)	Duration	Isotope Injection
Dipyridamole	142	4 min by hand infusion or pump	3 min after completion of infusion
Adenosine	140	6-min infusion by pump	At 3 min into infusion

Initial reports of intravenous adenosine testing described a protocol in which the dose was progressively increased. More commonly, adenosine is given now as an infusion starting with the maximum dose. This allows a shortened total infusion period of 4 minutes rather than 6 minutes, with radionuclide injected at 3 minutes into the 4-minute infusion. Published data (with thallium imaging) suggest that diagnostic sensitivity is maintained while decreasing the overall time of testing.[44]

Specific agonists of the adenosine A_{2a} receptor are under development to achieve arteriolar vasodilation and thus myocardial perfusion images similar to those obtained with adenosine or dipyridamole, accompanied by fewer or less severe side effects, because of lack of stimulation of the A_1, A_{2b}, and A_3 receptors. A bolus injection of the specific A_{2a} receptor agonist binodenoson achieves myocardial perfusion images that are concordant with adenosine MPI, with a significant reduction in the incidence and severity of side effects.[46]

DIFFERENCES BETWEEN VASODILATOR AND EXERCISE STRESS. The perfusion images obtained using vasodilator pharmacological stress are generally concordant with those obtained with maximal exercise stress in the same patient, but there are several important differences. *Higher levels of coronary flow are achieved during vasodilator pharmacological stress compared with exercise,* possibly because of the increased resistance to flow with exercise caused by higher subendocardial pressures (i.e., at the R3 level of resistance). Although theoretically this should result in increased sensitivity for detecting CAD with pharmacological stress, that has not been clearly demonstrated. The failure to demonstrate increased sensitivity may be due to the inability of the radionuclide tracers to reflect myocardial blood flow adequately at the highest levels of flow.[43-45]

Vasodilator pharmacological stress is less "physiological" than exercise, and symptoms during testing cannot be as clearly linked to the perfusion pattern. Optimal diagnostic performance of MPI during exercise is often dependent on the patient achieving a maximal level of stress, which does not always occur. In contrast, vasodilator pharmacological stress affords generally predictable coronary flow responses.[8,10,44]

Antiischemic medications may significantly affect the results of MPI during exercise.[10] The effect of background antiischemic medications on the results of pharmacological stress imaging is not as certain. Reports have now suggested that the extent and severity of myocardial perfusion defects may be affected in an important way by background medication during pharmacological stress.[49-51] Thus, antianginal medications should be withheld if possible prior to the study.

Dobutamine Stress to Induce Coronary Hyperemia

In some patients, vasodilator pharmacological stress is contraindicated because of reactive bronchospastic airways disease or background methylxanthines. In such situations, intravenous dobutamine hydrochloride may be used to induce coronary hyperemia.[8,10] Dobutamine has a relatively rapid onset of action, with a half-life of approximately 2 minutes. This agent is given starting at a dose of 5 μg/kg/min and increased in a stepwise fashion by 5 μg/kg/min every 3 minutes, to a maximum dose of 40 μg/kg/min. Dobutamine is a broad adrenergic receptor agonist, at varying doses stimulating the $beta_1$, $beta_2$, and $alpha_1$ receptors. At relatively low doses, the predominant effect is an increase in contractility through adrenergic receptors. As the dose is increased beyond 10 μg/kg/min, heart rate rises steadily, and the increase in oxygen demand stimulates an increase in myocardial blood flow.

The hemodynamic response to dobutamine generally involves a modest increase in systolic blood pressure with a modest decrease in diastolic blood pressure through doses up to 20 μg/kg/min, with only small further changes after that point. As the increase in myocardial blood flow is dependent on the increase in oxygen demand, optimal sensitivity for MPI based on optimizing heterogeneity of flow is dependent on achieving a high dose of dobutamine.

The increment in myocardial blood flow during maximal doses of dobutamine appears to be less than achieved during vasodilator pharmacological stress, and hence the degree of heterogeneity of coronary flow with a coronary stenosis is also less. Thus, vasodilator stress is the preferred pharmacological modality for MPI in patients who cannot exercise adequately. Dobutamine stress is reserved for cases in which vasodilator stress is contraindicated or cannot be performed because of background medications.[8,10,52]

Side effects during dobutamine are frequent and can be bothersome.[52] The most common side effects include palpitations and chest pain, and arrhythmias including ventricular extrasystoles and nonsustained ventricular tachycardia may be encountered. Hypotension occurs in approximately 10 percent of patients, possibly as a result of myocardial mechanoreceptor stimulation during increased contractility with resulting withdrawal of peripheral constrictor tone. Hypotension during dobutamine stress does not have the same prognostic implications as exercise-induced hypotension. Because of the relatively short half-life, side effects generally resolve within a few minutes of stopping the infusion and can be aborted more quickly with intravenous beta blockade.[8,10,52]

Assessment of Myocardial Cellular Metabolism and Physiology by Radionuclide Imaging

Myocardial Ischemia and Viability

Programmed Cell Survival. Imbalance between oxygen supply and demand results in myocardial ischemia. If the imbalance is transient (i.e., triggered by exertion), it represents reversible ischemia. However, if supply-demand imbalance is prolonged, high-energy phosphates are depleted, and regional contractile function progressively deteriorates. If the supply-demand balance is sufficiently prolonged, cell membrane rupture with cell death follows.

The myocardium has several mechanisms of acute and chronic adaptation to a temporary or sustained reduction in coronary blood flow (Fig. 13–26), known as stunning, hibernation, and ischemic preconditioning.[53] These responses to ischemia preserve sufficient energy to protect the structural and functional integrity of the cardiac myocyte. In contrast to programmed cell death, or apoptosis, the term "programmed cell survival" has been used to describe the commonality between myocardial stunning, hibernation, and ischemic preconditioning despite their distinct pathophysiology.[54] Radionuclide imaging has played an important role in understanding the changes in blood flow and metabolism in these states and clinically distinguishing their presence from regional infarct.[34]

Stunned and Hibernating Myocardium. In stunned and hibernating myocardium, *myocardial function is depressed at rest but myocytes remain viable.* Although LV dysfunction may be reversible in both stunning and hibernation, these states differ in the relationship between myocardial perfusion and function. *Stunned myocardium* is most commonly observed after a *transient period of ischemia followed by reperfusion* (depressed function at rest but preserved perfusion).[55] The ischemic episodes can be single or multiple, brief or prolonged, but never severe enough to result in injury. *Hibernating myocardium* refers to an adaptive response of the myocardium to *prolonged myocardial hypoperfusion at rest* (depressed function and perfusion at rest).[56] In the clinical setting, it is likely that the adaptive responses of hibernation and stunning coexist.

Myocardial Viability. Requirements for cellular viability include (1) sufficient myocardial blood flow, (2) cell membrane integrity, and (3) preserved metabolic activity. Myocardial blood flow has to be adequate to deliver substrate to the myocyte for metabolic processes and to remove the end products of metabolism.[57] If blood flow is severely reduced, metabolites accumulate, causing inhibition of the enzymes of the metabolic pathway, depletion of high-energy phosphates, cell membrane disruption, and cell death. Thus, with severe reduction in blood flow, perfusion tracers alone provide information regarding myocardial viability.[10] However, in regions in which the reduction in blood flow is of less severity, perfusion information alone may be an insufficient signal to identify clinically relevant viability, and additional data, such as metabolic indices, would be important.[10,57]

Membrane integrity to maintain electrochemical gradients across the myocyte is also a requirement for cell survival. Because cell membrane integrity is dependent on preserved intracellular metabolic activity to generate high-energy phosphates, tracers that reflect cation flux (thallium-201), electrochemical gradients (sestamibi or tetrofosmin), or metabolic processes (FDG) provide insight into myocardial viability (Fig. 13–27).[8,34,57]

Major Myocardial Fuels and Energetics in Normal and Ischemic Myocardium

High-energy phosphates, such as adenosine triphosphate (ATP), provide the fuel that powers the contractile proteins of the myocytes. ATP is generated in the myocardium by two different but integrated metabolic processes: *oxidative phosphorylation* and *glycolysis.*[58] Fatty acids, glucose, and lactate are the major sources of energy in the heart, and depending on the arterial concentration of each and the physiological condition, any one of these three substrates can be the principal provider of energy (Fig. 13–28). Increased uptake and utilization of one substrate leads to a decreased contribution by the others.

In the fasting state, long-chain free fatty acids are the preferred source of energy in the heart, with glucose accounting for only 15 to 20 percent of the total energy supply. The ATP yield is 130 per mole of free fatty acid and 38 per mole of glucose. When the oxygen supply is *normal*, high levels of ATP and tissue citrate formed by breakdown of fatty acids suppress the oxidation of glucose. When the oxygen supply is *decreased,* ATP and citrate levels fall, and the rate of glycolysis is accelerated. Anaerobic glycolysis can be maintained only if lactate and hydrogen ion (the byproducts of glycolysis) are removed and do not accumulate. In the setting of *severe* hypoperfusion, these end products of the glycolytic pathway accumulate, causing inhibition of the glycolytic enzymes and depletion of high-energy phosphates, resulting in cell membrane disruption and cell death.[59] Thus, to maintain anaerobic glycolysis, minimally sufficient blood flow is necessary.

IMAGING ALTERATIONS IN MYOCARDIAL METABOLISM

Imaging Fatty Acid Metabolism

[^{11}C]Palmitate. Because fatty acids are the primary source of myocardial energy production in the fasting state, early PET studies focused on characterizing the kinetics of long-chain fatty acids, such as [^{11}C]palmitate.[60] Measurement by dynamic PET imaging allows the observation of tracer inflow (by regional perfusion), peak accumulation, and release of the tracer within a region of interest. Once the tracer is in the cell, it either (1) enters the endogenous lipid pool or (2) moves to the mitochondria, where rapid degradation by beta-oxidation results in the generation of carbon dioxide. Depending on demand, about 80 percent of the extracted [^{11}C]palmitate is activated for transport from the lipid pool into the mitochondria for breakdown by beta-oxidation. Because of its complicated kinetic modeling and numerous confounding effects, [^{11}C]palmitate imaging has not gained wide clinical acceptance.

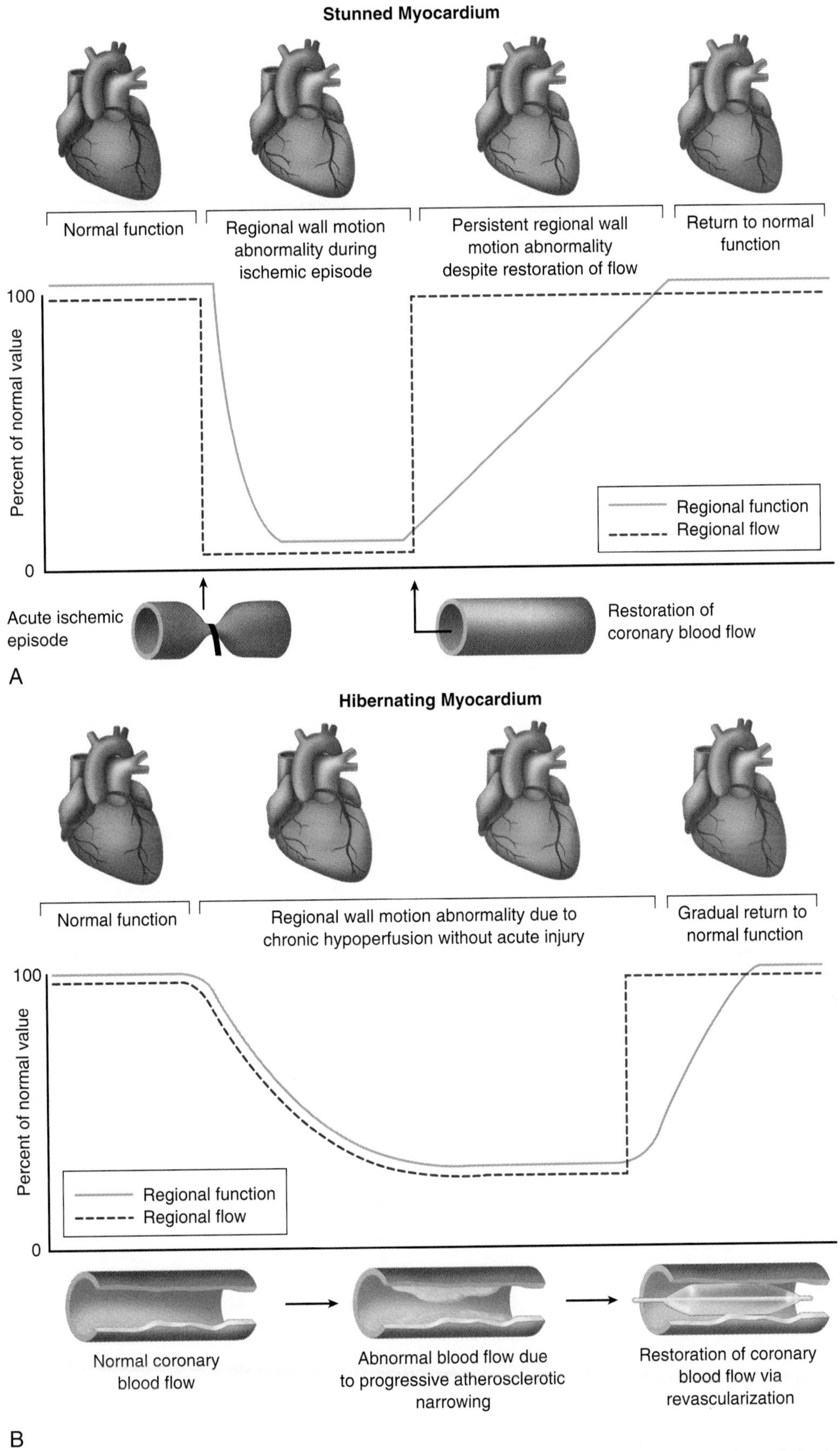

FIGURE 13–26 Pathophysiology of stunning and hibernation, representing different mechanisms of acute and chronic reversible left ventricular dysfunction. (Adapted from Dilsizian V: Myocardial viability: Reversible left ventricular dysfunction. *In* Dilsizian V, Narula J, Braunwald E [eds]: Atlas of Nuclear Cardiology. Philadelphia, Current Medicine, 2003, pp 131-145.)

[^{123}I]BMIPP. Fatty acid imaging with radioiodine-labeled fatty acid analogs such as iodine-123-beta-methyliodopentadecanoic acid (BMIPP) using SPECT is an investigational area for the assessment of *ischemic memory*.[61] After an ischemic episode, fatty acid metabolism may be suppressed for a prolonged time, and BMIPP imaging can demonstrate a regional metabolic defect even if perfusion has returned to normal.[62,63] This metabolic signal of recent ischemia has been termed "ischemic memory" and may be clinically useful, for example, in patients who report to an emergency department (ED) with chest pain that resolved hours earlier.[63] Although BMIPP is approved for clinical use in Japan, it has not yet received approval by the U.S. Food and Drug Administration.

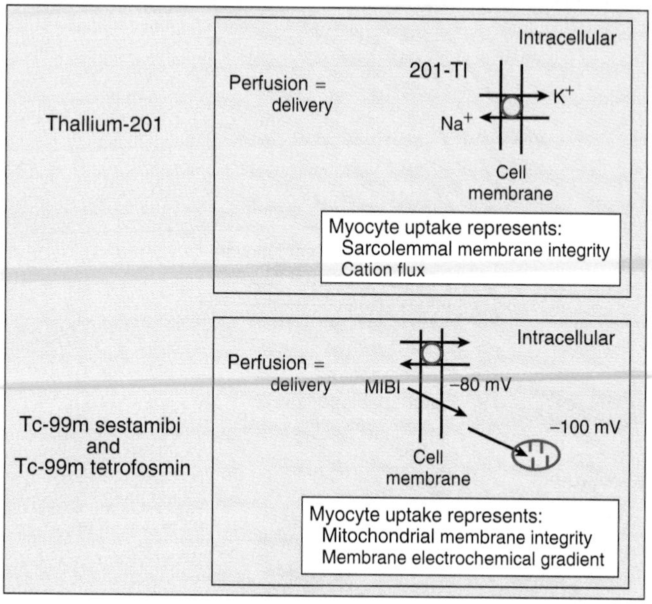

FIGURE 13–27 Mechanisms of uptake and retention of thallium-201 and technetium-99m perfusion tracers.

Imaging Glucose Metabolism

Whereas fatty acids are the primary source of fuel in the *fasting state*, increased arterial glucose concentration in the *fed state* results in an increase in insulin levels, stimulating glucose metabolism while inhibiting lipolysis.[31,32,64] The result is a switch in myocardial metabolism from predominantly fatty acid utilization to glucose utilization.

The principle of using a metabolic tracer that tracks glycolysis is based on the concept that glucose utilization may be preserved or increased relative to flow in hypoperfused but viable (hibernating) myocardium, termed *metabolism-perfusion mismatch*.[31,32,34,65] Myocardial glucose utilization is absent in scarred or fibrotic tissue, termed *metabolism-perfusion match* (Fig. 13-29). Although the amount of energy produced by glycolysis may be adequate to maintain myocyte viability and preserve the electrochemical gradient across the cell membrane, it may not be sufficient to sustain contractile function. This is the conceptual basis for hibernation, an adaptive response preserving myocardial viability in the absence of clinically evident ischemia.[34,53]

2-[^{18}F]Fluoro-2-Deoxyglucose. FDG is a glucose analog used to image myocardial glucose utilization with PET.[31,32,34,64,65] Following injection of 5 to 10 mCi, FDG rapidly exchanges across the capillary and cellular membranes. It is phosphorylated by hexokinase to FDG-6-phosphate (see Fig. 13-28) and not metabolized further or used in glycogen synthesis. Because the dephosphorylation rate of FDG is slow, it becomes trapped in the myocardium, permitting PET or SPECT imaging of regional glucose utilization (see Fig. 13-28). FDG uptake may be increased in hibernating but viable myocardium, and FDG uptake in asynergic myocardial regions with reduced blood flow at rest has become a scintigraphic marker of hibernation.

Diagnostic quality of FDG imaging is critically dependent on hormonal milieu and substrate availability. Most FDG clinical studies are performed after 50 to 75 gm of glucose loading in the form of oral dextrose approximately 1 to 2 hours before the FDG injection to increase glucose metabolism, increase FDG uptake, and improve image quality.[31,32] Although 90 percent of FDG images are of diagnostic quality in nondiabetic patients, the quality of FDG images after glucose loading alone is less certain in patients with clinical or subclinical diabetes, as the increase in plasma insulin levels may be attenuated, tissue lipolysis may not be inhibited, and free fatty acid levels may remain high. Standardization schemes to optimize FDG image quality in diabetic patients include[31,32] (1) intravenous insulin injections after glucose loading, (2) hyperinsulinemic-euglycemic clamping, and (3) use of nicotinic acid derivative.

Imaging Oxidative Metabolism and Mitochondrial Function

[^{11}C]Acetate. All oxidative fuels are metabolized in the tricarboxylic acid (TCA) cycle after conversion to acetyl coenzyme A (CoA). [^{11}C] Acetate is avidly extracted by the myocardium and metabolized predominantly by conversion to [^{11}C]acetyl-CoA in the cytosol and oxidation by the TCA cycle in the mitochondria to [^{11}C]carbon dioxide and water. Hence, the rapid myocardial turnover and clearance of [^{11}C]acetate in the form of [^{11}C]carbon dioxide may reflect myocardial oxidative metabolism and provide insight into mitochondrial function. In patients with recent MI and chronic stable angina, clearance rates of [^{11}C]acetate predict myocardial viability and functional recovery after revascularization. Despite encouraging data in the literature, [^{11}C]acetate remains an investigational tracer.[66]

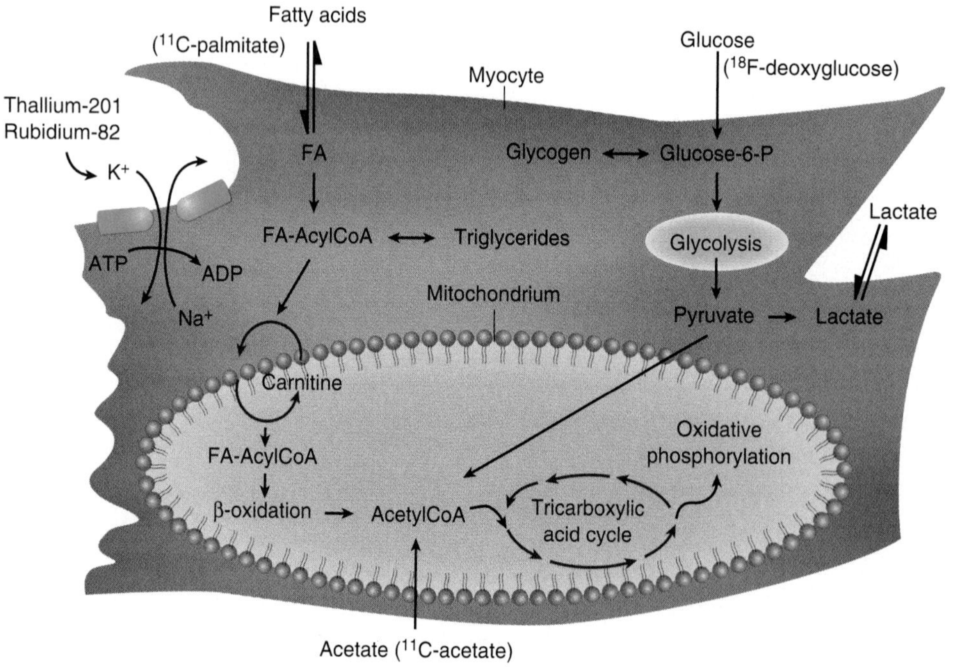

FIGURE 13–28 Mechanism of uptake and retention of positron-emission tomography agents tracing perfusion (rubidium-82) and oxidative and anaerobic metabolism (^{11}C-acetate, ^{11}C-palmitate, and ^{18}F-deoxyglucose). ADP = adenosine diphosphate; ATP = adenosine triphosphate; CoA = coenzyme A; FA = fatty acid. (Adapted from Dilsizian V: SPECT and PET techniques. *In* Dilsizian V, Narula J, Braunwald E [eds]: Atlas of Nuclear Cardiology. Philadelphia, Current Medicine, 2003, pp 19-46.)

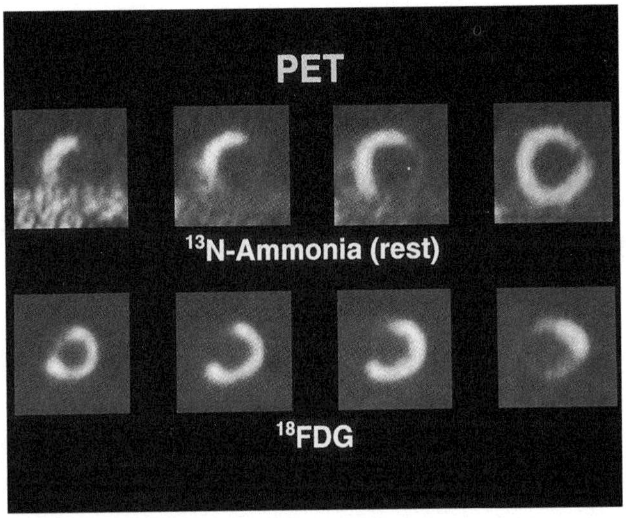

FIGURE 13–29 Assessment of viability by PET imaging. In the **top row,** ^{13}N-ammonia is used as a tracer of myocardial blood flow at rest in these short-axis images starting toward the apex (left) and moving toward the base of the heart (right). There is reduced resting blood flow in the anterolateral, lateral, and inferior walls (defects best seen on the first three images from the left). In the **bottom row,** ^{18}F-fluorodeoxyglucose (FDG) is used as a tracer of myocardial glucose metabolism. There is *enhanced* FDG uptake relative to blood flow in the anterolateral, lateral, and inferior walls, referred to as the "PET mismatch" pattern, indicative of viable myocardium in areas with diminished resting flow, or hibernation. (Adapted from Dilsizian V: Myocardial viability: Reversible left ventricular dysfunction. *In* Dilsizian V, Narula J, Braunwald E [eds]: Atlas of Nuclear Cardiology. Philadelphia, Current Medicine, 2003, pp 131-145.)

Assessment of Ventricular Function by Radionuclide Imaging

Assessing the Physiology of Ventricular Function

The EF is an index of global systolic LV performance influenced by many factors, including the intrinsic state of contractility, preload, and afterload as well as neurohormonal and inotropic influences. Despite its load dependence, EF as an index of ventricular performance has proved clinically quite useful. In the aftermath of acute MI, the postinfarction EF is among the most powerful indices predictive of subsequent mortality.[10,67] The radionuclide techniques used to image ventricular function, RVG and gated SPECT imaging, have provided substantial insight into the physiology of LV function and the response to disease states.

Assessing the Left Ventricular Response to Exercise. Equilibrium gated RVG and first-pass RVG are among the few noninvasive imaging techniques that can evaluate ventricular performance *during exercise.*[27,28] Most often, this is accomplished by imaging the patient during bicycle exercise, supine or semisupine for equilibrium RVG and upright for first-pass RVG bicycle exercise. EF measurements during exertion can then be compared with the resting EF.[27,28]

This technique has been used to study the response of LV function and volumes to exercise. For example, in younger normal subjects, the normal increase in EF and cardiac output is accomplished by decreasing end-systolic volume. In contrast, among older normal subjects, the increase in EF and cardiac output during exercise is accomplished by increasing end-diastolic volume (utilizing preload reserve). In healthy subjects, the normal EF response to exercise is an increase of more than five EF units. The underlying physiology of this increase changes as normal subjects age.[68]

The relative ease by which the EF response to exercise may be studied with RVG techniques led to many reports in the late 1970s and throughout the 1980s. However, evaluation of LV function during exercise by RVG has now been largely replaced by exercise echocardiography (see Chap. 11).

Evaluation of Left Ventricular Volumes. With the RVG technique, the counts detected from the LV region of interest are proportional to ventricular volume. The proportional relation can be estimated from a blood sample of known volume, in which the quantitative relationship between counts and volume can be determined after correction for attenuation.[69] The reader is referred to seminal publications for details.[70,71]

The major advantage of the RVG technique for evaluation of ventricular volumes (and function) over contrast ventriculographic and echocardiographic methods is that the radionuclide techniques *do not require assumptions about ventricular geometry.* Among patients with dilated left ventricles, particularly in the presence of multiple regional wall motion abnormalities, assumptions of ventricular shape, usually that of a prolate ellipsoid, may not be valid. Using RVG techniques, volumes are calculated from count rates over a region of interest involving the left or right ventricle, or both, and are based on photon emissions from the region of interest.[27] Thus, the radionuclide techniques are *not dependent on any assumption of ventricular geometry* and are suitable for the study of ventricular volumes when ventricular geometry is abnormal.

Serial studies of ventricular volumes have been useful in evaluating the process of LV remodeling after MI and in chronic heart failure,[72] in which there is a progressive increase in LV volume in the absence of neurohormonal blockade. Serial RVG studies have shown that the effect of angiotensin-converting enzyme (ACE) inhibition is an early reduction in LV volume, which is maintained over follow-up.[72]

LV volumes may also be calculated using *gated SPECT perfusion imaging,* and volumetric data have been validated against other quantitative techniques.[73,74] At this time, there is less experience using gated SPECT perfusion imaging for serial evaluation of LV volumes compared with equilibrium RVG volumetric techniques. Nonetheless, the ability to evaluate simultaneously LV function, perfusion, and volumes with gated SPECT perfusion imaging suggests that this technique will be increasingly used to study pathophysiological changes.

SERIAL EVALUATION OF LEFT VENTRICULAR FUNCTION

The quantitative nature of radionuclide analysis of ventricular function and the high reproducibility of the measurement make ECG-gated RVG or ECG-gated SPECT imaging well suited for serial follow-up of changes in LV systolic performance. There are many clinical situations in which serial changes in LV function are clinically relevant, such as in patients with heart failure,[75] those observed with valvular heart disease,[76,77] and those being treated with cardiotoxic chemotherapy.[78] Serial RVG studies demonstrating diminution in EF suggesting the early onset of myocardial dysfunction can herald the onset of a higher risk clinical course directing clinical management decisions.

The accuracy and reproducibility of the RVG technique for assessment of LV function make this technique particularly suitable for serial follow-up assessment of patients with regurgitant valvular heart disease. As an example, studies using RVGs have shown that patients being followed up with asymptomatic chronic severe aortic regurgitation who demonstrate the onset of LV dysfunction during follow-up, even when remaining asymptomatic, are at higher risk for adverse clinical outcomes than those with preserved LV performance.[76,77] On the basis of such RVG data, the onset of LV dysfunction in an asymptomatic patient with aortic regurgitation is an indication for surgery. Similarly, serial RVG follow-up of patients undergoing cardiotoxic chemotherapy[78] has demonstrated that a decline in EF as detected by RVG of 10 percent to a final level less than 50 percent indicates high risk for the development of subsequent heart failure.

EVALUATION OF DIASTOLIC FUNCTION WITH RADIONUCLIDE TECHNIQUES

Although the most important quantitative variable derived from RVG evaluation of LV function in the majority of cardiac diseases is the EF, numerous other quantitative variables, including indices describing LV diastolic performance, may also be derived.

Left Ventricular Diastolic Filling. Radionuclide assessment of LV filling properties is based on analysis of the LV time-activity curve, usually obtained using equilibrium RVG techniques,[68] which represents relative volume changes throughout the cardiac cycle (Fig. 13-30). With appropriate data acquisition methods and attention to technical considerations, several parameters of diastolic function may be computed from the time-activity curve, including the peak rate of rapid diastolic filling, the time to peak filling rate, and the relative contributions of the rapid filling period and of atrial systole to total LV stroke volume. Several studies have shown good correlation between various radionuclide and Doppler echocardiographic measures of filling, as both techniques assess physiological events during the filling period.[79]

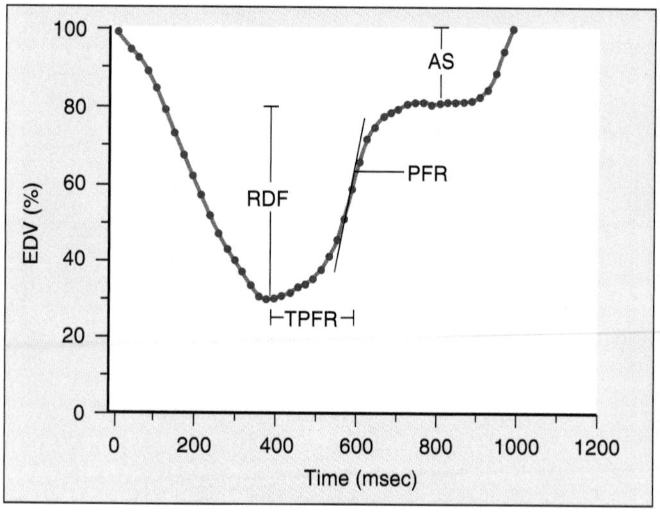

FIGURE 13–30 Quantitative analysis of systolic and diastolic events by radionuclide ventriculography. The x-axis represents time across one average cardiac cycle, and the y-axis represents count activity within the left ventricular region of interest, which is expressed as a percentage of end-diastolic volume (% EDV). The time-activity curve represents the relative change in volume within the ventricle during the cardiac cycle. In this high-temporal-resolution example, each point represents 20 milliseconds. Indices of diastolic function may be computed from analysis of the filling portion of the curve, including the peak rate of rapid filling (PFR), the time from end systole at which peak filling occurs (TPFR), and the relative contribution of rapid diastolic filling (RDF) and of atrial systole (AS) to total stroke volume. (Adapted from Udelson JE, Bonow RO: Radionuclide ventriculography in left ventricular diastolic dysfunction. *In* Gaasch WH, LeWinter M [eds]: Heart Failure and Diastolic Dysfunction. Philadelphia, Lea & Febiger, 1994, pp 167-191.)

COMBINED PRESSURE-VOLUME ANALYSIS OF LEFT VENTRICULAR FUNCTION. The influence of LV relaxation and distensibility on the rate, magnitude, and timing of diastolic filling may be studied in the context of the instantaneous relation between LV pressure and volume throughout the cardiac cycle. It is possible with equilibrium RVG techniques to obtain ventricular volume data in the catheterization laboratory, along with simultaneous acquisition of ventricular pressure measurements, to study the interplay between LV relaxation, filling, and pressure-volume relations (Fig. 13-31). LV distensibility or compliance may be studied by the contour, location, and slope of the pressure-volume relation during the filling phase of diastole.[68]

Evaluation of Diastolic Filling by Equilibrium Radionuclide Ventriculography Techniques in Disease States

Hypertrophic Cardiomyopathy. Abnormal diastolic properties of the hypertrophied ventricle are a characteristic feature of hypertrophic cardiomyopathy (HCM), contributing notably to clinical manifestations.[80] Studies using RVG evaluation of diastolic filling have demonstrated that the rate and extent of rapid filling are reduced in HCM, that the time to peak filling rate is prolonged, and that the contribution of atrial systole to total LV stroke volume is increased.[81]

Combined radionuclide and hemodynamic measurements indicate that enhanced LV filling after verapamil in HCM (effective in relieving symptoms in many patients) is associated with improved indices of LV relaxation and favorable shift in the diastolic pressure-volume relations (see Fig. 13-31).[68] Radionuclide studies have also demonstrated that enhanced LV filling after verapamil in HCM correlates with objective symptomatic improvement as measured by exercise treadmill time, suggesting that reversal of LV filling abnormalities is an important mechanism by which patients experience reduction of symptoms.[82]

Heart Failure. Radionuclide studies have provided evidence of an abnormal end-diastolic volume response to exercise in patients with heart failure and *preserved* systolic performance, supporting the concept of diastolic dysfunction as an underlying cause for symptoms.[83] Patients with heart failure but preserved systolic performance do not increase end-diastolic volume during exercise, associated with a substantial increase in wedge pressure (Fig. 13-32). In contrast, normal subjects demonstrate an increase in end-diastolic volume associated with no change in wedge pressure, recruiting preload despite no change in left atrial driving pressure. Patients with heart failure and normal systolic performance require higher filling pressures to maintain stroke volume, at the cost of an increased pulmonary wedge pressure, resulting in shortness of breath. Thus, abnormal diastolic performance, manifested by an ***impaired ability to recruit end-diastolic volume (preload reserve)***, as demonstrated by equilibrium RVG techniques, results in physiological abnormalities leading to heart failure in these patients with normal systolic function.

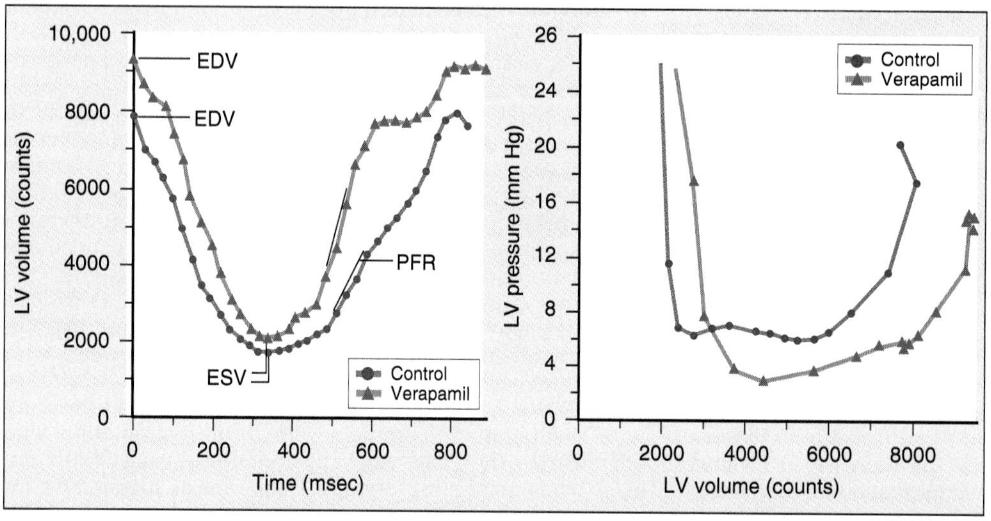

FIGURE 13–31 Pressure-volume analysis to study the effect of drug intervention in diastolic dysfunction. **Left,** Time-activity (volume) curves from a patient with hypertrophic cardiomyopathy under control conditions (magenta line) and after intravenous verapamil (blue line). There is an increase in left ventricular (LV) end-diastolic volume (EDV) and end-systolic volume (ESV) and an increase in peak filling rate (PFR) following verapamil administration. **Right,** Diastolic pressure-volume curves. Following verapamil, there is a favorable downward and rightward shift in diastolic pressure-volume relation, suggesting improved diastolic distensibility, as left ventricular volume is higher at any given pressure. In this example, volume data were acquired with radionuclide analysis of LV count changes and pressure data with a micronanometer catheter. (Adapted from Udelson JE, Bonow RO: Left ventricular diastolic function and the use of calcium channel blockers in hypertrophic cardiomyopathy. *In* Gaasch WH, LeWinter M [eds]: Heart Failure and Diastolic Dysfunction. Philadelphia, Lea & Febiger, 1994, pp 462-489.)

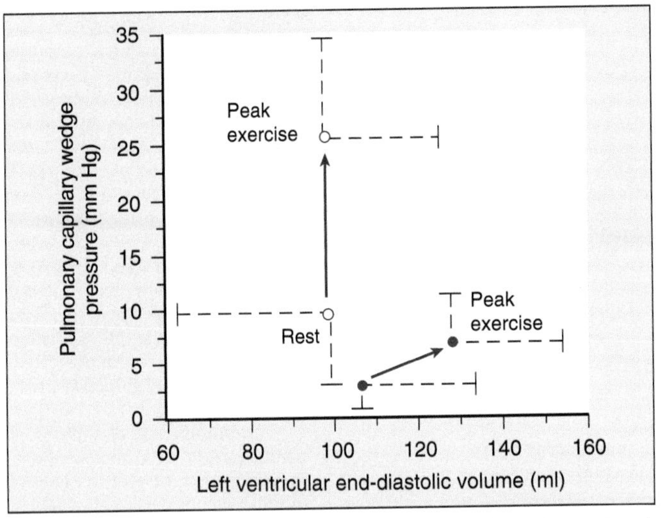

FIGURE 13–32 Use of radionuclide ventriculography to evaluate changes in end-diastolic volume (EDV) during exercise. In normal subjects (closed symbols), there is an increase in EDV during exercise (recruitment of preload reserve) with only minor change in pulmonary capillary wedge (PCW) pressure. In contrast, patients with heart failure and preserved systolic function (open symbols) manifest no change in EDV during exercise despite substantial increase in PCW pressure, to levels that would be associated with symptoms such as shortness of breath. (Adapted from Kitzman DW, Higginbotham MB, Cobb FR, et al: Exercise intolerance in patients with heart failure and preserved left ventricular systolic function: Failure of the Frank-Starling mechanism. J Am Coll Cardiol 17:1065, 1991.)

Disease Detection, Risk Stratification, and Clinical Decision-Making

Stable Chest Pain Syndromes

Application of Radionuclide Imaging: Answering the Clinical Questions

For patients with stable symptoms of suspected CAD who are referred for noninvasive testing, the two major goals of testing are (1) determination of whether CAD is present or absent (the "diagnostic" construct) and (2) determination of the longer term prognosis or risk of an adverse outcome over time (the "prognostic" construct). These goals of testing are linked to the treatment goals for any patients with suspected or known CAD. The two main goals of treatment are (1) minimization of symptoms in everyday life and (2) improvement in natural history.

Establishing the presence of or ruling out CAD is an important goal of testing. The performance characteristics of radionuclide imaging for this purpose are based on the detection of CAD, usually defined as greater than or equal to 50 or 70 percent stenosis in an individual epicardial vessel. This definition of CAD is in part based on seminal studies in animal models showing that a 50 percent stenosis begins to blunt coronary flow reserve.[84] However, over time a view has emerged that CAD is a more complex process than can be defined dichotomously by a 50 percent or even a 70 percent luminal stenosis. Throughout the progression of plaque growth, there is a risk of transformation from a stable plaque to an unstable plaque, with the potential for an acute coronary syndrome (ACS) that abruptly alters the natural history of the patient.[85] Plaque encroachment of the lumen occurs later in the process but has a potentially important impact on the patient's everyday quality of life by causing symptoms related to exertional ischemia.

PATIENT-RELATED OUTCOMES AS A "GOLD STANDARD." The evolution of preventive therapies, such as 3-hydroxy-3-methylglutaryl (HMG) CoA reductase inhibitors, to reduce cardiovascular risk has focused attention on the ability of global risk scores or noninvasive testing to *assess risk of future events* in order to best target strategies to reduce risk.[86,87] Thus, from the perspective of improving natural history, knowledge of whether or not a greater than 50 percent stenosis is present in a patient with stable anginal symptoms becomes less important than *knowledge of the patient's risk of a cardiovascular event, i.e., cardiac death or nonfatal MI.* After initial investigations of the performance of radionuclide imaging to detect or rule out CAD (sensitivity and specificity), the trajectory of the literature has been toward gaining more understanding of how noninvasive imaging results assess prognosis and stratify the risk of future cardiac events.[88] This has occurred in parallel with similar directions in primary prevention efforts, such as the use of a Framingham risk score, with a goal of life-style and treatment interventions to lower that risk.[86] In much the same way, risk stratification and assessment of prognosis by noninvasive imaging will inform clinical management decisions geared toward reducing risk of MI and cardiac death, and optimizing the selection of patients for revascularization and medical therapies.

Risk Stratification in Stable Chest Pain Syndromes

Definitions for Understanding the Literature. For prognostic assessment, an important goal is to detect patients at risk for "hard" cardiac events. This definition includes *nonfatal MI* as well as *cardiac death* or *all-cause mortality*, irreversible events that it is important to prevent.[89] "Soft" cardiac events include revascularization and hospital admission for unstable angina or heart failure. Such events occur more often than the hard cardiac events and thus contribute to a larger number of endpoints for data analysis. However, these events are not as important in terms of natural history and may be driven by subjective changes in symptoms and, in the case of revascularization, by the results of the imaging tests themselves.

Risk categories as described in the American College of Cardiology/American Heart Association (ACC/AHA) stable angina guidelines include (1) low risk, defined as a less than 1 percent per year risk of hard event; (2) intermediate risk, defined as a 1 to 3 percent per year risk, and (3) high risk, defined as a greater than 3 percent per year risk of hard cardiac events.[90] These definitions are conceptually linked to implied treatment strategies. Patients with greater than 3 percent per year risk would be most likely to benefit from a revascularization strategy, whereas those at low risk would be least likely to benefit from revascularization, in terms of natural history, and thus could be treated medically, with treatment directed against symptoms as well as risk factor modification.

The Relation Between the Extent of Perfusion Defect and Natural History Outcomes. Seminal studies in the 1980s demonstrated that the *extent of perfusion abnormality* by stress MPI has an important relationship with the *subsequent likelihood of an adverse natural history outcome* (cardiac death or nonfatal MI).[91,92] Among patients presenting with chest pain and *suspected* CAD (without any prior known CAD history, such as an MI or revascularization), the risk of cardiac death or MI increased as the number of reversible perfusion defects, i.e., the extent of inducible ischemia, increased (Fig. 13–33).

This concept has been confirmed many times by investigators around the world. Moreover, this robust concept not only applies to *exercise* stress MPI but also extends across the spectrum of procedural variation in nuclear cardiology, including different stressors (vasodilator pharmacological stress, dobutamine stress), isotopes (thallium-201 and ^{99m}Tc agents), and imaging protocols (including dual-isotope imaging).[10] An example of data on risk stratification implying therapeutic management strategies is demonstrated by the images shown in Figure 13–34A and B. In two older men with

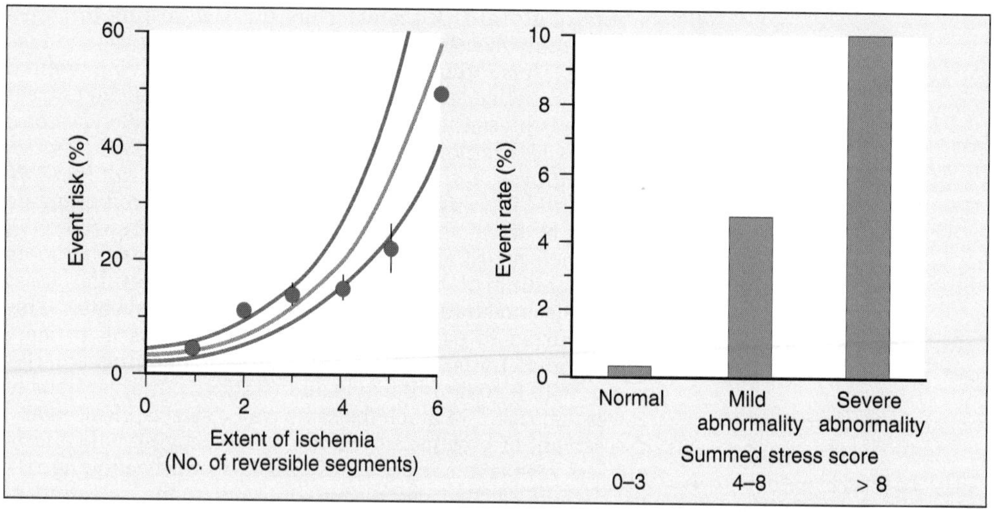

FIGURE 13–33 Prognostic implications of myocardial perfusion imaging. **A,** Cardiac event rate (risk of cardiac death or myocardial infarction [MI]) over long-term follow-up plotted as a function of the extent of inducible ischemia (the number of reversible perfusion defects). There is an exponential relationship between the extent of ischemia and the risk of a cardiac event (brown line = modeling of data points; magenta lines = confidence limits). **B,** Extent and severity of perfusion abnormality, expressed as the summed stress score, are related to the risk of subsequent cardiac death or MI. As the extent and severity of the perfusion abnormality increase, the event risk increases as well. (A, Adapted from Ladenheim ML, Pollock BH, Rozanski A, et al: Extent and severity of myocardial hypoperfusion as predictors of prognosis in patients with suspected coronary artery disease. J Am Coll Cardiol 7:464, 1986; B, adapted from Hachamovitch R, Berman DS, Kiat H, et al: Exercise myocardial perfusion SPECT in patients without known coronary artery disease: Incremental prognostic value and use in risk stratification. Circulation 93:905, 1996.)

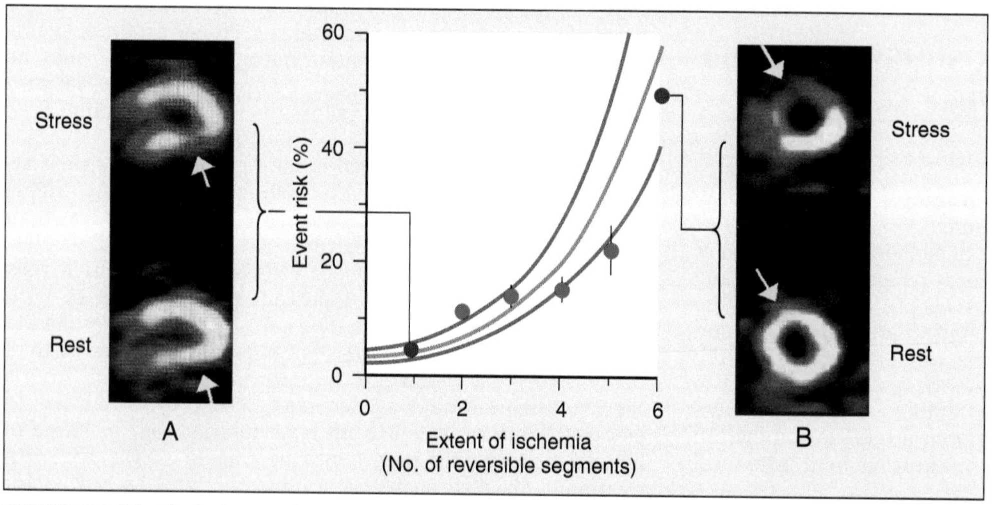

FIGURE 13–34 Single-photon emission computed tomography perfusion images in two patients with stable anginal symptoms. **A,** Small area of inferoapical ischemia (arrows). When this extent of ischemia is plotted on the graph from Figure 13–33A (line to red circle), the patient is placed in a low-risk category. **B,** In contrast, the large, severe area of anterior and septal ischemia in this patient places him in a high-risk group (line to red circle).

typical exertional angina, it would be predicted that the probability of CAD is very high, according to established guidelines. However, what is *not* established from that clinical information is the *natural history risk.* These examples demonstrate that patients presenting with similar symptoms might be identified as having distinct natural histories on the basis of perfusion imaging data, with distinct implications for subsequent management.

THE INCREMENTAL VALUE OF PERFUSION IMAGING. The term "incremental value" implies that perfusion imaging data provide information on natural history risk and outcomes that are *additive to* (incremental to) information from more available or less expensive tests, such as clinical data and stress ECG findings.[93,94]

Stress MPI data have been shown to have incremental prognostic value when added to prognostic stress ECG instruments such as the Duke Treadmill Score (DTS), a well-validated instrument incorporating symptoms, treadmill performance, and stress ECG findings to predict natural history outcomes (see Chap. 10). In a group of 2200 patients with suspected CAD referred for nuclear testing, the DTS was used to place patients in subgroups according to the risk of a hard event (Fig. 13-35).[95] When information from stress MPI studies was incorporated, incremental value to predict outcome was demonstrated within each of the three DTS risk categories.

The importance of this information in driving management decisions for patients can be illustrated by considering how clinicians would manage patients given certain amounts of information. Given the DTS information alone, the management of low-risk patients would probably be conservative and the management of high-risk patients would probably involve revascularization. The optimal management of intermediate-risk patients is unclear, but many would probably be referred for catheterization. However, almost 80 percent of the patients in the intermediate DTS category had a *normal* stress perfusion study (see Fig. 13-35A), associated with a very low risk natural history, implying that conservative management would be a safe and effective strategy.

These findings have been confirmed by other studies. In a large population of more than 4000 patients with an intermediate-risk DTS, normal stress MPI was associated with a very low risk of a hard cardiac event over multiple years of follow-up.[96]

Another method used to demonstrate the incremental value of MPI data over clinical, stress, and even angiographic data involves the creation of a multivariable model to measure the strength of association of individual factors with the natural history outcomes.[94,97,98] This is often illustrated by assessing the incremental chi-square value measuring the strength of the association of the factor with subsequent cardiac death and nonfatal MI (see Fig. 13-35B).

Identification of Treatment Benefit Following Risk Stratification. Although numerous studies have suggested that the extent and severity of perfusion abnormality are related to subsequent natural history risk, few studies have documented *reduction* in that risk associated with a particular therapy. Information is now available suggesting that more extensive ischemia determined by MPI identifies patients in whom revascularization would lead to an improvement in outcome. In a group of more than 10,000 patients with suspected CAD studied by stress MPI, the extent of ischemic myocardium predicted reduction in the risk of death with revascularization compared with medical therapy (Fig.

13–36), beginning at just over 10 percent of ischemic myocardium.[99] As the percentage of ischemic myocardium increased, the magnitude of benefit of revascularization increased as well. Thus, MPI data can predict the magnitude of a potential treatment benefit from revascularization, helping to guide management decisions.

The Prognostic Value of Normal Myocardial Perfusion Imaging. A consistent finding in studies assessing progno-sis has been the benign prognosis associated with a normal stress myocardial perfusion study. As summarized in the ACC/AHA/American Society for Nuclear Cardiology (ASNC) Radionuclide Imaging Guidelines,[10] data on outcomes associated with a normal stress MPI SPECT study now involve almost 21,000 patients. In patients with a normal study, the hard event rate occurring over an average follow-up of 2 years is 0.7 percent per year. This concept applies across a broad spectrum of isotopes, protocols, and stressors.[10,100] The prediction of low-risk outcome following a normal MPI extends approximately 2 years after testing (i.e., the "warranty period").[101] Patients who at baseline represent higher risk subsets (i.e., those with diabetes) have a slightly higher risk of an adverse outcome after a normal stress MPI,[102] consistent with Bayes' theorem; that is, given a certain MPI finding, the posttest probability (outcome risk) is related in part to the pretest risk.

Even when angiographic CAD is present with a stable symptom complex, a normal stress MPI study is associated with a low-risk outcome (~0.9 percent per year).[103] The mechanism for a normal MPI despite established CAD has not been conclusively demonstrated but may involve preserved endothelial function, allowing appropriate flow-mediated vasodilation during stress, reducing the impact of an angiographic stenosis on downstream myocardial perfusion. If this is true, such preserved endothelial function may identify a patient less susceptible to plaque fissuring or rupture and more likely to have a stable clinical course.

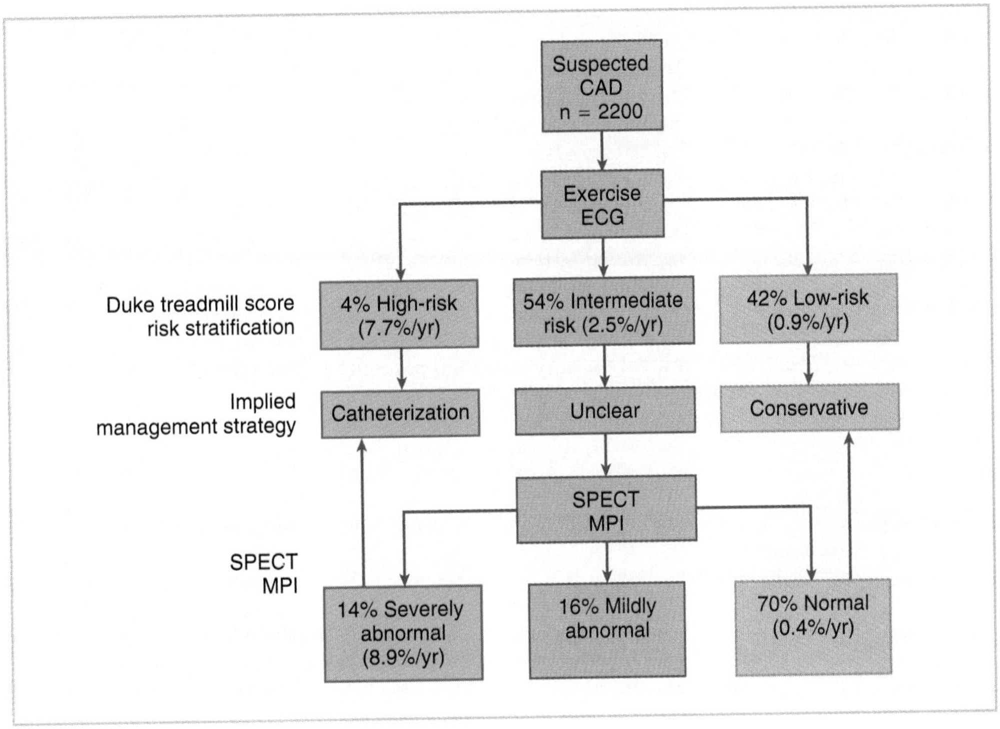

A

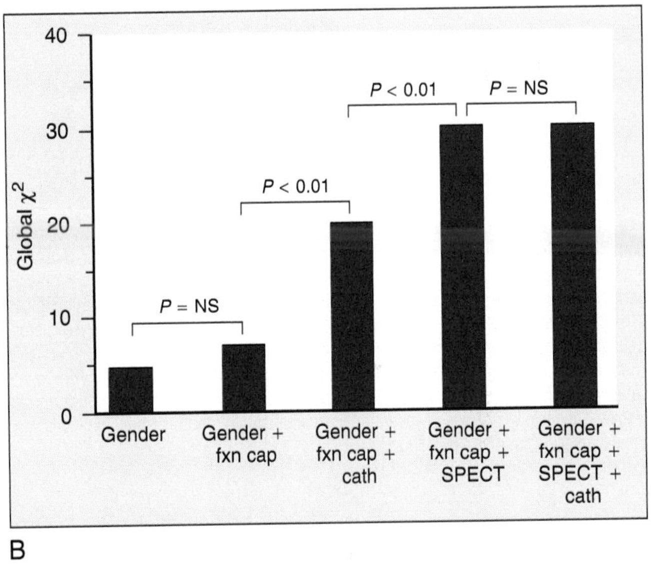

B

FIGURE 13–35 Incremental value of single-photon emission computed tomography (SPECT) perfusion imaging. **A,** Comparison with the Duke Treadmill Score (DTS). A large group of patients with suspected coronary artery disease (CAD) was initially risk stratified by the well-validated DTS. Figures in parentheses are the observed annual event rates. The majority of the population is classified as "intermediate risk" by DTS, and management strategy is not clear. High-risk patients may be managed aggressively, and low-risk patients may be managed conservatively. Among patients originally categorized as intermediate risk by the DTS, almost 70 percent had a normal SPECT perfusion study, associated with a very low event rate. Following SPECT myocardial perfusion imaging (MPI), more patients are classified at the "extremes" of risk (low or high), where management is more clearly implied by the risk prediction. Thus, the imaging data allowed further stratification and thus had incremental value over the DTS information. **B,** The incremental value of imaging data may be expressed as the incremental chi-square value, a statistical measure of the strength of the association of clinical, demographic, stress, or imaging factors to risk stratification. Among patients with known CAD who had undergone catheterization (cath), clinical information is added on the x-axis, with the global chi-square value associated with the information depicted on the y-axis. The larger the chi-square value, the stronger the relation between the combination of factors on the x-axis and the natural history outcome of cardiac death or myocardial infarction. Even when anatomical information is available, the physiological information provided by SPECT MPI adds significantly to risk prediction ability. fxn cap = functional capacity. (A, Adapted from Hachamovitch R, Berman DS, Kiat H, et al: Exercise myocardial perfusion SPECT in patients without known coronary artery disease: Incremental prognostic value and use in risk stratification. Circulation 93:905, 1996; B, adapted from Beller GA: First annual Mario S. Verani, MD, Memorial Lecture: Clinical value of myocardial perfusion imaging in coronary artery disease. J Nucl Cardiol 10:529, 2003.)

Dynamic Assessment of Prognosis by Serial Scintigraphic Studies: A New Paradigm?

Although there is an important correlation between the extent of ischemia and subsequent outcome, the specificity of such determinations is low. That is, among patients with high-risk scintigraphic signs, only a minority suffer an important cardiac event during follow-up and the majority of "high-risk" patients remain event-free. As most of these high-risk patients undergo catheterization and intervention, many patients who will not have an event are receiving interventions in order to prevent such events in the minority. Clinicians accept this trade-off, but evolving data suggest that the response of scintigraphic ischemia to medical therapy may allow more precise estimates of prognosis.

The Angioplasty Compared to Medicine (ACME) investigators[104] randomly assigned 328 patients with single- or double-vessel CAD and stable angina to medical therapy or percutaneous coronary intervention (PCI). Six months after randomization, exercise MPI was performed. The 6-month MPI data were strongly correlated with subsequent 5-year cardiac events.[104] Patients with a reversible perfusion defect 6 months after *either* PCI or medical therapy had a 3.6 percent annual mortality rate, compared with a 1.6 percent annual mortality rate among patients with no reversible defects, and the extent of ischemia was related to subsequent mortality.

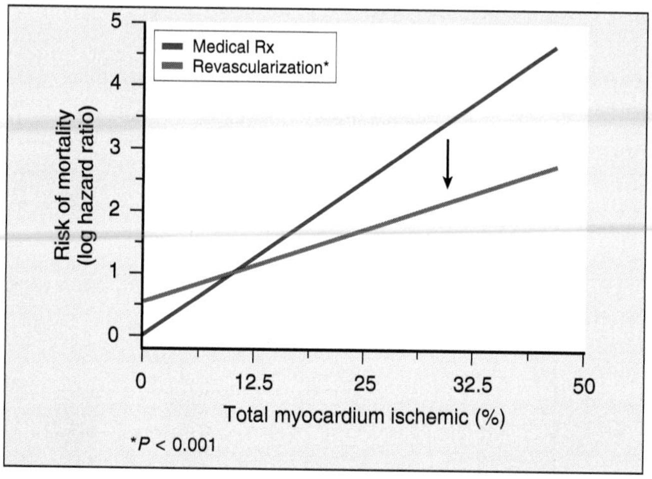

FIGURE 13–36 Predicting the magnitude of treatment benefit by revascularization. Risk of death is plotted as a function of the percent ischemic myocardium by single-photon emission computed tomography perfusion imaging. The solid lines represent patients treated with medical therapy (medical Rx, magenta) or revascularization (blue). When the magnitude of ischemia exceeds approximately 12 percent, there is a potential survival benefit with revascularization. (Adapted from Hachamovitch R, Hayes SW, Friedman JD, et al: Comparison of the short-term survival benefit associated with revascularization compared with medical therapy in patients with no prior coronary artery disease undergoing stress myocardial perfusion single photon emission computed tomography. Circulation 107:2900, 2003.)

Exercise ECG data were not predictive of late outcomes. Even if the 6-month MPI study was performed in patients receiving medical therapy alone in the absence of prior PCI, the outcome prediction was similar. These data suggest that follow-up MPI to assess the effect of medical therapy on the extent of ischemia may help to predict late outcomes more precisely and subcategorize patients more precisely within risk groups.

Similar results have been reported for patients who underwent PCI or medical therapy early after acute MI.[49] The extent of ischemia was similarly reduced with medical therapy compared with PCI on a follow-up SPECT perfusion study 6 weeks later. Event-free survival was significantly related to the reduction in perfusion defect size, independent of the intervention. Ongoing trials are testing this concept using contemporary aggressive secondary prevention therapies.

Studies using either PET or SPECT assessment of perfusion have concordantly demonstrated improvement in stress perfusion following statin therapy (Fig. 13–37).[105,106] As such therapy is unlikely to affect significantly the degree of luminal encroachment by a plaque, the data suggest that improvement in perfusion may be a result of statin-mediated improvement in endothelial function. Favorable changes in perfusion may identify cohorts of patients gaining most benefit from statin therapy in terms of vascular stability, a concept that requires longer term follow-up of such patients.

Detecting the Presence and Extent of Coronary Artery Disease

Noninvasive testing in patients with suspected CAD is commonly performed to determine the presence or absence of CAD. In this diagnostic construct, CAD is usually defined dichotomously, by a threshold degree of coronary stenosis in a major epicardial vessel, usually greater than or equal to 50 or 70 percent stenosis by angiography. In this paradigm, angiography is the gold standard to define the presence or absence of CAD, and performance of the noninvasive test is measured by its *sensitivity* (percentage of true-positive tests among those with CAD as defined by angiography) as well as its *specificity* (percentage of true-negative tests among those without CAD).[107] Published values of sensitivity for detecting CAD and specificity for ruling out CAD vary widely.[10] There are many factors influencing these performance characteristics that should be understood in order to incorporate imaging data appropriately into clinical decision-making. These include either methodological or physiological factors.

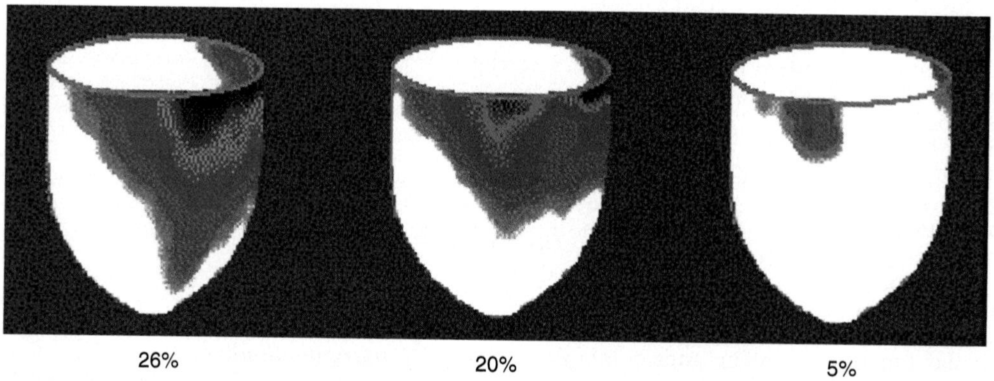

FIGURE 13–37 Improvement in perfusion after statin therapy. Three-dimensional surface-rendered models of myocardial perfusion before statin therapy (**left**) and after 6 weeks (**middle**) and 6 months (**right**) of therapy, viewed from the inferior surface of the heart. White areas represent normal perfusion, with red, blue, and black representing increasingly severe degrees of ischemia. The extent of ischemia is below each image, expressed as a percentage of total myocardium. There is a substantial improvement in the degree of inferior wall ischemia over the course of statin therapy. (Adapted from Schwartz RG, Pearson TA, Kalaria VG, et al: Prospective serial evaluation of myocardial perfusion and lipids during the first six months of pravastatin therapy: Coronary artery disease regression single photon emission computed tomography monitoring trial. J Am Coll Cardiol 42:600, 2003.)

METHODOLOGICAL INFLUENCES ON SENSITIVITY AND SPECIFICITY

Referral Bias. The *apparent* accuracy of any noninvasive test to detect CAD depends on the indications for coronary angiography. Accuracy of a new diagnostic test is usually determined initially in patients who are undergoing coronary angiography. As the test becomes implemented in routine diagnostic strategies, its results determine which patients are to be referred for coronary angiography (Fig. 13-38). For example, patients with abnormal MPI are more likely to undergo coronary angiography than those with normal MPI. This results in a phenomenon termed "posttest referral bias," in which the specificity of a diagnostic test declines over time as it is accepted into clinical practice and plays a gatekeeper role in determining which patients undergo angiography.[10,108] In its extreme form, in which only patients with an abnormal test are referred for angiography, the posttest referral bias drives the specificity to zero (all patients with normal coronary arteriograms have false-positive MPI results and there are no true-negatives). The same phenomenon artificially increases the sensitivity of the test and in its extreme drives the sensitivity to 100 percent (all patients with abnormal coronary arteriograms have true-positive MPI, with no false-negatives). This concept holds not only for MPI but also for any diagnostic test that might determine the indications for angiography.

The concept of "normalcy rate" has been developed in an attempt to compensate for this referral bias.[10] Normalcy is calculated in the same manner as specificity but includes only the imaging test results of patients with a clinically low or very low pretest likelihood of CAD, whether or not they are referred for cardiac catheterization. Normalcy rates tend to be greater than specificity.

Angiography as the Gold Standard. In humans, coronary atherosclerosis is a complex disease most often involving the coronary arteries diffusely and not merely focally. Moreover, whether a given discrete stenosis, imaged at rest during coronary angiography, results in a perfusion abnormality during stress is dependent on a number of factors besides the percent degree of stenosis. These factors include the dilatory or constrictor response of the vessel during stress (mediated by endothelial function) and the presence or absence of collaterals.[107,109] For example, a vessel with 70 percent stenosis but with preserved endothelial function and a well-developed collateral supply may *not* be associated with an abnormality on stress perfusion. In a diagnostic construct, such a result would be categorized as false-negative, reducing MPI sensitivity. However, the MPI data may be providing the *correct physiological information* regarding the functional significance of the angiographic finding, demonstrating that collateral flow during exercise or normal endothelial function or both were associated with preserved coronary blood flow reserve despite the coronary stenosis. This example illustrates the limitation of using angiography as a gold standard in evaluating a physiological modality.

Many published studies define CAD as greater than or equal to 50 percent stenosis, whereas others use a threshold of greater than or equal to 70 percent stenosis.[8,10] Using the former would decrease sensitivity (as some 50 to 70 percent stenoses are not hemodynamically significant) and increase specificity. In contrast, using the latter threshold would increase sensitivity, as more such stenoses are likely to be associated with perfusion abnormality, but decrease specificity, as any positive scan result with 50 to 70 percent stenosis would be considered false-positive.

PHYSIOLOGICAL INFLUENCES ON SENSITIVITY AND SPECIFICITY

A number of disease processes involving the coronary vasculature or the myocardium may result in abnormalities in myocardial perfusion in the *absence of a discrete coronary stenosis*. In a diagnostic construct for CAD, such abnormalities would be labeled false-positive, reducing specificity (i.e., the test is positive in the absence of epicardial CAD). However, MPI may actually be providing correct information regarding perfusion physiology.

Left Bundle Branch Block. Isolated reversible perfusion defects of the septum in patients with LBBB may be seen in the absence of stenosis of the left anterior descending (LAD) coronary artery.[8,10] This phenomenon may represent true heterogeneity of flow between the LAD and left circumflex territories, related to delayed relaxation of the septum in LBBB leading to reduced coronary flow reserve in early diastole, or reduced oxygen demand as a result of late septal contraction when wall stress is decreasing. The specificity and predictive value of a septal perfusion defect with LBBB are thus low. However, apical or anterior involvement in septal perfusion defects increases the specificity for CAD.[110] As a septal defect in LBBB is most commonly seen at high heart rates, pharmacological stress improves specificity, and vasodilator stress is recommended in the setting of LBBB.[10,110]

Hypertrophic Cardiomyopathy. The asymmetrical septal hypertrophy in many patients with HCM can lead to the appearance of a greater amount of tracer uptake in the hypertrophied septum relative to the lateral wall, creating the impression of a mild lateral wall perfusion defect, especially when polar maps are employed.

Many reports have demonstrated myocardial perfusion abnormalities in patients with HCM in the absence of epicardial CAD.[111,112] Such findings have important pathophysiological relevance: patients with fixed perfusion defects are likely to have thinned akinetic walls on echocardiography and diminished EF (Fig. 13-39).[113] Of asymptomatic patients

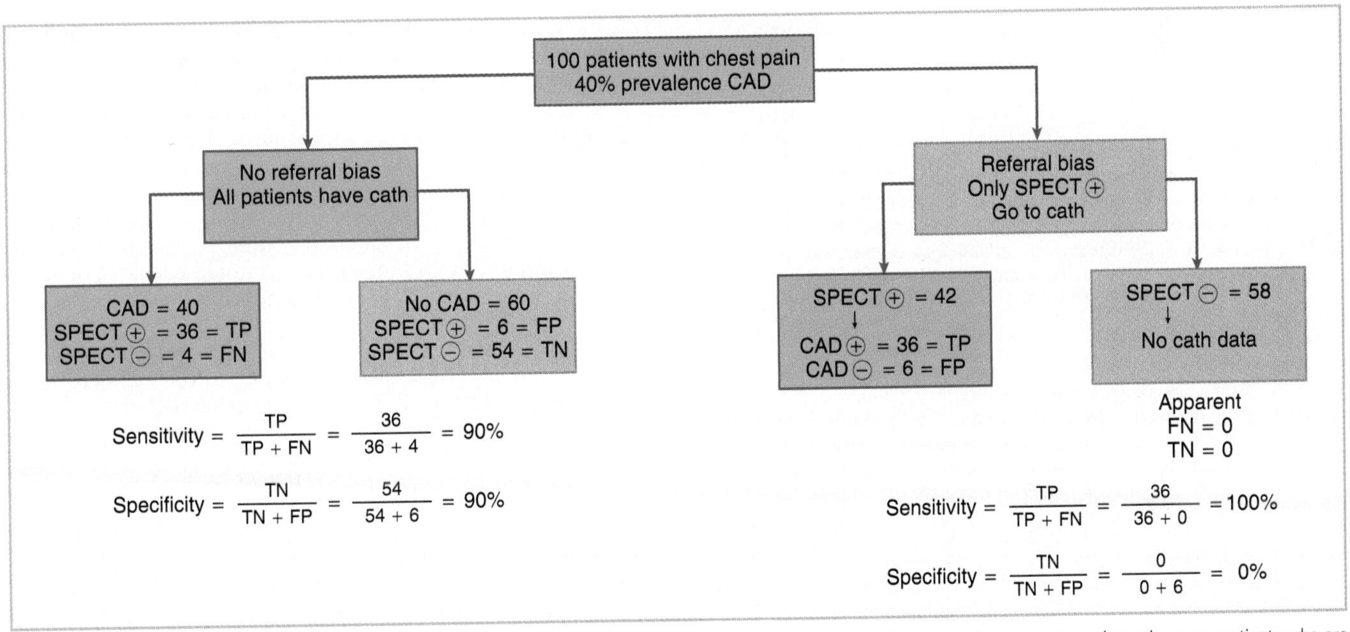

FIGURE 13-38 The effect of referral bias on specificity calculation. If the test being evaluated is used as the "gatekeeper" to coronary angiography, many patients who are true negatives (i.e., have a normal test and do not have coronary disease) will not undergo angiography and thus will not be included in the specificity calculations (right). This has an effect of artificially reducing the apparent specificity of the noninvasive test in question. CAD = coronary artery disease; FN = false negative; FP = false positive; TN = true negative; TP = true positive. (Adapted from Rozanski A, Diamond GA, Berman D, et al: The declining specificity of exercise radionuclide ventriculography. N Engl J Med.309:518, 1983.)

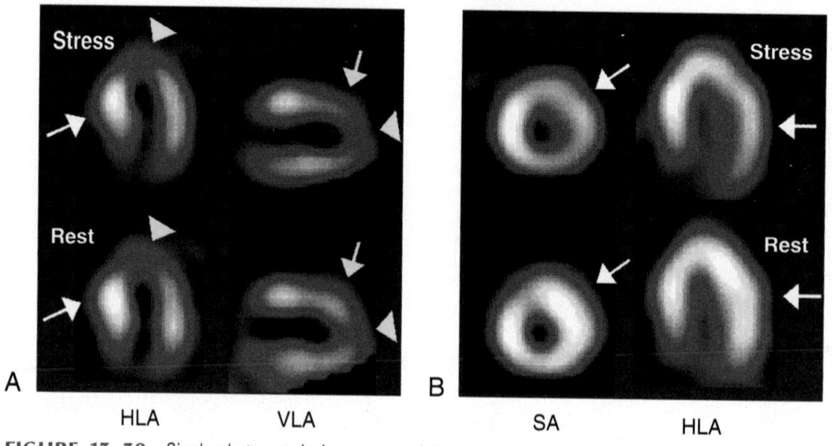

FIGURE 13–39 Single-photon emission computed tomography perfusion imaging in hypertrophic cardiomyopathy (HCM) in young asymptomatic patients with normal coronary arteries. **A,** Fixed perfusion defect of the apex consistent with infarction, indicated by yellow arrowheads in the horizontal (HLA) and vertical (VLA) long-axis images, with a reversible defect of the anterior wall (yellow arrows in the VLA images). The hypertrophied septum is evident (white arrows in the HLA images). **B,** Extensive inducible silent ischemia in the anterior, lateral, and inferior walls (white arrows). Transient ischemic cavity dilation is also present, possibly related to subendocardial ischemia.

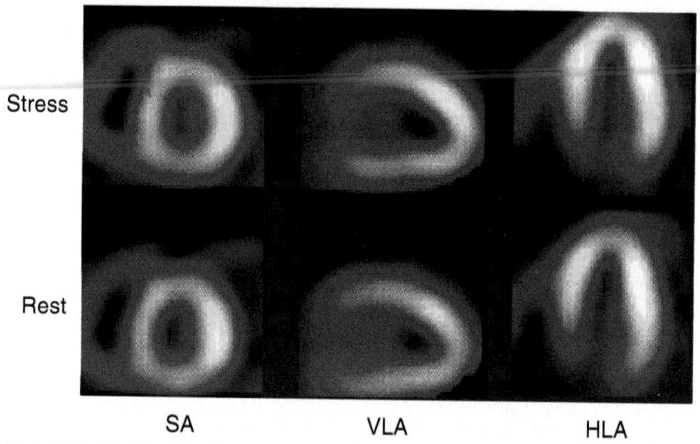

FIGURE 13–40 Single-photon emission computed tomography perfusion images at stress and rest from a patient with heart failure. The images depict a dilated left ventricle but with normal perfusion patterns, suggesting a low likelihood that coronary artery disease is the etiology of heart failure. HLA = horizontal long axis; SA = short axis; VLA = vertical long axis.

with HCM, approximately 50 percent have inducible, reversible perfusion abnormalities in the absence of CAD, typically involving the septum.[114] Such patients have more abnormal indices of diastolic function and demonstrate hemodynamic and metabolic abnormalities consistent with ischemia during atrial pacing tachycardia.[115] Thus, inducible perfusion defects in HCM represent inducible myocardial ischemia, possibly related to microvascular abnormalities, and as such have low specificity for CAD in patients with HCM. The blunted coronary flow reserve in patients with HCM is associated with a more unfavorable natural history.[112]

Left Ventricular Hypertrophy. As with the experience in HCM, inducible perfusion abnormalities may develop in patients with pressure overload LV hypertrophy (LVH) related to either hypertension or aortic stenosis.[116,117] In the absence of CAD, it is presumed that these abnormalities represent regional myocardial ischemia based on abnormal microcirculation and limited vasodilator reserve in patients with LVH. However, studies in patients with LVH by ECG criteria have generally demonstrated an accuracy of MPI for detecting CAD that is comparable to that in patients without LVH.[10] On the basis of such data, MPI is a class I indication for CAD detection when LVH is present on ECG according to ACC/AHA guidelines.[10] SPECT imaging data in patients with LVH also have a risk stratification value similar to that in patients without LVH.[118]

Dilated Cardiomyopathy. Abnormalities in myocardial perfusion are common in patients with dilated cardiomyopathy (DCM) despite normal epicardial coronary arteries.[119] Several studies have demonstrated abnormal coronary flow reserve in these patients, and as with data in HCM, blunted flow reserve identifies a cohort of patients with DCM with a more unfavorable natural history.[120,121] Such data support the relevance of the perfusion abnormalities rather than simply classifying them as false-positive if epicardial CAD is not present.

An important diagnostic consideration in patients with LV systolic dysfunction involves distinguishing those whose cardiomyopathy may be primarily due to CAD (many of whom have potentially reversible LV dysfunction) from those with idiopathic DCM. Although many patients with DCM may have perfusion abnormalities detected on MPI, the *absence* of perfusion abnormalities virtually excludes CAD as the etiology of the cardiomyopathy (Fig. 13–40).[122] *Extensive* perfusion abnormalities in the setting of LV dysfunction are virtually always associated with CAD rather than DCM, especially when the perfusion defects are segmental.

Endothelial Dysfunction. Abnormalities in myocardial perfusion detected by SPECT MPI in patients with coronary endothelial dysfunction, in the absence of "significant" epicardial vessel stenosis, have been demonstrated.[40] That these perfusion findings represent true abnormalities in coronary flow reserve is supported by studies showing *improvement* in perfusion on follow-up MPI after treatment with medical therapies directed at improving endothelial function.[123] Further support for this concept comes from cardiac magnetic resonance imaging studies demonstrating blunted subendocardial coronary flow reserve in patients with angina and normal coronary arteries.[124]

SENSITIVITY AND SPECIFICITY OF MYOCARDIAL PERFUSION IMAGING. The 2003 ACC/AHA/ASNC Radionuclide Imaging Guidelines summarize sensitivity and specificity data from 33 studies involving 4480 patients undergoing exercise SPECT imaging.[10] Sensitivity to detect CAD was 87 percent (range 71 to 97 percent) in this pooled analysis, and specificity to rule out CAD was 73 percent (range 36 to 100 percent). Few if any of these studies incorporated ECG-gated SPECT imaging of regional function or attenuation correction, techniques that appear to enhance specificity.[21] For example, in one study of women undergoing coronary angiography, specificity was improved from 76 to 96 percent when gated SPECT Tc 99m sestamibi imaging was used compared with non-gated SPECT thallium-201.[125]

Influence of Perfusion Tracer on Detection of Coronary Artery Disease. Despite the expectation of improved diagnostic accuracy with use of ^{99m}Tc-based agents, based on more favorable attributes as a radioisotope for gamma camera imaging compared with ^{201}Tl, studies comparing the widely used agents have not shown significant improvement in sensitivity or specificity. An exception is the demonstration of improved specificity in women with the use of ^{99m}Tc sestamibi compared with thallium,[125] as noted earlier. Thus, the choice of radiotracer for MPI does not notably affect the discrimination between the presence and absence of CAD. It is important to recognize that published studies often involve subjects who may not fully represent those who are most challenging to image. It would be expected that the ^{99m}Tc-based agents, with their greater photon energy, would offer improved performance in obese patients and those with large breasts as well as allow the option of higher quality gated images.

Influence of Automated Quantitation of Myocardial Perfusion Images in Detection of Coronary Artery Disease. There may be significant intra- and interobserver variability in the visual analysis of myocardial perfusion images. Several methods of quantitative analysis of MPI have been developed[10] to reduce the variability in reading by "objectifying" image analysis, by comparing regional uptake values with a normal data base.

Automated quantitative analysis systems are incorporated into most SPECT camera-computer equipment. Some of the most common are Emory Toolbox,[126] Cedars QPS,[127] and 4D MSPECT (Fig. 13–41).[128] Although published data do not clearly demonstrate improved sensitivity or specificity of these programs over visual analysis for CAD detection, such data arise from expert centers, often where the quantitative software was developed, and the visual analysis data are derived from experienced readers in laboratories with excellent quality control.

In practice, the use of contemporary quantitative programs can improve image acquisition quality as well as interpretation. Some programs incorporate motion-sensing algorithms that interrogate the raw data and alert the technologist that motion correction may be needed.

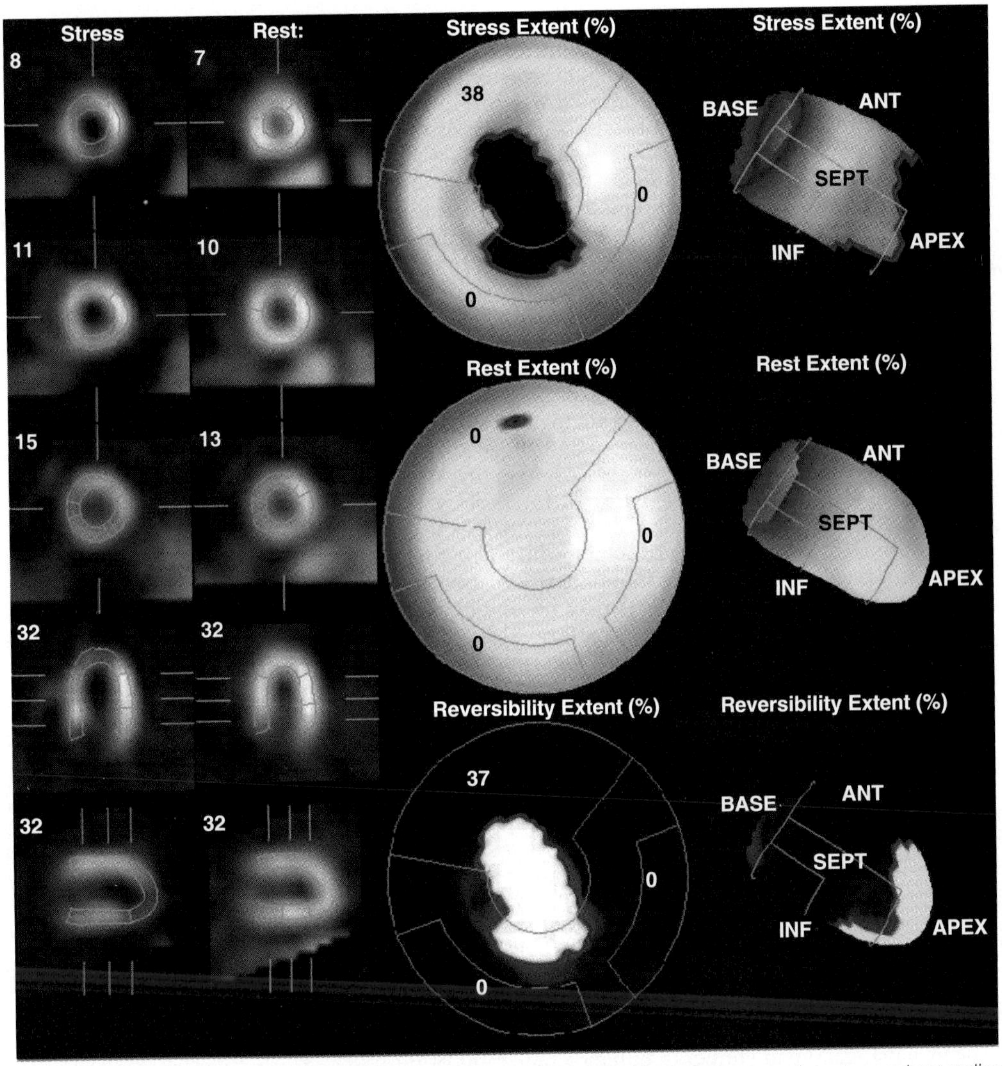

FIGURE 13–41 Automated quantitative analysis software. Selected short- and long-axis tomograms from stress and rest studies (two left columns) are automatically segmented and scored. Bull's-eye plots are created (third column) representing the stress (top) and rest (middle) data and demonstrate a large apical reversible defect. The bottom bull's-eye plot displays the extent of ischemic myocardium (white area), which measures 23 percent of the total myocardium. The bull's-eye information is also displayed in a three-dimensional format (right column, top, middle, and bottom, respectively). (Images courtesy of Guido Germano, Ph.D.)

PHARMACOLOGICAL STRESS TESTING FOR DETECTION OF CORONARY ARTERY DISEASE. Reports examining the sensitivity and specificity of vasodilator pharmacological stress combined with MPI for the detection of CAD have achieved results similar to those reported with exercise stress. A pooled analysis from the 2003 ACC/AHA/ASNC Radionuclide Imaging Guidelines involving 2465 catheterized patients in 17 studies[10] demonstrated sensitivity of 89 percent and specificity of 75 percent, similar to values from exercise SPECT MPI studies.

The more powerful hyperemic stress response achieved with vasodilator stress compared with exercise might be expected to result in improved sensitivity to detect CAD, particularly more moderate stenoses. This has not been demonstrated, possibly because of the "roll off" property of the common perfusion tracers, caused by diffusion limitation at hyperemic blood flow levels.[7] Thus, the more favorable hyperemic stress achieved with pharmacological stress is offset by the lack of linear tracer uptake in the areas with the highest flow.

The diagnostic ability of dobutamine stress imaging appears to be generally similar to that of other pharmacological and exercise stress modalities for the detection of CAD.[52] Relative to adenosine and dipyridamole, dobutamine results in a reduced hyperemic flow response, which may be exacerbated by an inadequate heart rate response. One study demonstrated that there is an increase in false-negative scans when patients with known positive dobutamine MPI are retested after receiving intravenous propranolol.[52] On the basis of these considerations, dobutamine is used only when adenosine or dipyridamole is contraindicated, such as in a patient with reactive airways disease.

EFFECT OF SUBMAXIMAL EXERCISE PERFORMANCE ON CORONARY ARTERY DISEASE DETECTION. The sensitivity of MPI to detect CAD is optimized by achieving the highest possible level of oxygen demand to stimulate the greatest increment in coronary flow reserve. In exercise ECG testing, sensitivity to detect CAD falls significantly if greater than 85 percent of maximum predicted heart rate for age is not achieved.[129] Because perfusion heterogeneity usually develops at a lower degree of supply-demand mismatch than ECG changes, the sensitivity of MPI to detect CAD is maintained at somewhat lower workloads. In one study, patients with CAD were stressed with MPI at a maximal workload and then again at a less than maximal workload.[130] There was no difference in sensitivity between the maximal and the submaximal tests. However, the extent and severity of reversible perfusion defects appear to be less at submaximal compared with maximal workloads, which may affect the prognostic value of the test.

Thus, the selection of a stress protocol can be summarized as follows[8,10]: exercise is the preferred stressor, as it allows the optimal potential association of symptoms with perfusion abnormalities. The use of exercise also allows incorporation of validated stress test criteria such as the DTS, heart rate reserve, or heart rate recovery with the MPI data.[42] For patients who cannot exercise adequately, vasodilator stress with adenosine or dipyridamole is the procedure of choice, with dobutamine used for patients with a contraindication to the vasodilators.[8,10] For patients who begin exercise but do not reach 85 percent of maximum predicted heart rate for age *or* who do not reach an appropriate symptomatic endpoint, isotope injection can be withheld, the exercise portion of the test terminated, and vasodilator stress performed to optimize diagnostic and risk stratification information.

DETECTING AND DEFINING THE EXTENT OF CORONARY ARTERY DISEASE. In formulating a management strategy for patients, it is important to determine the *extent* of disease rather than just the *presence or absence* of disease. The term "extensive CAD" refers to angiographic patterns of CAD that have prognostic significance and suggest treatment benefit from revascularization, such as left main or severe three-vessel CAD involving the proximal LAD artery.

SPECT MPI is limited by the relative nature of the perfusion information; if all areas are hypoperfused in the presence of three-vessel CAD, the least hypoperfused area appears normal and the true extent of CAD may be underestimated. However, although the perfusion pattern alone may not directly suggest the full extent of CAD, incorporation of other findings, including regional functional abnormalities, can be used to estimate more correctly the probability of disease extent.

Wall motion abnormalities on poststress gated SPECT imaging may be of benefit in the detection of extensive CAD. In one study,[131] incorporating the finding of poststress wall motion abnormality on gated SPECT imaging along with the degree of perfusion abnormality allowed improved sensitivity (85 to 91 percent) for detecting proximal 90 percent LAD lesions or multivessel disease related to 90 percent or greater proximal lesions. Similar findings have been reported for improving detection of three-vessel CAD.[132]

As noted previously, TID of the LV cavity and increased lung uptake of the perfusion tracer on poststress SPECT images have also been shown to enhance detection of multivessel CAD (see Fig. 13–8). Numerous reports suggest that the presence of TID raises the probability of multivessel CAD for any given extent of perfusion abnormality.[8,10]

Findings unrelated to imaging are also useful in enhancing the diagnosis of left main or three-vessel CAD. The development of greater than 2 mm of ST depression or hypotension on ECG treadmill testing increases the likelihood of left main or three-vessel CAD.[129]

DETECTION OF CORONARY ARTERY DISEASE IN WOMEN. The detection of CAD using exercise ECG testing is problematic in women.[90,129] A meta-analysis of 19 studies of exercise ECG testing in women revealed sensitivity and specificity of only 61 percent and 68 percent, respectively.[133] The use of ^{201}Tl for detecting CAD in women is limited by problems associated with breast attenuation. The use of ^{99m}Tc-labeled tracers should improve specificity as there is slightly less tissue attenuation, as demonstrated in a study comparing ^{201}Tl SPECT with ^{99m}Tc sestamibi gated SPECT for the detection of angiographic CAD.[125] With the incorporation of gated SPECT sestamibi imaging, a specificity of 92 percent was achieved compared with 67 percent with ^{201}Tl (see Fig. 13–10). A similar study confirmed these data in women, in whom a specificity of 91 percent was achieved using ^{99m}Tc sestamibi.[134]

DETECTION OF CORONARY ARTERY DISEASE IN VALVULAR HEART DISEASE. Several studies have evaluated the use of MPI in the assessment of the possible copresence of CAD in patients with valvular heart disease; most of the published studies involved patients with aortic stenosis. Sensitivity of MPI has ranged from 61 to 100 percent, with specificity 64 to 77 percent.[10] Although it is potentially useful in selected cases to assist in symptom evaluation, these performance characteristics are not sufficient to preclude the use of coronary angiography to define the presence of CAD in patients being considered for surgery.

RADIONUCLIDE ANGIOGRAPHY OR VENTRICULOGRAPHY FOR DETECTION OF CORONARY ARTERY DISEASE. Early reports of exercise RVG to detect CAD included predominantly patients with extensive CAD, resulting in high sensitivity. As the test was more widely applied to populations with less extensive disease, sensitivity values were lower. However, although the EF response to exercise may be a relatively insensitive marker of CAD, it is a powerful prognostic marker.[10,135]

As the LVEF response to exercise may be normal in many patients with less extensive CAD, a regional wall motion abnormality during exercise may be more sensitive for identifying CAD.[136] Radionuclide ventricular function data during exercise are usually acquired in only one view, the left anterior oblique "best septal" view.[27,28,135] Thus, the view of the inferior wall is limited, and regional wall motion abnormalities are insensitive for disease of the right coronary artery.

The normal range for an exercise EF response was initially defined by a group of young normal volunteers, a population that differs from those with chest pain and normal coronary arteriograms.[136] Posttest referral bias has also been invoked to explain the decline in specificity in exercise RVG.[137] However, as with a normal MPI study, a preserved ventricular response to exercise is associated with a good prognosis,[27,28,135] despite the presence of CAD.

In contrast to studies of MPI demonstrating little change in the ability to detect CAD at slightly submaximal workloads,[130] the sensitivity for detecting CAD by exercise RVG is impaired at submaximal workloads[137] A similar problem would be expected with stress echocardiographic studies of inducible regional wall motion abnormalities.

Exercise RVG is rarely used in contemporary practice for CAD detection. Sensitivity and specificity are modest, and visual image analysis of regional wall motion abnormalities is challenging. Nonetheless, the EF response to exercise or the absolute value of the exercise EF is a powerful prognostic indicator in suspected or known CAD, and these data have informed the contemporary use of poststress ECG-gated SPECT imaging as well as stress echocardiography.

Imaging in Patients with Established Coronary Artery Disease

There are several potential roles for SPECT MPI in patients who are known to have established CAD. Clinical questions may remain after angiography regarding the "physiological significance" of stenoses. The results of stress-rest SPECT MPI correlate generally with invasive measures of coronary flow reserve. Moreover, improvement of SPECT evidence of ischemia has been commonly documented after successful PCI, suggesting that SPECT MPI can identify the "culprit" ischemic lesion.[10]

Imaging after Coronary Artery Bypass Surgery. Studies of patients who develop recurrent symptoms after coronary artery bypass graft (CABG) surgery have demonstrated that SPECT MPI can accurately detect the presence and location of graft stenoses, even if the symptoms are atypical for ischemia.

A number of studies have concordantly demonstrated the risk stratification value of SPECT MPI in patients after CABG, especially late after CABG, even if symptoms are not present.[10] The extent of perfusion abnormality is related to the subsequent risk of cardiac death and nonfatal MI, and SPECT information has incremental predictive value over clinical and stress data (Fig. 13-42). As the outcome risk is generally low in the early years after CABG, *routine* assessment for the presence and extent of ischemia in an asymptomatic patient is not recommended by current guidelines. Nonetheless, in a study of almost 900 asymptomatic patients studied with SPECT MPI after CABG,[138] perfusion defects were common and were associated with significantly increased relative risk of death or

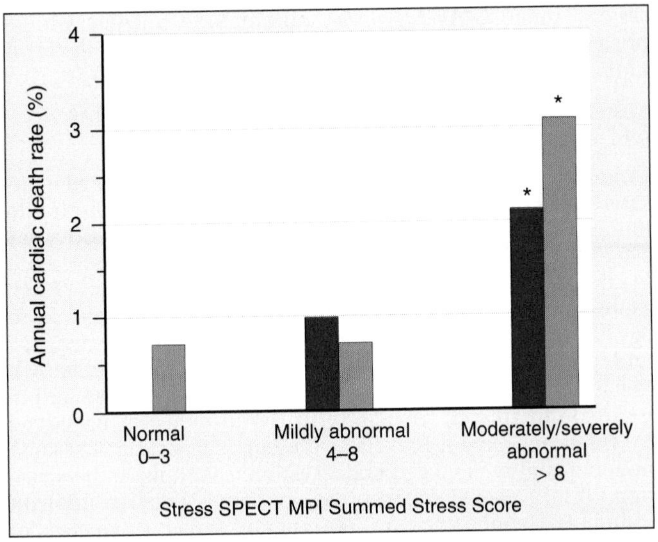

FIGURE 13–42 Annual cardiac death rate as a function of the extent of perfusion abnormality (as the summed stress score) in patients having coronary artery bypass graft (CABG) surgery within 5 years of testing (purple bars) or more than 5 years after CABG (blue bars). The risk of cardiac death increases significantly in both groups as the perfusion images become more abnormal, particularly with a moderate or severe abnormality (*$p < 0.05$ compared with other groups). MPI = myocardial perfusion imaging; SPECT = single-photon emission computed tomography. (Adapted from Zellweger M, Lewin H, Shenghan L, et al: When to stress patients after coronary artery bypass surgery? Risk stratification in patients early and late post-CABG using stress myocardial perfusion SPECT: Implications of appropriate clinical strategies. J Am Coll Cardiol 37:144, 2001.)

major events (as was impaired exercise capacity), even when controlling for time after CABG. In *symptomatic* post-CABG patients, such information can guide the need for catheterization and intervention. In *asymptomatic* patients, in whom aggressive secondary prevention strategies should be in place, the implications for clinical decision-making are less clear. In this situation, the *extent* of SPECT abnormality is important, as a more extensive perfusion abnormality is associated with a progressively higher risk of subsequent cardiac death or MI[139] and at some threshold would justify an invasive approach.

Imaging after Percutaneous Coronary Intervention. Exercise MPI is superior in detecting the presence and location of restenosis after PCI compared with exercise ECG, and current guidelines recommend stress imaging in symptomatic post-PCI patients.[10] In studies similar in concept to studies of patients with suspected CAD and those studied after CABG, the extent of SPECT MPI abnormality in patients studied after PCI is correlated with the subsequent risk of cardiac death or MI on long-term follow-up, even late after PCI, and this appears to hold true in patients even in the absence of symptoms.[140] Thus, although *routine* assessment of patients after PCI with SPECT MPI is not currently recommended, important information may be gleaned by imaging of symptomatic patients to guide decisions regarding reintervention and in selected high-risk asymptomatic patients late after PCI, to assess subsequent risk.[10]

Reports have suggested that very early after PCI, SPECT MPI may demonstrate a mild reversible defect in the territory of the treated vessel (although less severe than before PCI).[10] This may be due to delayed return of full coronary flow reserve after PCI, thus representing a true physiological phenomenon.

Left Ventricular Function During Exercise in Patients with Known Coronary Artery Disease. The EF response to exercise (as determined by exercise RVG) can be considered a reflection of the impact of regional ischemia on global ventricular performance. Even among patients with three-vessel disease by angiography, the EF response to exercise may be maintained.[136] This finding may be due to the possibility that only small areas of the LV become ischemic if some of the stenoses are not physiologically significant or if distal vessels are well collateralized. Patients with three-vessel disease who have an abnormal exercise EF response are at high risk for adverse events over follow-up and thus are more likely to benefit from revascularization.[136,141] In contrast, patients who manifest a more normal EF response to exercise have a more favorable natural history and thus are less likely to benefit from revacularization in terms of natural history.

Detection of Preclinical Coronary Artery Disease and Risk Stratification in Asymptomatic Subjects

As sudden cardiac death is too often the first manifestation of CAD, there is interest in screening populations for CAD or for CAD risk. On the basis of Bayesian principles, the low prevalence of CAD in the general asymptomatic population results in low predictive value of a positive test (for detection of CAD or determining risk of events), although negative predictive value is high. Current guidelines do not recommend routine stress MPI in asymptomatic populations.[10]

There may be circumstances, however, in which the baseline risk of a specific asymptomatic population may warrant testing with MPI. In a study of asymptomatic siblings of patients with known CAD, an abnormal SPECT MPI was associated with a fivefold increase in risk for cardiac events, with higher relative risk if both stress MPI and ECG were abnormal.[142] A key question in considering the use of testing such as SPECT MPI in asymptomatic populations is how the information will be used to manage or reduce risk. Current guidelines suggest aggressive risk factor reduction in those at high clinical risk for the development of vascular disease.[143] Whether further intensification of risk factor reduction in the setting of an abnormal imaging test, or diminished aggressiveness of risk factor reduction in the setting of a normal MPI study, results in improved outcomes is unproved and worthy of study.

Patients with diabetes are at significant risk for CAD development and cardiac events. An emerging literature suggests that a substantial proportion of *asymptomatic* diabetic patients have abnormal SPECT MPI studies and that such patients may be at even higher risk for events over time. Studies have suggested that 20 to 40 percent of asymptomatic diabetic patients have abnormal SPECT MPI studies, often with evidence of inducible, silent ischemia.[144-146] SPECT MPI has substantial risk stratification value in patients with diabetes, with risk being higher for any given perfusion abnormality than in nondiabetic patients. Moreover, similar risk stratification value has been demonstrated for diabetic patients who are *asymptomatic and without known CAD*.[146] Although guidelines at present do not suggest routine screening of asymptomatic diabetic patients with stress SPECT MPI, ongoing studies of prognosis and randomized trials in asymptomatic diabetic patients should clarify the role of SPECT MPI in diabetes.

Radionuclide Imaging in Acute Coronary Syndromes

Application of Radionuclide Imaging: Answering the Clinical Questions

For patients with *suspected* acute coronary syndromes (ACSs), radionuclide imaging techniques can both play a diagnostic role (is the clinical syndrome due to ischemia and CAD?) and provide prognostic information. Among patients who present with an ACS and ST segment depression or elevation, the typical role for imaging is in the stabilized patient, to provide risk stratification information to drive a management strategy aimed at improving natural history.

Acute Coronary Syndromes in the Emergency Department

Many patients present to EDs with symptoms suggestive of ACS but with nondiagnostic ECG findings and are often admitted to an observation unit for serial biomarker studies and possible stress testing. ^{99m}Tc- based perfusion agents may be administered to a patient in the ED with images acquired 45 to 60 minutes later,[147] and as there is minimal redistribution, images reflect myocardial blood flow *at the time of injection*.

In this setting, negative predictive value for ruling out MI has equaled or exceeded 99 percent in all observational series.[147] Patients with positive MPI have a higher risk of cardiac events during the index hospitalization as well as during follow-up (Fig. 13–43A and B). Thus, rest SPECT MPI provides information to assist triage decisions (admit or not admit) in the ED.

One study[148] found SPECT sestamibi imaging performed in the ED 92 percent sensitive for detecting acute MI, whereas

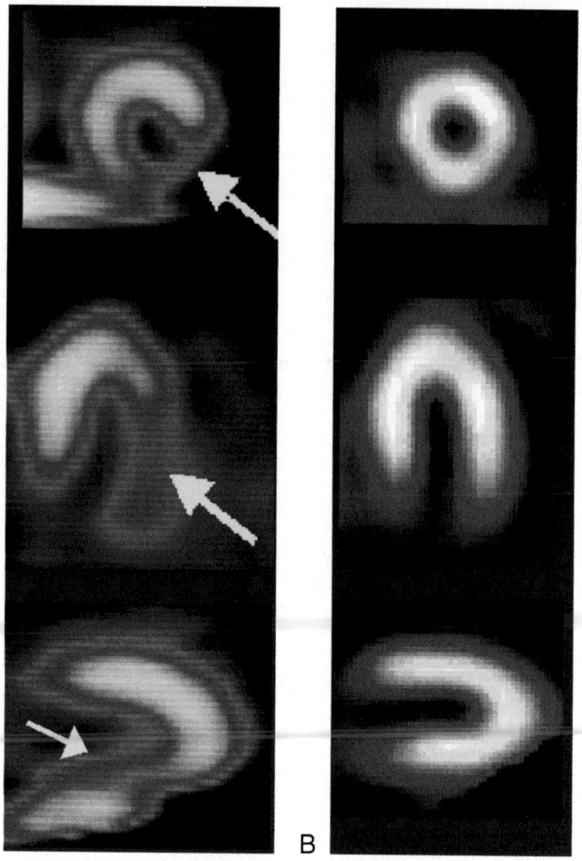

FIGURE 13–43 Examples of resting single-photon emission computed tomography (SPECT) images in patients evaluated in the emergency department with chest pain and nondiagnostic initial electrocardiographic findings. **A,** Patient with a severe inferolateral resting perfusion defect (arrows) suggestive of resting ischemia or infarction in that territory. Subsequent emergent angiography demonstrated an occluded left circumflex artery. **B,** Normal resting SPECT myocardial perfusion imaging study in a patient presenting with atypical chest pain and a nondiagnostic initial electrocardiogram in the emergency department. This normal study is associated with a very high negative predictive value for ruling out an acute coronary syndrome. HLA = horizontal long axis; SA = short axis; VLA = vertical long axis.

initial troponin I values in samples drawn at the same time had a sensitivity of only 39 percent. The maximum troponin I over the first 24 hours had a sensitivity similar to that of rest sestamibi imaging but at a distinctly later time point. Thus, acute MPI has the potential to identify ACS *earlier* than biomarkers. SPECT perfusion imaging data have been shown to provide incremental risk stratification value over clinical data for predicting unfavorable cardiac events.[149] One randomized study[150] of 46 ED patients with ongoing chest pain and a nondiagnostic ECG test found that an MPI-guided strategy incurred lower costs and resulted in shorter lengths of stay.

The Emergency Room Assessment of Sestamibi for Evaluation of (ERASE) Chest Pain Trial[151] randomly assigned 2475 patients with symptoms suggestive of ACS to a usual evaluation strategy or a strategy including acute rest SPECT MPI information. There was a significant 20 percent relative reduction in unnecessary admissions of patients ultimately found *not to have* ACS for those randomly assigned to the MPI strategy. The imaging data were among the most powerful factors associated with the decision to discharge the patient appropriately from the ED.

Thus, evidence from controlled, randomized trials suggests that incorporating SPECT MPI in ED patients with suspected ACS but no definitive ECG changes can improve triage decisions. The ACC/AHA/ASNC Radionuclide Imaging Guidelines classify MPI in this setting as a class I, level A indication.

Non-ST-Segment Elevation Myocardial Infarction and Unstable Angina

Guidelines suggest that patients with high-risk clinical characteristics in the setting of unstable angina (UA) should undergo direct catheterization.[89] Contemporary clinical trials suggest that patients with positive biomarkers, or those with a high-risk Thrombolysis in Myocardial Infarction (TIMI) score, benefit in terms of outcomes from an "invasive" strategy.[152] For patients with intermediate or low clinical risk, i.e., with "medically stabilized" UA, stress MPI has been shown to have substantial risk stratification value.[10] Patients without ischemia or infarct, especially in the presence of preserved LV function, have a low-risk outcome, suggesting that such patients can be managed conservatively without catheterization (Fig. 13–44),[153] whereas patients with significant inducible ischemia are at high-risk and thus are selected for intervention (see Fig. 13–44). The ACC/AHA/ASNC Radionuclide Imaging Guidelines[10] classify the use of stress MPI for detecting residual ischemia and the use of RVG or gated SPECT to assess LV function as class I indications.

Although the results of randomized clinical trials such as Treat Angina with Aggrastat and determine Cost of Therapy with an Invasive or Conservative Strategy (TACTICS)-TIMI 18 and others suggest slight superiority of an invasive approach in patients with UA or non–ST segment elevation MI (NSTEMI), subgroup analyses suggest that an important proportion of patients may be well managed by the conservative strategy of risk stratification by MPI followed by more selective catheterization and intervention. A retrospective analysis of the TIMI-III-B trial data has shown that by using a simple clinical score (based on age, creatine kinase with muscle and brain subunits, history of accelerated angina, and ST depression on the electrocardiogram), more than half of the population could be classified as at low risk with no outcome benefit after an early invasive strategy.[154] In TACTICS-TIMI 18, the troponin-positive subgroup, constituting 60 percent of the total population, had a larger reduction in death or MI with the early invasive strategy.[152] Therefore, patients of the TACTICS type without elevation of troponin or high TIMI risk score[155] may be optimally managed by a more conservative approach with risk stratification by using imaging techniques.

ST Segment Elevation Myocardial Infarction

Clinical variables such as recurrent ischemia, heart failure, and nonacute arrhythmias during hospitalization for acute ST segment elevation MI (STEMI) identify a subgroup of patients at high risk in whom early catheterization and intervention are indicated.[156] However, patients surviving the initial acute period may have a relatively stable course, and current guidelines suggest that noninvasive risk stratification prior to hospital discharge is appropriate.[10,156]

ASSESSMENT OF INDUCIBLE ISCHEMIA AFTER ACUTE MYOCARDIAL INFARCTION. Three major determinants of natural history risk following an acute MI include residual resting LV function; the extent of ischemic, jeopardized myocardium; and the susceptibility to ventricular arrhythmias. Thus, measures of LV function and the extent of inducible ischemia would be expected to provide important prognostic information in the aftermath of acute STEMI. Gated SPECT MPI, on the basis of the comprehensive ability to provide this information, has the potential to be the single most important test in the stable patient following STEMI.

In one of the earliest studies to examine the relation of MPI data to outcomes in stable patients following MI, thallium-

201 scintigraphic data contained the most robust information on stratifying post-MI risk. A "low-risk" thallium-201 image (no reversible defects and no lung uptake) was associated with a very low risk natural history outcome after MI.[157]

An important proportion of patients following uncomplicated MI are not able to exercise, even to a submaximal workload. Using pharmacological stress MPI in the post-MI setting, the presence of reversible defects has been reported as the only significant predictor of cardiac events on multivariable analysis,[158] whereas the absence of reversible defects identified a low-risk cohort. Subsequent reports[159] confirmed these findings.

Studies in the reperfusion era have reported generally similar results regarding the relation of stress-induced ischemia to post-MI outcomes. In a study of 134 consecutive patients within 14 days of an uncomplicated MI,[160] the extent of ischemia on the SPECT MPI was the only significant correlate of a future cardiac event on Cox regression analysis (Fig. 13–45). The extent of SPECT ischemia remained a strong correlate of a cardiac event in those who received thrombolytic therapy. The *quantitated* extent of ischemia on adenosine SPECT MPI was reported as an important predictor of post-MI cardiac events in another large study of post-MI risk stratification.[161]

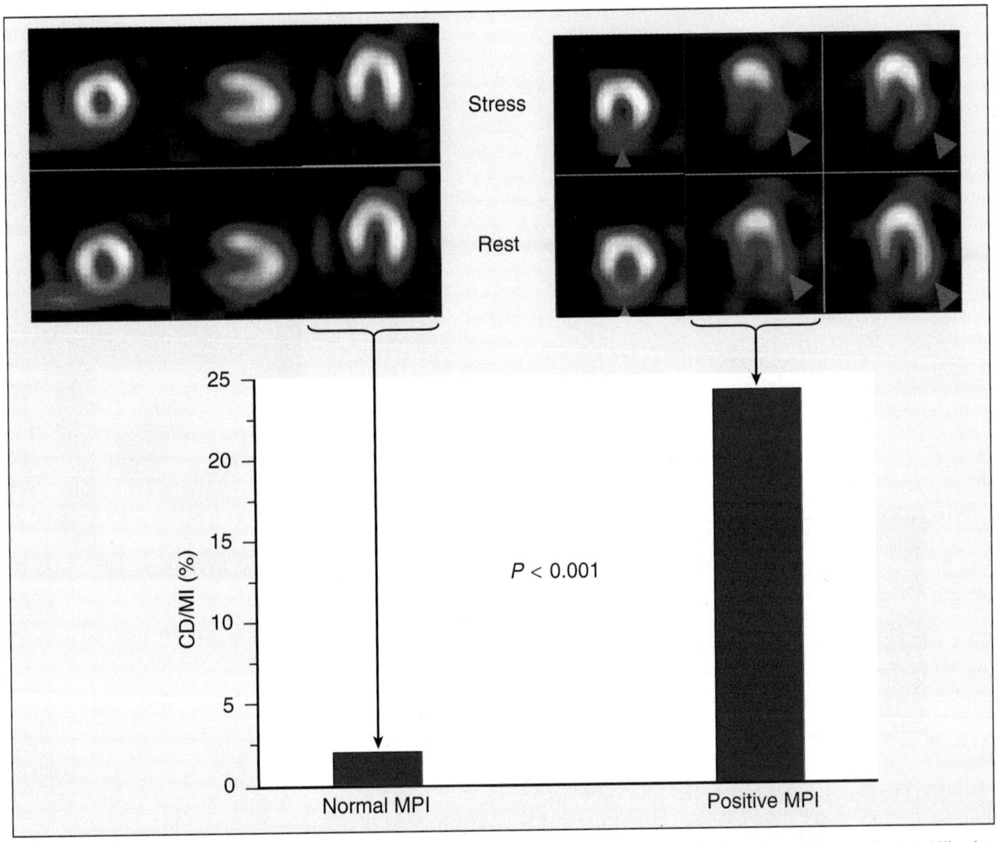

FIGURE 13–44 Single-photon emission computed tomography (SPECT) perfusion imaging in patients after medical stabilization of unstable angina. **Upper left,** Normal study, associated with a low risk of cardiac events during follow-up, suggesting that such a patient can be managed conservatively without catheterization, but with aggressive secondary preventive strategies. The bottom graph is a summary of predictive values of SPECT imaging in the aftermath of unstable angina from multiple studies. Similar to the concepts in populations with stable chest pain, the presence of abnormal perfusion imaging after unstable angina is associated with a substantial increase in the risk of cardiac death or myocardial infarction (CD/MI) during follow-up. **Upper right,** An example of a high-risk stress-rest SPECT myocardial perfusion imaging (MPI) study in the aftermath of unstable angina. Despite the stabilization of symptoms, extensive reversible perfusion abnormalities in the inferior and lateral walls suggest high risk of cardiac death or myocardial infarction, or both, during follow-up. Thus, this patient would be managed more aggressively with catheterization and intervention. (Adapted in part from Brown KA: Management of unstable angina: The role on noninvasive risk stratification. J Nucl Cardiol 4:S164,1997.)

These data are representative of the contemporary management of MI in large populations and suggest that there is an important role for post-MI gated SPECT MPI in the current era. By analogy with the data for stable outpatient populations, post-MI patients with extensive inducible ischemia are at high risk for future cardiac events, and interventional management is likely to result in improved outcome.

Clinical Trials Incorporating Results of Stress Testing Following Myocardial Infarction. The true utility of a risk-predictive test is best demonstrated insofar as it can be used not only to *predict* outcomes but also for clinical decision-making to *improve* outcomes. In this regard, several studies have been reported in which the presence of inducible ischemia following MI was used to guide clinical decisions.

The TIMI phase II trial[162] randomly assigned 3339 patients who received intravenous tissue plasminogen activator for acute MI to either an invasive strategy (catheterization at 18 to 48 hours after MI with angioplasty or CABG on the basis of angiographic findings) or a conservative arm in which catheterization was performed only in response to spontaneous or inducible ischemia (by stress RVG). The 1-year outcomes were similar with the two strategies, suggesting that a noninvasive strategy is associated with *similar outcomes* with less need for catheterization and revascularization compared with a direct catheterization strategy, implying cost-effectiveness.

The *absence* of scintigraphic ischemia has also been investigated for its influence on clinical decision-making after MI. In a study involving patients who had received thrombolytic therapy and had a *negative* functional test for ischemia in the setting of a residual infarct artery stenosis, patients were randomly assigned to medical therapy or to angioplasty of the residual stenosis.[163] Infarct-free survival was 98 percent at 12 months in the conservative therapy group and 91 percent in the group randomly assigned to PCI. These data suggest that patients with *no evidence of scintigraphic ischemia within the infarct zone on stress MPI*, even in the setting of a residual stenosis of the infarct-related artery, derive no benefit from angioplasty of the infarct-related artery.

These results suggest that testing for the presence and extent of myocardial ischemia in the aftermath of an acute MI can play an important role in clinical decision-making regarding the need for, and benefit of, catheterization and revascularization and can also identify a cohort of patients whose outcome is favorable *without* catheterization.

VERY EARLY POST-MYOCARDIAL INFARCTION RISK STRATIFICATION. Because pharmacological stress with

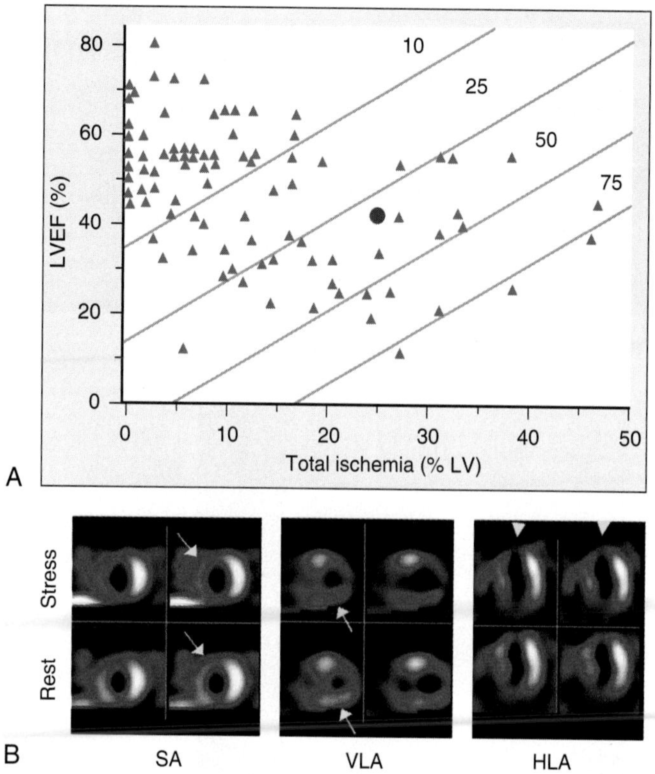

FIGURE 13–45 **A,** Risk of cardiac event during long-term follow-up after myocardial infarction (MI) is predicted by the combination of infarct size (represented by left ventricular ejection fraction [LVEF]) and the extent of reversible ischemia. As the extent of inducible ischemia increases (x-axis), and the LVEF decreases (y-axis), the outcome risk increases. The blue lines represent isobars of 10, 25, 50, and 75 percent risk of an adverse event during post-MI follow-up. The large red symbol refers to the images in panel B. **B,** Example of a patient studied several days after acute ST segment elevation MI and medical stabilization. Besides the fixed defect representing the MI in the anterior wall and apex (arrowhead), there is extensive inducible ischemia both within and remote from the infarct territory (septum and inferior walls, arrows), involving 25 percent of the ventricle. Gated single-photon emission computed tomography EF was 38 percent. On the basis of the data in A, there is an approximately 25 percent risk of post-MI adverse event (large red circle in A). HLA = horizontal long axis; SA = short axis; VLA = vertical long axis. (Adapted from Mahmarian JJ, Mahmarian AC, Marks GF, et al: Role of adenosine thallium-201 tomography for defining long term risk in patients after acute myocardial infarction. J Am Coll Cardiol 25:1333, 1995.)

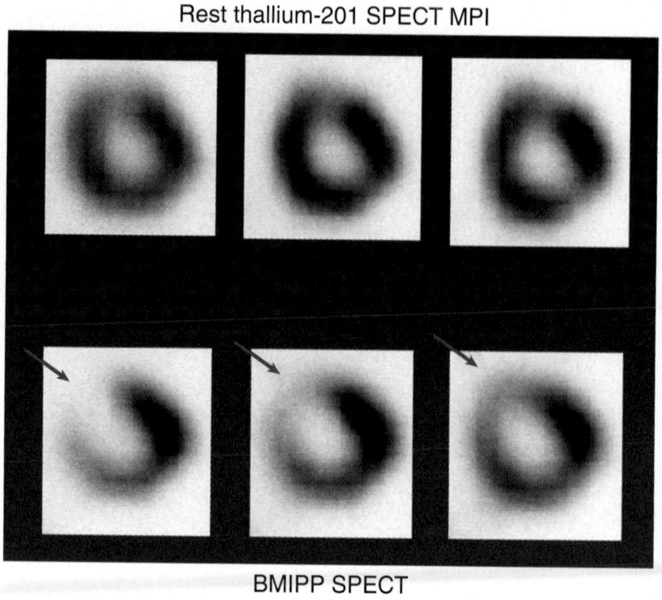

FIGURE 13–46 Iodine-123-beta-methyliodopentadecanoic acid (BMIPP) imaging of ischemic memory. In the top row, multiple short-axis tomograms of thallium-201 uptake at rest demonstrate near-homogeneous resting perfusion in a patient who presented to an emergency department and whose symptoms of chest pain had resolved many hours earlier. The BMIPP images in the same short-axis tomographic planes demonstrate a significant anteroseptal defect (arrows), suggesting prolonged postischemic suppression of fatty acid metabolism, referred to as "ischemic memory." MPI = myocardial perfusion imaging; SPECT = single-photon emission computed tomography. (Adapted from Kawai Y, Tsukamoto E, Nozaki Y, et al: Significance of reduced uptake of iodinated fatty acid analogues for the evaluation of patients with acute chest pain. J Am Coll Cardiol 38:1888, 2001.)

adenosine or dipyridamole induces coronary hyperemia with only minimal increments in oxygen demand, it may potentially be performed safely even very early after MI. This concept was examined[164] in a study of 451 patients randomly assigned to a standard post-MI evaluation strategy or to a strategy incorporating dipyridamole SPECT MPI *2 to 3 days* after uncomplicated MI. The testing was safe, and MPI supplied better risk stratification data predicting outcomes than the submaximal stress MPI data. Thus, pharmacological stress can safely allow management decisions to be made earlier in the post-MI course.

STUDIES EXAMINING BOTH PERFUSION IMAGING AND LEFT VENTRICULAR FUNCTION AFTER ACUTE MYOCARDIAL INFARCTION. As post-MI EF falls, there is a progressive increase in mortality risk. The availability of gated SPECT imaging to evaluate myocardial perfusion and LV function simultaneously raises an important question regarding the incremental information provided by combining the analysis of perfusion and function information within one test.

One study[165] comprehensively evaluated LV function and adenosine SPECT MPI in patients in relation to long-term cardiac events. Both the extent of perfusion defect and LVEF provided superior risk categorization compared with either variable alone. These data strongly suggest that perfusion abnormalities and LVEF following MI have complementary roles, and their measurement together powerfully categorizes patients' risk in the post-MI setting.

Radionuclide Imaging for Acute Coronary Syndromes: Research Directions

Imaging Ischemic Memory. A possible future approach to risk stratification in patients with *suspected* ACS involves the imaging of fatty acid metabolism. As noted earlier, following a regional ischemic insult, abnormalities in fatty acid metabolism may persist long after perfusion has returned to normal, a finding termed ischemic memory. Imaging fatty acid metabolism may therefore allow assessment of *recent* ischemia. The radiolabeled fatty acid analog 15-(*p*-[iodine-123] iodophenyl)-3-(*R,S*) methylpentadecanoic acid (BMIPP) was imaged with SPECT 1 to 5 days after presentation in patients with suspected ACS. The BMIPP images showed greater sensitivity than did rest MPI in identifying the presence and site of the culprit coronary stenosis (Fig. 13–46).[166] Future studies will determine whether such techniques can help guide management decisions.

Imaging of Potentially Unstable Atherosclerotic Plaques and Platelet Activation. Plaque rupture exposes the lipid core to platelet activation. ^{125}I-labeled low-density lipoprotein has been used to image atherosclerotic disease in carotid arteries. A radionuclide target for macrophages, ^{131}I-labeled monocyte chemoattractant protein-1, has been shown to accumulate in lipid-rich, macrophage-rich regions in animal models of atherosclerosis.[167,168] Whether these favorable results in animals can be translated to the clinical setting of patients with potentially unstable atherosclerosis is a subject of ongoing study.

Assessment of Heart Failure with Radionuclide Imaging

Is Coronary Artery Disease the Etiology of Heart Failure?

Determining whether LV dysfunction is due predominantly to the consequences of CAD or to one of the many other etiologies included in the term "nonischemic" cardiomyopathy is a critical early step in the management of patients with heart failure. Because CAD is the most common cause of heart failure in developed countries, noninvasive assessment of myocardial ischemia and viability would identify the subgroup of patients with heart failure who have a potentially *reversible* degree of LV dysfunction and may benefit from revascularization. Therapeutic interventions that improve dysfunctional but viable myocardium may significantly affect global LVEF, LV remodeling, and patients' survival. Furthermore, the identification of CAD in patients with heart failure has implications in secondary prevention strategies, as acute MI is a common mechanism of death in patients with heart failure.

A *normal* stress MPI scan in a patient with heart failure and LV dysfunction is highly predictive for the *absence* of CAD. Studies of MPI for detecting CAD in patients with LV dysfunction have shown high sensitivity but modest specificity (Fig. 13–47; see Fig. 13–40).[122] The modest specificity of MPI to rule out CAD is explained in part by pathological as well as cardiac magnetic resonance imaging studies[169] demonstrating that patients with "nonischemic" cardiomyopathy may have patchy or larger confluent territories of fibrosis or scarring, manifest as fixed defects on SPECT MPI. Invasive studies as well as PET imaging have demonstrated attenuated coronary blood flow at rest and during hyperemic stress in nonischemic cardiomyopathy,[121,170] which could be manifest as reversible defects. Hence, both fixed and reversible perfusion defects have been observed in patients with nonischemic cardiomyopathy, with important prognostic implications.[122,170]

Although the presence of *any* perfusion abnormality is not specific for ruling out CAD, the *pattern* of perfusion abnormality may assist in the differentiation between CAD and "nonischemic" etiology of heart failure. *More extensive* or *more severe* perfusion defects, or both, are more likely to represent CAD, whereas smaller and milder defects are more likely in patients with nonischemic cardiomyopathy.[10,122,171]

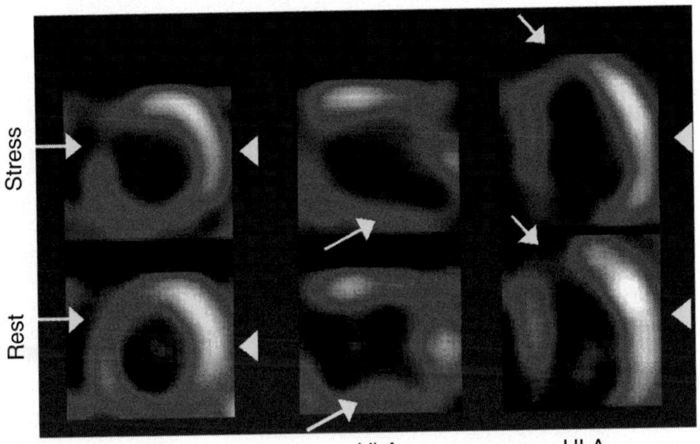

FIGURE 13–47 Single-photon emission computed tomography perfusion imaging demonstrating extensive severe fixed defects of the septum, apex, and inferior wall (arrows) suggestive of extensive prior myocardial infarction, as well as extensive inducible ischemia of the lateral wall (arrowheads). This strongly suggests that coronary artery disease is the etiology of the heart failure syndrome in this patient. HLA = horizontal long axis; SA = short axis; VLA = vertical long axis.

Hence, comprehensive early evaluation of patients with heart failure and LV systolic dysfunction includes an assessment of the underlying etiology (CAD or noncoronary causes). If CAD is identified as a causative factor in the heart failure syndrome, assessment of the extent of inducible ischemia and preserved viability within dysfunctional myocardium aids in determining the potential for reversal of LV dysfunction following revascularization.

Assessment of Myocardial Viability and the Potential Benefit of Revascularization

The goal of assessing viability is to optimize selection of patients with heart failure whose symptoms and natural history may improve following revascularization. Data suggest that hibernation and stress-induced ischemia are common in patients with stable heart failure, even in the absence of angina.[172] In a clinical trial of stable community-based patients with heart failure of whom only a minority had angina, hibernation or stress-induced ischemia, or both, were demonstrated by SPECT imaging in approximately 70 percent of patients, suggesting that an important subpopulation of patients with heart failure may benefit from a noninvasive search for viability and ischemia.

Studies have demonstrated that the *potential for improved heart failure symptoms* following revascularization correlates with the magnitude of the PET "mismatch" pattern (i.e., enhanced FDG uptake relative to perfusion).[173] In a meta-analysis of outcome studies after viability imaging, patients with evidence of preserved myocardial viability[174] who underwent revascularization had a substantial reduction in the *risk of cardiac death* during long-term follow-up (Fig. 13–48). Revascularization conferred no natural history advantage in patients without substantial myocardial viability. These data suggest that noninvasive imaging of viability and ischemia can play an important role in selecting patients for revascularization, with the expectation of improving symptoms and natural history.

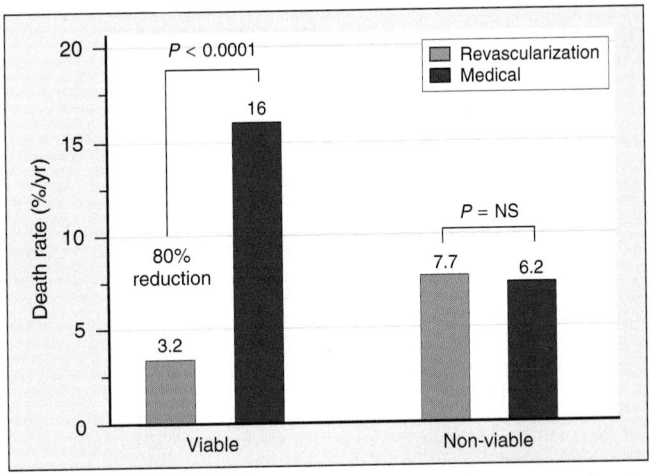

FIGURE 13–48 Outcome of patients with ischemic left ventricular dysfunction after viability testing. Among patients determined to have predominantly viable myocardium, treatment with medical therapy is associated with a 16 percent annual risk of cardiac death. Similar patients treated with revascularization have only a 3.2 percent annual risk of cardiac death, representing an 80 percent reduction in risk with revascularization. In contrast, patients with predominantly nonviable myocardium have no difference in outcome whether they are treated with medical therapy or revascularization. These data suggest that noninvasive interrogation of myocardial viability can identify treatment strategies associated with more favorable long-term outcomes. (Adapted from Allman K, Shaw L, Hachamovitch R, Udelson JE: Myocardial viability testing and impact of revascularization on prognosis in patients with coronary artery disease and left ventricular dysfunction: A meta-analysis. J Am Coll Cardiol 39:1151, 2002.)

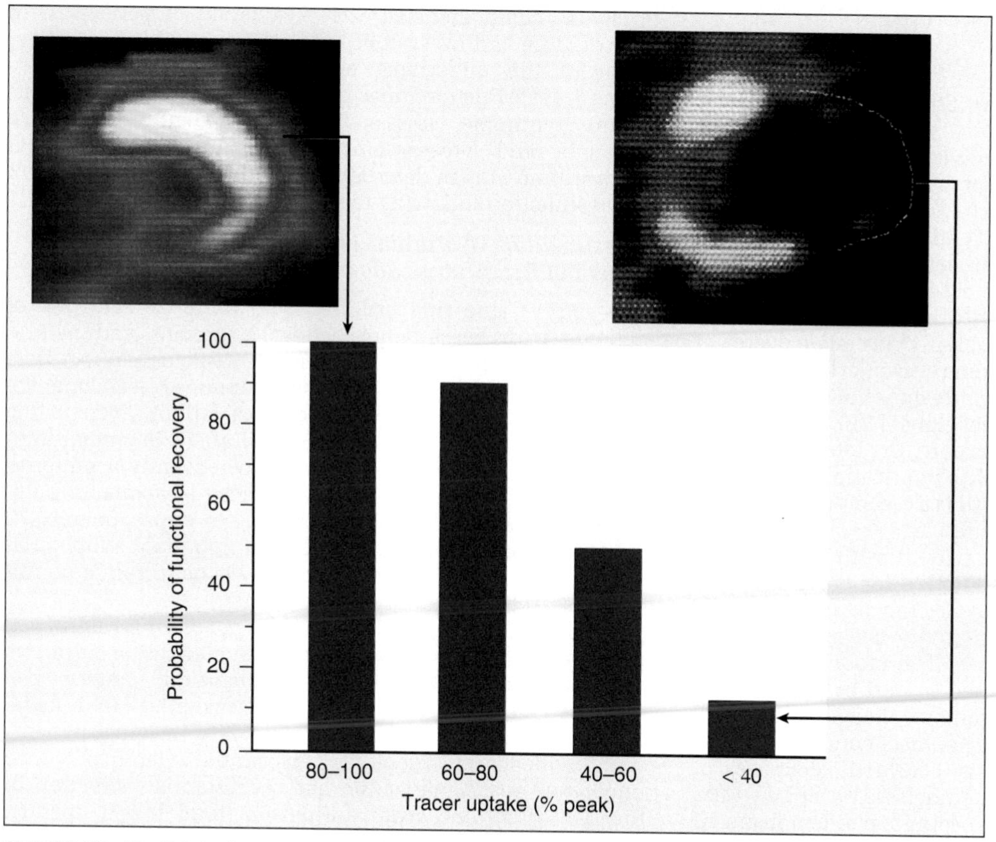

FIGURE 13–49 Relation between tracer uptake in a dysfunctional territory and the subsequent probability of functional recovery after revascularization. The probability of improved regional left ventricular function after revascularization is significantly related to the quantitative degree of tracer uptake. **Upper right,** A patient with a large, severe defect in the anterior and apical walls. The severity of the defect suggests that significant functional recovery would not be expected with revascularization. **Upper left,** Extensive myocardial viability in a patient with left ventricular dysfunction (ejection fraction 30 percent) and severe three-vessel coronary disease. There is substantial tracer uptake throughout the anterior wall and apex (arrow), territories with significant regional dysfunction. The retained degree of tracer uptake suggests extensive myocardial (myocyte) viability and high probability of functional recovery after revascularization. (Adapted from Bonow RO: Assessment of myocardial viability with thallium-201. *In* Zaret BL, Beller GA [eds]: Nuclear Cardiology: State of the Art and Future Directions. St. Louis, Mosby, 1999, pp 503-512; and Udelson JE: Assessment of myocardial viability with technetium-99m-labeled agents. *In* Zaret BL, Beller GA [eds]: Nuclear Cardiology: State of the Art and Future Directions. St. Louis, Mosby, 1999, pp 513-533.)

PRINCIPLES OF ASSESSING MYOCARDIAL VIABILITY BY RADIONUCLIDE TECHNIQUES

The radionuclide tracers and techniques most often used to assess viability have been evaluated for their relation to preserved tissue viability directly by correlating tracer uptake with histologically confirmed extent of tissue viability.[34] Quantitative analysis of tracer uptake correlates directly with the magnitude of preservation of tissue viability, and tracer uptake represents a *continuous variable*; i.e., the magnitude of tracer uptake directly reflects the magnitude of preserved tissue viability.[175,176] For a dysfunctional segment or territory, the probability of functional recovery after revascularization is related to the magnitude of tracer uptake, representing the degree of preserved myocardial viability (extent of hibernation or stunning) within that territory. A dysfunctional territory with normal or only mildly reduced tracer uptake thus has a high likelihood of improved function after revascularization. In contrast, a territory with a severe reduction in tracer uptake would represent predominant infarction, and the likelihood of improved function after revascularization would be low (Fig. 13–49). The magnitude of potential improvement of *global LV function* after revascularization is in turn determined by the extent of viable dysfunctional myocardium.

Imaging Protocols for Assessing Myocardial Viability

Thallium-201. The presence of thallium-201 after redistribution implies preserved myocyte cellular viability. However, as the *absence* of thallium-201 uptake on the redistribution images is not a sufficient sign of the *absence* of regional viability, iterations of the standard thallium-201 protocol have been investigated[175,177] in order to optimize the assessment of regional viability (Fig. 13–50A and B). After thallium-201 *reinjection*, approximately 50 percent of regions with "fixed" defects on stress-redistribution imaging show significant enhancement of thallium-201 uptake, predictive of improvement in regional LV function (see Fig. 13–50A). The presence of a severe thallium-201 defect after reinjection identifies areas with a very low probability of improvement in function.

Late redistribution imaging, 24 to 48 hours after the initial stress thallium-201 injection, allows more time for redistribution to occur and has good positive predictive value for improvement in function. The negative predictive value is suboptimal, as redistribution does not take place in some patients even after a prolonged time, and image quality may be suboptimal.[10,175]

With *rest-redistribution thallium-201 imaging,* images are obtained 15 to 20 minutes after tracer injection at rest, reflecting resting regional blood flow, and images obtained 3 to 4 hours following redistribution reflect preserved viability. The finding of a *reversible resting defect* may identify areas of myocardial hibernation (see Fig. 13–50B). This finding appears to be an insensitive although specific sign of potential improvement in regional function.[10,175,177]

Technetium 99m Sestamibi and Tetrofosmin. Studies have demonstrated that the performance of these agents for predicting improvement in regional function after revascularization is similar to that of thallium-201.[10,176] Administration of nitrates to improve resting blood flow prior to injection of sestamibi appears to improve slightly the ability of these tracers to detect myocardial viability.[10,176]

Positron-Emission Tomography. The extent of the PET mismatch pattern (enhanced FDG uptake relative to blood flow) correlates with improvement in LV function after revascularization as well as with the clinical course, magnitude of improvement in heart failure symptoms, and survival after revascularization (see Fig. 13–29).[10,32,173] Patients with heart failure and extensive PET match pattern (diminished blood flow and severe reduction in FDG uptake), representing predominant infarction, are unlikely to benefit clinically from revascularization.[173]

Comparison of Imaging Techniques for Viability Assessment. On the basis of a meta-analysis evaluating the ability of the various radionuclide techniques to predict improvements in regional function, all the radionuclide techniques (as well as low-dose dobutamine echocardiography) perform in a relatively similar manner regarding positive and negative predictive values for improvements in regional function.[178] SPECT techniques appear to be slightly more sensitive, dobutamine echocardiography slightly more specific, and PET techniques appear to have better accuracy. A randomized trial of patients with moderate LV dysfunction being considered for revascularization randomly allocated to have viability information supplied by either PET imaging or SPECT stress-rest sestamibi imaging found no difference in outcomes over long-term follow-up.[179] As noted previously, a meta-analysis of observational outcome studies related to myocardial viability demonstrated no difference between the techniques commonly used to assess viability (PET versus SPECT versus dobutamine echocardiography) with regard to reduction of mortality after revascularization.[174]

Selection of Patients with Heart Failure for Viability Assessment

Guidelines suggest that patients with heart failure *and* active angina benefit in terms of natural history from revascularization and thus should be referred directly for angiography.[180] In some situations, subsequent noninvasive definition of regional viability and ischemia may be important for planning the revascularization strategy when the anatomy is known.

For patients with heart failure and *no angina*, recommendations are less clear. Studies suggest that ischemia and viability may be present in a significant proportion of such patients, who have potential benefit from revascularization,[172] and for most patients with heart failure, a search for underlying ischemia and viability would be an appropriate clinical strategy at some point in their evaluation. If substantial ischemia or viability of dysfunctional territories is found in the setting of vessels technically amenable to revascularization, the literature would suggest a *clinical benefit* from revascularization.[10] In the *absence* of substantial ischemia or viability, such a benefit is less likely.The imaging data can be used in decision-making to help balance the *risks and benefits* of revascularization in a patient with heart failure and LV dysfunction, by supplying information on potential *benefit* of a revascularization strategy.

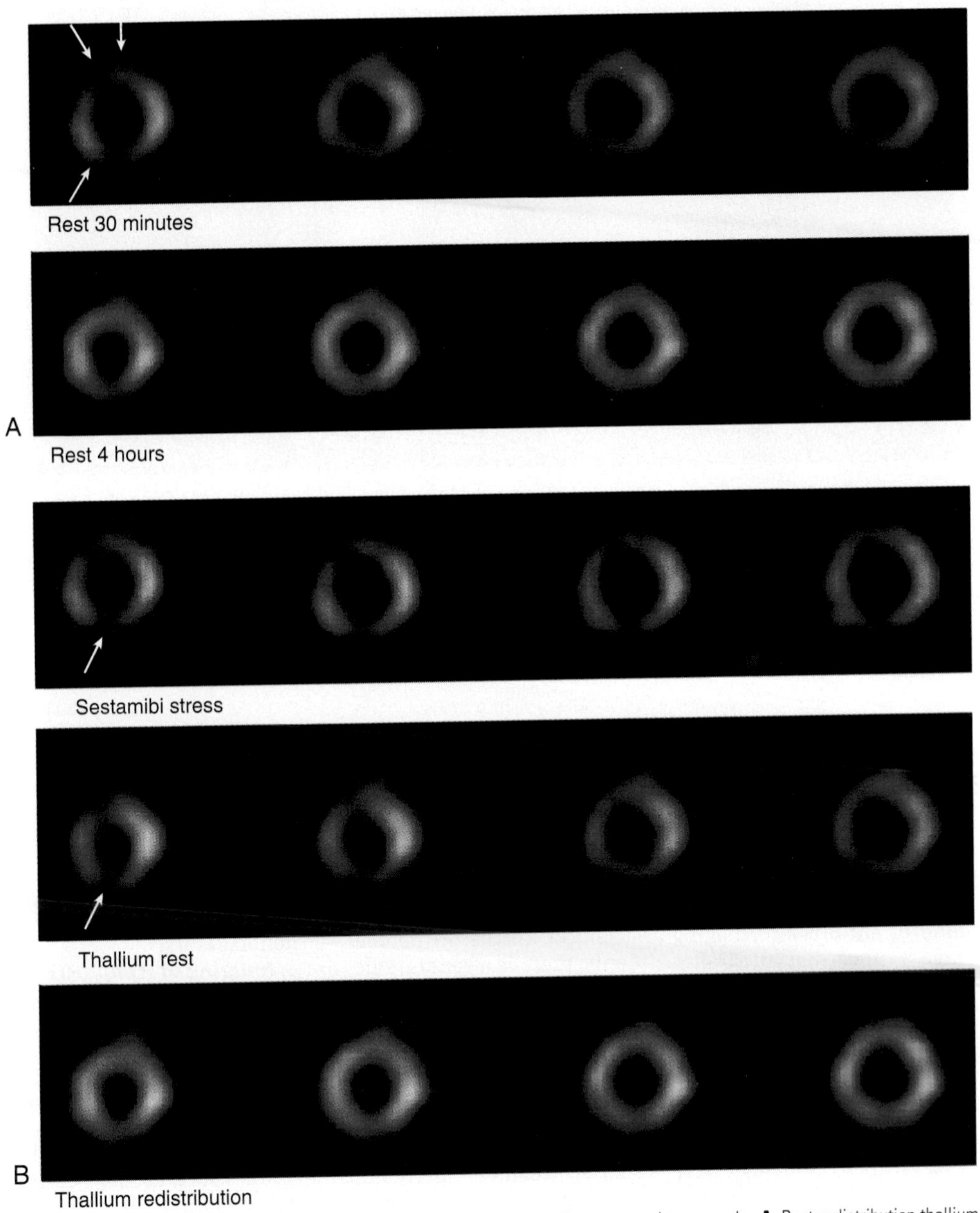

FIGURE 13–50 Myocardial viability imaging with single-photon emission computed tomography. **A,** Rest-redistribution thallium imaging, demonstrating redistribution in regions with initial reductions in thallium uptake, particularly the anterior wall, septum, and inferior walls (arrows), indicating resting hypoperfusion. **B,** Incorporation of rest-redistribution thallium imaging as part of a dual-isotope protocol using sestamibi with stress and thallium at rest. The irreversible defect of the inferior wall (arrow) between stress and rest images can be evaluated further by late imaging after decay of sestamibi to evaluate thallium redistribution kinetics.

Assessment of Left Ventricular Function in Heart Failure

For patients with the clinical syndrome of heart failure, the distinction between those with preserved and those with impaired systolic function has important clinical relevance. Clinical trials evaluating the use of such therapies as ACE inhibitors, angiotensin receptor blockers, and beta blockers have focused on the subpopulation of heart failure patients with impaired systolic function.[180] Less information is available from randomized trials for heart failure patients with preserved ventricular function, many of whom have abnormalities of diastolic function as the basis for symptoms. Thus, accurate determination of LV function in a patient with heart failure defines the evidence-based therapeutic approach that should be undertaken.

On the basis of the quantitative and reproducible nature of the EF results, equilibrium RVG techniques have been used in large clinical trials to identify systolic dysfunction.[10,180] In contemporary practice, the ECG-gated SPECT technique is often used for determination of systolic function. The *simultaneous* assessment of LV systolic function as well as stress and rest perfusion by gated SPECT imaging can provide a range of information relevant to the care and clinical decision-making for patients with heart failure, including the state of LV function, the probability of CAD as the etiology of heart failure, and the presence and extent of viability and ischemia.

Imaging in Inflammatory and Infiltrative Cardiomyopathies

MYOCARDITIS. Inflammatory injury to the myocardium by infective agents, postinfective immune processes (i.e., Chagas disease, rheumatic carditis), hypersensitivity, and autoimmune conditions can cause myocardial dysfunction. The clinical manifestation of such an inflammatory process is acute myocarditis and cardiac allograft rejection. As myocyte necrosis is an obligatory component of myocarditis (cellular infiltrates, predominantly lymphocytes and

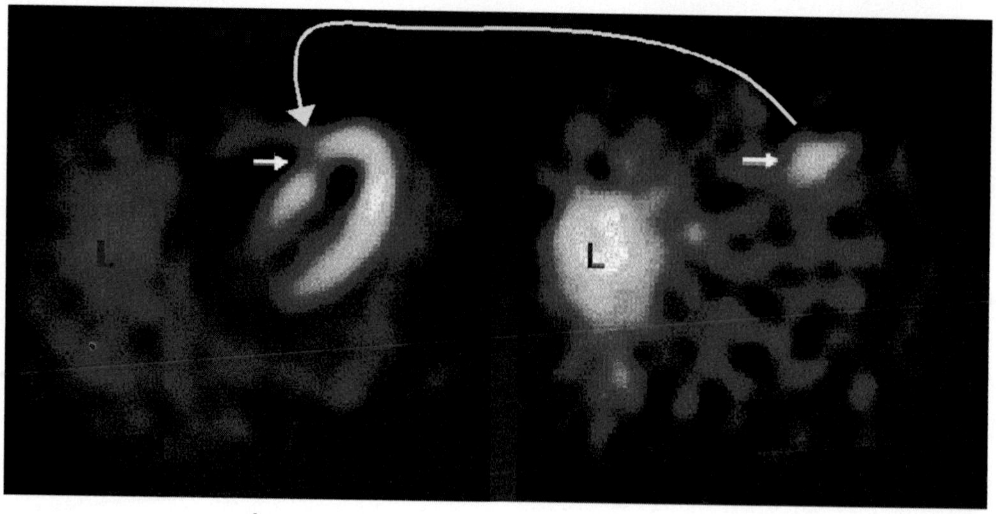

A B

FIGURE 13–51 Example of annexin imaging of apoptosis. **A,** Resting sestamibi study in a patient several days after myocardial infarction (MI), showing a defect in the septum, identifying the territory of the MI (white arrow). **B,** ^{99m}Tc-annexin imaging of apoptosis in the same tomographic plane. The area of uptake (white arrow) corresponds to the area of resting perfusion defect (yellow arrow), suggesting the presence of apoptosis in the MI territory. L = liver. (Adapted from Hofstra L, Liem IH, Dumont EA, et al: Visualization of cell death in vivo in patients with acute myocardial infarction. Lancet 356:209, 2000.)

macrophages, clustered around necrotic myocytes), ^{111}In-labeled antimyosin antibody, which specifically targets myosin heavy chain, has been used for the detection of necrosis associated with myocarditis and heart transplant rejection. In patients with biopsy-positive myocarditis, the sensitivity of an antimyosin scan is approximately 95 percent, with a negative predictive value of approximately 95 percent. However, the specificity and positive predictive value of antimyosin imaging are modest, in the 50 percent range.[181] In cardiac allograft recipients, there is a general relationship between the severity of transplant rejection by biopsy and the magnitude of antimyosin uptake by scintigraphy. However, the highly variable antimyosin uptake across the severity range of rejection precludes antimyosin imaging as a sufficiently reliable noninvasive test for detection of transplant rejection.[182] Observational studies with myocardial perfusion, gated blood pool, and ^{123}I metaiodobenzylguanidine (MIBG) imaging have reported regional perfusion defects, wall motion abnormalities, and sympathetic denervation in patients who present with myocarditis, in the absence of significant CAD.[10]

SARCOID HEART DISEASE. Cardiac involvement occurs in about 20 percent of patients with sarcoidosis. In patients presenting with advanced AV block, myocardial perfusion SPECT or gallium-67 imaging (a nonspecific indicator of inflammation) along with magnetic resonance imaging or chest computed tomography can localize myocardial involvement of sarcoidosis.[10] Focal fibromuscular dysplasia found in the small coronary arteries may provide an explanation for focal ischemic injuries and reversible defects described on myocardial perfusion SPECT. Perfusion defects involving the left ventricle have been associated with AV block and heart failure, and defects involving the right ventricle on SPECT have been associated with ventricular tachycardia of right ventricular origin.[183]

CARDIAC AMYLOIDOSIS. Cardiac involvement of amyloidosis involves the deposition of light chain amino acids into the myofibrils, which leads to impaired relaxation. Patients with amyloidosis may demonstrate abnormally prolonged LV diastolic filling and an increased atrial contribution to the total diastolic filling. These indices of abnormal diastolic filling pattern can be obtained from RNA as well as echocardiography. Although the hallmark of the clinical presentation is dyspnea and heart failure symptoms, advanced AV block can also be a presenting feature in cardiac amyloidosis. ^{123}I MIBG imaging has shown marked cardiac sympathetic denervation, providing insight into the pathogenesis of cardiac conduction disturbances in amyloidosis.[184] ^{99m}Tc pyrophosphate scintigraphy may be useful in identifying patients with cardiac amyloidosis, demonstrating diffuse uptake throughout the myocardium.[10]

Radionuclide Imaging in Heart Failure and Left Ventricular Dysfunction: Research Directions

Assessment of Cardiac Sympathetic Innervation. An emerging area of risk stratification involves the use of ^{123}I MIBG imaging of cardiac sympathetic innervation. In the post-MI setting, the territory of abnormal MIBG uptake (corresponding to sympathetic *denervation*) often exceeds the final infarct size, and such patients are at higher risk for subsequent ventricular arrhythmias.[122,185,186] Should this finding prove prognostic for outcomes in patients with LV dysfunction, as suggested by earlier studies, MIBG imaging may have a role in selecting post-MI patients who may optimally benefit from defibrillators.[186]

Imaging of Apoptosis. Another potential approach to evaluating patients with LV dysfunction after MI is the visualization of apoptosis, or programmed cell death, in humans using ^{99m}Tc-labeled annexin V, which localizes to apoptotic cells. In one study, positive uptake of this agent was seen in six of seven post-MI patients, localized to areas of resting perfusion defects (Fig. 13–51).[187] This agent may herald the onset of the ability to track this process noninvasively in syndromes such as heart failure and to study approaches to attenuate the unfavorable pathophysiology of apoptosis.

Radionuclide Imaging of Cell- or Gene-Based Regenerative Therapy. Local targeted gene delivery or implantation of autologous skeletal myoblasts, bone marrow stromal cells, or hematopoietic stem cells may functionally revitalize scarred, noncontractile myocardial regions. Noninvasive assessment of the fate of myogenic cell grafts and therapeutic genes in vivo may provide insight into the mechanism by which they improve cardiac function or prevent remodeling. In animal studies, transplanted cardiomyoblasts expressing a PET reporter gene have been imaged longitudinally to gain insight into the pattern of cell survival.[188] Using cardiac micro-PET imaging, detailed tomographic locations of transplanted cells were obtained (Fig. 13–52). This may become an important method to study regenerative therapies in human studies.

Imaging the Tissue Angiotensin-Converting Enzyme Receptor System. Radionuclide imaging has been used in experimental systems to study the tissue ACE receptor system directly. Using the radiotracer [^{18}F]fluorobenzyl-lisinopril,[189] preliminary observations have shown a relationship between ACE and collagen replacement, as ACE was absent in the collagen-stained areas and was increased in the juxtaposed areas of replacement fibrosis.[190,191] These data suggest that

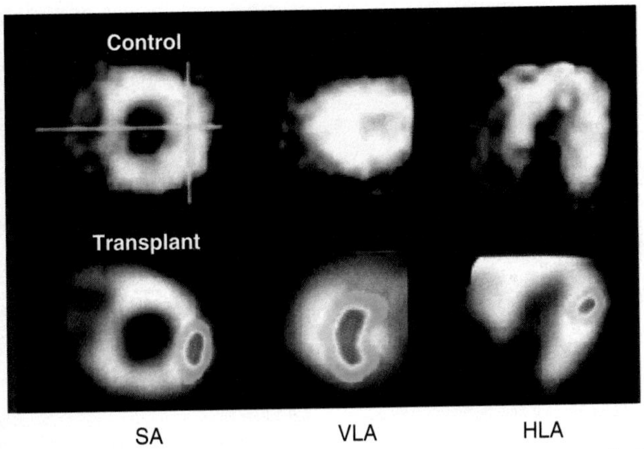

FIGURE 13–52 Cardiac micro-positron-emission tomography (PET) images in the short-axis (SA), vertical long-axis (VLA), and horizontal long-axis (HLA) views of a rat heart transplanted with cardiomyoblasts expressing a PET reporter gene. The gray/white uptake represents homogeneous perfusion by ^{13}N-NH_3, and the color uptake in the lateral wall represents the viable transplanted cardiomyoblasts studied in vivo (bottom row). There is no uptake in the control heart, with normal perfusion (top row). (Adapted from Wu JC, Chen IY, Sundaresan G, et al: Molecular imaging of cardiac cell transplantation in living animals using optical bioluminescence and positron emission tomography. Circulation 108:1302, 2003.)

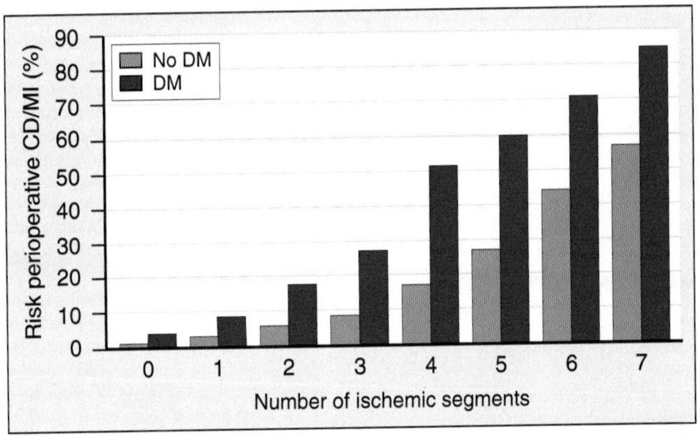

FIGURE 13–53 Relation between the extent of inducible ischemia (as the number of segments with ischemic defects, x-axis) and the risk of perioperative cardiac death (CD) or myocardial infarction (MI) in patients following peripheral vascular surgery undergoing preoperative pharmacological stress myocardial perfusion imaging. As the extent of preoperative reversible defect increases, the risk of a major perioperative event increases as well. Moreover, the presence of diabetes mellitus (DM) confers additional risk: for any given extent of preoperative ischemia, the event risk is higher if DM is present. (Adapted from Brown K: Prognostic value of myocardial perfusion imaging: State of the art and new developments. J Nucl Cardiol 3:516, 1996.)

increased ACE may be a stimulus for collagen replacement and remodeling. In the future, noninvasive imaging with PET in patients with heart failure may allow monitoring of changes in ACE patterns in vivo, possibly reflecting progression of disease and the effect of therapies before collagen replacement ensues.

Imaging to Assess Cardiac Risk Prior to Noncardiac Surgery

The clinical role of MPI for evaluating patients prior to elective noncardiac surgery has grown, as CAD represents an important perioperative and long-term risk in such patients. The ischemic burden from the stress of surgery and postoperative recovery can result in MI or cardiovascular death. Prospective identification of such patients has important prognostic and preventive implications.

Initial cardiac assessment of patients undergoing noncardiac surgery should be based on (1) the prevalence of CAD in a given surgical population, (2) the type of the surgical procedure and the institutional event rate, (3) cardiac history and risk factors, and (4) functional capacity.[192] Surgical procedures can be classified as high-risk procedures (cardiac risk of >5 percent), such as major vascular surgery, emergent major operations, and prolonged surgical procedures with large fluid shifts or blood loss. Intermediate-risk procedures have cardiac risks of 1 to 5 percent and include carotid endarterectomy, intraperitoneal and intrathoracic operations, and orthopedic operations. Low-risk (<1 percent) procedures include endoscopic procedures, cataract surgery, and breast surgery. If the institutional event rate for an elective operation is less than 2 to 3 percent, most screening studies are inefficient with regard to lowering the cardiac event rate in the perioperative period.

Clinical parameters of increased risk include advanced age (older than 70 years), diabetes, history of angina or recent ACS, heart failure, and ventricular arrhythmias. When added to the type of surgery and clinical parameters, the findings of exercise duration of less than 3 minutes and ST segment depression of greater than 1.5 to 2.0 mm indicate significant and independent risk for an adverse cardiac outcome.[192,193]

Patients with known prior CAD may be considered to have a low perioperative cardiac risk on the basis of their functional capacity and symptoms. Asymptomatic patients with known CAD who have had revascularization within the past 5 years require no further evaluation.[192] Patients with intermediate risk on the basis of clinical predictors, functional capacity, and type of surgery are optimal candidates for further stratification by imaging procedures.

Studies of MPI using pharmacological stress have uniformly shown that a normal MPI study predicts a low likelihood (~1 percent) for perioperative or longer term postoperative cardiac events.[193] Reversible perfusion defects predict an increased risk of cardiac events, and the magnitude of risk is related to the extent of ischemia (Fig. 13–53). Although fixed perfusion defects (infarct) portend a lower risk for perioperative cardiac events than ischemia, the risk is higher than that with a normal scan, and patients with infarct or LV dysfunction are at higher *long-term* risk for death or heart failure.[193]

In clinical practice, most patients in whom extensive ischemia is demonstrated preoperatively undergo catheterization with expectation of revascularization. Clinical trial evidence supporting this point is lacking, and the threshold of ischemia extent above which revascularization might *reduce* short- or long-term cardiac risk is not known. Clinical studies suggest that beta blockers, if appropriately administered, reduce perioperative ischemia and may reduce the risk for MI and death in high-risk patients.[194]

REFERENCES

Technical Aspects of Image Acquisition, Display, and Interpretation

1. Jain D, Strauss HW: Principles of cardiovascular nuclear imaging. *In* Dilsizian V, Narula J, Braunwald E (eds): Atlas of Nuclear Cardiology. Philadelphia, Current Medicine, 2003, pp 1-18.
2. Garcia EV: Physics and instrumentation of radionuclide imaging. *In* Braunwald E (ed): Cardiac Imaging: A Companion to Braunwald's Heart Disease. Philadelphia, WB Saunders, 1991, pp 977-1005.
3. Faber TL: Tomographic imaging: Methods. *In* Gerson MC (ed): Cardiac Nuclear Medicine. New York, McGraw-Hill, 1997.
4. Garcia E, Berman DS, Port SC, et al: American Society of Nuclear Cardiology. Imaging guidelines for nuclear cardiology procedures. Part 2. J Nucl Cardiol 6:G53, 1999.
5. Links JM, Becker LC, Rigo P, et al: Combined corrections for attenuation, depth-dependent blur, and motion in cardiac SPECT: A multicenter trial. J Nucl Cardiol 7:414, 2000.
6. Dilsizian V: SPECT and PET techniques. *In* Dilsizian V, Narula J, Braunwald E (eds): Atlas of Nuclear Cardiology. Philadelphia, Current Medicine, 2003, pp 19-46.

7. Kailasnath P, Sinusas AJ: Comparison of Tl-201 with Tc-99m-labeled myocardial perfusion agents: Technical, physiologic, and clinical issues. J Nucl Cardiol 8:482, 2001.
8. American Society of Nuclear Cardiology: Updated imaging guidelines for nuclear cardiology procedures, part 1. J Nucl Cardiol 8:G5, 2001.
9. DePuey EG: A stepwise approach to myocardial perfusion SPECT interpretation. *In* Gerson MC (ed): Cardiac Nuclear Medicine. New York, McGraw-Hill, 1997, pp 81-142.
10. Klocke FJ, Baird MG, Bateman TM, et al: ACC/AHA/ASNC guidelines for the clinical use of cardiac radionuclide imaging: A report of the American College of Cardiology/American Heart Association Task Force on Practice Guidelines (ACC/AHA/ASNC Committee to Revise the 1995 Guidelines for the Clinical Use of Radionuclide Imaging). 2003. American College of Cardiology Web Site. Available at: http://www.acc.org/clinical/ guidelines/radio/rni_fulltext.pdf.
11. Berman DS, Hachamovitch R, Germano G: Risk stratification and patient management. *In* Dilsizian V, Narula J, Braunwald E (eds): Atlas of Nuclear Cardiology. Philadelphia, Current Medicine, 2003, pp 97-114.
12. Cerqueira MD, Weissman NJ, Dilsizian V, et al: Standardized myocardial segmentation and nomenclature for tomographic imaging of the heart: A statement for healthcare professionals from the cardiac imaging committee of the council on clinical cardiology of the American Heart Association. Circulation 105:539, 2002.
13. Garcia EV, Van Train K, Maddahi J, et al: Quantification of rotational thallium-201 myocardial tomography. J Nucl Med 26:17, 1985.
14. Liu YH, Sinusas AJ, Deman P, et al: Quantification of SPECT myocardial perfusion images: Methodology and validation of the Yale-CQ method. J Nucl Cardiol 6:190, 1999.
15. Beller GA: Radionuclide perfusion imaging techniques for evaluation of patients with known or suspected coronary artery disease. Adv Intern Med 42:139, 1997.
16. McLaughlin MG, Danias PG: Transient ischemic dilation: A powerful diagnostic and prognostic finding of stress myocardial perfusion imaging. J Nucl Cardiol 9:663, 2002.
17. Mazzanti M, Germano G, Kiat H, et al: Identification of severe and extensive coronary artery disease by automatic measurement of transient ischemic dilation of the left ventricle in dual-isotope myocardial perfusion SPECT. J Am Coll Cardiol 27:1612, 1996.
18. Taillefer R, DePuey EG, Udelson JE, et al: Comparative diagnostic accuracy of Tl-201 and Tc-99m sestamibi SPECT imaging (perfusion and ECG-gated SPECT) in detecting coronary artery disease in women. J Am Coll Cardiol 29:69, 1997.
19. Kiat H, Van Train KF, Friedman JD, et al: Quantitative stress redistribution thallium-201 SPECT using prone imaging: Methodologic development and validation. J Nucl Med 33:1509, 1992.
20. DePuey EG: Artifacts clarified and caused by gated myocardial perfusion SPECT. *In* Germano G, Berman DS (eds): Clinical Gated Cardiac SPECT. Armonk, NY, Futura Publishing, 1999, pp 183-238
21. King MA, Tsui BMW, Pan T: Attenuation compensation for cardiac single-photon emission computed tomographic imaging: Part 2. Attenuation compensation algorithms. J Nucl Cardiol 3:55, 1996.
22. Hendel RC, Corbett JR, Cullom SJ, et al: The value and practice of attenuation correction for myocardial perfusion SPECT imaging: A joint position statement from the American Society of Nuclear Cardiology and the Society of Nuclear Medicine. J Nucl Cardiol 9:135, 2002.
23. Germano G, Berman DS: Acquisition and processing for gated SPECT: Technical aspects. *In* Germano G, Berman DS (eds): Clinical Gated Cardiac SPECT. Armonk, NY, Futura Publishing, 1999, pp 93-114.
24. Smith WH, Kastener RJ, Calnon DA, et al: Quantitative gated SPECT imaging: A counts-based method for display and measurement of regional and global ventricular systolic function. J Nucl Cardiol 4:451, 1997.
25. Bateman TM, Berman DS, Heller GV, et al: American Society of Nuclear Cardiology position statement on electrocardiographic gating of myocardial perfusion SPECT scintigrams. J Nucl Cardiol 6:470, 1999.
26. Gerson MC: Myocardial perfusion imaging: Planar methods. *In* Gerson MC (ed): Cardiac Nuclear Medicine. New York, McGraw-Hill, 1997, pp 29-52.
27. Wackers FJ: Equilibrium radionuclide angiography. *In* Gerson MC (ed): Cardiac Nuclear Medicine. New York, McGraw-Hill, 1997, pp 315-346.
28. Borer JS: First pass and equilibrium radionuclide angiography. *In* Dilsizian V, Narula J, Braunwald E (eds): Atlas of Nuclear Cardiology. Philadelphia, Current Medicine, 2003, pp 147-166.
29. Arrighi JA, Dilsizian V: Radionuclide angiography in coronary and noncoronary heart disease: Technical background and clinical applications. *In* Harbert JC, Eckelman WC, Neumann RD (eds): Nuclear Medicine. New York, Thieme Medical Publishers, 1996, pp 501-531.
30. Aggarwal, A, Brown KA, LeWinter MM: Diastolic dysfunction: Pathophysiology, clinical features, and assessment with radionuclide methods. J Nucl Cardiol 8:98, 2001.
31. Dilsizian V: SPECT and PET techniques. *In* Dilsizian V, Narula J, Braunwald E (eds): Atlas of Nuclear Cardiology. Philadelphia, Current Medicine, 2003, pp 131-146.
32. Bacharach SL, Bax JJ, Case J, et al: PET myocardial glucose metabolism and perfusion imaging: Part I—Guidelines for patient preparation and data acquisition. J Nucl Cardiol 10:543, 2003.

Assessment of the Physiology and Pathophysiology of Myocardial Blood Flow, Myocardial Metabolism, and Ventricular Function

33. Watson DD, Glover DK: Overview of kinetics and modeling. *In* Zaret BL, Beller GA (eds): Nuclear Cardiology: State of the Art and Future Directions. St. Louis, Mosby, 1999, pp 3-12.
34. Shirani J, Lee J, Quigg RJ, et al: Relation of thallium uptake to morphologic features of chronic ischemic heart disease: Evidence for myocardial remodeling in non-infarct myocardium. J Am Coll Cardiol 38:84, 2001.
35. Gibbons RJ, Miller TD, Christian TF: Infarct size measured by single photon emission computed tomographic imaging with ^{99m}Tc-sestamibi: A measure of the efficacy of therapy in acute myocardial infarction. Circulation 101:101, 2000.
36. Christian TF: The use of perfusion imaging in acute myocardial infarction. Application for clinical trials and clinical care. J Nucl Cardiol 2:423, 1995.
37. Kern MJ, Meier B: Evaluation of the culprit plaque and the physiological significance of coronary atherosclerotic narrowings. Circulation 103:3142, 2001.
38. Follansbee WP: Alternatives to leg exercise in the evaluation of patients with coronary artery disease: Functional and pharmacologic stress modalities. *In* Gerson MC (ed) Cardiac Nuclear Medicine. New York, McGraw-Hill, 1997, pp 193-236.
39. Gould KL, Nakagawa Y, Nakagawa K, et al: Frequency and clinical implications of fluid dynamically significant diffuse coronary artery disease manifest as graded, longitudinal, base-to-apex myocardial perfusion abnormalities by noninvasive positron emission tomography. Circulation 101:1931, 2000.
40. Hasdai D, Gibbons RJ, Holmes DR Jr, et al: Coronary endothelial dysfunction in humans is associated with myocardial perfusion defects. Circulation 96:3390, 1997.
41. He Z, Mahmarian JJ, Verani MS: Myocardial perfusion in patients with total occlusion of a single coronary artery with and without collateral circulation. J Nucl Cardiol 8:452, 2001.
42. Mark DB, Lauer MS: Exercise capacity: The prognostic variable that doesn't get enough respect. Circulation 108:1534, 2003.
43. Hendel RC: Diagnostic and prognostic applications for vasodilator stress myocardial perfusion imaging and the importance of radiopharmaceutical selection. J Nucl Cardiol 8:523, 2001.
44. Miller DD: Pharmacologic stressors in coronary artery disease. *In* Dilsizian V, Narula J, Braunwald E (eds): Atlas of Nuclear Cardiology. Philadelphia, Current Medicine, 2003, pp 47-62.
45. Verani MS: Pharmacologic stress myocardial perfusion imaging. Curr Probl Cardiol 18:481, 1993.
46. Udelson JE, Heller GV, Wackers FJ, et al: A randomized, controlled dose-ranging study of the selective adenosine A_{2A} receptor agonist binodenoson for pharmacologic stress as an adjunct to myocardial perfusion imaging. Circulation 109:457, 2004.
47. Thomas GS, Prill NV, Majmundar H, et al: Treadmill exercise during adenosine infusion is safe, results in fewer adverse reactions, and improves myocardial perfusion imaging quality. J Nucl Cardiol 7:439, 2000.
48. Elliott MD, Holly TA, Leonard SM, Hendel RC: Impact of abbreviated adenosine protocol incorporating adjunctive treadmill exercise on adverse effects and image quality in patients undergoing stress myocardial perfusion imaging. J Nucl Cardiol 7:584, 2000.
49. Dakik HA, Kleiman NS, Farmer JA, et al: Intensive medical therapy versus coronary angioplasty for suppression of myocardial ischaemia in survivors of acute myocardial infarction: A prospective randomized pilot study. Circulation 98:2017, 1998.
50. Sharir T, Rabinowitz B, Livschitz S, et al: Underestimation of extent and severity of coronary artery disease by dipyridamole stress thallium-201 single-photon emission computed tomographic myocardial perfusion imaging in patients taking antianginal drugs. J Am Coll Cardiol 31:1540, 1998.
51. Taillefer R, Ahlberg AW, Masood Y, et al: Acute beta-blockade reduces the extent and severity of myocardial perfusion defects with dipyridamole Tc-99m sestamibi SPECT imaging. J Am Coll Cardiol 42:1475, 2003.
52. Geleijnse M, Elhendy A, Fioretti P, et al: Dobutamine stress myocardial perfusion imaging. J Am Coll Cardiol 36:2017, 2000.
53. Wijns W, Vatner SF, Camici PG: Mechanisms of disease: Hibernating myocardium. N Engl J Med 339:173, 1998.
54. Taegtmeyer H: Modulation of responses to myocardial ischemia: Metabolic features of myocardial stunning, hibernation, and ischemic preconditioning. *In* Dilsizian V (ed): Myocardial Viability: A Clinical and Scientific Treatise. Armonk, NY, Futura Publishing, 2000, pp 25-36.
55. Braunwald E, Kloner RA: The stunned myocardium: Prolonged, postischemic ventricular dysfunction. Circulation 66:1146, 1982.
56. Rahimtoola SH: A perspective on the three large multicenter randomized clinical trials of coronary bypass surgery for chronic stable angina. Circulation 72(Suppl V):V-123, 1985.
57. Dilsizian V, Arrighi JA: Myocardial viability in chronic coronary artery disease: Perfusion, metabolism, and contractile reserve. *In* Gerson MC (ed): Cardiac Nuclear Medicine. New York, McGraw-Hill, 1997, pp 143-192.
58. Schelbert HR: Measurements of myocardial metabolism in patients with ischemic heart disease. Am J Cardiol 82:61K, 1998.
59. Tawakol A, Skopicki HA, Abraham SA, et al: Evidence of reduced resting blood flow in viable myocardial regions with chronic asynergy J Am Coll Cardiol 36:2146, 2000.
60. Feinendegen LE: Myocardial imaging of lipid metabolism with labeled fatty acids. *In* Dilsizian V (ed): Myocardial Viability: A Clinical and Scientific Treatise. Armonk, NY, Futura Publishing Company, 2000, pp 349-389.
61. Kudoh T, Tamaki N, Magata Y, et al: Metabolism substrate with negative myocardial uptake of iodine-123-BMIPP. J Nucl Med 38:548, 1997.
62. Hansen CL: Myocardial metabolic imaging with radiolabeled fatty acids. *In* Gerson MC (ed): Cardiac Nuclear Medicine. New York, McGraw-Hill, 1997, pp 239-258.
63. Udelson JE, Dilsizian V, Bateman TM, et al: Proof of principle study of β-methyl-*p*-[^{123}I]-iodophenyl-pentadecanoic acid (BMIPP) for ischemic memory following demand ischemia [abstract]. Circulation 108:IV-405, 2003.
64. Schelbert HR: Principles of positron emission tomography. *In* Skorton DJ, Schelbert HR, Wolf GL, Brundage BH (eds): Marcus Cardiac Imaging: A Companion to Braunwald's Heart Disease. 2nd ed. Philadelphia, WB Saunders, 1996, pp 1063-1092.
65. Dilsizian V, Bacharach SL, Maung KM, Smith MF: Fluorine-18-deoxyglucose SPECT and coincidence imaging for myocardial viability: Clinical and technological issues. J Nucl Cardiol 8:75, 2001.
66. Gropler RJ, Siegel BA, Sampathkumaran K, et al: Dependence of recovery of contractile function on maintenance of oxidative metabolism after myocardial infarction. J Am Coll Cardiol 19:989, 1992.
67. Jafary F, Udelson JE: Assessment of myocardial perfusion and left ventricular function in acute coronary syndromes: Implications for gated SPECT imaging. In Germano G,

Berman DS (eds): Clinical Gated Cardiac SPECT. Armonk, NY, Futura Publishing, 1999, pp 259-306.
68. Udelson JE, Bonow RO: Radionuclide ventriculography in left ventricular diastolic dysfunction. *In* Gaasch WH, LeWinter M (eds): Heart Failure and Diastolic Dysfunction. Philadelphia, Lea & Febiger, 1994, pp 167-191.
69. Gerson MC, Rohe R: Radionuclide ventriculography: Left ventricular volumes and pressure-volume relations. *In* Gerson MC (ed): Cardiac Nuclear Medicine. New York, McGraw-Hill, 1997, pp 347-370.
70. Links JM, Becker LC, Shindledecker JG, et al: Measurement of absolute left ventricular volumes from gated blood pool studies. Circulation 65:82, 1982.
71. Verani MS, Gaeta J, LeBlanc AD, et al: Validation of left ventricular volume measurements by radionuclide angiography. J Nucl Med 26:1394, 1985.
72. Anand IS, Florea VG, Solomon SD, et al: Noninvasive assessment of left ventricular remodeling: Concepts, techniques, and implications for clinical trials. J Card Fail 8:S452, 2002.
73. Iskandrian AE, Germano G, VanDecker W, et al: Validation of left ventricular volume measurements by gated SPECT 99mTc-labeled sestamibi imaging. J Nucl Cardiol 5:574, 1998.
74. Germano G, Berman DS: Quantitative gated perfusion SPECT. *In* Germano G, Berman DS (eds): Clinical Gated Cardiac SPECT. Armonk, NY, Futura Publishing, 1999, pp 115-146.
75. Metra M, Giubbini R, Nodari S, et al: Differential effects of ß-blockers in patients with heart failure: A prospective, randomized, double-blind comparison of the long-term effects of metoprolol versus carvedilol. Circulation 102:546, 2000.
76. Borer JS, Bonow RO: Contemporary approach to aortic and mitral regurgitation. Circulation 108:2432, 2003.
77. Bonow RO, Carabello B, de Leon AC Jr, et al: ACC/AHA guidelines for the management of patients with valvular heart disease: A report of the American College of Cardiology/American Heart Association Task Force on Practice Guidelines (Committee on Management of Patients with Valvular Heart Disease). J Am Coll Cardiol 32:1486, 1998.
78. Imitani I, Jain D, Joska TM, et al: Doxorubicin cardiotoxicity: Prevention of congestive heart failure with serial cardiac function monitoring with equilibrium radionuclide angiocardiography in the current era. J Nucl Cardiol 10:132, 2003.
79. Spirito P, Maron BJ, Bonow RO: Noninvasive assessment of left ventricular diastolic function: Comparative analysis of Doppler echocardiographic and radionuclide angiographic techniques. J Am Coll Cardiol 7:518, 1986.
80. Maron BJ: Hypertrophic cardiomyopathy: A systematic review. JAMA 287:1308, 2002.
81. Udelson JE, Bonow RO: Left ventricular diastolic function and the use of calcium channel blockers in hypertrophic cardiomyopathy. *In* Gaasch WH, LeWinter M (eds): Heart Failure and Diastolic Dysfunction. Philadelphia, Lea & Febiger, 1994, pp 462-489.
82. Bonow RO, Dilsizian V, Rosing DR, et al: Verapamil-induced improvement in left ventricular diastolic filling and increased exercise tolerance in patients with hypertrophic cardiomyopathy: Short- and long-term effects. Circulation 72:853, 1985.
83. Kitzman DW, Higginbotham MB, Cobb FR, et al: Exercise intolerance in patients with heart failure and preserved left ventricular systolic function: Failure of the Frank-Starling mechanism. J Am Coll Cardiol 17:1065, 1991.

Disease Detection, Risk Stratification, and Clinical Decision-Making

84. Gould KL: Noninvasive assessment of coronary stenoses by myocardial perfusion imaging during pharmacologic coronary vasodilatation: I. Physiologic basis and experimental validation. Am J Cardiol 41:267, 1978.
85. Libby P, Ridker PM, Maseri A: Inflammation and atherosclerosis Circulation 105:1135, 2002.
86. Expert Panel on Detection, Evaluation, and Treatment of High Blood Cholesterol in Adults: Executive Summary of the Third Report of the National Cholesterol Education Program (NCEP) Expert Panel on Detection, Evaluation and Treatment of High Blood Cholesterol in Adults (Adult Treatment Panel III). JAMA 285:2486, 2001.
87. Fletcher GF, Balady GJ, Vogel RA: Preventive cardiology: How can we do better? 33rd Bethesda Conference. J Am Coll Cardiol 40:579, 2002.
88. Gibbons RJ: Nuclear cardiology in hospital-based practice. J Nucl Cardiol 4:179, 1997.
89. Braunwald E, Antman EM, Beasley JW, et al: ACC/AHA 2002 guideline update for the management of patients with unstable angina and non-ST-segment elevation myocardial infarction: A report of the American College of Cardiology/American Heart Association Task Force on Practice Guidelines (Committee on the Management of Patients with Unstable Angina). 2002. Available at: http://www.acc.org/clinical/guidelines/unstable/incorporated/index.htm.
90. Gibbons RJ, Abrams J, Chatterjee K, et al: ACC/AHA 2002 guideline update for the management of patients with chronic stable angina—Summary article: A report of the American College of Cardiology/American Heart Association Task Force on Practice Guidelines (Committee on the Management of Patients with Chronic Stable Angina). Circulation 107:149, 2003.
91. Brown K: Prognostic value of myocardial perfusion imaging: State of the art and new developments. J Nucl Cardiol 3:516, 1996.
92. Ladenheim ML, Pollock BH, Rozanski A, et al: Extent and severity of myocardial hypoperfusion as predictors of prognosis in patients with suspected coronary artery disease. J Am Coll Cardiol 7: 464, 1986.
93. Shaw LJ, Hachamovitch R, Eisenstein EL: A primer of biostatistic and economic methods for diagnostic and prognostic modeling in nuclear cardiology: Part I. J Nucl Cardiol 3:538, 1996.
94. Pollock SG, Abbott RD, Boucher CA, et al: Independent and incremental prognostic value of tests performed in hierarchical order to evaluate patients with suspected coronary artery disease: Validation of models based on these tests. Circulation 85:237, 1992.
95. Hachamovitch R, Berman DS, Kiat H, et al: Exercise myocardial perfusion SPECT in patients without known coronary artery disease: Incremental prognostic value and use in risk stratification. Circulation 93:905, 1996.
96. Gibbons RJ, Hodge DO, Berman DS, et al: Long-term outcome of patients with intermediate-risk exercise electrocardiograms who do not have myocardial perfusion defects on radionuclide imaging. Circulation 100:2140, 1999.
97. Beller GA: First Annual Mario S. Verani, MD, Memorial Lecture: Clinical value of myocardial perfusion imaging in coronary artery disease. J Nucl Cardiol 10:529, 2003.
98. Vanzetto G, Ormezzano O, Fagret D, et al: Long-term additive prognostic value of thallium-201 myocardial perfusion imaging over clinical and exercise stress test in low to intermediate risk patients. Study in 1137 patients with 6-year follow-up. Circulation 100:1521, 1999.
99. Hachamovitch R, Hayes SW, Friedman JD, et al: Comparison of the short-term survival benefit associated with revascularization compared with medical therapy in patients with no prior coronary artery disease undergoing stress myocardial perfusion single photon emission computed tomography. Circulation 107: 2900, 2003.
100. Shaw LJ, Hendel R, Borges-Neto S, et al, for the Myoview Multicenter Registry: Prognostic value of normal exercise and adenosine 99mTc-tetrofosmin SPECT imaging: Results from the multicenter registry of 4,728 patients. J Nucl Med 44:134, 2003.
101. Hachamovitch R, Hayes S, Friedman JD, et al: Determinants of risk and its temporal variation in patients with normal stress myocardial perfusion scans. What is the warranty period of a normal scan? J Am Coll Cardiol 41:1329, 2003.
102. Giri S, Shaw LJ, Murthy DR, et al: Impact of diabetes on the risk stratification using stress single-photon emission computed tomography myocardial perfusion imaging in patients with symp toms suggestive of coronary artery disease. Circulation 105:32, 2002.
103. Brown K: Prognostic value of myocardial perfusion imaging: State of the art and new developments. J Nucl Cardiol 3:516, 1996.
104. Parisi AF, Hartigan PM, Folland ED, for the ACME Investigators: Evaluation of exercise thallium-201 scintigraphy versus exercise electrocardiography in predicting survival outcomes and morbid cardiac events in patients with single- and double-vessel disease. Findings from the angioplasty compared to medicine study. J Am Coll Cardiol 30:1256, 1997.
105. Schwartz RG, Pearson TA, Kalaria VG, et al: Prospective serial evaluation of myocardial perfusion and lipids during the first six months of pravastatin therapy: Coronary artery disease regression single photon emission computed tomography monitoring trial. J Am Coll Cardiol 42:600, 2003.
106. Baller D, Notohamiprodjo G, Gleichmann U, et al: Improvement in coronary flow reserve determined by positron emission tomography after 6 months of cholesterol-lowering therapy in patients with early stages of coronary atherosclerosis. Circulation 99:2871, 1999.
107. Beller GA, Zaret BL: Contributions of nuclear cardiology to diagnosis and prognosis of patients with coronary artery disease. Circulation 101:1465, 2000.
108. Rozanski A, Diamond GA, Berman D, et al: The declining specificity of exercise radionuclide ventriculography. N Engl J Med 309:518, 1983.
109. Gerson MC: Test accuracy, test selection, and test result interpretation in chronic coronary artery disease. *In* Gerson MC (ed): Cardiac Nuclear Medicine. New York, McGraw-Hill, 1997, pp 527-580.
110. Matzer L, Kiat H, Friedman JD, et al: A new approach to the assessment of tomographic thallium-201 scintigraphy in patients with left bundle branch block. J Am Coll Cardiol 17:1309, 1991.
111. Dilsizian V, Bonow RO, Epstein SE, Fananapazir L: Myocardial ischemia detected by thallium scintigraphy is frequently related to cardiac arrest and syncope in young patients with hypertrophic cardiomyopathy. J Am Coll Cardiol 22:796, 1993.
112. Cecchi F, Olivotto I, Gistri R, et al: Coronary microvascular dysfunction and prognosis in hypertrophic cardiomyopathy. N Engl J Med 349:1027, 2003.
113. O'Gara PT, Bonow RO, Maron BJ, et al: Myocardial perfusion abnormalities in patients with hypertrophic cardiomyopathy: Assessment with thallium-201 emission computed tomography. Circulation 76:1214, 1987.
114. Udelson JE, Bonow RO, O'Gara PT, et al: Verapamil prevents silent myocardial perfusion abnormalities during exercise in asymptomatic patients with hypertrophic cardiomyopathy. Circulation 79:1052, 1989.
115. Cannon RO, Dilsizian V, O'Gara PT, et al: Myocardial metabolic, hemodynamic, and electrocardiographic significance of reversible thallium-201 abnormalities in hypertrophic cardiomyopathy. Circulation 83:1660, 1991.
116. Schulman DS, Francis CK, Black HR, Wackers FJ: Thallium-201 stress imaging in hypertensive patients. Hypertension 10:16, 1987.
117. Tubau JF, Szlachcic J, Hollenberg M, Massie BM: Usefulness of thallium-201 scintigraphy in predicting the development of angina pectoris in hypertensive patients with left ventricular hypertrophy. Am J Cardiol 64:45, 1989.
118. Amanullah AM, Berman DS, Kang X, et al: Enhanced prognostic stratification of patients with left ventricular hypertrophy with the use of single-photon emission computed tomography. Am Heart J 140:3456, 2000.
119. Yamaguchi S, Tsuiki K, Hayasaka M, Yasui S: Segmental wall motion abnormalities in dilated cardiomyopathy: Hemodynamic characteristics and comparison with thallium-201 myocardial scintigraphy. Am Heart J 113:1123, 1987.
120. Doi YL, Chikamori T, Takata J, et al: Prognostic value of thallium-201 perfusion defects in idiopathic dilated cardiomyopathy. Am J Cardiol 67:188, 1991.
121. Neglia D, Michelassi C, Trivieri MG, et al: Prognostic role of myocardial blood flow impairment in idiopathic left ventricular dysfunction. Circulation 105:186, 2002.
122. Udelson JE, Shafer CD, Carrio I: Radionuclide imaging in heart failure: Assessing etiology and outcomes and implications for management. J Nucl Cardiol 9:S40, 2002.
123. Masoli O, Perez Baliño N, Sabaté D, et al: Effect of endothelial dysfunction on regional perfusion in myocardial territories supplied by normal and diseased vessels in patients with coronary artery disease. J Nucl Cardiol 7:199, 2000.
124. Panting JR, Gatehouse PD, Yang GZ, et al: Abnormal subendocardial perfusion in cardiac syndrome X detected by cardiovascular magnetic resonance imaging. N Engl J Med 346:1948, 2002.
125. Taillefer R, DePuey EG, Udelson JE, et al: Comparative diagnostic accuracy of Tl-201 and Tc-99m sestamibi SPECT imaging (perfusion and ECG-gated SPECT) in detecting coronary artery disease in women. J Am Coll Cardiol 29:69, 1997.

126. Faber TL, Cooke CD, Peifer JW, et al: Three-dimensional displays of left ventricular epicardial surface from standard cardiac SPECT perfusion quantification techniques. J Nucl Med 36:697, 1995.
127. Germano G, Berman DS: Quantitative gated SPECT. J Nucl Med 42:528, 2001.
128. Ficaro EP, Quaife RA, Kitzman JN, Corbett JR: Accuracy and reproducibility of 3D-MSPECT for estimating left ventricular ejection fraction in patients with severe perfusion abnormalities [abstract]. Circulation 100:I-26, 1999.
129. Gibbons RJ, Balady GJ, Timothy B, et al: ACC/AHA 2002 guideline update for exercise testing: Summary article. A report of the American College of Cardiology/American Heart Association Task Force on Practice Guidelines (Committee to Update the 1997 Exercise Testing Guidelines). J Am Coll Cardiol 40:1531, 2002.
130. Heller GV, Ahmed I, Tilkemeier PL, et al: Comparison of chest pain, electrocardiographic changes and thallium-201 scintigraphy during varying exercise intensities in men with stable angina pectoris. Am J Cardiol 68:569, 1991.
131. Sharir T, Bacher-Stier C, Dhar S, et al: Identification of severe and extensive coronary artery disease by postexercise regional wall motion abnormalities in Tc-99m sestamibi gated single-photon emission computed tomography. Am J Cardiol 86:1171, 2000.
132. Lima RSL, Watson, DD, Goode AR, et al: Incremental value of combined perfusion and function over perfusion alone by gated SPECT myocardial perfusion imaging for detection of severe three-vessel coronary artery disease. J Am Coll Cardiol 42:64, 2003.
133. Kwok Y, Kim C, Grady D, et al: Meta-analysis of exercise testing to detect coronary artery disease in women. Am J Cardiol 83:660, 1999.
134. Santana-Boado C, Candell-Riera J, Castell-Conesa J, et al: Diagnostic accuracy of technetium-99m-MIBI myocardial SPECT in women and men. J Nucl Med 39:751, 1998.
135. Garcia E, Berman DS, Port SC, et al: American Society of Nuclear Cardiology. Imaging guidelines for nuclear cardiology procedures. Part 2. J Nucl Cardiol 6:G53, 1999.
136. Borer JS: Measurement of ventricular volume and function. *In* Zaret BL, Beller GA (eds): Nuclear Cardiology: State of the Art and Future Directions. St. Louis, Mosby, 1999, pp 201-215.
137. Udelson JE, Rajendran V, Leppo JA: Detection of coronary disease by SPECT imaging and radionuclide angiography. *In* Murray IPC, Ell PJ, Van der Wall H (eds): Nuclear Medicine in Clinic Diagnosis and Treatment. 2nd ed. Edinburgh, Churchill Livingstone, 1998, pp 1389-1414.
138. Lauer MS, Lytle B, Pashkow F, et al: Prediction of death and myocardial infarction by screening with exercise-thallium testing after coronary-artery-bypass grafting. Lancet 351:615, 1998.
139. Zellweger M, Lewin H, Shenghan L, et al: When to stress patients after coronary artery bypass surgery? Risk stratification in patients early and late post-CABG using stress myocardial perfusion SPECT: Implications of appropriate clinical strategies. J Am Coll Cardiol 37:144, 2001.
140. Acampa W, Petretta M, Florimonte L, et al: Prognostic value of exercise cardiac tomography performed late after percutaneous coronary intervention in symptomatic and symptom-free patients. Am J Cardiol 9:259, 2003.
141. Bonow RO, Kent KM, Rosing DR: Exercise-induced ischemia in mildly symptomatic patients with coronary-artery disease and preserved left ventricular function. Identification of subgroups at risk of death during medical therapy. N Engl J Med 311:1339, 1984.
142. Blumenthal RS, Becker DM, Moy TF, et al: Exercise thallium tomography predicts future clinically manifest coronary heart disease in a high-risk asymptomatic population. Circulation 93:915, 1996.
143. Smith SC, Greenland P, Grundy SM: Prevention Conference V: Beyond secondary prevention: Identifying the high-risk patient for primary prevention: Executive summary. Circulation 101:111, 2000.
144. Wackers F, Young L, Inzucchi S, et al, and the DIAD Investigators: The prevalence of silent myocardial ischemia in asymptomatic patients with type 2 diabetes mellitus: Results of the DIAD study. Detection of Ischemia in Asymptomatic Diabetics [abstract]. Diabetes 52(Suppl 1):A56. 2003.
145. Miller TD, Rajagopalan N, Hodge DO, et al: The yield of screening stress myocardial perfusion imaging in asymptomatic diabetics [abstract]. J Am Coll Cardiol 39:163A, 2002.
146. De Lorenzo A, Lima RS, Siqueira-Filho AG, Pantoja MR: Prevalence and prognostic value of perfusion defects detected by stress technetium-99m sestamibi myocardial perfusion single-photon emission computed tomography in asymptomatic patients with diabetes mellitus and no known coronary artery disease. Am J Cardiol 90:827, 2002.
147. Wackers FJ, Brown KA, Heller GV, et al: American Society of Nuclear Cardiology position statement on radionuclide imaging in patients with suspected acute ischemic syndromes in the emergency department or chest pain center. J Nucl Cardiol 9:246, 2002.
148. Kontos MC, Jesse RL, Anderson P, et al: Comparison of myocardial perfusion imaging and cardiac troponin I in patients admitted to the emergency department with chest pain. Circulation 99:2073, 1999.
149. Heller GV, Stowers SA, Hendel RC, et al: Clinical value of acute rest technetium-99m tetrofosmin tomographic myocardial perfusion imaging in patients with acute chest pain and non diagnostic electrocardiogram. J Am Coll Cardiol 31:1011, 1998.
150. Stowers SA, Eisenstein EL, Wackers FJ, et al: An economic analysis of an aggressive diagnostic strategy with single photon emission computed tomography myocardial perfusion imaging and early exercise stress testing in emergency department patients who present with chest pain but non diagnostic electrocardiograms: Results from a randomized trial. Ann Emerg Med 35:17, 2000.
151. Udelson JE, Beshansky JR, Ballin DS, et al: Myocardial perfusion imaging for evaluation and triage of patients with suspected acute cardiac ischemia: A randomized controlled trial. JAMA 288:2693, 2002.
152. Cannon CP, Weintraub WS, Demopoulos LA, et al: Comparison of early invasive and conservative strategies in patients with unstable coronary syndromes treated with the glycoprotein IIb/IIIa inhibitor tirofiban. N Engl J Med 344:1879, 2001.
153. Brown KA: Management of unstable angina: The role of noninvasive risk stratification. J Nucl Cardiol 4:S164, 1997.
154. Solomon DH, Stone PH, Glynn RJ, et al: Use of risk stratification to identify patients with unstable angina likeliest to benefit from an invasive versus conservative management strategy. J Am Coll Cardiol 38:969, 2001.
155. Antman EM, Cohen M, Bernink PJ, et al: The TIMI risk score for unstable angina/non-ST elevation MI: A method for prognostication and therapeutic decision making. JAMA 284:835, 2000.
156. Ryan TJ, Antman EM, Brooks NH, et al: ACC/AHA guidelines for the management of patients with acute myocardial infarction. Circulation 100:1016, 1999.
157. Gibson RS, Watson DD, Craddock GB, et al: Prediction of cardiac events after uncomplicated myocardial infarction: Prospective study comparing predischarge exercise thallium-201 scintigraphy and coronary angiography. Circulation 68:321, 1983.
158. Leppo JA, O'Brien J, Rothendler JA, et al: Dipyridamole-thallium-201 scintigraphy in the prediction of future cardiac events after acute myocardial infarction. N Engl J Med 310:1014, 1984.
159. Miller DD, Stratman HG, Shaw LJ, et al: Dipyridamole technetium 99m sestamibi myocardial tomography as an independent predictor of cardiac event-free survival after acute ischemic events. J Nucl Cardiol 1:72, 1994.
160. Travin MI, Dessovki A, Cameron T, et al: Use of exercise technetium-99m sestamibi SPECT imaging to detect residual ischaemia and for risk stratification after acute myocardial infarction. Am J Cardiol 75:665, 1995.
161. Mahmarian JJ, Mahmarian AC, Marks GF, et al: Role of adenosine thallium-201 tomography for defining long term risk in patients after acute myocardial infarction. J Am Coll Cardiol 25:1333, 1995.
162. TIMI Study group: Comparison of invasive and conservative strategies after treatment with intravenous tPA in acute myocardial infarction: Results of the Thrombolysis in MI (TIMI) phase II trial. N Eng J Med 320:618, 1989:
163. Ellis SG, Mooney MR, George BS, et al: Randomised trial of late elective angioplasty versus conservative management for patients with residual stenoses after thrombolytic treatment for myocardial infarction (TOPS trial). Circulation 86:1400, 1992.
164. Brown KA, Heller GV, Landin RS, et al: Early dipyridamole ^{99m}Tc-sestamibi single photon emission computed tomographic imaging 2 to 4 days after acute myocardial infarction predicts in-hospital and postdischarge cardiac events: Comparison with submaximal exercise imaging. Circulation 100:2060, 1999.
165. Mahmarian JJ, Mahmarian AC, Marks GF, et al: Role of adenosine thallium-201 tomography for defining long-term risk in patients after acute myocardial infarction. J Am Coll Cardiol 25:1333, 1995.
166. Kawai Y, Tsukamoto E, Nozaki Y, et al: Significance of reduced uptake of iodinated fatty acid analogues for the evaluation of patients with acute chest pain. J Am Coll Cardiol 38:1888, 2001.
167. Narula J, Virmani R, Zaret BL: Radionuclide imaging of atherosclerotic lesions. *In* Dilsizian V, Narula J, Braunwald E (eds): Atlas of Nuclear Cardiology. Philadelphia, Current Medicine, 2003, pp 217-236.
168. Ohtsuki K, Hayase M, Akashi K, et al: Detection of monocyte chemoattractant protein-1 receptor expression in experimental atherosclerotic lesions: An autoradiographic study. Circulation 104:203, 2001.
169. McCrohon JA, Moon JCC, Prasad SK, et al: Differentiation of heart failure related to dilated cardiomyopathy and coronary artery disease using gadolinium-enhanced cardiovascular magnetic resonance. Circulation 108:54, 2003.
170. Bennett SK, Smith MF, Gottlieb SS, et al: Effect of metoprolol on absolute myocardial blood flow in patients with heart failure secondary to ischemic or non-ischemic cardiomyopathy. Am J Cardiol 89:1431, 2002.
171. Danias PG, Ahlberg AW, Clark BE 3rd, et al: Combined assessment of myocardial perfusion and left ventricular function with exercise technetium-99m sestamibi gated single-photon emission computed tomography can differentiate between ischemic and nonischemic dilated cardiomyopathy. Am J Cardiol 82:1253, 1998.
172. Cleland JG, Pennell DJ, Ray SG, et al: Myocardial viability as a determinant of the ejection fraction response to carvedilol in patients with heart failure (CHRISTMAS trial): Randomised controlled trial. Lancet 362:14, 2003.
173. Di Carli MF, Asgarzadie F, Schelbert HR, et al: Quantitative relation between myocardial viability and improvement in heart failure symptoms after revascularization in patients with ischemic cardiomyopathy. Circulation 92:3436, 1995.
174. Allman K, Shaw L, Hachamovitch R, Udelson JE: Myocardial viability testing and impact of revascularization on prognosis in patients with coronary artery disease and left ventricular dysfunction: A meta-analysis. J Am Coll Cardiol 39:1151, 2002.
175. Bonow RO: Assessment of myocardial viability with thallium201. *In* Zaret BL, Beller GA (eds): Nuclear Cardiology: State of the Art and Future Directions. St. Louis, Mosby, 1999, pp 503-512.
176. Udelson JE: Assessment of myocardial viability with technetium-99m-labeled agents. *In* Zaret BL, Beller GA (eds): Nuclear Cardiology: State of the Art and Future Directions. St. Louis, Mosby, 1999, pp 513-533.
177. Kitsiou AN, Srinivasan G, Quyyumi AA, et al: Stress-induced reversible and mild-to-moderate irreversible thallium defects: Are they equally accurate for predicting recovery of regional left ventricular function after revascularization? Circulation 98:501, 1998.
178. Bax JJ, Wijns W, Cornel JH, et al: Accuracy of currently available techniques for prediction of functional recovery after revascularization in patients with left ventricular dysfunction due to chronic coronary artery disease: Comparison of pooled data. J Am Coll Cardiol 30:1451, 1997.
179. Siebelink HM, Blanksma P, Crijns H, et al: No difference in cardiac event-free survival between positron emission tomography and single-photon emission computed tomography-guided patient management. J Am Coll Cardiol 37:81, 2001.
180. Hunt SA, Baker DW, Chin MH: ACC/AHA guidelines for the evaluation and management of chronic heart failure in the adult: Executive summary. J Am Coll Cardiol 38:2101, 2001.

181. Narula J, Khaw BH, Dec GW: Diagnostic accuracy of antimyosin scintigraphy in suspected myocarditis. J Nucl Cardiol 3:371, 1996.
182. Ballester M, Bordes R, Tazelaar HD, et al: Evaluation of biopsy classification for rejection: Relation to detection of myocardial damage by monoclonal antimyosin antibody imaging. J Am Coll Cardiol 31:1357, 1998.
183. Eguchi M, Tsuchihashi K, Hotta D, et al: Technetium-99m sestamibi/tetrofosmin myocardial perfusion scanning in cardiac and noncardiac sarcoidosis. Cardiology 94:193, 2000.
184. Hongo M, Urushibata K, Kai R, et al: Iodine-123 metaiodobenzylguanidine scintigraphic analysis of myocardial sympathetic innervation in patients with AL (primary) amyloidosis. Am Heart J 144:122, 2002.
185. Carrio I: Cardiac neurotransmission imaging. J Nucl Med 42:1062, 2001.
186. Arora R, Ferrick KJ, Nakata T, et al: 123-metaiodobenzylguanidine (MIBG) imaging and heart rate variability analysis to predict the need for an implantable cardioverter defibrillator. J Nucl Cardiol 10:121, 2003.
187. Hofstra L, Liem IH, Dumont EA, et al: Visualization of cell death in vivo in patients with acute myocardial infarction. Lancet 356:209, 2000.
188. Wu JC, Chen IY, Sundaresan G, et al: Molecular imaging of cardiac cell transplantation in living animals using optical bioluminescence and positron emission tomography. Circulation 108:1302, 2003.
189. Lee YHC, Kiesewetter DO, Lang L, et al: Synthesis of 4-[^{18}F]fluorobenzoyllisinopril: A radioligand for angiotensin converting enzyme (ACE) imaging with positron emission tomography. J Labelled Cpd Radiopharm 44:S268, 2001.
190. Dilsizian V, Shirani J, Lee YHC, et al: Specific binding of [^{18}F] fluorobenzoyl-lisinopril to angiotensin converting enzyme in human heart tissue of ischemic cardiomyopathy. Circulation 104:II-694, 2001.
191. Dilsizian V, Loredo ML, Ferrans VJ, et al: Evidence for increased angiotensin II type I receptor immunoreactivity in peri-infarct myocardium of human explanted hearts. J Am Coll Cardiol 39:365A, 2002.
192. Eagle KA, Berger PB, Calkins H, et al: ACC/AHA guideline update for perioperative cardiovascular evaluation for noncardiac surgery: Executive summary: A report of the American College of Cardiology/American Heart Association Task Force on Practice Guidelines (Committee to Update the 1996 Guidelines on Perioperative Cardiovascular Evaluation for Noncardiac Surgery). Circulation 105:1257, 2002.
193. Cohen MC, Eagle KA: Preoperative risk stratification: An overview. *In* Zaret BL, Beller GA (eds): Nuclear Cardiology: State of the Art and Future Directions. St. Louis, Mosby, 1999, pp 346-367.
194. Poldermans D, Boersma E, Bax JJ, et al: The effect of bisoprolol on perioperative mortality and myocardial infarction in high-risk patients undergoing vascular surgery. N Engl J Med 341:1789, 1999.

GUIDELINES *Thomas H. Lee and James E. Udelson*

Nuclear Cardiology

Guidelines for the use of cardiac radionuclide imaging were published by the American Heart Association (AHA), the American College of Cardiology (ACC), and the American Society of Nuclear Cardiology (ASNC) in 2003.[1] Other recent commentaries on the role of nuclear cardiology tests are included under guidelines for exercise testing published in 2002[2] and for the management of acute myocardial infarction in 1999.[3] These guidelines reaffirm the fundamental theme and recommendations of the 1995 ACC/AHA radionuclide imaging guidelines.[4] The consistent message is that radionuclide imaging should be used in situations in which the history, electrocardiographic changes, and other laboratory measurements do not provide reliable information to guide management.

As with most ACC/AHA guidelines, the indications for use of nuclear cardiology tests are classified into one of four classes:

Class I: Conditions for which there is evidence and/or general agreement that testing is useful and effective.

Class II: Conditions for which there is conflicting evidence and/or a divergence of opinion about the usefulness/efficacy of performing testing.

Class IIa: Weight of evidence/opinion is in favor of usefulness/efficacy.

Class IIb: Usefulness/efficacy is less well established by evidence/opinion.

Class III: Conditions for which there is evidence and/or general agreement that testing is not useful/effective and in some cases may be harmful.

Acute ST Segment Elevation Myocardial Infarction

The ACC/AHA/ASNC guidelines indicate that radionuclide imaging should have a limited role in the diagnosis of acute myocardial infarction. These technologies are not appropriate for routine diagnosis and should be used only when information from the history, electrocardiogram, and laboratory tests is not sufficient. The task force considered evidence to be supportive of the use of radionuclide imaging for the assessment of infarct size, for the diagnosis of right ventricular infarction, or for cases in which the diagnosis of myocardial infarction was unclear and the patient presented late (more than 24 hours and less than 7 days) after the onset of symptoms (Table 13G–1).

For evaluation of prognosis after acute myocardial infarction, stress myocardial perfusion imaging was considered appropriate to assess the presence and extent of stress-induced ischemia. The guidelines do not address settings in which radionuclide imaging is preferable to exercise electrocardiography, but the 1999 guidelines on care of acute myocardial infarction indicate that exercise electrocardiography should be the first test used for risk stratification after acute myocardial infarction; imaging studies should be reserved for cases in which the electrocardiogram is likely to be uninterpretable or when the exercise electrocardiograph is equivocal.[3] Radionuclide angiography was considered useful for assessment of ventricular function after acute myocardial infarction, but echocardiography is cited as a low-cost, convenient, widely accessible alternative technology for this purpose.[3]

Unstable Angina/Non-ST Segment Elevation Myocardial Infarction

The ACC/AHA/ASNC guidelines consider radionuclide imaging to be potentially useful for diagnosis and assessment of severity of ischemia in patients with unstable angina and for assessment of left ventricular function when angina is satisfactorily stabilized with medical therapy. Myocardial perfusion imaging was also considered potentially useful (class IIa) for patients with ongoing ischemia who undergo imaging at rest. For patients presenting to emergency departments with a possible acute coronary syndrome but with nondiagnostic initial ECG and biomarkers, the guidelines recommend perfusion imaging at rest as a class I indication, based in part on a randomized controlled trial that found that sestamibi imaging can improve emergency department triage decision making for patients with suspected acute cardiac ischemia.[5]

Chronic Ischemic Heart Disease

The ACC/AHA/ASNC guidelines consider exercise or pharmacological myocardial perfusion imaging to be appropriate (class I) for evaluation of the extent and severity of coronary artery disease in patients with chronic ischemic heart disease. The guidelines consider thallium-201 and technetium-99m to be sufficiently similar to be used interchangeably in this population. Review of data on the three most commonly used agents in pharmacological perfusion imaging (dipyridamole, adenosine, and dobutamine) led the task force to conclude that adenosine or dipyridamole is preferred for patients who cannot exercise adequately. The ACC/AHA guidelines

TABLE 13G–1 American College of Cardiology/American Heart Association/American Society of Nuclear Cardiology Guidelines for the Clinical Use of Cardiac Radionuclicle Imaging*

Indication	Class I (Indicated)	Class IIa (Good Supportive Evidence)	Class IIb (Weak Supportive Evidence)	Class III (Not Indicated)
Diagnosis of STE acute myocardial infarction		Right ventricular infarction Infarction not diagnosed by standard means—late presentation		Routine diagnosis with ischemia/necrosis already documented clinically
Risk assessment, prognosis, and assessment of therapy after STE acute myocardial infarction	Rest RV/LV function Presence/extent of stress-induced ischemia Detection of infarct size and residual viable myocardium			
Diagnosis, prognosis, and assessment of therapy in patients with unstable angina/NSTEMI	Identification of ischemia in the distribution of the culprit lesion or in remote areas Measurement of baseline LV function Identification of the severity/extent of disease in patients whose angina is satisfactorily stabilized with medical therapy	Identification of the severity/extent of disease in patients with ongoing ischemia but nondiagnostic ECG	Diagnosis of myocardial ischemia in patients when the combination of history and ECG changes is unreliable	
Suspected ACS in the emergency department with nondiagnostic ECG and initial biomarkers	Assessment of risk with rest MPI Stress MPI for diagnosis of CAD after negative biomarkers or normal rest MPI			
Diagnosis of chronic ischemic heart disease	Diagnosis of symptomatic and selected patients with asymptomatic myocardial ischemia Assessment of ventricular performance (rest or exercise) Planning PTCA—identifying lesions causing myocardial ischemia, if not otherwise known Risk stratification before noncardiac surgery in select patients			Screening of asymptomatic patients with low likelihood of disease
Assessment of severity/prognosis/risk stratification of chronic ischemic heart disease	Assessment of LV performance Identification of extent and severity of ischemia and localization of ischemia† Risk stratification in patients with an intermediate risk Duke Treadmill Score Assessment of functional significance of intermediate coronary stenosis	MPI as the initial test in patients with diabetes or with >20% 10-yr CHD risk	Redefining risk 1-3 yr after initial MPI in patients with stable symptoms	
Assessment of interventions in chronic ischemic heart disease	Assessment for restenosis after PCI (symptomatic) Assessment of ischemia in symptomatic patients after CABG	Assessment 3-5 yr after CABG or PCI in select, high-risk asymptomatic patients	Assessment of drug therapy for myocardial perfusion	Routine assessment of asymptomatic patients after PTCA or CABG
Heart failure	Determination of initial LV and RV performance in heart failure Initial evaluation of LV function in patients receiving chemotherapy with doxorubicin Assessment of myocardial viability in patients with CAD and LV dysfunction without angina	Assessment of the co-presence of CAD in patients without angina	Routine serial assessment of LV and RV function Detection of myocarditis Diagnosis of CAD in hypertrophic cardiomyopathy	
After cardiac transplantation	Assessment of ventricular performance		Detection and assessment of coronary angiopathy	
Valvular heart disease	Initial and serial assessment of LV and RV function		Detection and assessment of function significance of concomitant coronary artery disease	

*Table represents a compilation of recommendations from the 1995 and 2003 guidelines.

†Exercise MPI in patients with baseline ECG abnormalities, vasodilator pharmacologic stress MPI in patients who cannot exercise adequately or who have LBBB or paced rhythm.

ACS = acute coronary syndrome; CABG = coronary artery bypass graft; CAD = coronary artery disease; CHD = coronary heart disease; ECG = electrocardiographic; LBBB = left bundle branch block; LV = left ventricular; MPI = myocardial perfusion imaging; NSTEMI = non-ST segment elevation myocardial infarction; PCI = percutaneous coronary intervention; PTCA = percutaneous transluminal coronary angioplasty; RV = right ventricular; STE = ST segment elevation.

on exercise testing continue to assert that exercise electrocardiography remains the first-choice test for women as well as men, and the imaging technologies should be used when patients cannot exercise or when the electrocardiogram is likely to be uninterpretable.[2]

Asymptomatic Patients

The ACC/AHA/ASNC guidelines do not consider cardiac radionuclide imaging an appropriate routine test for diagnosis of coronary artery disease in patients who are not symptomatic. However, radionuclide imaging is considered potentially useful for determining the need for coronary angiography in patients with positive exercise electrocardiography tests.

Before Noncardiac Surgery

Most studies of the radionuclide imaging in patients undergoing noncardiac surgery have been performed in patients undergoing major vascular procedures. Such testing was considered appropriate (class I) in patients with chronic ischemic heart disease (see Table 13G–1). However, the guidelines discourage use of radionuclide imaging before noncardiac surgery in most patients undergoing nonvascular surgery because of the lower cardiac risk of these procedures.

Before and After Revascularization Procedures

Myocardial perfusion imaging is appropriate for planning for coronary revascularization procedures and for detection of ischemia in patients who are symptomatic after these procedures (see Table 13G–1). However, the guidelines discourage routine assessment of patients who are asymptomatic after revascularization because of lack of data supporting interventions in such patients. These conclusions are consistent with recent guidelines for exercise testing.[2]

Heart Failure

The ACC/AHA/ASNC guidelines consider radionuclide assessment of left and right ventricular function to be useful in the initial work-up for heart failure, although echocardiography provides additional information on valvular disease. The noninvasive assessment of the co-presence of coronary artery disease (CAD) by myocardial perfusion imaging in patients with heart failure without angina is considered a class IIa indication. The guidelines recommend radionuclide assessment of myocardial viability as a class I indication for consideration of revascularization in patients with known CAD and left ventricular systolic dysfunction who do not have active angina.

Other Conditions

Radionuclide angiography is considered to be useful for assessment of ventricular function in patients who have undergone cardiac transplantation or who have valvular heart disease. It is also considered to be useful for baseline and serial monitoring of left ventricular function during therapy with cardiotoxic drugs.

References

1. Klocke FJ, Baird MG, Bateman TM, et al: ACC/AHA/ASNC Guidelines for the Clinical Use of Cardiac Radionuclide Imaging: A Report of the American College of Cardiology/American Heart Association Task Force on Practice Guidelines, 2003. (http://www.acc.org/clinical/guidelines/radio/index.pdf)
2. Gibbons RJ, Balady GJ, Bricker JT, et al: ACC/AHA 2002 guideline update for exercise testing: Summary article: A report of the ACC/AHA Task Force on Practice Guidelines (Committee to Update the 1997 Exercise Testing Guidelines). Circulation 106:1883, 2002.
3. Ryan TJ, Antman EM, Brooks NH, et al: ACC/AHA guidelines for the management of patients with acute myocardial infarction: 1999 update: A report of the American College of Cardiology/American Heart Association Task Force on Practice Guidelines (Committee on Management of Acute Myocardial Infarction). (http:www.acc.org)
4. Guidelines for Clinical Use of Cardiac Radionuclide Imaging. A Report of the American College of Cardiology/American Heart Association Task Force on the Assessment of Cardiovascular Procedures (Committee on Nuclear Imaging). J Am Coll Cardiol 25:521, 1995.
5. Udelson JE, Beshansky JR, Ballis DS, et al: Myocardial perfusion imaging for evaluation and triage of patients with suspected acute cardiac ischemia: A randomized controlled trial. JAMA 288:2693, 2002.

CHAPTER 14

Cardiovascular Magnetic Resonance

Dudley Pennell

Introduction to Cardiovascular Magnetic Resonance

Magnetic resonance (MR) applied to the cardiovascular system has been termed *cardiovascular magnetic resonance*, or *CMR*, by the international scientific community. CMR has grown considerably in recent years and is now firmly established in clinical and research cardiovascular medicine in the larger centers. This growth and acceptance stem from a number of factors, including technical advancements (speed, reliability, ease of use, new applications), superb image quality and field of view, and the reporting of CMR-derived new insights into entrenched problem areas in cardiology. In addition, a recognition of the excellent reproducibility of CMR images has encouraged widespread adoption of its use by academic medicine and the pharmaceutical industry so that trials can be completed with considerable power but substantially reduced sample sizes, which hastens results and lower costs. It is also worth noting that in the modern climate of safety priority, radiowave technology shares with ultrasound an inescapable advant-age over x-ray and gamma-ray modalities, which suggests that these nonionizing technologies may be preferred in the future. Further strengthening this perspective is the appreciation that echocardiography is the faster and more portable modality, whereas CMR typically provides superior image quality at a higher entry price. Echocardiography and CMR are therefore powerful and complementary partners (see Chap. 11).

Fundamental Principles of Magnetic Resonance

This abbreviated physics background to MR is included to facilitate understanding of the technical terms used throughout this chapter; greater detail can be found in more specialized texts.[1] The physical interaction required for MR is at the level of the atomic nucleus and was first described in 1946, when it was also found that the frequency of radiowave absorption depends on the strength of the external magnetic field. These two key findings form the basis for modern clinical MR imaging. Because MR does not therefore interfere with electrons in the outer atomic shell, which are responsible for chemical binding, it is fundamentally safe, unlike ionizing radiation such as x-rays, which may interact with electron binding, damaging molecules such as DNA. MR occurs only in atomic nuclei with unpaired spin (nucleons). In clinical practice, this means hydrogen-1, which is abundant in water and fat. Since hydrogen is abundant in the human body and has good sensitivity to the phenomenon of magnetic resonance, images with a high signal-to-noise ratio can be obtained. Other important elements are useful for investigation in the laboratory to characterize biochemical processes (^{13}C, ^{17}O, ^{19}F, ^{23}Na, ^{39}K), but these are not used clinically. Human spectroscopy usually makes use of the phosphorus-31 nucleus, which is important because this occurs in compounds involved in energy metabolism, such as adenosine triphosphate (ATP) and phosphocreatine (PCr). MR spectra are rarely used to construct images, however; the data are usually used to quantify metabolite concentrations.

Hydrogen nuclei behave like magnets and align to an external magnetic field. At baseline, the nuclei precess randomly about a 1.5-T magnetic field at a resonance frequency of 63 MHz, which is in the radiowave range. A body region can be excited by a pulse of radiowaves at this frequency, which has the effect of causing all the excited hydrogen nuclei to rotate away from the direction of the main magnetic field axis (the flip angle) and precess in a coordinated manner, which causes a net magnetization. After the excitation pulse is finished, the net magnetization decays to its former position (relaxation), and energy is transmitted as a radio signal. Typically, this signal is formed into a radiowave echo by the scanner such that it can be used to form an image by a receiver antenna. The contrast between different tissues in the image depends on the delay between excitation and the signal read-out (TE, or echo time) and the time between repetitive radiowave excitations (TR, or repeat time). The different forms of contrast are derived from two principal relaxation processes that affect the net magnetization, which are decay in the longitudinal axis (T1) and the transverse plane (T2). Additional magnetic fields (gradient fields), which can be rapidly switched on and off, are required to localize the radiowaves coming from the body. An MR image therefore represents a spatially resolved map of radio signals.

THE CMR SCANNER. A modern CMR scanner consists of major components of hardware. The superconducting magnet produces the static magnetic field, which is highly homogeneous, stable over time, and large enough for chest examinations. The gradient fields are generated by gradient amplifiers with ultrafast capability, which rapidly drive large currents at high voltages through the resistive gradient coils within the bore of the magnet. The radiofrequency amplifier generates the excitation pulses, and a radiofrequency antenna receives the radio signals coming from the patient. A computer controls all the scanner components with complex software. It is also used to perform the Fourier transformation and other complex mathematical processes on the raw radio signal data matrix (known as k-space), which ultimately generates the images.

SEQUENCES

A CMR scanner can only generate useful images if the various component pieces of hardware are intricately coordinated. The timing and magnitude of radiowave and magnetic field pulses along with data collection form MR sequences, which are controlled by the scanner computer. Sequences have various components such as *preparation pulses* (used to alter contrast between tissues), *excitation pulses* (shape and location of the area of the body to be excited by radiowaves), *gradient* and *magnetic field pulses* (formation of a radiowave echo to generate a useful signal for image formation), and *signal read-out* (filling of the raw data matrix or k-space). There are a large variety of sequences, which can appear daunting at first. Fundamentally, however, it is a knowledge of the properties of the sequences rather than their exact nature that is required for medical interpretation.

For CMR, the majority of imaging is performed using two basic sequences known as *spin echo* and *gradient echo*. Spin-echo sequences are also known as "black blood" and gradient-echo sequences as "white blood," although this terminology is a simplification. Spin-echo sequences are routinely used for multislice anatomical imaging, whereas gradient-echo sequences are used for physiological assessment of function through cine acquisitions. The most common prepulse is known as *inversion recovery*, and this gives strong T1 weighting, which is valuable for infarct/viability imaging. Alternatively, T2 preparation is used for coronary imaging. The read-out of the signal can be achieved in many ways, leading to sequences with other names. Usually the read-out is modified for CMR to be as fast as possible so that images, or cines, can be acquired within single breath-holds, and the faster schemes include fast low angle shot (FLASH), steady state with free precession (SSFP, also known as FISP and FIESTA), spiral imaging, and echo-planar imaging (EPI). These fast sequences yield images during a 4- to 20-second breath-hold, which substantially reduces artifact from respiratory motion and also allows three-dimensional acquisitions.

Some other sequences are also very useful in examination of the cardiovascular system. *Velocity mapping* displays each pixel in the image as a pixel velocity rather than a signal magnitude.[2] This is derived from encoding of the phase of the radio signal by using modified gradient profiles. Higher pixel velocities cause a higher phase shift, and this information can be recovered during Fourier transformation of the signal read-out. This is invaluable for measurement of peak velocities through stenosis and true flow for shunt assessment, which is calculated from the integral over time throughout the cardiac cycle of the product of mean velocity and area of a vessel. For coronary CMR, some high resolution acquisitions cannot be completed within one breath-hold, and a specialized sequence called a *navigator echo* is used to greatly reduce respiratory motion. The diaphragm movement is monitored in real time and the scanning computer calculates the coronary position, corrected for the position in the breathing cycle. A sequence called *tagging* is being increasingly used to study myocardial contraction. In this sequence, a grid of dark lines is laid across the image in diastole. The lines of altered magnetization persist and deform throughout the cardiac cycle. Using computer analysis, the intersections of the lines can be used to calculate myocardial strain, which is a quantitative and observer-independent measure of myocardial contractility. CMR angiography is a rapidly growing technique in which three- or four-dimensional visualization of a vessel lumen is achieved, usually after intravenous injection of an MR contrast agent based on the element gadolinium.

CONTRAST AGENTS

A number of classes of contrast agents are used for MR, but for the cardiovascular system, only the gadolinium agents are currently in clinical use. Gadolinium has seven unpaired electrons in its outer shell, which allows it to couple efficiently with excited water spins such that their relaxation is hastened. This predominantly results in a shortening of T1, which increases signal on T1-weighted images. Gadolinium is a toxic element and is therefore chelated to other molecules for clinical use. The properties of the chelator determine the distribution of the gadolinium, and all current gadolinium contrast agents remain in the extracellular compartment. These agents have proven invaluable for arterial angiography and viability imaging. Many other MR contrast agents exist, and some are based on other elements such as iron, manganese, or dysprosium, which have dominant effects on shortening T2, thereby reducing the MR signal. Iron-based contrast agents have been evaluated in humans for angiography and perfusion and for showing macrophage activity in atherosclerotic plaque. Finally, a class of targeted contrast agents has been described that links large number of gadolinium atoms through an intermediary compound to antibody fragments, which in principle allows any biological epitope to be selectively imaged. This has been demonstrated for thrombus and may become a powerful CMR tool of the future.

Gating and Safety

All cardiac and many vascular CMR sequences rely on cardiac gating to prevent artifact from the periodic cardiac contraction cycle. In nearly all current scanners, this is achieved through gating to the R wave of the electrocardiogram. In some CMR scanners, gating is linked to the vector electrocardiogram (two-dimensional electrical activation over time), which may have advantages of reliability, more consistent timing to the R wave peak, and more effective arrhythmia rejection. Older scanners also used gating to the peripheral pulse, but this is now largely abandoned. Most recently, cardiac gating has been achieved without the electrocardiogram by gating the CMR image acquisition directly to bulk cardiac motion detected directly during imaging.

The safety of CMR is well described, and in comparison with x-ray–based techniques there are obvious advantages. However, there are two main problems with MR that must be considered. The first is the issue of flying projectiles in the magnet room, which have the potential to strike the patient. The problem items are iron-based with ferromagnetic properties. These include scissors, electrical items with power transformers such as injection pumps, and oxygen cylinders. Strict adherence to protocols restricting access into the magnet room to only fully trained staff is essential. The second major issue involves metallic implants or implanted electronic devices. Most metallic implants are MR compatible, including all prosthetic cardiac valves, vascular stents, and orthopedic implants. Although some stent manufacturers suggest abstinence from MR for a period after implantation, there are no published data to support this recommendation, and several reports concur with clinical experience that MR can be performed at any time after implantation with absence at 1.5 T of magnetic attraction,[3] heating,[4] or adverse clinical risk.[5] Problems remain with some neurological devices such as cerebrovascular clips, and a specialist's neurological advice is required in these patients. Electronic implants are more problematic for MR, and in principle the high magnetic field of MR will interfere with the electronics and programming of such devices. For CMR, the main implants in question are pacemakers and cardioverter-defibrillators, and their presence is a strong relative contraindication for CMR. An extra reason for caution is that the pacing wires can couple to the radiofrequency waves and heat significantly. Recent work, however, shows that there are strategies that will allow CMR in these patients, in particular if the device can be turned off for the duration of the scan, but until further evidence is available, this can only be considered in patients for whom benefit exceeds risk.

Clinical Applications

Coronary Artery Disease (see Chap. 50)

ASSESSMENT OF VENTRICULAR VOLUMES, MASS, AND FUNCTION. CMR is well validated for quantifying the volumes and mass of the ventricles, and it has become the clinical gold standard against which other techniques are measured because of its three-dimensional nature, which is not reliant on geometric assumptions. Comparisons with other techniques show wide variability in individual patients and are not greatly instructive, other than illustrating the difficulties of comparison of clinical techniques.[6] The accuracy and reproducibility of the measurements make CMR useful for the longitudinal follow-up of patients and for research using small sample sizes in hemodynamic and remodeling research.

The accuracy of CMR for measurement of global left ventricular volume has been established by comparing CMR images of ex vivo ventricles with the water displacement volume of casts of the ventricles.[7] In vivo, volume validation is more difficult to achieve, but the grounds for determining accuracy depend on comparing left ventricular stroke volume with the stroke volume of the right ventricle,[7] or with aortic flow measured using velocity mapping, [2] and showing their equivalence in normal human subjects. Right ventricular volumes have also been validated against water displacement of casts[8] and by comparing the right ventricular stroke volume with pulmonary artery flow. Left ventricular mass measurements have been validated against human autopsy hearts and in animals.[9] Right ventricular mass measurements have been validated against ex vivo animal hearts.[10]

An important feature of CMR is the excellent interstudy reproducibility of volume and mass measurements. Although other forms of reproducibility are often quoted for functional techniques (interobserver, intraobserver), they have little statistical import, whereas interstudy reproducibility can be directly used to quantify sample sizes in research studies and the minimum clinical difference observable, which represents a true clinical change. Interstudy reproducibility is measured as the standard deviation (SD) of the differences in two measurements of a parameter over a reasonable time period in which no clinical change is expected, but no substantial recollection is expected by the operator of patient positioning and other procedural factors. The SD is often expressed as a coefficient of variability by division into the parameter mean value. Sample sizes for trials are easily calculated from the technique interstudy SD, and low SDs are important because a reduction in SD between techniques leads to a squared reduction in sample size (i.e., half the SD equals one quarter the sample size). The interstudy SD for volumes and mass by CMR is excellent for both the left ventricle[11] and the right ventricle,[12] and is considerably superior to that of two-dimensional echocardiography.[11] Several drug trials have now used CMR as a primary or major endpoint.[13]

CMR is valuable for assessment of regional contractile function; clinically, this is usually achieved by visual inspection of cines in standard imaging planes. Quantification of wall motion and thickening using conventional techniques is possible for both the left ventricle and the right ventricle but is not widely used. A preferable CMR technique is tagging, which directly assesses myocardial strain and other deformations as a measure of contractility. Tagging CMR has been validated using sonomicrometer studies and can be applied for full three-dimensional myocardial analysis by collective modeling of the numerous small individual myocardial elements.[14] Recently, advanced tagging CMR acquisitions have greatly increased the spatial and temporal resolution and considerably simplified postprocessing. Clinical applications are just starting to emerge.

ASSESSMENT OF MYOCARDIAL INFARCTION AND VIABILITY. Myocardial infarction (MI) can be detected with high resolution using a protocol known as late gadolinium enhancement CMR. Gadolinium is given intravenously and CMR is performed after a delay using an inversion recovery sequence. Little gadolinium enters areas of normal myocardium, because there is uniform tightly packed muscle and gadolinium is an extracellular contrast agent. However, the extracellular compartment is expanded in areas of MI due to cellular rupture, and therefore differential distribution occurs. The kinetics of entry of gadolinium into the MI territory is delayed and the optimal time for imaging of the distribution of gadolinium is after 10 to 15 minutes. By nulling (forcing to near-zero) of the normal myocardial signal with adjustment of the inversion time, the area of infarction can be shown with extremely high contrast relative to the black normal myocardium. A simple but helpful mnemonic is that "bright is dead." The transmural distribution of MI can be visualized in vivo for the first time using this technique because of its high resolution. Validation has been performed in animal models (Fig. 14-1).[15] In humans, late gadolinium enhancement CMR detects Q wave and non-Q wave MI accurately[16] and with such high sensitivity that small MIs can be demonstrated that are not apparent using gated perfusion single-photon emission computed tomography (SPECT) (Fig. 14-2),[17] and microinfarcts can be shown after percutaneous coronary intervention.[18] In the acute setting, the extent of late gadolinium enhancement is related to the magnitude of cardiac enzyme release and the functional outcome after recovery. Late gadolinium enhancement CMR reveals a permanent record of MI (both acute and chronic) and is proving very useful clinically for the diagnosis of MI in cases of doubt, or when other techniques for detection are inconclusive. The technique has clarified the pathological significance of Q waves after MI.[19] It has good interstudy reproducibility,[20] suggesting a useful role in studies of therapies for limiting MI in the acute setting (see Chap. 47).

In the assessment of myocardial viability to determine the likely benefit from coronary bypass surgery, both conventional and late gadolinium CMR images are useful, and studies are ongoing to determine which technique yields more optimal results. An established approach is to measure myocardial wall thickness in areas of chronic transmural MI, using the premise from pathological studies that preserved thickness (>5 mm) indicates preserved viability. This simple criterion shows good correlation in cases of chronic MI to fluorodeoxyglucose positron emission tomography (FDG-PET).[21] In dysfunctional myocardium, improved thickening shown by low-dose dobutamine CMR is also in good agreement with FDG-PET findings.[21] More recently, the simple morphological measure of the transmural extent of late gadolinium enhancement by CMR has been shown to be highly predictive of viability,[22] with high likelihood of recovery when the transmural extent of infarction is less than 50 percent (Fig. 14-3).[23] Unlike wall thickness measurements, however, which can only be applied in cases of chronic MI, late gadolinium enhancement is also useful for prediction of functional recovery in cases of acute MI.[24] There is high concordance of late gadolinium enhancement CMR with PET,[25] and superior results have been shown in comparison with thallium 201 SPECT[26] (see Chap. 13).

STRESS VENTRICULOGRAPHY. Stress CMR using dobutamine is now clinically established for diagnosing obstructive coronary artery disease (CAD) through induction of new wall motion abnormalities (Fig. 14-4).[27] Pharmacological stress is preferred to dynamic exercise within the magnet to prevent motion artifacts. Stress CMR is superior to dobutamine stress echocardiography (see Chap. 11),[28] which is a function of higher image quality. Stress CMR is effective in the diagnosis of CAD in patients who are unsuitable for dobutamine echocardiography.[29] Outcome studies following normal stress CMR are limited but show a low event rate.[29-31] CMR has been used for preoperative risk assessment, and higher risk has been shown with demonstration of ischemia.[30] Real-time stress CMR may hasten the acquisition and make the study easier for the patient by eliminating the need for breath-holding.

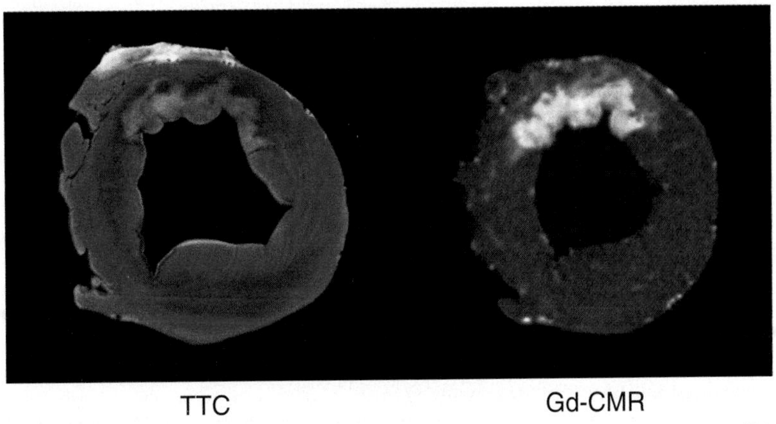

FIGURE 14–1 Validation of late gadolinium-enhanced cardiovascular magnetic resonance (Gd-CMR). A subendocardial infarct has been produced by ligation of a coronary artery in a dog, and gadolinium was injected shortly before sacrifice. On the **left,** the triphenyltetrazolium chloride (TTC)–negative area indicates the extent and shape of the infarct that is closely matched by the ex vivo CMR scan **(right).** Studies such as this have shown increased gadolinium concentration within the infarct zone and close correlation between the total infarct size by histology and CMR. Note the transmural resolution of the CMR scan and the similarity in shape of the infarctions. (Courtesy of Drs. R.J. Kim and R.M. Judd.)

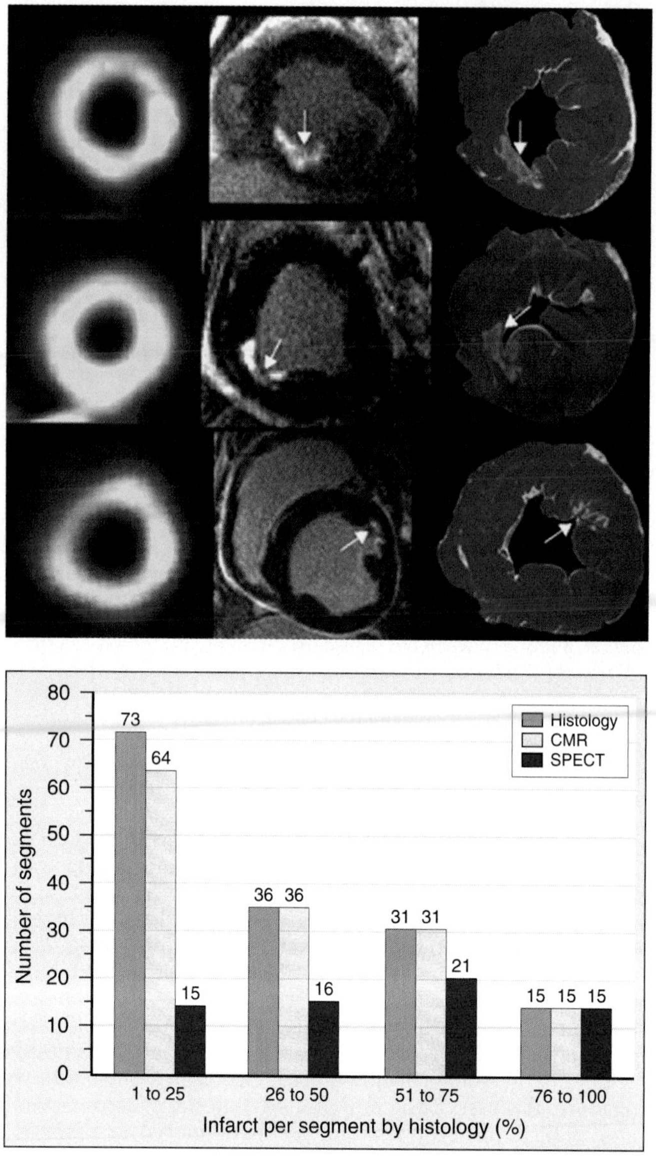

FIGURE 14–2 Comparison of cardiovascular magnetic resonance (CMR), ^{99m}Tc-sestamibi single-photon emission computed tomography (SPECT), and histologic findings in patients with subendocardial infarction. This figure shows a comparison between SPECT **(left),** late gadolinium-enhanced CMR **(middle),** and triphenyltetrazolium chloride histology **(right)** in three different dogs with experimentally induced subendocardial infarction. There is close similarity between histological and CMR findings, but in all three cases SPECT fails to demonstrate the infarction because of inadequate resolution. The effects of this are summarized in the graph, which shows excellent agreement between histology and CMR between the number of segments with infarction categorized by the percentage of infarction per segment. The agreement with SPECT, however, is only satisfactory in segments with greater than 75 percent infarction per segment. This shows that CMR is significantly more accurate in identifying small infarctions and the extent of infarction than SPECT. (From Wagner A, Mahrholdt H, Holly TA, et al: Contrast-enhanced MRI and routine single photon emission computed tomography [SPECT] perfusion imaging for detection of subendocardial myocardial infarcts: an imaging study. Lancet 361:374, 2003.)

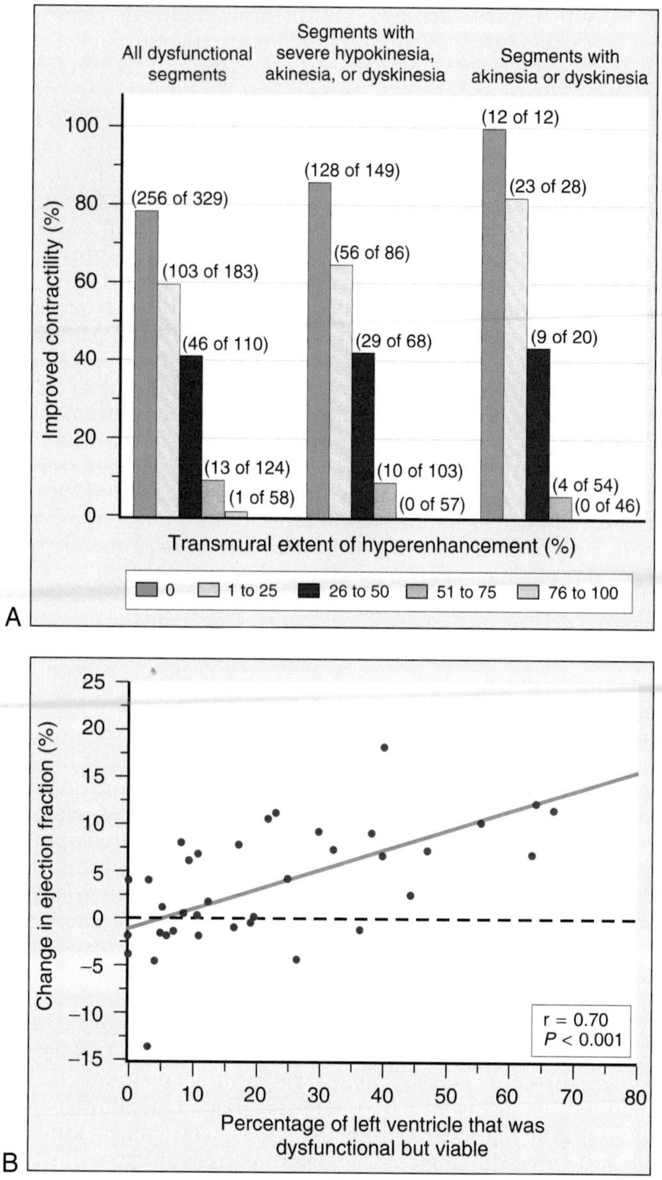

FIGURE 14–3 Assessment of myocardial hibernation by late gadolinium-enhanced cardiovascular magnetic resonance (CMR). There is a significant relationship between the likelihood of improvement of contraction in a segment that is dysfunctional, and the preoperative transmural extent of late gadolinium enhancement. **A,** Relation for all dysfunctional segments, those with at least severe hypokinesis, and those with at least akinesis. The discrimination is greatest for the most dysfunctional segments. The change in left ventricular ejection fraction was directly related to the percentage of the left ventricle, which was dysfunctional but viable using the late gadolinium-enhancement technique **(B)**. (From Kim RJ, Wu E, Rafael A, et al: The use of contrast-enhanced magnetic resonance imaging to identify reversible myocardial dysfunction. N Engl J Med 16:1445, 2000.)

A valuable adjunct to stress CMR would be the quantification of wall motion assessment, which would reduce the observer variability encountered with dobutamine-enhanced echocardiography. This has been approached in several ways, with early results. A center line method for assessing wall thickening during dobutamine-enhanced echocardiography, with comparison to normal ranges, improved the accuracy for detection of CAD in patients with single-vessel disease. Tagging CMR has also been applied, and this is expected to be more useful because of the independence of intrinsic strain measurements from endocardial motion.[32] Increased sensitivity with tagging has been shown,[31] but larger clinical trials and improved post-processing are needed to demonstrate clinical applicability. Other work in quantification has included assessment of stress diastolic function and stress global ventricular function measured with velocity mapping of aortic flow.[33] Further work is required to determine the clinical role of these techniques.

MYOCARDIAL PERFUSION. Myocardial perfusion CMR is in development but is close to achieving clinical utility. This has the potential for significant impact because of the combination of greatly enhanced resolution with no ionizing radiation. Full ventricular segmental coverage is achieved by using multiple contiguous short-axis slices or mixed short- and long-axis planes. A fast intravenous bolus (typically 5 to 7 ml/sec) of gadolinium contrast agent is given using a power injector, and the myocardial signal changes during the first pass are measured. Ideally, each slice is imaged with each cardiac cycle to maximize the quality of the analysis, although imaging on alternate cycles has been performed with good results.[34] Low signal areas representing reduced perfusion can be visualized directly. Alternatively, computer quantification of parameters such as the signal upslope can be used to generate parametric relative perfusion maps (Fig. 14–5)[34] or measures of perfusion index at rest and stress.[35] More complex analysis for quantification of myocardial perfusion or perfusion reserve includes preprocessing to remove respiratory motion and deconvolution of the myocardial signal curve with the input function taken from the left ventricular blood pool.[36] Perfusion CMR has been validated using microspheres in animal models[37,38] and in humans using PET.[34]

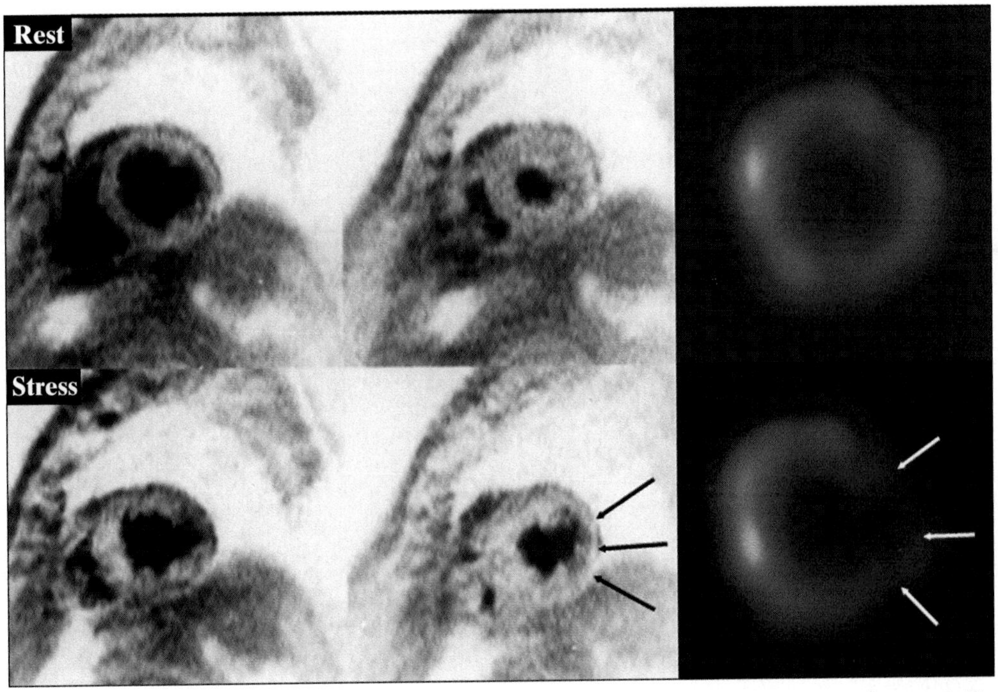

FIGURE 14–4 Cardiovascular magnetic resonance (CMR) stress ventriculography in a patient with left circumflex stenosis. The **left** and **middle panels** show end-diastolic and end-systolic frames, respectively, from CMR cines (the video scale is inverted, and blood therefore appears black), and the **right panels** show the corresponding slice by thallium single-photon emission computed tomography. The **upper row** is images taken at rest and the **lower row** is images taken during dobutamine stress. There is stress-induced wall motion abnormality; this is well shown in the end-systolic stress image (black arrows), which is similar in location and extent to the ischemia shown on the stress thallium scan (white arrows). (From Pennell DJ, Underwood SR, Manzara CC, et al: Magnetic resonance imaging during dobutamine stress in coronary artery disease. Am J Cardiol 70:34, 1992.)

For clinical application, several perfusion CMR protocols are being tested using adenosine as a pharmacological stress agent. One approach is to assess stress myocardial perfusion only[34] and define areas of nonviability using late gadolinium enhancement. A more conventional approach is to perform both stress and resting myocardial perfusion CMR to produce perfusion reserve measurements.[39] When both stress and resting studies are performed, however, the optimal order has not yet been defined, because residual gadolinium from the first injection has the potential to interfere with the subsequent study. The ideal CMR sequence is also not fully resolved, because superior coverage is obtained with a hybrid gradient-echo–echo-planar imaging sequence but higher signal is obtained with SSFP. Both techniques appear to give good results. A technique that does not require ultrafast imaging or gadolinium contrast has also been described called T2* blood oxygen level dependent (BOLD),[40] but the sensitivity of T2* to perfusion change may be quite low and its clinical role is not yet defined. There is general consensus that fast gadolinium injection is desirable for quantification, although for purely qualitative analysis this is not necessary. There is little difference among gadolinium contrast agents for perfusion CMR, because all currently distribute into the extracellular space, although those with lower viscosity can be injected at lower pressures, which has some patient safety advantages.

Myocardial perfusion CMR has shown very good results for the detection of CAD, in comparison with coronary angiography (see Chap. 18),[34] PET,[34] and SPECT (see Chap. 13). Improvements in myocardial perfusion reserve have been shown after coronary angioplasty.[41] The excellent resolution of perfusion CMR has also allowed visualization of perfusion abnormality not related to epicardial coronary artery in other conditions such as cardiac syndrome X (Fig. 14–6),[35] which agrees with results of CMR spectroscopy.[42] Perfusion CMR is likely to improve our understanding of the pathophysiology of these types of conditions and may have significant clinical application if the findings have diagnostic, therapeutic, or prognostic value.

CORONARY ANGIOGRAPHY AND FLOW. Coronary CMR angiography is still technically difficult for confident assignment of both presence and severity of coronary stenosis owing to small arterial size, tortuosity, complex anatomy, and cardiac and respiratory motion. Using highly optimized three-dimensional acquisitions, there has been gradual improvement in resolution and clinical robustness using both breath-hold and navigator techniques. The most significant clinical study, with multicenter participation, showed good results for the exclusion of multivessel proximal CAD requiring operative intervention.[43] However, current limitations of spatial resolution and rapid coronary motion during the acquisition allow only broad categorization of diameter stenosis, and distal run-off assessment is difficult for surgical planning.

These limitations of luminal stenosis imaging are not problematic, however, for the assessment of the course of anomalous coronary arteries, in which CMR plays a significant clinical role. The malignant course of some coronary arteries between the aorta and pulmonary artery is significantly better depicted by CMR than by x-ray coronary angiography because of the three-dimensional CMR tomograms in comparison with two-dimensional x-ray projections with overlapping structures.[44] Coronary CMR sequences can image coronary vein bypass grafts. Black and white blood approaches are approximately 90 percent accurate for identifying graft patency. This may prove useful in postoperative chest pain syndromes, but vein graft stenoses and the distal anastomoses cannot be assessed directly by luminal assessment. Although coronary imaging for luminal stenosis remains very challenging, some technical advances may prove valuable, such as high magnetic field scanners (Fig. 14–7),[45] intravascular contrast agents,[46] preoxygenation, and novel sequences.

Assessment of coronary function can also be achieved by measuring coronary flow velocities using CMR images. Adenosine stress coronary flow has been reported in animals and in humans, and the coronary flow

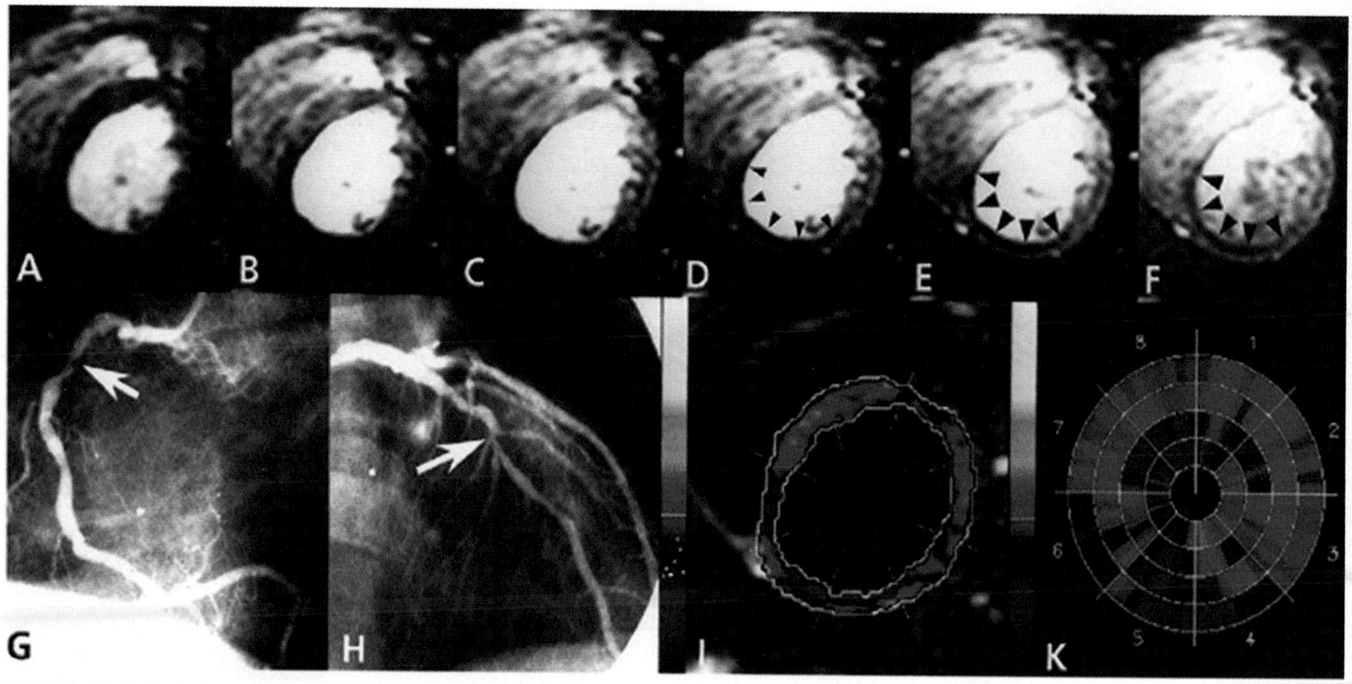

FIGURE 14–5 Perfusion cardiovascular magnetic resonance (CMR) images and parametric maps in a patient with stenosis of the right coronary and left anterior descending arteries (arrows in panels **G** and **H**). A single slice shown in panels **A** through **F** shows delayed wash-in the inferior wall of gadolinium-enhanced images during first pass (arrows). The parametric map in panel **I** shows this abnormality in blue. The polar map shown in panel **K** indicates areas of abnormal perfusion in blue in both the inferoseptal and the anteroseptal regions, corresponding to the right coronary and left anterior descending artery stenoses, respectively. (From Schwitter J, Nanz D, Kneifel S, et al: Assessment of myocardial perfusion in coronary disease by magnetic resonance: A comparison with positron emission tomography and coronary angiography. Circulation 103:2230, 2001.)

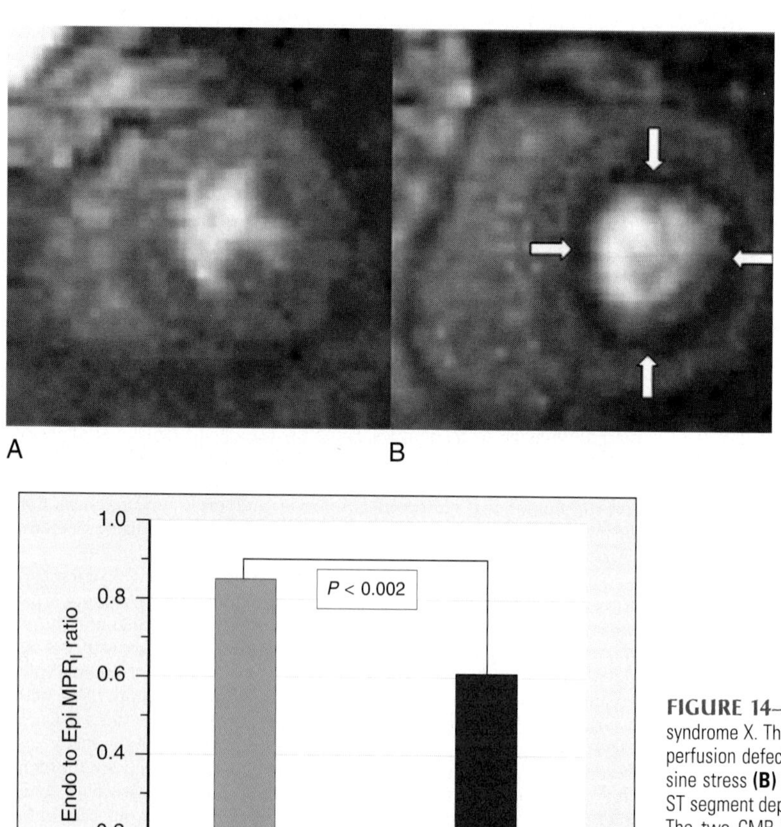

FIGURE 14–6 Perfusion cardiovascular magnetic resonance (CMR) in a patient with syndrome X. The high resolution of CMR allows the in vivo visualization of subendocardial perfusion defects for the first time. A perfusion CMR study at rest **(A)** and during adenosine stress **(B)** is shown in a patient with syndrome X (typical angina, greater than 2-mm ST segment depression during exercise electrocardiography, and normal coronary arteries). The two CMR images are from peak enhancement during the first pass of gadolinium enhancement. The image at baseline is normal but the image during adenosine enhancement shows subendocardial hypoperfusion. The graph **(C)** shows the myocardial perfusion reserve ratio between the endocardium and the epicardium in a group of syndrome X patients and control subjects. The ratio is significantly lower in patients with syndrome X, indicating reduced endocardial perfusion reserve. (From Panting JR, Gatehouse PD, Yang GZ, et al: Abnormal subendocardial perfusion in cardiac syndrome-X detected by cardiovascular magnetic resonance imaging. N Engl J Med 346:1948, 2002.)

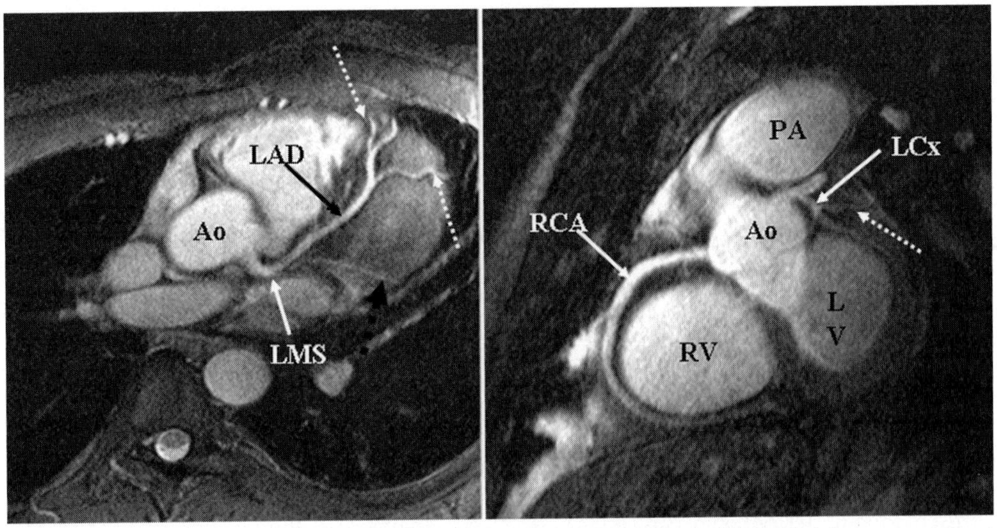

FIGURE 14–7 Coronary cardiovascular magnetic resonance (CMR) at 3 T. The **left panel** shows the left coronary artery and branches (dotted arrows) and the **right panel** shows the right coronary artery (RCA). Ao = aorta; LAD = left anterior descending artery; LMS = left main stem; LCx = left circumflex artery; LV = left ventricle; PA = pulmonary artery; RV = right ventricle. (From Stuber M, Botnar RM, Fischer SE, et al: Preliminary report on in vivo coronary MRA at 3 Tesla in humans. Magn Reson Med 48:425, 2002.)

reserve has been used to identify stenosis of the left anterior descending artery[47] and in-stent restenosis.[48] It has also been shown that reduced baseline flow and flow reserve in vein grafts are useful in identifying significant stenosis.[49]

ARTERIAL WALL: FUNCTION AND STRUCTURE. The arterial wall offers opportunities for assessment of atherosclerosis by CMR that have the potential to yield important additional information compared to luminal imaging, from endothelial dysfunction to arterial mechanical properties, total plaque burden, and plaque characterization, including vulnerability. Most CMR data are derived from work on the aorta and carotid and brachial arteries, but more recently coronary wall studies have been published (Fig. 14–8).

Endothelial function is considered one of the earliest triggers of atherosclerosis (see Chap. 35). As with ultrasonography, endothelial function can be examined noninvasively by CMR using stimuli that cause arterial vasodilation, such as flow-mediated dilation (endothelium dependent) and direct-acting drugs such as nitroglycerin (endothelium independent). Flow-mediated dilation is assessed by forearm cuff occlusion for a standard time period, followed by release, which induces increased endothelial shear, the release of nitric oxide, and arterial dilation. This technique has been performed using CMR on the brachial artery, but unlike ultrasonography, which measures arterial diameter, CMR measures arterial area and thus has significant advantages.[50] These include improved determination that the imaging is perpendicular to the vessel, greater immunity to arterial shape changes with transducer application and patient movement during the procedure, and increased sensitivity. Validation studies have been performed in humans using invasive techniques, and repeated measurements by CMR appear to have greater reproducibility than measurements by ultrasonography, suggesting smaller sample sizes for trials using CMR.[50] An additional advantage of CMR is that flow changes can also be measured directly in response to the standard stimuli.[51] Arterial dilation measurements have also been performed by CMR in the proximal coronary arteries, but more experience is needed in this area.

The mechanical properties of the arterial wall are significantly affected by sclerosis, and in the aorta this increases pulse pressure, afterload, and cardiac workload, resulting in reduced organ perfusion. Sclerosis of the vessel wall can be assessed in a number of ways, but CMR has usually been used to measure compliance in the ascending aorta (change of aortic sectional volume normalized to pulse pressure in μl/mm Hg) and pulse wave velocity around the aortic arch (rate of propagation of the flow wave in early systole in meters/sec). These measures have an age-dependent normal range, are abnormal in early atherosclerosis, and have been shown to be predictive of cardiac events.

Arterial wall CMR can also be used to identify total plaque burden within an imaging volume. Plaque burden is usually assessed on T1-weighted images with double or triple inversion to suppress blood signal in the lumen. Quantification of the vessel wall volume over the imaging stack is achieved by summation by planimetry of the difference in each image between the outer and inner vessel boundary.[52] This total vessel volume includes normal vessel wall and the atherosclerotic burden, which is dominant in cases of disease and dynamic for longitudinal studies of natural history and treatment. CMR studies show sufficient sensitivity to measure the effectiveness of antiatheroma therapy such as statin treatment over 12 months, showing a reduction in total wall volume.[53] More recently, the technique has been extended to the coronary wall, and wall thickening has been identified.[54]

Plaque constituents can be assessed using a combination of T1-, T2-, and proton density–weighted images, which allows assessment of plaque vulnerability.[55] Cholesterol pools are identified from low signal on T1 and T2 images,[56] and the fibrous cap can be identified overlying this.[57] Thin or disrupted caps on CMR have been strongly linked with cerebrovascular events.[58] Contrast agents have been used to further characterize

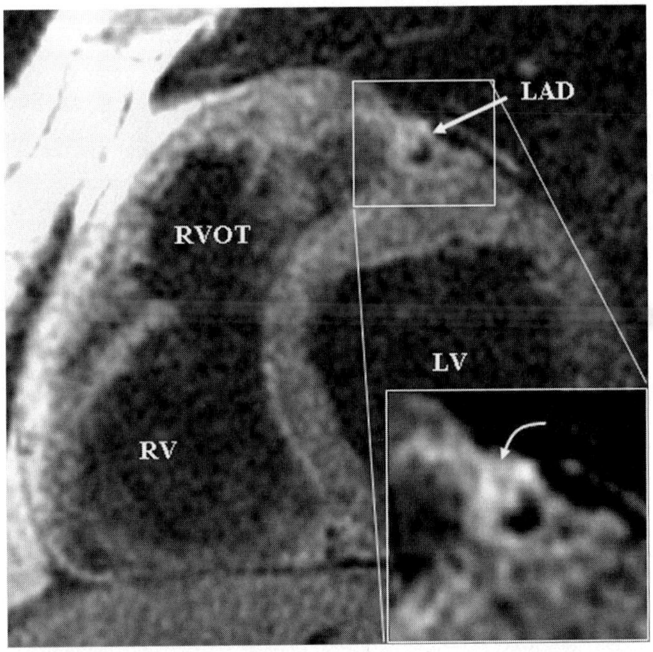

FIGURE 14–8 Coronary wall cardiovascular magnetic resonance (CMR). The **main panel** shows a short-axis cut of the ventricles at the base of the heart, and in the interventricular groove lies the left anterior descending artery (LAD). This is enlarged in the **inset** and a substantial eccentric plaque is identified (curved arrow). The lumen is still widely patent. RV = right ventricle; RVOT = right ventricular outflow tract; LV = left ventricle. (From Fayad ZA, Fuster V, Fallon JT, et al: Noninvasive in vivo human coronary artery lumen and wall imaging using black-blood magnetic resonance imaging. Circulation 102:506, 2000.)

plaque and show inflammation,[59] neovasculature,[60] and the fibrous cap.[61] Longitudinal study by CMR has followed the lipid pool.[62] Coronary plaque constituents have also been identified, but improved resolution would improve assessment in these small vessels.[54]

Evaluation of Acute Coronary Syndromes
(see Chaps. 47 and 49)

Cardiac myocardial resonance has been used for the assessment of acute chest pain.[63] CMR showed a sensitivity of 84 percent and a specificity of 85 percent, was the strongest predictor of an acute coronary syndrome, and added diagnostic value over the usual clinical parameters, including the electrocardiogram, troponin, and TIMI risk score. CMR also can be used to identify microvascular obstruction in cases of acute MI.[64] This is demonstrated approximately 1 to 2 minutes after intravenous injection of gadolinium during the vascular distribution phase of the contrast agent and well before late gadolinium-enhancement CMR is performed. Areas within the MI that have severely compromised perfusion appear black, indicating microvascular collapse. Microvascular obstruction detected by CMR is associated with ventricular remodeling[65] and an increased likelihood of cardiovascular events that is independent of the size of the MI.[66]

Cardiomyopathy (see Chap. 59)

DILATED CARDIOMYOPATHY. CMR clearly demonstrates the functional abnormalities associated with dilated cardiomyopathy (DCM), and ventricular volumetric analysis is useful for follow-up. The right ventricle is usually involved in DCM, which may be a useful diagnostic marker. The quantitative effects of therapy can be assessed.[13,67] A key clinical question in the diagnosis of DCM is its differentiation from heart failure resulting from CAD. In many centers, coronary angiography is routinely performed for this task. In those patients with unobstructed coronary arteries and no other etiological factor, the diagnosis of DCM is usually made. This differentiation is important clinically for several reasons in patients with CAD: they have a worse prognosis; they may benefit from revascularization and/or aneurysmectomy; and secondary preventive pharmacotherapy with statins and aspirin are typically used. Conversely, in DCM patients, secondary causes, such as excess alcohol ingestion or myocardial iron overload,[68] need to be excluded; as genetic studies of DCM begin to identify inherited abnormalities, accurate phenotyping and family screening are important for early diagnosis. Late gadolinium-enhanced CMR has been shown to be very useful in this respect. In a study of patients with the clinical label of DCM following normal coronary angiography, 59 percent showed no gadolinium enhancement, 28 percent showed patchy or longitudinal striae of midwall enhancement, clearly different than the distribution in CAD patients, and 13 percent had gadolinium enhancement indistinguishable from patients with CAD (Fig. 14–9).[69] These data suggest that using the coronary angiogram as the arbiter for the presence of left ventricular dysfunction due to CAD could have led to an incorrect assignment of DCM etiology in 13 percent of patients, possibly because of coronary recanalization after infarction. The midwall myocardial enhancement in DCM patients is similar to the fibrosis found at autopsy and has not been visualized in vivo with other techniques; it may have prognostic importance as a source of reentrant tachyarrhythmias. CMR may therefore become a useful alternative to routine coronary angiography in the diagnostic work-up of DCM by allowing direct and highly sensitive assessment of the myocardial substrate for CAD, rather than relying on the coronary angiogram, which yields problems with false-positive results (coincidental coronary disease in DCM that has not caused myocardial infarction) and false-negative results (normal coronary arteries despite previous myocardial damage due to arterial recanalization). Such accurate phenotyping is particularly useful for genotyping. Another CMR technique for assessing prognosis in DCM is spectroscopy, in which adverse outcomes are predicted by a low PCr/ATP ratio.[70]

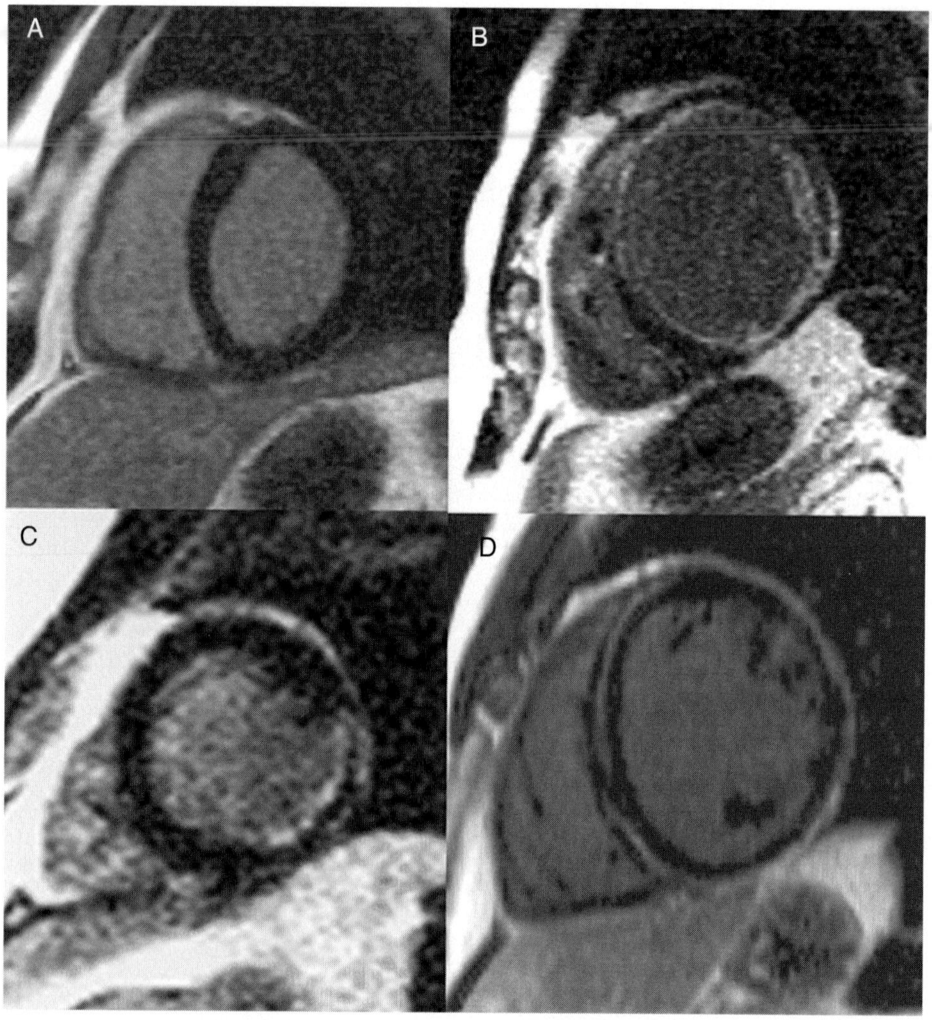

FIGURE 14–9 Late gadolinium-enhanced cardiovascular magnetic resonance (CMR) in patients with dilated cardiomyopathy (DCM). **A,** Patient with DCM and no gadolinium enhancement. **B,** Patient with known previous myocardial infarction resulting in heart failure in which late gadolinium enhancement is seen throughout the subendocardium causing thinning, particularly in the septum and inferolateral wall. **C,** Patient with the presumed clinical diagnosis of DCM because of the presence of a dilated heart with symptoms of heart failure but with normal coronary arteries by coronary angiography. Late gadolinium-enhanced CMR clearly shows an inferolateral infarction despite the normal coronary arteries, and it is likely that this patient's heart failure relates to coronary disease and not DCM. **D,** Patient with DCM who has late gadolinium enhancement of the midwall of the septum in the ventricular longitudinal fibers. This pattern of fibrosis is recognized by pathologists but has not been previously visualized in vivo. (From McCrohon JA, Moon JC, Prasad SK, et al: Differentiation of heart failure related to dilated cardiomyopathy and coronary artery disease using gadolinium-enhanced cardiovascular magnetic resonance. Circulation 108:54, 2003.)

HYPERTROPHIC CARDIOMYOPATHY. CMR is very useful in the diagnosis and assessment of hypertrophic cardiomyopathy (HCM), with ideal image quality covering both ventricles completely for localization of hypertrophy. CMR is used when echocardiography is questionable, particularly with apical hypertrophy.[71] Cines oriented in the plane of the left ventricular outflow tract show obstruction, and velocity mapping can be used to assess peak velocities. Systolic anterior motion of the mitral valve is also clearly seen. Improvement in obstruction after septal ablation or resection can be demonstrated, as can the location and size of the associated infarction, which are helpful for planning of repeat procedures. CMR myocardial tagging identifies abnormal patterns of strain, shear, and torsion in cases of HCM, demonstrating significant dysfunction in hypertrophic areas. CMR spectroscopy shows bioenergetic defects in HCM patients with varying genetic mutations, which supports the hypothesis that the underlying substrate for HCM might be inefficient energy utilization.[72] The accuracy of the phenotypic determination of HCM by CMR is helpful for family screening, and genetic linkage studies for causative mutations are improved in power. Late gadolinium enhancement occurs in HCM, which represents myocardial fibrosis.[73] Most patients have no gadolinium enhancement, and a common benign pattern is two stripes running along the junction of the right ventricular insertion into the left ventricle. More extensive gadolinium enhancement can be dense and plaque-like or diffuse. The greater the gadolinium enhancement, the higher the risk of heart failure or sudden death, presumably because of reentrant tachycardias and systolic failure from myocyte replacement (Fig. 14–10).[74] More work needs to be done in this promising area. CMR has also proved useful in differentiating causes of hypertrophy, which can mimic HCM. This includes Fabry disease (α-galactoside deficiency), which occurs in 4 percent of HCM populations and is an X-linked genetic disorder causing accumulation of glycosphingolipid in myocytes and endothelium, in which CMR shows unusual lateral wall gadolinium enhancement.[75] Other differential diagnoses, including amyloidosis and athletic heart, can be distinguished by CMR.

IRON OVERLOAD CARDIOMYOPATHY. Iron overload, or siderotic cardiomyopathy, occurs in patients with severe inherited anemia requiring regular blood transfusions from birth. The iron load of the transfusions can be combined with increased intestinal iron absorption, leading to iron deposition in the tissues because the body has no mechanism for iron excretion. The iron is toxic and causes oxidative cellular damage and organ dysfunction. The most important of these conditions is beta-thalassemia major; 71 percent of these patients die from heart failure at a young age. Beta-thalassemia major is a substantial worldwide health problem, with 60,000 affected children born annually who require long-term treatment. It has not been possible to measure cardiac iron except by myocardial biopsy, which is usually compromised because of sampling error due to patchy iron distribution. This has led to the usual clinical management being based on blood ferritin and liver iron levels, which is clearly not ideal because of the ongoing incidence of heart failure. Recently, CMR has been shown to be useful, with measurement of the myocardial relaxation parameter T2*. A low myocardial T2* indicates iron overload[68] and is related to left ventricular dysfunction and increased ventricular volumes and mass, providing clinical validation of the technique (Fig. 14–11). Further evidence for the value of the myocardial T2* measurement has come from evidence that T2* increases with left ventricular function recovery in thalassemia patients undergoing intensive iron chelation treatment for heart failure.[76] CMR has also shown the effects of different chelation regimens on myocardial

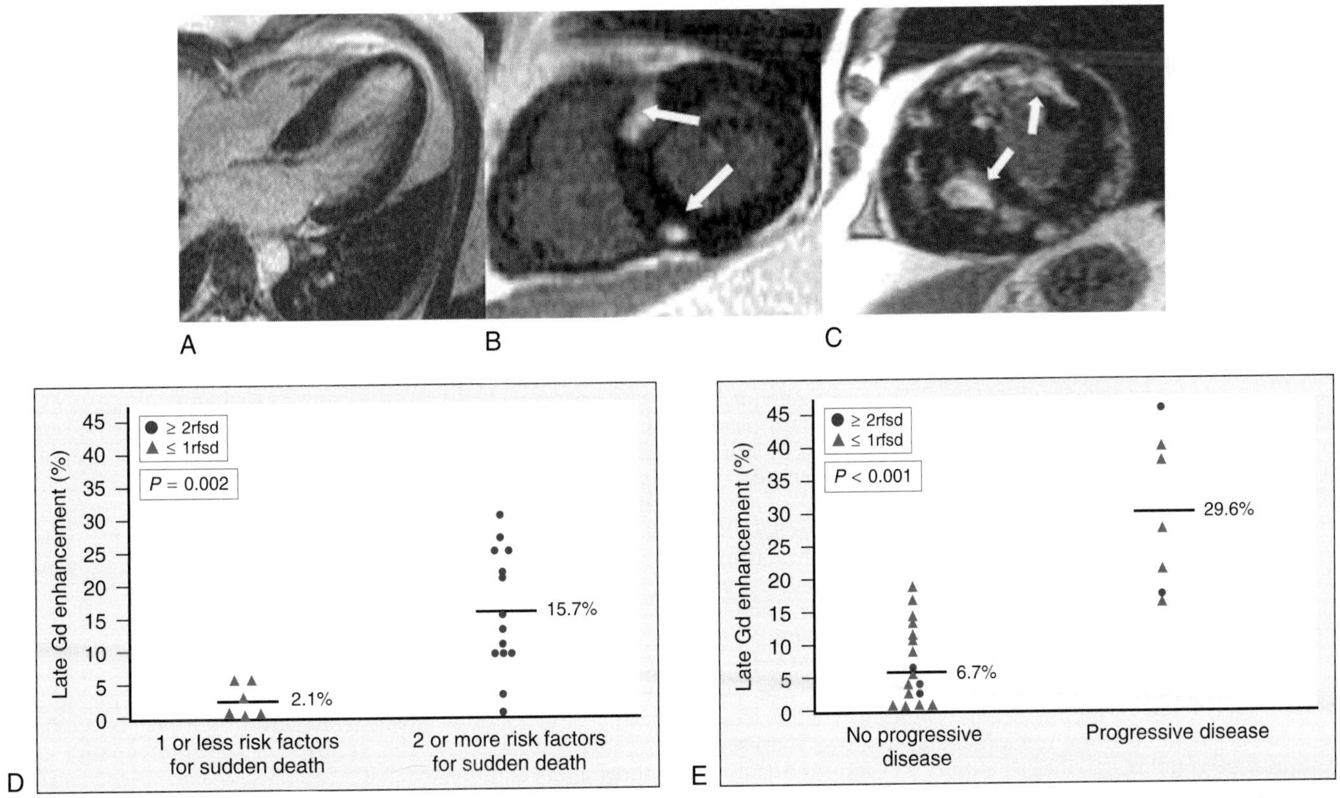

FIGURE 14–10 Late gadolinium enhancement and risk assessment in patients with hypertrophic cardiomyopathy (HCM). **A,** HCM patient with no gadolinium enhancement. **B,** HCM patient with longitudinal striae of late gadolinium enhancement at the insertion points of the right ventricle into the left ventricle (arrows). **C,** HCM patient with extensive plaque-like fibrosis (arrows). The relationship between the extent of late gadolinium enhancement and the number of risk factors for sudden death (rfsd) is shown in **D,** and documented progression of ventricular dilation toward heart failure is shown in **E.** In both cases, extensive gadolinium enhancement indicated a poor prognosis. (From Moon JCC, McKenna WJ, McCrohon JA, et al: Toward clinical risk assessment in hypertrophic cardiomyopathy with gadolinium cardiovascular magnetic resonance. J Am Coll Cardiol 41:1561, 2003.)

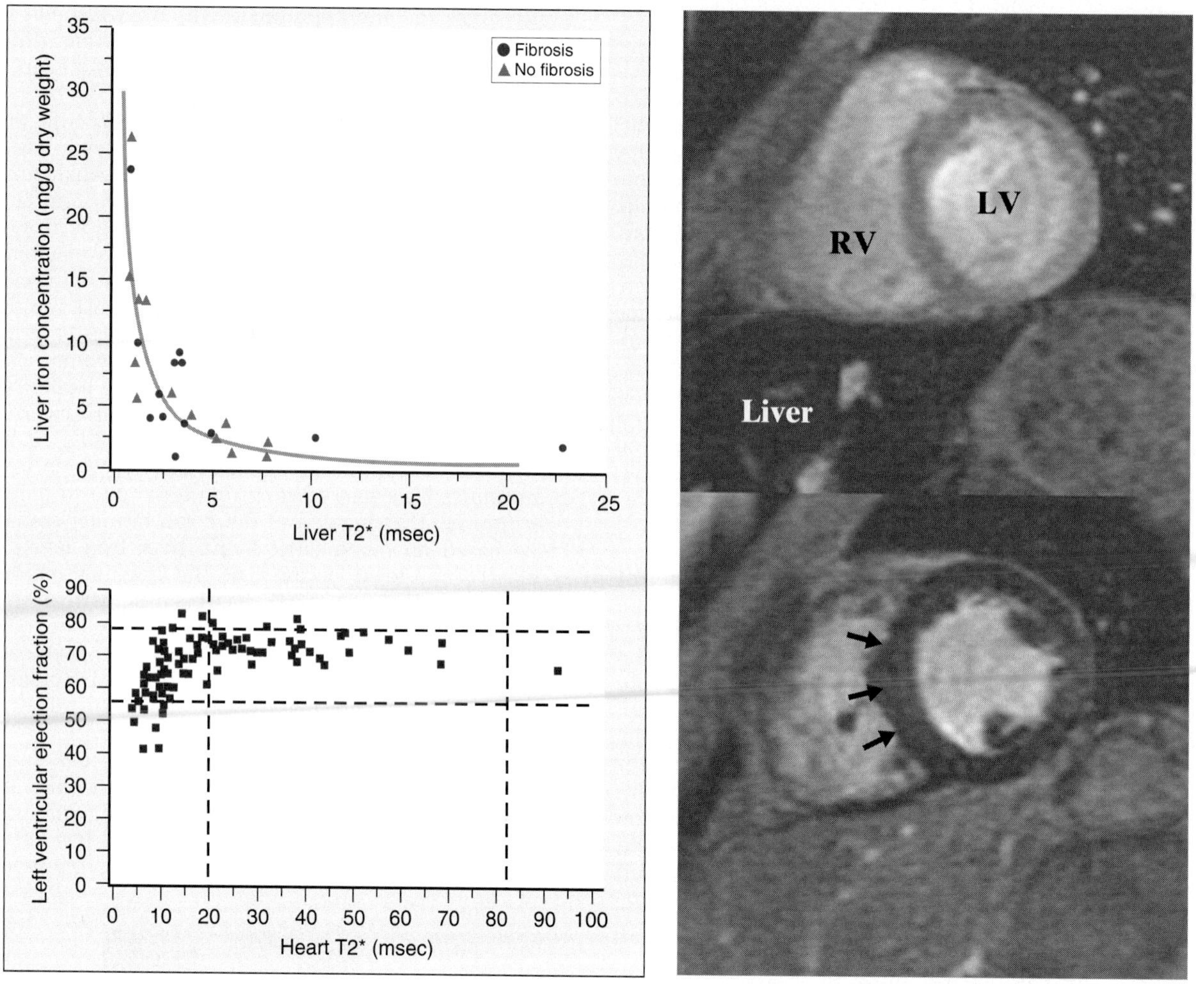

FIGURE 14–11 T2* cardiovascular magnetic resonance (CMR) in patients with iron overload cardiomyopathy. The **upper graph (left)** shows the tissue calibration between T2* of the liver and liver biopsy. The fit is best for the nonfibrotic liver samples, as expected. The curvilinear relationship is transformed into a linear relationship with a log-log plot. The **lower graph** shows the relationship between myocardial T2* and the left ventricular ejection fraction. Normal values for heart T2* are greater than 20 msec, and in this range the ejection fraction is normal. Below this range, there is a marked fall in ejection fraction related to iron toxicity. The two CMR scans **(right)** are short-axis cuts showing both the ventricular myocardium and the liver. The **upper panel** shows an iron-loaded liver (dark) but a normal heart appearance. If there were concern about this patient's heart iron status, liver biopsy would suggest iron loading, which could lead to an increase in chelation therapy with desferrioxamine and the risk of significant side effects. The **lower panel** shows the opposite scenario in which the liver has normal signal, but the heart is iron loaded (dark, arrows). Should this patient have a liver biopsy, the result would be falsely reassuring and chelation therapy would not be increased, and the patient would be at risk of death from heart failure and arrhythmias. These disparities in iron between the heart and liver help to explain why heart failure is the biggest cause of mortality in thalassemia patients. LV = left ventricle; RV = right ventricle. (From Anderson LJ, Holden S, Davies B, et al: Cardiovascular T2* (T2 star) magnetic resonance for the early diagnosis of myocardial iron overload. Eur Heart J 22:2171, 2001.)

iron.[77] On modern scanners, the T2* CMR sequence can be completed in a single breath-hold and may therefore prove to be cost-effective in areas of the world with large numbers of beta-thalassemia patients, such as in Asia and the Mediterranean.

ARRHYTHMOGENIC RIGHT VENTRICULAR CARDIOMYOPATHY. CMR depicts well the structural and functional abnormalities of the right ventricle, with no limitation from its retrosternal location. CMR is therefore widely used in expert centers for the investigation of arrhythmogenic right ventricular cardiomyopathy.[78] The diagnostic criteria of arrhythmogenic right ventricular cardiomyopathy are well defined, and CMR is helpful in ascertaining whether right ventricular regional wall motion abnormalities, increased volumes, morphological abnormalities, and fatty infiltration are present. Follow-up of the quantitative parameters over time can also be useful clinically. Problems occur if the scans are overinterpreted, because the right ventricle shows substantial normal variations, including reduced regional wall motion in the region of the moderator band insertion, highly variable trabeculation, and substantial fat around the coronary vessels and epicardium. Sufficient experience of the normal variants is therefore important. In addition, it is important to recognize the limitations of CMR, because poor-quality breath-holds with fast spin-echo images may lead to the misinterpretation of wall thinning, because epicardial fat may not be distinguished clearly from right ventricular myocardium, and artifacts may give rise to an increased right ventricular wall signal that mimics fat. Fatty infiltration is not considered a definitive sign of disease in any case, because it can occur in other circumstances.[79] An abnormal CMR scan has been linked to an adverse prognosis, but more work needs to be done in this area. Finally, patients with right ventricular outflow tract tachycardia that is not related to arrhythmogenic right ventricular cardiomyopathy may show abnormalities by CMR that are not seen by echocardiography.[80]

MYOCARDIAL SARCOIDOSIS. Myocardial sarcoidosis is relatively uncommon, but sudden death may be its initial clinical presentation. Standard imaging techniques suffer from low diagnostic accuracy, and the clinical diagnosis is difficult.[81] CMR may be of value, with gadolinium enhancement occurring in presumed areas of fibrosis.[82] Enhancement may reduce after steroid treatment and is therefore a potential therapeutic marker of myocardial activity. The use of T2-weighted sequences may also be helpful in identifying active myocardial inflammation. CMR requires further assessment in this area.

MYOCARDIAL AMYLOIDOSIS. CMR is useful in cases of restrictive cardiomyopathy, such as amyloidosis, which can be recognized by typical diastolic dysfunction, ventricular hypertrophy, and interatrial septum thickening.[83] Amyloid infiltration of the myocardium may show increased signal with late gadolinium enhancement. CMR can exclude with reasonable accuracy the differential diagnosis of constriction when the pericardial thickness is normal.

MYOCARDITIS (see Chap. 60). The diagnosis and investigation of myocarditis are often difficult. CMR shows focal increases of myocardial signal in patients with acute myocarditis using gadolinium-enhanced T1-weighted spin-echo CMR images with early imaging at 1 to 2 minutes and measurement of relative myocardial enhancement compared with skeletal muscle.[84] Abnormal myocardial signal is also seen with T2-weighted spin-echo CMR images. Normalization of signal intensity occurs with healing, unless cell death has occurred, in which case late gadolinium imaging may show patchy enhancement. Contrast enhancement 4 weeks after the onset of symptoms has been predictive for the functional and clinical long-term outcomes.[85] Although promising clinically, more experience is needed with this technique on various CMR scanners. A similar technique has been shown to predict anthracycline toxicity.[86]

HEART TRANSPLANTATION (see Chap. 26). Acute rejection results in an increase in myocardial mass, reduction in ventricular function, high myocardial signal intensity, and increased T2, which occur with myocardial edema or cellular infiltration. These changes are not reliable indicators of acute rejection, particularly in the early stages. In cases of early rejection, decreased PCr/ATP ratios are evident by CMR spectroscopy, although this has to be distinguished from ischemia. CMR can assess medical treatment on the remodeling process associated with long-term use of cyclosporine.[87]

Valvular Heart Disease (see Chap. 57)

CMR is useful in cases of valve disease but often plays a secondary role to echocardiography. However, in cases of difficulty in obtaining adequate echocardiography examinations, and for valvular regurgitation in particular, CMR has significant clinical utility.[88]

VALVE MORPHOLOGY. Normal heart valves are thin and rapidly moving, and only with the use of breath-hold sequences have the leaflets become well defined on CMR images on a routine basis. Abnormal valves are thicker and less mobile and are thus more easily visualized, but calcification causes local signal loss that may obscure valve pathology on black-blood images. Valve leaflet function throughout the cardiac cycle is well assessed using gradient-echo cines, especially with the latest SSFP techniques. Valve area can be assessed by direct planimetry using a cross-sectional plane immediately downstream from the valve, and plane-following techniques can be used to ensure tracking of the valve movement throughout the cycle, to eliminate through-plane motion errors.[89] Calcification has the potential to increase valve area on direct planimetry, but this is uncommon because calcifications are mainly located within the cusps. Bicuspid aortic valves or fused valve leaflets can be readily identified.

ASSESSMENT OF TURBULENCE AND JETS. Turbulence causes intravoxel dephasing with gradient-echo CMR cines, and this is useful clinically for the identification of regurgitation with signal loss in the receiving chamber (Fig. 14–12). The length and area of the signal loss are only semiquantitive measures of severity, however, because these measures depend on hemodynamic variables such as size and shape of the valve orifice, the pressure gradient, and technical parameters of the pulse sequence. Modern CMR systems now typically acquire cines using the SSFP technique, which is less sensitive to turbulence-related signal loss, so that comparison between cine types for the area of signal loss is not clinically useful. Real-time color flow CMR has been implemented, but its clinical utility has not yet been assessed. Therefore, flow and volumetric techniques are used to quantify regurgitation. For quantification of regurgitation, flow in the aorta and pulmonary artery at each time point through the cardiac cycle are measured by multiplying the vessel cross-sectional area by the mean flow; the results are displayed as flow curves. For stenotic jets, the peak velocity can be measured in plane or through plane using velocity mapping and related to the peak pressure gradient by the modified Bernoulli equation in the normal way. Using short echo time sequences, the jets appear coherent with high signal, although surrounding turbulence may cause signal loss (Fig. 14–13). The velocity-sensitivity should be set above the expected peak velocity, to avoid aliasing.

QUANTIFICATION OF REGURGITATION. Quantitative assessment of regurgitation can be obtained in a number of ways. If a single valve is affected on either side of the heart, the regurgitant volume can be calculated from the difference of right ventricular and left ventricular stroke volumes using the volumetric technique of contiguous short-axis cine slices spanning the ventricles.[90] If single valves on both sides of the heart are regurgitant, the method can be extended by subtracting great vessel flow, measured by CMR velocity mapping, from the ventricular stroke volumes measured with the volumetric technique. This method compares favorably with catheterization and Doppler echocardiography (see Chaps. 11 and 17).[91] Reversal of pulmonary vein flow indicates severe mitral regurgitation, as with echocardiography. Direct methods for measuring systolic regurgitant flow and ventricular inflow at the mitral annulus level are less satisfactory because of annulus motion and jet eccentricity. An alternative technique for pulmonary or aortic regurgitation is the direct assessment of regurgitation using flow mapping immediately downstream of the valve by measuring the retrograde volume flow after valve closure. This diastolic backflow is divided into the systolic forward flow to derive a regurgitant fraction. This simple technique has been used to identify responses to angiotensin-converting enzyme inhibition[92] and vasodilation.[93] It has high interstudy reproducibility, suggesting that it may be valuable for longitudinal follow-up of regurgitation severity over time.[94]

QUANTIFICATION OF STENOSIS. To quantify the velocity of a jet through a valve stenosis, it is necessary to adjust the imaging parameters so that signal is present in the jet core. For higher velocities, this requires a very short TE to prevent signal loss or other artifacts interfering with the measurement. Turbulence around the jet core is usual, appears dark on the cine, and does not interfere with measurements within the jet. There is good agreement between CMR and other techniques in evaluating mitral and aortic valve stenosis.[95] The valve area can also be directly

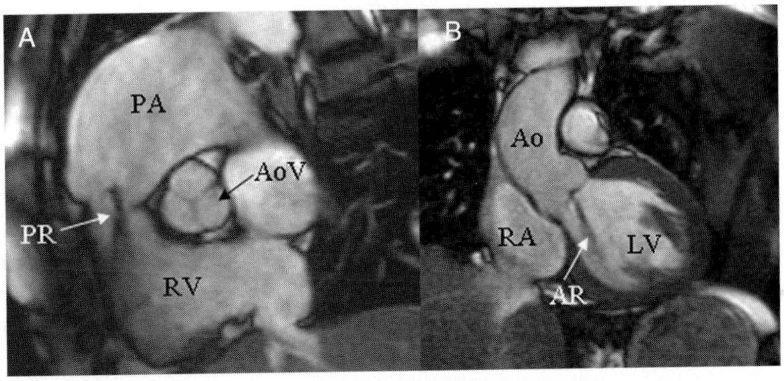

FIGURE 14–12 Cardiovascular magnetic resonance (CMR) of patients with valvular regurgitation. **A,** Patient with pulmonary hypertension with a dilated pulmonary artery. The images are from a steady state with free precession (SSFP) cine in diastole, and the aortic valve (AoV) is seen to be closed. A jet of pulmonary regurgitation (PR) can be seen entering the right ventricle. **B,** Patient with aortic regurgitation (AR) in the coronal plane. Ao = aorta; LV = left ventricle; PA = pulmonary artery; RA = right atrium; RV = right ventricle.

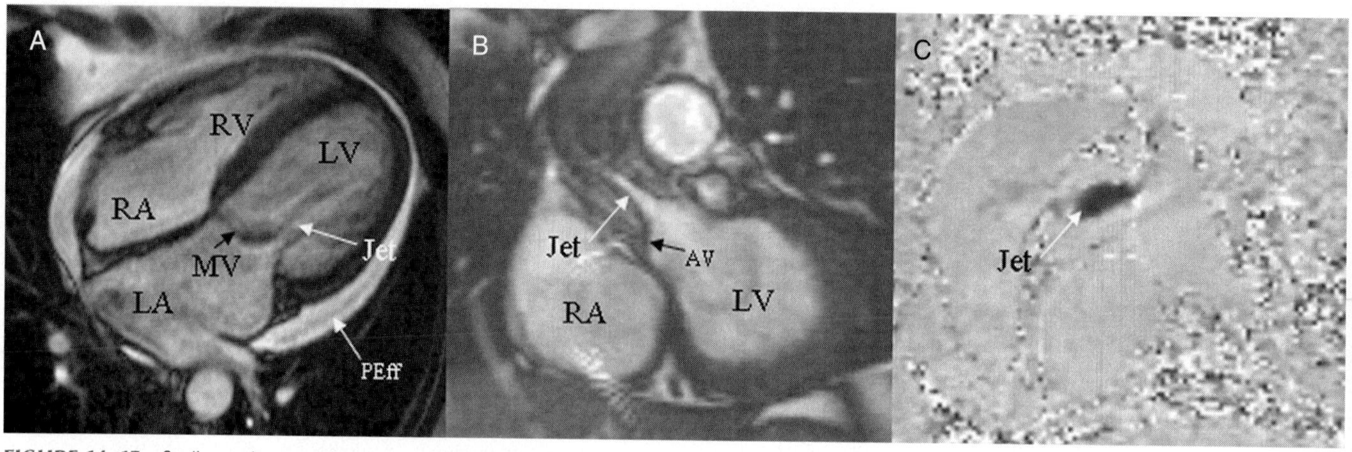

FIGURE 14–13 Cardiovascular magnetic resonance (CMR) of patients with valvular stenosis. **A,** Diastolic frame from a four-chamber steady state with free precession (SSFP) cine. The mitral valve (MV) is thickened, and there is poor opening with jet formation and surrounding signal loss from turbulence (Jet). The left atrium (LA) is enlarged and there is pericardial effusion (PEff). **B,** Aortic stenosis, with central bright jet formation and surrounding signal loss from turbulence. **C,** Velocity map taken through the aortic stenotic jet, with a measured velocity of 4.3 meters/sec, equal to a calculated pressure drop of 74 mm Hg. AV = aortic valve; LV = left ventricle; RA = right atrium; RV = right ventricle.

planimetered in patients with aortic stenosis.[96] Because echocardiography is the first-line clinical test to investigate valve stenosis, CMR is used when acoustic windows are poor or when discordant imaging and invasive results occur. Improved left ventricular and microvascular function and reduced hypertrophy,[97] as well as myocardial metabolism and diastolic function,[98] have been shown by CMR after aortic valve replacement for stenosis.

PROSTHETIC VALVES. CMR of all prosthetic heart valves at 1.5 T is safe, because there is no substantial magnetic interaction and heating is negligible.[99] Metallic valve components produce artifacts and signal loss, however, which are mild on spin-echo images but more apparent on gradient-echo cines. Small paravalvular jets can be obscured by the artifact, but velocity profiles close to aortic valve prostheses have been measured using valve tracking techniques.

Diseases of the Pericardium (see Chap. 64)

CMR is well suited to defining functional and anatomical abnormalities associated with the pericardium[100] but is mainly used when echocardiography yields incomplete information. CMR is very sensitive in the detection of pericardial effusion, which has high signal intensity with SSFP cine imaging and has clinical value when the effusion is loculated or complex. Signal from effusion is usually low on spin-echo images. Pericardial constriction is usually, but not invariably, associated with pericardial thickening, which is well depicted with both spin-echo and gradient-echo imaging (Fig. 14–14). The signal of the normal pericardium is low and appears as a thin dark line between fat outside the visceral and parietal layers. The thickness in normal subjects is 1 to 2 mm, but the upper range of normal for CMR is usually taken as 4 mm, which allows for chemical shift signal cancellation effects at the fat-pericardium border. Pericardial thickening is often inhomogeneous in cases of acute and chronic pericardial disease, and the signal characteristics can be variable. Acute inflammation may give rise to a pericardium with increased signal on spin-echo images, which enhances early after gadolinium administration. It is important to distinguish pericardial thickening from pericardial effusion, as both may appear dark on spin-echo images. The distinction is achieved by using cine sequences. Calcium is not seen directly by CMR but appears dark, and computed tomography should be used if information on calcium is clinically required. Other pericardial abnormalities can also be identified by CMR. Cysts have characteristic signal intensity, with low signal on T1-weighted spin-echo images but high signal with T2 weighting. Complete absence of the pericardium is indicated by a leftward shift of the long axis of the heart, and partial absence is seen as a protrusion of a portion of the heart.

Cardiac Tumors (see Chaps. 63 and 83)

Cardiac tumors are usually first diagnosed or suspected after transthoracic echocardiography, often as an incidental finding. Information can be obtained by echocardiography on the tumor localization, origin, extent, and resectability, but characterization may well be incomplete. CMR can then be very helpful.[101] The wide field of view of CMR allows significantly improved determination of the relationship of the tumor to adjacent structures for surgical planning, as well as identifying infiltration into the pericardium. CMR also offers a number of means of tumor characterization, which may have important clinical value. The most obvious example is that of a well-circumscribed, high signal intensity lesion that shows complete signal suppression using fat saturation techniques, which is diagnostic of lipoma (Fig. 14–15). A variant of this diagnosis, which is also very well demonstrated by CMR, is atrial lipomatous hypertrophy. Alternatively, an irregular tumor that shows signal increase during the first-pass bolus of

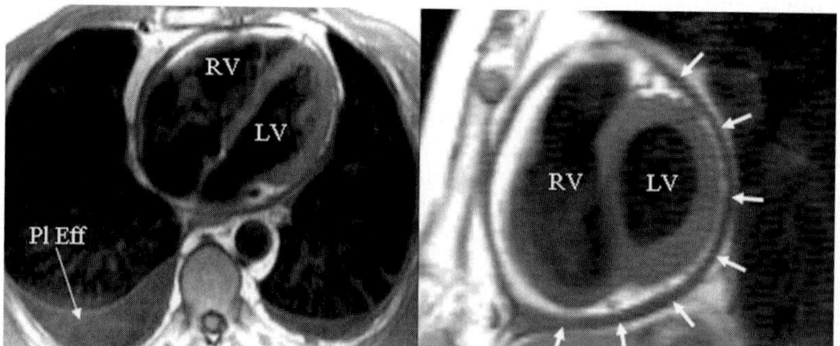

FIGURE 14–14 Cardiovascular magnetic resonance in a patient with constrictive pericarditis. On the **right** is a basal short-axis view of the ventricles showing a thickened pericardium encasing the heart (arrows). On the **left** is a transaxial view, again showing the thickened pericardium, particularly over the right heart, but also a pleural effusion (Pl Eff). LV = left ventricle; RV = right ventricle.

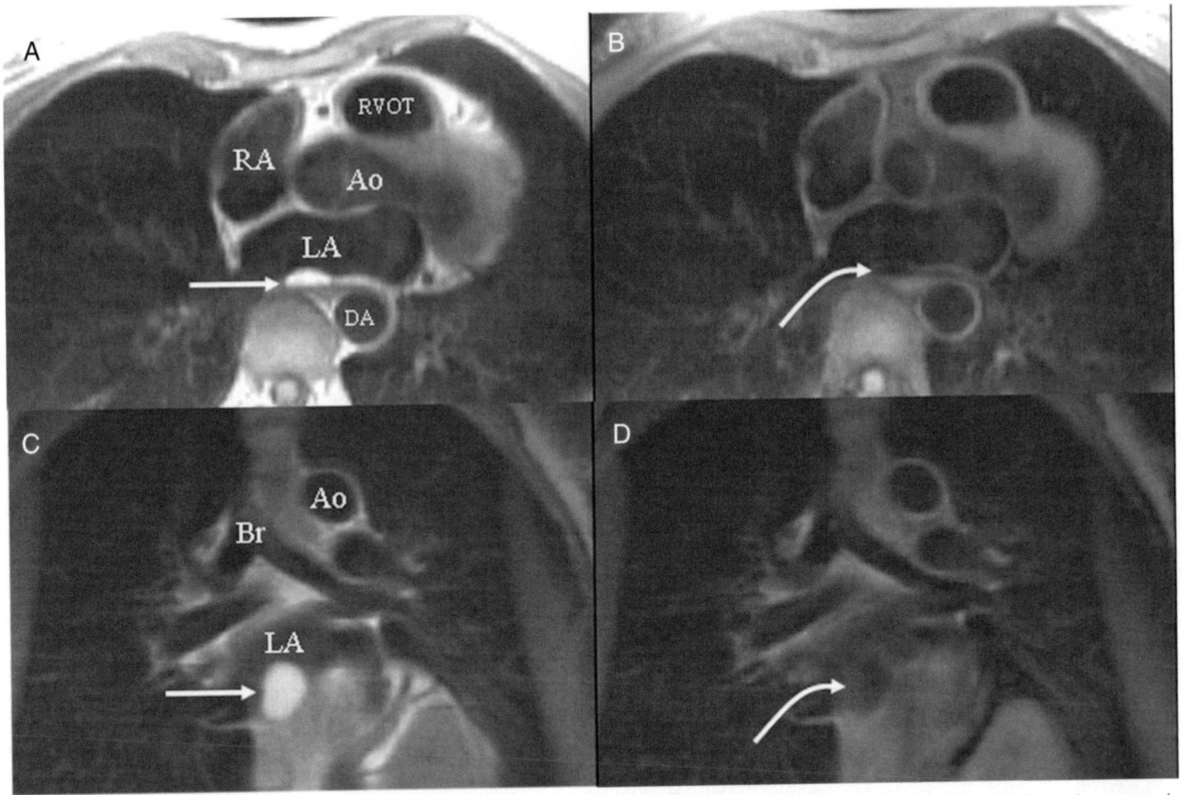

FIGURE 14–15 Cardiovascular magnetic resonance of a patient with retroatrial lipoma. **A** and **B,** Transaxial cuts through the heart. **C** and **D,** Coronal cuts posteriorly. A tumor is present posterior to the left atrium (straight arrow) in panels **A** and **C.** Panels **B** and **D** show the equivalent images with fat suppression turned on and abolition of signal within the tumor (curved arrows), therefore confirming the diagnosis of lipoma. Ao = aorta; Br = bronchus; DA = descending aorta; LA = left atrium; RA = right atrium; RVOT = right ventricular outflow tract.

gadolinium (perfusion), significant early tissue enhancement (increased vascularity), and significant late enhancement (fibrosis or necrosis) is typically an angiosarcoma (Fig. 14–16). Other useful signal characteristics include high T1-weighted signal in recent hemorrhage (due to the paramagnetic effects of the breakdown of hemoglobin), cysts with high protein content, and melanoma; low T1-weighted signal in low protein content cysts, calcified lesions, or air; high T2-weighted signal in cysts; high signal during the first pass of gadolinium in hemangioma (noninvasive) and angiosarcoma (invasive); necrotic areas highlighted against surrounding enhancement in malignant tumors 1 to 2 minutes after the intravenous administration of gadolinium; absence of early gadolinium enhancement in most benign tumors, with the exclusion of hemangioma and myxoma; and late gadolinium enhancement in fibrosis and its absence in cysts. The clinical setting and location of the tumor also yield important diagnostic information. Finally, CMR is excellent at identifying thrombus. Thrombus is usually hypointense on SSFP cines. On spin-echo images, thrombus is usually visible against the black blood pool and in the subacute phase may have areas of high signal intensity due to the paramagnetic effect of hemoglobin breakdown products. Thrombus is also identified with high accuracy using an inversion recovery technique with an inversion time 2 minutes after gadolinium injection. The thrombus has low vascularity and appears as a dark area surrounded by intense blood and myocardial signal.

Congenital Heart Disease (see Chap. 56)

CMR is ideally suited to the evaluation of congenital heart disease for several reasons: three-dimensional contiguous data sets are very effective for the complete depiction of anatomy; functional assessments are readily combined with the anatomical data; and CMR is less operator dependent than echocardiography. In addition, long-term follow-up is greatly facilitated by good reproducibility, noninvasiveness, access to relatively unrestricted fields of view, and freedom from ionizing radiation. The combination of CMR with transesophageal echocardiography has been particularly effective in patient evaluation because the two investigations often yield complementary information (see Chap. 11),[102] and the need, duration, and risks of invasive catheterization have diminished in recent years. However, the ease of use and value of CMR depend on the age and clinical condition of the patient. For small children, anesthesia or sedation is required for CMR, and monitoring may be demanding; for these patients, echocardiography is usually adequate. The contributions of CMR tend to increase in older children and adults. CMR is also relatively more effective in evaluating more complex anatomy and after surgery in the many patients now surviving to adult life, because scar tissue and limitations of acoustic access are increasing problems for echocardiography. CMR is thus the preferred technique for the serial evaluation of right ventricular volumes, mass, and function,[12,103] valvular regurgitation,[103] the pulmonary arteries, and extracardiac conduits. Expertise in CMR is highly recommended in centers specializing in the care of patients with congenital heart disease.[102] The range of congenital abnormalities is large, and a summary follows, but more detail can be found in specialized texts.[104,105]

GREAT VESSEL ABNORMALITIES. Coarctation usually occurs in the proximal descending aorta opposite the ductus arteriosus, just distal to the left subclavian artery. CMR is the optimal technique for assessment of coarctation (Fig. 14–17), especially in adults and after operative repair. CMR identifies the coarctation site and extent, any involvement of arch vessels, and poststenotic dilation. Velocity

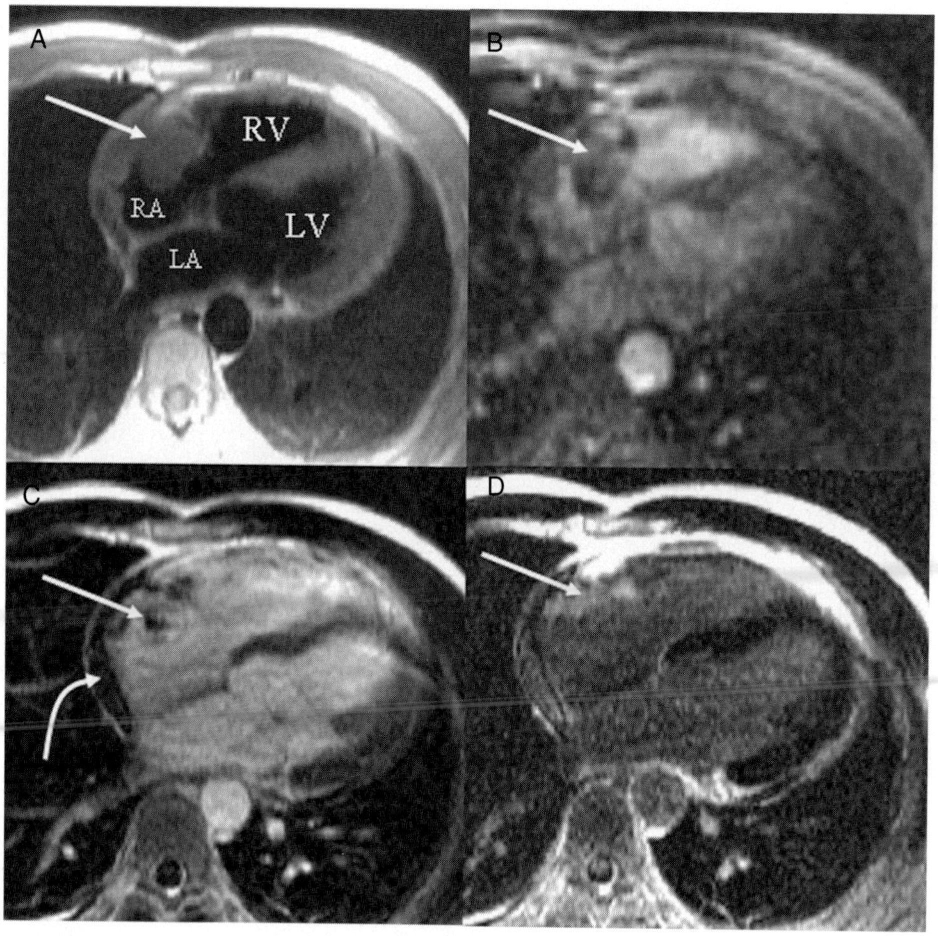

FIGURE 14–16 Cardiovascular magnetic resonance (CMR) of patients with right atrial angiosarcoma. All images are in the transaxial plane at the same level. **A,** T1-weighted spin-echo image showing a tumor (straight arrow) in the right atrial wall. For characterization, gadolinium was given intravenously as a bolus. **B,** CMR image taken during the first pass of gadolinium, showing considerable signal within the tumor, which indicates high vascularity (arrow). **C,** Inversion recovery image taken 1 to 2 minutes after injection, showing areas of absent signal within the tumor compatible with microvascular obstruction (straight arrow). There is also a pericardial effusion best seen in this image (curved arrow). **D,** Late gadolinium enhancement. The tumor has high signal, indicating fibrosis. All these feature taken together indicate a likely diagnosis of angiosarcoma, which was confirmed at surgery. LA = left atrium; LV = left ventricle; RA = right atrium; RV = right ventricle.

mapping of the coarctation jet yields a pressure gradient in most cases, and the jet duration into diastole is a useful guide to severity. Typically, CMR angiography is also performed to assess the size of collateral vessels, but flow mapping of upper and lower sites in the descending aorta can also be used to assess the volume of collateral flow. Long-term follow-up is advised in these patients because of the complications of restenosis and repair site aneurysms. Tortuosity of the isthmal region without significant obstruction has been termed *pseudocoarctation*. No significant narrowing or jet formation is present, however, and there is no collateral flow.

CMR displays vascular rings in detail, including the relationship between aortic arch anomalies and other structures. A double aortic arch may cause compression from encirclement of the trachea and esophagus. A vascular sling is also well demonstrated by CMR, in which an anomalous left pulmonary artery arises from the right pulmonary artery and courses between the trachea and esophagus back to the left lung, which can result in airway compression. In infants, patent ductus arteriosus is usually visualized by echocardiography, but CMR has a role in older patients. CMR is also useful for visualizing the aortopulmonary window. CMR is valuable for assessing anomalous pulmonary venous drainage, in which some or all of the pulmonary veins do not enter the left atrium. Anomalous pulmonary veins can be missed with conventional cardiological investigations, but the anatomy is easily visualized with standard CMR sequences or, more commonly, CMR angiography.[106] CMR correctly identifies anomalies of the systemic venous system (bilateral superior cava, interrupted inferior cava), including connection to the left heart in patients with occult arterial desaturation. Finally, pulmonary artery anatomy is very well depicted by CMR, including the presence of pulmonary arteries and their size, confluence, and relationship to other structures. Main and branch vessel stenosis can be detected, the pressure gradient assessed, and differential pulmonary flow measured. CMR angiography is very effective for demonstrating systemic to pulmonary collateral vessels.[107]

ATRIAL AND VENTRICULAR MORPHOLOGY. The morphological right atrium has a broad-based and triangular appendage, whereas the morphological left atrium has a narrow entrance to the appendage, with a tubular configuration. The right atrium is also connected to the inferior vena cava in virtually all cases. Furthermore, atrial situs is nearly always concordant with the visceral situs, and therefore the morphological right atrium is on the side of the short main bronchus and the liver. The morphological left atrium likewise is on the side of the long main bronchus and the aorta, spleen, and stomach. The morphological right ventricle is characterized by a prominent moderator band, a more apical insertion point of the tricuspid valve into the ventricular septum, and an infundibulum or conus separating the tricuspid and pulmonary valves. The morphological left ventricle is more smoothly contoured toward the apex and lacks a muscular infundibulum; therefore, it has a fibrous continuity between the mitral and aortic valves. In situs solitus, the normal atrial arrangement applies; the left pulmonary artery passes over the left main bronchus and the right pulmonary artery runs anterior and slightly inferior to the right bronchus. The atrial arrangement is reversed in cases of situs inversus. In atrial isomerism, both atria are alike and develop sidedness according to the thoracic and abdominal viscera. Left-sided isomerism is associated with polysplenia and right-sided isomerism with asplenia. Because CMR provides anatomical data that are easily related to the surrounding structures of the body, reliable diagnosis of situs is possible even in difficult cases.

ATRIOVENTRICULAR CONNECTION ABNORMALITIES. Because of the excellent ability to define the atrial and ventricular morphology, CMR demonstrates atrioventricular discordance well. Atrioventricular discordance is present in congenitally corrected transposition (combined with ventriculoarterial discordance), in which the left atrium drains into the right ventricle, which supplies the systemic arterial circulation. Other abnormalities of atrial connection include atrioventricular valve atresia, connection of both atria to a single ventricle, and connection of one valve to both ventricles. CMR also provides excellent visualization of crisscrossed atrioventricular connections, conditions in which ventricular positions are rotated with respect to the atria, with connections being either concordant or discordant.

VENTRICULOARTERIAL CONNECTION ABNORMALITIES. CMR demonstrates the anatomy of transposition of the great arteries (discordant ventriculoarterial connections) very well, with the connections between the ventricles and great vessels showing an anterior aorta arising from the morphological right ventricle and the posterior pulmonary artery arising from the morphological left ventricle. CMR is effective for assessing intraatrial baffles after atrial repair of transposition of the great arteries (Fig. 14–18).[108] After arterial switch repair, which has now become the operation of choice, CMR provides good views of the right ventricular outflow tract and pulmonary arteries, which may be stenosed. Double-outlet right ventricle is defined as an abnormal ventriculoarterial connection in which more than half of both the aorta and pulmonary artery arise from the morphological right ventricle. This condition typically presents with the aorta to the right of the pulmonary artery at the semilunar valve level. An additional feature is a complete muscle rim separating both semilunar valves from the anterior leaflet of the mitral valve. Truncus arteriosus is a failure of the embryonic truncus to separate into an individual aorta and a pulmonary artery. A single large artery arises above a ventricular septal defect from which the aorta, pulmonary, and coronary arteries arise, and this is well shown by CMR. Because of the problem with graft degeneration, CMR is valuable for assessing long-term postoperative conduit patency and stenosis, regurgitation, or aneurysm formation. Echocardiography can be limited in evaluating conduits by their retrosternal position and calcification.

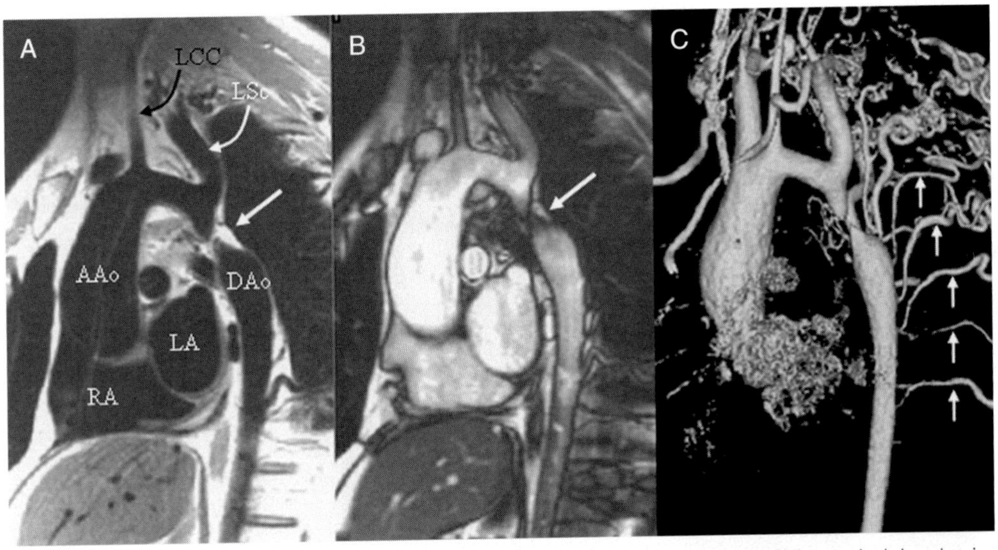

FIGURE 14–17 Cardiovascular magnetic resonance (CMR) in a patient with aortic coarctation. **A,** Oblique sagittal view showing the ascending aorta (AAo), which is dilated, giving rise to dilated left common carotid (LCC) and left subclavian (LSc) arteries. Immediately distal to the left subclavian artery is the coarctation (straight arrow), after which the descending aorta (DAo) is formed. **B,** Similar findings are seen in this image, one frame from a steady state with free precession (SSFP) cine. **C,** Projection from a three-dimensional CMR angiogram, showing multiple intercostal collateral arteries joining the descending aorta (small arrows), which can be responsible for rib notching on the chest x-ray. LA = left atrium; RA = right atrium. (From Babu-Narayan SV, Kilner PJ, Gatzoulis MA: When to order cardiovascular magnetic resonance in adults with congenital heart disease. Curr Cardiol Rep 5:324, 2003.)

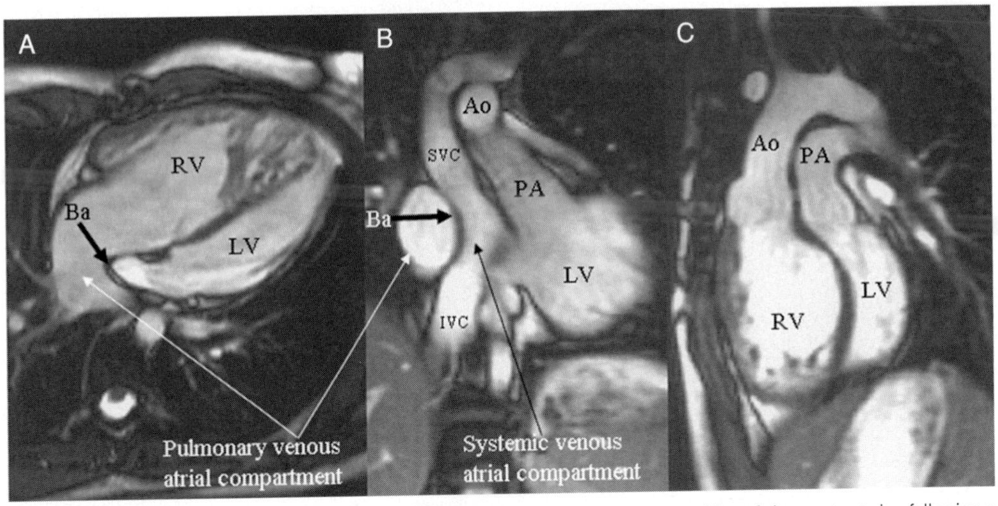

FIGURE 14–18 Cardiovascular magnetic resonance (CMR) in a patient with transposition of the great arteries following a Senning procedure, with insertion of atrial baffle, showing single frames from steady state with free precession (SSFP) cines. **A,** Oblique transaxial plane. **B,** Oblique coronal plane. **C,** Oblique sagittal plane. The atrial baffle (Ba) is seen in panels **A** and **B.** The pulmonary venous atrial compartment is unobstructed, as seen in panels **A** and **B,** and the systemic venous atrial compartment is likewise unobstructed, as seen in panel **B.** Panel **C** shows the aorta (Ao) arising from the right ventricle (RV) and the pulmonary artery (PA) arising from the left ventricle (LV). This is a good late postoperative result. IVC = inferior vena cava; SVC = superior vena cava.

SEPTAL DEFECTS. The anatomy of atrial and ventricular septal defects is usually well delineated using CMR, especially using SSFP sequences. The defect location and size can be determined directly and the systemic-to-pulmonary flow ratio measured,[109] all of which are useful for planning of intervention. The effects on right ventricular function can also be quantified. CMR is relatively more valuable than echocardiography in patients with more complex anatomy, especially those with additional abnormalities. In addition, CMR is valuable for excluding shunting from other sources, such as anomalous pulmonary venous drainage, in which echocardiography is problematic (Fig. 14–19).[110] This is important because partial anomalous venous return may coexist with atrial septal defect.

VALVULAR ABNORMALITIES. Simple (e.g., mitral stenosis) and complex (e.g., Ebstein anomaly of the tricuspid valve) congenital valve abnormalities can be assessed by CMR, but echocardiography has the significant primary role. CMR is particularly helpful in the assessment of valve regurgitation and the effects of valve pathology on the volumes and function of the associated ventricle. This has proved particularly useful for assessment of pulmonary regurgitation in patients with Fallot tetralogy[111] and surgical right ventricular to pulmonary artery conduits.[112]

TETRALOGY OF FALLOT. Tetralogy of Fallot is well assessed by CMR, both before intervention and in long-term follow-up. The full tetralogy includes an over-riding aorta with membranous ventricular septal defect, infundibular or pulmonary stenosis, and right ventricular hypertrophy, but additional features are common, such as stenosis of the pulmonary arteries and, in severe cases, aortopulmonary collateral vessels. As adults, most patients will have undergone corrective surgery, and CMR is ideal for monitoring right ventricular volumes and function as well as pulmonary regurgitation, which is common after correction. Right ventricular

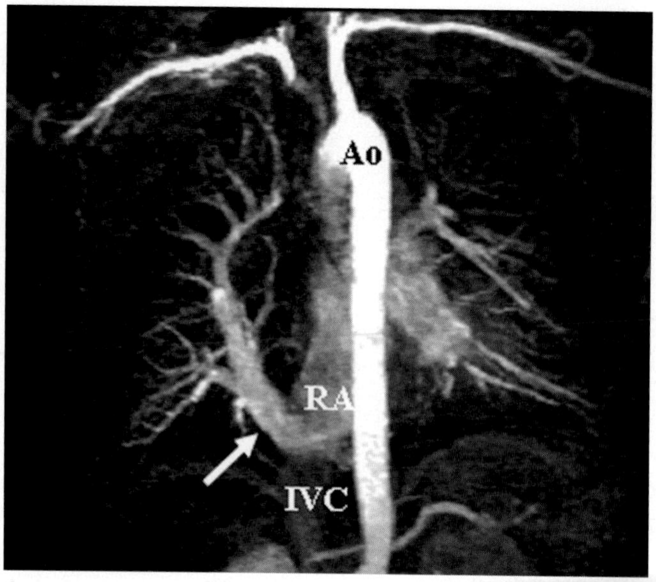

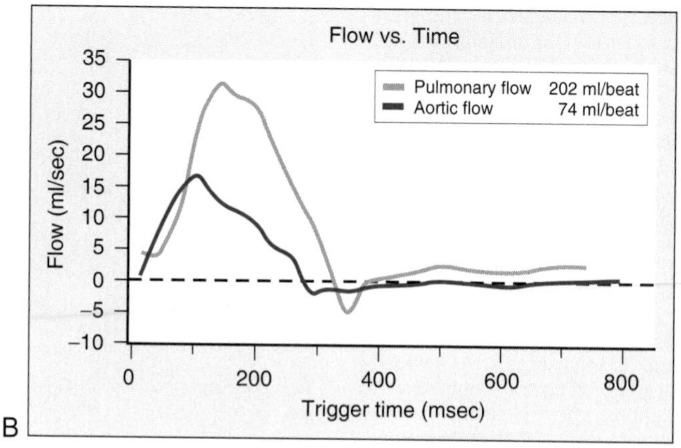

FIGURE 14–19 Cardiovascular magnetic resonance angiography in a patient with anomalous pulmonary venous drainage. **A,** The pulmonary venous angiogram showed the right upper and lower pulmonary veins draining into a common trunk (arrow) and into the inferior vena cava (IVC) and right atrium (RA). **B,** Direct flow measurements of the pulmonary artery and aorta (Ao) are shown in this graph, which yielded a Qp:Qs ratio of 2.7. (From Tan RS, Behr ER, McKenna WJ, Mohiaddin RH: Images in cardiovascular medicine. Occult anonymous pulmonary venous drainage: The clinical value of cardiac magnetic resonance imaging. Circulation 105:e25, 2002.)

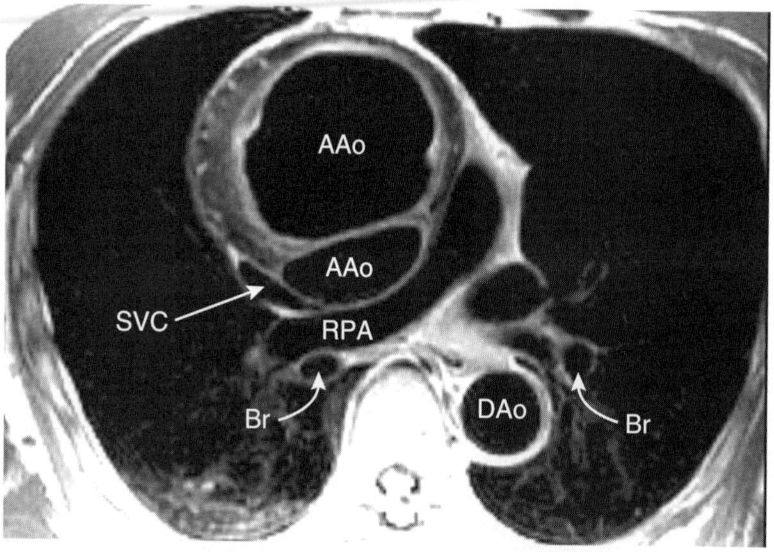

FIGURE 14–20 Cardiovascular magnetic resonance in a patient with type A aortic dissection. This transaxial spin-echo image shows a very dilated ascending aorta (AAo) with two lumina, intramural hematoma, and a compressed superior vena cava (SVC) and right pulmonary artery (RPA). Br = bronchus; Dao = descending aorta.

arrhythmias and failure are the most important causes of mortality.

SINGLE VENTRICLE. CMR is useful in determining the anatomical features of this condition, including the ventricular morphology, the atrioventricular and ventriculoarterial connections, situs, and the presence of associated anomalies. Compared with the dominant ventricle, a rudimentary right ventricle is usually anterosuperior and a rudimentary left ventricle is usually posteroinferior. In adults, a dominant left ventricle is most common. Some single ventricles have no characteristic morphological features and are termed *indeterminate*.

CORONARY ARTERY ANOMALIES. CMR is useful in defining congenital or inflammatory changes of the coronary arteries, as in Kawasaki disease.[113] In adults, the course of congenitally anomalous coronary arteries can be reliably depicted by CMR in patients with otherwise normal anatomy and in those with other congenital heart disease, in whom the prevalence of anomalies reaches 30 percent.[44] CMR has significant advantages over x-ray angiography in clarifying the spatial relationship of these arteries, most importantly whether the proximal portion runs between the aorta and the pulmonary artery, which is associated with sudden death. In other forms of congenital heart disease, the course and location of the coronary arteries can be important for surgical planning.

Acquired Disease of the Major Arteries

CMR angiography of the major central arteries has advanced rapidly in recent years and in experienced centers is replacing invasive x-ray techniques.[114] Substantial diagnostic information can often be gained in the larger vessels from conventional CMR images, but gadolinium-enhanced three-dimensional CMR angiography can now be completed in a few seconds and is now routinely used for large and small vessels. The older nongadolinium CMR angiographic techniques, such as time-of-flight angiography, are not commonly used in the central circulation but do have application elsewhere.

GREAT VESSELS. CMR is an ideal technique for assessing the aorta, because of the large field of view and ability of CMR angiography to image obliquely and in three dimensions. CMR accurately depicts aortic aneurysms showing cross-sectional diameter, the relation to branch vessels, and associated thrombus. Additional CMR angiography shows associated branch vessel occlusive disease and is useful to define the relationship of the aneurysm to smaller vessels. Inflammatory abdominal aortic aneurysms show enhancement with gadolinium. CMR can be used for stent planning and follow-up. Aortic dissection is a well-established indication for CMR,[115] and the diagnosis can be made rapidly (Fig. 14–20). The associated complications of dissection, such as extent, aortic regurgitation, pericardial effusion, and branch vessel involvement are all readily assessed by CMR. Other techniques, however, can be used in the acute setting, which largely reflects availability (see Chaps 11 and 15). In the chronic follow-up setting, CMR is the technique of choice. CMR is also useful for depiction of intramural hematoma and penetrating ulcer. CMR is ideal in the assessment and long-term follow-up of patients with Marfan syndrome. CMR angiography is also useful in the pulmonary arteries. Reasonable results have been obtained in patients with pulmonary embolism using three-dimensional contrast-enhanced CMR angiography,[116] but computed tomography remains the study of choice because of superior spatial resolution and a shorter breath-hold requirement (see Chap. 15). Pulmonary artery aneurysms and dissections are well evaluated by CMR.

ARTERIAL BRANCHES OF THE AORTA. CMR angiography of the internal carotid artery has proved valuable, and both three-dimensional time-of-flight and gadolinium-enhanced techniques have similar accuracy to invasive x-ray techniques,[117] although the gadolinium technique is faster and has improved coverage in the superior-inferior direction. Gadolinium CMR angiography is used for the renal (Fig. 14–21)[118] and mesenteric vessels. The lower spatial resolution of CMR compared with x-ray angiography limits quantitative assessment of the degree of stenosis and evaluation of accessory or branch vessels. For the arteries to the leg, three-dimensional gadolinium CMR angiography is very useful diagnostically[119] and has been used for interventional planning of limb-threatening ischemia. For the arms, there is less clinical experience, but gadolinium CMR angiography has been used with good results.

Intravascular and Interventional CMR

There is active research into the use of CMR for intravascular and interventional applications because of the whole-body imaging capability in any plane without exposure to x-rays. This requires the combination of a number of techniques, including real-time image acquisition and reconstruction, angiography, and image guidance. In addition, the instruments required must be safe to use in the MR environment, and magnet designs must allow sufficient patient access for the operator. For the cardiovascular system, a key component is the tracking of the catheter and guidewire. This can be achieved by incorporating a small receive-only coil in the tip of the device. The coil generates a signal that can be rapidly localized in three dimensions and shown on a previously acquired MR image, and different coils and receivers can be used for multiple devices. Technical advances are still in progress. Results have been reported for renal angiography,[120] femoral angioplasty, wall imaging, placement of stents, coronary angiography,[121] and assessment of radiofrequency ablation procedures.[122] Dual x-ray and CMR facilities have been proposed for more efficient diagnostic and interventional procedures during a single anesthesia session.[123] The future of this technology in uncertain at present, but there is considerable interest in its development.

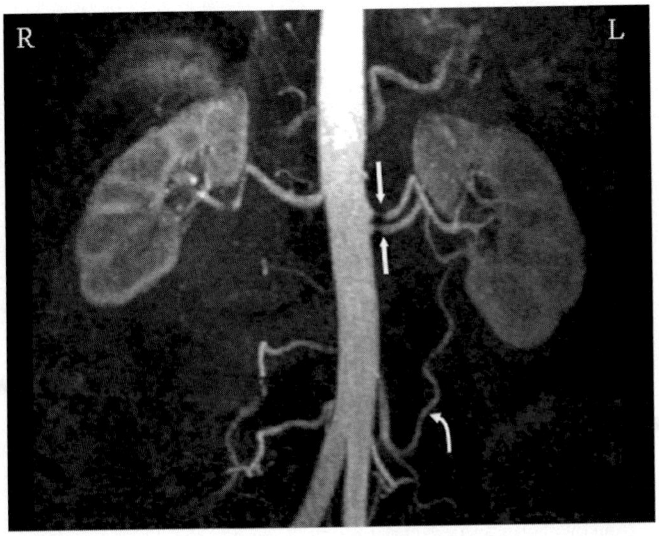

FIGURE 14–21 Cardiovascular magnetic resonance (CMR) renal angiography. The panels show a projection of a three-dimensional CMR angiogram of both kidneys from the thoracic aorta to beyond the bifurcation into the iliac arteries. The right kidney and renal artery are normal. There are three renal arteries supplying the left kidney. The upper pair, which are opposite the right renal artery, are both stenosed (straight arrows). Shortly before the bifurcation of the aorta, an accessory renal artery is seen, which is not stenosed (curved arrow).

REFERENCES

Properties of Magnetic Resonance

1. Manning WJ, Pennell DJ: Cardiovascular Magnetic Resonance. Philadelphia, Churchill Livingstone, 2002.
2. Firmin DN, Nayler GL, Klipstein RH, et al: In vivo validation of magnetic resonance velocity imaging. J Comput Assist Tomogr 11:751, 1987.
3. Scott NA, Pettigrew RI: Absence of movement of coronary stents after placement in a magnetic resonance imaging field. Am J Cardiol 73:900, 1994.
4. Strohm O, Kivelitz D, Gross W, et al: Safety of implantable coronary stents during H-1 magnetic resonance imaging at 1.0 and 1.5 T. J Cardiovasc Magn Reson 1:239, 1999.
5. Schroeder AP, Houlind K, Pedersen EM, et al: Magnetic resonance imaging seems safe in patients with intracoronary stents. J Cardiovasc Magn Reson 2:43, 2000.

Ventricular Volumes, Mass, and Function

6. Bellenger NG, Burgess M, Ray SG, et al, on behalf of the CHRISTMAS Steering Committee and Investigators: Comparison of left ventricular ejection fraction and volumes in heart failure by two-dimensional echocardiography, radionuclide ventriculography and cardiovascular magnetic resonance: Are they interchangeable? Eur Heart J 21:1387, 2000.
7. Longmore DB, Klipstein RH, Underwood SR, et al: Dimensional accuracy of magnetic resonance in studies of the heart. Lancet 1:1360, 1985.
8. Jauhainen T, Jarvinen VM, Hekali PE, et al: MR gradient echo volumetric analysis of human cardiac casts: Focus on the right ventricle. J Comput Assist Tomogr 22:899, 1998.
9. Myerson SG, Bellenger NG, Pennell DJ: Assessment of left ventricular mass by cardiovascular magnetic resonance. Hypertension 39:750, 2002.
10. Bloomgarden DC, Fayad ZA, Ferrari VA, et al: Global cardiac function using breath-hold MRI: Validation of new acquisition and analysis techniques. Magn Reson Med 37:683, 1997.
11. Grothues F, Smith GC, Moon JCC, et al: Comparison of interstudy reproducibility of cardiovascular magnetic resonance with two-dimensional echocardiography in normal subjects and in patients with heart failure or left ventricular hypertrophy. Am J Cardiol 90:29, 2002.
12. Grothues F, Moon JCC, Bellenger NG, et al: Interstudy reproducibility of right ventricular volumes, function and mass with cardiovascular magnetic resonance. Am Heart J 147:218, 2004.
13. Osterziel KJ, Strohm O, Schuler J, et al: Randomised, double-blind, placebo-controlled trial of human recombinant growth hormone in patients with chronic heart failure due to dilated cardiomyopathy. Lancet 351:1233, 1998.
14. Young AA, Axel L: Three dimensional motion and deformation of the heart wall: Estimation with spatial modulation of magnetisation—A model based approach. Radiology 185:241, 1992.

Myocardial Infarction and Viability

15. Kim RJ, Fieno DS, Parrish RB, et al: Relationship of MRI delayed contrast enhancement to irreversible injury, infarct age, and contractile function. Circulation 100:185, 1999.
16. Wu E, Judd RM, Vargas JD, et al: Visualisation of presence, location and transmural extent of healed Q-wave and non-Q-wave myocardial infarction. Lancet 357:21, 2001.
17. Wagner A, Mahrholdt H, Holly TA, et al: Contrast-enhanced MRI and routine single photon emission computed tomography (SPECT) perfusion imaging for detection of subendocardial myocardial infarcts: An imaging study. Lancet 361:374, 2003.
18. Ricciardi MJ, Wu E, Davidson CJ, et al: Visualization of discrete microinfarction after percutaneous coronary intervention associated with mild creatine kinase-MB elevation. Circulation 103:2780, 2001.
19. Moon JCC, Perez de Arenaza D, Elkington AG, et al: The pathological basis of Q wave and non-Q wave myocardial infarction: A cardiovascular magnetic resonance study. J Am Coll Cardiol 2003, in press.
20. Mahrholdt H, Wagner A, Holly TA, et al: Reproducibility of chronic infarct size measurement by contrast-enhanced magnetic resonance imaging. Circulation 106:2322, 2002.
21. Baer FM, Voth E, Schneider CA, et al: Comparison of low-dose dobutamine-gradient-echo magnetic resonance imaging and positron emission tomography with [18F]fluorodeoxyglucose in patients with chronic coronary artery disease. A functional and morphological approach to the detection of residual myocardial viability. Circulation 91:1006, 1995.
22. Ramani K, Judd RM, Holly TA, et al: Contrast magnetic resonance imaging in the assessment of myocardial viability in patients with stable coronary artery disease and left ventricular dysfunction. Circulation 98:2687, 1998.
23. Kim RJ, Wu E, Rafael A, et al: The use of contrast-enhanced magnetic resonance imaging to identify reversible myocardial dysfunction. N Engl J Med 16:1445, 2000.
24. Gerber BL, Garot J, Bluemke DA, et al: Accuracy of contrast-enhanced magnetic resonance imaging in predicting improvement of regional myocardial function in patients after acute myocardial infarction. Circulation 106:1083, 2002.
25. Klein C, Nekolla SG, Bengel FM, et al: Assessment of myocardial viability with contrast-enhanced magnetic resonance imaging: Comparison with positron emission tomography. Circulation 105:162, 2002.
26. Kitagawa K, Sakuma H, Hirano T, et al: Acute myocardial infarction: Myocardial viability assessment in patients early thereafter—Comparison of contrast enhanced MR imaging with resting 201-Tl SPECT. Radiology 226:138, 2003.
27. Nagel E, Lorenz C, Baer F, et al: Stress cardiovascular magnetic resonance: Consensus panel report. J Cardiovasc Magn Reson 3:267, 2001.
28. Nagel E, Lehmkuhl HB, Bocksch W, et al: Noninvasive diagnosis of ischemia induced wall motion abnormalities with the use of high dose dobutamine stress MRI. Comparison with dobutamine stress echocardiography. Circulation 99:763, 1999.

29. Hundley WG, Hamilton CA, Thomas MS, et al: Utility of fast cine magnetic resonance imaging and display for the detection of myocardial ischemia in patients not well suited for second harmonic stress echocardiography. Circulation 100:1697, 1999.
30. Hundley WG, Morgan TM, Neagle CM, et al: Magnetic resonance imaging determination of cardiac prognosis. Circulation 106:2328, 2002.
31. Kuijpers D, Ho KY, van Dijkman PR, et al: Dobutamine cardiovascular magnetic resonance for the detection of myocardial ischemia with the use of myocardial tagging. Circulation 107:1592, 2003.
32. Scott CH, St. John Sutton MG, Gusani N, et al: Effect of dobutamine on regional left ventricular function measured by tagged magnetic resonance imaging in normal subjects. Am J Cardiol 83:412, 1999.

Myocardial Perfusion

33. Pennell DJ, Firmin DN, Burger P, et al: Assessment of magnetic resonance velocity mapping of global ventricular function during dobutamine infusion in coronary artery disease. Br Heart J 74:163, 1995.
34. Schwitter J, Nanz D, Kneifel S, et al: Assessment of myocardial perfusion in coronary artery disease by magnetic resonance: A comparison with positron emission tomography and coronary angiography. Circulation 103:2230, 2001.
35. Panting JR, Gatehouse PD, Yang GZ, et al: Abnormal subendocardial perfusion in cardiac syndrome-X detected by cardiovascular magnetic resonance imaging. N Engl J Med 346:1948, 2002.
36. Jerosch-Herold M, Wilke N, Stillman AE, Wilson RF: Magnetic resonance quantification of the myocardial perfusion reserve with a Fermi function model for constrained deconvolution. Med Phys 25:73, 1998.
37. Wilke N, Simm C, Zhang J, et al: Contrast enhanced first pass myocardial perfusion imaging: Correlation between myocardial blood flow in dogs at rest and during hyperemia. Magn Reson Med 29:485, 1993.
38. Epstein FH, London JF, Peters DC, et al: Multislice first pass cardiac perfusion MRI: Validation in a model of myocardial infarction. Magn Reson Med 47:482, 2002.
39. Al-Saadi N, Nagel E, Gross M, et al: Noninvasive detection of myocardial ischemia from perfusion reserve based on cardiovascular magnetic resonance. Circulation 101:1379, 2000.
40. Wacker CM, Hartlep AW, Pfleger S, et al: Susceptibility-sensitive magnetic resonance imaging detects human myocardium supplied by a stenotic coronary artery without a contrast agent. J Am Coll Cardiol 41:834, 2003.
41. Al-Saadi N, Nagel E, Gross M, et al: Improvement of myocardial perfusion reserve early after coronary intervention: Assessment with cardiac magnetic resonance imaging. J Am Coll Cardiol 36:1557, 2000.
42. Buchtal SD, den Hollander JA, Merz NB, et al: Abnormal myocardial phosphorus-31 nuclear magnetic resonance spectroscopy in women with chest pain but normal coronary angiograms. N Engl J Med 342:829, 2000.

Imaging the Coronary Arteries

43. Kim WY, Danias PG, Stuber M, et al: Coronary magnetic resonance angiography for the detection of coronary stenosis. N Engl J Med 345:1863, 2001.
44. Taylor AM, Thorne SA, Rubens MB, et al: Coronary artery imaging in grown-up congenital heart disease: Complementary role of MR and x-ray coronary angiography. Circulation 101:1670, 2000.
45. Stuber M, Botnar RM, Fischer SE, et al: Preliminary report on in vivo coronary MRA at 3 Tesla in humans. Magn Reson Med 48:425, 2002.
46. Li D, Carr JC, Shea SM, et al: Coronary arteries: Magnetization-prepared contrast-enhanced three-dimensional volume-targeted breath-hold MR angiography. Radiology 219:270, 2001.
47. Hundley WG, Hamilton CA, Clarke GD, et al: Visualisation and functional assessment of proximal and middle left anterior descending coronary stenosis in humans with magnetic resonance imaging. Circulation 99:3248, 1999.
48. Nagel E, Thouet T, Klein C, et al: Noninvasive determination of coronary blood flow velocity with cardiovascular magnetic resonance in patients after stent deployment. Circulation 107:1738, 2003.
49. Langerak SE, Vliegen HW, Jukema JW, et al: Value of magnetic resonance imaging for the noninvasive detection of stenosis in coronary artery bypass grafts and recipient coronary arteries. Circulation 107:1502, 2003.
50. Sorenson MB, Collins P, Ong PJL, et al: Long term use of contraceptive depot medroxyprogesterone acetate in young women impairs arterial endothelial function assessed by cardiovascular magnetic resonance. Circulation 106:1646, 2002.
51. Silber HA, Bluemke DA, Ouyang P, et al: The relationship between vascular wall shear stress and flow-mediated dilation: Endothelial function assessed by phase-contrast magnetic resonance angiography. J Am Coll Cardiol 38:1859, 2001.
52. Yuan C, Beach KW, Smith LH, Hatsukami TS: Measurement of atherosclerotic carotid plaque size in-vivo using high resolution magnetic resonance imaging. Circulation 98:2666, 1998.
53. Corti R, Fuster V, Fayad ZA, et al: Lipid lowering by simvastatin induces regression of human atherosclerotic lesions: Two years' follow-up by high-resolution noninvasive magnetic resonance imaging. Circulation 106:2884, 2002.
54. Fayad ZA, Fuster V, Fallon JT, et al: Noninvasive in vivo human coronary artery lumen and wall imaging using black-blood magnetic resonance imaging. Circulation 102:506, 2000.

Acute Coronary Syndromes

55. Cai JM, Hatsukami TS, Ferguson MS, et al: Classification of human carotid atherosclerotic lesions with in vivo multicontrast magnetic resonance imaging. Circulation 106:1368, 2002.
56. Yuan C, Mitsumori LM, Ferguson MS, et al: In vivo accuracy of multispectral magnetic resonance imaging for identifying lipid-rich necrotic cores and intraplaque hemorrhage in advanced human carotid plaques. Circulation 104:2051, 2001.
57. Mitsumori LM, Hatsukami TS, Ferguson MS, et al: In vivo accuracy of multisequence MR imaging for identifying unstable fibrous caps in advanced human carotid plaques. J Magn Reson Imaging 17:410, 2003.
58. Yuan C, Zhang SX, Polissar NL, et al: Identification of fibrous cap rupture with magnetic resonance imaging is highly associated with recent transient ischemic attack or stroke. Circulation 105:181, 2002.
59. Ruehm SG, Corot C, Vogt P, et al: Magnetic resonance imaging of atherosclerotic plaque with ultrasmall superparamagnetic particles of iron oxide in hyperlipidemic rabbits. Circulation 103:415, 2001.
60. Kerwin W, Hooker A, Spilker M, et al: Quantitative magnetic resonance imaging analysis of neovasculature volume in carotid atherosclerotic plaque. Circulation 107:851, 2003.
61. Wasserman BA, Smith WI, Trout HH 3rd, et al: Carotid artery atherosclerosis: In vivo morphologic characterization with gadolinium-enhanced double-oblique MR imaging initial results. Radiology 223:566, 2002.
62. Zhao XQ, Yuan C, Hatsukami TS, et al: Effects of prolonged intensive lipid-lowering therapy on the characteristics of carotid atherosclerotic plaques in vivo by MRI: A case-control study. Arterioscler Thromb Vasc Biol 21:1623, 2001.
63. Kwong RY, Schussheim AE, Rekhraj S, et al: Detecting acute coronary syndrome in the emergency department with cardiac magnetic resonance imaging. Circulation 107:531, 2003.
64. Wu KC, Kim RJ, Bluemke DA, et al: Quantification and time course of microvascular obstruction by contrast-enhanced echocardiography and magnetic resonance imaging following acute myocardial infarction and reperfusion. J Am Coll Cardiol 32:1756, 1998.
65. Gerber BL, Rochitte CE, Melin JA, et al: Microvascular obstruction and left ventricular remodeling early after acute myocardial infarction. Circulation 101:2734, 2000.
66. Wu KC, Zerhouni EA, Judd RM, et al: Prognostic significance of microvascular obstruction by magnetic resonance imaging in patients with acute myocardial infarction. Circulation 97:765, 1998.

Cardiomyopathy

67. Groenning BA, Nilsson JC, Sondergaard L, et al: Antiremodeling effects on the left ventricle during beta-blockade with metoprolol in the treatment of chronic heart failure. J Am Coll Cardiol 36:2072, 2000.
68. Anderson LJ, Holden S, Davies B, et al: Cardiovascular T2* (T2 star) magnetic resonance for the early diagnosis of myocardial iron overload. Eur Heart J 22:2171, 2001.
69. McCrohon JA, Moon JC, Prasad SK, et al: Differentiation of heart failure related to dilated cardiomyopathy and coronary artery disease using gadolinium-enhanced cardiovascular magnetic resonance. Circulation 108:54, 2003.
70. Neubauer S, Horn M, Cramer M, et al: Myocardial phosphocreatine to ATP ratio is a predictor of mortality in patients with dilated cardiomyopathy. Circulation 96:2190, 1997.
71. Moon JCC, Fisher NG, McKenna WJ, Pennell DJ: Detection of apical hypertrophic cardiomyopathy by cardiovascular magnetic resonance in patients with non-diagnostic echocardiography. Heart 2004, in press.
72. Crilley JG, Boehm EA, Blair E, et al: Hypertrophic cardiomyopathy due to sarcomeric gene mutations is characterized by impaired energy metabolism irrespective of the degree of hypertrophy. J Am Coll Cardiol 41:1776, 2003.
73. Moon JCC, Reed E, Sheppard M, et al: The histological basis of myocardial enhancement by gadolinium cardiovascular magnetic resonance in hypertrophic cardiomyopathy. J Am Coll Cardiol 2004, in press.
74. Moon JCC, McKenna WJ, McCrohon JA, et al: Toward clinical risk assessment in hypertrophic cardiomyopathy with gadolinium cardiovascular magnetic resonance. J Am Coll Cardiol 41:1561, 2003.
75. Moon JCC, Sachdev B, Elkington AG, et al: Gadolinium enhanced cardiovascular magnetic resonance in Anderson-Fabry disease: Evidence for a disease specific abnormality of the myocardial interstitium. Eur Heart J 24:2151, 2003.
76. Anderson LJ, Bunce N, Davis B, et al: Reversal of siderotic cardiomyopathy: A prospective study with cardiac magnetic resonance. Heart 85(Suppl 1):33, 2001.
77. Anderson LJ, Wonke B, Prescott E, et al: Comparison of effects of oral deferiprone and subcutaneous desferrioxamine on myocardial iron levels and ventricular function in beta thalassemia. Lancet 360:516, 2002.
78. Blake LM, Scheinman MM, Higgins CB: MR features of arrhythmogenic right ventricular dysplasia. Am J Roentgenol 162:809, 1994.
79. Burke AP, Farb A, Tashko G, Virmani R: Arrhythmogenic right ventricular cardiomyopathy and fatty replacement of the right ventricular myocardium: Are they different diseases? Circulation 97:1571, 1998.
80. Proclemer A, Basadonna PT, Slavich GA, et al: Cardiac magnetic resonance imaging findings in patients with right ventricular outflow tract premature contractions. Eur Heart J 18:2002, 1997.
81. Danias PG: Gadolinium-enhanced cardiac magnetic resonance imaging: Expanding the spectrum of clinical applications. Am J Med 110:591, 2001.
82. Vignaux O, Dhote R, Duboc D, et al: Clinical significance of myocardial magnetic resonance abnormalities in patients with sarcoidosis: A 1-year follow-up study. Chest 122:1895, 2002.
83. Fattori R, Rocchi G, Celletti F, et al: Contribution of magnetic resonance imaging in the differential diagnosis of cardiac amyloidosis and symmetric hypertrophic cardiomyopathy. Am Heart J 136:824, 1998.
84. Friedrich MG, Strohm O, Schulz-Menger J, et al: Contrast media enhanced magnetic resonance imaging visualises myocardial changes in the course of viral myocarditis. Circulation 97:1802, 1998.
85. Wagner A, Schulz-Menger J, Dietz R, Friedrich MG: Long-term follow-up of patients with acute myocarditis by magnetic resonance imaging. MAGMA 16:17, 2003.
86. Wassmuth R, Lentzsch S, Erdbruegger U, et al: Subclinical cardiotoxic effects of anthracyclines as assessed by magnetic resonance imaging—A pilot study. Am Heart J 141:1007, 2001.

87. Schwitter J, De Marco T, Globits S, et al: Influence of felodipine on left ventricular hypertrophy and systolic function in orthotopic heart transplant recipients: Possible interaction with cyclosporine medication. J Heart Lung Transplant 18:1003, 1999.

Valvular Heart Disease

88. Mohiaddin RH, Kilner PJ: Valvular heart disease. *In* Manning WJ, Pennell DJ (eds): Cardiovascular Magnetic Resonance. Philadelphia, Churchill Livingstone, 2002, pp 387-404.
89. Kozerke S, Schwitter J, Pedersen EM, Boesiger P: Aortic and mitral regurgitation quantification using moving slice velocity mapping. J Magn Reson Imaging 14:106, 2001.
90. Globits S, Frank H, Mayr H, et al: Quantitative assessment of aortic regurgitation by magnetic resonance imaging. Eur Heart J 13:78, 1992.
91. Kizilbash AM, Hundley WG, Willett DL, et al: Comparison of quantitative Doppler with magnetic resonance imaging for assessment of the severity of mitral regurgitation. Am J Cardiol 81:792, 1998.
92. Globits S, Blake L, Bourne M, et al: Assessment of hemodynamic effects of ACE inhibitor therapy in chronic aortic regurgitation by using velocity encoded cine magnetic resonance imaging. Am Heart J 131:289, 1996.
93. Hoffmann U, Frank H, Stefenelli T, et al: Afterload reduction in severe aortic regurgitation. J Magn Reson Imaging 14:693, 2001.
94. Dulce MC, Mostbeck GH, O'Sullivan M, et al: Severity of aortic regurgitation: Interstudy reproducibility of measurements with velocity-encoded cine MR imaging. Radiology 185:235, 1992.
95. Kilner PJ, Manzara CC, Mohiaddin RH, et al: Magnetic resonance jet velocity mapping in mitral and aortic valve stenosis. Circulation 87:1239, 1993.
96. Friedrich MG, Schulz-Menger J, Poetsch T, et al: Quantification of valvular aortic stenosis by magnetic resonance imaging. Am Heart J 144:329, 2002.
97. Rajappan K, Rimoldi OE, Camici PG, et al: Functional changes in coronary microcirculatory function after valve replacement in patients with aortic stenosis. Circulation 107:3170, 2003.
98. Beyerbacht HP, Lamb HJ, van der Laarse A, et al: Aortic valve replacement in patients with aortic valve stenosis improves myocardial metabolism and diastolic function. Radiology 219:637, 2001.
99. Edwards MB, Taylor KM, Shellock FG: Prosthetic heart valves: Evaluation of magnetic field interactions, heating, and artifacts at 1.5 T. J Magn Reson Imaging 12:363, 2000.

Pericardial Disease and Cardiac Tumors

100. Vick GW, Rokey R: CMR evaluation of the pericardium in health and disease. *In* Manning WJ, Pennell DJ (eds): Cardiovascular Magnetic Resonance. Philadelphia, Churchill Livingstone, 2002, pp 355-363.
101. Frank H: Cardiac masses. *In* Manning WJ, Pennell DJ (eds): Cardiovascular Magnetic Resonance. Philadelphia, Churchill Livingstone, 2002, pp 342-354.

Congenital Heart Disease

102. Hirsch R, Kilner PJ, Connelly MS, et al: Diagnosis in adolescents and adults with congenital heart disease: Prospective assessment of indi-vidual and combined roles of magnetic resonance imaging and transesophageal echocardiography. Circulation 90:2937, 1994.
103. Niezen RA, Helbing WA, van der Wall EE, et al: Biventricular systolic function and mass studied with MR imaging in children with pulmonary regurgitation after repair for tetralogy of Fallot. Radiology 201:135, 1996.
104. Kilner PJ: Adult congenital heart disease. *In* Higgins CB, de Roos A (eds): Cardiovascular MRI and MRA. Philadelphia, Lippincott Williams & Wilkins, 2003, pp 353-366.
105. Higgins CB, Silverman NH, Kersting-Sommerhoff BA, Schmidt K: Congenital Heart Disease: Echocardiography and Magnetic Resonance Imaging. New York, Raven Press, 1990.
106. Prasad SK, Soukias N, Hornung T, et al: Role of MRA in the diagnosis of major aortopulmonary collateral arteries and partial anomalous pulmonary venous drainage. Circulation 109:207, 2004.
107. Geva T, Greil GF, Marshall AC, et al: Gadolinium-enhanced 3-dimensional magnetic resonance angiography of pulmonary blood supply in patients with complex pulmonary stenosis or atresia: Comparison with x-ray angiography. Circulation 106:473, 2002.
108. Chung KJ, Simpson IA, Glass RF, et al: Cine magnetic resonance imaging after surgical repair in patients with transposition of the great arteries. Circulation 77:104, 1988.
109. Hundley WG, Li HF, Lange RA, et al: Assessment of left-to-right intracardiac shunting by velocity-encoded, phase-difference magnetic resonance imaging: A comparison with oximetric and indicator dilution techniques. Circulation 91:2955, 1995.
110. Greil GF, Powell AJ, Gildein HP, Geva T: Gadolinium-enhanced three-dimensional magnetic resonance angiography of pulmonary and systemic venous anomalies. J Am Coll Cardiol 39:335, 2002.
111. Rebergen SA, Chin JG, Ottenkamp J, et al: Pulmonary regurgitation in the late postoperative follow-up of tetralogy of Fallot: Volumetric quantitation by nuclear magnetic resonance velocity mapping. Circulation 92:1123, 1993.
112. Holmqvist C, Oskarsson G, Stahlberg F, et al: Functional evaluation of extracardiac ventriculopulmonary conduits and of the right ventricle with magnetic resonance imaging and velocity mapping. Am J Cardiol 83:926, 1999.
113. Greil GF, Stuber M, Botnar RM, et al: Coronary magnetic resonance angiography in adolescents and young adults with Kawasaki disease. Circulation 105:908, 2002.

Diseases of the Major Arteries

114. Prince MR, Grist TM, Debatin JF (eds): 3D Contrast-Enhanced MR Angiography. Berlin, Springer-Verlag, 1997.
115. Nienaber CA, von Kodolitsch Y, Nicolas V, et al: The diagnosis of thoracic aortic dissection by noninvasive imaging procedures. N Engl J Med 328:1, 1993.
116. Oudkerk M, van Beek EJ, Wielopolski P, et al: Comparison of contrast-enhanced magnetic resonance angiography and conventional pulmonary angiography for the diagnosis of pulmonary embolism: A prospective study. Lancet 359:1643, 2002.
117. Fellner FA, Fellner C, Wutke R, et al: Fluoroscopically triggered contrast-enhanced 3D MR DSA and 3D time-of-flight turbo MRA of the carotid arteries: First clinical experiences in correlation with ultrasound, x-ray angiography, and endarterectomy findings. Magn Reson Imaging 18:575, 2000.
118. Schenberg SO, Rieger J, Johannson LO, et al: Diagnosis of renal artery stenosis with magnetic resonance angiography: Update 2003. Nephrol Dial Transplant 18:1252, 2003.
119. Ruehm SG, Goyen M, Barkhausen J, et al: Rapid magnetic resonance angiography for detection of atherosclerosis. Lancet 357:1086, 2001.

Intravascular and Interventional CMR

120. Wildermuth S, Debatin JF, Leung DA, et al: MR imaging-guided intravascular procedures: Initial demonstration in a pig model. Radiology 202:578, 1997.
121. Serfaty JM, Yang X, Foo TK, et al: MRI-guided coronary catheterization and PTCA: A feasibility study on a dog model. Magn Reson Med 49:258, 2003.
122. Lardo AC, McVeigh ER, Jumrussirikul P, et al: Visualization and temporal/spatial characterization of cardiac radiofrequency ablation lesions using magnetic resonance imaging. Circulation 102:698, 2000.
123. Kuehne T, Saeed M, Higgins CB, et al: Endovascular stents in pulmonary valve and artery in swine: Feasibility study of MR imaging-guided deployment and postinterventional assessment. Radiology 226:475, 2003.

CHAPTER 15

Computed Tomography of the Heart

Stephan Achenbach • Werner G. Daniel

Principles of Computed Tomography

Computed tomography (CT) imaging was introduced in 1972. The ability to obtain cross-sectional images of the body revolutionized medicine, and for the development of computer assisted tomography, Sir Geoffrey N. Hounsfield and Allan M. Cormack were awarded the Nobel Prize in Medicine in 1979. CT is an x-ray–based technique. An x-ray source that rotates on a circular path around the patient emits a fan-shaped beam of x-rays that passes through the body. Collimators are used to confine the x-ray beam to the slice that shall be imaged; its thickness can vary from less than one to several millimeters. Opposite to the x-ray source, extremely sensitive detectors record the intensity of x-rays that have passed through the body. Based on the x-ray attenuations obtained from a multitude of angles, a cross-sectional image of the body can be calculated. Each pixel of the reconstructed image is assigned an x-ray attenuation value (also called *CT number*), which is expressed in Hounsfield Units (HU). The Hounsfield scale is calibrated in a way that yields 0 HU for water and −1000 HU for air. CT numbers within one cross section of the body can thus range from close to −1000 HU (e.g., the lungs) to several thousand HU (e.g., bone or metal). Since the human eye cannot distinguish a gray scale over such a wide range, adjustments (window "width" and window "level" or "center") are made when displaying the reconstructed images. The width value represents the range of CT numbers that are displayed on a gray scale. Each value below that range will be displayed black, each value exceeding the range will be displayed white. The "level" or "center" value determines the CT number around which the "window" is centered (e.g., in an image displayed with a center of 500 HU and width of 400 HU, each pixel with a density of less than 300 HU will displayed black, and each pixel with a density greater than 700 HU will be displayed white). By convention, body images obtained by CT are displayed as if looking upward from the patient´s feet (Fig. 15–1).

Special Considerations for Cardiac Imaging

Due to technical limitations, the clinical value of cardiac CT has, for a long time, been very limited. Cardiac imaging requires a very high temporal resolution, because the heart is in constant, rapid motion. Conventional CT imaging, on the other hand, is an imaging modality with low temporal resolution: the heavy x-ray tube and the detector array must very accurately be moved in a circular pattern around the body, so centrifugal forces and the need to keep the geometry of source and detectors exactly aligned limit the rotation speed. Dedicated scanner designs therefore needed to be developed to increase acquisition speed.

Cardiac CT imaging requires one further prerequisite: to provide continuous cross-sectional images of the heart, every displayed image must be of the same heart phase. Otherwise, gaps may occur if adjacent images depict the heart in different phases of the cardiac cycle. Data acquisition must therefore either be triggered by the patient´s electrocardiogram (ECG) or, in case of continuous acquisition of x-ray data, image reconstruction must be synchronized to a function that is correlated to cardiac motion, such as the simultaneously recorded ECG ("retrospective ECG gating")

Lastly, the heart is subjected not only to intrinsic motion due to cardiac contraction, but also to motion caused by breathing. To avoid artifacts, CT imaging of the complete heart thus has to be performed within one single breath-hold and CT scanners have to provide for sufficiently fast volume coverage. In practice, image acquisition times of up to 35 seconds are usually tolerated by a cooperative patient.

The availability of CT techniques with high temporal resolution, the ability to obtain images in defined phases of the cardiac cycle, and progressive improvements in spatial resolution have continuously increased the clinical utility of cardiac CT imaging in recent years.

Electron Beam Tomography

The electron beam tomography (EBT) scanner was developed specifically for cardiac imaging. In contrast to conventional ("mechanical") CT scanners, x-rays are not created by a mechanically moving tube. Instead, a stationary high-voltage electron gun produces a beam of electrons at a substantial distance from the anode (Fig. 15–2). Within a large vacuum tube, a system of electromagnetic deflection coils focuses and steers the electron beam to sweep over tungsten targets, which constitute the anode and are arranged in a semicircular array under the patient table. Where the electron beam hits the anode, a fan of x-rays is created that penetrates the patient. Stationary detector arrays are mounted opposite the targets. Because of this design, cross-sectional images can be acquired without the constraints of mechanical motion: The electron beam can sweep across the target rings in as little as 33 msec. Typical scan speeds are 33, 50, or 100 msec for the newest generation of EBT scanners and 100 msec for previous generations of scanners. The two detector arrays permit simultaneous acquisition of two contiguous images of 1.5 mm, 3 mm, or 7 mm thickness. If desired, the electron beam can sweep up to four parallel targets in short succession. By combination of four targets with two detectors, up to eight images of 7 mm thickness each can be acquired without table motion.

Image acquisition by EBT can be prospectively triggered to the patient's ECG. X-rays

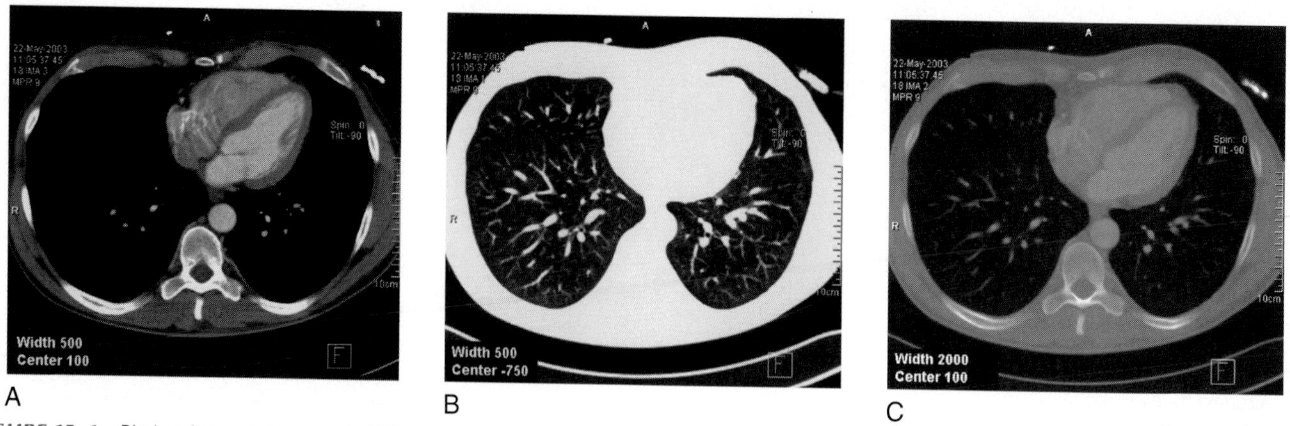

FIGURE 15–1 Display of computed tomography (CT) images. The same contrast-enhanced cross-sectional image of the chest is displayed in three different settings of window and level. **A,** Window width of 500 HU and center of 100 HU provides good soft-tissue contrast. Lungs (low CT attenuation) are displayed black, and bones (high attenuation) are displayed white. **B,** Same image, displayed with a window width of 500 HU and center of −750 HU. All structures with a CT number of −500 HU or more are now displayed in white, and low-density structures (e.g., the lungs) are displayed with good contrast. **C,** Window width of 2000 HU and center of 100 HU. The image has low contrast but displays all structures from very low (lungs) to high density (bones). By convention in CT, images are displayed as if looking up from the patient's feet.

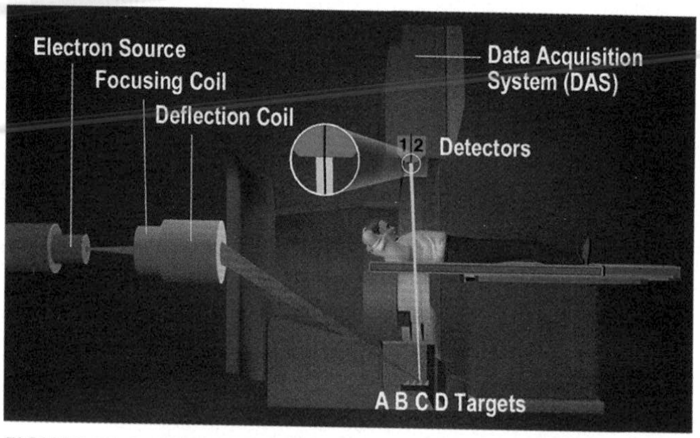

FIGURE 15–2 Principle of electron beam tomography (EBT). An electron beam is created by a high-voltage electron gun. In a large vacuum chamber, the electron beam is focused and deflected by electromagnetic coils to sweep over an anode that is arranged in a semicircular fashion below the patient. Where the electron beam hits the anode, x-rays are created. They penetrate the patient and are received by an array of detectors arranged on the opposite side. To create one image, the electron beam needs to perform a 210-degree sweep over the anodes, which in the usual scan modes requires 50 to 100 msec. By combining four parallel anode rings and two detector arrays, up to eight images can be obtained in rapid succession without movement of the patient table.

TABLE 15–1 Sample Image Acquisition Protocols for Cardiac Imaging by Electron Beam Tomography*

	Coronary Arteries	Coronary Calcium
Number of images	80	40
Slice collimation	2 × 1.5 mm	2 × 3.0 mm
Tube voltage	140 kV	130 kV
Electrocardiographic trigger	Prospective, one acquisition per cardiac cycle	Prospective, one acquisition per cardiac cycle
Temporal resolution	50 msec	50 msec
Contrast enhancement	Intravenous, iodinated contrast (~160 ml)	—
Approximate radiation dose†	~1.5-2.0 mSv[2] ~1.1 mSv[3]	~1.0-1.3 mSv[2] ~0.7 mSv[3]

*(The protocols are given for the newest generation of electron beam tomography scanners. Settings may vary for older generation scanners).

†Radiation doses are effective doses. As they are approximations and partly obtained from different sources than in Table 15–2, they are therefore not immediately comparable.

are emitted only at one or several predefined time points in the cardiac cycle. Table 15–1 lists typical image acquisition protocols for cardiac imaging by EBT.

Mechanical Computed Tomography

To use mechanical CT scanners for cardiac imaging, special measures had to be undertaken to improve temporal resolution. Modern multidetector CT (MDCT) scanners permit image acquisition in several parallel cross-sections (4 to 16) with slice collimations as low as 0.5 mm. Also, the time for one 360-degree tube rotation has been decreased to 500 msec or less. The scanners can be operated either in sequential ("step and shoot") mode or in spiral (or heli-cal) mode.

SEQUENTIAL AND SPIRAL SCAN MODES. In sequential mode, images are acquired at one level, and after enough data have been collected for image reconstruction, the table is advanced so that data can be acquired at another level (usually in the next cardiac cycle) (Fig. 15–3). Spiral mode offers faster coverage of large volumes. While the gantry is rotating and data are acquired continuously, the table is advanced at a constant speed. After the x-ray data set has been collected, images can retrospectively be reconstructed at any desired level. To reconstruct an image at a given level, a set of projections from numerous angles has to be obtained at that very plane. Since the tube does not perform a full rotation in any given plane, x-ray data for every projection angle are interpolated from the preceding and following tube rotation (see Fig. 15–3).

PARTIAL SCAN RECONSTRUCTION. One of the major prerequisites for cardiac imaging is high temporal resolution (short image acquisition times). Modern scanners have gantry rotation times of 500 msec or less, but due to the rapid cardiac motion, even reconstructing images with an acquisition window of 500 msec will not be fast enough to reliably suppress cardiac motion artifacts. However, it is not necessary to use x-ray data from a full rotation (360 degrees) to reconstruct one image. Parts of the data are redundant (for example, attenuation will be the same when an x-ray beam passes through the body from back to front or from front to back).

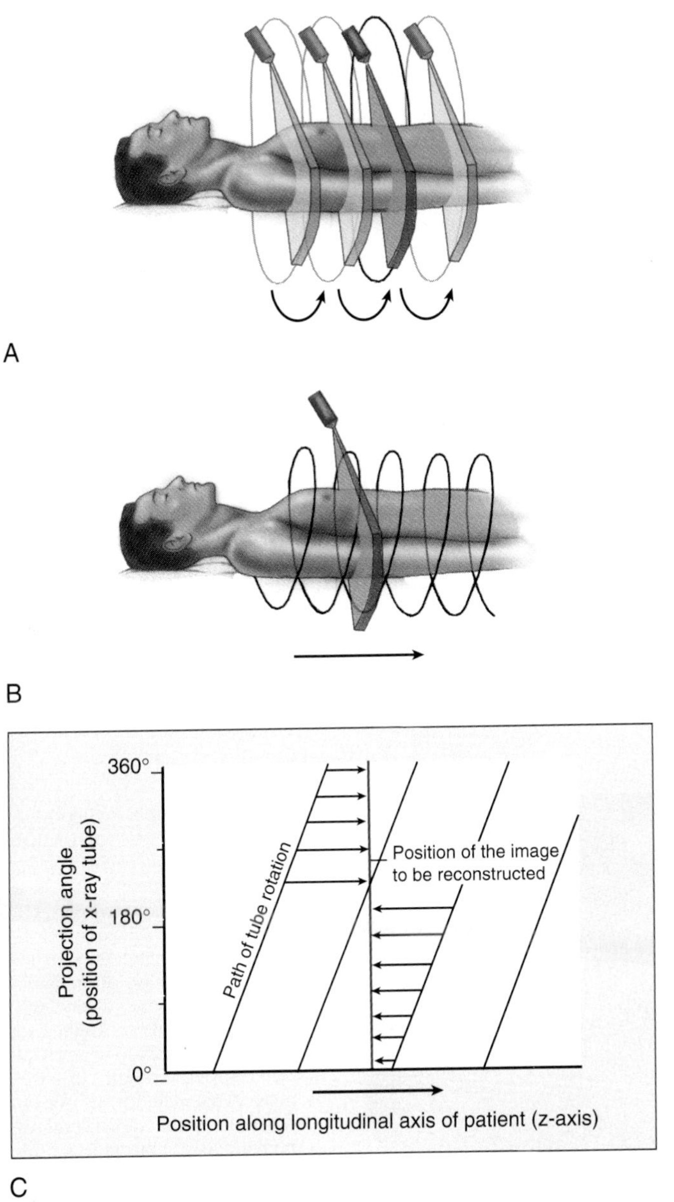

FIGURE 15–3 Principle of sequential and spiral scan modes. **A,** Sequential scanning. X-ray data are acquired at one table position with the x-ray source and detectors on a circular path. After enough data have been collected for image reconstruction, the x-ray tube is switched off and the table is advanced so that data can be acquired in another level. With multidetector computed tomography (CT), several (4 to 16) image slices can be acquired at each table position. Usually, table movement and image acquisition are triggered to the electrocardiogram so that every acquisition will be performed at the same instant in the cardiac cycle. **B,** Spiral scanning. X-ray data are continuously acquired with the x-ray tube and detectors in constant circular motion. Simultaneously, the patient table is advanced at a constant speed. The x-ray tube and detectors thus move on a spiral (or "helical") path relative to the patient. **C,** Image reconstruction in spiral CT. To reconstruct an image at a given level, a set of projections from numerous angles has to be obtained at that very plane. Since the tube does not perform a full rotation at any given imaging plane, x-ray data for every projection angle are interpolated from the preceding and following tube rotation.

To reconstruct one complete cross-sectional image, it is only necessary to use data from projections over 180 degrees plus the width of the fan angle emitted by the x-ray tube (approximately 50 degrees for most manufacturers). Image reconstruction algorithms that use projections covering less than 360 degrees are called *partial scan reconstruction algorithms.* The most commonly used algorithms for cardiac imaging use x-ray data from a single sweep over 180 degrees (plus the fan angle) and are usually referred to as *half-scan reconstruction algorithms.* With this reconstruction technique, a temporal resolution of half the gantry rotation time can be achieved in the center of the scan field.

For multidetector systems, more advanced partial scan reconstruction algorithms are available that make use of less than 180 degrees of tube rotation. To fill gaps and provide missing projection angles for reconstruction of an image at a given level, data are used that are acquired during a later heart beat by another detector and assigned to the correct heart phase by means of the simultaneously recorded ECG. Even though, theoretically, a better temporal resolution can be achieved by confining image reconstruction to shorter segments of the cardiac cycle, the necessity to combine data from several successive heart beats constitutes a major disadvantage. Since the heart may not return to exactly the same position from heart beat to heart beat, this may reduce image quality. A clear advantage of these techniques over half-scan reconstruction has so far not been shown.

ELECTROCARDIOGRAPHIC GATING. Another prerequisite for cardiac imaging by CT is the ability to synchronize the obtained images to the cardiac cycle. To achieve this, image acquisition can be triggered by the patient's ECG in sequential scan modes. In spiral scan mode, x-ray data are continuously acquired and modern CT systems permit simultaneous recording of the patient´s ECG with the x-ray data. Using the partial scan reconstruction methods described earlier, it is thus possible to reconstruct cross-sectional images at any given instant in the cardiac cycle. This technique can be used to minimize motion artifacts (by retrospectively selecting the cardiac phase with the fewest artifacts) or to provide data sets during systole and diastole, which permits dynamic analysis of cardiac function. Although the availability of data throughout the cardiac cycle thus represents an advantage of continuous data acquisition and retrospective ECG gating, this scanning mode is associated with a higher radiation dose than sequential scan modes.[1-4] Table 15–2 lists typical scan parameters for multidetector spiral CT of the heart.

VISUALIZATION OF THE HEART IN COMPUTED TOMOGRAPHY

NONENHANCED IMAGING. CT imaging of the heart can be performed with and without injection of a contrast agent. The x-ray attenuation of soft tissue (e.g., myocardium) and blood is almost identical. In cardiac images obtained without injection of contrast agent, it is therefore not possible to discern structures within the heart (Fig. 15–4). Epicardial fat has a lower CT attenuation value, so that the proximal coronary arteries, which are frequently surrounded by fat, can often be recognized (see Fig. 15–4). Nonenhanced CT studies of the heart are almost exclusively performed to assess calcified structures within the heart, most notably coronary artery calcification.

CONTRAST-ENHANCED IMAGING. To increase the CT attenuation of the blood pool, an iodinated contrast agent can be injected. During the time of CT data acquisition (15 to 35 seconds for a high-resolution MDCT or EBT scan, depending on scanner type and scan parameters), maximum enhancement of the blood pool should be maintained. To limit the amount of contrast agent that needs to be injected and to achieve good contrast, the correct timing of the actual CT scan relative to contrast injection is important. The CT scan should start when the contrast agent arrives in the ascending aorta. This is usually 15 to 25 seconds after the start of contrast injection into a peripheral vein. Individual determination of the contrast agent transit time is recommended for each patient. If only arterial structures (left ventricle, coronary arteries) are to be investigated, the duration of contrast injection should be approximately the same as the duration of the scan. If structures of the right heart and pulmonary circulation are also to be analyzed, contrast injection must be longer to maintain enhancement in the right heart until the end of the scan.

Contrast-enhanced CT studies permit delineation of the cardiac chambers, valves, great cardiac vessels, and, under the prerequisite of sufficient spatial resolution and successful suppression of motion artifacts, the coronary artery lumen (Fig. 15–5). Contrast enhancement in the right atrium is often inhomogeneous because blood saturated with contrast material from the superior vena cava mixes with nonenhanced blood

TABLE 15–2 Sample Image Acquisition Protocols for Cardiac Imaging by Multidetector Spiral Computed Tomography*

	Coronary Arteries	Coronary Calcium, Retrospective	Coronary Calcium, Prospective
Slice collimation	16 × 0.75 mm	16 × 1.5 mm	16 × 1.5 mm
Rotation time	420 ms	420 ms	420 ms
Tube voltage	120 kV	120 kV	120 kV
Electrocardiographic (ECG) gating†	Retrospective, half-scan reconstruction (temporal resolution 210 ms in center of scan field), individual positioning of reconstruction window in cardiac cycle	Retrospective, half-scan reconstruction (temporal resolution 200-250 ms in center of scan field), individual positioning of reconstruction window in cardiac cycle	Prospective, half-scan reconstruction (temporal resolution 210 ms in center of scan field)
Image reconstruction	1.0 mm slice thickness in 0.5 mm increments (~240 images)	3.0 mm slice thickness in 1.5 mm increments (~80 images)	3.0 mm slice thickness in 1.5 mm increments (~80 images)
Contrast enhancement	Intravenous, iodinated contrast (~80 ml)	—	—
Approximate radiation dose‡	~5-10 mSv[1]	~1-3 mSv [1]	~0.5-0.7 mSv[1] ~1.5-1.8 mSv[2] ~1.0 mSv[3]

*The protocols represent examples for a 16-slice scanner with 0.75 mm collimation (Siemens Sensation 16). Settings may vary for other manufacturers or older scanner generations.

†For retrospective ECG gated acquisitions, ECG-correlated tube current modulation may lead to a dose reduction of 30-50%[1,4].

‡Radiation doses represent effective doses. As they are approximations and partly obtained from different sources than in Table 15–1, they are not immediately comparable.

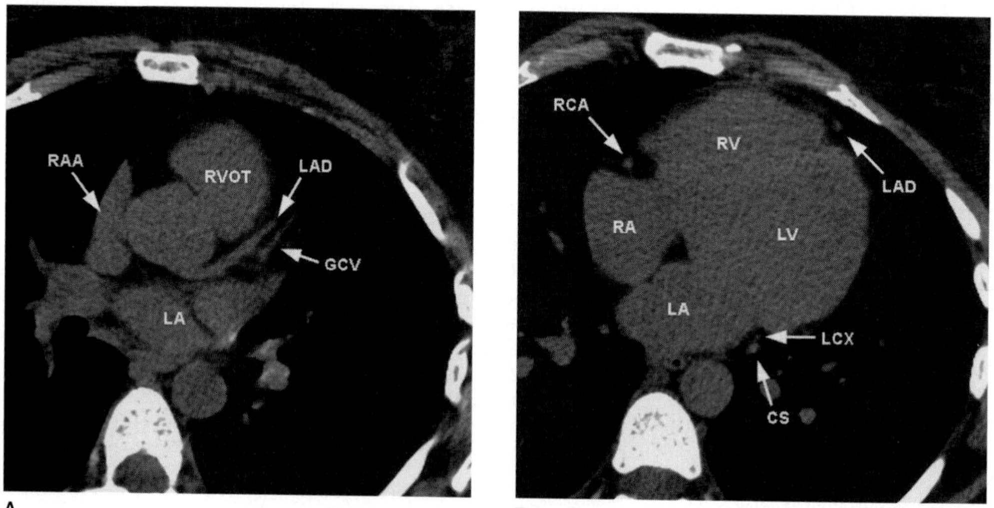

A B

FIGURE 15–4 Normal cardiac anatomy as depicted by nonenhanced computed tomography (CT). Images are in the axial (transverse) plane and displayed as if looking up from the patient's feet. Blood has a similar CT attenuation as connective tissue (e.g., the myocardium). It is therefore not possible to delineate the ventricular cavities or other structures within the heart. **A,** Level of the left coronary artery ostium from the aortic root. **B,** Level of the mid right coronary artery (RCA). CS = coronary sinus, GCV = great cardiac vein, LA = left atrium, LAD = left anterior descending coronary artery, LCX = left circumflex coronary artery, LV = left ventricle; RA = right atrium, RV = right ventricle, RVOT = right ventricular outflow tract.

from the inferior vena cava. The resulting artifacts can frequently impair visualization of structures in the right atrium, the interatrial septum, and the tricuspid valve.

TYPICAL ARTIFACTS. CT imaging of the heart is prone to artifacts, since it stretches the temporal and spatial resolution of CT scanners to their limits, and additional artifacts can be introduced by the partial scan reconstruction algorithms. It is important to recognize typical artifacts to avoid misinterpretation. Motion artifacts will typically blur the contours of the heart, especially of the coronary arteries (Fig. 15-6). Inconsistent triggering or arrhythmias may cause misalignment of adjacent slices (see Fig. 15-6). In combination with motion, partial scan reconstruction can cause streaks and low-density artifacts adjacent to regions of very high CT density (e.g., metal or calcium). Edge-enhancing reconstruction filters can lead to artifacts along borders between very low and high density (e.g., the interface between lung and cardiac tissue) by assigning artificially high CT numbers to pixels along that border (see Fig. 15-6). Finally, the partial volume effect is a general phenomenon in CT imaging: if an image pixel is only partially filled by a structure of very high attenuation (e.g., metal or bone), a very high CT number will be assigned to the complete pixel, which will thus appear bright on the image. This may lead to overestimation of the dimensions of high-intensity objects (e.g., calcifications within coronary arteries) and may cause difficulties in image interpretation.

Clinical Applications

Cardiac Morphology

Computed tomography imaging has a relatively high spatial resolution, and a high contrast between the blood pool and other tissues can be achieved after injection of contrast agent. CT imaging therefore has the ability to provide high-resolution morphologic imaging of the heart. Clinically, however, CT imaging does not play a very prominent role in evaluating cardiac morphology, because echocardiography or magnetic resonance imaging can provide all relevant information in most clinical situations (see Chaps. 11 and 14). Since echocardiography and magnetic resonance imaging neither expose the patient to radiation nor require the injection of potentially nephrotoxic contrast agents, echocardiography, possibly followed by magnetic resonance imaging, will usually be the preferred approach to imaging for assessment of cardiac morphology. However, cardiac CT imaging can be clinically helpful in a variety of situations, including the need for cross-sectional

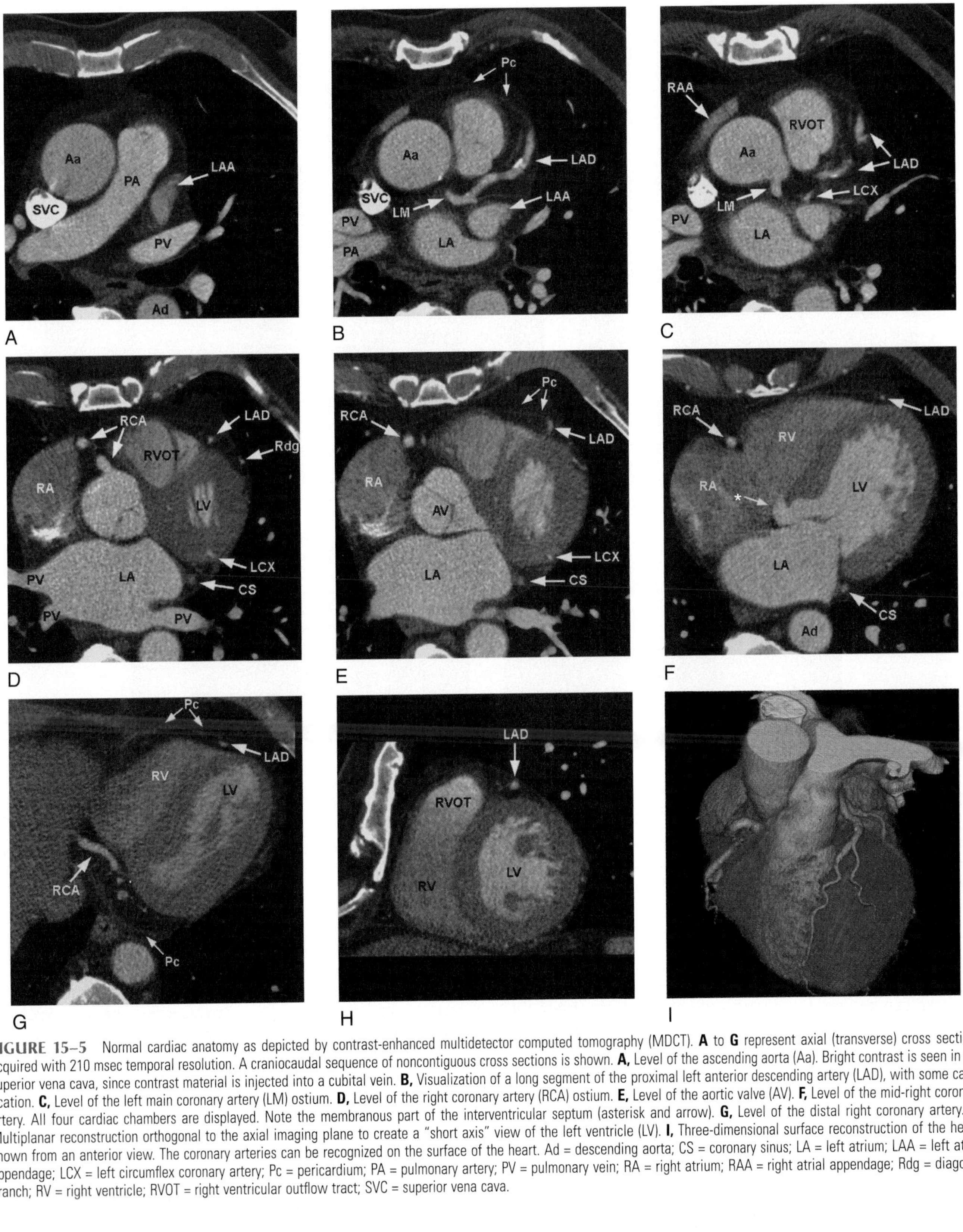

FIGURE 15–5 Normal cardiac anatomy as depicted by contrast-enhanced multidetector computed tomography (MDCT). **A** to **G** represent axial (transverse) cross sections acquired with 210 msec temporal resolution. A craniocaudal sequence of noncontiguous cross sections is shown. **A,** Level of the ascending aorta (Aa). Bright contrast is seen in the superior vena cava, since contrast material is injected into a cubital vein. **B,** Visualization of a long segment of the proximal left anterior descending artery (LAD), with some calcification. **C,** Level of the left main coronary artery (LM) ostium. **D,** Level of the right coronary artery (RCA) ostium. **E,** Level of the aortic valve (AV). **F,** Level of the mid-right coronary artery. All four cardiac chambers are displayed. Note the membranous part of the interventricular septum (asterisk and arrow). **G,** Level of the distal right coronary artery. **H,** Multiplanar reconstruction orthogonal to the axial imaging plane to create a "short axis" view of the left ventricle (LV). **I,** Three-dimensional surface reconstruction of the heart, shown from an anterior view. The coronary arteries can be recognized on the surface of the heart. Ad = descending aorta; CS = coronary sinus; LA = left atrium; LAA = left atrial appendage; LCX = left circumflex coronary artery; Pc = pericardium; PA = pulmonary artery; PV = pulmonary vein; RA = right atrium; RAA = right atrial appendage; Rdg = diagonal branch; RV = right ventricle; RVOT = right ventricular outflow tract; SVC = superior vena cava.

imaging after echocardiography in patients with pacemakers or other devices that preclude magnetic resonance imaging. Also, CT techniques have an extremely high accuracy for the depiction of calcified structures. Finally, cardiac CT imaging is increasingly applicable for coronary artery visualization.

Pericardial Disease (see Chap. 64)

Since the pericardium is usually embedded in epicardial and pericardial fat, it can, in most cases, be delineated in CT images. It usually appears as a thin line (see Fig. 15–5) and is best delineated on the anterior face of the heart. Congenital absence of the pericardium can be complete or partial. This condition is infrequent, and patients are usually asymptomatic. CT can be helpful in establishing the absence or presence of a segment of pericardium, but lack of visualization, especially on the posterior surface, is not a sufficient criterion to make the diagnosis.[5] Recent studies found the normal thickness of pericardium on high-resolution scans to

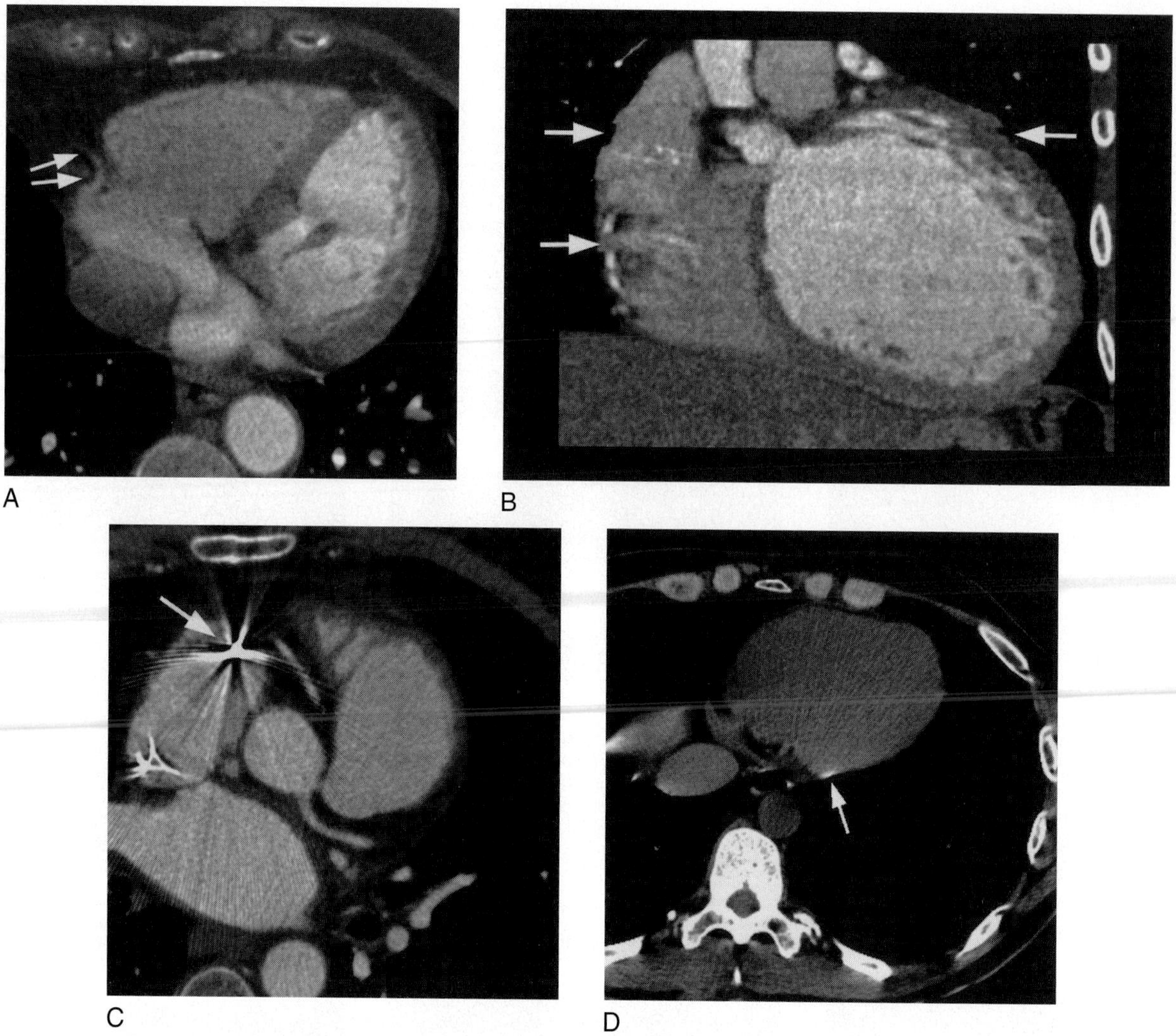

FIGURE 15–6 Examples of typical artifacts encountered in cardiac computed tomography (CT) imaging. Most artifacts are related to limited temporal resolution and partial scan reconstruction. **A,** Motion artifact of the right coronary artery. **B,** Trigger artifacts caused by irregular (ectopic) heart beats. Coronal multiplanar reconstruction of the heart. Arrows point at artifacts caused by ectopic beats, which result in parts of the imaging volume being acquired in an offset cardiac phase. **C,** Streaks and low-density artifacts caused by objects of very high density (here: pacemaker lead in right atrium). **D,** Edge-enhancement can cause artifacts at interfaces between tissues with a high difference in CT attenuation (here: interface of pericardium and lung; see arrow). Pixels along that interface may be assigned a higher intensity value than corresponds to their actual attenuation. In this case, this artifact could be misinterpretated as calcification.

range between 1 and 2 mm.[6] Pericardial thickening can be a helpful finding in cases of suspected constriction, but it does not prove any hemodynamic relevance. Thickened pericardium can be found in a multitude of situations, including the early postoperative period, uremia, rheumatic heart disease, and sarcoidosis or as a consequence of radiation therapy, and per se does not constitute proof of constriction. Similarly, a normal pericardial thickness can not rule out constriction.[5] CT imaging can clearly delineate pericardial calcification (Fig. 15–7) and in the clinical setting of suspected constriction, it should be considered a significant finding.[5]

PERICARDIAL FLUID. Pericardial fluid can reliably be detected by CT, and small amounts of fluid in pericardial recesses can frequently be observed in healthy individuals.[7] Although echocardiography has an excellent sensitivity to detect relevant pericardial effusion in the majority of clinical situations (see Chap. 11), its application can be limited in postoperative patients, and some localized effusions may be outside the echocardiographic acoustic windows. CT can clearly delineate the anatomical distribution of pericardial fluid (Fig. 15–8). CT attenuation numbers measured in the pericardial fluid may give some indication as to the genesis of the effusion. Densities higher than water (above approximately 10 HU) suggest high protein content (e.g., blood).

PERICARDIAL CYSTS AND NEOPLASMS. Pericardial cysts appear on CT images as paracardiac masses, typically in the right cardiophrenic angle. The cysts have a thin capsule that is not always visualized but that may occasionally be calcified. The cysts are usually filled with fluid of water-equivalent density (Fig. 15–9). Bronchiogenic cysts or teratomas may mimic pericardial cysts in location and appearance. Primary neoplasms of the pericardium are infrequent but can be the reason for thickened pericardium on CT scans. Both primary neoplasms and secondary involvement of the pericardium can be accompanied by hemorrhagic pericardial effusions.[8]

Myocardial Disease (see Chap. 59)

The role of CT in the assessment of myocardial disease is limited. Even though CT can clearly show left ventricular geometry, wall thickness, and also function, the diagnosis of dilated or hypertrophic cardiomyopathy does not require cross-sectional imaging. Except for occasional case reports, little is known about the value of CT in assessing infiltrative myocardial disease.[9,10] Typical findings in arrhythmogenic

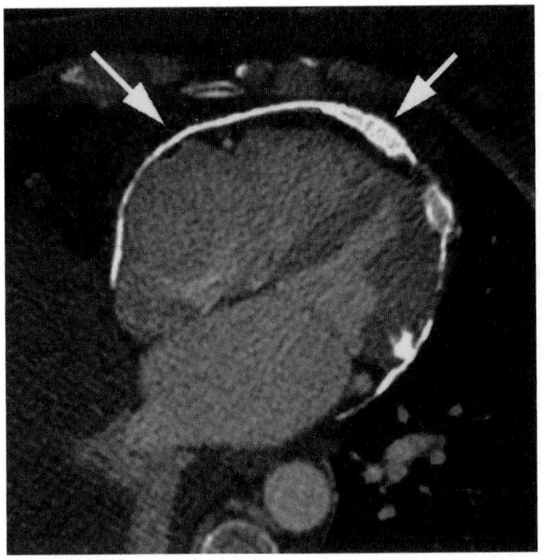

FIGURE 15–7 Severe pericardial calcification. (Courtesy of R. Rienmüller, MD, Interdisciplinary Cardiac Imaging Center, University Graz.)

right ventricular dysplasia include dilation of the right ventricle, infiltration of the myocardium with fatty tissue of low CT attenuation, and aneurysms and local bulging of the right ventricular free wall (Fig. 15–10).[11]

Valvular Disease (see Chap. 57)

Although visualization of the tricuspid and pulmonary valves is inconsistent, the mitral and aortic valves can reliably be depicted in contrast-enhanced cardiac CT scans (Fig. 15–11). Functional analysis is not possible, however, and CT plays no relevant role in the work-up of valvular lesions concerning their hemodynamic relevance. However, the unique ability of CT to detect and quantify calcification has recently been applied, especially to aortic valve disease (see Fig. 15–11). CT has shown high accuracy and reproducibility in quantifying aortic valve calcification and its progression.[12-15] This may develop into clinically relevant applications with respect to the prognostic relevance of aortic valve sclerosis[16] as well as the problem of bioprosthesis calcification.

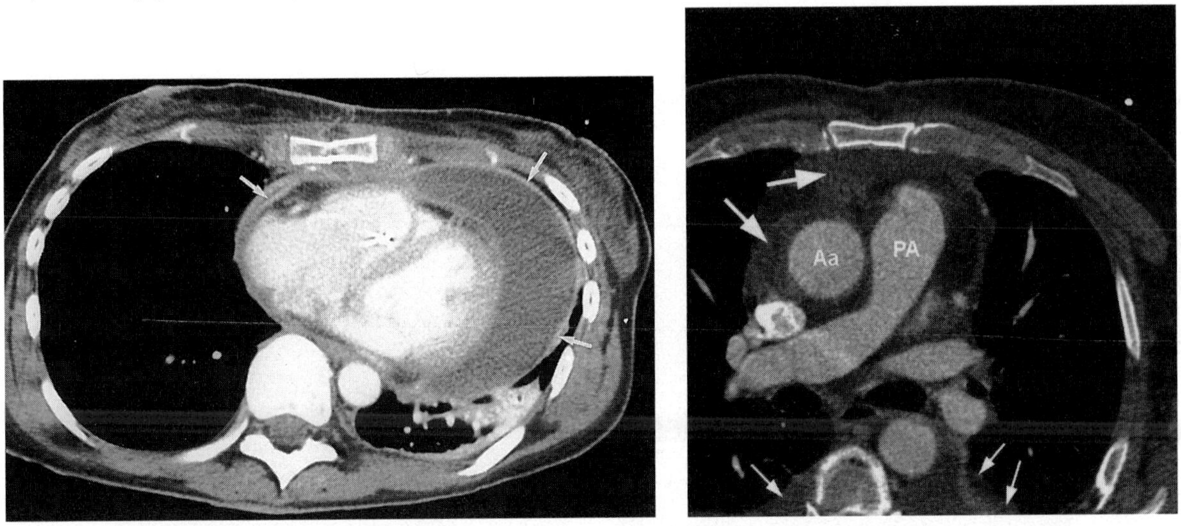

A B

FIGURE 15–8 Pericardial effusion. **A,** Large pericardial effusion with contrast enhancement of the pericardium (arrows), suggesting pericardial inflammation (Courtesy of GE Imatron). **B,** Localized pericardial effusion in the superior aortic recess in a patient 4 days after bypass surgery (large arrows). Bilateral pleural effusion is also present (small arrows). Aa = ascending aorta, PA = pulmonary artery.

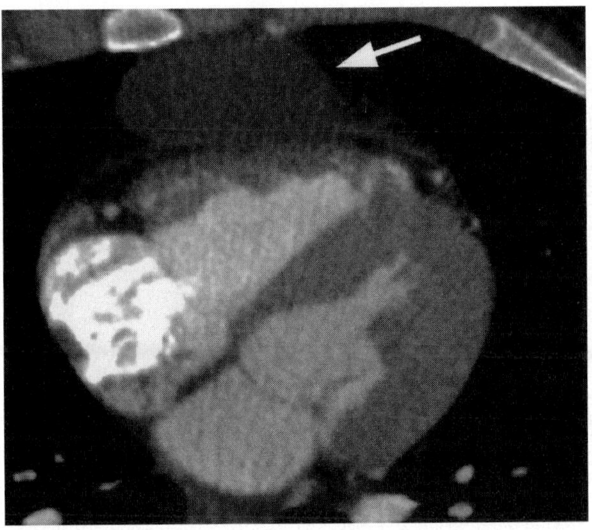

FIGURE 15–9 Pericardial cyst located anterior to the right ventricle in a contrast-enhanced scan (arrow).

Coronary Artery Disease (see Chap. 50)

Cardiac CT has several potential applications in patients with coronary artery disease. CT can demonstrate the morphological consequences of ischemic heart disease (Figs. 15–12 and 15–13),[17] can assess ventricular function and perfusion, and is applied with increasing success to visualizing coronary arteries. In addition, the assessment of coronary artery calcification, especially with EBT, has received considerable attention with respect to its potential role in the early detection of subclinical atherosclerosis. In the diagnostic work-up of coronary artery disease, the emerging abilities of CT imaging compete with a multitude of other well-established and readily available diagnostic modalities. In this context, the most appropriate clinical use of CT is made when limiting its application to situations in which clinical evidence shows advantages over other modalities.

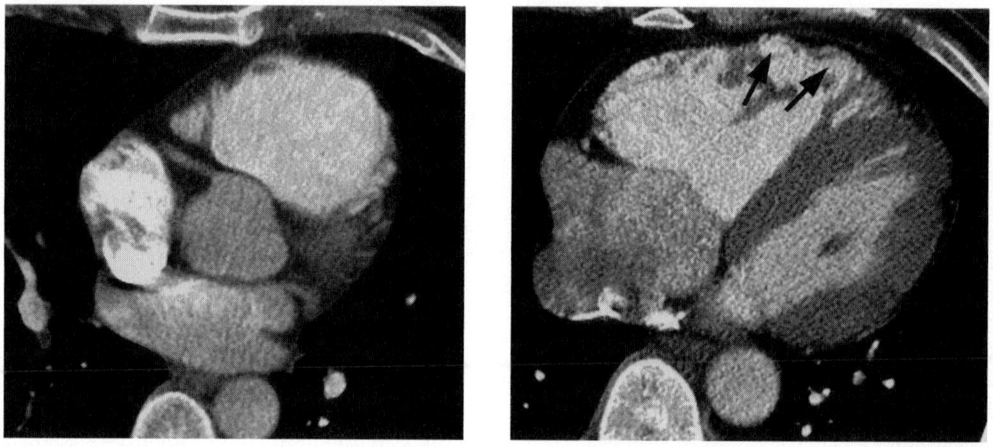

A B

FIGURE 15–10 Dilated right ventricle and aneurysmal bulging of the right ventricular free wall (arrows) in a patient with arrhythmogenic right ventricular dysplasia. (Courtesy of J. F. Breen, MD, Mayo Clinic, Rochester, MN.)

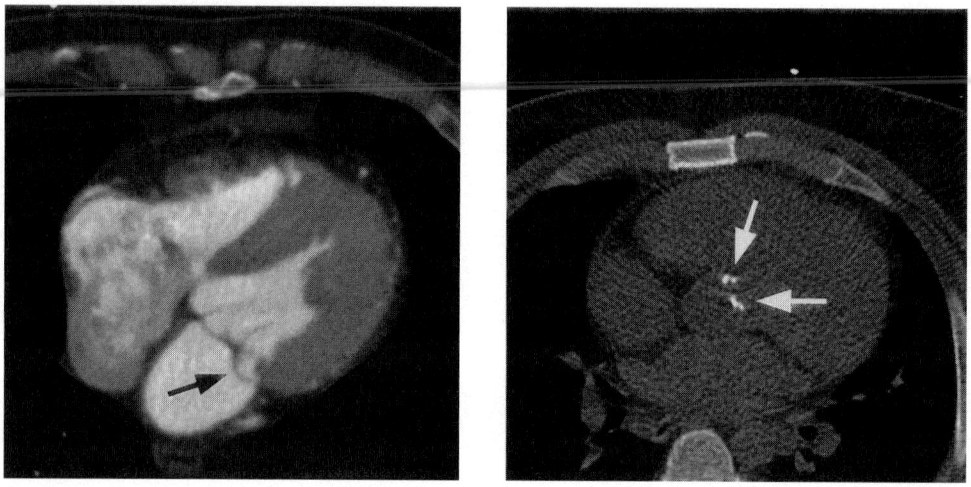

A B

FIGURE 15–11 Visualization of cardiac valves by computed tomography. **A,** Prolapse of the posterior mitral leaflet in a contrast-enhanced systolic image (arrow). **B,** Calcifications of the aortic valve (arrows) detected in a nonenhanced scan.

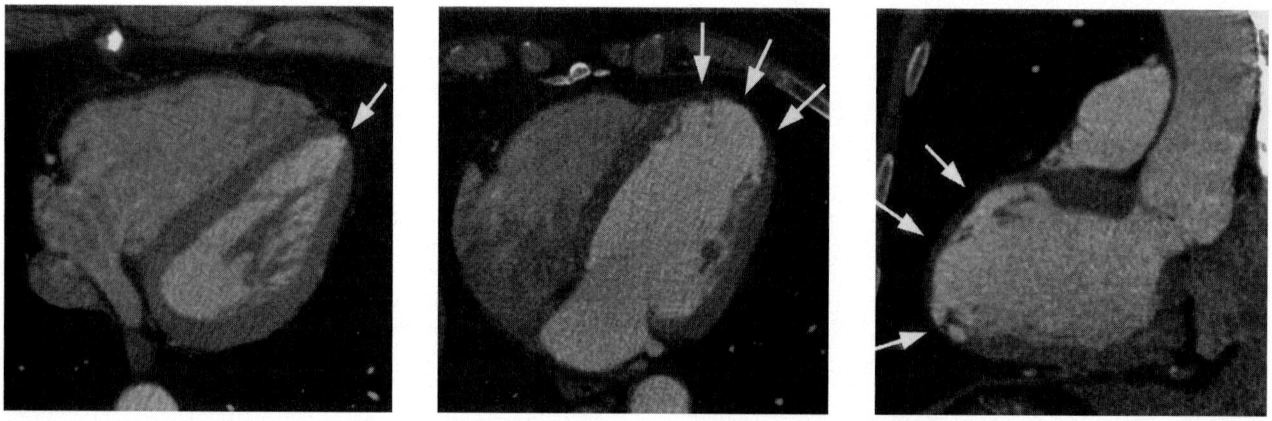

A B C

FIGURE 15–12 Computed tomography (CT) clearly depicts regional wall thinning as a consequence of myocardial infarction. It is important to note that in healthy subjects, the left ventricular wall in the very apical region can be paper-thin, which constitutes a frequent normal finding.[17] **A,** Normal tapering of the left ventricular apex as frequently observed in high-resolution CT scans (arrow). **B and C,** Infarction of the anterior wall (arrows) in an axial cross section **(B)** and multiplanar reformat **(C).**

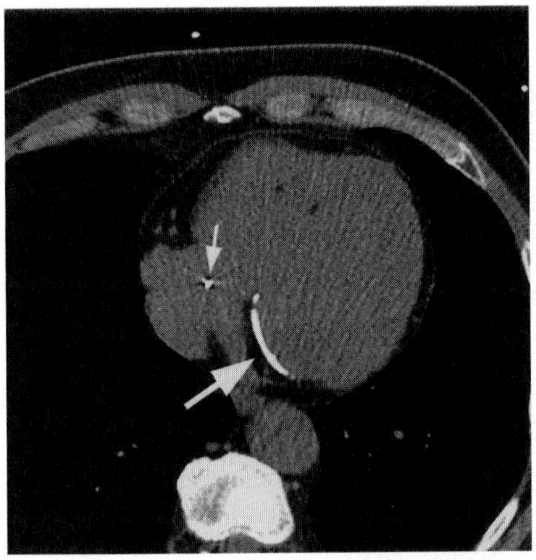

FIGURE 15–13 Calcified left ventricular aneurysm (large arrow) as a consequence of posterior myocardial infarction in a nonenhanced scan (small arrow = pacemaker lead).

CORONARY ARTERY CALCIFICATION

PATHOLOGY. Coronary calcium is a surrogate marker for coronary atherosclerotic plaque. In the coronary arteries, calcifications occur almost exclusively in the context of atherosclerotic changes.[18,19] Medial (nonatherosclerotic) calcification of the coronary artery wall is exceedingly rare. Within a coronary vessel or larger segment of the vessel, the quantity of coronary calcium correlates moderately closely with the extent of atherosclerotic plaque burden.[18,19] On the other hand, not every atherosclerotic coronary plaque is calcified. The presence or absence of calcium is not closely associated with the propensity of an individual atherosclerotic plaque to rupture, and calcification is a sign of neither stability nor instability of an individual plaque.[18] Plaques with healed ruptures almost invariably contain calcium, whereas plaque erosions are frequently not calcified. In the vast majority of patients with acute coronary syndromes, coronary calcium can be detected, and the amount of calcium in these patients is substantially greater than in matched control subjects without coronary artery disease.[20-22]

Although there is a strong quantitative relationship between coronary calcification and coronary plaque burden, there is only a weak, nonlinear correlation between the amount of coronary calcium and the angiographic severity of obstructive coronary artery disease.[19] The complete absence of coronary calcium makes the presence of significant coronary luminal obstruction highly unlikely, however.[19,23]

In patients with end-stage renal disease, the prevalence and extent of coronary calcification are high. However, the relationship of coronary calcium to coronary atherosclerosis is less well established in this patient group.[18,24]

DETECTION OF CORONARY CALCIUM. Electron beam tomography and ECG-gated spiral CT with subsecond rotation permit detection and quantification of coronary artery calcium.[25] Mechanical CT without ECG gating is unsuited for the reliable detection of coronary calcium.[26] The vast majority of existing data concerning histopathological validation and clinical evaluation of coronary calcium assessment has been obtained using EBT.

The usual protocol to detect and quantify coronary calcification by EBT consists of the acquisition of high-resolution axial cross-sections of the heart with a 100-msec acquisition time per image, 3.0 mm slice thickness, and no overlap (see Table 15-1). Some investigators propose a 0.5 mm overlap of consecutive images. The presence of calcifications is assumed if contiguous pixels with a density exceeding 130 HU are found within the coronary artery system (Fig. 15-14).[19] The so-called Agatston score has most frequently been used to quantify the amount of coronary calcium in EBT. The Agatston score is derived by measuring the area of each calcified coronary lesion and multiplying it by a coefficient that has a value of 1 to 4, depending on the maximum CT attenuation within the lesion. The sum of all lesions represents the Agatson score for the patient. Several large reference data sets are available that describe the distribution of Agatston scores found in the respective (usually self-referred) population, stratified by age and gender.[21,27]

By MDCT, prospectively triggered sequential scanning or retrospectively ECG-gated continuous spiral scanning can be applied for the detection of coronary calcium (see Table 15-2). Scan parameters have not been standardized and vary substantially according to scanner type and manufacturer. The best image quality is usually obtained with retrospectively gated scans and thin slice collimation, albeit at the expense of high radiation exposure.[28] Motion artifacts, especially in sequential scan mode, are more frequent than in EBT (Fig. 15-15). Similar to EBT, the presence of calcium is usually assumed if pixels above 130 HU are observed within the coronary arteries, and modified versions of the Agatston score are used for quantification.

The analysis of coronary calcification in coronary CT images is usually straightforward. Difficulties in interpretation can arise in the presence of motion artifacts (see Fig. 15-15). The close proximity of the left circumflex coronary artery to the mitral valve and annulus can sometimes lead to misinterpretation of mitral calcification as coronary calcium (see Fig. 15-15). The interobserver variability of coronary calcium quantification is low. Interscan variability can be high for patients with small amounts of calcium, but on average the latest technology provides for interscan variability of less than 10%. Alternative scoring methods, such as volumetric scores or determination of the calcium mass, have been proposed but have not been validated on a large scale.

CLINICAL SIGNIFICANCE OF CORONARY CALCIUM. Coronary calcium correlates with the presence and extent of coronary atherosclerosis. The absence of coronary calcium thus rules out the presence of significant coronary artery stenoses with high predictive value.[19,23] However, since even pronounced coronary atherosclerotic plaque burden is not necessarily associated with hemodynamically relevant luminal narrowings, the detection even of large amounts of calcium does not imply the presence of significant stenoses. Thus, the finding of pronounced calcifications by itself does not necessitate invasive coronary angiography.

Several cohort studies have shown that the presence of coronary calcium demonstrated by EBT in asymptomatic individuals is a prognostic parameter with high predictive power regarding the development of hard cardiac events during the following 3 to 5 years.[21,29-33] A meta-analysis demonstrated that a calcium score higher than the median was associated with an unadjusted odds ratio of 4.2 (95% CI, 1.6-11.3) for myocardial infarction or death.[34] It is currently assumed that individuals who seem to be at intermediate risk for coronary events (0.6-2.0 percent annual risk) based on traditional risk factor analysis will be most likely

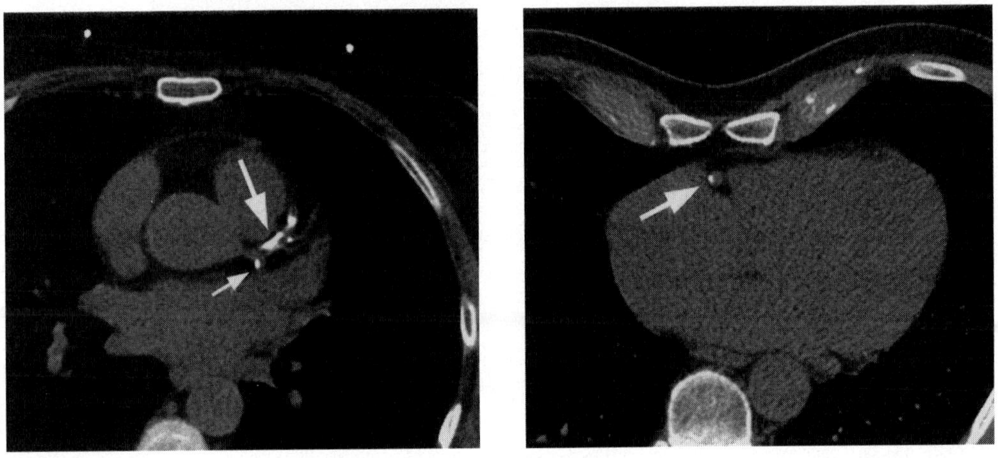

A B

FIGURE 15–14 Examples of coronary calcification. **A,** Calcification of the left anterior descending coronary artery (large arrow) and left circumflex coronary artery (small arrow). **B,** Calcification of the right coronary artery (arrow).

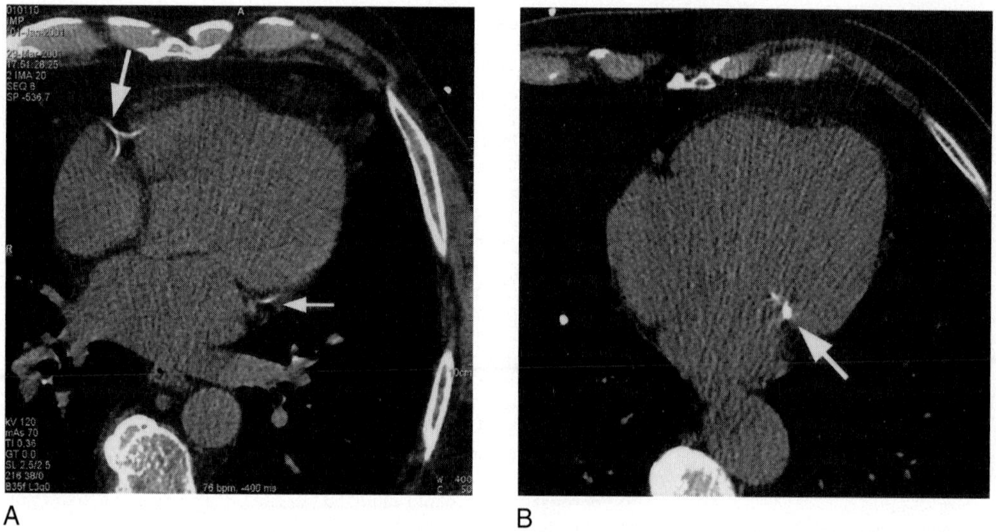

A B

FIGURE 15–15 Interpretation problems in coronary calcium scans. **A,** Motion artifacts of the right coronary artery (large arrow) and, to a lesser extent, of the left circumflex coronary artery (small arrow) in prospectively electrocardiographically triggered sequential multidetector computed tomography (four-slice scanner, 500 msec rotation, patient with a heart rate of 75/min). **B,** Calcification of the mitral annulus (arrow). Owing to the proximity of the course of the left circumflex coronary artery, mitral calcification can be misinterpreted as calcium in the left circumflex coronary artery.

to profit from noninvasive testing for subclinical atherosclerosis, such as the assessment of coronary calcification. Unselected "screening" or patient self-referral is uniformly not recommended.[19,35]

Coronary calcification has been found to be progressive over time.[36] Several studies have reported an influence of lipid levels and lipid-lowering therapy on the rate of progression of calcification.[37-39] Little is known, however, concerning the relationship between calcium progression and clinical events. Thus, recommendations for repeat scanning can currently not be made.[25]

VISUALIZATION OF THE CORONARY LUMEN. Electron beam tomography and multidetector spiral CT have been applied for visualization of the coronary artery lumen after intravenous injection of a contrast agent. Based on the axial cross sections of the heart, two- or three-dimensional reconstructions of the coronary arteries can be rendered (Figs. 15–16 and 15–17). Concerning the detection of coronary stenoses, two-dimensional "maximum intensity projections" provide the highest diagnostic accuracy. Three-dimensional reconstruction usually adds no further information but may be useful to document findings. Several investigators have compared the accuracy of EBT[40] and MDCT[41-45] for coronary stenosis detection to invasive coronary angiography. Given the small dimensions of the coronary arteries, it is obvious that high spatial resolution is critical for reliable assessment of the coronary lumen. Consequently, the best results so far have been obtained by 16-slice MDCT, with a sensitivity ranging from 92 to 95 percent and specificity of 86 to 93 percent for the detection of coronary stenoses of more than 50 percent diameter reduction.[44,45] However, MDCT is limited by its lower temporal resolution as compared to EBT, and several reports have shown that the patient should have a heart rate of 60 beats/min or less during the MDCT scan for good image quality to be reliably achieved. Hence, most investigators propose the administration of short-acting beta-blockers prior to the MDCT scan.[44,45] Heart rate is no limitation for the faster EBT scanner. Accurate grading of the severity of a coronary lesion (percentage of stenosis) is currently not possible, and even in optimally prepared patients, pronounced coronary calcifications, trigger artifacts due to arrhythmias, or high image noise can prevent analysis of coronary segments concerning the presence of stenoses. Owing to these limitations and the lack of larger clinical trials, EBT and MDCT coronary angiography currently cannot be considered routine clinical tools with broad applicability. However, clinical application, especially to rule out coronary stenoses in patients with low pretest likelihood of disease, is conceivable.

Imaging of coronary stents has been demonstrated (Fig. 15–18), but partial volume effects and artifacts caused by metal frequently prevent adequate visualization of the coronary lumen inside stents. Therefore, clinical application of CT for reliable assessment of in-stent restenosis is currently not possible. Patency and occlusion of bypass grafts can be established with very high accuracy[46,47] (Fig. 15–19), but limitations exist concerning the detection of stenoses at the site of the anastomosis to the coronary artery and in the peripheral run-off vessels. Clinical situations that may benefit from noninvasive assessment of bypass patency by CT are therefore limited.

The image quality of noninvasive coronary and bypass angiography by CT has rapidly improved during the last years. Technical developments toward faster

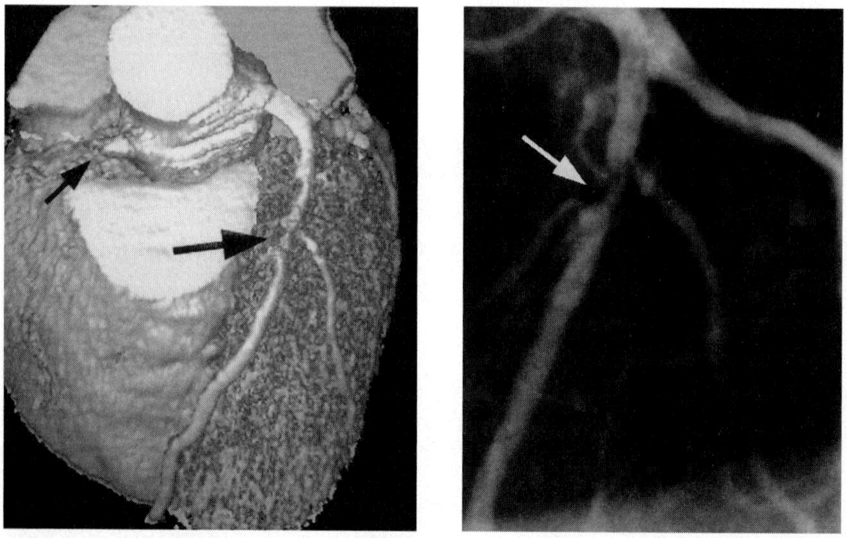

A B

FIGURE 15–16 Noninvasive coronary angiography by cardiac computed tomography. **A,** Three-dimensional reconstruction obtained by electron beam tomography in a patient with a high-grade stenosis of the left anterior descending coronary artery (large arrow). The right coronary artery is occluded (small arrow). **B,** Corresponding invasive angiogram of the left coronary artery.

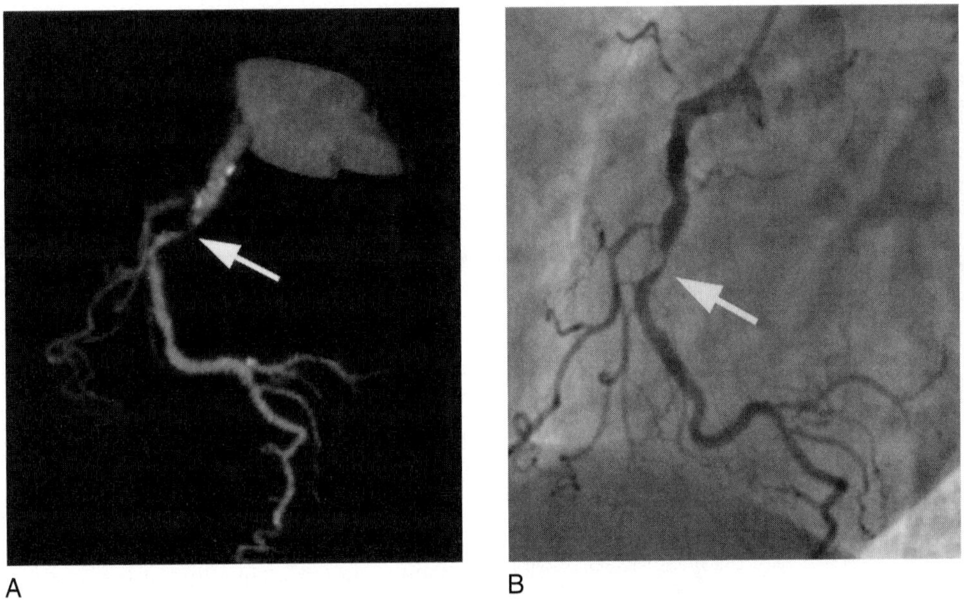

FIGURE 15–17 Patient with a high-grade right coronary artery stenosis (arrows). **A,** Two-dimensional reconstruction (maximum intensity projection) obtained by multidetector computed tomography. **B,** Corresponding invasive coronary angiogram.

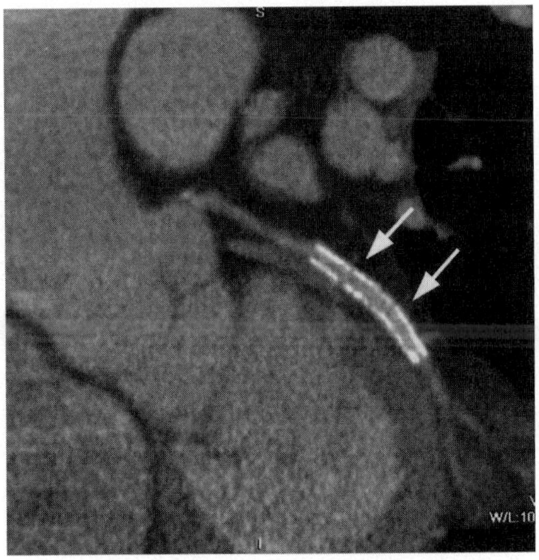

FIGURE 15–18 Visualization of a patent stent (arrows) in the left circumflex coronary artery. (Courtesy of M. Grover-McKay, MD, and S. Lipson, MD, Long Beach Memorial Medical Center, Long Beach, CA.)

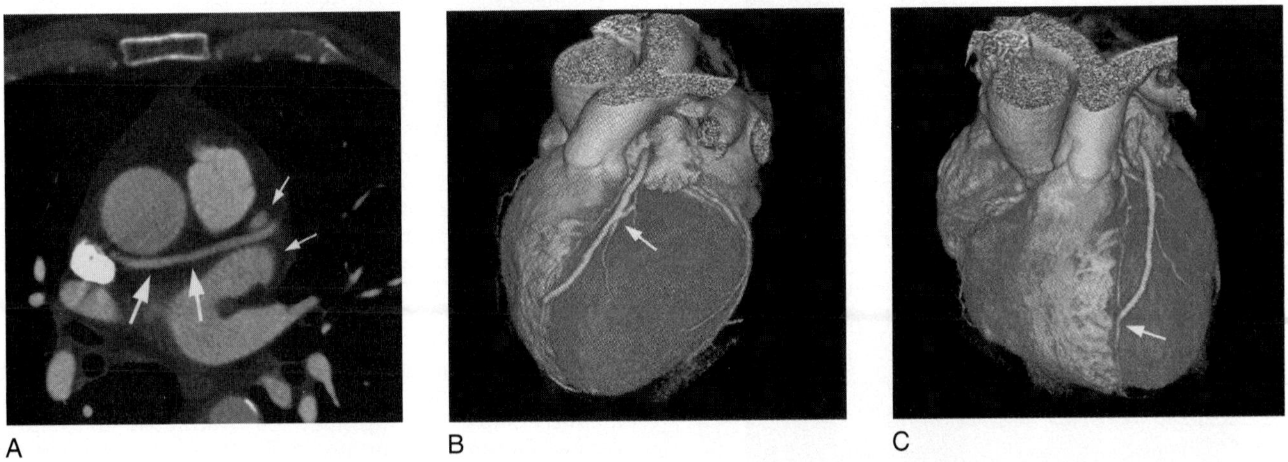

FIGURE 15–19 Patient with a single venous bypass graft to the diagonal branch and left anterior descending coronary artery. **A,** Axial contrast-enhanced image showing the bypass graft (large arrows), which follows a retroaortic course (small arrows = left atrial appendage). **B and C,** Three-dimensional reconstructions that show the bypass grafts and anastomoses to the diagonal branch and left anterior descending coronary artery (arrows).

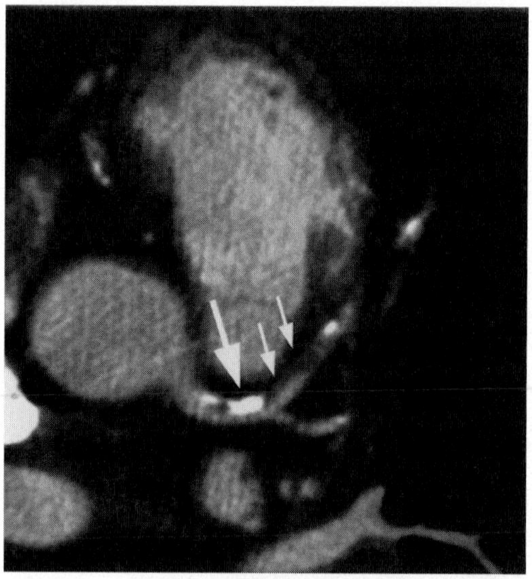

FIGURE 15–20 Visualization of calcified (large arrow) and noncalcified (small arrows) coronary atherosclerotic plaque by contrast-enhanced computed tomography.

scanners with higher resolution will continue. With increasing image quality, it can thus be anticipated that accuracy and clinical applicability of "noninvasive coronary angiography" by EBT and MDCT will continue to improve.

VISUALIZATION OF NONCALCIFIED CORONARY ARTERY PLAQUE. The observation that noncalcified coronary atherosclerotic plaque can be visualized in high-resolution, contrast-enhanced CT scans of the coronary arteries[48] has sparked intense interest in using CT imaging for the detection, quantification, and characterization of coronary plaque in the context of risk assessment (Fig. 15–20). A comparison of 21 patients with acute myocardial infarction to 19 patients with stable angina found that MDCT detected noncalcified coronary atherosclerotic plaque significantly more frequently in patients with acute infarction.[49] Sensitivity and specificity for plaque detection as well as the ability to quantify noncalcified plaque by CT have so far not been investigated systematically. Under the assumption that lipid-rich plaques have a higher risk of rupture with consequent thrombosis than fibrotic plaques, researchers have tried to use measurements of CT attenuation values to differentiate plaque types.[50-52] The clinical implications of these interesting initial findings, however, are currently unclear.[53]

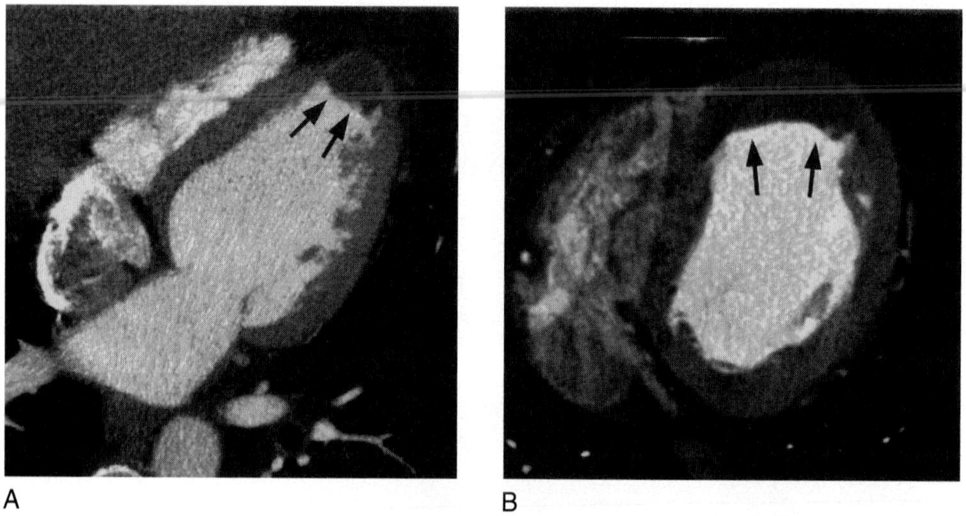

FIGURE 15–21 Left ventricular thrombi in contrast-enhanced computed tomography (CT) images. **A,** Spherical apical thrombus after myocardial infarction (arrows). **B,** Large mural thrombus (arrows) in a patient with a large anterior infarction. The CT attenuation of the thrombus is only a little less than the density of the adjacent myocardium.

Cardiac Masses (see Chap. 63)

Although echocardiography is the first-line diagnostic tool for cardiac masses, CT can provide helpful additional information due its high resolution and ability to clearly visualize cardiac morphology without the restriction of acoustic windows. CT provides less information concerning the tissue type than magnetic resonance imaging but may provide limited insight into the nature of a mass through measurement of the x-ray attenuation (CT numbers).[54] Lipomas have low CT numbers (typically <50 HU), whereas cysts have water-like density (0-10 HU). The CT numbers of intracardiac thrombi usually range from 20 to 90 HU,[55] but their density values may overlap with those of myocardium, and great care may thus be necessary to correctly delineate the extent of mural thrombi (Fig. 15–21). As they age, hematomas may develop calcifications or even take up contrast agent. Atrial myxomas are the most frequent primary intracardiac tumor. They have an average CT number of approximately 30 HU and may also contain calcification (Fig. 15–22).[56] Neoplasms can have an attenuation close to that of myocardium and if displaying a diffusely infiltrative pattern of growth, such as cardiac lymphoma, may be difficult to outline in CT images (Fig. 15–23). Both in primary cardiac neoplasms and in metastatic cardiac or pericardial involvement, pericardial effusion (often with above-water CT numbers) may be the only finding in CT.[8,54]

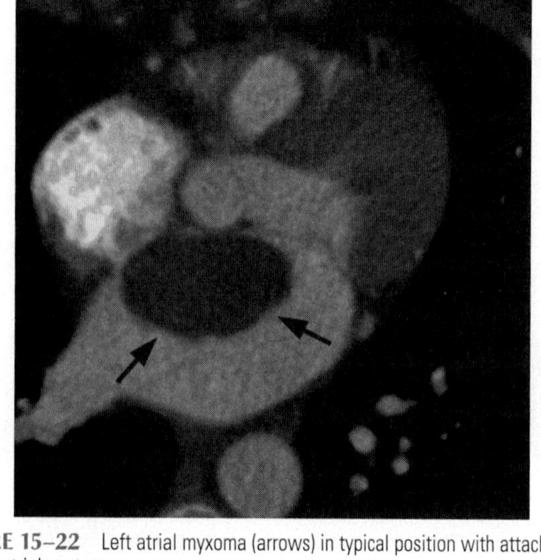

FIGURE 15–22 Left atrial myxoma (arrows) in typical position with attachment to the interatrial septum.

Congenital Heart Disease (see Chap. 56)

Although echocardiography constitutes the first-line diagnostic modality for patients with congenital heart disease, cross-sectional imaging may be warranted to delineate cardiac morphology and especially the anatomy of the great arteries, pulmonary veins, and anomalous coronary arteries. Newer EBT and MDCT scanner generations have the ability to cover a large imaging volume within one breath-hold and

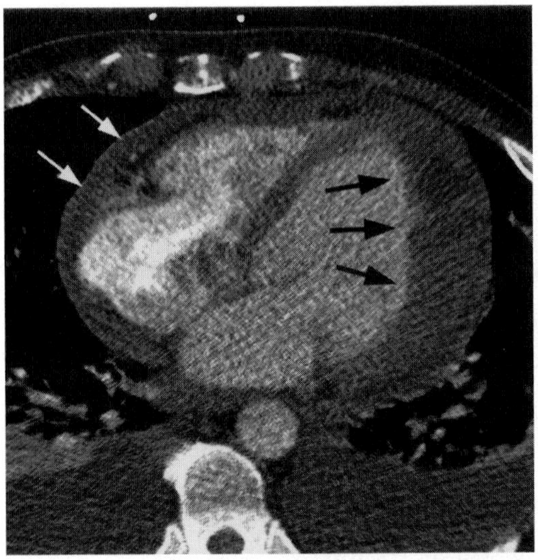

FIGURE 15–23 Primary cardiac lymphoma in a patient who presented with ventricular arrhythmias. Inhomogeneous thickening of the lateral left ventricular wall (black arrows) is caused by infiltrative growth of the lymphoma. Pericardial effusion (white arrows) and bilateral pleural effusion are present.

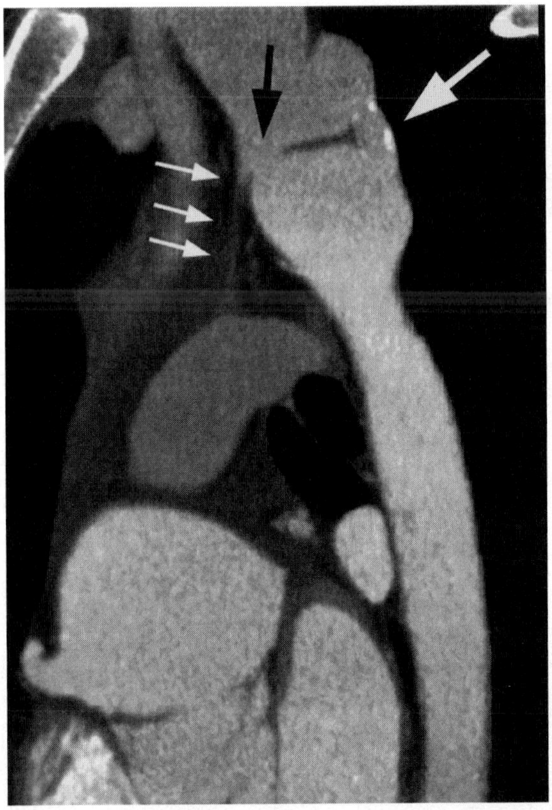

FIGURE 15–24 A 31-year-old patient with aortic coarctation. A sagitally reformatted multidetector computed tomography scan shows the descending aorta (black arrow = coarctation). A partly calcified, patent bypass conduit that was implanted at the age of 9 years can be seen (large white arrow). Note obliterated ductus arteriosus (small white arrows).

to acquire thin transaxial cross-sections that permit reformatting in any desired plane. This has substantially increased the diagnostic value of CT imaging in the setting of congenital heart disease. Limitations in obtaining information about flow or shunts and the necessity for contrast injection and radiation exposure constitute disadvantages of CT over magnetic resonance imaging (see Chap. 14). However, CT provides morphological analysis with very high resolution and is not limited by the presence of implanted devices such as pacemakers or ICDs, which are encountered with increasing frequency in adults with congenital heart disease. The systematic use of EBT and MDCT imaging has been described, especially for analysis of great vessels and pulmonary venous return[57,58] and for the exact delineation of the course of anomalous coronary arteries (Figs. 15–24 and 15–25).[59] The fact that detailed information about the dimensions and function of both ventricles can be obtained by CT may be important in the follow-up of adults with surgically corrected disease, since right ventricular assessment may be especially problematic by echocardiography.

Function and Perfusion

Computed tomography permits detailed and accurate analysis of left and right ventricular function. Using retrospective ECG gating, spiral CT data sets can be reconstructed at any desired phase of the cardiac cycle. EBT provides the option of prospectively acquiring high-resolution data sets at several predefined instances in the cardiac cycle. The high contrast between the ventricular cavity and myocardium in contrast-enhanced scans permits accurate measurements of ventricular volumes at systole and diastole, thus enabling exact analysis of global function and regional wall motion.[60,61] Thus, information about ventricular function can be obtained as a byproduct of contrast-enhanced data sets acquired for other reasons, such as coronary artery visualization or cardiac morphology in cases of congenital heart disease. In clinical reality, however, it is seldom necessary to resort to CT imaging to obtain information about global or regional wall motion.

Electron beam tomography is well suited to analyze myocardial perfusion after bolus injection of contrast agent with high resolution.[62] Studies can be performed at rest and during exercise. In fact, wall motion and perfusion analysis can be combined into one single scan. Owing to the ready availability of alternative imaging modalities (see Chap. 13), however, clinical applications have so far been limited.

Great Vessels

THORACIC AORTA. Computed tomography is extremely accurate for the diagnosis of aortic disease, including aneurysms, dissection, and intramural hematoma. Demonstration of the intimal flap (low CT attenuation within contrast-enhanced aortic lumen) is required for the diagnosis of aortic dissection (Fig. 15–26). A dissection with complete thrombosis of the false lumen may be difficult to differentiate from an aortic aneurysm with mural thrombus. Inward displacement of calcium toward the aortic lumen may help indicate dissection in this case. Higher temporal resolution and the availability of ECG triggering have substantially reduced pulsation artifacts that could cause misdiagnosis of dissection, especially in the ascending aorta,[63] and the accuracy of CT for establishing the diagnosis of dissection, assuming optimal technology, is close to 100 percent.[64,65] The individual clinical situation must dictate whether transesophageal echocardiography, magnetic resonance imaging, or computed tomography constitutes the optimal approach in a given patient (see Chaps. 11 and 14). Detailed visualization of the aorta and branch vessels and ready availability represent the advantages of CT, whereas the need for contrast injection is a drawback. The ability of CT to depict the lumen of metallic stents in the aorta and to detect leaks by demonstrating extravasation of contrast agent makes it a useful follow-up tool after interventional treatment of aortic aneurysms.[65]

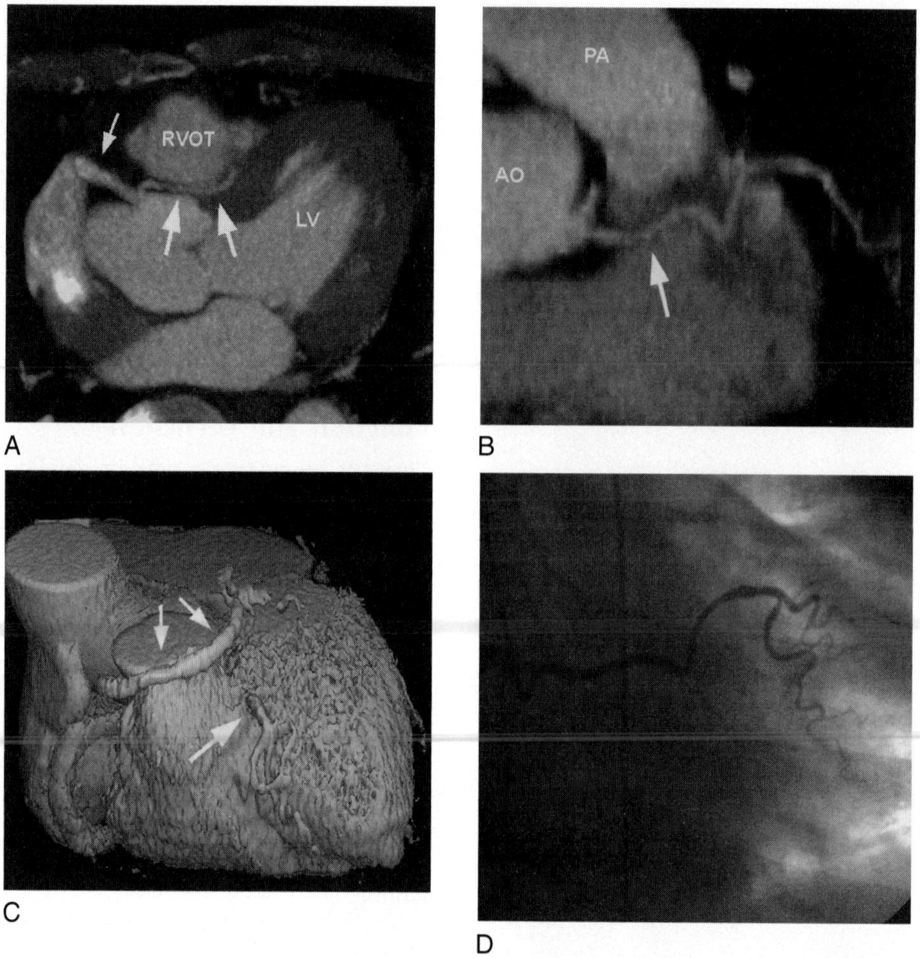

FIGURE 15–25 Patient with a complex anomaly of the coronary arteries. **A,** Axial maximum intensity projection shows the origin of the left anterior descending coronary artery (large arrows) from the right coronary ostium and course between the aortic root and right ventricular outflow tract (RVOT) toward the interventricular septum (small arrow = right coronary artery). **B,** Multiplanar reformat (sagittal view) shows passage of the left anterior descending coronary artery (arrow) through the interventricular septum. **C,** Three-dimensional reconstruction shows left anterior descending coronary artery surfacing in the anterior interventricular groove (large arrow). The left circumflex coronary artery also has an anomalous origin from the right sinus valsalvae and follows a course anterior to the pulmonary trunk (small arrows). **D,** Invasive angiogram of the left anterior descending coronary artery. AO = aortic root; LV = left ventricle; PA = pulmonary artery.

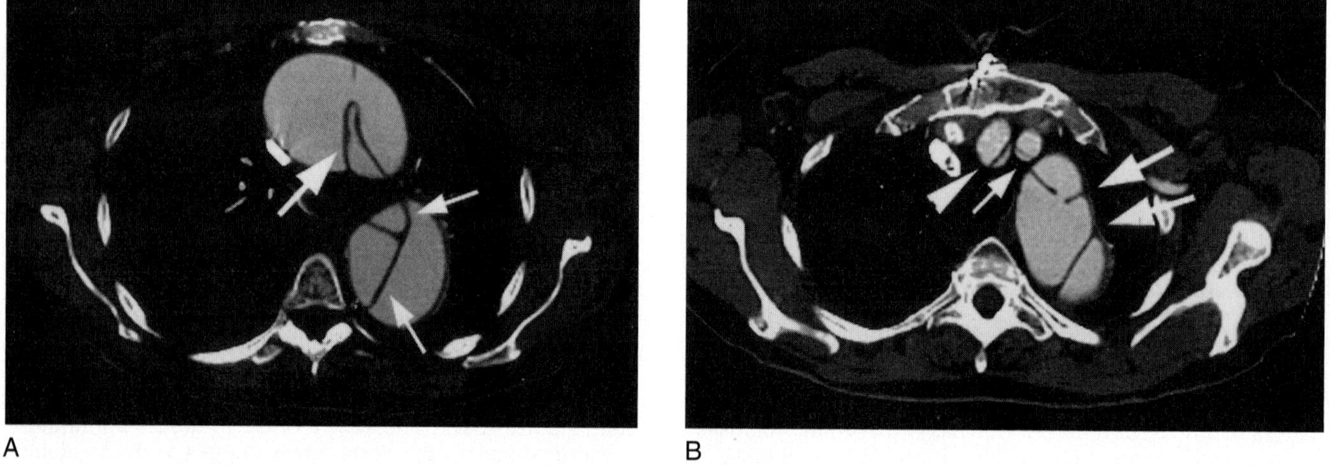

FIGURE 15–26 Aortic dissection. **A,** Dissection membranes clearly visualized in the ascending aorta (large arrow) and descending aorta (small arrows). **B,** Same patient. Dissection membrane, partially fenestrated, in the aortic arch (large arrows). The dissection extends into the left common carotid artery (small arrow) and innominate artery (arrowhead). (Courtesy of R. C. Gilkeson, MD, Case Western Reserve University, Cleveland, OH.)

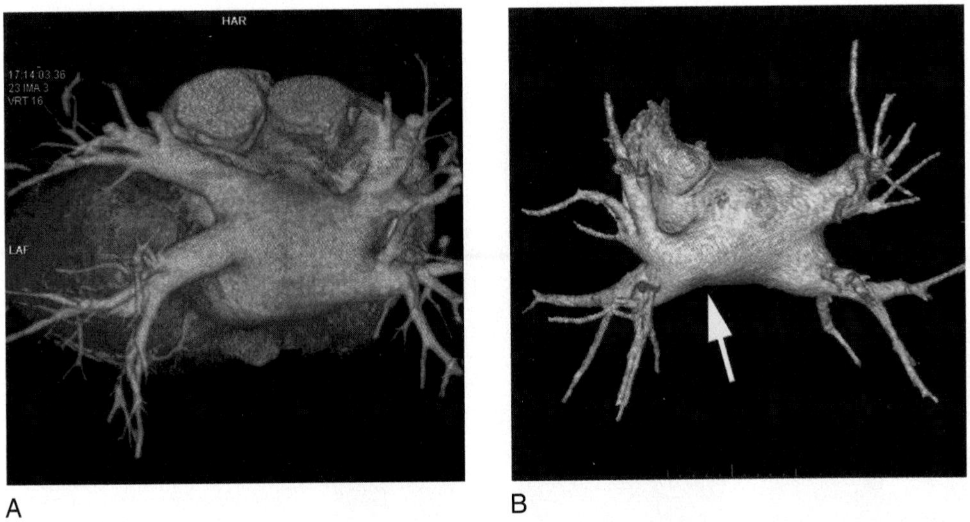

FIGURE 15–27 Three-dimensional visualization of pulmonary vein anatomy by computed tomography. **A,** Normal anatomy of the four pulmonary veins draining into the left atrium in a three-dimensional reconstructional view of the posterior face of the heart. **B,** Common ostium of the left inferior and superior pulmonary vein (arrow). (Courtesy of J. Lacomis, MD, University of Pittsburgh Medical Center, Pittsburgh, PA.)

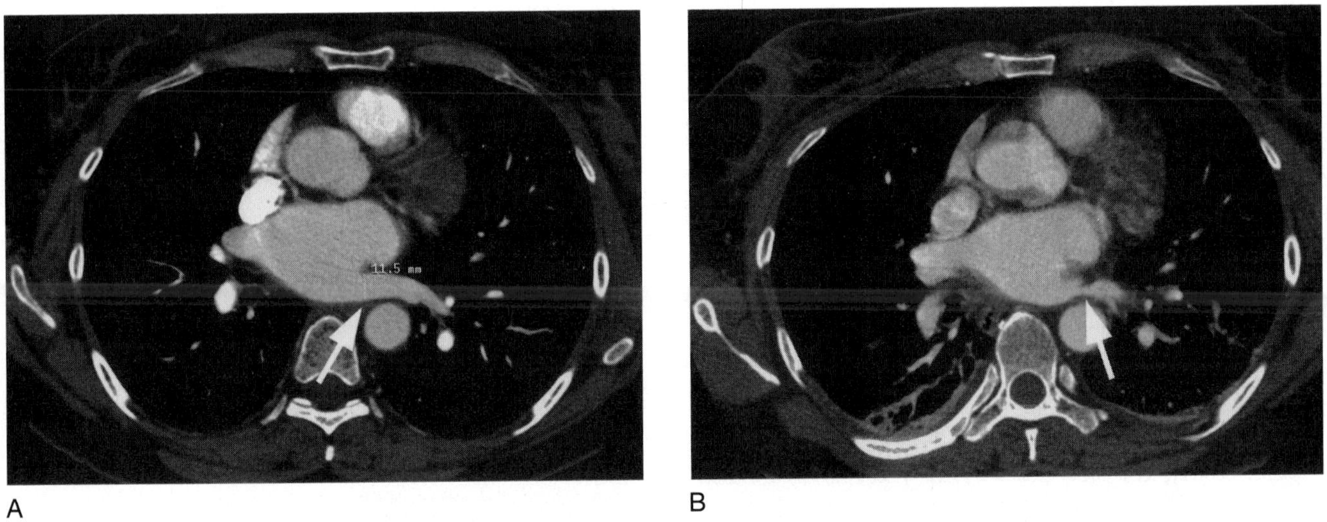

FIGURE 15–28 Visualization of pulmonary veins before and after ablation of the pulmonary vein ostium for atrial fibrillation. **A,** Transaxial cross section at the ostium of the left inferior pulmonary vein (arrow). Normal anatomy prior to ablation. **B,** Same patient 6 weeks after ablation. Severe stenosis can be seen at the ostium of the pulmonary vein (arrow). (Courtesy of J. F. Breen, MD, Mayo Clinic, Rochester, MN.)

PULMONARY VEINS. In the context of electrophysiology interventions, for example to electrically isolate the pulmonary veins for prevention of atrial fibrillation, visualization of the exact anatomy of pulmonary veins and detection of supernumerary veins are of clinical importance. Suitable imaging information can reduce the duration of the interventional procedure. In addition, pulmonary vein stenosis is a possible consequence of ablation and difficult to assess with echocardiography. Similar to magnetic resonance imaging, CT can provide two-dimensional and three-dimensional images that show the exact anatomy of pulmonary veins (Figs. 15–27 and 15–28).[66] Image quality may be degraded if the CT examination is performed during atrial fibrillation but usually remains sufficiently high. Anomalous pulmonary venous return can be present in congenital heart disease and is also clearly depicted by CT.

PULMONARY EMBOLISM (see Chap. 66). EBT[67] and MDCT[68] have been demonstrated to provide high diagnostic accuracy for the detection of pulmonary embolism. In contrast-enhanced scans, the thrombi appear as filling defects in the pulmonary arteries (Fig. 15–29). Approximately 60 to 120 ml of contrast agent are necessary to provide enhancement of the pulmonary vasculature during the scan. There is consensus that a thin-collimation CT scan of the thorax with 1 to 2 mm image reconstruction can be used as an alternative to $\dot{V}/\dot{Q}$ scan during the diagnostic evaluation of patients with suspected pulmonary embolism[69,70] and that a normal CT scan, possibly in combination with ultrasonography or CT venography of the lower extremity veins or other clinical findings, is sufficient to withhold anticoagulation therapy.[68-71] Current recommendations are based on the results of single-slice spiral CT. The accuracy of MDCT can be expected to be higher.[72-74] In patients with suspected pulmonary embolism, the individual clinical situation will drive the decision toward appropriate testing. In patients with acute right heart failure, the need to inject a relatively large amount of contrast

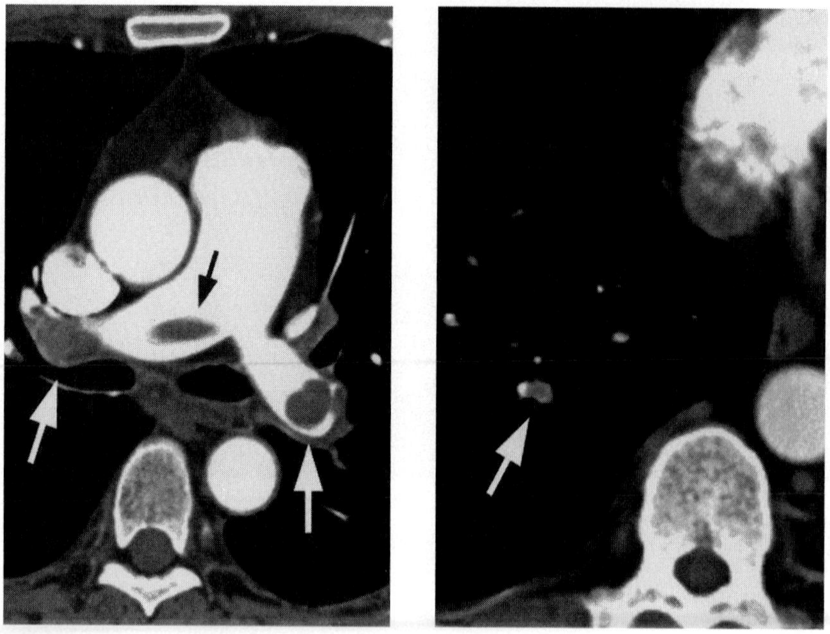

A B

FIGURE 15–29 Visualization of pulmonary embolism by contrast-enhanced computed tomography in central pulmonary arteries (**A**, arrows), and peripheral arteries (**B**, arrow). (Courtesy of U.J. Schoepf, MD, Brigham and Women's Hospital, Boston, MA.)

material constitutes a limitation of CT, but echocardiography will usually be sufficient to reach a treatment decision in these cases (see Chap. 11).

REFERENCES

Technical Principles

1. Flohr TG, Schoepf JU, Kuettner A, et al: Advances in cardiac imaging with 16-section CT systems. Acad Radiol 10:366, 2003.
2. Hunoldt P, Vogt FM, Schmermund A, et al: Radiation exposure during cardiac CT: Effective doses at multi-detector-row CT and electron beam CT. Radiology 226:145, 2003.
3. Morin RL, Gerber TC, McCollough CH: Radiation dose in computed tomography of the heart. Circulation 107:917, 2003.
4. Jakobs TF, Becker CR, Ohnesorge B, et al: Multislice helical CT of the heart with retrospective ECG gating: Reduction of radiation exposure by ECG-controlled tube current modulation. Eur Radiol 12:1081, 2002.

Diseases of the Pericardium and Myocardium

5. Breen JF: Imaging of the pericardium. J Thorac Imaging 16:47, 2001.
6. Bull RK, Edwards PD, Dixon AK: CT dimensions of the normal pericardium. Br J Radiol 71:923, 1998.
7. Groell R, Schaffler GJ, Rienmueller R: Pericardial sinuses and recesses: Findings at electrocardiographically triggered electron-beam CT. Radiology 212:69, 1999.
8. Chiles C, Woodard P, Gutierrez FR, et al: Metastatic involvement of the heart and pericardium: CT and MR imaging. Radiographics 21:439, 2001.
9. Funabashi N, Toyozaki T, Matsumoto Y, et al: Myocardial fibrosis in Fabry disease demonstrated by multislice computed tomography. Circulation 107:2519, 2003.
10. Scatarige JC, Fishman EK: Interventricular septal mass: An unusual manifestation of sarcoidosis demonstrated on helical computed tomography. Clin Imaging 24:344, 2000.
11. Kimura F, Sakai F, Sakomura Y, et al: Helical CT features of arrhythmogenic right ventricular cardiomyopathy. Radiographics 22:1111, 2002.

Valvular Heart Disease

12. Willmann JK, Weishaupt D, Lachat M, et al: Electrocardiographically gated multi-detector row CT for assessment of valvular morphology and calcification in aortic stenosis. Radiology 225:120, 2002.
13. Pohle K, Maffert R, Ropers D, et al: Progression of aortic valve calcification: Association with coronary atherosclerosis and cardiovascular risk factors. Circulation 104:1927, 2001.
14. Budoff MJ, Mao S, Takasu J, et al: Reproducibility of electron-beam CT derived measures of aortic valve calcification. Acad Radiol 9:1122, 2002.
15. Melina G, Scott MJ, Cunanan CM, et al: In-vitro verification of the electron beam tomography method for measurement of heart valve calcification. J Heart Valve Dis 11:402, 2002.
16. Otto CM, Lind BK, Kitzman DW, et al: Association of aortic-valve sclerosis with cardiovascular mortality and morbidity in the elderly. N Engl J Med 341:142, 1999.
17. Bradfield JW, Beck G, Vecht RJ: Left ventricular apical thin point. Br Heart J 39:806, 1977.

Coronary Artery Calcification

18. Burke AP, Virmani R, Galis Z, et al: Task Force #2—What is the pathologic basis for new atherosclerosis imaging techniques? J Am Coll Cardiol 41:1874, 2003.
19. O'Rourke RA, Brundage B, Froelicher VF, et al: ACC/AHA Expert Consensus Document on electron-beam computed tomography for the diagnosis and prognosis of coronary artery disease. Circulation 102:126, 2000.
20. Pohle K, Ropers D, Mäffert R, et al: Coronary calcifications in young patients with first, unheralded myocardial infarction: A risk factor matched analysis by electron beam tomography. Heart 89:625, 2003.
21. Raggi P, Callister TQ, Cooil B, et al: Identification of patients at increased risk of first unheralded acute myocardial infarction by electron-beam computed tomography. Circulation 101:850, 2000.
22. Schmermund A, Schwartz RS, Adamzik M, et al: Coronary atherosclerosis in unheralded sudden coronary death under age fifty: Histopathologic comparison with "healthy" subjects dying out of hospital. Atherosclerosis 155:499, 2001.
23. Haberl R, Becker A, Leber A, et al: Correlation of coronary calcification and angiographically documented stenoses in patients with suspected coronary artery disease: Results of 1,764 patients. J Am Coll Cardiol 37:451, 2001.
24. Schoenhagen P, Tuczu M: Coronary artery calcification and end-stage renal disease: Vascular biology and clinical implications. Cleve Clin J Med 69(Suppl 3):S12, 2002.
25. Redberg RF, Vogel RA, Criqui MH, et al: Task Force #3—What is the spectrum of current and emerging techniques for the noninvasive measurement of atherosclerosis? J Am Coll Cardiol 41:1886, 2003.
26. Goldin JG, Yoon HC, Greaser LE 3rd, et al: Spiral versus electron-beam CT for coronary artery calcium scoring. Radiology 221:213, 2001.
27. Hoff JA, Chomka EV, Krainik AJ, et al: Age and gender distribution of coronary artery calcium detected by electron beam tomography in 35246 adults. Am J Cardiol 87:1335, 2001.
28. Ulzheimer S, Kalender WA: Assessment of calcium scoring performance in cardiac computed tomography. Eur Radiol 13:484, 2003.
29. Arad Y, Spadaro LA, Goodman K, et al: Prediction of coronary events with electron beam computed tomography. J Am Coll Cardiol 36:1253, 2000.
30. Park R, Detrano R, Xiang M, et al: Combined use of computed tomography coronary calcium scores and C-reactive protein levels in predicting cardiovascular events in nondiabetic individuals. Circulation 106:2073, 2002.
31. Vliegenthart R, Oudkerk M, Song B, et al: Coronary calcification detected by electron-beam computed tomography and myocardial infarction. The Rotterdam Coronary Calcification Study. Eur Heart J 23:1596, 2002.
32. Wong ND, Hsu JC, Detrano RC, et al: Coronary artery calcium evaluation by electron beam computed tomography and its relation to new cardiovascular events. Am J Cardiol 86:495, 2000.
33. Kondos GT, Hoff JA, Sevrukov A, et al: Electron-beam tomography coronary artery calcium and coronary events: A 37-month follow-up of 5635 initially asymptomatic low- to intermediate-risk adults. Circulation 107:2571, 2003.
34. O'Malley PG, Taylor AJ, Jackson JL, et al: Prognostic value of coronary electron-beam computed tomography for coronary heart disease events in asymptomatic patients. Am J Cardiol 85:945, 2000.
35. Taylor AJ, Bairey Merz CN, Udelson JE: 34th Bethesda Conference. Executive Summary—Can atherosclerosis imaging techniques improve the detection of patients at risk for ischemic heart disease? J Am Coll Cardiol 41:1860, 2003.
36. Schmermund A, Baumgart D, Möhlenkamp S, et al: Natural history and topographic pattern of progression of coronary calcification in symptomatic patients. Arterioscler Thromb Vasc Biol 21:421, 2001.
37. Callister TQ, Raggi P, Cooil B, et al: Effect of HmG-CoA reductase inhibitors on coronary artery disease as assessed by electron-beam computed tomography. N Engl J Med 339:1972, 1998.
38. Achenbach S, Ropers D, Pohle K, et al: Influence of lipid-lowering therapy on the progression of coronary artery calcification: a prospective evaluation. Circulation 106:1077, 2002.
39. Budoff MJ, Lane KL, Bakhsheshi H, et al: Rates of progression of coronary calcium by electron beam tomography. Am J Cardiol 86:8, 2000.

Imaging the Coronary Artery Lumen

40. Achenbach S, Moshage W, Ropers D, et al: Value of electron-beam computed tomography for the detection of high-grade coronary artery stenoses and occlusions. N Engl J Med 339:1964, 1998.
41. Nieman K, Oudkerk M, Rensing BJ, et al: Coronary angiography with multi-slice computed tomography. Lancet 357:599, 2001.
42. Achenbach S, Giesler T, Ropers D, et al: Detection of coronary artery stenoses by contrast-enhanced, retrospectively ECG-gated, multi-slice spiral CT. Circulation 103:2535, 2001.
43. Kopp AF, Schroeder S, Kuettner A, et al: Non-invasive coronary angiography with high resolution multidetector-row computed tomography. Results in 102 patients. Eur Heart J 23:1714, 2002.

44. Nieman K, Cademartiri F, Lemos PA, et al: Reliable noninvasive coronary angiography with fast submillimeter multislice spiral computed tomography. Circulation 106:2051, 2002.
45. Ropers D, Baum U, Pohle K, et al: Detection of coronary artery stenoses with thin-slice multi-detector row spiral computed tomography and multiplanar reconstruction. Circulation 107:664, 2003.
46. Achenbach S, Moshage W, Ropers D, et al: Noninvasive, three-dimensional visualization of coronary artery bypass grafts by electron beam tomography. Am J Cardiol 79:856, 1997.
47. Ropers D, Ulzheimer S, Wenkel E, et al: Investigation of aortocoronary bypass grafts by multislice spiral computed tomography with electrocardiographic-gated image reconstruction. Am J Cardiol 88:792, 2001.

Coronary Artery Plaque Imaging

48. Becker CR, Knez A, Ohnesorge B, et al: Imaging of noncalcified coronary plaques using helical CT with retrospective ECG gating. AJR 175:423, 2000.
49. Leber AW, Knez A, White CR, et al: Composition of coronary atherosclerotic plaque in patients with acute myocardial infarction and stable angina pectoris determined by contrast-enhanced multislice computed tomography. Am J Cardiol 91:714, 2003.
50. Estes JM, Quist WC, Lo Gerfo FW, et al: Noninvasive characterization of plaque morphology using helical computed tomography. J Cardiovasc Surg (Torino) 39:527, 1998.
51. Schroeder S, Kopp AF, Baumbach A, et al: Noninvasive detection and evaluation of atherosclerotic coronary plaques with multislice computed tomography. J Am Coll Cardiol 37:1430, 2001.
52. Becker CR, Nikolaou K, Muders M, et al: Ex vivo coronary atherosclerotic plaque characterization with multi-detector-row CT. Eur Radiol 13:2094, 2003.
53. Fayad ZA, Fuster V, Nikolaou K, et al: Computed tomography and magnetic resonance imaging for noninvasive coronary angiography and plaque imaging: Current and potential future concepts. Circulation 106:2026, 2002.

Other Cardiac Applications

54. Araoz PA, Eklund HE, Welch TJ, et al: CT and MR imaging of primary cardiac malignancies. Radiographics 19:1421, 1999.
55. Kirchhof K, Welzel T, Mecke C, et al: Differentiation of white, mixed, and red thrombi: Value of CT in estimation of the prognosis of thrombolysis-Phantom study. Radiology 228:126, 2003.
56. Grebenc ML, Rosado-de-Christenson ML, Green CE, et al: Cardiac myxoma: Imaging features in 83 patients. Radiographics 22:673, 2002.
57. Gilkeson RC, Ciancibello L, Zahka K: Multidetector CT evaluation of congenital heart disease in pediatric and adult patients. AJR 180:973, 2003.
58. Haramati LB, Glickstein JS, Issenberg HJ, et al: MR imaging and CT of vascular anomalies and connections in patients with congenital heart disease: Significance in surgical planning. Radiographics 22:337, 2002.
59. Ropers D, Moshage W, Daniel WG, et al: Visualization of coronary artery anomalies and their course by contrast-enhanced electron beam tomography and three-dimensional reconstruction. Am J Cardiol 87:193, 2001.
60. Halliburton SS, Petersilka M, Schvartzman PR, et al: Evaluation of left ventricular dysfunction using multiphasic reconstructions of coronary multi-slice computed tomography data in patients with chronic ischemic heart disease: Validation against cine magnetic resonance imaging. Int J Cardiovasc Imaging 19:73, 2003.
61. Gerber TC, Behrenbeck T, Allison T, et al: Comparison of measurement of left ventricular ejection fraction by Tc-99m sestamibi first-pass angiography with electron beam computed tomography in patients with anterior wall acute myocardial infarction. Am J Cardiol 83:1022, 1999.
62. Mohlenkamp S, Lerman LO, Lerman A, et al: Minimally invasive evaluation of coronary microvascular function by electron beam computed tomography. Circulation 102:2411, 2000.

Great Vessels and the Pulmonary Circulation

63. Batra P, Bigoni B, Manning J, et al: Pitfalls in the diagnosis of thoracic aortic dissection at CT angiography. Radiographics 20:309, 2000.
64. Hartnell GG: Imaging of aortic aneurysms and dissection: CT and MRI. J Thorac Imaging 16:35, 2001.
65. Erbel R, Alfonso F, Boileau C, et al: Diagnosis and management of aortic dissection. Recommendations of the Task Force on Aortic Dissection, European Society of Cardiology. Eur Heart J 22:1642, 2001.
66. Schwartzman D, Lacomis J, Wigginton WG: Characterization of left atrium and distal pulmonary vein morphology using multidimensional computed tomography. J Am Coll Cardiol 41:1349, 2003.
67. Teigen CL, Maus TP, Sheedy PF, et al: Pulmonary embolism: Diagnosis with contrast-enhanced electron beam CT and comparison with pulmonary angiography. Radiology 194:313, 1995.
68. van Strijen MJ, de Monye W, Schiereck J, et al: Single-detector helical computed tomography as the primary diagnostic test in suspected pulmonary embolism: A multicenter clinical management study of 510 patients. Ann Intern Med 138:307, 2003.
69. American College of Chest Physicians: Clinical policy: Critical issues in the evaluation and management of adults presenting with suspected pulmonary embolism. Ann Emerg Med 41:257, 2003.
70. Kruip MJ, Leclercq MG, Heul CV, et al: Diagnostic strategies for excluding pulmonary embolism in clinical outcome studies: A systematic review. Ann Intern Med 138:941, 2003.
71. Katz DS, Loud PA, Bruce D, et al: Combined CT venography and pulmonary angiography: a comprehensive review. Radiographics 22:S3, 2002.
72. Raptopoulos V, Boiselle PM: Multi-detector row spiral CT pulmonary angiography: Comparison with single-detector row spiral CT. Radiology 221:606, 2001.
73. Schoepf JU, Holzknect N, Helmberger TK, et al: Subsegmental pulmonary emboli: Improved detection with thin-collimation multi-detector row spiral CT. Radiology 222:483, 2002.
74. Patel S, Kazerooni EA, Cascade PN: Pulmonary embolism: Optimization of small pulmonary artery visualization at multi-detector row CT. Radiology 227:455, 2003.

CHAPTER 16

Relative Merits of Cardiac Diagnostic Techniques

George A. Beller

The Spectrum of Cardiovascular Diagnostic Procedures

Noninvasive cardiovascular imaging can be used for the diagnostic and prognostic assessment of patients with suspected or known cardiovascular disease. The technologies supporting these techniques vary widely, are in constant evolution, and require significant training of physicians who supervise and interpret test results. The clinical indications for these imaging modalities are guided by practice guidelines emanating predominantly from specialty and subspecialty societies. Emerging technologies are initially evaluated in small single-center studies and later in multicenter trials. Use of technology in the practice setting is not only governed by evidence-based clinical science but also by reimbursement policies. Widespread clinical application of a given imaging technique is dependent on both evidence-based guidelines and reimbursement consideration by payers such as CMS. The confidence of requesting physicians who order tests based on these imaging technologies also relates to their own experience regarding the accuracy of test results in their patient populations from the laboratories to which such patients are referred. Although one test modality may have higher specificity for the detection of disease than a competing test aimed at identifying the same pathophysiology as reported from specialized centers of excellence, the specificity advantage may not apply in local settings because of issues related to quality control and/or experience of the test interpreter. It is always difficult to definitively declare superiority of one diagnostic test over another, since local instrumentation and expertise can substantially influence test results.

Most of the diagnostic imaging tests currently available are based on assessment of regional and global function (echocardiography [see Chap. 11], radionuclide angiography [see Chap. 13], magnetic resonance imaging [MRI] [see Chap. 14]), myocardial perfusion (single-photon emission computed tomography [SPECT], positron emission tomography [PET], contrast echocardiography, contrast-enhanced MRI), myocardial metabolism (PET [see Chap. 13]), or coronary anatomy (computed tomography [CT] angiography, magnetic resonance angiography, coronary angiography [see Chaps. 14, 15, and 18]) under resting conditions, stress conditions, or both. The cardiovascular system can be stressed by either exercise or pharmacological means, such as the infusion of a vasodilator or an inotropic agent. Combining low-level exercise with vasodilator stress for myocardial perfusion imaging enhances the quality of the images and reduces side effects of the vasodilator. The principle underlying nuclear and echocardiographic stress tests is uncovering abnormal flow reserve or an ischemic response in patients with physiologically significant luminal narrowing of one or more coronary arteries. The ischemic response can be identified as flow heterogeneity represented by a "defect" on a perfusion scan, abnormal regional systolic thickening or abnormal wall motion, or abnormal regional metabolism. Regional myocardial perfusion and metabolism are simultaneously assessed for the detection of myocardial viability in ischemic cardiomyopathy using nuclear techniques, particularly PET. Various other techniques used to distinguish viable from nonviable myocardium are inotropic reserve as assessed with dobutamine echocardiography or MRI, determination of the integrity of the microcirculation as evaluated with contrast echocardiography, evaluation of myocardial membrane transport as determined from imaging a radiolabeled monovalent cation such as thallium-201 (^{201}Tl), or delineation of the transmural extent of scar by contrast-enhanced MRI.

Diagnostic techniques such as electron beam CT (EBCT),[1] multislice cardiac CT scanning, and measurement of carotid intimal-medial thickness have emerged in recent years for detecting asymptomatic coronary or carotid atherosclerosis, respectively. These technologies are not aimed at identifying an ischemic response but at detecting occult vascular disease in the coronary or peripheral circulation.

SOURCES OF BIAS WHEN EVALUATING AND COMPARING DIAGNOSTIC TECHNIQUES

The "gold standard" used for comparing the sensitivity and specificity of the various noninvasive techniques for detecting coronary artery disease (CAD) remains the coronary angiogram, which can be obtained only with invasive means (see Chap. 18). However, the coronary angiogram can at times be misleading, and it often underestimates disease severity, particularly in segments with crescentic lumina and in the presence of diffuse disease rendering the reference diameter misleading. A high degree of intraobserver and interobserver variability in visually interpreting the degree and significance of coronary stenosis is well known. Quantitative angiography for measuring the minimal luminal diameter of a coronary lesion has greater predictive physiological significance with less intraobserver and interobserver variability. In recent years, the amount of information that can be obtained at the time of coronary angiography regarding the extent and severity of CAD has increased (see Chap. 18). Assessment of coronary flow reserve with Doppler-tipped catheters in conjunction with adenosine infusion adds value to the mere identification of coronary obstructive lesions. The use of intravascular ultrasonography has also provided important additional diagnostic and prognostic information in comparison with contrast angiography alone. Currently, the noninvasive techniques aimed at diagnosing CAD and assessing its functional and prognostic severity are being compared with physiological data obtained at cardiac catheterization using the flow wire or pressure wire and not with the degree of coronary anatomical narrowing alone.

Another significant limitation in determining the specificity of noninvasive techniques for detection of CAD is that most patients with normal noninvasive study findings (e.g., a normal stress perfusion scan or normal stress echocardiogram) are not referred for coronary angiography. Patients are referred for coronary angiography most often because of abnormal noninvasive test results, which leads to a *posttest referral bias,* whereby predominantly patients with true-positive or false-positive noninvasive test results (an abnormal perfusion scan or abnormal echocardiogram and normal coronary arteries) undergo angiography. Patients with true-negative noninvasive test results are usually not sent to cardiac catheterization. This trend has led to use of the normalcy rate as a surrogate for specificity in evaluating the accuracy of a noninvasive test for CAD diagnosis (see Chap. 13). The normalcy rate represents the percentage of normal scans in patients who have less than a 5 percent posttest likelihood of CAD when taking into account clinical information, the resting electrocardiogram (ECG), and exercise treadmill test results. When reviewing the literature, one should keep in mind this tendency of the posttest referral bias to lower the specificity if a normal coronary angiogram is required as the gold standard for a normal test result, particularly with reports following the introduction of a new test.

A critical observer should bear in mind that the sensitivity and specificity of a test for detecting a cardiovascular abnormality (e.g., significant CAD, resting left ventricular dysfunction) are always very high in the first few reports that are published for a newly introduced imaging methodology. These initial good results relate to many variables, including the inclusion of a highly selected patient population that may include normal volunteers on one end of the spectrum and patients with severe disease at the other end.

When evaluating the worth of a test for diagnosing cardiovascular disease or a complication of disease, cost should now also be considered.[2,3] One test may have a sensitivity that is a few percentage points higher than another test to which it is being compared, but the cost may be twice as high. Thus, the cost/benefit ratio should also be weighed when comparing the worth of two or more tests that are developed for the same clinical application.[4]

Table 16–1 summarizes the major clinical indications for noninvasive and invasive testing and lists various techniques applicable to each of these clinical indications. The remainder of this chapter sequentially addresses the headings provided in this table.

TABLE 16–1 Clinical Applications of Noninvasive and Invasive Techniques in Cardiovascular Disease

Assessment of left ventricular function
Two-dimensional or three-dimensional echocardiography
Contrast echocardiography
Radionuclide angiography
Gated SPECT
Gated MRI
Contrast ventriculography
Detection of coronary artery disease and assessment of prognosis
Exercise electrocardiographic stress testing
Exercise or pharmacological stress SPECT myocardial perfusion imaging
Exercise or dobutamine echocardiography
Contrast echocardiography with vasodilator stress
Pharmacological stress magnetic resonance perfusion imaging
Dobutamine stress MRI
Contrast-enhanced MRI
Magnetic resonance angiography
Magnetic resonance coronary lumen and plaque imaging
Electron beam computed tomography for calcium scoring and angiography
Multislice computed tomography angiography for calcium scoring and angiography
Selective intracoronary angiography, intravascular ultrasonography, and measurement of flow reserve
Assessment of myocardial viability
Resting SPECT perfusion imaging
Low-dose dobutamine echocardiography
Positron emission tomography
Contrast-enhanced MRI
Low-dose dobutamine MRI

MRI = magnetic resonance imaging; SPECT = single-photon emission computed tomography.

Assessment of Left Ventricular Function at Rest

Echocardiography (see Chap. 11)

Of all the noninvasive techniques available for the assessment of regional and global left ventricular function at rest, echocardiography is the most versatile overall, provides the most ancillary information, and has the lowest cost.[5] Two-dimensional echocardiography provides excellent images of the heart and great vessels, but it depends on obtaining satisfactory windows from the body surface to the area of interest in the heart. When good windows are obtained, echocardiography is superbly well suited for the evaluation of global and regional left ventricular systolic function because of its high spatial and temporal resolution and its ability to define both regional wall thickening and inward endocardial excursion. When compared with all other techniques, it should be the preferred initial test to diagnose heart muscle diseases of as yet unknown origin. These disease entities include ischemic cardiomyopathy, nonischemic dilated cardiomyopathy, hypertrophic cardiomyopathy, and restrictive myocardial disease (see Chap. 59). Resting echocardiographic technology not only allows a thorough assessment of cardiac morphology and function but also permits the simultaneous assessment of valvular, pericardial, intramyocardial, and extracardiac abnormalities.

Regional myocardial wall thickening is a better marker of regional function than is regional wall motion, and it is not influenced by either cardiac translation or the center of reference used. Regional thickening abnormalities cannot be well identified by radionuclide angiography or contrast ventriculography. The only other technique that perhaps permits a more accurate assessment of regional systolic thickening than echocardiography is gated MRI. This technique, however, is currently more expensive than two-dimensional echocardiography and cannot be performed at the bedside in critically ill patients. The advent of small portable echocardiographic apparatus could enhance only the bedside utility of this technique. A limitation of resting echocardiography in gauging the severity of regional or global left ventricular dysfunction is the lack of a reproducible quantitative technique to measure the left ventricular ejection fraction. A quantitative ejection fraction is better obtained by using alternative approaches such as left ventricular contrast angiography, radionuclide angiography, MRI, and quantitative gated SPECT imaging.

Echocardiography is invaluable in assisting in the detection of acute myocardial infarction and such mechanical complications as right ventricular infarction, acute mitral regurgitation from papillary muscle rupture or dysfunction, ventricular septal defect, a true or false left ventricular aneurysm, or pericardial effusion (see Chap. 11).[5] Thus, it is the noninvasive technique of choice for the comprehensive evaluation of regional and global left ventricular dysfunction and associated abnormalities in the setting of acute myocardial infarction. Transesophageal echocardiography can be performed at the bedside in an acutely ill patient with shock in the intensive care unit setting to help identify the cause of the hemodynamic disturbance. Echocardiography can also be performed in the emergency room in patients with chest pain and a possible acute ischemic syndrome. A defined regional wall motion abnormality in the absence of prior history of myocardial infarction lends support to a presumptive diagnosis that regional ischemia may be the cause of the chest pain syndrome.

Echocardiography is more sensitive than ECG for detecting left ventricular hypertrophy[6] and is an excellent technique for estimating left ventricular mass, which has been shown to independently predict cardiovascular morbidity and mortality.[7,8] The variability in left ventricular mass measurements and the reliability of serial measurements to assess regression of hypertrophy[9] have been reduced by the substitution of linear measurements of left ventricular wall thickness and internal dimension from the two-dimensional parasternal long-axis view whenever the two-dimensional directed M-mode beam is not ideally oriented for measuring thickness and cavity dimensions (see Chap. 11).[10] Further improvements in the echocardiographic measurement of left ventricular mass may be offered by three-dimensional localization of imaging slices.[11] Three-dimensional echocardiography with automatic edge detection software to identify endocardial borders permits measurement of left ventricular volumes with left ventricular ejection fraction calculated from volume-time loop curves for each frame. Tissue Doppler measurement of myocardial velocity displacement is another approach to better quantifying regional cardiac function.[12] Diastolic function can be evaluated by assessing transmitral flow velocities. Restrictive left ventricular filling patterns can be identified using pulsed Doppler echocardiography. Increased left atrial pressure from an increased left ventricular filling pressure can be assessed by measures of isovolumic relaxation time, E/A ratio, E-wave deceleration time, the ratio of systolic to diastolic pulmonary venous flow, and E/E′ ratio.[13]

Radionuclide Angiography (see Chap. 13)

First-pass radionuclide angiography and gated equilibrium blood pool radionuclide angiography are nuclear cardiology techniques that use a gamma camera and ECG gating for determining the changes in radioactivity in the left and right ventricular chambers over the cardiac cycle by generating time-activity curves. Quantitative ejection fraction measurements from both the right and left ventricles are highly accurate. Ventricular and pulmonary blood volumes and regional ventricular wall motion can also be assessed. As with echocardiography, resting radionuclide angiography is clinically useful for prognostication: the lower the resting left ventricular ejection fraction or the more global the left ventricular dysfunction, the worse the subsequent outcome with respect to survival. An advantage of radionuclide angiography over echocardiography is its ability to accurately quantitate the left and right ventricular ejection fractions by using a "count-based" technique and to obtain data in virtually all patients. Patients with arrhythmias can undergo radionuclide angiography, since windows for cycle length can be preset and all beats falling outside the window are rejected.

Chemotherapy with anthracycline agents can result in a dose-dependent deterioration in left ventricular function because of the toxic effects of the drug on cardiac myocytes (see Chap. 83). Radionuclide angiography is ideally suited to provide serial quantitative left ventricular ejection fraction measurements in patients who have received or are receiving doxorubicin therapy.[14] If doxorubicin administration is continued after objective evidence of reduced systolic function, significant symptomatic congestive heart failure and irreversible left ventricular dysfunction may ensue. Resting radionuclide angiography may provide a more quantitative assessment of left ventricular dysfunction after myocardial infarction, but it cannot provide other important information, such as the extent of infarction expansion, presence of left ventricular thrombus, development of mitral regurgitation, and extent of regional systolic thickening abnormalities. Radionuclide angiography provides significant prognostic information in patients with severe arrhythmias arising from the right ventricle in the setting of arrhythmogenic right ventricular cardiomyopathy.[15] Gated blood-pool imaging of left ventricular function can also be accomplished using SPECT technology, and left ventricular ejection fraction measurements using gated blood-pool SPECT correlate well with left ventricular ejection fraction measured by the standard planar technique.[16]

Gated Spect Imaging (see Chap. 13)

The emergence of technetium-99m (^{99m}Tc)-labeled myocardial perfusion agents led to the development of gated ^{99m}Tc-SPECT imaging, which permits simultaneous evaluation of regional systolic thickening, left ventricular volumes, global left ventricular function, and myocardial perfusion.[17,18] The introduction of gated ^{99m}Tc-SPECT imaging significantly enhanced the specificity of SPECT for the detection of CAD in patients with chest pain,[19,20] permitted measurement of regional wall thickening and detection of postischemic stunning,[21,22] and improved the ability to risk-stratify patients by providing information relevant to the global left ventricular ejection fraction.[23] New techniques using technology similar to that used for gated equilibrium blood pool imaging allow for automated determination of the left ventricular ejection fraction.[24] Thus, a quantitative global ejection fraction and percentage of thickening in various regions of the left ventricle can be reported with results of myocardial perfusion analysis under resting and stress conditions.

Severe perfusion abnormalities can limit quantitation of the left ventricular ejection fraction by the gated SPECT technique by interfering with detection of endocardial edges along the whole left ventricular volume on SPECT images. Manrique and colleagues found that gated SPECT underestimated the left ventricular ejection fraction when compared with equilibrium radionuclide angiography in patients with left ventricular dysfunction and large perfusion defects.[25] Other authors have reported accurate left ventricular ejection fraction measurements by gated SPECT in the presence of large perfusion defects.[26] Count-based techniques for assessing regional systolic thickening are not as adversely influenced by low regional radioactive counts in areas of severe defects.[24] Gated ^{99m}Tc-tetrofosmin SPECT imaging compared favorably with cine-MRI with respect to grading regional wall motion abnormalities in patients with an acute myocardial infarction.[27] Two methods of measuring left ventricular volumes by gated SPECT correlated well with MRI volumes, although the QGS (Quantitative Gated SPECT) technique underestimated the MRI values.[28] MRI cardiac images provide a complete three-dimensional portrayal of the heart with high spatial and temporal resolution.

Gated SPECT can also be performed with ^{201}Tl. He and associates[26] reported similar left ventricular ejection fraction measurements for ^{201}Tl-gated SPECT (54 ± 15 percent) and ^{99m}Tc-gated SPECT (54 ± 16 percent) in 63 patients who had left ventricular ejection fractions also determined by first-pass radionuclide angiography (54 ± 12 percent).

Gated fluorine-18 fluorodeoxyglucose (FDG) PET can accurately measure global left ventricular function and evaluate regional wall motion.[29] Global ejection fractions from FDG-PET were 29.3 ± 11.5 percent versus 31.1 ± 10.4 percent for radionuclide angiography.

Magnetic Resonance Imaging (see Chap. 14)

Cardiac MRI has emerged as a superb noninvasive technique for assessing left ventricular and right ventricular function.[30-32] Regional and global cardiac function can be evaluated at rest and under pharmacological stress with MRI, and high-speed MRI techniques allow for the simultaneous assessment of myocardial perfusion with magnetic resonance contrast agents. MRI is superior to other noninvasive imaging modalities in diagnosing congenital heart disease,[31,32] aortic disease, anomalous coronary arteries, and right ventricular dysplasia. At present, echocardiographic techniques appear to still have cost/benefit characteristics superior to those of MRI for assessing regional and global function. The major strength of MRI is its ability to provide high-resolution detail of cardiovascular anatomy. It can yield three-dimensional information on anatomy, function, and blood flow. It is accurate in determining wall thickness and may be the best technique for quantitating overall left ventricular mass. MRI tagging is an imaging modality that uses a grid overlying the full thickness of the myocardium on tomographic slices for assessment of progressive thickening of endocardial, midwall, and epicardial layers during the cardiac cycle. This technique measures intramyocardial function, which enhances measurement of the degree of regional myocardial dysfunction. Cardiac MRI is an excellent method for distinguishing ischemic from nonischemic cardiomyopathy and the assessment of patients with heart failure.[33] Serial assessment of left ventricular mass and volume is important in monitoring left ventricular remodeling after myocardial infarction, and this technique is being used in clinical trials to test certain pharmacological interventions for their effect on remodeling.

Contrast Left Ventriculography (see Chap. 17)

Left ventriculography has been available for many years for the assessment of left ventricular function in patients with a variety of pathological disorders. It has been used as the gold standard to which noninvasive techniques have been compared. Abnormal wall motion, but not abnormal thickening, can be assessed by contrast left ventriculography and quantitative measurements of left ventricular ejection fraction, and absolute volumes are highly reproducible and perhaps yield the most precise quantitative measurements of global function of all the noninvasive techniques discussed earlier. Limitations of contrast ventriculography include its invasive nature, high cost, potential nephrotoxicity of the dye, and the need to trace endocardial contours to quantitate ejection fraction and volume. Left ventricular hypertrophy and left ventricular mass are better quantitated by echocardiography or MRI. An advantage of contrast ventriculography is its ability to simultaneously measure intracavitary pressure and other hemodynamic variables such as stroke and end-diastolic volume, as well as performance of coronary angiography during the same cardiac catheterization procedure. Differentiation between dilated and ischemic cardiomyopathy can easily be made, and associated valvular lesions such as mitral or aortic regurgitation can be simultaneously diagnosed and semiquantitated. Left-to-right shunts at the atrial and ventricular levels are most accurately quantitated by cardiac catheterization measurements, although echocardiography and MRI can precisely localize atrial and ventricular septal defects.

THE UTILITY OF DIFFERENT APPROACHES TO THE ASSESSMENT OF LEFT VENTRICULAR FUNCTION

Overall, when all factors are considered, two-dimensional echocardiography with Doppler remains the most useful and convenient approach to assessment of resting left ventricular function. Its major limitation is an inability to visualize all regions of the left ventricle in every patient, and poor-quality images are acquired in certain patients, such as those with severe chronic obstructive pulmonary disease. The lack of a highly accurate and reproducible method for deriving a quantitative measurement of left ventricular ejection fraction also limits the utility of echocardiography. Contrast echocardiography improves visualization of myocardial walls and shows promise for the simultaneous assessment of regional perfusion at rest and during stress.[34] Echocardiographic contrast agents are capable of producing left ventricular cavity opacification, which helps in delineating endocardial borders, particularly in patients with poor acoustic windows.[35] Gated ^{99m}Tc-SPECT and gated MRI provide precise determinations of regional myocardial thickening and left ventricular ejection fraction, and MRI also allows for simultaneous assessment of perfusion and viability by using a contrast agent. Of course, patients with implanted pacemakers or automatic defibrillators are not candidates for MRI. Table 16–2 summarizes the strengths and limitations of the various techniques for assessment of regional and global left ventricular function.

Detection of Coronary Artery Disease

A number of noninvasive techniques are available to the clinician for detection of CAD in patients with chest pain. The techniques vary greatly in methodology but have as a fundamental principle the detection of myocardial ischemia or flow heterogeneity with exercise or pharmacological stress. The variables indicative of myocardial ischemia differ considerably and are specific for the test under consideration. The advent of myocardial imaging techniques using radionuclide tracers, echocardiography, or MRI methodology has provided enhanced accuracy for detection of CAD but at a higher cost than for the standard exercise treadmill test. Soon, noninvasive coronary angiography with multislice CT may become feasible, and plaque detection and characterization by MRI is on the horizon.[30,36,37] The strengths and limitations of the various noninvasive techniques used for the detection of CAD are described in the sections to follow.

Exercise Electrocardiography (see Chap. 10)

A review of the literature concerning the diagnostic accuracy of the standard exercise test was published by Gibbons and colleagues[38] and used as a basis for formulating guidelines for exercise testing by the American College of Cardiology/American Heart Association Practice Guidelines Task Force. Meta-analysis showed that the sensitivity and specificity of the exercise ECG stress test for the detection of CAD were 68 and 77 percent, respectively, in 147 consecutively published reports of patients who underwent both angiography and exercise testing.[39] However, bias from the selection of patients who agreed to undergo both treadmill testing and coronary angiography at the outset led to a 45 percent sensitivity for 1.0 mm of horizontal or downward ST segment depression but an 85 percent specificity.[40] Even when studies that included patients with resting ST segment depression were excluded, the sensitivity and specificity of the exercise test were only 67 and 84 percent, respectively.[38]

SENSITIVITY. The sensitivity of exercise ECG is very dependent on the level of exercise achieved. Sensitivity is reduced in patients who fail to achieve 85 percent of the age-adjusted maximum predicted heart rate or greater. Specificity of the ST segment depression response is markedly affected by variables such as left ventricular hypertrophy, hyperventilation, digoxin therapy, intraventricular conduction disturbances, preexcitation syndrome, hypokalemia, severe hypertension, and resting ST segment depression from a variety of causes. Many patients are precluded from undergoing treadmill testing alone because of nonspecific resting ST or T wave abnormalities, conduction abnormalities, or claudication. Interestingly, however, the specificity of the exercise test was only 69 percent in an analysis of 10 studies totaling 3548 patients who underwent exercise testing without digitalis therapy. Similarly, the specificity of the exercise test in studies excluding left ventricular hypertrophy only increased to 77 percent, which was just 8 percent higher than the 69 percent specificity of the ST segment response for CAD detection when studies including left ventricular hypertrophy were analyzed.

SPECIFICITY. The specificity of the exercise ECG response is also suboptimal in women, particularly those who are in the premenopausal age group with a low to intermediate pretest likelihood of CAD.[41] In contrast, the negative predictive value of a normal exercise ECG response in women

TABLE 16–2 Strengths and Limitations of the Various Diagnostic Techniques for Assessment of Left Ventricular Function

Technique	Strengths	Limitations
Echocardiography	Portability, immediate availability, versatility, repeatability Provides ancillary structural and physiological information High spatial and temporal resolution Accurately measures regional systolic thickening Sensitive for detecting LV hypertrophy and measuring LV mass Good for RV function assessment Excellent for detection of diastolic dysfunction LV volume with three-dimensional technique No ionizing radiation or contrast material needed Low cost	Poor acoustic windows in some patients Lack of quantitative ejection fraction High operator dependence
Radionuclide angiography	Accurate measurement of LV and RV ejection fractions Reproducibility Little operator dependency Serial monitoring of patients receiving cancer chemotherapy Quantitation of diastolic filling abnormalities	Regional systolic thickening not evaluated Radiation exposure Ancillary anatomical information not obtained Difficult to detect LV hypertrophy
Gated ^{99m}Tc SPECT imaging	Assessment of systolic thickening and wall motion Global LV ejection fraction and LV volumes accurately measured Simultaneous evaluation of perfusion and function Viability assessment Postischemic stunning identified	Decreased accuracy of LV ejection fraction assessment with large defects Lack of portability LV hypertrophy and mass not measured No ancillary structural information obtained Lower spatial resolution than ultrasonography and MRI
Magnetic resonance imaging	Absence of ionizing radiation Contrast agents not nephrotoxic Best technique for diagnosing congenital heart disease High-resolution anatomical detail Excellent for measuring wall thickness and LV mass Provides functional images in any desired imaging plane Can accurately assess regional and global LV function Gives three-dimensional information Proximal coronary arteries visualized Myocardial tagging permits analysis of subendocardial, midwall, and subepicardial function High-speed conrast-enhanced MRI permits perfusion imaging and viability assessment (delayed hyperenhancement)	Lack of portability Causes claustrophobia in some patients Need to correct for cardiac and respiratory motion Patients with metallic objects, pacemakers, and other devices excluded

LV = left ventricular; MRI = magnetic resonance imaging; RV = right ventricular; SPECT = single-photon emission computed tomography.

for excluding CAD is high. Women with a normal baseline resting ECG who achieve greater than 85 percent of the maximum predicted heart rate for age and have a normal peak stress ECG have an excellent prognosis and a low prevalence of underlying CAD. The negative predictive value of the exercise ECG response appears to be lower in men than in women, whereas the positive predictive value of the ST segment depression response is higher in men than women. Heart rate adjustment for the ST segment response may improve diagnostic accuracy of the exercise ECG.

EXTENT OF CAD. The extent of CAD affects the sensitivity of the exercise ECG. Its sensitivity is less than 50 percent for patients with single-vessel disease but exceeds 85 percent for patients with three-vessel disease. Horizontal or downsloping ST segment depression at low exercise heart rates has a higher positive predictive accuracy for CAD than does ST segment depression at very high heart rates or workloads. The administration of beta-blocking drugs certainly influences exercise test results, since these drugs prevent the patient from attaining the desired heart rate–blood pressure product at which ischemic ST segment depression would appear. This effect leads to an increased prevalence of false-negative responses. In addition, other antianginal drugs, such as nitrates given before testing, may prevent the appearance of abnormal ST segment changes. Slow upsloping ST segment depression has occasionally been used to increase the criteria for a positive test. Although such responses may enhance the sensitivity of the exercise ECG, specificity is lowered.[42]

In summary, although the exercise ECG is the least expensive of the noninvasive tests for detecting CAD, it has limited sensitivity and specificity in certain patient populations. Its main value may be as the initial test for excluding CAD in patients with a low pretest likelihood of CAD based on age and gender, in those who have a normal resting ECG, and in patients with nonanginal or very atypical chest pain.[43] If such patients achieve their maximum exercise heart rates with no ST segment depression and with normal hemodynamic responses, significant stenoses would not be likely to be the cause of their atypical chest pain syndrome. However, in most other populations, the exercise ECG is limited by suboptimal sensitivity and specificity for diagnosing CAD for the reasons outlined earlier.

Stress Radionuclide Myocardial Perfusion Imaging (see Chap. 13)

Exercise or pharmacological stress ^{201}Tl or ^{99m}Tc-sestamibi SPECT imaging in patients with chest pain yields a sensitivity for detecting CAD in the 85 to 90 percent range.[44,45] Specificity for excluding CAD is in the 90 percent range when gated SPECT imaging is used.[19] Exercise SPECT imaging and pharmacological SPECT imaging both yield sensitivities and specificities for CAD detection that are superior to those of exercise ECG testing alone.[44] Radionuclide stress perfusion imaging has particular value when compared with exercise ECG testing alone in (1) patients with resting ECG abnormalities, such as those seen with left ventricular hypertrophy, digitalis effect, preexcitation, and intraventricular conduction abnormalities, and (2) patients who fail to achieve greater than 85 percent of the maximum predicted heart rate and have no ST segment depression. Patients who fail to achieve a target heart rate and stop exercising at submaximal exercise levels demonstrate a higher sensitivity for CAD detection than when exercise ECG testing is performed alone because flow heterogeneity in response to stress appears earlier during the course of graded exercise stress. The ST segment depression response appears to require a higher rate-pressure product than that required to induce flow heterogeneity, which is demonstrated as a perfusion defect on scintigraphy.

The addition of stress perfusion imaging to the exercise ECG stress test greatly assists in differentiating true-positive from false-positive exercise ST segment depression responses. In patients with a low to intermediate pretest likelihood of CAD, approximately 40 percent with ST segment depression have no evidence of CAD (false-positive findings). Quantitative analysis of SPECT has resulted in a higher sensitivity and specificity than merely visual evaluation of SPECT images. The single-vessel disease detection rate with stress SPECT imaging is approximately 25 percent higher than the rate achieved with exercise ECG testing alone. The sensitivity for detecting three-vessel disease with exercise SPECT is in the range of 95 to 100 percent. A low percentage of patients with three-vessel disease, however, have inducible defects in all three vascular regions.[21,46]

LIMITATIONS OF PERFUSION IMAGING. A limitation of myocardial perfusion imaging is the difficulty in distinguishing false-positive defects due to attenuation artifacts from defects related to myocardial ischemia or scar. This high rate is predominantly attributed to image attenuation artifacts that are interpreted as defects secondary to CAD. Although quantitation of SPECT images improves specificity, the false-positive rate is higher than desirable, particularly with imaging of obese persons and women, who may demonstrate defects reflecting breast attenuation artifacts. Such artifacts are sometimes difficult to distinguish from myocardial perfusion abnormalities caused by inducible ischemia or from myocardial scarring (see Chap. 13). In the past decade, gated SPECT using ^{99m}Tc-labeled perfusion agents such as sestamibi and tetrofosmin has enhanced the specificity of SPECT. The quality of images obtained with ^{99m}Tc-labeled radionuclides is superior to that of images obtained with ^{201}Tl because of the more favorable physical characteristics of ^{99m}Tc for imaging with a gamma camera. The feasibility of using ^{99m}Tc doses approximately 10 to 20 times higher than the doses used with ^{201}Tl permits the acquisition of images with higher count density, less scatter and attenuation, and fewer artifacts than seen with ^{201}Tl imaging. Another limitation of exercise SPECT for detecting CAD is the influence of antiischemic medications administered at the time of testing.[47]

Electrocardiography-gated SPECT yields important information about regional and global left ventricular function that could previously be obtained only with a second test, such as radionuclide angiography, echocardiography, or contrast ventriculography. The ability to accurately measure the resting left ventricular ejection fraction with ^{99m}Tc-sestamibi or ^{99m}Tc-tetrofosmin adds supplementary value to the detection of reversible perfusion abnormalities alone.[23]

Since soft tissue attenuation causes nonuniformity of photon activity in the myocardium that results in artifacts often perceived as perfusion defects, attempts have been made to correct for attenuation by using certain algorithms emerging from advances in gamma camera instrumentation and software development.[48] Attenuation-corrected SPECT identified more left main CAD patterns (64 percent) than detected from uncorrected SPECT (7 percent) in a group of patients with 50 percent or greater left main stenoses.[49] Improvement in the normalcy rate can also be achieved by using attenuation/scatter-corrected images, thereby reducing the false-positive rate for CAD detection.[50] Attenuation correction and ECG gating in combination seems to provide the highest diagnostic accuracy for myocardial perfusion SPECT and enhance both sensitivity for multivessel disease detection and specificity for CAD detection.[51]

Some patients are less than ideal candidates for treadmill testing alone, and pharmacological stress with vasodilators such as dipyridamole or adenosine[52] or an inotropic agent such as dobutamine[53] is an alternative to exercise for detecting physiologically significant coronary artery stenosis. The basis for vasodilator perfusion imaging relates to the concept of coronary flow reserve (see Chap. 13). When coronary blood flow is maximally increased with an intravenously administered vasodilator, an impairment in flow reserve capacity in a stenotic artery simultaneous with a large flow increase in a normal vascular bed results in relative inhomogeneity of myocardial perfusion between normal and stenotic beds. If tracers such as ^{201}Tl or ^{99m}Tc-sestamibi are injected during peak vasodilation in the presence of a hemodynamically significant coronary stenosis with reduced flow reserve, heterogeneity in tracer uptake will be observed as defects on poststress images acquired soon after tracer injection. Sensitivity and specificity for CAD detection are comparable for dipyridamole and adenosine.[44] Dobutamine stress is preferred in patients who have bronchospasm or a history of asthma or in those who have consumed caffeine before testing. Dipyridamole or adenosine administration in these patients could result in severe bronchospasm. Vasodilator imaging is the scintigraphic method of choice for detection of CAD in patients with complete left bundle branch block. These patients are not candidates to undergo diagnostic exercise ECG testing alone.

Today, most laboratories use ^{99m}Tc perfusion imaging agents for detection of CAD in conjunction with exercise or pharmacological stress because of enhanced specificity for CAD detection and the ability to gate the images to the ECG to view regional systolic thickening. Mild nonreversible defects that represent attenuation artifacts usually show preserved systolic thickening, whereas if such areas of diminished tracer uptake represent scar, abnormal systolic thickening is observed. The dual-imaging approach involves performing rest ^{201}Tl imaging and stress imaging with one of the ^{99m}Tc-labeled perfusion agents.

Exercise and Dobutamine Stress Echocardiography (see Chap. 11)

Stress echocardiography can be performed with treadmill, upright bicycle, or supine bicycle exercise or by using pharmacological stressors such as dobutamine or dipyridamole.[5,54] Dobutamine stress has a higher sensitivity than does vasodilator stress. In a pooled analysis of data in the literature,[5] the weighted mean sensitivity, specificity, and overall accuracy for exercise echocardiography were 86 percent, 81 percent, and 85 percent, respectively. For dobutamine stress echocardiography, these values were 82 percent, 84 percent, and 83 percent, respectively. For the same reasons as outlined for SPECT perfusion imaging, stress echocardiography is more sensitive and specific for detecting inducible ischemia than is exercise ECG testing alone. Sensitivity is higher in multivessel-disease patients than in single-vessel disease patients and in patients with greater than 70 percent stenoses versus 50 percent to 70 percent stenoses.[5]

Variability exists in the literature with respect to sensitivity for CAD detection for stress echocardiography[5,55] and may be related to patient selection, including the percentage of patients in each study with previous infarction and/or multivessel disease, the definition of what constitutes a new stress-induced wall motion abnormality (a new wall motion abnormality versus failure to demonstrate hyperkinesis), the use of beta-blockers during testing, and pretest referral bias. The sensitivity of exercise echocardiography may be diminished if submaximal exercise heart rates are attained. Marwick and coauthors reported that when exercise heart rates were less than 85 percent of the maximum predicted heart rate, the sensitivity of exercise echocardiographic tests was only 42 percent.[56] The sensitivity of stress echocardiography in women is less than in men. Weighted mean sensitivity was 81 percent in 1000 women with suspected CAD, with a specificity of 86 percent.[5] Sensitivity was 89 percent in women with multivessel disease.

Digital imaging is advantageous for stress echocardiography for side-by-side comparison of regional function at rest and stress and for reviewing progression of contraction on a frame-by-frame basis.[54]

Side effects can be quite bothersome for patients undergoing dobutamine stress echocardiography. Secknus and Marwick reported premature termination of dobutamine stress echocardiography in 15 percent of 3000 patients.[57] Most of the episodes of premature test termination were due to cardiovascular side effects, including ventricular and supraventricular arrhythmias, severe hypertension, hypotension, severe ischemia by echocardiography, or severe chest pain.

COMPARISON OF EXERCISE SPECT PERFUSION IMAGING AND EXERCISE ECHOCARDIOGRAPHY

Stress echocardiography and stress perfusion imaging share common positive features that deserve emphasis before the value and limitations of each technique are compared. First, both are associated with a higher sensitivity and specificity for CAD detection than is exercise ECG testing alone. Second, both noninvasive techniques provide functional information for risk stratification, assessment of the area at risk, and determination of myocardial viability that is superior to that obtained with coronary angiography (see later).

Advantages of Stress Echocardiography. When compared with radionuclide perfusion imaging, advantages of stress echocardiography include the following: (1) The technique is totally noninvasive, safe, and repeatable; (2) no radiation exposure is involved; (3) the time to complete a full examination is short; (4) the technique is portable and requires no highly sophisticated instrumentation; (5) the cost is relatively low; (6) it has the ability to identify structural abnormalities of the heart, including coexisting valvular disease, left ventricular hypertrophy, and pericardial abnormalities; and (7) imaging quality is increased using contrast echocardiography versus conventional stress echocardiography to allow for simultaneous assessment of regional myocardial perfusion and regional systolic function. Contrast echocardiography with microbubbles performed in association with vasodilator stress permits the assessment of myocardial perfusion and can delineate the spatial extent and magnitude of stress-induced ischemia.[34,58]

Limitations of Stress Echocardiography. Limitations include the following: (1) Images are difficult to acquire at peak exercise because of exertional hyperapnea and cardiac excursion. (2) An ischemic response is required for the elucidation of regional abnormal wall motion, and inadequate heart rate responses, particularly with dobutamine echocardiography, reduce sensitivity. Atropine is often given to elevate the heart rate. (3) Rapid recovery of wall motion abnormalities can be seen with mild ischemia, particularly with single-vessel disease, which may lead to a false-negative test result if the images are not acquired rapidly after exercise. (4) Detection of residual ischemia within an infarct zone is difficult because of resting akinesis. (5) The technique is highly operator dependent for data collection and image analysis, and considerable interindividual variability in interpreting stress echocardiograms has been reported.[59] (6) Good-quality, complete images are acquired in only 70 percent of patients. An inability to image all of the left ventricular myocardium occurs in approximately 15 percent of patients. (7) A long training period is required to gain experience. (8) Quantitative assessment of inducible wall motion abnormalities and left ventricular ejection fraction is operator dependent. And (9), at present, myocardial contrast echocardiography can be difficult and is not ready for routine use. Intermittent imaging, in which microbubbles are destroyed and the time required for replenishment is measured by number of cardiac cycles, enhances the detection of flow heterogeneity using this technique.[58] Harmonic imaging has also increased the sensitivity of the technique. One multicenter phase II study showed a 93 percent concordance between dipyridamole ^{99m}Tc-sestamibi SPECT and dipyridamole stress myocardial contrast echocardiography for classifying patients as normal or abnormal and 74 percent concordance for location of perfusion defects.[60] For this study, intermittent harmonic power Doppler was performed to quantitate myocardial blood flow velocity. A limitation of assessment of myocardial perfusion imaging for CAD detection using this technique is the number of falsely abnormal results in the circumflex territory compared with ^{99m}Tc-sestamibi SPECT.[61]

Advantages of Stress Perfusion Imaging. When compared with conventional exercise echocardiography, the following advantages of exercise myocardial perfusion imaging for detection of CAD can be listed: (1) myocardial perfusion imaging detects abnormal flow reserve and does not require an ischemic response for a positive test result; (2) data relevant to abnormal myocardial perfusion are obtained at peak stress with treadmill exercise rather than after exercise, as required for echocardiography; (3) the sensitivity for detecting CAD is slightly higher (8 to 10 percent) with exercise perfusion imaging, chiefly because the sensitivity for detecting single-vessel disease and mild stenoses of 50 to 70 percent narrowing is lower with exercise echocardiography; (4) perfusion imaging appears to identify more ischemic regions than stress echocardiography does, perhaps because mere flow heterogeneity and not true ischemia causing systolic myocardial dysfunction produces defects on stress scintigrams; (5) infarct zone ischemia is more easily identified with perfusion imaging by demonstration of a partial reversible defect in an area that contains a mixture of scar and viable myocardium; (6) operator dependency is not nearly as much a factor with SPECT perfusion imaging for the acquisition of images as it is with echocardiography; (7) virtually 100 percent of patients can undergo adequate SPECT perfusion imaging in which all areas of the myocardium are visualized; (8) with ^{99m}Tc-sestamibi or ^{99m}Tc-tetrofosmin, simultaneous assessment of myocardial perfusion and function can be obtained, and the resting left ventricular ejection fraction, regional wall thickening, and ventricular volumes can be accurately measured from gated ^{99m}Tc SPECT; and (9) vasodilator stress SPECT imaging has a significantly higher sensitivity for CAD detection than does vasodilator stress echocardiography.

Limitations of Stress Perfusion Imaging. When compared with stress echocardiography, the limitations of stress SPECT imaging are (1) longer imaging protocols, which may take many hours; (2) greater equipment expense and the necessity of injecting radiopharmaceuticals with exposure to radiation; (3) less than desirable specificity for CAD detection in many laboratories because of failure to distinguish attenuation artifacts (e.g., breast, diaphragmatic) from scarring; (4) inability to visualize the heart in a real-time approach; (5) lower spatial resolution than seen with echocardiography; (6) higher cost to patients; (7) lower detection rate of three-vessel disease patients who have balanced ischemia or diffusely abnormal flow reserve yielding perfusion images with homogeneous tracer uptake; and (8) often difficulty in evaluating the inferior wall because of high visceral uptake of the ^{99m}Tc-labeled tracers.

COMPARATIVE STUDIES OF STRESS ECHOCARDIOGRAPHY VERSUS PERFUSION IMAGING

In seven comparative studies,[62] the overall sensitivity of myocardial perfusion imaging was 80 percent versus 74 percent for stress echocardiography. In contrast, the specificity for stress echocardiography was higher than that of myocardial perfusion imaging (88 percent versus 78 percent). When single-vessel disease detection was analyzed separately, the sensitivity of myocardial perfusion imaging was 76 percent, as compared with 67 percent for stress echocardiography. Another review of the literature by O'Keefe and colleagues that involved 11 studies and 808 patients reported an overall sensitivity and specificity for stress echocardiography of 78 and 86 percent, respectively, as compared with 83 and 77 percent for myocardial perfusion imaging.[63] Schinkel and colleagues[64] reviewed 17 direct comparisons comprising 1405 patients and confirmed a slightly higher overall sensitivity (84 percent versus 80 percent) for stress radionuclide perfusion imaging, but specificity was higher for echocardiography (86 percent versus 77 percent). Most of the nuclear studies analyzed did not employ gated SPECT, which enhances specificity.[65]

Fleischmann and associates reviewed 44 articles to compare the diagnostic performance of exercise echocardiography and exercise SPECT imaging for CAD detection.[66] These authors concluded that when exercise echocardiography was compared with exercise SPECT via a receiver operating characteristic model, exercise echocardiography yielded significantly better discriminatory power when adjusted for age, publication year, and a setting including known CAD than did SPECT studies. This review did not include some of the more recent studies using gated ^{99m}Tc SPECT in which the specificity for detection of CAD is higher than the specificity with ^{201}Tl.[19] Also, in the SPECT cohort, combination of different radionuclide imaging agents and reading techniques and inclusion of studies utilizing experimental techniques resulted in significant heterogeneity of sensitivity and specificity value.[55] A high prevalence of CAD in studies reported enhanced sensitivity in the meta-analysis.[67]

Few studies have compared multiple diagnostic techniques for CAD detection in the same patient population. In one study, 60 patients being evaluated for the first time for chest pain underwent exercise stress testing, dipyridamole and dobutamine stress echocardiography, and dipyridamole and dobutamine ^{99m}Tc-sestamibi imaging.[68] With greater than 70 percent coronary stenosis used as the criteria for CAD, the sensitivity was 58 percent for exercise ECG testing, 55 percent for dipyridamole echocardiography, 61 percent for dobutamine echocardiography, 97 percent for dipyridamole ^{99m}Tc-sestamibi, and 91 percent for dobutamine ^{99m}Tc-sestamibi. The specificities for these tests were 67, 96, 96, 89, and 81 percent, respectively. All tests yielded higher sensitivity values for multivessel disease than for single-vessel disease. Although dobutamine echocardiography had a lower sensitivity than reported by other groups, this result agrees with the observation in another study that approximately 25 percent of patients manifested dobutamine-induced perfusion abnormalities without reversible wall motion abnormalities on dobutamine echocardiography.[69] Smart and colleagues[70] reported comparable sensitivity (87 percent) for dobutamine-atropine echocardiography and dobutamine ^{99m}Tc-sestamibi SPECT, but dobutamine echocardiography was more specific (95 percent versus 76 percent). Gated SPECT was not performed, which may have influenced specificity. Diagnostic accuracy for single-vessel disease detection was not improved when dobutamine ^{99m}Tc-sestamibi imaging and dobutamine echocardiography were combined.[71] Quantitative gated SPECT correlates well with echocardiography for assessment of left ventricular volumes and left ventricular ejection fraction.

Magnetic Resonance Coronary Angiography
(see Chap. 14)

Magnetic resonance coronary angiography (MRCA) is a developing technique and can depict the major coronary arteries.[30,32,72,73] Obstacles to its clinical use include need for correction for cardiac and respiratory motion, for millimeter spatial resolution, and for suppression of signal from adjacent epicardial fat and myocardium. Avoiding the need for breath-holding with real-time tracking of diaphragmatic motion would be advantageous. Three-dimensional navigator-gated (to compensate for respiratory motion in the foot-to-head direction) and prospectively corrected free-breathing MRCA can provide more favorable signal-to-noise ratios but is limited by poor contrast between coronary blood and myocardium. Kim and colleagues[74] performed MRCA during free breathing and could evaluate 84 percent of proximal and middle coronary artery segments and found an accuracy of 72 percent in diagnosing CAD. It was highly accurate in ruling out left main CAD. Yang and colleagues[72] have reported the ability of a spiral high-resolution coronary imaging sequence for MRCA with rapid real-time localization. This technique achieved 0.7 to 0.9 mm resolution with 14-heartbeat breath-holds, good image quality in 78 percent of coronary segments, and a 76 percent sensitivity and a 91 percent specificity for CAD detection compared with x-ray angiography. Cardiac MRI can noninvasively measure coronary flow velocity reserve after stent deployment with values similar to those obtained with invasive intracoronary Doppler.[75] This method had an 83 percent sensitivity and 94 percent specificity for detecting restenosis (75 percent or greater stenoses). MRCA, using a high-resolution navigator-gated three-dimensional technique, was highly accurate in detecting vein graft disease.[76] The receiver-operating characteristic curve for detecting graft occlusion was 0.89.

Magnetic Resonance Perfusion Imaging
(see Chap. 14)

Magnetic resonance perfusion imaging can be used for CAD detection employing bolus injection of gadolinium after dipyridamole or adenosine administration. In 84 patients who also underwent coronary angiography, this technique employing a turbogradient echo/echo-planar imaging-hybrid sequence yielded a sensitivity of 88 percent, specificity of 90 percent, and accuracy of 89 percent.[77] A myocardial blood flow reserve index can be determined with vasodilator gadolinium MRI, which can assist in the identification of patients with abnormal flow reserve in areas remote from stenotic regions.[78] Resting MRI has been evaluated for detecting acute coronary syndromes in the emergency room and yields a sensitivity of 84 percent and a specificity of 85 percent.[79] This approach includes assessment of both perfusion and regional systolic function.

Dobutamine MRI is another approach to detecting myocardial ischemia. When used with myocardial tagging, dobutamine cardiac MRI was performed at rest and during increasing doses of dobutamine in 211 consecutive patients with chest pain. Patients with new wall motion abnormalities underwent coronary angiography, of whom 96 percent had significant CAD on angiography.[80] Compared with resting PET imaging, flow reserve indices by first-pass perfusion MRI underestimate flow reserve values but could represent a useful semiquantitative technique for detection and severity of regional stenotic lesions.[81] Myocardial perfusion imaging with cardiac MRI hypothetically should be more sensitive for detecting subendocardial ischemia compared with exercise or vasodilator SPECT imaging because of its enhanced resolution. Subendocardial ischemia can be separated from subepicardial ischemia with contrast MRI performed with hyperemia following vasodilator stress. In one study, receiver-operating characteristic analysis of subendocardial upslope data revealed a sensitivity of 91 percent and a specificity of 94 percent for detection of CAD as defined by PET and 87 percent and 85 percent, respectively, in comparison with quantitative coronary angiography.[82] Abnormal subendocardial perfusion has been detected in patients with cardiac syndrome X employing MRI with perfusion imaging.

Magnetic resonance imaging offers the potential of examining the atheromatous lesion as well as the lumen.[73] However, traditional selective x-ray coronary angiography currently offers higher resolution (0.1 mm). Arteries can be viewed by MRI in cross section, and plaques can be visualized and characterized.[83-85] High spatial resolution black-blood MRI, a method free of motion and blood flow artifacts, provides noninvasive images of the coronary artery lumen and wall. This technique might be useful for identifying asymptomatic coronary atherosclerosis.[86,87] Figure 16–1 shows an example of lipid-rich plaque identified by MRI.[87] Macrophages that accumulate in atherosclerotic plaques in carotid arteries have been detected with MRI enhanced by injection of ultrasmall superparamagnetic particles of iron oxide.[88] This may be a promising MRI approach for identifying rupture-prone atherosclerotic lesions in humans. In the future, real-time MRI-guided catheterization of coronary arteries using dilute contrast agents will be feasible.[89]

Noninvasive Intravenous Coronary Angiography Using Computed Tomography (see Chap. 15)

A new generation of multislice CT systems permits the simultaneous acquisition of up to 16 submillimeter slices with fast rotation, yielding

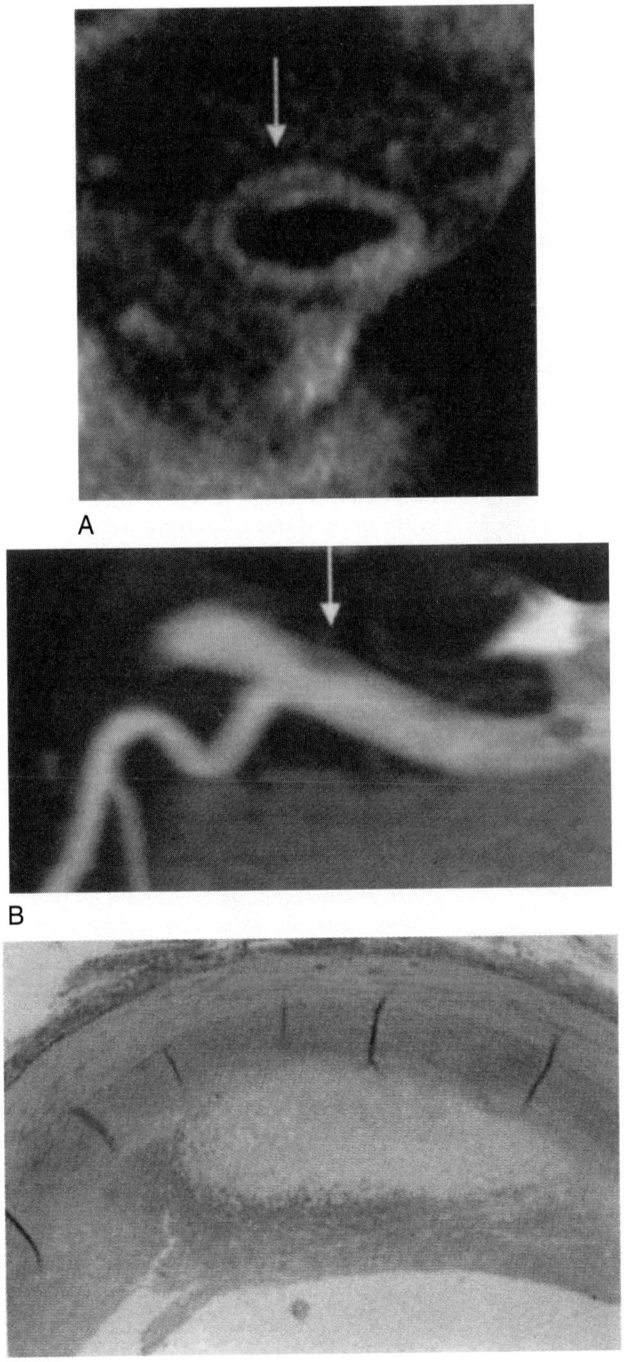

FIGURE 16–1 Magnetic resonance imaging and computed tomography (CT) plaque characterization. **A,** Cross-sectional ex vivo T2-weighted magnetic resonance image of the human left anterior descending artery with a lipid-rich lesion (arrow). **B,** Multislice CT image of the same lesion (arrow) showing a low-density area containing lipid-rich tissue. **C,** Corresponding histopathological section showing a significant lipid containing plaque. (From Fayad ZA, Fuster V, Nikolaou K, Becker C: Computed tomography and magnetic resonance imaging for noninvasive coronary angiography and plaque imaging: Current and potential future concepts. Circulation 106:2026, 2002.)

coronary CT angiograms of good quality when the heart rate is initially lowered to 60 beats/min employing beta blockade.[36] Figure 16–2 shows an example of a CT coronary angiogram showing an ostial stenosis of the left main coronary artery.[36] In comparison with invasive coronary angiography, multidetector spiral CT scanning correctly classified 85 percent of patients as having at least one coronary stenosis and correctly detected 73 percent of all coronary lesions. After excluding coronary arteries that were classified as unevaluable by noninvasive CT angiography, 57 of 62 lesions were detected, and absence of significant stenoses was correctly identified in 194 of 208 vessels. This yielded a 92 percent sensitivity and 93 percent specificity for detection of coronary artery stenoses. A limitation of contrast-enhanced, ECG-gated multislice spiral CT is that about 30 percent of coronary arteries are unevaluable, mainly because of artifacts caused by coronary motion. When only evaluable arteries are considered, this technique had a 91 percent sensitivity and an 84 percent specificity for detecting stenoses of 70 percent or greater.[90] EBCT can also be used for noninvasive coronary angiography.[91] Multislice CT angiography provides better image quality in more coronary segments than EBCT angiography because of its better contrast-to-noise ratio and higher spatial resolution.[91] One main reason for unevaluable arteries by multislice CT angiography is heavy coronary calcification that is seen in approximately 10 percent of plaques. Fortunately, breath-holding is reduced to 20 seconds in the 16-slice per second CT scanners. For the future, multislice CT must be done in real time with fast postprocessing techniques. Ultimately, its value could be greatest in imaging patients with a low probability of CAD to exclude a significant coronary stenosis.

Multidetector CT scanners or EBCT scanners can detect coronary atherosclerosis by the demonstration of coronary calcification (see Chap. 15).[1,92] Because the presence of coronary calcium is very specific for presence of atherosclerosis, any identifiable calcium on CT scanning is considered as evidence for CAD. The specificity of coronary calcification, however, for identifying flow-limiting stenoses is limited, since many patients can have a high coronary calcium score but no obstructive coronary stenoses that would produce an ischemic response on stress testing using other modalities. Sensitivity is, of course, very high, although some patients have lipid-laden, noncalcified plaques causing angina without demonstration of coronary calcification on scanning. Coronary calcification imaging with CT scanning has been chiefly employed for risk assessment in asymptomatic patients with data showing that the higher the calcium score, the greater the risk for subsequent coronary events. The relative risk of coronary events is in the range of 4.0 for patients with calcium scores above a certain threshold compared with those with scores below that threshold.[93] Figure 16–3 shows the risk of cardiac events relative to tertiles of calcium scores and low or high C-reactive protein values from the work of Park and associates.[94]

Assessment of Prognosis of Patients Evaluated for Coronary Artery Disease (see Chap. 50)

One of the chief applications of noninvasive stress testing in patients with suspected or known CAD is the identification of patients at either high or low risk for future ischemic cardiac events.[5,38] Prognostication using noninvasive stress ECG testing or stress imaging technology is based on the rationale that physiological alterations under stress conditions predict events better than does knowledge of coronary artery anatomy. Accurate risk stratification contributes importantly to clinical decision-making. For example, patients who are identified as being at low risk for future cardiac events on the basis of noninvasive test variables can be spared unnecessary or premature referral for invasive strategies unless symptoms are not adequately alleviated by antiischemic drugs. Conversely, patients with high-risk ECG stress test and/or imaging variables may benefit from early referral for invasive strategies, including revascularization, even if symptoms are mild.

Treadmill ECG Stress Testing for Evaluation of Prognosis (see Chap. 10)

Treadmill exercise ECG stress testing alone without the addition of an imaging procedure is useful for differentiating low- and high-risk patients with chest pain. The demonstration of 1.0 mm or more of horizontal or downsloping ST segment depression at low exercise heart rates or workloads is a significant predictor of an adverse outcome when using exercise ECG testing for prognostication. Perhaps the most powerful predictive variable on treadmill testing for identifying high-risk patients is functional capacity reflected by workload

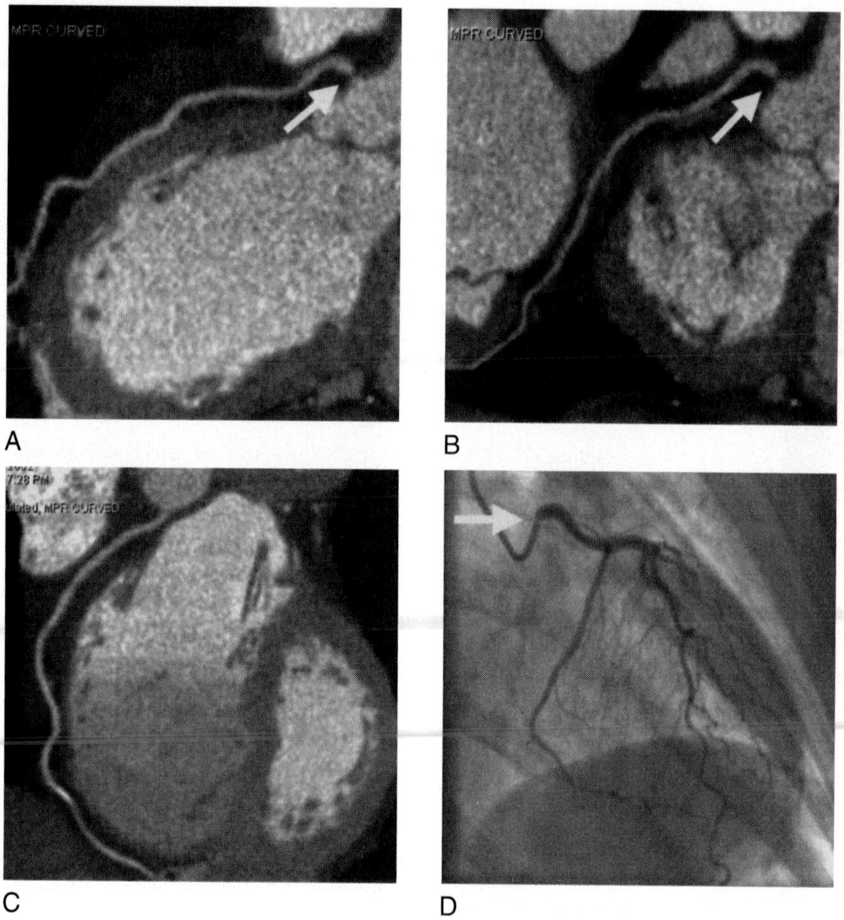

FIGURE 16–2 Thin-slice multidetector row spiral computed tomography scan showing an ostial stenosis of the left main coronary artery. **A,** Curved multiplanar reconstruction of the left main and left anterior descending coronary arteries showing the osteostenosis (arrow). **B,** Curved multiplanar reconstruction of the left main and circumflex coronary arteries with the same left main osteostenosis shown (arrow). **C,** Curved multiplanar reconstruction of the right coronary artery with no stenoses present. **D,** Contrast invasive coronary angiogram showing the severe left main osteostenosis (arrow). (From Ropers D, Baum U, Pohle K, et al: Detection of coronary artery stenoses with thin-slice multi-detector row spiral computed tomography and multiplanar reconstruction. Circulation 107:664, 2003.)

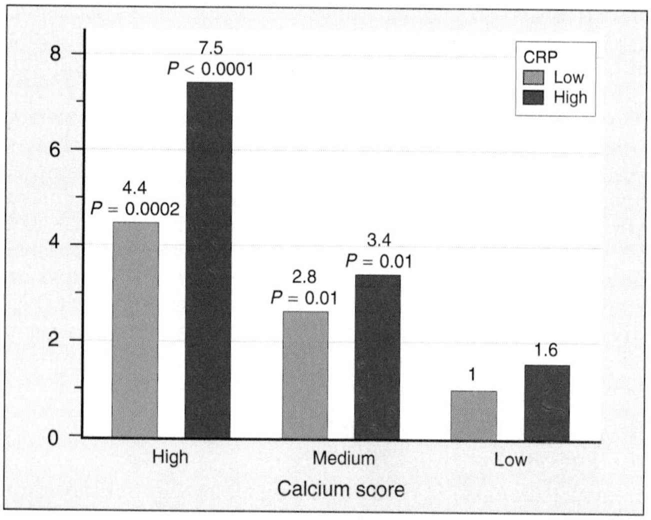

FIGURE 16–3 Risk ratios of nonfatal myocardial infarction, coronary death, percutaneous transluminal coronary angioplasty, coronary artery bypass grafting, or stroke associated with high (±75th percentile) and low levels of C-reactive protein (CRP) and high (>142.1), medium (3.7 to 142.1), and low (<3.7) tertiles of calcium scores. The highest risk of an event is in the patient group with a high calcium score and high CRP. (From Park R, Detrano R, Xiang M, et al: Combined use of computed tomography coronary calcium scores and C-reactive protein levels in predicting cardiovascular events in nondiabetic individuals. Circulation 106:2073, 2002.)

achieved.[95] Absolute peak exercise capacity is a stronger predictor of death than the percentage of age-predicted maximum heart rate achieved.[95] Each one metabolic equivalent (MET) increase in exercise capacity was associated with a 12 percent improvement in survival. Figure 16–4 shows the risk of death related to workload achieved on exercise testing in groups of patients with various risk factors.[95] Chronotropic incompetence, identified as an attenuated heart rate response to exercise, predicts increased mortality. A very rapid heart rate recovery immediately after exercise was associated with a lower risk of cardiovascular disease events in the Framingham study.[96] Poor exercise tolerance can be observed in patients with depressed resting left ventricular function with or without superimposed transient exercise-induced ischemia.

A treadmill score has been proposed for better separating high- and low-risk patients undergoing ECG stress testing (see Chap. 10). Perhaps the most popular of these scores, derived by the Duke University group, relies on the duration of exercise, the maximal ST segment deviation, and a treadmill angina index.[97] In a follow-up study from the Duke group,[98] patients with a low-risk Duke treadmill score who were treated medically had a 3.1 percent 5-year mortality rate, whereas those deemed at high risk had a 35 percent 5-year mortality rate. The low-risk group, which represented 36 percent of the cohort, had a 40 percent prevalence of any CAD and a 9 percent prevalence of severe CAD determined angiographically. The high-risk group, which represented only 9 percent of the entire cohort, had a 74 percent incidence of severe CAD, and all patients had at least one or more coronary stenoses.

The practical problem with the Duke treadmill score is that a substantial proportion of patients are classified as having intermediate or moderate risk after exercise ECG treadmill testing. In a study by Shaw and associates, 55 percent of the patients were classified as having moderate risk by the Duke treadmill score, and they had a 9.5 percent 5-year mortality rate and a 31 percent prevalence of severe CAD.[98] Perfusion imaging variables are useful in further risk-stratifying patients with intermediate-risk Duke treadmill scores.[99,100] A substantial number of these patients can be deemed to be at low risk if they show normal perfusion or only a mild posexercise defect.

LIMITATIONS. Exercise ECG stress tests have other important limitations in assessing prognosis. First, a strongly positive exercise ECG, which is defined as an early or low ischemic threshold, significant horizontal ST segment depression, and a prolonged ST depression recovery time, does not necessarily signify more severe CAD by either angiographic or scintigraphic criteria.[101] The extent of exercise ST segment depression poorly predicts the extent of CAD, and the maximum ST segment depression achieved at peak exercise correlates poorly with the extent of stress-induced hypoperfusion by scintigraphy. Also, a considerable portion of patients have an uninterpretable exercise ECG response.[102] For these patients, imaging variables provided substantial supplementary prognostic information over ECG stress test variables. Patients with normal exercise perfusion scans or exercise echocardiograms have an excellent outcome even if the ECG stress test is nondiagnostic or abnormal.

Exercise ECG testing alone has particular utility in the risk assessment of patients with a normal resting ECG who have nonanginal or very atypical chest pain. If these patients achieve an adequate exercise heart rate or workload without significant ST segment depression, the prognosis during follow-up is excellent. Stress imaging is not cost effective in patients with low-risk Duke treadmill scores unless they have a significant number of high-risk clinical variables (e.g., advanced age, diabetes). However, for improved diagnostic and prognostic value, an imaging technique should be performed in conjunction with treadmill testing in patients with an intermediate or a high pretest likelihood of CAD on the basis of age, gender, and type of chest pain.

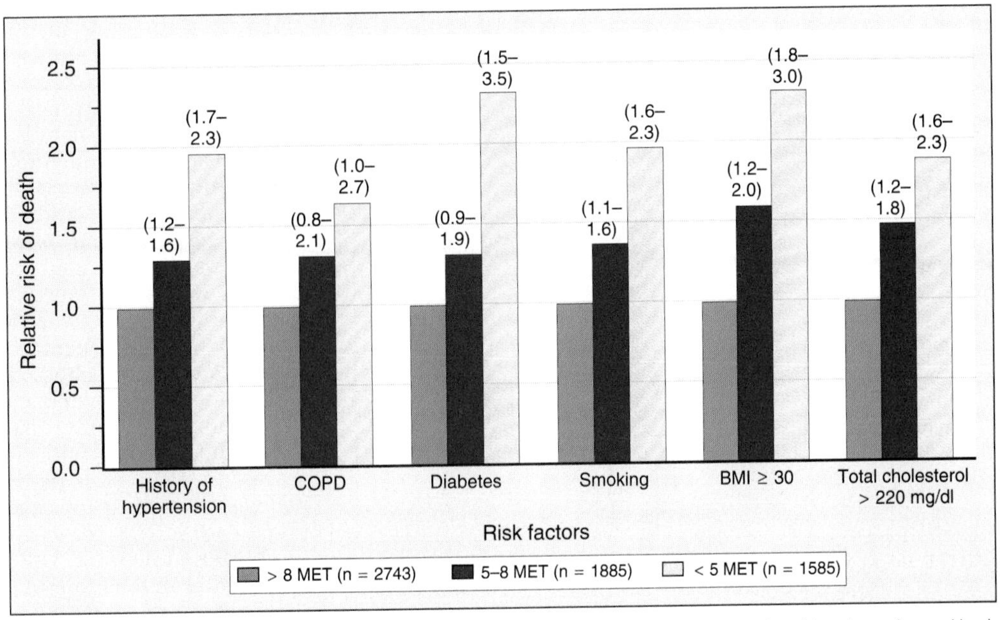

FIGURE 16–4 Relative risks of death from any cause among subjects with various risk factors who achieved exercise workloads of either less than 5 METs or 5 to 8 METs compared with subjects whose exercise capacity was more than 8 METs (first bar of each triad normalized to 1.0). The numbers within parentheses above the bars are 95% confidence intervals. BMI = body mass index; COPD = chronic obstructive pulmonary disease. (From Myers J, Prakash M, Froelicher V, et al: Exercise capacity and mortality among men referred for exercise testing. N Engl J Med 346:793, 2002. Copyright © 2002 Massachusetts Medical Society. All rights reserved.)

Stress Myocardial Perfusion Imaging for Evaluation of Prognosis (see Chap. 13)

The prognostic value of exercise and pharmacological stress myocardial perfusion imaging has been established in thousands of patients evaluated in multiple clinical studies.[44,45,103] The major prognostic variables on stress perfusion images predictive of future cardiac events are (1) a large defect size (>20 percent of the left ventricle); (2) multiple perfusion abnormalities in two or more coronary supply regions suggestive of multivessel CAD; (3) defect reversibility reflective of inducible ischemia in multiple myocardial segments, even in the distribution of one major coronary artery; (4) a large number of nonreversible defects; (5) transient left ventricular cavity dilation from stress to rest images; (6) increased ^{201}Tl lung uptake best assessed by quantitating the lung/heart ^{201}Tl ratio; and (7) a resting left ventricular ejection fraction of less than 40 percent measured on gated SPECT.[44,45] One of the most valuable features of exercise or pharmacological stress perfusion imaging with ^{201}Tl, ^{99m}Tc-sestamibi, or ^{99m}Tc-tetrofosmin is the ability to predict a low combined mortality and nonfatal myocardial infarction rate in patients with a totally normal scan. In a pooled analysis of 20,963 patients from 16 published studies in the literature with a follow-up of slightly more than 2 years, the combined annual cardiac death or nonfatal infarction rate in those with normal perfusion scans was 0.7 percent per year.[44] The annual hard cardiac event rate is in the range of 7.0 percent in patients with abnormal scans.[104]

INCREMENTAL VALUE OF PERFUSION IMAGING OVER ECG STRESS TESTING. Numerous published studies have demonstrated the incremental value of stress myocardial perfusion imaging over clinical and ECG treadmill stress test variables for prognostication. The event rate increases in proportion to the extent of stress-induced hypoperfusion or the extent or severity of reversible defects reflective of ischemia. With gated SPECT, the extent of regional wall motion or thickening abnormalities, the ejection fraction and end-systolic and end-diastolic volumes, and the extent of reversible regional dysfunction on poststress images indicative of stunning add to the high-risk assessment.[21-23,46,105,106] Patients at the highest risk for subsequent cardiac death or infarction are those with baseline left ventricular dysfunction with moderate to severe stress-induced reversible perfusion defects.[23] Patients at the lowest risk for subsequent cardiac events are those who demonstrate good exercise tolerance (e.g., achieving 85 percent or greater of maximum predicted heart rate) with normal perfusion on SPECT images.[107] As mentioned earlier, imaging variables on stress/rest SPECT imaging provide incremental prognostic information over clinical and exercise stress test variables, including the Duke treadmill score.[100,108] Figure 16–5 shows the death or myocardial infarction rate per year in patients with low, intermediate, or high Duke treadmill scores further risk stratified by the extent of the stress defect on exercise SPECT images.[100] It appears that variables on stress perfusion imaging might identify patients who have an excellent outcome with medical therapy even with the demonstration of mild ischemia.[109] In contrast, patients with extensive stress-induced hypoperfusion may have a better outcome with respect to cardiac mortality with revascularization strategies.[109]

COST-EFFECTIVENESS OF SPECT IMAGING. The use of myocardial perfusion imaging as an initial evaluation in patients with stable chest pain is highly cost-effective when compared with an initial invasive strategy. A large observational study consisting of 11,372 consecutive stable angina patients referred for stress myocardial perfusion SPECT imaging or direct catheterization revealed that costs were higher for the initial invasive strategy in clinical subsets with a low, intermediate, or high pretest likelihood of disease.[110] Diagnostic and follow-up costs of care were 30 to 41 percent higher for patients undergoing direct cardiac catheterization without any reduction in mortality or infarction. The diagnostic costs were, respectively, $1320, $1275, and $1229 greater for low-, intermediate-, and high-risk patients undergoing initial cardiac catheterization than for those having stress perfusion imaging as the initial test for CAD detection. The cardiac death rate and nonfatal infarction rate in the 5826 patients undergoing initial stress perfusion imaging for assessment of stable angina were both 2.8 percent as compared with 3.3 and 3.0 percent, respectively, for the 5423 patients who were referred directly for cardiac catheterization as the initial diagnostic strategy. The cost of screening women with myocardial perfusion imaging was shown in a separate analysis to be considerably lower than the cost of direct coronary angiography in a similar type of analysis.[111] Thus, stress myocardial perfusion imaging undertaken as the initial step in diagnosis and assessment of prognosis yields comparable outcomes at a lower cost than does direct referral for cardiac catheterization. This noninvasive strategy

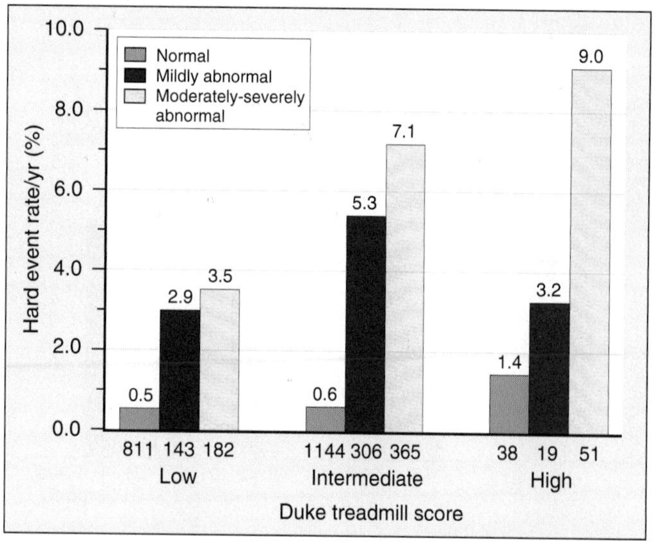

FIGURE 16–5 Rates of hard cardiac events per year as a function of the results of stress single-photon emission tomography (SPECT) in patients with low, intermediate, or high Duke treadmill scores; $P < 0.05$ across SPECT categories in all Duke treadmill score subgroups. (From Hachamovitch R, Berman DS, Kiat H, et al: Value of stress myocardial perfusion single photon emission computed tomography in patients with normal resting electrocardiograms: An evaluation of incremental prognostic value and cost-effectiveness. Circulation 105:823, 2002.)

is "ischemia driven" and should be applicable even to patients with angiographic disease and normal scans, since this group also has an excellent prognosis.[112]

CONCLUSIONS. Thus, taken together, data reported from the literature demonstrate that patients with normal regional myocardial perfusion and normal left ventricular function on gated SPECT scans have an excellent prognosis, whereas patients with abnormal scans have an increased rate of cardiac death and nonfatal infarction during follow-up. The greater the extent of stress-induced hypoperfusion and reversibility, the greater the probability of an event. It is apparent from the many studies cited that myocardial perfusion imaging variables provide supplementary prognostic information to exercise ECG testing alone, particularly in patients who have an intermediate risk of an adverse outcome estimated by clinical variables and exercise stress testing. Diabetic patients seem to significantly benefit from stress perfusion imaging for separating high and lower risk subsets.[113,114] Stress perfusion imaging variables appear to be equal or even superior to mere knowledge of coronary anatomical variables for assessing prognosis because the extent of hypoperfusion during stress and the magnitude and extent of stress-induced ischemia better predict subsequent cardiac death than does demonstration of the presence of one-, two-, or three-vessel disease alone. In fact, patients with three-vessel disease on angiography can be further risk-stratified by myocardial perfusion imaging performed after catheterization into low-, intermediate-, and high-risk groups.

Echocardiographic Assessment of Prognosis (see Chap. 11)

Evaluation of left ventricular function on the resting echocardiogram obtained before commencing the stress portion of the protocol offers considerable prognostic information by itself. A large area of asynergy is predictive of future cardiac events. The sensitivity of stress echocardiography to identify patients with severe CAD is good.

Heupler and coauthors reported that detection of exercise-induced wall motion abnormalities independently predicted cardiac events in 508 women monitored for 41 ± 10 months after exercise echocardiography.[115] Evidence of ischemia by echocardiography foretold future cardiac events better than did exercise capacity or inducible ST segment depression. The prognostic data provided by the exercise echocardiogram added to that provided by clinical and exercise ECG variables in patients with both undiagnosed and known CAD. In a study from the same institution consisting of both men and women, the presence of ischemia on exercise echocardiography predicted future cardiac events well and, in a multivariate model, was the strongest independent predictor of cardiac death, myocardial infarction, or unstable angina.[116]

Exercise echocardiography has been reported to provide incremental prognostic information in patients 65 years of age or older.[117] An abnormal left ventricular end-systolic volume response and exercise left ventricular ejection fraction were independent predictors of cardiac events. In patients with good exercise capacity, extent and severity of exercise-induced left ventricular dysfunction provided independent and incremental prognostic value.[118] Incremental values of exercise echocardiography are comparable in men and women.[119] Marwick and associates[120] showed that exercise echocardiography, like exercise SPECT, is particularly useful in patients with intermediate-risk Duke treadmill scores. In 5375 patients, the mortality rate was 1 percent per year in patients with normal exercise echocardiograms (Fig. 16–6).

COMPARISON WITH PERFUSION IMAGING

Few studies in the literature have compared exercise echocardiography with exercise perfusion imaging for long-term prediction of prognosis. Olmos and colleagues compared clinical, exercise, echocardiographic, and SPECT ^{201}Tl variables in 248 patients who underwent both stress imaging modalities simultaneously.[121] The clinical models characterized by exercise echocardiography with exercise ECG testing and ^{201}Tl SPECT with exercise ECG were comparable in the prediction of cardiac events. For the exercise echocardiography model, the exercise wall motion score index and induction of ischemia were the strongest predictors of events. For the model with exercise ^{201}Tl SPECT, the strongest predictor was the extent of the ischemic perfusion defect. Of interest, for the prediction of ischemic events and/or cardiac death, echocardiographic and ^{201}Tl variables were the only predictive variables.

One reason for the failure to predict some events by stress echocardiography is the inability to attain an adequate heart rate response. This limitation agrees with the finding of compromised sensitivity of stress echocardiography for detecting ischemia in the setting of inadequate heart rate responses.[56] Therefore, patients who are deemed unable to exercise

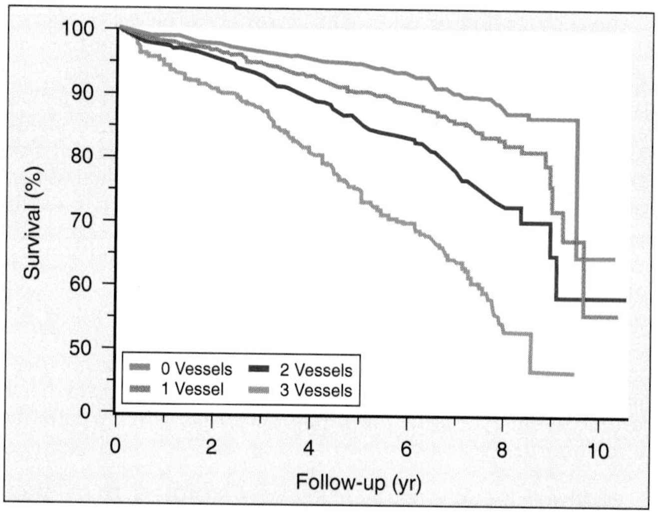

FIGURE 16–6 Survival free of death according to total extent of wall motion abnormalities at peak stress on exercise echocardiography. The extent of wall motion abnormality is reflected as a one-vessel, two-vessel, or three-vessel disease pattern. (From Marwick TH, Case C, Vasey C, et al: Prediction of mortality by exercise echocardiography: A strategy for combination with the Duke treadmill score. Circulation 103:2566, 2001.)

adequately should undergo dobutamine stress echocardiography for both diagnosis and prognosis indications.

With respect to the comparison of dobutamine echocardiography and simultaneously performed ^{99m}Tc-sestamibi SPECT imaging, Geleijnse and coauthors reported that any abnormality or ischemia on echocardiography or scintigraphy was associated with cardiac events.[122] Dobutamine-atropine echocardiography and ^{99m}Tc-sestamibi imaging provided comparable prognostic information. With respect to the negative predictive value of a normal study, patients with normal study results had equally very low event rates (0.4 percent by echocardiography and 0.5 percent by ^{99m}Tc-sestamibi). As with exercise perfusion imaging, patients with a normal exercise echocardiogram have a very low cardiac event rate.[5,123]

Dobutamine echocardiography also provides prognostic value in patients with suspected or known CAD. In the study by Poldermans and colleagues of 1737 patients with known or suspected CAD who underwent dobutamine-atropine stress echocardiography, a normal echocardiographic study was associated with an annual event rate of cardiac death or infarction of 1.3 percent over a 5-year period.[124] In that study, the rate of cardiac death or myocardial infarction in patients with new wall motion abnormalities or extensive resting wall motion abnormalities increased 3.6-fold and 2.5-fold, respectively. A negative echocardiographic response to pharmacological stress in women was associated with a less than 1 percent hard cardiac event rate over 3 years of follow-up.[125] Echocardiographic evidence of ischemia was found as the only independent predictor of hard cardiac events (odds ratio, 27.5) in this study. Marwick and colleagues[126] showed that dobutamine echocardiography is an independent predictor of death, and a normal study finding is associated with a 1 percent annual mortality risk. In a multicenter trial comprising 7333 patients who underwent either high-dose dipyridamole echocardiography or high-dose dobutamine echocardiography, Kaplan-Meier survival estimates showed a significantly better outcome for patients with normal pharmacological stress echocardiograms compared with those with abnormal studies during a mean follow-up of 2.6 years.[127]

Few studies have directly compared vasodilator stress and inotropic stress with echocardiography for prognostication.

Prediction of Perioperative Ischemic Events

A meta-analysis of 15 studies demonstrated the prognostic value of dipyridamole ^{201}Tl imaging and dobutamine echocardiography for predicting perioperative ischemic events in patients undergoing risk stratification before vascular surgery (see Chap. 77).[128] For dipyridamole ^{201}Tl studies, the cardiac death rate or myocardial infarction rate was 1, 7, and 9 percent for normal results, fixed defects, and reversible defects, respectively. For patients with a dobutamine-induced new or worsening wall motion response, 23.1 percent had a perioperative ischemic event as compared with 0.4 percent of patients with a normal stress echocardiographic response. Summary odds ratios were greater for dobutamine echocardiography than for dipyridamole ^{201}Tl, but the 95 percent confidence intervals were wider with echocardiography because of a smaller sample size. Late cardiac events after vascular surgery (average 19 ± 11 months) can also be predicted by stress-induced ischemia on dobutamine echocardiography.[129]

CONCLUSIONS: STRESS PERFUSION IMAGING VERSUS STRESS ECHOCARDIOGRAPHY

In summary, both stress perfusion imaging and stress echocardiography provide prognostic information supplemental to that of clinical and exercise ECG stress test variables. Both techniques have excellent negative predictive value for identifying low-risk patients. Such patients with either a normal perfusion study finding at peak stress or normal regional function have an excellent outcome with a cardiac death or infarction rate of less than 1 percent per year. The negative predictive value of a normal study result is perhaps slightly better with perfusion imaging than echocardiography because of its slightly higher sensitivity for identifying mild CAD. Patients with high-risk stress imaging findings on either perfusion imaging or echocardiography have a worse outcome with medical therapy, and the greater the degree of regional abnormalities (either perfusion or function), the higher the event rate. Either technique is superior to exercise ECG test variables alone. An abnormal workload and a suboptimal heart rate response are excellent prognostic variables derived from the ECG stress test for identifying high-risk patients. Ischemia occurring at low exercise heart rates and workloads should prompt evaluation with coronary angiography. Pharmacological stress imaging provides comparable prognostic information to exercise imaging for both nuclear cardiology and echocardiographic techniques, and either can be used for preoperative risk stratification in intermediate- or high-risk patients scheduled for vascular surgical procedures. Patients with normal vasodilator stress or dobutamine stress perfusion scans have a higher event rate than patients with normal exercise images. Improvement in ischemic perfusion abnormalities is observed with medical therapy for CAD, which improves endothelial function. Advances in contrast echocardiography and attenuation- and scatter-corrected SPECT with quantitation will improve accuracy of these imaging techniques.

MAGNETIC RESONANCE PERFUSION AND FUNCTION IMAGING (see Chap. 14)

Magnetic resonance perfusion imaging performed with gadolinium-based contrast agents and a stressor such as adenosine and assessment of regional left ventricular function with MRI during dobutamine stress are alternative approaches to detecting CAD and assessing prognosis. Few data are available with respect to the prognostic value of vasodilator stress myocardial perfusion MRI or dobutamine stress MRI. In one study, the cardiac event-free survival rate was 98.2 percent for patients with negative dobutamine cardiac MRI study at an average follow-up of 17.3 months.[80] The presence of inducible ischemia or a left ventricular ejection fraction of less than 40 percent on dobutamine/atropine MRI was associated with future cardiac death or myocardial infarction at 20 months of follow-up (hazard ratio 3.3).[130] Dipyridamole stress MRI had 85 percent agreement with ^{201}Tl scintigraphy in detection of CAD and a correlation of 0.86 in sizing perfusion defects.[131]

Stress MRI with contrast may ultimately be very clinically useful in that the technique provides high spatial resolution and has the capability of imaging in any desired plane without ionizing radiation. Images can be acquired with reproducible quality that is operator independent. Since no imaging window is required, images can be obtained in virtually all patients, including those with emphysema. The endocardial border can easily be defined and separated from the cavity blood volume.

Disadvantages of stress MRI techniques are an inability to image patients with pacemakers and implanted cardioverter-defibrillators and the need for prolonged breath-holding.

Table 16-3 summarizes the major strengths and limitations of the various techniques used for detection of CAD and assessment of prognosis.

Noninvasive Assessment of Myocardial Viability

Regional and global left ventricular dysfunction leading to depressed left ventricular ejection fractions in patients with CAD can result from myocardial necrosis or scarring, postischemic stunning, or myocardial hibernation (see Chaps. 44 and 50). *Hibernation* is defined as the state in which myocytes are chronically hypoperfused or repetitively

TABLE 16–3 Major Strengths and Limitations of Various Techniques for Detecting Coronary Artery Disease and Assessing Prognosis

Technique	Strengths	Limitations
Exercise ECG	Low cost, short duration Functional status evaluated High sensitivity in three-vessel or left main CAD Provides useful prognostic information (e.g., ischemia at low workload) Indicated as first test for patients at low probability of CAD	Suboptimal sensitivity Low detection rate of one-vessel disease Nondiagnostic with abnormal baseline ECG Poor specificity in certain patient populations (e.g., premenopausal women) Need to achieve ≥85 percent of maximum heart rate for maximizing accuracy
Exercise or pharmacological SPECT perfusion imaging	Simultaneous evaluation of perfusion and function with gated SPECT Higher sensitivity and specificity than exercise ECG High specificity with ^{99m}Tc-labeled agents Studies can be performed in almost all patients Significant additional prognostic value Comparable accuracy with pharmacological stress Viability and ischemia simultaneously assessed Quantitative image analysis	Suboptimal specificity because of artifacts Long procedure time when rest and stress both performed with ^{99m}Tc-labeled agents No standardized correction for attenuation and scatter Higher cost than exercise ECG Radiation exposure Poor-quality images in obese patients Absolute flow reserve not quantitated May underestimate three-vessel disease because of "balanced ischemia"
PET perfusion imaging	Accurate quantitation of blood flow in ml/g/min secondary to tracer kinetic modeling and attenuation correction using either rubidium-82 or nitrogen-13 ammonia	Use restricted to pharmacological stress High cost Low availability
Exercise or pharmacological stress echocardiography	Higher sensitivity and specificity than exercise ECG Additional prognostic value Comparable value with dobutamine stress Short time to complete examination Identification of coexisting structural cardiac abnormalities (e.g., valvular disease) Simultaneous evaluation of perfusion with contrast agents Relatively lower cost than other techniques No radiation	Decreased sensitivity for detection of one-vessel disease or mild stenosis with postexercise imaging Inability to image all of the left ventricle in some patients Highly operator dependent for image analysis No quantitative image analysis Poor acoustic window in some patients (e.g., chronic obstructive lung disease) Infarct zone ischemia less well detected False-positive defects in posterolateral wall with contract echo
Magnetic resonance imaging	High spatial resolution MRI coronary angiography promising Bypass grafts well seen Imaging of arterial wall and plaque Flow mapping with contrast Visualization of subendocardial perfusion Pharmacological stress procedure short No radiation	Inability to image patients with metal devices Difficult to image in setting of irregular heart rhythm Motion artifacts in absence of good breath-hold and respiratory gating Coronary motion No large clinical studies yet published
EBCT angiography and MSCT angiography	Noninvasive coronary angiography to rule out significant coronary stenoses	Radiation exposure Cardiac motion artifacts Beta blockers often required to reduce heart rate to <60 beats/min Artifacts caused by coronary motion Unevaluable arteries for lumen assessment with heavy calcification Prolonged breath-holding for scanners with <16-slice per sec Images not generated in real time MSCTA better contrast-to-noise ratio and spatial resolution compared with EBCTA but 3.5 times higher radiation exposure Slow acquisition time for MSCTA

CAD = coronary artery disease; EBCT = electron beam computed tomography; ECG = electrocardiogram; MSCT = multislice computed tomography; PET = positron emission tomography; SPECT = single-photon emission computed tomography; VD = vessel disease.

stunned but in which flow is sufficient to sustain structural integrity. Hibernating myocardium, by definition, demonstrates improved systolic function with improved resting perfusion after coronary revascularization.

An accurate noninvasive determination of myocardial viability that is capable of distinguishing irreversible myocardial cellular injury from hibernation is critically important for the clinical decision-making process. It allows for improved selection of patients with CAD and resting left ventricular dysfunction who will benefit most from revascularization strategies.[132] Patients with substantial zones of myocardial viability in asynergic myocardium reflective of hibernation demonstrate better function and overall improved outcomes after revascularization than do patients with left ventricular dysfunction predominantly caused by myocardial scarring. Such patients with extensive areas of viability have a better survival rate with revascularization than medical therapy (Fig. 16–7).[132]

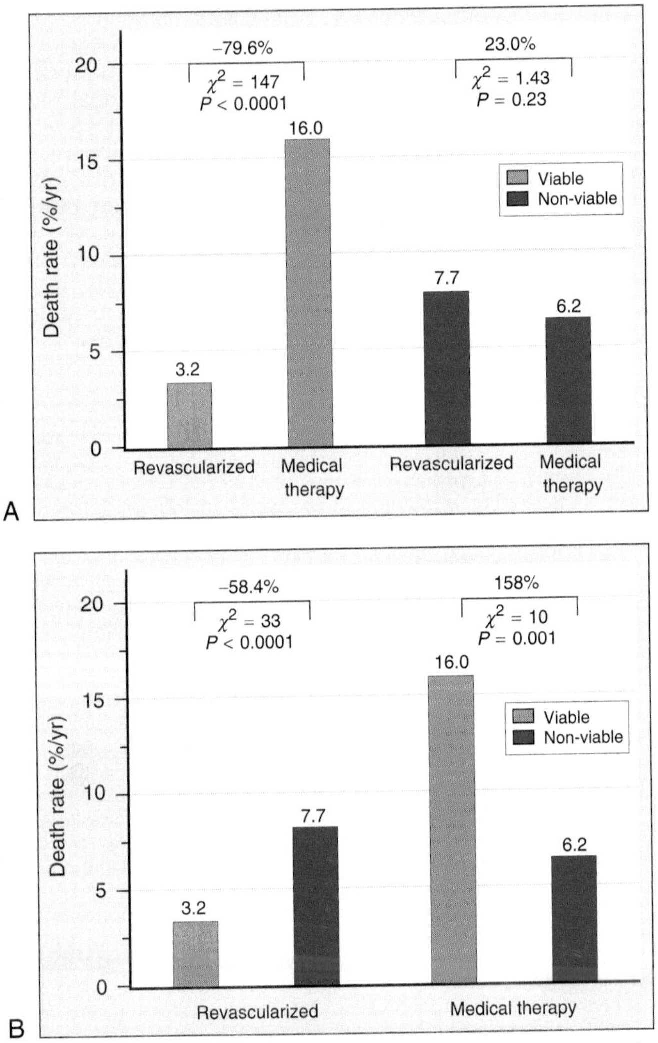

FIGURE 16–7 **A,** Death rates for patients with and without myocardial viability treated by revascularization or medical therapy. There is a 79.6 percent reduction in mortality for patients with viability treated by revascularization ($P < 0.001$). No significant difference in mortality with revascularization versus medical therapy was observed in patients with predominantly nonviable myocardium. **B,** Same data as in part A with comparison made on treatment strategy in patients with and without viability. Annual mortality was significantly higher in medically treated patients when viability was present versus absent. (From Allman KC, Shaw LJ, Hachamovitch R, Udelson JE: Myocardial viability testing and impact of revascularization on prognosis in patients with coronary artery disease and left ventricular dysfunction: A meta-analysis. J Am Coll Cardiol 39:1151, 2002. Copyright 2002, with permission from American College of Cardiology Foundation.)

Techniques Used for Myocardial Viability Assessment

Thallium-201 Imaging (see Chap. 13)

Thallium-201 rest and delayed redistribution imaging is the most commonly used radionuclide imaging modality for the assessment of myocardial viability. It is used for this purpose because the initial uptake of ^{201}Tl is related to both blood flow and myocardial membrane integrity. Several groups have shown that approximately 60 to 70 percent of asynergic myocardial segments showing greater than 50 or 60 percent ^{201}Tl uptake on resting ^{201}Tl scintigraphy will show improved systolic function after revascularization.[133] The most likely reason for the lack of enhanced systolic function after revascularization in zones judged to be viable before revascularization is the presence of subendocardial scar. That is, certain segments showing 20 to 30 percent subendocardial scarring may not demonstrate improved systolic thickening after revascularization, even if greater than 50 percent ^{201}Tl uptake is seen in those regions. However, such patients may benefit from revascularization by reducing stress-induced ischemic dysfunction or reinfarction. Other problems with ^{201}Tl include poor-quality images in obese patients, difficulty in distinguishing attenuation artifacts from scar, and the long imaging time to perform rest-redistribution studies (e.g., 4 hours).

Technetium-99m-Labeled Agents (see Chap. 13)

Technetium-99m-labeled perfusion agents do not show significant redistribution over time after being injected intravenously at rest. Nevertheless, several studies have shown comparable sensitivity and specificity for viability detection between these agents and ^{201}Tl.[134,135] The advantage of ^{99m}Tc-labeled agents is less attenuation and less scatter than noted with ^{201}Tl, which produces higher quality images. In addition, gated SPECT imaging can be undertaken with ^{99m}Tc-sestamibi or ^{99m}Tc-tetrofosmin to allow for simultaneous assessment of regional systolic thickening in myocardial perfusion. Demonstration of intact thickening at rest or when images are acquired during dobutamine infusion indicates viability. The detection of viability in asynergic regions is enhanced with nitrates given prior to ^{99m}Tc-sestamibi administration, as demonstrated by Sciagra and associates.[136] This study showed the prognostic value of nitrate ^{99m}Tc-sestamibi perfusion imaging in relation to medical versus revascularization therapy.

Positron Emission Tomography (see Chap. 13)

Positron emission tomography is considered by many to be the standard of reference for the noninvasive detection of myocardial viability by nuclear cardiology techniques because PET imaging can simultaneously assess myocardial perfusion and metabolism.[137] Nitrogen-13-labeled ammonia is the most often used perfusion tracer, and FDG is the metabolic tracer for assessing glucose utilization. Patients with a mismatch pattern, with reduced perfusion but preserved FDG uptake, will show improved regional and global left ventricular function after revascularization, whereas patients demonstrating a concordant reduction in perfusion and FDG uptake (a "match" pattern) have predominantly myocardial scar as the cause of asynergy, and segments showing this pattern have a significantly lower chance of improved function after revascularization. Preserved myocardial oxygen consumption estimated by carbon 11 (^{11}C)-acetate PET imaging is found in myocardial regions that are hibernating. Hence, ^{11}C-acetate PET imaging[138] is an alternative to FDG-PET imaging for detection of viability. From the practical standpoint relevant to clinical decision-making, no difference in cardiac event-free survival between PET-guided and SPECT-guided patient management has been observed.[139] Both techniques are associated with comparable outcomes with respect to patient survival after revascularization (Fig. 16–8).[132,139]

Dobutamine Echocardiography (see Chap. 11)

Low-dose dobutamine echocardiography is another useful modality for assessment of viability.[5,133] The rationale for inotropic stress is the identification of contractile reserve in zones of severe myocardial asynergy. This technique furnishes an alternative noninvasive approach to resting SPECT perfusion imaging or PET imaging. Enhanced systolic thickening with low-dose dobutamine predicts functional recovery well. A biphasic response in which systolic thickening increases at low doses and then deteriorates at high doses indicates both viability and ischemia and is the most sensitive criterion for improved function after revascularization.[140] End-diastolic wall thickness is also an important marker of

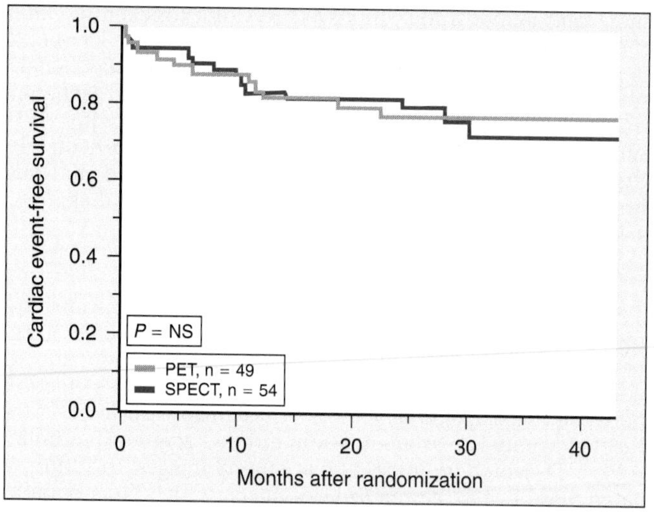

FIGURE 16–8 Cardiac event-free survival curves for patients randomized to ^{13}N-ammonia/^{18}FDG-PET or stress/rest ^{99m}Tc-sestamibi SPECT-based management (revascularization or medical therapy). All patients were potential candidates for revascularization. Note that there was no difference in survival with either the PET or the SPECT strategy in patient evaluation. (From Siebelink H-MJ, Blanksma PK, Crijns HJGM, et al: No difference in cardiac event-free survival between positron emission tomography-guided and single-photon emission computed tomography-guided patient management: A prospective, randomized comparison of patients with suspicion of jeopardized myocardium. J Am Coll Cardiol 37:81, 2001. Copyright 2001, with permission from American College of Cardiology Foundation.)

myocardial viability in patients with suspected hibernation and has been shown to predict recovery of function in a manner similar to that of ^{201}Tl scintigraphy after revascularization. The greater the number of viable segments detected by dobutamine echocardiography, the greater the chance is of survival after revascularization in patients with ischemic cardiomyopathy.

Contrast echocardiography with microbubbles for assessment of myocardial perfusion is a complementary technique to evaluating inotropic reserve for viability assessment in CAD patients with severe left ventricular dysfunction. This may be beneficial in predicting left ventricular contractile recovery in patients with acute myocardial infarction who have undergone reperfusion therapy.[141] The presence of preserved myocardial perfusion by myocardial contrast echocardiography before primary coronary stenting in acute myocardial infarction patients is associated with maintained or improved perfusion at 3 to 5 days and eventual recovery of resting wall motion of the infarct zone.[142] The greater the improvement in microcirculatory perfusion by intravenous contrast echocardiography, the greater the functional recovery in the zone of infarction. Myocardial contrast echocardiography can also be used to identify hibernating myocardium. In one study in 20 patients, the sensitivity of contrast echocardiography for prediction of recovery of function after revascularization was 90 percent, compared with 92 percent for ^{201}Tl SPECT and 80 percent for demonstration of dobutamine-induced contractile reserve.[143] A drawback of the contrast echocardiographic technique is artifacts in basal inferior segments, limiting interpretation in this area.[144]

Magnetic Resonance Imaging (see Chap. 14)

Contrast-enhanced MRI can accurately distinguish normal myocardium from myocardium with subendocardial or transmural scar based on the spatial extent of hyperenhancement.[145,146] With this technique, gadolinium is injected intravenously, and the agent concentrates in necrotic tissue in patients with acute infarction or in scar tissue 10 minutes later, whereas it has washed out of normally perfused and viable myocardium. The scarred area appears bright, and there is a close correlation between the volume of the signal enhancement and the transmural extent of nonviability. Wagner and colleagues reported that resting SPECT and contrast-enhanced MRI detect transmural myocardial infarctions at similar rates (Fig. 16–9), but MRI has significantly higher sensitivity for detecting subendocardial infarcts that are missed by SPECT.[147] In this study, cardiac MRI identified 92 percent of segments with subendocardial infarction characterized by less than 50 percent transmural extent of the full thickness of the left ventricular wall, whereas SPECT identified only 28 percent of these areas. Both techniques show comparable specificity (97 to 98 percent). MRI hyperenhancement, as a detector of myocardial scar, seems to identify scar tissue more frequently than PET (Fig. 16–10),[148] and MRI also differentiates between subendocardial scar and transmural scar better than PET.

The clinical reproducibility of contrast-enhanced MRI for infarct size assessment is excellent and compares favorably with that of clinical SPECT.[149] McCrohon and associates demonstrated that gadolinium-enhanced cardiac MRI may be a very useful technique to distinguish ischemic cardiomyopathy causing left ventricular dysfunction from dilated cardiomyopathy.[150] In that study, CAD patients had contrast enhancement primarily with a subendocardial or transmural pattern, whereas patients with dilated cardiomyopathy had either no enhancement (59 percent), patchy or midwall enhancement different from the distribution in CAD patients (28 percent), or enhancement patterns indistinguishable from those of patients with ischemic cardiomyopathy (13 percent). Finally, in a study looking at the ability of contrast MRI to predict improvement in left ventricular function after revascularization, Kim and associates[151] showed that the likelihood of improvement in regional contractility after revascularization decreased progressively as the transmural extent of hyperenhancement observed before revascularization increased. Approximately 80 percent of segments with no hyperenhancement improved function after revascularization, whereas if only 25 percent of the transmural tissue was normal, only a small percentage improved with revascularization.

Dobutamine MRI may also be employed for the assessment of viability and predicting myocardial functional recovery after revascularization.[152] Dobutamine-induced systolic wall thickening in zones of severe myocardial asynergy has an approximately 70 percent to 90 percent sensitivity and specificity for predicting functional recovery after revascularization. Dobutamine MRI with tagging and contrast-enhanced MRI have been shown to be complementary in assessing functional recovery after reperfused myocardial infarction.[153] A reduction in the transmural extent of a hyperenhancement by contrast-enhanced MRI early after myocardial infarction is associated with early restoration of flow and subsequent improvement in regional function.[154]

As previously cited for other applications with cardiac MRI, problems include patient claustrophobia in the closed scanner-designed instruments; inability to scan patients with implantable devices such as pacemakers, defibrillators, and cerebral aneurysm clips; and

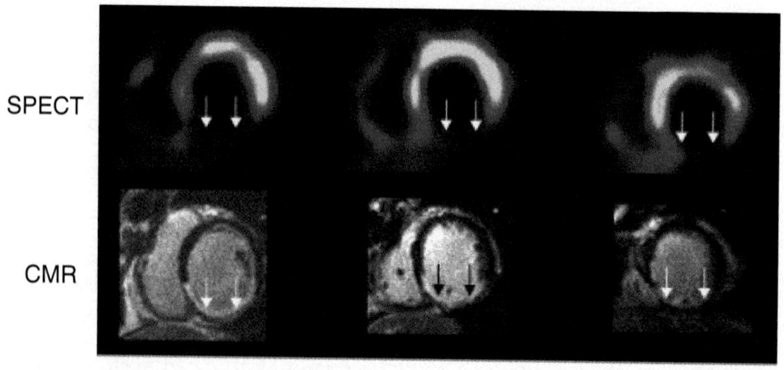

FIGURE 16–9 Short-axis views of resting thallium-201 single-photon emission computed tomography (^{201}Tl-SPECT) (top row) and contrast-enhanced cardiac magnetic resonance imaging (MRI) in a patient with a nearly transmural inferior wall infarction. Note that an area of delayed hyperenhancement on MRI scans (arrows) correlates well with the region of the severe perfusion abnormality on SPECT scan. (From Wagner A, Mahrholdt H, Holly TA, et al: Contrast-enhanced MRI and routine single photon emission computed tomography (SPECT) perfusion imaging for detection of subendocardial myocardial infarcts: An imaging study. Lancet 361:374, 2003.)

inability to obtain adequate images in patients with significantly irregular rhythms such as atrial fibrillation. Image artifact emanating from excessive respiratory motion may be a problem without good respiratory gating techniques such as navigator imaging. Long-term outcome studies in large numbers of patients with respect to the capability of contrast-enhanced MRI techniques to identify which patients have the best prognosis with revascularization versus medical therapy have not been undertaken as have been for the more conventional techniques employing radionuclide imaging or echocardiography.

STRENGTHS AND WEAKNESSES OF VARIOUS MODALITIES FOR ASSESSING VIABILITY

When compared with ^{201}Tl or ^{99m}Tc-sestamibi, dobutamine echocardiography is more specific but less sensitive. The positive predictive value of inotropic reserve for predicting improved regional systolic function with dobutamine echocardiography after revascularization is higher than that of ^{201}Tl scintigraphy when greater than 50 percent ^{201}Tl uptake is used as the criterion for myocardial viability. The number of asynergic segments exhibiting preserved ^{201}Tl uptake or showing rest ^{201}Tl redistribution exceeds the number of segments with residual capacity for systolic thickening as determined by dobutamine infusion.[155] Similarly, the number of severely asynergic segments with preserved FDG uptake significantly on PET imaging exceeds the number of segments with residual inotropic reserve on dobutamine echocardiography.[156]

The sensitivity of dobutamine echocardiography is lower than the sensitivity of SPECT imaging because certain regions that are severely underperfused and are akinetic at rest with no flow reserve can be viable but not demonstrate enhanced systolic thickening, even with the lowest doses of dobutamine.[157] Thus, SPECT imaging has a higher negative predictive value in terms of predicting which segments will *not* improve after revascularization. The combination of ^{201}Tl SPECT and dobutamine echocardiography provided higher accuracy than either technique alone for prediction of recovery of function after revascularization.[158]

Dobutamine echocardiography shows reduced sensitivity in predicting recovery of dysfunctional myocardium supplied by totally occluded vessels.[159] Despite the differences in sensitivity and specificity between SPECT or PET and dobutamine echocardiography for viability detection, the meta-analysis by Allman and associates[132] indicates that there is no measurable performance difference for predicting survival benefit from revascularization between the three imaging techniques. The decrease in mortality with revascularization of viable myocardium was 42.8 percent for ^{201}Tl and 40.5 percent for dobutamine echocardiography (see Fig. 16–7).[132] The lower the resting left ventricular ejection fraction is in patients with viable myocardium, the greater the survival benefit is after revascularization.

Summary of Approaches to Assessment of Viability

Taken together, all of the techniques for the assessment of myocardial viability have high accuracy in the noninvasive detection of viable but dysfunctional myocardium. All provide value in decision-making that is supplementary to clinical and coronary angiographic information alone with respect to the benefit of coronary revascularization in patients with ischemic cardiomyopathy. All the techniques show that the greater the number of viable segments preoperatively, the greater the improvement in ejection fraction and exercise tolerance after revascularization. A limitation of the published studies in the literature regarding the value of viability imaging is that patients were not randomized to medical therapy versus revascularization.[160] Referral bias may have been prevalent in the allocation of patients to either medical therapy or revascularization. Thus, the studies showing better outcomes with revascularization for patients with viability should be considered observational. A note of caution regarding viability imaging, in general, deserves mention. Increased left ventricular volumes and cavity size are predictors of poor prognosis in patients with ischemic cardiomyopathy even when viability is evident.[161] Progressive remodeling after infarction limits the value of revascularization in enhancing left ventricular function.

Table 16–4 summarizes the strengths and limitations of the various noninvasive techniques for the detection of myocardial viability. All have been shown to be clinically useful in identifying which patients with ischemic cardiomyopathy have the greatest chance of enhancement of regional and global left ventricular function, as well as improved survival, after revascularization. Contrast-enhanced MRI is emerging as one of the most promising techniques for assessment of myocardial viability and currently exhibits the greatest sensitivity for detecting subendocardial scar because of its superior spatial resolution compared with nuclear and echocardiographic techniques.

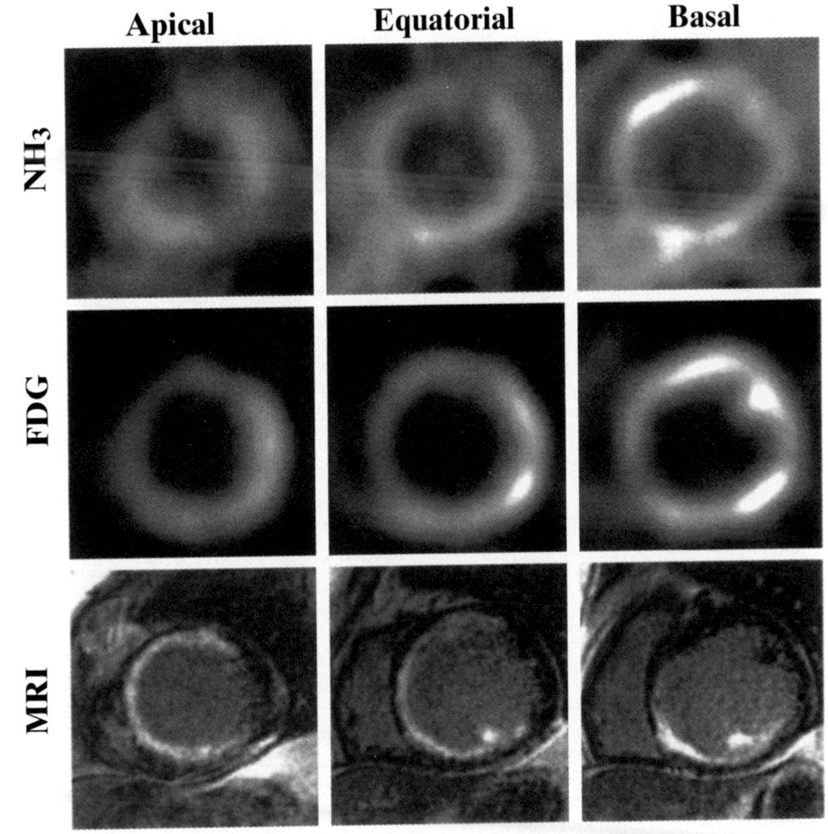

FOIGURE 16–10 Short-axis positron emission tomography (PET) images as part of a viability study employing nitrogen-13 ammonia (NH_3) for perfusion and fluorodeoxyglucose-18 (FDG) for metabolism compared with contrast magnetic resonance imaging (MRI) with evidence for delayed hyperenhancement shown on the bottom row. Note that in the areas showing reduced perfusion and metabolism, a corresponding increased MRI signal is observed. Because of better spatial resolution with MRI than with PET, the differentiation between subendocardial and transmural scans can be better identified. Often the border between hyperenhanced regions and normal areas is well delineated (see comparisons above). (From Klein C, Nekolla SG, Bengel FM, et al: Assessment of myocardial viability with contrast-enhanced magnetic resonance imaging: Comparison with positron emission tomography. Circulation 105:162, 2002.)

TABLE 16–4 Strengths and Limitations of Noninvasive Techniques for Assessment of Myocardial Viability

Technique	Strengths	Limitations
SPECT imaging	High sensitivity for predicting improved function after revascularization Uses quantitative objective criteria (e.g., ≥60 percent segmental uptake) FDG imaging with special collimator LVEF quantitated on ^{99m}Tc-sestamibi or ^{99m}TC-tetrofosmin imaging Predictive of clinical outcomes in a large number of studies	Reduced spatial resolution and sensitivity in comparison to PET Less quantitative than PET Areas of attenuation (e.g., inferior wall on ^{99m}Tc-sestamibi scans) misconstrued as nonviability Cannot differentiate endocardial from epicardial viability Lower specificity than dobutamine echocardiography for predicting improved function after revascularization but higher sensitivity
PET imaging	Simultaneous assessment of perfusion and metabolism More sensitive than other techniques Good specificity No attenuation problems Absolute blood flow can be measured Predictive of outcomes	Lower specificity than dobutamine echocardiography or MRI Cannot separate endocardial from epicardial viability High cost and highly sophisticated technology Limited availability
Dobutamine echocardiography	Higher specificity than nuclear techniques Viability assessed at low doses and ischemia at higher doses Evaluation of mitral regurgitation on baseline echocardiography Good spatial resolution Predictive of clinical outcomes Widely available Lower cost than dobutamine MRI	Poor windows in 30 percent of patients Lower sensitivity than nuclear techniques Viable regions with absent flow reserve will not show increased thickening during dobutamine stimulation Reliance on visual assessment of wall thickening
Contrast echocardiography	Microcirculatory integrity evaluated as well as systolic thickening Better estimation of extent of viability than functional assessment alone Precise delineation of area of necrosis Viability assessed in presence of total coronary occlusion Use of very long pulsing intervals Pulse inversion, power pulse inversion, and power modulation reduce attenuation artifacts	Difficult windows in 30 percent of patients Attenuation problems Scant clinical data available
Contrast-enhanced MRI and dobutamine MRI	Delayed hyperenhancement accurate for measuring extent of transmural scar Superior spatial resolution compared with nuclear and echo techniques More accurate detection of subendocardial infarction than echo or nuclear techniques Can evaluate inotropic reserve with tagging Measurement of wall thickness more accurate than with TEE Simultaneous assessment of perfusion, function, and viability Good imaging windows in all patients	Higher cost than echocardiography Limited availability Need better, faster automated techniques Imaging information not available in real time Patients with pacemakers or ICDs cannot be imaged No large outcome studies reported

FDG = ^{18}F-fluorodeoxyglucose; ICDs = implantable cardioverter-defibrillators; LVEF = left ventricular ejection fraction; MRI = magnetic resonance imaging; PET = positron emission tomography; SPECT = single-photon emission computed tomography; TEE = transesophageal echocardiography.

A PERSPECTIVE ON THE FUTURE OF CARDIAC IMAGING

The future appears bright for further progress in technology and clinical application of noninvasive imaging techniques. Advances in instrumentation and the emergence of new imaging agents will permit enhanced diagnostic and prognostic value of the methodologies reviewed in this chapter. With respect to nuclear cardiology, the widespread introduction of attenuation- and scatter-correction reconstruction algorithms with quantitative SPECT will be associated with fewer imaging artifacts and enhanced specificity and sensitivity for CAD detection. New SPECT camera design may provide higher resolution and sensitivity and ultimately the ability to measure absolute coronary flow reserve.[162] New radiopharmaceuticals on the horizon may allow molecular imaging of apoptosis, inflammation, and gene expression. Imaging of vulnerable atherosclerotic plaques and angiogenesis may soon be feasible. Receptor imaging of the adrenergic nervous system in the heart may have clinical utility in patients with heart failure.

With respect to contrast echocardiography, progress with microbubble contrast agents and imaging technology to enhance the microbubble signal-to-noise ratio will enable better assessment of myocardial perfusion and viability with intravenous injection of contrast material. Imaging of myocardial inflammation after ischemia-reperfusion, imaging with microbubbles targeted to *d*-integrins for evaluation of angiogenesis, detection of inflamed plaques, and imaging of acute cardiac transplant rejection have been shown to be feasible.[163-167] Microbubbles adhere to damaged endothelial cells and may thus furnish a way to assess areas of microvascular endothelial dysfunction in vivo. Microbubbles may ultimately prove useful for local drug delivery, since such bubbles can be destroyed in tissue by ultrasound in vivo.

We can expect continued advances in the field of cardiac MRI in the ensuing years. In addition to the noninvasive assessment of regional and global function, myocardial perfusion with first-pass gadolinium contrast with rest and stress, and viability assessment by quantitating the transmural extent of delayed hyperenhancement, cardiac magnetic resonance looks promising for imaging atherosclerotic plaques and determining its constituents, MRCA for detection of coronary stenoses, and molecular imaging using targeted contrast agents as with labeling of stem cells or macrophages with superparamagnetic iron oxide particles. In vivo characterization of molecular processes using nanoscale paramagnetic targeting agents (nanoparticles) for "hot spot" MRI has proved feasible.[168] Spectroscopic imaging using carbon-13-enhanced compounds may permit imaging of biochemical pathways in the heart.[30] The ability to visualize and track catheters will allow invasive MRCA that could replace x-ray angiography in the future.

Multislice CT is being perfected to achieve improved resolution and shorter acquisition times, which should allow for routine coronary lumen imaging and defining plaque composition. EBCT allows for rapid image acquisition in the time of 50 msec to 100 msec per slice and also has been used to perform contrast-enhanced coronary angiography. Its disadvantages compared with multislice CT are the poor signal-to-noise ratio and increased slice thickness, as well as the lack of general availability of EBCT. Compared with cardiac MRI, the radiation dose is a factor. With multislice CT, new scanners now permit 16 slices per rotation, which allows for greater coverage for a given acquisition time. The whole heart can be scanned with one breath-hold with a slice thickness of 1 mm.

REFERENCES

1. O'Rourke RA, Brundage BH, Froelicher VF, et al: American College of Cardiology/American Heart Association expert consensus document on electron beam computed tomography for the diagnosis and prognosis of coronary artery disease. J Am Coll Cardiol 36:326, 2000.
2. Maddahi J, Gambhir SS: Cost-effective selection of patients for coronary angiography. J Nucl Cardiol 4(Suppl):141, 1997.
3. Gibbons R: Nuclear cardiology in hospital-based practice. J Nucl Cardiol 4(Suppl):179, 1997.
4. Bax JJ, Wijns W, Cornel JH, et al: Accuracy of currently available techniques for prediction of functional recovery after revascularization in patients with left ventricular dysfunction due to chronic coronary artery disease: Comparison of pooled data. J Am Coll Cardiol 30:1451, 1997.

Assessment of Left Ventricular Function at Rest

5. Cheitlin MD, Armstrong WF, Aurigemma GP, et al: ACC/AHA/ASE 2003 guideline update for the clinical application of echocardiography: Summary article. A report of the American College of Cardiology/American Heart Association Task Force on Practice Guidelines (ACC/AHA/ASE Committee to Update the 1997 Guidelines on the Clinical Application of Echocardiography). J Am Coll Cardiol 42:954, 2003. Available at: www.acc.org/clinical/guidelines/echo/index.pdf.
6. Levy D, Labib SB, Anderson KM, et al: Determinants of sensitivity and specificity of electrocardiographic criteria for left ventricular hypertrophy. Circulation 81:815, 1990.
7. Bikkina M, Levy D, Evans JC, et al: Left ventricular mass and risk of stroke in an elderly cohort. The Framingham Heart Study. JAMA 272:33, 1994.
8. Quiñones MA, Greenberg BH, Kopelen HA, et al: Echocardiographic predictors of clinical outcome in patients with left ventricular dysfunction enrolled in the SOLVD registry and trials: Significance of left ventricular hypertrophy. J Am Coll Cardiol 35:1237, 2000.
9. Gardin J: How reliable are serial echocardiographic measurements in detecting regression in left ventricular hypertrophy and changes in function? J Am Coll Cardiol 34:1633, 1999.
10. Palmieri V, Dahlöf B, DeQuattro V, et al: Reliability of echocardiographic assessment of left ventricular structure and function: The PRESERVE study. J Am Coll Cardiol 34:1625, 1999.
11. Gopal AS, Schnellbaecher MJ, Shen Z, et al: Freehand three-dimensional echocardiography for determination of left ventricular volume and mass in patients with abnormal ventricles: Comparison with magnetic resonance imaging. J Am Soc Echocardiogr 10:853, 1997.
12. Cain P, Khoury V, Short L, et al: Usefulness of quantitative echocardiographic techniques to predict recovery of regional and global left ventricular function after acute myocardial infarction. Am J Cardiol 91:391, 2003.
13. Gibson DG, Francis DP: Clinical assessment of left ventricular diastolic function. Heart 89:231, 2003.
14. Mitani I, Jain D, Joska TM, et al: Doxorubicin cardiotoxicity: Prevention of congestive heart failure with serial cardiac function monitoring with equilibrium radionuclide angiocardiography in the current era. J Nucl Cardiol 10:132, 2003.
15. Le Guludec D, Gauthier H, Porcher R, et al: Prognostic value of radionuclide angiography in patients with right ventricular arrhythmias. Circulation 103:1972, 2001.
16. Groch MW, DePuey EG, Belzberg AC, et al: Planar imaging versus gated blood-pool SPECT for the assessment of ventricular performance: a multicenter study. J Nucl Med 42:1773, 2001.
17. Sharir T, Berman DS, Waechter PB, et al: Quantitative analysis of regional motion and thickening by gated myocardial perfusion SPECT: normal heterogeneity and criteria for abnormality. J Nucl Med 42:1630, 2001.
18. Nichols K, Santana CA, Folks R, et al: Comparison between ECTb and QGS for assessment of left ventricular function from gated myocardial perfusion SPECT. J Nucl Cardiol 9:285, 2002.
19. Taillefer R, DePuey EG, Udelson JE, et al: Comparative diagnostic accuracy of Tl-201 and Tc-99m sestamibi SPECT imaging (perfusion and ECG-gated SPECT) in detecting coronary artery disease in women. J Am Coll Cardiol 29:69, 1997.
20. Smanio PEP, Watson DD, Segalla DL, et al: Value of gating of technetium-99m sestamibi single-photon emission computed tomographic imaging. J Am Coll Cardiol 30:1687, 1997.
21. Shirai N, Yamagishi H, Yoshiyama M, et al: Incremental value of assessment of regional wall motion for detection of multivessel coronary artery disease in exercise ^{201}Tl gated myocardial perfusion imaging. J Nucl Med 43:443, 2002.
22. Emmett L, Iwanochko RM, Freeman MR, et al: Reversible regional wall motion abnormalities on exercise technetium-99m-gated cardiac single photon emission computed tomography predict high-grade angiographic stenoses. J Am Coll Cardiol 39:991, 2002.
23. Sharir T, Germano G, Kang X, et al: Prediction of myocardial infarction versus cardiac death by gated myocardial perfusion SPECT: Risk stratification by the amount of stress-induced ischemia and the poststress ejection fraction. J Nucl Med 42:831, 2001.
24. Calnon DA, Kastner RJ, Smith WH, et al: Validation of a new counts-based gated single photon emission computed tomography method for quantifying left ventricular systolic function: Comparison with equilibrium radionuclide angiography. J Nucl Cardiol 4:464, 1997.
25. Manrique A, Faraggi M, Vera P, et al: ^{201}Tl and ^{99m}Tc-MIBI gated SPECT in patients with large perfusion defects and left ventricular dysfunction: Comparison with equilibrium radionuclide angiography. J Nucl Med 40:805, 1999.
26. He ZX, Cwajg E, Preslar JS, et al: Accuracy of left ventricular ejection fraction determined by gated myocardial perfusion SPECT with Tl-201 and Tc-99m sestamibi: Comparison with first-pass radionuclide angiography. J Nucl Cardiol 6:412, 1999.
27. Vaduganathan P, He ZX, Vick GW 3rd, et al: Evaluation of left ventricular wall motion, volumes, and ejection fraction by gated myocardial tomography with technetium 99m-labeled tetrofosmin: A comparison with cine magnetic resonance imaging. J Nucl Cardiol 6:3, 1999.
28. Faber TL, Vansant JP, Pettigrew RI, et al: Evaluation of left ventricular endocardial volumes and ejection fractions computed from gated perfusion SPECT with magnetic resonance imaging: comparison of two methods. J Nucl Cardiol 8:645, 2001.
29. Saab G, Dekemp RA, Ukkonen H, et al: Gated fluorine 18 fluorodeoxyglucose positron emission tomography: determination of global and regional left ventricular function and myocardial tissue characterization. J Nucl Cardiol 10:297, 2003.
30. Forder JR, Pohost GM: Cardiovascular nuclear magnetic resonance: Basic and clinical applications. J Clin Invest 111:1630, 2003.
31. Manning WJ, Stuber M, Danias PG, et al: Coronary magnetic resonance imaging: Current status. Curr Probl Cardiol 27:275, 2002.
32. Pennell D: Cardiovascular magnetic resonance. Heart 85:581, 2001.
33. Prasad S, Pennell DJ: Magnetic resonance imaging in the assessment of patients with heart failure. J Nucl Cardiol 9:S60, 2002.
34. Lindner JR, Wei K: Contrast echocardiography. Curr Probl Cardiol 27:454, 2002.
35. Lang RM, Mor-Avi V, Zoghbi WA, et al: The role of contrast enhancement in echocardiographic assessment of left ventricular function. Am J Cardiol 90(suppl 10A):28J, 2002.

Detection of Coronary Artery Disease: General and Exercise ECG

36. Ropers D, Baum U, Pohle K, et al: Detection of coronary artery stenoses with thin-slice multi-detector row spiral computed tomography and multiplanar reconstruction. Circulation 107:664, 2003
37. de Feyter PJ, Nieman K, van Ooijen P, et al: Non-invasive coronary artery imaging with electron beam computed tomography and magnetic resonance imaging. Heart 84:442, 2000.
38. Gibbons RJ, Balady GJ, Bricker JT, et al: ACC/AHA 2002 guideline update for exercise testing: summary article: A report of the ACC/AHA Task Force on Practice Guidelines (Committee to Update the 1997 Exercise Testing Guidelines). Circulation 106:1883, 2002. Available at: www.acc.org/clinical/guidelines/exercise/dirIndex.htm.
39. Gianrossi R, Detrano R, Mulvihill D, et al: Exercise-induced ST depression in the diagnosis of coronary artery disease. A meta-analysis. Circulation 80:87, 1989.
40. Froelicher VF, Lehmann KG, Thomas R, et al: The electrocardiographic exercise test in a population with reduced workup bias: Diagnostic performance, computerized interpretation, and multivariable prediction. Veterans Affairs Cooperative Study in Health Services: 016 (QUEXTA) Study Group. Qualitative Exercise Testing and Angiography. Ann Intern Med 128:965, 1998.
41. Alexander KP, Shaw LJ, Shaw LK, et al: Value of exercise treadmill testing in women. J Am Coll Cardiol 32:1657, 1998 (published erratum appears in J Am Coll Cardiol 33:289, 1999).
42. Sansoy V, Watson DD, Beller GA: Significance of slow upsloping ST-segment depression on exercise stress testing. Am J Cardiol 79:709, 1997.
43. Gibbons RJ, Abrams J, Chatterjee K, et al: ACC/AHA 2002 guideline update for the management of patients with chronic stable angina-summary article: A report of the American College of Cardiology/American Heart Association Task Force on Practice Guidelines (Committee on the Management of Patients With Chronic Stable Angina). J Am Coll Cardiol 41:159, 2003.

Detection of Coronary Artery Disease: Perfusion Imaging

44. Klocke FJ, Baird MG, Bateman TM, et al: ACC/AHA/ASNC guidelines for the clinical use of cardiac radionuclide imaging: A report of the American College of Cardiology/American Heart Association Task Force on Practice Guidelines (ACC/AHA/ASNC Committee to Revise the 1995 Guidelines for the Clinical Use of Radionuclide Imaging). 2003. American College of Cardiology Web Site. Available at: http://www.acc.org/clinical/guidelines/radio/rni_fulltext.pdf.
45. Beller GA, Zaret BL: Contributions of nuclear cardiology to diagnosis and prognosis of patients with coronary artery disease. Circulation 101:1465, 2000.

46. Lima RSL, Watson DD, Goode AR, et al: Incremental value of combined perfusion and function over perfusion alone by gated SPECT myocardial perfusion imaging for detection of severe three-vessel coronary artery disease. J Am Coll Cardiol 42:64, 2003.
47. Berman DS, Kang X, Schisterman EF, et al: Serial changes on quantitative myocardial perfusion SPECT in patients undergoing revascularization or conservative therapy. J Nucl Cardiol 8:428, 2001.
48. Hendel RC, Corbett JR, Cullom SJ, et al: The value and practice of attenuation correction for myocardial perfusion SPECT imaging: A joint position statement from the American Society of Nuclear Cardiology and the Society of Nuclear Medicine. J Nucl Cardiol 9:135, 2002.
49. Duvernoy CS, Ficaro EP, Karabajakian MZ, et al: Improved detection of left main coronary artery disease with attenuation-corrected SPECT. J Nucl Cardiol 7:639, 2000.
50. Hendel RC, Berman DS, Cullom SJ, et al: Multicenter clinical trial to evaluate the efficacy of correction for photon attenuation and scatter in SPECT myocardial perfusion imaging. Circulation 99:2742, 1999.
51. Links JM, DePuey EG, Taillefer R, et al: Attenuation correction and gating synergistically improve the diagnostic accuracy of myocardial perfusion SPECT. J Nucl Cardiol 9:183, 2002.
52. Hendel RC: Diagnostic and prognostic applications for vasodilator stress myocardial perfusion imaging and the importance of radiopharmaceutical selection. J Nucl Cardiol 8:523, 2001.
53. Elhendy A, Bax JJ, Poldermans D: Dobutamine stress myocardial perfusion imaging in coronary artery disease. J Nucl Med 43:1634, 2002.

Detection of Coronary Artery Disease: Echocardiography

54. Marwick T: Stress echocardiography. Heart 89:113, 2003.
55. Kymes SM, Bruns DE, Shaw LJ, et al: Anatomy of a meta-analysis: A critical review of "exercise echocardiography or exercise SPECT imaging? A meta-analysis of diagnostic test performance." J Nucl Cardiol 7:599, 2000.
56. Marwick TH, Nemec JJ, Pashkow FJ, et al: Accuracy and limitations of exercise echocardiography in a routine clinical setting. J Am Coll Cardiol 19:74, 1992.
57. Secknus MA, Marwick TH: Evolution of dobutamine echocardiography protocols and indications: Safety and side effects in 3,011 studies over 5 years. J Am Coll Cardiol 29:1234, 1997.
58. Stewart MJ: Contrast echocardiography. Heart 89:342, 2003.
59. Hoffman R, Lethen H, Marwick T, et al: Analysis of interinstitutional observer agreement in interpretation of dobutamine stress echocardiograms. J Am Coll Cardiol 27:330, 1996.
60. Wei K, Crouse L, Weiss J, et al: Comparison of usefulness of dipyridamole stress myocardial contrast echocardiography to technetium-99m sestamibi single-photon emission computed tomography for detection of coronary artery disease (PB127 Multicenter Phase 2 Trial results). Am J Cardiol 91:1293, 2003.
61. Heinle SK, Noblin J, Goree-Best P, et al: Assessment of myocardial perfusion by harmonic power Doppler imaging at rest and during adenosine stress: Comparison with ^{99m}Tc-sestamibi SPECT imaging. Circulation 102:55, 2000.
62. Brown K: Diagnostic and prognostic use of noninvasive imaging in patients with known or suspected coronary artery disease. Comparison of stress myocardial perfusion imaging and echocardiography. Cardiol Rev 6:90, 1998.
63. O'Keefe JH Jr, Barnhart CS, Bateman TM: Comparison of stress echocardiography and stress myocardial perfusion scintigraphy for diagnosing coronary artery disease and assessing its severity. Am J Cardiol 75:25D, 1995.
64. Schinkel AF, Bax JJ, Geleijnse ML, et al: Noninvasive evaluation of ischaemic heart disease: Myocardial perfusion imaging or stress echocardiography? Eur Heart J 24:789, 2003.
65. Smanio PEP, Watson DD, Segalla DL, et al: Value of gating of technetium-99m sestamibi single-photon emission computed tomographic imaging. J Am Coll Cardiol 30:1687, 1997.
66. Fleischmann KE, Hunink MG, Kuntz KM, et al: Exercise echocardiography or exercise SPECT imaging? A meta-analysis of diagnostic test performance. JAMA 280:913, 1998.
67. Jacobs M: Review: Exercise ECHO is a more specific and discriminatory test than exercise SPECT for coronary artery disease. (Diagnosis.) ACP Journal Club 130:45, 1999. (Abstract and commentary for: Fleischmann KE, Hunink MG, Kuntz KM, et al: Exercise echocardiography or exercise SPECT imaging? A meta-analysis of diagnostic test performance. JAMA 280:913, 1998.)
68. Santoro GM, Sciagra R, Buonamici P, et al: Head-to-head comparison of exercise stress testing, pharmacologic stress echocardiography, and perfusion tomography as first-line examination for chest pain in patients without history of coronary artery disease. J Nucl Cardiol 5:19, 1998.
69. Elhendy A, Geleijnse ML, Roelandt JR, et al: Dobutamine-induced hypoperfusion without transient wall motion abnormalities: Less severe ischemia or less severe stress? J Am Coll Cardiol 27:323, 1996.
70. Smart SC, Bhatia A, Hellman R, et al: Dobutamine-atropine stress echocardiography and dipyridamole sestamibi scintigraphy for the detection of coronary artery disease: Limitations and concordance. J Am Coll Cardiol 36:1265, 2000.
71. Elhendy A, van Domburg RT, Bax JJ, et al: Accuracy of dobutamine technetium 99m sestamibi SPECT imaging for the diagnosis of single-vessel coronary artery disease: Comparison with echocardiography. Am Heart J 139:224, 2000.

Detection of Coronary Artery Disease: MRI and CT

72. Yang PC, Meyer CH, Terashima M, et al: Spiral magnetic resonance coronary angiography with rapid real-time localization. J Am Coll Cardiol 41:1134, 2003.
73. Worthley SG, Helft G, Fuster V, et al: Noninvasive in vivo magnetic resonance imaging of experimental coronary lesions in a porcine model. Circulation 101:2956, 2000.
74. Kim WY, Danias PG, Stuber M, et al: Coronary magnetic resonance angiography for the detection of coronary stenoses. N Engl J Med 345:1863, 2001.
75. Nagel E, Thouet T, Klein C, et al: Noninvasive determination of coronary blood flow velocity with cardiovascular magnetic resonance in patients after stent deployment. Circulation 107:1738, 2003.
76. Langerak SE, Vliegen HW, de Roos A, et al: Detection of vein graft disease using high-resolution magnetic resonance angiography. Circulation 105:328, 2002.
77. Nagel E, Klein C, Paetsch I, et al: Magnetic resonance perfusion measurements for the noninvasive detection of coronary artery disease. Circulation 108:432, 2003.
78. Doyle M, Fuisz A, Kortright E, et al: The impact of myocardial flow reserve on the detection of coronary artery disease by perfusion imaging methods: An NHLBI WISE study. J Cardiovasc Magn Reson 5:475, 2003.
79. Kwong RY, Schussheim AE, Rekhraj S, et al: Detecting acute coronary syndrome in the emergency department with cardiac magnetic resonance imaging. Circulation 107:531, 2003.
80. Kuijpers D, Ho KY, van Dijkman PR, et al: Dobutamine cardiovascular magnetic resonance for the detection of myocardial ischemia with the use of myocardial tagging. Circulation 107:1592, 2003.
81. Ibrahim T, Nekolla SG, Schreiber K, et al: Assessment of coronary flow reserve: Comparison between contrast-enhanced magnetic resonance imaging and positron emission tomography. J Am Coll Cardiol 39:864, 2002.
82. Schwitter J, Nanz D, Kneifel S, et al: Assessment of myocardial perfusion in coronary artery disease by magnetic resonance: A comparison with positron emission tomography and coronary angiography. Circulation 103:2230, 2001.
83. Murphy RE, Moody AR, Morgan PS, et al: Prevalence of complicated carotid atheroma as detected by magnetic resonance direct thrombus imaging in patients with suspected carotid artery stenosis and previous acute cerebral ischemia. Circulation 107:3053, 2003.
84. Kramer CM: Magnetic resonance imaging to identify the high-risk plaque. Am J Cardiol 90(suppl 3):15L, 2002.
85. Yuan C, Zhang SX, Polissar NL, et al: Identification of fibrous cap rupture with magnetic resonance imaging is highly associated with recent transient ischemic attack or stroke. Circulation 105:181, 2002.
86. Fayad ZA, Fuster V, Fallon JT, et al: Noninvasive in vivo human coronary artery lumen and wall imaging using black-blood magnetic resonance imaging. Circulation 102:506, 2000.
87. Fayad ZA, Fuster V, Nikolaou K, et al: Computed tomography and magnetic resonance imaging for noninvasive coronary angiography and plaque imaging: Current and potential future concepts. Circulation 106:2026, 2002.
88. Kooi ME, Cappendijk VC, Cleutjens KB, et al: Accumulation of ultrasmall superparamagnetic particles of iron oxide in human atherosclerotic plaques can be detected by in vivo magnetic resonance imaging. Circulation 107:2453, 2003.
89. Omary RA, Green JD, Schirf BE, et al: Real-time magnetic resonance imaging-guided coronary catheterization in swine. Circulation 107:2656, 2003.
90. Achenbach S, Giesler T, Ropers D, et al: Detection of coronary artery stenoses by contrast-enhanced, retrospectively electrocardiographically-gated, multislice spiral computed tomography. Circulation 103:2535, 2001.
91. Leber AW, Knez A, Becker C, et al: Non-invasive intravenous coronary angiography using electron beam tomography and multislice computed tomography. Heart 89:633, 2003.
92. Greenland P, Gaziano JM: Clinical practice. Selecting asymptomatic patients for coronary computed tomography or electrocardiographic exercise testing. N Engl J Med 349:465, 2003.
93. O'Malley PG, Taylor AJ, Jackson JL, et al: Prognostic value of coronary electron-beam computed tomography for coronary heart disease events in asymptomatic populations. Am J Cardiol 85:945, 2000.
94. Park R, Detrano R, Xiang M, et al: Combined use of computed tomography coronary calcium scores and C-reactive protein levels in predicting cardiovascular events in nondiabetic individuals. Circulation 106:2073, 2002.

Assessment of Prognosis of Patients Evaluated for Coronary Artery Disease

95. Myers J, Prakash M, Froelicher V, et al: Exercise capacity and mortality among men referred for exercise testing. N Engl J Med 346:793, 2002.
96. Morshedi-Meibodi A, Larson MG, Levy D, et al: Heart rate recovery after treadmill exercise testing and risk of cardiovascular disease events (The Framingham Heart Study). Am J Cardiol 90:848, 2002.
97. Mark DB, Shaw L, Harrell FE Jr, et al: Prognostic value of a treadmill exercise score in outpatients with suspected coronary artery disease. N Engl J Med 325:849, 1991.
98. Shaw LJ, Peterson ED, Shaw LK, et al: Use of a prognostic treadmill score in identifying diagnostic coronary disease subgroups. Circulation 98:1622, 1998.
99. Hachamovitch R, Berman DS, Kiat H, et al: Exercise myocardial perfusion SPECT in patients without known coronary artery disease: Incremental prognostic value and use in risk stratification. Circulation 93:905, 1996.
100. Hachamovitch R, Berman DS, Kiat H, et al: Value of stress myocardial perfusion single photon emission computed tomography in patients with normal resting electrocardiograms: An evaluation of incremental prognostic value and cost-effectiveness. Circulation 105:823, 2002.
101. Bogaty P, Guimond J, Robitaille NM, et al: A reappraisal of exercise electrocardiographic indexes of the severity of ischemic heart disease: Angiographic and scintigraphic correlates. J Am Coll Cardiol 29:1497, 1997 (published erratum appears in J Am Coll Cardiol 30:1416, 1997).
102. Berman DS, Hachamovitch R, Kiat H, et al: Incremental value of prognostic testing in patients with known or suspected ischemic heart disease: A basis for optimal utilization of exercise technetium-99m sestamibi myocardial perfusion single-photon emission computed tomography. J Am Coll Cardiol 26:639, 1995 (published erratum appears in J Am Coll Cardiol 27:756, 1996).

103. Beller GA: First Annual Mario S. Verani, MD, Memorial Lecture: Clinical value of myocardial perfusion imaging in coronary artery disease. J Nucl Cardiol 10:529, 2003.
104. Iskander S, Iskandrian AE: Risk assessment using single-photon emission computed tomographic technetium-99m sestamibi imaging. J Am Coll Cardiol 32:57, 1998.
105. Sharir T, Bacher-Stier C, Dhar S, et al: Identification of severe and extensive coronary artery disease by postexercise regional wall motion abnormalities in Tc-99m sestamibi gated single-photon emission computed tomography. Am J Cardiol 86:1171, 2000.
106. Yamagishi H, Shirai N, Yoshiyama M, et al: Incremental value of left ventricular ejection fraction for detection of multivessel coronary artery disease in exercise ^{201}Tl gated myocardial perfusion imaging. J Nucl Med 43:131, 2002.
107. Chatziioannou SN, Moore WH, Ford PV, et al: Prognostic value of myocardial perfusion imaging in patients with high exercise tolerance. Circulation 99:867, 1999.
108. Hachamovitch R, Berman DS, Shaw LJ, et al: Incremental prognostic value of myocardial perfusion single photon emission computed tomography for the prediction of cardiac death: Differential stratification for risk of cardiac death and myocardial infarction. Circulation 97:535, 1998 (published erratum appears in Circulation 98:190, 1998).
109. Hachamovitch R, Hayes SW, Friedman JD, et al: Comparison of the short-term survival benefit associated with revascularization compared with medical therapy in patients with no prior coronary artery disease undergoing stress myocardial perfusion single photon emission computed tomography. Circulation 107:2900, 2003.
110. Shaw LJ, Hachamovitch R, Berman DS, et al: The economic consequences of available diagnostic and prognostic strategies for the evaluation of stable angina patients: An observational assessment of the value of precatheterization ischemia. The Economics of Noninvasive Diagnosis (END) Multicenter Study Group. J Am Coll Cardiol 33:661, 1999.
111. Shaw LJ, Heller GV, Travin MI, et al: Cost analysis of diagnostic testing for coronary artery disease in women with stable chest pain. Economics of Noninvasive Diagnosis (END) study group. J Nucl Cardiol 6:559, 1999.
112. Brown KA, Rowen M: Prognostic value of a normal exercise myocardial perfusion imaging study in patients with angiographically significant coronary artery disease. Am J Cardiol 71:865, 1993.
113. Giri S, Shaw LJ, Murthy DR, et al: Impact of diabetes on the risk stratification using stress single-photon emission computed tomography myocardial perfusion imaging in patients with symptoms suggestive of coronary artery disease. Circulation 105:32, 2002.
114. Berman DS, Kang X, Hayes SW, et al: Adenosine myocardial perfusion single-photon emission computed tomography in women compared with men. Impact of diabetes mellitus on incremental prognostic value and effect on patient management. J Am Coll Cardiol 41:1125, 2003.

Assessment of Prognosis: Stress Echocardiography

115. Heupler S, Mehta R, Lobo A, et al: Prognostic implications of exercise echocardiography in women with known or suspected coronary artery disease. J Am Coll Cardiol 30:414, 1997.
116. Marwick TH, Mehta R, Arheart K, et al: Use of exercise echocardiography for prognostic evaluation of patients with known or suspected coronary artery disease. J Am Coll Cardiol 30:83, 1997.
117. Arruda AM, Das MK, Roger VL, et al: Prognostic value of exercise echocardiography in 2,632 patients ≥65 years of age. J Am Coll Cardiol 37:1036, 2001.
118. McCully RB, Roger VL, Mahoney DW, et al: Outcome after abnormal exercise echocardiography for patients with good exercise capacity: Prognostic importance of the extent and severity of exercise-related left ventricular dysfunction. J Am Coll Cardiol 39:1345, 2002.
119. Arruda-Olson AM, Juracan EM, Mahoney DW, et al: Prognostic value of exercise echocardiography in 5,798 patients: is there a gender difference? J Am Coll Cardiol 39:625, 2002.
120. Marwick TH, Case C, Vasey C, et al: Prediction of mortality by exercise echocardiography: A strategy for combination with the Duke treadmill score. Circulation 103:2566, 2001.

Comparison with Perfusion Imaging

121. Olmos LI, Dakik H, Gordon R, et al: Long-term prognostic value of exercise echocardiography compared with exercise ^{201}Tl, ECG, and clinical variables in patients evaluated for coronary artery disease. Circulation 98:2679, 1998.
122. Geleijnse ML, Elhendy A, van Domburg RT, et al: Cardiac imaging for risk stratification with dobutamine-atropine stress testing in patients with chest pain. Echocardiography, perfusion scintigraphy, or both? Circulation 96:137, 1997.
123. McCully RB, Roger VL, Mahoney DW, et al: Outcome after normal exercise echocardiography and predictors of subsequent cardiac events: Follow-up of 1,325 patients. J Am Coll Cardiol 31:144, 1998.
124. Poldermans D, Fioretti PM, Boersma E, et al: Long-term prognostic value of dobutamine-atropine stress echocardiography in 1737 patients with known or suspected coronary artery disease: A single-center experience. Circulation 99:757, 1999.
125. Cortigiani L, Dodi C, Paolini EA, et al: Prognostic value of pharmacological stress echocardiography in women with chest pain and unknown coronary artery disease. J Am Coll Cardiol 32:1975, 1998.
126. Marwick TH, Case C, Sawada S, et al: Prediction of mortality using dobutamine echocardiography. J Am Coll Cardiol 37:754, 2001.
127. Sicari R, Pasanisi E, Venneri L, et al: Echo Persantine International Cooperative (EPIC) Study Group; Echo Dobutamine International Cooperative (EDIC) Study Group: Stress echo results predict mortality: A large-scale multicenter prospective international study. J Am Coll Cardiol 41:589, 2003.
128. Shaw LJ, Eagle KA, Gersh BJ, et al: Meta-analysis of intravenous dipyridamole-thallium-201 imaging (1985 to 1994) and dobutamine echocardiography (1991 to 1994) for risk stratification before vascular surgery. J Am Coll Cardiol 27:787, 1996.
129. Poldermans D, Arnese M, Fioretti PM, et al: Sustained prognostic value of dobutamine stress echocardiography for late cardiac events after major noncardiac vascular surgery. Circulation 95:53, 1997.
130. Hundley WG, Morgan TM, Neagle CM, et al: Magnetic resonance imaging determination of cardiac prognosis. Circulation 106:2328, 2002.
131. Lauerma K, Virtanen KS, Sipila LM, et al: Multislice MRI in assessment of myocardial perfusion in patients with single-vessel proximal left anterior descending coronary artery disease before and after revascularization. Circulation 96:2859, 1997.

Noninvasive Assessment of Myocardial Viability

132. Allman KC, Shaw LJ, Hachamovitch R, et al: Myocardial viability testing and impact of revascularization on prognosis in patients with coronary artery disease and left ventricular dysfunction: A meta-analysis. J Am Coll Cardiol 39:1151, 2002.
133. Bax JJ, Poldermans D, Elhendy A, et al: Sensitivity, specificity, and predictive accuracies of various noninvasive techniques for detecting hibernating myocardium. Curr Probl Cardiol 26:141, 2001.
134. Udelson JE, Coleman PS, Metherall J, et al: Predicting recovery of severe regional ventricular dysfunction: Comparison of resting scintigraphy with ^{201}Tl and ^{99m}Tc-sestamibi. Circulation 89:2552, 1994.
135. Cuocolo A, Acampa W, Nicolai E, et al: Quantitative thallium-201 and technetium 99m sestamibi tomography at rest in detection of myocardial viability in patients with chronic ischemic left ventricular dysfunction. J Nucl Cardiol 7:8, 2000.
136. Sciagra R, Pellegri M, Pupi A, et al: Prognostic implications of Tc-99m sestamibi viability imaging and subsequent therapeutic strategy in patients with chronic coronary artery disease and left ventricular dysfunction. J Am Coll Cardiol 36:739, 2000.
137. Camici PG: Imaging techniques: Positron emission tomography and myocardial imaging. Heart 83:475, 2000.
138. Wolpers HG, Burchert W, van den Hoff J, et al: Assessment of myocardial viability by use of ^{11}C-acetate and positron emission tomography: Threshold criteria of reversible dysfunction. Circulation 95:1417, 1997.
139. Siebelink HM, Blanksma PK, Crijns HJ, et al: No difference in cardiac event-free survival between positron emission tomography-guided and single-photon emission computed tomography-guided patient management: A prospective, randomized comparison of patients with suspicion of jeopardized myocardium. J Am Coll Cardiol 37:81, 2001.
140. Rizzello V, Schinkel AF, Bax JJ, et al: Individual prediction of functional recovery after coronary revascularization in patients with ischemic cardiomyopathy: The scar-to-biphasic model. Am J Cardiol 91:1406, 2003.
141. Bandano LP, Werren M, Di Chiara A, et al: Contrast echocardiographic evaluation of early changes in myocardial perfusion after recanalization therapy in anterior wall acute myocardial infarction and their relation with early contractile recovery. Am J Cardiol 91:532, 2003.
142. Balcells E, Powers ER, Lepper W, et al: Detection of myocardial viability by contrast echocardiography in acute infarction predicts recovery of resting function and contractile reserve. J Am Coll Cardiol 41:827, 2003.
143. Shimoni S, Fragogiannis NG, Aggeli CJ, et al: Identification of hibernating myocardium with quantitative intravenous myocardial contrast echocardiography: Comparison with dobutamine echocardiography and thallium-201 scintigraphy. Circulation 107:538, 2003.
144. Senior R, Swinburn JM: Incremental value of myocardial contrast echocardiography for the prediction of recovery of function in dobutamine nonresponsive myocardium early after acute myocardial infarction. Am J Cardiol 91:397, 2003.
145. Ramani K, Judd RM, Holly TA, et al: Contrast magnetic resonance imaging in the assessment of myocardial viability in patients with stable coronary artery disease and left ventricular dysfunction. Circulation 98:2687, 1998.
146. Kim RJ, Fieno DS, Parrish TB, et al: Relationship of MRI delayed contrast enhancement to irreversible injury, infarct age, and contractile function. Circulation 100:1992, 1999.
147. Wagner A, Mahrholdt H, Holly TA, et al: Contrast-enhanced MRI and routine single photon emission computed tomography (SPECT) perfusion imaging for detection of subendocardial myocardial infarcts: An imaging study. Lancet 361:374, 2003.
148. Klein C, Nekolla SG, Bengel FM, et al: Assessment of myocardial viability with contrast-enhanced magnetic resonance imaging: Comparison with positron emission tomography Circulation 105:162, 2002.
149. Mahrholdt H, Wagner A, Holly TA, et al: Reproducibility of chronic infarct size measurement by contrast-enhanced magnetic resonance imaging. Circulation 106:2322, 2002.
150. McCrohon JA, Moon JC, Prasad SK, et al: Differentiation of heart failure related to dilated cardiomyopathy and coronary artery disease using gadolinium-enhanced cardiovascular magnetic resonance. Circulation 108:54, 2003.
151. Kim RJ, Wu E, Rafael A, et al: The use of contrast-enhanced magnetic resonance imaging to identify reversible myocardial dysfunction. N Engl J Med 343:1445, 2000.
152. Trent RJ, Waiter GD, Hillis GS, et al: Dobutamine magnetic resonance imaging as a predictor of myocardial functional recovery after revascularization. Heart 83:40, 2000.
153. Kramer CM, Rogers WJ Jr, Mankad S, et al: Contractile reserve and contrast uptake pattern by magnetic resonance imaging and functional recovery after reperfused myocardial infarction. J Am Coll Cardiol 36:1835, 2000.
154. Hillenbrand HB, Kim RJ, Parker MA, et al: Early assessment of myocardial salvage by contrast-enhanced magnetic resonance imaging. Circulation 102:1678, 2000.

Strengths and Weaknesses of Various Modalities for Assessing Viability

155. Perrone-Filardi P, Pace L, Prastaro M, et al: Assessment of myocardial viability in patients with chronic coronary artery disease: Rest-4-hour-24-hour ^{201}Tl tomography versus dobutamine echocardiography. Circulation 97:2712, 1996.

156. Bax JJ, Cornel JH, Visser FC, et al: Prediction of recovery of myocardial dysfunction after revascularization: Comparison of fluorine-18 fluorodeoxyglucose/thallium-201 SPECT, thallium-201 stress-reinjection SPECT and dobutamine echocardiography. J Am Coll Cardiol 28:558, 1996.
157. Skopicki HA, Abraham SA, Weissman NJ, et al: Factors influencing regional myocardial contractile response to inotropic stimulation: Analysis in humans with stable ischemic heart disease. Circulation 94:643, 1996.
158. Dellegrottaglie S, Perrone-Filardi P, Pace L, et al: Prediction of long-term effects of revascularization on regional and global left ventricular function by dobutamine echocardiography and rest Tl-201 imaging alone and in combination in patients with chronic coronary artery disease. J Nucl Cardiol 9:174, 2002.
159. Piscione F, Perrone-Filardi P, De Luca G, et al: Low dose dobutamine echocardiography for predicting functional recovery after coronary revascularisation. Heart 86:679, 2001.
160. Bourque JM, Velazquez EJ, Borges-Neto S, et al: Radionuclide viability testing: Should it affect treatment strategy in patients with cardiomyopathy and significant coronary artery disease? Am Heart J 145:758, 2003.
161. DiCarli MF, Hachamovitch R, Berman DS: The art and science of predicting postrevascularization improvement in left ventricular (LV) function in patients with severely depressed LV function. J Am Coll Cardiol 40:1744, 2002.

A Perspective on the Future of Cardiac Imaging

162. Schwaiger M: Future perspectives and conclusions. Eur Heart J Suppl 3(Suppl F):F, 2001.
163. Lindner JR, Coggins MP, Kaul S, et al: Microbubble persistence in the microcirculation during ischemia/reperfusion and inflammation is caused by integrin- and complement-mediated adherence to activated leukocytes. Circulation 101:668, 2000.
164. Lindner JR, Dayton PA, Coggins MP, et al: Noninvasive imaging of inflammation by ultrasound detection of phagocytosed microbubbles. Circulation 102:531, 2000.
165. Leong-Poi H, Christiansen J, Klibanov AL, et al: Noninvasive assessment of angiogenesis by ultrasound and microbubbles targeted to alpha(v)-integrins. Circulation 107:455, 2003.
166. Lindner JR: Detection of inflamed plaques with contrast ultrasound. Am J Cardiol 90(10C):32L, 2002.
167. Weller GE, Lu E, Csikari MM, et al: Ultrasound imaging of acute cardiac transplant rejection with microbubbles targeted to intercellular adhesion molecule-1. Circulation 108:218, 2003.
168. Wickline SA, Lanza GM: Molecular imaging, targeted therapeutics, and nanoscience. J Cell Biochem Suppl 39:90, 2002.

CHAPTER 17

Cardiac Catheterization

Charles J. Davidson • Robert O. Bonow*

Indications for Diagnostic Cardiac Catheterization

As with any procedure, the decision to recommend cardiac catheterization is based on an appropriate risk-benefit ratio. In general, diagnostic cardiac catheterization is recommended whenever it is clinically important to define the presence or severity of a suspected cardiac lesion that cannot be adequately evaluated by noninvasive techniques. Because the risk of a major complication from cardiac catheterization is less than 1 percent with a mortality of less than 0.08 percent, there are few patients who cannot be studied safely in an active laboratory. Intracardiac pressure measurements and coronary arteriography are procedures that can be performed with reproducible accuracy only by invasive catheterization. Noninvasive estimation of intracardiac pressures can be achieved with echocardiography (see Chap. 11), and magnetic resonance imaging and computed tomography show promise for assessment of coronary anatomy (see Chaps. 14 and 15).

The guidelines for diagnostic coronary angiography have been developed by a joint task force of the American College of Cardiology and the American Heart Association.[1] These guidelines describe a three-tiered priority classification for specific disease states. Class I indications apply to conditions in which there is general agreement that coronary angiography is justified, although this may not be the only appropriate diagnostic procedure. Class II indications apply to conditions in which coronary angiography is frequently performed but about which there is a divergence of opinion with respect to justification of the usefulness or efficacy of the procedure. Class IIa applies to situations in which the weight of evidence is in favor of usefulness. Class IIb indications are less well established by evidence or opinion. Class III conditions are those about which there is general agreement that cardiac catheterization is not ordinarily useful or effective and in some cases may be harmful. Diseases are grouped under several categories: known or suspected coronary heart disease, atypical chest pain, acute myocardial infarction, valvular heart disease, congenital heart disease, and other conditions. Table 17–1 summarizes the class I and IIa recommendations of the task force.

The indications for cardiac catheterization are likely to continue to evolve. Expansion of indications has been in two divergent directions. At one extreme, many critically ill and hemodynamically unstable patients are evaluated during acute myocardial ischemia, severe heart failure, or cardiogenic shock. At the other end of the spectrum, an increasing number of procedures are being performed in an outpatient setting. These settings include hospitals with or without cardiac surgery capability and freestanding or mobile laboratories.[2] The result has been the expansion of traditional indications for cardiac catheterization to include both critically ill patients and ambulatory patients.

Cardiac catheterization should be considered to be a diagnostic test used in combination with complementary noninvasive tests. For example, cardiac catheterization in patients with valvular or congenital heart disease is best done with full echocardiographic knowledge and any other functional information. The catheterization can be directed and simplified without obtaining redundant anatomical information.

Identification of coronary artery disease and assessment of its extent and severity are the most common indications for cardiac catheterization in adults (see Chap. 18). The information obtained by catheterization is crucial to optimize therapy for patients with various chest pain syndromes. In addition, the presence of dynamic coronary vascular lesions, such as spasm or thrombosis, can be identified. The consequences of coronary heart disease, such as ischemic mitral regurgitation or left ventricular dysfunction, can be defined. In the current era of acute percutaneous catheter intervention for acute coronary syndromes, patients are often studied during evolving acute myocardial infarction, unstable angina, or in the early period after acute myocardial injury (see Chaps. 48 and 49). The approach of individual centers in evaluating such patients often depends on local facilities and treatment philosophies as well as the availability of surgical support.

In patients with myocardial disease, cardiac catheterization may provide critical information (see Chap. 59). It can exclude coronary artery disease as the cause of symptoms and evaluate left ventricular dysfunction in patients with cardiomyopathy. Cardiac catheterization also permits quantification of the severity of both diastolic and systolic dysfunction, differentiation of myocardial restriction from pericardial constriction, assessment of the extent of valvular regurgitation, detection of active myocarditis by endomyocardial biopsy, and observation of the cardiovascular response to acute pharmacological intervention.

In patients with valvular heart disease, cardiac catheterization provides data both confirmatory and complementary to noninvasive echocardiography, magnetic resonance, and nuclear studies (see Chap. 57). The risk-benefit ratio of cardiac

*The authors would like to thank Robert Fishman, MD, for his contribution to a previous edition of this chapter.

TABLE 17–1 Indications for Coronary Angiography

Known or Suspected* Coronary Disease in Patients Who Are Currently Asymptomatic or Have Stable Angina (Known: Previous myocardial infarction, coronary bypass surgery, or PTCA. Suspected: Rest- or exercise-induced ECG abnormalities suggesting silent ischemia)

Asymptomatic or Stable Angina

Class I

1. Evidence of high risk on noninvasing testing.
2. Canadian Cardiovascular Society (CSS) class III or IV angina on medical treatment.
3. Patients resuscitated from sudden cardiac death or with sustained monomorphic VT or nonsustained polymorphic VT.

Class IIa

1. CCS class III or IV angina that improves to class I or II on medical therapy.
2. Serial noninvasive testing showing progressive abnormalities.
3. Patient with disability or illness that cannot be stratified by other means.
4. CCS class I or II with intolerance or failure to respond to medical therapy.
5. Individuals whose occupation involves safety of others (e.g., pilots, bus drivers) with abnormal stress test results or high-risk clinical profile.

Nonspecific Chest Pain

Class I

High-risk findings on noninvasive testing.

Class IIa

None.

Unstable Coronary Syndromes

Class I

1. High or intermediate risk for adverse outcome in patients with unstable angina refractory to initial adequate medical therapy or recurrent symptoms after initial stabilization. Emergent catheterization is recommended.
2. High risk for adverse outcome in patients with unstable angina. Urgent catheterization is recommended.
3. High- or intermediate-risk unstable angina that stabilizes after initial treatment.
4. Initially low short-term risk unstable angina that is subsequently high risk on noninvasive testing.
5. Suspected Prinzmetal variant angina.

Class IIa

None.

Patients with Postrevascularization Ischemia

Class I

1. Suspected abrupt closure or subacute stent thrombosis after percutaneous revascularization.
2. Recurrent angina or high-risk criteria on noninvasive evaluation within 9 mo of percutaneous revascularization.

Class IIa

1. Recurrent symptomatic ischemia within 12 mo of CABG.
2. Noninvasive evidence of high-risk criteria occurring at any time postoperatively.
3. Recurrent angina inadequately controlled by medical means after revascularization.

During the Initial Management of Acute MI (MI Suspected and ST Segment Elevation or Bundle Branch Block Present)

Coronary Angiography Coupled with the Intent to Perform Primary PTCA

Class I

1. As an alternative to thrombolytic therapy in patients who can undergo angioplasty of the infarct-related artery within 12 hr of the onset of symptoms or beyond 12 hr if ischemic symptoms persist, *if performed in a timely fashion by individuals skilled in the procedure and supported by experienced personnel in an appropriate laboratory environment.*
2. In patients who are within 36 hr of an acute ST elevation Q or new LBBB MI who develop cardiogenic shock, who are younger than 75 years, and in whom revascularization can be performed within 18 hr of the onset of the shock.

Class IIa

As a reperfusion strategy in patients who are candidates for reperfusion but who have a contraindication to fibrinolytic therapy, if angioplasty can be performed as outlined earlier in class I.

Early Coronary Angiography in the Patient with Suspected MI (ST Segment Elevation or Bundle Branch Block Present) Who Has Not Undergone Primary PTCA

Class I

None.

Class IIa

Cardiogenic shock or persistent hemodynamic instability.

Early Coronary Angiography in Acute MI (MI Suspected but No ST Segment Elevation)

Class I

1. Persistent or recurrent (stuttering) episodes of symptomatic ischemia, spontaneous or induced, with or without associated ECG changes.
2. The presence of shock, severe pulmonary congestion, or continuing hypotension.

Class IIa

None.

Coronary Angioplasty During the Hospital Management Phase (Patients with Q Wave and Non-Q-Wave Infarction)

Class I

1. Spontaneous myocardial ischemia or myocardial ischemia provoked by minimal exertion, during recovery from infarction.
2. Before definitive therapy of a mechanical complication of infarction such as acute mitral regurgitation, ventricular septal defect, pseudoaneurysm, or left ventricular aneurysm.
3. Persistent hemodynamic instability.

TABLE 17–1 Indications for Coronary Angiography—cont'd

Class IIa
1. When MI is suspected to have occurred by a mechanism other than thrombotic occlusion at an atheroslcerotic plaque (e.g., coronary embolism, arteritis, trauma, certain metabolic or hematological diseases or coronary spasm).
2. Survivors of acute MI with left ventricular EF < 0.40, CHF, prior revascularization, or malignant ventricular arrhythmias.
3. Clinical heart failure during the acute episode, but subsequent demonstration of preserved left ventricular function (left ventricular EF > 0.40).

During the Risk Stratification Phase (Patients with All Types of MI)

Class I
Ischemia at low levels of exercise with ECG changes (≥1-mm ST segment depression or other predicators of adverse outcome) and/or imaging abnormalities.

Class IIa
1. Clinically significant CHF during the hospital course.
2. Inability to perform an exercise test with left ventricular EF ≤ 0.45.

Perioperative Evaluation Before (or After) Noncardiac Surgery

Class I: Patients with suspected or known CAD
1. Evidence for high risk of adverse outcome based on noninvasive test results.
2. Angina unresponsive to adequate medical therapy.
3. Unstable angina, particularly when facing intermediate- or high-risk noncardiac surgery.
4. Equivocal noninvasive test result in high clinical risk patient undergoing high-risk surgery.

Class IIa
1. Multiple intermediate clinical risk markers and planned vascular surgery.
2. Ischemia on noninvasive testing but without high-risk criteria.
3. Equivocal noninvasive test result in intermediate clinical risk patient undergoing high-risk noncardiac surgery.
4. Urgent noncardiac surgery while convalescing from acute MI.

Patients with Valvular Heart Disease

Class I
1. Before valve surgery or balloon valvotomy in an adult with chest discomfort, ischemia by noninvasive imaging, or both.
2. Before valve surgery in an adult free of chest pain but with many risk factors for CAD.
3. Infective endocarditis with evidence of coronary embolization.

Class IIa
None.

Patients with Congenital Heart Disease

Class I
1. Before surgical correction of congenital heart disease when chest discomfort or noninvasive evidence is suggestive of associated CAD.
2. Before surgical correction of suspected congenital coronary anomalies such as congenital coronary artery stenosis, coronary arteriovenous fistula, and anomalous origin of the left coronary artery.
3. Forms of congenital heart disease frequently associated with coronary artery anomalies that may complicate surgical management.
4. Unexplained cardiac arrest in a young patient.

Class IIa
Before corrective open-heart surgery for congenital heart disease in an adult whose risk profile increases the likelihood of coexisting CAD.

Patients with Congestive Heart Failure

Class I
1. CHF due to systolic dysfunction with angina or with regional wall motion abnormalities and/or scintigraphic evidence or reversible myocardial ischemia when revascularization is being considered.
2. Before cardiac transplantation.
3. CHF secondary to postinfarction ventricular aneurysm or other mechanical complications of MI.

Class IIa
1. Systolic dysfunction with unexplained cause despite noninvasive testing.
2. Normal systolic function, but episodic heart failure raises suspicion if ischemically mediated left ventricular dysfunction.

Other Conditions

Class I
1. Diseases affecting the aorta when knowledge of the presence of extent of coronary artery involvement is necessary for management (e.g., aortic dissection or aneurysm with known CAD).
2. Hypertrophic cardiomyopathy with angina despite medical therapy when knowledge of coronary anatomy might affect therapy.
3. Hypertrophic cardiomyopathy with angina when heart surgery is planned.

Class IIa
1. High risk for CAD when other cardiac surgical procedures are planned (e.g., pericardiectomy or removal of chronic pulmonary emboli).
2. Prospective immediate cardiac transplant donors whose risk profile increases the likelihood of CAD.
3. Asymptomatic patients with Kawasaki disease who have coronary artery aneurysms on echocardiography.
4. Before surgery for aortic aneurysm/dissection in patients without known CAD.
5. Recent blunt chest trauma and suspicion of acute MI, without evidence of preexisting CAD.

CABG = coronary artery bypass graft; CAD = coronary artery disease; CHF = congestive heart failure; ECG = electrocardiographic; EF = ejection fraction; LBBB = left bundle branch block; MI = myocardial infarction; PTCA = percutaneous transluminal coronary angioplasty; VT = ventricular tachycardia.

From Scanlon PJ, Faxon DF, Auden AM, et al: ACC/AHA guidelines for coronary angiography: A report of the American College of Cardiology/American Heart Association Task Force on practice guidelines (Committee on Coronary Angiography). Developed in collaboration with the Society for Cardiac Angiography and Interventions. J Am Coll Cardiol 33:1756, 1999.

catheterization prior to valvular surgery is weighted heavily in favor of the cardiac catheterization. However, catheterization may be unnecessary in some preoperative situations, such as patients with an atrial myxoma or young patients with endocarditis or acute valvular regurgitation. Nevertheless, additional confirmation of the severity of the valvular lesion, identification of associated coronary disease or anomalies, quantification of the hemodynamic consequences of the valvular lesions (such as pulmonary hypertension), and occasionally quantification of the acute hemodynamic response to pharmacological therapy all provide useful preoperative information that fully defines the operative risk and permits a more directed surgical approach.

The current role of cardiac catheterization in certain congenital disease states is less well defined. Echocardiography with Doppler and cardiac magnetic resonance imaging often provides adequate information. Because gross cardiac anatomy can generally be well defined by these methods, catheterization is required only if certain hemodynamic information (e.g., shunt size or pulmonary vascular resistance) is important in determining the indications for surgical procedures, if percutaneous interventional methods are contemplated, or if coronary anomalies are suspected (see Chap. 56).

Technical Aspects of Cardiac Catheterization

CATHETERIZATION LABORATORY FACILITIES

Cardiac catheterization facilities have evolved to include traditional hospital-based laboratories with in-house cardiothoracic surgical programs, hospital-based laboratories without on-site surgical programs, freestanding laboratories, and mobile laboratories. The relative merits of each type of facility have been discussed in detail by a task force of the American College of Cardiology and Society for Cardiac Angiography and Interventions.[2] At present, about three quarters of cardiac catheterization laboratories have on-site surgical backup. The goals of the freestanding and mobile cardiac catheterization facilities are to reduce cost while offering services in a convenient location for low-risk patients. In one study evaluating the safety of mobile catheterization involving 1001 low-risk patients, no patient died, 0.9 percent required urgent referral for clinical instability, 0.6 percent had major complications, and 27 percent required further referral to a tertiary site for additional diagnostic or therapeutic procedures.[3] Recommendations for groups of patients who should be excluded from invasive procedures in settings without cardiac surgery are given in Table 17–2.

Because of cost containment considerations and the documented safety of diagnostic cardiac catheterization, there has been increasing utilization of catheterization on an outpatient basis.[2] Medicare data indicate that in 1986, catheterization was performed on an outpatient basis in 5 percent of total cases. This rate rose to 23 percent in 1993 and has increased further to 40 to 50 percent in most hospital-based practices today. In general, patients who require preprocedural hospitalization are uncommon. These cases include patients receiving continuous anticoagulation therapy in order to switch from warfarin to heparin, those with severe congestive heart failure, and those with renal insufficiency requiring prehydration. Noninvasive testing can identify patients who would be more appropriately evaluated in a setting where cardiac surgery is available, including those with severe ischemia discovered during stress testing, ischemia at rest, known or highly suspected severe left main or proximal three-vessel disease, critical aortic stenosis, and severe comorbid disease. Most patients can be discharged on the same day within 2 to 6 hours of their procedure.

The most common procedure-related complication necessitating hospitalization is hematoma formation requiring prolonged bed rest and observation. Also, findings from the procedures may require hospitalization, including left main or severe three-vessel coronary artery disease. Other considerations for hospitalization include New York Heart Association Class III or IV heart failure, unstable ischemic symptoms, recent myocardial infarction, severe aortic stenosis with left ventricular dysfunction, severe aortic insufficiency, renal insufficiency, or need for continuous anticoagulation.[2]

PERSONNEL

Personnel in the catheterization laboratory include the medical director, physicians, nurses, cardiology trainees (fellows), physician extenders including nurse practitioners and physician assistants, and radiological technologists. All members should be trained in cardiopulmonary resuscitation and preferably in advanced cardiac life support. It is desirable for facilities to be associated with a cardiothoracic surgical program. In

TABLE 17–2 General Exclusion Criteria for Invasive Cardiac Procedures in Settings Without Cardiac Surgery

Setting	Type of Patient	Diagnostic Procedures	Therapeutic Procedures
Hospital	Adult	• Age > 75 yr • NYHA Class III or IV heart failure • Acute, intermediate- or high-risk ischemic syndromes • Recent MI with postinfarction ischemia • Pulmonary edema thought to be caused by ischemia • Markedly abnormal noninvasive test indicating a high likelihood of left main or severe multivessel coronary disease • Known left main coronary artery disease • Severe valvular dysfunction, especially in the setting of depressed left ventricular performance • Patients at increased risk for vascular complications • Complex adult congenital heart disease	• All valvuloplasty procedures • Diagnostic pericardiocentesis when the effusion is small or moderate in size and there is no tamponade • Elective coronary interventions • Therapeutic procedures in adult congenital heart disease
	Pediatric	• No procedures approved	• No therapeutic procedures approved
Freestanding laboratory	Adult	• All of the above • Patients at high risk because of the presence of comorbid conditions, including the need for anticoagulation therapy, poorly controlled hypertension or diabetes, contrast agent allergy, or renal insufficiency	• No therapeutic procedures approved
	Pediatric	• No procedures approved	• No therapeutic procedures approved

NYHA = New York Heart Association.

From Bashore TM, Bates ER, Berger PB, et al: ACC/SCAI clinical expert consensus document on cardiac catheterization laboratory standards. J Am Coll Cardiol 37:2179, 2001.

general, high-risk diagnostic studies and all elective percutaneous interventions should be performed in laboratories with on-site surgical facilities. However, the American College of Cardiology/American Heart Association task force assessment of diagnostic and therapeutic cardiovascular procedures suggested that percutaneous coronary intervention in high-risk patients with acute myocardial infarction may be performed by trained physicians without on-site surgical backup if the patient cannot be transferred to a more traditional setting without additional risk.[4]

In order to maintain proficiency, laboratories for adult studies should perform a minimum of 300 procedures per year. Physicians training for diagnostic catheterization should perform a minimum of 300 procedures per year with 200 as a primary operator during 12 months of fellowship. However, the minimum caseload for established physicians in practice has not been established.[2,5] Regular evaluation with quality indicator assessment of laboratory and physician, nurse, and technology performance and outcomes is mandatory.[2]

EQUIPMENT

The physical requirements for the catheterization facility have been described in detail elsewhere.[2] Necessary equipment includes the radiographic system, physiological data monitoring and acquisition instrumentation, sterile supplies, and an emergency cart. Also included is support equipment consisting of a power injector, cineangiographic film with processing or digital archiving, and viewing equipment.

RADIOGRAPHIC EQUIPMENT. High-resolution x-ray imaging is required for optimal performance of catheterization procedures. The necessary equipment includes a generator, x-ray tube, image intensifier, video system, and either digital archiving or a cine camera.[6] Virtually all new facilities have made the transition from traditional film-based cineangiography to digital angiography, thus becoming "cinefilm-less" laboratories. There are many advantages of digital acquisition and archiving, including the ability to have immediate on-line review, elimination of film development, quantitative computer analysis, image manipulation capabilities, freeze frames, and flicker-free images at low frame rates, minimizing radiation exposure. With these technologies, transfer of images among cardiac catheterization laboratories, hospitals, and physician offices can be accomplished using a common network.[7,8] The development of Digital Imaging and Communications in Medicine (DICOM) standards for cardiac angiography has allowed compatibility among different systems. Compact disc read-only memory (CD-ROM) technology has been utilized to exchange information between providers. Digital image quality is superior to that of cinefilm and allows a telemedicine approach to cardiac catheterization. Increased computer storage capabilities have allowed storage and easy access to thousands of cases.

PHYSIOLOGICAL MONITORS. Continuous monitoring of blood pressure and the electrocardiogram (ECG) are required during cardiac catheterization. Systemic, pulmonary, and intracardiac pressures are generally recorded using fluid-filled catheters connected to strain-gauge pressure transducers and then transmitted to a monitor. Equipment for determination of thermodilution and Fick cardiac output and blood gas determination, as well as a standard 12-lead ECG machine, are necessary.

RADIATION SAFETY

The patient and catheterization laboratory personnel must be protected from the harmful effects of radiation. Installing and maintaining optimal x-ray imaging equipment reduce unnecessary radiation exposure. The amount of radiation exposure to the patient can be reduced by limiting fluoroscopic and image acquisition time, collimation of the beam to the anatomical region of interest, using low-intensity fluoroscopy, acquiring images at lower frame rates (i.e., 15 frames/sec), maintaining a minimum distance between the image intensifier and the x-ray tube, and using lead shielding when appropriate. Personnel in the laboratory can limit radiation exposure by minimizing acquisition and fluoroscopy times by using low-dose fluoroscopy and acquisition rates of 15 frames/sec. The most important factors are maximizing distance from the source of x-rays and using appropriate shielding (lead aprons, lead thyroid collars, lead eyeglasses, and movable leaded glass barriers). Severely angulated views, especially the left anterior oblique view, substantially increase the radiation exposure of the operators.

A method for measuring radiation exposure for personnel is required. It is recommended that two film badges be worn, one on the outside of the apron at the neck and another under the apron at the waist.[9] The latter monitors the effectiveness of the lead apron. The maximum allowable whole-body radiation dose per year for those working with radiation is 5 roentgen-equivalent-man (rem). A full discussion of radiation safety has been presented by the Society for Cardiac Angiography and Interventions and others.[2,9]

Catheterization Laboratory Protocol

PREPARATION OF THE PATIENT FOR CARDIAC CATHETERIZATION. Before arrival in the catheterization laboratory, the cardiologist responsible for the procedure should explain the procedure fully to patients, including the risks and benefits, and answer questions that the patient or family may have. Precatheterization evaluation includes the patient's history, physical examination, ECG, and laboratory evaluation (complete blood count, platelet count, and determinations of serum creatinine, serum electrolytes, blood glucose, prothrombin time, and partial thromboplastin time [in patients receiving heparin]). Important components of the history that need to be addressed include diabetes mellitus (insulin or non–insulin requiring), renal insufficiency, anticoagulation status, and peripheral vascular disease, as well as previous contrast medium or latex allergy. Full knowledge of any prior procedures, including cardiac catheterizations, percutaneous interventions, peripheral arterial interventions or surgery, and cardiac surgery, is necessary before the procedure. Patients should be fasting, and an intravenous line should be established.

Oral or intravenous sedation is usually administered (e.g., benzodiazepine). Pulse oximetry should be used to monitor respiratory status when these agents are used. Some laboratories routinely premedicate patients with antihistamines such as diphenhydramine (25 mg intravenous push) for its antiallergic properties and to prolong sedation. Oral anticoagulants should be discontinued and the prothrombin time international normalized ratio should be less than 1.8 to avoid increased risk of bleeding. Aspirin is not stopped prior to the procedure. Patients with diabetes receiving metformin should have the medication discontinued the morning of the procedure and not restarted until the creatinine is stable at least 48 hours after the procedure.[10] All patients should receive pre- and postprocedural hydration. The amount of hydration is dependent on the cardiac function but, if tolerated, at least 1 liter is recommended.

Those with a known history of contrast medium allergy need either oral or intravenous prophylaxis before the procedure.[11] A recommended regimen is administration of either prednisone 60 mg by mouth or hydrocortisone 100 mg intravenous push given 12 hours and immediately prior to the procedure. Cimetidine, a nonselective histamine antagonist, and diphenhydramine may also be given. A history of shellfish allergy does not predispose the patient to contrast medium reactions.

CATHETERIZATION PROTOCOL. Each physician should develop a routine for performing diagnostic catheterization to ensure efficient acquisition of all pertinent data. The particular technical approach and necessary procedures should be established individually for each patient so that the specific clinical questions can be addressed (Table 17–3). In general, hemodynamic measurements and cardiac output determination should be made before angiography to reflect basal conditions most accurately and to guide angiography. When angiography is performed, the vessel or chamber with most clinical importance should be visualized first in case an untoward reaction to the contrast medium or another complication of the procedure occurs.

Right-heart catheterization should not be performed in all patients undergoing routine coronary angiography. Despite limited risks, right-heart catheterization including screening oximetric analysis, measurement of pressures, and determination of cardiac output has a low yield in patients with suspected coronary artery disease without other known cardiac disease.[2] Right-heart catheterization is indicated when the clinical question cannot be answered by isolated left-heart catheterization or when a patient has left ventricular dysfunction, congestive heart failure, complicated acute myocardial infarction, valvular disease, suspected pulmonary

TABLE 17–3 Catheterization Protocol

Clinical Issue	LHC	RHC	CORO	LV	AO	RV	PA	BX	PROVO	IABP	PCI
Known or suspected coronary artery disease											
Stable angina	✓		✓	✓							
Positive stress test result	✓		✓	✓							
Preoperative evaluation	✓		✓	✓							
Atypical chest pain	✓		✓	✓					±		
Unstable or new-onset angina	✓		✓	✓							±
Acute myocardial infarction	✓	✓	✓	±						±	±
Failed thrombolysis	✓	✓	✓	±						±	±
Postinfarction angina	✓		✓	±						±	±
Cardiogenic shock	✓	✓	✓	±						±	±
Mechanical complications	✓	✓	✓	✓						±	±
Sudden cardiac death	✓	✓	✓	✓							
Valvular heart disease	✓	✓	✓	✓	✓						
Myocardial disease	✓	✓	✓	✓	✓			±			
Pericardial disease	✓	✓	✓	✓							
Congenital heart disease	✓	✓	✓	✓	±	±	±				
Aortic dissection	✓	±	✓	±	✓						
Pulmonary disease	✓	✓	✓	✓		±	±				

AO = aortogram; BX = biopsy; CORO = coronary angiography; IABP = intraaortic balloon pump; LHC = left-heart catheterization, including measurement of left ventricular end-diastolic pressure and aortic valve gradient; LV = left ventriculography; PA = pulmonary angiography or wedge pulmonary angiography; PROVO = provocative challenge (i.e., ergot alkaloids, acetylcholine); PCI = percutaneous coronary intervention; RHC = right-heart catheterization including pressure measurement, determination of cardiac output, oximetric analysis; RV = right ventriculography; ✓ = appropriate; ± = may be appropriate in certain clinical circumstances.

hypertension, a congenital anomaly, intracardiac shunts, or pericardial disease.

Although the use of a temporary pacemaker is not indicated for routine cardiac catheterization, operators should understand the techniques for proper insertion and setting of the pacemaker if needed. Even in patients with isolated left bundle branch block, right-heart catheterization can generally be safely performed with balloon flotation catheters without causing additional conduction disturbance.

CATHETERS AND ASSOCIATED EQUIPMENT. Physicians performing cardiac catheterization should be familiar with technical aspects of the equipment used during the procedure.[12] Catheters used for cardiac catheterization are available in various lengths, sizes, and shapes. The widely used balloon flotation catheter (Swan-Ganz) is shown in Figure 17–1. Typical catheter lengths vary between 50 and 125 cm, with 100 cm being the most commonly used length for adult left-heart catheterization by the femoral approach. The outer diameter of the catheter is specified using French units, where one French unit (F) = 0.33 mm. The inner diameter of the catheter is smaller than the outside diameter owing to the thickness of the catheter material. Guidewires used during the procedure must be small enough to pass through the inner diameters of both the introducer needle and the catheter. Guidewires are described by their length in centimeters, diameter in inches, and tip conformation. A commonly used wire is a 150-cm, 0.035-inch J-tipped wire. The introducer sheaths are specified by the French number of the largest catheter that passes freely through the inner diameter of the sheath, rather than its outer diameter. Therefore, a 7F introducer sheath accepts a 7F catheter but has an outer diameter of more than 7F or 2.31 mm.

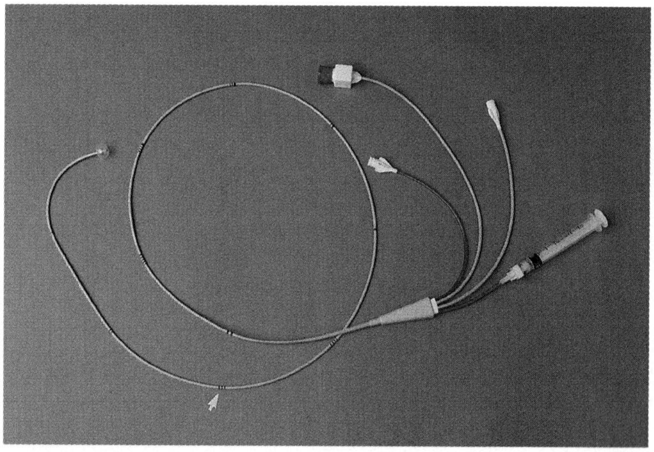

FIGURE 17–1 Typical Swan-Ganz catheter. Proximal ports, left to right, are proximal injection hub, thermistor connector, distal lumen hub, and balloon inflation valve with syringe. The distal end of the catheter has a balloon and a distal end-hole. The proximal injectate port exits at 30 cm from the distal lumen (arrow). The thermistor lies just proximal to the balloon.

The choice of the size of the catheters to be used is made by balancing the needs to opacify the coronary arteries and cardiac chambers adequately, to have adequate catheter manipulation, to limit vascular complications, and to permit early ambulation. Although the larger catheters (7 and 8F) allow greater catheter manipulation and excellent visualization, the smaller catheters (4 to 6F) permit earlier ambulation after catheterization. Catheter technology has advanced such that 4 to 6F systems are used for routine angiography without significant compromise of angiographic quality. The smaller catheters require greater technical skill of manipulation and have lower flow rates. Thus, their use in tortuous anatomy or patients with large body habitus is limited. The 6F diagnostic catheter is most widely used for routine angiography because this size appears to balance most appropriately the needs outlined earlier. The relationship between sheath size and vascular complications is not clear. Rather, anticoagulation status and operator experience are more important factors related to vascular complications.[13]

Techniques

Right-Heart Catheterization

Right-heart catheterization allows measurement and analysis of right-heart, pulmonary artery, and pulmonary capillary wedge pressures; measurement of cardiac output by thermodilution; screening for intracardiac shunts; temporary ventricular pacing; assessment of arrhythmias; and pulmonary wedge angiography. Right-heart catheterization is performed antegrade through either the inferior vena cava (IVC) or superior vena cava (SVC). Percutaneous entry is achieved through the femoral, subclavian, jugular, or antecubital vein. The anatomy of the major arteries and veins used for cardiac catheterization is shown in Figures 17–2 and 17–3. In the cardiac catheterization laboratory, the femoral venous access is used most often because the Judkins technique of left-heart catheterization is performed concurrently. However, when the catheter is to be left in place following the procedure, the internal jugular approach may be preferable. This approach allows the patient to sit up in bed rather than lying flat.

BALLOON FLOTATION CATHETERS. Balloon flotation catheters are the simplest and most widely used (see Fig. 17–1). If thermodilution cardiac outputs must be determined, catheters that contain thermistors, such as Swan-Ganz catheters, should be used. These catheters have balloon tips, proximal and distal ports, and thermistors. Therefore, both intracardiac pressures and oxygen saturation to evaluate intracardiac shunts can be obtained. They are both flexible and flow directed, but when the femoral approach is used, fluoroscopic guidance is almost always necessary to cannulate the pulmonary artery and to obtain pulmonary capillary wedge position. Although most right-heart catheters have a J-shaped curvature distally to facilitate passage from the SVC to the pulmonary artery, a catheter with an S-shaped distal end has been designed for femoral insertion. Despite limited manipulation, the balloon flotation catheters are the safest and most rapid method for obtaining right-heart pressures and blood samples. Other right-heart balloon flotation end-hole catheters are stiffer and allow passage of conventional 0.035- or 0.038-inch guidewires to improve manipulation. Although these lack the ability to obtain thermodilution cardiac outputs, they yield better pressure fidelity owing to less catheter whip artifact and a larger end hole.

There are two methods for advancing a balloon flotation catheter from the femoral vein. On many occasions, the catheter can be advanced directly through the right atrium and across the tricuspid valve. Once in the right ventricle, the catheter is manipulated to point superiorly and directly into the right ventricular outflow tract. This orientation can usually be achieved while the catheter is advanced with slight clockwise rotation. Once in the outflow tract, the balloon tip should allow flotation into the pulmonary artery and wedge positions (Fig. 17–4). When necessary, deep inspiration or cough can facilitate this maneuver and assist in crossing the pulmonic valve. If the catheter continues to point inferiorly toward the right ventricular apex, another technique should be used because further advancement can risk perforation of the right ventricular apex.

One such additional technique for performing right-heart catheterization with a balloon flotation catheter is shown in Figure 17–4. A loop is formed in the right atrium, with the catheter tip directed laterally. The loop can be created by hooking the catheter tip on the hepatic vein or by advancing the catheter while it is directed laterally in the right atrium. Once the loop is formed, the catheter should be advanced further, which directs the tip inferiorly and then medially across the tricuspid valve. Antegrade blood flow should then direct the catheter into the pulmonary artery. After the catheter is placed into the wedge position, the redundant loop should be removed by slow withdrawal.

Screening blood samples for oximetric analysis should be obtained from the SVC and the pulmonary artery to evaluate

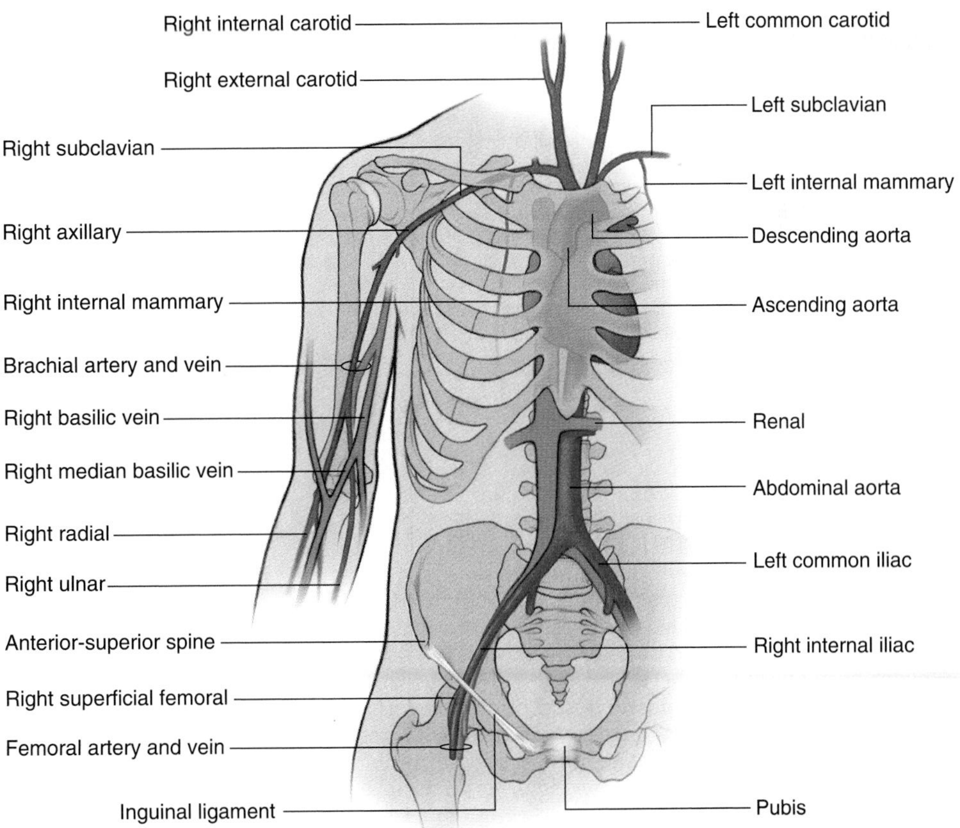

FIGURE 17–2 Principal arteries used for access during cardiac catheterization. Only the superficial veins are shown on the forearm. (Modified from Thibodeau GA, Patton KT [eds]: Anthony's Textbook of Anatomy and Physiology. 17th ed. St. Louis, CV Mosby, 2002.)

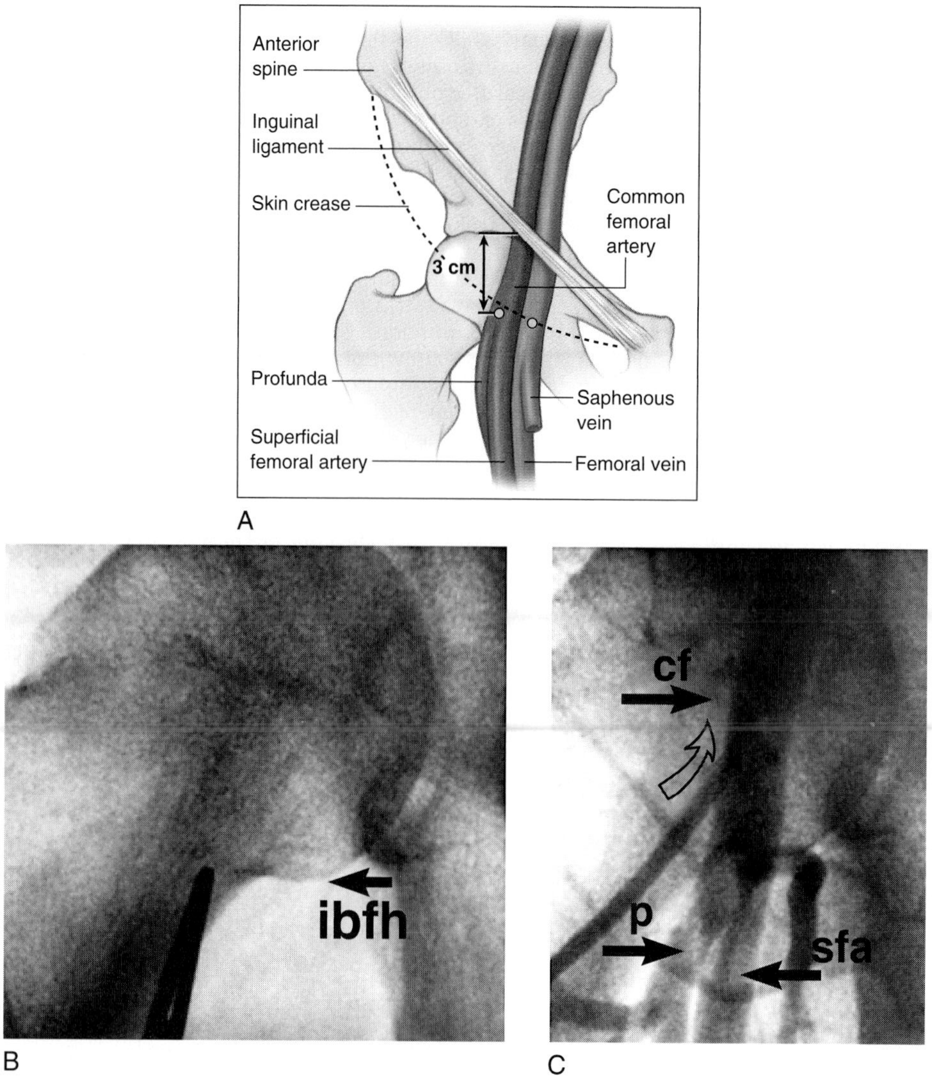

FIGURE 17–3 Regional anatomy relevant to percutaneous femoral arterial and venous catheterization. **A,** Schematic diagram showing the right femoral artery and vein coursing underneath the inguinal ligament, which runs from the anterior superior iliac spine to the pubic tubercle. The arterial skin nick should be placed approximately 3 cm below the ligament and directly over the femoral arterial pulsation, and the venous skin nick should be placed at the same level but approximately one fingerbreadth more medial. Although this level corresponds roughly to the skin crease in most patients, anatomical localization relative to the inguinal ligament provides a more constant landmark. **B,** Fluoroscopic localization of skin nick (marked by clamp tip) to the inferior border of the femoral head (ibfh). **C,** Catheter (open arrow) inserted through this skin nick has entered the common femoral artery (cf), above its bifurcation into the superficial femoral artery (sfa) and profunda (p) branches. (From Baim DS, Grossman W: Percutaneous approach, including transseptal and apical puncture. *In* Baim DS, Grossman W [eds]: Cardiac Catheterization, Angiography, and Intervention. 6th ed. Philadelphia, Lea & Febiger, 2000, p 71.)

for intracardiac shunts. Cardiac output can also be determined by thermodilution techniques.

NONFLOTATION CATHETERS. When an end-hole catheter (e.g., Cournand or multipurpose) that does not have a balloon tip is used, the technique for cannulating the pulmonary artery is markedly different. Manipulation and torquing of the nonflotation catheter are necessary to advance into the pulmonary artery. The catheter should be directed inferiorly across the tricuspid valve and then superiorly into the right ventricular outflow tract. It is generally recommended that one attempt be made to form a loop in the right atrium before advancement into the right ventricle in order to lessen the risk of perforation.

A probe-patent foramen ovale is present in about 30 percent of adult patients that allows access to the left atrium. It can be entered using a multipurpose catheter with the tip directed medially and slightly posterior. The catheter is withdrawn slowly from the SVC or high right atrium until a slight forward and medial motion is observed. The catheter then prolapses into the left atrium with mild pressure against the interatrial septum in patients with a probe-patent foramen ovale. Left atrial position can be verified by the pressure waveform, by blood samples demonstrating arterial saturation, or by hand contrast medium injection. If left atrial access is necessary and cannot be obtained with this technique, a transseptal catheterization should be undertaken (see Transseptal Catheterization).

COMPLICATIONS. The most common complications of right-heart catheterization are nonsustained atrial and ventricular arrhythmias. Major complications associated with right-heart catheterization are infrequent. These include pulmonary infarction, pulmonary artery or right ventricular perforation, and infection. Pulmonary artery rupture can be avoided by combined use of fluoroscopic guidance and constant evaluation of the pressure waveform. Confusion about the location of the distal end of the catheter may arise in the setting of large v waves in the pulmonary capillary wedge pressure tracing. The operator may mistake this waveform as a pulmonary artery waveform (Fig. 17–5). Careful attention to the timing of the peak pulmonary artery systolic pressure and the v wave with respect to the ECG, along with the use of fluoroscopy, prevents inadvertent inflation of the balloon in the wedged position, which can cause pulmonary artery rupture.

Left-Heart Catheterization and Coronary Arteriography

THE JUDKINS TECHNIQUE. Because of its relative ease, speed, reliability, and low complication rate,[1,2] the Judkins technique has become the most widely used method of left-heart catheterization and coronary arteriography. After local anesthesia with 1 percent lidocaine (Xylocaine), percutaneous entry of the femoral artery is achieved by puncturing the vessel 1 to 3 cm (or one to two fingerbreadths) below the inguinal ligament. The ligament can be palpated as it courses from the anterior superior iliac spine to the superior pubic ramus. This ligament, not the inguinal crease, should be used as the landmark. The inguinal crease can be misleading, particularly in the obese patient. A transverse skin incision is made over the femoral artery with a scalpel. A hemostatic clamp can be used under fluoroscopy to verify that the nick is made over the inferior edge of the femoral head. Using a modified Seldinger technique (Fig. 17–6), an 18-gauge thin-

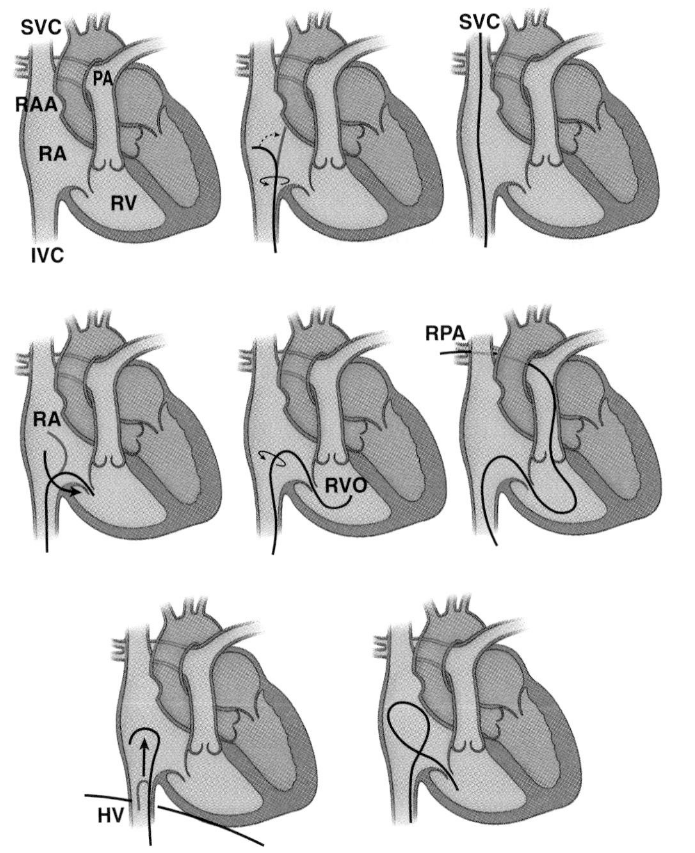

FIGURE 17–4 Right-heart catheterization from the femoral vein, shown in cartoon form. **Top row,** The right-heart catheter is initially placed in the right atrium (RA) aimed at the lateral atrial wall. Counterclockwise rotation aims the catheter posteriorly and allows advancement into the superior vena cava (SVC). Although not evident in the figure, clockwise catheter rotation into an anterior orientation would lead to advancement into the right atrial appendage (RAA), precluding SVC catheterization. **Center row,** The catheter is then withdrawn back into the right atrium and aimed laterally. Clockwise rotation causes the catheter tip to sweep anteromedially and cross the tricuspid valve. With the catheter tip in a horizontal orientation just beyond the spine, it is positioned below the right ventricular outflow (RVO) tract. Additional clockwise rotation causes the catheter to point straight up, allowing advancement into the main pulmonary artery and from there into the right pulmonary artery (RPA). **Bottom row,** Two maneuvers useful in catheterization of a dilated right heart. A larger loop with a downward-directed tip may be required to reach the tricuspid valve and can be formed by catching the catheter tip in the hepatic vein (HV) and advancing the catheter quickly into the right atrium. The reverse loop technique (bottom right) gives the catheter tip an upward direction, aimed toward the outflow tract. IVC = inferior vena cava; PA = pulmonary artery; RV = right ventricle. (From Baim DS, Grossman W: Percutaneous approach, including transseptal and apical puncture. *In* Baim DS, Grossman W [eds]: Cardiac Catheterization, Angiography, and Intervention. 6th ed. Philadelphia, Lea & Febiger, 2000, p 78.)

walled needle (Fig. 17–7) is inserted at a 30- to 45-degree angle into the femoral artery, and a 0.035- or 0.038-inch J-tip polytetrafluoroethylene (Teflon)-coated guidewire is advanced through the needle into the artery. The wire should pass freely up the aorta. After arterial access is obtained, a sheath at least equal in size to the coronary catheter is usually inserted into the femoral artery. Although it is generally recommended that the patient receive approximately 3000 U of heparin after access is obtained, its benefit has not been well proven. In patients receiving heparin prior to arrival in the laboratory, an activated clotting time should be obtained following access. Sheath removal is usually not recommended until the activated clotting time is less than 175 seconds unless a vascular closure device is being utilized.

Left ventricular systolic and end-diastolic pressures can be obtained by advancing a pigtail catheter into the left ventricle (Fig. 17–8). In assessing valvular aortic stenosis, left ventricular and aortic or femoral artery pressures should be recorded simultaneously. In suspected mitral stenosis, left ventricular and wedge or left atrial pressures should be obtained simultaneously. Left ventriculography is performed in the 30-degree right anterior oblique and 45- to 50-degree left anterior oblique views. A pigtail catheter is most commonly used for this purpose. Power injection of 30 to 40 ml of contrast medium into the ventricle is used to assess left ventricular function and the severity of mitral regurgitation. After ventriculography, left ventricular systolic and end-diastolic pressure measurements may be repeated and the systolic pressure recorded as the catheter is withdrawn from the left ventricle into the aorta. If an aortic transvalvular gradient is present, recording these pressures can detect it. For measurement of suspected intraventricular gradients, a multipurpose catheter with an end hole is desirable to localize the gradient in the left ventricle. Pigtail catheters contain side holes, which obscure the capacity to define whether the gradient is intraventricular, subvalvular, or transvalvular.

After coronary arteriography and left-heart catheterization have been completed, the catheters are removed and firm pressure is applied to the femoral area for 15 to 20 minutes, either by hand or by a mechanical clamp. The patient should be instructed to lie in bed for several hours, with the leg remaining straight to prevent hematoma formation. With 4 or 5F catheters, 2 hours of bed rest is usually sufficient, whereas use of 6F catheters usually involves at least 3 to 4 hours.

Alternatively, vascular closure devices may be used. Three types are currently available: collagen plugs, suture closure, and hemostatic patches. Each allows earlier ambulation of the patients, within 1 to 2 hours after the procedure.[14,15] They also permit early sheath removal in patients receiving anticoagulation. However, none has been shown to lower vascular complication rates compared with conventional hand compression.[16] The ultimate success of any means of achieving hemostasis relies on a single front wall puncture of the common femoral artery.

The main advantage of the Judkins technique is speed and ease of selective catheterization. These attributes do not, however, preclude the importance of extensive operator experience to ensure quality studies with acceptable safety. The main disadvantage of this technique is its use in patients with severe iliofemoral atherosclerotic disease, in whom retrograde passage of catheters through areas of extreme narrowing or tortuosity may be difficult or impossible. However, even passage through synthetic aortofemoral grafts has a low complication rate.[17]

BRACHIAL ARTERY TECHNIQUE—SONES TECHNIQUE. Sones and colleagues introduced the first technique for coronary artery catheterization by means of a brachial artery cutdown. The Sones technique is still popular in many centers and is described in Chapter 18.

PERCUTANEOUS BRACHIAL ARTERY TECHNIQUE

A modification of the Sones technique is the percutaneous brachial artery technique using preformed Judkins catheters. This technique uses the Seldinger method of percutaneous brachial artery entry. A 4 to 6F sheath is placed into the brachial artery, and 3000 to 5000 U of heparin is infused into the side port. A guidewire is then advanced to the ascending aorta under fluoroscopic control. Judkins left, right, and pigtail catheters are passed over the guidewire for routine arteriography and ventriculography. The guidewire may occasionally be necessary to direct the left coronary catheter into the left sinus of Valsalva and the ostium of the left main coronary artery. Alternatively, an Amplatz left 1 or 2 is used to intubate the coronary ostium. Following removal of the sheath, the arm should be maintained straight with an armband for 4 to 6 hours with observation of radial and brachial pulses.

The main advantage of the percutaneous brachial technique is that it avoids a brachial artery cutdown and repair. The main disadvantage is that manipulation of catheters can be difficult. When this technique was

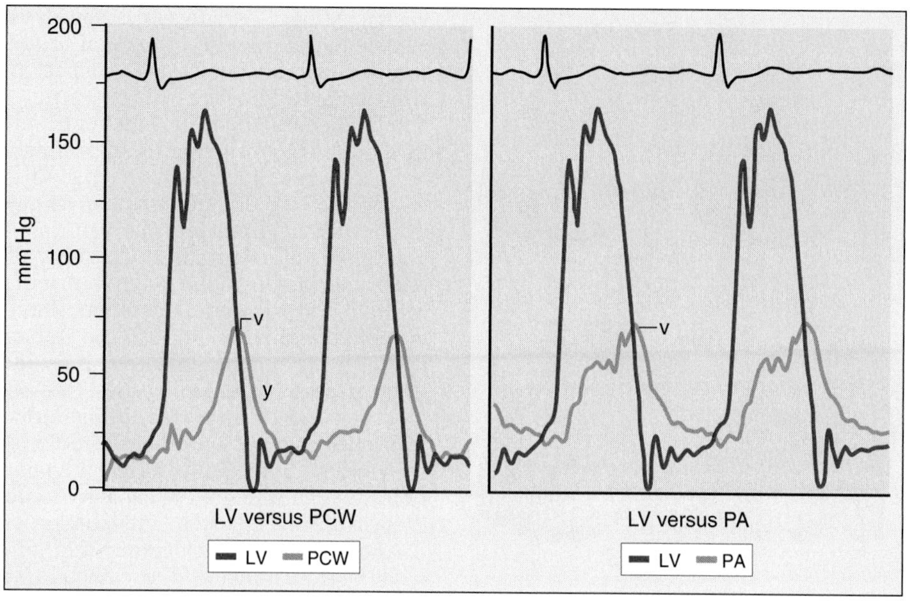

FIGURE 17–5 Acute mitral regurgitation with poor left atrial compliance. The left ventricle (LV) pressure versus the pulmonary capillary wedge (PCW) pressure is shown on the left. A large regurgitant v wave is seen. This v wave is transmitted through the pulmonary bed to the pulmonary arterial (PA) tracing and is superimposed in the right panel. (From Bashore TM, Harrison JK, Davidson CJ: Cardiac catheterization, angiography, and interventional techniques in valvular and congenital heart disease. *In* Sabiston DC, Spencer FC [eds]: Surgery of the Chest. 6th ed. Philadelphia, WB Saunders, 1995, p 1144.)

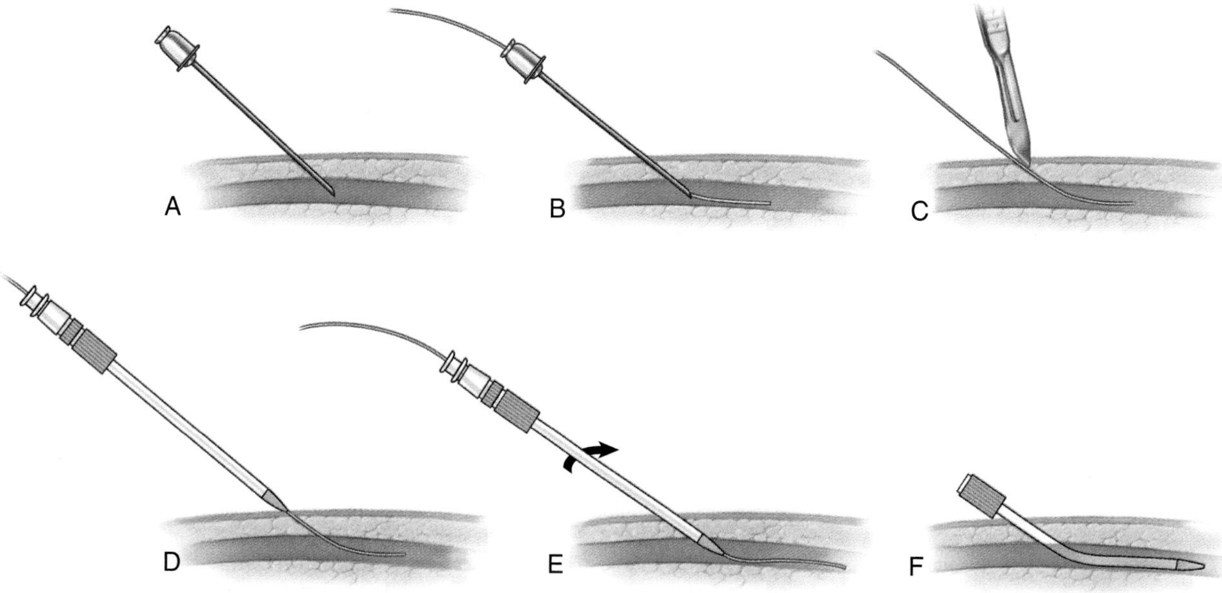

FIGURE 17–6 Modified Seldinger technique for percutaneous catheter sheath introduction. **A,** Vessel punctured by needle. **B,** Flexible guidewire placed into the vessel through the needle. **C,** Needle removed, guidewire left in place, and the hole in the skin around the wire enlarged with a scalpel. **D,** Sheath and dilator placed over the guidewire. **E,** Sheath and dilator advanced over the guidewire and into the vessel. **F,** Dilator and guidewire removed while the sheath remains in the vessel. (From Hill JA, Lambert CR, Vlietstra RE, Pepine CJ: Review of general catheterization techniques. *In* Pepine CJ, Hill JA, Lambert CR [eds]: Diagnostic and Therapeutic Cardiac Catheterization. 3rd ed. Baltimore, Williams & Wilkins, 1998, p 107.)

compared with the femoral technique, patients' comfort, hemostasis time, and time to ambulation favored the brachial technique, whereas procedural efficiency, time of radiation exposure, and diagnostic film quality were more favorable with the femoral approach.[18] Complication rates appear similar.

PERCUTANEOUS RADIAL ARTERY TECHNIQUE

Left-heart catheterization by the radial artery approach was developed as an alternative to the percutaneous transbrachial approach in an attempt to limit vascular complications. The inherent advantages of the transradial approach are that the hand has a dual arterial supply connected through the palmar arches and that there are no nerves or veins at the site of puncture. In addition, bed rest is unnecessary after the procedure, allowing more efficient outpatient angiography.

The procedure requires a normal Allen test result. After manual compression of both the radial and ulnar arteries during fist clenching, normal color returns to the opened hand within 10 seconds after releasing pressure over the ulnar artery, and significant reactive hyperemia is absent on releasing pressure over the radial artery.

The arm is abducted and the wrist hyperextended over a gauze roll. Routine skin anesthesia is used, a small incision is made just proximal to the styloid process of the radius, and the subcutaneous tissue is tunneled

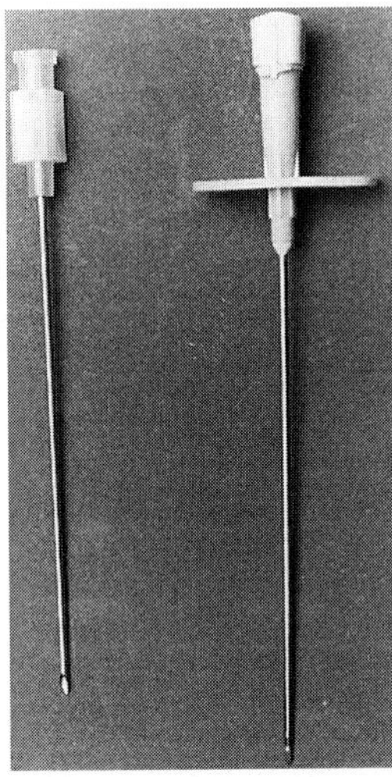

FIGURE 17–7 Two most commonly used needle types for vascular access. On the left, a single-piece, thin-walled "front-wall needle"; on the right, a two-component, thin-walled Seldinger needle. (From MacDonald RG: Catheters, sheaths, guidewires, needles, and related equipment. *In* Pepine CJ, Hill JA, Lambert CR [eds]: Diagnostic and Therapeutic Cardiac Catheterization. 3rd ed. Baltimore, Williams & Wilkins, 1998, p 130.)

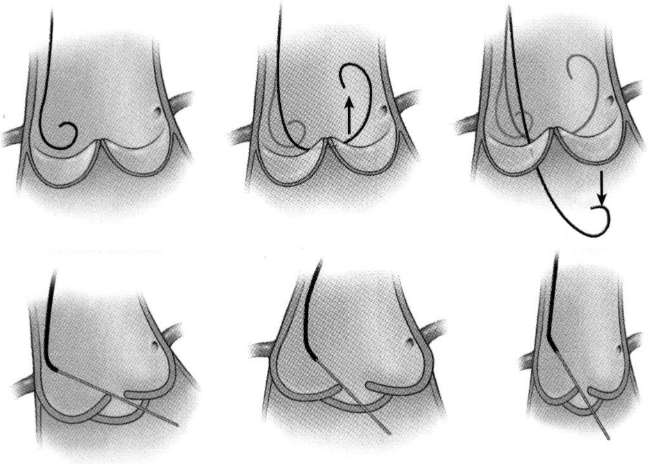

FIGURE 17–8 Technique for retrograde crossing of an aortic valve using a pigtail catheter. The upper row shows the technique for crossing a normal aortic valve. In the bottom row, the use of a straight guidewire and pigtail catheter in combination is shown. Increasing the length of protruding guidewire straightens the catheter curve and causes the wire to point more toward the right coronary ostium; reducing the length of protruding wire restores the pigtail contour and deflects the guidewire tip toward the left coronary artery. When the correct length of wire and the correct rotational orientation of the catheter have been found, repeated advancement and withdrawal of catheter and guidewire together allow retrograde passage across the valve. In a dilated aortic root, the angled pigtail catheter is preferable. In a small aortic root (bottom row, right), a right coronary Judkins catheter may have advantages. In patients with bicuspid valves, an Amplatz left catheter is often used as it directs the wire more superiorly. (From Baim DS, Grossman W: Percutaneous approach including transseptal and apical puncture. *In* Baim DS, Grossman W [eds]: Cardiac Catheterization, Angiography, and Intervention. 6th ed. Philadelphia, Lea & Febiger, 2000, p 86.)

using forceps. An 18-gauge needle is introduced at a 45-degree angle and an exchange-length 0.035- or 0.038-inch J-tip guidewire is inserted. A 23-cm-long 4 or 5F sheath is then introduced. Heparin, 5000 U, is administered through the side arm of the sheath. Coronary catheters are then advanced over the exchange wire into the ascending aorta. The left coronary artery is intubated in a manner similar to the brachial approach using either a left 4- or 5-cm tip Judkins (JL 4.0, 5.0), a left Amplatz, or a brachial Castillo type II catheter. The right coronary artery is intubated using a 4-cm right Judkins (JR 4.0), a left Amplatz, or a multipurpose catheter. Left ventriculography can be performed using a standard pigtail catheter. Hemostasis is obtained at the end of the procedure after sheath removal using direct pressure. It is recommended that the arterial puncture site be allowed to bleed for several beats before maintaining direct pressure. The radial pulse should be monitored regularly for several hours after the procedure.

The potential limitations of this procedure include the inability to cannulate the radial artery owing to its smaller size and propensity to develop spasm, poor visualization of the coronary arteries resulting from the small-caliber catheters with limited manipulation potential, and risk of radial arterial occlusion caused by dissection or thrombus formation. In addition, when right-heart catheterization is required, additional approaches are necessary. If intervention is contemplated, device selection may be limited by guide catheter size. Although there is little debate that the femoral approach is the simplest and probably the safest technique for left-heart catheterization, the transradial approach for left-heart catheterization has gained in popularity.[19]

Transseptal Catheterization

Transseptal left-heart catheterization has received renewed interest with the advent of percutaneous balloon mitral commissurotomy as a viable option to surgical commissurotomy, with electrophysiological procedures requiring access to pulmonary veins, and with increasing use of disc-type prosthetic valves in the aortic position. This type of mechanical prosthetic valve cannot be crossed safely and prohibits retrograde left-heart catheterization. When performed by experienced operators, the technique has a low complication rate of less than 2 percent.[20]

The transseptal catheter is a short, curved catheter with a tapered tip (Fig. 17–9). Alternatively, an 8F Mullins sheath and dilator combination is used. The Brockenbrough needle is 18 gauge that tapers to 21 gauge at the distal tip. One commonly used approach is to place a 0.032-inch guidewire through the femoral vein, through the right atrium, and into the SVC. The Mullins transseptal sheath and dilator are then advanced over the wire into the SVC. The guidewire is removed and replaced with a Brockenbrough needle, and the distal port is connected to a pressure manifold. With the needle tip just proximal to the Mullins sheath tip, the entire catheter system is withdrawn. The catheter is simultaneously rotated from a 12 o'clock to a 5 o'clock position. The operator observes two abrupt rightward movements. The first occurs as the catheter descends from the SVC to the right atrium. The second occurs as the Mullins dilator tip passes over the limbic edge into the fossa ovalis. The curve of the sheath and needle should be oriented slightly anteriorly. The dilator and needle can then be advanced gently as a unit. Steady gentle pressure is often adequate to advance the system through the fossa ovalis into the left atrium. If not, the needle should be advanced across the interatrial septum while holding the Mullins sheath in place. In cases in which transseptal puncture is technically difficult because of a large right atrium, postsurgical condition, or anatomical variant, intracardiac echocardiography can be useful to localize the fossa ovalis and interatrial septum. (See Intracardiac Echocardiography.)

Left atrial position can be confirmed by the overall increase in pressure with left atrial a and v waveforms, hand injection of contrast medium, or measurement of arterial oxygen saturation. When the position is confirmed, the catheter should be rotated toward 3 o'clock and the dilator and sheath safely advanced 2 to 3 cm into the left atrium. The sheath is held firmly, and the dilator and needle are removed. Left atrial pressure measurements should then be repeated. If measurement of left ventricular pressure or left ventriculography, or both, is necessary, the catheter can usually be advanced easily into the left ventricle after slight counterclockwise rotation. The major risk of transseptal catheterization lies in inadvertent puncture of atrial structures, such as the atrial free wall, left atrial appendage, or coronary sinus, or entry into the aortic root or pulmonary artery.

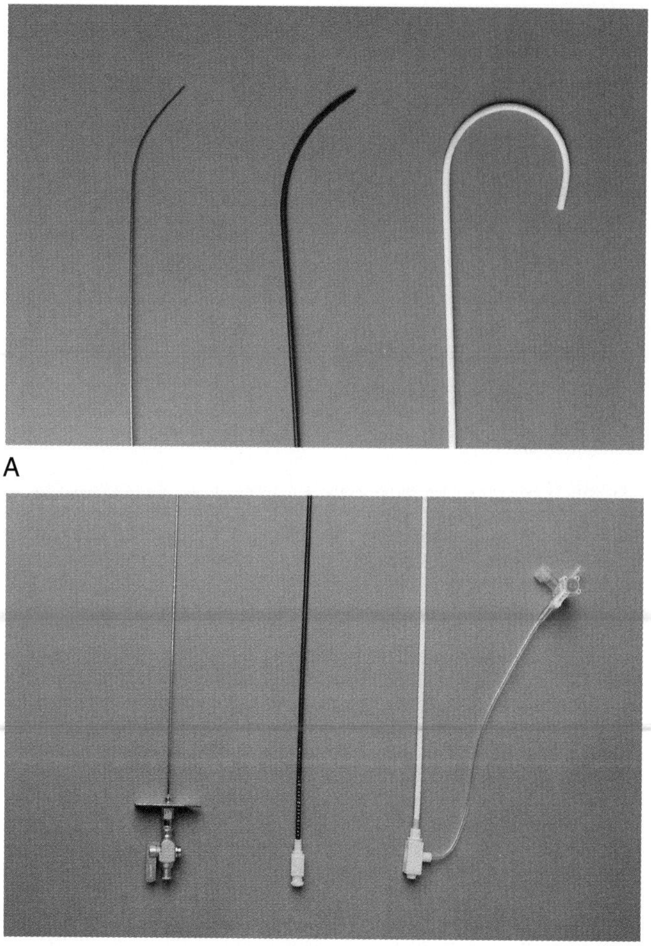

A

B

FIGURE 17–9 Transseptal catheters. **A,** Distal catheter. **B,** Proximal catheter. Left, Mullins transseptal sheath. Middle, Introducer (dilator) that is placed inside sheath to add stiffness to the catheter. Right, Brockenbrough transseptal needle that is placed inside the sheath and is used to penetrate the septum.

Direct Transthoracic Left Ventricular Puncture

The sole indication for direct left ventricular puncture is to measure left ventricular pressure and to perform ventriculography in patients with mechanical prosthetic valves in both the mitral and aortic positions, preventing retrograde arterial and transseptal catheterization. Crossing tilting-disc valves with catheters should be avoided because it may result in catheter entrapment, occlusion of the valve, or possible dislodgment of the disc with embolization.

The procedure is performed after localizing the left ventricular apex by palpation or, preferably, by using echocardiography.[21] After local anesthesia is administered, an 18- or 21-gauge 6-inch Teflon catheter system is inserted at the upper rib margin and directed slightly posteriorly and toward the right second intercostal space until the impulse is encountered. The needle and sheath are advanced into the left ventricle The stylet and needle are removed, and the sheath is connected for pressure measurement.

The risks of this procedure include cardiac tamponade, hemothorax, pneumothorax, laceration of the left anterior descending coronary artery, embolism of left ventricular thrombus, vagal reactions, and ventricular arrhythmias. The risk of pericardial tamponade, however, is limited in patients who have undergone prior cardiac surgery because mediastinal fibrosis is present. However, with current noninvasive imaging techniques including transesophageal echocardiography, this procedure is infrequently indicated.

ENDOMYOCARDIAL BIOPSY

Endomyocardial biopsy can be performed using various disposable or reusable bioptomes. Disposable bioptomes have become the more commonly used devices because of the difficulty in maintaining and adequately resterilizing the reusable varieties.The most popular devices used for the internal jugular vein approach include the reusable stiff-shaft Caves-Schulz Stanford bioptome and the floppy-shaft King bioptome. Right ventricular biopsy may be performed using the internal jugular vein,[22] the subclavian vein, or the femoral vein. Left ventricular biopsy may be performed using the femoral arterial approach.

When performing right ventricular biopsy through the right internal jugular vein, a 7 to 9F sheath is introduced using the usual Seldinger technique. A 7 to 9F bioptome is advanced under fluoroscopic guidance to the lateral wall of the right atrium. Using counterclockwise rotation, the device is advanced across the tricuspid valve and toward the interventricular septum. Position of the bioptome against the interventricular septum is confirmed using 30-degree right anterior oblique and 60-degree left anterior oblique fluoroscopic projections. Alternatively, two-dimensional echocardiography has been used to guide the position of the bioptome with good results. Contact with the myocardium is confirmed by the presence of premature ventricular contractions, lack of further advancement, and transmission of the ventricular impulse to the operator.The bioptome is then slightly withdrawn from the septum, the forceps jaws are opened, the bioptome is readvanced to make contact with the myocardium, and the forceps closed. A slight tug is felt on removal of the device.Approximately four to six samples of myocardium are required for adequate pathological analysis. Consultation with a pathologist should be obtained to ensure appropriate specimen collection and processing.

Right ventricular biopsy from the femoral vein requires insertion of a long 6 or 7F sheath directed toward the portion of the ventricle to be sampled. Various configurations of sheaths are used for right ventricular biopsy. The conventional sheath has a 45-degree angle on its distal end to allow access to the right ventricle. However, newer designs including the Daig biopsy sheath have dual curves. This catheter possesses the usual 180-degree Mullins curve and an additional distal perpendicular septal plane curve of 90 degrees, which allows improved manipulation and positioning toward the interventricular septum.

An angled pigtail or balloon flotation catheter and long guidewire system can be used to enter the right ventricle. The sheath is then advanced over the pigtail catheter into the right ventricle, the catheter is withdrawn, the sheath is flushed, and pressure is measured. The bioptome is advanced through the sheath. The biopsy sheath should be visualized in both the 30-degree right anterior oblique and 40-degree left anterior oblique views. The right anterior oblique view ensures that the catheter is in the midventricle away from the apex. The left anterior oblique view verifies that the sheath tip is oriented toward the interventricular septum. Contrast medium infusion through the side port of the sheath can be confirmatory. Samples of myocardium are taken in a manner similar to that described earlier.

If left ventricular biopsy is to be performed, the biopsy sheath is generally inserted through the femoral artery and positioned over a multipurpose or pigtail catheter that has been placed in the ventricle. The sheath is advanced below the mitral apparatus and away from the posterobasal wall. The catheter is then withdrawn, and either a long King bioptome or the Stanford left ventricular bioptome is inserted. Care must be taken when left ventricular biopsy is performed to prevent air embolism while introducing the bioptome into the sheath. A constant infusion of flush solution through the sheath minimizes the risk of air or thrombus embolism.

Complications of endomyocardial biopsy include cardiac perforation with cardiac tamponade, emboli (air, tissue, or thromboembolus), arrhythmias, electrical conduction disturbances, injury to heart valves, vasovagal reactions, and pneumothorax. The overall complication rate is between 1 and 2 percent, with the risk of cardiac perforation with tamponade generally reported as less than 0.05 percent.[23] Systemic embolization and ventricular arrhythmias are more common with left ventricular biopsy. Left ventricular biopsy should generally be avoided in patients with right bundle branch block because of the potential for developing complete atrioventricular block as well as in patients with known left ventricular thrombus.

The indications for endomyocardial biopsy remain controversial.[24] Generally agreed is that endomyocardial biopsy is indicated to monitor cardiac allograft rejection and that it may also be useful to monitor for anthracycline cardiotoxicity. However, considerable persistent controversy surrounds the use of endomyocardial biopsy to evaluate the cause of dilated cardiomyopathy.[24] Other possible indications for endomyocardial biopsy include differentiation between restrictive and constrictive myopathies,[25] determination of whether myocarditis is the cause of ventricular arrhythmias, and assessment of patients with left ventricular dysfunction associated with human immunodeficiency virus infection.[26]

Percutaneous Intraaortic Balloon Pump Insertion

The intraaortic balloon counterpulsation devices available for adults are positioned in the descending thoracic aorta. They have a balloon volume of 30 to 50 ml, use helium as the inflation gas, and are timed to inflate during diastole and deflate during systole. Details of the technique of balloon insertion have been well described.[27] Briefly, the device is inserted through the femoral artery using the standard Seldinger technique. The device is placed so that the tip is just below the level of the left subclavian artery. Optimal positioning requires fluoroscopic guidance. Timing of the balloon is adjusted during 1:2 (one inflation for each two beats) pumping so that inflation of the balloon occurs at the aortic dicrotic notch and deflation occurs immediately before systole. This timing ensures maximal augmentation of diastolic flow and maximal systolic unloading.

Favorable hemodynamic effects include reduction in left ventricular afterload and improvement in myocardial oxygenation.[28] Intraaortic balloon pump (IABP) insertion is indicated for patients with angina refractory to medical therapy, cardiogenic shock, or mechanical complications of myocardial infarction (including severe mitral regurgitation, ventricular septal defect) or for those who have severe left main coronary artery stenosis and will be undergoing cardiac surgery. IABP may also be valuable in patients undergoing high-risk percutaneous coronary intervention or after primary angioplasty in the setting of acute myocardial infarction.[29,30] IABP insertion is contraindicated in patients with moderate or severe aortic regurgitation, aortic dissection, aortic aneurysm, patent ductus arteriosus, severe peripheral vascular disease, bleeding disorders, or sepsis.

Complications of IABP insertion include limb ischemia requiring early balloon removal or vascular surgery, balloon rupture, balloon entrapment, hematomas, and sepsis.[29] The incidence of vascular complications ranges from 12 to greater than 40 percent.[29] Most patients in whom limb ischemia develops after insertion of a balloon pump device have resolution of the ischemia on balloon removal and do not require surgical intervention (thrombectomy, vascular repair, fasciotomy, or amputation). The risk of limb ischemia is heightened in patients with diabetes or peripheral vascular disease, in women, and in patients with a postinsertion ankle-brachial index of less than 0.8. However, with the development of smaller catheters (8 to 9.5F) and the advent of the sheathless insertion techniques, vascular complications have been reduced.[29-31]

Hemodynamic Data

The hemodynamic component of the cardiac catheterization procedure focuses on pressure measurements, the measurement of flow (e.g., cardiac output, shunt flows, flow across a stenotic orifice, regurgitant flows, and coronary blood flow), and the determination of vascular resistances. Simply stated, flow through a blood vessel is determined by the pressure difference within the vessel and the vascular resistance as described by Ohm's law: $Q = \Delta P/R$.

Pressure Measurements

Accurate recording of pressure waveforms and correct interpretation of physiological data derived from these waveforms are major goals of cardiac catheterization. A pressure wave is the cyclical force generated by cardiac muscle contraction, and its amplitude and duration are influenced by various mechanical and physiological parameters. The pressure waveform from a particular cardiac chamber is influenced by the force of the contracting chamber and its surrounding structures, including the contiguous chambers of the heart, the pericardium, the lungs, and the vasculature. Physiological variables of heart rate and the respiratory cycle also influence the pressure waveform. An understanding of the components of the cardiac cycle is essential to the correct interpretation of hemodynamic data obtained in the catheterization laboratory.

Pressure Measurement Systems

FLUID-FILLED SYSTEMS. Intravascular pressures are typically measured using a fluid-filled catheter that is attached to a pressure transducer. The pressure wave is transmitted from the catheter tip to the transducer by the fluid column within the catheter. The majority of pressure transducers used currently are disposable electrical strain gauges. The pressure wave distorts the diaphragm or wire within the transducer. This energy is then converted to an electrical signal proportional to the pressure being applied using the principle of the Wheatstone bridge. This signal is then amplified and recorded as an analog signal.[32]

There are a number of sources of error when pressures are measured using a fluid-filled catheter-transducer system. Distortion of the output signal occurs as a result of the frequency response characteristics and damping characteristics of the system. The frequency response of the system is the ratio of the output amplitude to input amplitude over a range of frequencies of the input pressure wave. The natural frequency is the frequency at which the system oscillates when it is shock-excited in the absence of friction. Dissipation of the energy of the system, such as by friction, is called *damping*. To ensure a high-frequency response range, the pressure measurement system should have the highest possible natural frequency and optimal damping. With optimal damping the energy is dissipated gradually, thus maintaining the frequency response curve as close as possible to an output/input ratio of 1 as it approaches the system's natural frequency. Optimal damping is achieved by using a short, wide-bore, noncompliant catheter-tubing system that is directly connected to the transducer using a low-density liquid from which all air bubbles have been removed.[32]

The pressure transducer must be calibrated against a known pressure, and the establishment of a zero reference must be undertaken at the start of the catheterization procedure. To "zero" the transducer, the transducer is placed at the level of the atria, which is approximately midchest. If the transducer is attached to the manifold and is therefore at variable positions during the procedure, a second fluid-filled catheter system should be attached to the transducer and positioned at the level of the midchest. All transducers being used during the procedure should be zeroed and calibrated simultaneously. Because of possible variable drift during the procedure, all transducers should be rebalanced immediately prior to obtaining simultaneous recordings for transvalvular gradient determinations.

Potential sources of error include catheter whip artifact (motion of the tip of the catheter within the measured chamber), end-pressure artifact (an end-hole catheter measures an artificially elevated pressure because of streaming or high velocity of the pressure wave), catheter impact artifact (when the catheter is struck by the walls or valves of the cardiac chambers), and catheter tip obstruction within small vessels or valvular orifices occurring because of the size of the catheter itself. The operator must be aware of the many sources of potential error, and when there is a discrepancy between the observed data and the clinical scenario, the system should be examined for errors or artifacts.

MICROMANOMETER CATHETERS. The use of these catheters, which have the pressure transducer mounted at their tip, greatly reduces many of these errors in measurement. However, their utility is limited by the additional cost and time needed for properly calibrating and using the system. These catheters have higher natural frequencies and more optimal damping characteristics because the interposing fluid column is eliminated. In addition, there is a decrease in catheter whip artifact. The pressure waveform is less distorted and is without the 30- to 40-millisecond delay seen in the fluid-filled catheter-transducer system. Commercially available high-fidelity micromanometer systems have both an end hole and side holes to allow over-the-wire insertion into the circulation while also permitting angiography. Catheters that have two transducers separated by a short distance are useful for accurate measurement of gradients across valvular structures and within ventricular chambers. The micromanometer system has been used for research purposes to assess the rate of ventricular pressure rise (dP/dt), wall stress, the rate of ventricular pressure decay (−dP/dt), the time constant of relaxation, and ventricular pressure-volume relationships (see Chap. 20).

The micromanometer catheter systems have several disadvantages, including their expense, fragility, and added procedural time. In addition, the zero level of these systems may drift after the pressure is zeroed to the fluid-filled lumen within the catheter.

Normal Pressure Waveforms

An understanding of the normal pressure waveform morphologies is necessary for comprehending the abnormalities that characterize certain pathological conditions. Normal pressures in the cardiac chambers and great vessels are listed in Table 17–4. Simply stated, whenever fluid is added to a chamber or compressed within a chamber, the pressure usually rises; conversely, whenever fluid exits from a chamber or the chamber relaxes, the pressure usually falls. One exception to this rule is the early phase of ventricular diastolic filling, when ventricular volume increases after mitral valve opening but ventricular pressure continues to decrease because of active relaxation.[33] Examples of normal pressure waveforms are shown in Figure 17–10.

TABLE 17–4 Normal Pressures and Vascular Resistances

Pressures	Average (mm Hg)	Range (mm Hg)
Right atrium		
a wave	6	2-7
v wave	5	2-7
mean	3	1-5
Right ventricle		
peak systolic	25	15-30
end-diastolic	4	1-7
Pulmonary artery		
peak systolic	25	15-30
end-diastolic	9	4-12
mean	15	9-19
Pulmonary capillary wedge		
mean	9	4-12
Left atrium		
a wave	10	4-16
v wave	12	6-21
mean	8	2-12
Left ventricle		
peak systolic	130	90-140
end-diastolic	8	5-12
Central aorta		
peak systolic	130	90-140
end-diastolic	70	60-90
mean	85	70-105
Vascular Resistances	**Mean (dyne-sec · cm^{-5})**	**Range (dyne-sec · cm^{-5})**
Systemic vascular resistance	1100	700-1600
Total pulmonary resistance	200	100-300
Pulmonary vascular resistance	70	20-130

ATRIAL PRESSURE. The *right atrial pressure waveform* has three positive deflections, the a, c, and v waves. The a wave is due to atrial systole and follows the P wave of the ECG. The height of the a wave depends on atrial contractility and the resistance to right ventricular filling. The *x* descent follows the a wave and represents relaxation of the atrium and downward pulling of the tricuspid annulus by right ventricular contraction. The *x* descent is interrupted by the c wave, which is a small positive deflection caused by protrusion of the closed tricuspid valve into the right atrium. Pressure in the atrium rises after the *x* descent owing to passive atrial filling. The atrial pressure then peaks as the v wave, which represents right ventricular systole. The height of the v wave is related to atrial compliance and the amount of blood returning to the atrium from the periphery. The right atrial v wave is generally smaller than the a wave. The *y* descent occurs after the v wave and reflects tricuspid valve opening and right atrial emptying into the right ventricle. During spontaneous respiration, right atrial pressure declines during inhalation as intrathoracic pressure falls. Right atrial pressure rises during exhalation as intrathoracic pressures increase. The opposite effect is seen when patients are mechanically ventilated.

The *left atrial pressure waveform* is similar to that of the right atrium, although normal left atrial pressure is

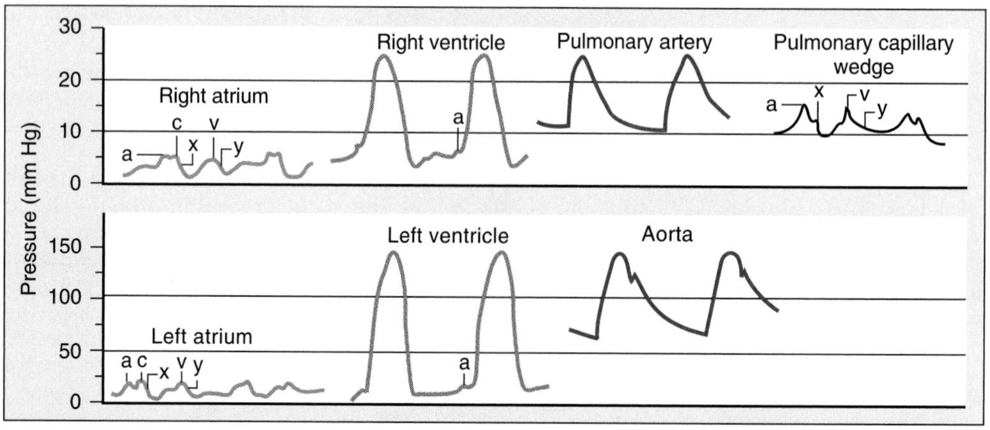

FIGURE 17–10 Normal right- and left-heart pressures recorded from fluid-filled catheter systems in a human. (From Pepine C, Hill JA, Lambert CR [eds]: Diagnostic and Therapeutic Cardiac Catheterization. 3rd ed. Baltimore, Williams & Wilkins, 1998.)

higher, reflecting the high-pressure system of the left side of the heart. In the left atrium, as opposed to the right atrium, the v wave is generally higher than the a wave. This difference occurs because the left atrium is constrained posteriorly by the pulmonary veins, whereas the right atrium can easily decompress throughout the IVC and SVC. The height of the left atrial v wave most accurately reflects left atrial compliance.

PULMONARY CAPILLARY WEDGE PRESSURE. The pulmonary capillary wedge pressure waveform is similar to the left atrial pressure waveform but is slightly damped and delayed as a result of transmission through the lungs. The a and v waves with both *x* and *y* descents are visible, but c waves may not be seen. In the normal state, the pulmonary artery diastolic pressure is similar to the mean pulmonary capillary wedge pressure because the pulmonary circulation has low resistance. In certain disease states that are associated with elevated pulmonary vascular resistance (hypoxemia, pulmonary embolism, and chronic pulmonary hypertension), and occasionally after mitral valve surgery, the pulmonary capillary wedge pressure may overestimate true left atrial pressure. In this circumstance, accurate measurement of the mitral valve gradient may require obtaining direct left atrial pressure.[34,35]

VENTRICULAR PRESSURE. Right and left ventricular waveforms are similar in morphology. They differ mainly with respect to their magnitudes. The durations of systole and isovolumic contraction and relaxation are longer and the ejection period shorter in the left than in the right ventricle. There may be a small (5 mm Hg) systolic gradient between the right ventricle and the pulmonary artery. Ventricular diastolic pressure is characterized by an early rapid filling wave during which most of the ventricle fills, a slow filling phase, and the a wave denoting atrial systolic activity. End-diastolic pressure is generally measured at the C-point, which is the rise in ventricular pressure at the onset of isovolumic contraction. When the C-point is not well seen, a line is drawn from the R wave on the simultaneous ECG to the ventricular pressure waveform, and this is used as the end-diastolic pressure.

GREAT VESSEL PRESSURES. The contour of the *central aortic pressure* and the *pulmonary artery pressure* tracing consists of a systolic wave, the incisura (indicating closure of the semilunar valves), and a gradual decline in pressure until the following systole. The pulse pressure reflects the stroke volume and compliance of the arterial system. The mean aortic pressure more accurately reflects peripheral resistance. As the systemic pressure wave is transmitted through the length of the aorta, the systolic wave increases in amplitude and becomes more triangular, and the diastolic wave decreases until it reaches the midthoracic aorta and then increases. The mean aortic pressures, however, are usually similar, with the mean *peripheral arterial pressure* typically equal to or less than 5 mm Hg lower than the mean central aortic pressure. The difference in systolic pressures between the central aorta and the periphery (femoral, brachial, or radial arteries) is greatest in younger patients owing to their increased vascular compliance. These potential differences between proximal aorta and peripheral artery must be considered in order to measure and interpret the peak systolic pressure gradient between the left ventricle and systemic arterial system in patients with suspected aortic stenosis. When a transvalvular gradient is present, the most accurate measure of the aortic pressure is obtained at the level of the coronary arteries. This measurement avoids the effect of pressure recovery, which is defined as the variable increase in lateral pressure downstream from a stenotic orifice (see Chap. 57). This approach can become clinically important in cases of mild to moderate aortic stenosis, particularly when the aorta is small.[36,37]

ABNORMAL PRESSURE CHARACTERISTICS. Abnormal pressure waveforms may be diagnostic of specific pathological conditions. Table 17–5 summarizes the more commonly encountered waveforms.

Cardiac Output Measurements

There is no totally accurate method of measuring cardiac output, but it can be estimated on the basis of various assumptions. The two most commonly used methods are the Fick method and thermodilution method. For comparison among patients, cardiac output is often corrected for the patient's size on the basis of the body surface area and expressed as cardiac index.

INDICATOR-DILUTION TECHNIQUES. The indicator-dilution method was the original clinical method used to measure cardiac output since its introduction by Stewart in 1897 and subsequent modification by Hamilton in 1932. The basic equation, commonly referred to as the Stewart-Hamilton equation, follows:

$$\text{Cardiac output (liter/min)} = \frac{\text{amount of indicator injected (mg)} \cdot 60 \text{ sec/min}}{\text{mean indicator concentration (mg/ml)} \cdot \text{curve duration}}$$

The assumption is made that after the injection of a certain quantity of an indicator into the circulation, the indicator appears and disappears from any downstream point in a manner commensurate with the cardiac output. For example, if the indicator rapidly appears at a specific location downstream and then washes out quickly, the assumption is that the cardiac output is high. Although variation can occur, the site of injection is usually a systemic vein or the right side of the heart, and the sampling site is generally a systemic artery. The normal curve itself has an initial rapid upstroke followed by a slower downstroke and eventual appearance of recirculation of the tracer. In practice, this recirculation creates some uncertainty on the tail of the curve, and assumptions are required to correct for this distortion.

There are several sources of error in this determination. Because the dye is unstable over time and can be affected by light, fresh preparations of indocyanine green dye are necessary. The exact amount of dye must be accurately measured. After injection, the indicator must mix well before reaching the sampling site, and the dilution curve must have an exponential decay over time so that extrapolation can be performed. If, for example, there is severe valvular regurgitation or a low cardiac output state in which the washout of the indicator is prolonged and recirculation begins well before an adequate decline in the indicator curve occurs, determinations are erroneous. Intracardiac shunts may also greatly affect the shape of the curve.

THERMODILUTION TECHNIQUES. Because of the rather tedious and time-consuming nature of the indicator-dilution method, it has been replaced by thermodilution techniques in many laboratories. The development of balloon flotation (e.g., Swan-Ganz) catheters with a proximal port and distal thermistor (see Fig. 17–1) has greatly expanded the ability to obtain thermodilution cardiac outputs in many clinical settings.

The thermodilution procedure requires injection of a bolus of liquid (saline or dextrose) into the proximal port of the catheter. The resultant change in temperature in the liquid is measured by a thermistor mounted in the distal end of the catheter. The change in temperature versus time can be plotted in a manner similar to that in the dye-dilution method described earlier (in which the indicator is now the cooler liquid). The cardiac output is then calculated using an equation that considers the temperature and specific gravity of the injectate and the temperature and specific gravity of the blood

TABLE 17–5 Pathological Waveforms

I. Right atrial pressure waveforms
  A. Low mean atrial pressure
    1. Hypovolemia
    2. Improper zeroing of the transducer
  B. Elevated mean atrial pressure
    1. Intravascular volume overload states
    2. Right ventricular failure due to valvular disease (tricuspid or pulmonic stenosis or regurgitation)
    3. Right ventricular failure due to myocardial disease (right ventricular ischemia, cardiomyopathy)
    4. Right ventricular failure due to left-sided heart failure (mitral stenosis/regurgitation, aortic stenosis/regurgitation, cardiomyopathy, ischemia)
    5. Right ventricular failure due to increased pulmonary vascular resistance (pulmonary embolism, chronic obstructive pulmonary disease, primary pulmonary hypertension)
    6. Pericardial effusion with tamponade physiology
    7. Obstructive atrial myxoma
  C. Elevated a wave (any increase to ventricular filling)
    1. Tricuspid stenosis
    2. Decreased ventricular compliance due to ventricular failure, pulmonic valve stenosis, or pulmonary hypertension
  D. Cannon a wave
    1. Atrial-ventricular asynchrony (atria contract against a closed tricuspid valve, as during complete heart block, following premature ventricular contraction, during ventricular tachycardia, with ventricular pacemaker)
  E. Absent a wave
    1. Atrial fibrillation or atrial standstill
    2. Atrial flutter
  F. Elevated v wave
    1. Tricuspid regurgitation
    2. Right ventricular heart failure
    3. Reduced atrial compliance (restrictive myopathy)
  G. a wave equal to v wave
    1. Tamponade
    2. Constrictive pericardial disease
    3. Hypervolemia
  H. Prominent *x* descent
    1. Tamponade
    2. Subacute constriction and possibly chronic constriction
    3. Right ventricular ischemia with preservation of atrial contractility
  I. Prominent *y* descent
    1. Constructive pericarditis
    2. Restrictive myopathies
    3. Tricuspid regurgitation
  J. Blunted *x* descent
    1. Atrial fibrillation
    2. Right atrial ischemia
  K. Blunted *y* descent
    1. Tamponade
    2. Right ventricular ischemia
    3. Tricuspid stenosis
  L. Miscellaneous abnormalities
    1. Kussmaul sign (aspiratory rise or lack of decline in right atrial pressure): constrictive pericarditis, right ventricular ischemia
    2. Equalization (≤5 mm Hg) of mean right atrial ventricular diastolic, pulmonary artery diastolic, pulmonary capillary wedge, and pericardial pressures in tamponade
    3. M or W patterns: right ventricular ischemia, pericardial constriction, congestive heart failure
    4. Ventricularization of the right atrial pressure: severe tricuspid regurgitation
    5. Sawtooth pattern: atrial flutter
    6. Dissociation between pressure recording and intracardiac electrocardiogram: Ebstein anomaly

II. Left atrial pressure/pulmonary capillary wedge pressure waveforms
  A. Low mean pressure
    1. Hypovolemia
    2. Improper zeroing of the transducer
  B. Elevated mean pressure
    1. Intravascular volume overload states
    2. Left ventricular failure due to valvular disease (mitral or aortic stenosis or regurgitation)
    3. Left ventricular failure due to myocardial disease (ischemia or cardiomyopathy)
    4. Left ventricular failure due to systemic hypertension
    5. Pericardial effusion with tamponade physiology
    6. Obstructive atrial myxoma
  C. Elevated a wave (any increase to ventricular filling)
    1. Mitral stenosis
    2. Decreased ventricular compliance due to ventricular failure, aortic valve stenosis, or systemic hypertension
  D. Cannon a wave
    1. Atrial-ventricular asynchrony (atria contract against a closed mitral valve, as during complete heart block, following premature ventricular contraction, during ventricular tachycardia, or with ventricular pacemaker)
  E. Absent a wave
    1. Atrial fibrillation or atrial standstill
    2. Atrial flutter

TABLE 17–5 Pathological Waveforms—cont'd

F. Elevated v wave
  1. Mitral regurgitation
  2. Left ventricular heart failure
  3. Ventricular septal defect
G. a wave equal to v wave
  1. Tamponade
  2. Constrictive pericardial disease
  3. Hypervolemia
H. Prominent *x* descent
  1. Tamponade
  2. Subacute constriction and possibly chronic constriction
I. Prominent *y* descent
  1. Constrictive pericarditis
  2. Restrictive myopathies
  3. Mitral regurgitation
J. Blunted *x* descent
  1. Atrial fibrillation
  2. Atrial ischemia
K. Blunted *y* descent
  1. Tamponade
  2. Ventricular ischemia
  3. Mitral stenosis
L. Pulmonary capillary wedge pressure not equal to left ventricular end-diastolic pressure
  1. Mitral stenosis
  2. Left atrial myxoma
  3. Cor triatriatum
  4. Pulmonary venous obstruction
  5. Decreased ventricular compliance
  6. Increased pleural pressure
  7. Placement of catheter in a nondependent zone of the lung

III. Pulmonary artery pressure waveforms
  A. Elevated systolic pressure
    1. Primary pulmonary hypertension
    2. Mitral stenosis or regurgitation
    3. Congestive heart failure
    4. Restrictive myopathies
    5. Significant left-to-right shunt
    6. Pulmonary disease (pulmonary embolism, hypoxemia, chronic obstructive pulmonary disease)
  B. Reduced systolic pressure
    1. Hypovolemia
    2. Pulmonary artery stenosis
    3. Subvalvular or supravalvular stenosis
    4. Ebstein anomaly
    5. Tricuspid stenosis
    6. Tricuspid atresia
  C. Reduced pulse pressure
    1. Right-heart ischemia
    2. Right ventricular infarction
    3. Pulmonary embolism
    4. Tamponade
  D. Bifid pulmonary artery waveform
    1. Large left atrial v wave transmitted backward (i.e., mitral regurgitation)
  E. Pulmonary artery diastolic pressure greater than pulmonary capillary wedge pressure
    1. Pulmonary disease
    2. Pulmonary embolus
    3. Tachycardia

IV. Ventricular pressure waveforms
  A. Systolic pressure elevated
    1. Pulmonary or systemic hypertension
    2. Pulmonary valve or aortic stenosis
    3. Ventricular outflow tract obstruction
    4. Supravalvular obstruction
    5. Right ventricular pressure elevation with significant:
      a. Atrial septal defect
      b. Ventricular septal defect
    6. Right ventricular pressure elevation due to factors that increase pulmonary vascular resistance (see factors that increase right atrial pressure)
  B. Systolic pressure reduced
    1. Hypovolemia
    2. Cardiogenic shock
    3. Tamponade
  C. End-diastolic pressure elevated
    1. Hypervolemia
    2. Congestive heart failure
    3. Diminished compliance
    4. Hypertrophy
    5. Tamponade
    6. Regurgitant valvular disease
    7. Pericardial constriction
  D. End-diastolic pressure reduced
    1. Hypovolemia
    2. Tricuspid or mitral stenosis
  E. Diminished or absent a wave
    1. Atrial fibrillation or flutter
    2. Tricuspid or mitral stenosis
    3. Tricuspid or mitral regurgitation when ventricular compliance is increased
  F. Dip and plateau in diastolic pressure wave
    1. Constrictive pericarditis
    2. Restrictive myopathies
    3. Right ventricular ischemia
    4. Acute dilation associated with:
      a. Tricuspid regurgitation
      b. Mitral regurgitation
  G. Left ventricular end-diastolic pressure > right ventricular end-diastolic pressure
    1. Restrictive myopathies

V. Aortic pressure waveforms
  A. Systolic pressure elevated
    1. Systemic hypertension
    2. Arteriosclerosis
    3. Aortic insufficiency
  B. Systolic pressure reduced
    1. Aortic stenosis
    2. Heart failure
    3. Hypovolemia
  C. Widened pulse pressure
    1. Systemic hypertension
    2. Aortic insufficiency
    3. Significant patent ductus arteriosus
    4. Significant ruptures of sinus of Valsalva aneurysm
  D. Reduced pulse pressure
    1. Tamponade
    2. Congestive heart failure
    3. Cardiogenic shock
    4. Aortic stenosis
  E. Pulsus bisferiens
    1. Aortic insufficiency
    2. Obstructive hypertrophic cardiomyopathy
  F. Pulsus paradoxus
    1. Tamponade
    2. Chronic obstructive airway disease
    3. Pulmonary embolism
  G. Pulsus alternans
    1. Congestive heart failure
    2. Cardiomyopathy
  H. Pulsus parvus et tardus
    1. Aortic stenosis
  I. Spike-and-dome configuration
    1. Obstructive hypertrophic cardiomyopathy

along with the injectate volume. A calibration factor is also used. The cardiac output is inversely related to the area under a thermodilution curve, plotted as a function of temperature versus time, with a smaller area indicative of a higher cardiac output. The use of two thermistors can significantly improve the accuracy of this technique.[38]

The thermodilution method has several advantages. It obviates the need for withdrawal of blood from an arterial site and is less affected by recirculation. Perhaps its greatest advantage is the rapid display of results using computerized methods (Fig. 17–11). However, a significant error occurs in patients with severe tricuspid regurgitation. Also, in patients with low outputs (especially <2.5 liter/min), thermodilution tends to overestimate the cardiac output.

FICK METHOD

The Fick principle assumes that the rate at which oxygen is consumed is a function of the rate of blood flow times the rate of oxygen pickup by the red blood cells. The basic assumption is that the flow of blood in a given period of time is equal to the amount of substance entering the stream of flow in the same period of time divided by the difference between the concentrations of the substance in the blood upstream and downstream from its point of entry into the circulation (Fig. 17–12). The same number of red blood cells that enter the lung must leave the lung if no intracardiac shunt is present. Thus, if certain parameters were known (the number of oxygen molecules that were attached to the red blood cells entering the lung, the number of oxygen molecules that were attached to the red blood cells leaving the lung, and the number of oxygen molecules consumed during travel through the lung), the rate of flow of these red blood cells as they pass through the lung could be determined. This can be expressed in the following terms:

$$\text{Cardiac output (liter/min)} = \frac{O_2 \text{ consumption (ml/min)}}{\text{A-V}O_2 \text{ difference (vol \%)} \cdot 10}$$

where A-VO_2 is the arteriovenous oxygen difference.

Measurements must be made in the steady state. Automated methods can accurately determine the oxygen content within the blood samples. Thus, the greatest source of measurement variability is the oxygen consumption. In traditional Fick determinations, expiratory gas samples were collected in a large bag over a specified period. By measuring the expiratory oxygen concentration and by knowing the concentration of oxygen in room air, the quantity of oxygen consumed over time could be determined. Techniques that allow measurement of the expired oxygen concentration are quantified by using a polarograph. This device can be connected to the patient by use of a plastic hood or by a mouthpiece and tubing.

The advantage of the Fick method is that it is the most accurate method in patients with low cardiac output and thus is preferred over the thermodilution method in these circumstances. It is also independent of the factors that affect curve shape and cause errors in thermodilution cardiac output. The Fick method suffers primarily from the difficulty in obtaining accurate oxygen consumption measurements and the inability to obtain a steady state under certain conditions. Because the method assumes mean flow over a period of time, it is not suitable during rapid change in flow. It requires additional time and effort in the catheterization laboratory to obtain the appropriate data. Many laboratories use an "assumed" Fick method in which the oxygen consumption index is assumed on the basis of the patient's age, gender, and body surface area or an estimate is made (125 ml/m^2) on the basis of body surface area. The inaccuracy of oxygen consumption measurements results in up to 10 percent variability in the calculated cardiac output, which may be even greater when assumed oxygen consumption, rather than measured oxygen consumption, is used.

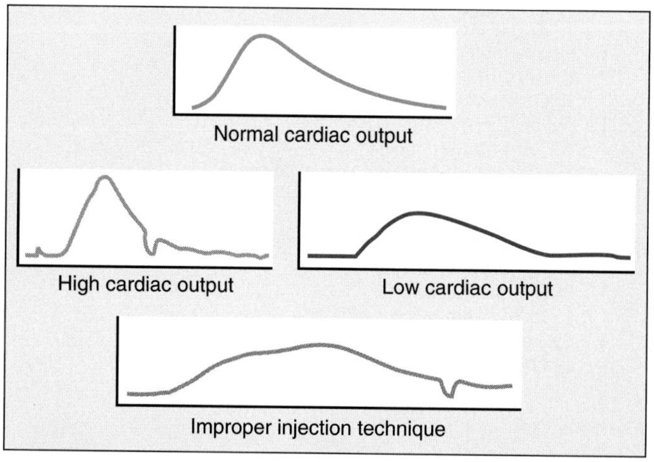

FIGURE 17–11 Thermodilution cardiac output curves. A normal curve has a sharp upstroke following an injection of saline. A smooth curve with a mildly prolonged downslope occurs until it is back to baseline. The area under the curve is inversely related to the cardiac output. At low cardiac output, a prolonged period is required to return to baseline. Therefore, there is a larger area under the curve. In a high cardiac output state, the cooler saline injectate moves faster through the right side of the heart and temperature returns to baseline more quickly. The area under the curve is smaller and the output is higher.

ANGIOGRAPHIC CARDIAC OUTPUT. Angiographic stroke volume can be calculated by tracing the end-diastolic and end-systolic images. Stroke volume is the quantity of blood ejected with each beat. End-diastolic volume is the maximum left ventricular volume and occurs immediately before the onset of systole. It occurs immediately after atrial contraction in patients in sinus rhythm. End-systolic volume is the minimum volume during the cardiac cycle. Calibration of the images with grids or ventricular phantoms is necessary to obtain accurate ventricular volumes. Angiographic cardiac output and stroke volume are derived from the following equations:

$$\text{Stroke volume} = \text{EDV} - \text{ESV}$$
$$\text{Cardiac output} = (\text{EDV} - \text{ESV}) \cdot \text{heart rate}$$

where EDV = end-diastolic volume and ESV = end-systolic volume. The inherent inaccuracies of calibrating angiographic volumes often make this method of measurement unreliable. In cases of valvular regurgitation or atrial fibrillation, angiographic cardiac output does not accurately measure true systemic outputs. However, the angiographic or thermodilution cardiac output is preferred over the Fick or thermodilution output for calculation of stenotic valve areas in patients with significant aortic or mitral regurgitation.

Determination of Vascular Resistance

Vascular resistance calculations are based on hydraulic principles of fluid flow, in which resistance is defined as the ratio of the decrease in pressure between two points in a vascular

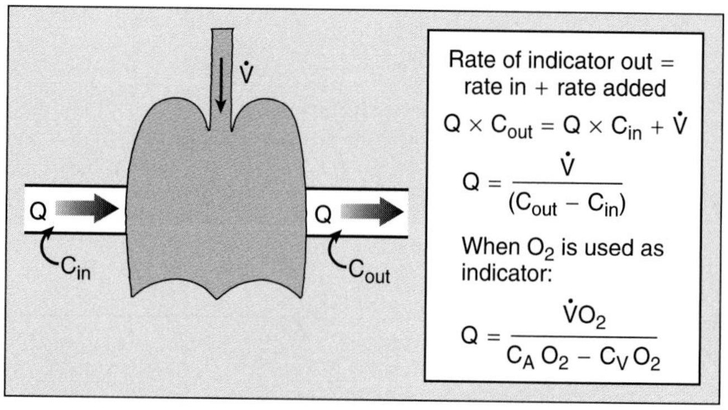

FIGURE 17–12 Schematic illustration of flow measurement using the Fick principle. Fluid containing a known concentration of an indicator (C_{in}) enters a system at flow rate Q. As the fluid passes through the system, indicator is continuously added at rate $\dot{V}$, raising the concentration in the outflow to C_{out}. In a steady state, the rate of indicator leaving the system (QC_{out}) must equal the rate at which it enters (QC_{in}) plus the rate at which it is added ($\dot{V}$). When oxygen is used as the indicator, cardiac output can be determined by measuring oxygen consumption ($\dot{V}O_2$), arterial oxygen content (C_AO_2), and mixed venous oxygen content (C_VO_2). (From Winniford MD, Kern MJ, Lambert CR: Blood flow measurement. *In* Pepine CJ, Hill JA, Lambert CR [eds]: Diagnostic and Therapeutic Cardiac Catheterization. 3rd ed. Baltimore, Williams & Wilkins, 1998, p 400.)

segment and the blood flow through the segment. Although this straightforward analogy to Ohm's law represents an oversimplification of the complex behavior of pulsatile flow in dynamic and diverse vascular beds, the calculation of vascular resistance based on these principles has proven to be of value in a number of clinical settings.

Determination of the resistance in a vascular bed requires measurement of the mean pressure of the proximal and distal ends of the vascular bed and accurate measurement of cardiac output. Vascular resistance (R) is usually defined in absolute units (dyne-sec · cm^{-5}) and is defined as R = [mean pressure gradient (dyne/cm^2)]/[mean flow (cm^3/sec)]. Hybrid units (Wood units) are less often used.[39]

Systemic vascular resistance in absolute units is calculated using the following equation:

$$SVR = 80(Ao_m - RA_m)/Q_s$$

where Ao_m and RA_m are the mean pressures (in mm Hg) in the aorta and right atrium, respectively, and Q_s is the systemic cardiac output (in liter/min). The constant 80 is used to convert units from mm Hg/liter/min (Wood units) to the absolute resistance units dyne-sec · cm^{-5}. If the right atrial pressure is not known, the term RA_m can be dropped, and the resulting value is called the *total peripheral resistance* (TPR).

$$TPR = 80(Ao_m)/Q_s$$

Similarly, the pulmonary vascular resistance is derived from the following equation:

$$PVR = 80(PA_m - LA_m)/Q_p$$

where PA_m and LA_m are the pulmonary artery and left atrial pressures, respectively, and Q_p is the pulmonary blood flow. Mean pulmonary capillary wedge pressure is commonly substituted for mean left atrial pressure if the latter has not been measured directly, although errors can occur because of this substitution. In the absence of an intracardiac shunt, Q_p is equal to the systemic cardiac output. Normal values are listed in Table 17–4.

Elevated resistances in the systemic and pulmonary circuits may represent reversible abnormalities or may be fixed owing to irreversible anatomical changes. In several clinical situations, such as congestive heart failure, valvular heart disease, primary pulmonary hypertension, and congenital heart disease with intracardiac shunting, determination of whether elevated systemic or pulmonary vascular resistance can be lowered transiently in the catheterization laboratory may provide important insights into potential management strategies. Interventions that may be used in the laboratory for this purpose include administration of vasodilating drugs (e.g., sodium nitroprusside), exercise, and (in patients with pulmonary hypertension) oxygen inhalation or intravenous epoprostenol (Flolan), a pulmonary and systemic vasodilator (see Chap. 67).

Vascular impedance measurements account for blood viscosity, pulsatile flow, reflected waves, and arterial compliance. Hence, vascular impedance has the potential to describe the dynamic relation between pressure and flow more comprehensively than is possible using the simpler calculations of vascular resistance. However, because the simultaneous pressure and flow data required for the calculation of impedance are complex and difficult to obtain, the concept of impedance has failed to gain widespread acceptance, and vascular impedance has not been adopted as a routine clinical index.

Evaluation of Valvular Stenosis (see Chap. 57)

Determining the severity of valvular stenosis on the basis of the pressure gradient and flow across the valve is one of the most important aspects of evaluation of patients with valvular heart disease. In many patients, the magnitude of the pressure gradient alone is sufficient to distinguish clinically significant from insignificant valvular stenosis.

DETERMINATION OF PRESSURE GRADIENTS

In patients with *aortic stenosis*, the transvalvular pressure gradient is best measured with a catheter in the left ventricle and another in the proximal aorta. Although it is convenient to measure the gradient between the left ventricle and the femoral artery, downstream augmentation of the pressure signal and delay in pressure transmission between the proximal aorta and femoral artery may alter the pressure waveform substantially and introduce errors into the measured gradient.[37,38]

Left ventricular-femoral artery pressure gradients may suffice in many patients as an estimate of the severity of aortic stenosis to confirm the presence of a severely stenotic valve. If the side port of the arterial introducing sheath is used to monitor femoral pressure, the inner diameter of the sheath should be at least 1F size larger than the outer diameter of the left ventricular catheter.

The operator should obtain simultaneous ascending aortic and femoral artery pressures in order to verify similarity between the two sites. The left ventricular-femoral artery pressure gradient may not always be relied on in the calculation of valve orifice area in patients with moderate valve gradients. A careful single catheter pull-back from left ventricle to aorta is often preferable to simultaneous measurement of left ventricular and femoral artery pressures. Alternatively, a single catheter with distal and proximal lumen or a micromanometer catheter with distal and proximal transducers may be used for simultaneous measurement of left ventricular pressure and central aortic pressure. Another method is to place two arterial catheters, one in the aorta and the second in the left ventricle. However, this requires punctures of both femoral arteries and is rarely used.

In patients with very severe aortic stenosis, the left ventricular catheter itself may reduce the effective orifice area, resulting in an artifactual increase in the measured pressure gradient. This overestimation of the severity of aortic stenosis is rarely an important clinical issue because the diagnosis of severe aortic stenosis is already apparent in such patients.

The mean pressure gradient across the aortic valve is determined by planimetry of the area separating the left ventricular and aortic pressures using multiple beats (Fig. 17-13), and it is this gradient that is applied to calculation of the valve orifice area. The peak-to-peak gradient, measured as the difference between peak left ventricular pressure and peak aortic pressure, is commonly used to quantify the valve gradient because this measurement is rapidly obtained and can be estimated visually. However, there is no physiological basis for the peak-to-peak gradient because the maximum left ventricular and aortic pressures rarely occur

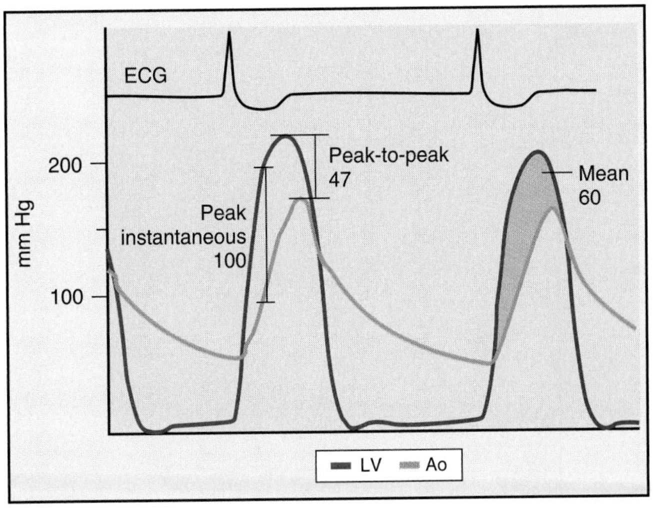

FIGURE 17–13 Various methods of describing an aortic transvalvular gradient. The peak-to-peak gradient (47 mm Hg) is the difference between the maximal pressure in the aorta (Ao) and the maximal left ventricle (LV) pressure. The peak instantaneous gradient (100 mm Hg) is the maximal pressure difference between the Ao and LV when the pressures are measured in the same moment (usually during early systole). The mean gradient (green shaded area) is the integral of the pressure difference between the LV and Ao during systole (60 mm Hg). ECG = electrocardiogram. (From Bashore TM: Invasive Cardiology: Principles and Techniques. Philadelphia, BC Decker, 1990.)

simultaneously. The peak-to-peak gradient measured in the catheterization laboratory is generally lower than the peak instantaneous gradient measured in the echocardiography laboratory. It is lower because the peak instantaneous gradient represents the maximum pressure difference between the left ventricle and aorta when measured simultaneously. This maximum pressure difference occurs on the upslope of the aortic pressure tracing (see Fig. 17–13). Mean aortic transvalvular gradient and aortic valve area are well correlated with both techniques.[40]

In patients with *mitral stenosis,* the most accurate means of determining the mitral valve gradient is measurement of left atrial pressure using the transseptal technique with simultaneous measurement of left ventricular pressure and with planimetry of the area bounded by the left ventricular and left atrial pressures in diastole using several cardiac cycles (Fig. 17–14). In most laboratories, the pulmonary capillary wedge pressure is substituted for the left atrial pressure, as the pulmonary wedge pressure is more readily obtained. The pulmonary wedge pressure tracing must be realigned with the left ventricular tracing for accurate mean gradient determination. Although it has been generally accepted that pulmonary capillary wedge pressure is a satisfactory estimate of left atrial pressure, some studies indicate that the pulmonary wedge pressure may systematically overestimate the left atrial pressure by 2 to 3 mm Hg, thereby increasing the measured mitral valve gradient.[34] In addition, accurate wedge tracings may be difficult to obtain in patients with mitral stenosis because of pulmonary hypertension or dilated right-sided heart chambers. Improperly wedged catheters, resulting in damped pulmonary artery pressure recordings, further overestimate the severity of mitral stenosis. If there is doubt about accurate positioning of the catheter in the wedge position, the position can be confirmed by slow withdrawal of blood for oximetric analysis. An oxygen saturation equal to that of the systemic circulation confirms the wedge position.

In *pulmonic stenosis,* the valve gradient is usually obtained by a catheter pull-back from the pulmonary artery to the right ventricle or by placing separate catheters in the right ventricle and pulmonary artery. Multilumen catheters are also available for simultaneous pressure recordings. *Tricuspid valve gradients* should be assessed with simultaneous recording of right atrial and right ventricular pressures.

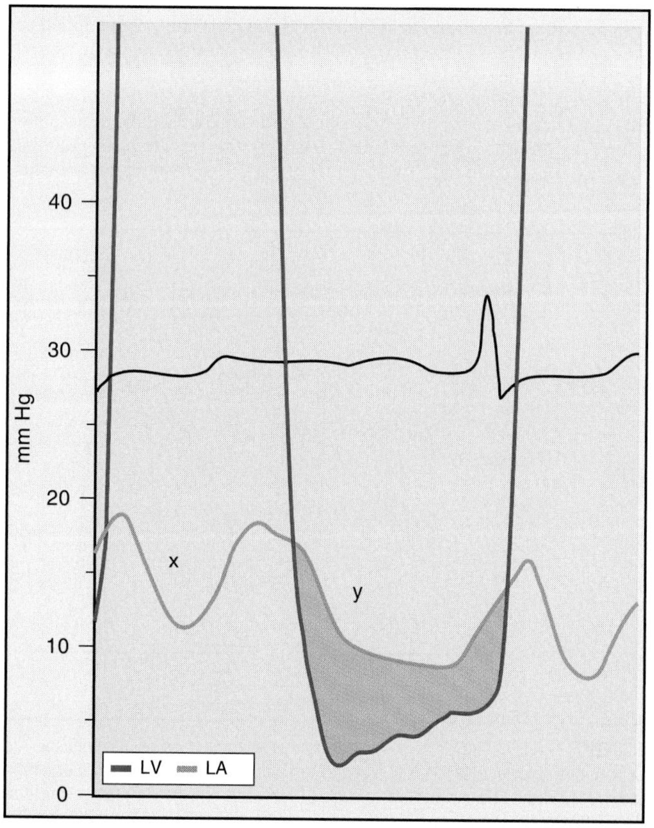

FIGURE 17–14 Pressure gradient in a patient with mitral stenosis. The pressure in the left atrium (LA) exceeds the pressure in the left ventricle (LV) during diastole, producing a diastolic pressure gradient (green shaded area). (From Bashore TM: Invasive Cardiology: Principles and Techniques. Philadelphia, BC Decker, 1990.)

CALCULATION OF STENOTIC VALVE ORIFICE AREAS. The stenotic orifice area is determined from the pressure gradient and cardiac output using the formula developed by Gorlin and Gorlin from the fundamental hydraulic relationships linking the area of an orifice to the flow and pressure drop across the orifice. Flow (F) and orifice area (A) are related by the fundamental formula

$$F = cAV$$

where V is velocity of flow and c is a constant accounting for central streaming of fluid through an orifice, which tends to reduce the effective orifice size. Hence,

$$A = F/cV$$

Velocity is related to the pressure gradient through the relation $V = k\sqrt{(2g\Delta P)}$, where k is a constant accounting for frictional energy loss, g is the acceleration due to gravity (980 cm/sec^2), and ΔP is the mean pressure gradient (mm Hg). Substituting for V in the orifice area equation and combining c and k into one constant C,

$$A = FC\sqrt{(1960\Delta P)} = F\,44.3C\sqrt{\Delta P}$$

Gorlin and Gorlin determined the value of the constant C by comparing the calculated valve area with actual valve area measured at autopsy or at surgery in 11 mitral valves. The maximal discrepancy between the actual mitral valve area and calculated values was only 0.2 cm^2 when the constant 0.85 was used. No data were obtained for aortic valves, a limitation noted by the Gorlins, and a constant of 1.0 was assumed. Because flow across the aortic valve occurs only in systole, the flow value for calculating aortic valve area (cm^2) is the cardiac output in milliliters per minute divided by the systolic ejection period (SEP) in seconds per beat times the heart rate (HR) in beats per minute. The systolic ejection period is defined from aortic valve opening to closure. Hence, the aortic valve area is calculated from the Gorlin formula using the following equation:

$$\text{Aortic value area} = \frac{\text{cardiac output}}{44.3(\text{SEP})(\text{HR})\sqrt{\text{mean gradient}}}$$

Similarly, as mitral flow occurs only in diastole, the cardiac output is corrected for the diastolic filling period (DFP) in seconds per beat in the equation for mitral valve area, where the diastolic filling period is defined from mitral valve opening to mitral valve closure:

$$\text{Mitral valve area} = \frac{\text{cardiac output}}{37.7(\text{DFP})(\text{HR})\sqrt{\text{mean gradient}}}$$

The normal aortic valve area is 2.6 to 3.5 cm^2 in adults. Valve areas of 0.8 cm^2 or less represent severe aortic stenosis. The normal mitral valve area is 4 to 6 cm^2, and severe mitral stenosis is present with valve areas less than 1.3 cm^2.

The calculated valve area is often crucial in management decisions for patients with aortic stenosis or mitral stenosis. Hence, it is essential that accurate and simultaneous pressure gradient and cardiac output determinations be made, especially in patients with borderline or low pressure gradients.

Limitations of the Orifice Area. As the square root of the mean gradient is used in the Gorlin formula, the valve area calculation is more strongly influenced by the cardiac output than the pressure gradient. Thus, errors in measuring cardiac output may have profound effects on the calculated valve area, particularly in patients with low cardiac outputs, in whom the calculated valve area is often of greatest importance.

The Fick method of determining cardiac output is the most accurate for assessing cardiac output, especially in low-output states. As noted previously, both the dye-dilution technique and the thermodilution technique may provide inaccurate cardiac output data when cardiac output is reduced or when concomitant aortic, mitral, or tricuspid regurgitation is present. In patients with mixed valvular disease (stenosis and regurgitation) of the same valve, the use of forward flow as determined by the Fick method or thermodilution technique overestimates the severity of the valvular stenosis. This overestimation occurs because the Gorlin formula depends on total forward flow across the stenotic valve, not net forward flow. If valvular regurgitation is present, the angiographic cardiac output is the most appropriate measure of flow. If both aortic and mitral regurgitation are present, flow across a single valve cannot be determined and neither aortic valve area nor mitral valve area can be assessed accurately.

Other potential errors and limitations are inherent in the use of the Gorlin formula, related both to inaccuracies in measurement of valve gradients and to more fundamental issues regarding the validity of the assumptions underlying the formula. In low-output states, the Gorlin formula may systematically predict smaller valve areas than are actually present. Several lines of evidence indicate that the aortic valve area from the Gorlin formula increases with increases in cardiac output.[41] Although this may represent an actual greater opening of stenotic valves by the higher proximal opening pressures that result from increases in transvalvular flow, the flow dependence of the calculated valve area may also reflect inherent errors in the assumptions underlying the Gorlin formula, particularly with respect to the aortic valve.[41,42] Tricuspid aortic valve stenosis determinations appear particularly influenced by flow.[42]

A study was performed to compare simultaneous aortic valve area determinations by transesophageal echocardiographic planimetry and the Gorlin formula.[43] The study demonstrated that with increases in transvalvular flow, the Gorlin valve area also increased. This finding was not associated with alterations in direct planimetry of the aortic valve area. These results suggest that flow-related variation in the Gorlin aortic valve area is due to disproportional flow dependence of the formula and not a true change in the valve area.

An alternative simplified formula for determining valve areas has been proposed but is not well validated. The effects of the systolic ejection period and the diastolic filling period are relatively constant at normal heart rates, and these terms can be eliminated from the equation. This assumes that (HR · SEP · 44.3) ≈ 1000 in most circumstances. In this modified approach, the aortic valve area can be quickly estimated from the following formula:

$$\text{Aortic valve area} = \frac{\text{cardiac output (liter/min)}}{\sqrt{\text{mean gradient (mm Hg)}}}$$

One approach to patients with a low aortic transvalvular gradient and low cardiac output is to calculate the aortic valve resistance using the following formula:

$$\text{Aortic valve resistance} = \frac{\text{mean gradient}}{\text{flow}} = \frac{1.33(\text{mean gradient})(\text{HR})(\text{SEP})}{\text{cardiac output}}$$

where HR is heart rate, SEP is systolic ejection period, and valve resistance is expressed in dyne-sec · cm^{-5}.[41,44] The limited data available using aortic valve resistance suggest that this measure may be a helpful adjunct in distinguishing the patients with borderline aortic valve areas (0.8 to 1.0 cm^2) who have severe versus mild aortic stenosis. Despite its theoretical limitations, however, the Gorlin formula has proved to be an excellent clinical determination for evaluating patients with suspected aortic stenosis.[45]

Measurement of Intraventricular Pressure Gradients

The demonstration of an intracavitary pressure gradient is among the most interesting and challenging aspects of diagnostic catheterization. Simultaneous pressure measurements are usually obtained in either the central aorta or femoral artery and from within the ventricular cavity. Pull-back of the catheter from the ventricular apex to a posterior position just beneath the aortic valve demonstrates an intracavitary gradient. An erroneous intracavitary gradient may be seen if the catheter becomes entrapped by the hypertrophic myocardium.

The intracavitary gradient is distinguished from aortic valvular stenosis related to the loss of the aortic–left ventricular gradient when the catheter is still within the left ventricle yet proximal to the myocardial obstruction. In addition, careful analysis of the upstroke of the aortic pressure waveform distinguishes a valvular from a subvalvular stenosis, as the aortic pressure waveform demonstrates a slow upstroke in aortic stenosis. Other methods for localizing intracavitary gradients include the use of a dual-lumen catheter, a double-sensor micromanometer catheter, or placement of an end-hole catheter in the left ventricular outflow tract while a transseptal catheter is advanced into the left ventricle, with pressure measured simultaneously. An intracavitary gradient may be increased by various provocative maneuvers including the Valsalva maneuver, inhalation of amyl nitrate, introduction of a premature ventricular beat, or isoproterenol infusion (see Physiological and Pharmacological Maneuvers).

ASSESSMENT OF VALVULAR REGURGITATION

The severity of valvular regurgitation is generally graded by visual assessment, although calculation of the regurgitant fraction is used occasionally.

VISUAL ASSESSMENT OF REGURGITATION. Valvular regurgitation may be assessed visually by determining the relative amount of radiographic contrast medium that opacifies the chamber proximal to its injection. The estimation of regurgitation depends on the regurgitant volume as well as the size and contractility of the proximal chamber. The original classification scheme devised by Sellers and colleagues remains the standard in most catheterization laboratories:

- \+ Minimal regurgitant jet seen. Clears rapidly from proximal chamber with each beat.
- ++ Moderate opacification of proximal chamber, clearing with subsequent beats.
- +++ Intense opacification of proximal chamber, becoming equal to that of the distal chamber.
- ++++ Intense opacification of proximal chamber, becoming more dense than that of the distal chamber. Opacification often persists over the entire series of images obtained.

REGURGITANT FRACTION. A gross estimate of the degree of valvular regurgitation may be obtained by determining the regurgitant fraction (RF). The difference between the angiographic stroke volume and the forward stroke volume can be defined as the regurgitant stroke volume. The RF is that portion of the angiographic stroke volume that does not contribute to the net cardiac output.

$$\text{Regurgitant stroke volume} = \text{angiographic stroke volume} - \text{forward stroke volume}$$

$$\text{RF} = \frac{(\text{angiographic stroke volume} - \text{forward stroke volume})}{\text{angiographic stroke volume}}$$

Forward stroke volume is the cardiac output determined by the Fick or thermodilution method divided by the heart rate. Thermodilution cardiac output cannot be used if there is significant concomitant tricuspid regurgitation.

As detected visually, 1+ regurgitation is roughly equivalent to an RF less than or equal to 20 percent, 2+ regurgitation to an RF of 21 to 40 percent, 3+ to an RF of 41 to 60 percent, and 4+ to an RF of more than 60 percent.

The assumption underlying the determination of RF is that the angiographic and forward cardiac outputs are accurate and comparable, a state requiring similar heart rates, stable hemodynamic states between measurements, and only a single regurgitant valve. Given these conditions, the equation yields only a gross approximation of regurgitant flow.

Shunt Determinations

Normally, pulmonary blood flow and systemic blood flow are equal. With an abnormal communication between intracardiac chambers or great vessels, blood flow is shunted either from the systemic circulation to the pulmonary circulation (left-to-right shunt), from the pulmonary circulation to the systemic circulation (right-to-left shunt), or in both directions (bidirectional shunt). Although many shunts are suspected before cardiac catheterization, physicians performing the procedure should be vigilant in determining the cause of unexpected findings. For example, an unexplained pulmonary artery oxygen saturation exceeding 80 percent should raise the operator's suspicion of a left-to-right shunt, whereas unexplained arterial desaturation (<93 percent) may indicate a right-to-left shunt.[46] Arterial desaturation commonly results from alveolar hypoventilation and associated "physiological shunting," the causes of which include oversedation from premedication, pulmonary disease, pulmonary venous congestion, pulmonary edema, and cardiogenic shock. If arterial desaturation persists after the patient takes several deep breaths, coughs, or after administration of 100 percent oxygen, a right-to-left shunt must be highly suspected.

Several noninvasive and invasive methods are available for detection of intracardiac shunts. Noninvasive methods include echocardiographic, radionuclide, and magnetic resonance imaging techniques. The most commonly used method in the cardiac catheterization laboratory is the oximetric method.

OXIMETRIC METHOD. The oximetric method is based on blood sampling from various cardiac chambers for the determination of oxygen saturation. A left-to-right shunt is detected when a significant increase in blood oxygen saturation is found between two right-sided vessels or chambers.

A screening oxygen saturation measurement for any left-to-right shunt is often performed with right-heart catheterization by sampling blood in the SVC and the pulmonary artery. If the difference in oxygen saturation between these samples is 8 percent or more, a left-to-right shunt may be present, and an oximetry "run" should be performed. This run includes obtaining blood samples from all right-sided locations including the SVC, IVC, right atrium, right ventricle, and pulmonary artery. In cases of interatrial or interventricular shunts, it may be helpful to obtain multiple samples from the high, middle, and low right atrium or the right ventricular inflow tract, apex, and outflow tract in order to localize the level of the shunt. One may miss a small left-to-right shunt using the right atrium for screening purposes rather than the SVC because of incomplete mixing of blood in the right atrium, which receives blood from the IVC, SVC, and coronary sinus. Oxygen saturation in the IVC is higher than in the SVC because the kidneys use less oxygen relative to their blood flow than do other organs, whereas coronary sinus blood has very low oxygen saturation. Mixed venous saturation is most accurately measured in the pulmonary artery after complete mixing has occurred.

A full saturation run involves obtaining samples from the high and low IVC; high and low SVC; high, middle, and low right atrium; right ventricular inflow and outflow tracts and midcavity; main pulmonary artery; left or right pulmonary artery; pulmonary vein and left atrium if possible; left ventricle; and distal aorta. When a right-to-left shunt must be localized, oxygen saturation samples must be taken from the pulmonary veins, left atrium, left ventricle, and aorta. Although the major weakness of the oxygen step-up method is its lack of sensitivity, clinically significant shunts are generally detected by this technique. Obtaining multiple samples from each chamber can improve sampling error and variability. Most instruments analyze samples with a measurement error ranging from 2.5 to 1 percent saturation or better.[47] Another method of oximetric determination of intracardiac shunts uses a balloon-tipped fiberoptic catheter that allows continuous registration of oxygen saturation as it is withdrawn from the pulmonary artery through the right-heart chambers into the SVC and IVC.

Shunt Quantification. The principles used to determine Fick cardiac output are also used to quantify intracardiac shunts. To determine the size of a left-to-right shunt, pulmonary blood flow (PBF) and systemic blood flow (SBF) determinations are required. PBF is simply oxygen consumption divided by the difference in oxygen content across the pulmonary bed, whereas SBF is oxygen consumption divided by the difference in oxygen content across the systemic bed. The effective blood flow (EBF) is the fraction of mixed venous return received by the lungs without contamination by the shunt flow. In the *absence* of a shunt, PBF, SBF, and EBF all are equal. These equations are as follows:

$$\text{PBF} = \frac{\text{O}_2 \text{ consumption (ml/min)}}{(\text{P}\bar{\text{v}}\text{O}_2 - \text{PaO}_2)}$$

$$\text{SBF} = \frac{\text{O}_2 \text{ consumption (ml/min)}}{(\text{SaO}_2 - \text{M}\bar{\text{v}}\text{O}_2)}$$

$$\text{EBF} = \frac{\text{O}_2 \text{ consumption (ml/min)}}{(\text{P}\bar{\text{v}}\text{O}_2 - \text{M}\bar{\text{v}}\text{O}_2)}$$

where $\text{P}\bar{\text{v}}\text{O}_2$, PaO_2, SaO_2, and $\text{M}\bar{\text{v}}\text{O}_2$ are the oxygen contents (in milliliters of oxygen per liter of blood) of pulmonary venous, pulmonary arterial, systemic arterial, and mixed venous bloods, respectively. The oxygen content is determined as outlined in the section on Fick cardiac output.

If a pulmonary vein is not sampled, systemic arterial oxygen content may be substituted, assuming systemic arterial saturation is 95 percent or more. As discussed earlier, if systemic arterial saturation is less than 95 percent, a right-to-left shunt may be present. If arterial desaturation is present but not secondary to a right-to-left shunt, systemic arterial oxygen content is used. If a right-to-left shunt is present, pulmonary venous oxygen content is calculated as 98 percent of the oxygen capacity.

The mixed venous oxygen content is the average oxygen content of the blood in the chamber proximal to the shunt. When assessing a left-to-right shunt at the level of the right atrium, one must calculate mixed venous oxygen content on the basis of the contributing blood flow from the IVC, SVC, and coronary sinus. The most common method used is the Flamm formula:

$$\text{Mixed venous oxygen content} = \frac{3(\text{SVC O}_2 \text{ content}) + 1(\text{IVC O}_2 \text{ content})}{4}$$

Assuming conservation of mass, the size of a left-to-right shunt, when there is no associated right-to-left shunt, is simply

$$\text{L}\rightarrow\text{R shunt} = \text{PBF} - \text{SBF}$$

When there is evidence of a right-to-left shunt in addition to a left-to-right shunt, the approximate left-to-right shunt size is

$$\text{L}\rightarrow\text{R shunt} = \text{PBF} - \text{EBF}$$

and the approximate right-to-left shunt size is

$$\text{R}\rightarrow\text{L shunt} = \text{SBF} - \text{EBF}$$

The flow ratio PBF/SBF (or Q_p/Q_s) is used clinically to determine the significance of the shunt. A ratio of less than 1.5 indicates a small left-to-right shunt, and a ratio of 1.5 to 2.0, a moderate-sized shunt. A ratio of 2.0 or more indicates a large left-to-right shunt and generally requires percutaneous or surgical repair to prevent future pulmonary or right ventricular complications, or both. A flow ratio of less than 1.0 indicates a net right-to-left shunt. If oxygen consumption is not measured, the pulmonic/systemic blood flow ratio may be calculated as follows:

$$\frac{PBF}{SBF} = \frac{(SaO_2 - M\bar{v}O_2)}{(P\bar{v}O_2 - PaO_2)}$$

where SaO_2, $M\bar{v}O_2$, $P\bar{v}O_2$, and PaO_2 are systemic arterial, mixed venous, pulmonary venous, and pulmonary arterial blood oxygen saturations, respectively.

INDICATOR-DILUTION METHOD

Although the indicator-dilution method is more sensitive than the oximetric method in detection of small shunts, it cannot be used to localize the level of a left-to-right shunt (Fig. 17-15). An indicator such as indocyanine green dye is injected into a proximal chamber while a sample is taken from a distal chamber using a densitometer, and the density of dye is displayed over time. To detect a left-to-right shunt, dye is injected into the pulmonary artery and sampling is performed in a systemic artery. Presence of a shunt is indicated by early recirculation of the dye on the downslope of the curve. The presence of aortic or mitral regurgitation may distort the downslope of the curve, yielding a false-positive result. In adults, the indocyanine green method provides estimates of shunt magnitude that are somewhat smaller than those of the oximetric method, although they are in general agreement with one another concerning the PBF/SBF.[48,49] To detect a right-to-left shunt, dye is injected into the right side of the heart proximal to the presumed shunt and sampling is performed in a systemic artery. If there is a right-to-left shunt, a distinct early peak is seen on the upslope of the curve. The level of the right-to-left shunt may be localized by injecting more distally until the early peak disappears. Shunts may also be quantified using this technique.

MISCELLANEOUS TECHNIQUES

A sensitive method for detection and localization of a left-to-right shunt is to check systematically within the various right-heart chambers for the early appearance of an indicator that is injected distal to the presumed shunt. Indicators that have been used for this purpose include indocyanine green dye, inhaled hydrogen, hydrogen dissolved in saline, and ascorbic acid. Platinum-tipped electrodes are used for detection when hydrogen and ascorbic acid are used. These techniques may also be used to detect small right-to-left shunts by altering the sites of injection and sampling.

Selective injection of radiographic contrast medium (angiocardiography) can detect both left-to-right and right-to-left shunts, although these cannot be quantified. Angiocardiography is a useful adjunct to transesophageal echocardiography as part of a preoperative evaluation. It is also useful in detecting pulmonary arteriovenous fistulas that may not be detected by other methods.

Physiological and Pharmacological Maneuvers

Potentially significant cardiac abnormalities may be absent in the resting condition but may be unmasked by stress. Therefore, if the physician performing a cardiac catheterization procedure cannot elucidate the cause of a patient's symptoms at rest, various physiological and pharmacological maneuvers can be considered.

DYNAMIC EXERCISE

Dynamic exercise in the catheterization laboratory is most commonly performed using supine bicycle ergometry, although straight leg raises or arm or upright bicycle exercise may be used. Upright treadmill exercise may also be performed outside the catheterization laboratory, using a balloon flotation catheter inserted through an antecubital vein to measure pulmonary artery and wedge pressures and cardiac output. The associated changes in the heart rate, cardiac output, oxygen consumption, and intracardiac pressures are monitored at steady state during progressive stages of exercise. Normally, the increased oxygen requirements of exercise are met by an increase in cardiac output and an increase in oxygen extraction from arterial blood. Patients with cardiac dysfunction are unable to increase their cardiac output appropriately in response to exercise and must meet the demands of the exercising muscle groups by increasing the extraction of oxygen from arterial blood, thereby increasing the arteriovenous oxygen difference. The relationship between cardiac output and oxygen consumption is linear, and a regression formula can be used to calculate the predicted cardiac index at a given level of oxygen consumption. The actual cardiac index divided by the predicted cardiac index is defined as the *exercise index*. A value of 0.8 or more indicates a normal cardiac output response to exercise. The *exercise factor* is another method of describing the same relationship

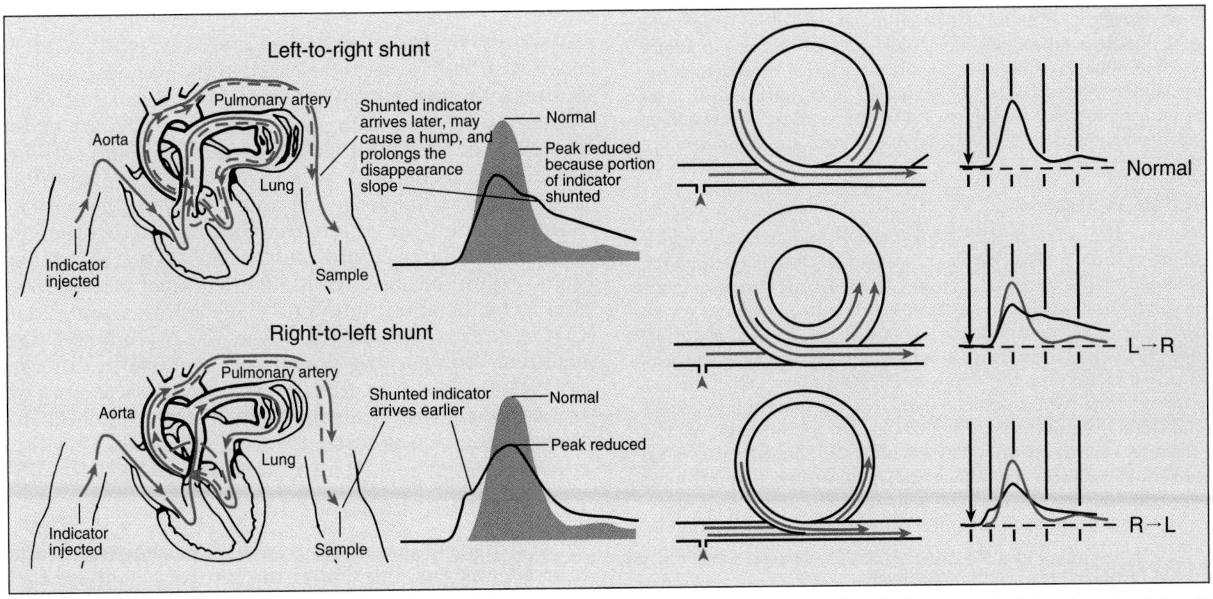

FIGURE 17-15 **Top,** Left-to-right shunt (increased pulmonic flow). Indicator is not cleared rapidly but recirculates through the central circulation through a defect. Depending on the magnitude of the shunt, a constant fraction leaves the central pool with each circulation. Maximal deflection is reduced, and the disappearance is prolonged as a result of slow clearance. **Bottom,** Right-to-left shunt (decreased pulmonic flow). A portion of the indicator passes directly to the arterial circulation through the defect without passing through the lungs and arrives at the arterial sampling site before the portion that did traverse the pulmonary circulation. (From Kern MJ, Deligonul U, Donohue T, et al: Hemodynamic data. *In* Kern MI [ed]: The Cardiac Catheterization Handbook. 2nd ed. St. Louis, Mosby–Year Book, 1995, p 142.)

between the cardiac output and oxygen consumption. The exercise factor is the increase in cardiac output divided by the increase in oxygen consumption. Normally, for every 100 ml/min increase in oxygen consumption with exercise, the cardiac output should increase by at least 600 ml/min. Therefore, a normal exercise factor should be 0.6 or more.[50]

Supine exercise normally causes a rise in mean arterial and pulmonary pressures. There is a proportionately greater decrease in systemic vascular resistance compared with pulmonary vascular resistance and an increase in heart rate. Myocardial contractility increases owing to both increased sympathetic tone and the increase in heart rate. Left ventricular ejection fraction rises. During early levels of exercise, increased venous return augments left ventricular end-diastolic volume, leading to an increase in stroke volume. At progressively higher levels of exercise, both left ventricular end-systolic and end-diastolic volumes decrease so that there is a negligible rise in stroke volume. Thus, the augmentation in cardiac output during peak supine exercise in the catheterization laboratory is generally caused by an increase in heart rate. For this reason, all agents that may impair the chronotropic response should be discontinued before catheterization if exercise is contemplated during the procedure.

Exercise may provoke symptoms in a patient who had been found to have valvular disease of borderline significance in the resting state (see Chap. 57). Exercise increases the gradient across the mitral valve and pulmonary artery pressures in mitral stenosis and may provoke symptoms not experienced at rest. The hemodynamic response to exercise is also useful in evaluating regurgitant valvular lesions. Clinically important valvular regurgitation exists if an increase occurs in left ventricular end-diastolic pressure, pulmonary capillary wedge pressure, and systemic vascular resistance, in conjunction with a reduced exercise index and abnormal exercise factor. Simultaneous echocardiographic data may also be useful in equivocal cases. Patients with myocardial disease, ischemic or otherwise, may have pronounced increases in left ventricular end-diastolic pressure with exercise.

ISOMETRIC EXERCISE

Isometric handgrip exercise causes an increase in heart rate, mean arterial pressure, and cardiac output. Because the systemic vascular resistance does not increase, the elevation in arterial pressure is due to the rise in cardiac output rather than a vasoconstrictor response. Patients with left ventricular dysfunction respond abnormally to isometric exercise (i.e., significant increase in left ventricular end-diastolic pressure, a failure to increase stroke work appropriately, and a blunted rise in left ventricular peak dP/dT).[50]

PACING TACHYCARDIA

Rapid atrial or ventricular pacing increases myocardial oxygen consumption and myocardial blood flow. With pacing, in contradistinction to dynamic or isometric exercise, left ventricular end-diastolic volume decreases and there is little change in cardiac output.[51] This method may be used to determine the significance of coronary artery disease or valvular abnormalities. For example, the gradient across the mitral valve increases with rapid atrial pacing owing to the increase in heart rate. Pacing has the advantage of allowing greater control and rapid termination of the induced stress.

PHYSIOLOGICAL STRESS

Various physiological stresses alter the severity of obstruction in hypertrophic cardiomyopathy. The *Valsalva maneuver* (forcible expiration against a closed glottis) increases the systolic subaortic pressure gradient in the strain phase, during which there is a decrease in venous return and decreased left ventricular volume. This maneuver is often abnormal in patients with heart failure. The *Müller maneuver* (forced inspiration against a closed glottis) has the opposite effect. Another useful maneuver in patients with hypertrophic obstructive cardiomyopathy is the introduction of a *premature ventricular beat* (Brockenbrough maneuver). Premature ventricular contractions normally increase the pulse pressure of the subsequent ventricular beat. In obstructive hypertrophic cardiomyopathy, the outflow gradient is increased during the postpremature beat with a decrease in the pulse pressure of the aortic contour. A premature ventricular beat may also accentuate the spike-and-dome configuration of the aortic pressure waveform.

Rapid volume loading may reveal occult pericardial constriction, when atrial and ventricular filling pressures are relatively normal under baseline conditions owing to hypovolemia, and may help distinguish pericardial constriction from myocardial restriction. The *Kussmaul sign* occurs in pericardial constriction. It is demonstrated when, with inspiration, right atrial pressure fails to decrease or actually increases in relation to impaired right ventricular filling.[52]

PHARMACOLOGICAL MANEUVERS

Isoproterenol infusion may be used to simulate supine dynamic exercise, although untoward side effects may limit its applicability. This drug's positive inotropic and chronotropic effects may increase the gradients in obstructive hypertrophic cardiomyopathy and mitral stenosis. *Nitroglycerin* and *amyl nitrate* decrease preload and accentuate the systolic gradient in patients with obstructive hypertrophic cardiomyopathy. Amyl nitrate is generally inhaled, and its onset and offset of action are very rapid. Agents that increase systemic vascular resistance, such as *phenylephrine*, reduce the gradient in obstructive hypertrophic cardiomyopathy. Afterload reduction or an intravenous inotropic agent may clarify the precise severity of aortic stenosis in patients with low cardiac outputs and low transvalvular gradients.[53] Infusion of *sodium nitroprusside* may improve the cardiac output and filling pressures in patients with dilated cardiomyopathies and in patients with mitral regurgitation by lowering systemic and pulmonary vascular resistances. A favorable response to sodium nitroprusside infusion may predict a good clinical outcome.

Methylergonovine maleate has replaced ergonovine as a safer and more specific provocation test for coronary artery spasm. Small intracoronary increments of 5 to 10 μg are given. Total dose should not exceed 50 μg. Intracoronary acetylcholine is also as effective and safe as methylergonovine.[54]

Adjunctive Diagnostic Techniques

Coronary Pressure and Blood Flow Determinations

Five methods are available for measuring human coronary blood flow in the cardiac catheterization laboratory: thermodilution, digital subtraction angiography, electromagnetic flowmeters, Doppler velocity probes, and pressure wires.[55] Although most current methods measure relative changes in coronary blood flow, useful information about the physiological significance of stenosis, cardiac hypertrophy, and pharmacological interventions can be obtained. Doppler FloWires and translesional gradients are the most commonly used clinical techniques (see Chap. 44).

Left Ventricular Electromechanical Mapping

Advances in catheter design and navigational technology have resulted in catheter-based three-dimensional mapping systems for evaluating regional and global left ventricular function. By integrating measurements of local endocardial electrical activity and wall motion during the cardiac cycle, the electromechanical mapping system provides information about myocardial ischemia and viability. The ability of the electromechanical left ventricular maps to distinguish viable from nonviable myocardium and ischemic from nonischemic myocardium has been validated in animal models of myocardial ischemia and infarction.[56,57] The clinical experience with this system is limited. However, the preliminary data indicate that the mapping system has promise in differentiating normal myocardium from myocardial fibrosis and ischemic from infarcted myocardium and has the potential to guide transendocardial therapeutic administration.[58-60]

Intracardiac Echocardiography

Intracardiac echocardiography (ICE) has become available for transvenous imaging within the cardiac chambers. It consists of a 10F, 90-cm-long device that permits two planes of bidirectional steering in the anterior-posterior and left-right direction. The transducers have variable frequencies of 5 to 10 MHz with multiple phased array features including two-dimensional imaging, color, and spectral Doppler.

ICE can provide imaging of interatrial or interventricular septum and left-heart structures from either the right atrium or ventricle, with penetration up to 15 cm. Current applications include guidance of percutaneous atrial septal defect and patent foramen ovale closures, thus mitigating the need for transesophageal echocardiography and anesthesia (Fig. 17–16). In patients undergoing transseptal puncture, ICE can facilitate localization of the fossa ovalis. ICE can also be used to guide electrophysiological procedures with identification of anatomical structures difficult to view by fluoroscopy (e.g., pulmonary veins or fossa ovalis for transseptal puncture).

Complications Associated with Cardiac Catheterization (Table 17–6)

Cardiac catheterization is a relatively safe procedure but has a well-defined risk of morbidity and mortality.[1,61,62] The potential risk of major complications during cardiac catheterization may be difficult to ascertain owing to the confounding aspects of comorbid disease and disparities in methods used to collect complication data. Advances including the use of low-osmolar and isosmolar contrast media, lower profile diagnostic catheters, and extensive operator experience all serve to reduce further the incidence of complications. Several large studies provide insight into the incidence of major events and delineate cohorts of patients that are at increased risk.[1,61-63]

Death related to diagnostic cardiac catheterization occurs in 0.08 to 0.75 percent of patients, depending on the population studied. Data from the Society for Cardiac Angiography identified subsets of patients with an increased mortality rate.[62] In an analysis of 58,332 patients, multivariate predictors of significant complications were moribund status, advanced New York Heart Association functional class, hypertension, shock, aortic valve disease, renal insufficiency, unstable angina, mitral valve disease, acute myocardial infarction within 24 hours, congestive heart failure, and cardiomyopathy. The risk of cardiac catheterization appears to be further increased in octogenarians.[63] Although the overall mortality is approximately 0.8 percent in this cohort, the risk of nonfatal major complications, which are primarily peripheral vascular, is about 5 percent.

The risk of myocardial infarction varies from 0.03 to 0.06 percent, of neurological complications from 0.03 to 0.2 percent, and of significant bradyarrhythmias or tachyarrhythmias from 0.56 to 1.3 percent.[62] One study utilizing serial cranial magnetic resonance imaging demonstrated a 22 percent incidence of focal acute cerebral embolic events following retrograde crossing of stenotic aortic valves. Three percent demonstrated clinically apparent neurological deficits.[64] This preliminary study is in direct contradistinc-

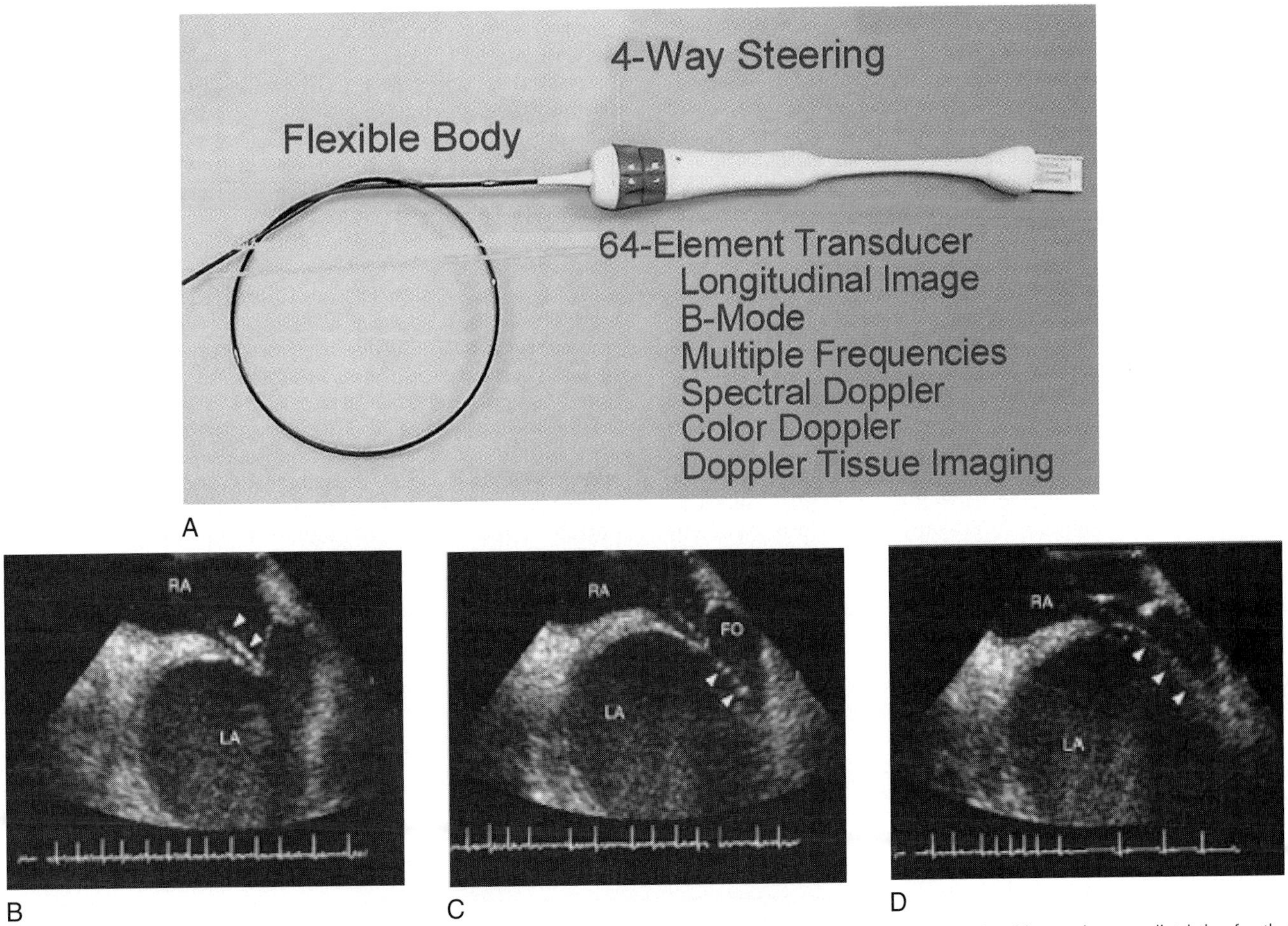

FIGURE 17–16 **A,** Intracardiac echo disposable transducer (Acuson, Inc.). Steering apparatus on proximal end and flexible body with transducer on distal tip of catheter. **B,** Tenting of the membranous fossa by the dilator-needle assembly. The transseptal needle assembly (arrowheads) is advanced to indent the fossal membrane. **C,** Advancements of the transseptal needle across the membranous fossa. Here the needle (arrowheads) is seen near the posterosuperior left atrial wall. The membrane remains tented because the dilator has not yet crossed the septum. **D,** Dilator and sheath passage across the interatrial septum. The dilator and sheath assembly has now advanced into the left atrium, releasing the tenting of the membranous fossa. FO = fossa ovalis; LA = left atrium; RA = right atrium. (From Johnson SB, Seward JB, Packer DL. Phased-array intracardiac echocardiography for guiding transseptal catheter placement: Utility and learning curve. Pacing Clin Electrophysiol 25:402, 2002.)

TABLE 17–6 Risk of Cardiac Catheterization and Coronary Angiography*

Complication	Risk (%)
Mortality	0.11
Myocardial infarction	0.05
Cerebrovascular accident	0.07
Arrhythmia	0.38
Vascular complications	0.43
Contrast reaction	0.37
Homodynamic complications	0.26
Perforation of heart chamber	0.03
Other complications	0.28
Total of major complications	1.70

From Scanlon PJ, Faxon DP, Audet AM, et al: ACC/AHA guidelines for coronary angiography: A report of the American College of Cardiology/American Heart Association Task Force on Practice Guidelines (Committee on Coronary Angiography). J Am Coll Cardiol 33:1760, 1999.
*No. of patients = 59,792.

tion to previously published large clinical series and requires additional validation.

Reports of the incidence of major vascular complications have varied widely, with most series suggesting a slightly higher frequency when the Sones brachial approach is used. The incidence of major vascular complications has been reported as approximately 0.40 percent.[62] Major vascular complications include occlusion requiring arterial repair or thrombectomy, retroperitoneal bleeding, hematoma formation, pseudoaneurysm, arteriovenous fistula formation, and infection. The risk of requiring surgical repair for vascular injury is related to advanced age, congestive heart failure, and larger body surface area.[65]

Systemic complications can vary from mild vasovagal responses to severe vagal reactions that lead to cardiac arrest. Prolonged hypotension during the procedure may also occur as a result of various mechanisms that include the vasodepressor vagal response, contrast medium–induced vasodilation or osmotic diuresis, cardiac tamponade caused by myocardial perforation or coronary laceration, myocardial infarction, and an acute anaphylactoid reaction to the contrast medium. Minor complications occur in approximately 4 percent of patients undergoing routine cardiac catheterization.[66] The most common untoward effects are transient hypotension and brief episodes of angina lasting less than 10 minutes. With the use of low-osmolar contrast media, however, bradycardia is infrequent and usually responds to cough. Rarely, administration of intravenous atropine is necessary.

Contrast Media–Induced Nephropathy

After the procedure, diuresis from the radiographic contrast load and subsequent hypotension can occur. Intravenous hydration given before and after the procedure can usually restore the intravascular volume to compensate for the anticipated diuresis. A prospective trial evaluated the effects of saline, mannitol, and furosemide in preventing nephropathy induced by contrast media.[67] It was concluded that saline hydration alone without forced diuresis was the most effective in reducing nephropathy. The incidences of acute renal dysfunction in patients with baseline renal insufficiency were 28 and 40 percent with mannitol and furosemide, respectively, compared with 11 percent with saline hydration alone.

The various classes of contrast agents are given in Table 17–7. High-osmolar ionic contrast media produce various adverse hemodynamic and electrophysiological effects during coronary angiography. Most of these adverse events are clearly related to the osmolality, sodium content, and calcium-binding characteristics of the ionic contrast solutions. Low-osmolar contrast agents clearly reduce acute adverse hemodynamic and electrophysiological reactions. The selection of contrast media, particularly for high-risk patients including those with preexisting renal impairment, is unsettled. Several studies have demonstrated that contrast media–related toxicity occurs in 1.4 to 2.3 percent of patients receiving ionic contrast media.[66,68] Patients with diabetes and those with preexisting renal insufficiency are at higher risk, with up to 48 percent of patients experiencing an increase in creatinine greater than 0.5 mg/dL.[68]

Clinical studies reveal no advantage of low-osmolar contrast over ionic contrast media in the prevention of nephrotoxicity in patients with normal renal function.[66,69] However, the risk of contrast media–induced nephropathy is significantly reduced in patients with baseline renal insufficiency with or without diabetes mellitus if nonionic low-osmolar contrast medium is used (odds ratio = 3.3 [1.6 to 6.6]).[68]

Baseline renal insufficiency has been consistently shown to be the most important independent predictor of subsequent contrast media–induced nephrotoxicity.[69] Contrast media–induced renal dysfunction can be minimized if the dose of contrast medium is kept below 30 ml for the entire study. Several studies have suggested that acetylcysteine, an antioxidant, can be orally administered in the periprocedural period to reduce the incidence of contrast media–induced nephropathy.[70,71] However, other investigators have not confirmed this effect.[72,73] Larger trials are necessary to define the potential role of this agent.

TABLE 17–7 Classification of Contrast Media

	Osmolality (mOsm/kg)			
Property	*High osmolar (1800-2100)*	*Low osmolar (600)*	*Low osmolar (700-840)*	*Isosmolar (280)*
Ionicity	Ionic	Ionic	Nonionic	Nonionic
Benzene rings	Monomer	Dimer	Monomer	Dimer
Iodine-to-particle ratio	1.5	3	3	6
Generic names (brand names)	Diatrizoate (Renografin, Hypaque)	Ioxaglate (Hexabrix)	Iohexol (Omnipaque) Iopamidol (Isovue) Ioversol (Optiray)	Iodixanol (Visipaque)
Viscosity at 37°C	8.4	7.5	8-10.5	12

TABLE 17–8	Recommendations for Management of Patients with Renal Insufficiency
1.	Administer at least 1 liter of 0.9% NS over 12-24 hr before and after the procedure.[67] Adjust for patients with history of CHF. *Avoid dehydration.*
2.	Limit contrast dose to <30 ml for diagnostic studies and <100 ml for PCI. Use biplane angiography if available.
3.	If PCI is complex, stage PCI at least 48 hr after diagnositic procedure.
4.	Administer low osmolar contrast media.[68] Consider isosmolar contrast media.[75]
5.	Discontinue nonsteroidal antiinflammatory medications, if possible.
6.	Discontinue metformin for at least 48 hr after procedure or until creatinine returns to baseline.[10]
7.	Avoid repeated contrast exposure during the recovery phase of acute tabular necrosis.
8.	Consider administering acetylcysteine 300 mg PO b.i.d. × 2 d.[70-73]

NS = normal saline; PCI = percutaneous coronary intervention.

A prospective multicenter trial has demonstrated that an isosmolar nonionic contrast agent, iodixanol, produced fewer major adverse cardiac events during percutaneous coronary interventions than the low-osmolar ionic contrast medium ioxaglate.[74] Data also indicate that the isosmolar agent can reduce the incidence of contrast media–induced nephropathy in patients with preexisting renal insufficiency (3 percent versus 26 percent, $p = 0.002$).[75] Thus, clinical studies evaluating both cardiovascular and renal effects of contrast media indicate that the pharmacological properties can have a salutary effect on local thrombogenicity and nephrotoxicity within the coronary vasculature, particularly in high-risk patients. Table 17–8 outlines clinical recommendations for prevention of contrast media–induced nephropathy in patients with renal impairment presenting for invasive cardiac procedures.

REFERENCES

Indications for Cardiac Catheterization

1. Scanlon PJ, Faxon DP, Audet AM, et al: ACC/AHA guidelines for coronary angiography: A report of the American College of Cardiology/American Heart Association Task Force on Practice Guidelines (Committee on Coronary Angiography). J Am Coll Cardiol 33:1756, 1999.
2. Bashore, TM, Bates ER, Berger PB, et al: ACC/SCAI clinical expert consensus document on cardiac catheterization laboratory standards. J Am Coll Cardiol 37:2170, 2001.

Technical Aspects of Cardiac Catheterization

3. Bersin RM, Elliott CM, Fedor JM, et al: Mobile cardiac catheterization registry: Report of the first 1,001 patients. Cathet Cardiovasc Diagn 31:1, 1994.
4. Smith SC, Dove JT, Jacobs AK, et al: ACC/AHA Guidelines for percutaneous coronary intervention—Executive summary. J Am Coll Cardiol 37:2215, 2001.
5. Jacobs AK, Faxon DP, Hirshfeld JW, Holmes DR: Task force 3: Training in diagnostic cardiac catheterization and interventional cardiology. Revision of the 1995 COCATS training statement. J Am Coll Cardiol 39:1242, 2002.
6. Holmes DR Jr, Wondrow MS, Tulsrud PR: Radiographic techniques used in cardiac catheterization. *In* Pepine CJ, Hill JA, Lambert CR (eds): Diagnostic and Therapeutic Cardiac Catheterization. 2nd ed. Baltimore, Williams & Wilkins, 1998, p 162.
7. Cusma JT, Wondrow MA, Holmes DR: Replacement of cinefilm with a digital archive and review network. Int J Card Imaging 14:293,1998.
8. American College of Cardiology, American College of Radiology and industry develop standard for digital transfer of Angiographic images. ACC/ACR/NEMA Ad Hoc Group. J Am Coll Cardiol 25:800,1995.
9. Limacher MC, Douglas PS, Germano G, et al: Radiation safety in the practice of cardiology. J Am Coll Cardiol 31:892, 1998.
10. Heupler FA Jr: Guidelines for performing angiography in patients taking metformin. Members of the Laboratory Performance Standards Committee of the Society for Cardiac Angiography and Interventions. Cathet Cardiovasc Diagn 43:121, 1998.
11. Goss JE, Chambers CE, Heupler FA: Systemic anaphylactoid reactions to iodinated contrast media during cardiac catheterization procedures: Guidelines for prevention, diagnosis, and treatment. Laboratory Performance Standards Committee for the Society for Cardiac Angiography and Interventions. Cathet Cardiovasc Diagn 34:99, 1995.
12. Baim DS: Percutaneous approach, including transseptal and apical puncture. *In* Baim DS, Grossman W (eds). Cardiac Catheterization, Angiography, and Intervention. 6th ed. Philadelphia, Lippincott Williams & Wilkins, 2000, p 69.
13. Piper WD, Malenka DJ, Ryan TR Jr: Predicting vascular complications in percutaneous coronary interventions. Am Heart J 145:1022, 2003.
14. Kussmaul WG, Buchbinder M, Whitlow P, et al: Rapid arterial hemostasis after cardiac catheterization and percutaneous transluminal angioplasty—Results of a randomized trial of a novel hemostatic device. J Am Coll Cardiol 25:1685, 1995.
15. Baim DS, Knopf WDD, Hinohara T, et al: Suture mediated closure of the femoral access site after cardiac catheterization. Am J Cardiol 85:864, 2000.
16. Ward SR, Casale P, Raymond R, et al: Efficacy and safety of a hemostatic puncture closure device with early ambulation after coronary angiography. Am J Cardiol 81:569, 1998.
17. Lesnefsky EJ, Carrea FP, Groves BM: Safety of cardiac catheterization via peripheral vascular grafts. Cathet Cardiovasc Diagn 29:113, 1993.
18. Lefevre T, Morice MC, Bonan R, et al: Coronary angiography using 4 or 6 French diagnostic catheters: A prospective, randomized study. J Invasive Cardiol 13:674, 2001.
19. Kiemeneij F, Laarman GH, Odekerken D, et al: A randomized comparison of percutaneous transluminal coronary angioplasty by the radial, brachial, and femoral approaches: The ACCESS study. J Am Coll Cardiol 29:1269, 1997.
20. Roelke M, Smith AJC, Palacios IF: The technique and safety of transseptal left heart catheterization—The Massachusetts General Hospital experience with 1279 procedures. Cathet Cardiovasc Diagn 32:332, 1994.
21. Ommen SR, Higano ST, Nishimura RA, Holmes DR: Summary of the Mayo Clinic experience with direct left ventricular puncture. Cathet Cardiovasc Diagn 44:175, 1998.
22. Anderson AS, Levin TN, Feldman T: External jugular vein approach for percutaneous right ventricular biopsy. J Heart Lung Transplant 16:576, 1997.
23. Wu LA, Lapeyre AC 3rd, Cooper LT: Current role of endomyocardial biopsy in the management of dilated cardiomyopathy and myocarditis. Mayo Clin Proc 76:1030, 2001.
24. Hunt SA, Baker DW, Chin MH: ACC/AHA Guidelines for the evaluation and management of chronic heart failure in the adult. J Am Coll Cardiol 38:2101, 2001.
25. Mehta A, Mehta M, Jain AC: Constrictive pericarditis. Clin Cardiol 22:334, 1999.
26. Barbaro G, DiLorenzo G, Grisorio B, et al: Incidence of dilated cardiomyopathy and detection of HIV in myocardial cells in HIV-positive patients. N Engl J Med 339:1093, 1998.
27. Cohen M, Ferguson JJ 3rd, Freedman RJ Jr, et al: Comparison of outcomes after 8 vs. 9.5 French size intra-aortic balloon counterpulsation catheters based on 9,332 patients in the prospective Benchmark registry. Cathet Cardiovasc Interv 56:200, 2002.
28. O'Rourke MF: Augmentation of coronary blood flow with intra-aortic balloon pump counter-pulsation. Circulation 103:E129, 2001.
29. Ferguson JJ, Cohen M, Freedman RJ: The current practice of intra-aortic balloon counterpulsation: Results from the Benchmark registry. J Am Coll Cardiol 38:1456, 2001.
30. Stone GW, Ohman EM, Miller MF: Contemporary utilization and outcomes of intra-aortic balloon counterpulsation in acute myocardial infarction: The Benchmark registry. J Am Coll Cardiol 41:1940, 2003.
31. Winters KJ, Smith SC, Cohen M: Reduction in ischemic vascular complications with a hydrophilic-coated intra-aortic balloon catheter. Cathet Cardiovasc Interv 46:357, 1999.

Hemodynamic Data

32. Grossman W: Pressure measurement. *In* Grossman W, Baim DS (eds): Cardiac Catheterization, Angiography, and Intervention. 6th ed. Philadelphia, Lea & Febiger, 2000, p 139.
33. Ruzumna P, Gheorghiade M, Bonow RO: Mechanisms and management of heart failure due to diastolic dysfunction. Curr Opin Cardiol 11:269, 1996.
34. Nishimura RA, Rihal CS, Tajik AJ, Holmes DR: Accurate measurements of the transmitral gradient in patients with mitral stenosis: A simultaneous catheterization and Doppler echocardiographic study. J Am Coll Cardiol 24:152, 1994.
35. Hildick-Smith DJ, Walsh JT, Shapiro LM: Pulmonary capillary wedge pressure in mitral stenosis accurately reflects mean left atrial pressure but overestimates transmitral gradient. Am J Cardiol 85:512, 2000.
36. Schobel WA, Voelker W, Haase KK: Extent, determinants and clinical importance of pressure recovery in patients with aortic valve stenosis. Eur Heart J 20:1355, 1999.
37. Niederberger J, Schima H, Maurer G, Baumgartner H: Importance of pressure recovery for the assessment of aortic stenosis by Doppler ultrasound. Circulation 94:1934, 1996.
38. Lehmann, KG, Platt MS: Improved accuracy and precision of thermodilution cardiac output measurement using a dual thermistor catheter system. J Am Coll Cardiol 33:883, 1999.
39. Nichols WW, O'Rourke MF (eds): McDonald's Blood Flow in Arteries. 4th ed. New York, Oxford University Press, 1998.
40. Otto CM: Cardiac catheterization and angiography. *In* Otto CM (ed): Valvular Heart Disease. Philadelphia, WB Saunders, 1999, pp 87-92.
41. Tardif JC, Rodrigues AG, Hardy JF: Simultaneous determination of aortic valve area by the Gorlin formula and by transesophageal echocardiography under different transvalvular flow conditions. Evidence that anatomic aortic valve area does not change with variations in flow in aortic stenosis. J Am Coll Cardiol 29:1296, 1997.
42. Shively BK, Charlton GA, Crawford MH, Chaney RK: Flow dependence of valve area in aortic stenosis: Relation to valve morphology. J Am Coll Cardiol 31:654, 1998.
43. Tardif JC, Rodrigues AG, Hardey JF, et al: Simultaneous determination of aortic valve area by the Gorlin formula and by transesophageal echocardiography under different transvalvular flow conditions. J Am Coll Cardiol 29:1296, 1997.
44. ACC/AHA guidelines for the management of patients with valvular heart disease. A report of the American College of Cardiology/American Heart Association Task Force on Practice Guidelines (Committee on Management of Patients with Valvular Heart Disease). J Am Coll Cardiol 32:1486, 1998.

45. Voelker W, Reul H, Nienhaus G, et al: Comparison of valvular resistance, stroke work loss, and Gorlin valve area for quantification of aortic stenosis. Circulation 91:1196, 1995.
46. Grossman W: Shunt detection and measurement. *In* Grossman W, Baim DS (eds): Cardiac Catheterization, Angiography, and Intervention. 6th ed. Philadelphia, Lea & Febiger, 2000, p 179.
47. Shepherd AP, McMahon CA: Role of oximeter error in the diagnosis of shunts. Cathet Cardiovasc Diagn 37:435, 1996.
48. Daniel WC, Lange RA, Willard JE, et al: Oximetric versus indicator dilution techniques for quantitating intracardiac left-to-right shunting in adults. Am J Cardiol 75:199, 1995.
49. Dehmer GJ, Rutala WA: Current use of green dye curves. Am J Cardiol 75:170, 1995.
50. Grossman W: Stress testing during cardiac catheterization: Exercise and pacing tachycardia. *In* Grossman W, Baim DS (eds): Cardiac Catheterization, Angiography, and Intervention. 6th ed. Philadelphia, Lea & Febiger, 2000, p 325.
51. Udelson JE, Bacharach SL, Cannon RO, Bonow RO: Minimum left ventricular pressure during beta-adrenergic stimulation in human subjects: Evidence for elastic recoil and diastolic "suction" in the normal heart. Circulation 82:1174, 1990.
52. Higano ST, Azrak E, Tahirkheli NK, Kern MJ: Hemodynamic rounds series II: Hemodynamics of constrictive physiology: Influence of respiratory dynamics on ventricular pressures. Cathet Cardiovasc Interv 46:473, 1999.
53. Carabello BA, Crawford FA: Valvular heart disease. N Engl J Med 337:32, 1997.
54. Baim DS, Grossman W: Coronary angiography. *In* Grossman W, Baim DS (eds): Cardiac Catheterization, Angiography, and Intervention. 6th ed. Philadelphia, Lea & Febiger, 2000, p 211.

Adjunctive Diagnostic Techniques

55. Kern MJ: Curriculum in interventional cardiology: Coronary pressure and flow measurements in the cardiac catheterization laboratory. Cathet Cardiovasc Interv 54:378, 2001.
56. Kornowski R, Hong MK, Gepstein L, et al: Preliminary animal and clinical experiences using an electro-mechanical endocardial mapping procedure to distinguish infarcted from healthy myocardium. Circulation 98:1116, 1998.
57. Gepstein L, Goldin A, Lessick I, et al: Electromechanical characterization of chronic myocardial infarction in the canine coronary occlusion model. Circulation 98:2055, 1998.
58. Kornowski R, Hong MK, Leon MB: Comparison between left ventricular electromechanical mapping and radionuclide perfusion imaging for detection of myocardial viability. Circulation 98:1837, 1998.
59. Kornowski R, Baim DS, Moses JW: Short and intermediate term clinical outcomes from direct myocardial laser revascularization guided by biosense left ventricular electromechanical mapping. Circulation 102:1120, 2000.
60. Vale PR, Losordo DW, Milliken CE, et al: Left ventricular electromechanical mapping to assess efficacy of phVEGF$_{165}$ gene transfer for therapeutic angiogenesis in chronic myocardial ischemia. Circulation 102:965, 2000.

Complications Associated with Cardiac Catheterization

61. Davidson CJ, Mark DB, Pieper KS, et al: Thrombotic and cardiovascular complications related to nonionic contrast media during cardiac catheterization. Analysis of 8517 patients. Am J Cardiol 65:1481, 1990.
62. Laskey W, Boyle J, Johnson LW, and the Registry Committee of the Society for Cardiac Angiography and Interventions: Multivariable model for prediction of risk of significant complication during diagnostic cardiac catheterization. Cathet Cardiovasc Diagn 30:185, 1993.
63. Clark VL, Khaja F: Risk of cardiac catheterization in patients aged >80 years without previous cardiac surgery. Am J Cardiol 74:1076, 1994.
64. Omran H, Schmidt H, Hackenbroch M, et al: Silent and apparent cerebral embolism after retrograde catheterisation of the aortic valve in valvular stenosis: A prospective, randomised study. Lancet 361:1241, 2003.
65. McCann RL, Schwartz LB, Pieper KS: Vascular complications of cardiac catheterization. J Vasc Surg 14:375, 1991.
66. Davidson CJ, Hlatky M, Morris GG, et al: Cardiovascular and renal toxicity of a nonionic radiographic contrast agent after cardiac catheterization. Ann Intern Med 110:119, 1989.

Contrast Media–Induced Nephropathy

67. Solomon R, Werner C, Mann D, et al: Effects of saline, mannitol, and furosemide on acute decreases in renal function induced by radiocontrast agents. N Engl J Med 331:1416, 1994.
68. Rudnick MR, Goldfarb S, Wexler L, et al: Nephrotoxicity of ionic and nonionic contrast media in 1,196 patients: A randomized trial. The Iohexol Cooperative Study. Kidney Int 47:254, 1995.
69. Erdogan A, Davidson CJ: Recent trials with iodixanol. Rev Cardiovasc Med 4:543, 2003.
70. Tepel M, Von Der Giet M, Schwarzfeld C, et al: Prevention of radiographic contrast agent induced reactions in renal function by acetylcysteine. N Engl J Med 343:180, 2000.
71. Kay J, Chow W, Chan TM, et al: Acetylcysteine for prevention of acute deterioration of renal function following elective coronary angiography and intervention. JAMA 289:553, 2003.
72. Briguori C, Maganelli F, Scarpato P, et al: Acetylcysteine and contrast agent–associated nephrotoxicity. J Am Coll Cardiol 40:298, 2002.
73. Durham JD, Caputo C, Dokko J, et al: A randomized controlled trial of *N*-acetylcysteine to prevent contrast nephropathy in cardiac angiography. Kidney Int 62:2202, 2002.
74. Davidson CJ, Laskey WK, Hermiller JB, et al: Randomized trial of contrast media utilization in high-risk PTCA: The COURT Trial. Circulation 101:2172, 2000.
75. Aspelin P, Aubry P, Fransson SG, et al, the NEPHRIC study investigators: Nephrotoxic effects in high-risk patients undergoing angiography. N Engl J Med 348:491, 2003.

CHAPTER 18

Coronary Angiography and Intravascular Ultrasound Imaging

Jeffery J. Popma*

Coronary arteriography remains the "gold standard" for identifying the presence or absence of arterial narrowings related to atherosclerotic coronary artery disease (CAD) and provides the most reliable anatomical information for determining the appropriateness of medical therapy, percutaneous coronary intervention (PCI), or coronary artery bypass graft (CABG) surgery in patients with ischemic CAD. First performed by Sones in 1959, coronary arteriography has subsequently become one of the most widely used invasive procedures in cardiovascular medicine. It is performed by directly injecting radiopaque contrast material into the coronary arteries and recording radiographic images on 35-mm cinefilm or digital recordings. More than 2 million patients will undergo coronary arteriography in the United States this year alone, and coronary arteriography is now available in 25 percent of acute care hospitals in this country.

The methods used to perform coronary arteriography have evolved substantially since 1959. Smaller (5 to 6 French [5 to 6F]), high-flow injection catheters have replaced larger (8F), thick-walled catheters, and the reduced sheath size has allowed same-day coronary arteriography, ambulation, and discharge. Complication rates associated with coronary arteriography have fallen due to a better understanding of the periprocedural management of patients undergoing cardiac catheterization. The number of "filmless" digital laboratories increases steadily because of advances in digital image acquisition, storage, and data transfer.[1] New adjunct invasive imaging modalities that can be performed at the time of coronary arteriography, such as intravascular ultrasonography (IVUS), can now provide the clinician with more precise characterization of the vessel wall and extent of atherosclerosis.

This chapter reviews the indications for and techniques of coronary arteriography, the normal coronary anatomy and pathological coronary variants, the qualitative and quantitative angiographic methods for assessing severity of stenoses, and the advantages and limitations of IVUS for characterizing atherosclerotic plaque.

Indications for Coronary Arteriography

Coronary arteriography can establish the presence or absence of coronary stenoses, define therapeutic options, and determine the prognosis of patients with symptoms or signs of ischemic CAD.[2] Coronary arteriography can also be utilized as a research tool to evaluate serial changes that occur after PCI or pharmacological therapy. The American College of Cardiology/American Heart Association (ACC/AHA) Task Force has established indications for coronary arteriography in patients with known or suspected CAD (Table 18–1).[2]

Patients with suspected CAD who have severe stable angina (Canadian Cardiovascular Society [CCS] class III or IV) or those who have less severe symptoms or are asymptomatic but demonstrate "high-risk" criteria for an adverse outcome on noninvasive testing should undergo coronary arteriography. High-risk features include resting or exercise-induced left ventricular dysfunction (left ventricular ejection fraction [LVEF] < 35 percent) or a standard exercise treadmill test demonstrating hypotension or 1 to 2 mm or more ST segment depression associated with decreased exercise capacity.[2] Stress imaging that demonstrates a moderate or large perfusion defect (particularly in the anterior wall), multiple defects, a large fixed perfusion defect with left ventricular dilation or increased lung uptake, or extensive stress or dobutamine-induced wall motion abnormalities also indicate high risk for an adverse outcome. Patients resuscitated from sudden cardiac death, particularly those with residual ventricular arrhythmias, are also candidates for coronary arteriography, given the favorable outcomes associated with revascularization in these patients. In the absence of symptoms and signs of ischemia, the presence of coronary calcification on fluoroscopy and a high calcium score by ultrafast computed tomographic scanning are not indications for coronary arteriography.

Patients with unstable angina who develop recurrent symptoms despite medical therapy or who are at intermediate or high risk for subsequent death or myocardial infarction (MI) are also candidates for coronary arteriography.[2,3] High-risk features include prolonged ongoing (>20 minutes) chest pain, pulmonary edema, worsening mitral regurgitation, dynamic ST segment depression of 1 mm or more, and hypotension.[2] Intermediate-risk features include

*The author acknowledges the contributions of Dr. John Bittl, a coauthor of this chapter in previous editions of this book.

TABLE 18–1 Indications for Coronary Arteriography

Class I	Class IIa	Class IIb	Class III
Asymptomatic or stable angina			
CCS class III and IV on medical therapy High-risk criteria on noninvasive testing irrespective of angina Successfully resuscitated from sudden cardiac death with sustained monomorphic VT or nonsustained polymorphic VT	CCS class III or IV which improves to class I or II with medical therapy Worsening noninvasive testing Patients with angina and severe illness that precludes risk stratification CCS class I or II angina with intolerance to medical therapy Individuals whose occupation affects the safety of others	CCS class I or II angina with demonstrable ischemia but no high-risk criteria on noninvasive testing Asymptomatic men or postmenopausal women with > two major clinical risks with low-risk noninvasive testing and no prior CAD Asymptomatic patients with prior MI, normal LV function, and not-high-risk noninvasive testing	Angina in patients who prefer to avoid revascularization Angina in patients who are not candidates for revascularization or in whom it will not improve QOL As a screening test for CAD After CABG when there is no evidence of ischemia on noninvasive testing Coronary calcification on fluoroscopy or EBCT
Unstable angina			
High or intermediate risk for adverse outcome in patients refractory to medical therapy High or intermediate risk that stabilizes after initial treatment Initially low short-term risk that is high risk on noninvasive testing Suspected Prinzmetal variant angina	None	Low short-term risk unstable angina without high-risk criteria on noninvasive testing	Recurrent chest discomfort suggestive of unstable angina but without objective signs of ischemia and with a normal coronary angiogram within the past 5 years Unstable angina in patients who are not candidates for revascularization
Postrevascularization ischemia			
Suspected abrupt closure or subacute stent thrombosis after PCI Recurrent angina and high-risk criteria on noninvasive evaluation within 9 months of PCI	Recurrent symptomatic ischemia within 12 months of CABG Noninvasive evidence of high-risk criteria occurring anytime after CABG Recurrent angina inadequately controlled by medications	Asymptomatic post-PCI patient suspected of having restenosis within the first months after PCI because of an abnormal but not high-risk noninvasive test Recurrent angina without high-risk criteria on noninvasive testing occurring >1 year postoperatively Asymptomatic post-CABG patient in whom a deteriorating noninvasive test is found	Symptoms in a post-CABG patient who is not a candidate for revasascularization Routine angiography after PCI or CABG unless part of an approved research protocol
After QWMI or NQWMI			
Spontaneous myocardial ischemia or ischemia provoked with minimal exertion Before surgical therapy for acute MR, VSD, true or pseudoaneurysm Persistent hemodynamic instability	Suspected MI due to coronary embolism, arteritis, trauma, certain metabolic diseases, or coronary spasm Survivors of acute MI with LVEF < 0.40, CHF, prior PCI or CABG, or malignant ventricular arrhythmias	For a suspected persistent occlusion of the IRA to perform delayed PCI Coronary arteriography performed without risk stratification to identify the presence of left main or three-vessel CAD All patients after NQWMI Recurrent ventricular tachycardia despite antiarrhyhtmic therapy without ongoing ischemia	Patients who are not a candidate for or refuse revascularization
Nonspecific chest pain			
High-risk features on noninvasive testing	None	Patients with recurrent hospitalizations for chest pain who have abnormal or equivocal findings on noninvasive testing	All other patients with nonspecific chest pain

Class I: Conditions for which there is agreement that the procedure is useful and effective; Class IIa: Weight of the evidence is in favor of usefulness and efficacy; Class IIb: Weight of the evidence is less well established by evidence and opinion; Class III: Conditions for which there is general agreement that the procedure is not useful and effective and in some cases may be harmful.

CABG = coronary artery bypass graft surgery; CAD = coronary artery disease; CCS = Canadian Cardiovascular Society; CHF = congestive heart failure; EBCT = electron beam computed tomography; IRA = infarct-related artery; LV = left ventricular; MI = myocardial infarction; MR = mitral regurgitation; NQWMI = non-Q-wave MI; PCI = percutaneous coronary intervention; QOL = quality of life; VSD = ventricular septal defect; VT = ventricular tachycardia.

From Scanlon P, Faxon D, Audet A, et al: ACC/AHA guidelines for coronary angiography. J Am Coll Cardiol 33:1756, 1999.

angina at rest (>20 minutes) relieved with rest or sublingual nitroglycerin, angina associated with dynamic electrocardiographic changes, recent-onset angina with a high likelihood of CAD, pathological Q waves or ST segment depression less than 1 mm in multiple leads, and age older than 65 years.[2]

Patients with an ST segment elevation myocardial infarction (STEMI), a non-ST segment elevation myocardial infarction (NSTEMI), or unstable angina who develop spontaneous ischemia; or with ischemia at a minimal workload; or who have MI complicated by congestive heart failure (CHF), hemodynamic instability, cardiac arrest, mitral regurgitation, or ventricular septal rupture should undergo coronary arteriography. Patients with angina or provocable ischemia after MI should also undergo coronary arteriography because revascularization may reduce the high risk of reinfarction in these patients.

Patients who present with chest pain of unclear etiology, particularly those who have high-risk criteria on noninvasive testing, may benefit from coronary arteriography to diagnose or exclude the presence of significant CAD.[2,4] Patients who have undergone prior revascularization should undergo coronary arteriography if there is suspicion of abrupt vessel closure or when recurrent angina develops that meets high-risk noninvasive criteria.

Coronary arteriography should also be performed in patients scheduled to undergo noncardiac surgery who demonstrate high-risk criteria on noninvasive testing, have angina unresponsive to medical therapy, develop unstable angina, or have equivocal noninvasive test results and are scheduled to undergo high-risk surgery (see also Chap. 77). Coronary arteriography is also recommended for patients scheduled to undergo surgery for valvular heart disease or congenital heart disease, particularly those with multiple cardiac risk factors and those with infective endocarditis and evidence of coronary embolization.[2]

Coronary arteriography should be performed annually in patients after cardiac transplantation in the absence of clinical symptoms because of the characteristically diffuse and often asymptomatic nature of graft atherosclerosis. Coronary arteriography is useful in potential donors for cardiac transplantation whose age or cardiac risk profile increases the likelihood of CAD. The arteriogram often provides important diagnostic information about the presence of CAD in patients with intractable arrhythmias before electrophysiological testing or in patients who present with a dilated cardiomyopathy of unknown etiology.

CONTRAINDICATIONS. Although there are no absolute contraindications for coronary arteriography, relative contraindications include unexplained fever, untreated infection, severe anemia with hemoglobin less than 8 gm/dl, severe electrolyte imbalance, severe active bleeding, uncontrolled systemic hypertension, digitalis toxicity, previous contrast reaction but no pretreatment with corticosteroids, and ongoing stroke.[2] Other disease states that are relative contraindications to coronary arteriography include acute renal failure; decompensated CHF; severe intrinsic or iatrogenic coagulopathy (international normalized ratio [INR] > 2.0); and active endocarditis.[2] Risk factors for significant complications after catheterization include advanced age as well as several general medical, vascular, and cardiac characteristics (Table 18–2).

Given that the majority of these conditions are self-limited, deferral of coronary arteriography until important comorbidities have been stabilized is generally preferred unless there is evidence of ongoing myocardial necrosis. It is recognized that coronary arteriography performed under emergency conditions is associated with a higher risk of procedural complications, and the risks and benefits of the procedure and its alternatives should be carefully reviewed with the patient and family in all circumstances before undertaking coronary arteriography in the presence of relative contraindications.

TABLE 18–2 Patients at Increased Risk for Complications after Coronary Arteriography

Increased general medical risk
Age > 70 years
Complex congenital heart disease
Morbid obesity
General debility or cachexia
Uncontrolled glucose intolerance
Arterial oxygen desaturation
Severe chronic obstructive lung disease
Renal insufficiency with creatinine greater than 1.5 mg/dl
Increased cardiac risk
Three-vessel coronary artery disease
Left main coronary artery disease
Functional class IV
Significant mitral or aortic valve disease or mechanical prosthesis
Ejection fraction less than 35%
High-risk exercise treadmill testing (hypotension or severe ischemia)
Pulmonary hypertension
Pulmonary artery wedge pressure greater than 25 mm Hg
Increased vascular risk
Anticoagulation or bleeding diathesis
Uncontrolled systemic hypertension
Severe peripheral vascular disease
Recent stroke
Severe aortic insufficiency

Adapted from Scanlon P, Faxon D, Audet A, et al: ACC/AHA guidelines for coronary angiography. J Am Coll Cardiol 33:1756, 1999.

Complications of Coronary Arteriography

Major complications are uncommon (<1 percent) after coronary arteriography (Table 18–3)[5] and include death (0.10 to 0.14 percent), MI (0.06 to 0.07 percent), contrast agent reactions (0.23 percent), and local vascular complications (0.24 to 0.1 percent).[6,7] More recent series have shown no change in the major complication rates associated with coronary arteriography, despite increased morbidity of patients and lesion complexity.[5,8,9]

The incidence of death during coronary arteriography is higher in the presence of left main coronary artery (LMCA) disease (0.55 percent), with LVEF less than 30 percent (0.30 percent), and with New York Heart Association functional Class IV disease (0.29 percent). Stroke is uncommon (0.07 to 0.14 percent) after coronary arteriography[10] but may develop due to embolization of atherosclerotic debris into the cerebral circulation or embolization of clot that formed on the injection catheters, particularly in patients with prior CABG who have a diseased ascending aorta.[9,11] Embolic stroke related to atherothrombotic embolization is generally reversible.

Air embolus is an uncommon occurrence (0.1 percent) during diagnostic coronary arteriography and is generally preventable with meticulous flushing and elimination of air within the manifold. If an air embolus and air lock do occur, 100 percent oxygen should be administered, which allows resorption of smaller amounts of air within 2 to 4 minutes. Morphine sulfate may be given for pain relief. Ventricular arrhythmias associated with air embolus can be treated with lidocaine and direct-current cardioversion. Cholesterol embolization is a rare but important complication that can occur during coronary arteriography.[12] Cholesterol embolization occurs more often in the presence of catheter manipulation within an abdominal aortic aneurysm that has diffuse atherosclerosis (see also Chap. 54).[13] Nerve pain after diagnostic catheterization occurs rarely.[14,15] Although there was initial concern about the occurrence of lactic acidosis after coronary angiography in diabetic patients taking metformin, this complication has been minimized when metformin is discontinued after coronary arteriography until renal function has recovered.[16]

With the expanded use of complex PCI, patients may now return for multiple procedures over their lifetime that may subject them to the risk of cumulative radiation injury. Scattered reports of radiodermatitis related to prolonged x-ray exposure[17,18] have led to the recommendation that patients who receive fluoroscopy for more than 60 minutes be counseled about the delayed effects of radiation injury to the skin. Radiation-induced lesions are generally identified by their location in the region of the x-ray tube and are manifest by an acute erythema, delayed pigmented telangiectasia, and indurated or ulcerated plaques in the upper back or below the axilla.[17]

TABLE 18–3 Risk of Cardiac Catheterization

Complication	SCAI Registry (%)
Mortality	0.11
Myocardial infarction	0.05
Cerebrovascular accident	0.07
Arrhythmias	0.38
Vascular complications	0.43
Contrast reaction	0.37
Hemodynamic complications	0.26
Perforation of heart chamber	0.03
Other complications	0.28
Total of major complications	1.70

SCAI = Society for Cardiac Angiography and Intervention.
Adapted from Scanlon P, Faxon D, Audet A, et al: ACC/AHA guidelines for coronary angiography. J Am Coll Cardiol 33:1756, 1999.

Technique of Coronary Arteriography

PREPARATION OF THE PATIENT. Elective coronary arteriography should be performed alone or in conjunction with right-heart catheterization or contrast left ventriculography (see Chap. 17) when comorbid conditions, such as CHF, diabetes mellitus, or renal insufficiency, are stable. A baseline electrocardiogram (ECG), electrolyte and renal function tests, complete blood cell count, and coagulation panel should be reviewed before coronary arteriography. Patients who may undergo PCI should receive aspirin, 80 to 325 mg, at least 2 hours before the procedure if PCI is planned. Warfarin should be discontinued 2 days before elective coronary arteriography, and the INR should be less than 2.0 before arterial puncture. Patients at increased risk for systemic thromboembolism on withdrawal of warfarin, such as those with atrial fibrillation, mitral valve disease, or a prior history of systemic thromboembolism, may be treated with intravenous unfractionated heparin or subcutaneous low-molecular-weight heparin in the periprocedural period.

VASCULAR ACCESS. A variety of vascular approaches are available for coronary arteriography. The selection of the vascular access depends on the operator's and patient's preferences, anticoagulation status, and presence of peripheral vascular disease.

Femoral Artery Approach. The right or left femoral arteries are the most commonly used access sites for coronary arteriography. The common femoral artery courses medially to the femoral head and the bifurcation of the common femoral artery into its branches is generally distal to the middle third of the femoral head, which can be localized by fluoroscopy before arterial puncture (Fig. 18–1A). The anterior wall of the common femoral artery should be punctured several centimeters below the inguinal ligament but proximal to the bifurcation of the superficial femoral and profunda arterial branches (see Fig. 18–1B). If the puncture site is proximal to the inguinal ligament, hemostasis after the procedure may be difficult with manual compression, leading to an increased risk of retroperitoneal hemorrhage. If the puncture site is at or distal to the femoral bifurcation, there is a higher risk of pseudoaneurysm formation after sheath removal. Ipsilateral cannulation of the femoral artery and femoral vein also increases the risk of arteriovenous fistula formation.

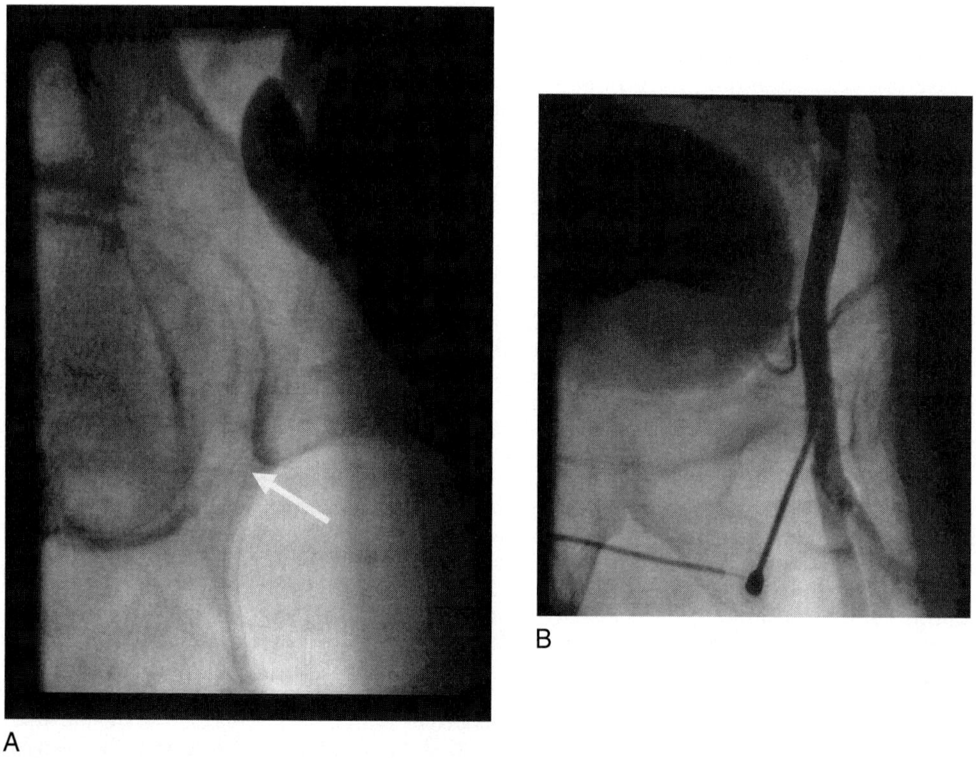

FIGURE 18–1 Radiographic landmarks can be used to identify the course of the common femoral artery. **A,** The middle third of the right femoral head identifies the usual course of the common femoral artery (arrow). **B,** The arterial sheath is shown placed proximally to the bifurcation of the femoris superficial femoral artery and the profunda femoris.

Brachial and Radial Artery Approaches. Although Sones first introduced the cutdown approach to the brachial artery for coronary arteriography, access to the brachial and radial arteries is now most often obtained percutaneously. These approaches are preferred to the femoral approach in the presence of severe peripheral vascular disease[19] and morbid obesity.[20] Systemic anticoagulation with intravenous heparin, use of hydrophilic sheath, and administration of intraarterial verapamil and nitroglycerin have reduced the occurrence of vascular complications with the radial approach. Saphenous vein grafts (SVGs) can be engaged using either brachial or radial artery, but cannulation of the internal mammary artery (IMA) is best performed from the left brachial or radial artery. Engagement of the left IMA from the right brachial or radial artery is technically challenging but may be performed using a "headhunter" or another shaped catheter for selective entry into the left subclavian artery. A 0.035-inch angled hydrophilic guidewire is the most useful guidewire for access to the subclavian artery.

The brachial artery easily accommodates an 8F (1 French = 0.33 mm in diameter) sheath, whereas the radial artery is smaller and generally limited to 6 or 7F catheters. Before radial artery access is attempted, an Allen test should be carried out to ensure that the ulnar artery is patent in the event of radial artery occlusion.

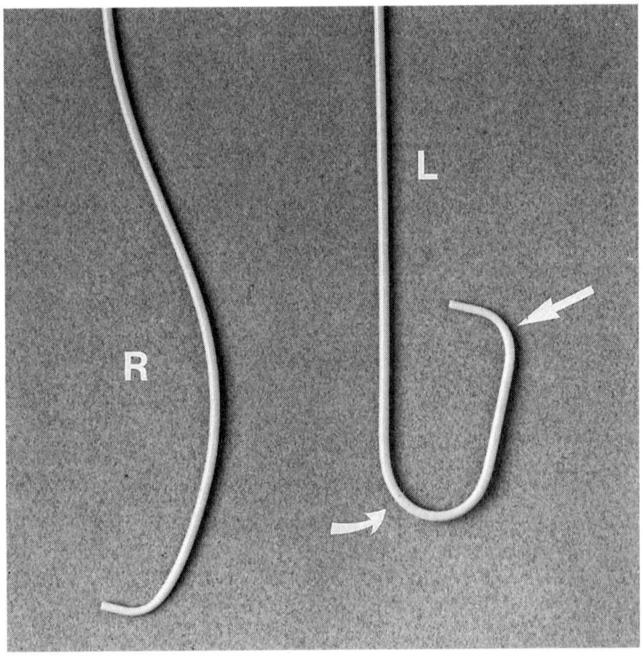

FIGURE 18–2 Right (R) and left (L) Judkins catheters. The primary (straight arrow) and secondary (curved arrow) curves of the left Judkins catheter are shown. (Courtesy of Cordis Corporation.)

Catheters

A number of injection catheters have been developed for coronary arteriography. Diagnostic catheters are generally constructed of polyethylene or polyurethane with a fine wire braid within the wall to allow advancement and directional control (torquability) and to prevent kinking. The outer diameter size of the catheters ranges from 4 to 8F, but 5 and 6F catheters are used most commonly for diagnostic arteriography.

JUDKINS CATHETERS. The left Judkins catheter is preshaped to allow entry into the left coronary ostium from the femoral approach with minimal catheter manipulation (Figs. 18–2 and 18–3). A preformed left Judkins catheter can also be used from the left brachial or radial artery, but a catheter with 0.5 cm less curvature than required for the femoral approach is generally better suited for coronary cannulation. The right Judkins catheter is shaped to permit entry into the right coronary artery (RCA) with a small amount of rotational (clockwise) catheter manipulation from any vascular approach.

Selection of Judkins catheter shape is based on the body habitus of the patient and size of the aortic root. The left coronary artery (LCA) is easily engaged with the Judkins left 4.0 catheter from the femoral approach in most patients, whereas patients with a dilated ascending aorta (e.g., in the setting of congenital aortic stenosis and poststenotic dilation) may require the use of a Judkins left 5.0 or 6.0 catheter. Patients with large ascending aortic aneurysms may require arteriography with heat-modified catheters to achieve Judkins left 7.0 to 10.0 shapes. Use of a Judkins shape that is too small for the ascending aorta often leads to folding of the catheter within the aortic root. The best technique for removing a folded Judkins left catheter from the body involves withdrawing the folded catheter into the descending aorta and advancing a guidewire anterograde in the contralateral common iliac artery. On withdrawal of the catheter and guidewire together, the catheter straightens and can be removed safely from the body without disrupting the arterial access site.

AMPLATZ CATHETERS. Amplatz catheters can be used for the femoral or brachial approach to coronary arteriography (Fig. 18–4). The Amplatz catheters are an excellent alternative in cases in which the Judkins catheter is not appropriately shaped to enter the coronary arteries. The Amplatz L-1 or L-2 catheter may be used for coronary angiography from the right brachial or radial approach. A modified right Amplatz catheter (AR-1 or AR-2) can be used for engagement of a horizontal or upward takeoff RCA or SVG.

OTHER CATHETERS. Other catheters used for coronary arteriography include the left IMA catheter with an angulated tip that allows engagement of the IMA or an upward takeoff RCA. Catheter shapes that permit engagement of SVGs include the multipurpose catheter (Fig. 18–5), right Judkins, modified right Amplatz, and hockey stick catheters. Specially designed catheters for engagement of the coronary arteries from the radial artery have also been developed.

Drugs Used During Coronary Arteriography

ANALGESICS. The goal of analgesic use is to achieve a state of conscious sedation, defined by a minimally depressed level of consciousness that allows a patient to respond appropriately to verbal commands and to maintain a patent airway.[21-23] Several different sedation regimens are recommended, but depending on the patient's comorbid conditions, most use diazepam, 2.5 to 10 mg orally, and diphenhydramine, 25 to 50 mg orally, 1 hour before the procedure. Intravenous midazolam, 0.5 to 2 mg, and fentanyl, 25 to 50 μg, are useful agents to provide sedation during the procedure. Patients undergoing conscious sedation should have continuous hemodynamic, ECG, and oximetry monitoring and access to oxygen and suction ports and a resuscitation cart.

ANTICOAGULANTS. Intravenous unfractionated heparin is no longer required during routine coronary arteriography. Patients at increased risk for thromboembolic complications, including those with severe aortic stenosis, critical peripheral arterial disease, or arterial atheroembolic disease or those undergoing procedures in which there is a need for prolonged (>1 to 2 minutes) use of guidewires in the central circulation may be given intravenous heparin, 2000 to 5000 units. Patients undergoing brachial or radial artery catheterization should also receive systemic anticoagulation with unfractionated heparin or bivalirudin. Frequent flushing of all diagnostic and guiding catheters with heparinized saline prevents the formation of microthrombi within the catheter tip. A continuous flush through the arterial access sheath may also lower the occurrence of distal thromboembolism.

The anticoagulant effect of unfractionated heparin can be reversed with protamine, 1 mg for every 100 units of heparin. Protamine causes anaphylaxis or serious hypotensive episodes in approximately 2 percent of patients, and protamine should not be administered to patients with prior exposure to NPH insulin, in those with a history of unstable angina or high-risk coronary anatomy, or in patients who have undergone coronary arteriography by means of the brachial or radial arteries. Femoral sheaths can be removed

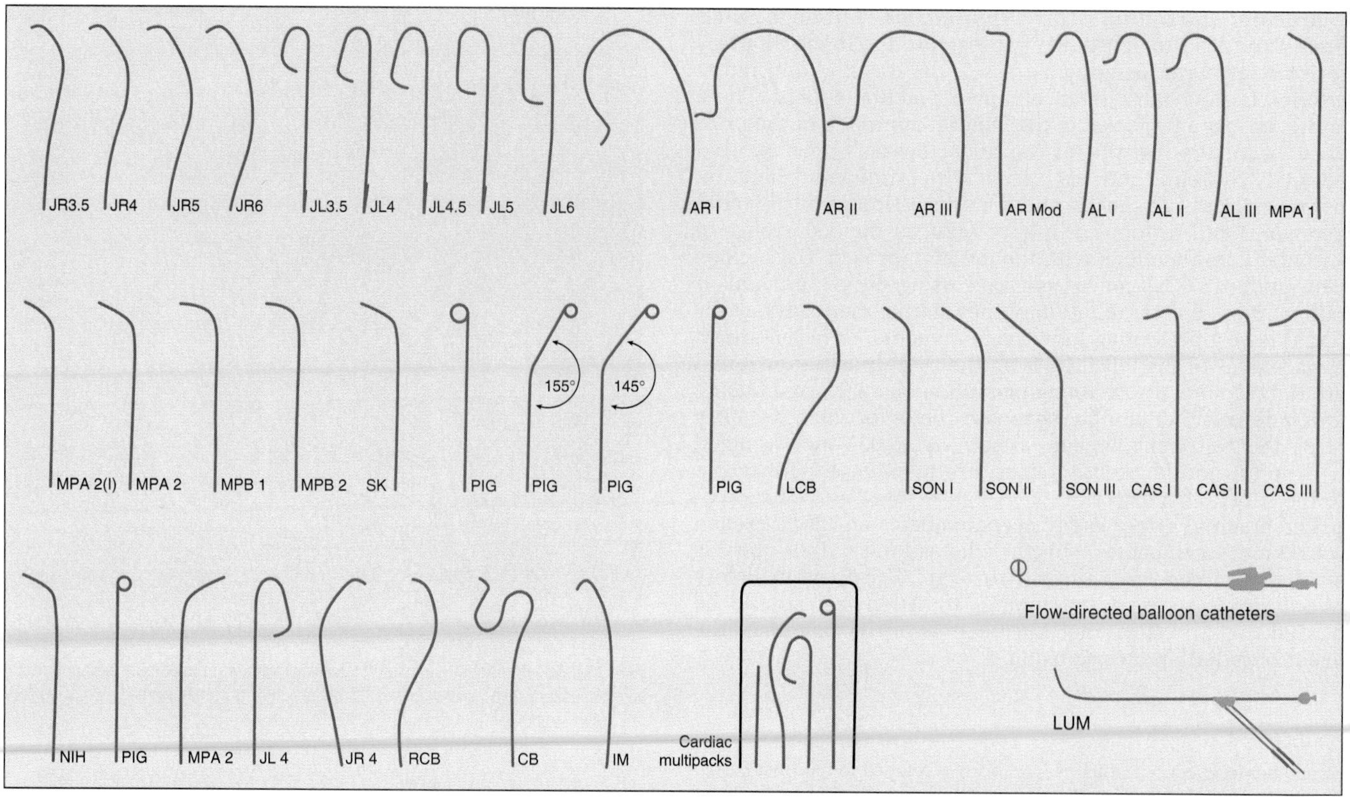

FIGURE 18–3 Tip configurations for several catheters useful in coronary arteriography. JR = Judkins right; JL = Judkins left; AR = Amplatz right; Mod = modified; AL = Amplatz left; MP = multipurpose; PIG = pigtail; LCB = left coronary bypass graft; SON = Sones; CAS = Castillo; NIH = National Institutes of Health; RCB = right coronary bypass graft; CB = coronary bypass catheter; IM = internal mammary; LUM = lumen. (Courtesy of Cordis Corporation.)

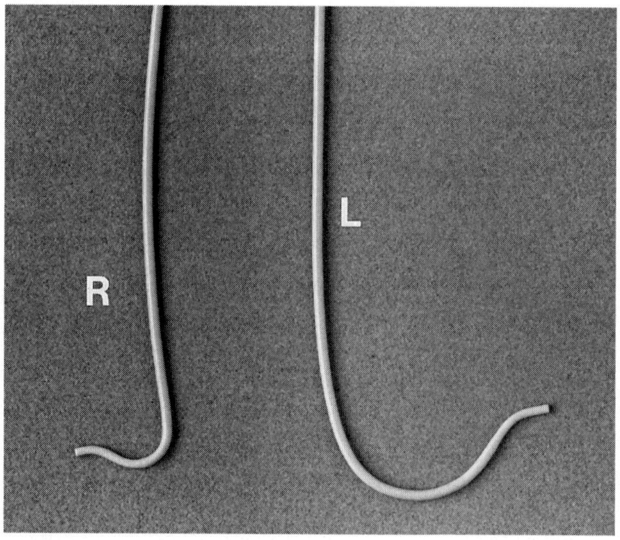

FIGURE 18–4 Right (R) and left (L) Amplatz catheters. (Courtesy of Cordis Corporation.)

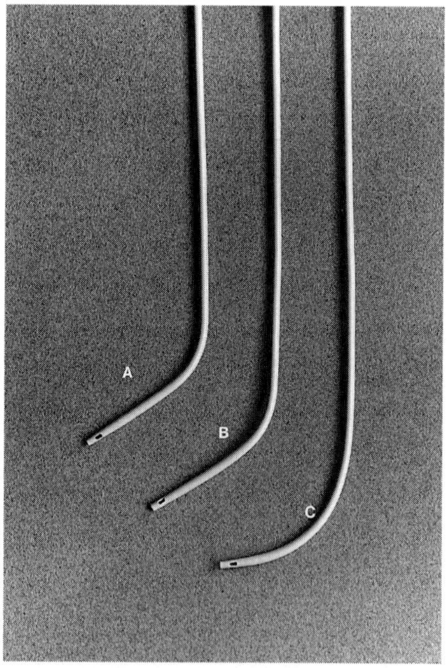

FIGURE 18–5 Multipurpose A, B, and C type catheters. (Courtesy of Cordis Corporation.)

after the anticoagulant effect of unfractionated heparin has dissipated, as assessed by an activated clotting time less than 150 to 180 seconds.

TREATMENT OF PERIPROCEDURAL ISCHEMIA. Patients may develop angina during coronary arteriography because of ischemia induced by tachycardia, hypertension, contrast agents, microembolization, coronary spasm or enhanced vasomotor tone, or dynamic platelet aggregation. Sublingual (0.3 mg), intracoronary (50 to 200 μg), or intravenous (10 to 25 μg/min) nitroglycerin can be given in patients with a systolic blood pressure greater than 100 mm Hg. Patients without contraindications to beta blockers, such as bradycardia, bronchospasm, or left ventricular dysfunction, can be given intravenous metoprolol, 2.5 to 5.0 mg, or

TABLE 18–4 Characteristics of Radiocontrast Agents

Compound	Brand Name	Osmolality mOsm/kg H_2O	Viscosity at 37°C	Iodine (mg/ml)	Sodium (mEq/liter)	Additives	Side Effects Profile
High osmolar ionic agents							
Sodium diatrizoate	Hypaque	1690	9.0	370	160	Calcium disodium EDTA	Electophysiologic (++++) Hemodynamic (++++) Anticoagulant (++++) Nephrotoxicity (+++) Allergic (+++)
Sodium meglumine diatrizoate	Renografin	1940	8.4	370	160	Sodium citrate, disodium EDTA	
Nonionic or low osmolar							
Ioxaglate	Hexabrix	600	7.5	320	150	Calcium disodium EDTA	Electophysiologic (+) Hemodynamic (+) Anticoagulant (+) Nephrotoxicity (++) Allergic (+)
Iohexol	Omnipaque	844	10.4	350	5	Tromethamine calcium disodium EDTA	
Iopamidol	Isovue	790	9.4	370	2	Tromethamine calcium disodium EDTA	
Ioversol	Optiray	702	5.8	320	2	Tromethamine calcium disodium EDTA	
Iodixanol	Visipaque	290	11.8	320	19	Tromethamine calcium disodium EDTA + 0.15 mEq/liter calcium	

++++ = common; +++ = occasional; ++ = infrequent; + = rare; EDTA = ethylene diaminetetraacetic acid (a divalent cation chelating agent).
Modified from Hill J, Lambert C, Pepine C: Radiographic contrast agents. *In* Pepine C, Hill J, Lambert C (eds): Diagnostic and Therapeutic Cardiac Catheterization. Baltimore, Williams & Wilkins, 1994, pp 182-194.

propranolol, 1 to 4 mg. Intraaortic balloon counterpulsation is also a useful adjunct in patients with coronary ischemia and left main CAD, cardiogenic shock, or refractory pulmonary edema.

Contrast Agents

All radiographic contrast agents contain iodine, which effectively absorbs x-rays in the energy range of the angiographic imaging system. Radiographic contrast agents currently used for coronary arteriography may also produce a number of adverse hemodynamic, electrophysiological, and renal effects. The frequency of these side effects varies among the different radiocontrast agents because of differences in their ionic content, osmolality, and viscosity (Table 18–4).

IONIC CONTRAST AGENTS. The monomeric ionic contrast agents initially used for coronary arteriography were the high-osmolar meglumine and sodium salts of diatrizoic acid. These substances dissociated into cations and iodine-containing anions that have a higher serum osmolality (>1500 mOsm) than human plasma (300 mOsm). The hypertonicity of these compounds produced sinus bradycardia, heart block, QT interval and QRS prolongation, ST segment depression, giant T wave inversion, decreased left ventricular contractility, decreased systolic pressure, and increased left ventricular end-diastolic pressure, owing, in part, to the calcium-chelating properties of these agents. Ventricular tachycardia and fibrillation occurred in 0.5 percent of cases and developed more often when ionic contrast agents were injected into a damped coronary catheter, were given too rapidly, or were administered in too great a volume. Because of the availability of other less toxic contrast agents, ionic contrast agents are now rarely used for coronary arteriography. When ionic agents are selected, additional precautions are needed to avoid complications. Patients should be counseled about coughing, which helps clear contrast material from within the coronary artery, before the first selective coronary arteriogram is performed and the minimal amount of contrast agent needed to fill the entire coronary artery should be given.

NONIONIC AND LOW-OSMOLAR CONTRAST AGENTS. Nonionic agents do not ionize in solution and provide more iodine-containing particles per milliliter of contrast material than ionic agents. Their osmolality is substantially reduced (<850 mOsm) because these agents exist in solution as single neutral molecules and do not chelate calcium, potentially leading to fewer side effects.

Side Effects. Unwanted reactions may also occur after use of nonionic radiocontrast agents, related in part to the hyperosmolality of these agents (Table 18–5). These reactions include hot flushing, nausea, vomiting, and arrhythmia. Hypotension after contrast medium administration may be due to an anaphylactoid reaction, a direct toxic effect, or a vasovagal reaction. Ionic radiocontrast agents may inhibit clot formation when mixed with blood. Although nonionic agents exhibit less of an anticoagulant effect, potentially leading to clots within the manifold where low-osmolar and nonionic contrast agents and blood are in direct contact with one another, the clinical effects of this finding related to embolization of thrombus into the coronary arteries are not known. The low-osmolality ionic dimer methylglucamine-sodium ioxaglate retains most of the anticoagulant properties of diatrizoate sodium, but has more complications than the

TABLE 18–5 Toxicities Associated with Radiocontrast Agents

Side Effect
Allergic (anaphylactoid) reactions
Grade I: Single episode of emesis, nausea, sneezing, or vertigo
Grade II: Hives, multiple episodes of emesis, fevers, or chills
Grade III: Clinical shock, bronchospasm, laryngospasm or edema, loss of consciousness, hypotension, hypertension, cardiac arrhythmia, angioedema, or pulmonary edema
Cardiovascular toxicity
Electrophysiologic
Bradycardia (asystole, heart block)
Tachycardia (sinus, ventricular)
Ventricular fibrillation
Hemodynamic
Hypotension (cardiac depression, vasodilation)
Heart failure (cardiac depression, increased intravascular volume)
Nephrotoxicity
Discomfort
Nausea, vomiting
Heat and flushing
Hyperthyroidism

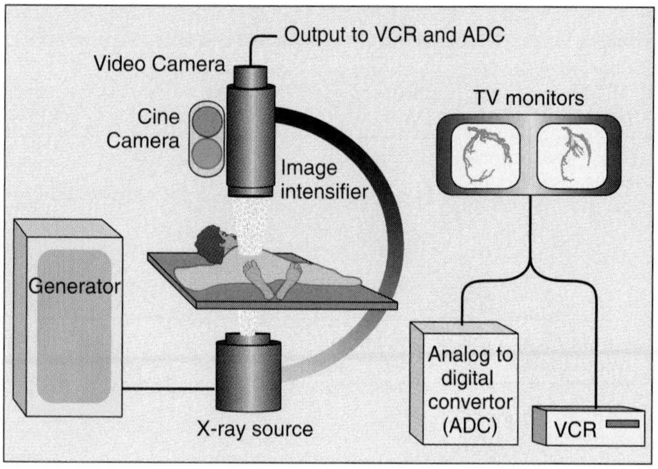

FIGURE 18–6 Cineangiographic equipment. The major components include a generator, x-ray tube, image intensifier attached to a positioner such as a C-arm, optical system, cine camera, video camera, videocassette recorder (VCR), analog-to-digital converter (ADC), and television monitors. The x-ray tube is the source of the x-ray beam, which passes superiorly through the patient.

isosmolar, nonionic dimer contrast agent iodixanol.[24] Iodixanol may also be the preferred contrast agent in diabetic patients with underlying renal insufficiency.[25]

CONTRAST-INDUCED NEPHROPATHY (see also Chap. 86). Worsening of renal function may occur after contrast agent administration in 13 to 20 percent of patients, particularly in those with prior renal insufficiency, diabetes mellitus, dehydration before the procedure, CHF, larger volumes of contrast material, and recent (<48 hour) contrast exposure.[26-30] The incidence, pathogenesis, and preventive measures for the treatment of contrast-induced nephropathy are reviewed in detail in Chapter 86. Fluid administration is recommended in all patients.[31-34] Periprocedural aminophylline appears to be of limited value.[35] Although the clinical data have been mixed,[36] a weighted analysis of the preprocedural use of *N*-acetylcysteine, particularly in patients with underlying renal insufficiency, appears to indicate a benefit for reduction of the occurrence of contrast-induced nephropathy (see Chap. 86).[37-42] Despite encouraging initial results,[43-45] use of felodipine does not appear to lessen the occurrence of nephropathy after contrast agent administration.[46] Randomized trials have shown a benefit with hemofiltration[47,48] but not hemodialysis[49] for the prevention of contrast-induced renal insufficiency in high-risk patients.

CONTRAST REACTION PROPHYLAXIS. Reactions to radiocontrast agents are classified as mild (grade I: single episode of emesis, nausea, sneezing, or vertigo), moderate (grade II: hives, multiple episodes of emesis, fevers, or chills), or severe (grade III: clinical shock, bronchospasm, laryngospasm or edema, loss of consciousness, hypotension, hypertension, cardiac arrhythmias, angioedema, or pulmonary edema). Although mild or moderate reactions occur in approximately 9.0 percent of patients, severe reactions are uncommon (0.15 to 0.7 percent). Contrast reactions may be more difficult to manage in patients receiving beta blocker therapy. Recurrence rates may approach 50 percent on reexposure to contrast agents, and prophylactic use of H_1 and H_2 histamine blocking agents and aspirin therapy has been advocated. Patients treated with corticosteroids (methylprednisolone, 32 mg) 12 hours and 2 hours before contrast agent exposure had a lower (6.4 percent) incidence of allergic reactions than patients treated with a single dose of methylprednisolone 2 hours before contrast agent exposure (9.4 percent) or placebo (9.0 percent) ($p < 0.001$).[50] On the basis of these findings, patients with a prior history of radiocontrast reactions should receive two doses of prednisone, 60 mg (or its equivalent) the night before and again at 2 hours before the procedure. Diphenhydramine, 50 mg, and cimetidine, 300 mg, may also be given before the procedure.

Anatomy and Variations of the Coronary Arteries

The basic principle of radiographic coronary imaging is that radiation produced by the x-ray tube is attenuated as it passes through the body and detected by the image intensifier (Fig. 18–6). Iodinated contrast medium injected into the coronary arteries enhances the absorption of x-rays and produces a sharp contrast with the surrounding cardiac tissues. The x-ray shadow is then converted into a visible light image by an image intensifier, displayed on fluoroscopic monitors, and stored on 35-mm cinefilm or digital storage systems. Although 35-mm cinefilm has better image resolution (4 line pairs/mm) than digital imaging (2.5 line pairs/mm) archived in a standard DICOM3 512 × 512 × 8 bit pixel matrix format, digital imaging has largely replaced 35-mm cinefilm for coronary angiography due to its versatility with respect to image transfer, low-cost acquisition and storage, and capability for image enhancement after image acquisition.

The major epicardial branches and their second- and third-order branches can be visualized using coronary arteriography. The network of smaller intramyocardial branches generally are not seen because of their size, cardiac motion, and limitations in resolution of cineangiographic systems. These fourth-order and higher "resistance" vessels play a major role in autoregulation of coronary blood flow, may limit myocardial perfusion during stress, and contribute to ischemia in patients with left ventricular hypertrophy or systemic hypertension. Coronary perfusion within these smaller branch vessels can be quantitatively assessed using the myocardial blush score.[51]

ARTERIAL NOMENCLATURE AND EXTENT OF DISEASE. The Coronary Artery Surgery Study (CASS) inves-

TABLE 18–6 Classification System for Coronary Segments

Number	Map Location	Number	Map Location	Number	Map Location
Right coronary artery		**Left main coronary artery**		**Left circumflex**	
1	Proximal RCA	11	Left main coronary artery	18	Proximal LCx
2	Mid RCA	**Left anterior descending**		19	Distal LCx
3	Distal RCA	12	Proximal LAD	20	1st obtuse marginal
4	Right posterior descending branch	13	Mid LAD	21	2nd obtuse marginal
5	Right posterior atrioventricular	14	Distal LAD	22	Third obtuse marginal
6	First right posterolateral	15	1st diagonal	23	LCx atrioventricular groove
7	Second right posterolateral	16	2nd diagonal	24	1st left posterolateral branch
8	Third right posterolateral	17	LAD septal perforators	25	2nd left posterolateral branch
9	Posterior descending septals	29	3rd diagonal	26	3rd left posterolateral branch
10	Acute marginal segment			27	Left posterior descending branch
				28	Ramus intermedium branch

LAD = left anterior descending; LCx = left circumflex; RCA = right coronary artery.

From CASS Principal Investigators and their Associates: Coronary Artery Surgery Study (CASS): A randomized trial of coronary artery surgery: Survival data. Circulation 68:939, 1983.

tigators established the nomenclature most commonly used to describe the coronary anatomy, defining 27 segments in three major coronary arteries (Table 18–6). The Bypass Angioplasty Revascularization Investigators (BARI) modified these criteria by addition of two segments for the ramus intermedius and the third diagonal branch. In this system, the three major coronary arteries include the left anterior descending (LAD), left circumflex (LCx), and RCA with a right-dominant, balanced, or left-dominant circulation (see later). CAD is defined as a more than 50 percent diameter stenosis in one or more of these vessels, although it is clear that stenoses of less than 50 percent have major prognostic implications because these lesions most commonly lead to plaque rupture and acute MI. Subcritical stenoses of less than 50 percent are best characterized as nonobstructive CAD; obstructive CAD is classified as one-, two-, or three-vessel disease.

A number of "jeopardy scores" were developed to quantitate plaque burden, predict patient-based clinical outcomes, and identify risk factors for the presence of atherosclerosis and its progression. The Califf scoring system divided the coronary circulation into six segments with two points allotted for each coronary stenosis of 75 percent or more (score range: 0 to 12). The Gensini scoring system used an ordinal ranking based on stenosis severity in 11 coronary segments (score range: 0 to 72). The Candell-Riera scoring system used an ordinal ranking (from 1 to 5) of 13 coronary segments (score range: 0 to 65). Differences between these scoring systems were primarily related to definitions rather than to their ability to provide unique prognostic information, as one comparative study found that 80 percent of the prognostic information in one jeopardy index was obtained with other indices using subtly different methodologies. In CASS, the major determinants of 6-year outcome included the number of diseased vessels, the number of diseased proximal segments, and the global left ventricular function; these three factors alone accounted for 80 percent of the prognostic information.

ANGIOGRAPHIC PROJECTIONS. The major coronary arteries traverse the interventricular and atrioventricular grooves, aligned with the long and short axes of the heart, respectively. Because the heart is oriented obliquely in the thoracic cavity, the coronary circulation is generally visualized in the right anterior oblique (RAO) and left anterior oblique (LAO) projections to furnish true posteroanterior and lateral views of the heart (Figs. 18–7 and 18–8), but these views are limited by vessel foreshortening and superimposition of branches. Simultaneous rotation of the x-ray beam in the sagittal plane provides a better view of the major coronary arteries and their branches. A simple nomenclature has evolved for the description of these sagittal views, which characterizes the relationship between the image intensifier and the patient. Assuming that the x-ray tube is under the patient's table and the image intensifier is over the patient's table, the projection is referred to as the "cranial" view if the image intensifier is tilted toward the head of the patient. The projection is referred to as "caudal" if the image intensifier is tilted down toward the feet of the patient.

It is difficult to predict which angulated views will be most useful for any particular patient because the "optimal" angiographic projection depends largely on body habitus, variation in the coronary anatomy, and location of the lesion. It is recommended that the coronary arteries be visualized in both the LAO and RAO projections using both cranial and caudal angulation.

Left Coronary Artery

CANNULATION. The Judkins left 4.0 coronary catheter is used most often to engage the LCA (Fig. 18–9). If the Judkins left catheter begins to turn out of profile (so that one or both curves of the catheter are no longer visualized en face), it can be rotated clockwise very slightly and advanced slowly to enter the left sinus of Valsalva, permitting the catheter tip to engage the ostium of the LCA. When the ascending aorta is dilated or the aortic arch is unfolded, advancement of the Judkins left 4.0 coronary catheter may result in the formation of an acute secondary angle of the catheter, pointing the tip of the catheter upward, away from the left coronary ostium. Further advancement of the left Judkins catheter in this position should be avoided because the catheter then prolapses upon itself and becomes folded in the ascending aortic arch. In the event this occurs, a guidewire can be temporarily reinserted into the catheter to straighten the secondary bend and permit the catheter to be advanced to the left sinus of Valsalva. If the ascending aorta is significantly dilated, the Judkins left 4.0 catheter should be exchanged for a larger size (e.g., Judkins left 5.0 or 6.0). If the tip of the Judkins left catheter advances beyond the ostium of the LCA without engagement, the primary bend of the catheter can be reshaped within the patient's body by further careful advancement and prompt withdrawal of the catheter, allowing the tip to "pop into" the ostium of the LCA. This maneuver, along with gentle clockwise or counterclockwise rotation, frequently permits selective engagement of the LCA when the initial attempt has failed. If the catheter tip is located below the origin of the LCA, as in the case of a smaller aortic root, a shorter Judkins 3.5 catheter can be used to allow coaxial engagement of the LCA.

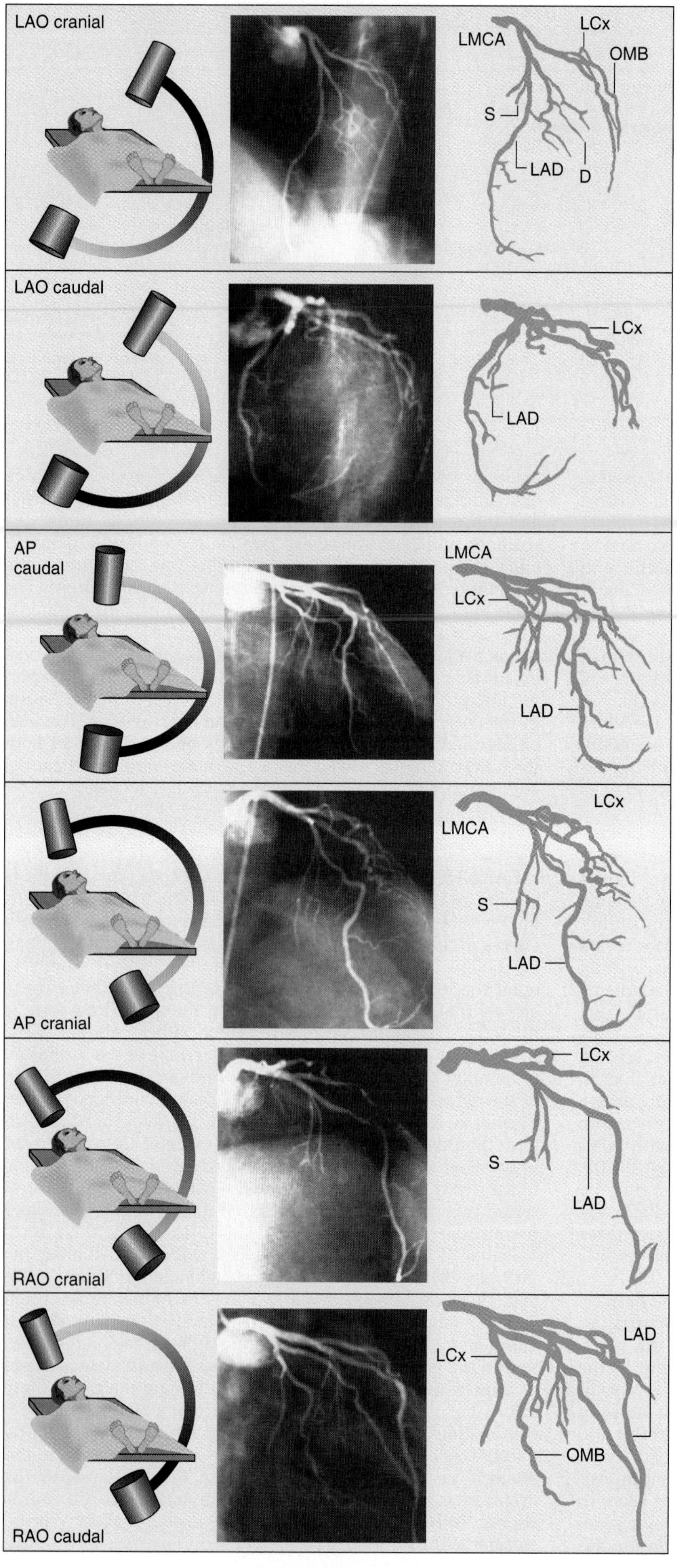

FIGURE 18–7 Angiographic views of the left coronary artery. The approximate positions of the x-ray tube and image intensifier are shown for each of the commonly used angiographic views. The 60-degree left anterior oblique view with 20 degrees of cranial angulation (LAO cranial) shows the ostium and distal portion of the left main coronary artery (LMCA), the middle and distal portions of the left anterior descending artery (LAD), septal perforators (S), diagonal branches (D), and the proximal left circumflex (LCx) and superior obtuse marginal branch (OMB). The 60-degree left anterior oblique view with 25 degrees of caudal angulation (LAO caudal) shows the proximal LMCA and the proximal segments of the LAD and LCx. The anteroposterior projection with 20 degrees of caudal angulation (AP caudal) shows the distal LMCA and proximal segments of the LAD and LCx. The anteroposterior projection with 20 degrees of cranial angulation (AP cranial) also shows the midportion of the LAD and its septal (S) branches. The 30-degree right anterior oblique projection with 20 degrees of cranial angulation (RAO cranial) shows the course of the LAD and its septal (S) and diagonal branches. The 30-degree right anterior oblique projection with 25 degrees of caudal angulation (RAO caudal) shows the LCx and obtuse marginal branches (OMB).

Use of the Amplatz left catheters to cannulate the LCA requires more catheter manipulation than with the standard Judkins left catheter. In this circumstance, the broad secondary curve of the Amplatz left 1 or 2 catheter is positioned so that it rests on the right aortic cusp with its tip pointing toward the left aortic cusp. Alternating advancement and retraction of the catheter with slight clockwise rotation allows the catheter tip to advance slowly and superiorly along the left sinus of Valsalva to enter the left coronary ostium. When the tip enters the ostium, the position of the catheter can usually be stabilized with slight retraction of the catheter. After the left coronary ostium has been cannulated, the pressure at the tip of the catheter should be checked immediately to ensure that there is no damping or "ventricularization" of the pressure contour. If a damped or ventricularized pressure tracing is obtained, the catheter should be removed immediately from the LCA and an attempt at repositioning should be made. If abnormal pressure recording persists, the catheter should be withdrawn from the coronary artery and a nonselective injection of contrast medium into the LCA should be performed in the anteroposterior (AP) view to evaluate the LMCA. If the pressure measured at the catheter tip is normal and a test injection of contrast agent suggests the absence of LMCA disease, left coronary arteriography is then performed using standard techniques. To remove the Amplatz left catheter from the coronary artery, the catheter should be advanced forward in the body to disengage the catheter tip superiorly from the coronary ostium. Simply withdrawing the Amplatz left catheter results in deep seating of the catheter tip within the coronary artery, potentially resulting in catheter-induced arterial dissection.

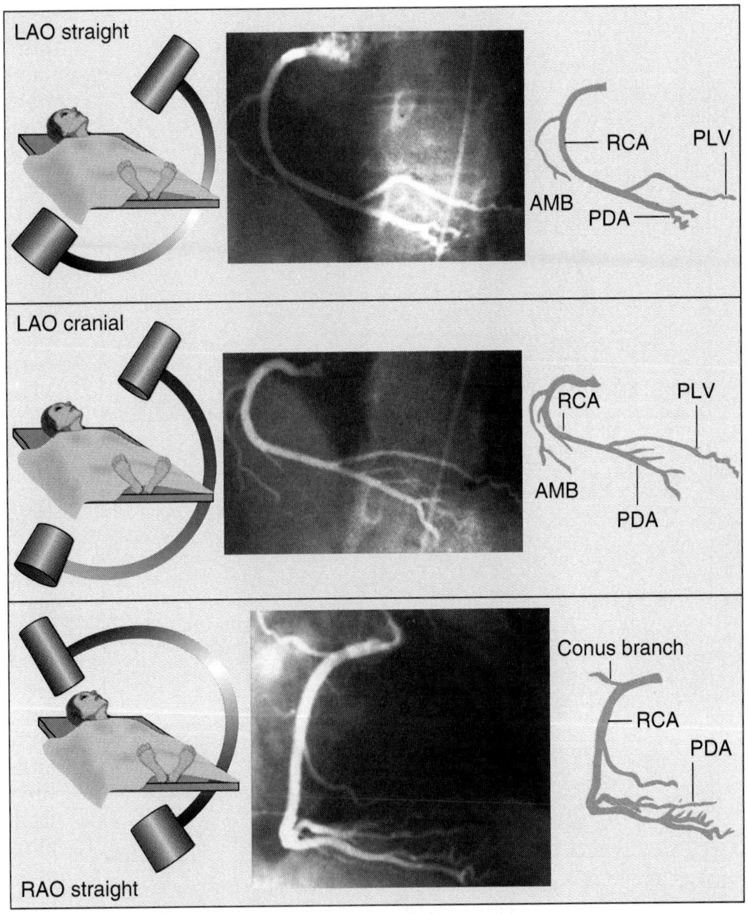

FIGURE 18–8 Angiographic views of the right coronary artery. The approximate positions of the x-ray tube and image intensifier are shown for each of the commonly used angiographic views. The 60-degree left anterior oblique view (LAO straight) shows the proximal and midportions of the right coronary artery (RCA) as well as the acute marginal branches (AMB) and termination of the RCA in the posterior left ventricular branches (PLV). The 60-degree left anterior oblique view with 25 degrees of cranial angulation (LAO cranial) shows the midportion of the RCA and the origin and course of the posterior descending artery (PDA). The 30-degree right anterior oblique view (RAO) shows the midportion of the RCA, the conus branch, and the course of the PDA.

LEFT MAIN CORONARY ARTERY. The LMCA arises from the superior portion of the left aortic sinus, just below the sinotubular ridge of the aorta, which defines the border separating the left sinus of Valsalva from the smooth (tubular) portion of the aorta. The LMCA ranges from 3 to 6 mm in diameter and may be up to 10 to 15 mm in length. The LMCA courses behind the right ventricular outflow tract and usually bifurcates into the LAD artery and LCx branches. Rarely, the LMCA is absent, and there are separate ostia of the LAD and LCx arteries. The LMCA is best visualized in the AP projection with slight (0 to 20 degrees) caudal angulation, but it should be viewed in several projections with the vessel off the spine to exclude LMCA stenosis (Figs. 18–10 to 18–12).

LEFT ANTERIOR DESCENDING ARTERY. The LAD courses along the epicardial surface of the anterior interventricular groove toward the cardiac apex. In the RAO projection, it extends along the anterior aspect of the heart; in the LAO projection, it passes down the cardiac midline, between the right and left ventricles (see Fig. 18–7).

The major branches of the LAD are the septal and diagonal branches. The septal branches arise from the LAD at approximately 90-degree angles and pass into the interventricular septum, varying in size, number, and distribution. In some cases there is a large first septal branch that is vertically oriented and divides into a number of secondary "pitch forking" branches that ramify throughout the septum. In other cases, a more horizontally oriented, large first septal branch is present that passes parallel to the LAD itself within the myocardium. In still other cases, a number of septal arteries are roughly comparable in size. These septal branches interconnect with similar septal branches passing upward from the posterior descending branch of the RCA to produce a network of potential collateral channels. The interventricular septum is the most densely vascularized area of the heart.

The diagonal branches of the LAD pass over the anterolateral aspect of the heart. Although virtually all patients have a single LAD in the anterior interventricular groove, there is wide variability in the number and size of diagonal branches. Most patients (90 percent) have one to three diagonal branches, and acquired atherosclerotic occlusion of the diagonal branches should be suspected if no diagonal branches are seen, particularly if there are unexplained contraction abnormalities of the anterolateral left ventricle. Visualization of the origin of the diagonal branches often requires very steep (50 to 60 degrees) LAO and angulated cranial (20 to 40 degrees) skews.

In some patients, the LMCA trifurcates into the LAD, LCx, and ramus intermedius. When present, the ramus intermedius arises between the LAD and LCx arteries. This vessel is analogous to either a diagonal branch or an obtuse marginal branch, depending on its anterior or posterior course along the lateral aspect of the left ventricle. In most patients (80 percent), the LAD courses around the left ventricular apex and terminates along the diaphragmatic aspect of the left ventricle. In the remaining patients, the LAD fails to reach the diaphragmatic surface, terminating instead either at or before the cardiac apex. In this circumstance, the posterior descending branch (PDA) of the RCA or LCx is larger and longer than usual and supplies the apical portion of the ventricle.

The best angiographic projections for viewing the course of the LAD are the cranially angulated LAO, AP, and RAO views. The LAO cranial view displays the midportion of the LAD and separates the diagonal and septal branches. The RAO cranial view displays the proximal, middle, and distal segment of the LAD and allows separation of the diagonal branches superiorly and the septal branches inferiorly. The AP view requiring cranial (20 to 40 degrees) skew often projects the midportion of the LAD,

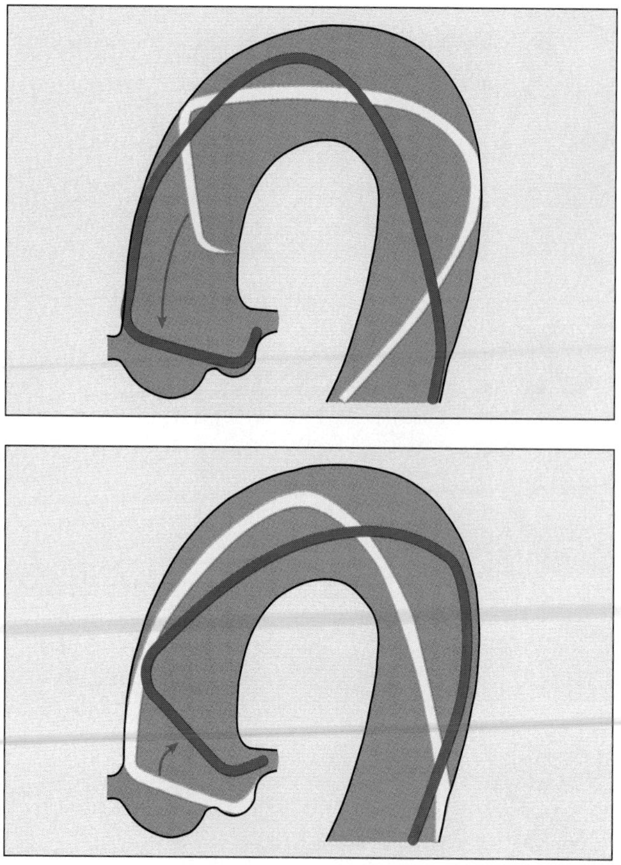

FIGURE 18–9 Push-pull technique for catheterizing the left coronary artery with the Judkins left catheter. In the left anterior oblique view, the coronary catheter is positioned in the ascending aorta over a guidewire and the guidewire is removed. The catheter is advanced so that the tip enters the left sinus of Valsalva. If the catheter does not selectively engage the ostium of the left coronary artery, further slow advancement into the left sinus of Valsalva imparts a temporary acute angle at the catheter. Prompt withdrawal of the catheter allows easy entry into the left coronary artery.

separating the vessel from its diagonal and septal branches. The LAO caudal view also displays the origin of the LAD in a horizontally oriented heart, and the AP caudal or shallow RAO caudal view visualizes the proximal LAD as it arises from the LMCA. The RAO caudal projection is also useful for visualizing the distal LAD and its apical termination.

In some patients with no LMCA but separate ostia for the LAD and LCx, the LAD generally has a more anterior origin than the LCx. The LAD can be engaged with the left Judkins catheter in this setting with paradoxical counterclockwise rotation, which rotates the secondary bend of the catheter to a posterior position in the aorta and turns the primary bend and tip of the catheter to an anterior position. The opposite maneuver may be used to engage the LCx selectively in the setting of separate LAD and LCx ostia. A Judkins catheter, such as a Judkins left 5.0 with a larger curve, selectively engages the downward coursing LCx, and a catheter with shorter curve, such as a Judkins left 3.5, tends to engage selectively the more anterior and superior LAD.

LEFT CIRCUMFLEX ARTERY. The LCx artery originates from the LMCA and courses within the posterior (left) atrioventricular groove toward the inferior interventricular groove (see Fig. 18–7). The LCx artery is the dominant vessel in 15 percent of patients, supplying the left PDA from the distal continuation of the LCx. In the remaining vessels, the distal LCx varies in size and length, depending on the number of posterolateral branches supplied by the distal RCA. The LCx usually gives off one to three large obtuse marginal branches as it passes down the atrioventricular groove. These are the principal branches of the LCx because they supply the lateral free wall of the left ventricle. Beyond the origins of the obtuse marginal branches, the distal LCx tends to be small. The actual position of the LCx can be determined on the late phase of a left coronary injection when the coronary sinus becomes opacified with diluted contrast material.

The RAO caudal and LAO caudal projections are best for visualizing the proximal and middle LCx and obtuse marginal branches. The AP (or 5- to 15-degree RAO) caudal projections also show the origins of the obtuse marginal branches. More severe rightward angulation often superimposes the origins of the obtuse marginal branches on the LCx. If the LCA is dominant, the optimal projection for the left PDA is the LAO cranial view. The LCx also gives rise to one or two left atrial circumflex branches. These branches supply the lateral and posterior aspects of the left atrium.

Right Coronary Artery

Cannulation of the origin of the RCA is also performed in the LAO position but requires different maneuvers than cannulation of the LCA. Whereas the left Judkins catheter naturally seeks the ostium of the LCA, the right Judkins or modified Amplatz catheters must be rotated to engage the vessel. This is usually accomplished by first passing the catheter to a point just superior to the aortic valve in the left sinus of Valsalva with the tip of the catheter facing rightward and then rotating the catheter clockwise while withdrawing the catheter slightly, which forces the tip to move anteriorly from the left sinus of Valsalva to the right sinus of Valsalva along the sinotubular ridge (Fig. 18–13). Sudden rightward and downward movement of the catheter tip signifies the entry into the right coronary ostium. If the ostium of the RCA is not easily located, the most common reason is that the ostium has a more superior and anterior origin than anticipated. Repeated attempts to engage the RCA should be made at a level slightly more distal to the aortic valve. Nonselective contrast agent injections in the right sinus of Valsalva may reveal the site of the origin of the RCA. Positioning a left Amplatz catheter in the ostium of the RCA requires a technique similar to that used with the right Judkins catheter. If a gentle attempt to withdraw the Amplatz catheter results in paradoxical deep entry into the coronary artery, removal of the catheter can be achieved by clockwise or counterclockwise rotation and advancement to prolapse the catheter into the aortic sinus.

An abnormal pressure tracing showing damping or ventricularization may suggest the presence of an ostial stenosis or spasm, selective engagement of the conus branch, or deep intubation of the RCA. If an abnormal pressure tracing has been encountered, the catheter tip should be gently rotated counterclockwise and withdrawn slightly in an effort to free the tip of the catheter. If persistent damping occurs, a very small amount of contrast medium (<1 ml) can be injected carefully and the catheter immediately withdrawn in a "shoot-and-run" maneuver, which may allow the cause of damping to be identified. The frequency of ventricular fibrillation and iatrogenic coronary dissection are higher when the RCA is injected in the presence of a damped pressure tracing. If the pressure tracing is normal on entry into the RCA, the vessel should be imaged in at least two projections. The initial injection should be gentle because of the possibility that forceful injection through a catheter whose tip is immediately adjacent to the vessel wall may also lead to dissection. Coronary spasm of the RCA ostium may also occur as a result of catheter intubation. When an ostial stenosis of the RCA is seen, intracoronary nitroglycerin or calcium channel antagonists may be useful in excluding catheter-induced spasm as a cause of the coronary artery narrowing.

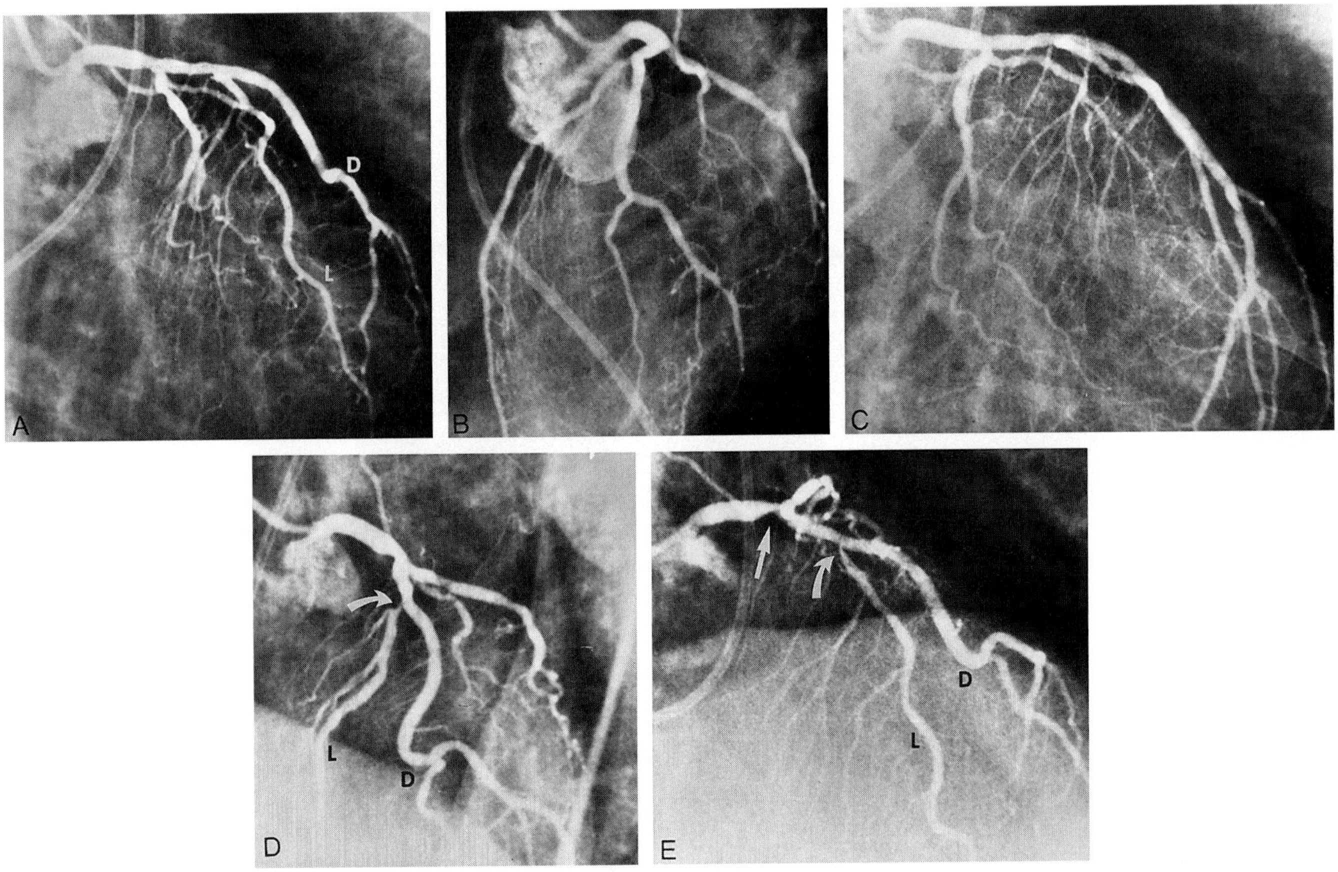

FIGURE 18–10 Missed left main coronary artery (LMCA) stenosis. **A** to **C,** Left coronary arteriography in the standard right anterior oblique, left anterior oblique, and right anterior oblique caudal views fails to demonstrate significant stenoses of the LMCA or left anterior descending (LAD) artery. **D,** Left anterior oblique cranial view shows severe stenosis (curved arrow) for the LAD (L) immediately beyond the origin of the diagonal branch. **E,** Right anterior oblique cranial view shows the LAD stenosis (curved arrow) but also shows a severe stenosis of the LMCA (straight arrow) at its bifurcation.

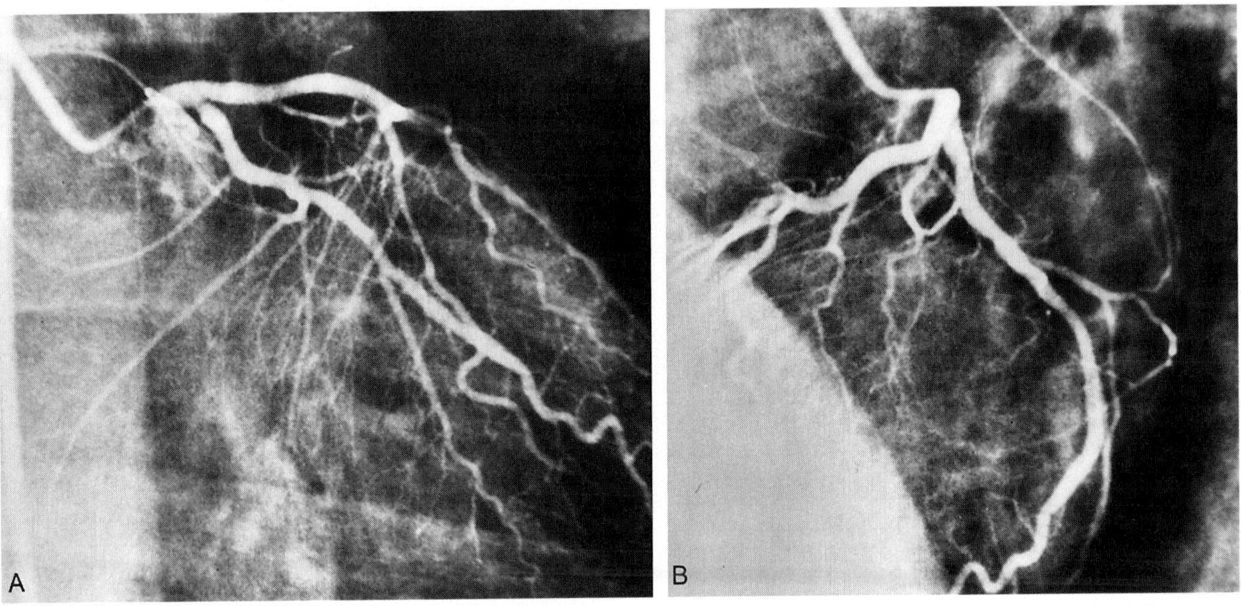

FIGURE 18–11 Difficulty in detecting ostial left main coronary artery (LMCA) stenosis. **A,** Shallow right anterior oblique view of the left anterior descending artery with the catheter not well seated in the vessel results in poor visualization of the ostial stenosis of the LMCA. **B,** Left anterior oblique cranial view shows the catheter tip selectively positioned in the LMCA without reflux of contrast medium around the tip.

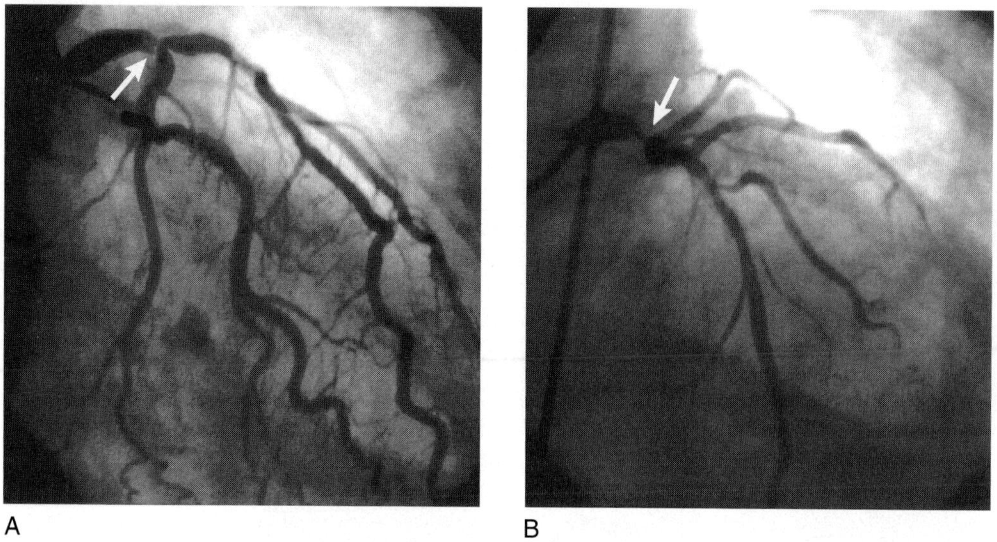

FIGURE 18–12 Severe stenosis of the distal left main coronary artery. **A,** Right anterior oblique projection with caudal angulation demonstrates a severe ulcerated stenosis in the distal portion of the left main coronary artery (arrow). **B,** An anteroposterior view with cranial angulation demonstrates this stenosis in a second view. Limited coronary arteriography should be performed when severe left main stenosis (arrow) has been demonstrated.

The RCA originates from the right anterior aortic sinus somewhat inferior to the origin of the LCA (see Fig. 18–8). It passes along the right atrioventricular groove toward the crux (a point on the diaphragmatic surface of the heart where the anterior atrioventricular, the posterior atrioventricular groove, and the inferior interventricular groove coalesce. The first branch of the RCA is generally the conus artery, which arises at the right coronary ostium or within the first few millimeters of the RCA in about 50 percent of patients. In the remaining patients, the conus artery arises from a separate ostium in the right aortic sinus just above the right coronary ostium. The second branch of the RCA is usually the sinoatrial node artery. It has been found that this vessel arises from the RCA in just under 60 percent of patients, from the LCx in just under 40 percent, and from both arteries with a dual blood supply in the remaining cases. The midportion of the RCA usually gives rise to one or several medium-sized acute marginal branches. These branches supply the anterior wall of the right ventricle and may provide collateral circulation in patients with LAD occlusion. The RCA terminates in a PDA and one or more right posterolateral branches.

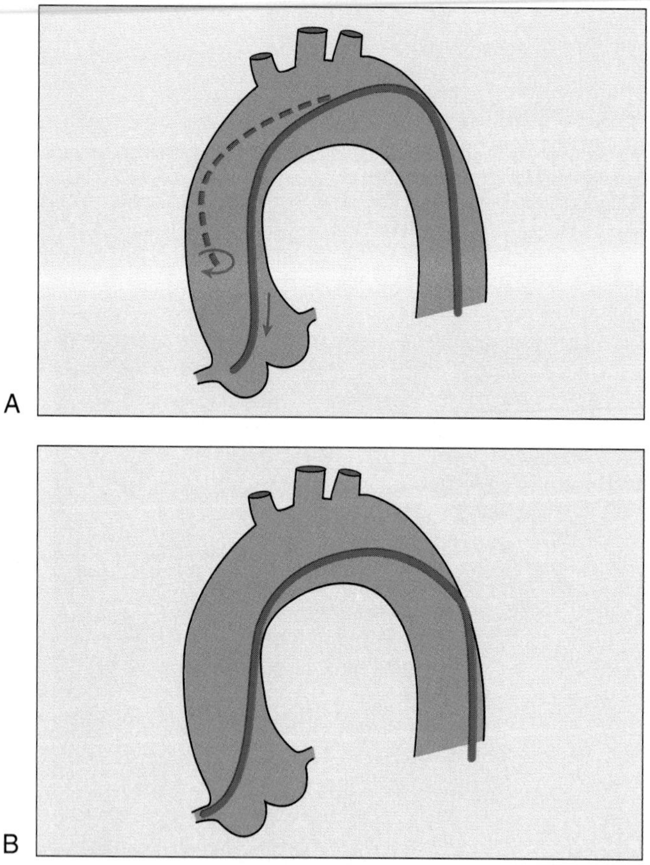

FIGURE 18–13 Cannulation of the right coronary artery using the right Judkins catheter. **A,** The catheter is advanced to a point just superior to the aortic valve in the left sinus of Valsalva with the tip of the catheter facing rightward, and then the catheter is rotated clockwise while withdrawing the catheter slightly. **B,** Sudden rightward and downward movement of the catheter tip signifies the entry into the right coronary ostium.

Because the RCA traverses both the atrioventricular and the interventricular grooves, multiple angiographic projections are needed to visualize each segment of the RCA. The ostium of the RCA is best evaluated in the LAO views, with or without cranial or caudal angulation. The left lateral is also useful for visualizing the ostium of the RCA in difficult cases. The ostium is identified by the reflux of contrast material from the RCA that also delineates the aortic root with swirling of contrast in the region of the ostium. The proximal RCA is generally evaluated in the LAO cranial or LAO caudal projections but is markedly foreshortened in the RAO projections. The midportion of the RCA is best seen in the LAO cranial, RAO, and left lateral projections. The origin of the PDA and the posterolateral branches are best evaluated in the LAO cranial or AP cranial views, whereas the midportion of the PDA can be shown in the AP cranial or RAO projection.

RIGHT CORONARY ARTERY DOMINANCE. The RCA is dominant in 85 percent of patients, supplying the PDA and at least one posterolateral branch (right dominant) (Figs. 18–14 to 18–16). The PDA courses in the inferior interventricular groove and gives rise to a number of small inferior septal branches, which pass upward to supply the lower portion of the interventricular septum and interdigitate with superior septal branches passing down from the LAD. After giving rise to the PDA, the dominant RCA continues beyond the crux cordis (the junction of the atrioventricular and interventricular grooves) as the right posterior atrioventricular branch along the distal portion of the posterior (left) atrioventricular groove, terminating in one or several posterolateral branches that supply the diaphragmatic surface of the left ventricle. The RCA is nondominant in 15 percent of patients. One-half of these patients have a left PDA and left posterolateral branches that are provided by the distal LCx artery (left dominant circulation). In these cases, the RCA is very small, terminates before reaching the crux, and does not supply any blood to the left ventricular myocardium. The remaining patients have an RCA that gives rise to the PDA with the LCx artery providing all the posterolateral branches (balanced or codominant circulation). In about 25 percent of patients with RCA dominance, there are significant anatomical variations in the origin of the PDA. These variations include partial supply of the PDA territory by acute marginal branches, double PDA, and early origin of the PDA proximal to the crux. At or near the crux, the dominant artery gives rise to a small atrioventricular node artery, which passes upward to supply the atrioventricular node.

CORONARY BYPASS GRAFTS. Selective cannulation of bypass grafts may be more challenging than cannulation of

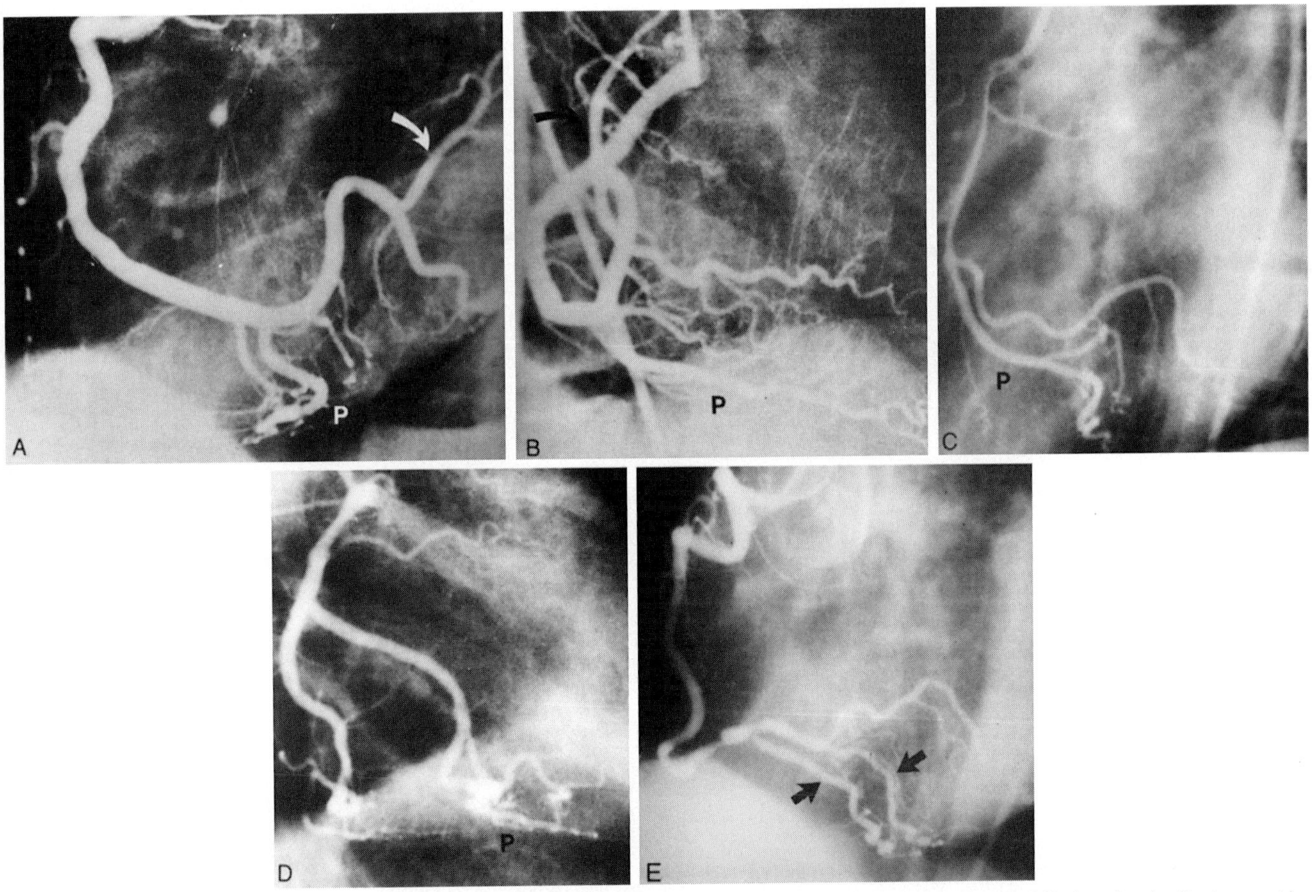

FIGURE 18–14 Strongly dominant right coronary artery (RCA). **A** and **B,** Left anterior oblique and right anterior oblique views of the RCA show that the distal segment (arrows) extends to the left atrioventricular groove. After giving rise to the posterior descending artery, the RCA gives rise to multiple posterior left ventricular branches. **C,** A variation in the origin of the posterior descending artery, which originates early from the RCA, runs parallel to it, and enters the posterior interventricular groove. **D,** Right anterior oblique right coronary arteriogram showing the posterior descending artery (P) arising from a right ventricular branch of the RCA. **E,** Left anterior oblique right coronary arteriogram showing duplicated posterior descending arteries (arrows). (From Levin DC, Baltaxe HA: Angiographic demonstration of important anatomic variations of the posterior descending artery. AJR 116:41, 1972.)

the native coronary arteries because the locations of graft ostia are more variable, even when surgical clips or ostia markers are used. Knowledge of the number, course, and type of bypass grafts obtained from the operative report is invaluable for the identification of the location of the bypass grafts during arteriography.

SAPHENOUS VEIN GRAFTS. SVGs from the aorta to the distal RCA or PDA originate from the right anterolateral aspect of the aorta approximately 5 cm superior to the sinotubular ridge. SVGs to the LAD originate from the anterior portion of the aorta about 7 cm superior to the sinotubular ridge. SVGs to the obtuse marginal branches arise from the left anterolateral aspect of the aorta 9 to 10 cm superior to the sinotubular ridge. In most patients, all SVGs can be engaged with a single catheter, such as a Judkins right 4.0 or a modified Amplatz right 1 or 2. Other catheters useful for engaging SVGs include the right and left bypass graft catheters. Amplatz left 1 to 2 catheters are useful for superiorly oriented SVGs (see Fig. 18–4). A multipurpose catheter may also be useful for the cannulation of the downward takeoff SVG to the RCA or PDA.

Viewed in the LAO projection, the Judkins right 4 or Amplatz right 2 catheters rotate anteriorly from the leftward position as the catheter is rotated in a clockwise direction. The relation between the movement of catheter shaft at the femoral artery and the response of catheter tip on fluoroscopy immediately indicates whether the catheter tip is anteriorly positioned in the aorta and likely to enter an SVG ostium or posteriorly positioned and unlikely to engage an SVG. Steady advancement and withdrawal of the catheter tip proximal and distal in the ascending aorta, 5 to 10 cm above the sinotubular ridge, with varying degrees of rotation, usually result in entry into the SVG. Entry into the SVG is associated with abrupt outward motion of the tip of the catheter. When this occurs, a small test injection of contrast material verifies that the catheter is in the SVG. A well-circumscribed "stump" is almost always present if the SVG is occluded. Each SVG or stump must be viewed in nearly orthogonal views. The relation between the origin of the SVGs and surgical clips confirms whether all targeted SVGs have been visualized. If neither a patent SVG nor a stump can be located, it may be necessary to perform an ascending aortogram (preferably in biplane) in an attempt to visualize all SVGs and their course to the coronary arteries.

The goal of SVG angiography is to assess the ostium of the SVG, its entire course, and the distal insertion ("touchdown") site at the anastomosis between the bypass SVG and the native coronary vessel. The ostium of a SVG must be evaluated by achieving a coaxial engagement of the catheter tip and the origin of the SVG. The midportion (body) of the SVG must be evaluated with complete contrast filling of the SVG because inadequate opacification produces an angiographic artifact suggestive of friable filling defects. It is critical to assess the SVG insertion or anastomotic site in full profile without any overlap of the distal SVG or the native vessel. Angiographic assessment of the native vessels beyond SVG

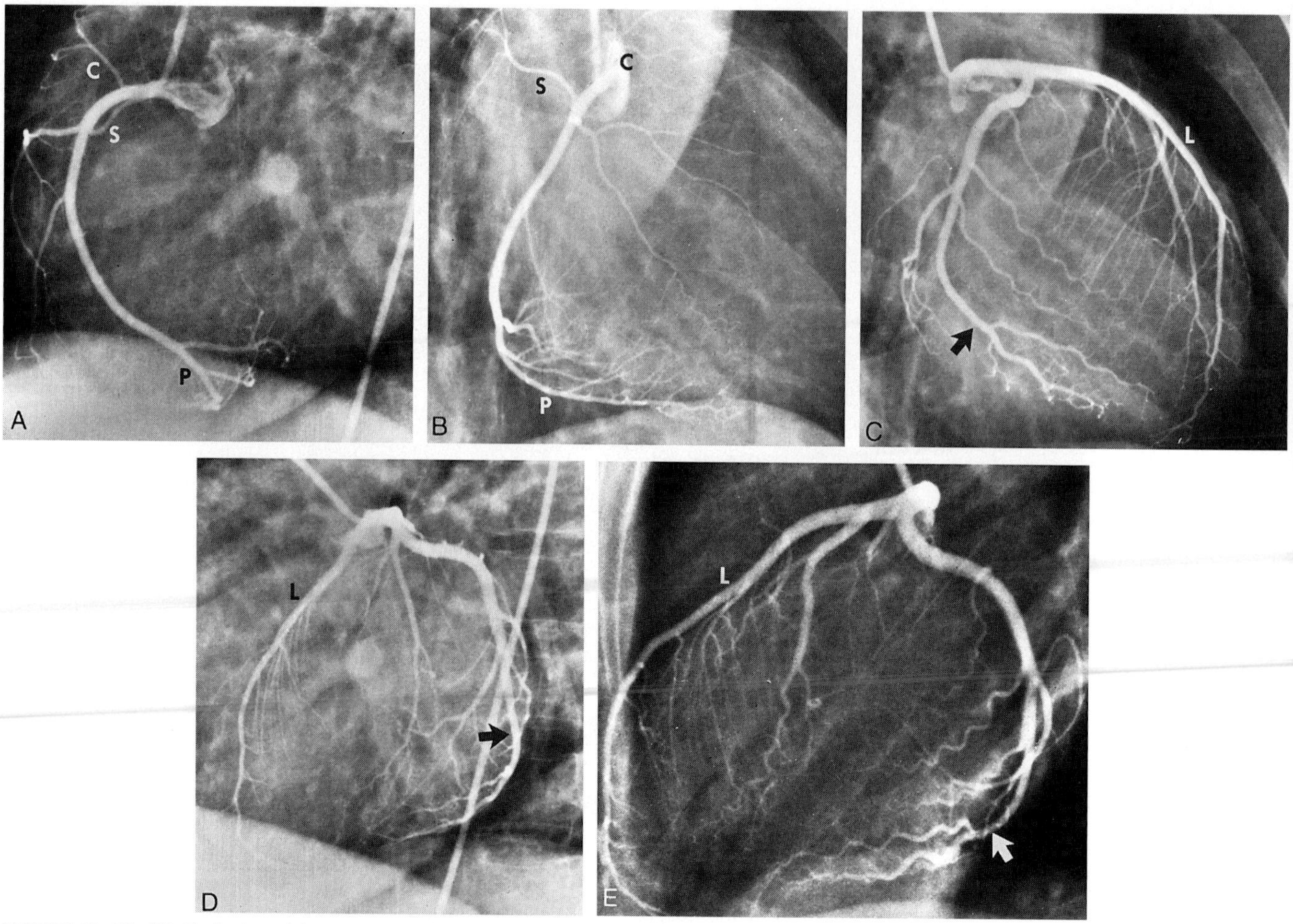

FIGURE 18–15 Weakly dominant right coronary artery (RCA). **A** and **B,** Left anterior oblique and right anterior oblique views of the RCA. Both the conus and sinoatrial node artery arise from the RCA. The distal portion of the RCA beyond the origin of the posterior descending artery is short and gives rise to a single small posterior left ventricular branch. **C** to **E,** Left coronary artery in the right anterior oblique, left anterior oblique, and left lateral projections. Note that the circumflex artery gives rise to four obtuse marginal branches, the most distal of which (arrow) supplies some of the diaphragmatic surface of the left ventricle. The left anterior descending artery gives rise to two small and one medium-sized diagonal branches. C = conus branch; L = left anterior descending artery; P = posterior descending artery; S = sinoatrial nodal artery.

anastomotic sites requires views that are conventionally used for the native segments themselves.

INTERNAL MAMMARY ARTERY. The left IMA arises inferiorly from the left subclavian artery approximately 10 cm from its origin. Catheterization of the left IMA is performed with a specially designed J-tip IMA catheter (see Fig. 18–3, bottom row). The catheter is advanced into the aortic arch distal to the origin of the left subclavian artery in the LAO projection and then rotated counterclockwise and is gently withdrawn with the tip pointing in a cranial direction, allowing entry into the left subclavian artery (Fig. 18–17). A 0.035 J or angled Terumo guidewire is advanced to the left subclavian artery under fluoroscopy, and the catheter is advanced into the subclavian artery. The RAO or AP projections then can be used to cannulate the IMA selectively by withdrawing and slightly rotating the catheter anteriorly (counterclockwise) with tip down. The right IMA can also be cannulated with the IMA catheter. The innominate artery is entered in the LAO projection, and the guidewire is advanced cautiously to avoid entry into the right common carotid artery. When the guidewire is positioned in the distal right subclavian artery, the IMA catheter is advanced to a point distal to the expected origin of the right IMA. The catheter is withdrawn in the LAO view and rotated to cannulate the right IMA.

The IMA itself is rarely affected by atherosclerosis. Angiographic studies of the IMAs should assess not only the patency of the graft itself but also the distal anastomosis, where most IMA graft compromise occurs. Although the LAO cranial view may be limited in its ability to demonstrate the anastomosis of the IMA and the LAD because of vessel overlap, the left lateral or AP cranial projection usually provides adequate visualization of the LIMA-LAD anastomotic site. The risk of catheter-induced dissection of the origin of the IMA can be reduced by careful manipulation of the catheter tip and avoidance of forceful advancement without the protection of the guidewire. If the IMA cannot be selectively engaged because of tortuosity of the subclavian artery, nonselective arteriography can be enhanced by placing a blood pressure cuff on the ipsilateral arm and inflating it to a pressure above systolic arterial pressure. Alternatively, the ipsilateral brachial or radial artery may be used to facilitate coaxial IMA engagement. IMA spasm can be treated with 50 to 200 μg of intraarterial nitroglycerin or 50 to 100 μg of intraarterial verapamil. The patient may feel chest warmth or discomfort with contrast injection due to injection into small IMA branches supplying the chest wall.

GASTROEPIPLOIC ARTERY. The right gastroepiploic artery (GEA) is the largest terminal artery of the gastroduodenal artery and was briefly used as an alternative in situ

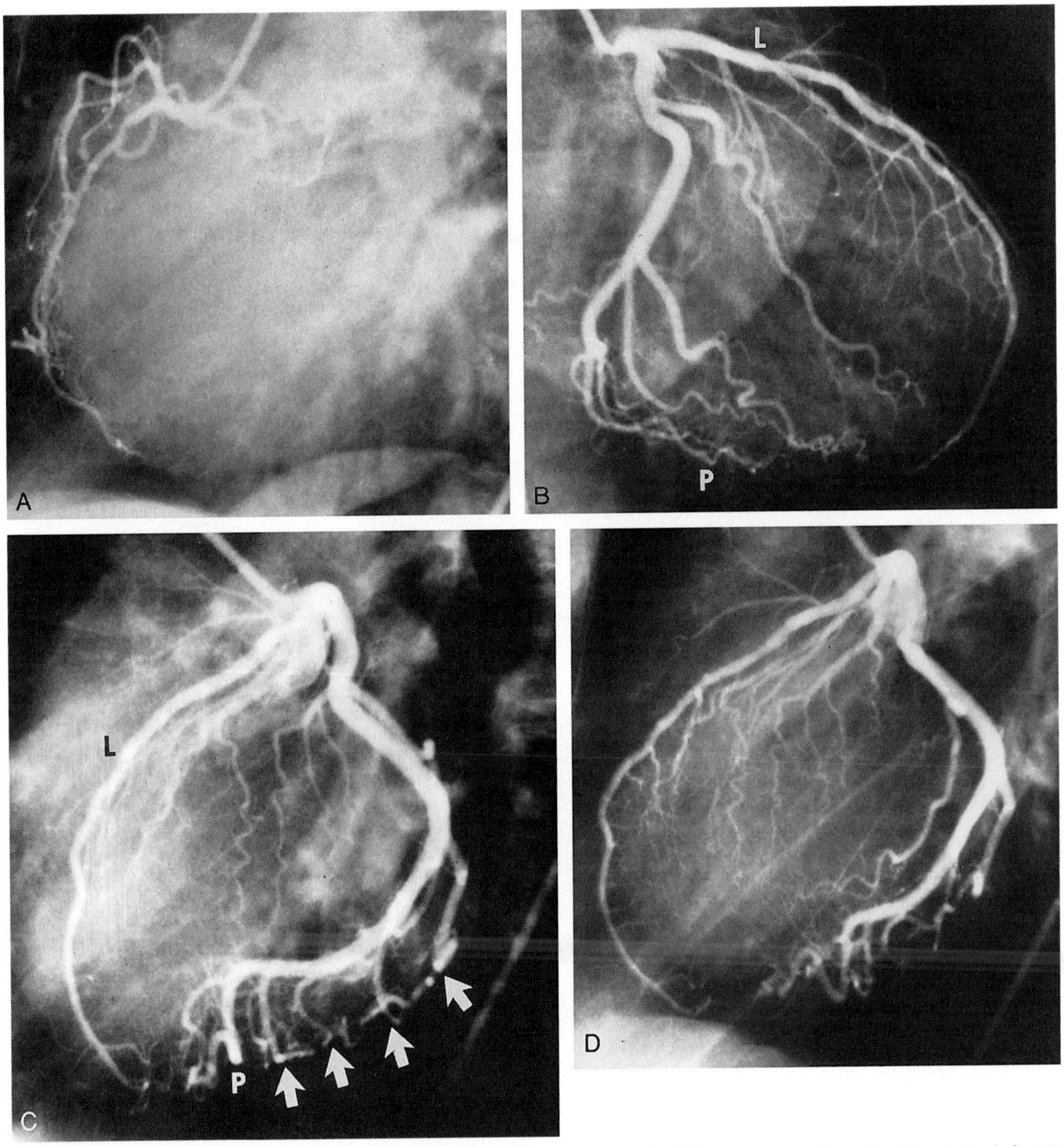

FIGURE 18–16 Dominant left coronary system. **A,** The left anterior oblique projection shows that the right coronary artery is small and terminates before reaching the crux. **B** to **D,** The right anterior oblique, left anterior oblique, and left lateral projections show that the left circumflex artery is large and gives rise to the posterior descending artery (PDA) at the crux of the heart and to several posterior descending arteries. L = left anterior descending coronary artery; P = posterior descending artery.

arterial conduit to the PDA in patients undergoing CABG. The gastroduodenal artery arises from the common hepatic artery in 75 percent of cases, but it may also arise from the right or left hepatic artery or the celiac trunk. Catheterization of the right GEA is carried out by first entering the common hepatic artery with a cobra catheter (Fig. 18–18). A torquable, hydrophilic-coated guidewire is advanced to the gastroduodenal artery and then to the right GEA. The cobra catheter is then exchanged for a multipurpose or Judkins right coronary catheter, which then permits selective arteriography of the right GEA.

STANDARDIZED PROJECTION ACQUISITION. Although general recommendations can be made for sequences of angiographic image acquisition that are applicable to most patients, tailored views may be needed to accommodate individual variations in anatomy. As a general rule, each coronary artery should be visualized with a number of different projections that minimize vessel foreshortening and overlap (Figs. 18–19 to 18–21). An AP view with shallow caudal angulation is often performed first to evaluate the possibility of LMCA disease. Other important views include (1) the LAO cranial view used to evaluate the middle and distal LAD, which should have sufficient leftward positioning of the image intensifier to allow separation of the LAD, diagonal, and septal branches; (2) the LAO caudal view to evaluate the LMCA, origin of the LAD, and proximal segment of the LCx; (3) the RAO caudal view to assess the LCx and marginal branches; and (4) a shallow RAO or AP cranial view to evaluate the midportion and distal portion of the LAD. The RCA should be visualized in at least two views, including an LAO cranial view that demonstrates the RCA and origin of the PDA and posterolateral branches and an RAO view that demonstrates the mid-RCA and proximal, middle, and distal termination of the PDA. An AP cranial projection may also be useful for the demonstration of the distal termination of the RCA, and a left lateral view is useful to visual the ostium of the RCA and midportion of the RCA with separation of the RCA and its right ventricular branches.

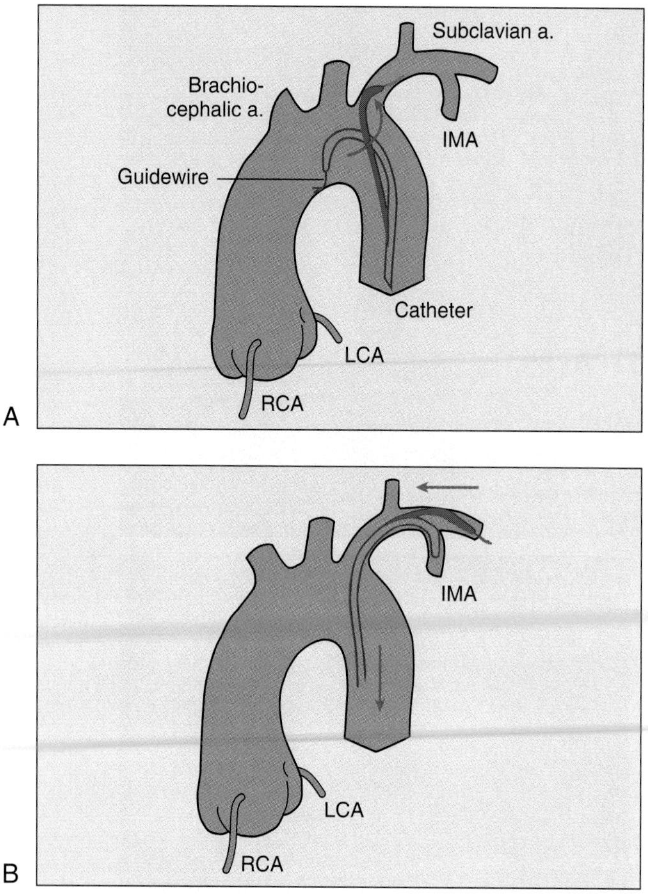

FIGURE 18–17 Catheterization of the left internal mammary artery (IMA). The internal mammary catheter is positioned in the aortic arch and visualized in the left anterior oblique position. The catheter tip is rotated so that it engages the origin of the left subclavian artery immediately subjacent to the head of the clavicle **(A)**. This is followed by gentle advancement of the guidewire into the left subclavian artery to a point distal to the origin of the left internal mammary artery. After the guidewire is removed, the left subclavian artery is visualized in the right anterior oblique projection, the catheter is withdrawn, and the catheter tip engages the ostium of the left internal mammary artery selectively **(B)**. (From Judkins MW: Coronary arteriography. *In* Douglas JS Jr, King SB III [eds]: Coronary Arteriography and Intervention. New York, McGraw-Hill, 1985, p 231.)

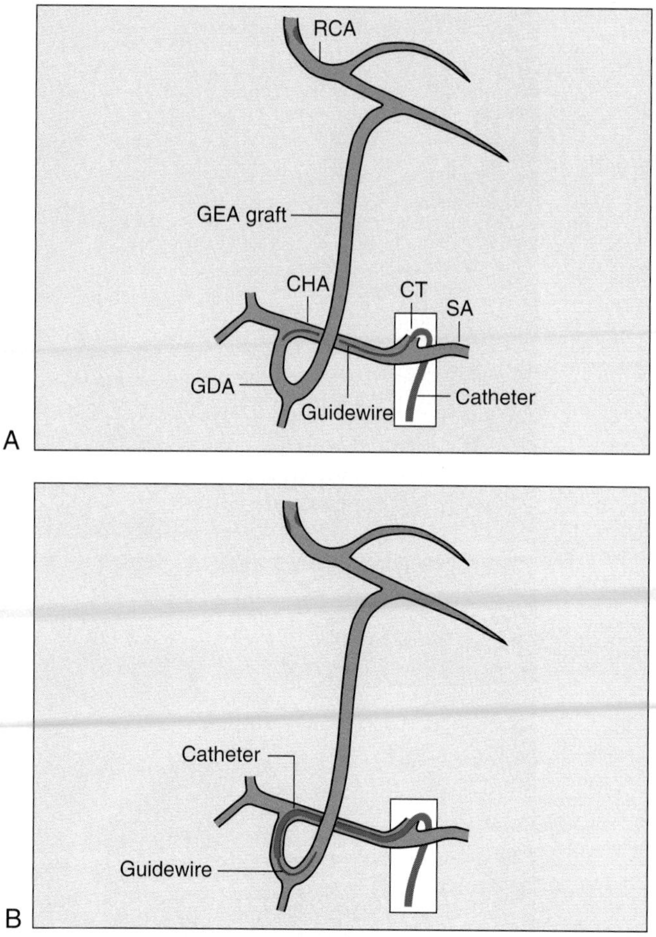

FIGURE 18–18 Catheterization of the right gastroepiploic artery (GEA) graft. The celiac trunk (CT) is selectively engaged with a cobra catheter, and a guidewire is gently advanced to the gastroduodenal artery (GDA) and the GEA. The catheter is advanced over the guidewire for selective arteriography of the GEA graft. CHA = common hepatic artery; RCA = right coronary artery; SA = splenic artery.

Congenital Anomalies of the Coronary Circulation

Anomalous origins of the coronary arteries are present in approximately 0.5 percent of patients undergoing coronary arteriography.[52] The most common anomaly is a separate origin of the LAD and LCx coronary arteries (35.3 percent), followed by an origin of the RCA from the left coronary sinus (20.6 percent) and origin of the LCx from the right coronary sinus (20 percent). A single coronary artery was seen in fewer cases (8.8 percent).[52] Other anomalies occurred much less commonly. Coronary artery anomalies are divided into those that cause and those that do not cause myocardial ischemia.[53,54]

ANOMALIES THAT CAUSE MYOCARDIAL ISCHEMIA

CORONARY ARTERY FISTULAS. Coronary artery fistulas are a common hemodynamically significant abnormality of the coronary arteries.[55] Although half of the patients with a coronary artery fistula remain asymptomatic, the other half develop CHF, infective endocarditis, myocardial ischemia, or rupture of an aneurysm. Fistulas arise from the RCA or its branches in about half of the cases; the remaining fistulas arise from the LAD or LCx arteries or their branches, or they have multiple origins (Fig. 18–22). Drainage occurs into the right ventricle in 41 percent, right atrium in 26 percent, pulmonary artery in 17 percent, left ventricle in 3 percent, and superior vena cava in 1 percent. A left-to-right shunt exists in more than 90 percent. Coronary arteriography is the best method for demonstrating the origin of these fistulas.

ORIGIN OF THE LEFT CORONARY ARTERY FROM THE PULMONARY ARTERY. Most infants with the origin of the LCA from the main pulmonary artery manifest CHF and myocardial ischemia in the first 4 months of life.[56] About 25 percent survive to adolescence or adulthood but develop mitral regurgitation, angina, or CHF. Aortography typically shows a large RCA with absence of a left coronary ostium in the left aortic sinus. During the late phase of the aortogram, patulous LAD and LCx branches fill by means of collateral circulation from RCA branches. Still later in the filming sequence, retrograde flow from the LAD and LCx opacifies the LMCA and its origin from the main pulmonary artery (Fig. 18–23). The clinical course of the patient tends to be more favorable if extensive collateral circulation exists. In rare instances, the RCA rather than the LCA may arise from the pulmonary artery.

CONGENITAL CORONARY STENOSIS OR ATRESIA. Congenital stenosis or atresia of a coronary artery can occur as an isolated lesion or in association with other congenital diseases, such as calcific coronary sclerosis, supravalvular aortic stenosis, homocystinuria, Friedreich ataxia, Hurler syndrome, progeria, and rubella syndrome. In these cases, the atretic vessel usually fills by means of collateral circulation from the contralateral side.[57]

ANOMALOUS ORIGIN OF EITHER CORONARY ARTERY FROM THE CONTRALATERAL SINUS. Origin of the LCA from the proximal RCA or the right aortic sinus with subsequent passage between the aorta and the right ventricular outflow tract has been associated with

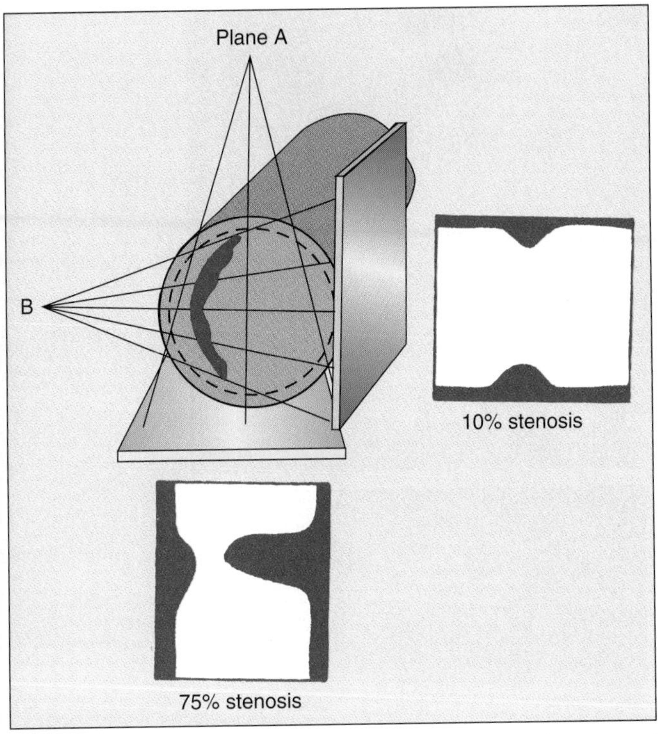

FIGURE 18–19 Importance of orthogonal projections. Each vascular segment of the coronary artery must be recorded in two orthogonal or nearly orthogonal views to avoid missing important diagnostic information about eccentric stenoses. In plane A the image is associated with 75 percent stenosis, but in plane B the image results in 10 percent stenosis.

sudden death during or shortly after exercise in young persons (see Fig. 18–23).[58-60] The increased risk of sudden death may be due to a slit-like ostium with acute takeoff angles of the aberrant coronary arteries or possible compression between the pulmonary trunk and aorta. After its aberrant origin, the LCA takes an abrupt leftward turn and tunnels between the aorta and the right ventricular outflow tract. Sudden death is thought to result from transient occlusion of the anomalous LCA, caused by an increase in blood flow through the aorta and pulmonary artery that occurs during exercise and creates either a kink at the sharp leftward bend or a pinchcock mechanism in the tunnel. Origin of the RCA from the LCA or left aortic sinus with passage between the aorta and the right ventricular outflow tract is somewhat less dangerous (Figs. 18–24 and 18–25).[61-63] This anomaly, however, has also been associated with myocardial ischemia or sudden death, presumably through the same mechanism. In rare cases of anomalous origin of the LCA from the right aortic sinus, myocardial ischemia may occur even if the LCA passes anterior to the right ventricular outflow tract or posterior to the aorta (i.e., not through a tunnel between the two great vessels).

The course of the anomalous coronary arteries is easily assessed by angiography in the RAO view (Fig. 18–26). The four common courses for the anomalous LCA arising from the right sinus of Valsalva include a septal, anterior, interarterial, or posterior course.[64,65] The posterior course of the anomalous LCA arising from the left sinus of Valsalva is similar to the course of the anomalous LCx arising from the right sinus of Valsalva (Fig. 18–27), whereas the common interarterial course of the anomalous RCA from the left sinus of Valsalva is similar to the interarterial course of the anomalous LCA arising from the right sinus of Valsalva.

When either the LCA or the LAD arises anomalously from the right aortic sinus, another angiographic method to identify the course of the anomalous vessel is to pass a catheter into the main pulmonary artery and then perform an arteriogram of the aberrant coronary artery in the steep AP caudal projection. This places the aberrant coronary artery, the rightward and anterior pulmonary valve, and the leftward and posterior aortic valve all in one plane (see Fig. 18–27). From this "laid-back" aortogram, which can be used even in mapping the course of anomalous coronary arteries in transposition of the great vessels, it is usually possible to confirm whether the course of the aberrant coronary artery is between the great vessels. Although angiography is useful for establishing the presence of anomalous coronary arteries, transesophageal echocardiography may also be an important adjunctive diagnostic tool for establishing the course of the vessels.

SINGLE CORONARY ARTERY. Although there are numerous variations of this anomaly, it assumes hemodynamic significance when a major branch passes between the aorta and the right ventricular outflow tract.[66]

ANOMALIES NOT CAUSING MYOCARDIAL ISCHEMIA

In this category of anomalies, the coronary arteries originate from the aorta, but their origins are in unusual locations. Although myocardial perfusion is normal, cannulation of the origin of these vessels may be problematic. These anomalies occur in about 0.5 to 1.0 percent of adult patients undergoing coronary arteriography.

ORIGIN OF THE LEFT CIRCUMFLEX ARTERY FROM THE RIGHT AORTIC SINUS. Anomalous origin of the circumflex artery from the right aortic sinus is the most common of these anomalies (see Fig. 18–27). In a series of nearly 3000 patients, this anomaly was found in 0.67 percent. The anomalous LCx generally arises posterior to the RCA and courses inferiorly and posteriorly to the aorta to enter the left atrioventricular groove. An interarterial course for an anomalous LCx originating from the right sinus of Valsalva is extremely uncommon.

HIGH ANTERIOR ORIGIN OF THE RIGHT CORONARY ARTERY. This anomaly is commonly encountered but of no hemodynamic significance. The inability to engage the ostium of the RCA selectively by conventional catheter manipulation raises the question of this superior origin of the RCA above the sinotubular ridge. Forceful, nonselective injection of contrast medium into the right sinus of Valsalva may reveal the anomalous takeoff of the RCA, which can then be selectively engaged with a Judkins right 5.0 catheter or Amplatz left 1.0 or 2.0 catheter.

Coronary Artery Spasm (see also Chap. 50)

Coronary artery spasm is defined as a dynamic and reversible occlusion of an epicardial coronary artery because of focal constriction of the smooth muscle cells within the arterial wall.[67] It was first described as a clinical syndrome in 1959 by Prinzmetal and colleagues ("Prinzmetal" or "variant" angina), who described an unusual or variant form of angina in which the onset of chest pain was not provoked by the usual factors, such as exercise, emotional upset, cold, or ingestion of a meal. Patients considered to have variant angina are those in whom chest pain commences at rest or both at rest and during exertion, occurs in a cyclical pattern at the same time every day, and is accompanied by ST segment elevation if an ECG is recorded. Coronary artery spasm can be invoked by cigarette smoking, cocaine use, alcohol, intracoronary radiation, and administration of catecholamines during general anesthesia. Although the ST segment elevation is often striking, it rapidly reverts to normal when the pain disappears spontaneously or is terminated by the administration of nitroglycerin. Coronary artery spasm may be accompanied by atrioventricular block, ventricular ectopic activity, ventricular tachycardia, or ventricular fibrillation. MI and death are rare manifestations of coronary artery spasm. Coronary artery spasm can be superimposed on the presence of an intramyocardial bridge.[68]

Coronary arteriography is useful in patients with suspected coronary artery spasm, both to exclude the presence of concomitant CAD and to document an episode of coronary artery spasm using provocative intravenous medications. Angiographic studies have shown that coronary spasm is superimposed on areas of fixed stenosis in about 60 percent of patients, and it occurs in segments of coronary arteries that appear angiographically normal in about 40 percent of patients. MI in the presence of normal epicardial coronary arteries is often attributed to the presence of coronary artery spasm, but other conditions such as cocaine abuse, coronary embolism, hypercoagulable states, coronary trauma, and anemia must first be excluded.

Three provocative tests can be performed to detect the presence of coronary artery spasm. Intravenous ergonovine maleate was introduced in the late 1970s to provoke spasm

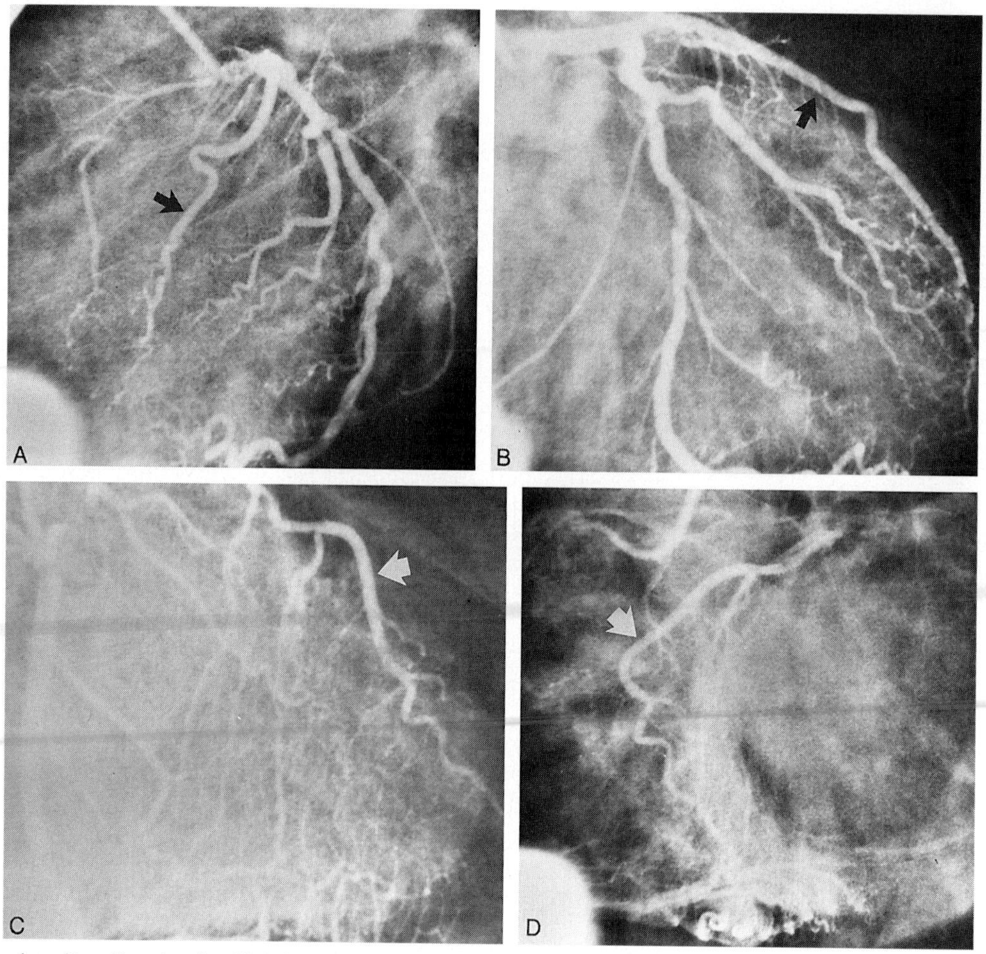

FIGURE 18–20 Superimposition of branches. **A** and **B,** Left anterior oblique and right anterior oblique views of the left coronary arteriogram show that the left anterior descending artery (LAD) is totally occluded, although the point of occlusion is not visualized. There is a large diagonal branch (black arrows) that closely parallels the LAD in both projections and could be mistaken for the LAD. Late-phase frames from a right anterior oblique **(C)** and left anterior oblique **(D)** right coronary arteriogram show filling of the LAD (white arrows) by means of septal collaterals.

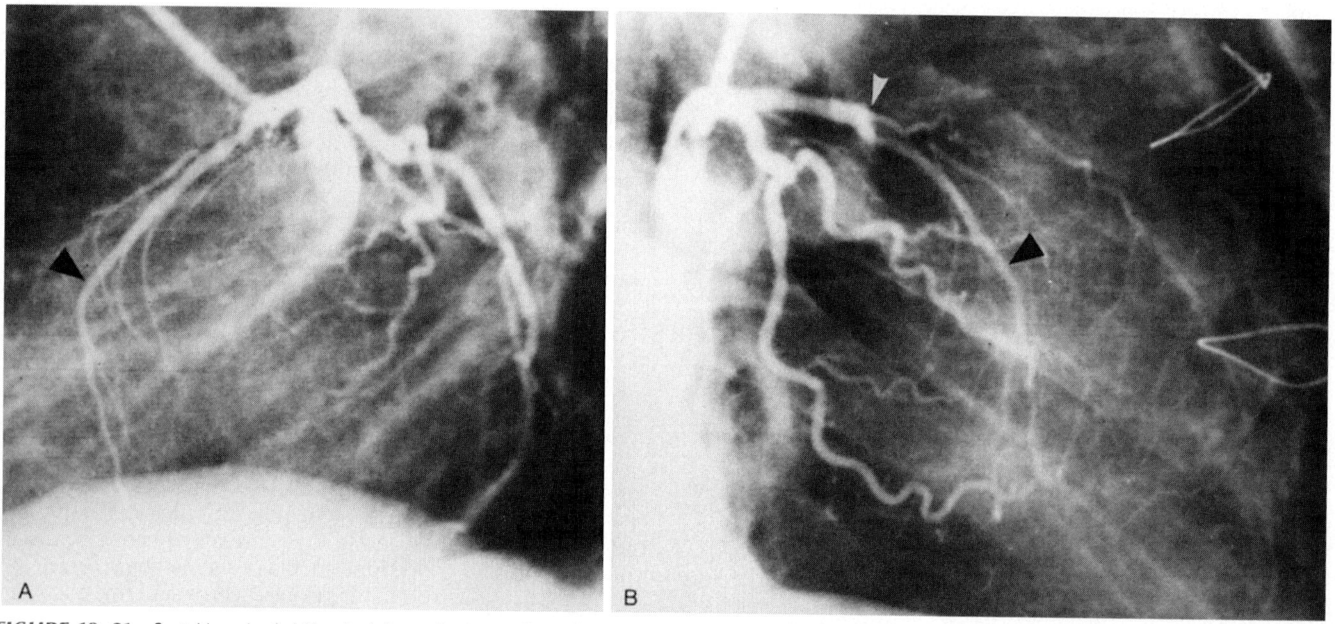

FIGURE 18–21 Septal branch mimicking the left anterior descending artery (LAD). **A,** Left anterior oblique left coronary arteriogram shows an enlarged septal branch (arrowhead) occupying the expected course of the LAD. **B,** The right anterior oblique view shows that the LAD is totally occluded (white arrowhead). The septal branch (black arrowhead) runs in a course approximately parallel to the LAD but below it and within the interventricular septum. (From Levin DC, Baltaxe HA, Sos TA: Potential sources of error in coronary arteriography: II. Interpretation of the study. AJR 124:386, 1975.)

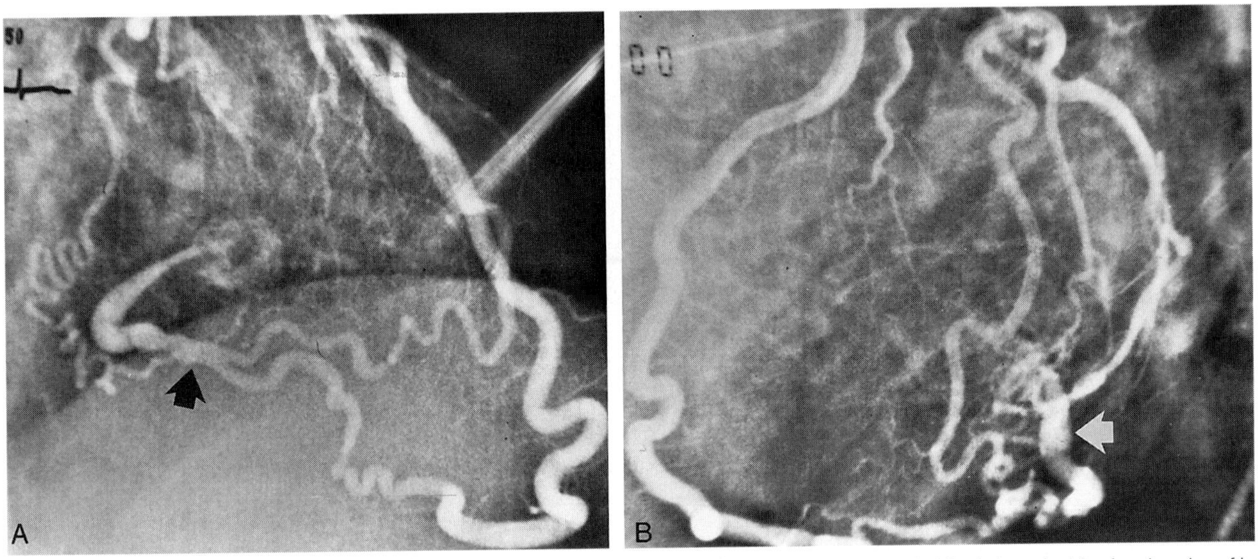

FIGURE 18–22 Congenital fistula. **A,** Right anterior oblique cranial view of the left coronary arteriogram shows a congenital fistula (arrow) arising from branches of both the left anterior descending and left circumflex arteries and draining into the left ventricle. **B,** Left anterior oblique view of the left coronary arteriogram shows the fistula (arrow).

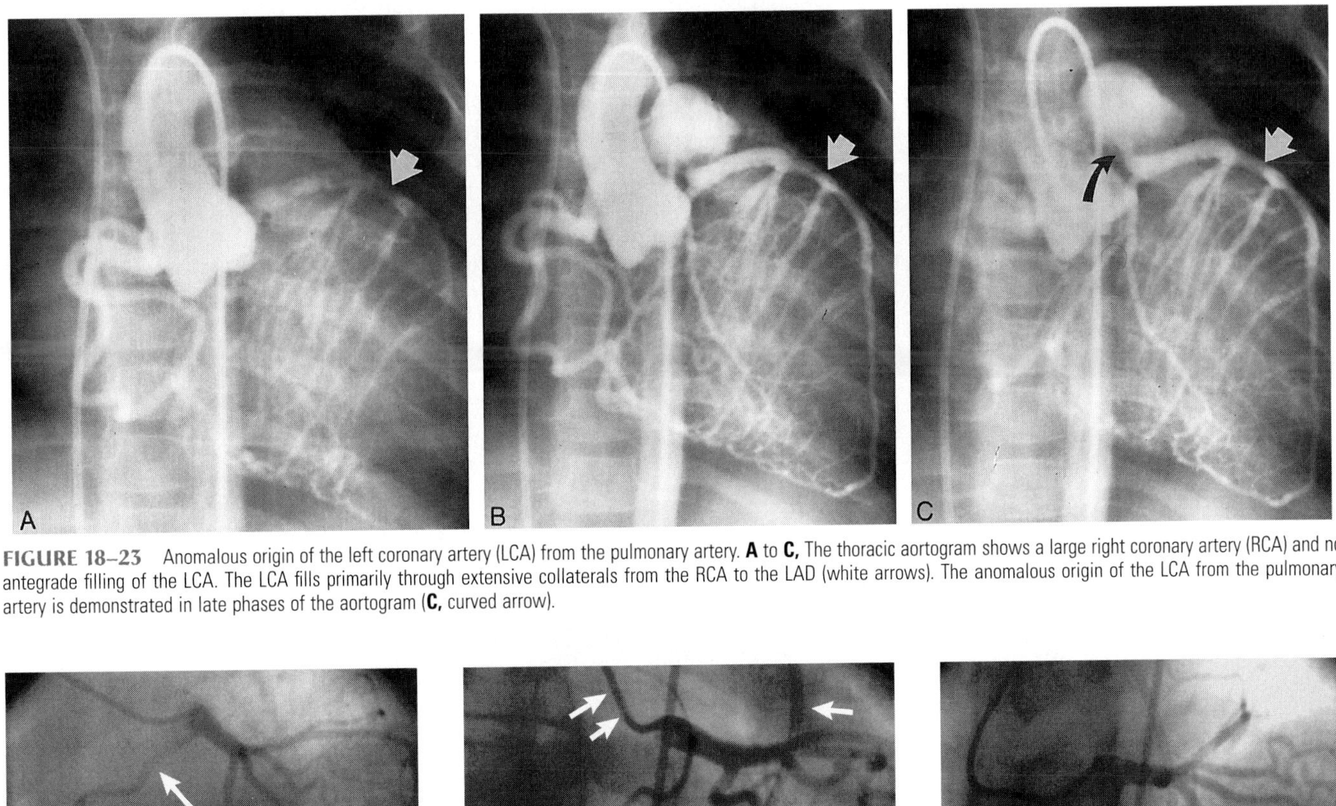

FIGURE 18–23 Anomalous origin of the left coronary artery (LCA) from the pulmonary artery. **A** to **C,** The thoracic aortogram shows a large right coronary artery (RCA) and no antegrade filling of the LCA. The LCA fills primarily through extensive collaterals from the RCA to the LAD (white arrows). The anomalous origin of the LCA from the pulmonary artery is demonstrated in late phases of the aortogram (**C,** curved arrow).

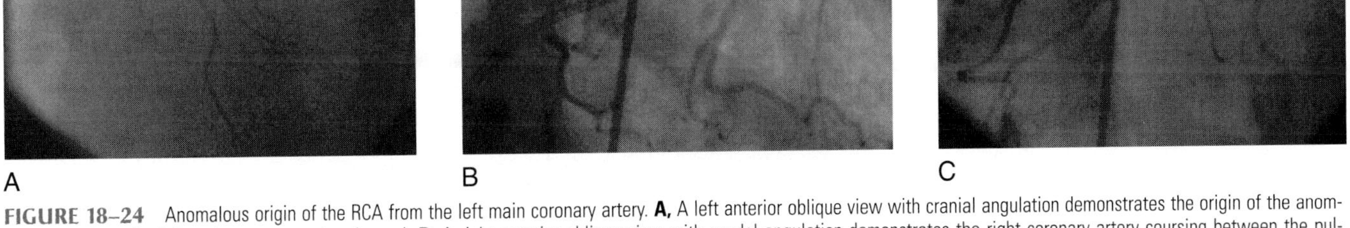

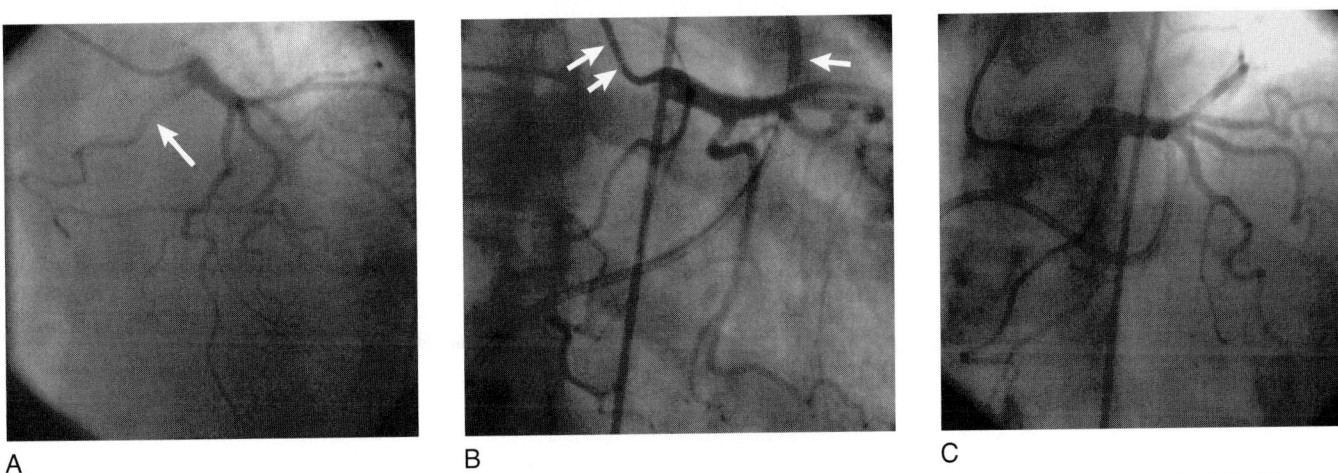

FIGURE 18–24 Anomalous origin of the RCA from the left main coronary artery. **A,** A left anterior oblique view with cranial angulation demonstrates the origin of the anomalous RCA from the left main coronary artery (arrow). **B,** A right anterior oblique view with caudal angulation demonstrates the right coronary artery coursing between the pulmonary artery (noted by the arrow with the pulmonary artery catheter) and aorta (noted by the double arrow of the injection catheter). **C,** The relationship of the RCA to the pulmonary artery and aorta is confirmed in the anteroposterior view with cranial angulation.

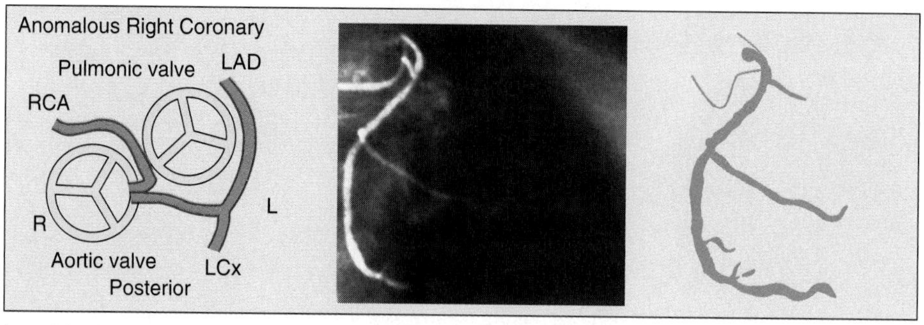

FIGURE 18–25 Anomalous origin of the right coronary artery (RCA). Right anterior oblique coronary arteriogram shows an anomalous RCA arising from the left sinus of Valsalva. The origin of the aberrantly arising artery, which is engaged with a left Judkins catheter, arises immediately anterior to the origin of the left coronary artery (not shown in the arteriogram). The anomalous right coronary follows an interarterial course opposite but analogous to that for the anomalous left coronary artery arising from the right sinus of Valsalva.

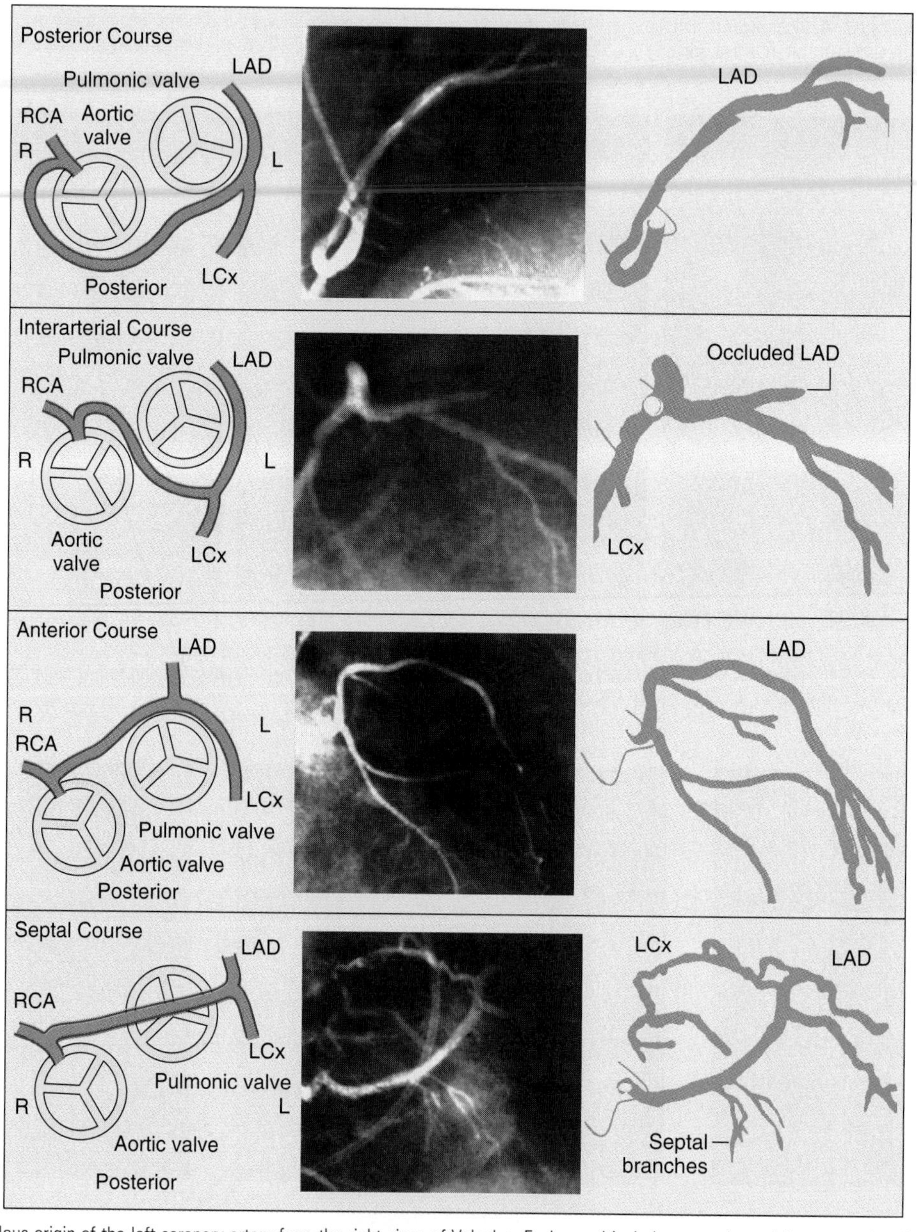

FIGURE 18–26 Anomalous origin of the left coronary artery from the right sinus of Valsalva. Each panel includes a caudocranial cross-sectional schematic representation at the level of the semilunar valves, showing the course of the anomalous coronary. The right anterior oblique angiograms and bitmaps show examples of each of the four most common courses of the anomalous left coronary artery aberrantly arising from the right sinus of Valsalva: posterior (retroaortic), interarterial, anterior, and septal (subpulmonic) courses. LAD = left anterior descending; LCx = left circumflex; RCA = right coronary artery.

in patients with suspected variant angina who were undergoing coronary arteriography.[69] Two types of angiographic responses can be expected with escalating dosages of intravenous ergonovine. A diffuse coronary vasoconstriction may occur in all the epicardial arteries that may be associated with angina symptoms. This physiological response to ergonovine is not diagnostic of coronary artery spasm. The second response to ergonovine is a focal, occlusive spasm of the epicardial artery that is associated with chest pain and ST segment elevation. Nitroglycerin should be administered directly into the coronary artery to relieve the coronary spasm. This response is diagnostic for coronary artery spasm. Ergonovine-induced coronary spasm may be found in 85 percent of patients with primarily rest angina who are observed to have spontaneous episodes of ST segment elevation. Intravenous acetylcholine may also be used to detect the presence of coronary artery spasm.[70] Although it is more sensitive, it may be less specific because of the positive response in patients with atherosclerotic CAD. In a study of 685 consecutive patients who were injected with incremental doses of acetylcholine, 20, 50, and 80 µg into the RCA and 20, 50, and 100 µg into the LCA, coronary vasospasm was found in 32.3 percent of patients.[70] Coronary artery spasm occurred in 49 percent of patients with effort and rest angina, in 34 percent of patients with exertional angina, and in 67 percent of patients with rest angina. It also occurred in 9 percent of patients with nonischemic heart disease. The third test is hyperventilation during coronary arteriography, which is less sensitive but highly specific for the presence of coronary artery spasm.

In the absence of a positive stimulation test, the diagnosis of coronary artery spasm must rely instead on clinical features and response to treatment with nitrates and calcium channel blockers. Sole therapy with beta blockers should be avoided because it can worsen the occurrence of coronary artery spasm. Coronary artery spasm that is refractory to conventional therapy with long-acting calcium channel blockers and nitrates can be treated with coronary stenting.[71]

Angiographic Morphology of Atherosclerotic Lesions

Heterogeneity of the composition, distribution, and location of atherosclerotic plaque within the native coronary artery results in unique patterns of stenosis morphology in patients with CAD. These unique atherosclerotic patterns have been used to identify risk factors for procedural outcome and complications after PCI and to assess the risk for recurrent events in patients who present with an acute coronary syndrome.[72,73] Criteria established by a joint ACC/AHA task force (Table 18–7) were prospectively tested in a series of 350 patients undergoing multivessel PCI; it was found that procedural success and complication rates after balloon angioplasty were 92 and 2 percent, respectively, for type A lesions; 76 and 10 percent, respectively, for type B lesions; and 61 and 21 percent, respectively, for type C lesions. Lesions with two or more type B lesion characteristics (modified ACC/AHA B2) had a risk intermediate between those of lesions with one type B characteristic (modified ACC/AHA B1) and type C lesions.[74] Certain lesion characteristics were associated with

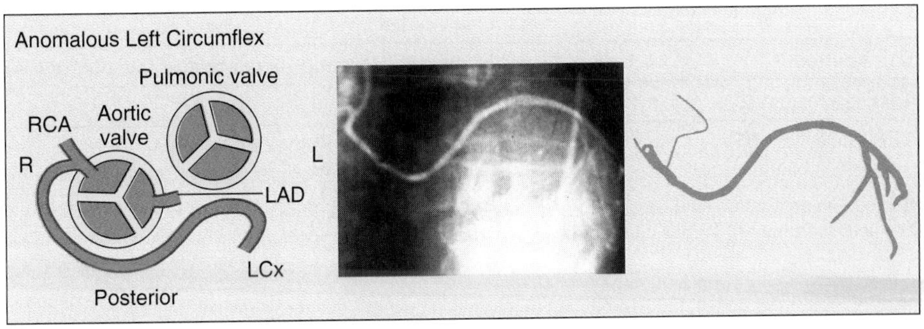

FIGURE 18–27 Anomalous origin of the left circumflex artery. The caudocranial cross-sectional view at the level of the semilunar valves shows the common course of the left circumflex coronary artery aberrantly arising from the right sinus of Valsalva. The left circumflex artery passes behind the aortic root and runs to the left atrioventricular groove following an initial course identical to that for the anomalous left coronary artery arising from the right sinus of Valsalva that follows a posterior, retroaortic course. LAD = left anterior descending; LCx = left circumflex; RCA = right coronary artery.

TABLE 18–7 Characteristics of Type A, B, and C Coronary Lesions

Lesion-Specific Characteristics	
Type A lesions (high success, > 85%; low risk)	
Discrete (<10 mm)	Little or no calcium
Concentric	Less than totally occlusive
Readily accessible	Not ostial in locations
Nonangulated segment, < 45 degree	No major side branch involvement
Smooth contour	Absence of thrombus
Type B lesions (moderate success, 60-85%; moderate risk)	
Tubular (10 to 20 mm length)	Moderate to heavy calcification
Eccentric	Total occlusions < 3 mo old
Moderate tortuosity of proximal segment	Ostial in location
Moderately angulated segment, ≥ 45 degrees, < 90 degrees	Bifurcation lesion requiring double guidewire
Irregular contour	Some thrombus present
Type C lesions (low success, < 60%; high risk)	
Diffuse (≥2 cm length)	Total occlusion > 3 mo old
Excessive tortuosity of proximal segment	Inability to protect major side branches
Extremely angulated segments, ≥ 90 degrees	Degenerated vein grafts with friable lesions

From Ryan TJ, Bauman WB, Kennedy JW, et al: Guidelines for percutaneous coronary angioplasty. A report of the American Heart Association/American College of Cardiology Task Force on Assessment of Diagnostic and Therapeutic Cardiovascular Procedures (Subcommittee on Percutaneous Transluminal Coronary Angioplasty). Circulation 88:2987, 1993.

TABLE 18–8 Definitions of Preprocedural Lesion Morphology

Feature	Frequency (%)	Definition
Eccentricity	48.0	Stenosis that is noted to have one of its luminal edges in the outer one-quarter of the apparent normal lumen.
Irregularity	17.9	Characterized by lesion ulceration, intimal flap, aneurysm, or sawtooth pattern
Ulceration	12.1	Lesions with a small crater consisting of a discrete luminal widening in the area of the stenosis
Intimal flap	3.22	A mobile, radiolucent extension of the vessel wall into the arterial lumen
Aneurysm	5.49	Segment of arterial dilation larger than the dimensions of the normal arterial segment
"Sawtooth"	0.84	Multiple, sequential stenosis irregularities
Length		Measured "shoulder to shoulder" in an unforeshortened view
Discrete	55.0	Lesion length < 10 mm
Tubular	34.8	Lesion length 10-20 mm
Diffuse	10.2	Lesion length ≥ 20 mm
Ostial location	10.0	Origin of the lesion within 3 mm of the vessel origin
Angulation		Vessel angle formed by the centerline through the lumen proximal and distal to the stenosis
Moderate	15.3	Lesion angulation ≥ 45 degrees
Severe	0.93	Lesion angulation ≥ 90 degrees
Bifurcation stenosis	6.05	Stenosis involving the parent and daughter branch if a medium or large branch (>1.5 mm) originates within the stenosis and if the side branch is completely surrounded by stenotic portions of the lesion to be dilated
Proximal tortuosity		
Moderate	15.3	Lesion is distal to two bends ≥ 75 degrees
Severe	NR	Lesion is distal to three bends ≥ 75 degrees
Degenerated SVG	7.1	Graft characterized by luminal irregularities or ectasia constituting > 50% of the graft length
Calcification	34.3	Readily apparent densities noted within the apparent vascular wall at the site of the stenosis
Total occlusion	6.4	TIMI 0 or 1 flow
Thrombus	3.4	Discrete, intraluminal filling defect is noted with defined borders and is largely separated from the adjacent wall. Contrast staining may or may not be present.

NR = not reported; SVG = saphenous vein graft; TIMI = Thrombolysis in Myocardial Infarction.
Data obtained from 846 lesions undergoing qualitative angiographic analysis at the Washington Hospital Center Angiographic Core Laboratory.

higher risk, including chronic total occlusions, high-grade stenoses, stenoses on a bend of 60 degrees or more, and lesions located in vessels with proximal tortuosity.

Specific Lesion Characteristics

Estimation of procedural risk may be more usefully based on the presence of one or more specific adverse morphological features rather than use of a composite scoring system (see Chap. 52) (Table 18–8).

IRREGULAR LESIONS. Lesion irregularity, including lesions with ulceration, aneurysm formation, a "sawtooth" pattern, or an intimal flap, suggests a friable surface, correlating pathologically with plaque fissuring, rupture, and platelet and fibrin aggregation. Complex, irregular plaques have been associated with unstable coronary syndromes and progression to total occlusion, whereas smooth lumen contours are more suggestive of stable angina. Other surface morphology features associated with unstable angina and infarction include lesions with sharply angulated leading or trailing borders, multiple serpiginous channels, and discrete intraluminal filling defects.

LESION LENGTH. Estimates of axial lesion length have been obtained using a number of methods, including measurement of the "shoulder-to-shoulder" extent of atherosclerotic narrowing greater than 20 percent and determination of the lesion length with a more than 50 percent visual diameter stenosis. In clinical practice, the lesion length is often estimated by the distance between the proximal and distal angiographically "normal" segments. The ACC/AHA criteria categorize lesions as discrete (<10 mm), tubular (10 to 20 mm), and diffuse (>20 mm). Diffuse lesions are associated with reduced procedural success. Lesion length is also an important predictor of restenosis after PCI, potentially related to the more extensive plaque burden in long lesions. The prognosis of patients with long lesions has been markedly improved with the availability of drug-eluting stents (see Chap. 52).

OSTIAL LOCATION. Ostial lesions are defined as those arising within 3 mm of origin of the vessel or branch. Balloon angioplasty of aortoostial lesions and ostial lesions of LAD or LCx coronary arteries has been associated with reduced procedural success and high recurrence rates owing to smooth muscle and eccentric intimal proliferation noted pathologically in ostial lesions. Technical factors may also account for the suboptimal success rates, such as difficulty with guide catheter support, lesion inelasticity precluding maximal balloon inflation, and the need for multiple balloon exchanges.

ANGULATED LESIONS. Balloon angioplasty of highly angulated (>45 degrees) lesions carries an increased risk of procedural complications (13 versus 3.5 percent in nonangulated stenoses; $p < 0.001$). Complications are most often due to coronary dissection, with the risk of dissection related to the severity of the angulation.[75] Vessel curvature should be measured in the most unforeshortened projection using a length of curvature that approximates the balloon or stent length used for coronary dilation. Devices that are relatively rigid (e.g., directional atherectomy) are less useful in angulated lesions. Coil stents appear better able to conform to an angulated segment than tubular slotted or multicellular designs.

BIFURCATION LESIONS. The risk of side branch occlusion ranges from 14 to 27 percent in bifurcation lesions, related to the extent of atherosclerotic involvement within the origin of the side branch. The risk of side branch compromise has been reduced using advanced angioplasty methods, including guidewire protection, "kissing balloon" techniques, branch vessel stent placement, and lesion angulation, but calcification or vessel size may preclude adequate side branch protection in some cases. Side branch occlusion during PCI is a frequent cause of periprocedural cardiac enzyme elevation.

DEGENERATED SAPHENOUS VEIN GRAFTS. The procedural success rate after balloon angioplasty of SVG lesions ranges from 84 to 92 percent, depending, in part, on the presence of SVG friability or degeneration, lesion location, and SVG age of 36 months or more. Few criteria have been proposed for classifying the degree of SVG degeneration, although such a definition should include an estimate of the percentage of SVG irregularity and ectasia, friability, presence of thrombus, and number of discrete or diffuse lesions (>50 percent stenosis) located within the SVG. The major periprocedural risk for PCI is the occurrence of distal embolization of thrombus and plaque contents, often associated with the "no-reflow" phenomenon.

LESION CALCIFICATION. Coronary artery calcium is an important marker for coronary atherosclerosis. With IVUS as a reference standard, conventional angiography is moderately sensitive for the detection of extensive lesion calcium (sensitivity 60 and 85 percent for three- and four-quadrant calcium, respectively) but is less sensitive for the presence of milder degrees of lesion calcification. The presence of angiographic coronary artery calcium has also been related to reduced procedural success rates after balloon angioplasty and directional coronary atherectomy (DCA). Higher (90 percent) procedural success rates have been reported after rotational atherectomy in heavily calcified lesions.

THROMBUS. Conventional angiography is a relatively insensitive method for detecting coronary thrombus, although complex lesion morphology has been associated with clinical findings of "high-risk" unstable angina. When it is present, angiographic thrombus, defined as discrete, intraluminal filling defects within the arterial lumen, has also been associated with a variably higher (range: 6 to 73 percent) incidence of ischemic complications after PCI. Large, intracoronary thrombi may be treated with a combination of pharmacological agents (e.g., glycoprotein IIb/IIIa inhibitors) and mechanical devices (e.g., rheolytic thrombectomy) (see Chap. 52).

TOTAL OCCLUSION. Total coronary occlusion is identified on the cineangiogram as an abrupt termination of the epicardial vessel; anterograde and retrograde collaterals may be present and are helpful in quantifying the length of the totally occluded segment. Primary success rates for balloon angioplasty of total occlusions remain suboptimal (66 to 83 percent), lower than the 94.2 percent primary success rates for subtotal occlusions. The risk of an unsuccessful procedure depends on the duration of the occlusion and certain lesion morphological features, such as bridging collaterals, occlusion length greater than 15 mm, and the absence of a "nipple" to guidewire advancement.

CORONARY PERFUSION. Perfusion distal to a coronary stenosis can occur anterograde by means of the native vessel, retrograde through collaterals, or through a coronary bypass graft. The rate of anterograde coronary flow is influenced by both the severity and complexity of the stenosis and the status of the microvasculature. The Thrombolysis in Myocardial Infarction (TIMI) study group established criteria to assess the degree of anterograde coronary reperfusion in patients with acute MI (Table 18–9). Successful reperfusion was present with TIMI flow 2 or 3, whereas TIMI 0 or 1 flow was deemed failed reperfusion. It is now clear that TIMI 2 flow may also be insufficient for myocardial perfusion, associated with increased mortality in patients with acute MI compared with those with normal TIMI 3 perfusion.[51] The TIMI frame count was subsequently introduced to quantify the coronary artery perfusion rates in patients with acute MI that have been correlated with mortality rates.[51] With this method, the number of cinefilm frames required for opacification of the involved vessel is counted by means of an automated frame counter, which is present on most cine projectors. Flow delayed more than 60 frames (approximately two cardiac cycles at 30 frames/sec) and 90 frames (approximately three cardiac cycles at 30 frames/sec) may be associated with increased risks for cardiac morbidity.

Coronary Collateral Circulation

In the normal human heart, networks of tiny anastomotic branches interconnect the major coronary arteries and are precursors for the development of a collateral circulation.[76] These anastomotic arteries cannot be visualized in patients with normal or mildly diseased coronary arteries because they carry only minimal flow and their small (<200 μm) caliber is well beyond the spatial resolution capabilities of coronary imaging systems, yet recruitable collaterals can be identified in up to 30 percent of patients with nonobstructive CAD or normal coronary arteries.[77] As atherosclerosis progresses and coronary artery obstructions develop, a pressure

TABLE 18–9 Thrombolysis in Myocardial Infarction (TIMI) Flow

TIMI Flow	
Grade 3 (complete reperfusion)	Anterograde flow into the terminal coronary artery segment through a stenosis is as prompt as anterograde flow into a comparable segment proximal to the stenosis. Contrast material clears as rapidly from the distal segment as from an uninvolved, more proximal segment.
Grade 2 (partial reperfusion)	Contrast material flows through the stenosis to opacify the terminial artery segment. However, contrast material enters the terminal segment perceptibly more slowly than more proximal segments. Alternatively, contrast material clears from a segment distal to a stenosis noticeably more slowly than from a comparable segment not preceded by a significant stenosis.
Grade 1 (penetration with minimal perfusion)	A small amount of contrast material flows through the stenosis but fails to opacity fully the artery beyond.
Grade 0 (no perfusion)	No contrast flow through the stenosis.

Modified from Sheehan F, Braunwald E, Canner P, et al: The effect of intravenous thrombolytic therapy on left ventricular function: A report on the tissue-type plasminogen activator and streptokinase from the Thrombolysis in Myocardial Infarction (TIMI) phase 1 trial. Circulation 72:817, 1989.

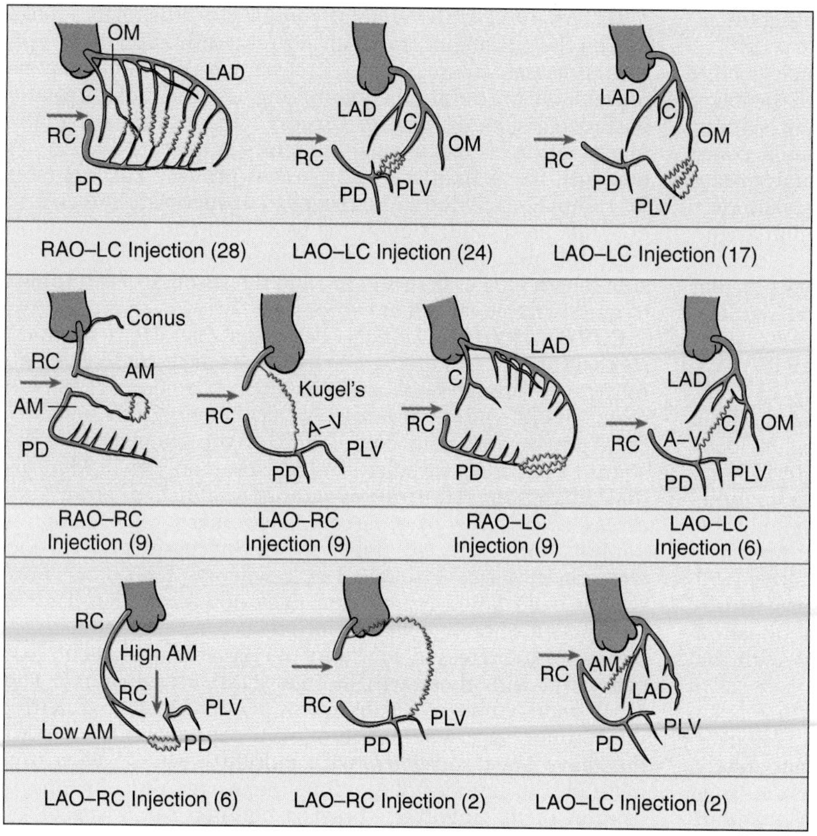

FIGURE 18–28 Coronary collaterals seen with right coronary artery occlusion and common collateral pathways seen with right coronary artery occlusion. The arrows point to the site of obstruction. The small tortuous channels represent the collateral connections. Numbers in parentheses refer to the frequency with which each pathway was visualized in a series of 200 patients with significant coronary disease. AM = acute marginal branch of the right coronary artery; A-V = artery to the atrioventricular node; C = circumflex artery; LAD = left anterior descending; LAO = left anterior oblique; OM = obtuse marginal branch of the circumflex artery; PD = posterior descending branch of the RCA; RAO = right anterior oblique; RC = right coronary artery. (From Levin DC: Pathways and functional significance of the coronary collateral circulation. Circulation 50:831, 1974. Copyright 1974, American Heart Association.)

gradient is generated within anastomotic vessels connecting the distal hypoperfused segment with the proximal artery or the adjacent anastomotic channels of other vessels. The transstenosis pressure gradient facilitates blood flow through the anastomotic vessels, which progressively dilate and eventually become visible as collateral channels.

Angiographically apparent coronary collaterals are usually not seen until the coronary obstruction is greater than 90 percent, at which point the coronary perfusion pressure falls substantially and the blood flow through the collateral increases. A number of collateral pathways exist in patients with severe CAD (Figs. 18–28 to 18–30). The visible collateral channels arise either from the contralateral coronary artery or from the ipsilateral coronary artery through intracoronary collateral channels or through "bridging" channels that have a serpiginous course from the proximal coronary artery to the coronary artery distal to the occlusion. The collateral circulation may provide up to 50 percent of anterograde coronary flow in chronic total occlusions. A considerable fraction of collateral flow is immediately lost after recanalization, indicating that chronic occlusion may not remain protected from future ischemic events by a well-developed collateral function.[78]

It is not entirely clear why some patients develop effective collateral vessels distal to a severe stenosis and others do not; a gradual rate of obstruction formation may allow enlargement of preexisting channels or growth of new ones by angiogenesis.[79] This may allow the development of a "protected" region of myocardial perfusion that does not develop ischemia during enhanced myocardial oxygen demands. Collateral circulation may be severely compromised in patients who have a limited degree of spontaneous myocardial angiogenesis and arteriogenesis, resulting in ischemia during stress in the compromised zone. One study identified the clinical characteristics associated with angiographically apparent collaterals and myocardial blush score in a consecutive group of 112 patients with a native artery chronic total coronary occlusion.[80] Ejection fraction tended to be higher in patients with better collateral grades (grades 1 to 4: 46, 48, 51, and 54 percent, respectively; $p = 0.052$). Hypercholesterolemia was a predictor of a better angiographic collateral grade (odds ratio = 1.3), and diabetes mellitus was correlated with a lower perfusion grade (odds ratio = 0.72).[80]

Recruitment of collateral channels may occur quickly in patients who develop an acute ST segment elevation MI because of a sudden thrombotic occlusion. Among patients studied within 6 hours of MI, about half show angiographically visible collateral vessels. When angiography was performed more than 24 hours after MI, virtually all patients had visible collaterals. This suggests that recruited collateral flow may develop rapidly, potentially within hours after an abrupt vessel occlusion. Accordingly, it appears that collateral circulation results from the utilization of already existing vessels that carried little blood flow because of adequate distal perfusion before the occlusion rather than from the formation of new blood vessels after the occlusion occurs. Other factors that affect collateral development are patency of the arteries supplying the collateral and the size and vascular resistance of the segment distal to the stenosis. A classification system is used for the grading of coronary collaterals (Table 18–10).[81]

Coronary collateral vessels have a number of functional roles. In patients with total occlusions, regional left ventricular contraction is better in segments supplied by adequate collateral circulation than in segments supplied by inadequate or no collateral circulation. In patients with acute MI undergoing emergency coronary arteriography without antecedent thrombolytic therapy, those with adequate collaterals had significantly lower left ventricular end-diastolic pressures, higher cardiac index, higher ejection fraction, and lower percentage of area dyssynergy than patients without collaterals.[79] Patients with stress-induced myocardial perfusion defects have insufficient collaterals more often than those with an intact collateral circulation. During balloon occlusion, patients with well-developed collateral vessels experience less pain, have better distal coronary perfusion pressures, and have less left ventricular asynergy and summed ST segment elevation than those with poorly developed collateral vessels. The presence of well-developed coronary collaterals reduced the risk for subsequent unstable cardiac events.[82] In a series of 403 patients with stable angina pectoris undergoing PCI and quantitative collateral assessment using Doppler measurements, the occurrence of cardiac death, MI, unstable angina pectoris, and stable angina pectoris was only 2.2 percent in patients with good collateral flow compared with 9.0 percent in patients with poorly developed collaterals ($p = 0.01$).[82] The incidence of stable angina pectoris (compared with unstable angina) was

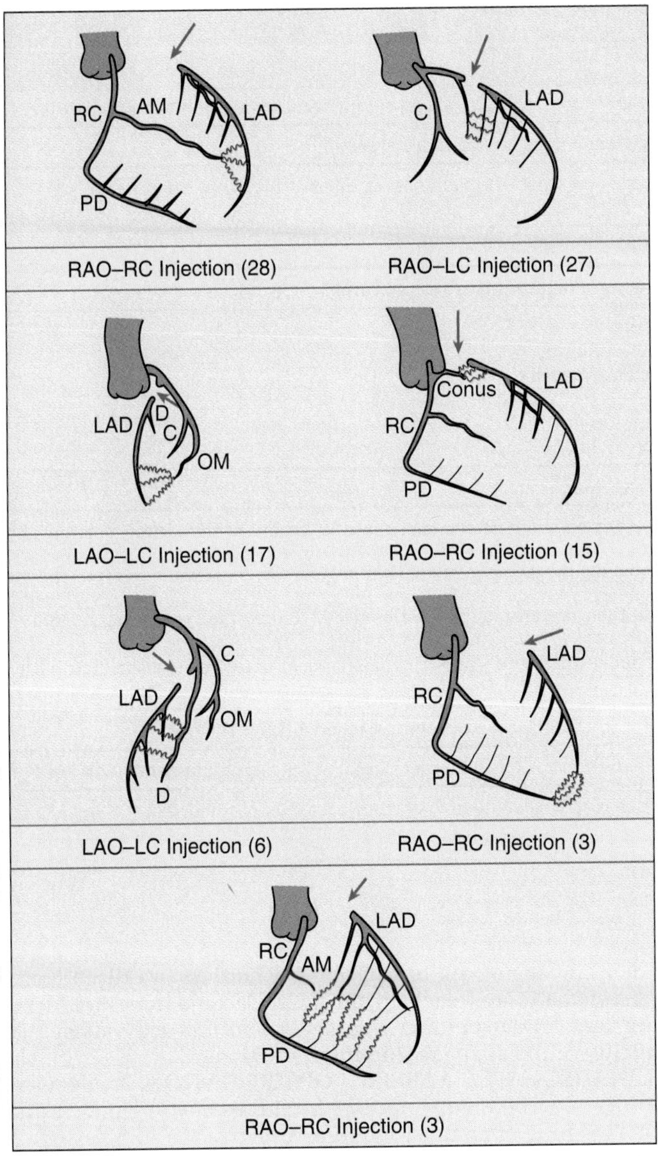

FIGURE 18–29 Common collateral pathways seen with left anterior descending artery occlusion. AM = acute marginal branch of the right coronary artery; A-V = artery to the atrioventricular node; C = circumflex artery; LAO = left anterior oblique; OM = obtuse marginal branch of the circumflex artery; PD = posterior descending branch of the RCA; RAO = right anterior oblique; RC = right coronary artery. (From Levin DC: Pathways and functional significance of the coronary collateral circulation. Circulation 50:831, 1974. Copyright 1974, American Heart Association.)

significantly higher in patients with well-developed collaterals than in those with poorly developed collaterals (21 versus 12 percent; $p = 0.01$).[82]

QUANTITATIVE ANGIOGRAPHY

Both qualitative and quantitative angiographic measures can be used to assess procedural outcome after PCI (Table 18-11). The development of quantitative angiography as a research tool emerged from the recognized limitations of visual estimation of stenosis severity, which include observer variability, overestimation of the stenosis severity before PCI and underestimation of the stenosis severity after PCI, and provision of some visual estimates (>90 percent) that are physiologically untenable. It does seem clear that once the inherent limitations of visual estimation

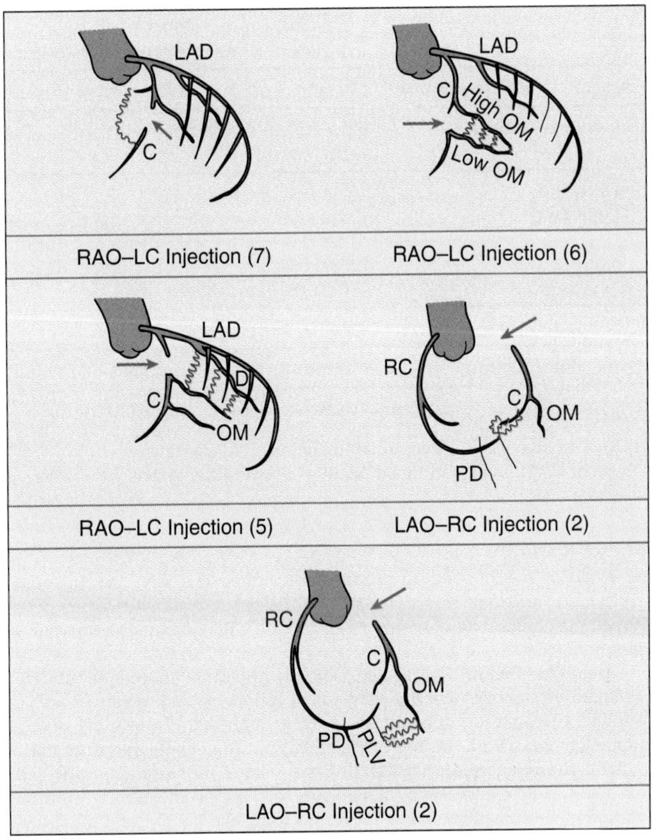

FIGURE 18–30 Common collateral pathways seen with left circumflex artery occlusion. AM = acute marginal branch of the right coronary artery; A-V = artery to the atrioventricular node; C = circumflex artery; LAO = left anterior oblique; OM = obtuse marginal branch of the circumflex artery; PD = posterior descending branch of the RCA; RAO = right anterior oblique; RC = right coronary artery. (From Levin DC: Pathways and functional significance of the coronary collateral circulation. Circulation 50:831, 1974. Copyright 1974, American Heart Association.)

TABLE 18–10 Perfusion Grades Distal to a Coronary Stenosis

Grade	TIMI	Collateral Flow	Rentrop Collateral Grade
3	Prompt anterograde flow and rapid clearing	Excellent	Complete perfusion. Contrast material enters and completely opacifies the target epicardial vessel.
2	Slow distal filling but full opacification of distal vessel	Good	Partial collateral flow. Contrast material enters but fails to opacify the target epicardial vessel completely.
1	Small amount of flow but incomplete opacification of distal vessel	Poor	Barely detectable collateral flow. Contrast medium passes through collateral channels but fails to opacify the epicardial vessel at any time.
0	No contrast flow	No visible flow	No collaterals present

Modified from Alderman E, Stadius M: The angiographic definitions of the Bypass Angioplasty Revascularization Investigation. Coron Artery Dis 3:1189, 1992.

TABLE 18–11 Standardized Criteria for Postprocedural Lesion Morphology

Feature	Definition
Abrupt closure	Obstruction of contrast flow (TIMI 0 or 1) in a dilated segment with previously documented anterograde flow.
Ectasia	A lesion diameter greater than the reference diameter in one or more areas.
Luminal irregularities	Arterial contour that has a "sawtooth" pattern consisting of opacification but not fulfilling the criteria for dissection or intracoronary thrombus
Intimal flap	A discrete filling defect in apparent continuity with the arterial wall
Thrombus	Discrete, mobile angiographic filling defect with or without contrast staining
Dissection,* A	Small radiolucent area within the lumen of the vessel
B	Linear, nonpersisting extravasation of contrast material
C	Extraluminal, persisting extravasation of contrast material
D	Spiral-shaped filling defect
E	Persistent lumen defect with delayed anterograde flow
F	Filling defect accompanied by total coronary occlusion
Dissection, length (in mm)	Measure end to end for type B through F dissections
Dissection, staining	Persistence of contrast within the dissection after washout of contrast material from the remaining portion of the vessel
Perforation	
Localized	Extravasation of contrast material confined to the pericardial space immediately surrounding the artery and not associated with clinical tamponade
Nonlocalized	Extravasation of contrast material with a jet not localized to the pericardial space, potentially associated with clinical tamponade
Side branch loss	TIMI 0, 1, or 2 flow in a side branch > 1.5 mm in diameter that previously had TIMI 3 flow
Distal embolization	Migration of a filling defect or thrombus to distally occlude the target vessel or one of its branches
Coronary spasm	Transient or permanent narrowing > 50% when a < 25% stenosis has been previously noted

TIMI = Thrombolysis in Myocardial Infarction.
*National Heart, Lung and Blood Institute classification system for coronary dissection.

of stenosis severity are understood, the clinician's eye can become "retrained," and one series has shown that visual estimates by experienced observers may correlate more closely with quantitative measurements.

DIGITAL CALIPERS. Digital calipers provide a more quantitative estimate of stenosis severity than visual estimates, and, when properly applied, this method appears to correlate with automated edge detection algorithms. With the use of digital calipers, cineangiograms are magnified and projected onto a wall or flat surface. Calibration is performed by measuring the known dimensions of the diagnostic or guiding catheter. The lumen border is measured using the caliper, and a calibration factor is obtained to determine quantitative dimensions.

AUTOMATED EDGE DETECTION ALGORITHMS. On the basis of early work using hand-drawn arterial contours that corrected for pincushion distortion and reconstructed a three-dimensional representation of the arterial contour, computer-assisted methods for automated arterial contour detection were developed. Quantitative angiographic analysis is divided into several distinct processes, including film digitization, image calibration, and arterial contour detection. The contrast agent–filled diagnostic or guiding catheter can be used as a scaling device for determining absolute vessel dimensions, yielding a calibration factor in millimeters per pixel. Catheter and arterial contours are obtained by drawing a centerline through the segment of interest. Linear density profiles are then constructed perpendicular to the centerline, and a weighted average of the first and second derivative function is used to define the catheter or arterial edges. Individual edge points are then connected using an automated algorithm, and outliers are discarded and the edges smoothed. The automated algorithm is then applied to a selected arterial segment, and absolute coronary dimensions and percent diameter stenosis are obtained.

Pitfalls of Coronary Arteriography

Errors in image acquisition and interpretation can have a profound impact on management strategies, particularly when the angiographic and clinical findings are discordant. A systematic approach to the image acquisition should be pursued, understanding that several factors may affect the quality of the angiographic interpretation.

INADEQUATE VESSEL OPACIFICATION. Inadequate filling of the coronary artery with contrast medium may result in streaming of contrast medium and give the impression of ostial stenoses, missing side branches, or thrombus. Superselective injection of contrast medium into the LCx through a short LMCA may give the impression of total occlusion of the LAD. Adequate filling of the coronary arteries and bypass grafts is required to overcome the native flow of unopacified blood and produce high-quality coronary arteriograms. Streaming of contrast medium, admixed with unopacified blood, leads to an artifactual impression of filling defects and incomplete assessment of stenosis severity. The causes of incomplete filling include competition from increased native coronary blood flow in the setting of left ventricular hypertrophy associated with aortic insufficiency or anemia and inadequate placement of the diagnostic catheter with subselection of the LCx through a short LCMA. The problem of underfilling can be overcome by more forceful contrast agent injection as long as catheter tip position and pressure recording confirm the safety of such a maneuver. Under some conditions, switching to an angioplasty-guiding catheter with a soft, short tip and a larger lumen than a diagnostic catheter may allow more complete opacification of the target coronary artery or bypass graft.

ECCENTRIC STENOSES. Coronary atherosclerosis more often leads to eccentric or slit-like atherosclerotic narrowings than concentric narrowings. If the long axis of the lumen is projected, the vessel may appear to have a normal or near-normal caliber. Only if the short axis of the stenotic lumen is projected is the narrowing visible. For this reason, coronary arteries must be viewed in at least two projections approximately 90 degrees apart.

A related problem is that of the band-like or membranous stenosis. Such lesions may be exceedingly difficult to detect. It is not clear whether these peculiar lesions represent pure atherosclerotic stenosis or are caused in some instances by congenital membranous bands. Aside from the difficulty in detecting these lesions, it is difficult to ascertain their hemodynamic significance. Measurement of the pressure gradient across the lesion using a micromanometer-tip guidewire during intracoronary or intravenous adenosine may be useful to identify significant narrowings.

UNRECOGNIZED OCCLUSIONS. Flow disturbances associated with branch points predispose to the development of atherosclerosis and total occlusions of major arteries at this location. Because of this fact and the variability of the number and distribution of side branches in the normal coronary circulation, it is possible for flush occlusions at branch origins to escape detection. In some cases, occlusion of a branch can be recognized only by late filling of the distal segment of this branch by means of collateral circulation.

SUPERIMPOSITION OF BRANCHES. Superimposition of major branches of the left coronary tree in the LAO and RAO projections can result in failure to detect stenoses or total occlusions of these branches. Although this problem most commonly affects the LAD and parallel diagonal branches, it is alleviated by the use of cranial and caudal angulation. Septal branches may mimic the LAD in the LAO cranial projection. When the LAD is occluded beyond the origin of the first septal branch, this branch often becomes quite enlarged in an attempt to provide collateral circulation to the vascular bed of the distal LAD.

MYOCARDIAL BRIDGING. The major coronary arteries generally pass over the epicardial surface of the heart. In some cases, however, short segments descend into the myocardium for a variable distance. This occurs in 5 to 12 percent of patients and is almost always confined to the LAD. Because a "bridge" of myocardial fibers passes over the involved segment of the LAD, each systolic contraction of these fibers can cause narrowing of the artery. Myocardial bridging has a characteristic appearance on cineangiography. The bridged segment is of normal caliber during diastole but abruptly narrows with each systole. Systolic narrowing caused by myocardial bridging should not be confused with an atherosclerotic plaque. Although bridging is not thought to have any hemodynamic significance in most cases, some have suggested that when it produces severe systolic narrowing, ischemia or infarction may result. The presence of myocardial bridging has important implications for interventional cardiovascular therapy because bridges do not respond to balloon dilation or other interventions.

RECANALIZATION. Although a narrowed segment of a coronary artery seen on arteriography is usually considered a "stenosis," such lesions may actually be a segment that was once totally occluded but has recanalized. Pathological studies suggest that approximately one-third of totally occluded coronary arteries ultimately recanalize. The arteriographic appearances of stenosis and recanalization may be indistinguishable. Recanalization usually results in the development of multiple tortuous channels, which are quite small and close to one another, creating an impression on cineangiography of a single, slightly irregular channel. Cineangiography lacks sufficient spatial resolution to demonstrate this degree of detail in most patients with recanalized total occlusions, but this has important implications for interventional cardiovascular treatments because they are unlikely to be successful in the setting of multiple microscopic channels.

Intravascular Ultrasonography

(see also Chap. 11)

Contrast coronary arteriography is limited in its ability to quantify the extent or distribution of atherosclerosis or to identify changes within the vessel wall over time. IVUS is a safe, accurate, and reproducible method of detecting vessel wall structure and disease and lends insight into the dynamic changes before, after, and late after PCI. The two-dimensional tomographic images provided by IVUS also permit 360-degree characterization of arterial lumen dimensions in regions that are difficult to assess using conventional angiography, such as the LMCA and the ostia of the LAD, LCx, and RCA. When a mechanized pullback of the IVUS catheter is performed at a fixed rate, a three-dimensional reconstruction of the arterial wall and its lumen can be obtained.

TECHNICAL ISSUES. IVUS has evolved substantially since the early 1990s, resulting in the commercial availability of rapid exchange, mechanical, or dynamic array imaging catheters, ranging in size from 2.6 to 3.2F, compatible with 6 to 7F guiding catheters, and yielding a 30-MHz imaging frequency for enhanced tissue characterization. Longitudinal or three-dimensional display of the arterial wall is best performed using an automated pullback device, which uses side branches and other anatomical landmarks to ascertain the plaque location along the axial length of the vessel.

VESSEL WALL COMPOSITION. In nondiseased arteries, IVUS differentiates the vessel wall into three components: (1) the intima, which is composed of endothelial cells, subjacent smooth muscle cells, and extracellular matrix, is 150 to 200 μm in diameter and partitioned from the media by the internal elastic lamina; (2) the media, which is composed of smooth muscle cells, elastin, and collagen, is 100 to 350 μm in diameter and encircled by the external elastic membrane (EEM); and (3) the adventitia, which contains fibrous tissue, is 300 to 500 μm in diameter and encased by perivascular stroma and epicardial fat.[83] Differences in acoustic impedance between the cell layers generally account for the "three-layer" appearance seen in the normal vessel wall of most patients by IVUS. A "two-layer" coronary artery is seen in some patients, depending on the IVUS transducer frequency (<30 MHz), intimal thickness (<160 μm), and collagen content of the media.

In diseased arteries, the differentiation between vessel wall components becomes more obscure and, depending on the cellular composition of the atherosclerotic plaque, at least three plaque types can be described.[83] Hypoechoic, or soft, plaques are echolucent compared with the EEM and indicate a high lipid content present in a pool (Fig. 18–31).[83] IVUS has also been used to assess the changes in plaque volume after lipid-lowering therapy[84] and has demonstrated that multiple plaques may develop simultaneous rupture in patients with acute MI.[85]

Thrombus within the vessel lumen often can be mistaken for soft plaque, but it can be distinguished from soft plaque by its mobility, lobular edges, and movement away from the vessel wall during the cardiac cycle.[83] Fibrous plaques have brightness similar to that of the adventitia and consistent with a higher content of collagen and elastin.[83] Calcified plaques are identified by their bright, echogenic components with acoustic shadowing of the underlying vascular structures.[83] A calcified plaque may be characterized as superficial or deep and quantified by its circumferential extent (from 0 to 360 degrees) and by its axial length (in millimeters).[83] Comparative studies with IVUS show that fluoroscopy is relatively insensitive for the detection of vessel wall calcium. In one study of 110 patients undergoing PCI, IVUS detected calcium in 76 percent of target lesions, whereas fluoroscopy identified calcium in only 48 percent ($p < 0.001$).

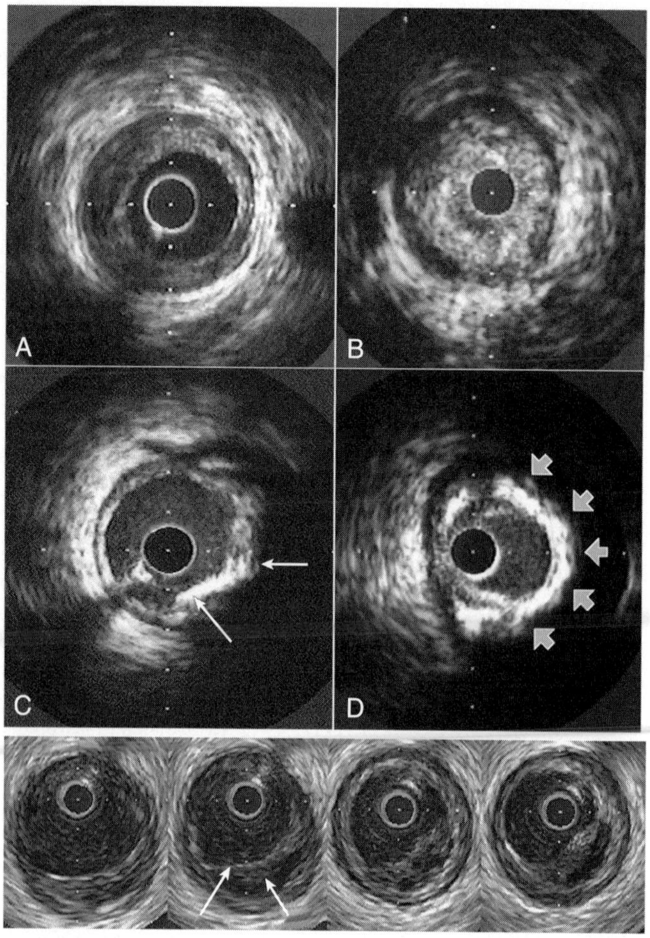

E

FIGURE 18–31 Intravascular ultrasound (IVUS) characterization of plaque morphology. **A,** A concentric "soft" plaque with concentric vessel wall involvement is less echogenic than a fibrous plaque that presumably contains more collagenous components. **B,** Calcification within the vessel is characterized by a bright leading edge with echo dropout (acoustic shadowing) behind the calcification, and may be focal **(C)** (arrows) or extensive **(D)** (arrows). (Courtesy of Steven Nissen, MD.) **E,** Adjacent IVUS cross sections of a "vulnerable" plaque show a thin fibrous cap (thick arrow) and a large lipid core (thin arrow). (Courtesy of Gary Mintz, MD.)

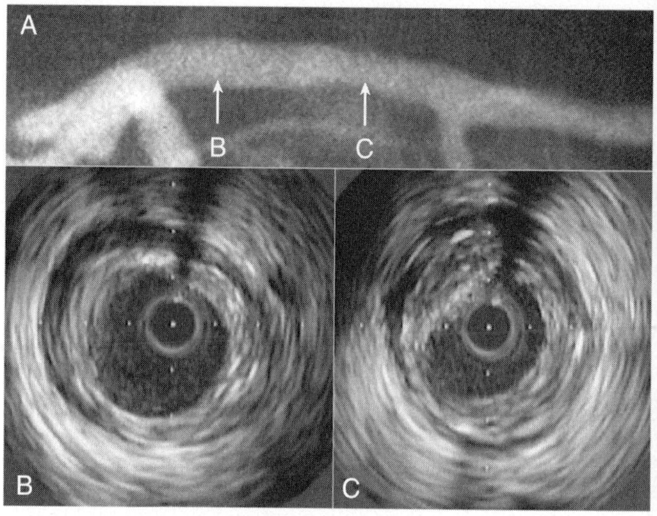

FIGURE 18–32 Discordance between angiographic and intravascular ultrasound (IVUS) findings. **A,** Angiographic imaging of the midportion of the LAD shows only minor lumen irregularities within the vessel. The arrows show the sites imaged in cross section by IVUS below. IVUS imaging of the angiographically normal site **(B)** and the most normal aspect **(C)** of the LAD. Note the substantial atherosclerotic plaque within the wall of the coronary artery that is not appreciated by angiography. (Courtesy of Steven Nissen, MD.)

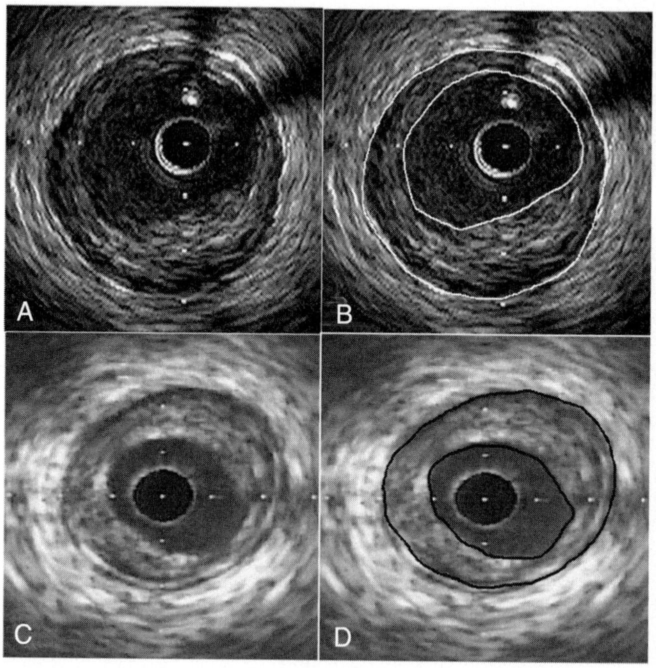

FIGURE 18–33 Quantitative intravascular ultrasound (IVUS) measurements. **A,** IVUS image obtained using a mechanical imaging transducer. **B,** The external elastic membrane is identified by the outer circle and the lumen cross-sectional area is demonstrated by the inner circle. (Courtesy of Gary Mintz, MD.) **C,** IVUS cross-sectional image obtained using a phased-array catheter. **D,** The external elastic membrane is identified by the outer circle and the lumen cross-sectional area is demonstrated by the inner circle. (Courtesy of Steven Nissen, MD.)

Fluoroscopic detection of calcium increased to 74 percent in lesions with two or more quadrants of calcium by IVUS and 86 percent in lesions with calcium 6 mm or more in length or with a circumferential arc of calcium of 180 degrees or more by IVUS. The presence of lesion calcification has also been correlated with the overall plaque burden.

IVUS studies in patients undergoing PCI have also demonstrated that coronary atherosclerosis is more diffuse than appreciated using conventional angiography (Fig. 18–32). In an IVUS series of 884 angiographically "normal" reference segments, only 6.8 percent were free of atherosclerosis, with an average 51 percent cross-sectional plaque area found proximal or distal to the target lesion. IVUS studies have also confirmed an earlier pathological finding of Glagov and colleagues, suggesting that the coronary artery undergoes "adaptive" remodeling, or vessel expansion, in most patients in the early stages of atherosclerosis, maintaining a nonobstructive coronary lumen diameter (Figs. 18–33 and 18–34; see also Chap. 35). Once the EEM has expanded by 40 percent, further accumulation of plaque encroaches on the arterial lumen. Arterial constriction does occur in some patients, particularly diabetic patients, owing to "negative" arterial remodeling.[86]

USE OF INTRAVASCULAR ULTRASONOGRAPHY DURING PERCUTANEOUS CORONARY INTERVENTION. IVUS may be used for several purposes during PCI: (1) to characterize baseline plaque composition, vessel size, and lesion accessibility to select the best single device or combination of devices for PCI; (2) to confirm (or refute) angiographic estimates of stenosis severity, particularly in regions

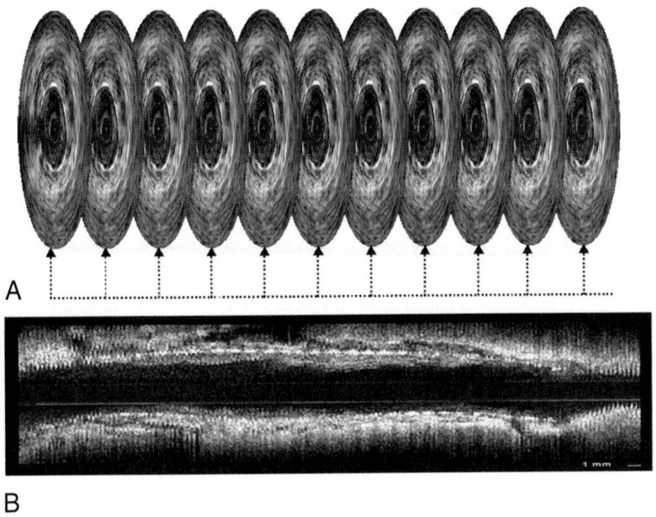

FIGURE 18–34 Longitudinal intravascular ultrasound (IVUS) imaging. Motorized "pullback" IVUS allows reconstruction of the individual two-dimensional cross-sectional images **(A)** into a longitudinal display that characterizes the coronary artery in three dimensions **(B)**. (Courtesy of Peter Fitzgerald, MD.)

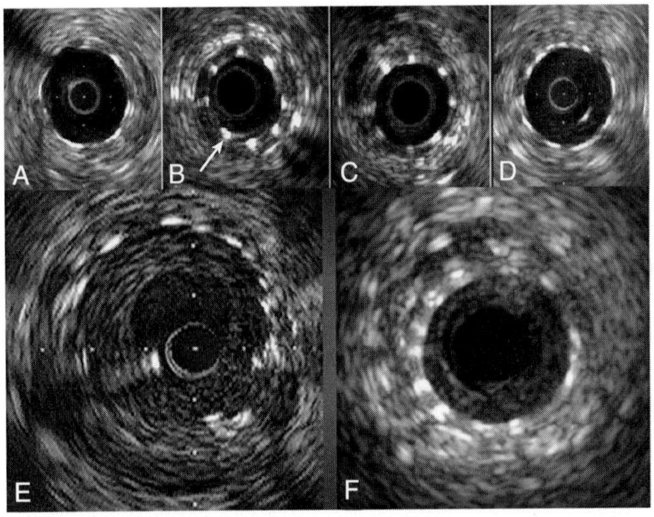

FIGURE 18–35 Stent deployment and in-stent restenosis assessed by intravascular ultrasound (IVUS). **A–D,** Coronary stent apposed against the vessel wall (**B,** arrow). **E,** Obtained in a patient who developed in-stent restenosis, as assessed by the soft-shadowed intimal hyperplasia that obstructs the lumen. **F,** Complete catheter entrapment with the soft intimal hyperplasia that results in stent restenosis. (Courtesy of Gary Mintz, MD, and Neil Weissman, MD.)

difficult to visualize using conventional methods; and (3) to assess anatomical results and detect complications, including dissections and residual minimal cross-sectional area, after PCI.[87] One study of 144 patients with long lesions found that IVUS guidance resulted in lower restenosis rates (23 percent) than in patients treated with angiography alone (45 percent; $p = 0.008$).[88] At 12 months, target lesion revascularization and the combined endpoint occurred in 10 and 12 percent of the IVUS group and 23 and 27 percent of the angiography group ($p = 0.018$ and $p = 0.026$), respectively.[88]

VESSEL WALL CHANGES AFTER PERCUTANEOUS CORONARY INTERVENTION. IVUS provides unique insight into the dynamic changes that occur within the vessel wall after PCI.[89] Sequential IVUS studies show that lumen renarrowing after balloon angioplasty and atherectomy is related to both arterial remodeling and, to a lesser extent, intimal hyperplasia. In the Serial Ultrasound Restenosis (SURE) trial involving a registry of 61 lesions treated with balloon angioplasty or DCA, performing angiography and IVUS at baseline, after PCI, and 24 hours, 1 month, and 6 months later. Lumen cross-sectional area by IVUS improved from 6.81 mm^2 after PCI to 8.22 mm^2 at 1 month ($p = 0.0001$) but decreased to 4.88 mm^2 6 months later ($p = 0.0001$). Vessel, or EEM, cross-sectional area enlarged from 17.32 mm^2 after PCI to 19.39 mm^2 at 1 month ($p = 0.0001$) but decreased to 16.33 mm^2 at 6 months ($p = 0.0001$). Intimal hyperplasia, as assessed by the plaque plus media cross-sectional area, increased from 10.51 mm^2 after PCI to 10.96 mm^2 at 24 hours ($p = 0.001$) and 11.45 mm^2 ($p = 0.03$) 6 months later. Changes in lumen cross-sectional area in each study interval correlated more closely with changes in vessel cross-sectional area than with changes in intimal hyperplasia cross-sectional area. In contrast to these findings, IVUS studies have also shown that lumen renarrowing after stent implantation is virtually all due to intimal hyperplasia within the axial length of the stent or its border.

IVUS has also been used to evaluate the magnitude of intimal hyperplasia in patients treated with drug-eluting stents (Fig. 18–35).[90] In the RAndomized study with the sirolimus-eluting VElocity balloon-expandable stent in the treatment of patients with de novo native coronary artery Lesions (RAVEL) trial, 238 patients were randomly assigned to receive either an 18-mm sirolimus-eluting or an uncoated

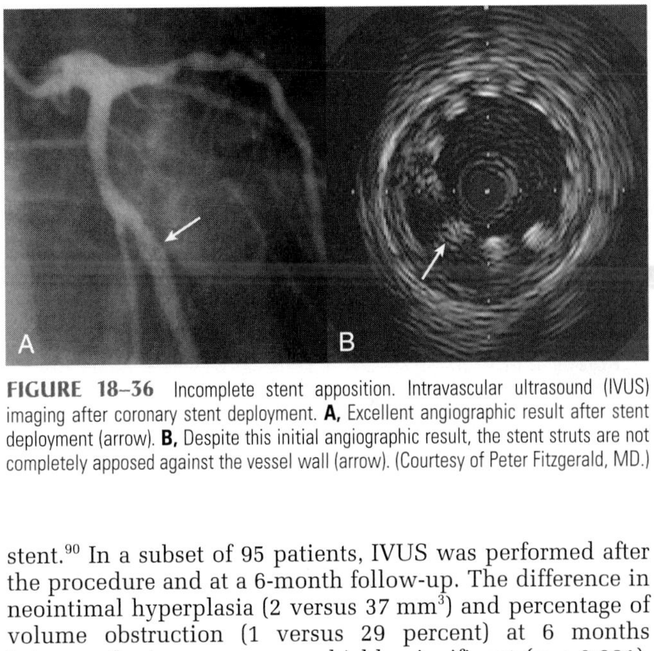

FIGURE 18–36 Incomplete stent apposition. Intravascular ultrasound (IVUS) imaging after coronary stent deployment. **A,** Excellent angiographic result after stent deployment (arrow). **B,** Despite this initial angiographic result, the stent struts are not completely apposed against the vessel wall (arrow). (Courtesy of Peter Fitzgerald, MD.)

stent.[90] In a subset of 95 patients, IVUS was performed after the procedure and at a 6-month follow-up. The difference in neointimal hyperplasia (2 versus 37 mm^3) and percentage of volume obstruction (1 versus 29 percent) at 6 months between the two groups was highly significant ($p < 0.001$), emphasizing the nearly complete abolition of the proliferative process inside the drug-eluting stent.[90] Although there was a higher incidence of incomplete stent apposition in the sirolimus group compared with the uncoated stent group ($p < 0.05$), it was not associated with any adverse clinical events at 1 year (Fig. 18–36).[90]

LIMITATIONS OF INTRAVASCULAR ULTRASONOGRAPHY. A number of factors have limited the widespread use of IVUS during PCI, including its cost, its cumbersome setup for occasional IVUS users, the steep "learning curve" for "on-line" IVUS interpretation, and the improved outcomes associated with routine use of stents. Current catheter-based IVUS systems are also limited by their inability to assess lumen diameters less than 1.0 mm owing to the catheter size and "ring-down" artifact, and the limited spatial resolution of a 30-MHz imaging transducer (theoretical spatial resolution, 80 μm; usual spatial resolution, 120 to 150 μm) makes IVUS detection of a "vulnerable" plaque somewhat problematic. Radiofrequency backscatter analysis may provide better insights into plaque morphology than standard IVUS image analysis.[91,92] Other invasive imaging techniques, such as optical coherence tomography, may provide higher spatial resolution (20 to 50 μm) for the characterization of vulnerable plaque.[93] Nevertheless, IVUS will remain useful for lesions difficult to assess using conventional angiography as these limitations are addressed with newer IVUS designs. Nonetheless, IVUS provides a powerful research tool for clinical trials, taking advantage of its ability to visualize the vessel wall as well as the lumen. Insights into the efficacy of therapeutic interventions have already emerged from application of this tool to clinical trials.

REFERENCES

Guidelines for Coronary Arteriography

1. Oetgen M, New G, Moussa I, et al: Procedural costs of digital vs. analog archiving of diagnostic cardiac catheterizations. Catheter Cardiovasc Interv 49:246, 2000.
2. Scanlon P, Faxon D, Audet A, et al: ACC/AHA guidelines for coronary angiography. J Am Coll Cardiol 33:1756, 1999.
3. Braunwald E, Antman E, Beasley J, et al: ACC/AHA 2002 guideline update for the management of patients with unstable angina and non-ST-segment elevation myocardial infarction—Summary article: A report of the American College of Cardiology/American Heart Association task force on practice guidelines (Committee on the Management of Patients With Unstable Angina). J Am Coll Cardiol 40:1366, 2002.
4. Wright R, Monnahan R, Kopecky S, et al: Cardiac catheterization reduces resource utilization in patients with chronic chest pain. Catheter Cardiovasc Interv 49:363, 2000.

Complications

5. Ammann P, Brunner-La Rocche HP, Angehrn W, et al: Procedural complications following diagnostic coronary angiography are related to the operator's experience and the catheter size. Catheter Cardiovasc Interv 59:13, 2003.
6. Samal A, White C: Percutaneous management of access site complications. Catheter Cardiovasc Interv 57:12, 2002.
7. Witz M, Cohen Y, Lehmann J: Retroperitoneal haematoma—A serious vascular complication of cardiac catheterisation. Eur J Vasc Endovasc Surg 18:364, 1999.
8. Chandrasekar B, Doucet S, Bilodeau L, et al: Complications of cardiac catheterization in the current era: A single-center experience. Catheter Cardiovasc Interv 52:289, 2001.
9. Jackson J, Meyer G, Pettit T: Complications from cardiac catheterization: Analysis of a military database. Mil Med 165:298, 2000.
10. Segal A, Abernethy W, Palacios I, et al: Stroke as a complication of cardiac catheterization: Risk factors and clinical features. Neurology 56:975, 2001.
11. Hinchey J, Sweeney P: Transient cortical blindness after coronary angiography. Lancet 351:1513,. 1998.
12. Fukumoto Y, Tsutsui H, Tsuchihashi M, et al: The incidence and risk factors of cholesterol embolization syndrome, a complication of cardiac catheterization: A prospective study. J Am Coll Cardiol 42:211, 2003.
13. Blanco V, Moris C, Barriales V, et al: Retinal cholesterol emboli during diagnostic cardiac catheterization. Catheter Cardiovasc Interv 51:323, 2000.
14. Butler R, Webster M: Meralgia paresthetica: An unusual complication of cardiac catheterization via the femoral artery. Catheter Cardiovasc Interv 56:69, 2002.
15. Kuruvilla A, Kuruttukulam G, Francis B: Femoral neuropathy following cardiac catheterization for balloon mitral valvotomy. Int J Cardiol 71:197, 1999.
16. Heupler F: Guidelines for performing angiography in patients taking metformin. Members of the Laboratory Performance Standards Committee of the Society for Cardiac Angiography and Interventions. Cathet Cardiovasc Diagn 43:121, 1998.
17. Dehen L, Vilmer C, Humiliere C, et al: Chronic radiodermatitis following cardiac catheterisation: A report of two cases and a brief review of the literature. Heart 81:308, 1999.
18. Schecter A, Lewis M, Robinson-Bostom L, et al: Cardiac catheterization–induced acute radiation dermatitis presenting as a fixed drug eruption. J Drugs Dermatol 2:425, 2003.
19. Cooper C, El-Shiekh R, Cohen D, et al: Effect of transradial access on quality of life and cost of cardiac catheterization: A randomized comparison. Am Heart J 138:430, 1999.
20. McNulty P, Ettinger S, Field J, et al: Cardiac catheterization in morbidly obese patients. Catheter Cardiovasc Interv 56:174, 2002.

Conscious Sedation

21. Scheinman M, Calkins H, Gillette P, et al: NASPE policy statement on catheter ablation: Personnel, policy, procedures, and therapeutic recommendations. Pacing Clin Electrophysiol 26:789, 2003.
22. Goodwin S: Pharmacologic management of patients undergoing conscious sedation. Clin Nurse Spec 15:269, 2001.
23. Venneman I, Lamy M: Sedation, analgesia and anesthesia for interventional radiological procedures in adults. Part II. Recommendations for interventional radiologists. JBR-BTR 83:116, 2000.

Radiocontrast Agents

24. Davidson CJ, Laskey WK, Hermiller JB, et al: Randomized trial of contrast media utilization in high-risk PTCA: The Court Trial. Circulation 101:2172, 2000.
25. Aspelin P, Aubry P, Fransson S-G, et al: Nephrotoxic effects in high-risk patients undergoing angiography. N Engl J Med 348:491, 2003.
26. Agrawal M, Stouffer G: Cardiology grand rounds from The University of North Carolina at Chapel Hill. Contrast induced nephropathy after angiography. Am J Med Sci 323:252, 2002.
27. Curhan G: Prevention of contrast nephropathy. JAMA 289:606, 2003.
28. Gomes V, Blaya P, de Figueiredo, CE, et al: Contrast-media induced nephropathy in patients undergoing coronary angiography. J Invasive Cardiol 15:304, 2003.
29. Huber W, Schipek C, Ilgmann K, et al: Effectiveness of theophylline prophylaxis of renal impairment after coronary angiography in patients with chronic renal insufficiency. Am J Cardiol 91:1157, 2003.
30. Solomon R: Radiocontrast-induced nephropathy. Semin Nephrol 18:551, 1998.
31. Bailey S: Past and present attempts to prevent radiocontrast nephropathy. Rev Cardiovasc Med 2(Suppl 1):S14, 2001.
32. Baker C: Prevention of radiocontrast-induced nephropathy. Catheter Cardiovasc Interv 58:532, 2003.
33. Stevens M, McCullough P, Tobin K, et al: A prospective randomized trial of prevention measures in patients at high risk for contrast nephropathy: Results of the P.R.I.N.C.E. Study. Prevention of Radiocontrast Induced Nephropathy Clinical Evaluation. J Am Coll Cardiol 33:403, 1999.
34. Mueller C, Buerkle G, Buettner H, et al: Prevention of contrast media–associated nephropathy: Randomized comparison of 2 hydration regimens in 1620 patients undergoing coronary angioplasty. Arch Intern Med 162:329, 2002.
35. Shammas N, Kapalis M, Harris M, et al: Aminophylline does not protect against radiocontrast nephropathy in patients undergoing percutaneous angiographic procedures. J Invasive Cardiol 13:738, 2001.
36. Allaqaband S, Tumuluri R, Malik A, et al: Prospective randomized study of *N*-acetylcysteine, fenoldopam, and saline for prevention of radiocontrast-induced nephropathy. Catheter Cardiovasc Interv 57:279, 2002.
37. Baker C, Wragg A, Kumar S, et al: A rapid protocol for the prevention of contrast-induced renal dysfunction: The RAPPID study. J Am Coll Cardiol 41:2114, 2003.
38. Diaz-Sandoval L, Kosowsky B, et al: Acetylcysteine to prevent angiography-related renal tissue injury (the APART trial). Am J Cardiol 89:356, 2002.
39. Durham J, Caputo C, Dokko J, et al: A randomized controlled trial of *N*-acetylcysteine to prevent contrast nephropathy in cardiac angiography. Kidney Int 62:2202, 2002.
40. Kay J, Chow W, Chan T, et al: Acetylcysteine for prevention of acute deterioration of renal function following elective coronary angiography and intervention: A randomized controlled trial. JAMA 289:553, 2003.
41. Shyu K, Cheng J, Kuan P: Acetylcysteine protects against acute renal damage in patients with abnormal renal function undergoing a coronary procedure. J Am Coll Cardiol 40:1383, 2002.
42. Vaitkus P: Does *N*-acetylcysteine prevent contrast-induced nephropathy? Am J Cardiol 90:1424; author reply 1424, 2002.
43. Kini A, Sharma S: Managing the high-risk patient: Experience with fenoldopam, a selective dopamine receptor agonist, in prevention of radiocontrast nephropathy during percutaneous coronary intervention. Rev Cardiovasc Med 2(Suppl 1):S19, 2001.
44. Madyoon H: Clinical experience with the use of fenoldopam for prevention of radiocontrast nephropathy in high-risk patients. Rev Cardiovasc Med 2(Suppl 1):S26, 2001.
45. Mathur V: Pathophysiology of radiocontrast nephropathy and use of fenoldopam for its prevention. Rev Cardiovasc Med 2(Suppl 1):S4, 2001.
46. Stone GW, McCullough PA, Tumlin JA, et al: Fenoldopam mesylate for the prevention of contrast-induced nephropathy: A randomized controlled trial. JAMA 290:2284, 2003.
47. Marenzi G, Bartorelli A, Lauri G, et al: Continuous veno-venous hemofiltration for the treatment of contrast-induced acute renal failure after percutaneous coronary interventions. Catheter Cardiovasc Interv 58:59, 2003.
48. Marenzi G, Marana I, Lauri G, et al: The prevention of radiocontrast-agent-induced nephropathy by hemofiltration. N Engl J Med 349:1333, 2003.
49. Frank H, Werner D, Lorusso V, et al: Simultaneous hemodialysis during coronary angiography fails to prevent radiocontrast-induced nephropathy in chronic renal failure. Clin Nephrol 60:176, 2003.
50. Lasser ED, Berry CC, Talner LB, et al: Participants. Pretreatment with corticosteroids to alleviate reactions to intravenous contrast material. N Engl J Med 317:845, 1987.
51. Gibson C, Cannon C, Murphy S, et al: Relationship of TIMI myocardial perfusion grade to mortality after administration of thrombolytic drugs. Circulation 101:125, 2000.

Coronary Anomalies

52. Harikrishnan S, Jacob S, Tharakan J, et al: Congenital coronary anomalies of origin and distribution in adults: A coronary arteriographic study. Indian Heart J 54:271, 2002.
53. Angelini P: Coronary artery anomalies—Current clinical issues: definitions, classification, incidence, clinical relevance, and treatment guidelines. Tex Heart Inst J 29:271, 2002.
54. Rapp A, Hillis L: Clinical consequences of anomalous coronary arteries. Coron Artery Dis 12:617, 2001.
55. Burma O, Rahman A, Ilkay E: Coronary arteriovenous fistulas from both coronary arteries to pulmonary artery. Eur J Cardiothorac Surg 21:86, 2002.
56. Kandzari D, Harrison J, Behar V: An anomalous left coronary artery originating from the pulmonary artery in a 72-year-old woman: Diagnosis by color flow myocardial blush and coronary arteriography. J Invasive Cardiol 14:96, 2002.
57. McConnell S, Collins K: Sudden unexpected death resulting from an anomalous hypoplastic left coronary artery. J Forensic Sci 43:708, 1998.
58. Altun A, Erdogan O: Stent implantation to the stenosed right coronary artery in a patient whose right and left coronary arteries originate from a single ostium in the right sinus of Valsalva. Cardiol Rev 11:101, 2003.
59. Fineschi M, Del SM, Leosco D, et al: A rare anatomic variation of the anomalous origin of all three major coronary arteries from the right sinus of Valsalva. G Ital Cardiol 28:564, 1998.

60. Wong C, Schreiber T: Stenting of an anomalous left circumflex coronary artery arising from the right sinus of Valsalva. Tex Med 94:64, 1998.
61. Cohen M, Tolleson T, Peter R, et al: Successful percutaneous coronary intervention with stent implantation in anomalous right coronary arteries arising from the left sinus of Valsalva: A report of two cases. Catheter Cardiovasc Interv 55:105, 2002.
62. Doorey A: Anomalous origin of the right coronary artery from the left coronary sinus. Tex Heart Inst J 29:232, 2002.
63. Garcia-Rinaldi R: Right coronary arteries that course between aorta and pulmonary artery. Ann Thorac Surg 74:973; author reply 974, 2002.
64. Serota H, Barth CW III, Seuc CA, et al: Rapid identification of the course of anomalous coronary arteries in adults: The "dot and eye" method. Am J Cardiol 65:891, 1990.
65. Rentoukas E, Alpert M, Deftereos S, et al: Anomalous left coronary artery arising from the right sinus of Valsalva in a man with unstable angina pectoris and right coronary artery stenosis. Am J Med Sci 323:223, 2002.
66. Turkay C, Golbasi I, Bayezid O: A single coronary artery from the right sinus of Valsalva associated with atherosclerosis. Acta Cardiol 57:377, 2002.

Coronary Artery Spasm

67. Auch-Schwelk W: [Coronary spasm—A clinically relevant problem?]. Herz 23:106, 1998.
68. Rozenberg V, Nepomnyashchikh L: Pathomorphology of myocardial bridges and their role in the pathogenesis of coronary disease. Bull Exp Biol Med 134:593, 2002.
69. Yoshitomi Y, Kojima S, Sugi T, et al: Coronary vasoreactivity to ergonovine after angioplasty: Difference between the infarct-related coronary artery and the noninfarct-related coronary artery. Coron Artery Dis 9:105, 1998.
70. Sueda S, Ochi N, Kawada H, et al: Frequency of provoked coronary vasospasm in patients undergoing coronary arteriography with spasm provocation test of acetylcholine. Am J Cardiol 83:1186, 1999.
71. Jeong M, Park J, Rhew J, et al: Successful management of intractable coronary spasm with a coronary stent. Jpn Circ J 64:897, 2000.

Lesion Morphology

72. Krone R, Kimmel S, Laskey W, et al: Evaluation of the Society for Coronary Angiography and Interventions' lesion classification system in 14,133 patients with percutaneous coronary interventions in the current stent era. Catheter Cardiovasc Interv 55:1, 2002.
73. Krone R, Laskey W, Johnson C, et al: A simplified lesion classification for predicting success and complications of coronary angioplasty. Registry Committee of the Society for Cardiac Angiography and Intervention. Am J Cardiol 85:1179, 2000.
74. Smith S, Dove J, Jacobs A, et al: ACC/AHA guidelines of percutaneous coronary interventions (revision of the 1993 PTCA guidelines)—Executive summary. A report of the American College of Cardiology/American Heart Association Task Force on Practice Guidelines (committee to revise the 1993 guidelines for percutaneous transluminal coronary angioplasty). J Am Coll Cardiol 37:2215, 2001.
75. Ellis SG, Vandormael MG, Cowley MJ, et al, for the Multivessel Angioplasty Prognosis Study Group: Coronary morphologic and clinical determinants of procedural outcome with angioplasty for multivessel coronary disease: Implications for patient selection. Circulation 82:1193, 1990.
76. Koerselman J, van der Graaf Y, de Jaegere PP, et al: Coronary collaterals: An important and underexposed aspect of coronary artery disease. Circulation 107:2507, 2003.
77. Wustmann K, Zbinden S, Windecker S, et al: Is there functional collateral flow during vascular occlusion in angiographically normal coronary arteries? Circulation 107:2213, 2003.
78. Werner GS, Richartz BM, Gastmann O, et al: Immediate changes of collateral function after successful recanalization of chronic total coronary occlusions. Circulation 102:2959, 2000.
79. Werner GS, Ferrari M, Betge S, et al: Collateral function in chronic total coronary occlusions is related to regional myocardial function and duration of occlusion. Circulation 104:2784, 2001.
80. Kornowski R: Collateral formation and clinical variables in obstructive coronary artery disease: The influence of hypercholesterolemia and diabetes mellitus. Coron Artery Dis 14:61, 2003.
81. Werner GS, Ferrari M, Heinke S, et al: Angiographic assessment of collateral connections in comparison with invasively determined collateral function in chronic coronary occlusions. Circulation 107:1972, 2003.
82. Billinger M, Kloos P, Eberli FR, et al: Physiologically assessed coronary collateral flow and adverse cardiac ischemic events: A follow-up study in 403 patients with coronary artery disease. J Am Coll Cardiol 40:1545, 2002.

Intravascular Ultrasound

83. Uren N, Yock P, Fitzgerald P: Intravascular ultrasound image interpretation: Normal arteries, abnormal vessels, and atheroma types pre- and post-intervention. *In* Siegel R (ed): Intravascular Ultrasound Imaging in Coronary Artery Disease. New York, Marcel Dekker, 1998, pp 19-37.
84. Matsuzaki M, Hiramori K, Imaizumi T, et al: Intravascular ultrasound evaluation of coronary plaque regression by low density lipoprotein-apheresis in familial hypercholesterolemia: The Low Density Lipoprotein-Apheresis Coronary Morphology and Reserve Trial (LACMART). J Am Coll Cardiol 40:220, 2002.
85. Mintz G, Maehara A, Bui A, et al: Multiple versus single coronary plaque ruptures detected by intravascular ultrasound in stable and unstable angina pectoris and in acute myocardial infarction. Am J Cardiol 91:1333, 2003.
86. Kornowski R, Mintz GS, Lansky AJ, et al: Paradoxic decreases in atherosclerotic plaque mass in insulin-treated diabetic patients. Am J Cardiol 81:1298, 1998.
87. Dangas G, Ambrose J, Rehmann D, et al: Balloon optimization versus stent study (BOSS): Provisional stenting and early recoil after balloon angioplasty. Am J Cardiol 85:957, 2000.
88. Oemrawsingh P, Mintz G, Schalij M, et al: Intravascular ultrasound guidance improves angiographic and clinical outcome of stent implantation for long coronary artery stenoses: Final results of a randomized comparison with angiographic guidance (TULIP Study). Circulation 107:62, 2003.
89. Ahmed J, Mintz G, Castagna M, et al: Intravascular ultrasound assessment of the mechanism of lumen enlargement during cutting balloon angioplasty treatment of in-stent restenosis. Am J Cardiol 88:1032, 2001.
90. Serruys P, Degertekin M, Tanabe K, et al: Intravascular ultrasound findings in the multicenter, randomized, double-blind RAVEL (RAndomized study with the sirolimus-eluting VElocity balloon-expandable stent in the treatment of patients with de novo native coronary artery Lesions) trial. Circulation 106:798, 2002.
91. Stahr P, Hofflinghaus T, Voigtlander T, et al: Discrimination of early/intermediate and advanced/complicated coronary plaque types by radiofrequency intravascular ultrasound analysis. Am J Cardiol 90:19, 2002.
92. Nair A, Kuban B, Tuzcu E, et al: Coronary plaque classification with intravascular ultrasound radiofrequency data analysis. Circulation 106:2200, 2002.
93. MacNeill BD, Hayase M, Jang I: The comparison between optical coherence tomography and intravascular ultrasound. Minerva Cardioangiol 50:497, 2002.

PART III

Heart Failure

CHAPTER 19

Mechanisms of Cardiac Contraction and Relaxation

Lionel H. Opie

Microanatomy of Contractile Cells and Proteins

Ultrastructure of Contractile Cells

The major function of myocardial muscle cells *(cardiomyocytes* or *myocytes)* is to execute the cardiac contraction-relaxation cycle. The contractile proteins of the heart lie within these myocytes, which constitute about 75 percent of the total volume of the myocardium although only about one-third in number of all the cells. About half of each ventricular cell is occupied by myofibers and about one-quarter to one-third by mitochondria (Table 19–1). A *myofiber* is a group of myocytes (Fig. 19–1) held together by surrounding collagen connective tissue, the latter being the major component of the extracellular matrix. Further strands of collagen connect myofibers to each other. Excess collagen, one cause of left ventricular (LV) diastolic dysfunction, accumulates as part of the growth response to LV pressure overload.

The individual contractile myocytes that account for more than half of the heart's weight are roughly cylindrical in shape. Those in the atrium are quite small, being less than 10 μm in diameter and about 20 μm in length. Relative to atrial cells, human ventricular myocytes are large, measuring about 17 to 25 μm in diameter and 60 to 140 μm in length (see Table 19–1).

When examined under the light microscope, the atrial and ventricular myocytes have cross striations and are branched. Each myocyte is bounded by a complex cell membrane, the *sarcolemma* (*sarco* = flesh; *lemma* = thin husk), and is filled with rod-like bundles of *myofibrils* (see Fig. 19–1). The latter are the contractile elements. The sarcolemma of the myocyte invaginates to form an extensive tubular network (the *T tubules*) that extends the extracellular space into the interior of the cell (Fig. 19–2; see Fig. 19–1). The nucleus, which contains almost all of the cell's genetic information, is often centrally located. Some myocytes have several nuclei. Interspersed between the myofibrils and immediately beneath the sarcolemma are many mitochondria, the main function of which is to generate the energy in the form of adenosine triphosphate (ATP) needed to maintain the heart's contractile function and the associated ion gradients. Of the other organelles, the *sarcoplasmic reticulum* (SR) is most important (see Fig. 19–1).

When the wave of electrical excitation reaches the closely approximated T tubules, the tubular calcium channels open to admit a relatively small amount of calcium to trigger the release of much more calcium from the calcium release channels of the SR. This is the calcium that initiates myocardial contraction. When the calcium is once again taken up into the SR, relaxation ensues.

Anatomically, the SR is a fine network spreading throughout the myocytes, demarcated by its lipid bilayer, which is rather similar to that of the sarcolemma. The *calcium release channels* (also called the *ryanodine receptors*) are found in the expanded parts of the SR that lie in very close apposition to the T tubules. These are called *subsarcolemmal cisternae* (boxes or baskets, Latin) or the *junctional SR*. The second part of the SR, the *longitudinal or network SR*, consists of ramifying tubules (see Fig. 19–1) and is concerned with the uptake of calcium that initiates relaxation. This uptake is achieved by the ATP-requiring calcium pump, also called *SERCA* (sarcoendoplasmic reticulum Ca^{2+}-adenosine triphosphatase [ATPase]), which increases its activity in response to beta-adrenergic stimulation. Calcium taken up into the SR is then stored at high concentration in a number of storage proteins including *calsequestrin* before being released again in response to the next wave of depolarization.

TABLE 19–1 Characteristics of Cardiac Cells, Organelles, and Contractile Proteins

	Microanatomy of Heart Cells		
Characteristic	***Ventricular Myocyte***[a]	***Atrial Myocyte***	***Purkinje Cells***
Shape	Long and narrow	Elliptical	Long and broad
Length, μm	60-140	About 20	150-200
Diameter, μm	About 20	5-6	35-40
Volume, μm^3	15,000-45,000	About 500	135,000-250,000
T-tubules	Plentiful	Rare or none	Absent
Intercalated disc	Prominent end-to-end transmission	Side-to-side as well as end-to-end transmission	Very prominent abundant gap junctions. Fast; end-to-end transmission
General appearance	Mitochondria and sarcomeres very abundant. Rectangular branching bundles with little interstitial collagen	Bundles of atrial tissue separated by wide areas of collagen	Fewer sarcomeres, paler
	Composition and Function of Ventricular Cell		
Organelle	***% of Cell Volume***	***Function***	
Myofibril	About 50-60	Interaction of thick and thin filaments during contraction cycle	
Mitochondria	16 in neonate 33 in adult rat 23 in adult human	Provide adenosine triphosphate chiefly for contraction	
T system	About 1	Transmission of electrical signal from sarcolemma to cell interior	
Sarcoplasmic reticulum (SR)	33 in neonate 2 in adult	Takes up and releases Ca^{2+} during contraction cycle	
Terminal cisternae of SR	0.33 in adult	Site of calcium storage and release	
Rest of network of SR	Rest of volume	Site of calcium uptake en route to cisternae	
Sarcolemma	Very low	Control of ionic gradients; channels for ions (action potential); maintenance of cell integrity; receptors for drugs and hormones	
Nucleus	About 5	Protein synthesis	
Lysosomes	Very low	Intracellular digestion and proteolysis	
Sarcoplasm (= cytoplasm) (+ nuclei + other structures)	About 12 in adult rat 18 in humans	Provides cytosol in which rise and fall of ionized calcium occur; contains other ions and small molecules	

The *cytoplasm* is the intracellular fluid and proteins therein, contained within the sarcolemma but excluding the contents of organelles such as mitochondria and the SR. The fluid component of the cytoplasm, minus the proteins, is called the *cytosol.* It is in the cytosol that the concentrations of calcium ions rise and fall to cause cardiac contraction and relaxation. The proteins of the sarcoplasm include myriads of specialized molecules, the *enzymes* that accelerate the conversion of one chemical form to another, thereby stimulating crucial metabolic or signaling paths and eventually promoting energy production.

SUBCELLULAR MICROARCHITECTURE. The molecular signal systems that convey messages from surface receptors to intracellular organelles may be directed to specific sites by molecules that "anchor" components of the internal messenger chain to specific organelles, as when the beta-adrenergic chain must link up with the calcium pump of the SR (see later). *Scaffolding proteins* bring interacting molecules closely together as in the case of the signaling chain leading to myocyte growth. An example of physiological subcellular compartmentation is the local unloading of ATP where it is needed by the exact location of the enzyme creatine kinase, which converts creatine phosphate to ATP. "In the world of intracellular real estate, location, location, and location are the key determinants of in vivo function."[1]

Contractile Proteins

The major molecules involved in the contraction-relaxation cycle are the two chief contractile proteins, the thin actin filament and the thick myosin filament (see Fig. 19–1). Calcium ions initiate the contraction cycle by interacting with troponin C to relieve the inhibition otherwise exerted by troponin I (Fig. 19–3). Titin is a newly discovered large elastic molecule that supports myosin (Fig. 19–4). During contraction, the filaments slide over each other without the individual molecules of actin or myosin actually shortening. As they slide, they pull together the two ends of the fundamental contractile unit called the *sarcomere.* On electron microscopy, the sarcomere is limited on either side by the *Z line* (Z, abbreviation for German *Zückung*, contraction) to which the actin filaments are attached (see Fig. 19–2). Conversely, the myosin filaments extend from the center of the sarcomere in either direction toward but not actually reaching the Z lines (see Fig. 19–1).

The interaction of the myosin heads with actin filaments when sufficient calcium arrives from the SR (see Fig. 19–1) is called *cross-bridge cycling.* As the actin filaments move inward toward the center of the sarcomere, they draw the Z lines closer together so that the sarcomere shortens. The energy for this shortening is provided by the breakdown of ATP, chiefly made in the mitochondria.

TITIN AND LENGTH SENSING. Titin is a giant molecule, the largest protein yet described. It is an extraordinarily long, flexible, and slender myofibrillar protein (see Fig. 19–4). Titin acts as a third filament to provide elasticity. Being between 0.6 and 1.2 mm in length, the titin molecule extends from the Z line stopping just short of the M line (see Fig. 19–1). It has two distinct segments: an inextensible anchoring segment and an extensible elastic segment that stretches as sarcomere length increases.

Titin has multiple functions. First, it tethers the myosin molecule to the Z line (see Fig. 19–2), thereby stabilizing the contractile proteins. Second, as it stretches and relaxes, its elasticity explains the stress-strain relation of cardiac and skeletal muscle. At short sarcomere lengths, the elastic domain is folded on itself to generate restoring forces (see Fig. 19–4). These changes in titin help to explain the *series elastic element*, the postulate being that there is elasticity in series between the contractile elements and the ends of the muscle. Third, increased diastolic stretch of titin as the sarcomere length of cardiac muscle is increased causes the enfolded part of the titin molecule to straighten. This stretched molecular spring then contracts more vigorously in systole.[2] Such enhanced systolic contraction helps to explain the Frank-Starling mechanism (see later). Fourth, titin may transduce mechanical stretch into growth signals. In sustained diastolic stretch as in volume overload, the elastic segment of titin is constantly under strain and transmits this mechanical signal to the muscle LIM (Lin-11 and mec-3) protein (MLP) that is attached to the terminal part of titin that forms part of the Z disc complex.[3] The MLP is proposed as the stretch sensor that transmits the signals that result in the myocyte growth pattern characteristic of volume overload.[3] This signal system may be defective in a subset of human dilated cardiomyopathy.[3]

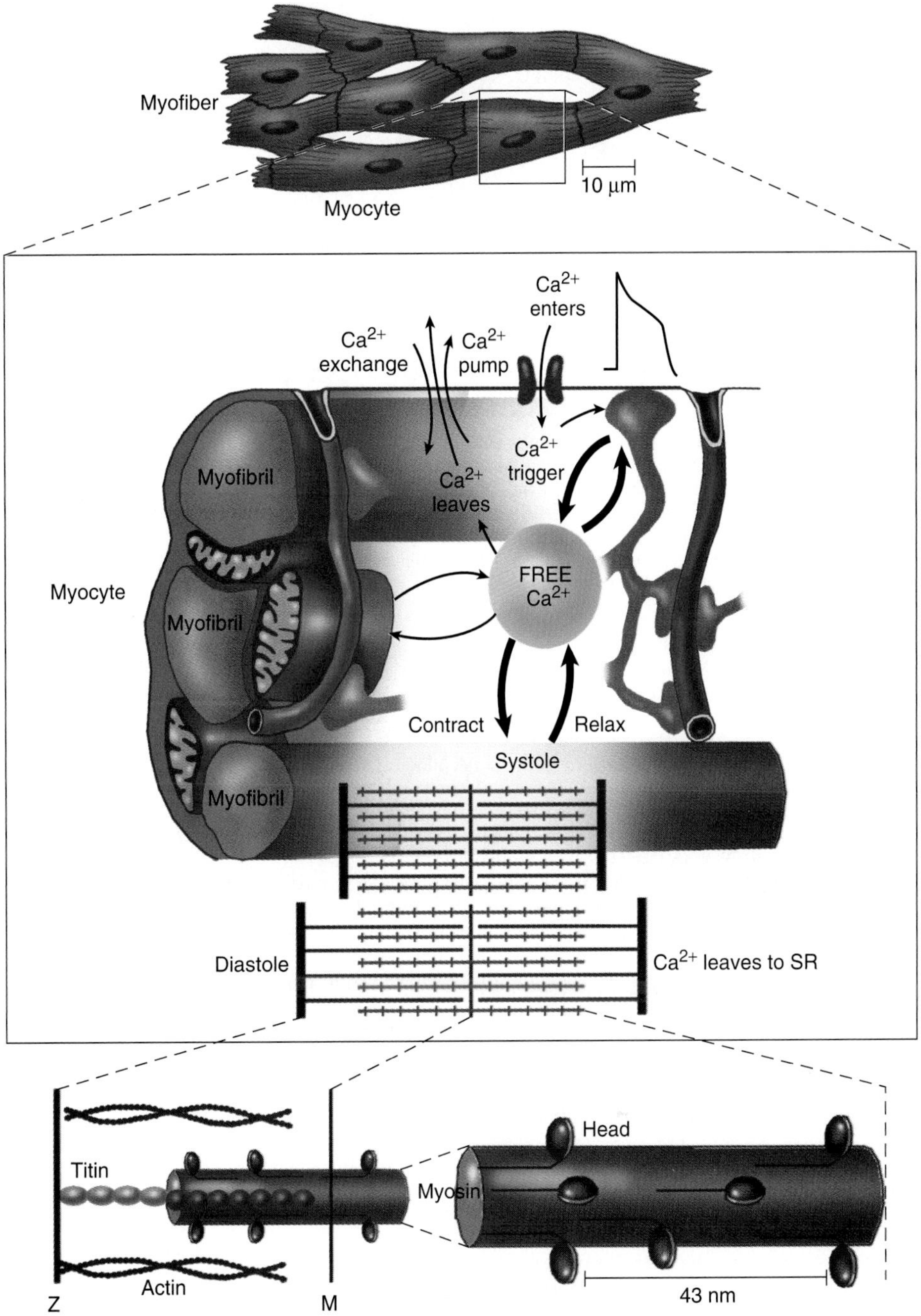

FIGURE 19–1 The crux of the contractile process lies in the changing concentrations of Ca^{2+} ions in the myocardial cytosol. Ca^{2+} ions are schematically shown as entering through the calcium channel that opens in response to the wave of depolarization that travels along the sarcolemma. These Ca^{2+} ions "trigger" the release of more calcium from the sarcoplasmic reticulum (SR) and thereby initiate a contraction-relaxation cycle. Eventually, the small amount of calcium that has entered the cell leaves predominantly through an Na^+/Ca^{2+} exchanger with a lesser role for the sarcolemmal calcium pump. The varying actin-myosin overlap is shown for systole, when calcium ions arrive, and diastole, when calcium ions leave. The myosin heads, attached to the thick filaments, interact with the thin actin filaments, as shown in Figure 19–6. For the role of titin, see Figure 19–4. The upper panel shows the difference between the myocardial cell or myocyte and the myofiber, composed of many myocytes. MITO = mitochondria. (The upper panel is from Braunwald E, Ross J, Sonnenblick EH: Mechanisms of Contraction of the Normal and Failing Heart. 2nd ed. Boston, Little Brown, 1976. The other panels are from Opie LH: Heart Physiology, from Cell to Circulation. Philadelphia, Lippincott Williams & Wilkins, 2004. Copyright L. H. Opie, © 2004.)

STRONG AND WEAK BINDING STATES. Although at a molecular level the events underlying the cross-bridge cycle are exceedingly complex, one simple current hypothesis is that the cross bridges exist in either a strong or a weak binding state.[4] The arrival of calcium ions at the contractile proteins is a crucial link in the series of events known as *excitation-contraction coupling*. The ensuing interaction of calcium with troponin C and the deinhibition of troponin I put the cross bridges in the strong binding state. As long as enough calcium ions are present, the strong binding state potentially dominates. If, however, the strong binding state were continuously present, the contractile proteins could never relax. Thus, the proposal is that the binding of ATP to the myosin head puts the cross bridges into a weak binding state even when calcium is high.[4]

Conversely, when ATP is hydrolyzed to adenosine diphosphate (ADP) and inorganic phosphate (P_i), the strong binding state again predominates (Fig. 19-5). Thus, the ATP-induced changes in the molecular

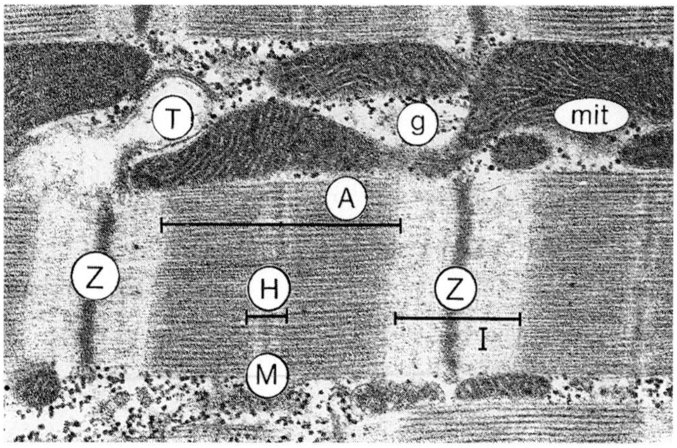

FIGURE 19–2 The sarcomere is the distance between the two Z lines. Note the presence of numerous mitochondria (mit) sandwiched between the myofibrils and the presence of T tubules (T), which penetrate into the muscle at the level of the Z lines. This two-dimensional picture should not disguise the fact that the Z line is really a "Z disc," as is the M line (M), also shown in Figure 19–1. A = band of actin-myosin overlap; g = glycogen granules; H = central clear zone containing only myosin filament bodies and the M line; I = band of actin filaments, titin, and Z line. Rat papillary muscle, ×32,000. (Courtesy of Dr. J. Moravec, Dijon, France.)

configuration of the myosin head result in corresponding variations in the physical properties (a similar concept is common in metabolic regulation). Length activation also promotes the strong binding state (see Length-Dependent Activation). Conversely, the weak binding state predominates when cytosolic calcium levels fall at the start of diastole. As the calcium ions leave troponin C, a master switch is turned off and tropomyosin again assumes the inhibitory configuration.

ACTIN AND TROPONIN COMPLEX. Although calcium ions provide the essential switch-on signal to the cross-bridge cycle by binding to troponin C, current evidence suggests more than an "on-off" signaling process. Rather, the arrival of calcium initiates a series of interactions between the troponin components of the thin filament to allow movement of the tropomyosin molecule, which in turn promotes the strong binding state so that contraction takes place. To understand the role of calcium first requires a brief description of the molecular structure of actin and the troponin complex. Thin filaments are composed of two actin units, which intertwine in a helical pattern, both being carried on a heavier tropomyosin molecule that functions as a "backbone" (see Fig. 19-5A). At regular intervals of 38.5 nm along this twisting structure is a closely bound group of three regulatory proteins called the *troponin complex*. Of these three, it is troponin C that responds to the calcium ions that are released in large amounts from the SR to start the cross-bridge cycle.

Schematically, when the cytosolic calcium level is low, the tropomyosin molecule is twisted in such a way that the myosin heads cannot interact with actin (see Fig. 19-3D). Thereby most cross bridges are in the "blocked position," although some are still in the weakly binding state.[5] As calcium ions increasingly arrive at the start of the contractile cycle and interact with troponin C, the activated troponin C binds tightly to the inhibitory molecule, troponin I. The latter moves to a new position on the thin filament, thereby weakening the interaction between troponin T and tropomyosin (see Fig. 19-3D). Ultimately, tropomyosin is repositioned on the thin filament,[5] thereby removing most of the inhibition exerted by tropomyosin on the actin-myosin interaction. Thus, weakly bound or blocked cross bridges enter the strongly bound state, and the cross-bridge cycle is initiated. As the strong cross bridges form, they activate "near neighbors" and thereby spread the activation process.[5] They also promote further tropomyosin movement to cause more forceful cross-bridge interaction.

MYOSIN AND MOLECULAR BASIS OF MUSCULAR CONTRACTION. Each myosin head is the terminal part of a heavy chain. The bodies of two of these chains intertwine, and each terminates in a short "neck" that carries the elongated myosin head (see Fig. 19–3B). According to the model of Rayment and colleagues,[6] it is the base of the head, also sometimes called the neck, that changes configuration in the contractile cycle. Together with the "bodies" of all the other heads, the myosin thick filament is formed. Each lobe of the bilobed head has an *ATP-binding pocket* (also called nucleotide pocket) and a narrow cleft that extends from the base of this pocket to the actin-binding face.[6] ATP and its breakdown products ADP and P_i bind to the nucleotide pocket in close proximity to the myosin ATPase activity that breaks down ATP to its products (see Fig. 19–3B).

Currently, there is controversy about the role in the contractile cycle of the narrow *actin-binding cleft* that splits the central 50-kDa segment of the myosin head. According to the revised Rayment model,[7] this cleft responds to the binding of ATP or its breakdown products to the nucleotide pocket in such a way that the conformational changes necessary for movement of the head are produced. According to Dominguez and colleagues,[8] the cleft is closed in the weakly attached states before the power stroke (see Fig. 19–5) but opens when P_i is released through the cleft, whereupon the myosin head attaches strongly to actin to induce the power stroke (see Fig. 19–5D and E).

Starting with the rigor state (see Fig. 19–5A), the binding of ATP to its pocket changes the molecular configuration of the myosin head so that the head detaches from actin to terminate the rigor state (see Fig. 19–5B). Next, the ATPase activity of the myosin head splits ATP into ADP and P_i and the head flexes (see Fig. 19–5C). As ATP is hydrolyzed, the myosin head binds to an adjacent actin unit. Then P_i is released from the head through the cleft, and there is strong binding of the myosin head to actin (see Fig. 19–5D). Next, the head extends, i.e., straightens. A power stroke takes place, the actin molecule moves by about 10 nm,[8] and the myosin head is now in the rigor state. The pocket then releases ADP, ready for acceptance of ATP and repetition of the cycle.

The Rayment model[6] postulates straightening and not flexion of the light chain region of the head (i.e., the neck) that produces the power stroke. The lever-arm model[9] is more applicable to many cells and organelles that depend on movement of myosin rather than of actin, for example, for intracellular transport. By contrast, in contracting cardiomyocytes, myosin is fixed and tethered by titin and myosin binding protein C. The lever-arm model proposes that movements of the neck, which is the lever arm, produce large displacements that translate into movement of the whole myosin molecule. This model provides evolutionary data that reinforce the crucial nature of movements of the myosin neck (shown as the flexible domain in Fig. 19–5C).

MYOSIN ATPase ACTIVITY. This activity normally responds to calcium in such a way that increases in calcium concentrations that are associated with the contraction cycle in the whole heart result in a severalfold increase in the myosin ATPase activity besides increasing calcium binding to troponin C and force development.[10]

MYOSIN HEAVY CHAIN ISOFORMS. These isoforms help regulate myosin ATPase activity. Each myosin filament consists of two heavy chains, the bodies of which are intertwined and each ending in one head, and four light chains, two in apposition to each head. The heavy chains, containing the myosin ATPase activity on the heads, occur in two isoforms, beta and alpha, of the same molecular weight but with substantially different ATPase activities. The beta myosin heavy chain (beta-MHC) isoform has lower ATPase activity and is the predominant form in the adult human. The faster alpha-MHC component decreases and the slower beta-MHC pattern increases in human heart failure.[11]

MYOSIN HEADS: TWO ARE BETTER THAN ONE. The double-headed structure is required to produce the full displacement of actin, about 10 nm, versus only 6 nm with single-headed myosin.[12]

THE MYOSIN NECK. The myosin neck is chiefly formed by long alpha helix (see Fig. 19-3B), surrounded by two *light chains* (four per bilobed head) that act as a cervical collar. The light chain that is more proximal to the myosin head, the *essential light chain* (myosin light chain-1 [MLC-1]), may inhibit the contractile process by interaction with actin. The other *regulatory light chain* (MLC-2) is a potential site for phosphorylation, for example, in response to beta-adrenergic stimulation. Such phosphorylation (i.e., the gaining of a phosphate grouping) may promote cross-bridge cycling by increasing the affinity of myosin for actin.[13] Mutation of this light chain in one type of human cardiomyopathy impairs the contractile response to tachycardia.[14] In vascular smooth muscle, the phosphorylation that occurs under the influence of the enzyme myosin light chain kinase (MLCK) is an obligatory step in the initiation of the contractile process.

MYOSIN BINDING PROTEIN C. This protein runs at approximate right angles to the myosin molecules to tether myosin molecules by linking the structures that lie around subfragments of the myosin heads. This binding protein stabilizes the myosin head as it flexes and extends at the level of the light chains. Defects in binding protein C may be involved in some types of hypertrophic cardiomyopathy.

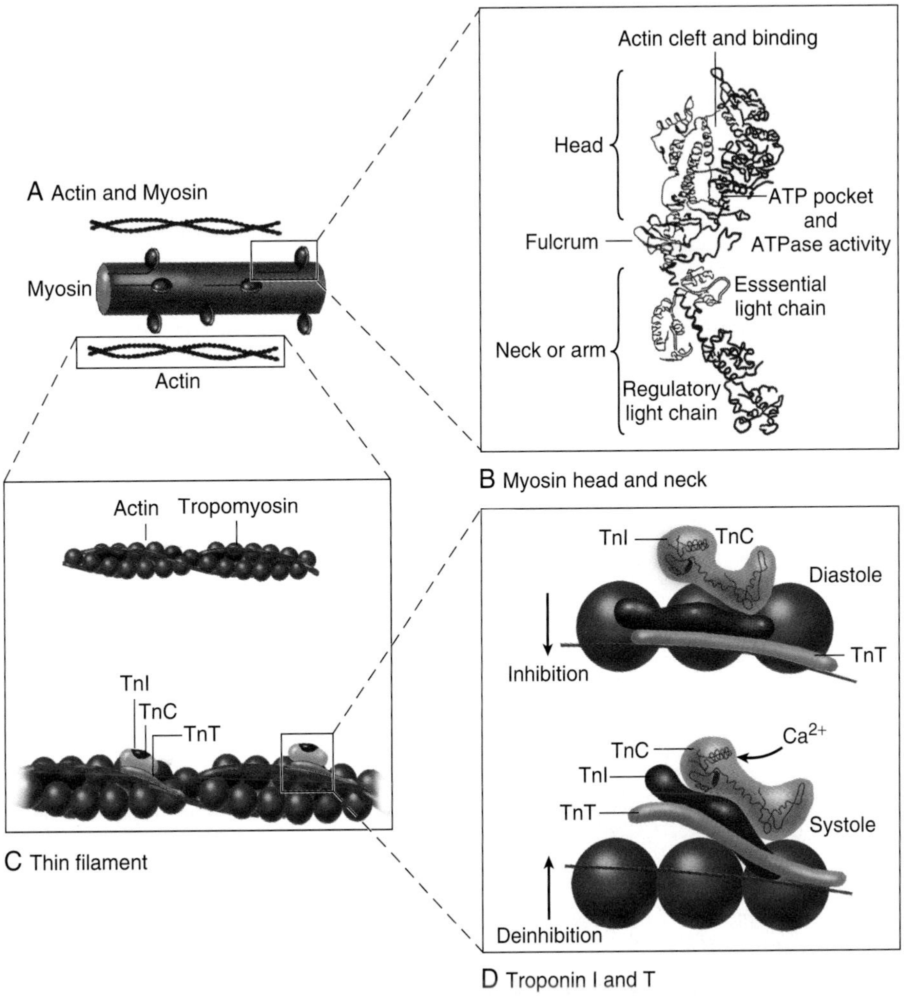

FIGURE 19–3 The major molecules of the contractile system. The thin actin filament **(A)** interacts with the myosin head **(B)** when Ca^{2+} ions arrive at troponin C (TnC) **(C)**. A complex interaction between TnC and the other troponins moves tropomyosin to "uncover" an actin site to which a myosin head can attach (see Fig. 19–5). The molecular aspects are as follows. **A,** The thin actin filament contains TnC and its Ca^{2+} binding sites. When TnC is not activated by Ca^{2+}, troponin I (TnI) inhibits the actin-myosin interaction. Troponin T (TnT) may also participate in the activation cycle **(D)**. **B,** Myosin head molecular structure, based on Rayment and colleagues,[6] is composed of heavy and light chains. The heavy head chain in turn has two major domains: one of 70 kDa (i.e., molecular weight 70,000) that interacts with actin at the actin cleft and has an ATP-binding pocket. The "neck" domain of 20 kDa, also called the "lever," is an elongated alpha helix that extends and bends and has two light chains surrounding it as a collar. The essential light chain is part of the structure. The other regulatory light chain may respond to phosphorylation to influence the extent of the actin-myosin interaction. **C,** TnC with sites in the regulatory domain for activation by calcium and for interaction with TnI. **D,** Calcium binding to TnC induces a conformational change in TnC that elongates (compare systole with diastole). TnI closes up to TnC, and the normal inhibition of TnI on actin-tropomyosin is lessened. There is a strengthening of the interaction between TnC and TnT. These changes allow repositioning of tropomyosin in relation to actin, with lessening of its normal inhibitory effects, as shown in the bottom panel. Now the contractile cycle can start. ATP = adenosine triphosphate; ATPase = adenosine triphosphatase. (Modified from Opie LH: Heart Physiology, from Cell to Circulation. Philadelphia, Lippincott Williams & Wilkins, 2004. Copyright L. H. Opie, © 2004. **D,** Modified from Solaro RJ, Van Eyk J: Altered interactions among thin filament proteins modulate cardiac function. J Mol Cell Cardiol 28:217, 1999.)

GRADED EFFECTS OF INCREASED CYTOSOLIC CALCIUM LEVELS ON THE CROSS-BRIDGE CYCLE. Calcium ions play a crucial role in linking external neurohumoral control of the heart to stimulation of the contractile process by acting at multiple control sites[5,10]; calcium interaction with troponin C is essential for cross-bridge cycling. Does calcium act as an on-off switch to regulate the total number of cycling cross bridges? According to this proposal, the enhanced force development in response to a greater calcium ion concentration must be due to recruitment of additional cross bridges. Alternatively, to explain the graded model, there may be (1) a graded response of troponin C to calcium ions, including altered rates of calcium binding and release; (2) a graded response of myosin ATPase to calcium; (3) near-neighbor self-activation whereby the actin-myosin interaction activates additional cross bridges even in the absence of increased binding of calcium to the troponin C of those cross bridges[5]; or (4) alterations in the extent of myosin light chain phosphorylation.[13] Of specific interest is the proposal that tightly bound cross bridges act to spread activation to near-neighbor units to achieve full activation.[5] By such mechanisms, one calcium-troponin complex could turn on as many as 14 actin molecules.

LENGTH-DEPENDENT ACTIVATION. Besides the cytosolic calcium concentration, the other major factor influencing the strength of contraction is the length of the muscle fiber at the end of diastole, just before the onset of systole. Starling observed that the greater the volume of the heart in diastole, the more forceful the contraction. The increased heart volume translates into an increased muscle length, which acts by a length-sensing mechanism (Fig. 19–6). Previously, this relation was ascribed to a more optimal overlap between actin and myosin. The current view is that an increased sarcomere length leads to greater sensitivity of the contractile apparatus to the prevailing cytosolic calcium ion concentration.[5] A plausible mechanism for this regulatory change may reside in the decreasing interfilament spacing as the heart muscle is stretched.[5] This rather satisfactory lattice-dependent explanation for the Frank-Starling relationship has been dealt a setback by the careful x-ray diffraction studies of de Tombe's group.[15] Reducing sarcomere lattice spacing by osmotic compression failed to influence calcium sensitivity. Alternatively, sarcomere stretch increases the passive forces built up by titin,[16] which could in turn hypothetically influence the position of myosin heads. Another proposal, that troponin C is the length sensor, is currently less favored.[5] Probably several mechanisms are at work.

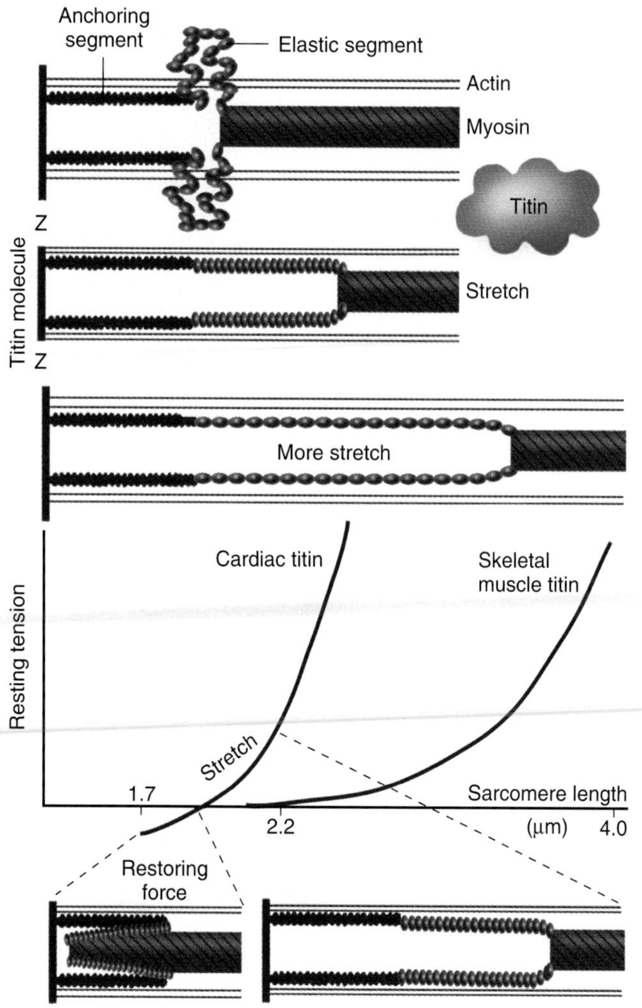

FIGURE 19–4 Titin, a very large elongated protein with elasticity, binds myosin to the Z line. It may act as a bidirectional spring that develops passive forces in stretched sarcomeres and resting forces in shortened sarcomeres. As the sarcomere is stretched to its maximum physiological diastolic length of 2.2 mm (Fig. 19–23), titin first undergoes straightening (up to 2 μm) and then elongation, the latter rapidly increasing the passive forces generated. At low sarcomere lengths, when sarcomeres are slack at about the diastolic limit of 1.85 mm (Fig. 19–23), the mechanically active elastic domain is folded on top of itself. At even shorter lengths, which may not be physiological in the intact heart, substantial restoring forces are generated. (Modified with permission of the American Heart Association from Trombitas K, Jian-Ping J, Granzier H: The mechanically active domain of titin in cardiac muscle. Circ Res 77:856, 1995, and Helmes M, Trombitas K, Granzier H: Titin develops restoring force in rat cardiac myocytes. Circ Res 79:619, 1996.)

CROSS-BRIDGE CYCLING DIFFERS FROM CARDIAC CONTRACTION-RELAXATION CYCLE. The cardiac cycle of Wiggers (see Fig. 19-19) must be distinguished from the cross-bridge cycle. The former reflects the overall pressure changes in the left ventricle, whereas the latter cycle is the repetitive interaction between myosin heads and actin. According to the Rayment model, the binding of ATP or ADP regulates in part whether the cross bridges are weak or strong in nature (see Fig. 19-5). As long as enough calcium ions are bound to troponin C, many repetitive cycles of this nature occur. Thus, at any given moment, some myosin heads are flexing or flexed, some are extending or extended, and some are attached to actin and some detached from actin. Numerous such cross-bridge cycles, each lasting only a few microseconds, actively move the thin actin filaments toward the central bare area of the thick myosin filaments, thereby shortening the sarcomere. The sum total of all the shortening sarcomeres leads to systole, which is the contraction phase of the cardiac cycle. When calcium ions depart from their binding sites on troponin C, cross-bridge cycling cannot occur, and the diastolic phase of the cardiac cycle sets in.

MYOFILAMENT RESPONSE TO HEMODYNAMIC DEMANDS. Solaro and Rarick[5] hypothesized that myofilament activity is coupled to the prevailing hemodynamic demands of the circulation. Besides length-dependent activation, there are two chief mechanisms. First, there may be variable rates of calcium binding and release from troponin C (as discussed in a previous section). Second, phosphorylation and dephosphorylation of the contractile proteins may help to control the extent of activation of the myofilaments. Thus, increased beta-adrenergic-dependent phosphorylation of troponin I *reduces* the myofilament sensitivity to calcium and thereby leads to an *increased* rate of relaxation during beta-adrenergic stimulation.[13] Hypothetically, this mechanism enhances the relaxant (lusitropic) effect of increased uptake rates of calcium into the SR. The effects of phosphorylation of other proteins such the myosin essential light chains and C protein, still imperfectly understood, may also be important.[5]

FORCE TRANSMISSION. Volume overload and pressure overload may owe their different effects on myocardial growth to different patterns of force transmission. Whereas increased diastolic forces are transmitted longitudinally through titin to reach the postulated sensor, the MLP (see earlier, Titin and Length Sensing), increased systolic forces may be transmitted laterally (that is, at right angles) through the Z disc and cytoplasmic actin to reach the proteins of the cell-to-matrix junctions such as the focal adhesion complex. How these mechanical forces become translated into signals that activate the growth pathways such as those leading to mitogen-activated protein (MAP) kinase still remains to be discovered.

CONTRACTILE PROTEINS AND CARDIOMYOPATHY (see Chap. 59). The concept is that genetically based hypertrophic and dilated cardiomyopathies not only produce hearts that look and behave very differently but also have diverse molecular etiologies. Hypertrophic cardiomyopathy is, in general, linked to mutant genes that cause abnormalities in the force-generating system, such as beta-MHC. Less commonly, there may be defects in the genes encoding troponin T, myosin light chain isoforms, troponin I and C isoforms, myosin binding protein C, and alpha-tropomyosin. In some human familial cases, there are abnormalities in the enzyme that functions as the "fuel gauge of the cell," adenosine monophosphate (AMP)–activated protein kinase, giving rise to the current hypothesis that the mutations all impair the contractile response, with less force generated per ATP expenditure. This defect is postulated to induce a compensatory hypertrophy in the remaining fibers.[17]

In contrast, dilated cardiomyopathy can be related to mutations in non-force-generating cytoskeletal proteins, such as dystrophin, nuclear lamin, cytoplasmic actin, and titin. This distinction between the two types of cardiomyopathy remains useful but not totally true. For example, abnormal actin and titin have been found in hypertrophic cardiomyopathy and abnormal myosin in dilated cardiomyopathy. Chien's group postulated that at least in some cases of dilated cardiomyopathy, there is a defect of the length sensor.[3] The Seidman group found a family with dilated cardiomyopathy and early death from heart failure related to enhanced activity of phospholamban, the proposed mechanism being inhibition of the calcium uptake pump of the SR and limitation of normal calcium cycling.[18]

Calcium Ion Fluxes in Cardiac Contraction-Relaxation Cycle

Calcium Movements and Excitation-Contraction Coupling

Calcium has a crucial role in regulating the contraction and relaxation phases of the cardiac cycle. The details of the associated calcium ion fluxes that link contraction to the wave of excitation (*excitation-contraction coupling*) are now reasonably well clarified.[19] The generally accepted hypothesis is based on the crucial role of *calcium-induced calcium release* from the SR. Relatively small amounts of calcium ions, the *trigger calcium ions*, actually enter and leave the cardiomyocyte during each cardiac cycle, whereas much larger amounts move in and out of the SR (Fig. 19–7). The basic proposal is that each wave of depolarization traveling down the T tubules opens the L-type calcium channels that are physically closely approximated to the part of the SR lying close to the T tubule to activate the calcium release channels, collectively called the *ryanodine receptors*. Depolarization thereby releases relatively large amounts of calcium ions into the cytosol in response to the much smaller amounts entering the cardiomyocyte.[19] This process elevates by about 10-fold the concentration of calcium ions in the cytosol. The result is the increasing interaction of calcium ions with troponin C to trigger the contractile process.

This theory has received strong support from several sources: (1) the tight proximity of the ryanodine receptors on the SR to the L-type calcium channels of the T tubules; (2) the molecular characterization of the calcium-releasing ryanodine receptor on the SR (Fig. 19–8); (3) proof of the control of this receptor not only by calcium ions but also by beta-adrenergic-mediated phosphorylation and by binding proteins of the FK506 binding protein (FKBP) family[20]; and (4) electrophysiological evidence closely linking the duration of the action potential with the extent of Ca^{2+} release.[19]

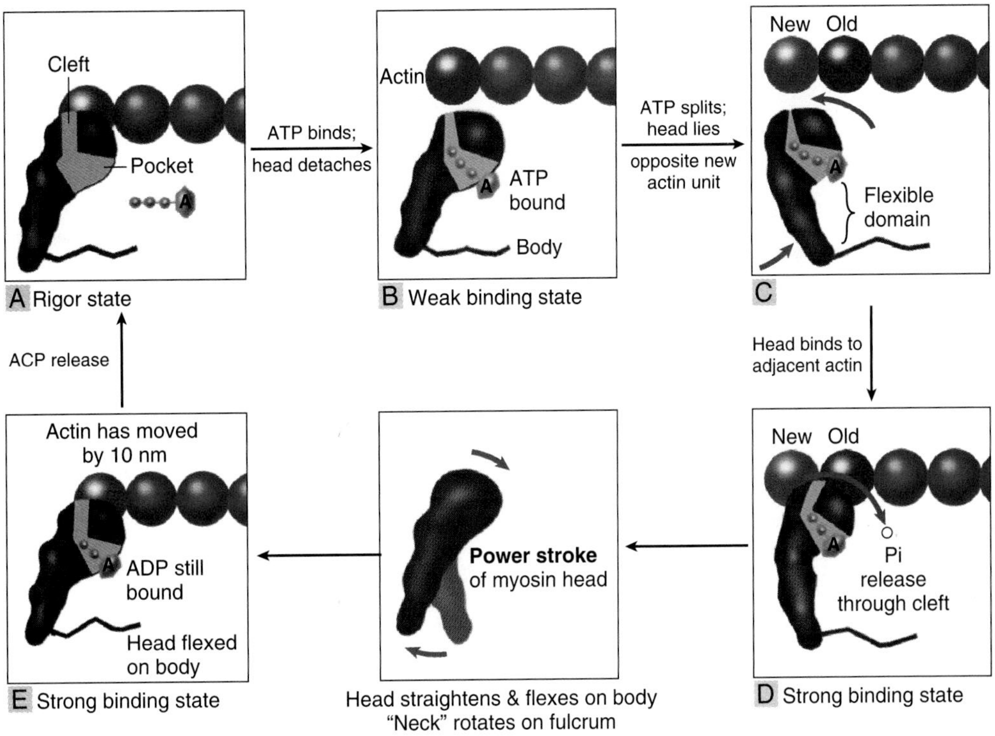

FIGURE 19–5 Cross-bridge cycling molecular model updated by the present author from the five-step model of Rayment and colleagues[6] for interaction between the myosin head and the actin filament, taking into account other models.[8,139,140] The cross bridge (only one myosin head depicted) is pear shaped and consists of the catalytic motor domain that interacts with the actin molecule and an extended alpha helical "neck region" acting as a lever arm.[8] The nucleotide pocket receiving and binding adenosine triphosphate (ATP) is a depression near the center of the catalytic domain. The actin-binding cleft bisects the catalytic motor domain. During the cross-bridge cycle, the width of the actin-binding cleft changes in size, although details remain controversial. Starting with the rigor state **(A)**, the binding of ATP to the pocket **(B)** is followed by ATP hydrolysis **(C)** that partly closes the actin-binding cleft. The cleft opens when phosphate is released (through the cleft rather than through the pocket) and the myosin head strongly attaches to actin to induce the power stroke **(D, E)**. During the power stroke, the latter rotates about a fulcrum in the region where the helix terminates within the catalytic motor domain.[8] As the head flexes, the actin filament is displaced by about 10 nm **(E)**. In the process adenosine diphosphate is also released so that the binding pocket becomes vacant. Finally, the rigor state is reached again **(A)** when the myosin head is again ready to receive ATP to reinitiate the cross-bridge cycle. Throughout, the actin monomer with which the myosin head is interacting is shown in orange. Pi = inorganic phosphate. (Professor J. C. Rüegg of Heidelberg University, Germany, is thanked for valuable comments.)

Calcium Release Channels of the Sarcoplasmic Reticulum

RYANODINE RECEPTORS. Each L-type calcium channel of the sarcolemma controls a cluster of possibly 6 to 20 SR release channels by virtue of close anatomical proximity of the calcium channels on the T tubules to the calcium release channels, situated on the SR. The calcium release channel is part of the complex structure known as the *ryanodine receptor*, so called because it coincidentally binds the potent insecticide ryanodine and is often abbreviated to RyR2 to indicate the cardiac isoform.

Ryanodine receptors have a dual function, containing the calcium release channels of the SR and acting as scaffolding proteins that localize numerous key regulatory proteins to the junctional complexes.[19] These proteins include those that respond to phosphorylation by protein kinase A (PKA) and its anchoring protein, AKAP, to enhance channel opening (see Figs. 19-8 and 19-11), phosphatases that work in the opposite direction, and binding proteins (technical term: FKBP-506 and others) that are thought to coordinate opening of neighboring ryanodine calcium channels by the process of *coupled gating*.

The anatomical basis of the scaffolding function is that part of the ryanodine receptor extends from the membrane of the SR toward the T tubule to constitute the *junctional calcium release complex* that bridges the gap between the SR and the T tubule. Here the ryanodine receptors are packed in large organized arrays of perhaps 50 to 300 per junction. The ryanodine receptor is very large, and four of them link to form a megacomplex containing one calcium release channel (see Fig. 19-8) Added to this are all the proteins adhering to the complex through their binding sites so that the total megacomplex has a molecular weight approximating that of titin. After the wave of depolarization has reached the T tubule and opened the voltage-operated L-type calcium channels, the trigger calcium ions enter the cardiomyocyte to reach the junctional regions of the SR with their ryanodine receptors. The result is a change in the molecular configuration of the ryanodine receptor that opens the calcium release channel of the SR to discharge calcium ions into the subsarcolemmal space between the foot and the T tubule and thence into the cytosol.

TURN-OFF OF CALCIUM RELEASE. The rise of cytosolic calcium that triggers contraction comes to an end as the wave of excitation passes, no more calcium ions enter, and the release of calcium from the SR ceases. This turn-off of release is not as well understood as control of calcium release from the SR but is important in avoiding cytosolic calcium overload with potentially serious consequences such as arrhythmias and impaired contraction-relaxation cycles. There are several proposals to explain turn-off, as follows: (1) the rising cytosolic calcium ion concentration inhibits the release process; (2) the rising cytosolic calcium ion concentration can activate the calcium uptake pump of the SR; (3) the SR becomes locally depleted of calcium; or (4) the ryanodine receptor is inactivated so that it becomes resistant to the prevailing calcium concentration.[19] The overall effect of these mechanisms is that the cytosolic calcium ion concentration starts to fall and diastole is initiated. As the cytosolic calcium decreases, calcium binding to troponin C lessens, tropomyosin again starts to inhibit the interaction between actin and myosin, and relaxation proceeds.

CALCIUM SPARKS. These are the very small amounts of calcium spontaneously and locally released from the SR even in the absence of L-channel opening. Hypothetically, the spark represents the spontaneous opening of one or at the most a cluster of calcium release channels. There is so little calcium diffusing away from a spark, that it fails to activate the neighboring calcium release channels and contraction is not initiated. When the calcium channels of the T tubules open, several thousand

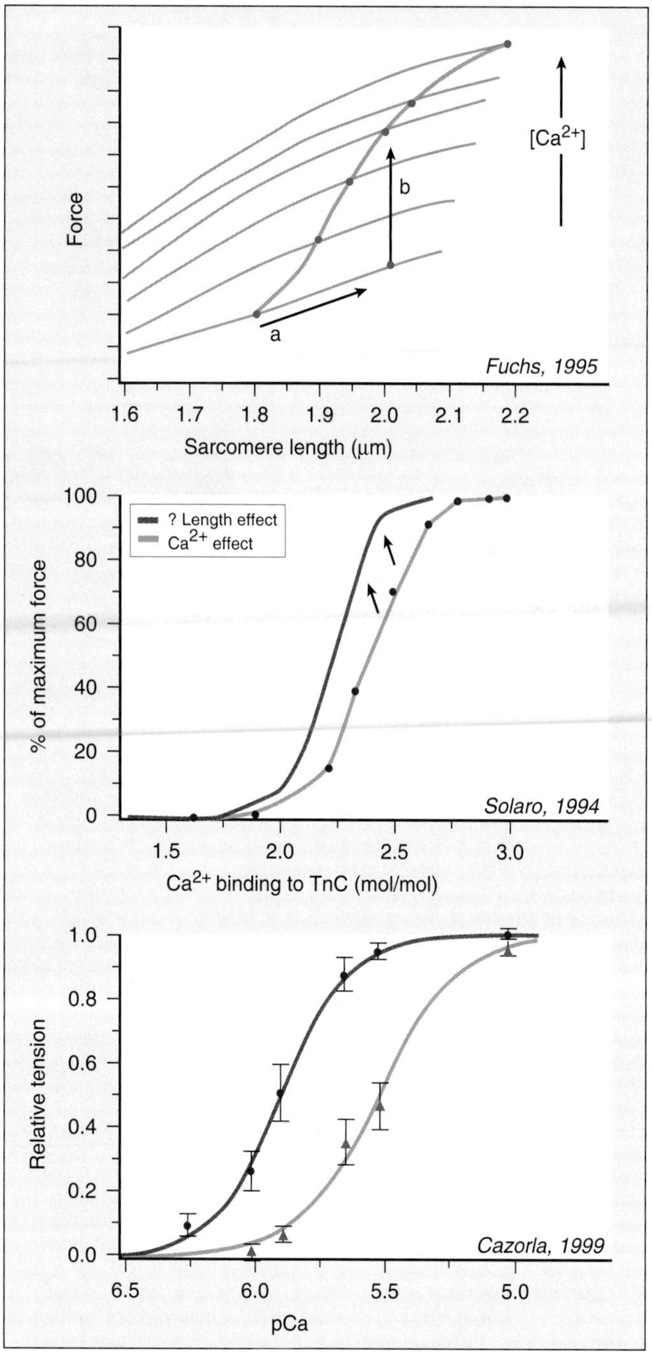

FIGURE 19–6 The proposed explanation for the Starling effect, whereby a greater end-diastolic fiber length develops a greater force. **Top,** How the steep ascending limb of the cardiac force-length curve is explained by an interaction between sarcomere length and calcium ions. Light lines show a family of hypothetical force-length curves for increasing free Ca^{2+} concentrations, each drawn on the assumption that the shape of the curve is determined solely by the degree of overlap of thin and thick filaments (see Fig. 19–1). It is postulated that an increase in end-diastolic fiber length (a) at any given free Ca^{2+} concentration would increase force by a small amount on the basis of the change in filament overlap. In addition, length-dependent activation explains how the sarcomere can "upgrade itself" (b) to a higher force-length curve. **Middle,** Proposal that the effects of Ca^{2+} and length can be explained by the properties of troponin C (TnC) and the binding of calcium to TnC. As more Ca^{2+} ions bind to TnC in a skinned-fiber preparation, more force is developed. There is a steep relation, similar to that shown in the top panel. When the fiber is stretched and the sarcomere length increased, it is postulated that for any given number of Ca^{2+} ions binding to TnC there is greater force development. **Bottom,** How the Ca^{2+} concentration influences the development of tension at long (filled circles) and shorter (open circles) sarcomere lengths. (**Top,** Modified from Fuchs F: Mechanical modulation of the Ca^{2+} regulatory protein complex in cardiac muscle. News Physiol Sci 10:6, 1995; **Middle,** modified from Solaro RJ, Wolska BM, Westfall M: Regulatory proteins and diastolic relaxation. *In* Lorell BH, Grossman W [eds]: Diastolic Relaxation of the Heart. Norwell, Mass, Kluwer Academic Publishers, 1994, pp 53-53; **Bottom,** modified from Cazorla O, Vassort G, Garnier D, LeGuennec J-Y: Length modulation of active force in rat cardiac myocytes: Is titin the sensor? J Mol Cell Cardiol 31:1215, 1995.)

calcium sparks can unite in time and space to become a subsarcolemmal calcium wave that triggers excitation-contraction coupling.[21] This model predicts that the graded response in calcium release can be explained by both an increased number of channels that are opened and an increased amount of calcium released by each channel. When the SR is overloaded with calcium as in pathological conditions such as catecholamine toxicity or during early reperfusion, calcium sparks can lead to propagated calcium waves with risk of serious arrhythmias or impaired contractile activity.

CALCIUM UPTAKE BY THE CALCIUM ATPASE OF THE SARCOPLASMIC RETICULUM (see also Chap. 21). Calcium ions are taken up into the SR by the activity of the calcium pump called SERCA that constitutes nearly 90 percent of the protein component of the SR. Its molecular weight is about 115 kDa, and it straddles the SR membrane in such a way that part of it actually protrudes into the cytosol. It exists in several isoforms, of which the dominant cardiac form is SERCA2a. For each mole of ATP hydrolyzed by this enzyme, two calcium ions are taken up to accumulate within the SR (Fig. 19–9). The source of the energy is at least in part cytosolic generation of ATP through glycolysis.[22] Important links between SERCA and cardiac contractile activity are found in a variety of genetic models. For example, in heart failure the activity of SERCA is decreased, whereas gene transfer of SERCA2a improves survival and high-energy phosphate metabolism.[23]

Phospholamban was so named by its discoverers, Tada and Katz, to mean "phosphate receiver."[24] The activity of phospholamban is governed by a state of phosphorylation, a process that alters the molecular configuration of SERCA to promote its activity (see Fig. 19–9). Two major protein kinases are involved, one activated by PKA in response to beta-adrenergic stimulation and cyclic AMP and the other by calcium ions and calmodulin, and these act at two different phosphorylation sites.[25] When phospholamban responds to beta-adrenergic stimulation of the cardiomyocyte by enhancing the uptake of calcium by SERCA into the SR, thus increasing the rate of relaxation,[19] the major activation is phosphorylation of the PKA site.[25] A further proposal is that the enhanced store of calcium in the SR correspondingly increases the amount of calcium released by the ryanodine receptor in response to subsequent waves of depolarization to give an increased rate and force of contraction.[26] This sequence is strongly supported by a model of transgenic mice, totally deficient in phospholamban, with hyperdynamic hearts in which rates of contraction and relaxation are maximal with attenuated responses to added beta-adrenergic stimulation by isoproterenol.[25] Conversely, in hearts overexpressing phospholamban, cardiac function is depressed.[25]

Calcium, taken up into the SR by the calcium uptake pump, is stored within the SR prior to further release. The highly charged storage protein, *calsequestrin*, is found in the part of the SR that lies near the T tubules. Calcium stored with calsequestrin becomes available for the release process as calsequestrin discharges Ca^{2+} into the inner mouth of the calcium release channel. This process replaces the calcium ions liberated from the outer mouth into the cytosol. *Calreticulin* is another Ca^{2+}-storing protein, similar in structure to calsequestrin and probably similar in function. Hypothetically, calsequestrin and two other proteins located in the SR

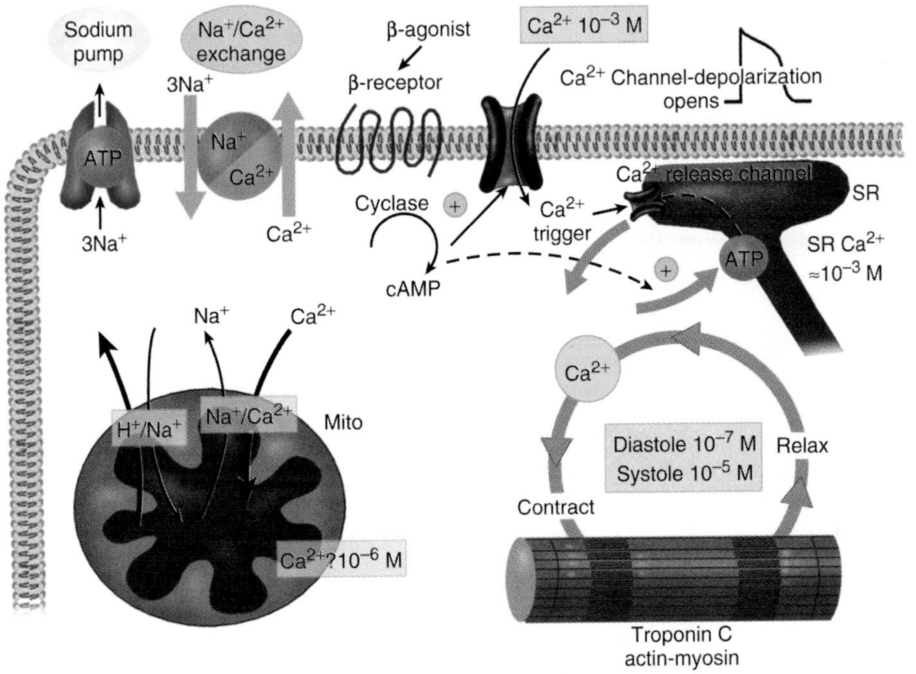

FIGURE 19–7 Calcium fluxes in the myocardium. Crucial features are (1) entry of Ca^{2+} ions through the voltage-sensitive L-type Ca^{2+} channels, acting as a trigger for the release of Ca^{2+} ions from the sarcoplasmic reticulum (SR); (2) the effect of beta-adrenergic stimulation with adenylate cyclase forming cyclic adenosine monophosphate (cAMP), the latter helping both to open the Ca^{2+} channel and to increase the rate of uptake of Ca^{2+} into the SR; and (3) exit of Ca^{2+} ions chiefly through Na^+/Ca^{2+} exchange, with the sodium pump thereafter extruding the Na^+ ions thus gained. The latter process requires adenosine triphosphate. Note the much higher extracellular (10^{-3} M) than intracellular cytosolic Ca^{2+} values, with much higher calcium values in the SR because of its storage function, and a hypothetical mitochondrial value of about 10^{-6} M. The mitochondria can act as a buffer against excessive changes in the free cytosolic calcium concentration. MITO = mitochondria. (From Opie LH: Heart Physiology, from Cell to Circulation. Philadelphia, Lippincott Williams & Wilkins, 2004. Copyright L. H. Opie, © 2004.)

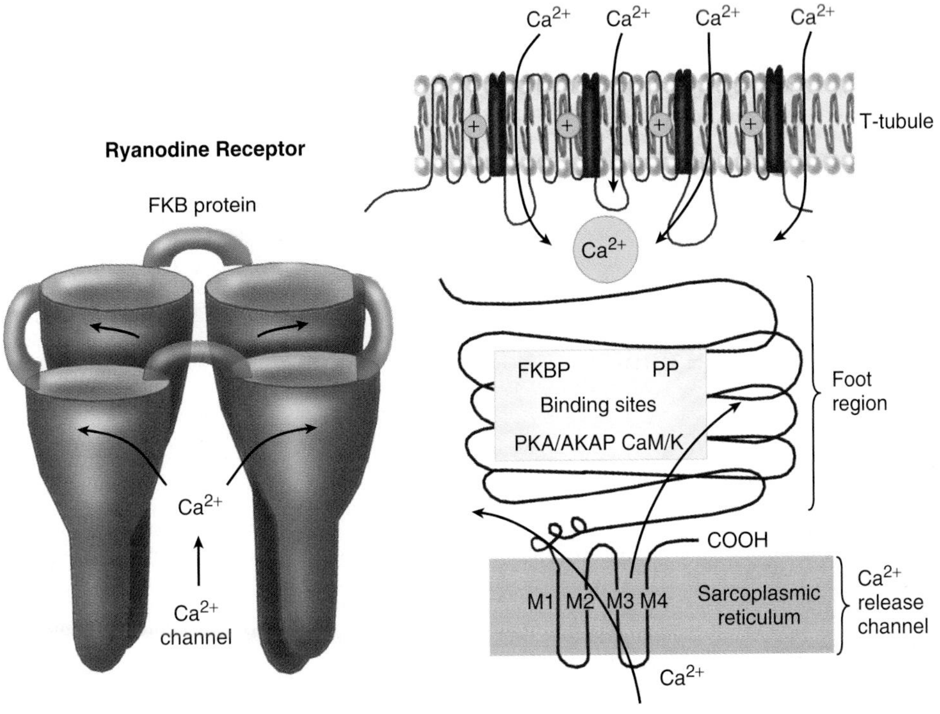

FIGURE 19–8 Role of ryanodine receptor (RyR) in calcium-induced calcium release. The RyR protein forms a link between the T tubule and the SR and is a scaffolding protein (which binds other proteins such as kinases and phosphatases). The result is a macromolecular complex, also called the "foot" region. One high-affinity RyR is composed of four RyR monomer proteins. The molecular model of one RyR is shown schematically at the right. The four RyR proteins make a single calcium release channel, in a manner similar to the formation of some other ion channels (schematic, left). Depolarization stimulates the L-type calcium channel of the T tubule to allow calcium ion entry. The incoming calcium binds to the RyR to cause molecular conformational changes that result in opening of the calcium release channel and calcium release from the SR. AKAP = anchoring protein for PKA; CaM/K = calmodulin or calmodulin kinase; FKBP = FK506 binding protein; PKA = protein kinase A; PP = protein phosphatases. (From Opie LH: Heart Physiology, from Cell to Circulation. Philadelphia, Lippincott Williams & Wilkins, 2004. Copyright L. H. Opie, © 2004.)

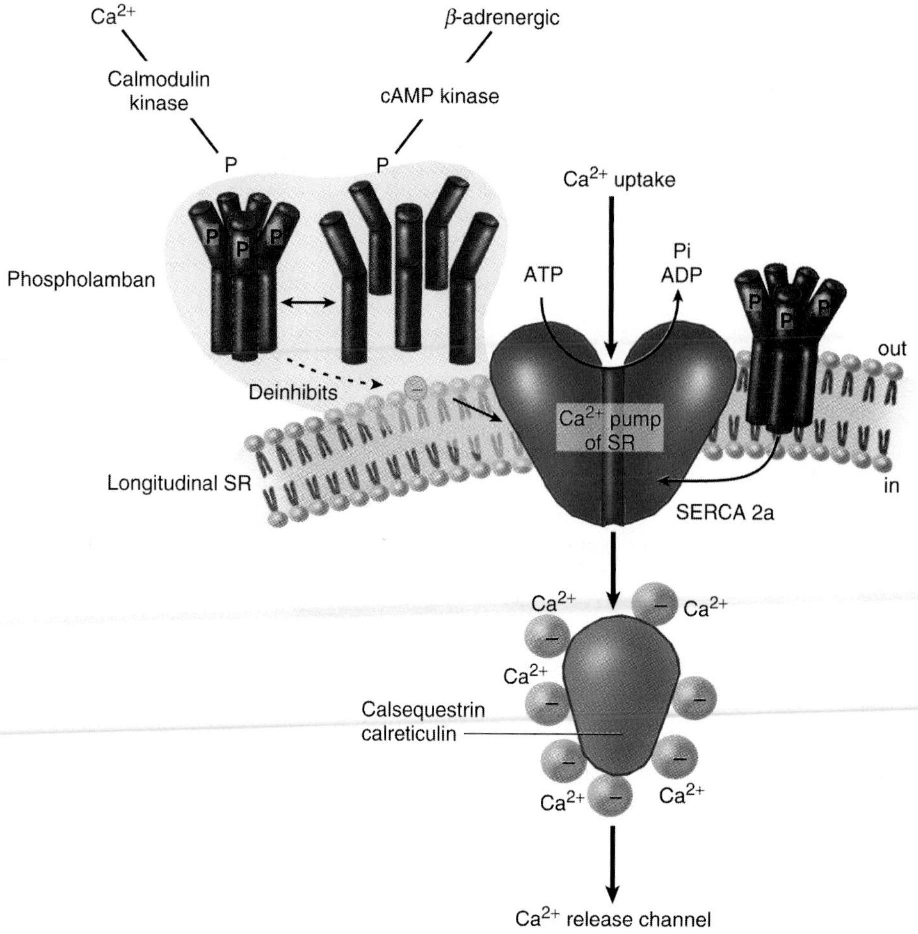

FIGURE 19–9 Lusitropic mechanism of calcium uptake into the sarcoplasmic reticulum (SR) by the energy-requiring calcium pump sarcoendoplasmic reticulum Ca^{2+}-adenosine triphosphatase ($SERCA_{2a}$). Phospholamban can be phosphorylated (P) to remove the inhibition exerted by its dephosphorylated form (positive charges) on the calcium pump. Thereby, calcium uptake is increased in response to either enhanced cytosolic calcium or beta-adrenergic stimulation. Thus, there are two phosphorylations activating phospholamban at two distinct sites and their effects are additive. An increased rate of uptake of calcium into the SR enhances the rate of relaxation (*lusitropic effect*). cAMP = cyclic adenosine monophosphate; P_i = inorganic phosphate. (Modified from Opie LH: Heart Physiology, from Cell to Circulation. Philadelphia, Lippincott Williams & Wilkins, 2004. Copyright L. H. Opie, © 2004.)

membrane (junctin and triadin) may help regulate the properties of the ryanodine receptor.[27]

Sarcolemmal Control of Calcium and Sodium Ions

Calcium Channels

All current models of excitation-contraction coupling ascribe a crucial role to the voltage-induced opening of the sarcolemmal L-type calcium channels in the initiation of the contractile process. Channels are pore-forming macromolecular proteins that span the sarcolemmal lipid bilayer to allow a highly selective pathway for ion transfer into the heart cell when the channel changes from a closed to an open state. Ion channels have two major properties: gating and permeation. Guarding each channel are two or more hypothetical gates that control its opening. Ions can permeate through the channel only when both gates are open. In the case of the sodium and calcium channels, which are best understood, the activation gate is shut at the normal resting membrane potential and the inactivation gate is open so that the channels are *voltage gated.* Depolarization opens the activation gate.

MOLECULAR STRUCTURE OF L-TYPE CALCIUM CHANNELS. There is a superfamily of voltage-gated ion channels that includes both the sodium and calcium channels and some of the potassium channels.[27] The potassium channels have a simpler structure from which it is thought that the more complex sodium and calcium channels evolved. Both sodium and calcium channels contain a major alpha subunit with four transmembrane subunits or domains that are similar to each other in structure. In addition, both sodium and calcium channels include in their overall structure a number of other subunits whose function is less well understood, such as the alpha subunit. Each of the four transmembrane domains of the alpha subunit is made up of six helices and is folded in on itself so that the four S5-S6 spans combine structurally to form the single functioning *pore* of each calcium channel (Fig. 19–10).[28]

Activation is now understood in molecular terms as the change in charge on the fourth transmembrane segment, S4, called the *voltage sensor*, of each of the four subunits of the sodium or calcium channel.[28] *Inactivation* is the process whereby the current initially elicited by depolarization decreases with time despite continuation of the original stimulus. Channels are not simply open or closed. Rather, the open state is the last of a sequence of many molecular states, varying from a fully closed to a fully open configuration. Therefore, it is more correct to speak of the *probability of channel opening*.

CURRENT ACTIVATION AND DEACTIVATION. Having been activated by depolarization, the L-type calcium current is inactivated by (1) the rising voltage during depolarization, at a more positive potential than for activation; and (2) the rising internal calcium ion concentration. Especially the calcium flowing from the ryanodine receptor pushes up the subsarcolemmal internal calcium ion concentration near the mouth of the L channels of the T tubules to help terminate current flow.[29]

CALCIUM CHANNEL PHOSPHORYLATION. The $alpha_1$ subunit (the organ-specific subunit) of the sarcolemmal calcium channel can be phosphorylated at several sites especially in the C-terminal tail.[27] During beta-adrenergic stimulation, cyclic AMP increases within the cell and phosphate groups are transferred from ATP to the $alpha_1$ subunit. Thereby, the electrical charges near the inner mouth of the nearby pores are altered to induce changes in the molecular conformation of the pores so that there is an increased probability of opening of the calcium channel.

T- AND L-TYPE CALCIUM CHANNELS. There are two major subpopulations of sarcolemmal calcium channels relevant to the cardiovascular system, namely the T channels and the L channels. The T (transient) channels open at a more negative voltage, have short bursts of opening, and do not interact with conventional calcium antagonist drugs.[28] The T channels presumably account for the earlier phase of the opening of the calcium channel, which may also give them a special role in the early electrical depolarization of the sinoatrial node and hence initiation of the heartbeat. Although T channels are found in atrial cells, their existence in normal ventricular cells is controversial. T channels are not found in T tubules despite the coincidental sharing of the T.[19] Rather, the sarcolemmal L (long-lasting) channels are the standard calcium channels found in the myocardium and the T tubules; they are involved in calcium-induced calcium release and are inhibited by calcium channel blockers such as verapamil, diltiazem, and the dihydropyridines.

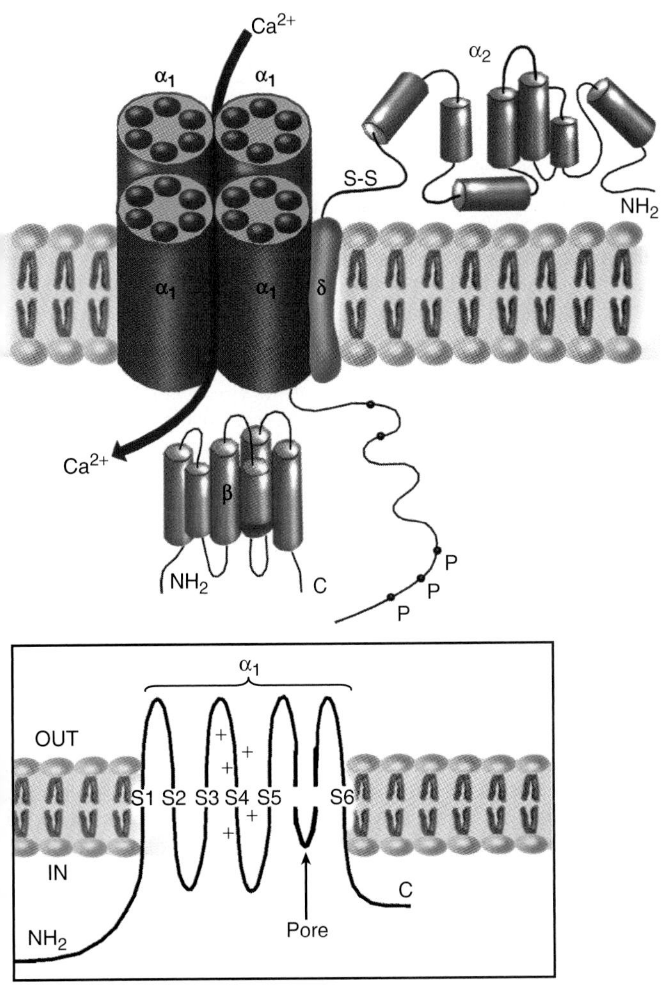

FIGURE 19–10 Simplified model of Ca^{2+} channel showing the alpha$_1$ subunit (α_1) forming the central pore, the regulatory beta-subunit (β), and alpha$_2$ and delta subunits of unknown function. Beta-adrenergic stimulation, by means of cyclic adenosine monophosphate, promotes phosphorylation (P) and the opening probability of the Ca^{2+} channel. The proposal is that four domains, each similar to that shown at the bottom and composed of six spanning segments, combine to form the alpha$_1$ subunit. Segment S4 is thought to respond to voltage depolarization (+ = positive charges) by altering the molecular configuration of the loop between S5 and S6 (part of the pore) so that there is a greater probability of Ca^{2+} ions entering (channel opens). (**Top,** modified from Varadi G, Mori Y, Mikala G, Schwartz A: Molecular determinants of Ca^{2+} channel function and drug action. Trends Pharmacol Sci 16:43, 1995; **Bottom,** modified from Tomaselli GF, Backx PH, Marban E: Molecular basis of permeation in voltage-rated ion channels. Circ Res 72:491, 1993. Copyright 1993, American Heart Association.)

Ion Exchangers and Pumps

To balance the small amount of calcium ions entering the heart cell with each depolarization, a similar quantity must leave the cell by one of two processes. First, calcium can be exchanged for sodium ions entering by Na^+/Ca^{2+} exchange, and, second, an ATP-consuming sarcolemmal calcium pump can transfer calcium into the extracellular space against a concentration gradient.

SODIUM-CALCIUM EXCHANGER. During relaxation, the sarcoplasmic calcium uptake pump and the Na^+/Ca^{2+} exchanger compete for the removal of cytosolic calcium, with the SR pump normally being dominant.[19] Restitution of calcium balance takes place by the activity of a series of transsarcolemmal exchangers, the chief of which is the Na^+/Ca^{2+} exchanger (see Fig. 19–17). The exchanger (molecular weight 108 kDa) consists of 970 amino acids and does not have substantial homology to any other known protein. The direction of ion exchange is responsive to the membrane potential and to the concentrations of sodium and calcium ions on either side of the sarcolemma. Because sodium and calcium ions can exchange either inward or outward in response to the membrane potential, there must be a specific membrane potential, called the *reversal* or *equilibrium potential*, at which the ions are so distributed that they can move as easily one way as the other. The reversal potential may lie about halfway between the resting membrane potential and the potential of the fully depolarized state.

The other major factor influencing the exchanger is the concentration of sodium and calcium ions on either side of the sarcolemma. Changing the membrane potential from the resting value of, say, −85 mV to +20 mV in the phase of rapid depolarization of the action potential and entry of sodium ions therefore briefly reverse the direction of Na^+/Ca^{2+} exchange. Thus, the sodium ions that have just entered during the opening of the sodium channel tend to leave, and calcium ions tend to enter. This process, thought to occur more in larger mammals with slow heart rates and long action potential durations, contrasts with the standard "forward mode" (Na^+ in, Ca^{2+} out) and is called "reverse mode" exchange. Such transsarcolemmal calcium entry may participate in calcium-induced calcium release.[19] In myocytes from the failing human heart, enhanced reversed exchange contributes to the slow decline of the Ca^{2+} transient,[30] which may explain delayed diastolic relaxation (see Impaired Relaxation and Cytosolic Calcium). Prolongation of the action potential duration also provokes reverse mode exchange, with risk of ventricular arrhythmias.[19]

Heart Rate and Na^+/Ca^{2+} Exchange. This exchanger may participate in the force-frequency relationship (treppe or Bowditch phenomenon). According to the "sodium pump lag" hypothesis, the rapid accumulation of calcium ions during fast stimulation of the myocardium outstrips the ability of the Na^+/Ca^{2+} exchanger and the sodium pump to achieve return to ionic normality. The result is an accumulation of calcium ions within the SR and an increased force of contraction.

SODIUM PUMP (Na^+,K^+-ATPase). The sarcolemma becomes highly permeable to Na^+ only during the opening of the Na^+ channel during early depolarization, and Na^+ also enters during the exit of Ca^{2+} by Na^+/Ca^{2+} exchange. Most of this influx of Na^+ across the sarcolemma must be corrected by the activity of the Na^+/K^+ pump, also called the Na^+, K^+-ATPase pump or simply the Na^+ pump. The pump is activated by internal Na^+ or external K^+.[31] One ATP molecule is used per transport cycle. The ions are first secluded within the pump protein and then extruded to either side. Although there has been some dispute about the exact ratio of Na^+ to K^+ ions that are pumped, a generally accepted model is that for each three Na^+ exported, two K^+ are imported. During this process, one positive charge must leave the cell. Hence, the pump is electrogenic and is also called the electrogenic Na^+ pump.[31] The current induced by sustained activity of the pump may contribute about −10 mV to the resting membrane potential.[28] Because the pump must extrude Na^+ ions entering by either Na^+/Ca^{2+} exchange or by the Na^+ channel, its sustained activity is essential for the maintenance of normal ion balance.

Beta-Adrenergic Signal Systems

Families of Receptors Coupled to G Proteins

The autonomic nervous system can initiate signal systems that profoundly alter the fluxes of calcium and other ions. Both adrenergic and cholinergic receptors belong to the family of seven transmembrane-spanning receptors, also called the G protein–coupled receptors.[32] The sum total of these processes converting an extracellular hormonal or neural stimulus to an intracellular physiological change is called *signal transduction*, which typically starts with the agonist binding to a receptor site. Thus, adrenergic or cholinergic stimulation of the sarcolemmal receptors inaugurates the activity of a complex system of sarcolemmal and cytosolic messengers. Occupancy of the beta-adrenergic receptor is coupled by a G protein complex (Figs. 19–11 and 19–12) to activation of a sarcolemmal enzyme, *adenylyl cyclase* (also called adenylate cyclase or shortened to adenyl cyclase), that sets in motion a series of signals that terminate with activation by phosphorylation of certain crucial proteins, such as those of the calcium channel (see Fig. 19–12).

Other cardiac receptors, such as the alpha-adrenergic receptor, have an alternative dual messenger system involving inositol triphosphate (IP_3) and diacylglycerol, with the latter activating protein kinase C (PKC). Such signals are of established importance in controlling calcium flux in vascular smooth muscle, thereby regulating vascular tone and indirectly the blood pressure. In the case of cardiac myocytes, it is now appreciated that receptors coupled to PKC, such as angiotensin II, may play a major role in the regulation of cardiac myocyte growth and sometimes may have inotropic effects. Yet other messenger systems exist to convey different signals. For example, in blood vessels, nitric oxide (NO) formed in the inner endothelial layer stimulates the formation of cyclic guanosine monophosphate (GMP) in the smooth muscle layer, thereby causing relaxation (vasodilation).

Beta-Adrenergic Receptor Subtypes

Cardiac beta-adrenergic receptors are chiefly the $beta_1$ subtype, whereas most noncardiac receptors are $beta_2$. There are also $beta_2$ receptors in the human heart, about 20 percent of the total beta receptor population in the left ventricle and about twice as high a percentage in the atria. $Beta_3$ receptors have also been identified and are probably of major importance only in heart failure. Whereas the $beta_1$ receptors are linked to the stimulatory G protein, G_s, component of the G protein–adenylyl cyclase system, $beta_2$ receptors are linked to both G_s and the inhibitory G_i, so that controversially their signaling pathway bifurcates at the first postreceptor step.[33] Hypothetically, $beta_2$ receptors are normally more strongly coupled to G_s, but in heart failure this coupling is weakened and that to G_i is strengthened.[33] The beta-adrenergic receptor site is highly stereospecific, the best fit among catecholamines being obtained with the synthetic agent isoproterenol (ISO) rather than with the naturally occurring catecholamines norepinephrine (NE) and epinephrine (E). In the case of $beta_1$ receptors, the order of agonist activity is ISO > E = NE, whereas in the case of $beta_2$ receptors, the order is ISO > E > NE. Human $beta_1$ and $beta_2$ receptors have now been cloned.[34] The transmembrane domains are held to be the site of agonist and antagonist binding, whereas the cytoplasmic domains interact with G proteins. One of the phosphorylation sites on the terminal COOH tail may be involved in desensitization (see next section).

G Proteins

THE STIMULATORY G PROTEIN G_S. G proteins are a superfamily of proteins that bind guanosine triphosphate (GTP) and other guanine nucleotides. G proteins are crucial in carrying the signal onward from the first messenger and its receptor to the activity of the membrane-bound enzyme system that produces the second messenger (see Fig. 19–12).[35] The triple combination of the beta receptor, the G protein complex, and adenylate cyclase is termed the *beta-adrenergic system*. The G protein itself is a heterotrimer composed of G_α, G_β, and G_γ, which upon receptor stimulation splits into the alpha subunit that is bound to GTP and the beta-gamma subunit. Either of these subunits may regulate different effectors such as adenylate cyclase, phospholipase C, and ion channels. The activity of adenylate cyclase is controlled by two different G protein complexes, namely G_s, which stimulates, and G_i, which inhibits. The alpha subunit of G_s ($alpha_s$) combines with GTP and then separates off from the other two subunits to enhance the activity of adenylate cyclase. The beta and gamma subunits (beta-gamma) appear to be linked structurally and in function.

THE INHIBITORY G PROTEIN, G_I. In contrast, a second trimeric GTP-binding protein, G_i, is responsible for inhibition of adenylate cyclase.[35] During cholinergic signaling, the muscarinic receptor is stimulated and GTP binds to the inhibitory alpha subunit ($alpha_i$). The latter then dissociates from the other two components of the G protein complex, which are, as in the case of G_s, the combined beta-gamma subunits.

The beta-gamma subunits act as follows. By stimulating the enzyme GTPase, they

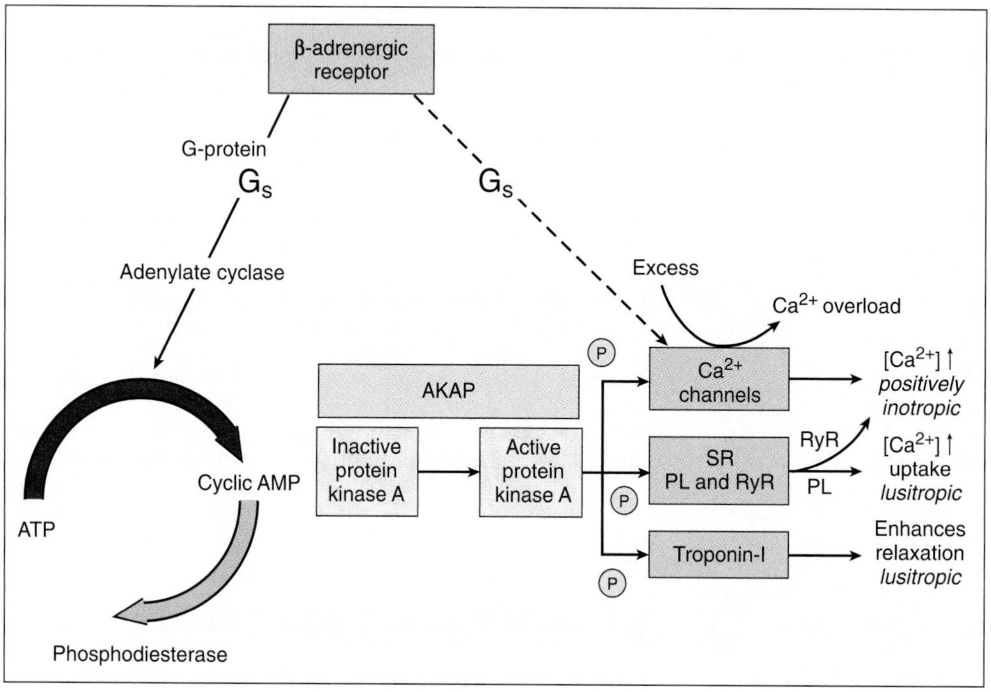

FIGURE 19–11 Key role of protein kinase A (PKA) in the beta-adrenergic response. The major intracellular effects of beta-agonist catecholamines occur by formation of cyclic adenosine monophosphate (Cyclic AMP), which increases the activity of the cAMP-dependent PKA. The latter achieves its optimal intracellular site by localizing to the scaffolding protein, A-kinase anchoring protein (AKAP), whereupon PKA phosphorylates various proteins concerned with contraction and relaxation. PL = phospholamban; RyR = ryanodine receptor; SR = sarcoplasmic reticulum. For inotropic and lusitropic mechanisms, see Figure 19–12. (Modified from Opie LH: Heart Physiology, from Cell to Circulation. Philadelphia, Lippincott Williams & Wilkins, 2004. Copyright L. H. Opie, © 2004.)

break down the active alpha$_s$ subunit (alpha$_s$-GTP) so that the activation of adenylate cyclase in response to alpha stimulation becomes less. Furthermore, the beta-gamma subunit activates the K_{ACh} channel, which, in turn, can inhibit the sinoatrial node to contribute to the bradycardiac effect of cholinergic stimulation. The alpha$_i$ subunit activates another potassium channel (K_{ATP}) whose physiological function in the myocardium is still unclear. Pathophysiologically, preconditioning may link to this channel (see later).

THE THIRD G PROTEIN, G_Q. G_q links a group of heptahelical (*hepta* = seven) myocardial receptors, including the alpha-adrenergic receptor and those for angiotensin II and endothelin, to another membrane-associated enzyme, phospholipase C, and thence to PKC (see later). G_q has at least four isoforms, of which two have been found in the heart. This G protein, unlike G_i, is not susceptible to inhibition by the pertussis toxin. Overexpression of G_q in mice induced a dilated cardiomyopathy,[36] which is of interest because angiotensin II and endothelin, which act through Gq, are overactive in human heart failure. Conversely, when the activity of G_q is genetically inhibited, the hypertrophic response to pressure overload is attenuated, and wall stress increases, but cardiac function is relatively well maintained.[37]

CYCLIC ADENOSINE MONOPHOSPHATE AND PROTEIN KINASE A

Adenylyl Cyclase. Adenylyl cyclase is a transmembrane enzyme system, also called adenylate or adenyl cyclase, that responds to input from G proteins. When stimulated by G_s, adenylyl cyclase produces the second messenger cyclic AMP, which then acts through a further series of intracellular signals and specifically the third messenger PKA to increase cytosolic calcium transients. In contrast, cholinergic stimulation exerts inhibitory influences, largely on the heart rate but also on contraction, acting at least in part by decreasing the rate of formation of cyclic AMP.

Adenylyl cyclase is the only enzyme system producing cyclic AMP and specifically requires low concentrations of ATP (and magnesium) as substrate. Surprisingly, the proposed molecular structure resembles that of certain channel proteins, such as that of the calcium channel. Most of the protein is located on the cytoplasmic side, the presumed site of interaction with the G protein. Another cyclic nucleotide, cyclic GMP, acts as a second messenger for some aspects of vagal activity. In vascular smooth muscle, cyclic GMP is the second messenger of the NO messenger system. These messenger chemicals are present in the heart cell in minute concentrations, that of cyclic AMP being roughly about 10^{-9} M and that of cyclic GMP about 10^{-11} M.

Cyclic AMP has very rapid turnover as a result of a constant dynamic balance between its formation by adenylate cyclase and removal by another enzyme, phosphodiesterase. In general, directional changes in the tissue content of cyclic AMP can be related to directional changes in cardiac contractile activity. For example, beta-adrenergic stimulation increases both, whereas beta blockade inhibits the increases induced by beta agonists. *Forskolin*, a direct stimulator of adenylate cyclase, increases cyclic AMP and contractile acivity. Adenosine, acting through A_1 receptors, inhibits adenylate cyclase, decreases cyclic AMP, and lessens contractile activity. A number of hormones or peptides can couple to myocardial adenylate cyclase independently of the beta-adrenergic receptor. These are glucagon, thyroid hormone, prostacyclin (prostaglandin I_2), and the calcitonin gene–related peptide.

INHIBITION OF ADENYLYL CYCLASE. The major physiological stimulus to G_i is thought to be vagal muscarinic receptor stimulation. In addition, adenosine, by interaction with A_1 receptors, couples to G_i to inhibit contraction and heart rate. The adenosine A_2 receptor paradoxically increases cyclic AMP. The latter effect, only of ancillary significance in the myocardium, is of major importance in vascular smooth muscle, where it induces vasorelaxation. Pathologically, inhibitory G_i is increased in experimental postinfarct heart failure[38] and in donor hearts prior to cardiac transplantation.[39]

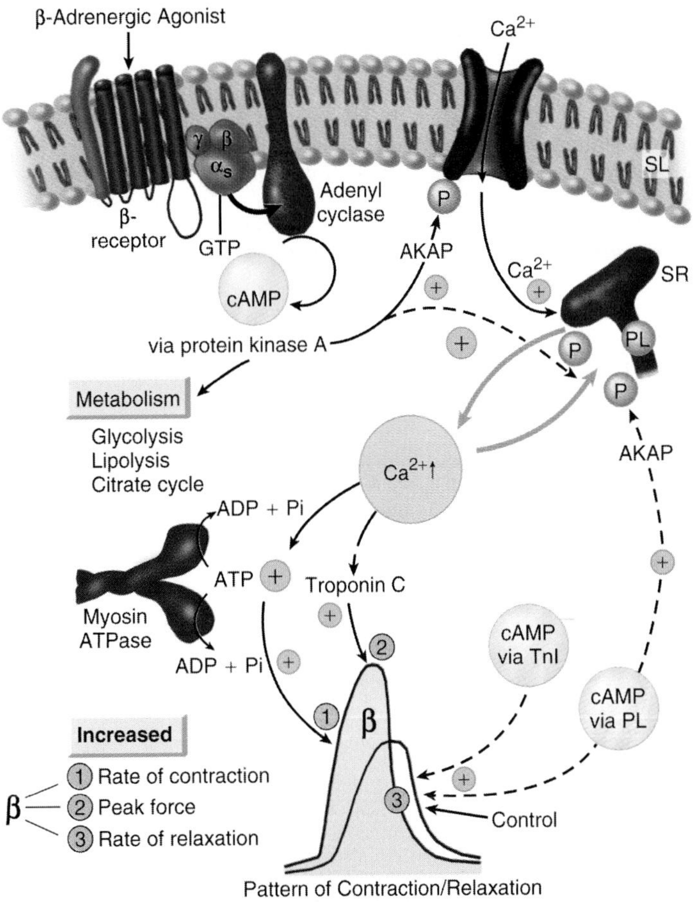

FIGURE 19–12 Signal systems involved in positive inotropic and lusitropic (enhanced relaxation) effects of beta-adrenergic stimulation. When the beta-adrenergic agonist interacts with the beta receptor, a series of G protein–mediated changes (see Fig. 19–11) lead to activation of adenylate cyclase and formation of cyclic adenosine monophosphate (cAMP). The latter acts through protein kinase A to stimulate metabolism (on the left) and to phosphorylate the calcium channel protein. The result is an enhanced opening probability of the calcium channel, thereby increasing the inward movement of Ca^{2+} ions through the sarcolemma (SL) of the T tubule. These Ca^{2+} ions release more calcium from the sarcoplasmic reticulum (SR) (see Fig. 19–7) to increase cytosolic calcium and to activate troponin C. Calcium ions also increase the rate of breakdown of ATP to ADP and inorganic phosphate (P_i). Enhanced myosin adenosine triphosphatase (ATPase) activity explains the increased rate of contraction with increased activation of troponin C explaining increased peak force development. An increased rate of relaxation is explained because cAMP also activates the protein phospholamban, situated on the membrane of the SR that controls the rate of uptake of calcium into the SR (see Fig. 19–9). The latter effect explains enhanced relaxation (lusitropic effect). AKAP = A-kinase anchoring protein; P = phosphorylation; PL = phospholamban. For TnI see Fig. 19–3. (Modified from Opie LH: Heart Physiology, from Cell to Circulation. Philadelphia, Lippincott Williams & Wilkins, 2004. Copyright L. H. Opie, © 2004.)

CYCLIC AMP–DEPENDENT PROTEIN KINASES. It is now clear that most, if not all, of the effects of cyclic AMP are ultimately mediated by PKA, which phosphorylates various key proteins and enzymes (see Fig. 19–11).[40] *Phosphorylation* is the donation of a phosphate group to the enzyme concerned, acting as a fundamental metabolic switch that can extensively amplify the signal.

Each protein kinase is composed of two subunits, regulatory (R) and catalytic (C). When cyclic AMP (cAMP) interacts with the inactive protein kinase, it binds to the R subunit to liberate the active kinase, which is the C subunit:

$$(R_2 + C_2) + 2cAMP \rightarrow 2RcAMP + 2C$$

At a molecular level, this active kinase catalyzes the transfer of the terminal phosphate of ATP to serine and threonine residues of the protein substrates, leading to phosphorylation and modification of the properties of the proteins concerned and thereby promoting further key reactions. PKA occurs in different cells in two isoforms: PKA-II predominates in cardiac cells. The proposed anchorage of this kinase by *A-kinase anchoring proteins* (AKAPs) to specific organelles such as the SR explains the phenomenon of cyclic AMP compartmentation[40] because anchored PKA requires focal elevation of cyclic AMP even at an unchanged cytosolic concentration. In addition, the G protein system may not be evenly spread throughout the sarcolemma but may be localized to certain focal areas. Thus, it is likely that there is only a specific subcompartment of cyclic AMP available to increase contractile activity.

PHYSIOLOGICAL BETA$_1$-ADRENERGIC EFFECTS. The probable sequence of events describing the positive inotropic effects of catecholamines is as follows (Fig. 19–13).

Catecholamine stimulation → beta receptor → molecular changes → binding of GTP to alpha$_s$ subunit of G protein → GTP alpha$_s$ subunit stimulates adenylyl cyclase → formation of cyclic AMP from ATP → activation of cyclic AMP–dependent protein kinase (PKA), locally bound by an A-kinase anchoring protein (AKAP) → phosphorylation of a sarcolemmal protein p27 → increased entry of calcium ion through increased opening of the voltage-dependent L-type calcium channels → greater calcium-induced calcium release through ryanodine receptor of SR, coupled with phosphorylation of the ryanodine receptor → greater and more rapid rise of intracellular free calcium ion concentration → increased calcium-troponin C interaction with deinhibition of tropomyosin effect on actin-myosin interaction → increased rate and number of cross bridges interacting with increased myosin ATPase activity → increased rate and peak of force development.

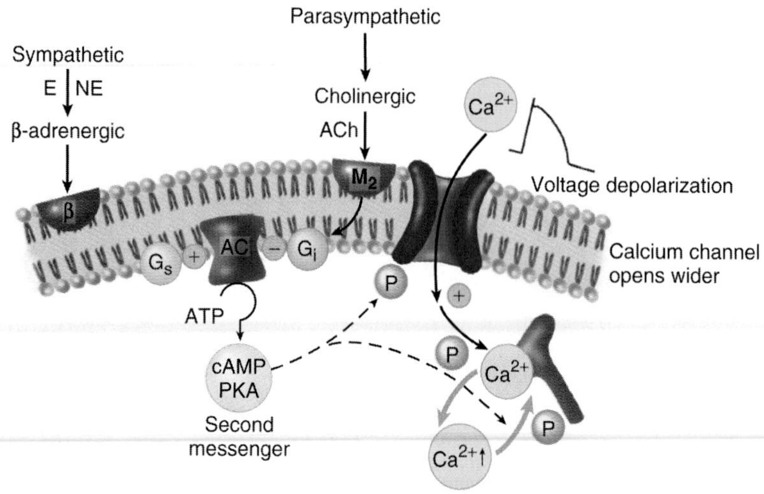

FIGURE 19–13 Interaction between sympathetic and parasympathetic systems could best be explained by the inhibitory effect on the formulation of cyclic adenosine monophosphate (cAMP), including formation of inhibitory G protein G_i in response to M_2 receptor stimulation. AC = adenylyl cyclase; ACh = acetylcholine; E = epinephrine; NE = norepinephrine; PKA = protein kinase A. (Modified from Opie LH: Heart Physiology, from Cell to Circulation. Philadelphia, Lippincott Williams & Wilkins, 2004. Copyright L. H. Opie, © 2004.)

The increased *lusitropic (relaxant)* effect is the consequence of increased PKA-mediated phosphorylation of phospholamban (see Fig. 19–12). Also, increased phosphorylation of troponin I may help to desensitize the contractile apparatus to calcium ions.

Physiological Switch-Off, Beta-Agonist Receptor Kinase, and Arrestin

There is a potent feedback mechanism whereby the degree of postreceptor response to a given degree of beta-adrenergic receptor stimulation can be muted (Fig. 19–14). Sustained beta-agonist stimulation rapidly induces the activity of the beta-agonist receptor kinase (βARK) that is involved in the transfer of the phosphate group to the phosphorylation site on the terminal COOH tail of the receptor, a process that of itself does not markedly affect the signaling properties. Rather, βARK increases the affinity of the beta receptor for another protein family, the *arrestins*, which cause the uncoupling. Beta-arrestin is a scaffolding protein that links to one of the cytoplasmic loops of the G protein–coupled beta-adrenergic receptor,[41] thus uncoupling receptor occupancy from G_s and activation of adenylyl cyclase, and thereby inhibiting the functioning of this receptor. Resensitization of the receptor occurs if the phosphate group is split off by a phosphatase and the receptor may then be more readily linked to G_s.

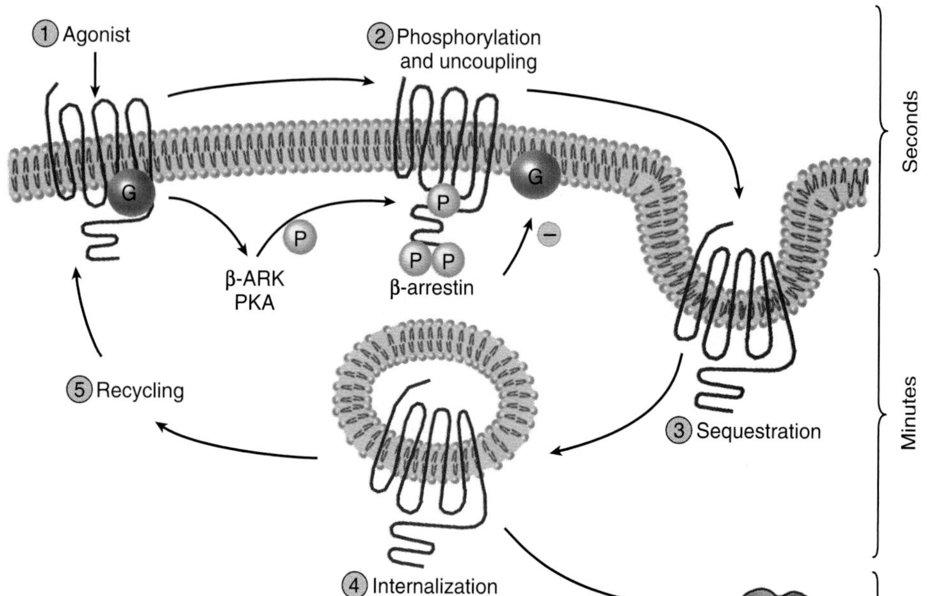

FIGURE 19–14 Mechanisms of beta-adrenergic receptor desensitization and internalization. Note links between the internalized receptor complex with growth stimulation through mitogen-activated protein (MAP) kinase. βARK = beta-agonist receptor kinase; PKA = protein kinase A. (Modified from Hein L, Kobilka BK: Adrenergic receptors. From molecular structures to in vivo function. Trends Cardiovasc Med 7:137, 1997.)

Physiologically, the βARK-arrestin mechanism helps to terminate the beta receptor signal by a rapid *desensitization of the beta receptor* within minutes to seconds (see Fig. 19-14). This mechanism also plays a role in long-term desensitization of the beta-adrenergic receptor in heart failure. Because beta-arrestin is a scaffolding protein, it simultaneously activates other systems[41] such as the tyrosine kinases, leading to growth by ultimately linking to MAP kinase.[42] Thus, prolonged beta receptor stimulation may have growth as an end result rather than conventional inotropic and lusitropic endpoints. Although the βARK-arrestin effects are best described for the $beta_2$ receptor, they also occur to a lesser extent with the $beta_1$ receptor.[43] These changes in postreceptor signaling may help to explain some of the harm of excess beta stimulation and relative upregulation of the $beta_2$ receptor in heart failure.

ISCHEMIC INACTIVATION OF βARK. As outlined, βARK regulates beta-adrenergic activity by phosphorylation of the target receptor. Following ischemia, there is a decrease in βARK activity and loss of the ability of increased beta stimulation to be desensitized.[44] Following coronary ligation, this loss of regulatory ability coincides with a phase of increased fatal ventricular arrhythmias,[44] presumably the result of increased beta-adrenergic activity.

BETA$_2$ AND BETA$_3$ ADRENERGIC EFFECTS. In the normal ventricle, about 20 percent of the receptors are $beta_2$ in nature; yet in heart failure this percentage of the whole can double because of $beta_1$ receptor downregulation (see Heart Failure). The $beta_2$ postreceptor signaling involves both the stimulatory and the inhibitory G proteins.[45] In humans, the positive inotropic response to $beta_2$ stimulation by salbutamol occurs, at least in part, through $beta_2$ receptors on the terminal neurons of the cardiac sympathetic nerves, thereby releasing norepinephrine, which in turn exerts dominant $beta_1$ effects.[46] Indirect evidence suggests that the G_i inhibitory path is relatively augmented in heart failure, whereas the strength of the stimulatory G_s path is lessened because of uncoupling of G_s from the $beta_2$ receptor.

Regarding *$beta_3$-adrenergic receptors*, their stimulation results in a negative inotropic effect through NO and formation of inhibitory cyclic GMP.[47] These effects resemble those of cholinergic stimulation (see next section). Physiologically, the role of the $beta_3$ receptor system could be pictured as opposing adverse effects of excess $beta_1$ stimulation such as too rapid a heart rate. In heart failure the $beta_3$ receptors are relatively upregulated (see later) and may contribute to the overall spectrum of adversely altered beta-adrenergic stimulation rather than promoting contraction (Fig. 19-15).

Cholinergic and Nitric Oxide Signaling

Cholinergic Signaling

Parasympathetic stimulation reduces heart rate and is negatively inotropic. The key features of its signaling system are similar to that of the $beta_1$-adrenergic system. There are again an extracellular first messenger (acetylcholine), a receptor system (the cholinergic muscarinic receptor), a sarcolemmal signaling system (the G protein system, specifically the inhibitory G_i), and a second messenger (cyclic GMP). The myocardial *muscarinic receptor* (M_2) is associated specifically with the activity of the vagal nerve endings. Receptor stimulation produces a negative chronotropic response that is inhibited by atropine. NO facilitates cholinergic signaling at two levels, the nerve terminal and the activity of the enzyme system that produces cyclic GMP.

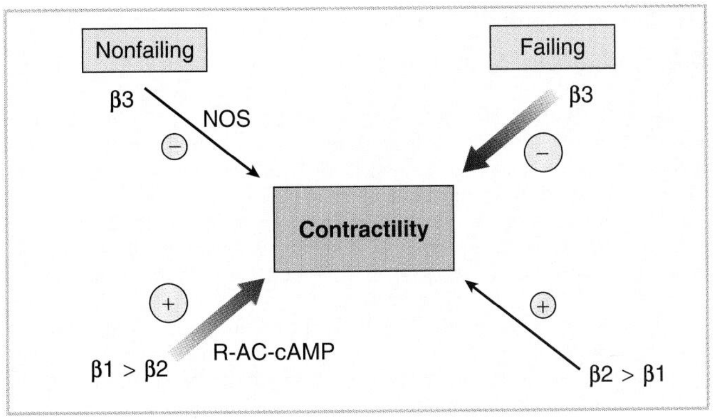

FIGURE 19–15 Proposed role of $beta_3$-adrenergic receptors. Normally, beta-adrenergic stimulation increases contractility, acting largely through the $beta_1$ receptors with backup from the $beta_2$ receptors. The $beta_3$-adrenergic receptors mediate cardioinhibitory signals that may counterbalance excess adrenergic stimulation, through nitric oxide and cyclic guanosine monophosphate (see Fig. 19–17), according to the proposals of Moniotte and colleagues.[120] In heart failure, the $beta_1$ receptors are downregulated (see Fig. 19–34) and the $beta_2$ receptors uncoupled so that their combined inotropic input is diminished. Conversely, $beta_3$ receptors are upregulated with a manifest negative inotropic effect despite some nitric oxide downregulation.[120] AC = adenylyl cyclase; cAMP = cyclic adenosine monophosphate; NOS = endothelial nitric oxide synthase; R = receptor.

THE MECHANISM OF VAGAL HEART RATE LOWERING. Cyclic GMP acts as a second messenger to vagal stimulation just as cyclic AMP does to beta-adrenergic stimulation. Of note, cell-permeable analogs of cyclic GMP have antiadrenergic effects. Cholinergic stimulation of the M_2 receptor activates guanylyl (= guanylate = guanyl) cyclase to form cyclic GMP, with consequent stimulation of protein kinase G that results in inhibitory cardiac effects such as a decreased heart rate and negative inotropic response.[48] These effects are largely achieved by modulation of calcium ion entry through the L calcium channel and through inhibition of internal calcium cycling.[49] In addition, muscarinic M_2 stimulation acts through G_i to lessen the G_s activation that results from beta receptor occupation. Thus, the vagus has a dual effect on second messengers, inhibiting the formation of cyclic AMP and increasing that of cyclic GMP, thereby providing one of several explanations for *sympathetic-parasympathetic interaction.*

Regarding the *negative inotropic effect of vagal stimulation* (see Fig. 19–16), the mechanism includes (1) heart rate slowing (negative treppe phenomenon), (2) inhibition of the formation of cyclic AMP, and (3) a direct negative inotropic effect mediated by cyclic GMP. It has been controversial whether ventricular tissue is as responsive to muscarinic agonists as atrial tissue, although the receptor populations are similar in density. However, using pressure-volume loops and the slope of the pressure-volume relationship (see E_s in Fig. 19–26) as an index of contractility, vagal stimulation in humans markedly decreased this load-independent measure.[50]

The sympathetic terminal neurons are another site of parasympathetic-sympathetic interaction (see Fig. 19–17). There the presynaptic muscarinic M_2 receptor inhibits the release of norepinephrine. In addition, both adrenergic and cholinergic stimuli exert important and often opposing effects on ion channels and cardiac function (Table 19–2). The presence of such multiple mechanisms for the inhibitory effects of vagal stimulation on the heart rate, the inotropic state, and arrhythmogenicity, suggests that "braking" of beta-adrenergic stimulation is desirable. Otherwise, the risk may be that intense beta-adrenergic stimulation would excessively increase the heart rate or inotropic state or provoke potentially fatal arrhythmias.

Nitric Oxide, the Ubiquitous Messenger
(Figs. 19–16, 19–17)

NO, the focus of a Nobel Prize for 1998, is a unique messenger in that it is formed in so many tissues, is a gas, and is a physiological free radical that should more correctly (but infrequently) be written as •NO. Nonetheless, the standard abbreviation is NO. It is generated in the heart by one of three isoenzymes.[49] Vasodilatory NO is generated in the vascular endothelium by endothelial nitric oxide synthase (eNOS, also called NOS-3) in response to increased blood flow, increased cardiac load, or bradykinin. It is induced in cardiomyocytes in disease states such as cardiogenic or septic shock by the inducible enzyme (iNOS, also called NOS-2). Generation of NO by neuronal NOS (nNOS, also called NOS-1), the form of the synthase found in vagal nerve terminals, enhances the release of acetylcholine.[51] Exercise training leads to increased formation of NO through iNOS in animals[51] and through

TABLE 19–2 Ionic Effects of Adrenergic and Cholinergic Stimulation: Relation to Heart Rate and Contractile Activity

Agonist	Ionic Current	Effect
Beta-adrenergic stimulation*,†	I_{Ca} increased	+Inotropic
	I_K increased	↓APD, ↑filling time
	I_{Ks} increased‡	↓APD, ↑filling time
	I_{to} increased	↓APD, ↑filling time
	I_f increased	↑Heart rate
	I_{Na} increased	↑Contraction, ↑conduction
Acetylcholine (ACh) during beta stimulation*,§	I_{Ca} decreased	–Inotropic
	I_{Na} decreased	–Dromotropic
	I_f decreased	–Chronotropic
ACh direct effect on K^+ currents‖	I_{kACh} and I_{kATP} increased	Heart rate↓
Alpha-adrenergic stimulation¶	I_{to} decreased	+Inotropic
	I_k decreased	+Inotropic
	I_{kACh} decreased	Atrial current, effects not clear

*Data from Matsuda et al.[130]
†Data from Matsuda et al.[131]
‡Data from Volders et al.[135]
§Data from Chang and Cohen[132]
‖Data from Kurachi.[133]
¶Data from Fedida.[134]
– = negative; + = positive; ↑ = increased; ↓ = decreased; APD = action potential duration; ATP = adenosine triphosphate.

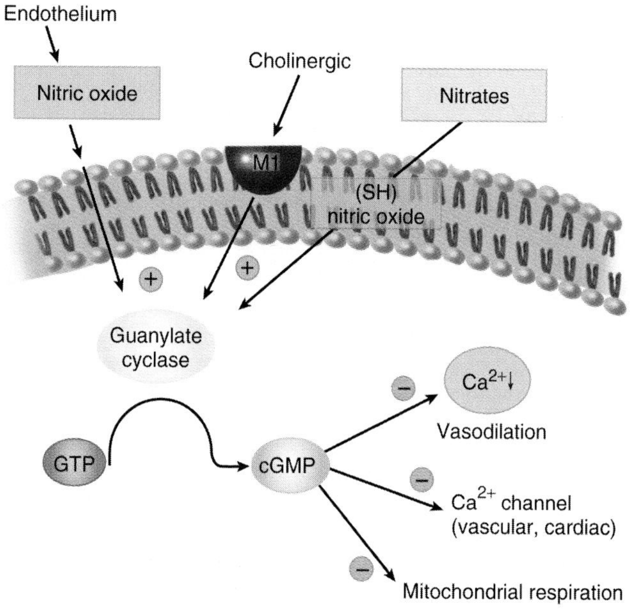

FIGURE 19–16 Nitric oxide messenger system. Proposed role of nitric oxide in stimulating soluble guanylate cyclase to form cyclic guanosine monophosphate (cGMP) to cause vasodilation and a negative inotropic effect. Antianginal nitrates also cause coronary vasodilation by this mechanism. GTP = guanosine triphosphate; M1 = muscarinic receptor, subtype 1. (Modified from Opie LH: Heart Physiology, from Cell to Circulation. Philadelphia, Lippincott Williams & Wilkins, 2004. Copyright L. H. Opie, © 2004.)

eNOS in humans with coronary disease.[52] Because the activity of guanylyl cyclase, promoted by cholinergic stimulation, is sensitive to and enhanced by NO,[48] previous concepts are revised in that NO is now seen as augmenting parasympathetic simulation both upstream and downstream from acetylcholine.

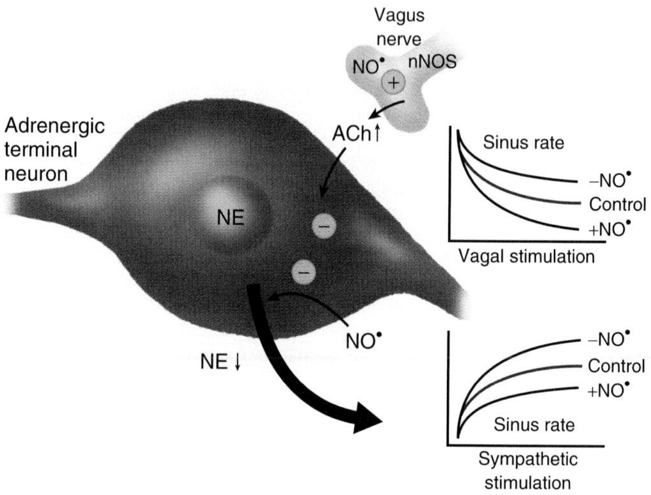

FIGURE 19–17 Nitric oxide (NO) mediates release of acetylcholine (ACh) from vagal nerve terminals. NO, produced in the terminal vagal nerve endings, increases the release of ACh and decreases that of norepinephrine (NE). Thus, the sinus rate response to either vagal or sympathetic stimulation is changed accordingly. For concept, see Paterson.[51] nNOS = neuronal nitric oxide synthase. (Modified from Opie LH: Heart Physiology, from Cell to Circulation. Philadelphia, Lippincott Williams & Wilkins, 2004. Copyright L. H. Opie, © 2004.)

Protective Role of Nitric Oxide. NO contributes to both early and late phases of preconditioning (see later), either as part of the protective messenger systems invoked by ischemia or by inhibition of mitochondrial calcium uptake.[53]

Adverse Effects of Excess Nitric Oxide. Whereas physiological amounts of NO are cardioprotective, substantial evidence indicates that excess NO is harmful. The free radical peroxynitrite ($ONOO^-$), formed from NO and superoxide, leads to the conversion product nitrotyrosine, both with toxic myocardial effects. Examples occur in septic or cardiogenic shock[54] or during prolonged nitrate therapy when peroxynitrite inhibits the formation of cyclic GMP to contribute to nitrate tolerance. Whereas physiological NO suppresses cell death through apoptosis, higher levels promote it.

Does Nitric Oxide Regulate Contractility? This role of NO is controversial. "Puffs" of NO may be formed in diastole to prolong diastole and ventricular filling.[55] Yet any effects on contractility are probably not direct but occur through the autonomic modulation of heart rate.[56]

Other Inhibitory Signal Systems

ADENOSINE SIGNALING. Adenosine, like NO, is a physiological vasodilator. It is formed from the breakdown of ATP both physiologically (as during an increased heart load) and pathologically (as in ischemia). Adenosine can diffuse from myocardial cells to act on coronary arterial smooth muscle to cause vasodilation. The mechanism of the latter effect is reasonably well understood and involves the stimulation of vascular adenylate cyclase and cyclic AMP formation. A_2 receptors mediate such vasodilation. Although A_2 receptors have also been identified in cardiomyocytes, stimulation of such receptors does not have functional consequences.[57] Therefore, it is only the A_1 receptors that are coupled to adenylate cyclase by the inhibitory G protein (alpha$_i$ subunit) that are functional in the myocardium.

Other signal systems and other receptor subtypes are also involved. First, A_1 receptors couple to the acetylcholine-sensitive potassium channel (current I_{KACh}) to stimulate channel opening and thereby to exert inhibitory effects on the sinus and atrioventricular nodes. The latter inhibition is the basis for the use of adenosine in the treatment of supraventricular nodal reentry arrhythmias. Second, A_1 receptors may couple to the PKC system, and thence to the ATP-sensitive potassium channel, thereby hypothetically explaining their role in preconditioning (see Preconditioning). Third, A_3 receptors also precondition through PKC but without the obvious hemodynamic effects of A_1 receptor stimulation.[58]

OPIOID RECEPTORS. Opioids released in the central nervous system are known to participate in cardiovascular regulation by inhibiting sympathetic and promoting parasympathetic outflow. Such endogenous opiates, called *endorphins*, may be involved in the benefits of cardiovascular training. In congestive heart failure, opioid activity may limit adrenergic activation. In animals, opioid receptor stimulation may help to explain the phenomenon of hibernation.[59] In addition, opioid drugs such as morphine are often used in cardiovascular medicine and may have effects beyond pain relief. Opioid effects may be mediated, in part, through local cardiovascular opioid receptors that respond to stimulation of the opioid system in response to conditions of physiological or psychosocial stress. There are three opioid receptors, delta, kappa, and mu, of which the first two are found in the human heart, whereas the mu receptors mediate signals that dampen the pain response. In the heart, the delta receptors inhibit the adrenergic system by coupling to G_i to inhibit the activation of adenylyl cyclase by beta-adrenergic stimulation. In addition, by stimulation of the PKC pathway (see later), they mediate preconditioning.[60]

Vasoconstrictive Signaling

VASCULAR G PROTEIN–COUPLED RECEPTORS. Agonists with vasoconstriction as their major physiological role are $alpha_1$-adrenergic catecholamines, angiotensin II, and endothelin (Fig. 19–18). By regulating the degree of vasoconstriction, the peripheral vascular resistance can be tuned to the needs of the circulation, with, for example, vasoconstriction occurring in response to $alpha_1$-adrenergic stimulation during the stress of blood loss. Each of these agonists is coupled to its appropriate seven-transmembrane-spanning receptor, linked through the G protein G_q to effectors different from those of adrenergic and cholinergic signaling. Specifically, a different calcium release signal system is involved to achieve vasoconstrictive calcium release in vascular tissue. The myocardial ryanodine receptor is replaced by that for IP_3. This IP_3 receptor has a high degree of molecular homology with the ryanodine receptor but is only about half its size. The IP_3 messenger system is of fundamental importance in regulating the release of calcium from the SR and thereby regulating arterial tone and hence the afterload against which the heart must work. In cardiac muscle, the role of IP_3 is still sufficiently controversial to question its role in the inotropic response.

VASOCONSTRICTIVE PATHS AND MYOCARDIAL GROWTH. IP_3 is one of two major signaling molecules produced by the G_q-mediated activation of phospholipase C that converts phosphatidylinositol to IP_3 and diacylglycerol. The latter activates PKC, once PKC has been translocated from the cytosol to the sarcolemma, for example, during the preconditioning sequence (see later). PKC is also implicated as a key activator of the MAP kinase path that leads to increased myocardial growth and LV hypertrophy, especially in response to receptor stimulation by angiotensin II. In addition, mechanically induced cytoskeletal distortion, acting through integrins and other structural proteins, can activate the MAP kinase cascade.[61] Whether the vasoconstrictive agonists can also act as backup positive inotropic agents for the myocardium remains controversial.

Cytokine Signaling

TUMOR NECROSIS FACTOR-ALPHA. Tumor necrosis factor-alpha (TNF-α) is one of the family of peptide cytokines that form part of the innate immune system. Such cytokines mediate local events and are distinct from circulating neurotransmitters or hormones. TNF-α stimulation has bifunctional effects, mediating both protective signals as a component of preconditioning[62] and adverse cardiodepressant signaling in response to diffuse myocardial ischemia as in embolization.[63] The signaling paths involved are complex, starting with two surface receptors for TNF-α leading through sphingolipids to apparently bifurcating paths. One path is adaptive and sends further signals through nuclear factor kappa B to the nucleus for the manufacture of protective molecules. The other maladaptive path leads to apoptosis through activation of caspases. These paths are neither simple nor well understood. For example, NO can act both upstream and downstream from TNF-α.[63] Currently, it is not known why the intracellular signaling paths activated by TNF-α sometimes lead to beneficial effects such as preconditioning and cell survival and at other times lead to depressed myocardial function and apoptosis. Two proposals are (1) that there are short-term adaptive and long-term maladaptive effects of TNF-α and (2) that low concentrations are adaptive and high concentrations maladaptive.[64]

Contractile Performance of the Intact Heart

There are three main determinants of myocardial mechanical performance, namely the Frank-Starling mechanism, the contractile state, and the heart rate. This section describes the cardiac cycle and then the determinants of LV function.

The Cardiac Cycle

The cardiac cycle, fully assembled by Lewis[65] but first conceived by Wiggers,[66] yields important information on the temporal sequence of events in the cardiac cycle. The three basic events are (1) LV contraction, (2) LV relaxation, and (3) LV filling (Table 19–3). Although similar mechanical events occur in the right side of the heart, it is those on the left side that are focused on.

LEFT VENTRICULAR CONTRACTION. LV pressure starts to build up when the arrival of calcium ions at the contractile proteins starts to trigger actin-myosin interaction (Fig. 19–19). On the electrocardiogram, the advance of the wave of depolarization is indicated by the peak of the R wave. Soon after, LV pressure in the early contraction phase builds up and exceeds that in the left atrium (normally 10 to 15 mm Hg) followed about 20 milliseconds later by M_1, the mitral component of the first heart sound. The exact relation of M_1 to mitral valve closure is open to dispute. Although mitral valve closure is often thought to coincide with the crossover point at which the LV pressure starts to exceed the left atrial pressure,[67] in reality mitral valve closure is delayed because the valve is kept open by the inertia of the blood flow. Shortly thereafter, pressure changes in the right ventricle, similar in pattern to those in the left ventricle but of lesser magnitude, cause the tricuspid valve to close, thereby creating T_1, which is the second component of the first heart sound. During this phase of contraction between mitral valve and aortic valve opening, the LV volume is fixed (*isovolumic contraction*) because both aortic and mitral valves are shut. As more and

TABLE 19–3 The Cardiac Cycle

Left Ventricular Contraction
Isovolumic contraction (b)
Maximal ejection (c)
Left Ventricular Relaxation
Start of relaxation and reduced ejection (d)
Isovolumic relaxation (e)
LV filling: rapid phase (f)
Slow LV filling (diastasis) (g)
Atrial systole or booster (a)

The letters a to g refer to the phases of the cardiac cycle shown in Wiggers' diagram (Fig. 19–19). These letters are arbitrarily allocated so that atrial systole (a) coincides with the A wave and (c) with the C wave of the jugular venous pressure.

LV = left ventricular.

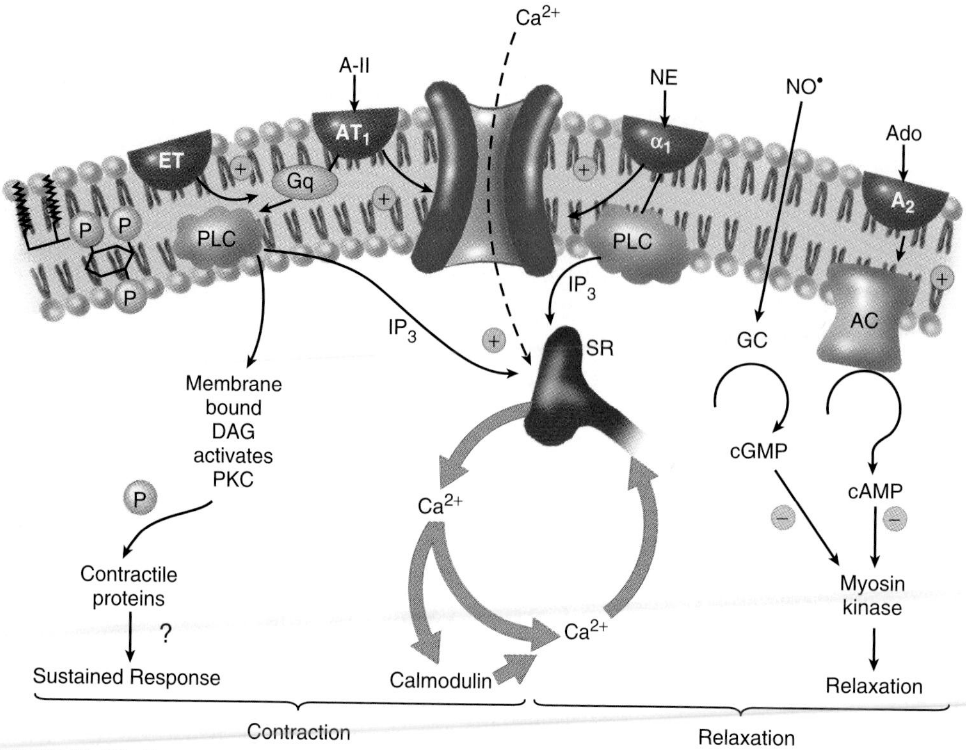

FIGURE 19–18 Patterns of contraction and relaxation in vascular smooth muscle. For example, the angiotensin II (A-II) signaling system is coupled through a G protein to phospholipase C (PLC), which breaks down phosphatidylinositol (PIP_2) to 1,2-diacylglycerol (DAG) and inositol triphosphate (IP_3). DAG translocates protein kinase C from cytosol to the sarcolemma, thereby activating PKC. Signals beyond PKC are not clear. It may phosphorylate ion channels to give the sustained vasoconstrictive response. IP_3 releases calcium from the sarcoplasmic reticulum to initiate vascular smooth muscle contraction. Other vasoconstrictors such as endothelin (ET receptor) act by the same signal system. In response to norepinephrine (NE), an alpha$_1$-agonist, a similar sequence of events occurs to promote contraction. Relaxation is achieved by inhibition of myosin kinase when either cyclic guanosine monophosphate (cGMP) or cyclic adenosine monophosphate (cAMP) is formed in response, respectively, to nitric oxide (NO•) or adenosine (A). AC = adenylyl cyclase; GC = guanylyl cyclase. (Modified from Opie LH: Heart Physiology, from Cell to Circulation. Philadelphia, Lippincott Williams & Wilkins, 2004. Copyright L. H. Opie, © 2004.)

more myofibers enter the contracted state, pressure development in the left ventricle proceeds. The interaction of actin and myosin increases, and cross-bridge cycling is augmented. When the pressure in the left ventricle exceeds that in the aorta, the aortic valve opens, usually a clinically silent event. Opening of the aortic valve is followed by the phase of *rapid ejection.* The rate of ejection is determined not only by the pressure gradient across the aortic valve but also by the elastic properties of the aorta and the arterial tree, which undergoes systolic expansion. LV pressure rises to a peak and then starts to fall.

LEFT VENTRICULAR RELAXATION. As the cytosolic calcium ion concentration starts to decline because of uptake of calcium into the SR under the influence of activated phospholamban, more and more myofibers enter the state of relaxation and the rate of ejection of blood from the left ventricle into the aorta falls (*phase of reduced ejection*). During this phase, blood flow from the left ventricle to the aorta rapidly diminishes but is maintained by aortic recoil—the Windkessel effect. The pressure in the aorta exceeds the falling pressure in the left ventricle. The aortic valve closes, creating the first component of the second sound, A_2 (the second component, P_2, results from closure of the pulmonary valve as the pulmonary artery pressure exceeds that in the right ventricle). Thereafter, the ventricle continues to relax. Because the mitral valve is closed during this phase, the LV volume cannot change (*isovolumic relaxation*). When the LV pressure falls to below that in the left atrium, the mitral valve opens (normally silent) and the filling phase of the cardiac cycle restarts (see Fig. 19–19).

LEFT VENTRICULAR FILLING PHASES. As LV pressure drops below that in the left atrium, just after mitral valve opening, the *phase of rapid or early filling* occurs to account for most of ventricular filling.[68] Active diastolic relaxation of the ventricle may also contribute to early filling (see section on ventricular suction). Such rapid filling may cause the physiological third heart sound (S_3), particularly when there is a hyperkinetic circulation.[69] As pressures in the atrium and ventricle equalize, LV filling virtually stops (*diastasis,* separation). Renewed filling requires that the pressure gradient from the atrium to the ventricle increase. This is achieved by *atrial systole* (or the *left atrial booster*), which is especially important when a high cardiac output is required as during exercise or when the left ventricle fails to relax normally as in LV hypertrophy.[68]

Definitions of Systole and Diastole

In Greek, *systole* means contraction and *diastole* means "to send apart." The start of systole can be regarded as either (1) the beginning of isovolumic contraction when LV pressure exceeds the atrial pressure or (2) mitral valve closure (M_1). These correspond reasonably well because mitral valve closure actually occurs only about 20 milliseconds after the crossover point of the pressures. Thus, in practice the term isovolumic contraction often also includes this brief period of early systolic contraction even before the mitral valve shuts, when the heart volume does not change substantially. *Physiological systole* lasts from the start of isovolumic contraction (at which LV pressure crosses over atrial pressure, see Fig. 19–19) to the peak of the ejection phase, so that physiological diastole commences as the LV pressure starts to fall (Table 19–4).

TABLE 19–4 Physiological Versus Cardiologic Systole and Diastole

Physiological Systole	**Cardiologic Systole**
Isovolumic contraction Maximal ejection	From M_1 to A_2, including: Major part of isovolumic contraction* Maximal ejection Reduced ejection
Physiological Diastole	**Cardiologic Diastole**
Reduced ejection Isovolumic relaxation Filling phases	A_2-M_1 interval (filling phases included)

*Note that M_1 occurs with a definite albeit short delay after the start of LV contraction.

This concept fits well with the standard pressure-volume curve. *Physiological diastole* commences as calcium ions are taken up into the SR, so that myocyte relaxation dominates over contraction, and the LV pressure starts to fall as shown on the pressure-volume curve. In contrast, *cardiological systole* is demarcated by the interval between the first and second heart sounds, lasting from the first heart sound (M_1) to the closure of the aortic valve (A_2). The remainder of the cardiac cycle automatically becomes *cardiological diastole*. Thus, cardiological systole, demarcated by heart sounds rather than physiological events, starts fractionally later than physiological systole and ends significantly later. For the cardiologist, *protodiastole* is the early phase of rapid filling, the time when the third heart sound (S_3) can be heard. This sound probably reflects ventricular wall vibrations during rapid filling and becomes audible with an increase in LV diastolic pressure or wall stiffness or rate of filling.

In contrast stands another physiological concept, promulgated by Brutsaert and colleagues,[70] who argued that diastole starts much later, only when the whole of the contraction-relaxation cycle is over. According to this minority view, diastole would occupy only a short portion of the cardiac cycle.[70] This definition of diastole, although seldom used in cardiological practice, does give a reminder that abnormalities of LV contraction often underlie defective relaxation.

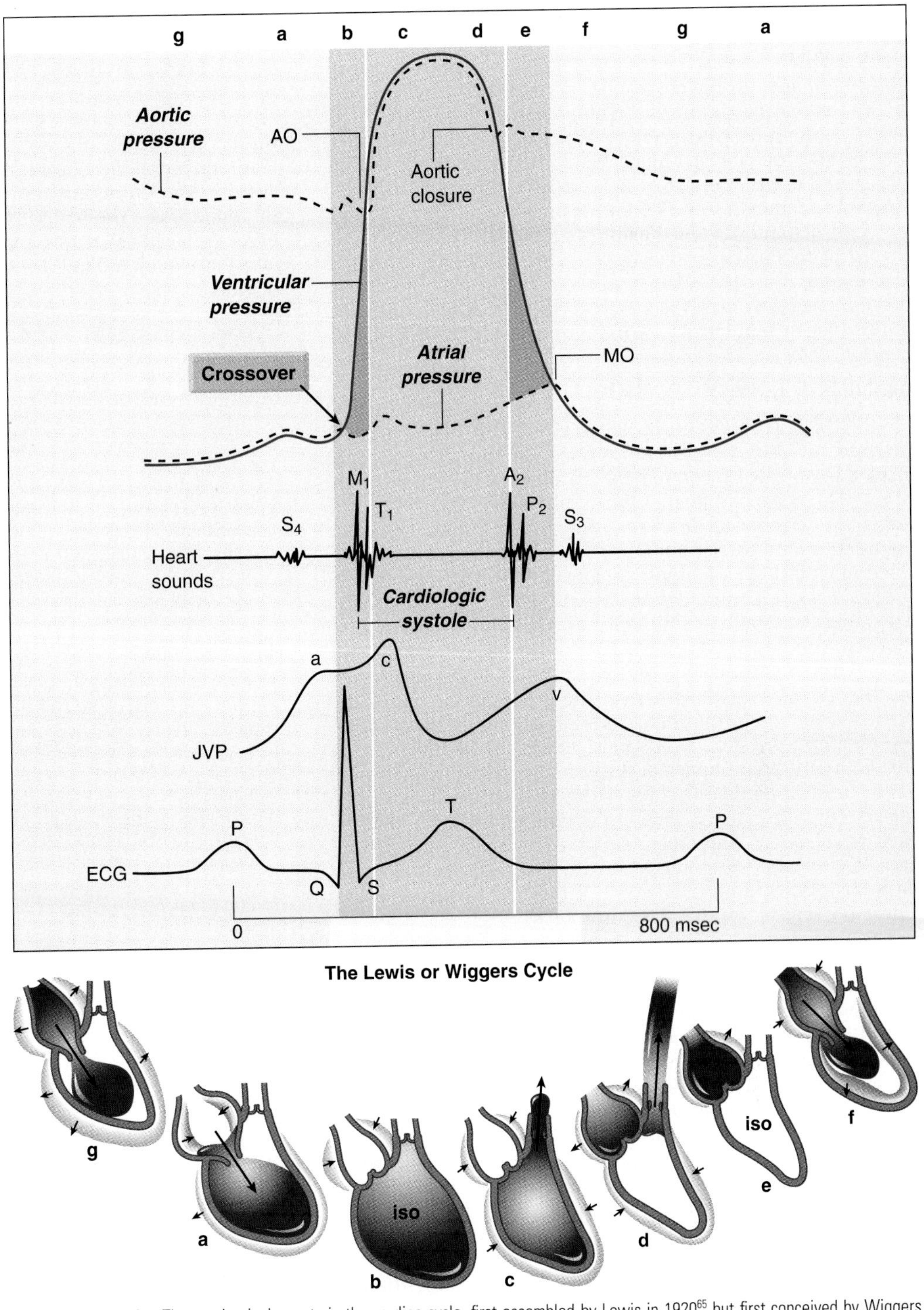

FIGURE 19–19 The mechanical events in the cardiac cycle, first assembled by Lewis in 1920[65] but first conceived by Wiggers in 1915.[66] Note that mitral valve closure occurs *after* the crossover point of atrial and ventricular pressures at the start of systole. For an explanation of phases a to g, see Table 19–3. Cycle length of 800 milliseconds for 75 beats/min. A_2 = aortic valve closure, aortic component of second sound; AO = aortic valve opening, normally inaudible; ECG = electrocardiogram; JVP = jugular venous pressure; M_1 = mitral component of first sound at time of mitral valve closure; MO = mitral valve opening, may be audible in mitral stenosis as the opening snap; P_2 = pulmonary component of second sound, pulmonary valve closure; S_3 = third heart sound; S_4 = fourth heart sound; T_1 = tricuspid valve closure, second component of first heart sound; a = wave produced by right atrial contraction; c = carotid wave artifact during rapid left ventricular ejection phase; v = venous return wave, which causes pressure to rise while tricuspid valve is closed. (Visual phases of the ventricular cycle at the bottom modified from Shepherd JT, Vanhoutte PM: The Human Cardiovascular System. New York: Raven Press, 1979, p 68. Modified from Opie LH: Heart Physiology, from Cell to Circulation. Philadelphia, Lippincott Williams & Wilkins, 2004.)

Contractility Versus Loading Conditions

CONTRACTILITY. *Contractility is the inherent capacity of the myocardium to contract independently of changes in the preload or afterload.* It is a key word in our cardiological language. At a molecular level, an increase in contractility can be explained by enhanced interaction between calcium ions and the contractile proteins. Increased contractility means a greater rate of contraction to reach a greater peak force. Often, an increased contractility is associated with enhanced rates of relaxation, called the *lusitropic effect*. Alternative names for contractility are the *inotropic state* (*ino*, fiber; *tropos*, to move) and the *contractile state*. Contractility is an important regulator of the myocardial oxygen uptake. Factors that increase contractility include exercise, adrenergic stimulation, digitalis, and other inotropic agents.

PRELOAD AND AFTERLOAD. It is important to stress that any change in the contractile state should be independent of the loading conditions. The *preload* is the load present before contraction has started, at the end of diastole (the afterload is discussed later). The preload reflects the venous filling pressure that fills the left atrium, which in turn fills the left ventricle during diastole. When the preload increases, the left ventricle distends during diastole, and the stroke volume rises according to Starling's law (see next section). The heart rate is also increased by stimulation of the atrial mechanoreceptors that enhance the rate of discharge of the sinoatrial node. Thus, the cardiac output (stroke volume times heart rate) rises.

Starling's Law of the Heart

VENOUS FILLING PRESSURE AND HEART VOLUME. Starling in 1918 related the venous pressure in the right atrium to the heart volume in the dog heart-lung preparation.[28] He proposed that, within physiological limits, the larger the volume of the heart, the greater the energy of its contraction and the amount of chemical change at each contraction. Starling did not, however, measure sarcomere length. He could only relate *LV volume* to cardiac output. This relationship holds in normal, compliant hearts. One modern version of Starling's law is that stroke volume is related to the end-diastolic volume. The LV volume can now be directly measured with two-dimensional echocardiography. Yet the value found depends on a number of simplifying assumptions such as a spherical LV shape and neglects the confounding influence of the complex anatomy of the left ventricle. In practice, therefore, the LV volume is not often measured; rather, use is made of a variety of surrogate measures such as LV end-diastolic pressure or the pulmonary capillary wedge pressure. Yet the relation between LV end-diastolic volume and LV end-diastolic pressure is curvilinear depending on the LV compliance.

The venous filling pressure can be measured in humans albeit indirectly by the technique of *Swan-Ganz catheterization*, as can the stroke volume. The LV pressure and volume are, however, not linearly related because of variations in the compliance of the myocardium. Therefore, a jump from pressure to volume is required to apply the Starling concept to the hemodynamic management of those who are critically ill and receiving a Swan-Ganz catheter.

FRANK AND ISOVOLUMIC CONTRACTION. If a larger heart volume increases the initial length of the muscle fiber, to increase the stroke volume and hence the cardiac output, then diastolic stretch of the left ventricle actually increases contractility. Frank in 1895 had already reported that the greater the initial LV volume, the more rapid the rate of rise, the greater the peak pressure reached, and the faster the rate of relaxation.[28] He described both a positive *inotropic effect* and an increased lusitropic effect. These complementary findings of Frank and Starling are often combined into the *Frank-Starling law.* Between them, they could account for two of the mechanisms underlying the increased stroke volume of exercise, namely both the increased diastolic filling (Starling's law) and the increased inotropic state (Frank's findings).

AFTERLOAD. The afterload is the systolic load on the left ventricle after it has started to contract. In the nonfailing heart, the left ventricle can overcome any physiological acute increase in load. Chronically, however, the left ventricle must hypertrophy to overcome sustained arterial hypertension or significant aortic stenosis. In clinical practice, the arterial blood pressure is often taken to be synonymous with the afterload while ignoring the *aortic compliance*—the extent to which the aorta can "yield" during systole. A stiff aorta, as in isolated systolic hypertension of elderly people, increases the afterload.

PRELOAD AND AFTERLOAD ARE INTERLINKED. The preceding distinctions between preload and afterload do not allow for the situations in which the two change concurrently. By the Frank-Starling law, an increased LV volume leads to increased contractility, which in turn increases the systolic blood pressure and hence the afterload. Nonetheless, in general, the preload is related to the degree to which the myocardial fibers are stretched at the end of diastole, and the afterload is related to the wall stress generated by those fibers during systole.

FORCE-LENGTH RELATIONSHIPS AND CALCIUM TRANSIENTS. Proof that there is no increase in the calcium transient as the sarcomere length increases is provided by direct measurements (Fig. 19-20). The favored explanation for the steep length-tension relation of cardiac muscles is *length-dependent activation,* whereby an increase in calcium sensitivity is the major factor explaining the steep increase of force development as the initial sarcomere length increases. This change may be explained by stretch of the titin molecule (see Fig. 19-4). Is the degree of overlap of actin and myosin also involved? Whereas the overlap theory explains the force-length relationship in skeletal muscle, in cardiac muscle the situation is different (Fig. 19-21). In cardiac muscle, even at 80 percent of the maximal length, only 10 percent or less of the maximal force is developed. Thus, it can be predicted that cardiac sarcomeres must function near the upper limit of their maximal length (L_{max}). Rodriguez and colleagues[71] have tested this prediction by relating sarcomere length changes to volume changes of the intact heart. By implanting small radiopaque beads in only about 1 cm^3 of the LV free wall and using biplane cineradiography, the motion of the markers could be tracked through various cardiac cycles with allowances made for local myocardial deformation. Thus, the change in sarcomere length from approximately 85 percent of L_{max} to L_{max} itself is able to effect physiological LV volume changes (Fig. 19-22). This estimate is remarkably close to the normal fiber shortening of 15 percent in the human heart in situ.[72]

ANREP EFFECT: ABRUPT INCREASE IN AFTERLOAD. When the aortic pressure is elevated abruptly, a positive inotropic effect follows within 1 or 2 minutes. This effect used to be called homeometric autoregulation (*homeo*, the same; *metric*, length) because it was apparently independent of muscle length and by definition a true inotropic effect. A reasonable speculation would be that increased LV wall tension could act on myocardial stretch receptors to increase cytosolic sodium and then, by Na^+/Ca^{2+} exchange, the cytosolic calcium. Thus, this effect would be different from that of an increase in preload (which acts by length activation).

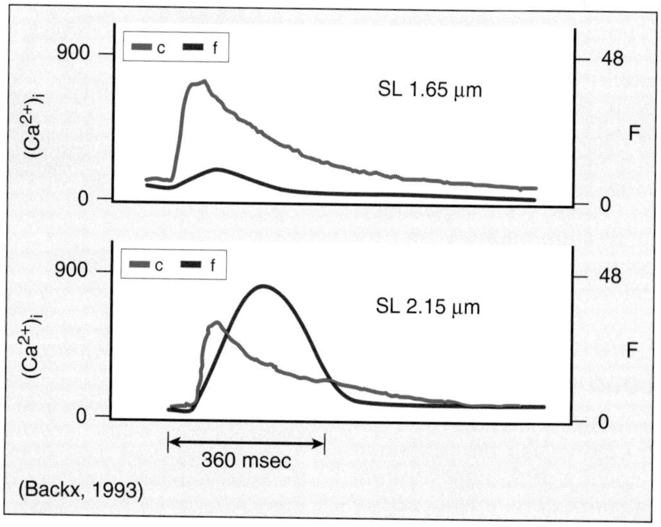

FIGURE 19–20 Length sensitization of the sarcomere. **Top,** The sarcomere length (SL) is 1.65 μm, which gives very little force (f) development (see Fig. 19–7). **Bottom,** At a near-maximum sarcomere length (see Fig. 19–7), the same Ca^{2+} transient (c) with the same peak value and overall pattern causes much greater force development. Therefore, there has been length-induced calcium sensitization. (Modified from Backx PH, ter Keurs HEDJ: Fluorescent properties of rat cardiac trabeculae microinjected with fura-2 salt. Am J Physiol 264:H1098, 1993.)

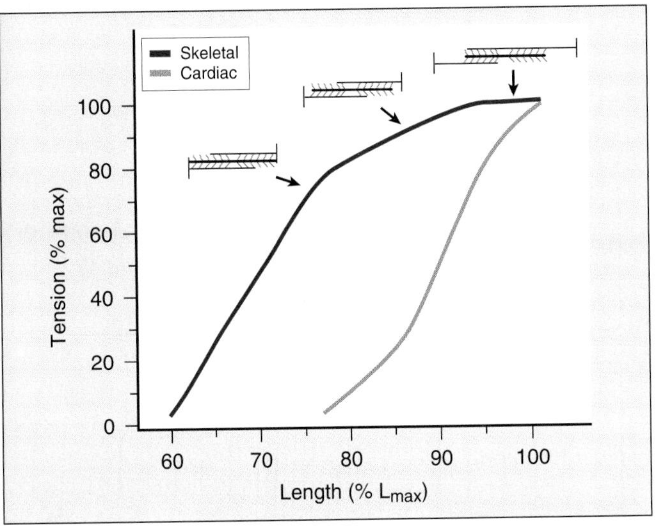

FIGURE 19–21 Force-length relationship. Schematic drawing illustrating general shape of ascending limb in skeletal (A) and cardiac (B) muscle. Normalized force is plotted as a function of normalized length, that is, length relative to the length at which maximum force is generated (L_{max}). Also shown is the approximate disposition of thick and thin filaments at different points along the physiologically relevant portion of the ascending limb. The maximum length (L_{max} 100%) corresponds to the situation at maximum sarcomere lengths, 2.2 mm (Fig. 19–22) or 2.15 mm (Fig. 19–20). (Modified from Fuchs F: Mechanical modulation of the Ca^{2+} regulatory protein complex in cardiac muscle. News Physiol Sci 10:6, 1995.)

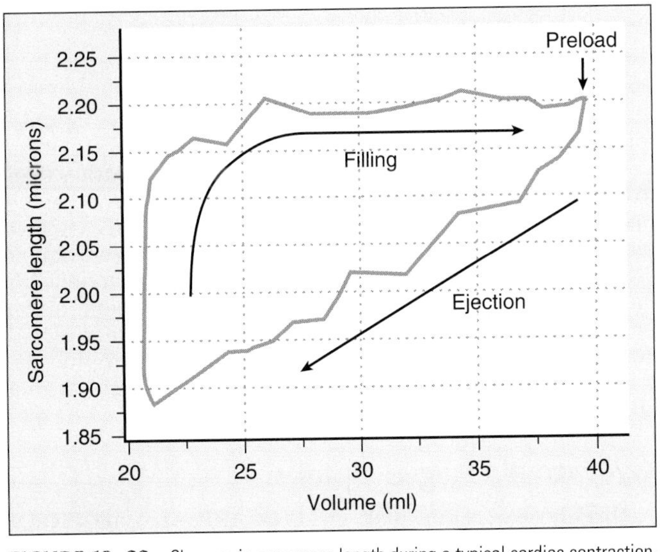

FIGURE 19–22 Changes in sarcomere length during a typical cardiac contraction-relaxation cycle. During diastole the sarcomere length is 2.2 μm, decreasing to 1.90 μm during systole in the intact dog heart. Starting at the top right, the *preload* is the maximum sarcomere length just before the onset of contraction. As ejection decreases the left ventricular volume, by somewhat more than half, sarcomere length falls from 2.20 to 1.90 μm. Then, during the rapid phase of filling (see Fig. 19–19), the sarcomere length increases from 1.90 to 2.15 mm to be followed by the phase of constant sarcomere length (diastasis). (Modified from Rodriguez EK, Hunter WC, Royce MJ, et al: A method to reconstruct sarcomere lengths and orientations to transmural sites in beating canine hearts. Am J Physiol 263:H293, 1992, with permission of the American Physiological Society.)

Wall Stress

Stress develops when tension is applied to a cross-sectional area, and the units are force per unit area. According to the Laplace law (Fig. 19–23):

$$\text{Wall stress} = \frac{\text{pressure} \times \text{radius}}{2 \times \text{wall thickness}}$$

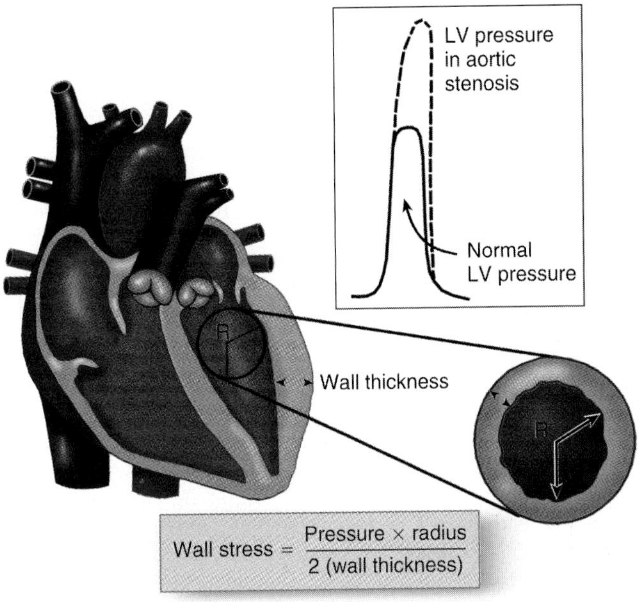

FIGURE 19–23 Wall stress increases as the afterload increases. The formula shown is derived from the Laplace law. The increased left ventricular (LV) pressure in aortic stenosis is compensated for by LV wall hypertrophy, which decreases the denominator on the right side of the equation. (Modified from Opie LH: Heart Physiology, from Cell to Circulation. Philadelphia, Lippincott Williams & Wilkins, 2004. Copyright L. H. Opie, © 2004.)

This equation, although an oversimplification, emphasizes two points. First, the bigger the left ventricle and the greater its radius, the greater the wall stress. Second, at any given radius (LV size), the greater the pressure developed by the left ventricle, the greater the wall stress. An increase in wall stress achieved by either of these two mechanisms (LV size or intraventricular pressure) increases myocardial oxygen uptake because a greater rate of ATP use is required as the myofibrils develop greater tension.

In cardiac hypertrophy, Laplace's law explains the effects of changes in wall thickness on wall stress (see Fig. 19–23). The increased wall thickness related to hypertrophy balances the increased pressure, and the wall stress remains unchanged during the phase of compensatory hypertrophy. This change, previously regarded as compensatory and beneficial, has been seriously challenged by a mouse model in which the process of hypertrophy was genetically inhibited so that wall stress increased in response to a pressure load, yet these mice had better cardiac mechanical function than the wild type that developed compensatory hypertrophy (see Chap. 21).[37] Despite this "mighty mouse" challenge, it is difficult to see how a patient with significant aortic stenosis could develop the intraventricular pressure required to eject blood through the stenosed valve without the development of LV hypertrophy. Another clinically useful concept is that in congestive heart failure, the heart dilates so that the increased radius elevates wall stress. Furthermore, because ejection of blood is inadequate, the radius stays too large throughout the contractile cycle, and both end-diastolic and end-systolic tensions are higher. Reduction of heart size decreases wall stress and improves LV function.

WALL STRESS, PRELOAD, AND AFTERLOAD. *Preload* can now be defined more exactly as the wall stress at the end of diastole and therefore at the maximal resting length of the sarcomere (see Fig. 19–22). Measurement of wall stress in vivo is difficult because the radius of the left ventricle (see preceding sections) neglects the confounding influence of the complex anatomy of the left ventricle. Surrogate measurements of the indices of preload include LV end-diastolic pressure or dimensions (the latter being the major and minor axes of the heart in a two-dimensional echocardiographic view). The *afterload*, being the load on the contracting myocardium, is also the wall stress during LV ejection. Increased afterload means that an increased intraventricular pressure has to be generated first to open the aortic valve and then during the ejection phase. These increases translate into an increased myocardial wall stress, which can be measured either as an average value or at end systole. *End-systolic wall stress* reflects the three major components of the afterload, namely the peripheral resistance, the arterial compliance, and the peak intraventricular pressure. Decreased arterial compliance and increased afterload can be anticipated when there is aortic dilation as in severe systemic hypertension or in elderly persons. Generally, in clinical practice, it is a sufficient approximation to take the systolic blood pressure as an indirect measure of the afterload (reflecting both peripheral resistance and peak intraventricular pressure), provided there is neither significant aortic stenosis nor change in arterial compliance.

AORTIC IMPEDANCE. Also termed *arterial input impedance*, aortic impedance gives another accurate measure of the afterload. The aortic impedance is the aortic pressure divided by the aortic flow at that instant, so that this index of the afterload varies at each stage of the contraction cycle. Factors that reduce aortic flow, such as high arterial blood pressure or aortic stenosis or loss of aortic compliance, increase impedance and hence the afterload. During systole, when the aortic valve is open, an increased afterload communicates itself to the ventricles by increasing wall stress. In LV failure, aortic impedance is augmented not only by peripheral vasoconstriction but also by decreases in aortic compliance. The problem with the clinical measurement of aortic impedance is that invasive instrumentation is required. An approximation can be found by using transesophageal echocardiography to determine aortic blood flow at, for example, the time of maximal increase of aortic flow just after aortic valve opening.

Heart Rate And Force-Frequency Relation

TREPPE OR BOWDITCH EFFECT. An increased heart rate progressively enhances the force of ventricular contraction, even in an isolated papillary muscle preparation (Bowditch staircase phenomenon). Alternative names are the *treppe* (steps, German) phenomenon or positive inotropic effect of activation or force-frequency relationship (Fig. 19–24). Conversely, a decreased heart rate has a negative staircase effect. When stimulation becomes too rapid, force decreases. The proposal is that during rapid stimulation, more sodium and calcium ions enter the myocardial cell than can be handled by the sodium pump and the mechanisms for calcium exit. Opposing the force-frequency effect is the negative contractile influence of the decreased duration of ventricular filling at high heart rates. The longer the filling interval, the better the ventricular filling and the stronger the subsequent contraction. This phenomenon can be shown in patients with atrial fibrillation with a variable filling interval.

Post-extrasystolic potentiation and the inotropic effect of paired pacing can be explained by the same model, again assuming an enhanced contractile state after the prolonged interval between beats. Nonetheless, the exact cellular mechanism remains to be clarified.

FORCE-FREQUENCY RELATIONSHIP AND OPTIMAL HEART RATE. Normally, peak contractile force at a fixed muscle length (isometric contraction) increases and a peak is reached at about 150 to 180 stimuli per minute.[73] This is the human counterpart of the treppe phenomenon. In situ, the optimal heart rate not only is the rate that would give maximal mechanical performance of an isolated muscle strip but also is determined by the need for adequate time for diastolic filling. In normal humans, it is not possible to attach exact values to the heart rate required to decrease rather than to increase cardiac output or to keep it steady. Atrial pacing rates of up to 150 per minute can be tolerated, whereas higher rates cannot because of the development of atrioventricular block. In contrast, during exercise, indices of LV function still increase up to a maximum heart rate of about 170 per minute, presumably because of enhanced contractility and peripheral vasodilation.[74] In patients with severe LV hypertrophy, the critical heart rate is between 100 and 130 per minute, with a fall-off in LV function at higher rates.[75]

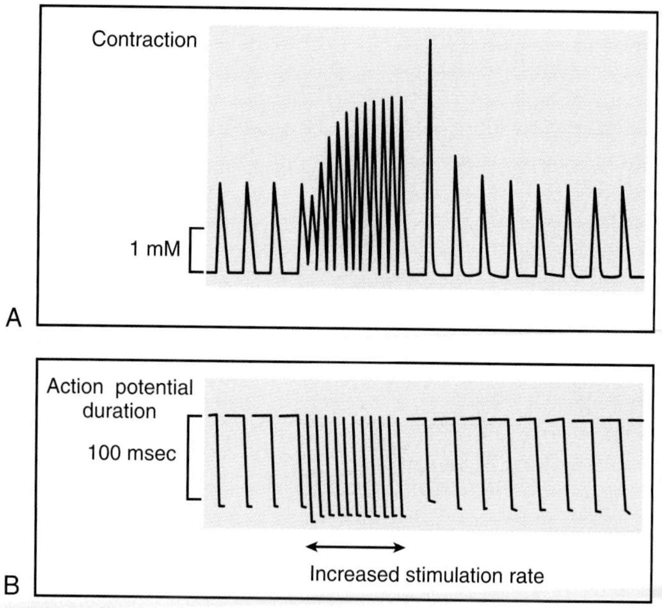

FIGURE 19–24 Bowditch or treppe phenomenon. An increased stimulation rate **(B)** increases the force of contraction **(A)**. The stimulus rate is shown as the action potential duration on an analog analyzer where ms equals milliseconds. The tension developed by papillary muscle contraction is shown in mN (millinewtons). On cessation of rapid stimulation, the contraction force gradually declines. Hypothetically, the explanation for the increased contraction during the increased stimulation is repetitive Ca^{2+} entry with each depolarization and, hence, an accumulation of cytosolic calcium. (From Noble MIM: Excitation-contraction coupling. *In* Drake-Holland AJ, Noble MIM [eds]: Cardiac Metabolism. Chichester, England, John Wiley, 1983, pp 49-71.)

Myocardial Oxygen Uptake

DETERMINANTS OF MYOCARDIAL OXYGEN DEMAND. Myocardial oxygen demand can be increased by heart rate, preload, or afterload (Fig. 19–25), factors that can all precipitate myocardial ischemia in those with coronary artery disease. The O_2 uptake can be augmented by increased contractility as during beta-adrenergic stimulation. Because myocardial O_2 uptake ultimately reflects the rate of mitochondrial metabolism and of ATP production, any increase of ATP requirement is reflected in increased O_2 uptake. In general, factors that increase wall stress increase the O_2 uptake. An increased afterload causes an increased systolic wall stress, which requires greater O_2 uptake. An increased diastolic wall stress, resulting from an increased preload, also requires more O_2 because the greater stroke volume must be ejected against the afterload. In states of enhanced contractility, the rate of change of wall stress is increased. Thus, thinking in terms of wall stress provides a comprehensive approach to the problem of myocardial O_2 uptake. Because the systolic blood pressure is an important determinant of the afterload, a practical index of the O_2 uptake is systolic blood pressure × heart rate, the *double product*. In addition, there

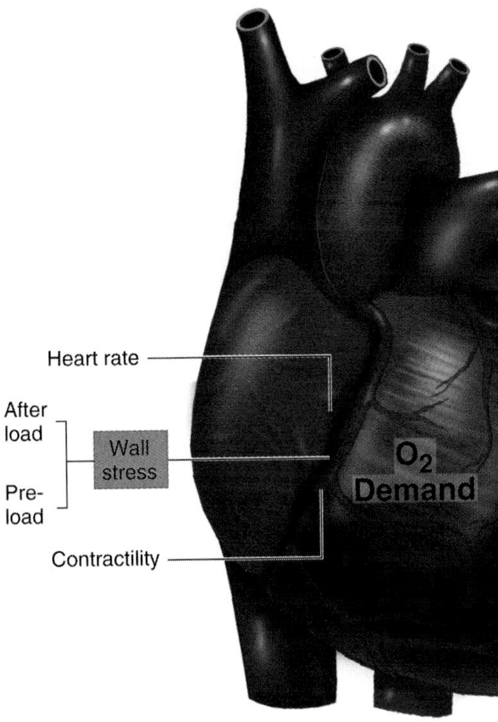

FIGURE 19–25 Major determinants of the oxygen demand of the normal heart. These are heart rate, wall stress, and contractility. For use of pressure-volume area as index of oxygen uptake, see Figure 19–26. (Modified from Opie LH: The Heart, Physiology, from Cell to Circulation. Philadelphia, Lippincott Raven, 1998. Copyright L. H. Opie, © 1998.)

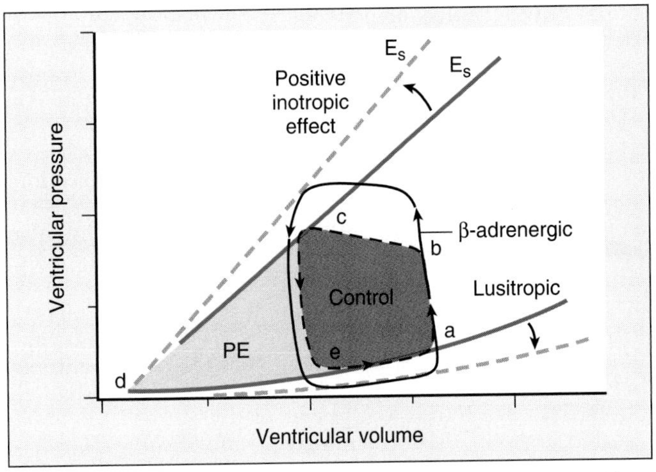

FIGURE 19–26 Pressure-volume loop of left ventricle. Note the effects of beta-adrenergic catecholamines with both positive inotropic (increased slope of line E_s) and increased lusitropic (relaxant) effects. E_s is the slope of the pressure-volume relationship. The total pressure-volume area (for control area, see a, b, c, d) is closely related to the myocardial oxygen uptake. The area c, d, e is the component of work spent in generating potential energy (PE). (Modified from Opie LH: Heart Physiology, from Cell to Circulation. Philadelphia, Lippincott Williams & Wilkins, 2004. Copyright L. H. Opie, © 2004.)

may be a metabolic component of the oxygen uptake that is usually small but may be prominent in certain special conditions, such as the "oxygen wastage" found with abnormally high circulating free fatty acid values. The concept of wall stress in relation to O_2 uptake also explains why heart size is such an important determinant of the myocardial O_2 uptake (because a larger radius increases wall stress).

WORK OF THE HEART. External work is done when, for example, a mass is lifted a certain distance. In terms of the heart, the cardiac output is the mass moved, and the resistance against which it is moved is the blood pressure. Because volume work requires less oxygen than pressure work, it might be supposed that external work is not an important determinant of the myocardial O_2 uptake. However, three determinants of the myocardial O_2 uptake are involved: preload (because it helps determine the stroke volume), afterload (in part determined by the blood pressure), and heart rate, as can be seen from the following formula:

$$\text{Minute work} = \text{SBP} \times \text{SV} \times \text{heart rate}$$

where SBP = systolic blood pressure and SV = stroke volume. Thus, it is not surprising that heart work is related to oxygen uptake. The *pressure-work index* takes into account both the double product (SBP × HR) and the HR × stroke volume, i.e., cardiac output. The *pressure-volume area* is another index of myocardial O_2 uptake, requiring invasive monitoring for accurate measurements. External cardiac work can account for up to 40 percent of the total myocardial O_2 uptake.

Internal Work (Potential Energy). The total oxygen consumption is related to the total work of the heart (area a, b, c, d in Fig. 19–26), meaning both the external work (the area a, b, c, e) and the volume-pressure triangle joining the end-systolic volume-pressure point to the origin (the area c, d, e; marked PE).[76] Although this area has been called internal work, more strictly it should be called *potential energy* that is generated within each contraction cycle but not converted to external work. Such potential energy at the end of systole (point c) may be likened to the potential energy of a compressed spring.

Kinetic Work. In strict terms, the work performed *(power production)* needs to take into account not only pressure but also kinetic components. It is the pressure work that has been discussed (product of cardiac output and peak systolic pressure). The kinetic work is the component required to move the blood against the afterload. Normally, kinetic work is less than 1 percent of the total. In aortic stenosis, kinetic work increases sharply as the cross-sectional area of the aortic valve narrows, whereas pressure work increases as the gradient across the aortic valve rises. Noninvasive measures of peak power production are being assessed as indices of cardiac contractility.

Efficiency of Work. The efficiency of work is the relation between the work performed and the myocardial oxygen uptake. Exercise increases the efficiency of external work, an improvement that offsets any metabolic cost of the increased contractility.[77] Metabolically, efficiency is increased by promotion of glucose rather than fatty acids as the major myocardial fuel.[78] Conversely, heart failure decreases the efficiency of work, possibly by beta-adrenergically promoted fatty acid metabolism.[79] The subcellular basis for changes in efficiency of work is not fully understood. Because as little as 12 to 14 percent of the oxygen uptake may be converted to external work,[77] it is probably the "internal work" that becomes more or less demanding. Internal ion fluxes ($Na^+/K^+/Ca^{2+}$) account for about 20 to 30 percent of the ATP requirement of the heart, so that most ATP is spent on actin-myosin interaction and much of that on generation of heat rather than on external work. An increased initial muscle length sensitizes the contractile apparatus to calcium (see Fig. 19–20), thereby theoretically increasing the efficiency of contraction by diminishing the amount of calcium flux required.

Measurements of Contractility

(see also Chap. 20)

FORCE-VELOCITY RELATIONSHIP AND MAXIMUM CONTRACTILITY IN MUSCLE MODELS. If the concept of contractility is truly independent of the load and the heart rate, unloaded heart muscle stimulated at a fixed rate should have a maximum value of contractility for any given magnitude of the cytosolic calcium transient. This value, the V_{max} of muscle contraction, is defined as the *maximal velocity of contraction* when there is no load on the isolated muscle or no afterload to prevent maximal rates of cardiac ejection. Beta-adrenergic stimulation increases V_{max}, and converse changes are found in the failing myocardium. V_{max} is also termed V_0 (the maximum velocity at zero load). The problem with this relatively simple concept is that V_{max} cannot be measured directly but is extrapolated from the peak rates of force development in unloaded muscle obtained from the intercept on the velocity axis. In another extreme condition, there is no muscle shortening at all (zero shortening), and all the energy goes into development of pressure (P_0) or force (F_0). This situation is an example of *isometric shortening* (*iso*, the same; *metric*, length). Because the peak velocity is obtained at zero load when there is no external force development, the relationship is usually termed the *force-velocity relationship*.

The concept of V_{max} has been subject to much debate over many years, chiefly because of the technical difficulties in obtaining truly unloaded conditions. Braunwald and coworkers[80] used cat papillary muscle to define a hyperbolic force-velocity curve, with V_{max} relatively independent of the initial muscle length but increased by the addition of norepinephrine. Another preparation used to examine force-velocity relations involves single cardiac myocytes isolated by enzymatic digestion of the rat myocardium and then permeabilized with a staphylococcal toxin. Again, the force-velocity relation is hyperbolic, suggesting the existence of intracellular *passive elastic elements* that contribute to the load on the isolated myocyte. In fact, the more hyperbolic and increased curvilinear nature of the force-velocity relationship in isolated myocytes than in the papillary muscle suggests that internal passive forces such as those generated by titin (see Fig. 19–4) are greater than expected in the isolated myocytes. In the intact heart, the noncontractile components contribute relatively little to overall mechanical behavior, at least in physiological circumstances.[81] Data from both papillary muscle and sarcomeres suggest that in unloaded conditions the intrinsic contractility as assessed by V_{max} does not change with initial fiber or sarcomere length.

MECHANISM OF BETA-ADRENERGIC EFFECTS ON FORCE-VELOCITY RELATIONSHIP. The data on papillary muscles showing that norepinephrine can increase V_{max} could be explained by either an effect of beta-adrenergic stimulation on enhancing calcium ion entry or a direct effect on the contractile proteins, or both. Strang and coworkers[82] showed that either isoproterenol (beta stimulant) or PKA (intracellular messenger) increased V_{max} by about 40 percent concurrently with phosphorylation of troponin I and of C protein in an isolated ventricular myocyte preparation. The overall concept would be that beta-adrenergic stimulation mediates the major component of its inotropic effect through increasing the cytosolic calcium transient and the factors controlling it, such as the rate of entry of calcium ions through the sarcolemmal L-type channels, the rate of calcium uptake under the influence of phospholamban into the SR, and the rate of calcium release from the ryanodine receptor in response to calcium entry in association with depolarization.

ISOMETRIC VERSUS ISOTONIC CONTRACTION. Despite the similarities in the force-velocity patterns in the data obtained on papillary muscle and isolated myocytes, it should be considered that a number of different types of muscular contraction may be involved. For example, data for P_0 are obtained under isometric conditions (length unchanged). When muscle is allowed to shorten against a steady load, the conditions are *isotonic* (*iso*, same; *tonic*, contractile force). Thus, the force-velocity curve may be a combination of initial isometric conditions followed by isotonic contraction and then followed by the abrupt and total unloading to measure V_{max}. Although isometric conditions can be found in the whole heart as an approximation during isovolumic contraction, isotonic conditions cannot prevail because the load is constantly changing during the ejection period, and complete unloading is impossible. Therefore, the application of force-velocity relations to the heart in vivo is limited.

PRESSURE-VOLUME LOOPS. Accordingly, measurements of pressure-volume loops are among the best of the current approaches to the assessment of the contractile behavior of the intact heart. Major criticisms arise when it is assumed that E_s is necessarily linear (it may be curvilinear) or when E_s is used as an index of "absolute" contractility (for E_s, see Fig. 19–26). Also, in clinical practice, the need to change the loading conditions and the requirement for invasive monitoring, required for the full loop, lessen the usefulness of this index. To measure LV volume adequately and continuously throughout the cardiac cycle is not easy. During a positive inotropic intervention, the pressure-volume loop reflects a smaller end-systolic volume and a higher end-systolic pressure, so that the slope of the pressure-volume relationship (E_s) has moved upward and to the left (see Fig. 19–26). When the positive inotropic intervention is by beta-adrenergic stimulation, enhanced relaxation (lusitropic effect) results in a lower pressure-volume curve during ventricular filling than in controls.

CONTRACTILITY

Defects in the Concept. Despite all the foregoing procedures that can be adopted to attempt to measure true contractility, the concept has at least two serious defects: (1) the absence of any potential index that can be measured in situ and that is free of significant criticism and, in particular, the absence of any acceptable noninvasive index, and (2) the impossibility of separating the cellular mechanisms of contractility changes from those of load or heart rate. Thus, an increased heart rate through the sodium pump lag mechanism gives rise to increased cytosolic calcium, which is thought to explain the treppe phenomenon. An increased preload involves increased fiber stretch, which in turn causes length activation, explicable by sensitization of the contractile proteins to the prevailing cytosolic calcium concentration. An increased afterload may increase cytosolic calcium through stretch-sensitive channels. Thus, there is a clear overlap between contractility, which should be independent of load or heart rate, and the effects of load and heart rate on the cellular mechanisms. Hence, the traditional separation of inotropic state from load or heart rate effects as two independent regulators of cardiac muscle performance is no longer simple now that the underlying cellular mechanisms have been uncovered. An example of this dilemma arises in humans with atrial fibrillation and a constantly varying force-frequency relationship. Contractility as measured in situ by pressure-volume loops constantly changes from beat to beat, and the explanation could be either a "true" change in contractility or the operation of the Frank-Starling mechanism because of varying diastolic filling times.[83]

The Concept Is Essential and the Search Continues. Whatever the defects of the concept and the problems of measuring it, contractility remains an essential cardiac concept to separate the effects of a primary change in loading conditions or heart rate from an intrinsic change in the force of contraction. An analogy could be that the rate at which a truck travels is determined not only by external "loading" factors such as the weight of the goods carried on the back and the slope of the road but also by "internal" factors such as the horsepower of the engine and the gear used. Hence, the quest for the perfect index of contractility continues. Currently, tissue Doppler imaging is being assessed to provide indices such as the rate of myocardial acceleration during the phase of isovolumic contraction.[84]

Ventricular Relaxation and Diastolic Dysfunction (see also Chaps. 20 and 21). Diastolic dysfunction and diastolic heart failure are frequently discussed but controversial topics.[85,86] Among the many complex physiological and pathological factors influencing relaxation, four are of chief interest. First, the cytosolic calcium level must fall to cause the relaxation phase, a process requiring ATP and phosphorylation of phospholamban for uptake of calcium into the SR (see Fig. 19–27). Second, the inherent viscoelastic properties of the myocardium are of importance. In the hypertrophied heart with increased fibrosis, relaxation occurs more slowly. Particularly in the early stages of the hypertrophied heart of hypertension and aortic stenosis, a situation arises in which systolic function is relatively well preserved but diastolic relaxation is impaired. The probable explanation is that hypertrophy is accompanied by increasing fibrosis.[87] Third, increased phosphorylation of troponin I enhances the rate of relaxation.[88] Fourth, relaxation is influenced by the systolic load.[86] Thus, the history of contraction affects cross-bridge relaxation. Within limits, the greater the systolic load, the faster the rate of relaxation.

This complex relationship has been explored in detail by Brutsaert and colleagues[70] but could perhaps be simplified as follows. When the workload is high, peak cytosolic calcium is also high. Thus, the rate of fall of calcium is also greater provided that the diastolic uptake mechanisms function effectively. In this way, a systolic pressure load and the rate of diastolic relaxation can be related. Furthermore, a greater muscle length (when the workload is high) at the end of systole should produce a more rapid rate of relaxation by the opposite of length-dependent sensitization. When the afterload exceeds a certain limit, relaxation is delayed[86] with diastolic dysfunction. Thus, in congestive heart failure caused by an excess systolic load, relaxation becomes increasingly afterload dependent, so that therapeutic reduction of the systolic load should improve LV relaxation.

IMPAIRED RELAXATION AND CYTOSOLIC CALCIUM. For these purposes, this chapter uses the clinical definition of diastole according to which diastole extends from aortic valve closure to the start of the first heart sound. The first phase of diastole is the isovolumic phase, which, by definition, does not contribute to ventricular filling. The second phase of rapid filling provides most of ventricular filling. The third phase of slow filling or diastasis accounts for only 5 percent of the total filling. The final atrial booster phase accounts for the remaining 15 percent.

Isovolumic relaxation is energy dependent, requiring ATP for the uptake of calcium ions by the SR (Fig. 19–27), which is an active, not a passive process. Impaired relaxation is an early event in angina pectoris. A proposed metabolic explanation is that there is impaired generation of energy, which diminishes the supply of ATP required for the early diastolic uptake of calcium by the SR. The result is that the cytosolic calcium level, at a peak in systole, has a delayed return to normal in the early diastolic period. In other conditions, too, there is a relationship between the rate of diastolic decay of the calcium transient and diastolic relaxation, with a relation to impaired function of the SR.[89] When the relaxation is prolonged by hypothyroidism, the return of the systolic calcium elevation is likewise delayed, whereas opposite changes occur in hyperthyroidism. In congestive heart failure, diastolic relaxation is also delayed and irregular, as is the rate of decay of the cytosolic calcium elevation. Most patients with coronary artery disease have a variety of abnormalities of diastolic filling, probably related to those also found in angina pectoris. Theoretically, such abnormalities of relaxation are potentially reversible because they depend on changes in patterns of calcium ion movement. Indices of the

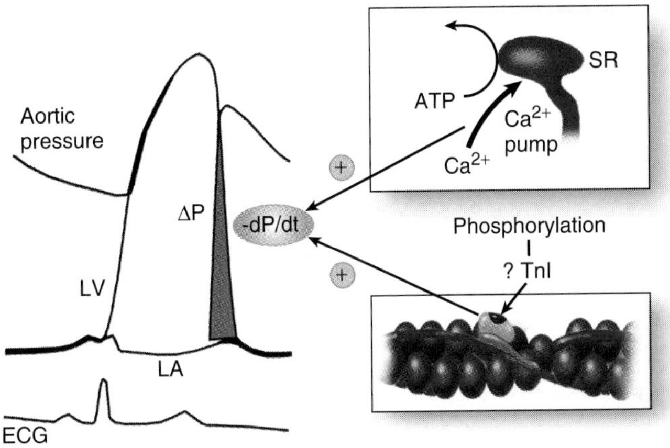

FIGURE 19–27 Factors governing the isovolumic relaxation phase of the cardiac cycle. This period of the cycle extends from the aortic second sound (A_2) to the crossover point between the left ventricular and left atrial pressures (see Fig. 19–20). The maximum negative rate of pressure development ($-dP/dt_{max}$), which gives the isovolumic relaxation rate, is measured either invasively or by a continuous-wave Doppler velocity spectrum in aortic regurgitation. Isovolumic relaxation is increased (+ sign) when the rate of calcium uptake into the sarcoplasmic reticulum (SR) is enhanced, for example during beta-adrenergic stimulation (see Fig. 19–15). Isovolumic relaxation may also be enhanced when phosphorylation of troponin I (TnI), as in response to beta-adrenergic stimulation, may decrease the affinity of the contractile system for calcium. ECG = electrocardiogram; LA = left atrium; LV = left ventricle. (Modified from Opie LH: Heart Physiology, from Cell to Circulation. Philadelphia, Lippincott Williams & Wilkins, 2004. Copyright L. H. Opie, © 2004.)

isovolumic phase and other indices of diastolic function are shown in Table 19–5.

IS THERE VENTRICULAR SUCTION DURING EARLY FILLING? Whether the LV suction by active relaxation could increase the pressure gradient from left atrium to left ventricle during the early filling phase remains controversial although well supported by data. An LV suction effect can be found by carefully comparing LV and left atrial pressures, and it occurs especially in the early diastolic phase of rapid filling. The sucking effect may be of most importance in mitral stenosis when the mitral valve does not open as it otherwise should in response to diastolic suction. During catecholamine stimulation, the rate of relaxation may increase to enhance the sucking effect and to prolong the period of filling. The currently proposed mechanism of sucking is as follows. In early diastole, myosin is pulled into the space between the two anchoring segments of titin (see Fig. 19–4) to lower the intraventricular pressure to below that in the atrium.[90]

ATRIAL FUNCTION. The left atrium, besides its well-known function as a blood-receiving chamber, helps to complete LV filling by presystolic contraction and the atrial booster function. The atrial pressure-volume loop is very different in shape from that of the ventricles. There are two parts, the overall loop somewhat resembling a figure of 8. The first phase of volume increase (v loop) reflects atrial filling and passive emptying, followed by atrial work (a loop) done during presystolic atrial contraction.[91] During atrial pacing, the preload is increased and the atria are distended so that the volume part of the loop is small and the contraction part of the loop is much enlarged.[91]

Two additional functions of the atria are as follows. First, it is the volume sensor of the heart, releasing atrial natriuretic peptide in response to intermittent stretch and several other stimuli including angiotensin II and endothelin. Second, the atrium contains receptors for the afferent arms of various reflexes including mechanoreceptors that increase the sinus discharge rate, thereby contributing to the tachycardia of exercise as the venous return increases (Bainbridge reflex). The atria have a number of differences in structure and function from the ventricles, having smaller myocytes with a shorter action potential duration as well as a more fetal type of myosin (in both heavy and light chains). The more rapid atrial repolarization is thought to be due to increased outward potassium currents, such as I_{to} and I_{kACh}. In general, these histological and physiological changes can be related to the decreased need for the atria to generate high intrachamber pressures, rather being sensitive to volume changes, while retaining enough contractile action to help with LV filling and to respond to inotropic stimuli.

MEASUREMENT OF ISOVOLUMIC RELAXATION. The rate of isovolumic relaxation is best measured by negative

TABLE 19–5 Some Indices of Diastolic Function

Isovolumic Relaxation
(−)dP/dt$_{max}$ (Fig. 19–28)
Aortic closing–mitral opening interval
Peak rate of LV wall thinning
Time constant of relaxation (τ)
Early Diastolic Filling
Relaxation kinetics on ERNA (rate of volume increase)
Early filling phase (E phase) on Doppler transmitral velocity trace
Diastasis
Pressure-volume relation indicates compliance
Atrial Contraction
Invasive measurement of atrial and ventricular pressures
Doppler transmitral pattern (E to A ratio)

A = atrial contraction phase; E = early filling phase; ERNA = equilibrated radionuclide angiography; LV = left ventricular.

dP/dt$_{max}$ at invasive catheterization. *Tau*, the time constant of relaxation, describes the rate of fall of LV pressure during isovolumic relaxation and also requires invasive techniques for precise determination. Tau is increased as the systolic LV pressure rises. Other indices of isovolumic relaxation can be obtained echocardiographically or from tissue Doppler measurements to monitor the peak rate of wall thinning.

DIASTOLIC DYSFUNCTION AND MYOCARDIAL MECHANICAL PROPERTIES. In hypertrophic hearts, as in chronic hypertension or severe aortic stenosis, abnormalities of diastole are common and may precede systolic failure (see Chap. 21). But the existence of "pure" diastolic dysfunction and heart failure is challenged by tissue Doppler measurements that show subtle but evident systolic abnormalities.[92,93] Experimentally, there are several defects in early hypertensive hypertrophy, including decreased rates of contraction and relaxation and decreased peak force development. The mechanism of diastolic dysfunction is not clear, although it is thought to be related to the fibrosis that occurs with ventricular hypertrophy or indirectly to a stiff left atrium. Impaired relaxation is associated with an increase of the late (atrial) filling phase so that E/A ratios (see Table 19–5) on the mitral Doppler pattern decline (see also Chap. 20).

Effects of Ischemia and Reperfusion on Contraction and Relaxation

Contractile Impairment in Ischemia

HIGH-ENERGY PHOSPHATES. These are reviewed by Opie and Heusch.[94] Early contractile failure (Fig. 19–28) can occur even when calcium transients are normal or even increased; therefore, a metabolic cause must be sought. The latter could be either decreased sensitivity of the contractile proteins to calcium, such as caused by acidosis, or inhibition of the cross-bridge cycle, such as from the early rise in P_i. As creatine phosphate falls, the activity of the creatine phosphate shuttle decreases so that "local" ATP, required for calcium movements in the contractile cycle, falls. In addition, the free energy of hydrolysis of ATP decreases during ischemia. The large increase in P_i that results from creatine phosphate breakdown decreases the free energy of hydrolysis, as do the smaller decreases in ATP and increases in ADP. The creatine phosphate decrease can also indirectly inhibit contractility by accumulation of P_i, which decreases the contractile effects of any given cytosolic calcium level. P_i may act by promotion of formation of weak rather than strong cross bridges. *Accumulation of neutral lactate* can promote mitochondrial damage, decrease the action potential

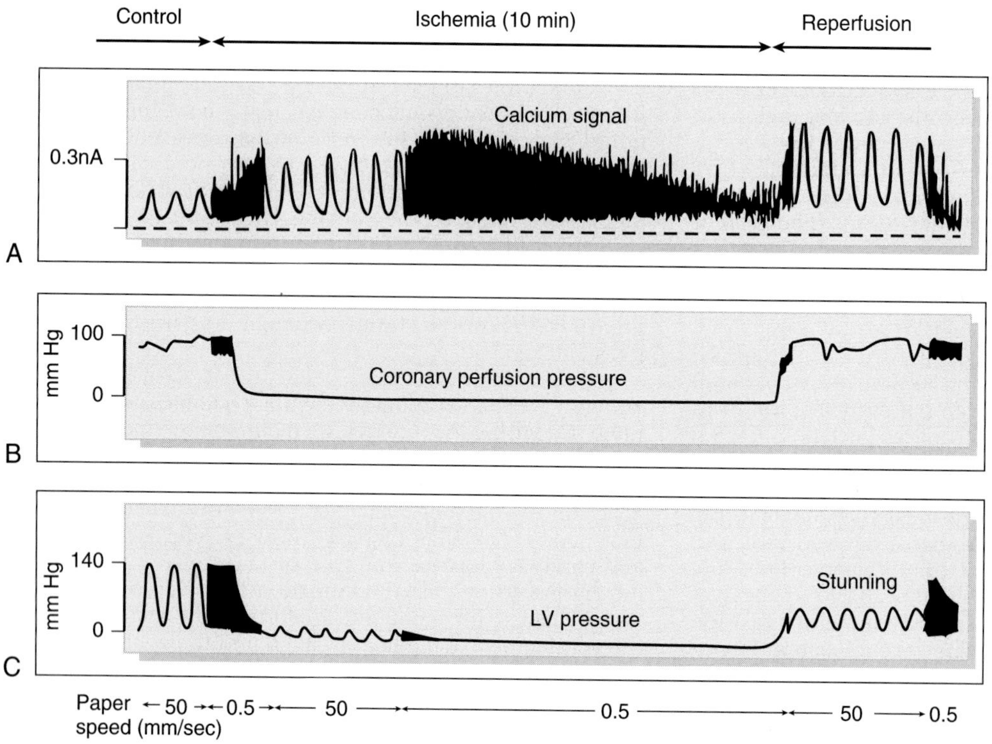

FIGURE 19–28 Can left ventricular (LV) mechanical failure during severe ischemia be explained by changes in the cytosolic calcium? These data show that when there is abrupt ischemic LV failure (LV pressure falls to zero in **C**), the calcium signal **(A)** increases before it falls. Ischemia is designated by the abrupt fall of coronary perfusion pressure to zero in this isolated rat heart preparation **(B)**. During reperfusion there is also a dissociation between the cytosolic calcium oscillations, which are augmented (right side of **A**), in contrast to LV contraction, which is decreased (right side of **C**), so that there is mechanical stunning. It is thought that excess calcium oscillations damage the contractile proteins. (From Meisner A, Morgan JP: Contractile dysfunction and abnormal Ca^{2+} modulation during postischemic reperfusion in rat heart. Am J Physiol. 268:H100, 1995.)

duration, and inhibit glyceraldehyde-3-phosphate dehydrogenase. The mechanism of these lactate effects may include extracellular acidosis with Na^+/H^+ exchange, a subsequent gain in cell Na^+, and then Na^+/Ca^{2+} exchange with gain of harmful Ca^{2+}.

POTASSIUM EFFLUX. Major early potassium efflux in ischemia occurs as the ATP-inhibited potassium channel (K_{ATP}) opens, as shown in a mouse model in which this channel is genetically inactivated.[95] In addition, other potassium channels such as those activated by sodium or by fatty acids may play a role. Second, inhibition of the sodium-potassium pump has long been suspected; the onset of such inhibition is probably too late to explain early potassium egress, although it probably contributes to the later phase of potassium loss. The importance of potassium loss is that because the action potential duration is shortened, calcium influx diminishes, which is one of the several factors causing early loss of contractile function after the onset of ischemia.

Response to Ischemia

The myocardium is now known to have a diverse and flexible response to ischemia, varying from rapid contractile arrest to delayed stimulation of potentially protective synthetic pathways involving signals similar to those inducing growth. Three specific new entities identified are preconditioning, hibernation, and stunning. All three have in common that they are different responses to ischemia and reperfusion. Ischemia-reperfusion injury is a well-recognized experimental entity, varying from reversible damage with mild transient ischemia to irreversible cell death with severe ischemia followed by reperfusion. Adverse effects associated with reperfusion include arrhythmias, mechanical dysfunction, degradation of contractile proteins such as troponin I, and apoptosis.[96] The proposal is that these adverse effects are at least to some extent offset by *a repertoire of myocardial protective events resulting from activation of a variety of signaling and metabolic pathways.*

Preconditioning

Preconditioning is the chief among these protective mechanisms. Contrary to expectations, many repetitive episodes of ischemia do not produce cumulative damage if each is short lived and followed by reperfusion. Rather, an endogenous myocardial protective mechanism is invoked, namely, preconditioning as first described by Jennings and colleagues in a seminal paper.[97] The final result is that when a prolonged ischemic episode occurs that would normally give rise to lethal myocardial damage, the heart is largely, but not totally, protected. This protection comes in two phases; the first window of early or "classical" preconditioning lasts only a few hours, whereas the second window of protection lasts for several days.

MECHANISMS OF PRECONDITIONING. Even after extensive research, the full mechanism of preconditioning is not clarified, and several different paths appear to be involved. The current consensus of opinion[98] is that the first window results from the liberation of a number of compounds from the ischemic myocardium, including adenosine, bradykinin, and opioids. Adenosine preconditioning is best understood and involves the A_1 and A_3 receptors acting through the inhibitor G_i protein to increase the activity of PKC (Fig. 19–29). Further signaling steps are not clear but might involve activation of MAP kinase. The mitochondria also play an important role with increased activity of the ATP-dependent potassium channel (K_{ATP}), which in turn decreases the calcium load of the ischemic mitochondria and increases ATP production. Mitochondria also produce reactive oxygen species that help to activate PKC. NO may play a role by generation of free radicals but is not a direct activator of preconditioning.[99]

SECOND WINDOW OF PROTECTION. This phase may be a "universal response of the heart to stress in general."[100] The mechanism involves at least two pathways leading to nuclear protein synthesis (Fig.

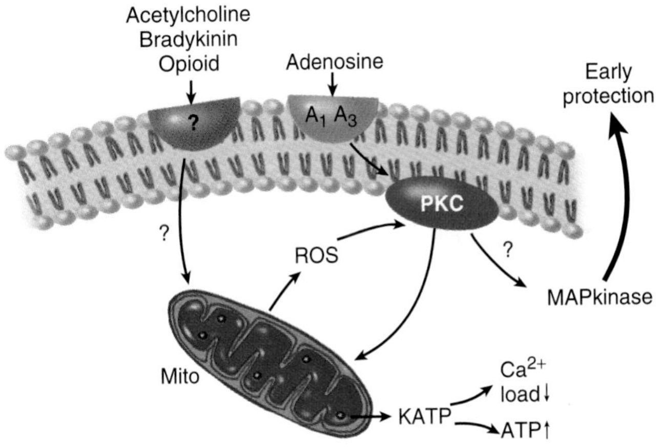

FIGURE 19–29 Early phase preconditioning. Adenosine, liberated during the brief ischemic period that triggers preconditioning and acting chiefly by myocardial A_1 and A_3 receptors, is thought to play a crucial role. A crucial event is activation of protein kinase C (PKC), particularly the epsilon isoform. Further steps leading to opening of the mitochondrial ATP-sensitive potassium channel (KATP) are not clear. Other effects could occur through the inhibitory protein G_i or the mitogen-activated protein (MAP) kinase cascade. In response to other mediators of preconditioning such as acetylcholine, liberation of reactive oxygen species (ROS), possibly from the mitochondria, is a key event and probably upstream from PKC. (Modified from Opie LH: Heart Physiology, from Cell to Circulation. Philadelphia, Lippincott Williams & Wilkins, 2004. Copyright L. H. Opie, © 2004.)

19–30) One involves the epsilon isoform of PKC (PKC-ε) that activates nuclear factor kappa B, which in turn increases nuclear synthesis of a variety of protective proteins such as cyclooxygenase-2 and iNOS. At present, much attention has been focused on the role of the mitochondria in both windows of preconditioning.[101] The mitochondrial permeability transition pore (PTP) is activated by ischemia-reperfusion injury and mitochondrial calcium overload results. Bcl-2 is an antiapoptotic protein found in the outer mitochondrial membrane that inhibits PTP opening and the release of cytochrome *c* that promotes apoptotic cell death. The second window of protection may be associated with increased Bcl-2 expression and, hence, with closing of the PTP.[102] Clearly, much more work needs to be done before the mechanisms underlying preconditioning, a powerful protective mechanism, have definite clinical application.

PRECONDITIONING VERSUS CARDIOPROTECTION

Protein Kinase C Isoforms. These are not the same entities in that preconditioning is only one form of cardioprotection. PKC is a key kinase with multiple functions and plays an important role in both. First, it is linked to the phospholipase signaling system, which is of prime importance in vascular contraction and possibly acts as an inotropic backup system in the myocardium (see Fig. 19–18). Second, PKC may be a key molecular switch in the "hypertrophic signal system," responding to stretch and to neurohormonal input[103] such as the angiotensin II released during stretch. Third, it plays a pivotal role in preconditioning, receiving stimuli from a number of G protein–linked receptors and ultimately activating the mitochondrial ATP-sensitive potassium channels (see Fig. 19–29). Such multiple functions may be mediated by different isoforms of PKC, of which there are at least 10, the functions of which are still poorly understood. The isoforms are divided into three groups, the conventional (which respond to calcium in vitro), the novel (which respond to diacylglycerol but not to calcium), and the atypical isoforms (which respond to neither calcium nor diacylglycerol but rather to phospholipids). The conventional beta isoforms, increased in the failing human heart, may be linked to enhanced growth.[103]

Current attention is focused on the delta and epsilon isoforms.[104] Each isoform becomes active when localized to a specific subcellular site by binding to its selective anchoring protein or RACK (receptor for activated C kinase). By inhibiting and activating, respectively, delta- and epsilon-specific forms of RACK, infarct size in rat hearts was markedly reduced,[104] showing that these two isoforms have opposite effects in this model. Concordant studies with overexpression of activated PKC-ε also showed cardioprotection.[105] In preconditioning, PKC-ε is translocated, consonant with its cardioprotective role.

PRECONDITIONING IN HUMANS. Does preconditioning occur in humans? Early preconditioning explains why during balloon angioplasty the manifestations of ischemia including chest pain become less with repeated balloon inflations.[98] Early preconditioning may be part of the explanation for the phenomenon of "walk-through" or "warm-up" angina, in which the severity of the initial anginal attack is lessened during subsequent exercise.[98] Exercise can also induce late preconditioning in those with coronary artery disease.[106] This effect could contribute to the clinical benefit of exercise training. Patients with preinfarction angina may suffer from a less severe infarct than those thought to undergo sudden coronary occlusion without the opportunity for preconditioning.[98] Pharmacologically, a number of adenosine analogs have been used to test the effects of preconditioning in humans but thus far without consistent success. One antianginal compound, nicorandil, besides having nitrate-like qualities, opens the mitochondrial ATP-dependent potassium channel and thereby potentially invokes preconditioning in humans. Whether this property expands the antianginal protection is not clear.

Hibernation

The hibernating myocardium, like the hibernating animal, is temporarily asleep and can wake up to function normally when the blood supply is fully restored (Table 19–6). Rahimtoola[107] proposed that the fall of myocardial function to a lower level copes with the reduced myocardial oxygen supply and leads to self-preservation so that the myocardium is "exquisitely regulated" and successfully adapted to the prevailing circumstances. The alternative and now dominant point of view is that hibernation can occur even when the resting coronary flow is normal or low normal despite the presence of coronary disease. The basic problem lies in a critical stenosis that limits coronary vascular reserve[108] so that episodes of tachycardia must precipitate ischemia. Such recurrent episodes of ischemia would then leave behind a repetitively stunned myocardium. Thus, chronic hibernation, according to this proposal, is no more than cumulative stunning. The mandatory need for revascularization remains.

CELLULAR EVENTS IN HIBERNATION. Heusch and Schulz[108] related the loss of contractile function to signaling by inflammatory-like processes involving TNF-α, known to depress myocardial function.[109] In humans, too, there is increased gene expression of both TNF-α and NOS, both inhibitory to contraction.[110] In addition, there are complex defects in calcium cycling and excitation-contraction coupling[108] and decreased beta-adrenergic receptor density.[110] The hypocontractile segments that still have sustained glucose extraction, as shown by positron-emission tomography (PET), have a high chance of recovery after coronary artery bypass surgery. "Mismatch" refers to the increased glucose extraction of the viable myocardium that can be visibly contrasted with the poor coronary blood flow (ammonia signal on PET). In one series, up to 27 percent of patients with ischemic cardiomyopathy could have enough viable segments to benefit from revascularization.[111] Postoperative recovery of contractile function may vary from rapid, within hours or even minutes, to long delays over weeks or even months. Thus, hibernation, like stunning, is a "syndrome."

Stunning

The first observation was that the recovery of mechanical function following transient coronary occlusion was not instant but delayed. Thereafter, Braunwald and Kloner[112] defined the "stunned myocardium" as one characterized by prolonged postischemic myocardial dysfunction with eventual return of normal contractile activity. Stunning is now thought to occur in many clinical situations,[113] including hibernation, delayed recovery from effort angina, unstable angina, early thrombolytic reperfusion, ischemic cardioplegia, cardiac transplantation, cardiac arrest, and coronary angioplasty. Interactive mechanisms are increased cytosolic calcium (Fig. 19–31; see Fig. 19–28) and the formation of oxygen-derived free radicals upon reperfusion.[113] The hydroxyl ion is "one of the most aggressive species of oxygen free radicals"[114] and is the key mediator of stunning.[115] Direct measurements of cytosolic calcium in stunned myocardium show that antioxidants decrease cytosolic calcium levels and increase the force of contraction.[116]

TUMOR NECROSIS FACTOR-ALPHA AND POSTISCHEMIC CONTRACTILE DEPRESSION. Following ischemia, production of TNF-α by both interstitial cells and human cardiomyocytes increases.[109] Theoretically, TNF-α may promote stunning by several mechanisms such as desensitization of the contractile proteins to calcium, induction of other cardiodepressant agents such as NO or interleukin-1, or formation of free radicals.

TABLE 19–6 Characteristics of Stunning, Hibernation, and Ischemia

Parameter	Stunning	Hibernation	True Ischemia
Myocardial mechanical function	Reduced	Reduced	Reduced
Coronary blood flow	Postischemic: normal/high	Modestly reduced or low normal; reduced coronary vascular reserve	Most severely reduced
Myocardial energy metabolism	Harmful effects of fatty acid fuels versus glucose	Reduced or low normal; in steady state with intermittent ischemia-reperfusion	Reduced; increasingly severe as ischemia proceeds
Duration	Hours to days; merges with delayed recovery from ischemia over weeks	Days to hours to months; occasionally longer	Minutes to hours; then lethal
Outcome	Full spontaneous recovery	Variable recovery if revascularized	Myocyte necrosis if severe ischemia persists
Proposed change in metabolic regulation of calcium	Cytosolic overload of calcium in early reperfusion with damage to contractile proteins	Hypothetically enough glycolytic ATP to prevent contracture (glucose mismatch)	Insufficient glycolytic ATP to prevent calcium overload and irreversibility

ATP = adenosine triphosphate.

Modified from Opie L, Heusch G: Lack of blood flow: Ischemia and angina. *In* Opie LH (ed): Heart Physiology, from Cell to Circulation. 4th ed. Philadelphia, Lippincott Williams & Wilkins, 2004, pp 525-552.

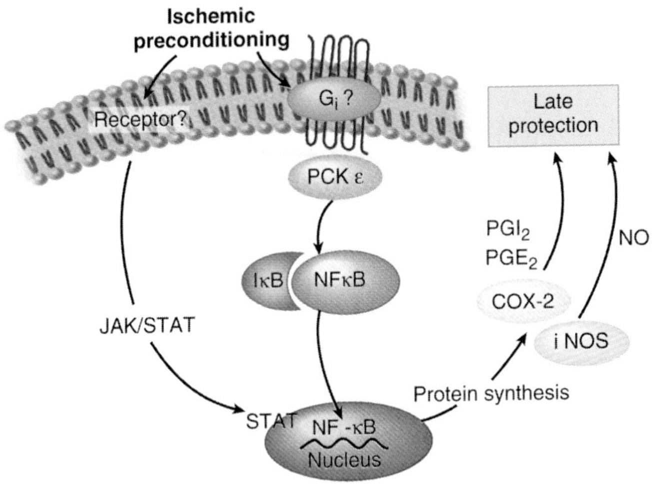

FIGURE 19–30 Late phase preconditioning. Note that preconditioning occurs in two phases, early and late, the latter probably involving nuclear protein synthesis. Figure based on the concepts of Bolli and colleagues.[141] COX-2 = cyclooxygenase-2; IκB = inhibitor of nuclear factor kappa B; iNOS = inducible nitric oxide synthase; JAK = Janus kinase; NFκB = nuclear factor kappa B; NO = nitric oxide; PG = prostaglandin; STAT = signal transducer and activator of transcription. (Modified from Opie LH: Heart Physiology, from Cell to Circulation. Philadelphia, Lippincott Williams & Wilkins, 2004. Copyright L. H. Opie, © 2004.)

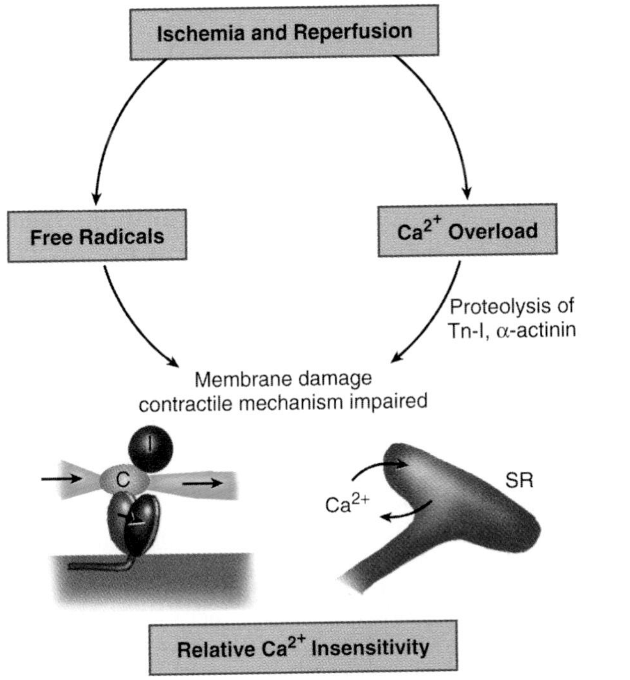

FIGURE 19–31 Mechanisms of ischemic reperfusion damage. The major three, probably with interactive effects, involve oxygen-derived free radicals, calcium overload, and relative insensitivity of the contractile protein troponin C (C) to calcium released from the sarcoplasmic reticulum (SR). For role of proteolysis of troponin I (Tn-I), see Bolli and Marban.[113] (Copyright L.H. Opie © 2001.)

ATRIAL STUNNING. After cessation of atrial fibrillation, atrial contractility may be reduced or absent up to several weeks despite normal electrical activity. Such stunning is clinically relevant and potentially harmful because it predisposes to the formation of atrial thrombosis with risk of stroke. Atrial stunning is part of the complex process of atrial remodeling that occurs during and after atrial fibrillation.[91]

CONCURRENT ISCHEMIA-RELATED EVENTS. Because the human heart with advanced coronary artery disease is known to suffer from intermittent ischemia, ischemia-reperfusion injury and its consequences may all be occurring at the same time. Thus, the same heart may concurrently manifest one or more components of the newly emphasized ischemic syndromes, namely stunning, hibernation, and preconditioning, as well as ischemic damage. When one episode of severe ischemia is followed by clinical reperfusion, as in thrombolysis, the extent of postischemic dysfunction could be determined by a combination of ischemic and reperfusion pathology, the former depending on how long the myocardium has been ischemic and the latter potentially causing a spectrum of ischemic syndromes.

Heart Failure (see also Chap. 21)

Human heart failure is a complex phenomenon at both clinical and cellular levels, the end result of several disparate disease processes that have been subject to a variety of therapies. There is poor contractile performance with systolic impairment and delayed diastolic relaxation. In human tissue obtained at cardiac transplantation, there are major disturbances in the force-frequency relationship, in gene programming, in beta-adrenergic activity, and in calcium cycling.

Force-Frequency Relationship

Muscle strips prepared from patients with severe LV failure behave very differently from normal muscle in that there is hardly any response to an increased stimulation frequency (Fig. 19–32). Whereas in strips from normal hearts, optimal force development is reached at rates of about 150 to 180 beats/min, in patients with cardiomyopathy an increased heart rate produces a decreased twitch tension (Fig. 19–33) In addition, the diastolic tension rises markedly with the stimulation frequency,[117] compatible with a rate-induced cytosolic calcium overload causing diastolic dysfunction. This complex picture is at least in part related to changes in gene expression and to downregulated beta-adrenergic receptor activity.

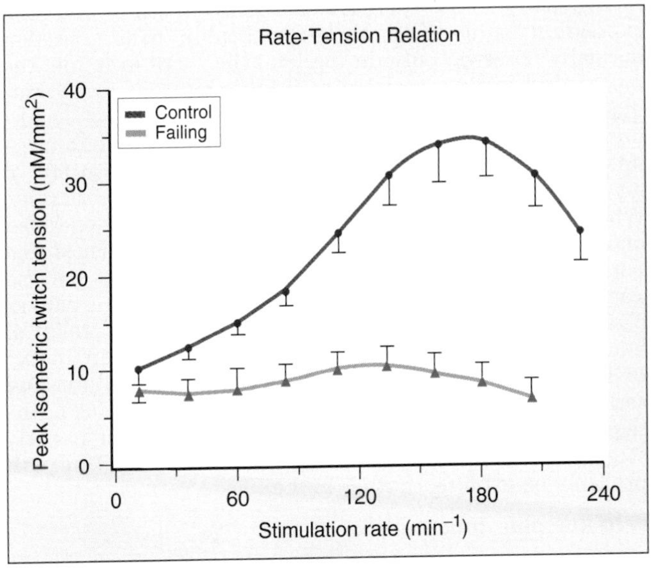

FIGURE 19–32 Force-frequency relationship in humans, comparing nonfailing control hearts with failing hearts with mitral regurgitation. Plots of average steady-state isometric twitch tension versus stimulation frequency. Each point represents the mean ± standard error of the mean of eight control or mitral regurgitation preparations at 37°C. (Data from Mulieri LA, Leavitt BJ, Martin BJ: Myocardial force-frequency defect in mitral regurgitation heart failure is reversed by forskolin. Circulation 88:2700, 1993. Copyright 1993, American Heart Association.)

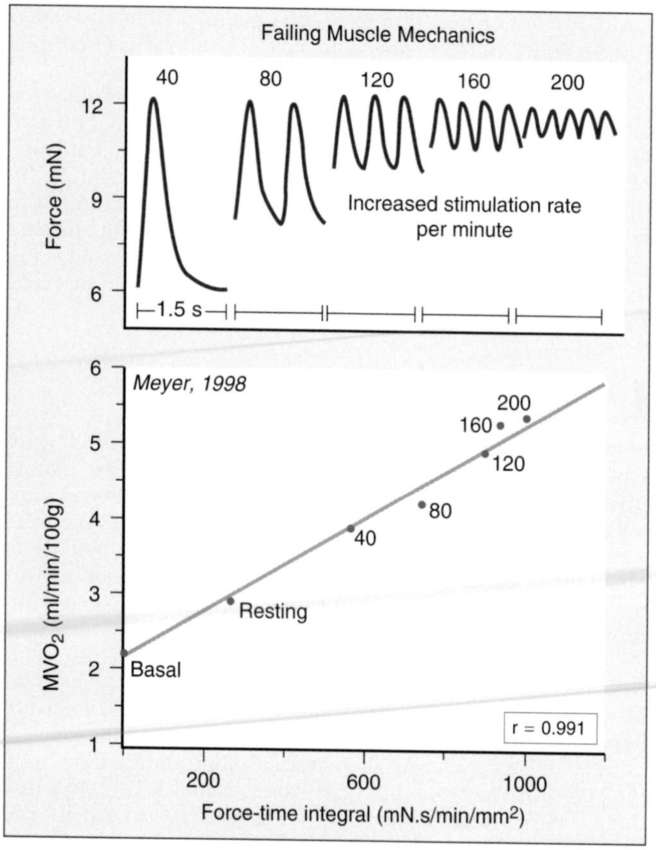

FIGURE 19–33 Diastolic tension markedly increased during pacing of a muscle strip from a patient with advanced heart failure. Note, at the bottom, the increased myocardial oxygen uptake (MVO_2) with increased force (measured as the force-time integral). The combination of decreased cardiac force development and increased oxygen uptake indicates decreased efficiency of cardiac work. (Modified from Meyer M, Keweloh B, Guth K, et al: Frequency-dependence of myocardial energetics in failing human myocardium as quantified by a new method for the measurement of oxygen consumption in muscle strip preparations. J Mol Cell Cardiol 30:1459, 1998.)

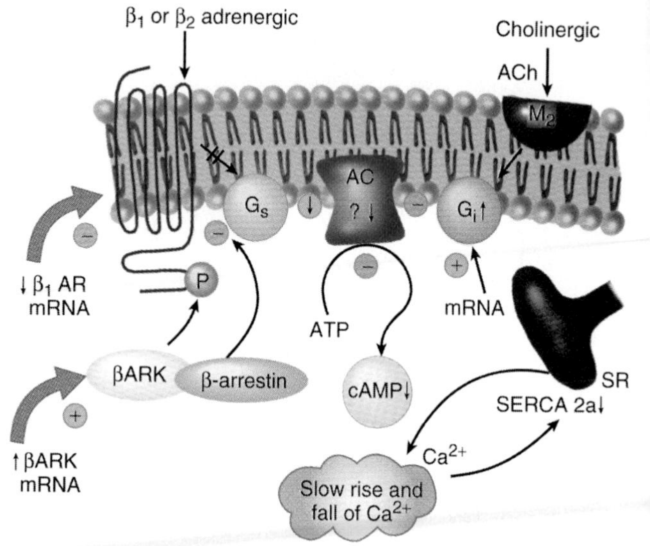

FIGURE 19–34 Proposed changes in beta-adrenergic receptor signal system and sarcoplasmic reticulum (SR) in severe congestive heart failure (CHF). AC = adenylate cyclase; ACh = acetylcholine; β_1AR = beta$_1$-adrenergic receptor; β_2AR = beta$_2$-adrenergic receptor; βARK = beta-adrenergic receptor kinase; G_i = inhibitory G protein; G_s = stimulatory G protein; M_2 = muscarinic receptor; mRNA = messenger ribonucleic acid. For SERCA2, see Figure 19–9. (From Opie LH: Heart Physiology, from Cell to Circulation. Philadelphia, Lippincott Williams & Wilkins, 2004. Copyright L. H. Opie, © 2004.)

Fetal Gene Program

As the ventricle fails, there is a change in the ventricular gene expression pattern from the normal adult pattern to that normally observed only during fetal life.[11] For example, the mechanical forces associated with LV failure lead to myocardial expression of atrial natriuretic peptide and brain natriuretic peptide (BNP). There is downregulation of the calcium uptake pump (SERCA2) and of the fast-contracting isoform of myosin heavy chain that has the greater ATPase activity. What activates the fetal program? Cytosolic calcium overload may be basic, by adding phosphate groups to enzymes that normally inhibit the fetal program.[118] There is, as yet, no known means of reverting a fetal to a normal adult pattern besides nonspecific treatment of heart failure with relief of biomechanical stress on the left ventricle. Thus, circulating BNP levels drop during the treatment of heart failure, and serial decreases of BNP levels should mirror lessening of the severity of LV failure. Metabolic therapies, as yet at an early stage, include inhibition of fatty acid metabolism and will probably be explored further in the future.[11]

Beta Receptor Abnormalities

BETA-ADRENERGIC SIGNALING IN HEART FAILURE. In congestive heart failure (Fig. 19–34), changes in the beta-adrenergic system include downregulation of the receptors and G proteins that stimulate the contraction cycle (beta$_1$ and beta$_2$, both through G_s) and upregulation of the inhibitory paths (beta$_2$ through G_i and beta$_3$ through NO). In more detail, (1) there is major beta$_1$ receptor downregulation[119] with moderate uncoupling from the stimulatory G protein, (2) beta$_2$ receptor density is unchanged but modestly uncoupled from G_s, and (3) inhibitory beta$_3$ receptors, linked to NO, are upregulated.[120] Adenylate cyclase activity decreases and levels of the inhibitory G_i proteins increase.[120] *Uncoupling* of the beta$_1$ and beta$_2$ receptors from the G_s signaling system may be explained by the increased activity of the βARK mechanism and of arrestin (see Fig. 19–14). Note the dual effect of beta$_2$ receptors on both stimulatory and inhibitory G proteins. The downregulation of G_s should decrease the stimulatory effect of beta$_2$ receptors through G_s on formation of cyclic AMP, yet the effect of arrestin is to uncouple these receptors from adenyl cyclase. Thus, overall, the upregulated G_i gives an increased inhibitory effect. According to this scheme, beta blockade can be expected to lessen the degree of hyperphosphorylation of the ryanodine receptor, thereby improving calcium channel release function toward normal.[121] The consequence would be improved calcium cycling as reflected in the better calcium transients found in transplant recipients who received prior beta blockade.[122] In addition, some nonselective blockers could be expected to block the beta$_3$-mediated inhibitory stimuli.

METABOLIC EFFECTS OF BETA-BLOCKADE ON MYOCARDIAL OXYGEN UPTAKE. Beta blockade might also be beneficial in heart failure by increasing the efficiency of work. This measure compares the myocardial oxygen uptake with the work performance. In experimental heart failure there is a marked fall-off in myocardial efficiency, which can be remedied by inhibition of fatty acid metabolism.[123] The hypothesis may be that excess fatty acid mobilization occurs as part of the increased catecholamine stimulation in heart failure and that this mobilization increases the uptake of fatty acids by the myocardium with a detrimental uncoupling effect on the mitochondria. The increased efficiency of work achieved when beta blockade is given to patients with heart failure may be related to inhibition of fatty acid oxidation.[79,124]

Calcium Cycling, Contractile Heart Failure, and Arrhythmias

CALCIUM CYCLING. Changes in the calcium cycle are fundamental to the impaired contractile performance of the

TABLE 19–7 Abnormalities of Calcium Cycling in Heart Failure

Subcellular	Organelle	Whole Heart	Reference
SERCA2a$\downarrow$	SR Ca depleted	Negative FFR	127
RyR hyperphosphorylated	SR Ca release$\downarrow$ Diastolic leak	Rate of contraction$\downarrow$ Diastolic tension$\uparrow$	126 136
Na/Ca exchange $\uparrow$	Released Ca extruded	Negative FFR	137
Prolonged APD and RyR changes	Cytosolic Ca$\uparrow$	Diastolic tension$\uparrow$ with pacing	138

APD = action potential duration; FFR = force-frequency relationship; RyR = ryanodine receptor; SERCA = sarcoendoplasmic reticulum Ca^{2+}-adenosine triphosphatase; SR = sarcoplasmic reticulum.

failing heart (Table 19–7). The SR calcium stores are severely depleted because of the combined effects of (1) depressed calcium uptake into the SR resulting from decreased SERCA activity, both downregulated and inhibited,[125] and (2) the diastolic calcium leak associated with hyperphosphorylation and abnormal functioning of the ryanodine receptor.[126] Thus, the calcium ions entering with depolarization are unable to trigger release of enough calcium to generate a normal calcium transient (see Fig. 19–34). There is a close relationship between the depression of SERCA in human heart failure and the depressed force-frequency relationship.[127] Paradoxically, the diastolic calcium level is higher than normal, a probable result of the diastolic leak through the defective ryanodine receptor and the prolonged action potential. Starting from this higher level, the proposed events as the heart rate increases could be that calcium ions enter more rapidly through the calcium channels of the T tubules than can be extruded through the Na/Ca exchange so that the diastolic levels rise, as does the diastolic tension.

ELECTRICAL ALTERNANS IN HEART FAILURE AND MYOCARDIAL ISCHEMIA. Ventricular fibrillation is probably the major cause of sudden death in patients with severe heart failure. An important mechanism of ventricular fibrillation is the subcellular phenomenon of *cardiac transient alternans,*[128] which is increased in cardiovascular disease and particularly in ischemic or failing hearts, or both. Alternans describes a fluctuation in any signal from beat to beat. Electrical alternans is the beat-to-beat variation in the electrocardiographic pattern. Calcium transient alternans is the fluctuation in peak amplitude of the cytosolic calcium transient from beat to beat. Such transient alternans is the cause of mechanical alternans.[128] Transient alternans may not be uniform throughout the cell but may occur in different subcellular patterns.[129] Such subcellular alternans appears to be commonly associated with depressed RyR function, even before measurable electrical or mechanical alternans occurs. In heart failure, the RyR is abnormal with dissociation of the binding protein FKBP12.6 that increases the diastolic calcium leak from the SR and depresses the triggered release of calcium from the SR. Conversely, genetic overexpression of this protein improves calcium handling and keeps the RyR in the closed stable conformation.[129]

Defective RyR function predisposes to calcium transient alternans in a manner not fully clarified. Hypothetically, cytosolic calcium overload and SR calcium "underload" mean that the trigger calcium is unable to elicit more than feeble calcium release from the SR. However, more calcium has entered the cytosol with the wave of depolarization and more is taken up by the SR. Thus, the next wave of depolarization elicits more calcium release from the SR with a larger calcium transient. Thereafter the pattern is repeated, with electrical inhomogeneity and risk of ventricular tachycardia and fibrillation. Thus, a currently provocative hypothesis is that abnormal subcellular patterns of calcium ion movement are found in both myocardial ischemia and heart failure and predispose to serious ventricular arrhythmias.[129]

REFERENCES

Microanatomy of Contractile Cells and Proteins

1. Zuker CZ, Ranganathan R: The path to specificity. Science 283:650, 1999.
2. Sutko JL, Publicover NG, Moss RL: An elastic link between length and active force production in myocardium. Circulation 104:1585, 2001.
3. Knoll R, Hoshijima M, Hoffman HM, et al: The cardiac mechanical stretch sensor machinery involves a Z disc complex that is defective in a subset of human dilated cardiomyopathy. Cell 111:943, 2002.
4. Solaro RJ, Wolska BM, Westfall M: Regulatory proteins and diastolic relaxation. *In* Lorell BH, Grossman W (eds): Diastolic Relaxation of the Heart. Boston, Kluwer Academic Publishers, 1994, pp 43-53.
5. Solaro RJ, Rarick HM: Troponin and tropomyosin: Proteins that switch on and tune in the activity of cardiac myofilaments. Circ Res 83:471, 1998.
6. Rayment I, Holden HM, Whittaker M: Structure of the actin-myosin complex and its implications for muscle contraction. Science 261:58, 1993.
7. Fisher AJ, Smith CA, Thoden J: Structural studies of myosin: A revised model for the molecular basis of muscle contraction. Biophys J 68:19s, 1995.
8. Dominguez R, Freyzon Y, Trybus KM, Cohen C: Crystal structure of a vertebrate smooth muscle myosin motor domain and its complex with the essential light chain: Visualization of the prepower stroke state. Cell 94:559, 1998.
9. Geeves M: Stretching the lever-arm theory. Nature 415:129, 2002.
10. Bers DM: Calcium fluxes involved in control of cardiac myocyte contraction. Circ Res 87:275, 2000.
11. Bristow M: Etomoxir: A new approach to treatment of chronic heart failure. Lancet 356:1621, 2000.
12. Tyska MJ, Dupuis DE, Guilford WH, et al: Two heads of myosin are better than one for generating force and motion. Proc Natl Acad Sci U S A 96:4402, 1999.
13. Solaro RJ: Modulation of cardiac myofilament activity by protein phosphorylation. *In* Fozzard H, Solaro RJ (eds): Handbook of Physiology. Sec 2: The Cardiovascular System. New York, Oxford University Press, 2002, pp 264-300.
14. Vemuri R, Lankford EB, Poetter K, et al: The stretch-activation response may be critical to the proper functioning of the mammalian heart. Proc Natl Acad Sci U S A 96:1048, 1999.
15. Konhilas JP, Irving TC, de Tombe PP: Myofilament calcium sensitivity in skinned rat cardiac trabeculae. Role of interfilament spacing. Circ Res 90:59, 2002.
16. Cazorla O, Vassort G, Garnier D, Le Guennec J-Y: Length modulation of active force in rat cardiac myocytes: Is titin the sensor? J Mol Cell Cardiol 31:1215, 1999.
17. Blair E, Redwood C, Ashrafian H, et al: Mutations of the G_2 subunit of AMP-activated protein kinase cause familial hypertrophic cardiomyopathy: Evidence for the central role of energy compromise in disease pathogenesis. Hum Mol Genet 10:1215, 2001.
18. Schmitt JP, Kamisago M, Asahi M, et al: Dilated cardiomyopathy and heart failure caused by a mutation in phospholamban. Science 299:1410, 2003.

Calcium Ion Fluxes in Cardiac Contraction-Relaxation Cycle

19. Bers DM: Cardiac excitation-contraction coupling. Nature 415:198, 2002.
20. Marx SO, Reiken S, Hisamatsu Y, et al: PKA phosphorylation dissociates FKBP12.6 from the calcium release channel (ryanodine receptor): Defective regulation in failing hearts. Cell 101:365, 2000.
21. Wier WG, Balke CW: Ca^{2+} release mechanisms, Ca^{2+} sparks, and local control of excitation-contraction coupling in normal heart muscle. Circ Res 85:770, 1999.
22. Boehm E, Ventua-Clapier R, Mateo P, et al: Glycolysis supports calcium uptake by the sarcoplasmic reticulum in skinned ventricular fibres of mice deficient in mitochondrial and cytosolic creatinine kinase. J Mol Cell Cardiol 32:891, 2000.
23. del Monte F, Williams E, Lebeche D, et al: Improvement in survival and cardiac metabolism after gene transfer of sarcoplasmic reticulum Ca^{2+}- ATPase in a rat model of heart failure. Circulation 104:1424, 2001.
24. Tada M, Katz AM: Phosphorylation of the sarcoplasmic reticulum and sarcolemma. Annu Rev Physiol 44:401, 1982.
25. Brittsan AG, Kranias EG: Phospholamban and cardiac contractile function. J Mol Cell Cardiol 32:2131, 2000.
26. Li Y, Kranias EG, Mignery GA, Bers DM: Protein kinase A phosphorylation of the ryanodine receptor does not affect calcium sparks in mouse ventricular myocytes. Circ Res 90:309, 2002.
27. Bers DM, Perez-Reyes E: Ca channels in cardiac myocytes: Structure and function in Ca influx and intracellular Ca release. Cardiovasc Res 42:339, 1999.
28. Opie LH: Heart Physiology, from Cell to Circulation. 4th ed. Philadelphia, Lippincott Williams & Wilkins, 2004.
29. Carmeliet E: Cardiac ionic currents and acute ischemia: from channels to arrhythmias. Physiol Rev 79:917, 1999.
30. Dipla K, Mattiello JA, Margulies KB, et al: The sarcoplasmic reticulum and the Na^+/Ca^{2+} exchanger both contribute to the Ca^{2+} transient of failing human ventricular myocytes. Circ Res 84:435, 1999.
31. Glitsch HG: Electrophysiology of the sodium-potassium-ATPase in cardiac cells. Physiol Rev 81:1781, 2001.

32. Rockman HA, Koch WJ, Lefkowitz RJ: Seven-transmembrane-spanning receptors and heart function. Nature 415:206, 2002.
33. Xiao RP, Cheng H, Zhou YY, et al: Recent advances in cardiac β_2-adrenergic signal transduction. Circ Res 85:1092, 1999.
34. Smith C, Teitler M: Beta-blocker selectivity at cloned human beta$_1$- and beta$_2$-adrenergic receptors. Cardiovasc Drugs Ther 13:123, 1999.
35. Lefkowitz RJ: Clinical implications of basic research. G proteins in medicine. N Engl J Med 332:186, 1995.
36. Roth DM, Gao MH, Lai C, et al: Cardiac-detected adenylyl cyclase expression improves heart function in murine cardiomyopathy. Circulation 99:3099, 1999.
37. Esposito G, Rapacciuolo A, Prasad SVN, et al: Genetic alterations that inhibit in vivo pressure-overload hypertrophy prevent cardiac dysfunction despite increased wall stress. Circulation 105:85, 2002.
38. Kompa AR, Gu X-H, Evans BA, Summers RJ: Desensitization of cardiac β-adrenoreceptor signaling with heart failure produced by myocardial infarction in the rat. Evidence for the role of G_i but not G_s phosphorylating proteins. J Mol Cell Cardiol 31:1185, 1999.
39. Owen VA, Burton PBJ, Michel MC, et al: Myocardial dysfunction in donor hearts. A possible etiology. Circulation 99:2565, 1999.
40. Bers DM, Ziolo M: When is cAMP not cAMP? Effects of compartmentalization [editorial]. Circ Res 89:373, 2001.
41. Hall RA, Lefkowitz RJ: Regulation of G protein–coupled receptor signaling by scaffold proteins. Circ Res 91:672, 2002.
42. Luttrell LM, Ferguson SSG, Kaaka Y, et al: β-Arrestin-dependent formation of β_2 adrenergic receptor–Src protein kinase complexes. Science 283:655, 1999.
43. Rohrer DK: Molecular organisation of the β-adrenergic system. *In* Böhm M, Laragh J, Zehender M (eds): From Hypertension to Heart Failure. Berlin, Springer, 1998, pp 129-158.
44. Yu X, Zhang M, Kyker K, et al: Ischemic inactivation of G protein–coupled receptor kinase and altered desensitization of canine cardiac β-adrenergic receptors. Circulation 102:2535, 2000.
45. Xiao R-P, Avdonin P, Zhou U-Y, et al: Coupling of β_2-adrenoreceptor to G_i proteins and its physiological relevance in murine cardiac myocytes. Circ Res 84:43, 1999.
46. Newton GE, Azevedo ER, Parker JD: Inotropic and sympathetic responses to the intracoronary infusion of a β_2-receptor agonist. A human in vivo study. Circulation 99:2402, 1999.
47. Varghese P, Harrison RW, Lofthouse RA, et al: β_3-Adrenorecptor deficiency blocks nitric oxide–dependent inhibition of myocardial contractility. J Clin Invest 106:697, 2000.

Cholinergic and Nitric Oxide Signaling

48. Friebe A, Koesling D: Regulation of nitric oxide–sensitive guanylyl cyclase. Circ Res 93:96, 2003.
49. Ziolo MT, Bers DM: The real estate of NOS signaling. Location, location, location. Circ Res 92:1279, 2003.
50. Lewis ME, Al-Khalidi AH, Bonser RS, et al: Vagus nerve stimulation decreases left ventricular contractility in vivo in the human and pig heart. J Physiol (Lond) 534:547, 2001.
51. Paterson DJ: Nitric oxide and the autonomic regulation of cardiac excitability. Exp Physiol 86:1, 2001.
52. Hambrecht R, Adams V, Erbs S, et al: Regular physical activity improves endothelial function in patients with coronary artery disease by increasing phosphorylation of endothelial nitric oxide synthase. Circulation 107:3152, 2003.
53. Rakhit RD, Mojet MH, Marber MS, Duchen MR: Mitochondria as targets for nitric oxide–induced protection during simulated ischemia and reoxygenation in isolated neonatal cardiomyocytes. Circulation 103:2617, 2001.
54. Hochman JS: Cardiogenic shock complicating acute myocardial infarction. Expanding the paradigm. Circulation 107:2998, 2003.
55. Pinsky DJ, Patton S, Mesaros S, et al: Mechanical transduction of nitric oxide synthesis in the beating heart. Circ Res 81:372, 1997.
56. Chowdhary S, Nuttall SL, Coote JH, Townend JN: L-Arginine augments cardiac vagal control in healthy human subjects. Hypertension 39:51, 2002.
57. Shyrock J, Song Y, Wang D, et al: Selective A_2-adenosine receptor agonists do not alter action potential duration, twitch shortening, or cAMP accumulation in guinea pig, rat or rabbit isolated ventricular myocytes. Circ Res 72:194, 1993.
58. Tracey WR, Magee W, Masamune H, et al: Selective activation of adenosine A_3 receptors with N^6-(3-chlorobenzyl)-5′-*N*-methylcarboxamidoadenosine (CB-MECA) provides cardioprotection via K_{ATP} channel activation. Cardiovasc Res 40:138, 1998.
59. Kevelaitis E, Peynet J, Mouas C, et al: Opening of potassium channels. The common cardioprotective link between preconditioning and natural hibernation. Circulation 99:3079, 1999.
60. Gross GJ: Role of opioids in acute and delayed preconditioning. J Mol Cell Cardiol 35:709, 2003.
61. Bishop JE, Lindahl G: Regulation of cardiovascular synthesis by mechanical load. Cardiovasc Res 42:27, 1999.
62. Lecour S, Smith RM, Woodward B, et al: Identification of a novel role for sphingolipid signalling in TNF-α and ischemic preconditioning mediated protection. J Mol Cell Cardiol 34:509, 2002.
63. Thielmann M, Dorge H, Martin C, et al: Myocardial dysfunction with coronary microembolization. Signal transduction through a sequence of nitric oxide, tumour necrosis factor-α, and sphingosine. Circ Res 90:807, 2002.
64. Sack MN, Smith RM, Opie LH: Tumour necrosis factor in myocardial hypertrophy and ischaemia—An anti-apoptotic perspective. Cardiovasc Res 45:688, 1999.

Contractile Performance of the Intact Heart

65. Lewis T: The Mechanism and Graphic Registration of the Heart Beat. London, Shaw and Sons, 1920.
66. Wiggers CJ: Modern Aspects of Circulation in Health and Disease. Philadelphia, Lea & Febiger, 1915.
67. Rhodes J, Udelson JE, Marx GR, et al: A new noninvasive method for the estimation of peak dP/dt. Circulation 88:2693, 1993.
68. Ohno M, Cheng CP, Little WC: Mechanism of altered patterns of left ventricular filling during the development of congestive heart failure. Circulation 89:2241, 1994.
69. Glower DD, Murrah RL, Olsen CO, et al: Mechanical correlates of the third heart sound. J Am Coll Cardiol 19:450, 1992.
70. Brutsaert DL, Sys SU, Gilbert TC: Diastolic failure: Pathophysiology and therapeutic implications. J Am Coll Cardiol 22:318, 1993.
71. Rodriguez EK, Hunter WC, Royce MJ: A method to reconstruct myocardial sarcomere lengths and orientations at transmural sites in beating canine hearts. Am J Physiol 263:H293, 1992.
72. MacGowan GA, Shapiro EP, Azhari H, et al: Noninvasive measurement of shortening in the fiber and cross-fiber directions in the normal human left ventricle and in idiopathic dilated cardiomyopathy. Circulation 96:535, 1997.
73. Mulieri LA, Leavitt BJ, Martin BJ: Myocardial force-frequency defect in mitral regurgitation heart failure is reversed by forskolin. Circulation 88:2700, 1993.
74. Pierard LA, Serruys PW, Roelandt J, Melzer RS: Left ventricular function at similar heart rates during tachycardia induced by exercise and atrial pacing: An echocardiographic study. Br Heart J 57:154, 1987.
75. Inagaki M, Yokota M, Izawa H, et al: Impaired force-frequency relations in patients with hypertensive left ventricular hypertrophy. Circulation 99:1822, 1999.
76. Suga H, Hisano R, Hirata S, et al: Mechanism of higher oxygen consumption rate: Pressure-loaded vs volume-loaded heart. Am J Physiol 242:H942, 1982.
77. Nozawa T, Cheng C-P, Noda T, Little WC: Effect of exercise on left ventricular mechanical efficiency in conscious dogs. Circulation 90:3047, 1994.
78. Chavez PN, Stanley WC, McElfresh TA, et al: Effect of hyperglycemia and fatty acid oxidation inhibition during aerobic conditions and demand-induced ischemia. Am J Physiol 284:H1521, 2003.
79. Beanlands RSB, Nahmias C, Gordon E, et al: The effects of β_1-blockade on oxidative metabolism and the metabolic cost of ventricular work in patients with left ventricular dysfunction. Circulation 102:2070, 2000.
80. Braunwald E, Sonnenblick EH, Ross J: Normal and abnormal circulatory function. *In* Braunwald E (ed): Heart Disease. A Textbook of Cardiovascular Medicine. 4th ed. Philadelphia, WB Saunders, 1992, pp 351–392.
81. Campbell KB, Kirkpatrick RD, Tobias AH: Series coupled non-contractile elements are functionally unimportant in the isolated heart. Cardiovasc Res 28:242, 1994.
82. Strang KT, Sweitzer NK, Greaser ML, Moss RL: β-Adrenergic receptor stimulation increases unloaded shortening velocity of skinned single ventricular myocytes from rats. Circ Res 74:542, 1994.
83. Brookes CIO, White PA, Staples M, et al: Myocardial contractility is not constant during spontaneous atrial fibrillation in patients. Circulation 98:1762, 1998.
84. Vogel M, Cheung MH, Li J, et al: Noninvasive assessment of left ventricular force-frequency relationships using tissue Doppler-derived isovolumic acceleration. Circulation 107:1647, 2003.
85. Zile MR, Brutsaert DL: New concepts in diastolic dysfunction and diastolic heart failure: Part 1. Circulation 105:1387, 2002.
86. Leite-Moreira AF, Correia-Pinto J, Gillebert TC: Afterload induced changes in myocardial relaxation: A mechanism for diastolic dysfunction. Cardiovasc Res 43:344, 1999.
87. Hein S, Amon E, Kostin S, et al: Progression from compensated hypertrophy to failure in the pressure-overloaded human heart. Structural deterioration and compensatory mechanisms. Circulation 107:984, 2003.
88. Zhang R, Zhao J, Mandveno A, Potter JD: Cardiac troponin I phosphorylation increases the rate of cardiac muscle relaxation. Circ Res 76:1028, 1995.
89. Cory CR, Grange RW, Houston ME: Role of sarcoplasmic reticulum in loss of load-sensitive relaxation in pressure overload cardiac hypertrophy. Am J Physiol 266:H68, 1994.
90. Bell SP, Nyland L, Tischler MD, et al: Alterations in the determinants of diastolic suction during pacing tachycardia. Circ Res 87:235, 2000.
91. Schotten U, Duytschaever M, Ausma J, et al: Electrical and contractile remodeling during the first days of atrial fibrillation go hand in hand. Circulation 107:1433, 2003.
92. Yu C-M, Lin H, Yang H, et al: Progression of systolic abnormalities in patients with "isolated" diastolic heart failure and diastolic dysfunction. Circulation 105:1195, 2002.
93. Nagueh SF, Middleton KJ, Kopelen HA, et al: Doppler tissue imaging: A noninvasive technique for evaluation of left ventricular relaxation and estimation of filling pressures. J Am Coll Cardiol 30:1527, 1997.

Effects of Ischemia and Reperfusion on Contraction and Relaxation

94. Opie L, Heusch G: Lack of blood flow: Ischemia and angina. *In* Opie LH (ed): Heart Physiology, from Cell to Circulation. 4th ed. Philadelphia, Lippincott Williams & Wilkins, 2004, pp 525–552.
95. Li RA, Leppo M, Miki T, et al: Molecular basis of electrocardiographic ST-segment elevation. Circ Res 87:837, 2000.
96. McDonough JL, Arrell K, Van Eyk JE: Troponin I degradation and covalent complex formation accompanies myocardial ischemia/reperfusion injury. Circ Res 84:9, 1999.
97. Murry CE, Jennings RB, Reimer KA: Preconditioning with ischemia: A delay of lethal cell injury in ischemic myocardium. Circulation 74:1124, 1986.
98. Yellon DM, Downey JM: Preconditioning the myocardium: From cellular physiology to clinical cardiology. Physiol Rev 83:1113, 2003.
99. Nakano A, Liu GS, Heusch G, et al: Exogenous nitric oxide can trigger a preconditioned state through a free radical mechanism, but endogenous nitric oxide is not a trigger of classical ischemic preconditioning. J Mol Cell Cardiol 32:1159, 2000.
100. Bolli R: Cardioprotective function of inducible nitric oxide synthase and role of nitric oxide in myocardial ischemia and preconditioning: An overview of a decade of research. J Mol Cell Cardiol 33:1897, 2001.

101. Minners J, McLeod C, Sack MN: Mitochondrial plasticity in classical ischemic preconditioning—Moving beyond the mitochondrial K_{ATP} channel. Cardiovasc Res 59:1, 2003.
102. Rajesh KG, Sasaguri S, Zhitian Z, et al: Second window of ischemic preconditioning regulates mitochondrial permeability transition pore by enhancing Bcl-2 expression. Cardivasc Res 59:297, 2003.
103. Simpson PC: β-Protein kinase C and hypertrophic signaling in human heart failure. Circulation 99:334, 1999.
104. Inagaki K, Hahn HS, Dorn GW 2nd, Mochly-Rosen D: Additive protection of the ischemic heart ex vivo by combined treatment with δ-protein kinase C inhibitor and ε-protein kinase C activator. Circulation 108:869, 2003.
105. Cross HR, Murphy E, Bolli R, et al: Expression of activated PKC epsilon (PKC_{ε}) protects the ischemic heart, without attenuating ischemic H^+ production. J Mol Cell Cardiol 34:361, 2002.
106. Lambiase PD, Edwards RJ, Cusack MR, et al: Exercise-induced ischemia initiates the second window of protection in humans independent of collateral recruitment. J Am Coll Cardiol 41:1174, 2003.
107. Rahimtoola S: Myocardial hibernation: Current clinical perspectives. *In* Yellon DM, Rahimtoola SH, Opie LH (eds): New Ischemic Syndromes. New York, Lippincott-Raven, 1997, pp 215-234.
108. Heusch G, Schulz R: Hibernating myocardium. New answers, still more questions! Circ Res 91:863, 2002.
109. Cain BS, Harken AH, Meldrum DR: Therapeutic strategies to reduce TNF-α medicated cardiac contractile depression following ischemia and reperfusion. J Mol Cell Cardiol 31:931, 1999.
110. Kalra DK, Zhu X, Ranchandani MK, et al: Increased myocardial gene expression of tumour necrosis factor-alpha and nitric oxide synthase-2: A potential mechanism for depressed myocardial function in hibernating myocardium in humans. Circulation 105:1537, 2002.
111. Auerbach MA, Scholder H, Hoh C, et al: Prevalence of myocardial viability as detected by position emission tomography in patients with ischemic cardiomyopathy. Circulation 99:2921, 1999.
112. Braunwald E, Kloner RA: The stunned myocardium: Prolonged, postischemic ventricular dysfunction. Circulation 66:1146, 1982.
113. Bolli R, Marban E: Molecular and cellular mechanisms of myocardial stunning. Physiol Rev 79:609, 1999.
114. Zeitz O, Maass E, Van Nguyen P, et al: Hydroxyl radical–induced acute diastolic dysfunction is due to calcium overload via reverse-mode Na^+-Ca^{2+} exchange. Circ Res 90:988, 2002.
115. Kloner RA, Jennings RB: Consequences of brief ischemia: Stunning, preconditioning, and their clinical implications. Part 1. Circulation 104:2981, 2001.
116. Perez NG, Gao WD, Marban E: Novel myofilament Ca^{2+}-sensitizing property of xanthine oxidase inhibitors. Circ Res 83:423, 1998.

Heart Failure

117. Meyer M, Keweloh B, Guth K, et al: Frequency-dependence of myocardial energetics in failing human myocardium as quantified by a new method for the measurement of oxygen consumption in muscle strip preparations. J Mol Cell Cardiol 30:1459, 1998.
118. Marx J: How to subdue a swelling heart. Science 300:1492, 2003.
119. Maurice JP, Shah AS, Kypson AP, et al: Molecular beta-adrenergic signaling abnormalities in failing rabbit hearts after infarction. Am J Physiol 276:H1853, 1999.
120. Moniotte S, Kobzik L, Feron O, et al: Upregulation of $beta_3$-adrenoreceptors and altered contractile response to inotropic amines in human failing myocardium. Circulation 103:1649, 2001.
121. Reiken S, Wehrens XHT, Vest JA, et al: β-Blockers restore calcium release channel function and improve cardiac muscle performance in human heart failure. Circulation 107:2459, 2003.
122. Kubo H, Margulies K, Piacentino V 3rd, et al: Patients with end-stage congestive heart failure treated with β-adrenergic receptor antagonists have improved ventricular myocyte calcium regulatory protein abundance. Circulation 104:1012, 2001.
123. Chandler MP, Stanley WC, Morita H, et al: Short-term treatment with ranolazine improves mechanical efficiency in dogs with chronic heart failure. Circ Res 91:278, 2002.
124. Wallhaus TR, Taylor M, Degrado TR, et al: Myocardial free fatty acid and glucose use after carvedilol treatment in patients with congestive heart failure. Circulation 103:2441, 2001.
125. Münch G, Bolck B, Karczewski P, Schwinger RHG: Evidence for calcineurin-mediated regulation of SERCA 2a activity in human myocardium. J Mol Cell Cardiol 34:321, 2002.
126. Marks AR, Reiken S, Marx SO: Progression of heart failure: Is protein kinase a hyperphosphorylation of the ryanodine receptor a contributing factor. Circulation 105:272, 2002.
127. Münch G, Bolck B, Brixius K, et al: SERCA2a activity correlates with the force-frequency relationship in human myocardium. Am J Physiol 278:H1924, 2000.
128. Clusin WT: Calcium and cardiac arrhythmias: DADs, EADs and alternans. Crit Rev Clin Lab Sci 40:337, 2003.
129. Pieske B, Kockskämper J: Alternans goes subcellular. A "disease" of the ryanodine receptor? Circ Res 91:553, 2002.
130. Matsuda JJ, Lee H-C, Shibata EF: Acetylcholine reversal of isoproterenol-stimulated sodium currents in rabbit ventricular myocytes. Circ Res 72:517, 1993.
131. Matsuda JJ, Lee H, Shibata EF: Enhancement of rabbit cardiac sodium channels by β-adrenergic stimulation. Circ Res 74:369, 1992.
132. Chang F, Cohen IS: Mechanism of acetylcholine action on pacemaker current (I_f) in canine Purkinje fibers. Pflugers Arch 420:389, 1992.
133. Kurachi Y: G-protein control of cardiac potassium channels. Trends Cardiovasc Med 4:64, 1994.
134. Fedida D: Modulation of cardiac contractility by α_1-adrenoreceptors. Cardiovasc Res 27:1735, 1993.
135. Volders PGA, Stengl M, van Opstal JM, et al: Probing the contribution of I_{KS} to canine ventricular repolarization. Circulation 107:2753, 2003.
136. Shannon TR, Ginsburg KS, Bers DM: Quantitative assessment of the SR Ca^{2+} leak-load relationship. Circ Res 91:594, 2002.
137. Pieske B, Maier LS, Bers DM, Hasenfuss G: Ca^{2+} handling and sarcoplasmic reticulum Ca^{2+} content in isolated failing and nonfailing human myocardium. Circ Res 85:38, 1999.
138. Piacentino V 3rd, Weber CR, Chen X, et al: Cellular basis of abnormal calcium transients of failing human ventricular myocytes. Circ Res 92:651, 2003.
139. Cooke R: Actomyosin interactions in striated muscle. Physiol Rev 77:671, 1997.
140. Holmes KC: The swinging lever-arm hypothesis of muscle contraction. Curr Biol 7:R112, 1997.
141. Bolli R, Shinmura K, Tang X-L, et al: Discovery of a new function of cyclooxygenase (COX)-2: COX-2 is a cardioprotective protein that alleviates ischemia/reperfusion injury and mediates the late phase of preconditioning. Cardiovasc Res 55:506, 2002.

CHAPTER 20

Assessment of Normal and Abnormal Cardiac Function

John D. Carroll • Otto M. Hess

The history of the study of cardiac function has been a progression from a description of cardiac anatomy, from this deducing function, to quantifying physiology, and now to the unraveling of molecular pathways.[1] The phenotype and genotype of disease states in patients provide a comprehensive understanding of pathophysiology, yielding answers to the question of why alterations in cardiac function occur. On the other hand, it is the clinical assessment of cardiac function that is necessary to determine the prognosis and the impact of therapy (Table 20–1).

New Relevance of Assessment of Cardiac Function

The rapid introduction and dissemination of novel therapies for cardiac dysfunction (see Chaps. 23 and 24) have characterized clinical cardiology in the last decade. Many of these new approaches and therapies have called on, resurrected, and extended a large reservoir of prior art in the field of assessment of cardiac function. The five examples that follow illustrate how contemporary investigators and clinicians require an in-depth understanding of the assessment of the relations between cardiac function, the quantification of reverse remodeling, and clinical outcomes.

RESYNCHRONIZATION THERAPY (see Chaps. 24 and 31). The mechanical and metabolic inefficiencies consequent to the loss of synchronous contraction and relaxation were topics confined to laboratory investigators of ventricular function until the advent of resynchronization therapy in heart failure with biventricular pacing.[2] Now there is a broad need for tools to quantify asynchrony and its modification by various modes of pacing (see Fig. 20–5).

VENTRICULAR ASSIST DEVICES (see Chap. 25). New mechanical cardiac assist devices may be implanted surgically or placed percutaneously and require a high level of sophistication in assessing cardiac function.[3] Distinguishing between the right and left ventricular components of a clinical syndrome of severe heart failure is important for proper patient selection. Management issues that involve assessment of preload and afterload in a two-pump environment, i.e., the native heart and the mechanical assist device, are common. Finally, the evaluation of therapeutic endpoints including reverse remodeling, as well as the serial assessment of cardiac function during weaning from the ventricular assist device, are critical to patient management.

ANGIOGENESIS AND STEM CELL TRANSPLANTATION (see Chap. 69). Transplantation of skeletal myoblasts and hematopoietic stem cells into regions of damaged myocardium is currently a field of active investigation.[4] Some cell lines enhance angiogenesis with the potential for ending the hibernating status of native myocytes. Others may become functional components of the myocardial syncytium. Both approaches present investigators with challenges in clarifying mechanisms of altered cardiac mechanical function and bring the need to assess serially regional and global chamber function.

PERCUTANEOUS VALVE REPAIR AND REPLACEMENT (see Chap. 57). Percutaneous approaches to reducing mitral regurgitation by either a coronary venous approach of annular reduction or a leaflet attachment approach provide a more comprehensive understanding of the complexities of valvular function that are linked to chamber size and function. Instantaneous changes in annular size, the severity of mitral regurgitation, and left ventricular function need to be assessed acutely and followed serially noninvasively.

VENTRICULAR PASSIVE CONSTRAINT DEVICES. Another novel therapeutic approach is the surgical or percutaneous insertion of passive ventricular restraining devices that prevent ventricular distention.[5] This approach focuses on prevention of deleterious remodeling after acute events such as large myocardial infarctions. A large body of knowledge on pericardial mechanics and restraining forces on the normal heart has now become timely to understand device design and to anticipate the changes of systolic and diastolic function occurring after implantation. As shown in Figure 20–1, a variety of tools is needed to evaluate the therapeutic effect of a restraining device as well as to monitor for unwanted effects.

Left Ventricular Systolic Function

Concepts

The fundamental task of the cardiovascular system is to supply adequate quantities of oxygenated blood to the peripheral tissues. The performance of the heart that is required to perform this task requires the complex interplay between the properties of the myocardium, the influences of neural and humoral factors, the circulating blood volume, and peripheral vascular compliance and resistance. An important determinant of cardiac performance is left ventricular systolic function, which in turn is determined by (1) preload, (2) afterload, (3) myocardial contractility, and (4) heart rate.

These four determinants allow the heart to adapt its performance to the changing requirements of the peripheral organs, as well as to compensate for a loss of myocardial mass and/or function. Cardiac performance is evaluated primarily by assessing left ventricular systolic function. Systole begins with the onset of depolarization and contraction and ends at the cessation of muscle contraction (Fig. 20–2).

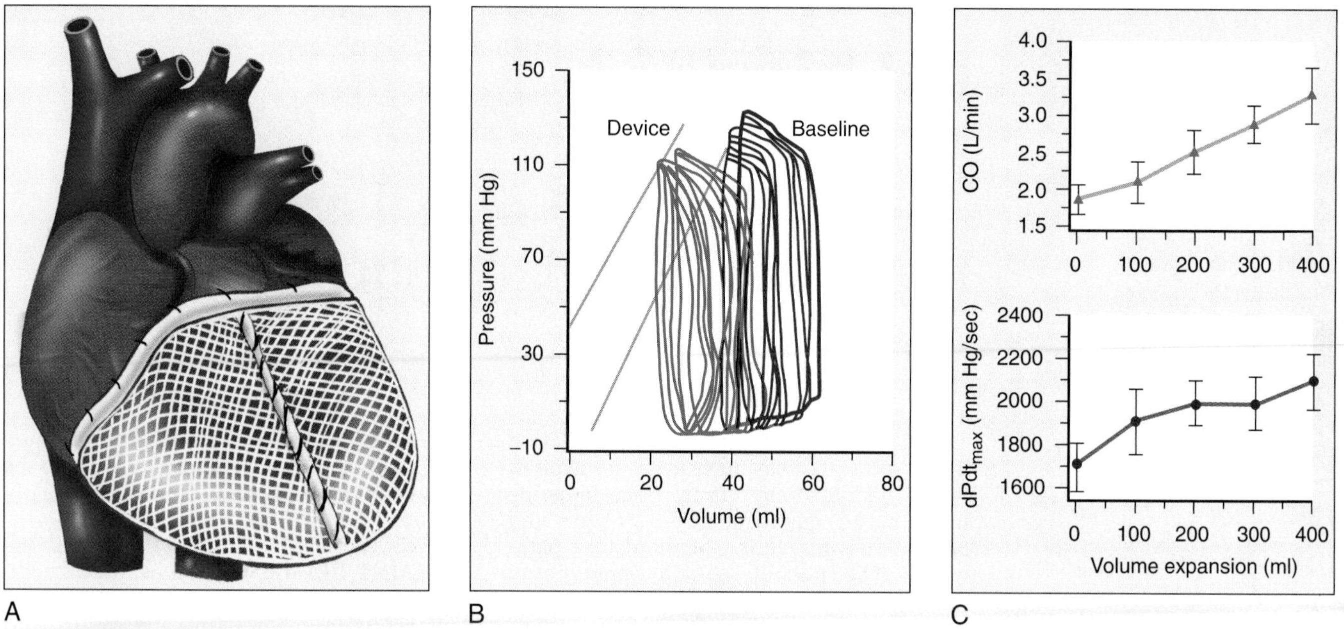

FIGURE 20–1 **A,** Passive ventricular restraining device. **B,** Device-induced reduction in chamber size and enhanced systolic performance accompanying this reverse remodeling. **C,** Preservation of recruitable preload with volume expansion. The pressure-volume loops generated under different loading states **(B)** demonstrate end-systolic pressure-volume relationships as well as diastolic chamber properties. Data in **C** show the systolic augmentation with volume expansion that was not compromised by the device. These data were obtained in an animal model. (Adapted from Saavedra WF, Tunin RS, Paolocci N, et al: Reverse remodeling and enhanced adrenergic reserve from passive external support in experimental dilated heart failure. J Am Coll Cardiol 39:2069, 2002.)

TABLE 20–1 Uses of Cardiac Function Assessment

Diagnosis
Prognostication
Timing of intervention
Mechanism of therapy
Assessment of therapy
Detection of complications
Surrogate for clinical outcomes

Definitions (Table 20–2)

PRELOAD. The stretch of the individual sarcomere regulates the performance of the heart. In the words of physiologists in the 19th century, preload is the property of cardiac muscle such that "the larger the quantity of blood which reaches the ventricles . . . the larger the quantity will be which it throws out."[6] Surrogates of the degree of sarcomere stretch at the onset of contraction include the ventricular end-diastolic volume, diameter, and end-diastolic pressure. Table 20–2 contrasts the differences between acute and chronic alterations in ventricular end-diastolic volume and pressure. The former enhance cardiac performance (adaptive mechanisms), whereas the latter ultimately impair performance (maladaptive mechanisms) (Table 20–3).

AFTERLOAD. This is the force against which muscle contracts. It is more challenging to quantify afterload in the intact circulation than in isolated cardiac muscle. Two approaches have been followed. The first focuses on the vascular load and uses descriptors such as peripheral vascular resistance or the more complex input impedance (see later) that includes the pulsatile load. The second focuses on the tension in the ventricular wall and considers pressure and cavity size in a more complex formulation, Laplace's law, which considers wall tension to be the product of pressure and radius, whereas the force (or tension) per unit of muscle is expressed in three dimensions, i.e., circumferential, meridional, and radial (Fig. 20–3).

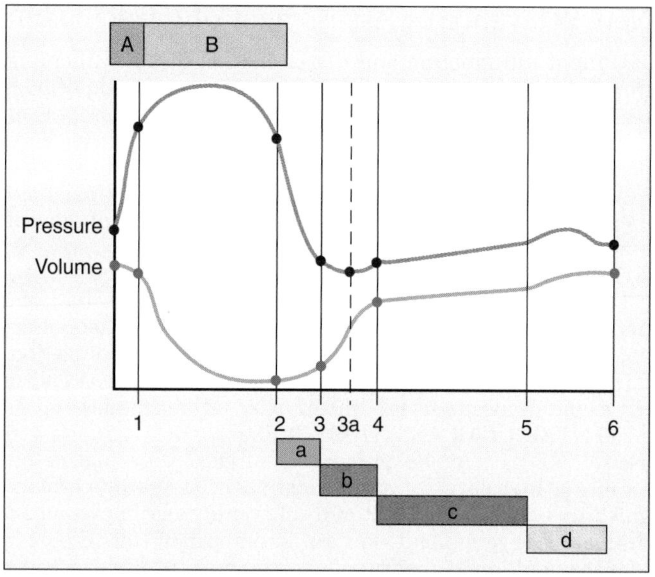

FIGURE 20–2 The cardiac cycle is shown in this schematic with both the left ventricular pressure waveform and a plot of left ventricular volume. The time landmarks during the cardiac cycle include the following: 1, aortic valve opening and the beginning of ejection; 2, aortic valve closure; 3, mitral valve opening; 3a, pressure nadir; 4, end of rapid early diastolic filling; 5, onset of atrial contraction; and 6, end-diastole. The phases of the cardiac cycle are denoted with the shaded rectangles displaying the timing of each phase. The two systolic phases are noted above the waveforms, where A = isovolumic contraction and B = ejection. The four diastolic phases are noted below the waveforms, where a = isovolumic relaxation; b = early diastolic filling; c = diastasis; and d = atrial filling.

CONTRACTILITY. This is the intrinsic ability of heart muscle to generate force and to shorten. In the intact circulation it is manifest as the rate of pressure development and of shortening from any given preload. Contractility is normally modulated by a variety of factors including the neurohumoral milieu. Measures of systolic function and

TABLE 20–2 Definitions of Terms Used to Describe Systolic and Diastolic Function

Term	Definition
Preload	Distending force of the ventricular wall, which is highest at end-diastole and is responsible for sarcomere length at the beginning of systolic contraction
Afterload	Resisting force of the ventricular wall during systolic ejection, which is necessary to overcome peripheral vascular resistance or impedance; measures of afterload are peak-systolic, mean-systolic, or end-systolic wall stress
Contractility	Intrinsic ability of the myocardium to generate force at a certain rate and time (controlled for loading conditions)
Cardiac output	Stroke volume multiplied by heart rate
Stroke work	Mean systolic blood pressure multiplied by stroke volume
Stroke force	Stroke work per ejection time
Stress	Force per area
Wall stress	Pressure multiplied by radius, divided by wall thickness × 2
Compliance or distensibility	Change in volume per change in pressure (dV/dP)
Elastance	Slope of the end-systolic pressure-volume relation
Elasticity	Property of a material to restore its initial length or geometry after distending force has been removed
Strain	Length change in percent of initial length; two definitions are used: LaGrangian strain $e = (l - l_o)l_o$ and natural strain $e = \ln(l/lo)$
Stiffness	Pressure per volume change (dP/dV). *Ventricular stiffness* is a measure for changes of the ventricle as a whole; *myocardial stiffness* is a measure for changes of the myocardium itself. Ventricular properties are characterized by instantaneous pressure-volume relations, whereas myocardial properties are best described by stress-strain relations.
Creep	Time-dependent lengthening of a material in the presence of a constant force
Stress relaxation	Time-dependent decrease of stress in the presence of a constant length
Viscoelasticity	Resistance of a material to length changes (strain) or the velocity of length changes (strain rate)

TABLE 20–3 Two Pathways of Ventricular Dilation and Increased Filling Pressure

Hemodynamic (Acute)
Dilation and increased end-diastolic pressure caused when increased venous return or decreased ejection increases end-diastolic volume. This form of dilation occurs when physiological (functional) signaling increases sarcomere length, which increases the heart's ability to perform work (Starling law of the heart)

Architectural (Chronic)
Dilation and increased filling pressures caused when hypertrophy increases cardiac myocyte length and alters passive muscle properties. By increasing wall stress, this growth response increases the energy demands of the heart and decreases cardiac efficiency, initiating a vicious circle that worsens heart failure. This form of dilation occurs when abnormal transcriptional (proliferative) signaling causes eccentric hypertrophy (systolic dysfunction), and it tends to progress (remodeling)

Adapted from Katz A: Ernest Henry Starling, his predecessors, and the "law of the heart." Circulation 106:2986, 2002.

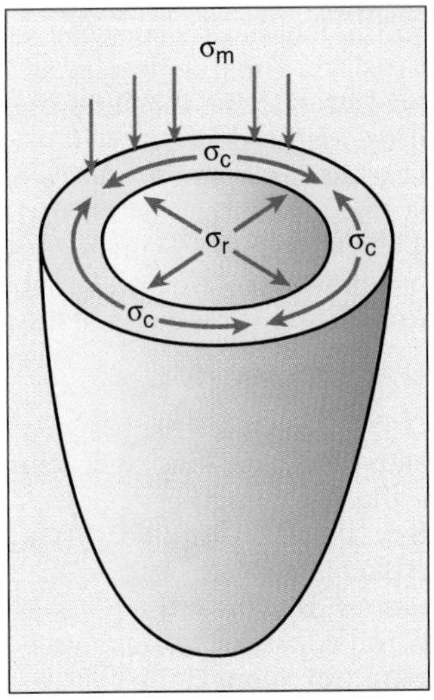

FIGURE 20–3 Circumferential (σ_c), meridional (σ_m), and radial (σ_r) components of left ventricular wall stress from an ellipsoid model. The three components of wall stress are mutually perpendicular. (From Fifer MA, Grossman W: Measurement of ventricular volumes, ejection fraction, mass, and wall stress. In Grossman W [ed]: Cardiac Catheterization and Angiography. 5th ed. Philadelphia, Lea & Febiger, 1996, p 34.)

contractility are often considered together and include stroke volume, ejection fraction, the maximum rate of pressure increases during isovolumic contraction, and a variety of more sophisticated measurements that attempt to control for loading conditions (Table 20–4).[1]

FILLING PRESSURES. The determination of systolic function should be placed in the framework of the ventricular filling pressure that reflects preload; the latter, in turn, is influenced importantly by the status of the circulating blood volume. Filling pressures are also related to both the contractility and diastolic properties of the ventricle (see later). Filling pressures such as ventricular end-diastolic pressure, atrial pressure, and pulmonary capillary wedge pressure (for the left ventricle) and central venous pressure (for the right

TABLE 20–4 Characteristics of Selected Indices of Global Ventricular Function

Index	Sensitive to Inotropic Changes	Dependence On Preload	Dependence On Afterload	Dependence On Ventricular Volume or Mass	Ease of Application
Ejection fraction; fractional shortening	++	++	+++	++	++++
End-systolic volume or dimension	+	0	+++	++	++++
VCF	+++	0	+++	++	+++
Afterload-corrected VCF	+++	0	0	0	+
ESPVR	++++	0	0	+++	+
End-systolic stiffness	++++	0	0	0	+
Preload recruitable stroke work	+++	0	0	++	+
Left ventricular dP/dt	++++	++	++	++	++

ESPVR = slope of end-systolic pressure-volume relation; VCF = velocity of circumferential fiber shortening; dP/dt = rate of ventricular pressure rise.
Adapted from Carabello B: Evolution of the study of left ventricular function: Everything old is new again. Circulation 105:2701, 2002.

ventricle) provide valuable clinical information that aids in the differentiation between disparate conditions causing hypotension, e.g., hypovolemia versus myocardial failure.

Left ventricular end-diastolic pressure (LVEDP) is measured routinely in the cardiac catheterization laboratory during retrograde left heart catheterization (see Chap. 17). It may be difficult to measure LVEDP precisely at rapid heart rates using fluid-filled catheters, especially when there is not a distinctive plateau after atrial contraction. The measurement of LVEDP during invasive and interventional procedures provides a simple and often useful indicator of cardiac function. Several common clinical examples demonstrate the utility of this measurement. An elevated LVEDP in the presence of a normal left ventricular ejection fraction (LVEF) suggests the presence of diastolic dysfunction (see later). A low LVEDP after a percutaneous coronary intervention suggests volume depletion that should be corrected before the development of hypotension. A markedly elevated LVEDP may be a strong contraindication to the injection of contrast dye and suggests that diuresis is needed.

Central venous pressure is a poor indicator of left ventricular filling pressure, since it may be normal in the presence of an abnormally elevated LVEDP. Tricuspid regurgitation and pericardial disease may elevate central venous pressure and confound it as an indicator of volume status.

Calculations and Measurements of Systolic Function

Clinical parameters for assessing left ventricular systolic function include the following:

- Cardiac index (liter/min/m^2): heart rate × stroke volume per body surface area
- Stroke volume index (ml/m^2)
- Stroke work index: stroke volume index × mean systolic blood pressure (ml × mm Hg/m^2)
- Stroke force index: stroke work index per ejection period in seconds
- Preload recruitable stroke work = relationship between stroke work and end-diastolic volume

CARDIAC OUTPUT AND RELATED MEASURES. Cardiac output is commonly measured by the thermodilution technique (see Chap. 17). Saline injected into the right atrium is detected as a temperature change at a thermistor at the tip of a catheter in the pulmonary artery. The thermodilution catheter transmits the temperature data to a small computer that calculates cardiac output. To improve accuracy, the determination is usually repeated several times and the results are averaged. This technique is less accurate when flow is severely reduced, especially in the presence of tricuspid regurgitation, which leads to dissipation of the "temperature bolus." The presence of intracardiac shunts also introduces potential errors and misinterpretation since right- and left-sided flows are not equal. The Fick method of measuring cardiac output has greater accuracy than the thermodilution method when oxygen consumption is actually measured, rather than assumed. However measured, cardiac output is usually expressed relative to body size, i.e., cardiac index, which is calculated as cardiac output divided by body surface area, expressed in square meters.

Cardiac output (and index) can be divided by the heart rate to yield stroke volume (and index). An alternative method of deriving stroke volume is by calculating the difference between left ventricular volume at end-diastole and end-systole. This approach is limited by the accuracy of the imaging modality in determining chamber volumes. Accuracy is greatest with a three-dimensional (3D) determined volume with high-resolution imaging, but it may be impaired by the normal beat-to-beat variation in chamber size that occurs during respiration and is accentuated in atrial fibrillation and other arrhythmias. The product of pressure generation and stroke volume equals stroke work; when related to the time interval during which the stroke volume is ejected from the left ventricle (i.e., the ejection time) stroke force may be derived.

VENTRICULAR FUNCTION CURVES. Reduced values of stroke parameters (volume, work, force, and their indices, i.e., corrected for body surface area) are often associated with depressed myocardial contractility, but since these parameters are highly dependent on the loading conditions (preload and afterload), these two variables must also be assessed. The dependency of stroke volume on preload was described more than 100 years ago by Otto Frank and E. H. Starling, and since then has been called the Frank-Starling mechanism.[6] Using this relationship between preload and stroke volume or stroke work, a *ventricular function curve* can be constructed by plotting stroke work at various levels of preload; the latter may be expressed as ventricular end-diastolic volume, end-diastolic pressure, or end-diastolic wall stress. Preload can be altered by volume loading (leg elevation, volume infusion) and unloading (vena caval balloon occlusion). Left ventricular afterload can be estimated from the mean or end systolic arterial or ventricular pressure or, more accurately, by calculating mean systolic, peak systolic, or end-systolic wall stress. The most reliable method for determination of left ventricular contractility represents the end-systolic pressure-volume relationship (ESPVR; maximum elastance), which is nearly

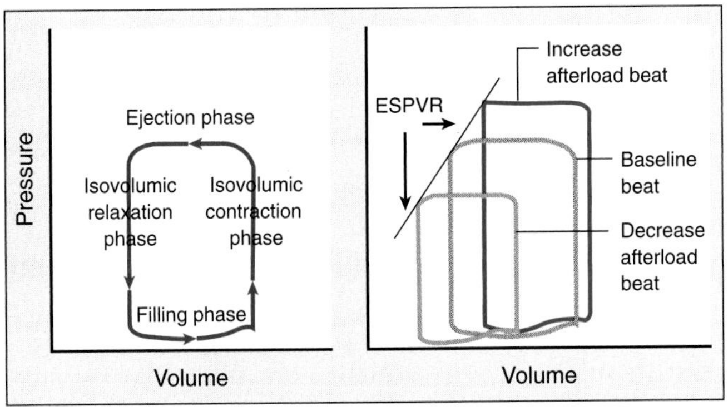

FIGURE 20–4 **Left,** Left ventricular pressure-volume relationship is shown, with the four phases of the cardiac cycle. **Right,** The graph shows how two additional pressure-volume loops appear with an acute increase and decrease in afterload. Changes in preload can also be used to generate the coordinates. In the clinical setting it is difficult to generate the end-systolic pressure-volume relationship (ESPVR) free of changes in reflex-mediated variations in contractility. It also requires a means to measure pressure and volume accurately and simultaneously. The end-systolic pressure-volume coordinates form a linear relationship, ESPVR. The slope of the ESPVR line is end-systolic elastance.

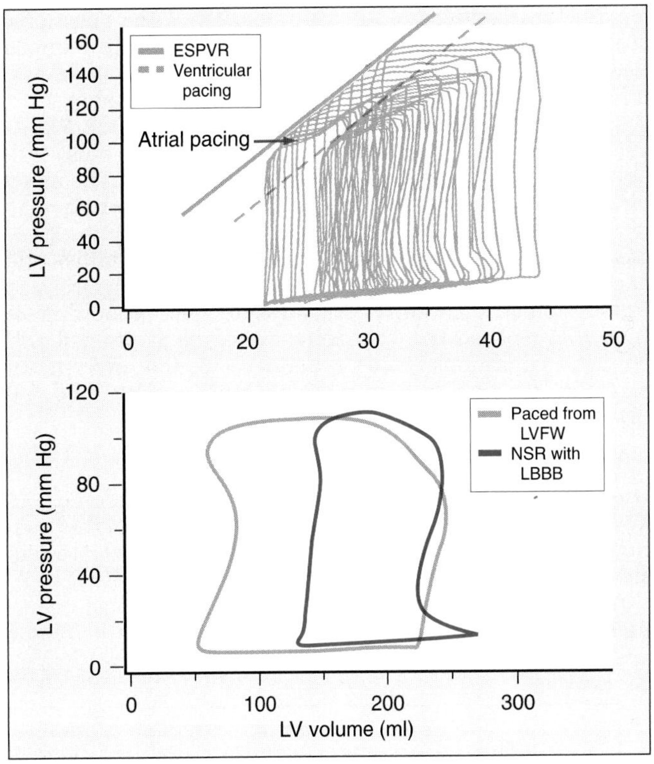

FIGURE 20–5 **Top,** Left ventricular (LV) pressure-volume loops in an experimental animal during transient caval occlusions. The upper left corners of the loops define the LV end-systolic pressure-volume relation (ESPVR). During atrial pacing producing normal LV activation, the ESPVR is shifted leftward in a parallel fashion, compared with ventricular pacing that produces dyssynchronous LV activation and contraction. **Bottom,** Steady-state LV pressure-volume loop recorded using the conductance catheter in a patient with dilated cardiomyopathy and dyssynchronous LV activation due to left bundle branch block (LBBB). A decrease in dyssynchronous contraction produced by LV free wall (LVFW) pacing produced loops with greater width (stroke volume) as the end-systolic pressure-volume point shifted toward the left. NSR = normal sinus rhythm. (**Top,** From Park RC, Little WC, O'Rourke RA: Effect of alteration of left ventricular activation sequence on the left ventricular end-systolic pressure-volume relation in closed-chest dogs. Circ Res 57:711, 1985; and **Bottom,** Kass DA, Chen DH, Curry C, et al: Improved left ventricular mechanics from acute VDD pacing in patients with dilated cardiomyopathy and ventricular conduction delay. Circulation 99:1570, 1999.)

independent of preload and afterload. The slope of this relationship is a measure of left ventricular contractility (Figs. 20–4 and 20–5; see also Fig. 20–1).

The use of ventricular function curves in assessing left ventricular function is limited by variability dependent on gender, age, and afterload. Furthermore, changes in right ventricular filling pressure can affect the position of the interventricular septum and thereby alter left ventricular diastolic pressure and thereby alter the position of the ventricular function curve as well.

Specific Indices

There are several indices of global left ventricular systolic function and contractility.[1] As shown in Table 20–4, each index is variably dependent on preload and afterload and can be modified by ventricular volume and myocardial mass. The ease of application to the clinical setting is an important feature.

EJECTION FRACTION. The *ejection fraction* is defined as the ratio of stroke volume to end-diastolic volume. It is most often computed as follows:

$$EF = EDV - ESV/EDV \times 100\ (\%)$$

where EF = ejection fraction, EDV = end-diastolic volume, and ESV = end-systolic volume.

Normal values of LVEF are 0.55 to 0.75 when determined by angiocardiography and echocardiography but may be lower when determined by radionuclide angiography (0.50 to 0.65). There are no gender differences, but ejection fraction normally declines with age. An acute increase in afterload, such as occurs during acute pressure loading, may decrease ejection fraction to 0.45 or 0.50 in normal subjects. However, a reduction of LVEF below 0.45 indicates impaired myocardial function, independent of loading conditions.

The widespread utility of the ejection fraction in clinical practice is a result of multiple factors including the conceptual simplicity of its derivation, the ability to determine it easily and reproducibly, using a variety of different imaging techniques, and an extensive documentation of its clinical utility.[1] This parameter has been shown to be of great prognostic value both short-term and long-term in patients with a variety of heart diseases. However, its limitation is its dependency not only on myocardial contractility but also on preload and afterload, as well as heart rate and synchronicity of contraction. Therefore, it measures much more than contractility.

END-SYSTOLIC VENTRICULAR VOLUME OR DIMENSION. The clinical utility of end-systolic volume or dimension is its relative *independence* of preload. Although strongly afterload dependent, it is of particular value in assessing left ventricular function in patients with valvular regurgitation.

VELOCITY OF CIRCUMFERENTIAL FIBER (VCF) SHORTENING. This ejection phase index of systolic function has been used primarily in research studies. Typically, the changes in the left ventricular volume or circumference during systole (corrected to the end-diastolic value) are divided by ejection time to yield the mean velocity of ejection or fiber shortening.

AFTERLOAD-CORRECTED VCF. Since ejection phase indices such as VCF are highly afterload dependent, they become more accurate indicators of ventricular function by correcting with some measure of afterload. Further correction for left ventricular geometry is made by using stress instead of pressure. There are several methods for calculating wall stress; the most common model of Sandler and Dodge has been used (circumferential wall stress):

$$P \times b/h \times (1 - b^2/[a^2 + 2b + h])$$

where P = pressure, h = left ventricular wall thickness, b = short half-axis, and a = long half-axis. Patients with reduced left ventricular contractility have a downward shift of the systolic shortening–mean systolic wall stress relationship.

SLOPE OF END-SYSTOLIC PRESSURE-VOLUME RELATIONSHIP (END SYSTOLIC ELASTANCE). The most reliable index for assessing myocardial contractility in the intact circulation is the ESPVR, which is almost *insensitive* to changes in preload, afterload, and heart rate (see Figs. 20–1, 20–4, and 20–5). This is widely used in animal studies and occasionally clinically. This relationship can be determined from instantaneous end-systolic pressure-volume coordinates from different cardiac contractions at varying preload and afterload conditions. Using a linear regression analysis for assessing the end-systolic pressure-volume curve, the following equation is used:

$$E(t) = P(t)/V(t) - V_o(t)$$

where E = maximum elastance, P = pressure, V = volume, and V_o = extrapolated volume at pressure 0. The slope of this relationship represents the end-systolic elastance, which is a sensitive parameter for assessing myocardial contractility.

Assessment of elastance is difficult under clinical conditions, because it requires simultaneous pressure-volume relations, as well as changes in preload or afterload for construction of the ESPVR. However, this measurement is facilitated by the use of techniques such as radionuclide angiography or the use of conductance catheters, which allow continuous measurements of left ventricular volume while left ventricular volume is changed, e.g., by caval occlusion.

END-SYSTOLIC STIFFNESS. This index of contractile function is derived from the exponential constant of the end-systolic relation between wall stress and the natural logarithm of the reciprocal of wall thickness.[1]

PRELOAD RECRUITABLE STROKE WORK. The relation between left ventricular stroke work and left ventricular end-diastolic volume is a representation of systolic function.[7] Like the end-systolic elastance, it is difficult to assess this parameter in patients because preload needs to be varied to generate this parameter.

MAXIMUM RATE OF PRESSURE RISE. The maximal rate of ventricular pressure rise (maximum dP/dt) is analogous to the maximal rate of tension development of isolated cardiac muscle, a well-established index of myocardial contractility. However, the concept of a true isovolumic contraction period in the intact heart is no longer correct, since it has been shown with myocardial tagging that during isovolumic contraction there is systolic rotation (reflecting myocardial shortening) without a change in volume (see Fig. 20–12). As a further limitation, maximum dP/dt is dependent not only on left ventricular contractility but also on heart rate, preload, and afterload (Fig. 20–6), synchronicity of contraction, and myocardial hypertrophy. Since this isovolumic index of systolic function is preload dependent, the relationship between ventricular end-diastolic volume and dP/dt is a more accurate index of contractility than dP/dt alone.

Regional Indices of Left Ventricular Function

Global measures of left ventricular function, such as those described earlier, lose accuracy when the disease process affects regions of the ventricle differentially; this occurs most notably in coronary artery disease. Chronic myocardial ischemia, i.e., stunning or hibernation (see Chap. 19), and acute or old myocardial infarction may be associated with regional wall motion abnormalities with hypokinesis (reduced shortening) and akinesis (absent shortening) or dyskinesis (systolic elongation or bulging). Often the nonischemic portion of the ventricle is hypercontractile, leading to a normal *global* left ventricular function in the presence of impairment of regional function.

The most widely used technique for assessing regional wall motion is the centerline method (Fig. 20–7), which demonstrates that shortening at the apex normally is less than at the base. For normalization, systolic shortening may be divided by ejection time. This approach to quantifying regional left ventricular function was initially used in contrast angiograms and then extended to echocardiograms. These measures of endocardial motion and

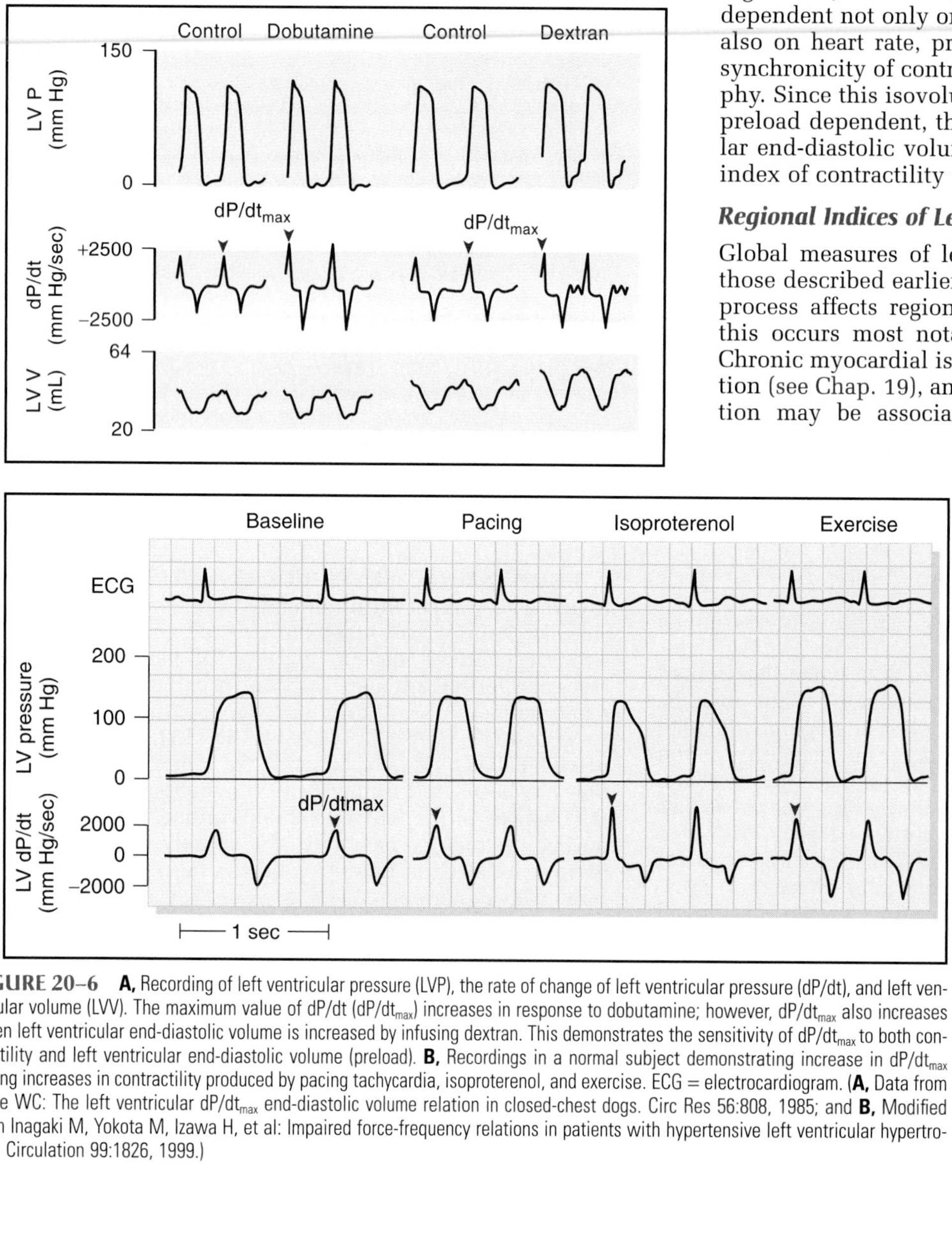

FIGURE 20–6 **A,** Recording of left ventricular pressure (LVP), the rate of change of left ventricular pressure (dP/dt), and left ventricular volume (LVV). The maximum value of dP/dt (dP/dt_{max}) increases in response to dobutamine; however, dP/dt_{max} also increases when left ventricular end-diastolic volume is increased by infusing dextran. This demonstrates the sensitivity of dP/dt_{max} to both contractility and left ventricular end-diastolic volume (preload). **B,** Recordings in a normal subject demonstrating increase in dP/dt_{max} during increases in contractility produced by pacing tachycardia, isoproterenol, and exercise. ECG = electrocardiogram. (**A,** Data from Little WC: The left ventricular dP/dt_{max} end-diastolic volume relation in closed-chest dogs. Circ Res 56:808, 1985; and **B,** Modified from Inagaki M, Yokota M, Izawa H, et al: Impaired force-frequency relations in patients with hypertensive left ventricular hypertrophy. Circulation 99:1826, 1999.)

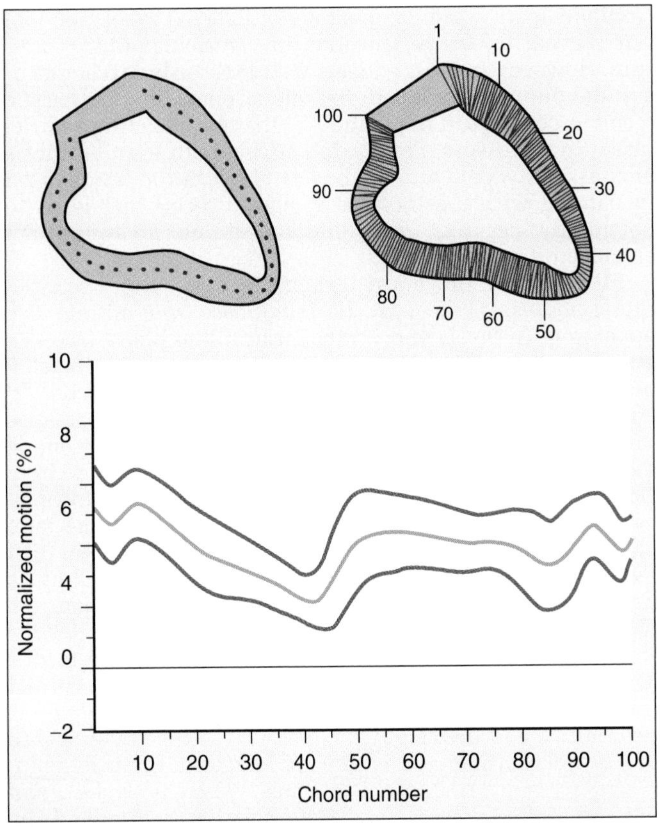

FIGURE 20–7 Assessment of regional left ventricular function using the centerline method. Regional wall motion is determined along 100 chords drawn perpendicular to a centerline constructed midway between the end-diastolic and end-systolic contours. Calculated wall motion of the 100 chords **(bottom)** is normalized for heart size by dividing each chord by the length of the end-diastolic perimeter. The normal range is indicated by the dotted lines (mean ± 1 SD). (From Sheehan FH, Bolson EL, Dodge HT, et al: Advantages and applications of the centerline method for characterizing regional ventricular function. Circulation 74:293, 1986.)

changes in wall thickness are afterload dependent but do allow comparisons of different regions of the ventricle. As discussed later, nuclear magnetic resonance imaging with tagging provides the most comprehensive assessment of regional wall motion, and more recently tissue Doppler strain rates (see Chap. 11) have been used experimentally and clinically.

Diastolic Function

(see Chaps. 19, 21, and 22)

Assessment of cardiac performance has focused traditionally on systolic function, whereas diastole was considered of secondary importance. More recently, however, diastolic function has been found to play an important role in cardiac morbidity and mortality and to influence both preload and afterload. Diastolic function is influenced importantly by ventricular structure and composition.[8-10] Diastole begins with the isovolumic relaxation period that starts after aortic valve closure (see Fig. 20–2). Because relaxation is an active, energy-consuming process, some authors consider relaxation in a strict sense to be a part of systole.[9,10] However, from a clinical standpoint, four separate phases of diastole need to be distinguished: (1) isovolumic relaxation; (2) early (rapid) diastolic filling; (3) slow ventricular filling (diastasis); and (4) atrial filling.

Definitions (see Table 20–2)

Diastolic function is influenced by several factors, e.g., myocardial relaxation, ventricular filling, and the ventricle's passive elastic properties, but one of the major determinants is heart rate, which determines how much time is available for ventricular filling. An increase in heart rate shortens the diastolic filling time interval disproportionately. This reduction must be compensated for by an increase in the rate of relaxation and an augmentation of elastic recoil with enhanced diastolic suction. Thus, impaired diastolic function can be aggravated by tachycardia and can be improved simply by a reduction in heart rate, which allows the heart to fill over a longer period.

In the normal left ventricle, the end-systolic volume is smaller than its elastic equilibrium and it thus generates *elastic recoil,* which varies inversely with the end-systolic volume. The elastic recoil causes diastolic suction that fills the ventricle at a low pressure and induces a potential for negative left ventricular pressure in early diastole. This filling mechanism is important during exercise and allows the normal ventricle to reduce minimal diastolic pressure and to maintain end-diastolic pressure constant despite a threefold to fivefold increase in cardiac output.[8-10] A loss of elastic recoil occurs during acute ischemia with a reduction in early diastolic filling accompanied by an increase in left atrial filling pressure and heart rate.[11,12]

Another important determinant of diastolic function is the *atrioventricular pressure gradient,* which is dependent on atrial pressure, relaxation rate, viscous forces in the myocardium, and ventricular filling rates.[8-11] An increase in the rate of relaxation can maintain left atrial pressure at normal levels, despite an increase in cardiac output. However, a reduction in ventricular filling rate can be compensated for by an increase in left atrial pressure, as occurs in patients with left ventricular hypertrophy or myocardial infarction.

ABNORMALITIES OF DIASTOLIC FUNCTION. From a clinical standpoint, a number of abnormalities of diastolic function have been described.[13-17] They are variously termed *diastolic abnormalities, diastolic dysfunction,* and *diastolic heart failure,* in ascending order of severity.

Diastolic abnormalities are characterized by abnormal filling indices, are commonly identified by echocardiography, and known to have a reduced early diastolic filling rate or a prolonged isovolumic relaxation period, but without clinical symptoms. In this situation the ventricle is able to compensate for abnormal diastolic function and to maintain a normal level of left ventricular filling pressure. *Diastolic dysfunction* is characterized by an increase in diastolic filling pressure, which may be responsible for the occurrence of dyspnea. This symptom may occur during exercise ("latent" diastolic dysfunction) or may be present also at rest ("manifest" diastolic dysfunction). Many patients with moderate to severe left ventricular hypertrophy may suffer from diastolic dysfunction. *Diastolic heart failure* is associated with the clinical signs of heart failure, such as paroxysmal nocturnal dyspnea, orthopnea, and edema. The clinical differentiation between systolic and diastolic dysfunction is important, because prognosis and therapeutic interventions are different in these two forms of heart failure (see Chap. 22).[9,10,13-17]

RELAXATION. Isovolumic relaxation begins with aortic valve closure and ends with mitral valve opening. The timing and the rate of relaxation are dependent on preload and afterload, myocardial inactivation, and synchrony of cardiac contraction.[8-10] The important determinants of relaxation are maximal systolic pressure, end-systolic fiber stretch, coronary flow ("erectile effect"), and stored energy (elastic recoil). A delayed or incomplete relaxation (>3.5 time constants) can retard and/or delay the onset of diastolic filling (Fig. 20–8).

This is typically the case in patients with left ventricular hypertrophy or myocardial ischemia and, when sufficiently severe, leads to an increase in diastolic filling pressure. An increase in myocardial contractility and an augmentation of elastic recoil, as occurs in patients with hypertrophic cardiomyopathy, can compensate for delayed relaxation and can prevent excessive elevation of ventricular filling pressure. However, in most patients with myocardial ischemia or systolic pump failure, both the rate of relaxation and elastic recoil are decreased in parallel,[18,19] thereby elevating ventricular filling pressure. Finally, in patients with mitral stenosis or constrictive pericarditis, the rate of relaxation is enhanced in parallel with the increase in elastic recoil that leads to potentially negative early diastolic filling pressures and enhanced diastolic suction.

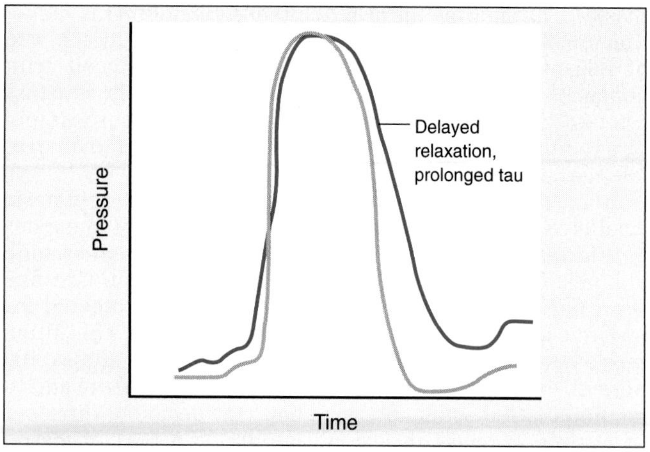

FIGURE 20–8 Two left ventricular pressure waveforms show a normal contour and then a waveform with delayed relaxation producing a prolonged time constant of relaxation (tau). The pressure coordinates from aortic valve closing to mitral valve opening, i.e., during the isovolumic relaxation period, can be plotted and the negative reciprocal of the log plot is the calculated relation value (tau).

FILLING. In the normal ventricle there are two rapid filling phases: (1) the early diastolic phase from mitral valve opening to diastasis and (2) the atrial filling phase (see Fig. 20–2).[8-10] Rapid diastolic filling is dependent on four mechanisms: (1) rate of relaxation, (2) elastic ventricular recoil, (3) atrioventricular pressure gradient, and (4) passive elastic properties of the atrium and the ventricle. Assessment of diastolic filling can be obtained most conveniently from Doppler echocardiography (see Chap. 11), which allows an assessment of maximal filling velocities as well as the ratio between early (E wave) and late (A wave) filling velocity (E/A ratio) (Fig. 20–9) (see Chap. 21). Late diastolic filling is dependent on the strength of left atrial contraction and the diastolic stiffness of the left ventricle.

PASSIVE ELASTIC PROPERTIES. It is necessary to distinguish between ventricular (chamber) and myocardial (muscle) properties (Fig. 20–10).[8-10,20] *Ventricular stiffness* is determined and defined by the pressure-volume relationship of the left ventricle and is directly related to clinical symptoms, whereas *myocardial stiffness* is determined by the stress-strain relationship of the left ventricle, which is a function of the structural composition of the myocardium.[8-10,21-25] Ventricular stiffness reaches its nadir at the lowest diastolic pressure but increases progressively during diastolic filling and is maximal at end-diastole. Myocardial stiffness impedes myocardial lengthening. Since wall stress and myocardial fiber length increase during diastolic filling, they reach maximal levels at end-diastole (i.e., the preload), which according to the Frank-Starling principle is an important determinant of the extent of systolic myocardial fiber shortening.

CHAMBER PROPERTIES. The diastolic properties of the left ventricle can be described by the diastolic pressure-volume or pressure-dimension relationships (Fig. 20–11; see also Fig. 20–10). These relations can be described mathematically by an exponential equation, the constant of chamber stiffness, defined by the slope of this relationship. The slope and position of the pressure-volume relationship represent *ventricular stiffness,*

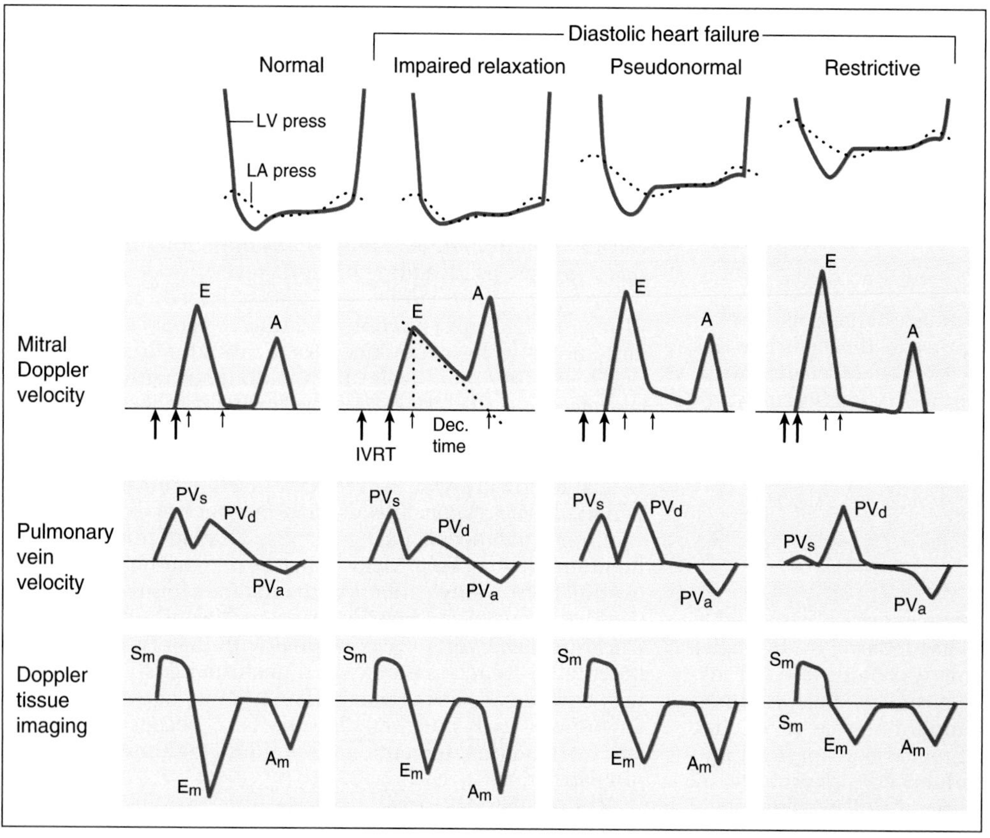

FIGURE 20–9 The techniques of assessing diastolic function include direct pressure measurement of the small diastolic, physiological gradients between the left atrium (LA) and the left ventricle (LV) (**first panel** [top]), transmitral inflow Doppler velocity profile (**second panel,** IVRT = isovolumic relaxation time; Dec. time = deceleration time of e wave; E = early LV filling velocity; A = velocity of LV filling contributed by atrial contraction), pulmonary vein Doppler velocity (**third panel,** PV_s = systolic pulmonary vein velocity; PV_d = diastolic pulmonary vein velocity; PV_a = pulmonary vein velocity resulting from atrial contraction), and Doppler tissue velocity (**fourth panel,** S_m = myocardial velocity during systole; E_m = myocardial velocity during early filling; A_m = myocardial velocity during filling produced by atrial contraction). (Adapted from Zile M, Brutsaert D: New concepts in diastolic dysfunction and diastolic heart failure: I. Diagnosis, prognosis, and measurements of diastolic function. Circulation 105:1387, 2002.)

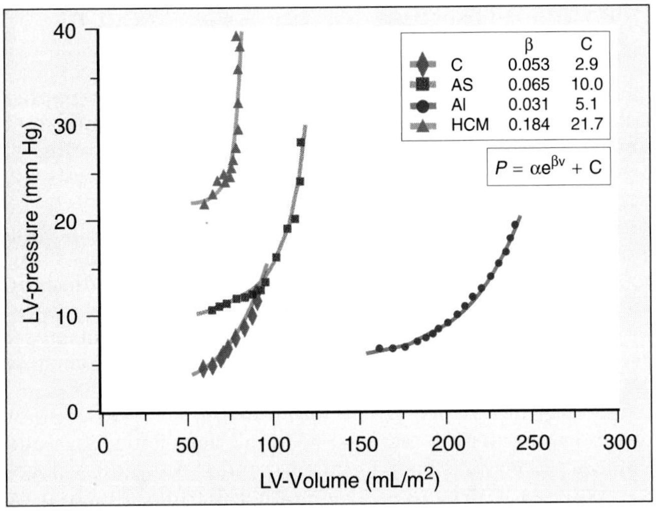

FIGURE 20–10 Left ventricular (LV) pressure-volume relationship during diastole in a control subject (C) and patients with aortic stenosis (AS), aortic regurgitation (AI), and hypertrophic cardiomyopathy (HCM). There is a parallel upward shift in the HCM and a small upward shift in the AS patient due to the increase in diastolic stiffness. The constant of chamber stiffness (β) is 0.184 in HCM and 0.065 in AS compared with 0.053 in the control patient. However, there is a rightward shift in the AI patient due to the increase in LV diastolic volume with a minimal increase in diastolic filling pressure (i.e., due to a low diastolic chamber stiffness). β is 0.031 in this patient. (From Mandinov L, Eberli FR, Seiler C, Hess OM: Diastolic heart failure. Cardiovasc Res 45:814, 2000.)

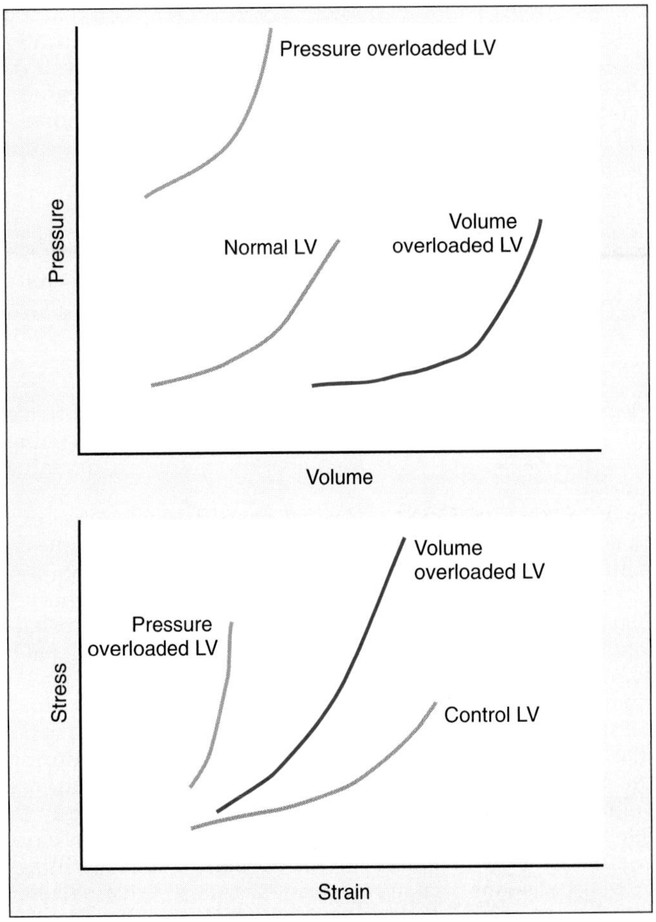

FIGURE 20–11 Schematic representation of the diastolic left ventricular (LV) pressure-volume **(top)** and LV stress-strain relationship **(bottom)**. The pressure-volume relationship is dependent on changes of the left ventricle as a whole associated with chronic pressure (upward shift) or volume-overload (rightward shift), whereas the LV stress-strain relationship represents changes of the myocardium. The slope of the stress-strain relationship has been called *stiffness constant of the myocardium*, i.e., the steeper the slope, the stiffer the muscle. Muscle stiffness is influenced by the composition of the myocardium, i.e., the ratio of the muscular tissue to the extracellular matrix.

which is dependent on intrinsic and extrinsic factors.[8-10] The intrinsic factors include left ventricular chamber size, left ventricular muscle mass, coronary perfusion, collagen tissue, and collagen orientation. The extrinsic factors include right/left ventricular interaction, pericardial pressure, intrathoracic pressure, and intravascular volume.

MYOCARDIAL PROPERTIES. Myocardial stiffness is represented by the passive elastic properties of the myocardium that are influenced by the cardiac interstitium and by the structural composition of the myocytes themselves.[20,21,24] Histomorphometric examinations have shown that disorientation of the collagen fibers in experimental heart failure contributes to the increase in myocardial stiffness. The slope of the diastolic stress-strain relationship has been termed the *constant of myocardial stiffness* (see Figs. 20–10 and 20–11). This constant is dependent on the properties, quantity, and orientation of the collagen fibers, as well as on myocardial perfusion and temperature.[8-10,20-25]

PERICARDIAL PROPERTIES. The pericardium forms a strong, purely elastic sac with extensions that enclose the origins of the ascending aorta, venae cavae, as well as the proximal and distal ends of the pulmonary artery and veins (see Chap. 64). The pericardium consists of two layers—the fibrous outer and the serous inner—with up to 30 ml of fluid normally. The pericardium acts as a barrier to reduce friction between the heart and the surrounding organs. The normal pericardium is relatively stiff,[26,27] and the relationship between intrapericardial volume and pressure is a steep, monoexponential curve. A small increase in intrapericardial volume leads to a rapid augmentation of intrapericardial pressure and, thereby, intracavitary diastolic pressures. Normal intrapericardial pressure is zero or negative. However, when the volume of the heart increases and exceeds the elastic limit of the pericardial sac, intracavitary pressures in all four chambers of the heart increase. An acute increase in the right- or left-sided volume affects the filling of the contralateral chamber by increasing its diastolic pressure (i.e., through ventricular interaction). The pericardium contributes to diastolic coupling of the atria and ventricles such that right and left ventricular filling pressures are closely correlated in the presence of an intact pericardium but are lower in the absence of the pericardium. Cardiac distensibility without the pericardium is influenced primarily by the properties of the myocardium. Chronic elevations of intrapericardial volume lead to an increase in the volume of the pericardial sac. If the intrapericardial volume increases slowly and persists over days or weeks, the pericardium slowly stretches and pericardial constraint may remain.[26,27] The volume of intrapericardial fluid may be as high as 1000 to 1200 ml in chronic pericardial effusion with little constraint on cardiac chambers.

Assessment

Several noninvasive techniques may be useful tools for the diagnosis of diastolic dysfunction, but cardiac catheterization with simultaneous pressure and volume measurements still represents the gold standard for quantitative studies.

LEFT VENTRICULAR RELAXATION. The most commonly used parameter to evaluate left ventricular relaxation is the time constant of isovolumic pressure decay (τ, expressed in milliseconds), which has been shown to be exponential under most circumstances but may deviate from a true monoexponential decay in the presence of aortic regurgitation or myocardial ischemia. Originally, a logarithmic pressure-time relation was used with the assumption that the asymptote of the pressure decline is zero. However, recently it has been shown that, in the transiently nonfilling ventricle, left ventricular pressure declines to negative values. Thus, a nonzero asymptote was added to the monoexponential model or a two-sequential monoexponential, polynomial or logistic model has been proposed[18]:

$$P = Ae^{-\alpha t} + Pb$$

where P = pressure, A = pressure at peak negative dP/dt, e = base of natural logarithm, α = slope of pressure time relationship, t = time, and Pb = pressure asymptote.

The time constant τ is calculated as

$$\tau = -1/\alpha$$

In normal subjects, τ averages 48 milliseconds, with a range from 40 to 60 milliseconds.[8-10] Relaxation is defined as being complete at 3.5 times the time constant τ after aortic valve closure.[18]

DIASTOLIC FILLING. The left ventricular chamber can be assessed angiographically from a frame-by-frame analysis, which may be accurate but has a lower temporal resolution (20 to 40 milliseconds) in comparison to Doppler echocardiography. Several indices of diastolic filling can be calculated, including the instantaneous filling rate, time to peak filling rate (PFR) (i.e., the time from end-systole to peak positive dV/dt), the fraction of filling that occurs during the rapid filling phase, as well as acceleration and deceleration of early diastolic filling. The most rapid rate of filling occurs during the first half of diastole and is termed the *early PFR* (normal value 300 ± 70 ml/sec). This index and the ratio of early to late diastolic filling (PFR1/PFR2 or E/A ratio) are the most commonly used parameters to describe left ventricular filling. Filling parameters calculated using a conductance catheter may be more useful than angiographic filling parameters due to their higher temporal resolution.

PASSIVE ELASTIC PROPERTIES. Calculation of *left ventricular chamber stiffness* is carried out by plotting left ventricular diastolic filling pressure against left ventricular diastolic volume from the minimal diastolic pressure to the end-diastolic pressure (see Figs. 20-10 and 20-11).

The most commonly used equation for assessing chamber stiffness is

$$P = \alpha e^{\beta V} + C$$

where P = pressure, α = intercept, e = base of the natural logarithm, β = slope of the pressure-volume relationship (chamber stiffness constant), V = volume, and C = pressure asymptote. A nonlinear curve-fitting procedure is employed. Normal values for the chamber stiffness constant average 0.05 ml^{-1}, and they range between 0.01 and 0.09 ml^{-1}.[8-10,12,19]

Left ventricular myocardial stiffness is calculated by plotting instantaneous left ventricular wall stress against left ventricular midwall strain from the lowest diastolic to end-diastolic pressure or from the end of the rapid filling phase to the peak of the a wave (see Fig. 20–11). The calculation of stress involves a geometric model of the left ventricle, whereas the calculation of strain requires some assumption of the unstressed left ventricular volume. The most commonly used equation for assessing myocardial stiffness is

$$S = \alpha e^{\beta V} + C$$

where S = wall stress, α = intercept, e = base of the natural logarithm, β = slope of the stress-strain relationship (muscle stiffness constant), V = strain, and C = stress asymptote. Again, a nonlinear curve-fitting procedure is employed. *Muscle stiffness* is the slope of the myocardial stress-strain relation. Average normal values for the muscle stiffness constant are 12, ranging between 5 and 20.

Imaging Techniques for the Assessment of Diastolic Function

Although the intraventricular pressure and angiographic volume measurements remain the gold standard, a number of noninvasive techniques have been used for the clinical assessment of diastolic function in patients with coronary, valvular, or myocardial heart disease.

DOPPLER ECHOCARDIOGRAPHY (Table 20–5). This technique (see Chap. 11) has emerged as an important clinical tool that provides reliable and useful data on diastolic function. Three different approaches are used routinely in the assessment of diastolic function: measurement of transmitral and pulmonary venous flow as well as intraventricular flow patterns (Doppler-flow propagation) (see Fig. 20–9).[28-31]

The *transmitral velocity pattern* remains the starting point of echocardiographic assessment of left ventricular diastolic function, since it is easy to acquire and can rapidly categorize patients with normal or abnormal diastolic function by E/A ratio (early to late filling velocity). In healthy young individuals, most diastolic filling occurs in early diastole so that the E/A ratio exceeds 1.0.[4] When relaxation is impaired, early diastolic filling decreases progressively and a vigorous compensatory atrial contraction ("atrial kick") occurs. This results in a reversed E/A ratio (E/A < 1 = *delayed relaxation pattern*), increased deceleration time, and increased isovolumic relaxation time (IVRT).[8-10] With further disease progression, left ventricular compliance becomes reduced and filling pressures begin to increase, leading to compensatory augmentation of left atrial pressure with increase in early filling despite impaired relaxation, so that the filling pattern becomes relatively normal (*pseudonormalization pattern* = E/A ratio > 1). This pattern, however, represents abnormalities of both relaxation and compliance and is distinguished from normal filling by a shortened early deceleration time. Finally, in patients with severe decrease in left ventricular compliance, left atrial pressure is markedly elevated and drives vigorous early diastolic filling despite impaired relax-

TABLE 20–5 Normal Values of Parameters of Left Ventricular Diastolic Filling Measured by Doppler Echocardiography

Parameters	Adults <41 yr	Adults >55 yr
Peak mitral flow velocity (E) (cm/sec)	76 ± 13	63 ± 11
Peak mitral filling rate (A) (cm/sec)	38 ± 8	52 ± 9
Mitral E/A	2.1 ± 0.6	1.3 ± 0.3
Mitral E deceleration time	184 ± 24	—
Mitral E deceleration rate (m/sec²)	5.6 ± 2.7	—
Isovolumetric relaxation time (msec)	74 ± 26	—
Peak pulmonary venous AR wave (cm/sec)	18 ± 3	25 ± 5
Peak pulmonary venous S wave (cm/sec)	41 ± 10	60 ± 10
Peak pulmonary venous D wave (cm/sec)	53 ± 10	38 ± 10

E/A = E wave/A wave ratio.

Data from Little WC. Downes TR: Clinical evaluation of left ventricular diastolic performance. Prog Cardiovasc Dis 32:273, 1990; and Rakowski H, et al: Canadian consensus recommendations for the measurements and reporting of diastolic dysfunction by echocardiography. J Am Soc Echocardiogr 9:745, 754, 1996.

TABLE 20–6 Left Atrial and Ventricular Function Influences on the Pulmonary Venous Flow Velocity Profile

Pulmonary Venous Wave	Left Atrial Function	LV Function
First systolic wave	Atrial relaxation	
Second systolic wave	Reservoir function Atrial compliance	LV contraction RV contraction
Early diastolic wave	Conduit function	Ventricular relaxation Ventricular chamber stiffness
Atrial reversal wave	Booster pump function Atrial compliance	Ventricular chamber stiffness

LV = left ventricular; RV = right ventricular.
Adapted from Tabata T, Thomas JD, Klein AL: Pulmonary venous flow by Doppler echocardiography: Revisited 12 years later. J Am Coll Cardiol 41:1243-1250, 2003.

ation. This *restrictive filling pattern* (E/A >> 1) is consistent with an abnormal rise in left ventricular diastolic pressure and an abrupt deceleration of flow with little additional filling during mid-diastole and atrial contraction. In extreme cases the dP/dT overshoots left atrial pressure so that mitral regurgitation in mid-diastole may occur.

The *IVRT* represents the time interval from closure of the aortic to opening of the mitral valve (see Fig. 20–2). The IVRT (normal range, 60 to 90 milliseconds) reflects the rate of myocardial relaxation but is dependent on afterload and heart rate.[8-10] It is probably the most sensitive Doppler index to detect impaired relaxation because it is the first to become abnormal. The deceleration time (see Fig. 20–9), which is affected by ventricular stiffness and atrial and ventricular pressure, can be used to derive the rapid filling rate. The normal value of this parameter is 193 ± 23 milliseconds; when prolonged, this index permits distinction between a normal and pseudonormal E/A ratio.[28]

Analysis of the *pulmonary venous filling patterns* (Table 20–6) provides a second window into left ventricular diastolic function.[29,30] The S wave, occurring during systole, depends on atrial relaxation and mitral annular motion. The D wave occurring during diastole reflects left ventricular filling, and the A wave, which is opposite to the other waves and occurs during atrial contraction, reflects left ventricular compliance. One indication for examining the pulmonary venous flow pattern is to distinguish the truly normal filling pattern from pseudonormalization. The main difference between these is the forward A wave of the transmitral flow and the reversed A wave in the pulmonary veins (see Fig. 20–9). In the presence of pseudonormalization, the atrium contracts against an increased afterload due to an elevated diastolic filling pressure or a stiff left ventricle. Accordingly, blood is preferentially ejected into the pulmonary veins, resulting in a high and prolonged pulmonary venous A wave.

Color M-mode Doppler echocardiography is a useful technique for examining the dynamics of blood flow across the mitral valve.[31] The velocity of inflow is enhanced with rapid relaxation and left ventricular suction. Clinical and experimental studies have demonstrated that the inverse correlation to τ (the time constant of relaxation [see earlier]) is relatively independent of left atrial pressure. Furthermore, combined evaluation of flow propagation velocity and early diastolic annular velocity can be used for estimation of filling pressure.[32] In normal persons the mitral annular motion is almost a mirror image of the transmitral flow pattern, but in patients with a pseudonormal or restrictive filling pattern, annular motion is abnormally low, implying that it is relatively independent of preload.[33-36]

Doppler tissue imaging (see Chap. 11) yields information on intramyocardial velocity, providing a unique insight into left ventricular mechanics during isovolumic contraction and relaxation (see Fig. 20–9).[9,37,38] It has been shown that relaxation velocities in the myocardium are inversely correlated with τ, so that calculation of the time constant of relaxation may be possible. Furthermore, this preload-independent peak negative myocardial velocity gradient may be used as a noninvasive index of left ventricular diastolic function.

Through the integrated use of Doppler echocardiography and Doppler tissue imaging, it is possible to obtain a fairly precise picture of left ventricular systolic and diastolic function. However, atrial fibrillation or frequent ectopic beats introduce major limitations of these techniques.

MAGNETIC RESONANCE IMAGING (see Chap. 14). This technique has been shown to be of considerable use in the morphological and functional assessment of the heart. Additional information may be gained from newer techniques such as magnetic resonance (MR) myocardial tagging, which allows the labeling of specific myocardial regions (Fig. 20–12).[39-43] From these tags the rotational and translational motion of the left ventricle can be determined; it is characterized by a systolic twisting motion with a clockwise rotation at the base and a counterclockwise rotation at the apex during systole. This motion can best be described by the wringing out of a wet towel. The untwisting motion occurs very early in diastole and is directly related to myocardial relaxation. Untwisting may be used as a measure of the rate and completeness of relaxation and may serve as an estimate of early diastolic filling. In the normal left ventricle, systolic rotation commences during isovolumic contraction (see Fig. 20–12) and continues during systolic ejection after the aortic valve has opened. Diastolic back rotation starts at end-systole and continues during isovolumic relaxation, whereas diastolic lengthening begins with mitral valve opening and ends with the next end-diastole.

Thus, the normal left ventricle performs a rectangular twisting-shortening (i.e., systole) and untwisting-lengthening (i.e., diastole) loop that occurs in opposite directions at the apex and base (Fig. 20–13) and is determined by the orientation of the muscle fibers within the myocardium. The relationship between myocardial rotation or twisting and changes in chamber size provide a unique insight into left ventricular systolic and diastolic function and their interaction.

A loss of myocardial tissue, as in myocardial infarction, or the occurrence of left ventricular asynchrony, as occurs in left bundle branch block, leads to a loss of the normal rotation-relaxation pattern that is associated with an increase in myocardial energy requirements. The normal systolic wringing motion allows the heart to work economically at a low-energy threshold because the wringing motion requires less energy than the "squeezing" motion. The traditional physiological concept of an isovolumic contraction and relaxation period has to be revised because the concept of an isometrically contracting or isometrically relaxing muscle is no longer valid. The shortening of the muscle fibers within the left ventricular wall induces systolic rotation during isovolumic contraction and diastolic untwisting during isovolumic relaxation. Athletes (with physiological hypertrophy) have a normal rotation–diastolic relaxation pattern, whereas patients with aortic stenosis (with pathologic hypertrophy) show a delayed systolic rotation–diastolic relaxation pattern (Fig. 20–14).

RADIONUCLIDE ANGIOGRAPHY (see Chap. 13). This technique may be used to study the rapid filling phase of diastole, the duration of the isovolumic relaxation phase, the relative contribution of rapid filling to total diastolic filling, and

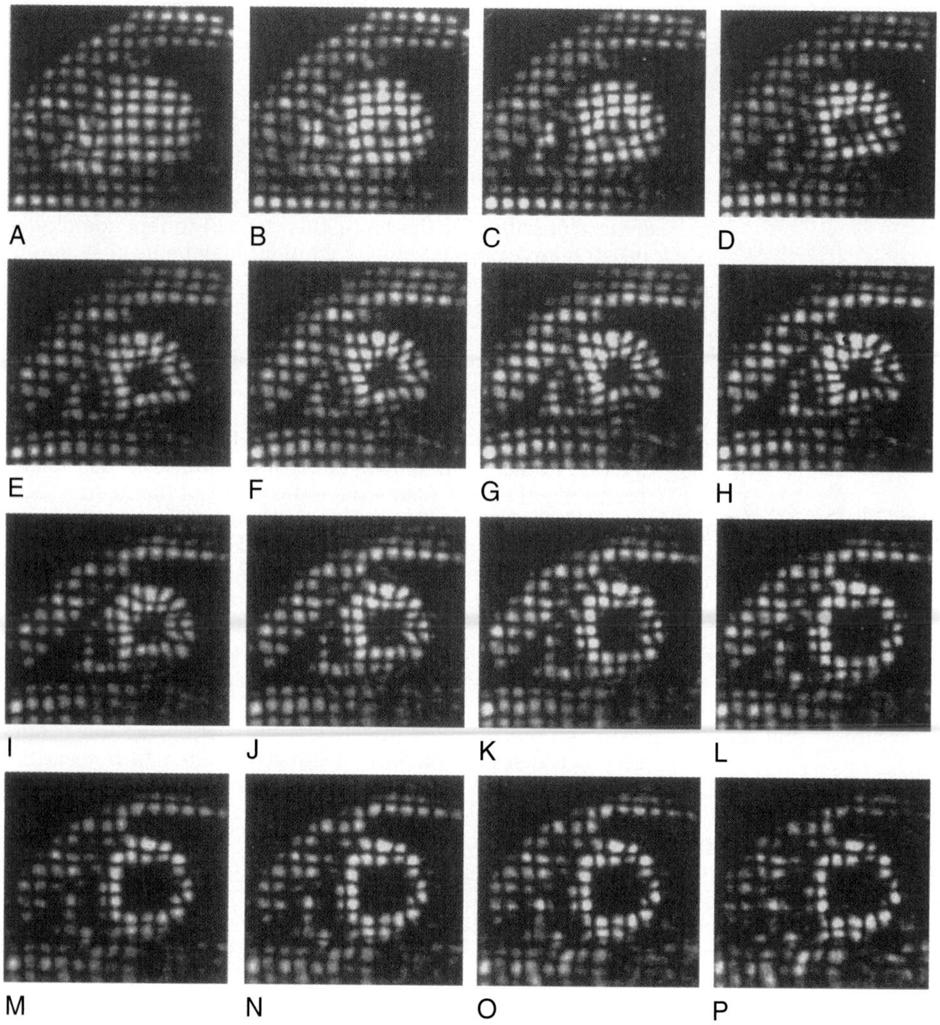

FIGURE 20–12 **A-P,** Series of MR images in a control patient with normal left ventricular function (temporal resolution 35 milliseconds). The MR images show horizontal and vertical lines (myocardial tags) that are superimposed on the conventional MR image. From the movement of the grid crossing points, the contraction and relaxation behavior of the left ventricle can be determined. During isovolumic contraction there is a counterclockwise rotation at the apex followed by systolic shortening. During isovolumic relaxation there is a clockwise rotation ("untwisting") followed by diastolic lengthening. This systolic-diastolic contraction-relaxation behavior is altered in patients with diastolic dysfunction with prolongation of diastolic back-rotation. (From Lazar-Mandinov L, Eberli F, Seiler C, Hess OM: Diastolic heart failure. Cardiovasc Res 45:813-825, 2000.)

the relation between regional nonuniformity of left ventricular function and global filling properties.[44] However, radionuclide angiography does *not* permit assessment of the left atrial–left ventricular pressure gradient or the simultaneous evaluation of changes in left ventricular pressure and volume during relaxation and filling. Therefore, complete clinical interpretation of "abnormal" left ventricular filling indices or changes in these indices after interventions is not possible. However, despite its inherent limitations, radionuclide evaluation of left ventricular filling may provide clinically useful insights.

COMPUTED TOMOGRAPHY (see Chap. 15). Computed tomography (CT) scanning of the heart permits rapid and accurate investigation of the heart and the adjacent vessels. Three techniques are currently used to evaluate cardiac anatomy and function.

Spiral CT scanning uses multiple rotations of the CT gantry while the table is moved continuously through the x-ray source. Computer reconstructions allow determination of multiple transaxial scans, 4 to 10 mm in thickness, of the entire heart and the adjacent vessel during a single breath-hold period. Usually, 80 to 100 ml of contrast medium is injected intravenously to study intravascular volumes and myocardial perfusion.

Ultrafast electron-beam tomography uses an electron gun that produces a stream of electrons that are magnetically focused and directed into different target rings, each of which emits two x-ray beams. This technology allows complete cardiac imaging in 50 milliseconds without the need for electrocardiographic gating or breath-holding. Contrast enhancement by intravenous injection of contrast medium permits accurate delineation of intracardiac chambers and vessels at end-diastole and end-systole. However, the infrastructure of this technique is expensive and radiation exposure is relatively high. Therefore, electron-beam tomography has not gained wide application.

Multislice CT scanning has gained a lot of interest in the recent years. This technique uses 8 to 64 image planes for assessing cardiac dimensions and function. Quantification of regional myocardial wall thickening and noninvasive representation of the coronary arteries have been done in normal patients and in patients with coronary artery disease.

Right Ventricular Function

PATHOPHYSIOLOGY. Right ventricular function plays a central role in the clinical outcome in a wide variety of cardiopulmonary disorders. The right ventricle is pivotal in many specific congenital cardiac malformations, and this importance continues into adulthood. Examples are the adaptation to chronic volume overloading from residual pulmonary regurgitation in repaired tetralogy of Fallot and to left-to-right shunting from an untreated atrial septal defect. In addition, acquired diseases such as primary and secondary pulmonary hypertension produce a remodeling of the right ventricle that resembles the remodeling of the left ventricle with pressure overload.

The right ventricle differs from the left ventricle regarding the type of work performed. Stroke volume is, of course, equal for the two ventricles, but the left ventricle must generate a high pressure to overcome gravitation effects and allow appropriate distribution of flow to multiple beds with differences in local resistance. The right ventricle, on the other hand, ejects into a more uniform and compliant pulmonary vascular bed and, therefore, has a thinner wall than the left ventricle to generate this lower pressure. The right ventricle also fills differently. It takes in systemic venous return at very low pressures, including the inspiratory creation of negative intrathoracic pressures that further sucks venous return into this chamber.

Although the prognostic significance of right ventricular adaptation to pressure or volume overload is widely recognized, the methods for studying this chamber have been slow to develop. A central problem has been in the imaging of this unusually shaped chamber that normally wraps around the interventricular septum, which functions primarily as a component of the left ventricle (Fig. 20–15). The thin-walled right ventricular free wall reduces the feasibility of studying wall thickening during systole and thinning during diastole, as is done in the assessment of left ventricular function.

ASSESSMENT OF RIGHT VENTRICULAR FUNCTION. Traditional 2D echocardiography allows assessment of right ventricular shape, size, and changes in size during the cardiac cycle. More recently, MR imaging has advanced the study of right ventricular function by providing images of this eccentric chamber and information on blood flow, regional function, and wall characteristics. A summary of the parameters assessed by MR imaging and ultrasonography is provided in Table 20–7. Contrast angiography, nuclear angiography, and the conductance catheter have their roles in special focused applications in assessing right ventricular function.

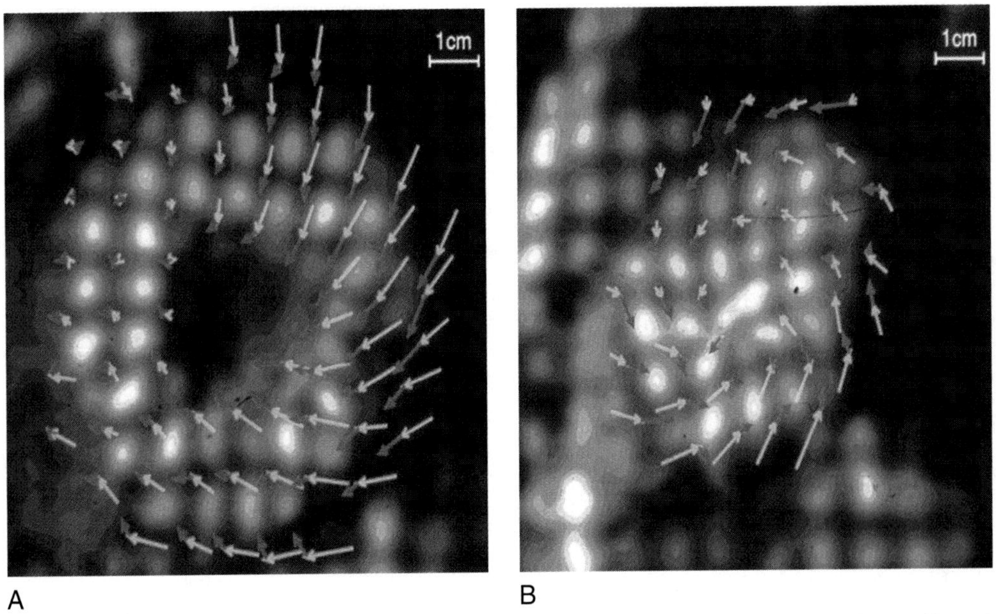

FIGURE 20–13 Ejection phase of the left ventricle at the apex **(A)** and at the base **(B)** of a healthy subject. End-systolic acquisitions are overlaid with corresponding local trajectories. There is a clockwise rotation at the base and counterclockwise rotation at the apex. This motion pattern has been described as a systolic wringing motion and provides a more sophisticated approach to quantifying regional left ventricular systolic function versus the traditional methods of endocardial shortening and simple wall thickening. (From Stuber M, Schedegger MB, Fischer SE, et al: Alterations in the local myocardial motion pattern in patients suffering from pressure overload due to aortic stenosis. Circulation 100:361-368, 1999.)

Function and Remodeling of the Right Ventricle: Four Paradigms

An understanding of right ventricular function is best illustrated by considering four examples of the response of this chamber to different pathophysiological conditions, as discussed in the following sections.

CHRONIC VOLUME OVERLOAD. Tricuspid regurgitation from damage to the valve apparatus by frequent endomyocardial biopsy in heart transplantation patients provides a model of the evolution of right ventricular volume overload.[45] Two-dimensional echocardiography (see Fig. 20–15) allows quantification of the progressive enlargement of the right ventricular end-diastolic cavity area with a change toward a more spherical chamber as reflected in an increased ratio of midchamber minor dimension to long axis of 0.5 to 0.7.

Atrial septal defect before and after closure provides another example of the chronic remodeling of the right ventricle and the extent of reversal following percutaneous closure.[46] Within 1 month of closure, the right ventricle undergoes important electrical-mechanical remodeling with a subsequent plateau at 6 months. The four-chamber 2D echocardiographic views of the right ventricular inflow and outflow tracts demonstrate that all patients have a decrease in chamber size, but 29 percent have some residual chamber enlargement at 1 year. Accompanying this structural remodeling is a significant reduction in QRS duration.[46]

Both right ventricular and left ventricular function, including chamber compliance, are major determinants of the degree and direction of shunting through the atrial septal defect and ultimately may influence right ventricular remodeling after closure.[47] Left-to-right shunting may increase in adulthood as the left ventricle becomes less compliant from acquired diseases. Shunting can, on the other hand, become bidirectional as the right ventricle loses its more compliant nature or develops frank failure.

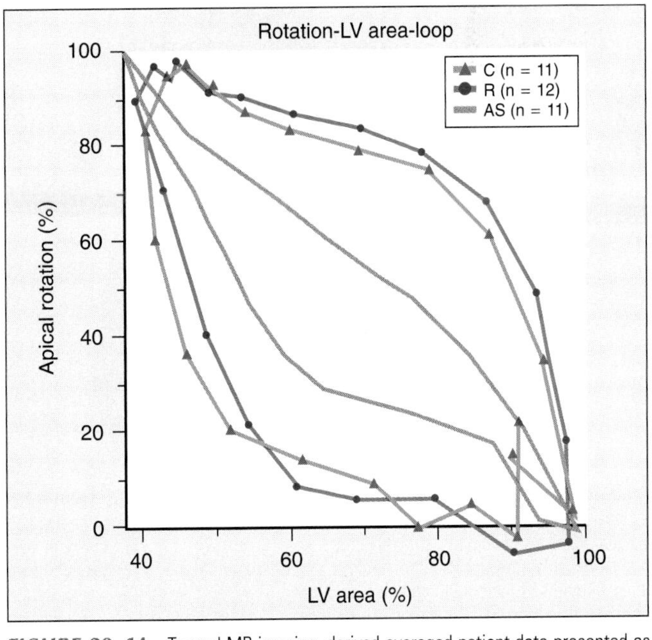

FIGURE 20–14 Tagged MR imaging–derived averaged patient data presented as rotation-area loop in controls (C; $n = 11$), professional rowers (R; $n = 12$), and patients with severe aortic stenosis (AS; $n = 11$). In the rowing athletes the rotation-area loop has a rectangular shape, as in controls, but in patients with severe hypertrophy (AS), delayed systolic rotation and relaxation are observed. This abnormal rotation-relaxation behavior in pathologic hypertrophy reflects changes in left ventricular (LV) afterload and myocardial hypertrophy. (From Stuber M, Schedegger MB, Fischer SE, et al: Alterations in the local myocardial motion pattern in patients suffering from pressure overload due to aortic stenosis. Circulation 100:361-368, 1999.)

CHRONIC PRESSURE OVERLOAD. The right ventricle undergoes extensive hypertrophy in primary pulmonary hypertension and leads to progressive right ventricular dilation, reduced systolic performance, secondary tricuspid regurgitation, and overt right ventricular failure with

TABLE 20–7 Echo/Doppler Assessment and MR Imaging of Right Ventricular Size, Shape, and Function

Parameter	Echo/Doppler	MR imaging
RV volume	Standard 2D views allow measurement of multiple dimensions (Fig. 20-15). The parasternal long-axis view shows the outflow tract diameter	Segmentation of individual slices provides chamber size. Adjacent areas are then summated to provide volume and shape measurements
Regional wall motion	Free RV wall and interventricular septum are imaged and paradoxical motion can easily be detected	Cine MR imaging provides contrast between the blood pool and the myocardial wall. RV wall motion is assessed using RVOT cines in the sagittal and short-axis cine images
RV mass	Approximated by wall thickness determinations along with chamber size measurements	Myocardium from the junction between the RV free wall and the interventricular septum can be traced on each slice from the base to the apex, including trabeculations. Myocardial volume computed from summated multiple slices is multiplied by 1.05 to give the mass in grams
RV wall composition	Not well studied in transthoracic images. Intracardiac ultrasound provides higher resolution data	MR imaging is potentially useful to distinguish fat from muscle
Regurgitant fraction	Doppler profiles provide semiquantitative approach	True regurgitant volumes can be measured from phase velocity maps in the main pulmonary artery and aortic root

RV = right ventricular; RVOT = RV outflow tract; 2D = two-dimensional.

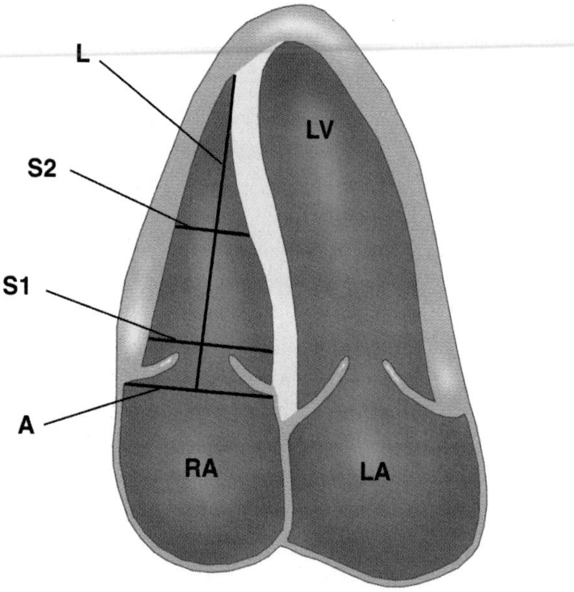

FIGURE 20–15 The right ventricle is schematically illustrated as seen in the echocardiographic apical four-chamber view. From this view right ventricular size can be quantified along its major axis (L) and two minor axes (S1 and S2) of the right ventricle. Tricuspid annular diameter (A) may also be measured. The important additional measurements of the outflow tract are not shown. The two-dimensional images of the right ventricle from echocardiography are suboptimal in assessing chamber volume and function and provide an impetus for three-dimensional techniques based on ultrasound or other modalities such as MR imaging and CT scanning. LV = left ventricle; RA = right atrium; LA = left atrium. (From Reynertson S, Kundur R, Mullen G, et al: Asymmetry of right ventricular enlargement in response to tricuspid regurgitation. Circulation 100:465, 1999.

peripheral edema and ascites (see Chap. 67).[48] Although regression of right ventricular hypertrophy has been described as a result of vasodilator therapy, the progressive nature of the primary disease process is unremitting. Direct (catheter-based) measurement of pressure and cardiac output is an important complement to noninvasive imaging.

A more reversible form of pressure overload hypertrophy of the right ventricle is seen in pulmonary hypertension secondary to chronic thromboembolism.[49] After surgical thromboembolectomy, 2D echocardiography quantified a significant reduction in end-diastolic (30 ± 7 to 21 ± 5 cm^2) and end-systolic (24 ± 6 to 14 ± 4 cm^2) cavity area in the four-chamber view.[50] Right ventricular fractional shortening increased and tricuspid regurgitation decreased. Furthermore, there was a resultant normalization of interventricular septal motion, improved diastolic filling, and rise in cardiac output.

Valvular pulmonic stenosis produces right ventricular hypertrophy that appears reversible after successful balloon valvuloplasty.[47] The secondary relief of a subvalvular pressure gradient in the right ventricular outflow tract also occurs, presumably from regression of infundibular hypertrophy.[51]

ACUTE ISCHEMIC DYSFUNCTION (see Chap. 46). The acute deterioration in right ventricular function during acute myocardial infarction has been studied by 2D echocardiography and invasively determined pressures and cardiac output.[52,53] Motion of the right ventricular free wall may be dramatically decreased with chamber dilation and an acute elevation of right-sided filling pressures resulting from increased chamber stiffness, mediated in part by an acute pericardial restraining influence. Enlargement of the right ventricular cavity may develop rapidly with a reversal of septal curvature and paradoxical movement during systole. The derangement of right ventricular function, if severe enough, can result in right-sided heart failure, clear lung fields, and a low cardiac output despite nearly normal left ventricular function.

CHRONIC VENTRICULAR DYSFUNCTION. Preliminary studies have shown that resynchronization with right ventricular pacing improves function in patients with chronic right ventricular dysfunction, as reflected in right ventricular maximum positive dP/dt and cardiac output.[1,54]

THE LEFT ATRIUM

In the last decade Doppler echocardiography has provided a large experience in functional assessment of the left atrium while MR imaging and CT scanning now provide in-depth 3D anatomical assessment of this chamber. A variety of new interventional techniques require more intensive study of the left atrium. For example, catheter-based treatment of atrial fibrillation, left atrial appendage occlusion devices, atrial septal closure devices, and a variety of emerging mitral valve interventions have stimulated an interest in the left atrium, whereas there also has been a new appreciation of the importance of left atrial size and function in a broad spectrum of cardiac disease states.[55-57]

LEFT ATRIAL APPENDAGE. Pulsed-Doppler interrogation of left atrial appendage flow is a major component of the functional assessment of this chamber. The function of the left atrial appendage is determined by factors well studied in the past for left ventricular function.[58-61] Removal of the appendage as well as insertion of devices into the left atrial appendage to block thrombus formation may make the remaining left atrial chamber less compliant.[60]

LEFT ATRIAL CHAMBER SIZE AND SHAPE. The relations between body size, gender, age, and left atrial volume have been detailed in a reference population using ultrasound techniques.[62] The normal left atrial volume is 42 ± 12 ml. The 3D reconstruction of the left atrium has been developed with ultrasound.[63] CT scanning and MR imaging have been applied to both left atrial size and shape. Images of the left atrium and distal pulmonary veins using multidetector helical CT with multidimensional reconstruction provide accurate, detailed information of these structures.[64]

LEFT ATRIAL FUNCTION. Conceptually, left atrial function can be described as having three components: (1) a distensible reservoir during ventricular systole as blood enters this chamber from the pulmonary veins, while the mitral valve is closed; (2) a passive conduit of blood in early ventricular diastole after mitral valve opening; and (3) a booster pump function occurring during late ventricular diastole and involving atrial contraction.

To understand its function, the volume of the left atrium is determined at three points in time during the cardiac cycle. Immediately before mitral valve opening the left atrium is at its maximal volume, reflecting its reservoir function. With mitral valve opening, the left atrium decompresses rapidly, in part due to a suction effect from the normal left ventricle during early diastole. The second time point is reached immediately before atrial systole, when the left atrial pre-A volume is determined. With subsequent atrial contraction there is further emptying of the left atrium until ventricular end-diastole is reached, and this minimum left atrial volume is measured immediately after atrial contraction. Hoit and Gabel have shown that left atrial conduit function represented 35 percent of all flow through the chamber.[65] The relative roles of active atrial contraction versus atrial conduit function have been clarified in animal studies demonstrating that the conduit function can compensate for atrial myocardial failure as long as left ventricular function is normal.

Left atrial function studied by transmitral flow as well as pulmonary venous flow patterns and left atrial appendage emptying flow are Doppler-based techniques that are widely available and can be applied clinically. Multiple factors influence the triphasic and quadriphasic pattern of pulmonary venous flow pattern (see Table 20-6).[29] The systolic or booster pump function of the left atrium can be characterized in many ways that are parallel to left ventricular systolic function assessment.[66-70]

CLINICAL APPLICATIONS OF ASSESSMENTS OF THE LEFT ATRIUM. Doppler-based techniques have been applied to understand better the timing and extent of left atrial myocardial dysfunction, or stunning, after conversion to sinus rhythm from atrial fibrillation[71] and the return of left atrial contractile function following the Maze operation.[72] Pharmacological modification of left ventricular diastolic properties that enhance chamber distensibility can augment the atrial contribution to left ventricular filling.[73] A reduction in left atrial size and an increase in left atrial-mediated passive filling of the left ventricle have been observed after modification of left ventricular systolic and diastolic properties following alcohol septal ablation in obstructive hypertrophic cardiomyopathy.[74]

Exercise (see Chap. 17)

Physical exercise is associated with increases in heart rate, venous return, cardiac output, stroke volume, and systolic pressure. Arterial diastolic pressure remains relatively unchanged or decreases slightly and, thus, pulse pressure increases during exercise, while the ejection period shortens. Hemodynamic adaptation depends largely on the type of exercise, i.e., dynamic or isometric exercise, as well as the severity of exercise and the mass of exercising muscles. Exercise capacity is determined by many factors, such as body position; gender; age; body mass; level of exercise training; and environmental factors, such as temperature, humidity, and ambient oxygen concentration. Adaptation of cardiac function is largely dependent on the level of exercise and the response of the cardiovascular system as well as the magnitude of adrenergic stimulation. For instance, dynamic exercise (e.g., running, swimming, cycling) is associated with a large increase in cardiac output achieved mainly by increases in heart rate and in stroke volume,[75] whereas isometric exercise (e.g., handgrip, weight lifting, bodybuilding) is associated with a moderate increase in cardiac output but a large increase in arterial pressure consequent to enhanced sympathetic stimulation (*pressure loading*). In daily living, both forms of exercise are frequently used.

Definition of Abnormal Cardiac Function During Exercise

Most noninvasive exercise studies are carried out in the upright position (treadmill, bicycle ergometer), but invasive (catheter-based) studies are usually performed in the supine position. Since venous return is increased in the supine position, diastolic filling pressure, stroke volume, and cardiac output in the resting state are higher in the supine than in the upright position. Assessment of cardiac function during dynamic or isometric exercise has been carried out by hemodynamic monitoring of the right heart using Swan-Ganz catheters or with fluid-filled catheters in the left heart and left ventricular angiography. However, most data on exercise have been obtained from right heart catheterization in the supine position. However, higher cardiac outputs are reached during maximal exercise in the erect position, but due to technical limitations of most measuring techniques, submaximal exercise has been preferred, to allow a short steady state for measuring hemodynamic data. Increasingly, noninvasive techniques, including 2D echocardiography, radionuclide angiography, and MR imaging, have been employed to study the response to exercise.

Abnormal cardiac function during *maximal* exercise has been based on pulmonary capillary wedge pressure or LVEDP exceeding 20 mm Hg, the cardiac output failing to reach 15 liters per minute, and the ejection fraction failing to rise.

SYSTOLIC FUNCTION. Hemodynamic adaptation of the ventricles to exercise is regulated by the increase in sympathetic activity and the resultant increases in heart rate and cardiac contractility. In the normal heart, when exercise is carried out in the supine position, both left and right ventricular end-diastolic volumes increase slightly, whereas end-systolic volumes decrease significantly. Both stroke volume and systolic ejection fraction increase and contribute to the augmentation of cardiac output. Since end-diastolic volume exhibits little change during exercise, the Frank- Starling mechanism does not play a major role in cardiac adaptation during exercise in the healthy heart. Increases in the ventricular filling pressures during exercise and volume occur only when the increase in the heart rate rise during exercise is blunted, as occurs in patients with atrioventricular block or in those treated with a beta-adrenergic blocker.

The increase in cardiac output during mild exercise is achieved by an augmentation of both stroke volume and heart rate, whereas the further increases in output during severe exercise result primarily from an increase in heart rate. Normal aging is associated with a decline in cardiac output that is mainly due to the reduction in the maximal heart rate.

DIASTOLIC FUNCTION. Most studies of the effects of exercise have focused on systolic function; less is known about diastolic function of the normal heart during exercise. There is general agreement that left ventricular end-systolic volume is smaller during exercise due to the enhanced contractile state. At the same time, the rate of relaxation is increased, which allows more rapid filling. These two mechanisms lead to an increase in elastic recoil that enhances ventricular filling at high heart rates when diastolic filling time is abbreviated.[76] These mechanisms maintain stroke volume and prevent undue elevation of ventricular diastolic pressures even at very high workloads and, thus, preload reserve is not needed in the normal heart to achieve maximal cardiac output.

In summary, left ventricular diastolic function during exercise is characterized by the following:

1. Enhanced elastic recoil with a small left ventricular end-systolic volume
2. Rapid left ventricular relaxation due to enhanced inotropic stimulation
3. Low early diastolic pressures (even negative pressures may occur) due to enhanced diastolic suction
4. Rapid diastolic filling that starts after mitral valve opening; one third of the stroke volume enters the left ventricle when its pressure is still falling

COUPLING OF CARDIAC CHAMBERS AND THE VASCULAR SYSTEM (Table 20–8)

The interplay between the left ventricle and the properties of the vascular bed is described by the term *ventriculoarterial coupling* and has been studied with a variety of tools such as Fourier analysis of arterial waveforms, ESPVRs, and calculations of power.[77] An additional form of analysis can be applied to the vascular systems themselves.[78] The computation of vascular resistance is commonly performed (see Chap. 17) and is clinically useful for a variety of purposes. More sophisticated measurements of vascular properties involve assessments of the pressure and vessel size, including the impact of different degrees of vascular tone. The measurement of pulse wave velocity provides insight into vascular properties, including the composition of the vessel wall and vascular tone and the relationships between wave velocity and distending pressure. With normal aging, arterial pulse pressure and pulse wave velocity rise while arterial compliance falls. Age-related differences in pulse wave velocity are differentially modified by vasodilators such as nitroprusside.

The arterial system has been traditionally modeled using a Windkessel model with the more recent addition of wave reflections into the conceptual framework. Total arterial compliance is calculated from the arterial diastolic pressure decay either measured directly or estimated from tonometry. Estimated arterial compliance, C, can be calculated by the formula

$$C = A_d/R(P_s - P_d)$$

where A_d = area under the diastolic pressure waveform computed from P_s (the maximum pressure after the dicrotic notch) to P_d (minimum pressure near end-diastole), and R = the systemic vascular resistance calculated from cardiac output and mean aortic pressure.

TABLE 20–8 Age-Related Differences in LV and Arterial Coupling in Patients with Dilated Cardiomyopathy

Parameters	Young Patients <35 yr	Intermediate-Aged Patients 35-50 yr	Older Patients >50 yr
Maximum + dP/dt (mm Hg/sec)	1011 ± 160	1170 ± 159	1147 ± 374
Stroke work (g-m/m²)	19 ± 10	20 ± 10	19 ± 10
Pulse pressure (mm Hg)	26 ± 8	30 ± 11	38 ± 10
Pulse wave velocity (m/sec)	4.7 ± 0.4	6.5 ± 0.9	7.9 ± 0.6
Systemic vascular resistance (dyn-sec · cm⁻⁵)	1872 ± 789	2373 ± 762	2440 ± 770
Arterial compliance (ml/mm Hg)	1.33 ± 0.63	0.72 ± 0.40	0.51 ± 0.17

LV = left ventricular.

Adapted from Carroll JD, Shroff S, Arand P, et al: Arterial mechanical properties in dilated cardiomyopathy. J Clin Invest 87:1002-1009, 1991.

NEUROHUMORAL ASSESSMENT OF CARDIAC FUNCTION (see Chap. 21)

The use of neurohumoral assays to complement and potentially replace direct assessment of cardiac function has emerged in the last decade.[79,80] This development follows our understanding of the neurohumoral response as an important part of the pathophysiology of cardiovascular dysfunction as well as a target of treatment. The activation of the neurohumoral system occurs in a variety of forms of heart failure including systolic and diastolic dysfunction but also in patients with valvular disease. Activation of the adrenergic and renin-angiotensin systems have been well characterized. Theoretically whenever a cardiac condition produces elevated pressures, activation of intramyocardial stretch receptors and other hemodynamic and mechanical perturbations may lead to a release of natriuretic peptides. The results of these assays can provide insights and direction for the clinician in a broad range of circumstances, including the differential diagnosis of dyspnea as being of cardiac or noncardiac origin, as an early warning sign of disease progression, as a correlate of functional class, as a surrogate of the magnitude of the cardiac function abnormality, and as an independent determinant of the patient's prognosis and response to therapy.[81,82]

The complex interplay between cardiac mechanical function, neurohumoral function, and modification in hemostatic control is also apparent in the left atrium. Left atrial mechanical function is specifically linked to the release of atrial natriuretic peptide release. This interplay is illustrated in patients converted from atrial fibrillation.[83] Left atrial enlargement is also an independent risk factor for the development of left atrial thrombi. The reduced velocity of blood motion within the fibrillating, dilated left atrium is suggested by the presence of "smoke" on transesophageal and intracardiac echocardiographic visualization of the left atrium.[84]

Abnormal hemodynamics may cause other biochemical effects. Recent attention has been given to understanding how von Willebrand factor circulating in the blood as a large protein is altered by cardiac conditions with pathologically high fluid shear stress such as aortic stenosis, ventricular septal defect, and patent ductus arteriosus.[85] Acquired defects occur as a consequence of damage to von Willebrand factor during passage through the stenotic orifice and then contribute to the known association of severe aortic stenosis and bleeding, especially from preexisting lesions such as gastrointestinal angiodysplasia. The correlation between the hemostatic defect and the hemodynamic severity of aortic stenosis is strong and may in the future help determine the timing of valve intervention.

These recent insights emphasize that cardiac function can be quantified from different perspectives. The biology of cardiac function is an area that will advance rapidly during the next decade.

REFERENCES

1. Carabello B: Evolution of the study of left ventricular function: Everything old is new again. Circulation 105:2701, 2002.
2. Abraham WT, Fisher WG, Smith AL, et al: Cardiac resynchronization in chronic heart failure. N Engl J Med 346:1845, 2002.
3. Delgado D, Rao V, Ross H, et al: Mechanical circulatory assistance: State of art. Circulation 106:2046, 2002.
4. Perin E, Geng Y, Willerson J: Adult stem cell therapy in perspective. Circulation 107:935, 2003.
5. Sabbah H: The cardiac support device and the Myosplint: Treating heart failure by targeting left ventricular size and shape. Ann Thorac Surg 75:S13, 2003.
6. Katz A: Ernest Henry Starling: His predecessors, and the "law of the heart." Circulation 106:2986, 2002.
7. Karunanithi M, Feneley M: Single-beat determination of preload recruitable stroke work relationship: Derivation and evaluation in conscious dogs. J Am Coll Cardiol 35:502, 2000.

Diastolic Function

8. Hess OM: Diastolic Function of the Left Ventricle. Stuttgart, Georg Thieme Verlag, 1982.
9. Zile M, Brutsaert D: New concepts in diastolic dysfunction and diastolic heart failure: I. Diagnosis, prognosis, and measurements of diastolic function. Circulation 105:1387, 2002.
10. Zile M, Brutsaert D: New concepts in diastolic dysfunction and diastolic heart failure: II. Causal mechanisms and treatment. Circulation 105:1503, 2002.
11. Bell SP, Nyland L, Tischler MD, et al: Alterations in the determinants of diastolic suction during pacing tachycardia. Circ Res 87:235, 2000.
12. Hess OM, Osakada G, Lavelle J, et al: Diastolic myocardial wall stiffness and ventricular relaxation during partial and complete coronary occlusion in the conscious dog. Circ Res 52:387, 1983.
13. Angeja B, Grossmann W: Evaluation and management of diastolic heart failure. Circulation 107:659, 2003.
14. Zile MR, Gaasch WH, Carroll JD, et al: Heart failure with a normal ejection fraction: Is measurement of diastolic function necessary to make the diagnosis of diastolic heart failure? Circulation 104:779-782, 2001.

15. Paulus WJ, for the European Study Group on Diastolic Heart Failure: How to diagnose diastolic heart failure. European Study Group on Diastolic Heart Failure. Eur Heart J 19:990-1003, 1998.
16. Kass DA: Assessment of diastolic dysfunction: Invasive modalities. Cardiol Clin 18:571-586, 2000.
17. Paulus WJ, Vantrimpont PJ, Rousseau MF: Diastolic function of nonfilling human left ventricle. J Am Coll Cardiol 20:1524, 1992.
18. Mandinov L, Eberli FR, Seiler C, Hess OM: Diastolic heart failure. Cardiovasc Res 45:813, 2000.
19. Carroll JD, Hess OM, Hirzel HO, Krayenbuehl HP: Exercise-induced ischemia: The influence of altered relaxation on early diastolic pressures. Circulation 67:521, 1983.
20. Nagel E, Hess OM: Ventrikelfunktion: Systolische und diastolische funktion. *In* Hess OM, Simon RWR (eds): Herzkatheter-Einsatz in Diagnostik und Therapie. Berlin, Springer Verlag 2000.
21. Neumann T, Vollmer A, Schaffner T, et al: Diastolic dysfunction and collagen structure in canine pacing-induced heart failure. J Am Coll Cardiol 31:179, 1999.
22. Spinale FG, Coker ML, Thomas CV, et al: Time-dependent changes in matrix metalloproteinase activity and expression during the progression of congestive heart failure: Relation to ventricular and myocyte function. Circ Res 82:482, 1998.
23. Javier Díez J, Querejeta R, López B, et al: Losartan-dependent regression of myocardial fibrosis is associated with reduction of left ventricular chamber stiffness in hypertensive patients. Circulation 105:2512, 2002.
24. Hein S, Gaasch W, Schaper J: Giant molecule titin and myocardial stiffness. Circulation 106:1303, 2002.
25. Weber KT: Targeting pathological remodeling: Concepts of cardioprotection and reparation. Circulation 102:1342, 2000.
26. Hess OM, Bhargava V, Ross J, Shabetai R: The role of the pericardium in interactions between the cardiac chambers. Am Heart J 106:1377, 1983.
27. Hoit B: Management of effusive and constrictive pericardial heart disease. Circulation 105:2939, 2002.
28. Rakowski H, Appleton C, Chan KL, et al: Canadian consensus recommendations for the measurement and reporting of diastolic dysfunction by echocardiography. The Investigators of Consensus on Diastolic Dysfunction by Echocardiography. J Am Soc Echocardiogr 9:736, 1999.
29. Tabata T, Thomas JD, Klein AL: Pulmonary venous flow by Doppler echocardiography: Revisited 12 years later. J Am Coll Cardiol 41:1243, 2003.
30. Jensen JL, Williams FE, Beilby BJ, et al: Feasibility of obtaining pulmonary venous flow velocity in cardiac patients using transthoracic pulsed wave Doppler technique. J Am Soc Echocardiogr 10:60, 1997.
31. Takatsuji H, Mikami T, Urasawa K, et al: A new approach for evaluation of left ventricular diastolic function: Spatial and temporal analysis of left ventricular filling flow propagation by color M-mode Doppler echocardiography [see comments]. J Am Coll Cardiol 27:365, 1996.
32. Nagueh SF, Lakkis NM, Middleton KJ, et al: Doppler estimation of left ventricular filling pressure in patients with hypertrophic cardiomyopathy. Circulation 99:254, 1999.
33. Sohn DW, Chai IH, Lee DJ, et al: Assessment of mitral annulus velocity by Doppler tissue imaging in the evaluation of left ventricular diastolic function. J Am Coll Cardiol 30:474, 1997.
34. Lindstrom L, Wranne B: Pulsed tissue Doppler evaluation of mitral annulus motion: A new window to assessment of diastolic function. Clin Physiol 19:1, 1999.
35. Sohn DW, Kim YJ, Kim HC, et al: Evaluation of left ventricular diastolic function when mitral E and A waves are completely fused: role of assessing mitral annulus velocity. J Am Soc Echocardiogr 12:203, 1999.
36. Blomstrand P, Kongstad O, Broqvist M, et al: Assessment of left ventricular diastolic function from mitral annulus motion: A comparison with pulsed Doppler measurements in patients with heart failure. Clin Physiol 16:483, 1996.
37. Oki T, Tabata T, Yamada H, et al: Clinical application of pulsed Doppler tissue imaging for assessing abnormal left ventricular relaxation .Am J Cardiol 79:921, 1997.
38. Shimizu Y, Uematsu M, Shimizu H, et al: Peak negative myocardial velocity gradient in early diastole as a noninvasive indicator of left ventricular diastolic function: Comparison with transmitral flow velocity indices. J Am Coll Cardiol 32:1418, 1998.
39. Kudelka AM, Turner DA, Liebson PR, et al: Comparison of cine magnetic resonance imaging and Doppler echocardiography for evaluation of left ventricular diastolic function. Am J Cardiol 80:384, 1997.
40. Stuber M, Schedegger MB, Fischer SE, et al: Alterations in the local myocardial motion pattern in patients suffering from pressure overload due to aortic stenosis. Circulation 100:361, 1999.
41. Maier SE, Fischer SE, McKinnon GC, et al: Evaluation of left ventricular segmental wall motion in hypertrophic cardiomyopathy with myocardial tagging. Circulation 86:1919, 1992.
42. Fischer SE, McKinnon GC, Maier SE, Boesiger P: Improved myocardial tagging contrast. Magn Reson Med 31:401, 1994.
43. Briguori C, Betocchi S, Losi MA, et al: Noninvasive evaluation of left ventricular diastolic function in hypertrophic cardiomyopathy. Am J Cardiol 81:180, 1998.
44. Bonow RO: Radionuclide angiographic evaluation of left ventricular diastolic function. Circulation 84:I208, 1991.

Right Ventricular Function

45. Reynertson S, Kundur R, Mullen G, et al: Asymmetry of right ventricular enlargement in response to tricuspid regurgitation. Circulation 100:465, 1999.
46. Veldtman G, Razack V, Siu S, et al: Right ventricular form and function after percutaneous atrial septal defect device closure. J Am Coll Cardiol 37:2108, 2001.
47. Brickner M, Hillis L, Lang R: Congenital heart disease in adults: I. N Engl J Med 342:256, 2000.
48. Rubin L: Primary pulmonary hypertension. N Engl J Med 336:111, 1997.
49. Fedullo P, Auger W, Kerr K, Rubin L: Chronic thromboembolic pulmonary hypertension. N Engl J Med 345:1465, 2001.
50. Menzel T, Wagner S, Kramm T, et al: Pathophysiology of impaired right and left ventricular function in chronic embolic pulmonary hypertension: Changes after pulmonary thromboendarterectomy. Chest 118:897, 2000.
51. Chen C, Cheng T, Huang T, et al: Percutaneous balloon valvuloplasty for pulmonic stenosis in adolescents and adults. N Engl J Med 335:21, 1996.
52. Goldstein J: Pathophysiology and management of right heart ischemia. J Am Coll Cardiol 40:841, 2002.
53. Bowers T, O'Neill W, Pica M, Goldstein J: Patterns of coronary compromise resulting in acute right ventricular ischemic dysfunction. Circulation 106:1104, 2002.
54. Dubin A, Feinstein J, Reddy M, et al: Electrical resynchronization: A novel therapy for the failing right ventricle. Circulation 107:2287, 2003.
55. Grigioni F, Avierinos JF, Ling LH, et al: Atrial fibrillation complicating the course of degenerative mitral regurgitation. J Am Coll Cardiol 40:84-92, 2002.
56. Rossi A, Cicoira M, Zanolla L, et al: Determinants and prognostic value of left atrial volume in patients with dilated cardiomyopathy. J Am Coll Cardiol 40:142, 2002.
57. Moller J, Hillis GS, Oh JK, et al: Left atrial volume: A powerful predictor of survival after acute myocardial infarction. Circulation 107:2207, 2003.
58. Hoit BD, Shao Y, Gabel M: Influence of acutely altered loading conditions on left atrial appendage flow velocities. J Am Coll Cardiol 24:1117, 1994.
59. Hondo T, Okamoto M, Yamane T, et al: The role of the left atrial appendage: A volume loading study in open-chest dogs. Jpn Heart J 36:225, 1995.
60. Hoit BD, Shao Y, Tsai LM, et al: Altered left atrial compliance after atrial appendectomy: Influence on left atrial and ventricular filling. Circ Res 72:167, 1993.
61. Agmon Y, Khanderia K, Gentile F, Seward JB: Echocardiographic assessment of the left atrial appendage. J Am Coll Cardiol 34:1867, 1999.
62. Pritchett AM, Jacobsen SJ, Mahoney DW, et al: Left atrial volume as an index of left atrial size: A population-based study. J Am Coll Cardiol 41:1036, 2003.
63. Szili-Torok T, Kimman GJ, Scholten HF, et al: Interatrial septum pacing guided by three-dimensional intracardiac echocardiography. J Am Coll Cardiol 40:2139, 2002.
64. Schwartzman D, Lacomis J, Wigginton W: Characterization of left atrium and distal pulmonary vein morphology using multidimensional computed tomography. J Am Coll Cardiol 41:1349, 2003.
65. Hoit BD, Gabel M: Influence of left ventricular dysfunction on the role of atrial contraction: An echocardiographic-hemodynamic study in dogs. J Am Coll Cardiol 36:1713, 2000.
66. Manning WJ, Silverman DI, Katz SE, Douglas PS: Atrial ejection force: A noninvasive assessment of atrial systolic function. J Am Coll Cardiol 22:221, 1993.
67. Alexander J Jr, Sunagawa K, Chang N, Sagawa K: Instantaneous pressure-volume relation of the ejecting canine left atrium. Circ Res 61:209 , 1987.
68. Hoit BD, Shao Y, Gabel M, Walsh RA: In vivo assessment of left atrial contractile performance in normal and pathological conditions using a time-varying elastance model. Circulation 89:1829, 1994.
69. Stefanadis C, Dernellis J, Tsiamis E, Toutouza P: Effects of pacing-induced and balloon coronary occlusion ischemia on left atrial function in patients with coronary artery disease. J Am Coll Cardiol 33:687, 1999.
70. Nakatani S, Garcia MJ, Firstenberg MS, et al: Noninvasive assessment of left atrial maximum dP/dt by a combination of transmitral and pulmonary venous flow. J Am Coll Cardiol 34:795, 1999.
71. Sparks P, Jayaprakash S, Mond Hg, et al: Left atrial mechanical function after brief duration atrial fibrillation. J Am Coll Cardiol 33:342, 1999.
72. Yuda S, Nakatani S, Kosakai Y, et al: Long-term follow-up of atrial contraction after the Maze procedure in patients with mitral valve disease. J Am Coll Cardiol 37:1622, 2001.
73. Sakai H, Kunichika H, Murata K, et al: Improvement of afterload mismatch of left atrial booster pump function with positive inotropic agent. J Am Coll Cardiol 37:270, 2001.
74. Nagueh S, Lakkis NM, Middleton KJ, et al: Changes in left ventricular filling and left atrial function six months after nonsurgical septal reduction therapy for hypertrophic obstructive cardiomyopathy. J Am Coll Cardiol 34:1123, 1999.

Exercise

75. Weber KT, Janicki JS, McElroy PA, Reddy HK: Concepts and applications of cardiopulmonary exercise testing. Chest 93:843, 1988.
76. Nonogi H, Hess OM, Ritter M, Krayenbuehl HP: Diastolic properties of the normal left ventricle during supine exercise. Br Heart J 60:30-38, 1988.
77. Kawaguchi M, Hay I, Fetics B, Kass D: Combined ventricular systolic and arterial stiffening with heart failure and preserved ejection fraction: Implications for systolic and diastolic reserve. Circulation 107:714, 2003.
78. Nichols WW, O'Rourke W: McDonald's Blood Flow in Arteries. 4th ed. London, Arnold, 1998.
79. Francis GS, Cohn JN, Johnson G, et al. Plasma norepinephrine, plasma renin activity, and congestive heart failure: Relations to survival and the effects of therapy in V-HeFT II. Circulation 87:V140, 1993.
80. Lubien E, DeMaria A, Krishnaswamy P, et al: Utility of B-natriuretic peptide in detecting diastolic dysfunction: Comparison with Doppler velocity recordings. Circulation 105:595, 2002.
81. de Lemos JA, McGuire DK, Drazner MH: B-type natriuretic peptide in cardiovascular disease. Lancet 362:316, 2003.
82. Bozkurt B, Mann DL: Use of biomarkers in the management of heart failure: Are we there yet? Circulation 107:1231, 2003.
83. Wozÿkowska-Kaplon B, Opolski G: Concomitant recovery of atrial mechanical and endocrine function after cardioversion in patients with persistent atrial fibrillation. J Am Coll Cardiol 41:1716 , 2003.
84. Peverill RE, Harris G, Gelman J, et al: Effect of warfarin on regional left atrial coagulation activity in mitral stenosis. Am J Cardiol 79:339, 1997.
85. Vincentelli A, Susen S, Le Tourneau T, et al: Acquired von Willebrand syndrome in aortic stenosis. N Engl J Med 349:343, 2003.

CHAPTER 21

Pathophysiology of Heart Failure

Wilson S. Colucci • Eugene Braunwald

Heart (or cardiac) failure is the pathophysiological state in which the heart is unable to pump blood at a rate commensurate with the requirements of the metabolizing tissues or can do so only from an elevated filling pressure. The American College of Cardiology/American Heart Association Guidelines for the Evaluation and Management of Chronic Heart Failure in the Adult defined heart failure as a "complex clinical syndrome that can result from any structural or functional cardiac disorder that impairs the ability of the ventricle to fill with or eject blood."[1] It is often, but not always, caused by a defect in myocardial contraction, that is, by *myocardial failure.*[2,3] However, in some patients with heart failure a similar clinical syndrome is present without a detectable abnormality of *myocardial* function. In many such cases, heart failure is caused by conditions in which the normal heart is suddenly presented with a load that exceeds its capacity[4] or in which ventricular filling is impaired.[1]

Heart failure may be caused by myocyte death, myocyte dysfunction, ventricular remodeling, or some combination. Abnormal energy utilization, ischemia, and neurohormonal disturbances can lead to the progression of heart failure (see also Chap. 23).[2,5-8] *Heart failure* should be distinguished from *circulatory failure,* in which an abnormality of some component of the circulation—the heart, the blood volume, the concentration of oxygenated hemoglobin in the arterial blood, or the vascular bed—is responsible for the inadequate cardiac output.

Thus, the terms myocardial failure, heart failure, and circulatory failure are *not* synonymous but refer to progressively more inclusive entities. Myocardial failure, when sufficiently severe, always causes heart failure, but the converse is not necessarily the case because a number of conditions in which the heart is suddenly overloaded (e.g., acute aortic regurgitation secondary to acute infective endocarditis) can cause heart failure in the presence of normal myocardial function, at least early in the course of the illness. Myocardial failure may be associated with systolic dysfunction, diastolic dysfunction, or most commonly both. Also, conditions such as tricuspid or mitral stenosis and constrictive pericarditis, which interfere with cardiac filling, can cause heart failure without myocardial failure. Heart failure, in turn, always causes circulatory failure, but again the converse is not necessarily the case because a variety of noncardiac conditions (e.g., hypovolemic shock) can produce circulatory failure at a time when cardiac function is normal or only modestly impaired.

The hemodynamic, contractile, and wall motion disorders in heart failure are discussed in the chapters on echocardiography (see Chap. 11), cardiac catheterization (see Chap. 17), radionuclide imaging (see Chap. 13), assessment of cardiac function (see Chap. 20), and clinical features (see Chap. 22). In this chapter, we focus on the physiological, neurohumoral, biochemical, molecular, and cellular changes characteristic of heart failure.

Short-Term Adaptive Mechanisms

In the presence of a primary disturbance in myocardial contractility or an excessive hemodynamic burden placed on the ventricle, or both, the heart depends on a number of adaptive mechanisms for maintenance of its pumping function (Fig. 21–1, Table 21–1).[9] Most important among these are (1) the Frank-Starling mechanism, in which an increased preload helps to sustain cardiac performance; (2) activation of neurohumoral systems, especially the release of the neurotransmitter norepinephrine (NE) by adrenergic cardiac nerves, which augments myocardial contractility, and activation of the renin-angiotensin-aldosterone system as well as other neurohumoral adjustments that act to maintain arterial pressure and perfusion of vital organs; and (3) myocardial remodeling with or without cardiac chamber dilatation, in which the mass of contractile tissue is augmented. The first two of these adaptations occur rapidly, within several cardiac cycles after the onset of severe myocardial dysfunction, and may be adequate to maintain the overall pumping performance of the heart at relatively normal levels. Myocardial remodeling and hypertrophy develop more slowly, over weeks to months, and play an important role in long-term adaptation to hemodynamic overload. However, each of these mechanisms has a finite capacity to sustain cardiac performance in the presence of hemodynamic overload and, when chronically maintained, becomes maladaptive.

HEMODYNAMIC AND CIRCULATORY CONSEQUENCES OF HEART FAILURE. *Cardiac output* is often depressed, and the arterial–mixed venous oxygen difference is widened in the basal state in patients with the common forms of chronic heart failure secondary to ischemic heart disease, hypertension, primary myocardial disease, valvular disease, and pericardial disease (so-called low-output, systolic heart failure). Arterial pressure is maintained and systemic vascular resistance is elevated. In mild heart failure, the cardiac output may be normal at rest but fails to rise normally

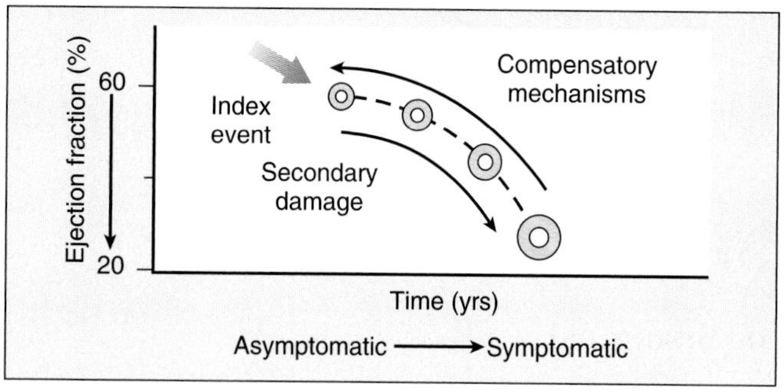

FIGURE 21–1 Pathogenesis of heart failure. Heart failure begins after an "index event" produces an initial decline in pumping capacity of the heart. After this initial decline in pumping capacity of the heart, a variety of compensatory mechanisms are activated, including the adrenergic nervous system, the renin-angiotensin system, and the cytokine system. In the short term, these systems are able to restore cardiovascular function to a normal hemostatic range and the patient remains asymptomatic. However, with time the sustained activation of these systems can lead to secondary end-organ damage within the ventricle, with worsening left ventricular remodeling and subsequent cardiac decompensation. As a result of worsening left ventricular remodeling and cardiac decompensation, patients undergo the transition from asymptomatic to symptomatic heart failure. (From Mann DL: Mechanisms and models in heart failure: A combinatorial approach. Circulation 100:99, 1999.)

during exercise. When the volume of blood delivered into the systemic arterial bed is chronically reduced or when one or both ventricles have an elevated filling pressure, or both, a complex sequence of adjustments occurs that ultimately results in the *retention of sodium and water* in the intravascular and interstitial compartments. Many of the clinical manifestations of heart failure such as dyspnea and edema are secondary to this excessive retention of fluid in the pulmonary and systemic venous beds (see Chap. 22).

Interaction Between the Frank-Starling Mechanism and the Adrenergic Nervous System

It is useful to consider the function of the normal and failing heart within the framework of the Frank-Starling mechanism, in which an increase in preload, reflected in an elevation of end-diastolic volume, augments ventricular performance.[4] The normal relationship between ventricular end-diastolic volume and performance is shown in Figure 21–2, curve 1. During exercise and other stresses, the increases in adrenergic nerve impulses to the myocardium, increases in the concentration of circulating catecholamines, and tachycardia all augment myocardial contractility with a shift from curve 1 to curve 2. Ventricular performance, as reflected in stroke work or cardiac output, increases with little change in end-diastolic pressure and volume. This is represented by a shift from point A to point B in Figure 21–2. Vasodilation occurs in the exercising skeletal muscles as a consequence of their heightened metabolism, reducing peripheral vascular resistance and aortic impedance. This combination of augmented myocardial contractility and vasodilatation enhances ventricular emptying and allows achievement of a greatly elevated cardiac output during exercise, at an arterial pressure only slightly higher than in the resting state. During intense exercise in a normal subject, cardiac output can rise 5-fold (and total body O_2 10-fold) if use is also made of the Frank-Starling mechanism, as reflected in modest increases in the left ventricular end-diastolic volume and pressure (point B to point C).

In moderately severe systolic heart failure, as represented by curve 3, cardiac output and external ventricular performance at rest are within normal limits but are maintained at these levels only because the end-diastolic fiber length and the ventricular end-diastolic volume (ventricular preload) are elevated (i.e., through the operation of the Frank-Starling mechanism). The elevations of left ventricular diastolic pressure are associated with abnormally high levels of pulmonary capillary pressure, contributing to the dyspnea experienced by patients with heart failure, sometimes even at rest (point D).

Heart failure is characterized by generalized adrenergic activation and parasympathetic withdrawal (Fig. 21–3).[4,10,11] This condition leads to stimulation of myocardial contractility, tachycardia, sodium retention, activation of the renin-angiotensin-aldosterone system, and generalized systemic vasoconstriction. Heart failure is frequently accompanied by

TABLE 21–1 Short-Term and Long-Term Responses to Impaired Cardiac Performance

Response	Short-Term Effects*	Long-Term Effects†
Salt and water retention	Augments preload	Causes pulmonary congestion, anasarca
Vasoconstriction	Maintains blood pressure for perfusion of vital organs (brain, heart)	Exacerbates pump dysfunction (after-load mismatch); increases cardiac energy expenditure
Sympathetic stimulation	Increases heart rate and ejection	Increases energy expenditure
Sympathetic desensitization		Spares energy
Hypertrophy	Unloads individual muscle fibers	Leads to deterioration and death of cardiac cells; cardiomyopathy of overload
Capillary deficit		Leads to energy starvation
Mitochondrial density	Increase in density helps meet energy demands	Decrease in density leads to energy starvation
Appearance of slow myosin		Increases force, decreases shortening velocity and contractility; is energy sparing
Prolonged action potential		Increases contractility and energy expenditure
Decreased density of sarcoplasmic reticulum calcium pump sites		Slows relaxation; may be energy sparing
Increased collagen	May reduce dilatation	Impairs relaxation

From Katz AM: Cardiomyopathy of overload: A major determinant of prognosis in congestive heart failure. N Engl J Med 322:100, 1990. Copyright 1990, Massachusetts Medical Society.

*Short-term effects are mainly adaptive and occur after hemorrhage and in acute heart failure.

†Long-term effects are mainly deleterious and occur in chronic heart failure.

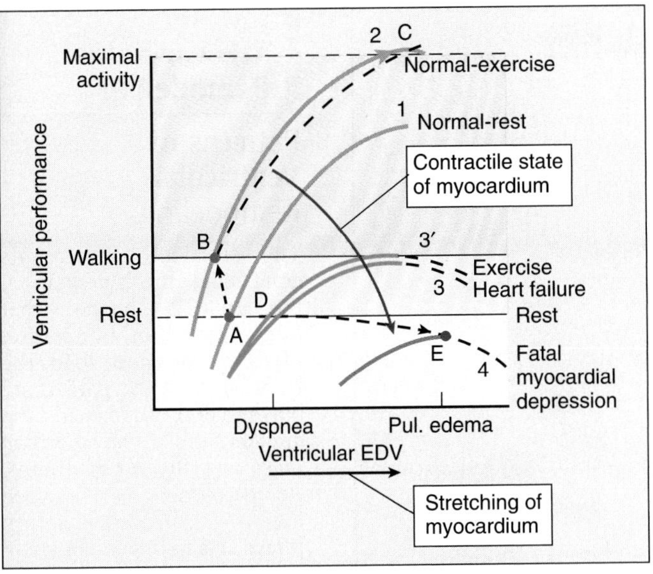

FIGURE 21–2 Diagram showing the interrelationship of influences on ventricular end-diastolic volume (EDV) through stretching of the myocardium and the contractile state of the myocardium. Levels of ventricular EDV associated with filling pressures that result in dyspnea and pulmonary edema are shown on the abscissa. Levels of ventricular performance required during rest, walking, and maximal activity are designated on the ordinate. The dashed lines are the descending limbs of the ventricular performance curves, which are rarely seen during life but that show what the level of ventricular performance would be if EDV could be elevated to very high levels. (Modified from Braunwald E, Ross J Jr, Sonnenblick EH: Mechanisms of Contraction of the Normal and Failing Heart. Boston, Little, Brown, 1979.)

reductions in NE stores and myocardial beta adrenoceptor density. As a consequence, ventricular function (performance) curves cannot be elevated to normal levels by the adrenergic nervous system and the normal enhancement of contractility that takes place during physical activity is attenuated (see Fig. 21–2, curves 3 to 3′). The factors that tend to augment ventricular filling during exertion push the failing ventricle even farther along its flattened, depressed function curve. There are marked elevations of ventricular end-diastolic volume and pressure and therefore of pulmonary capillary pressure. The elevation of the latter intensifies dyspnea and plays an important role in limiting the intensity of exertion that can be performed. Left ventricular failure becomes fatal when the left ventricular function curve becomes depressed (curve 4) to the point at which either cardiac output is insufficient to satisfy the requirements of the peripheral tissue at rest or the left ventricular end-diastolic and pulmonary capillary pressures are elevated to levels that result in pulmonary edema or both (point E).

Vascular Redistribution of Left Ventricular Output

Maintenance of arterial pressure in the presence of a reduced cardiac output is a primitive but effective compensatory mechanism. In both hypovolemia and severe heart failure, this important mechanism is brought into play to allow the limited cardiac output to be most useful for survival. Thus, vasoconstriction occurs earliest and is most intense in areas that are not vital for immediate survival, such as the skin, skeletal muscle, gut, and kidney.

INCREASED VASOCONSTRICTOR ACTIVITY

The major mechanism of increased vascular tone is an increase in the activity of vasoconstrictor systems, in particular the sympathetic nervous system, the renin-angiotensin-aldosterone system, and endothelin. In patients with moderately severe heart failure, in whom the cardiac output at rest is normal, abnormal vasoconstriction in selected vascular beds occurs when an additional burden (such as exertion) is imposed on the circulation and the cardiac output fails to rise normally to meet the peripheral demands. As cardiac performance declines, left ventricular output is ultimately redistributed, even at rest. This redistribution maintains the delivery of oxygen to vital organs such as the brain and heart, whereas blood flow to less critical areas is reduced.[12,13]

This underperfusion of skeletal muscle leads to anaerobic metabolism,[14] lactic acidosis, an excess oxygen debt, weakness, and fatigue. Occasionally, serious complications can result from the redistribution of cardiac output and the resulting regional reductions of blood flow. These include marked sodium and nitrogen retention as a consequence of diminished renal perfusion, hepatic dysfunction, and, in extreme cases, gangrene of the tips of the phalanges and mesenteric infarction.

With heart failure there is a generalized increase in sympathetic activity. Neurograms obtained from adrenergic nerves to the limbs display increased traffic in patients with heart failure.[11] Substantial changes also occur in the function of the adrenergic nerves that innervate splanchnic and renal vessels.[15] Although direct neurograms of the nerves to these beds are not feasible in humans, it has been shown that exercise induces a much more marked reduction in mesenteric blood flow and elevation of mesenteric vascular resistance in dogs with experimental heart failure than in normal dogs.[16] Similar changes during exercise were observed in other major visceral vascular beds, such as the renal bed. Evidence that this intense vasoconstriction during exercise is mediated by the adrenergic nervous system is provided by observations on dogs with experimentally produced heart failure in which one kidney was denervated. Blood flow through the innervated kidney declined precipitously during exercise, and calculated renal vascular resistance increased markedly. In contrast, little change in renal blood flow and calculated renal vascular resistance occurred in the denervated kidney.[16] This intense visceral vasoconstriction during exercise helps to divert the limited cardiac output to exercising muscle but contributes to hypoperfusion of the gut and kidneys.

The renin-angiotensin system and endothelin also contribute to the increased systemic vascular tone in heart failure. These potent vasoconstrictor systems are activated in patients with heart failure (see Renin-Angiotensin-Aldosterone System, later), in whom their contribution to systemic vasoconstriction has been demonstrated by the ability of specific inhibitors for angiotensin[17] and endothelin[18] receptors to cause vasodilation in patients with heart failure. Vasopressin is released in very advanced stages.

ENDOTHELIAL DYSFUNCTION. Both ischemia-induced and exercise-induced vasodilations in the extremities are attenuated in patients with heart failure, and this attenuation impairs the normal exercise-induced blood flow response.[19] The attenuation is related in part to endothelial dysfunction. The response of blood flow to infused acetylcholine and methacholine, which are endothelium-dependent vasodilators, is reduced in heart failure. The vasodilator response can be restored by the administration of L-arginine, a precursor of endothelium-derived nitric oxide (NO), which is synthesized in vascular endothelial cells by endothelial cell NO synthase (eNOS). These findings suggest that defective endothelial function contributes to the impaired vasodilator capacity in heart failure. The mechanisms potentially responsible include impaired endothelial cell receptor function, deficiency of L-arginine substrate, and abnormal expression of eNOS resulting in the impaired release and rapid degradation of NO by superoxide anion.[20] Activation of the renin-angiotensin-aldosterone system may contribute to endothelial dysfunction as well. Impaired endothelial function is improved in patients by regular exercise.[21]

CHANGES IN THE VASCULAR WALL. The sodium content of the vascular wall is increased in heart failure, and this contributes to the stiffening, thickening, and compression of blood vessel walls, which raises vascular resistance and also prevents normal vasodilation during exercise. It has been postulated that angiotensin II causes proliferation of smooth muscle and other elements of the vascular wall, causing vascular stiffening. Reduced density of skeletal muscle capillaries may contribute as well. The venous system in the extremities of patients with heart failure is also constricted by the activity of the adrenergic nervous system as well as by circulating and locally acting venoconstrictors (NE, angiotensin, and endothelin). This venoconstriction results in displacement of blood to the heart and lungs.

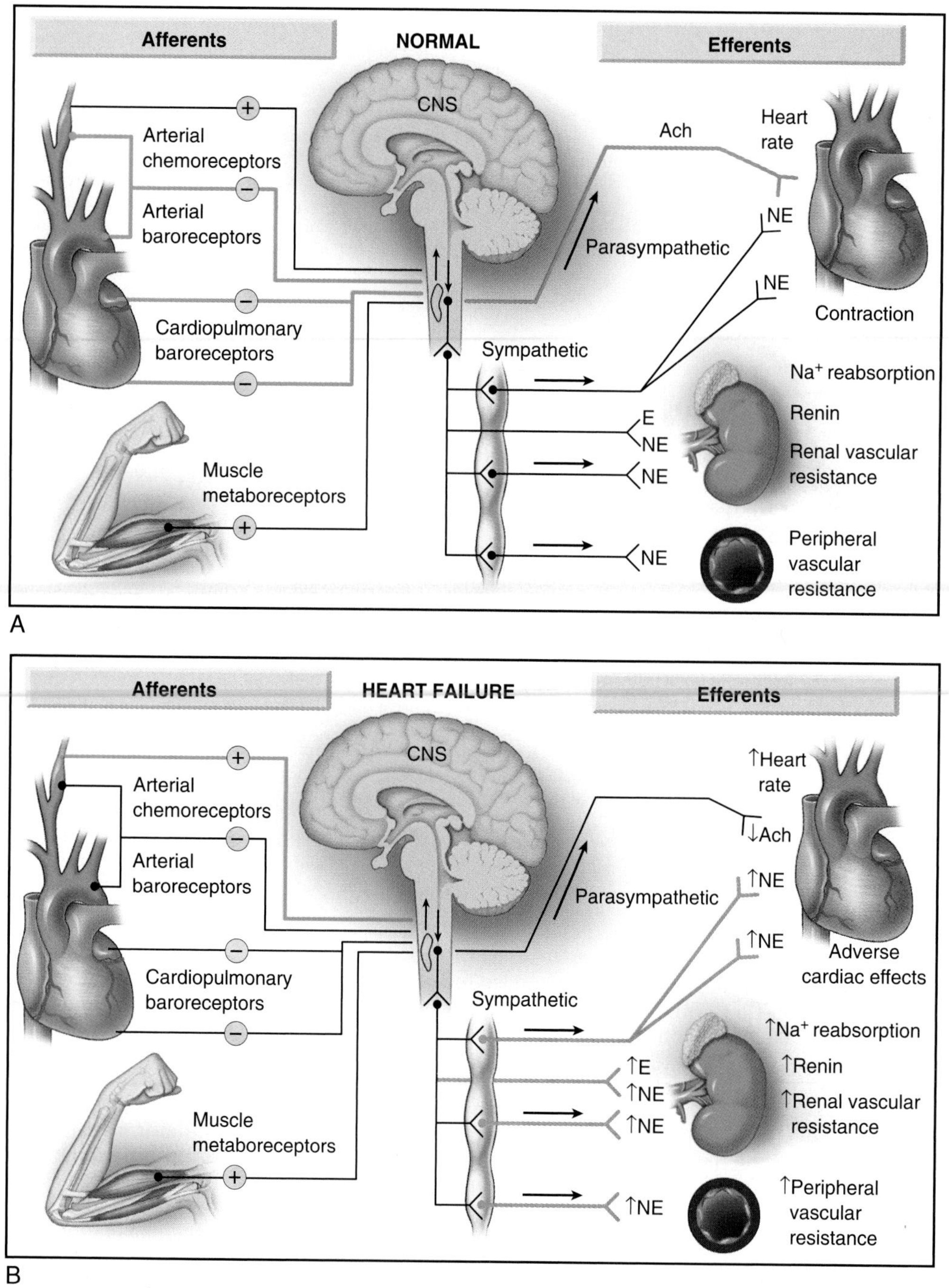

FIGURE 21–3 Mechanisms for generalized sympathetic activation and parasympathetic withdrawal in heart failure. **A,** Under normal conditions, inhibitory (–) inputs from arterial and cardiopulmonary baroreceptor afferent nerves are the principal influence on sympathetic outflow. Parasympathetic control of heart rate is also under potent arterial baroreflex control. Efferent sympathetic traffic and arterial catecholamines are low, and heart rate variability is high. **B,** As heart failure progresses, inhibitory input from arterial and cardiopulmonary receptors decreases and excitatory (+) input increases. The net response to this altered balance includes a generalized increase in sympathetic nerve traffic, blunted parasympathetic and sympathetic control of heart rate, and impairment of the reflex sympathetic regulation of vascular resistance. Anterior wall ischemia has additional excitatory effects on efferent sympathetic nerve traffic. See text for details. Ach = acetylcholine; CNS = central nervous system; E = epinephrine; Na^+ = sodium; NE = norepinephrine. (From Floras JS: Alterations in the sympathetic and parasympathetic nervous system in heart failure. *In* Mann DL [ed]: Heart Failure: A Companion to Braunwald's Heart Disease. Philadelphia, Elsevier, 2004, pp 247-278.)

2,3-DIPHOSPHOGLYCERATE. A progressive decline in the affinity of hemoglobin for oxygen caused by an increase in 2,3-diphosphoglycerate (DPG) also occurs in heart failure.[22] The rightward shift in the oxygen-hemoglobin dissociation curve represents a compensatory mechanism that facilitates oxygen transport; the increased DPG, tissue acidosis, and slowed circulation characteristic of heart failure act synergistically to maintain the delivery of oxygen to the metabolizing tissues in the presence of reduced cardiac output.

Chronic Myocardial Remodeling

Patterns of Ventricular Remodeling

The classical experiments conducted by Meerson in the 1960s[23] showed that immediately on imposition of a large pressure load, the increase in work performed by the ventricle exceeds the augmentation of cardiac mass and the heart dilates. As discussed earlier (see Fig. 21–1), a compensatory phase sets in as the ventricle remodels and the contractile function returns to approximately normal levels. If the compensatory response is adequate to "match" the work demands, a period of relative stability ensues. However, if the extent or form of myocardial remodeling is insufficient or if the magnitude of the overload increases further, regardless of the initial cause, there is further deterioration in myocardial function as a consequence of "afterload mismatch"; that is, the hypertrophy is insufficient to normalize mechanical stress on the myocyte and a vicious circle is created. Later, in what Meerson termed the "exhaustion" phase, several macroscopic events take place; there may be myofibrillar lysis, an increase in the number of lysosomes (presumably to digest worn-out cell constituents), distortion of the sarcoplasmic reticulum (SR), a reduction in the surface density of the key tubular system, and fibrous replacement of cardiac cells. This combination of changes leads to failure of the cardiac pump.

Ventricular remodeling, comprising changes in mass, volume, shape, and composition, constitutes one of the principal mechanisms by which the heart compensates for an increased load (Fig. 21–4).[24] Grossman and associates examined systolic and diastolic wall stresses in normal subjects and in patients with chronic pressure- and volume-overloaded left ventricles who were compensated and not in heart failure.[25] Left ventricular mass was increased approximately equally in both the pressure- and volume-overloaded groups. There was a substantial

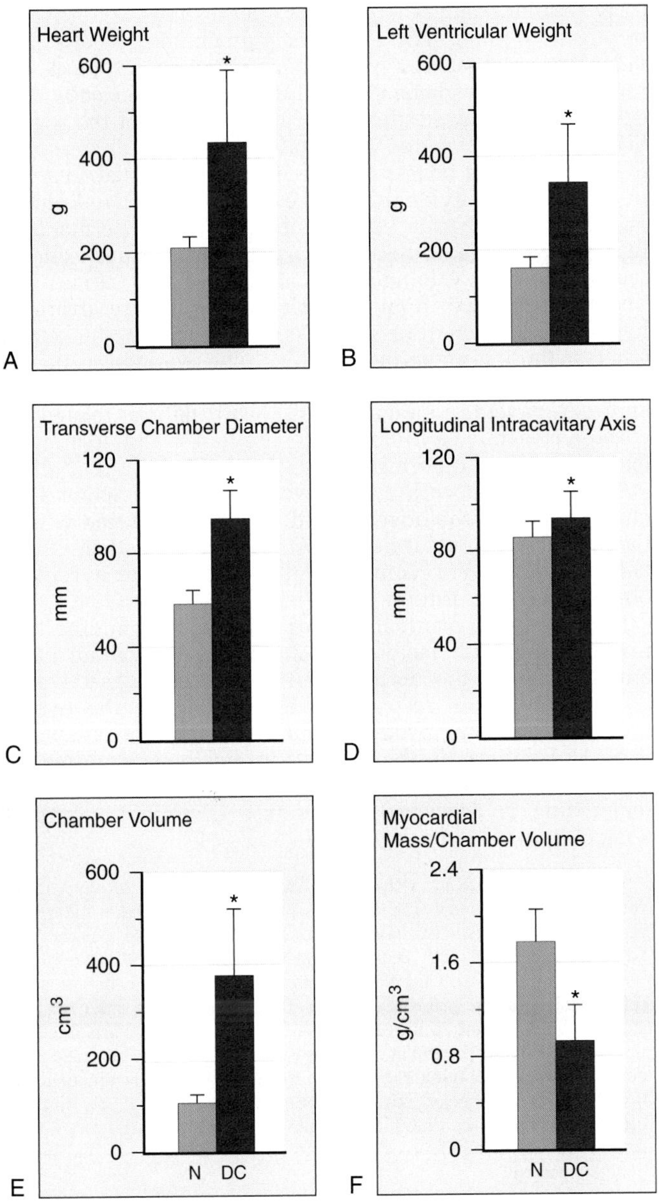

FIGURE 21–4 Cardiac characteristics of human dilated cardiomyopathy. Results are presented as mean + SD. N = normal hearts; DC = dilated cardiomyopathy; $*p < 0.05$) (From Mann DL [ed]: Heart Failure: A Companion to Braunwald's Heart Disease: A Textbook of Cardiovascular Medicine. Philadelphia, Elsevier, 2004. Data adapted from Beltrami CA, Finato N, Roco M, et al: The cellular basis of dilated cardiomyopathy in humans. J Mol Cell Cardiol 27:291, 1995.)

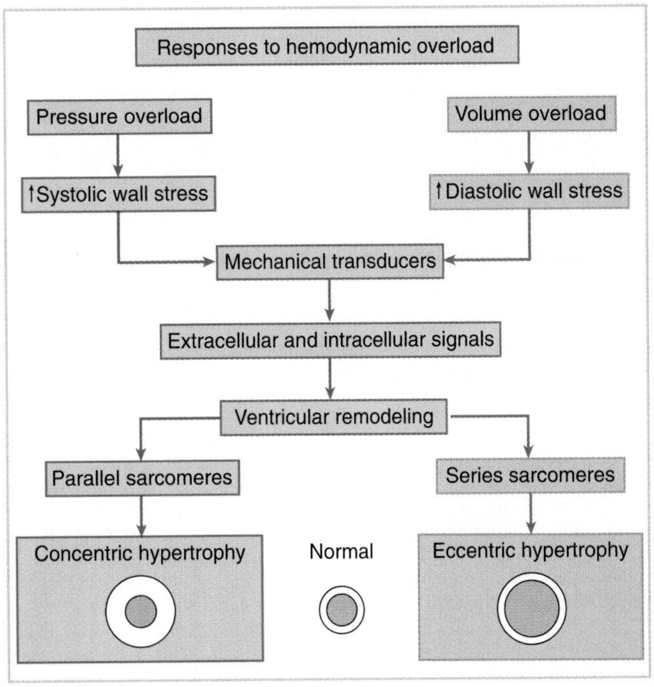

FIGURE 21–5 The morphological response to a hemodynamic overload depends on the nature of the stimulus. When the overload is predominantly due to an increase in pressure (e.g., with systemic hypertension or aortic stenosis), the increase in systolic wall stress leads to the parallel addition of sarcomeres and widening of the cardiac myocytes, resulting in concentric hypertrophy of the ventricle. When the overload is predominantly due to an increase in ventricular volume, the increase in diastolic wall stress leads to the series addition of sarcomeres, lengthening of cardiac myocytes, and eccentric chamber hypertrophy. (From Colucci WS [ed]: Heart Failure: Cardiac Function and Dysfunction. 2nd ed. Philadelphia, Current Medicine, 1999, p 4.2.)

increase in wall thickness in the pressure-overloaded ventricles but only a mild increase in wall thickness in the volume-overloaded ventricles (Fig. 21–5). The latter was just sufficient to counterbalance the increased radius so that the ratio of wall thickness to radius remained normal for the patients with volume-overload hypertrophy. However, this ratio was substantially increased in patients with pressure-overload hypertrophy, in whom there was disproportionate thickening of the ventricular wall.

These observations suggest that myocardial hypertrophy develops in a manner that maintains or returns systolic stress to normal limits. Thus, when the primary stimulus to hypertrophy is *pressure overload*, the resultant increase in systolic wall stress leads to parallel replication of myofibrils, thickening of individual myocytes, which at the organ level is referred to as "concentric" hypertrophy. A small increase in cell number (hyperplasia) has also been documented.[26] On the other hand, when the primary stimulus is ventricular *volume overload*, increased diastolic wall stress leads to replication of sarcomeres in series, elongation of myocytes, and ventricular dilatation. This effect, in turn, results in a modest increase in systolic stress (by the Laplace relationship), which causes proportional wall thickening that (as in pressure overload) returns systolic stress toward normal (Fig. 21–6). The chronically volume-overloaded ventricle becomes more spherical, and this change in shape can distort papillary muscle geometry and thereby cause functional mitral regurgitation.

In compensated subjects, both volume overload and pressure overload alter ventricular geometry and wall thickness so that systolic stress does not change greatly. Pressure overload and volume overload result in distinct cellular phenotypes at the molecular level with different patterns of activation of genes for several peptide growth factors.[27] This heterogeneity at the molecular level presumably reflects differences in the way the two types of hemodynamic overload activate signaling pathways.

Left ventricular wall thickness is a critical determinant of ventricular performance in patients with pressure overload hypertrophy related to aortic stenosis or hypertension. Impaired performance in such patients may be secondary to inadequate hypertrophy, leading to increased wall stress (afterload), which in turn may be responsible for inadequate muscle shortening. This condition has been termed afterload mismatch by Ross,[28] whose group found that when the aorta in conscious dogs was suddenly constricted and left ventricular systolic pressure rose, the left ventricle dilated and the left ventricular wall thinned; this effect was associated with a large increase in wall stress and a reciprocal reduction in the extent and velocity of shortening. During the next few weeks, the left ventricle became hypertrophied and left ventricular wall stress and shortening both returned toward normal. When the constriction was

	Normal	Acute load	Compensatory hypertrophy	Cardiac failure
LV systolic pressure	N	+	+	+
LV radius	N	+	+	+
LV wall thickness	N	N	+	+
LV diastolic volume	N	+	±	++
Systolic wall stress	N	+	N	+
Diastolic wall stress	N	+	N	+

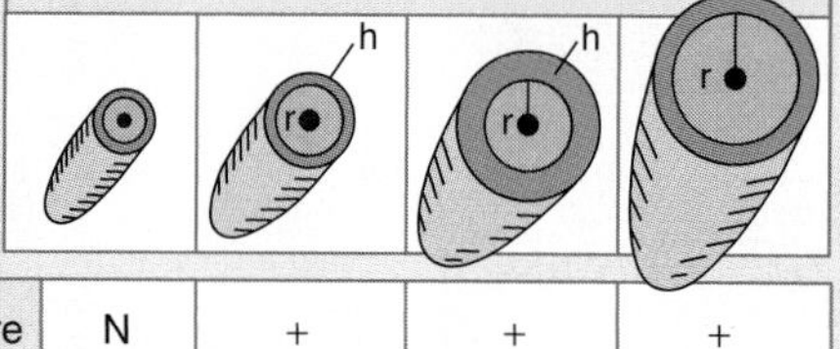

FIGURE 21–6 The normal (N) relationship between left ventricular wall thickness (h) and chamber radius (r) is shown (first panel). An acute increase in systolic pressure (acute load) causes an increase in systolic wall stress, which can be approximated by the equation P × r/h, where P is left ventricular (LV) systolic pressure. Diastolic wall stress is also increased when there is chamber dilation or when diastolic pressure is elevated (second panel). If sufficient compensatory hypertrophy occurs, the increase in ventricular wall thickness may normalize the systolic and diastolic wall stresses (third panel). However, if additional chamber dilation occurs or the increase in wall thickness is insufficient, systolic and diastolic wall stresses remain abnormally elevated. In this situation, further chamber dilation may occur in association with hemodynamic failure (fourth panel). (From Colucci WS [ed]: Heart Failure: Cardiac Function and Dysfunction. 2nd ed. Philadelphia, Current Medicine, 1999, p 4.2.)

suddenly released, wall stress declined and shortening became supernormal. (More recent experiments have challenged these traditional concepts but require confirmation.)

Prolonged athletic training causes a moderate increase in myocardial mass (see also Chap. 75). Isotonic exercise, such as long-distance running or swimming, resembles volume overload and causes an increase in left ventricular diastolic volume with only mild thickening of the wall. Isometric exercise, such as weightlifting or wrestling, causes intermittent pressure overload and can result in an increase in wall thickness. Neither form of hypertrophy appears to be deleterious in the absence of heart disease, and the hypertrophy rapidly disappears when training is discontinued.

CELLULAR CHANGES IN MYOCARDIAL REMODELING. The synthesis of additional mitochondria is one of the early cellular changes that occurs after a stimulus for hypertrophy is applied. The expanded mitochondrial mass provides the high-energy phosphates required to meet the increased energy demands of the hypertrophied cell. This synthesis is followed closely by an expansion of the myofibrillar mass. After the neonatal period, the increase in myocardial mass is associated with a proportional increase in the size of individual cells (i.e., hypertrophy) and only a minor increase in the number of cells (i.e., hyperplasia).[26] Intense, prolonged stress can cause some cardiac cells to reenter the cell cycle and replicate (see Chaps. 69 and 71). Myocytes isolated from animals with pressure overload hypertrophy related to aortic constriction are thickened, whereas those from animals with volume overload related to an aortocaval fistula are elongated.[29] Myocytes from patients and experimental animals with heart failure related to chronic ischemic cardiomyopathy are longer and, to a lesser extent, wider than normal cells (Fig. 21–7).

These changes within the myocyte are accompanied by changes in both the quantity and quality of collagen within the extracellular matrix (ECM).[30] Taken together, these changes in myocyte geometry and the ECM result in remodeling of the myocardium.

Hemodynamic overload causes gene reprogramming that reactivates growth factors present in the embryonic heart but dormant in the normal adult heart. These reactivated growth factors are responsible for stimulating the hypertrophy of cardiac myocytes and regulating the synthesis and degradation of the ECM. Current understanding of the funda-mental mechanisms responsible for myocardial remodeling is described earlier (see Chronic Myocardial Remodeling).

ULTRASTRUCTURAL CHANGES. Structural features of hypertrophied human myocytes (Fig. 21–8) include abnormal Z-band patterns, multiple intercalated discs, and prominent collagen fibrils connecting adjacent myocardial cells. Nuclei are enlarged and lobulated and contain well-developed nucleoli; there is an abundance of ribosomes, presumably reflecting enhanced protein synthesis. However, electron microscopic studies of myocardium removed from overloaded, dilated hearts fixed at the elevated filling pressures that existed during life have revealed sarcomere lengths averaging 2.2 μm—no longer than those at the apex of the length–active tension curve of normal cardiac muscle. This finding indicates that the depressed contractility of failing heart muscle is *not* due to the disengagement of actin and myosin filaments, as had once been suggested.

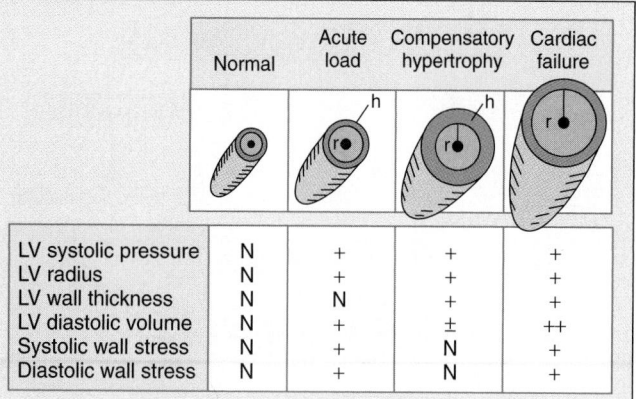

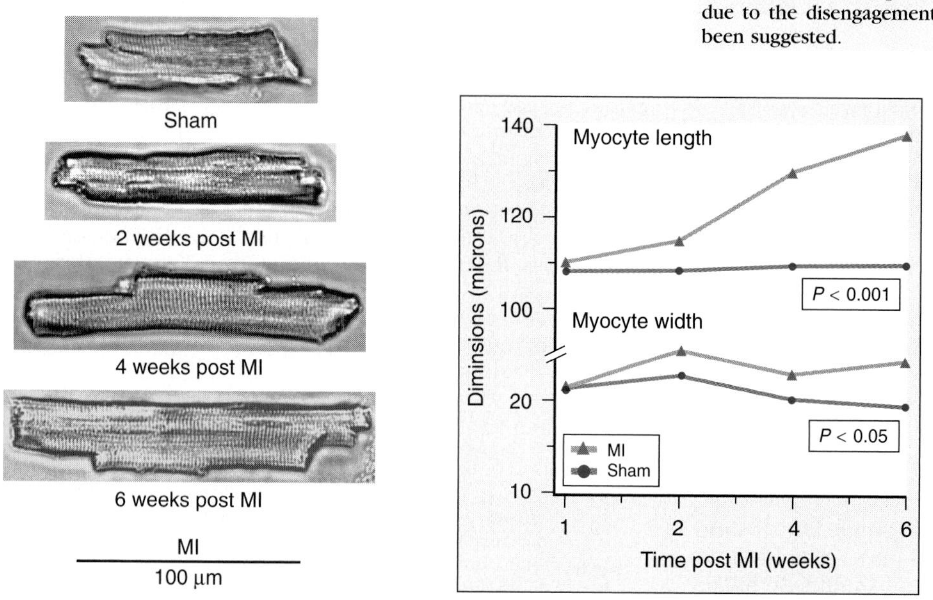

FIGURE 21–7 Cardiac myocyte remodeling in the rat infarct model. Myocyte length and width from rats at 2, 4, and 6 weeks after myocardial infarction are compared with those from a sham-operated animal. Note the predominant increase in myocyte length as the major determinant of the increase in ventricular volume. MI = myocardial infarction. (From Anand IS, Liu D, Chugh SS, et al: Isolated myocyte contractile function is normal in postinfarct remodeled rat heart with systolic dysfunction. Circulation 96:3974, 1997.)

Mechanical Performance of Remodeled Myocardium

Myocardial remodeling provides one of the aforementioned key compensatory mechanisms that permits the ventricle to sustain an increased load (as in hypertension or valvular disease) or to sustain a normal load in the presence of a loss of myocytes (as following myocardial infarction). However, as described later, a ventricle subjected to an abnormally elevated load for a prolonged period may fail to maintain compensation despite the presence of remodeling, and pump failure may ultimately occur. The widely held notion that hypertrophy is a compensatory, albeit insufficient, response to hemodynamic overload has been challenged by exper-

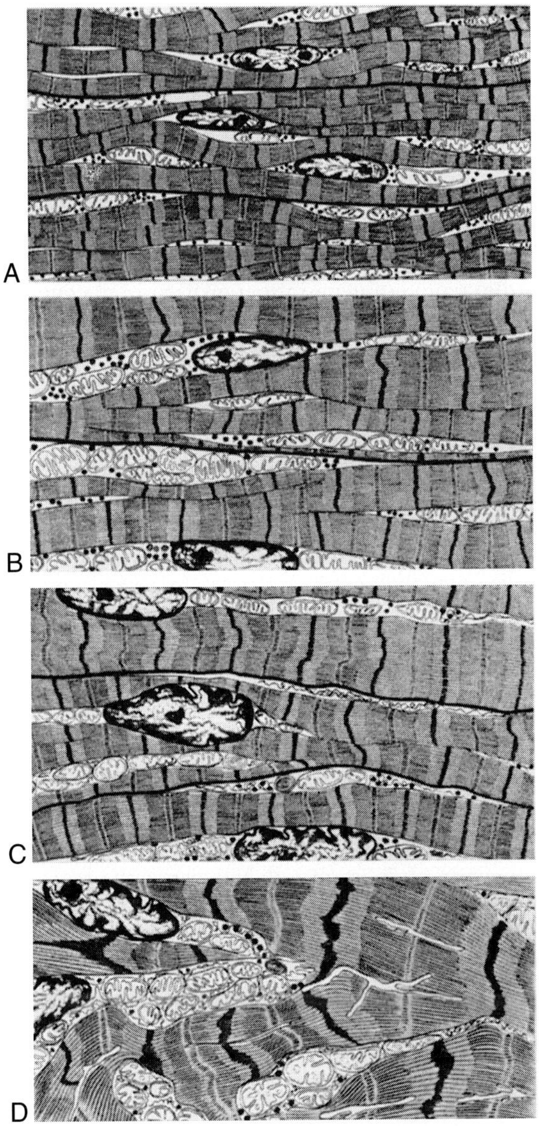

FIGURE 21–8 The early stage of cardiac hypertrophy **(A)** is characterized morphologically by increases in the number of myofibrils and mitochondria as well as enlargement of mitochondria and nuclei. Muscle cells are larger than normal, but cellular organization is largely preserved. At a more advanced stage of hypertrophy **(B)**, preferential increases in the size or number of specific organelles, such as mitochondria, as well as irregular addition of new contractile elements in localized areas of the cell, result in subtle abnormalities of cellular organization and contour. Adjacent cells may vary in their degree of enlargement. Cells subjected to longstanding hypertrophy **(C)** show more obvious disruptions in cellular organization, such as markedly enlarged nuclei with highly lobulated membranes, which displace adjacent myofibrils and cause breakdown of normal Z-band registration. The early preferential increase in mitochondria is supplanted by a predominance by volume of myofibrils. The late stage of hypertrophy **(D)** is characterized by loss of contractile elements with marked disruption of Z bands, severe disruption of the normal parallel arrangement of the sarcomeres, deposition of fibrous tissue, and dilation and increased tortuosity of T tubules. (From Ferrans VJ: Morphology of the heart in hypertrophy. Hosp Pract 18:69, 1983. Copyright 1983, McGraw-Hill Companies, Inc.)

iments in which transgenic mice that overexpress an inhibitor to G_q were exposed to pressure overload caused by aortic constriction.[31] In these mice, the usual hypertrophic response did *not* occur, and yet the progression to failure was delayed, suggesting that the hypertrophic response to a pathological stimulus need not be compensatory. These new ideas require confirmation.

ISOLATED CARDIAC MUSCLE. Cardiac muscle isolated from animals in which the heart had been subjected to a controlled stress has been studied by many investigators. One convenient experimental model of ventricular pressure overload is the cat (or ferret) with pulmonary artery constriction. Papillary muscles are then removed from the right ventricles in which either hypertrophy or overt failure has developed, and the excised muscles are studied in vitro. Both right ventricular hypertrophy and failure reduce the maximum velocity of (unloaded) shortening (V_{max}) of excised muscle below the values observed in muscles obtained from normal cats.[32-34] These changes are more marked in animals in which heart failure has been present than in those with hypertrophy alone (Fig. 21–9). Because the depression of myocardial contractility is evident in vitro and when the muscle's physical and chemical milieu is controlled, it is considered to be *intrinsic* and not the result of any humoral or neural stimuli or abnormal loading conditions that are present in vivo.

In this model, the depression of contractility in hypertrophied myocardium is less marked or even absent when the stress is imposed slowly and when the measurements are made during a stable phase of the ventricular response to overload. The force and rate of force development are also

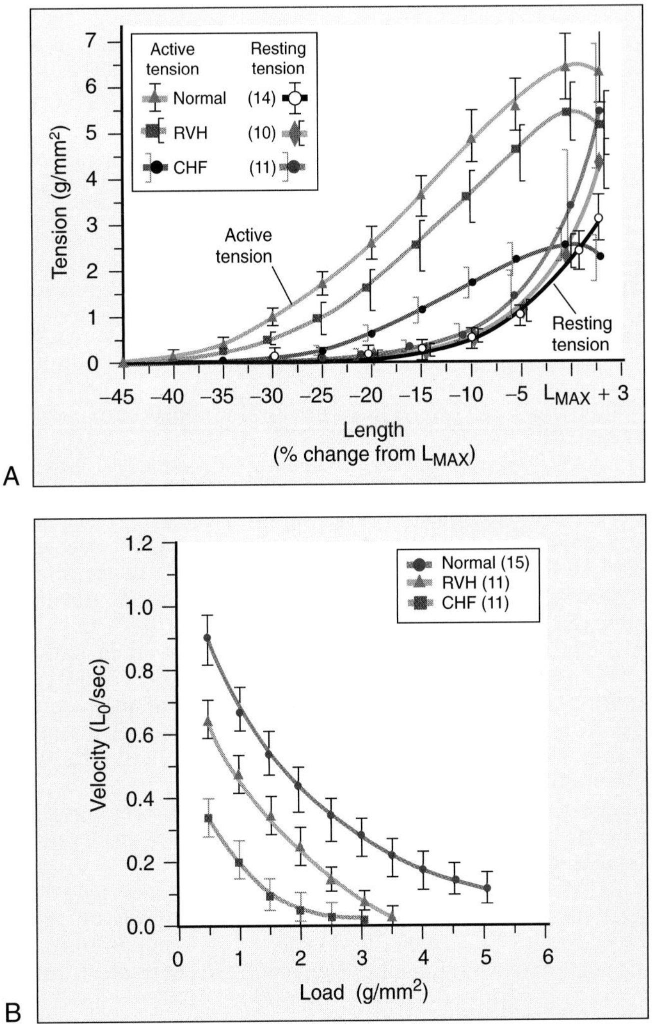

FIGURE 21–9 **A,** Relation between muscle length and tension of papillary muscles from normal (blue), hypertrophied (RVH, brown), and failing (CHF, black) right ventricles. Resting tension and actively developed tension is shown. Tension is corrected for cross-sectional area (g/mm^2). Numbers in parentheses = number of animals. **B,** Force-velocity relations of the three groups of cat papillary muscles. Average values ± SEM are given for each point. Velocity has been corrected to muscle lengths per second (L_0/sec). RVH = right ventricular hypertrophy; CHF = congestive heart failure. (From Spann JF Jr, Buccino RA, Sonnenblick EH, Braunwald E: Contractile state of cardiac muscle obtained from cats with experimentally produced ventricular hypertrophy and heart failure. Circ Res 21:341, 1967. Copyright 1967, American Heart Association.)

depressed in isometrically contracting myocardium obtained from hearts with totally different forms of heart failure (e.g., Syrian hamsters with hereditary cardiomyopathy) as well as papillary muscles removed from the left ventricles of patients with heart failure related to chronic valvular disease. Also in the failing heart, the inotropic effects of adrenergic stimulation are reduced.[34,35] Thus, the "contractile reserve" of the failing heart is usually greatly reduced.

INTACT HEART. Changes in performance of the intact heart subjected to abnormal hemodynamic loads are, in general, similar to those in isolated cardiac tissue. Thus, the right ventricles of cats with pulmonary artery constriction exhibit a marked depression paralleling that observed in the isolated papillary muscles removed from these ventricles. When compared with normal values, the active tension developed by the right ventricle at equivalent end-diastolic fiber lengths is markedly reduced in cats with heart failure produced by pressure overload.[36]

Immediately after the imposition of a *volume* overload (e.g., the opening of a large arteriovenous fistula), the contractility of the ventricle, as reflected in the end-systolic stress-circumference relationship, may actually increase, perhaps as a consequence of adrenergic stimulation. However, it then declines while overall hemodynamic performance (i.e., cardiac work) is sustained. Later in the course of a large volume overload, overt clinical heart failure develops, accompanied by increases in left ventricular end-diastolic volume and in the ratio of left ventricular weight to body weight and by depressed indices of left ventricular contractility (see Chap. 19). As the ventricle fails, it moves to the right along a depressed performance (function) curve (see Fig. 21–2) so that it requires an abnormally elevated end-diastolic volume (and often an elevation of end-diastolic pressure as well) to generate a level of tension equal to that achieved by the normal heart at a normal end-diastolic volume.[36]

Transition to Heart Failure

When the ventricle is stressed, cardiac performance is initially maintained by the acute adaptive (compensatory) mechanisms summarized in Table 21–1. However, when the hemodynamic overload is severe and prolonged, myocardial contractility becomes depressed. In an animal model of pressure overload hypertrophy produced by gradually tightening a hydraulic constrictor around the ascending aorta, there was depression of myocardial contractility, as assessed by *load-independent* contractility indices, suggesting that the cardiac dysfunction in this model was due not entirely to insufficient hypertrophy causing afterload mismatch but also to a depression of the myocardium's *intrinsic* contractility.[37] Impaired myocardial contractility has also been observed in patients with hypertension and fully compensatory ventricular hypertrophy, normal myocardial stress, and apparently normal pump function. Such patients have displayed reduction of intramural myocardial shortening, as determined by spatial modulation of magnetization, using magnetic resonance imaging techniques[38]; this reduction indicates a depression of myocardial contractility in the presence of apparently normal loading conditions.

In its mildest form, this depression is manifested by a reduction in the velocity of shortening of unloaded myocardium (V_{max}) (see Fig. 21–9)[32] or by a reduction in the rate of force development during isometric contraction but by little if any reduction in the development of maximal isometric force or in the extent of shortening of afterloaded isotonic contractions. As myocardial contractility becomes further depressed, V_{max} is further reduced, now accompanied by a decline in isometric force development and shortening. At this point, circulatory compensation may still be provided by ventricular remodeling, dilation, and an increase in muscle mass—which tend to maintain systolic tension development while maintaining wall stress at normal levels. Although cardiac output and stroke volume are sustained in the resting state, the ejection fraction at rest as well as the maximal cardiac output that can be attained during stress decline. As contractility falls farther, overt congestive heart failure, reflected in a depression of cardiac output and work or an elevation of ventricular end-diastolic volume and pressure at rest, or both, supervenes.

Molecular Mechanisms of Myocardial Remodeling and Failure

Myocardial remodeling and the transition from compensated hypertrophy to failure of the myocardium involve a complex of events at the molecular and cellular level.[37-41] These events include (1) myocyte growth or hypertrophy; (2) changes in myocyte phenotype resulting from reexpression of fetal gene programs and decreased expression of adult gene programs; (3) alterations in the expression or function, or both, of proteins involved in excitation-contraction coupling and contraction; (4) myocyte death caused by necrosis and apoptosis; (5) changes in the ECM; and (6) abnormalities in energetics (Fig. 21–10). Together, these events result in changes in myocardial structure (e.g., increase in myocardial mass, chamber dilation, greater sphericity) and function (e.g., impaired systolic or diastolic function, or both) that often lead to further pump dysfunction and hemodynamic overload. Stimuli for these changes include mechanical strain on the myocyte, neurohormones (e.g., NE, angiotensin II), inflammatory cytokines (e.g., tumor necrosis factor-alpha [TNF-α]), other peptides and growth factors (e.g., endothelin), and reactive oxygen species (e.g., superoxide, NO).[41-44] These stimuli occur both systemically and in the myocardium in response to circulatory failure and hemodynamic overload. They serve as an important link between pathological factors in the environment and the inter- and intracellular signaling pathways that mediate changes in the structure and function of the cellular elements in the myocardium.[41,45]

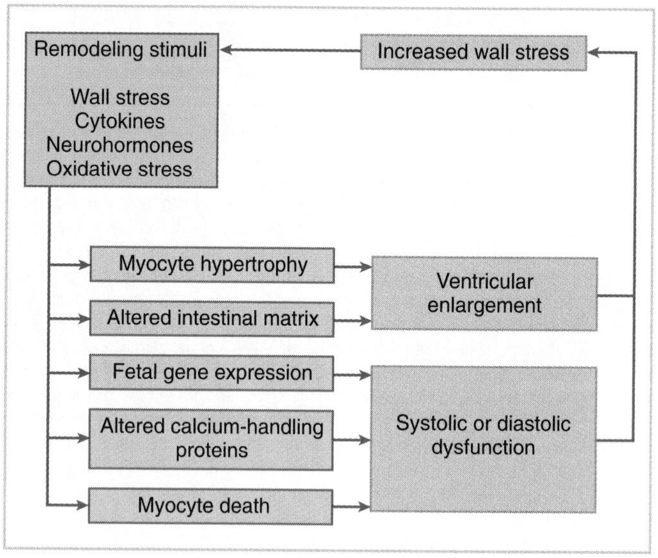

FIGURE 21–10 Overview of the pathophysiology of myocardial remodeling. Remodeling stimuli such as increased mechanical wall stress and neuroendocrine activation lead to a complex of molecular and cellular events, including hypertrophy of cardiac myocytes, changes in gene expression with a reexpression of fetal programs and decreased expression of adult programs, changes in the quantity and nature of the interstitial matrix, and cell death. These events lead to changes in the structure and function of the ventricle, which may result in further pump dysfunction and increased wall stresses, thereby promoting further pathological remodeling. (From Sawyer DB, Colucci WS: Molecular and cellular events in myocardial hypertrophy and failure. *In* Colucci WS [ed]: Heart Failure: Cardiac Function and Dysfunction. Vol 4. Philadelphia, Current Medicine, 1999, p 4.2.)

Myocyte Loss

Impaired myocardial contractile function may reflect a decrease in the number of viable, fully functional myocytes, a decrement in the function of viable myocytes, or a combination of these mechanisms. Myocyte loss may occur by one of two major mechanisms—necrosis or apoptosis. In most instances, myocyte death is caused by a (variable) combination of these two mechanisms.

NECROSIS. Necrosis occurs when myocytes are deprived of oxygen or energy, leading to the loss of cellular membrane integrity, the influx of extracellular fluid, cellular swelling, and the release of proteolytic enzymes that cause cellular disruption. Myocyte necrosis may be localized, as in myocardial infarction, or diffuse, as in dilated cardiomyopathy (see Chap. 59), myocardial damage by toxic agents such as daunorubicin (see Chap. 62), or myocarditis (see Chap. 60). In addition, capillary density and coronary reserve are reduced in remodeled myocardium and may result in diffuse ischemia, which is most severe in the subendocardium. Thus, a diminished response of endocardial blood flow to adenosine and exercise-induced vasodilation has been demonstrated in dogs with pressure overload hypertrophy. This diminished response is caused in part by hypertrophy and in part by an exercise-induced increase in left ventricular subendocardial wall stress. The reduced subendocardial perfusion in turn may cause subendocardial ischemic cell death and replacement fibrosis, which impair both systolic and diastolic function, accelerating the development of heart failure (see Chap. 44)

APOPTOSIS (see Chap. 71). In contrast to necrosis, apoptosis (programmed cell death) is an energy-dependent process in which a specific genetic program leads to the activation of a molecular cascade that causes the degradation of nuclear deoxyribonucleic acid (DNA) (Fig. 21–11). Also in contrast to necrosis, apoptosis is marked by the involution of the myocyte, resulting in phagocytosis by neighboring cells (Fig. 21–12).[46] Apoptosis is a common cellular mechanism during organogenesis and in adult cells that have rapid turnover, such as blood cells and gut epithelium. Because cardiac myocytes were uniformly considered to be terminally differentiated, it was not generally believed that they would undergo apoptosis. However, there have now been several reports demonstrating the presence of apoptotic myocytes in failing human myocardium (Fig. 21–13)[46] as well as in models of myocardial failure, hemodynamic overload, and myocardial infarction.[47,48]

Several factors known to be present or increased in the failing myocardium have been shown to cause apoptosis of

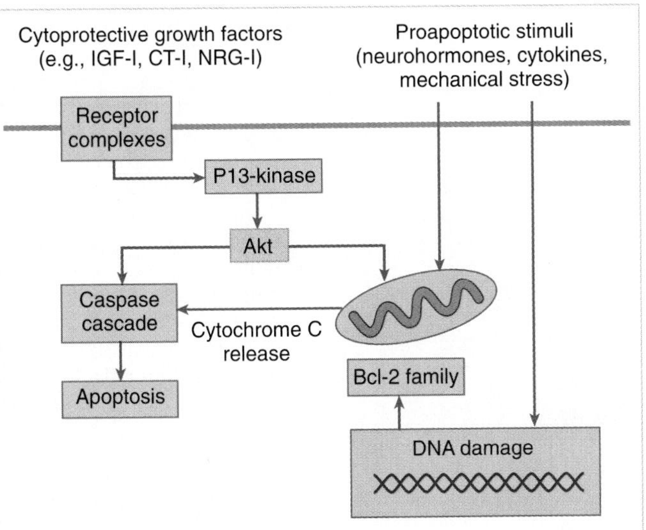

FIGURE 21–11 Regulation of myocyte survival in heart failure. The proapoptotic effects of chronic neurohormonal, inflammatory cytokine, mechanical stress, and other stimuli are counterbalanced by prosurvival pathways. The fate of any single myocyte is a function of the *net* effect of these influences. Antiapoptotic influences in the myocardium are mediated in part by cytoprotective growth factors, including insulin-like growth factor-1 (IGF-1), cardiotrophin-1 (CT-1), and neuregulin-1 (NRG-1), that suppress the apoptotic cascade at multiple levels at least in part through the activation of phosphoinositol-3kinase and Akt as depicted. (From Sawyer DB, Colucci WS: Molecular and cellular events in myocardial hypertrophy and failure. *In* Colucci WS [ed]: Atlas of Heart Failure: Cardiac Function and Dysfunction. 3d ed. Philadelphia, Current Medicine, 2002.)

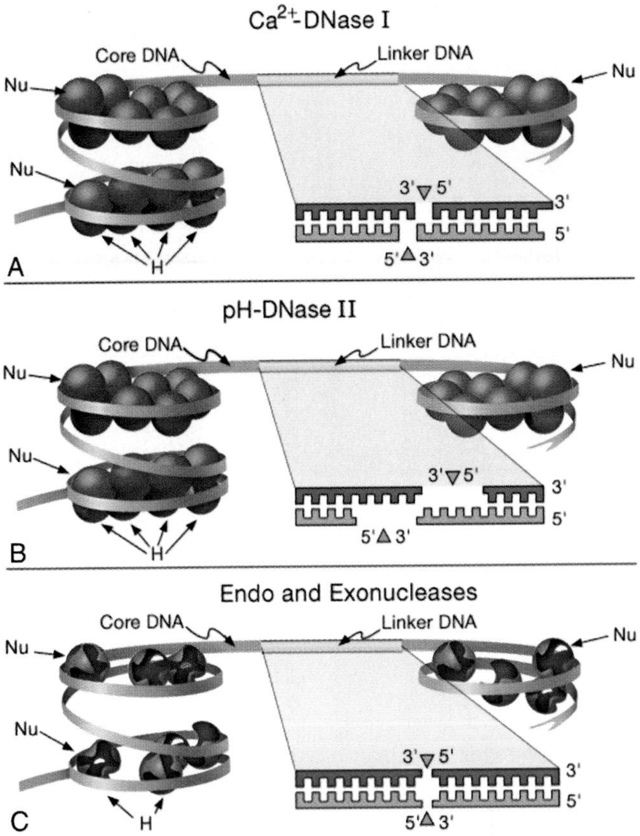

FIGURE 21–12 Schematic representation of chromatin structure and DNA damage associated with apoptosis **(A** and **B)** and necrosis **(C)**. Panels **A** to **C** each illustrate three nucleosomes (Nu) connected by linker DNA. Each nucleosome consists of a histone (H) core surrounded by two full turns of double-stranded DNA (Core DNA). A sequence of nucleotides present in the linker DNA is shown in the lower part of **A** and **B.** A similar sequence of nucleotides pertaining to the linker or core DNA is depicted in the lower part of **C. A,** DNA damage mediated by activation of Ca^{2+}-dependent DNase I characterized by staggered ends in the DNA with single-base 3′ overhangs (solid arrows in the sequence of the nucleotides). This type of DNA injury is identified by a polymerase chain reaction (PCR)–generated *Taq* polymerase probe, which processes complementary structures; this probe interacts only with damaged DNA exhibiting single-base 3′ overhangs. **B,** DNA damage mediated by activation of pH-dependent DNase II characterized by staggered ends in the DNA with one or more, up to four, base 3′ overhangs (solid arrows in the sequence of nucleotides). This type of DNA injury is identified by the terminal deoxynucleotidyl transferase (TdT) assay that links labeled nucleotides to 3′ overhangs, and the generated sequence can be visualized by fluorescence. **C,** DNA damage associated with cell necrosis. Loss of plasma membrane integrity and the release of lysosomal proteases lead to degradation of histones in the nucleosomes (Nu), which results in the loss of DNA protection and its exposure to endonucleases and exonucleases. Endonucleases produce double-strand cleavage of the DNA with recessed 3′ ends or 3′ overhangs, whereas exonucleases remove terminal nucleotides leading to a form of damage with blunt DNA ends (solid arrows in the sequence of nucleotides). This type of DNA injury is identified by a PCR-generated *Pfu* polymerase probe, which possesses complementary structures; this probe interacts only with damaged DNA exhibiting blunt ends. (From Anversa P: Myocyte apoptosis in the development of heart failure. *In* Braunwald E [ed]: Harrison's Advances in Cardiology. New York, McGraw Hill, 2003, pp 446-450.)

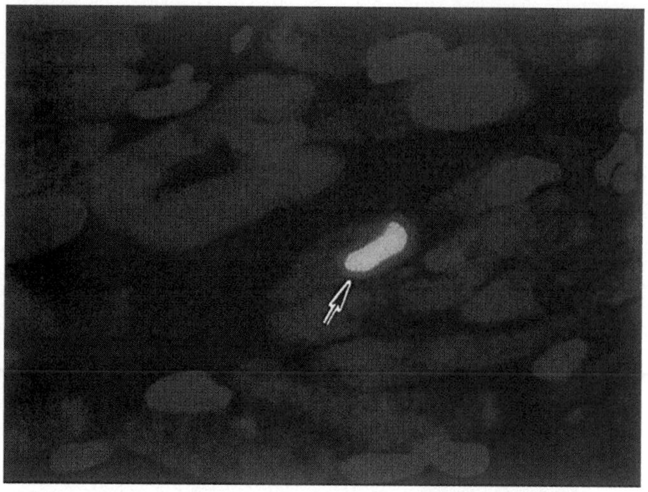

FIGURE 21–13 Human heart affected by end-stage ischemic cardiomyopathy. Confocal image illustrating an apoptotic myocyte by yellow fluorescence (arrow). The myocyte nucleus shows positive staining for terminal deoxynucleotidyl transferase assay. Red fluorescence of nuclei corresponds to propidium iodide staining, and red fluorescence of the myocyte cytoplasm corresponds to sarcomeric actin antibody labeling. Confocal microscopy, 800×. (From Anversa P: Myocyte apoptosis in the development of heart failure. *In* Braunwald E [ed]: Harrison's Advances in Cardiology. New York, McGraw Hill, 2003, pp 446-450.)

cardiac myocytes in vitro, including catecholamines acting through beta-adrenergic receptors,[49,50] angiotensin II,[51] reactive oxygen species (Fig. 21–14),[52] NO,[53] inflammatory cytokines, and mechanical strain.[54] Although the role of apoptosis in the transition to heart failure is not known, it appears likely that it represents an important cause of cell death in the failing heart.[9] Because both angiotensin II and catecholamines promote apoptosis, the therapeutic success of angiotensin-converting enzyme (ACE) inhibitors and beta-adrenergic antagonists in the treatment of heart failure suggests that this may be an important mechanism for myocardial failure.

Dropout of individual myocytes has also been observed in the senescent rat and human heart.[55] Olivetti and colleagues reported a loss of an average of 38 million nuclei per year in aging persons without cardiovascular disease. This loss in myocyte number was accompanied by a reciprocal increase in myocyte cell volume per nucleus, thereby preserving ventricular wall thickness.[56] This process, which appears to reflect myocyte death by both necrosis and apoptosis, may contribute to cardiac dysfunction and, when there is an additional stress such as hypertension, to the development of heart failure in elderly persons.

Alterations in Excitation-Contraction Coupling (see Chap. 20)

In addition to reducing the absolute number of myocytes, as already described, hemodynamic overload may cause a decrease in the *intrinsic* contractility of individual myocytes.[2] Several functional abnormalities involving excitation-contraction coupling, contractile proteins, and energetics have been identified in hypertrophied and failing myocardium.

Role of Calcium in Excitation-Contraction Coupling

Ca^{2+} plays a central role in the regulation of myocardial contraction and relaxation,[2,3,9,34,39] and there is increasing evidence that disturbances in Ca^{2+} handling play a central role in the disturbed contractile function in myocardial failure.

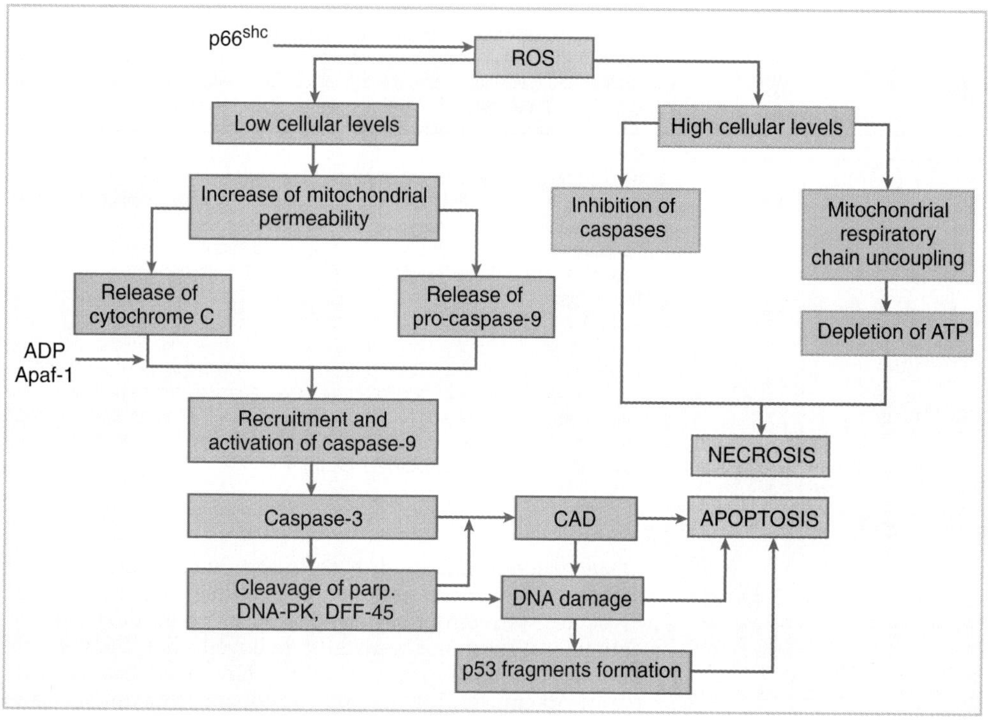

FIGURE 21–14 Scheme illustrating the effects of different levels of reactive oxygen species (ROS) on the activation of cell apoptosis and necrosis. Apaf-1 = apoptotic protease activating factor; ADP = adenosine diphosphate; ATP = adenosine triphosphate; CAD = caspase-activated deoxyribonuclease; DFF-45 = DNA fragmentation factor; DNA-PK = DNA-dependent protein kinase; parp = poly(ADP-ribose) polymerase. (From Anversa P: Myocardial basis for heart failure. Role of cell death. *In* Mann DL [ed]: Heart Failure: A Companion to Braunwald's Heart Disease. Philadelphia, Elsevier, 2004.)

Hypocalcemia, secondary to hypoparathyroidism and to a variety of other conditions, can cause heart failure that is responsive to the infusion of calcium. Elevation of serum ionized Ca^{2+} has been shown to augment contractility in patients with renal failure undergoing dialysis and in patients with severe heart failure secondary to cardiomyopathy who have downregulation of beta-adrenergic receptors.

Myocardium obtained at the time of cardiac transplantation from patients with end-stage heart failure exhibits abnormal prolongation of the action potential and developed force and impaired relaxation.[34] Observations using the Ca^{2+} indicator aequorin in myocardium have shown that these alterations in electrical and contractile properties are associated with a prolonged elevation of the intracellular Ca^{2+} transient during relaxation. Likewise, in myocytes obtained from patients with end-stage heart failure, the action potential is prolonged. The intracellular Ca^{2+} transient, as assessed by the fluorescent indicator fura-2, demonstrates a blunted rise with depolarization, reflecting slower delivery of Ca^{2+} to the contractile apparatus (causing slower activation) and a slowed rate of fall during repolarization (causing slowed relaxation) (Fig. 21–15).[57] These two abnormalities could explain both systolic and diastolic dysfunction.

Additional evidence of abnormal myocardial Ca^{2+} handling is provided by the observation that there is a reduction in the amount of tension-independent heat produced in myocardium from patients with heart failure.[58] Tension-independent heat, which is believed to reflect the energy expended for Ca^{2+} transport, can be used to estimate the amount of Ca^{2+} cycled per heartbeat. With this approach, it was shown that Ca^{2+} cycling is reduced by approximately 50 percent in failing human myocardium.[58]

FORCE-FREQUENCY RELATIONSHIP. In nonfailing myocardium, the force of contraction and rate of tension development rise with increased stimulation frequency, the so-called *positive force-frequency relationship* (see Chap. 19). However, there is evidence of an abnormal (negative) force-frequency relationship in failing human myocardium.[2] The mechanism responsible for this response appears to be impaired reuptake of calcium into the SR because of a decrease in Ca^{2+} adenosine triphosphatase (ATPase) (SERCA2) activity in failing myocardium.[34,39] Excitation-contraction coupling can also be assessed by examination of the force-frequency response. In normal myocardium, contractile force increases with increasing rates of stimulation, whereas in myocardium obtained from patients with end-stage heart failure the force-frequency response is markedly attenuated.[2,33] A similar phenomenon is observed in intact patients with heart failure studied at the time of catheterization. In patients with normal ventricular function, left ventricular contractility (as measured by +dP/dt or the end-systolic pressure-volume ratio) increases progressively as heart rate is increased by atrial pacing. By comparison, in patients with severe heart failure there is little or no increase in either contractile index. The normal force-frequency relationship depends on the cycling of Ca^{2+} between the SR and cytoplasm with each beat, an event that is accomplished by several enzymes and channels located in the sarcolemma, and SR (see Chap. 19). The expression or function, or both, of a number of these proteins may be altered in hypertrophied and failing myocardium,[59,60] leading to dysfunction of otherwise viable myocytes. Observations on the altered force-frequency relation in failing heart muscle are consistent with the suggestion that the quantity of Ca^{2+} released from the SR is reduced at more rapid heart rates.[61] There is evidence that Ca^{2+} release from the SR by the inward Ca^{2+} current during depolarization is reduced.

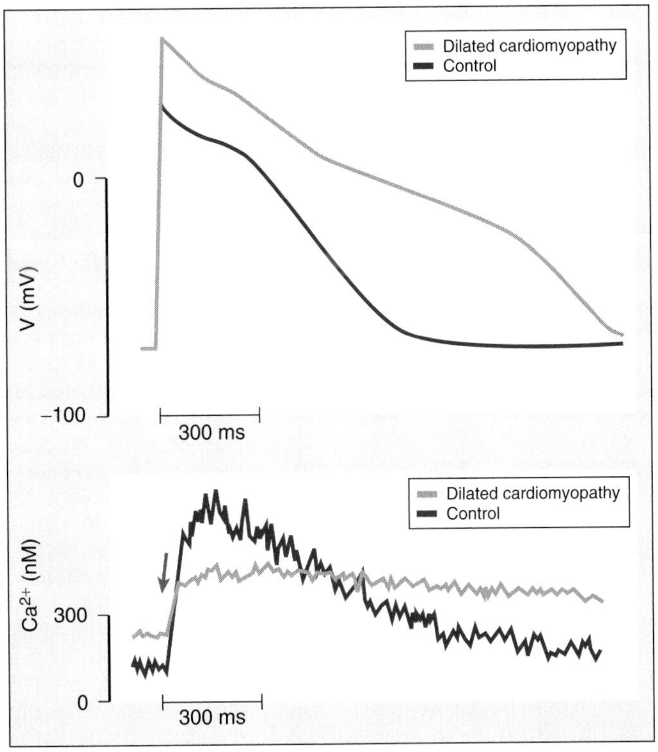

FIGURE 21–15 Abnormal action potential and intracellular calcium transient in failing cardiac myocytes. **Top,** The action potential recorded in a myocyte isolated from the heart of a patient with dilated cardiomyopathy is markedly prolonged compared with that in a myocyte from a normal heart (control). Such abnormalities could contribute to both the generation of arrhythmias and the abnormal diastolic relaxation. **Bottom,** The intracellular calcium transient measured with the fluorescent calcium indicator fura-2 is also markedly abnormal in myocytes isolated from the myocardium of patients with dilated cardiomyopathy. Compared with a normal myocyte (control), the myocyte from a patient with dilated cardiomyopathy shows an attenuated rise with depolarization (arrow) and a markedly delayed return to baseline. These abnormalities reflect the altered expression or function of key calcium-handling proteins (e.g., Ca^{2+}-adenosine triphosphatase) and probably contribute to the abnormal action potential in the top illustration. (Modified from Beuckelmann DJ, Nabauer M, Erdmann E: Intracellular calcium handling in isolated ventricular myocytes from patients with terminal heart failure. Circulation 85:1046, 1992. Copyright 1992, American Heart Association.)

SARCOPLASMIC RETICULUM Ca^{2+}-ATPASE AND PHOSPHOLAMBAN. A number of alterations in the SR in the failing heart have been described (Table 21–2). Ca^{2+} reuptake by the SR is mediated primarily by SERCA2. The activity of SERCA2 is inhibited by the associated protein phospholamban, and this inhibition is relieved by cyclic adenosine monophosphate (AMP)–mediated (e.g., by beta-adrenergic receptor stimulation) phosphorylation of phospholamban, thereby resulting in increased Ca^{2+} reuptake into the SR and the acceleration of diastolic relaxation (see Fig. 19–10). The reuptake of Ca^{2+} by the SR is equally important for normal systolic function, which requires that ample SR Ca^{2+} be available for release during systole to mediate contraction.

Several (but not all) reports indicate that the levels of SERCA2 messenger ribonucleic acid (mRNA) and protein are reduced in myocardium obtained from patients with end-stage heart failure as well as in the animal model of tachycardia-induced heart failure.[60] The decrease in SERCA2, which is part of an "adult" gene program in cardiac muscle, correlates inversely with the reexpression of fetal genes such as atrial natriuretic peptide (ANP) (Fig. 21–16). This shift in SERCA2 expression was associated with a corresponding

TABLE 21–2 Sarcoplasmic Reticulum Alterations in the Failing Heart

Protein	Change in Human Heart Failure
Sarcoplasmic Reticulum	
Calcium pump ATPase (SERCA)	Normal or decreased
Phospholamban	Normal or decreased
Calcium release channel (ryanodine receptor)	Normal or decreased
Calsequestrin	Normal
Calreticulin	Normal
Plasma Membrane	
L-type calcium channels	?Increased channel opening
Sodium/calcium exchanger	Increased
Sodium pump	Reexpression of fetal isoforms

ATPase = adenosine triphosphatase.

From Katz AM: Heart Failure. Philadelphia, Lippincott Williams & Wilkins, 2000.

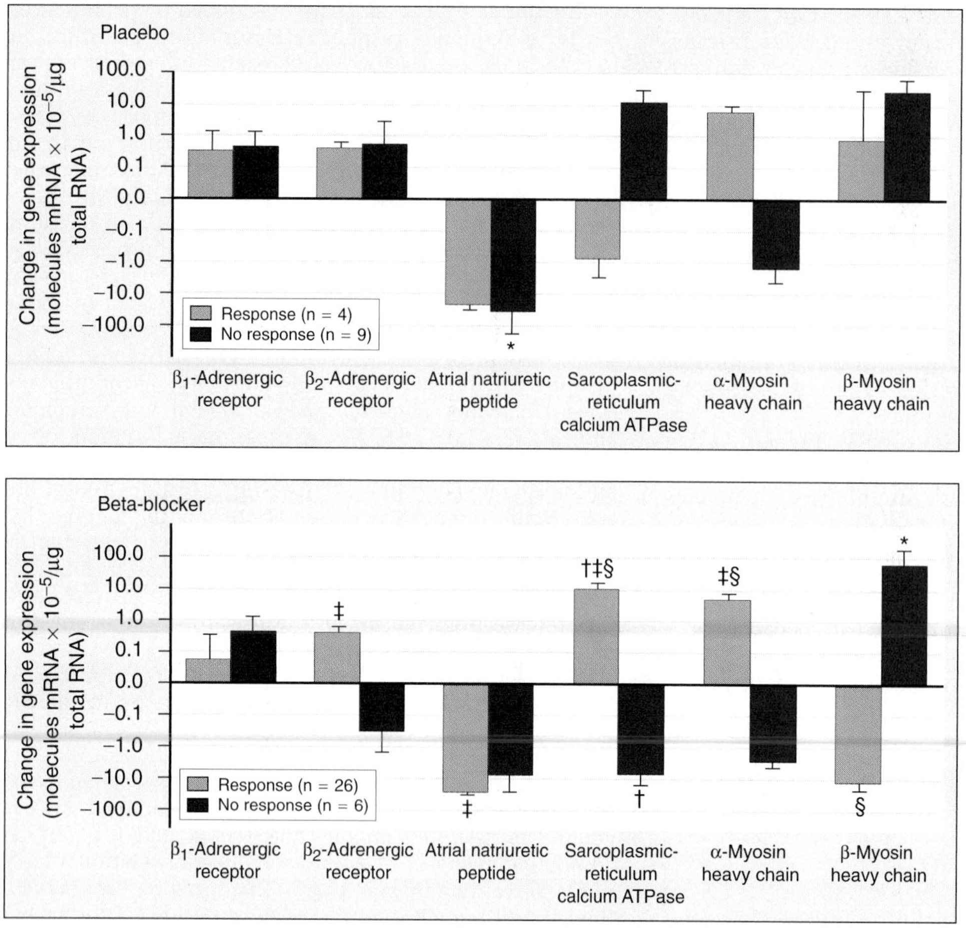

FIGURE 21–16 Changes in myocardial messenger RNA (mRNA) expression and beta-adrenergic receptor protein levels. **A** and **B,** Changes between baseline and the end of the 6-month study in the abundance of myocardial mRNA for six contractility-regulating or hypertrophy-regulating proteins in patients who received placebo or a beta blocker. The changes in patients who had an improvement in left ventricular ejection fraction (a "response," defined as an increase by at least five ejection fraction [EF] units) were compared with the changes in patients who did not have such a response. Gene expression is shown as molecules of mRNA per microgram of total RNA on a logarithmic scale; The asterisk indicates $p < 0.10$ for the change between the baseline value and the value measured at 6 months by the paired t-test, the daggers $p < 0.05$ for the comparison with the placebo group by the test for interaction, the double daggers $p < 0.05$ for the change between the baseline value and the value measured at 6 months by the paired t-test, and the section marks $p < 0.05$ for the comparison with patients who did not have a response. Each panel shows results for patients with complete data for the indicated mRNA and receptor protein measurements. (From Lowes BD, Gilbert EM, Abraham WT, et al: Myocardial gene expression in dilated cardiomyopathy treated with beta blocking agents. N Engl J Med 346:1357, 2002.)

reduction in SR Ca^{2+} reuptake in some[62-64] (but not all) studies of human myocardium from patients with severe failure. Furthermore, the decreases in SERCA2 protein and Ca^{2+}-ATPase activity have been shown to correlate inversely with the force-frequency relationship,[63] suggesting that reduced expression of SERCA2 contributes to intrinsic myocyte dysfunction. In vitro, mechanical strain and several agonists such as NE and angiotensin II downregulate the expression of SERCA2 in cardiac myocytes. It has been proposed that the reduced activity of SERCA2 alters Ca^{2+} release from the SR; this alteration impairs both contraction and relaxation and is responsible for the transition from compensation to heart failure.[65]

Because phospholamban activity inhibits SERCA2, the net activity of SERCA2 depends on the ratio of SERCA2 to phospholamban.[66] The expression of phospholamban is decreased in failing human myocardium,[62] as is its phosphorylation,[2,3,9] and this may interfere with SR function. Viral expression vectors have been used to express SERCA2 and phospholamban in cultured cardiac myocytes.[67] SERCA2 has also been expressed in transgenic mice[68] and in rat hearts after direct injection of an adenovirus carrying the gene.[69] These or similar approaches might allow the use of SERCA2 or inhibitors of phospholamban to augment myocyte function in patients. It has been suggested that induced changes in the ratio of SERCA2 to its inhibitor phospholamban can alter Ca^{2+} handling by the failing heart.

Na^+/Ca^{2+} EXCHANGER. The Na^+/Ca^{2+} exchanger in the cell membrane accounts for approximately 20 percent of the removal of Ca^{2+} from the cytoplasm during diastole. Abnormalities in Na^+/Ca^{2+} exchange have been demonstrated in heart failure.[2,3,9] The mRNA and protein levels of the Na^+/Ca^{2+} exchanger were found to be increased in myocardium obtained from patients with heart failure related to both ischemic and idiopathic dilated cardiomyopathy and correlated inversely with the decrease in SERCA2 mRNA levels.[69] This augmentation in Na^+/Ca^{2+} exchange activity might be a compensatory response to the reduction in Ca^{2+} reuptake caused by a decrease in SERCA2. In animals with experimental heart failure, impaired cytosolic Ca^{2+} removal caused by reduced SERCA2 was partially compensated for by an increase in the Na^+/Ca^{2+} exchanger.[69,70] Although this compensation would facilitate diastolic Ca^{2+} removal, it might do so at the expense of increased arrhythmogenicity because Ca^{2+} efflux by this mechanism is associated with an influx of Na^+ that can prolong depolarization and cause afterdepolarizations.

THE Ca^{2+} RELEASE CHANNEL. The Ca^{2+} release channel (CRC), located on the SR, mediates the release of Ca^{2+} from the SR into the myoplasm during systole and is therefore critical to the activation of the contractile elements of the myocyte. Some[71] (but not all[72]) studies of failing human myocardium have shown decreases in the mRNA level for the CRC. In addition, in myocardium from patients with heart failure the CRC is hyperphosphorylated by protein kinase A, resulting in a high rate of Ca^{2+} "leakage" from the SR. This leakage can reduce the SR Ca^{2+} content, release, and net uptake,[2,73-75] and treatment with beta blockers has been shown to restore CRC function toward normal[76]

VOLTAGE-DEPENDENT Ca^{2+} CHANNEL. The mRNA and protein levels of the voltage-dependent Ca^{2+} channel have also been shown to be decreased in failing human myocardium obtained from patients with both ischemic heart disease and dilated cardiomyopathy, which may contribute to a depressed calcium transient[77] leading to impaired excitation-contraction coupling.

CALSEQUESTRIN. This is the major protein in the SR that binds Ca^{2+} and thereby serves a storage function. Several studies have found calsequestrin mRNA levels to be unchanged in failing human myocardium.

Alterations in the Contractile Apparatus

Patients with aortic stenosis without heart failure exhibit a normal fraction of myofibrils per cell, whereas those with left ventricular failure show a significant reduction in cell volume occupied by myofibrils, suggesting that this reduction in the quantity of the contractile machinery may play a role in the development of cardiac decompensation. In end-stage heart failure in the human, electron microscopic observations likewise show a reduction of ventricular myofibrillar protein (Table 21–3).

Reduction of Myosin Adenosine Triphosphatase Activity

Considerable data suggest that qualitative, as well as quantitative, alterations of contractile proteins occur in heart failure. First, the finding that the reduced velocity of contraction of failing myocardium occurs in chemically skinned ventricular fibers suggests that this change reflects intrinsic alterations in the contractile apparatus. Early studies showed that the activity of myofibrillar ATPase was reduced in the hearts of patients who died of heart failure.[9,78] Furthermore, reductions in the activities of myofibrillar ATPase, actomyosin ATPase, or myosin ATPase have been demonstrated in several animal models of heart failure. These depressions of enzymatic activity could occur if an altered subunit of the myosin molecule (i.e., the portion of the molecule responsible for the ATPase activity) were produced in the overloaded heart and reduced contractility by lowering the rate of interaction between actin and myosin filaments. A reduction in the Mg^{2+}-ATPase activity (which expresses the response of myofibrils to Ca^{2+}) has been demonstrated in myofibrils obtained from patients with end-stage heart failure at the time of transplantation and in less sick patients undergoing valve replacement.[79]

MYOSIN ISOFORM CHANGES. Animal studies have indicated that when the adult heart hypertrophies, fetal and neonatal forms of contractile proteins (termed isoforms) and other proteins (such as ANP) reappear, signifying reexpression of the genes for these fetal and neonatal isoforms.[80] Thus, hemodynamic overload leads to enhanced overall protein synthesis[9] and alters the proteins qualitatively as well (i.e., it leads to the synthesis of protein isoforms that were present during fetal and neonatal life when protein synthesis in the heart was also rapid).

TABLE 21–3 Contractile Protein Alterations in the Failing Heart

Protein	Experimental Heart Failure	Human Heart Failure
Myosin heavy chain	Reversion to fetal phenotype	Reversion to fetal phenotype
Myosin light chains	Reversion to fetal phenotype	Reversion to fetal phenotype
Actin	Reversion to fetal phenotype	No change
Troponin I	Reversion to fetal phenotype	Reversion to fetal phenotype
Troponin T	Reversion to fetal phenotype	Reversion to fetal phenotype
Troponin C	No change	No change
Tropomyosin	No change	No change

From Katz AM: Heart Failure. Philadelphia, Lippincott Williams & Wilkins, 2000.

Altered isoforms of cardiac proteins may arise from the expression of different members of a multigene family or from the assembly of the same gene in a different pattern. In rodents the predominant myosin heavy chain (MHC) is the "fast" V_1 isoform (high ATPase activity, encoded by the alpha-MHC gene). With pressure-induced hypertrophy or myocardial failure after myocardial infarction in the rat, there is reexpression of the "slow" V_3 isoform (low ATPase activity, encoded by the beta-MHC gene) and deinduction of the V_1 isoform.[80] A shift in MHC isoforms would provide an attractive explanation for the reduction in myofibrillar ATPase activity observed in failing human myocardium. However, the predominant MHC isoform in humans is the slower V_3 isoform (encoded by the beta-MHC gene) and the V_1 isoform (encoded by the alpha-MHC mRNA) has been difficult to detect, making it appear unlikely that a shift in myosin isoforms is responsible for the observed decrease in myosin ATPase activity in failing human myocardium. However, the use of more refined methodology has demonstrated that alpha-MHC accounts for about 33 percent of MHC mRNA in normal human myocardium and is markedly reduced to about 2 percent in failing myocardium.[81,82] It remains to be determined whether the decrease in alpha-MHC mRNA translates into a comparable decrease in the ratio of the beta- to alpha-MHC protein isoforms and, thus, a decrease in ATPase activity.

Bristow and colleagues measured the expression of mRNA for alpha- and beta-MHC in right ventricular biopsy specimens from patients with idiopathic dilated cardiomyopathy at 6-month intervals.[80,83] In patients with an improvement in left ventricular function there were reciprocal changes in the levels of alpha-MHC (increase) and beta-MHC (decrease) mRNA but no consistent changes in the mRNA levels for SERCA2, the $beta_1$- or $beta_2$-adrenergic receptors, or ANP. They further showed that patients who had a good hemodynamic response to beta blocker therapy had a similar increase in the alpha-/beta-MHC ratio. These observations support the thesis that a decrease in the expression of alpha-MHC plays a significant role in the pathophysiology of dilated cardiomyopathy.

ALTERED REGULATORY PROTEINS. Another possible cause of a decrease in cardiac contractile function is an alteration in the expression or activity, or both, of regulatory proteins. In animals with experimental heart failure, there are changes in the myosin light chain and the troponin-tropomyosin complex.[84] Changes in myosin light chain isoforms have been observed in the atria and ventricles of patients whose hearts have been subjected to mechanical overload; and the expression of troponin T, a component of the troponin complex that regulates the interaction of myosin and actin, was found to be altered in failing human myocardium. In normal myocardium, troponin T is expressed as a single isoform (T_1), which accounts for approximately 98 percent of the troponin T. In myocardium from patients with end-stage heart failure, a second isoform (T_2) was found to be expressed at increased levels, and its level of expression was related to the severity of heart failure.[85]

Mice with deletion of the troponin I gene are born normally but express a fetal isoform of troponin that takes the place of the absent adult isoform. Over time, the expression of the fetal isoform decreases and the mice develop lethal heart failure.[86] Likewise, the transgenic overexpression of a mutant tropomyosin results in increased calcium sensitivity and decreased rate of relaxation.[87] Although the clinical significance of changes in the expression of troponin and other regulatory proteins remains to be determined, these observations suggest that important functional changes in contractile proteins could be due to changes in regulatory proteins and need not reflect alterations in the contractile proteins themselves.[88]

Alterations in the Cardiac Matrix

The structural properties of the ventricle are determined not only by its myocytes but also by the interstitial connective tissue, which is rich in type I and type III fibrillar collagen (Fig. 21–17).[89,90] The latter provides struts along which the myocytes are aligned. Branches of collagen fibers course at right angles to connect and align muscle bundles. A depletion of these struts may lead to chamber dilation, and an excess may interfere with ventricular relaxation and filling. Thus, the quantity and type of ECM can have profound effects on the diastolic properties of the myocardium by affecting its elasticity and physical disposition.[90,91]

REGULATION OF INTERSTITIAL COLLAGEN. The quantity and nature of the collagen in the ECM are determined by the balance between synthesis and degradation. The latter is regulated by the opposing actions of matrix metalloproteinases (MMPs), a family of enzymes that degrade matrix proteins, and tissue inhibitors of metalloproteinases (TIMPs), a family of enzymes that inhibit the activity of MMPs (Fig. 21–18).[91] The ECM is a dynamic system. It changes with and contributes to ventricular remodeling in the presence of pressure and volume overload, myocardial infarction, and cardiomyopathy (Table 21–4).[89]

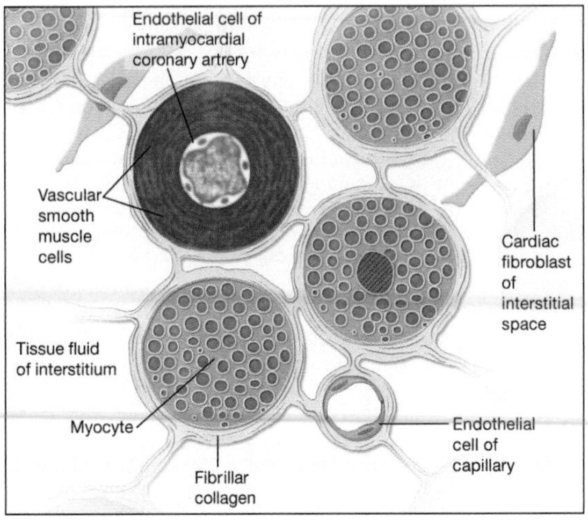

FIGURE 21–17 Myocyte and nonmyocyte constituents of the heart. Although myocytes are the major components of the heart on the basis of mass, they represent only a minority of the cells on the basis of number. Nonmyocyte cellular constituents of the myocardium include fibroblasts, smooth muscle cells, and endothelial cells. Myocytes and nonmyocytes are interconnected by a complex of connective tissue and extracellular matrix. Components of the extracellular matrix include collagens, proteoglycans (such as fibronectin), several peptide growth factors, and proteases (such as plasminogen activators). There is increasing appreciation that by regulating the nature and quantity of the extracellular matrix, nonmyocytes in the heart play an important role in determining the response of the myocardium to pathologic stimuli, such as hemodynamic overload. (From Colucci WS [ed]: Atlas of Heart Failure: Cardiac Function and Dysfunction. 3rd ed. Philadelphia, Current Medicine, 2002, p 7.7. Adapted from Weber KT, Brilla CG: Pathological hypertrophy and cardiac interstitium. Fibrosis and renin-angiotensin-aldosterone system. Circulation 83:1849, 1991.)

COLLAGEN STRUT DEPLETION. In myocardium from humans and animal models of systolic failure, ultrastructural observations have shown a depletion of the fibrillar collagen struts that help to maintain the alignment of myocytes. It has been proposed that *depletion* of the collagen struts may contribute to chamber dilation by allowing "slippage" of myocytes.[91] This thesis is consistent with the observation that the activity of MMPs is increased in myocardium obtained from patients with end-stage heart failure[92] and in animal models of heart failure.[93] Likewise, the activity of TIMPs is decreased in myocardium from patients with end-stage heart failure.[94] A role for MMPs is supported by the demonstration that an MMP inhibitor partially protected against the loss of collagen struts in an animal model of heart failure.[95] It has been shown that post-myocardial infarction remodeling is exacerbated in mice deficient in TIMP-1,[96] whereas it is ameliorated in mice with the targeted deletion of MMP9.[97] In patients with dilated cardiomyopathy, reduced fibrillar collagen and its cross-linking have been reported.

INTERSTITIAL MATRIX ACCUMULATION. On the other hand, in experimentally induced chronic pressure overload hypertrophy, as well as in patients with hypertension, there is an *increase* in the quantity of interstitial collagen, which may contribute to the characteristic abnormalities of diastolic function.[91] The spontaneously hypertensive rat develops progressive myocardial hypertrophy and failure with age. Papillary muscles from these animals have increased passive stiffness that is associated with increased left ventricular collagen concentration, interstitial fibrosis,[98] and expression of mRNAs for collagen and transforming growth factor-alpha (TGF-α).[99] Treatment with an ACE inhibitor prevented the increases in muscle stiffness, interstitial fibrosis, and the induction of collagen and TGF-α mRNAs.[100] Thus, it seems likely that pathways leading to increased collagen accumulation are involved in the pathogenesis of diastolic dysfunction.

Myocardial Energetics in Heart Failure

The heart is an aerobic organ requiring substantial energy. Energy is required for myofibrillar contraction and relaxation, the uptake (against a concentration gradient) of Ca^{2+} into the SR, and the restoration of ion concentrations between the

TABLE 21–4 Extracellular Myocardial Remodeling Events During the Progression of Heart Failure: A Summary of Potential Global Extracellular Matrix Changes in the Left Ventricular Remodeling Process

Disease Process	Myocardial Infarction	Hypertrophy	Cardiomyopathy
Early adaptive phase	ECM proteolysis in MI region Activation of MMPs Rapid ECM turnover MI scar formation	ECM turnover to facilitate myocyte growth ECM biosynthesis rates favor accumulation Diminished MMP activity	Biophysical stress induces MMPs Proteolysis of normal ECM
Compensatory phase	Scar maturation ECM accumulation in viable myocardium Persistent ECM turnover in MI border zone	ECM reaches steady state Continued downregulation of MMPs	Induction of "MMP portfolio" and continued ECM turnover Diminished ECM support of myocytes
Transition to failure	Continued ECM proteolysis in MI border and infarct expansion LV wall remodeling and dilation Increased MMPs and acceleration of LV remodeling and dilation	Increased myocardial stiffness due to ECM accumulation and impairment of diastolic function	Increased MMP activation and reduced inhibitory control Accelerated proteolysis of normal ECM structure and loss of structural support LV dilation and diminished transduction of myocyte shortening

ECM = extracellular matrix; LV = left ventricular; MI = myocardial infarction; MMP = matrix metalloproteinase.
From Gunasinghe SK, Spinale FG: Myocardial basis for heart failure. *In* Mann DL (ed): Heart Failure. Philadelphia, Elsevier, 2004, p 66.

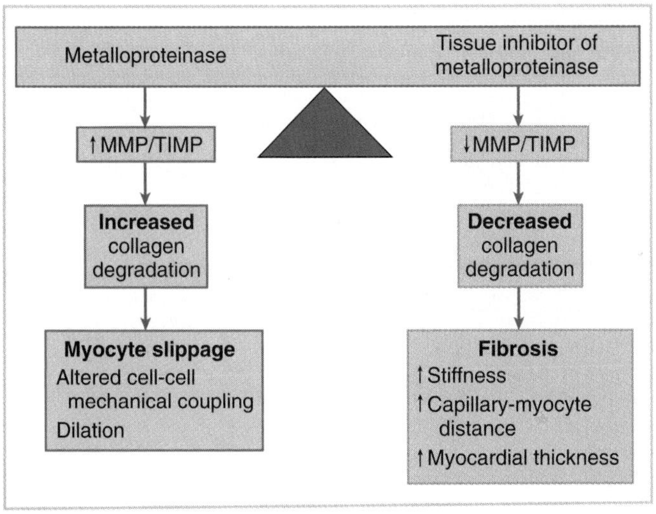

FIGURE 21–18 The regulation of extracellular matrix degradation is determined by the balance between the activity of matrix metalloproteinases (MMPs) and their tissue inhibitors (TIMPs). Both an increase in MMP activity and a decrease in TIMP activity have been observed in failing myocardium from patients. Theoretically, such an increase in the MMP/TIMP ratio could contribute to depletion of the fibrillar collagen struts that tether myocytes together and might thus contribute to chamber dilation. Conversely, an increase in extracellular matrix accumulation, which might occur as the result of a decrease in the MMP/TIMP ratio or an increase in matrix synthesis, could contribute to chamber stiffness and abnormal relaxation. (From Sawyer DB, Colucci WS: Molecular and cellular events in myocardial hypertrophy and failure. *In* Colucci WS [ed]: Atlas of Heart Failure: Cardiac Function and Dysfunction. 3rd ed. Philadelphia, Current Medicine, 2002, p 7.8.)

extracellular and intracellular spaces in diastole. Although acutely induced energy deficiency, as occurs in severe ischemia, can interfere with cardiac contraction and relaxation, heart failure frequently occurs in the presence of adequate myocardial perfusion, oxygen, and substrate. When contractility is acutely depressed in experimental preparations, myocardial oxygen consumption of the intact ventricle also declines.[101] However, in chronic heart failure myocardial O_2 consumption is normal or increased.[102]

MYOCARDIAL ENERGY PRODUCTION. Lactate is a more important fuel for energy generation in heart failure than in the normal state.[102] Considerable dispute has centered on the question of whether mitochondrial oxidative phosphorylation (i.e., ATP production) is abnormal in heart failure. The cytochromes are located in the inner mitochondrial membrane and are constituents of the respiratory chain that couples oxidation to the synthesis of chemical energy. In one study in human dilated cardiomyopathy, a reduction in cytochrome *a* content and in cytochrome-dependent enzyme activity was reported.[103] Mitochondria obtained from failing human cardiac muscle have also shown reduced oxygen consumption during active phosphorylation and reduced rates of reduced nicotinamide adenine dinucleotide (NADH)–linked respiratory activity. These and other observations have led to the thesis that myocardial failure in the setting of hemodynamic overload may be related to an inability of oxidative phosphorylation (i.e., ATP production by mitochondria) to keep pace with the needs of the contractile apparatus. Katz has proposed that the mitochondrial abnormalities observed in the failing heart may be the result of damage to these structures and that the resultant mitochondrial abnormalities reduce the high-energy phosphates available for contraction and thereby contribute to the development of heart failure.[9]

The nucleotide-transporting protein located on the inner mitochondrial membrane, the so-called adenosine diphosphate (ADP)-ATP carrier, has been identified as an autoantigen in viral myocarditis and in dilated cardiomyopathy. In guinea pigs immunized to this carrier protein, both myocardial oxygen flux (i.e., O_2 production and consumption) and cardiac work fell.[104] These findings are compatible with the hypothesis that the impaired cardiac performance in some cases of myocarditis (and dilated cardiomyopathy) may be secondary to an imbalance between energy delivery and demand.

MYOCARDIAL ENERGY RESERVES. Observations on myocardial ATP concentration in compensated *hypertrophy* have shown no consistent change.[105] However, in myocardium from dogs with heart failure related to rapid pacing or chronic ischemia and from humans with end-stage cardiomyopathy, ATP, the total adenine nucleotide pool (ATP, AMP, and AMP), creatine kinase (CK) activity (required for synthesis of ATP), the concentrations of creatine phosphate (CrP), and the CPr/ATP ratio were all decreased[102,105-107] whereas the ATP/AMP and ATP/ADP ratios were maintained as the total adenine pool declined.[102] ATP synthesis and utilization were both reduced and, because the latter may exceed the former, ATP concentration declined. These observations have led to the hypothesis that myocardial failure may be the consequence of decreased energy reserve or at least that such decreased reserve contributes to the development of heart failure (Fig. 21–19). The measurement of CK flux provides a sensitive measure of myocardial energy reserves and may detect abnormalities in the absence of changes in ATP and CrP concentrations. By studying high-energy flux in vivo using nuclear magnetic resonance (NMR) technology, it has been demonstrated that CK activity is markedly reduced in the myopathic Syrian hamster. This abnormality was almost completely corrected by treatment with an ACE inhibitor. Likewise, in turkeys with furazolidone-induced heart failure, contractile failure was associated with a reduction in ATP, CrP, and CK activity.[102]

The mechanism responsible for the decrease in CK activity is not understood, but it is associated with alterations in the isoforms of CK. In failing myocardium, there was a decrease in the adult (MM) isoform and an increase or no change in the fetal isoform (MB).[105] The effect of

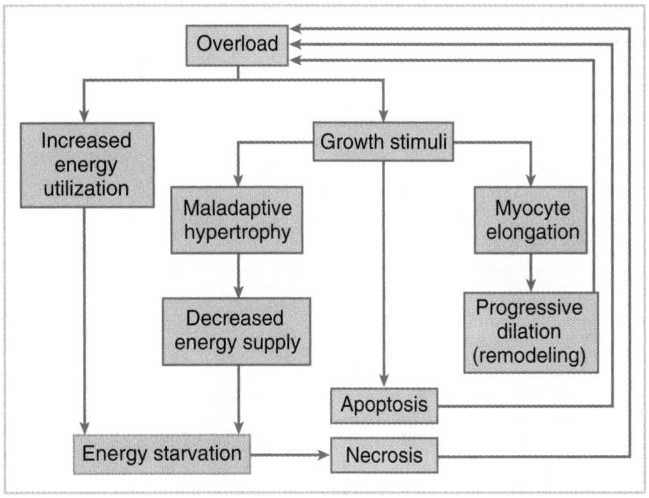

FIGURE 21–19 Some of the vicious circles that operate in the overloaded heart. Overload both increases energy utilization and stimulates growth. The former contributes directly to a state of energy starvation, which is made worse by several consequences of maladaptive hypertrophy that decrease energy supply. The latter include myocyte elongation, which causes remodeling, a progressive dilation that increases wall tension so as to increase the overload. Growth stimuli also promote apoptosis, which by decreasing the number of viable cardiac myocytes increases the load on those that survive. Hypertrophy also causes architectural changes that reduce the energy supply to working cardiac myocytes. (From Katz AM: Heart Failure. Philadelphia, Lippincott Williams & Wilkins, 2000.)

decreased CK activity on myocardial function and energetics was tested in mice with genetic deficiencies of the CK M isoform, the mitochondrial isoform, or both. The mice lacking both isoforms had a greater increase in ADP and a more pronounced decrease in the free energy released from ATP, suggesting that cardiac work was more costly energetically. In studies of rat hearts hypertrophied consequent to aortic bounding, increase in ADP and inorganic phosphate (P_i) were associated with slowing of cross-bridge cycling as well as cardiac relaxation.[102]

NMR spectroscopy with phosphorus-31, a noninvasive technique (see Chap. 13), has been employed to study the CrP-to-ATP ratio (CrP/ATP) in normal subjects and in patients. Reductions have been described in patients with severe aortic valve disease, cardiomyopathy, and myocardial ischemia.[108,109] In patients with chronic mitral regurgitation, the reduction in CrP/ATP has been found to be related to the severity of the hemodynamic impairment as reflected in the left ventricular end-systolic diameter. The extent of reduction of the ratio has been shown to correlate with the clinical severity of the heart failure and with the prognosis (Fig. 21-20).[110] These changes in CrP/ATP may be caused by the previously mentioned reduction in the phosphorylation of creatine and of CK activity.[102,105-107,111]

One unusual form of heart failure that is primarily related to a reduction of myocardial energy stores is that caused by phosphate deficiency. Chronic hypophosphatemia induced by dietary means is associated with reversible depression of myocardial performance in isolated muscle as well as in the intact heart of animals and humans, presumably as a consequence of reduced ATP stores.[112]

In the final analysis, the reduction of high-energy phosphates in the failing heart results in a decrease in the quantity of energy made available by the hydrolysis of ATP. When severe, the reduction in the energy available to the SR for Ca^{2+} uptake impairs relaxation (diastolic failure) and in that available to the contractile apparatus impairs cross-bridge cycling (systolic failure).[102]

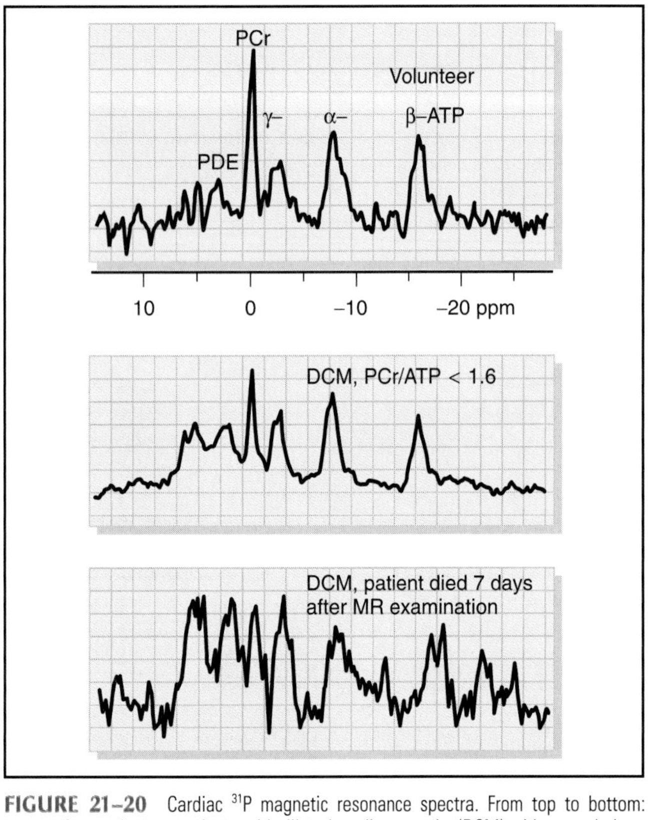

FIGURE 21–20 Cardiac ^{31}P magnetic resonance spectra. From top to bottom: spectra from volunteer patients with dilated cardiomyopathy (DCM) with normal phosphocreatine/ATP ratio and severely reduced phosphocreatine/ATP ratio; the latter patient died 7 days after the magnetic resonance examination. (From Neubauer S, Horn M, Cramer M, et al: Myocardial phosphocreatine-to-ATP ratio is a predictor of mortality in patients with dilated cardiomyopathy. Circulation 96:2190, 1997. Copyright 1997, American Heart Association.)

Pathophysiology of Diastolic Heart Failure (see also Chaps. 19 and 20)

Alterations in Diastolic Properties

Approximately one-third of patients with heart failure have predominantly diastolic heart failure (see Chap. 22), which may be defined as pulmonary (or systemic) venous congestion, and the symptoms consequent thereto in the presence of normal or almost normal systolic function.[113-116] Several mechanisms may be operative (Fig. 21–21). Approximately one third have predominantly disordered systolic function, and the remainder exhibit impairment of both systolic and diastolic function. Left ventricular pressure-volume loops displaying the difference between systolic and diastolic heart failure are shown in Figure 22–3. Among patients with the clinical diagnosis of congestive heart failure in the Framingham Heart Study population, 51 percent had a left ventricular ejection fraction greater than or equal to 0.50.[115]

ALTERED VENTRICULAR RELAXATION (see also Sarcoplasmic Reticulum Ca^{2+}-ATPase and Phospholamban, earlier). Although two aspects of the heart's diastolic characteristics (i.e., relaxation and wall stiffness) are often considered together, they actually describe two different properties.[113,114] Relaxation (inactivation of contraction) is a dynamic process that begins at the termination of contraction and occurs during isovolumetric relaxation and early ventricular filling (Fig. 21–22; see Fig. 19–19). The rate of ventricular relaxation is controlled primarily by the uptake of Ca^{2+} by the SR but also by the efflux of Ca^{2+} from the myocyte. These processes are regulated by SERCA2 as well as by sarcolemmal calcium pumps (see Table 21–2). Because these Ca^{2+} movements are against concentration gradients, they are energy consuming. Therefore, reductions in ATP concentration due to ischemia-induced ATP depletion interfere with these processes and slow myocardial relaxation (see Fig. 21–22A). Increases in cytoplasmic P_i contribute to this effect.[102] On the other hand, beta-adrenergic receptor stimulation, by increasing cyclic AMP and cyclic AMP–dependent protein kinase activity, causes the phosphorylation of phospholamban (see Chap. 19), which accelerates Ca^{2+} uptake by the SR and thereby enhances relaxation.

Impaired relaxation can also be caused by abnormalities in the sarcolemmal channels through which Ca^{2+} is extruded from the cytoplasm, in the Na^+/Ca^{2+} exchanger (see Na^+/Ca^{2+} Exchanger, earlier), as well as in the phosphorylation of proteins that affect SERCA2 such as phospholamban.[116] Cardiac relaxation requires hydrolysis of ATP for detachment of

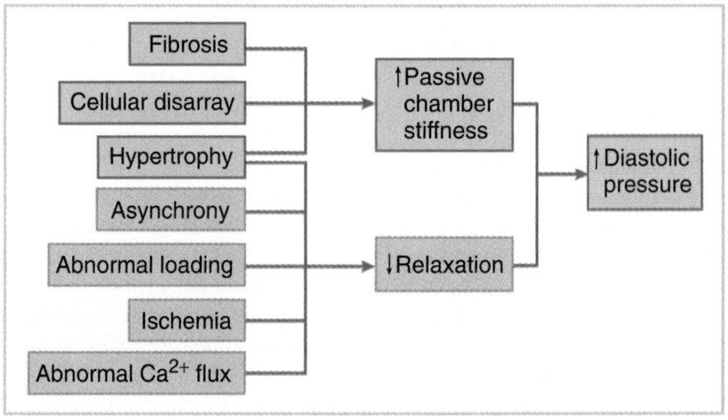

FIGURE 21–21 Factors responsible for diastolic dysfunction and increased left ventricular diastolic pressure. (From Gaasch WH, Izzi G: Clinical diagnosis and management of left ventricular diastolic dysfunction. *In* Hori M, Suga H, Baan J, Yellin EL [eds]: Cardiac Mechanics and Function in the Normal and Diseased Heart. New York, Springer-Verlag, 1989, p 296.)

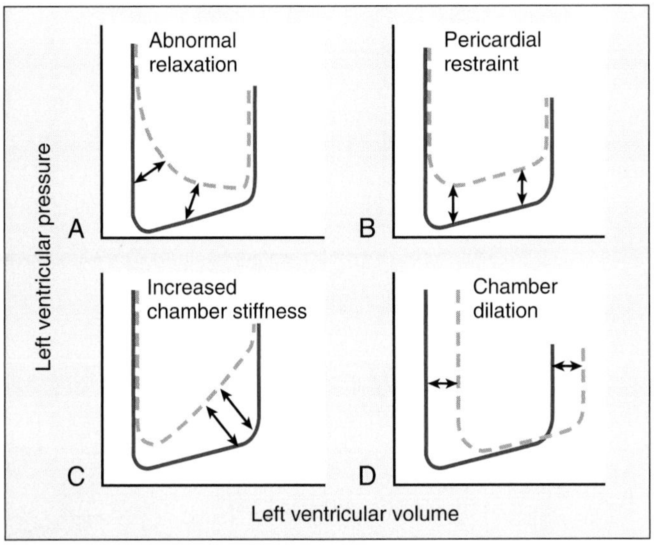

FIGURE 21–22 Mechanisms that cause diastolic dysfunction. Only the bottom half of the pressure-volume loop is depicted. Solid lines represent normal subjects; dashed lines represent patients with diastolic dysfunction. (From Zile MR: Diastolic dysfunction: Detection, consequences, and treatment: II. Diagnosis and treatment of diastolic function. Mod Concepts Cardiovasc Dis 59:1, 1990. Copyright 1990, American Heart Association.)

myosin from actin. Ischemia (or any process including heart failure; see earlier) that reduces myocyte ATP concentration can interfere with this process as well.

ALTERED VENTRICULAR FILLING. During early ventricular filling, the myocardium normally lengthens rapidly and homogeneously. Regional variation in the onset, rate, and extent of myocardial lengthening is referred to as *ventricular heterogeneity* or *diastolic asynergy.* Temporal dispersion of relaxation, with some fibers lengthening later than others, is referred to as *diastolic asynchrony.*[117] Both diastolic asynergy and asynchrony interfere with early diastolic filling. In contrast to these early diastolic events, myocardial *elasticity* (i.e., the change in muscle length for a change in force), ventricular *compliance* (i.e., the change in ventricular volume for a given change in pressure), and ventricular *stiffness* (i.e., the inverse of compliance) are generally measured in the relaxed ventricle at end diastole.

These diastolic properties of the ventricle are described by its curvilinear pressure-volume relation (see Fig. 21–22D). The slope of a tangent to this curvilinear relation (dP/dv) defines the chamber compliance at any level of filling pressure. An increase in chamber stiffness may occur secondary to any one or a combination of these three mechanisms:

1. *A rise in filling pressure* (i.e., movement of the ventricle up along its pressure-volume [stress-strain] curve to a steeper portion) (see Fig. 21–22D). This rise may occur in conditions such as volume overload secondary to acute valvular regurgitation and in acute left ventricular failure caused by myocarditis.
2. *A shift to a steeper ventricular pressure-volume* (see Fig. 21–22C) *or stress-strain curve.* Such an increase in stiffness results most commonly from an increase in ventricular mass and wall thickness. Thus, although hypertrophy constitutes a principal compensatory mechanism to sustain systolic emptying of the overloaded ventricle, it may simultaneously interfere with the ventricle's diastolic properties and impair ventricular filling. This shift to a steeper pressure-volume curve can also be caused by an increase in *intrinsic* myocardial stiffness (the stiffness of a unit of the cardiac wall regardless of the total mass or thickness of the myocardium), as occurs with disorders in which there is myocardial infiltration (e.g., amyloidosis), myocardial or endomyocardial fibrosis, or myocardial ischemia.
3. *A parallel upward displacement of the diastolic pressure-volume curve.* This effect is generally referred to as a *decrease in ventricular distensibility* and is usually caused by extrinsic compression of the ventricles, as occurs in cardiac tamponade or constrictive pericarditis (see Chap. 64) (see Fig. 21–22B).

Chronic Changes in Ventricular Diastolic Pressure-Volume Relationships

The compliance (inverse of stiffness) of the ventricle, reflected in the end-diastolic pressure-volume relationship, is altered in a variety of cardiac disorders, reflecting one or more basic mechanisms (see Fig. 21–21) (see Chap. 20). Substantial shifts in the diastolic pressure-volume curve of the left ventricle can be demonstrated during sustained volume overload.[118] For example, dogs with large chronic arteriovenous fistulas exhibit a rightward displacement of the entire diastolic pressure-volume curve, whereby ventricular volume is greater at any end-diastolic pressure but the slope of this curve is steeper, indicating increased chamber stiffness.[119] Patients with severe volume overloading related to chronic aortic or mitral regurgitation, or both, demonstrate similar shifts of the diastolic left ventricular pressure-volume relationship. Similar changes frequently occur in patients with dilated or ischemic cardiomyopathy or after large transmural myocardial infarction (see later).

In contrast, concentric left ventricular hypertrophy, as occurs in aortic stenosis, hypertension, and hypertrophic cardiomyopathy, shifts the pressure-volume relation of the ventricle to the left along its volume axis so that at any diastolic volume ventricular diastolic pressure is abnormally elevated (see Fig. 21–22C).[113,114] In contrast to the changes in the diastolic properties of the ventricular *chamber,* the stiffness of *each unit of myocardium* may or may not be altered in the presence of myocardial hypertrophy secondary to pressure overload. In the presence of concentric left ventricular hypertrophy, there is an inverse relationship between the thickness of the posterior wall of the ventricle and its peak thinning rate during early diastole; a higher than normal diastolic ventricular pressure is required to fill the hypertrophied ventricle. Patients with hypertension have demonstrated slowing of ventricular filling even when systolic function is normal.

Chronic changes in ventricular diastolic pressure-volume relations can also result from alterations in the cytoskeleton of the myocyte. For example, experimental cardiomyopathy with an increase in ventricular stiffness has been found to be associated with changes in titin isoforms and their distribution.[120] Changes in the *extracellular* matrix, especially in fibrillar collagen, can affect ventricular stiffness.[121] Collagen synthesis can be influenced by preload and afterload, as well as by activation of the adrenergic nervous system and of the renin-angiotensin-aldosterone system, and by the activities of MMPs and their inhibitors.[121]

ISCHEMIC HEART DISEASE. Marked changes in the diastolic properties of the left ventricle can occur in the presence of ischemic heart disease. First, acute myocardial ischemia slows ventricular relaxation (see Fig. 21–22A) and increases myocardial wall stiffness.[122] Myocardial infarction causes more complex changes in ventricular pressure-volume relationships, depending on the size of the infarct and the time after infarction at which the measurements are made. Infarcted muscle tested very early exhibits reduced stiffness. Subsequently, the development of myocardial contracture, interstitial edema, fibrocellular infiltration, and scar contributes to increased chamber stiffness, with a steeper ventricular pressure-volume curve (a greater increase in pressure for any increase in volume).[123] Later still, in the case of large infarcts, left ventricular remodeling and dilatation cause a rightward displacement of the pressure-volume curve,[124] resembling that observed in volume overload.

The subendocardial ischemia that is characteristic of severe concentric hypertrophy (even in the presence of a normal coronary circulation) intensifies the failure of relaxation; and when coronary artery obstruction accompanies severe hypertrophy, this abnormality may be particularly severe. Tachycardia, by reducing the duration of diastole and thereby intensifying ischemia, exaggerates this diastolic abnormality and may raise ventricular diastolic pressure even while reducing diastolic ventricular volume, whereas bradycardia has the opposite effect. Successful treatment of ischemia improves diastolic relaxation and lowers ventricular diastolic and pulmonary venous pressures, thereby reducing dyspnea.

CARDIOMYOPATHY AND PERICARDIAL DISEASE. The restrictive cardiomyopathies, especially those such as amyloid heart disease with intracardiac infiltration, the transplanted heart during rejection, and endomyocardial fibrosis (see Chap. 59), are all characterized by upward and leftward displacement of the diastolic pressure-volume relation, with a higher pressure at any volume and a greater increase in diastolic pressure for any increase in volume. Pericardial tamponade and constrictive pericarditis also change the apparent diastolic properties of the heart (see Chap. 50). Early filling is unimpaired because the myocardium is normal. However, filling is abruptly halted in mid-diastole by the constricted or tamponading pericardium, which imposes its mechanical properties on those of the ventricle in the latter half of diastole (see Fig. 21–22B).

Neurohormonal, Autocrine, and Paracrine Adjustments

In response to the reduction of cardiac output, the inadequate arterial volume that is characteristic of systolic heart failure, and atrial hypertension, a complex series of neurohormonal changes takes place (see Table 21–1). In the early stages of severe, acute systolic failure, these changes—heightened adrenergic drive, activation of the renin-angiotensin-aldosterone axis, and augmented release of vasopressin and endothelin—compensate and act to maintain perfusion to vital organs and to expand the inadequate arterial blood volume and via renal retention of sodium and water (Figs. 21–23 and 21–24). However, each of these mechanisms may be thought of as a "double-edged sword." As heart failure becomes chronic, several of these compensatory mechanisms can cause undesirable effects, such as excessive vasoconstriction, increased afterload, excessive retention of salt and water,[125] electrolyte abnormalities, arrhythmias, and direct effects on cardiac myocytes leading to cell death or changes in protein expression and functions (see Table 21–1). In contrast, other responses, such as the release of ANP and brain natriuretic peptide (BNP) in response to distention of the atria and ventricles, may oppose these adverse effects by causing vasodilation, increased excretion of salt and water, and inhibition of sympathetic activity.[126]

Several mediators are involved in control of the cardiovascular system in heart failure. Some are circulating hormones (endocrine effect). Some act on neighboring cells of another type (paracrine effect) or on the cell of origin (autocrine effect). These include peptides that act primarily locally in the vicinity of their production, such as endothelin, peptide growth factors (e.g., TGF-α), and inflammatory cytokines (e.g., interleukin-1 beta [IL-1β] and TNF-α). These and other local mediators act in concert with the autonomic nervous system and circulating hormones to modulate cardiovascular organ function. In addition, many if not all of these mediators have effects on the growth, death, and phenotype of cardiovascular tissues and may thereby play an important role in the remodeling of myocardium and its progression to failure (see Fig. 21–10).[41]

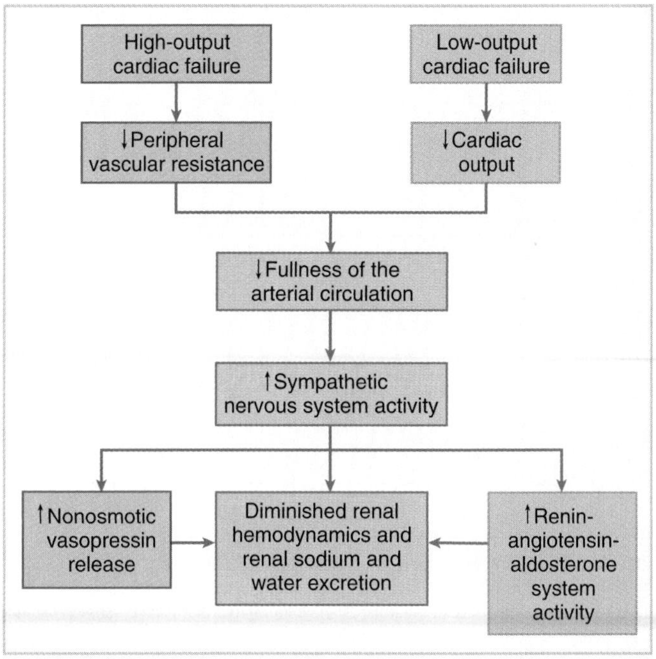

FIGURE 21–23 Mechanisms by which high-output or low-output heart failure leads to the activation of neurohumoral vasoconstrictor systems and renal sodium and water retention. (From Schrier RW, Abraham WT: Hormones and hemodynamics in heart failure. N Engl J Med 341:577, 1999; adapted from Schrier RW: Pathogenesis of sodium and water retention in high-output and low output cardiac failure, nephrotic syndrome, cirrhosis, and pregnancy. N Engl J Med 319:1065, 1988.)

Autonomic Nervous System

INCREASED SYMPATHETIC ACTIVITY (see Figs. 21–23 and 21–24). Activation of the sympathetic (adrenergic) nervous system is a hallmark of heart failure. Measurements of the concentration of the adrenergic neurotransmitter NE in arterial blood provide a crude index of the activity of this system, which is critical to the normal regulation of cardiac performance. At rest, in patients with advanced heart failure, the circulating NE concentration is elevated, generally two to three times the level found in normal subjects,[127] and this elevation is accompanied by elevation of circulating dopamine and sometimes by epinephrine as well; the latter reflects increased adrenomedullary activity. Measurement of 24-hour urinary NE excretion also reveals marked elevations in patients with heart failure.[128] Plasma NE may be elevated, even in asymptomatic patients with left ventricular dysfunction, and is a predictor of mortality in heart failure. During comparable levels of exercise, much greater elevations in circulating NE occur in patients with heart failure than in normal subjects, presumably reflecting greater activation of the adrenergic nervous system during exercise in these patients.

The elevation of circulating NE may result from a combination of increased release of NE from adrenergic nerve endings and its consequent "spillover" into the plasma as well as reduced uptake of NE by adrenergic nerve endings.[129] Patients with heart failure demonstrate increased adrenergic nerve outflow, as measured by microneurography of the peroneal nerve, and the level of nerve activity correlates with the concentration of plasma NE.[130] The level of adrenergic nerve activity also correlates directly with the levels of left and right ventricular filling pressures. Whereas the normal heart usually extracts NE from the arterial blood, in patients with heart failure the coronary sinus NE concentration exceeds the arterial concentration, indicating increased adrenergic activation of the heart. Drugs such as the alpha$_2$-agonist moxonidine (which reduces adrenergic nerve impulse traffic) reduce plasma NE, indicating that presynaptic control of adrenergic nervous activity is intact in patients with heart failure.[131] It has been suggested that treatment with such agents might be useful in the treatment of heart failure. However, this general concept has been challenged by the results of a large clinical trial in which moxonidine was associated with a substantial decrease in plasma NE but an *increase* in morbidity and mortality.[132] Perhaps in this trial the dose of the drug was too high and the reduction in adrenergic support too profound, analogous to the hazardous effects of rapidly escalating doses of beta-adrenergic blockers in patients with advanced heart failure.

Increased adrenergic activation results in an increase in Ca^{2+} influx into the myocytes, an increase in Ca^{2+} storage (and release) by the SR, phosphorylation and therefore reduced inhibition of SERCA2 by phospholamban, as well as a decreased Ca^{2+} binding affinity of troponin.[2] Although NE enhances both contraction and relaxation, myocardial energy requirements are augmented, which could intensify ischemia when myocardial O_2 delivery is restricted. The augmented adrenergic outflow from the central nervous system in patients with heart failure may trigger ventricular tachycardia or even sudden cardiac death, particularly in the presence of myocardial ischemia, as well as myocyte apoptosis.

In addition to activation of beta-adrenergic receptors in the heart, the heightened activity of the adrenergic nervous system leads to stimulation of myocardial $alpha_1$-adrenergic receptors, which elicits a modest positive inotropic effect.[133] Stimulation of myocardial $alpha_1$-adrenergic receptors may also cause myocyte hypertrophy, changes in phenotype characterized by the reexpression of a fetal gene program, and the induction of peptide growth factors.[134] $Alpha_1$-adrenergic receptors are of low density in the human heart; however, in contrast to $beta_1$-adrenergic receptors, which are downregulated, $alpha_1$-adrenergic receptors appear to be unchanged in number in failing human myocardium.

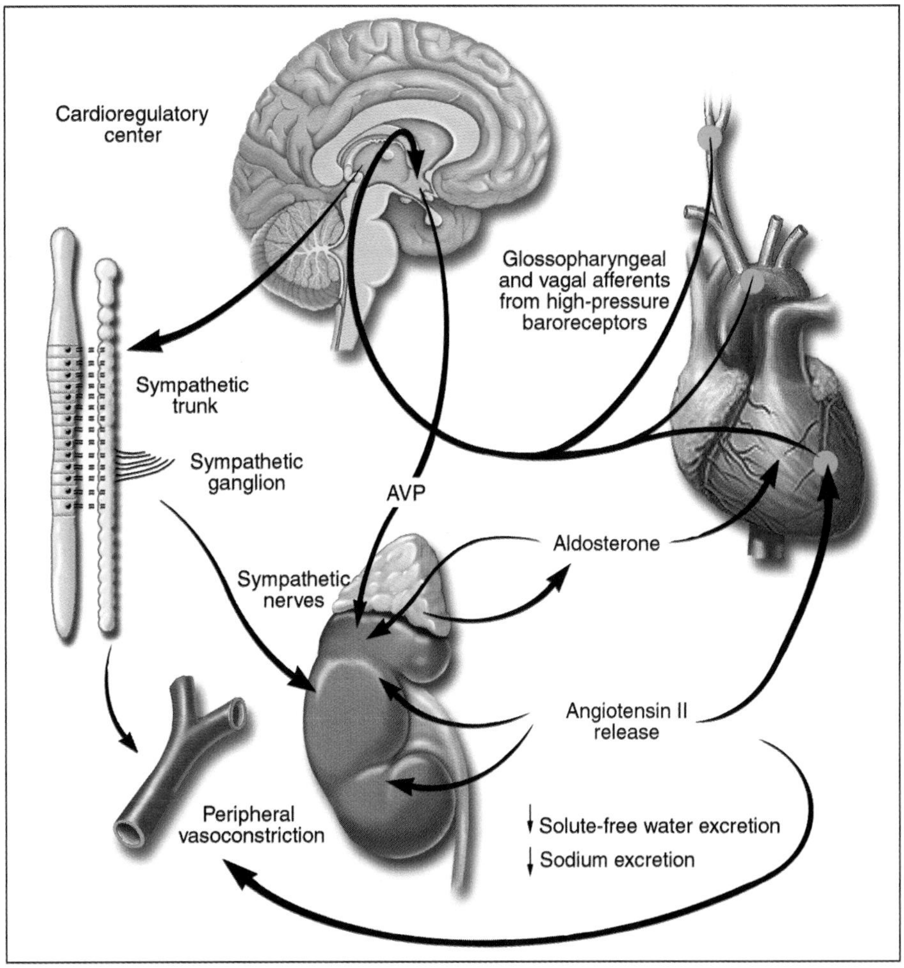

FIGURE 21–24 Unloading of high-pressure baroceptors (circles) in the left ventricle, carotid sinus, and aortic arch generates afferent signals that stimulate cardioregulatory centers in the brain, resulting in the activation of efferent pathways in the sympathetic nervous system. The sympathetic nervous system appears to be the primary integrator of the neurohumoral vasoconstrictor response to arterial underfilling. Activation of renal sympathetic nerves stimulates the release of arginine vasopressin (AVP). Sympathetic activation also causes peripheral and renal vasoconstriction, as does angiotensin II. Angiotensin II constricts blood vessels and stimulates the release of aldosterone from the adrenal gland, and it also increases tubular sodium reabsorption and causes remodeling of cardiac myocytes. Aldosterone may also have direct cardiac effects, in addition to increasing the reabsorption of sodium and the secretion of potassium and hydrogen ions in the collecting duct. The lines designate circulating hormones. (Modified from Schrier RW, Abraham WT: Hormones and hemodynamics in heart failure. N Engl J Med 341:577, 1999.)

CARDIAC NOREPINEPHRINE DEPLETION. The concentration of NE in atrial and ventricular tissue removed at operation from patients with heart failure is extremely low.[127,128,134] In patients, cardiac NE content determined from endomyocardial biopsies correlates directly with the ejection fraction and inversely with plasma epinephrine concentration. NE concentrations are also markedly depressed in the ventricles of dogs with right ventricular failure produced by the creation of pulmonary stenosis and tricuspid regurgitation.[135] Local cardiac NE stores do not appear to play any role in the *intrinsic* contractile state of cardiac muscle. Thus, no differences were found in the length-tension or force-velocity relationships displayed by papillary muscles removed from normal cats and from cats with NE depletion produced by chronic cardiac denervation or reserpine pretreatment.[136] However, the reduction in cardiac NE stores represents a depletion of the adrenergic neurotransmitter in adrenergic nerve endings, and, as a consequence, the response to activation of the sympathetic nervous system is blunted (see Fig. 21-2).

The mechanism responsible for cardiac NE depletion in severe heart failure is not clear; it may be an "exhaustion" phenomenon resulting from the prolonged adrenergic activation of the cardiac adrenergic nerves in heart failure. Reductions in the activity of tyrosine hydroxylase, which catalyzes the rate-limiting step in the biosynthesis of NE, and in the rate at which noradrenergic vesicles can take up dopamine have also been incriminated. In patients with cardiomyopathy, iodine-131-labeled metaiodobenzylguanidine (MIBG), a radiopharmaceutical that is taken up by adrenergic nerve endings, is not taken up normally,[137] suggesting that NE reuptake is impaired in heart failure. Treatment with the beta-adrenergic antagonist metoprolol was associated with correction of MIBG uptake.[138]

ABNORMAL BAROREFLEX CONTROL IN HEART FAILURE. Increased adrenergic activity in heart failure is due, in part, to abnormal baroreflex control of adrenergic outflow from the central nervous system (see Fig. 21-24). In dogs with experimental heart failure, carotid occlusion elicited a blunted reflex response of heart rate, arterial pressure, and vascular resistance.[139]

The possibility of defective adrenergic control of heart rate in patients with heart failure has been studied by observing the reflex hemodynamic responses to stimuli such as upright tilt and vasodilator-induced hypotension. An inadequate increase in heart rate in patients with heart failure was observed when arterial pressure was reduced by a vasodilator.[140] Although the changes in mean arterial pressure

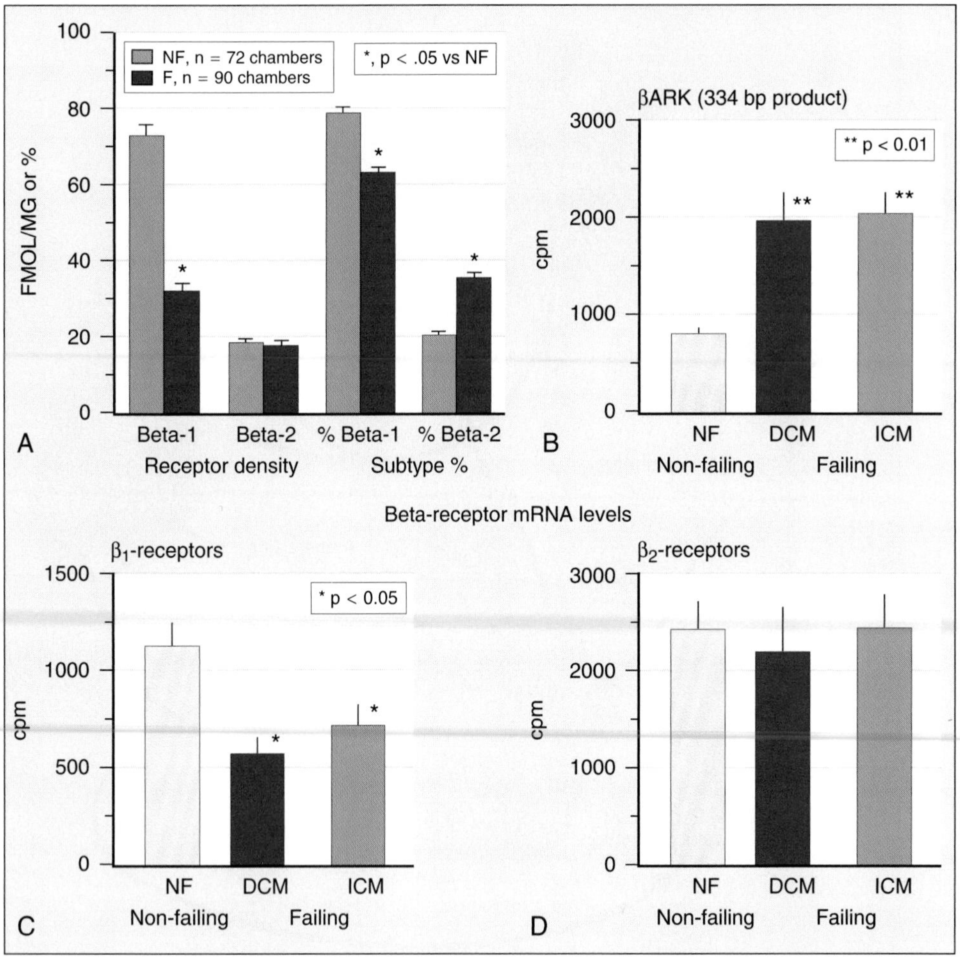

FIGURE 21–25 Downregulation of beta-adrenergic receptors in myocardium from patients with heart failure. Although human ventricular myocardium expresses both beta$_1$- and beta$_2$-adrenergic receptor subtypes, only the beta$_1$ subtype is significantly downregulated in failing myocardium **(A)**. Downregulation of beta$_1$ receptors is associated with upregulation of beta-adrenergic receptor kinase (βARK), an enzyme that phosphorylates beta-adrenergic receptors and thereby contributes to their uncoupling from second messenger pathways **(B)**. In addition, the messenger RNA (mRNA) level for beta$_1$-, but not beta$_2$-, adrenergic receptors is decreased in failing human myocardium **(C** and **D)**. NF = nonfailure; F = congestive heart failure; DCM = dilated cardiomyopathy; ICM = ischemic cardiomyopathy. (Data from Bristow MR: Changes in myocardial and vascular receptors in heart failure. J Am Coll Cardiol 22:61A, 1993; and Ungerer M, Bohm M, Elce JS, et al: Altered expression of beta-adrenergic receptor kinase and beta$_1$-adrenergic receptors in the failing human heart. Circulation 87:454, 1993. Copyright 1993, American Heart Association.)

observed in response to the vasodilators were similar in patients with heart failure and in normal subjects, the changes in heart rate after vasodilators correlated significantly with the changes in concentration of circulating NE and with the sum of circulating NE and epinephrine. In normal individuals, both heart rate and NE concentrations rose, whereas in patients with heart failure, in whom resting catecholamine levels were already increased, cardiac acceleration was blunted and NE concentration failed to rise normally. Similarly, during upright tilt, patients with heart failure exhibited a blunting of the normal increases in plasma NE and forearm vascular resistance.[141]

Some patients with heart failure exhibit a major reduction in arterial pressure during tilting, analogous to what is observed in idiopathic orthostatic hypotension. Further evidence for impairment of baroreflex control of the systemic circulation comes from investigations in which lower body negative pressure failed to cause normal reflex augmentation of forearm vascular resistance.[142]

ATRIAL STRETCH RECEPTORS. Abnormal baroreflex control of the circulation also contributes to the reduced ability of patients with heart failure to excrete salt and water. Under normal circumstances, elevated left atrial pressure stimulates atrial stretch receptors. The increased activity of both myelinated and nonmyelinated (C-fiber) afferents inhibits the release of antidiuretic hormone, thereby increasing water excretion, which in turn reduces plasma volume and thereby restores left atrial pressure to normal. In addition, enhanced activation of left atrial stretch receptors depresses renal efferent sympathetic nerve activity and increases renal blood flow and glomerular filtration rate, thereby enhancing the ability of the kidney to reduce plasma volume.

With the prolonged elevation of left atrial pressure in heart failure, there is desensitization of atrial (and arterial) baroreceptors. This desensitization may be responsible for the inappropriately high plasma antidiuretic hormone levels in severe heart failure and may contribute to the renal vasoconstriction, peripheral edema, ascites, and hyponatremia characteristic of this condition. With chronic heart failure and its attendant cardiac distention and decreased sensitivity of cardiac receptors, the reflex inhibition of adrenergic activity disappears. The adrenergic drive to the peripheral vascular bed and the adrenal medulla is enhanced, contributing to the vasoconstriction, tachycardia, and sodium retention state characteristic of heart failure.

There is evidence that blunted baroreflex responsiveness is associated with increased activity of Na^+,K^+-ATPase in the baroreceptors; digitalis glycosides, which inhibit Na^+,K^+-ATPase, can partially correct this abnormality. This ability of digitalis to correct baroreflex function and thereby suppress adrenergic nerve activity may play a significant role in its clinical efficacy (see Chap. 23). NO also increases baroreflex sensitivity, whereas angiotensin II decreases it, and exogenous NO and blockade of angiotensin receptors can correct the reduced baroreceptor sensitivity characteristic of experimental heart failure.[143]

Beta-Adrenergic Receptor–G Protein–Adenylyl Cyclase Pathway

BETA-ADRENERGIC RECEPTORS (see also Chap. 19). Ventricles obtained from patients with heart failure demonstrate a marked reduction in NE content, beta-adrenergic receptor density, isoproterenol-mediated adenylyl cyclase stimulation, and the contractile response to beta-adrenergic agonists.[144] It is generally believed that the downregulation of beta-adrenergic receptors is mediated by increased levels of NE in the vicinity of the receptor. In patients with dilated cardiomyopathy, this reduction in receptor density is proportional to the severity of heart failure and involves primarily beta$_1$, but not beta$_2$, receptors, thus reducing the ratio of beta$_1$ to beta$_2$ receptors (Fig. 21–25A). The beta$_2$ receptor, although not downregulated, becomes partially "uncoupled" from its effector enzyme (adenylyl cyclase), producing a similar effect.

In isolated cardiac myocytes, the proapoptotic effect of beta-adrenergic receptor stimulation is mediated by the beta$_1$

receptor subtype, whereas the beta$_2$ subtype exerts an opposing antiapoptotic effect.[145] Although this observation might lead to the prediction that clinically beta$_1$-selective blockade would be superior to nonselective blockade in the treatment of heart failure, such superiority has not been observed in clinical trials,[146] probably reflecting other adverse actions of the beta$_2$ subtype such as facilitation of NE release from presynaptic sympathetic neuron.

In myocardium from patients with heart failure the level of beta$_1$-adrenergic receptor mRNA is decreased, indicating that the downregulation of beta$_1$-adrenergic receptors is mediated, at least in part, by a decrease in receptor synthesis, whereas the level of beta$_2$-adrenergic receptor mRNA is unchanged (see Fig. 21–25). In addition, there are increases in the expression of beta-adrenergic receptor kinase (βARK) and its mRNA level in failing human myocardium (see Fig. 21–25B). βARK is an enzyme that phosphorylates both beta$_1$- and beta$_2$-adrenergic receptors and thereby plays a central role in uncoupling of the receptor from its G protein (Fig. 21–26).[147] Increased βARK activity may therefore contribute to the uncoupling of both beta$_1$- and beta$_2$-adrenergic receptors in patients with heart failure.

Downregulation of beta$_1$ receptors in patients with heart failure may be reversed by the administration of metoprolol, a relatively specific beta$_1$ antagonist. The long-term clinical benefit of beta blockade in heart failure (see Chap. 23) has been reported to be associated with both a restoration of myocardial beta receptor density and the contractile response to administered catecholamines.[148]

The relative importance of beta-adrenergic receptor downregulation versus receptor uncoupling may depend on the cause of heart failure. In myocardium obtained from patients with heart failure secondary to ischemic heart disease, there is a relatively greater degree of receptor desensitization than in myocardium from patients with dilated cardiomyopathy. This observation, together with apparent differences in the regulation of G protein function, has led to the suggestion that there are differences in the behavior of the beta-adrenergic receptor–G protein complex in these two forms of heart failure.

Genetic differences related to polymorphisms or mutations that affect the function of beta- or alpha-adrenergic receptors may contribute to the pathophysiology of myocardial failure. Patients with heart failure with a Thr-to-Ile polymorphism at amino acid 164 of the beta$_2$ receptor have a decrease in receptor function that is associated with a decrease in survival.[149] Likewise, black patients who have a polymorphism in the beta$_1$ receptor resulting in increased function combined with a polymorphism in the alpha$_{2C}$ receptor resulting in decreased function were found to have an increased risk of heart failure (Fig. 21–27).[150] Because the alpha$_2$ receptor inhibits NE release from sympathetic nerve endings, whereas the beta$_1$ receptor mediates the proapoptotic effect on the cardiac myocyte, these polymorphisms may exert synergistic adverse effects by providing higher levels of NE to a hyperresponsive beta$_1$ receptor on the cardiac myocyte.

G PROTEINS AND ADENYLYL CYCLASE (see also Chap. 20). G proteins play a critical role in coupling receptors, including beta-adrenergic receptors, to effector enzymes such as adenylyl cyclase (see Fig. 19–12).[151] Cardiac cells contain at least three types of G proteins: (1) G_s, which mediates the *stimulation of adenylyl cyclase* (and thereby causes a rise in intracellular cyclic AMP, which in turn stimulates Ca^{2+} influx into the myocyte through Ca^{2+} channels in the sarcolemmal membrane and accelerates the uptake of Ca^{2+} by the SR); (2) G_i, which mediates the *inhibition of adenylyl cyclase* and has the opposite effect on the movements of Ca^{2+}; and (3) G_q, which mediates the *stimulation of phospholipase C,* thereby leading to an activation of protein kinase C by several receptors generally associated with myocyte hypertrophy including those for angiotensin II, alpha-adrenergic receptors for NE, and endothelin.[152]

Heart failure secondary to dilated cardiomyopathy is associated with an increase in G_i activity and protein level in heart muscle, which appears to be mediated at the post-transcriptional level. G_s appears normal in failing human myocardium. However, the functional consequences of an increase in G_i activity remain to be established. In mice, the cardiac-specific overexpression of G_s led to cardiac failure that was associated with apoptosis of cardiac myocytes and with myocardial fibrosis and hypertrophy.[153] Mice with overexpression of cardiac G_q exhibited myocardial hypertrophy and, with higher levels of G_q expression, developed dilated cardiomyopathy associated with myocyte apoptosis.[154] Although the effects of overexpression studies such as

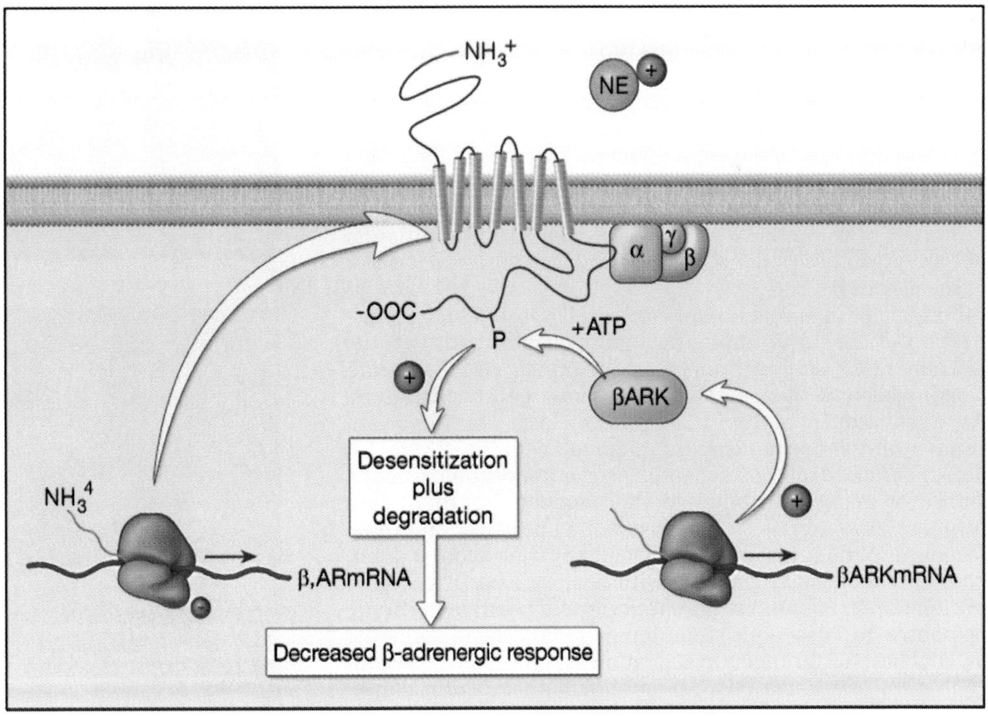

FIGURE 21–26 Alterations in beta-adrenergic pathways in the failing heart. A characteristic physiological abnormality in patients with heart failure is a reduction in the inotropic and chronotropic responses to exercise and other types of sympathetic stimulation. The molecular basis for this appears to involve multiple changes in the beta$_1$-adrenergic receptor coupling that are a response to the chronic increase in adrenergic stimulation. In myocardium from patients with end-stage heart failure, compared with control tissue from patients without failure, the level of beta-adrenergic receptor kinase (ßARK) messenger RNA (mRNA) is increased and the level of beta$_1$-adrenergic receptor mRNA is reduced. This leads not only to reduction in transcription of new beta$_1$-adrenergic receptors but also to increased phosphorylation of receptors leading to desensitization and degradation of receptors. (From Colucci WS [ed]: Atlas of Heart Failure: Cardiac Function and Dysfunction. 3rd ed. Philadelphia, Current Medicine, 2002, p 7.9.)

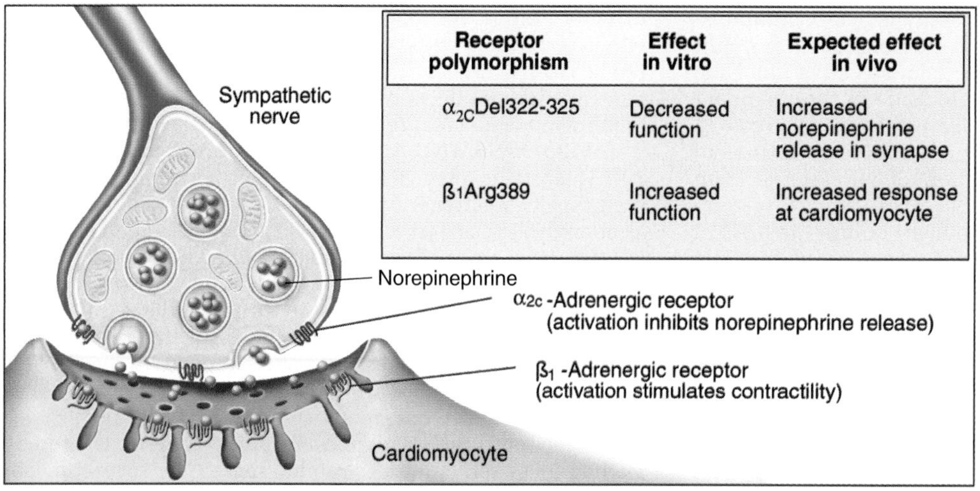

FIGURE 21–27 Basis of the hypothesis that the α_{2c}Del322-325 and β_1Arg389 receptors act synergistically as risk factors for heart failure. The α_{2c}-adrenergic receptor (along with the α_{2a}-adrenergic receptor) inhibits norepinephrine release at cardiac presynaptic nerve endings through negative feedback. The presence of the dysfunctional α_{2c}Del322-325 receptor would be expected to result in enhanced norepinephrine release. The β_1-adrenergic receptor is the receptor for norepinephrine on the cardiomyocyte, and the presence of the hyperfunctional β_1Arg389 receptor would be expected to increase contractile response at the myocytes. The combination of increased norepinephrine release and increased responsiveness of the receptor was hypothesized to be a risk factor for heart failure. (From Small KM, Wagoner LE, Levin AM, et al: Synergistic polymorphisms of β_1 and α_{2c}-adrenergic receptors and the risk of congestive heart failure. N Engl J Med 347:1135, 2002.)

these need to be interpreted with caution, they suggest that receptors coupled to G_s and G_q play an important role in the pathophysiology of myocardial hypertrophy and failure.

REDUCED ADRENERGIC SUPPORT OF THE FAILING HEART. The importance of the adrenergic nervous system in maintaining ventricular contractility when myocardial function is depressed in heart failure is demonstrated by the effects of adrenergic blockade. *Acute* pharmacological blockade of the adrenergic nervous system may cause intensification of heart failure as well as sodium and water retention.[155,156] The *acute* administration of beta blockers to patients with heart failure results in reductions in both systolic and diastolic myocardial function. Despite the long-term very salutary effects of beta-blocker therapy in patients with heart failure (see Chaps. 23 and 24), caution should be exercised in using these agents, particularly at the initiation of therapy and in patients in whom heart failure is severe or of recent onset.

Because of the depletion of cardiac NE stores and desensitization of the postsynaptic beta adrenoceptor pathway, the capacity of the myocardium to produce cyclic AMP is diminished, sometimes profoundly, in patients with heart failure. As a consequence, the failing heart loses an important compensatory mechanism. In patients with heart failure, downregulation of postsynaptic beta adrenoceptors in the sinoatrial node contributes to the attenuated chronotropic response to exercise. Likewise, the positive inotropic response to the infusion of the beta-adrenergic agonist dobutamine is reduced in patients with heart failure. The degree of attenuation of both the chronotropic and positive inotropic responses to adrenergic stimulation is correlated with the level of baseline adrenergic activation as reflected by the concentration of plasma NE. An important therapeutic consequence of the alterations of the beta-adrenergic pathway described earlier is that the positive inotropic response to beta adrenoceptor agonists, and to a lesser extent to phosphodiesterase inhibitors, is reduced in myocardium obtained from patients with end-stage heart failure.

ADVERSE EFFECTS OF ADRENERGIC STIMULATION. Increased adrenergic nerve activity may influence the chronic remodeling of the myocardium by affecting the progression of myocardial failure through direct harmful effects of NE on adrenergic receptors located on several cardiac cell types, including cardiac myocytes and fibroblasts. The tonic stimulation of beta-adrenergic receptors, or the downstream cyclic AMP pathway to which they are coupled, resulted in death of cardiac myocytes by apoptosis.[157] In vitro, tonic exposure to NE caused apoptosis of adult rat cardiac myocytes that was mediated through the beta-adrenergic receptor adenylyl cyclase and cyclic AMP (Fig. 21–28).[49] A similar effect was seen in neonatal rat cardiomyocytes.[49] Likewise, the chronic infusion of isoproterenol to rats caused myocardial failure associated with apoptosis,[158] and transgenic mice that overexpressed either the beta$_1$-adrenergic receptor or G_s[153,154,159] developed myocardial failure associated with myocyte

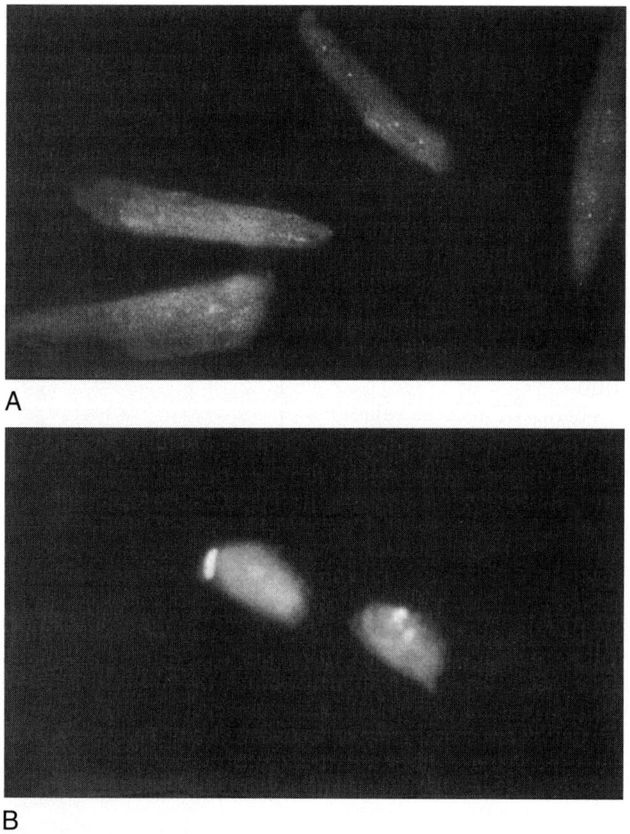

FIGURE 21–28 Effect of norepinephrine (NE) on myocyte apoptosis. Adult rat cardiac myocytes in tissue culture were exposed to control media **(A)** or NE **(B)** for 24 hours and apoptosis was measured by the terminal deoxynucleotidyl transferase-mediated-VTP nick end labeling (TUNEL) staining for fragmented DNA shown in two nuclei in this panel. NE caused an approximately fourfold increase in TUNEL-positive myocytes (From Sawyer DB, Colucci WS: Molecular and cellular events in myocardial hypertrophy and failure. *In* Colucci WS [ed]: Heart Failure: Cardiac Function and Dysfunction. 3rd ed. Philadelphia, Current Medicine, 2002, p 4.12.)

apoptosis. When viewed from this perspective, the desensitization of the beta-adrenergic pathway, although impairing short-term myocardial function, may protect the myocardium from excessive adrenergic activation.

In addition, NE, acting on both alpha$_1$-adrenergic and beta-adrenergic receptors located on cardiac myocytes and fibroblasts, can increase and alter the composition of the interstitial matrix, which may play an important role in the pathophysiology of myocardial dysfunction (see Interstitial Matrix Accumulation, earlier).

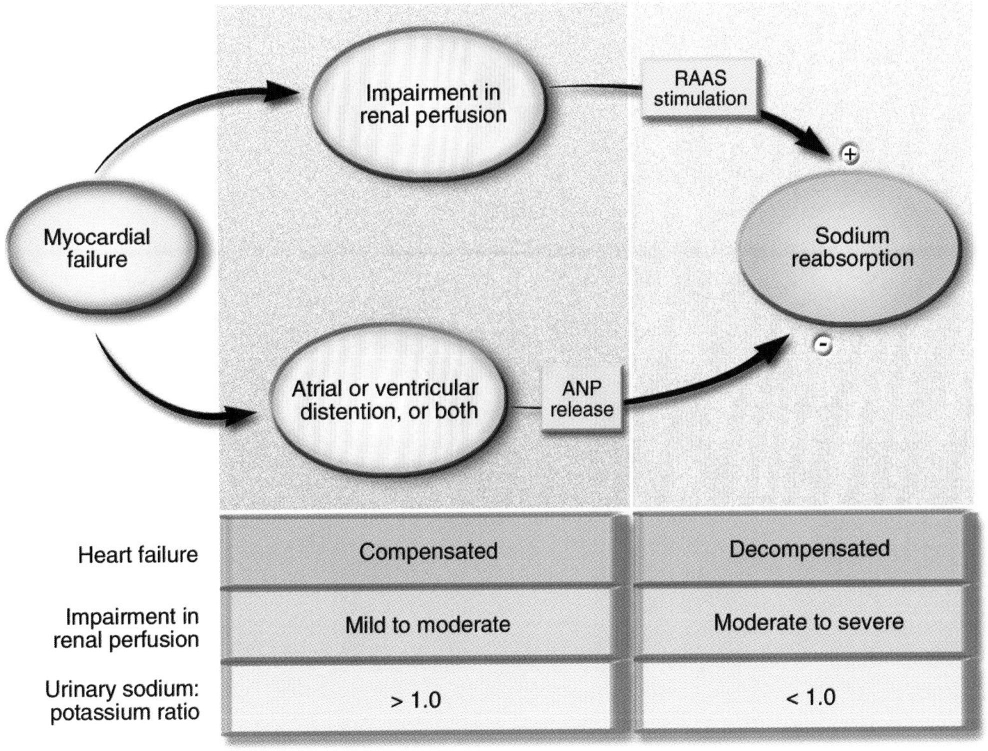

FIGURE 21–29 Compensated and decompensated heart failure, as indicated by the presence or absence of urinary sodium retention, together with symptoms and signs of expanded intravascular and extravascular volume. In compensated heart failure with mild to moderate reductions in renal perfusion, natriuretic peptides, such as atrial natriuretic peptide (ANP) released by distended atria, stimulate sodium excretion (decreasing reabsorption, minus sign) so that the urinary sodium/potassium ratio is greater than 1.0. In decompensated heart failure, moderate to severe reductions in renal perfusion activate the renin-angiotensin-aldosterone system (RAAS), overriding the action of natriuretic peptides to stimulate nearly complete urinary sodium reabsorption (plus sign), resulting in a urinary sodium/potassium ratio less than 1.0. (From Weber KT: Aldosterone in congestive heart failure. N Engl J Med 345:1689, 2001, and Weber KT, Villareal D: Aldosterone and antialdosterone therapy in congestive heart failure. Am J Cardiol 71[Suppl 3A]:11A, 1993.)

PARASYMPATHETIC FUNCTION IN HEART FAILURE

Cardiac enlargement, with or without heart failure, is associated with marked disturbances of parasympathetic as well as sympathetic function. The parasympathetic restraint on sinoatrial node automaticity was markedly reduced in patients with heart failure (see Fig. 21-3), who exhibited less heart rate slowing for any given elevation of systemic arterial pressure than did normal subjects.[160] The aforementioned reduction in the sensitivity of the baroreceptor reflex, which is notably dependent on parasympathetic outflow, has also been shown to be significantly reduced in dogs with heart failure. Measurements of heart rate variability, which indirectly reflect autonomic nervous system function, indicated that parasympathetic activity in patients with heart failure is abnormal both at rest and in response to exercise.[161]

Abnormal parasympathetic function may also be altered at the level of the peripheral nerve and the postsynaptic receptor. Cardiomyopathic hamster hearts display a reduction in the activity of choline acetyltransferase, an enzyme that provides an estimate of the density of parasympathetic innervation, and there is evidence that the density of high-affinity muscarinic receptors is reduced in the hearts of dogs with experimental heart failure.

Renin-Angiotensin-Aldosterone System

In low–cardiac output states, there is activation of the renin-angiotensin-aldosterone system, which operates in concert with the activated adrenergic nervous–adrenal medullary system to maintain arterial pressure and to retain sodium and water (Figs. 21–24 and 21–29). These two systems are clearly coupled. Heightened adrenergic drive stimulates beta$_1$ adrenoceptors in the juxtaglomerular apparatus of the kidneys. This process is a principal mechanism responsible for the release of renin in acute heart failure. Activation of the baroreceptors in the renal vascular bed by a reduction of renal blood flow is also responsible for the release of renin, and in patients with severe chronic heart failure after salt restriction and diuretic treatment, reduction of the sodium presented to the macula densa contributes to the release of renin. Elevated plasma renin activity is a common, although not universal, finding in heart failure. In the Studies of Left Ventricular Dysfunction (SOLVD) study of heart failure, plasma angiotensin II was significantly elevated even in asymptomatic patients and was further elevated in patients with symptomatic heart failure.[162]

ADVERSE EFFECTS OF RENIN-ANGIOTENSIN-ALDOSTERONE SYSTEM ACTIVATION. Angiotensin II is a potent peripheral vasoconstrictor and contributes, along with increased adrenergic activity, to the excessive elevation of systemic vascular resistance and the vicious circle already referred to (see Increased Vasoconstrictor Activity, earlier) in patients with heart failure. Angiotensin II also enhances the adrenergic nervous system's release of NE as well as the release of aldosterone from the adrenal cortex. Aldosterone has potent sodium-retaining properties and contributes to the development of edema (see later). Therefore, it is not surprising that interruption of the renin-angiotensin-aldosterone axis by means of ACE inhibition reduces system vascular resistance, diminishes afterload, and thereby elevates cardiac output in heart failure. In some patients ACE inhibitors also exert a mild diuretic action, presumably by lowering the angiotensin II–stimulated production of aldosterone.[163-165]

Angiotensin II may also play a direct role in modifying myocardial structure and function.[166] Angiotensin II has been shown to cause cellular hypertrophy, the induction of fetal gene programs, and apoptosis in cultured cardiac myocytes (Fig. 21–30).[167] Angiotensin II also appears to play a role in mediating the apoptotic effect of mechanical strain on the myocardium and is a potent stimulator of several signaling pathways, including those involved in oxidative stress, inflammation, and the regulation of the ECM.[168]

TISSUE RENIN-ANGIOTENSIN SYSTEM. The major portion (90 to 99 percent) of ACE in the body is found in tissues, and the remaining 1 to 10 percent circulates. All of

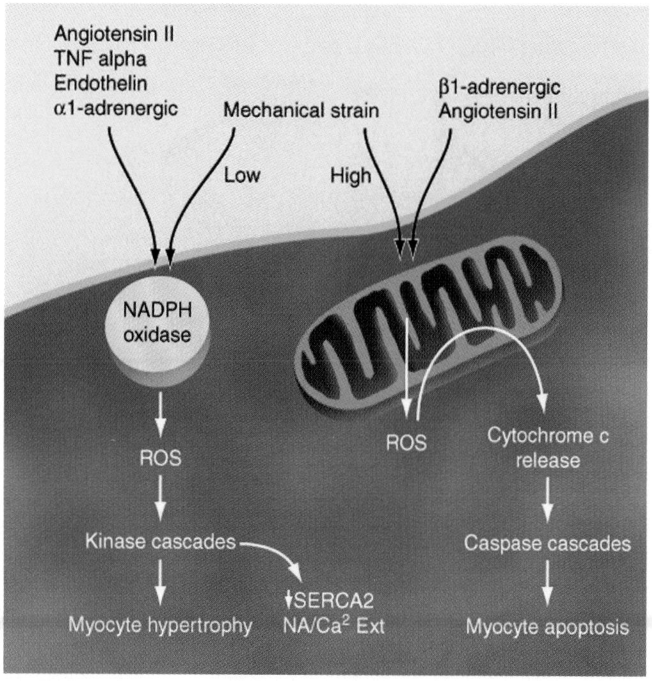

FIGURE 21–30 Schematic of the effects of reactive oxygen species (ROS) on myocyte phenotype. Through activation of kinase cascades such as mitogen activated protein kinase (MAPK), ROS can induce myocyte hypertrophy. ROS can also alter the activity and expression of Ca^{2+}-handling proteins including SERCA2 and the Na^+/Ca^{2+} exchanger to alter myocardial contractility. Mitochondrial ROS may be particularly prone to induce apoptosis by stimulating the mitochondrial release of cytochrome *c*, which is necessary for the activation of caspase cascades. NADPH = reduced nicotinamide adenine dinucleotide phosphate; TNF = tumor necrosis factor. (From Mann DL [ed]: Heart failure: A Companion to Braunwald's Heart Disease. Philadelphia, Elsevier, 2004. Adapted from Sawyer DB, Siwik DA, Xiao L, et al: Role of oxidative stress in myocardial hypertrophy and failure. J Mol Cell Cardiol 34:379, 2002.)

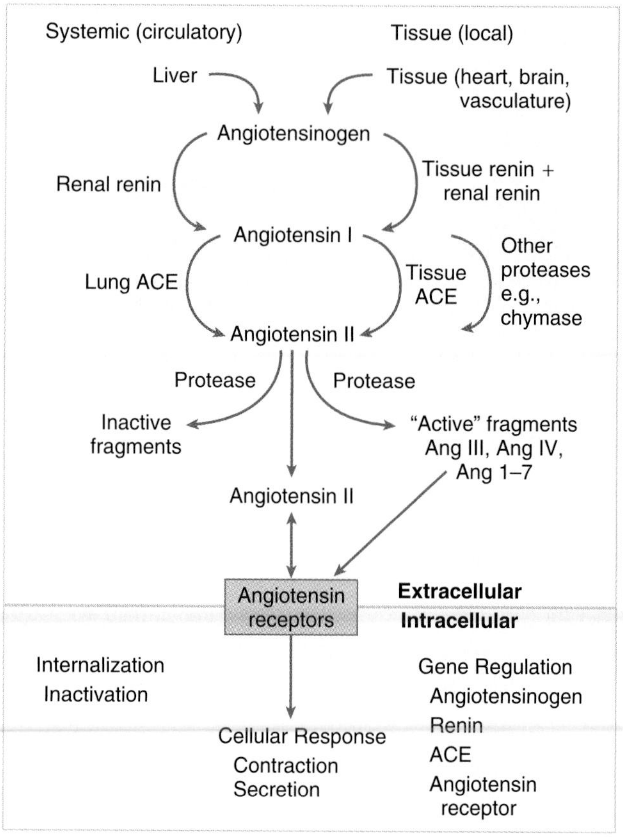

FIGURE 21–31 The systemic and tissue components of the renin-angiotensin system. Several tissues, including myocardium, vasculature, kidney, and brain, have the capacity to generate angiotensin II independent of the circulating renin-angiotensin system. Angiotensin II produced at the tissue level may play an important role in the pathophysiology of heart failure. ACE = angiotensin-converting enzyme. (Modified from Timmermans PB, Wong PC, Chiu AT, et al: Angiotensin II receptors and angiotensin II receptor antagonists. Pharmacol Rev 45:205, 1993.)

the necessary components of the renin-angiotensin system (RAS) (Fig. 21–31) are likewise present in several organs and tissues, including the vasculature, heart, and kidneys. In myocardium from animals with experimental myocardial hypertrophy or failure, there is increased expression of ACE and angiotensinogen, the substrate for angiotensin I production by renin. It has been suggested that the tissue RAS may be activated during compensated heart failure at a time when activity of the circulating system can be relatively normal (Fig. 21–32). The tissue production of angiotensin II may also occur by a pathway not dependent on ACE (the chymase pathway). This pathway may be of major importance in the myocardium, particularly when the levels of renin and angiotensin I are increased by the use of ACE inhibitors. The density of ACE binding sites is increased in myocardium from patients with end-stage heart failure related to idiopathic cardiomyopathy.[169]

ANGIOTENSIN RECEPTORS. The predominant angiotensin receptor in the vasculature is the angiotensin$_1$ subtype (AT_1). Both AT_1 and AT_2 receptor subtypes are present in human myocardium with the AT_2 receptor predominating in a ratio of 2:1. The number of AT_1 and AT_2 receptors is normal in patients with moderate heart failure, but both are downregulated in patients with end-stage heart failure. Downregulation of the AT_1 subtype has been observed in myocardium from patients with both ischemic and idiopathic dilated cardiomyopathy and is associated with a decrease in the mRNA level for the receptor.[9]

Aldosterone

Beyond its action to increase renal sodium retention, aldosterone may exert direct adverse effects on both the vascula-

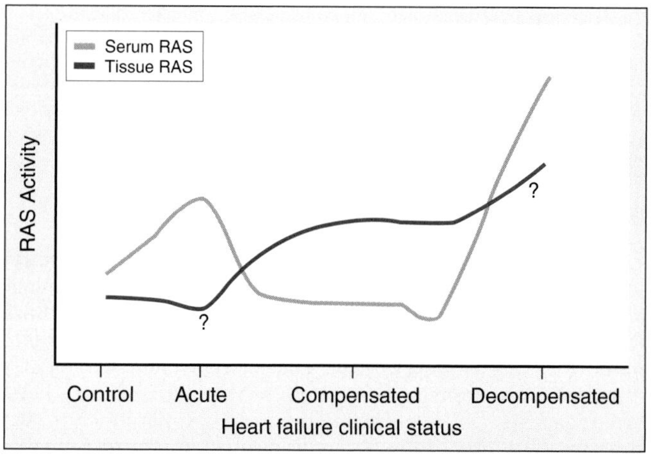

FIGURE 21–32 Relative roles of the circulating and tissue renin-angiotensin systems (RASs) postulated in patients with heart failure. The tissue system may have alternative pathways for the production of angiotensin II that do not depend on converting enzyme (e.g., chymase) and that therefore are not suppressed by converting enzyme inhibitors. It has been proposed that activation of the tissue RAS may follow a different time course than that of the circulating system, particularly during the compensated phase of heart failure when the circulating RAS may be relatively quiescent and during treatment with converting enzyme inhibitors that may increase the activity of the tissue system by elevating circulating renin levels. (Modified from Dzau VJ: Tissue renin-angiotensin system in myocardial hypertrophy and failure. Arch Intern Med 153:937, 1993. Copyright 1993, American Medical Association.)

ture and myocardium (Fig. 21–33) leading to hypertrophy and fibrosis and thereby contribute to reduced vascular compliance and ventricular diastolic dysfunction.[170] These direct effects on the cardiovascular system appear to involve inflammation and oxidative stress in target tissues.[171] Transgenic mice with a selective increase in activation of the aldosterone receptors in cardiac myocytes develop myocardial hypertrophy and interstitial fibrosis leading to progressive left ventricular dilation, heart failure, and death: All of these events are prevented by treatment with the aldosterone receptor antagonist eplerenone.[172]

The importance of aldosterone, independent of angiotensin II, was demonstrated by two large clinical trials. The randomized aldactone evaluation study (RALES) trial found that low-dose spironolactone increased the survival of patients with chronic heart failure related to systolic dysfunction.[173] This effect could not be attributed to changes in volume or electrolyte status. The EPlerenone's neuroHormonal Efficacy and SUrvival Study (EPHESUS) trial likewise found that early administration of the selective aldosterone receptor antagonist eplerenone improved survival after myocardial infarction.[174]

ARGININE VASOPRESSIN

Arginine vasopressin (AVP) is a pituitary hormone that plays a central role in the regulation of free water clearance and plasma osmolality (see Fig. 21-24). Circulating AVP is elevated in many patients with heart failure, even after correction for plasma osmolality. Patients with acute heart failure secondary to massive myocardial infarction may have particularly elevated levels, which are usually associated with elevated concentrations of catecholamines and renin. The plasma AVP concentration was significantly elevated in asymptomatic patients in the prevention arm of the SOLVD study and was elevated further in patients with symptomatic heart failure.[162] Control of circulating AVP concentration is abnormal in patients with heart failure who fail to show the normal reduction of AVP with a reduction of osmolality. This abnormal control may contribute to their inadequate ability to excrete free water and hence to the plasma hypoosmolarity in some patients with heart failure. Decreased sensitivity of atrial stretch receptors, which normally inhibit AVP release with atrial distention, may contribute to the elevation of circulating AVP. In addition, patients with heart failure exhibit failure of the normal suppression of AVP after administration of ethanol.

Two types of AVP receptors (V_1 and V_2) have been identified in a variety of tissues. In dogs with pacing-induced heart failure, the selective inhibition of V_1 receptors increased cardiac output without affecting electrolytes or hormone levels.[175] In contrast, inhibition of V_2 receptors increased serum sodium concentration, plasma renin activity, and plasma AVP levels but did not affect hemodynamics. When the two inhibitors were combined, the hemodynamic effects were potentiated. These results suggest that in heart failure, in addition to regulating free water clearance through the V_2 receptor, AVP may contribute to systemic vasoconstriction through the V_1 receptor.

Natriuretic Peptides

Three natriuretic peptides—ANP, BNP, and C-natriuretic peptide (CNP)—have been identified. ANP is stored mainly in the right atrium and is released in response to an increase in atrial distending pressure. This peptide causes vasodilation and natriuresis and counteracts the water-retaining effects of the adrenergic, renin-angiotensin-aldosterone, and AVP systems. BNP is stored mainly in cardiac ventricular myocardium and may be responsive—albeit less so than ANP—to changes in ventricular filling pressures. BNP has a high level of homology with ANP at the structural level and, like ANP, causes natriuresis and vasodilation. CNP is located primarily in the vasculature. Although the physiological role of CNP is not yet clarified, it appears to play an important regulatory role in juxtaposition to the RAS system.

At least three receptors for natriuretic peptides (A, B, and C) have been identified. The A and B receptors mediate the vasodilatory and natriuretic effects of the peptides. The C-type receptor appears to act primarily as a clearance receptor, which, along with neutral endopeptidase, regulates available levels of the peptides.

Circulating levels of both ANP and BNP are elevated in the plasma of patients with heart failure.[176] In normal human hearts, ANP predominates in the atria, where there is also a low level of expression of BNP and CNP. In patients with heart failure, the atrial content of ANP is unchanged and the contents of BNP and CNP increase 10-fold and 2- to 3-fold, respectively.[176] In the SOLVD study, the level of plasma ANP was elevated even in asymptomatic patients and was further elevated in patients with symptoms.[162] Although the atrial peptides are present only in very low levels in normal ventricular myocardium, in patients with heart failure all three peptides are markedly elevated, and ventricular production contributes significantly to the circulating levels.[177] The secretion of ANP and BNP appears to be regulated mainly by wall tension. The N-terminal of the ANP free hormone (N-terminal pro-ANP) has a longer half-life and greater stability than ANP and has been shown to be a powerful and independent predictor of cardiovascular mortality and the development of heart failure. ANP levels become normal after cardiac transplantation.

Because plasma BNP release is less affected by atrial filling pressures, it provides a better reflection of myocardial disease. Plasma BNP has been shown to be useful in distinguishing cardiac from noncardiac causes of dyspnea[178] and provides prognostic information in patients with chronic heart failure[179] and following acute coronary syndromes.[180] Changes in plasma BNP may also reflect beneficial effects of drug therapy.[181] As with ANP, the N-terminal peptide frag-

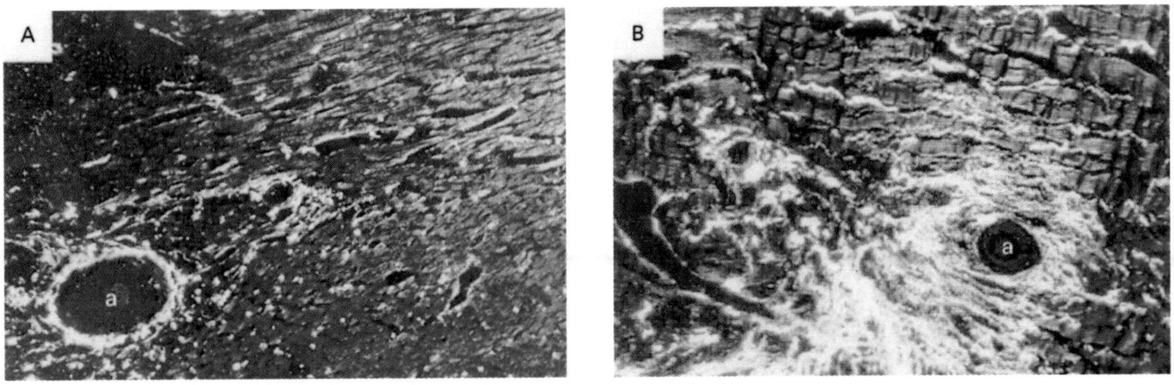

FIGURE 21–33 Coronary vascular remodeling caused by hyperaldosteronism in rats. **A,** A section from a normal heart with a normal intramural coronary artery (a) surrounded by yellow-stained fibrillar collagen. A small amount of collagen is also present between the muscle fibers. **B,** A section from the heart of a rat given aldosterone (plus salt) shows marked perivascular fibrosis of coronary vessels (a) and the contiguous interstitial space between muscle fibers. (Sirius red staining and polarized light, 40×). (From Weber KT: Aldosterone in congestive heart failure. N Engl J Med 345:1689, 2001.)

ment (N-terminal pro-BNP), which is cleaved to form the active hormone, may be more stable than BNP and thus provide more reliable information.

Studies using an ANP receptor antagonist in dogs with pacing-induced heart failure showed that despite attenuated hemodynamic and renal effects, the peptide continues to exert an important suppressive effect on the activity of the RAS and NE levels.[182] One approach that attempts to capitalize on the beneficial effects of the natriuretic peptides is to inhibit their degradation through the use of neutral endopeptidase inhibitors. The infusion of the endopeptidase inhibitor candoxatrilat into patients with heart failure mimics the action of infused ANP; it causes a reduction in left- and right-sided filling pressures associated with suppression of plasma NE levels and a transient reduction in plasma vasopressin, aldosterone, and renin activity. Likewise, the infusion of a human BNP exerts beneficial hemodynamic effects characterized by decreases in arterial and venous pressures, an increase in cardiac output, and suppression of neurohormonal activation,[183] and it has been approved by the Food and Drug Administration for the short-term treatment of patients with decompensated heart failure (see Chap. 23). In addition to the beneficial effect of natriuretic peptides on neurohormones, renal function, and hemodynamics, there is evidence that the natriuretic peptides may directly inhibit myocyte and vascular smooth muscle hypertrophy and interstitial fibrosis.

Natriuretic peptides are degraded by neutral endopeptidase. Vasopeptidase inhibitors such as omapatrilat inhibit both neutral endopeptidase and ACE and thereby combine the effects of ACE inhibition with increased levels of natriuretic peptides chronically. Although some early trials suggested that neutral endopeptidase inhibition would have a greater benefit than ACE inhibition, more recent trials have found the two classes of drug to exert similar effects on survival.[184]

ENDOTHELIN AND OTHER PEPTIDES

Endothelin is a potent peptide vasoconstrictor released by endothelial cells throughout the circulation. Like angiotensin II, endothelin can also be synthesized and released by a variety of other cell types such as cardiac myocytes. Three endothelin peptides (endothelin-1, endothelin-2, and endothelin-3), all of which are potent constrictors, have been identified.[185] At least two subtypes of endothelin receptors (types A and B) have been identified in human myocardium.[186]

The release of endothelin from endothelial cells in vitro can be enhanced by several vasoactive agents (e.g., NE, angiotensin II, thrombin) and cytokines (e.g., TGF-β and IL-1β). Several reports have documented an increase in circulating levels of endothelin-1 in patients with heart failure.[187] Plasma endothelin concentration correlates directly with pulmonary artery pressure, pulmonary vascular resistance, and the ratio of pulmonary to systemic vascular resistance. This has led to the suggestion that endothelin plays a pathophysiological role in mediating pulmonary hypertension in patients with heart failure. In normal subjects, plasma endothelin levels rise with orthostatic stress. However, in patients with heart failure, endothelin levels are already elevated and show no further increase with orthostatic stress, similar to the pattern of response seen with a variety of other vasoconstrictor substances, including angiotensin II and NE. Plasma endothelin levels have been shown to be increased in patients with acute myocardial infarction and to correlate with the Killip class in these patients.

Antagonists of endothelin receptors have been used to demonstrate the physiological effects of endothelin. When administered to rats with heart failure after myocardial infarction, the endothelin antagonist bosentan, which blocks both endothelin$_A$ and endothelin$_B$ receptors, decreased arterial pressure and exerted an effect additive to that of an ACE inhibitor.[188] Endothelin causes hypertrophy of cardiac myocytes in vitro, and the endothelin$_A$ receptor antagonist BQ123 inhibited myocardial hypertrophy in rats with pressure overload–induced hypertrophy caused by aortic banding. In rats with myocardial infarction, chronic administration of endothelin antagonists resulted in a reduction in left ventricular chamber remodeling and enlargement; it also improved hemodynamic function and improved survival.[189] This beneficial effect of endothelin receptor blockade on left ventricular dilation is associated with inhibition of MMPs, which may be involved in chamber dilation.[190] Likewise, endothelin$_A$ receptor blockade improved hemodynamic function in pigs with rapid pacing-induced heart failure.[191] These observations suggest that endothelin receptor antagonists may be of value in both the acute and chronic treatment of patients with heart failure.[192] Although administration of endothelin antagonists to patients has been shown to improve hemodynamic function,[193,194] long-term clinical beneficial effects on disease progression and survival have not been shown.

Several other peptides, including acidic fibroblast growth factor, basic fibroblast growth factor, TGF-β1, and platelet-derived growth factor, have been shown to affect the growth and phenotype of cardiac myocytes or fibroblasts in vitro. The expression of these and other peptides is increased in myocardium after myocardial infarction[195] or with hemodynamic overload, suggesting that they play a role in the orchestration of myocardial remodeling.

INFLAMMATORY CYTOKINES, INCLUDING TNF-α. Inflammatory cytokines, including TNF-α and IL-1β, may play an important role in the pathogenesis of myocardial failure.[196,197] In vitro, these and other inflammatory cytokines can regulate growth and gene expression in cardiac myocytes and other cells present in the myocardium. The circulating levels of proinflammatory cytokines including TNF-α and interleukin-6 (IL-6) are increased in patients with heart failure. The level of TNF-α correlated with depressed heart rate variability, an index of integrated autonomic nervous system function.[198] Conversely, the plasma concentrations of antiinflammatory cytokines such as IL-10 are reduced in patients with heart failure and are decreased more in patients with severe than with mild disease.[199] The failing myocardium, itself, may be a source of inflammatory cytokines, which might thus be present in high concentrations locally.[200]

Inflammatory cytokines have protean effects on the myocardium (Table 21–5). TNF-α can induce immediate myocardial dysfunction and has been shown to attenuate intracellular calcium transients in vitro.[201] In cultured cardiac myocytes, TNF-α and IL-1β can stimulate hypertrophy and

TABLE 21–5 Inflammatory Mediators

Cardiac Pathophysiologic Conditions Associated with Inflammatory Mediators
Acute viral myocarditis
Cardiac allograft rejection
Myocardial infarction
Unstable angina
Myocardial reperfusion injury
Hypertrophic cardiomyopathy*
Heart failure*
Cardiopulmonary bypass*
Magnesium deficiency*
Pressure overload*
Effects of Inflammatory Mediators on Left Ventricular Remodeling
Alterations in the biology of the myocyte
Myocyte hypertrophy
Contractile abnormalities
Fetal gene expression
Alteration in the extracellular matrix
MMP activation
Degradation of the matrix
Fibrosis
Progressive myocyte loss
Necrosis
Apoptosis

MMP = matrix metalloproteinase.

From Mann DL: Activation of inflammatory mediators in heart failure. *In* Mann DL (ed): Heart Failure. Philadelphia, Elsevier, 2004, pp 159, 164.

*Indicates conditions not traditionally associated with immunologiclly mediated inflammation.

reexpression of a fetal gene program[202] and can cause apoptosis,[203] which may be mediated, in part, by NO.[53] The chronic systemic infusion of TNF-α in rats resulted in left ventricular failure,[204] and mice that overexpressed TNF-α in the myocardium developed a dilated cardiomyopathy that was associated with increased myocyte apoptosis. Although pilot clinical trials with soluble TNF-α receptors that reduce the level of TNF-α available to the tissues have suggested that this may a feasible form of therapy for patients,[205] the results of a large clinical trial failed to demonstrate benefit with regard to hospitalization and survival.[206] The results of another trial that used infliximab, an antibody directed against TNF-α, found an increase in hospitalizations and mortality.[207] Likewise, observations from the Food and Drug Administration MedWatch program have suggested that the use of anti-TNF-α therapy may be associated with the new onset of heart failure.[208] It remains to be determined whether this lack of benefit is a reflection of the basic premise, the mode of drug action, or the complexity of the immune response. Other drugs that decrease plasma TNF-α levels, thalidomide[209] and pentoxifylline,[210] have shown promise in small clinical trials.

Nitric Oxide

At least two of the three known isoforms of nitric oxide synthase (NOS), termed NOS1, NOS2, and NOS3, are expressed in human myocardium. NOS2 is an inducible isoform that is not normally expressed in the myocardium but is synthesized de novo in response to inflammatory cytokines, thereby causing high levels of NO production. The expression and activity of NOS2 are increased in myocardium from animals with experimental heart failure[211] and patients with severe heart failure,[211] possibly as a result of stimulation by inflammatory cytokines.

The actions of NO on the myocardium are complex, involving both short-term alterations in function and energetics and longer term effects on structure.[212,213] It has been shown that NO mediates the inhibitory effect of inflammatory cytokines on the contractile response to beta-adrenergic stimulation in cardiac myocytes and myocardium by the induction of NOS2.[212-214] In normal human subjects, intracoronary infusion of nitroprusside, an NO donor, improved left ventricular distensibility,[215] whereas inhibition of NO synthesis by intracoronary infusion of an NOS inhibitor potentiated the positive inotropic response to dobutamine in patients with left ventricular dysfunction.[216] NO also appears to play a role in the regulation of myocardial energetics.[217] In addition to these short-term effects on myocardial function, NO may lead to longer term alterations in myocardial structure and function through its direct actions on myocytes to cause apoptosis[53,218] and modulate the response to hypertrophic stimuli such as NE and angiotensin. In transgenic mice deficient in NOS2, left ventricular remodeling was ameliorated and survival improved after myocardial infarction,[219] and beta-adrenergic responsiveness was improved in mice with dilated cardiomyopathy related to cardiac-specific overexpression of TNF-α.[213] Conversely, overexpression of NOS3 resulted in improved remodeling after myocardial infarction.[220] These contrasting effects of NOS2 (inducible) and NOS3 (endothelial) may reflect the differences in amount of NO produced, which is much higher with NOS2.

Oxidative Stress

There is evidence that oxidative stress is increased both systemically and in the myocardium of patients with heart failure.[221] Increased oxidative stress may be due to reduced antioxidant capacity or the increased production of reactive oxygen species, which may be a consequence of mechanical strain on the myocardium or stimulation by neurohormones and inflammatory cytokines. Possible sources of increased production of reactive oxygen species include the mitochondria, xanthine oxidase, and NADPH oxidase.[222] Reactive oxygen species can stimulate myocyte hypertrophy (see Fig. 21–30), reexpression of fetal gene programs, and apoptosis in cardiac myocytes in culture.[223] Mice with knockout of the antioxidant enzyme manganese superoxide dismutase (MnSOD) developed dilated cardiomyopathy and died at a young age.[224] Conversely, in animal models of hemodynamic overload–induced remodeling and failure, treatment with antioxidants prevented the progression to myocardial failure.[224-226] Although these observations have led to the suggestion that antioxidants might be of therapeutic value in patients, clinical trials to test this thesis are not available.

REFERENCES

Short-Term Adaptive Mechanisms

1. Hunt SA, Baker, DW, Chin ML, et al: Report of the ACC/AHA Guidelines for the Evaluation and Management of Chronic Heart Failure in the Adult. Circulation 104:2996, 2001.
2. Houser SR, Margulies KB: Is depressed myocyte contractility centrally involved in heart failure? Circ Res 92:350, 2003.
3. Hasenfuss G, Pieske B: Calcium cycling in congestive heart failure. J Mol Cell Cardiol 34:951, 2002.
4. Braunwald E, Ross J Jr, Sonnenblick EH: Mechanisms of Contraction of the Normal and Failing Heart. 2nd ed. Boston, Little, Brown, 1976, p 417.
5. Francis GS: Pathophysiology of chronic heart failure. Am J Med 110:37S, 2001.
6. Braunwald E, Bristow MR: Congestive heart failure: Fifty years of progress. Circulation 102:IV-14, 2000.
7. Konstam MA, Mann DL: Contemporary medical options for treating patients with heart failure. Circulation 105:2244, 2002.
8. Alpert NR, Mulieri LA, Warshaw D: The failing human heart. Cardiovasc Res 54:1, 2002.
9. Katz AM: Heart Failure. Philadelphia, Lippincott Williams & Wilkins, 2000.
10. Floras JS: Alterations in the sympathetic and parasympathetic nervous system in heart failure. *In* Mann DL (ed): Heart Failure: A Companion to Braunwald's Heart Disease: A Textbook of Cardiovascular Medicine. Philadelphia, WB Saunders, 2004, pp 247-278.
11. Leier CV, Brinkley PF, Cody RJ: Alpha adrenergic component of the sympathetic nervous system in congestive heart failure. Circulation 82:168, 1990.
12. Zelis R, Mason DT, Braunwald E: A comparison of the effects of vasodilator stimuli on peripheral resistance vessels in normal subjects and in patients with congestive heart failure. J Clin Invest 47:960, 1968.
13. Zelis R, Mason DT, Braunwald E: Partition of blood flow to the cutaneous and muscular beds of the forearm at rest and during leg exercise in normal subjects and in patients with heart failure. Circ Res 24:799, 1969.
14. Mancini DM, Coyle E, Coggan A, et al: Contribution of intrinsic skeletal muscle changes to ^{31}P NMR skeletal muscle metabolic abnormalities in patients with chronic heart failure. Circulation 80:1338, 1989.
15. Leier CV, Binkley PF, Cody RJ: Alpha-adrenergic component of the sympathetic nervous system in congestive heart failure. Circulation 82:168, 1990.
16. Higgins CB, Vatner SF, Millard RW, et al: Alterations in regional hemodynamics in experimental heart failure in conscious dogs. Trans Assoc Am Physicians 85:267, 1972.
17. Newby DE, Goodfield NE, Flapan AD, et al: Regulation of peripheral vascular tone in patients with heart failure: Contribution of angiotensin II. Heart 80:134, 1998.
18. Muders F, Luchner A, Friedrich EB, et al: Modulation of renal blood flow by endogenous endothelin-1 in conscious rabbits with left ventricular dysfunction. Am J Hypertens 12:835, 1999.
19. Wilson JR, Mancini DM: Factors contributing to the exercise limitation of heart failure. J Am Coll Cardiol 22(Suppl A):93a, 1993.
20. Hirooka Y, Imaizumi T, Tagawa T, et al: Effects of L-arginine on impaired acetylcholine-induced and ischemic vasodilation of the forearm in patients with heart failure. Circulation 90:658, 1994.
21. Hambrecht R, Fiehn E, Weigl C, et al: Regular physical exercise corrects endothelial dysfunction and improves exercise capacity in patients with chronic heart failure. Circulation 98:2709, 1998.
22. Bersin RM, Kwasman M, Lau D, et al: Importance of oxygen-haemoglobin binding to oxygen transport in congestive heart failure. Br Heart J 70:443, 1993.

Chronic Myocardial Remodeling

23. Meerson FZ: The myocardium in hyperfunction, hypertrophy, and heart failure. Circ Res 25(Suppl 2):1, 1969.
24. Cohn JN, Ferrari R, Sharpe N: Cardiac remodeling—Concepts and clinical implications: A consensus paper from an international forum on cardiac remodeling. J Am Coll Cardiol 35:569, 2000.
25. Grossman W, Jones D, McLaurin LP: Wall stress and patterns of hypertrophy in the human left ventricle. J Clin Invest 56:56, 1975.
26. Anversa P, Kajstura J: Ventricular myocytes are not terminally differentiated in the adult mammalian heart. Circ Res 83:1, 1998.
27. Calderone A, Takahashi N, Izzo NJ Jr, et al: Pressure- and volume-induced left ventricular hypertrophies are associated with distinct myocyte phenotypes and differential induction of peptide growth factor mRNAs. Circulation 92:2385, 1995.

28. Ross J Jr: Afterload mismatch and preload reserve: A conceptual framework for the analysis of ventricular function. Prog Cardiovasc Dis 18:255, 1976.
29. Gerdes AM: Cardiac myocyte remodeling in hypertrophy and progression to failure. J Card Fail 8:S264, 2002.
30. Spinale FG: Matrix metalloproteinases: Regulation and dysregulation in the failing heart. Circ Res 90:520, 2002.
31. Esposite G, Rapacciuolo A, Naga PSV, et al: Genetic alterations that inhibit in vivo pressure-overload hypertrophy prevent cardiac dysfunction despite increased wall stress. Circulation 105:85, 2002.
32. Spann JF Jr, Buccino RA, Sonnenblick EH, Braunwald E: Contractile state of cardiac muscle obtained from cats with experimentally produced ventricular hypertrophy and heart failure. Circ Res 21:341, 1987.
33. Pieske B, Maier LS, Piacentino V 3rd, et al: Rate dependence of $[Na^+]_i$ contractility in nonfailing and failing human myocardium. Circulation 106:447, 2002.
34. Piacentino V III, Weber CR, Chen X, et al: Cellular basis of abnormal calcium transients of failing human ventricular myocytes. Circ Res 92:651, 2003.
35. Lefkowitz RJ, Rockman HA, Koch WJ: Catecholamines, cardiac β adrenergic receptors, and heart failure. Circulation 101:1634, 2000.
36. Spann JF Jr, Covell JW, Eckberg DL et al: Contractile performance of the hypertrophied and chronically failing cat ventricle. Am J Physiol 223:1150, 1972.
37. Aoyagi T, Fujii AM, Flanagan MF, et al: Transition from compensated hypertrophy to intrinsic myocardial dysfunction during development of left ventricular pressure-overload hypertrophy in conscious sheep: Systolic dysfunction precedes diastolic dysfunction. Circulation 88:2415, 1993.
38. Palmon LC, Reichek N, Yeon SB, et al: Intramural myocardial shortening in hypertensive left ventricular hypertrophy with normal pump function. Circulation 89:122, 1994.

Molecular Mechanisms of Myocardial Remodeling and Failure

39. Monte FD, Hajjar RJ: Targeting calcium cycling proteins in heart failure through gene transfer. J Physiol (Lond) 546:49, 2003.
40. Sawyer DB, Colucci WS: Molecular and cellular events in myocardial hypertrophy and failure. *In* Colucci WS (ed): Atlas of Heart Failure: Cardiac Function and Dysfunction. 3rd ed. Philadelphia, Current Medicine, 2002, pp 65-85.
41. Maytin M, Colucci WS: Molecular and cellular mechanisms of myocardial remodeling. J Nucl Cardiol 9:319, 2002.
42. Givertz MM, Colucci WS: New targets for heart-failure therapy: Endothelin, inflammatory cytokines, and oxidative stress. Lancet 352(Suppl 1):SI34, 1998.
43. Hunter JJ, Chien KR: Signaling pathways for cardiac hypertrophy and failure. N Engl J Med 341:1276, 1999.
44. Sawyer DB, Siwik DA, Xiao L, et al: Role of oxidative stress in myocardial hypertrophy and failure. J Mol Cell Cardiol 34:379, 2002.
45. Dorn GW, Mann DL: Signaling pathways involved in left ventricular remodeling: Summation. J Card Fail 8:S387, 2002.
46. Kang PM, Yue P, Izumo S: New insights into the role of apoptosis in cardiovascular disease. Circ J 66:1, 2002.
47. Olivetti G, Abbi R, Quaini F, et al: Apoptosis in the failing human heart. N Engl J Med 336:1131, 1997.
48. Kajstura J, Liu Y, Baldini A, et al: Coronary artery constriction in rats: Necrotic and apoptotic myocyte death. Am J Cardiol 82(5A):30K, 1998.
49. Communal C, Singh K, Pimentel DR, Colucci WS: Norepinephrine stimulates apoptosis in adult rat ventricular myocytes by activation of the β-adrenergic pathway. Circulation 98:1329, 1998.
50. Iwai-Kanai E, Hasegawa K, Araki M, et al: Alpha- and beta-adrenergic pathways differentially regulate cell type–specific apoptosis in rat cardiac myocytes. Circulation 100:305, 1999.
51. Leri A, Claudio PP, Li Q, et al: Stretch-mediated release of angiotensin II induces myocyte apoptosis by activating p53 that enhances the local renin-angiotensin system and decreases the Bcl-2-to-Bax protein ratio in the cell. J Clin Invest 101:1326, 1998.
52. Siwik DA, Tzortzis JD, Pimental DR, et al: Inhibition of copper-zinc superoxide dismutase induces cell growth, hypertrophic phenotype, and apoptosis in neonatal rat cardiac myocytes in vitro. Circ Res 85:147, 1999.
53. Ing DJ, Zang J, Dzau VJ, et al: Modulation of cytokine-induced cardiac myocyte apoptosis by nitric oxide, Bak, and Bcl-x. Circ Res 84:21, 1999.
54. Pimentel DR, Amin JK, Xiao L, et al: Reactive oxygen species mediate amplitude-dependent hypertrophic and apoptotic responses to mechanical stretch in cardiac myocytes. Circ Res 89:453, 2001.
55. Pollack M, Phaneuf S, Dirks A, Leeuwenburgh C: The role of apoptosis in the normal aging brain, skeletal muscle, and heart. Ann NY Acad Sci 959:93, 2002.
56. Olivetti G, Melissari M, Capasso JM, Anversa B: Cardiomyopathy of the aging human heart: Myocyte loss and reactive cellular hypertrophy. Circ Res 68:1560, 1991.

Role of Calcium in Excitation-Contraction Coupling

57. Beuckelmann DJ, Nabauer M, Erdmann E: Intracellular calcium handling in isolated ventricular myocytes from patients with terminal heart failure. Circulation 85:1046, 1992.
58. Hasenfuss G, Mulieri LA, Leavitt BJ, et al: Alteration of contractile function and excitation-contraction coupling in dilated cardiomyopathy. Circ Res 70:1225, 1992.
59. Shorofsky SR, Aggarwal R, Corretti M, et al: Cellular mechanisms of altered contractility in the hypertrophied heart: Big hearts, big sparks. Circ Res 84:424, 1999.
60. Winslow RL, Rice J, Jafri S, et al: Mechanisms of altered excitation-contraction coupling in canine tachycardia-induced heart failure: II. Model studies. Circ Res 84:571, 1999.
61. Margulies KB, Houser SR: Myocyte abnormalities in human heart failure. *In* Mann DL (ed): Heart Failure: A Companion to Braunwald's Heart Disease: A Textbook of Cardiovascular Medicine. Philadelphia, WB Saunders, 2004, pp 41-56.
62. Flesch M, Schwinger RH, Schnabel P, et al: Sarcoplasmic reticulum Ca^{2+} ATPase and phospholamban mRNA and protein levels in end-stage heart failure due to ischemic or dilated cardiomyopathy. J Mol Med 74:321, 1996.
63. Frank K, Bolck B, Bavendiek U, Schwinger RH: Frequency dependent force generation correlates with sarcoplasmic calcium ATPase activity in human myocardium. Basic Res Cardiol 93:405, 1998.
64. Hobai IA, O'Rourke B: Decreased sarcoplasmic reticulum calcium content is responsible for defective excitation-contraction coupling in canine heart failure. Circulation 103:1577, 2001.
65. Li S, Margulies KB, Cheng H, Houser SR: Calcium current and calcium transients are depressed in failing human ventricular myocytes and recover in patients supported with left ventricular assist devices [abstract]. Circulation 100:160, 1999.
66. Meyer M, Bluhm WF, He H, et al: Phospholamban-to-SERCA2 ratio controls the force-frequency relationship. Am J Physiol 276:H779, 1999.
67. Giordano FJ, He H, McDonough P, et al: Adenovirus-mediated gene transfer reconstitutes depressed sarcoplasmic reticulum Ca^{2+}-ATPase levels and shortens prolonged cardiac myocyte Ca^{2+} transients. Circulation 96:400, 1997.
68. He H, Giordano FJ, Hilal-Dandan R, et al: Overexpression of the rat sarcoplasmic reticulum Ca^{2+} ATPase gene in the heart of transgenic mice accelerates calcium transients and cardiac relaxation. J Clin Invest 100:380, 1997.
69. Studer R, Reinecke H, Bilger J, et al: Gene expression of the cardiac Na^+-Ca^{2+} exchanger in end-stage human heart failure. Circ Res 75:443, 1994.
70. Weber CR, Piacentino V III, Margulies KB, et al: Calcium influx via I(NCX) is favored in failing human ventricular myocytes. Ann NY Acad Sci 976:478, 2002.
71. Brillantes A-M, Allen P, Takahasi T, et al: Differences in cardiac calcium release channel (ryanodine receptor) expression in myocardium from patients with end-stage heart failure caused by ischemic versus dilated cardiomyopathy. Circ Res 71:18, 1992.
72. Schumacher C, Konigs B, Sigmund M, et al: The ryanodine binding sarcoplasmic reticulum calcium release channel in nonfailing and in failing human myocardium. Naunyn Schmiedebergs Arch Pharmacol 353:80, 1995.
73. Marks AR, Reiken S, Marx SO: Progression of heart failure: Is protein kinase a hyperphosphorylation of the ryanodine receptor a contributing factor? Circulation 105:272, 2002.
74. Prestle J, Janssen PM, Janssen AP, et al: Overexpression of FK506-binding protein FKBP12.6 in cardiomyocytes reduces ryanodine receptor-mediated Ca^{2+} leak from the sarcoplasmic reticulum and increased contractility. Circ Res 88:188, 2001.
75. Marx SO, Marks AR. Regulation of the ryanodine receptor in heart failure. Basic Res Cardiol 97(Suppl 1):I49, 2002.
76. Reiken S, Wehrens XH, Vest JA, et al: Beta-blockers restore calcium release channel function and improve cardiac muscle performance in human heart failure. Circulation 107:2459, 2003.
77. Chen X, Piacentino V III, Furukawa S, et al: L-type Ca^{2+} channel density and regulation are altered in failing human ventricular myocytes and recover after support with mechanical assist devices. Circ Res 91:517, 2002.

Reduction of Myosin ATPase Activity

78. Izumo S, Pu WT: The molecular basis of heart failure. *In* Mann DL (ed): Heart Failure: A Companion to Braunwald's Heart Disease: A Textbook of Cardiovascular Medicine. Philadelphia, Saunders, 2004, pp 10-40.
79. Solaro RJ, Powers FM, Gao L, Gwathmey JK: Control of myofilament activation in heart failure. Circulation 87:VII-38, 1993.
80. Abraham WT, Gilbert EM, Lowes BD, et al: Coordinate changes in myosin heavy chain isoform gene expression are selectively associated with alterations in dilated cardiomyopathy phenotype. Mol Med 8:750, 2002.
81. Nakao K, Minobe W, Roden R, et al: Myosin heavy chain gene expression in human heart failure. J Clin Invest 100:2362, 1997.
82. Lowes BD, Minobe W, Abraham WT, et al: Changes in gene expression in the intact human heart: Downregulation of alpha myosin heavy chain in hypertrophied, failing ventricular myocardium. J Clin Invest 100:2315, 1997.
83. Lowes BD, Gilbert EM, Abraham WT, et al: Myocardial gene expression in dilated cardiomyopathy treated with beta-blocking agents. N Engl J Med 346:1357, 2002.
84. Solaro RJ, Rarick HM: Troponin and tropomyosin: Proteins that switch on and tune in the activity of cardiac myofilaments. Circ Res 83:471, 1998.
85. Anderson PA, Malouf NN, Oakeley AE, et al: Troponin T isoform expression in the normal and failing human left ventricle: A correlation with myofibrillar ATPase activity. Basic Res Cardiol 87:117, 1992.
86. Huang X, Pi Y, Lee KJ, et al: Cardiac troponin I gene knockout: A mouse model of myocardial troponin I deficiency. Circ Res 84:1, 1999.
87. Fatkin D, McConnell BK, Mudd JO, et al: An abnormal Ca^{2+} response in mutant sarcomere protein-mediated familial hypertrophic cardiomyopathy. J Clin Invest 106:1351, 2000.
88. Kamisago M, Sharman SD, DePalma SR, et al: Mutations in sarcomere protein genes as a cause of dilated cardiomyopathy. N Engl J Med 343:1688, 2000.
89. Gunasinghe SK, Spinale FG: Myocardial basis for heart failure: Role of cardiac interstitium. *In* Mann DL (ed): Heart Failure: A Companion to Braunwald's Heart Disease: A Textbook of Cardiovascular Medicine. Philadelphia, WB Saunders, 2004, pp 57-70.
90. Mann DL, Spinale FG: Activation of matrix metalloproteinases in the failing human heart: Breaking the tie that binds [editorial]. Circulation 98:1699, 1998.
91. Burlew BS, Weber KT: Cardiac fibrosis as a cause of diastolic dysfunction. Herz 27:92, 2002.
92. Thomas CV, Coker ML, Zellner JL, et al: Increased matrix metalloproteinase activity and selective upregulation in LV myocardium from patients with end-stage dilated cardiomyopathy. Circulation 97:1708, 1998.
93. Coker ML, Thomas CV, Clair MJ, et al: Myocardial matrix metalloproteinase activity and abundance with congestive heart failure. Am J Physiol 274:H1516, 1998.
94. Li YY, Feldman AM, Sun Y, McTiernan CF: Differential expression of tissue inhibitors of metalloproteinases in the failing human heart. Circulation 98:1728, 1998.

95. Spinale FG, Coker ML, Krombach SR, et al: Matrix metalloproteinase inhibition during the development of congestive heart failure: Effects on left ventricular dimensions and function. Circ Res 85:364, 1999.
96. Creemers EE, Davis JN, Parkhurst AM, et al: Deficiency of TIMP-1 exacerbates LV remodeling after myocardial infarction in mice. Am J Physiol 284:H364, 2003.
97. Ducharme A, Frantz S, Aikawa M, et al: Targeted deletion of matrix metalloproteinase-9 attenuates left ventricular enlargement and collagen accumulation after experimental myocardial infarction. J Clin Invest 106:55, 2000.
98. Conrad CH, Brooks WW, Hayes JA, et al: Myocardial fibrosis and stiffness with hypertrophy and heart failure in the spontaneously hypertensive rat. Circulation 91:161, 1995.
99. Boluyt MO, O'Neill L, Meredith AL, et al: Alterations in cardiac gene expression during the transition from stable hypertrophy to heart failure: Marked upregulation of genes encoding extracellular matrix components. Circ Res 75:23, 1994.
100. Brooks WW, Bing OH, Robinson KG, et al: Effect of angiotensin-converting enzyme inhibition on myocardial fibrosis and function in hypertrophied and failing myocardium from the spontaneously hypertensive rat. Circulation 96:4002, 1997.
101. Graham TP Jr, Ross J Jr, Covell JW: Myocardial oxygen consumption in acute experimental cardiac depression. Circ Res 21:123, 1967.
102. Ingwall JS: Energetic basis for heart failure. *In* Mann DL (ed): Heart Failure: A Companion to Braunwald's Heart Disease: A Textbook of Cardiovascular Medicine. Philadelphia, WB Saunders, 2004, pp 91-108.
103. Buchwald A, Till H, Unterberg C, et al: Alterations of the mitochondrial respiratory chain in human dilated cardiomyopathy. Eur Heart J 11:509, 1990.
104. Schulze K, Becker BF, Schauer R, Schultheiss HP: Antibodies to ADP-ATP carrier—An autoantigen in myocarditis and dilated cardiomyopathy impairs cardiac function. Circulation 81:959, 1990.
105. Ingwall JS: Is cardiac failure a consequence of decreased energy reserve? Circulation 87:VII-58, 1993.
106. Conway MA, Allis J, Ouwerkerk R, et al: Detection of low phosphocreatine to ATP ratio in failing hypertrophied human myocardium by ^{31}P magnetic resonance spectroscopy. Lancet 338:973, 1991.
107. Hardy CJ, Weiss RG, Bottomley PA, Gerstenblith G: Altered myocardial high-energy phosphate metabolites in patients with dilated cardiomyopathy. Am Heart J 122:795, 1991.
108. Bottomley PA: NMR spectroscopy of the human heart: The status and the challenges. Radiology 191:593, 1994.
109. Conway MA, Bottomley PA, Ouwerkerk R, et al: Mitral regurgitation: Impaired systolic function, eccentric hypertrophy, and increased severity are linked to lower phosphocreatine/ATP ratios in humans. Circulation 97:1716, 1998.
110. Neubauer S, Horn M, Cramer M, et al: Myocardial phosphocreatine-to-ATP ratio is a predictor of mortality in patients with dilated cardiomyopathy. Circulation 96:2190, 1997.
111. Liao R, Nascimben L, Friedrich J, et al: Decreased energy reserve in an animal model of dilated cardiomyopathy: Relationship to contractile performance. Circ Res 78:893, 1996.
112. Davis SV, Olichwier KK, Chakko SC: Reversible depression of myocardial performance in hypophosphatemia. Am J Med Sci 295:183, 1988.

Pathophysiology of Diastolic Heart Failure

113. Zile MR, Brutsaert DL: New concepts in diastolic dysfunction and diastolic heart failure: Part I: Diagnosis, prognosis, and measurements of diastolic function. Circulation 105:1387, 2002.
114. Zile MR, Brutsaert DL: New concepts in diastolic dysfunction and diastolic heart failure: Part II: Causal mechanisms and treatment. Circulation 105:1503, 2002.
115. Vasan RS, Larson MG, Benjamin EJ, et al: Congestive heart failure in subjects with normal versus reduced left ventricular ejection fraction: Prevalence and mortality in a population-based cohort. J Am Coll Cardiol 33:1948, 1999.
116. Zile MR, Baicu CF: Alterations in ventricular function: Diastolic heart failure. *In* Mann DL (ed): Heart Failure: A Companion to Braunwald's Heart Disease: A Textbook of Cardiovascular Medicine. Philadelphia, WB Saunders, 2004, pp 209-228.
117. Heyndrickx GR, Paulus WJ: Effect of asynchrony on left ventricular relaxation. Circulation 81(Suppl III):41, 1990.
118. Corin WJ, Murakami T, Monrad ES, et al: Left ventricular passive diastolic properties in chronic mitral regurgitation. Circulation 83:797, 1991.
119. McCullagh WH, Covell JW, Ross J Jr: Left ventricular dilatation and diastolic compliance changes during chronic volume overloading. Circulation 45:943, 1972.
120. Cazolla O, Freiburg A, Helmes M, et al: Differential expression of cardiac titin isoforms and modulation of cellular stiffness. Circ Res 86:59, 2000.
121. Burlew BS, Weber KT: Connective tissue and the heart. Functional significance and regulatory mechanisms. Cardiol Clin 18:435, 2000.
122. Hess OM, Osakada G, Lavelle JF, et al: Diastolic myocardial wall stiffness and ventricular relaxation during partial and complete coronary occlusions in the conscious dog. Circ Res 52:387, 1983.
123. Diamond C, Forrester JS: Effect of coronary artery disease and acute myocardial infarction on left ventricular compliance in man. Circulation 45:11, 1972.
124. Fletcher PJ, Pfeffer JM, Pfeffer MA, Braunwald E: Left ventricular diastolic pressure-volume relations in rats with healed myocardial infarction: Effects on systolic function. Circ Res 49:618, 1981.

Neurohormonal, Autocrine, and Paracrine Adjustments

125. Schrier RW, Abraham WT: Hormones and hemodynamics in heart failure. N Engl J Med 341:577, 1999.
126. Abramson BL, Ando S, Notarius CF, et al: Effect of atrial natriuretic peptide on muscle sympathetic activity and its reflex control in human heart failure. Circulation 99:1810, 1999.
127. Chidsey CA, Harrison DC, Braunwald E: Augmentation of plasma norepinephrine response to exercise in patients with congestive heart failure. N Engl J Med 267:650, 1962.
128. Chidsey CA, Braunwald E, Morrow AG: Catecholamine excretion and cardiac stores of norepinephrine in congestive heart failure. Am J Med 39:442, 1965.
129. Esler M, Kaye D, Lambert G, et al: Adrenergic nervous system in heart failure. Am J Cardiol 80:71, 1997.
130. Leimbach WN, Wallin BG, Victor HG, et al: Direct evidence from intraneural recordings for increased central sympathetic outflow in patients with heart failure. Circulation 73:913, 1986.
131. Swedberg K, Bristow MR, Cohn JN, et al: Effects of sustained-release moxonidine, an imidazoline agonist, on plasma norepinephrine in patients with chronic heart failure. Circulation 105:1797, 2002.
132. Jones CG, Cleland JG: Meeting report—The LIDO, HOPE, MOXCON and WASH studies. Heart Outcomes Prevention Evaluation. The Warfarin/Aspirin Study of Heart Failure. Eur J Heart Fail 1:425, 1999.
133. Landzberg JS, Parker JD, Gauthier DF, Colucci WS: Effects of myocardial alpha$_1$-adrenergic receptor stimulation and blockade on contractility in humans. Circulation 84:1608, 1991.
134. Satoh N, Suter TM, Liao R, Colucci WS: Chronic alpha-adrenergic receptor stimulation modulates the contractile phenotype of cardiac myocytes in vitro. Circulation 102:2249, 2000.
135. Chidsey CA, Sonnenblick EH, Morrow AG, Braunwald E: Norepinephrine stores and contractile force of papillary muscle from the failing human heart. Circulation 33:43, 1966.
136. Spann JF Jr, Sonnenblick E, Cooper EH, Braunwald E: Cardiac norepinephrine stores and the contractile state of heart muscle. Circ Res 19:317, 1966.
137. Merlet P, Benvenuti C, Moyse D, et al: Prognostic value of MIBG imaging in idiopathic dilated cardiomyopathy. J Nucl Med 40:917, 1999.
138. Merlet P, Pouillart F, Dubois-Rande JL, et al: Sympathetic nerve alterations assessed with ^{123}I-MIBG in the failing human heart. J Nucl Med 40:224, 1999.
139. Higgins CB, Vatner SF, Eckberg DL, Braunwald E: Alterations in the baroreceptor reflex in conscious dogs with heart failure. J Clin Invest 51:715, 1972.
140. Levine TB, Francis GS, Goldsmith SR, Cohn JN: The neurohumoral and hemodynamic response to orthostatic tilt in patients with congestive heart failure. Circulation 67:1070, 1983.
141. Goldsmith SR, Francis GS, Levine TB, Cohn JN: Regional blood flow response to orthostasis in patients with congestive heart failure. J Am Coll Cardiol 1:1391, 1983.
142. Kubo SH, Cody RJ: Circulatory autoregulation in chronic congestive heart failure: Responses to head-up tilt in 41 patients. Am J Cardiol 52:512, 1983.
143. Liu JL, Zucker IH: Regulation of sympathetic nerve activity in heart failure: A role for nitric oxide and angiotensin II. Circ Res 84:417, 1999.
144. Bristow MR: Beta adrenergic receptor blockade in chronic heart failure. Circulation 101:558, 2000.
145. Communal C, Singh K, Sawyer DB, Colucci WS: Opposing effects of beta (1)- and beta (2)-adrenergic receptors on cardiac myocyte apoptosis: Role of pertussis toxin–sensitive G protein. Circulation 100:2210, 1999.
146. Poole-Wilson PA, Swedberg K, Cleland JG, et al: A comparison of carvedilol and metoprolol on clinical outcomes in patients with chronic heart failure in the Carvedilol Or Metoprolol European Trial (COMET): Randomised controlled trial. Lancet 362:7, 2003.
147. Eckhart AD, Ozaki T, Tevaearai H, et al: Vascular-targeted overexpression of G protein–coupled receptor kinase-2 in transgenic mice attenuates beta-adrenergic receptor signaling and increases resting blood pressure. Mol Pharmacol 61:749, 2002.
148. Gilbert EM, Abraham WT, Olsen S, et al: Comparative hemodynamic, left ventricular functional, and antiadrenergic effects of chronic treatment with metoprolol versus carvedilol in the failing heart. Circulation 94:2817, 1996.
149. Ligett SB, Wagoner LE, Craft LL, et al: The Ile164 beta2-adrenergic receptor polymorphism adversely affects the outcome of congestive heart failure. J Clin Invest 102:1534, 1998.
150. Small KM, Wagoner LE, Levin AM, et al: Synergistic polymorphisms of beta1- and alpha2C-adrenergic receptors and the risk of congestive heart failure. N Engl J Med 347:1135, 2002.
151. Zolk O, Kouchi I, Schnabel P, Bohm M: Heterotrimeric G proteins in heart disease. Can J Physiol Pharmacol 78:187, 2000.
152. Dorn GW, Brown JH: Gq signaling in cardiac adaptation and maladaptation. Trends Cardiovasc Med 9:26, 1999.
153. Geng YJ, Ishikawa Y, Vatner DE, et al: Apoptosis of cardiac myocytes in Gs-alpha transgenic mice. Circ Res 84:34, 1999.
154. Iwase M, Uechi M, Vatner DE, et al: Cardiomyopathy induced by cardiac Gs alpha overexpression. Am J Physiol 272:H585, 1997.
155. Gaffney TE, Braunwald E: Importance of the adrenergic nervous system in the support of circulatory function in patients with congestive heart failure. Am J Med 34:320, 1963.
156. Epstein SE, Braunwald E: The effect of beta-adrenergic blockade on patterns of urinary sodium excretion: Studies in normal subjects and in patients with heart disease. Ann Intern Med 75:20, 1966.
157. Singh K, Xiao L, Remondino A, et al: Adrenergic regulation of cardiac myocyte apoptosis. J Cell Physiol 189:257, 2001.
158. Shizukuda Y, Buttrick PM, Geenen DL, et al: Beta-adrenergic stimulation causes cardiocyte apoptosis: Influence of tachycardia and hypertrophy. Am J Physiol 275:H961, 1998.
159. Bisognano JD, Weinberger HD, Bohlmeyer TJ, et al: Myocardial-directed overexpression of the human beta$_1$-adrenergic receptor in transgenic mice. J Mol Cell Cardiol 32:817, 2000.
160. Eckberg DL, Drabinsky M, Braunwald E: Defective cardiac parasympathetic control in patients with heart disease. N Engl J Med 285:877, 1971.

161. Grassi G, Esler M: How to assess sympathetic activity in humans. J Hypertens 17:719, 1999.
162. Francis GS, Benedict C, Johnstone DE, et al: Comparison of neuroendocrine activation in patients with left ventricular dysfunction with and without congestive heart failure: A substudy of the Studies of Left Ventricular Dysfunction (SOLVD). Circulation 82:1724, 1990.
163. Yusuf S, Sleight P, Pogue J, et al: Effects of an angiotensin-converting-enzyme inhibitor, ramipril, on cardiovascular events in high-risk patients. The Outcomes Prevention Evaluation Study. N Engl J Med 342:145, 2000.
164. Farquharson CA, Struthers AD: Spironolactone increases nitric oxide bioactivity, improves endothelial vasodilator dysfunction, and suppresses vascular angiotensin I/angiotensin II conversion in patients with chronic heart failure. Circulation 101:1594, 2000.
165. van Veldhuisen DJ, Voors AA: Blockade of the renin angiotensin system in heart failure: The potential place of angiotensin II receptor blockers. Eur Heart J 21:14, 2000.
166. Kim S, Iwao H: Molecular and cellular mechanisms of angiotensin II–mediated cardiovascular and renal diseases. Pharmacol Rev 52:11, 2000.
167. Kajstura J, Cigola E, Malhotra A, et al: Angiotensin II induces apoptosis of adult ventricular myocytes in vitro. J Mol Cell Cardiol 29:859, 1997.
168. Kawano H, Do YS, Kawano Y, et al: Angiotensin II has multiple profibrotic effects in human cardiac fibroblasts. Circulation 101:1130, 2000.
169. Zisman LS, Asano K, Dutcher DL, et al: Differential regulation of cardiac angiotensin converting enzyme binding sites and AT1 receptor density in the failing human heart. Circulation 98:1735, 1998.
170. Weber KT: Aldosterone in congestive heart failure. N Engl J Med 345:1689, 2001.
171. Sun Y, Zhang J, Lu L, et al: Aldosterone-induced inflammation in the rat heart: Role of oxidative stress. Am J Pathol 161:1773, 2002.
172. Qin W, Rudolph AE, Bond BR, et al: Transgenic model of aldosterone-driven cardiac hypertrophy and heart failure. Circ Res 93:69, 2003.
173. Pitt B, Zannand F, Remme WJ, et al: The effect of spironolactone on morbidity and mortality in patients with severe heart failure. Randomized Aldactone Evaluation Study Investigators. N Engl J Med 341:709, 1999.
174. Pitt B, Remme W, Zannad F, et al: Eplerenone, a selective aldosterone blocker, in patients with left ventricular dysfunction after myocardial infarction. N Engl J Med 348:1309, 2003.
175. Naitoh M, Suzuki H, Murakami M, et al: Effects of oral AVP receptor antagonists OPC-21268 and OPC-31260 on congestive heart failure in conscious dogs. Am J Physiol 267:H2245, 1994.
176. Talwar S, Siebenhofer A, Williams B, Ng L: Influence of hypertension, left ventricular hypertrophy, and left ventricular systolic dysfunction on plasma N terminal proBNP. Heart 83:278, 2000.
177. Wei CM, Heublein DM, Perrella MA, et al: Natriuretic peptide system in human heart failure. Circulation 88:1004, 1993.
178. Morrison LK, Harrison A, Krishnaswamy P, et al: Utility of rapid B-natriuretic peptide assay in differentiating congestive heart failure from lung disease in patients presenting with dyspnea. J Am Coll Cardiol 39:202, 2002.
179. Sugimoto Y, Kinoshita M: Attenuation of compensation of endogenous cardiac natriuretic peptide system in chronic heart failure: Prognostic role of plasma brain natriuretic peptide concentration in patients with chronic symptomatic left ventricular dysfunction. Circulation 96:509, 1997.
180. Morrow DA, deLemos JA, Sabatine MS, et al: Evaluation of B-type natriuretic peptide for risk assessment in unstable angina/non-ST-elevation myocardial infarction: B-type natriuretic peptide and prognosis in TACTICS-TIMI 18. J Am Coll Cardiol 41:1264, 2003.
181. Anand IS, Fisher LD, Chiang YT, et al: Changes in brain natriuretic peptide and norepinephrine over time and mortality and morbidity in the Valsartan Heart Failure Trial (Val-HeFT). Circulation 107:1278, 2003.
182. Wada A, Tsutamoto T, Matsuda Y, Kinoshita M: Cardiorenal and neurohumoral effects of endogenous atrial natriuretic peptide in dogs with severe congestive heart failure using a specific antagonist for guanylate cyclase–coupled receptors. Circulation 89:2232, 1994.
183. Colucci WS: Nesiritide for the treatment of decompensated heart failure. J Card Fail 7:92, 2001.
184. Packer M, Califf RM, Konstam MA, et al: Comparison of omapatrilat and enalapril in patients with chronic heart failure: The Omapatrilat Versus Enalapril Randomized Trial of Utility in Reducing Events (OVERTURE). Circulation 106:920, 2002.
185. Sam F, Colucci WS: Role of endothelin-1 in myocardial failure. Proc Assoc Am Physicians 111:417, 1999.
186. Zolk O, Quattek J, Sitzler G, et al: Expression of endothelin-1, endothelin-converting enzyme, and endothelin receptors in chronic heart failure. Circulation 99:2118, 1999.
187. Serneri GG, Cecioni I, Vanni S, et al: Selective upregulation of cardiac endothelin system in patients with ischemic but not idiopathic dilated cardiomyopathy: Endothelin-1 system in the human failing heart. Circ Res 86:377, 2000.
188. Teerlink JR, Loffler BM, Hess P, et al: Role of endothelin in the maintenance of blood pressure in conscious rats with chronic heart failure: Acute effects of the endothelin receptor antagonist Ro 47-0203 (bosentan). Circulation 90:2510, 1994.
189. Fraccarollo D, Hu K, Galuppo P, et al: Chronic endothelin receptor blockade attenuates progressive ventricular dilation and improves cardiac function in rats with myocardial infarction: Possible involvement of myocardial endothelin system in ventricular remodeling. Circulation 96:3963, 1997.
190. Podesser BK, Siwik DA, Eberli FR, et al: ET(A)-receptor blockade prevents matrix metalloproteinase activation late postmyocardial infarction in the rat. Am J Physiol 280:H984, 2001.
191. Saad D, Mukherjee R, Thomas PB, et al: The effects of endothelin-A receptor blockade during the progression of pacing-induced congestive heart failure. J Am Coll Cardiol 32:1779, 1998.
192. Colucci WS: Myocardial endothelin: Does it play a role in myocardial failure? Circulation 93:1069, 1996.

193. Kiowski W, Sutsch G, Hunziker P, et al: Evidence for endothelin-1–mediated vasoconstriction in severe chronic heart failure. Lancet 346:732, 1995.
194. Sutsch G, Bertel O, Kiowski W: Acute and short-term effects of the nonpeptide endothelin-1 receptor antagonist bosentan in humans. Cardiovasc Drugs Ther 10:717, 1997.
195. Ono K, Matsumori A, Shioi T, et al: Cytokine gene expression after myocardial infarction in rat hearts: Possible implication in left ventricular remodeling. Circulation 98:149, 1998.
196. Mann DL: Inflammatory mediators and the failing heart: Past, present, and the foreseeable future. Circ Res 91:988, 2002.
197. Mann DL: Activation of cytokine systems in heart failure. *In* Mann DL (ed): Heart Failure: A Companion to Braunwald's Heart Disease: A Textbook of Cardiovascular Medicine. Philadelphia, Elsevier, 2004, pp 159-180.
198. Malave HA, Taylor AA, Nattama J, et al: Circulating levels of tumor necrosis factor correlate with indexes of depressed heart rate variability: A study in patients with mild-to-moderate heart failure. Chest 123:716, 2003.
199. Stumpf C, Lehner C, Yilmaz A, et al: Decrease of serum levels of the anti-inflammatory cytokine interleukin-10 in patients with advanced chronic heart failure. Clin Sci (Lond) 105:45, 2003.
200. Torre-Amione G, Kapadia S, Lee J, et al: Tumor necrosis factor-alpha and tumor necrosis factor receptors in the failing human heart. Circulation 93:704, 1996.
201. Janczewski AM, Kadokami T, Lemster B, et al: Morphological and functional changes in cardiac myocytes isolated from mice overexpressing TNF-alpha. Am J Physiol 284:H960, 2003.
202. Thaik CM, Calderone A, Takahashi N, Colucci WS: Interleukin-1 beta modulates the growth and phenotype of neonatal rat cardiac myocytes. J Clin Invest 96:1093, 1995.
203. Krown KA, Page MT, Nguyen C, et al: Tumor necrosis factor alpha–induced apoptosis in cardiac myocytes: Involvement of the sphingolipid signaling cascade in cardiac cell death. J Clin Invest 98:2854, 1996.
204. Bozkurt B, Kribbs SB, Clubb FJ Jr, et al: Pathophysiologically relevant concentrations of tumor necrosis factor-alpha promote progressive left ventricular dysfunction and remodeling in rats. Circulation 97:1382, 1998.
205. Deswal A, Bozkurt B, Seta Y, et al: Safety and efficacy of a soluble P75 tumor necrosis factor receptor (Enbrel, etanercept) in patients with advanced heart failure. Circulation 99:3224, 1999.
206. Krum H: Tumor necrosis factor-alpha blockade as a therapeutic strategy in heart failure (RENEWAL and ATTACH): Unsuccessful, to be specific. J Card Fail 8:365, 2002.
207. Chung ES, Packer M, Lo KH, et al: Randomized, double-blind, placebo-controlled, pilot trial of infliximab, a chimeric monoclonal antibody to tumor necrosis factor-alpha, in patients with moderate-to-severe heart failure: Results of the anti-TNF Therapy Against Congestive Heart Failure (ATTACH) trial. Circulation 107:3133, 2003.
208. Kwon HJ, Cote TR, Cuffe MS, et al: Case reports of heart failure after therapy with a tumor necrosis factor antagonist. Ann Intern Med 138:807, 2003.
209. Gullestad L, Semb AG, Holt E, et al: Effect of thalidomide in patients with chronic heart failure. Am Heart J 144:847, 2002.
210. Sliwa K, Woodiwiss A, Candy G, et al: Effects of pentoxifylline on cytokine profiles and left ventricular performance in patients with decompensated congestive heart failure secondary to idiopathic dilated cardiomyopathy. Am J Cardiol 90:1118, 2002.
211. Orus J, Heras M, Morales-Ruiz M, et al: Nitric oxide synthase II mRNA expression in cardiac tissue of patients with heart failure undergoing cardiac transplantation. J Heart Lung Transplant 19:139, 2000.
212. Hare JM, Colucci WS: Role of nitric oxide in the regulation of myocardial function. Prog Cardiovasc Dis 38:155, 1995.
213. Funakoshi H, Kubota T, Kawamura N, et al: Disruption of inducible nitric oxide synthase improves beta-adrenergic inotropic responsiveness but not the survival of mice with cytokine-induced cardiomyopathy. Circ Res 90:959, 2002.
214. Gealekman O, Abassi Z, Rubinstein I, et al: Role of myocardial inducible nitric oxide synthase in contractile dysfunction and beta-adrenergic hyporesponsiveness in rats with experimental volume-overload heart failure. Circulation 105:236, 2002.
215. Paulus WJ, Vantrimpont PJ, Shah AM: Acute effects of nitric oxide on left ventricular relaxation and diastolic distensibility in humans: Assessment by bicoronary sodium nitroprusside infusion. Circulation 89:2070, 1994.
216. Hare JM, Loh E, Creager MA, Colucci WS: Nitric oxide inhibits the positive inotropic response to beta-adrenergic stimulation in humans with left ventricular dysfunction. Circulation 92:2198, 1995.
217. Chen Y, Traverse JH, Du R, et al: Nitric oxide modulates myocardial oxygen consumption in the failing heart. Circulation 106:273, 2002.
218. Bishopric NH: A thousand times NO. J Mol Cell Cardiol 34:601, 2002.
219. Sam F, Sawyer DB, Xie Z, et al: Mice lacking inducible nitric oxide synthase have improved left ventricular contractile function and reduced apoptotic cell death late after myocardial infarction. Circ Res 89:351, 2001.
220. Scherrer-Crosbie M, Ullrich R, Bloch KD, et al: Endothelial nitric oxide synthase limits left ventricular remodeling after myocardial infarction in mice. Circulation 104:1286, 2001.
221. Mallat Z, Philip I, Lebret M, et al: Elevated levels of 8-iso-prostaglandin F2alpha in pericardial fluid of patients with heart failure: A potential role for in vivo oxidant stress in ventricular dilatation and progression to heart failure. Circulation 97:1536, 1998.
222. Li JM, Gall NP, Grieve DJ, et al: Activation of NADPH oxidase during progression of cardiac hypertrophy to failure. Hypertension 40:477, 2002.
223. Hare JM: Oxidative stress and apoptosis in heart failure progression. Circ Res 89:198, 2001.
224. Li Y, Huang T-T, Carlson EJ, et al: Dilated cardiomyopathy and neonatal lethality in mutant mice lacking manganese superoxide dismutase. Nat Genet 11:376, 1995.
225. Dhalla AK, Hill MF, Singal PK: Role of oxidative stress in transition of hypertrophy to heart failure. J Am Coll Cardiol 28:506, 1996.
226. Kinugawa S, Tsutsui H, Hayashidani S, et al: Treatment with dimethylthiourea prevents left ventricular remodeling and failure after experimental myocardial infarction in mice: Role of oxidative stress. Circ Res 87:392, 2000.

CHAPTER 22

Clinical Aspects of Heart Failure; Pulmonary Edema, High-Output Failure

Michael M. Givertz • Wilson S. Colucci • Eugene Braunwald

Definition

Heart failure is a principal complication of virtually all forms of heart disease. An American College of Cardiology/American Heart Association (ACC/AHA) Task Force on Practice Guidelines described this condition as follows.

Heart failure is a complex clinical syndrome that can result from any structural or functional cardiac disorder that impairs the ability of the ventricle to fill with or eject blood. The cardinal manifestations of heart failure are dyspnea and fatigue, which may limit exercise tolerance, and fluid retention, which may lead to pulmonary congestion and peripheral edema. Both abnormalities can impair the functional capacity and quality of life of affected individuals, but they do not necessarily dominate the clinical picture at the same time. Because not all patients have volume overload at the time of initial or subsequent evaluation, the term "heart failure" is preferred over the older term "congestive heart failure."[1]

Myocardial failure, a term used to denote abnormal systolic or diastolic function, may be asymptomatic or progress to heart failure. *Circulatory failure* is not synonymous with heart failure because a variety of noncardiac conditions (e.g., hemorrhagic shock) can lead to circulatory collapse while cardiac function is preserved. *Cardiomyopathy* and *left ventricular dysfunction* are more general terms that describe abnormalities of cardiac structure or function, or both, which may lead to heart failure.

The clinical manifestations of heart failure vary enormously and depend on a variety of factors, including the age of the patient, the extent and rate at which cardiac performance becomes impaired, and the ventricle initially involved in the disease process. A broad spectrum of severity of impairment of cardiac function is ordinarily included within the definition of heart failure, ranging from the mildest, which is manifest clinically only during stress, to the most advanced form, in which cardiac pump function is unable to sustain life without external support. Useful criteria for the diagnosis of heart failure, which emerged from the Framingham Study (Table 22–1),[2] emphasize that heart failure is, in the final analysis, a clinical diagnosis.

To emphasize the evolution and progression of heart failure, the ACC/AHA guidelines on the evaluation and management of heart failure set forth a staging system (Table 22–2).[1] This staging system recognizes that there are established risk factors and structural prerequisites for the development of heart failure, that therapeutic interventions that are initiated before the onset of left ventricular dysfunction or symptoms can reduce morbidity and mortality, that patients generally progress from one stage to the next unless disease progression is slowed or stopped by treatment, and that all patients benefit from risk factor modification including blood pressure control, lipid management, exercise training, and smoking and alcohol cessation.

Prevalence and Incidence

Heart failure is a relatively common disorder. It is estimated that 4.9 million persons in the United States are being treated for heart failure, with 550,000 new cases diagnosed each year.[3,4] The prevalence of heart failure increases dramatically with age, occurring in 1 to 2 percent of persons aged 45 to 54 years and up to 10 percent of individuals older than 75 years (Fig. 22–1).[2,3] For individuals free of heart failure at age 40, the remaining lifetime risk for developing heart failure is 21 percent for men and 20.3 percent for women.[5] Approximately 80 percent of all heart failure admissions occur in patients older than 65; as a result, heart failure is the leading discharge diagnosis in persons aged 65 years or older in the United States with an average length of stay of 5.3 days.[6] Between 1979 and 2000, the number of heart failure hospitalizations rose from 377,000 to 999,000, an increase of 165 percent (Fig. 22–2).[3] In the United States, approximately 56,000 deaths each year are primarily caused by heart failure and heart failure was listed as a contributing cause in 262,000 deaths.[7] The U.S. mortality rate related to heart failure is estimated at 20.2 deaths per 100,000 population. The trend toward increased morbidity and mortality related to heart failure may be due in part to the aging of the population and in part to the improved survival of patients with cardiovascular disease.

Heart failure has an enormous economic impact on the U.S. health care system, owing to direct medical costs, disability, and loss of employment. In 2000, $3.5 billion was spent on Medicare beneficiaries for the in-hospital management of heart failure.[8] Estimated treatment costs for all inpatients with heart failure in 2003 were $24.3 billion. The cost of hospitalizations for heart failure is twice that for all forms of cancer and myocardial infarctions combined.[9]

Forms and Causes of Heart Failure

Forward Versus Backward Heart Failure

Focusing on cardiovascular hemodynamics, early investigators postulated that the

TABLE 22–1 Framingham Criteria for Heart Failure*

Major Criteria
Paroxysmal nocturnal dyspnea
Neck vein distention
Rales
Radiographic cardiomegaly
Acute pulmonary edema
S_3 gallop
Increased central venous pressure > 16 cm H_2O
Circulation time ≥ 25 sec
Hepatojugular reflux
Pulmonary edema, visceral congestion, or cardiomegaly at autopsy
Weight loss ≥ 4.5 kg in 5 days in response to treatment of heart failure
Minor Criteria
Bilateral ankle edema
Nocturnal cough
Dyspnea on ordinary exertion
Hepatomegaly
Pleural effusion
Decrease in vital capacity by one third from maximal value recorded
Tachycardia (rate ≥ 120 beats/min)

From Ho KL, Pinsky JL, Kannel WB, Levy D: The epidemiology of heart failure: The Framingham Study. J Am Coll Cardiol 22(Suppl A):6A, 1993.

*The diagnosis of heart failure in this study required that two major or one major and two minor criteria be present concurrently. Minor criteria were acceptable only if they could not be attributed to another medical condition.

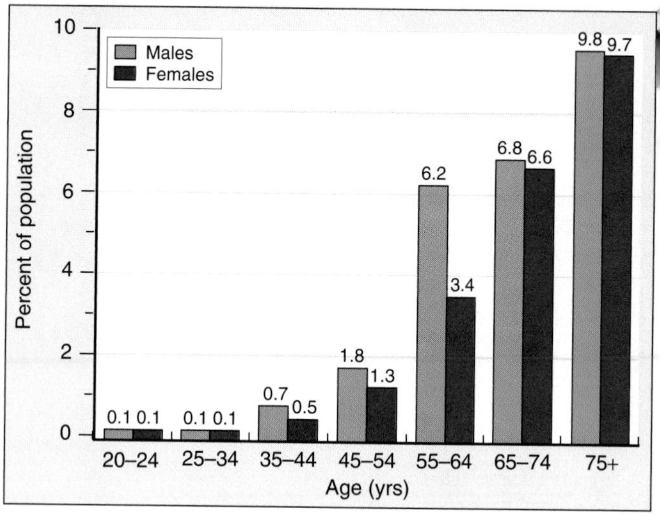

FIGURE 22–1 Prevalence rates of heart failure by gender and age in the United States between 1988 and 1994: the Third National Health and Nutrition Examination Survey (NHANES III). Among men (blue), the prevalence increased from 18 cases per 1000 in those aged 45 to 54 years to 98 cases per 1000 in those aged 75 years and older. Among women (purple), the prevalence increased from 13 cases per 1000 in those aged 45 to 54 years to 97 cases per 1000 in those aged 75 years and older. (Data from American Heart Association: Heart Disease and Stroke Statistics—2003 Update. Dallas, American Heart Association, 2002.)

clinical manifestations of heart failure arose as a consequence of inadequate cardiac output or damming up of blood behind one or both ventricles, or both. These two principal mechanisms were the basis of the forward and backward pressure theories of heart failure. The *backward failure hypothesis*, first proposed by James Hope in 1832, contends that when the ventricle fails to discharge its contents, blood accumulates and pressure rises in the atrium and the venous system emptying into it. As discussed in Chapter 19, the inability of cardiac muscle to shorten against a load alters the relationship between ventricular end-systolic pressure and volume so that end-systolic volume rises. The following sequence then occurs, which at first maintains cardiac output at a normal level but ultimately leads to clinical decompensation: (1) ventricular end-diastolic volume and pressure increase, (2) the volume and pressure rise in the atrium behind the failing ventricle, (3) the atrium contracts more vigorously (a manifestation of Starling's law, operating on the atrium), (4) the pressure in the venous and capillary beds behind the failing ventricle rises, and (5) transudation of fluid from the capillary bed into the interstitial space (pulmonary or systemic) increases. Many of the symptoms characteristic of heart failure can be traced to this sequence of events and the resultant increase in fluid in the interstitial spaces of the lungs, liver, subcutaneous tissues, and serous cavities.

An important extension of the backward failure theory is the development of right ventricular failure as a consequence of left ventricular failure. According to this concept, the

TABLE 22–2 Stages of Heart Failure

Stage	Description	Examples
A	At high risk for developing HF because of the presence of conditions that are strongly associated with the development of HF No identified structural or functional abnormalities of the pericardium, myocardium, or cardiac valves No history of signs or symptoms of HF	Systemic hypertension Coronary artery disease Diabetes mellitus History of cardiotoxic drug therapy History of alcohol abuse Family history of cardiomyopathy
B	Presence of structural heart disease that is strongly associated with the development of HF No history of signs or symptoms of HF	Left ventricular hypertrophy or fibrosis Left ventricular dilation or dysfunction Asymptomatic valvular heart disease Previous myocardial infarction
C	Current or prior symptoms of HF associated with underlying structural heart disease	Dyspnea or fatigue due to left ventricular systolic dysfunction Asymptomatic patients receiving treatment for prior symptoms of HF
D	Advanced structural heart disease and marked symptoms of HF at rest despite maximal medical therapy Require specialized interventions	Frequent HF hospitalizations and cannot be discharged In the hospital awaiting heart transplant At home with continuous inotropic or mechanical support In hospice setting for management of HF

HF = heart failure.

Adapted from Hunt SA, Baker DW, Chin MH, et al: ACC/AHA guidelines for the evaluation and management of chronic heart failure in the adult: Executive summary. A report of the American College of Cardiology/American Heart Association Task Force on Practice Guidelines (Committee to Revise the 1995 Guidelines for the Evaluation and Management of Heart Failure). Circulation 104:2996, 2001.

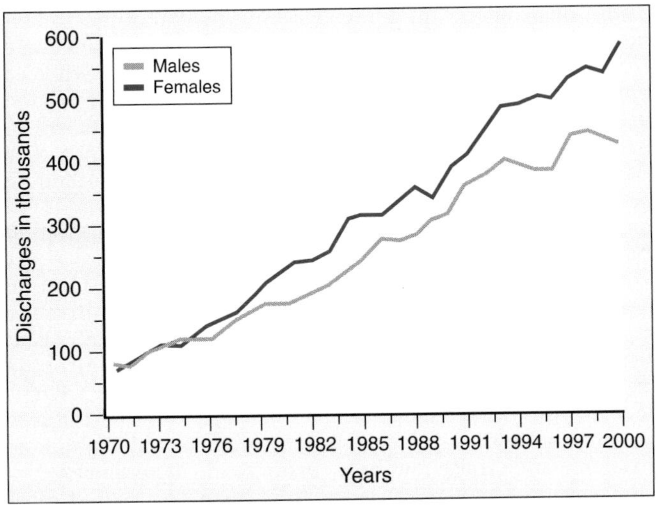

FIGURE 22–2 Hospital discharges for heart failure by gender in the United States between 1970 and 2000. Among men (blue), the number of discharges increased from 90,000 per year in 1970 to 410,000 per year in 2000. Among women (magenta), the number of discharges increased from 90,000 per year in 1970 to 580,000 per year in 2000. Source: Centers for Disease Control and Prevention, National Center for Health Statistics. (Data from American Heart Association: Heart Disease and Stroke Statistics—2003 Update. Dallas, American Heart Association, 2002.)

elevation of left ventricular diastolic, left atrial, and pulmonary venous pressures results in backward transmission of pressure into the pulmonary arterial circulation and leads to pulmonary hypertension, which ultimately causes right ventricular failure. It is now recognized that changes in the structure and function of the pulmonary vasculature play an important role in the development of secondary pulmonary hypertension associated with heart failure.[10]

Eighty years after the publication of Hope's work, Mackenzie proposed the *forward failure hypothesis*, which relates clinical manifestations of heart failure to inadequate delivery of blood into the arterial system. According to this hypothesis, the principal clinical manifestations of heart failure are due to reduced cardiac output, which results in diminished perfusion of vital organs, including the brain, leading to mental confusion; skeletal muscles, leading to weakness; and kidneys, leading to sodium and water retention. Sodium and water retention occurring through a series of complex neurohormonal mechanisms[11,12] in turn augment extracellular fluid volume and ultimately lead to symptoms of heart failure.

Although these two seemingly opposing views concerning the pathogenesis of heart failure led to lively controversy during the first half of the 20th century, neither theory takes into account the full spectrum of pathophysiological changes that contribute to ventricular remodeling and disease progression in patients with chronic heart failure.

RIGHT-SIDED VERSUS LEFT-SIDED HEART FAILURE

Implicit in the backward failure theory is the idea that fluid localizes behind the specific cardiac chamber that is *initially* affected. Thus, symptoms secondary to pulmonary congestion initially predominate in patients with left ventricular infarction, hypertension, or aortic or mitral valve disease; that is, they manifest *left-sided heart failure*. With time, however, fluid accumulation becomes generalized, and ankle edema, congestive hepatomegaly, ascites, and pleural effusion occur; thus, the patients subsequently exhibit *right-sided heart failure* as well.

FLUID RETENTION

Fluid retention in heart failure is due in part to reduction in glomerular filtration rate and in part to activation of neurohormonal systems, including the renin-angiotensin-aldosterone system and sympathetic nervous system.[12] Reduced cardiac output is associated with a lowered glomerular filtration rate and an increased elaboration of renin, which, through the activation of angiotensin, results in the release of aldosterone (see Chap. 21). The combination of impaired hepatic function, owing to hepatic venous congestion, and reduced hepatic blood flow interferes with the metabolism of aldosterone, further raising its plasma concentration and augmenting the retention of sodium and water. Arginine vasopressin is also elevated in patients with chronic heart failure and contributes to systemic vasoconstriction and free water retention.

Cardiac output (and glomerular filtration rate) may be normal in many patients with heart failure, particularly when they are at rest. However, during stress, such as physical exercise, the cardiac output fails to rise normally, the glomerular filtration rate declines, and the renal mechanisms for salt and water retention described earlier come into play. In addition, ventricular filling pressure and therefore pressures in the atrium and systemic veins behind the ventricle may be normal at rest, only to rise abnormally during stress. This effect, in turn, may cause transudation and symptoms of tissue congestion (e.g., pulmonary congestion in the case of the left ventricle) during exercise. For this reason, rest may induce diuresis and relieve symptoms in many patients with mild to moderate heart failure.

ACUTE VERSUS CHRONIC HEART FAILURE

The clinical manifestations of heart failure depend importantly on the *rate* at which the syndrome develops and specifically on whether sufficient time has elapsed for compensatory mechanisms to become operative and for fluid to accumulate in the interstitial space. For example, when a previously normal individual suddenly develops a serious anatomical or functional abnormality of cardiac function, such as a massive myocardial infarction, tachyarrhythmia with a very rapid rate, or rupture of a valve secondary to infective endocarditis, a marked reduction in cardiac output occurs, associated with symptoms related to inadequate organ perfusion or acute congestion of the venous bed behind the affected ventricle, or both. If the same anatomical abnormality develops gradually, or if the patient survives the acute insult, a number of adaptive mechanisms become operational, including cardiovascular remodeling and neurohormonal activation (see Chap. 21), and these allow the patient to adjust to and tolerate not only the anatomical abnormality but also a reduction in cardiac output with less difficulty.

LOW-OUTPUT VERSUS HIGH-OUTPUT HEART FAILURE

Low cardiac output at rest, or in milder cases during exertion and other stresses, characterizes heart failure occurring in many forms of cardiovascular disease (i.e., congenital, valvular, rheumatic, hypertensive, coronary, and cardiomyopathic). A variety of high-cardiac output states, including thyrotoxicosis, arteriovenous fistulas, beriberi, Paget disease of bone, and anemia (discussed later in this chapter), may lead to heart failure as well. Low-output heart failure is characterized by clinical evidence of systemic vasoconstriction with cold, pale, and sometimes cyanotic extremities. In advanced forms of low-output failure, marked reduction in the stroke volume is reflected by a narrowing of the pulse pressure.[13] In contrast, in high-output heart failure, the extremities are usually warm and flushed and the pulse pressure is widened or at least normal.

The ability of the heart to deliver the oxygen required by the metabolizing tissues is reflected in the arterial-mixed venous oxygen difference, which is abnormally widened (i.e., >50 ml/liter in the resting state) in patients with systemic hypoperfusion or low-output heart failure. This difference may be normal or even reduced in high-output states owing to elevation of the mixed venous oxygen saturation by the admixture of blood that has been shunted away from metabolizing tissues.

Systolic Versus Diastolic Heart Failure

Heart failure has been defined in physiological terms to occur when an abnormality of cardiac function causes the heart to fail to pump blood at a rate required by the metabolizing tissues or to do so only with an elevated filling pressure.[14] Implicit in this definition is the observation that heart failure can be caused by an abnormality in systolic function leading to a defect in the expulsion of blood (i.e., *systolic heart failure*) or by an abnormality in diastolic function leading to a defect in ventricular filling (i.e., *diastolic heart failure*) (Fig. 22–3). The former is the classic form of heart failure associated with an impaired inotropic state. Equally important is diastolic heart failure (also termed heart failure with normal

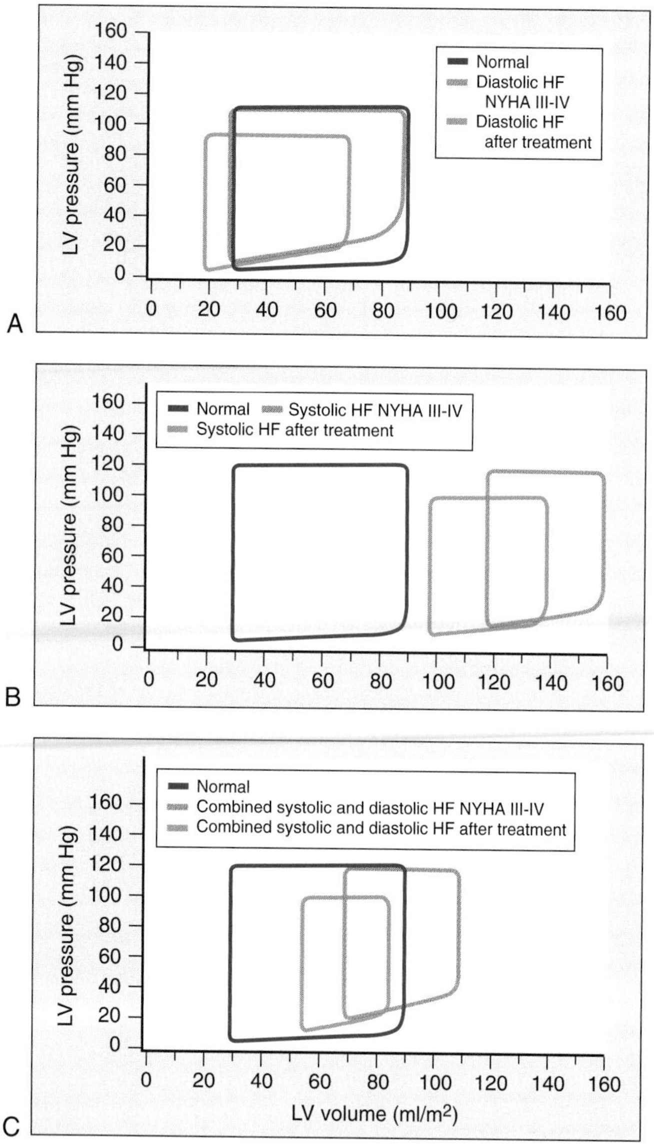

FIGURE 22–3 Pressure-volume loops contrasting isolated diastolic heart failure **(A)** with systolic heart failure **(B)** and combined systolic and diastolic heart failure **(C)**. In each panel, a normal subject (magenta) is compared with a patient with heart failure before (gold) and after (blue) treatment. **A,** Isolated diastolic heart failure is characterized by increased diastolic pressures with normal diastolic volumes (i.e., an upward shift of the diastolic pressure-volume relationship). Contractile performance is normal. When diastolic pressures are markedly elevated, patients are symptomatic with minimal exertion or at rest. With treatment, diastolic volumes and pressures can be reduced and the patient is less symptomatic, but the diastolic pressure-volume relationship remains abnormal. **B,** Systolic heart failure is characterized by abnormalities of the systolic pressure-volume relationship with decreases in ejection fraction and stroke volume. In addition, the diastolic pressure-volume relationship is shifted to the right. The increase in diastolic pressures and abnormal relaxation reflect diastolic dysfunction. With treatment, systolic and diastolic pressures are reduced, resulting in either no change or an increase in stroke volume. **C,** Combined systolic and diastolic heart failure typical of patients with ischemic heart disease is characterized by a modest decrease in contractile function and a modest increase in end-diastolic volume but a marked increase in end-diastolic pressure reflecting decreased left ventricular compliance. HF = heart failure; LV = left ventricular; NYHA = New York Heart Association. (From Zile MR, Brutsaert DL: New concepts in diastolic dysfunction and diastolic heart failure: Part I. Circulation 105:1387, 2002.)

systolic function or preserved ejection fraction), in which the ability of the ventricle or ventricles to accept blood is impaired.[15-18] This may be due to slowed or incomplete ventricular relaxation, which may be transient, as occurs in acute ischemia, or sustained, as in myocardial hypertrophy or restrictive cardiomyopathy secondary to infiltrative conditions such as amyloidosis. The principal clinical manifestations of systolic heart failure result from an inadequate cardiac output or salt and water retention, or both, whereas the major consequences of diastolic heart failure are related to elevation of the ventricular filling pressure leading to pulmonary or systemic venous congestion, or both. Studies also suggest that systolic ventricular and arterial stiffening beyond that associated with aging or hypertension is an important contributor to heart failure with normal systolic function.[19,20]

There are many examples of isolated systolic or diastolic heart failure. Examples of the former are patients with acute massive myocardial infarction or pulmonary embolism, whereas examples of the latter are patients with hypertrophic or restrictive cardiomyopathy. Community-based epidemiological studies have demonstrated that diastolic heart failure is common and is particularly prevalent in older patients, women, and those with a history of hypertension.[21-23] However, in many patients, systolic heart failure and diastolic heart failure coexist. The most common form of heart failure, that caused by chronic ischemic heart disease, is an example of combined systolic and diastolic heart failure. In this condition, systolic heart failure is caused by both the chronic loss of contracting myocardium secondary to prior myocardial infarction and the acute loss of myocardial contractility induced by transient ischemia. Diastolic heart failure is due to the ventricle's reduced compliance caused by replacement of normal, distensible myocardium with nondistensible fibrous scar tissue and by the acute reduction of diastolic distensibility during ischemia. A number of clinical features and laboratory findings characterize these two forms of heart failure (Table 22–3). However, it is important to recognize that the clinical features of heart failure may be similar whether left ventricular systolic function is normal or depressed, underscoring the need for evaluation of ventricular function in all patients with heart failure. Vasan and Levy have proposed diagnostic criteria for diastolic heart failure (Table 22–4) that consider the clinical presentation as well as documentation of systolic and diastolic function.[24]

Underlying Causes of Heart Failure

From a clinical viewpoint, it is useful to classify the causes of heart failure into two broad categories: (1) *underlying causes*, comprising the structural abnormalities—congenital or acquired—that affect the peripheral and coronary vessels, pericardium, myocardium, or cardiac valves and lead to the increased hemodynamic burden, increased myocardial stress, or coronary insufficiency responsible for heart failure (see Fig. 22–4), and (2) *precipitating causes*, including the specific causes or incidents that precipitate worsening heart failure in 50 to 90 percent of episodes of clinical heart failure.[25,26] *Underlying mechanisms* comprise the neurohormonal, biochemical, and genetic pathways through which either an increased hemodynamic burden or a reduction in myocardial oxygen delivery results in abnormal myocardial structure and function (see Chap. 21). Population-based epidemiological studies have also recognized *risk factors* for the development of heart failure,[27,28] including hypertension, smoking, diabetes mellitus, and obesity (Fig. 22–4).

It is helpful for the clinician to identify both the underlying and the precipitating causes of heart failure. Appropriate management of the underlying heart disease (e.g., surgical correction of a congenital defect or an acquired valvular abnormality or pharmacological management of hypertension) may prevent the development or progression of heart failure. Similarly, treatment of a precipitating cause such as an infection often results in a significant improvement in the clinical status of a patient with heart failure and may be life

TABLE 22–3 Systolic Versus Diastolic Heart Failure*

Parameters	Systolic	Diastolic
History		
Coronary artery disease	+++†	++
Hypertension	++	++++
Diabetes	++	++
Valvular heart disease	++++	+
Paroxysmal dyspnea	++	+++
Physical Examination		
Cardiomegaly	+++	+
Soft heart sounds	++++	+
S_3 gallop	+++	+
S_4 gallop	+	+++
Hypertension	++	++++
Mitral regurgitation	+++	+
Rales	++	+
Edema	+++	+
Jugular venous distention	+++	+
Chest Radiograph		
Cardiomegaly	+++	+
Pulmonary congestion	+++	+++
Electrocardiogram		
Left ventricular hypertrophy	++	++++
Q waves	++	+
Low voltage	+++	−
Echocardiogram		
Left ventricular hypertrophy	++	++++
Left ventricular dilation	++	−
Left atrial enlargement	++	++
Reduced ejection fraction	++++	−

Adapted from Young JB: Assessment of heart failure. *In* Colucci WS (ed): Heart Failure: Cardiac Function and Dysfunction. 3rd ed. *In* Braunwald E (series ed): Atlas of Heart Diseases. Philadelphia, Current Medicine, 2002, pp 127–143.

*Certain aspects of the history and physical examination, along with clinical measurements, may help to distinguish diastolic from systolic heart failure. For example, patients with hypertensive heart disease and severe left ventricular hypertrophy often experience heart failure because of diastolic dysfunction.

†*Plus signs* indicate "suggestive" (the number reflects relative weight). *Minus signs* indicate "not very suggestive."

saving. More important, *avoidance* of a precipitating cause can *prevent* worsening heart failure.

Decompensated heart failure may also be precipitated by the progression of the underlying heart disease. A previously stable, compensated patient may develop heart failure that is apparent clinically for the first time when the intrinsic process has advanced to a critical point, such as with further narrowing of a stenotic aortic valve or progressive obliteration of the pulmonary vascular bed in a patient with cor pulmonale. Alternatively, decompensation may occur as a result of failure or exhaustion of the compensatory mechanisms, but without any change in the load on the heart, in patients with chronic severe pressure or volume overload.

Precipitating Causes of Heart Failure

In one study of 435 patients admitted nonelectively to an urban university hospital with the diagnosis of heart failure, precipitating factors could be identified in 66 percent.[25]

INAPPROPRIATE REDUCTION OF THERAPY. Perhaps the most common cause of decompensation in a previously compensated patient with heart failure is inappropriate reduction in the intensity of treatment, be it dietary sodium and fluid restriction, pharmacological therapy, or both. *Dietary excesses of sodium*, incurred frequently on vacations or holidays or during any change in home cooking routine, are frequent causes of cardiac decompensation. Education of the patient and family, including referral to a nutritionist when indicated, is a simple and effective measure to prevent this common clinical problem. Self-discontinuation or physician withdrawal of effective pharmacotherapy such as angiotensin-converting enzyme (ACE) inhibitors, diuretics, or digoxin can precipitate heart failure.[26]

ARRHYTHMIAS. Cardiac arrhythmias are common in patients with underlying structural heart disease and commonly precipitate or worsen heart failure. The development of arrhythmias may precipitate heart failure through several mechanisms:

1. *Tachyarrhythmias*, most commonly atrial fibrillation, reduce the time available for ventricular filling. When there is already an impairment of ventricular filling, as in mitral stenosis, or reduced ventricular compliance, as in left ventricular hypertrophy, tachycardia raises atrial pressure and reduces cardiac output further. In addition, tachyarrhythmias increase myocardial oxygen demands and, in a patient with obstructive coronary artery disease, may induce or intensify myocardial ischemia, thereby raising left atrial pressure and causing pulmonary congestion. Tachycardia may also directly impair contractility in failing human myocardium, owing in part to a negative force-frequency relationship (see Chap. 19), and, if persistent, may cause a reversible dilated cardiomyopathy.[29]
2. *Marked bradycardia* in a patient with underlying heart disease usually depresses cardiac output because stroke volume may already be maximal and cannot rise further to maintain cardiac output.
3. *Dissociation between atrial and ventricular contraction*, which occurs in many arrhythmias, results in loss of the atrial booster pump mechanism, which impairs ventricular filling, lowers cardiac output, and raises atrial pressure. This loss is particularly deleterious in patients with impaired ventricular filling related to cardiac hypertrophy (e.g., in systemic hypertension, aortic stenosis, and hypertrophic cardiomyopathy).
4. *Abnormal intraventricular conduction*, which occurs in many arrhythmias such as ventricular tachycardia, impairs myocardial performance because of loss of the normal mechanical synchrony of ventricular contraction. In addition to precipitating heart failure, arrhythmias, which may be fatal, may be *caused* by heart failure.

TABLE 22–4 Diagnostic Criteria for Diastolic Heart Failure

Criterion	Possible Diastolic Heart Failure	Probable Diastolic Heart Failure	Definite Diastolic Heart Failure
Definitive evidence of HF	Signs and symptoms of HF, supporting laboratory tests,* and response to diuretics	Signs and symptoms of HF, supporting laboratory tests,* and response to diuretics	Signs and symptoms of HF, supporting laboratory tests,* and response to diuretics
Objective evidence of normal LV systolic function	LVEF ≥ 50% but not at the time of HF event	LVEF ≥ 50% within 72 hr of HF event	LVEF ≥ 50% within 72 hr of HF event
Objective evidence of LV diastolic dysfunction	No conclusive information	No conclusive information	Abnormal LV relaxation, filling, and/or distensibility at cardiac catheterization

*Chest radiograph, B-type natriuretic peptide level.
HF = heart failure; LV = left ventricular; LVEF = LV ejection fraction.
Adapted from Vasan RS, Levy D: Defining diastolic heart failure: A call for standardized diagnostic criteria. Circulation 101:2118, 2000.

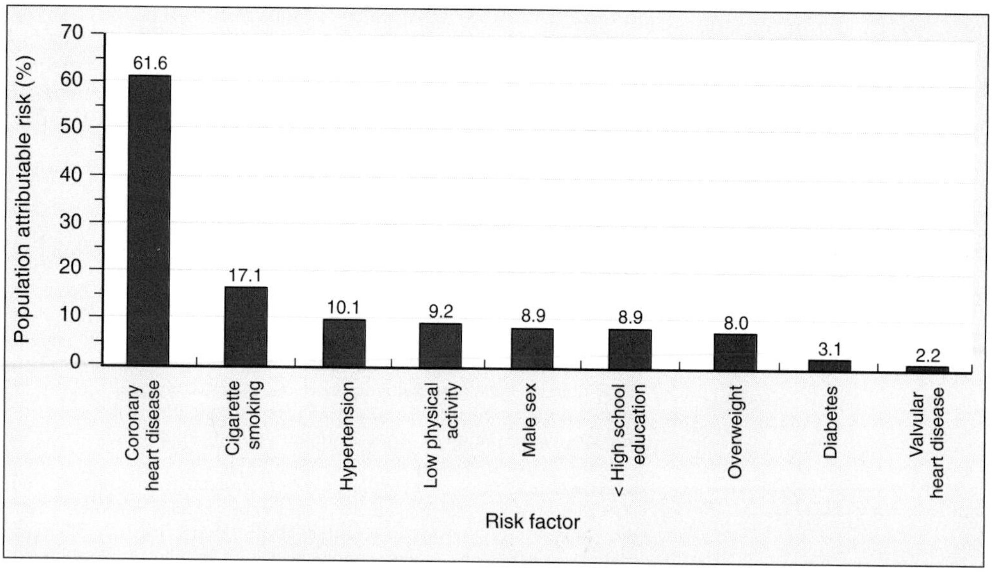

FIGURE 22–4 Estimates of the population attributable risk of heart failure related to various risk factors in 5545 men and 8098 women participating in the First National Health and Nutrition Examination Survey (NHANES I) Epidemiologic Follow-up Study. In the general population, coronary heart disease was the major cause of heart failure in 61.6 percent of all cases, followed by cigarette smoking (17.1 percent) and hypertension (10.1 percent). Obesity accounted for 8.0 percent of cases, and diabetes accounted for only 3.1 percent. (From He J, Ogden LG, Bazzano LA, et al: Risk factors for congestive heart failure in US men and women: NHANES I Epidemiologic Follow-up Study. Arch Intern Med 161:996, 2001.)

MYOCARDIAL ISCHEMIA OR INFARCTION. In patients with ischemic heart disease, acute myocardial infarction (see Chap. 46), unstable angina (see Chap. 49), or silent ischemia (see Chap. 50) can precipitate heart failure. Reduced myocardial oxygen delivery may be exacerbated by the increase in myocardial oxygen demand resulting from tachycardia and hypertension. Mitral regurgitation related to ischemic papillary muscle dysfunction may contribute to heart failure and lead to acute pulmonary edema.[30]

SYSTEMIC INFECTION. Any serious infection may precipitate cardiac failure. The mechanisms include increased total body metabolism as a consequence of fever, discomfort, and cough, which increases the hemodynamic burden on the heart; the accompanying sinus tachycardia plays an additional adverse role. Patients with advanced heart failure are particularly susceptible to pulmonary infections,[26] presumably because of the diminished ability of congested lungs to expel respiratory secretions. Furthermore, it is postulated that increased circulating levels of proinflammatory cytokines, such as tumor necrosis factor-α and interleukin-1β, which impair myocardial function in sepsis, may precipitate heart failure in the setting of non–life-threatening bacterial or viral infections.[31]

PULMONARY EMBOLISM (see also Chap. 66). Patients with heart failure, particularly when confined to bed, are at high risk for the development of venous thromboembolism. Other thromboembolic risk factors in heart failure include low cardiac output with intracardiac stasis and atrial fibrillation.[32] Pulmonary emboli may increase the hemodynamic burden on the right ventricle by elevating pulmonary artery pressure and pulmonary vascular resistance further and may cause fever, tachypnea, hypoxemia, and tachycardia.

PHYSICAL, EMOTIONAL, AND ENVIRONMENTAL STRESS. Intense, prolonged exertion or marked fatigue, such as may result from prolonged travel or emotional crises, are relatively common precipitants of cardiac decompensation. Severe climatic change (e.g., to a hot, humid environment) may also precipitate worsening heart failure.

CARDIAC INFECTION AND INFLAMMATION. Myocarditis as a consequence of a variety of inflammatory, allergic, or infectious processes, including viral myocarditis (see Chap. 60), may impair myocardial function directly and exacerbate existing heart disease. The anemia, fever, and tachycardia that frequently accompany these processes are also deleterious. In patients with infective endocarditis (see Chap. 58), valvular damage may also precipitate cardiac decompensation.

DEVELOPMENT OF AN UNRELATED ILLNESS. Heart failure may be precipitated in patients with compensated cardiovascular disease when an unrelated illness develops. For example, the development of acute or acute-on-chronic renal failure[33] may further impair the ability of patients with heart failure to excrete sodium or free water and thus may exacerbate fluid retention (see Chap. 86). Similarly, blood transfusion or the administration of sodium-containing fluid during and after noncardiac surgery may result in acute heart failure in patients with underlying structural heart disease.

ADMINISTRATION OF MYOCARDIAL DEPRESSANT OR SALT-RETAINING DRUGS. A number of drugs depress myocardial function; among these are nondihydropyridine calcium antagonists (verapamil and diltiazem), many antiarrhythmic agents, inhalation and intravenous anesthetics (see Chap. 50), and antineoplastic drugs such as doxorubicin and cyclophosphamide (see Chap. 83). Beta-adrenergic antagonists, which are now mainstays of therapy for chronic heart failure (see Chap. 23), can decrease cardiac contractility and must be initiated at low doses and titrated slowly in patients with heart failure. Other medications, such as estrogens, corticosteroids, and nonsteroidal antiinflammatory agents,[34] may cause salt and water retention. Cyclooxygenase-2 (COX-2)-specific inhibitors have been implicated in causing renal insufficiency and fluid retention.[35] Any of these drugs, when administered to a patient with already impaired cardiac function, can precipitate or worsen heart failure.

CARDIAC TOXINS. Alcohol is a potent myocardial depressant and may be responsible for the development of cardiomyopathy (see Chap. 59), arrhythmias, and sudden death.[36] In patients with asymptomatic or mildly symptomatic left ventricular dysfunction, excessive alcohol consumption may precipitate heart failure, either directly by an acute depression of myocardial contractility or indirectly through the development of tachyarrhythmias. Illicit use of cocaine may precipitate acute heart failure by a number of mechanisms, including myocardial ischemia or infarction (see Chap. 62), severe hypertension, arrhythmias, myocarditis, or, in the case of injection drug users, acute infective endocarditis.

HIGH-OUTPUT STATES. Acute heart failure may be precipitated in patients with underlying heart disease, such as valvular heart disease, or by the development of one of the hyperkinetic circulatory states, such as pregnancy or anemia (see High-Output Heart Failure). Anemia may also contribute to disease progression and clinical decompensation in patients with chronic heart failure.[37]

It is essential to search for these precipitating causes systematically in all patients with heart failure. In most instances, the precipitant can be treated effectively, after which appropriate measures should be instituted to avoid recurrence.

Clinical Manifestations

Symptoms

Respiratory Distress

Breathlessness, a cardinal manifestation of left ventricular failure, may arise with progressively increasing severity as (1) exertional dyspnea, (2) orthopnea, (3) paroxysmal nocturnal dyspnea, (4) dyspnea at rest, and (5) acute pulmonary edema.

EXERTIONAL DYSPNEA (see also Chap. 7). The principal difference between exertional dyspnea in normal subjects and that in patients with heart failure is the degree of activity necessary to induce the symptom. As left ventricular failure progresses, the intensity of exercise resulting in breathlessness declines progressively. However, there is no close correlation between subjective exercise tolerance and objective measures of left ventricular performance.[38] Exertional dyspnea may be absent in patients with heart failure who are sedentary for a variety of reasons, such as angina pectoris, intermittent claudication, or a noncardiovascular condition (e.g., osteoarthritis).

ORTHOPNEA. This symptom may be defined as dyspnea that develops in the recumbent position and is relieved by elevation of the head with pillows or by use of an electric adjustable bed. In the recumbent position, blood is displaced from the extrathoracic to the thoracic compartment. The failing left ventricle cannot accept and pump out the extra blood volume delivered to it by the competent right ventricle without dilating. Pulmonary venous and capillary pressures rise further, causing interstitial pulmonary edema, reduced pulmonary compliance, increased airway resistance, and dyspnea.[39] Orthopnea occurs rapidly, often within a minute or two of assuming recumbency, and develops when the patient is awake. It is a nonspecific symptom and may occur in *any* condition in which vital capacity is low. Marked ascites or a large pleural effusion, for example, whatever their cause, may cause orthopnea. *Trepopnea* is a rare form of orthopnea limited to one lateral decubitus position. In patients with advanced heart failure, trepopnea is related to impaired left ventricular filling and may explain the preference for sleeping in the right lateral decubitus position.[40]

The patient with orthopnea generally elevates his or her head and chest on several pillows to prevent nocturnal breathlessness and subsequently the development of paroxysmal nocturnal dyspnea. In advanced left ventricular failure, orthopnea may be so severe that the patient cannot lie down and must spend the night in the sitting position.

COUGH. Cough may be caused by pulmonary congestion, occurs under the same circumstances as dyspnea (i.e., during exertion or on recumbency), and is relieved by treatment of heart failure. Thus, a nonproductive cough in patients with heart failure is often a "dyspnea equivalent," whereas a cough on recumbency may be considered an "orthopnea equivalent."

PAROXYSMAL NOCTURNAL DYSPNEA. Attacks of paroxysmal dyspnea in resting patients usually occur at night. The patient awakens, often quite suddenly and with a feeling of severe anxiety and suffocation, sits bolt upright, and gasps for breath. Bronchospasm, which may be caused by congestion of the bronchial mucosa and by interstitial pulmonary edema compressing the small airways, increases ventilatory difficulty and the work of breathing and is a common complicating factor. The associated wheezing is responsible for the alternative name of this condition, *cardiac asthma*. In contrast to orthopnea, which may be relieved immediately by sitting upright at the side of the bed with the legs dependent, attacks of paroxysmal nocturnal dyspnea may require 30 minutes or longer in this position for relief.

Paroxysmal nocturnal dyspnea is a common clinical feature associated with Cheyne-Stokes respiration in patients with heart failure (see later).[41] Cardiac asthma may be exacerbated by downregulation of pulmonary beta receptors leading to attenuation of cyclic adenosine monophosphate–mediated airway relaxation.

MECHANISMS OF DYSPNEA

Increased awareness of respiration or difficulty in breathing is commonly associated with pulmonary venous hypertension caused by an elevation of left atrial or left ventricular filling pressure. This is particularly true in patients with acute heart failure in whom activation of J receptors in the lung by elevated pulmonary pressures and hypoxemia is the main stimulus for dyspnea.[42] Patients with chronic left ventricular failure typically exhibit a restrictive ventilatory defect, characterized by a reduction of vital capacity as a consequence of the replacement of the air in the lungs with blood or interstitial fluid or both. Consequently, the lungs become stiffer, air trapping occurs because of earlier than normal closure of dependent airways, and the work of breathing is increased because higher intrapleural pressures are needed to distend the stiff lungs.[39] Tidal volume is reduced, and respiratory frequency rises in a compensatory fashion. Engorgement of blood vessels may reduce the caliber of the peripheral airways, increasing airway resistance.

Thus, dyspnea and orthopnea in heart failure are clinical expressions of pulmonary venous and capillary congestion. In addition, there are alterations in the distribution of ventilation and perfusion, resulting in widened alveolar-arterial differences for oxygen, hypoxemia, and an increased ratio of dead space to tidal volume. Paroxysmal nocturnal dyspnea reflects the presence primarily of *interstitial* edema, whereas pulmonary edema, in which there is transudation and expectoration of blood-tinged fluid, is often a manifestation of *alveolar* edema.

There is an increased ventilatory drive as a consequence of the stimulation of stretch receptors in the pulmonary vessels and interstitium as well as of hypoxemia and metabolic acidosis. The increased work of breathing, combined with a low cardiac output and resulting impaired perfusion of the respiratory muscles, causes fatigue and ultimately the sensation of dyspnea.[43]

Dyspnea at rest may also occur in end-stage heart failure when low cardiac output, hypoxemia, and acidosis combine to reduce the delivery of oxygen to the respiratory and peripheral muscles.

Differentiation Between Cardiac and Pulmonary Dyspnea

In most patients with dyspnea there is obvious clinical evidence of disease of either the heart *or* the lungs, but in some the differentiation between cardiac and pulmonary dyspnea may be difficult. Like patients with heart failure, those with chronic obstructive pulmonary disease also may awaken at night with dyspnea, but it is usually associated with sputum production; the dyspnea is relieved after patients rid themselves of secretions by coughing rather than specifically by sitting up. When the dyspnea arises after a history of intensified cough and expectoration, it is often primarily pulmonary in origin. *Acute cardiac asthma* (paroxysmal nocturnal dyspnea with prominent wheezing) usually occurs in patients who have obvious clinical evidence of heart disease and may be further differentiated from acute bronchial asthma by diaphoresis and bubblier airway sounds and the more common occurrence of cyanosis.

Airway obstruction and dyspnea that respond to bronchodilators or smoking cessation favor a pulmonary origin of the dyspnea, whereas symptomatic improvement with diuretics or nitrates supports heart failure as the cause of dyspnea. The availability of a rapid point-of-care assay for measuring plasma levels of B-type natriuretic peptide (BNP), a cardiac neurohormone that is elevated in heart failure (see Chap. 21), may help to differentiate heart failure from lung disease in patients presenting with dypnea.[44] Dyspnea that persists despite appropriate cardiovascular or respiratory pharmacotherapy may be related to psychosocial factors (e.g., anxiety, emotional stress).[45]

Pulmonary Function Testing

Pulmonary function testing should be carried out in patients in whom the etiology of dyspnea is unclear despite detailed clinical evaluation. The major alterations in pulmonary function in heart failure are reductions of vital capacity, total lung capacity, pulmonary diffusion capacity, and pulmonary compliance; resistance to air flow is moderately increased; residual volume and functional residual volume are normal.[46] Expiratory flows are further reduced by smoking.[46] Often there is hyperventilation at rest and during exercise, an increase in dead space, and some abnormalities of ventilation-perfusion relations with slight reductions in arterial carbon dioxide partial pressure (Pco_2) and Po_2. With pulmonary capillary hypertension, pulmonary compliance decreases and there is air trapping because of earlier than normal closure of dependent airways.

Rarely, it may be difficult, on clinical examination, to differentiate between cardiac dyspnea, dyspnea based on *malingering,* and dyspnea caused by *anxiety.*[47,48] Careful observation for the appearance of effortless or irregular respiration during exercise testing often helps to identify the patient in whom dyspnea is related to the latter two noncardiac causes. Patients whose anxiety focuses on the heart may exhibit sighing respiration and difficulty in taking a deep breath as well as dyspnea at rest. Their breathing patterns are not rapid and shallow, as in cardiac dyspnea. Rarely a "therapeutic test" is helpful, and amelioration of dyspnea, accompanied by a weight loss exceeding 2 kg induced by administration of a diuretic, supports a cardiac origin for the dyspnea. Conversely, failure of these measures to achieve such weight reduction and to diminish dyspnea argues against a cardiac origin. Other noninvasive tools to assess cardiac size, such as echocardiography, and cardiac filling pressures in heart failure, such as thoracic bioimpedance[49] and BNP levels,[50] may help to clarify the cause of dyspnea in some patients.

Reduced Exercise Capacity

MECHANISMS OF EXERCISE INTOLERANCE. Exercise capacity may be limited for a variety of reasons in patients with heart failure, including abnormalities in central and peripheral cardiovascular function.[51] The primary central limitations to exercise in patients with heart failure include the development of dyspnea related to pulmonary vascular congestion and the failure of the cardiovascular system to provide sufficient blood flow to exercising muscles. The latter reflects primarily an inadequate cardiac output response to exercise[52] and in some instances worsening functional mitral regurgitation (Fig. 22–5).[53] Secondary pulmonary hypertension[54] and right ventricular dysfunction may also contribute to the reduced cardiac output response to exercise in patients with advanced heart failure.

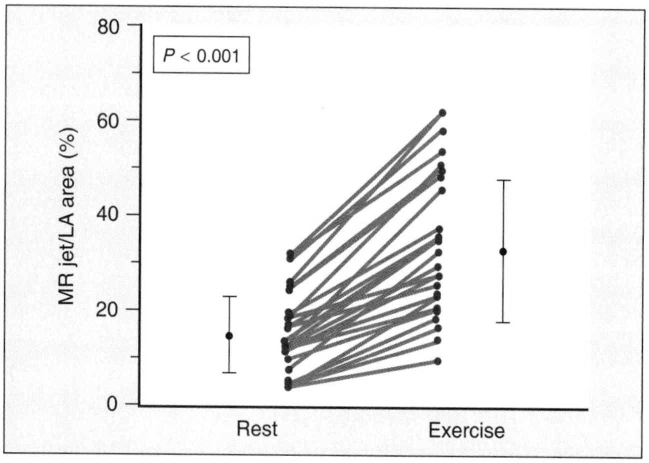

FIGURE 22–5 Functional mitral regurgitation increases with dynamic exercise in heart failure. In this study, 25 patients with chronic heart failure (mean age 53 ± 12 years; New York Heart Association Class 2.6 ± 0.6; left ventricular end-diastolic dimension 73 ± 7 mm; fractional shortening 17 ± 4 percent) underwent symptom-limited bicycle exercise testing with gas-exchange analysis and echocardiography. Individual changes in mitral regurgitation (MR) jet/left atrium (LA) areas are shown. On average, MR was mild to moderate at baseline (MR jet/LA area 15 ± 8 percent) and increased with exercise (MR jet/LA area 33 ± 15 percent). (Data from Lapu-Bula R, Robert A, Van Craeynest D, et al: Contribution of exercise-induced mitral regurgitation to exercise stroke volume and exercise capacity in patients with left ventricular dysfunction. Circulation 106:1342, 2002.)

Other factors that may contribute to reduced exercise capacity in patients with heart failure[51] include anemia,[55] attenuated peripheral vascular response,[56] abnormal skeletal muscle metabolism,[57] and deconditioning of skeletal and respiratory muscles.[58] A rapid improvement in the peripheral vascular response to exercise after intensive, hemodynamically guided therapy has been demonstrated.[59]

There is evidence that the judicious use of cardiac rehabilitation can improve functional capacity,[60] quality of life,[60] and clinical outcomes[61] in patients with heart failure, possibly by (1) improving chronotropic responsiveness, diastolic function, autonomic control of the circulation, and peripheral blood flow[62,63]; (2) reducing neurohormonal activation,[64] proinflammatory cytokines[65] and oxidative stress[66]; (3) reversing abnormalities of skeletal muscle metabolism[67] and respiratory muscle function; and (4) improving patients' perceptions of their quality of life and symptom severity.

To determine the long-term safety and efficacy of exercise training in heart failure,[68] the National Heart, Lung and Blood Institute has initiated a large, multicenter randomized controlled trial of exercise training in patients with New York Heart Association (NYHA) functional Class II to IV heart failure (HF-ACTION).

Exercise Testing (see also Chap. 10)

MAXIMAL EXERCISE CAPACITY. Exercise stress testing may be an exceedingly useful adjunct in the *clinical assessment* of patients with suspected or known heart failure. With use of a bicycle ergometer or treadmill and a progressively increasing load, the maximum level of exercise that can be achieved can be determined; the latter correlates closely with the total oxygen uptake ($\dot{V}o_2$). Close observation of the patient during an exercise test may disclose obvious difficulty in breathing at a low level of exercise (or the opposite). Thus, this simple test may be considered an extension of the clinical examination.

A more formal assessment, in which $\dot{V}o_2$ is measured at each stage of exercise or preferably in which $\dot{V}o_2$ and $\dot{V}co_2$ are measured continuously, allows determination of maximum $\dot{V}o_2$. It also permits measurement of the anaerobic threshold (i.e., the point during the exercise test at which the respiratory quotient rises as a consequence of the production of excess lactate). A progressive exercise test is carried out until (1) $\dot{V}o_2$ fails to rise with further increases in activity or (2) the patient is limited by severe dyspnea or fatigue, or both. When the $\dot{V}o_2$ is less than 25 ml/kg/min and the reduction is caused by a cardiac abnormality (rather than by pulmonary disease, anemia, peripheral vascular disease, osteoarthritis, an orthopedic disability, marked obesity, or severe deconditioning), it may be used to classify the severity of heart failure. It may also be used to follow the progress of the patient, assess the efficacy of therapeutic maneuvers, and determine prognosis.[69,70] The percentage achieved of predicted maximum $\dot{V}o_2$,[71] the hyperventilatory response to exercise as measured by the $\dot{V}e/\dot{V}co_2$ slope,[72] and the cardiac output response to exercise measured directly with a pulmonary artery catheter[52] also provide important independent prognostic information in ambulatory patients with heart failure.

SUBMAXIMAL EXERCISE CAPACITY. Because usual daily activities generally require much less than maximal exercise capacity, the measurement of submaximal exercise capacity may provide information that is complementary to that provided by maximal exercise testing.[73] Submaximal exercise capacity can be assessed by measuring the duration of exercise at a constant workload that is generally chosen to be at or below the patient's anaerobic threshold.[74] The 6-minute walk test, most common of the fixed-time tests, measures the distance walked on level ground in 6 minutes.[75] In this test, the patient is asked to walk along a level corridor as far as he or she can in 6 minutes. The patient can slow down or even stop, may be given a carefully controlled level of encouragement, and is told when 3 and 5 minutes have elapsed. The 6-minute walk test and other similar submaximal tests are moderately predictive of maximal oxygen consumption, and, as noted later, the 6-minute walk test independently predicts morbidity and mortality in heart failure.[75,76]

OTHER SYMPTOMS

FATIGUE AND WEAKNESS. These symptoms, which are often accompanied by a feeling of heaviness in the limbs, are generally related to poor perfusion of the skeletal muscles in patients with a reduced cardiac output. They may be associated with impaired flow-mediated vasodilation and altered metabolism in skeletal muscle,[56,57] activation of inflammatory cytokines, and poor nutrition.[77] However, fatigue and weakness are nonspecific symptoms and may be caused by a variety of noncardiopulmonary diseases.

URINARY SYMPTOMS. *Nocturia* may occur relatively early in the course of heart failure. Urine formation is suppressed during the day when the patient is upright and active. When the patient rests in the recumbent position at night, renal vasoconstriction diminishes, and urine formation increases. Nocturia may be troublesome in that it prevents the patient with heart failure from obtaining much-needed rest. *Oliguria* is a sign of advanced heart failure and is related to the suppression of urine formation as a consequence of severely reduced cardiac output.

CEREBRAL SYMPTOMS. Confusion, memory loss, anxiety, headache, insomnia, nightmares, and, rarely, psychosis with disorientation, delirium, and even hallucinations may occur in elderly patients with advanced heart failure,[78] particularly in those with underlying cerebrovascular disease.

SYMPTOMS OF PREDOMINANT RIGHT-SIDED HEART FAILURE. Breathlessness is not as prominent in isolated right ventricular failure as it is in left-sided heart failure because pulmonary congestion is usually absent. Congestive hepatomegaly may produce discomfort, generally described as a dull ache or heaviness, in the right upper quadrant or epigastrium. This discomfort, which is caused by stretching of the hepatic capsule, may be severe when the liver enlarges rapidly, as in *acute* right-sided heart failure. Other gastrointestinal symptoms, including anorexia, nausea, bloating, a sense of fullness after meals, and constipation, are due to congestion of the liver and gastrointestinal tract.

Functional Classification

A classification of patients with heart disease on the basis of the relation between symptoms and the amount of effort required to provoke them was developed by the NYHA.[79] Although there are obvious limitations to assigning numerical values to subjective findings, this classification is nonetheless useful in comparing groups of patients as well as the same patient at different times. In addition, NYHA class has proved to be a strong, independent predictor of survival in patients with chronic heart failure.[80]

As discussed in Chapter 7, the accuracy and reproducibility of this classification are limited. To overcome these limitations, Goldman and associates developed a useful classification based on the estimated metabolic cost of various activities (see Table 7–7). This Specific Activity Scale (SAS) has been used in chronic heart failure trials to assess clinical response to pharmacotherapy.[81]

QUALITY OF LIFE. The three main goals of treatment for heart failure are to reduce symptoms, prolong survival, and improve quality of life. A good "quality of life" implies the ability to live as one wants, free of physical, social, emotional, and economic limitations. Heart failure can have an enormous deleterious impact on the quality of life. Although a number of generic instruments are available to assess health-related quality of life,[82,83] the Minnesota Living with Heart Failure (MLHF) questionnaire[83] and the Kansas City Cardiomyopathy Questionnaire (KCCQ)[84] were designed specifically for use in these patients.

The MLHF consists of 21 brief questions, each of which is answered on a scale of 0 to 5. Eight questions have a strong relationship to the symptoms of dyspnea and fatigue and are referred to as *physical dimension measures.* Five other questions that are strongly related to emotional issues are referred to as *emotional dimension measures.* The test is self-administered and takes only 5 to 10 minutes to complete. For each question, the patient selects a number from 0 to 5. Zero indicates that heart failure had no effect, and 5 indicates a very large effect.

The KCCQ is a self-administered, 23-item questionnaire developed to provide a better description of health-related quality of life in patients with heart failure. It quantifies physical limitation, symptoms, quality of life, social interference, and self-efficacy. The survey requires 4 to 6 minutes to complete and is scored by assigning each response an ordinal value, beginning and summing items within each domain. A clinical summary score is calculated by combining the functional status with the quality of life and social limitation domains.

Although such questionnaires have little role in routine clinical management of patients, they have provided valuable information in clinical investigation by providing prognostic information independent of clinical variables[85] and allowing the response to various pharmacological and device therapies to be quantified.[86] Quality of life instruments have also been used to assess response to cardiac rehabilitation (Fig. 22–6) and multidisciplinary, disease management programs.[87]

Physical Findings (see also Chap. 8)

GENERAL APPEARANCE. Patients with mild or moderate heart failure appear to be in no distress after a few minutes of rest. However, they may be obviously dyspneic during and immediately after moderate activity. Patients with left ventricular failure may become uncomfortable if they lie flat without elevation of the head for more than a few minutes. Those with severe heart failure appear anxious and may exhibit signs of air hunger in this position. Patients with heart failure of recent onset appear acutely ill but are usually well nourished, whereas those with chronic heart failure often appear malnourished and sometimes even cachectic. Chronic, marked elevation of systemic venous pressure may produce severe tricuspid regurgitation and may lead to visible systolic pulsation of the eyes and of the neck veins. Cyanosis, icterus, a malar flush, and abdominal distention caused by ascites may be evident in patients with severe heart failure or adults with chronic heart failure related to uncorrected congenital heart disease.

In *severe* heart failure, stroke volume is reduced, which is reflected in a diminished pulse pressure and dusky discoloration of the skin. With severe unstable heart failure,

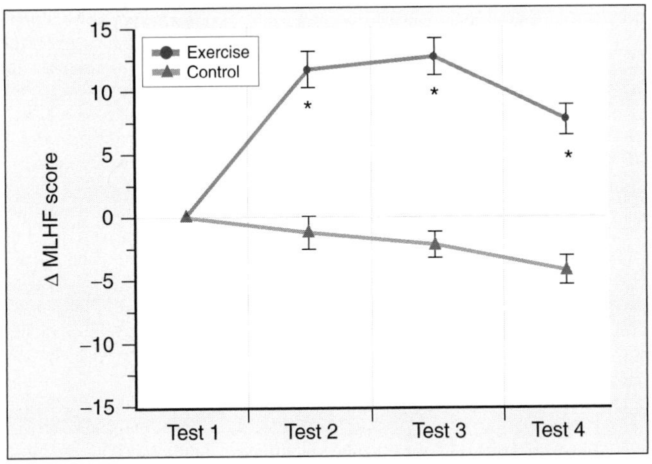

FIGURE 22–6 Changes in the Minnesota Living with Heart Failure (MLHF) questionnaire scores for stable heart failure patients enrolled in a 14-month exercise training program (magenta) compared with untrained control subjects (blue) at baseline (test 1) and after 2, 14, and 24 months (tests 2, 3, and 4). MLHF scores improved significantly in trained patients after 2 months and remained stable after the subsequent 12-month exercise-training program and during follow-up (*$P < 0.001$ for all comparisons). Exercise training was associated with an increase in peak total oxygen uptake ($\dot{V}O_2$) and reductions in both mortality and hospital readmission for heart failure. (Data from Belardinelli R, Georgiou D, Cianci G, Purcaro A: Randomized, controlled trial of long-term moderate exercise training in chronic heart failure: Effects on functional capacity, quality of life, and clinical outcome. Circulation 99:1173, 1999.)

particularly if the cardiac output has declined acutely, systolic arterial pressure may be reduced. The pulse may be rapid, weak, and thready. The proportional pulse pressure (pulse pressure/systolic pressure) shows some correlation with the cardiac output, especially in patients with pulmonary congestion.[88] In one study, when the proportional pulse pressure was less than 25 percent, it usually reflected a cardiac index of less than 2.2 liters/min/m^2.

INCREASED ADRENERGIC ACTIVITY. This is responsible for pallor and coldness of the extremities and cyanosis of the digits, diaphoresis, sinus tachycardia, and distention of the peripheral veins secondary to venoconstriction. Diastolic arterial pressure may be slightly elevated.

PULMONARY RALES. Moist rales result from the transudation of fluid into the alveoli and then into the airways. Rales heard over the lung bases are characteristic of left ventricular failure of at least moderate severity. They are usually heard at both lung bases, but if unilateral they occur more commonly on the right side and may be related to unilateral pleural effusion.[89] In acute pulmonary edema, coarse, bubbling rales and wheezes are heard over both lung fields and are accompanied by the expectoration of frothy, blood-tinged sputum (see Cardiogenic Pulmonary Edema). However, the absence of rales does not exclude considerable elevation of pulmonary capillary pressure. With congestion of the bronchial mucosa, excessive bronchial secretions or bronchospasm or both may give rise to rhonchi and wheezes.

SYSTEMIC VENOUS HYPERTENSION. This can be detected more readily by inspection of the jugular veins, which provides a useful index of right atrial pressure.[90] The upper limit of normal of the jugular venous pressure is approximately 4 cm above the sternal angle when the patient is examined at a 45-degree angle, corresponding to a right atrial pressure of less than 10 cm H_2O. When tricuspid regurgitation is present, the v wave and y descent are most prominent. The jugular venous pressure normally declines on inspiration, but in patients with heart failure (and in those with constrictive pericarditis; see Chap. 64) it rises, a finding known as the *Kussmaul sign.* Elevated jugular venous pressure independently predicts adverse outcomes including death or hospitalization for heart failure.[91]

HEPATOJUGULAR REFLUX. In patients with mild right-sided heart failure, the jugular venous pressure may be normal at rest but rises to abnormal levels with compression of the right upper quadrant, a sign known as the *hepatojugular (or abdominojugular) reflux.*[92] To elicit this sign, the right upper quadrant or epigastrium should be compressed firmly, gradually, and continuously for up to 1 minute while the veins of the neck are observed. The patient should be advised to avoid straining, holding the breath, or carrying out a Valsalva maneuver. A positive test (i.e., expansion of the jugular veins, or increase in jugular venous pressure greater than 3 cm, during and immediately after compression) usually reflects the combination of a congested abdomen and inability of the right side of the heart to accept or eject the transiently increased venous return.

CONGESTIVE HEPATOMEGALY. The liver often enlarges *before* overt edema develops, and it may remain so even after other symptoms of right-sided heart failure have disappeared. If hepatomegaly has occurred rapidly and relatively recently, the liver is usually tender owing to rapid stretching of its capsule. In longstanding heart failure this tenderness disappears, even though the liver remains enlarged. In patients with advanced heart failure, hepatomegaly has been associated with systemic hypoperfusion in the absence of congestion (e.g., the "cold/dry" hemodynamic profile).[88]

Splenomegaly may also occur in severe chronic heart failure or in the presence of severe congestive hepatomegaly in patients with tricuspid valve disease or constrictive pericarditis.[93]

EDEMA. Although a cardinal manifestation of heart failure, edema does not correlate well with the level of systemic venous pressure. In patients with chronic left ventricular failure and a low cardiac output, extracellular fluid volume may be sufficiently expanded to cause edema in the presence of only slight elevations of systemic venous pressure. A substantial gain of extracellular fluid volume, a minimum of 4 liters in adults, must usually take place before peripheral edema is manifested.

Edema in heart failure is usually symmetrical and pitting and generally occurs first in the dependent portions of the body. Accordingly, cardiac edema in ambulatory patients is usually first noted in the feet or ankles at the end of the day and generally resolves overnight. In bedridden patients it is most commonly found over the sacrum. Late in the course of heart failure, edema may become massive and generalized (anasarca), and weight gain associated with anasarca correlates with attenuation of electrocardiographic (ECG) voltage.[94] Longstanding edema results in pigmentation, reddening, and induration of the skin of the lower extremities, usually the dorsum of the feet and the pretibial areas.

HYDROTHORAX (PLEURAL EFFUSION). Because the pleural veins drain into both the systemic and the pulmonary venous beds, hydrothorax is observed most commonly in patients with hypertension involving both venous systems; it may also occur when there is marked elevation of pressure in either venous bed.[95] Effusions occur as increased amounts of fluid in the lung interstitial spaces exit across the visceral pleura, which in turn overwhelm the capacity of the lymphatics in the parietal pleura to resorb the fluid. An increase in capillary permeability probably also plays a role in the pathogenesis of cardiac hydrothorax. Hydrothorax is usually bilateral, but when unilateral it is usually confined to the right side.[89,96] When hydrothorax develops, dyspnea usually intensifies, owing to a further reduction in vital capacity and stimulation of J receptors. Although the excess fluid in hydrothorax is usually resorbed as heart failure improves, loculated interlobar effusions may persist and may require therapeutic thoracentesis.

ASCITES. This finding occurs in patients with increased pressure in the hepatic veins and in the veins draining the peritoneum. Ascites usually reflects longstanding systemic venous hypertension. In patients with organic tricuspid valve disease and chronic constrictive pericarditis,[97] ascites may be more prominent than subcutaneous edema. As in the case of hydrothorax, there is increased capillary permeability because the protein content is similar to that of hepatic lymph (i.e., four to six times that of edema fluid). Protein-losing enteropathy may rarely occur in patients with visceral congestion[98] or end-stage congenital heart disease, and the resultant reduced plasma oncotic pressure may lower the threshold for the development of ascites.

Cardiac Findings (see also Chap. 8)

The presence of cardiac disease is usually readily evident on clinical examination of patients with chronic heart failure.

CARDIOMEGALY. This finding is nonspecific and occurs in the majority of patients with chronic systolic heart failure. Notable exceptions include diastolic heart failure, heart failure associated with chronic constrictive pericarditis or restrictive cardiomyopathy, and acute forms of heart failure.

GALLOP SOUNDS. Protodiastolic sounds, generally emanating from the left ventricle (but occasionally from the right) and occurring 0.13 to 0.16 second after the second heart sound, are common findings in healthy children and young adults. Such physiological sounds are seldom audible in healthy persons after age 40 but occur in patients of all ages with heart failure and are referred to as *protodiastolic,* or *S_3, gallops.*[90] A study showed that the third heart sound is an independent predictor of death and heart failure hospitalizations.[91]

PULSUS ALTERNANS. This sign is characterized by a regular rhythm with alternating strong and weak ventricular contractions.[99] It should be distinguished from the alternation of strong and weak beats that occurs in pulsus bigeminus, in which the weak beat follows the strong beat by a shorter time interval than the strong beat follows the weak. In pulsus alternans, the beats are equally spaced. Severe pulsus alternans may be detected either by palpation of the peripheral pulses (the femoral more readily than the brachial, radial, or carotid) or by sphygmomanometry. As the cuff is slowly deflated, only alternate beats are audible for a variable number of millimeters of mercury below the systolic level, depending on the severity of the alternans, and then all beats are heard. Rarely, the weak beat is so small that the aortic valve is not opened, and this results in an apparent halving of the pulse rate, a condition referred to as *total alternans.* Pulsus alternans may be accompanied by alternation in the intensity of the heart sounds and of existing heart murmurs.

Pulsus alternans occurs most commonly in systolic heart failure and is usually associated with a ventricular protodiastolic gallop sound (S_3). It signifies advanced myocardial disease and often disappears with treatment of heart failure. Pulsus alternans can often be elicited by assumption of the erect posture, tends to be present during tachycardia, and is often initiated by a premature beat.

Pulsus alternans is attributed to an alternation in the stroke volume ejected by the left ventricle and, ultimately, to a deletion in the number of contracting cells in every other cycle, presumably owing to incomplete myocardial recovery. Rarely, pulsus alternans is accompanied by *electrical alternans;* however, the latter condition is usually due not to mechanical alternans but to alternating positions of the heart within the fluid-filled pericardial sac.

ACCENTUATION OF P_2 AND SYSTOLIC MURMURS. With the development of left ventricular failure, pulmonary artery pressure rises and P_2 becomes accentuated (often louder than A_2) and more widely transmitted. *Systolic murmurs* are common in heart failure owing to the functional mitral or tricuspid regurgitation that may occur secondary to ventricular and annular dilation. Often, these murmurs diminish or disappear when compensation is restored with pharmacological[100] or device therapies.[101]

ABNORMAL RESPONSE TO THE VALSALVA MANEUVER. Performance of this maneuver—forced expiration against a closed glottis—is helpful in the diagnosis of heart failure. The test has been standardized as follows. The patient is asked to blow against an aneroid manometer and to maintain a pressure of 40 mm Hg for 30 seconds. Intrathoracic pressure rises, venous return to the heart diminishes, stroke volume falls, and venous pressure rises. Arterial pressure tracings normally show four distinct phases: (1) an initial rise in arterial pressure, which represents transmission to the periphery of the increased intrathoracic pressure; (2) with continuation of the strain and the accompanying reduction of venous return, reductions in systolic, diastolic, and pulse pressures accompanied by a reflex increase in heart rate; (3) on release of the strain, a sudden drop of arterial pressure equivalent to the fall in intrathoracic pressure; and (4) an overshoot of arterial pressure to above control levels, with a wide pulse pressure and bradycardia, caused by a transient rise in cardiac output as blood pooled in the venous system returns to the heart with the release of the strain.

In heart failure, phases 1 and 3 are normal; that is, there is normal transmission of the elevated intrathoracic pressure into the arterial tree during phase 1 and sudden loss of this with the release of the strain during phase 3. However, because the heart operates on the flat portion of its Starling curve, the impedance of venous return during phase 2 does not affect stroke volume. Therefore, the baroreceptor reflex is not activated, and there is no overshoot on release of the strain. This results in a "square-wave" appearance of the tracing. An intermediate response (the so-called absent overshoot response) to the Valsalva maneuver has been demonstrated in patients with moderate depression of left ventricular systolic function.

Experienced clinicians may use bedside sphygmomanometric determination of arterial blood pressure with the Valsalva maneuver to detect elevated left-sided filling pressure.[102] Automated devices are being developed for the same purpose.[103]

FEVER. A low-grade fever (38°C), which results from cutaneous vasoconstriction and therefore impairment of heat loss, may occur in severe heart failure. Fever usually subsides when compensation is restored. Greater elevations of temperature usually signify the presence of infection, pulmonary infarction, or infective endocarditis.

CARDIAC CACHEXIA. Long-standing severe heart failure, particularly right ventricular failure, may lead to anorexia as a consequence of hepatic and intestinal congestion and mesenteric hypoperfusion. Occasionally, there is impaired intestinal absorption of fat[104] and, rarely, protein-losing enteropathy.[98] An association between celiac disease and cardiac cachexia has been described.[105]

Patients with heart failure may also exhibit increased total metabolism secondary to (1) an augmentation of myocardial oxygen consumption, as occurs in patients with aortic stenosis and hypertension; (2) excessive work of breathing; (3) low-grade fever; (4) increased activity of the sympathetic nervous system; and (5) elevated levels of circulating tumor necrosis factor-α.[106] This proinflammatory cytokine is produced by monocytes and contributes to cachexia and anorexia. There is also evidence that inflammatory cytokines, including tumor necrosis factor-α, may depress myocardial contractility and contribute to ventricular remodeling by stimulating myocyte apoptosis and turnover of the extracellular matrix.[107,108]

Other metabolic pathways that cause catabolic-anabolic imbalance and that have been implicated in wasting associated with heart failure include the growth hormone–insulin-like growth factor-1 system and the pituitary-thyroid hormone axis.[109] The combination of reduced caloric intake and increased caloric expenditure may lead to a reduction of tissue mass and, in severe cases, to cardiac cachexia. In some patients, the cachexia may be severe enough to suggest the presence of disseminated malignant disease. In others, the loss of lean body mass may be masked by the accumulation of edema. Cardiac cachexia is an independent risk factor for increased mortality in heart failure.[110]

CHEYNE-STOKES RESPIRATION. Also known as *periodic* or *cyclic respiration,* Cheyne-Stokes respiration is characterized by the combination of depression in the sensitivity of the respiratory center to carbon dioxide and left ventricular failure (Fig. 22–7).[41,111] During the apneic phase, arterial P_{O_2} falls and P_{CO_2} rises; this combination excites the depressed respiratory center, resulting in hyperventilation and, subsequently, hypocapnia, followed by another period of apnea. The principal causes of depression of the respiratory center in patients with Cheyne-Stokes respiration are cerebral arteriosclerosis, stroke, and head injury. These causes are often exaggerated by sleep, barbiturates, and narcotics, all of which further depress the sensitivity of the respira-

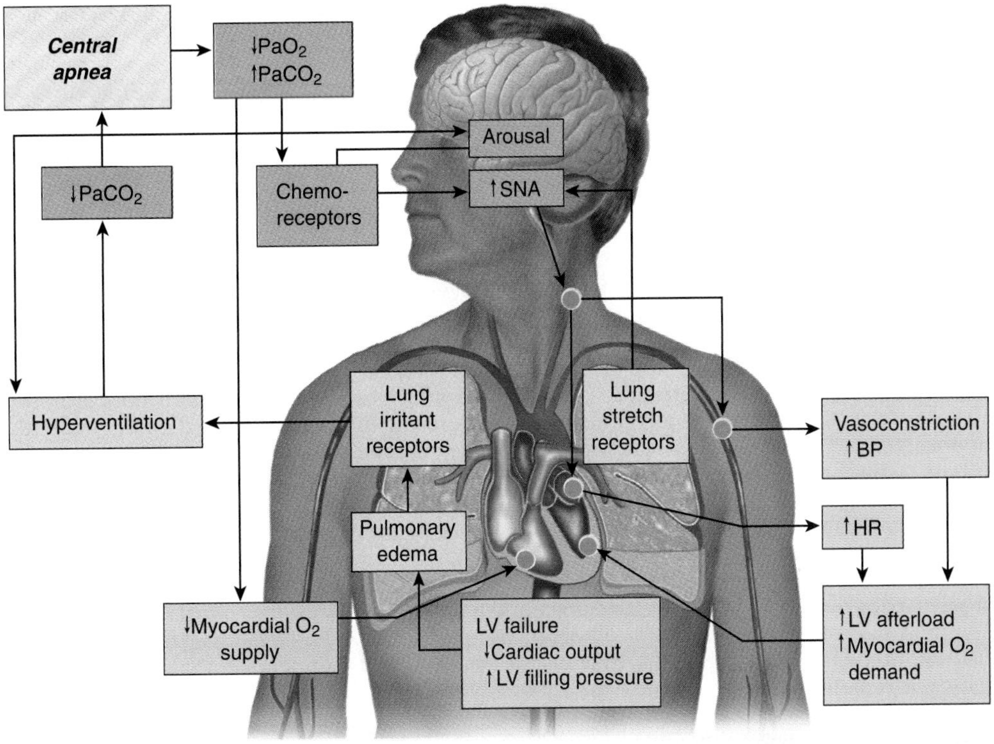

FIGURE 22–7 Pathophysiology of central sleep apnea and Cheyne-Stokes respiration in heart failure (HF). HF leads to increased left ventricular (LV) filling pressure. The resulting pulmonary congestion activates lung vagal irritant receptors, which stimulate hyperventilation and hypocapnia. Superimposed arousals cause further abrupt increases in ventilation and drive the partial pressure of carbon dioxide in arterial blood (Pa_{CO_2}) below the threshold for ventilation, triggering a central apnea. Central sleep apneas are sustained by recurrent arousal resulting from apnea-induced hypoxia and the increased effort to breathe during the ventilatory phase because of pulmonary congestion and reduced lung compliance. Increased sympathetic activity causes increases in blood pressure (BP) and heart rate (HR) and increases myocardial oxygen (O_2) demand in the presence of reduced supply. SNA = sympathetic nervous system activity; Pa_{O_2} = partial pressure of oxygen in arterial blood. (Redrawn from Bradley TD, Floras JS: Sleep apnea and heart failure. Part II: Central sleep apnea. Circulation 107:1822, 2003.)

tory center. Left ventricular failure, which prolongs the circulation time from the lung to the brain, results in a sluggish response of the system and is responsible for the oscillations between apnea and hyperpnea that prevent return to a steady state of ventilation and blood gases. Cheyne-Stokes respiration is also associated with enhanced cardiac sympathetic activity,[112] decreased heart rate variability, and increased peripheral chemosensitivity.[111]

Cheyne-Stokes respiration is seen in up to 40 percent of patients with heart failure and is typically associated with more advanced symptoms.[111] Usually, patients are not aware of Cheyne-Stokes respiration. However, it can be readily observed in a sleeping patient or a history can be elicited from the patient's bed partner. Cheyne-Stokes respiration may contribute to daytime sleepiness, insomnia, and snoring.

PATHOLOGICAL FINDINGS

LUNGS. In patients who have died of left ventricular failure, the lungs are enlarged, firm, and dark and may be filled with bloody fluid. With long-standing pulmonary congestion, they are brown with deposition of hemosiderin and usually do not seep edematous fluid. On microscopic examination, the capillaries are engorged, and there is thickening of the alveolar septa as well as extravasation of large mononuclear cells containing red blood cells or hemosiderin granules or both. Often, the pulmonary vessels show medial hypertrophy and intimal hyperplasia.

LIVER. In acute right-sided heart failure, the liver is slightly enlarged, tense, and cyanotic with rounded edges. On microscopic examination, the central hepatic veins and sinusoids are dilated. With chronic right-sided heart failure, the liver returns to normal size, subsequently atrophies, and becomes "nutmeg" in appearance as a consequence of the dark red areas of central venous congestion and the lighter, fatty area in the periphery of the lobule. Cardiac cirrhosis, also termed *cardiac sclerosis*, is a result of sustained, chronic severe heart failure and is characterized by centrilobular necrosis and atrophy as well as extensive or patchy fibrous retraction. In addition, there may be fibrosis and thrombosis of the hepatic veins.[113]

Liver biopsy specimens of patients with acute cardiomyopathy and fulminant hepatic failure show bridging centrilobular necrosis. Presumably, the hypoxia caused by hypoperfusion produces hepatocyte necrosis; erythrocytes may then enter the space of Disse between damaged endothelial cells.

Laboratory Findings

SERUM ELECTROLYTES. In severe heart failure, prolonged sodium restriction, coupled with intensive diuretic therapy and the inability to excrete free water, may lead to dilutional hyponatremia.[12] Hypervolemic hyponatremia occurs because of substantial expansion of extracellular fluid volume and a normal or only slightly increased level of total body sodium. It may be accompanied by, and presumably is caused in part by, elevated circulating levels of arginine vasopressin.[114] Serum potassium levels are usually normal, although prolonged administration of kaliuretic diuretics, such as the thiazides or loop diuretics, may result in hypokalemia.[115] Secondary hyperaldosteronism may also contribute to hypokalemia. Hyperkalemia may occur in patients with severe heart failure who show marked reductions in glomerular filtration rate and inadequate delivery of sodium to the distal tubular sodium-potassium exchange sites,[116] particularly if they are also receiving ACE inhibitors,[117] potassium-sparing diuretics,[117,118] or potassium supplements. Other common electrolyte abnormalities observed in heart failure include hypophosphatemia and hypomagnesemia[119] (commonly associated with alcohol use and poor nutrition) and hyperuricemia,[120] which may precipitate gout.

RENAL FUNCTION. Proteinuria and a high urine specific gravity are common findings in heart failure. Blood urea nitrogen and creatinine levels are often moderately elevated secondary to reductions in renal blood flow and glomerular filtration rate.[121] Other contributing factors include altered balance of vasoconstrictor and vasodilating hormones and comorbidities such as diabetes and hypertension. In patients with advanced heart failure, the *cardiorenal syndrome*[13] may be exacerbated by several commonly used classes of drugs including ACE inhibitors, angiotensin receptor antagonists, diuretics, nonsteroidal antiinflammatory agents, and COX-2 inhibitors.

LIVER FUNCTION TESTS. Congestive hepatomegaly and cardiac cirrhosis are often associated with impaired hepatic function, characterized by abnormal values of aspartate aminotransferase (AST), alanine aminotransferase (ALT), lactate dehydrogenase (LDH), and other liver enzymes.[122,123] Hyperbilirubinemia, both direct and indirect, is common, and in severe cases of acute (right or left) ventricular failure, frank jaundice may occur. *Acute* hepatic venous congestion can result in severe jaundice with a bilirubin level as high as 15 to 20 mg/dl, elevation of AST to more than 10 times the upper limit of normal, and elevation of the serum alkaline phosphatase level, as well as prolongation of the prothrombin time. The impairment of hepatic function is rapidly ameliorated by successful treatment of heart failure.[124] In patients with longstanding cardiac cirrhosis, albumin synthesis may be impaired, with resultant hypoalbuminemia intensifying the accumulation of fluid. In advanced heart failure, hypoalbuminemia may contribute to and be exacerbated by cardiac cachexia.[77]

HEMATOLOGICAL STUDIES. Anemia is common in heart failure[37,125] and may be due to increased plasma volume (hemodilution) or decreased red cell mass (true anemia). Contributing factors include malnutrition with iron deficiency, bone marrow suppression from activation of proinflammatory cytokines or ACE inhibitors, and chronic renal insufficiency. In a population-based cohort of over 12,000 patients with heart failure, 17 percent had anemia, 58 percent of whom had anemia of chronic disease.[126] Anemia may contribute to ventricular remodeling and disease progression in heart failure by stimulating neurohormonal and cytokine activation and promoting left ventricular hypertrophy.[127] When moderate to severe anemia is present, it may exacerbate underlying ischemic heart disease by causing myocardial and peripheral hypoxia. Rarely, severe anemia may cause high-output failure. Erythropoietin may improve symptoms, exercise tolerance, and cardiac function in anemic patients with chronic heart failure,[55] although the effect of erythropoietin on morbidity and mortality remains to be determined.[128]

Leukocytosis may occur following acute myocardial infarction. In patients presenting with acute heart failure or hemodynamic instability, leukocytosis may suggest the presence of infective endocarditis (see Chap. 58) or pulmonary embolism (see Chap. 66). The erythrocyte sedimentation rate may be low or normal in advanced heart failure because of impaired fibrinogen synthesis and decreased fibrinogen concentration, but more commonly it is elevated because of cytokine activation.[129] A marked increase in sedimentation rate, when present with fever or leukocytosis, should prompt an investigation for infective endocarditis or Takayasu or giant cell arteritis (see Chap. 54).

Chest Radiography (see also Chap. 12)

Two principal features of the chest radiograph are useful in the evaluation of patients with heart failure.[130] The *size and shape of the cardiac silhouette* provide important information concerning the precise nature of the underlying heart disease. Both the cardiothoracic ratio and the heart volume determined on the plain film are relatively specific but insensitive indicators of increased left ventricular end-diastolic volume.

In the presence of normal pulmonary capillary and venous pressure, the lung bases are better perfused than the apices in the erect position, and the vessels supplying the lower lobes are significantly larger than those supplying the upper lobes. With elevation of left atrial and pulmonary capillary pressures, interstitial and perivascular edema develops and is most prominent at the lung bases because hydrostatic pressure is greater there. When pulmonary capillary pressure is slightly elevated (i.e., 13 to 17 mm Hg), the resultant compression of pulmonary vessels in the lower lobes causes equalization in size of the vessels at the apices and bases. With greater pressure elevation (18 to 23 mm Hg), actual pulmonary vascular redistribution occurs (i.e., further constriction of vessels leading to the lower lobes and dilation of vessels leading to the upper lobes) (see Figs. 12–5A and 12–17A). When pulmonary capillary pressures exceed 20 to 25 mm Hg, interstitial pulmonary edema occurs. This edema may be of several varieties: (1) *septal*, producing Kerley lines (i.e., sharp, linear densities of interlobular interstitial edema); (2) *perivascular,* producing loss of sharpness of the central and peripheral vessels; and (3) *subpleural,* producing spindle-shaped accumulations of fluid between the lung and adjacent pleural surface. When pulmonary capillary pressure exceeds 25 mm Hg, alveolar edema, with a cloud-like appearance and concentration of the fluid around the hili in a "butterfly" pattern, and large pleural effusions may occur (see Fig. 12–15). With elevation of systemic venous pressure, the azygos vein and superior vena cava may enlarge.

In patients with *chronic* left ventricular failure, higher pulmonary capillary pressures can be accommodated with fewer clinical and radiological signs of congestion, presumably because of enhanced lymphatic drainage. Pleural effusions are also commonly seen on the chest radiograph in patients with chronic heart failure and, if necessary, can be better defined by thoracic ultrasonography.[131]

Prognosis

Survival is markedly shortened in patients with heart failure, which accounts for a substantial portion of all deaths from cardiovascular diseases. The overall 5-year mortality for all patients with heart failure is approximately 50 percent,[3,132] and the 1-year mortality in patients with end-stage heart failure may be as high as 75 percent.[133] In the United States alone, approximately 260,000 patients die of heart failure each year.[7] The Framingham Heart Study found that between the years 1948 and 1988, patients with a diagnosis of heart failure had a median survival of 1.7 years for men and 3.2 years for women despite the fact that the patients with the poorest prognosis—that is, those dying within 90 days of the diagnosis—were excluded from the analysis.[134] More recent data from the Framingham Study looking at long-term trends in the survival of patients with heart failure demonstrate improved survival in both men and women.[132] Survival of patients with heart failure and preserved systolic function may be better than that of patients with reduced systolic function.[21] More than 90 percent of deaths of patients with heart failure are due to cardiovascular causes, most commonly progressive heart failure and sudden cardiac death.

A large number of factors have been found to correlate with mortality in patients with heart failure.[80,135,136] These fall into four major categories, as follows.

CLINICAL. In general, male gender,[132,137] the presence of coronary artery disease as the etiology of heart failure,[138] the presence of an audible S_3 or elevated jugular venous pressure (Fig. 22–8),[91] low pulse and systolic arterial pressures, a high NYHA class (Fig. 22–9), and reduced exercise capacity (Fig. 22–10)[52,70,139] have each been shown to be associated with increased mortality. When the NYHA class is integrated with the maximal O_2 consumption ($\dot{V}O_{2max}$) determined during exercise, the mortality is 20 percent per year in patients in Class III with a $\dot{V}O_{2max}$ of 10 to 15 ml/kg/min and rises to 60 percent in patients in Class IV with a $\dot{V}O_{2max}$ of less than 10 ml/kg/min. Submaximal exercise also carries important prognostic information in ambulatory patients with heart failure.[75] The distance walked in 6 minutes predicted both morbidity and mortality in the Studies of Left Ventricular Dysfunction (SOLVD) trial (Fig. 22–11)[76] and the Digitalis Investigation Group (DIG) trial. Other exercise parameters associated with impaired survival in heart failure include enhanced ventilatory response to exercise,[140] reduced anaerobic threshold,[141] inspiratory muscle dysfunction,[142] and impaired peripheral chemosensitivity.[143] Additional clinical predictors of mortality in chronic heart failure include important comorbidities such as diabetes mellitus[144] and chronic renal insufficiency (Fig. 22–12),[33] Cheyne-Stokes respiration,[145] sleep apnea,[146,147] cardiac cachexia,[110] and depression.[148] Obesity may confer a more favorable prognosis in patients with advanced heart failure.[149]

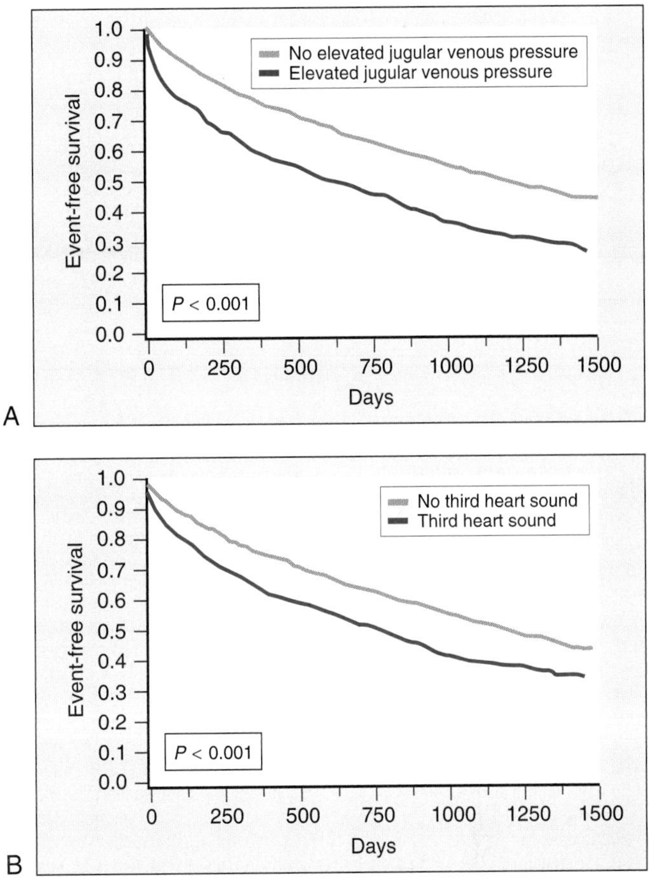

FIGURE 22–8 Event-free survival according to the presence or absence of elevated jugular venous pressure **(A)** and a third heart sound **(B)** in 2569 patients with heart failure enrolled in the Studies of Left Ventricular Dysfunction (SOLVD) treatment trial. **A,** The 280 patients with an elevated jugular venous pressure had a rate of death or hospitalization for heart failure significantly higher than that of the 2199 patients without elevated jugular venous pressure (38.1 events per 100 person-years versus 22.0 events per 100 person-years, $P < 0.001$ by the log rank test). **B,** The 597 patients with a third heart sound had a rate of death or hospitalization for heart failure significantly higher than that of the 1882 patients without a third heart sound (30.9 events per 100 person-years versus 21.4 events per 100 person-years, $P < 0.001$ by log rank test). (From Drazner MH, Rame JE, Stevenson LW, Dries DL: Prognostic importance of elevated jugular venous pressure and a third heart sound in patients with heart failure. N Engl J Med 345:574, 2001.)

STRUCTURAL. The cardiothoracic ratio as measured by chest radiography carries strong independent prognostic information. Other structural variables that can be assessed by two-dimensional echocardiography and that have been associated with increased risk of arrhythmias or death include left ventricular volumes, ventricular mass and sphericity index,[150] secondary mitral or tricuspid regurgitation[151] and left atrial enlargement.[152]

HEMODYNAMIC. Variables such as cardiac index, stroke work index, and both left and right ventricular ejection fractions[153-155] have been shown to correlate directly with survival in patients with heart failure, whereas heart rate, systemic and pulmonary vascular resistances, pulmonary artery pressures, and pulmonary capillary wedge pressure correlate inversely.[156] Combinations of hemodynamic abnormalities, such as depression of stroke work associated with elevation of filling pressure and systemic vascular resistance, are associated with a poor prognosis. Studies have examined the impact of exercise hemodynamics on survival and found that the stroke work index[139] and cardiac output[52] responses to

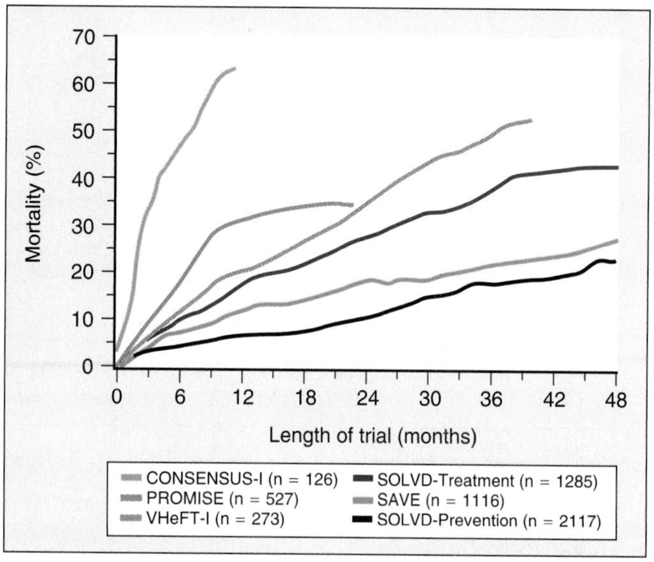

FIGURE 22–9 Clinical correlates of survival in heart failure. On the basis of data from several contemporary, placebo-controlled clinical trials, it can be estimated that the 1-year mortality is on the order of 50 to 60 percent in patients with New York Heart Association (NYHA) functional Class IV symptoms, 15 to 30 percent in patients with Class II to III symptoms, and 5 to 10 percent in asymptomatic patients with left ventricular dysfunction. Patients in CONSENSUS I were in NYHA Class IV and were treated with digitalis and diuretics; patients in SOLVD (Prevention) and SAVE had reduced left ventricular ejection fractions (35 and 40 percent, respectively) but no or mild limitation (NYHA Classes I or II). Patients in PROMISE, SOLVD (Treatment), and VHeFT-I had moderate heart failure (NYHA Class II or III). CONSENSUS = Cooperative North Scandinavian Enalapril Survival Study; PROMISE = Prospective Randomized Milrinone Survival Evaluation; SAVE = Survival And Ventricular Enlargement; SOLVD = Studies of Left Ventricular Dysfunction; VHeFT = Vasodilator Heart Failure Trial. (From Young JB: Assessment of heart failure. *In* Colucci WS [ed]: Heart Failure: Cardiac Function and Dysfunction. 3rd ed. *In* Braunwald E [series ed]: Atlas of Heart Diseases. Philadelphia, Current Medicine, 2002, pp 127-143.)

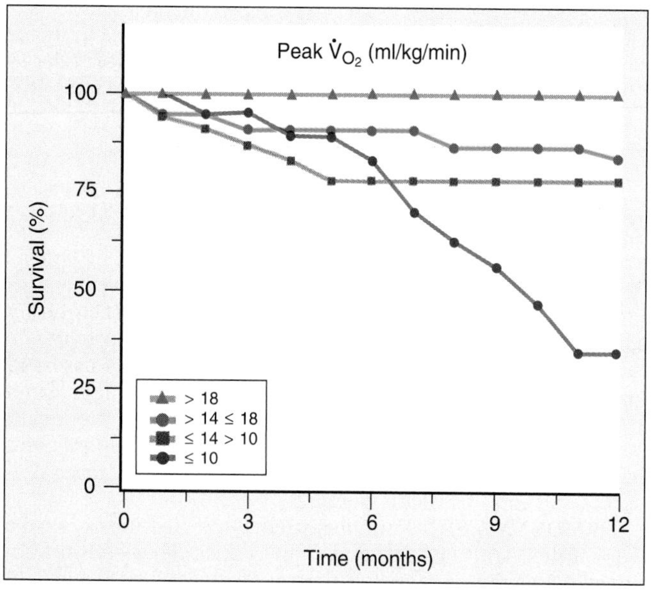

FIGURE 22–10 Kaplan-Meier survival analysis in patients with severe left ventricular dysfunction stratified by peak oxygen consumption ($\dot{V}O_2$) as measured by cardiopulmonary exercise testing during evaluation for cardiac transplantation. Patients with a peak $\dot{V}O_2$ of 10 ml/kg/min or less had significantly reduced survival rates compared with patients with peak $\dot{V}O_2$ greater than 14 ml/kg/min. (From Mancini DM, Eisen H, Kussmaul W, et al: Value of peak exercise oxygen consumption for optimal timing of cardiac transplantation in ambulatory patients with heart failure. Circulation 83:778, 1991.)

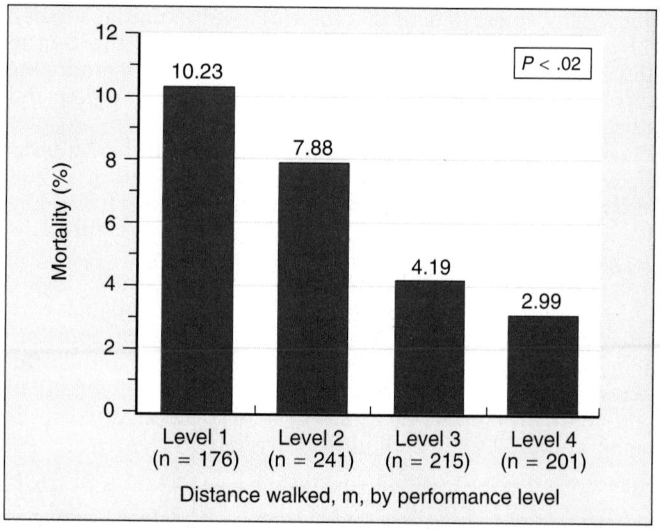

FIGURE 22–11 Mortality (percent) as a function of performance level (based on distance walked in 6 minutes). Mortality decreased as performance on the 6-minute walk test improved. (From Bittner V, Weiner DH, Yusuf S, et al: Prediction of mortality and morbidity with a 6-minute walk test in patients with left ventricular dysfunction. JAMA 270:1702, 1993.)

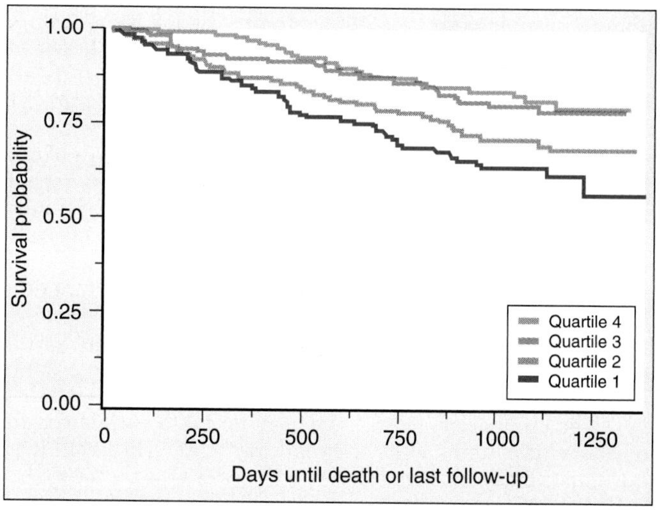

FIGURE 22–12 The prognostic value of baseline renal function was determined in 585 participants in an exercise substudy of the Digitalis Investigation Group (DIG) trial. Baseline characteristics of these patients were similar to those of the main trial (age 65 ± 12 years, ejection fraction 35 ± 13 percent). Mortality by increasing quartiles of estimated creatinine clearance using the Cockcroft-Gault equation was 37 percent (18 to 48 ml/min), 29 percent (47 to 64 ml/min), 18 percent (64 to 86 ml/min), and 21 percent (86 to 194 ml/min) with corresponding hazard ratios relative to the top quartile of 2.1, 1.6, and 0.9, respectively. (From Mahon NG, Blackstone EH, Francis GS, et al: The prognostic value of estimated creatinine clearance alongside functional capacity in ambulatory patients with chronic congestive heart failure. J Am Coll Cardiol 40:1106, 2002.)

exercise provide valuable independent prognostic information. In one study, patients with reduced cardiac output response to exercise and $\dot{V}O_{2max}$ less than or equal to 10 ml/kg/min had an extremely poor prognosis (i.e., 1-year survival rate of 38 percent).[52] Others have shown that $\dot{V}O_{2max}$ is superior to hemodynamic measurements in predicting outcome in severe heart failure.[157] In patients with idiopathic dilated cardiomyopathy, a significant reduction in myocardial blood flow as assessed by positron emission tomography was associated with an increased risk of death or progression of heart failure.[154]

Studies using Doppler echocardiography to assess the pattern of mitral valve inflow have demonstrated an association between *diastolic* dysfunction and impaired survival in patients with chronic *systolic* heart failure.[158] In a prospective study of 331 patients with impaired left ventricular function (ejection fraction < 40 percent), a restrictive filling pattern added incremental value to $\dot{V}O_{2max}$ in determining the risk of death or transplantation.[158]

BIOCHEMICAL. The observation that there is activation of the neurohormonal axis in heart failure has prompted examination of the relationships between a variety of biochemical measurements and clinical outcome. Strong inverse correlations have been reported between survival and plasma levels of norepinephrine (Fig. 22–13),[159,160] renin,[159] arginine vasopressin,[161] aldosterone,[162] atrial and B-type natriuretic peptides (Fig. 22–14),[160,163-165] and endothelin-1.[166] The concentrations of these substances reflect the severity of the underlying impairment of cardiovascular function. In addition, some may exert adverse hemodynamic effects; norepinephrine, angiotensin II, arginine vasopressin, and endothelin-1 are potent vasoconstrictors, augmenting ventricular afterload and thereby reducing the shortening of myocardial fibers. Furthermore, they may be directly responsible for adverse biochemical effects on the myocardium. For example, the elevated norepinephrine concentration may be responsible for ventricular tachyarrhythmias, as may hypokalemia and reduction of total-body potassium stores

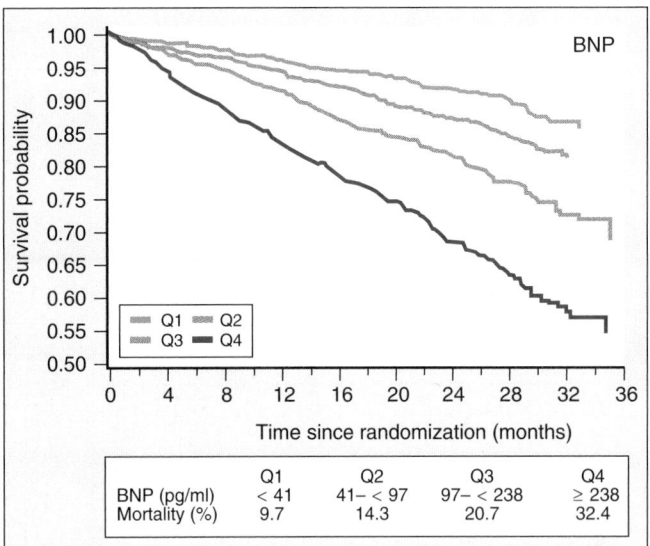

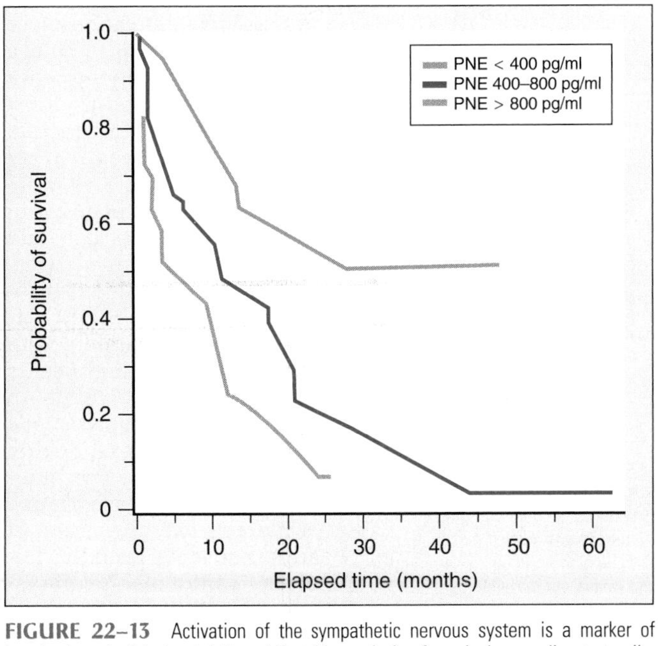

FIGURE 22–13 Activation of the sympathetic nervous system is a marker of impaired survival in heart failure. Life table analysis of survival, according to tercile, based on level of plasma norepinephrine (PNE). Group 1 (<400 pg/ml) contained 27 patients, group 2 (400 to 800 pg/ml) had 49 patients, and group 3 (>800 pg/ml) had 30 patients. The probability of survival in each group was significantly different from the probabilities in the other two groups. (From Cohn JN, Levine TB, Olivari MT, et al: Plasma norepinephrine as a guide to prognosis in patients with chronic congestive heart failure. N Engl J Med 311:819, 1984.)

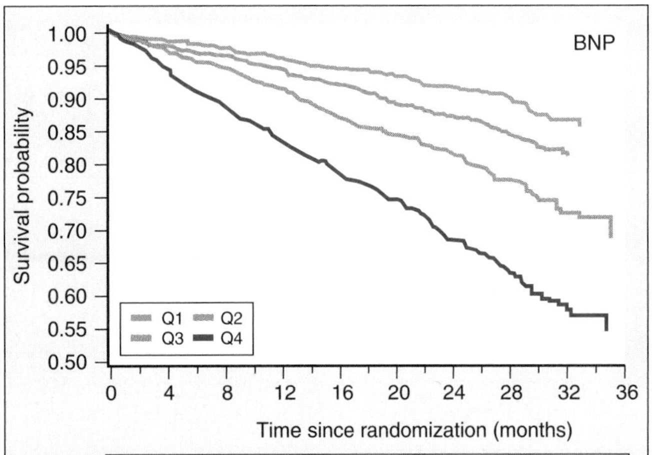

	Q1	Q2	Q3	Q4
BNP (pg/ml)	< 41	41– < 97	97– < 238	≥ 238
Mortality (%)	9.7	14.3	20.7	32.4

FIGURE 22–14 Plasma B-type natriuretic peptide (BNP) was measured before randomization and during follow-up in approximately 4300 patients in the Valsartan Heart Failure Trial. The baseline values for BNP in quartiles were less than 41, 41 to less than 97, 97 to less than 238, and greater than or equal to 238 pg/ml. Kaplan-Meier curves show a significant quartile-dependent increase in mortality and first morbid events. (From Anand IS, Fisher LD, Chiang YT, et al: Changes in brain natriuretic peptide and norepinephrine over time and mortality and morbidity in the Valsartan Heart Failure Trial (Val-HeFT). Circulation 107:1278, 2003.)

resulting from the activation of the renin-angiotensin-aldosterone system (and the administration of potassium-losing diuretics). Norepinephrine also exerts direct toxic effects on the myocardium, including stimulation of cellular hypertrophy, apoptosis, and changes in extracellular matrix regulation, and thus contributes directly to ventricular remodeling and disease progression.[167] Like norepinephrine, endothelin-1 is a potent vasoconstrictor peptide that exerts growth-promoting effects on the myocardium and vascular smooth muscle cells.[10,31] Hyponatremia also correlates well with increased mortality,[168] but it is likely that this variable reflects activation of the renin-angiotensin-aldosterone axis.

MULTIVARIATE ANALYSIS. In many studies, the aforementioned variables have been assessed in a univariate manner (i.e., independently of one another) and there is disagreement regarding which provides *independent* prognostic information. However, Rector and Cohn have shown that although left ventricular function appears to have the most profound effect on survival in patients with advanced heart failure, exercise tolerance (as reflected in peak oxygen consumption during a progressive exercise test) and activation of the sympathetic nervous system (as reflected in the plasma norepinephrine concentration) *each* provide important independent information.[135] More recent studies of patients with heart failure receiving neurohormonal antagonists (e.g., ACE inhibitors and beta blockers) have identified pro-BNP and BNP levels as strong independent predictors of sudden cardiac death[169] and all-cause mortality.[80,160,163,164]

It is important to note that most of these studies measured biomarkers at baseline and assessed their relationship to subsequent clinical events. Only recently have investigators sought to determine the relationship between the *change* in biomarkers over time and outcomes. An analysis of more than 4000 patients observed in the Valsartan Heart Failure Trial (Val-HeFT) demonstrated that the percentage changes in norepinephrine and BNP over 12 months are independently associated with corresponding changes in morbidity and mortality.[160] Data such as these may allow clinicians to use biomarkers to manage chronic heart failure.[170]

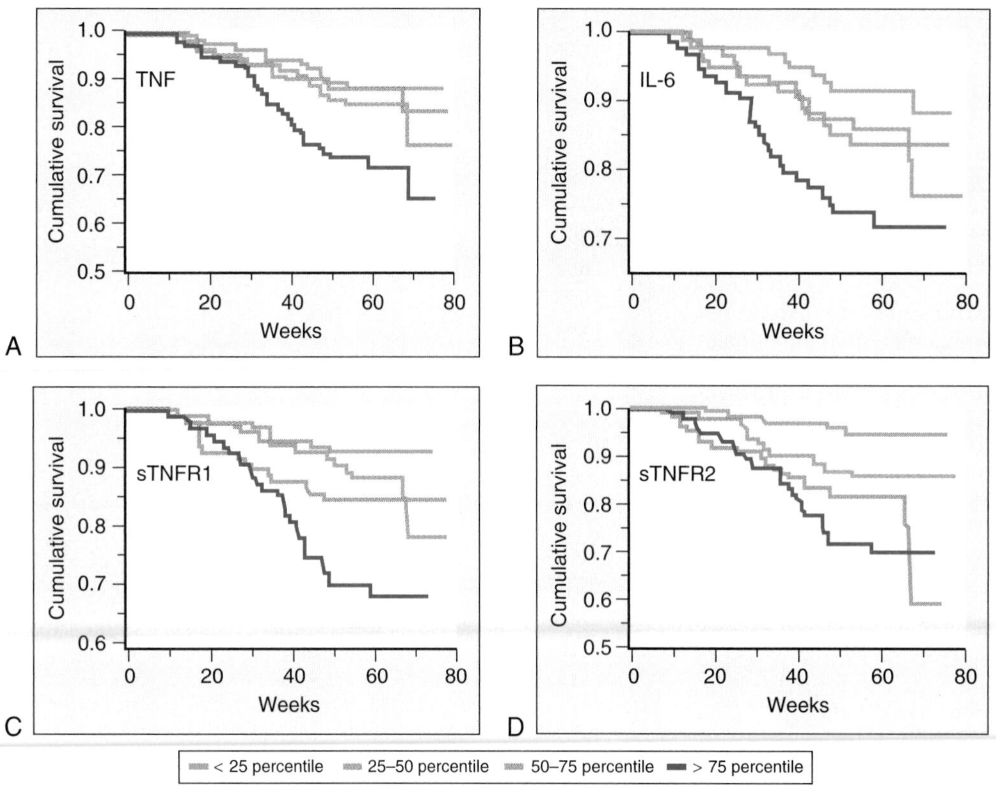

FIGURE 22–15 Kaplan-Meier survival analysis in 1200 consecutive subjects who were enrolled in a multicenter, randomized, placebo-controlled trial of vesnarinone in patients with advanced heart failure (VEST study). Circulating levels of **(A)** tumor necrosis factor (TNF), **(B)** interleukin-6 (IL-6), **(C)** soluble TNF receptor 1 (sTNFR1), and **(D)** soluble TNF receptor 2 (sTNFR2) were examined in relation to patients' survival during a mean follow-up of 55 weeks. Plasma levels of cytokines and cytokine receptors were divided into quartiles, with increasing levels associated with worse survival. (From Deswal A, Petersen NJ, Feldman AM, et al: Cytokines and cytokine receptors in advanced heart failure: an analysis of the cytokine database from the Vesnarinone Trial (VEST). Circulation 103:2055, 2001.)

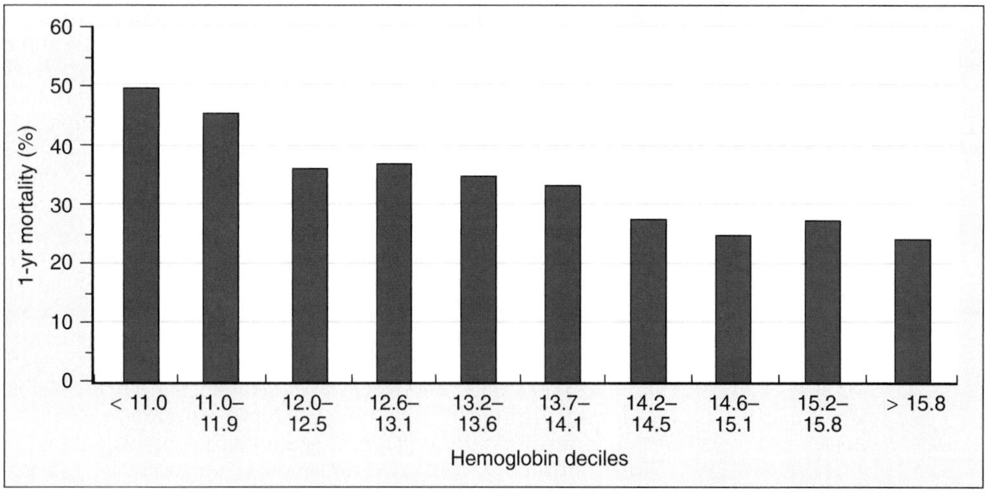

FIGURE 22–16 Anemia is associated with increased mortality in heart failure. In this single-center study, 1061 patients with advanced heart failure were evaluated for cardiac transplantation between 1983 and 1999. At initial presentation, mean hemoglobin (Hb) was 13.5 ± 1.9 gm/dl, and Hb ranged from 7.1 to 19.0 gm/dl. Lower hemoglobin levels were associated with greater symptoms, reduced exercise capacity, and impaired renal function. One-year mortality rates in the entire cohort divided by decile of Hb level are shown. (From Horwich TB, Fonarow GC, Hamilton MA, et al: Anemia is associated with worse symptoms, greater impairment in functional capacity and a significant increase in mortality in patients with advanced heart failure. J Am Coll Cardiol 39:1780, 2002.)

OTHER MARKERS OF PROGNOSIS. In addition to traditional neurohormones, several other biological mediators have been shown to carry important prognostic information in heart failure. Plasma levels of proinflammatory cytokines, including tumor necrosis factor-α[171,172] and interleukin-6[165,173] and their cognate receptors (Fig. 22–15), are elevated in relation to disease severity and predict adverse outcomes. Cytokines exert direct negative effects on cardiac myocytes and the extracellular matrix and have been implicated in ventricular remodeling and disease progression.[107] Markers of oxidative stress, such as oxidized low-density lipoprotein[174] and serum uric acid,[175] have also been associated with worsening clinical status and impaired survival in patients with chronic heart failure. Like inflammation, oxidative stress probably plays an important role in the pathophysiology of heart failure. In patients with stable chronic heart failure, the erythrocyte sedimentation rate correlates with inflammatory cytokines, and high erythrocyte sedimentation rates indicate a poor prognosis independent of NYHA class, ejection fraction, and $\dot{V}O_{2max}$.[129] Cardiac troponin T, a sensitive marker of myocyte damage (see Chap. 46), may be elevated in patients with nonischemic heart failure and predict adverse cardiac outcomes.[176]

A strong association between chronic heart failure and anemia has been demonstrated that carries important prognostic implications (see Laboratory Findings).[125] In a study of 1061 patients with NYHA Class III or IV heart failure and ejection fraction less than 40 percent, lower hemoglobin quartiles were associated with worse symptoms, lower $\dot{V}O_{2max}$, and increased mortality (Fig. 22–16).[125]

ELECTROPHYSIOLOGICAL. Death in patients with severe heart failure occurs either by progressive pump failure or, in as many as one half of all patients, suddenly and unexpectedly, presumably from an arrhythmia. When present, a variety of arrhythmias, especially frequent ventricular extrasystoles,[177] ventricular tachycardia,[178] left bundle branch block[179] and atrial fibrillation,[180] have been shown to be predictors of mortality and sudden death. What is not yet clear is whether these arrhythmias are simply indicators of the severity of left ventricular dysfunction or whether they are responsible for and trigger fatal arrhythmias. Although there is some evidence that ventricular arrhythmias confer independent adverse prognostic effects,[177] this may not hold true after adjusting for other variables, especially ejection fraction.[178] Furthermore, the routine treatment of patients with heart failure–associated arrhythmias with antiarrhythmic drugs has not been shown to exert a protective effect and reduce mortality.[181] Preliminary data from a large trial of cardiac resynchronization therapy (see Chap. 24) suggest a significant survival benefit when biventricular pacing is combined with an implantable cardioverter-defibrillator in patients with ischemic or nonischemic cardiomyopathy.[182]

Other electrophysiological parameters that have been associated with increased mortality or sudden death in heart failure, or both, include increased QT interval[183] and QT dispersion,[184] T wave alternans,[185] abnormal signal-averaged ECG, and decreased heart rate variability.[177]

Pulmonary Edema

Mechanism of Pulmonary Edema

ALVEOLAR-CAPILLARY MEMBRANE. Pulmonary edema develops when the movement of liquid from the blood to the interstitial space, and in some instances to the alveoli, exceeds the return of liquid to the blood and its drainage through the lymphatics.[186] The barrier between pulmonary capillaries and alveolar gas, the alveolar-capillary membrane, consists of three anatomical layers with distinct structural characteristics: (1) cytoplasmic projections of the capillary endothelial cells that join to form a continuous cytoplasmic tube; (2) the interstitial space, which varies in thickness and may contain connective tissue fibrils, fibroblasts, and macrophages between the capillary endothelium and the alveolar epithelium, terminal bronchioles, small arteries and veins, and lymphatic channels; and (3) the lining of the alveolar wall, which is continuous with the bronchial epithelium and is composed predominantly of large squamous cells (type I) with thin cytoplasmic projections.

There is normally a continuous exchange of liquid, colloid, and solutes between the vascular bed and interstitium.[187] A pathological state exists only when there is an increase in the net flux of liquid, colloid, and solutes from the vasculature into the interstitial space. Experimental studies have confirmed that the basic principles outlined in the classic Starling equation apply to the lung as well as to the systemic circulation.

$$Q_{(iv\text{-}int)} = K_f[(P_{iv} - P_{int}) - \sigma_f(\Pi_{iv} - \Pi_{int})]$$

where $Q_{iv\text{-}int}$ = net rate of transudation (flow of liquid from blood vessels to interstitial space), P_{int} = interstitial hydrostatic pressure, P_{iv} = intravascular hydrostatic pressure, Π_{int} = interstitial colloid osmotic pressure, Π_{iv} = intravascular colloid osmotic pressure, σ_f = reflection coefficient for proteins, and K_f = filtration coefficient.

LYMPHATICS. These vessels serve to remove solutes, colloid, and liquid derived from the blood vessels. Because of a more negative pressure in the peribronchial and perivascular interstitial spaces and the increased compliance of this nonalveolar interstitium, liquid is more likely to increase here when the pumping capacity of the lymphatic channels is exceeded. As a consequence of the development of interstitial edema, small airways and blood vessels may become compressed.

The lymphatics play a key role in removing liquid from the interstitial space, and if the pumping capacity of the lymphatic channels is exceeded, pulmonary edema occurs. With chronic elevations of left atrial pressure, the pulmonary lymphatic system hypertrophies and is able to transport greater quantities of capillary filtrate, thereby protecting the lungs from edema. By contrast, a sudden marked increase in pulmonary capillary pressure can be rapidly fatal in a patient not preconditioned by growth of the lymphatic drainage system.

SEQUENCE OF FLUID ACCUMULATION DURING PULMONARY EDEMA. Whether initiated by an imbalance of Starling forces or by primary damage to the various components of the alveolar-capillary membranes, the sequence of liquid exchange and accumulation in the lungs is the same and can be represented in three stages. In *stage 1,* there is an increase in mass transfer of liquid and colloid from blood capillaries through the interstitium. Despite the increased filtration, there is no measurable increase in interstitial volume because there is an equal increase in lymphatic outflow. *Stage 2* occurs when the filtered load from the pulmonary capillaries is sufficiently large that the pumping capacity of the lymphatics is approached or exceeded, and liquid and colloid begin to accumulate in the more compliant interstitial compartment surrounding bronchioles, arterioles, and venules. In *stage 3,* further increments in filtered load exceed the volume limits of the loose interstitial spaces, causing distention of the less compliant interstitial space of the alveolar-capillary septum and resulting in alveolar flooding.

Classification of Pulmonary Edema

The two most common forms of pulmonary edema are those initiated by an imbalance of Starling forces and those initiated by disruption of one or more components of the alveolar-capillary membrane (Table 22–5).[186,188] Less often, lymphatic insufficiency can be involved as a predisposing, if not initiating, factor in the genesis of edema.

IMBALANCE OF STARLING FORCES

INCREASED PULMONARY CAPILLARY PRESSURE. Pulmonary edema occurs only when the pulmonary capillary pressure rises to values exceeding the plasma colloid osmotic pressure, which is approximately 28 mm Hg in the human. Because the normal pulmonary capillary pressure is 8 to 12 mm Hg, there is a substantial margin of safety in the development of pulmonary edema. Although pulmonary capillary pressures must be abnormally high to increase the flow of interstitial fluid, at a time when edema is clearly present these pressures may not correlate with the severity of pulmonary edema. In fact, pulmonary capillary wedge pressures may have returned to normal at a time when there is still considerable pulmonary edema because time is required for removal of both interstitial and alveolar edema. Other factors obscure the relationship between the severity of edema and measured pulmonary capillary pressures in addition to slower rates of removal after edema has collected. The rate of increase in lung liquid at any given elevation of capillary pressure is related to the functional capacity of lymphatics, which may vary from patient to patient, and to variations in interstitial oncotic and hydrostatic pressures.

HYPOALBUMINEMIA. Pulmonary edema does not develop with hypoalbuminemia alone. However, hypoalbuminemia may alter the fluid conductivity of the interstitial space so that liquid moves more easily between capillaries and lymphatics. Therefore, in addition to hypoalbuminemia, there must be some elevations of pulmonary capillary pressure, but only small increases are necessary before pulmonary edema ensues in the presence of hypoalbuminemia.

INCREASED NEGATIVE INTERSTITIAL PRESSURE. Pulmonary edema may result from the rapid removal of pleural air to relieve a pneumothorax—so-called reexpansion pulmonary edema. Risk factors include young age and a large pneumothorax.[189] Usually, the pneumothorax has been present for several hours to days, allowing time for alterations in surfactant so that large negative pressures are necessary to open collapsed alveoli. In these instances, the edema is unilateral and is most often only a radiographic finding, with few clinical findings. In rare cases, reexpansion pulmonary edema may be severe and require rapid and extensive clinical treatment. Studies using radiolabeled transferrin suggest that an abnormality in microvascular permeability contributes to the development of localized pulmonary edema, possibly related to hypoxic injury[190] and local production of proinflammatory cytokines.[191] Hemodynamic studies have also demonstrated an increase in cardiac output immediately prior to the development of pulmonary edema.[192]

PRIMARY ALVEOLAR-CAPILLARY BARRIER DAMAGE

Many diverse medical and surgical conditions are associated with pulmonary edema that is due to damage of the alveolar-capillary barrier rather than to a primary alteration in Starling forces.[186] These conditions include acute pulmonary infections and pulmonary effects of gram-negative sepsis and nonthoracic trauma, as well as any condition associated with disseminated intravascular coagulation. Despite the diversity of underlying causes, when diffuse alveolar-capillary injury has occurred, the pathophysiological and clinical sequence of events are quite similar in most patients. Because of the resemblance of the clinical picture to that seen with respiratory distress of the neonate, these conditions have been referred to as the *acute respiratory distress syndrome* (ARDS).[193,194]

TABLE 22–5 Classification of Pulmonary Edema on the Basis of Initiating Mechanism

Imbalance of Starling Forces
Increased pulmonary capillary pressure
1. Increased pulmonary venous pressure without left ventricular failure (e.g., mitral stenosis)
2. Increased pulmonary venous pressure secondary to left ventricular failure
3. Increased pulmonary capillary pressure secondary to increased pulmonary arterial pressure (so-called overperfusion pulmonary edema)*

Decreased plasma oncotic pressure: hypoalbuminemia secondary to renal, hepatic, protein-losing enteropathic, or dermatological disease or nutritional causes†

Increased negativity of interstitial pressure
1. Rapid removal of pneumothorax with large applied negative pressures
2. Large negative pressures due to acute airway obstruction along with increased end-expiratory volumes (asthma)*

Increased interstitial oncotic pressure: no known clinical or experimental example

Alveolar-Capillary Barrier Damage (Acute Respiratory Distress Syndrome)
Direct lung injury
1. Pneumonia—bacterial, viral, parasitic
2. Aspiration of gastric contents
3. Inhaled toxins (e.g., phosgene, ozone, chlorine, nitrogen dioxide, smoke)
4. Pulmonary contusion
5. Fat emboli
6. Near-drowning
7. Radiation pneumonitis

Indirect lung injury
1. Sepsis
2. Nonthoracic trauma with shock and multiple transfusions
3. Disseminated intravascular coagulation
4. Hypersensitivity pneumonitis due to drugs (e.g., nitrofurantoin), leukoagglutinins
5. Acute pancreatitis
6. Endogenous vasoactive substances (e.g., histamine, kinins*)
7. Circulating foreign substances (e.g., snake venom, alloxan,† alpha-naphthyl thiourea‡)

Lymphatic Insufficiency
After lung transplantation
Lymphangitic carcinomatosis
Fibrosing lymphangitis (e.g., silicosis)

Unknown or Incompletely Understood
High-altitude pulmonary edema
Neurogenic pulmonary edema
Narcotic overdose
Pulmonary embolism
Preeclampsia-eclampsia
After cardioversion
After anesthesia
After cardiopulmonary bypass

*Not certain to exist as a clinical entity.
† Not certain that this, as a single factor, leads to pulmonary edema.
‡ Predominantly an experimental technique.

Direct evidence for increased permeability of the alveolar-capillary barrier in ARDS, leading to influx of protein-rich fluid into the air spaces,[195] has come mainly from experimental studies. It is likely that epithelial injury leading to increased permeability of the alveolar-capillary barrier is a critical initiating event in most cases of ARDS.[193] The loss of integrity of the alveolar epithelium results in impaired removal of edema fluid from the alveolar space, reduced production of surfactant, increased risk of septic shock, and disorganized epithelial repair. Although it remains unclear whether neutrophil-mediated inflammation is a cause or the result of lung injury, evidence suggests that an imbalance between proinflammatory cytokines and antiinflammatory mediators contributes to both the initiation and amplification of injury.[186]

Cardiogenic Pulmonary Edema

PATHOPHYSIOLOGY. Cardiogenic pulmonary edema is characterized by the transudation of protein-poor fluid into the lungs secondary to an increase in left atrial and subsequently pulmonary capillary pressure. This transudation occurs in the absence of an alteration in the permeability or integrity of the alveolar-capillary membrane and results in decreased diffusing capacity, hypoxemia, and shortness of breath.

During *stage 1*, the distention and recruitment of small pulmonary vessels secondary to elevation of left atrial pressure may actually improve gas exchange in the lung and augment slightly the diffusing capacity for carbon monoxide. Exertional dyspnea accompanies these abnormalities, and inspiratory rales related to opening of closed airways may be present.

With progression to *stage 2*, *interstitial edema* attributable to increased liquid in the loose interstitial space contiguous with the perivascular tissue of larger vessels may cause a loss of the normally sharp radiographic definition of pulmonary vascular markings, haziness and loss of demarcation of hilar shadows, and thickening of interlobular septa (Kerley B lines). Competition for space between vessels, airways, and increased liquid within the loose interstitium may compromise small airway lumina, particularly in the dependent portions of the lungs, and there may be reflex bronchoconstriction. A mismatch exists between ventilation and perfusion that results in hypoxemia and more wasted ventilation. Indeed, in the setting of acute myocardial infarction, the degree of hypoxemia correlates with the degree of elevation of the pulmonary capillary wedge pressure. Tachypnea is a frequent finding with interstitial edema and has been attributed to stimulation of J-type receptors or stretch receptors in the interstitium rather than to hypoxemia, which is rarely of sufficient magnitude to stimulate breathing. There are few changes in the standard spirometric indices.

With the development of alveolar flooding, or *stage 3* edema, gas exchange is quite abnormal, with severe hypoxemia and often hypocapnia. Alveolar flooding can proceed to such a degree that many large airways are filled with blood-tinged foam that may be expectorated. Vital capacity and other lung volumes are markedly reduced. A right-to-left intrapulmonary shunt develops as a consequence of perfusion of the flooded alveoli. Although hypocapnia is the rule, hypercapnia with acute respiratory acidemia can occur in more severe cases or in patients with concomitant chronic obstructive pulmonary disease. It is in such instances that morphine, with its well-known respiratory depressant effects, should be used with caution.

ROLE OF LYMPHATICS. As discussed earlier, the rate of accumulation of lung liquid at a given elevation in pulmonary capillary pressure is related to the functional capacity of the pulmonary lymphatic vessels to remove excess fluid. With acute increases in pulmonary capillary pressure, lymphatic vessels in the lungs lack the capacity to increase rapidly the rate of fluid removal. As a result, patients with acute heart failure develop pulmonary edema at pulmonary capillary pressures as low as 18 mm Hg. In contrast, patients with chronic heart failure usually do not develop pulmonary edema until pulmonary capillary pressures have increased to 25 mm Hg or higher, presumably because of increased lymphatic capacity.

ETIOLOGY AND DIAGNOSIS. Acute cardiogenic pulmonary edema is the most dramatic symptom of left-sided heart failure.[196,197] It may be caused by impairment of left atrial outflow, left ventricular systolic or diastolic dysfunction, left ventricular volume overload, or left ventricular outflow obstruction. Elevated left atrial and pulmonary capillary wedge pressures lead to cardiogenic pulmonary edema, which, in turn, interferes with oxygen transfer in the lungs and depresses arterial oxygen tension. Simultaneously, the sensation of suffocation and oppression in the chest intensifies the patient's fright, elevates heart rate and blood pressure, and further restricts ventricular filling. The increased discomfort and work of breathing place an additional load on the heart, and cardiac function becomes depressed further by the hypoxia. If this vicious circle is not interrupted, it may lead rapidly to death.

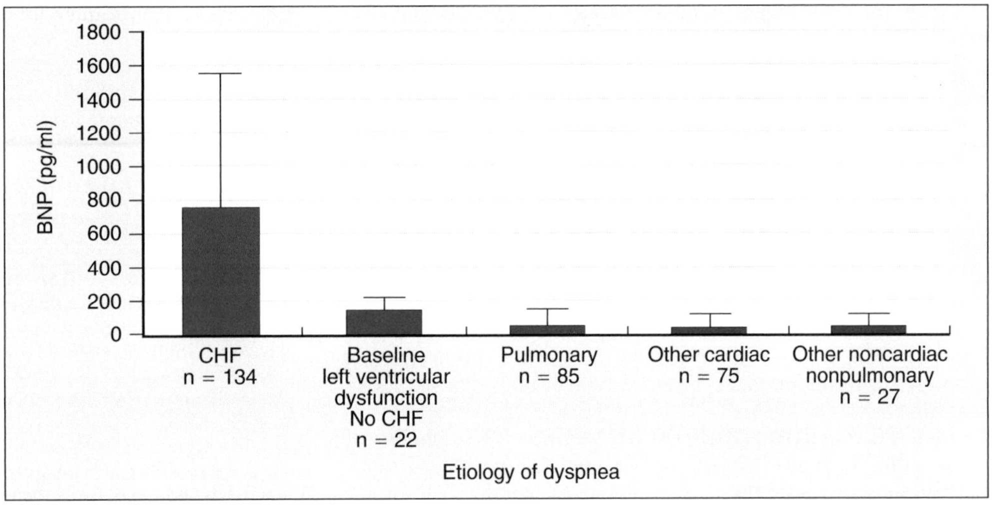

FIGURE 22–17 B-type natriuretic peptide (BNP) levels in 321 patients presenting to the emergency room with acute dyspnea and diagnosed with congestive heart failure (CHF), left ventricular dysfunction without CHF, pulmonary disease, other cardiac disease (e.g., angina, atypical chest pain), or other noncardiac nonpulmonary disease (e.g., anxiety, gastroesophageal reflux). In patients with pulmonary disease ($n = 85$), BNP levels were highest in the small groups of patients with pulmonary embolism or lung cancer. (From Morrison LK, Harrison A, Krishnaswamy P, et al: Utility of a rapid B-natriuretic peptide assay in differentiating congestive heart failure from lung disease in patients presenting with dyspnea. J Am Coll Cardiol 39:202, 2002.)

CLINICAL MANIFESTATIONS. Acute cardiogenic pulmonary edema differs from orthopnea and paroxysmal nocturnal dyspnea in the more rapid and extreme development of pulmonary capillary hypertension. Acute pulmonary edema is a terrifying experience for the patient and often the bystander as well. Usually, extreme breathlessness develops suddenly and the patient becomes extremely anxious, coughs, and expectorates pink, frothy liquid with a feeling of drowning. The patient sits bolt upright or may stand, exhibits air hunger, and may thrash about. The respiratory rate is elevated, the alae nasi are dilated, and there is inspiratory retraction of the intercostal spaces and supraclavicular fossae that reflects the large negative intrapleural pressures required for inspiration. The patient often grasps the sides of the bed to allow use of the accessory muscles of respiration. Respiration is noisy, with loud inspiratory and expiratory gurgling sounds that are often easily audible across the room. Sweating is profuse, and the skin is usually cold, ashen, and cyanotic, reflecting low cardiac output and increased sympathetic drive.

On *auscultation*, there are many adventitious lung sounds, with rhonchi, wheezes, and moist and fine crepitant rales that appear at first over the lung bases but then extend upward to the apices as the condition worsens. Cardiac auscultation may be difficult because of the respiratory sounds, but a third heart sound and an accentuated pulmonic component of the second heart sound are frequently present. In patients with ischemic heart disease, a holosystolic murmur of mitral regurgitation may also be heard at the cardiac apex or axilla.

The patient may suffer from intense precordial pain if the pulmonary edema is secondary to acute myocardial infarction (see Chap. 46). Unless cardiogenic shock is present, arterial pressure is usually elevated above the patient's baseline as a result of anxiety and discomfort, which cause adrenergically mediated vasoconstriction. Because of the presence of systemic hypertension, it may be suspected (inappropriately) that the pulmonary edema is due to hypertensive heart disease. However, it should be noted that hypertensive crises[198] are now uncommon (Chap. 37), and if arterial pressure is elevated, funduscopic examination usually indicates whether or not hypertensive heart disease is actually present.

DIFFERENTIATION FROM ASTHMA. It may be difficult to differentiate severe asthma[199] from acute pulmonary edema because both conditions may be associated with extreme dyspnea, pulsus paradoxus, demands for an upright posture, and diffuse wheezes that interfere with cardiac auscultation. In asthma, there is usually a history of previous similar episodes and the patient is aware of the diagnosis. During the acute attack, the asthmatic patient does not usually sweat profusely, and arterial hypoxemia, although present, is not usually of sufficient magnitude to cause cyanosis. In addition, the chest is hyperexpanded and hyperresonant and use of accessory muscles is most prominent during expiration. Although nonspecific, wheezes are higher pitched and more musical than in pulmonary edema, and other adventitious sounds such as rhonchi and rales are less prominent.

The patient with acute cardiogenic pulmonary edema usually perspires profusely and is frequently cyanotic owing to desaturation of arterial blood and decreased cutaneous blood flow. The chest is often dull to percussion, there is no hyperexpansion, accessory muscle use is less prominent than in asthma, and moist, bubbly rales and rhonchi are heard in addition to wheezes. Chest radiography shows interstitial or alveolar edema. As the patient recovers, the radiological appearance of pulmonary edema usually resolves more slowly than the elevated pulmonary capillary wedge pressure.

Other diagnostic tests have been evaluated in this setting. Rapid measurement of plasma BNP levels may help to distinguish acute cardiogenic pulmonary edema from severe asthma in patients presenting to an emergency room with dyspnea (Fig. 22–17).[44,50] Alternatively, in patients with intermediate BNP levels and nonspecific radiological findings, a "restrictive" pattern of mitral valve inflow as assessed by Doppler echocardiography may suggest the diagnosis of heart failure.[200]

PULMONARY CAPILLARY WEDGE PRESSURE. Measurement of pulmonary capillary wedge pressure by means of a flow-directed catheter (see Chap. 17) may be critical in distinguishing between pulmonary edema secondary to an imbalance of Starling forces (i.e., cardiogenic pulmonary edema) and that secondary to alterations of the alveolar-capillary barrier. Specifically, a pulmonary capillary wedge or pulmonary artery diastolic pressure greater than 20 mm Hg in a patient without previous pulmonary capillary pressure elevation (or greater than 30 mm Hg in a patient with chronic pulmonary capillary hypertension) and with the clinical features of pulmonary edema strongly suggests that the edema is cardiogenic. However, the use of a pulmonary artery catheter to measure pulmonary capillary wedge pressure is generally reserved for hospitalized patients with decompensated heart failure, leaving only noninvasive means of estimating left heart pressures in the majority of patients. Unfortunately, the routine clinical evaluation of patients with chronic systolic heart failure lacks the sensitivity and specificity needed for accurate assessment of left atrial pressure. Noninvasive methods that can reliably predict left-sided filling pressures and may have clinical application in the ambulatory setting are being investigated.[102] These include newer echocardiographic techniques such as Doppler tissue imaging and measurement of pulmonary venous inflow, thoracic bioimpedence, and a noninvasive Valsalva response recorder.

ELECTROCARDIOGRAPHIC CHANGES. ECG changes of myocardial ischemia or infarction (see Chap. 9) are commonly seen in patients with acute cardiogenic pulmonary edema. In patients presenting with hypertensive crises, the electrocardiogram may reveal left ventricular hypertrophy with a "strain" pattern that is exaggerated compared with the baseline tracing. In patients with cardiogenic but nonischemic pulmonary edema, large inverted T waves with marked QT prolongation may evolve within 24 hours of clinical stabilization and resolve within 1 week.[201] The cause of these "nonischemic" changes is unknown but may include subendocardial ischemia related to increased wall stress, acute increase in cardiac sympathetic tone, or increased electrical heterogeneity exacerbated by metabolic changes or catecholamines.

PROGNOSIS. After effective treatment of the pulmonary edema (see Chaps. 23 and 24), patients are often restored rapidly to the condition that existed before the attack, although they usually feel exhausted. Between attacks of pulmonary edema, there may be few symptoms or signs of heart failure. The long-term prognosis after an episode of acute pulmonary edema depends on the underlying cause of pulmonary edema (e.g., acute myocardial infarction) and the presence of comorbidities such as diabetes or end-stage renal disease. In a study of 150 consecutive patients hospitalized with acute pulmonary edema, the in-hospital mortality rate was 12 percent, with more than 80 percent of deaths attributed to cardiac failure.[202] Predictors of in-hospital mortality included diabetes, left ventricular dysfunction, hypotension or shock, and need for mechanical ventilation.

Pulmonary Edema of Unknown or Incompletely Defined Pathogenesis

HIGH-ALTITUDE PULMONARY EDEMA. High-altitude pulmonary edema (HAPE) is a noncardiogenic pulmonary edema that occurs most commonly in healthy young adults who ascend rapidly to altitudes in excess of 2500 meters and who then engage in strenuous exercise at those altitudes before they have become acclimated.[203,204] Estimates place the incidence of HAPE at 6.4 clinically apparent cases per 100 exposures to high altitude in persons younger than 21 years of age and 0.4 cases per 100 exposures in those older than 21 years. In addition to age, the major factors that determine the occurrence of HAPE are the altitude achieved (although HAPE may occur at altitudes of less than 2400 meters[205]), the speed of ascent, the level of exertion, and individual susceptibility. Affected individuals complain of dry cough, exertional dyspnea, and fatigue, usually within 1 to 2 days of ascent. As pulmonary edema worsens, these symptoms may progress rapidly (i.e., to dyspnea at rest) and may be associated with chest pain, orthopnea, and pink frothy sputum. Headache, drowsiness, and confusion may occur secondary to hypoxemia and the development of acute mountain sickness or high-altitude cerebral edema. Clinical evaluation reveals tachypnea, tachycardia, bilateral moist rales, and cyanosis, accompanied by marked arterial hypoxemia and respiratory alkalosis. Fever may also be present. The electrocardiogram reveals sinus tachycardia and evidence of right heart strain, and the chest radiograph shows discrete, patchy pulmonary infiltrates. As HAPE progresses and then resolves, pulmonary infiltrates often become diffuse and homogeneous.

A central abnormality in the pathophysiology of HAPE is an abnormal rise in pulmonary artery pressures and pulmonary vascular resistance in response to hypoxia (Fig. 22–18).[206] Possible mechanisms underlying the exaggerated hypoxic pulmonary vascular response in susceptible individuals include a decreased hypoxic ventilatory response, exaggerated sympathetic activation,[207] and endothelial dysfunction related to decreased pulmonary production of nitric oxide,[208] augmented release or decreased clearance of endothelin-1, or both.[209] The association of HAPE with the major histocompatibility human leukocyte antigens HLA-DR6 and HLA-DQ4 also suggests an immunogenetic susceptibility.[210] Uneven pulmonary vasoconstriction during hypoxia or exercise,[206] resulting in overperfused areas and "stress failure" of the pulmonary capillaries,[211] is believed to contribute to the development of pulmonary edema. Analysis of bronchoalveolar lavage fluid from subjects with HAPE revealed normal levels of leukocytes and proinflammatory cytokines, suggesting that inflammation does not play a primary role in the pathogenesis of HAPE.[212]

TREATMENT. Early recognition of this syndrome is critical. HAPE is reversed rapidly (i.e., in less than 48 hours) by returning the patient to a lower altitude or by administering a high inspiratory concentration of oxygen, or both. Bed rest, fluid restriction, and continuous positive airway pressure should also be considered.[205] Sleeping below 2500 meters, slow ascent with gradual acclimatization, and avoidance of heavy exertion for the first 2 or 3 days at high altitude are thought to be preventive. Nifedipine has been used successively both in

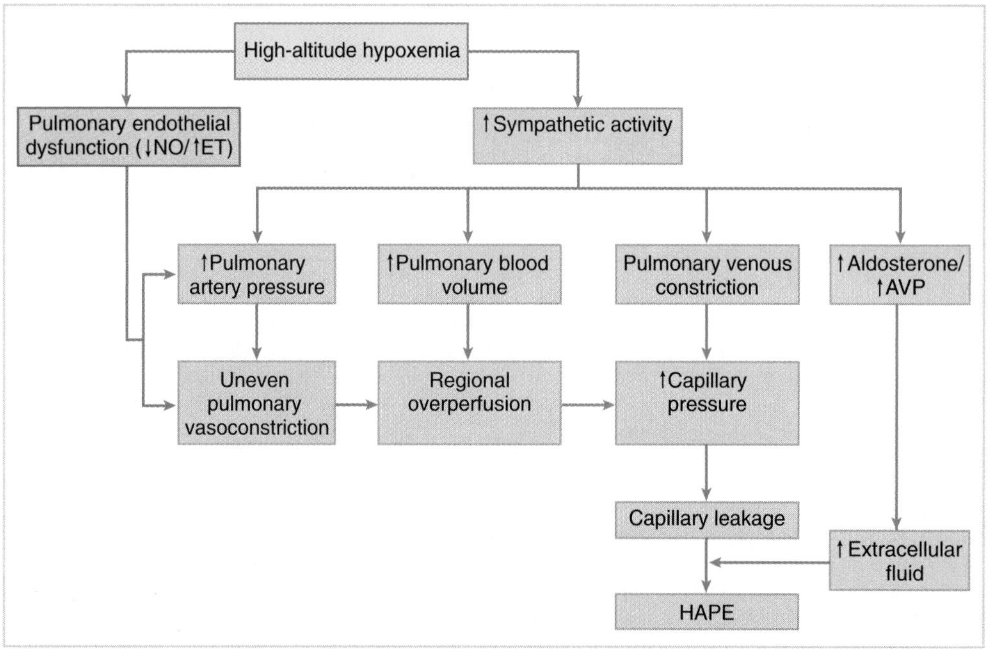

FIGURE 22–18 Diagram showing the sequence of events in the pathogenesis of high-altitude pulmonary edema (HAPE). AVP = arginine vasopressin; ET = endothelin-1; NO = nitric oxide. (Modified from Hackett PH, Roach RC: High-altitude illness. N Engl J Med 345:107, 2001.)

the treatment of HAPE and as prophylaxis[203,213] but is necessary only when oxygen is unavailable or descent is impossible. Prophylactic inhalation of salmeterol, a beta-adrenergic agonist, has been shown to reduce the incidence of HAPE by about 50 percent in susceptible individuals.[214] When HAPE has developed, inhaled nitric oxide, either alone or in combination with supplemental oxygen, can lower pulmonary vascular resistance and improve arterial oxygenation, although its availability is limited.[215] The improvement in gas exchange with inhaled NO may be due to a shift in blood flow away from edematous segments of the lung toward nonedematous segments. Although death caused by HAPE is rare, HAPE is responsible for the majority of deaths related to high-altitude illness.

NEUROGENIC PULMONARY EDEMA. A variety of central nervous system disorders including head trauma, seizures, stroke, and subarachnoid hemorrhage can be associated with acute pulmonary edema (without detectable left ventricular dysfunction).[216,217] Neurogenic pulmonary edema can also occur after surgical craniotomy. It is believed that sympathetic overactivity with massive catecholamine surges shifts blood from the systemic to the pulmonary circulation, with secondary elevations of left atrial and pulmonary capillary pressures. The resulting imbalance of Starling forces (i.e., a hydrostatic mechanism[218]) may therefore be the basis for this form of pulmonary edema. Pulmonary capillary leak caused by pressure-induced mechanical injury or direct nervous system control over capillary permeability, or both, may also play a contributory role. Although inhibition of nitric oxide production in the central nervous system has been shown to worsen neurogenic pulmonary edema in a rat model, the therapeutic implications of this finding remain unclear.[219] Symptom onset tends to be rapid (i.e., within 4 hours of the neurological event), and chest radiography shows diffuse bilateral infiltrates.

Treatment of neurogenic pulmonary edema, usually in an intensive care setting, consists of ventilatory support and maneuvers to reduce intracranial pressure. A reversible impairment in left ventricular systolic function resulting in hypotension may accompany neurogenic pulmonary edema. Mortality rates of 10 percent have been reported, but surviving patients usually recover quickly.

NARCOTIC OVERDOSE PULMONARY EDEMA. First described by Osler in 1880, acute pulmonary edema is a well-recognized sequela of heroin overdose.[220,221] Risk factors include male gender and shorter duration of heroin use, and concomitant use of cocaine and alcohol is common.[221] The onset of dyspnea and hypoxemia is usually rapid, occurring immediately or within hours of heroin overdose. Chest radiography typically shows diffuse fluffy infiltrates, although unilateral or patchy lung involvement has been described. Treatment consists of naloxone, supplemental oxygen, and in approximately one third of patients temporary mechanical ventilatory support.[220] Complete resolution of hypoxemia in 1 to 2 days is the rule. Because of the illicit traffic in this drug, which is given by the intravenous route, the syndrome was initially thought to be due to injected impurities rather than to the heroin itself. However, because oral methadone and dextropropoxyphene can also be associated with pulmonary edema, the syndrome cannot be attributed entirely to injected impurities. The fact that edema fluid contains protein concentrations nearly identical to those found in plasma and that pulmonary capillary wedge pressures, when measured, are normal argues for an alveolar-capillary membrane leak as the initiating cause.

PULMONARY EMBOLISM (see Chap. 66). Acute pulmonary edema in association with either a massive embolus or multiple smaller emboli has been well described and most often attributed to concomitant left ventricular dysfunction related to a combination of hypoxemia and encroachment of the interventricular septum on the left ventricular cavity.[222] It has been suggested that in the pulmonary edema related to pulmonary microthrombi an increase in permeability of the alveolar-capillary membrane occurs.

ECLAMPSIA (see Chap. 74). Acute pulmonary edema is a well-recognized complication of preeclampsia-eclampsia, occurring with an overall frequency of 3 to 5 percent.[223] In a retrospective review of 16,800 deliveries at a large, urban medical center, pulmonary edema occurred in 0.5 percent of all obstetrical cases.[224] The incidence of pulmonary edema is higher in women who are older, who are multiparous, and who have preexisting chronic hypertension. The majority of cases, approximately 70 percent, occur post partum. Multiple factors including cerebral dysfunction with massive sympathetic discharge, left ventricular dysfunction secondary to acute systemic hypertension, hypervolemia caused by excessive colloid and crystalloid infusions or transfusions, hypoalbuminemia secondary to renal losses, and disseminated intravascular coagulation may play a role in the pathogenesis.

Patients present with acute dyspnea and arterial hypoxemia, and chest radiography reveals extensive airspace consolidation. The average time to resolution of pulmonary edema is 2 to 3 days, and a minority of patients (approximately 15 percent) require mechanical ventilatory support. Risk factors for prolonged intubation include infection and fetal surgery.[224] Pulmonary artery catheterization is safe and commonly reveals elevated right- and left-sided cardiac filling pressures, elevated cardiac index, and normal systemic vascular resistance, although hemodynamics consistent with pulmonary capillary leak have also been reported.[225] Echocardiography may show normal, hyperdynamic, or depressed left ventricular systolic function with or without diastolic filling abnormalities.[226] The occurrence of pulmonary edema in obstetrical patients is associated with high maternal and perinatal morbidity and mortality.

AFTER CARDIOVERSION. Acute pulmonary edema is an uncommon albeit well-recognized complication of cardioversion, occurring in less than 0.5 percent of cases.[227] The mechanisms underlying postcardioversion pulmonary edema are poorly understood. Ineffective left atrial function immediately after cardioversion resulting in decreased cardiac output has been suggested as a contributing factor,[227] yet left ventricular diastolic dysfunction related to direct current shock and neurogenic mechanisms are also possible. Additional contributory factors may include underlying cardiac disease, cardiodepressant anesthetic agents, and pulmonary or cardiac emboli or both. One half of cases occur within 3 hours after cardioversion.

AFTER ANESTHESIA. Pulmonary edema has been described in the early postoperative period in previously healthy subjects, without a clear relationship to fluid overload or any subsequent evidence of left ventricular dysfunction.[228] The basis for this disorder is unknown, but proposed mechanisms include postanesthesia laryngospasm with marked negative intrathoracic pressure ("postobstructive" or "negative pressure" pulmonary edema), hypoxia, and a hyperadrenergic state. In a retrospective analysis of 8195 major operations, pulmonary edema occurred in 7.6 percent of cases, with a mortality rate of 12 percent.[228] Patients with fatal postoperative pulmonary edema retained an average of 67 ml/kg of fluid within the first 24 hours following surgery and presented with cardiopulmonary arrest, arterial hypoxemia, and metabolic acidosis. Pulmonary artery pressures were normal.

AFTER CARDIOPULMONARY BYPASS. Although all patients who undergo cardiopulmonary bypass have significant heart disease, the development of pulmonary edema has been associated with normal left atrial pressures.[229] Alterations of surfactant related to prolonged collapse of the lung during the procedure, with subsequent need to apply high negative intrapleural pressures for reexpansion, and release of toxic substances including thromboxane have been suggested as mechanisms. Increased pulmonary vascular resistance and intrapulmonary shunting contribute to hypoxemia. Cardiopulmonary bypass also causes a systemic inflammatory response[229] with activation of complement, cytokines, and reactive oxygen species, which may contribute to the development of noncardiogenic pulmonary edema. Some data suggest that allergic reactions to fresh frozen plasma or protamine may account for some episodes. The increasing use of off-pump coronary artery bypass (OPCAB)[230] in high-risk elderly patients with reduced left ventricular function or chronic renal insufficiency would be expected to reduce the incidence of this already rare entity.

TRANSFUSION-RELATED ACUTE LUNG INJURY. A clinical syndrome that includes fever, dyspnea, hypotension, and bilateral pulmonary edema may occur following transfusion of blood products.[231] The pathogenesis is poorly understood, and affected individuals often have other acute or chronic illnesses that may contribute to the development of cardiogenic or noncardiogenic pulmonary edema. Data suggest that this syndrome is underdiagnosed and underreported.[231]

HANTAVIRUS PULMONARY SYNDROME. In Asia, hantaviruses are associated with hemorrhagic fever and renal disease. In 1993, an outbreak of severe respiratory illness occurred in the southwestern United States and was attributed to a newly described hantavirus.[232] The majority of patients affected were Native American. Prodromal symptoms included fever, myalgia, cough, dyspnea, and gastrointestinal symptoms. Most infected patients developed rapidly progressive noncardiogenic pulmonary edema associated with profound hypotension, with a case-fatality rate of 76 percent. The pathogenesis of hantavirus pulmonary syndrome remains unknown. It has been suggested that local T cells acting on the infected pulmonary vascular endothelium result in the production of cytokines, including interferon-gamma and tumor necrosis factor-α, which may play an important role in the reversible increase in vascular permeability.[233]

OTHER VIRAL INFECTIONS. Enteroviruses can cause outbreaks of hand-foot-and-mouth disease or herpangina, which are usually self-limiting. In 1998, an outbreak of enterovirus 71 infection in Taiwan

TABLE 22–6 Initial Differentiation of Cardiogenic from Noncardiogenic Pulmonary Edema

Parameters	Cardiogenic Pulmonary Edema	Noncardiogenic Pulmonary Edema
History		
Acute cardiac event	Usually present	Uncommon (but possible)
Physical Examination		
Cardiac output state	Low-flow state (cool periphery)	High-flow state (warm periphery, bounding pulses)
S_3 gallop	Present	Absent
Jugular venous distention	Present	Absent
Crackles	Wet	Dry
Underlying noncardiac disease (e.g., sepsis)	Usually absent	Present
Laboratory Tests		
Electrocardiogram	Ischemia/infarction	Usually normal
Chest radiograph	Perihilar distribution	Peripheral distribution
Cardiac enzymes	May be elevated	Usually normal
Pulmonary capillary wedge pressure	≥18 mm Hg	<18 mm Hg
Intrapulmonary shunting	Small	Large
Edema fluid/serum protein	<0.5	>0.7

From Sibbald WJ, Cunningham DR, Chin DN: Noncardiac or cardiac pulmonary edema? A practical approach to clinical differentiation in critically ill patients. Chest 84:460, 1983.

resulted in severe infection in more than 400 patients with a case-fatality rate of 19 percent.[234] Complications of severe disease, which were commonly seen in children younger than 6 years, included meningoencephalitis, flaccid paralysis, pulmonary edema or hemorrhage, and myocarditis. Of the patients who died, 83 percent had pulmonary edema or hemorrhage.

Several outbreaks of severe acute respiratory syndrome (SARS) have been reported in China, Vietnam, Canada, and Germany.[235,236] Common symptoms include fever, chills, myalgias, and cough. Peripheral airspace consolidation leading to respiratory failure and death have occurred, and postmortem examination of the lungs revealed pulmonary edema with hyaline membrane formation suggestive of the early phase of ARDS.[235] Using virus isolation techniques, electron microscopic and histological studies, and molecular and serological assays, investigators have identified a novel coronavirus as the causative agent.[236]

Differential Diagnosis of Pulmonary Edema

The differentiation between the two principal forms of pulmonary edema—that is, cardiogenic (hemodynamic) and noncardiogenic (caused by alterations in the alveolar-capillary barrier)—can usually be made through assessment of the clinical context in which it occurs and through examination and consideration of the clinical data as shown in Table 22–6. Although this approach suggests an either/or situation, this may not be the case in clinical practice. For example, sudden and large increases in intravascular pressure may disrupt the capillary and alveolar membranes, leading to interstitial edema and alveolar loading with macromolecules that produce an edema liquid more compatible with noncardiogenic causes.[188] Thus, a primary hemodynamic event can cause "stress failure" of the alveolar-capillary barrier. Furthermore, only mild elevations in capillary hydrostatic pressures in the presence of alveolar capillary damage can cause an increase in the rate and extent of edema formation. Therefore, hemodynamic factors can and do play a role in increasing and perpetuating increased permeability.

High-Output Heart Failure

High–cardiac output states (Table 22–7) by themselves are seldom responsible for heart failure, but their development in the presence of underlying heart disease often precipitates heart failure. In these conditions, which are often characterized by arteriovenous shunting, the requirements of the peripheral tissues for oxygen can be met only by an increase in cardiac output. Although the normal heart is capable of augmenting its output on a long-term basis, this may not be true of the diseased heart.

TABLE 22–7 High-Cardiac Output States

Anemia
Acquired arteriovenous fistulas Traumatic Iatrogenic Infectious Surgical (hemodialysis) Atherosclerotic Malignancy
Congenital arteriovenous fistulas Hemangiomas Hereditary hemorrhagic telangiectasia Hepatic hemangioendothelioma
Thyrotoxicosis
Beriberi heart disease
Paget disease of bone
Fibrous dysplasia
Multiple myeloma
Polycythemia vera
Carcinoid syndrome
Acromegaly
Pregnancy

Anemia

Chronic anemia is associated with high cardiac output when hemoglobin is equal to or less than approximately 8 gm/dl. Reduced systemic vascular resistance, which results from decreased arteriolar tone and decreased blood viscosity, plays an important role in the pathophysiology of this high-output state (Fig. 22–19). Enhanced basal production of endothelium-derived nitric oxide may be responsible, in part, for the low systemic vascular resistance in patients with anemia.[237] Impaired renal excretion of sodium and water leading to volume overload may be due to decreased renal blood flow,

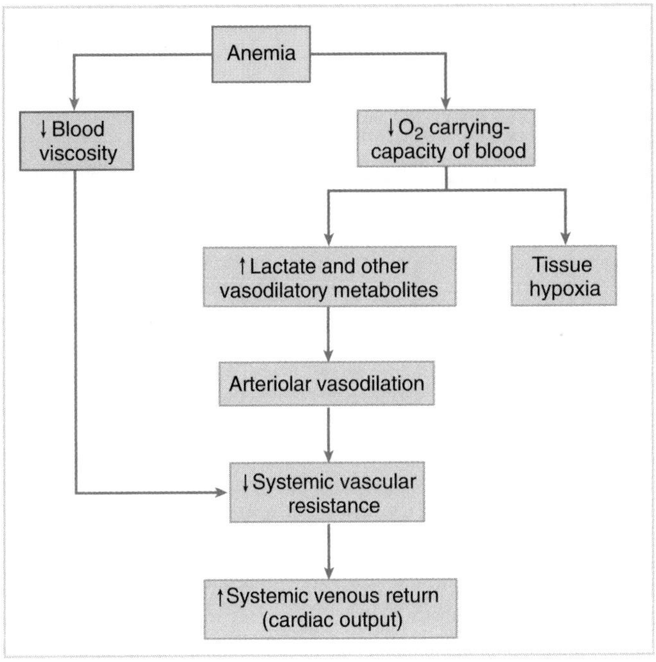

FIGURE 22–19 Diagram showing the pathophysiological mechanisms underlying the high–cardiac output state associated with anemia. Decreased blood viscosity and a reduction in arteriolar tone resulting from tissue hypoxia and lactic acidosis contribute to reduced systemic vascular resistance, which in turn increases cardiac output. In addition, chronic anemia is associated with increased endothelium-derived nitric oxide, which contributes to enhanced vasodilation. O_2 = oxygen. (From Hassapoyannes CA, Nelson WP, Hopkins CB, et al: Other causes and contributing factors to congestive heart failure. *In* Hosenpud JD, Greenberg BH [eds]: Congestive Heart Failure. New York, Springer-Verlag, 1994, pp 281-300.)

reduced glomerular filtration rate, and neurohormonal activation.[238] In animal models of high-output heart failure, blunted cardiac secretion of natriuretic peptides in response to a volume challenge and decreased renal responsiveness to their actions have also been demonstrated.[239]

Anemia, even when severe, rarely causes heart failure or angina pectoris in patients with normal hearts; when these problems occur, it is likely that the high cardiac output is superimposed on some specific cardiac abnormality, such as valvular or ischemic heart disease.

PHYSICAL EXAMINATION. Physical findings secondary to anemia are often superimposed on those of an underlying cardiovascular disorder. The anemic patient often has a pale, "pasty" appearance; in blacks, the findings of paleness of the conjunctivae, mucous membranes, and palmar creases are helpful. Arterial pulses are bounding, "pistol shot" sounds can be heard over the femoral arteries (Traube sign), and subungual capillary pulsations (Quincke pulse) are present, as in patients with aortic regurgitation (see Chap. 57). A medium-pitched, midsystolic murmur along the left sternal border, generally grade 1/6 to 3/6 in intensity (seldom accompanied by a thrill), is common. Heart sounds are accentuated, and the pulmonic component of the second heart sound may be particularly prominent in patients with sickle cell anemia and pulmonary hypertension; in such patients, a right ventricular lift can usually be palpated. A mid-diastolic flow murmur secondary to augmented blood flow across the mitral orifice, holosystolic murmurs resulting from tricuspid and mitral regurgitation secondary to ventricular dilation, and, rarely, diastolic murmurs resulting from aortic and pulmonic valve incompetence secondary to dilation of these vessels may be heard. A protodiastolic gallop sound (S_3) is frequently audible at the cardiac apex. Jugular venous distention is uncommon and, although peripheral edema and hepatomegaly are occasionally present, they may be due not only to heart failure but also to accompanying abnormalities such as hypoalbuminemia and nutritional deficiency.

DIAGNOSTIC TESTING. In patients with severe chronic anemia without underlying heart disease, the chest radiograph usually demonstrates mild to moderate cardiomegaly. The electrocardiogram often does not show any specific changes but may reveal tachycardia and T wave inversions in the lateral precordial leads. The echocardiogram generally shows a modest and symmetrical increase in the size of all chambers, with large systolic excursions of the septal and posterior left ventricular walls. In addition, an attenuated increase in the fractional shortening in response to exercise, abnormal ventricular filling, valvular regurgitation, pericardial thickening with or without effusion, and pulmonary hypertension may be seen.[240] These findings are superimposed on those resulting from the underlying heart disease. Hematological and blood chemistry findings reflect the specific type of anemia present.

MANAGEMENT. Treatment of heart failure associated with severe anemia should be specific for the anemia (e.g., iron, folate, vitamin B_{12}). When heart failure is present, diuretics and cardiac glycosides are advisable, although some believe that the latter drugs are not helpful in this condition. ACE inhibitors or angiotensin receptor antagonists may improve the renal response to natriuretic peptides and facilitate diuresis[239] but may cause systemic hypotension from excessive vasodilation.

When both heart failure and anemia are severe, treatment must be carried out on an urgent basis and presents a difficult challenge. On the one hand, correction of the anemia is desirable to increase oxygen delivery to metabolizing tissues and thereby decrease the need for a sustained high cardiac output. On the other hand, rapid expansion of the blood volume may intensify the manifestations of heart failure.

The diagnostic steps for determining the etiology of the anemia should be taken immediately (e.g., blood drawn for serum iron, folate, and vitamin B_{12} and reticulocyte count, review of peripheral smear, and stool guaiac). The patient should be placed at bed rest and given supplementary oxygen. *Packed red blood cells* should then be transfused slowly (250 to 500 ml per 24 hours), preceded or accompanied, or both, by vigorous diuretic therapy (e.g., furosemide, 40 mg intravenously every 8 to 12 hours), and the patient should be observed closely for the development or exacerbation of dyspnea and pulmonary rales. If worsening heart failure occurs, the transfusion should be discontinued or slowed to avoid precipitating pulmonary edema. Vasodilator therapy is seldom helpful because impedance to left ventricular emptying is already markedly reduced in most cases.

Systemic Arteriovenous Fistulas

Systemic arteriovenous fistulas may be congenital or acquired; the latter are usually posttraumatic or iatrogenic. Increased cardiac output associated with such fistulas depends on the size of the communication and the magnitude of the resultant reduction in systemic vascular resistance.

The *physical findings* depend on the underlying disease and the location and size of the shunt. In general, a widened pulse pressure, brisk carotid and peripheral arterial pulsations, and mild tachycardia are present. The extremities are often warm and flushed. The *Branham sign* (also called the *Nicoladoni-Branham sign*), which consists of slowing of the heart rate after manual compression of the fistula,[241] is present in the majority of cases; this maneuver also raises arterial and lowers venous pressure. It appears to result from the operation of a cardioaccelerator reflex with both afferent and efferent pathways in the vagus nerves. The decrease in heart rate after fistula occlusion correlates with the flow in the fistula.

The skin overlying the fistula is warmer than normal, and a continuous "machinery" murmur and thrill are usually present over the lesion. Third and fourth heart sounds are commonly heard, as well as a precordial midsystolic murmur secondary to increased cardiac output. The ECG changes of left ventricular hypertrophy are often seen. Rarely, the fistula may become infected, leading to bacterial endarteritis, or cause major bleeding.

ACQUIRED ARTERIOVENOUS FISTULAS. These occur most frequently after such injuries as gunshot wounds and stab wounds and may involve any part of the body, most frequently the thigh.[242] Blood flow in the affected limb distal to the fistula diminishes after the creation of the fistula but then returns to normal and often increases with the passage of time. As a consequence, the affected limb is usually larger than its opposite member and the overlying skin is warmer. Cellulitis, venostasis, edema, and dermatitis with pigmentation frequently occur, in part as a consequence of chronically elevated venous pressure. Surgical repair or excision is generally advisable in fistulas that develop after gunshot wounds or trauma.[242]

Femoral arteriovenous fistulas following diagnostic or interventional cardiac catheterization are uncommon (0.11 to 0.16 percent of cases) but may result in high-output cardiac failure.[243,244] These may occur when a needle track crosses both the femoral artery and vein and is then dilated during the catheterization. Although the traditional approach to management of catheterization-related femoral artery injuries has been surgical repair,[245] newer techniques include ultrasound-guided compression and percutaneous stent placement or coil embolization.[243,246] Late stent thrombosis has been reported.

A rare form of acquired arteriovenous fistula results from spontaneous rupture of an aortic aneurysm into the inferior vena cava.[247] This event usually produces an enormous arteriovenous shunt, renal insufficiency, and rapidly progressive left ventricular failure. On physical examination, a pulsating mass can be readily palpated superficially in the abdomen and a continuous bruit is audible. Severe lower extremity and scrotal edema may be present. Survival depends on prompt diagnosis by ultrasonography or angiography and surgical closure with aortic reconstruction. Aortocaval fistulas may rarely occur after blunt or penetrating abdominal trauma.[248] Massive arteriovenous fistulas have been associated with Wilms tumors of the kidney and can cause high-output cardiac failure in children. Renal arteriovenous fistulas complicating pregnancy have also been reported.[249]

High-output heart failure resulting from the arteriovenous shunts surgically constructed for vascular access in patients undergoing long-term hemodialysis is uncommon.[250] Cardiac outputs as high as 10 liters/min, which decrease substantially during temporary occlusion of the shunt, are found. These values also reflect the chronic anemia present in many of these patients, but it is clear that it is the added hemodynamic burden[251] imposed by the shunt that precipitates heart failure in patients who had previously tolerated chronic anemia without apparent impairment of cardiac function. It is usually possible to revise or band the fistula to reduce it to the appropriate size for dialysis without compromising cardiac function. If this approach is ineffective, the shunt should be surgically closed and a new arteriovenous fistula created.

CONGENITAL ARTERIOVENOUS FISTULAS

Congenital arteriovenous fistulas result from arrest of the normal embryonic development of the vascular system and are structurally similar to embryonic capillary networks. When fistulas are large, patients generally complain of disfigurement as well as swelling and pain in the limb. On physical examination, erythema and cyanosis are often present, as are venous varices, a continuous murmur, and thrill. Examination also shows hemangiomatous changes associated with venous distention, deformity, and increased limb length. The fistulous connection may involve any vascular bed, including an internal mammary artery–pulmonary artery connection. *Left-sided heart failure* occurs particularly in patients with larger lesions that involve the pelvis as well as the extremities. Angiography is useful in confirming the diagnosis and in determining the physical extent of the anomaly.

Surgical excision is the ideal treatment,[252] but in many instances the lesions are not sufficiently localized to permit this. Embolization of absorbable gelatin (Gelfoam) pellets delivered through a catheter has been reported to obliterate multiple systemic arteriovenous fistulas and thereby diminish high-output heart failure.

HEREDITARY HEMORRHAGIC TELANGIECTASIA. Also known as *Osler-Weber-Rendu disease,* this autosomal dominant disorder is characterized by angiodysplastic lesions involving the skin, gastrointestinal tract, and brain. In addition, in 15 to 30 percent of cases, arteriovenous fistulas are present in the lungs[253] or liver.[254] Involvement of the liver, in particular, can produce a hyperdynamic circulation, with heart failure as well as hepatomegaly, liver bruits, manifestations of severe portal hypertension such as ascites and variceal bleeding, or biliary disease.

The congenital arteriovenous communications resulting from *infantile hepatic hemangioendothelioma* are commonly associated with marked increases in cardiac output, sometimes as high as 10 liters/min, and heart failure.[255] Other common presenting features include an abdominal mass, coagulopathy, and anemia. The hepatic lesions may be quite large, increase in size with time, and lead to heart failure, even in infancy. Treatment strategies include medical management with corticosteroids or interferon alfa or, in cases of failed medical therapy, use of percutaneous or surgical intervention, including hepatic artery ligation or embolization, surgical resection, or orthotopic liver transplantation.

Hyperthyroidism (see also Chap. 79)

In addition to enhancing sympathetic activation, increased circulating levels of thyroid hormone exert direct effects on the cardiovascular system including an increase in heart rate and cardiac contractility and a reduction in systemic vascular resistance. The principal findings on the physical examination of the cardiovascular system are resting tachycardia, systolic hypertension with a widened pulse pressure, brisk carotid and peripheral arterial pulsations, a hyperkinetic cardiac apex, and loud first heart sound. A midsystolic murmur along the left sternal border, secondary to increased flow, is common; occasionally, this murmur has an unusual scratchy component (the so-called Means-Lerman scratch), thought to be due to the rubbing together of normal pleural and pericardial surfaces by the hyperdynamic heart. Rarely, systolic murmurs of mitral and tricuspid regurgitation, secondary to papillary muscle dysfunction or ventricular dilation, may occur.

As in many other high-output states, the hyperkinetic state of hyperthyroidism does not usually lead to heart failure in the absence of underlying cardiovascular disease.[256] The normal heart appears capable of tolerating the burden imposed by hyperthyroidism simply by means of dilation and hypertrophy. However, heart failure may be precipitated when the elevated flow load of hyperthyroidism is superimposed on a reduced cardiovascular reserve (i.e., a patient with heart disease who is compensated).[257] Similarly, in patients with ischemic heart disease who are asymptomatic or who have only mild evidence of ischemia in the euthyroid state, the demand for increased coronary blood flow with hyperthyroidism frequently leads to an exacerbation of angina, often with the sensation of palpitations. The high-output cardiac failure of hyperthyroidism is frequently accompanied by and exacerbated by atrial fibrillation and a rapid ventricular rate.[258] Atrial fibrillation occurs in about 10 percent of hyperthyroid patients. In addition, respiratory muscle weakness may contribute to exertional dyspnea.

It is particularly important to recognize *apathetic hyperthyroidism,*[259] a condition in elderly people in which the usual clinical manifestations of thyrotoxicosis, such as palpitations, tachycardia, and moist skin, are not present. In such patients, the first clinical signs of hyperthyroidism may be unexplained heart failure, an exacerbation of angina, or new-onset atrial fibrillation,[260] usually but not always with a rapid ventricular rate.

BERIBERI HEART DISEASE

PATHOGENESIS AND CLINICAL CONSIDERATIONS. Thiamine pyrophosphate (TPP), the most abundant thiamine ester found in tissues, is essential for carbohydrate metabolism. Deficiency leads to impaired oxidative metabolism through inhibition of the citric acid cycle and the hexose monophosphate shunt and results in lactic acidosis.[261] Beriberi heart disease is due to severe thiamine deficiency persisting for at least 3 months.[262-264] Clinical beriberi is found most frequently in the Far East,[263,264] although even in that part of the world it is far less prevalent now than in the past. It occurs predominantly in individuals whose staple diet consists of polished rice, which is deficient in thiamine but high in carbohydrates, or foods containing thiaminases. The presence of thiamine in the enriched flour used in white bread has virtually eradicated this disease in the United States and Western Europe, where beriberi is found most commonly in diet faddists and alcoholics. Like polished rice, alcohol is low in vitamin B_1 but has a high carbohydrate content. In the West, alcoholics may become thiamine deficient not only because of low intake and impaired absorption and storage of the vitamin but also because they eat "junk" foods or drink large quantities of beer. The high carbohydrate content of these foods leads to a greater requirement for thiamine. Beriberi heart disease has also been reported in Western countries in elderly persons and in patients with malnutrition associated with advanced human immunodeficiency virus disease or those receiving total parenteral nutrition.[265]

Patients in Asia present with edema, ranging from peripheral edema to anasarca, as well as general malaise and fatigue. The elevation of cardiac output[263,266] is presumably secondary to the reduced systemic vascular resistance and augmented venous return (Fig. 22-20).

PHYSICAL FINDINGS. In most cases in Western countries, physical findings of the high-output state and usually of severe generalized malnutrition and vitamin deficiency are present. Evidence of peripheral polyneuropathy with sensory and motor deficits is common ("dry beriberi"), as is the presence of nutritional "cirrhosis" characterized by paresthesias of the extremities, absent or decreased knee and ankle jerks, painful glossitis, the anemia of combined iron and folate deficiency, and hyperkeratinized skin lesions.

Beriberi heart disease[262,263] is characterized by biventricular heart failure, sinus rhythm, and marked edema ("wet beriberi"). There is arteriolar vasodilation and the cutaneous vessels may be dilated, or in later cases with heart failure they may be constricted. A third heart sound and an apical systolic murmur are heard almost invariably, and there is a wide pulse pressure characteristic of the hyperkinetic state.

Heart failure may develop explosively in beriberi, and some patients succumb to the illness within 48 hours of the onset of symptoms. *Shoshin* (Japanese for "acute damage to the heart") *beriberi,* found most frequently in Asia and Africa, is a fulminant form of thiamine deficiency[267] characterized by hypotension, tachycardia, and lactic acidosis. If left untreated, patients with this disorder die within hours of cardiogenic shock and pulmonary edema. Thus, because the course of the disease may advance rapidly, treatment must be begun immediately once the diagnosis has been established. In the Western world, this fulminant form of the disease is uncommon.

LABORATORY FINDINGS. The electrocardiogram characteristically exhibits low voltage of the QRS complex, prolongation of the QT interval, and low voltage or inversion of T waves, most commonly in the right precordial leads. The chest radiograph usually shows cardiomegaly, pulmonary vascular congestion, and pleural effusions. In alcoholics with beriberi heart disease, the left ventricular ejection fraction and peak rate of rise of left ventricular pressure are usually reduced. The role played by alcoholic cardiomyopathy[36] (see Chap. 59) in this hemodynamic picture is not clear. The cardiac output falls, and the peripheral resistance rises acutely when thiamine is administered in the catheterization laboratory (see Fig. 22-20).[263]

Laboratory diagnosis of thiamine deficiency can be made by demonstration of increased serum pyruvate and lactate levels in the presence of a low red blood cell transketolase level.[262] Enhancement in transketolase activity resulting from added TPP is referred to as the TPP effect. A TPP effect greater than 15 percent suggests thiamine deficiency. The thiamine concentration may be determined in biological fluids to confirm the diagnosis. If specific laboratory tests are unavailable or impractical, an objective clinical and hemodynamic response to thiamine administration (see later) is considered diagnostic.

At *postmortem examination,* the heart usually shows chamber dilation without other changes. On microscopic examination, there is sometimes edema and fatty degeneration of the muscle fibers. Nonspecific histological and electron microscopic abnormalities have been found in cardiac biopsy specimens.

TREATMENT. Patients with beriberi heart disease fail to respond adequately to digitalis and diuretics alone. However, improvement after the administration of thiamine (up to 100 mg intravenously followed by 25 mg/d orally for 1 to 2 weeks) may be dramatic (see Fig. 22-20). Marked diuresis, decreases in heart rate and left ventricular size, and clearing of pulmonary congestion may occur within 12 to 48 hours. However, acute reversal of vasodilation induced by correction of the deficiency may cause the unprepared left ventricle to go into low-output failure. Therefore, patients should receive a glycoside and diuretic therapy along with thiamine. Thiamine replacement also results in improvement in the polyneuropathy caused by thiamine deficiency.

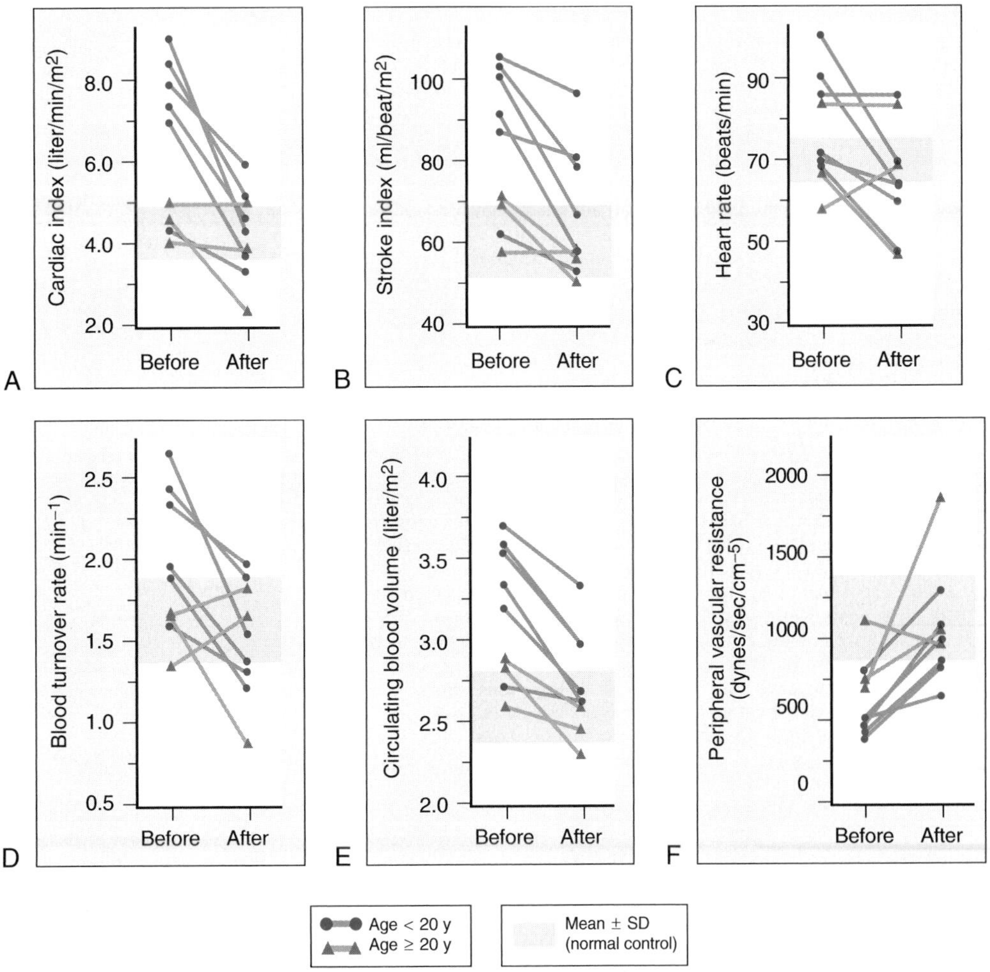

FIGURE 22-20 Hemodynamic changes in beriberi heart disease before and after treatment with intravenous thiamine in patients younger than or older than or equal to 20 years of age. Wet beriberi is characterized by increases in cardiac index **(A)**, stroke index **(B)**, heart rate **(C)**, blood turnover rate **(D)**, and circulating blood volume **(E)** and a decrease in peripheral vascular resistance **(F)**, particularly in younger patients. Thiamine replacement results in a rapid reversal of the high-output state. (From Kawai C, Nakamura Y: The heart in nutritional deficiencies. *In* Abelmann WH [ed]: Cardiomyopathies, Myocarditis, and Pericardial Disease. *In* Braunwald E [series ed]: Atlas of Heart Diseases. Vol 2. Philadelphia, Current Medicine, 1995, pp 7.1-7.18.)

In endemic areas, effective management of beriberi heart disease also involves disease prevention. Recommendations include (1) ingestion of germ-retaining polished rice, undermilled rice, or rice enriched with thiamine; (2) avoidance of excessive intake of carbonated beverages and strenuous exercise during hot summer months; (3) baking or boiling foods that contain thiaminase, such as clams or raw fish; and (4) avoidance of chronic diuretic therapy.

PAGET DISEASE

PATHOGENESIS. Paget disease of bone (osteitis deformans) is an asymmetrical skeletal disorder characterized by excessive resorption of bone followed by replacement of normal marrow with vascular, fibrous connective tissue and of resorbed bone with coarse, trabecular bone.[268] The cause of Paget disease is unknown, although genetic factors or viral infection, or both, may play an important role. Paget disease is most commonly asymptomatic and is diagnosed on a plain radiograph obtained for other reasons or because of a high serum alkaline phosphatase level noted on a routine chemistry screen.

CLINICAL FINDINGS. The two main clinical manifestations of Paget disease are pain and skeletal deformities most commonly affecting the pelvis, skull, spine, and long bones. Traumatic and pathological fractures, bone tumors including malignant osteosarcomas and benign giant cell tumors, and cranial neuropathies may also occur. There appears to be a linear relationship between the amount of skeletal involvement and the increase in cardiac output. Involvement of at least 15 percent of the skeleton by Paget disease in an active stage, accompanied by a high alkaline phosphatase level, is necessary before a clinically significant augmentation of cardiac output is observed.[269] Such a high-output state may be well tolerated for years with the patient remaining asymptomatic. However, if a specific cardiac disorder (e.g., valvular or ischemic heart disease) is present, the combination may cause rapid clinical deterioration.

The cardiovascular findings are not distinguishable from those in other conditions with high-output states. However, metastatic calcifications are characteristic and, if they involve the heart, may lead to sclerosis and calcification of the valve rings, with extension into the interventricular septum. The electrocardiogram may show atrioventricular conduction disturbance or bundle branch block. Echocardiograms often demonstrate aortic sclerosis or stenosis as well as left ventricular dilation, hypertrophy, and mild systolic dysfunction.[270] Successful treatment of the underlying bone disease with bisphosphonates or calcitonin,[271] as reflected by decreases in serum alkaline phosphatase levels or the urinary excretion of hydroxyproline, may normalize the cardiac output over several months.

OTHER CAUSES OF HIGH-OUTPUT CARDIAC FAILURE

FIBROUS DYSPLASIA. This condition, in which there is proliferation of fibrous tissue in bone, may also be associated with an elevated cardiac output, especially when multiple bones are involved.[272] Approximately one quarter of patients with polyostotic fibrous dysplasia have more than half the skeleton affected by disease, most commonly the limbs and craniofacial bones. Calcitonin may be an effective treatment in widespread disease. Bisphosphonates (e.g., pamidronate) have also been used to decrease bone pain and serum alkaline phosphatase levels.

MULTIPLE MYELOMA. Increased cardiac output and less commonly high-output heart failure have been described in this condition.[273,274] The mechanism is not clear, but it may be due to the associated anemia or hyperperfusion of the neoplastic tissue, or both, especially in patients with extensive bone disease.[275] Arteriovenous shunting has been demonstrated in involved bones, especially the femur, using intraarterial injection of radiolabeled albumin, and correlates with cardiac index.[273]

OTHER CONDITIONS. During normal pregnancy (see Chap. 74), cardiac output is elevated secondary to increases in blood volume, heart rate, and metabolic demands as well as the presence of the placenta acting as an arteriovenous shunt. If pregnancy is complicated by marked anemia, high-output heart failure may rarely develop, requiring bed rest and diuretic therapy in addition to transfusions. High-output heart failure also occurs in renal disease, especially glomerulonephritis (see Chap. 86), cor pulmonale (see Chap. 67), polycythemia vera (see Chap. 83), the carcinoid syndrome,[276] acromegaly[277] and marked obesity.[278] In patients with widespread psoriasis or exfoliative dermatitis, increased cardiac output related to marked cutaneous dilation may precipitate heart failure when underlying structural heart disease is present.

REFERENCES

Forms and Causes of Heart Failure

1. Hunt SA, Baker DW, Chin MH, et al: ACC/AHA guidelines for the evaluation and management of chronic heart failure in the adult: Executive summary. A Report of the American College of Cardiology/American Heart Association Task Force on Practice Guidelines (Committee to Revise the 1995 Guidelines for the Evaluation and Management of Heart Failure). Circulation 104:2996, 2001.
2. Ho KK, Pinsky JL, Kannel WB, Levy D: The epidemiology of heart failure: The Framingham Study. J Am Coll Cardiol 22:6A, 1993.
3. American Heart Association: Heart Disease and Stroke Statistics—2004 Update. Dallas, American Heart Association, 2003.
4. Massie BM, Shah NB: Evolving trends in the epidemiologic factors of heart failure: Rationale for preventive strategies and comprehensive disease management. Am Heart J 133:703, 1997.
5. Lloyd-Jones DM, Larson MG, Leip EP, et al: Lifetime risk for developing congestive heart failure: The Framingham Heart Study. Circulation 106:3068, 2002.
6. Rich MW, Nease RF: Cost-effectiveness analysis in clinical practice: The case of heart failure. Arch Intern Med 159:1690, 1999.
7. Minino AM, Arias E, Kochanek KD, et al: Deaths: Final Data for 2000. National Vital Statistics Reports. Vol 50, No 15. Hyattsville, Md, National Center for Health Statistics, 2002.
8. Centers for Medicare and Medicaid Services: 2002 Data Compendium. Baltimore, 2002.
9. O'Connell JB, Bristow MR: Economic impact of heart failure in the United States: Time for a different approach. J Heart Lung Transplant 13:S107, 1994.
10. Moraes DL, Colucci WS, Givertz MM: Secondary pulmonary hypertension in chronic heart failure: The role of the endothelium in pathophysiology and management. Circulation 102:1718, 2000.
11. Winaver J, Abassi Z, Green J, Skorecki KL: Control of extracellular fluid volume and the pathophysiology of edema formation. *In* Brenner BM, Rector FC (eds): Brenner and Rector's The Kidney. Philadelphia, WB Saunders, 2000, pp 795-865.
12. Schrier RW, Abraham WT: Hormones and hemodynamics in heart failure. N Engl J Med 341:577, 1999.
13. Nohria A, Lewis E, Stevenson LW: Medical management of advanced heart failure. JAMA 287:628, 2002.
14. Braunwald E: Report of the Task Force on Research in Heart Failure. Bethesda, Md, National Heart, Lung and Blood Institute, 1994.
15. Hogg K, Swedberg K, McMurray J: Heart failure with preserved left ventricular systolic function: Epidemiology, clinical characteristics, and prognosis. J Am Coll Cardiol 43:317, 2004.
16. Zile MR, Brutsaert DL: New concepts in diastolic dysfunction and diastolic heart failure: Part II: Causal mechanisms and treatment. Circulation 105:1503, 2002.
17. Zile MR, Brutsaert DL: New concepts in diastolic dysfunction and diastolic heart failure: Part I: Diagnosis, prognosis, and measurements of diastolic function. Circulation 105:1387, 2002.
18. Angeja BG, Grossman W: Evaluation and management of diastolic heart failure. Circulation 107:659, 2003.
19. Hundley WG, Kitzman DW, Morgan TM, et al: Cardiac cycle–dependent changes in aortic area and distensibility are reduced in older patients with isolated diastolic heart failure and correlate with exercise intolerance. J Am Coll Cardiol 38:796, 2001.
20. Kawaguchi M, Hay I, Fetics B, Kass DA: Combined ventricular systolic and arterial stiffening in patients with heart failure and preserved ejection fraction: Implications for systolic and diastolic reserve limitations. Circulation 107:714, 2003.
21. Vasan RS, Larson MG, Benjamin EJ, et al: Congestive heart failure in subjects with normal versus reduced left ventricular ejection fraction: Prevalence and mortality in a population- based cohort. J Am Coll Cardiol 33:1948, 1999.
22. Senni M, Redfield MM: Heart failure with preserved systolic function. A different natural history? J Am Coll Cardiol 38:1277, 2001.
23. Masoudi FA, Havranek EP, Smith G, et al: Gender, age, and heart failure with preserved left ventricular systolic function. J Am Coll Cardiol 41:217, 2003.
24. Vasan RS, Levy D: Defining diastolic heart failure: A call for standardized diagnostic criteria. Circulation 101:2118, 2000.
25. Chin MH, Goldman L: Factors contributing to the hospitalization of patients with congestive heart failure. Am J Public Health 87:643, 1997.
26. Tsuyuki RT, McKelvie RS, Arnold JM, et al: Acute precipitants of congestive heart failure exacerbations. Arch Intern Med 161:2337, 2001.
27. He J, Ogden LG, Bazzano LA, et al: Risk factors for congestive heart failure in US men and women: NHANES I epidemiologic follow-up study. Arch Intern Med 161:996, 2001.
28. Levy D, Larson MG, Vasan RS, et al: The progression from hypertension to congestive heart failure. JAMA 275:1557, 1996.
29. Shinbane JS, Wood MA, Jensen DN, et al: Tachycardia-induced cardiomyopathy: A review of animal models and clinical studies. J Am Coll Cardiol 29:709, 1997.
30. Bentancur AG, Rieck J, Koldanov R, Dankner RS: Acute pulmonary edema in the emergency department: Clinical and echocardiographic survey in an aged population. Am J Med Sci 323:238, 2002.
31. Givertz MM, Colucci WS: New targets for heart-failure therapy: Endothelin, inflammatory cytokines, and oxidative stress. Lancet 352(Suppl 1):S134, 1998.
32. Koniaris LS, Goldhaber SZ: Anticoagulation in dilated cardiomyopathy. J Am Coll Cardiol 31:745, 1998.
33. Dries DL, Exner DV, Domanski MJ, et al: The prognostic implications of renal insufficiency in asymptomatic and symptomatic patients with left ventricular systolic dysfunction. J Am Coll Cardiol 35:681, 2000.
34. Page J, Henry D: Consumption of NSAIDs and the development of congestive heart failure in elderly patients: An underrecognized public health problem. Arch Intern Med 160:777, 2000.

35. Brater DC: Anti-inflammatory agents and renal function. Semin Arthritis Rheum 32:33, 2002.
36. Piano MR: Alcohol and heart failure. J Card Fail 8:239, 2002.
37. Felker GM, Gattis WA, Leimberger JD, et al: Usefulness of anemia as a predictor of death and rehospitalization in patients with decompensated heart failure. Am J Cardiol 92:625, 2003.

Clinical Manifestations

38. Wilson JR, Rayos G, Yeoh TK, et al: Dissociation between exertional symptoms and circulatory function in patients with heart failure. Circulation 92:47, 1995.
39. Duguet A, Tantucci C, Lozinguez O, et al: Expiratory flow limitation as a determinant of orthopnea in acute left heart failure. J Am Coll Cardiol 35:690, 2000.
40. Leung RS, Bowman ME, Parker JD, et al: Avoidance of the left lateral decubitus position during sleep in patients with heart failure: Relationship to cardiac size and function. J Am Coll Cardiol 41:227, 2003.
41. Quaranta AJ, D'Alonzo GE, Krachman SL: Cheyne-Stokes respiration during sleep in congestive heart failure. Chest 111:467, 1997.
42. Mancini DM: Pulmonary factors limiting exercise capacity in patients with heart failure. Prog Cardiovasc Dis 37:347, 1995.
43. Nanas S, Nanas J, Kassiotis C, et al: Respiratory muscles performance is related to oxygen kinetics during maximal exercise and early recovery in patients with congestive heart failure. Circulation 100:503, 1999.
44. Morrison LK, Harrison A, Krishnaswamy P, et al: Utility of a rapid B-natriuretic peptide assay in differentiating congestive heart failure from lung disease in patients presenting with dyspnea. J Am Coll Cardiol 39:202, 2002.
45. Rietveld S, van Beest I, Everaerd W: Stress-induced breathlessness in asthma. Psychol Med 29:1359, 1999.
46. Johnson BD, Beck KC, Olson LJ, et al: Pulmonary function in patients with reduced left ventricular function: Influence of smoking and cardiac surgery. Chest 120:1869, 2001.
47. Weisman IM, Zeballos RJ: Clinical evaluation of unexplained dyspnea. Cardiologia 41:621, 1996.
48. Coats AJ: Origin of symptoms in patients with cachexia with special reference to weakness and shortness of breath. Int J Cardiol 85:133, 2002.
49. Rosenberg P, Yancy CW: Noninvasive assessment of hemodynamics: An emphasis on bioimpedance cardiography. Curr Opin Cardiol 15:151, 2000.
50. Maisel AS, Krishnaswamy P, Nowak RM, et al: Rapid measurement of B-type natriuretic peptide in the emergency diagnosis of heart failure. N Engl J Med 347:161, 2002.
51. Pina IL, Apstein CS, Balady GJ, et al: Exercise and heart failure: A statement from the American Heart Association Committee on exercise, rehabilitation, and prevention. Circulation 107:1210, 2003.
52. Chomsky DB, Lang CC, Rayos GH, et al: Hemodynamic exercise testing. A valuable tool in the selection of cardiac transplantation candidates. Circulation 94:3176, 1996.
53. Lapu-Bula R, Robert A, Van Craeynest D, et al: Contribution of exercise-induced mitral regurgitation to exercise stroke volume and exercise capacity in patients with left ventricular systolic dysfunction. Circulation 106:1342, 2002.
54. Butler J, Chomsky DB, Wilson JR: Pulmonary hypertension and exercise intolerance in patients with heart failure. J Am Coll Cardiol 34:1802, 1999.
55. Mancini DM, Katz SD, Lang CC, et al: Effect of erythropoietin on exercise capacity in patients with moderate to severe chronic heart failure. Circulation 107:294, 2003.
56. Shoemaker JK, Naylor HL, Hogeman CS, Sinoway LI: Blood flow dynamics in heart failure. Circulation 99:3002, 1999.
57. Mancini DM, Wilson JR, Bolinger L, et al: In vivo magnetic resonance spectroscopy measurement of deoxymyoglobin during exercise in patients with heart failure. Demonstration of abnormal muscle metabolism despite adequate oxygenation. Circulation 90:500, 1994.
58. Cicoira M, Zanolla L, Franceschini L, et al: Skeletal muscle mass independently predicts peak oxygen consumption and ventilatory response during exercise in noncachectic patients with chronic heart failure. J Am Coll Cardiol 37:2080, 2001.
59. Johnson W, Lucas C, Stevenson LW, Creager MA: Effect of intensive therapy for heart failure on the vasodilator response to exercise. J Am Coll Cardiol 33:743, 1999.
60. Gottlieb SS, Fisher ML, Freudenberger R, et al: Effects of exercise training on peak performance and quality of life in congestive heart failure patients. J Card Fail 5:188, 1999.
61. Belardinelli R, Georgiou D, Cianci G, Purcaro A: Randomized, controlled trial of long-term moderate exercise training in chronic heart failure: Effects on functional capacity, quality of life, and clinical outcome. Circulation 99:1173, 1999.
62. Keteyian SJ, Brawner CA, Schairer JR, et al: Effects of exercise training on chronotropic incompetence in patients with heart failure. Am Heart J 138:233, 1999.
63. Linke A, Schoene N, Gielen S, et al: Endothelial dysfunction in patients with chronic heart failure: Systemic effects of lower-limb exercise training. J Am Coll Cardiol 37:392, 2001.
64. Braith RW, Welsch MA, Feigenbaum MS, et al: Neuroendocrine activation in heart failure is modified by endurance exercise training. J Am Coll Cardiol 34:1170, 1999.
65. Adamopoulos S, Parissis J, Karatzas D, et al: Physical training modulates proinflammatory cytokines and the soluble Fas/soluble Fas ligand system in patients with chronic heart failure. J Am Coll Cardiol 39:653, 2002.
66. Ennezat PV, Malendowicz SL, Testa M, et al: Physical training in patients with chronic heart failure enhances the expression of genes encoding antioxidative enzymes. J Am Coll Cardiol 38:194, 2001.
67. Pu CT, Johnson MT, Forman DE, et al: Randomized trial of progressive resistance training to counteract the myopathy of chronic heart failure. J Appl Physiol 90:2341, 2001.
68. Whellan DJ, O'Connor CM: The state of exercise training: A need for action. Am Heart J 144:1, 2002.
69. Wasserman K, Hansen JE, Sue D, et al: Principles of Exercise Testing and Interpretation. 3rd ed. Philadelphia, Lippincott Williams & Wilkins, 1999.
70. Pardaens K, Van Cleemput J, Vanhaecke J, Fagard RH: Peak oxygen uptake better predicts outcome than submaximal respiratory data in heart transplant candidates. Circulation 101:1152, 2000.
71. Stelken AM, Younis LT, Jennison SH, et al: Prognostic value of cardiopulmonary exercise testing using percent achieved of predicted peak oxygen uptake for patients with ischemic and dilated cardiomyopathy. J Am Coll Cardiol 27:345, 1996.
72. Arzt M, Harth M, Luchner A, et al: Enhanced ventilatory response to exercise in patients with chronic heart failure and central sleep apnea. Circulation 107:1998, 2003.
73. Larsen AI, Aarsland T, Kristiansen M, et al: Assessing the effect of exercise training in men with heart failure; comparison of maximal, submaximal and endurance exercise protocols. Eur Heart J 22:684, 2001.
74. Faggiano P, D'Aloia A, Gualeni A, Giordano A: Hemodynamic profile of submaximal constant workload exercise in patients with heart failure secondary to ischemic or idiopathic dilated cardiomyopathy. Am J Cardiol 81:437, 1998.
75. Cahalin LP, Mathier MA, Semigran MJ, et al: The six-minute walk test predicts peak oxygen uptake and survival in patients with advanced heart failure. Chest 110:325, 1996.
76. Bittner V, Weiner DH, Yusuf S, et al: Prediction of mortality and morbidity with a 6-minute walk test in patients with left ventricular dysfunction. SOLVD Investigators. JAMA 270:1702, 1993.
77. Anker SD, Rauchhaus M: Insights into the pathogenesis of chronic heart failure: Immune activation and cachexia. Curr Opin Cardiol 14:211, 1999.
78. Zuccala G, Cattel C, Manes-Gravina E, et al: Left ventricular dysfunction: A clue to cognitive impairment in older patients with heart failure. J Neurol Neurosurg Psychiatry 63:509, 1997.
79. The Criteria Committee of the New York Heart Association: Nomenclature and Criteria for Diagnosis of Diseases of the Heart and Great Vessels. 9th ed. Boston, Little, Brown, 1994.
80. Bettencourt P, Ferreira A, Dias P, et al: Predictors of prognosis in patients with stable mild to moderate heart failure. J Card Fail 6:306, 2000.
81. Australia/New Zealand Heart Failure Research Collaborative Group: Randomised, placebo-controlled trial of carvedilol in patients with congestive heart failure due to ischaemic heart disease. Lancet 349:375, 1997.
82. Bennet SJ, Oldridge NB, Eckert GJ, et al: Discriminant properties of commonly used quality of life measures in heart failure. Qual Life Res 11:349, 2002.
83. al Kaade S, Hauptman PJ: Health-related quality of life measurement in heart failure: Challenges for the new millennium. J Card Fail 7:194, 2001.
84. Green CP, Porter CB, Bresnahan DR, Spertus JA: Development and evaluation of the Kansas City Cardiomyopathy Questionnaire: A new health status measure for heart failure. J Am Coll Cardiol 35:1245, 2000.
85. Konstam V, Salem D, Pouleur H, et al: Baseline quality of life as a predictor of mortality and hospitalization in 5,025 patients with congestive heart failure. SOLVD Investigations. Studies of Left Ventricular Dysfunction Investigators. Am J Cardiol 78:890, 1996.
86. Abraham WT, Fisher WG, Smith AL, et al: Cardiac resynchronization in chronic heart failure. N Engl J Med 346:1845, 2002.
87. Kasper EK, Gerstenblith G, Hefter G, et al: A randomized trial of the efficacy of multidisciplinary care in heart failure outpatients at high risk of hospital readmission. J Am Coll Cardiol 39:471, 2002.
88. Shah MR, Hasselblad V, Stinnett SS, et al: Hemodynamic profiles of advanced heart failure: Association with clinical characteristics and long-term outcomes. J Card Fail 7:105, 2001.
89. Kataoka H: Pericardial and pleural effusions in decompensated chronic heart failure. Am Heart J 139:918, 2000.
90. Perloff JK: The jugular venous pulse and third heart sound in patients with heart failure. N Engl J Med 345:612, 2001.
91. Drazner MH, Rame JE, Stevenson LW, Dries DL: Prognostic importance of elevated jugular venous pressure and a third heart sound in patients with heart failure. N Engl J Med 345:574, 2001.
92. Wiese J: The abdominojugular reflux sign. Am J Med 109:59, 2000.
93. O'Reilly RA: Splenomegaly in 2,505 patients at a large university medical center from 1913 to 1995. 1963 to 1995: 449 patients. West J Med 169:88, 1998.
94. Madias JE, Bazaz R, Agarwal H, et al: Anasarca-mediated attenuation of the amplitude of electrocardiogram complexes: A description of a heretofore unrecognized phenomenon. J Am Coll Cardiol 38:756, 2001.
95. Light RW: Clinical practice. Pleural effusion. N Engl J Med 346:1971, 2002.
96. Johnson JL: Pleural effusions in cardiovascular disease. Pearls for correlating the evidence with the cause. Postgrad Med 107:95, 2000.
97. Van der Merwe S, Dens J, Daenen W, et al: Pericardial disease is often not recognised as a cause of chronic severe ascites. J Hepatol 32:164, 2000.
98. Chan FK, Sung JJ, Ma KM, et al: Protein-losing enteropathy in congestive heart failure: Diagnosis by means of a simple method. Hepatogastroenterology 46:1816, 1999.
99. Kodama M, Kato K, Hirono S, et al: Mechanical alternans in patients with chronic heart failure. J Card Fail 7:138, 2001.
100. Capomolla S, Pozzoli M, Opasich C, et al: Dobutamine and nitroprusside infusion in patients with severe congestive heart failure: Hemodynamic improvement by discordant effects on mitral regurgitation, left atrial function, and ventricular function. Am Heart J 134:1089, 1997.
101. Linde C, Leclercq C, Rex S, et al: Long-term benefits of biventricular pacing in congestive heart failure: Results from the MUltisite STimulation in cardiomyopathy (MUSTIC) study. J Am Coll Cardiol 40:111, 2002.
102. Sanders GP, Mendes LA, Colucci WS, Givertz MM: Noninvasive methods for detecting elevated left-sided cardiac filling pressure. J Card Fail 6:157, 2000.
103. Givertz MM, Slawsky MT, Moraes DL, et al: Noninvasive determination of pulmonary artery wedge pressure in patients with chronic heart failure. Am J Cardiol 87:1213, 2001.
104. King D, Smith ML, Chapman TJ, et al: Fat malabsorption in elderly patients with cardiac cachexia. Age Ageing 25:144, 1996.
105. Peracchi M, Trovato C, Longhi M, et al: Tissue transglutaminase antibodies in patients with end-stage heart failure. Am J Gastroenterol 97:2850, 2002.

106. Torre-Amione G, Kapadia S, Benedict C, et al: Proinflammatory cytokine levels in patients with depressed left ventricular ejection fraction: A report from the studies of left ventricular dysfunction (SOLVD). J Am Coll Cardiol 27:1201, 1996.
107. Feldman AM, Combes A, Wagner D, et al: The role of tumor necrosis factor in the pathophysiology of heart failure. J Am Coll Cardiol 35:537, 2000.
108. Mann DL, Spinale FG: Activation of matrix metalloproteinases in the failing human heart: Breaking the tie that binds. Circulation 98:1699, 1998.
109. Anker SD, Chua TP, Ponikowski P, et al: Hormonal changes and catabolic/anabolic imbalance in chronic heart failure and their importance for cardiac cachexia. Circulation 96:526, 1997.
110. Anker SD, Negassa A, Coats AJ, et al: Prognostic importance of weight loss in chronic heart failure and the effect of treatment with angiotensin-converting enzyme inhibitors: An observational study. Lancet 361:1077, 2003.
111. Ponikowski P, Anker SD, Chua TP, et al: Oscillatory breathing patterns during wakefulness in patients with chronic heart failure: Clinical implications and role of augmented peripheral chemosensitivity. Circulation 100:2418, 1999.
112. Mansfield D, Kaye DM, Brunner La Rocca H, et al: Raised sympathetic nerve activity in heart failure and central sleep apnea is due to heart failure severity. Circulation 107:1396, 2003.
113. Giallourakis CC, Rosenberg PM, Friedman LS: The liver in heart failure. Clin Liver Dis 6:947, 2002.
114. Palm C, Reimann D, Gross P: The role of V2 vasopressin antagonists in hyponatremia. Cardiovasc Res 51:403, 2001.
115. Laragh JH, Sealey JE: K(+) depletion and the progression of hypertensive disease or heart failure. The pathogenic role of diuretic-induced aldosterone secretion. Hypertension 37:806, 2001.
116. Obialo CI, Ofili EO, Mirza T: Hyperkalemia in congestive heart failure patients aged 63 to 85 years with subclinical renal disease. Am J Cardiol 90:663, 2002.
117. Schepkens H, Vanholder R, Billiouw JM, Lameire N: Life-threatening hyperkalemia during combined therapy with angiotensin-converting enzyme inhibitors and spironolactone: An analysis of 25 cases. Am J Med 110:438, 2001.
118. Bozkurt B, Agoston I, Knowlton AA: Complications of inappropriate use of spironolactone in heart failure: When an old medicine spirals out of new guidelines. J Am Coll Cardiol 41:211, 2003.
119. Milionis HJ, Alexandrides GE, Liberopoulos EN, et al: Hypomagnesemia and concurrent acid-base and electrolyte abnormalities in patients with congestive heart failure. Eur J Heart Fail 4:167, 2002.
120. Doehner W, Schoene N, Rauchhaus M, et al: Effects of xanthine oxidase inhibition with allopurinol on endothelial function and peripheral blood flow in hyperuricemic patients with chronic heart failure: Results from 2 placebo-controlled studies. Circulation 105:2619, 2002.
121. Ruilope LM, van Veldhuisen DJ, Ritz E, Luscher TF: Renal function: The Cinderella of cardiovascular risk profile. J Am Coll Cardiol 38:1782, 2001.
122. Batin P, Wickens M, McEntegart D, et al: The importance of abnormalities of liver function tests in predicting mortality in chronic heart failure. Eur Heart J 16:1613, 1995.
123. Naschitz JE, Slobodin G, Lewis RJ, et al: Heart diseases affecting the liver and liver diseases affecting the heart. Am Heart J 140:111, 2000.
124. Wiesen S, Reddy KR, Jeffers LJ, Schiff ER: Fulminant hepatic failure secondary to previously unrecognized cardiomyopathy. Dig Dis 13:199, 1995.
125. Horwich TB, Fonarow GC, Hamilton MA, et al: Anemia is associated with worse symptoms, greater impairment in functional capacity and a significant increase in mortality in patients with advanced heart failure. J Am Coll Cardiol 39:1780, 2002.
126. Ezekowitz JA, McAlister FA, Armstrong PW: Anemia is common in heart failure and is associated with poor outcomes: Insights from a cohort of 12 065 patients with new-onset heart failure. Circulation 107:223, 2003.
127. Levin A, Thompson CR, Ethier J, et al: Left ventricular mass index increase in early renal disease: Impact of decline in hemoglobin. Am J Kidney Dis 34:125, 1999.
128. SoRelle R: Erythropoietin—Not at the Olympics but maybe for anemic heart failure patients. Circulation 107:e9004, 2003.
129. Sharma R, Rauchhaus M, Ponikowski PP, et al: The relationship of the erythrocyte sedimentation rate to inflammatory cytokines and survival in patients with chronic heart failure treated with angiotensin-converting enzyme inhibitors. J Am Coll Cardiol 36:523, 2000.
130. Davidson C: Can heart failure be diagnosed in primary care? Chest radiography is still useful. BMJ 321:1414, 2000.
131. Kataoka H, Takada S: The role of thoracic ultrasonography for evaluation of patients with decompensated chronic heart failure. J Am Coll Cardiol 35:1638, 2000.

Prognosis

132. Levy D, Kenchaiah S, Larson MG, et al: Long-term trends in the incidence of and survival with heart failure. N Engl J Med 347:1397, 2002.
133. Rose EA, Gelijns AC, Moskowitz AJ, et al: Long-term mechanical left ventricular assistance for end-stage heart failure. N Engl J Med 345:1435, 2001.
134. Ho KK, Anderson KM, Kannel WB, et al: Survival after the onset of congestive heart failure in Framingham Heart Study subjects. Circulation 88:107, 1993.
135. Rector TS, Cohn JN: Prognosis in congestive heart failure. Annu Rev Med 45:341, 1994.
136. Deedwania PC: The key to unraveling the mystery of mortality in heart failure: An integrated approach. Circulation 107:1719, 2003.
137. Simon T, Mary-Krause M, Funck-Brentano C, Jaillon P: Sex differences in the prognosis of congestive heart failure: Results from the Cardiac Insufficiency Bisoprolol Study (CIBIS II). Circulation 103:375, 2001.
138. Bart BA, Shaw LK, McCants CB Jr, et al: Clinical determinants of mortality in patients with angiographically diagnosed ischemic or nonischemic cardiomyopathy. J Am Coll Cardiol 30:1002, 1997.
139. Metra M, Faggiano P, D'Aloia A, et al: Use of cardiopulmonary exercise testing with hemodynamic monitoring in the prognostic assessment of ambulatory patients with chronic heart failure. J Am Coll Cardiol 33:943, 1999.
140. Ponikowski P, Francis DP, Piepoli MF, et al: Enhanced ventilatory response to exercise in patients with chronic heart failure and preserved exercise tolerance: Marker of abnormal cardiorespiratory reflex control and predictor of poor prognosis. Circulation 103:967, 2001.
141. Gitt AK, Wasserman K, Kilkowski C, et al: Exercise anaerobic threshold and ventilatory efficiency identify heart failure patients for high risk of early death. Circulation 106:3079, 2002.
142. Meyer FJ, Borst MM, Zugck C, et al: Respiratory muscle dysfunction in congestive heart failure: Clinical correlation and prognostic significance. Circulation 103:2153, 2001.
143. Ponikowski P, Chua TP, Anker SD, et al: Peripheral chemoreceptor hypersensitivity: An ominous sign in patients with chronic heart failure. Circulation 104:544, 2001.
144. Dries DL, Sweitzer NK, Drazner MH, et al: Prognostic impact of diabetes mellitus in patients with heart failure according to the etiology of left ventricular systolic dysfunction. J Am Coll Cardiol 38:421, 2001.
145. Sin DD, Logan AG, Fitzgerald FS, et al: Effects of continuous positive airway pressure on cardiovascular outcomes in heart failure patients with and without Cheyne-Stokes respiration. Circulation 102:61, 2000.
146. Bradley TD, Floras JS: Sleep apnea and heart failure: Part I: Obstructive sleep apnea. Circulation 107:1671, 2003.
147. Bradley TD, Floras JS: Sleep apnea and heart failure: Part II: Central sleep apnea. Circulation 107:1822, 2003.
148. Vaccarino V, Kasl SV, Abramson J, Krumholz HM: Depressive symptoms and risk of functional decline and death in patients with heart failure. J Am Coll Cardiol 38:199, 2001.
149. Horwich TB, Fonarow GC, Hamilton MA, et al: The relationship between obesity and mortality in patients with heart failure. J Am Coll Cardiol 38:789, 2001.
150. Naqvi TZ, Goel RK, Forrester JS, et al: Usefulness of left ventricular mass in predicting recovery of left ventricular systolic function in patients with symptomatic idiopathic dilated cardiomyopathy. Am J Cardiol 85:624, 2000.
151. Koelling TM, Aaronson KD, Cody RJ, et al: Prognostic significance of mitral regurgitation and tricuspid regurgitation in patients with left ventricular systolic dysfunction. Am Heart J 144:524, 2002.
152. Dini FL, Cortigiani L, Baldini U, et al: Prognostic value of left atrial enlargement in patients with idiopathic dilated cardiomyopathy and ischemic cardiomyopathy. Am J Cardiol 89:518, 2002.
153. Cohn JN, Johnson GR, Shabetai R, et al: Ejection fraction, peak exercise oxygen consumption, cardiothoracic ratio, ventricular arrhythmias, and plasma norepinephrine as determinants of prognosis in heart failure. The V-HeFT VA Cooperative Studies Group. Circulation 87:VI-5, 1993.
154. Neglia D, Michelassi C, Trivieri MG, et al: Prognostic role of myocardial blood flow impairment in idiopathic left ventricular dysfunction. Circulation 105:186, 2002.
155. Zornoff LA, Skali H, Pfeffer MA, et al: Right ventricular dysfunction and risk of heart failure and mortality after myocardial infarction. J Am Coll Cardiol 39:1450, 2002.
156. Rickenbacher PR, Trindade PT, Haywood GA, et al: Transplant candidates with severe left ventricular dysfunction managed with medical treatment: Characteristics and survival. J Am Coll Cardiol 27:1192, 1996.
157. Myers J, Gullestad L, Vagelos R, et al: Clinical, hemodynamic, and cardiopulmonary exercise test determinants of survival in patients referred for evaluation of heart failure. Ann Intern Med 129:286, 1998.
158. Hansen A, Haass M, Zugck C, et al: Prognostic value of Doppler echocardiographic mitral inflow patterns: Implications for risk stratification in patients with chronic congestive heart failure. J Am Coll Cardiol 37:1049, 2001.
159. Francis GS, Cohn JN, Johnson G, et al: Plasma norepinephrine, plasma renin activity, and congestive heart failure. Relations to survival and the effects of therapy in V-HeFT II. The V-HeFT VA Cooperative Studies Group. Circulation 87:VI-40, 1993.
160. Anand IS, Fisher LD, Chiang YT, et al: Changes in brain natriuretic peptide and norepinephrine over time and mortality and morbidity in the Valsartan Heart Failure Trial (Val-HeFT). Circulation 107:1278, 2003.
161. Goldsmith SR: Vasopressin: A therapeutic target in congestive heart failure? J Card Fail 5:347, 1999.
162. Jessup M: Aldosterone blockade and heart failure. N Engl J Med 348:1380, 2003.
163. Stanek B, Frey B, Hulsmann M, et al: Prognostic evaluation of neurohumoral plasma levels before and during beta-blocker therapy in advanced left ventricular dysfunction. J Am Coll Cardiol 38:436, 2001.
164. Berger R, Stanek B, Frey B, et al: B-type natriuretic peptides (BNP and PRO-BNP) predict longterm survival in patients with advanced heart failure treated with atenolol. J Heart Lung Transplant 20:251, 2001.
165. Maeda K, Tsutamoto T, Wada A, et al: High levels of plasma brain natriuretic peptide and interleukin-6 after optimized treatment for heart failure are independent risk factors for morbidity and mortality in patients with congestive heart failure. J Am Coll Cardiol 36:1587, 2000.
166. Hulsmann M, Stanek B, Frey B, et al: Value of cardiopulmonary exercise testing and big endothelin plasma levels to predict short-term prognosis of patients with chronic heart failure. J Am Coll Cardiol 32:1695, 1998.
167. Cohn JN, Ferrari R, Sharpe N: Cardiac remodeling—Concepts and clinical implications: A consensus paper from an international forum on cardiac remodeling. Behalf of an International Forum on Cardiac Remodeling. J Am Coll Cardiol 35:569, 2000.
168. Saxon LA, Stevenson WG, Middlekauff HR, et al: Predicting death from progressive heart failure secondary to ischemic or idiopathic dilated cardiomyopathy. Am J Cardiol 72:62, 1993.
169. Berger R, Huelsman M, Strecker K, et al: B-type natriuretic peptide predicts sudden death in patients with chronic heart failure. Circulation 105:2392, 2002.
170. Bozkurt B, Mann DL: Use of biomarkers in the management of heart failure: Are we there yet? Circulation 107:1231, 2003.
171. Deswal A, Petersen NJ, Feldman AM, et al: Cytokines and cytokine receptors in advanced heart failure: An analysis of the cytokine database from the vesnarinone trial (VEST). Circulation 103:2055, 2001.

172. Rauchhaus M, Doehner W, Francis DP, et al: Plasma cytokine parameters and mortality in patients with chronic heart failure. Circulation 102:3060, 2000.
173. Tsutamoto T, Hisanaga T, Wada A, et al: Interleukin-6 spillover in the peripheral circulation increases with the severity of heart failure, and the high plasma level of interleukin-6 is an important prognostic predictor in patients with congestive heart failure. J Am Coll Cardiol 31:391, 1998.
174. Tsutsui T, Tsutamoto T, Wada A, et al: Plasma oxidized low-density lipoprotein as a prognostic predictor in patients with chronic congestive heart failure. J Am Coll Cardiol 39:957, 2002.
175. Hare JM, Johnson RJ: Uric acid predicts clinical outcomes in heart failure: Insights regarding the role of xanthine oxidase and uric acid in disease pathophysiology. Circulation 107:1951, 2003.
176. Sato Y, Yamada T, Taniguchi R, et al: Persistently increased serum concentrations of cardiac troponin t in patients with idiopathic dilated cardiomyopathy are predictive of adverse outcomes. Circulation 103:369, 2001.
177. La Rovere MT, Pinna GD, Maestri R, et al: Short-term heart rate variability strongly predicts sudden cardiac death in chronic heart failure patients. Circulation 107:565, 2003.
178. Singh SN, Fisher SG, Carson PE, Fletcher RD: Prevalence and significance of nonsustained ventricular tachycardia in patients with premature ventricular contractions and heart failure treated with vasodilator therapy. Department of Veterans Affairs CHF STAT Investigators. J Am Coll Cardiol 32:942, 1998.
179. Iuliano S, Fisher SG, Karasik PE, et al: QRS duration and mortality in patients with congestive heart failure. Am Heart J 143:1085, 2002.
180. Dries DL, Exner DV, Gersh BJ, et al: Atrial fibrillation is associated with an increased risk for mortality and heart failure progression in patients with asymptomatic and symptomatic left ventricular systolic dysfunction: A retrospective analysis of the SOLVD trials. Studies of Left Ventricular Dysfunction. J Am Coll Cardiol 32:695, 1998.
181. Moss AJ, Zareba W, Hall WJ, et al: Prophylactic implantation of a defibrillator in patients with myocardial infarction and reduced ejection fraction. N Engl J Med 346:877, 2002.
182. Bristow MR, Feldman AM, Saxon LA: Heart failure management using implantable devices for ventricular resynchronization: Comparison of Medical Therapy, Pacing, and Defibrillation in Chronic Heart Failure (COMPANION) trial. COMPANION Steering Committee and COMPANION Clinical Investigators. J Card Fail 6:276, 2000.
183. Vrtovec B, Delgado R, Zewail A, et al: Prolonged QTc interval and high B-type natriuretic peptide levels together predict mortality in patients with advanced heart failure. Circulation 107:1764, 2003.
184. Pinsky DJ, Sciacca RR, Steinberg JS: QT dispersion as a marker of risk in patients awaiting heart transplantation. J Am Coll Cardiol 29:1576, 1997.
185. Klingenheben T, Zabel M, D'Agostino RB, et al: Predictive value of T-wave alternans for arrhythmic events in patients with congestive heart failure. Lancet 356:651, 2000.

Pulmonary Edema

186. Flick MR, Matthay MA: Pulmonary edema and acute lung injury. *In* Murray JF, Nadel JA (eds): Textbook of Respiratory Medicine. Philadelphia, WB Saunders, 2000, pp 1575-1629.
187. Guyton AC, Hall JE: Pulmonary circulation; pulmonary edema; pleural fluid. Textbook of Medical Physiology. Philadelphia, WB Saunders, 2000, pp 444-451.
188. West JB, Mathieu-Costello O: Structure, strength, failure, and remodeling of the pulmonary blood-gas barrier. Annu Rev Physiol 61:543, 1999.
189. Sherman SC: Reexpansion pulmonary edema: A case report and review of the current literature. J Emerg Med 24:23, 2003.
190. Woodring JH: Focal reexpansion pulmonary edema after drainage of large pleural effusions: Clinical evidence suggesting hypoxic injury to the lung as the cause of edema. South Med J 90:1176, 1997.
191. Nakamura M, Fujishima S, Sawafuji M, et al: Importance of interleukin-8 in the development of reexpansion lung injury in rabbits. Am J Respir Crit Care Med 161:1030, 2000.
192. Tan HC, Mak KH, Johan A, et al: Cardiac output increases prior to development of pulmonary edema after re-expansion of spontaneous pneumothorax. Respir Med 96:461, 2002.
193. Ware LB, Matthay MA: The acute respiratory distress syndrome. N Engl J Med 342:1334, 2000.
194. Herridge MS, Cheung AM, Tansey CM, et al: One-year outcomes in survivors of the acute respiratory distress syndrome. N Engl J Med 348:683, 2003.
195. Pugin J, Verghese G, Widmer MC, Matthay MA: The alveolar space is the site of intense inflammatory and profibrotic reactions in the early phase of acute respiratory distress syndrome. Crit Care Med 27:304, 1999.
196. Edoute Y, Roguin A, Behar D, Reisner SA: Prospective evaluation of pulmonary edema. Crit Care Med 28:330, 2000.
197. Gandhi SK, Powers JC, Nomeir AM, et al: The pathogenesis of acute pulmonary edema associated with hypertension. N Engl J Med 344:17, 2001.
198. Phillips RA, Greenblatt J, Krakoff LR: Hypertensive emergencies: Diagnosis and management. Prog Cardiovasc Dis 45:33, 2002.
199. McFadden ER Jr, Warren EL: Observations on asthma mortality. Ann Intern Med 127:142, 1997.
200. Logeart D, Saudubray C, Beyne P, et al: Comparative value of Doppler echocardiography and B-type natriuretic peptide assay in the etiologic diagnosis of acute dyspnea. J Am Coll Cardiol 40:1794, 2002.
201. Littmann L: Large T wave inversion and QT prolongation associated with pulmonary edema: A report of nine cases. J Am Coll Cardiol 34:1106, 1999.
202. Roguin A, Behar D, Ben Ami H, et al: Long-term prognosis of acute pulmonary oedema—An ominous outcome. Eur J Heart Fail 2:137, 2000.
203. Hackett PH, Roach RC: High-altitude illness. N Engl J Med 345:107, 2001.
204. Bartsch P, Swenson ER, Maggiorini M: Update: High altitude pulmonary edema. Adv Exp Med Biol 502:89, 2001.
205. Gabry AL, Ledoux X, Mozziconacci M, Martin C: High-altitude pulmonary edema at moderate altitude (<2,400 m; 7,870 feet): A series of 52 patients. Chest 123:49, 2003.
206. Grunig E, Mereles D, Hildebrandt W, et al: Stress Doppler echocardiography for identification of susceptibility to high altitude pulmonary edema. J Am Coll Cardiol 35:980, 2000.
207. Duplain H, Vollenweider L, Delabays A, et al: Augmented sympathetic activation during short-term hypoxia and high-altitude exposure in subjects susceptible to high-altitude pulmonary edema. Circulation 99:1713, 1999.
208. Busch T, Bartsch P, Pappert D, et al: Hypoxia decreases exhaled nitric oxide in mountaineers susceptible to high-altitude pulmonary edema. Am J Respir Crit Care Med 163:368, 2001.
209. Sartori C, Vollenweider L, Loffler BM, et al: Exaggerated endothelin release in high-altitude pulmonary edema. Circulation 99:2665, 1999.
210. Hanaoka M, Tanaka M, Ge RL, et al: Hypoxia-induced pulmonary blood redistribution in subjects with a history of high-altitude pulmonary edema. Circulation 101:1418, 2000.
211. West JB: Invited review: Pulmonary capillary stress failure. J Appl Physiol 89:2483, 2000.
212. Swenson ER, Maggiorini M, Mongovin S, et al: Pathogenesis of high-altitude pulmonary edema: Inflammation is not an etiologic factor. JAMA 287:2228, 2002.
213. Hackett P, Rennie D: High-altitude pulmonary edema. JAMA 287:2275, 2002.
214. Sartori C, Allemann Y, Duplain H, et al: Salmeterol for the prevention of high-altitude pulmonary edema. N Engl J Med 346:1631, 2002.
215. Scherrer U, Vollenweider L, Delabays A, et al: Inhaled nitric oxide for high-altitude pulmonary edema. N Engl J Med 334:624, 1996.
216. Ayus JC, Varon J, Arieff AI: Hyponatremia, cerebral edema, and noncardiogenic pulmonary edema in marathon runners. Ann Intern Med 132:711, 2000.
217. Fontes RB, Aguiar PH, Zanetti MV, et al: Acute neurogenic pulmonary edema: Case reports and literature review. J Neurosurg Anesthesiol 15:144, 2003.
218. Smith WS, Matthay MA: Evidence for a hydrostatic mechanism in human neurogenic pulmonary edema. Chest 111:1326, 1997.
219. Hamdy O, Maekawa H, Shimada Y, et al: Role of central nervous system nitric oxide in the development of neurogenic pulmonary edema in rats. Crit Care Med 29:1222, 2001.
220. Sporer KA, Dorn E: Heroin-related noncardiogenic pulmonary edema: A case series. Chest 120:1628, 2001.
221. Sterrett C, Brownfield J, Korn CS, et al: Patterns of presentation in heroin overdose resulting in pulmonary edema. Am J Emerg Med 21:32, 2003.
222. Goldhaber SZ, Elliott CG: Acute pulmonary embolism: Part I: Epidemiology, pathophysiology, and diagnosis. Circulation 108:2726, 2003.
223. Mattar F, Sibai BM: Eclampsia. VIII. Risk factors for maternal morbidity. Am J Obstet Gynecol 182:307, 2000.
224. DiFederico EM, Burlingame JM, Kilpatrick SJ, et al: Pulmonary edema in obstetric patients is rapidly resolved except in the presence of infection or of nitroglycerin tocolysis after open fetal surgery. Am J Obstet Gynecol 179:925, 1998.
225. Gilbert WM, Towner DR, Field NT, Anthony J: The safety and utility of pulmonary artery catheterization in severe preeclampsia and eclampsia. Am J Obstet Gynecol 182:1397, 2000.
226. Desai DK, Moodley J, Naidoo DP, Bhorat I: Cardiac abnormalities in pulmonary oedema associated with hypertensive crises in pregnancy. Br J Obstet Gynaecol 103:523, 1996.
227. Upshaw CB Jr: Hemodynamic changes after cardioversion of chronic atrial fibrillation. Arch Intern Med 157:1070, 1997.
228. Arieff AI: Fatal postoperative pulmonary edema: Pathogenesis and literature review. Chest 115:1371, 1999.
229. Asimakopoulos G, Smith PL, Ratnatunga CP, Taylor KM: Lung injury and acute respiratory distress syndrome after cardiopulmonary bypass. Ann Thorac Surg 68:1107, 1999.
230. Nathoe HM, van Dijk D, Jansen EW, et al: A comparison of on-pump and off-pump coronary bypass surgery in low-risk patients. N Engl J Med 348:394, 2003.
231. Kopko PM, Marshall CS, MacKenzie MR, et al: Transfusion-related acute lung injury: Report of a clinical look-back investigation. JAMA 287:1968, 2002.
232. Duchin JS, Koster FT, Peters CJ, et al: Hantavirus pulmonary syndrome: A clinical description of 17 patients with a newly recognized disease. The Hantavirus Study Group. N Engl J Med 330:949, 1994.
233. Peters CJ, Khan AS: Hantavirus pulmonary syndrome: The new American hemorrhagic fever. Clin Infect Dis 34:1224, 2002.
234. Ho M, Chen ER, Hsu KH, et al: An epidemic of enterovirus 71 infection in Taiwan. Taiwan Enterovirus Epidemic Working Group. N Engl J Med 341:929, 1999.
235. Lee N, Hui D, Wu A, et al: A major outbreak of severe acute respiratory syndrome in Hong Kong. N Engl J Med 348:1986, 2003.
236. Ksiazek TG, Erdman D, Goldsmith CS, et al: A novel coronavirus associated with severe acute respiratory syndrome. N Engl J Med 348:1947, 2003.

High-Output Heart Failure

237. Anand IS, Chandrashekhar Y, Wander GS, Chawla LS: Endothelium-derived relaxing factor is important in mediating the high output state in chronic severe anemia. J Am Coll Cardiol 25:1402, 1995.
238. Anand IS, Chandrashekhar Y, Ferrari R, et al: Pathogenesis of oedema in chronic severe anaemia: Studies of body water and sodium, renal function, haemodynamic variables, and plasma hormones. Br Heart J 70:357, 1993.
239. Willenbrock R, Scheuermann M, Thibault G, et al: Angiotensin inhibition and atrial natriuretic peptide release after acute volume expansion in rats with aortocaval shunt. Cardiovasc Res 42:733, 1999.
240. Aessopos A, Farmakis D, Karagiorga M, et al: Cardiac involvement in thalassemia intermedia: A multicenter study. Blood 97:3411, 2001.
241. Wattanasirichaigoon S, Pomposelli FB Jr: Branham's sign is an exaggerated Bezold-Jarisch reflex of arteriovenous fistula. J Vasc Surg 26:171, 1997.

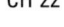

242. Ilijevski N, Radak D, Radevic B, et al: Popliteal traumatic arteriovenous fistulas. J Trauma 52:739, 2002.
243. Thalhammer C, Kirchherr AS, Uhlich F, et al: Postcatheterization pseudoaneurysms and arteriovenous fistulas: Repair with percutaneous implantation of endovascular covered stents. Radiology 214:127, 2000.
244. Nasser TK, Mohler ER III, Wilensky RL, Hathaway DR: Peripheral vascular complications following coronary interventional procedures. Clin Cardiol 18:609, 1995.
245. Toursarkissian B, Allen BT, Petrinec D, et al: Spontaneous closure of selected iatrogenic pseudoaneurysms and arteriovenous fistulae. J Vasc Surg 25:803, 1997.
246. Waigand J, Uhlich F, Gross CM, et al: Percutaneous treatment of pseudoaneurysms and arteriovenous fistulas after invasive vascular procedures. Catheter Cardiovasc Interv 47:157, 1999.
247. Davidovic LB, Kostic DM, Cvetkovic SD, et al: Aorto-caval fistulas. Cardiovasc Surg 10:555, 2002.
248. Sigler L, Gutierrez-Carreno R, Martinez-Lopez C, et al: Aortocava fistula: Experience with five patients. Vasc Surg 35:207, 2001.
249. Korn TS, Thurston JM, Sherry CS, Kawalsky DL: High-output heart failure due to a renal arteriovenous fistula in a pregnant woman with suspected preeclampsia. Mayo Clin Proc 73:888, 1998.

250. Young PR Jr, Rohr MS, Marterre WF Jr: High-output cardiac failure secondary to a brachiocephalic arteriovenous hemodialysis fistula: Two cases. Am Surg 64:239, 1998.
251. Ori Y, Korzets A, Katz M, et al: Haemodialysis arteriovenous access—A prospective haemodynamic evaluation. Nephrol Dial Transplant 11:94, 1996.
252. McCarthy RE, Lytle JO, Van Devanter S: The use of total circulatory arrest in the surgery of giant hemangioma and Klippel-Trenaunay syndrome in neonates. Clin Orthop (289):237, 1993.
253. Pollak Y, Katzen BT, Pollak W: High-output congestive failure in a patient with pulmonary arteriovenous malformations. Cardiol Rev 10:188, 2002.
254. Hisamatsu K, Ueeda M, Ando M, et al: Peripheral arterial coil embolization for hepatic arteriovenous malformation in Osler-Weber-Rendu disease; useful for controlling high output heart failure, but harmful to the liver. Intern Med 38:962, 1999.
255. Daller JA, Bueno J, Gutierrez J, et al: Hepatic hemangioendothelioma: Clinical experience and management strategy. J Pediatr Surg 34:98, 1999.
256. Kahaly GJ, Kampmann C, Mohr-Kahaly S. Cardiovascular hemodynamics and exercise tolerance in thyroid disease. Thyroid 12:473, 2002.
257. Biondi B, Palmieri EA, Lombardi G, Fazio S: Effects of subclinical thyroid dysfunction on the heart. Ann Intern Med 137:904, 2002.
258. Shimizu T, Koide S, Noh JY, et al: Hyperthyroidism and the management of atrial fibrillation. Thyroid 12:489, 2002.
259. Kahaly GJ, Nieswandt J, Mohr-Kahaly S: Cardiac risks of hyperthyroidism in the elderly. Thyroid 8:1165, 1998.
260. Krahn AD, Klein GJ, Kerr CR, et al: How useful is thyroid function testing in patients with recent-onset atrial fibrillation? The Canadian Registry of Atrial Fibrillation Investigators. Arch Intern Med 156:2221, 1996.
261. Witte KK, Clark AL, Cleland JG: Chronic heart failure and micronutrients. J Am Coll Cardiol 37:1765, 2001.
262. Blanc P, Boussuges A: Cardiac beriberi. Arch Mal Coeur Vaiss 93:371, 2000.
263. Kawai C, Wakabayashi A, Matsumura T, Yui Y: Reappearance of beriberi heart disease in Japan. A study of 23 cases. Am J Med 69:383, 1980.
264. Chen KT, Chiou ST, Chang YC, et al: Cardiac beriberi among illegal mainland Chinese immigrants. J Int Med Res 29:37, 2001.
265. Kitamura K, Yamaguchi T, Tanaka H, et al: TPN-induced fulminant beriberi: A report on our experience and a review of the literature. Surg Today 26:769, 1996.
266. Gabrielli A, Caruso L, Stacpoole PW: Early recognition of acute cardiovascular beriberi by interpretation of hemodynamics. J Clin Anesth 13:230, 2001.
267. Shivalkar B, Engelmann I, Carp L, et al: Shoshin syndrome: Two case reports representing opposite ends of the same disease spectrum. Acta Cardiol 53:195, 1998.
268. Reddy SV, Kurihara N, Menaa C, Roodman GD: Paget's disease of bone: A disease of the osteoclast. Rev Endocr Metab Disord 2:195, 2001.
269. Lyles KW, Siris ES, Singer FR, Meunier PJ: A clinical approach to diagnosis and management of Paget's disease of bone. J Bone Miner Res 16:1379, 2001.
270. Hultgren HN: Osteitis deformans (Paget's disease) and calcific disease of the heart valves. Am J Cardiol 81:1461, 1998.
271. Roux C, Dougados M: Treatment of patients with Paget's disease of bone. Drugs 58:823, 1999.
272. Krane SM, Shiller AL: Paget's disease and other dysplasias of bone. *In* Braunwald E, Fauci AS, Kasper DL, et al (eds): Harrison's Principles of Internal Medicine. New York, McGraw-Hill, 2001, pp 2237-2245.
273. Inanir S, Haznedar R, Atavci S, Unlu M: Arteriovenous shunting in patients with multiple myeloma and high-output failure. J Nucl Med 39:1, 1998.
274. Kuribayashi N, Matsuzaki H, Hata H, et al: Multiple myeloma associated with serum amino acid disturbance and high output cardiac failure. Am J Hematol 57:77, 1998.
275. McBride W, Jackman JD Jr, Grayburn PA: Prevalence and clinical characteristics of a high cardiac output state in patients with multiple myeloma. Am J Med 89:21, 1990.
276. Yun D, Heywood JT: Metastatic carcinoid disease presenting solely as high-output heart failure. Ann Intern Med 120:45, 1994.
277. Damjanovic SS, Neskovic AN, Petakov MS, et al: High output heart failure in patients with newly diagnosed acromegaly. Am J Med 112:610, 2002.
278. Alpert MA, Terry BE, Mulekar M, et al: Cardiac morphology and left ventricular function in normotensive morbidly obese patients with and without congestive heart failure, and effect of weight loss. Am J Cardiol 80:736, 1997.

CHAPTER 23

Drugs in the Treatment of Heart Failure

Michael R. Bristow • Stuart Linas • J. David Port

Pharmacological therapy for heart failure (HF) is divided into two distinct settings and approaches: treatment of *decompensated HF* and treatment of *chronic stable HF* (Table 23–1). The goals of these two types of treatment are different, and part of the challenge of treating individual patients with HF is the art of converting patients in the former category to the latter. In the treatment of patients with decompensated HF, the goals are to stabilize the patient, restore organ perfusion, return filling pressure to optimal levels, and begin the conversion to chronic therapy. In contrast, the goals of treatment of patients with chronic stable HF are to enhance survival, minimize symptoms and disability, improve functional capacity, and delay disease progression. As discussed here, diuretics, vasodilators, and positive inotropic agents are used to minimize symptoms and improve functional capacity, and neurohormonal inhibitors are used primarily to enhance survival and delay disease progression.

Diuretics

The importance of diuretics in the treatment of HF is related to the central role of the kidney as the target organ of many of the neurohumoral and hemodynamic changes that occur in response to a failing heart.[1–4] The net effect of these physiological responses is an increase in salt and water retention, which results in expansion of the extracellular fluid volume. This effect is highlighted in Figure 23–1, where the adrenergic system and the renin-angiotensin-aldosterone system (RAAS), two important compensatory neurohormonal mechanisms that are activated in concert early in the course of HF, produce volume expansion. In the case of adrenergic mechanisms, volume expansion may occur through adrenergic receptor (alpha and beta)[5]-mediated nonosmotic release or beta receptor-mediated increase in gene expression of vasopressin. For RAAS mechanisms, volume expansion occurs through angiotensin II-mediated increases in aldosterone and vasopressin secretion and stimulation of thirst.[5] In the short term, volume expansion serves to sustain cardiac output and tissue perfusion by allowing the heart to operate higher on its ventricular function (Frank-Starling) curve (Fig. 23–2). However, these physiological adaptations also result in higher end-diastolic filling pressure and increased wall stress in diastole and systole, which contributes to hypertrophy and remodeling (see Chap. 21) and may cause dyspnea or even pulmonary edema.

With the exception of the aldosterone antagonists, diuretics do not influence the natural history of chronic HF. However, diuretics improve congestive symptoms and may also slow the progression of ventricular remodeling by reducing ventricular filling pressure and wall stress. The acute effect of diuretics in patients with HF-related volume overload is to decrease left ventricular (LV) filling pressure without much change in cardiac output because of the depressed and flat Frank-Starling curve in these subjects as depicted in Figure 23–2. However, it should also be emphasized that in situations of very high filling pressures diuretics can actually increase organ perfusion, because decreasing markedly elevated venous pressures can increase flow across capillary beds.

Renal Adaptation to Heart Failure (see also Chap. 86)

Increased salt and water retention by the kidney is due primarily to characteristic alterations in intrarenal hemodynamics that occur in response to decreased cardiac output. In addition, salt and water retention activates the adrenergic nervous system and several hormonal and cytokine systems (see Chap. 21). A decrease in cardiac output results in increased peripheral and intrarenal vascular resistance, activation of intrarenal and other tissue vasoconstrictor systems such as angiotensin II and endothelin-1, and release of vasopressin from the posterior pituitary gland. Angiotensin II-mediated increased adrenal cortical activity promote aldosterone synthesis and release, and increased intraatrial and intraventricular pressure promote the production and secretion of atrial natriuretic peptide (ANP) and brain natriuretic peptide (BNP) in cardiac muscle.

INTRARENAL HEMODYNAMICS IN HEART FAILURE. The changes in intrarenal hemodynamics that occur early in the course of HF result in preservation of the glomerular filtration rate (GFR) despite a decline in cardiac output and renal blood flow.[1–4] Although increases in adrenergic activity and local release of angiotensin II act to increase resistance in both the afferent and efferent glomerular arterioles, preservation of the GFR is due in large part to a greater increase in efferent than in afferent arteriolar tone. Pressure differences across the glomerulus (P_{GC}) and across the glomerular capillary membrane and Bowman's space (P_t) are two major determinants of single-nephron GFR. The other main determinants of single-nephron GFR are the glomerular membrane ultrafiltration coefficient (K_f), which tends to decline in HF, and differences between glomerular capillary and proximal tubular colloid osmotic pressure, which are usually unchanged in HF.

NEUROHORMONAL ACTIVATION. In addition to hemodynamic changes in the proximal nephron, increased renal sympathetic nerve activity activates the intrarenal renin-angiotensin system (RAS) and has direct tubular effects that result in augmented salt retention along the nephron.[2] Activation of a local endothelin-1 generating system also occurs.[6]

TABLE 23–1 Classes of Drugs (Noninvestigational Agents Only) Used to Treat Heart Failure

Drug Class	Use
Diuretics	
"Loop" diuretics ($Na^+/K^+/2Cl^-$ cotransporter inhibitors)	DHF (IV); CSHF (PO) stage 2-4*
Thiazides (Na^+/Cl^- cotransporter inhibitors)	DHF (IV); CSHF (PO) stage 2-4
K^+ sparing (epithelial Na^+ channel inhibitors)	CSHF (PO) stage 2-4
Type I (mineralocorticoid) receptor antagonists	CSHF (PO) stage 3, 4
Carbonic anhydrase inhibitors (acetazolamide)	DHF (IV)
Vasodilators	
Nitrovasodilators	DHF (IV); CSHF (PO) stage 2-4
"Direct-acting" or unknown mechanism vasodilators	DHF (IV); CSHF (PO) stage 2-4
Calcium channel blockers (vasoselective agents only)	Angina or persistent HTN in setting of HF DHF (IV)
Natriuretic peptides (nesiritide)	
Positive Inotropic Agents	
Digitalis derivatives	CSHF (PO), stage 2-4
Beta-adrenergic receptor agonists	DHF (IV), stage 4
Phosphodiesterase inhibitors	DHF (IV)
Phosphodiesterase inhibitors with calcium sensitizer action	DHF (IV)
Neurohormonal Inhibitors	
Angiotensin-converting enzyme inhibitors (ACEIs)	CSHF (PO) stage 1-4
Angiotensin receptor blockers (ARBs)	CSHF (PO) stage 2, 3
Beta-adrenergic receptor blocking compounds	CSHF (PO) stage 2, 3

CSHF = chronic stable heart failure; DHF = decompensated heart failure; HTN = hypertension.

*For definitions of the stages of heart failure, see Table 24–3.

As a result of renal vasoconstrictor influences, renal blood flow is directed away from superficial cortical nephrons to the more efficient solute-resorbing juxtamedullary nephrons. These nephrons rely on the high capacity of the ion transport carriers in the loop of Henle and the countercurrent mechanism of the medulla to allow the formation of concentrated urine. Elevated arginine vasopressin (AVP) levels cause further reductions in free water clearance by the kidney. This reduced clearance of free water, coupled with the increased thirst of many patients with advanced HF (perhaps caused by higher intracerebral angiotensin II levels), often leads to a hypotonic edematous state. As with other complex biological systems, countervailing intrarenal and humoral responses also occur, including increased prostaglandin E_2 and prostacyclin levels within the kidney and the release of humoral natriuretic factors, including ANP and BNP.[1,4]

Mechanisms of Action of Diuretics

By definition, a diuretic is any drug that increases urine flow. However, the term "diuretic" is commonly used to refer to agents that enhance the delivery of sodium chloride, other small ions, and water into urine. In this context, agents such as cardiac glycosides and dopamine may indirectly increase urine production by enhancing renal blood flow and the GFR, which promotes a fall in the glomerular filtration fraction and thereby diminishes water and solute resorption by the proximal tubule. Furthermore, endogenous substances such as ANP or BNP, when administered as drugs, may have salutary effects on cardiovascular function as well as on intrarenal hemodynamics and tubular sodium resorption.

Most diuretics, however, act directly on the kidney to inhibit solute and water reabsorption. A number of classification schemes for diuretics have been proposed on the basis of their mechanism of action, their anatomical locus of action within the nephron, and the form of diuresis that they elicit. Diuretics can be classified according to whether they induce a "solute" or "water" diuresis. Of the latter ("aquaretics"), only three agents are of clinical relevance: demeclocycline, lithium, and vasopressin V_2 receptor antagonists, each of which, by different mechanisms, inhibits the action of AVP on the collecting duct, thereby increasing free water clearance. Drugs that cause solute diuresis are subdivided into two types: osmotic diuretics, which are nonresorbable solutes that osmotically retain water and other solutes in the tubular lumen, and drugs that selectively inhibit ion transport pathways across tubular epithelia, which constitute the majority of potent, clinically useful diuretics.

Now that many of the specific ion transport proteins that are the molecular targets for diuretics have been cloned and their intrarenal distribution characterized, a new classification of these drugs on the basis of their molecular pharmacology has been advocated. However, a more traditional and familiar scheme of classification, employing a combination of chemical (e.g., "thiazide" diuretic), site of action (e.g., "loop" diuretics), or clinical outcome (e.g., "potassium-sparing" diuretics), is used throughout this chapter. The sites of action of commonly used diuretics and those in clinical development are given in Table 23–2.

Classes of Diuretics

Classes of diuretics and individual class members are listed in Table 23–2, and their renal sites of action are depicted in Figure 23–3.

Loop Diuretics

The agents traditionally classified as loop or high-ceiling diuretics, including furosemide, bumetanide, and torsemide, have been known for more than a decade to inhibit reversibly the $Na^+/K^+/2Cl^-$ symporter (cotransporter) when applied to the luminal but not the basolateral membranes of epithelial cells of the thick ascending limb of the loop of Henle (Fig. 23–3; see Table 23–2). Agents in a second functional class of these drugs, typified by ethacrynic acid, are also effective only from the tubular lumen but exhibit a slower onset of action and delayed and only partial reversibility. Individual agents that act as $Na^+/K^+/2Cl^-$ cotransporter inhibitors[7] are listed in Table 23–2.

MECHANISMS OF ACTION. The molecular targets of these drugs have been cloned and sequenced and were found to encompass a family of cation chloride symporters that have now been described in a number of cell types and tissues.[7] Inhibition of this cotransporter results in a marked increase in the fractional excretion of Na^+ and Cl^- and indirectly results in the fractional excretion of Ca^{2+} and Mg^{2+}. By inhibiting the concentration of solute within the medullary interstitium, these drugs also reduce the driving force for water resorption in the collecting duct, regardless of the presence of AVP; the decreased resorption of water in turn results in the production of urine that is nearly isotonic with plasma at the height of the diuresis. The delivery of large amounts of Na^+ and fluid to the distal nephron increases both K^+ and H^+ secretion, a process that is accelerated by aldosterone and that results in hypokalemia and metabolic alkalosis.

HEMODYNAMIC EFFECTS. Loop diuretics also exhibit several characteristic effects on intracardiac pressure and systemic hemodynamics. An increase in venous capacitance and lowering of pulmonary capillary wedge pressure within minutes of a bolus infusion of intravenous furosemide (0.5 to 1.0 mg/kg) have been well documented in patients with congestive symptoms following acute myocardial infarction or in those with valvular heart disease.[8] Some increase in pulmonary venous compliance probably occurs as well. Similar data, although not as extensive, have accumulated for bumetanide and torsemide.[9] Despite the fall in LV end-diastolic filling pressure, systemic vascular resistance often increases acutely in response to loop diuretics, an effect that has been attributed to transient activation of the systemic or intravascular RAS. The net effect of these actions on cardiac function may contribute to some improvement in HF symptoms. However, the potentially deleterious rise in LV afterload reinforces the importance of initiating vasodilator therapy with diuretics in patients with acute pulmonary edema and adequate blood pressure.

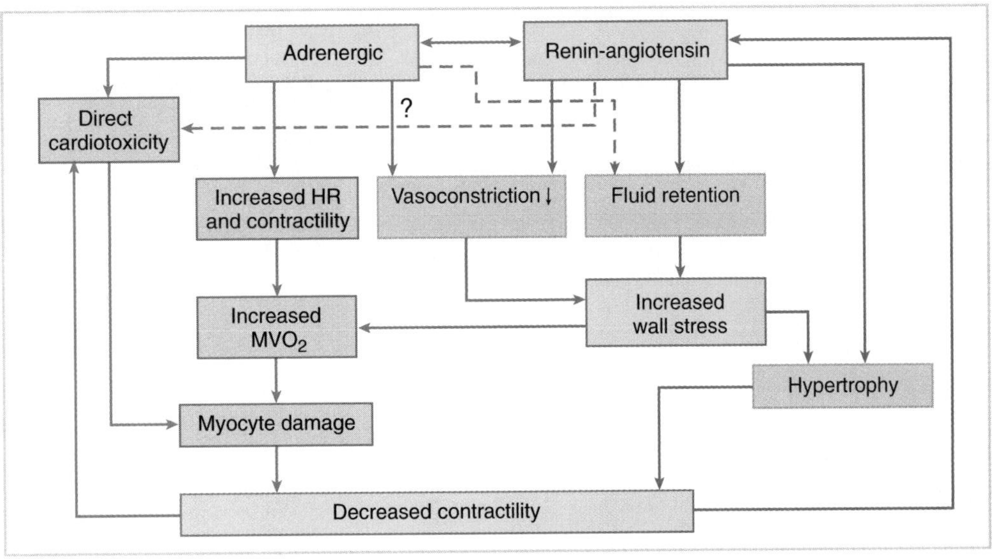

FIGURE 23–1 Hemodynamic and biological consequences of coordinated activation of the adrenergic and renin-angiotensin systems in heart failure. HR = heart rate; MVO_2 = myocardial oxygen consumption. Solid lines = established mechanisms.

All the rapid hemodynamic actions of loop diuretics are attenuated in patients with chronic HF. Although most of these effects have been attributed in the past to activation of the RAS by the kidney in response to loop diuretics, with subsequent release of renal and intravascular prostaglandins, more recent evidence indicates that these drugs have direct effects on endothelial cells and vascular smooth muscle. In in vitro experiments, furosemide stimulated the release of prostacyclin and nitric oxide by increasing the release of vasoactive kinins, presumably after inhibition of $Na^+/K^+/2Cl^-$ cotransporter function in endothelial cells in vitro.[10] Furosemide has also been shown to relax precontracted pulmonary venous rings by a direct effect on smooth muscle that was dependent on inhibition of vascular smooth muscle $Na^+/K^+/2Cl^-$ cotransporter function in these cells.[11]

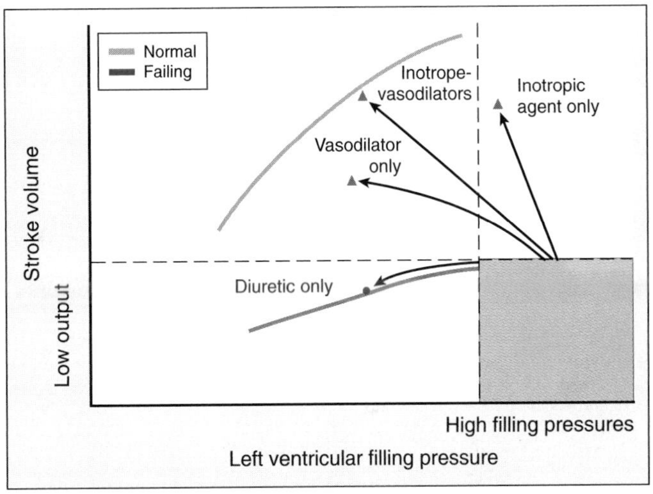

FIGURE 23–2 Frank-Starling relationship for ventricular function in heart failure. In patients with heart failure, the normal relationship between cardiac output (y-axis) and filling pressure (x-axis) is shifted lower and to the right such that a low-output state and congestive symptoms may be coincident. At one extreme, the addition of a pure inotropic agent, such as digoxin, primarily increases stroke volume with minimal impact on filling pressure. Conversely, the addition of a diuretic primarily decreases filling pressure without having an impact on cardiac output. Clinically, it is common to use multiple classes of agents, or agents with combined effects, to produce both increased cardiac output and decreased filling pressure. (Adapted from Cohn JN, Franciosa JA: Vasodilator therapy of cardiac failure [first of two parts]. N Engl J Med 297:27, 1977.)

Thiazide and Thiazide-Like Diuretics

This class of diuretic, of which chlorothiazide is the prototype, includes the first effective orally bioavailable diuretics with acceptable safety profiles to become widely used in clinical practice, supplementing the much more toxic mercurial diuretics of the 1950s. A number of these agents are available for clinical use in the United States (Table 23–2). Although not all are technically benzothiadiazine derivatives, they are often collectively referred to as "thiazide" diuretics. The site of action of these drugs within the distal convoluted tubule has been identified at a molecular level as being the Na^+/Cl^- cotransporter of the distal convoluted tubule. This cotransporter has 12 membrane-spanning domains and shares 60 percent amino acid homology with the $Na^+/K^+/2Cl^-$ cotransporter of the ascending limb of the loop of Henle; however, it is insensitive to the effects of furosemide. This cotransporter (or related isoforms) is also present on cells within the vasculature and many cell types within other organs and tissues and may contribute to some of the other actions of these agents, such as their utility as antihypertensive agents.

By blocking solute uptake in the distal convoluted tube, Na^+/Cl^- cotransporter inhibitors prevent maximal dilution of urine, decrease the kidney's ability to increase free water clearance, and may contribute to the development of hyponatremia. Thiazides increase Ca^{2+} resorption in the distal nephron (Fig. 23–3) by several mechanisms, occasionally resulting in a small increase in serum Ca^{2+} levels. In contrast, Mg^{2+} resorption is diminished and hypomagnesemia may occur with prolonged use. Increased delivery of NaCl and fluid into the collecting duct directly enhances K^+ and H^+

TABLE 23–2 Diuretic Classes Used in the Treatment of Chronic Heart Failure

Diuretic	Brand Name	Principal Site and Mechanism of Action	Effects on Urinary Electrolytes	Effects on Blood Electrolytes and Acid-Base Balance	Extrarenal Effects	Usual Dosage*	Drug Interactions
Loop Diuretics ($Na^+/K^+/2Cl^-$/ Cotransporter Inhibitors)							
Furosemide	Lasix	Thick ascending limb of the loop of Henle; inhibition of the $Na^+/K^+/2Cl^-$ cotransporter	↑Na^+ ↑Cl^- ↑K^+	Hypochloremic alkalosis ↑HCO_3^- ↓K^+, ↓Na^+ ↓Cl^- ↑Uric acid	Acute: ↑venous capacitance ↑Systemic vascular resistance when given IV, secondary to neurohormonal activation Chronic: ↓cardiac preload, ototoxicity	10-360 mg/d	Tubular secretion delayed by competing organic acids (renal failure) and some drugs Effectiveness reduced by prostaglandin inhibitors Additive ototoxicity with aminoglycosides Longer duration of action that furosemide
Bumetanide	Bumex					0.5-20 mg/d	
Piretanide[†]	Arelix, Diumax, Tauliz					6-20 mg/d	
Ethacrynic acid	Edecrin					50-200 mg/d	
Torsemide	Demadex					2.5-200 mg/d	
Thiazide and Thiazide-like Diuretics (Na^+/Cl^- Cotransporter Inhibitors)							
Chlorothiazide	Diuril	Distal tubule: inhibits Na^+/Cl^- cotransporter	↑Na^+, ↑Cl^-, ↑K^+ ↑Mg^{2+}, ↓Ca^{2+}	↓Na^+, particularly in elderly patients ↓Cl^-, ↑HCO_3^- (mild alkalosis) ↑Uric acid, ↑Ca^{2+} ↓K^+, ↓Mg^{2+}	↑Glucose ↑LDL/triglycerides (may be dose related) Extrarenal effects less marked with indapamide	50-100 mg/d	Efficacy reduced by prostaglandin inhibitors Reduces renal lithium clearance Additive effect on NaCl and K^+ excretion with loop diuretics
Hydroclorothiazide	HydroDIURIL					25-50 mg/d	
Trichlormethiazide	Metahydrin					2-8 mg/d	
Chlorthalidone	Hygroton					25-100 mg/d	
Metolazone	Mykrox, Zaroxolyn					0.5-10 mg/d 5-10 mg/d	
Quinethazone	Hydromox					50-100 mg/d	
Indapamide	Lozol					2.5-5 mg/d	
K^+-Sparing Diuretics (Epithelial Na^+ Channel Inhibitors)							
Triamterene	Dyrenium	Collecting duct; inhibits apical membrane Na^+ conductance	↓K^+ ↑Na^+	Metabolic acidosis ↑Mg^{2+}		100-300 mg/d	Useful when used with K^+ wasting diuretics; may induce hyperkalemia with ACE inhibitors/ARBs
Amiloride	Midamor					5-10 mg/d	
Type I Mineralocorticoid Receptor Antagonists (also K^+-Sparing Diuretics)							
Spironolactone	Aldactone	Collecting duct: aldosterone antagonists	↓K^+, ↑Na^+, ↑Cl^-	↑K^+, metabolic acidosis	Gynecomastia for spironolactone, not for eplerenone	12.5-25 mg/d	Useful adjunct to K^+ wasting diuretics; ↑K^+ may be worse in presence of other RAAS inhibitors
Eplerenone	Inspra					25-50 mg/d	
Carbonic Anhydrase Inhibitors							
Acetazolamide	Diamox	Proximal tubule Carbonic anhydrase inhibition	↑Na^+, ↑K^+, ↑HCO_3^-	Metabolic acidosis	↑Ventilatory drive ↓Intraocular pressure	250-500 mg/d	May be useful in alkalemia related to other diuretics; may cause severe K^+ wasting
Dichlorphenamide	Doranide					10-20 mg/d	
Methazolamide	Neptazane					25-100 mg/d	
Vasopressin Antagonists							
Tolvaptan (V_2 RA)[†]	TBD	Collecting duct, inhibits recruitment of aquaporin H_2O channels	↓Na^+, ↑free H_2O	Hypernatremia, ↑ osmolarity	?	TBD	May cause diabetes insipidus
Lixivaptan (V_2 RA)[†]							
Conivaptan (V_1/V_2 RA)[†]							

ACE = angiotensin-converting enzyme; ARB = angiotensin receptor blocker; LDL = low-density lipoprotein; RA = receptor antagonist; TBD = to be determined; RAAS = renin-angiotensin-aldosterone system.
*Dosages are approximate (PO).
[†]Not yet approved in the United States.

secretion by this segment of the nephron and may lead to clinically important hypokalemia.

Potassium-Sparing Diuretics

The apical (luminal) membranes of the principal cells of the late distal convoluted tubule and the cortical collecting duct contain Na^+-selective channels that permit Na^+ entry from within the tubular lumen, driven by the electrochemical gradient established by Na^+,K^+-adenosine triphosphatase (ATPase) in the basolateral membranes of these cells (Fig. 23–3).[12] The number of epithelial Na^+ channels available for entry into tubular epithelial membranes is regulated in part by mineralocorticoid levels. The activity (conductance) of these Na^+ channels appears to be regulated by both protein kinase A-mediated phosphorylation and guanosine triphosphate (GTP) binding proteins (i.e., $G_{\alpha i}$). Na^+ conductance by these channels is inhibited by *amiloride* and by *triamterene* (Table 23–2), which subsequently diminishes the electrochemical potential for K^+ secretion into the urine. Thus, these agents, along with mineralocorticoid inhibitors (see later), are commonly referred to as "potassium-sparing" diuretics.

Because Na^+ retention in HF occurs in more proximal nephron sites, neither amiloride nor triamterene is effective in achieving a net negative Na^+ balance when given alone. Amiloride and its congeners also inhibit Na^+/H^+ antiporters in renal epithelial cells and in many other cell types, but only at concentrations that are higher than those used clinically. Both amiloride and triamterene affect cardiac repolarization, possibly by inhibiting delayed rectifier K^+ currents (I_K), and may exaggerate the prolonged repolarization observed with Na^+ channel blocker antiarrhythmics (e.g., quinidine).[13,14]

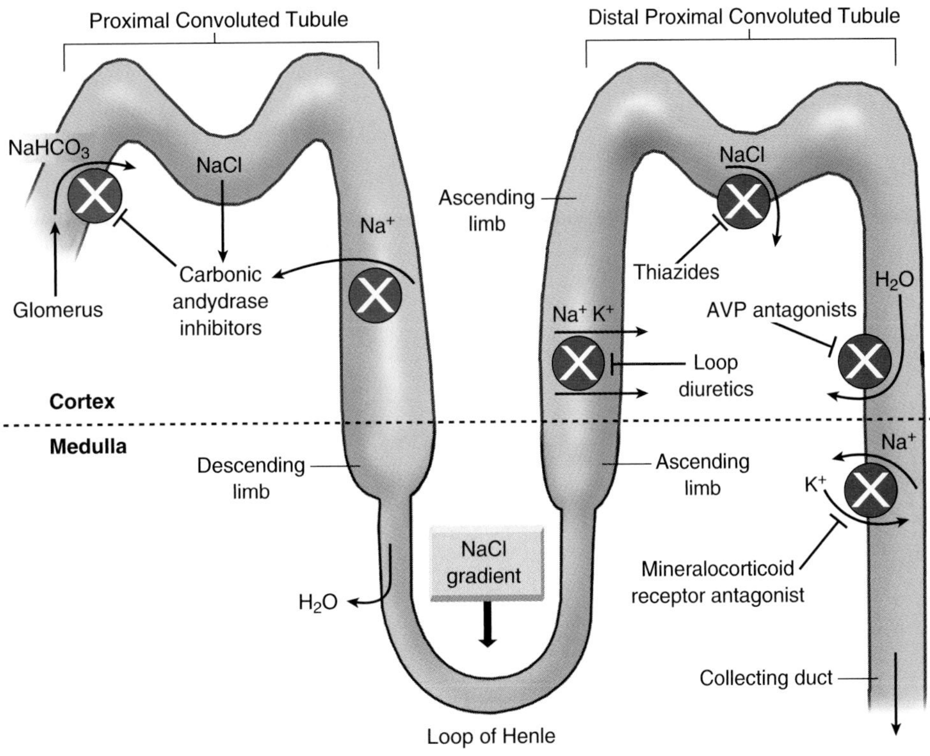

FIGURE 23–3 Sites of action of diuretics in the kidney. AVP = arginine vasopressin.

Aldosterone Type I or Mineralocorticoid Receptor Antagonists

Spironolactone (see Table 23–2) and its active metabolites canrenone and potassium canrenoate have been known for more than two decades to inhibit competitively the binding of aldosterone to mineralocorticoid or type I receptors in many tissues, including epithelial cells of the distal convoluted tubule and collecting duct. These cytosolic receptors are members of a "superfamily" of cytosolic proteins that are ligand-dependent transcription factors, which upon ligand binding translocate to the cell nucleus, where they bind to specific DNA sequences and regulate the transcription and synthesis of a number of gene products, including apical membrane Na^+ channels, H^+,K^+-ATPase, and Na^+,K^+-ATPase, among others.[15] The spironolactone-bound type I receptor complex is inactive and prevents Na^+ resorption as well as K^+ and H^+ secretion by this portion of the nephron, particularly in patients with high plasma aldosterone levels, as in HF.[16] Hyperkalemia and metabolic acidosis may result from the use of these drugs. The molecular pharmacology of steroid receptors is complex and relatively poorly understood. Endogenous glucocorticoids appear to be the principal ligand for the type I "mineralocorticoid" receptor in most cell types,[17] but in the cortical collecting tubule, the enzyme 11β-hydroxysteroid dehydrogenase protects the receptor from contact with high circulating levels of glucocorticoids so that aldosterone binding is facilitated. As discussed in Chapter 24, and shown in Table 23–7, spironolactone reduces mortality in patients with Class III and IV (stage 3) HF when administered on a background of angiotensin-converting enzyme (ACE) inhibition.[18] However, spironolactone or its metabolites, or both, have antiandrogenic and progestational activities, which may cause side effects that include gynecomastia or impotence in men and menstrual irregularities in women.

Eplerenone is another competitive inhibitor of the mineralocorticoid receptor. It was developed by replacing the 17α-thioacetyl group of spironolactone with a carbomethoxy group.[19] Because of this modification, eplerenone has greater selectivity for the mineralocorticoid receptor than for steroid receptors.[20] The sex hormone side effects associated with spironolactone are not observed with eplerenone.[21] Eplerenone has been shown to lower mortality when administered after myocardial infarction in patients with LV dysfunction when added to background therapy of ACE inhibition and beta blockers (Fig. 23–4).[21] Eplerenone is also an effective antihypertensive agent and produces regression of LV hypertrophy that is additive with ACE inhibitors (ACEIs).[22]

VASOPRESSIN ANTAGONISTS

Increased levels of circulating vasopressin (AVP, antidiuretic hormone) contribute to the increased systemic vascular resistance and positive solute and water balance in patients with advanced HF.[23] Physiologically, the primary site of action of vasopressin is the renal collecting duct (see Fig. 23–3), where it acts to increase water permeability (see later); however, it is clear that vasopressin has a number of nonrenal effects on the cardiovascular and central nervous system and on blood coagulation.

VASOPRESSIN RECEPTORS. These have been divided into V_1 and V_2 receptor subtypes, which exhibit different ligand-binding specificities. V_{1a} (vascular/hepatic/myocardial) and V_{1b} (pituitary) receptors, like angiotensin II (AT_1) and alpha$_1$-adrenergic receptors, are coupled through the $G_{\alpha q}$ subtype of G proteins to activation of phospholipase C in the plasma membranes of vascular smooth muscle cells and other tissues. Stimulation of V_1 receptors results in vasoconstriction, platelet activation, glycogenolysis, and adrenocorticotropic hormone release as well as stimulation of the transcription factors c-fos and c-jun, which ultimately results in cell growth. In contrast, V_2 receptors, found largely in distal nephron segments within the kidney, are coupled through stimulatory $G_{\alpha s}$ proteins to the stimulation of adenylyl cyclase activity, increased production of the second messenger cyclic adenosine monophosphate (cAMP), and activation of protein kinase A. By interrupting this phosphorylation cascade, V_2-selective receptor antagonists inhibit recruitment of aquaporin-CD water channels,[24] amiloride-sensitive Na^+ channels, and urea transporters into the apical membranes of collecting duct epithelial cells. Therefore, the ability of the collecting duct to resorb water is reduced.

The prototypical orally bioavailable nonpeptide V_2-selective antagonist is OPC-31260.[24] In general, this agent increases free water clearance, thereby increasing plasma osmolality as well as increasing the serum Na^+ concentration. A general consensus from studies in animal models with both the V_1-selective antagonist, OPC-21268,[25] and OPC-31260[26] suggests that vasopressin contributes to the development of HF more through the actions of V_2 receptor-mediated fluid retention and less so through alterations in systemic hemodynamics.[27] An analog of OPC-31260, OPC-41061 (tolvaptan),[27] is in clinical development and has shown efficacy as an aquaretic in HF.[28] Another V_2-selective antagonist, WAY-VPA-985 (lixivaptan),[29] has also shown dose-related aquaretic efficacy in HF. In addition, nonselective vasopressin antagonists such as YM087 (conivaptan)[30] have been developed. In a clinical trial in patients with HF, conivaptan, a V_{1a}/V_2 antagonist delivered intravenously, acutely reduced pulmonary wedge

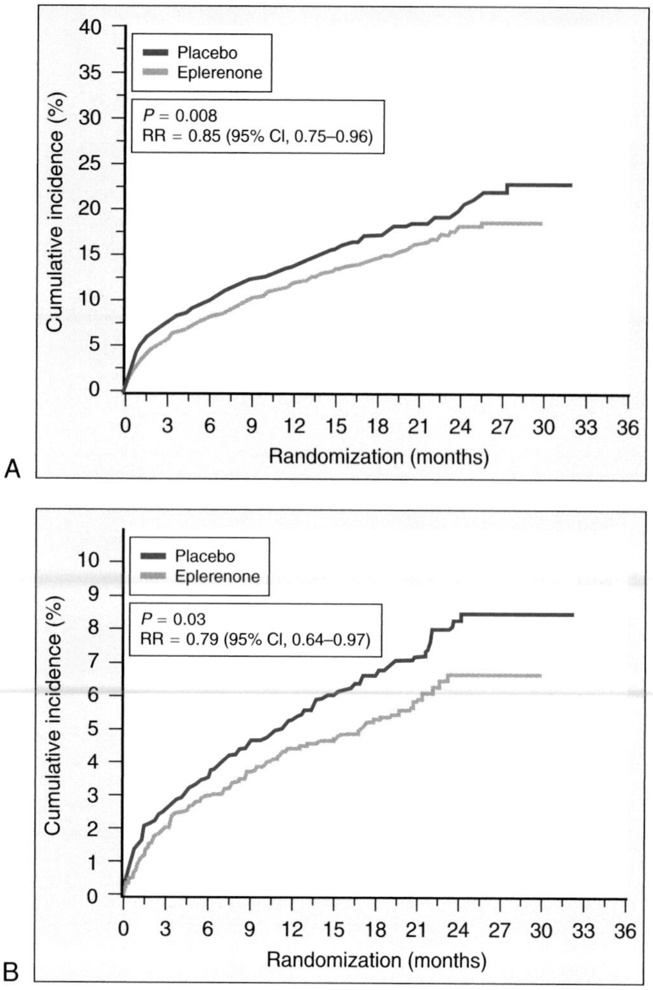

FIGURE 23–4 Kaplan-Meier estimates of the rate of death from any cause **(A)** and the rate of sudden death from cardiac causes **(B)** in the Eplerenone Post-Acute Myocardial Infarction Heart Failure Efficacy and Survival Study (EPHESUS) trial. This trial involved 6632 patients with acute myocardial infarction complicated by heart failure and left ventricular systolic dysfunction. CI = confidence interval; RR = relative risk. (Modified from Pitt B, Remme W, Zannad F, et al, Eplerenone Post-Acute Myocardial Infarction Heart Failure Efficacy and Survival Study Investigators: Eplerenone, a selective aldosterone blocker, in patients with left ventricular dysfunction after myocardial infarction. N Engl J Med 348:1309, 2003.)

and right atrial mean pressures while increasing free water excretion,[31] and this agent is undergoing additional testing in the setting of chronic HF.[32] This agent could have an advantage in long-term use in view of the fact that V_{1a} antagonism but not V_2 prevented remodeling in the infarct rat model.[33]

Although the use of these drugs (see Table 23-2) will undoubtedly present challenges in patients with HF, most of whom receive other vasodilators and natriuretic aquatic drugs and in whom vasopressin levels vary as a function of plasma osmolality and cardiac output, among other factors, vasopressin antagonists may ultimately prove to be valuable adjuncts to the treatment of HF.

CARBONIC ANHYDRASE INHIBITORS

At least two isoenzymes (types II and IV) of carbonic anhydrase are abundantly expressed in proximal tubular epithelial cells, in the luminal and basolateral membranes (see Fig. 23-3). These isoforms are inhibited by acetazolamide, whose use as a diuretic in patients with HF is confined to temporary administration to correct the metabolic alkalosis that occurs as a "contraction" phenomenon in response to the administration of other diuretics. When used repeatedly, acetazolamide (see Table 23-2) can cause metabolic acidosis as well as severe hypokalemia. The latter effect may occur in HF because increases in distal nephron HCO_3^- delivery favor K^+ secretion when aldosterone levels are elevated.

Diuretic Resistance and Management

Loop diuretics are the only class of diuretics that are effective as single agents in moderate and advanced HF. The rationale for this assumption was the magnitude of their maximal ("ceiling") natriuretic effect and the fact that the natriuretic effect of more distally acting drugs may be limited by the increased resorption of solute and water by proximal nephron segments in individuals with HF. However, even the effectiveness of potent loop diuretics can decrease with worsening HF. Although the bioavailability of these drugs is not generally decreased in HF, the potential delay in their rate of absorption may result in peak drug levels within the tubular lumen in the ascending loop of Henle that are insufficient to induce maximal natriuresis.[34] Resorting to an intravenous formulation typically obviates this problem. However, even with intravenous dosing, a rightward shift of the dose-response curve is observed between the diuretic concentration in the tubular lumen and its natriuretic effect in HF; in addition, the maximal effect or ceiling is lower. This rightward shift has been termed "diuretic resistance" and can be due to several contributing factors. A point of distinction is that diuretic resistance should be distinguished from "diuretic adaptation" or the "braking" phenomenon that is observed even in normal subjects given multiple doses of a short-acting loop diuretic.[35]

Mechanisms

Diuretic-induced alterations in intrarenal hemodynamics, caused by tubuloglomerular feedback and increased sympathetic nerve activity, among other possible mechanisms (see later), result in avid renal sodium retention by all nephron segments as intraluminal drug levels decline. If dietary salt intake is sufficiently high, as in many Western diets, a daily net negative sodium balance may not be achieved despite several daily intravenous doses of a loop diuretic. These data imply that salt intake must be restricted in normal subjects and particularly in patients with HF to obtain a negative sodium balance. They also indicate that short-acting diuretics, particularly furosemide and bumetanide, must be administered several times per day to obtain consistent daily salt and water loss unless dietary sodium intake is severely restricted.

An alternative strategy in hospitalized patients is to administer the same daily parenteral dose of a loop diuretic by continuous intravenous infusion, which leads to sustained natriuresis because of the continuous presence of high drug levels within the tubular lumen. This approach requires the use of a constant-infusion pump but permits more precise control of the natriuretic effect achieved over time, particularly in carefully monitored patients. It also diminishes the potential for a too rapid decline in intravascular volume and hypotension as well as the risk of ototoxicity in patients given large bolus intravenous doses of a loop diuretic. A typical continuous furosemide infusion is initiated with a 20- to 40-mg intravenous loading dose as a bolus injection, followed by a continuous infusion of 5 to 10 mg/hr for a patient who had been receiving 200 mg of oral furosemide (or 100 mg of intravenous drug) per day in divided doses.

Even in normal subjects with an Na^+-restricted diet, the natriuretic effect of diuretics declines with time; that is, a rightward and downward shift is seen in the sigmoidal concentration-effect relationship as a result of the braking phenomenon. This effect is now known to be due in large part to compensatory hypertrophy of the tubular epithelium distal to the site of action of the $Na^+/K^+/2Cl^-$ cotransporter inhibitor, which increases the solute resorptive capacity of the kidney, as well as other adaptive mechanisms.[36] In this context,

Morsing and colleagues[36] demonstrated that chronic and perhaps even acute treatment with loop diuretics causes rapid (within 60 minutes) upregulation of the thiazide-sensitive Na^+/Cl^- cotransporter in the distal tubule (as measured by increased ^3H-metolazone binding). In addition, many patients with HF manifest some degree of renal impairment, which also shifts the diuretic concentration-effect relationship downward and to the right. Although the maximum effect expressed as the fractional excretion of sodium may be unchanged in patients with some degree of intrinsic renal disease, the absolute natriuretic effect is limited by the reduced filtered load of sodium into the remaining functional nephrons.

The cause of apparent resistance to diuretics in patients who initially achieve an acceptable natriuretic and diuretic response may be multifactorial, as indicated. In the absence of an abrupt decline in cardiac or renal function or noncompliance with either the drug regimen or dietary salt restriction, the usual reason for diuretic resistance is the concurrent administration of other drugs. In this regard, one of the biggest offending classes of agents is nonsteroidal antiinflammatory drugs (NSAIDs), which reduce renal function by decreasing the renal synthesis of vasodilator prostaglandins.[36] The same effects occur with cyclooxygenase-2 inhibitors. All NSAIDs, including aspirin, can diminish diuretic efficacy. Rarely, drugs such as probenecid or high plasma concentrations of some antibiotics may compete with the organic ion transporters in the proximal tubule responsible for the transfer of most diuretics from the recirculation into the tubular lumen.

The use of increasing doses of vasodilators, with or without a marked decline in intravascular volume as a result of concomitant diuretic therapy, is a common cause of diuretic resistance. It is often difficult to distinguish clinically between intravascular volume depletion following aggressive diuretic and vasodilator therapy and a decrease in cardiac output caused by primary HF, although a more marked decline in urea clearance than in creatinine clearance suggests intravascular volume depletion. Pulmonary arterial and venous or left atrial pressure monitoring may be required to make this distinction. In addition, all vasodilators commonly used as afterload-reducing agents in HF dilate a number of central and peripheral vascular beds. Therefore, renal blood flow may be reduced despite an increase in cardiac output, and the effectiveness of the diuretic declines. Vasodilator therapy also may lower renal perfusion pressure below that necessary to maintain normal autoregulation and glomerular filtration in patients with renal artery stenosis from atherosclerotic disease.

Management

Among the vasodilators, RAS antagonists can uniquely augment the effectiveness of diuretics by mechanisms that are independent of their ability to reduce systemic vascular resistance (see later).[38] However, by reducing efferent arteriolar tone, these drugs may also diminish diuretic effectiveness by reducing the transglomerular perfusion pressure to the point that the GFR declines abruptly. This response is most commonly observed in patients with decreased renal arterial perfusion pressure caused either by renal artery stenosis or by limited cardiac output; in these patients, high efferent arteriolar tone mediated by angiotensin II is necessary to maintain glomerular filtration. This cause of diuretic resistance is usually characterized by an abrupt rise in the serum creatinine concentration and should be distinguished from the more common, limited increases in serum creatinine levels that often accompany initiation of ACEI therapy. In addition to ACEIs, the $alpha_1$-adrenergic antagonist prazosin has been shown to have direct tubular action in reducing sodium resorption at doses below those necessary to lower arterial pressure (e.g., 0.50 mg).

With a cardiac output and mean arterial pressure adequate to sustain autoregulation of glomerular filtration, diuretic resistance can be managed by increasing the frequency of loop diuretic dosing or by switching to a continuous intravenous infusion. If this treatment is ineffective, concomitant administration of a more distally acting diuretic, usually an Na^+/Cl^- symport inhibitor (e.g., a thiazide or thiazide-like diuretic such as intravenous chlorothiazide or oral metolazone), usually results in substantial natriuresis.[39] Although effective, this diuretic combination may cause profound intravascular volume depletion, hypotension, renal potassium wasting, hyponatremia, and eventually a fall in cardiac output and GFR. Accordingly, this combination should be used cautiously and with careful monitoring of renal function and serum potassium and sodium, especially in outpatients. A mineralocorticoid receptor antagonist (e.g., spironolactone) may also increase diuretic effectiveness of more proximally acting diuretics, although patients are at increased risk for hyperkalemia if they concomitantly receive another RAAS antagonist. Despite this possibility, most subjects receiving large doses of loop diuretics or loop diuretics plus thiazides benefit from a potassium-sparing diuretic. If tolerated, spironolactone or eplerenone should be the potassium-sparing diuretics used because of their mortality-reducing effects.

In hospitalized patients, dopamine administered at doses that cause selective dopaminergic receptor stimulation may increase renal blood flow and decrease tubular solute resorption (i.e., ≤ 2 μg/kg/min, based on estimated lean body weight). In some subjects, a short-term infusion of nesiritide (human BNP [hBNP]) may be beneficial in improving renal hemodynamics and enhancing the effects of diuretics (see Natriuretic Peptides). In addition, selective V_1 and V_2 vasopressin receptor antagonists, once approved, may individually or in combination increase the efficacy of $Na^+/K^+/2Cl^-$ symporter inhibitors as indicated by experimental animal data and preliminary evidence in humans. Finally, mechanical circulatory support may become necessary in patients with marginal cardiac output for diuretics to be effective, particularly in patients recovering from cardiac surgery or myocarditis or as a "bridge" to transplantation. Discrete renal arterial stenoses that limit renal blood flow and systemic vasodilator therapy may be amenable to percutaneous angioplasty in patients with adequate cardiac output and diuretic resistance from marginal renal perfusion.

Electrolyte and Metabolic Disorders in Heart Failure: Complications of Diuretic Therapy

POTASSIUM HOMEOSTASIS. All of the diuretics discussed in this chapter, with the exceptions of V_2 vasopressin receptor antagonists and hBNP, affect renal K^+ handling.[39] In patients with chronic HF, both hypokalemia caused by K^+-wasting diuretics and hyperkalemia caused by K^+ supplements administered with a K^+-sparing diuretic or an RAS antagonist may contribute to morbidity and mortality. Renal K^+ losses from diuretic use can be exacerbated by the hyperaldosteronism characteristic of patients with untreated HF and by the marked increases in distal nephron Na^+ delivery that follow use of either loop or distal nephron diuretics. The level of dietary salt intake may also contribute to the extent of renal K^+ wasting with diuretics. High-salt diets increase delivery of NaCl to distal tubular K^+ secretory sites, and very low-salt diets may stimulate aldosterone-induced K^+ secretion. Extrarenal regulators of the serum K^+ concentration may also produce effects additive to renal loss of K^+. K^+ is shifted from extra- to intracellular sites after the release of epinephrine in response to stress, myocardial ischemia, pulmonary edema, or the administration of insulin. Long-term infusion of either low-molecular-weight or unfractionated heparin, conversely, reduces aldosterone synthesis and may cause hyperkalemia, particularly in patients with insulin-dependent diabetes and in patients receiving potassium replacement or potassium-sparing drugs, or both.[51] Any beta-agonist or phosphodiesterase inhibitor (PDEI) lowers potassium levels by shifting potassium into skeletal muscle through a beta$_2$-adrenergic or cAMP pathway effect.[40,41]

Despite the absence of conclusive data to determine whether routine administration of K supplements or K-sparing diuretics, or both, reduces serious morbidity or mortality in the treatment of patients with primary hypertension, it is recommended that serum K^+ be maintained between 3.5 and 5.0 mEq/liter.[42] However, for patients with HF, the recommendation is to maintain serum K^+ between 4.3 and 5.0 mEq/liter. One of the reasons for the higher serum K^+ is that subjects with HF are often being treated with agents in which the proarrhythmic effects are exacerbated by hypokalemia, including digoxin, type III antiarrhythmics, beta-agonists, or PDEIs. Because patients with chronic HF are at a much higher risk for malignant ventricular arrhythmias and sudden death than patients with hypertension, it is sound clinical practice to monitor K^+ levels frequently and maintain them well up in the normal range.

If supplementation is necessary, oral K supplements in the form of KCl extended-release tablets or liquid concentrate should be used whenever possible. Intravenous K is potentially hazardous and should be avoided except in emergencies. The routine use of "sliding scales" for intravenous K administration in hospitalized patients is also potentially dangerous and should be discouraged.

OTHER METABOLIC AND ELECTROLYTE DISTURBANCES. Diuretics may be associated with multiple other metabolic and electrolyte disturbances, including hypomagnesemia, hyponatremia, metabolic alkalosis, hyperglycemia, hyperlipidemia, and hyperuricemia.[43] None of these disturbances are limiting in the usual patient with HF. Hypomagnesemia can be caused by both loop and thiazide diuretics, but its detection (because of the poor correlation of total serum magnesium levels with either ionized levels or total-body stores) is difficult and its impact is uncertain. Magnesium replacement should be given for signs or symptoms that could be due to hypomagnesemia (arrhythmias, muscle cramps), and it can be routinely given (with uncertain benefit) to all subjects receiving large doses of diuretics or requiring large amounts of K^+ replacement.

Hyponatremia. This is usually a manifestation of advanced HF with very high degrees of activation of the vasopressin system or inadequate RAS inhibition, or both. Hyponatremia can typically be treated by more stringent water restriction or an increase in RAS inhibition. When V_2 receptor antagonists are available as diuretics, this problem will probably be eliminated.

Metabolic Alkalosis. This complication can generally be treated by increasing KCl supplementation, lowering diuretic doses, or transiently treating with acetazolamide, as discussed earlier. The small level of glucose intolerance or hyperlipidemia produced by thiazide diuretics is not usually clinically important, and blood glucose and lipids should be controlled according to standard guidelines regardless of the presence of any perceived diuretic effect. Hyperuricemia from thiazide diuretics is occasionally a problem and may precipitate gout, particularly in predisposed subjects or in the presence of renal dysfunction. If a thiazide diuretic is absolutely necessary in such patients, allopurinol can be administered to reduce uric acid synthesis.

Vasodilators

Rationale and Mechanism of Action

The rationale for the use of vasodilators grew out of experience with parenteral sympatholytic agents and nitroprusside in patients with severe HF. Cohn and Franciosa, in an influential article in 1977, reviewed the evidence and advocated the use of these drugs in decompensated HF.[44] As originally conceived, the pharmacological rationale for the use of vasodilators in HF was purely hemodynamic and based on the application of Ohm's law to blood flow: flow = $\Delta P/R$, where ΔP is the difference between arterial and venous pressure and R is resistance across the vascular bed. Because systemic vascular resistance is usually increased in HF as a result of neurohormonal activation, vasodilation of resistance vessels increases central cardiac output and flow to some organs. Figure 23–1 illustrates this point: activation of the adrenergic and RAS systems results in multiple effects that are detrimental to the natural history of HF, including vasoconstriction. The hemodynamic consequences of alterations in preload and afterload by vasodilators are shown in Figure 23–2, and the vasodilator profiles of individual agents or classes are given in Table 23–3.

TABLE 23–3 Profile of Various Vasodilator Classes for Producing Venous or Arteriolar Dilation

Class/Compound	Venodilation	Arteriolar Dilation
Nitrovasodilators	+++	+
Direct acting (hydralazine)	+	+++
Flosequinan	++	+++
Calcium channel blockers	+	+++
K^+ channel activators (e.g., diazoxide, minoxidil)	++	+++
Vasodilator prostaglandins (prostacyclin)	+++	++
Natriuretic peptides (BNP)	+++	+
ACEIs, ARBs	++	+

ACEI = angiotensin-converting enzyme inhibitor; ARB = angiotensin receptor blocker; BNP = brain natriuretic peptide.

VENTRICULAR-VASCULAR COUPLING. As described in Chapters 19 and 20, myocardial function is dependent on loading conditions. From the point of view of the ventricles, *afterload* is the force opposing contraction and *preload* is the amount of stretch applied to ventricular myocardium before contraction. Vasodilator-mediated arteriolar relaxation reduces vascular resistance, which is a major component of afterload.[44] From a biomechanical point of view, the circulatory system is defined by *ventricular-vascular coupling*.[45] The force ejecting blood from the ventricle is known as end-systolic elastance, a load-independent measure of contractility, and the force resisting ejection of blood is termed vascular elastance. When end-systolic elastance overcomes vascular elastance, blood is ejected as stroke volume. For a given end-diastolic volume, the major determinants of the size of the stroke volume are the velocity of shortening of ventricular contraction and the amount of vascular elastance.[45] For the left ventricle, systemic vascular resistance is a major component of vascular elastance.[44,45] From these relationships it is clear that stroke volume can be increased by increasing the velocity of shortening (positive inotropic effect) or by decreasing systemic vascular resistance (vasodilator effect) to overcome the abnormal respective decreases and increases in these parameters inherent in HF resulting from systolic dysfunction.

EFFECTS ON DIFFERENT VASCULAR BEDS. An important aspect of vasodilator use in chronic HF is that the potential exists to affect different types of vascular beds. The original concept of vasodilator use was based on small arteriolar dilation because this is the biggest contribution to systemic vascular resistance. However, perhaps even more important is the ability of certain classes of agents to effect venodilation of "capacitance" vessels. This effect reduces venous return by enlarging the effective blood volume reservoir and therefore reduces end-diastolic, pulmonary, and systemic venous pressures. The clinical consequence of this reduction in preload is to reduce pulmonary and hepatic congestion and, more important, diastolic wall stress. As described in Chapter 21, increased wall stress is a major signaling pathway for hypertrophy and other changes in gene expression that are important in producing the dilated cardiomyopathy phenotype of ventricular dilatation and systolic dysfunction. Because a chronically failing heart is usually operating on a flat portion of the preload-performance relationship (see Fig. 23–2), pharmacological reduction in preload does not ordinarily reduce cardiac output in that setting, but it may do so in acute situations.

Studies of vasodilators in the 1980s demonstrated that they were well tolerated and effective in improving symptoms in patients with HF. These short-term trials eventually led to the first mortality-based clinical trial in chronic HF, the Vasodilator HF Trial (V-HeFT-I).[46] V-HeFT-I was a comparison of the alpha$_1$-adrenergic receptor blocking agent prazosin, the combination of isosorbide dinitrate and hydralazine, and placebo for their effects on total mortality.[47] In this trial, prazosin was not different from placebo, but isosorbide dinitrate–hydralazine reduced mortality at 2 years by 34 percent ($p < 0.03$) but did not reduce mortality over the entire period of follow-up by the log-rank test ($p = 0.09$). On the basis of these statistically marginal results (because of a relatively underpowered sample size as opposed to an inadequate effect size), the Food and Drug Administration (FDA) has not approved the hydralazine–isosorbide dinitrate combination for the treatment of HF.

V-HeFT-I introduced the idea that the natural history of HF could be favorably influenced by medical therapy, and it also provided strong support to the vasodilator approach to treating HF. However, subsequent clinical trials with "pure" vasodilating agents (i.e., those that are not also neurohumoral inhibitors) have not demonstrated a reduction in mortality, and, in fact, the powerful vasodilators flosequinan[48] and epoprostenol[49] markedly (by respective values of 43 and 29 percent) *increased mortality* despite salutary effects on exercise tolerance in earlier, smaller studies. Therefore, vasodilation per se is not a particularly effective method for improving the natural history of chronic HF, but it is an important strategy for dealing with acute, decompensated HF.

Nitrovasodilators

Despite the fact that nitrovasodilators are among the oldest vasodilators in common clinical practice, the cellular mechanisms by which these drugs lead to the relaxation of vascular smooth muscle have only become apparent since 1990. It is now understood that these drugs mimic the activity of nitric oxide and its congeners. These autocrine and paracrine signaling autacoids are formed in endothelial and smooth muscle cells throughout the vasculature as well as in many other cell types, including cardiac muscle cells (see also Chap. 19).[50,51] Nitrogen oxides were originally identified as the bioactive factor (endothelium-derived relaxing factor [EDRF]) responsible for endothelium-dependent relaxation of blood vessels. Their primary mechanism of action in vascular smooth muscle cells is based on their ability to bind to a heme moiety in soluble guanylyl cyclase, with a subsequent increase in intracellular cyclic guanosine monophosphate. The pharmacological activity of each of the nitrovasodilators depends on their biotransformation into nitrogen oxides within the blood and vascular tissue.[50]

Organic Nitrates

The organic nitrates are powerful venodilators and mild arteriolar vasodilators and produce the most extensive epicardial coronary vasodilation of any class of vasodilator. Because of their relatively selective vasodilating effects on the epicardial coronary vasculature, organic nitrates may directly increase systolic and diastolic ventricular function by improving coronary blood flow in patients with ischemic cardiomyopathy, in addition to their activity in reducing ventricular filling pressure, wall stress, and myocardial oxygen consumption.[52] In acute myocardial infarction, however, the effect of the routine use of nitrovasodilators on mortality remains controversial.

Experience with the newer nitrovasodilators, including isosorbide mononitrate, in the treatment of HF, is limited in comparison with their use in the treatment of angina. The spectrum of activity of 5-isosorbide mononitrate would not be expected to differ from that of isosorbide dinitrate in HF. Although isosorbide mononitrate's greater bioavailability and longer elimination half-life may provide a convenient pharmacokinetic profile, only isosorbide dinitrate among the nitrate formulations has been shown to increase exercise tolerance[53] and, in combination with hydralazine, may have prolonged survival in patients with HF.[46]

Although it has never been approved for this purpose by the FDA, intravenous nitroglycerin or glyceryl trinitrate (TNG) is widely used to lower filling pressures and increase cardiac output in decompensated HF. When administered at doses ranging from 10 to 100 μg/min intravenously, TNG is effective in this regard (Fig. 23–5)[54] and in particular should be considered when there is any question of active myocardial ischemia. The main problem with longer term (>24 hours) use of organic nitrates is the development of tolerance (see Chap. 50).

Most of the data on the efficacy of intermittent versus continuous NTG have been obtained in patients with angina rather than chronic congestive HF.[55] Indeed, it is somewhat controversial whether patients with HF should be exposed to a long nitrate-free period. Nevertheless, it seems prudent to recommend nitrate-free intervals in patients receiving chronic doses of isosorbide dinitrate, which can usually be achieved by providing the last dose of isosorbide dinitrate in the early evening. In addition, there is some evidence that the simultaneous administration of hydralazine (see later) can attenuate nitrate tolerance.[56]

Nitroprusside

Intravenous nitroprusside is an effective venous and arterial vasodilator that acts to reduce both ventricular preload and afterload. Because of the fact that it is quickly metabolized to cyanide and nitric oxide, its onset of action is rapid and upward titration can usually be achieved expeditiously to produce an optimal and predictable hemodynamic effect. For these reasons, nitroprusside is commonly used in intensive care settings for the management of acutely decompensated

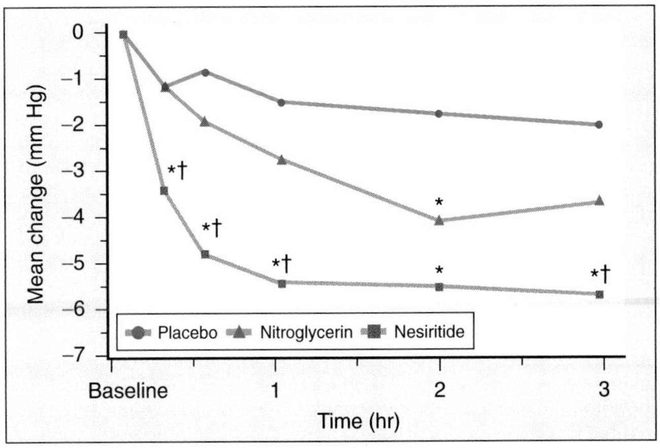

FIGURE 23–5 Changes from baseline in pulmonary capillary wedge pressure in patients in decompensated heart failure treated with placebo, nitroglycerin, or nesiritide. (From Publication Committee for the VMAC Investigators: Intravenous nesiritide vs nitroglycerin for treatment of decompensated congestive heart failure. A randomized controlled trial. JAMA 287:1531, 2002.)

HF when blood pressure is adequate to maintain cerebral, coronary, and renal perfusion. Nitroprusside has balanced effects on afterload and preload, and ventricular filling pressures are rapidly reduced by an increase in venous compliance.[57]

Nitroprusside is among the most effective afterload-reducing agents because of its spectrum of vasodilating activity on different vascular beds. It reduces systemic vascular resistance, increases aortic wall compliance, and, at optimal doses, improves ventricular-vascular coupling. Nitroprusside also decreases pulmonary vascular resistance and improves other components of right ventricular afterload, including the amplitude and timing of reflected pressure waves during ejection.[58]

Nitroprusside should not be used in active ischemia because its powerful intramyocardial afterload-reducing effects may "steal" coronary blood flow from segments of myocardium supplied by epicardial vessels with high-grade lesions. This phenomenon is probably the reason why nitroprusside increased mortality in a study of acute myocardial infarction.[59] In the setting of ischemia, any indicated vasodilator therapy should be delivered by organic nitrates, which are less powerful intramyocardial afterload-reducing agents than nitroprusside and which produce greater epicardial vasodilation.

"Directly Acting" and Other Vasodilators

HYDRALAZINE

Hydralazine, an effective afterload-reducing agent whose cellular mechanism of action remains poorly understood, is best used in chronic HF when combined with isosorbide dinitrate to provide more effective venodilation.[46] This combination produces a more balanced form of vasodilation; in addition, some evidence indicates that hydralazine can attenuate nitrate tolerance by acting as a reducing agent.[56] In HF, hydralazine reduces right and LV afterload by reducing systemic as well as pulmonary artery input impedance and vascular resistance.[60] Unlike the results when hydralazine is used to treat hypertension, the reduction in afterload is usually accompanied by only minor reflex increases in sympathetic nervous system activity, unless symptomatic hypotension occurs. These hemodynamic changes result in an increase in forward stroke volume and reductions in ventricular systolic wall stress and the regurgitant fraction in mitral or aortic regurgitation. Hydralazine's effect on regional blood flow consists of an increase in renal and skeletal muscle blood flow.[61]

One of the problems with the use of hydralazine is its short half-life, which necessitates dosing four times daily. In addition, side effects that may necessitate dose adjustment or withdrawal of hydralazine therapy are common. For example, in V-HeFT-I,[46] 20 percent of patients complained of symptoms that could have been related to hydralazine. The most common complaints—headache and dizziness—could also have been due to the concomitantly administered nitrates. However, with time, the symptoms diminish or respond to a reduction in dose.

Hydralazine metabolism is primarily through hepatic acetylation, although many additional potential metabolic pathways have been described.[62] Therefore, patients with a "slow acetylator" phenotype have a prolonged elimination half-life of the drug. At the usual doses and dosing intervals of hydralazine, these patients are at greater risk for arthritis or other components of a lupus-like syndrome.

Because of the somewhat equivocal results obtained with hydralazine-isosorbide dinitrate in V-HeFT-I[46] and the superiority of the ACEI enalapril to this combination in V-HeFT-II,[63] hydralazine-isosorbide dinitrate is reserved for subjects who cannot tolerate ACEIs or who have need for additional afterload reduction (blood pressure remaining high normal or greater in the presence of full-dose ACE inhibition). Another potential use for hydralazine-isosorbide dinitrate is in American blacks, who in V-HeFT-II had better clinical responses to the combination than to enalapril.[64] A trial evaluating the effects of combination therapy with nitrates and hydralazine in African American patients (A-HeFT) is being conducted.

Natriuretic Peptides

The contribution of the natriuretic peptides ANP, BNP, and related proteins, including urodilatin and fragments of the pro-ANP protein, to the physiological adaptations that accompany HF and their potential role in pharmacotherapy for this syndrome have been the subject of intensive research efforts by cardiovascular and renal pharmacologists for more than a decade.[65] Apart from C-type natriuretic peptide, which is synthesized in endothelial (and other) cells in a number of organs and tissues and has limited natriuretic activity, plasma levels of these peptides are increased in most patients with HF (see Chap. 21) and exhibit both vasodilator effects and a direct natriuretic effect on the kidney.[66]

The natriuretic peptides act at both particulate (i.e., membrane-bound) guanylyl cyclase–linked (GC-A and GC-B or NPR-A [natriuretic peptide receptor A] and NPR-B) receptors and so-called clearance receptors (NPR-C) that are linked through inhibitory GTP-binding proteins to adenylyl cyclase or through stimulatory GTP-binding proteins to phospholipase C. Aside from actions that indirectly affect renal function, such as inhibition of AVP release by the pituitary, inhibition of aldosterone synthesis by adrenal zona glomerulosa cells, sympathoinhibitory effects, and relaxant effects on systemic vascular resistance and venous capacitance, natriuretic peptides directly affect renal solute and water homeostasis. Acting predominantly through guanylyl cyclase (GC-A and GC-B)–linked receptors, natriuretic peptides alter the hemodynamic forces regulating glomerular filtration and tubular Na^+ resorption, particularly in the distal nephron.

Infusions of ANP have been shown to cause afferent arteriolar dilation and efferent arteriolar constriction, which results in an increase in GFR.[5] Even when infused at concentrations that do not affect the GFR, ANP induces natriuresis by inhibiting the resorptive capacity of the proximal tubular epithelium largely by inhibiting the actions of locally acting antinatriuretic agents such as angiotensin II and by augmenting the activity of intrarenal dopamine. In the distal nephron, particularly in the medullary portion of the collecting duct, there is evidence that natriuretic peptides, acting through GC-A receptors, decrease Na^+ influx from the tubular lumen through amiloride-sensitive epithelial Na^+ channels. The result is a natriuresis with minimal effect on urinary potassium excretion. ANP, which is likewise synthesized and released by vascular endothelial cells,[67] may also be important in regulating blood pressure, particularly during physiological stress. For example, the blood pressure of mice that have had their pro-ANP gene disrupted by gene-targeting techniques—and therefore have no detectable circulating ANP—is very sensitive to dietary salt intake.[68] Little evidence has been presented for any clinically significant direct effect of ANP[69] or BNP on ventricular function.

Nesiritide (Human Brain Natriuretic Peptide)

Although ANP has a favorable pharmacological profile in HF, therapeutic trials with ANP have been disappointing because of its short biological half-life, end-organ resistance, the development of pharmacological tolerance, and undesirable hemodynamic effects.[70] Results with BNP have been much more promising.[71-73] When infused continuously into patients with HF, recombinant hBNP (nesiritide) produced vasodilator and cardiac output–increasing effects.[54,71-74] The vasodilation was not accompanied by neurohormonal activation, apparently because of sympathoinhibition.[75] Although BNP was natriuretic and diuretic in one study,[71] in another study, approximately half of the subjects were resistant to the natriuretic effects of BNP.[72] In clinical trials involving patients hospitalized for decompensated HF, nesiritide has been shown to improve hemodynamics and clinical status.[54,73,74] Moreover, nesiritide is less arrhythmogenic than dobutamine.[76] Compared with intravenous nitroglycerin, when administered at a dose of 2 μg/kg as a bolus followed by an infusion of 0.01 μg/kg/min, nesiritide produced faster relief of dyspneic symptoms and quicker reductions in elevated pulmonary capillary wedge pressure (see Fig. 23–5).[54]

Another approach to the use of natriuretic peptides is to deliver them subcutaneously, whereby they could then be used to treat chronic HF. This approach works in animal models of HF,[77] and initial studies in humans are promising.[78]

NEUTRAL ENDOPEPTIDASE INHIBITORS

Because receptor-mediated clearance and metabolism by the zinc metallopeptidase neutral endopeptidase (NEP) are the two predominant mechanisms for natriuretic peptide inactivation and removal, two approaches have been taken to lengthening the biological half-life of endogenous and exogenously infused natriuretic peptides.[79] Analogs of ANP have been developed that bind to ANP-R_2 receptors with high affinity but exhibit little biological activity. Several classes of NEP inhibitors have also been developed that alone or in combination with ANP-R_2 antagonists induce natriuresis and delay the clearance of exogenously infused ANP. NEP antagonists have been shown to increase plasma ANP levels and induce natriuresis with little effect on potassium excretion in patients with HF. However, in limited clinical trials in patients with HF, NEP inhibitors had relatively little efficacy.[80]

NEUTRAL ENDOPEPTIDASE–ANGIOTENSIN-CONVERTING ENZYME (VASOPEPTIDASE) INHIBITION

The combination of an NEP antagonist with an ACEI has been shown to result in more sustained natriuretic effects than an NEP antagonist alone in experimental animal models of HF, in part because of the inhibition of angiotensin II–mediated effects but also because of the fact that both NEP and ACE degrade bradykinin, a vasodilatory and natriuretic peptide.[81]

There is some evidence that ACE inhibition in HF patients may favorably affect the release or clearance, or both, of endogenous ANP, but not BNP, by resetting the relationship between ANP levels and atrial pressure.[82] With these actions in mind, single agents with dual metalloproteinase inhibitor activity (i.e., NEP and ACE inhibition) have been developed that address the mechanisms contributing to both pharmacological tolerance and end-organ resistance to natriuretic peptides in HF.[84] Indeed, both renal (natriuresis) and humoral (decrease in renin) responses to omapatrilat are superior to those to an ACEI in subjects with HF.[83] When omapatrilat was compared with the ACEI lisinopril in two phase II trials, the results were quite promising.[84] Unfortunately, large clinical trials with omapatrilat in HF have failed to demonstrate a clear benefit of NEP-ACE inhibition over ACE inhibition alone.[85] In addition, omapatrilat was associated with a slightly higher incidence of angioedema than enalapril alone.[86]

CALCIUM ANTAGONISTS

Although all three classes of calcium channel antagonists (i.e., phenylalkylamines such as verapamil, benzothiazepines such as diltiazem, and dihydropyridines such as nifedipine, nitrendipine, felodipine, nicardipine, isradipine, or amlodipine) are effective arteriolar vasodilators, none has been shown to produce sustained improvement in symptoms or natural history in patients with HF with predominant systolic ventricular dysfunction. Indeed, some of these agents appear to worsen symptoms and may increase mortality in patients with systolic dysfunction.[86] The reason for these adverse effects or lack of efficacy of calcium channel blockers in HF is unclear. It may be related to the known negative inotropic effects of these drugs, to reflex neurohumoral activation, or a combination of these and other effects.

Second-generation calcium channel antagonists of the dihydropyridine class, such as amlodipine, nicardipine, and felodipine, have fewer negatively inotropic effects than earlier drugs of this class as a result of their higher degrees of vasoselectivity. All three have been evaluated in medium- or large-scale randomized trials,[83–88] where they have not shown efficacy but have had acceptable adverse event profiles. Therefore, highly vasoselective dihydropyridine calcium antagonists can be used in patients with ischemic cardiomyopathy to treat angina that is uncontrolled by beta blockers and nitrates.

Positive Inotropic Agents

Cardiac Glycosides

Cardiac glycosides are used to treat chronic HF in patients in sinus rhythm and to control the response of the ventricular rate to supraventricular arrhythmias, including atrial fibrillation.[89] Digoxin is the most commonly prescribed cardiac glycoside because of its convenient pharmacokinetics, alternative routes of administration, and the widespread availability of serum drug level measurements.

Mechanisms of Action

Digoxin is a complex agent in that its mode of action, inhibition of Na^+,K^+-ATPase, affects multiple cellular processes, including several critical to cardiac myocyte function (see Chap. 19).[89] Digoxin is also extremely toxic, not surprising in view of its apparent role in nature as a toxin evolved by plants to kill mammals. Cardiac glycosides bind to a specific high-affinity site on the extracytoplasmic face of the alpha subunit of Na^+,K^+-ATPase, the enzymatic equivalent of the cellular "sodium pump."[89] The affinity of the subunit for cardiac glycosides varies among species and among the three known mammalian subunit isoforms, each of which is encoded by a separate gene.[89]

Cardiac glycoside binding to and inhibition of the Na^+,K^+-ATPase sodium pump are reversible and entropically driven. Under physiological conditions, these drugs preferentially bind to the enzyme after phosphorylation of a beta-aspartate on the cytoplasmic face of the alpha subunit, thus stabilizing what is known as the E_2P conformation.[89,90] Extracellular K^+ promotes dephosphorylation at this site, resulting in a decrease in the cardiac glycoside binding affinity for the enzyme.[90] This action presumably explains why increased extracellular K^+ tends to reverse some manifestations of digitalis toxicity.

POSITIVE INOTROPIC EFFECT. Cardiac glycosides increase the velocity and extent of shortening of cardiac muscle, thereby resulting in an upward and leftward shift of the ventricular function curve (Frank-Starling) relating cardiac performance to filling volume or pressure (see Fig. 23–2). This process occurs in normal as well as failing myocardium and in atrial as well as ventricular muscle. The effect appears to be sustained for periods of weeks or months without evidence of desensitization or tolerance.[91]

The positive inotropic effect is due to an increase in the availability of cytosolic Ca^{2+} during systole, thus increasing the velocity and extent of sarcomere shortening. The increase in intracellular $[Ca^{2+}]$ is a consequence of cardiac glycoside–induced inhibition of sarcolemmal Na^+,K^+-ATPase.[89,90] Inhibition of Na^+,K^+-ATPase causes an increase in intracellular Na^+, which is then exchanged for extracellular Ca^{2+} through the Na^+/Ca^{2+} exchanger.[92] The net effect of these adjustments is to increase intracellular Ca^{2+} during systole, which increases systolic function.

In part because cardiac glycosides produce an increase in contractile function without increasing the heart rate, the positive inotropic effects are more energetically efficient than the effects of beta-adrenergic agonists and higher doses of PDEIs.[93] This difference may be one of the reasons why low-dose digoxin does not increase mortality in patients with HF.[92]

ANTIADRENERGIC PROPERTIES. Na^+,K^+-ATPase is involved in baroreflex afferent signaling and may be upregulated in the carotid sinus in HF.[94] Decreased baroreflex control is one of the mechanisms responsible for an increase in generalized and cardiac[95] adrenergic activity in HF. Inhibition of Na^+,K^+-ATPase by ouabain modulates baroreflex function toward normal in animal models of HF,[94] which is likely to be the mechanism by which cardiac glycosides inhibit adrenergic activity in HF.

ELECTROPHYSIOLOGICAL ACTIONS. Cardiac glycosides have complex electrophysiological effects that are a combination of indirect, parasympathetic, and direct effects on specialized cardiac pacemaker and conduction tissues.[96] At low to moderate therapeutic serum concentrations (0.5 to 1.9 ng/ml), digoxin usually decreases automaticity and increases maximal diastolic resting membrane potential in atrial and atrioventricular (AV) nodal cells as a result of augmented vagal tone and decreased sympathetic nervous system activity. These effects are accompanied by prolongation of the effective refractory period and decreased AV nodal conduction velocity. At higher, toxic digoxin levels or in the presence of underlying disease, patients are susceptible to sinus bradycardia or arrest, prolongation of AV conduction, or heart block. At toxic levels, cardiac glycosides can also increase sympathetic nervous system activity, potentially contributing to the generation of arrhythmias.

Increased intracellular Ca^{2+} loading and increased sympathetic tone both contribute to an increased rate of spontaneous (phase 4) diastolic depolarization and also to delayed afterdepolarizations that may reach threshold and generate propagated action potentials. The combination of increased automaticity and depressed conduction in the His-Purkinje network predisposes to arrhythmias, including ventricular tachycardia and fibrillation. Data from the Digitalis Investigation Group (DIG) Trial[97] suggest that the increase in ventricular arrhythmia manifested in chronic HF as an increase in sudden death extends down to digoxin serum levels of 1.0 ng/ml, inasmuch as higher concentrations were associated with an increase in mortality.

Clinical Observations

Despite the use of cardiac glycosides for more than 200 years in the treatment of HF, the debate over their use in chronic HF continues. Small and medium-sized trials conducted in the 1970s and 1980s yielded equivocal results. However, in the early 1990s, two relatively large digoxin withdrawal studies, the Randomized Assessment of Digoxin and Inhibitors of Angiotensin-Converting Enzyme (RADIANCE)[98,99] and the Prospective Randomized Study of Ventricular Function and Efficacy of Digoxin (PROVED),[99,100] provided strong support for clinical benefit from digoxin. In these studies,[98-100] worsening HF and HF hospitalizations developed in more patients withdrawn from digoxin to placebo treatment than patients maintained with a therapeutic regimen of digoxin. However, because withdrawal studies are difficult to interpret, a large placebo-controlled mortality trial, the DIG trial, was conducted.[92]

The DIG trial had all-cause mortality as its primary endpoint and had secondary endpoints of hospitalization and worsening HF.[92] This trial enrolled 6800 patients with Classes I to III HF with an average LV ejection fraction of 28 percent, and patients were monitored for an average of 37 months. Remarkably, the DIG trial finished with a relative risk ratio of 1.00 (confidence intervals of 0.91 and 1.07, $p = 0.80$), which indicates that at the doses (0.125 to 0.375 mg/d, with 70 percent receiving 0.25 mg/d) and serum levels of digoxin studied, this positive inotropic agent does *not* increase mortality in chronic HF. The data indicated a strong trend ($p = 0.06$) toward a decrease in deaths assigned to a progressive pump failure etiology, balanced by an increase in sudden and other non–pump failure cardiac deaths ($p = 0.04$).[92] The number of patients hospitalized was statistically significantly reduced (by 4 percent) by digoxin therapy, and the total number of hospitalizations per subject was significantly reduced by 6 percent.[93] Therefore, evidence of efficacy was seen in the DIG trial, but in view of its large size and power, this evidence is modest.

One of the most important findings to emerge from the DIG trial was that mortality was directly related to the digoxin serum level.[97] In addition, data from other studies have demonstrated that the beneficial effects of digoxin on ventricular function[101] and neurohormonal activation[101,102] occur at the "safe" lower serum levels of 0.5 to 1.0 ng/ml. Moreover, in men in the DIG trial, trough levels between 0.6 and 0.8 ng/ml actually reduced mortality.[97] This information means that if digoxin is used in subjects with HF, *trough levels should be kept between 0.5 and 1.0 ng/ml.*

Overall, clinical trial results support the routine use of digoxin in patients in sinus rhythm who have mild to moderate HF, which is why most HF practice guidelines recommend the use of digoxin. Because the DIG trial,[92] as well as RADIANCE[98] and PROVED,[100] were conducted in patients with Class II to III (stage 2) HF, no firm recommendation is possible for patients with more advanced HF in sinus rhythm. In addition, digoxin is indicated in all patients with HF with atrial fibrillation in whom ventricular response slowing is required. However, in both the sinus rhythm and atrial fibrillation settings, digoxin must be used in such a way as to avoid overt toxicity or an increase in sudden death without obvious toxicity. There is some evidence that digoxin is less efficacious in women than men,[103] but this is probably based on higher serum levels and more toxicity in the former when patients in the DIG trial were prescribed doses on the basis of a nomogram rather than trough levels. Although the numbers were too small to derive statistical significance in the DIG trial, women exhibited a trend for higher (>1.0 ng/ml) levels to be associated with increased mortality and lower levels for lower mortality than in placebo-treated patients.[97]

Pharmacokinetics and Dosing

Orally administered digoxin is variably absorbed, depending on the preparation, but Lanoxin is 60 to 80 percent absorbed. Digoxin is approximately 25 percent protein bound in plasma, has a large volume of distribution (4 to 7 liter/kg), and crosses both the blood-brain barrier and the placenta. Digoxin is eliminated primarily by renal mechanisms, both glomerular filtration and tubular secretion. Tubular excretion is through the energy-dependent membrane-bound efflux pump/transport enzyme, P-glycoprotein, which is modulated by many other drugs. Digoxin is largely excreted in the urine unchanged with a clearance rate proportional to the GFR, which results in the excretion of approximately one-third of body stores daily. The half-life for digoxin elimination of 36 to 48 hours in patients with normal or near-normal renal function permits once-daily or every-other-day dosing.[104]

In the presence of an elevated blood urea nitrogen/creatinine ratio (i.e., "prerenal azotemia"), digoxin clearance more closely parallels urea clearance, indicating that under these circumstances some of the drug filtered through the glomerulus undergoes tubular reabsorption.[104] In patients with HF, increased cardiac output and renal blood flow in response to treatment with vasodilators or sympathomimetic agents may increase renal digoxin clearance and necessitate dosage adjustment.

Digoxin can be loaded at a dose of 0.75 to 1.25 mg orally (or intravenously at doses 25 percent lower) over a 24-hour period in three to four divided doses and then given at a maintenance dose, or a daily maintenance dose of 0.0625 to 0.25 mg/d orally can be started, depending on renal function, body size, and the presence or absence of coadministered drugs causing pharmacokinetic interactions. In the absence of loading doses, nearly steady-state blood levels are achieved in four to five half-lives, or about 1 week after initiation of maintenance therapy if normal renal function is present. If given intravenously, administration should be carried out over at least 15 minutes to avoid vasoconstrictor responses to a more rapid injection. Intramuscular digoxin is absorbed unpredictably, causes local pain, and is not recommended.

Patients with HF usually have a reduced volume of distribution and reduced renal function, and both may be influenced by other treatment and by the ebb and flow of the HF. Although nomograms on digoxin dosing have been published, these nomograms should not be used in patients with HF because of the narrow therapeutic index and the unpredictability of the numerous factors that can alter digoxin pharmacokinetics. Instead, patients should be started on a dose as just described and trough levels (see later) measured 1 to 2 weeks later and at frequent intervals (every 1 to 3 months) thereafter.

DRUG INTERACTIONS WITH DIGOXIN. Multiple drugs interact with digoxin at multiple levels, including reduced renal tubular excretion by drugs inhibiting P-glycoprotein renal tubular transport,[105] induction of gut P-glycoprotein,[106] alterations in gut flora by antibiotics causing less gut metabolism of digoxin before absorption, displacement from plasma protein-binding sites, or reduction in renal function. A partial list of these interactions is given in Table 23–4. Among these interactions are drugs that are routinely used in patients with HF, including carvedilol and amiodarone, in whose presence digoxin doses should be lowered.

TABLE 23–4 Partial List of Drugs Interacting with Digoxin

Drug	Effect on Serum Digoxin Level	Mechanism
Amiodarone	Increases	? ↓ Renal clearance
Verapamil	Increases	↓ Renal clearance
Nifedipine	Increases	↓ Renal clearance
Diltiazem	Increases	↓ Renal clearance
Quinidine	Increases	Displacement of protein binding, ↓ renal clearance
Propafenone	Increases	↓ Renal clearance
Captopril	? Increases	? Renal clearance
Carvedilol	Increases	↑ Oral bioavailability
Spironolactone	Increases	↓ Renal clearance
Amiloride	Increases	↓ Renal clearance
Triamterene	Increases	↓ Renal clearance
Salbutamol	Decreases	Unknown
Macrolide antibiotics (erythromycin, clarithromycin)	Increases	Altered gut flora, ↓ renal clearance
Tetracycline	Increases	Altered gut flora
Indomethacin	Increases	↓ Renal clearance
Alprazolam	Increases	? ↓ Renal clearance
Itraconazole	Increases	↓ Renal clearance
Rifampin	Decreases	Induction of gut P-glycoprotein
Sucralfate	Decreases	Decreased gut absorption
Cholestyramine	Decreases	Decreased gut absorption
Cyclosporine	Increases	↓ Renal clearance
St. John's wort	Increases	↓ Renal clearance

THERAPEUTIC DRUG MONITORING

Digoxin has an extremely low therapeutic index, and its use should be carefully monitored by serum blood levels. The various clinical conditions and drug interactions that can alter digoxin's pharmacokinetics are also reflected in the serum digoxin level. As discussed earlier, on the basis of the dose range of the positive inotropic effects,[101] the neurohormonal inhibition effects,[102] and the DIG trial mortality data,[97] the optimal trough digoxin serum level is 0.5 to 1.0 ng/ml. This concentration range is also the one that should be used to control the ventricular rate response to atrial fibrillation in patients with HF, particularly because digoxin is not a very effective agent in this regard in the setting of high amounts of adrenergic activity.[107] Blood samples for measurement of serum digoxin levels should be taken at least 6 to 8 hours following the last digoxin dose, and patients should be instructed to take their digoxin in the evening so that any level determined during the day is a trough measurement.

DIGITALIS TOXICITY

In patients with HF, overt clinical toxicity tends to emerge at serum concentrations greater than 2.0 ng/ml, but substantial overlap in serum levels exists among patients exhibiting symptoms and signs of toxicity and those with no clinical evidence of intoxication. Disturbances in cardiac impulse formation, conduction, or both are the hallmarks of digitalis toxicity. Among the common electrocardiographic manifestations are ectopic beats of AV junctional or ventricular origin, first-degree AV block, an excessively slow ventricular rate response to atrial fibrillation, or an accelerated AV junctional pacemaker. These manifestations may require only dosage adjustment and monitoring. Sinus bradycardia, sinoatrial arrest or exit block, and second- or third-degree AV conduction delay often respond to atropine, but temporary ventricular pacing is sometimes necessary and should be available.

MANAGEMENT. Oral potassium administration is often useful for atrial, AV junctional, or ventricular ectopic rhythms, even when the serum potassium is in the normal range, unless high-grade AV block is also present. However, [K^+] must be monitored carefully to avoid hyperkalemia, especially in patients with renal failure. Magnesium may be useful in patients with atrial fibrillation in an accessory pathway in whom digoxin administration has facilitated a rapid accessory pathway-mediated ventricular response; again, careful monitoring is required to avoid hypermagnesemia.[108] Neurological or gastrointestinal complaints can also be manifestations of digitalis toxicity. Occasionally, gynecomastia results from digoxin administration, apparently because of the similarity of the glycoside structure to that of estrogens.

ANTIDIGOXIN IMMUNOTHERAPY. Potentially life-threatening digoxin or digitoxin toxicity can be reversed by antidigoxin immunotherapy. Purified Fab fragments from digoxin-specific antisera are available at most poison control centers and larger hospitals in North America and Europe. Clinical experience in adults and children has established the effectiveness and safety of antidigoxin Fab in treating life-threatening digoxin toxicity, including cases of massive ingestion with suicidal intent.[109] Doses of Fab are calculated by using a simple formula based on either the estimated dose of drug ingested or the total-body digoxin burden and are administered intravenously in saline over a period of 30 to 60 minutes.

Adrenergic Agonists

Mechanism of Action

The most powerful way to increase contractility in the human heart is by the use of a beta-adrenergic receptor agonist. Beta-agonists operate through the mechanism that regulates contractility and heart rate on a beat-to-beat basis in the intact heart (see also Chap. 19).[110] As depicted in Figure 23–6, this system is composed of two cell surface membrane receptors ($beta_1$ and $beta_2$); two G proteins (the stimulatory G protein, $G_{\alpha s}$, and the inhibitory G protein, $G_{\alpha i}$); the adenylyl cyclase enzyme (which converts Mg-ATP to cAMP); cAMP-activated protein kinase (protein kinase A); compartmentalized phosphodiesterases, which modulate cAMP levels to produce selective signaling; and target structures whose phosphorylation leads to a positive inotropic effect by changes in Ca^{2+} handling (phospholamban, the ryanodine release channel, and slow inward current calcium channels). An important point in the function of beta-adrenergic pathways is that they are not all cAMP dependent[110]; in Figure 23–6 the $beta_1$ receptor is depicted with direct activation of voltage-sensitive Ca^{2+} channels as well as cAMP-dependent activation. The end result is a powerful positive inotropic as well as positive chronotropic effect.

In the failing human heart, beta-adrenergic pathways undergo *desensitization*, a pharmacological term encompassing the regulatory changes that occur in receptors, G proteins, and adenylyl cyclase.[111,112] In advanced HF, the degree of beta-adrenergic receptor desensitization approaches 50 to 60 percent of the maximum capacity of signal transduction,[113,114] and in severe HF, beta-agonists may no longer be able to support myocardial function.[115] However, the vast majority of patients with advanced HF still exhibit a substantial inotropic response to beta-agonists,[114] which is the basis for their usefulness as inotropic agents in the treatment of decompensated HF.

All beta-agonists are given intravenously for short-term support of decompensated HF. They are all arrhythmogenic to some extent through direct mechanisms as well as through increasing the skeletal muscle deposition of potassium[40] and decreasing serum magnesium. Their administration should be carefully monitored and the lowest possible effective doses used. In addition, all beta-agonists are subject to the development of desensitization phenomena when used continuously, another reason to keep the doses low and use short term or intermittently. Beta-agonists all have short (in minutes) half-lives, which is an advantage for powerful inotropes that may have adverse effects. As shown in Table 23–5,[116,117] from a therapeutic standpoint, it is important to understand how beta-agonists differ from one another with respect to intrinsic activity; affinity for binding to $beta_1$, $beta_2$, and $alpha_1$ receptors; and affinity for the cardiac adrenergic neuronal reuptake system ($uptake_1$). Neuronal reuptake is an important consideration in the heart, which has the most active $uptake_1$ system of any organ and uses neuronal reuptake to terminate the majority of the action of released norepinephrine.

Although $beta_1$- and $beta_2$-adrenergic receptors are coupled to positive inotropic and chronotropic responses through cAMP-dependent and -independent mechanisms, these two receptors have important differences. For one thing, $beta_1$ receptors are positioned inside or near the synaptic cleft area to mediate the effects of released norepinephrine, which also means that catecholamines that have high affinity for neuronal reuptake do not reach myocardial $beta_1$ receptors unless neuronal reuptake is functionally decreased (as it is in myocardial failure) or absent (as it is in a recently [<2 years] transplanted heart). In addition, a growing body of evidence indicates that chronic $beta_1$ receptor agonist occupancy or pathway activation, or both, is more deleterious than $beta_2$ receptor activation.[110,118] However, from an acute support standpoint, both receptors can be used in supporting cardiac function in decompensated patients.

NEURONAL REUPTAKE AFFINITIES FOR SYMPATHOMIMETIC AMINES. Table 23–5 lists the adrenergic receptor and neuronal reuptake ($uptake_1$) affinities for catecholamines that are used therapeutically to increase cardiac performance or increase systemic vascular resistance or blood pressure. Although the primary action of $uptake_1$ is to terminate the action of norepinephrine, the functional status of $uptake_1$ is also an important determinant of catecholamine therapeutic action when these agents are administered exogenously. For

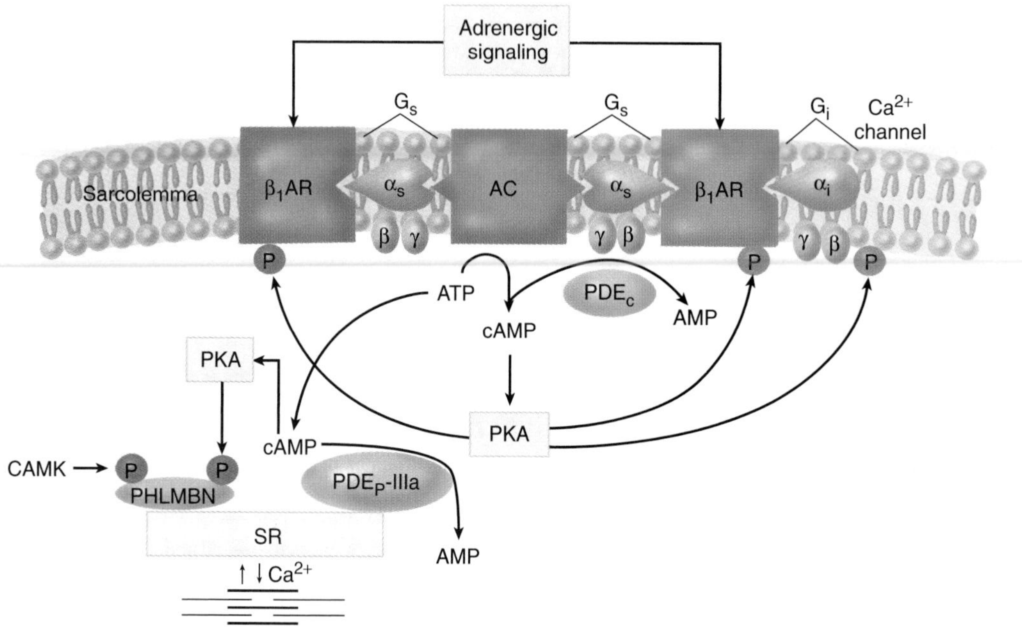

FIGURE 23–6 Schematic representation of selected components of the cardiac myocyte $beta_1$- and $beta_2$-adrenergic receptor pathways. The $beta_1$-adrenergic receptor is illustrated with direct coupling through $G_{\alpha s}$ to voltage-sensitive Ca^{2+} channels as well as to Ca^{2+} channels by cyclic adenosine monophosphate (cAMP)-dependent protein kinase A (PKA) phosphorylation. AC = adenylyl cyclase; AR = adrenergic receptor; ATP = adenosine triphosphate; CAMK = calmodulin-activated kinase; PDE = phosphodiesterase; PHLMBN = phospholamban; SR = sarcoplasmic reticulum.

TABLE 23–5 Pharmacological Characteristics of Various Adrenergic Agonists Used to Treat Decompensated Heart Failure

Agent	$Beta_1$-Receptor Affinity (K_d, nM)	$Beta_2$-Receptor Affinity (K_d, nM)	$Alpha_1$-Receptor Affinity (K_d, nM)	$Uptake_1$ Affinity (nM)	Intrinsic Activity* for Human $Beta_1$ Receptors
Dobutamine	470	570	130	190,330	0.5
Dopamine	25,000	100,000	36,000	130,230	0.2
Epinephrine	20	20	160	1,400	1.0
Isoproterenol	20	20	>10,000	9,000	1.0
Norepinephrine	20	400	200	500,670	1.0
Phenylephrine	>10,000	>10,000	1,000	>10,000	0

Median inhibitory concentration (IC_{50}) data were converted to affinity constants using the Cheng-Prusoff equation.

Some data from Iverson LL (ed): The Uptake and Storage of Noradrenaline in Sympathetic Nerves. Cambridge, UK, Cambridge University Press, 1967.

*Relative to isoproterenol = 1.0 in nonfailing isolated human RV trabeculae. Affinity data are based on radioligand-cold ligand competition curves in (1) human ventricular myocardial membrane preparations ($beta_1$, $beta_2$, $alpha_1$ in nonfailing hearts, norepinephrine, epinephrine, isoproterenol), (2) human recombinant $beta_2$ receptors in COS cell membranes (isoproterenol, norepinephrine, and epinephrine), (3) DTT_1 cell membranes ($beta_2$, dobutamine, and dopamine), and rat heart membranes ($alpha_1$, dobutamine). Additional $alpha_1$-agonist affinity data are derived from irreversible dibenamine antagonism in rabbit aorta, with relative affinities corrected for human/rabbit $alpha_1$ receptor–norepinephrine K values (dopamine, phenylephrine, epinephrine). $Uptake_1$ data are from the human recombinant protein cloned from SK-N-SH neuroblastoma cells (norepinephrine, dopamine),[119] rabbit brain synaptosomes (dobutamine, dopamine, isoproterenol),[120] or the original data for rat heart (epinephrine, norepinephrine, phenylephrine).

example, epinephrine, which has an affinity for $uptake_1$ that is slightly lower than that of norepinephrine, is a much more potent therapeutic catecholamine when administered to denervated cardiac transplant hearts than to innervated hearts.[119,120] When the heart is innervated, $uptake_1$ removes much of the systemically administered epinephrine before it can reach myocardial $beta_1$-adrenergic receptors, which are preferentially located within the synaptic cleft area. In contrast, isoproterenol, which has essentially no affinity for $uptake_1$, is equally effective in innervated and denervated hearts.[121,122]

The failing human heart has a functional impairment in $uptake_1$ that essentially creates functional denervation, which in the case of catecholamines with higher affinity for $uptake_1$ can offset some of the postsynaptic desensitization changes. Another way in which $uptake_1$ can influence drug action is to compete with neurotransmitter norepinephrine for neuronal reuptake, which increases the amount of norepinephrine available in the synaptic cleft area. As can be observed in Table 23–5, the substituted synthetic catecholamine, dobutamine, and the endogenous catecholamine, dopamine, have even higher affinity for $uptake_1$ than does norepinephrine, and at least in the case of dopamine, this higher affinity contributes to its predominant inotropic action, which is to potentiate norepinephrine release.

Dobutamine

Dobutamine is a very useful inotropic agent for moderately decompensated HF.[127] As available clinically, dobutamine is a racemic mixture that stimulates both $beta_1$- and $beta_2$-adrenergic receptor subtypes (binding at an approximately 3:1 ratio)[124] and either binds to but does not activate alpha-adrenergic receptors ([+] enantiomer) or stimulates $alpha_1$ and $alpha_2$ receptor subtypes ([–] enantiomer). As discussed earlier, dobutamine also has a relatively high affinity for $uptake_1$. The affinity constants for racemic dobutamine binding to $beta_1$, $beta_2$, and $alpha_{1B}$ receptors are given in Table 23–5, where it can seen that dobutamine is relatively nonselective for binding to $beta_1$ versus $beta_2$ receptors and binds to $alpha_1$ receptors and $uptake_1$ at a slightly higher affinity. When compared with isoproterenol, in human cardiac preparations, dobutamine is a partial beta-agonist with an intrinsic activity of approximately 0.5.[125] The binding to alpha receptors by each isomer of dobutamine results in a mixture of antagonist and agonist action that, when coupled with some peripheral vascular $beta_2$-agonism, usually produces a net mild degree of vasodilation at lower (≤5 μg/kg/min) doses. At these doses, dobutamine reduces aortic impedance and systemic vascular resistance, thus reducing afterload and improving ventricular-vascular coupling by reducing aortic impedance.[126,127] In contrast, dopamine (see later) may either have no effect or increase ventricular afterload by increasing systemic vascular resistance and by causing a more rapid return of reflected aortic pressure waves, depending on the infusion rate. Therefore, dobutamine is preferable to dopamine for most patients with advanced decompensated HF who have not responded adequately to intravenous diuretics.

The neuronal reuptake inhibition of dobutamine means that in subjects with preserved neuronal uptake mechanisms, dobutamine may increase synaptic cleft area norepinephrine concentrations in the heart in addition to its intrinsic receptor-mediated actions. Dobutamine does not stimulate dopaminergic receptors and, unlike dopamine, does not selectively alter renal blood flow.[128] The importance of the vascular effects of dobutamine has been demonstrated by experiments in animals with artificial hearts.[129,130] Even in the presence of a mechanical heart, dobutamine increased cardiac output by 10 to 15 percent and decreased systemic vascular resistance. Interestingly, dobutamine also decreases venous capacitance and increases right atrial pressure, possibly as a result of $alpha_1$-adrenergic agonism of the (–) enantiomer.[130] These experiments also demonstrated that the (+) enantiomer is responsible for the racemic drug's favorable effects on aortic input impedance, wave reflectance, and systemic vascular resistance.[129] The LV afterload–reducing effects are also responsible for the reduction in functional mitral regurgitation often observed concomitantly with dobutamine infusions in patients with large dilated ventricles and high LV end-diastolic pressure.[131] Dobutamine also causes a mild decline in pulmonary vascular resistance that is present regardless of chronic background vasodilator therapy.

At higher doses, the (–) isomer of dobutamine begins to exert $alpha_1$-adrenergic agonist action, thereby preventing progressive vasodilation and usually leading to minimal changes in preload and afterload. The advantage of this alpha-adrenergic effect of dobutamine is that because preload and afterload do not change dramatically, dobutamine can be administered without pulmonary artery catheter monitoring of LV filling pressure. Another advantage of the relative lack of vasodilation coupled to the partial agonist action is that dobutamine does not produce much increase in the heart rate at doses of 10 μg/kg/min or less. Because of its partial agonist activity, desensitization to prolonged infusions of dobutamine is not pronounced.[132] Dobutamine infusions are initiated at 2 to 3 μg/kg/min and are titrated upward according to the patient's hemodynamic response (usually not higher than 20 μg/kg/min).[127,128]

The limitations of dobutamine are that it (1) is a relatively weak beta-agonist,[125] (2) only modestly lowers elevated pulmonary artery pressure, (3) eventually produces desensitization phenomena when used chronically,[132,133] and (4) cannot be effectively used in the presence of high levels of beta-adrenergic receptor blockade.[119,120] The first three of these limitations can be overcome by combining dobutamine with a phosphodiesterase inhibitor (see below), which results in additive effects on myocardial performance,[134] substantial reductions in pulmonary wedge and pulmonary artery pressure,[134] and a protective effect on desensitization[133] related to being able to lower the dobutamine dose. The fourth limitation is best dealt with by avoiding dobutamine and using a PDEI alone in patients receiving carvedilol or high doses of $beta_1$-blocking agents; in the presence of carvedilol, dobutamine produces little or no increase in stroke volume and increases systemic vascular resistance.[119,120] On the other hand, favorable hemodynamic responses to the PDEIs, enoximone or milrinone, are enhanced by either carvedilol[119,120] or metoprolol.[120]

Dopamine

Dopamine is an endogenous catecholamine that is the precursor to norepinephrine in the catecholamine synthetic pathway. When administered therapeutically, dopamine is a complex agent. Dopamine, through its direct effects, is a weak partial beta-agonist. When initially administered, it releases norepinephrine through a tyramine-like effect.[135] It is a potent (relative to its receptor affinities) neuronal uptake inhibitor and by direct action acts as an agonist at dopamine D_1 postsynaptic vasodilator receptors[136] and D_2 presynaptic receptors on blood vessels and in the kidney.[137] The affinities for $beta_1$, $beta_2$, and $alpha_{1B}$ receptors are shown in Table 23–5, where it can be seen that dopamine has extremely low affinity for all three adrenergic receptors.

At lower doses (≤2 μg/kg/min), dopamine causes a relatively selective dilation of splanchnic and renal arterial beds. This effect may be useful in promoting renal blood flow and maintaining GFR in selected patients who become refractory to diuretics, especially when caused by marginal renal perfusion. Dopamine also has direct renal tubular effects that promote natriuresis. At intermediate (2 to 10 μg/kg/min) infusion rates, dopamine, by virtue of its tyramine and neuronal uptake-inhibiting properties, enhances norepinephrine release from vascular and myocardial adrenergic neurons, thereby resulting in increased cardiac beta-adrenergic receptor activation and an increase in peripheral vascular resistance. In patients with advanced HF, who often have depleted intracardiac norepinephrine stores, dopamine is a less effective positive inotropic drug than are other "directly" acting inotropes.[128,129] At higher infusion rates (5 to 20 μg/kg/min), peripheral vasoconstriction occurs as a result of direct alpha-adrenergic receptor stimulation. Increases in systemic vascular resistance are common even at intermediate infusion rates. On initial administration, tachycardia and arrhythmia tend to be more pronounced than with dobutamine[128] and are related to cardiac norepinephrine release.[135,138]

In patients with advanced, decompensated HF, dopamine should not be used as a positive inotropic agent but rather should be used in low doses for renal perfusion and in intermediate to high doses to increase peripheral resistance. The latter property is often necessary for a variety of reasons, including sepsis, iatrogenic overvasodilation, and brain injury.

OTHER ADRENERGIC AGONISTS

EPINEPHRINE. Epinephrine is an endogenous full beta-agonist catecholamine that, like dobutamine, produces relatively balanced effects between vasodilation and vasoconstriction. This balance between vasodilation and vasoconstriction occurs because epinephrine has relatively equal high affinities for $beta_1$, $beta_2$, and $alpha_1$ receptors (see Table 23–5). Epinephrine has a moderately high affinity for neuronal reuptake, which means that the majority of administered drug may not reach $beta_1$-adrenergic receptors in the normal heart. However, neuronal reuptake is markedly reduced in the failing heart,[139,140] which allows epinephrine to reach more $beta_1$-adrenergic receptors in this setting. Epinephrine is an excellent positive inotropic agent in the denervated, transplanted heart[121,122] because neuronal reuptake is no longer a factor. The dose of epinephrine usually ranges from 0.05 to 0.50 μg/kg/min.

When cardiogenic shock is profound, calcium is often added to an epinephrine infusion to produce synergistic increases in contractility[141] and an increase in vascular tone. This combination, made by adding 1 gm of $CaCl_2$ to 250 ml of intravenous solution containing epinephrine and called Epi-Cal, has never been subjected to a clinical trial and should be used in resuscitative settings only.

ISOPROTERENOL. Isoproterenol is a full, nonselective beta-agonist that produces powerful positive chronotropic, inotropic, and vasodilator responses. At therapeutic doses, isoproterenol does not bind to the neuronal uptake system (see Table 23–5). As a therapeutic inotrope, isoproterenol has only one indication—postoperatively, after heart transplantation. Isoproterenol is useful in this setting because an increase in heart rate is not a problem in the presence of normal coronary arteries and the chronotropic stimulation is useful in the newly transplanted heart, which often has a sluggish sinus node mechanism. The pulmonary vasodilator properties of isoproterenol are also useful in this setting, in which pulmonary artery pressure and pulmonary vascular resistance are usually elevated. The dose of isoproterenol ranges from 0.005 to 0.05 μg/kg/min.

NOREPINEPHRINE. As shown in Table 23–5, norepinephrine is a moderately (10- to 30-fold) $beta_1$ versus $beta_2$ receptor-selective agonist with relatively high affinity for $alpha_1$ receptors and for $uptake_1$. This constellation of properties means that norepinephrine is a powerful vasoconstrictor but not a very powerful inotrope in hearts with functioning neuronal uptake. Norepinephrine does not have any recommended uses in subjects with cardiac decompensation; subjects who need peripheral vascular resistance support (such as in sepsis, iatrogenic overvasodilation, or brain injury) are served better by dopamine or dopamine plus phenylephrine administration.

Phosphodiesterase Inhibitors (PDEI)

MECHANISMS OF ACTION. The enzyme phosphodiesterase type IIIa is associated with the sarcoplasmic reticulum (SR) in human cardiac myocytes (see Fig. 23–6),[142,143] platelets, and vascular smooth muscle, where it breaks down cAMP into AMP. Type IIIa phosphodiesterase has an SR-anchoring moiety[143] that accounts for its compartmentalization in cardiac myocytes and vascular smooth muscle. Elevations in cAMP in the vicinity of the SR can then activate locally compartmentalized protein kinase A, which phosphorylates phospholamban and relieves this molecule's inhibition of SR function (see Chap. 19).[144] Thus, specific type III PDEIs, particularly at low doses, may have a relatively selective effect on phospholamban phosphorylation[145] and SR function, which explains why they lower diastolic Ca^{2+} and increase systolic Ca^{2+} in cultured cardiac myocytes. This SR-selective effect is probably the reason why highly type III–specific PDEIs increase contractile function without as much of an increase in heart rate. This is similar to the phenotype of transgenic mice with phospholamban knockout, which exhibit an increase in contractility without an increase in heart rate.[146] However, PDEIs also increase the calcium channel current,[147] and higher doses increase the phosphorylation of phosphoproteins other than phospholamban,[145] similar in effect to beta-agonists.[148]

Type III PDEIs are also potent vasodilators, particularly on venous capacitance and pulmonary vascular beds. The vasodilator properties of PDEIs substantially exceed that of beta-agonists,[119,120,134] including isoproterenol. The reason for this superior vasodilation effect appears to be that, in vascular smooth muscle, PDEI-induced elevations in cAMP activate protein kinase G,[149] which leads to prominent vasodilation that is not unlike a nitrovasodilator effect in its regional distribution. PDEIs are among the best agents for lowering pulmonary artery pressure and pulmonary vascular resistance, which is one of the reasons why they have assumed an important role in postoperative cardiac surgical regimens, including cardiac transplantation.[150-152] The effect of PDEIs on LV function curves is shown in Figure 23–2; PDEIs as inotrope-vasodilators move the LV function curve both upward and leftward.

As with beta-agonists, a PDEI's inotropic response is blunted in failing versus nonfailing hearts (Fig. 23–7).[134,153] In the failing human heart, the reason for blunting of the response to PDEIs is not an alteration in myocardial type III phosphodiesterase[142] but rather upregulation of the inhibitory G protein, G_α,[154-156] because a decrease in $G_{\alpha i}$[157] leads to augmentation of the PDEI response.[158] However, by comparison with beta-agonists, little or no subsensitivity develops to the inotrope-vasodilator effects of more potent type III PDEIs such as milrinone[159] and enoximone.[119,159,160]

As discussed previously, the substantial preload- and pulmonary artery pressure–reducing properties of PDEIs are both a strength and a weakness of this class of agents, inasmuch as before their acute intravenous administration, it is necessary to be certain of an elevated LV filling pressure. Therefore, in the absence of elevated right-sided venous pressure in a subject with biventricular failure, pulmonary artery catheter–determined documentation of a pulmonary wedge mean pressure greater than 15 mm Hg is desirable before administering a PDEI intravenously. Otherwise, a precipitous drop in blood pressure may accompany drug administration.

PDEIs are absorbed orally, and their attractive hemodynamic profile has led to multiple clinical trials in chronic HF. The increase in cardiac output from PDEIs is preferentially distributed to skeletal muscle,[161] which should theoretically increase maximum exercise responses. Such does appear to be the case.[160,162] In addition, in a dilated, failing heart, PDEIs have a favorable energetic effect,[163] and PDEIs improve diastolic[164,165] as well as systolic[166] function. All these observations suggest that PDEIs would be useful in the long-term treatment of chronic HF.

CLINICAL OBSERVATIONS. In placebo-controlled clinical trials, selective type III PDEIs given in doses that produce large hemodynamic effects are associated with increased mortality.[166-168] Moreover, agents with PDEI activity and K^+ channel antagonism (vesnarinone),[169] as well as PDEI activity and Ca^{2+} sensitization (pimobendan, see later),[170] are also associated with increased mortality. The basis for the increase in mortality is increased sudden death,[168,171] presumably on an arrhythmic basis.

Despite these discouraging results, PDEIs continue in development for the treatment of chronic HF through two new approaches. One is a "low-dose" approach[172] that takes advantage of the fact that doses that are one-sixth to one-third those used in earlier clinical trials are hemodynamically active,[173] increase exercise tolerance,[160] do not increase the heart rate,[160] are not proarrhythmic,[160] and apparently do not increase mortality.[133,160] That a positive inotropic agent can increase mortality at higher doses but be safely given at low doses has been established by the DIG trial,[92,97] but it remains to be seen whether the same is true for PDEIs. The second approach to the safe, long-term use of PDEIs in chronic HF is to combine them with a beta-blocking agent.[175,176] This combination is possible because the site of action of PDEIs is beyond the beta-adrenergic receptor (see Fig. 23–6), and the combination appears to produce additive efficacy and subtractive adverse effects.[174] Treatment with beta-blocking agents actually enhances the hemodynamic effects of PDEIs[119,120,158] because of a beta blocker–related reduction in upregulated $G_{\alpha i}$.[157] As discussed earlier, one practical consequence of these findings and realizations is that subjects receiving beta-blocking agents chronically who decompensate to the point of needing positive inotropic support should be treated with a PDEI rather than dobutamine or some other beta-agonist.[119,120]

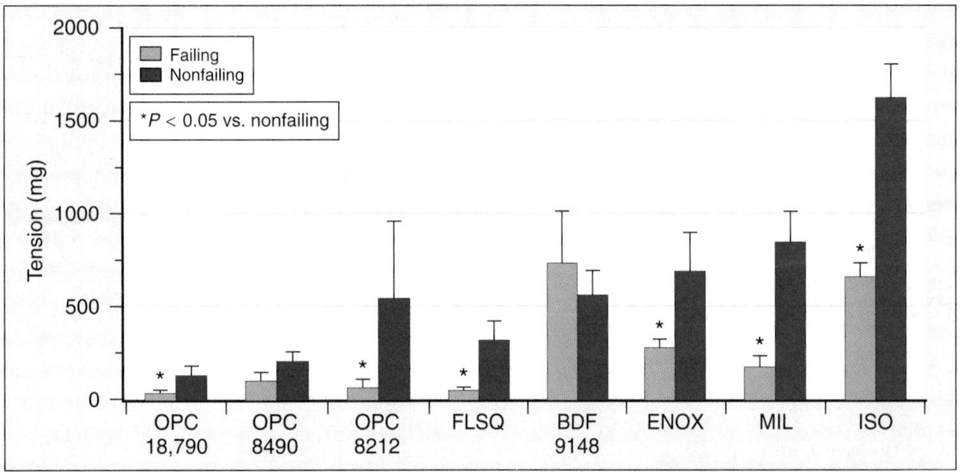

FIGURE 23–7 Effects of various inotropic agents on the systolic tension response in nonfailing and failing human right ventricular trabeculae, mean + standard error of the mean. ENOX = enoximone; FLSQ = flosequinan; ISO = isoproterenol; MIL = milrinone; OPC 8212 = vesnarinone.

Individual Agents

AMRINONE. Amrinone was the first type III PDEI approved for the treatment of decompensated HF.[176] Because amrinone causes thrombocytopenia and may be associated with rapid subsensitivity in subjects with advanced HF,[177] it is no longer widely used to treat decompensated HF.

MILRINONE. Unlike amrinone, milrinone rarely causes thrombocytopenia.[178] Although milrinone is a highly selective type III PDEI, other actions capable of producing an inotropic effect have been described, including stimulation of the Ca^{2+} release channel,[179] Ca^{2+} channel agonism, and effects on sarcolemmal Ca^{2+}-ATPase.[180]

Milrinone produces sustained inotropic and vasodilator effects when administered intravenously.[181] The elimination half-life is 2.3 hours, and milrinone is usually administered as a 25- to 75-μg/kg bolus over a 10- to 20-minute period, followed by a continuous infusion of 0.25 to 0.75 μg/kg/min.[182] Development of oral milrinone has been abandoned because of the increase in mortality in the Prospective Randomized Milrinone Survival Evaluation (PROMISE) trial,[166] which was conducted at doses that are at least four times higher than the minimum effective hemodynamic dose.[182] Milrinone is mostly (80 percent) excreted by the kidney unchanged, and in renal failure the continuous-infusion dose should be decreased by 50 percent.

ENOXIMONE. Enoximone is approved for intravenous use in Europe and is in development in the United States for oral use as low-dose enoximone alone and in combination with $beta_1$-selective blockade. Enoximone is a highly selective type III PDEI with no other known pharmacological actions at therapeutic plasma concentrations. Enoximone rarely causes thrombocytopenia and produces sustained hemodynamic effects with intravenous[183] or oral[160] administration.

Enoximone is about one-tenth as potent as milrinone for inhibiting type III phosphodiesterase, which translates to oral and intravenous doses of enoximone being approximately 10 times those of milrinone. The intravenous loading dose is 0.25 to 0.75 mg/kg, with the continuous infusion rate being 1.25 to 7.5 μg/kg/min. Enoximone is extensively metabolized by the liver to sulfoxide derivatives, including at least one active metabolite.[184] Sulfoxide metabolites (about 75 percent within 24 hours in subjects with HF) are eliminated by the kidney, and dose reductions in renal failure are the same as with milrinone.[185] Enoximone doses should also be reduced in patients with hepatic failure.

PHOSPHODIESTERASE INHIBITORS WITH CALCIUM SENSITIZER ACTIVITY

MECHANISM OF ACTION. These positive inotropic agents act in part by increasing the sensitivity of troponin C or some other part of the myofibrillar Ca^{2+}-binding apparatus to ionized calcium. This property alone would prolong contraction time and decrease diastolic function, which would not be desirable in an inotropic agent. However, all agents that have gone on to clinical development are also PDEIs, and this property "cancels" the increased contraction time and provides favorable effects on diastolic function.[186,187] Under these circumstances, the advantage of Ca^{2+} sensitization is that the pharmacological effect of the drug does not rely on increasing systolic calcium concentrations, although this action occurs if the compound also has PDEI activity. Another advantage would be in not increasing the heart rate, but again, PDEI activity would lead to a chronotropic effect at higher doses. The combination of not increasing intracellular Ca^{2+} or the heart rate would confer an energetic advantage to Ca^{2+} sensitizers.

The mixed-action Ca^{2+} sensitizers levosimendan and pimobendan have undergone the most clinical experience, and their hemodynamic profiles,[186,188] including increasing the heart rate at higher doses, do not differ from those of milrinone and enoximone. This similarity occurs because, as discussed subsequently, the dominant pharmacological action of both compounds is type III phosphodiesterase inhibition.

PIMOBENDAN. This agent is available in oral form for the treatment of HF, but only in Japan. Pimobendan has weak Ca^{2+}-sensitizing properties through facilitating the interaction of Ca^{2+} with troponin C,[189] its major mechanism of action being phosphodiesterase inhibition.[190] In several medium-sized trials, pimobendan increased exercise performance or improved quality of life, or both,[191] but its development in the United States and Europe was put on hold when a strong trend (relative risk 1.8, confidence interval 0.9 to 3.5) toward an increase in mortality was noted in the Pimobendan in Congestive Heart Failure (PICO) trial, which was conducted in subjects with mild to moderate HF.[170]

LEVOSIMENDAN. This drug is available in some European countries in intravenous form. Levosimendan was discovered as part of a screening strategy for identifying compounds that bind to a troponin C affinity column,[192] and levosimendan does bind to free troponin C. However, other data indicate that levosimendan does not bind to the human troponin C-troponin I complex,[193] which is the natural state of the regulatory thin filament proteins.

Levosimendan is in clinical development in the United States in intravenous form. Intravenous levosimendan has been evaluated in two clinical trials. In an acute myocardial infarction study conducted in Russia, patients were randomly assigned to receive levosimendan or a placebo.[194] Not surprisingly, the positive inotropic agent produced better circulatory support, with the secondary endpoints of death, worsening HF, or development of HF being lower in prevalence during the 6-hour infusion period and at 24 hours as well.[194] Only the highest dose (0.4 μg/kg/min) of levosimendan exacerbated myocardial ischemia.[194] In another study in which approximately 40 percent of the subjects were taking beta blockers, levosimendan performed better than dobutamine in terms of hemodynamic response.[195] This result is also expected because by virtue of their respective sites of action, beta blockade would inhibit the response to dobutamine but not to levosimendan. In this study, the statistical advantage of levosimendan over dobutamine was confined to patients receiving beta blockade.[195] These studies do not provide evidence that levosimendan is superior to other PDEI-positive inotropic agents currently available in intravenous form.

In the studies with levosimendan, the hemodynamic and even clinical benefits have extended beyond the duration of the infusion period.[194,195] The explanation for this is a hemodynamically active metabolite with an elimination half-life of 70 to 80 hours.[196] Sustained action beyond the duration of infusion could be an advantage for levosimendan as an intermittently administered agent delivered to outpatients but could be a disadvantage in terms of short-term use when drug action of an inotropic agent is not required or desired beyond a brief period of support.

Neurohormonal Inhibitors

Without question, the greatest advance in the treatment of chronic HF has been the application of agents that inhibit harmful neurohormonal systems that are activated to support the failing heart (see Chaps. 19 and 21). This generally useful paradigm had multiple origins, including work done in the late 1970s and early 1980s that documented the nature and extent of neurohormonal activation in chronic HF,[197] the association of systemic neurohormonal activation with adverse outcomes,[198] observations in the failing human heart that excessive adrenergic activation produces harmful biological effects,[113,199] and astute clinical observations regarding the degree of improvement effected by inhibitors of the adrenergic[200-202] and renin-angiotensin[203,204] systems. By the middle to late 1980s, influential commentaries on the validity of the "neurohormonal hypothesis" were being articulated,[197,205] and all of these developments ultimately culminated in the performance of large-scale clinical trials that demonstrated that inhibition of the renin-angiotensin[206,207] (see Fig. 24–6) and adrenergic[208-212] (see Fig. 24–5) systems improved the natural history of chronic HF caused by primary or secondary cardiomyopathies.

The general mechanisms by which neurohormonal activation worsens and neurohormonal inhibition improves the natural history of myocardial dysfunction and remodeling are discussed in Chapter 21. In essence, multiple neurohormonal signaling pathways, such as β_1-, β_2-, and α_1-adrenergic receptor,[118] angiotensin II AT_1 receptor,[213] endothelin-1 ET_A receptor,[214] and tumor necrosis factor-alpha receptor pathways,[215] are activated in the failing heart and promote maladaptive growth, remodeling, and progressive myocardial dysfunction.[216] Inhibition of these systems may prevent or reverse these adverse biological processes, thereby leading to improvement in the natural history of HF. Therapy targeting individual neurohormonal or cytokine systems is now discussed.

Inhibitors of the Renin-Angiotensin-Aldosterone System (see also Chap. 38)

Angiotensin-Converting Enzyme Inhibitors

ACEIs were the first consistent and substantial success story of medical therapy improving the natural history of chronic HF, and this class of neurohormonal inhibitors remains a mainstay in HF treatment. ACEIs were originally developed within the vasodilator paradigm, but when their clinical results proved to be out of proportion to their relatively weak vasodilator effects, it became apparent that another mechanism was operative. That general mechanism, as elucidated by the Pfeffers' laboratory in elegant studies in animal models of myocardial infarction [217,218] and then in humans[203,204] including those with chronic HF,[219] is the prevention of angiotensin II–mediated remodeling.[216]

RATIONALE AND MECHANISM OF ACTION. Figure 23–8 shows the pathways for angiotensin II formation, which occurs systemically as well as locally in cardiac and vascular tissues. Note that generation of angiotensin II is accomplished by two pathways, one that uses converting enzyme found in high abundance in endothelium and one that uses the protease chymase, which is found in interstitial cells. Transmyocardial studies in the intact human heart have indicated that more than 80 percent of the generation of angiotensin II is by the ACE pathway,[220] but studies in isolated human heart preparations[221] and in model systems[222] have emphasized the contribution of the chymase pathway. If the chymase pathway is important in producing ventricular remodeling in the failing heart, angiotensin receptor-blocking agents (ARBs) would be more effective than ACEIs in decreasing angiotensin II signaling. If, on the other hand, ACEIs are just as effective clinically as ARBs, by inference, the ACE pathway is the dominant mechanism for generating angiotensin II in the failing heart. Finally, if ACEIs are superior to ARBs, additional properties of ACEIs, such as increasing bradykinin,[223] are presumably responsible. From the results of clinical trials with ACEIs and ARBs in chronic HF (see later), it appears that ACEIs are at least as effective as ARBs, supporting the idea that the ACE pathway is dominant in angiotensin II formation in the failing human heart.

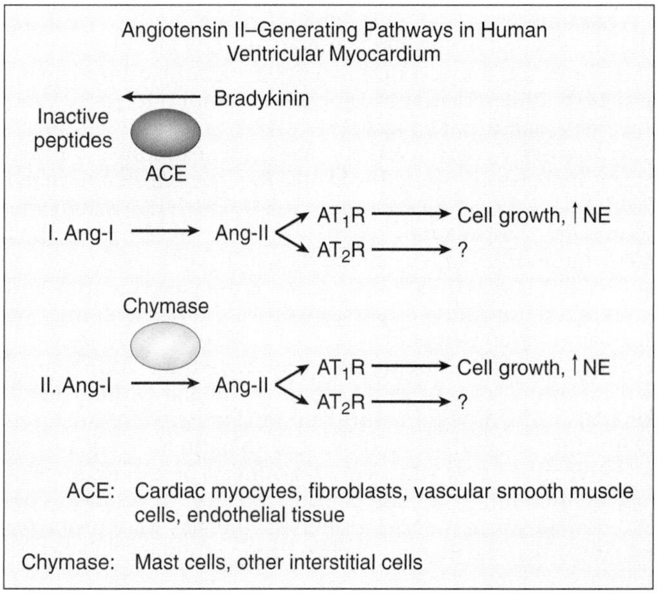

FIGURE 23–8 Pathways of angiotensin II formation. ACE = angiotensin-converting enzyme; Ang-1 = angiotensin I; AT_1R = angiotensin II type 1 receptor; AT_2R = angiotensin II type 2 receptor; NE = norepinephrine.

As shown in Table 23–6, increased levels of angiotensin II have several adverse effects on the cardiovascular system, including cardiac myocyte hypertrophy, myocyte apoptosis, prejunctional facilitation of norepinephrine release, and mitogenic effects on fibroblasts. Most, if not all, of these effects are mediated by the AT_1 subtype. In addition, most of these biological effects of angiotensin II contribute to the development of hypertrophy and remodeling.

CLINICAL OBSERVATIONS. Two types of studies demonstrate the consistent efficacy of ACEIs in HF: post-myocardial infarction studies and clinical trials in chronic HF. As shown in Table 23–7, more of the former types of studies than the latter types have been conducted. All placebo-controlled chronic HF trials, with the exception of the "asymptomatic" Studies of Left Ventricular Dysfunction (SOLVD) Prevention Study,[224] demonstrated a reduction in mortality. As can be observed in Table 23–7, the Class IV Cooperative North Scandinavian Enalapril Survival Study (CONSENSUS I) had a much larger effect size than the SOLVD Treatment Trial, which in turn had a larger effect size than the SOLVD Prevention Trial. Although only these three placebo-controlled mortality trials have been conducted in patients with chronic HF, it seems obvious that ACEIs reduce mortality in direct relation to the degree of severity of chronic HF. Although not placebo controlled, the V-HeFT-II trial provided evidence that ACEIs improve the natural history of HF through mechanisms other than vasodilation, inasmuch as subjects treated with enalapril had significantly lower mortality than subjects treated with the nonneurohormonal inhibitor-vasodilator combination of hydralazine plus isosorbide dinitrate.[63] Although only one ACEI, enalapril, has been used in placebo-controlled mortality trials in chronic HF, as can be observed in Table 23–7, multiple ACEIs have proven to be more or less equally effective when administered in oral form within the first week of the ischemic event in post-myocardial infarction trials.[225-227] ACEIs also have a proven track record in preventing HF in two settings: enalapril in asymptomatic LV dysfunction (see Table 23–7)[224] and ramipril in cardiovascular at-risk patients without LV dysfunction.[228] These observations support the conclusion that the effects of ACE inhibition on the natural history of chronic HF, post-myocardial infarction LV dysfunction, or

TABLE 23–6 Biological Responses Mediated by Angiotensin II Receptors in the Human Cardiovascular System

Biologic Response	Receptor Mediation
Cardiac myocyte growth	AT_1
Positive inotropic response (minimal)	AT_1
Myocyte apoptosis	AT_1, AT_2
Aldosterone release	AT_1
Norepinephrine release	AT_1
Cardiac myocyte toxicity	Beta-adrenergic via norepinephrine release
Fibroblast proliferation	AT_1
Smooth muscle proliferation	AT_1
Vasoconstriction	AT_1

TABLE 23–7 Crude, Annualized Mortality Rates in Renin-Angiotensin-Aldosterone System Inhibitor Placebo-Controlled Trials Conducted in Chronic Heart Failure (HF) from Systolic Dysfunction, Left Ventricular (LV) Dysfunction after Myocardial Infarction, or in Patients Without LV Dysfunction at Risk for HF*

Trial Name	Agent	NYHA Class	No. of Subjects Enrolled	12-Month Placebo Mortality (%)	12-Month Effect Size (%)	*P* Value 12 Months (Full F/U)
ACEIs						
CHF						
CONSENSUS-I[217]	Enalapril	IV	253	52	↓31	0.01 (0.003)
SOLVD-Rx[218]	Enalapril	I-III	2569	15	↓21	0.02 (0.004)
SOLVD-Asx[235]	Enalapril	I, II	4228	5	0	0.82 (0.30)
Totals		I-IV	7050	11	↓16	0.02
POST-MI						
SAVE[236]	Captopril	—	2231	12	↓18	0.11 (0.02)
AIRE[237]	Ramipril	—	1986	20	↓22	0.01 (0.002)
TRACE[238]	Trandolapril	—	1749	26	↓16	0.046 (0.001)
Totals			5966	19	↓18	0.001
ARBs						
CHF						
Val-HeFT[253]	Valsartan	II-IV	5010	9	0	NS
CHARM-Alternative[254]	Candesartan	II-IV	2028	8	↓14	NS
CHARM-Added[255]	Candesartan	II-IV	2548	8	↓12	NS
Totals		II-IV	9586	9	↓6	NS
Aldosterone Antagonists						
CHF						
RALES[18]	Spironolactone	III, IV	1663	24	↓25	(<0.001)
POST-MI						
EPHESUS[21]	Eplerenone	I	6632	12	↓15	(0.005)

AIRE = Acute Infarction Ramipril Efficacy; CHARM = candesartan in heart failure—assessment of reduction in mortality and morbidity; CHF = congestive heart failure; CONSENSUS = Cooperative North Scandinavian Enalapril Survival Study; EPHESUS = Eplerenone Post-Acute Myocardial Infarction Heart Failure Efficacy and Survival Study; MI = myocardial infarction; RALES = Randomized Aldactone Evaluation Study; SAVE = Survival and Ventricular Enlargement; SOLVD = Studies of Left Ventricular Dysfunction; TRACE = Trandolapril Cardiac Evaluation; Val-HeFT = Valsartan Heart Failure Trail.

*Twelve-month mortality rates are taken from survival curves when data not directly available in published material.

TABLE 23–8 Properties of Widely Used Angiotensin-Converting Enzyme Inhibitors

Agent	Half-Life (hr)	Recommended Starting Dose (mg)	Recommended Target Dose (mg)	Relative Tissue Binding
Captopril	3	6.25	50 t.i.d.	+
Enalapril	11	2.5-5	10 b.i.d.	+
Lisinopril	12	5	20 qd	+
Ramipril	9-18	2.5	5 b.i.d.	++
Quinapril	2 (25)	5	20 b.i.d.	+++
Trandolapril	6	1	1-2 b.i.d.	NA

NA = not available.

HF prevention in cardiovascular at-risk patients are class effects.

In summary, an ACEI is considered mandatory treatment in chronic HF, asymptomatic LV systolic dysfunction, or in the setting of cardiovascular disease with any risk factor for the development of HF. The doses employed should be at least the average dose used to lower mortality in HF or post-myocardial infarction trials (Table 23–8). The only consistent adverse effect noted with ACEIs is a low-level (5 percent greater than placebo) increase in cough. In such patients, an angiotensin II AT_1 receptor–blocking agent can be substituted.

Angiotensin II AT_1 Receptor-Blocking Agents

RATIONALE AND MECHANISM OF ACTION. It has been shown in numerous studies that ACEIs do not completely inhibit tissue-based RAASs[229] and that after several months of treatment, "escape" can occur with an increase in systemic angiotensin II[230] or aldosterone levels (see Fig. 23–8).[231] These observations set the stage for additional RAAS inhibitor strategies, including the use of ARBs and aldosterone antagonists.

Multiple ARBs approved for the treatment of hypertension are now on the market in the United States (Table 23–9). Three of these, losartan, valsartan, and candesartan, have been extensively evaluated in the setting of HF. The rationale for the use of these agents in HF is derived from information presented in Table 23–6, showing that virtually all the adverse biological effects relevant to a failing, remodeled heart are mediated by the AT_1 receptor. Moreover, ARBs antagonize the effects of angiotensin II regardless of its origin (through the ACE or chymase pathway; see Fig. 23–8). All these compounds are selective, high-affinity antagonists of AT_1 receptors.

Hemodynamic studies and studies with ARBs in HF have demonstrated effects that are similar to those of ACEIs; that is, these agents reduce pulmonary wedge and pulmonary artery pressure moderately, are mild preload reducers, and increase cardiac output.[232-234] Heart rate is not affected unless baroreflexes are excessively activated by hypotension. Maximum exercise time is also improved to a similar degree with each type of RAS inhibitor.[235,236] The combination of an ACEI and an ARB produces additive hemodynamic effects[237,238] as well as additive effects on prevention of remodeling.[239]

CLINICAL OBSERVATIONS. Clinical trial data on ARBs have, on balance, demonstrated that (1) in HF populations not treated with ACEIs, they are about as effective as ACEIs in reducing mortality[240-243] or mortality and morbidity, including patients intolerant of ACEIs (see Fig. 24–6)[242,243]; (2) on a background of ACEIs, they reduce HF hospitalizations[242,243]; (3) when given in addition to ACEIs in general cohorts of patients with symptomatic HF, they have a modest beneficial[244] or no[242] effect on mortality (Table 23–7); and (4) in subgroups of patients receiving ACEIs and beta blockers they have been reported either to increase mortality[242] or to decrease HF hospitalizations and mortality.[244] In addition, in diastolic dysfunction the ARB candesartan has reduced hospitalizations for HF.[245] ARBs are well tolerated in HF populations and do not produce the most common side effect associated with ACEIs, cough.[240,241] In a large trial comparing the ACEI captopril and the ARB valsartan (the valsartan in acute myocardial infarction [VALIANT] trial) in patients with impaired LV function following acute myocardial infarction, no difference in mortality was observed.[246] Furthermore, the combination of these drugs produced no further reduction in mortality, although the number of adverse events increased.

As discussed in Chapter 24, the clinical trial data for ARBs in HF from systolic dysfunction currently support their use in ACE-intolerant patients, added to ACEIs in patients not treated with beta-blocking agents, and added to ACEIs and beta blockers in patients with preserved blood pressures. With regard to the last use, there may be a drug- or dose-specific aspect of ARB use,[242,244] and only candesartan has demonstrated benefit.[244]

Aldosterone Receptor Antagonists

RATIONALE AND MECHANISM OF ACTION. As discussed previously, aldosterone levels are not reduced by long-term treatment with ACEIs.[231] There are numerous lines of evidence that aldosterone produces harmful myocardial effects, including the promotion of fibrosis[247] and ventricular arrhythmias.[248] These effects are probably mediated through the mineralocorticoid receptor, which is supported by evidence in transgenic mice overexpressing an enzyme that leads to increased aldosterone receptor occupancy of this receptor.[249] In these experiments, mice developed a cardiomyopathy with increased interstitial fibrosis.[249] These observations provide the rationale for the use of aldosterone receptor antagonists as therapy in addition to ACE inhibition in HF.

CLINICAL OBSERVATIONS. The first evidence that this approach could produce a major clinical benefit was provided by the Randomized Aldactone Evaluation Study (RALES) trial,[18] which evaluated the addition of the competitive aldosterone antagonist spironolactone versus placebo to standard HF therapy in stage 3 (New York Heart Association [NYHA] Class III or IV) patients, the primary endpoint being all-cause mortality. As can be seen in Table 23–7, in RALES,[18] spironolactone produced a 30 percent reduction in total mortality when compared with placebo ($p = 0.001$). The beneficial effect of spironolactone appeared to be on both

TABLE 23–9 Properties of Widely Used Angiotensin Receptor Blockers

Agent	Half-Life (hr)	Recommended Starting Dose (mg)	Recommended Target Dose (mg)
Losartan	2	25	50-100 qd
Valsartan	6	40	80-160 b.i.d.
Irbesartan	11-15	75	150 qd
Candesartan	9	4	16-32 qd
Telmisartan†	24	20	80 qd
Eprosartan	5-9	200	400 b.i.d.

*Indicates half-life of the active metabolite.
†Decreases digoxin clearance.

sudden and pump failure–related deaths. Although the mechanism behind the benefit of spironolactone has not been fully elucidated, prevention of extracellular matrix remodeling[247] and prevention of increasing potassium levels are leading contenders. In RALES, serum potassium levels were 0.3 mEq/liter higher in the spironolactone group than in the placebo group ($p = 0.001$),[18] which could have played a major role in reducing sudden or even pump failure–related deaths.

Although spironolactone was well tolerated in RALES,[18] it has antiandrogenic and progesterone-like effects and is associated with a small incidence of gynecomastia, impotence, and menstrual irregularities, which may lead to discontinuation. Newer generation aldosterone antagonists are associated with a much lower incidence of these adverse effects and should be considered for patients intolerant of spironolactone. Eplerenone[19,20] is a selective aldosterone inhibitor that has been evaluated in the Eplerenone Post-Acute Myocardial Infarction Heart Failure Efficacy and Survival Study (EPHESUS) (see Fig. 23–4).[21] Patients with LV ejection fractions less than 40 percent were randomly assigned 3 to 14 days after myocardial infarction to therapy with eplerenone or placebo. During a mean follow-up of 16 months, eplerenone significantly improved mortality (relative risk 0.85, 95 percent confidence interval 0.75 to 0.96, $p = 0.008$) (see Table 23–7). Gynecomastia, impotence, and breast tenderness were not increased by eplerenone.

Both spironolactone and eplerenone can produce hyperkalemia, particularly in patients with advanced HF with compromised renal function when administered on a background of ACE inhibition or in patients receiving potassium supplementation. For that reason, when initiating aldosterone antagonist therapy in a patient with HF, it is prudent to lower the level of potassium supplementation and check the potassium serum level frequently until a steady state of potassium balance has been achieved. In addition, in HF there is inadequate information regarding the efficacy of aldosterone antagonists when added to background therapy of ACEIs and beta blockers. It is likely that the presence of a beta blocker, because of its antirenin effects, further reduces the tolerability of aldosterone antagonists in patients with advanced HF; for example, in a clinical trial in which spironolactone was mandated background therapy along with ACEIs or ARBs and beta blockers, the proportion of patients who could tolerate spironolactone was only 55 percent.[250]

From the results of RALES[18] and EPHESUS,[21] a case can be made for all patients with HF related to systolic dysfunction being treated with an aldosterone antagonist, with eplerenone being used if endocrine-related side effects of spironolactone are observed.

TABLE 23–10 Biological Responses Mediated by Adrenergic Receptors in the Human Heart

Biological Response	Adrenergic Receptor Mediation
Positive inotropic response	β_1, β_2, α_1 (minimal)
Positive chronotropic response	β_1, β_2
Myocyte toxicity	$\beta_1 >> \beta_2$
Myocyte apoptosis	β_1
Cardiac myocyte growth	$\beta_1 >> \beta_2$, α_1
Fetal gene induction	$\beta_1 >> \beta_2$, α_1
Proarrhythmic	β_1, β_2, α_1

Antiadrenergic Agents

Rationale and Mechanism of Action

Adrenergic Dysfunction in the Failing Human Heart (see also Chaps. 19 and 21)

The failing human heart is adrenergically activated to maintain cardiac performance over the short term by increasing contractility[251] and heart rate. In contrast, in the resting state, no adrenergic support occurs in normally functioning human left ventricles.[251] Multiple lines of evidence[252-255] indicate that it is increased cardiac adrenergic drive rather than an increase in circulating norepinephrine that is both ini-tially supportive and then ultimately damaging to the failing human heart. Norepinephrine, the adrenergic neurotransmitter, is a beta$_1$-selective agonist[256] with an affinity for beta$_1$ receptors that is approximately 20-fold greater than for beta$_2$ receptors and 10-fold greater than for alpha$_1$ receptors (see Table 23–5).

As shown in Table 23–10, human cardiac myocytes have three adrenergic receptors (beta$_1$, beta$_2$, and alpha$_1$) that are coupled to both beneficial and to harmful biological responses.[111,112,118,257] Beta-adrenergic receptors are coupled through the stimulatory G protein G_s to the effector enzyme adenylyl cyclase (see Fig. 23–6), which converts the substrate Mg-ATP to cAMP. cAMP is a positive inotropic and chronotropic second messenger and is also strongly growth promoting. In younger (<50 years) nonfailing human left or right ventricles, the beta$_1$/beta$_2$ ratio is 70 to 80:30 to 20,[257] but in failing[111,257] or older[258] human ventricles, 35 to 40 percent of the total number of beta receptors are beta$_2$ as a result of selective downregulation in the beta$_1$ subtype. Alpha$_1$ receptors are coupled through a different G protein (G_q) to the effector enzyme phospholipase C, which through the second messenger diacylglycerol activates the growth-promoting protein kinase C family. Because alpha$_1$ receptors are upregulated in the failing heart,[259,260] the cardiac myocyte adrenergic receptor profile changes from predominantly (>70 percent of the total adrenergic receptor population) beta$_1$ to more of a mixed, 2:1:1 (beta$_1$/beta$_2$/alpha$_1$) ratio in end-stage HF.[111,112,118] Beta$_2$ receptors are also present on adrenergic nerve terminals in the heart, where they facilitate norepinephrine release.[261] The beta$_3$ receptor may also be present in the human heart as a counterregulatory receptor coupled to the inhibitory G protein G_i,[262] and some evidence also existed for a beta$_4$ receptor[263]; however, this now appears to be discounted.

Cardiac Damage Induced by Receptor Activation

Norepinephrine is an exceptionally cardiotoxic substance that produces cardiac myocyte injury in concentrations found in the failing human heart. As shown in Table 23–5, norepinephrine is mildly beta$_1$ receptor selective (10- to 30-fold compared with the binding affinity to beta$_2$ receptors, 10-fold compared with alpha$_1$), and its cytotoxicity appears to be mediated through beta- rather than alpha-adrenergic receptors.[264] In transgenic mice, cardiac overexpression of human beta$_1$ receptors,[264-266] beta$_2$ receptors,[267,268] $G_{\alpha s}$,[269] or $G_{\alpha q}$[270] can produce an overtly cardiomyopathic phenotype and, ultimately, chamber dilation and systolic dysfunction. Although direct comparisons have yet to be made, it appears that approximately 10-fold higher levels of expression of human beta$_2$ versus beta$_1$ receptors are required to produce histopathology.[264,265,268] Overexpression of $G_{\alpha s}$ is also associated with increased markers of apoptosis, which can be produced in cardiac myocytes by norepinephrine exposure.[271,272] Norepinephrine-mediated apoptosis is mediated through beta$_1$ receptors,[272] and apoptosis is prominent in cardiac beta$_1$ receptor–overexpressing mice.[265] Finally, cardiac expression of a constitutively activated alpha$_1$ receptor produces concentric hypertrophy,[273] and cardiac overexpression of alpha$_{1C}$ receptors produces a cardiomyopathy.[274] These data from model systems incontrovertibly indicate that chronic adrenergic signaling is a harmful compensatory mechanism in the failing human heart. The data are quite convincing for chronic beta$_1$ receptor signaling and less convincing but likely for chronic beta$_2$ and alpha$_1$ receptor pathway activation. The compensatory as well as adverse effects of adrenergic signaling pathways are summarized in Figure 23–1 and Table 23–10.

Interestingly, when components of the beta-adrenergic–adenylyl cyclase–phospholamban phosphorylation pathway are transgenically manipulated beyond the level of $G_{\alpha s}$, no overt pathology is apparent despite marked and sustained increases in contractility.[146,266,275] This finding may mean that $G_{\alpha s}$-coupled cAMP-independent pathways that include calcium channel activation[276] may mediate the majority of myocardial damage in beta-adrenergic receptor– and $G_{\alpha s}$-overexpressing animals.

In the failing heart, beta-adrenergic signal transduction is reduced secondary to desensitization changes at the level of beta$_1$ and beta$_2$ receptors, the inhibitory G protein ($G_{\alpha i}$), and an enzyme responsible for modulating receptor activity by phosphorylation (beta-adrenergic receptor kinase) as well as by changes in expression of the adenylyl cyclase enzyme itself.[111,118,154-156,258,277,278] In an end-stage failing heart, 50 to 60 percent of the total signal-transducing potential is lost, but substantial signaling capacity remains.[116] These and other data from model systems[279] suggest that the beta-adrenergic receptor pathway desensitization changes present in the failing human heart are adaptive changes and that a potentially effective therapeutic strategy would be to add to this endogenous antiadrenergic strategy by inhibiting receptor signal transduction.[111,118,199,205,280]

Thus, the chronically increased adrenergic drive present in the failing human heart delivers adverse biological signals to the cardiac myocyte through beta$_1$-, beta$_2$-, and possibly alpha$_1$-adrenergic receptors. Elimination of these adverse signals is the fundamental reason for using antiadrenergic agents in the treatment of chronic HF.[118]

Beta-Adrenergic Receptor–Blocking Agents

Because of their clinical availability, beta-adrenergic blocking agents were the first antiadrenergic agents used to treat chronic HF.[200] Although three classes of beta blockers are now available for clinical use, only the "second-generation" beta$_1$ receptor–selective antagonists or the "third-generation" beta blocker-vasodilators are tolerated to an acceptable degree by subjects with chronic HF.[281] Second-generation compounds are tolerated because they do not block cardiac pre- or postjunctional beta$_2$ receptors,[118,261,281,282] and third-generation compounds are tolerated because their afterload-reducing properties mitigate the cardiac output–reducing effects of beta-adrenergic withdrawal.[118,281,283] The receptor-binding profiles of beta-blocking agents that have been used successfully to treat HF are given in Table 23–11.

Regardless of the type of beta-blocking agent used, the treatment approach that must be taken in subjects with chronic HF is to start with extremely low doses (1/8 to 1/16 of the target dose) (Table 23–12) and gradually increase the dose every 1 to 2 weeks until full beta-blocking doses are achieved.[281] When this approach is taken, more than 90 percent of subjects with mild to moderate (stage 2) and more than 70 percent of subjects with advanced (stage 3) HF can tolerate beta blockade. The general mechanism of action of beta blockade in the failing and adversely remodeled heart has been reviewed extensively.[112,118,216,284] Both second- and third-generation beta-blocking agents improve intrinsic systolic function and reverse remodeling in primary or secondary cardiomyopathy in a time-dependent fashion that begins after an initial period of myocardial depression related to withdrawal of beta-adrenergic support.[112,115,216] However, these effects are not uniform across all treated subjects, and

TABLE 23–11 Adrenergic Receptor Blocking Affinities of Beta-Blocking Agents in Human Receptors*

Generation/ Class	Compound	K(beta$_1$)† (nM)	K(beta$_2$) (nM)	Beta$_1$/Beta$_2$ Selectivity	K(alpha$_1$) (nM)	Beta$_1$/Alpha$_1$ Selectivity
First/nonselective	Propranolol‡	4.1	8.5	2.1	—	—
Second/selective beta$_1$	Metoprolol	45	3,345	74	—	—
	Bisoprolol	121	14,390	119	—	—
Third/beta blocker–vasodilator	Carvedilol‡	4.0	29	7.3	9.4	2.4
	Bucindolol‡	3.6	5.0	1.4	238	66 (19)*
	Nebivolol	0.7	225	352	330	471

*Beta receptors are the average of data from radiological binding data in myocardial membranes and recombinant receptors, and inhibition in functional assays; alpha$_1$ receptors are from myocardial membranes. Metoprolol and bisoprolol data are from radiological binding data in myocardial membranes. Nebivolol data are from another laboratory, in guinea pig receptor preparations.[4]

†K(beta$_1$) = average of high-affinity dissociation constant determined from ^{125}I-CYP competition curves in human ventricular myocardial membranes, dissociation constant determined from competition curves in transfected cells expressing recombinant human beta$_1$ receptors, and dissociation constant determined from inhibition of isoproterenol-mediated stimulation of muscle contraction in preparations of nonfailing human heart. K(beta$_2$) = average of low-affinity dissociation constant determined from ^{125}I-CYP competition curves, dissociation constant determined from simple curve fitting in transfected cells expressing recombinant human beta$_2$ receptors, and dissociation constant determined from inhibition of isoproterenol-mediated stimulation of adenylyl cyclase in membrane preparations of human heart. K(alpha$_1$) = dissociation constant determined from ^{125}I-BE2254 competition curves in human ventricular myocardial membranes.

‡Based on an alpha$_1$ K_i of 69 nM in human saphenous vein ring segments (Tackett RL, personal communication, 1999).

TABLE 23–12 Starting and Target Doses for Beta Blockers

Agent	Starting Dose	Target Dose <75-85 kg	Target Dose ≥75-85 kg
Metoprolol CR/XL	12.5 or 25 mg PO qd*	200 mg PO qd	200 mg PO qd
Bisoprolol†	1.25 mg PO qd	5 mg PO qd	10 mg PO qd
Carvedilol	3.125 mg PO b.i.d.	25 mg PO b.i.d.	50 mg PO b.i.d.

*Starting dose should be half of above if disease is Class III or IV or if the patient has severe right-sided heart failure or is tenuous.

†Not approved by the Food and Drug Administration for heart failure in the United States.

some subjects may deteriorate and have an adverse clinical response to beta blockade.[285] The specific mechanism by which beta blockers produce a time-dependent improvement in systolic function and reversal of remodeling has also been investigated.[286,287] In the failing, remodeled human heart, both second- and third-generation beta-blocking agents produce changes in myocardial gene expression that would be expected to increase systolic function and reverse remodeling.[286] These changes in gene expression fall within a family of genes that constitute the so-called fetal gene program, shown several years ago to be associated with the development of pathological hypertrophy and systolic dysfunction in rodent models of cardiomyopathy.[288]

As discussed earlier and shown in Table 23–10, the $beta_1$ receptor pathways have much greater pathological potential than the $beta_2$ or $alpha_1$ pathways, and as shown in Table 23–5, norepinephrine, the adrenergic neurotransmitter, is a $beta_1$-selective agonist. These two realities mean that $beta_1$-selective blocking agents have equal or nearly equal therapeutic potential compared with agents that block $beta_1$, $beta_2$, and $alpha_1$ receptor pathways.[256] Accordingly, a study that compared gene expression changes between equal $beta_1$-blocking doses of the second-generation compound metoprolol and the third-generation beta blocker carvedilol found no difference in their respective abilities to reverse partially fetal gene induction.[286]

Unlike members of the ACEI, ARB, and aldosterone antagonist classes of neurohormonal inhibitors, beta-blocking agents are more diverse in their pharmacological effects and they are therefore discussed individually. However, as shown in Table 23–11, all beta blockers have in common the property of competitive antagonism of $beta_1$-adrenergic receptors.

Metoprolol

Metoprolol is a second-generation $beta_1$ receptor–selective blocking agent with an approximately 75-fold higher affinity for human $beta_1$- than $beta_2$-adrenergic receptors. Metoprolol, in its long-acting, controlled-release form (metoprolol succinate, CR/XL), is approved for the treatment of HF in the United States. Metoprolol is also approved for hypertension and ischemic heart disease indications.

The first placebo-controlled multicenter trial with a beta-blocking agent was the Metoprolol in Dilated Cardiomyopathy (MDC) trial, which used the shorter acting tartrate preparation at a target dose of 50 mg three times a day.[208] The MDC trial compared metoprolol tartrate with placebo in subjects with symptomatic HF caused by idiopathic dilated cardiomyopathy. The sample size estimate was based on an expected 50 percent reduction by metoprolol in the combined endpoint of all-cause mortality and deterioration of the patient to the point of requiring listing for heart transplantation. The MDC trial had in addition numerous prespecified secondary endpoints, including mortality alone, number of hospitalizations, LV function, quality of life, and exercise tolerance.[208] In the MDC trial, metoprolol at an average dose of 108 mg/d reduced the prevalence of the primary endpoint by 34 percent, which was not quite statistically significant ($p = 0.058$).[208] The benefit was due entirely to a reduction by metoprolol in the morbidity component of the primary endpoint (a reduction of 90 percent), with no favorable trends in the mortality component of the primary endpoint. In addition, when compared with placebo, metoprolol improved LV function, quality of life, number of hospitalizations, and exercise tolerance at 12 months.[208]

THE MERIT-HF TRIAL. Despite the salutary clinical effects demonstrated for metoprolol tartrate in MDC,[288] this agent was not selected by at least two trial steering committees (BEST and MERIT-HF) for use in a phase III, placebo-controlled mortality trial, primarily because of its pharmacokinetic properties. Metoprolol tartrate given at a 50-mg dose has relatively short elimination and pharmacological half-lives in non–slow metabolizer subjects (respectively 3 to 4 hours and 6 hours), which ideally necessitates dosing three times a day. Although it is possible to increase the metoprolol tartrate dose to attain twice-daily $beta_1$ receptor blockade,[286] higher (100 mg) doses produce large peak blood levels that may produce adverse effects. At lower doses (≤50 mg twice a day), the short pharmacological half-life and rapid receptor offset kinetics[289] of metoprolol tartrate mean that a "beta blocker withdrawal" syndrome is more likely to occur, especially if doses are missed or delayed, a situation that could predispose patients with HF to sudden death. Thus, a more efficacious formulation of metoprolol was developed, metoprolol CR/XL, which because of its controlled-release profile has operational elimination and pharmacological half-lives of 12 to 15 hours plus very shallow, near-plateau plots of plasma concentration versus time.[290]

The steering committee of the Metoprolol CR/XL Randomized Interventional Trial in Congestive Heart Failure (MERIT-HF) therefore selected the succinate continuous release, coated metoprolol succinate pellet formulation for use in a placebo-controlled mortality trial.[291] MERIT-HF was stopped prematurely because of a 34 percent reduction in mortality in the metoprolol arm (Table 23–13; see Fig. 24–5).[292] MERIT-HF enrolled 3991 subjects with ischemic and nonischemic dilated cardiomyopathy who had Classes II to IV HF.[292] The average dose of metoprolol achieved in MERIT-HF was larger than in the MDC trial, 159[212] versus 108[208] mg. The majority (97 percent) of patients enrolled in MERIT-HF were categorized as having Class II or III HF, and on the basis of the annualized mortality rate of 11 percent in the placebo group and the baseline LV ejection fraction of 28 percent, this landmark clinical trial[212] enrolled subjects with mild to moderate HF and moderate to severe systolic dysfunction. Notably, in MERIT-HF, mortality from sudden death or progressive pump failure was reduced.[212] In addition, mortality was reduced across most demographic groups, including older versus younger subjects, nonischemic versus ischemic etiology, and lower versus higher ejection fractions.[212] However, almost no mortality reduction was noted in the relatively small number of female subjects enrolled (23 percent of the total),[212] which suggests that gender may influence the response to beta blockade in HF populations.

The CR/XL preparation used in MERIT-HF produces a relatively constant blood level of metoprolol for 24 hours, but the bioavailability of the CR preparation is approximately 70 percent that of the conventional formulation. However, when compared with 50 mg twice daily of the conventional formulation, 100 mg/d of the CR preparation produces similar trough levels and average degrees of reduction in exercise heart rate, indicating bioequivalence of the two preparations. The reduced fluctuation in blood levels for the CR versus the conventional formulation provides the potential for improved tolerability of the CR formulation in patients with HF. In addition, as discussed previously, the much more shallow slope of the CR plasma concentration curve at the end of the dosing interval would theoretically reduce the potential of producing a beta blocker withdrawal effect. Although these differences in pharmacokinetics could account for greater efficacy of the CR preparation in reducing mortality, a direct comparison of metoprolol tartrate with the CR succinate preparation in subjects with chronic HF indicated no obvious difference in LV function or clinical improvement between the two preparations.[292]

A mortality trial (Carvedilol or Metoprolol European Trial [COMET] comparing metoprolol tartrate with carvedilol demonstrated 17 percent greater mortality reduction in favor of carvedilol, with respective mean daily doses of the two beta blockers being 85 and 42 mg.[293] This

TABLE 23–13 Beta Blocker Trials Conducted in Chronic Heart Failure, with 12-Month Mortality Rates Taken from Survival Curves When Data Not Directly Available in Published Material

Trial Name	Agent	NYHA Class	Heart Failure Stage, 1-4*	No. of Subjects Enrolled	12-Month Placebo Mortality (%)	12-Month Effect Size (%)
Stage 2 Populations of Patients						
CIBIS-I	Bisoprolol	"III,IV"	2	641	11	↓20
Carvedilol U.S.	Carvedilol	II,III	2	1,094	10	↓66
CIBIS-II	Bisoprolol	"III,IV"	2	2,647	13	↓33
MERIT-HF	Metoprolol CR	II-IV	2	3,991	11	↓35
Stage 3 Populations of Patients						
BEST	Bucindolol	III,IV	3	2,708	17	↓10†
COPERNICUS	Carvedilol	"Severe HF"	3	2,289	18	↓38
Beta blocker totals		II-IV	2-3	13,370	14	↓32
Post-MI Populations of Patients						
CAPRICORN	Carvedilol	I	1	1,959	11	↓23
BEAT	Bucindolol	I	1	343	21	↓12

BEAT = bucindolol evaluation in acute myocardial infarction trial; BEST = Beta Blocker Evaluation of Survival Trial; CAPRICORN = Carvedilol Post-Infarct Survival Control in Left Ventriular Dysfunction; CIBIS = Cardiac Insufficiency Bisoprolol Study; COPERNICUS = Carvedilol Prospective Randomized Cumulative Survival; MERIT-HF = Metoprolol CR/XL Randomized Interventional Trial in Congestive Heart Failure; NYHA = New York Heart Association.

*See Chapter 21.

†Effect size at 2 years.

relatively low average dose of metoprolol also produced less heart rate or blood pressure reduction than carvedilol.[293] In view of the fact that in MERIT-HF the degree of mortality reduction produced by metoprolol CR/XL in the entire cohort[212] as well as in a subpopulation with "severe HF" [294] was essentially identical to that produced by carvedilol in the Carvedilol Prospective Randomized Cumulative Survival (COPERNICUS)[295] trial (see Table 23–13 and Fig. 24–9), at least some of the differential efficacy of carvedilol and metoprolol in COMET was probably due to the lower beta$_1$-blocking doses of immediate-release metoprolol tartrate rather than to an absolute difference in efficacy between metoprolol and carvedilol.[256]

Bisoprolol

Bisoprolol is a second-generation beta$_1$ receptor–selective blocking agent with approximately 120-fold higher affinity for human beta$_1$ versus beta$_2$ receptors (see Table 23–12). Bisoprolol has long elimination (9 to 12 hours in healthy subjects, probably longer in patients with HF) and pharmacological (12 to 14 hours) half-lives, making it suitable for once-daily dosing.[296] Bisoprolol is approved for the treatment of hypertension in the United States and for HF or hypertension in Europe.

The first trial performed with bisoprolol was the Cardiac Insufficiency Bisoprolol Study I (CIBIS-I) trial,[297] which was a placebo-controlled trial of the effects of bisoprolol on mortality in subjects with symptomatic ischemic or nonischemic cardiomyopathy treated for an average follow-up of 22.8 months (see Table 23–13). This trial, sample sized on an unrealistically high expected event rate in the control group, ended up with a statistically insignificant, 20 percent mortality reduction.[297] In addition, the benefit in this trial was confined to subjects with nonischemic cardiomyopathy.[297] Despite the lack of overall statistical significance in CIBIS-I, the reduction in mortality was similar to what has been accomplished with ACEIs and was viewed as encouraging. The results prompted a follow-up trial, CIBIS-II,[211] with more conservative effect size estimates and sample size calculations.

The CIBIS-II trial was stopped by the Data and Safety Monitoring Committee 18 months early because of a 32 percent reduction ($p < 0.001$) in all-cause mortality (see Table 23–13) in the bisoprolol-treated group (see Fig. 24–5).[211] CIBIS-II enrolled 2647 patients with Class III or IV HF caused by ischemic and nonischemic cardiomyopathy; the median follow-up was 1.3 years. In addition to the reduction in mortality, bisoprolol reduced the number of hospitalizations (by 20 percent) and cardiovascular deaths (by 29 percent).[211] In CIBIS-II,[211] deaths classified as sudden were statistically reduced (by 44 percent) in the bisoprolol group, whereas pump failure deaths were nonsignificantly reduced by 26 percent.

This trend toward a greater reduction in sudden versus pump failure deaths was opposite to that obtained in CIBIS-I.[211,297] Another difference between CIBIS-I and CIBIS-II was the effect on ischemic versus nonischemic cardiomyopathy, which also demonstrated opposite trends. In CIBIS-I,[297] the reduction in mortality in the nonischemic group was 47 percent ($p = 0.01$), whereas in patients with a history of myocardial infarction, a trend toward an increase in mortality (by 11 percent) was noted in the bisoprolol group. One possible explanation for the differences between the CIBIS-I and CIBIS-II trials is the average dose of bisoprolol used; in CIBIS-II the target dose was 10 mg/d,[211] whereas in CIBIS-I it was 5 mg/d.[297]

Although CIBIS-II enrolled patients with Class III (>90 percent of the total) or Class IV symptoms, the annualized placebo mortality was only 13.2 percent (see Table 23-13).[211] This mortality rate is similar to that found in the enalapril arm of the SOLVD Treatment Trial[207] (see Table 23-7), which was composed of 68 percent Class I and II patients. In addition, the average blood pressure of patients enrolled in CIBIS-II was 130/80 mm Hg, which is higher than the blood pressures of the SOLVD patients[207] or the patients enrolled in the U.S. carvedilol trials,[209] who were approximately 50:50 Class II and III. A relatively large proportion of CIBIS-II patients were enrolled in Eastern Europe and Russia, where practice patterns, HF etiology, or symptom interpretation may not be comparable to that in Western Europe and the United States. Nevertheless, the results of CIBIS-II were internally consistent through all major demographic groups,[211] and the impressive results constitute a landmark clinical trial in the development of beta blockade as therapy for chronic HF.

Carvedilol

Carvedilol is currently approved for the treatment of chronic HF in the United States; it is also approved in most other countries. As noted in Table 23–11, carvedilol is a minimally beta$_1$ receptor–selective beta-blocking agent that has high affinity for alpha$_1$-adrenergic receptors as well as ancillary antioxidant action.[298] Because carvedilol is a potent vasodilator, its side effect profile on initiation of therapy and during uptitration is different from that of highly beta$_1$-selective second-generation agents, with orthostatic symptoms being more prominent.[281] At low doses (≤6.25 mg twice daily), carvedilol may exhibit some beta$_1$ selectivity in humans with HF.[299] At higher target doses, carvedilol blocks all three adrenergic receptors coupled to hypertrophy and other adverse biological effects (beta$_1$, beta$_2$, and alpha$_1$ receptors; see Table 23–11) that contribute to remodeling and myocardial dysfunction in the failing human heart.

In addition, because it blocks prejunctional beta$_2$ receptors, carvedilol mildly reduces cardiac adrenergic drive.[300] Perhaps because of its comprehensive antiadrenergic action, the beneficial effects of carvedilol on myocardial function and reversal of remodeling are consistent and substantial.[300-306]

PHARMACODYNAMICS. Carvedilol is a highly lipophilic beta blocker that is stereospecifically metabolized by the liver. The preferential metabolism of the *S* isomer means that *R* isomer concentrations are approximately 2.5 times higher in plasma, and this effect may be even greater in slow metabolizers.[118] The *S* isomer of carvedilol has an affinity constant (K_D) for human cardiac beta$_1$ receptors of 0.4 nM, and the *R* isomer has a K_D of 26 nM (unpublished data) and a net (directly measured) K_D of the racemate of 4 nM (see Table 23-11). The *S* and *R* isomers have comparable K_D values for the human cardiac alpha$_1$ receptor of 9.4 nM. This means that at 2.5-fold higher plasma and presumably myocardial levels of the *R* versus the *S* isomer, the degrees of beta$_1$ and alpha$_1$ receptor blockade are approximately equal, which is what is observed clinically. Carvedilol has an elimination half-life of 4 to 6 hours in normal volunteers or hypertensive subjects, which necessitates twice-daily dosing.[307] However, carvedilol has very slow receptor offset kinetics,[289] the likely explanation for a third compartment with a 14.5-hour elimination half-life observed after intravenous administration. As a result, carvedilol is less prone to beta receptor withdrawal phenomena on dose interruption.

DOSE-RESPONSE RESULTS. Unlike the case of other beta-blocking agents approved for the treatment of HF, there is extensive dose-response information on the efficacy and safety of carvedilol. The Multicenter Oral Carvedilol Heart Failure Assessment (MOCHA) trial[210] demonstrated LV functional and clinical superiority of 25 mg of carvedilol twice daily over 6.25 mg twice daily but clearly defined efficacy of 6.25 mg twice daily compared with placebo. In addition, most,[308-310] but not all,[311] studies comparing carvedilol with beta$_1$-selective antagonists have found at least trends in favor of quantitatively greater effects for carvedilol. On the other hand, in these studies the degree of beta$_1$ receptor blockade, as assessed by exercise heart rate inhibition, has generally been greater with carvedilol.[310] Even if carvedilol does produce a slightly greater degree of improvement in myocardial function and reversal of remodeling, as discussed earlier, it is not yet clear whether this superiority translates into better clinical results in view of the excellent results of beta$_1$-selective compounds in the MERIT-HF[212] and CIBIS-II[211] trials. The COMET trial described previously did show a small advantage (by 17 percent) for carvedilol versus immediate-release metoprolol tartrate for mortality reduction, but heart rate data also indicated a greater degree of beta$_1$ blockade by carvedilol,[293] and so this trial cannot be interpreted as demonstrating superior efficacy of carvedilol versus metoprolol. Data from the MOCHA trial[210] and from CIBIS I[297] and CIBIS II[211] strongly suggest that the responses to beta blockade in terms of survival and improvements in LV ejection fraction are dependent on dose and degree of beta blockade, and the COMET results are probably another example of this.[256]

CLINICAL TRIALS. The database of placebo-controlled clinical trials for carvedilol is the most extensive for any beta blocker in chronic HF. To date, 4037 patients have been enrolled in nine randomized, placebo-controlled phase II and III clinical trials in chronic HF,[209,210,295,300-302,312-316] plus one trial involving 1959 patients after myocardial infarction or LV dysfunction (see Table 23–13).[317] The phase III U.S. Carvedilol Trials Program, composed of four individual trials managed by single Steering and Data and Safety Monitoring committees, was stopped prematurely by the Data and Safety Monitoring Committee because of a highly significant ($p <$ 0.0001) 65 percent reduction in mortality by carvedilol versus placebo across all four trials.[209] In addition, one individual trial (MOCHA) demonstrated a highly statistically significant, 73 percent reduction in mortality.[210] However, because these trials were relatively short term and the number of events was small, the data from MOCHA or the rest of the U.S. Carvedilol Trials Program were not considered by the FDA to be conclusive for an indication of mortality reduction. Carvedilol was originally approved by the FDA for delaying progression of the myocardial disease process and lowering the combined risk of morbidity plus mortality on the basis of data from the carvedilol U.S. trials[210,312-314] and then later approved for mortality reduction on the basis of the COPERNICUS trial[295] results.

The COPERNICUS trial investigated "severe" HF with no documentation of NYHA functional class.[295] Patients qualifying by symptoms had to be clinically euvolemic and have an LV ejection fraction less than 25 percent. Compared with placebo, carvedilol reduced the mortality risk at 12 months by 38 percent (see Table 23–13)[295] and the risk of death or HF hospitalization by 31 percent (see Fig. 24–5).[317]

Carvedilol has also been evaluated in a post-myocardial infarction trial in which patients had to exhibit LV dysfunction, the CAPRICORN trial.[316] Although carvedilol did not reduce the primary endpoint of mortality plus cardiovascular hospitalization, it did reduce total mortality (by 23 percent, $p = 0.03$), cardiovascular mortality (by 25 percent, $p < 0.05$), and nonfatal myocardial infarction (by 41 percent, $p = 0.014$).[316]

BUCINDOLOL*

PHARMACOLOGICAL PROPERTIES. Bucindolol is a completely nonselective third-generation beta-blocking agent with mild vasodilator activity that is probably due to weak alpha$_1$ receptor–blocking properties.[118] The pharmacokinetic properties of bucindolol are similar to those of carvedilol, except that there is no stereospecific metabolism. The mild vasodilator properties of bucindolol coupled with its low "inverse agonist" profile[118,318,319] make this beta blocker extremely well tolerated in HF patients,[281] including those with advanced HF.[320] Inverse agonism is the ability of a receptor antagonist to inactivate "active-state" receptors that are precoupled to G proteins and capable of transducing signals without agonist occupancy.[112] In the human heart, the percentage of such precoupled beta-adrenergic receptors identified by high-affinity agonist binding is on the order of 10 to 30 percent of the total. Antagonists with high degrees of inverse agonist activity such as metoprolol have a greater ability than bucindolol to inactivate these active-state receptors, which is probably why bucindolol is associated with less intrinsic myocardial depression and lowers 24-hour Holter-monitored heart rates less than metoprolol or carvedilol.[283] The latter property translates into less symptomatic bradycardia with bucindolol, which is why the BEST trial had a much lower heart rate exclusion criterion (50 beats/min)[320] than other beta blocker HF trials (typically 68 beats/min). Thus, a low inverse agonist profile is a property that increases the tolerability of a beta blocker in subjects with HF.

Although bucindolol has intrinsic sympathomimetic activity in some smaller animal species,[321] because of differences in the stoichiometry of receptor–G protein coupling between animal models and humans, bucindolol has no intrinsic sympathomimetic activity in failing[322-326] or nonfailing[326] functioning human myocardial preparations or in the intact failing human heart.[201,283] Finally, because of its potent beta$_2$ receptor–blocking properties coupled with only mild vasodilation, bucindolol is the only beta-blocking agent that has been shown to lower systemic adrenergic activity in subjects with HF.[210,320,327] Thus, the unique pharmacological

*Not approved by the FDA.

profile of bucindolol allows an agent with comprehensive antiadrenergic activity to be given to patients with advanced, stage 3 HF.

CLINICAL OBSERVATIONS. Bucindolol was the first beta-blocking agent shown to improve LV function in a placebo-controlled trial,[201] and it was the first beta-blocking agent shown to improve load-independent, intrinsic systolic function.[202] In those and subsequent phase II trials,[328,329] bucindolol was well tolerated, in marked contrast to previous[330,331] and subsequent[332] experience with the nonselective first-generation agent propranolol. Bucindolol was the second beta-blocking agent to be evaluated in a multicenter trial, in which bucindolol produced a dose-related improvement in LV function and a dose-unrelated prevention of deterioration in LV function in subjects with symptomatic ischemic and nonischemic cardiomyopathy treated for a 12-week period.[329] On the basis of these data, doses of bucindolol with very high degrees of beta blockade[329] (100 mg twice daily for subjects heavier than 75 kg, 50 mg twice daily for subjects less than 75 kg) were chosen for use in phase III trials.

THE BEST TRIAL. The largest of these phase III trials, the Beta Blocker Evaluation of Survival Trial (BEST),[320] randomly assigned 2708 subjects with advanced (Class III or IV) HF to placebo or bucindolol. As can be observed from the 12-month placebo mortality rates in Table 23-13, BEST[320] was conducted in subjects with advanced HF comparable to that investigated in COPERNICUS.[295] In the BEST subject population as a whole, bucindolol produced a statistically nonsignificant (p = 0.10), 10 percent reduction in total mortality that was heterogeneous with respect to race.[320] That is, the 76 percent of subjects in BEST who were not black had a statistically significant (p = 0.01), 19 percent reduction in mortality, whereas the 24 percent who were black had a nonsignificant trend for an increase (by 17 percent) in mortality (interaction p value < 0.05). Because BEST was the first beta blocker mortality trial to enroll a substantial percentage of black patients and is the first reported beta blocker study in advanced HF, it is uncertain whether the demographically heterogeneous findings can be extrapolated to other beta-blocking agents or to less advanced HF.

Of note is that in the U.S. Carvedilol Trials conducted in mild to moderate HF, an agent with a similar pharmacological profile produced a similar degree of improvement in LV function and clinical parameters in blacks and nonblacks.[333] In addition, in a small single-center experience[334] and in the small number of black subjects investigated in MERIT-HF,[335] metoprolol appeared to improve LV function[334] or reduce HF hospitalizations[325] in blacks to a similar degree as in whites. Therefore, the apparent lack of favorable effect of bucindolol in blacks in BEST may be due to the more advanced nature of HF investigated in BEST or the unique characteristics of the population of black patients in this trial. However, there are also potential drug-specific explanations for the bucindolol versus carvedilol or metoprolol data in blacks, including the greater degree of vasodilation with carvedilol being beneficial in an HF population with a high incidence of a history of hypertension, the beta$_1$ selectivity of metoprolol, or the norepinephrine-lowering property of bucindolol producing too much withdrawal of adrenergic support (see later for moxonidine) in the black population of BEST.

Norepinephrine lowering is a beta$_2$ receptor blockade–mediated response, and the black population of BEST had higher baseline systemic norepinephrine levels than nonblacks.[320] In addition, 67 percent of blacks in BEST were homozygous for an alpha$_{2C}$-adrenergic receptor loss-of-function polymorphism that is associated with an increased risk for developing HF, presumably because of increased adrenergic activity (Liggett S, Bristow MR, unpublished observations). This would could have predisposed black patients to being susceptible to the adverse sympatholytic effects of bucindolol.[327] From previous trials it is known that black hypertensives respond less well to beta-blocking agents or ACEIs[336] than nonblacks and that blacks with HF also do not respond well to ACEIs.[337] Thus, the most beneficial therapy for favorably affecting the natural history of HF, ACEIs and beta-blocking agents, may be less effective or even ineffective in a population group that represents 12 percent of the U.S. population.

In the BEST population as a whole, bucindolol produced statistically favorable effects on multiple secondary endpoints, including cardiovascular deaths, HF hospitalizations, the combined endpoint of mortality plus hospitalization, the need for cardiac transplantation, left and right ventricular function, and the incidence of myocardial infarction.[320,337] Bucindolol is the first beta blocker to demonstrate reduction in myocardial infarction in a population with chronic HF or ischemic cardiomyopathy.[337] In addition, in an immediate post-myocardial infarction trial, a study that was ended early by the sponsor, bucindolol did not significantly reduce mortality (reduction by 12 percent, p = not significant) but substantially (by at least 30 percent, $p < 0.05$) reduced all myocardial reinfarction–related endpoints and was well tolerated.[338] These data suggest that the sympatholytic and comprehensive antiadrenergic effects of bucindolol may have had heightened efficacy in certain subpopulations with LV dysfunction, such as those with active ischemia or even adrenergic receptor polymorphisms in which more powerful antiadrenergic action is desired.[339]

NEBIVOLOL*

Nebivolol is another third-generation beta blocker–vasodilator in development, which is approved in Europe for the treatment of hypertension. Nebivolol has limited but favorable experience[340,341] in HF trials. As can be observed in Table 23-12, nebivolol is markedly beta$_1$ selective and, as such, it is unique among third-generation compounds available or in development for HF. Another unique feature of nebivolol is that its vasodilatory action appears to be due to the generation of nitric oxide.[342] Interestingly, in a small study comparing nebivolol and placebo, nebivolol improved intrinsic systolic function and resulted in regression of hypertrophy in South African blacks with mild to moderate HF.[340] Although it is likely that the populations of patients differ substantially (such as more subjects with a history of hypertension in the carvedilol U.S. data), it is worth noting that carvedilol and nebivolol, both of which have substantial vasodilator properties, have shown some success in black populations with mild to moderate HF.

Class Recommendations for the Use of Beta-Blocking Agents in Chronic Heart Failure

Table 23–14 summarizes the class effects of beta-blocking agents, related to competitive antagonism of beta$_1$-adrenergic receptors, that have been observed in large, placebo-controlled HF clinical trials. Doses are shown in Table 23–11. Patients with mild to moderate compensated HF from nonischemic or ischemic dilated cardiomyopathy and NYHA Class II to III symptoms (stage 2 subjects) who are receiving standard treatment, including diuretics and ACEIs, and who do not have a contraindication to beta blockade, are candidates for treatment with a beta-blocking agent.[118,134,343,344] For the present, this group would include black patients, although the data supporting use in such patients are not extensive.

Euvolemic patients with advanced, Class III or IV (stage 3) HF should also be routinely treated with a beta blocker on the basis of data from the COPERNICUS[295] and MERIT-HF trials.[294] For patients with decompensated Class III or IV HF, beta blockers remain contraindicated, but this position could change pending the outcome of current trials such as Enoximone Plus Metoprolol in Subjects With Advanced Chronic Heart Failure (EMPOWER), which combines a type III PDEI with a beta blocker, on the basis of encouraging phase II data.[175]

When patients with HF reach a maintenance dose of a beta blocker, treatment should be maintained indefinitely because of the risk of deterioration after drug withdrawal.[345] As discussed earlier (see Positive Inotropic Agents) if it is necessary to treat a decompensated patient receiving maintenance beta blockade with a positive inotropic agent, a PDEI rather than a beta-agonist should be used because the hemodynamic effects of PDEIs are not antagonized by beta blockade.[119,120,158,174]

Which Beta-Blocker Should Be Used to Treat Chronic Heart Failure?

From the preceding discussions, it is apparent that beta-blocking agents are more pharmacologically diverse in mechanism of action than ACEIs or even ARBs. On the other hand, the predominance of the beta$_1$ receptor over other adrenergic receptor pathways in protein abundance, binding affinity for norepinephrine, and pathological potential leads to a thera-

*Not approved by the FDA.

TABLE 23–14 Class Clinical Effects of Beta-Adrenergic Blocking Agents in Chronic Heart Failure

Effect	Studies	Beta Blockers
Reduction in total mortality	CIBIS-II, MERIT-HF, COPERNICUS	Metoprolol CR/XL, bisoprolol, carvedilol
Reduction in CV mortality	CIBIS-II, MERIT-HF, COPERNICUS, BEST	Metoprolol CR/XL, bisoprolol, carvedilol, bucindolol
Reduction in CV or HF hospitalizations	MDC, MERIT-HF, CIBIS-II, U.S. Carvedilol, BEST	Metoprolol tartrate, metoprolol CR/XL, bisoprolol, carvedilol, bucindolol
Improved HF symptoms	MDC, MERIT-HF, CIBIS-II, U.S. Carvedilol	Metoprolol tartrate, metoprolol CR/XL, bisoprolol, carvedilol
Reduced need for cardiac transplantation	MDC, BEST	Metoprolol tartrate, bucindolol
Reduction in myocardial infarction	BEST	Bucindolol

BEST = Beta Blocker Evaluation of Survival Trial; CIBIS = Cardiac Insufficiency Bisoprolol Study; COPERNICUS = Carvedilol Prospective Randomized Cumulative Survival; CV = cardiovascular; HF = heart failure; MDC = Metoprolol in Dilated Cardiomyopathy; MERIT-HF = Metoprolol CR/XL Randomized Interventional Trial in Congestive Heart Failure.

peutic class effect for any competitive antagonist that binds with high affinity to beta$_1$-adrenergic receptors without possessing intrinsic sympathomimetic activity. Although data indicating that carvedilol is superior to metoprolol have been generated in direct comparison trials,[293,300] these trials were flawed by the use of a lower beta$_1$-blocking dose of the formulation of metoprolol in comparison with carvedilol.[256] However, the COMET trial[293] has demonstrated that lower beta$_1$-blocking doses of immediate-release metoprolol given twice daily are inferior to higher beta$_1$ receptor–blocking doses of carvedilol. Therefore, lower doses of shorter acting beta$_1$-selective blocking agents such as metoprolol tartrate or atenolol (for which there is no controlled experience in HF) *cannot be* recommended as equivalent to therapy with higher doses of carvedilol, controlled-release (CR/XL) metoprolol, or bisoprolol. Of course, there remains the possibility that carvedilol is truly superior to beta$_1$-selective agents delivered to the same degree of beta$_1$ receptor blockade, but no study demonstrating this has been conducted.

Because of the pharmacological heterogeneity among beta-blocking agents, the degree of polymorphic variation in key components of adrenergic mechanisms, and the clinical diversity of HF subpopulations, there remains an excellent possibility that antiadrenergic therapy with beta-blocking agents will evolve to a more tailored and targeted approach involving individual types of agents being more effective for subsets of polymorphic receptor variants or other determinants of antiadrenergic response, or both.[338]

Limitations of Beta Blocker Therapy in Chronic Heart Failure

Despite their proven efficacy in HF in patients with primary or secondary dilated cardiomyopathy, it is important to emphasize that beta blockers have limitations to general application in HF populations. First and foremost is that many patients with HF have contraindications to beta blockade, such as reactive airway disease, sinus node or conduction system disease with bradycardia, and advanced HF with hemodynamic decompensation. Another problem is that even in mild to moderate HF, initiation of therapy and uptitration of beta-blocking agents can be difficult and require both persistence and a knowledge of management maneuvers[281] that allow target doses to be achieved. A third problem is that for reasons that are not yet clear, some patients do not respond to beta blockade in terms of favorable effects on myocardial function, and these individuals may have a worse outcome than patients treated with placebo.[285] Some, but not all, of these problems might be overcome by the development of more efficacious or better tolerated compounds; the use of other, more effective types of antiadrenergic therapy; or the use of a combination of beta blockers with positive inotropic agents.[174,175] The importance of the beta blocker data set is not that it demonstrates a "cure" for chronic HF but rather that it has now been shown that in some patients, the prognosis can be substantially improved by medical therapy. This observation should provide an impetus to develop further types of treatment that improve the biological properties of the failing heart.

OTHER ANTIADRENERGIC AGENTS

The success of beta-blocking agents and the realization that many subjects have contraindications to them have prompted attempts to develop antiadrenergic approaches other than beta receptor blockade. An obvious approach would be to inhibit norepinephrine synthesis or release, but these approaches have not produced much success. In small studies conducted in less advanced HF, clonidine, which inhibits norepinephrine release through alpha$_2$ receptor agonist activity, has been well tolerated and has produced some evidence of clinical benefit.[346,347] In a medium-sized trial, the imidazoline receptor agonist moxonidine powerfully lowered norepinephrine in a dose-related fashion and produced evidence of reverse remodeling at higher doses.[348] However, in this trial, moxonidine also produced dose-related increases in adverse events that were greater than in the placebo group.[348] In addition, a phase III trial of high-dose moxonidine (MOXCON) had to be stopped because of a marked (by >50 percent) increase in mortality.[349] These data indicate that a drug that powerfully lowers adrenergic activity in a potentially insurmountable manner is not a good strategy in the treatment of chronic stable HF.

THE NEXT GENERATION OF HEART FAILURE TREATMENT

As can be observed by the effects of ACEIs, aldosterone antagonists, and beta blocker therapy (see Tables 23–7 and 23–13), medical therapy of HF has improved substantially over the past 15 years. This neurohormonal inhibitor approach to HF has been remarkably successful and has resulted in cumulated reductions in mortality of 30 to 40 percent. Unfortunately, we appear to have reached a limit in further antagonism of neurohormonal-cytokine systems inasmuch as most recent trials attempting to add additional neurohormonal-cytokine inhibition to background therapy of ACE inhibition and beta blockade have been unsuccessful. This list of failures includes certain endothelin antagonists, tumor necrosis factor-alpha inhibitors, and an NEP-ACEI. This experience indicates the limits of neurohormonal inhibition and strongly signals that different drug development approaches are now needed. Fortunately, these approaches are under way, with new small molecules, cell replacement therapy, gene therapy, and new devices all being examined. From the standpoint of small-molecule drug or gene therapy, major developmental programs exist targeting fetal gene induction, metabolism, apoptosis, and SR dysfunction. These are all novel approaches that target correction of maladaptive mechanisms, and it is likely that some of them will be successful in the near term.

Diuretics

1. Rouse D, Suki WN: Effects of neural and humoral agents on the renal tubules in congestive heart failure. Semin Nephrol 14:412, 1994.
2. Abassi Z, Winawer J, Skorecki KL: Control of extracellular fluid volume and the pathophysiology of edema formation. *In* Brenner BM (ed): Brenner and Rector's the Kidney. 7th ed. Philadelphia, WB Saunders, 2004, pp 777-856.
3. Maddox DA, Brenner BM: Glomerular ultrafiltration. *In* Brenner BM (ed): Brenner and Rector's the Kidney. 7th ed. Philadelphia, WB Saunders, 2004, pp 353-412.
4. Schrier RW, Abraham WT: Hormones and hemodynamics in heart failure. N Engl J Med 341:577, 1999.
5. Sladek CD, Kapoor JR: Neurotransmitter/neuropeptide interactions in the regulation of neurohypophyseal hormone release. Exp Neurol 171:200, 2001.
6. Benigni A, Perico N, Remuzzi G: Endothelin antagonists and renal protection. J Cardiovasc Pharmacol 35(4 Suppl 2):S75, 2000.
7. Haas M: The Na-K-Cl cotransporters. Am J Physiol 267:C869, 1994.
8. Raftery EB: Hemodynamic effects of diuretics in heart failure. Br Heart J 72:44, 1994.
9. Dunn CJ, Fitton A, Brogden RN: Torsemide. An update of its pharmacological properties and therapeutic efficacy. Drug Eval 49:121, 1995.
10. Wiemer G, Fink E, Linz W, et al: Furosemide enhances the release of endothelial kinins, nitric oxide and prostacyclin. J Pharmacol Exp Ther 271:1611, 1994.
11. Greenberg S, McGowan C, Xie J, Summer WR: Selective pulmonary and venous smooth muscle relaxation by furosemide: A comparison with morphine. J Pharmacol Exp Ther 270:1077, 1994.
12. Canessa C, Schild L, Buell G, et al: Amiloride-sensitive epithelial Na^+ channel is made of three homologous subunits. Nature 367:463, 1994.
13. Daleau P, Turgeon J: Triamterene inhibits the delayed rectifier potassium current (K_K) in guinea pig ventricular myocytes. Circ Res 74:1114, 1994.
14. Wang L, Sheldon RS, Mitchell B, et al: Amiloride-quinidine interaction: Adverse outcomes. Clin Pharmacol Ther 56:659, 1994.
15. Wingo CS, Cain BD: The renal H-K-ATPase: Physiological significance and role in potassium homeostasis. Annu Rev Physiol 55:323, 1993.
16. Farquharson CA, Struthers AD: Spironolactone increases nitric oxide bioactivity, improves endothelial vasodilator dysfunction, and suppresses vascular angiotensin I/angiotensin II conversion in patients with chronic heart failure. Circulation 101:594, 2000.
17. Funder JW: Aldosterone action. Annu Rev Physiol 55:115, 1993.
18. Pitt B, Zannad F, Remme WJ, et al: The effect of spironolactone on morbidity and mortality in patients with severe heart failure. Randomized Aldactone Evaluation Study Investigators. N Engl J Med 341:709, 1999.
19. Delyani JA: Mineralocorticoid receptor antagonists: The evolution of utility and pharmacology. Kidney Int 57:1408, 2000.
20. Hameedi A, Chadow HL: The promise of selective aldosterone receptor antagonists for the treatment of hypertension and congestive heart failure. Curr Hypertens Rep 2:378, 2000.
21. Pitt B, Remme W, Zannad F, et al, Eplerenone Post-Acute Myocardial Infarction Heart Failure Efficacy and Survival Study Investigators: Eplerenone, a selective aldosterone blocker, in patients with left ventricular dysfunction after myocardial infarction. N Engl J Med 348:1309, 2003.
22. White WB, Duprez D, St Hillaire R, et al: Effects of the selective aldosterone blocker eplerenone versus the calcium antagonist amlodipine in systolic hypertension. Hypertension 41:1021, 2003.
23. Schrier RW, Martin PY: Recent advances in the understanding of water metabolism in heart failure. Adv Exp Med Biol 449:415, 1998.
24. Burrell LM, Phillips PA, Stephenson JM, et al: Vasopressin and a nonpeptide antidiuretic hormone receptor antagonist (OPC-31260). Blood Press 3:137, 1994.
25. Naitoh M, Suzuki H, Murakami M, et al: Effects of oral AVP receptor antagonists OPC-21268 and OPC-31260 on congestive heart failure in conscious dogs. Am J Physiol 267:H2245, 1994.
26. Yamamura Y, Ogawa H, Yamashita H, et al: Characterization of a novel aquaretic agent, OPC-31260, as an orally effective, nonpeptide vasopressin V_2 receptor antagonist. Br J Pharmacol 105:787, 1992.
27. Hirano T, Yamamura Y, Nakamura S, et al: Effects of the V(2)-receptor antagonist OPC-41061 and the loop diuretic furosemide alone and in combination in rats. J Pharmacol Exp Ther 292:288, 2000.
28. Gheorghiade M, Niazi I, Ouyang J, et al, Tolvaptan Investigators: Vasopressin V2-receptor blockade with tolvaptan in patients with chronic heart failure: Results from a double-blind, randomized trial. Circulation 107:2690, 2003.
29. Abraham WT, Oren RM, Crisman TS, et al: Effects of an oral, non-peptide, selective V_2 receptor vasopressin antagonist in patients with chronic heart failure. J Am Coll Cardiol 29:169A, 1997.
30. Tahara A, Tomuira Y, Wada KI, et al: Pharmacological profile of YM087, a novel potent nonpeptide vasopressin V1A and V2 receptor antagonist, in vitro and in vivo. J Pharmacol Exp Ther 282:301, 1997.
31. Udelson JE, Smith WB, Hendrix GH, et al: Acute hemodynamic effects of conivaptan, a dual V(1A) and V(2) vasopressin receptor antagonist, in patients with advanced heart failure. Circulation 104:2417, 2001.
32. Russell SD, Selaru P, Pyne DA, et al: Rationale for use of an exercise end point and design for the ADVANCE (A Dose evaluation of a Vasopressin ANtagonist in CHF patients undergoing Exercise) trial. Am Heart J 145:179, 2003.
33. Van Kerckhoven R, Lankhuizen I, van Veghel R, et al: Chronic vasopressin V(1A) but not V(2) receptor antagonism prevents heart failure in chronically infarcted rats. Eur J Pharmacol 49:135, 2002.
34. Brater DC: Diuretic resistance: Mechanisms and therapeutic strategies. Cardiology 84:57, 1994.
35. Wilcox CS: Diuretics. *In* Brenner BM (ed): Brenner and Rector's the Kidney. 7th ed. Philadelphia, WB Saunders, 2004, pp 2345-2381.
36. Morsing P, Velazquez H, Wright FS, Ellison DH: Adaptation of distal convoluted tubule of rats. II. Effects of chronic thiazide infusion. Am J Physiol 261:F137, 1991.
37. Dzau VJ, Packer M, Lilly LS, et al: Prostaglandins in severe congestive heart failure. Relation to activation of the renin-angiotensin system and hyponatremia. N Engl J Med 310:347, 1984.
38. Good JM, Brady AJB, Noormohamed FH, et al: Effect of intense angiotensin II suppression on the diuretic response to furosemide during chronic ACE inhibition. Circulation 90:220, 1994.
39. Bailey MA, Giebisch G: Control of renal potassium excretion. *In* Brenner BM (ed): Brenner and Rector's the Kidney. 7th ed. Philadelphia, WB Saunders, 2004, pp 453-496.
40. Brown MJ, Brown DC, Murphy MB: Hypokalemia from beta2-receptor stimulation by circulating epinephrine. N Engl J Med 309:1414, 1983.
41. Haffner CA, Kendall MJ: Metabolic effects of beta 2-agonists. J Clin Pharm Ther 17:155, 1992.
42. Siscovick DS, Raghunathan TE, Psaty BM, et al: Diuretic therapy for hypertension and the risk of primary cardiac arrest. N Engl J Med 330:1852, 1994.
43. Ramsay LE, Yeo WW, Jackson PR: Metabolic effects of diuretics. Cardiology 84:48, 1994.

Vasodilators

44. Cohn JN, Franciosa JA: Vasodilator therapy of cardiac failure. N Engl J Med 297:27, 1977.
45. Kass DA, Kelly RP: Ventriculo-arterial coupling: Concepts, assumptions, and applications. Ann Biomed Eng 20:41, 1992.
46. Cohn JN, Archibald DG, Ziesche S, et al: Effect of vasodilator therapy on mortality in chronic congestive heart failure. Results of a Veterans Administration Cooperative Study. N Engl J Med 314:1547, 1986.
47. Cohn JN: Effect of vasodilator therapy on mortality in chronic congestive heart failure. Eur Heart J 9(Suppl A):171, 1988.
48. Packer M, Rouleau J, Swedberg K, et al: Effect of flosequinan on survival in chronic heart failure: Preliminary results of the PROFILE study [abstract]. Circulation 88(Suppl 1):301, 1993.
49. Califf RM, Adams KF, McKenna WJ, et al: A randomized controlled trial of epoprostenol therapy for severe congestive heart failure: The Flolan International Randomized Survival Trial (FIRST). Am Heart J 134:44, 1997.
50. Harrison DG, Bates JN: The nitrovasodilators. New ideas about old drugs. Circulation 87:1461, 1993.
51. Hare JM, Keaney JF Jr, Balligand JL, et al: Role of nitric oxide in parasympathetic modulation of β-adrenergic myocardial contractility in normal dogs. J Clin Invest 95:360, 1995.
52. Fallen EL, Nahmias C, Scheffel A, et al: Redistribution of myocardial blood flow with topical nitroglycerin in patients with coronary artery disease. Circulation 91:1381, 1995.
53. Leier CV, Huss P, Magouin RD, Unverferth DV: Improved exercise capacity and differing arterial and venous tolerance during chronic isosorbide dinitrate therapy for congestive heart failure. Circulation 67:817, 1983.
54. Publication Committee for the VMAC Investigators (Vasodilatation in the Management of Acute CHF): Intravenous nesiritide vs nitroglycerin for treatment of decompensated congestive heart failure: A randomized controlled trial. JAMA 287:1531, 2002.
55. Parker JD, Parker AB, Farrell B, et al: Intermittent transdermal nitroglycerin therapy. Decreased anginal threshold during the nitrate-free interval. Circulation 91:973, 1995.
56. Munzel T, Kurz S, Rajagopalan S, et al: Hydralazine prevents nitroglycerin tolerance by inhibiting activation of a membrane-bound NADH oxidase. A new action for an old drug. J Clin Invest 98:1465, 1996.
57. Risoe C, Simonsen S, Rootwelt K, et al: Nitroprusside and regional vascular capacitance in patients with severe congestive heart failure. Circulation 85:997, 1992.
58. Kussmaul WG, Altschuler JA, Matthai WH, et al: Right ventricular-vascular interaction in congestive heart failure. Importance of low-frequency impedance. Circulation 88:1010, 1993.
59. Cohn JN, Franciosa JA, Francis GS, et al: Effect of short-term infusion of sodium nitroprusside on mortality rate in acute myocardial infarction complicated by left ventricular failure: Results of a Veterans Administration cooperative study. N Engl J Med 306:1129, 1982.
60. Ginks WR, Redwood DR: Hemodynamic effects of hydralazine at rest and during exercise in patients with chronic heart failure. Br Heart J 44:259, 1980.
61. Leier CV: Regional blood flow responses to vasodilators and inotropes in congestive heart failure. Am J Cardiol 62:86E, 1988.
62. Hofstra AH: Metabolism of hydralazine: Relevance to drug-induced lupus. Drug Metab Rev 26:485, 1994.
63. Cohn JN, Johnson G, Ziesche S, et al: A comparison of enalapril with hydralazine-isosorbide dinitrate in the treatment of chronic congestive heart failure. N Engl J Med 325:303, 1991.
64. Carson P, Ziesche S, Johnson G, et al: Racial differences in response to therapy for heart failure: Analysis of the vasodilator-heart failure trials. Vasodilator-Heart Failure Trial Study Group. J Card Fail 5:178, 1999.
65. Vesely DL, Douglass MA, Dietz JR, et al: Three peptides from the atrial natriuretic factor prohormone amino terminus lower blood pressure and produce diuresis, natriuresis, and/or kaliuresis in humans. Circulation 90:1129, 1994.
66. Nakamura M, Arakawa N, Yoshida H, et al: Vasodilatory effects of C-type natriuretic peptide on forearm resistance vessels are distinct from those of atrial natriuretic peptide in chronic heart failure. Circulation 90:1210, 1994.
67. Suga SI, Nakao K, Itoh H, et al: Endothelial production of C-type natriuretic peptide and its marked augmentation by transforming growth factor-β. Possible existence of "vascular natriuretic peptide system." J Clin Invest 90:1145, 1992.

68. John SWM, Krege JH, Oliver PM, et al: Genetic decreases in atrial natriuretic peptide and salt-sensitive hypertension. Science 267:679, 1995.
69. Semigran MJ, Aroney CN, Herrmann HC, et al: Effects of atrial natriuretic peptide on myocardial contractile and diastolic function in patients with heart failure. J Am Coll Cardiol 20:98, 1992.
70. Connelly TP, Francis GS, Williams KJ, et al: Interaction of intravenous atrial natriuretic factor with furosemide in patients with heart failure. Am Heart J 127:392, 1994.
71. Marcus LS, Hart D, Packer M, et al: Hemodynamic and renal excretory effects of human brain natriuretic peptide infusion in patients with congestive heart failure: A double-blind, placebo-controlled, cross-over trial. Circulation 94:3184, 1996.
72. Abraham WT, Lowes BD, Ferguson DA, et al: Systemic hemodynamic, neurohormonal, and renal effects of a steady-state infusion of human brain natriuretic peptide in patients with advanced hemodynamically decompensated heart failure. J Card Fail 4:37, 1998.
73. Colucci WS, Elkayam U, Horton DP, et al: Intravenous nesiritide, a natriuretic peptide, in the treatment of decompensated congestive heart failure. Nesiritide Study Group. N Engl J Med 343:246, 2000.
74. Mills RM, Hobbs RE, Young JB: "BNP" for heart failure: Role of nesiritide in cardiovascular therapeutics. Congest Heart Fail 8:270, 2002.
75. Abramson BL, Ando S, Notarius CF, et al: Effect of atrial natriuretic peptide on muscle sympathetic activity and its reflex control in human heart failure. Circulation 99:1810, 1999.
76. Burger AJ, Horton DP, LeJemtel T, et al, Prospective Randomized Evaluation of Cardiac Ectopy with Dobutamine or Natrecor Therapy: Effect of nesiritide (B-type natriuretic peptide) and dobutamine on ventricular arrhythmias in the treatment of patients with acutely decompensated congestive heart failure: The PRECEDENT study. Am Heart J 44:1102, 2002.
77. Chen HH, Grantham JA, Schirger JA, et al: Subcutaneous administration of brain natriuretic peptide in experimental heart failure. J Am Coll Cardiol 36:1706, 2000.
78. Chen HH, Nordstrom LJ, Redfield MM, et al: Subcutaneous BNP administration in symptomatic human heart failure: A novel therapeutic strategy for congestive heart failure [abstract]. J Am Coll Cardiol 35:240, 2000.
79. Kentsch M, Otter W: Novel neurohormonal modulators in cardiovascular disorders. The therapeutic potential of endopeptidase inhibitors. Drugs R D 1:331, 1999.
80. Margulies KB, Burnett JC Jr: Neutral endopeptidase 24.11: A modulator of natriuretic peptides. Semin Nephrol 13:71, 1993.
81. Trippodo NC, Panchal BC, Fox M: Repression of angiotensin II and potentiation of bradykinin contribute to the synergistic effects of dual metalloprotease inhibition in heart failure. J Pharmacol Exp Ther 272:619, 1995.
82. Vera WG, Fournie-Zaluski MC, Pham I, et al: Hypotensive and natriuretic effects of RB 105, a new dual inhibitor of angiotensin converting enzyme and neutral endopeptidase in hypertensive rats. J Pharmacol Exp Ther 272:343, 1995.
83. Chen HH, Lainchbury JG, Harty G, Burnett JC: The superior renal and humoral actions of acute dual NEP/ACE inhibition by vasopeptidase inhibitor versus ACE inhibition alone in experimental mild heart failure: Properties mediated via potentiation of endogenous cardiac natriuretic peptides [abstract]. J Am Coll Cardiol 35:270, 2000.
84. Kostis JB, Rouleau JL, Pfeffer MA, et al: Beneficial effects of vasopeptidase inhibition on mortality and morbidity in heart failure: Evidence from the omapatrilat heart failure program [abstract]. J Am Coll Cardiol 35:240, 2000.
85. Packer M, Califf RM, Konstam MA, et al: Comparison of omapatrilat and enalapril in patients with chronic heart failure: The Omapatrilat Versus Enalapril Randomized Trial of Utility in Reducing Events (OVERTURE). Circulation 106:920, 2002.
86. Elkayam U: Calcium channel blockers in heart failure. Cardiology 89:38, 1998.
87. Cohn JN, Ziesche S, Smith R, et al: Effect of the calcium antagonist felodipine as supplementary vasodilator therapy in patients with chronic heart failure treated with enalapril: V-HeFT III. Vasodilator-Heart Failure Trial (V-HeFT) Study Group. Circulation 96:856, 1997.
88. Packer M, O'Connor CM, Ghali JK, et al: Effect of amlodipine on morbidity and mortality in severe chronic heart failure. Prospective Randomized Amlodipine Survival Evaluation Study (PRAISE) Group. N Engl J Med 335:1107, 1996.

Positive Inotropic Agents

89. Hauptman PJ, Kelly RA: Digitalis. Circulation 99:1265, 1999.
90. Blaustein MP: Physiological effects of endogenous ouabain: Control of intracellular Ca^{2+} stores and cell responsiveness. Am J Physiol 264:C1367, 1993.
91. Schmidt TA, Allen PD, Colucci WS, et al: No adaptation to digitalization as evaluated by digitalis receptor (Na,K-ATPase) quantification in explanted hearts from donors without heart disease and from digitalized recipients with end-stage heart failure. Am J Cardiol 70:110, 1992.
92. The Digitalis Investigation Group: The effect of digoxin on mortality and morbidity in patients with heart failure. N Engl J Med 336:525, 1997.
93. Holubarsch C, Hasenfuss G, Just H, Alpert NR: Positive inotropism and myocardial energetics: Influence of β receptor agonist stimulation, phosphodiesterase inhibition, and ouabain. Cardiovasc Res 28:994, 1994.
94. Wang W, Chen JS, Zucker IH: Carotid sinus baroreceptor sensitivity in experimental heart failure. Circulation 81:1959, 1990.
95. Esler M, Kaye D, Lambert G, et al: Adrenergic nervous system in heart failure. Am J Cardiol 80(11A):7L, 1997.
96. Kelly RA, Smith TW: Pharmacologic treatment of heart failure. *In* Hardman JG, Limbird LT (eds): Goodman and Gilman's Pharmacological Basis of Therapeutics. 9th ed. New York, McGraw-Hill, 1996, pp 809-838.
97. Rathore SS, Curtis JP, Wang Y, et al: Serum digoxin concentration and the efficacy of digoxin therapy in the treatment of heart failure: An analysis of the Digitalis Investigation Group (DIG) trial. JAMA 289:871, 2003.
98. Packer M, Gheorghiade M, Young JB, et al: Withdrawal of digoxin from patients with chronic heart failure treated with angiotensin-converting-enzyme inhibitors. RADIANCE study. N Engl J Med 329:1, 1993.
99. Young JB, Gheorghiade M, Uretsky BF, et al: Superiority of "triple" drug therapy in heart failure: Insights from the PROVED and RADIANCE trials. Prospective Randomized Study of Ventricular Function and Efficacy of Digoxin. Randomized Assessment of Digoxin and Inhibitors of Angiotensin-Converting Enzyme. J Am Coll Cardiol 32:686, 1998.
100. Uretsky BF, Young JB Shahidi FE, et al: Randomized study assessing the effect of digoxin withdrawal in patients with mild to moderate chronic congestive heart failure: Results of the PROVED trial. PROVED Investigative Group. J Am Coll Cardiol 22:955, 1993.
101. Slatton ML, Irani WN, Hall SA, et al: Does digoxin provide additional hemodynamic and autonomic benefit at higher doses in patients with mild to moderate heart failure and normal sinus rhythm? J Am Coll Cardiol 29:1206, 1997.
102. Gheorghiade M, Hall VB, Jacobsen G, et al: Effects of increasing maintenance dose of digoxin on left ventricular function and neurohormones in patients with chronic heart failure treated with diuretics and angiotensin-converting enzyme inhibitors. Circulation 92:1801, 1995.
103. Rathore SS, Wang Y, Krumholz HM: Sex-based differences in the effect of digoxin for the treatment of heart failure. N Engl J Med 347:1403, 2002.
104. Magnani B, Malini PL: Cardiac glycosides. Drug interactions of clinical significance. Drug Saf 12:97, 1995.
105. Fromm MF, Kim RB, Stein CM, et al: Inhibition of P-glycoprotein-mediated drug transport: A unifying mechanism to explain the interaction between digoxin and quinidine. Circulation 99:552, 1999.
106. Greiner B, Eichelbaum M, Fritz P, et al: The role of intestinal P-glycoprotein in the interaction of digoxin and rifampin. J Clin Invest 104:147, 1999.
107. Goldman S, Probst P, Selzer A, Cohn K: Inefficacy of "therapeutic" serum levels of digoxin in controlling the ventricular rate in atrial fibrillation. Am J Cardiol 35:651, 1975.
108. Merrill JJ, DeWeese G, Wharton JM: Magnesium reversal of digoxin-facilitated ventricular rate during atrial fibrillation in the Wolff-Parkinson-White syndrome Am J Med 97:25, 1994.
109. Bosse GM, Pope TM: Recurrent digoxin overdose and treatment with digoxin-specific Fab antibody fragments. J Emerg Med 12:179, 1994.
110. Port JD, Bristow MR: Altered beta-adrenergic receptor gene regulation and signaling in chronic heart failure. J Mol Cell Cardiol 33:887, 2001.
111. Bristow MR: Changes in myocardial and vascular receptors in heart failure. J Am Coll Cardiol 22(Suppl A):61, 1993.
112. Bristow MR: Mechanism of action of beta-blocking agents in heart failure. Am J Cardiol 80(11A):261, 1997.
113. Bristow MR, Ginsburg R, Minobe WA, et al: Decreased catecholamine sensitivity and β-adrenergic-receptor density in failing human hearts. N Engl J Med 307:205, 1982.
114. Fowler MB, Laser JA, Hopkins GL, et al: Assessment of the β-adrenergic receptor pathway in the intact failing human heart: Progressive receptor down-regulation and subsensitivity to agonist response. Circulation 74:1290, 1986.
115. Ginsburg R, Esserman L, Bristow MR: Myocardial performance and extracellular ionized calcium in a severely failing human heart. Ann Intern Med 98:603, 1983.
116. Pacholczyk T, Blakely RD, Amara SG: Expression cloning of a cocaine- and antidepressant-sensitive human noradrenaline transporter. Nature 350:350, 1991.
117. Mitchell PD, Smith GW, Wells E, West PA: Inhibition of $uptake_1$ by dopexamine hydrochloride in vitro. Br J Pharmacol 92:265, 1987.
118. Bristow MR: β-Adrenergic receptor blockade in chronic heart failure. Circulation 101:558, 2000.
119. Lowes BD, Tsvetkova T, Eichhorn EJ, et al: Milrinone vs. dobutamine in heart failure subjects treated chronically with carvedilol. Int J Cardiol 81:141, 2001.
120. Metra M, Nodari S, D'Aloia A, et al: Beta-blocker therapy influences the hemodynamic response to inotropic agents in patients with heart failure. A randomized comparison of dobutamine and enoximone before and after chronic treatment with metoprolol or carvedilol. J Am Coll Cardiol 40:1248, 2002.
121. Gilbert EM, Eiswirth CC, Mealey PC, et al: β-Adrenergic supersensitivity of the transplanted human heart is presynaptic in origin. Circulation 79:344, 1989.
122. von Scheidt W, Bohm M, Schneider B, et al: Isolated presynaptic inotropic beta-adrenergic supersensitivity of the transplanted denervated human heart in vivo. Circulation 85:1056, 1992.
123. Scrutinio D, Napoli V, Passantino A, et al: Low-dose dobutamine responsiveness in idiopathic dilated cardiomyopathy: Relation to exercise capacity and clinical outcome. Eur Heart J 21:927, 2000.
124. Maccarrone C, Malta E, Raper C: β-Adrenoceptor selectivity of dobutamine: In vivo and in vitro studies. J Cardiovasc Pharmacol 6:132, 1984.
125. Wollmering MM, Wiechmann RJ, Port JD, et al: Dobutamine is a partial agonist with an intrinsic activity of 0.5 in human myocardium [abstract]. J Am Coll Cardiol 17:283, 1991.
126. Binkley PF, VanFossen DV, Nunziata E, et al: Influence of positive inotropic therapy on pulsatile hydraulic load and ventricular-vascular coupling in congestive heart failure. J Am Coll Cardiol 15:1127, 1990.
127. Leier CV: Current status of non-digitalis positive inotropic drugs. Am J Cardiol 69:120G, 1992.
128. Leier CV, Heban PT, Huss P, et al: Comparative systemic and regional hemodynamic effects of dopamine and dobutamine in patients with cardiomyopathic heart failure. Circulation 58:466, 1978.
129. Binkley PF, Murray KD, Watson KM, et al: Dobutamine increases cardiac output of total artificial heart. Implications for vascular contribution of inotropic agents to augmented ventricular function. Circulation 84:1210, 1991.
130. Cork RC, Gallo JA Jr, Copeland JG: Acute effects of dobutamine and isoproterenol after implantation of a total artificial heart. J Heart Lung Transplant 11:253, 1992.
131. Keren G, Laniado S, Sonnenblick EH, LeJemtel LH: Dynamics of functional mitral regurgitation during dobutamine therapy in patients with severe congestive heart failure. A Doppler echocardiographic study. Am Heart J 118:748, 1989.

132. Gilbert EM, Larrabee PA, Volkman AK, et al: Does dobutamine tolerance result from myocardial β-receptor down-regulation [abstract]? J Am Coll Cardiol 19:253, 1992.
133. Lee HR, Hershberger RE, Port JD, et al: Low-dose enoximone in subjects awaiting cardiac transplantation: Clinical results and effects on β-adrenergic receptors. J Thorac Cardiovasc Surg 102:246, 1991.
134. Gilbert EM, Hershberger RE, Wiechmann RJ, et al: Pharmacologic and hemodynamic effects of combined β-agonist stimulation and phosphodiesterase inhibition in the failing human heart. Chest 108:1524, 1995.
135. Port JD, Gilbert EM, Larrabee P, et al: Neurotransmitter depletion compromises the ability of indirect-acting amines to provide inotropic support in the failing human heart. Circulation 81:929, 1990.
136. Nichols AJ, Ruffolo RR Jr, Brooks DP: The pharmacology of fenoldopam. Am J Hypertens 3(Suppl):116, 1990.
137. Lokhandwala MF, Amenta F: Anatomical distribution and function of dopamine receptors in the kidney. FASEB J 5:3023, 1991.
138. Anderson FL, Port JD, Reid BB, et al: Effect of therapeutic dopamine administration on myocardial catecholamine and neuropeptide Y concentrations in the failing ventricles of patients with idiopathic dilated cardiomyopathy. J Cardiovasc Pharmacol 20:800, 1992.
139. Abraham WT, Lowes BD, Roden RL, et al: Mechanism of increased cardiac adrenergic activity in heart failure: Evidence for decreased cardiac neuronal norepinephrine reuptake. Circulation 96(Suppl 1):92, 1997.
140. Rundqvist B, Elam M, Eisenhofer G, Friberg P: Increased cardiac adrenergic drive precedes generalized sympathetic activation human heart failure. Circulation 95:516, 1997.
141. Bristow MR, Daniels JR, Kernoff RS, Harrison DC: Effect of compound D600, practolol and alterations in magnesium on ionized calcium relationships in the intact dog heart. Circ Res 41:574, 1977.
142. Movsesian MA, Smith CJ, Krall J, et al: Sarcoplasmic reticulum-associated cyclic adenosine 5′-monophosphate phosphodiesterase activity in normal and failing human hearts. J Clin Invest 88:15, 1991.
143. Leroy M-J, Degerman E, Taira M, et al: Characterization of two recombinant PDE_3 (cGMP-inhibited cyclic nucleotide phosphodiesterase) isoforms, RcGIP1 and HcGIP2, expressed in NIH 3006 murine fibroblasts and Sf9 cells. Biochemistry 35:10194, 1996.
144. Koss KL, Kranias EG: Phospholamban: A prominent regulator of myocardial contractility. Circ Res 79:1059, 1996.
145. Edes I, Kiss E, Kitada Y, et al: Effects of levosimendan, a cardiotonic agent targeted to troponin C, on cardiac function and on phosphorylation and Ca^{2+} sensitivity of cardiac myofibrils and sarcoplasmic reticulum in guinea pig hearts. Circ Res 77:107, 1995.
146. Luo W, Grupp IL, Ponniah S, et al: Targeted ablation of the phospholamban gene is associated with markedly enhanced myocardial contractility and loss of β-agonist stimulation. Circ Res 75:401, 1994.
147. Kajimoto K, Hagiwara N, Kasanuki H, Hosoda S: Contribution of phosphodiesterase isozymes to the regulation of the L-type calcium current in human cardiac myocytes. Br J Pharmacol 121:1549, 1997.
148. Walaas SI, Czernik AJ, Olstad OK, et al: Protein kinase C and cyclic AMP-dependent protein kinase phosphorylate phospholemman, an insulin and adrenaline-regulated membrane phosphoprotein, at specific sites in the carboxy terminal domain. Biochem J 304:635, 1994.
149. Jiang H, Colbran JL, Francis SH, Corbin JD: Direct evidence for cross-activation of cGMP-dependent protein kinase by cAMP in pig coronary arteries. J Biol Chem 267:1015, 1992.
150. Kikura M, Levy JH, Michelsen LG, et al: The effect of milrinone on hemodynamics and left ventricular function after emergence from cardiopulmonary bypass. Anesth Analg 85:16, 1997.
151. Paulus S, Lehot JJ, Bastien O, et al: Enoximone and acute left ventricular failure during weaning from mechanical ventilation after cardiac surgery. Crit Care Med 22:74, 1994.
152. Chen EP, Bittner HB, Davis RD, Van Tright P: Hemodynamic and inotropic effects of milrinone after heart transplantation in the setting of recipient pulmonary hypertension. J Heart Lung Transplant 17:669, 1998.
153. Feldman MD, Copelas L, Gwathmey JK, et al: Deficient production of cyclic AMP: Pharmacologic evidence of an important cause of contractile dysfunction in patients with end-stage heart failure. Circulation 75:331, 1987.
154. Feldman AM, Cates AE, Veazey WB, et al: Increase of the 40,000-mol wt pertussis toxin substrate (G protein) in the failing human heart. J Clin Invest 82:189, 1988.
155. Neumann J, Schmitz W, Scholz H, et al: Increase in myocardial G_i-proteins in heart failure. Lancet 2:936, 1988.
156. Bristow MR, Anderson FL, Port JD, et al: Differences in β-adrenergic neuroeffector mechanisms in ischemic versus idiopathic dilated cardiomyopathy. Circulation 84:1024, 1991.
157. Sigmund M, Jakob H, Becker H, et al: Effects of metoprolol on myocardial β-adrenoceptors and G_α-proteins in patients with congestive heart failure. Eur J Clin Pharmacol 51:127, 1996.
158. Böhm M, Deutsch HJ, Hartmann D, et al: Improvement of postreceptor events by metoprolol treatment in patients with chronic heart failure. J Am Coll Cardiol 30:992, 1997.
159. Shipley JB, Tolman D, Hastillo A, Hess ML: Milrinone: Basic and clinical pharmacology and acute and chronic management. Am J Med Sci 311:286, 1996.
160. Lowes B, Higginbotham M, Petrovich L, et al: Low dose enoximone improves exercise capacity in chronic heart failure. J Am Coll Cardiol 36:501, 2000.
161. Leier CV, Meiler SEL, Matthews S, Unverferth DV: A preliminary report of the effects of orally administered enoximone on regional hemodynamics in congestive heart failure. Am J Cardiol 60:27C, 1987.
162. Dibianco R, Shabetai R, Kostuk W, et al: A comparison of oral milrinone, digoxin, and their combination in the treatment of patients with chronic heart failure. N Engl J Med 320:677, 1989.
163. Monrad ES, Baim DS, Smith HS, et al: Effects of milrinone on coronary hemodynamics and myocardial energetics in patients with congestive heart failure. Circulation 71:972, 1985.
164. Monrad ES, McKay RG, Baim DS, et al: Improvement in indexes of diastolic performance in patients with congestive heart failure treated with milrinone. Circulation 70:1030, 1984.
165. Ludmer PL, Wright RF, Arnold JM, et al: Separation of the direct myocardial and vasodilator actions of milrinone administered by an intracoronary infusion technique Circulation 73:130, 1986.
166. Packer M, Carver JR, Chesebro JH, et al: Effect of oral milrinone on mortality in severe chronic heart failure. PROMISE Study Research Group. N Engl J Med 325:1468, 1991.
167. Uretsky BF, Jesup M, Konstam MA, et al: Multicenter trial of oral enoximone in patients with moderate to moderately severe congestive heart failure: Lack of benefit compared to placebo. Enoximone Multicenter Trial Group. Circulation 82:774, 1990.
168. Cowley AJ, Skene AM, on behalf of the Enoximone Investigators: Treatment of severe heart failure: Quantity or quality of life? A trial of enoximone. Br Heart J 72:226, 1994.
169. Cohn JN, Goldstein SO, Greenberg BH, et al: A dose-dependent increase in mortality with vesnarinone among patients with severe heart failure. N Engl J Med 339:1810, 1998.
170. Lubsen J, Just H, Hjalmarsson AC, et al: Effect of pimobendan on exercise capacity in patients with heart failure: Main results from the Pimobendan in Congestive Heart Failure (PICO) trial. Heart 76:223, 1996.
171. Teerlink JR, Jalaluddin M, Anderson S, et al: Ambulatory ventricular arrhythmias in patients with heart failure do not specifically predict an increased risk of sudden death. PROMISE (Prospective Randomized Milrinone Survival Evaluation) Investigators. Circulation 101:40, 2000.
172. Bristow MR, Lowes BD: Low-dose inotropic therapy of ambulatory heart failure. Coron Artery Dis 5:112, 1994.
173. Gilbert EM, Bristow MR, Mason JW: The acute hemodynamic response to low dose enoximone (MDL 17,043): An oral dose-range study. Am J Cardiol 82:57C, 1987.
174. Lowes BD, Simon MA, Tsekova TO, Bristow MR: Inotropes in the β-blocker era. Clin Cardiol 23(Suppl 3):11, 2000.
175. Shakar SF, Abraham WT, Gilbert EM, et al: Combined oral positive inotropic and beta-blocker therapy for the treatment of refractory Class IV heart failure. J Am Coll Cardiol 31:1336, 1998.
176. Benotti JR, Grossman W, Braunwald E, et al: Hemodynamic assessment of amrinone: A new inotropic agent. N Engl J Med 299:1373, 1978.
177. Maisel AS, Wright CM, Carter SM, et al: Tachyphylaxis with amrinone therapy: Association with sequestration and down-regulation of lymphocyte beta-adrenergic receptors. Ann Intern Med 110:195, 1989.
178. Kikura M, Lee MK, Safon RA, et al: The effects of milrinone on platelets in patients undergoing cardiac surgery. Anesth Analg 81:44, 1995.
179. Holmberg SR, Williams AJ: Phosphodiesterase inhibitors and the cardiac sarcoplasmic reticulum calcium release channel: Differential effects of milrinone and enoximone. Cardiovasc Res 25:537, 1991.
180. Cody V, Wojtczak A, Davis FB, et al: Structure-activity relationships of milrinone analogues determined in vitro in a rabbit heart membrane Ca^{2+}-ATPase model. J Med Chem 38:1990, 1995.
181. Siostrzonek P, Koreny M, Delle-Karth G, et al: Milrinone therapy in catecholamine-dependent critically ill patients with heart failure. Acta Anaesth Scand 44:403, 2000.
182. Seino Y, Takano T, Hayakawa H, et al: Hemodynamic effects and pharmacokinetics of oral milrinone for short-term support in acute heart failure. Cardiology 86:34, 1995.
183. Gibeline P, Dadoun-Dybal M, Candito M, et al: Hemodynamic effects of prolonged enoximone infusion (7 days) in patients with severe chronic heart failure. Cardiovasc Drugs Ther 7:333, 1993.
184. Okerholm RA, Chan KY, Lang JF, et al: Biotransformation and pharmacokinetic overview of enoximone and its sulfoxide metabolite. Am J Cardiol 60:21C, 1987.
185. Burns AM, Park GR: Prolonged action of enoximone in renal failure. Anaesthesia 46:864, 1991.
186. Boknik P, Neumann J, Kaspereit G, et al: Mechanisms of the contractile effects of levosimendan in the mammalian heart. J Pharmacol Exp Ther 280:277, 1997.
187. Remme WJ, Kruijssen DA, van Hoogenhuyze DC, et al: Hemodynamic, neurohumoral, and myocardial energetic effects of pimobendan, a novel calcium-sensitizing compound, in patients with mild to moderate heart failure. J Cardiovasc Pharmacol 24:730, 1994.
188. Lilleberg J, Sundberg S, Nieminen MS: Dose-range study of a new calcium sensitizer, levosimendan, in patients with left ventricular dysfunction. J Cardiovasc Pharmacol 26(Suppl):63, 1995.
189. Hagemeijer F: Calcium sensitization with pimobendan: Pharmacology, haemodynamic improvement, and sudden death in patients with chronic congestive heart failure. Eur Heart J 14:551, 1993.
190. Bethke T, Eschenhagen T, Klimkiewicz A, et al: Phosphodiesterase inhibition by enoximone in preparations from nonfailing and failing human hearts. Arzneimittelforschung 42:437, 1992.
191. Kubo SH, Gollub S, Bourge R, et al: Results of a multicenter trial. The Pimobendan Multicenter Research Group. Circulation 85:942, 1992.
192. Haikala H, Kaivola J, Nissinen E, et al: Cardiac troponin C as a target protein for a novel calcium sensitizing drug, levosimendan. J Mol Cell Cardiol 27:1859, 1995.
193. Kleerekoper Q, Putkey JA: Drug binding to cardiac troponin C. J Biol Chem 274:23932, 1999.
194. Moiseyev VS, Poder P, Andrejevs N, et al: Safety and efficacy of a novel calcium sensitizer, levosimendan, in patients with left ventricular failure due to an acute myocardial infarction. A placebo-controlled, double-blind study (RUSSLAN). Eur Heart J 23:1422, 2002.
195. Follath F, Cleland JG, Just H, et al: Efficacy and safety of intravenous levosimendan compared with dobutamine in severe low-output heart failure (the LIDO study): A randomized double-blind trial. Lancet 360:196, 2002.
196. Kivikko M, Lehtonen L, Colucci WS: Sustained hemodynamic effects of intravenous levosimendan. Circulation 107:81, 2003.

Neurohormonal Inhibitors

197. Francis GS, Goldsmith SR, Levine TB, et al: The neurohumoral axis in congestive heart failure. Ann Intern Med 101:370, 1984.
198. Packer M, Lee WH, Kessler PD, et al: Role of neurohormonal mechanisms in determining survival in patients with severe chronic heart failure. Circulation 75(Suppl 4):80, 1987.
199. Bristow MR, Kantrowitz NE, Ginsburg R, Fowler MB: β-Adrenergic function in heart muscle disease and heart failure. J Mol Cell Cardiol 17(Suppl 2):41, 1985.
200. Waagstein F, Hjalmarson A, Varnauskas E, Wallentin I: Effect of chronic beta-adrenergic receptor blockade in congestive cardiomyopathy. Br Heart J 37:1022, 1975.
201. Gilbert EM, Anderson JL, Deitchman D, et al: Long-term β-blocker vasodilator therapy improves cardiac function in idiopathic dilated cardiomyopathy: A double-blind, randomized study of bucindolol versus placebo. Am J Med 88:223, 1990.
202. Eichhorn EJ, Bedotto JB, Malloy CR, et al: Effect of beta-adrenergic blockade on myocardial function and energetics in congestive heart failure: Improvements in hemodynamic, contractile, and diastolic performance with bucindolol. Circulation 82:473, 1990.
203. Pfeffer MA, Lamas GA, Vaughan DE, et al: Effect of captopril on progressive ventricular dilation after anterior myocardial infarction. N Engl J Med 319:80, 1988.
204. Sharpe N, Smith H, Murphy J, Hannan S: Treatment of patients with symptomless left ventricular dysfunction after myocardial infarction. Lancet 365:255, 1988.
205. Fowler MB, Bristow MR: Rationale for beta-adrenergic blocking drugs in cardiomyopathy. Am J Cardiol 55:D120, 1985.
206. The CONSENSUS Trial Study Group: Effects of enalapril on mortality in severe congestive heart failure. Results of the Cooperative North Scandinavian Enalapril Survival Study (CONSENSUS). N Engl J Med 316:429, 1987.
207. The SOLVD Investigators: Effect of enalapril on survival in patients with reduced left ventricular ejection fractions and congestive heart failure. N Engl J Med 325:293, 1991.
208. Waagstein F, Bristow MR, Swedberg K, et al: Beneficial effects of metoprolol in idiopathic dilated cardiomyopathy. Metoprolol in Dilated Cardiomyopathy (MDC) Trial Study Group. Lancet 342:1441, 1993.
209. Packer M, Bristow MR, Cohn JN, et al: Effect of carvedilol on morbidity and mortality in patients with chronic heart failure. U.S. Carvedilol Heart Failure Study Group. N Engl J Med 334:1349, 1996.
210. Bristow MR, Gilbert EM, Abraham WT, et al: Carvedilol produces dose-related improvements in left ventricular function and survival in subjects with chronic heart failure. MOCHA Investigators. Circulation 94:2807-2816, 1996.
211. The Cardiac Insufficiency Bisoprolol Study II (CIBIS-II): A randomised trial. Lancet 353:9, 1999.
212. MERIT-HF Study Group: Effect of metoprolol CR/XL in chronic heart failure: Metoprolol CR/XL Randomized Intervention Trial in Congestive Heart Failure (MERIT-HF). Lancet 353:2001, 1999.
213. Inagami T: Molecular biology and signaling of angiotensin receptors: An overview. J Am Soc Nephrol 10(Suppl 11):2, 1999.
214. Mulder P, Richard V, Bouchart F, et al: Selective ET_A receptor blockade prevents left ventricular remodeling and deterioration of cardiac function in experimental heart failure. Cardiovasc Res 39:600, 1998.
215. Torre-Amione G, Bozkurt B, Deswal A, Mann DL: An overview of tumor necrosis factor alpha and the failing human heart. Curr Opin Cardiol 14:206, 1999.
216. Eichhorn EJ, Bristow MR: Medical therapy can improve the biologic properties of the chronically failing heart: A new era in the treatment of heart failure. Circulation 94:2285, 1996.

Inhibitors of the Renin-Angiotensin-Aldosterone System

217. Pfeffer JM, Pfeffer MA, Braunwald E: Hemodynamic benefits and prolonged survival with long-term captopril therapy in rats with myocardial infarction and heart failure. Circulation 75:1149, 1987.
218. Pfeffer JM, Pfeffer MA, Mirsky I, Braunwald E: Regression of left ventricular hypertrophy and prevention of left ventricular dysfunction by captopril in the spontaneously hypertensive rat. Proc Natl Acad Sci USA 79:3310, 1982.
219. Greenberg B, Quinones MA, Koilpillai C, et al: Effects of long-term therapy on cardiac structure and function in patients with left ventricular dysfunction. Results of the SOLVD echocardiography substudy. Circulation 91:2573, 1995.
220. Zisman LS, Abraham WT, Meixell GE, et al: Angiotensin II formation in the intact human heart: Predominance of the angiotensin-converting enzyme pathway. J Clin Invest 96:1490, 1995.
221. Urata H, Hoffmann S, Ganten D: Tissue angiotensin II system in the human heart. Eur Heart J 15(Suppl):68, 1994.
222. Wei CC, Meng QC, Palmer R, et al: Evidence for angiotensin-converting enzyme and chymase-mediated angiotensin II formation in the interstitial fluid space of the dog heart in vivo. Circulation 99:2583, 1999.
223. Liu YH, Yang XP, Mehta D, et al: Role of kinins in chronic heart failure and in the therapeutic effect of ACE inhibitors in kininogen-deficient rats. Am J Physiol 278:H507, 2000.
224. The SOLVD Investigators: Effect of enalapril on mortality and the development of heart failure in asymptomatic patients with reduced left ventricular ejection fractions. N Engl J Med 327:685, 1992.
225. Pfeffer MA, Braunwald E, Moye LA, et al: Effect of captopril on mortality and morbidity in patients with left ventricular dysfunction after myocardial infarction. Results of the survival and ventricular enlargement trial. The SAVE Investigators. N Engl J Med 327:669, 1992.
226. The Acute Infarction Ramipril Efficacy (AIRE) Study Investigators: Effect of ramipril on mortality and morbidity of survivors of acute myocardial infarction with clinical evidence of heart failure. Lancet 342:821, 1993.
227. Kober L, Torp-Pedersen C, Carlsen JE, et al: A clinical trial of the angiotensin-converting-enzyme inhibitor trandolapril in patients with left ventricular dysfunction after myocardial infarction. Trandolapril Cardiac Evaluation (TRACE) Study Group. N Engl J Med 333:1670, 1995.
228. Arnold JMO, Yusuf S, Young J, et al: Prevention of heart failure in patients without known left ventricular dysfunction: The Heart Outcomes Prevention Study (HOPE). Circulation 107:1284, 2003.
229. Ruzicka M, Leenen FHH: Relevance of blockade of cardiac and circulatory angiotensin-converting enzyme for the prevention of volume overload-induced cardiac hypertrophy. Circulation 91:16, 1995.
230. Borghi C, Boschi S, Ambrosioni E, et al: Evidence of a partial escape of renin-angiotensin-aldosterone blockade in patients with acute myocardial infarction treated with ACE inhibitors. J Clin Pharmacol 33:40, 1993.
231. Pitt B: "Escape" of aldosterone production in patients with left ventricular dysfunction treated with an angiotensin converting enzyme inhibitor: Implications for therapy. Cardiovasc Drugs Ther 9:145, 1995.
232. Gottlieb SS, Kickstein K, Fleck E, et al: Hemodynamic and neurohormonal effects of the angiotensin II antagonist losartan in patients with congestive heart failure. Circulation 88:1602, 1993.
233. Havranek EP, Thomas I, Smith WB, et al: Dose-related beneficial long-term hemodynamic and clinical efficacy of irbesartan in heart failure. J Am Coll Cardiol 33:1174, 1999.
234. Mazayev VP, Fomina IG, Kazkov EN, et al: Valsartan in heart failure patients previously untreated with an ACE inhibitor. Int Cardiol 65:239, 1998.
235. Guazzi M, Palermo P, Pontone G, et al: Synergistic efficacy of enalapril and losartan on exercise performance and oxygen consumption at peak exercise in congestive heart failure. Am J Cardiol 84:1038, 1999.
236. Riegger GA, Bouzo H, Petr P, et al: Improvement in exercise tolerance and symptoms of congestive heart failure during treatment with candesartan cilexetil. Symptom, Tolerability, Response to Exercise Trial of Candesartan Cilexetil in Heart Failure (STRETCH) Investigators. Circulation 100:2224, 1999.
237. Hamroff G, Katz SD, Mancini D, et al: Addition of angiotensin II receptor blockade to maximal angiotensin-converting enzyme inhibition improves exercise capacity in patients with severe congestive heart failure. Circulation 99:990, 1999.
238. Baruch L, Anand I, Cohen IS, et al: Augmented short- and long-term hemodynamic and hormonal effects of an angiotensin receptor blocker added to angiotensin converting enzyme inhibitor therapy in patients with heart failure. Vasodilator Heart Failure Trial (V-HeFT) Study Group. Circulation 99:2658, 1999.
239. McKelvie RS, Yusuf S, Pericak D, et al: Comparison of candesartan, enalapril, and their combination in congestive heart failure: Randomized evaluation of strategies for left ventricular dysfunction (RESOLVD) pilot study. The RESOLVD Pilot Study Investigators. Circulation 100:1056, 1999.
240. Pitt B, Segal R, Martinez FA, et al: Randomized trial of losartan versus captopril in patients over 65 with heart failure (Evaluation of Losartan in the Elderly Study, ELITE). Lancet 349:747, 1997.
241. Pitt B, Poole-Wilson PA, Segal R, et al: Effect of losartan compared with captopril on mortality in patients with symptomatic heart failure: Randomised trial—The Losartan Heart Failure Survival Study ELITE II. Lancet 355:1582, 2000.
242. Cohn JN, Tognoni G, Valsartan Heart Failure Trial Investigators: A randomized trial of the angiotensin-receptor blocker valsartan in chronic heart failure. N Engl J Med 345:1667, 2001.
243. Granger CB, McMurray JJV, Yusuf S, et al, for the CHARM Investigators. Effects of candesartan in patients with chronic heart failure and reduced left ventricular systolic function intolerant to angiotensin-converting-enzyme inhibitors: The CHARM-Alternative Trial. Lancet 362:772, 2003.
244. McMurray JJV, Ostergren J, Swedberg K, et al, for the CHARM Investigators: Effects of candesartan in patients with chronic heart failure and reduced left ventricular systolic function taking angiotensin-converting-enzyme inhibitors: The CHARM-Added Trial. Lancet 362:767, 2003.
245. Yusuf S, Pfeffer MA, Swedberg K, et al, for the CHARM Investigators. Effects of candesartan in patients with chronic heart failure and preserved left-ventricular ejection fraction: The CHARM-Preserved Trial. Lancet 362:777, 2003.
246. Pfeffer MA, McMurray JJV, Velazquez EJ, et al: Valsartan, captopril, or both in myocardial infarction complicated by heart failure, left ventricular dysfunction, or both. N Engl J Med 349:1893, 2003
247. Weber KT, Brilla CG, Campbell SE, et al: Myocardial fibrosis: Role of angiotensin II and aldosterone. Basic Res Cardiol 8:107, 1998.341.
248. Ramires FJ, Mansor A, Coelho O, et al: Effect of spironolactone on ventricular arrhythmias in congestive heart failure secondary to idiopathic dilated or to ischemic cardiomyopathy. Am J Cardiol 85:1207, 2000.
249. Qin W, Rudolph AE, Bond BR, et al: Transgenic model of aldosterone-driven cardiac hypertrophy and heart failure. Circ Res 93:69, 2003.
250. Bristow MR, Saxon LA, Boehmer J, et al: Cardiac resynchronization therapy with or without an implantable defibrillator in advanced chronic heart failure: The COMPANION trial. N Engl J Med 350:2140, 2004.

Antiadrenergic Agents

251. Haber HL, Christopher LS, Gimple LW, et al: Why do patients with congestive heart failure tolerate the initiation of β-blocker therapy? Circulation 88:1610, 1993.
253. Goldsmith SR, Francis GS, Cohn JN: Norepinephrine infusions in congestive heart failure. Am J Cardiol 56:802, 1985.
254. Bristow MR, Minobe W, Rasmussen R, et al: β-Adrenergic neuroeffector abnormalities in the failing human heart are produced by local, rather than systemic mechanisms. J Clin Invest 89:803, 1992.
255. Kaye DM, Lefkovits J, Jennings GL, et al: Adverse consequences of high sympathetic nervous activity in the failing human heart. J Am Coll Cardiol 26:1257, 1995.

256. Bristow MR, Feldman AM, Adams KF, Goldstein S: Selective versus nonselective β-blockade for heart failure therapy—Are there lessons to be learned from the COMET Trial? J Card Fail 9:444, 2003.
257. Bristow MR, Ginsburg R, Fowler M, et al: β_1 and β_2-adrenergic receptor subpopulations in normal and failing human ventricular myocardium: Coupling of both receptor subtypes to muscle contraction and selective β_1 receptor down-regulation in heart failure. Circ Res 59:297, 1986.
258. White M, Roden R, Minobe W, et al: Age-related changes in β-adrenergic neuroeffector systems in the human heart. Circulation 90:1225, 1994.
259. Vago T, Bevilacqua M, Norbiato G, et al: Identification of α_1-adrenergic receptors on sarcolemma from normal subjects and patients with idiopathic dilated cardiomyopathy: Characteristics and linkage to GTP-binding protein. Circ Res 64:474, 1989.
260. Bristow MR, Port JD, Gilbert EM: The role of adrenergic receptor regulation in the treatment of heart failure. Cardiovasc Drugs Ther 3:971, 1989.
261. Newton GE, Parker JD: Acute effects of β_1-selective and nonselective β-adrenergic receptor blockade on cardiac sympathetic activity in congestive heart failure. Circulation 94:353, 1996.
262. Gauthier C, Tavernier G, Charpentier F, et al: Functional β_3-adrenoceptor in the human heart. J Clin Invest 98:556, 1996.
263. Kaumann AJ, Molenaar P: Modulation of human cardiac function through 4 beta-adrenergic populations. Naunyn Schmiedebergs Arch Pharmacol 355:667, 1997.
264. Engelhardt S, Hein L, Wiesman F, Lohse MJ: Progressive hypertrophy and heart failure in β_1-adrenergic receptor transgenic mice. Proc Natl Acad Sci USA 96:7059, 1999.
265. Bisognano JD, Weinberger HD, Bohlmeyer TJ, et al: Myocardial-directed overexpression of the human β_1-adrenergic receptor in transgenic mice. J Mol Cell Cardiol 32:817, 2000.
266. Perez JM, Rathz DA, Petrashevskaya NN, et al: β_1-Adrenergic receptor polymorphisms confer differential function and predisposition to heart failure. Nat Med 10:1300, 2003.
267. Freeman K, Lerman I, Kranias EG, et al: Alterations in cardiac adrenergic signaling and calcium cycling differentially affect the progression of cardiomyopathy. J Clin Invest 107:967, 2001.
268. Liggett SB, Tepe NM, Lorenz JN, et al: Early and delayed consequences of β_2-adrenergic receptor overexpression in mouse hearts: Critical role for expression level. Circulation 101:1707, 2000.
269. Iwase M, Bishop SP, Uechi M, et al: Adverse effects of chronic endogenous sympathetic drive induced by cardiac $G_{s\alpha}$ overexpression. Circ Res 78:517, 1996.
270. D'Angelo DD, Sakatra Y, Lorenz JN, et al: Transgenic $G\alpha q$ overexpression induces cardiac contractile failure in mice. Proc Natl Acad Sci USA 94:8121, 1997.
271. Communal C, Singh K, Pimental DR, Colucci WS: Norepinephrine stimulates apoptosis in adult rat ventricular myocytes by activation of the β-adrenergic receptor. Circulation 98:1329, 1998.
272. Communal C, Singh K, Sawyer DB, Colluci WS: Opposing effects of β_1- and β_2-adrenergic receptors on cardiac myocyte apoptosis. Role of a pertussis-toxin sensitive G protein. Circulation 100:2210, 1999.
273. Milano CA, Dolber PC, Rockman HA, et al: Myocardial expression of a constitutively active α_{1B}-adrenergic receptor in transgenic mice induces cardiac hypertrophy. Proc Natl Acad Sci USA 91:10109, 1994.
274. Lemire I, Ducharme A, Tardif JC, et al: Cardiac-directed overexpression of wild-type alpha1B-adrenergic receptor induces dilated cardiomyopathy. Am J Physiol 281:H931, 2001.
275. Gao MH, Lai C, Roth DM, et al: Adenylylcyclase increases responsiveness to catecholamine stimulation in transgenic mice. Circulation 99:1618, 1999.
276. Kim SJ, Yatani A, Vatner DE, et al:. Differential regulation of inotropy and lusitropy in overexpressed Gsalpha myocytes through cAMP and Ca^{2+} channel pathways. J Clin Invest 103:1089, 1999.
277. Bristow MR, Hershberger RE, Port JD, et al: β_1- and β_2-adrenergic receptor mediated adenylate cyclase stimulation in nonfailing and failing human ventricular myocardium. Mol Pharmacol 35:295, 1989.
278. Ungerer M, Parruti G, Bohm M, et al: Expression of β-arrestins and β-adrenergic receptor kinases in the failing human heart. Circ Res 74:206, 1994.
279. Tan LB, Benjamin IJ, Clark WA: β-Adrenergic receptor desensitization may serve a cardioprotective role. Cardiovasc Res 26:608, 1992.
280. Bristow MR: Pathophysiologic and pharmacologic rationales for clinical management of chronic heart failure with beta-blocking agents. Am J Cardiol 71:12C, 1993.
281. Eichhorn EJ, Bristow MR: Practical guidelines for initiation of beta-adrenergic blockade in patients with chronic heart failure. Am J Cardiol 79:794, 1997.
282. Newton GE, Azevedo ER, Parker JD: Inotropic and sympathetic responses to the intracoronary infusion of a beta2-receptor agonist: A human in vivo study. Circulation 99:2402, 1999.
283. Bristow MR, Roden RL, Lowes BD, et al: The role of third generation β-blocking agents in chronic heart failure. Clin Cardiol 21(Suppl 1):I3, 1998.
284. Bristow MR, Gilbert EM: Improvement in cardiac myocyte function by biologic effects of medical therapy: A new concept in the treatment of heart failure. Eur Heart J 16(Suppl F):20, 1995.
285. Lechat P, Escolano S, Golmard JL, et al: Prognostic value of bisoprolol-induced hemodynamic effects in heart failure during the Cardiac Insufficiency Bisoprolol Study (CIBIS). Circulation 96:2197, 1997.
286. Lowes BD, Gilbert EM, Abraham WT, et al: Myocardial gene expression in dilated cardiomyopathy treated with beta-blocking agents. N Engl J Med 346:1357, 2002.
287. Abraham WT, Gilbert EM, Lowes BD, et al: Coordinate changes in myosin heavy chain isoform gene expression are selectively associated with alterations in dilated cardiomyopathy phenotype. Mol Med 8:750, 2002.
288. Nadal-Ginard B, Mahdavi V: Molecular basis of cardiac performance. Plasticity of the myocardium generated through protein isoform switches. J Clin Invest 84:1693, 1989.
289. Asano K, Zisman LS, Yoshikawa T, et al: Bucindolol, a nonselective β_1- and β_2-adrenergic receptor antagonist, decreases β-adrenergic receptor density in cultured embryonic chick cardiac myocyte membranes. J Cardiovasc Pharmacol 37:678, 2001.
290. Sandberg A, Abrahamsson B, Regardh C-G, et al: Pharmacokinetic and biopharmaceutic aspects of once daily treatment with metoprolol CR/ZOK: A review article. J Clin Pharm 30:S2, 1990.
291. The International Steering Committee: Rationale, design, and organization of the Metoprolol CR/XL Randomized Intervention Trial in Heart Failure (MERIT-HF). Am J Cardiol 80(9B):54J, 1997.
292. Kukin ML, Mannino MM, Freudenberger RS, et al: Hemodynamic comparison of twice daily metoprolol tartrate with once daily metoprolol succinate in congestive heart failure. J Am Coll Cardiol 35:45, 2000.
293. Poole-Wilson PA, Swedberg K, Cleland JGF, et al, for the COMET Investigators: Comparison of carvedilol and metoprolol on clinical outcomes in patients with chronic heart failure in the Carvedilol Or Metoprolol European Trial (COMET): Randomised controlled trial. Lancet 362:7, 2003.
294. Goldstein S, Fagerberg B, Hjalmarson A, et al, for the MERIT-HF Study Group: Metoprolol controlled release/extended release in patients with severe heart failure. J Am Coll Cardiol 38:932, 2001.
295. Packer M, Fowler MB, Roecker EB, et al, for the Carvedilol Prospective Randomized Cumulative Survival (COPERNICUS) Study Group: Effect of carvedilol on the morbidity of patients with severe chronic heart failure: Results of the Carvedilol Prospective Randomized Cumulative Survival (COPERNICUS) study. Circulation 106:2194, 2002.
296. Le Coz F, Sauleman P, Poirier JM, et al: Oral pharmacokinetics of bisoprolol in resting and exercising healthy volunteers. J Cardiovasc Pharmacol 18:28, 1991.
297. CIBIS Investigators and Committees: A randomized trial of beta-blockade in heart failure: The Cardiac Insufficiency Bisoprolol Study (CIBIS). Circulation 90:1765, 1994.
298. Noguchi N, Nishino K, Niki E: Antioxidant action of the antihypertensive drug, carvedilol, against lipid peroxidation. Biochem Pharmacol 59:1069, 2000.
299. Lindenfeld JA, Lowes BD, Bristow MR: Hypotension with dobutamine. Beta-adrenergic antagonist selectivity at low doses of carvedilol. Ann Pharmacother 33:1266, 1999.
300. Metra M, Nardi M, Giubbini R, Dei Cas L: Effects of short- and long-term carvedilol administration on rest and exercise hemodynamic variables, exercise capacity and clinical conditions in patients with idiopathic dilated cardiomyopathy. J Am Coll Cardiol 24:1678, 1994.
301. Olsen SL, Gilbert EM, Renlund DG, et al: Carvedilol improves left ventricular function and symptoms in heart failure: A double-blind randomized study. J Am Coll Cardiol 25:1225, 1995.
302. Krum H, Sakner-Bernstein JD, Goldsmith RL, et al: Double-blind, placebo-controlled study of the long-term efficacy of carvedilol in patients with severe chronic heart failure. Circulation 92:1499, 1995.
303. Lowes BD, Gill EA, Abraham WT, et al: The effect of carvedilol on left ventricular mass, chamber geometry and mitral regurgitation in chronic heart failure. Am J Cardiol 83:1201, 1999.
304. Doughty RN, Whalley GA, Gamble G, et al: Left ventricular remodeling with carvedilol in patients with congestive heart failure due to ischemic heart disease. J Am Coll Cardiol 29:1060, 1997.
305. Doughty RN, Whalley GA, Gamble G, et al: Effects of carvedilol on left ventricular regional wall motion in patients with heart failure caused by ischemic heart disease. J Card Fail 6:11, 2000.
306. O'Keefe JH Jr, Magalski A, Stevens TL, et al: Predictors of improvement in left ventricular ejection fraction with carvedilol for congestive heart failure. J Nucl Cardiol 7:3, 2000.
307. McTavish D, Campoli-Richards D, Sorkin EM: Carvedilol: A review of its pharmacodynamic and pharmacokinetic properties, and therapeutic efficacy. Drugs 45:232, 1993.
308. Gilbert EM, Abraham WT, Olsen S, et al: Comparative hemodynamic, left ventricular functional, and antiadrenergic effects of chronic treatment with metoprolol versus carvedilol in the failing heart. Circulation 94:2817, 1996.
309. Bristow MR, Abraham WT, Yoshikawa T, et al: Second- and third-generation beta-blocking drugs in chronic heart failure. Cardiovasc Drugs Ther 11:291, 1997.
310. Metra M, Nodari S, Giubbini R, et al: Differential effects of beta-blockers in patients with heart failure. A prospective, randomized, double-blind comparison of the long-term effects of metoprolol versus carvedilol. Circulation 102:546, 2000.
311. Kukin ML, Kalman J, Charney RH, et al: Prospective, randomized comparison of effect of long-term treatment with metoprolol or carvedilol on symptoms, exercise, ejection fraction, and oxidative stress in heart failure. Circulation 99:2645, 1999.
312. Packer M, Colucci WS, Sackner-Bernstein JD, et al: Double-blind, placebo-controlled study of the effects of carvedilol in patients with moderate to severe heart failure: The PRECISE Trial. Circulation 94:2793, 1996.
313. Colucci WS, Packer M, Bristow MR, et al: Carvedilol inhibits clinical progression in patients with mild symptoms of heart failure. Circulation 94:2800, 1996.
314. Cohn JN, Fowler MB, Bristow MR, et al: Effect of carvedilol in severe chronic heart failure J Card Fail 3:173, 1997.
315. Australia-New Zealand Heart Failure Research Collaborative Group: Effects of carvedilol, a vasodilator-β-blocker, in patients with congestive heart failure due to ischemic heart disease. Circulation 92:212, 1995.
316. Australia/New Zealand Heart Failure Research Collaborative Group: Randomised, placebo-controlled trial of carvedilol in patients with congestive heart failure due to ischaemic heart disease. Lancet 349:375, 1997.
317. Packer M, Fowler MB, Roecker EB, et al: Carvedilol Prospective Randomized Cumulative Survival (COPERNICUS) Study Group: Effect of carvedilol on the morbidity of patients with severe chronic heart failure: Results of the carvedilol prospective randomized cumulative survival (COPERNICUS) study. Circulation 106:2194, 2002.
318. Lowes BD, Chidiac P, Olsen S, et al: Clinical relevance of inverse agonism and guanine nucleotide modulatable binding properties of adrenergic receptor blocking agents. Circulation 90(Suppl 1):543, 1994.

319. Yoshikawa T, Port JD, Asano K, et al: Cardiac adrenergic receptor effects of carvedilol. Eur Heart J 17(Suppl B):8, 1996.
320. BEST Trial Investigators: A trial of the beta-adrenergic blocker bucindolol in patients with advanced heart failure. N Engl J Med 344:1659, 2001.
321. Willette RN, Mitchell MP, Ohlstein EH, et al: Evaluation of intrinsic sympathomimetic activity of bucindolol and carvedilol in rat heart. Pharmacology 56:30, 1998.
322. Hershberger RE, Wynn JR, Sundberg L, Bristow MR: Mechanism of action of bucindolol in human ventricular myocardium. J Cardiovasc Pharmacol 15:959, 1990.
323. Maack C, Cremers B, Flesch M, et al: Different intrinsic activities of bucindolol, carvedilol and metoprolol in human failing myocardium. Br J Pharmacol 130:1131, 2000.
324. Brixius K, Bundkirchen A, Bolck B, et al: Nebivolol, bucindolol, metoprolol and carvedilol are devoid of intrinsic sympathomimetic activity in human myocardium. Br J Pharmacol 133:1330, 2001.
325. Bristow MR, Larrabee P, Minobe W, et al: Receptor pharmacology of carvedilol in the human heart. J Cardiovasc Pharmacol 19(Suppl 1):68, 1992.
326. Sederberg J, Wichman WE, Lindenfeld J, et al: Bucindolol has no intrinsic sympathomimetic activity in nonfailing human ventricular preparations [abstract]. J Am Coll Cardiol 35:207, 2000.
327. Bristow MR, Krause-Steinrauf H, Nuzzo R, et al: Effect of baseline changes in adrenergic activity on clinical outcomes in the Beta-blocker Evaluation of Survival Trial (BEST). Circulation (in press).
328. Pollock SG, Lystash J, Tedesco C, et al: Usefulness of bucindolol in congestive heart failure. Am J Cardiol 66:603, 1990.
329. Bristow MR, O'Connell JB, Gilbert EM, et al: Dose-response of chronic β-blocker treatment in heart failure from either idiopathic dilated or ischemic cardiomyopathy. Circulation 89:1632, 1994.
330. Stephen SA: Unwanted effects of propranolol. Am J Cardiol 18:463, 1966.
331. Epstein SE, Braunwald E: The effect of beta adrenergic blockade on patterns of urinary sodium excretion: Studies in normal subjects and in patients with heart disease. Ann Intern Med 65:20, 1968.
332. Talwar KK, Bhargava B, Upasani PT, et al: Hemodynamic predictors of early intolerance and long-term effects of propranolol in dilated cardiomyopathy. J Card Fail 2:273, 1996.
333. Yancy C, Fowler MB, Colucci WS, et al: Race and the response to adrenergic blockade with carvedilol in patients with chronic heart failure. N Engl J Med 344:1358, 2001.
334. Freudenberger R, Kalman J, Mannino M, et al: Effect of race in the response to metoprolol in patients with congestive heart failure secondary to idiopathic dilated or ischemic cardiomyopathy. Am J Cardiol 80:1372, 1997.
335. Goldstein S, Deedwania P, Gottlieb S, Wikstrand J; MERIT-HF Study Group: Metoprolol CR/XL in black patients with heart failure (from the metoprolol CR/XL randomized intervention trial in chronic heart failure). Am J Cardiol 92:478, 2003.
336. Carson P, Ziesche S, Johnson G, Cohn J: Racial differences in response to therapy for heart failure: Analysis of the vasodilator-heart failure trials. J Card Fail 5:178, 1999.
337. Domanski M, Krause-Steinrauf H, Deedwania P, et al: The effect of diabetes on outcome of advanced heart failure patients in the BEST Trial. J Am Coll Cardiol 42:914, 2003.
338. Torp-Pedersen C, Kober L, Ball S, et al: The incomplete bucindolol evaluation in acute myocardial infarction trial (BEAT). Eur J Heart Fail 4:495, 2002.
339. Bristow MR: Anti-adrenergic therapy of chronic heart failure: Surprises and new opportunities. Circulation 107:1100, 2003.
340. Wisenbaugh T, Katz I, Davis J, et al: Long-term (3 month) effects of a new beta-blocker (nebivolol) on cardiac performance in dilated cardiomyopathy. J Am Coll Cardiol 21:1094, 1993.
341. Uhlir O, Dvorak I, Gregor P, et al: Nebivolol in the treatment of cardiac failure: A double-blind controlled clinical trial. J Card Fail 3:271, 1997.
342. Cockcroft JR, Chowienczyk PJ, Brett SE, et al: Nebivolol vasodilates human forearm vasculature: Evidence for an L-arginine/NO-dependent mechanism. J Pharmacol Exp Ther 274:1067, 1995.
343. Abraham WT: Beta blockers; the new standard of therapy for mild heart failure. Arch Intern Med 160:1237, 2000.
344. Metra M, Nodari S, D'Aloia A, et al: A rationale for the use of beta blockers as standard treatment for heart failure. Am Heart J 139:511, 2000.
345. Swedberg K, Hjalmarson A, Waagstein F, Wallentin I: Adverse effects of beta-blockade withdrawal in patients with congestive cardiomyopathy. Br Heart J 44:134, 1980.
346. Manolis AJ, Olympios C, Sifaki M, et al: Chronic sympathetic suppression in the treatment of chronic congestive heart failure. Clin Exp Hypertens 20:717, 1998.
347. Zhang YH, Zhu J, Song YC: Suppressing sympathetic activation with clonidine on ventricular arrhythmias in congestive heart failure. Int J Cardiol 65:233, 1998.
348. Swedberg K, Bristow MR, Cohn JN, et al, for the MOXSE Investigators: The effects of moxonidine SR, an imidazoline agonist, on plasma norepinephrine in patients with congestive heart failure. Circulation 105:1797, 2002.
349. Cohn JN, Pfeffer MA, Rouleau J, et al, for the MOXCON Investigators: Adverse mortality effect of central sympathetic inhibition with sustained-release moxonidine in patients with heart failure (MOXCON). Eur J Heart Fail 5:659, 2003.

CHAPTER 24

Management of Heart Failure

Michael R. Bristow • Brian D. Lowes

Heart failure (HF) is a specific term used to define the clinical syndrome that ensues when the heart is unable to pump enough blood to supply the metabolic needs of the body (see Chaps. 19 and 21). The clinical syndrome of HF is caused by *cardiac failure*, a term used to define the various types of pump dysfunction that may cause HF. Cardiac failure may be produced by processes involving the pericardium, heart valves, coronary circulation, or myocardium (Table 24–1). Of these etiologies, the most common cause of chronic HF is myocardial dysfunction, termed *myocardial failure*. Myocardial failure is usually divided into two general types, *systolic dysfunction* and *diastolic dysfunction*, to reflect the dominant abnormalities of contraction and relaxation, respectively. Subjects with myocardial failure can have symptomatic HF or asymptomatic ventricular dysfunction.

As typically used, HF generally refers to the chronic syndrome, or *chronic HF*. The qualifier "congestive" should not be used in association with HF inasmuch as many HF patients receiving modern medical treatment do not manifest congestive symptoms or signs. Rather, HF symptoms usually relate to impaired exercise tolerance, plus or minus symptoms related to fluid overload. Symptoms of exercise intolerance are typically assessed by the New York Heart Association (NYHA) functional classification (see Chap. 7),[1] where

I = no symptoms
II = symptoms with moderate or marked levels of activity
III = symptoms with mild activity
IV = symptoms at rest

Because of its high prevalence (~2 percent of the adult population,[2,3] lifetime risk for men or women ~20 percent)[4] and frequent hospitalizations, the clinical syndrome of HF is among the most costly medical problems in the United States (see Chap. 22).[5] Despite improvements in the treatment of HF introduced since the early 1980s, including the general availability of cardiac transplantation and better medical treatment, clinical outcome following the onset of symptoms remains characterized by high mortality, morbidity, and progression of symptoms. For example, even in recent clinical trials showing benefit of new agents superimposed on successful older treatment, annualized mortality (percentage) and hospitalization rates (number of hospitalizations per patient per year) in the active treatment groups have been, respectively, 5 to 9 percent and 0.3 to 0.4 in Classes II and III[6-8] and 14 to 18 percent and 0.6 to 0.8 in Classes III and IV HF.[9,10] Furthermore, HF is the only cardiovascular disorder in the United States that is increasing in prevalence,[11] and since the prevalence is directly related to age,[12] the incidence and prevalence of HF will continue to increase on the basis of population demographics (Fig. 24–1). At present, an estimated 4.5 million patients have HF in the United States,[11] plus at least as many additional subjects with asymptomatic left ventricular dysfunction.[13] As can be observed in Figure 24–1, by 2050 the number of subjects with symptomatic HF will increase to more than 7 million on the basis of an increase in the number of persons older than 65 years,[14] in whom the prevalence of HF is 6 percent.[2]

Pathophysiology of Heart Failure due to Primary or Secondary Dilated Cardiomyopathies

The discussion of pathophysiology here is confined to primary and secondary dilated cardiomyopathy (see Chap. 59), the cause of the majority of cases of HF, as it may relate to medical therapy. More detailed discussion of the pathophysiology of myocardial failure is given in Chapter 21. HF caused by pericardial (see Chap. 64), valvular (see Chap. 57), and ischemic (see Chap. 50) heart disease is discussed elsewhere.

As depicted in Figure 24–2, two interrelated processes, chamber remodeling and myocardial systolic dysfunction, are thought to play critical roles in the development and progression of primary and secondary dilated cardiomyopathy.[15,16] Although both are the products of changes that occur at the cardiac myocyte level, changes in the interstitium also contribute.[17] In the remodeling process, cardiac myocytes become longer without a proportional increase in transverse diameter, which explains the increase in chamber diameter without an increase in wall thickness.[18] Factors known to contribute to the cellular and chamber remodeling process are activation of "compensatory mechanisms" that include the renin-angiotensin-aldosterone system (RAAS) and the adrenergic nervous system.[16] Although the remodeling process does increase the number of contractile elements as new sarcomeres are laid down in series, the law of Laplace dictates that diastolic wall stress will be markedly increased (see Chap. 19). Also, the elongated and remodeled cardiac myocyte is poorly contractile,[19] in part due to the activation of a "fetal" gene program that can directly cause contractile dysfunction.[20] The end result of these processes is a poorly contractile, dilated ventricular chamber that at some point can no longer adequately support the circulatory requirements of daily living. These processes are progressive in most patients with established chronic HF,[21] and the pace[22] and degree[23] of this progression are directly related to prognosis. This is why the pharmacological therapy of HF, discussed in detail in Chapter 23, is aimed at inhibiting the mechanistic processes that promote systolic dysfunction and remodeling.[16,20,21]

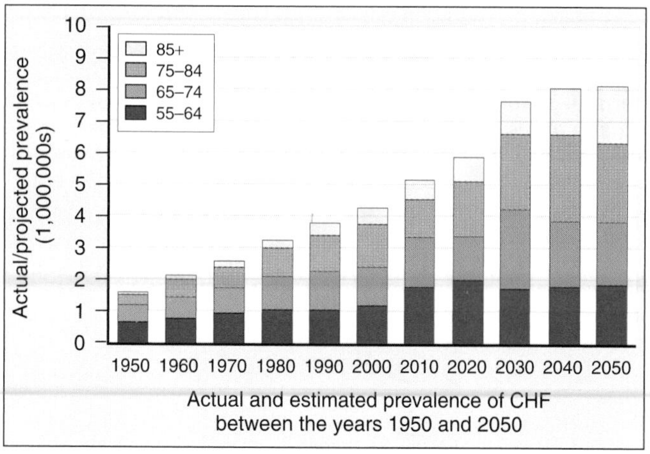

FIGURE 24–1 Effect of the aging population on the prevalence of heart failure, based on data from the National Heart, Lung, and Blood Institute (www.nhlbi.nih.gov/health/public/heart/other/CHF) and the U.S. Bureau of the Census. CHF = congestive heart failure.

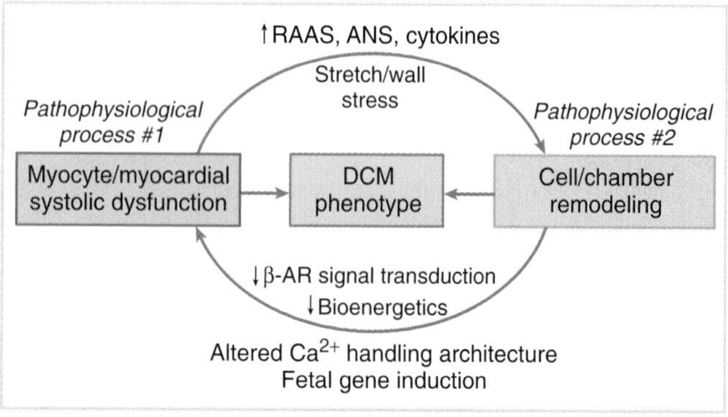

FIGURE 24–2 Relationship between contractile dysfunction and remodeling. RAAS = renin-angiotensin-aldosterone system; ANS = adrenergic nervous system; DCM = dilated cardiomyopathy; β-AR = beta-adrenergic receptor.

TABLE 24–1 General Etiologies of Cardiac Failure

General Cause	Specific Examples
Pericardial	Tamponade, pericardial constriction
Valvular	Aortic or mitral regurgitation
Myocardial	Idiopathic dilated cardiomyopthy, familial dilated cardiomyopathy, ischemic cardiomyopathy, valvular cardiomyopathy
Coronary vascular	Acute ischemic episodes
Rhythm disturbances	Tachycardia-induced heart failure

Diagnosis of Heart Failure: Determination of Etiology and Prognosis

One of the major problems in HF is its initial diagnosis, since the earliest symptoms of HF are often mistaken for other medical problems, including bronchial asthma, chronic obstructive pulmonary disease, pneumonia, and other pulmonary and nonpulmonary problems (see Chap. 22). Numerous studies have documented the lack of sensitivity and specificity of HF signs and symptoms,[24] and the initial diagnosis is often first made by the radiologist from a chest radiograph demonstrating pulmonary edema and cardiomegaly. Because of these realities, alternative means of initially diagnosing HF have and are being developed, such as point-of-care blood tests. Two of these tests, brain natriuretic peptide (BNP)[25] and N-terminal pro-BNP,[26] have been shown to improve the accuracy of HF diagnosis in an urgent care setting. The utility of these tests would appear to markedly improve the sensitivity of the diagnosis of HF, while at the same time reducing costs by limiting the number of unnecessary diagnostic echocardiograms.[27,28]

DETECTION OF SYSTOLIC DYSFUNCTION (see Chap. 20). An algorithm for diagnosing and evaluating HF is given in Figure 24-3. If HF is suspected because of symptoms (dyspnea, dyspnea on exertion, paroxysmal nocturnal dyspnea, orthopnea, peripheral edema, easy fatigability), radiographic or biochemical data, or a high natriuretic peptide concentration, an echocardiogram needs to be obtained. In the limited number of subjects who cannot be imaged by ultrasound for technical reasons, radionuclide ventriculography or magnetic resonance imaging (MRI) can be used to detect ventricular systolic dysfunction. An echocardiogram is the initial test of choice because it evaluates valvular and pericardial causes of HF, as well as being able to detect systolic dysfunction, and it may also be able to detect diastolic dysfunction. An echocardiogram (see Chap. 11) provides immediate information about whether the etiology is a pericardial, valvular, or myocardial process. HF needs to be diagnosed as early as possible so that mortality- and morbidity-lowering treatment can be initiated.

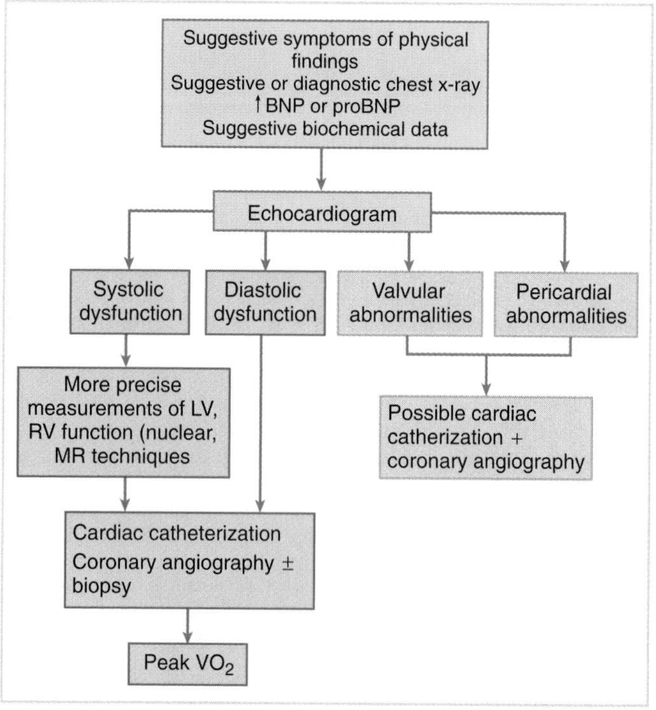

FIGURE 24–3 Algorithm for establishing the diagnosis of heart failure and determining etiology and prognosis. LV = left ventricular; MR = magnetic resonance; RV = right ventricular; BNP = brain natriuretic peptide; VO_2 = oxygen consumption.

If impaired left ventricular systolic function is detected by echocardiography, more precise measurement of the function of both ventricles may be indicated via radionuclide ventriculography (see Chap. 13). This imaging modality is able to measure left ventricular systolic function more precisely, which is important from a prognostic standpoint,[22,23] and for monitoring the response to beta blocker therapy, a treatment that favorably affects systolic function (see later).[16] Radionuclide ventriculography can also measure right ventricular function, which is another prognostic index in chronic HF.[29] When right ventricular structural abnormalities are suspected, cardiac MRI is indicated (see Chap. 14) because this modality is currently the best available imaging method for visualizing right ventricular pathology and function.

DIASTOLIC DYSFUNCTION (see Chap. 20). The diagnosis of diastolic dysfunction is largely one of exclusion. That is, to make the diagnosis of diastolic dysfunction, two pieces of data are required: documentation of normal or near-normal systolic function and unequivocal evidence of HF. The latter may be provided by unambiguous documentation of acute episodes of decompensation (e.g., pulmonary edema on a chest radiograph plus symptoms of breathlessness or right-sided failure) or chronic myocardial dysfunction resulting in high filling pressure, decreased cardiac output, and impaired functional capacity. Although echocardiographic and radionuclide ventriculographic data can contribute to a diagnosis of diastolic dysfunction, neither are considered sufficiently definitive to establish the diagnosis on the basis of isolated measurements. Importantly, diastolic dysfunction as the cause of HF in a relatively young (<60-year-old) patient suggests an infiltrative process, and an endomyocardial biopsy may be indicated.

Once the diagnosis of HF has been established, additional data need to be gathered. In general, the goals of this additional work-up are to determine the etiology and establish a general prognosis. The diagnostic work-up of HF should seek to determine the etiology, as outlined in Figure 24-3, unless the patient is so infirm that no form of intervention would be possible. Cardiac catheterization is often indicated to eliminate the possibility of coronary artery disease and other processes for whom specific management is required. Examples of indications for cardiac catheterization in a patient with newly diagnosed HF and various echocardiographic data are given in Table 24-2.

ENDOMYOCARDIAL BIOPSY. Perhaps the most controversial diagnostic test in the work-up of heart muscle disease is endomyocardial biopsy (see Chap. 17). This procedure in inexperienced hands can be associated with complications, including death in rare cases (<1 percent). On the other hand, in the presence of unexplained heart muscle disease, endomyocardial biopsy yields important diagnostic and prognostic information in 11 percent of patients,[30] a figure high enough to justify biopsy provided that experienced personnel are available to perform it and interpret the results.

In cases of systolic dysfunction caused by a primary or secondary dilated cardiomyopathy, precise determination of the degree of left and right ventricular dysfunction has important prognostic value. Additional clinical characteristics that may have an impact on the prognosis are the degree of pulmonary hypertension, the presence or absence of high-grade ventricular arrhythmia, and the extent of coronary artery disease. Valuable prognostic information can be gained by measuring peak oxygen consumption, which in chronic HF correlates with prognosis independently of left ventricular function.[31]

Management of Acute, New-Onset Heart Failure

TRANSIENT HEART FAILURE. (Management of episodes of acute decompensation in patients with chronic HF is discussed later.) Although chronic HF is the most commonly encountered form of symptomatic myocardial dysfunction, HF may also be acute and not superimposed on chronic pump dysfunction. Such manifestations can occur in the postoperative state following cardiac surgery,[32] in the setting of severe brain injury,[33] secondary to ischemic insults, or after the sudden onset of an inflammatory process or any pathophysiological mechanism that rapidly produces myocardial injury. The general pathophysiological mechanism involved is either some form of "stunning" of functional myocardium (see Chap. 19) or abrupt loss of functioning tissue that occurs before compensatory mechanisms can stabilize function. In both of these situations, myocardial function is adequate to support the circulation once recovery has occurred, and in the case of mechanisms that may produce stunning, such as cardiopulmonary bypass, other ischemic insults, and severe brain injury (where the stunning is probably related to massive release of catecholamines),[31] myocardial function may be completely normal on recovery.

TABLE 24–2 Indications for Cardiac Catheterization after Evaluation for Heart Failure and Performance of an Echocardiogram

Echo, Clinical Findings	Cardiac Catheterization or Other Procedure
Significant pericardial effusion, evidence of tamponade	Right heart catheterization, pericardiocentesis
Thickened pericardium, evidence of cardiac compression	Right and left heart catheterization ± endomyocardial biopsy if restriction suspected
Severe aortic or mitral regurgitation, LVE with decreased systolic function	Right and left heart catheterization, coronary angiography in anticipation of possible surgery
Aortic stenosis	Right heart catheterization, coronary angiography in anticipation of surgery
Mitral stenosis	Right and left heart catheterization, coronary angiography in anticipation of possible surgery or balloon valvuloplasty
LVE, decreased systolic function with valvular abnormalities < severe	Right and left heart catheterization, coronary angiography, possible endomyocardial biopsy if coronary arteries normal
Normal LV size, function	Right and left heart catheterization, coronary angiography, possible endomyocardial biopsy if coronary arteries normal, to rule out an infiltrative process
Hypertrophic cardiomyopathy with ASH, ± mitral regurgitation	Coronary angiography if surgery (myectomy, ± mitral valve replacement) contemplated
Normal LV size, decreased systolic function, no history of anthracyclines	Right and left heart catheterization, coronary angiography, endomyocardial biopsy if coronary arteries normal to rule out inflammatory heart disease
RV dysfunction, arrhythmia	MRI (to rule out ARVC)
RV dysfunction, isolated	Right heart catheterization (to rule out PAH)

ARVC = arrhythmic RV cardiomyopathy; ASH = asymmetrical septal hypertrophy; Echo = echocardiogram; LV = left ventricular; LVE = LV enlargement; PAH = pulmonary arterial hypertension; RV = right ventricular.

Management of episodes of acute HF caused by an evanescent process depressing myocardial function is therapy with diuretics, support of pump function with positive inotropic agents (see Chap. 23) and/or, if extremely severe, with mechanical devices (see Chap. 25) to the extent necessary to provide adequate perfusion of critical organs. Once function has recovered, no further treatment may be necessary. In the case of ischemia caused by coronary artery disease or another mechanism that may persist to cause recurrent problems, treatment of the underlying process is the management goal. Further details of the treatment of transient myocardial failure are given later in the section on the treatment of decompensated chronic HF.

NEW-ONSET, PERSISTENT HEART FAILURE. The most common manifestation of acute, new-onset HF is superimposition on a chronic process that has previously been subclinical and in which myocardial function has been supported by the compensatory mechanisms depicted in Figure 24–2. Therefore, most episodes of new-onset HF are actually the first episode of decompensation, similar to what occurs in established chronic HF.

How much myocardial functional loss can be countered by compensatory mechanisms? The quantitative relationship between degree of myocardial loss and development of myocardial pump dysfunction has been examined in two settings: following myocardial infarction[34] and after individual cardiac myocyte "dropout" from anthracycline cardiotoxicity.[35] The experimental model data from acute myocardial infarction[34] are more relevant to acute-onset HF superimposed on previously normal cardiac function, whereas the anthracycline data generated in patients[35] represent decompensation superimposed on a chronic myocardial process that has previously been stabilized by compensatory mechanisms. The conclusion from the myocardial infarction studies conducted in animal models was that loss of 30 percent or less of the left ventricle in rats[34] and 25 percent or less in dogs is relatively well tolerated, whereas in rats, infarcts in excess of 46 percent were associated with severe hemodynamic compromise.

ANTHRACYCLINE-INDUCED CARDIOMYOPATHY. Investigation of the structure-function relationship in anthracycline-induced cardiomyopathy (see Chap. 83) was conducted in the intact human heart in patients receiving the antitumor agent doxorubicin (Adriamycin).[35-37] Myocardial damage in this unique form of drug-induced heart disease consists of vacuolization and myofibrillar loss in individual cardiac myocytes, which are typically surrounded by myocytes that are unaffected.[35,36] By morphometrically counting the number of affected myocytes relative to the total in a field of endomyocardial biopsy material, it is possible to determine the percentage of cells that are nonfunctional because of the anthracycline process.[36,37] The degree of myocardial damage can then be related to the degree of myocardial dysfunction, as assessed by right-heart catheterization performed at rest and with exercise.[35-37] In anthracycline cardiomyopathy it is not until more than 15 percent of cells are damaged that detectable myocardial dysfunction develops, and moderate dysfunction does not develop until more than 25 percent of cardiac myocytes are involved.[35-37] In other words, as in myocardial infarction, in anthracycline-associated cardiomyopathy a certain amount of myocardial damage can be tolerated with the aid of compensatory mechanisms. In anthracycline cardiomyopathy, these compensatory mechanisms rely heavily on adrenergic stimulation, since hypertrophy is inhibited by the effects of anthracyclines on myocardial protein synthesis.[38,39]

Therefore, data from these model systems suggest that the initial, sudden onset of HF occurs when compensatory mechanisms can no longer sustain normal myocardial function. Consequently, myocardial function and structural measurements usually indicate a chronic remodeling process at the initial evaluation for HF.

Management of Chronic Heart Failure

Pharmacological Therapy for Chronic Heart Failure Caused by Systolic Dysfunction

The pharmacological treatment of chronic HF is best understood by subdividing the patient population into four groups

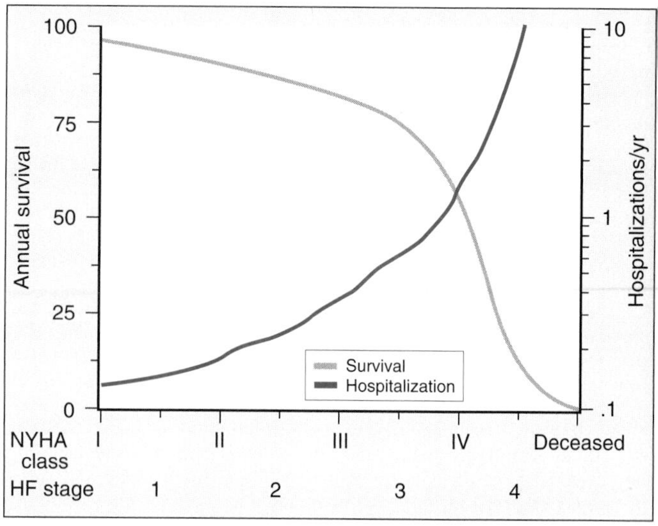

FIGURE 24–4 Plot of the relationship between survival or hospitalization frequency and New York Heart Association (NYHA) class or heart failure (HF) stage in chronic HF.

as described in Table 24–3. This "HF stage" classification system reflects the average symptomatic status of the patient inasmuch as patients typically move from one NYHA class to another within the stage groups, and is not the same as the American College of Cardiology/American Heart Association (ACC/AHA) Task Force stage classification that begins with stage A being an at-risk patient without HF or myocardial dysfunction.[40] In general, the average symptomatic status is directly related to hospitalization frequency and is also related to mortality risk as demonstrated in Figure 24–4. Important differences between the HF stage–ordered classification and the NYHA functional class are that the stage classification (1) begins with some level of disability as opposed to asymptomatic status, (2) ends with a more advanced level of disability than is generally reflected by the NYHA Class IV category, and (3) recognizes the reality that patients with HF often move from one level of symptoms to another, for example, typically exhibiting Class III symptoms that transiently increase to Class IV depending on medical management and other factors.

As outlined in Table 24–3, the goals of treatment for chronic HF are to (1) relieve symptoms and improve functional capacity, (2) reduce disability and hospitalizations, (3) delay progression of or reverse remodeling and myocardial dysfunction, and (4) reduce mortality. Depending on the stage that a particular HF patient is in, one or more of these goals may be more important than the others and dictate the type of agent to be developed or used once efficacy and safety are established.

STAGE 1 (MYOCARDIAL DYSFUNCTION WITH NO OR MILD HEART FAILURE, NYHA CLASS I/II SYMPTOMS). As for any chronic disease process, the most effective way to deal with the HF problem is to treat it early, before irreversible damage has developed. The goals of treatment of stage 1 HF (see Table 24–3) are to prevent progression of the underlying pathophysiological processes of remodeling and dysfunction and thereby prevent disease progression and overt development of the HF syndrome. However, only limited data actually support this generally accepted belief. Clinical trial experience is confined to one study—the Studies of Left Ventricular Dysfunction (SOLVD) Prevention Trial (see Table 23–7).[41] That trial demonstrated that the angiotensin-converting enzyme (ACE) inhibitor enalapril reduced the probability of development of overt HF by 37 percent and reduced the combined endpoint of mortality plus HF hospitalizations by 20 percent.[41]

TABLE 24–3 Goals and Pharmacological Treatment for Various Stages of Heart Failure

Stage	Goals (in order of importance)	Treatment
1 (asymptomatic–mild)	Reverse or prevent progressive remodeling and dysfunction	ACE inhibitors ? Beta-blocking agents ? ARBs
	Prevent overt heart failure or progressive symptoms	ACE inhibitors ? Beta-blocking agents ? ARBs
2 (mild–moderate)	Reverse or prevent progressive remodeling and dysfunction	ACE inhibitors Beta-blocking agents ARBs
	Improve symptoms and functional capacity	Diuretics ACE inhibitors ARBs Digoxin
	Reduce disability and hospitalizations	Diuretics ACE inhibitors Beta-blocking agents ARBs Digoxin
	Reduce mortality	ACE inhibitors Beta-blocking agents
3 (advanced)	Reduce mortality	ACE inhibitors Spironolactone Beta-blocking agents
	Reduce disability and hospitalizations	Diuretics ACE inhibitors Beta-blocking agents Spironolactone ? Positive inotropic agents, including digoxin
	Improve symptoms and functional capacity	Diuretics ACE inhibitors Spironolactone ? Positive inotropic agents, including digoxin
4 (severe)	Reduce disability and hospitalizations	Diuretics ACE inhibitors Positive inotropic agents, for periods of decompensation
	Improve symptoms and functional capacity	Diuretics ACE inhibitors Positive inotropic agents, for periods of decompensation
	Reduce mortality	ACE inhibitors ? Beta-blocking agents + positive inotropes

ACE = angiotensin-converting enzyme; ARB = angiotensin receptor blocker.

Although it is likely that beta-adrenergic blocking agents will reduce mortality in stage 1 HF, because of the sample size and therefore the cost considerations of performing placebo-controlled trials in this patient population, to date no beta blocker clinical trial has examined this patient population. Similarly, trials with other neurohormonal antagonists will probably not be performed until efficacy has been demonstrated in later-stage HF.

STAGE 2 (MILD TO MODERATE HEART FAILURE, NYHA CLASS II/III SYMPTOMS). This is the HF stage in which the majority of clinical trial data are available, because of the prevalence and relative stability of these patients. As a result, recommendations for medical therapy for Class II to III or stage 2 HF can be given with a high degree of certainty, as outlined in Table 24–3. The goals of therapy in this stage are, similar to stage 1, centered around reversal or prevention of progression of remodeling and dysfunction because the potential for reversibility of the dilated cardiomyopathy phenotype still exists. As remodeling/dysfunction is attenuated or reversed, the other treatment goals outlined in Table 24–3 will be realized, and all are important in stage 2 HF.

ACE inhibitors[42-44] (see Table 23–7) and beta-blocking agents[6-8,45] (Fig. 24–5) have been shown to reduce mortality and hospitalizations in patients with stage 2 HF. ACE inhibitors also improve symptoms and tend to improve functional capacity in this stage of HF,[44] whereas beta-blocking agents have produced variable results on symptoms and functional capacity.[45] Angiotensin-receptor blockers (ARBs) can reduce the combined endpoint of cardiovascular mortality and HF hospitalizations when administered on top of an ACE inhibitor in stage 2 patients with preserved blood pressures (average systolic blood pressure >120 mm Hg),[46,47] mostly by reducing HF hospitalizations. However, in one of these trials (Val-Heft)[46] there was an increase in mortality in patients treated with the ARB valsartan on top of ACE inhibition and beta blockade. This adverse effect was not found in the CHARM-Added Trial, which investigated the ARB candesartan.[47] In both trials ARBs were effective in lowering mortality and HF morbidity in patients intolerant of ACE inhibitors (Fig. 24–6).[46,48]

On balance, digoxin has generally improved symptoms and functional capacity in patients in sinus rhythm with mild to moderate HF,[49] slightly reduces hospitalizations but does not reduce mortality.[50] Other, nonapproved positive inotropic agents have also improved functional capacity.[51,52] However, positive inotropic agents other than digoxin have been associated with increased mortality when used chronically in HF, and it is unclear whether newer

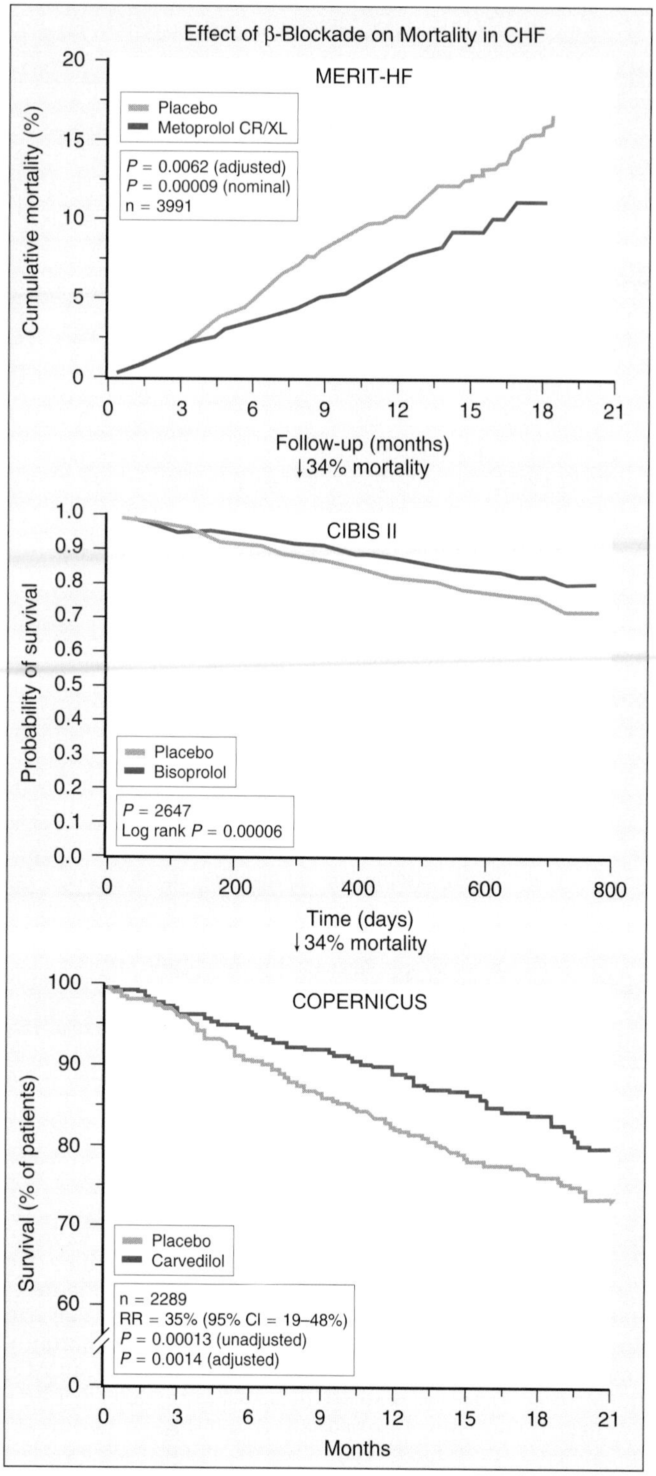

FIGURE 24–5 Kaplan-Meier analysis of the probability of survival among patients in the placebo and beta-blocker groups in the MERIT-HF **(top)**, CIBIS II **(middle)**, and COPERNICUS **(bottom)** trials. CHF = chronic heart failure; CI = confidence interval. (Data from The Cardiac Insufficiency Bisoprolol Study II [CIBIS II]. Lancet 353:9-13, 1999; Metoprolol CR/XL randomized intervention trial in congestive heart failure [MERIT-HF]. Lancet 353:2001-2007, 1999; and Packer M, Coats AJ, Fowler MB, et al, for The Carvedilol Prospective Randomized Cumulative Survival Study Group: Effect of carvedilol on survival in severe chronic heart failure. N Engl J Med. 344:1651-1658, 2001.)

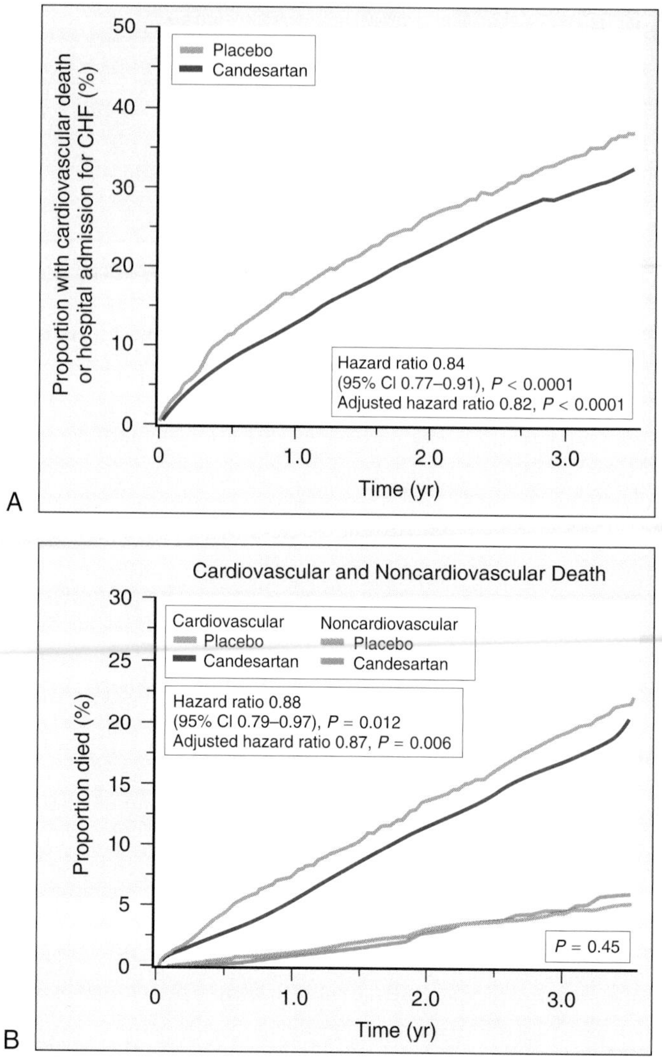

FIGURE 24–6 **A,** Effect of candesartan on cardiovascular mortality or hospital admission for congestive heart failure (CHF) in the CHARM trials. Three groups of patients include (1) patients with left ventricular ejection fraction less than 0.40 who could not tolerate angiotensin-converting enzyme (ACE) inhibitors; (2) patients in whom angiotensin-receptor blocker was given in addition to the ACE inhibition; and (3) patients with HF and preserved ejection fraction. **B,** Kaplan-Meier curves of cardiovascular or noncardiovascular deaths. (From Pfeffer MA, Swedberg K, Granger CB, et al: Effects of candesartan on mortality and morbidity in patients with chronic heart failure. The CHARM-Overall programme. Lancet 362:759-766, 2003.)

strategies such as low-dose administration[52,53] or combination with beta-blocking agents[54] will mitigate theses adverse effects.

If digoxin is used, the trough serum level should be kept at or below 1.0 ng/ml,[55] because levels above that are associated with increased mortality. Keeping digoxin levels low also mitigates adverse effects on women,[55,56] which at least in part are due to higher levels related to smaller volumes of distribution compared to men given the same fixed doses.

Although never subjected to large-scale trials, loop diuretics are a cornerstone of symptomatic HF treatment beginning in stage 2.[57] The goals of diuretic therapy are to reduce congestive symptoms, reduce wall stress, and attenuate the harmful signaling of remodeling/dysfunction mechanisms outlined in Table 24–3. In stage 2, a loop diuretic alone usually suffices, along with potassium replacement to maintain serum levels well into the normal range. Diuretics should be used in conjunction with dietary salt restriction, initially avoiding added salt and then avoiding foods prepared with salt such as canned foods and processed foods.

The aldosterone antagonist, K^+-sparing minimal diuretic spironolactone, has been shown to lower mortality in stage 3 patients (see later), and results with the newer aldosterone antagonist eplerenone in a post-myocardial infarction setting[58] (see Fig. 23–4) suggest that aldosterone inhibition added to an ACE inhibitor would be effective in lowering mortality and morbidity in stage 2 HF.

In summary, patients in stage 2 should be treated with an ACE inhibitor, a beta-adrenergic blocker, a diuretic, and sodium restriction; digoxin is optional. If patients cannot tolerate an ACE inhibitor, typically because of cough, they can be treated with an ARB. If blood pressure is relatively preserved (≥120 mm Hg), an ARB can be added to an ACE inhibitor or an ACE inhibitor and a beta blocker. For lower blood pressures an ARB should be added with caution, particularly on top of a beta blocker and an ACE inhibitor. Another option is the addition of an aldosterone antagonist to an ACE inhibitor and beta blocker, although in stage 2 HF this is not yet supported by clinical trial data.

STAGE 3 (ADVANCED HEART FAILURE, NYHA CLASS III/IV SYMPTOMS). As shown in Figure 24–4, in stage 3 HF the hospitalization rate and mortality begin to increase markedly. Therefore, the main goal of therapy in advanced, stage 3 HF is to lower the probability of HF-related hospitalization and mortality. ACE inhibitors (see Table 23–7) and the aldosterone antagonist spironolactone[9] have been shown to be effective in this regard. Beta-blocking agents, which are quantitatively more effective than ACE inhibitors in stage 2 HF, appear to be less effective in reducing mortality and hospitalizations in more advanced HF.[8] However, if patients with advanced HF and severe left ventricular dysfunction (left ventricular ejection fraction [LVEF] < 0.25) are carefully selected (compensated, no fluid overload) they can benefit substantially from beta blockade, with annualized mortality reductions in the 30 to 40 percent range (see Fig. 24–5).[59,60]

In terms of symptom relief and improvement of functional capacity in stage 3 patients, inhibitors of the RAAS, diuretics, and possibly positive inotropic agents have had some success in controlled trials. For diuretics, in stage 3 HF it is often necessary to add the powerful thiazide-like diuretic metolazone plus a K^+-sparing compound (spironolactone if it is tolerated) to control fluid retention. Dietary salt restriction should be intensified. Trials of inotropic agents in this patient population have not prolonged survival thus far,[61-63] but promising low-dose and combined beta blocker–inotrope approaches are currently being evaluated.[52-54]

STAGE 4 (SEVERE HEART FAILURE, NYHA CLASS III/IV SYMPTOMS WITH FREQUENT OR SUSTAINED DECOMPENSATION). When subjects progress to stage 4, i.e., severe HF despite optimal medical management, as shown in Table 24–3, the goals of therapy change to include palliation of symptoms, reducing rates of hospitalization, and in subjects who are eligible, bridging to cardiac transplantation (see also Chap. 26). In general, reversal of the intrinsic biological processes of remodeling and dysfunction are not possible in this stage. The only treatment shown to be effective in lowering mortality in this stage of HF is ACE inhibition,[64] but despite this treatment, when subjects reach stage 4 HF, the possibility of salvage by medical therapy is indeed remote.

Although for ethical reasons no randomized study has provided convincing proof, in subjects who periodically decompensate to incipient or overt cardiogenic shock, the administration of non–glycoside-positive inotropic agents appear to be life saving. Currently, no orally administered positive inotropic agents are approved for palliation of advanced HF, but investigational agents[52,53,65] have shown enough promise to initiate Phase III clinical trials in this regard. Until an oral agent is available, the standard treatment for palliation of advanced HF will remain intermittent or continuous administration of intravenous inotropic agents such as dobutamine,[66] milrinone,[67] enoximone,[68] or levosimendan (see Chap. 23).[69]

SUMMARY OF PLACEBO CONTROLLED PHASE III CLINICAL TRIALS MEASURING MORTALITY AS A PRIMARY ENDPOINT. Tables 23–7 and 23–13 list the clinical trials discussed earlier, with all data expressed as 12-month event rate rates and event rate reductions. As successful therapy is developed, the next generation of clinical trials is conducted on a background of that therapy, and as a result any efficacy signal must be detected as one that is additive with the background therapy. By adding the risk reductions given in these tables, it is possible to estimate the cumulative degree of reduction in mortality ("combined mortality reduction") referenced back to placebo. Only therapies that have produced a statistically significant reduction in mortality have the cumulative risk reduction calculated. Compared to placebo, 12 months of treatment with ACE inhibitors produces an average reduction in mortality of 17 percent. Beta blockers, whose trials were conducted on a background of ACE inhibitors, lowered mortality further, by an average of 32 percent. This figure yields a cumulative reduction in mortality, referenced back to placebo, of 44 percent. Spironolactone, also evaluated on a background of ACE inhibitors, produces a reduction in mortality of 25 percent and a cumulative reduction of 38 percent.

PHARMACOLOGICAL THERAPY IN SPECIALIZED SUBGROUPS

THE BLACK POPULATION. Some HF demographic groups have exhibited responses to pharmacological treatment that appears to be different from that of other groups or the population as a whole. One of them is American blacks, who in the Beta-Blocker Evaluation of Survival Trial[10] (BEST) exhibited a worse response to beta blockade than did the rest of the population. American blacks treated with bucindolol had a statistically insignificant 17 percent increase in mortality as compared with a statistically significant 19 percent reduction in mortality in the rest of the population.[10]

However, blacks treated with carvedilol in the U.S. Carvedilol Trials fared as well as the remainder of the population,[70] perhaps because they had only stage 2 HF as opposed to the stage 3 subjects in BEST. Another possibility for the difference in response to beta blockade in BEST and the U.S. Carvedilol Trials is that the more powerful vasodilator properties of carvedilol were beneficial in a population enriched in hypertensive heart disease.[10,70] What is certain is that blacks with HF have quite different associated demographics, including a lower prevalence of ischemic cardiomyopathy, more hypertension by history, a higher prevalence of diabetes, and a younger subject population.[10,70,71]

Another likely factor influencing therapeutic response of blacks is gene polymorphisms enriched in the black population compared to nonblacks. An example of this is the alpha$_{2C}$-receptor deletion polymorphism α_{2C}Del322-325, which leads to loss of function[72] in a receptor that ordinarily inhibits norepinephrine release. This polymorphism is present in the homozygous state in more than 50 percent of the American black population but in fewer than 10 percent of American whites.[73] How this relates to an increased adrenergic drive in blacks is not yet clear, but this polymorphism is associated with an approximate fivefold increase in the risk of developing HF.[73] Thus, it is not clear whether genetic modifier mechanisms or race-associated demographic conditions account for the difference in response to beta blockers and ACE inhibitors that has been noted in clinical trials. The scientific basis for these differences needs to be further elucidated, and more effective treatment of blacks with HF needs to be developed. For the present, it is prudent to carefully utilize beta blockers in black patients with stage 3 HF and to consider the alternative of hydralazine/isosorbide dinitrate instead of ACE inhibitor treatment.[74]

WOMEN. Gender may also influence pharmacological treatment.[75-77] Women with HF have a better prognosis than men,[12] greater functional incapacity for the same degree of left ventricular dysfunction,[75] a higher prevalence of diastolic dysfunction,[76,77] and a higher percentage of elderly individuals.[76] Some or all of these factors may contribute to the tendency for lower effect sizes in women versus men in the few clinical trials that have enrolled enough women to report differences in response versus men.[8,10] However, based on currently available data, there is no reason to treat women with HF any different than men. This includes the use of digoxin, as long as trough long serum levels are kept at or below 1.0 ng/ml.[55]

DIABETICS. Another common subgroup in HF populations is patients with diabetes. Diabetes mellitus is a risk factor for developing HF,[4] and most HF cohorts have a prevalence of diabetes that is higher than 20 percent. In addition, the presence of diabetes in patients with systolic dysfunction confers a greater risk of mortality, but only in patients who have coronary artery disease.[78,79] Pharmacological therapy for the diabetic patient with HF should be the same as for nondiabetics, with extra attention paid to tight control of hyperglycemia. Medical therapy of diabetic HF patients should include beta-blocking agents, which have clinical effects that are at least as beneficial as in nondiabetics, with acceptable safety profiles.[79,80]

Pharmacological Therapy for Chronic Heart Failure Caused by Diastolic Dysfunction

As many as 30 to 50 percent of patients with symptomatic HF exhibit diastolic rather than systolic dysfunction (see Chaps. 20 and 21).[3,77,81] Diastolic dysfunction is more common in women[73] and the elderly,[80] and in the latter it may be the dominant form of HF.[82] Additional risk factors for diastolic dysfunction include a history of hypertension[83] and diabetes mellitus.[84] Most studies indicate that patients with diastolic dysfunction as the primary cause of HF have a better prognosis than do control subjects with systolic dysfunction. As discussed earlier, predominantly diastolic dysfunction in a younger (<60-year-old) patient suggests an infiltrative cardiomyopathic process.

Unlike systolic dysfunction, no medical treatment that reduces mortality in diastolic dysfunction is available. The cornerstone of treatment is careful regulation of ventricular filling pressure by diuretics, in a range that prevents excessive dyspnea and liver congestion but allows for adequate cardiac output. ACE inhibitors and/or spironolactone may make diuretic management easier by preventing excessive activation of the RAAS. In addition, some evidence indicates that ACE inhibitors improve ventricular relaxation,[85] but this improvement does not seem to be translated into benefit in subjects with diastolic HF. A large clinical trial (CHARM-Preserved)[86] comparing an angiotensin receptor–blocking agent (candesartan) to placebo demonstrated a small (18 percent) reduction in HF hospitalizations, without a beneficial effect on the primary endpoint (cardiovascular death or HF hospitalizations) or on mortality. In patients with tachycardia (resting heart rates > 90 beats/min) beta blockers may be used to slow the heart rate and prolong filling time, and beta blockers or amiodarone may be required to control and prevent supraventricular arrhythmias. Finally, phosphodiesterase inhibitors (PDEIs) have been shown to improve diastolic function acutely,[87] but there has been no controlled experience with these agents in chronic therapy.

Adjunctive Pharmacological Therapy

ANTIARRHYTHMIC AGENTS (see Chap. 30). In general, antiarrhythmic therapy in HF patients is reserved for symptomatic arrhythmias or for control of ventricular responses to atrial fibrillation. With regard to treatment of ventricular arrhythmias, the Cardiac Arrhythmia Suppression Trial (CAST),[88,89] which was conducted not in a HF population but in subjects with left ventricular dysfunction after myocardial infarction, convincingly demonstrated that type 1 antiarrhythmic agents (i.e., sodium-channel blockers) increase mortality when used to suppress ventricular premature contractions. The Electrophysiological Study Versus Electrocardiographic Monitoring (ESVEM)[90] extended the evidence for adverse effects of type 1 agents in subjects with left ventricular dysfunction and Holter monitor–documented ventricular arrhythmias or inducible sustained ventricular tachycardia. In the ESVEM trial, sotalol, a beta-blocking agent with type III antiarrhythmic properties, was the most effective agent. However, ESVEM had no placebo control, so it was not possible to precisely measure the efficacy and adverse effects of sotalol.

The antiarrhythmic agent that has undergone the most extensive evaluation for efficacy and safety in populations with HF or left ventricular dysfunction is amiodarone. Similar to sotalol, amiodarone is a type III antiarrhythmic with antiadrenergic properties. In controlled clinical trials in HF or asymptomatic left ventricular dysfunction, amiodarone either has been associated with reduced mortality[91] or has been equivalent to placebo.[92] In other words, amiodarone is the one antiarrhythmic agent that appears to be safe in patients with left ventricular dysfunction and HF. However, amiodarone has pulmonary, thyroid, liver, and other toxicities, and its use should be accompanied by careful surveillance for adverse effects. Additionally, as for all antiarrhythmic agents, amiodarone has negative inotropic effects and may be poorly tolerated by patients with advanced HF.

Treatment of arrhythmias has evolved to catheter-based ablation and implantable defibrillators (see Chap. 31). Current indications for device therapy for ventricular arrhythmias are given later.

ANTICOAGULATION (see Chap. 80). The use of anticoagulation in the form of warfarin in patients with normal sinus rhythm and severe left ventricular dysfunction is an area of considerable controversy. In controlled clinical trials, the risk of arterial thromboembolic events, most of which are stroke, ranges from 0.9 to 5.5 per 100 patient-years.[93,94] Since warfarin convincingly lowers thromboembolism and stroke risk in atrial fibrillation,[95] it is logical that this benefit would extend to subjects with severe left ventricular dysfunction. Such benefit may be particularly true in nonischemic cardiomyopathies, which are associated with a relatively high incidence of left ventricular thrombus.[96] A few small studies generally support a benefit of oral anticoagulation. On the basis of these considerations, many, but not all HF centers routinely administer anticoagulants to all patients with moderate or severe left ventricular dysfunction who do not have a contraindication. However, anticoagulation with warfarin is not without risk, and it must be carefully monitored. In chronic HF, a firm indication for anticoagulation can be made in patients with atrial fibrillation, those with a visualized left ventricular thrombus, and those with a history of a thromboembolic event.[97] Anticoagulation in left ventricular dysfunction with normal sinus rhythm should be considered optional, with the issue to be settled by ongoing clinical trials.

Device Therapy

Implantable Cardioverter-Defibrillators

Implantable cardioverter-defibrillators (ICDs) (see Chap. 31) are now the treatment of choice in patients with left ventricular dysfunction who have survived sudden cardiac death,[98] have symptomatic sustained ventricular tachycardia,[99] have asymptomatic nonsustained but inducible ventricular tachycardia,[9,100] or have an ischemic cardiomyopathy with an LVEF less than 30 percent.[101] Data supporting these recommendations are derived from the Antiarrhythmic Versus Implantable Defibrillator (AVID) Trial,[98] the Multicenter Automatic Defibrillator Implantation Trial (MADIT),[99] the Multicenter Unsustained Tachycardia Trial (MUSTT),[100] and the Multicenter Automatic Defibrillator Implantation Trial II (MADIT II) (Fig. 24–7).[101] The benefit of ICD implantation was most striking in patients with a QRS wider than 0.12 seconds (Fig. 24–7B).

At this point, a major question is whether ICDs can reduce mortality in other left ventricular dysfunction or HF populations, such as patients with nonsustained and noninducible ventricular tachycardia, nonischemic cardiomyopathies,

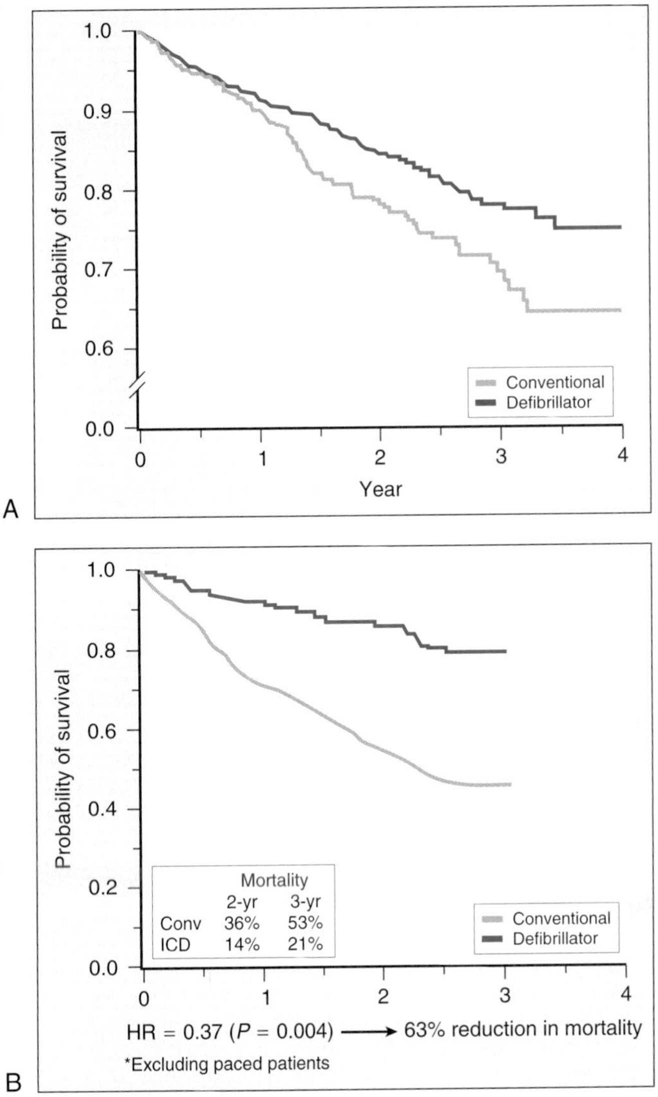

FIGURE 24–7 MADIT II Trial. **A,** Kaplan-Meier estimates of the probability of survival in post-myocardial infarction patients with ejection fraction less than 0.30 assigned to receive an implantable cardioverter-defibrillator (ICD) and the group assigned to receive conventional medical therapy. The difference in survival between the two groups was significant (nominal $p = 0.007$, by the log rank test). **B,** Survival in MADIT II patients with QRS wider than 0.12 seconds. HR = heart rate. (**A,** From Moss AJ, Zareba W, Hall WJ, et al: Prophylactic implantation of a defibrillator in patients with myocardial infarction and reduced ejection fraction. N Engl J Med 346:877, 2002; **B,** Courtesy of Dr. A. J. Moss.)

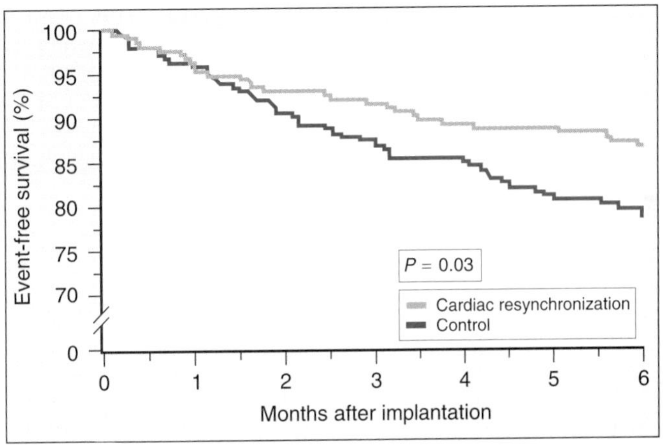

FIGURE 24–8 Kaplan-Meier estimates of the time to death or hospitalization for worsening heart failure in the control and resynchronization groups in the MIRACLE Trial, which enrolled 453 patients with heart failure, an ejection fraction less than 0.35, and a QRS wider than 130 milliseconds. The risk of an event was 40 percent lower in the resynchronization group (95 percent confidence interval, 4 to 63 percent; $p = 0.03$). (Data from Abraham WT, Fisher WG, Smith AL, et al: Cardiac resynchronization in chronic heart failure. N Engl J Med 346:1845-1853, 2002.)

large numbers of premature ventricular contractions, intraventricular conduction delays, and abnormal signal-averaged electrocardiograms, or even in subjects with no evidence of electrophysiological abnormalities. In this regard, the Comparison of Medical Therapy, Pacing and Defibrillation in Chronic Heart Failure (COMPANION) Trial recently evaluated patients with a lengthened QRS (>120 milliseconds), left ventricular dysfunction (LVEF < 0.35), and a HF hospitalization within the past year.[102] In this trial patients were randomized between optimal medical therapy (OPT), OPT + biventricular pacing to provide cardiac resynchronization therapy (CRT), or OPT + CRT and an ICD (CRT-D). The primary endpoint in this trial was time to all-cause death or any hospitalization. In this patient population, the combination of biventricular pacing and an ICD substantially reduced mortality in nonischemic cardiomyopathy patients, by 50 percent ($p < 0.01$) compared to 27 percent in the ischemic cardiomyopathy group.[103] In contrast, in the biventricular pacing without ICD arm, mortality was reduced by only 9 percent (p = NS).[103] These data indicate that the addition of an ICD to biventricular pacing in patients with intraventricular conduction defects and other enrollment criteria used in the COMPANION Trial can reduce mortality in nonischemic cardiomyopathy patients.

Biventricular Pacing

One of the more interesting recent developments in HF is the concept that left ventricular or biventricular pacing (see Chap. 31) may be beneficial in a subset of subjects with intraventricular conduction delay, which may include 15 to 30 percent of subjects with advanced left ventricular dysfunction (Fig. 24–8).[104-106] The biventricular pacing strategy is based on the fact that most subjects with intraventricular conduction delay have dyssynchronous left ventricular contraction, which results in a reduction in ventricular performance and unfavorable myocardial energetics.[107] There is no question that, acutely, biventricular or left ventricular pacing can, by synchronizing left ventricular contraction, improve left ventricular rate of pressure increase (dP/dT)[107,108] and ejection fraction,[109] cardiac index,[108] and myocardial energetics.[107] These favorable myocardial functional effects contribute to a short-term reduction in neurohormonal activation[110] and to an improvement in functional capacity and quality of life over a several-month period.[103,111-113] Moreover, the improvement in systolic function discussed earlier is translated by 6 months into reverse remodeling, with a sustained increase in ejection fraction and a reduction in left ventricular size.[114-116]

The COMPANION Trial, mentioned above, was designed to determine if CRT can improve major clinical outcomes in advanced HF patients with intraventricular conduction defects.[100] CRT or CRT + CRT-D was compared to optimal pharmacological therapy for effects on survival and hospitalizations.[103] In this study both CRT and CRT-D reduced the incidence of the primary endpoint of all-cause mortality or all-cause hospitalization by 19 to 20 percent ($p < 0.02$), secondary to an favorable effects on mortality and HF hospitalizations.[103] CRT alone reduced mortality by 24 percent (p = 0.06), whereas, as mentioned earlier, CRT-D reduced mortality by 36 percent ($p < 0.01$).[103] Thus in advanced HF patients with intraventricular conduction defects CRT produces a major reduction (by 35 to 40 percent) in HF hospitalizations and a moderate reduction in mortality; the addition of an

ICD adds an additional increment of mortality reduction, to a degree (by 36 percent) that statistical significance is achieved and the clinical impact is substantial. Thus patients with LVEFs less than 0.35 and QRS durations wider than 120 milliseconds should be considered for CRT or CRD-D therapy, as an adjunct to optimal background pharmacological treatment.

Ventricular Assist Devices (see Chap. 25)

Ventricular assist devices have emerged as a potential treatment of chronic HF, beyond their traditional role as a bridge to transplantation. A randomized, controlled clinical trial (the Randomized Evaluation of Mechanical Assistance for the Treatment of Congestive Heart Failure [REMATCH] Trial)[117] was conducted to evaluate one device (Heartmate vented electric device) in patients who were not transplant eligible. This trial randomized patients with an LVEF less than 0.25, NYHA Class IV symptoms, and the continued need for inotropic therapy to continued medical therapy or an assist device.[117] Patients randomized to an assist device had a 48 percent reduction in death from any cause as well as an improved quality of life (see Fig. 25–12).[118] Unfortunately, long-term survival with this device was still poor (1 year, 52 percent, and 2 years, 25 percent).[118] The frequency of serious adverse events including serious bleeding, infection, and neurological dysfunction was also 2.35 times that noted in the medical therapy group.[118] Despite these limitations, left ventricular assist devices will likely have an expanding role in the treatment of a subset of ultraadvanced HF patients.

OTHER DEVICES. Several other devices in development may have a role in the treatment of HF. For example, external pneumatic counterpulsation, shown to be effective in treating angina,[119] may have a role in treating HF.[120] One of the more interesting approaches to preventing progressive remodeling is a device (the "Acorn" device) that physically prevents ventricular dilation in animal models (see Fig. 20–1).[121] Clearly, devices of various types will increasingly contribute to HF treatment in the future.

Surgical Therapy

CARDIAC TRANSPLANTATION (see Chap. 26). This procedure was the first definitive treatment developed for HF, that is, the first treatment that lowered mortality.[122] The treatment is so successful in advanced or severe stage 3 or 4 HF that to this point no randomized study could have been ethically justified. Survival curves for severe HF (stage 4) subjects from the enalapril arm of the Cooperative New Scandinavian Enalapril Survival (CONSENSUS) Trial,[64] a cohort of stage 3 subjects from 1980 prior to ACE inhibitor treatment, the beta-blocker arms of the Carvedilol Prospective Randomized Cumulative Survival Study (COPERNICUS)[59] and BEST[10] Trials conducted in stage 3 patients, the CRT-D arm of the COMPANION Trial representing the current best available medical and device therapy in stage 3 HF, and cardiac transplantation for stage 3 or 4 patients are shown in Figure 24–9. Survival after transplantation is superior to that with pharmacological or pharmacological + device therapy. However, as can be observed in the COMPANION Trial CRT-D patients,[103] survival with the combination of pharmacological and device therapy is improving and with another incremental improvement it will rival transplantation for outcomes in at least stage 3 patients.

The biggest limitation of cardiac transplantation is not efficacy or safety but rather the limited supply of donors available to apply the treatment. It has been estimated that less than 10 percent of subjects who would benefit from cardiac transplantation can actually receive it on the basis of the upward limit of 2500 usable donors per year in the United

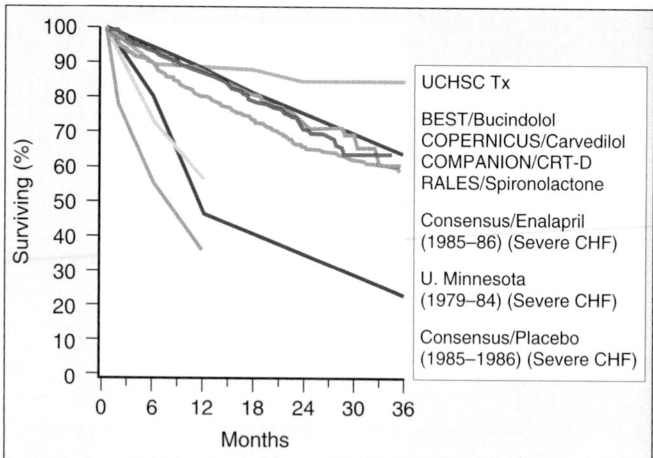

FIGURE 24–9 Survival curves in stage 3 or 4 heart failure, patients treated medically (see text for description of trials) or with cardiac transplantation (UCHSC Tx).

States.[123] Therefore, transplantation is reserved for subjects who have reached stage 4 or late stage 3 HF and are progressing despite application of all medical therapy of proven benefit.

CORONARY ARTERY BYPASS GRAFTING (see Chap. 50). More than 15 years ago, the Coronary Artery Surgery Study (CASS)[124] demonstrated that coronary artery bypass grafting (CABG) is superior to medical therapy from a survival standpoint in subjects with symptomatic triple-vessel coronary artery disease and reduced but not severely depressed LVEFs. In recent years, the benefit of CABG has been extended to patients with LVEFs lower than the 0.35 cutoff in CASS. Many centers have successfully extended CABG therapy to stage 3 HF subjects with LVEFs less than 0.30,[125,126] but no large controlled trials have compared CABG with current recommended standard medical therapy, including beta blockers. One such trial, also including investigation of the addition of surgical anterior ventricular restoration (a form of surgical reshaping of the ventricle without removal of viable myocardium)[127] to CABG (the STICH Trial) is currently being conducted.

MITRAL VALVE RECONSTRUCTION IN LEFT VENTRICULAR DYSFUNCTION (see Chap. 57). Mitral regurgitation occurs to a greater or lesser degree in the remodeled, dilated ventricle. During the past decade surgical approaches to correction of mitral regurgitation without valve replacement have been applied to the failing, remodeled ventricle with low operative mortality and impressive early clinical outcomes.[128] However, no prospective controlled, randomized studies have compared mitral valve reconstruction with the best available medical therapy, which itself can reverse remodeling in patients with mitral regurgitation. Thus, the role of mitral valve reconstruction in the setting of remodeling and mitral regurgitation is somewhat unclear and at the moment should be conservatively confined to cases of severe mitral regurgitation with some preservation of left ventricular function, i.e., with ejection fractions greater than 0.30.

Management of Episodes of Acute Decompensation

As discussed earlier, acute manifestations of HF can either be in the context of new onset or be in subjects with established chronic HF. Treatment of acute episodes of HF are similar in these two scenarios, with the exception that a diagnostic work-up potentially leading to definitive therapy should be done in new cases. Since multiple-treatment modalities may be brought to bear on acute HF episodes, the discussion is

TABLE 24–4 Pharmacological Therapy for Acute, Decompensated Heart Failure

Treatment Modality	Specific Examples
Intravenous diuretics	Furosemide, bumetatide, torsemide
Intravenous positive inotropic agents	Dobutamine, milrinone, enoximone
Intravenous vasodilators	Nitroprusside, nitroglycerine, nesiritide
Blood pressure, renal perfusion support	Intravenous dopamine, intravenous vasopressin

TABLE 24–5 Nonpharmacological Therapy for Acute, Decompensated Heart Failure

Treatment Modality	Specific Examples
Oxygenation	Supplemental oxygen, mechanical ventilation
Balloon counterpulsation	Intraaortic balloon pump
VAD	Pulsatile-flow LVAD
Pacing	AV sequential pacemaker; biventricular pacing
Urgent cardiac catheterization	PTCA, mitral valvuloplasty, pericardiocentesis
Urgent cardiac surgery	CABG, AVR, MV repair or replacement, transplantation

AV = atrioventricular; AVR = aortic valve replacement; CABG = coronary artery bypass grafting; LVAD = left ventricular assist device; MV = mitral valve; PTCA = percutaneous transluminal coronary angioplasty; VAD = ventricular assist device.

divided into pharmacological and nonpharmacological forms of therapy.

PHARMACOLOGICAL THERAPY (see Chap. 23). Table 24–4 gives the standard treatment modalities typically used to treat acute episodes of HF with advanced, Class IV symptoms. In general, treatment begins with intravenous diuretics, which in subjects with adequate organ perfusion often suffice to produce diuresis accompanied by a prompt drop in preload and relief of symptoms related to pulmonary edema. If peripheral perfusion is compromised or diuresis does not ensue, intravenous dobutamine, an inotropic beta/alpha-adrenergic agonist that produces an increase in cardiac output without substantially dropping preload or blood pressure,[129] or nesiritide (BNP)[130] (see Fig. 23–5), a vasodilator, can be added via a well-secured peripheral line. A PDEI such as milrinone[131,132] or enoximone[133,134] can also be used to treat decompensated HF but should not be administered without pulmonary artery pressure monitoring unless it is certain that left ventricular filling pressure is high (>15 mm Hg). The reason for this precaution is that PDEIs are such potent venodilators that in patients with normal or low filling pressure, they can drop preload to undesirably low levels. Finally, in decompensated subjects who are still receiving beta-blocking agents, a PDEI rather than a beta blocker is the treatment of choice because PDEIs retain full or even have enhanced activity in the presence of beta blockade.[135]

If the situation has not stabilized, additional inotropic support with or without supplemental afterload reduction is indicated and best delivered with the aid of pulmonary artery catheter monitoring. The combination of dobutamine and a PDEI is additive for effects on cardiac output and, via the PDEI, will produce a reduction in pulmonary artery and left ventricular filling pressure.[136,137] The latter may provide welcome unloading of the right ventricle inasmuch as high pulmonary artery pressure can produce limiting right ventricular dysfunction in some patients.

Once optimal inotropic therapy is being delivered, pure vasodilators can be additionally administered to subjects with persistently high systemic or pulmonary vascular resistance. Vasodilators such as nitroprusside or nitroglycerin can also be used in lieu of a positive inotropic agent, particularly in patients with higher systemic vascular resistance. As a vasodilator, nesiritide has the unique property of preferentially increasing renal blood flow[138,139] and theoretically may be of value in patients with compromised renal function; however, nesiritide may also precipitate renal failure and must be used cautiously in this setting.

Finally, in patients with blood pressure so low that renal perfusion is compromised, dopamine may be added to increase perfusion pressure and renal blood flow via this agent's alpha-adrenergic and dopaminergic properties. However, dopamine should not be considered an effective positive inotropic agent because the majority of its weak, partial beta-agonist effect is mediated by norepinephrine release,[140] which results in tachyphylaxis within 12 hours of administration.[135]

NONPHARMACOLOGICAL THERAPY. Table 24–5 lists some nonpharmacological therapies that can be used to treat acute episodes of HF. In general, nonpharmacological therapy is used only if drug therapy does not stabilize the patient. Although its effectiveness has never been demonstrated in a controlled clinical trial, use of an intraaortic balloon pump (IABP) can increase cardiac output modestly while increasing effective coronary perfusion pressure. This benefit and the ease of use of this device make it an attractive adjunct in myocardial failure occurring in the context of ischemia. The IABP is also helpful in nonischemic myocardial failure. However, contraindications to IABP use include significant aortic regurgitation and severe peripheral vascular disease. If pharmacological therapy plus IABP does not stabilize the patient, a ventricular assist device should be used in selected individuals, as discussed in Chapter 25.

Because of the success of treating acute myocardial infarction by primary angioplasty[141] with stenting,[142] percutaneous coronary intervention techniques (see Chap. 48) have assumed an important role in treating the most common cause of new-onset acute HF, that arising in the setting of myocardial infarction. In general, the primary goal of treating myocardial failure in the setting of infarction is to establish and maintain patency of the infarct artery in the most expeditious manner possible. The catheterization laboratory is also an ideal setting in which to initiate adjunctive treatment such as an IABP, mechanical ventilation, and optimal pharmacological support guided by hemodynamic monitoring. Other techniques that can be applied in the catheterization laboratory used to treat acute HF treatment include pericardiocentesis for tamponade (see Chap. 64) and relief of severe mitral stenosis by balloon valvuloplasty (see Chap. 57).

Occasionally, urgent cardiac surgery is required for the treatment of acute HF. These procedures include CABG in acute ischemic disorders involving disease of the left main coronary artery or in patients in whom percutaneous coronary intervention is not a technical option, acute aortic or mitral valve surgery, and on rare occasion, transplantation. In general, it is neither desirable nor feasible to perform cardiac transplantation on someone during the initial HF decompensation.

Health Care Delivery Strategies

HEART FAILURE CENTERS. The number of therapeutic options for the care of HF patients is extensive, and access to investigational agents or complex approaches limited to specialized centers, such as transplantation, is often required. Numerous outcomes studies[143-145] have documented the utility of such centers, and there is strong argument[146] for federal support of such a center analogous to what was done in the United States in the early 1970s for cancer. However, it must be appreciated that most patients are cared for by primary care physicians rather than HF specialists or general cardiologists.[147] The sheer number of HF patients dictates that primary care physicians will continue to care for these patients, but it is likely that specialized centers will have an increasing role as treatment becomes even more complex.

HEART FAILURE CLINICS FOR DISEASE MANAGEMENT. It has become evident that a substantial and perhaps a majority of HF patients are not being optimally treated with medications that are clearly indicated, much less given more aggressive treatment options such as some of the surgical and device approaches described earlier. For example, estimates of the percentage of HF patients in the United States being treated with ACE inhibitors are between 50 percent[148] and 71 percent,[149] whereas on the basis of what is achieved in controlled clinical trials, it should be higher than 90 percent.[6,9,10] For beta blockers, the results are even worse, with estimates of 25 percent of the HF population receiving therapy[144,146] as compared with the ideal figure of more than 60 percent.[103] Inadequate medical treatment of HF no doubt extends beyond the appropriate use of ACE inhibitors or beta blockers and probably includes failure to consistently adhere to a low-salt diet, suboptimal use of diuretics, failure to maintain digoxin levels lower than 1.0 ng/ml,[55] inadequate interval follow-up, and numerous other important factors.

The failure to deliver optimal medical care to HF patients is multifactorial. As for other medical conditions, optimal care includes a health care provider with knowledge and the ability to communicate that knowledge, a method of ensuring that the patient has received and understood the knowledge, a system of encouraging adherence to the recommended regimen, and patient compliance. The elderly nature of many HF patients and the incapacitating nature of the HF disease syndrome present special challenges to caregivers. However, many of the challenges to delivering optimal care to HF patients can be met through an integrated specialized clinic approach that uses nurse and physician extenders to deliver and ensure the implementation of care. This disease management approach has been shown to reduce hospitalizations and increase the percentage of patients receiving ideal, guideline-recommended therapy.[150] The end result is lowered cost of HF treatment and likely improved survival.[151]

The biggest challenge to this obvious solution to the delivery of HF care is how to support the additional personnel required in the disease management model. In specialized centers, the costs are usually supported by sponsored research, and in the community, some health care maintenance organizations or hospitals have seen the wisdom of this cost-reducing approach. This model will probably be adopted in direct relation to the availability of financial support for it, which in turn is dependent on the health care system.

Exercise

Until recently, HF patients were instructed to avoid exercise, and at one point, bed rest was offered as a treatment of HF.[152] Bed rest is no longer prescribed, and in fact, exercise now appears to be promising as a treatment of HF. It is not surprising that an exercise regimen can increase functional capacity in subjects with HF, as documented in numerous studies.[153-158] What is surprising is that in small controlled studies, various other aspects of HF thought to be important in prognosis, such as neurohormonal activation,[153-155] symptoms,[157] resting cardiac function,[158] and quality of life,[153] appear to be improved by exercise. What is lacking is a large, well-controlled clinical outcomes trial to test the hypothesis that moderate levels of exercise improve the natural history of HF. Such a trial is currently ongoing (the Anticoagulation Consortium to Improve Outcomes Nationally [ACTION] Trial). Until results are available, it appears prudent to suggest to patients that they maintain at least some level of conditioning with mild to moderate regimens of aerobic exercise in view of the lack of evidence that such exercise is harmful and the potential beneficial effect on symptoms and individual psychology.

Investigational Treatment and Future Directions

In the last 10 years, major progress has been made in the medical treatment of HF. In clinical trials conducted in mild to moderate stage 2 HF, the use of ACE inhibitors and beta-adrenergic blocking agents has reduced mortality by more than 40 percent,[45] and in patients with intraventricular conduction defects the addition of CRT-D to optimal background pharmacological therapy further reduces mortality by more than 60 percent.[103] This progress is beginning to be manifest in improved clinical outcomes in community-based studies.[159] The enormous magnitude of the challenge that remains and the growing number of patients with HF will ensure that efforts to improve pharmacological and device therapy will continue. However, to attain such progress, subjects with HF will need to continue to be enrolled in investigational protocols, typically available at larger, well-organized HF centers. More important, the advances in HF treatment need to be more rapidly translated into application in community practice. This requires a strong cooperative effort among the various components of the health care industry, including pharmaceutical and device companies, academic medical centers, health care delivery organizations, as well as individual physicians.

REFERENCES

1. New York Heart Association: Nomenclature and Criteria for Diagnosis of Diseases of the Heart and Blood Vessels. New York, New York Heart Association, 1963.
2. Schocken DD, Arrieta MI, Leaverton PE, Ross EA: Prevalence and mortality of congestive heart failure in the United States. J Am Coll Cardiol 20:301-306, 1992.
3. Redfield MM, Jacobsen SJ, Burnett JC Jr, et al: Burden of systolic and diastolic ventricular dysfunction in the community: Appreciating the scope of the heart failure epidemic. JAMA 289:194-202, 2003.
4. Lloyd-Jones DM, Larson MG, Leip EP, et al: Lifetime risk for developing congestive heart failure: The Framingham Heart Study. Circulation 106:3068-3072, 2002.
5. O'Connell JB: The economic burden of heart failure. Clin Cardiol 23:II-I6–II-20, 2000.
6. Packer M, Bristow MR, Cohn JN, et al: Effect of carvedilol on morbidity and mortality in patients with chronic heart failure. N Engl J Med 334:1349-1355, 1996.
7. CIBIS-II Investigators and Committees: The Cardiac Insufficiency Bisoprolol Study II (CIBIS-II): A randomised trial. Lancet 353:9-13, 1999.
8. MERIT-HF Study Group: Effect of metoprolol CR/XL in chronic heart failure: Metoprolol CR/XL Randomized Intervention Trial in Congestive Heart Failure (MERIT-HF). Lancet 353:2001-2006, 1999.
9. Pitt B, Zannad F, Remme WJ, et al: The effect of spironolactone on morbidity and mortality in patients with severe heart failure. N Engl J Med 341:709-717, 1999.
10. BEST Trial Investigators: Effect of β-adrenergic blockade on mortality in patients with advanced chronic heart failure: The β-blocker Evaluation of Survival Trial. New Engl J Med 344:1659-1667, 2001.
11. American Heart Association: 2004 Heart and Stroke Statistical Update. Dallas, American Heart Association, 2004.
12. Ho KKL, Anderson KM, Kannel WB, et al: Survival after the onset of congestive heart failure in Framingham Heart Study subjects. Circulation 88:107-115, 1993.
13 Wang TJ, Evans JC, Benjamin EJ, et al: Natural history of asymptomatic left ventricular systolic dysfunction in the community. Circulation 108:977-982, 2003.
14. Hayflick L: How and Why We Age. New York, Ballantine, 1994.

Pathophysiology of Heart Failure due to Primary or Secondary Dilated Cardiomyopathies

15. Bristow MR: Why does the myocardium fail? New insights from basic science. Lancet 352(Suppl 1):8-14, 1998.

16. Eichhorn EJ, Bristow MR: Medical therapy can improve the biologic properties of the chronically failing heart: A new era in the treatment of heart failure. Circulation 94:2285-2296, 1996.
17. Weber KT: Extracellular matrix remodeling in heart failure: A role for de novo angiotensin II generation. Circulation 96:4065-4082, 1997.
18. Gerdes AM, Kellerman SE, Moore JA, et al: Structural remodeling of cardiac myocytes from patients with chronic ischemic heart disease. Circulation 86:426-430, 1992.
19. Davies CH, Davia K, Bennett JG, et al: Reduced contraction and altered frequency response of isolated ventricular myocytes from patients with heart failure. Circulation 92:2540-2549, 1995.
20. Lowes BD, Gilbert EM, Abraham WT, et al: Myocardial gene expression in dilated cardiomyopathy treated with beta-blocking agents. New Engl J Med 346:1357-1365, 2002.
21. Cohn JN: Structural basis for heart failure: Ventricular remodeling and its pharmacological inhibition. Circulation 91:2504-2507, 1995.
22. Cintron C, Johnson G, Francis G, et al: Prognostic significance of serial changes in left ventricular ejection fraction in patients with congestive heart failure. Circulation 87(Suppl 6):17-23, 1993.
23. Cohn JN, Johnson GR, Shabetai R, et al: Ejection fraction, peak exercise oxygen consumption, cardiothoracic ratio, ventricular arrhythmias, and plasma norepinephrine as determinants of prognosis in heart failure. Circulation 87(Suppl 6):5-16, 1993.

Diagnosis of Heart Failure

24. Cleland JGF, Habib F: Assessment and diagnosis of heart failure. J Intern Med 239:317-325, 1996.
25. Maisel AS, Krishnaswamy P, Nowak RM, et al, for The Breathing Not Properly Multinational Study Investigators: Rapid measurement of B-type natriuretic peptide in the emergency diagnosis of heart failure. N Engl J Med. 347:161-167, 2002.
26. Groenning BA, Nilsson JC, Sondergaard L, et al: Detection of left ventricular enlargement and impaired systolic function with plasma *N*-terminal pro brain natriuretic peptide concentration. Am Heart J 143:923-929, 2002.
27. Sim V, Hampton D, Phillips C, et al: The use of brain natriuretic peptide as a screening test for left ventricular systolic dysfunction: Cost-effectiveness in relation to open access echocardiography. Fam Pract 20:570-574, 2003.
28. Lainchbury JG, Campbell E, Frampton CM, et al: Brain natriuretic peptide and *N*-terminal brain natriuretic peptide in the diagnosis of heart failure in patients with acute shortness of breath. J Am Coll Cardiol 42:728-735, 2003.
29. de Groote P, Millaire A, Foucher-Hossein C, et al: Right ventricular ejection fraction is an independent predictor of survival in patients with moderate heart failure. J Am Coll Cardiol 32:948-954, 1998.
30. Felker GM, Hu W, Hare LM, et al: The spectrum of dilated cardiomyopathy: The Johns Hopkins experience with 1278 patients. Medicine (Baltimore) 78:270-283, 1999.
31. Myers J, Gullestad L, Vagelos R, et al: Clinical, hemodynamic, and cardiopulmonary exercise test determinants of survival in patients referred for evaluation of heart failure. Ann Intern Med 129:286-293, 1998.

Management of Acute, New-Onset Heart Failure

32. Hannen EL, Kilburn H, O'Donnell JF, et al: Adult open heart surgery in New York State: An analysis of risk factors and hospital mortality rates. JAMA 264:2768-1774, 1990.
33. White M, Wiechmann RJ, Roden RL, et al: Cardiac β-adrenergic neuroeffector systems in acute myocardial dysfunction related to brain injury: Evidence for catecholamine-mediated myocardial damage. Circulation 92:2183-2189, 1995.
34. Pfeffer MA, Pfeffer JM, Fishbein MC, et al: Myocardial infarct size and ventricular function in rats. Circ Res 44:503-512, 1979.
35. Bristow MR, Mason JW, Billingham ME, Daniels JR: Dose-effect and structure function relationships in doxorubicin cardiomyopathy. Am Heart J 102:709-718, 1981.
36. Billingham ME, Mason JW, Bristow MR, Daniels JR: Anthracycline cardiomyopathy monitored by morphological changes. Cancer Treat Rep 62:865-872, 1978.
37. Bristow MR, Lopez MB, Mason JW, et al: Efficacy and cost of cardiac monitoring in patients receiving doxorubicin. Cancer 50:32-41, 1982.
38. Lewis W, Gonzalez B: Actin isoform synthesis by cultured cardiac myocytes: Effects of doxorubicin. Lab Invest 56:295-301, 1987.
39. Bristow MR: Is too much or too little hypertrophy of individual cardiac myocytes the problem in the failing heart? Heart Fail 10:162-165, 1994.

Management of Chronic Heart Failure

40. Hunt SA, Baker DW, Chin MH, et al: ACC/AHA guidelines for the evaluation and management of chronic heart failure in the adult. Circulation 104:2996-3007, 2001.
41. The SOLVD Investigators: Effect of enalapril on mortality and the development of heart failure in asymptomatic patients with reduced left ventricular ejection fractions. N Engl J Med 327:685-691, 1992.
42. The SOLVD Investigators: Effect of enalapril on survival in patients with reduced left ventricular ejection fractions and congestive heart failure. N Engl J Med 325:293-302, 1991.
43. Packer M, Poole-Wilson PA, Armstrong PW, et al: Comparative effects of low and high doses of the angiotensin-converting enzyme inhibitor, lisinopril, on morbidity and mortality in chronic heart failure. ATLAS Study Group. Circulation 100:2312-2318, 1999.
44. Pfeffer MA: Angiotensin-converting enzyme inhibition in congestive heart failure: Benefit and perspective. Am Heart J 126:789-793, 1993.
45. Bristow MR: β-Adrenergic receptor blockade in chronic heart failure. Circulation 101:558-569, 2000.
46. Cohn JN, Tognoni G, Valsartan Heart Failure Trial Investigators: A randomized trial of the angiotensin-receptor blocker valsartan in chronic heart failure. N Engl J Med 345:1667-1675, 2001.
47. McMurray JJV, Ostergren J, Swedberg K, et al, for The CHARM Investigators: Effects of candesartan in patients with chronic heart failure and reduced left ventricular systolic function taking angiotensin-converting-enzyme inhibitors: The CHARM-Alternative Trial. Lancet 362:772-776, 2003.
48. Granger CB, McMurray JJV, Yusuf S, et al, for The CHARM Investigators: Effects of candesartan in patients with chronic heart failure and reduced left ventricular systolic function taking angiotensin-converting-enzyme inhibitors: The CHARM-Added Trial. Lancet 362:767-761, 2003.
49. Hauptman PJ, Kelly RA: Digitalis. Circulation 99:1265-1270, 1999.
50. Digitalis Investigation Group: The effect of digoxin on mortality and morbidity in patients with heart failure. N Engl J Med 336:525-533, 1997.
51. DiBianco R, Shabetai R, Kostak W, et al: A comparison of oral milrinone, digoxin, and their combination in the treatment of patients with chronic heart failure. N Engl J Med 320:677-683, 1989.
52. Lowes BD, Higginbotham M, Petrovich L, et al: Low-dose enoximone improves exercise capacity in chronic heart failure. J Am Coll Cardiol 36:501-508, 2000.
53. Bristow MR, Lowes BD: Low-dose inotropic therapy of ambulatory heart failure. Coron Artery Dis 5:112-118, 1994.
54. Shakar SF, Abraham WT, Gilbert EM, et al: Combined oral positive inotropic and beta-blocker therapy for the treatment of refractory Class IV heart failure. J Am Coll Cardiol 31:1336-1340, 1998.
55. Rathore SS, Curtis JP, Wang Y, et al: Association of serum digoxin concentration and outcomes in patients with heart failure. JAMA 289:871-878, 2003.
56. Rathore SS, Wang Y, Krumholz HM: Sex-based differences in the effect of digoxin for the treatment of heart failure. N Engl J Med 347:1403-1411, 2002.
57. Taylor HS: Diuretic therapy in congestive heart failure. Cardiol Rev 8:104-114, 2000.
58. Pitt B, Remme W, Zannad F, et al, for The Eplerenone Post-Acute Myocardial Infarction Heart Failure Efficacy and Survival Study Investigators: Eplerenone, a selective aldosterone blocker, in patients with left ventricular dysfunction after myocardial infarction. N Engl J Med 348:1309-1321, 2003.
59. Packer M, Coats AJ, Fowler MB, et al, for The Carvedilol Prospective Randomized Cumulative Survival Study Group: Effect of carvedilol on survival in severe chronic heart failure. N Engl J Med. 344:1651-1658, 2001.
60. Goldstein S, Fagerberg B, Hjalmarson A, et al, for The MERIT-HF Study Group: Metoprolol controlled release/extended release in patients with severe heart failure: Analysis of the experience in the MERIT-HF study. J Am Coll Cardiol. 38:932-938, 2001.
61. Packer M, Carver JR, Chesebro JH, et al: Effect of milrinone on mortality in severe chronic heart failure: The prospective randomized milrinone survival evaluation (PROMISE). N Engl J Med 325:1468-1475, 1991.
62. Cohn JN, Goldstein SO, Greenberg BH, et al: A dose-dependent increase in mortality with vesnarinone among patients with severe heart failure. Vesnarinone Trial Investigators. N Engl J Med 339:1810-1816, 1998.
63. Uretsky BF, Jesup M, Konstam M, et al: Multicenter trial of oral enoximone in patients with moderate to moderately severe congestive heart failure: Lack of benefit compared to placebo. Circulation 82:774-780, 1990.
64. The CONSENSUS Trial Study Group: Effects of enalapril on mortality in severe congestive heart failure. N Engl J Med 316:1429-1435, 1987.
65. Lee HR, Hershberger RE, Port JD, et al: Low-dose enoximone in subjects awaiting cardiac transplantation: Clinical results and effects on beta-adrenergic receptors. J Thorac Cardiovasc Surg 102:246-258, 1991.
66. Sindone AP, Keogh AM, Macdonald PS, et al: Continuous home ambulatory intravenous inotropic therapy in severe heart failure: Safety and cost efficacy. Am Heart J 134:889-900, 1997.
67. Milfred-LaForest SK, Shubert J, Mendoza B, et al: Tolerability of extended-duration intravenous milrinone in patients hospitalized for advanced heart failure and the usefulness of uptitration of oral angiotensin-converting enzyme inhibitors. Am J Cardiol 84:894-899, 1999.
68. Gibelein P, Dadoun-Dybal M, Candito M, et al: Hemodynamic effects of prolonged enoximone infusion (7 days) in patients with severe chronic heart failure. Cardiovasc Drugs Ther 7:333-336, 1993.
69. Follath F, Cleland JG, Just H, et al, for The Steering Committee and Investigators of the Levosimendan Infusion versus Dobutamine (LIDO) Study: Efficacy and safety of intravenous levosimendan compared with dobutamine in severe low-output heart failure (the LIDO study): A randomised double-blind trial. Lancet 360:196-202, 2002.
70. Yancy C, Fowler MB, Colluci WS, et al: Response of black heart failure patients to carvedilol [abstract]. J Am Coll Cardiol 29:84, 1997.
71. Dries DL, Exner DV, Gersh BJ, et al: Racial differences in the outcome of left ventricular dysfunction. N Engl J Med 340:609-616, 1999.
72. Small KM, Forbes SL, Rahman FF, et al: A four-amino acid deletion polymorphism in the third intracellular loop of the human alpha$_{2C}$-adrenergic receptor confers impaired coupling to multiple effectors. J Biol Chem 275:23059-23064, 2000.
73. Small KM, Wagoner LE, Levin AM, et al: Synergistic polymorphisms of beta$_1$- and alpha$_{2C}$-adrenergic receptors and the risk of congestive heart failure. New Engl J Med 347:1135-1142, 2002.
74. Carson P, Ziesche S, Johnson G, Cohn J: Racial differences in response to therapy for heart failure: Analysis of the vasodilator-heart failure trials. Vasodilator-Heart Failure Trial Study Group. J Card Fail 5:178-187, 1999.
75. Daida H, Allison TJ, Johnson BD, et al: Comparison of peak exercise oxygen uptake in men versus women in chronic heart failure secondary to ischemic or idiopathic dilated cardiomyopathy. Am J Cardiol 80:85-88, 1997.
76. Vaccarino V, Chen YT, Wang Y, et al: Sex differences in the clinical care and outcomes of congestive heart failure. Am Heart J 138:835-842, 1999.
77. Bonow RO, Udelson JE: Left ventricular diastolic dysfunction as a cause of congestive heart failure: Mechanisms and management. Ann Intern Med 117:502-510, 1992.
78. Dries D, Sweitzer N, Drazner M, et al: Prognostic impact of diabetes mellitus in patients with heart failure according to the etiology of left ventricular dysfunction. J Am Coll Cardiol 38:421-428, 2001.

79. Domanski M, Krause-Steinrauf H, Deedwania P, et al: The effect of diabetes on outcome of advanced heart failure patients in the BEST Trial. J Am Coll Cardiol 42:914-922, 2003.
80. Bristow MR, Gilbert, EM, Abraham WT, et al: Effect of carvedilol on LV function and mortality in diabetic versus non-diabetic patients with ischemic or nonischemic dilated cardiomyopathy. Circulation 94(Suppl): I-664, 1996.
81. Diller PM, Smucker DR, David B, Graham RJ: Congestive heart failure due to diastolic dysfunction: Frequency and patient characteristics in an ambulatory setting. Arch Fam Med 8:414-420, 1999.
82. Rich MW: Epidemiology, pathophysiology, and etiology of congestive heart failure in older adults. J Am Geriatr Soc 45:968-974, 1997.
83. Iriarte M, Murga N, Sagastagoitia D, et al: Congestive heart failure from left ventricular diastolic dysfunction in systemic hypertension. Am J Cardiol 71:308-312, 1993.
84. Spector KS: Diabetic cardiomyopathy. Clin Cardiol 21:885-887, 1998.
85. Friedrich SP, Lorrell BH, Rousseau MF, et al: Intracardiac angiotensin-converting enzyme inhibition improves diastolic function in patients with left ventricular hypertrophy due to aortic stenosis. Circulation 90:2761-2771, 1994.
86. Yusuf S, Pfeffer MA, Swedberg K, et al, for The CHARM Investigators: Effects of candesartan in patients with chronic heart failure and preserved left-ventricular ejection fraction. The CHARM-Preserved Trial. Lancet 362:767-771, 2003.
87. Mitrovic V, Strasser R, Berwig K, et al: Acute effects of enoximone after intracoronary administration on hemodynamics, myocardial perfusion, and regional wall motion. Z Kardiol 85:856-867, 1996.
88. Echt DS, Liebson PR, Mitchell LB, et al: Mortality and morbidity in patients receiving encainide, flecainide, or placebo. The Cardiac Arrhythmia Suppression Trial. N Engl J Med 324:781-788, 1991.
89. The Cardiac Arrhythmia Suppression Trial Investigators: Effect of the antiarrhythmic agent moricizine on survival after myocardial infarction. N Engl J Med 327:227-233, 1992.
90. Mason JW: A comparison of seven antiarrhythmic drugs in patients with ventricular tachyarrhythmias. Electrophysiologic Study Versus Electrocardiographic Monitoring Investigators. N Engl J Med 329:452-458, 1993.
91. Doval HC, Nul DR, Grancelli HO, et al: Randomised trial of low-dose amiodarone in severe congestive heart failure. Grupo de Estudio de la Sobrevida en la Insufficiencia Cardiaca en Argentina. Lancet 344:493-498, 1994.
92. Singh SN, Fletcher RD, Fisher SG, et al: Amiodarone in patients with congestive heart failure and asymptomatic ventricular arrhythmia. Survival Trial of Antiarrhythmic Therapy in Congestive Heart Failure. N Engl J Med 333:77-82, 1995.
93. Dunkman WB, Johnson GR, Carson PE, et al: Incidence of thromboembolic events in congestive heart failure. The V-HeFT VA Cooperative Studies Group. Circulation 87(Suppl 6):94-101, 1993.
94. Baker DW, Wright RF: Management of heart failure: IV. Anticoagulation for patients with heart failure due to left ventricular dysfunction. JAMA 272:1614-1618, 1994.
95. Hart RG, Haperin JL: Atrial fibrillation and thromboembolism: A decade of progress in stroke prevention. Ann Intern Med 131:688-695, 1999.
96. Falk RH, Foster E, Coats MH: Ventricular thrombi and thromboembolism in dilated cardiomyopathy: A prospective follow-up. Am Heart J 123:136-142, 1992.
97. Garg RK, Gheorghiade M, Jafri SM: Antiplatelet and anticoagulant therapy in the prevention of thromboemboli in chronic heart failure. Prog Cardiovasc Dis 41:225-236, 1998.
98. AVID Investigators: A comparison of antiarrhythmic drug therapy with implantable defibrillators in patients resuscitated from near-fatal ventricular arrhythmias. N Engl J Med 337:1576-1583, 1997.
99. MADIT Investigators: Improved survival with an implanted defibrillator in patients with coronary disease at high risk for ventricular arrhythmia. N Engl J Med 335:1933-1940, 1996.
100. Buxton AE, Lee KL, Fisher JD, et al: A randomized study of the prevention of sudden death in patients with coronary artery disease. N Engl J Med 341:1882-1890, 1999.
101. Moss AJ, Zareba W, Hall WJ, et al, for The Multicenter Automatic Defibrillator Implantation Trial II Investigators: Prophylactic implantation of a defibrillator in patients with myocardial infarction and reduced ejection fraction. N Engl J Med 346:877-883, 2002.
102. Bristow MR, Feldman AM, Saxon L, for the COMPANION Steering Committee: Heart failure management with biventricular pacing: The Comparison of Medical Therapy, Pacing and Defibrillation in Chronic Heart Failure (COMPANION) Trial. J Card Fail 6:276-285, 2000.
103. Bristow MR, Saxon LA, Boehmer J, et al: Cardiac resynchronization therapy with or without an implantable defibrillator in advanced chronic heart failure: The COMPANION Trial. N Engl J Med 350:2140, 2004.
104. Shamim W, Francis DP, Yousufuddin M, et al: Intraventricular conduction delay: A prognostic marker in chronic heart failure. Int J Cardiol 70:171-178, 1999.
105. Baldasseroni S, Opasich C, Gorini M, et al: Left bundle branch block is associated with increased 1-year sudden and total mortality rate in 5517 outpatients with congestive heart failure: A report from the Italian Network on Congestive Heart Failure. Am Heart J 143:398-405, 2002.
106. Werling C, Weisse U, Siemon G, et al. Biventricular pacing in patients with ICD: How many patients are possible candidates? Thorac Cardiovasc Surg 50:67-70, 2002.
107. Kass DA, Chen CH, Curry C, et al: Improved left ventricular mechanics from acute VDD pacing in patients with dilated cardiomyopathy and ventricular conduction delay. Circulation 99:1567-1573, 1999.
108. Leclercq C, Cazeau S, LeBreton H, et al: Acute hemodynamic effects of biventricular DDD pacing in patients with end-stage heart failure. J Am Coll Cardiol 32:1825-1831, 1998.
109. Kerwin WF, Botvinick EH, O'Connell JW, et al: Ventricular contraction abnormalities in dilated cardiomyopathy: Effect of biventricular pacing to correct interventricular dyssynchrony. J Am Coll Cardiol 35:1221-1227, 2000.
110. Saxon L, DeMarco T, Chatterjee K, et al: Chronic biventricular pacing decreases serum norepinephrine in dilated heart failure patients with the greatest sympathetic activation at baseline. Pacing Clin Electrophysiol 22:830, 1999.
111. Cazeau S, Leclercq C, Lavergne T, et al, for The Multisite Stimulation in Cardiomyopathies (MUSTIC) Study Investigators: Effects of multisite biventricular pacing in patients with heart failure and intraventricular conduction delay. N Engl J Med 344:873-880, 2001.
112. Auricchio A, Stellbrink C, Sack S, et al, for The Pacing Therapies in Congestive Heart Failure (PATH-CHF) Study Group: Long-term clinical effect of hemodynamically optimized cardiac resynchronization therapy in patients with heart failure and ventricular conduction delay. J Am Coll Cardiol 39:2026-2033, 2002.
113. Abraham WT, Fisher WG, Smith AL, et al, for The MIRACLE Study Group: Multicenter InSync Randomized Clinical Evaluation: Cardiac resynchronization in chronic heart failure. N Engl J Med 346:1845-1853, 2002.
114. Lau CP, Yu CM, Chau E, et al: Reversal of left ventricular remodeling by synchronous biventricular pacing in heart failure. Pacing Clin Electrophysiol 231722-1725, 000.
115. Saxon LA, De Marco T, Schafer J, et al, for The VIGOR Congestive Heart Failure Investigators: Effects of long-term biventricular stimulation for resynchronization on echocardiographic measures of remodeling. Circulation 105:1304-1310, 2002.
116. St. John Sutton MG, Plappert T, Abraham WT, et al, for The Multicenter InSync Randomized Clinical Evaluation (MIRACLE) Study Group: Effect of cardiac resynchronization therapy on left ventricular size and function in chronic heart failure. Circulation 107:1985-1990, 2003.
117. Rose EA, Moskowitz AJ, Packer M, et al: The REMATCH trial: Rationale, design, and end points. Randomized Evaluation of Mechanical Assistance for the Treatment of Congestive Heart Failure. Ann Thorac Surg 67:723-730, 1999.
118. Rose EA. Gelijns AC. Moskowitz AJ, et al, for The Randomized Evaluation of Mechanical Assistance for the Treatment of Congestive Heart Failure (REMATCH) Study Group: Long-term mechanical left ventricular assistance for end-stage heart failure. N Engl J Med 345:1435-1443, 2001.
119. Arora RR, Chou TM, Jain D, et al: The Multicenter Study of Enhanced External Counterpulsation (MUST-EECP): Effect of EECP on exercise-induced myocardial ischemia and anginal episodes. J Am Coll Cardiol 33:1833-1840, 1999.
120. Soran O, Fleishman B, Demarco T, et al: Enhanced external counterpulsation in patients with heart failure: A multicenter feasibility study. Congest Heart Fail 8:204-208, 227, 2002.
121. Chaudhry PA, Anagnostopouls PV, Mishima T, et al: Acute ventricular reduction with the acorn cardiac support device: Effect on progressive left ventricular dysfunction and dilation in dogs with chronic heart failure. J Card Surg 16:118-126, 2001.
122. Miniati DN, Robbins RC: Heart transplantation: A thirty-year perspective. Annu Rev Med 53:189-205, 2002.
123. Zaroff JG, Rosengard BR, Armstrong WF, et al: Consensus conference report: Maximizing use of organs recovered from the cadaver donor—cardiac recommendations, March 28-29, 2001, Crystal City, Va. Circulation 106:836-841, 2002.
124. Passamani E, Davis KB, Gillespie MJ, Killip T: A randomized trial of coronary artery bypass surgery. Survival of patients with a low ejection fraction. N Engl J Med 312:1665-1671, 1985.
125. Elefteriades JA, Morales DL, Gradel C, et al: Results of coronary artery bypass grafting by a single surgeon in patients with left ventricular ejection fractions ≤ 30 percent. Am J Cardiol 79:1573-1578, 1997.
126. Bax JJ, Poldermans D, Elhendy A, et al: Improvement of left ventricular ejection fraction, heart failure symptoms, and prognosis after revascularization in patients with chronic coronary artery disease and viable myocardium detected by dobutamine stress echocardiography. J Am Coll Cardiol 34:163-169, 1999.
127. Athanasuleas CL, Buckberg GD, Menicanti L, Gharib M, for the RESTORE Group: Optimizing ventricular shape in anterior restoration. Semin Thorac Cardiovasc Surg 13:459-467, 2001.
128. Bolling SF, Pagani FD, Deeb GM, Bach DS: Intermediate-term outcome of mitral reconstruction in cardiomyopathy. J Thorac Cardiovasc Surg 115:381-386, 1998.

Management of Episodes of Acute Decompensation

129. Leier CV, Ebel J, Bush CA: The cardiovascular effects of the continuous infusion of dobutamine in patients with severe cardiac failure. Circulation 56:468-472, 1977.
130. Publication Committee for the VMAC Investigators (Vasodilatation in the Management of Acute CHF): Intravenous nesiritide versus nitroglycerin for treatment of decompensated congestive heart failure: A randomized controlled trial. JAMA 287:1531-1540, 2002.
131. Likoff MJ, Weber KT, Andrews V, et al: Milrinone in the treatment of chronic cardiac failure: A controlled trial. Am Heart J 110:1035-1042, 1985.
132. Biddle TL, Benotti JR, Creager MA, et al: Comparison of intravenous milrinone and dobutamine for congestive heart failure secondary to either ischemic or dilated cardiomyopathy. Am J Cardiol 59:1345-1350, 1987.
133. Gilbert E, for the Enoximone Working Group: Double-blind, placebo-controlled comparison of enoximone and dobutamine infusions in moderate to severe heart failure patients (NYHA III-IV) [abstract]. J Am Coll Cardiol 17:274, 1991.
134. Berti S, Palmieri C, Ravani M, et al: Acute enoximone effect on systemic and renal hemodynamics in patients with heart failure. Cardiovasc Drugs Ther 10:81-87, 1996.
135. Lowes BD, Simon MA, Tsvetkova TO, Bristow MR: Inotropes in the β-blocker era. Clin Cardiol 23(Suppl 3):11-16, 2000.
136. Gage J, Rutman H, Lucido D, LeJemtel TH: Additive effects of dobutamine and amrinone on myocardial contractility and ventricular performance in patients with severe heart failure. Circulation 74:367-373, 1986.
137. Gilbert EM, Hershberger RE, Wiechmann RJ, et al: Pharmacologic and hemodynamic effects of combined β-agonist stimulation and phosphodiesterase inhibition in the failing human heart. Chest 108:1524-1532, 1995.
138. Marcus LS, Hart D, Packer M, et al: Hemodynamic and renal excretory effects of human brain natriuretic peptide infusion in patients with congestive heart failure: A double-blind, placebo-controlled, cross-over trial. Circulation 94:3184-3189, 1996.
139. Abraham WT, Lowes BD, Ferguson DA, et al: Systemic hemodynamic, neurohormonal, and renal effects of a steady-state infusion of human brain natriuretic peptide in

patients with advanced hemodynamically decompensated heart failure. J Card Fail 4:37-44, 1998.
140. Port JD, Gilbert EM, Larrabee P, et al: Neurotransmitter depletion compromises the ability of indirect-acting amines to provide inotropic support in the failing human heart. Circulation 81:929-938, 1990.
141. Grines CI, Browne KF, Marco J, et al: A comparison of immediate angioplasty with thrombolytic therapy for acute myocardial infarction. The Primary Angioplasty in Myocardial Infarction Study Group. N Engl J Med 328:673-679, 1993.
142. Grines CI, Cox DA, Stone GW, et al: Coronary angioplasty with or without stent implantation for acute myocardial infarction. Stent Primary Angioplasty in Myocardial Infarction Study Group. N Engl J Med 341:1949-1956, 1999.

Health Care Delivery Strategies

143. Hanumanthu S, Butler J, Chomsky D, et al: Effect of a heart failure program on hospitalization frequency and exercise tolerance. Circulation 96:2842-2848, 1997.
144. Chapman DB, Torpy J: Development of a heart failure center: A medical center and cardiology practice join forces to improve care and reduce costs. Am J Managed Care 3:431-437, 1997.
145. Nohria A, Chen YT, Morton DJ, et al: Quality of care for patients hospitalized at academic medical centers. Am Heart J 137:1028-1034, 1999.
146. Bristow MR, Abraham WT: Specialized centers for heart failure management. Circulation 96:2755-2757, 1997.
147. Croft JB, Giles WH, Roegner RH, et al: Pharmacologic management of heart failure among older adults by office-based physicians in the United States. J Fam Pract 44:382-390, 1997.
148. Schmedtje JF Jr, Evans GW, Byerly W, et al: Treatment of chronic heart failure in a managed care setting: Baseline results from the Achieving Cardiac Excellence Project. N C Med J 64:4-10, 2003.
149. Roe CM, Motheral BR, Teitelbaum F, Rich MW: Angiotensin-converting enzyme inhibitor compliance and dosing among patients with heart failure. Am Heart J 138:818-825, 1999.
150. Balk AH: The "heart failure nurse" to help us close the gap between what we can and what we do achieve. Eur Heart J 20:632-633, 1999.
151. Stromberg A, Martensson J, Fridlund B, et al: Nurse-led heart failure clinics improve survival and self-care behaviour in patients with heart failure: Results from a prospective, randomised trial. Eur Heart J 24:1014-1023, 2003.

Exercise

152. Burch GE, Giles TD: Prolonged bed rest in the management of patients with cardiomyopathy. Cardiovasc Clin 4:375-387, 1972.
153. Coats AJ, Adamopoulos S, Radaelli A, et al: Controlled trial of physical training in chronic heart failure: Exercise performance, hemodynamics, ventilation, and autonomic function. Circulation 85:2119-2131, 1992.
154. Kiilavuaori K, Naveri H, Leinonen H, Harkonen M: The effect of physical training on hormonal status and exertional response in patients with congestive heart failure. Eur J Cardiol 20:456-464, 1999.
155. Keteyian SJ, Brawner CA, Schairer, et al: Effects of exercise training on chronotropic incompetence in patients with heart failure. Am Heart J 138:233-240, 1999.
156. Braith RW, Welsch MA, Feigenbaum MS, et al: Neuroendocrine activation in heart failure is modified by endurance exercise training. J Am Coll Cardiol 34:1170-1175, 1999.
157. Coats AJ, Adamopoulous S, Meyer TE, et al: Effects of physical training in chronic heart failure. Lancet 335:63-66, 1990.
158. Willenheimer R, Erhardt L, Cline C, et al: Exercise training in heart failure improves quality of life and exercise capacity. Eur Heart J 19:774-781, 1998.
159. Levy D, Kenchaiah S, Larson MG, et al: Long-term trends in the incidence of and survival with heart failure. N Engl J Med 347:1397-1402, 2002.

GUIDELINES *Thomas H. Lee*

Management of Heart Failure

Guidelines for the evaluation and management of heart failure (HF) were published by a joint task force of the American College of Cardiology and the American Heart Association (ACC/AHA) in 2001.[1] These guidelines updated previous sets of recommendations issued by the ACC/AHA in 1995,[2] as well as guidelines from the Agency for Health Care Policy and Research in 1994[3] and the Heart Failure Society of America in 1999.[4]

Reflecting growing appreciation for the importance of prevention of HF, the updated ACC/AHA guidelines classified patients according to four stages, as follows:

Stage A patients are at high risk for developing HF but have no structural disorder of the heart.

Stage B patients have a structural disorder of the heart but have never developed symptoms of HF.

Stage C patients are those with past or current symptoms of HF associated with underlying structural heart disease.

Stage D patients have end-stage disease and require specialized treatment strategies such as mechanical circulatory support, continuous inotropic infusions, cardiac transplantation, or hospice care.

The traditional New York Heart Association (NYHA) functional classification system primarily gauges the severity of symptoms in patients who are in stage C or D. The usefulness of the four-stage system is that it recommends interventions for asymptomatic patients with the goal of preventing signs or symptoms of HF. Figure 24G-1 summarizes the guideline recommendations for therapy by stage.

As with other ACC/AHA guidelines, these recommendations classify interventions into one of three classes as follows, including two levels of the intermediate group:

Class I: conditions for which there is evidence and/or general agreement that a given procedure/therapy is useful and effective

Class II: conditions for which there is conflicting evidence and/or a divergence of opinion about the usefulness/efficacy of performing the procedure/therapy

Class IIa: weight of evidence and opinion in favor of usefulness/efficacy

Class IIb: usefulness/efficacy is less well established by evidence and opinion

Class III: conditions for which there is evidence and/or general agreement that a procedure or therapy is not useful or effective and in some cases may be harmful

The ACC/AHA guidelines also adopted a convention for rating levels of evidence on which recommendations have been based. *Level A* recommendations were derived from data from multiple randomized clinical trials; *level B* recommendations were derived from a single randomized trial or nonrandomized studies; and *level C* recommendations were based on the consensus opinion of experts. The guidelines emphasize that the strength of evidence does not necessarily reflect the strength of a recommendation. A treatment may be controversial despite having been evaluated in controlled clinical trials; conversely, a strong recommendation may be supported only by historical data or by no data at all.

Initial Evaluation of Patient

The ACC/AHA guidelines state that a complete history and physical examination should be the first step in the evaluation of patients with HF (Table 24G-1). This evaluation may provide insight into the cause of the patient's HF and the presence or absence of structural cardiovascular abnormalities. Other issues to be addressed include presence or absence of history of diabetes, rheumatic fever, chest radiation, and exposure to cardiotoxic drugs. The patient's functional and hemodynamic status should also be evaluated to assess prognosis and guide management.

The guidelines recommend that the initial evaluation should include a complete blood count; urinalysis; serum electrolytes, renal and hepatic function, calcium, and magnesium; thyroid function tests; blood lipids; a chest radiograph; and a 12-lead electrocardiogram. Measurement of serum ferritin level and transferrin saturation was considered potentially useful for the detection of hemochromatosis, since this condition is a treatable cause of HF. Only weak support was found for routine screening for human immunodeficiency virus, connective tissue diseases, or pheochromocytoma unless other clinical data suggest that these diagnoses should be suspected.

Echocardiography to assess left ventricular function and detect underlying myocardial, valvular, or pericardial disease was considered

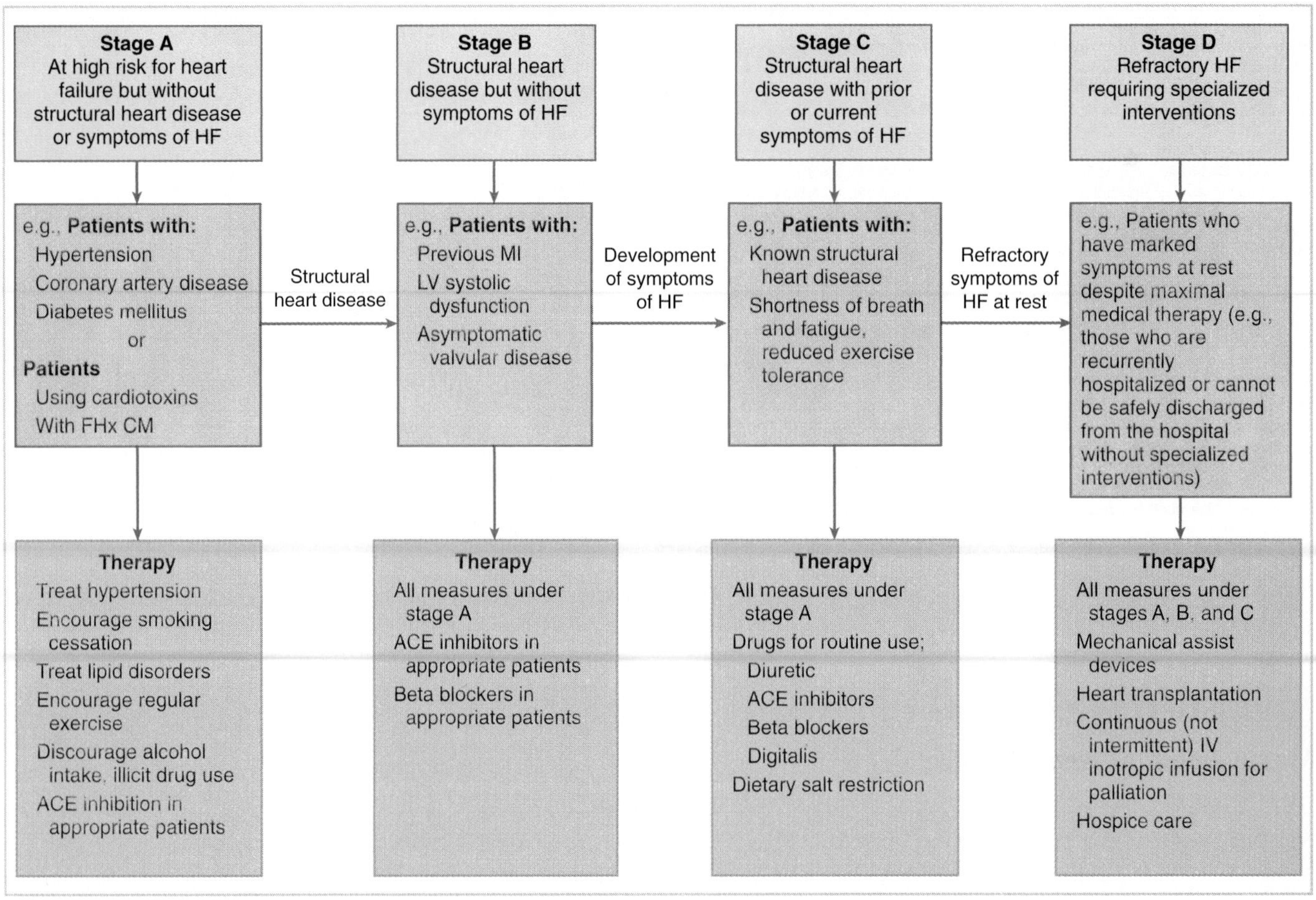

FIGURE 24G–1 Stages in the evolution of heart failure and recommended therapy by stage. FHx CM = family history of cardiomyopathy; HF = heart failure; ACE = angiotensin-converting enzyme; MI = myocardial infarction; LV = left ventricular; IV = intravenous. (From Hunt SA, Baker DW, Chin MH, et al: ACC/AHA guidelines for the evaluation and management of chronic heart failure in the adult: A report of the American College of Cardiology/American Heart Association Task Force on Practice Guidelines [Committee to Revise the 1995 Guidelines for the Evaluation and Management of Heart Failure]. American College of Cardiology, 2001. [http://www.acc.org/ clinical/guidelines/failure/hf_index.htm])

a more valuable initial test than radionuclide ventriculography or magnetic resonance imaging. The guidelines were noncommittal about routine measurement of brain natriuretic peptide; considerable data on this topic have been published since release of these guidelines, and future updates can be expected to offer recommendations on use of this test.

Screening for and assessment of coronary artery disease in patients with HF were given considerable attention in these guidelines, reflecting the frequent coexistence of these conditions and the survival benefit of revascularization of patients with severe coronary disease and left ventricular dysfunction. Coronary angiography was recommended (Class I indication) for patients with angina and HF who would be candidates for revascularization. For patients who have chest pain and HF, the guidelines provide support for bypassing the step of noninvasive testing and proceeding directly to coronary angiography (Class IIa indication). For patients without chest pain, the guidelines consider coronary angiography "reasonable" in younger patients with HF to exclude the diagnosis of coronary disease. However, the guidelines did not support routine coronary angiography in older HF patients without chest pain syndromes and found only weak support (Class IIb) for noninvasive testing for ischemia in such patients.

The guidelines did not recommend routine use of endomyocardial biopsy or ambulatory monitoring to detect arrhythmia.

Ongoing Assessment of Patients with Heart Failure

Although the guidelines support routine assessment of functional and volume status in patients with HF, they recommend restraint in the use of noninvasive testing with the exception of serum electrolytes and renal function. They specifically discourage routine serial measurement of ejection fraction at regular intervals. Instead, they recommend that ejection fraction be reassessed if patients have had a change in clinical status, recovered from a significant clinical event, or received treatment that might affect left ventricular function. Similarly, routine invasive or noninvasive assessment of hemodynamic function is discouraged.

Treatment of Patients at High Risk of Developing Heart Failure (Stage A)

The ACC/AHA guidelines provide strong recommendations (Class I) for control of risk factors for coronary disease and other causes of cardiomyopathy, including hypertension, hyperlipidemia, diabetes, alcohol abuse, cigarette smoking, and hyperthyroidism (Table 24G–2). Patients at risk for HF should also be assessed frequently for evidence that they are developing this condition, and a low threshold for use of angiotensin-converting enzyme (ACE) inhibitors is recommended. The ACC/AHA task force did not find evidence to support life-style interventions for prevention of HF in this population, including exercise, salt restriction, or routine use of nutritional supplements.

Restraint in the use of noninvasive testing was urged in patients without signs or symptoms of HF or structural heart disease. Noninvasive evaluation of left ventricular function was considered probably reasonable (Class IIa) in patients with a strong family history of cardiomyopathy or who were receiving cardiotoxic interventions.

TABLE 24G–1 ACC/AHA Guidelines for Evaluation of Heart Failure

Class	Indication	Level of Evidence*
I (indicated)	1. Thorough history and physical examination to identify cardiac and noncardiac disorders that might lead to the development of heart failure or accelerate the progression of heart failure	C
	2. Initial and ongoing assessment of a patient's ability to perform routine and desired activities of daily living	C
	3. Initial and ongoing assessment of volume status	C
	4. Initial measurement of complete blood count, urinalysis, serum electrolytes (including calcium and magnesium), blood urea nitrogen, serum creatinine, blood glucose, liver function tests, and thyroid-stimulating hormone	C
	5. Serial monitoring of serum electrolytes and renal function	
	6. Initial 12-lead electrocardiogram and chest radiograph	C
	7. Initial two-dimensional echocardiography with Doppler or radionuclide ventriculography to assess left ventricular systolic function	C
	8. Cardiac catheterization with coronary arteriography in patients with angina who are candidates for revascularization	B
IIa (good supportive evidence)	1. Cardiac catheterization with coronary arteriography in patients with chest pain who have not had evaluation of their coronary anatomy and who have no contraindications to coronary revascularization	C
	2. Cardiac catheterization with coronary arteriography in patients with known or suspected coronary artery disease but without angina who are candidates for revascularization	C
	3. Noninvasive imaging to detect ischemia and viability in patients with known coronary artery disease and no angina who are being considered for revascularization	C
	4. Maximal exercise testing with measurement of respiratory gas exchange and/or blood oxygen saturation to help determine whether heart failure is the cause of exercise limitation when the contribution of heart failure is uncertain	C
	5. Maximal exercise testing with measurement of respiratory gas exchange to identify high-risk patients who are candidates for cardiac transplantation or other advanced treatments	B
	6. Echocardiography in asymptomatic first-degree relatives of patients with idiopathic dilated cardiomyopathy	C
	7. Repeat measurement of ejection fraction in patients who have had a change in clinical status or who have experienced or recovered from a clinical event or received treatment that might have had a significant effect on cardiac function	C
	8. Screening for hemochromatosis	C
	9. Measurement of serum antinuclear antibody, rheumatoid factor, urinary vanillylmandelic acid, and metanephrines in selected patients	C
IIb (weak supportive evidence)	1. Noninvasive imaging to define the likelihood of coronary artery disease in patients with left ventricular dysfunction	C
	2. Maximal exercise testing with measurement of respiratory gas exchange to facilitate prescription of an appropriate exercise program	C
	3. Endomyocardial biopsy in patients in whom an inflammatory or infiltrative disorder of the heart is suspected	C
	4. Assessment of HIV status	C
III (not indicated)	1. Endomyocardial biopsy in the routine evaluation of patients with heart failure	C
	2. Routine Holter monitoring or signal-averaged electrocardiography	C
	3. Repeat coronary arteriography or noninvasive testing for ischemia in patients for whom coronary artery disease has previously been excluded as the cause of left ventricular dysfunction	C
	4. Routine measurement of circulating levels of norepinephrine or endothelin	C

ACC = American College of Cardiology; AHA = American Heart Association; HIV = human immunodeficiency virus.
*See guidelines text for definition of level of evidence categories.

Treatment of Patients with Left Ventricular Dysfunction Who Have Not Developed Symptoms (Stage B)

In this population, the goal of therapy is to reduce the risk of further damage to the left ventricle and to minimize the rate of progression of left ventricular dysfunction. The same risk factor modifications supported for stage A patients are also recommended for stage B patients (Table 24G-3). As was true with stage A patients, no evidence was found to support use of exercise and other life-style modifications for this population.

The two major pharmacological interventions that warrant consideration in all stage B patients are ACE inhibitors and beta blockers. In the absence of contraindications, medications in these two classes are recommended for all patients with histories of myocardial infarction, regardless of ejection fraction, and for all patients with diminished ejection fraction, regardless of history of myocardial infarction. In contrast, the guidelines discourage use of digoxin in this population.

Because tachyarrhythmias may hasten the progression of left ventricular dysfunction, the guidelines urge interventions to control ventricular response to supraventricular tachyarrhythmias. They also support surgery to correct valvular disease that causes HF, but note the absence of evidence providing support for the use of vasodilators in patients with aortic insufficiency.

TABLE 24G–2 ACC/AHA Guidelines for Treatment of Patients at High Risk of Developing Heart Failure (Stage A)

Class	Indication	Level of Evidence*
I (indicated)	1. Control of systolic and diastolic hypertension in accordance with recommended guidelines	A
	2. Treatment of lipid disorders, in accordance with recommended guidelines	B
	3. Avoidance of patient behaviors that may increase the risk of heart failure (e.g., smoking, alcohol consumption, and illicit drug use)	C
	4. ACE inhibition in patients with a history of atherosclerotic vascular disease, diabetes mellitus, or hypertension and associated cardiovascular risk factors	B
	5. Control of ventricular rate in patients with supraventricular tachyarrhythmias	B
	6. Treatment of thyroid disorders	C
	7. Periodic evaluation for signs and symptoms of heart failure	C
IIa (good supportive evidence)	Noninvasive evaluation of left ventricular function in patients with a strong family history of cardiomyopathy or in those receiving cardiotoxic interventions	C
IIb (weak supportive evidence)	None	
III (not indicated)	1. Exercise to prevent the development of heart failure	C
	2. Reduction of dietary salt beyond that which is prudent for healthy individuals in patients without hypertension or fluid retention	C
	3. Routine testing to detect left ventricular dysfunction in patients without signs or symptoms of heart failure or evidence of structural heart disease	C
	4. Routine use of nutritional supplements to prevent the development of structural heart disease	C

ACC = American College of Cardiology; AHA = American Heart Association; ACE = angiotensin-converting enzyme.
*See guidelines text for definition of level of evidence categories.

TABLE 24G–3 ACC/AHA Guidelines for Treatment of Asymptomatic Left Ventricular Systolic Dysfunction (Stage B)

Class	Indication	Level of Evidence*
I (indicated)	1. ACE inhibition in patients with a recent or remote history of myocardial infarction regardless of ejection fraction	A
	2. ACE inhibition in patients with a reduced ejection fraction, whether or not they have experienced a myocardial infarction	B
	3. Beta blockade in patients with a recent myocardial infarction regardless of ejection fraction	A
	4. Beta blockade in patients with a reduced ejection fraction, whether or not they have experienced a myocardial infarction	B
	5. Valve replacement or repair for patients with hemodynamically significant valvular stenosis or regurgitation	B
	6. Regular evaluation for signs and symptoms of heart failure	C
	7. Measures listed as Class I recommendations for patients in stage A (see Table 23G–2)	
IIa (good supportive evidence)	None	
IIb (weak supportive evidence)	1. Long-term treatment with systemic vasodilators in patients with severe aortic regurgitation	B
III (not indicated)	1. Treatment with digoxin in patients with left ventricular dysfunction who are in sinus rhythm	C
	2. Reduction of dietary salt beyond that which is prudent for healthy individuals in patients without hypertension or fluid retention	C
	3. Exercise to prevent the development of heart failure	C
	4. Routine use of nutritional supplements to treat structural heart disease or prevent the development of symptoms of heart failure	C

ACC = American College of Cardiology; AHA = American Heart Association; ACE = angiotensin-converting enzyme.
*See guidelines text for definition of level of evidence categories.

Treatment of Patients with Left Ventricular Dysfunction and Current or Prior Symptoms (Stage C)

The measures recommended to prevent or minimize progression of left ventricular dysfunction for stage A and B patients are also supported for stage C patients, who have current or prior symptoms attributable to left ventricular dysfunction (Table 24G-4). However, in contrast with the recommendations for stage B patients, the guidelines support use of moderate sodium restriction as well as daily measurement of weight. Immunization with influenza and pneumococcal vaccines is also encouraged.

Physical activity is also recommended for stage C patients in the 2001 ACC/AHA guidelines, although they also stipulate that most patients should not engage in heavy labor or exhaustive sports. More

TABLE 24G–4 ACC/AHA Guidelines for Treatment of Symptomatic Left Ventricular Systolic Dysfunction (Stage C)

Class	Indication	Level of Evidence*
I (indicated)	1. Diuretics in patients who have evidence of fluid retention	A
	2. ACE inhibition in all patients, unless contraindicated	A
	3. Beta-adrenergic blockade in all stable patients, unless contraindicated. Patients should have no or minimal evidence of fluid retention and should not have required treatment recently with an intravenous positive inotropic agent	A
	4. Digitalis for the treatment of symptoms of heart failure, unless contraindicated	A
	5. Withdrawal of drugs known to adversely affect the clinical status of patients (e.g., nonsteroidal antiinflammatory drugs, most antiarrhythmic drugs, and most calcium-channel blocking drugs)	B
	6. Measures listed as Class I recommendations for patients in stages A and B (see Tables 24G–2 and 24G–3)	
IIa (good supportive evidence)	1. Spironolactone in patients with recent or current Class IV symptoms, preserved renal function, and a normal potassium concentration	B
	2. Exercise training as an adjunctive approach to improve clinical status in ambulatory patients	A
	3. Angiotensin-receptor blockade in patients who are being treated with digitalis, diuretics, and a beta blocker and who cannot be given an ACE inhibitor because of cough or angioedema	A
	4. A combination of hydralazine and a nitrate in patients who are being treated with digitalis, diuretics, and a beta blocker and who cannot be given an ACE inhibitor because of hypotension or renal insufficiency	B
IIb (weak supportive evidence)	1. Addition of an angiotensin-receptor blocker to an ACE inhibitor	B
	2. Addition of a nitrate (alone or in combination with hydralazine) to an ACE inhibitor in patients who are also being given digitalis, diuretics, and a beta blocker	B
III (not indicated)	1. Long-term intermittent use of an infusion of a positive inotropic drug	C
	2. Use of an angiotensin-receptor blocker instead of an ACE inhibitor in patients with heart failure who have not been given or who can tolerate an ACE inhibitor	B
	3. Use of an angiotensin-receptor blocker before a beta blocker in patients with heart failure who are taking an ACE inhibitor	A
	4. Use of a calcium-channel blocking drug as a treatment for heart failure	B
	5. Routine use of nutritional supplements (coenzyme Q10, carnitine, taurine, and antioxidants) or hormonal therapies (growth hormone or thyroid hormone) for the treatment of heart failure	C

ACC = American College of Cardiology; AHA = American Heart Association; ACE = angiotensin-converting enzyme.
*See guidelines text for definition of level of evidence categorises.

detailed recommendations were subsequently provided in an AHA Scientific Statement on Exercise and Heart Failure published in 2003.[5] This Scientific Statement noted the absence of large randomized trials of the impact of exercise on outcome for patients with HF and observed that most available data on this topic preceded the era of treatment of HF with beta blockers. Nevertheless, the authors considered the likely benefit sufficient to support exercise training using an individualized approach. This statement supported use of technologies including gas exchange measurements to provide an objective assessment of functional capacity and direct monitoring (including telemetry monitoring), particularly for initial training sessions. Even fewer data are available on the risks of resistive training in this population, but the Scientific Statement observed that such training seems to offer some physiological benefits and supported the use of small free weights and exercises aimed at strengthening the upper body.

The 2001 ACC/AHA guidelines support use of ACE inhibitors and beta blockers for all stage C patients, in the absence of contraindications, and use of diuretics for patients with fluid overload and digitalis for symptomatic patients (see Table 24G-4). Of note is that these guidelines preceded data published in 2002 indicating worse prognosis for women treated with digoxin[6]; hence, it is possible that support for use of digoxin may be tempered in future revisions. The risks of initiation of beta blockers are considered in detail in these guidelines, but these agents are recommended for "all patients with stable [HF] due to left ventricular systolic dysfunction unless they have a contraindication to their use or have been shown to be unable to tolerate treatment with these drugs."

The guidelines offer qualified support (Class IIa) for use of spironolactone in patients with Class IV HF symptoms based on its effectiveness in one large-scale, long-term trial.[7] They also offer support for use of angiotensin-receptor blockade and hydralazine/nitrate combinations in patients who cannot tolerate an ACE inhibitor, although as a second choice after ACE inhibitors. The recommendations regarding use of angiotensin-receptor blockers will likely be revised to reflect findings from the Valsartan Heart Failure Trial (Val-HeFT).[8]

They recommend withdrawal of drugs from three classes that are known to exacerbate HF or worsen prognosis: nonsteroidal antiinflammatory agents, most antiarrhythmic drugs, and most calcium-channel blocking drugs. Of the latter two classes of drugs, the guidelines observed that only amiodarone and amlodipine had not been shown to adversely affect survival. The guidelines also explicitly discourage use of intermittent infusions of positive inotropic agents and of routine use of nutritional supplements or hormonal therapies.

Treatment of Patients With Refractory End-Stage Heart Failure (Stage D)

Stage D HF patients typically have symptoms at rest, have severely limited functional capacity, and often have frequent hospitalizations for management of symptoms. The ACC/AHA guidelines emphasize the importance of meticulous application of the measures listed as Class I recommendations for patients in stages A, B, and C (see Tables

TABLE 24G–5 ACC/AHA Guidelines for Treatment of Patients with Refractory End-Stage Heart Failure (Stage D)

Class	Indication	Level of Evidence*
I (indicated)	1. Meticulous identification and control of fluid retention	B
	2. Referral for cardiac transplantation in eligible patients	B
	3. Referral to a heart failure program with expertise in the management of refractory heart failure	A
	4. Measures listed as Class I recommendations for patients in stages A, B, and C (see Tables 24G–2 to 24G–4)	
IIa (good supportive evidence)	None	
IIb (weak supportive evidence)	1. Pulmonary artery catheter placement to guide therapy in patients with persistently severe symptoms	C
	2. Mitral valve repair or replacement for severe secondary mitral regurgitation	C
	3. Continuous intravenous infusion of a positive inotropic agent for palliation of symptoms	C
III (not indicated)	1. Partial left ventriculectomy	C
	2. Routine intermittent infusions of positive inotropic agents	B

ACC = American College of Cardiology; AHA = American Heart Association.
*See guidelines text for definition of level of evidence categories.

TABLE 24G–6 ACC/AHA Guidelines: Indications for Cardiac Transplantation

Absolute Indications

- For hemodynamic compromise due to heart failure
  - Refractory cardiogenic shock
  - Documented dependence on IV inotropic support to maintain adequate organ perfusion
  - Peak V_{O_2} < 10 ml/kg/min with achievement of anaerobic metabolism
- Severe symptoms of ischemia that consistently limit routine activity and are not amenable to coronary artery bypass surgery or percutaneous coronary intervention
- Recurrent symptomatic ventricular arrhythmias refractory to all therapeutic modalities

Relative Indications

- Peak V_{O_2} 11–14 ml/kg/min (or 55% predicted) and major limitation of the patient's daily activities
- Recurrent unstable ischemia not amenable to other intervention
- Recurrent instability of fluid balance/renal function not due to patient noncompliance with medical regimen

Insufficient Indications

- Low left ventricular ejection fraction
- History of functional Class III or IV symptoms of heart failure
- Peak V_{O_2} > 15 ml/kg/min (and >55% predicted) without other indications

ACC = American College of Cardiology; AHA = American Heart Association.
From Hunt SA, Baker DW, Chin MH, et al: ACC/AHA guidelines for the evaluation and management of chronic heart failure in the adult: A report of the American College of Cardiology/American Heart Association Task Force on Practice Guidelines (Committee to Revise the 1995 Guidelines for the Evaluation and Management of Heart Failure). American College of Cardiology, 2001. (http://www.acc.org/clinical/guidelines/failure/hf_index.htm)

24G–2 to 24G–4) and consider these patients candidates for specialized treatment strategies, such as mechanical circulatory support, continuous intravenous positive inotropic therapy, referral for cardiac transplantation, or hospice care (Table 24G–5). The guidelines also endorse the use of team management approaches such as HF programs. Detailed specifications of the components of such HF programs were provided in an AHA Scientific Statement published in 2000.[9]

The 2001 ACC/AHA guidelines include explicit cautionary notes about the use of ACE inhibitors and beta blockers for this population. Although consideration of these agents is supported, the guidelines state that "treatment with either agent should not be initiated in patients with systolic blood pressures less than 80 mm Hg or who have signs of peripheral hypoperfusion. In addition, patients should not be started on a beta-blocker if they have significant fluid retention or if they recently required treatment with an intravenous positive inotropic agent." When these medications are used, very low doses should be prescribed at initiation, and patients should be monitored closely for evidence of intolerance. The guidelines note that spironolactone has been shown to be beneficial in patients with advanced HF, but they emphasize that these data are derived from patients with preserved renal function[7] and that spironolactone may induce hyperkalemia in patient with impaired renal function.

The ACC/AHA guidelines recognized the value of continuous intravenous inotropic support for some patients who require a "bridge" strategy while awaiting cardiac transplantation or who cannot otherwise be discharged from hospital. However, the guidelines directly discouraged routine intermittent intravenous infusion of inotropic agents. Similarly, the guidelines did not encourage use of partial left ventriculectomy.

The guidelines also include a summary of indications for cardiac transplantation (Table 24G–6). These indications make explicit that low

TABLE 24G–7 ACC/AHA Guidelines for Management of Concomitant Diseases in Patients with Heart Failure

Class	Indication	Level of Evidence*
I (indicated)	1. Control of systolic and diastolic hypertension in patients with heart failure in accordance with recommended guidelines	A
	2. Nitrates and beta blockers (in conjunction with diuretics) for the treatment of angina in patients with heart failure	B
	3. Coronary revascularization in patients who have both heart failure and angina	A
	4. Anticoagulants in patients with heart failure who have paroxysmal or chronic atrial fibrillation or a previous thromboembolic event	A
	5. Control of the ventricular response in patients with heart failure and atrial fibrillation with a beta blocker (or amiodarone, if the beta blocker is contraindicated or not tolerated)	A
	6. Beta-adrenergic blockade (unless contraindicated) in patients with heart failure to reduce the risk of sudden death. Patients should have no or minimal fluid retention and should not have recently required treatment with an intravenous positive inotropic agent	A
	7. Implantable cardioverter-defibrillator (alone or in combination with amiodarone) in patients with heart failure who have a history of sudden death, ventricular fibrillation, or hemodynamically destabilizing ventricular tachycardia	A
IIa (good supportive evidence)	1. Antiplatelet agents for prevention of myocardial infarction and death in patients with heart failure who have underlying coronary artery disease	B
	2. Digitalis to control the ventricular response in patients with heart failure and atrial fibrillation	A
IIb (weak supportive evidence)	1. Coronary revascularization in patients who have heart failure and coronary artery disease but no angina	B
	2. Restoration of sinus rhythm by electrical cardioversion in patients with heart failure and atrial fibrillation	C
	3. Amiodarone to prevent sudden death in patients with heart failure and asymptomatic ventricular arrhythmias	B
	4. Anticoagulation in patients with heart failure who do not have atrial fibrillation or a previous thromboembolic event	B or C
III (not indicated)	1. Routine use of an implantable cardioverter-defibrillator in patients with heart failure	C
	2. Class I or III antiarrhythmic drugs (except amiodarone) in patients with heart failure for the prevention or treatment of asymptomatic ventricular arrhythmias	A
	3. Ambulatory electrocardiographic monitoring for the detection of asymptomatic ventricular arrhythmias	A

ACC = American College of Cardiology; AHA = American Heart Association.
*See guidelines text for definition of level of evidence categories.

left ventricular ejection fraction and poor functional status are insufficient indications in the absence of demonstrated peak oxygen consumption less than 15 ml/kg/min.

Special Populations and Concomitant Disorders

The ACC/AHA guidelines support consideration of patient-specific needs and coexisting medical conditions. Clinicians are reminded that women, minorities, and the elderly are less likely to receive interventions supported by clinical trials and that differences in the natural history of HF and response to treatment exist among various patient subsets. Specific clinical recommendations (Table 24G-7) emphasize the importance of meticulous management of hypertension, ischemic heart disease, anticoagulation, and supraventricular and ventricular arrhythmias.

The guidelines do not support routine use of implantable cardioverter-defibrillators or use of Class I or III antiarrhythmic drugs except amiodarone. Since these guidelines were issued, additional trials have been published providing insight into the potential beneficial impact of implantable cardioverter-defibrillators for primary prevention of sudden death in patients with dilated cardiomyopathy with or without acute myocardial infarction,[10,11] so future revisions of these guidelines may offer support for these devices in a wider population. Because of the absence of effective therapies other than implantable cardioverter-defibrillators, the guidelines do not support screening for asymptomatic ventricular arrhythmias with ambulatory electrocardiographic monitoring.

Diastolic Dysfunction

Recommendations for management of patients with HF in the absence of left ventricular systolic dysfunction reflect the lack of conclusive data on effective therapies. The major strategies are control of hypertension, control of ventricular rate in patients with atrial fibrillation, and use of diuretics to control pulmonary congestion (Table 24G-8). Because myocardial ischemia can cause diastolic dysfunction, the guidelines offer support for consideration of use of coronary revascularization in patients with coronary disease (Class IIa indication).

TABLE 24G–8 ACC/AHA Guidelines for Management of Heart Failure and Preserved Systolic Function

Class	Indication	Level of Evidence*
I (indicated)	1. Control of systolic and diastolic hypertension, in accordance with published guidelines	A
	2. Control of ventricular rate in patients with atrial fibrillation	C
	3. Diuretics to control pulmonary congestion and peripheral edema	C
IIa (good supportive evidence)	Coronary revascularization in patients with coronary artery disease in whom symptomatic or demonstrable myocardial ischemia is judged to be having an adverse effect on diastolic function	C
IIb (weak supportive evidence)	1. Restoration of sinus rhythm in patients with atrial fibrillation	C
	2. Use of beta-adrenergic blocking agents, ACE inhibitors, angiotensin-receptor blockers, or calcium antagonists in patients with controlled hypertension to minimize symptoms of heart failure	C
	3. Digitalis to minimize symptoms of heart failure	C
III (not indicated)	None	

ACC = American College of Cardiology; AHA = American Heart Association; ACE = angiotensin-converting enzyme.
*See guidelines text for definition of level of evidence categories.

References

1. Hunt SA, Baker DW, Chin MH, et al: ACC/AHA guidelines for the evaluation and management of chronic heart failure in the adult: A report of the American College of Cardiology/American Heart Association Task Force on Practice Guidelines (Committee to Revise the 1995 Guidelines for the Evaluation and Management of Heart Failure). American College of Cardiology, 2001. (http://www.acc.org/clinical/guidelines/failure/ hf_index.htm)
2. Williams JF Jr, Hlatky MA, Bristow MR, et al: Guidelines for the Evaluation and Management of Heart Failure: Report of the American College of Cardiology/American Heart Association Task Force on Practice Guidelines (Committee on Evaluation and Management of Heart Failure). J Am Coll Cardiol 26:1376-1398, 1996.
3. Konstam M, Dracup K, Baker, D, et al: Heart Failure: Evaluation and Care of Patients with Left-Ventricular Systolic Dysfunction. Clinical Practice Guidelines No. 11. AHCPR Publication No. 94-0612. Rockville, MD, Agency for Health Care Policy and Research and the National Heart, Lung, and Blood Institute; Public Health Service, U.S. Department of Health and Human Services, June 1994.
4. Baughman KL, Dec WB, Uklayam U, et al: HFSA guidelines for management of patients with heart failure caused by left ventricular systolic dysfunction–pharmacological approaches. J Card Fail 5:357-382, 1999.
5. Pina IL, Apstein CS, Balady GJ, et al: Exercise and heart failure: A statement from the American Heart Association Committee on Exercise, Rehabilitation, and Prevention. Circulation 107:1210-1225, 2003.
6. Rathore SS, Wang Y, Krumholz HM: Sex-based differences in the effect of digoxin for the treatment of heart failure. N Engl J Med 347:1403-1411, 2002.
7. Pitt B, Zannad F, Remme WJ, et al: The effect of spironolactone on morbidity and mortality in patients with severe heart failure. Randomized Aldactone Evaluation Study Investigators. N Engl J Med 341:709-717, 1999.
8. Cohn JN, Tognoni G: A randomized trial of the angiotensin receptor blocker valsartan in chronic heart failure. N Engl J Med 345:1667-1675, 2001.
9. Grady KL, Dracup K, Kennedy G, et al: Team management of patients with heart failure: A statement for healthcare professionals from the Cardiovascular Nursing Council of the American Heart Association. Circulation 102:2443-2456, 2000.
10. Moss AJ, Zareba W, Hall WJ, et al: Prophylactic implantation of a defibrillator in patients with myocardial infarction and reduced ejection fraction. N Engl J Med 346:877-883, 2002.
11. Bansch D, Antz M, Boczor S, et al: Primary prevention of sudden death in idiopathic dilated cardiomyopathy: The Cardiomyopathy Trial (CAT). Circulation 105:1453-1458, 2002.

CHAPTER 25

Assisted Circulation in the Treatment of Heart Failure

Yoshifumi Naka • Jonathan M. Chen • Eric A. Rose

Although advanced medical therapy benefits increasing numbers of patients with progressive heart failure (see Chap. 24), the overall survival and quality of life for these patients remains limited. Cardiac transplantation has traditionally represented the only treatment to provide substantial individual benefit in this setting. However, with donor availability limited to only 3000 annually worldwide, the overall impact of transplantation on heart failure has been described as "epidemiologically trivial."[1] Improving the survival and quality of life of patients with end-stage heart disease remains the ultimate goal of mechanical circulatory assistance.

Since their inception in the late 1960s, mechanical circulatory assist devices have evolved substantially, with widespread availability today of intraaortic balloon pumps (IABPs) in even small hospitals, to a broad array of sophisticated univentricular, biventricular, short, long-term, and permanent assist devices accessible at designated specialized centers. With this evolution has developed a better understanding of the technological drawbacks limiting current device design as well as a growing comprehension of appropriate indications for insertion and management. The dream of a completely implantable device, a total artificial heart, or a device whose design specifications allow its use for neonates, infants, and children is not only likely to be attainable but also expected to reach clinical trial and application in the near future.

History

The year 2003 marked the 50th anniversary of the first clinical application of the heart-lung machine, introduced by John Gibbon to repair an atrial septal defect in a young woman.[2] Revolutionizing the field of cardiac surgery, the heart-lung machine quickly had broad application in the treatment of pulmonary embolus, cardiogenic shock, and intracardiac defects by Cooley, Stuckey, and DeBakey and their colleagues.[3-5] DeBakey later modified a concept first reported by Dennis in 1962, using left-heart bypass as a means of support for patients who could not be weaned intraoperatively.[6]

Development of the theory of counterpulsation as an adjunct allowing systolic unloading and diastolic augmentation ultimately resulted in the report by Kantrowitz and coworkers in 1968 of clinical application of IABP counterpulsation.[7] Initiatives from the National Heart, Lung, and Blood Institute (NHLBI) helped to develop a family of mechanical assist devices, later versions of which enjoyed refinement in design, materials, and indications through the 1970s and 1980s. Today, ventricular assist devices (VADs) exist for a wide variety of conditions, requiring the clinician to enunciate clearly the needs of the given patient—does the patient need right-sided support, left-sided support, or both? Is recovery of myocardial function anticipated? Can the patient be sent home safely? Is the patient a transplant candidate? As experience with mechanical assistance has grown, the indications for insertion of the devices have become more specific. Only with continued collaboration between industry and clinical investigators, with preliminary application in patients, will incremental progress in this field be made.

Intraaortic Balloon Counterpulsation

Intraaortic balloon counterpulsation (the IABP) represents one of the most commonly used and widely available methods of mechanical circulatory support, employing the concepts of systolic unloading and diastolic augmentation proposed initially by Moulopolous and associates in 1962.[8] Bregman and Casarella[9] modified these concepts for percutaneous use in 1980, and between 1996 and 2001 more than 22,000 IABPs were inserted worldwide.[10]

The IABP, which is an intravascular, catheter-based device with a balloon volume of 30 to 50 ml, is generally positioned within the thoracic aorta distal to the left subclavian artery and proximal to the renal arteries (Fig. 25–1). The balloon itself may be inserted percutaneously or through direct arterial cannulation from the femoral artery, the axillary artery, or, in cases of postcardiotomy shock, directly through a purse-string suture in the thoracic aorta. When used percutaneously, the balloon may be inserted either through the lumen of a larger sheath (between 8 and 9 French) or alone ("sheathless").

With appropriate synchronization, by arterial blood pressure tracing or electrocardiogram, a set volume of gas (usually helium) is injected into the balloon from a bedside console during cardiac diastole and withdrawn during systole. Balloon inflation thus increases diastolic pressure, thereby augmenting coronary blood flow and myocardial oxygen supply; deflation reduces the afterload component of cardiac work during ventricular contraction and thereby decreases myocardial oxygen consumption. The frequency with which the balloon inflates can be timed to each, every other, or every third cardiac cycle, and balloon support may be adjusted by this method.

Whereas IABP assistance affects the myocardial supply/demand ratio considerably, it has only modest effects on cardiac output, limited naturally to the overall contractility and reserve of the ventricular

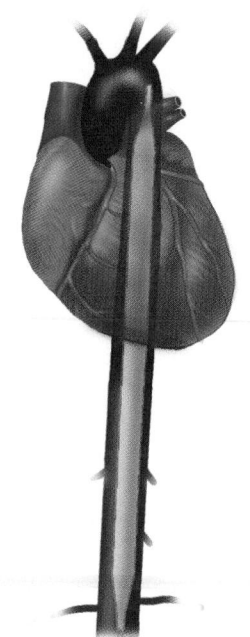

FIGURE 25–1 Schematic representing proper positioning of the intraaortic balloon. (Courtesy of Datascope, Inc.)

TABLE 25–1 Indications for Intraaortic Balloon Counterpulsation

Cardiogenic shock
Postcardiotomy
Associated with acute myocardial infarction
Mechanical complications of myocardial infarction
Mitral regurgitation
Ventricular septal defect
In association with coronary artery bypass surgery
Preoperative insertion
Patients with severe left ventricular dysfunction
Patients with intractable ischemic arrhythmias
Postoperative insertion
Postcardiotomy cardiogenic shock
In association with nonsurgical revascularization
Hemodynamically unstable infarct patients
High-risk coronary angioplasty
Patients with severe left ventricular dysfunction
Complex coronary artery disease
Stabilization of cardiac transplant recipient before insertion of ventricular assist device
Postinfarction angina
Ventricular arrhythmias related to ischemia

myocardium. A common misconception is that the institution of IABP counterpulsation should result in an immediate increase in systemic blood pressure; although this event may occur as a net result of the preceding effects, systemic blood pressure is not a parameter by which the efficacy of IABP assistance should be gauged.

Clinical Applications

IABP counterpulsation has traditionally been used in a variety of surgical and nonsurgical patients in the setting of cardiogenic shock and low-output state or unstable angina (Table 25–1). Some have even advocated its use as a bridge to cardiac transplantation, although this strategy has largely been discarded as the waiting time for transplantation has increased substantially. It has been estimated that of the patients who experience cardiogenic shock refractory to medical therapy in the setting of an acute myocardial infarction (AMI), as many as three-quarters may improve with IABP use (see Chap. 47).[11] The goal of IABP application in this setting is to stabilize the patient for either revascularization (catheter based or operative) or insertion of a more durable VAD. For those undergoing insertion intraoperatively as an adjunct to aid in weaning from cardiopulmonary bypass, IABP counterpulsation is used to offset temporary, reversible myocardial dysfunction.

In a cohort of patients undergoing IABP placement for AMI, in-hospital mortality rates varied significantly depending on the indication for insertion. Patients receiving IABP support for refractory angina had 6.4 percent mortality, those receiving IABP support intraoperatively had 7.7 percent mortality, those requiring IABP support to aid in weaning from cardiopulmonary bypass had 25.9 percent mortality, and those receiving IABP support for cardiogenic shock (without percutaneous or operative intervention) had 38.7 percent mortality.[10]

It is estimated that IABP is used in the setting of coronary artery bypass surgery in as many as 5 to 13 percent of cases nationwide, and of the IABP recipients listed in the international registry, 17 percent underwent pump insertion for perioperative indications.[12] Here, preoperative IABP insertion may be especially helpful for those with profound left ventricular dysfunction, and postoperative IABP use may counterbalance the effects of postcardiotomy cardiogenic shock from a variety of causes. Although the efficacy of IABP use in the setting of unstable or postinfarction angina is controversial, generally its use for those with ongoing ischemia, unstable angina, deteriorating hemodynamics, or ischemic ventricular tachyarrhythmias refractory to medical management is well supported.

The use of IABP is absolutely *contraindicated* in the setting of aortic insufficiency and aortic dissection. Relative contraindications for use through a femoral arterial approach are related to the vascular consequences of cannulation: significant aortoiliac or iliofemoral disease and abdominal or descending thoracic aortic aneurysms. In addition, some advocate avoiding the femoral approach in the setting of a recent groin incision at the insertion site or in the setting of morbid obesity, in which transperitoneal cannulation may occur because of anatomical distortion.[13]

INSERTION TECHNIQUE

Before device insertion, accurate examination and documentation of pedal pulses are essential. A balloon should be selected according to the height of the patient. The common femoral artery is then cannulated, a guidewire placed using the Seldinger technique, and a series of dilators placed and withdrawn until either the balloon itself (sheathless) or a larger introducer sheath is finally inserted. In some systems, prior to insertion, the balloon must be purged of any residual air; however, the balloon should not be tested (inflated) before insertion. We have found it easiest to "size" the balloon to the patient by aseptically holding the tip of the balloon above the suprasternal notch and noting the distance to the femoral cannulation site. The balloon is then inserted so that the tip may be seen just below the left subclavian artery (approximately the 2nd or 3rd intercostal space), a location that may be confirmed echocardiographically or on a routine chest radiograph, where the radiopaque tip of the IABP may be seen just at the level of the carina. Counterpulsation should *not* be employed before confirmation of accurate balloon placement.

Alternatively, the balloon may be inserted in the femoral artery or axillary artery using a side-arm graft of polyethylene terephthalate (Dacron) or polytetrafluoroethylene (Gore-Tex) sewn end to side to the artery through which the balloon is passed and secured. At the conclusion of IABP support, the balloon may be withdrawn and the graft closed with a vascular stapler (leaving the artery-graft anastomosis intact). Although more complicated in its approach, this technique maintains the advantage that it reduces impairment to antegrade flow through the artery during and after support and thus minimizes the risk of limb ischemia. The balloon may also be inserted directly through the femoral artery or antegrade through the thoracic aorta through concentric purse-string sutures.

When accurate location has been confirmed, the balloon is connected to the bedside console and synchronized to either the patient's arterial blood pressure tracing or electrocardiogram; in patients with frequent premature contractions, adjusting the timing to arterial blood pressure may be more efficacious. Inflation and deflation must be adjusted assiduously to effect the greatest augmentation. Absolute indications for immediate balloon removal include blood in the gas line leading to the balloon (indicating balloon rupture), inability to adjust the balloon, or ongoing limb ischemia and impending limb threat.

REMOVAL TECHNIQUE

The patient may be weaned slowly from balloon support by adjusting the frequency with which the balloon inflates (e.g., 1 : 1 to 1 : 3). The patient's coagulation profile and platelet count should be normalized with exogenous blood products, if necessary, prior to balloon removal. When hemodynamic stability with minimal support is confirmed, balloon inflation is discontinued and the balloon aspirated of any residual gas. Manual pressure is held on the distal femoral artery, and the balloon and sheath are removed. The proximal femoral artery is allowed to exsanguinate for 2 to 4 seconds to clear any debris, pressure is transferred to the proximal artery, and the distal artery is allowed to purge its debris. Pressure is then applied to the insertion site for at least 30 minutes. Removal under direct vision with potential patch angioplasty is recommended in cases of limb ischemia or in obese patients in whom manual compression may not be adequate.

COMPLICATIONS

The frequency of complications of IABP insertion ranges from 1 to 14 percent (Table 25-2).[10] Over the years, although the overall *rate* of complications has not decreased significantly, the *severity* of complications has diminished. Most of the major morbidities are related to the sequelae of vascular compromise or problems encountered with insertion. The incidence of ischemia has diminished slightly with the advent of smaller introducer sheaths and the development of a sheathless balloon technique. Unfortunately, irreversible limb ischemia resulting from IABP insertion renders most such affected patients poor candidates for later VAD insertion or transplantation and thus represents a condition for which ongoing vigilance in its earlier, potentially reversible, stages is mandatory.

Ventricular Assist Devices

The clinical application of VADs grew from experience with their application in the operating room. Unlike the IABP, VADs function to reduce myocardial work by completely unloading the ventricle while maintaining its output. They may be employed for right ventricular, left ventricular, or biventricular support for short-term (<1 week) or longer term support and for permanent ("destination therapy") use. The device may be completely extracorporeal, paracorporeal, implantable but with percutaneous power support, or totally implantable, and it may provide continuous or pulsatile flow.

TABLE 25–2 Complications of Intraaortic Balloon Counterpulsation

Minor	
	Bleeding at the insertion site
	Superficial wound infection
	Lymphocele
	Peritoneal perforation
Major	
	Limb ischemia requiring thrombectomy, revascularization, or amputation
	Aortic dissection
	Aortoiliac laceration
	Femoral artery pseudoaneurysm
	Retroperitoneal hemorrhage
	Renal ischemia from malposition
	Myocardial ischemia from poor timing of balloon augmentation
	Deep wound infection requiring operative débridement

BASIC RATIONALE AND TREATMENT GOALS. Hemodynamic eligibility criteria for mechanical cardiac assistance have traditionally been those representative of cardiogenic shock, namely a cardiac index less than 2.0 liter/min/m^2, a systolic blood pressure less than 90 mm Hg, left or right atrial pressures greater than 20 mm Hg, and a systemic vascular resistance greater than 2100 dyne-sec·cm^{-1}.[14] In addition, those with intractable cardiac arrhythmias are considered candidates. The population of patients has expanded from patients in decompensated chronic heart failure to include a large proportion of patients with acute heart failure in cardiogenic shock. Although some reports have demonstrated better outcomes in stable patients awaiting transplantation, favorable results have also been obtained in this emerging population of patients.[15-18]

There are essentially four groups of patients for whom support with different types of VADs is appropriate (Table 25–3). The first group consists of those in whom reversibility of ventricular insult is anticipated, the so-called *bridge-to-recovery* group. Here, patients who may be experiencing postcardiotomy shock despite reasonable preoperative myocardial reserve or who may suffer from a potentially reversible process (e.g., acute myocarditis) benefit from short- to medium-term device support. The management of these patients (even if implantation took place elsewhere) should be continued at a specialized center experienced in weaning. After a short period of myocardial rest with VAD support, the device is weaned at the bedside or in the operating room with guidance from transesophageal echocardiography. Resumption of native myocardial function in this setting may allow device removal (sometimes presaged by myocardial viability as evidenced by positron emission tomography [see Chap. 13]). If hemodynamic decompensation ensues after device removal, a more long-term device or permanent device should be considered.

The second, the *bridge-to-bridge* cohort, consists of patients who experience acute cardiogenic shock, after cardiotomy or without an operation, at a center that does not offer transplantation or long-term assist devices. For these patients, the efficacious institution of short-term assistance and rapid transfer to a center specialized in longer term ventricular assist support are warranted. We have described the success of this strategy, which we call the "hub and spoke" design.[16]

The third group is the traditional *bridge-to-transplantation* cohort, who meet criteria for transplantation and undergo VAD insertion to improve their overall candidacy for transplantation.[17] This decision by necessity limits the cohort to patients younger than 65 years and often involves delineation by blood group; a transplant candidate who is blood type O has a protracted waiting time and thus a lower threshold for device insertion while waiting. Because of concerns regarding infection and the potential need for long-term support, these patients require a more long-term device, preferably implantable, for bridging.

Finally, patients are selected who are *destination therapy* candidates. Several prospective randomized trials including the Randomized Evaluation of Mechanical Assistance for the Treatment of Congestive Heart Failure (REMATCH)[1] and currently the *non*randomized Investigation of Non-Transplant-Eligible Patients who are Inotrope Dependent (INTrEPID) have examined the efficacy of permanent implantable left ventricular assist device (LVAD) insertion for patients who are not transplant candidates (destination therapy).[1] REMATCH demonstrated clear advantages in overall survival and quality of life; INTrEPID is still ongoing. Such long-term expectations, however, challenge the extended durability of

TABLE 25–3 Indications for Ventricular Assist Device Implantation

			Outcomes		
Intended Use	**Therapeutic Goal**	**Devices**	***Quality of Life***	***Short-Term Survival*** **(days to weeks)**	***Long-Term Survival*** **(months)**
Bridge to recovery	Temporary support	IABP	+	++	0
		Centrifugal pump	+	+	0
		ECMO	+	+	0
		Abiomed	+	+	0
		HeartMate	+++	+++	+++
		Novacor	+++	+++	+++
Bridge to bridge	Stabilization to LVAD/BiVAD	Abiomed	+	++	0
		Centrifugal pump	+	+	0
		ECMO	+	+	0
Bridge to transplantation	Support to transplantation	HeartMate	+++	+++	+++
		Novacor	+++	+++	+++
		Thoratec BiVAD	++	++	++
		Abiocor/TAH	++	+	+
		Axial flow pump	+++	++	++
Destination	Permanent support	HeartMate	+++	+++	+++
		Novacor	+++	Undocumented →	
		Abiocor/TAH	+++	Undocumented →	
		LionHeart	+++	Undocumented →	

BiVAD = biventricular assist device; ECMO = extracorporeal membrane oxygenator; IABP = intraaortic balloon pump; LVAD = left ventricular assist device; TAH = total artificial heart.

device design, currently the limiting factor to extended use for this indication. At present, only those who are not transplant candidates are eligible for destination therapy.

Indications for Ventricular Assist Device Support

The indications for VAD insertion are in flux. With further experience, the spectrum of disease for which VADs are implanted continues to expand while our understanding of the timing of implementation and the specific cohorts for which it is appropriate becomes more refined. Broadly speaking, patients in profound shock with end-organ dysfunction and biventricular heart failure need early, efficacious support to avoid permanent end-organ damage and increase their chances of survival. The preferred devices in such a scenario are ones that may provide full ventricular support reestablishing nearly normal hemodynamics and potentially allowing myocardial recovery. If a prolonged support period is expected, a longer term biventricular device may be implanted or, if preferred, a longer term LVAD may be used with concomitant utilization of a short-term right ventricular assist device (RVAD).

POSTCARDIOTOMY SHOCK. Patients undergoing cardiac surgical procedures are at risk for myocardial injury owing to myocardial stunning and ischemia, insufficient myocardial protection, reperfusion injury, and cardiac arrhythmias. These patients may be categorized into two groups: (1) those who had persistent or significant dysfunction prior to surgery (and are unlikely to be weaned from device support) and (2) those who had adequate myocardial reserve prior to surgery (and who may require only a few days of temporary support). In general, for patients who cannot be weaned from cardiopulmonary bypass who maintain otherwise reasonable end-organ function, the best strategy is often the placement of a temporary VAD that may stabilize the patient long enough for transfer to a center with more experience and more choices of long-term devices should the patient be deemed unweanable (*bridge-to-bridge,* see earlier).

Patients undergoing high-risk cardiac surgery may need mechanical ventricular support if the surgical procedure is not successful. Ideally, such patients should be screened for transplant candidacy preoperatively and cardiac surgery scheduled with LVAD back-up in the event that LVAD support and subsequent heart transplantation are needed.

Although postcardiotomy shock represented the indication for which early clinical application of VADs was approved, increasing experience with device support in this population has been discouraging. Conservative estimates at our center support only a 25 percent hospital survival for these patients, refuting the concept of widespread use of VADs for this indication alone.

CARDIOGENIC SHOCK AFTER ACUTE MYOCARDIAL INFARCTION (see also Chap. 47)**.** The survival of patients in cardiogenic shock related to AMI often depends upon the timely institution of circulatory support.[19] Cardiogenic shock is thought to occur when more than 40 percent of ventricular mass is lost to infarction; without some form of cardiac assistance, this condition is associated with 80 percent mortality.[19,20] Even with early revascularization, 1-year survival of these patients remains less than 50 percent.[21] Although it is controversial, it has been our contention that coronary artery bypass grafting (CABG) may be detrimental to those who suffer AMI with cardiogenic shock. Although LVAD support allows myocardial rest, in this setting it is highly unlikely that myocardial recovery sufficient to allow LVAD weaning and explantation would develop. Thus, we advocate early institution of VAD support without CABG for this subset of patients for the reasons described as well as to avoid both another operation involving cardiopulmonary bypass (for the CABG) and additional technical problems of inserting an LVAD with CABG grafts already in place.

DECOMPENSATED CHRONIC HEART FAILURE—TRANSPLANT ELIGIBLE. Because of the increase in waiting times, some patients awaiting cardiac transplantation deteriorate hemodynamically and require increasing doses of intravenous inotropic support. These patients may not have been listed for transplantation at the time of failure, although often they are observed at transplantation centers. Acute decompensation can be triggered by several etiologies, including new ischemic injuries, arrhythmias, and infections. In the absence of an immediately available donor organ, VAD support for this indication allows establishment of hemodynamic stability, improvement in end-organ function, and the opportunity for nutritional support and rehabilitation before transplantation. For these patients, long-term support must be considered.

Some patients are not deemed candidates for transplantation at the time of LVAD implantation for reasons of marginal end-organ function, most commonly renal impairment. For these patients, LVAD support often reverses the injury and allows full recovery of end-organ function, rendering such patients good candidates for transplantation provided that other impaired end-organ function improves as well.

DECOMPENSATED CHRONIC HEART FAILURE—TRANSPLANT INELIGIBLE. Other patients are not candidates for transplantation at the time of LVAD implantation on the basis of age or other absolute criteria. When these patients decompensate, LVAD implantation is performed with the anticipation of permanent use for destination therapy. The precise indications and contraindications for LVAD insertion in this cohort require further study and refinement.

ACUTE MYOCARDITIS AND VENTRICULAR ARRHYTHMIAS. LVAD implantation for acute myocarditis, particularly in young patients, may sometimes be used as a bridge to recovery rather than to transplantation. Unfortunately, it is difficult to determine which patients will benefit from short-term support and which will require long-term devices with subsequent transplantation; thus, we feel that one should prepare for long-term support.[22] We advocate initial insertion of a long-term device to allow expeditious extubation and rehabilitation. After a sufficient degree of rehabilitation has taken place, cardiac function may be evaluated carefully and the device may be explanted if recovery sufficient to sustain reasonable hemodynamics is documented; if no appreciable recovery is demonstrated, the device may be a bridge to transplantation.

Patients with ventricular arrhythmias represent a unique population in that, aside from the arrhythmia, their native cardiac function may not be compromised significantly. If pharmacological therapy and defibrillators have failed, VAD support may be warranted, and it has been successfully implemented in these cases.[23,24] Further, although ventricular decompression often helps to diminish the arrhythmias, if they persist after LVAD insertion, ventricular arrhythmias are generally well tolerated.[25]

Preoperative Risk Assessment

The selection process for VAD implantation must reach a balance between too liberal listing of highest risk patients who have unacceptably high mortality rates and too conservative an approach that overlooks patients who would otherwise have benefited from VAD support. Indeed, judicious use of this resource is essential, as VAD implantation involves a significant social and financial investment.

In 1995 we, in conjunction with investigators from the Cleveland Clinic Foundation, devised a scoring system to predict which patients would have successful outcomes after LVAD implantation.[26,27] This scoring scheme relied upon five clinical factors weighted to determine post-LVAD outcome: urine output, central venous pressure, prothrombin time, the need for mechanical ventilation, and prior median sternotomy. However, as our perioperative management improved, our cohort of potential LVAD patients expanded, and the old score was revised in 2001 to better reflect the current LVAD-eligible population.[28]

The revised score was based on 130 patients receiving vented electric HeartMate devices from 1996 to 2001 (Table 25–4). Interestingly, with the new scoring scale, unlike the old system, preoperative renal insufficiency was not demonstrated to affect survival. After multivariable analysis, the five factors included in the new scoring system are ventilatory support, reoperative surgery, previous LVAD insertion, central venous pressure greater than 16 mm Hg, and prothrombin time greater than 16 seconds. After adding up the scores of these risk factors, a sum greater than five corresponds to 47 percent post-LVAD mortality as opposed to 9 percent mortality for a score less than five.[28]

Perhaps not surprisingly, the urgency of device placement has also been demonstrated to be a factor in survival. In a study by Schmid and colleagues,[15] patients receiving LVADs emergently because of acute heart failure such as AMI, acute myocarditis, and postcardiotomy low-output syndrome had a lower survival to transplantation than those receiving devices for chronic failure or those who did not need devices while awaiting transplantation.[15] In contrast, other data from our institution have suggested that those receiving an LVAD as a bridge to transplantation have a posttransplantation survival comparable to that of patients who did not have an LVAD as a bridge. Clearly, both groups (transplantation with or without prior LVAD) are heterogeneous, and posttransplantation outcome may be in fact best reflective of the relative pretransplantation acuity and comorbidity of the patient (regardless of whether an LVAD bridge was used). Certainly, more data are required to establish the full effect of pretransplantation LVAD support on posttransplantation survival.

CONTRAINDICATIONS. Although the list of contraindications to VAD insertion has diminished substantially in the past decade, several important factors still exist. First, patients with irreversible end-organ failure are poor device candidates. In particular, those with longstanding renal impairment (whose likelihood of improvement with VAD support is small) have prohibitively high morbidity and mortality after VAD insertion because of difficulties in fluid management and the infectious risks of long-term dialysis access. These patients are also unlikely to be candidates for transplantation.

Irreversible neurological injury represents an *absolute* contraindication to VAD insertion. Although this condition may be difficult to assess in the immediate postcardiotomy or acute cardiogenic shock setting, it is important to evaluate prior to VAD insertion (e.g., reduce sedation to help assess even gross neurological function). Because of the very poor outcomes after VAD insertion of patients who experience

TABLE 25–4 Revised Risk Factor Summation Score "LVAD Screening Score"[28]

Variable	Relative Risk	Weight
Mechanical ventilation	5.3	4
Postcardiotomy	3.3	2
Prior LVAD	3.3	2
Central venous pressure >16 mm Hg	2.1	1
Prothrombin time >16 sec	2.1	1
Excluded by multivariable analysis:		
Prior RVAD	3.2	
Coronary artery disease	2.0	
Acute myocardial infarction	1.7	
Urine output <30 ml/hr	1.2	
Reoperative surgery	1.2	

LVAD = left ventricular assist device; RVAD = right ventricular assist device.

severe neurological insults, we aggressively employ a strategy that involves preoperative family consent to discontinue support in the event of catastrophic neurological impairment.[29]

Overwhelming infection and sepsis are also *absolute* contraindications to insertion. Bacteremia may lead to device infection with the potential for device endocarditis, prolonged sepsis, and multiorgan failure and certainly should be treated before LVAD insertion. Once established, however, LVAD infections are often treatable. In a review of our experience with device infection (defined as the presence of a positive culture from the inflow, outflow, diaphragm, pocket, or driveline with leukocytosis or LVAD endocarditis), we demonstrated 15 to 20 percent of patients infected whose survival to transplantation and long-term survival after transplantation were identical to those of noninfected patients.[25,30]

Device Selection

Device selection is invariably influenced by both availability and physicians' experiences. Although much has been published on individual devices, few studies have compared assist devices at a single institution. The Food and Drug Administration (FDA) has approved several assist devices, in addition to the IABP, for these various indications. These devices include (1) the Abiomed biventricular system (BVS) 5000i for postcardiotomy and post-AMI cardiogenic shock; (2) the Thoratec paracorporeal device, the Novacor left ventricular assist system (LVAS), and both the implantable pneumatic (IP) and vented electric (VE) HeartMate LVADs for bridge to transplantation; (3) the HeartMate LVAD for destination therapy; and (4) a variety of investigational implantable devices, including the Arrow LionHeart, the Jarvik, HeartMate II, and MicroMed DeBakey axial flow pumps, and the Cor-Aide centrifugal device for acute cardiogenic shock. In addition to the FDA-approved devices, there are several other VADs in development and clinical use that are discussed later.

Important clinical issues to consider when choosing a device include the expected duration of support, the need for biventricular support, cost, device-related risks (such as the need for anticoagulation and device failure rates), patients' characteristics (especially the size and blood type of the patient), and United Network of Organ Sharing (UNOS) classification rules. Institutional standards of care, ranging from community practice to tertiary heart failure-transplant centers, also influence device selection. With regard to the size of the patient, the implantable HeartMate and Novacor LVADs require the patient's body surface area (BSA) to be greater than 1.5 m^2. Patients whose BSA is less than 1.5 m^2 require support with the Abiomed BVS, a centrifugal pump, the Thoratec paracorporeal device, or other devices in development (see later), depending upon the estimated period of support.

Short-Term Devices

EXTRACORPOREAL CENTRIFUGAL PUMPS. Centrifugal pumps were first introduced as alternatives to roller pumps for cardiopulmonary bypass and have been available since the late 1970s for use as short-term cardiac support. These pumps are widely available, relatively inexpensive, and simple. They may be used for right, left, or biventricular support and require systemic anticoagulation.

One of the most commonly used is the BioMedicus Biopump (Medtronic-BioMedicus, Eden Prairie, MN), which consists of an acrylic pump head with inlet and outlet ports oriented at right angles. An impeller composed of parallel cones is driven by an external motor and, with rotation, creates a vortex that drives blood in proportion to rotational speed. The pump is versatile and may be used as an RVAD (from right atrium or right ventricle to pulmonary artery), as an LVAD (from left atrium or left ventricular apex to aorta), or as part of an extracorporeal membrane oxygenation (ECMO) circuit.

This device has several disadvantages. First, the need for systemic anticoagulation to an activated clotting time of 200 seconds increases the possibility of bleeding complications. Second, there is an appreciable amount of interstitial edema potentially created by increased capillary permeability as part of a systemic inflammatory response. In this setting, fluid management can be extremely difficult, as this device is significantly preload dependent. Finally, the device requires continuous supervision by specially trained personnel, a constraint that can cost as much as $1000 per day.

SHORT-TERM SYSTEMS: EXTRACORPOREAL MEMBRANE OXYGENATION. ECMO provides mechanical cardiac support (univentricular or biventricular) as well as pulmonary support. Although its success has been extensively documented in the neonatal and infant population, the outcomes of its use for adults have been less promising.[31]

The main indications for ECMO are the need for mechanical assistance in the presence of combined pulmonary failure or pure respiratory failure. When it was initially used for postcardiotomy cardiogenic shock, survival was low (25 percent). With experience and improved circuits, survival increased to 40 percent. ECMO's benefits include potential peripheral cannulation and the versatility of small consoles, which together allow potential implementation for both cardiac and pulmonary support in areas outside the operating room. Major limitations, however, include a requirement for sedation or paralysis to effect immobilization and full systemic heparinization. As with the centrifugal pumps (many of which are used in the ECMO circuit), full-time trained personnel are also necessary to manage the ECMO circuit continuously. Complications are common, including leg ischemia, renal failure, bleeding, and oxygenator failure. Overall, the successful use of ECMO in adults has been limited to selected centers.[31]

ABIOMED BVS 5000i. The Abiomed BVS 5000i (Abiomed Cardiovascular, Danvers, MA) is a short-term uni- or biventricular support system composed of external pumps driven by a computer-controlled drive console (Fig. 25–2). Since its initial FDA approval in the setting of postcardiotomy failure, the indications for its use have expanded to include AMI, myocarditis, right ventricular support in conjunction with a long-term left ventricular support device, bridge to recovery, and bridge to transplantation. As a result, the device has become one of the most commonly used means of short-term mechanical cardiac support.[19,32]

The device is an extracorporeal dual-chamber device composed of two 100-ml polyurethane blood sacs, the inlet and outlet portions of which are guarded by polyurethane valves. Although the device fills passively, it ejects blood from a pneumatic drive console that adjusts the duration of systole and diastole to maintain a stroke volume of approximately 80 ml. One advantage of the BVS 5000i system is its weanability; a hand dial on the console allows the device flow to be weaned manually to off. When used in conjunction with transesophageal echocardiography and measures of hemodynamics, this feature allows easy bedside assessment of return of myocardial function.

Other advantages that have made the BVS system popular are ease of insertion and simplicity in operation, obviating the need for a full-time perfusionist at the bedside. The system functions reliably for several days and has even been used as long as 90 days. However, such use commits a patient to systemic anticoagulation for the duration of support. We tend not to use the device for more than 5 to 7 days because if there is no evidence of recovery after this time, we feel its development is unlikely and a more long-term device should be inserted or the support withdrawn. Because of its ease in placement, the 5000i has been particularly helpful in hospitals where there may be a need to transfer the patient to a transplant center for further treatment.[16,32]

Disadvantages of this device include the requirement for continuous anticoagulation, limited mobility compared with implantable devices, and the requirement of intensive care unit (ICU) monitoring and management. Flow rates are also limited compared with those of other devices, with the BVS maximum flow rate of 6 liter/min at times being insufficient to support fully larger or septic patients.

MAJOR CONCERNS FOR LONG-TERM DEVICES. Several key characteristics govern the development of long-term device design and are helpful in considering the advantages and disadvantages of these devices. First, all pulsatile long-term devices require inflow and outflow valves. In some, these are tissue valves; in others, they are mechanical valves and require long-term anticoagulation. The blood contact surface of the device must also be addressed with regard to anticoagulation. To overcome the need for anticoagulation, the HeartMate device employs an innovative textured surface, which ultimately becomes lined with a pseudoneointima less likely to promote thrombus.[33] The disadvantage is that its neointima may also act as an immunologically active entity, which can itself promote a form of autoimmunity and immunological reactivity that limits the ultimate eligibility of its recipients for transplantation.[33-35] Finally, device durability remains a concern for devices expected to function beyond 1 year.[1] The only study to date comparing directly the Novacor and Thoratec HeartMate devices demonstrated these findings; the Novacor patients had a higher rate of neurological disorders despite anticoagulation, and the HeartMate patients demonstrated a higher rate of infectious complications and device malfunction.[36]

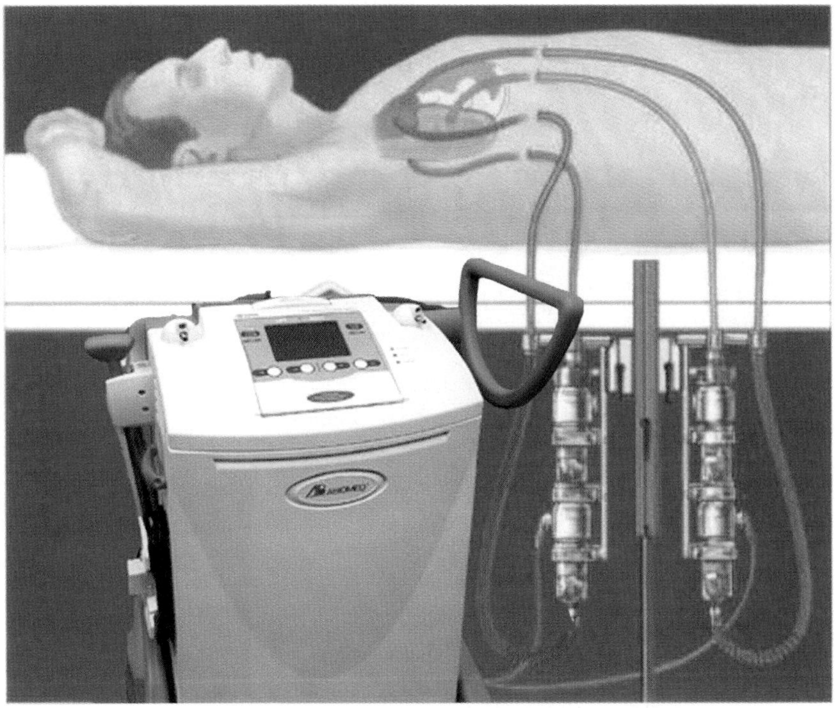

FIGURE 25–2 The Abiomed biventricular system (BVS) 5000i. (Courtesy of Abiomed, Inc.)

Pulsatile Devices

HEARTMATE LEFT VENTRICULAR ASSIST DEVICE (IMPLANTABLE). The HeartMate LVAD (Thoratec Corporation, Pleasanton, CA) was designed in 1975 (Fig. 25–3). The system was originally a pneumatic vented (IP) system requiring a large console that limited patients' mobility outside the hospital. In 1991, a clinical trial of the VE model was begun that allowed greater mobility, with portable battery units worn in a holster.[37] Since then, both models have been associated with a 60 to 70 percent rate of survival to transplantation.[38,39] The worldwide average implant duration is 80 to 100 days, and maximum duration of support has exceeded 2 years. However, of note, in the REMATCH trial, the probability of device failure was demonstrated to be 35 percent at 2 years.[1]

The HeartMate has a titanium alloy external housing, with inflow and outflow conduits that utilize porcine xenograft valves (25 mm). The unique characteristic of the device is its internal blood contact surface, which is made of textured titanium on one side and textured polyurethane on the other (Fig. 25–4). This textured surface results in the deposition of a fibrin-cellular matrix that forms a pseudoneointima. The formation of this surface decreases the need for anticoagulation, as thrombus formation is greatly reduced. Patients with these devices take aspirin (for antiinflammation but not primarily for anticoagulation) with a remarkably low rate of thromboembolic complications and without the need for warfarin (Coumadin).

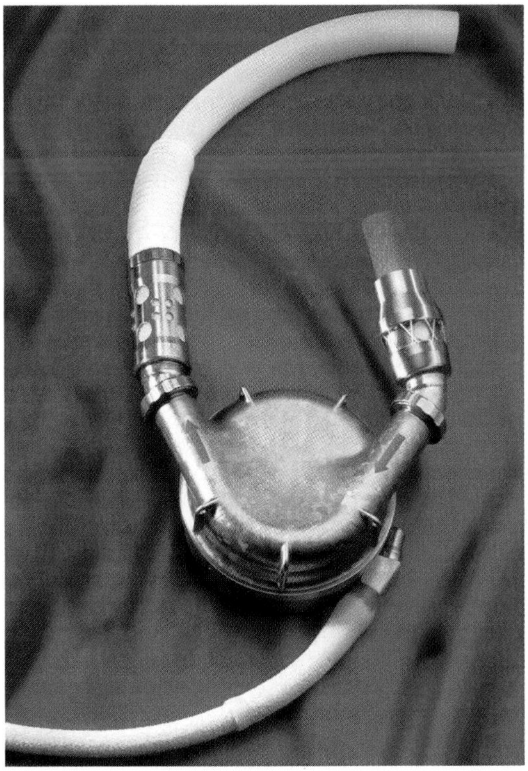

FIGURE 25–3 The HeartMate left ventricular assist device. (Courtesy of Thoratec, Inc.)

The device has a pumping capacity in excess of 9 liter/min, a maximal stroke volume of 83 ml, and pulsatile flow is created using a pusher-plate system. The device is operated in either a fixed-rate or automatic mode; in automatic mode, the pump senses when the chamber is full and activates the pusher plate. The pump is inserted into the left upper quadrant of the abdomen either pre- or intraperitoneally. The driveline, consisting of an air vent and power cables, is tunneled subcutaneously and brought out of the skin in the right upper quadrant. Small battery units, worn in a harness, are connected to the cables; battery life is between 4 and 6 hours, depending on the patient's activity level. In case of an

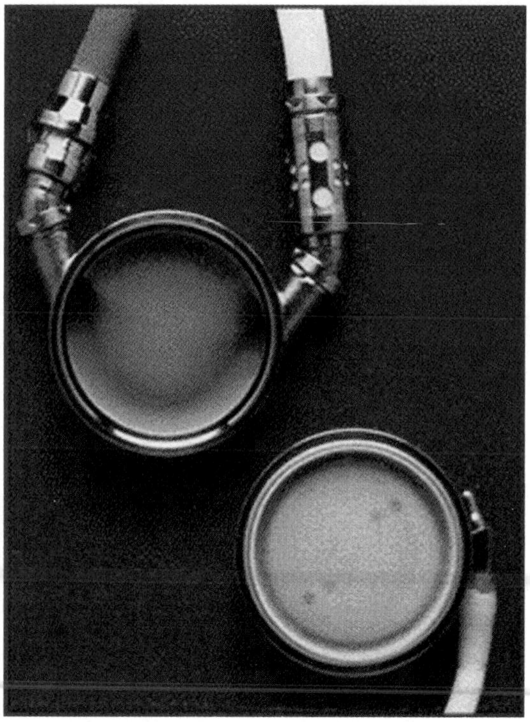

FIGURE 25–4 The inside surface of the HeartMate left ventricular assist device. (Courtesy of Thoratec, Inc.)

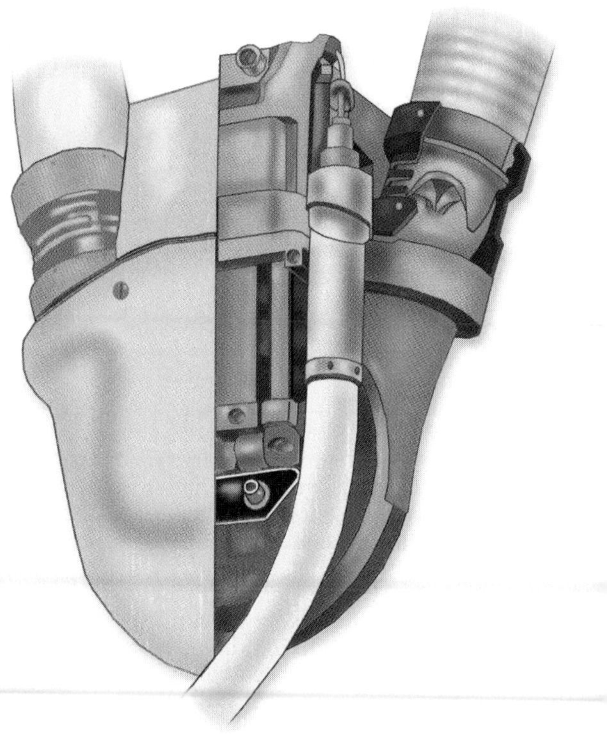

FIGURE 25–5 The Novacor left ventricular assist device. (Courtesy of World Heart Corporation.)

emergency, a portable hand pump can be used to activate the device.

The patient's body size is an important factor in allowing device placement. Because of the size of the device and flow limitations to avoid thromboembolic complications caused by blood stagnation, patients are required to have a BSA greater than 1.5 m^2 for successful implantation.

NOVACOR (IMPLANTABLE). The Novacor (World Heart Corporation, Ottawa, Ontario, Canada) LVAS was first successfully used in 1984 as a bridge to transplantation (Fig. 25–5). Initially, it was designed as a console-based controller system, but since 1993 it has been available with a wearable controller. This system has proved to be reliable, with about 55 to 65 percent of patients surviving to transplantation.[40] The worldwide mean time of LVAS support using this system is 85 days, with the device lasting as long as 962 days.[40]

The device is similar to the overall design of the HeartMate. The pump works using dual pusher plates that compress a polyurethane sac. Twenty-five millimeter bioprosthetic valves are used in both the inflow and outflow tracts. As with the HeartMate device, the pump is placed in the left upper abdominal quadrant, the inflow tract connected to the left ventricular apex and the outflow tract to the ascending aorta. The percutaneous driveline is brought out in the right upper quadrant of the abdomen and connected to a controller worn on a belt system.

However, unlike patients with the HeartMate system, those with the Novacor LVAS require anticoagulation with warfarin to avoid embolic events. The prevalence of embolic cerebrovascular events is estimated as between 27 and 41 percent.[40,41] However, comparison of the HeartMate and Novacor devices in this realm is particularly difficult owing to variation in the definition of "embolism" utilized in the literature.[41] A new inflow cannula made with Gore-Tex was introduced with the hope that it will reduce the rate of cerebrovascular events. Preliminary reports suggest that the Vascutek inflow conduit reduced embolic events to 12 percent.[42]

PARACORPOREAL PULSATILE DEVICES: THORATEC. The Thoratec paracorporeal VAD (Thoratec Corporation, Pleasanton, CA) is a commonly used system for biventricular support (Fig. 25–6). Unlike the Novacor and HeartMate, it is a paracorporeal system that can be applied for univentricular or biventricular support. Because the actual pump chamber is outside the body, this device can be used on patients with body sizes too small to house the HeartMate or Novacor devices (i.e., <1.5 m^2). However, a paracorporeal system also limits mobility and thus presents an obstacle for patients in a long-term setting.

The pump consists of a prosthetic ventricle with a maximum stroke volume of 65 ml and cannulas for ventricular or atrial inflow and arterial outflow. Currently, a large pneumatic drive console is available and a smaller briefcase-sized power driver unit is in trial.[43] Pneumatic drivers provide alternating air pressure to fill and empty the blood pump, and the pump flow rate ranges from 1.3 to 7.2 liter/min. Although inflow cannula placement can occur in either an atrial or ventricular position, ventricular cannula placement is preferred for left-sided support as it allows greater flow rates than does atrial cannulation. Anticoagulation with warfarin is necessary, as in patients with mechanical valves.[43]

This device has been used in more than 1000 patients for uni- and biventricular support for both bridge to transplantation and postcardiotomy recovery. Survival to transplantation has been between 60 and 80 percent, depending upon which ventricle was supported.[43] As with the BVS 5000i, the biggest advantage of this system is its versatility; it is easy to place with less surgical dissection, can be used for patients of various sizes, can be attached to either the atrium or ventricle, and can be used for right- and left-heart support. However, its paracorporeal location potentially limits the patient's activity and thus its use as a permanent device.

THORATEC INTRACORPOREAL VENTRICULAR ASSIST DEVICE. The Thoratec intracorporeal VAD (Thoratec Corporation, Pleasanton, CA) is being designed by the same firm that developed the paracorporeal device and clinical trials are currently anticipated. The intracorporeal

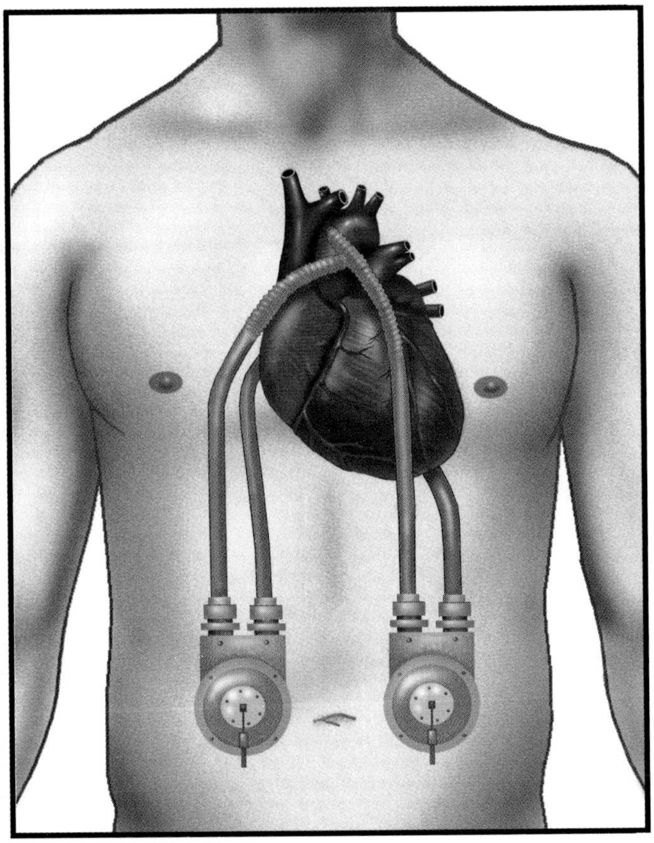

FIGURE 25–6 The Thoratec paracorporeal ventricular assist device. (Courtesy of Thoratec, Inc.)

system is the same size as the external system but is encased in a titanium alloy housing, and its pumps will be placed intracorporeally (not paracorporeally); two drivelines still exit the skin. The advantages of this system are its small size; reliability; implantable right, left, and biventricular support; and technology similar to that of the currently used Thoratec system. It is targeted toward patients who would benefit from long-term support and the benefits of an implanted device.

Total Artificial Heart

CARDIOWEST TOTAL ARTIFICIAL HEART. The CardioWest total artificial heart (TAH) (Syncardia, Tucson, AZ) began as the Jarvik-7 TAH used in the 1980s and is a pneumatic, biventricular, orthotopically implanted TAH with an externalized driveline to its console.[17,44,45] It consists of two spherical polyurethane chambers with polyurethane diaphragms. Inflow and outflow conduits are constructed of Dacron and contain Medtronic Hall (Medtronic, Minneapolis, MN) valves. Despite early obstacles, a new investigational device exemption study began in 1993 and demonstrated support durations of 12 to 186 days with a 93 percent survival to transplantation.[44]

The TAH benefits from the ability to provide complete support and, unlike the other devices, it obviates the presence of the native heart. This is particularly useful in situations in which leaving the native heart in place would be detrimental or impossible (e.g., cardiac tumors).

However, adequate intrathoracic space is required to accommodate the TAH. Fitting criteria include BSA greater than 1.7 m^2, cardiothoracic ratio greater than 0.5, LV diastolic dimension greater than 66 mm, anterior-posterior distance greater than 10 cm, and combined ventricular volume greater than 1500 ml. Careful intraoperative fitting is critical. In addition to size requirements, strict anticoagulation with warfarin, aspirin, and pentoxifylline is needed. As with the Thoratec paracorporeal system, rehabilitation and hospital discharge are unfortunately limited because of the current design of the large console.

ABIOCOR. The AbioCor TAH (Abiomed Cardiovascular, Danvers, MA) consists of an internal thoracic pump, an internal rechargeable battery, internal electronics, and an external battery pack (Fig. 25–7). External power is delivered through a transcutaneous energy transmission coil located under the skin of the chest wall. The AbioCor TAH is an electrohydraulically actuated device implanted in the pericardial space after excision of the native heart. The pump chambers are sutured to atrial tissue and the great vessels by textured Dacron (E.I. du Pont de Nemours, Wilmington, DE) atrial cuffs and grafts. Two polyurethane blood pump chambers with a 60-ml stroke volume produce flow at 8 liter/min. A centrifugal pump moves hydraulic fluid between the ventricles, providing alternate left and right ventricular pulsatile flow. In addition, there is an atrial "balance chamber" that adjusts for left and right atrial pressures. Anticoagulation is maintained with warfarin and clopidogrel.

After extensive animal testing starting in 1998 at the University of Louisville and the Texas Heart Institute, the device received FDA approval for a multicenter limited human testing trial involving patients requiring total heart support who did not qualify for heart transplantation. As of May 2003, 11 patients have been enrolled in the AbioCor clinical trial; 2 patients died in the immediate perioperative period, and 9 survived from 53 to 512 days, with an average support of 5 months. Four patients experienced neurological events significant enough to lead to withdrawal of support. Two patients are currently alive and remain hospitalized.

Axial Flow Pumps

Axial flow pumps represent one of the newest generations of assist devices. They can provide full cardiac support in a much smaller pump with fewer moving parts and a smaller blood contact surface than pusher-plate devices. Their small size allows implantation into smaller patients than most pulsatile pumps and also makes placement and explantation easier. With fewer moving parts, there are fewer points of

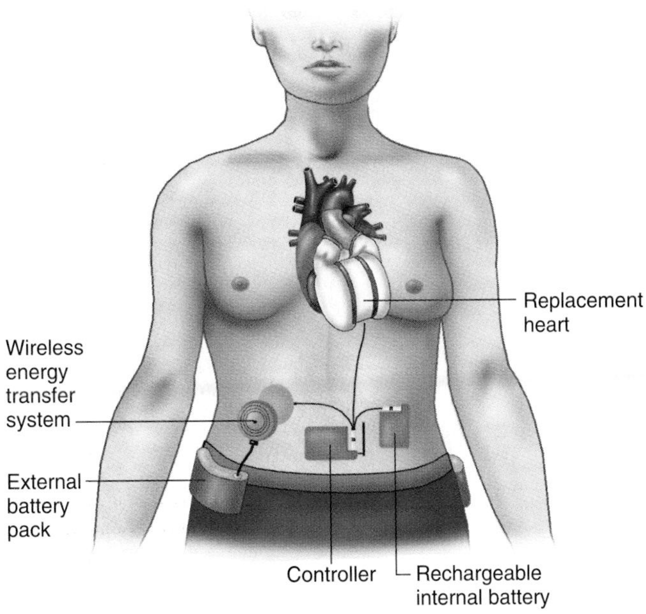

FIGURE 25–7 The AbioCor total artificial heart. (Courtesy of Abiomed, Inc.)

friction; therefore, expected durability is increased. In addition, because of their small size, these pumps represent the most likely candidates for development as pediatric assist devices in the near future. However, the bearings of these devices are lubricated with blood, a characteristic that may ultimately limit durability. In addition, shear rates with resultant hemolysis remain a concern.

In addition to their small size, axial flow pumps are notable for nonpulsatile flow. Metabolic and neurohumoral changes in organ perfusion with nonpulsatile flow have been demonstrated.[46-50] However, both clinical and long-term animal studies have failed to demonstrate significant differences in morbidity and mortality with axial flow pumps (Figs. 25–8 and 25–9).[51,52] Also, many patients maintain some native cardiac function during axial pump support and therefore continue to have pulsatile patterns of blood flow, unlike the situation with many of the pumps previously described (which completely unload the ventricle). Conversely, in the event of a device failure, few options or back-up mechanisms exist for axial flow pumps other than replacement, and because these pumps lack valves, if device malfunction does occur, the patient experiences hemodynamic perturbations equivalent to those seen with severe aortic insufficiency.

Finally, most axial flow pumps generate such negative pressure continuously that there is a potential risk of collapsing the ventricle and causing transient pump cessation (and therefore thrombus formation) and air entrainment (and therefore air emboli). To counteract this, many have device inflow cannulas that have a long tract to stent open the middle of the ventricle and allow more reliable continuous flow throughout the cardiac cycle.[53] Because of this phenomenon, both ventricular preload and cannula placement are of paramount importance with these pumps.

MICROMED DEBAKEY VENTRICULAR ASSIST DEVICE. This pump unit is 1.2 inches in diameter, 3 inches long, and weighs 95 gm (see Fig. 25-8). It is made of titanium casing with an impeller-inducer capable of pumping 10 liter/min. The rest of the pump consists of a titanium inflow cannula, a flowmeter, a Dacron outflow graft (Sulzer, Austin, TX), and a percutaneous cable connecting to a wearable battery-control console.[54] The inflow cannula is inserted into the left ventricular apex, the pump is placed into a small abdominal pocket, and the outflow graft is anastomosed to the ascending or descending aorta. Patients require chronic anticoagulation with warfarin and an antiplatelet agent.[54] A pump index greater than 2.0 to 2.5 liter/min/m^2 is recommended and the pump is started at 7500 rpm and adjusted for an average pump flow of 3.9 to 5.4 liter/min; flow is preload dependent. This pump also has a flow probe on its outflow graft that allows continuous flow monitoring, enabling pump speed adjustment as well as detection of extreme suction (and thus ventricular collapse). The major complication of this device in European clinical trials was late bleeding probably related to the level of anticoagulation (which has since been decreased to a target International Normalized Ratio [INR] of 2.0 to 2.5).[55] Follow-up of patients with the device has demonstrated improved exercise tolerance and the ability to be discharged home with the device while awaiting transplantation.[56]

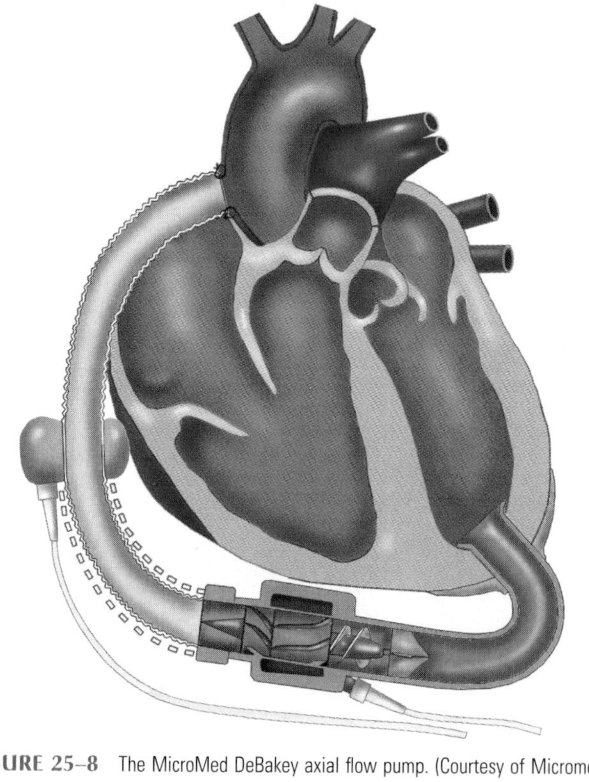

FIGURE 25–8 The MicroMed DeBakey axial flow pump. (Courtesy of Micromed, Inc.)

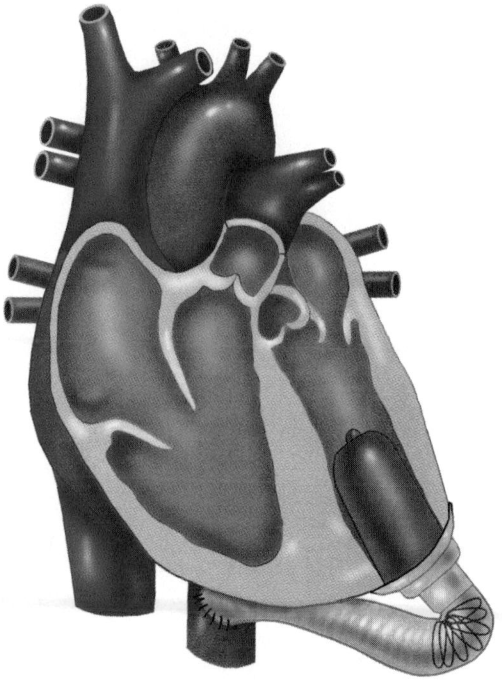

FIGURE 25–9 The Jarvik 2000 axial flow pump. (Courtesy of THI.)

HEARTMATE II. This is an axial flow rotary LVAD made of titanium with a rotor capable of producing flow rates greater than 10 liter/min at speeds greater than 10,000 rpm. As with the DeBakey VAD, the inflow cannula is joined to the apex of the left ventricle with the outflow graft connected to the ascending aorta.[53] Anticoagulation is at present required to keep the INR between 1.5 and 2.5. The pump has a volume of 124 ml and is inserted preperitoneally or within the abdominal musculature. Power and control are supplied by a percutaneous lead that attaches to either a power base unit or portable rechargeable batteries. This system similarly may be operated in either manual or automatic mode.

JARVIK 2000. The titanium Jarvik 2000 pump measures 2.5 cm in diameter, displaces 25 ml, and weighs 90 gm (see Fig. 25-9).[57] The rotor includes titanium impeller blades and is held in place by two ceramic bearings. The impeller rotates at 8000 to 12,000 rpm, producing a flow rate of 7 liter/min. Unlike the DeBakey VAD or the HeartMate II, this pump is positioned inside the ventricle with the outflow graft anastomosed to the descending aorta. The pump can operate in either a fixed-rate or variable mode and has manual rate adjustment capabilities. Two different control and energy systems are currently available: (1) a percutaneous model that, like most other LVAD systems, has a power lead that exits the patient's skin and (2) a modified percutaneous system that uses a titanium pedestal screwed into the skull with a transcutaneous connector that attaches to an external cable (for more permanent use). The fixed skull implantation is thought to provide a low level of repeated trauma and minimize the risk of infection owing to high vascularity of the scalp.

Unlike the other systems, which require a sternotomy, the Jarvik 2000 is implanted through a left thoracotomy incision. The pump is mainly used as a partial decompression device, allowing the aortic valve to open. However, if full decompression is achieved (and the aortic valve remains closed), because the outflow graft is anastomosed to the descending aorta, thrombus can form in areas of stagnation in the ascending aorta more proximally. Similarly to other systems, the pump provides a low pulsatile flow with a narrowing of pulse pressure at higher speeds.[57]

Totally Implantable Pulsatile Devices

ARROW LIONHEART LVD-2000. The Arrow LionHeart LVD-2000 is the first system designed specifically with destination support in mind.[58] It is a completely implantable system with a transcutaneous energy transmission system and a compliance chamber that allows complete implantation with no percutaneous lines or connections (Fig. 25–10). The pump is made of a titanium casing with pumping activated by a pusher plate. Unidirectional blood flow is maintained by two Derlin disc monostrut valves (27-mm inlet; 25-mm outlet). The inflow and outflow tracts are positioned in the ventricular apex and aorta, respectively. Maximum pump flow is 8 liter/min with a stroke volume of 64 ml. The controller is housed in a titanium casing, which also houses rechargeable batteries. The compliance chamber consists of a circular polymer sac (placed in the pleural space) and an attached subcutaneous port infusion system (this chamber loses gas through the polymer and requires replenishment once a month).[58] Recharging of the battery is accomplished through a transcutaneous system with a wand overlying the recharging coil. Patients may be completely disconnected from the external power supply for a short period of time and during that time rely on internal back-up batteries. The internal coil must be positioned under the skin so as to allow no more than 1 cm of tissue thickness between the coil and skin surface.[58]

NOVACOR II. Novacor II (World Heart Corporation, Ottawa, ON, Canada) is a totally implantable pump for the definitive treatment of heart failure. Its unique dual-chamber, four-valve pump requires no volume compensator. The pusher plate is suspended and magnetically driven, thus providing a system with few moving parts (the magnetic drive obviates the need for bearings, cams, or linkages).[59] The two chambers fill alternately, creating pulsatile flow. The system also uses transcutaneous energy transfer technology to supply power. It is currently in preclinical testing.[59]

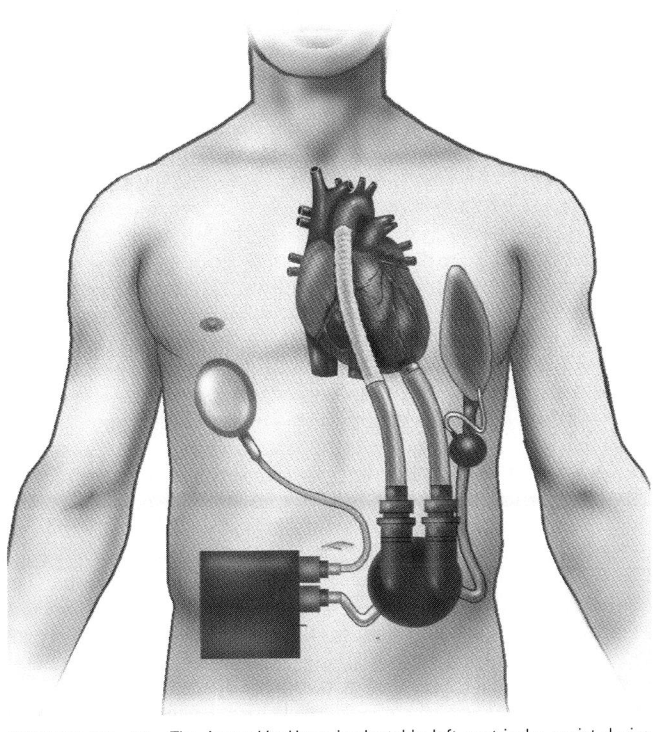

FIGURE 25–10 The Arrow LionHeart implantable left ventricular assist device. (Courtesy of Arrow, Inc.)

Postoperative Management

EARLY POSTOPERATIVE PERIOD. Several factors are important in the postoperative management of patients with mechanical support. Antibiotic prophylaxis is started preoperatively and continues for at least 3 days after implantation. Right-sided heart failure is immediately or prophylactically treated with milrinone and inhaled nitric oxide.[60] In addition, vasodilatory hypotension is treated with intravenous arginine vasopressin.[61] Aprotinin is continued in the postoperative period until bleeding has stopped.[62] Arrhythmias are managed with appropriate pharmacological agents and cardioversion if necessary. Aspirin is used for patients with all devices. Anticoagulation with heparin and, subsequently, warfarin is used in all patients except those receiving the HeartMate device. Physical therapy and nutrition are addressed early.

LATE POSTOPERATIVE PERIOD. Late postoperative care focuses on rehabilitation and monitoring of the immunological changes induced by the LVAD during the wait for heart transplantation.[63] Patients with the vented electric Thoratec LVAD and the Novacor LVAD are eligible for discharge home while awaiting transplantation. General criteria for discharge include physical rehabilitation, echocardiographic evidence of marginal heart function (to keep the patient alive in cases of device failure), and a training course in use and care of the device. Support from the family is very important. When these criteria are met, patients undergo a gradual program with longer trips outside the hospital and final discharge with weekly follow-up visits.[64] Panel-reactive antibody levels are measured in patients with LVADs biweekly to monitor immunological sensitization during device support.

LEFT VENTRICULAR ASSIST DEVICE EXPLANT VERSUS TRANSPLANT. The profound ventricular unloading provided by LVAD support can lead to reverse remodeling evident at genetic, biochemical, and histological levels.[65,66] Long-term LVAD explantation is considered at our institution only if there is significant myocardial recovery as evidenced by improvement of parameters on an exercise testing protocol. LVAD flow is reduced to 2 liter/min as the patient exercises on a treadmill, and right-heart catheterization and echocardiography are performed to determine the adequacy of ventricular function.[67] Although functional recovery allowing LVAD explantation has been reported, our experience has demonstrated that only a minority of patients can be successfully weaned from their devices.[48,68-70] The question of which patients are suitable for bridge to recovery and device explantation requires further clinical evaluation.

COMPLICATIONS AND ADVERSE EVENTS

BLEEDING. Bleeding is a major complication after implantation of LVADs and can occur both in the immediate perioperative period and later postoperatively. Immediate postoperative bleeding occurs in 20 to 40 percent of patients who receive assist devices. Preoperative heart failure leading to hepatic dysfunction, preoperative anticoagulation, coagulopathy caused by blood-device surface interaction, extensive surgical dissection, and prolonged cardiopulmonary bypass time all contribute to higher rates of bleeding after device implantation. In the immediate postoperative period, coagulation parameters as well as complete blood counts must be monitored closely, and deficiencies in platelet count and coagulation factors must be replaced as necessary. Because excessive transfusion of blood products can cause volume overload and subsequently exacerbate right-sided heart failure, care must be taken to avoid unnecessary transfusion. Although meticulous surgical technique is the mainstay of hemostasis, several medications can be used to prevent postoperative bleeding.

It is well established that aprotinin reduces blood loss and blood use in patients receiving assist devices.[62] Desmopressin (DDAVP) may also be used as an adjunct for uremic patients or those taking aspirin. Reexploration for bleeding should be performed in a timely fashion if needed. However, if excessive bleeding is noted at the time of chest closure, the chest may be left open and packed and the patient taken to the ICU, stabilized, and the chest closed when coagulation is normalized.

Bleeding can also occur late postoperatively. All devices except the HeartMate require heparin and subsequently warfarin to achieve an INR of 2.5 to 3.5 postoperatively. Aspirin is added to this regimen as an anti-inflammatory agent in all cases. Care must be taken to maintain adequate levels of anticoagulation. Because LVADs can activate both coagulation and fibrinolytic pathways, there is potential to exacerbate either bleeding or thrombotic complications even late postoperatively.[33] Therefore, clinical signs of late bleeding need to be carefully monitored in those patients.

INFECTION. Infection is one of the most serious complications common after LVAD implantation, affecting short- and long-term survival for patients receiving mechanical circulatory support. Although the definition of device-related infection varies among publications, LVAD infection, in general, can be manifest as driveline, pocket, or bloodstream infections or, ultimately, as device endocarditis.[30] In addition to device-related infections, these patients are susceptible to the common infections seen in critically ill patients such as pneumonia, line sepsis (with multiple catheters and intravenous lines), and urinary tract infections. For these reasons, it is sometimes difficult to identify the source of infection when a patient with LVAD support has positive blood cultures.

The reported infection rates in these patients are from 12 to 55 percent.[30,49] Pocket infection rates have been reported to be 11 to 24 percent for the HeartMate and Novacor systems; the driveline infection rate is even higher and in the range of 18 to 30 percent for the two devices.[30] Again, there is much variability in these data because definitions for these infections have not been standardized. Sepsis accounts for 21 to 25 percent of LVAD deaths and occurs at a rate of 11 to 26 percent.[30]

A variety of microorganisms are responsible for VAD infections. Gram-positive cocci are most commonly seen, but gram-negative bacilli and fungi can be identified. If organisms are identified, timely and appropriate systemic and topical management of infection is necessary. Infection itself is not a contraindication to transplantation in this population, and transplantations have been accomplished successfully in infected patients.[49,50] Topical treatments of driveline infections include immobilization of the exit site, local sterilization, drainage, and, if necessary, surgical débridement. Appropriate drainage of the cavity is needed for an LVAD pocket infection. Device endocarditis can be treated with systemic antibiotics as well as emergent heart transplantation, device explantation, or device replacement.[30]

The interaction between device and human that occurs after VAD implantation is a topic of much interest and is discussed later. LVAD implantation is accompanied by progressive defects in cellular immunity caused by an aberrant state of T-cell activation and apoptosis. These defects together predispose LVAD patients toward susceptibility to infections.[34,35]

THROMBOEMBOLIC EVENTS. Thromboembolism is a major concern in any patient with mechanical circulatory support because of the blood-device interface. The prevalence of embolism varies from 2 to 47 percent, with the majority of events occurring in cerebral distribution in 25 percent, although the definition of embolism varies among publications.[71,72] The HeartMate has the lowest thromboembolic rate of all the devices despite the fact that these patients do not receive warfarin (probably because of the device's promotion of formation of a neointimal surface that reduces thrombus formation).[73] All other devices require heparin in the immediate postoperative period and, subsequently, warfarin as well as antiplatelet agents such as aspirin or clopidogrel.

DEVICE FAILURE. Device failure is also a major concern because the number of heart transplantations is declining and, according to a new UNOS rule, the status of patients awaiting heart transplantation who receive mechanical assist devices changes from 1A to 1B after 30 days of implantation.

Device failure involves a variety of events, although the definition and therefore the reported event rate also vary among publications. Major failures, such as disconnection of the outflow assembly from the pump body or pump diaphragm rupture, require emergent device replacement.[55] Minor failures, such as controller or battery malfunction, usually do not require emergency surgery but do require appropriate treatment such as replacement of controllers.[74]

The HeartMate IP and VE devices are reported to have a failure rate of approximately 10 percent, including major and minor failures.[38,55] Of note, although no system failed within 12 months of implantation, the probability of device failure was 35 percent at 24 months in the REMATCH trial, in which the device was used as destination therapy. However, modifications of the system are aimed at reducing this incidence substantially.[55]

For example, repeated pulsatile flow, especially in the setting of significant afterload (hypertension), can lead to inflow valve damage and regurgitation. Modifications in valve mounting and flow algorithms to reduce intracavitary pressures have been adopted and, it is hoped, will have a significant impact on long-term device durability. In the event of electronic failure, the HeartMate device can be operated by a pneumatic console, and the overall reported survival rate to heart transplantation with the HeartMate is comparable (72 percent) to that of other devices even when back-up components are used.[55]

According to publications in 1999 and 2000, the Novacor LVAS has better durability than the HeartMate, with a failure rate between 0 and 2 percent and devices replaced after 3 to 4 years of support.[36,40] The main failure mode is bearing wear, which can be monitored periodically in vivo. If signs of wear are detected, the patient can be upgraded to UNOS status 1A or device replacement can be scheduled on a nonemergency basis. The Thoratec paracorporeal device is reported to have a lower incidence (3.5 percent) of major failures.[74]

RIGHT-SIDED HEART FAILURE. This complication is reported in 10 to 30 percent of patients who received either HeartMate or Novacor implantable LVADs, and an RVAD was used in 1 to 11 percent of all cases.[55,60,75] In patients with Thoratec paracorporeal devices, the incidence of RVAD use was as high as 38 to 42 percent.[71,74] However, this difference may be related to differences in device selection criteria and device availability among institutions. We reviewed our institutional experience in this area and demonstrated no difference in posttransplantation survival between those who received an RVAD as a bridge and those who did not. Of interest, however, was the fact that there was a significant survival advantage for those who received their RVAD within 24 hours after LVAD insertion compared with those who received it after 24 hours.

In patients with end-stage heart failure, pulmonary vascular resistance is usually elevated because of longstanding left-sided heart failure and is further increased in the early postoperative period by the effects of cardiopulmonary bypass and extensive blood product transfusion.[76] These factors, individually or in combination, can lead to impaired RV contractility, increased RV afterload, and subsequent RV dysfunction.[60] In most cases, unloading and supporting the LV help to reduce pulmonary vascular resistance and improve RV performance. However, it must be noted that complete LV decompression can also reduce the septal contribution to RV function by causing the interventricular septum to bulge toward the left.[77] In this setting, RV contractility may be impaired further by the enhanced preload to the RV from the superlative LVAD output. Interestingly, two independent analyses elucidated low preoperative RV stroke work index and low preoperative mean pulmonary artery pressure as risk factors for either postoperative development of right-sided heart failure or postoperative use of an RVAD, indicating that, in this setting, the failing RV may be unable to generate high pulmonary artery pressures (making the pulmonary artery pressures appear fictitiously low).[60,75]

Because the perioperative use of blood transfusions can contribute to right-sided heart failure, the intraoperative use of aprotinin is strongly recommended.[62] Perioperatively, if there is any indication of right-sided heart failure, such as increased central venous pressure or decreased LVAD flow with appropriate LV decompression and without tamponade, treatment of right-sided heart failure must be initiated immediately with pulmonary vasodilators (inhaled nitric oxide) and inotropic agents to enhance RV contractility.[60] If the RV function does not improve and the LVAD flow still remains suboptimal (<2.4 liter/min/m^2 with central venous pressure >16 mm Hg), RVAD insertion may be required.

MULTISYSTEM ORGAN FAILURE. Multisystem organ failure is another frequent complication in the LVAD population. Because of the significant amount of preoperative end-organ dysfunction and the number of comorbid conditions, some patients with LVADs do not recover fully after device implantation. In many situations, multiple organ failure is the end result of a long cascade of complications including sepsis, bleeding, and other events. At other times, multisystem organ failure may be the result of significant preoperative multiorgan dysfunction that deteriorates after the insult of surgery. In all of these scenarios, multisystem organ failure accounts for 11 to 29 percent of deaths with the device.

IMMUNOLOGICAL PERTURBATION. Itescu and colleagues at out institution have extensively analyzed the immunological interaction of patients with the HeartMate LVAD and demonstrated several important findings.[34,35] First significant T-cell activation was noted, both on the LVAD surface and in the circulation, albeit with defective proliferative responses to stimulation. Second, the circulating T cells demonstrated susceptibility to activation-induced cell death after T-cell receptor engagement. Third, the LVAD recipients demonstrated significant B-cell hyperreactivity. Together, it is thought that these phenomena are responsible for both (1) a progressive defect in cellular immunity (and thus produce an increased risk of infection) and (2) an increased rate of allosensitization.[34]

Few comparable studies have been performed with recipients of other types of devices. Immunological evaluation of the patient-device interaction with the DeBakey axial flow pump (which does not promote a neointimal layer) demonstrated an initial finding of increased markers of apoptosis. However, these markers declined to normal levels after 7 weeks and did not appear to confer an increased risk of infection in this cohort. Clearly, more data are necessary to evaluate these effects fully and to determine whether such findings may be attributable specifically to these devices.

SENSITIZATION. LVAD implantation is thus associated with an increased risk of developing circulating anti-human leukocyte antigen (HLA) class I and II antibodies (sensitization), causing as many as 66 percent of patients with an LVAD to be sensitized prior to transplantation.[34,35] This increased antibody level is associated with a significant risk for early graft failure and poorer survival of patients as a result of complement-mediated humoral rejection.[34] Thus, all efforts are made to reduce the number of necessary blood product (especially platelet) transfusions where possible.[34]

If the patient has become sensitized, donor-specific crossmatching is mandatory prior to transplantation, resulting in an increased waiting time for these patients.[34] Studies have demonstrated that pretransplantation immunomodulatory therapy with intravenously administered cyclophosphamide together with intravenous immunoglobulin successfully diminishes serum alloreactivity and reduces waiting list times and the risk of acute rejection in many LVAD recipients.[35]

Destination Therapy

Because of the constant shortage of available donor organs, the large group of patients who would benefit from circulatory assistance, and the encouraging results from the use of current LVADs as long-term support, a multicenter trial was conducted to evaluate the use of LVADs as permanent devices in the treatment of heart failure. REMATCH was undertaken in 1998 and included 129 patients in 20 centers using the HeartMate VE LVAD (see Figs. 25–3 and 25–4) as the study device. Eligible patients were adults with end-stage heart failure with contraindications to transplantation.[1]

The patients in the study were randomly assigned to receive either an LVAD or maximal medical therapy, with death as the primary endpoint and several secondary endpoints assessing quality of life, complications, and hospitalizations. The study ended in July 2001 and demonstrated a 48 percent reduction in the risk of death in the group treated with LVADs compared with the medically treated group (Fig. 25–11), with superior quality of life measurements demonstrated in the LVAD treatment group. However, patients with devices were more than twice as likely to develop an adverse event and had a higher median number of days spent in and out of the hospital.[1]

The INTrEPID trial is a nonrandomized study currently near completion that assesses destination therapy using the Novacor LVAD. INTrEPID assesses all-cause 6-month mortality as its primary endpoint, and 6-month cardiac mortality and health-related quality of life as its secondary endpoint. To date, enrollment of patients has been completed.

Further analysis of the REMATCH data after study completion has demonstrated improved outcomes across several "eras" of the study (Figs. 25–12 and 25–13).[78] Notably, survival in the LVAD cohort was significantly higher for those

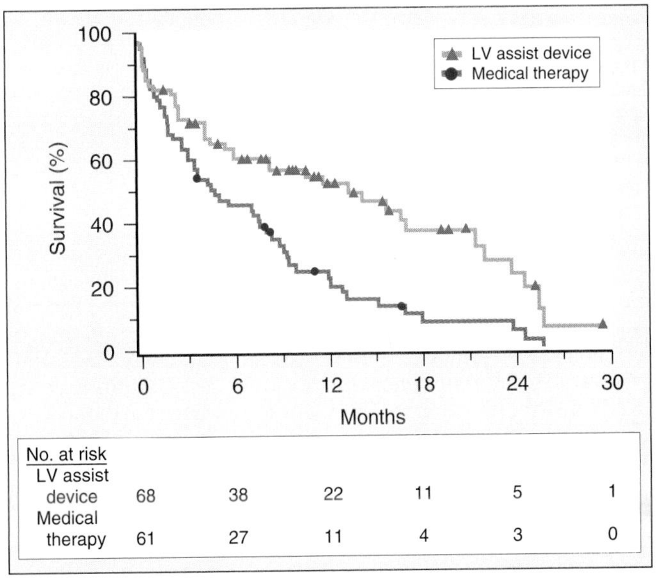

FIGURE 25–11 Comparison of actuarial survival curves from the Randomized Evaluation of Mechanical Assistance for the Treatment of Congestive Heart Failure (REMATCH). LV = left ventricular. (From Rose EA, Gelijns AC, Moskowitz AJ, et al: Long-term mechanical left ventricular assistance for end-stage heart failure. N Engl J Med 345:1435, 2001.)

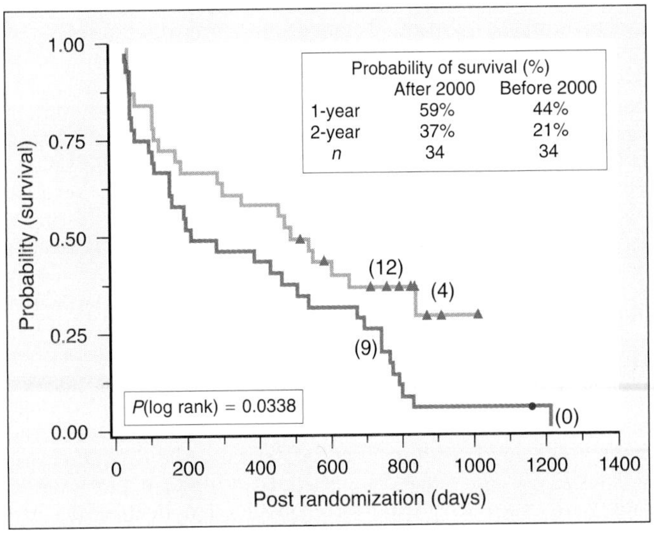

FIGURE 25–12 Randomized Evaluation of Mechanical Assistance for the Treatment of Congestive Heart Failure (REMATCH) left ventricular (LV) assist device "learning curve": comparison of actuarial survival curves of those enrolled in REMATCH before and after 2000. Upper line (blue) denotes those enrolled after 2000, lower line (magenta) denotes those enrolled prior to 2000.[78]

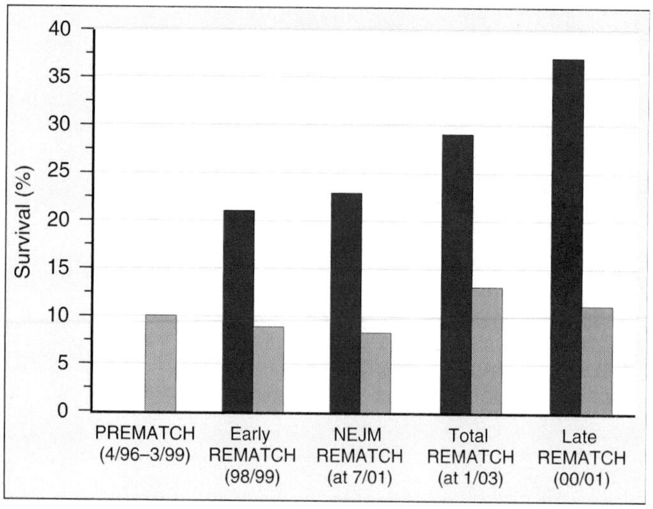

FIGURE 25–13 Comparison of 2-year survival among patients enrolled in the Randomized Evaluation of Mechanical Assistance for the Treatment of Congestive Heart Failure (REMATCH) during different "eras" of study. OMM = optimal medical management cohort; NEJM REMATCH = New England Journal of Medicine reference REMATCH data. *Includes three crossover patients with ventricular assist devices, accounting for 5 percent of OMM patients.[78]

enrolled after 2000, and 2-year survival demonstrated incremental improvement despite little change in the optimal medical management cohort. Certainly, with the advent of more durable devices, other design improvements, and greater clinical experience, the survival benefit conferred by LVAD destination therapy is likely to improve further.

Future Development

Long-term mechanical circulatory support continues to be a source of intense research and development. The obstacles of thrombogenicity (and embolization), device infection, and immunological sensitization remain a target of ongoing research for the currently available VADs. The potential of VADs as destination therapy has further tested the limits of device durability. Finally, the increasing desire to miniaturize pump design to allow complete implantability and pediatric applications continues to drive development.

MINIATURIZED CENTRIFUGAL PUMPS. Years after the invention of centrifugal pumps, researchers are re-evaluating these pumps as the third generation of implantable circulatory assist devices. The Levitronix LVAS (Levitronix, Waltham, MA) is one such pump built on the "maglev" (magnetic levitation) concept, which allows the motor to levitate the rotor magnetically so that rotation is achieved without friction, with less thrombogenicity, with minimal noise and vibration, and with anticipated long-term durability because of lack of metal-to-metal contact. The DuraHeart (Terumo, Ann Arbor, MI) is based on a similar concept and design and may be implemented in patients whose BSA is as low as 1.1 m^2, with flows from 2 to 10 liter/min. It, like the Cor-Aide device (Cor-Aide, Cleveland, OH), has been operated without anticoagulation in animal trials. Whether this strategy will be feasible in clinical applications remains unknown.

PEDIATRIC ASSIST DEVICES. Children with end-stage heart failure are at particular risk for dying while awaiting transplantation owing to the relative unavailability of donor organs in pediatric size ranges. Most clinical experience to date with isolated ventricular assistance has been with children larger than 6 kg; the largest experience in smaller children and neonates has been with ECMO.

Several specific requirements for a pediatric assist device make its development difficult. First, the device must be versatile; children with complex heart disease often require biventricular support or alternatively have only a single functional ventricle. In addition, the ability to include an oxygenator in the support circuit may be required. Second, the cannulas must be small enough to allow ventricular decompression without generating excessive negative pressure (and air entrainment). Third, the device itself must be small enough to be used potentially as an implantable device in larger children and not be cumbersome as a paracorporeal device in smaller infants. Finally, the device must be able to run at flows that are considered low by adult standards but would fully support children (e.g., 0.5 to 1.5 liter/min).

Worldwide, only the Berlin Heart and the Medos pumps have enjoyed significant application in children. Both are essentially miniaturized versions of the Pierce-Donachy paracorporeal biventricular assist device (similar to the Thoratec).[79,80] However, a directive from the NHLBI has been issued to address this need, with expectations of clinical trials in 5 years.

Conclusion

Mechanical circulatory assistance has evolved over the past 20 years from an investigational strategy for the moribund to a standard therapy supporting patients in cardiogenic shock and decompensated heart failure. Although medical therapy has advanced significantly during this time and had a considerable impact on moderate heart failure, its lasting influence on severe heart failure has been less substantial.[81] Today, a wide variety of devices are available for short-, medium-, and long-term and permanent support at a variety of centers worldwide. Indeed, the consistent results with VAD use in this setting have advanced beyond those of pharmacotherapy to the point at which randomly assigning patients between VAD use and medical therapy alone has been questioned as ethically inappropriate.

As experience with device implantation and management has grown, so too has the interest in outcome shifted from mere postoperative survival and safety to more subtle parameters of quality of life.[1] Only with the persistent introduction and trial of new VADs, with sufficient registries to document efficacy, adverse events, and quality of life measures, will innovative therapies continue to develop. The dream of the ideal device—completely implantable, requiring no anticoagulation, available across a wide variety of patients' sizes, and endlessly durable—continues to evade current technology but remains a target of design for the future.

REFERENCES

1. Rose EA, Gelijns AC, Moskowitz AJ, et al: Long term use of a left ventricular assist device for end-stage heart failure. N Eng J Med 345:1435, 2001.
2. Gibbon JH Jr: Application of a mechanical heart and lung apparatus to cardiac surgery. Minn Med 37:171, 1954.
3. Cooley DA, Beall AC Jr, Alexander JK: Acute massive pulmonary embolism: Successful surgical treatment using temporary cardiopulmonary bypass. JAMA 177:283, 1961.
4. Stuckey JH, Newman MM, Dennis C, et al: The use of the heart-lung machine in selected cases of acute myocardial infarction. Surg Forum 8:342, 1957.
5. DeBakey ME: Left ventricular bypass pump for cardiac assistance. Clinical experience. Am J Cardiol 27:3, 1971.
6. Dennis C, Carlens E, Senning A, et al: Clinical use of a cannula for left heart bypass without thoracotomy. Ann Surg 156:623, 1962.
7. Kantrowitz AM, Tjønneland S, Freed PS, et al: Initial clinical experience with intra-aortic balloon pumping in cardiogenic shock. JAMA 203:135, 1968.

Intraaortic Balloon Counterpulsation

8. Moulopoulos SD, Topaz S, Kolff WJ: Diastolic balloon pumping (with carbon dioxide) in the aorta—A mechanical assistance to the failing circulation. Am Heart J 63:669, 1962.
9. Bregman D, Casarella WJ: Percutaneous intraaortic balloon pumping: Initial clinical experience. Ann Thorac Surg 29:153, 1980.
10. Stone GW, Ohman EM, Miller MF, et al: Contemporary utilization and outcomes of intra-aortic balloon counterpulsation in acute myocardial infarction. J Am Coll Cardiol 41:1940, 2003.

11. Pae WE Jr, Pierce WS, Sapirstein JS: Intra-aortic balloon counterpulsation, ventricular assist pumping and the artificial heart. *In* Baue AE, Geha AS, Hammond GL, et al (eds): Glenn's Thoracic and Cardiovascular Surgery. Stamford, Conn, Appleton & Lange, 1996, p 1825.
12. Ghali WA, Ash AS, Hall RE, Moskowitz MA: Variation in hospital rates of intraaortic balloon pump use in coronary artery bypass operations. Ann Thorac Surg 67:441, 1999.
13. Reichenbacher WE, Pierce WS: Treatment of heart failure: Assisted circulation. *In* Braunwald E, Zipes DP, Libby P (eds): Heart Disease: A Textbook of Cardiovascular Medicine. Philadelphia, WB Saunders, 2001, p. 602.
14. Normal JC, Cooley DA, Igo SR, et al: Prognostic indices for survival during postcardiotomy intra-aortic balloon pumping: Methods of scoring and classification, with implications for LVAD utilization. J Thorac Cardiovasc Surg 74:709, 1977.
15. Schmid C, Deng M, Hammel D, et al: Emergency versus elective/urgent left ventricular assist device implantation. J Heart Lung Transplant 17:1024, 1998.
16. Helman DN, Morales DL, Edwards NM, et al: Left ventricular assist device bridge-to-transplant network improves survival after failed cardiotomy. Ann Thorac Surg 68:1187, 1999.
17. Copeland JG, Smith RG, Arabia FA, et al: The CardioWest total artificial heart as a bridge to transplantation. Semin Thorac Cardiovasc Surg 12:238, 2000.
18. Hendry PJ, Masters RG, Mussivand TV, et al: Circulatory support for cardiogenic shock due to acute myocardial infarction: A Canadian experience. Can J Cardiol 15:1090, 1999.
19. Chen JM, DeRose JJ, Slater JP, et al: Improved survival rates support left ventricular assist device implantation early after myocardial infarction. J Am Coll Cardiol 33:1903, 1999.
20. Hands ME, Rutherford JD, Muller JE, et al: The in-hospital development of cardiogenic shock after myocardial infarction: Incidence, predictors of occurrence, outcome and prognostic factors. J Am Coll Cardiol 14:40, 1989.
21. Hochman JS, Sleeper LA, White HD, et al: One-year survival following early revascularization for cardiogenic shock. JAMA 285:190, 2001.
22. Houel R, Vermes E, Tixier DB, et al: Myocardial recovery after mechanical support for acute myocarditis: Is sustained recovery predictable? Ann Thorac Surg 68:2177, 1999.
23. Swartz MT, Lowdermilk GA, McBride LR: Refractory ventricular tachycardia as an indication for ventricular assist device support. J Thorac Cardiovasc Surg 118:1119, 1999.
24. Oz MC, Rose EA, Slater J, et al: Malignant ventricular arrhythmias are well tolerated in patients receiving long-term left ventricular assist devices. J Am Coll Cardiol 24:1688, 1994.
25. Morgan JA, John R, Rao V, et al: Bridging to transplant with the HeartMate left ventricular assist device: The Columbia-Presbyterian experience. J Thorac Cardiovasc Surg 127:1309, 2004.
26. Oz MC, Rose EA, Levin HR: Selection criteria for placement of left ventricular assist devices. Am Heart J 129:173, 1995.
27. Oz MC, Goldstein DJ, Pepino P, et al: Screening scale predicts patients successfully receiving long-term implantable left ventricular assist devices. Circulation 92:II169, 1995.
28. Rao V, Oz MC, Flannery MA, et al: Revised screening scale to predict survival after insertion of a left ventricular assist device. J Thorac Cardiovasc Surg 125:855, 2003.
29. Oz M, Prager KM: Proposed policy for VAD removal. Ann Thorac Surg 73:1688, 2002.
30. Sinha P, Chen JM, Rajasinghe HR, et al: Infections during left-ventricular assist device support do not affect post-transplant outcomes. Circulation 102:III194, 2000.
31. Smedira NG, Moazami N, Golding CM, et al: Clinical experience with 202 adults receiving extracorporeal membrane oxygenation for cardiac failure: Survival at five years. J Thorac Cardiovasc Surg 122:92, 2001.
32. Wassenberg PA: The Abiomed BVS 5000 biventricular support system. Perfusion 15:369, 2000.
33. Spanier T, Oz MC, Levin H, et al: Activation of coagulation and fibrinolystic pathways in patients with left ventricular assist devices. J Thorac Cardiovasc Surg 112:1090, 1996.
34. John R, Lietz K, Schuster M: Immunologic sensitization in recipients of left ventricular assist devices. J Thorac Cardiovasc Surg 125:578, 2003.
35. Itescu S, John R: Interactions between the recipient immune system and the left ventricular assist device surface: Immunological and clinical implications. Ann Thorac Surg 75:S58, 2003.
36. El-Banayosy A, Arusoglu L, Kizner L, et al: Novacor left ventricular assist system versus HeartMate vented electric left ventricular assist system as a long-term mechanical circulatory support device in bridging patients: A prospective study. J Thorac Cardiovasc Surg 119:581, 2000.
37. Frazier OH: First use of an untethered, vented electric left ventricular assist device for long-term support. Circulation 89:2908, 1994.
38. Sun BC, Catanese KA, Spanier TB, et al: 100 long-term implantable left ventricular assist devices: The Columbia Presbyterian interim experience. Ann Thorac Surg 68:688,1999.
39. Poirier VL: Worldwide experience with the TCI HeartMate system: Issues and future perspective. Thorac Cardiovasc Surg 49:316, 1999.
40. Murali S: Mechanical circulatory support with Novacor LVAS: World-wide clinical results. Thorac Cardiovasc Surg 47:321, 1999.
41. Pasque MK, Rogers JG: Adverse events in the use of the HeartMate vented electric and Novacor left ventricular assist devices: Comparing apples and oranges. J Thorac Cardiovasc Surg 124:1063, 2002.
42. Portner PM, Jansen PGM, Oyer PE: Improved outcomes with an implantable left ventricular assist system: A multicenter study. Ann Thorac Surg 71:205, 2001.
43. Farrar DJ: The Thoratec ventricular assist device: A paracorporeal pump for treating acute and chronic heart failure. Semin Thorac Cardiovasc Surg 12:243, 2000.
44. Copeland JG, Arabia FA, Banchy ME, et al: The CardioWest total artificial heart bridge to transplantation: 1993 to 1996 national trial. Ann Thorac Surg 66:1662,1998.
45. Arabia FA, Copeland JG, Smith RG, et al: International experience with the CardioWest total artificial heart as a bridge to heart transplantation. Eur J Cardiothorac Surg 11:S5, 1997.
46. Sezai A, Shiono M, Orime Y, et al: Comparison studies of major organ microcirculations under pulsatile- and nonpulsatile-assisted circulations. Artif Organs 20:139, 1996.
47. Reddy RC, Goldstein AH, Pacella J, et al: End organ function with prolonged nonpulsatile circulatory support. ASAIO J 41:M547, 1995.
48. Yacoub MH: A novel strategy to maximize the efficacy of left ventricular assist devices as a bridge to recovery. Eur Heart J 22:534, 2001.
49. Holman WL, Rayburn BK, McGiffin DC: Infection in ventricular assist devices: Prevention and treatment. Ann Thorac Surg 75:S48, 2003.
50. Nurozler F, Argenziano M, Oz MC, Naka Y: Fungal left ventricular assist device endocarditis. Ann Thorac Surg 71:614, 2001.
51. Macha M, Litwak P, Yamazaki K, et al: Survival for up to six months in calves supported with an implantable axial flow ventricular assist device. ASAIO J 43:311, 1997.
52. Kawahito K, Damm G, Benkowski R, et al: Ex vivo phase 1 evaluation of the DeBakey/NASA axial flow ventricular assist device. Artif Organs 20:47, 1996.
53. Griffith BP, Kormos RL, Borovetz HS, et al: HeartMate II left ventricular assist system: From concept to first clinical use. Ann Thorac Surg 71:S116, 2001.
54. Noon GP, Morley DL, Irwin S, et al: Clinical experience with the MicroMed DeBakey ventricular assist device. Ann Thorac Surg 71:S133, 2001.
55. Frazier OH, Rose EA, Oz MC, et al: HeartMate LVAS Investigators. Left ventricular assist system, multicenter clinical evaluation of the HeartMate vented electric left ventricular assist system in patients awaiting heart transplantation. J Thorac Cardiovasc Surg 122:1186, 2001.
56. Wieselthaler GM, Schima H, Dworschak M, et al: First experience with outpatient care of patients with implanted axial flow pumps. Artif Organs 25:331, 2001.
57. Frazier OH, Myers TJ, Jarvik RK, et al: Research and development of an implantable, axial-flow left ventricular assist device: The Jarvik 2000 Heart. Ann Thorac Surg 71:S125, 2001.
58. Mehta SM, Pae WE, Rosenberg G, et al: The LionHeart LVD-2000: A completely implanted left ventricular assist device for chronic circulatory support. Ann Thorac Surg 71:S156, 2001.
59. Robbins RC, Kown MH, Portner PM, et al: The totally implantable Novacor left ventricular assist system. Ann Thorac Surg 71:S162, 2001.
60. Kavarana MN, Pessin-Minsley MS, Urtecho J, et al: Right ventricular dysfunction and organ failure in left ventricular assist device recipients: A continuing problem. Ann Thorac Surg 73:745, 2002.
61. Argenziano M, Choudhri AF, Oz MC, et al: A prospective randomized trial of arginine vasopressin in the treatment of vasodilatory shock after left ventricular assist device placement. Circulation 96:II-90, 1997.
62. Goldstein DJ, Seldomridge JA, Chen JM, et al: Use of aprotinin in LVAD recipients reduces blood loss, blood use, and perioperative mortality. Ann Thorac Surg 59:1063, 1995.
63. Morrone TM, Buck LA, Catanese KA, et al: Early progressive mobilization of left ventricular assist device patients is safe and optimizes recovery before heart transplantation. J Heart Lung Transplant 15:423, 1996.
64. El-Banayosy A, Fey O, Sarnowski P, et al: Midterm follow-up of patients discharged from hospital under left ventricular assistance. J Heart Lung Transplant 20:53, 2001.
65. Levin HR, Oz MC, Chen JM, et al: Reversal of chronic ventricular dilation in patients with end-stage cardiomyopathy by prolonged mechanical unloading. Circulation 91:2717, 1995.
66. Frazier OH, Benedict CR, Radovancevic B, et al: Improved left ventricular function after chronic left ventricular unloading. Ann Thorac Surg 62:675, 1996.
67. Foray A, Williams D, Reemtsma K, et al: Assessment of submaximal exercise capacity in patients with left ventricular assist devices. Circulation 94:II222, 1996.
68. Mueller J, Wallukat G, Weng Y, et al: Predictive factors for weaning from a cardiac assist device. An analysis of clinical, gene expression, and protein data. J Heart Lung Transplant 20:202, 2001.
69. Helman DN, Maybaum SW, Morales DL, et al: Recurrent remodeling after ventricular assistance: Is long-term myocardial recovery attainable? Ann Thorac Surg 70:1255, 2000.
70. Hetzer R, Muller JH, Weng YG, et al: Midterm follow-up of patients who underwent removal of a left ventricular assist device after cardiac recovery from end-stage dilated cardiomyopathy. J Thorac Cardiovasc Surg 120:843, 2000.
71. McBride LR, Naunheim KS, Fiore AC, et al: Clinical experience with 111 Thoratec ventricular assist devices. Ann Thorac Surg 67:1233, 1999.
72. Thomas CE, Jichici D, Petrucci R, et al: Neurologic complications of the Novacor left ventricular assist device. Ann Thorac Surg 72:1311, 2001.
73. Rafii S, Oz MC, Seldomridge JA, et al: Characterization of hematopoietic cells arising on the textured surface of left ventricular assist devices. Ann Thorac Surg 60:1627, 1995.
74. Korfer R, El-Banayosy A, Arusoglu L, et al: Single-center experience with the Thoratec ventricular assist device. J Thorac Cardiovasc Surg 119:596, 2000.
75. Fukamachi K, McCarthy PM, Smedira NG, et al: Preoperative risk factors for right ventricular failure after implantable left ventricular assist device insertion. Ann Thorac Surg 68:2181, 1999.
76. Cave AC, Manche A, Derias NW, et al: Thromboxane A_2 mediates pulmonary hypertension after cardiopulmonary bypass in the rabbit. J Thorac Cardiovasc Surg 106:959, 1993.
77. Chen JM, Levin HR, Rose EA, et al: Experience with right ventricular assist devices for perioperative right sided circulatory failure. Ann Thorac Surg 61:305, 1996.
78. Park SJ, Frazier OH, Piccioni W, et al: LVAD destination therapy: An extended follow-up of outcomes. J Thorac Cardiovasc Surg (in press).
79. Konertz W, Reul H: Mechanical circulatory support in children. Int J Artif Organs 20:657, 1997.
80. Warnecke H, Berdijs F, Lange P, et al: Mechanical left ventricular support as a bridge to cardiac transplantation in childhood. Eur J Cardiothorac Surg 5:300, 1991.
81. Stevenson LW, Kormos KL: Mechanical cardiac support 2000: Current applications and future trial design. J Am Coll Cardiol 37:341, 2001.

CHAPTER 26

Heart Transplantation

Sharon A. Hunt • Peter C. Kouretas • Leora B. Balsam • Robert C. Robbins

History

Clinical heart transplantation has become a mature clinical science in the last 15 years or so, but its maturation was preceded by several decades of preclinical and preliminary clinical work involving a variety of scientific disciplines. The earliest work defining the optimum surgical methods for excision of the donor heart and implantation of the heart in the orthotopic position happened in the 1950s, and the technique with use of cardiopulmonary bypass and topical hypothermia for donor heart preservation was published as a two-page report by the Shumway group in 1960. The basic surgical technique has changed little since that time and is outlined in this chapter.

The first clinical heart transplant was performed in South Africa in December 1967 and was greeted with much publicity and followed by much surgical enthusiasm for the next year, with just over 100 procedures being performed in 1968. This enthusiasm was soon tempered, however, by the observation of very poor survival rates in these early patients (~15 percent at 1 year) and by 1970 essentially only two centers (Stanford and the Medical College of Virginia) continued to pursue programs in clinical heart transplantation. Working virtually alone in the decade of the 1970s, these programs gradually evolved recipient and donor acceptance criteria, introduced the endomyocardial biopsy as a means to detect the presence of and the adequacy of therapy for rejection, and outlined what have come to be the expected posttransplant complications.

In the 1980s, general advances in the field of immunosuppression, prominently including the clinical introduction of the calcineurin inhibitor cyclosporine, led to a gradual resurgence of interest and clinical activity in the field of heart transplantation. In 1982 an international registry of heart transplantation data was begun by the International Society for Heart and Lung Transplantation (ISHLT) and continues to accrue data today. In 1994, this registry was merged with the overall organ transplant registry in the United States supervised by the United Network for Organ Sharing (UNOS). In the United States reporting of data is mandatory; it is voluntary for the rest of the world, but completeness of reporting is quite good. The data are updated and published annually in the *Journal of Heart and Lung Transplantation* and are available online at the UNOS website (www.UNOS.org).

By the decade of the 1990s, the demand for heart transplantation began to exceed the supply of available donor hearts, and since then the annual numbers of transplants performed has been strictly limited by the numbers of donor hearts available. The annual numbers seem to have plateaued at approximately 4000 procedures worldwide per year.[1]

Heart Transplantation: The Operation

DONOR OPERATIVE TECHNIQUE

Retrieval of the donor heart in the modern era typically occurs as a part of a multiorgan procurement effort. The cardiothoracic team works in conjunction with an abdominal team, which procures the liver and/or kidneys, and communication between the two teams is critical for optimum management of the donor during the retrieval process.

The donor operation is performed via a median sternotomy. The heart and great vessels are carefully inspected for any signs of contusion, infarction, congenital anomalies, and aneurysmal disease and for overall ventricular function. The coronary arteries are palpated to evaluate coronary artery disease. Substantial abnormalities identified in this manner preclude the use of the donor heart for transplantation.

When the abdominal team has completed their dissection, heparin is administered to the donor and the aorta is cannulated for infusion of cardioplegic solution., The left heart is decompressed by incising one of the pulmonary veins; the heart is then allowed to empty and the aortic cross clamp is applied. Cold crystalloid cardioplegia is administered via the aortic root. When the infusion is completed, the heart is rapidly excised by dividing the superior vena cava (SVC), the four pulmonary veins, the aorta, and the pulmonary artery at its bifurcation.

RECIPIENT OPERATIVE TECHNIQUE

The recipient operation for heart transplantation proceeds in two phases. The first step is the excision of the recipient's native organ and the second step is the implantation of the allograft. The recipient is brought to the operating room and appropriate monitoring lines are placed. After induction of general anesthesia and endotracheal intubation, a median sternotomy is performed and the pericardium is opened and reflected laterally. The ascending aorta, SVC, and inferior vena cava (IVC) are dissected free and encircled with tapes. After the recipient is fully heparinized, the high ascending aorta and both venae cavae are cannulated separately, cardiopulmonary bypass (CPB) is instituted, and the patient is cooled to 28°C. Once the donor heart has been delivered to the operating room, the recipient cardiectomy is performed. The aorta is cross-clamped just proximal to the aortic cannulation site. The right and left atrial walls, atrial septum, pulmonary artery, and aorta are divided. Division of the pulmonary artery and aorta is performed just above the semilunar valves (Fig. 26–1).

The donor heart is then brought onto the operative field and prepared for implantation into the recipient. The tissue between the orifices of the four pulmonary veins is excised, leaving a single large opening (Fig. 26–2). The right atrium is opened beginning from the lateral aspect of the IVC and extending into the base of the right atrial appendage (Fig. 26–3). The heart is carefully examined for any valvular or congenital anomalies. The standard or biatrial technique, as originally described by Lower and Shumway, proceeds with anastomoses of the left atrium, right atrium, pulmonary artery, and aorta (Figs. 26–4 and 26–5).

After at least 30 minutes of reperfusion, the patient is gradually weaned from CPB with implementation of the appropriate inotropic support. The cannulas are removed and protamine is administered slowly to reverse the effect of heparin. Temporary atrial and ventricular pacing wires are placed as well as mediastinal and pleural drainage tubes. The sternum is then closed in the standard fashion. Induction immunosuppressive therapy is administered at this time.

In recent years, the bicaval technique for orthotopic heart transplantation has become the preferred approach at most transplant centers.[2,3] Several modifications distinguish the bicaval approach from the standard biatrial technique. First, the recipient SVC is cannulated just below the innominate vein junction and the IVC is cannulated at the diaphragm. Recipient cardiectomy is performed as a two-step procedure. In the first step, the heart is transected at the midatrial level, the aorta and pulmonary artery are divided, and the heart is removed. In the second step, the posterior walls of both atria are removed; on the right side, the SVC and IVC are transected at their junction with the right atrium, and on the left side, the left atrium is trimmed, leaving a cuff of tissue around the pulmonary vein orifices (Fig. 26–6). The donor heart left atrium is trimmed, leaving a single orifice where the pulmonary vein entry sites had been, and the right atrium remains intact. In the bicaval approach, the typical sequence of anastomoses is left atrium, IVC, SVC, pulmonary arteries, and aorta (Figs. 26–7 and 26–8). The left atrial, pulmonary artery, and aortic anastomoses are performed as described in the standard biatrial technique.

The standard biatrial technique is still used in some transplant centers because of the advantage of shorter operative times and avoidance of the potential complications of SVC and IVC thromboses and stenoses. There are several disadvantages of the biatrial technique, however, which has prompted a shift to the bicaval technique in many transplant centers.[3,4] The biatrial technique distorts the atrioventricular geometry, which can result in atrial enlargement, atrioventricular valve insufficiency, impaired atrial function, atrial thromboses, and a propensity toward sinoatrial node dysfunction.[5] Several studies have demonstrated improved atrial function and ventricular function and decreased atrioventricular valvular insufficiency as well as a decreased incidence of arrhythmias and heart block with the bicaval technique.[3,6,7] A reported disadvantage of the bicaval technique is the risk of SVC stenosis, particularly when there is a size mismatch between the donor and recipient. A recent series from Stanford reported a 2.4 percent incidence of this complication.[8]

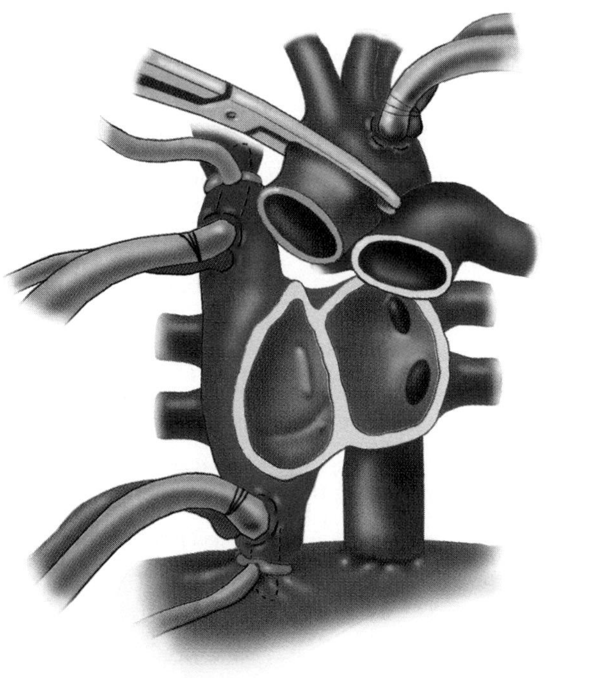

FIGURE 26–1 Completed recipient cardiectomy in preparation for standard orthotopic transplantation.

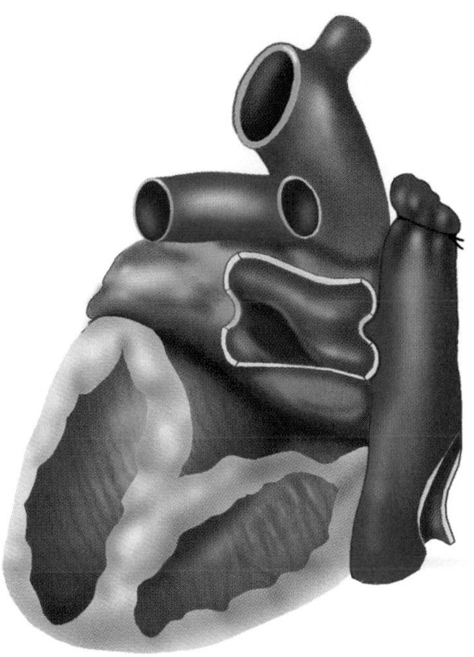

FIGURE 26–2 Creation of donor heart left atrial cuff by incising through the pulmonary vein orifices.

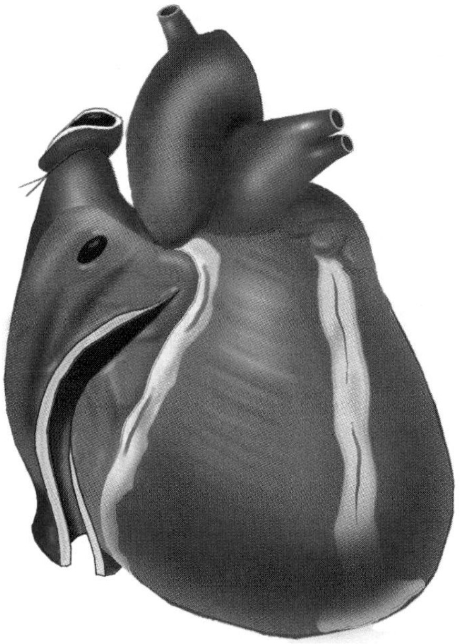

FIGURE 26–3 Creation of the donor heart right atrial cuff.

Recipient Selection

Cardiac recipient selection criteria aim to identify the patients with end-stage heart disease who are most likely to

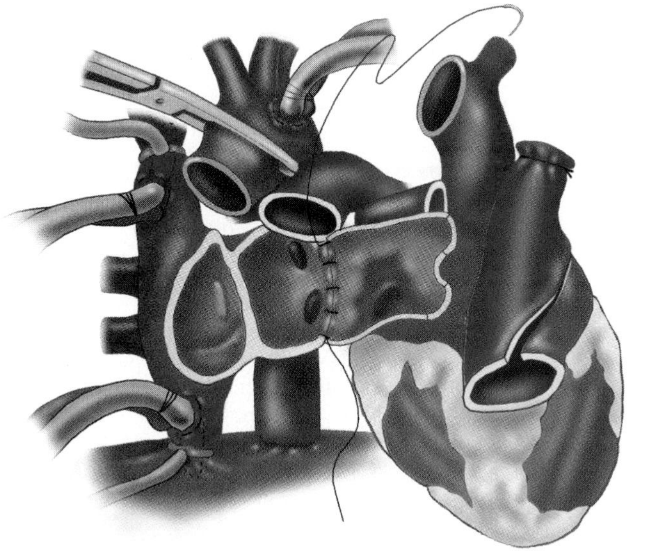

FIGURE 26–4 Commencement of the left atrial anastomosis.

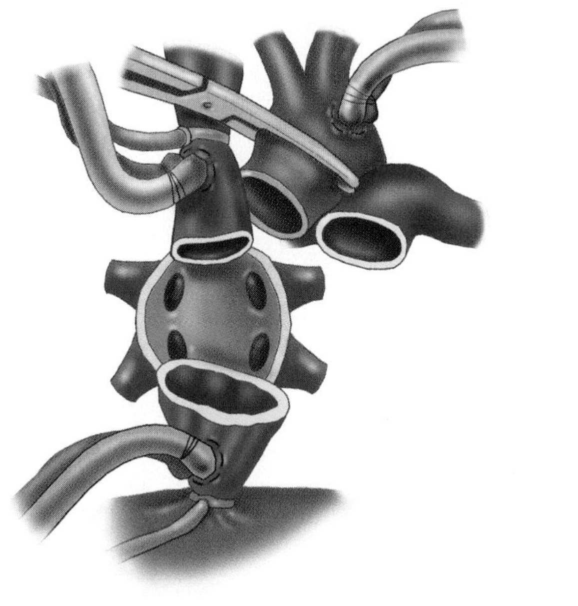

FIGURE 26–6 Creation of superior and inferior vena caval cuffs in preparation for bicaval technique.

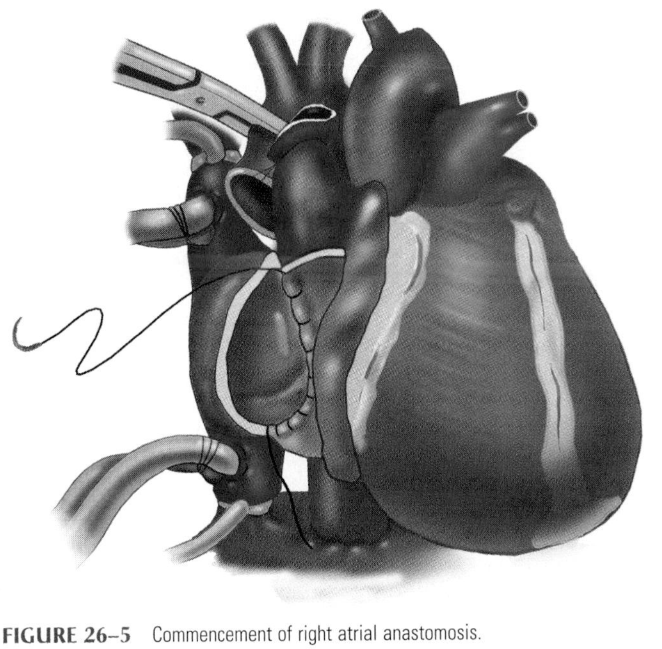

FIGURE 26–5 Commencement of right atrial anastomosis.

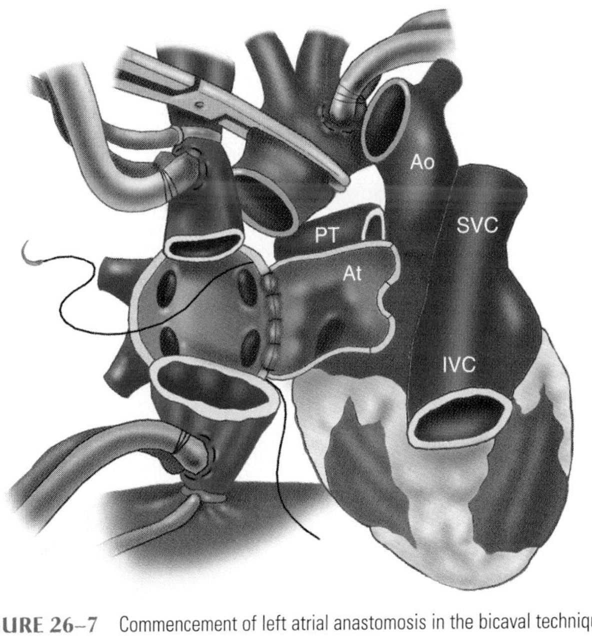

FIGURE 26–7 Commencement of left atrial anastomosis in the bicaval technique.

have the greatest benefit from the scarce societal resource of the donor heart (Table 26–1). The criteria have evolved a great deal over time and continue to do so as experience and expertise at dealing with issues limiting postoperative survival accrue. The most fundamental criterion remains the presence of advanced heart disease that is irremediable by any more conservative forms of therapy. As medical therapy for heart failure has improved over the years, the designation of truly "end-stage" heart disease has become a "moving target" since many patients who are referred for heart transplantation end up improving their clinical status with judicious use of newer therapies.

Most patients eventually accepted for transplantation in the current era have failed aggressive medical management at a heart failure center and usually have required recurrent hospitalizations for heart failure management. Many are hospital-bound with requirement for intravenous inotropic support and/or mechanical support of the circulation. In ambulatory patients the goal is to select those with the very worst prognosis.[9] In this context the measurement of peak oxygen consumption with exercise to anaerobic threshold (VO_2 max) has been shown to be one of the best predictors of prognosis.[10-12] Patients with a VO_2 max less than 15 ml/kg/min have a poor prognosis and a level of 14 ml/kg/min is often considered a basic threshold for transplant eligibility in ambulatory patients.

The other criteria listed in Table 26–1 all are open to interpretation.[13]

Advanced Age

Age criteria for eligibility were initially rigid, but it became apparent that chronological and physiological age could be quite discrepant, and there have been a number of single-

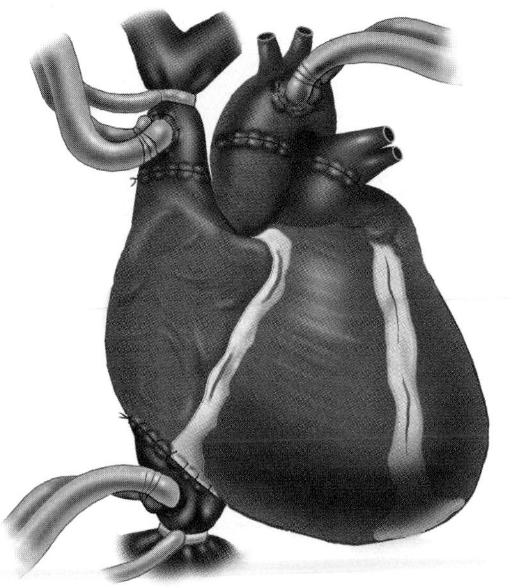

FIGURE 26–8 Completion of bicaval transplant technique, showing the inferior vena caval, superior vena caval, aortic, and pulmonary artery anastomoses.

TABLE 26–1 Cardiac Recipient Selection Criteria

End-stage heart disease not remediable by more conservative measures
Absence of Advanced age Severe peripheral or cerebrovascular disease Irreversible dysfunction of another organ (kidney, liver, lung) unless being considered for multiorgan transplantation History of malignancy with probability of recurrence Inability to comply with complex medical regimen Irreversible pulmonary hypertension (>4 Wood units) Active systemic infection

center reports of excellent post heart transplant survival in carefully selected older recipients. Most programs currently do not have fixed upper age limits, but patients older than 65 years of age are very highly selected for lack of comorbidities.

Severe Peripheral or Cerebrovascular Disease

Since systemic vascular disease contributes to both poor prognosis for survival as well as poor quality of life on a noncardiac basis, and since risk factors contributing to the disease are also major risk factors for development of vascular disease in the allograft, advanced noncardiac vascular disease is a major comorbidity that can preclude eligibility for cardiac transplantation. It would be difficult to design an exact description of the extent of disease that would disqualify a patient, however.

Irreversible Organ Dysfunction

Coexisting disease in other organs that might separately limit a patient's survival has generally been considered a contraindication to heart transplantation, and this has applied primarily to disease of the lungs, kidneys, and liver. With advances in the general area of solid-organ transplantation, some centers have commenced programs in multiorgan transplantation in highly selected patients and referral of patients in need of more than one organ to such a center can be considered.

History of Malignancy

The institution of chronic immunosuppression, a form of therapy known to be associated with a higher-than-usual incidence of malignancy, might favor recurrence of or more aggressive behavior of a prior or current malignancy. There are many reports, however, of long-term successful heart transplantation in patients with a remote history of malignancy that is considered to have essentially no probability of recurrence. Many of these patients have developed their end-stage heart disease as a direct consequence of the chemotherapy and/or radiation therapy that cured their malignancy. In cases in which the malignancy is less remote in history or probability of recurrence less certain, consultation with an oncologist regarding prognosis can be quite helpful.

Inability or Unwillingness to Comply with a Complex Medical Regimen

Psychosocial criteria, including history of compliance with medical regimens and medical follow-up and quality of family or social support structure, have a long history of being considered as factors for transplant eligibility. They are, however, the most difficult ones to quantify or defend. Certainly, the existence of active substance abuse or refusal to take medications should be a major consideration; however, more vague measures of "social worth" (including incarceration status, level of mental retardation, health care coverage status, family support or lack thereof) cannot be considered as major factors.

Irreversible Pulmonary Hypertension

It was discovered in the early days of clinical heart transplantation that a normal donor right ventricle faced with high recipient pulmonary vascular resistance (PVR) and the demand to increase its external workload acutely often failed abruptly, frequently as early as on the operating table. Subsequently, pulmonary hypertension in excess of about 4 Wood units became an exclusion to transplant candidacy. In recent years the concept of reversibility of the pulmonary hypertension seen in some patients with chronic heart failure has been recognized, and it is believed that if reversibility can be demonstrated acutely with pharmacological maneuvers either in the cardiac catheterization laboratory or in the intensive care unit setting with hemodynamic monitoring, a patient can be expected to do well with a transplant since the same reversal could presumably be accomplished in the postoperative setting.[14,15] Thus, the cardiologist often becomes in a sense a patient advocate in the cardiac catheterization laboratory, devising combinations of inotropes and vasodilators to try and demonstrate reversibility of elevated PVR while maintaining adequate systemic pressures.[16,17] Irreversible pulmonary hypertension remains an exclusion from transplant candidacy in most centers unless combined heart and lung transplantation is considered.

Active Systemic Infection

As discussed in the section on malignancy, there is a general and intuitive feeling that the institution of systemic immunosuppression is also contraindicated in the presence of significant active systemic infection since the state of immunosuppression would be expected to be deleterious to defense mechanisms against infection. The existence of a systemic infection is thus considered a (sometimes temporary) contraindication to transplant eligibility. Some infections that are not considered "temporary" include human immunodeficiency virus (HIV) infection and disseminated tuberculosis, although some clinical experience has actually been reported with organ transplantation in HIV-positive patients.

Donor Selection and Management

The selection of donors for heart transplantation is a stepwise process coordinated by the organ procurement organization, the transplant physicians, and the procuring surgeons. A primary screen is performed by a specialist from the organ procurement organization who collects information regarding the medical history, cause of death, body size, ABO blood type, serologies (including HIV, hepatitus B virus [HBV], and hepatitus C virus [HCV]), and clinical course of the potential donor. A secondary screen is performed by a transplant physician who reviews relevant history, physical findings, and test results, including the baseline electrocardiogram, chest radiograph, laboratory data, and echocardiogram. A final screen is performed by the procuring surgeon, who directly inspects the organ, usually at a site distant from the transplant hospital, and works in concert with procurement teams for the donor's other organs.

Guidelines for Donor Selection

Standard guidelines have been established for cardiac donor selection (Table 26–2).[18,19] Potential donors must meet legal requirements for brain death. Donor age younger than 55 years is preferred, although on occasion older donors are considered. Donors with a history of cardiac disease, including prior myocardial infarction or significant valvular or other structural disease or arrhythmia, are usually excluded. In addition, donors with a history of severe chest trauma are excluded because of concern about cardiac contusion. Donors must meet established hemodynamic criteria, including a mean arterial pressure (MAP) higher than 60 mm Hg and a central venous pressure (CVP) of 8 to 12 mm Hg, either on initial evaluation or after appropriate resuscitation maneuvers as described later. Prolonged cardiac arrest, arterial hypoxemia, hypotension, and/or high-dose inotropic support are reasons for exclusion. Donors with a history of active malignancy (excluding basal cell and squamous cell carcinomas of the skin and some isolated brain tumors) are excluded because there is a high probability of transferring malignant cells to the immunosuppressed recipient. Coronary angiography is recommended for most male donors older than 45 years and female donors older than 50 years to evaluate coronary artery stenoses. Serologies for HIV, HBV, and HCV should be negative, although some centers "match" donors who have positive hepatitis serology with seropositive recipients.

In response to the donor organ shortage, there has been a trend toward liberalizing donor selection criteria. Expansion of the cardiac donor pool has involved accepting hearts of older donors, tolerating longer organ ischemic times, and accepting hearts with some structural abnormalities, including mild left ventricular hypertrophy, mild valvular anomalies, or mild coronary artery disease. Limited information is available regarding the long-term durability of organs derived from this expanded donor pool, though there is some evidence that certain donor factors, such as older age and prolonged ischemic time, may act synergistically to increase recipient mortality risk.[20]

TABLE 26–2 Cardiac Donor Selection Criteria

Age < 55 yr
No history of chest trauma or cardiac disease
No prolonged hypotension or hypoxemia
Meets hemodynamic criteria MAP > 60 mm Hg CVP 8-12 mm Hg Inotropic support < 10 μg/kg/min dopamine or dobutamine
Normal ECG
Normal echocardiogram
Normal cardiac angiography*
Negative HBsAg, HCV, and HIV serologies

CVP = central venous pressure; ECG = electrocardiogram; HBsAg = hepatis B surface antigen; HCV = hepatitis C virus; HIV = human immunodeficiency virus; MAP = mean arterial pressure.
*Performed as indicated by donor age and history.

Donor Management

Aggressive hemodynamic and metabolic management of donors has been shown to result in higher organ retrieval rates.[21,22] Brain-injured patients often suffer from hemodynamic instability due to neurogenic shock, excessive fluid loss, and bradycardia. Typical management should include correction of volume deficits, metabolic derangements, and hormonal abnormalities. Fluid should be administered to maintain a CVP between 5 and 10 mm Hg and blood transfusions given sparingly to maintain a hematocrit of 30 percent. When available, cytomegalovirus (CMV)-negative and leukocyte-filtered blood is preferred. Inotropic support should be used as little as possible. Metabolic derangements, including acidosis, hypoxemia, and hypercarbia, should be corrected. Because hormonal abnormalities are common in brain-injured patients, hormonal replacement with arginine vasopressin, triiodothyronine, methylprednisolone, and/or insulin may be necessary.

The Crystal City Guidelines are a consensus statement formulated in 2002 with a goal of improving cardiac donor management and organ utilization.[18] A management strategy for potential organ donors is described in this document. The algorithm begins with conventional management (volume replacement, correction of acidosis, hypoxemia, and anemia, and weaning of inotropes), followed by an initial echocardiogram to identify any structural abnormalities and to evaluate left ventricular function. If the left ventricular ejection fraction (LVEF) is 0.45 or higher, the heart is considered appropriate for transplantation. If the LVEF is less than 0.45, recommendations include hormonal therapy with arginine vasopressin, triiodothyronine, methylprednisolone, and insulin and placement of a pulmonary artery catheter to guide hemodynamic management. The heart should be considered for transplantation only if appropriate hemodynamic criteria are reached (MAP > 60 mm Hg, pulmonary capillary wedge pressure 8 to 12 mm Hg, CVP 4 to 12 mm Hg, SVR 800 to 1200 $dyne \cdot sec^{-1} \cdot cm^{-5}$, cardiac index > 2.4 $liter \cdot min^{-1} \cdot m^{-2}$, and dopamine or dobutamine < 10 $\mu g/kg \cdot min^{-1}$).

Donor and Recipient Matching

Donor/recipient matching parameters for heart transplantation include only ABO compatibility and body size.[19] ABO compatibility is an absolute requirement, because hyperacute rejection may occur within minutes when transplantation is performed across ABO barriers. For reasons involving the limitations on ischemic times as well as laboratory availability, human leukocyte antigen (HLA) matching is not considered to be practical in this field. For cardiac transplantation, height and weight differences up to 20 percent may be tolerated; however, in potential recipients with elevated PVR, a donor whose body size is at least equal to that of the recipient should be chosen to decrease the likelihood of acute right ventricular failure. For potential recipients with an elevated panel reactive antibody (PRA) titer, indicating a high level of presensitization to HLA (often due to prior transfusions or pregnancies), a prospective crossmatch with donor lymphocytes is also necessary. A positive crossmatch occurs if the recipient harbors antibodies against donor HLA. In such an instance, hyperacute rejection is likely, and the donor organ cannot be accepted for that recipient.

Adoption of allocation schemes has facilitated equitable distribution of donor organs. In the United States, the UNOS contracts with the federal government to oversee organ allocation. Under UNOS policy, thoracic organs are distributed based on blood type, medical urgency, and time on the waiting list. Distribution occurs first locally and then regionally. Allocation policies are reviewed and updated on a regular basis with input from transplant physicians as well as organ procurement specialists, patient organizations, and scientists involved in the field of transplantation.

Organ Procurement

Improved techniques in organ preservation have allowed longer safe ischemic times and thus more distant procurement, thereby increasing the donor organ pool.[23] For heart grafts, cold ischemic periods up to 4 to 6 hours are currently considered permissible. As described earlier, donor organ retrieval usually occurs as part of a multiorgan procurement, and often thoracic and abdominal surgical teams will be working simultaneously on the same donor.

Immunosuppression

Postoperative management of the cardiac transplant recipient is similar to that for other postoperative heart surgery, with the important exception of the need to institute immunosuppression. Regimens used to provide suppression of the normal recipient immune response to an allograft vary at different centers and what is considered "state of the art" evolves, seemingly more rapidly over time. All currently used regimens are nonspecific, however, providing general hyporeactivity to foreign antigens rather than donor-specific hyporeactivity. For this reason, current regimens all lead to an unwanted susceptibility to infections and malignant complications in the recipient.

Most cardiac transplantation centers currently introduce immunosuppression with a three-drug regimen commencing immediately at the time of transplant. Most include a calcineurin inhibitor (cyclosporine or tacrolimus), an inhibitor of T-lymphocyte proliferation or differentiation (azathioprine or mycophenolate mofetil or sirolimus), and at least a short course of corticosteroids. Many also include in the perioperative period "induction" therapy with polyclonal (antithymocyte preparations) or monoclonal (mouse CD3 monoclonal antibodies such as Orthoclone OKT3) anti-T cell antibodies to decrease the frequency or severity of early posttransplant rejection. Most recently introduced have been monoclonal antibodies (daclizumab and basiliximab) that block the interleukin-2 receptor and may provide prevention of allograft rejection without additional global immunosuppression.[24] The "tapering" or adjustment of the immunosuppressive regimen after the perioperative period is a process that is highly individualized for each patient and determined by the patient's rejection history and tolerance to and complications from the drugs or modalities used. The following section details the methods for surveillance and therapy for acute allograft rejection.

Physiology of the Transplanted Heart

The cardiac allograft is functionally and anatomically denervated and relies on atypical adaptive mechanisms to meet varying demands for cardiac output. Having no direct neural stimulus to acutely increase heart rate in response to exercise, the allograft responds with the intrinsic Frank-Starling mechanism (the property of cardiac muscle that causes it to increase the force of its contraction in response to increased stretch or tension) to increase cardiac output in response to increased venous return at the onset of exercise. Circulating catecholamine levels later rise and provide a delayed chronotropic response to exercise. Slowing of the heart rate occurs in a likewise delayed fashion as catecholamine levels decline, but cardiac output drops mainly in response to a reduction in venous return and the reverse of the Frank-Starling mechanism.

Despite the theoretical adequacy of these atypical adaptive mechanisms, heart transplant recipients have subnormal capacity for exercise, although they have normal hemodynamic function at rest.[25-27] However, heart transplant recipients have sufficient capacity to perform activities of daily living and at least moderate exercise and generally enjoy an excellent quality of life. A number of lines of evidence suggest that reinnervation may occur in some patients late posttransplant, and a recent study suggested that reinnervation may lead to functional improvement of the transplanted heart.[28]

Since the transplanted heart lacks not only efferent but also afferent innervation, patients are classically unable to experience the sensation of angina pectoris in response to cardiac ischemia or infarction. They may experience symptoms related to the sequelae of ischemia such as dyspnea due to heart failure or arrhythmias or low cardiac output. Clinicians caring for these patients, especially late postoperatively, need to be sensitive to the subtle signs or symptoms that may signal ischemic heart disease.

Expected Postoperative Complications

Rejection

As is the case with any organ graft, the transplanted heart is subject to normal immune responses that, left unchecked, destroy the graft. The immunosuppression described earlier mitigates this reaction to variable extents in individual patients. Detection of cardiac allograft rejection and the attendant need for augmented immunosuppression are generally accomplished in some part on clinical and echocardiographic grounds but usually also with the use of the right ventricular endomyocardial biopsy. Histological grading of biopsy specimens is done with an internationally accepted grading scale[29] and this grade, when integrated with clinical and echocardiographic indices, determines the aggressiveness of augmentation of immunosuppression (Fig. 26–9). Most centers pursue serial biopsies on a surveillance basis during the first year or so after transplant and infrequently thereafter, or as clinically indicated. The endomyocardial biopsy is usually performed under fluoroscopic guidance with the use of a bioptome using a percutaneous approach from the right internal jugular vein (see previous editions of this text for details of this procedure).

Infection

All of the nonspecific immunosuppressive regimens currently used heighten susceptibility of the allograft recipient to infectious complications, particularly with opportunistic organisms. The degree of susceptibility correlates with the ntensity of immunosuppression and thus is greatest during the early postoperative period. For this reason, available expertise in the specialty of infectious disease is generally considered an important aspect of institutional qualifications for an excellent transplant program.

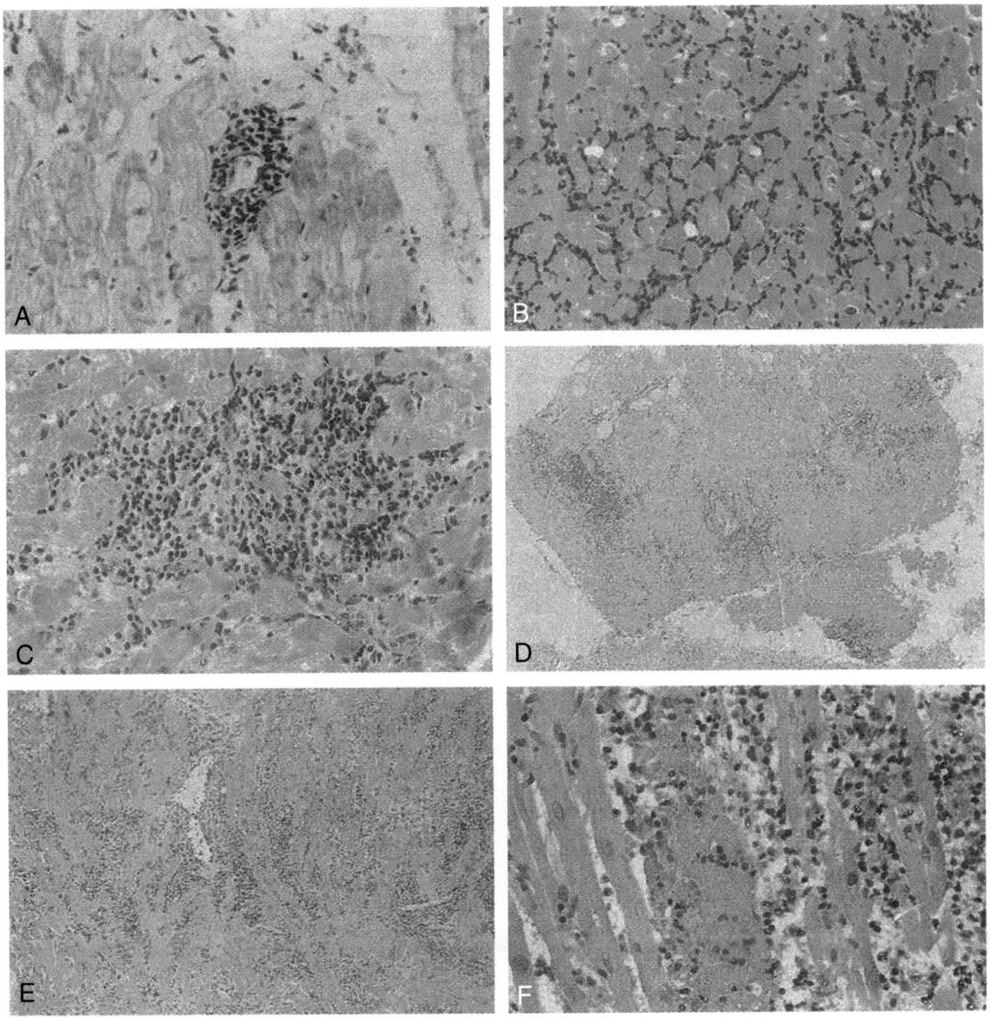

FIGURE 26–9 International Society for Heart and Lung Transplantation (ISHLT) grades of rejection. **A,** Grade 1A: Focal perivascular lymphocytic infiltrate without damage to adjacent myocytes. **B,** Grade 1B: Diffuse interstitial lymphocytic infiltrate without damage to adjacent myocytes. **C,** Grade 2: One focus of dense lymphocytic infiltrate with associated myocyte damage. **D,** Grade 3A: Multiple foci of dense lymphocytic infiltrates with associated myocyte damage. There are intervening areas of uninvolved myocardium. **E,** Grade 3B: Diffuse infiltrate with associated myocyte damage. **F,** Grade 4: Polymorphous infiltrate with extensive myocyte damage, edema, and hemorrhage. (Hematoxylin & eosin.) (From Winters GL, Schoen FJ: Pathology of cardiac transplantation. *In* Silver MD, Gotlieb AI, Schoen FJ [eds]: Cardiovascular Pathology. 3rd ed. Philadelphia, WB Saunders, 2001, pp 725-762.)

Malignancy

The tendency to develop an incidence of malignancy in excess of that seen in the general population is yet another consequence of the current nonspecific forms of immunosuppression, or the "price of immunotherapy" to use the words of the patriarch of the field, Israel Penn. The need to recognize and treat malignancy has become a standard part of the set of clinical skills required for physicians caring for organ transplant recipients. For many years the Cincinnati Transplant Tumor Registry, under the direction of Dr. Penn, maintained a database of de novo malignancies reported in organ transplant recipients.[30] This registry has amply documented that transplant recipients tend to have cancers that are common in the general population with a normal incidence but have a markedly increased incidence of both lymphoproliferative malignancy and carcinomas of the skin.

The lymphoproliferative malignancies occurring in the context of transplantation (commonly known as *posttransplant lymphoproliferative disorder*) consist mostly of abnormal proliferations of B lymphocytes, and most appear to be driven by the Epstein-Barr virus. The clinical presentations are quite heterogeneous and differ from the well-recognized clinical patterns seen with other lymphomas, with more than 70 percent involving extranodal sites. Reduction of immunosuppression can lead to durable tumor regression in these patients, but this maneuver is truly a "double-edged sword" when used with a life-sustaining allograft such as the heart. Traditional cytotoxic chemotherapy does not have a good response rate with these malignancies, and newer targeted antibody approaches, currently with the anti-CD20 monoclonal antibody rituximab, have been encouraging.[31-33]

Graft Coronary Artery Disease

The development of a chronologically premature and anatomically quite diffuse and often rapidly progressive obliterative pattern of coronary artery disease, a vascular disease that is limited to the allograft, is currently the major complication limiting truly long-term survival in cardiac transplant recipients (see also Chap. 35). Its etiology is likely complex and is thought to involve an interplay of immunologic (HLA and other mismatches), infectious (CMV and others), and more usual (lipid status, diabetes, and other) factors.

Some angiographic evidence of this disease is present by 1 year posttransplant in 10 percent of patients, and 50 percent have some evidence by 5 years (Fig. 26–10). In recent years the use of intravascular ultrasound has provided earlier and more sensitive diagnosis of the intimal thickening that characterizes the disease, and the technique has provided a surrogate endpoint for clinical trials of newer immunosuppressive agents designed to evaluate changes in the incidence of the disease consequent to changed immunosuppression (Fig. 26–11).[34]

As noted earlier, as transplant recipients generally have a high degree of both afferent and efferent denervation, they often do not experience the subjective sensation of angina pectoris. Ischemic sequelae in these patients can include arrhythmias leading to sudden death as well as ischemic left ventricular dysfunction leading to the clinical syndrome of heart failure. The very diffuseness of the disease makes the use of standard revascularization with percutaneous or surgical interventions palliative at best. The prognosis once graft

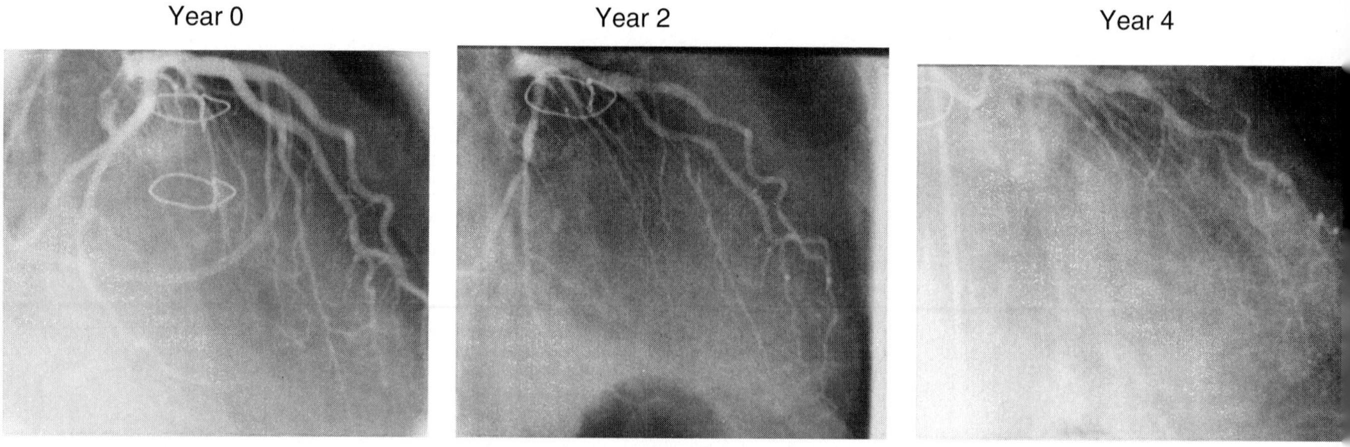

FIGURE 26–10 Graft coronary artery disease—progression by angiography. Serial angiograms obtained at time of transplantation (year 0) and at years 2 and 4 following engraftment show progressive "pruning" of the distal vessels and, by year 4, segmental stenoses of the proximal epicardial coronary arteries. (Courtesy of James C. Fang, Brigham and Women's Hospital, Boston, MA.)

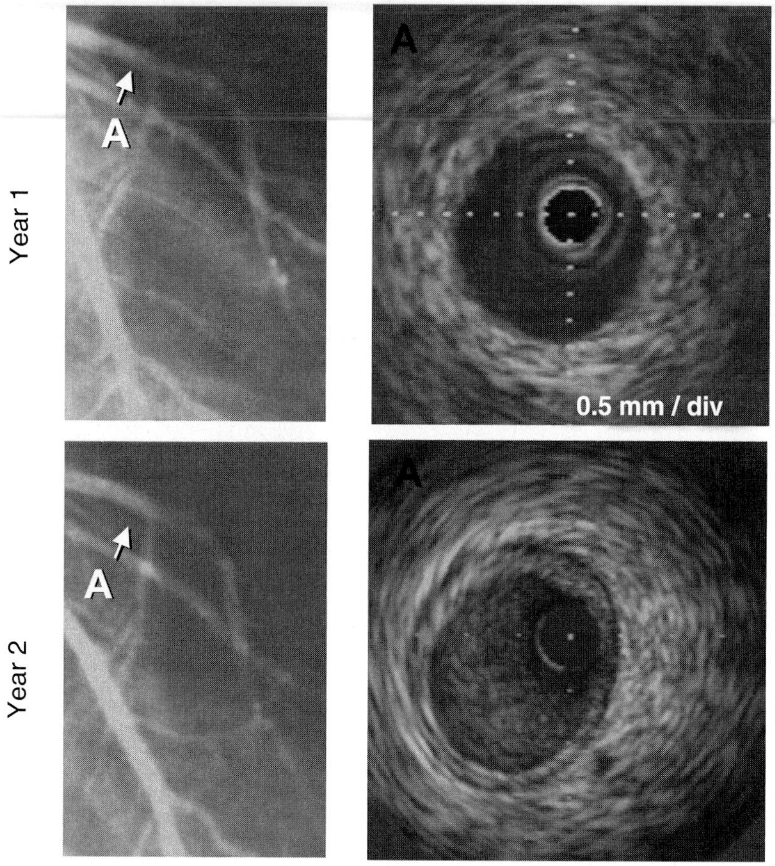

FIGURE 26–11 Graft coronary artery disease—appearance by angiography and intravascular ultrasound. The **left** panels show angiograms obtained on a transplanted heart at years 1 and 2 following engraftment. The **right** panels show intravascular ultrasound images obtained at the same time at the points labeled A in the angiogram. Note the progression of concentric intimal thickening that produces narrowing but not the appearance of a focal stenosis on the angiogram. These paired images show that the angiogram can underestimate the degree of intimal thickening in allograft coronary artery disease owing to the concentric nature of the intimal expansion. (From Lee RT, Braunwald E [eds]: Atlas of Cardiac Imaging. Philadelphia, Churchill Livingstone, 1998.

vasculopathy has led to clinical events is poor, with one study finding only 18 to 20 percent survival in heart transplant recipients 1 year after an ischemic clinical event. No drug or agent has been shown to reverse this disease, and the only definitive therapy available is retransplantation. The overall survival rates reported after retransplantation late after a first transplant are slightly inferior to those after the first transplant, and the use of scarce donor hearts for this purpose is a somewhat contentious issue in the transplant community.

Drug-Related Toxicity

Each of the drugs used in the immunosuppressive regimen comes with its inherent toxicity profile and set of drug interactions. The class of drugs now known as *calcineurin inhibitors* (cyclosporine and tacrolimus) was introduced into clinical heart transplantation in 1980, and the introduction was followed by marked improvement in survival. The class has subsequently provided the cornerstone of otherwise variable immunosuppressive regimens. These drugs have potent inherent nephrotoxicity and have led to the development of end-stage renal disease in many patients despite meticulous monitoring of drug levels. Newer drugs with less nephrotoxicity (but, of course, other toxicities) may eventually replace calcineurin inhibitors.

Overall Results

ISHLT maintains a registry of information regarding nearly 63,000 heart transplants that have been performed worldwide; every year, an annual report is presented containing data regarding survival, risk factors for mortality, and posttransplant functional status.[1] The number of reported heart transplants continues to decline for the past several years (Fig. 26–12). This decline results almost entirely from a decrease in transplants reported by non-U.S. centers. The age distribution of heart transplant recipients has changed in recent years (Fig. 26–13). The proportion of recipients in the 50- to 64-year and greater than 65-year age ranges has increased whereas the proportion in the 35- to 49-year age range has decreased. The age distribution of heart transplant donors, however, has remained relatively stable during the past several years. The major diagnoses in adult heart transplants continue to be idiopathic cardiomyopathy and ischemic cardiomyopathy (Fig. 26–14).

Over the past 20 years, survival after heart transplantation has improved, with 1-year, 5-year, 10-year, and 20-year survival rates of 80, 66, 29, and 16 percent, respectively (Fig. 26–15). Patient half-life (i.e., time to 50 percent survival)

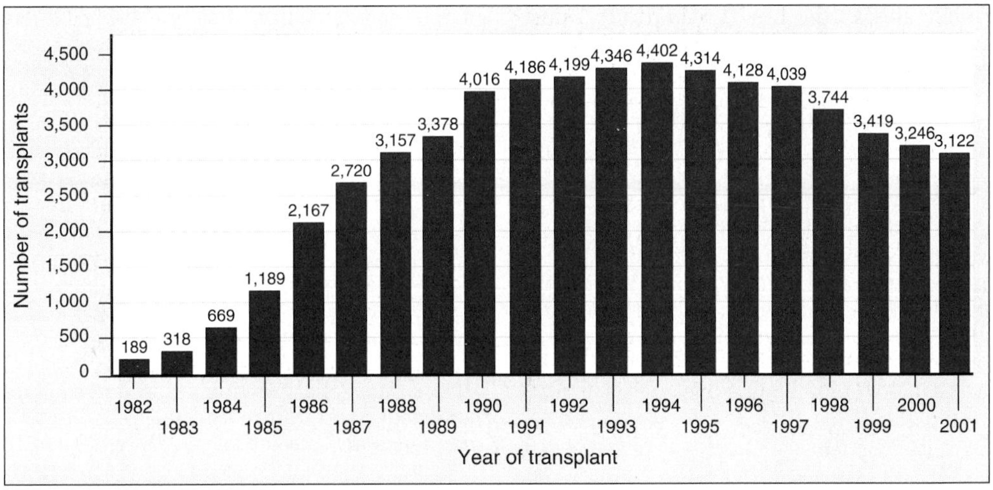

FIGURE 26–12 Number of heart transplants by year. (From Taylor DO, Edwards LB, Mohacsi PJ, et al: The registry of The International Society for Heart and Lung Transplantation: Twentieth official adult heart transplant report—2003. J Heart Lung Transplant 22:616, 2003.)

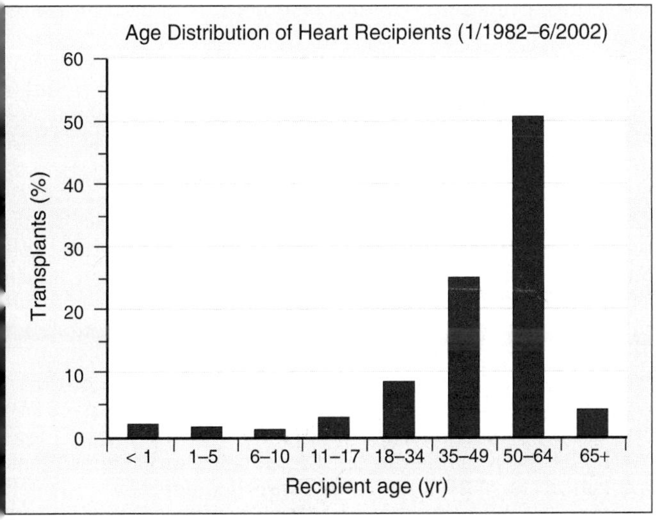

FIGURE 26–13 Age distribution of heart transplant recipients as reported between January 1982 and June 2002. (From Taylor DO, Edwards LB, Mohacsi PJ, et al: The registry of The International Society for Heart and Lung Transplantation: Twentieth official adult heart transplant report—2003. J Heart Lung Transplant 22:616, 2003.)

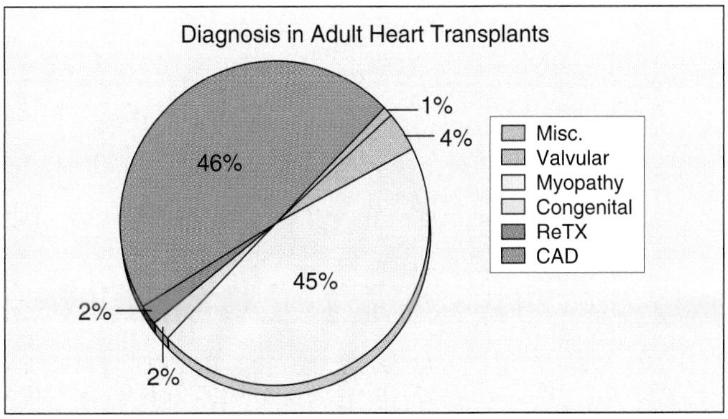

FIGURE 26–14 Diagnoses of adult heart transplant recipients. CAD = coronary artery disease; ReTX = retransplant. (From Taylor DO, Edwards LB, Mohacsi PJ, et al: The registry of The International Society for Heart and Lung Transplantation: Twentieth official adult heart transplant report—2003. J Heart Lung Transplant 22:616, 2003.)

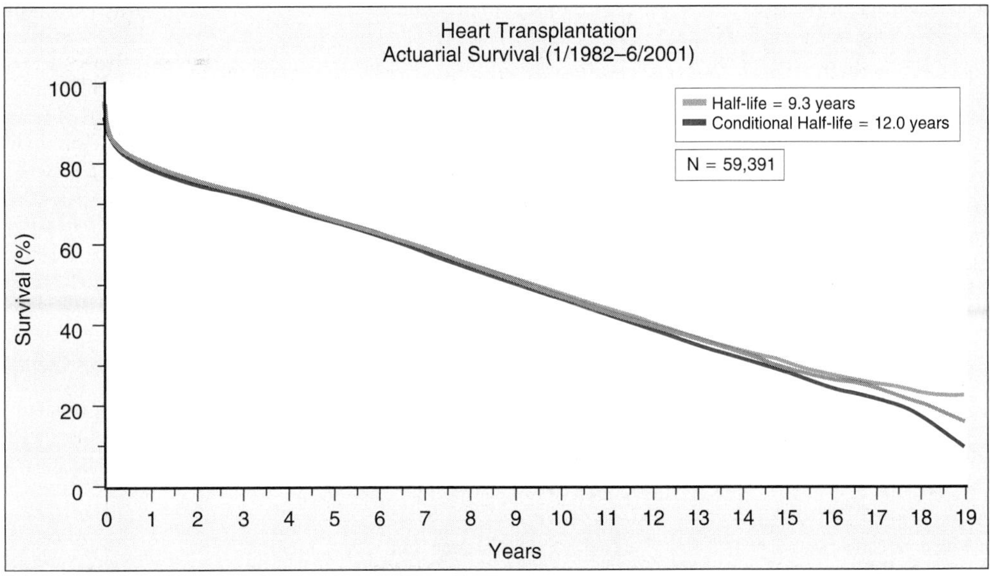

FIGURE 26–15 Actuarial survival for heart transplants performed between January 1982 and June 2001. (From Taylor DO, Edwards LB, Mohacsi PJ, et al: The registry of The International Society for Heart and Lung Transplantation: Twentieth official adult heart transplant report—2003. J Heart Lung Transplant 22:616, 2003.)

is 9.3 years. Survival rates in the first 2 years after transplantation have improved over the last 20 years, but late survival has changed little. When patients transplanted after 1982 are grouped into arbitrary 4- to 5-year eras, survival improves with each successive era (Fig. 26–16).

The ISHLT lists the following as major risk factors for 1-year mortality: underlying diagnosis of congenital heart disease, patient in hospital and/or on ventilator before transplant, PRA >10 percent, and dialysis. Additional risk factors include older donor age, older recipient age, increased donor heart ischemic time, and elevated recipient bilirubin or creatinine. While in the past, an underlying diagnosis of coronary artery disease, retransplantation, the presence of an intra-aortic balloon pump or ventricular assist device at the time of transplant, or a history of malignancy were risk factors for 1-year mortality, they are not risk factors in the most recent cohort of patients. Five-year mortality risk factors include graft coronary artery disease within the first posttransplant year, infection prior to transplant discharge or during the first posttransplant year, cerebrovascular disease at transplant, insulin-dependent diabetes, and underlying diagnosis of coronary artery disease.

Approximately 40 percent of patients are hospitalized in the first posttransplant year, often for treatment of rejection or infection. By the second posttransplant year, only 20 percent are hospitalized. The vast majority report good functional status after transplantation. Nevertheless, less than 40 percent of heart transplant recipients return to work after transplantation. Thus, despite the lack of sufficient donor organs, and the growing importance of device therapy for end-stage heart failure, cardiac transplantation can offer independence and a relatively high quality of life to many.

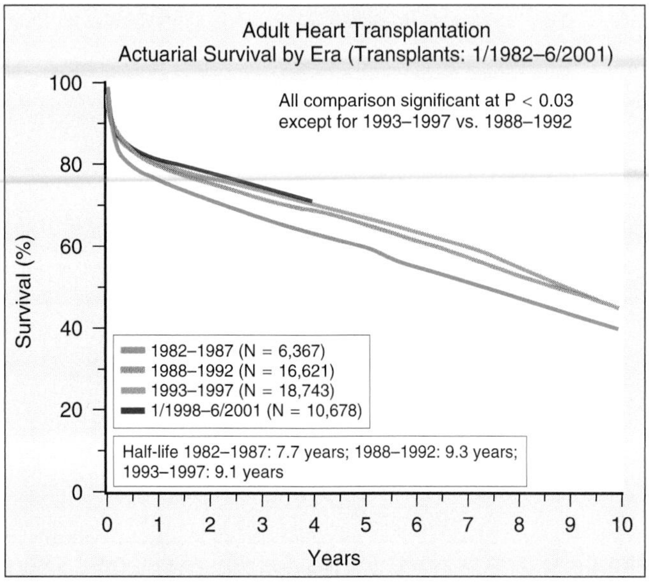

FIGURE 26–16 Actuarial survival for heart transplants performed between January 1982 and June 2001 by era of transplantation. (From Taylor DO, Edwards LB, Mohacsi PJ, et al: The registry of The International Society for Heart and Lung Transplantation: Twentieth official adult heart transplant report—2003. J Heart Lung Transplant 22:616, 2003.)

Heart-Lung Transplantation

Since the initial clinical transplants performed by Reitz and associates at Stanford in 1981, the field of heart-lung transplantation has evolved dramatically, particularly over the last several years. Heart-lung transplantation was developed initially for patients suffering from severe pulmonary vascular disease, specifically primary pulmonary hypertension and Eisenmenger syndrome secondary to congenital heart disease. A total of 2190 heart-lung transplants were performed between January 1992 and June 2002 (Fig. 26–17). The diagnostic profile of heart-lung transplant recipients reported to the Registry of the ISHLT through 2002 lists pulmonary hypertension secondary to congenital heart disease as the most frequent diagnosis, accounting for 32 percent of these procedures ($n = 705$). Primary pulmonary hypertension associated with irreversible right heart failure is the second most common indication for heart-lung transplantation, with 24 percent of recipients carrying this diagnosis ($n = 526$). Despite the widespread use of bilateral lung transplantation, cystic fibrosis remains the third most common diagnosis, the indication for 16 percent of these patients ($n = 341$).[35] However, the trend over the past few years has been to reserve combined heart and lung transplantation for patients who are not candidates for double-lung transplantation and cardiac repair because of concomitant end-stage pulmonary and cardiac disease processes.

The technique of heart-lung transplantation has also evolved over the last several years. The standard biatrial technique for the heart transplant has been converted to the bicaval technique (see Figs. 26–6 through 26–8). The physiological advantages of the bicaval technique have already been discussed in the heart transplant section and apply to heart-lung transplantation as well. The second major change in the operative technique is the positioning of the pulmonary hila anterior to the phrenic nerve pedicle.[36] This modification requires less posterior mediastinal dissection, which decreases the rates of phrenic and vagus nerve injury. It also affords

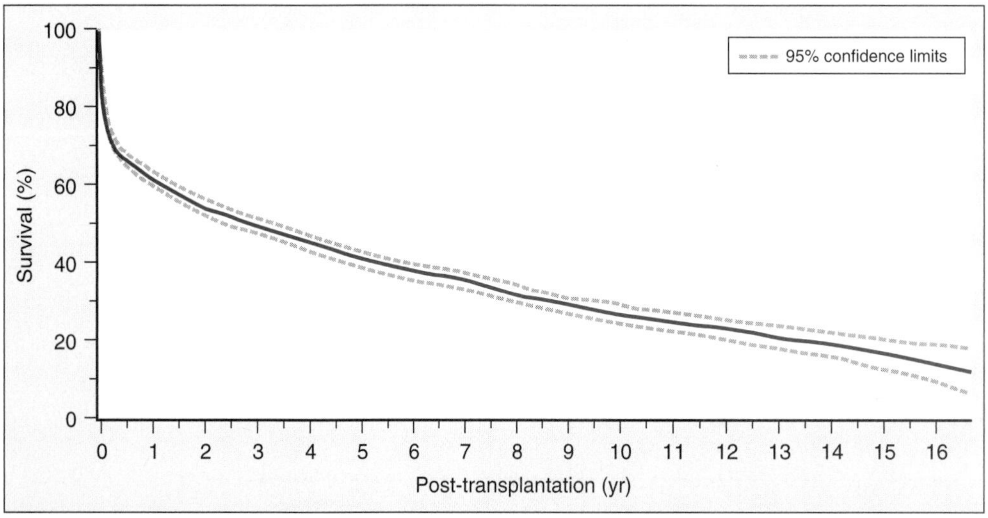

FIGURE 26–17 Actuarial curve showing survival rate after heart-lung transplantation (January 1992 to June 2002).(From Taylor Do, Edwards LB, Mohacsi PJ, et al: The registry of The International Society for Heart and Lung Transplantation: Twentieth official adult heart transplant report—2003. J Heart Lung Transplant 22:616, 2003.)

easier access to the posterior mediastinum for inspection of bleeding while still on CPB.

The actuarial survival for adult heart-lung transplant recipients at 1, 5, and 10 years were 61, 40, and 25 percent, respectively (see Fig. 26–17).[35] Recipients with Eisenmenger syndrome have had significantly better survival rates than those with other congenital anomalies or primary pulmonary hypertension. The cause of early mortality include graft failure, non-CMV infection, and technical complications, together accounting for 80 percent of the deaths. After the first year of transplantation, the most common cause of death is chronic rejection manifested as obliterative bronchiolitis (OB). The overall prevalence of OB in patients surviving heart-lung transplantation longer than 3 months was 64 percent, with an overall mortality greater than 70 percent after 5 years of follow-up.[37] The incidence and severity of transplant coronary artery disease are significantly less when compared with the heart transplantation population but affect approximately 10 percent of patients within 5 years following transplantation.

Heart-lung transplantation continues to be an accepted therapy for selected patients with end-stage cardiopulmonary disease. The goal of restoring the function of heart-lung transplantation without significant long-term morbidity and mortality will require considerable advances in immunosuppression and immunotolerance.

REFERENCES

1. Taylor DO, Edwards LB, Mohacsi PJ, et al: The registry of the International Society for Heart and Lung Transplantation: Twentieth Offiicial Adult Heart Transplant Report 2003. J Heart Lung Transplant 22:616-624, 2003.

Heart Transplantation: The Operation

2. Aziz TM, Burgess MI, El Gamel A, et al: Orthotopic cardiac transplantation technique: A survey of current practice. Ann Thorac Surg 68:1242-1246, 1999.
3. Aziz T, Burgess M, Khafagy R, et al: Bicaval and standard techniques in orthotopic heart transplantation: Medium-term experience in cardiac performance and survival. J Thorac Cardiovasc Surg 118:115-122, 1999.
4. Traversi E, Pozzoli M, Grande A, et al: The bicaval anastomosis technique for orthotopic heart transplantation yields better atrial function than the standard technique: An echocardiographic automatic boundary detection study. J Heart Lung Transplant 17:1065-1074, 1998.
5. Miniati DN, Robbins RC: Techniques in orthotopic cardiac transplantation: A review. Cardiol Rev 9:131-136, 2001.
6. Aziz TM, Saad RA, Burgess MI, et al: Clinical signifiicance of tricuspid valve dysfuntion after orthotopic heart transplantation. J Heart Lung Transplant 21:1101-1108, 2002.
7. Aziz TM, Burgess MI, Rahman AN, et al: Risk factors for tricuspid valve regurgitation after orthotopic heart transplantation. Ann Thorac Surg 68:1247-1251, 1999.
8. Sze DY, Robbins RC, Semba CP, et al: Superior vena cava syndrome after heart transplantation: Percutaneous treatment of a complication of bicaval anastomoses. J Thorac Cardiovasc Surg 116:253-261, 1998.

Recipient Selection

9. Aaronson KD, Schwartz JS, Chen T-M, et al: Development and prospective validation of a clinical index to predict survival in ambulatory patients referred for cardiac transplant evaluation. Circulation 95:2660-2667, 1997.
10. Mancini DM, Eisen H, Kussmaul W, et al: Value of peak exercise consumption for optimal timing of cardiac transplantation in ambulatory patients with heart failure. Circulation 83:778-786, 1991.
11. Osada N, Chaitman BR, Miller LW, et al: Cardiopulmonary exercise testing identifiie low-risk patients with heart failure and severely impaired exercise capacity considered for heart transplantation. J Am Coll Cardiol 31:577-582, 1998.
12. Myers J, Gullestad L, Vagelos R, et al: Clinical, hemodynamic, and cardiopulmonary exercise test determinants of survival in patients referred for evaluation of heart failure. Ann Intern Med 129:286-293, 1998.
13. Cimato TR, Jessup M: Recipient selection in cardiac transplantation: Contraindications and risk factors for mortality. J Heart Lung Transplant 21:1161-1173, 2002.
14. Costard-Jackle, Fowler MB: Inflluence of preoperative pulmonary artery pressure on motality after heart transplantation: Test of potential reversibility of pulmonary hypertension with nitroprusside is useful in defiining a high-risk group. J Am Coll Cardio 19:48-54, 1992.
15. Natale ME, Pina I: Evaluation of pulmonary hypertension in heart transplant candidates. Curr Opin Cardiol 18:136-140, 2003.
16. Haraldsson A, Kieler-Jensen N, Nathorst-Westfelt U, et al: Comparison of inhaled nitric oxide and inhaled aerosolized prostacyclin in the evaluation of heart transplant candidates with elevated pulmonary vascular resistance. Chest 114:780-786, 1998.
17. Sablotzki A, Hentschel T, Gruenig I, et al: Hemodynamic effects of inhaled aerosolized iloprost and inhaled nitric oxide in heart transplant candidates with elevated pulmonary vascular resistance. Eur J Cardiothorac Surg 22:746-752, 2002.
18. Zaroff JG, Rosengard BR, Armstrong WF, et al: Consensus conference report: Maximizing Use of Organs Recovered from the Cadaver Donor—Cardiac Recommendations, March 28-29, 2001, Crystal City, VA. Circulation 106:836-841, 2002.
19. Harringer W, Haverich A: Heart and heart-lung transplantation: Standards and improvements. World J Surg 26:218-225, 2002.
20. Del Rizzo DF, Menkis AH, Pfllugfelder PW, et al: The role of donor age and ischemi time on survival following orthotopic heart transplantation. J Heart Lung Transplant 18:310-319, 1999.
21. Wheeldon DR, Potter CD, Oduro A, et al: Transforming the "unacceptable" donor: Outcomes from the adoption of a standardized donor management technique. J Heart Lung Transplant 14:734-742, 1995.
22. Stoica SC, Satchithananda DK, Charman S, et al: Swan-Ganz catheter assessment of donor hearts: Outcome of organs with borderline hemodynamics. J Heart Lung Transplant 21:615-622, 2002.
23. Jahania MS, Sanchez JA, Narayan P, et al: Heart preservation for transplantation: Principles and strategies. Ann Thorac Surg 68:1983-1987, 1999.
24. Beniaminovitz A, Itescu S, Lietz K, et al: Prevention of rejection in cardiac transplantation by blockade of the interleukin-2 receptor with a monoclonal antibody. N Engl J Med 342:613-619, 2000.

Physiology of the Transplanted Heart

25. Givertz MM, Hartley LH, Colucci W: Long-term sequential changes in exercise capacity and chronotropic responsiveness after cardiac transplantation. Circulation 96:232-237, 1997.
26. Osada N, Chaitman BR, Donohue TJ, et al: Long-term cardiopulmonary exercise performance after heart transplantation. Am J Cardiol 79:451-456, 1997.
27. Mettauer B, Zhao QM, Epailly E, et al: Vo_2 kinetics reveal a central limitation at the onset of subthreshold exercise in heart transplant recipients. J Appl Physiol 88:1228-1238, 2000.
28. Bengel FM, Ueberfuhr P, Schiepel N, et al: Effect of sympathetic reinnervation on cardiac performance after heart transplantation. N Engl J Med 345:731-738, 2001.
29. Billingham ME, Cary NR, Hammond ME, et al: A working formulation for the standardization of nomenclature in the diagnosis of heart and lung rejection: Heart Rejection Study Group. The International Society for Heart Transplantation. J Heart Transplant 9:587-593, 1990.
30. Penn I: Occurrence of cancers in immunosuppressed organ transplant recipients. Clin Transpl 11:147-158, 1998.
31. Cook RC, Connors JM, Gascoyne RD, et al: Treatment of post-transplant lymphoproliferative disease with rituximab monoclonal antibody after lung transplantation. Lancet 354:1698-1699, 1999.
32. Zilz ND, Olson LJ, McGregor CG: Treatment of post-transplant lymphoproliferative disorder with monoclonal CD20 antibody (rituximab) after heart transplantation. J Heart Lung Transplant 20:770-772, 2001.
33. Dotti G, Rambaldi A, Fiocchi R, et al: Anti-CD20 antibody (rituximab) administration in patients with late-occurring lymphomas after solid organ transplant. Haematologica 86:618-623, 2001.
34. Kobashigawa JA: First-year intravascular ultrasound results as a surrogate marker for outcomes after heart transplantation. J Heart Lung Transplant 22:711-714, 2003.

Heart-Lung Transplantation

35. Trulock EP, Edwards LB, Taylor DO, et al: The registry of the International Society for Heart and Lung Transplantation: Twentieth Offiicial Adult Lung and Heart-Lung Transplant Report—2003. J Heart Lung Transplant 22:625-635, 2003.
36. Lick SD, Copeland JG, Rosado LJ, et al: Simplifiied technique of heart-lung transplanttion. Ann Thorac Surg 59:1592-1593, 1995.
37. Reichenspurner H, Girgis RE, Robbins RC, et al: Stanford experience with obliterative bronchiolitis after lung and heart-lung transplantation. Ann Thorac Surg 62:1467-1472, 1996.

PART IV

Arrhythmias, Sudden Death, and Syncope

CHAPTER 27

Genesis of Cardiac Arrhythmias: Electrophysiological Considerations

Michael Rubart • Douglas P. Zipes

Anatomy of the Cardiac Conduction System

Sinus Node

In humans, the sinus node is a spindle-shaped structure composed of a fibrous tissue matrix with closely packed cells. It is 10 to 20 mm long, 2 to 3 mm wide, and thick, tending to narrow caudally toward the inferior vena cava. It lies less than 1 mm from the epicardial surface, laterally in the right atrial sulcus terminalis at the junction of the superior vena cava and right atrium (Figs. 27–1 and 27–2). The artery supplying the sinus node branches from the right (55 to 60 percent of the time) or the left (40 to 45 percent) circumflex coronary artery and approaches the node from a clockwise or counterclockwise direction around the superior vena caval–right atrial junction.

CELLULAR STRUCTURE. Cells from the sinoatrial node region exhibit a wide variety of morphologies, including spindle- and spider-shaped cells, rod-shaped atrial cells with clear striations, and small round cells corresponding to endothelial cells.[1] Only the spindle- and spider-shaped cells exhibit the typical electrophysiological characteristics of pacemaker cells, including the presence of the hyperpolarization-activated current, I_f,[2] and absence of the inwardly rectifying potassium current, I_{K1}, as well as spontaneous beating under physiological conditions.[3,4]

GAP JUNCTIONS AND SINOATRIAL COUPLING. The sinoatrial node requires a delicate balance of intercellular electrical coupling in order to maintain its function as a pacemaker. Excess electrical coupling depresses sinus node automaticity because the sinus node membrane potential is damped by the surrounding atrial myocardium to a more negative potential than the normal maximal diastolic potential, thereby inhibiting spontaneous diastolic depolarization (see Fig. 27–14). Too little coupling may prevent impulse transmission to the adjacent atrial muscle. Restriction of the hyperpolarizing influence of the atrial muscle on the sinus node while maintaining impulse exit into the crista terminalis is achieved by the composition and spatial organization of connexins, proteins that form gap junction channels responsible for intercellular current fluxes (see under Intercalated Discs). Connexin40 and connexin45, but not connexin43, are expressed in the central sinus node (Fig. 27–3). The major part of the crista terminalis–sinus node border exhibits a sharp demarcation boundary of connexin43-expressing atrial myocytes and connexin40/connexin45-expressing myocytes. On the endocardial site a transitional zone between the crista terminalis and the peripheral node exists in which connexin45 and connexin43 are colocalized.[5] This colocalization of different connexin isoforms raises the possibility that individual gap junctional channels in the transitional zone are formed by more than one connexin isoform.[1] These disparate connexin phenotypes may create specific types of hybrid channels with rectifying electrical properties that ensure the maintenance of sinus node pacemaker activity but diminish electrotonic interference from the atrial muscle.[1,6,7]

FUNCTION. Very probably, no single cell in the sinus node serves as *the* pacemaker. Rather, sinus nodal cells function as electrically coupled oscillators that discharge synchronously because of mutual entrainment. Thus, faster discharging cells are slowed by cells firing more slowly, and they themselves are sped so that a "democratically derived" discharge rate occurs.[8] The interaction depends on the degree of coupling and the electrophysiological characteristics of the individual sinoatrial node cell. The resulting rate is not just a simple average of each of the cells. With an individual pacemaker cell coupled to an average of five other cells,[8] each with potentially different electrophysiological properties, the resulting discharge rate is not obvious. In humans, sinus rhythm may result from impulse origin at widely separated sites, with two or three individual

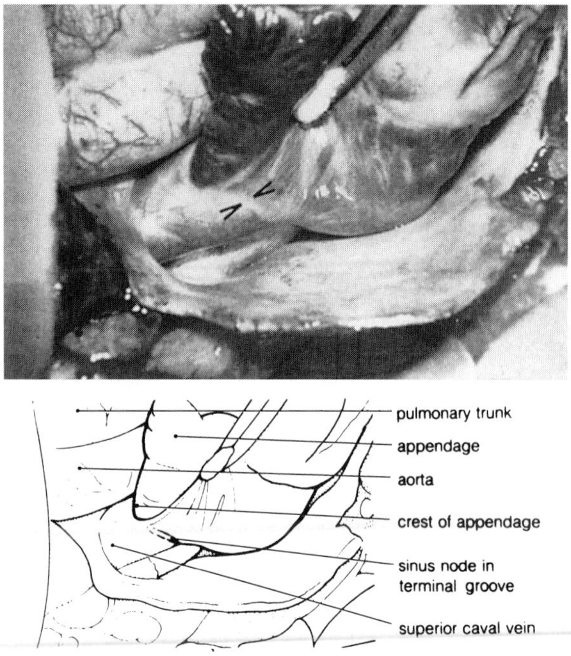

FIGURE 27–1 The human sinus node. This photograph, taken in the operating room, shows the location of the normal cigar-shaped sinus node along the lateral border of the terminal groove at the superior vena cava–atrial junction (arrowheads). (From Anderson RH, Wilcox BR, Becker AE: Anatomy of the normal heart. *In* Hurst JW, Anderson RH, Becker AE, Wilcox BR [eds]: Atlas of the Heart. New York, Gower, 1988, p 1.2.)

wave fronts created that merge to form a single, widely disseminated wave front.[8] Modulated parasystole can occur.

INNERVATION. The sinus node is densely innervated with postganglionic adrenergic and cholinergic nerve terminals.[9] Discrete vagal efferent pathways innervate both the sinus and atrioventricular (AV) regions of the dog and nonhuman primate. Most efferent vagal fibers to the atria appear to converge first at a single fat pad that is located between the medial portion of the superior vena cava and the aortic root, superior to the right pulmonary artery; the fibers then project onto two other fat pads found at the inferior vena cava-left atrial junction and the right pulmonary vein-atrial junction and subsequently project to both atria. Vagal fibers to the sinus and AV nodes also converge at the superior vena cava-aortic root fat pad before projection to the right pulmonary vein and inferior vena cava fat pads.[9] The concentration of norepinephrine is two to four times higher in atrial than in ventricular tissue in canine and guinea pig hearts. Although the sinus nodal region contains amounts of norepinephrine equivalent to those in other parts of the right atrium, acetylcholine, acetylcholinesterase, and choline acetyltransferase (the enzyme necessary for the synthesis of acetylcholine) have all been found in greatest concentration in the sinus node, with the next highest concentration in the right and then the left atrium. The concentration of acetylcholine in the ventricles is only 20 to 50 percent of that in the atria.

Neurotransmitters modulate the sinus node discharge rate by stimulation of beta-adrenergic and muscarinic receptors. Both beta$_1$ and beta$_2$ adrenoceptor subtypes are present in the sinoatrial node. Human sinoatrial nodes contain a more than threefold greater density of beta-adrenergic and muscarinic cholinergic receptors than adjacent atrial tissue.[8] The functional significance of beta adrenoceptor subtype diversity in the sinus node is unclear. Binding of receptor agonists released from sympathetic nerve terminals causes a positive chronotropic response through a beta$_1$ receptor-activated pathway involving the stimulatory guanosine triphosphate (GTP) regulatory protein (G_s), activation of adenylyl cyclase, intracellular accumulation of cyclic adenosine monophosphate (cAMP), stimulation of cAMP-dependent protein kinase A, and phosphorylation of target proteins (including the L-type Ca^{2+} channel, the channels underlying I_f, and the ryanodine-sensitive Ca^{2+} release channel [ryanodine receptor] in the sarcoplasmic reticulum membrane[10]). The second messenger pathway underlying beta$_2$ receptor activation–induced heart rate increase and the key target proteins are currently unknown but most likely involve an inhibitory GTP regulatory protein (G_i).[11] The negative chronotropic response of vagal stimulation is mediated by acetylcholine binding to and ensuing activation of M2 muscarinic receptors. Membrane currents regulated by muscarinic receptor activation include the acetylcholine- and adenosine-sensitive K^+ current ($I_{K(Ach,Ado)}$; see Table 22–3), $I_{Ca,L}$, and I_f. The effect of muscarinic receptor agonist in activating $I_{K(Ach,Ado)}$ is mediated by direct interaction of a G-protein subunit with the $K_{(Ach,Ado)}$ channel and does not require second messengers.[12] Activation of $I_{K(Ach,Ado)}$ causes hyperpolarization of the sinoatrial node cell membrane, resulting in a reduced rate of diastolic depolarization. Muscarinic receptor activation–mediated effects on $I_{Ca,L}$ and I_f are primarily due to a reduction in the intracellular cAMP level, thereby antagonizing the positive chronotropic effects of beta adrenoceptor stimulation.

Besides its negative chronotropic effect, acetylcholine also prolongs intranodal conduction time, at times to the point of sinus nodal exit block. Acetylcholine increases whereas norepinephrine decreases refractoriness in the center of the sinus node. The phase (timing) in the cardiac cycle at which vagal discharge occurs and the background sympathetic tone importantly influence vagal effects on the sinus rate and conduction (see later). After cessation of vagal stimulation, sinus nodal automatically may accelerate transiently (postvagal tachycardia). The neurotransmitters neuropeptide Y (NPY) and vasoactive intestinal peptide (VIP) are localized in sympathetic and parasympathetic nerve terminals, respectively. VIP reversibly increases I_f, whereas NPY reversibly decreases I_f.[13] The role of other peripheral neurotransmitters (such as calcitonin gene-related peptide, substance P) in controlling sinus node electrophysiology is unclear.

Internodal and Intraatrial Conduction

Whether impulses travel from the sinus to the AV node over preferentially conducting pathways has been contested. Anatomical evidence has been interpreted to indicate the presence of three intraatrial pathways. The *anterior internodal pathway* begins at the anterior margin of the sinus node and curves anteriorly around the superior vena cava to enter the anterior interatrial band, called the *Bachmann bundle.* This band continues to the left atrium, with the anterior internodal pathway entering the superior margin of the AV node. The *Bachmann bundle* is a large muscle bundle that appears to conduct the cardiac impulse preferentially from the right to the left atrium. The *middle internodal tract* begins at the superior and posterior margins of the sinus node, travels behind the superior vena cava to the crest of the interatrial septum, and descends in the interatrial septum to the superior margin of the AV node. The *posterior internodal tract* starts at the posterior margin of the sinus node and travels posteriorly around the superior vena cava and along the crista terminalis to the eustachian ridge and then into the interatrial septum above the coronary sinus, where it joins the posterior portion of the AV node. Some fibers from all three tracts bypass the crest of the AV node and enter its more distal segment. These groups of internodal tissue are best referred to as *internodal atrial myocardium,* not tracts, because they do not appear to be histologically discrete specialized tracts, only plain atrial myocardium.

Preferential internodal conduction, that is, higher conduction velocity between the nodes in some parts of the atrium than in other parts, does exist and may be due to fiber orientation, size, geometry, or other factors rather than to specialized tracts located between the nodes. Impulse propagation from the atrium to the AV node occurs through multiple preferential input pathways. On the basis of their conduction velocities, these inputs are divided into fast, slow, and intermediate pathways. Notably, the atrial anterosuperior and posteroinferior inputs or approaches to the AV node are the anatomical substrates constituting the fast and slow pathways of AV nodal reentry.[14,15] The reentrant circuit of the slow/fast type begins counterclockwise with block in the fast pathway located at the apex of the Koch triangle, delay in the slow pathway located near the coronary sinus, then exit from the AV node to the fast pathway and return to the slow pathway through atrial tissue along the base of Koch's triangle. The reentrant circuit of the fast/slow type is clockwise. The term "triangle of Koch," however, has to be used with caution because histological studies of anatomically normal adult hearts demonstrated that the tendon of Todaro, which forms one side of the triangle of Koch, is absent in about two-thirds of hearts.[16]

The Atrioventricular Junctional Area and Intraventricular Conduction System

The normal AV junctional area (Figs. 27–4 and 27–5) can be divided into distinct regions: the transitional cell zone, also called nodal approaches; the compact portion, or the AV node itself; and the penetrating part of the AV bundle (His bundle), which continues as a nonbranching portion.

TRANSITIONAL CELL ZONE. In the rabbit AV node, the transitional cells or nodal approaches are located in posterior, superficial, and deep groups of cells. They differ histologically from atrial myocardium and connect the latter with the compact portion of the AV node. Some fibers may pass from the posterior internodal tract to the distal portion of the AV node or His bundle and provide the anatomical substrate for conduction to bypass AV nodal slowing. However, the importance of this structure is unclear.

The Atrioventricular Node

The compact portion of the AV node is a superficial structure lying just beneath the right atrial endocardium, anterior to the ostium of the coronary sinus, and directly above the insertion of the septal leaflet of the tricuspid valve. It is at the apex of a triangle formed by the tricuspid annulus and the tendon of Todaro, which originates in the central fibrous body and passes posteriorly through the atrial septum to continue with the eustachian valve (see Figs. 27–4 and 27–5; however, see previous comments on the triangle of Koch).[14,15] The compact portion of the AV node is divided from and becomes the penetrating portion of the His bundle at the point where it enters the central fibrous body. In 85 to 90 percent of human hearts, the arterial supply to the AV node is a branch from the right coronary artery that originates at the posterior intersection of the AV and interventricular grooves (crux). A branch of the circumflex coronary artery provides the AV nodal artery in the remaining hearts. Fibers in the lower part of the AV node may exhibit automatic impulse formation. The main function of the AV node is modulation of atrial impulse transmission to the ventricles, thereby coordinating atrial and ventricular contractions (Fig. 27–6).

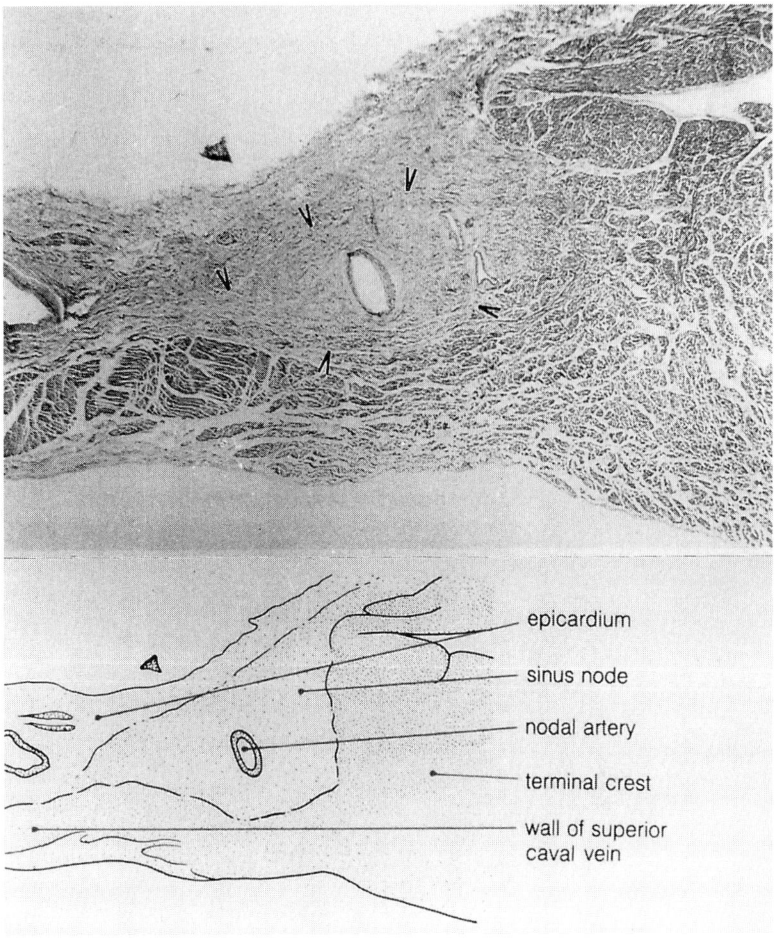

FIGURE 27–2 Histological section taken at right angles to the cigar-shaped sinus node shows that in short axis, the node is a wedge-shaped structure located between the wall of the superior vena cava and the terminal crest. Discrete boundaries between the sinus node and atrial muscle are noted (arrowheads). The node is penetrated by the sinus nodal artery. (From Anderson RH, Wilcox BR, Becker AE: Anatomy of the normal heart. *In* Hurst JW, Anderson RH, Becker AE, Wilcox BR [eds]: Atlas of the Heart. New York, Gower, 1988, p 1.2.)

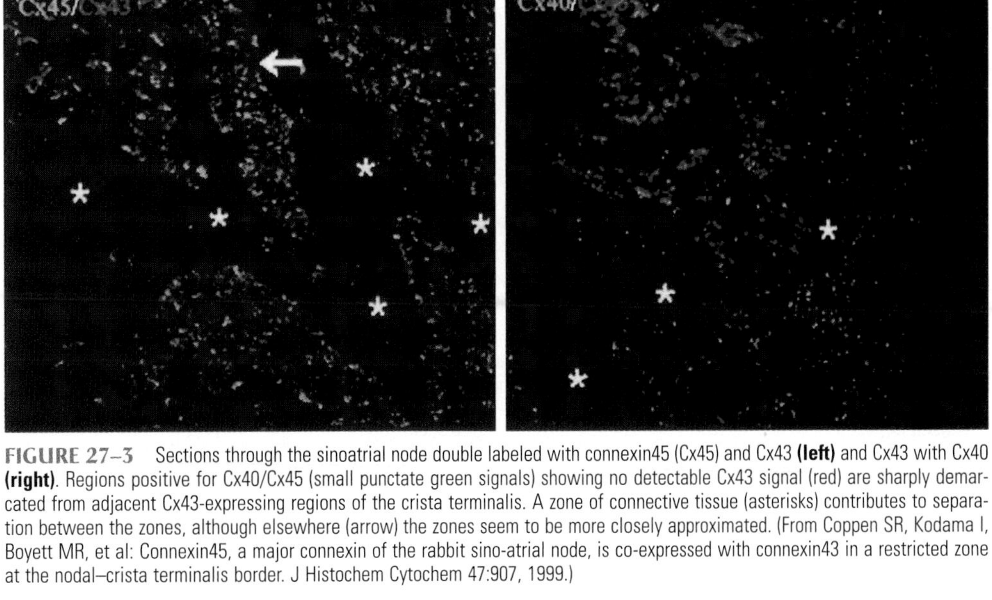

FIGURE 27–3 Sections through the sinoatrial node double labeled with connexin45 (Cx45) and Cx43 **(left)** and Cx43 with Cx40 **(right)**. Regions positive for Cx40/Cx45 (small punctate green signals) showing no detectable Cx43 signal (red) are sharply demarcated from adjacent Cx43-expressing regions of the crista terminalis. A zone of connective tissue (asterisks) contributes to separation between the zones, although elsewhere (arrow) the zones seem to be more closely approximated. (From Coppen SR, Kodama I, Boyett MR, et al: Connexin45, a major connexin of the rabbit sino-atrial node, is co-expressed with connexin43 in a restricted zone at the nodal–crista terminalis border. J Histochem Cytochem 47:907, 1999.)

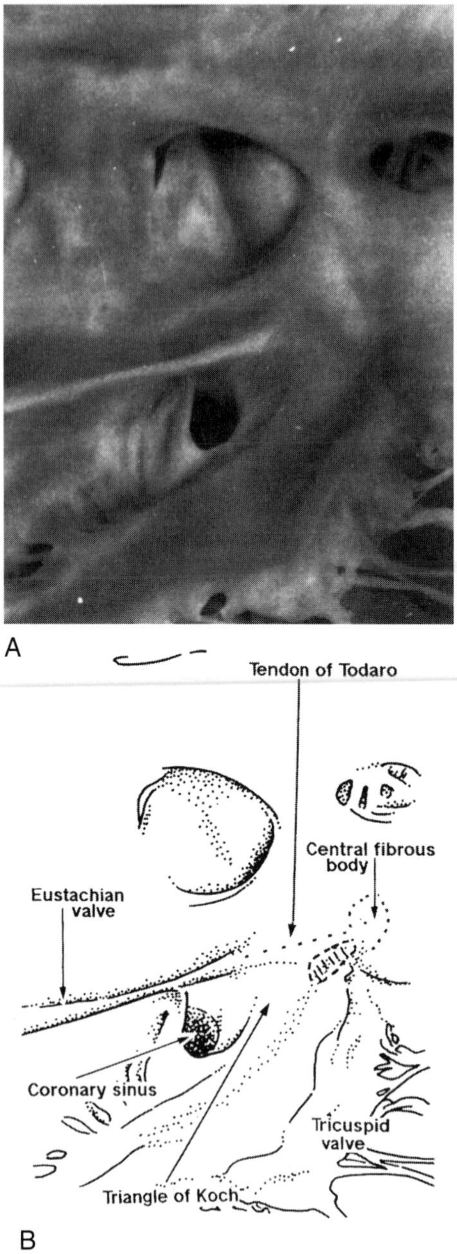

FIGURE 27–4 **A,** hotograph of a normal human heart showing the anatomical landmarks of the triangle of Koch. This triangle is delimited by the tendon of Todaro superiorly, which is the fibrous commissure of the flap guarding the openings of the inferior vena cava and coronary sinus, by the attachment of the septal leaflet of the tricuspid valve inferiorly, and by the mouth of the coronary sinus at the base. **B,** The stippled area adjacent to the central fibrous body is the approximate site of the compact atrioventricular node. (From Janse MJ, Anderson RH, McGuire MA, et al: "AV nodal" reentry: I. "AV nodal" reentry revisited. J Cardiovasc Electrophysiol 4:561, 1993.)

The Bundle of His, or Penetrating Portion of the Atrioventricular Bundle

This structure connects with the distal part of the compact AV node, perforates the central fibrous body, and continues through the annulus fibrosis, where it is called the nonbranching portion as it penetrates the membranous septum (see Fig. 27–5). Proximal cells of the penetrating portion are heterogeneous and resemble those of the compact AV node; distal cells are similar to cells in the proximal bundle branches. Connective tissue of the central fibrous body and membranous septum encloses the penetrating portion of the AV bundle, which may send out extensions into the central fibrous body.[17] However, large well-formed fasciculoventricular connections between the penetrating portion of the AV bundle and the ventricular septal crest are rarely found in adult hearts. Branches from the anterior and posterior descending coronary arteries supply the upper muscular interventricular septum with blood, which makes the conduction system at this site more impervious to ischemic damage unless the ischemia is extensive.

The Bundle Branches, or Branching Portion of the Atrioventricular Bundle

These structures begin at the superior margin of the muscular interventricular septum, immediately beneath the membranous septum, with the cells of the left bundle branch cascading downward as a continuous sheet onto the septum beneath the noncoronary aortic cusp (Fig. 27–7). The AV bundle may then give off other left bundle branches, sometimes constituting a true bifascicular system with an anterosuperior branch, in other hearts giving rise to a group of central fibers, and in still others appearing more as a network without a clear division into a fascicular system. The right bundle branch continues intramyocardially as an unbranched extension of the AV bundle down the right side of the interventricular septum to the apex of the right ventricle and base of the anterior papillary muscle. In some human hearts, the His bundle traverses the right interventricular crest and gives rise to a right-sided narrow stem origin of the left bundle branch. The anatomy of the left bundle branch system may be variable and may not conform to a constant bifascicular division. However, the concept of a trifascicular system remains useful to both the electrocardiographer and the clinician (see Fig. 27–7).

Terminal Purkinje Fibers

These fibers connect with the ends of the bundle branches to form interweaving networks on the endocardial surface of both ventricles that transmit the cardiac impulse almost simultaneously to the entire right and left ventricular endocardium. Purkinje fibers tend to be less concentrated at the base of the ventricle and at the papillary muscle tips. They penetrate the myocardium for varying distances depending on the animal species: In humans, they apparently penetrate only the inner third of the endocardium, whereas in the pig they almost reach the epicardium. Such variations could influence changes produced by myocardial ischemia, for example, because Purkinje fibers appear to be more resistant to ischemia than ordinary myocardial fibers are.

CELLULAR COMPOSITION OF THE ATRIOVENTRICULAR JUNCTIONAL AREA AND THE INTRAVENTRICULAR CONDUCTION SYSTEM. Transitional cells in the rabbit are elongated and smaller than atrial cells, stain more palely, and are separated by numerous strands of connective tissue.They merge at the entrance of the compact portion of the AV node, where the cells are small and spherical, not separated by muscle or connective tissue, and have very few nexuses.They interweave in interconnecting whorls of fasciculi.The AV node is divided on the basis of electrophysiological characteristics into AN, N, and NH regions.[18] In the rabbit, the AN region corresponds to the transitional cell groups of the posterior portion of the node, the NH region to the anterior portion of the bundle of lower nodal cells, and the N region to the small enclosed node where transitional cells merge with midnodal cells. *Dead-end pathways*—groups of cells that form an apparent electrophysiological cul-de-sac that does not contribute to overall conduction in the node—are also found at several sites. Cells in the penetrating bundle remain similar to compact AV nodal cells.

Purkinje cells are found in the His bundle and bundle branches, cover much of the endocardium of both ventricles, and align to form multicellular bundles in longitudinal strands separated by collagen. Although conduction of the cardiac impulse appears to be their major function, free-running Purkinje fibers, sometimes called *false tendons,* which are

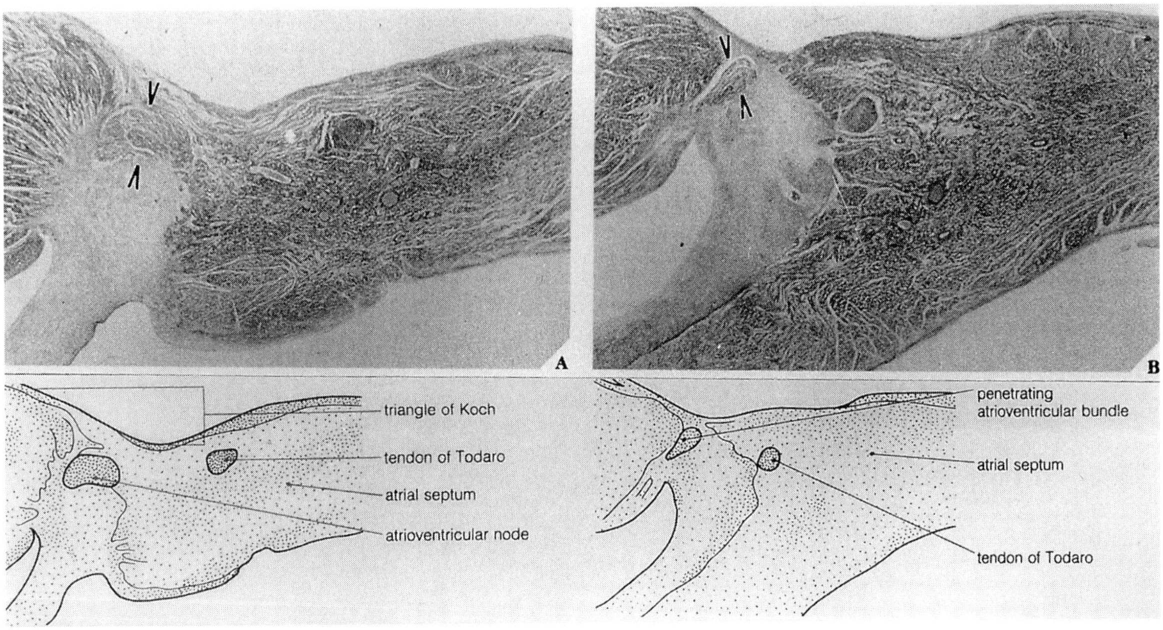

FIGURE 27–5 Sections through the atrioventricular (AV) junction show the position of the AV node (arrowhead) within the triangle of Koch **(A)** and the penetrating AV bundle of His (arrowheads) within the central fibrous body **(B)**. (From Anderson RH, Wilcox BR, Becker AE: Anatomy of the normal heart. *In* Hurst JW, Anderson RH, Becker AE, Wilcox BR [eds]. Atlas of the Heart. New York, Gower, 1988, p 1.2.)

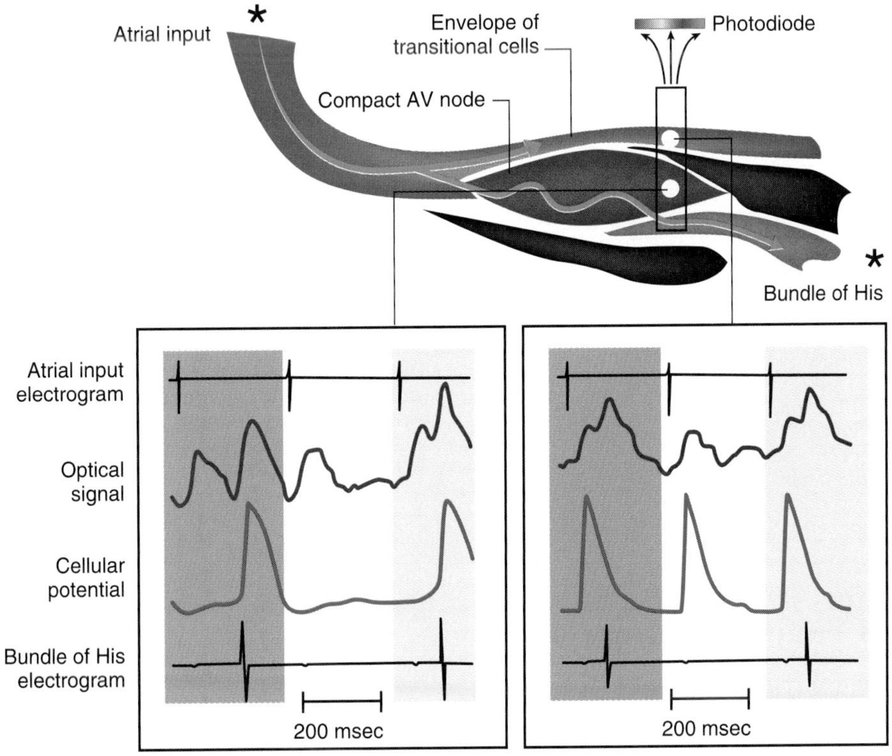

FIGURE 27–6 Multilayer conduction pattern in the atrioventricular (AV) node. Diagram of a cross section through the rabbit AV junction perpendicular to the endocardial atrial surface. The compact node (red) is covered with a superficial layer of transitional cells (blue), providing a connection between the atrial tissue and the compact node. The compact node, in turn, connects to the bundle of His (orange). Connective tissue protrusions are shown in black. Optical recordings of membrane potential changes obtained with a photodiode from the underlying tissue were accompanied by local electrograms from the atrial input to the AV node and from the bundle of His (asterisks). In addition, a microelectrode was used to measure transmembrane potentials at different AV node layers (circles). Each of the **lower panels** illustrates three consecutive heartbeats with simultaneously acquired atrial input and His electrograms, along with optical and microelectrode signals. In the time interval between an atrial input activation and ensuing activation of the bundle of His, two distinct optical action potentials can be identified. The first component corresponds to the depolarization of cells located in the superficial transitional cell layer, whereas the second component reflects the depolarization of cells in the distal portion of the compact AV node. The second beats (white strips) are blocked in the AV node, as indicated by the absence of the signal from the distal portion of the AV node but continued presence of the signal obtained from the transitional cell layer. (From Efimov IR, Mazgalev TN: High resolution three-dimensional fluorescent imaging reveals multiplayer conduction pattern in the atrioventricular node. Circulation 98:54, 1998. By permission of the American Heart Association.)

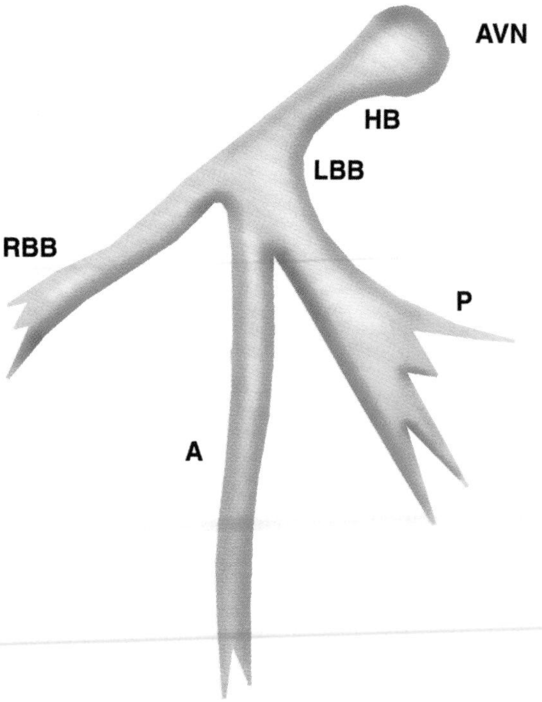

FIGURE 27–7 Schematic representation of the trifascicular bundle branch system. A = anterosuperior fascicle of the left bundle; AVN = atrioventricular node; HB = His bundle; LBB = main left bundle branch; P = posteroinferior fascicle of the left bundle branch; RBB = right bundle branch. (Modified from Rosenbaum MB, Elizari MV, Lazzari JO: The Hemiblocks. Oldsmar, Fla, Tampa Tracings, 1970, cover illustration.)

composed of many Purkinje cells in a series, are capable of contraction. Direct visualization of impulse conduction within the specialized conduction system using high-resolution optical mapping illustrated that action potentials propagate within thin Purkinje fiber bundles from base to apex before activation of the surrounding myocytes occurs.[19] Action potential propagation within the His-Purkinje system and the working myocardium is mediated by connexins. Ventricular myocytes express mainly connexin43 and Purkinje fibers express connexin40 and connexin45.[19,20] The molecular identity of the connexin type that enables impulse transmission at the Purkinje fiber-myocyte junction (PMJ) is unclear. It is also still not clear how the small amount of depolarizing current provided by the thin bundle of Purkinje fibers can activate a much larger mass of ventricular muscle (current-to-load mismatch).[21] It is possible that individual gap junctional channels at the PMJ are formed by more than one connexin isoform.[20] These disparate connexin phenotypes may create specific types of hybrid channels with unique properties that ensure safe conduction at the PMJ. Because Purkinje cells have markedly longer repolarization times than surrounding myocytes (see Fig. 27-15), these connexin hybrids could also decrease entrainment of repolarization at the PMJ and thereby increase repolarization gradients.

Innervation of the Atrioventricular Node, His Bundle, and Ventricular Myocardium

PATHWAYS OF INNERVATION. The AV node and His bundle region are innervated by a rich supply of cholinergic and adrenergic fibers with a density exceeding that found in the ventricular myocardium. Ganglia, nerve fibers, and nerve nets lie close to the AV node. Parasympathetic nerves to the AV node region enter the canine heart at the junction of the inferior vena cava and the inferior aspect of the left atrium, adjacent to the coronary sinus entrance. Nerves in direct contact with AV nodal fibers have been noted, along with agranular and granular vesicular processes, presumably representing cholinergic and adrenergic processes. Acetylcholine release may be concentrated around the N region of the AV node.[9]

In general, autonomic neural input to the heart exhibits some degree of "sidedness," with the right sympathetic and vagal nerves affecting the sinus node more than the AV node and the left sympathetic and vagal nerves affecting the AV node more than the sinus node. The distribution of the neural input to the sinus and AV nodes is complex because of substantial overlapping innervation. Despite the overlap, specific branches of the vagal and sympathetic nerves can be shown to innervate certain regions preferentially, and sympathetic or vagal nerves to the sinus node can be interrupted discretely without affecting AV nodal innervation. Similarly, vagal or sympathetic neural input to the AV node can be interrupted without affecting sinus innervation. Supersensitivity to acetylcholine follows vagal denervation. Stimulation of the right stellate ganglion produces sinus tachycardia with less effect on AV nodal conduction, whereas stimulation of the left stellate ganglion generally produces a shift in the sinus pacemaker to an ectopic site and consistently shortens AV nodal conduction time and refractoriness but inconsistently speeds the sinus nodal discharge rate. Stimulation of the right cervical vagus nerve primarily slows the sinus nodal discharge rate, and stimulation of the left vagus primarily prolongs AV nodal conduction time and refractoriness when sidedness is present. Although neither sympathetic nor vagal stimulation affects normal conduction in the His bundle, either can affect abnormal AV conduction. The negative dromotropic response of the heart to vagal stimulation is mediated by activation of $I_{K(Ach,Ado)}$, which results in hyperpolarization of the AV nodal cells, thereby influencing the conductive properties of the node. The positive dromotropic effect of sympathetic stimulation arises as a consequence of activation of the L-type Ca^{2+} current, $I_{Ca.L}$ (see Table 27-3).

Most efferent sympathetic impulses reach the canine ventricles over the ansae subclaviae, branches from the stellate ganglia. Sympathetic nerves then synapse primarily in the caudal cervical ganglia and form individual cardiac nerves that innervate relatively localized parts of the ventricles. On the right side, the major route to the heart is the recurrent cardiac nerve, and on the left, the ventrolateral cardiac nerve. In general, the right sympathetic chain shortens refractoriness primarily of the anterior portion of the ventricles and the left affects primarily the posterior surface of the ventricles, although overlapping areas of distribution occur.

The intraventricular route of sympathetic nerves generally follows coronary arteries. Functional data suggest that afferent and efferent sympathetic nerves travel in the superficial layers of the epicardium and dive to innervate the endocardium, and anatomical observations support this conclusion. Vagal fibers travel intramurally or subendocardially and rise to the epicardium at the AV groove (Fig. 27-8).[9]

EFFECTS OF VAGAL STIMULATION. The vagus modulates cardiac sympathetic activity at prejunctional and postjunctional sites by regulating the amount of norepinephrine released and by inhibiting cAMP–induced phosphorylation of cardiac proteins such as phospholamban. The latter inhibition occurs at more than one level in the series of reactions constituting the adenylate cyclase-, AMP-dependent protein kinase system. Neuropeptides released from nerve fibers of both autonomic limbs also modulate autonomic responses. For example, NPY released from sympathetic nerve terminals inhibits cardiac vagal effects.[22]

Tonic vagal stimulation produces a greater absolute reduction in sinus rate in the presence of tonic background sympathetic stimulation, a sympathetic-parasympathetic interaction termed *accentuated antagonism.* In contrast, changes in AV conduction during concomitant sympathetic and vagal stimulation are essentially the *algebraic sum* of the individual AV conduction responses to tonic vagal and sympathetic stimulation alone. Cardiac responses to brief vagal bursts begin after a short latency and dissipate quickly; in contrast, cardiac responses to sympathetic stimulation commence and dissipate slowly. The rapid onset and offset of responses to vagal stimulation allow dynamic beat-to-beat vagal modulation of heart rate and AV conduction, whereas the slow temporal response to sympathetic stimulation precludes any beat-to-beat regulation by sympathetic activity. Periodic vagal bursting (as may occur each time a systolic pressure wave arrives at the baroreceptor regions in the aortic and carotid sinuses) induces phasic changes in sinus cycle length and can entrain the sinus node to discharge faster or slower at periods that are identical to those of the vagal burst. In a similar phasic manner, vagal bursts prolong AV nodal conduction time and are influenced by background levels of sympathetic tone. Because the peak vagal effects on sinus rate and AV nodal conduction occur at different times in the

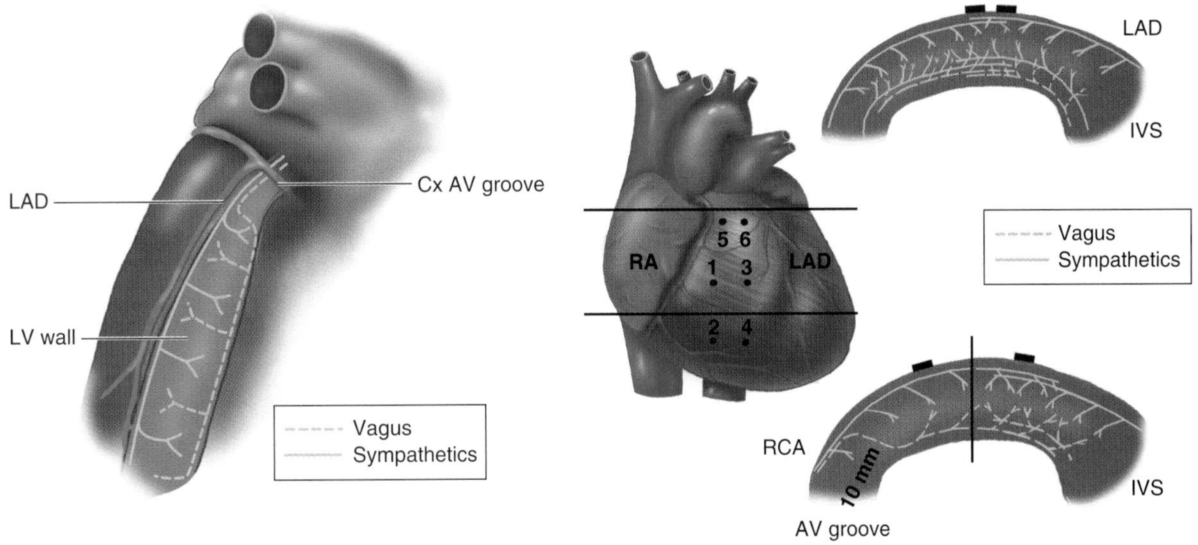

FIGURE 27–8 **Left,** Intraventricular route of sympathetic and vagal nerves to the left ventricle. **Right,** Schematic of the transverse views of the right ventricular (RV) wall showing functional pathways of the efferent sympathetic and vagal nerves. **Top right,** Transverse view of the RV outflow tract at the upper horizontal line on the left. **Bottom right,** Transverse view of the anterolateral wall at the lower horizontal line on the left. The vertical solid line indicates the center of the RV anterolateral wall. Closed circles indicate positions of plunge electrodes labeled 1 to 6. IVS = interventricular septum; LAD = left anterior descending coronary artery; RA = right atrium; RCA = right coronary artery. (From Ito M, Zipes DP: Efferent sympathetic and vagal innervation of the canine right ventricle. Circulation 90:1459, 1994. By permission of the American Heart Association.)

cardiac cycle, a brief vagal burst can slow the sinus rate without affecting AV nodal conduction or can prolong AV nodal conduction time and not slow the sinus rate.[22]

EFFECTS OF SYMPATHETIC STIMULATION. Stimulation of sympathetic ganglia shortens the refractory period equally in the epicardium and underlying endocardium of the left ventricular free wall, although dispersion of recovery properties occurs; that is, different degrees of shortening of refractoriness occur when measured at different epicardial sites. Nonuniform distribution of norepinephrine may, in part, contribute to some of the nonuniform electrophysiological effects because the ventricular content of norepinephrine is greater at the base than at the apex of the heart, with greater distribution to muscle than to Purkinje fibers. Afferent vagal activity appears to be greater in the posterior ventricular myocardium, which may account for the vagomimetic effects of inferior myocardial infarction.[9]

The vagi exert minimal but measurable effects on ventricular tissue: decreasing the strength of myocardial contraction and prolonging refractoriness. Under some circumstances, acetylcholine can cause a positive inotropic effect. It is now clear that the vagus (acetylcholine) can exert direct effects on some types of ventricular fibers as well as exert indirect effects by modulating sympathetic influences.[9]

Arrhythmias and the Autonomic Nervous System

Alterations in vagal and sympathetic innervation can influence the development of arrhythmias and sudden cardiac death from ventricular tachyarrhythmias.[9,23-25] Damage to nerves extrinsic to the heart, such as the stellate ganglia, as well as to intrinsic cardiac nerves from diseases that may affect nerves primarily, such as viral infections, or secondarily, from diseases that cause cardiac damage, may produce cardioneuropathy. Such neural changes may create electrical instability through a variety of electrophysiological mechanisms. For example, myocardial infarction can interrupt afferent and efferent neural transmission and create areas of sympathetic supersensitivity that may be conducive to the development of arrhythmias.[9] Mutations in genes encoding cardiac ion channel subunits also affect channel function in the central autonomic nervous system,[26] resulting in abnormal firing properties of affected neurons.[27] This observation may partially explain the clinical finding that sudden cardiac death in some variants of the long QT syndrome (see Chaps. 28 and 32) is typically preceded by a sympathetic arousal.

Basic Electrophysiological Principles

Physiology of Ion Channels

Electrical signaling in the heart involves the passage of ions through ionic channels. The Na^+, K^+, Ca^{2+}, and Cl^- ions are the major charge carriers, and their movement across the cell membrane creates a flow of current that generates excitation and signals in cardiac myocytes. Ion channels are macromolecular pores that span the lipid bilayer of the cell membrane (Fig. 27–9). Conformational transitions change (gate) a single ion channel from closed to open, which allows selected ions to flow passively down the electrochemical activity gradient at a very high rate (>10^6 ions per second). The high transfer rates and restriction to "downhill" fluxes not stoichiometrically coupled to the hydrolysis of energy-rich phosphates distinguish ionic channel mechanisms from those of other ion-transporting structures such as the sarcolemmal Na^+,K^+-adenosine triphosphatase (ATPase) or the sarcoplasmic reticular Mg^{2+},Ca^{2+}-ATPase. Ion channels may be gated by extracellular and intracellular ligands, changes in transmembrane voltage, or mechanical stress (see Table 27–3). Gating of single ion channels can best be studied by means of the patch-clamp technique (see, e.g., reference 28).

Ion channels are usually named after the strongest permeant ion—Na^+, Ca^{2+}, K^+, Cl^-—but some channels are less or not selective, as in gap junctional channels. Channels have also been named after neurotransmitters, as in acetylcholine-sensitive K^+ channels, $I_{K.Ach}$.

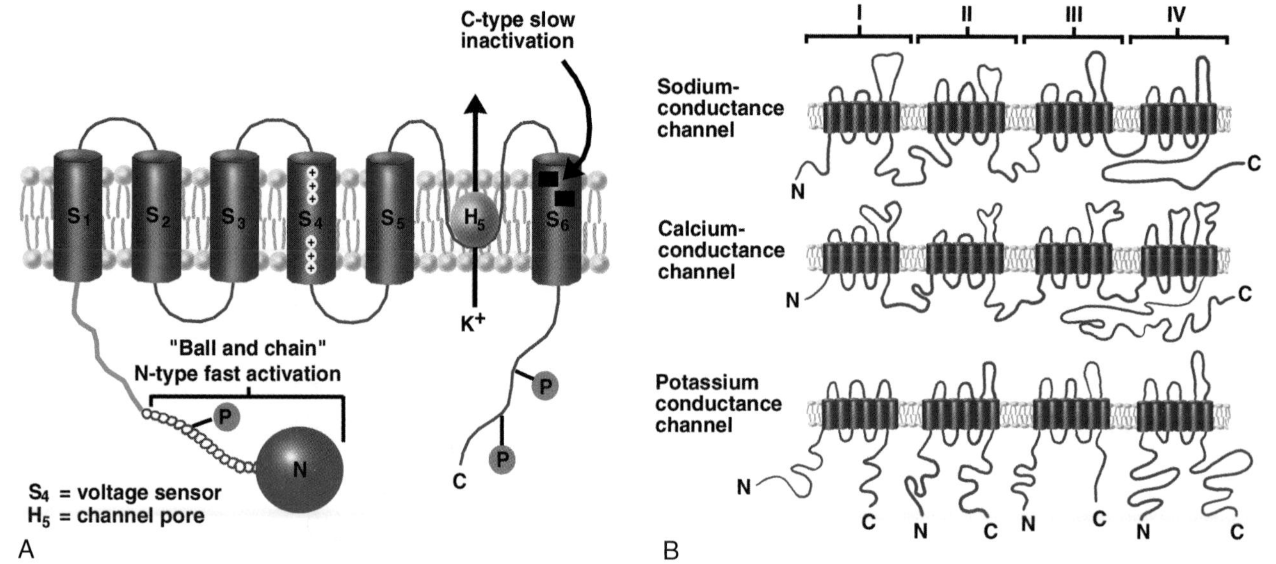

FIGURE 27–9 Structure of ion channels. **A,** Subunit of a voltage-gated potassium channel containing six membrane-spanning domains (S_1 through S_6) linked by intracellular and extracellular sequences of hydrophilic amino acids. One of the subunits (S_4) has positively charged lysine and arginine residues, and this region is thought to form the voltage sensor of the channel. Transmembrane segments S_5 and S_6, along with the intervening peptide chain (H), line the pore through which ions pass into the lipid bilayer. Voltage-dependent "fast" or N-type inactivation is mediated by an N-terminal particle that binds to the activated channel and plugs the permeation pathway. C-type or "slow" inactivation requires conformational changes at the outer side of the channel pore. Both the COOH terminus and the NH_2 terminus have phosphorylation sites (P) that are potential targets for a variety of protein kinases and protein phosphatases. A change in phosphorylation status may then result in altered gating and/or permeation properties of the channel. **B,** Voltage-gated Na^+ and Ca^{2+} channels are composed of a *single* tetramer consisting of four covalently linked repeats of the six-transmembrane-spanning motifs, whereas voltage-gated K^+ channels are composed of four *separate* subunits, each containing a single six-transmembrane-spanning motif. (Modified from Katz AM: Molecular biology in cardiology, a paradigmatic shift. J Mol Cell Cardiol 20:355, 1988.)

The ionic permeability ratio is a commonly used quantitative index of a channel's selectivity. It is defined as the ratio of the permeability of one ion type to that of the main permeant ion type. Permeability ratios of voltage-gated K^+ and Na^+ channels for monovalent and divalent (e.g., Ca^{2+}) cations are usually less than 1:10. Voltage-gated Ca^{2+} channels exhibit a more than thousandfold discrimination against Na^+ and K^+ ions (e.g., $P_K/P_{Ca} = 1/3000$) and are impermeable to anions.

Because ions are charged, net ionic flux through an open channel is determined by both the concentration and electrical gradient across the membrane (electrodiffusion). The potential at which the passive flux of ions along the chemical driving force is exactly balanced by the electrical driving force is called the reversal or Nernst potential of the channel. In the case of a channel that is perfectly selective for one ion species, the reversal potential equals the thermodynamic equilibrium potential of that ion, E_S, which is given by the Nernst equation in the form

$$E_S = RT/zF \ln([S_o]/[S_i])$$

where S_i and S_o are the intracellular and extracellular concentrations of the permeant ion, respectively, z is the valence of the ion, R is the gas constant, F is the Faraday constant, T is the temperature in kelvins, and ln is the logarithm to the base e. At membrane voltages more positive to the reversal potential of the channel, passive ion movement is outward, whereas it is inward at membrane potentials that are more negative to the Nernst potential of that channel. If the current through an open channel is carried by more than one permeant ion, the reversal potential becomes a weighted mean of all Nernst potentials.

As shown in Figures 27-13, 27-14, and 27-15 and Table 27-2, membrane voltages during a cardiac action potential are in the range of −95 to +30 mV. With physiological external K^+ (4 mM; see Table 27-1), E_K is approximately −91 mV, and passive K^+ movement during an action potential is out of the cell. On the other hand, because the calculated reversal potential of a cardiac Ca^{2+} channel is +64 mV (assuming $P_K/P_{Ca} = 1/3000$, K_i = 150 mM, K_o = 4 mM, Ca_i = 100 nM, Ca_o = 2 mM), passive Ca^{2+} flux is into the cell. With physiological internal and external chloride concentrations (Table 27-1), E_{Cl} is −80 to −35 mV, and passive movement of Cl^- ions through open chloride channels can be both inward and outward at membrane potentials typically occurring during a cardiac action potential. In more general terms, the direction and magnitude of passive ion flux through a single open channel at any given transmembrane voltage are governed by the reversal potential of that ion and its concentration on the two sides of the membrane, with the net flux being larger when ions move from the more concentrated side.

TABLE 27–1 Intracellular and Extracellular Ion Concentrations in Cardiac Muscle

Ion	Extracellular Concentration (mM)	Intracellular Concentration	Ratio of Extracellular to Intracellular Concentration	E_I (mV)
Na	145	15 mM	9.7	+60
K	4	150 mM	0.027	−94
Cl	120	5-30 mM	4-24	−83 to −36
Ca	2	10^{-7} M	2×10^4	+129

Athough intracellular Ca content is about 2 mM, most of this Ca is bound or sequestered in intracellular organelles (mitochondria and sarcoplasmic reticulum).

E_I = equilibrium potential for a particular ion at 37°C.

Modified after Sperelakis N: Origin of the cardiac resting potential. *In* Berne RM, Sperelakis N, Geiger SR (eds): Handbook of Physiology, The Cardiovascular System. Bethesda, Md, American Physiological Society, 1979, p. 193.

ION FLUX THROUGH VOLTAGE-GATED CHANNELS

Changes in transmembrane potential determine ion flux through voltage-gated channels not only through the voltage dependence of the electrochemical driving force on the permeant ion but also through the voltage dependence of channel activation; that is, the fraction of time that a channel permits ions to permeate is determined by the membrane voltage. If the probability of a channel being activated (i.e., the open-state probability of that channel) exhibits voltage dependence, as is the case with the fast Na^+ channel or voltage-dependent K^+ channels in cardiac myocytes, activation increases with membrane depolarization. Note that channels do not have a sharp voltage threshold for opening. The dependence of channel activation on membrane potential is rather a continuous function of voltage and follows a sigmoidal curve (Fig. 27-10). The potential at which activation is half-maximal and the steepness of the activation curve determine the channel's activity during changes in membrane potential. Shifting the activation curve to potentials positive to the midpoint of activation or reducing the steepness of the channel's acti-

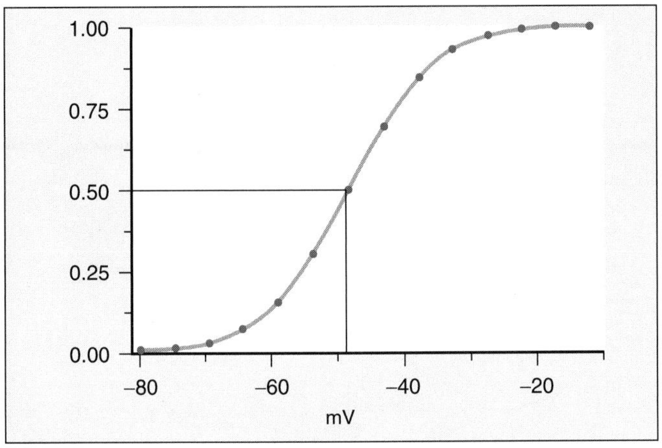

FIGURE 27–10 Voltage dependence of fast Na^+ current activation. Fractional activation (y-axis) is plotted as a function of membrane potential. Voltage at which activation is half-maximal is demarked by a vertical line.

vation curve or both are two possible mechanisms by which ion channel blockers can inhibit ion channel activity.

As indicated in Figure 27–11, open channels enter a nonconducting conformation after a depolarizing change in membrane potential, a process termed *inactivation.*[29] If membrane depolarization persists, the channel remains inactivated and cannot reopen. This steady-state inactivation increases with membrane depolarization in a sigmoidal fashion. Inactivation curves of the various voltage-gated ion channel types in the heart differ in their slopes and midpoints of inactivation. For example, sustained cardiomyocyte membrane depolarization to −50 mV (as may occur in acutely ischemic myocardium) causes almost complete inactivation of the fast, voltage-gated Na^+ channel, whereas the L-type Ca^{2+} channel exhibits only little inactivation at this membrane potential.[30] Activation and inactivation curves can overlap, in which case a steady-state or non-inactivating current flows. The existence of such a "window" current has been verified for both the voltage-gated Na^+ current[31] and the L-type Ca^{2+} current.[32] The L-type window current has been implicated in the genesis of triggered activity arising from early afterdepolarizations (EADs).

Channels recover from inactivation and then enter the closed state from which they can be reactivated (see Fig. 27–11). Rates of recovery from inactivation vary among the different types of voltage-dependent channels and usually follow monoexponential or multiexponential time courses, with the longest time constants ranging from a few milliseconds, as, for example, for the fast sodium channel,[33] to several seconds, as for some subtypes of K^+ channels (see Table 27–3).[34] Together, the activity of voltage-dependent ion channels in cardiomyocytes over the course of an action potential is tightly regulated by the orchestrated interplay of a number of time- and voltage-dependent gating mechanisms, including activation, inactivation, and recovery from inactivation. All of these mechanisms represent potential targets for pharmacological interventions.

PRINCIPLES OF IONIC CURRENT MODULATION

The whole-cell current amplitude, I, is the product of the number of functional channels in the membrane available for opening (N), the probability that a channel will open (P_o), and the single-channel current amplitude (i), or $I = N \cdot P_o \cdot i$. Modulation of current amplitudes in single

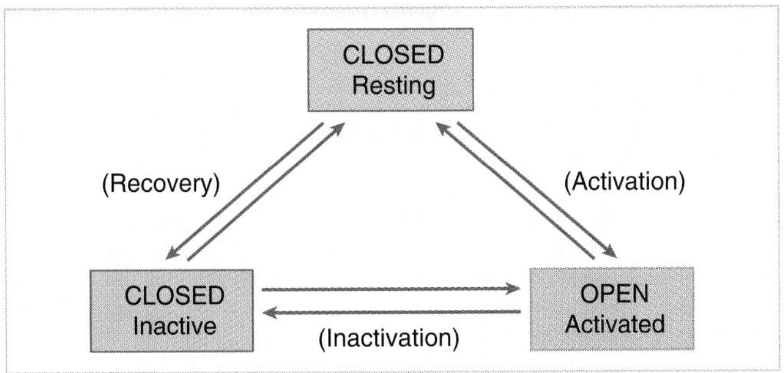

FIGURE 27–11 Simplest scheme for gating of voltage-gated ion channels.

cardiomyocytes therefore results from alterations in N, P_o, i, or any combination of these. Changes in the number of available channels in the cell membrane may result from changes in the expression of ion channel-encoding genes.[35] The magnitude of the single-channel current amplitude is dependent, among other factors, on the ionic concentration gradient across the membrane. For example, an increase in the extracellular Ca^{2+} concentration increases current through a single Ca^{2+} channel. Changes in channel activation can result from phosphorylation/dephosphorylation of the channel protein by second messenger–mediated activation of protein kinases and protein phosphatases, respectively (see also Fig. 27–9).[36] Channel phosphorylation/dephosphorylation causes a shift in the membrane potential dependence of a channel's activation or availability curve, or both, or modification of the sensitivity of channel activation/inactivation to changes in membrane potential. For example, protein kinase A–mediated potentiation of the cardiac sodium current is partially due to a shift of the sodium channel activation curve to more negative potentials.[37]

Molecular Structure of Ion Channels

Voltage-gated potassium channels are composed of four *separate* subunits, each containing six regions of hydrophobic amino acids (S1 through S6) that are thought to form membrane-spanning domains, and these hydrophobic regions are linked by sequences of hydrophilic amino acids that are exposed to the intracellular or extracellular space (see Fig. 27–9A). One of the membrane-spanning subunits (S4) is positively charged, having a cluster of basic amino acids (lysine or arginine), and this region is thought to be part of the voltage sensor. The peptide chain linking S5 and S6 (H5 loop) lines the water-filled pore. Voltage-dependent "fast" inactivation of the channel is mediated by a tethered N-terminal particle ("inactivation ball") that binds to the activated channel and occludes the intracellular mouth of the permeation pathway (see Fig. 27–9A). In contrast to this "tethered ball" mechanism of N-type inactivation, C-type (or "slow") inactivation involves relatively localized changes in conformation of amino acid residues near the external mouth of the channel pore.[29] The rate of C-type inactivation and its recovery strongly determine refractoriness and can be modulated by binding of drugs, for example, dofetilide. Voltage-gated Na^+ and Ca^{2+} channels have a basic structure similar to that of voltage-dependent potassium channels, although, unlike K^+ channels, each Ca^{2+} or Na^+ channel consists of a single (alpha) subunit containing the four repeats of the six transmembrane-spanning domains (see Fig. 27–9B).

A structurally different family of potassium channels is that containing the inwardly rectifying potassium-selective channels (Kir). Kir channels in cardiac myocytes, as in other cells, conduct inward current at membrane potentials negative to E_K and smaller outward currents at membrane potentials positive to E_K. The activity of Kir channels is a function of both the membrane potential and the extracellular K^+ concentration ($[K^+]_o$). As $[K^+]_o$ changes, the channel conducts inward current at potentials negative to the new E_K while a small outward current within a certain potential range positive to the new E_K remains. Structurally, Kir channels resemble voltage-gated K^+ channels, but the subunits lack the S1 to S4 domains, whereas the pore-forming domains and the H5 region are conserved. Kir channel subunits can form heteromultimeric complexes with other proteins, which adds considerable complexity to the behavior of Kir channels. For example, the ATP-sensitive K^+ channel $I_{K.ATP}$ is a heteromeric complex of inwardly rectifying potassium channel subunits and the sulfonylurea receptor. Drugs such as nicorandil, pinacidil, and diazoxide open ATP-sensitive K^+ channels, whereas sulfonylurea compounds (such as glibenclamide) inhibit the activity of $I_{K.ATP}$. Opening of cardiac sarcolemmal K_{ATP} channels underlies electrocardiographic ST segment elevation during acute myocardial ischemia.[38]

The molecular basis of the acetylcholine-activated potassium channel $I_{K.Ach}$ is a heteromultimer of two inwardly rectifying potassium channel subunits. This channel is activated after direct binding of the beta-gamma subunits of G protein. Stimulation of $I_{K.Ach}$ by vagally secreted acetylcholine decreases spontaneous depolarization in the sinus node and slows the velocity of conduction in the AV node.[39] Adenosine, through type 1 purinergic receptor–mediated G protein activation, also increases $I_{K.Ach}$ activity in atrial, sinoatrial node, and AV node cells, thus making this compound a treatment of choice for AV reentry tachycardia.

Intercalated Discs

Another family of ion channel proteins is that containing the gap junctional channels. These dodecameric channels are found in the intercalated discs between adjacent cells. Three types of specialized junctions make up each intercalated disc. The macula adherens or desmosome and fascia adherens form areas of strong adhesion between cells and may provide a linkage for the transfer of mechanical energy from one cell to the next. The *nexus,* also called the *tight* or *gap junction,* is a region in the intercalated disc where cells are in functional contact with each other. Membranes at these junctions are separated by only about 10 to 20 Å and are connected by a series of hexagonally packed subunit bridges. Gap junctions provide low-resistance electrical coupling between adjacent cells by establishing aqueous pores that directly link the cytoplasm of these adjacent cells. Gap junctions allow movement of ions and small molecules between cells, thereby linking the interiors of adjacent cells.

Gap junctions permit a multicellular structure such as the heart to function electrically like an orderly, synchronized, interconnected unit and are probably responsible in part for the fact that conduction in the myocardium is *anisotropic*; that is, its anatomical and biophysical properties vary according to the direction in which they are measured. Usually, conduction velocity is two to three times faster longitudinally, in the direction of the long axis of the fiber, than it is transversely, in the direction perpendicular to this long axis.[40,41] Resistivity is lower longitudinally than transversely. Interestingly, the safety factor for propagation is greater transversely than horizontally. Conduction delay or block occurs more commonly in the longitudinal direction than it does transversely. Cardiac conduction is discontinuous because of resistive discontinuities created by the gap junctions, which have an anisotropic distribution on the cell surface.[42] Because of anisotropy, propagation is discontinuous and can be a cause of reentry.

Gap junctions may also provide "biochemical coupling" that might permit cell-to-cell movement of ATP or other high-energy phosphates. Gap junctions can also change their electrical resistance. When intracellular calcium rises, as in myocardial infarction, the gap junction may close to help "seal off" the effects of injured from noninjured cells. Acidosis increases and alkalosis decreases gap junctional resistance. Increased gap junctional resistance tends to slow the rate of action potential propagation, a condition that could lead to conduction delay or block.[43] Cardiac restricted inactivation of gap junctions decreases transverse conduction velocity to a greater degree than longitudinal conduction, resulting in an increased anisotropic ratio that may play a role in premature sudden death from ventricular arrhythmias.[44]

Connexins are the proteins that form the intercellular channels of gap junctions. An individual channel is created by two hemichannels (connexons), each located in the plasma membrane of adjacent cells and composed of six integral membrane protein subunits (connexins). The hemichannels surround an aqueous pore and thereby create a transmembrane channel (Fig. 27–12). Connexin43, a 43-kDa polypeptide, is the most abundant cardiac connexin, with connexin40 and connexin45 found in smaller amounts. Ventricular muscle expresses connexin43 and connexin45, whereas atrial muscle and components of the specialized conduction system express connexin43, connexin45, and connexin40. Individual cardiac connexins form gap junctional channels with characteristic unitary conductances, voltage sensitivities, and ionic permeabilities.[45] Tissue-specific connexin expression and spatial distribution of gap junctions determine the disparate conduction properties of cardiac tissue. The functional heterogeneity of cardiac gap junctions is further enhanced by the ability of different connexin isoforms to form hybrid gap junctional channels with unique electrophysiological properties. These channel chimeras appear to have a major function in controlling impulse transmission at the sinus node–atrium border, the atrium–AV node transitional zone, and the Purkinje-myocyte border.[7,20]

Phases of the Cardiac Action Potential

The cardiac transmembrane potential consists of five phases: phase 0, upstroke or rapid depolarization; phase 1, early rapid repolarization; phase 2, plateau; phase 3, final rapid repolarization; and phase 4, resting membrane potential and diastolic depolarization (see Fig. 27–14). These phases are the result of passive ion fluxes moving down electrochemical gradients established by active ion pumps and exchange

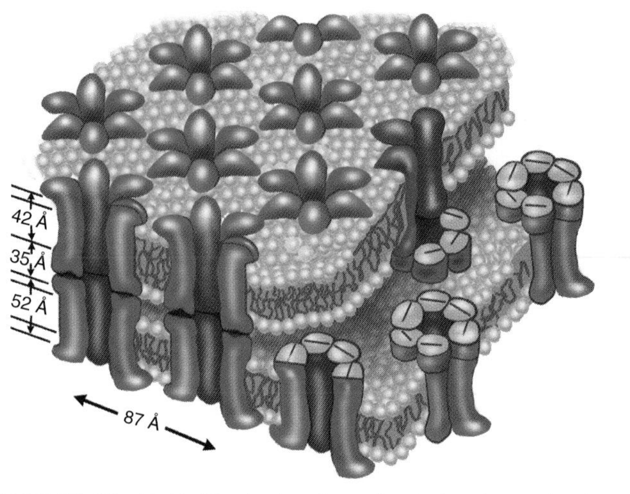

FIGURE 27–12 Model of the structure of a gap junction based on results of x-ray diffraction studies. Individual channels are composed of paired hexamers that travel in the membranes of adjacent cells and adjoin in the extracellular gap to form an aqueous pore that provides continuity of the cytoplasm of the two cells. (From Saffitz JE: Cell-to-cell communication in the heart. Cardiol Rev 3:86, 1995.)

mechanisms. Each ion moves primarily through its own ion-specific channel. Impulses spread from one cell to the next without requiring neural input. The transplanted heart dramatically demonstrates this fact. The following discussion explains the electrogenesis of each of these phases. For in-depth coverage, the reader is referred to other reference sources.[46]

General Considerations

Ionic fluxes regulate membrane potential in cardiac myocytes in the following fashion. When only one type of ion channel opens, assuming that this channel is perfectly selective for that ion, the membrane potential of the entire cell would equal the Nernst potential of that ion. Solving the Nernst equation for the four major ions across the plasma membrane, one obtains the following equilibrium potentials: sodium, +60 mV; potassium, −94 mV; calcium, +129 mV; and chloride, −80 to −35 mV. Therefore, if a single K^+-selective channel opens, such as the inwardly rectifying K^+ channel, the membrane potential approaches E_K (−94 mV). If a single Na^+-selective channel opens, the transmembrane potential becomes E_{Na} (+60 mV). A quiescent cardiac myocyte (phase 4) has many more open potassium than sodium channels, and the cell's transmembrane potential is close to E_K (Table 27–2). When two or more types of ion channel open simultaneously, each type tries to make the membrane potential go to the equilibrium potential of that channel. The contribution of each ion type to the overall membrane potential at any given moment is determined by the instantaneous permeability of the plasma membrane to that ion. For example, deviation of the measured resting membrane potential from E_K (see Table 27–1) would predict that other ion types with equilibrium potentials positive to E_K contribute to the resting membrane potential in cardiac myocytes. If it is assumed that Na^+, K^+, and Cl^- are the permeant ions at resting potential, their individual contributions to the resting membrane potential V can be quantified by the GHK *voltage* equation of the form

$$V = RT/F \ln[(P_K\,[K]_o + P_{Na}\,[Na]_o + P_{Cl}[Cl]_i)/(P_K[K]_I + P_{Na}[Na]P_{Cl}[Cl]_o)]$$

where the symbols have the meanings outlined previously. With only one permeant ion, V becomes the Nernst potential for that ion. With several permeant ion types, V is a weighted mean of all the Nernst potentials.

Intracellular electrical activity can be recorded by inserting a glass microelectrode filled with an electrolyte solution and having a tip diameter less than 0.5 μm into a single cell. The electrode produces minimal damage, its entry point apparently being sealed by the cell. The transmembrane potential is recorded by using this electrode in reference to an extracellular ground electrode placed in the tissue bath near the cell membrane and represents the potential difference between intracellular and extracellular voltage (Fig. 27–13). Alternatively, the patch-clamp technique in current clamp mode can be used to measure transmembrane potentials.

TABLE 27–2 Properties of Transmembrane Potentials in Mammalian Hearts

Property	Sinus Nodal Cell	Atrial Muscle Cell	AV Nodal Cell	Purkinje Fiber	Ventricular Muscle Cell
Resting potential (mV)	−50 to −60	−80 to −90	−60 to −70	−90 to −95	−80 to −90
Action potential					
Amplitude (mV)	60-70	110-120	70-80	120	110-120
Overshoot (mV)	0-10	30	5-15	30	30
Duration (msec)	100-300	100-300	100-300	300-500	200-300
V_{max} (V/S)	1-10	100-200	5-15	500-700	100-200
Propagation velocity (m/sec)	<0.05	0.3-0.4	0.1	2-3	0.3-0.4
Fiber diameter (μm)	5-10	10-15	1-10	100	10-16

Modified from Sperelakis N: Origin of the cardiac resting potential. *In* Berne RM, Sperelakis N, Geiger SR (eds): Handbook of Physiology. The Cardiovascular System. Bethesda, Md, American Physiological Society, 1979, p. 190.

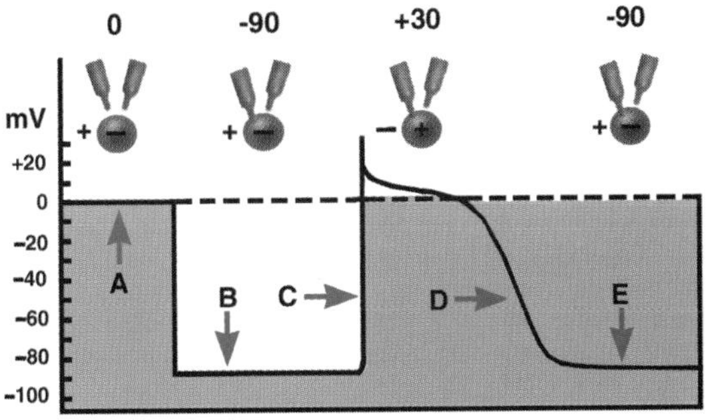

FIGURE 27–13 Demonstration of action potentials recorded during impalement of a cardiac cell. The **upper row** of diagrams shows a cell (circle), two microelectrodes, and stages during impalement of the cell and its activation and recovery. A, Both microelectrodes are extracellular, and no difference in potential exists between them (0 potential). The environment inside the cell is negative and the outside is positive because the cell is polarized. B, One microelectrode has pierced the cell membrane to record the intracellular resting membrane potential, which is −90 mV with respect to the outside of the cell. C, The cell has depolarized and the upstroke of the action potential is recorded. At its peak voltage, the inside of the cell is about +30 mV with respect to the outside of the cell. D, Phase of repolarization, with the membrane returning to its former resting potential (E). (From Cranefield PF: The Conduction of the Cardiac Impulse. Mt Kisco, NY, Futura, 1975.)

Phase 4—The Resting Membrane Potential

The intracellular potential during electrical quiescence in diastole is −50 to −95 mV, depending on the cell type (see Table 27–2). Therefore, the inside of the cell is 50 to 95 mV negative relative to the outside of the cell because of the distribution of ions such as K^+, Na^+, and Cl^-.

Because cardiac myocytes have an abundance of open K^+ channels at rest, the cardiac transmembrane potential (in phase 4) is close to E_K. Potassium outward current through open, inwardly rectifying K^+ channels, I_{K1}, mainly contributes to the resting membrane potential in atrial and ventricular myocytes, as well as in Purkinje cells, under normal conditions. Deviation of the resting membrane potential from E_K is due to movement of monovalent ions with an equilibrium potential greater than the E_K, for example, Cl^- efflux through activated chloride channels, such as $I_{Cl.cAMP}$, $I_{Cl.Ca}$, and $I_{Cl.swell}$.[47] Calcium does not contribute directly to the resting membrane potential, but changes in intracellular free calcium concentration can affect other membrane conductance values. For instance, an increase in sarcoplasmic reticulum Ca^{2+} load can cause spontaneous intracellular Ca^{2+} waves,[48] which in turn activate the Ca^{2+}-dependent chloride conductance $I_{Cl.Ca}$ and thereby lead to spontaneous transient inward currents and concomitant membrane depolarization. Increases in $[Ca^{2+}]_i$ can also stimulate the Na^+/Ca^{2+} exchanger $I_{Na/Ca}$. This protein exchanges three Na^+ ions for one Ca^{2+} ion, the direction being dependent on the sodium and calcium concentrations on the two sides of the membrane and the transmembrane potential difference. At resting membrane potential and during a spontaneous sarcoplasmic reticulum Ca^{2+} release event, this exchanger would generate a net Na^+ influx, possibly causing transient membrane depolarizations (see Fig. 27–23).[49,50] $[Ca^{2+}]_i$ has also been shown to activate I_{K1} in cardiac myocytes, thereby indirectly contributing to cardiac resting membrane potential.[51] Because of the Na-K pump, which pumps Na^+ out of the cell against its electrochemical gradient and simultaneously pumps K^+ into the cell against its chemical gradient, the intracellular K^+ concentration remains high and the intracellular Na^+ concentration remains low. This pump, fueled by an Na^+,K^+-ATPase enzyme that hydrolyzes ATP for energy, is bound to the membrane. It requires both Na^+ and K^+ to function and can transport three Na^+ ions outward for two K^+ ions inward. Therefore, the pump can be electrogenic and generate a net outward movement of positive charges. The rate of Na^+–K^+ pumping to maintain the same ionic gradients must increase as the heart rate increases because the cell gains a slight amount of Na^+ and loses a slight amount of K^+ with each depolarization. Cardiac glycoside–induced block of the Na^+,K^+-ATPase increases contractility through an increase in intracellular Na^+ concentration, which in turn reduces Ca^{2+} extrusion through the Na^+/Ca^{2+} exchanger (see later), ultimately increasing myocyte contractility.[52]

Phase 0—Upstroke or Rapid Depolarization

A stimulus delivered to excitable tissue evokes an action potential characterized by a sudden voltage change caused by transient depolarization followed by repolarization. The action potential is conducted throughout the heart and is responsible for initiating each "heartbeat." Electrical changes in action potential follow a relatively fixed time and voltage relationship that differs according to specific cell types (Figs. 27–14 and 27–15). In nerve, the entire process takes several milliseconds, whereas action potentials in human cardiac fibers last several hundred milliseconds. Normally, the action potential is independent of the size of the depolarizing stimulus if the latter exceeds a certain threshold potential. Small subthreshold depolarizing stimuli depolarize the membrane in proportion to the strength of the stimulus. However, when the stimulus is sufficiently intense to reduce membrane potential to a threshold value in the range of −70 to −65 mV for normal Purkinje fibers, more intense stimuli do not produce larger action potential responses, and an "all-or-none" response results. In contrast, hyperpolarizing pulses, stimuli that render the membrane potential more negative, elicit a response proportional to the strength of the stimulus.

MECHANISM OF PHASE 0. The upstroke of the cardiac action potential in atrial and ventricular muscle and His-Purkinje fibers is due to a sudden increase in membrane

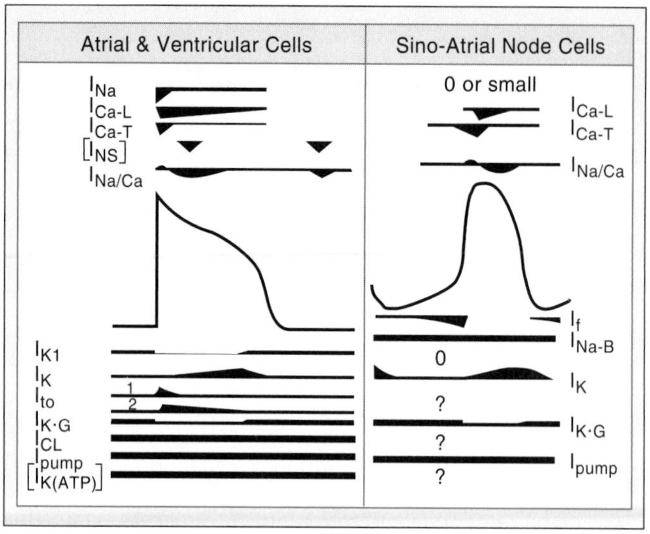

FIGURE 27–14 Currents and channels involved in generating resting and action potentials. The time course of a stylized action potential of atrial and ventricular cells is shown on the left, and that of sinoatrial node cells is on the right. Above and below are the various channels and pumps that contribute the currents underlying the electrical events. See Table 27–3 for identification of the symbols and description of the channels or currents. Where possible, the approximate time courses of the currents associated with the channels or pumps are shown symbolically without an effort to represent their magnitudes relative to each other. I_K incorporates at least two currents, $I_{K\text{-}R}$ and $I_{K\text{-}S}$. There appears to be an ultrarapid component as well, designated $I_{K\text{-}UR}$. The heavy bars for I_{Cl}, I_{pump}, and $I_{K(ATP)}$ indicate only the presence of these channels or pump without implying magnitude of currents because that would vary with physiological and pathophysiological conditions. The channels identified by brackets (I_{NS} and $I_{K(ATP)}$) are active only under pathological conditions. I_{NS} may represent a swelling-activated cation current. For the sinoatrial node cells, I_{NS} and I_{K1} are small or absent. Question marks indicate that experimental evidence is not yet available to determine the presence of these channels in sinoatrial cell membranes. Although it is likely that other ionic current mechanisms exist, they are not shown here because their roles in electrogenesis are not sufficiently well defined. (From Members of the Sicilian Gambit: Antiarrhythmic Therapy: A Pathophysiologic Approach. Mt Kisco, NY, Futura, 1994, p 13.)

conductance to Na^+. An externally applied stimulus or a spontaneously generated local membrane circuit current in advance of a propagating action potential depolarizes a sufficiently large area of membrane at a sufficiently rapid rate to open the Na^+ channels and depolarize the membrane further. When the stimulus activates enough Na^+ channels, Na^+ ions enter the cell, down their electrochemical gradient. The excited membrane no longer behaves like a K^+ electrode, that is, exclusively permeable to K^+, but more closely approximates a Na^+ electrode, and the membrane moves toward the Na^+ equilibrium potential.

The rate at which depolarization occurs during phase 0, that is, the maximum rate of change of voltage over time, is indicated by the expression dV/dt_{max} or $\dot{V}_{max}$ (see Table 27–2), which is a reasonable approximation of the rate and magnitude of Na^+ entry into the cell and a determinant of conduction velocity for the propagated action potential. The transient increase in sodium conductance lasts 1 to 2 milliseconds. The action potential, or more properly the Na^+ current (I_{Na}), is said to be regenerative; that is, intracellular movement of a little Na^+ depolarizes the membrane more, which increases conductance to Na^+ more, which allows more Na^+ to enter, and so on. As this process is occurring, however, $[Na^+]_i$ and positive intracellular charges increase and reduce the driving force for Na^+. When the equilibrium potential for Na^+ (E_{Na}) is reached, Na^+ no longer enters the cell; that is., when the driving force acting on the ion to enter the cell balances the driving force acting on the ion to exit the cell, no current flows. In addition, Na^+ conductance is time dependent, so that when the membrane spends some time at voltages less negative than the resting potential, Na^+ conductance decreases (inactivation; see earlier). Therefore, an intervention that reduces membrane potential for a time (acute myocardial ischemia)—but not to threshold—partially inactivates Na^+ channels, and if threshold is now achieved, the magnitude and rate of Na^+ influx are reduced, causing the conduction velocity to slow.

In cardiac Purkinje fibers and to a lesser extent in ventricular muscle, two different populations of Na^+ channels, or two different modes of operation of the same Na^+ channel, exist. One is responsible for the brief Na^+ current of phase 0, and the other, which is longer lasting, participates in the action potential plateau (steady-state or window current).[31] Tetrodotoxin (TTX) and local anesthetics block both types of channels,

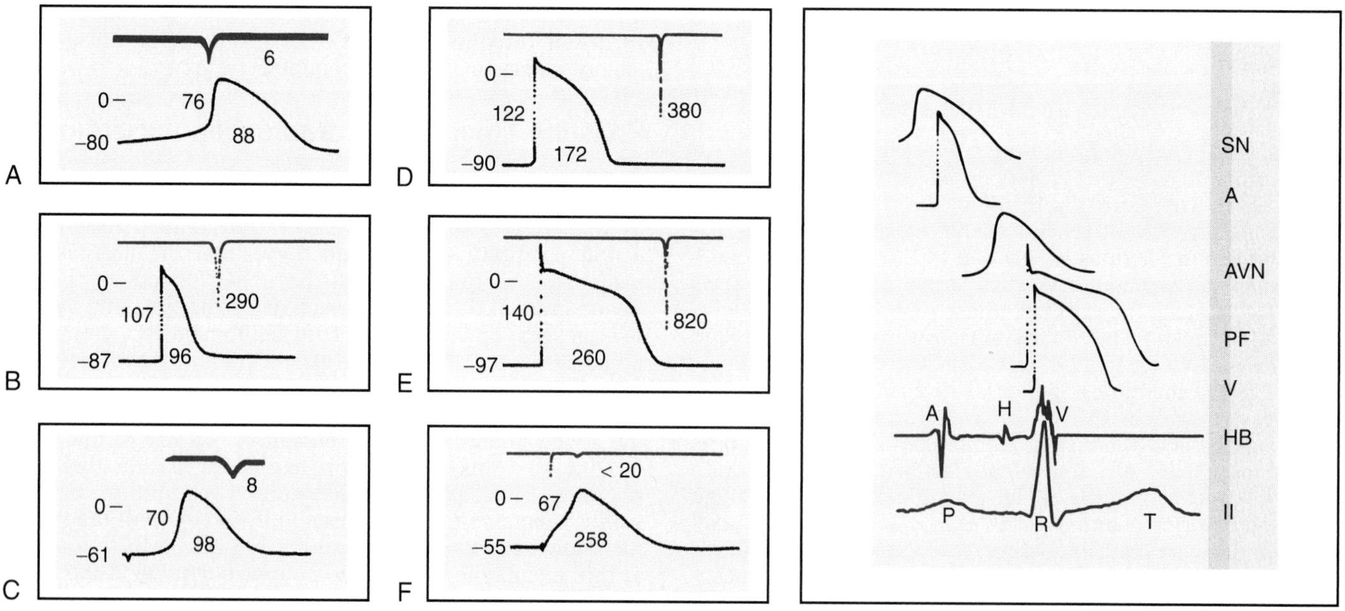

FIGURE 27–15 Action potentials recorded from different tissues in the heart **(left)** remounted along with a His bundle recording and scalar electrocardiogram from a patient **(right)** to illustrate the timing during a single cardiac cycle. In panels **A to F,** the top tracing is dV/dt of phase 0 and the second tracing is the action potential. For each panel the numbers (from left to right) indicate maximum diastolic potential (mV), action potential amplitude (mV), action potential duration at 90 percent of repolarization (milliseconds), and $\dot{V}_{max}$ of phase 0 (V/sec). Zero potential is indicated by the short horizontal line next to the zero on the upper left of each action potential. **A,** Rabbit sinoatrial node. **B,** Canine atrial muscle. **C,** Rabbit atrioventricular node. **D,** Canine ventricular muscle. **E,** Canine Purkinje fiber. **F,** Diseased human ventricle. Note that the action potentials recorded in **A, C,** and **F** have reduced resting membrane potentials, amplitudes, and $\dot{V}_{max}$ when compared with the other action potentials. In the right panel, A = atrial muscle potential; AVN = atrioventricular nodal potential; HB = His bundle recording; II = lead II; PF = Purkinje fiber potential; SN = sinus nodal potential; V = ventricular muscle potential. Horizontal calibration on the left: 50 milliseconds for A and C, 100 milliseconds for B, D, E, and F; 200 milliseconds on the right. Vertical calibration on the left: 50 mV. Horizontal calibration on the right: 200 milliseconds. (Modified from Gilmour RF Jr, Zipes DP: Basic electrophysiology of the slow inward current. *In* Antman E, Stone PH [eds]: Calcium Blocking Agents in the Treatment of Cardiovascular Disorders. Mt Kisco, NY, Futura, 1983, pp 1-37.)

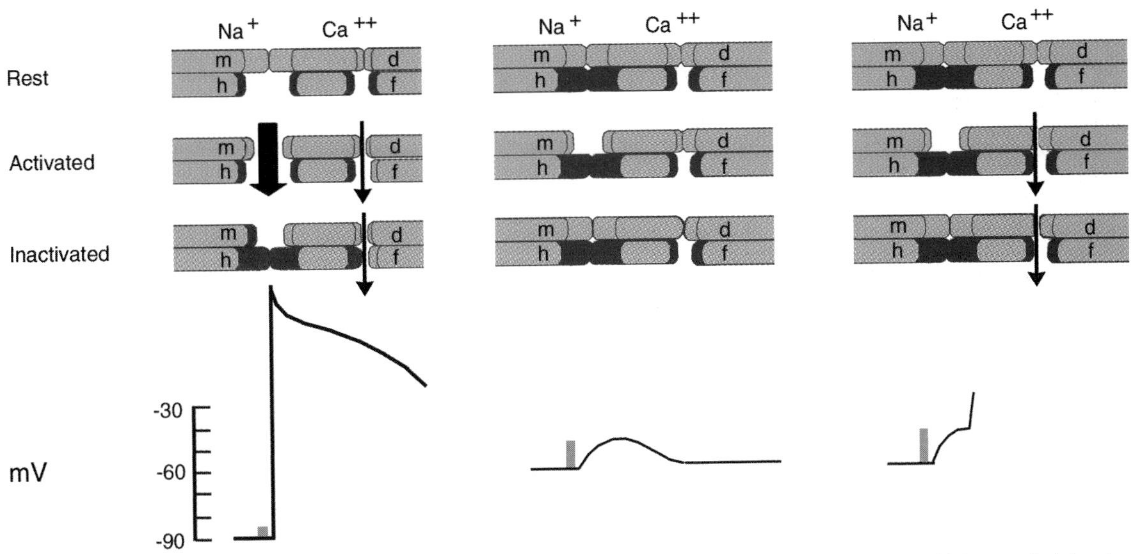

FIGURE 27–16 Schematic representation of membrane channels for rapid and slow inward currents at resting membrane potential **(top row)**, during the activated state **(middle row)**, and during the inactivated state **(bottom row)**. Vertically separated panels depict fibers with a normal resting potential of −90 mV **(left)**, with resting membrane potential reduced to less than −60 mV **(middle)**, and after stimulation of the cell with catecholamines **(right)**. The activation (m) and inactivation (h) gates of the fast channel and the activation (d) and inactivation (f) gates of the slow channel are depicted. During the resting state **(left)**, the activation gates of both channels are closed while the inactivation gates are open. When the cell is stimulated, the m gates of the fast channel open, and for a brief period, the open m gates and h gates allow inward sodium current to flow, depolarize the cell, and produce its upstroke. The action potential is depicted below. The h gates then close the channel and inactivate sodium conductance. Membrane depolarization also activates voltage-gated Ca^{2+} channels (d gates open), allowing influx of Ca^{2+} that contributes to the plateau phase of the action potential. The inactivation gates of the slow Ca^{2+} channel are both voltage and $[Ca^{2+}]_i$ dependent. High and low levels of intracellular free calcium ions, respectively, accelerate and slow inactivation, thereby functioning as a negative feedback mechanism to control intracellular calcium content. When the upstroke of the action potential exceeds the threshold for activation of the slow inward current, the d gates open and allow ingress of the slow inward current that contributes to the plateau phase of the action potential. The f gates of the slow channel close more slowly than the h gates. Although the slow inward channel remains open longer than the fast channel does, less total current flows. When the resting membrane potential is reduced below −60 mV by increasing $[K]_o$ from 4.0 to 14.0 mm **(middle)**, the cell depolarizes to −60 mV and the fast channel becomes inactivated because the h gates remain closed. Even though the m gate may open during activation, the amount of sodium current is too small to elicit an action potential. The inactivation gates of the slow channel (f gates) remain open, and when the cell is excited after the addition of catecholamine **(right)**, the d gates open and permit flow of a slow inward current that causes a slow-response action potential. This action potential resembles those in panels A, C, and F of Figure 27–15. (From Wit AL, Bigger JT Jr: Possible electrophysiological mechanisms for lethal arrhythmias accompanying myocardial ischemia and infarction. Circulation 52[Suppl 3]:96, 1975.)

thereby diminishing the rate of rise of phase 0 and shortening the action potential duration. Furthermore, there may be a background Na^+ current ($I_{Na\text{-}B}$) through a voltage-independent channel in sinus nodal cells that contributes to pacemaker behavior.[8]

GATING OF VOLTAGE-DEPENDENT FAST SODIUM CHANNELS. In this model, three m (activation) gates and one h (inactivation) gate can be considered to be lined up in series in the membrane Na^+ channel (Fig. 27–16), with the m gate on the extracellular side and the h gate on the intracellular side of the membrane. When the membrane is in a resting polarized state, the m gates are almost completely closed, the h gate is open, and no Na^+ can cross the membrane. Although depolarization of the membrane opens the m gates and closes the h gate, the m gates open faster than the h gate closes; that is, activation of the channel proceeds faster than inactivation can occur, and Na^+ flows through the Na^+ channel for about 1 millisecond while both gates are open simultaneously (see Fig. 27–16, left, thick arrow).

When the membrane repolarizes to fairly high negative values, that is, the membrane potential becomes more negative than about −60 mV, the m gates shut rapidly, the h gate opens more slowly (reactivation or recovery from inactivation), and the membrane is once again capable of depolarization. Until that time, the cell is absolutely refractory; that is, no stimulus, regardless of intensity, can activate the cell. If the membrane is activated a second time before reaching a large negative value, all the h gates have not yet reopened and the maximum number of Na^+ channels that can open is reduced. The resulting action potential has reduced $\dot{V}_{max}$, amplitude, duration, and conduction velocity. The state of the gates at any time depends on the membrane potential and the length of time that the potential has been maintained.

A cluster of positively charged arginine and lysine residues in the S4 domain is thought to function as the voltage sensor (m gate), and the peptide loop connecting repeats S3 and S4 binds to the activated channel and occludes the intracellular mouth of the channel pore (h gate; Fig. 27–17). This loop could be regarded as analogous to the N-terminal peptide chain of inactivating voltage-gated potassium channels (see Fig. 27–9A).

The Hodgkin-Huxley theory has been used to describe the voltage dependence of single-channel permeability to sodium, with four hypothetical gating particles making independent transitions between con-

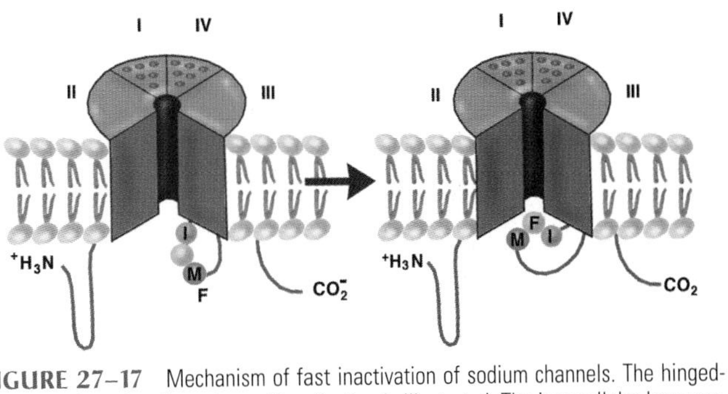

FIGURE 27–17 Mechanism of fast inactivation of sodium channels. The hinged-lid mechanism of sodium channel inactivation is illustrated. The intracellular loop connecting domains III and IV of the sodium channel is depicted as forming a hinged lid. The critical residue (Phe1489F) is shown as occluding the intracellular mouth of the pore. (From Catteral WA: Molecular analysis of voltage gated sodium channels in the heart and other tissues. *In* Zipes DP, Jalife J [eds]: Cardiac Electrophysiology: From Cell to Bedside. 2nd ed. Philadelphia, WB Saunders, 1994, p 1.)

ducting and nonconducting positions to control ion flux. Three m particles control activation and one h particle controls inactivation. The probability that they are all in a position where the channel conducts is m^3h, and for the Na^+ channel,

$$P_{Na} = m^3 \cdot h \cdot P_{Na,max}$$

where P_{Na} is the permeability of the sodium channel at a given voltage, $P_{Na,max}$ is the maximal possible permeability of the channel, m^3 represents the probability that all three activation particles are in a position to make up an open channel (m = 1, gate is permissive; m = 0, gate is nonpermissive), whereas h represents the probability that the Na^+ channel is not inactivated (h = 1, gate is open; h = 0, gate is shut). Because opening and closing of the gates are voltage *and* time dependent, the permeability of the channel (P_{Na}) is some fraction of the maximum possible permeability ($P_{Na,max}$), depending on membrane potential and the period for which the membrane has been at that voltage.

UPSTROKE OF THE ACTION POTENTIAL. In normal atrial and ventricular muscle and in fibers in the His-Purkinje system, action potentials have very rapid upstrokes with a large $\dot{V}_{max}$ and are called *fast responses.* Action potentials in the normal sinus and AV nodes and many types of diseased tissue have very slow upstrokes with a reduced $\dot{V}_{max}$ and are called *slow responses* (Table 27–3; see Fig. 27–15). Upstrokes of slow responses are mediated by a slow inward, predominantly Ca^{2+} current (I_{Ca}) rather than the fast inward I_{Na} (Table 27–4). These potentials received the name *slow response* because the time required for activation and inactivation of the slow inward current ($I_{Ca.L}$) is approximately an order of magnitude slower than that for the fast inward Na^+ current (I_{Na}). Recovery from inactivation also takes longer. Calcium entry and $[Ca^{2+}]_i$ help promote inactivation. Thus, the slow channel opens (activation gates d) and closes (inactivation gates f) more slowly than the fast channel does, remains open for a longer time, and requires more time following a stimulus to be reactivated (see Fig. 27–16). In fact, recovery of excitability outlasts full restoration of maximum diastolic potential, which means that even though the membrane potential has returned to normal, the cell has not recovered excitability completely because the latter depends on elapse of a certain amount of time (i.e., is time dependent) and not just on recovery of a particular membrane potential (i.e., voltage dependence), a phenomenon termed postrepolarization refractoriness.

The threshold for activation of $I_{Ca.L}$, that is, the voltage that the cell must reach to "turn on" the slow inward current, is about −30 to −40 mV. In fibers of the fast response type, $I_{Ca.L}$ is normally activated during phase 0 by the regenerative depolarization caused by the fast sodium current. Current flows through both fast and slow channels during the latter part of the action potential upstroke. However, $I_{Ca.L}$ is much smaller than the peak Na^+ current and therefore contributes little to the action potential until the fast Na^+ current is inactivated, after completion of phase 0. Thus, $I_{Ca.L}$ affects mainly the plateau of action potentials recorded in atrial and ventricular muscle and His-Purkinje fibers. When the fast Na^+ current is inactivated rapidly, such as in frog ventricle, $I_{Ca.L}$ may contribute noticeably to the peak of phase 0. In addition, $I_{Ca.L}$ may play a prominent role in partially depolarized cells in which the fast Na^+ channels have been inactivated, if conditions are appropriate for slow-channel activation.[30,53]

At least two types of calcium current exist in human cardiac myocytes: a slowly inactivating dihydropyridine-sensitive current $I_{Ca.L}$ and a rapidly inactivating dihydropyridine-insensitive current $I_{Ca.T}$. $I_{Ca.L}$ produces depolarization and propagation in sinus and AV nodal cells and contributes to the plateau of atrial and ventricular myocytes. Calcium channel blockers block this channel, which is strongly modulated by neurotransmitters. $I_{Ca.T}$ is activated at membrane potentials intermediate between I_{Na} and $I_{Ca.L}$ and probably contributes inward current to the later stages of phase 4 depolarizations in the sinus node and His-Purkinje cells.[54] A functional role of $I_{Ca.T}$ in normal atrial and ventricular myocytes is less certain. Whether Ca^{2+} influx through open T-type channels provides a sufficient trigger for Ca^{2+} release from the sarcoplasmic reticulum is controversial. The density of T-type Ca^{2+} channels has been found to be increased in myocytes from hearts with experimentally induced hypertrophy,[54] but the role of enhanced T-type channel density under these conditions remains to be determined.

Other significant differences exist between the fast and slow channels (see Table 27–4). Drugs that elevate cAMP levels, such as beta adrenoceptor agonists, phosphodiesterase inhibitors such as theophylline, and the lipid-soluble derivative of cAMP dibutyryl cAMP, increase $I_{Ca.L}$. Binding of the beta adrenoceptor agonist to specific sarcolemmal receptors facilitates the dissociation of two subunits of a regulatory protein (G protein, see Chap. 19), one of which (G_s) activates adenylate cyclase and thus increases intracellular levels of cAMP. The latter binds to a regulatory subunit of a cAMP-dependent protein kinase that promotes phosphorylation of specific phosphorylation sites on the channel protein (see Fig. 27–9A), ultimately resulting in enhanced open-state probability of the channel.

Acetylcholine reduces $I_{Ca.L}$ by decreasing adenylate cyclase activity. However, acetylcholine stimulates cyclic guanosine monophosphate (cGMP) accumulation. cGMP has negligible effects on basal $I_{Ca.L}$ but decreases $I_{Ca.L}$ levels that have been elevated by beta adrenoceptor agonists. This effect is mediated by cAMP hydrolysis through a cGMP-stimulated cyclic nucleotide phosphodiesterase.[55]

DIFFERENCES BETWEEN CHANNELS. Fast and slow channels can be differentiated on the basis of their pharmacological sensitivity. Drugs that block the slow channel with a *fair* degree of specificity include verapamil, nifedipine, diltiazem, and D-600 (a methoxy derivative of verapamil). Antiarrhythmic agents such as lidocaine, quinidine, procainamide, and disopyramide (see Chap. 30) affect the fast channel and not the slow channel. The puffer fish poison TTX, which is too toxic to be used clinically, blocks the fast channel with considerable specificity (see Table 27–4).

Normal action potentials recorded from the sinus node and the N region of the AV node have a reduced resting membrane potential, action potential amplitude, overshoot, upstroke, and conduction velocity compared with action potentials in muscle or Purkinje fibers (see Fig. 27–15).

Slow-channel blockers, but not TTX, suppress sinus and AV nodal action potentials. The prolonged time for reactivation of $I_{Ca.L}$ probably accounts for the fact that sinus and AV nodal cells remain refractory longer than the time that it takes for full voltage repolarization to occur. Thus, premature stimulation immediately after the membrane potential reaches full repolarization leads to action potentials with reduced amplitudes and upstroke velocities. Therefore, slow conduction and prolonged refractoriness are characteristic features of nodal cells. These cells also have a reduced "safety factor for conduction," which means that the stimulating efficacy of the propagating impulse is low and conduction block occurs easily. Membranes of nodal cells probably do have Na channels that are inactivated by the relatively depolarized range of potentials over which activity takes place. Hyperpolarization exposes a fast TTX-sensitive sodium current in nodal cells.

INWARD CURRENTS. Thus, I_{Na} and I_{Ca} represent two important inward currents. Another important inward current is I_f, also called the *pacemaker current.*[2] This current is activated by hyperpolarization and is carried by Na^+ and K^+. It generates phase 4 diastolic depolarization in the sinus node. I_f modulation is one major mechanism by which beta-adrenergic and cholinergic neurotransmitters regulate cardiac rhythm under physiological conditions. Catecholamines increase the probability of channel opening, with no change in single-channel amplitude, and increase the discharge rate, with cholinergic action, in general, having an opposite effect.

A variety of manipulations, including those that block or inactivate I_{Na} (such as administration of TTX or sustained depolarization of the cell membrane with external Ba^{2+} to block K^+ efflux through I_{kl} channels), combined with those that increase $I_{Ca.L}$ (such as administration of catecholamines), can transform a fast channel–dependent fiber (e.g., a Purkinje fiber) to a slow channel–dependent fiber. Whether these artificial in vitro alterations have clinical relevance is not known.

The electrophysiological changes accompanying *acute* myocardial ischemia may represent a depressed form of a fast response in the center of the ischemic zone and a slow response in the border area. Probable slow-response activity has been shown in myocardium resected from patients undergoing surgery for recurrent ventricular tachyarrhythmias (see Fig. 27–15F). Whether and how slow responses play a role in the genesis of ventricular arrhythmias in these patients have not been established.

Phase 1—Early Rapid Repolarization

Following phase 0, the membrane repolarizes rapidly and transiently to nearly 0 mV (early notch), partly because of inactivation of I_{Na} and concomitant activation of several outward currents:

I_{to}. The 4-aminopyridine–sensitive transient outward K^+ current, commonly termed I_{to} (or I_{to1}), is turned on rapidly by depolarization and then rapidly inactivates. Both the density and recovery of I_{to} from inactivation exhibit transmural gradients in the left ventricular free wall, with the density decreasing and reactivation becoming progressively prolonged from epicardium to endocardium.[56] It is currently unknown whether these nonuniformities in I_{to} recovery reflect transmural differences in channel subunit composition or in posttranslational modification of channel proteins that are thought to underlie I_{to} (Kv4.2 and Kv4.3). Gradients in I_{to} channel density and reactivation kinetics give rise to regional differences in action potential shape, with increasingly slower phase 1 restitution kinetics and diminution of the notch along the transmural axis (Fig. 27–18). These regional differences might create transmural voltage gradients, specifically at higher rates, thereby increasing

TABLE 27–3 Synopsis of Ionic Currents in Mammalian Cardiac Myocytes

I_{Na}	Tetrodotoxin-sensitive voltage-gated Na^+ current
$I_{Na\text{-}B}$	Proposed background Na^+ current through a voltage-independent channel in sinus nodal cells
$I_{Ca.L}$	L-type (*l*ong lasting, *l*arge conductance) Ca^{2+} currents through voltage-gated channels blocked by dihydropyridine-type antagonists (e.g., nifedipine), phenylalkylamines (e.g., verapamil), benzothiazepines (e.g., diltiazem), and a variety of divalent ions (e.g., Cd^{2+}), activated by dihydropyridine-type agonists (e.g., Bay K 8644), responsible for phase 0 depolarization and propagation in sinoatrial and AV nodal tissue, and contributing to the plateau of atrial, His-Purkinje, and ventricular cells; main trigger of Ca^{2+} release from the sarcoplasmic reticulum (Ca^{2+}-induced Ca^{2+} release); a noninactivating or "window" component may underlie early afterdepolarizations
$I_{Ca.T}$	T-type (*t*ransient current, *t*iny conductance) Ca^{2+} currents through voltage-gated channels blocked by mibefradil but insensitive to dihydropyridines; may contribute inward current to the later phase of phase 4 depolarization in pacemaker cells
I_f	Hyperpolarization-activated current carried by Na^+ and K^+ in sinoatrial and AV nodal cells and His-Purkinje cells and involved in generating phase 4 depolarization; increases rate of impulse initiation in pacemaker cells
I_{K1}	Inward rectifier K^+ current, voltage-dependent block by Ba^{2+} at micromolar concentrations: responsible for maintaining resting membrane potential in atrial, His-Purkinje, and ventricular cells; channel activity is a function of both membrane potential and $[K^+]_0$; inward rectification appears to result from depolarization-induced internal block by Mg^{2+}
$I_{K.G}$ ($I_{K.Ach}$, $I_{K.Ade}$)	Inwardly rectifying K^+ current activated by muscarinic [M_2] and purinergic (type 1) receptor stimulation via GTP regulatory (G) protein signal transduction; expressed in sinoatrial and AV nodal cells and atrial cells, where it causes hyperpolarization and action potential shortening; activation causes negative chronotropic and dromotropic effects
I_K	K^+ current carried by a voltage-gated K^+ channel (delayed rectifier K^+ channel); composed of the rapid (I_{Kr}) and slow (I_{Ks}) component. I_{Kr} is specifically blocked by dofetilide and sotalol in a reverse-use–dependent manner; inward rectification of I_{Kr} result from depolarization-induced fast inactivation; plays a major role in determining action potential duration
$I_{K.ur}$	K^+ current through a voltage-gated channel with ultrarapid activation, but ultraslow inactivation kinetics; expressed in atrial myocytes; determines action potential duration
I_{to} (I_{to1}, I_A)	Transient outward K^+ current through voltage-gated channels; exhibits fast activation and inactivation kinetics; blocked by 4-aminopyridine in a reverse-use–dependent manner; determines time course of phase 1 repolarization
$I_{Cl.Ca}$ (I_{to2})	4-Aminopyridine–resistant transient outward current carried by Cl^- ions; activated by rises in intracellular calcium; blocked by stilbene derivatives (SITS, DIDS); determines time course of phase 1 repolarization; may underlie spontaneous transient inward currents under conditions of Ca^{2+} overload
$I_{Cl.cAMP}$	Time-independent chloride current regulated by the cAMP/adenylate cyclase pathway; slightly depolarizes resting membrane potential and significantly shortens action potential duration; antagonizes action potential prolongation associated with β-adrenergic stimulation of $I_{Ca,L}$
$I_{Cl.swell}$	Outwardly rectifying, swelling-activated Cl^- current; inhibited by 9-anthracene carboxylic acid; activation causes resting membrane depolarization and action potential shortening
$I_{K.ATP}$	Time-independent K^+ current through channels activated by a fall in intracellular ATP concentration; inhibited by sulfonylurea drugs, such as glibenclamide; activated by pinacidil, nicorandil, cromakalim; causes shortening of action potential duration during myocardial ischemia or hypoxia
$I_{Cir.swell}$	Inwardly rectifying, swelling-activated cation current; permeable to Na^+ and K^+ ($P_{Na}/P_K = 8$); inhibited by Gd^{3+}; depolarizes resting membrane potential and prolongs terminal (phase 3) repolarization
$I_{Na/Ca}$	Current carried by the Na/Ca exchanger; causes a net Na^+ outward current and a Ca^{2+} inward current (reverse mode) or a net Na^+ inward and Ca^{2+} outward current (3 Na^+ for 1 Ca^{2+}), the direction of Na^+ flux being dependent on membrane potential and intracellular and extracellular concentrations of Na^+ and Ca^{2+}; Ca^{2+} influx mediated by $I_{Na/Ca}$ can trigger SR Ca^{2+} release; underlies I_{ti} (transient inward current) under conditions of intracellular Ca^{2+} overload
$I_{Na/K}$	Na^+ outward current generated by Na^+, K^+-ATPase (stoichiometry: 3 Na^+ leave and 2 K^+ enter); inhibited by digitalis
Electroneutral Ion-Exchanging Proteins	
Ca^{2+}-ATPase	Extrudes cytosolic calcium
Na/H	Exchanges intracellular H^+ for extracellular Na^+; cardiac myocytes express isoform NHE 1; specifically inhibited by the benzoylguanidine derivatives HOE 694 and HOE 642; inhibition causes intracellular acidification
Cl^--HCO_3^-	Exchanges intracellular HCO_3^- for external Cl^-; inhibited by SITS
Na^+-K^+-$2Cl^-$	Cotransporter blocked by amiloride

ATP = adenosine triphosphate; AV = atrioventricular; cAMP = cyclic adenosine monophosphate; DIDS = 4,4′-diisothiocyanatostilbene-2,2′-disulfonic acid; GTP = guanosine triphosphate; SITS = 4-acetamido-4′-isothiocyanatostilbene-2,2′-disulfonic acid; SR = sarcoplasmic reticulum.

TABLE 27–4 Characteristics of Fast and Slow Inward Currents in Cardiac Tissue

Characteristic	Fast	Slow
Primary charge carrier	Na	Ca (Na)
Activation threshold* (mV)	−70 to −55	−55 to −30
Magnitude (μA)	1-30	0.1-3.0
Time constant of		
Activation (msec)	<1	<5
Inactivation (msec)	<1	3-80
Inhibitors	Tetrodotoxin, local anesthetics, sustained depolarization at less than −40 mV	Verapamil, D-600, nifedipine, diltiazem, Mn, Co, Ni, La, Ca^{2+}
Resting membrane potential (mV)	−80 to −95	−40 to −70
Conduction velocity (m/sec)	0.3-3.0	0.01-0.10
Rate of rise ($\dot{V}_{max}$) of action potential upstroke (V/sec)	200-1000	1-10
Action potential amplitude (mV)	100-130	35-75
Response to stimulus	All or none	Affected by characteristics of stimulus
Recovery of excitability	Prompt, ends with repolarization	Delayed, outlasts full repolarization
Safety factor for conduction	High	Low
Major current of action potential upstroke in the following:		
SA node	−	+
Atrial myocardium	+	−
AV node (N region)	−	+
His-Purkinje system	+	−
Ventricular myocardium	+	−
Neurotransmitter influence		
Beta-adrenergic	−	↑↑
Alpha-adrenergic	−	↑
Muscarinic, cholinergic	−	↓ In atrium ↓ In ventricle

AV = atrioventricular; SA = sinoatrial.

*Note that the term "threshold" does not stand for a sharp voltage threshold for channel opening but a threshold for reversal of the net membrane current. This situation occurs when the membrane potential reaches a range where just enough Na^+ (or Ca^{2+}) channels open to make an inward current that opposes the sum of outward currents carried by K^+ and other ions.

CH 27

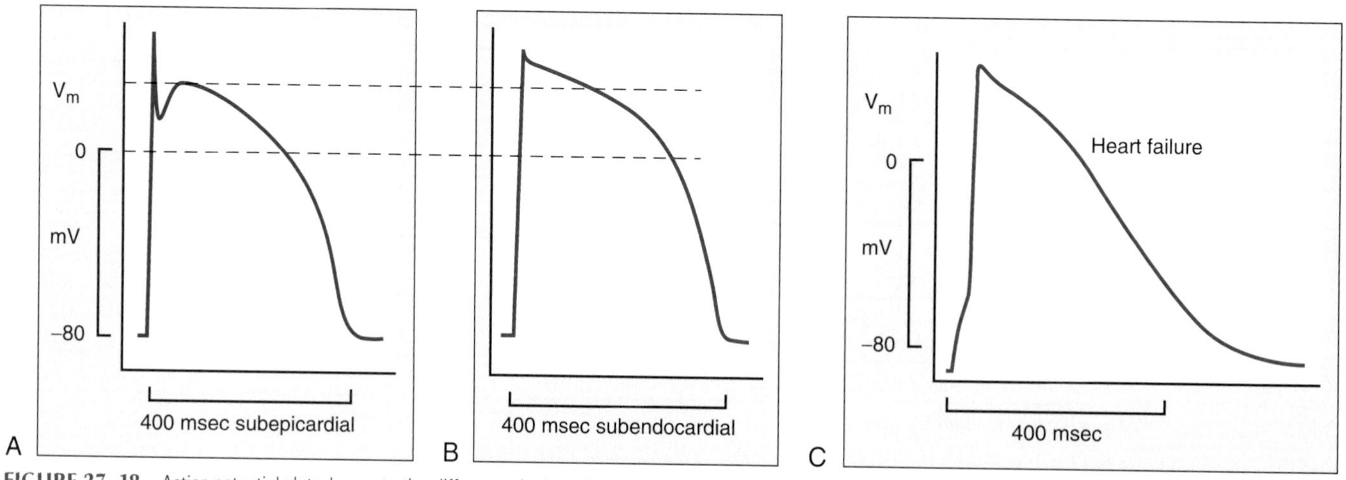

FIGURE 27–18 Action potential plots demonstrating differences in the action potential shape of human ventricular myocytes of subepicardial **(A)** and subendocardial **(B)** origin. Subepicardial myocytes present a prominent notch during phase 1 repolarization of the action potential, most likely caused by a larger I_{to} in these cells. The notch is absent in subendocardial cells. The peak plateau potential is higher in subendocardial than in subepicardial myocytes, and the action potential duration tends to be shorter in subepicardial cells. Recording temperature = 35°C; V_m = membrane potential. **C,** Transmembrane action potential in a human ventricular cardiomyocyte of a failing heart. Note loss of the prominent phase 1 notch and delayed repolarization. (**A** and **B,** From Näbauer M, Beuckelmann DJ, Uberfuhr P, Steinbeck G: Regional differences in current density and rate-dependent properties of the transient outward current in subepicardial and subendocardial myocytes of human left ventricle. Circulation 93:168, 1996. By permission of the American Heart Association. **C,** From Priebe L, Beuckelmann DJ: Simulation studies of cellular electrical properties in heart failure. Circ Res 82:1206-1223, 1998.)

dispersion of repolarization, a putative arrhythmogenic factor (see Brugada syndrome in Chap. 32). Because I_{to} overlaps I_{Na}, changes in I_{to} density or properties can also affect cellular excitability. Downregulation of I_{to} is at least partially responsible for slowing of phase 1 repolarization in failing human myocytes.[57] Studies have demonstrated that these changes in the phase 1 notch of the cardiac action potential cause a reduction in the kinetics and peak amplitude of the action potential-evoked intracellular Ca^{2+} transient because of failed recruitment and synchronization of the sarcoplasmic reticulum Ca^{2+} release through $I_{Ca,L}$. Thus, modulation of I_{to} appears to play a significant physiological role in controlling cardiac excitation-contraction coupling,[58,59] and it remains to be determined whether transmural differences in phase 1 repolarization translate into similar differences in regional contractility.

$I_{Cl.Ca}$. The 4-aminopyridine-resistant, Ca^{2+}-activated chloride current $I_{Cl.Ca}$ (or I_{to2}) also contributes a significant outward current during phase 1 repolarization.[60] This current is activated by the action potential-evoked intracellular Ca^{2+} transient. Therefore, interventions that augment the amplitude of the Ca^{2+} transient associated with the twitch (such as beta-adrenergic receptor stimulation) also enhance outward $I_{Cl.Ca}$. It is not currently known whether human cardiac myocytes express Ca^{2+}-activated chloride channels. Other, time-*in*dependent chloride currents may also play a role in determining the time course of early repolarization, such as the cAMP- or swelling-activated chloride conductances $I_{Cl.cAMP}$ and $I_{Cl.swell}$.[47]

Na/Ca EXCHANGER. A third current contributing to early repolarization is Na^+ outward movement through the Na/Ca exchanger operating in reverse mode (see Fig. 27–14).[61] Overexpression of the exchanger in transgenic mice caused accentuation of the early "notch" in left ventricular myocytes.[62]

Sometimes, a transient depolarization follows phase 1 repolarization. This notch is well defined and separated from phase 2 in Purkinje fibers and left ventricular epicardial and midmyocardial myocytes (see Fig. 27–18).

Phase 2—Plateau

During the plateau phase, which may last several hundred milliseconds, membrane conductance to all ions falls to rather low values. Thus, less change in current is required near plateau levels than near resting potential levels to produce the same changes in transmembrane potential. The plateau is maintained by the competition between outward current carried by K^+ and Cl^- ions and inward current carried by Ca^{2+} moving through open L-type Ca^{2+} channels and Na^+ being exchanged for internal Ca^{2+} by the Na^+/Ca^{2+} exchanger operating in forward mode. After depolarization, potassium conductance falls to plateau levels as a result of inward rectification in spite of the large electrochemical driving force on K^+ ions.

Rectification simply means that membrane conductance changes with voltage. Specifically, inward rectification means that K^+ channels are open at negative potentials but shut at less negative or positive voltages. Membrane depolarization-induced internal block by intracellular ionized magnesium is thought to underlie inward rectification of cardiac I_{K1} channels. The mechanism underlying rectification of the rapid component of the delayed rectifier K^+ current (I_{Kr}) in cardiac cells is the inactivation that channels rapidly undergo during depolarizing pulses. More I_{Kr} channels enter the inactivated state with stronger depolarizations, thereby causing inward rectification. This fast inactivation mechanism is sensitive to changes in extracellular K^+ in the physiological range, with inactivation more accentuated at low extracellular K^+ concentrations.[63] Thus, hypokalemia would decrease outward I_{Kr}, thereby prolonging action potential duration.

Outward K^+ movement carried by the slow component of the delayed rectifier K^+ current (I_{Ks}) also contributes to plateau duration. (1) I_{Ks} density has been shown to be correlated with action potential duration[57] and (2) isolated defects in the KvLQT1 subunit, which in combination with the IsK subunit (minK) reconstitutes the cardiac I_{Ks} current, are associated with abnormally prolonged ventricular repolarization (long QT syndrome type 1; see Chaps. 28 and 32). Although I_{Ks} activates slowly compared with action potential duration, it is only slowly inactivated. Therefore, increases in heart rate can cause this activation to accumulate during successive depolarizations. Thus, cumulative activation can determine the contribution to repolarization of K^+ currents that are active during the plateau of the action potential.[29] In conditions of reduced intracellular ATP concentration (hypoxia, ischemia), K^+ efflux through activated K_{ATP} channels is enhanced, thereby shortening the plateau phase of the action potential. Other ionic mechanisms that control plateau potential and duration include the kinetics of inactivation of the L-type Ca^{2+} current. Reduced efficiency of intracellular free Ca^{2+} to induce Ca^{2+}-dependent inactivation, such as in myocytes from hypertrophic hearts, can result in delayed repolarization. Steady-state components of both I_{Na} and $I_{Ca.L}$ (window currents) can shape the plateau phase.

One type of the long QT syndrome, LQT3, is caused by a defective sodium channel gene, *SCN5A*. One mutation in patients with LQT3 involves a deletion of three amino acids in the S3-S4 cytoplasmic linker loop (see Fig. 27–17 and Chap. 28), which is thought to mediate inactivation. The mutant sodium channel is inactivated only incompletely, which results in prolonged depolarizations. Na^+,K^+-ATPase generates a net outward current by pumping out three Na^+ ions in exchange for two K^+. Noninactivating chloride currents, such as $I_{Cl.swell}$ and $I_{Cl.cAMP}$, may produce significant outward currents during the plateau phase under certain conditions, thereby significantly shortening action potential duration. A nonselective, swelling-induced cation current has been shown to cause action potential prolongation in myocytes from failing ventricles.[64]

Phase 3—Final Rapid Repolarization

In this portion of the action potential, repolarization proceeds rapidly owing at least in part to two currents: time-dependent inactivation of $I_{Ca.L}$, with a decrease in the intracellular movement of positive charges, and activation of repolarizing K^+ currents, including the slow and rapid components of the delayed rectifier K^+ current I_{Ks} and I_{Kr} and the inwardly rectifying K^+ currents I_{K1} and $I_{K.Ach}$, all causing an increase in the movement of positive charges out of the cell. The net membrane current becomes more outward, and the membrane potential shifts to the resting potential. Mutations in the human ether-a-go-go–related gene (*HERG*), which is responsible for I_{Kr}, prolong phase 3 repolarization, thereby predisposing to the development of torsades de pointes. Macrolide antibiotics such as erythromycin, antihistamines such as terfenadine, and antifungal drugs such as ketoconazole all inhibit I_{Kr} and have been implicated in the acquired form of long QT syndrome (see Chaps. 28 and 32). A decrease in I_{K1} activity, as is the case in left ventricular myocytes from failing hearts,[57] causes action potential prolongation by slowing of phase 3 repolarization and resting membrane depolarization (Fig. 27–19). Reduction in the outward

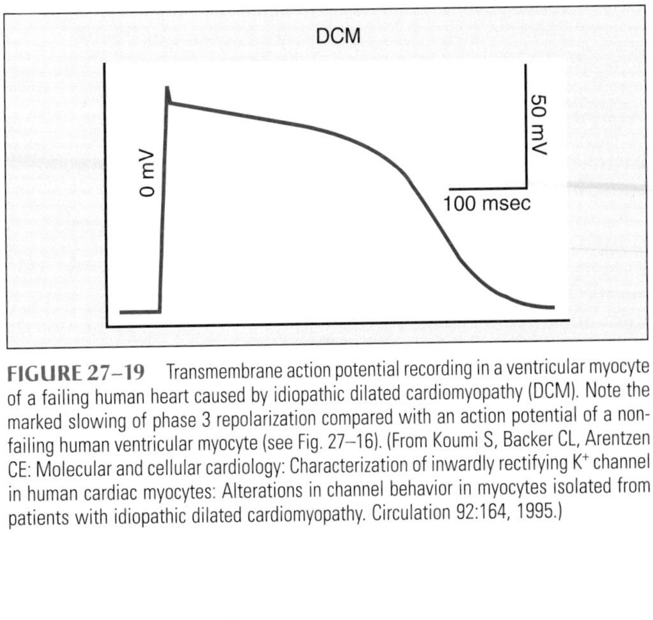

FIGURE 27–19 Transmembrane action potential recording in a ventricular myocyte of a failing human heart caused by idiopathic dilated cardiomyopathy (DCM). Note the marked slowing of phase 3 repolarization compared with an action potential of a nonfailing human ventricular myocyte (see Fig. 27–16). (From Koumi S, Backer CL, Arentzen CE: Molecular and cellular cardiology: Characterization of inwardly rectifying K^+ channel in human cardiac myocytes: Alterations in channel behavior in myocytes isolated from patients with idiopathic dilated cardiomyopathy. Circulation 92:164, 1995.)

potassium current through open inward rectifier K^+ channels renders the failing cardiomyocyte more susceptible to the induction of delayed afterdepolarizations triggered by spontaneous intracellular Ca^{2+} release events and therefore plays a major role in arrhythmogenesis in the failing heart (see Fig. 27–23).

Phase 4—Diastolic Depolarization

Under normal conditions, the membrane potential of atrial and ventricular muscle cells remains steady throughout diastole. I_{K1} is the current responsible for maintaining the resting potential near the K^+ equilibrium potential in atrial, His-Purkinje, and ventricular cells. I_{K1} is the inward rectifier and shuts off during depolarization. It is absent in sinus nodal and AV nodal cells. In other fibers found in certain parts of the atria, in the muscle of the mitral and tricuspid valves, in His-Purkinje fibers, and in the sinus node and distal portion of the AV node, the resting membrane potential does not remain constant in diastole but gradually depolarizes (see Fig. 27–15A). If a propagating impulse does not depolarize the cell or group of cells, it can reach threshold by itself and produce a spontaneous action potential. The property possessed by spontaneously discharging cells is called *phase 4 diastolic depolarization*; when it leads to initiation of action potentials, automaticity results. The discharge rate of the sinus node normally exceeds the discharge rate of other potentially automatic pacemaker sites and thus maintains dominance of the cardiac rhythm. The discharge rate of the sinus node is normally more sensitive to the effects of norepinephrine and acetylcholine than the discharge rate of ventricular muscle cells. Normal or abnormal automaticity at other sites can cause discharge at rates faster than the sinus nodal discharge rate and can usurp control of the cardiac rhythm for one cycle or many (see Chap. 32).

Normal Automaticity

The ionic basis of automaticity is explained by a net gain in intracellular positive charges during diastole. Contributing to this change is a voltage-dependent channel activated by potentials negative to −50 to −60 mV, that is, a hyperpolarization-activated inward pacemaker current. At this potential I_f becomes activated and is carried by a channel relatively nonselective for monovalent cations. Hyperpolarization increases its rate of activation, and at −70 mV the time constant of activation ranges from 2 to 4 seconds. I_f probably underlies the slow diastolic depolarization that occurs between −90 and −60 mV in Purkinje fibers. Although either K^+ or Na^+ ions can serve as ion transporters, I_f carries largely Na^+ at the more negative intracellular voltages. Extracellular K^+ ions activate I_f, but $[Na^+]_o$ does not influence its conductance.

Automaticity in Sinus Nodal Cells

At the reduced membrane potentials of sinus nodal cells, I_f contributes only about 20 percent of the pacemaker current, and automaticity is primarily dependent on I_K and $I_{Ca.L}$. However, sinus nodal cells exhibit significant I_f current if they are hyperpolarized in the range of −50 to −100 mV. Conversely, I_K in normally polarized Purkinje fibers adds little to the pacemaker current. Deactivation of I_K, the presence of an unidentified background inward current, deactivation of $I_{Ca.T}$, and activation of $I_{Ca.L}$ are the essential processes governing the rate of pacemaker depolarization in sinus and AV nodal cells and in Purkinje fibers whose membrane potential has been depolarized to voltages largely positive to the activation range of I_f.

The sinus nodal discharge rate maintains dominance over latent pacemaker sites because it depolarizes more rapidly and because of the mechanism called *overdrive suppression*, a phenomenon characterized by prolonged suppression of normal pacemakers in proportion to the duration and rate of stimulation by a more rapidly discharging pacemaker. The mechanism may be related to active Na extrusion during the more rapid rate that maintains diastolic depolarization of latent pacemakers at a level more negative than the threshold potential for automatic discharge.

The rate of sinus nodal discharge can be varied by several mechanisms in response to autonomic or other influences. The pacemaker locus can shift within or outside the sinus node to cells discharging faster or more slowly. If the pacemaker site remains the same, alterations in the slope of the diastolic depolarization, maximum diastolic potential, or threshold potential can speed or slow the discharge rate. For example, if the slope of diastolic depolarization steepens and if the resting membrane potential becomes less negative or the threshold potential more negative (within limits), discharge rate increases. Opposite changes slow the discharge rate.

Acetylcholine activates K^+ efflux through acetylcholine-sensitive inward rectifier K^+ channels, which are expressed in both sinus nodal and AV nodal cells, thereby shifting the maximum diastolic potential to more negative values. The same mechanism reduces input resistance at diastolic potentials, which means that a greater depolarizing current would be required to achieve "threshold" for firing an action potential.

Studies using fluorescent calcium-sensitive indicators, combined with imaging and simultaneous measurement of transmembrane action potential, suggest that cyclic variations in submembrane Ca^{2+} concentration coupled to activation of the Na^+/Ca^{2+} exchange current modulate sinoatrial node cell beating rate and are a factor in establishing dominance of the sinoatrial node cell pacemaker function (Fig. 27-20).[65]

Passive Membrane Electrical Properties

We have just discussed many of the features of active membrane properties. In addition, it is important to be aware of some features of the passive membrane properties of cardiac myocytes, such as membrane resistance, capacitance, and cable properties.

Although the cardiac cell membrane is resistant to current flow, it also has capacitative properties, which means that it behaves like a battery and can store charges of opposite sign on its two sides: an excess of negative charges inside the membrane balanced by equivalent positive charges outside the membrane. These resistive and capacitative properties cause the membrane to take a certain amount of time to respond to an applied stimulus, rather than responding instantly, because the charges across the capacitative membrane must be altered first. A subthreshold rectangular current pulse applied to the membrane produces a slowly rising and decaying membrane voltage change rather than a rectangular voltage change. A value called the *time constant of the membrane* reflects this property. The time constant tau is equal to the product of membrane resistance R_m and cell capacitance C_m,

$$\text{tau} = R_m \bullet C_m$$

and is the time taken by the membrane voltage to reach 63 percent of its final value after application of a steady current.

When aligned end to end, cardiac cells, particularly the His-Purkinje system, behave like a long cable in which current flows more easily inside the cell and to the adjacent cell across the gap junction than it does across the cell membrane to the outside. When current is injected at a point, most of it flows along inside the cell, but some leaks out. Because of this loss of current, the voltage change of a cell at a site distant from the point of applied current is less than the change in membrane voltage where the stimulus was given. A measure of this property of a cable is called the space or length constant *lambda* (λ), which is the distance along the cable from the point of stimulation at which the voltage at steady state is $1/e$ (37 percent) of its value at the point of introduction.

Restated, λ describes how far current flows before leaking passively across the surface membrane to a value about one-third of its initial value. This distance is normally about 2 mm for Purkinje fibers, 0.5 mm for the sinus node, and 0.8 mm for ventricular muscle fibers. λ is about 10 times the length of an individual cell. As an example, if e is about 2.7 and a hyperpolarizing current pulse in a Purkinje fiber produces a membrane voltage change of 15 mV at the site of current injection, the membrane potential change one space constant (2 mm) away would be 15/2.7 = 5.5 mV.

Because the current loop in any circuit must be closed, current must flow back to its point of origin. Local circuit currents pass across gap junctions between cells and exit across the sarcolemmal membrane to

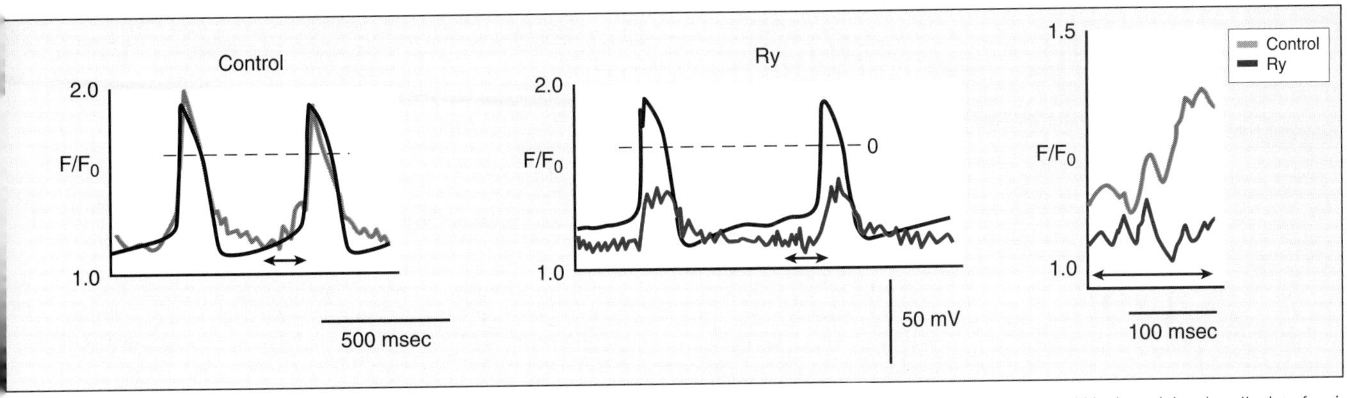

FIGURE 27–20 Ca^{2+} release from the sarcoplasmic reticulum through ryanodine receptors during diastolic depolarization in an isolated rabbit sinoatrial node cell; plot of variations in intracellular calcium concentration (in blue and magenta, respectively) with simultaneously recorded membrane potential. In the control state, the Ca^{2+} waveform exhibits an increase, during the later part of the spontaneous diastolic depolarization, that precedes the rapid upstroke of the action potential (bracketed by arrows and shown at greater resolution in the rightmost panel). This increase is abolished by the specific blocker of the sarcoplasmic reticulum Ca^{2+} release channel, ryanodine (Ry), concurrent with a slowing of the beating rate by this drug. (From Lakatta EG, Maltsev VA, Bogdanov KY, et al: Cyclic variation in intracellular calcium. A critical factor for cardiac pacemaker cell dominance. Circ Res 92:e45, 2003.)

close the loop and complete the circuit. Inward excitation currents in one area (carried by Na^+ in most regions) flow intracellularly along the length of the tissue (carried mostly by K^+), escape across the membrane, and flow extracellularly in a longitudinal direction. The outside local circuit current is the current recorded in an electrocardiogram (ECG; see Chap. 9). Through these local circuit currents the transmembrane potential of each cell influences the transmembrane potential of its neighbor because of the passive flow of current from one segment of the fiber to another across the low-resistance gap junctions.

As discussed earlier, the speed of conduction depends on active membrane properties such as the magnitude of the Na^+ current, a measure of which is $\dot{V}_{max}$. Passive membrane properties also contribute to conduction velocity and include excitability threshold, which influences the capability of cells adjacent to the one that has been discharged to reach threshold; the intracellular resistance of the cell, which is determined by the free ions in the cytoplasm; the resistance of the gap junction; and the cross-sectional area of the cell. Direction of propagation is crucial because of the influence of anisotropy, as mentioned earlier.

Loss of Membrane Potential and Arrhythmia Development

Many acquired abnormalities of cardiac muscle or specialized fibers that result in arrhythmias produce a loss of membrane potential; that is, maximum diastolic potential becomes less negative. This change should be viewed as a symptom of an underlying abnormality, analogous to fever or jaundice, rather than as a diagnostic category in and of itself because both the ionic changes resulting in cellular depolarization and the more fundamental biochemical or metabolic abnormalities responsible for the ionic alterations are probably multicausal. Cellular depolarization can result from elevated $[K^+]_o$ or decreased $[K^+]_i$, an increase in membrane permeability to Na^+ (P_{Na} increases), or a decrease in membrane permeability to K^+ (P_K decreases). Reference to the GHK equation for V (see Phases of the Cardiac Action Potential, General Considerations) illustrates that these changes alone or in combination make membrane diastolic voltage less negative.

Normal cells perfused by an abnormal milieu (e.g., hyperkalemia), abnormal cells perfused by a normal milieu (e.g., healed myocardial infarction), or abnormal cells perfused by an abnormal milieu (e.g., acute myocardial ischemia and infarction) can exist alone or in combination and reduce resting membrane voltage. Each of these changes can have one or more biochemical or metabolic causes. For example, acute myocardial ischemia results in decreased $[K^+]_i$[66] and increased $[K^+]_o$[67], norepinephrine release, and acidosis that may be related to an increase in intracellular Ca^{2+} and Ca^{2+}-induced transient inward currents and accumulation of amphipathic lipid metabolites and oxygen free radicals. All these changes can contribute to the development of an abnormal electrophysiological environment and arrhythmias during ischemia and reperfusion. Knowledge of these changes may provide insight into therapy that actually reverses basic defects and restores membrane potential or other abnormalities to normal.

EFFECTS OF REDUCED RESTING POTENTIAL. The reduced resting membrane potential alters the depolarization and repolarization phases of the cardiac action potential. For example, partial membrane depolarization causes a decrease in the steady-state availability of fast sodium channels, thereby reducing the magnitude of peak I_{Na} during phase 0 of the action potential. The subsequent reduction in $\dot{V}_{max}$ and action potential amplitude prolongs the conduction time of the propagated impulse, at times to the point of block.[30]

Action potentials with reduced upstroke velocity resulting from partial inactivation of I_{Na} are called depressed fast responses (see Fig. 27–15F). Their contours often resemble and can be difficult to distinguish from slow responses, in which upstrokes are due to $I_{Ca.L}$ (see Fig. 27–15F). Membrane depolarization to levels of −60 to −70 mV can inactivate half the Na^+ channels, and depolarization to −50 mV or less can inactivate all the Na^+ channels. At membrane potentials positive to −50 mV, $I_{Ca.L}$ can be activated to generate phase 0 if conditions are appropriate. These action potential changes are likely to be heterogeneous, with unequal degrees of Na^+ inactivation that create areas with minimally reduced velocity, more severely depressed zones, and areas of complete block. These uneven changes are propitious for the development of arrhythmias (Fig. 27–21).

In these cells with reduced membrane potential, refractoriness can outlast voltage recovery of the action potential; that is, the cell can still be refractory or partially refractory after the resting membrane potential returns to its most negative value. Furthermore, if block of the cardiac impulse occurs in a fairly localized area without significant slowing of conduction proximal to the site of block, cells in this proximal zone exhibit short action potentials and refractory periods because unexcited cells distal to the block (still in a polarized state) electrotonically speed recovery in cells proximal to the site of block.

If conduction slows gradually proximal to the site of block, the duration of these action potentials and their refractory periods can be prolonged. Some cells can exhibit abnormal electrophysiological properties even though they have a relatively normal resting membrane potential.

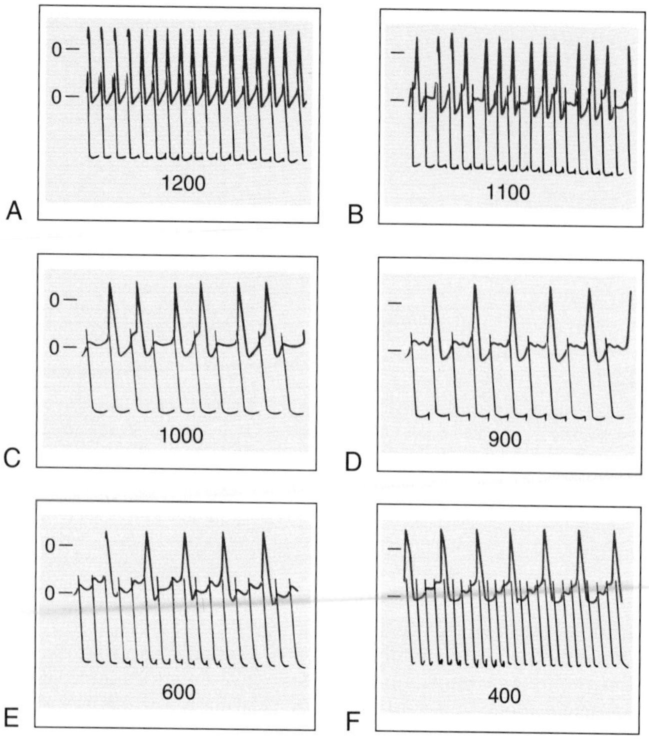

FIGURE 27–21 Rate-dependent conduction from the normal zone into the abnormal zone. When the pacing cycle length in the normal zone was shortened from 1200 to 400 milliseconds (**A** to **F**), increasing degrees of entrance block into the abnormal area occurred and progressed from 1:1 conduction at a cycle length of 1200 milliseconds to 4:3 conduction at 1100 milliseconds, 3:2 conduction at 1000 milliseconds, 2:1 conduction at 900 milliseconds, 3:1 conduction at 600 milliseconds, and 4:1 conduction at 400 milliseconds. Pacing the abnormal zone (not shown) resulted in block to the normal zone (unidirectional propagation). Vertical calibration: 50 mV. Horizontal calibration: 4 seconds in A and B and 2 seconds in C to F. (From Gilmour RF Jr, Heger JJ, Prystowsky EN, et al: Cellular electrophysiologic abnormalities of diseased human ventricular myocardium. Am J Cardiol 51:137, 1983.)

Mechanisms of Arrhythmogenesis

The mechanisms responsible for cardiac arrhythmias (Table 27–5) are generally divided into categories of disorders of impulse formation, disorders of impulse conduction, or combinations of both.[46] It is important to realize, however, that our present diagnostic tools do not permit unequivocal determination of the electrophysiological mechanisms responsible for many clinically occurring arrhythmias or their ionic bases. This is especially true for ventricular arrhythmias. It may be difficult to separate micro-reentry from automaticity clinically, and often one is left with a postulate that a particular arrhythmia is "most consistent with" or "best explained by" one or the other electrophysiological mechanism. Some tachyarrhythmias can be started by one mechanism and perpetuated by another. An episode of tachycardia caused by one mechanism can precipitate another episode caused by a different mechanism. For example, an initiating tachycardia or premature complex caused by abnormal automaticity can precipitate an episode of tachycardia sustained by reentry. However, by using the features of entrainment (see later), arrhythmias caused by macro-reentry circuits can be identified.

TABLE 27–5 Mechanisms of Arrhythmogenesis

Disorders of Impulse Formation
- Automaticity
  - Normal automaticity
    - Experimental examples—Normal in vivo or in vitro in sinus node. Purkinje fibers, others
    - Clinical examples—Sinus tachycardia or bradycardia inappropriate for the clinical situation, possibly ventricular parasystole
  - Abnormal automaticity
    - Experimental example—Depolarization-induced automaticity in Purkinje fibers or ventricular muscle
    - Clinical example—Possibly accelerated ventricular rhythms after myocardial infarction
- Triggered activity
  - Early afterdepolarizations
    - Experimental examples—EADs produced by barium, hypoxia, high concentrations of catecholamines, drugs such so sotalol, *N*-acetylprocainamide, cesium
    - Clinical examples—Possibly idiopathic and acquired long QT syndromes and associated ventricular arrhythmias
  - Delayed afterdepolarizations
    - Experimental example—DADs produced in Purkinje fibers by digitalis
    - Clinical example—Possibly some digitalis-induced arrhythmias

Disorders of Impulse Conduction
- Block
  - Bidirectional or unidirectional without reentry
    - Experimental example—SA, AV, bundle branch, Purkinje-muscle, others
    - Clinical examples—SA, AV, bundle branch, others
  - Unidirectional block with reentry
    - Experimental examples—AV node, Purkinje-muscle junction, infarcted myocardium, others
    - Clinical examples—Reciprocating tachycardia in WPW syndrome, AV nodal reentry, VT due to bundle branch reentry, others
- Reflection
  - Experimental example—Purkinje fiber with area of inexcitability
  - Clinical example—Unknown

Combined Disorders
- Interactions between automatic foci
  - Experimental examples—Depolarizing or hyperpolarizing subthreshold stimuli speed or slow automatic discharge rate
  - Clinical examples—Modulated parasystole
- Interactions between automaticity and conduction
  - Experimental examples—Deceleration-dependent block, overdrive suppression of conduction, entrance and exit block
  - Clinical examples—Similar to experimental

AV = atrioventricular; DAD = delayed afterdepolarization; EAD = early afterdepolarization; SA = sinoatrial; WPW = Wolfe-Parkinson-White.

Disorders of Impulse Formation

Disorders in this category are characterized by an inappropriate discharge rate of the normal pacemaker, the sinus node (e.g., sinus rates too fast or too slow for the physiological needs of the patient), or discharge of an ectopic pacemaker that controls atrial or ventricular rhythm. Pacemaker discharge from ectopic sites, often called *latent* or *subsidiary pacemakers*, can occur in fibers located in several parts of the atria, the coronary sinus and pulmonary veins, AV valves, portions of the AV junction, and the His-Purkinje system. Ordinarily kept from reaching the level of threshold potential because of overdrive suppression by the more rapidly firing sinus node or electrotonic depression from contiguous fibers, ectopic pacemaker activity at one of these latent sites can become manifest when the sinus nodal discharge rate slows or block occurs at some level between the sinus node and the ectopic pacemaker site and permits *escape* of the latent pacemaker at the latter's normal discharge rate. A clinical example would be sinus bradycardia to a rate of 45 beats/min that permits an AV junctional escape complex to occur at a rate of 50 beats/min.

Alternatively, the discharge rate of the latent pacemaker can speed up inappropriately and usurp control of cardiac rhythm from the sinus node, which has been discharging at a normal rate. A clinical example would be interruption of normal sinus rhythm by a premature ventricular complex or a burst of ventricular tachycardia. It is important to remember that such disorders of impulse formation can be due to speeding or slowing of a *normal* pacemaker mechanism (e.g., phase 4 diastolic depolarization that is ionically normal for the sinus node or for an ectopic site such as a Purkinje fiber but occurs inappropriately fast or slow) or due to an ionically *abnormal* pacemaker mechanism.

A patient with persistent sinus tachycardia at rest or sinus bradycardia during exertion exhibits inappropriate sinus nodal discharge rates, but the ionic mechanisms responsible for sinus nodal discharge may still be normal, although the kinetics or magnitude of the currents may be altered. Conversely, when a patient experiences ventricular tachycardia during an acute myocardial infarction, ionic mechanisms ordinarily not involved in formation of spontaneous impulses for this fiber type may be operative and generate the tachycardia. For example, although pacemaker activity is not generally found in ordinary working myocardium, the effects of myocardial infarction can perhaps depolarize these cells to membrane potentials at which inactivation of I_K and activation of $I_{Ca.L}$ cause automatic discharge. Because the maximum rate that can be achieved by adrenergic stimulation of normal automaticity is generally less than 200 beats/min, it is likely that episodes of faster tachycardia are not due to enhanced normal automaticity.

Abnormal Automaticity

Mechanisms responsible for *normal* automaticity were described earlier. *Abnormal* automaticity can arise from cells that have reduced maximum diastolic potentials, often at membrane potentials positive to −50 mV, when I_K and $I_{Ca.L}$ may be operative.

Automaticity at membrane potentials more negative than −70 mV may be due to I_f. When the membrane potential is between −50 and −70 mV, the cell may be quiescent. Electrotonic effects from surrounding normally polarized or more depolarized myocardium influence the development of automaticity. Abnormal automaticity has been found in Purkinje fibers removed from dogs subjected to myocardial infarction, in rat myocardium damaged by epinephrine, in human atrial samples, and in ventricular myocardial specimens from patients undergoing aneurysmectomy and endocardial resection for recurrent ventricular tachyarrhythmias.

Abnormal automaticity can be produced in normal muscle or Purkinje fibers by appropriate interventions such as current passage that reduces diastolic potential. An automatic discharge rate speeds up with progressive depolarization, and hyperpolarizing pulses slow the spontaneous firing. It is possible that partial depolarization and failure to reach normal maximal diastolic potential can induce automatic discharge in most if not all cardiac fibers. Although this type of spontaneous automatic activity has been found in human atrial and ventricular fibers, its relationship to the genesis of clinical arrhythmias has not been established.

Rhythms resulting from automaticity may be slow atrial, junctional, and ventricular escape rhythms; certain types of atrial tachycardias (such as those produced by digitalis or perhaps those coming from the pulmonary veins); accelerated junctional (nonparoxysmal junctional tachycardia) and idioventricular rhythms; and parasystole (see Chap. 32).

Triggered Activity

Automaticity is the property of a fiber to initiate an impulse *spontaneously,* without need for prior stimulation, so that electrical quiescence does not occur. *Triggered activity* is initiated by afterdepolarizations, which are depolarizing oscillations in membrane voltage induced by one or more preceding action potentials. Thus, triggered activity is pacemaker activity that results *consequent* to a preceding impulse or series of impulses, without which electrical quiescence occurs (Fig. 27–22). This triggering activity is not caused by an automatic self-generating mechanism, and the term *triggered automaticity* is therefore contradictory. These depolarizations can occur before or after full repolarization of the fiber and are best termed *early afterdepolarizations* (EADs) when they arise from a reduced level of membrane potential during phases 2 (type 1) and 3 (type 2) of the cardiac action potential and called *late* or *delayed afterdepolarizations*

A

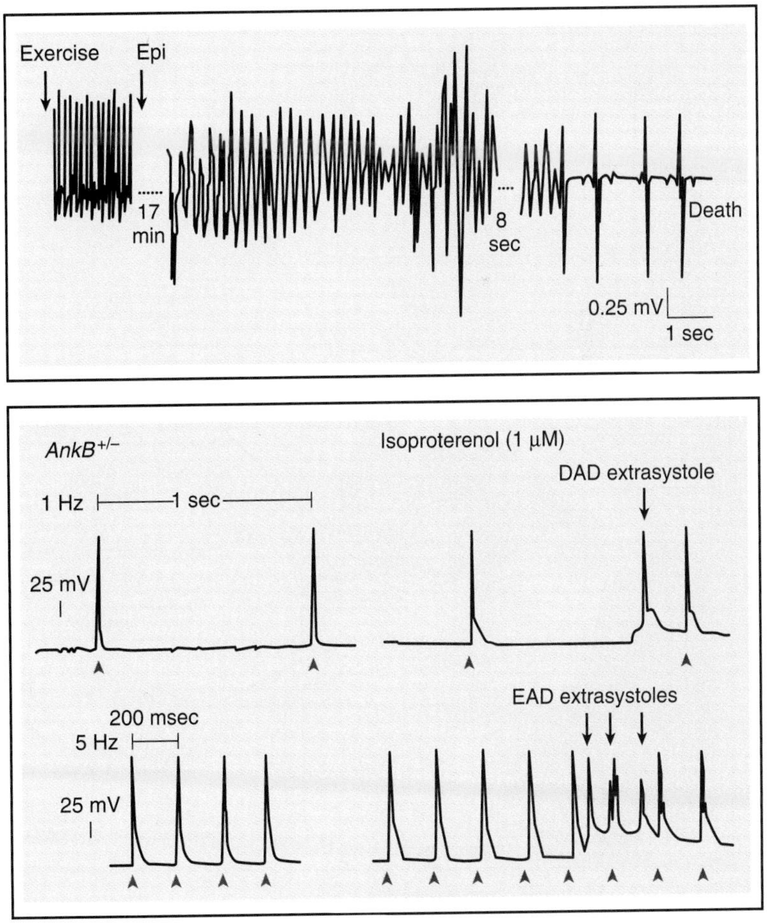

B

FIGURE 27–22 Polymorphic ventricular tachycardia and sudden death in an animal model of type 4 long QT syndrome. **A,** Electrocardiogram after exercise and administration of epinephrine in a mouse heterozygous for a loss-of-function mutation in the gene encoding ankyrin-B (*AnkB*$^{+/-}$). Polymorphic ventricular tachycardia (torsades de pointes) occurred within about 17 minutes of epinephrine administration, followed by marked bradycardia and death 2 minutes after the arrhythmia. **B,** Transmembrane action potentials in single cardiomyocytes from *AnkB*$^{+/-}$ mice at the frequencies indicated. Acute exposure to isoproterenol induced both delayed and early afterdepolarizations that led to extra beats. (From Mohler PJ, Schott J, Gramolini AO, et al: Ankyrin-B mutation causes type 4 long-QT cardiac arrhythmia and sudden cardiac death. Nature 421:634, 2003.)

TABLE 27–6 Determinants of the Amplitude of Afterdepolarizations

Intervention	Effect on Amplitude of EADs	DADs
Long cycles (basic and premature)	↑	↓
Long action potential duration	↑	↑
Reduced membrane potential	↑	↓
Na channel blockers	No effect	↓
Ca channel blockers	↓	↓
Catecholamines	↑	↑

↑ = increase amplitude; ↓ = decrease amplitude; DADs = delayed afterdepolarizations; EADs = early afterdepolarizations.

(DADs) when they occur after completion of repolarization (phase 4), generally at a more negative membrane potential than that from which EADs arise (Table 27–6). Not all afterdepolarizations may reach threshold potential, but if they do, they can trigger another afterdepolarization and thus self-perpetuate.

EARLY AFTERDEPOLARIZATIONS

A variety of interventions, each of which results in an increase in intracellular positivity, can cause EADs. EADs may be responsible for the lengthened repolarization time and ventricular tachyarrhythmias in several clinical situations, such as the acquired and congenital forms of the long QT syndrome (see Fig. 27–22; see Chap. 32).[68,68a] Left ansa subclavian stimulation increases the amplitude of cesium-induced EADs in dogs and the prevalence of ventricular tachyarrhythmias more than does right ansa subclavian stimulation, possibly because of a greater quantitative effect of the left than the right stellate ganglion on the left ventricle.

Patients with the heritable long QT syndrome have abnormally prolonged cardiac action potential duration and are at increased risk for sudden cardiac death from ventricular tachyarrhythmias. The genesis of long QT syndrome–associated ventricular tachycardia or fibrillation is uncertain. There is mounting evidence that increased intracellular Ca^{2+} concentration related to spontaneous Ca^{2+} release from the sarcoplasmic reticulum in cardiomyocytes coupled with dispersion of repolarization plays a causative role in long QT syndrome–associated cardiac arrhythmia and sudden cardiac death (Fig. 27–23; see Fig. 27–22). Action potential prolongation may increase Ca^{2+} influx through L-type Ca^{2+} channels during a cardiac cycle, causing excessive Ca^{2+} accumulation in the sarcoplasmic reticulum and spontaneous sarcoplasmic reticular Ca^{2+} release. The ensuing elevation of intracellular free calcium may depolarize cardiomyocyte membrane potential by activation of Ca^{2+}-dependent chloride currents or the electrogenic Na^+/Ca^{2+} exchange current, or both, thereby evoking EADs. EADs can trigger a propagated response and thereby elicit an extra beat, potentially launching a tachycardia.

Experimental observations[69] also suggest an important role of transmural or longitudinal heterogeneity of repolarization, or both.[70] Marked transmural dispersion of repolarization can create a vulnerable window for the development of reentry. Multiple studies of isolated ventricular myocytes or tissue preparations have demonstrated spatial dispersion of repolarization along the transmural axes of the left and right ventricular free wall. A prominent spike and dome is apparent in myocytes from epicardium and the M region but not in myocytes from endocardium. Action potential duration-rate relationships are considerably more pronounced in cells isolated from the M region.[69] The ionic basis for electrophysiologi-

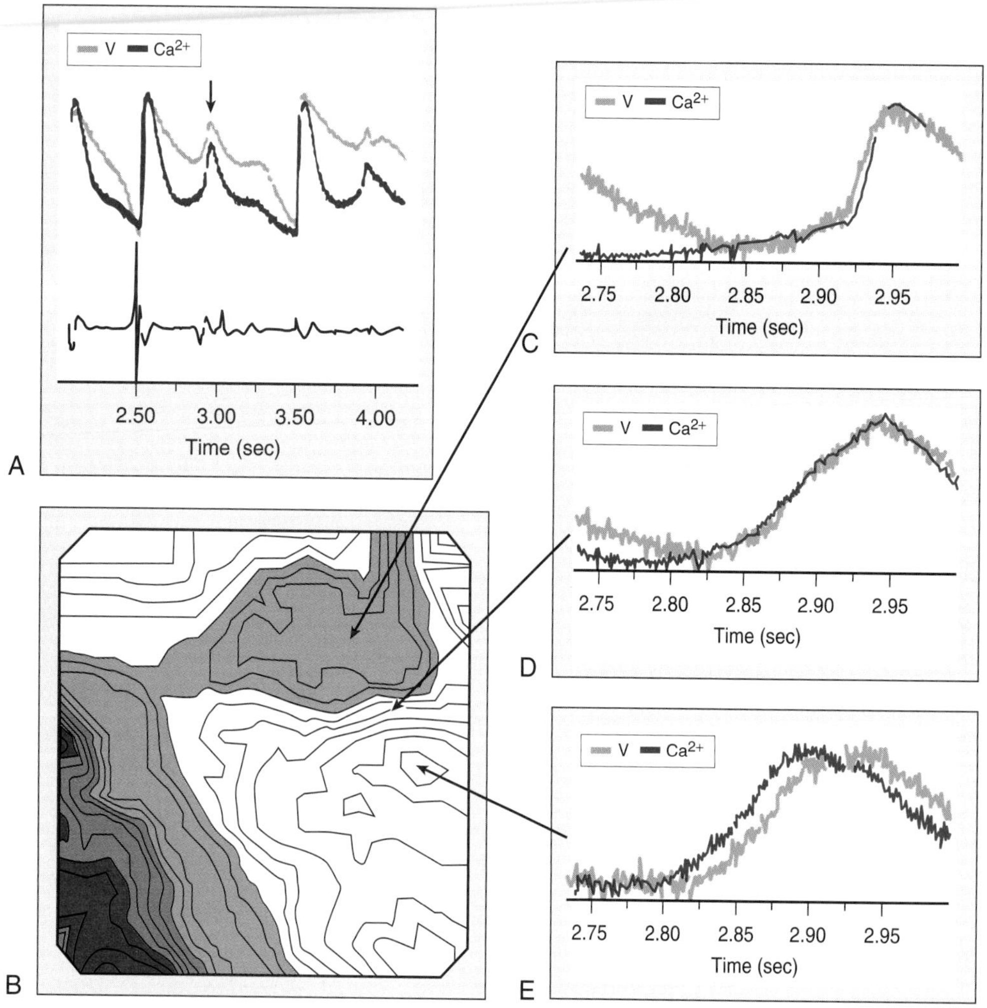

FIGURE 27–23 Primary role of spontaneous increases in intracellular Ca^{2+} $[Ca^{2+}]_i$ in triggering early afterdepolarizations (EADs) in an animal model of type 2 long QT syndrome. Simultaneous mapping of membrane potential (V_m) and intracellular Ca^{2+} concentration using voltage- and Ca^{2+}-sensitive fluorescent dyes, respectively, from the epicardial surface of a Langendorff-perfused isolated rabbit heart exposed to the I_{Kr} inhibitor E4031 and low extracellular concentrations of K^+ and Mg^{2+}. Under these conditions, action potentials are markedly prolonged and spontaneous EADs develop causing polymorphic ventricular tachycardia (torsades de pointes). **A,** Recording of V_m and $[Ca^{2+}]_i$ during an EAD (arrow) and the corresponding depolarizations recorded with bipolar electrogram (bottom trace). **B,** Activation map of the EAD labeled with an arrow in panel A. **C** and **D,** Superimposition of V_m and $[Ca^{2+}]_i$ traces measured at sites remote from the site of origin of the EAD. At those sites, V_m changes precede or are synchronous with those in $[Ca^{2+}]_i$. **E,** Voltage and $[Ca^{2+}]_i$ traces at the first site to fire an EAD. Here, the rise in $[Ca^{2+}]_i$ precedes the rise of V_m. (From Choi B, Burton F, Salama G: Cytosolic Ca^{2+} triggers early afterdepolarizations and torsade de pointes in rabbit hearts with type 2 long QT syndrome. J Physiol (Lond) 543.2:615, 2002.)

cal distinctions among epicardial, midmyocardial, and endocardial myocytes is a large gradient in both the density- and rate-dependent properties of the transient outward K^+ current[56] and a smaller density of the slow component of the delayed rectifier K^+ current I_{Ks} as well as larger late Na^+ currents and inward $I_{Na/Ca}$[71,72] in midmyocardial cells than in myocytes of endocardial and epicardial origin.[56]

Sympathetic stimulation, primarily left, could increase the EAD amplitude to provoke ventricular tachyarrhythmias. Alpha adrenoceptor stimulation also increases the amplitude of cesium-induced EADs and the prevalence of ventricular tachyarrhythmias, both of which are suppressed by magnesium.

In patients with the acquired long QT syndrome and torsades de pointes from drugs such as quinidine, *N*-acetylprocainamide, cisapride, erythromycin, and some class III antiarrhythmic agents, EADs can also be responsible. Such drugs easily elicit EADs experimentally and clinically, whereas magnesium suppresses them. It is possible that multiple drugs can cause summating effects to provoke EADs and torsades de pointes in patients. Activators of ATP-dependent potassium channels, such as pinacidil and nicorandil, can eliminate EADs.[73]

DELAYED AFTERDEPOLARIZATIONS

DADs and triggered activity have been demonstrated in Purkinje fibers, specialized atrial fibers and ventricular muscle fibers exposed to digitalis preparations, pulmonary veins,[74] normal Purkinje fibers exposed to Na-free superfusates from the endocardium of the intact heart, ventricular myocardial cells from failing hearts (Fig. 27–24)[50] and hearts with ankyrin-B mutations (see Fig. 27–22)[68] during beta-adrenergic stimulation, and endocardial preparations 1 day after a myocardial infarction. When fibers in the rabbit, canine, simian, and human mitral valves and in the canine tricuspid valve and coronary sinus are superfused with norepinephrine, they exhibit the capacity for sustained triggered rhythmic activity.

Triggered activity caused by DADs has also been noted in diseased human atrial and ventricular fibers studied in vitro. Left stellate ganglion stimulation can elicit DADs in canine ventricles. In vivo, atrial and ventricular arrhythmias apparently caused by triggered activity have been reported in the dog and possibly in humans. It is tempting to ascribe certain clinical arrhythmias to DADs, such as some arrhythmias precipitated by digitalis or some atrial fibrillations arising from DADs in pulmonary veins. The accelerated idioventricular rhythm 1 day after experimental canine myocardial infarction may be due to DADs, and some evidence suggests that certain ventricular tachycardias, such as those arising in the right ventricular outflow tract, may be due to DADs whereas other data suggest that EADs are responsible.[75]

IONIC BASIS OF DELAYED AFTERDEPOLARIZATIONS. DADs appear to be caused by a transient inward current (I_{ti}) that is small or absent under normal physiological conditions.

When intracellular Ca^{2+} overload occurs, as is the case during adrenergic stimulation, elevated extracellular Ca^{2+} levels, prolonged action potentials, and rapid repetitive stimulation or after large doses of digitalis, spontaneous release of Ca^{2+} from the sarcoplasmic reticulum can activate Cl^- currents[60] or the Na/Ca exchanger[50] and result in transient inward currents and brief membrane depolarizations (see Fig. 27–24). Compounds that reduce the sarcoplasmic Ca^{2+} load (L-type Ca^{2+} channel antagonists, beta-adrenergic receptor blocker) or inhibit sarcoplasmic Ca^{2+} release (thapsigargin, ryanodine, cyclopiazonic acid) suppress DADs. Inhibitors of calmodulin kinase eliminated I_{ti} carried by inward $I_{Na/Ca}$ in isolated rabbit ventricular myocytes,[49] indicating that activation of this enzyme appears to play an important role in cardiac arrhythmogenesis. In addition, drugs that reduce I_{Na} also reduce I_{ti}, relieve Ca^{2+} overload, and

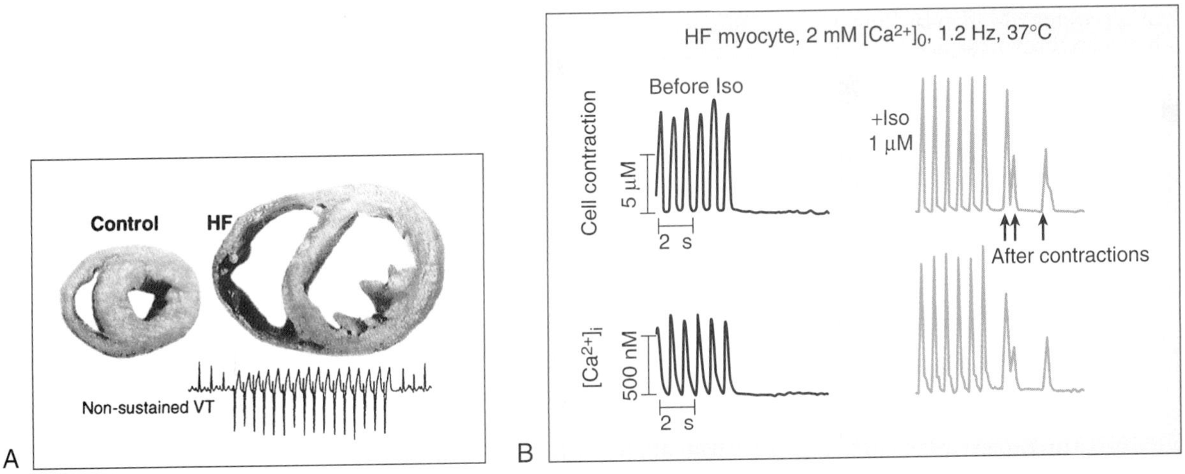

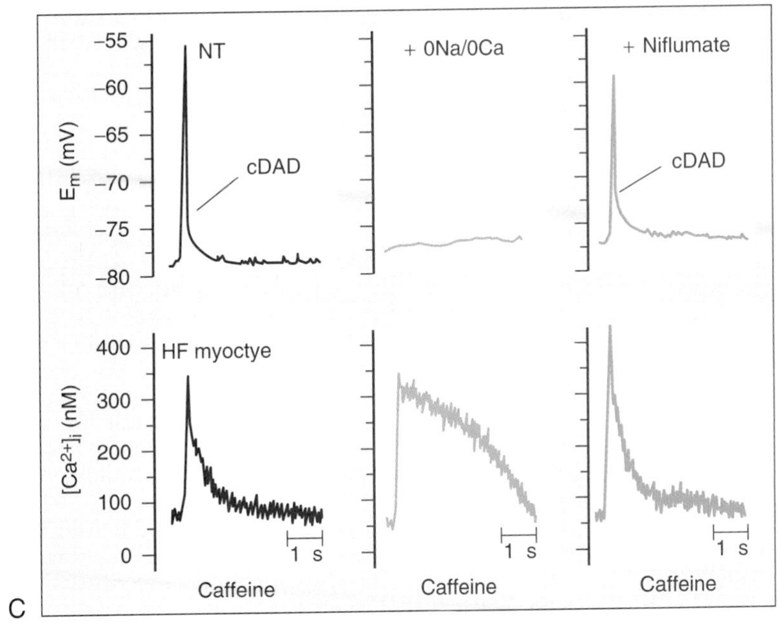

FIGURE 27–24 Ventricular arrhythmia in an animal model of heart failure (aortic constriction-insufficiency in rabbit). **A,** Cross sections of a control and failing heart (HF) and Holter recording of nonsustained ventricular tachycardia (VT) seen in a failing heart. **B,** Spontaneous aftercontractions and increases in $[Ca^{2+}]_i$ in a failing cardiomyocyte after exposure to isoproterenol. **C,** Induction of a delayed afterdepolarization (DAD) by application of caffeine (cDAD) in a cardiomyocyte isolated from a failing rabbit heart. In normal Tyrode's (NT) solution, caffeine causes rapid release of Ca^{2+} from the sarcoplasmic reticulum that leads to increases in intracellular free calcium concentration **(bottom trace),** which in turn causes membrane depolarization. Blocking the Na^+/Ca^{2+} exchange current in Na^+-free and Ca^{2+}-free solution (0Na/0Ca) abolished DADs despite similar increase in $[Ca^{2+}]_i$, whereas blocking the Ca^{2+}-activated Cl^- current with niflumate did not prevent DADs. E_m = membrane voltage. (From Pogwizd SM, Schlotthauer K, Li L, et al: Arrhythmogenesis and contractile dysfunction in heart failure. Circ Res 88:1159, 2001. With permission by the American Heart Association.)

can abolish DADs. DADs most likely play a causative role in arrhythmogenesis in the failing heart. It was found that a given sarcoplasmic reticular Ca^{2+} release produced greater arrhythmogenic inward current in failing cardiomyocytes (because of upregulation of the Na/Ca exchange current), and approximately 50 percent less Ca^{2+} release was required to trigger an action potential in failing myocytes.[50] In addition, downregulation of the inward rectifier K^+ current, I_{K1}, in heart failure allows greater depolarization for a given Na/Ca exchange current. Thus, increased $I_{Na/Ca}$ in concert with reduced I_{K1} (see also Table 27–6) creates a strongly proarrhythmogenic milieu in the failing heart.

Short coupling intervals or pacing at rates more rapid than the triggered activity rate (overdrive pacing) increases the amplitude and shortens the cycle length of the DAD following cessation of pacing (overdrive acceleration) rather than suppressing and delaying the escape rate of the afterdepolarization, as in normal automatic mechanisms. Premature stimulation exerts a similar effect; the shorter the premature interval, the larger the amplitude and shorter the escape interval of the triggered event.

The clinical implication might be that tachyarrhythmias caused by DAD-triggered activity may not be suppressed easily or, indeed, may be precipitated by rapid rates, either spontaneous (such as a sinus tachycardia) or pacing induced. Finally, because a single premature stimulus can both initiate and terminate triggered activity, differentiation from reentry (see later) becomes quite difficult. The response to overdrive pacing may help separate triggered arrhythmias from reentrant ones.

Parasystole

Classically, parasystole has been likened to the function of a fixed-rate asynchronously discharging pacemaker: Its timing is not altered by the dominant rhythm, it produces depolarization when the myocardium is excitable, and the intervals between discharges are multiples of a basic interval (see Chap. 32). Complete *entrance block*, constant or intermittent, insulates and protects the parasystolic focus from surrounding electrical events and accounts for such behavior. Occasionally, the focus can exhibit *exit block*, during which it may fail to depolarize excitable myocardium. In fact, the dominant cardiac rhythm may modulate parasystolic discharge to speed up or slow down its rate. Experimental simulations of parasystole demonstrate that the discharge rate of an isolated, "protected" focus can be modulated by electrotonic interactions with the dominant rhythm across an area of depressed excitability. Brief subthreshold depolarizations induced during the first half of the cardiac cycle of a spontaneously discharging pacemaker delay the subsequent discharge, whereas similar depolarizations induced in the second half of the cardiac cycle accelerate it (Fig. 27–25).

The ionic basis for these rate changes is not totally established, but it is probable that early depolarizing stimuli reactivate outward potassium currents and retard depolarization and late stimuli contribute depolarizing current that enables the cell to reach threshold more quickly. Early hyperpolarizing subthreshold stimuli accelerate and late hyperpolarizing stimuli retard discharge. Similar examples have been noted in human ventricular tissue, and interactions may be predicted according to the general rules of biological oscillators. Numerous clinical examples have been published to support these experimental observations.

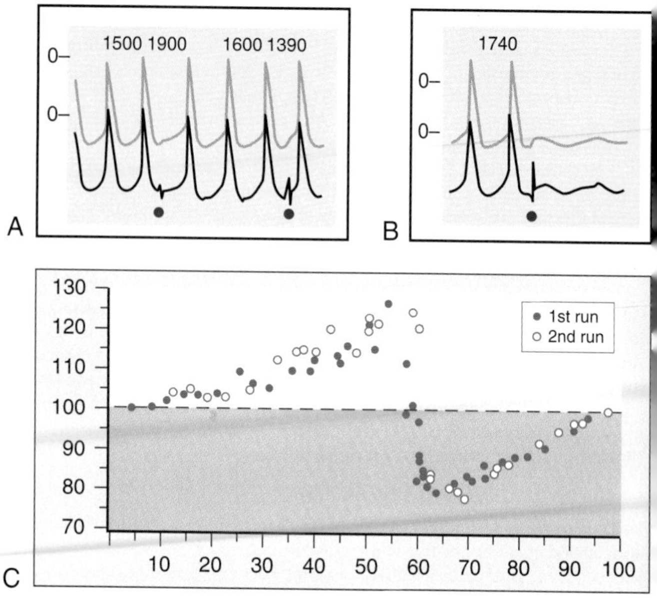

FIGURE 27–25 Modulation of pacemaker activity by subthreshold current pulses in diseased human ventricle. **A,** Two recording sites along the same trabecula in a spontaneously active preparation. Current pulses (indicated by the red dots) 30 milliseconds in duration were injected through the lower microelectrode at various times. The interval between the spontaneous action potentials is given in milliseconds above each cycle. Injection of a subthreshold current pulse through the lower microelectrode relatively early in the spontaneous cycle (about 680 milliseconds after initiation of the rapid portion of the preceding action potential upstroke) produced a subthreshold depolarization in the upper recording and delayed the next spontaneous discharge by 400 to 1900 milliseconds. This response curve would fall in the first half of the curve indicated in C. A current pulse of the same intensity and duration delivered later in the spontaneous cycle (950 milliseconds after the preceding upstroke) accelerated the next discharge by 210 to 1390 milliseconds relative to the previous two action potentials. The response to this current injection falls in the second half of the graph depicted in C. **B,** A stimulus at a precise interval in the cardiac cycle (called the singular point; in this example, 930 milliseconds after the preceding action potential upstroke) abolishes pacemaker activity. **C,** Phase-response curves from experimental data obtained in canine Purkinje fibers in a manner similar to the human experiment shown in A and B. Two different runs are shown. Ordinate = percent increase or decrease in spontaneous cycle length of the "parasystolic focus" (control cycle length equals 100 percent); abscissa = percentage of the "parasystolic focus" spontaneous cycle length during which stimulation was performed. The spontaneous cycle length was maximally prolonged (by 26 percent) or shortened (by 20 percent) by subthreshold depolarizations that entered the parasystolic focus after approximately 50 and 60 percent of the cycle had elapsed, respectively. Very similar curves can be plotted for patients with parasystole (for example, see Figs. 9 and 10 from Zipes DP: Plenary lecture. Cardiac electrophysiology: Promises and contributions. J Am Coll Cardiol 13:1329, 1989). (**A** and **B,** From Gilmour RF Jr, Heger JJ, Prystowsky EN, et al: Cellular electrophysiological abnormalities of diseased human ventricular myocardium. Am J Cardiol 51:137, 1983; **C,** From Jalife J, Moe GK: Effect of electronic potentials on pacemaker activity of canine Purkinje fibers and relation to parasystole. Circ Res 39:801, 1976, By permission of the American Heart Association.)

Disorders of Impulse Conduction

Conduction delay and block[76] can result in bradyarrhythmias or tachyarrhythmias, the former when the propagating impulse is blocked and is followed by asystole or a slow escape rhythm and the latter when the delay and block produce reentrant excitation (see later). Various factors involving both active and passive membrane properties determine the conduction velocity of an impulse and whether conduction is successful. Among these factors are the stimulating efficacy of the propagating impulse, which is related to the amplitude and rate of rise of phase 0, the excitability of the tissue into which the impulse is conducted,[77] and the geometry of the tissue.[30,53]

DECELERATION-DEPENDENT BLOCK. Diastolic depolarization has been suggested as a cause of conduction block at slow rates, so-called bradycardia- or deceleration-dependent block (see Chap. 32). Yet excitability *increases* as the membrane depolarizes until about −70 mV, despite a reduction in action potential amplitude and $\dot{V}_{max}$. Evidently, depolarization-induced inactivation of fast Na^+ channels is offset by other factors such as reduction in the difference between membrane potential and threshold potential and increase in membrane excitability.

PHASE 3 OR TACHYCARDIA-DEPENDENT BLOCK. More commonly, impulses are blocked at rapid rates or short cycle lengths as a result of incomplete recovery of refractoriness caused by incomplete time- or voltage-dependent recovery of excitability (see Chap. 32). For example, such incomplete recovery is the usual mechanism responsible for a nonconducted premature P wave or one that conducts with a functional bundle branch block.

DECREMENTAL CONDUCTION. Decremental conduction is used commonly in the clinical literature but is often misapplied to describe any Wenckebach-like conduction block, that is, responses similar to block in the AV node during which progressive conduction delay precedes the nonconducted impulse. Correctly used, *decremental conduction* refers to a situation in which the properties of the fiber change along its length so that the action potential loses its efficacy as a stimulus to excite the fiber ahead of it. Thus, the stimulating efficacy of the propagating action potential diminishes progressively, possibly as a result of its decreasing amplitude and $\dot{V}_{max}$.

Reentry

Electrical activity during each normal cardiac cycle begins in the sinus node and continues until the entire heart has been activated. Each cell becomes activated in turn, and the cardiac impulse dies out when all fibers have been discharged and are completely refractory. During this absolute refractory period, the cardiac impulse has "no place to go." It must be extinguished and restarted by the next sinus impulse. If, however, a group of fibers not activated during the initial wave of depolarization recover excitability in time to be discharged before the impulse dies out, they may serve as a link to reexcite areas that were just discharged and have now recovered from the initial depolarization. Such a process is given various names, all meaning approximately the same thing: reentry, reentrant excitation, circus movement, reciprocal or echo beat, or reciprocating tachycardia.

ANATOMICAL REENTRY. The earliest studies on reentry were with models that had anatomically defined separate pathways in which it could be shown that they had (1) an area of unidirectional block, (2) recirculation of the impulse to its point of origin, and (3) elimination of the arrhythmia by cutting the pathway. In models with anatomically defined pathways, because the two (or more) pathways have different electrophysiological properties (e.g., a refractory period longer in one pathway than the other), the impulse (1) is blocked in one pathway (site A in Fig. 27–26A) and (2) propagates slowly in the adjacent pathway (serpentine arrow, D to C, Fig. 27–26A). If conduction in this alternative route is sufficiently depressed, the slowly propagating impulse excites tissue beyond the blocked pathway (horizontal lined area in Fig. 27–26A) and returns in a reversed direction along the pathway initially blocked (B to A in Fig. 27–26A) to (3) reexcite tissue proximal to the site of block (A to D in Fig. 27–26A). A clinical arrhythmia caused by anatomical reentry is most likely to have a monomorphic contour.

For reentry of this type to occur, the time for conduction within the depressed but unblocked area and for excitation of the distal segments must exceed the refractory period of the initially blocked pathway (A in Fig. 27–26A) and the tissue proximal to the site of block (D in Fig. 27–26A). Stated another way, continuous reentry requires the anatomical length of the circuit traveled to equal or exceed the reentrant wavelength. The latter is equal to the mean conduction velocity of the impulse multiplied by the longest refractory period of the elements in the circuit. Both values can be different at different points along the reentry pathway, and thus the wavelength value is somewhat contrived.

Conditions for Reentry. The length of the pathway is fixed and determined by the anatomy. Conditions that depress conduction velocity or abbreviate the refractory period promote the development of reentry in this model, whereas prolonging refractoriness and speeding conduction velocity can hinder it. For example, if conduction velocity (0.30 m/sec) and refractoriness (350 milliseconds) for ventricular muscle were normal, a pathway of 105 mm (0.30 m/sec × 0.35 seconds) would be necessary for reentry to occur. However, under certain conditions, conduction velocity in ventricular muscle and Purkinje fibers can be very slow (0.03 m/sec), and if refractoriness is not greatly prolonged (600 milliseconds), a pathway of only 18 mm (0.03 m/sec × 0.60 seconds) may be necessary. Such reentry frequently exhibits an excitable gap, that is, a time interval between the end of refractoriness from one cycle and the beginning of depolarization in the next, when tissue in the circuit is excitable. This condition results because the wavelength of the reentrant circuit is less than the pathway length. Electrical stimulation during this time period can invade the reentrant circuit and reset its timing or terminate the tachycardia.

Rapid pacing can entrain the tachycardia, that is, continuously reset it by entering the circuit and propagating around it in the same way as the reentrant impulse, which increases the tachycardia rate to the pacing rate without terminating the tachycardia (see Fig. 27–28). In reentrant circuits with an excitable gap, conduction velocity determines the revolution time of the impulse around the circuit and, hence, the rate of the tachycardia. Prolongation of refractoriness, unless it is great enough to eliminate the excitable gap and make the impulse propagate in relatively refractory tissue, does not influence the revolution time around the circuit or the rate of the tachycardia. Anatomical reentry occurs in patients with the Wolff-Parkinson-White syndrome, in AV nodal reentry, in some atrial flutters, and in some ventricular tachycardias.

FUNCTIONAL REENTRY. Functional reentry lacks confining anatomical boundaries and can occur in contiguous fibers that exhibit functionally different electrophysiological properties caused by local differences in transmembrane action potential. Dispersion of excitability or refractoriness, or both, as well as anisotropic distributions of intercellular resistance permit initiation and maintenance of reentry.[78] A clinical arrhythmia caused by functional reentry is most likely to be polymorphic because of changing circuits.

Leading Circle Reentry. Leading circle reentry, important in atrial fibrillation (AF), is reentrant excitation during which the reentrant circuit propagates around a functionally refractory core and follows a course along fibers that have a shorter refractory period so that the impulse is blocked in one direction in fibers with a longer refractory period (Fig. 27–27). The maintenance of leading circle reentry is due to repetitive centripetal wavelets that keep the core in a constant state of refractoriness. In addition to refractoriness, the wave front curvature is important in maintaining functional reentry. The curvature of a wave front progressively increases from the periphery to the core. When a critical curvature is reached, propagation fails despite the presence of excitable tissue, forming a central core of reentry.[79]

The pathway length of a functional circuit is determined by the smallest circuit in which the leading wave front is just able to excite tissue ahead that is still relatively refractory. If these parameters change, the size of the circuit can also change and alter the rate of the tachycardia. Shorter wavelengths can predispose to fibrillation. No or a very short excitable gap exists, and the duration of the refractory period of the tissue in the circuit primarily determines the cycle length of the tachycardia because the stimulating efficacy of the head of the next impulse is just sufficient to excite the relatively refractory tissue in the wake of the preceding impulse. Propagating impulses originating outside the circuit cannot easily enter the circuit to reset, entrain, or terminate the reentry.[78]

Theoretically, drugs that prolong refractoriness and do not delay conduction would slow tachycardia as a result of the leading circle mechanism and not affect tachycardia with an excitable gap until the prolongation of refractoriness exceeded the duration of the excitable gap. Drugs that primarily slow conduction would have major effects on tachycardia with an excitable gap and not on tachycardias resulting from the leading circle concept. Mixed circuits with both anatomical and functional pathways obfuscate these differences.

RANDOM REENTRY. Random reentry, also important in AF, occurs when the reentry propagates continuously and randomly and reexcites areas that were excited shortly before by another wavelet.

ANISOTROPIC REENTRY. Anisotropic reentry is due to the structural features responsible for variations in conduction velocity and the time course of repolarization, such as a density of gap junctions at the ends rather than on the side of cells, which can result in block and slowed conduction with subsequent reentry (see Fig. 27–27).[80,81] Even in normal cardiac tissue showing normal transmembrane potentials and uniform refractory periods, conduction can be blocked in the direction parallel to the long axis of fiber orientation, propagate slowly in the direction transverse to the long axis of fiber orientation, and reenter the area of block. Spatial differences in refractoriness may not be necessary for reentry to occur. Such anisotropic reentry has been shown in atrial and ventricular muscle and may be responsible for ventricular tachycardia in epicardial muscle surviving myocardial infarction. An excitable gap may be present.[81]

SPIRAL WAVE REENTRY. Spiral waves of excitation have been demonstrated in cardiac muscle and represent a two-dimensional form of reentry; in three dimensions, spiral waves may be represented by scroll

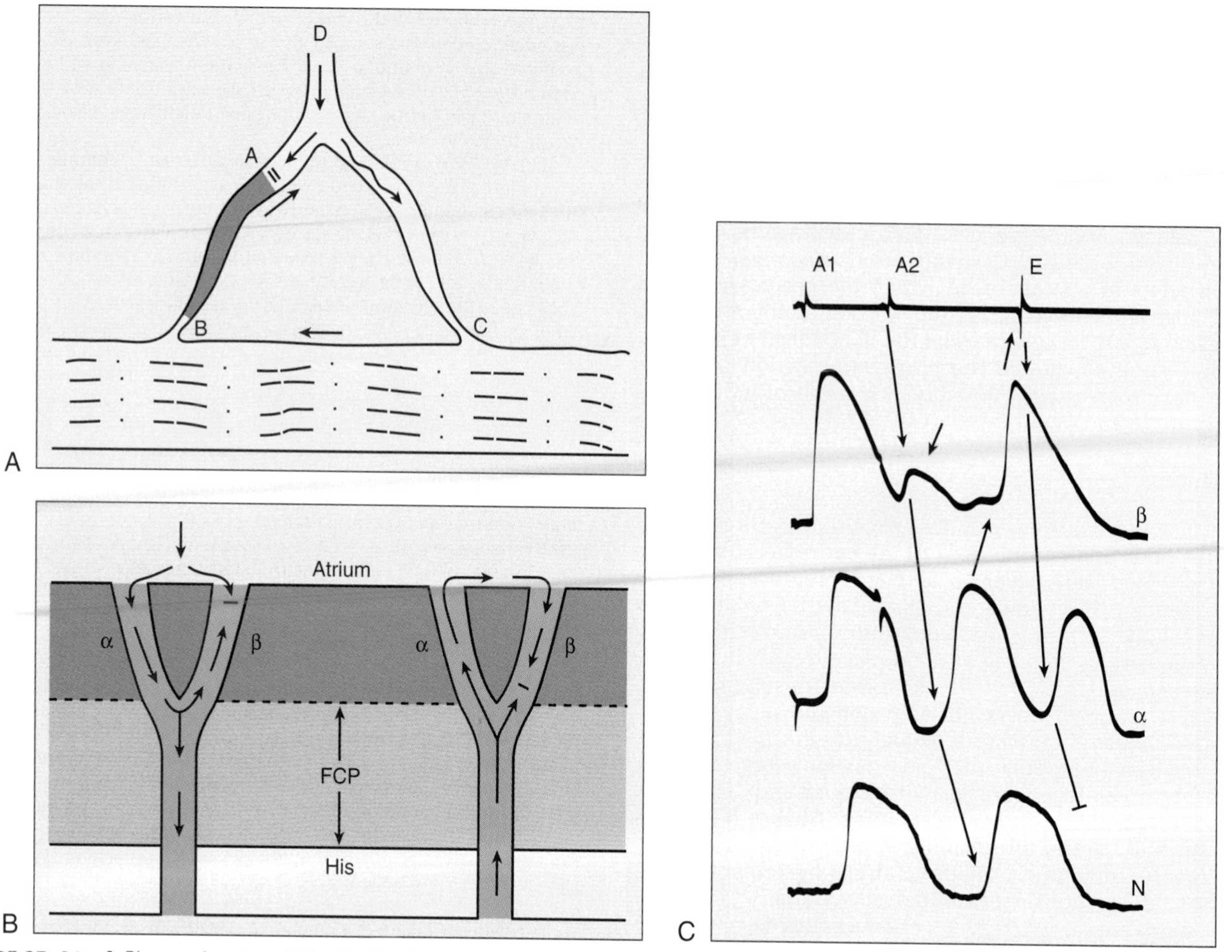

FIGURE 27–26 **A,** Diagram of reentry published by Schmitt and Erlanger in 1928. A Purkinje fiber (D) divides into two pathways (B and C), both of which join ventricular muscle. It is assumed that the original impulse travels down D, is blocked in its anterograde direction at site A (arrow followed by a double bar), but continues slowly down C (serpentine arrow) to excite ventricular muscle. The impulse then reenters the Purkinje twig at B and retrogradely excites A and D. If the impulse continues to propagate through D to the ventricular myocardium and elicits ventricular depolarization, a reentrant ventricular extrasystole results. Continued reentry of this type would produce ventricular tachycardia. **B,** Schematic representation of intranodal dissociation responsible for an atrial echo **(left diagram).** A premature atrial response fails to penetrate the beta (β) pathway, which exhibits a unidirectional block but propagates anterogradely through the alpha (α) pathway. Once the final common pathway (FCP) is engaged, the impulse may return to the atrium through the now-recovered beta pathway to produce an atrial echo. The neighboring **(right)** diagram illustrates the pattern of propagation during generation of a ventricular echo. A premature response in the His bundle traverses the FCP, encounters a refractory beta pathway (unidirectional block), reaches the atrium over the alpha pathway, and returns through a now-recovered beta pathway to produce a ventricular echo. **C,** Actual recordings from the atrium **(top tracing),** with cells impaled in the beta region **(second tracing),** alpha region **(third tracing)**, and N portion of the atrioventricular (AV) node **(bottom tracing)** in an isolated rabbit preparation. The basic response to A1 activated both alpha and beta pathways and the N cell (first tier of action potentials). The premature atrial response A2 caused only a local response in the beta cell (short arrow), was delayed in transmission to the alpha cell, and was further delayed in propagation to the N cell. Following the alpha response, a retrograde spontaneous response occurred in the beta cell and propagated to the atrium (E). This atrial response represents an atrial echo. The echo returned to stimulate the alpha cell but was not propagated to the N cell. It is important that although intranodal reentry has been shown to occur within the rabbit AV node, AV nodal reentry in humans probably occurs over extranodal pathways. (From Mendez C, Moe GK: Demonstrations of a dual AV nodal conduction system in the isolated rabbit heart. Circ Res 19:378, 1966. By permission of the American Heart Association.)

waves. Spiral waves may be stationary when the shape, size, and location of the arc remain unchanged throughout the episode, drifting when the arc migrates away from its site of origin, or anchoring when the drifting core becomes anchored to some small obstacle, such as a blood vessel. One can speculate that a stationary spiral wave could be responsible for a monomorphic tachycardia, a drifting spiral wave responsible for rhythm with changing contours such as torsades de pointes, and an anchoring spiral wave responsible for the transition from a polymorphic to a monomorphic tachycardia (see Fig. 27–27).[82,83] The use of voltage-sensitive probes in combination with high-resolution video imaging to record electrical wave propagation on the surface of the heart has provided experimental evidence for the role of spiral wave reentry in cardiac fibrillation. Experiments in isolated perfused hearts[84] demonstrate that a single rapidly moving rotor or a small number of coexisting but short-lived rotors give rise to ECG patterns of activity indistinguishable from ventricular fibrillation (VF). The rotors can drift and interact with each other and with boundaries in the heart and result in annihilation or formation of new but also short-lived rotors, or both.[84]

REFLECTION. Reflection can be considered a special subclass of reentry. As in reentry, an area of conduction delay is required, and the total time for the impulse to leave and return to its site of origin must exceed the refractory period of the proximal segment. Reflection differs from reentry in that the impulse does not require a circuit but appears to travel along the *same* pathway in both directions.

Tachycardias Caused by Reentry

Reentry is probably the cause of many tachyarrhythmias, including various kinds of supraventricular and ventricular tachycardias, flutter, and fibrillation (see Chap. 32). However, in complex preparations, such as large pieces of tissue in vitro or the intact heart, it becomes much more difficult to prove unequivocally that reentry exists.

Brugada Syndrome

A reentry mechanism has been implicated in the genesis of ventricular tachycardia-fibrillation associated with the inheritable Brugada syndrome, which is characterized by ST segment elevation (unrelated to ischemia, electrolyte abnormalities, or structural heart disease) in the right precordial (V_1 to V_3) ECG leads, often but not always accompanied by an apparent right bundle branch block. The Brugada syndrome appears to be a congenital ion channel disorder because mutations in the cardiac sodium channel gene *SCN5A* have been reported (see Chap. 28).[85] The gene defect causes either acceleration of recovery of the sodium channel from inactivation or a nonfunctional sodium channel. Inhibition of the sodium channel current causes heterogeneous loss of the action potential dome during the plateau phase (phase 2) in the right ventricular epicardium, which leads to a marked dispersion of repolarization and refractoriness and the potential for phase 2 reentry.[86] Whether transmural heterogeneity in Na^+ channel recovery in the right ventricular free wall causes arrhythmia by a similar mechanism remains to be determined.

In addition, many other factors such as stretch, autonomic stimulation, and a host of modulating influences can act on these electrophysiological mechanisms and obscure the cause of many arrhythmias. Initiation or termination of tachycardia by pacing stimuli, the demonstration of electrical activity bridging diastole, fixed coupling, and a variety of other clinically used techniques such as entrainment and resetting curves, although consistent with reentry, do not constitute absolute proof of its existence. The most compelling evidence for reentry is probably provided by entrainment.[87]

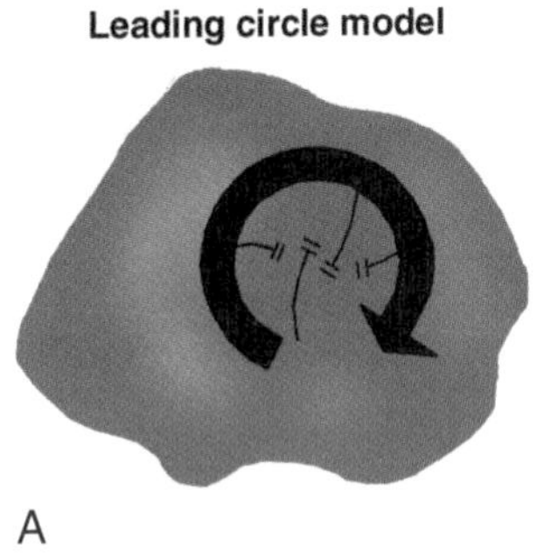

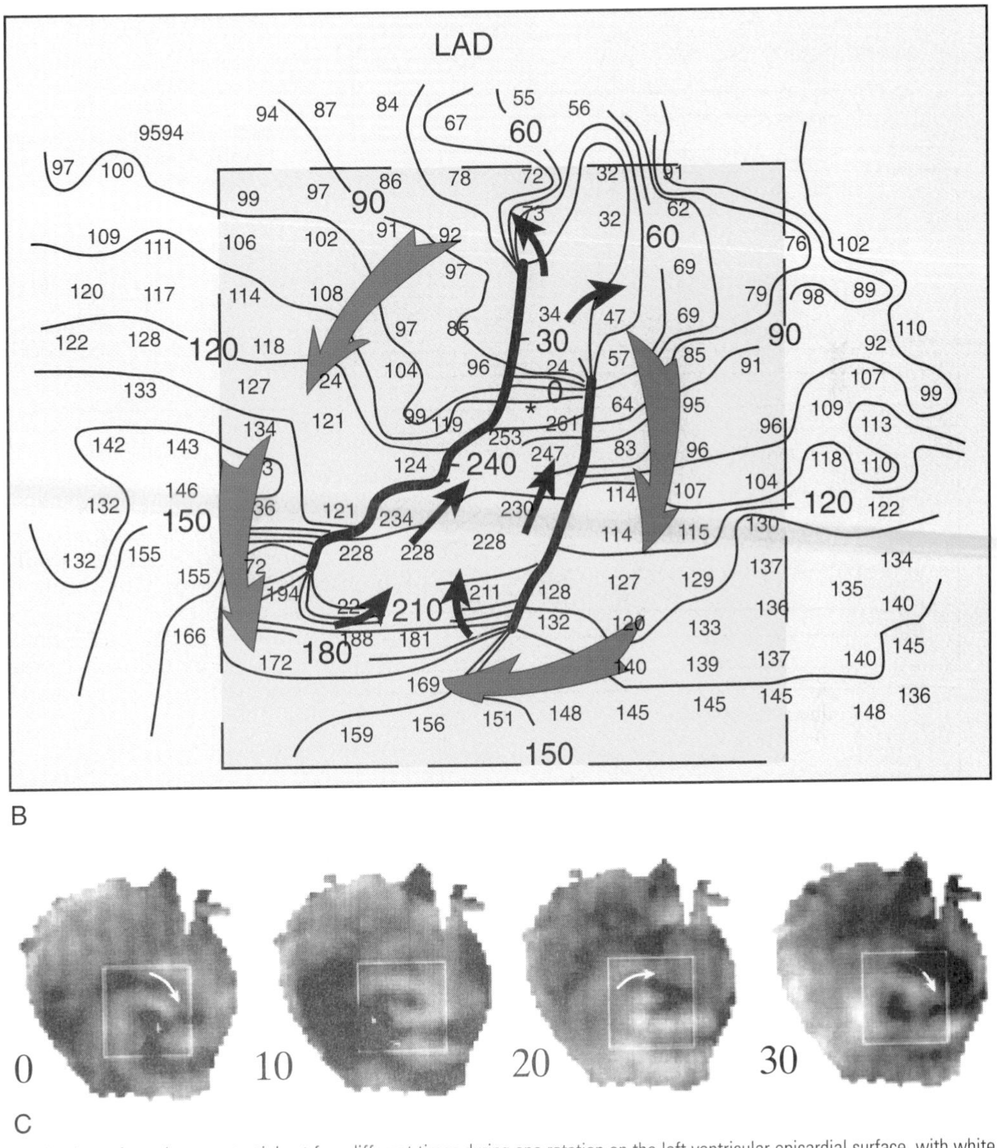

FIGURE 27-27 Functional models of reentry. **A,** *Leading circle model,* a diagrammatic representation of the leading circle model of reentry in isolated left atrium of the rabbit. The central area is activated by converging centripetal wavelets. **B,** *Figure-8-reentry in anisotropic myocardium.* Maps of activation times of a stable reentrant circuit during ventricular tachycardia in the epicardial border zone of a 4-day-old anterior infarct in a dog. The activation times (in milliseconds, small numbers) are shown, as are lines of isochronal activation, at 10-millisecond intervals (larger numbers). The lines of functional block are shown in bold. The circuit consists of clockwise and counterclockwise wave fronts around two functional arcs of block that merge into a central common pathway that usually represents the slow zone of the reentrant circuit. The localization of the functional arcs of block coincides with the spatial disarray of connexin43 gap junctions **C,** *Spiral wave model.* Recording of spiral wave reentry during ventricular fibrillation in a Langendorff-perfused guinea pig heart using a potentiometric fluorophore. Shown are the distributions of membrane potentials at four different times during one rotation on the left ventricular epicardial surface, with white and black being the most positive and most negative membrane potentials, respectively. Numbers are time in milliseconds. Arrows denote direction of wave front propagation. (**A,** From Allessie MA, Bonke FIM, Schopman FJG: Circus movement in rabbit atrial muscle as a mechanism of tachycardia: III. The "leading circle" concept: A new model of circus movement in cardiac tissue without the involvement of an anatomical obstacle. Circ Res 41:9, 1977. By permission of the American Heart Association. **B,** From Peters NS, Coromilas J, Severs NJ, et al: Disturbed connexin43 gap junction distribution correlates with the location of reentrant circuits in the epicardial border zone of healing canine infarcts that cause ventricular tachycardia. Circulation 95:988, 1997. By permission of the American Heart Association. **C,** From Samie FH, Berenfeld O, Anumonwo J, et al: Background potassium current. A determinant of rotor dynamics in ventricular fibrillation. Circ Res 1216, 2001. By permission of the American Heart Association.)

Entrainment

It has been shown that if one could entrain the tachycardia, that is, increase the rate of the tachycardia by pacing, with resumption of the intrinsic rate of the tachycardia when pacing was stopped, the presence of reentry could be established. (Fig. 27–28A). Entrainment represents capture or continuous resetting of the reentrant circuit of the tachycardia by the pacing-induced activation. Each pacing stimulus creates a wave front that travels in an anterograde direction (orthodromic) and resets the tachycardia to the pacing rate. A wave front propagating retrogradely in the opposite direction

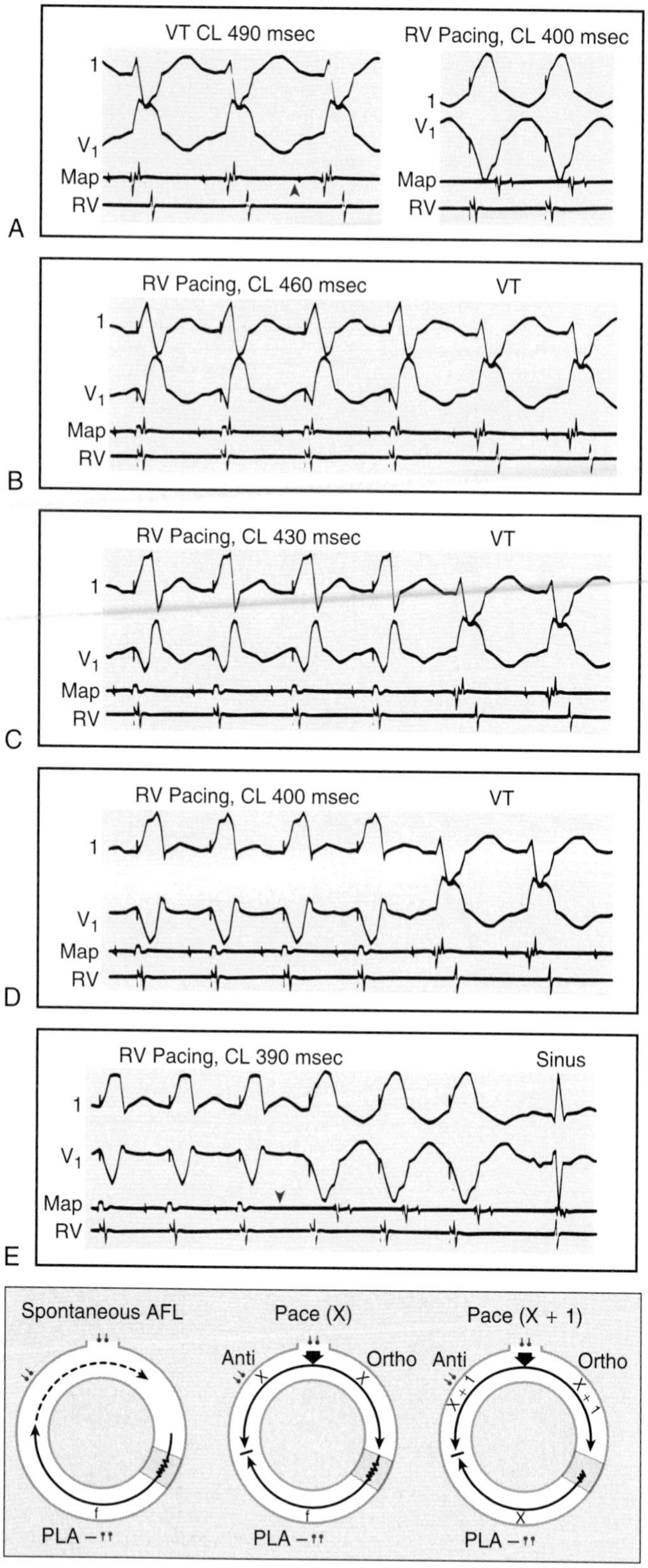

FIGURE 27–28 **Top:** Illustrated criteria for entrainment exemplified in a case of postinfarct ventricular tachycardia (VT). **A, left,** Two electrocardiographic (ECG) leads of a VT and intracardiac recordings from a mapping catheter (Map) at a left ventricular site critical for VT continuation, as well as from the right ventricular apex (RV). Note the diastolic potential (red arrow) during VT. Recordings are similarly arranged in all subsequent panels. **A, right,** RV pacing in the setting of sinus rhythm. **B,** RV pacing at a cycle length (CL) slightly shorter than VT produces a QRS complex that is a blend between fully VT and fully paced ("fusion") complexes. All recordings are accelerated to the paced CL, and after pacing ceases, the same VT resumes. Each fused QRS complex is identical and the last beat is entrained, but surface fusion is absent. **C** and **D,** The same phenomena, but at shorter paced CLs. Note that the fused QRS complex appears more similar to pacing than it does to VT as the pacing CL shortens. B through D thus illustrate a progressive degree of ECG fusion. The Map recording of B through D also shows a progression of fusion, with both the morphology and timing of a portion of the electrogram changing with faster pacing. **E,** Finally, a still shorter paced CL results in a sudden change in both the Map electrogram (block in the small diastolic potential, red arrow) and the surface ECG, which is now fully paced. When pacing ceases, VT has been interrupted. **Bottom:** Diagrammatic representation of the reentrant circuit during spontaneous atrial flutter (AFL) and during transient entrainment of the AFL. **Left,** The reentrant circuit during spontaneous type I AFL. f = circulating wave front of the AFL. **Center,** Introduction of the first pacing impulse (X) during rapid pacing from a high atrial site during AFL. The large arrow indicates entry of the pacing impulse into the reentrant circuit, whereupon it is conducted orthodromically (Ortho) and antidromically (Anti). The antidromic wave front of the pacing impulse (X) collides with the previous beat, in this case the circulating wave front of the spontaneous AFL (f), which results in an atrial fusion beat and, in effect, terminates the AFL. However, the orthodromic wave front from the pacing impulse (X) continues the tachycardia and resets it to the pacing rate. **Right,** Introduction of the next pacing impulse (X + 1) during rapid pacing from the same high atrial site. The large arrow again indicates the entry of the pacing impulse into the reentrant circuit, whereupon it is conducted orthodromically and antidromically. Once again, the antidromic wave front from the pacing impulse (X + 1) collides with the orthodromic wave front of the previous beat. In this case, it is the orthodromic wave front of the previous paced beat (X), and an atrial fusion beat results. The orthodromic wave front from the pacing impulse (X + 1) continues the tachycardia and resets it to the pacing rate. In all three parts, arrows indicate the direction of spread of the impulses; the serpentine line indicates slow conduction through a presumed area of slow conduction (stippled region) in the reentrant circuit, and the red dots with tails indicate bipolar electrodes at the high atrial pacing site, the posteroinferior portion of the left atrium (PLA), and another atrial site. (**Top,** From Zipes DP: A century of cardiac arrhythmia: In search of Jason's golden fleece. J Am Coll Cardiol 34:959, 1999; **Bottom,** from Waldo AL: Atrial flutter. Entrainment characteristics. J Cardiovasc Electrophysiol 8:337, 1997.)

(antidromic) collides with the orthodromic wave front of the previous beat (Fig. 27–28B). These wave front interactions create ECG and electrophysiological features that can be explained only by reentry. Therefore, the criteria of entrainment can be used to prove the reentrant mechanism of a clinical tachycardia and form the basis for localizing the pathway traveled by the tachycardia wave front. Such localization is essential for ablation therapy.[88]

Atrial Flutter (see also Chap. 32)

Reentry is the most likely cause of the usual form of atrial flutter, with the reentrant circuit confined to the right atrium, where it usually travels counterclockwise, in a caudocranial direction in the interatrial septum and in a craniocaudal direction in the right atrial free wall. An area of slow conduction is present in the posterolateral to posteromedial inferior area of the right atrium with a central area of block that can include an anatomical (inferior vena cava) and functional component. It is possible that several different reentrant circuits exist in patients with some types of atrial flutter. However, this area of slow conduction is rather constant and represents the site of successful ablation of atrial flutter. Ablation results are consistent with a macro-reentry circuit.[87-89]

Ventricular Fibrillation (see also Chap. 32)

ELECTRICAL RESTITUTION AND CRITICAL MASS. Substantial experimental support has accumulated in favor of the concept that the onset of VF involves the disintegration of a single spiral wave into many self-perpetuating waves.[84,90] It has been proposed that the breakup of spiral waves is precipitated by oscillations of action potential duration that are of sufficiently large amplitude to cause conduction block along the spiral wave front.

Experimental support for this idea comes from studies demonstrating that if action potential duration restitution (which relates action potential duration to the preceding diastolic interval) contains a region of slope greater than 1, action potential duration alternans is possible and can lead to the formation of reentrant waves.[91,92] Reduction of the slope of the restitution relationship prevented the induction of VF, indicating that the kinetics of electrical restitution appears to be a key determinant of VF. The mass of the tissue appears to be another important factor in the development of fibrillation. In an isolated swine model, it was shown that tissue mass reduction resulted in the termination of VF when a critical mass (19 gm) was reached.[93] In humans, this value appears to be much greater (>111 gm).[92] Similarly, partitioning the atrium into its small segments prevents AF, a concept that has led to a corrective surgical[94] and ablation[95] procedure (see Chap. 30).

LOWER AND UPPER LIMITS OF VULNERABILITY. The cardiac response to electrical stimulation depends on the strength and timing of the stimulus relative to cardiac recovery (coupling interval). A vulnerable zone is present in the T wave during which a stimulus with appropriate strength can induce VF. When the heart is beating spontaneously (e.g., during sinus rhythm), the timing of the vulnerable period corresponds to the T wave on the surface ECG, more precisely, to the latter part of its upslope and its peak.[96] The strength of a stimulus may not be either too low or too high. There is a lower limit of stimulus strength that can induce VF, as well as an upper limit of vulnerability, defined as a current strength at or above which VF cannot be induced.

Propagated graded responses may underlie the mechanisms of ventricular vulnerability to a single premature stimulus. A stimulus delivered during incomplete recovery evokes a gradual response that propagates slowly to neighboring recovered cells and, if its amplitude is large enough, can induce an all-or-none response. This all-or-none response spreads in all directions except into regions near the site of stimulus because of a graded response-induced increase in effective refractory period at the latter site, which results in unidirectional block and reentry (propagated graded-response hypothesis of ventricular vulnerability). When the extrastimulus strength and thus the magnitude of gradual responses increase beyond a critical level, the increase in refractoriness at the site of the stimulus becomes so long that the unidirectional block becomes bidirectional and prevents the formation of reentry (upper limit of vulnerability).[96]

Atrial Fibrillation

SPATIOTEMPORAL ORGANIZATION AND FOCAL DISCHARGE (see also Chap. 32). According to the multiple-wavelet hypothesis, AF is characterized by fragmentation of the wave front into multiple daughter wavelets that wander randomly throughout the atrium and give rise to new wavelets that collide with each other and are mutually annihilated or that give rise to new wavelets in a perpetual activity (for a demonstration of wave front dynamics during fibrillation, see enclosed movie from Samie and colleagues[84]).

The randomness of the irregular electrical activity during AF has been disputed on the basis of both statistical methods and experimental studies. A combination of high-resolution video imaging, ECG recordings, and spectral analysis was used to demonstrate that reentry in anatomically or functionally determined circuits forms the basis of spatiotemporal periodicity during acute AF.[97-99] The cycle length of the source in the left atrium determines the dominant peak in the frequency spectra. The underlying periodicity may stem from a repetitive focal source of activity propagated from an individual pulmonary vein to the remainder of the atrium as fibrillating waves.[100] If a single repetitive focal source of activity that undergoes fractionation underlies maintenance of AF, ablation of this focal source should interrupt AF. Indeed, delivery of radiofrequency energy to discrete sites in the distal pulmonary veins in humans has been shown to eliminate or reduce recurrence of AF.[101]

ELECTRICAL REMODELING OF THE ATRIA. Electrical remodeling of the atria appears to be a key determinant for maintenance of AF.[102] Prolonged rapid atrial pacing in goats and dogs causes electrophysiological alterations of the atria, including shortening and loss of the physiological rate adaptation of refractoriness and decrease in conduction velocity. Because abbreviation of the atrial refractory period is disproportionally larger than reduction of conduction velocity, the wavelength of the reentrant wavelets shortens and thereby promotes reentrant activity (the wavelength is the distance traveled by the depolarization wave front during the duration of its refractory period and equals conduction velocity times refractoriness). The rapid atrial rate also remodels the sinus node.[103]

The ionic basis of shortening of the refractory period and slowing of conduction may be due to a significant reduction in the density of both the L-type Ca^{2+} and the fast Na^{+} currents.[104,105] The electrophysiological changes are paralleled by similar decreases in messenger ribonucleic acid (mRNA) levels of Ca^{2+} and Na^{+} channel genes, which suggests alterations in gene expression as the underlying molecular mechanisms of atrial electrical remodeling.[106] Changes in the density or spatial distribution, or both, of various connexin types may also cause alterations in atrial impulse propagation.[107] Autonomic remodeling also appears to play a key role in both triggering and maintaining AF. Long-term selective vagal denervation of the atria and sinus and AV nodes prevents induction of AF.[108] Heterogeneous sympathetic denervation of the atria favors the development of sustained AF.[109,110]

A variety of interventions attenuate atrial electrical remodeling resulting from short-term rapid atrial pacing, including administration of L-type Ca^{2+} channel blockers,[111] inhibition of reverse mode Na/Ca exchange current[112] and Na/H exchange,[113] and treatment with ascorbate.[114] Digoxin, in contrast, increases tachycardia-induced electrical remodeling of the atria.[115] These findings support the idea that disturbances of the intracellular ionic homeostasis and oxidative stress may electrically remodel the atria by as yet unknown signaling pathways. The signaling pathways underlying long-term tachycardia-fibrillation–induced electrical remodeling, specifically the molecular mechanisms responsible for altered ion channel gene expression, are unknown.

Sinus Reentry (see also Chap. 32)

The sinus node shares with the AV node electrophysiological features such as the potential for *dissociation of conduction*; that is, an impulse can conduct in some nodal fibers but not in others, thereby permitting reentry to occur.[116] The reentrant circuit can be located entirely within the sinus node or involve both the sinus node and atrium. Supraventricular tachycardias caused by sinus node reentry are generally less symptomatic than other supraventricular tachycardias because of slower rates. Ablation of the sinus node may be necessary in an occasional refractory tachycardia.[116]

Atrial Reentry (see also Chap. 32)

Reentry within the atrium, unrelated to the sinus node, can be a cause of supraventricular tachycardia in humans.[117] Atrial reentry appears to be less frequently encountered than other types of supraventricular tachycardia. It has been shown to be due to reentry, automaticity, and afterdepolarizations causing triggered activity. Distinguishing atrial tachycardia caused by automaticity from atrial tachycardia sustained by reentry over quite small areas, that is, microreentry of the leading circle type, is difficult. Multiple foci can be present.

Atrioventricular Nodal Reentry (see also Chap. 32)

Studies employing optical mapping coupled with microelectrode recording have provided detailed insight into the localization and properties of AV nodal conduction and reentrant pathways underlying AV nodal reentrant tachycardia (AVNRT) (Figs. 27–29 and 27–30).[14,15,118] On the basis of conductive properties, multiple, nondiscrete AV nodal input pathways exist, which can be arbitrarily divided into fast, intermediate, and slow pathways (Fig. 27–29). Impulse propagation occurs rapidly over the atrial tissue (red zone in Fig. 27–29D) and slowly toward the AV node through the transi-

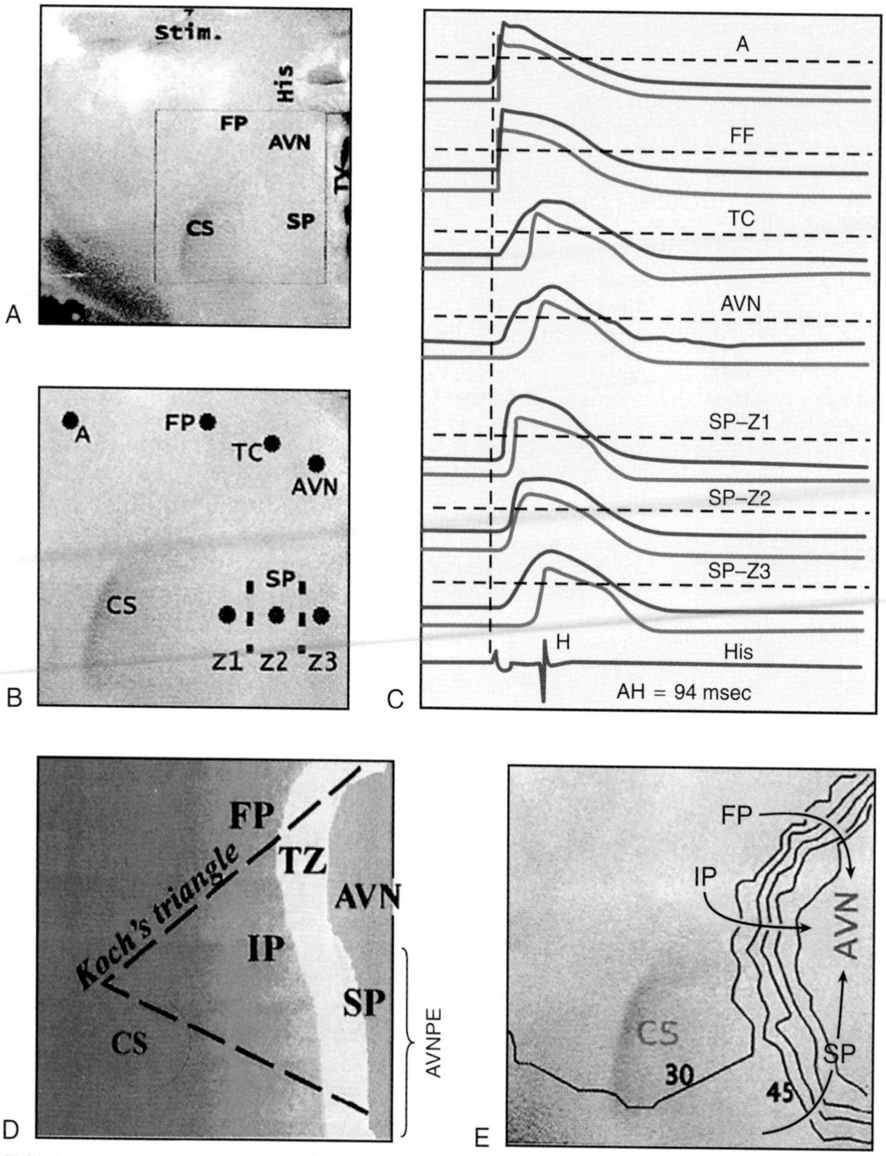

FIGURE 27–29 Atrioventricular (AV) nodal conduction in an isolated, arterially perfused canine preparation. Optical mapping of a potentiometric fluorophore combined with the conventional microelectrode technique were used to delineate the conduction pathways across the AV node. **A,** Endocardial aspect of the preparation. The stimulation electrode (Stim.) and bipolar electrode recording His bundle electrogram (His) are located in the top portion of the picture. The square box next to the tricuspid valve (TV) represents the optical mapping area. AVN = AV node; CS = coronary sinus; FP = fast pathway; SP = slow pathway. **B,** Enlarged picture of optical mapping area to illustrate the sites of microelectrode impalements (dark circles) in atrium (A), fast pathway (FP), transitional cells (TC), AV node (AVN), and three zones (Z1 to Z3) of the slow pathway (SP). **C,** Optical (top, red) and intracellular action potentials (bottom, blue) recorded from different anatomical regions are superimposed and displayed at fast sweep. **D,** Distribution of atrial (red), transitional (yellow), and AV nodal (green) cells in relation to AV nodal inputs (fast [FP], intermediate [IP], and slow [SP] pathways) and posterior extension (AVNPE). **E,** Sketch of the nondiscrete AV nodal input pathways as shown in the optical activation map. (From Wu J, Zipes DP: Mechanisms underlying atrioventricular nodal conduction and the reentrant circuit of atrioventricular nodal reentrant tachycardia using optical mapping. J Cardiovasc Electrophysiol 13:831, 2002.)

tional zone (yellow in Fig. 27–29D) surrounding the AV node. All of the atrial tissue enveloping Koch's triangle (see Fig. 27–29) delivered impulses to the AV node, providing direct evidence to support the concept that slow pathway conduction is present in all normal hearts with or without AVNRT. As seen in Figure 27–29C, conduction delay is associated with a progressive decrease in the upstroke velocity of transmembrane action potentials as well as a progressive lengthening of action potential duration as the impulse approaches the AV node area, suggesting that spatial heterogeneity in the passive (density, cellular distribution, and characteristics of gap junctional channels[118]) or active membrane properties (density or characteristics of ion channels, or both) in the transitional zone underlies AV conduction delay. Optical mapping during echo beats reveals the reentrant pathways underlying the various types of AVNRT (see Fig. 27–30). The reentrant pathway of the slow/fast type starts counterclockwise with block in the fast pathway, delay in conduction across the slow pathway to the compact AV node, then exit from the AV node to the fast pathway and rapid return to the slow pathway through atrial tissue located at the base of Koch's triangle. The reentrant circuit of the fast/slow type is clockwise. In the slow/slow type, anterograde conduction is over the intermediate pathway and retrograde conduction is over the slow pathway. Because slow pathway conduction is involved in each type of AVNRT, this observation explains why ablation of the slow pathway is effective in all types of AVNRT. These results also demonstrate that atrial tissue surrounding Koch's triangle is clearly involved in all three types of AV nodal reentry in these examples (see also Fig. 27–26).

Preexcitation Syndrome

(see also Chap. 32)

In most patients who have reciprocating tachycardias associated with Wolff-Parkinson-White syndrome, the accessory pathway conducts more rapidly than the normal AV node but takes a longer time to recover excitability; that is, the anterograde refractory period of the accessory pathway exceeds that of the AV node at long cycles.[119] Consequently, a premature atrial complex that occurs sufficiently early is blocked anterogradely in the accessory pathway and continues to the ventricle over the normal AV node and His bundle. After the ventricles have been excited, the impulse is able to enter the accessory pathway retrogradely and return to the atrium. A continuous conduction loop of this kind establishes the circuit for the tachycardia. The usual (orthodromic) activation wave during such a reciprocating tachycardia in a patient with an accessory pathway occurs anterogradely over the normal AV node–His-Purkinje system and retrogradely over the accessory pathway, which results in a normal QRS complex (Fig. 27–31).

Because the circuit requires both atria and ventricles, the term *supraventricular tachycardia* is not precisely correct, and the tachycardia is more accurately called *atrioventricular reciprocating tachycardia* (AVRT). The reentrant loop can be interrupted by ablation of the normal AV node–His bundle pathway *or* the accessory pathway.[119,120] Occasionally, the activation wave travels in a reverse (antidromic) direction to the ventricles over the accessory pathway and to the atria retrogradely up the AV node.[119,120] Two accessory pathways can form the circuit in some patients with antidromic AVRT. In

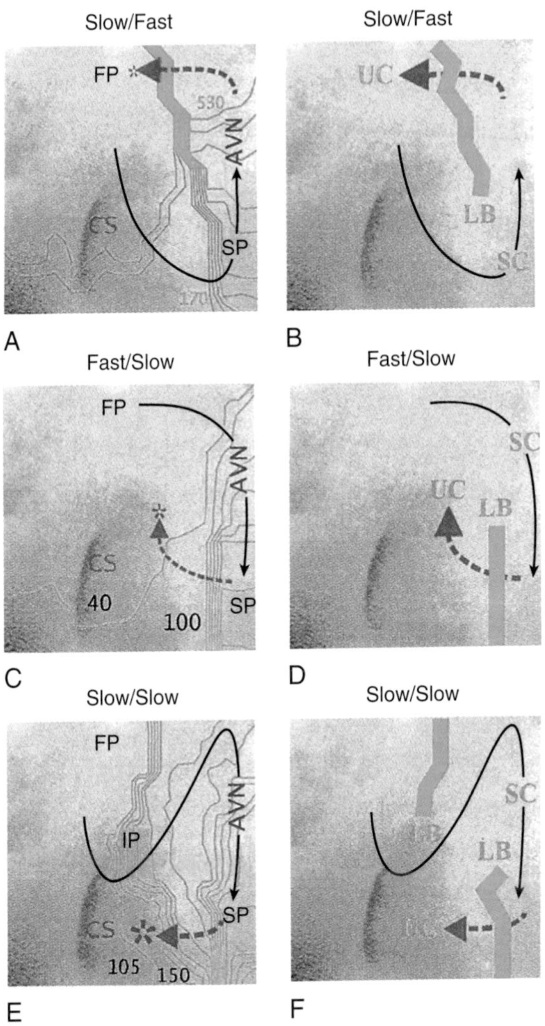

FIGURE 27–30 Reentrant circuits of different types of AV nodal reentrant tachycardia. Pictures of the optical activation maps of A2 obtained from three different experiments at A2 coupling intervals of 190, 220, and 190 milliseconds were merged with the pictures of the mapping area to show the initiation of echo beats in **A** (slow/fast), **C** (fast/slow), and **E** (slow/slow), respectively. The numbers in the maps indicate the activation times in reference to the A2 stimulus. The interrupted black arrow indicates anterograde conduction, and the star and the dashed red arrow represent the site of earliest retrograde atrial activation. The corresponding locations of the lines of block (LB, green), slow anterograde conduction (SC, black arrow), and unidirectional conduction (UC, red) are shown in **B, D,** and **F,** respectively. (From Wu J, Zipes DP: Mechanisms underlying atrioventricular nodal conduction and the reentrant circuit of atrioventricular nodal reentrant tachycardia using optical mapping. J Cardiovasc Electrophysiol 13:831, 2002.)

some patients, the accessory pathway may be capable of only retrograde conduction ("concealed"), but the circuit and mechanism of AVRT remain the same. Less commonly, the accessory pathway can conduct only anterogradely. The pathway can be localized by analysis of the scalar ECG.[121] Patients can have AF as well as AVRT.

Unusual accessory pathways with AV node–like electrophysiological properties, that is, nodofascicular or nodoventricular fibers, can constitute the circuit for reciprocating tachycardias in patients who have some form of the Wolff-Parkinson-White syndrome. Tachycardia in patients with nodoventricular fibers can be due to reentry with these fibers used as the anterograde pathway and the His-Purkinje fibers and a portion of the AV node used retrogradely. In the so-called Lown-Ganong-Levine syndrome (short PR interval and normal QRS complex), conduction over a James fiber that connects the atrium to the distal portion of the AV node and His bundle has been *proposed*, although little functional evidence exists to support the presence of this entity.

Ventricular Tachycardia Caused by Reentry

(see also Chap. 32)

Reentry in the ventricle, both anatomical and functional, as a cause of sustained ventricular tachycardia has been supported by many animal[81] and clinical[122,123] studies (Fig. 27–32). Reentry in ventricular muscle, with or without contribution from specialized tissue, is responsible for many or most ventricular tachycardias in patients with ischemic heart disease. The area of micro-reentry appears to be quite small, and, less uncommonly, a macro-reentry is found around the infarct scar. Surviving myocardial tissue separated by connective tissue provides serpentine routes of activation traversing infarcted areas that can establish reentry pathways. Bundle branch reentry can cause sustained ventricular tachycardia, particularly in patients with dilated cardiomyopathy.[123]

Both figure-of-8 (see Fig. 27–27) and single-circle (see Fig. 27–32) reentrant loops have been described as circulating around an area of functional block in a manner consistent with the leading circle hypothesis or conducting slowly across an apparent area of block created by anisotropy.[81] When intramural myocardium survives, it can form part of the reentrant loop. Structural discontinuities that separate muscle bundles, for example, as a result of naturally occurring myocardial fiber orientation and anisotropic conduction, as well as collagen matrices formed from the fibrosis after a myocardial infarction, establish the basis for slowed conduction, fragmented electrograms, and continuous electrical activity that can lead to reentry. After the infarction, the surviving epicardial border zone undergoes substantial electrical remodeling,[124] including reduced conduction velocity and increased anisotropy associated with the occurrence of reentrant circuits and ventricular tachycardia. Conduction slowing arises from alterations in the spatial distribution[81] and electrophysiological properties of connexin43 gap junctions[125] as well as from reduced sodium current.[126] During acute ischemia, a variety of factors, including elevated $[K]_o$ and reduced pH, combine to create depressed action potentials in ischemic cells that retard conduction and can lead to reentry.[67]

Ventricular Tachycardias Caused by Nonreentrant Mechanisms

In some instances of ventricular tachycardia related to coronary artery disease, but especially in patients without coronary artery disease, nonreentrant mechanisms are important causes of ventricular tachycardias. However, in many patients the mechanism of the ventricular tachycardia remains unknown.

TRIGGERED ACTIVITY. A group of probably nonreentrant ventricular tachycardias occurring in the absence of structural heart disease can be initiated and terminated by programmed stimulation. They are catecholamine dependent and are terminated by the Valsalva maneuver, adenosine, and verapamil. These ventricular tachycardias are generally, but not exclusively, located in the right ventricular outflow tract and may be due to triggered activity, possibly DADs that are cAMP dependent.[75] EADs have been recorded in this tachycardia as well. Left ventricular fascicular tachycardias can be suppressed by verapamil but not generally by adenosine, and some may be due to triggered activity and others to reentry.[75] EADs and triggered activity may be responsible for torsades de pointes.[68,70]

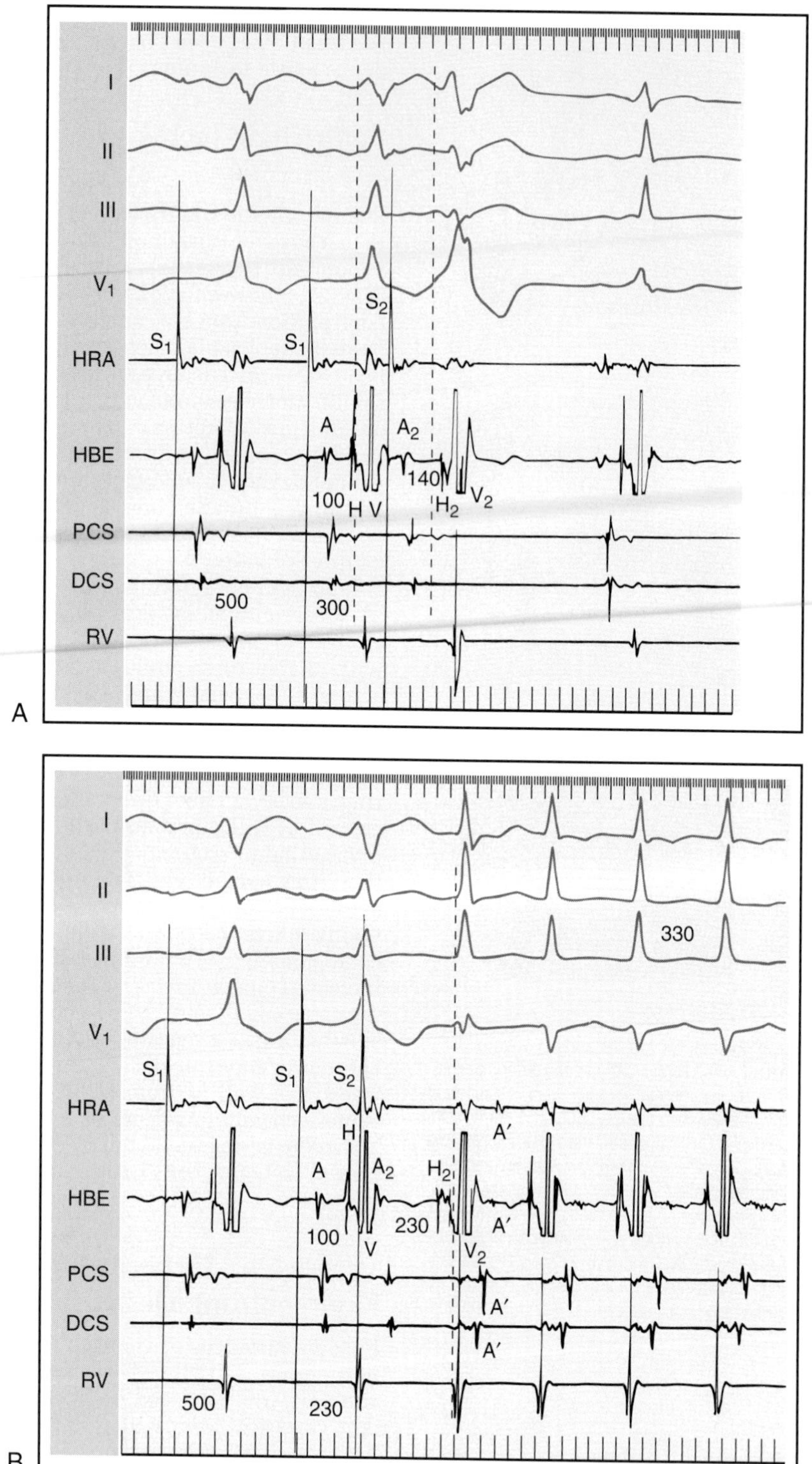

FIGURE 27–31 **A,** Wolff-Parkinson-White syndrome. Following high right atrial pacing at a cycle length of 500 milliseconds (S_1-S_1), premature stimulation at a coupling interval of 300 milliseconds (S_1-S_2) produces physiological delay in atrioventricular (AV) nodal conduction resulting in an increase in the A-H interval from 100 to 140 milliseconds but no delay in the AV interval. Consequently, activation of the His bundle occurs following activation of the QRS complex (second interrupted line), and the QRS complex becomes more anomalous in appearance because of increased ventricular activation over the accessory pathway. I, II, III, and V_1 indicate scalar ECG leads. DCS = distal coronary sinus electrogram; HBE = His bundle electrogram; HRA = high right atrium; PCS = proximal coronary sinus electrogram; RV = right ventricular electrogram. Time lines are in 50- and 10-millisecond intervals. S_1, stimulus of the drive train; S_2, premature stimulus. A, H-V, atrial His bundle, and ventricular activation during the drive train; A_2, H_2, V_2, atrial His bundle, and ventricular activation during the premature stimulus. **B,** Induction of reciprocating atrioventricular tachycardia. Premature stimulation at a coupling interval of 230 milliseconds prolongs the A-H interval to 230 milliseconds and results in anterograde block in the accessory pathway and normalization of the QRS complex (a slight functional aberrancy in the nature of incomplete right bundle branch block occurs). Note that H_2 precedes onset of the QRS complex (interrupted line). Following V_2, the atria are excited retrogradely (A′) beginning in the distal coronary sinus, followed by atrial activation in leads recording from the proximal coronary sinus, His bundle, and high right atrium. A supraventricular tachycardia is initiated at a cycle length of 330 milliseconds. Conventions are as in panel A. (From Zipes DP, Mahomed Y, King RD, et al: Wolff-Parkinson-White syndrome: Cryosurgical treatment. Indiana Med 89:432, 1986.)

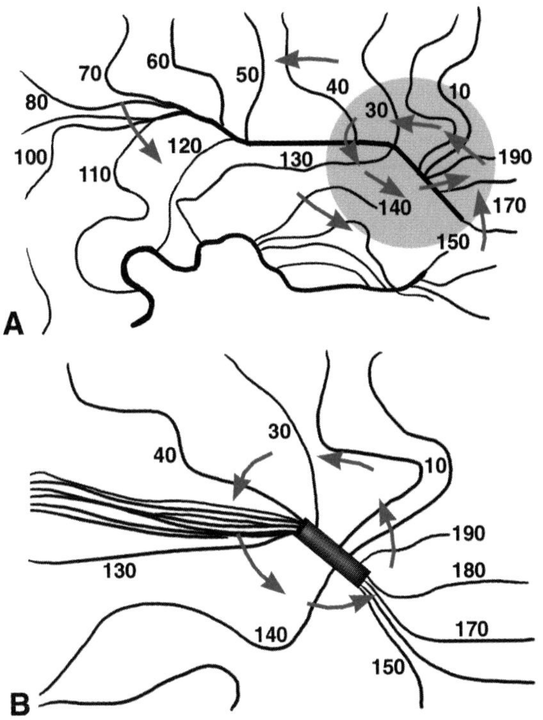

FIGURE 27–32 Model of anisotropic reentry in the epicardial border zone. **A,** The activation map of the single reentrant circuit is shown. The arrows point out the general activation pattern; activation appears to occur around a long line of block. However, parallel isochrones adjacent to the line (isochrones 130 and 140) suggest that activation is also occurring across the line and thereby results in the smaller circuit shown by the arrows in the shaded area. **B,** This circuit is shown enlarged. Rapid activation occurs parallel to the long axis of the fiber orientation (isochrones 10 to 40 and 130 to 150), whereas very slow activation (closely bunched isochrones 50 to 120) occurs transverse to fiber orientation in the circuit. The dark black rectangle is an area of either functional or anatomical block that forms the fulcrum of the circuit. (From Wit AL, Dillon SM: Anisotropic reentry. *In* Zipes DP, Jalife J [eds]: Cardiac Electrophysiology: From Cell to Bedside. Philadelphia, WB Saunders, 1990.)

AUTOMATICITY. Automatic discharge can be responsible for some ventricular tachycardias and does not appear to be suppressed by adenosine. Unless invasive studies are undertaken, mechanisms of ventricular tachycardia can only be conjectured.

REFERENCES

Anatomy of the Cardiac Conduction System

1. Honjo H, Boyett MR, Coppen SR, et al: Heterogeneous expression of connexins in rabbit sinoatrial node cells: Correlation between connexin isotype and cell size. Cardiovasc Res 53:89, 2002.
2. Altomare C, Terragni B, Brioschi C, et al: Heteromeric HCN1-HCN4 channels: A comparison with native pacemaker channels from the rabbit sinoatrial node. J Physiol (Lond) 549:347, 2003.
3. Boyett MR, Honjo H, Kodama I: The sinoatrial node, a heterogeneous pacemaker structure. Cardiovasc Res 47:658, 2000.
4. Lei M, Honjo H, Kodama I, et al: Characterization of the outward K+ current in rabbit sinoatrial node cells. Cardiovasc Res 46:431, 2000.
5. Coppen SR, Kodama I, Boyett MR, et al: Connexin45, a major connexin of the rabbit sino-atrial node, is co-expressed with connexin43 in a restricted zone at the nodal–crista terminalis border. J Histochem Cytochem 47:907, 1999.
6. Martinez AD, Hayrapetyan V, Moreno AP, et al: Connexin43 and connexin45 form heteromeric gap junction channels in which individual components determine permeability and regulation. Circ Res 90:1100, 2002.
7. Bukauskas FF, Bukaukien A, Verselis VH, et al: Coupling asymmetry of heterotypic connexin 45/ connexin 43-EGFP gap junctions: Properties of fast and slow gating mechanisms. Proc Natl Acad Sci USA 99:7113, 2002.
8. Schuessler RB, Boineau JP, Saffitz JE, et al: Cellular mechanisms of sinoatrial activity. *In* Zipes DP, Jalife J (eds): Cardiac Electrophysiology: From Cell to Bedside. 3rd ed. Philadelphia, WB Saunders, 1999, pp 187-195.
9. Schwartz PJ, Zipes DP: Autonomic modulation of cardiac arrhythmias. *In* Zipes DP, Jalife J (eds): Cardiac Electrophysiology: From Cell to Bedside. 3rd ed. Philadelphia, WB Saunders, 1999, pp 300-314.
10. Lakatta EG, Maltsev VA, Bogdanov KY, et al: Cyclic variation of intracellular calcium: A critical factor for cardiac pacemaker cell dominance. Circ Res 92:45, 2003.
11. Steinberg SF: The molecular basis for distinct ß-adrenergic receptor subtype actions in cardiomyocytes. Circ Res 85:1101, 1999.
12. Ackerman MJ, Clapham DE: G proteins and ion channels. *In* Zipes DP, Jalife J (eds): Cardiac Electrophysiology: From Cell to Bedside. 3rd ed. Philadelphia, WB Saunders, 1999, pp 112-118.
13. Chang F, Yu H, Cohen IS: Actions of vasoactive intestinal peptide and neuropeptide Y on the pacemaker current in canine Purkinje fibers. Circ Res 74:157, 1994.
14. Wu J, Wu J, Olgin J, et al: Mechanisms underlying the reentrant circuit of atrioventricular nodal reentry tachycardia in isolated canine nodal preparations using optical mapping. Circ Res 88:1189, 2001.
15. Nikolski V, Efimov IR: Fluorescent imaging of a dual-pathway atrioventricular nodal conduction system. Circ Res 88:e23, 2001.
16. James TN: The tendons of Todaro and the "triangle of Koch": Lessons from eponymous hagiolatry. J Cardiovasc Electrophysiol 10:1478, 1999.
17. Wu J, Zipes DP: Mechanisms underlying atrioventricular nodal conduction and the reentrant circuit of atrioventricular nodal reentrant tachycardia using optical mapping. J Cardiovasc Electrophysiol 13:831, 2002.
18. Mazgalev TN, Van Wagoner DR, Efimov IR: Mechanisms of AV nodal excitability and propagation. *In* Zipes DP, Jalife J (eds): Cardiac Electrophysiology: From Cell to Bedside. 3rd ed. Philadelphia, WB Saunders, 1999, pp 196-205.
19. Tamaddon HS, Vaidya D, Simon AM, et al: High-resolution optical mapping of the right bundle branch in connexin40 knockout mice reveals slow conduction in the specialized conduction system. Circ Res 87:929, 2000.
20. Connen SR, Dupont E, Rothery S, et al: Connexin45 expression is preferentially associated with the ventricular conduction system in mouse and rat heart. Circ Res 82:232, 1998.
21. Rohr S, Kucera JP, Fast VG, et al: Paradoxical improvement of impulse conduction in cardiac tissue by partial uncoupling. Science 275:841, 1997.
22. Levy MN: Time dependency of the autonomic interactions that regulate heart rate and rhythms. *In* Zipes DP, Jalife J (eds): Cardiac Electrophysiology: From Cell to Bedside. 2nd ed. Philadelphia, WB Saunders, 1994, p 454.
23. Olgin JE, Sih HJ, Hanish S, et al: Heterogeneous atrial denervation creates substrate for sustained atrial fibrillation. Circulation 98:2608, 1998.
24. Liu Y, Wu C, Lu L, et al: Sympathetic nerve sprouting, electrical remodeling, and increased vulnerability to ventricular fibrillation in hypercholesterolemic rabbits. Circ Res 92:1145, 2003.
25. Cao J, Chen LS, KenKnight BH, et al: Nerve sprouting and sudden cardiac death. Circ Res 86:816, 2000.
26. Hartmann HA, Colom LV, Sutherland ML, Noebels JL: Selective localization of cardiac SCN5A sodium channels in limbic regions of rat brain. Nat Neurosci 2:593, 1999.
27. Shamsuzzaman ASM, Ackerman MJ, Kara T, et al: Sympathetic nerve activity in the congenital long-QT syndrome. Circulation 107:1844, 2003.

Basic Electrophysiological Principles

28. Inoue M, Bridge JHB: Ca^{2+} sparks in rabbit ventricular myocytes evoked by action potentials. Involvement of clusters of L-type Ca^{2+} channels. Circ Res 92:532, 2003.
29. Rasmusson RL, Morales MJ, Wang S, et al: Inactivation of voltage-gated cardiac K^+ channels. Circ Res 82:739, 1998.
30. Rohr S, Kucera JP, Kléber AG: Slow conduction in cardiac tissue, I. Circ Res 83:781, 1998.
31. Sakmann BFAS, Spindler AJ, Bryant SM, et al: Distribution of a persistent sodium current across the ventricular wall in guinea pigs. Circ Res 87:910, 2000.
32. Kamp TJ, Zhou Z, Zhang S, et al: Pharmacology of L- and T-type calcium channels in the heart. *In* Zipes DP, Jalife J (eds): Cardiac Electrophysiology: From Cell to Bedside. 3rd ed. Philadelphia, WB Saunders, 1999, pp 141-156.
33. Gaspo R, Bosch RF, Bou-Abboud E, at el: Tachycardia-induced changes in Na^+ current in a chronic dog model of atrial fibrillation. Circ Res 81:1045, 1997.
34. Wang Z, Feng J, Shi H, et al: Potential molecular basis of different physiological properties of the transient outward K^+ current in rabbit and human atrial myocytes. Circ Res 84:551, 1999.
35. Yue L, Melnik P, Gaspo R, et al: Molecular mechanisms underlying ionic remodeling in a dog model of atrial fibrillation. Circ Res 87:776, 1999.
36. Antos CL , Frey N, Marx SO, et al: Dilated cardiomyopathy and sudden death resulting from constitutive activation of protein kinase A. Circ Res 89:997, 2001.
37. Zhou J, Shin H, Ji Y, et al: Phosphorylation and ER retention signals are required for protein kinase A–mediated potentiation of cardiac sodium current. Circ Res 91:540, 2002.
38. Li RA, Leppo M, Miki T, et al: Molecular basis of electrocardiographic ST-segment elevation. Circ Res 87:837, 2000.
39. Martynuyk AE, Morey TE, Belardinelli L, et al: Hyperkalemia enhances the effect of adenosine on $I_{K,Ado}$ in rabbit isolated AV nodal myocytes and on AV nodal conduction in guinea pig isolated heart. Circulation 99:312, 1999.
40. Baker LC, London B, Choi B, et al: Enhanced dispersion of repolarization and refractoriness in transgenic mouse hearts promotes ventricular tachycardia. Circ Res 86:396, 2000.
41. Spach MS, Heidlage JF, Dolber PC, et al: Electrophysiological effects of remodeling cardiac gap junctions and cell size. Circ Res 86:302, 2000.
42. Kléber AG, Fast VG, Rohr S: Continuous and discontinuous propagation. *In* Zipes DP, Jalife J (eds): Cardiac Electrophysiology: From Cell to Bedside. 3rd ed. Philadelphia, WB Saunders, 1999, pp 205-213.
43. Morley GE, Vaidya D, Samie FH, et al: Characterization of conduction in the ventricles of normal and heterozygous Cx43 knockout mice using optical mapping. J Cardiovasc Electrophysiol 10:1361, 1999.
44. Gutstein DE, Morley GE, Tamaddon H, et al: Conduction slowing and sudden arrhythmic death in mice with cardiac-restricted inactivation of connexin43. Circ Res 88:333, 2001.

45. Saffitz JE, Yamada KA: Gap junction distribution in the heart. *In* Zipes DP, Jalife J (eds): Cardiac Electrophysiology: From Cell to Bedside. Philadelphia, WB Saunders, 1999, pp 179-187.
46. Zipes DP, Jalife J (eds): Cardiac Electrophysiology: From Cell to Bedside. 3rd ed. Philadelphia, WB Saunders, 2000.
47. Clemo HF, Stambler BS, Baumgarten CM: Swelling-activated chloride current is persistently activated in ventricular myocytes from dogs with tachycardia-induced congestive heart failure. Circ Res 84:157, 1999.
48. Kaneko T, Tanaka H, Oyamada M, et al: Three distinct types of Ca^{2+} waves in Langendorff-perfused rat heart revealed by real-time confocal microscopy. Circ Res 86:1093, 2000.
49. Wu Y, Roden DM, Anderson ME: Calmodulin kinase inhibition prevents development of the arrhythmogenic transient inward current. Circ Res 84:906, 1999.
50. Pogwizd SM, Schlotthauer K, Li L, et al: Arrhythmogenesis and contractile dysfunction in heart failure. Circ Res 88:1159, 2001.
51. Zaza A, Rocchetti M, Brioschi A, et al: Dynamic Ca^{2+}-induced inward rectification of K^+ current during the ventricular action potential. Circ Res 82:947, 1998.
52. Reuter H, Henderson SA, Han T, et al: The Na^+-Ca^{2+} exchanger is essential for the action of cardiac glycosides. Circ Res 90:305, 2002.
53. Kucera JP, Kléber AG, Rohr S: Slow conduction in cardiac tissue, II. Circ Res 83:795, 1998.
54. Balke CW, Marbán E, O'Rourke B: Calcium channels: structure, function, and regulation. *In* Zipes DP, Jalife J (eds): Cardiac Electrophysiology: From Cell to Bedside. Philadelphia, WB Saunders, 1999, pp 8-21.
55. Belardinelli L, Song Y, Shryock JC: Cholinergic control of cardiac electrical activity. *In* Zipes DP, Jalife J (eds): Cardiac Electrophysiology: From Cell to Bedside. Philadelphia, WB Saunders, 1999, pp 294-300.
56. Snyders DJ: Molecular biology of potassium channels. *In* Zipes DP, Jalife J (eds): Cardiac Electrophysiology: From Cell to Bedside. Philadelphia, WB Saunders, 1999, pp 21-31.
57. Priebe L, Beuckelmann DJ: Simulation studies of cellular electrical properties in heart failure. Circ Res 82:1206, 1998.
58. Sah R, Ramirez RJ, Backx PH: Modulation of Ca^{2+} release in cardiac myocytes by changes in repolarization rate. Circ Res 90:165, 2002.
59. Sah R, Ramirez RJ, Oudit GY, et al: Regulation of cardiac excitation-contraction coupling by action potential repolarization: Role of the transient outward potassium current (I_{to}). J. Physiol (Lond) 546:5, 2003.
60. Zygmunt AC, Goodrow RJ, Weigel CM: I_{NaCa} and $I_{Cl(Ca)}$ contribute to isoproterenol-induced delayed afterdepolarizations in midmyocardial cells. Am J Physiol 275:H1979, 1998.
61. Weber CR, Ginsburg KS, Bers DM: Cardiac submembrane $[Na^+]$ transients sensed by Na^+-Ca^{2+} exchange current. Circ Res 92:950, 2003.
62. Yao A, Su Z, Nonaka A, et al: Effects of overexpression of the Na^+-Ca^{2+} exchanger on $[Ca^{2+}]_i$ transients in murine ventricular myocytes. Circ Res 82:657, 1998.
63. Yang T, Snyders DJ, Roden DM: Rapid inactivation determines the rectification and $[K^+]_o$ dependence of the rapid component of the delayed rectifier K^+ current in cardiac cells. Circ Res 80:782, 1997.
64. Clemo HF, Stambler BS, Baumgarten CM: Persistent activation of a swelling-activated cation current in ventricular myocytes from dogs with tachycardia-induced congestive heart failure. Circ Res 83:147, 1998.
65. Lakatta EG, Maltsev VA, Bogdanov KY, et al: Cyclic variation in intracellular calcium. A critical factor for cardiac pacemaker cell dominance. Circ Res 92:e45, 2003.
66. Shivkumar K, Deutsch NA, Lamp ST, et al: Mechanism of hypoxic K loss in rabbit ventricle. J Clin Invest 100:1782, 1997.
67. Kanda A, Watanabe I, Williams ML, et al: Unanticipated lessening of the rise in extracellular potassium during ischemia by pinacidil. Circulation 95:1937,1997.

Mechanisms of Arrhythmogenesis

68. Mohler PJ, Schott J, Gramolini AO, et al: Ankyrin-B mutation causes type 4 long-QT cardiac arrhythmia and sudden cardiac death. Nature 421:634, 2003.
68a. Kass RS, Moss AJ: Long QT syndrome: Novel insights into the mechanisms of cardiac arrhythmias. J Clin Invest 112:810-815, 2003.
69. Antzelevitch C, Shimizu W, Yan G, et al: The M cell: Its contribution to the ECG and to normal and abnormal electrical function of the heart. J Cardiovasc Electrophysiol 10:1124, 1999.
70. Choi B, Burton F, Salama G: Cytosolic Ca^{2+} triggers early afterdepolarizations and torsade de pointes in rabbit hearts with type 2 long QT syndrome. J Physiol (Lond) 543.2:615, 2002.
71. Zygmunt AC, Eddlestone GT, Thomas GP, et al: Larger late sodium conductance in M cells contributes to electrical heterogeneity in canine ventricle. Am J Physiol 281:H689, 2001.
72. Zygmunt AC, Goodrow RJ, Antzelevitch C: I_{NaCa} contributes to electrical heterogeneity within the ventricle. Am J Physiol 278:H2671, 2000.
73. Shimizu W, Kurita T, Matsuo K, et al: Improvement of repolarization abnormalities by a K^+ channel opener in the LQT1 of congenital long-QT syndrome. Circulation 97:1581, 1998.
74. Hwang C, Karagueuzian HS, Chen PS: Idiopathic paroxysmal atrial fibrillation induced by a focal discharge mechanism in the left superior pulmonary vein: Possible roles of the ligament of Marshall. J Cardiovasc Electrophysiol 10:636, 1999.
75. Lerman BB, Stein KM, Markowitz SM, et al: Ventricular tachycardia in patients with structurally normal hearts. *In* Zipes DP, Jalife J (eds): Cardiac Electrophysiology: From Cell to Bedside. Philadelphia, WB Saunders, 1999, pp 640-656.
76. Zipes DP, Jalife J: Atrioventricular block and dissociation. *In* Zipes DP, Jalife J (eds): Cardiac Electrophysiology: From Cell to Bedside. 4th ed. Philadelphia, WB Saunders, 2003, pp 451-458.
77. Hund TJ, Rudy Y: Determinants of excitability in cardiac myocytes: Mechanistic investigation of memory effect. Biophys J 79:3095, 2000.
78. Krinsky V: Qualitative theory of reentry. *In* Zipes DP, Jalife J (eds): Cardiac Electrophysiology: From Cell to Bedside. 3rd ed. Philadelphia, WB Saunders, 1999, pp 320-326.
79. Athill CH, Ikeda T, Kim Y, et al: Transmembrane potential properties at the core of functional reentrant wavefronts in isolated canine atria. Circulation 98:1556, 1998.
80. Uzzaman M, Honjo H, Takagishi Y, et al: Remodeling of gap junctional coupling in hypertrophied right ventricles of rats with monocrotaline-induced pulmonary hypertension. Circ Res 86:871, 2000.
81. Peters NS, Coromilas J, Severs NJ, et al: Disturbed connexin43 gap junction distribution correlates with the location of reentrant circuits in the epicardial border zone of healing canine infarcts that cause ventricular tachycardia. Circulation 95:988, 1997.
82. Beaumont J, Jalife J: Rotors and spiral waves in two dimensions. *In* Zipes DP, Jalife J (eds): Cardiac Electrophysiology: From Cell to Bedside. 3rd ed. Philadelphia, WB Saunders, 1999, pp 327-335.
83. Pertsov AM, Jalife J: Three-dimensional vortex-like reentry. *In* Zipes DP, Jalife J (eds): Cardiac Electrophysiology: From Cell to Bedside. 3rd ed. Philadelphia, WB Saunders, 1999, pp 336-344.
84. Samie FH, Berenfeld O, Anumonwo J, et al: Background potassium current. A determinant of rotor dynamics in ventricular fibrillation. Circ Res 89:1216, 2001.
85. Chen Q, Glenn E, Zhang D, et al: Genetic basis and molecular mechanism for idiopathic ventricular fibrillation. Nature 392:293, 1998.
86. Antzelevitch C, Brugada P, Brugada J, et al: Brugada syndrome. A decade of progress. Circ Res 91:1114, 2002.
87. Waldo AL: Atrial flutter: Mechanisms, clinical features, and management. *In* Zipes DP, Jalife J (eds): Cardiac Electrophysiology: From Cell to Bedside. 3rd ed. Philadelphia, WB Saunders, 1999, pp 468-475.
88. Zipes DP: 50th anniversary historical article. A century of cardiac arrhythmias: In search of Jason's golden fleece. J Am Coll Cardiol 34:959, 1999.
89. Uno K, Kumagai K, Khrestian CM, et al: New insights regarding the atrial flutter reentrant circuit. Circulation 100:1354, 1999.
90. Witkowski FX, Leon LJ, Penkoske PA, et al: Spatiotemporal evolution of ventricular fibrillation. Nature 392:78, 1998.
91. Riccio ML, Koller ML, Gilmour RF: Electrical restitution and spatiotemporal organization during ventricular fibrillation. Circ Res 84:955, 1999.
92. Wu TJ, Yashima M, Doshi R, et al: Relation between cellular repolarization characteristics and critical mass for human ventricular fibrillation. J Cardiovasc Electrophysiol 10:1077, 1999.
93. Kim YH, Garfinkel A, Ikeda T, et al: Spatiotemporal complexity of ventricular fibrillation revealed by tissue mass reduction in isolated swine right ventricle. J Clin Invest 100:2486, 1997.
94. Pagé PL: Surgery for atrial fibrillation and other supraventricular tachyarrhythmias. *In* Zipes DP, Jalife J (eds): Cardiac Electrophysiology: From Cell to Bedside. 3rd ed. Philadelphia, WB Saunders, 1999, pp 1065-1077.
95. Haïssaguerre M, Jaïs P, Shah DC, et al: Catheter ablation for atrial fibrillation: clinical electrophysiology of linear lesions. *In* Zipes DP, Jalife J (eds): Cardiac Electrophysiology: From Cell to Bedside. 3rd ed. Philadelphia, WB Saunders, 1999, pp 994-1008.
96. Chen PS, Swerdlow CD, Hwang C, Karagueuzian HS: Current concepts of ventricular defibrillation. J Cardiovasc Electrophysiol 9:553, 1998.
97. Skanes AC, Manapati R, Berenfeld O, et al: Spatiotemporal periodicity during atrial fibrillation in the isolated sheep heart. Circulation 98:1236, 1998.
98. Manapati R, Skanes AC, Chen J, et al: Stable microreentrant sources as a mechanism of atrial fibrillation in the isolated sheep heart. Circulation 101:194, 2000.
99. Sih HJ, Zipes DP, Berbari EJ, et al: Differences in organization between acute and chronic atrial fibrillation in dogs. J Am Coll Cardiol 36:924, 2000.
100. Jaïs P, Haïssaguerre M, Shah DC, et al: A focal source of atrial fibrillation treated by discrete radiofrequency ablation. Circulation 95:572, 1997.
101. Haissaguerre M, Jais P, Shah DC, et al: Spontaneous initiation of atrial fibrillation by ectopic beats originating in the pulmonary veins. N Engl J Med 339:659, 1998.
102. Olgin JE, Rubart M: Remodeling of the atria and ventricles due to rate. *In* Zipes DP, Jalife J (eds): Cardiac Electrophysiology: From Cell to Bedside. 3rd ed. Philadelphia, WB Saunders, 1999, pp 364-378.
103. Hadian D, Zipes DP, Olgin JE, et al: Short-term rapid atrial pacing produces electrical remodeling of sinus node function in humans. J Cardiovasc Electrophysiol 13:584, 2002.
104. Yue L, Feng J, Gaspo R, et al: Ionic remodeling underlying action potential changes in a canine model of atrial fibrillation. Circ Res 81:512, 1997.
105. Gaspo R, Bosch RF, Bou-Abboud E, Nattel S: Tachycardia-induced changes in Na^+ current in a chronic dog model of atrial fibrillation. Circ Res 81:1045, 1997.
106. Yue L, Melnyk P, Gaspo R, et al: Molecular mechanisms underlying ionic remodeling in a dog model of atrial fibrillation. Circ Res 84:776, 1999.
107. Elvan A, Huang XD, Pressler ML, Zipes DP: Radiofrequency catheter ablation of the atria eliminates pacing-induced sustained atrial fibrillation and reduces connexin 43 in dogs. Circulation 96:1675, 1997.
108. Chio CW, Eble JN, Zipes DP: Efferent vagal innervation of the canine atria and sinus and atrioventricular nodes. The third fat pad. Circulation 9:2573, 1997.
109. Olgin JE, Sih HJ, Hanish S, et al: Heterogeneous atrial denervation creates substrate for sustained atrial fibrillation. Circulation 98:2608, 1998.
110. Jayachandran JV, Sih HJ, Winkle W, et al: Atrial fibrillation produced by prolonged rapid atrial pacing is associated with heterogeneous changes in atrial sympathetic innervation. Circulation 101:1185, 2000.
111. Yu WC, Chen SA, Lee SH, et al. Tachycardia-induced change of atrial refractory period in humans: Rate dependency and effects of antiarrhythmic drugs. Circulation 97:2331, 1998.
112. Miyata A, Hall SD, Zipes DP, et al: KB-R7943 prevents acute, atrial fibrillation-induced shortening of atrial refractoriness in anesthetized dogs. Circulation 106:1410, 2002.

113. Jayachandran JV, Zipes DP, Weksler J, et al: Role of the Na^+/H^+ exchanger in short-term atrial electrophysiological remodeling. Circulation 101:1861, 1999.
114. Carnes CA, Chung MK, Nakayma T, et al: Ascorbate attenuates atrial pacing-induced peroxynitrite formation and electrical remodeling and decreases the incidence of post-operative atrial fibrillation. Circ Res 89:e32, 2001.
115. Sticherling C, Oral H, Horrocks J, et al: Effects of digoxin on acute, atrial fibrillation–induced changes in atrial refractoriness. Circulation 102:2503, 2000.
116. Olgin JE: Sinus tachycardia and sinus node reentry. *In* Zipes DP, Jalife J (eds): Cardiac Electrophysiology: From Cell to Bedside. 3rd ed. Philadelphia, WB Saunders, 1999, pp 459-468.
117. Lesh MD: Catheter ablation of atrial flutter and tachycardia. *In* Zipes DP, Jalife J (eds): Cardiac Electrophysiology: From Cell to Bedside. 3rd ed. Philadelphia, WB Saunders, 1999, pp 1009-1027.
118. Nikolski VP, Jones SA, Lancaster MK, et al: Cx43 and dual-pathway electrophysiology of the atrioventricular node and atrioventricular nodal reentry. Circ Res 92:469, 2003.
119. Miles WM, Zipes DP: Atrioventricular reentry and variants: Mechanisms, clinical features, and management. *In* Zipes DP, Jalife J (eds): Cardiac Electrophysiology: From Cell to Bedside. 3rd ed. Philadelphia, WB Saunders, 1999, pp 488-504.
120. Yee R, Klein GJ, Prystowsky E: The Wolff-Parkinson-White syndrome and related variants. *In* Zipes DP, Jalife J (eds): Cardiac Electrophysiology: From Cell to Bedside. 3rd ed. Philadelphia, WB Saunders, 1999, pp 845-861.
121. Maury P, Metzger J, Zimmermann M: Intermittent anterograde conduction in an accessory pathway during atrial pacing: What is the mechanism? J Cardiovasc Electrophysiol 9:1394, 1998.
122. Callans DJ, Josephson ME: Ventricular tachycardias in the setting of coronary artery disease. *In* Zipes DP, Jalife J (eds): Cardiac Electrophysiology: From Cell to Bedside. 3rd ed. Philadelphia, WB Saunders, 1999, pp 530-536.
123. Galvin JM, Ruskin JN: Ventricular tachycardia in patients with dilated cardiomyopathy. *In* Zipes DP, Jalife J (eds): Cardiac Electrophysiology: From Cell to Bedside. 3rd ed. Philadelphia, WB Saunders, 1999, pp 537-546.
124. Cabo C, Boyden PA: Electrical remodeling of the epicardial border zone in the canine infarcted heart: A computational analysis. Am J Physiol 284:H372, 2002.
125. Yao J, Hussain W, Patel P, et al: Remodeling of gap junctional channel function in epicardial border zone of healing canine infarcts. Circ Res 92:437, 2003.
126. Pu J, Balser JR, Boyden PA: Lidocaine action on Na^+ currents in ventricular myocytes from the epicardial border zone of infarcted hearts. Circ Res 83:431, 1998.

CHAPTER 28

Genetics of Cardiac Arrhythmias

Silvia G. Priori • Carlo Napolitano • Peter J. Schwartz

Cardiac arrhythmias most often occur in the presence of an abnormal substrate that is responsible for a derangement in impulse initiation and conduction. Ischemic heart disease is the primary cause for the development of ventricular fibrillation, and other structural heart diseases (such as hypertrophic and dilated cardiomyopathies) account for most of the remaining cases (see Chaps. 50 and 59). In most postmortem series of cardiac arrest victims, structural abnormalities were absent in approximately 5 to 8 percent[1] of cases, which, for many years, were referred to as cases of idiopathic ventricular fibrillation (IVF).[2] Now, with the help of molecular biology, the substrate of IVF has been partially defined. In little more than a decade, substantial evidence has been collected to demonstrate that genetically determined abnormalities of proteins that control the electrical activity of the heart can cause cardiac arrest in the structurally intact heart. At least nine genes (Table 28–1) have been associated with inherited arrhythmogenic diseases, and it is expected that several more genes will be identified and linked to sudden death in persons with an apparently normal heart (Fig. 28–1).

In this chapter we review the clinical and genetic characteristics of the three most common inherited arrhythmogenic diseases predisposing to arrhythmias and sudden death, the long QT syndrome, Brugada syndrome, and catecholaminergic polymorphic ventricular tachycardia.

Long QT Syndrome

The long QT syndrome (LQTS) is an inherited arrhythmogenic disease characterized by susceptibility to life-threatening ventricular arrhythmias. Two major forms of LQTS have been identified, one transmitted as an autosomal dominant trait (Romano-Ward syndrome) and the second transmitted as an autosomal recessive disease in which the cardiac phenotype is associated with neurosensory deafness (Jervell and Lange-Nielsen syndrome). The electrocardiographic (ECG) marker of LQTS consists of prolonged repolarization (i.e., prolonged QT interval), abnormal morphology of the T wave (Fig. 28–2), and a characteristic polymorphic ventricular tachycardia called torsades de pointes that is most often induced by activation of the sympathetic nervous system.[3]

Clinical Manifestations

Syncope and fainting are the typical manifestations of LQTS, and their occurrence is often precipitated by physical or emotional stress (e.g., fear, anger, loud noises, sudden awakening).[4] Onset of symptoms is typically in the first two decades of life, including the neonatal period, when LQTS can be misdiagnosed as sudden infant death syndrome,[5] but the first symptoms can appear later in life, especially among females.[4] The severity of the clinical manifestations of LQTS is highly variable, ranging from full-blown disease with a markedly prolonged QT interval and recurrent syncope to subclinical forms with borderline QT interval prolongation and no arrhythmias or syncopal events.[6] Thus, risk stratification becomes a crucial step for clinical management.

Clinical Management of Long QT Syndrome (see Chap. 30)

The link between the onset of cardiac events and increased sympathetic activity suggested the use of beta blockers in the treatment of the disease.[3] The efficacy of beta blockade in patients with LQTS has been reassessed in a large collaborative study that showed a significant residual risk for sudden death.[7] Left cardiac sympathetic denervation is also used for patients unresponsive to, or not tolerating, beta-blocking therapy.[3] Because cardiac arrest survivors represent the subset of LQTS patients at higher risk for sudden death despite treatment, prophylactic implantation of an implantable cardioverter defibrillator (ICD) is recommended for them. Permanent pacemaker implantation is indicated in selected LQTS patients who have atrioventricular block or bradycardia- or pause-dependent tachyarrhythmias. The implantation of a pacemaker is not an alternative to beta blocker treatment.

GENETIC BASIS OF LONG QT SYNDROME

The discovery of the genetic basis of LQTS accelerated in the early 1990s with linkage analysis studies performed in large affected kindreds that allowed the mapping of four LQTS loci on chromosomes 11, 3, and 7 (Online Mendelian Inheritance in Man [OMIM] identification numbers 192500, 152427, and 603830). The gene on chromosome 11 (LQT1), *KCNQ1*, was identified in 1996 using positional cloning, and the candidate gene approach allowed the identification of the genes located on chromosomes 7 (LQT2) and 3 (LQT3) as *KCNH2* and *SCN5A*, respectively. Subsequently, the candidate gene approach allowed identification of mutations in two additional genes both located on chromosome 21 and called *KCNE1* (LQT5; OMIM 176261) and *KCNE2* (LQT6; OMIM 603796). All the genes associated with LQT1 to 3 and LQT5 and 6 encode cardiac ion channel subunits.[8] On the basis of this evidence, LQTS was initially considered a "channelopathy." A locus on chromosome 4 was identified in 1995 as responsible for LQT4 (OMIM 600919). The responsible gene was identified as *ANKB*; at variance with the other genes, however,

TABLE 28–1 Genetic Bases of Inherited Arrhythmogenic Diseases

Disease	Inheritance	Locus	Gene	Protein
LQT3	AD	3p21-p23	*SCN5A*	Nav 1.5
LQT4	AD	4q25-q27	*ANKB*	Ankyrin
LQT2	AD	7q35-q36	*KCNE2*	HERG
LQT1	AD	11p15.5	*KCNQ1*	KvLQT1
LQT5	AD	21q22.1-p22.2	*KCNE1*	MinK
LQT6	AD	21q22.1-p22.2	*KCNE2*	MiRP1
JLN1	AR	11p15.5	*KCNQ1*	KvLQT1
JLN2	AR	21q22.1-q22.2	*KCNE1*	MinK
Brugada	AD	3p21-p23	*SCN5A*	Nav1.5
CPVT	AD	1q42-43	*RyR2*	RyR2
CPVT	AR	1p11-13.3	*CASQ2*	CASQ2

AD = autosomal dominant; AR = autosomal recessive; Brugada = Brugada syndrome; CPVT = catecholaminergic polymorphic ventricular tachycardia; JLN = Jervell and Lange-Nielsen type of long QT syndrome; LQT = long QT syndrome.

ANKB encodes not a cardiac ion channel but a structural protein called ankyrin that is most likely implicated in ion channel anchoring to the cellular membrane.[9]

***KCNQ1* (LQT1) AND *KCNE1* (LQT5).** The cardiac delayed rectifier current (I_K) is a major determinant of phase 3 of the cardiac action potential. It comprises two independent components: one rapid (I_{Kr}) and one slow and catecholamine sensitive (I_{Ks}) (see Chap. 27).

The *KCNQ1* gene and the *KCNE1* gene encode, respectively, the alpha (KVLQT1) and beta (MinK) subunits of the potassium channel conducting the I_{Ks} current. *KCNQ1* mutations are found in the LQT1 variant of the disease, which is also the most prevalent genetic form of LQTS. Approximately half of genotyped patients have a mutation on this gene (see Fig. 28–1).

More than 130 different *KCNQ1* mutations (mainly single amino acid substitutions) have been described (see http://pc4.fsm.it:81/cardmoc). Homozygous or compound heterozygous mutations of *KCNQ1* have been associated with the recessive Jervell and Lange-Nielsen form of LQTS (JLN1). LQT5 is a rather uncommon variant of LQTS caused by mutations in the *KCNE1* gene; it accounts for approximately 2 to 3 percent of all genotyped LQTS patients. Mutations in the *KCNE1* gene cause both Romano-Ward (LQT5) and Jervell and Lange-Nielsen (JLN2) syndromes.

Expression studies of mutated proteins suggest multiple mechanisms of functional failure. Defective proteins can coassemble with wild-type protein and exert a dominant negative effect. Other mutations lead to defective proteins that do not assemble with wild-type peptides, resulting in a loss of function that reduces the I_{Ks} current by 50 percent (haploinsufficiency). Finally, defective peptides may not even reach the membrane of the cardiac cell because the mutations interfere with intracellular protein trafficking.[8,10]

***KCNH2* (LQT2) AND *KCNE2* (LQT6).** The *KCNH2* and *KCNE2* genes encode, respectively, the alpha (HERG) and beta (MIRP) subunits of the potassium channel conducting the I_{Kr} current (see Fig. 28–1). Approximately 100 *KCNH2* mutations have been reported (http://pc4.fsm.it:81/cardmoc), suggesting that this is the second most common variant of LQTS, accounting for 35 to 40 percent of mutations in LQTS genotyped patients. Functional expression studies have demonstrated that mutations in the *KCNH2* gene cause a reduction of the I_{Kr} current. *KCNH2* mutants have reduced function compared with the wild-type peptides; therefore, I_{Kr} channels that incorporate mutated subunits carry a reduced I_{Kr} repolarizing current. Defective proteins can have a dominant negative effect on the wild-type subunits or may not interfere with the function of the normal subunits, thus causing haploinsufficiency. Trafficking abnormalities have also been reported as a consequence of *KCNH2* mutations.[11]

Mutations in the *KCNE2* gene are found in the LQT6 variant of LQTS. This gene encodes MiRP1 (MinK-related peptide 1), a small peptide that coassembles with the HERG protein to form the I_{Kr} channel. In the literature worldwide there are only a few examples of *KCNE2* mutations associated with LQTS (http://pc4.fsm.it:81/cardmoc). Accordingly, LQT6 seems the rarest variant of the disease.

***SCN5A* (LQT3).** The *SCN5A* gene encodes the protein of the cardiac sodium channel. This gene was cloned in 1992 and mapped to chromosome 3p21 in 1995. The Na^+ channel protein is a relatively large molecule that folds onto itself to surround the channel pore (see Fig. 28–1).

The first *SCN5A* mutations were clustered in the regions that regulate the inactivation of the channel (delKPQ, R1623Q, N1325S). In vitro expression studies showed that these mutations cause an increased late inward sodium current (I_{Na}). It was concluded that Na^+ channel mutations originate the LQTS phenotype by inducing a gain of function leading to an increase in the Na^+ inward current that prolongs the action potential duration.

Approximately 25 mutations have been reported so far in the literature (http://pc4.fsm.it:81/cardmoc), and the prevalence of LQT3 among LQTS patients is estimated to be 10 to 15 percent.

***ANKB* (LQT4).** Only one family linked to this locus (4q25-q27) has been reported so far. Interestingly, the phenotype of the LQT4 patients differs from the typical LQTS phenotype. In addition to QT interval prolonga-

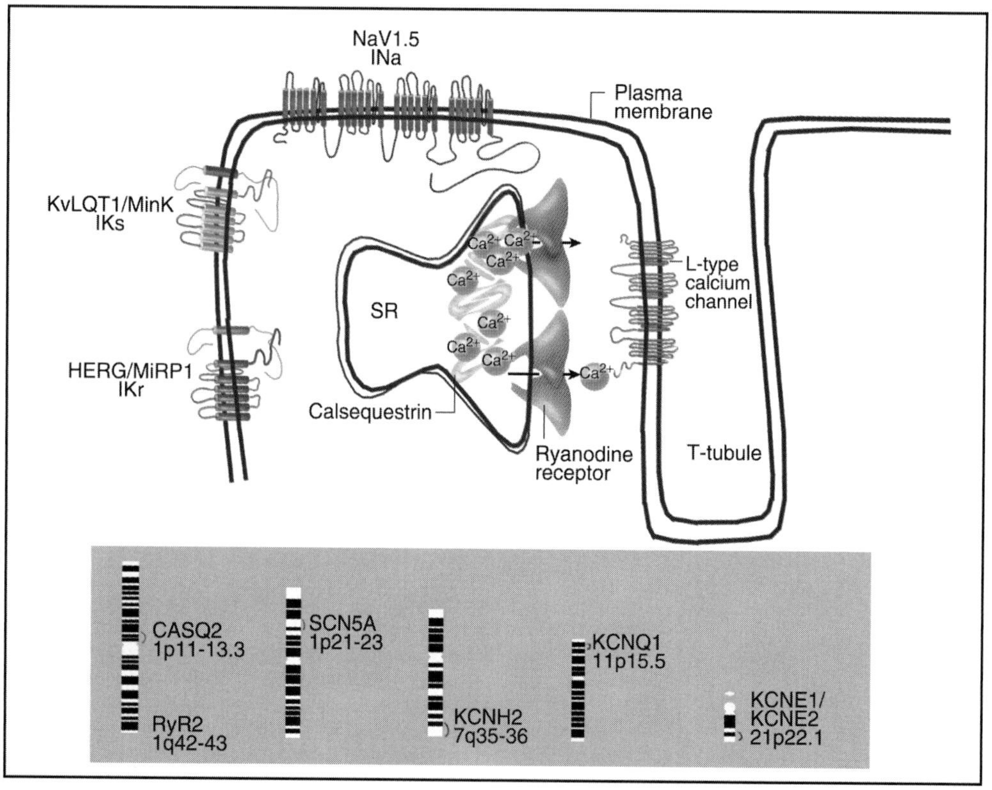

FIGURE 28–1 Genes and proteins in inherited arrhythmogenic diseases: the chromosomal locations of the genes known to cause cardiac inherited disorders. The proteins encoded by each gene are schematically drawn in the figure.

tion, most of the affected individuals present with severe sinus bradycardia, paroxysmal atrial fibrillation (detected in more than 50 percent of the patients), and biphasic T waves. Experimental data for ankyrin knockout mice suggested that this protein, located in the LQT4 critical region, was a plausible candidate gene for LQT4. Subsequently, a missense mutation in the *ANKB* gene was identified in the family linked to the critical region on chromosome 4, confirming that the gene for LQT4 is the *Ankyrin* gene.[9]

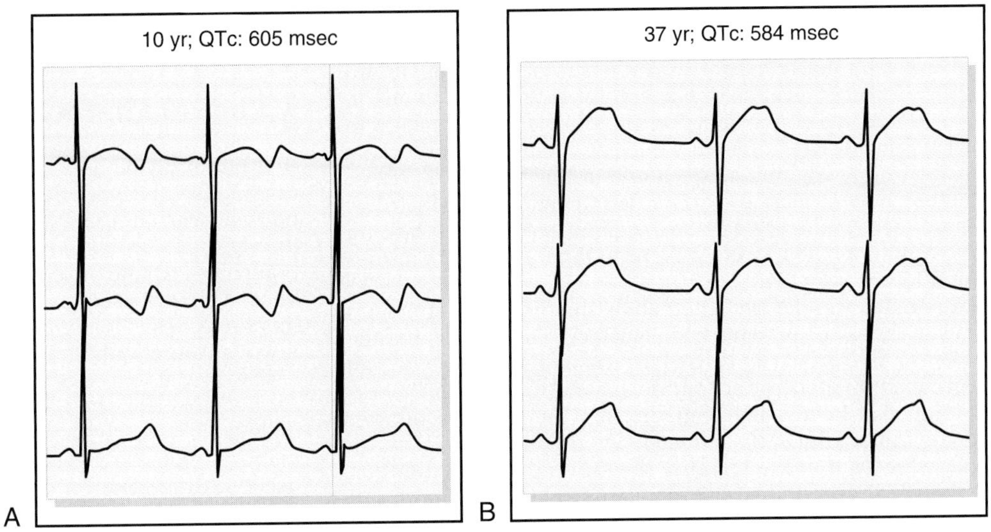

FIGURE 28–2 Electrocardiograms in long QT syndrome (LQTS). Typical electrocardiograms of two LQTS patients, 10 **(A)** and 37 **(B)** years old, showing QT interval prolongation and T wave morphological abnormalities. The genetic defect is LQTS *KCNH2* mutation (HERG) A561V.

GENOTYPE-PHENOTYPE CORRELATION STUDIES. The distinguishing features of the three most common genetic variants of LQTS, namely LQT1, LQT2, and LQT3, have been outlined.[12] Analysis of the ECG patterns revealed a gene-specific morphology of the ST-T wave complex,[13] which may guide genotyping.

Schwartz and coworkers[4] have provided evidence that the triggers for cardiac events differ among the genetic variants of LQTS. This difference is particularly evident for lethal events. LQT1 patients have an increased risk during physical or emotional stress. They experience 90 percent of lethal events in this setting, whereas LQT3 patients experience most of their events (64 percent) at rest or while asleep and only 4 percent do so during exercise. LQT2 patients are at higher risk for lethal events during arousal or emotional states (49 percent) but are also at risk during sleep and at rest (29 percent) and not at all at risk during exercise. There are also triggers that appear highly specific. Indeed, 99 percent of cardiac events that occur while swimming involve LQT1 patients and 80 percent of events related to acoustic stimuli involve LQT2 patients.[4,12]

Natural History and Risk Stratification

The increased availability of data collected for genotyped LQTS patients has allowed the development of risk stratification models based on the genetic substrate. Priori and colleagues have reported information on 647 LQTS patients from 193 genotyped families.[14]

This study showed that a lower cumulative event-free survival was observed among LQT2 versus LQT1 patients, and a similar trend was present among LQT3 versus LQT1 patients. Gender had a different effect across different genotypes. It had no influence in LQT1 patients, whereas a higher risk was present for LQT2 females and LQT3 males. It was also observed that the percentage of genetically affected patients with a normal QT interval ("silent mutation carriers") differed strikingly among genotypes, being much greater ($P < 0.001$) in LQT1 (36 percent) than in LQT2 (19 percent) and especially than in LQT3 (10 percent) patients. Quartiles of QTc distribution were determined within each genetic subgroup and permitted recognition that among LQT1 and LQT2 patients, those with a QTc in the upper quartile had respectively a 5.3- and 8.4-fold risk increase compared with those in the first quartile. In contrast, QTc duration did not differentiate risk among LQT3 patients.

These data were incorporated in a risk quantification model by comparing the event-free survival in 12 categories including, for each genetic locus, the four combinations of gender and QTc below or above 500 milliseconds. This analysis provided the identification of a differential risk within these 12 categories (Fig. 28–3).

In this study, it was assumed that patients with mutations on the same gene share a common risk profile. Risk stratification, however, may be further refined when the location of a mutation is also taken into consideration. In 1997 Donger and colleagues observed in a small subset of patients that mutations located in the carboxyl terminus of the *KCNQ1* gene were associated with a mild clinical phenotype.[14a] In 2002 Moss and associates[15] studied 201 LQT2 patients and showed that individuals with mutations in the pore region were at considerably greater risk for cardiac events than patients with nonpore mutations even though the difference in the incidence of aborted cardiac arrest and sudden death was not statistically significant.

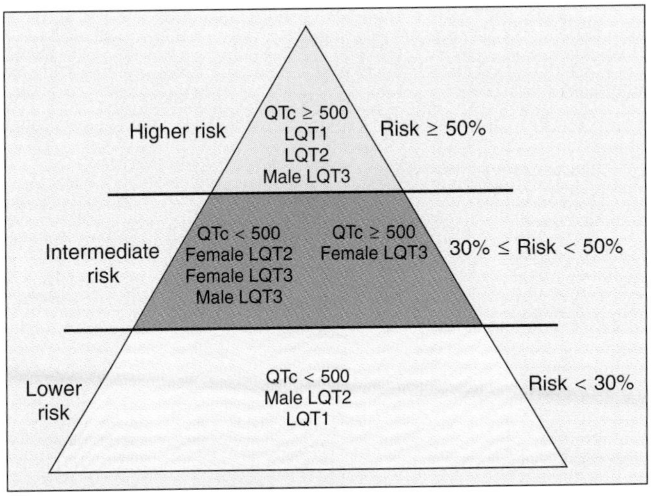

FIGURE 28–3 Risk stratification in the long QT (LQT) syndrome. Shown here is the risk stratification scheme for patients with long QT syndrome according to genotype and gender. The risk groups have been defined on the basis of the probability of experiencing a first cardiac event (syncope, cardiac arrest, or sudden death) by age 40 years. A 50 percent or higher probability of events constitutes the higher risk subgroup, a risk between 30 and 50 percent the intermediate risk group, and a risk less than 30 percent the lower risk group. (Modified from Priori SG, Schwartz PJ, Napolitano C, et al: Risk stratification in the long-QT syndrome. N Engl J Med 348:1866, 2003.)

GENE-SPECIFIC THERAPY. Data collected from small cohorts of LQT3 patients[7,16] have raised concern that beta blockers may not be effective in this subset of patients with LQTS. However, available data are not sufficiently robust to allow definitive conclusions on the role of beta blockers in LQT3. Specifically, it remains unclear whether beta blockers are ineffective and therefore should not be used in LQT3 or whether they at least provide a partial reduction of cardiac events. The main obstacle in reaching conclusive data on this issue is related to the limited number of LQT3 families identified worldwide.

Attempts to devise alternative therapeutic strategies specific for LQT3 patients have emerged. On the basis of the evidence that LQT3 is caused by an increased late I_{Na}, an experimental preparation mimicking LQT3 and LQT2 was developed.[17] In this LQT3 model, the Na^+ channel blocker mexiletine significantly reduced the action potential duration, whereas it did not modify the action potential duration in the LQT2 model. In 1995 the feasibility of this pharmacological intervention was tested in a few genotyped patients, and indeed sodium channel blockade with mexiletine shortened the QT interval among LQT3 patients but not among LQT2 patients.[16] Other authors later confirmed that QT was also shortened in response to another sodium channel blocker, flecainide. However, concerns exist about the use of flecainide in LQT3 patients as Priori and colleagues demonstrated that intravenous flecainide may induce ST segment elevation in the right precordial leads (Brugada-like electrocardiogram).[18]

A gene-specific therapy for LQT2 patients was proposed in 1996 by Compton and associates,[18a] who suggested that one could compensate for the reduced I_{Kr} current by increasing the potassium plasma concentration with exogenous administration of potassium salts and potassium-sparing diuretics.

It is important to remember that, despite the appeal of gene-specific therapy, its place is still in research studies rather than in clinical practice as there is no evidence that it can affect mortality or reduce the number of cardiac events.

Brugada Syndrome

Clinical Characteristics

In 1992, Brugada and Brugada described a novel autosomal dominant inherited disease occurring in the structurally normal heart and characterized by ST segment elevation in the right precordial leads (V_1 to V_3) (Fig. 28–4), right bundle branch block, and susceptibility to ventricular tachyarrhythmias. This disease is now referred to as Brugada syndrome. Its prevalence is not known, but the disease seems to be more prevalent in countries in the Far East (see Chap. 32).

The age at onset of clinical manifestations (syncope or cardiac arrest) is the third to fourth decade of life, although malignant forms with earlier onset and even with neonatal manifestations have been reported.[19] Cardiac events typically occur during sleep or at rest.[20] Even though the disease is inherited as an autosomal dominant trait, there is a striking male-to-female ratio of 8:1 in clinical manifestations.

Diagnosis

The diagnosis of Brugada syndrome is complicated by the intermittent nature of the ECG pattern. Concealed forms may be unmasked only after performing provocative drug testing with selected Class IC drugs such as ajmaline, flecainide or procainamide.[21] It has been suggested that the autonomic nervous system can modify the ECG phenotype because intravenous administration of isoproterenol attenuates whereas acetylcholine accentuates the ECG abnormalities in affected patients.

Prognostic Indicators and Management

Initial data from Brugada and colleagues published in 1992 and data subsequently published in 1998 provided an alarming estimate of the lethality of the disease when they suggested that the risk of sudden death within 3 years from the time of the clinical diagnosis was close to 30 percent in both asymptomatic and symptomatic patients. Because no drug therapy is effective in preventing arrhythmic events in Brugada syndrome, the only prophylactic treatment to prevent cardiac arrest is the ICD (see Chap. 31). It is therefore reassuring to observe that with the collection of larger groups of patients, the estimated lethality of the disease is much lower than initially feared.[22] In a study by Priori and coworkers,[22] assessment of the natural history of Brugada syndrome showed that 28 percent of patients had a cardiac arrest from birth to age 60. Later, they proposed a novel risk stratification scheme (Fig. 28–5) based on retrospective analysis of the event-free survival in 200 individuals,[23] the

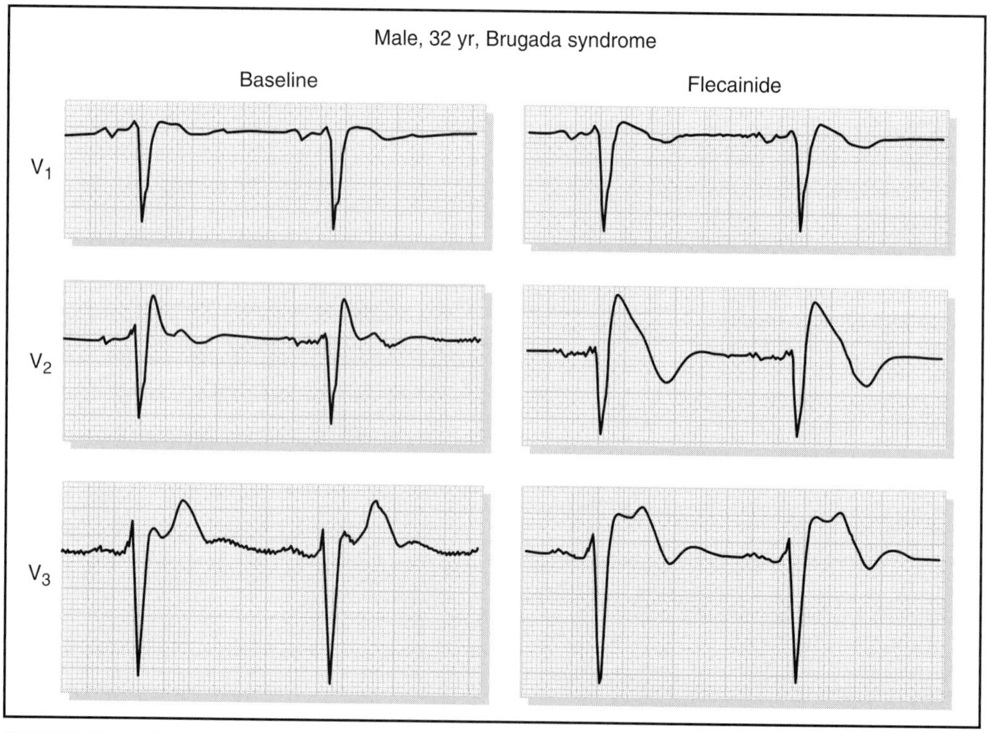

FIGURE 28–4 Electrocardiograms in Brugada syndrome. V_1 to V_3 leads show a mild ST segment elevation and an incomplete right bundle branch block, possibly indicating Brugada syndrome. The typical and conclusively diagnostic pattern is unmasked in the same patient by the intravenous administration of flecainide (2 mg/kg). The genetic defect is Brugada *SCN5A* mutation R526H.

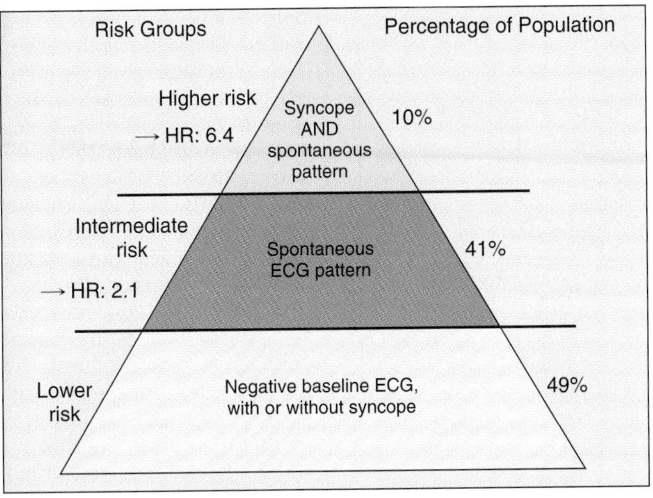

FIGURE 28–5 Risk stratification in Brugada syndrome using the history of syncope and the presence of a spontaneously diagnostic electrocardiographic pattern as the clinical variables for quantification of risk. Hazard ratios are calculated using the lower risk group as a reference. ECG = electrocardiogram; HR = hazard ratio. (From Priori SG, Napolitano C, Gasparini M, et al: Clinical and genetic heterogeneity of right bundle branch block and ST-segment elevation syndrome: A prospective evaluation of 52 families. Circulation 2000; 102:2509, 2000.).

severity of the ECG signs (spontaneously present ST elevation versus ST elevation unmasked only by drug testing), and the occurrence of syncopal events. The latest data from Brugada and colleagues included a larger proportion of asymptomatic individuals and also showed that individuals with the spontaneous ECG pattern are at higher risk for cardiac events.[24]

One area of persistent disagreement in the risk stratification for patients with Brugada syndrome concerns the role of programmed electrical stimulation (PES) to identify individuals at higher risk for cardiac arrest. Brugada and associates[25] showed that PES is highly sensitive in predicting the risk of major cardiac events, whereas Priori,[23] Gasparini,[26] and Eckardt[27] and their coworkers failed to show that it is a good indicator of risk for cardiac events. As a consequence, the use of PES in Brugada syndrome has received a Class IIb recommendation by the Task Force on Sudden Cardiac Death of the European Society of Cardiology.[1]

GENETIC BASIS OF BRUGADA SYNDROME

The understanding of the molecular basis of Brugada syndrome is still limited; so far, only one gene has been identified and it accounts for no more than 20 percent of clinical cases.[10]

In 1998, the gene responsible for some of the cases of Brugada syndrome was identified as the cardiac sodium channel gene (*SCN5A*), the same gene responsible for the LQT3 variant of LQTS.[28] Mutations identified in Brugada syndrome are either missense mutations, in-frame deletions, or mutations (insertions or deletions) leading to frameshifts and early truncation of the protein of the cardiac sodium channel. In vitro functional characterization of *SCN5A* mutations showed that several distinct electrophysiological mechanisms can lead to the clinical phenotype of Brugada syndrome but the overall effect of all the mutations identified leads to a "reduction " in the sodium current (loss of function). This finding is at variance with the effect of *SCN5A* mutations identified in LQT3, in which mutations lead to an excess of sodium inward current (gain of function). Interestingly, overlapping phenotypes of LQT3 and Brugada syndrome have been reported by Bezzina and colleagues,[29] who described the simultaneous presence of QT prolongation and ST segment elevation in a family in which an *SCN5A* mutation (InsD1795) was present. Grant and coworkers[29a] also reported a family with ECG features of both diseases.

Catecholaminergic Polymorphic Ventricular Tachycardia

Catecholaminergic polymorphic ventricular tachycardia (CPVT)[30] was initially described in 1978. It was reported that the disease is characterized by ventricular tachycardia (VT), syncope, and sudden death occurring in familial or in sporadic cases in the absence of structural abnormalities of the heart and in the absence of any ECG abnormality. Three distinguishing features of CPVT were highlighted: (1) a direct relationship between adrenergic activation (physical or emotional stress) and the onset of arrhythmias, (2) a typical pattern of bidirectional VT with an unremarkable resting electrocardiogram (Fig. 28–6), and (3) a structurally normal heart. CPVT (OMIM 604772) has now been recognized as a genetically determined arrhythmogenic disease and its pathophysiological mechanisms are being progressively unveiled (see Chap. 32).

Clinical Features

ELECTROCARDIOGRAPHIC CHARACTERISTICS. The resting electrocardiogram of patients with CPVT is unremarkable with the exception of a sinus bradycardia reported in some patients; atrioventricular conduction is within normal limits and no significant abnormalities are identified by signal-averaging electrocardiography.

Physical activity and acute emotions are the specific triggers for arrhythmias in CPVT patients. The complexity of arrhythmias progressively increases with increase in workload, from isolated premature beats to bigeminy and to runs of nonsustained VT. If the patients continue to exercise, the duration of VT runs progressively increases and the arrhythmia can become sustained. A 180-degree alternating QRS axis on a beat-to-beat basis, the so-called bidirectional VT, is often the distinguishing presentation of CPVT-related arrhythmias. However, later observations have pointed to the fact that CPVT patients can also show irregular polymorphic VT without a "stable" QRS vector alternans. At variance with LQTS, exercise-induced runs of nonsustained supraventricular tachycardia are a relatively common finding among CPVT patients. Triggered activity has been suggested as the most likely arrhythmogenic mechanism in CPVT.

CARDIAC EVENTS AND CLINICAL MANIFESTATIONS. Syncope, triggered by exercise or acute emotion, is often the first manifestation of CPVT even though sudden cardiac death can occur in previously asymptomatic subjects. In approximately 30 percent of cases, the family history reveals one or multiple premature sudden deaths that usually occurred during childhood, even if later onset (after age 20 years) events have been reported. Often, unheralded sudden death occurring in individuals without cardiac structural abnormalities can lead to the postmortem diagnosis of IVF.

GENETIC BASIS

AUTOSOMAL DOMINANT CPVT. Evidence supporting a familial distribution of CPVT has been provided since the initial description of the disease. The distribution of the phenotype in the first reported familial cases was consistent with an autosomal dominant pattern of inheritance.[31] The availability of two large kindreds allowed Swan and coworkers to perform genome-wide linkage analysis and to map the disease locus to chromosome 1q42-43 with a significant logarithm of odds (LOD) score of 4.74.[32]

On the basis of these findings and the evidence that the gene encoding the human cardiac ryanodine receptor (*RyR2*) maps to the CPVT critical region, Priori and colleague performed molecular screening of this gene in families with stress-induced bidirectional VT and successfully identified *RyR2* mutations in four probands, demonstrating that *RyR2* is

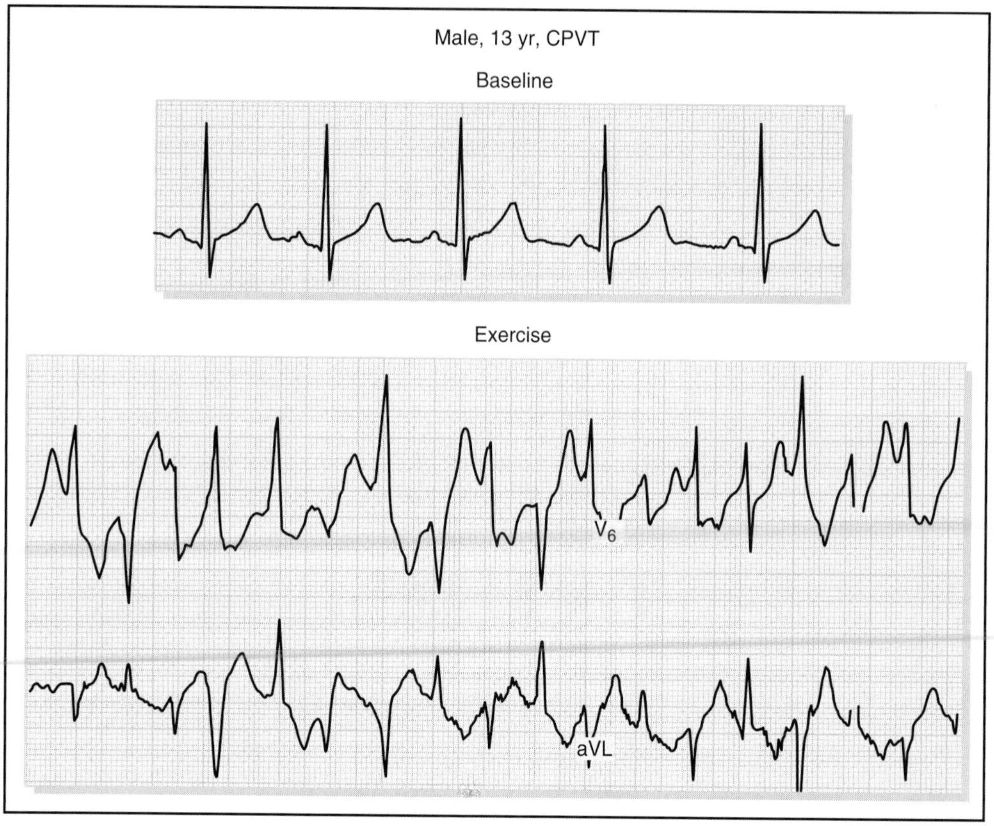

FIGURE 28–6 Electrocardiograms in catecholaminergic polymorphic ventricular tachycardia (CPVT). The findings in a young teenager with CPVT show an unremarkable electrocardiogram at rest **(upper panel)** and the onset of polymorphic or bidirectional ventricular tachycardia during an exercise stress test **(lower panel).** The genetic defect is CPVT *RyR2* mutation 52246L.

the gene for autosomal dominant CPVT.[33] The involvement of the cardiac ryanodine receptor in the genesis of CPVT was shortly afterward confirmed by other groups and by functional characterization of the defective proteins.[34]

RyR2 plays a major role in the regulation of intracellular calcium fluxes and excitation-contraction coupling. This large tetrameric protein is localized across the membrane of the sarcoplasmic reticulum (SR), and it releases Ca^{2+} ions from the SR in response to Ca^{2+} entry through the L-type channels during phase 2 of the action potential. The identification of *RyR2* mutations in CPVT patients constitutes the first demonstration of the involvement of an intracellular ion channel in an inherited arrhythmia and points to the pivotal role of intracellular Ca^{2+} handling in arrhythmogenesis.[35]

An increasing number of *RyR2* mutations is being reported (http://pc4.fsm.it:81/cardmoc), and abnormal variants of this gene have also been linked to an atypical or "concealed" form of arrhythmogenic right ventricular dysplasia (ARVD2) characterized by exercise-induced bidirectional VT.[36]

AUTOSOMAL RECESSIVE CPVT. Lahat and associates in 2001 provided the first evidence for a variant of CPVT inherited as an autosomal dominant trait. They mapped the disease in seven consanguineous Bedouin families in a 16-cM interval on chromosome 1p23-21 with a LOD score of 8.24. Subsequently, they identified *CASQ2* as the gene for this variant of CPVT.[37,38] *CASQ2* encodes calsequestrin, a protein highly expressed in the heart. It serves as a major Ca^{2+} binding protein localized in the terminal cisternae of the SR of cardiac muscle cells, and it binds Ca^{2+} with high capacity and moderate affinity. Thus, calsequestrin is a Ca^{2+} storage protein in the lumen of the SR. CPVT patients of different ethnic backgrounds have been successfully genotyped as carriers of *CASQ2* mutations, suggesting that patients with CPVT should be screened for this gene when an autosomal recessive pattern of inheritance is suspected.

Clinical Management

GENOTYPE-PHENOTYPE CORRELATION IN *RYR2*-CPVT. *RyR2* mutations are found in approximately 50 percent of patients who have a clinical diagnosis of CPVT. Thus, the disease is genetically heterogeneous, and at present no additional genes have been linked to the autosomal dominant variant of CPVT. This lack of knowledge limits the definition of gene-specific therapeutic strategies and risk stratification schemes. The evidence so far collected in small cohorts of patients supports the view that the age of onset of the disease is greater among patients not harboring *RyR2* genetic defects than among RyR2 mutation carriers (20 ± 12 versus 8 ± 2 years) and that among carriers of *RyR2* mutations, males seem to be at higher risk (relative risk = 4.2) of cardiac events at a young age.[39] Furthermore, it has been shown that *RyR2* mutations are not always associated with typical bidirectional VT, because polymorphic VT is present in approximately 40 percent of genotyped probands.[39] The incidence of cardiac events from birth is not different when patients with and without *RyR2* mutations are compared. Both groups present with the majority of cardiac events during childhood, and by age 20, more than 60 percent of the patients experience a first cardiac event (syncope or cardiac arrest).

GENOTYPE-PHENOTYPE CORRELATION IN *CASQ2*-CPVT. Because of the limited number of *CASQ2* genotyped patients, it is not yet possible to compare *CASQ2*- and *RyR2*-related CPVT. Lahat and colleagues reported a mild QT interval prolongation in their initial paper,[37] but it was not confirmed in their subsequent report.

Risk Stratification and Therapy in Catecholaminergic Polymorphic Ventricular Tachycardia

Antiadrenergic treatment with beta blockers is the cornerstone of therapy for CPVT patients.[39] Despite the limited experience available, amiodarone and Class I antiarrhythmic agents appear ineffective (see Chap. 30).

PES is not useful for diagnosis and risk stratification because CPVT patients usually do not have inducible arrhythmias.[39] On the other hand, the highly reproducible pattern of arrhythmia during exercise among CPVT patients allows diagnosis, dose titration, and monitoring. Overall, chronic treatment with full-dose beta-blocking agents can prevent recurrences of syncope in some patients.[39] Nonetheless, Priori and colleagues reported that in approximately 40 percent of their cases, the control of arrhythmias was unsatisfactory despite optimization of therapy with repeated exercise stress testing.[39] They concluded that the use of an ICD may be indicated when exercise stress testing and repeated Holter monitoring suggest that only incomplete protection from arrhythmias is obtained with beta blockers.

REFERENCES

Long QT Syndrome

1. Priori SG, Aliot E, Blomstrom-Lundqvist C, et al: Task Force on Sudden Cardiac Death of the European Society of Cardiology. Eur Heart J 22:1374, 2001.
2. Survivors of out-of-hospital cardiac arrest with apparently normal heart. Need for definition and standardized clinical evaluation. Consensus Statement of the Joint Steering Committees of the Unexplained Cardiac Arrest Registry of Europe and of the Idiopathic Ventricular Fibrillation Registry of the United States. Circulation 95:265, 1997.
3. Schwartz PJ, Priori SG, Napolitano C: The long QT syndrome. *In* Zipes DP, Jalife J (eds): Cardiac Electrophysiology: From Cell to Bedside. Philadelphia, WB Saunders, 2000, pp 597-615.
4. Schwartz PJ, Priori SG, Spazzolini C, et al: Genotype-phenotype correlation in the long-QT syndrome: Gene-specific triggers for life-threatening arrhythmias. Circulation 103:89, 2001.
5. Schwartz PJ, Priori SG, Dumaine R, et al: A molecular link between the sudden infant death syndrome and the long-QT syndrome. N Engl J Med 343:262, 2000.
6. Priori SG, Napolitano C, Schwartz PJ: Low penetrance in the long-QT syndrome: Clinical impact. Circulation 99:529, 1999.
7. Moss AJ, Zareba W, Hall WJ, et al: Effectiveness and limitations of beta-blocker therapy in congenital long-QT syndrome. Circulation 101:616, 2000.
8. Keating MT, Sanguinetti MC: Molecular and cellular mechanisms of cardiac arrhythmias. Cell 104:569, 2001.
9. Mohler PJ, Schott JJ, Gramolini AO, et al: Ankyrin-B mutation causes type 4 long-QT cardiac arrhythmia and sudden cardiac death. Nature 421:634, 2003.
10. Priori SG, Rivolta I, Napolitano C: Genetics of long QT, Brugada and other channelopathies. *In* Zipes DP, Jalife J (eds): Cardiac Electrophysiology. 4th ed. Philadelphia, Elsevier (in press).
11. Zhou Z, Gong Q, Epstein ML, January CT: HERG channel dysfunction in human long QT syndrome. Intracellular transport and functional defects. J Biol Chem 273:21061, 1998.
12. Schwartz PJ, Priori SG: Long QT syndrome—Phenotype genotype considerations. *In* Zipes DP, Jalife J (eds): Cardiac Electrophysiology. 4th ed. Philadelphia, Elsevier (in press).
13. Zhang L, Timothy KW, Vincent GM, et al: Spectrum of ST-T-wave patterns and repolarization parameters in congenital long-QT syndrome: ECG findings identify genotypes. Circulation 102:2849, 2000.
14. Priori SG, Schwartz PJ, Napolitano C, et al: Risk stratification in the long-QT syndrome. N Engl J Med 348:1866, 2003.

14a. Donger C, Denjoy I, Berthet M, et al: KVLQT1 C-terminal missense mutation causes a forme fruste long-QT syndrome. Circulation 96:2778, 1997.

15. Moss AJ, Zareba W, Kaufman ES, et al: Increased risk of arrhythmic events in long-QT syndrome with mutations in the pore region of the human ether-a-go-go-related gene potassium channel. Circulation 105:794, 2002.
16. Schwartz PJ, Priori SG, Locati EH, et al: Long QT syndrome patients with mutations of the *SCN5A* and *HERG* genes have differential responses to Na^+ channel blockade and to increases in heart rate. Implications for gene-specific therapy. Circulation 92:3381, 1995.
17. Priori SG, Napolitano C, Cantu F, et al: Differential response to Na^+ channel blockade, beta-adrenergic stimulation, and rapid pacing in a cellular model mimicking the SCN5A and HERG defects present in the long-QT syndrome. Circ Res 78:1009, 1996.
18. Priori SG, Napolitano C, Schwartz PJ, et al: The elusive link between LQT3 and Brugada syndrome: The role of flecainide challenge. Circulation 102:945, 2000.

18a. Compton SJ, Lux RL, Ramsey MR, et al: Genetically defined therapy of inherited long QT syndrome. Correction of abnormal repolarization by potassium. Circulation 94:1018, 1996.

Brugada Syndrome

19. Priori SG, Napolitano C, Giordano U, et al: Brugada syndrome and sudden cardiac death in children. Lancet 355:808, 2000.
20. Brugada J, Brugada P, Brugada R: The syndrome of right bundle branch block ST segment elevation in V1 to V3 and sudden death—The Brugada syndrome. Europace 1:156, 1999.
21. Brugada R, Brugada J, Antzelevitch C, et al: Sodium channel blockers identify risk for sudden death in patients with ST-segment elevation and right bundle branch block but structurally normal hearts. Circulation 101:510, 2000.
22. Priori SG, Napolitano C, Gasparini M, et al: Clinical and genetic heterogeneity of right bundle branch block and ST-segment elevation syndrome: A prospective evaluation of 52 families. Circulation 102:2509, 2000.
23. Priori SG, Napolitano C, Gasparini M, et al: Natural history of Brugada syndrome. Insights for risk stratification and management. Circulation 105:1342, 2002.
24. Brugada J, Brugada R, Antzelevitch C, et al: Long-term follow-up of individuals with the electrocardiographic pattern of right bundle-branch block and ST-segment elevation in precordial leads V1 to V3. Circulation 105:73, 2002.
25. Brugada P, Geelen P, Brugada R, et al: Prognostic value of electrophysiologic investigations in Brugada syndrome. J Cardiovasc Electrophysiol 12:1004, 2001.
26. Gasparini M, Priori SG, Mantica M, et al: Programmed electrical stimulation in Brugada syndrome: How reproducible are the results? J Cardiovasc Electrophysiol 13:880, 2002.
27. Eckardt L, Kirchhof P, Schulze-Bahr E, et al: Electrophysiologic investigation in Brugada syndrome; yield of programmed ventricular stimulation at two ventricular sites with up to three premature beats. Eur Heart J 23:1394, 2002.
28. Chen Q, Kirsch GE, Zhang D, et al: Genetic basis and molecular mechanism for idiopathic ventricular fibrillation. Nature 392:293, 1998.
29. Bezzina C, Veldkamp MW, van Den Berg MP, et al: A single Na(+) channel mutation causing both long-QT and Brugada syndromes. Circ Res 85:1206, 1999.

29a. Grant AO, Carboni MP, Nipliovera V, et al: Long QT syndrome, Brugada syndrome, and conduction system disease are linked to a single sodium channel mutation. J Clin Invest 110:1201, 2002.

Catecholaminergic Polymorphic Ventricular Tachycardia

30. Napolitano C, Priori SG: Catecholaminergic polymorphic ventricular tachycardia. *In* Zipes DP, Jalife J (eds); Cardiac Electrophysiology. 4th ed. Philadelphia, Elsevier (in press).
31. Fisher JD, Krikler D, Hallidie-Smith KA: Familial polymorphic ventricular arrhythmias: A quarter century of successful medical treatment based on serial exercise-pharmacologic testing. J Am Coll Cardiol 34:2015, 1999.
32. Swan H, Piippo K, Viitasalo M, et al: Arrhythmic disorder mapped to chromosome 1q42-q43 causes malignant polymorphic ventricular tachycardia in structurally normal hearts. J Am Coll Cardiol 34:2035, 1999.
33. Priori SG, Napolitano C, Tiso N, et al: Mutations in the cardiac ryanodine receptor gene (*hRyR2*) underlie catecholaminergic polymorphic ventricular tachycardia. Circulation 103:196, 2001.
34. Wehrens XH, Lehnart SE, Huang F, et al: FKBP12.6 deficiency and defective calcium release channel (ryanodine receptor) function linked to exercise-induced sudden cardiac death. Cell 113:829, 2003.
35. Marks AR, Priori S, Memmi M, et al: Involvement of the cardiac ryanodine receptor/calcium release channel in catecholaminergic polymorphic ventricular tachycardia. J Cell Physiol 190:1, 2002.
36. Tiso N, Stephan D, Nava A: Identification on mutations in the cardiac ryanodine receptor gene in families affected with arrhythmogenic right ventricular cardiomyopathy type 2 (ARVD2). Hum Mol Genet 10:189, 2001.
37. Lahat H, Pras E, Olender T, et al: A missense mutation in a highly conserved region of CASQ2 is associated with autosomal recessive catecholamine-induced polymorphic ventricular tachycardia in Bedouin families from Israel. Am J Hum Genet 69:1378, 2001.
38. Lahat H, Eldar M, Levy-Nissenbaum E, et al: Autosomal recessive catecholamine- or exercise-induced polymorphic ventricular tachycardia. Circulation 103:2822, 2001.
39. Priori SG, Napolitano C, Memmi M, et al: Clinical and molecular characterization of patients with catecholaminergic polymorphic ventricular tachycardia. Circulation 106:69, 2002.

CHAPTER 29

Diagnosis of Cardiac Arrhythmias

John M. Miller • Douglas P. Zipes

Diagnosis of Cardiac Arrhythmias

In the management of clinical arrhythmias, the physician must evaluate and treat the whole patient, not just the rhythm disturbance.[1] Some arrhythmias are hazardous to the patient regardless of the clinical setting (e.g., ventricular fibrillation, VF), whereas others are hazardous because of the clinical setting (e.g., rapidly conducted atrial fibrillation in a patient with severe coronary artery stenoses). Some arrhythmias, such as premature ventricular complexes (PVCs), may be highly symptomatic yet are not associated with any adverse outcome, whereas some patients with atrial fibrillation have no symptoms at all but may still be at significant risk of stroke. Evaluation of the patient begins with a careful history and physical examination and should usually progress from the simplest to the most complex test, from the least invasive and safest to the most invasive and risky, and from the least expensive out-of-hospital evaluations to those that require hospitalization and sophisticated, costly procedures. Occasionally, depending on the clinical circumstances, the physician may wish to proceed directly to a high-risk, expensive procedure, such as an electrophysiological study (EPS), before obtaining a 24-hour electrocardiographic (ECG) recording.

History

Patients with cardiac rhythm disturbances can present with a variety of complaints, but commonly symptoms such as palpitations, syncope, presyncope, or congestive heart failure cause them to seek a physician's help. Their awareness of palpitations and of a regular or irregular cardiac rhythm varies greatly.[2] Some patients perceive slight variations in their heart rhythm with uncommon accuracy, whereas others are oblivious even to sustained episodes of ventricular tachycardia (VT); still others complain of palpitations when they actually have regular sinus rhythm.

In assessing a patient with known or suspected arrhythmia, several key pieces of information should be obtained that can help determine a diagnosis or guide further diagnostic testing. The *mode of onset* of an episode may give clues about the type of arrhythmia or preferred treatment option. For example, palpitations that occur in the setting of exercise, fright, or anger are often caused by catecholamine-sensitive automatic or triggered tachycardias that may respond to adrenergic blocking agents; palpitations that occur at rest or that awaken the patient may be due to vagal initiation, such as atrial fibrillation. Lightheadedness or syncope occurring in the setting of a tightly fitting collar, shaving the neck, or turning the head suggests carotid sinus hypersensitivity. The *mode of termination* of episodes may also be helpful: if palpitations can be reliably terminated by breath-holding, Valsalva, or other vagal maneuvers, it is likely that the atrioventricular (AV) node comprises an integral part of a tachycardia circuit; occasionally, focal atrial tachycardias or VTs terminate with vagal maneuvers. Patients should be asked *how frequently episodes occur, how long they last,* and *how severe their symptoms.* These features can help guide how aggressively and quickly the physician needs to pursue a diagnostic or therapeutic plan (a patient with daily episodes associated with near-syncope or severe dyspnea warrants a more expeditious evaluation than one with infrequent episodes of mild palpitations and no other symptoms). Patients can sometimes report the heart rate during an episode (either rapid or slow, regular or irregular) by counting their pulse directly or using an automatic blood pressure or heart rate monitor. Characteristics of mode of onset and frequency of episodes can guide the choice of diagnostic tests (see later).

A careful drug and dietary history should also be sought; some nasal decongestants can provoke tachycardia episodes, whereas beta-adrenergic blocking eye drops for treatment of glaucoma can drain into tear ducts, be absorbed systemically, and precipitate syncope due to bradycardia. Dietary supplements, particularly those containing ephedrine, can cause arrhythmias. A growing list of drugs can directly or indirectly affect ventricular repolarization and produce long-QT interval–related tachyarrhythmias (see Chaps. 5 and 32). The patient should be questioned about the presence of systemic illnesses that may be associated with arrhythmias such as chronic obstructive pulmonary disease, thyrotoxicosis, pericarditis, or congestive heart failure. A family history of rhythm disturbances is often present in long-QT syndrome, hypertrophic cardiomyopathy, and muscular or myotonic dystrophies.

Physical Examination

Examination of the patient during a symptomatic episode can be revealing. Clearly, heart rate and blood pressure are key measurements to make. Assessment of the jugular venous pressure and waveform can disclose the rapid oscillations of atrial flutter or "cannon" A waves indicative of contraction of the right atrium against a closed tricuspid valve in patients with AV dissociation in disorders such as complete heart block or VT. Variation in the intensity of the first heart sound has the same implications.

Physical maneuvers during a tachycardia can have diagnostic and therapeutic value. The Valsalva maneuver or carotid sinus massage causes a transient increase in vagal tone; tachyarrhythmias that depend on the AV node for continuation can terminate or slow with these maneuvers but may also show no change. Focal atrial tachycardias occasionally terminate in response to vagal stimulation, as do rare VTs. Sinus tachycardia slows slightly following vagal stimulation, returning to its original rate soon thereafter; the ventricular response during atrial flutter and fibrillation and other atrial tachycardias can slow briefly. During wide-QRS tachycardias with a 1:1 relationship between P waves and QRS complexes, vagal influence may terminate or slow a supraventricular tachycardia (SVT) with aberrant interventricular conduction that depends on the AV node for perpetuation; on the other hand, vagal effects on the AV node may transiently block retrograde conduction and thus establish the diagnosis of VT by demonstrating AV dissociation. The effect of either of these physical maneuvers typically lasts only seconds; the physician must be ready to observe or record any changes in rhythm on an ECG when the maneuver is performed or they may not be appreciated.

Carotid massage is performed with the patient supine and comfortable, with the head tipped away from the side being stimulated. Careful auscultation for carotid bruits must always precede any attempt at carotid massage since there have been reports of embolic events associated with massage. The area of the carotid sinus, at the artery's bifurcation, is palpated with two fingers at the angle of the jaw until a good pulse is felt. Even this minimal amount of pressure may induce a hypersensitive response in affected individuals. If there is no initial effect, a side-to-side or rotating motion of the fingers over the site is performed for up to 5 seconds. A negative response is lack of ECG effect after 5 seconds of pressure adequate to cause mild discomfort. Because responses to carotid massage may differ on the two sides, the maneuver can be repeated on the opposite side; both sides should never be stimulated simultaneously.

Physical findings can suggest the presence of structural heart disease (and, thus, generally a clinically more serious situation with worse overall prognosis) even in the absence of an arrhythmia episode. For instance, a laterally displaced or dyskinetic apical impulse, a regurgitant or stenotic murmur, or a third heart sound in an older adult can denote significant myocardial or valvular dysfunction or damage.

Electrocardiogram

The ECG is the primary tool in arrhythmia analysis (see Chap. 9); only an EPS, in which intracardiac catheters are used to record activity from several regions of the heart at one time, is more definitive. Initially, a 12-lead ECG is recorded. In addition, a long continuous recording using the lead that shows distinct P waves is often quite helpful for closer analysis; most commonly, this is one of the inferior leads (2, 3, aVF) and occasionally V_1 or aVR. The ECG obtained during an episode of arrhythmia may be diagnostic by itself, obviating the need for further diagnostic testing. Figure 29–1 depicts an algorithm for diagnosing specific tachyarrhythmias from the 12-lead ECG. A major branch point in the differential diagnosis concerns the QRS duration: Wide-QRS (>0.12-second) tachycardias are often VT, and narrow-QRS (≤0.12-second) tachycardias are almost always SVT, but there is some overlap (Table 29–1).[3] The next most important questions to answer, regardless of QRS width, concern characteristics of P waves. If P waves are not clearly visible, atrial activity can sometimes be recorded by placing the right and left arm leads in various anterior chest positions to discern P waves (so-called Lewis leads) or by applying esophageal electrodes or intracavitary right atrial recordings; the latter methods are not readily available in most clinical situations.

TABLE 29–1 Electrocardiographic Distinctions for Diagnosis of Wide QRS Complex Tachycardia

Favor Supraventricular Tachycardia	Favor Ventricular Tachycardia
Initiation with premature P wave	Initiation with premature QRS complex
"Long-short" sequence preceding initiation	Tachycardia beats identical to PVCs during sinus rhythm
Changes in P-P interval precede changes in R-R interval	Changes in R-R interval precede changes in P-P interval
QRS contours consistent with aberrant conduction (V_1, V_6)	QRS contours inconsistent with aberrant conduction (V_1, V_6)
Slowing or termination with vagal maneuvers	AV dissociation or other non-1:1 AV relationship Fusion beats, capture beats QRS duration >0.14 sec Left axis deviation (especially −90 to 180 degrees) Concordant R wave progression pattern Absence of "rS" complex in any precordial lead

AV = atrioventricular; PVC = premature ventricular complex.

An echocardiogram showing atrial contraction can be helpful. The long rhythm strip may yield important clues by revealing P waves if perturbations occur during the arrhythmia (changes in rate, premature complexes, sudden termination, effect of physical maneuvers, as noted earlier).

Each arrhythmia should be approached in a systematic manner to answer the several key questions; as suggested earlier, many of these relate to P wave characteristics and underscore the importance of assessing the ECG carefully for these. If P waves are visible, are the atrial and ventricular rates identical? Are the P-P and R-R intervals regular or irregular? If irregular, is it a consistent, repeating irregularity? Is there a P wave related to each QRS complex? Does the P wave seem to precede ("long-RP" interval) or follow ("short-RP" interval) the QRS complex (Fig. 29–2)? Are the resultant RP and PR intervals constant? Are all P waves and QRS complexes identical? Is the P wave vector normal or abnormal? Are P, PR, QRS, and QT durations normal? Once these questions are addressed, one needs to assess the significance of the arrhythmia in view of the clinical setting. Should it be treated, and, if so, how? For SVTs with a normal QRS complex, a branching decision tree such as Figure 29–1 may be useful.

THE LADDER DIAGRAM. The ladder diagram, derived from the ECG, is used to depict depolarization and conduction schematically to aid understanding of the rhythm. Straight or slightly slanting lines drawn on a tiered framework beneath an ECG represent electrical events occurring in the various cardiac structures (Fig. 29–3). Since the ECG and therefore the ladder diagram represent electrical activity against a time base, conduction is indicated by the lines of the ladder diagram sloping in a left-to-right direction. A steep line represents rapid conduction, with more slanting lines depicting slower conduction. A short bar drawn perpendicular to a sloping line represents blocked conduction. Activity originating in an ectopic site such as the ventricle is indicated by lines emanating from that tier. Sinus nodal discharge and conduction and, under certain circumstances, AV junctional discharge and conduction can only be inferred; their activity is not directly recorded on a scalar ECG.

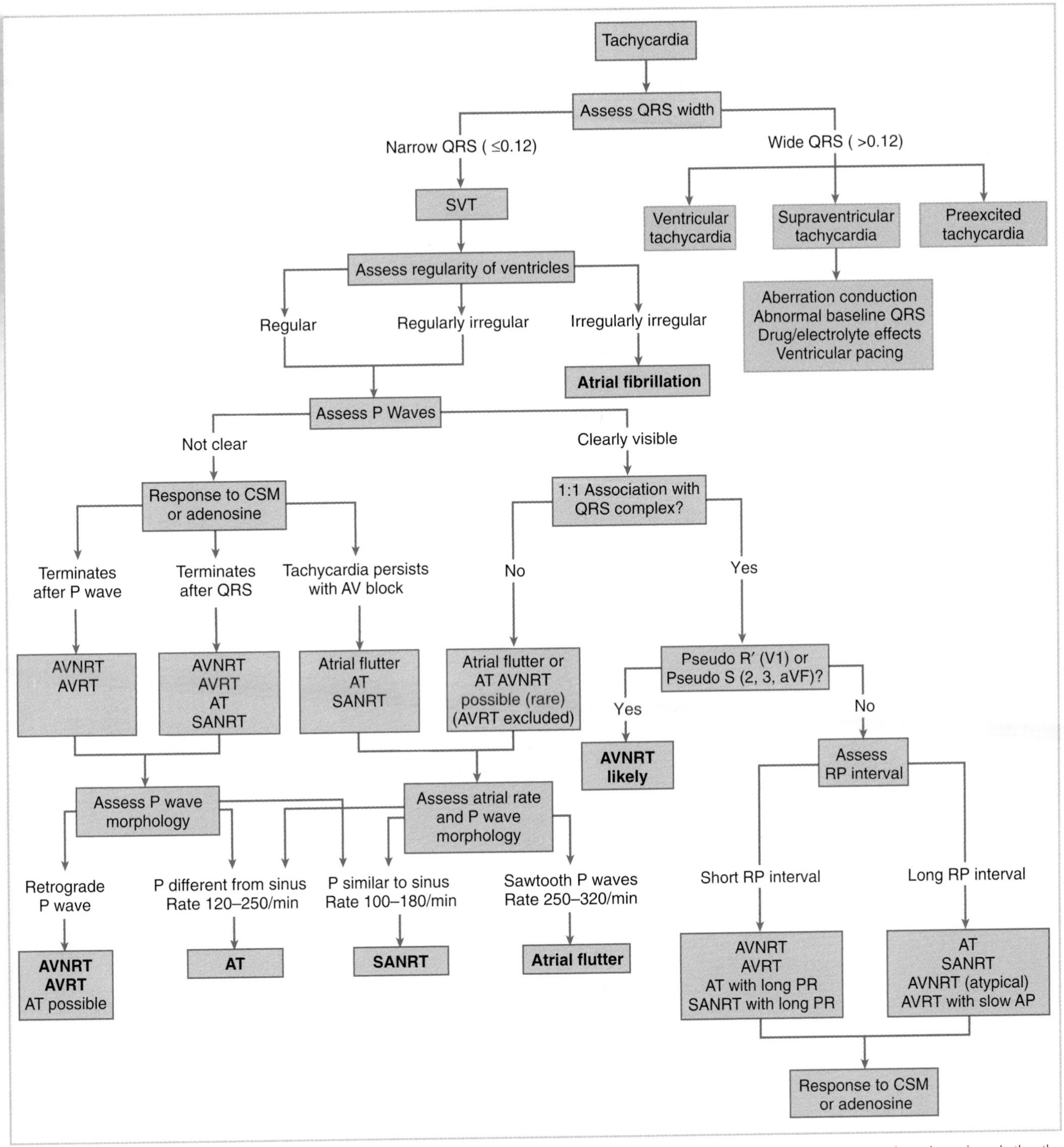

FIGURE 29–1 Stepwise approach to diagnosis of type of tachycardia based on 12-lead electrocardiogram during the episode. The initial step is to determine whether the tachycardia has a wide or narrow QRS complex. For wide-complex tachycardia, see Table 29–1; the remainder of the algorithm is helpful in diagnosing the type of narrow-complex tachycardia. SVT = supraventricular tachycardia; CSM = carotid sinus massage; AV = atrioventricular; AVNRT = AV nodal reentrant tachycardia; AVRT = AV reciprocating tachycardia; AT = atrial tachycardia; SANRT = sinoatrial nodal reentry tachycardia; AP = accessory pathway.

Additional Tests

The following additional tests can be used to evaluate patients who have cardiac arrhythmias. The physician's choice of which test to use depends on the clinical circumstances. For instance, a patient with multiple daily episodes of presyncope is likely to have an event recorded on a 24-hour ambulatory ECG (Holter) monitor, whereas in a patient who complains of infrequent anxiety- or exercise-induced palpitations, exercise stress testing may be more likely to provide a diagnosis.

Exercise Testing (see also Chap. 10)

Exercise can induce various types of supraventricular and ventricular tachyarrhythmias and, uncommonly, bradyarrhythmias.[4] About one third of normal subjects develop ventricular ectopy in response to exercise testing. Ectopy is

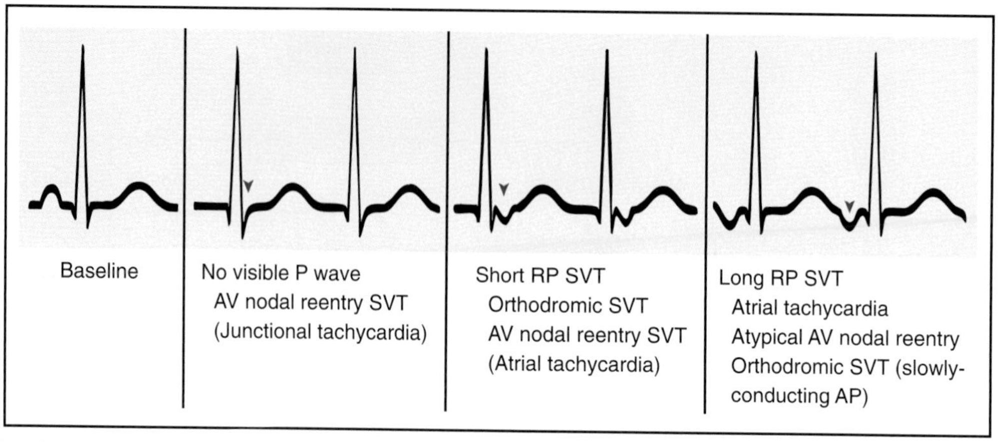

FIGURE 29–2 Differential diagnosis of different types of supraventricular tachycardia (SVT) based on timing of atrial activity (RP and PR intervals). A normal beat is shown at left; different types of tachycardia are listed below the representative electrocardiographic patterns they can produce, categorized by P wave position relative to the QRS complex. Arrow shows the location of the P wave in each example. AV = atrioventricular; AP = accessory pathway.

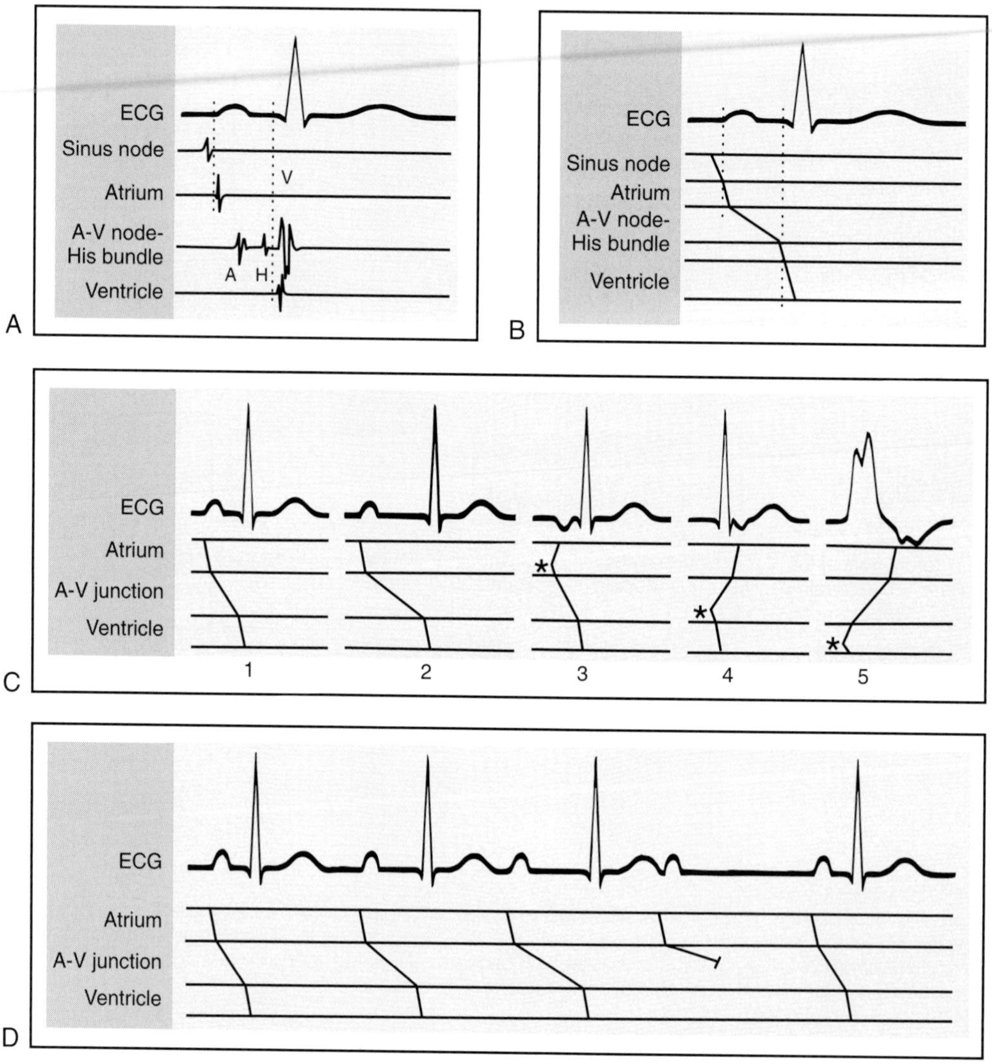

FIGURE 29–3 Intracardiac signals and ladder diagrams. **A,** A single beat is shown with accompanying intracardiac signals from the sinus node, right atrium, atrioventricular (AV) nodal and His bundle regions, and right ventricle. **B,** The same beat is shown with accompanying ladder diagram below. Cardiac regions have been divided into tiers separated by horizontal lines. Vertical dotted lines denote onset of P wave and QRS complexes. Note the relatively steep lines (rapid conduction through atrium, His bundle, and ventricular muscle) and more gently sloping lines as the impulse traverses the sinus and AV nodes (signifying slow conduction). **C,** Several different situations are depicted with accompanying explanatory ladder diagrams. Beat 1 is normal, as in **B**; beat 2 shows first-degree AV delay, with a more gradual slope than normal in the AV nodal tier, signifying very slow conduction in this region. In beat 3, an atrial premature complex is shown (starting in atrial tier as asterisk) producing an inverted P wave on electrocardiogram. In beat 4, an ectopic impulse arises in the His bundle (*) and propagates to the ventricle as well as retrogradely through the AV node to the atrium. In beat 5, a ventricular ectopic complex (*) conducts retrogradely through the His bundle and AV node and eventually to the atrium. **D,** A Wenckebach AV cycle (type 1 second-degree block) is shown. As the PR interval progressively increases from left to right in the figure, the slope of the line in the AV nodal region is progressively less steep until it fails to propagate at all after the fourth P wave (small line perpendicular to sloping AV nodal conduction line), after which the cycle repeats. A = atrial recording; ECG = electrocardiograph; H = His recording; V = ventricular recording.

more likely to occur at faster heart rates, usually in the form of occasional PVCs of constant morphology, or even pairs of PVCs, and is often not reproducible from one stress test to the next. Three to six beats of nonsustained VT can occur in normal patients, especially the elderly, and its occurrence does not establish the existence of ischemic or other forms of heart disease or predict increased cardiovascular morbidity or mortality. Premature supraventricular complexes are often more common during exercise than at rest and increase in frequency with age; their occurrence does not suggest the presence of structural heart disease. A persistent elevation of heart rate after the end of exercise (delay in return to baseline) is associated with a worse cardiovascular prognosis.[5]

Approximately 50 percent of patients who have coronary artery disease develop PVCs in response to exercise testing. Ventricular ectopy appears in these patients at lower heart rates (<130 beats/min) than in the normal population and often occurs in the early recovery period as well. Frequent (>7 PVCs/min) or complex ectopy is associated with a worse prognosis.[6] Exercise reproduced sustained VT or VF in only about 10 percent of patients with spontaneous VT or VF late after myocardial infarction, but those who had it experienced a worse outcome. The relation of exercise to ventricular arrhythmia in patients with structurally normal hearts has no prognostic implications. Stress testing with Holter recording has been used to assess antiarrhythmic drug efficacy.[7]

Patients who have symptoms consistent with an arrhythmia induced by exercise (e.g., syncope, sustained palpitations) should be considered for stress testing. Stress testing may be indicated to uncover more complex grades of ventricular arrhythmia, to provoke supraventricular arrhythmias, to determine the relationship of the arrhythmia to activity, to aid in choosing antiarrhythmic therapy and uncovering proarrhythmic responses, and possibly to provide some insight into the mechanism of the tachycardia. The test can be performed safely and appears more sensitive than a standard 12-lead resting ECG to detect ventricular ectopy. However, prolonged ambulatory recording is more sensitive than exercise testing in detecting ventricular ectopy. Because either technique can uncover serious arrhythmias that the other technique misses, both examinations may be indicated for selected patients.

Long-Term Electrocardiographic Recording

Prolonged ECG recording in patients engaged in normal daily activities is the most useful noninvasive method to document and quantitate the frequency and complexity of an arrhythmia, correlate the arrhythmia with the patient's symptoms, and evaluate the effect of antiarrhythmic therapy on spontaneous arrhythmia.[8] For example, recording normal sinus rhythm during the patient's typical symptomatic episode effectively excludes cardiac arrhythmia as a cause. In addition, some recorders can document alterations in QRS, ST, and T contours (Fig. 29–4).

AMBULATORY ECG (HOLTER) RECORDING. Continuous ECG tape recorders represent the traditional Holter monitor and typically record (on analog tape or digital cards) two or three ECG channels for 24 hours.[9] Interpretative accuracy of long-term recordings varies with the system used, but most computers that scan the recording media are sufficiently accurate to meet clinical needs. All systems can potentially record more information than the physician needs or can assimilate. As long as the system detects important episodes of ectopic activity, VT, or asystolic intervals and semiquantitates these abnormalities, the physician probably receives all the clinical information that is needed. Twenty-five to 50 percent of patients experience a complaint during a 24-hour

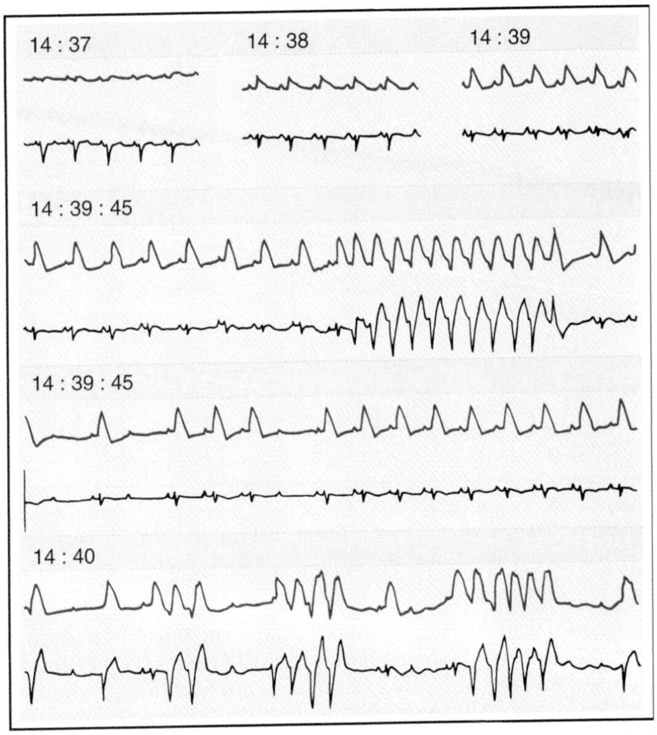

FIGURE 29–4 Long-term electrocardiographic recording in a patient with atypical angina. The top channel reflects an inferior lead, and the bottom channel records an anterior lead. Note progressive ST segment elevation in the inferior lead, eventually resembling a monophasic action potential. Bursts of nonsustained ventricular tachycardia result. Then, sinus slowing and Wenckebach atrioventricular (AV) block occur from a vasodepressor reflex response elicited by ischemia of the inferior myocardial wall or possibly caused by ischemia of the sinus and AV nodes. In the bottom tracing, both AV block and ventricular arrhythmias are apparent. Numbers indicate time (e.g., 2:37 P.M.). (Courtesy of D. A. Chilson, MD.)

recording, caused by an arrhythmia in 2 to 15 percent (see Fig. 29–4). The ability to temporally correlate symptoms with ECG abnormalities is one of the strengths of this technique.

Significant rhythm disturbances are fairly uncommon in healthy young persons. However, sinus bradycardia with heart rates of 35 to 40 beats/min, sinus arrhythmia with pauses exceeding 3 seconds, sinoatrial exit block, type 1 (Wenckebach) second-degree AV block (often during sleep), a wandering atrial pacemaker, junctional escape complexes, and premature atrial complexes (PACs) and PVCs are not necessarily abnormal. Frequent and complex atrial and ventricular rhythm disturbances are less commonly observed, however, and type II second-degree AV conduction disturbances (see Chap. 32) are not recorded in normal patients. Elderly patients may have a greater prevalence of arrhythmias, some of which may be responsible for neurological symptoms (Fig. 29–5). The long-term prognosis in asymptomatic healthy subjects with frequent and complex PVCs resembles that of the healthy U.S. population without an increased risk of death.

Most patients who have ischemic heart disease, particularly those after myocardial infarction, exhibit PVCs when monitored for 6 to 24 hours. The frequency of PVCs progressively increases over the first several weeks, decreasing at about 6 months after infarction. Frequent and complex PVCs constitute an independent risk factor and are associated with a twofold to fivefold increased risk of cardiac or sudden death in patients after myocardial infarction. Evidence from the Cardiac Arrhythmia Suppression Trial (CAST) raises the possibility that the ventricular ectopy is a marker identifying the patient at risk rather than being causally related to sudden death, because PVC suppression with flecainide, encainide,

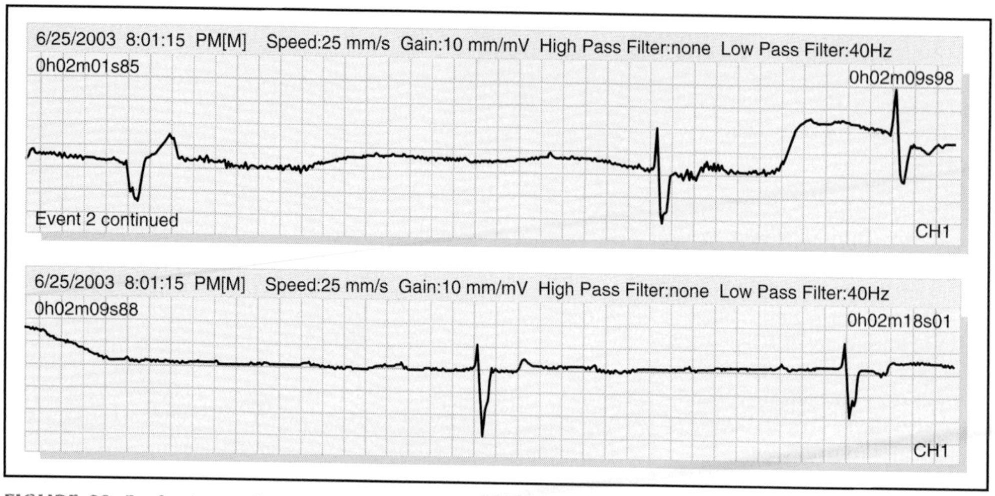

FIGURE 29–5 Continuous electrocardiographic recording from a patient-activated event monitor during an episode of lightheadedness. Sinus rhythm at 75 beats/min with sudden atrioventricular block is present with pauses of longer than 4 seconds and, in the bottom strip, there is an effective heart rate of about 8 beats/min.

or moricizine was associated with increased mortality compared with placebo.[10] Thus, the PVC may be an "innocent bystander," unrelated to the tachyarrhythmia producing sudden death. Although the mechanism responsible for the drug-induced exacerbation of mortality is not clear, it may relate to an increase in ischemia-produced conduction delay due to sodium-channel blocking drugs.

Holter recordings have been used to determine antiarrhythmic drug efficacy. In one study, Holter recordings led to predictions of antiarrhythmic drug efficacy more often than did electrophysiological testing in patients with sustained ventricular tachyarrhythmias, and there was no significant difference in the success of drug therapy as selected by the two methods.[7] The beneficial results of noninvasive compared with invasive assessment of drug efficacy in this study have been challenged.

Long-term ECG recording also has exposed potentially serious arrhythmias and complex ventricular ectopy in patients with left ventricular hypertrophy; in those with mitral valve prolapse; in those who have otherwise unexplained syncope or transient vague cerebrovascular symptoms; in those with conduction disturbances, sinus node dysfunction, bradycardia-tachycardia syndrome, Wolff-Parkinson-White syndrome, increased QT dispersion, and pacemaker malfunction; and after thrombolytic therapy. It has shown that asymptomatic atrial fibrillation occurs far more often than symptomatic atrial fibrillation in patients with that arrhythmia.[11] This has important implications for deciding whether a patient needs chronic anticoagulation based only on recurrent symptoms or a single ECG recording.

Variations of Holter recording have been used for particular applications. Repeated 24-hour recording periods may be needed to obtain enough episodes of PAC triggering atrial fibrillation to warrant proceeding to an EPS and catheter ablation. Some monitoring systems are able to "reconstruct" a full 12-lead ECG from a seven-electrode recording system. This is especially useful when trying to document the ECG morphology of VT before an ablation procedure or a consistent morphology of PACs that may arise from an ablatable focus of atrial fibrillation. Most Holter recording and analysis systems have the ability to place a clearly recognizable deflection on the recording when a pacemaker stimulus is detected. This greatly facilitates diagnosis of potential pacemaker malfunction. Occasionally, ECG artifacts due to alterations in tape recording or playback speed can mimic bradycardias or tachycardias and lead to erroneous therapy. Newer digital Holter systems are less subject to this phenomenon. Finally, most systems can also provide heart rate variability data (see later).

EVENT RECORDING. In many patients, the 24-hour "snapshot" provided by the Holter recording is incapable of documenting the cause of the patient's symptoms. Longer term monitoring is necessary in these cases, which occur frequently, such as with an event recorder.[12] These devices are about the size of a pager and are kept by the patient for 30 days. During that time, digital recordings can be made during symptomatic episodes and transmitted to a receiving station over standard telephone lines at the patient's convenience (see Fig. 29–5). Some of these recorders store more than 30 seconds of ECG before the time when the patient activates the recording. These "loop" recorders record continuously, but only a small window of time is present in memory at any time; when the event button is pressed by the patient, the current window is "frozen" while the device continues recording for another 30 to 60 seconds, depending on how it is configured. Event recorders are highly effective in documenting infrequent events, but the quality of the recordings is more variable than Holter recorders and usually only one channel can be recorded. Using some systems, the patient must be able to press the event button to begin recording; if syncope occurs without warning and the patient is not able to actuate the device, it cannot provide diagnostic information. With other systems, the device automatically begins recording the rhythm when the heart rate falls outside predetermined parameters.

Some pacemakers and implantable defibrillators are capable of providing Holter-like data on occurrence of premature beats or tachycardia episodes and can even store electrograms of these events from the implanted leads. The device can then be interrogated later and the electrograms printed for analysis.

IMPLANTABLE LOOP RECORDER. For patients with infrequent and transient symptoms, neither Holter recorders nor 30-day event recorders may yield diagnostic information. In such patients, implantable loop recorders may be used. This device (about the size of a pack of chewing gum) is inserted under the skin at about the second rib on the left front of the chest and is activated by passing a special magnet over the device.[13] It is capable of recording up to 42 minutes of a single ECG channel that can be partitioned for 1 to 7 episodes, with up to 20 minutes of preactivation ECG saved for subsequent downloading to a programming unit for analysis. Both P waves and QRS complexes can usually be identified. The device can be configured to store patient-activated episodes, automatically activated recordings (heart rate outside preset parameters), or a combination of these (Fig. 29–6). In one report, this device was implanted in 24 patients with recurrent syncope who had undergone extensive evaluation without determining a cause of syncope. Over a mean 5-month period after implant, 21 patients had recurrent syncope; the device was instrumental in establishing the diagnosis in 18 patients.[13]

Heart Rate Variability

Heart rate variability is used to evaluate vagal and sympathetic influences on the sinus node (inferring that the same

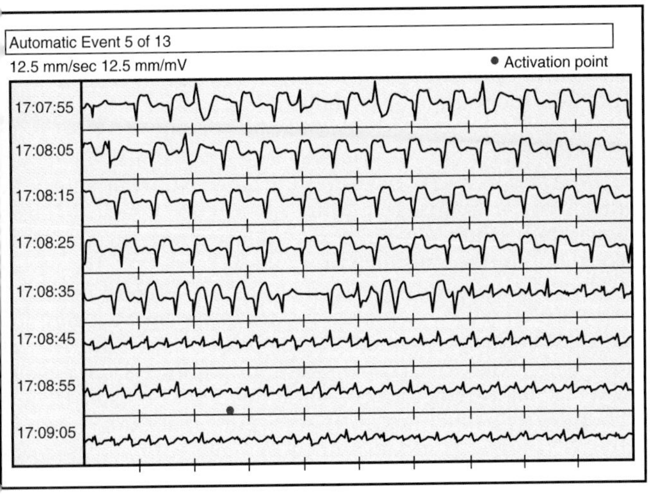

FIGURE 29–6 Recordings from an implantable loop recorder. Each line contains 10 seconds of continuous electrocardiogram from the implanted device. The first four lines show sinus rhythm with premature ventricular complexes; during the fifth line, short runs of atrial tachycardia precede an episode of a faster tachycardia with a different complex (ventricular tachycardia). This episode triggered an automatic activation (red circle) of the device recording (no symptoms associated with the episode).

activity is occurring in the ventricles also) and to identify patients at risk for a cardiovascular event or death.[14] Frequency domain analysis resolves parasympathetic and sympathetic influences better than does time domain analysis, but both types of analysis are useful. R-R variability predicts all-cause mortality as well as does left ventricular ejection fraction or nonsustained VT in patients after myocardial infarction and can be added to other measures of risk to enhance predictive accuracy. Similar results have been obtained in patients with dilated cardiomyopathy.[15] High-frequency components of R-R interval variability reflect vagal activity. Reduced RR interval variability, the marker of increased risk, indicates loss or reduction of the physiological periodic sinus node fluctuations, which can be due to many different influences and may not necessarily represent a particular shift in autonomic modulation. Some investigators have determined that simple heart rate measurement contains as much prognostic information as heart rate variability.[16]

QT Dispersion

Heterogeneity in refractoriness and conduction velocity is a hallmark of reentrant arrhythmias. One index of heterogeneity of ventricular refractoriness can be found in differences in length of the QT interval in surface ECG leads. The most commonly used index to calculate this QT dispersion has been the difference between the longest and shortest QT intervals on the 12-lead ECG, which is often adjusted for heart rate as well as number of leads sampled (when the T wave is flat in some). Other indices have been developed. Abnormally high QT dispersion has been correlated with risk of arrhythmic death in a variety of disorders,[17] although results are not consistent. QT dispersion has been correlated with efficacy and proarrhythmic potential of drug therapy. Different techniques exist for determining dispersion (including automated algorithms), and the results of one study are often difficult to compare with those of another; in addition, seasonal variation in QT dispersion has been shown.[18] It remains to be seen whether QT dispersion measured on a scalar ECG will be a useful clinical tool.[19,20]

Late Potentials

Signal averaging is a method that improves signal-to-noise ratio when signals are recurrent and the noise is random.[21] In conjunction with appropriate filtering and other methods of noise reduction, signal averaging can detect cardiac signals of a few microvolts in amplitude, reducing noise amplitude, such as muscle potentials that are typically 5 to 25 μV, to less than 1 μV. With this method, very low-amplitude electrical potentials generated by the sinus and AV nodes, His bundle, and bundle branches are detectable at the body surface.

One of the constituents of reentrant ventricular arrhythmias in patients with prior myocardial damage is slow conduction. Direct cardiac mapping techniques can record myocardial activation from damaged areas that occurs after the end of the surface ECG QRS complex during sinus rhythm. These delayed signals have very low amplitude that cannot be discerned on routine ECG and correspond to the delayed and fragmented conduction in the ventricles recorded with direct mapping techniques (Fig. 29–7). Signal averaging has been applied clinically most often to detect such late ventricular potentials of 1 to 25 μV. Criteria for late potentials are (1) filtered QRS complex duration greater than 114 to 120 milliseconds, (2) less than 20 μV of root-mean-square signal amplitude in the last 40 milliseconds of the filtered QRS complex, and (3) the terminal filtered QRS complex remains below 40 μV for longer than 39 milli-

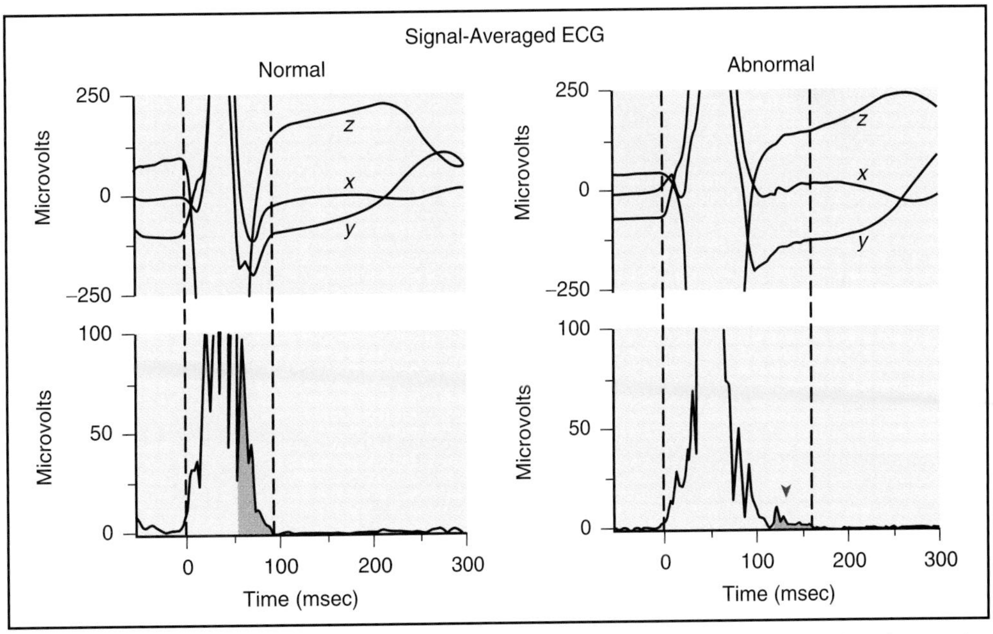

FIGURE 29–7 Signal-averaged electrocardiogram (ECG). Normal **(left)** and abnormal **(right)** results are shown from a patient with prior myocardial infarction and venticular tachycardia. **Bottom panels:** Shaded blue areas at the end of each tracing represent voltage content of last 40 milliseconds of the filtered QRS integral. The small shaded area in the abnormal study denotes prolonged, slow conduction and suggests the potential for reentrant ventricular arrhythmias.

seconds. These late potentials have been recorded in 70 to 90 percent of patients with spontaneous sustained and inducible VT after myocardial infarction, in only 0 to 6 percent of normal volunteers, and in 7 to 15 percent of patients after myocardial infarction who do not have VT. Late potentials can be detected as early as 3 hours after the onset of chest pain, increase in prevalence in the first week after myocardial infarction, and disappear in some patients after 1 year. If not present initially, late potentials usually do not appear later. Early use of thrombolytic agents may reduce the prevalence of late potentials after coronary occlusion. Patients with bundle branch block or paced ventricular rhythms have wide QRS complexes already, rendering the technique less useful in these cases.

Late potentials also have been recorded in patients with VT not related to ischemia, such as dilated cardiomyopathies. Successful surgical resection of the VT can eliminate late potentials but is not necessary to cause tachycardia suppression. The presence of a late potential is a sensitive, but not specific, marker of arrhythmic risk and thus its prognostic use is limited.[22] In specific situations, it can be helpful; for instance, a patient with a prior inferior wall myocardial infarction (normally the last portion of the heart to be activated) who has no late potential has a very low likelihood of having VT episodes.

The high-pass filtering used to record late potentials meeting the criteria just noted is called *time domain analysis* because the filter output corresponds in time to the input signal. Because late potentials are high-frequency signals, Fourier transform can be applied to extract high-frequency content from the signal-averaged ECG, called *frequency domain analysis*. Some data suggest that frequency domain analysis provides useful information not available in the time domain analysis.

Signal averaging has been applied to the P wave to determine risk for developing atrial fibrillation as well as maintenance of sinus rhythm after cardioversion. The overall use of the technique remains limited at present.

T Wave Alternans

Beat-to-beat alternation in the amplitude and/or morphology of the ECG measurement of ventricular repolarization, the ST segment and T wave, has been found in conditions favoring the development of ventricular tachyarrhythmias such as ischemia and long-QT interval syndrome and in patients with ventricular arrhythmias.[23] The electrophysiological basis appears to be the alternation of repolarization of ventricular myocytes.[24] In the presence of a long QT interval, the cellular basis of alternation has been shown to be due to beat-to-beat repolarization changes in midmyocardial cells (M cells).[25] Whether this mechanism applies to different disease states is not known. T wave alternans testing requires exercise or atrial pacing to achieve a heart rate of 100 to 120 beats/min with relatively little atrial or ventricular ectopic activity. The test is less useful in patients with a wide QRS complex (>120 milliseconds). A positive T wave alternans test is associated with a worse arrhythmic prognosis in a variety of disorders, including ischemic heart disease[26] and nonischemic cardiomyopathy.[27] T wave alternans may represent a fundamental marker of an electrically unstable myocardium prone to developing VT or VF, and, as such, ST-T wave analysis for alternans may be useful in the future as a method to risk-stratify patients (Fig. 29–8).

Baroreceptor Reflex Sensitivity Testing
(see Chap. 87)

Acute blood pressure elevation triggers a baroreceptor reflex that augments vagal "tone" to the heart and slows the sinus rate. The increase in sinus cycle length per millimeter of mercury systolic blood pressure increase is a measure of the sensitivity of the baroreceptor reflex and, when reduced, identifies patients susceptible to developing VT and VF.[28,29] The mechanism of the reduction in baroreceptor reflex

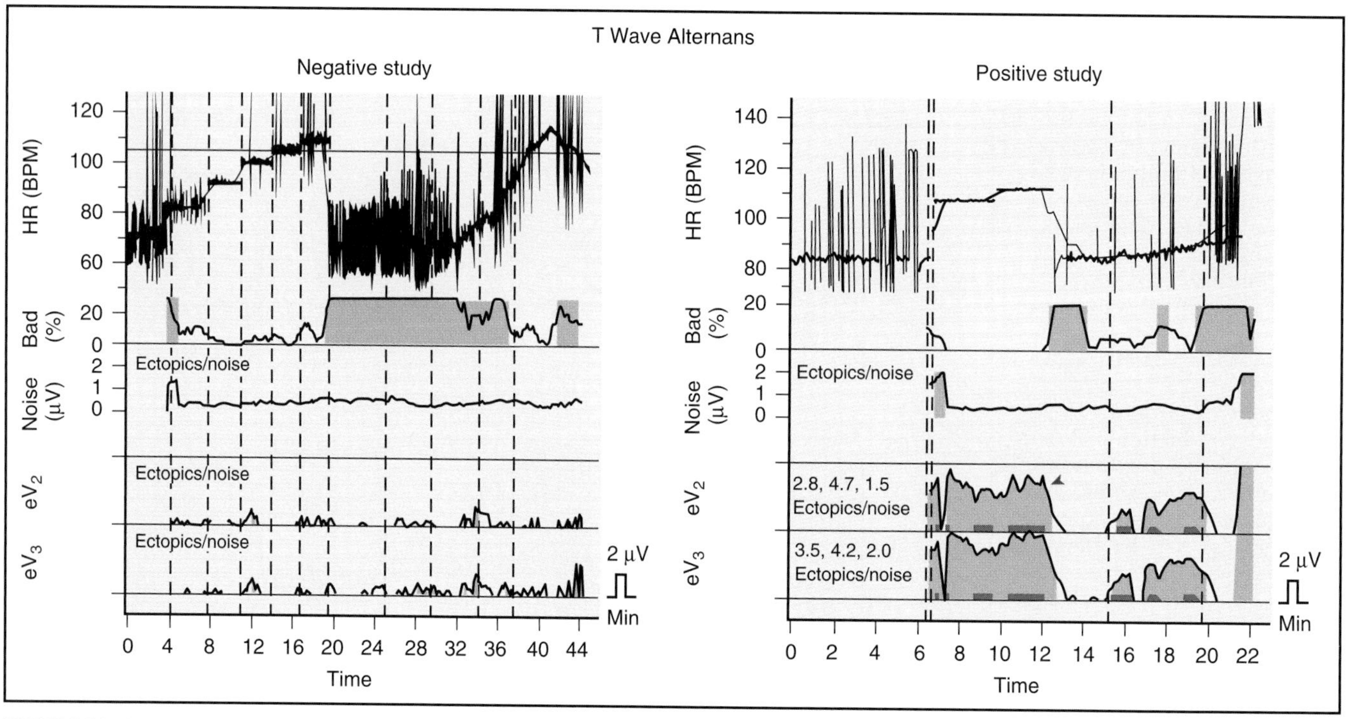

FIGURE 29–8 T wave alternans. Reports of T wave alternans analysis from two patients are shown, displaying heart rate (HR) in beats per minute (BPM), proportion of beats rejected from analysis (% Bad), electrocardiogram noise level (in microvolts), and selected precordial leads (V_2 and V_3) as a function of time. Records in the left panel are from a patient with no structural heart disease; the amplitude of T wave alternans was minimal. The study in the right panel, from a patient hospitalized for sustained ventricular tachycardia after myocardial infarction, shows T wave alternans (blue shaded area, arrow).

sensitivity is not certain. However, this test may be useful to identify patients at risk for developing a serious ventricular arrhythmia after myocardial infarction.

Body Surface Mapping

Isopotential body surface maps are used to provide a complete picture of the effects of the currents from the heart on the body surface. The potential distributions are represented by contour lines of equal potential, and each distribution is displayed instant by instant throughout activation or recovery, or both.[30]

Body surface maps have been used clinically to localize and size areas of myocardial ischemia, localize ectopic foci or accessory pathways, differentiate aberrant supraventricular conduction from ventricular origin, recognize the patient prone to developing arrhythmias, and possibly understand the mechanisms involved. Although these procedures are of interest, their clinical utility has not yet been established. In addition, the technique is cumbersome and the analysis is complex.

Upright Tilt-Table Testing

The tilt-table test is used to identify patients who have a vasodepressor and/or a cardioinhibitory response as a cause of syncope.[31] Patients are positioned on a tilt table in the supine position and are tilted upright to a maximum of 60 to 80 degrees for 20 to 45 minutes, or longer if necessary (Fig. 29–9). Isoproterenol, as a bolus or an infusion, may provoke syncope in patients whose initial upright tilt-table testing shows no abnormalities or after just several minutes of tilt to shorten the time of the test necessary to produce a positive response. An initial intravenous isoproterenol dose of 1 μg/min can be increased in 0.5-μg/min steps until symptoms occur or a maximum of 4 μg/min is given. Isoproterenol induces a vasodepressor response in upright, susceptible patients generally consisting of a decrease in heart rate and blood pressure along with near-syncope or syncope. Intravenous edrophonium chloride, nitroglycerin, and esmolol withdrawal have also been used. Atropine can block the early bradycardia but not the hypotension; beta blockers can inhibit the latter. Tilt-table test results are positive in two thirds to three fourths of patients susceptible to neurally mediated syncope and are reproducible in about 80 percent, but have a 10 to 15 percent false-positive response rate. Repeating an initially negative tilt-table test on a subsequent day rarely yields a positive result. A positive test result is more meaningful when it reproduces symptoms that have occurred spontaneously. Positive responses can be divided into cardioinhibitory, vasodepressor, and mixed categories. Therapy with beta blockers, disopyramide, theophylline, selective serotonin reuptake inhibitors, midodrine, and salt loading or fludrocortisone have each been reported to be successful, as has "tilt training" (in which the patient leans against a wall for prolonged periods to increase tolerance to this body position).

MECHANISM[32]

Vasodepressor reactions, which are thought to be caused by activation of unmyelinated left ventricular vagal C fibers, can be triggered by a variety of events, including increased left ventricular pressure (see Chap. 34). Stimulation of C fibers from vigorous left ventricular contraction on a relatively empty cavity reduces efferent sympathetic tone while increasing efferent vagal tone, possibly producing vasodepression and paradoxical bradycardia. Isoproterenol increases left ventricular contractility while reducing left ventricular volume. A passive upright tilt exaggerates these responses because the tilt also reduces venous return and prevents isoproterenol from increasing cardiac output. Some patients may experience profound bradycardia, whereas others may have a prominent vasodepressor component. Dual-chamber pacing has been shown to benefit some patients with refractory neurocardiogenic syncope.[33] Before pacemaker implantation, some investigators have advocated performing a tilt-table test with temporary pacing catheters in place to simulate how a permanent pacing system would perform; however, correlation between this type of acute testing and long-term pacing results has not been proven.

A variant of the neurocardiogenic response, the postural orthostatic tachycardia syndrome, is characterized by dramatic increases in heart rate during the first 10 minutes of tilt-table testing.[34] This syndrome appears to be distinct from simple orthostatic hypotension as well as standard neurocardiogenic responses and is thought to be due to various forms of autonomic imbalance. Relief of symptoms has been effected with fludrocortisone, beta blockers, or combinations.

ESOPHAGEAL ELECTROCARDIOGRAPHY

Esophageal electrocardiography is a useful noninvasive technique to diagnose arrhythmias. The esophagus is located immediately behind the left atrium, between the left and right pulmonary veins. An electrode in the lumen of the esophagus can record atrial potentials. Bipolar recording is superior to unipolar recording because far-field ventricular events

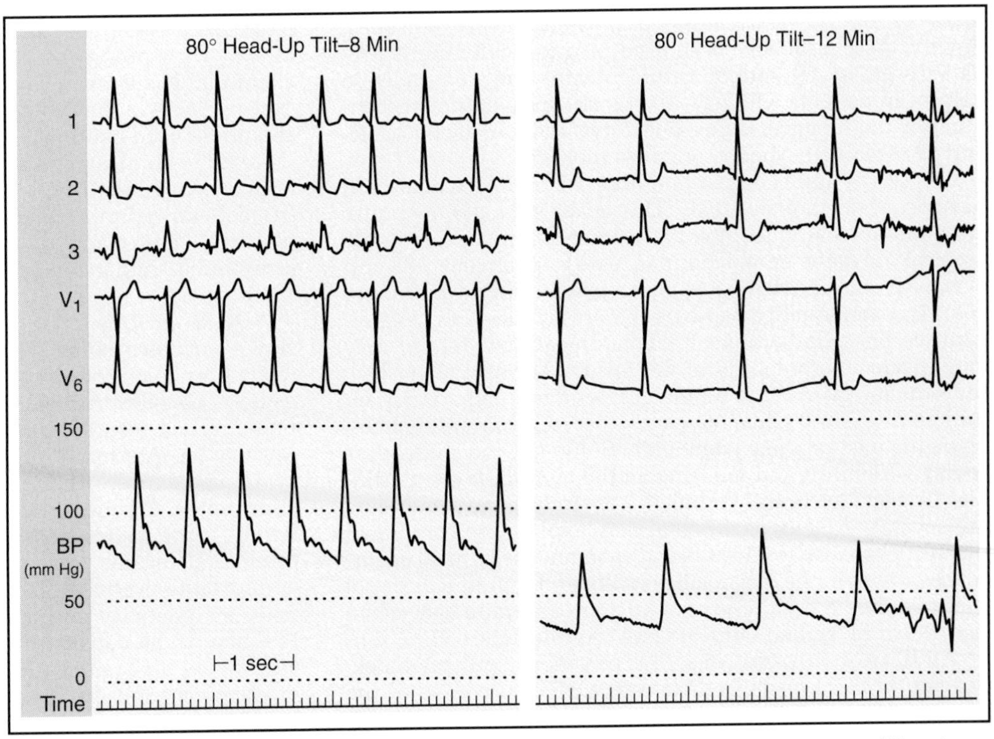

FIGURE 29–9 Head-up tilt-table testing. Surface electrocardiogram (ECG) leads and an arterial blood pressure (BP) tracing are shown. After 8 minutes of head-up tilt at 80 degrees (left), heart rate and BP were normal and the patient was asymptomatic. Four minutes later (right), systolic BP dropped precipitously to 80 mm Hg, the heart rate fell to 50 beats/min, and the patient lost consciousness. ECG artifact at right is seizure activity.

with the former method can lead to possible diagnostic confusion. In addition, atrial and occasionally ventricular pacing can be performed by means of a catheter electrode inserted into the esophagus, and initiation and termination of tachycardias can be accomplished. Optimal electrode position for atrial pacing correlates with patient height and is within about 1 cm of the site at which the maximum amplitude of the atrial electrogram is recorded. When recorded simultaneously with the surface ECG, the esophageal atrial electrogram can be used to differentiate SVT with aberrancy from VT and to define the mechanism of SVTs. For example, if atrial and ventricular depolarizations occur simultaneously during a narrow QRS tachycardia, reentry using an accessory AV pathway (Wolff-Parkinson-White syndrome) can be excluded, and AV nodal reentry is the most likely mechanism for the tachycardia. Complications of transesophageal recording and pacing are uncommon, but the technique is not comfortable for most patients and it is thus not commonly applied.

Invasive Electrophysiological Studies

An invasive EPS involves introducing multipolar catheter electrodes into the venous and/or arterial system and positioning the electrodes at various intracardiac sites to record and/or stimulate cardiac electrical activity. Assessment of AV conduction at rest is made by positioning the catheter along the septal leaflet of the tricuspid valve and measuring the atrial-His interval (an estimate of AV nodal conduction time; normally 60 to 125 milliseconds) and the His-ventricular (HV) interval (a measure of infranodal conduction; normally 40 to 55 milliseconds). The heart is stimulated from portions of the atria or ventricles and from the region of the His bundle, bundle branches, accessory pathways, and other structures. Such studies are performed diagnostically to provide information on the type of clinical rhythm disturbances and insight into its electrophysiological mechanism. They are used therapeutically to terminate a tachycardia by electrical stimulation or electroshock; to evaluate the effects of therapy by determining whether a particular intervention modifies or prevents electrical induction of a tachycardia or whether an electrical device properly senses and terminates an induced tachyarrhythmia; and to ablate myocardium involved in the tachycardia to prevent further episodes. Finally, these tests have been used prognostically to identify patients at risk for sudden cardiac death. The study may be helpful in patients who have AV block, intraventricular conduction disturbance, sinus node dysfunction, tachycardia, and unexplained syncope or palpitations.[35]

The EPS is quite good at initiating VT or SVT when these have occurred spontaneously. This enables the use of similar stimulation techniques after an intervention (drug therapy or surgical or catheter ablation) to assess treatment efficacy. However, false-negative responses (not finding a particular electrical abnormality known to be present) as well as false-positive ones (induction of a nonclinical arrhythmia) may complicate interpretation of the results, because many lack reproducibility. Altered autonomic tone in a supine patient undergoing study, hemodynamic or ischemic influences, changing anatomy (e.g., new infarction) after the study, day-to-day variability, and the fact that the test employs an artificial "trigger" (electrical stimulation) to induce the arrhythmia are several of many factors that may explain the occasional disparity between test results and spontaneous clinical occurrences. Overall, the diagnostic validity and reproducibility of these studies are quite good, and they are quite safe when performed by skilled clinical electrophysiologists.

AV BLOCK (see also Chap. 32). In patients with AV block, the site of block usually dictates the clinical course of the patient and whether a pacemaker is needed. Generally, the site of AV block can be determined from an analysis of the scalar ECG. When the site of block cannot be determined from such an analysis, and when knowing the site of block is imperative for patient management, an invasive EPS is indicated. Candidates include symptomatic patients in whom His-Purkinje block is suspected but not established and patients with AV block treated with a pacemaker who continue to be symptomatic in whom a causal ventricular tachyarrhythmia is sought. Possible candidates are those with second- or third-degree AV block in whom knowledge of the site of block or its mechanism may help direct therapy or assess prognosis and patients suspected of having concealed His bundle extrasystoles. Patients with block in the His-Purkinje system more commonly become symptomatic because of periods of bradycardia or asystole and more commonly require pacemaker implantation than do patients who have AV nodal block.[36] Type I (Wenckebach) AV block in older patients may have clinical implications similar to type II AV block. The results of EPS for evaluating the conduction system must be interpreted with caution, however. In rare cases, the process of recording conduction intervals alters their values. For instance, catheter pressure on the AV node or His bundle can cause a prolongation of the atrial-His or HV interval and lead to erroneous diagnosis and therapy.

INTRAVENTRICULAR CONDUCTION DISTURBANCE. For patients with an intraventricular conduction disturbance, an EPS provides information on the duration of the HV interval, which can be prolonged with a normal PR interval or normal with a prolonged PR interval. A prolonged HV interval (>55 milliseconds) is associated with a greater likelihood of developing trifascicular block (but the rate of progression is slow, 2 to 3 percent annually), having structural disease, and higher mortality. Finding very long HV intervals (>80 to 90 milliseconds) identifies patients at increased risk of developing AV block. The HV interval has a high specificity (~80 percent) but low sensitivity (~66 percent) for predicting the development of complete AV block. During the study, atrial pacing is used to uncover abnormal His-Purkinje conduction. A positive response is provocation of distal His block during 1:1 AV nodal conduction. Once again, sensitivity is low but specificity is high. Functional His-Purkinje block due to normal His-Purkinje refractoriness is not a positive response. Drug infusion, such as that with procainamide or ajmaline, sometimes exposes abnormal His-Purkinje conduction (Fig. 29–10). Ajmaline (not available in the United States) can cause arrhythmias and should be used cautiously.

An EPS is indicated in the patient with symptoms (syncope or presyncope) that appear to be related to a bradyarrhythmia or tachyarrhythmia when no other cause of symptoms is found. For many of these patients, ventricular tachyarrhythmias rather than AV block can be the cause of their symptoms.

SINUS NODE DYSFUNCTION. The demonstration of slow sinus rates, sinus exit block, or sinus pauses temporally related to symptoms suggests a causal relationship and usually obviates further diagnostic studies. Carotid sinus pressure that results in several seconds of complete cardiac asystole or AV block and reproduces the patient's usual symptoms exposes the presence of a hypersensitive carotid sinus reflex. Carotid sinus massage must be done cautiously. Rarely, carotid sinus massage can precipitate a stroke. Neurohumoral agents, adenosine, or stress testing can be employed to evaluate the effects of autonomic tone on sinus node automaticity and sinoatrial conduction time (SACT). EPS should be considered in patients who have symptoms attributable to bradycardia or asystole, such as presyncope or syncope, and for whom noninvasive approaches have provided no explanation for the symptoms.

Sinus Node Recovery Time. Sinus node recovery time (SNRT) is a technique that can be useful to evaluate sinus node function. The interval between the last paced high right atrial response and the first spontaneous (sinus) high right atrial response after termination of pacing is measured to determine the SNRT. Because the spontaneous sinus rate influences the SNRT, the value is corrected by subtracting the spontaneous sinus node cycle length (before pacing) from the SNRT (Fig. 29–11). This value, the CSNRT, is generally less than 525 milliseconds. Prolonged CSNRT has been found in patients suspected of having sinus node dysfunction. Direct recordings of the sinus node electrogram have documented that SNRT is influenced by prolongation of sinoatrial conduction time (the time from the onset of the sinus impulse to the onset of activation of surrounding atrial myocardium), as well as by changes in sinus node automaticity, especially in the first beat after cessation of pacing. After cessation of pacing, the first return sinus cycle can be normal and can be followed by secondary pauses. Secondary pauses appear to be more common in patients whose sinus node dysfunction is caused by sinoatrial exit block (a potential cause of ECG sinus pauses). Finally, it is important to evaluate AV node and His-Purkinje function in patients with sinus node dysfunction, because many also exhibit impaired AV conduction.

Sinoatrial Conduction Time. SACT can be estimated using simple pacing techniques based on the assumptions that (1) conduction times into and out of the sinus node are equal, (2) no depression of sinus node automaticity occurs, and (3) the pacemaker site does not shift after premature stimulation (see Chap. 32). These assumptions can be erroneous, particularly in patients with sinus node dysfunction. SACT can also be measured directly with extracellular electrodes placed in the region of the sinus node. This direct measurement correlates well with the SACT measured indirectly in patients with normal sinus node function. The sensitivity of the SACT and SNRT tests is only about 50 percent for each test alone and about 65 percent when combined. The specificity, when combined, is about 88 percent, with a low predictive value. Thus, if these tests are abnormal, the likelihood of the patient having sinus node dysfunction is great. However, normal results do not exclude the possibility of sinus node disease.

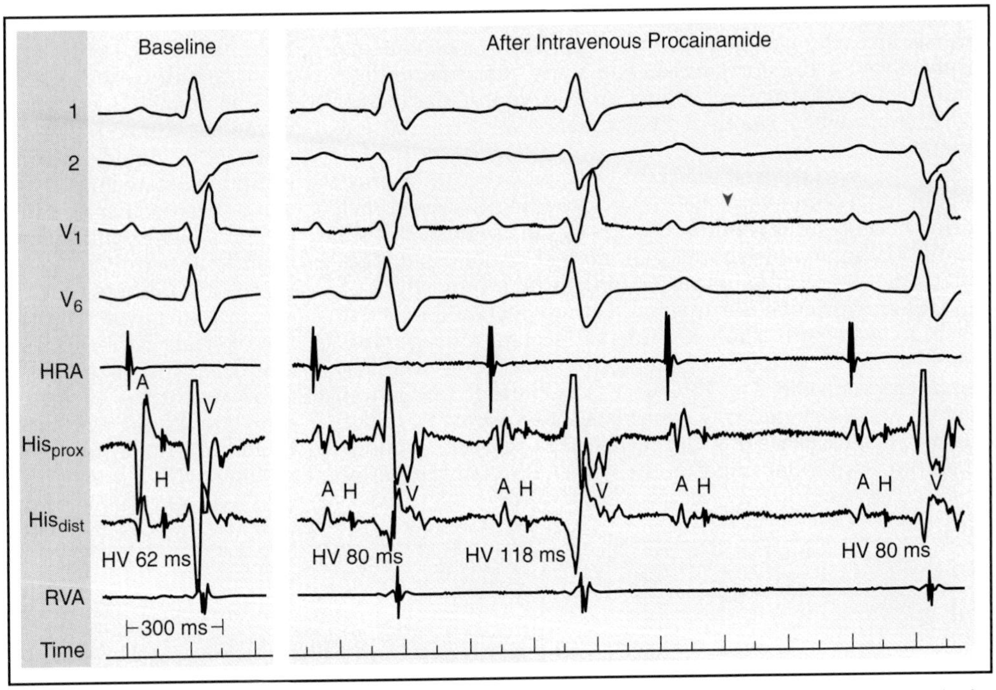

FIGURE 29–10 Testing the His-Purkinje system. A 43-year-old woman with sarcoid underwent electrophysiological study after a syncopal episode. Surface leads 1, 2, V_1, and V_6 are shown with intracardiac recordings from catheters in the high right atrium (HRA), proximal (His_{prox}), and distal (His_{dist}) electrode pairs of a catheter at the atrioventricular junction to record the His potential, and right ventricular apex (RVA). During baseline recording, the HV interval is only slightly prolonged (62 milliseconds). After infusion of intravenous procainamide, the HV interval is longer and infra-His Wenckebach block is present. Arrow denotes "missing" QRS complex due to infra-His block. A = atrial electrogram; H = His potential; V = ventricular electrogram.

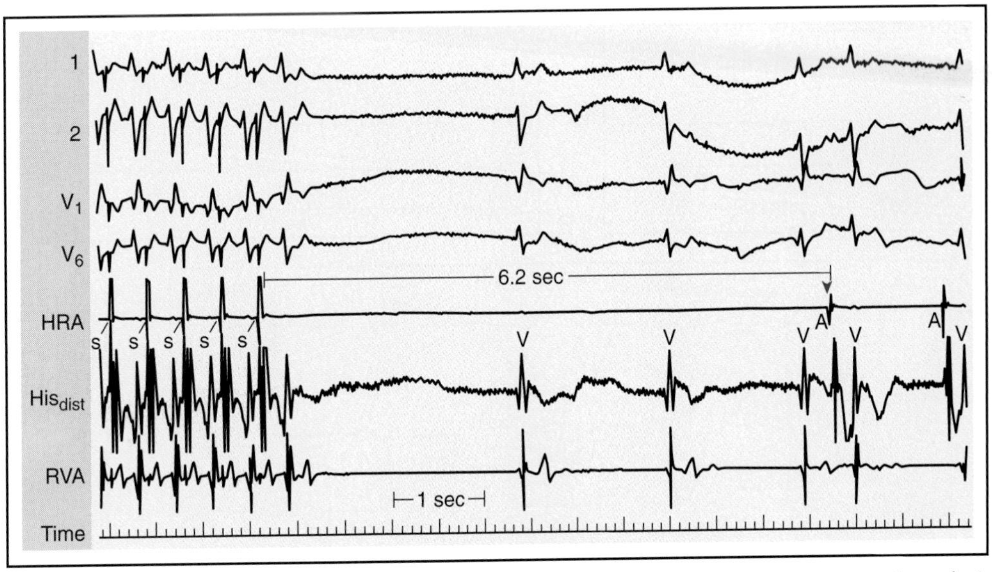

FIGURE 29–11 Abnormal sinus node function. Recordings are similar to those in Figure 23-3. The last five complexes of a 1-minute burst of atrial pacing (S) at a cycle length of 400 milliseconds are shown, after which pacing is stopped. The sinus node does not spontaneously discharge (sinus node recovery time) until 6.2 seconds later (arrow). Three junctional escape beats occurred before this time.

Candidates for invasive EPS to evaluate sinus node function are symptomatic patients in whom sinus node dysfunction has not been established as a cause of the symptoms. Potential candidates are those requiring pacemakers to determine the pacing modality, patients with sinus node dysfunction to determine the mechanism and response to therapy, and patients in whom other causes of symptoms (e.g., tachyarrhythmias) are to be excluded.

TACHYCARDIA. In patients with tachycardias, an EPS can be used to diagnose the arrhythmia, determine and deliver therapy, determine the anatomical site(s) involved in the tachycardia, identify patients at high risk for developing serious arrhythmias, and gain insights into mechanisms responsible for the arrhythmia. The study can differentiate aberrant supraventricular conduction from ventricular tachyarrhythmias when standard ECG criteria fail to make the differentiation.

An SVT is recognized electrophysiologically by the presence of an HV interval equaling or exceeding that recorded during normal sinus rhythm (Fig. 29–12). In contrast, during VT, the HV interval is shorter than normal or the His deflection cannot be recorded clearly owing to superimposition of the larger ventricular electrogram. Only two situations exist when a consistently short HV interval occurs: during retrograde activation of the His bundle from activation originating in the ventricle (i.e., PVC or VT) or during conduction over an accessory pathway (preexcitation syndrome). Atrial pacing at rates exceeding the tachycardia rate can demonstrate the ventricular origin of the wide QRS tachycardia by producing fusion and capture beats and normalization of the HV interval. The only VT that exhibits an HV interval equal to or slightly exceeding the normal sinus HV interval is bundle branch reentry, but His activation will be in the retrograde direction.

An EPS should be considered (1) in patients who have symptomatic, recurrent, or drug-resistant supraventricular or ventricular tachyarrhythmias to help select optimal therapy; (2) in patients with tachyarrhythmias occurring too infrequently to permit adequate diagnostic or therapeutic assessment; (3) to differentiate SVT and aberrant conduction from VT; (4) whenever nonpharmacological therapy such as the use of electrical devices, catheter ablation, or surgery is contemplated; (5) in patients surviving an episode of cardiac arrest (occurring 48 hours after an acute myocardial infarction or without evidence of an acute Q-wave myocardial infarction); and (6) in assessing risk of sustained VT in patients with a prior myocardial infarction, ejection fraction

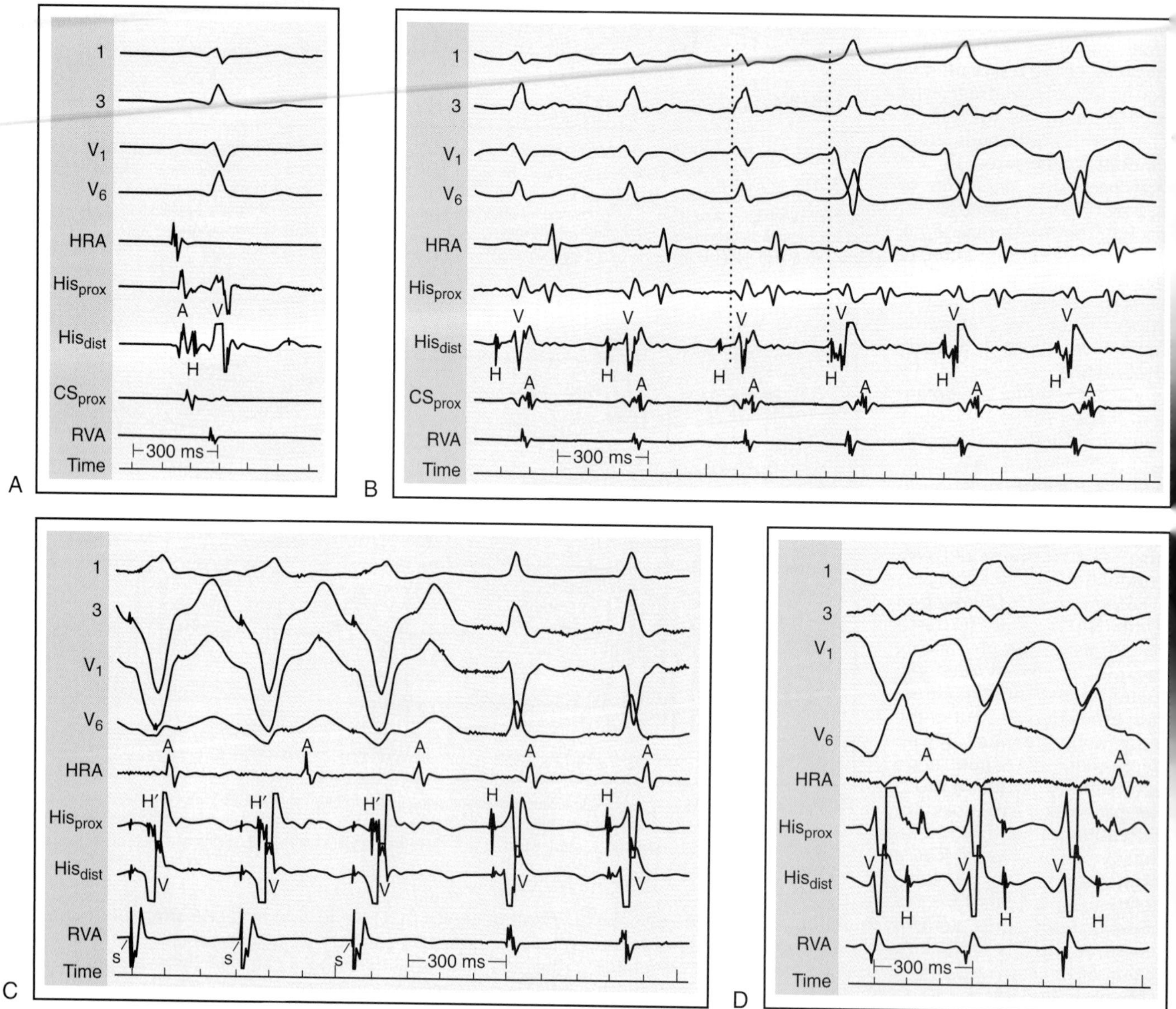

FIGURE 29–12 Bundle of His recordings in different situations similar to those in prior figures (see Figs. 29–10 and 29–11). **A,** Baseline sinus rhythm with normal atrioventricular (AV) conduction. **B,** Orthodromic supraventricular tachycardia with retrograde conduction over a left-sided accessory pathway throughout the tracing. The first three beats have a narrow QRS complex with a normal HV interval; the last three QRS complexes represent a fusion of conduction over the AV node-His and a slowly conducting right-sided accessory pathway. The His potential occurs after the onset of the wide QRS complex (dashed lines). In **C,** three paced ventricular beats are shown with a retrograde His potential (H′), followed by initiation of AV node reentrant supraventricular tachycardia (atrial depolarization near the end of the QRS complex, as seen in HRA tracing). **D,** Ventricular tachycardia with delayed activation of the His potential and complete retrograde AV node block (dissociated atrial complexes). CS_{prox} = proximal coronary sinus; His_{dis} = distal electrode pair; His_{prox} = proximal electrode pair; HRA = high right atrium; RVA = right ventricular apex.

of 0.3 to 0.4, and nonsustained VT on ECG.[37,38] Generally, EPS is not indicated in patients with long-QT syndrome and torsades de pointes.

The process of initiation and termination of SVT or VT with programmed electrical stimulation to test the potential efficacy of pharmacological, electrical, or surgical therapy represents an important application of EPS in patients with tachycardia. The role of drug therapy in clinically significant arrhythmias continues to diminish; although EPS was widely used at one time to predict the efficacy of drug therapy in suppressing spontaneous tachycardia recurrences, the technique is now rarely used for this purpose. Noninvasive stimulation from an implanted pacemaker or defibrillator can be used to test the effects of drug therapy given to try to decrease arrhythmia frequency.

UNEXPLAINED SYNCOPE (see Chap. 34). The three common arrhythmic causes of syncope include sinus node dysfunction, AV block, and tachyarrhythmias. Of the three, tachyarrhythmias are most reliably initiated in the electrophysiology laboratory, followed by sinus node abnormalities and then His-Purkinje block.[39]

The cause of syncope remains uncertain in up to 50 percent of patients, depending in part on the extent of the evaluation. A careful, accurately performed history and physical examination begin the evaluation,[1] followed by noninvasive tests, including a 12-lead ECG, and can lead to a diagnosis in half or more of the patients.[40,41] A small percentage (<5 percent) of patients develops an arrhythmia coincident with syncope or presyncope during a 24-hour ECG recording, whereas a larger percentage (15 percent) have symptoms without an arrhythmia, excluding an arrhythmic cause. Prolonged ECG monitoring with patient-activated transtelephonic event recorders that have memory loops may increase the yield. Signal averaging has a high sensitivity (~75 percent) and specificity (~90 percent) for predicting patients with syncope in whom VT can be induced at EPS.[22] Tilt-table and stress testing can be useful in some patients, as can long-term ECG recordings.

The EPS helps explain the cause of syncope or palpitations when it induces an arrhythmia that replicates the patient's symptoms. Syncopal patients with a nondiagnostic EPS have a low incidence of sudden death and 80 percent remission rate. In those with recurrent syncope, the test is falsely negative in 20 percent, owing to failure to find AV block or sinus node dysfunction. On the other hand, in many patients with structural heart disease, several abnormalities that could account for syncope can be diagnosed at EPS. Deciding which among these abnormalities is responsible for syncope and therefore requires therapy can be difficult. Mortality and incidence of sudden cardiac death are mainly determined by the presence of underlying heart disease.[42]

Syncopal patients considered for EPS are those whose spells remain undiagnosed despite general, neurological, and noninvasive cardiac evaluation, particularly if the patient has structural heart disease. The diagnostic yield is about 70 percent in that group but only about 12 percent in patients without structural heart disease.[43] Therapy for a putative cause found during EPS prevents recurrence of syncope in about 80 percent of patients. Among arrhythmic causes of syncope, intermittent conduction disturbances are the most difficult to diagnose. EPS is poor at establishing this diagnosis despite an array of provocative tests that can be applied. When tachyarrhythmias have been thoroughly sought and excluded and the clinical suspicion of intermittent heart block is high (e.g., bundle branch block or long HV interval), empirical permanent pacing may be justified.

PALPITATIONS. An EPS is indicated in patients with palpitations who have had a pulse documented by medical personnel to be inappropriately rapid without ECG recording or in those suspected of having clinically significant palpitations without ECG documentation.

In patients with syncope or palpitations, the sensitivity of the EPS may be low but may be increased at the expense of specificity. For example, more aggressive pacing techniques (e.g., using three or four premature stimuli), administration of drugs (e.g., isoproterenol), or left ventricular pacing can increase the success rate of ventricular arrhythmia induction, but by precipitating nonclinical ventricular tachyarrhythmias such as nonsustained polymorphic or monomorphic VT or VF. Similarly, aggressive techniques during atrial pacing can induce nonspecific episodes of atrial flutter or atrial fibrillation. A diagnostic dilemma arises when the patient's clinical, symptom-producing arrhythmia is one of these nonspecific arrhythmias that can be produced in the normal patient who has no arrhythmia. In most patients, these arrhythmias are regarded as "nonclinical" (i.e., nonspecific responses to intense stimulation). In other patients, such as those with hypertrophic or dilated nonischemic cardiomyopathy, these may be clinically relevant arrhythmias. However, induction of sustained SVT (e.g., AV nodal reentry, AV reciprocating tachycardia) or monomorphic VT is never an artifact of intense stimulation. Initiation of these arrhythmias in patients who have not had known spontaneous episodes of these tachycardias is uncommon and provides important information that the induced tachyarrhythmia may be clinically significant and responsible for the patient's symptoms. Generally, other abnormalities, such as prolonged sinus pauses after overdrive atrial pacing or His-Purkinje AV block, are not induced in patients who do not or may not experience these abnormalities spontaneously. Induction of these arrhythmias has a high degree of specificity.

COMPLICATIONS OF ELECTROPHYSIOLOGICAL STUDIES. The risks of undergoing only an EPS are small. Because most procedures do not involve left-sided heart access, risk of stroke, systemic embolism, or myocardial infarction is less than that of coronary arteriography. Myocardial perforation with cardiac tamponade, pseudoaneurysms at arterial access sites, and provocation of nonclinical arrhythmias can occur, each with less than 1/500 incidence. Adding therapeutic maneuvers (e.g., ablation) to the procedure increases the incidence of complications. In a European survey[44] based on 4398 patients reported from 68 institutions, procedure-related complications ranged from 3.2 to 8 percent. Five deaths occurred within the perioperative period of the ablation. In a North American Society of Pacing and Electrophysiology (NASPE) survey[45] of 164 hospitals reporting in 1998 on more than 3300 patients who received radiofrequency ablation, complications ranged from 1 to 3 percent, with procedure-related deaths of about 0.2 percent. In a study of 1050 patients undergoing temperature-controlled ablation for supraventricular arrhythmias, 32 (3%) had a major complication. Predictors of major complications were ejection fraction less than 0.35 and multiple ablation targets.[46] The improvement in the complication rate probably reflects the learning curve for radiofrequency ablation. In many centers, diagnostic EPS and even ablation procedures are performed on an outpatient basis. With the increasing use of extensive ablation in the left atrium to treat atrial fibrillation, an increase in systemic thromboembolic complications may be observed.

DIRECT CARDIAC MAPPING: RECORDING POTENTIALS DIRECTLY FROM THE HEART

Cardiac mapping is a method whereby potentials recorded directly from the heart are spatially depicted as a function of time in an integrated manner (Fig. 29-13). The location of recording electrodes (epicardial, intramural, or endocardial) and the recording mode used (unipolar versus bipolar) as well as the method of display (isopotential versus isochronal maps) depend on the problem under consideration. Special electrodes can record monophasic action potentials.

Direct cardiac mapping by means of catheter electrodes (or, less commonly, at the time of cardiac surgery) can be used to identify and localize the areas responsible for rhythm disturbances in patients with

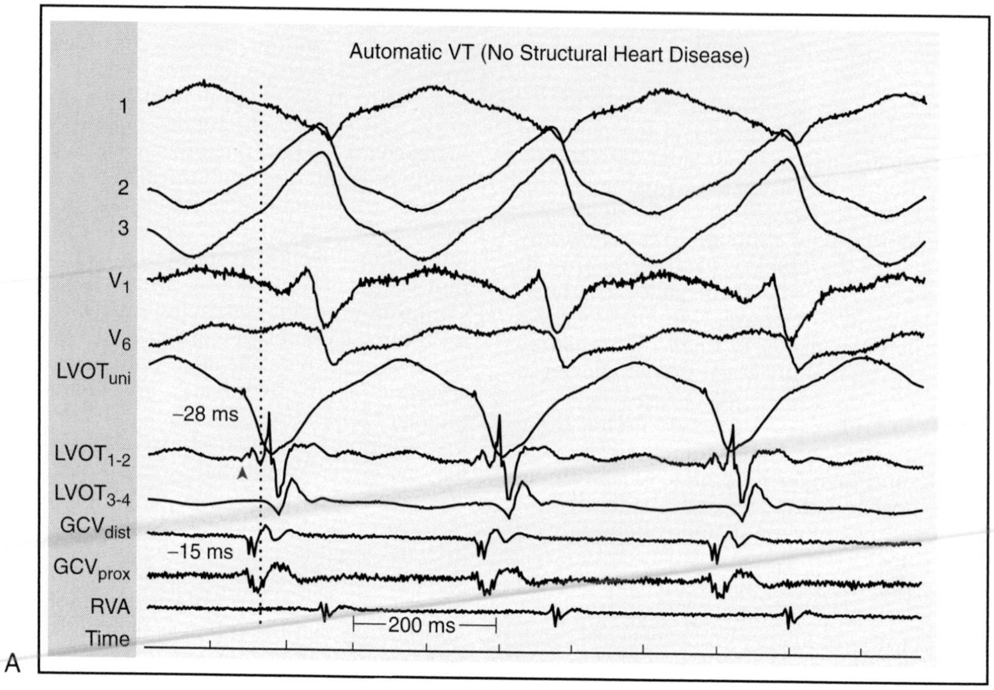

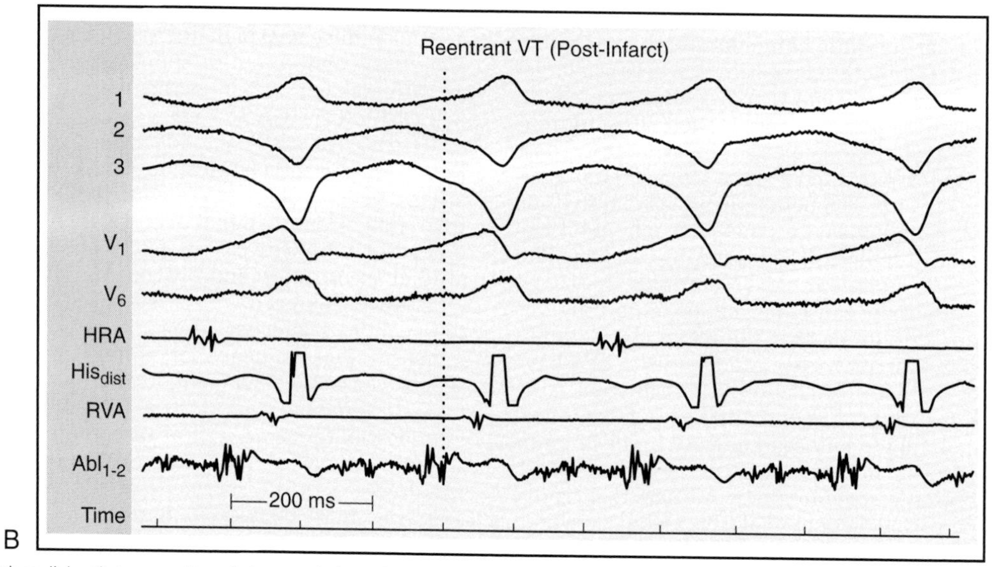

FIGURE 29–13 Endocardial catheter recordings during ventricular tachycardia (VT) in two patients. Dotted lines denote onset of QRS complexes. **A,** A woman without structural heart disease had a sustained VT arising from the left ventricular outflow tract (LVOT). Note unipolar (uni) electrogram with a sharp "QS" complex and the onset (arrow) distal bipolar recording ($LVOT_{1-2}$) preceding right ventricular recordings. They also precede recordings from a multielectrode catheter advanced along the coronary sinus and down the great cardiac vein (GCV_{dist} and GCV_{prox}) on the epicardial surface opposite the endocardial recording. Retrograde 1:1 conduction is present. Ablation at this site (LVOT) terminated the VT. **B,** A patient with reentrant VT due to a prior inferior wall infarction underwent mapping. The ablation catheter on the inferomedial wall shows a very prolonged, fragmented electrogram indicative of slow conduction. The electrogram spans all of the diastolic interval between QRS complexes. Ablation at this site eliminated the VT.

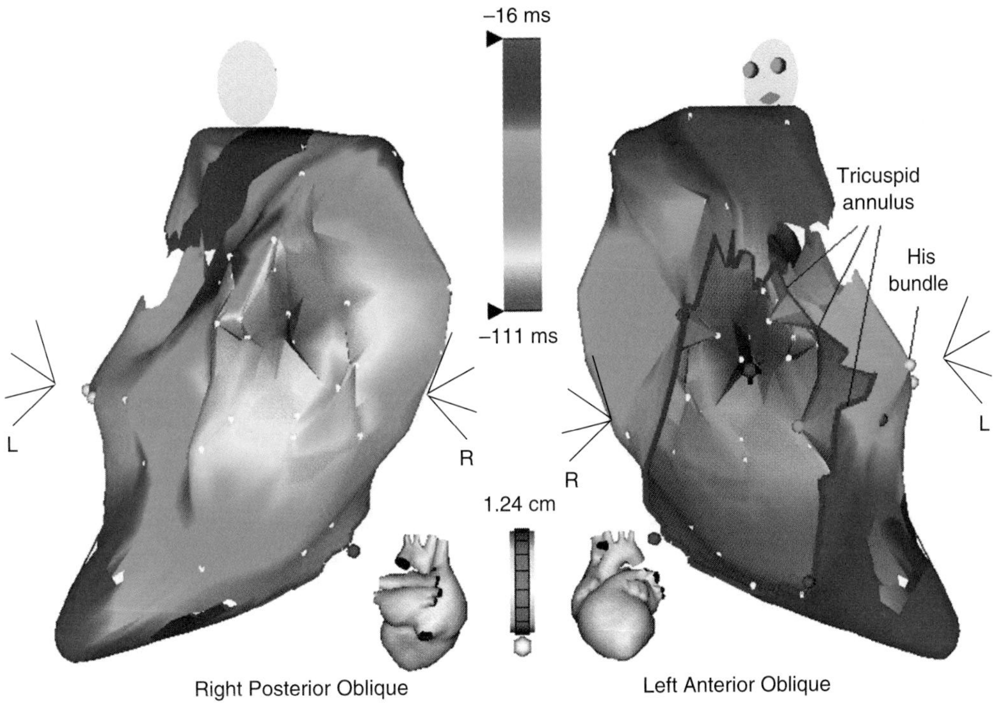

FIGURE 29–14 Electroanatomical map of focal atrial tachycardia. The right atrium is shown in two views (small gray icons at bottom center help with orientation). A color-coded time scale of activation is shown at top center; red indicates earliest activation, purple latest. A distance scale is below. This atrial tachycardia arose in the posterolateral right atrium (red spot) with all other areas activated centrifugally. Ablation at this site eliminated the tachycardia.

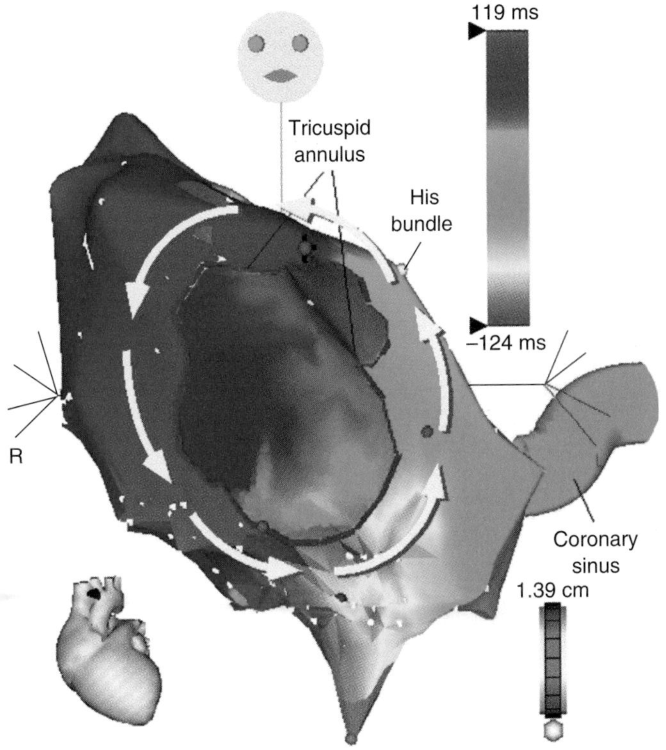

FIGURE 29–15 Electroanatomical map of reentrant atrial flutter. A left anterior oblique view of the right atrium is shown along with a depiction of the coronary sinus. See Figure 29-14 for other details. The electrical wave front propagates around the tricuspid annulus in a counterclockwise direction; in this complete circuit, "early" activation (in red) abuts "late" activation (purple) near the bottom of the tricuspid annulus. The cycle length of the tachycardia was 250 milliseconds, almost completely described by the points shown in the figure (from –124 to +119 milliseconds, a total of 243 milliseconds).

supraventricular and ventricular tachyarrhythmias for catheter or surgical ablation, isolation, or resection. Disorders amenable to this approach include accessory pathways associated with Wolff-Parkinson-White syndrome, the pathway(s) in AV node reentry, AV node/His bundle ablation, sites of origin of atrial tachycardia and VTs, isolated pathways essential for maintenance of reentrant atrial tachycardia or VTs, and various substrates responsible for episodes of atrial fibrillation. Mapping can also be used to delineate the anatomical course of the His bundle to avoid injury during open-heart surgery (usually for congenital heart surgery or septal accessory pathway ablation).

Early efforts at mapping involved moving an electrode from location to location, acquiring data from a single point at a time, and comparing the timing of local activation with some reference recording as well as other mapped sites. Obtaining enough data points to determine where ablation should be performed relied heavily on the memory of the operator. Specialized mapping systems have been developed that use computers to log not only the activation times at various points in the heart but the physical locations from which these were obtained. The mapping information thus acquired can be displayed on a screen showing relative activation times in a color-coded sequence. Using such systems, dozens or even hundreds of sites can be sampled relatively quickly, leading to a clear picture of cardiac activation and potential target sites for ablation (Figs. 29-14 and 29-15). Other mapping systems can acquire data from several thousand points simultaneously using a multipolar electrode array. This is particularly useful in hemodynamically unstable tachycardias or those that terminate spontaneously within just seconds, precluding detailed point-to-point mapping.

REFERENCES

1. Zipes DP, Miles WM: Assessment of the patient with a cardiac arrhythmia. *In* Zipes DP, Jalife J (eds): Cardiac Electrophysiology: From Cell to Bedside. 3rd ed. Philadelphia, WB Saunders, 1999, pp 706-709.
2. Barsky AJ: Palpitations, arrhythmias, and awareness of cardiac activity. Ann Intern Med 134:832-837, 2001.

Electrocardiogram

3. Miller JM, Rothman SA, Hsia HH, Buxton AE: Ventricular tachycardia versus supraventricular tachycardia: ECG recognition. *In* Zipes DP, Jalife J (eds): Cardiac Electrophysiology: From Cell to Bedside. 3rd ed. Philadelphia, WB Saunders, 1999, pp 696-705.

4. Lauer MR, Sung RJ: Exercise-induced cardiac arrhythmias. *In* Zipes DP, Jalife J (eds): Cardiac Electrophysiology: From Cell to Bedside. 3rd ed. Philadelphia, WB Saunders, 1999, pp 710-715.
5. Cole CR, Blackstone EH, Pashkow FJ, et al: Heart-rate recovery immediately after exercise as a predictor of mortality. N Engl J Med 341:1351-1357, 1999.
6. Frolkis JP, Pothier CE, Blackstone EH, Lauer MS: Frequent ventricular ectopy after exercise as a predictor of death. N Engl J Med 348:781-790, 2003.
7. Mason JW: A comparison of electrophysiologic testing with Holter monitoring to predict antiarrhythmic-drug effiicacy for ventricular tachyarrhythmias. Electrophysiologic Stud Versus Electrocardiographic Monitoring Investigators. N Engl J Med 329:445-451, 1993.
8. Crawford MH, Bernstein SJ, Deedwania PC, et al: ACC/AHA Guidelines for Ambulatory Electrocardiography: A report of the American College of Cardiology/American Heart Association Task Force on Practice Guidelines (Committee to Revise the Guidelines for Ambulatory Electrocardiography). Developed in collaboration with the North American Society for Pacing and Electrophysiology. J Am Coll Cardiol 34:912-948, 1999.
9. Kennedy HL: Use of long-term (Holter) electrocardiography recordings. *In* Zipes DP, Jalife J (eds): Cardiac Electrophysiology: From Cell to Bedside. 3rd ed. Philadelphia, WB Saunders, 1999, pp 716-729.
10. Investigators TC: Preliminary report: Effect of encainide and fllecainide on mortality i a randomized trial of arrhythmia suppression after myocardial infarction. N Engl J Med 321:406-412, 1989.
11. Page RL, Tilsch TW, Connolly SJ, et al: Asymptomatic or "silent" atrial fiibrillation: Frquency in untreated patients and patients receiving azimilide. Circulation 107:1141-1145, 2003.
12. Zimetbaum PJ, Josephson ME: The evolving role of ambulatory arrhythmia monitoring in general clinical practice. Ann Intern Med 130:848-856, 1999.
13. Krahn AD, Klein GJ, Yee R, Manda V: The high cost of syncope: Cost implications of a new insertable loop recorder in the investigation of recurrent syncope. Am Heart J 137:870-877, 1999.

Heart Rate Variability

14. Stein PK: Assessing heart rate variability from real-world Holter reports. Card Electrophysiol Rev 6:239-244, 2002.
15. Karcz M, Chojnowska L, Zareba W, Ruzyllo W: Prognostic signifiicance of heart rate variability in dilated cardiomyopathy. Int J Cardiol 87:75-81, 2003.
16. Abildstrom SZ, Jensen BT, Agner E, et al: Heart rate versus heart rate variability in risk prediction after myocardial infarction. J Cardiovasc Electrophysiol 14:168-173, 2003.
17. Zabel M, Klingenheben T, Franz MR, Hohnloser SH: Assessment of QT dispersion for prediction of mortality or arrhythmic events after myocardial infarction: Results of a prospective, long-term follow-up study. Circulation 97:2543-2550, 1998.
18. Voon WC, Wu JC, Lai WT, Sheu SH: Seasonal variability of the QT dispersion in healthy subjects. J Electrocardiol 34:285-288, 2001.
19. Zabel M, Malik M: Predictive value of T-wave morphology variables and QT dispersion for postmyocardial infarction risk assessment. J Electrocardiol 34(Suppl):27-35, 2001.
20. Rautaharju PM: Why did QT dispersion die? Card Electrophysiol Rev 6:295-301, 2002.
21. Berbari EJ. High-resolution electrocardiography. *In* Zipes DP, Jalife J (eds): Cardiac Electrophysiology: From Cell to Bedside. 3rd ed. Philadelphia, WB Saunders, 1999, pp 730-736.
22. Kudaiberdieva G, Gorenek B, Goktekin O, et al: Combination of QT variability and signal-averaged electrocardiography in association with ventricular tachycardia in postinfarction patients. J Electrocardiol 36:17-24, 2003.

T Wave Alterans

23. Gold MR, Spencer W: T wave alternans for ventricular arrhythmia risk stratifiication Curr Opin Cardiol 18:1-5, 2003.
24. Rosenbaum DS: T wave alterans: A mechanism of arrhythmogenesis comes of age after 100 years. J Cardiovasc Electrophysiol 12:196-206, 2001.
25. Shimizu W, Antzelevitch C: Cellular and ionic basis for T wave alternans under long-QT conditions. Circulation 99:1499-1507, 1999.
26. Pruvot EJ, Rosenbaum DS: T wave alternans for risk stratifiication and prevention o sudden cardiac death. Curr Cardiol Rep 5:350-357, 2003.
27. Hohnloser SH, Klingenheben T, Bloomfiield D, et al: Usefulness of microvolt T wav alternans for prediction of ventricular tachyarrhythmic events in patients with dilate cardiomyopathy: Results from a prospective observational study. J Am Coll Cardio 41:2220-2224, 2003.
28. Hoffmann J, Grimm W, Menz V, et al: Heart rate variability and baroreflex sensitivity i idiopathic dilated cardiomyopathy. Heart 83:531-538, 2000.
29. La Rovere MT, Pinna GD, Hohnloser SH, et al: Baroreflex sensitivity and heart rate var ability in the identifiication of patients at risk for life-threatening arrhythmias: Implic-tions for clinical trials. Circulation 103:2072-2077, 2001.
30. Flowers NC, Horan LG: Body surface potential mapping. *In* Zipes DP, Jalife J (eds) Cardiac Electrophysiology: From Cell to Bedside. 3rd ed. Philadelphia, WB Saunders 1999, pp 737-745.
31. Benditt DG: Head-up tilt-table testing: Rationale, methodology and applications. *I* Zipes DP, Jalife J (eds): Cardiac Electrophysiology: From Cell to Bedside. 3rd ed Philadelphia, WB Saunders, 1999, pp 746-752.
32. Atiga W, Calkins H: Management of vasovagal syncope. J Cardiovasc Electrophysio 10:874-886, 1999.
33. Connolly SJ, Sheldon R, Roberts RS, Gent M: The North American Vasovagal Pacemake Study (VPS): A randomized trial of permanent cardiac pacing for the prevention of vaso vagal syncope. J Am Coll Cardiol 33:16-20, 1999.
34. Shen WK, Low PA, Jahangir A, et al: Is sinus node modifiication appropriate for ina-propriate sinus tachycardia with features of postural orthostatic tachycardia syndrome? Pacing Clin Electrophysiol 24:217-230, 2001.

Invasive Electrophysiological Studies

35. Zipes DP, DiMarco JP, Gillette PC, et al: Guidelines for clinical intracardiac electro-physiological and catheter ablation procedures: A report of the American College of Cardiology/American Heart Association Task Force on Practice Guidelines (Committee on Clinical Intracardiac Electrophysiologic and Catheter Ablation Procedures), developed in collaboration with the North American Society of Pacing and Electrophysiology. J Am Coll Cardiol 26:555-573, 1995.
36. Rardon DP, Miles WM, Zipes DP: Atrioventricular block and dissociation. *In* Zipes DP, Jalife J (eds): Cardiac Electrophysiology: From Cell to Bedside. 3rd ed. Philadelphia, WB Saunders, 1999, pp 451-458.
37. Moss AJ, Hall WJ, Cannom DS, et al: Improved survival with an implanted defiibrill-tor in patients with coronary disease at high risk for ventricular arrhythmias. N Engl J Med 335:1933-1940, 1996.
38. Buxton AE, Lee KL, Fisher JD, et al: A randomized study of the prevention of sudden death in patients with coronary artery disease. Multicenter Unsustained Tachycardia Trial Investigators. N Engl J Med 341:1882-1890, 1999.
39. Calkins H: Syncope. *In* Zipes DP, Jalife J (eds): Cardiac Electrophysiology: From Cell to Bedside. 3rd ed. Philadelphia, WB Saunders, 1999, pp 873-881.
40. Linzer M, Yang EH, Estes NA III, et al: Diagnosing syncope: I. Value of history, physical examination, and electrocardiography. Clinical Effiicacy Assessment Project of th American College of Physicians. Ann Intern Med 126:989-996, 1997.
41. Linzer M, Yang EH, Estes NA III, et al: Diagnosing syncope: II. Unexplained syncope. Clinical Effiicacy Assessment Project of the merican College of Physicians. Ann Intern Med 127:76-86, 1997.
42. Kapoor WN: Current evaluation and management of syncope. Circulation 106:1606-1609, 2002.
43. Goldschlager N, Epstein AE, Grubb BP, et al: Etiologic considerations in the patient with syncope and an apparently normal heart. Arch Intern Med 163:151-162, 2003.
44. Hindricks G: The Multicentre European Radiofrequency Survey (MERFS): Complications of radiofrequency catheter ablation of arrhythmias. The Multicentre European Radiofrequency Survey (MERFS) Investigators of the Working Group on Arrhythmias of the European Society of Cardiology. Eur Heart J 14:1644-1653, 1993.
45. Scheinman MM, Huang S: The 1998 NASPE Prospective Catheter Ablation Registry. Pacing Clin Electrophysiol 23:1020-1028, 2000.
46. Calkins H, Yong P, Miller JM, et al: Catheter ablation of accessory pathways, atrioventricular nodal reentrant tachycardia, and the atrioventricular junction: Final results of a prospective, multicenter clinical trial. The Atakr Multicenter Investigators Group. Circulation 99:262-270, 1999.

CHAPTER 30

Therapy for Cardiac Arrhythmias

John M. Miller • Douglas P. Zipes

The treatment of patients with cardiac arrhythmias has evolved dramatically in the last 40 years. In the mid-1960s, patients with bradyarrhythmias could be treated with bulky implantable pacemakers with a battery life less than 5 years and fixed-rate pacing; patients with tachyarrhythmias had a limited number of drugs as their only treatment option. In the late 1960s, surgical therapy—and the prospect for cure, not just suppression of tachyarrhythmias—became a reality. It was first applied to Wolff-Parkinson-White syndrome and then extended to other forms of supraventricular tachycardia (SVT) and ventricular tachycardia (VT). Catheter ablation (at first with direct current, delivered from an external defibrillator, and then with radiofrequency current) for cure of tachyarrhythmias was first performed in the 1980s and underwent refinement in subsequent decades. This form of therapy has largely replaced surgical and drug therapy for patients who need treatment for SVT and VT in the absence of structural heart disease and has employed other forms of energy as well. Finally, the implantable cardioverter-defibrillator (ICD) was also developed in the early 1980s and has become standard therapy for patients with serious ventricular arrhythmias in the presence of structural heart disease. Some patients require a combination of these forms of treatment ("hybrid" therapy, such as an ICD and antiarrhythmic drugs or surgery and an ICD).[1] Drug therapy of arrhythmias, at one time the only option, now plays a supporting role in most cases.

Pharmacological Therapy

Principles of clinical pharmacokinetics and pharmacodynamics are covered in Chapter 5.

General Considerations Regarding Antiarrhythmic Drugs

Most of the available antiarrhythmic drugs (Table 30–1) can be classified according to whether they exert blocking actions predominantly on sodium, potassium, or calcium channels and whether they block beta adrenoceptors. The commonly used Vaughan Williams classification is limited because it is based on the electrophysiological effects exerted by an arbitrary concentration of the drug, generally on normal cardiac tissue. Actually, the actions of these drugs are quite complex and depend on tissue type, species, the degree of acute or chronic damage, heart rate, membrane potential, the ionic composition of the extracellular milieu, age (see Chap. 72), and other factors (see Table 30–1). Many drugs exhibit actions that belong in multiple categories or operate indirectly, such as by altering hemodynamics, myocardial metabolism, or autonomic neural transmission. Some drugs have active metabolites that exert effects different from those produced by the parent compound. Not all drugs in the same class have identical effects (e.g., bretylium, sotalol, and amiodarone). Whereas all class III agents are dramatically different, some drugs in different classes have overlapping actions (e.g., classes IA and IC drugs). In vitro studies on healthy fibers usually establish the properties of antiarrhythmic agents rather than their actual antiarrhythmic properties.

Despite these limitations, the Vaughan Williams classification[2] is widely known and provides a useful communication shorthand. It is listed here, but the reader is cautioned that drug actions are more complex than those depicted by the classification. A more realistic view of antiarrhythmic agents is provided by the "Sicilian gambit."[3] This approach to drug classification is an attempt to identify the mechanisms of a particular arrhythmia, determine the vulnerable parameter of the arrhythmia most susceptible to modification, define the target most likely to affect the vulnerable parameter, and then select a drug that will modify the target. This concept provides a framework in which to consider antiarrhythmic drugs (Table 30–2; see Table 30–1).[4]

DRUG CLASSIFICATION (Table 30–3). According to the Vaughan Williams classification, class I drugs predominantly block the fast sodium channel (they can also block potassium channels). They, in turn, are divided into three subgroups:

TABLE 30–1 Actions of Drugs Used in Treatment of Arrhythmias

Drug	Channels: Na*: Fast	Med	Slow	Ca	K_r	K_s	Receptors: α	β	M_2	P	Pumps: Na^+, K^+-ATPase	Clinical Effects: LV Function	Sinus Rate	Extracardiac
Quinidine		●A			⊙		○		○			—	↑	⊙
Procainamide		●A			⊙							↓	—	⊙
Disopyramide		●A			⊙				○			↓	—	●
Lidocaine	○											—	—↓	○
Mexiletine	○											—	—	○
Phenytoin	○											—	—	⊙
Flecainide			●A		○							↓	—	○
Propafenone		●A			○			⊙				↓	↓	○
Moricizine	●I											↓	—	○
Propranolol	○							●				↓	↓	○
Nadolol								●				↓	↓	○
Amiodarone	○			⊙	●	⊙	⊙	⊙				—	↓	●
Bretylium					●		⊡	⊡				—	↓	○
Sotalol					●			●				↓	↓	○
Ibutilide					○							—	↓	○
Dofetilide					●							—	—	○
Azimilide					⊙	⊙	○					—	—	○
Verapamil	○			●			⊙					↓	↓	○
Diltiazem				⊙								↓	↓	○
Adenosine										□		—	↓	⊙
Digoxin									○		●	↑	↓	⊙
Atropine									●			—	↑	⊙

Relative potency of blockade or extracardiac side effect: ○ = low; ⊙ = moderate; ● = high. □ = agonist; ⊡ = agonist-antagonist; A = activated state blocker; I = inactivated state blocker; — = minimal effect; ↑ = increase; ↓ = decrease; K_r = rapid component of delayed rectifier K^+ current; K_s = slow component of delayed rectifier K^+ current; M_2 = muscarinic receptor subtype 2; P = A_1 purinergic receptor.

Adapted from Schwartz PJ, Zaza A: Eur Heart J 13:26, 1992. Copyright © 1992, reproduced by permission of Elsevier.

*Fast, med (medium), and slow refer to kinetics of recovery from sodium channel blockade.

Class IA. Drugs that reduce $\dot{V}_{max}$ (rate of rise of action potential upstroke [phase 0]) and prolong action potential duration (see Chap. 77): quinidine, procainamide, disopyramide; kinetics of onset and offset in blocking the Na^+ channel are of intermediate rapidity (<5 seconds).

Class IB. Drugs that do not reduce $\dot{V}_{max}$ and that shorten action potential duration: mexiletine, phenytoin, and lidocaine; fast onset and offset kinetics (<500 milliseconds).

Class IC. Drugs that reduce $\dot{V}_{max}$, primarily slow conduction, and can prolong refractoriness minimally: flecainide, propafenone, and moricizine; slow onset and offset kinetics (10 to 20 seconds).

Class II. Drugs that block beta-adrenergic receptors and include propranolol, timolol, metoprolol, and others.

Class III. Drugs that predominantly block potassium channels (such as I_{Kr}) and prolong repolarization. They include sotalol, amiodarone, and bretylium.

Class IV. Drugs that predominantly block the slow calcium channel ($I_{Ca\text{-}L}$) and include verapamil, diltiazem, nifedipine, and others (felodipine blocks $I_{Ca\text{-}T}$).

A newer model suggests that antiarrhythmic drugs cross the cell membrane and interact with receptors in the membrane channels when the latter are in the rested, activated, or inactivated state (see Table 30–1) and that each of these interactions is characterized by different association and dissociation rate constants. Such interactions are voltage and time dependent. Transitions among rested, activated, and inactivated states are governed by standard Hodgkin-Huxley–type equations. When the drug is bound (associated) to a receptor site at or very close to the ionic channel (the drug probably does not actually "plug" the channel), the latter cannot conduct, even in the activated state.

USE-DEPENDENCE. Some drugs exert greater inhibitory effects on the upstroke of the action potential at more rapid rates of stimulation and after longer periods of stimulation, a characteristic called use-dependence. Use-dependence means that depression of $\dot{V}_{max}$, is greater after the channel has been "used" (i.e., after action potential depolarization rather than after a rest period). It is possible that this use-dependence results from preferential interaction of the antiarrhythmic drug with either the open or the inactive channel, and there is little interaction with the resting channels of the unstimulated cell. Agents in class IB exhibit fast kinetics of onset and offset or use-dependent block of the fast channel; that is, they bind and dissociate quickly from the receptors. Class IC drugs have slow kinetics, and class IA drugs are intermediate. With increased time spent in diastole (slower rate), a greater proportion of receptors become drug free, and the drug exerts less effect. Cells with reduced membrane potentials recover more slowly from drug actions than cells with more negative membrane potentials.

REVERSE USE-DEPENDENCE. Some drugs exert greater effects at slow rates than at fast rates, a property known as reverse use-dependence. This is particularly true for drugs that lengthen repolariza-

TABLE 30–2 Classification of Drug Actions on Arrhythmias Based on Modification of Vulnerable Parameter

Mechanism	Arrhythmia	Vulnerable Parameter (Effect)	Drugs (Effect)
Automaticity			
Enhanced normal	Inappropriate sinus tachycardia Some idiopathic ventricular tachycardias	Phase 4 depolarization (decrease)	Beta-adrenergic blocking agents Na^+ channel blocking agents
Abnormal	Atrial tachycardia	Maximum diastolic potential (hyperpolarization) Phase 4 depolarization (decrease)	M_2 agonist Ca^{2+} or Na^+ channel blocking agents
			M_2 agonist
	Accelerated idioventricular rhythms	Phase 4 depolarization (decrease)	Ca^{2+} or Na^+ channel blocking agents
Triggered activity			
EAD	Torsades de pointes	Action potential duration (shorten)	Beta-adrenergic agonists; vagolytic agents (increase rate)
		EAD (suppress)	Ca^{2+} channel blocking agents; Mg^{2+}; beta-adrenergic blocking agents
DAD	Digitalis-induced arrhythmias	Calcium overload (unload) DAD (suppress)	Ca^{2+} channel blocking agents Na^+ channel blocking agents
	RV outflow tract ventricular tachycardia	Calcium overload (unload) DAD (suppress)	Beta-adrenergic blocking agents Ca^{2+} channel blocking agents; adenosine
Reentry—Na^+ channel dependent			
Long excitable gap	Typical atrial flutter	Conduction and excitability (depress)	Type IA, IC Na^+ channel blocking agents
	Circus movement tachycardia in WPW	Conduction and excitability (depress)	Type IA, IC Na^+ channel blocking agents
	Sustained uniform ventricular tachycardia	Conduction and excitability (depress)	Na^+ channel blocking agents
Short excitable gap	Atypical atrial flutter	Refractory period (prolong)	K^+ channel blocking agents
	Atrial fibrillation	Refractory period (prolong)	K^+ channel blocking agents
	Circus movement tachycardia in WPW	Refractory period (prolong)	Amiodarone, sotalol
	Polymorphic and uniform ventricular tachycardia	Refractory period (prolong)	Type IA Na^+ channel blocking agents
	Bundle branch reentry	Refractory period (prolong)	Type IA Na^+ channel blocking agents; bretylium
	Ventricular fibrillation	Refractory period (prolong)	
Reentry—Ca^{2+} channel dependent			
	AV nodal reentrant tachycardia	Conduction and excitability (depress)	Ca^{2+} channel blocking agents
	Circus movement tachycardia in WPW	Conduction and excitability (depress)	Ca^{2+} channel blocking agents
	Verapamil-sensitive ventricular tachycardia	Conduction and excitability (depress)	Ca^{2+} channel blocking agents

AV = atrioventricular; DAD = delayed afterdepolarization; EAD = early afterdepolarization; RV = right ventricular; WPW = Wolff-Parkinson-White.

Data from Task Force of the Working Group on Arrhythmias of the European Society of Cardiology: The Sicilian gambit: A new approach to the classification of antiarrhythmic drugs based on their actions on arrhythmogenic mechanisms. Circulation 84:1831, 1991. Copyright 1991, American Heart Association.

tion. The QT interval becomes prolonged more at slow than fast rates. This effect is opposite to what the ideal antiarrhythmic agent would do because prolongation of refractoriness should be increased at fast rates so as to interrupt or prevent a tachycardia and should be minimal at slow rates to avoid precipitating torsades de pointes.

MECHANISMS OF ARRHYTHMIA SUPPRESSION (see Table 30–2). Given the fact that enhanced automaticity, triggered activity, or reentry can cause cardiac arrhythmias (see Chaps. 27 and 32), mechanisms by which antiarrhythmic agents suppress arrhythmias can be postulated. Antiarrhythmic agents can slow the spontaneous discharge frequency of an automatic pacemaker by depressing the slope of diastolic depolarization, shifting the threshold voltage toward zero, or hyperpolarizing the resting membrane potential. Mechanisms by which different drugs suppress normal or abnormal automaticity may not be the same. In general, however, most antiarrhythmic agents in therapeutic doses depress the automatic firing rate of spontaneously discharging ectopic sites while minimally affecting the discharge rate of the normal sinus node. Slow-channel blockers such as verapamil, beta blockers such as propranolol, and some antiarrhythmic agents such as amiodarone also depress spontaneous discharge of the sinus node, whereas drugs that exert vagolytic effects, such as disopyramide or quinidine, can increase the sinus discharge rate. Drugs can also suppress early or delayed afterdepolarizations and eliminate triggered arrhythmias related to these mechanisms.

As mentioned earlier, reentry depends critically on the timing interrelationships between refractoriness and conduction velocity, the presence of unidirectional block in one of the pathways, and other factors that influence refractoriness and conduction, such as excitability. An antiarrhythmic agent can stop reentry that is already present or prevent it from starting if the drug improves or depresses conduction. For example, improved conduction can (1) eliminate the unidirectional block so that reentry cannot begin or (2) facilitate conduction in the reentrant loop so that the returning wave front reenters too quickly, encroaches on fibers that are still refractory, and extinguishes. A drug that depresses conduction can transform the unidirectional block to a bidirectional block and thus terminate reentry or prevent it from

TABLE 30–3 In Vitro Electrophysiological Characteristics of Antiarrhythmic Drugs

Drug	APA	APD	dV/dt	MDP	ERP	CV	PF Phase 4	SN Auto	Memb Res	ET	VFT	Contr	SI Curr	Autonomic Nervous System	Local Anesth.
Quinidine	↓	↑	↓	0	↑	↓	↓	0	↓	↑	↑	0	0	Antivagal; alpha blocker	Yes
Procainamide	↓	↑	↓	0	↑	↓	↓	0	↓	↑	↑	0	0	Slight antivagal	Yes
Disopyramide	↓	↑	↓	0	↑	↓	↓	↓0↑	↓	↑	↑	↓	0	Central: antivagal, antisympathetic	Yes
Lidocaine	0↓	↓	0↓	0	↓	0↓	↓	0	0↓	0↑	↑	0	0	0	Yes
Mexiletine	0	↓	0↓	0	↓	↓	↓	0	↓	↑	↑	↓	0	0	Yes
Phenytoin	0	↓	↓0↑	0	↓	0	↓	0	0↑	0			0	0	No
Flecainide	↓	0↑	↓	0	↑	↓↓	↓	0	↓			↓	0	0	Yes
Propafenone	↓	0↑	↓	0	↑	↓↓	↓	0	↓	↑	↑	↓	0↓	Antisympathetic	Yes
Moricizine	↓	↓	↓	0	↓	↓	0	0	↓	↑	0		0	0	No
Propranolol	0↓	0↓	0↓	0	↓	0	↓*	↓	↓			↓	0↓	Antisympathetic	No
Amiodarone	0	↑	0↓	0	↑	↓	↓	↓	0	0	↑	0↑	0	Antisympathetic	Yes
Bretylium	0	↑	0	0	↑	0	0↓*	0↓	0↑	0	0↑	↓	0	Antisympathetic	Yes
Sotalol	0↓	↑	0↓	0	↑	0	0↓	↓	0↓	0	0	↓	0↓	Antisympathetic	No
Ibutilide	0	↑	0	0	↑	0	0	↓	0	0		0	0	0	No
Dofetilide	0	↑	0	0	↑	0	0	0	0	0		0	0	0	No
Azimilide	0	↑	0	0	↑	0	0	0	0	0		0	0	0	No
Verapamil	0	↓	0	0	0	0	↓*	↓	0	0	0	↓	↓↓	? Block alpha receptors; enhance vagal	Yes
Adenosine	0	↑	0↓	0	↑	0	0↓	↓	0	0	0	0	↓	Vagomimetic	No

APA = action potential amplitude; APD = action potential duration; dV/dt = rate of rise of action potential; MDP = maximum diastolic potential; ERP = effective refractory period (longest S_1-S_2 interval at which S_2 fails to produce a response); CV = conduction velocity; PF = Purkinje fiber; SN Auto = sinus nodal automaticity; Memb Res = membrane responsiveness; ET = excitability threshold; VFT = ventricular fibrillation threshold; Contr = contractility; SI Curr = slow inward current; Local Anesth. = local anesthetic effect.

*With a background of sympathetic activity.

occurring by creating an area of complete block in the reentrant pathway. Conversely, a drug that slows conduction without producing block or lengthening refractoriness significantly can promote reentry. Finally, most antiarrhythmic agents share the ability to prolong refractoriness relative to their effects on action potential duration (APD); that is, the ratio of effective refractory period (ERP) to APD exceeds 1.0. If a drug prolongs refractoriness of fibers in the reentrant pathway, the pathway may not recover excitability in time to be depolarized by the reentering impulse and the reentrant propagation ceases. The different types of reentry (see Chap. 27) influence the effects and effectiveness of a drug.

When considering the properties of a drug, it is important that the situation or model, or both, from which conclusions are drawn be defined with care. Electrophysiological, hemodynamic, autonomic, pharmacokinetic, and adverse effects may all differ in normal subjects compared with patients, in normal tissue compared with abnormal tissue, in cardiac muscle compared with specialized conduction fibers, in atrium as opposed to ventricular muscle, and in different species (Table 30–4).

STEREOSELECTIVITY. Drug interactions with a channel, receptor, or enzyme may depend on the three-dimensional geometry of the drug. Many drugs have stereoisomers (molecules with the same atomic composition but different spatial arrangement) that can influence drug effects, metabolism, binding, clearance, and excretion. Most drugs of this type are prescribed as 50:50 mixtures of their two forms (racemates), which may make 50 percent of the dose ineffective for some drugs. Except for timolol, virtually all beta blockers are racemates. *d*-Propranolol exerts antiarrhythmic actions unrelated to beta adrenoceptor blockade, whereas *l*-propranolol blocks the beta receptor. Both enantiomers (mirror images) of sotalol block the potassium channel to prolong APD and suppress arrhythmias equally, but *d*-sotalol does not block the beta adrenoceptor and, alone, can be arrhythmogenic. Racemic propafenone exhibits beta-blocking actions related to the *S* enantiomer. Other drugs with notable stereoselective differences include disopyramide, with one form (*S* [+]) prolonging repolarization and having greater antiarrhythmic effects than *R* (–), which shortens repolarization. The latter form has fewer anticholinergic effects. The (–) enantiomer of verapamil exerts much more negative inotropic and dromotropic effects than the (+) form and may have more potent antiarrhythmic actions. Stereoselectivity affects sodium channel blocking drugs less than it affects beta adrenoceptor, potassium, and calcium blockers.

DRUG METABOLITES. Drug metabolites may add to or alter the effects of the parent compound by exerting similar actions, competing with the parent compound, or mediating drug toxicity. Quinidine has at least four active metabolites but none with a potency exceeding that of the parent drug and none preliminarily implicated in causing torsades de pointes. About 50 percent of procainamide is metabolized to *N*-acetylprocainamide (NAPA). Only the parent drug blocks cardiac sodium channels and slows impulse propagation in the His-Purkinje system. NAPA prolongs repolarization and is a less effective antiarrhythmic drug but competes with procainamide for renotubular secretory sites and can increase the parent drug's elimination half-life. Lidocaine's metabolite can compete with lidocaine for sodium channels and partially reverse block produced by lidocaine.

PHARMACOGENETICS (see Chap. 5). Genetically determined metabolic pathways account for many of the differences in patients' responses to some drugs. The genetically determined activity of hepatic *N*-acetyltransferase regulates the development of antinuclear antibodies and development of the lupus syndrome in response to procainamide. Slow acetylator phenotypes appear more prone to develop lupus than rapid acetylators. About 7 percent of subjects lack debrisoquin 4-hydroxylase. This enzyme (termed $P450_{dbl}$) is needed to metabolize debrisoquin (an antihypertensive drug) and propafenone, to hydroxylate several beta blockers, and to biotransform flecainide. Lack of this enzyme reduces metabolism of the parent compound, leading to increased plasma concentrations of the parent drug and reduced concentrations of metabolites. Propafenone is metabolized by this enzyme to a compound with slightly less antiarrhythmic and beta-adrenergic blocking effects as well as fewer central nervous system side effects. Thus, poor metabolizers may experience more heart rate slowing and neurotoxicity than extensive metabolizers. Quinidine in low doses can inhibit this enzyme and thereby alter concentrations of the drugs and metabolites given in combination that are affected by the $P450_{dbl}$ enzyme, such as propafenone or flecainide.

Understanding stereoselectivity and pharmacogenetics can provide major clues to understanding differences in drug efficacy and toxicity from one patient to the next. Cimetidine and ranitidine also affect drug metabolism, probably by inhibiting hepatic P450-metabolizing enzymes. Other commonly used noncardiovascular medications affect this important metabolic pathway. Drugs such as rifampin, phenobarbital, and phenytoin induce synthesis of larger amounts of cytochrome $P450_{dbl}$, leading to lower concentrations of parent drugs that are extensively metabolized, whereas erythromycin, clarithromycin, fluoxetine, and grapefruit juice inhibit enzyme activity, leading to accumulation of the parent compound. This effect is thought to explain why cisapride, an agent that had been used to increase gastric motility, could cause QT interval prolongation and torsades de pointes in isolated cases. Cisapride blocked the delayed rectifier current I_{Kr} but did not prolong the QT interval significantly in the majority of patients, presumably owing to extensive metabolism. In patients who take an inhibitor of cytochrome P450 (such as erythromycin) along with cisapride, the latter drug can accumulate, leading to QT prolongation and torsades de pointes.

SIDE EFFECTS. Antiarrhythmic drugs produce one group of side effects related to excessive dosage and plasma concentrations, resulting in both noncardiac (e.g., neurological defects) and cardiac (e.g., heart failure, some arrhythmias) toxicity, and another group of side effects unrelated to plasma concentrations, which is termed idiosyncratic. Examples of the latter include procainamide-induced lupus syndrome and some arrhythmias such as quinidine-induced torsades de pointes. The latter phenomenon can occur in individuals with a "forme fruste" of the long QT syndrome (i.e., normal QT interval at rest but markedly prolonged interval in the presence of certain medications).[5] In the future, it is likely that genetic differences will explain many "idiosyncratic" reactions.[6-11]

Proarrhythmia. Drug-induced or drug-exacerbated cardiac arrhythmias (proarrhythmia) constitute a major clinical problem.[12] Proarrhythmia can be manifested as an increase in frequency of a preexisting arrhythmia, sustaining of a previously nonsustained arrhythmia (even making it incessant), or development of arrhythmias the patient has not previously experienced. Electrophysiological mechanisms are probably related to prolongation of repolarization, the development of early afterdepolarizations to cause torsades de pointes, and alterations in reentry pathways to initiate or sustain ventricular tachyarrhythmias. Proarrhythmic events can occur in as many as 5 to 10 percent of patients receiving antiarrhythmic agents. Heart failure increases proarrhythmic risk. Patients with atrial fibrillation treated with antiarrhythmic agents had a relative risk of cardiac death of 4.7 if they had a history of heart failure compared with patients not so treated, who had a relative risk of arrhythmic death of 3.7. Patients without a history of congestive heart failure had no increased risk of cardiac mortality during antiarrhythmic drug treatment.[13] Reduced left ventricular function, treatment with digitalis and diuretics, and longer pretreatment QT interval characterize patients who experience drug-induced ventricular fibrillation (VF). The more commonly known proarrhythmic events occur within several days of beginning drug therapy or changing dosage and are represented by such developments as incessant VT, long QT syndrome, and torsades de pointes. However, in the Cardiac Arrhythmia Suppression Trial (CAST),[14] researchers found that encainide and flecainide reduced spontaneous ventricular arrhythmias but were associated with a total mortality of 7.7 percent, in comparison with 3.0 percent in the group receiving placebo. Deaths were equally distributed throughout the treatment period, raising the important consideration that another kind of proarrhythmic response can occur some time after the beginning of drug therapy. Such late proarrhythmic effects may be related to drug-induced exacerbation of regional myocardial conduction delay caused by ischemia and heterogeneous drug concentrations that can promote reentry. Moricizine also increased mortality, leading to termination of CAST II.

Until the 1970s, when separate surgical treatments were developed to treat Wolff-Parkinson-White syndrome and VT (see later), antiarrhythmic drugs were the only form of treatment for patients with tachyarrhythmias. The availability of catheter ablation (see later) and ICDs (see Chap. 31) to treat a wide variety of arrhythmias has relegated drug therapy to a secondary role. Drugs are still useful to prevent or decrease frequency of recurrences in patients who have relatively infrequent episodes of benign tachycardias, those who have had incomplete success with catheter ablation procedures, and patients with an ICD who have frequent episodes of ventricular arrhythmia resulting in shocks.

Class IA Antiarrhythmic Agents

Quinidine

Quinidine and quinine are isomeric alkaloids isolated from cinchona bark. Although quinidine shares the antimalarial, antipyretic, and vagolytic actions of quinine, the latter lacks the significant electrophysiological and antiarrhythmic effects of quinidine.

ELECTROPHYSIOLOGICAL ACTIONS (Table 30-5; see Tables 30-1, 30-2, and 30-3). Quinidine exerts little effect on automaticity of the isolated or denervated normal sinus node but suppresses automaticity in normal Purkinje fibers, especially in ectopic pacemakers, by decreasing the slope of phase 4 diastolic depolarization and shifting the threshold voltage toward zero. In patients with the sick sinus syndrome, quinidine can depress sinus node automaticity. It does not affect abnormal automaticity in partially depolarized Purkinje fibers. Quinidine produces early afterdepolarizations in experimental preparations and in humans, which may be responsible for torsades de pointes.[15] Because of its significant anticholinergic effect and reflex sympathetic stimulation resulting from alpha-adrenergic blockade that causes peripheral vasodilation, quinidine can increase sinus node discharge rate and can improve atrioventricular (AV) nodal conduction. Direct myocardial effects can prolong AV nodal and His-Purkinje conduction times and refractoriness in an AV accessory pathway. Quinidine slightly prolongs the APD of atrial and ventricular muscle and Purkinje fibers while also prolonging the ERP without significantly changing resting membrane potential. Prolongation of repolarization is more prominent at slow heart rates (reverse use-dependence) owing to block of I_{Kr}. Action potential amplitude, overshoot, and $\dot{V}_{max}$ of phase 0 are reduced, more so during ischemia, hypoxia, and in partially depolarized fibers, especially at fast rates. The open channel has a high affinity for quinidine, resulting in block of a fraction of sodium channels with each action potential upstroke. The time for unblocking by class IA drugs (about 4 seconds) is longer than for class IB drugs but shorter than for class IC drugs. For the duration of the plateau of the action potential (inactivated state) or in depolarized fibers, the rate of unblocking is slow, but it is much faster in polarized fibers. Therefore, faster rates result in more block of sodium channels and less unblocking because of a smaller percentage of time spent in a polarized state (use-dependence). Isoproterenol can modulate the effects of quinidine on reentrant circuits in humans. Quinidine's effect on I_{to} (but not I_{K}) varies according to the patient's age and may account for its lower efficacy in children than adults.

TABLE 30–4 Clinical Usage Information for Antiarrhythmic Agents*

Drug	Usual Dosage Ranges: Intravenous (mg) Loading	Intravenous (mg) Maintenance	Oral (mg) Loading	Oral (mg) Maintenance
Quinidine	6 to 10 mg/kg at 0.3 to 0.5 mg/kg/min	—	800 to 1000	300 to 600 q6hr
Procainamide	6 to 13 mg/kg at 0.2 to 0.5 mg/kg/min	2 to 6 mg/min	500 to 1000	250 to 1000 q4-6hr
Disopyramide	1 to 2 mg/kg over 15 to 45 min[‡]	1 mg/kg/hr		100 to 300 q6-8hr
Lidocaine	1 to 3 mg/kg at 20 to 50 mg/min	1 to 4 mg/min	N/A	N/A
Mexiletine	500 mg[‡]	0.5 to 1.0 gm/24 hr	400 to 600	150 to 300 q8-12hr
Phenytoin	100 mg q5min for ≤1000 mg		1000	100 to 400 q12-24hr
Flecainide	2 mg/kg[‡]	100 to 200 q12hr		50 to 200 q12hr
Propafenone	1 to 2 mg/kg[‡]		600 to 900	150 to 300 q8-12hr
Moricizine	N/A	N/A	300	100 to 400 q8hr
Propranolol	0.25 to 0.5 mg q5min to ≤0.20 mg/kg			10 to 200 q6-8hr
Amiodarone	15 mg/min for 10 min, 1 mg/min for 3 hr, 0.5 mg/min thereafter	1 mg/min	800 to 1600 qd for 7-14 days	200 to 600 qd
Bretylium	5 to 10 mg/kg at 1 to 2 mg/kg/min	0.5 to 2 mg/min	N/A	4 mg/kg/d
Sotalol	10 mg over 1 to 2 min[‡]			80 to 320 q12hr
Ibutilide	1 mg over 10 min	N/A	N/A	N/A
Dofetilide	2 to 5 µg/kg infusion[‡]	N/A	N/A	0.125 to 0.5 q12hr
Azimilide	N/A	N/A	N/A	100 to 200 qd
Verapamil	5 to 10 mg over 1 to 2 min	0.005 mg/kg/min		80 to 120 q6-8hr
Adenosine	6 to 18 mg (rapidly)	N/A	N/A	N/A
Digoxin	0.5 to 1.0 mg	0.125 to 0.25 qd	0.5 to 1.0	0.125 to 0.25 qd

N/A = not applicable.
*Results presented may vary according to doses, disease state, and intravenous or oral administration.
†Pregnancy class: A, controlled studies show no fetal risk; B, no controlled studies, but no evidence of fetal risk; fetal harm unlikely; C, fetal risk cannot be excluded; drug should be used only if potential benefits outweigh potential risk; D, definite fetal risk; drug should be avoided unless in a life-threatening situation or safer alternatives do not exist; X, contraindicated in pregnancy.
‡Intravenous use investigational.
§Investigational only.

HEMODYNAMIC EFFECTS. Quinidine decreases peripheral vascular resistance and can cause significant hypotension because of its alpha-adrenergic receptor blocking effects. Concomitant administration of vasodilators can exaggerate the potential for hypotension. In some patients, quinidine can increase cardiac output, possibly by reducing afterload and preload. No significant direct myocardial depressant action occurs with orally administered quinidine.

PHARMACOKINETICS (aee Table 30–4). Although orally administered quinidine sulfate and quinidine gluconate exhibit similar degrees of systemic availability, plasma quinidine concentrations peak at about 90 minutes after oral administration of quinidine sulfate and at 3 to 4 hours after oral administration of quinidine gluconate. Intramuscular administration should be avoided because of incomplete absorption and tissue necrosis. Quinidine can be given intravenously if it is infused slowly. Approximately 80 percent of plasma quinidine is protein bound, especially to $alpha_1$-acid glycoprotein, which increases in heart failure. Both the liver and the kidneys remove quinidine, and dose adjustments may be made according to the creatinine clearance. Metabolism is by means of the cytochrome P450 system. Approximately 20 percent is excreted unchanged in the urine. Because congestive heart failure, hepatic disease, or poor renal function can reduce quinidine elimination and increase plasma concentration, the dosage should probably be reduced and the drug given cautiously to patients with these disorders while serum quinidine concentration is monitored. Elimination half-life is 5 to 8 hours after oral administration. Quinidine's effect on repolarization and overall efficacy vary directly with left ventricular function; for the same serum concentration, the QT interval is longer in women and with higher degrees of sympathetic tone.[16,17]

DOSAGE AND ADMINISTRATION (see Table 30–4). The usual oral dose of quinidine sulfate for an adult is 300 to 600 mg four times daily, which results in a steady-state level within about 24 hours. A loading dose of 600 to 1000 mg produces an earlier effective concentration. Similar doses of quinidine gluconate are used intramuscularly, whereas the intravenous (IV) dose of quinidine gluconate is about 10 mg/kg given at a rate of about 0.5 mg/kg/min as blood pressure and electrocardiographic (ECG) parameters are checked frequently. Oral doses of the gluconate are about 30 percent greater than those of sulfate. Important interactions with other drugs occur.

INDICATIONS. Quinidine is a versatile antiarrhythmic agent, useful for treating premature supraventricular and ventricular complexes and sustained tachyarrhythmias. It may prevent spontaneous recurrences of AV nodal reentrant tachycardia (AVNRT) by prolonging atrial and ventricular

Time to Peak Plasma Concentration (Oral) (hr)	Effective Serum or Plasma Concentration (μg/ml)	Half-Life (hr)	Bioavailability (%)	Major Route of Elimination	Pregnancy Class†
1.5 to 3.0	3 to 6	5 to 9	60 to 80	Liver	C
1	4 to 10	3 to 5	70 to 85	Kidneys	C
1 to 2	2 to 5	8 to 9	80 to 90	Kidneys	C
N/A	1 to 5	1 to 2	N/A	Liver	B
2 to 4	0.75 to 2	10 to 17	90	Liver	C
8 to 12	10 to 20	18 to 36	50 to 70	Liver	D
3 to 4	0.2 to 1.0	20	95	Liver	C
1 to 3	0.2 to 3.0	5 to 8	25 to 75	Liver	C
1 to 3	0.1	2	40	Liver	B
4	1 to 2.5	3 to 6	35 to 65	Liver	C
	0.5 to 1.5	56 days	25	Kidneys	D
2 to 4	0.04 to 0.90	8 to 14	20 to 50	Liver	C
2.5 to 4	2.5	12	90 to 100	Kidneys	B
N/A	N/A	6		Kidneys	C
		7 to 13	90	Kidneys	C
	200 to 1000		90 to 100	Kidneys	—
1 to 2	0.10 to 0.15	3 to 8	10 to 35	Liver	C
N/A					C
2 to 6	0.0008 to 0.002	36 to 48	60 to 80	Kidneys	C

refractoriness and depressing conduction in the retrograde fast pathway. In patients with the Wolff-Parkinson-White syndrome, quinidine prolongs the ERP of the accessory pathway and, by so doing, can prevent reciprocating tachycardias and slow the ventricular response from conduction over the accessory pathway during atrial flutter or atrial fibrillation. Quinidine and other antiarrhythmic agents can also prevent recurrences of tachycardia by suppressing the "trigger" (i.e., the premature atrial complex [PAC] or premature ventricular complex [PVC] that initiates a sustained tachycardia).[6]

Quinidine successfully terminates atrial flutter or atrial fibrillation in 20 to 60 percent of patients, with higher success rates if the arrhythmia is of more recent onset and if the atria are not enlarged. Before quinidine is administered to these patients, the ventricular response should be slowed sufficiently with digitalis, propranolol, or verapamil because quinidine-induced slowing of the atrial flutter rate (e.g., from 300 to 230 beats/min) and its vagolytic effect on AV nodal conduction can convert a 2:1 AV response (ventricular rate 150 beats/min) to a 1:1 AV response, with an increase in the ventricular rate (to 230 beats/min).[18] If quinidine is going to be used to try to maintain sinus rhythm after elective cardioversion of patients with atrial fibrillation, it probably should be given for 1 to 2 days before planned cardioversion because this regimen restores sinus rhythm in some patients (thus obviating the need for direct-current cardioversion) and helps maintain sinus rhythm once it is achieved. In addition, early toxicity or patient's intolerance of the drug may be observed and changes made in drug therapy before attempting cardioversion. However, a meta-analysis of six studies testing the effects of quinidine versus control in maintaining sinus rhythm in patients with atrial fibrillation showed that quinidine-treated patients remained in sinus rhythm longer than the control group but had an increased total mortality over the same period.

Quinidine has prevented sudden death in some patients resuscitated after out-of-hospital cardiac arrest and may be combined with other antiarrhythmic agents for increased efficacy in suppressing serious ventricular tachyarrhythmias; however, the majority of these patients have ICDs and drug therapy is strictly adjunctive (i.e., used to decrease the frequency of arrhythmia episodes). It is important to stress that no published data from controlled, randomized studies indicate improved survival in quinidine-treated patients after myocardial infarction and cardiac arrest can occur despite quinidine therapy. Because it crosses the placenta, quinidine can be used to treat arrhythmias in the fetus.

ADVERSE EFFECTS. The most common adverse effects of chronic oral quinidine therapy are gastrointestinal and include nausea, vomiting, diarrhea, abdominal pain, and anorexia. Gastrointestinal side effects may be milder with the gluconate form. Central nervous system toxicity includes tinnitus, hearing loss, visual disturbances, confusion, delirium, and psychosis. Cinchonism is the term usually applied to these side effects. Allergic reactions may be manifested as rash, fever, immune-mediated thrombocytopenia, hemolytic anemia, and, rarely, anaphylaxis. Thrombocytopenia is due to the presence of antibodies to quinidine-platelet complexes, causing platelets to agglutinate and lyse. In patients

TABLE 30–5 In Vivo Electrophysiological Characteristics of Antiarrhythmic Drugs*

	Electrocardiographic Measurements					Electrophysiologic Intervals					
Drug	***Sinus Rate***	***PR***	***QRS***	***QT***	***JT***	***ERP-AVN***	***ERP-HPS***	***ERP-A***	***ERP-V***	***AH***	***HV***
Quinidine	0 ↑	↓ 0 ↑	↑	↑	↑	0 ↑	↑	↑	↑	0 ↓	↑
Procainamide	0	0 ↑	↑	↑	↑	0 ↑	↑	↑	↑	0 ↑	↑
Disopyramide	0 ↑	↓ 0 ↑	↑	↑	↑	↑ 0	↑	↑	↑	↓ 0 ↑	↑
Lidocaine	0	0	0	0 ↓	↓	0 ↓	0 ↑	0	0	0 ↓	0 ↑
Mexiletine	0	0	0	0 ↓	↓	0 ↑	0 ↑	0	0	0 ↑	0 ↑
Phenytoin	0	0	0	0	0	0 ↓	↓	0	0	0 ↑	0
Flecainide	0 ↓	↑	↑	0 ↑	0	↑	↑	↑	↑	↑	↑
Propafenone	0 ↓	↑	↑	0 ↑	0	0 ↑	0 ↑	0 ↑	↑	↑	↑
Moricizine	0 ↓	0 ↑	0 ↑	0	↓	0	0	0 ↑	0 ↑	↑	↑
Propranolol	↓	0 ↑	0	0 ↓	0	↑	0	0	0	0	0
Amiodarone	↓	0 ↑	↑	↑	↑	↑	↑	↑	↑	↑	↑
Bretylium	↓ 0 ↑	0	0	0 ↑	↑	0	↑	↑	↑	↓ 0 ↑	0
Sotalol	↓	0 ↑	0	↑	↑	↑	↑	↑	↑	↑	0
Ibutilide	↓	0 ↓	0	↑	↑	0	0	↑	↑	0	0
Dofetilide	0	0	0	↑	↑	0	0	↑	↑	0	0
Azimilide	0	0	0	↑	↑	0	0	↑	↑	0	0
Verapamil	0 ↓	↑	0	0	0	↑	0	0	0	↑	0
Adenosine	↓ then ↑	↑	0	0	0	↑	0	↓	0	↑	0
Digoxin	↓	↑	0	0	↓	↑	0	↓	0	↑	0

↑ = increase; ↓ = decrease; 0 = no change; 0 ↑ or 0 ↓ = slight or inconsistent increase or decrease; A = atrium; AH = atrio-His interval (an index of atrioventricular nodal conduction); AVN = atrioventricular node; ERP = effective refractory period (longest S_1-S_2 interval at which S_2 fails to produce a response); HPS = His-Purkinje system; HV = His-ventricular interval (an index of His-Purkinje conduction); V = ventricle.

*Results presented may vary according to tissue type, drug concentration, and autonomic tone.

receiving oral anticoagulants, quinidine can cause bleeding. Side effects may preclude long-term administration of quinidine in 30 to 40 percent of patients.

Quinidine can slow cardiac conduction, sometimes to the point of block, manifested as prolongation of the QRS duration or sinoatrial (SA) or AV nodal conduction disturbances. Quinidine-induced cardiac toxicity can be treated with molar sodium lactate. Quinidine can produce syncope in 0.5 to 2.0 percent of patients, most often the result of a self-terminating episode of torsades de pointes. Torsades de pointes may be due to the development of early afterdepolarizations, as noted earlier. Quinidine prolongs the QT interval in most patients, whether or not ventricular arrhythmias occur, but significant QT prolongation (QT interval of 500 to 600 milliseconds) is often a characteristic of patients with quinidine syncope. Many of these patients are also receiving digitalis or diuretics or have hypokalemia; women are more susceptible than men.[17,18] Syncope is unrelated to plasma concentrations of quinidine or duration of therapy, although the majority of episodes occur within the first 2 to 4 days of therapy (often after conversion of atrial fibrillation to sinus rhythm) (see Table 72–3).

Therapy for quinidine syncope requires immediate discontinuation of the drug and avoidance of other drugs that have similar pharmacological effects, such as disopyramide, because cross-sensitivity exists in some patients. Magnesium given intravenously (2 gm over 1 to 2 minutes, followed by an infusion of 3 to 20 mg/min) is the initial drug treatment of choice. Atrial or ventricular pacing can be used to suppress the ventricular tachyarrhythmia and may act by suppressing early afterdepolarizations. For some patients, drugs that do not prolong the QT interval, such as lidocaine or phenytoin, can be tried. When pacing is not available, isoproterenol can be given with caution. The arrhythmia gradually dissipates as quinidine is cleared and the QT interval returns to baseline.

Drugs that induce hepatic enzyme production, such as phenobarbital and phenytoin, can shorten the duration of quinidine's action by increasing its rate of elimination. Quinidine can increase plasma concentrations of flecainide by inhibiting the P450 enzyme system. Quinidine may elevate serum digoxin and digitoxin concentrations by decreasing total-body clearance of digitoxin and by decreasing the clearance, volume of distribution, and affinity of tissue receptors for digoxin.

Procainamide

ELECTROPHYSIOLOGICAL ACTIONS (see Tables 30–1, 30–2, 30–3, and 30–5). The cardiac actions of procainamide on automaticity, conduction, excitability, and membrane responsiveness resemble those of quinidine. Procainamide predominantly blocks the inactivated state of I_{Na}. It also blocks I_{Kr} and I_{KATP}. Like quinidine, procainamide usually prolongs the ERP more than it prolongs the APD and thus may prevent reentry. Compared with disopyramide and quinidine, procainamide exerts the least anticholinergic effects. It does not affect normal sinus node automaticity. In vitro, procainamide decreases abnormal automaticity, with less effect on triggered activity or catecholamine-enhanced normal automaticity.

The electrophysiological effects of NAPA, procainamide's major metabolite, differ from those of the parent compound. NAPA (10 to 40 mg/liter) does not suppress the rate of phase 4 diastolic depolarization of Purkinje fibers and does not alter resting membrane potential, action potential amplitude, or $\dot{V}_{max}$ of phase 0 of the action potential of Purkinje fibers or ventricular muscle. However, NAPA, a K^+ channel blocker (I_{Kr}), exerts a class III action and prolongs the APD of ventricular muscle and Purkinje fibers in a dose-dependent manner. Toxic doses produce early afterdepolarizations, triggered activity, and ventricular tachyarrhythmias, including torsades de pointes. Procainamide appears to exert greater electrophysiological effects than NAPA.

HEMODYNAMIC EFFECTS. Procainamide can depress myocardial contractility in high doses. It does not produce alpha blockade but can result in peripheral vasodilation, possibly through antisympathetic effects on brain or spinal cord that can impair cardiovascular reflexes.

PHARMACOKINETICS (see Table 30–4). Oral administration produces a peak plasma concentration in about 1 hour. Approximately 80 percent of oral procainamide is bioavailable, with 20 percent bound to serum proteins. The overall elimination half-life for procainamide is 3 to 5 hours, with 50 to 60 percent of the drug eliminated by the kidney and 10 to 30 percent eliminated by hepatic metabolism. Prolonged-release forms of procainamide given every 6 hours provide steady-state plasma levels of the drug equivalent to those from an equal total daily dose of short-acting procainamide given every 4 hours.

The drug is acetylated to NAPA, which is excreted almost exclusively by the kidneys. As renal function decreases and in patients with heart failure, procainamide levels—particularly NAPA levels—increase and, because of the risk of serious cardiotoxicity, need to be carefully monitored in such situations. NAPA has an elimination half-life of 7 to 8 hours, but the half-life exceeds 10 hours if high doses of procainamide are used. Small amounts of NAPA are converted back to procainamide by deacetylation. Increased age, congestive heart failure, and reduced creatinine clearance lower the procainamide clearance and necessitate a reduced dosage.

DOSAGE AND ADMINISTRATION (see Table 30–4). Procainamide can be given by the oral, IV, or intramuscular route to achieve plasma concentrations in the range of 4 to 10 mg/ml that produce an antiarrhythmic effect. Occasionally, plasma concentrations exceeding 10 mg/ml have been required, but the probability of adverse effects at these higher plasma concentrations generally precludes long-term administration. Several IV regimens have been used to administer procainamide. Twenty-five to 50 mg can be given over a 1-minute period and then repeated every 5 minutes until the arrhythmia is controlled, hypotension results, or the QRS complex is prolonged more than 50 percent. Doses of 10 to 15 mg/kg at 50 mg/min can also be used. Using this method, plasma concentration falls rapidly during the first 15 minutes after the loading dose, with parallel effects on refractoriness and conduction. A constant-rate IV infusion of procainamide can be given at a dose of 2 to 6 mg/min. The upper limits regarding total IV dose are flexible and range between 1000 and 2000 mg, depending on the patient's response.

Oral administration of procainamide requires a 3- to 4-hour dosing interval at a total daily dose of 2 to 6 gm, with a steady state reached within 1 day. When a loading dose is used, it should be twice the maintenance dose. Frequent dosing is required because of the short elimination half-life in normal subjects. For the prolonged-release forms of procainamide, dosing is at 6- to 12-hour intervals. Although a longer half-life may be seen in some cardiac patients, allowing longer intervals between drug administration, this needs to be documented for the individual patient. Procainamide is well absorbed after intramuscular injection, with virtually 100 percent of the dose bioavailable.

INDICATIONS. Procainamide is used to treat both supraventricular and ventricular arrhythmias in a manner comparable with that of quinidine. Although both drugs have similar electrophysiological actions, either drug can effectively suppress a supraventricular or ventricular arrhythmia that is resistant to the other drug.[7]

Procainamide can be used to convert atrial fibrillation of recent onset to sinus rhythm. As with quinidine, prior treatment with digitalis, propranolol, or verapamil is recommended to prevent acceleration of the ventricular response during atrial fibrillation after procainamide therapy. Procainamide's effect on conduction and refractoriness in the "flutter isthmus" of the right atrial free wall (see later) varies depending on the direction of wave front propagation in the isthmus.[19] Procainamide can block conduction in the accessory pathway of patients with the Wolff-Parkinson-White syndrome and may be used in patients with atrial fibrillation and a rapid ventricular response related to conduction over the accessory pathway. It can produce His-Purkinje block (see Fig. 29–10) and is sometimes administered during electrophysiology study (EPS) to "stress" the His-Purkinje system in evaluating the need for a pacemaker. However, it should be used with caution in patients with evidence of His-Purkinje disease (bundle branch block) in whom a ventricular pacemaker is not readily available.

Procainamide is more effective than lidocaine in acutely terminating sustained VT. Most consistently, procainamide slows the VT rate, a change correlated with the increase in QRS duration.[20] The electrophysiological response to procainamide given intravenously appears to predict the response to the drug given orally. Procainamide appears to affect preferentially the reentrant circuit of the VT compared with other areas of myocardium. The antiarrhythmic response to procainamide does not predict the response to NAPA.

ADVERSE EFFECTS. Multiple adverse noncardiac effects have been reported with procainamide administration and include rashes, myalgias, digital vasculitis, and the Raynaud phenomenon. Fever and agranulocytosis may be due to hypersensitivity reactions, and white blood cell and differential blood cell counts should be performed at regular intervals. Gastrointestinal side effects are less frequent than with quinidine, and adverse central nervous system side effects are less frequent than with lidocaine (although it can cause giddiness, psychosis, hallucinations, and depression). Toxic concentrations of procainamide can diminish myocardial performance and promote hypotension. A variety of conduction disturbances or ventricular tachyarrhythmias can occur that are similar to those produced by quinidine, including prolonged QT syndrome and polymorphic VT. NAPA can also cause QT prolongation and torsades de pointes (see Table 72–3). In the absence of sinus node disease, procainamide does not adversely affect sinus node function. In patients with sinus node dysfunction, procainamide tends to prolong corrected sinus node recovery time and can worsen symptoms in some patients who have the bradycardia-tachycardia syndrome. Procainamide does not increase the serum digoxin concentration.

Arthralgia, fever, pleuropericarditis, hepatomegaly, and hemorrhagic pericardial effusion with tamponade have been described in a systemic lupus erythematosus (SLE)–like syndrome related to procainamide administration. The syndrome occurs more frequently and earlier in patients who are slow acetylators of procainamide and is genetically influenced. Acetylating an aromatic amino group on procainamide to form NAPA appears to block the SLE-inducing effect. Sixty to 70 percent of patients who receive procainamide on a chronic basis develop antinuclear antibodies, with clinical symptoms in 20 to 30 percent, but this is reversible when procainamide is stopped. When symptoms occur, SLE cell preparations are often positive. Positive serological tests are not necessarily a reason to discontinue drug therapy; however, the development of symptoms or a positive anti-

DNA antibody is, unless it is the only effective treatment of a life-threatening arrhythmia (which would be very rare). Corticosteroid administration in these patients may eliminate the symptoms. In this syndrome, in contrast to naturally occurring SLE, the brain and kidney are spared and there is no predilection for females.

Disopyramide

Disopyramide has been approved in the United States for oral but not IV administration to treat patients with ventricular arrhythmias.

ELECTROPHYSIOLOGICAL ACTIONS (see Tables 30–1, 30–2, 30–3, and 30–5). Although structurally different from quinidine and procainamide, disopyramide produces similar electrophysiological effects in vitro. It causes use-dependent block of I_{Na} and non–use-dependent block of I_{Kr}. Along with quinidine, low concentrations tend to prolong APD and induce early afterdepolarizations just as do higher concentrations.[9] Disopyramide also inhibits I_{KATP}. It decreases the slope of phase 4 diastolic depolarization in Purkinje fibers, produces a rate-dependent depression of $\dot{V}_{max}$ of phase 0, prolongs the ERP more than it prolongs the APD, and lengthens conduction time in normal and depolarized Purkinje fibers; it does not affect calcium-dependent action potentials, except possibly at very high concentrations. Disopyramide, like procainamide, reduces the differences in APD between normal and infarcted tissue by lengthening the action potential of normal cells more than that of cells from infarcted regions.

Disopyramide is a muscarinic blocker and can increase the sinus node discharge rate and shorten AV nodal conduction time and refractoriness when the nodes are restrained by cholinergic (vagal) influences. Disopyramide can also slow the sinus node discharge rate by a direct action when given in high concentration and can significantly depress sinus node activity in patients with sinus node dysfunction. Disopyramide exerts greater anticholinergic effects than quinidine and does not appear to affect alpha or beta adrenoceptors.

Disopyramide prolongs atrial and ventricular refractory periods, but its effect on AV nodal conduction and refractoriness is not consistent. Disopyramide prolongs His-Purkinje conduction time, but infra-His block rarely occurs. Disopyramide can be administered safely to patients who have first-degree AV delay and narrow QRS complexes.

HEMODYNAMIC EFFECTS. Disopyramide suppresses ventricular systolic performance and is a mild arterial vasodilator. Patients who have abnormal ventricular function tolerate disopyramide's negative inotropic effects quite poorly. In these patients, the drug should generally be avoided.

PHARMACOKINETICS (see Table 30–4). Disopyramide is 80 to 90 percent absorbed, with a mean elimination half-life of 8 to 9 hours in healthy volunteers but almost 10 hours in patients with heart failure and sometimes longer in some patients with ventricular arrhythmias. Total-body clearance and volume of distribution are lower and mean serum concentration is higher in patients than in normal subjects. Renal insufficiency prolongs the elimination time. Thus, in patients who have renal, hepatic, or cardiac insufficiency, loading and maintenance doses need to be reduced. Peak blood levels after oral administration result in 1 to 2 hours, and bioavailability exceeds 80 percent. The fraction of disopyramide bound to serum protein varies inversely with the total plasma concentration of the drug but may be more stable (30 to 40 percent) at clinically relevant concentrations of 3 μg/ml. It is bound to alpha$_1$-acid glycoprotein and passes through the placenta. About half an oral dose is recovered unchanged in the urine, with about 30 percent as the mono-*N*-dealkylated metabolite. The metabolites appear to exert less effect than the parent compound. Erythromycin inhibits its metabolism.

DOSAGE AND ADMINISTRATION (see Table 30–4). Doses are generally 100 to 200 mg orally every 6 hours, with a range of 400 to 1200 mg/d. A controlled-release preparation can be given as 200 to 300 mg every 12 hours. The IV (investigational) dose is 1 to 2 mg/kg as an initial bolus given over 5 to 10 minutes, which may be followed by an infusion of 1 mg/kg/hr.

INDICATIONS. Disopyramide appears comparable to quinidine and procainamide in reducing the frequency of PVCs and effectively preventing recurrence of VT in selected patients. Disopyramide has been combined with other drugs such as mexiletine to treat patients who do not respond or only partially respond to one drug.

Disopyramide helps prevent recurrence of atrial fibrillation after successful cardioversion as effectively as quinidine and may terminate atrial flutter. In treating patients with atrial fibrillation, particularly atrial flutter, the ventricular rate must be controlled before administering disopyramide, or the combination of a decrease in atrial rate vagolytic effects on the AV node can result in 1:1 AV conduction during atrial flutter. Disopyramide may be useful in preventing episodes of neurally mediated syncope. It has been used in patients with hypertrophic cardiomyopathy (see Chap. 59).

ADVERSE EFFECTS. Three categories of adverse effects follow disopyramide administration. The most common effects are related to the drug's potent parasympatholytic properties and include urinary hesitancy or retention, constipation, blurred vision, closed-angle glaucoma, and dry mouth. Symptoms are less with the sustained-release form. Second, disopyramide can produce ventricular tachyarrhythmias that are commonly associated with QT prolongation and torsades de pointes[8] (see Table 72–3). Some patients can have "cross-sensitivity" to both quinidine and disopyramide and develop torsades de pointes while receiving either drug. When drug-induced torsades de pointes occurs, agents that prolong the QT interval should be used cautiously or not at all. Finally, disopyramide can reduce contractility of the normal ventricle, but the depression of ventricular function is much more pronounced in patients with preexisting ventricular failure. Occasionally, cardiovascular collapse can result.

Class IB Antiarrhythmic Agents

Lidocaine

ELECTROPHYSIOLOGICAL ACTIONS (see Tables 30–1, 30–2, 30–3, and 30–5). Lidocaine blocks I_{Na}, predominantly in the open or possibly inactivated state. It has rapid onset and offset kinetics and does not affect normal sinus node automaticity in usual doses but does depress other normal as well as abnormal forms of automaticity, as well as early and late afterdepolarizations in Purkinje fibers in vitro. Lidocaine has only a modest depressant effect on $\dot{V}_{max}$ and has no effect on maximal diastolic potential of normal muscle and specialized tissue in concentrations of about 1.5 μg/ml. However, faster rates of stimulation, reduced pH,[21] increased extracellular K^+ concentration, and reduced membrane potential—all changes that can result from ischemia—increase the ability of lidocaine to block I_{Na}. Lidocaine reduces the magnitude of the transient inward current responsible for some forms of afterdepolarization. Intracellular calcium activity may be reduced because of the sodium-calcium exchange mechanism. Lidocaine can convert areas of unidirectional block into bidirectional block during ischemia and prevent development of VF by preventing fragmentation of organized large wave fronts into heterogeneous wavelets. Lidocaine may be arrhythmogenic if it depresses conduction but not to the point of bidirectional block, but this does not appear to be an important clinical problem.

Except in very high concentrations, lidocaine does not affect slow channel–dependent action potentials despite its moderate suppression of the slow inward current. In fact, its depressant effect on electrical potentials from ischemic myocardium supports the idea that these ischemic potentials are depressed fast responses rather than slow responses. Lidocaine significantly reduces the APD and the ERP of Purkinje fibers and ventricular muscle because of blockade of sodium channels and decreasing entry of sodium into the cell. It has little effect on atrial fibers and does not affect conduction in accessory pathways. In some in vitro preparations, lidocaine can improve conduction by hyperpolarizing tissues depolarized as a result of stretch or low external potassium concentration.

In vivo, lidocaine has a minimal effect on automaticity or conduction except in unusual circumstances. Patients with preexisting sinus node dysfunction, abnormal His-Purkinje conduction, or junctional or ventricular escape rhythms can develop depressed automaticity or conduction. Part of its effects may be to inhibit cardiac sympathetic nerve activity.

HEMODYNAMIC EFFECTS. Clinically significant adverse hemodynamic effects are rarely noted at usual drug concentrations unless left ventricular function is severely impaired.

PHARMACOKINETICS (see Table 30–4). Lidocaine is used only parenterally because oral administration results in extensive first-pass hepatic metabolism and unpredictable, low plasma levels with excessive metabolites that can produce toxicity. Hepatic metabolism of lidocaine depends greatly on hepatic blood flow, so that clearance of this drug almost equals (and can be approximated by) measurements of this flow. Severe hepatic disease or reduced hepatic blood flow, as in heart failure or shock, can markedly decrease the rate of lidocaine metabolism. Beta adrenoceptor blockers can decrease hepatic blood flow and increase lidocaine serum concentration. Prolonged infusion can reduce lidocaine clearance. Its elimination half-life averages 1 to 2 hours in normal subjects, more than 4 hours in patients after relatively uncomplicated myocardial infarction, more than 10 hours in patients after myocardial infarction complicated by cardiac failure, and even longer in the presence of cardiogenic shock. Maintenance doses should be reduced by one third to one half for patients with low cardiac output. Lidocaine is 50 to 80 percent protein bound and binds to alpha$_1$-acid glycoprotein, which may increase in heart failure and myocardial infarction. A two-compartment model accurately predicts serum concentrations.

DOSAGE AND ADMINISTRATION (see Table 30–4). Although lidocaine can be given intramuscularly, the IV route is most commonly used. Intramuscular lidocaine is given in doses of 4 to 5 mg/kg (250 to 350 mg), resulting in effective serum levels at about 15 minutes and lasting for about 90 minutes. Intravenously, lidocaine is given as an initial bolus of 1 to 2 mg/kg of body weight at a rate of 20 to 50 mg/min, with a second injection of one half of the initial dose 20 to 40 minutes later. Patients treated with an initial bolus followed by a maintenance infusion may experience transient subtherapeutic plasma concentrations at 30 to 120 minutes after initiation of therapy. A second bolus of about 0.5 mg/kg without increasing the maintenance infusion rate reestablishes therapeutic serum concentrations.[9]

If recurrence of arrhythmia appears after a steady state has been achieved (e.g., 6 to 10 hours after starting therapy), a similar bolus should be given and the maintenance infusion rate increased. Increasing the maintenance infusion rate alone without an additional bolus results in a very slow increase in plasma lidocaine concentrations, reaching a new plateau in over 6 hours (four elimination half-lives), and is therefore not recommended. Another recommended IV dosing regimen is 1.5 mg/kg initially and 0.8 mg/kg at 8-minute intervals for three doses. Doses are reduced by about 50 percent for patients with heart failure.

If the initial bolus of lidocaine is ineffective, up to two more boluses of 1 mg/kg may be administered at 5-minute intervals. Patients who require more than one bolus to achieve a therapeutic effect have arrhythmias that respond only to higher lidocaine plasma concentrations, and a greater maintenance dose may be necessary to sustain these higher concentrations. Patients requiring only a single initial bolus of lidocaine should probably receive a maintenance infusion of 30 mg/kg/min, whereas those requiring two or three boluses may need infusions of 40 to 50 mg/kg/min.

Loading doses may also be administered by rapid infusion, and a constant-rate IV infusion may be used to maintain an effective concentration. Maintenance infusion rates in the range of 1 to 4 mg/min produce steady-state plasma levels of 1 to 5 μg/ml in patients with uncomplicated myocardial infarction, but these rates must be reduced during heart failure or shock because of concomitant reduced hepatic blood flow. A loading dose of approximately 75 mg followed by an initial infusion rate of 5.33 mg/min that declines exponentially to 2 mg/min with a half-life of 25 minutes has also been recommended.

INDICATIONS. Lidocaine demonstrates efficacy against ventricular arrhythmias of diverse etiology, the ability to achieve effective plasma concentrations rapidly, and a fairly wide toxic-to-therapeutic ratio with a low incidence of hemodynamic complications and other side effects. However, its first-pass hepatic effect precludes oral use, and it is generally ineffective against supraventricular arrhythmias. In patients with the Wolff-Parkinson-White syndrome, for whom the ERP of the accessory pathway is relatively short, lidocaine generally has no significant effect and may even accelerate the ventricular response during atrial fibrillation.

Lidocaine is used primarily for patients with recurrent ventricular tachyarrhythmias; although once a common usage, lidocaine prophylaxis in patients with acute myocardial infarction is currently not recommended because its ability to reduce the incidence of VF in hospitalized patients with acute myocardial infarction has not been clearly established and it can produce side effects and a possible increase in the risk of developing asystole. It has been effective in patients after coronary revascularization and in patients resuscitated from out-of-hospital VF, although amiodarone has been shown to yield higher rates of survival to hospital admission.[22]

ADVERSE EFFECTS. The most commonly reported adverse effects of lidocaine are dose-related manifestations of central nervous system toxicity: dizziness, paresthesias, confusion, delirium, stupor, coma, and seizures. Occasional sinus node depression and His-Purkinje block have been reported. In patients with atrial tachyarrhythmias, ventricular rate acceleration has been noted. Rarely, lidocaine can cause malignant hyperthermia. Both lidocaine and procainamide can elevate defibrillation thresholds.

Mexiletine

Mexiletine, a local anesthetic congener of lidocaine with anticonvulsant properties, is used for oral treatment of patients with symptomatic ventricular arrhythmias.

ELECTROPHYSIOLOGICAL ACTIONS (see Tables 30–1, 30–2, 30–3, and 30–5). Mexiletine is similar to lidocaine in many of its electrophysiological actions. In vitro, mexiletine shortens the APD and ERP of Purkinje fibers and, to a lesser extent, of ventricular muscle. It depresses $\dot{V}_{max}$ of phase 0 by blocking I_{Na}, especially at faster rates, and depresses automaticity of Purkinje fibers but not of the normal sinus node. Its onset and offset kinetics are rapid. Hypoxia or ischemia can increase its effects on $\dot{V}_{max}$.

Mexiletine can result in severe bradycardia and abnormal sinus node recovery time in patients with sinus node disease but not in patients with a normal sinus node. It does not affect AV nodal conduction and can depress His-Purkinje conduction, but not greatly, unless conduction was abnormal initially. Mexiletine does not appear to affect the ERP of human atrial and ventricular muscle. The duration of the QT interval does not increase. Because of its rate-dependent effects, theoretically, mexiletine might be expected to suppress closely coupled rather than late-coupled ventricular extrasystoles or faster tachycardias.

HEMODYNAMIC EFFECTS. Mexiletine exerts no major hemodynamic effects. It does not depress myocardial performance when given orally, although IV administration can produce hypotension.

PHARMACOKINETICS (see Table 30–4). Mexiletine has been reported to be rapidly and almost completely absorbed after oral ingestion by volunteers, with peak plasma concentrations attained in 2 to 4 hours. Elimination half-life in healthy subjects is approximately 10 hours, and in patients after myocardial infarction it is 17 hours. Therapeutic plasma levels of 0.5 to 2 μg/ml are maintained by oral doses of 200 to 300 mg every 6 to 8 hours. Absorption with less than a 10 percent first-pass hepatic effect occurs in the upper small intestine and is delayed and incomplete in patients who have myocardial infarction and in patients receiving narcotic analgesics, antacids, or atropine-like drugs that retard gastric emptying. Bioavailability of orally administered mexiletine is approximately 90 percent, and about 70 percent of the drug is protein bound. The apparent volume of distribution is large, reflecting extensive tissue uptake. Normally, mexiletine is eliminated metabolically by the liver, with less than 10 percent excreted unchanged in the urine. Doses probably should be reduced in patients with cirrhosis and those with left ventricular failure. Renal clearance of mexiletine decreases as urinary pH increases. Known metabolites exert no electrophysiological effects. Metabolism can be increased by phenytoin, phenobarbital, and rifampin and reduced by cimetidine. It is influenced by the genotype for the *CYP206* gene.

DOSAGE AND ADMINISTRATION (see Table 30–4). The recommended starting dose is 200 mg orally every 8 hours when rapid arrhythmia control is not essential. Doses may be increased or decreased by 50 to 100 mg every 2 to 3 days and are better tolerated when given with food. Total daily dose should not exceed 1200 mg. In some patients, administration every 12 hours can be effective. For rapid loading, 400 mg followed in 8 hours by a 200-mg dose is suggested.

INDICATIONS. Mexiletine is an effective antiarrhythmic agent for treating patients with both acute and chronic ventricular tachyarrhythmias but not with SVTs. Success rates vary from 6 to 60 percent and can be increased in some patients if mexiletine is combined with other drugs such as procainamide, beta blockers, quinidine, disopyramide, or amiodarone. Most studies show no clear superiority of mexiletine over other class I agents. Mexiletine may be very useful in children with congenital heart disease and serious ventricular arrhythmias. In treating patients with a long QT interval, mexiletine may be safer than drugs such as quinidine that increase the QT interval further. Limited experience in treating subsets of patients with long QT syndrome (LQT3, which is related to the *SCN5A* gene for the cardiac sodium channel) suggests a beneficial role (see Chap. 28). It does not appear to alter the prognosis of patients with inducible ventricular tachyarrhythmias after myocardial infarction. It may be effectively combined with propafenone or amiodarone.[23]

ADVERSE EFFECTS. Thirty to 40 percent of patients may require a change in dose or discontinuation of mexiletine therapy as a result of adverse effects, including tremor, dysarthria, dizziness, paresthesia, diplopia, nystagmus, mental confusion, anxiety, nausea, vomiting, and dyspepsia. Cardiovascular side effects are seen most often after IV dosing and include hypotension, bradycardia, and exacerbation of arrhythmia. Adverse effects of mexiletine appear to be dose related, and toxic effects occur at plasma concentrations only slightly higher than therapeutic levels. Therefore, effective use of this antiarrhythmic drug requires careful titration of dose and monitoring of plasma concentration. Lidocaine should be avoided, or the dose reduced, in patients also receiving lidocaine congeners such as mexiletine.

Phenytoin

Phenytoin was employed originally to treat seizure disorders. Its value as an antiarrhythmic agent remains limited.

ELECTROPHYSIOLOGICAL ACTIONS (see Tables 30-1, 30-2, 30-3, and 30-5). Phenytoin effectively abolishes abnormal automaticity caused by digitalis-induced delayed afterdepolarizations in cardiac Purkinje fibers and suppresses certain digitalis-induced arrhythmias in humans. The rate of rise of action potentials initiated early in the relative refractory period is increased, as is membrane responsiveness, possibly reducing the chance for impaired conduction and block. Phenytoin minimally affects sinus discharge rate and AV conduction in humans. As with other class IB agents, phenytoin has little effect on $\dot{V}_{max}$ in normally polarized fibers at slow rates and shows use-dependence and rapid kinetics for onset and termination of effects. Some of phenytoin's antiarrhythmic effects may be neurally mediated because it can modulate both sympathetic and vagal efferent activity. It has no peripheral cholinergic or beta-adrenergic blocking actions. Phenytoin exerts minimal hemodynamic effects.

PHARMACOKINETICS (See Table 30–4). The pharmacokinetics of phenytoin are less than ideal. Absorption after oral administration is incomplete and varies with the brand of drug. Plasma concentrations peak 8 to 12 hours after an oral dose. Ninety percent of the drug is protein bound. Phenytoin has limited solubility at physiological pH, and intramuscular administration is associated with pain, muscle necrosis, sterile abscesses, and variable absorption. Therapeutic serum concentrations of phenytoin (10 to 20 μg/ml) are similar for treating both cardiac arrhythmias and epilepsy. Lower concentrations can suppress certain digitalis-induced arrhythmias or other arrhythmias when decreased plasma protein binding occurs (as in uremia) because a larger fraction of drug is free and pharmacologically active.

METABOLISM. Over 90 percent of a dose is hydroxylated in the liver to presumably inactive compounds; significant genetically determined variation can occur. Elimination half-time is about 24 hours and can be slowed in the presence of liver disease or when phenytoin is administered concomitantly with drugs such as phenylbutazone, warfarin, isoniazid, chloramphenicol, and phenothiazines that compete with phenytoin for hepatic enzymes. Because of the large number of medications that can increase or decrease phenytoin levels during chronic therapy, phenytoin plasma concentration should be determined frequently when changes are made in other medications. Phenytoin has concentration-dependent kinetics for elimination that can cause unexpected toxicity because disproportionately large changes in plasma concentration can follow dose increases.

DOSAGE AND ADMINISTRATION (see Table 30–4). To achieve a therapeutic plasma concentration rapidly, 100 mg of phenytoin should be administered intravenously every 5 minutes until the arrhythmia is controlled, about 1 gm has been given, or adverse side effects result. Generally, 700 to 1000 mg controls the arrhythmia. A large central vein should be used to avoid pain and development of phlebitis produced by the extremely alkalotic (pH 11.0) vehicle in which phenytoin is dissolved. Orally, phenytoin is given as a loading dose of approximately 1000 mg the first day, 500 mg on the second and third days, and 300 to 400 mg daily thereafter. All maintenance doses can be given once or twice daily, depending on the brand, because of the long half-life of elimination.

INDICATIONS. Phenytoin has been used successfully to treat atrial and ventricular arrhythmias caused by digitalis toxicity but is much less effective in treating ventricular arrhythmias in patients with ischemic heart disease or with atrial arrhythmias not due to digitalis toxicity. It may be useful in some patients with the long QT syndrome.

ADVERSE EFFECTS. The most common manifestations of phenytoin toxicity are central nervous system effects of nystagmus, ataxia, drowsiness, stupor, and coma. Progression of such symptoms can be correlated with increases in plasma drug concentration. Nausea, epigastric pain, and anorexia are also relatively common effects of phenytoin. Long-term administration can result in hyperglycemia, hypocalcemia, rashes, megaloblastic anemia, gingival hypertrophy, lymph node hyperplasia (a syndrome resembling malignant lymphoma), peripheral neuropathy, pneumonitis, and drug-induced SLE. Birth defects can also result.[24]

Class IC Antiarrhythmic Agents

Flecainide

Flecainide is approved by the U.S. Food and Drug Administration (FDA) to treat patients with life-threatening ventricular arrhythmias as well as a variety of supraventricular arrhythmias.

ELECTROPHYSIOLOGICAL ACTIONS (see Tables 30–1, 30–2, 30–3, and 30–5). Flecainide exhibits marked use-dependent depressant effects on the rapid sodium channel, decreasing $\dot{V}_{max}$ with slow onset and offset kinetics. Drug dissociation from the sodium channel is very slow, with time constants of 10 to 30 seconds (compared with 4 to 8 seconds for quinidine and less than 1 second for lidocaine).Thus, marked drug effects can occur at physiological heart rates. Flecainide shortens the duration of the Purkinje fiber action potential but prolongs it in ventricular muscle, actions that, depending on the circumstances, could enhance or reduce electrical heterogeneity and create or suppress arrhythmias. Flecainide profoundly slows conduction in all cardiac fibers and, in high concentrations, inhibits the slow Ca^{2+} channel. Conduction time in the atria, ventricles, AV node, and His-Purkinje system is prolonged. It can terminate experimental atrial reentry by causing conduction block in the reentry pathway and eliminate atrial tachycardia (AT) by producing exit block from the focus. Flecainide can also promote reentry. Minimal increases in atrial or ventricular refractoriness or in the QT interval result. Anterograde and retrograde refractoriness in accessory pathways can increase significantly in a use-dependent fashion. Sinus node function remains unchanged in normal subjects but may be depressed in patients with sinus node dysfunction. Pacing and defibrillation thresholds are characteristically slightly increased.

HEMODYNAMIC EFFECTS. Flecainide depresses cardiac performance, particularly in patients with compromised ventricular systolic function. Left ventricular ejection fraction decreases after oral (single dose of 200 to 250 mg) or IV (1 mg) administration. Flecainide should be used cautiously, or not at all, in patients with moderate or severe ventricular systolic dysfunction.

PHARMACOKINETICS (see Table 30–4). Flecainide is at least 90 percent absorbed, with peak plasma concentrations in 3 to 4 hours. Elimination half-life in patients with ventricular arrhythmias is 20 hours, with 85 percent of the drug being excreted unchanged or as an inactive metabolite in urine. Two major metabolites exert fewer effects than the parent drug. Elimination is slower in patients with renal disease and heart failure, and doses should be reduced in these situations. Therapeutic plasma concentrations range from 0.2 to 1.0 μg/ml. About 40 percent of the drug is protein bound. Increases in serum concentrations of digoxin (15 to 25 percent) and propranolol (30 percent) result during coadministration with flecainide. Propranolol, quinidine, and amiodarone may increase flecainide serum concentrations. Five to 7 days of dosing may be required to reach steady state in some patients.

DOSAGE AND ADMINISTRATION (see Table 30–4). The starting dose is 100 mg every 12 hours, increased in increments of 50 mg twice daily, no sooner than every 3 to 4 days, until efficacy is achieved, an adverse effect is noted, or to a maximum of 400 mg/d. Cardiac rhythm and QRS duration should be monitored.

INDICATIONS. Flecainide is indicated for the treatment of life-threatening ventricular tachyarrhythmias, SVTs, and paroxysmal atrial fibrillation. Some experts suggest that therapy should begin in the hospital while the electrocardiogram is being monitored because of the possibility of proarrhythmic events (see later). Serum concentration should not exceed 1.0 μg/ml. Flecainide is particularly effective in almost totally suppressing PVCs and short runs of nonsustained VT, although the importance of such a response to the subsequent outcome of the patient has not been established. As with other class I antiarrhythmic drugs, there are no data from controlled studies to indicate that the drug favorably affects survival or sudden cardiac death, and data from CAST (see later) indicate increased mortality in patients with coronary artery disease. Flecainide produces a use-dependent prolongation of VT cycle length that improves hemodynamic tolerance.

Flecainide is also useful in a variety of SVTs such as atrial flutter and atrial fibrillation,[10] in Wolff-Parkinson-White syndrome, and for AT. Isoproterenol can reverse some of these effects. Flecainide may be more effective than procainamide in the acute termination of atrial fibrillation. It is important to slow the ventricular rate before treating with flecainide to avoid 1:1 AV conduction. Flecainide has been used to treat fetal arrhythmias and arrhythmias in children.[25] It may increase defibrillation thresholds. Flecainide administration may produce ST elevation in lead V_1 characteristic of Brugada syndrome (see Chap. 32) and has been used as a diagnostic tool in patients suspected of having this disorder.

ADVERSE EFFECTS. Proarrhythmic effects are some of the most important adverse effects of flecainide. Its marked slowing of conduction precludes its use in patients with second-degree AV block without a pacemaker and warrants cautious administration in patients with intraventricular conduction disorders. Worsening of existing ventricular arrhythmias or onset of new ventricular arrhythmias can occur in 5 to 30 percent of patients, with the increased percentage in patients with preexisting sustained VT, cardiac decompensation, and higher doses of the drug. Failure of the flecainide-related arrhythmia to respond to therapy, including electrical cardioversion-defibrillation, may result in mortality as high as 10 percent in patients who develop proarrhythmic events. Negative inotropic effects can cause or worsen heart failure. Patients with sinus node dysfunction may experience sinus arrest, and those with pacemakers may develop an increase in pacing threshold. In CAST, patients treated with flecainide had 5.1 percent mortality or nonfatal cardiac arrest compared with 2.3 percent in the placebo group over 10 months.[14] Mortality was highest in those with non-Q-wave infarction, frequent PVCs, and faster heart rates, raising the possibility of drug interaction with ischemia and electrical instability. Exercise can amplify the conduction slowing in the ventricle produced by flecainide and in some cases can precipitate a proarrhythmic response. Therefore, exercise testing has been recommended to screen for proarrhythmia. Central nervous system complaints, including confusion and irritability, represent the most frequent noncardiac adverse effects. The safety of flecainide during pregnancy has not been determined although, as noted previously, it is occasionally used to treat fetal arrhythmias. It is concentrated in breast milk to levels 2.5- to 4-fold higher than in plasma.

Propafenone

Propafenone has been approved by the FDA for treatment of patients with life-threatening ventricular tachyarrhythmias.

ELECTROPHYSIOLOGICAL ACTIONS (see Tables 30-1, 30-2, 30-3, and 30-5). Propafenone blocks the fast sodium current in a use-dependent manner, as well as at rest, in Purkinje fibers and to a lesser degree in ventricular muscle. Use-dependent effects contribute to its ability to terminate experimental atrial fibrillation. The dissociation constant from the receptor is slow, like that of flecainide. Effects are greater in ischemic than normal tissue and at reduced membrane potentials. Propafenone decreases excitability and suppresses spontaneous automaticity and triggered activity. It terminates experimental VT by producing conduction block or by collision of the impulse with an echo wave. Propafenone is a weak blocker of I_{Kr}[26] and beta-adrenergic receptors. Although ventricular refractoriness increases, conduction slowing is the major effect. The active metabolites of propafenone exert important actions, reducing $\dot{V}_{max}$, action potential amplitude and duration in canine Purkinje fibers. Propafenone depresses sinus node automaticity. In patients, the AH, HV, PR, and QRS intervals increase, as do refractory periods of the atria, ventricles, AV node, and accessory pathways. The corrected QT interval increases only as a function of increased QRS duration.

HEMODYNAMIC EFFECTS. Propafenone and 5-hydroxypropafenone exhibit negative inotropic properties at high concentrations in vitro, and large doses depress left ventricular function in vivo. In patients with ejection fractions exceeding 40 percent, the negative inotropic effects are well tolerated, but patients with preexisting left ventricular dysfunction and congestive heart failure may have symptomatic worsening of their hemodynamic status.

PHARMACOKINETICS (see Table 30–4). With more than 95 percent of the drug absorbed, propafenone's maximum plasma concentration occurs in 2 to 3 hours. Systemic bioavailability is dose dependent and ranges from 3 to 40 percent because of variable presystemic clearance. Bioavailability increases as the dose increases, and plasma concentration is therefore nonlinear. A threefold increase in dosage (300 to 900 mg/d) results in a 10-fold increase in plasma concentration, presumably because of saturation of hepatic metabolic mechanisms. Propafenone is 97 percent bound to alpha$_1$-acid glycoprotein, with an elimination half-life of 5 to 8 hours. Maximum therapeutic effects occur at serum concentrations of 0.2 to 1.5 μg/ml. Marked interpatient variability of pharmacokinetics and pharmacodynamics may be due to genetically determined differences in metabolism. About 93 percent of the population are extensive metabolizers and exhibit shorter elimination half-lives (5 to 6 hours), lower plasma concentrations of the parent compound, and higher concentrations of metabolites. Poor metabolizers, because of diminished capacity of the hepatic microsomal cytochrome P450 enzyme system, exhibit an elimination half-life of 15 to 20 hours for the parent compound and virtually no 5-hydroxypropafenone. The (+) enantiomer provides nonspecific beta-adrenergic receptor blockade with 2.5 to 5 percent of the potency of propranolol. Because plasma propafenone concentrations may be 50 times or more higher than propranolol levels, these beta-blocking properties may be relevant. Poor metabolizers have a greater beta-adrenergic receptor blocking effect than extensive metabolizers. Propafenone also blocks the slow calcium channel to a degree about 1 percent that of verapamil.

DOSAGE AND ADMINISTRATION (see Table 30–4). Most patients respond to oral doses of 150 to 300 mg every 8 hours, not exceeding 1200 mg/d. Doses are similar for patients of both metabolizing phenotypes. Concomitant food administration increases bioavailability, as does hepatic dysfunction. No good correlation between plasma propafenone concentration and arrhythmia suppression has been shown. Doses should not be increased more often than every 3 to 4 days. Propafenone increases plasma concentrations of warfarin, digoxin, and metoprolol.

INDICATIONS. Propafenone is indicated for the treatment of SVTs,[11] paroxysmal atrial fibrillation, and life-threatening ventricular tachyarrhythmias and effectively suppresses spontaneous PVCs and nonsustained and sustained VT. Propafenone has also been approved for use in patients with AT, AV node reentry, AV reentry, and atrial flutter or fibrillation. Acute termination of atrial fibrillation episodes was effected with a single 600-mg oral dose of propafenone in 76 percent of patients given the drug (twice the rate of those given placebo).[27] It has been used effectively in the pediatric age group. Propafenone increases the pacing threshold but minimally affects the defibrillation threshold. Sinus rate during exercise is reduced. Propafenone use is associated with higher mortality in cardiac arrest survivors than use of an implantable defibrillator. Sotalol was more effective than propafenone in the Electrophysiology Study Versus Electrocardiographic Monitoring (ESVEM) trial. Propafenone has been combined effectively with mexiletine.

ADVERSE EFFECTS. Minor noncardiac effects occur in about 15 percent of patients, with dizziness, disturbances in taste, and blurred vision the most common and gastrointestinal side effects next. Exacerbation of bronchospastic lung disease can occur because of mild beta-blocking effects. Cardiovascular side effects occur in 10 to 15 percent of patients, including conduction abnormalities such as AV block, sinus node depression, and worsening of heart failure. Proarrhythmic responses, which occur more often in patients with a history of sustained VT and decreased ejection fractions, appear less commonly than with flecainide and may be in the range of 5 percent. The applicability of data from CAST about flecainide to propafenone is not clear, but limiting propafenone's application in a manner similar to that of other class IC drugs seems prudent at present until more information is available. Its beta-blocking actions may make it different, however. The safety of propafenone administration during pregnancy has not been established.

Moricizine (Ethmozine)

Moricizine is a phenothiazine derivative indicated for treatment of patients with ventricular tachyarrhythmias; it has also been used for atrial fibrillation.[28] It was formerly discussed as a class IB antiarrhythmic drug because it shortens Purkinje fiber action potential. However, the intensity of its effect on the Na^+ channel is more like that of a class IA antiarrhythmic drug, whereas the time constants for onset and offset resemble those of class IC agents.

ELECTROPHYSIOLOGICAL ACTIONS. Moricizine decreases I_{Na} predominantly in the inactivated state, with a resultant decrease in $\dot{V}_{max}$ of phase 0 and action potential amplitude (see Tables 30-1, 30-2, 30-3, and 30-5). Maximum diastolic potential is not changed. Moricizine blocks $I_{Ca\text{-}L}$ and I_K and prolongs AV node and His-Purkinje conduction times and QRS duration. The JT interval shortens slightly, whereas the QTc is prolonged 5 percent owing to QRS prolongation. Ventricular refractoriness is prolonged slightly, with no consistent atrial change. No alterations in sinus node automaticity result. Moricizine minimally raises the defibrillation threshold.

HEMODYNAMIC EFFECTS. Moricizine exerts minimal effects on cardiac performance in patients with impaired left ventricular function; an occasional patient with significant left ventricular dysfunction may have worsening of heart failure.

PHARMACOKINETICS (see Table 30–4). After oral ingestion, moricizine undergoes extensive first-pass metabolism, resulting in absolute bioavailability of 35 to 40 percent. Peak plasma concentrations are reached in 0.5 to 2 hours and later if the drug is taken after meals. Protein binding is 95 percent to alpha$_1$-acid glycoprotein and albumin. Antiarrhythmic and electrophysiological actions do not relate to plasma concentrations or to any of its more than 20 metabolites. Plasma elimination half-life is 1.5 to 3.5 hours, with slightly more than half the drug excreted in the feces and slightly less than half excreted in the urine.

DOSAGE AND ADMINISTRATION (see Table 30–4). The usual adult dose is 600 to 900 mg/d, given every 8 hours in divided doses, with increments of 150 mg/d at 3-day intervals. Some patients may be treated every 12 hours. Dosage should be reduced in patients with hepatic or neural disease, AV conduction disturbances, or sinus node dysfunction without a pacemaker and with significant congestive heart failure.

INDICATIONS. Moricizine is indicated for prevention of life-threatening ventricular arrhythmias and has an efficacy about comparable to those of quinidine and disopyramide. Moricizine can have proarrhythmic effects; in CAST, it caused an increase in mortality compared with placebo during initial treatment of patients who had symptomatic or minimally symptomatic ventricular arrhythmias after myocardial infarction.[29] Risk was greater in patients taking diuretics.

ADVERSE EFFECTS. Usually, the drug is well tolerated. Noncardiac adverse effects primarily involve the nervous system and include tremor, mood changes, headache, vertigo, nystagmus, and dizziness. Gastrointestinal side effects include nausea, vomiting, and diarrhea. Worsening of congestive heart failure may rarely occur. Proarrhythmic effects have been reported in 3 to 15 percent of patients, more commonly in patients with severe ventricular arrhythmias. Advancing age increases the susceptibility to adverse effects. Moricizine appears to be relatively safe to use during pregnancy (class B) and is present in small amounts in breast milk.

Class II Antiarrhythmic Agents

Beta Adrenoceptor Blocking Agents

Although many beta adrenoceptor blocking drugs have been approved for use in the United States, acebutolol (PVCs), esmolol (SVT), metoprolol (post-myocardial infarction), atenolol (post-myocardial infarction), propranolol (post-myocardial infarction, SVT, VT), and timolol (post-myocardial infarction) have been approved to treat arrhythmias or to prevent sudden death after myocardial infarction.[30] It is generally considered that no beta blocker offers distinct advantages over others and that, when titrated to the proper dose, all can be used effectively to treat cardiac arrhythmias, hypertension, or other disorders. However, differences in pharmacokinetic or pharmacodynamic properties that confer safety, reduce adverse effects, or affect dosing intervals or drug interactions influence the choice of agent. Also, some beta blockers such as sotalol, pindolol, and carvedilol exert unique actions.

Beta receptors can be separated into those that affect predominantly the heart ($beta_1$) and those that affect predominantly blood vessels and the bronchi ($beta_2$). In low doses, selective beta blockers can block $beta_1$ receptors more than they block $beta_2$ receptors and might be preferable for treating patients with pulmonary or peripheral vascular diseases. In high doses, the "selective" $beta_1$ blockers also block $beta_2$ receptors. Carvedilol also exerts alpha blocking effects and is used primarily in patients with heart failure (see Chap. 23).

Some beta blockers exert intrinsic sympathomimetic activity; that is, they slightly activate the beta receptor. These drugs appear to be as efficacious as beta blockers without intrinsic sympathomimetic actions and may cause less slowing of heart rate at rest and less prolongation of AV nodal conduction time. They have been shown to induce less depression of left ventricular function than beta blockers without intrinsic sympathomimetic activity. Only nonselective beta blockers without intrinsic sympathomimetic activity have been demonstrated to reduce mortality in patients after myocardial infarction (Fig. 30–1).

The following discussion concentrates on the use of propranolol as a prototypical antiarrhythmic agent, generally applicable to other beta blockers.

ELECTROPHYSIOLOGICAL ACTIONS. Beta blockers exert an electrophysiological action by competitively inhibiting catecholamine binding at beta adrenoceptor sites, an effect almost entirely due to the (−)-levorotatory stereoisomer, or by their quinidine-like or direct membrane-stabilizing action (see Tables 30–1, 30–2, 30–3, and 30–5). The latter is a local anesthetic effect that depresses I_{Na} and membrane responsiveness in cardiac Purkinje fibers, occurs at concentrations generally 10 times that necessary to produce beta blockade, and most likely plays an insignificant antiarrhythmic role. Thus, beta blockers exert their major effects in cells most actively stimulated by adrenergic actions. At beta-blocking concentrations, propranolol slows spontaneous automaticity in the sinus node or in Purkinje fibers that are being stimulated by adrenergic tone, producing block of I_f (see Chap. 27). Beta blockers also block $I_{Ca\text{-}L}$ stimulated by beta agonists. In the absence of adrenergic stimulation, only high concentrations of propranolol slow normal automaticity in Purkinje fibers, probably by a direct membrane action.

Concentrations that cause beta receptor blockade but no local anesthetic effects do not alter the normal resting membrane potential, maximum diastolic potential amplitude, $\dot{V}_{max}$, repolarization, or refractoriness of atrial, Purkinje, or ventricular muscle cells in the absence of catecholamine stimulation. However, in the presence of isoproterenol, a pure beta receptor stimulator, beta blockers reverse isoproterenol's accelerating effects on repolarization; in the presence of norepinephrine, beta blockade permits unopposed alpha adrenoceptor stimulation to prolong APD in Purkinje fibers. Propranolol (2×10^{-6} M) reduces the amplitude of digitalis-induced delayed afterdepolarizations and suppresses triggered activity in Purkinje fibers. Propranolol upregulates beta adrenoceptors in part by externalizing receptors from a light vesicle fraction to the sarcolemma.

Concentrations exceeding 3 mg/ml are required to depress $\dot{V}_{max}$ action potential amplitude, membrane responsiveness, and conduction in normal atrial, ventricular, and Purkinje fibers without altering resting membrane potential. These effects probably result from depression of I_{Na}. Propranolol shortens the APD of Purkinje fibers and, to a lesser extent, of atrial and ventricular muscle fibers. Long-term administration of propranolol may lengthen APD. As with the effects of lidocaine, acceler-

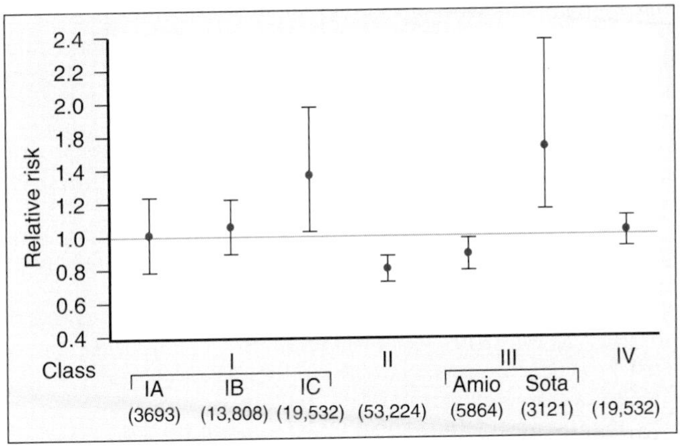

FIGURE 30–1 Meta-analytical data from randomized clinical trials of antiarrhythmic drugs in survivors of acute myocardial infarction. The relative risk is compared with placebo therapy (mean and 95 percent confidence interval) for death during therapy with various electrophysiological classes of compounds. Class I agents, particularly IC, and sotalol increase mortality, whereas beta blockers and amiodarone decrease mortality. Numbers under each drug class refer to number of patients involved in the trials. Amio = amiodarone; Sota = sotalol. (Modified from Teo KK, Yusuf S: *In* Singh BN, Dzau VJ, Vanhoutte PM, Woosley RL [eds]: Cardiovascular Pharmacology and Therapeutics. New York, Churchill Livingstone, 1994, pp 631-643; and Waldo AL, Camm AJ, deRuyter H, et al: Effect of *d*-sotalol on mortality in patients with left ventricular dysfunction after recent and remote myocardial infarction: The SWORD Investigators. Survival With Oral *d*-Sotalol. Lancet 348:7, 1996.)

ation of repolarization of Purkinje fibers is most marked in areas of the ventricular conduction system in which the APD is greatest. At least one beta blocker, sotalol, markedly increases the time course of repolarization in Purkinje fibers and ventricular muscle. Smaller doses of propranolol are required to prevent sympathetically induced shortening of ventricular refractoriness than are required to prevent sympathetically induced sinus acceleration.

Propranolol slows the sinus discharge rate in humans by 10 to 20 percent, although severe bradycardia occasionally results if the heart is particularly dependent on sympathetic tone or if sinus node dysfunction is present. The PR interval lengthens, as do AV nodal conduction time and effective and functional refractory periods (if the heart rate is maintained constant), but refractoriness and conduction in the normal His-Purkinje system remain unchanged even after high doses of propranolol. Therefore, therapeutic doses of propranolol in humans do not exert a direct depressant or "quinidine-like" action but influence cardiac electrophysiology through a beta-blocking action. Beta blockers do not affect conduction in normal ventricular muscle, as evidenced by their lack of effect on the QRS complex, and they insignificantly prolong the uncorrected QT interval.

Because administration of beta blockers that do not have direct membrane action prevents many arrhythmias resulting from activation of the autonomic nervous system, it is thought that the beta-blocking action is responsible for their antiarrhythmic effects. Nevertheless, the possible importance of the direct membrane effect of some of these drugs cannot be discounted totally because beta blockers with direct membrane actions can affect transmembrane potentials of diseased cardiac fibers at much lower concentrations than are needed to affect normal fibers directly. However, indirect actions on arrhythmogenic effects of ischemia are probably most important. Beta blockers reduce myocardial injury during experimental cardiopulmonary resuscitation.

HEMODYNAMIC EFFECTS. Beta blockers exert negative inotropic effects and can precipitate or worsen heart failure. However, beta blockers clearly improve survival in patients with heart failure (see Chap. 23). By blocking beta receptors, these drugs may allow unopposed alpha-adrenergic effects to cause peripheral vasoconstriction and exacerbate coronary artery spasm or pain from peripheral vascular disease in some patients.

PHARMACOKINETICS (see Table 30–4). Although various types of beta blockers exert similar pharmacological effects, their pharmacokinetics differ substantially. Propranolol is almost 100 percent absorbed, but the effects of first-pass hepatic metabolism reduce bioavailability to about 30 percent and produce significant interpatient variability of plasma concentration for a given dose. Reduction in hepatic blood flow, as in patients with heart failure, decreases the hepatic extraction of propranolol; in these patients propranolol may further decrease its own elimination rate by reducing cardiac output and hepatic blood flow. Beta blockers eliminated by the kidney tend to have longer half-lives and exhibit less interpatient variability of drug concentration than beta blockers metabolized by the liver.

DOSAGE AND ADMINISTRATION (see Table 30–4). The appropriate dose of propranolol is best determined by a measure of the patient's physiological response, such as changes in resting heart rate or in the prevention of exercise-induced tachycardia, because wide individual differences exist between the observed physiological effect and plasma concentration. For example, IV dosing is best achieved by titrating the dose to a clinical effect, beginning with doses of 0.25 to 0.50 mg, increasing to 1.0 mg if necessary, and administering doses every 5 minutes until either a desired effect or toxicity is produced or a total of 0.15 to 0.20 mg/kg has been given. In many instances, the short-acting effects of esmolol are preferred. Orally, propranolol is given in four divided doses, usually ranging from 40 to 160 mg/d to more than 1 gm/d. A once-daily long-acting propranolol preparation is available, to which patients may be switched after dosage titration with the short-acting form if needed. Generally, if one agent in adequate doses proves to be ineffective, other beta blockers are also ineffective.

INDICATIONS. Arrhythmias associated with thyrotoxicosis, pheochromocytoma, and anesthesia with cyclopropane or halothane or arrhythmias largely related to excessive cardiac adrenergic stimulation, such as those initiated by exercise, emotion, or cocaine, often respond to beta blocker therapy. Beta-blocking drugs usually do not convert chronic atrial flutter or atrial fibrillation to normal sinus rhythm but may do so if the arrhythmia is of recent onset and in patients who have recently undergone cardiac surgery.[31-34] The atrial rate during atrial flutter or fibrillation is not changed, but the ventricular response decreases because beta blockade prolongs AV nodal conduction time and refractoriness. Esmolol combined with digoxin has been useful. In the absence of heart failure, beta blockers can be more effective than digoxin to control the rate. For reentrant SVTs using the AV node as one of the reentrant pathways, such as AVNRT and orthodromic reciprocating tachycardias in the Wolff-Parkinson-White syndrome or inappropriate sinus tachycardia, or for ATs, beta blockers can slow or terminate the tachycardia and be used prophylactically to prevent a recurrence. Combining beta blockers with digitalis, quinidine, or a variety of other agents may be effective when the beta blocker as a single agent fails. Metoprolol and esmolol may be useful in patients with multifocal AT. These agents must be used with caution in this arrhythmia, however, because a common setting for it is advanced lung disease, often with a bronchospastic component.

Beta blockers may be effective for digitalis-induced arrhythmias such as AT, nonparoxysmal AV junctional tachycardia, PVCs, or VT. If a significant degree of AV block is present during a digitalis-induced arrhythmia, lidocaine or phenytoin may be preferable to propranolol. Beta blockers may also be useful to treat ventricular arrhythmias associated with the prolonged QT interval syndrome and with mitral valve prolapse. For patients with ischemic heart disease, beta blockers generally do not prevent episodes of recurrent monomorphic VT that occur in the absence of acute ischemia but may be effective in some patients, usually at a beta-blocking concentration. It is well accepted that propranolol, timolol, and metoprolol reduce the incidence of overall death and sudden cardiac death after myocardial infarction. The mechanism of this reduction in mortality is not entirely clear and may be related to reduction of the extent of ischemic damage, autonomic effects, a direct antiarrhythmic effect, or combinations of these factors. Beta blockers may have been protective against proarrhythmic responses in CAST and may be more effective in some patients than electrophysiologically guided antiarrhythmic drug therapy for ventricular tachyarrhythmias.

Labetalol, an alpha$_1$- and beta-blocking drug, has been used for ventricular arrhythmias in eclampsia. *Carvedilol,* another alpha- and beta-blocking agent, has been shown to improve survival in moderate to severe heart failure. *Esmolol* is an ultra-short-acting (elimination half-life, 9 minutes), cardioselective beta adrenoceptor blocker that is useful for the rapid control of the ventricular rate in patients with atrial flutter or fibrillation.

ADVERSE EFFECTS. Adverse cardiovascular effects from beta blockers include unacceptable hypotension, bradycardia, and congestive heart failure. The bradycardia may be due to sinus slowing or AV block. Sudden withdrawal of propranolol in patients with angina pectoris can precipitate or worsen angina and cardiac arrhythmias and cause an acute myocardial infarction, possibly owing to heightened sensitivity to beta agonists caused by previous beta blockade (receptor upregulation). Heightened sensitivity may begin several days after cessation of beta blocker therapy and may last 5 or 6 days. Other adverse effects of beta blockers include worsening of asthma or chronic obstructive pulmonary disease, intermittent claudication, Raynaud phenomenon, mental depression, increased risk of hypoglycemia among insulin-dependent diabetic patients, easy fatigability, disturbingly vivid dreams or insomnia, and impaired sexual function. Many of these side effects were noted less frequently when using $beta_1$-selective agents, but even so-called cardioselective beta blockers can exacerbate asthma or diabetic control in individual patients.

Class III Antiarrhythmic Agents

Amiodarone

Amiodarone is a benzofuran derivative approved by the FDA for the treatment of patients with life-threatening ventricular tachyarrhythmias when other drugs are ineffective or are not tolerated. Dronedarone, a noniodinated derivative of amiodarone, is being studied as a potentially less toxic alternative to amiodarone. As of this writing, it has not been approved for use in the United States.[32-34]

ELECTROPHYSIOLOGICAL ACTIONS (see Tables 30–1, 30–2, 30–3, and 30–5). When chronically given orally, amiodarone prolongs APD and refractoriness of all cardiac fibers without affecting resting membrane potential. When acute effects are evaluated, amiodarone and its metabolite, desethylamiodarone, prolong the APD of ventricular muscle but shorten the APD of Purkinje fibers. Injected into the sinus and AV node arteries, amiodarone reduces sinus and junctional discharge rates and prolongs AV nodal conduction time. It decreases the slope of diastolic depolarization of the sinus node and markedly depresses $\dot{V}_{max}$ in guinea pig papillary muscle in a rate- or use-dependent manner. Such depression of $\dot{V}_{max}$ is caused by blocking of inactivated sodium channels, an effect that is accentuated by depolarized and reduced by hyperpolarized membrane potentials. Amiodarone also inhibits depolarization-induced automaticity. Amiodarone depresses conduction at fast rates more than at slow rates (use-dependence), not only by depressing $\dot{V}_{max}$ but also by increasing resistance to passive current flow. It does not prolong repolarization more at slow than fast rates (i.e., does not demonstrate reverse use-dependence) but does exert time-dependent effects on refractoriness, which may in part explain the low incidence of torsades de pointes and high efficacy.

Desethylamiodarone has relatively greater effects on fast-channel tissue and probably contributes notably to antiarrhythmic efficacy. The delay to build up adequate concentrations of this metabolite may explain in part the delay in amiodarone's antiarrhythmic action.

In vivo, amiodarone noncompetitively antagonizes alpha and beta receptors and blocks conversion of thyroxine (T_4) to triiodothyronine (T_3), which may account for some of its electrophysiological effects. Amiodarone exhibits slow-channel blocking effects, and chronic oral therapy slows the spontaneous sinus node discharge rate in anesthetized dogs even after pretreatment with propranolol and atropine. With oral administration it slows the sinus rate by 20 to 30 percent and prolongs the QT interval, at times changing the contour of the T wave and producing U waves.

ERPs of all cardiac tissues are prolonged. His-Purkinje conduction time increases and QRS duration lengthens, especially at fast rates. Amiodarone given intravenously modestly prolongs the refractory period of atrial and ventricular muscle. The PR interval and AV nodal conduction time lengthen. The duration of the QRS complex lengthens at increased rates but less than after oral amiodarone. Thus, far less increase in prolongation of conduction time (except for the AV node), duration of repolarization, and refractoriness occur after IV administration compared with the oral route. Considering these actions, it is clear that amiodarone has class I (blocks I_{Na}), class II (antiadrenergic), and class IV (blocks $I_{Ca\text{-}L}$) actions in addition to class III effects (blocks I_K). Amiodarone's actions approximate those of a theoretically ideal drug that exhibits use-dependent Na^+ channel blockade with fast diastolic recovery from block and use-dependent prolongation of APD. It does not increase and may decrease QT dispersion. Catecholamines can partially reverse some of the effects of amiodarone.

HEMODYNAMIC EFFECTS. Amiodarone is a peripheral and coronary vasodilator. When administered intravenously (150 mg over 10 min, then 1 mg/min infusion) amiodarone decreases heart rate, systemic vascular resistance, left ventricular contractile force, and left ventricular dP/dt. Oral doses of amiodarone sufficient to control cardiac arrhythmias do not depress left ventricular ejection fraction, even in patients with reduced ejection fractions, and ejection fraction and cardiac output may increase slightly. However, because of antiadrenergic actions of amiodarone and because it does exert some negative inotropic action, it should be given cautiously, particularly intravenously, to patients with marginal cardiac compensation.

PHARMACOKINETICS (see Table 30–4). Amiodarone is slowly, variably, and incompletely absorbed, with systemic bioavailability of 35 to 65 percent. Plasma concentrations peak 3 to 7 hours after a single oral dose. There is a minimal first-pass effect, indicating little hepatic extraction. Elimination is by hepatic excretion into bile with some enterohepatic recirculation. Extensive hepatic metabolism occurs with desethylamiodarone as a major metabolite. The plasma concentration ratio of parent to metabolite is 3:2. Both accumulate extensively in the liver, lung, fat, "blue" skin, and other tissues. Myocardium develops a concentration 10 to 50 times that found in the plasma. Plasma clearance of amiodarone is low, and renal excretion is negligible. Doses need not be reduced in patients with renal disease. Amiodarone and desethylamiodarone are not dialyzable. Volume of distribution is large but variable, averaging 60 liter/kg. Amiodarone is highly protein bound (96 percent), crosses the placenta (10 to 50 percent), and is found in breast milk.

The onset of action after IV administration is generally within 1 to 2 hours. After oral administration, the onset of action may require 2 to 3 days, often 1 to 3 weeks, and, on occasion, even longer. Loading doses reduce this time interval. Plasma concentrations relate well to oral doses during chronic treatment, averaging about 0.5 μg/ml for each 100 mg/d at doses between 100 and 600 mg/d. Elimination half-life is multiphasic with an initial 50 percent reduction in plasma concentration 3 to 10 days after cessation of drug ingestion (probably representing elimination from well-perfused tissues) followed by a terminal half-life of 26 to 107 days (mean, 53 days), with most patients in the 40- to 55-day range. To achieve steady state without a loading dose takes about 265 days. Interpatient variability of these pharmacokinetic parameters mandates close monitoring of the patient. Therapeutic serum concentrations range from 1 to 2.5 μg/ml. Greater suppression of arrhythmias may occur up to 3.5 μg/ml, but the risk of side effects increases.

DOSAGE AND ADMINISTRATION (see Table 30–4). An optimal dosing schedule for all patients has not been achieved. One recommended approach is to treat with 800 to 1600 mg/d for 1 to 3 weeks, reduced to 800 mg/d for the next 2 to 4 weeks, then 600 mg/d for 4 to 8 weeks, and finally, after 2 to 3 months of treatment, a maintenance dose of 300 mg or less per day. Maintenance drug can be given once or twice daily and should be titrated to the lowest effective dose to minimize the occurrence of side effects. Doses as low as 100 mg/d can be effective in some patients. Regimens must be individualized for a given patient and clinical situation. Amiodarone may be administered intravenously to achieve more rapid loading and an effect in emergencies at initial doses of 15 mg/min for 10 minutes, followed by 1 mg/min for 6 hours and then 0.5 mg/min for the remaining 18 hours and for the next several days, as necessary. Supplemental infusions of 150 mg over 10 minutes can be used for breakthrough VT or VF. IV infusions can be continued safely for 2 to 3 weeks. IV amiodarone is generally well tolerated even in patients with left ventricular dysfunction. Patients with depressed ejection fractions should receive IV amiodarone with great caution because of hypotension. High-dose oral loading (800 to 2000 mg two or three times a day to maintain trough serum concentrations of 2 to 3 mg/ml) may suppress ventricular arrhythmias in 1 to 2 days.

INDICATIONS. Amiodarone has been used to suppress a wide spectrum of supraventricular and ventricular tachyarrhythmias in utero, in adults, and in children, including AV node and AV entry, junctional tachycardia, atrial flutter and fibrillation, VT and VF associated with coronary artery disease, and hypertrophic cardiomyopathy. Success rates vary widely depending on the population of patients, arrhythmia, underlying heart disease, length of follow-up, definition and determination of success, and other factors. In general, however, amiodarone's efficacy equals or exceeds that of all other antiarrhythmic agents and may be in the range of 60 to 80 percent for most supraventricular tachyarrhythmias and 40 to 60 percent for ventricular tachyarrhythmias. Amiodarone may be useful in improving survival in patients with hypertrophic cardiomyopathy, nonischemic dilated cardiomyopathy,[35] asymptomatic ventricular arrhythmias after myocardial infarction, and ventricular tachyarrhythmia during and after resuscitation from cardiac arrest. Amiodarone given before open-heart surgery,[36] as well as postoperatively, has been shown to decrease the incidence of postoperative atrial fibrillation. Amiodarone is superior to class I antiarrhythmic agents and sotalol in maintaining sinus rhythm in patients with recurrent atrial fibrillation.

Patients who have an ICD receive fewer shocks if they are treated with amiodarone compared with conventional drugs.[37] Amiodarone has little effect on pacing threshold but typically increases the electrical defibrillation threshold slightly.

A number of prospective, randomized, controlled trials have demonstrated improved survival with amiodarone therapy compared with placebo or metoprolol in patients after myocardial infarction. Amiodarone was found to improve survival in patients resuscitated from VF compared with conventional drugs. In patients with congestive heart failure, amiodarone therapy improved survival in one study (in which heart failure was mainly due to nonischemic cardiomyopathy), whereas no benefit was observed in another (primarily ischemic cardiomyopathy patients). The Antiarrhythmics Versus Implantable Defibrillator (AVID) trial was designed to compare mortality between patients treated with antiarrhythmic drugs (empirical amiodarone or EPS- or Holter-guided sotalol) versus an ICD in patients with ejection fraction less than 0.40 who had suffered spontaneous hypotensive VT or cardiac arrest. This study was stopped prematurely when an interim analysis showed that ICD-treated patients survived better after 1 year of treatment.[38]

Some controversy exists regarding the ability to predict the effectiveness of amiodarone in patients with ventricular tachyarrhythmias. Clinical assessment, suppression of spontaneous ventricular arrhythmias as documented by 24-hour ECG recordings, and response to EPS have served as endpoints to judge therapy. In the patient with a history of sustained VT or VF and minimal spontaneous ventricular arrhythmias in between symptomatic episodes, an invasive EPS is indicated to judge drug efficacy. The answer to when, after amiodarone therapy is started, such a study should be done is still not entirely resolved, but the interval should probably be 1 week or longer. In the 10 to 20 percent of patients whose electrically induced, clinical, ventricular tachyarrhythmias become no longer inducible while they are receiving amiodarone, the chances for a spontaneous recurrence of the arrhythmias are low while the patients are taking amiodarone, probably less than 5 to 10 percent at 1 year. For patients whose ventricular tachyarrhythmias are still inducible, the recurrence rate is 40 to 50 percent at 1 year. Patients' hemodynamic responses to the induced arrhythmia may also predict how they tolerate a spontaneous recurrence. Amiodarone slows the VT rate, but it is important to remember that the supine patient in the electrophysiology laboratory may tolerate the same tachycardia better than the patient in an erect position. An ejection fraction greater than 0.4 may predict a good response to amiodarone in patients with VT or VF.

Because of the serious nature of the arrhythmias being treated, the unusual pharmacokinetics of the drug, and its adverse effects, amiodarone therapy should be started with the patient hospitalized and monitored for at least several days. Combining other antiarrhythmic agents with amiodarone may improve efficacy in some patients.

ADVERSE EFFECTS. Adverse effects are reported by about 75 percent of patients treated with amiodarone for 5 years but compel stopping the drug in 18 to 37 percent. The most frequent side effects requiring drug discontinuation involve pulmonary and gastrointestinal complaints. Most adverse effects are reversible with dose reduction or cessation of treatment. Adverse effects are more common when therapy is continued in the long term and at higher doses. Of the noncardiac adverse reactions, pulmonary toxicity is the most serious; in one study it occurred between 6 days and 60 months of treatment in 33 of 573 patients, with 3 deaths. The mechanism is unclear but may involve a hypersensitivity reaction or widespread phospholipidosis, or both. Dyspnea, nonproductive cough, and fever are common symptoms, with crackles on examination, hypoxia, a positive gallium scan, reduced diffusion capacity, and radiographic evidence of pulmonary infiltrates.[39,40] Amiodarone must be discontinued if such pulmonary inflammatory changes occur. Corticosteroids can be tried, but no controlled studies have been done to support their use. A 10 percent mortality results in patients with pulmonary inflammatory changes, often in patients with unrecognized pulmonary involvement that is allowed to progress. Chest radiographs and pulmonary function tests, including carbon monoxide diffusion capacity (DLCO), at 3-month intervals for the first year and then twice a year for several years have been recommended. At maintenance doses less than 300 mg/d, pulmonary toxicity is uncommon. Advanced age, high drug maintenance dose, and reduced predrug diffusion capacity are risk factors for developing pulmonary toxicity. An unchanged DLCO on therapy may be a negative predictor of pulmonary toxicity.

Although asymptomatic elevations of liver enzymes are found in most patients, the drug is not stopped unless values exceed two or three times normal in a patient with initially abnormal values. Cirrhosis occurs uncommonly but may be fatal. Neurological dysfunction, photosensitivity (perhaps minimized by sunscreens), bluish skin discoloration, gastroenterological disturbances, and hyperthyroidism[41] (1 to 2 percent) or hypothyroidism (2 to 4 percent) can occur. Amiodarone appears to inhibit the peripheral conversion of T_4 to T_3 so that chemical changes result, which are characterized by a slight increase in T_4, reverse T_3 and thyroid-stimulating hormone (TSH), and a slight decrease in T_3. Reverse T_3 concentration has been used as an index of drug efficacy. During hypothyroidism, TSH increases greatly, whereas T_3 increases in hyperthyroidism. Thyroid function tests should be obtained approximately every 3 months for the first year while amiodarone is taken and once or twice yearly thereafter, sooner if symptoms develop that are consistent with thyroid dysfunction. Corneal microdeposits occur in almost 100 percent of adults receiving the drug more than 6 months. More serious ocular reactions, including optic neuritis or atrophy with visual loss, or both, have been reported but are rare and causality by amiodarone has not been established.[42]

Cardiac side effects include symptomatic bradycardias in about 2 percent; worsening of ventricular tachyarrhythmias (with occasional development of torsades de pointes)[40] in 1 to 2 percent, possibly higher in women (see Table 72–3); and worsening of congestive heart failure in 2 percent. Possibly because of interactions with anesthetics, complications after open-heart surgery, including pulmonary dysfunction, hypotension, hepatic dysfunction, and low cardiac output, have been noted by some, but not all, investigators.

In general, the lowest possible maintenance dose of amiodarone that is still effective should be used to avoid significant adverse effects. Many supraventricular arrhythmias can be successfully managed with daily doses of 200 mg or less, whereas ventricular arrhythmias generally require higher doses. Adverse effects are uncommon at doses of 200 mg/d or less but still occur. Because of potential toxicity in a variety of organ systems, special multidisciplinary amiodarone clinics have been used by some to attempt to prevent adverse outcomes when using the drug.

Important interactions with other drugs occur, and when they are given concomitantly with amiodarone, the doses of warfarin, digoxin, and other antiarrhythmic drugs should be reduced by one third to one half and the patient observed closely. Drugs with synergistic actions, such as beta blockers or calcium channel blockers, must be given cautiously. Amiodarone's safety during pregnancy has not been established, and it should be used in the pregnant patient only if no alternatives exist.

Bretylium Tosylate

Bretylium is a quaternary ammonium compound that is approved by the FDA for parenteral use only in patients with life-threatening ventricular tachyarrhythmias.

ELECTROPHYSIOLOGICAL ACTIONS (see Tables 30–1, 30–2, 30–3, and 30–5). Bretylium is selectively concentrated in sympathetic ganglia and their postganglionic adrenergic nerve terminals. After initially causing norepinephrine release, bretylium prevents norepinephrine release by depressing sympathetic nerve terminal excitability without depressing preganglionic or postganglionic sympathetic nerve conduction, impairing conduction across sympathetic ganglia, depleting the adrenergic neuron of norepinephrine, or decreasing the responsiveness of adrenergic receptors. It produces a state resembling chemical sympathectomy. During chronic bretylium treatment, the beta-adrenergic responses to circulating catecholamines are increased. The initial release of catecholamines results in several transient electrophysiological responses, such as an increase in the discharge rates of the isolated, perfused sinus node and of in vitro Purkinje fibers, often making quiescent fibers automatic.

Bretylium initially increases conduction velocity and excitability and decreases refractoriness in the rabbit atrium, and partially depolarized fibers may hyperpolarize. Pretreatment with propranolol prevents these early changes. Initial catecholamine release can exacerbate some arrhythmias, such as those caused by digitalis excess or myocardial infarction. Prolonged drug administration lengthens the duration of the action potential and refractoriness of atrial and ventricular muscle and Purkinje fibers, possibly by blocking one or more repolarizing potassium currents. The ratio of ERP to APD does not change, nor do membrane responsiveness and conduction velocity. Bretylium exerts little effect on diastolic excitability. It has little if any effect on sustained VT but can prevent recurrences of VF. It is not clear whether the chemical sympathectomy-like state alone or together with other actions exerts the antifibrillatory effect. Reduced disparity between APD and ERP in regions of normal and infarcted myocardium may account for some of its antifibrillatory effects. Bretylium has no effect on vagal reflexes and does not alter the responsiveness of cholinergic receptors in the heart.

HEMODYNAMIC EFFECTS. Bretylium does not depress myocardial contractility. After an initial increase in blood pressure, the drug can cause significant hypotension by blocking the efferent limb of the baroreceptor reflex. Hypotension results most commonly when patients are sitting or standing but can also occur in the supine position in seriously ill patients. Bretylium reduces the extent of the vasoconstriction and tachycardia reflexes during standing. Orthostatic hypotension can persist for several days after the drug has been discontinued.

PHARMACOKINETICS (see Table 30–4). Bretylium is effective orally as well as parenterally, but it is absorbed poorly and erratically from the gastrointestinal tract and thus is practically useful only intravenously. Bioavailability may be less than 50 percent, and elimination is almost exclusively by renal excretion without significant metabolism or active metabolites being recognized. Elimination half-life is 5 to 10 hours but with fairly wide variability. Doses should be reduced in patients with renal insufficiency. In survivors of VT or VF, bretylium had an elimination half-life of 13.5 hours after single IV dosing, which was similar to previous results in normal subjects. Renal clearance accounted for virtually all elimination. Onset of action after IV administration occurs within several minutes, but full antiarrhythmic effects may not be seen for 30 minutes to 2 hours.

DOSAGE AND ADMINISTRATION (see Table 30–4). Bretylium can be given intravenously in doses of 5 to 10 mg/kg of body weight diluted in 50 to 100 ml of 5 percent dextrose in water and administered over 10 to 20 minutes or more quickly in a life-threatening state. This dose can be repeated in 1 to 2 hours if the arrhythmia persists. The total daily dose probably should not exceed 30 mg/kg. A similar initial dose, but undiluted, can be given intramuscularly. The maintenance IV dose is 0.5 to 2.0 mg/min. Intramuscular injection during cardiopulmonary resuscitation from cardiac arrest and in shock states should be avoided because of unreliable absorption during reduced tissue perfusion. In this situation, bretylium should be given intravenously.

INDICATIONS. Bretylium is used in patients who are in an intensive care setting and who have life-threatening, recurrent ventricular tachyarrhythmias that have not responded to other antiarrhythmic drugs. Bretylium has been effective in treating some patients with drug-resistant tachyarrhythmias and in treating victims of out-of-hospital VF.

ADVERSE EFFECTS. Hypotension, most prominently orthostatic but also supine, appears to be the most significant side effect and can be prevented with tricyclic drugs such as protriptyline. Transient hypertension, increased sinus rate, and worsening of arrhythmias, often those related to digitalis excess or ischemia, may follow initial drug administration and may be due to initial release of catecholamines. Bretylium should be used cautiously or not at all in patients who have a relatively fixed cardiac output, such as those with severe aortic stenosis. Vasodilators or diuretics can enhance these hypotensive effects. Nausea and vomiting can occur after parenteral administration.

Sotalol

Sotalol is a nonspecific beta adrenoceptor blocker without intrinsic sympathomimetic activity that prolongs repolarization.[43] It was approved in 1992 by the FDA to treat patients with life-threatening ventricular tachyarrhythmias and in 1998 for atrial fibrillation.

ELECTROPHYSIOLOGICAL ACTIONS (see Tables 30–1, 30–2, 30–3, and 30–5). Both *d* and *l* isomers have similar effects on prolonging repolarization, whereas the *l* isomer is responsible for virtually all the beta-blocking activity. Sotalol does not block alpha adrenoceptors and does not block the sodium channel (no membrane-stabilizing effects) but does prolong atrial and ventricular repolarization times by reducing I_{Kr}, thus prolonging the plateau of the action potential. Action potential prolongation is greater at slower rates (reverse use-dependence). Resting membrane potential, action potential amplitude, and $\dot{V}_{max}$ are not significantly altered. Sotalol prolongs atrial and ventricular refractoriness, AH and QT intervals, and sinus cycle length. It shortens the excitable gap in reentrant VT.

HEMODYNAMICS. Sotalol exerts a negative inotropic effect only through its beta-blocking action. It can increase the strength of contraction by prolonging repolarization, which occurs maximally at slow heart rates. In patients with reduced cardiac function, sotalol can cause a decrease in cardiac index, an increase in filling pressure, and overt heart failure. Therefore, it must be used cautiously in patients with marginal cardiac compensation but appears to be well tolerated in patients with normal cardiac function.

PHARMACOKINETICS (see Table 30–4). Sotalol is completely absorbed and not metabolized, making it 90 to 100 percent bioavailable. It is not bound to plasma proteins, is excreted unchanged primarily by the kidneys, and has an elimination half-life of 10 to 15 hours. Peak plasma concentrations occur 2.5 to 4.0 hours after oral ingestion, with steady state attained after five or six doses. Effective antiarrhythmic plasma concentration is in the range of 2.5 μg/ml. There is little intersubject variability in plasma levels. Over the dose range of 160 to 640 mg, sotalol displays dose proportionality with plasma concentration. The dose must be reduced in patients with renal disease. The beta-blocking effect is half maximal at 80 mg/d and maximal at 320 mg/d. Significant beta-blocking action occurs at 160 mg/d.

DOSAGE (see Table 30–4). The typical oral dose is 80 to 160 mg every 12 hours, allowing 2 to 3 days between dose adjustments to attain steady state and monitor the electrocardiogram for arrhythmias and QT prolongation. Doses exceeding 320 mg/d can be used in patients when the potential benefits outweigh the risk of proarrhythmia.

INDICATIONS. Approved by the FDA to treat patients with ventricular tachyarrhythmias and atrial fibrillation, sotalol is also useful to prevent recurrence of a wide variety of SVTs, including atrial flutter, AT, AV node reentry, and AV reentry. It also slows the ventricular response to atrial tachyarrhythmias. It appears to be more effective than conventional antiarrhythmic drugs and may be comparable to amiodarone in treating patients with ventricular tachyarrhythmias. Sotalol has been shown to be superior to lidocaine for acute termination of sustained VT and is useful in patients with arrhythmogenic right ventricular dysplasia. Sotalol may be effective in pediatric patients. Unlike most other antiarrhythmic drugs, it may decrease the frequency of ICD discharges[44] and reduce the defibrillation threshold.

ADVERSE EFFECTS. Proarrhythmia is the most serious adverse effect. Overall, new or worsened ventricular tachyarrhythmias occur in about 4 percent, and this response is due to torsades de pointes in about 2.5 percent. The incidence of torsades de pointes increases to 4 percent in patients with a history of sustained VT and is dose related, reportedly only 1.6 percent at 320 mg/d but 4.4 percent at 480 mg/d (see Table 72–3). This proarrhythmic effect was probably the cause of excess mortality in patients given *d*-sotalol (the enantiomer lacking a beta-blocking effect) after an acute myocardial infarction in the Survival With Oral *d*-Sotalol (SWORD) trial. Other adverse effects commonly seen with other beta blockers also apply to sotalol. Sotalol should be used with caution or not at all in combination with other drugs that prolong the QT interval. However, such combinations have been used successfully.

Ibutilide

Ibutilide is an agent released for use in acutely terminating episodes of atrial flutter and fibrillation.

ELECTROPHYSIOLOGICAL ACTIONS (see Tables 30–1, 30–2, 30–3, and 30–5). Like other class III agents, ibutilide prolongs repolarization. Although it is like other class III agents that block outward potassium currents such as I_{Kr}, ibutilide is unique in that it also appears to activate a slow inward sodium current. Administered intravenously, ibutilide causes mild slowing of the sinus rate and has minimal effects on AV conduction or QRS duration, but the QT interval is characteristically prolonged. Ibutilide has no significant effect on hemodynamics.

PHARMACOKINETICS (see Table 30–4). Ibutilide is administered intravenously and has a large volume of distribution. Clearance is predominantly renal, with a drug half-life averaging 6 hours (but with considerable interpatient variability). Protein binding is approximately 40 percent. One of the drug's metabolites has weak class III effects.

DOSAGE AND ADMINISTRATION (see Table 30–4). Ibutilide is given as a rapid IV infusion of 1 mg over 10 minutes. It should not be given in the presence of a QTc interval greater than 440 milliseconds or other drugs that prolong the QT interval or when uncorrected hypokalemia or bradycardia exists. A second 1-mg dose may be given after the first dose is finished if the arrhythmia persists. Patients must have continuous ECG monitoring throughout the dosing period and for 6 to 8 hours thereafter because of the risk of ventricular arrhythmias. Up to 60 percent of patients with atrial fibrillation and 70 percent of those with atrial flutter convert to sinus rhythm after 2 mg of ibutilide.[45]

INDICATIONS. Ibutilide is indicated for termination of an established episode of atrial flutter or fibrillation. It should not be used in patients with frequent, short paroxysms of atrial fibrillation because it merely terminates episodes and is not useful for prevention. Patients whose condition is hemodynamically unstable should proceed to direct-current cardioversion. Ibutilide has been administered at the time of transthoracic electrical cardioversion to increase the likelihood of termination of atrial fibrillation. In one study, all 50 patients given ibutilide before attempted electrical cardioversion achieved sinus rhythm, whereas only 34 of 50 who did not receive the drug converted to sinus rhythm.[46] Of note, all 16 patients who did not respond to electrical cardioversion without ibutilide were successfully electrically cardioverted to sinus rhythm when a second attempt was made after ibutilide pretreatment.

Ibutilide prolongs accessory pathway refractoriness and can temporarily slow the ventricular rate during preexcited atrial fibrillation. The drug can also terminate episodes of sustained uniform morphology VT.

ADVERSE EFFECTS. The most significant adverse effects of ibutilide are QT prolongation and torsades de pointes, which occur in approximately 2 percent of patients given the drug. The adverse effect occurs within the first 4 to 6 hours of dosing, after which the risk is negligible. Thus, patients in whom the drug is used must undergo ECG monitoring for up to 8 hours after dosing. This requirement can make ibutilide's use in emergency departments or private offices problematic. Ibutilide's safety during pregnancy is not well studied. Its use should be restricted to cases in which no safer alternative exists (see Table 72–3).

Dofetilide

Dofetilide is approved for acute conversion of atrial fibrillation to sinus rhythm as well as chronic suppression of recurrent atrial fibrillation.[47]

ELECTROPHYSIOLOGICAL ACTIONS (see Tables 30–1, 30–2, 30–3, and 30–5). The sole electrophysiological effect of dofetilide appears to be block of the rapid component of the delayed rectifier potassium current (I_{Kr}), which is important in repolarization (see Chap. 27). This effect is more prominent in the atria than in the ventricles (30 percent increase in atrial refractory periods versus 20 percent in the ventricles). Dofetilide's effect on I_{Kr} prolongs refractoriness without slowing conduction, which is believed to be largely responsible for its antiarrhythmic effect. It is also responsible for the prolongation of the QT interval on the electrocardiogram, which averages 11 percent but can be much greater. This effect on the QT interval is dose dependent and linear. No other important ECG changes are observed with the drug. It has no significant hemodynamic effects. Dofetilide is more effective than quinidine at converting atrial fibrillation to sinus rhythm.

PHARMACOKINETICS (see Table 30–4). Orally administered dofetilide is absorbed well, with over 90 percent bioavailability. Fifty to 60 percent of the drug is excreted unchanged in urine, with a mean elimination half-life of 7 to 13 hours. The remainder of the drug undergoes hepatic metabolism to inert compounds. Significant drug-drug interactions have been reported in patients using dofetilide; cimetidine, verapamil, ketoconazole, and trimethoprim (alone or in combination with sulfamethoxazole) cause significant elevation in dofetilide serum concentration and should not be used with this drug.

DOSAGE AND ADMINISTRATION (see Table 30–4). Dofetilide is available only as an oral preparation. Dosing is from 0.125 to 0.5 mg twice daily and must be initiated in a hospital setting with continuous ECG monitoring to ensure that inordinate QT prolongation and torsades de pointes do not develop. Physicians must be certified to prescribe the drug. Dosage must be decreased in the presence of impaired renal function or increase in QT interval of more than 50 percent. The drug should not be given to patients with a creatinine clearance less than 20 ml/min or a baseline corrected QT interval greater than 440 milliseconds.

INDICATIONS. IV dofetilide has been used on an investigational basis for termination of an established episode of atrial flutter, fibrillation, or other types of SVT. Oral dofetilide is indicated for prevention of episodes of supraventricular tachyarrhythmias, particularly atrial flutter and fibrillation. Dofetilide's role in therapy for ventricular arrhythmias is less clear. Dofetilide has been shown to have a neutral effect on mortality when given to patients after myocardial infarction.[48]

ADVERSE EFFECTS. The most significant adverse effect of dofetilide is QT interval prolongation with torsades de pointes, occurring in 2 to 4 percent of patients given the drug. Risk is highest in patients with a baseline prolonged QT interval, those who are hypokalemic, those taking some other agent that prolongs repolarization, and after conversion from atrial fibrillation to sinus rhythm (see Table 72–3). The drug is otherwise well tolerated with few side effects. Its use in pregnancy (class C) has not been studied extensively, and it should probably be avoided in this setting if possible.

Azimilide

Azimilide is a new agent (not yet approved by the FDA at the time of this writing) for use in the treatment of atrial flutter and fibrillation.[49]

ELECTROPHYSIOLOGICAL ACTIONS (see Tables 30–1, 30–2, 30–3, and 30–5). Unlike dofetilide, which blocks the rapid component of the delayed rectifier potassium current, azimilide produces a more balanced blockade of both rapid and slow components of I_K. It is presumed that this effect is responsible for the lower rate of proarrhythmia as well as better preservation of drug efficacy at higher heart rates with this agent compared with pure I_{Kr} blockers. Azimilide produces a mild prolongation of the QT interval but no other meaningful ECG changes. Unlike dofetilide and sotalol, which have greater effects on atrial than ventricular refractoriness, azimilide exerts a similar effect on each.[50]

PHARMACOKINETICS (see Table 30–4). Azimilide's pharmacokinetic profile is relatively simple and predictable. It can be taken orally once a day, and its absorption is nearly complete and unaffected by food intake. Few drug interactions have been reported. Azimilide is cleared by the kidney; some metabolism of the drug to inactive compounds occurs. The drug has no significant adverse hemodynamic effects.

DOSAGE AND ADMINISTRATION (see Table 30–4). Azimilide can be taken by mouth once a day at a dose of 100 to 200 mg. The drug is well tolerated, and dosing need not be adjusted in the presence of renal or hepatic disease.

INDICATIONS. Azimilide is indicated for IV administration to terminate an established episode of atrial flutter or fibrillation, as well as orally for long-term prevention of these arrhythmias. Studies are under way to evaluate its efficacy in ventricular arrhythmias.

ADVERSE EFFECTS. The drug is generally well tolerated. As with other class III agents, the most significant adverse effect of azimilide is torsades de pointes, although this arrhythmia appears to be less common with this agent than with other class III medications (occurring in approximately 1 percent of patients given the drug) (see Table 72–3). Azimilide's safety in pregnancy is not known; its use should probably be avoided if possible.

Class IV Antiarrhythmic Agents

Calcium Channel Antagonists: Verapamil and Diltiazem

Verapamil, a synthetic papaverine derivative, is the prototype of a class of drugs that block the slow calcium channel and reduce $I_{Ca\text{-}L}$ in cardiac muscle. Diltiazem has electrophysiological actions similar to those of verapamil. Nifedipine exhibits minimal electrophysiological effects at clinically used doses; felodipine blocks the T-type calcium current (see Chap. 27), and its clinical application has not been established. Neither of these drugs is discussed here.

ELECTROPHYSIOLOGICAL ACTIONS (see Tables 30–1, 30–2, 30–3, and 30–5). By blocking $I_{Ca\text{-}L}$ in all cardiac fibers, verapamil reduces the plateau height of the action potential, slightly shortens muscle action potential, and slightly prolongs total Purkinje fiber action potential. It does not appreciably affect the action potential amplitude, $\dot{V}_{max}$ of phase 0, or resting membrane voltage in cells that have fast-response characteristics related to I_{Na} (atrial and ventricular muscle, the His-Purkinje system). Verapamil suppresses slow responses elicited by a variety of experimental methods as well as triggered sustained rhythmic activity and early and late afterdepolarizations. Verapamil and diltiazem suppress electrical activity in the normal sinus and AV nodes in concentrations that do not suppress action potentials of fast channel-dependent cells. Verapamil depresses the slope of diastolic depolarization in sinus node cells, $\dot{V}_{max}$ of phase 0, maximum diastolic potential, and action potential amplitude in sinus node and AV node cells and prolongs conduction time and the effective and functional refractory periods of the AV node. The AV node blocking effects of verapamil and diltiazem are more apparent at faster rates of stimulation (use-dependence) and in depolarized fibers (voltage dependence). Verapamil slows the activation and delays recovery from inactivation of the slow channel. Unbinding of the drug from its receptor occurs more rapidly in tissue that is hyperpolarized.

Verapamil does exert some local anesthetic activity because the dextrorotatory stereoisomer of the clinically used racemic mixture exerts slight blocking effects on I_{Na}. The levorotatory stereoisomer blocks the slow inward current carried by calcium, as well as other ions, traveling through the slow channel. Verapamil does not modify calcium uptake, binding, or exchange by cardiac microsomes, nor does it affect calcium-activated adenosine triphosphatase. Verapamil does not block beta receptors but may block alpha receptors and potentiate vagal effects on the AV node. Verapamil may also cause other effects that indirectly alter cardiac electrophysiology, such as decreasing platelet adhesiveness or reducing the extent of myocardial ischemia.

In humans, verapamil prolongs conduction time through the AV node (the AH interval) without affecting the P wave or QRS duration or HV interval and lengthens the anterograde and retrograde functional refractory periods and ERPs of the AV node. Spontaneous sinus rate may decrease slightly, an effect only partially reversed by atropine. More commonly, the sinus rate does not change significantly because verapamil causes peripheral vasodilation, transient hypotension, and reflex sympathetic stimulation that mitigates any direct slowing effect verapamil exerts on the sinus node. If verapamil is given to a patient who is also receiving a beta blocker, the sinus node discharge rate may slow because reflex sympathetic stimulation is blocked. Verapamil does not exert a significant direct effect on atrial or ventricular refractoriness or on antero-grade or retrograde properties of accessory pathways. However, reflex sympathetic stimulation following IV verapamil administration may increase the ventricular response over the accessory pathway during atrial fibrillation in patients with the Wolff-Parkinson-White syndrome.

HEMODYNAMIC EFFECTS. Because verapamil interferes with excitation-contraction coupling, it inhibits vascular smooth muscle contraction and causes marked vasodilation in coronary and other peripheral vascular beds. Propranolol does not block the vasodilation produced by verapamil. Reflex sympathetic effects may reduce in vivo the marked negative inotropic action of verapamil on isolated cardiac muscle, but the direct myocardial depressant effects of verapamil may predominate when the drug is given in high doses. In patients with well-preserved left ventricular function, combined therapy with propranolol and verapamil appears to be well tolerated, but beta blockade can accentuate the hemodynamic depressant effects produced by oral verapamil. Patients who have reduced left ventricular function may not tolerate the combined blockade of beta receptors and slow channels, and thus in these patients verapamil and propranolol should be used in combination either cautiously or not at all. Verapamil decreases myocardial oxygen demand while decreasing coronary vascular resistance and reduces the extent of ischemic damage in experimental preparations. Such changes may be antiarrhythmic. Diltiazem also reduces ventricular arrhythmias during coronary occlusion in the dog, possibly by preventing calcium overload.

Peak alterations in hemodynamic variables occur 3 to 5 minutes after completion of a verapamil injection, with the major effects dissipating within 10 minutes. Systemic resistance and mean arterial pressure decrease, as does left ventricular dP/dt_{max}, and left ventricular end-diastolic pressure increases. Heart rate, cardiac index, left ventricular minute work, and mean pulmonary artery pressure do not change significantly. Thus, afterload reduction produced by verapamil significantly minimizes its negative inotropic action so that the cardiac index may not be reduced. In addition, when verapamil slows the ventricular rate in a patient with a tachycardia, cardiac slowing may also improve hemodynamics. Nevertheless, caution should be exercised when giving verapamil to patients with severe myocardial depression or those receiving beta blockers or disopyramide because hemodynamic deterioration may progress in some patients.

PHARMACOKINETICS (see Table 30–4). After single oral doses of verapamil, measurable prolongation of AV nodal conduction time occurs in 30 minutes and lasts 4 to 6 hours. After IV administration, AV nodal conduction delay occurs within 1 to 2 minutes and AH interval prolongation is still detectable after 6 hours. Effective plasma concentrations necessary to terminate SVT are in the range of 125 ng/ml after doses of 0.075 to 0.150 mg/kg. After oral administration, absorption is almost complete, but an overall bioavailability of 20 to 35 percent suggests substantial first-pass metabolism in the liver, particularly of the *l*-isomer. The elimination half-life of verapamil is 3 to 7 hours, with up to 70 percent of the drug excreted by the kidneys. Norverapamil is a major metabolite that may contribute to verapamil's electrophysiological actions. Serum protein binding is approximately 90 percent. With diltiazem, the percentage of heart rate reduction in atrial fibrillation is related to plasma concentration.

DOSAGE AND ADMINISTRATION (see Table 30–4). The most commonly used IV dose of verapamil is 10 mg infused over 1 to 2 minutes while cardiac rhythm and blood pressure are monitored. A second injection of equal dose may be given 30 minutes later. The initial effect achieved with the first bolus injection, such as slowing of the ventricular response during atrial fibrillation, may be maintained by a continuous infusion of the drug at a rate of 0.005 mg/kg/min. The oral dose is 240 to 480 mg/d in divided doses. Diltiazem is given intravenously at a dose of 0.25 mg/kg as a bolus over 2 minutes, with a second dose in 15 minutes if necessary; because it is generally better tolerated (less hypotension) for long-term administration, such as for control of ventricular rate during atrial fibrillation, diltiazem is preferred over verapamil in this setting. Orally, doses must be adjusted to the patient's needs, with a 120- to 360-mg range. Various long-acting preparations exist for verapamil and diltiazem.

INDICATIONS. After simple vagal maneuvers have been tried and adenosine given, IV verapamil or diltiazem is the next treatment of choice for terminating sustained sinus node reentry, AV node reentry, or orthodromic AV reciprocating tachycardia associated with an accessory pathway. Verapamil is as effective as adenosine for termination of these arrhythmias. Verapamil should definitely be tried before attempting termination by digitalis administration, pacing, electrical direct-current cardioversion, or acute blood pressure elevation with vasopressors. Verapamil and diltiazem terminate 60 to 90 percent or more episodes of paroxysmal SVTs within several minutes. Verapamil may be of use in some fetal SVTs as well. Although IV verapamil has been given along with IV propranolol, this combination should be used only with great caution.

Verapamil and diltiazem decrease the ventricular response over the AV node during atrial fibrillation or atrial flutter, possibly converting a small number of episodes to sinus rhythm, particularly if the atrial flutter or fibrillation is of recent onset. In addition, verapamil may prevent early recurrence of atrial fibrillation after cardioversion.[51] Some patients who exhibit atrial flutter may develop atrial fibrillation after verapamil administration. As noted earlier, in patients with preexcited ventricular complexes during atrial fibrillation associated with the Wolff-Parkinson-White syndrome, IV verapamil may accelerate the ventricular response; therefore, the IV route is contraindicated in this situation. Verapamil can terminate some ATs. Even though verapamil terminates a left septal VT, hemodynamic collapse can occur if IV verapamil is given to patients with the more common forms of VT because they generally occur in the setting of decreased left ventricular systolic function. A general rule to avoid complications, however, is not to administer IV verapamil to any patient with wide QRS tachycardia unless one is absolutely certain of the nature of the tachycardia and its response to verapamil.

Orally, verapamil or diltiazem can prevent the recurrence of AV node reentrant and orthodromic AV reciprocating tachycardias associated with the Wolff-Parkinson-White syndrome as well as help maintain a decreased ventricular response during atrial flutter or atrial fibrillation in patients without an accessory pathway. In this regard, the effectiveness of verapamil appears to be enhanced when given concomitantly with quinidine, and that of diltiazem is enhanced when given with digoxin. Verapamil generally has not been effective in treating patients who have recurrent ventricular tachyarrhythmias, although it may suppress some forms of VT, such as a left septal VT, as noted earlier. It may also be useful in about two thirds of patients with idiopathic VT that has a left bundle branch block morphology, in patients with hypertrophic cardiomyopathy who have experienced cardiac arrest, in patients with a short-coupled variant of torsades de pointes, in patients with right ventricular dysplasia, and in patients with ventricular arrhythmias related to coronary artery spasm. Whereas data from animal models suggest that verapamil may be useful in reducing or preventing ventricular arrhythmias related to acute myocardial ischemia, calcium antagonists have not been shown to reduce mortality or prevent sudden cardiac death in patients after acute myocardial infarction, except for diltiazem in patients with non-Q-wave infarctions. Verapamil abolishes the wall motion abnormality found in patients with the long QT syndrome.

ADVERSE EFFECTS. Verapamil must be used cautiously in patients with significant hemodynamic impairment or in those receiving beta blockers, as previously noted. Hypotension, bradycardia, AV block, and asystole are more likely to occur when the drug is given to patients who are already receiving beta-blocking agents. Hemodynamic collapse has been noted in infants, and verapamil should be used cautiously in patients younger than 1 year. Verapamil should also be used with caution in patients with sinus node abnormalities because marked depression of sinus node function or asystole can result in some of these patients. Isoproterenol, calcium, glucagon infusion, dopamine, or atropine (which may be only partially effective) or temporary pacing may be necessary to counteract some of the adverse effects of verapamil. Isoproterenol may be more effective for treating bradyarrhythmias and calcium may be used for treating hemodynamic dysfunction secondary to verapamil. AV node depression is common in overdoses. Contraindications to the use of verapamil and diltiazem include the presence of advanced heart failure, second- or third-degree AV block without a pacemaker in place, atrial fibrillation and anterograde conduction over an accessory pathway, significant sinus node dysfunction, most VTs, cardiogenic shock, and other hypotensive states. Although the drugs probably should not be used in patients with overt heart failure, if the latter is due to one of the supraventricular tachyarrhythmias noted earlier, verapamil or diltiazem may restore sinus rhythm or significantly decrease the ventricular rate, leading to hemodynamic improvement. Finally, it is important to note that verapamil can decrease the excretion of digoxin by about 30 percent. Hepatotoxicity may occur on occasion. Verapamil crosses the placental barrier; its use in pregnancy has been associated with impaired uterine contraction, fetal bradycardia, and, possibly, fetal digital defects. It should thus be used only if no good alternatives exist.

Other Antiarrhythmic Agents

Adenosine

Adenosine is an endogenous nucleoside present throughout the body and has been approved by the FDA to treat patients with SVTs.

ELECTROPHYSIOLOGICAL ACTIONS (see Tables 30–1, 30–2, 30–3, and 30–5). Adenosine interacts with A_1 receptors present on the extracellular surface of cardiac cells, activating K^+ channels ($I_{K\,Ach}$, $I_{K\,Ado}$) in a fashion similar to that produced by acetylcholine. The increase in K^+ conductance shortens atrial APD, hyperpolarizes the membrane potential, and decreases atrial contractility. Similar changes occur in the sinus and AV nodes. In contrast to these direct effects mediated through the guanine nucleotide regulatory proteins G_i and G_o, adenosine antagonizes catecholamine-stimulated adenylate cyclase to decrease cyclic adenosine monophosphate accumulation and to decrease $I_{Ca\text{-}L}$ and the pacemaker current I_f in sinus node cells, along with a decrease in $\dot{V}_{max}$. Shifts in pacemaker site within the sinus node and sinus exit block may occur. Adenosine slows the sinus rate in humans, which is followed by a reflex increase in sinus rate. In the N region of the AV node, conduction is depressed, along with decreases in action potential amplitude, duration, and $\dot{V}_{max}$. Transient prolongation of the AH interval results, often with transient first-, second-, or third-degree AV node block. Delay in AV nodal conduction is rate dependent. His-Purkinje conduction is generally not directly affected. Adenosine does not affect conduction in normal accessory pathways. Conduction may be blocked in accessory pathways that have long conduction times or decremental conduction properties. Patients with heart transplants exhibit a supersensitive response to adenosine. Adenosine may mediate the phenomenon of ischemic preconditioning.

PHARMACOKINETICS (see Table 30–4). Adenosine is removed from the extracellular space by washout, enzymatically by degradation to inosine, by phosphorylation to adenosine monophosphate, or by reuptake into cells through a nucleoside transport system. The vascular endothelium and the formed blood elements contain these elimination systems, which result in very rapid clearance of adenosine from the circulation. Elimination half-life is 1 to 6 seconds. Most of adenosine's effects are produced during its first passage through the circulation. Important drug interactions occur: methylxanthines are competitive antagonists, and therapeutic concentrations of theophylline totally block the exogenous adenosine effect. Dipyridamole is a nucleoside transport blocker that blocks reuptake of adenosine, delaying its clearance from the circulation or interstitial space and potentiating its effect. Smaller adenosine doses should be used in patients receiving dipyridamole.

DOSAGE AND ADMINISTRATION (see Table 30–4). To terminate tachycardia, a bolus of adenosine is rapidly injected intravenously at doses of 6 to 12 mg followed by a flush. Pediatric dosing should be 0.1 to 0.3 mg/kg. When given into a central vein and in patients after heart transplantation or in patients receiving dipyridamole, the initial dose should be reduced to 3 mg. Transient sinus slowing or AV node block results, lasting less than 5 seconds.

INDICATIONS. Adenosine has become the drug of first choice to terminate acutely an SVT such as AV node or AV reentry. It is useful in pediatric patients and to judge the effectiveness of ablation of accessory pathways. Adenosine can produce AV block or terminate ATs and sinus node reentry. It results in only transient AV block during atrial flutter or fibrillation and is thus useful only in their diagnosis (not therapy). Adenosine terminates a group of VTs whose maintenance depends on adrenergic drive, which is most often located in the right ventricular outflow tract but found at other sites as well. Adenosine has less potential than verapamil for lowering the blood pressure should tachycardia persist after injection.

Doses as low as 2.5 mg terminate some tachycardias; doses of 12 mg or less terminate 92 percent of SVTs, usually within 30 seconds. Successful termination rates with adenosine are comparable to those achieved with verapamil. Because of its effectiveness and extremely short duration of action, adenosine is preferable to verapamil in most instances, particularly in patients who previously received IV beta adrenoceptor blockers, in those having poorly compensated heart failure or severe hypotension, and in neonates. Verapamil might be chosen first in patients receiving drugs such as theophylline, which is known to interfere with adenosine's actions or metabolism; in patients with active bronchoconstriction; and in those with inadequate venous access.

Adenosine may be useful to help differentiate among causes of wide QRS tachycardias because it terminates many SVTs with aberrancy or reveals the underlying atrial mechanism, and it does not block conduction over an accessory pathway or terminate most VTs. Adenosine in rare cases terminates some VTs (characteristically those of right ventricular outflow tract origin), and therefore tachycardia termination is not completely diagnostic for an SVT. This agent may predispose to the development of atrial fibrillation and possibly can increase the ventricular response in patients with atrial fibrillation conducting over an accessory pathway. Adenosine may also be useful in differentiating conduction over the AV node from that over an accessory pathway during ablative procedures designed to interrupt the accessory pathway. However, this distinction is not absolute because adenosine can block conduction in slowly conducting accessory pathways and does not always effect block in the AV node. Endogenously released adenosine may be important in ischemia and hypoxia-induced AV node block and in post-defibrillation bradyarrhythmias.

ADVERSE EFFECTS. Transient side effects occur in almost 40 percent of patients with SVT given adenosine and are most commonly flushing, dyspnea, and chest pressure. These symptoms are fleeting, lasting less than 1 minute, and are well tolerated. PVCs, transient sinus bradycardia, sinus arrest, and AV block are common when an SVT abruptly terminates. Atrial fibrillation is occasionally observed (12 percent in one study) with adenosine administration,[52] perhaps owing to the drug's effect in shortening atrial refractoriness. Induction of atrial fibrillation can be problematic in patients with the Wolff-Parkinson-White syndrome and rapid AV conduction over the accessory pathway.

Digoxin

Cardiac actions of digitalis glycosides have been recognized for centuries. Digoxin is used for control of supraventricular arrhythmias, mainly control of ventricular rate during atrial fibrillation. The use of digoxin has decreased owing to the availability of agents with greater potency and a wider therapeutic-to-toxic drug concentration range.

ELECTROPHYSIOLOGICAL ACTIONS (see Tables 30-1, 30-2, 30-3, and 30-5). Digoxin acts mainly through the autonomic nervous system, in particular by enhancing both central and peripheral vagal tone. These actions are largely confined to slowing the sinus node discharge rate, shortening atrial refractoriness, and prolonging AV nodal refractoriness. Electrophysiological effects on the His-Purkinje system and ventricular muscle are minimal except in toxic concentrations. In studies of denervated hearts, digoxin has relatively little effect on the AV node and causes a mild increase in atrial refractoriness. Digoxin has a mild antiadrenergic effect in low doses but may enhance central sympathetic tone at higher concentrations, which may be important in the development of digitalis-toxic arrhythmias.

The sinus rate and P wave duration are minimally changed in most patients taking digoxin. The sinus rate may decrease in patients with heart failure whose left ventricular performance is improved by the drug; individuals with significant underlying sinus node disease also have slower sinus rates or even sinus arrest. Similarly, the PR interval is generally unchanged except in patients with underlying AV node disease. QRS and QT intervals are unaffected. The characteristic ST and T wave abnormalities seen with digoxin use do not represent toxicity.

PHARMACOKINETICS (see Table 30–4). Intravenously administered digoxin yields some electrophysiological effect within minutes, with a peak effect occurring after 1.5 to 3 hours. After oral dosing, the peak effect occurs in 4 to 6 hours. The extent of digoxin absorption after oral administration varies depending on the preparation: tablet forms are 60 to 75 percent absorbed, whereas encapsulated gel forms are almost completely absorbed. Ingestion of cholestyramine or an antacid preparation at the same time as digoxin ingestion decreases its absorption. The serum half-life of digoxin is 36 to 48 hours, and the drug is excreted unchanged by the kidneys.

DOSAGE AND ADMINISTRATION (see Table 30–4). In acute loading doses of 0.5 to 1.0 mg, digoxin may be given intravenously or by mouth. Chronic daily oral dosing should be adjusted on the basis of clinical indications and the extent of renal dysfunction. Most patients require from 0.125 to 0.25 mg/d as a single dose; however, as little as 0.125 mg every other day is needed in some patients receiving renal dialysis, whereas young patients may require as much as 0.5 mg/d. Serum digoxin levels may be used to monitor compliance with therapy as well as to determine whether digitalis toxicity is the cause of new symptoms compatible with the diagnosis. However, routine monitoring of digoxin levels is not warranted in patients whose ventricular rate is controlled during atrial fibrillation and who have no symptoms of toxicity.

A large number of pharmacokinetic interactions have been described for digoxin, the most important being with quinidine (which increases serum digoxin concentrations by displacing the drug from tissue binding sites and decreasing renal clearance).

INDICATIONS. Digoxin can be used intravenously to slow the ventricular rate during atrial fibrillation and flutter; it has been used in the past to attempt to convert SVTs to sinus rhythm, but its onset of action is much slower and its success rate less than that of adenosine, verapamil, or beta blockers; thus, it is rarely used in this way at present. Digoxin is more commonly used orally to control the ventricular rate in chronic atrial fibrillation. When the patient with atrial fibrillation is at rest and vagal tone predominates, the ventricular rate can be maintained between 60 and 100 beats/min in 40 to 60 percent of cases. However, when the patient begins to exercise, the decrease in vagal tone and increase in adrenergic tone combine to diminish digoxin's beneficial effects on AV nodal conduction. Patients may experience a marked increase in ventricular rate with even mild exertion. Thus, digoxin is rarely used as a single agent to control the ventricular rate in chronic atrial fibrillation. The drug has little capacity to prevent episodes of paroxysmal atrial fibrillation or to control ventricular rate during episodes. Finally, digoxin is no more effective than placebo at terminating episodes of acute- or recent-onset atrial fibrillation.

ADVERSE EFFECTS. One of the main reasons why digoxin use has decreased is the potential for serious adverse effects and the narrow window between therapeutic and toxic concentrations. Digitalis toxicity produces a variety of symptoms and signs, including headache, nausea and vomiting, altered color perception, halo vision, and generalized malaise. More serious than these are digitalis-related arrhythmias. These include bradycardias related to a markedly enhanced vagal effect (sinus bradycardia or arrest, AV node block) and tachyarrhythmias that may be due to delayed afterdepolarization–mediated triggered activity (atrial, junctional, and fascicular or ventricular tachycardia). Worsening renal function, advanced age, hypokalemia, chronic lung disease, hypothyroidism, and amyloidosis increase the patient's sensitivity to digitalis-related arrhythmias. The diagnosis can be confirmed using serum digoxin levels. Therapy for most bradycardias consists of withdrawal of digoxin; atropine or temporary pacing may be needed in symptomatic patients. Phenytoin can be used for control of atrial tachyarrhythmias, whereas lidocaine has been successful in treating infranodal tachycardias. Life-threatening arrhythmias can be treated with digoxin-specific antibody fragments. Electrical direct-current cardioversion should be performed only when absolutely necessary in the digitalis-toxic patient because life-threatening VT or VF can result, which can be very difficult to control.

Electrotherapy of Cardiac Arrhythmias

Direct-Current Electrical Cardioversion

Electrical cardioversion offers obvious advantages over drug therapy in terminating tachycardia. Under conditions optimal for close supervision and monitoring, a precisely regulated "dose" of electricity can restore sinus rhythm immediately and safely. The distinction between supraventricular and ventricular tachyarrhythmias—crucial to the proper medical management of arrhythmias—becomes less significant, and the time-consuming titration of drugs with potential side effects is obviated.

MECHANISMS. Electrical cardioversion appears to terminate most effectively the tachycardias related to reentry, such as atrial flutter and many cases of atrial fibrillation, AV node reentry, reciprocating tachycardias associated with the Wolff-Parkinson-White syndrome, most forms of VT, ventricular flutter, and VF. The electrical shock, by depolarizing all excitable myocardium and possibly by prolonging refractoriness, interrupts reentrant circuits and establishes electrical homogeneity that terminates reentry. The mechanism by which a shock successfully terminates VF has not been completely explained. If the precipitating factors are no longer present, interrupting the tachyarrhythmia for only the brief time produced by the shock may prevent its return for long periods even though the anatomical and electrophysiological substrates required for the tachycardia are still present.

Tachycardias thought to be due to disorders of impulse formation (automaticity) include parasystole, some forms of AT, ectopic junctional tachycardia (with or without digitalis toxicity), accelerated idioventricular rhythm, and rare forms of VT. An attempt to cardiovert these tachycardias electrically is not indicated in most instances because they typically recur within seconds after the shock. It has not been established whether cardioversion can terminate tachycardias caused by enhanced automaticity or triggered activity.

TECHNIQUE. Before *elective* cardioversion, a careful physical examination, including palpation of all pulses, should be performed. A 12-lead electrocardiogram is obtained before and after cardioversion, as well as a rhythm strip during the electroshock. The patient, who should be informed completely about what to expect, is in a fasting state and "metabolically balanced"; that is, blood gases, pH, and electrolytes should be normal with no evidence of drug toxicity. Withholding digitalis for several days before elective cardioversion in patients without clinical evidence of digitalis toxicity is not necessary, although patients in whom digitalis toxicity is suspected should not be electrically cardioverted until this situation is corrected. Maintenance antiarrhythmic drug administration 1 to 2 days before electrical cardioversion of patients with atrial fibrillation can revert some patients to sinus rhythm, help prevent recurrence of atrial fibrillation once sinus rhythm is restored, and help determine the patient's tolerance for the drug.

Self-adhesive pads applied in the standard apicoanterior or apicoposterior paddle positions have transthoracic impedances similar to those of paddles and are useful in elective cardioversions or other situations in which there is time for their application. Paddles 12 to 13 cm in diameter can be used to deliver maximum current to the heart, but the benefits of these paddles compared with those of paddles 8 to 9 cm in diameter have not been clearly established. Larger paddles may distribute the intracardiac current over a wider area and may reduce shock-induced myocardial necrosis.

A synchronized shock (i.e., one delivered during the QRS complex) is used for all cardioversions except for very rapid ventricular tachyarrhythmias, such as ventricular flutter or VF (Fig. 30–2). Although generally minimal, shock-related myocardial damage increases directly with increases in applied energy, and thus the minimum effective energy should be used. Therefore, shocks are "titrated" when the clinical situation permits. Except for atrial fibrillation, shocks in the range of 25 to 50 joules successfully terminate most SVTs and should be tried initially. If unsuccessful, a second shock of higher energy can be delivered. The starting level to terminate atrial fibrillation with older monophasic machines should be no less than 100 joules, but with newer biphasic systems, energies as little as 25 joules may succeed.[53] Delivered energy can be increased in a stepwise fashion; up to 360 joules can be used safely. Anteroposterior pads may have a higher efficacy rate by placing more of the atrial mass in the shock vector than is the case for apicoanterior pads. If a shock of 360 joules fails to convert the rhythm, repeated shocks at the same energy may succeed by decreasing chest wall impedance; reversing pad polarity can occasionally help as well. Administration of ibutilide has been shown to facilitate electrical cardioversion of atrial fibrillation to sinus rhythm. Intracardiac defibrillation can be tried if all attempts at external cardioversion fail. For patients with stable VT, starting levels in the range of 25 to 50 joules can be employed. If there is some urgency to terminate the tachyarrhythmia, one can begin with higher energies. To terminate VF, 100 to 200 joules (biphasic; 200 to 360 joules with monophasic machines) is generally used, although much lower energies (<50 joules) terminate VF when the shock is delivered at the onset of the arrhythmia, using adhesive pads in the electrophysiology laboratory, for example.

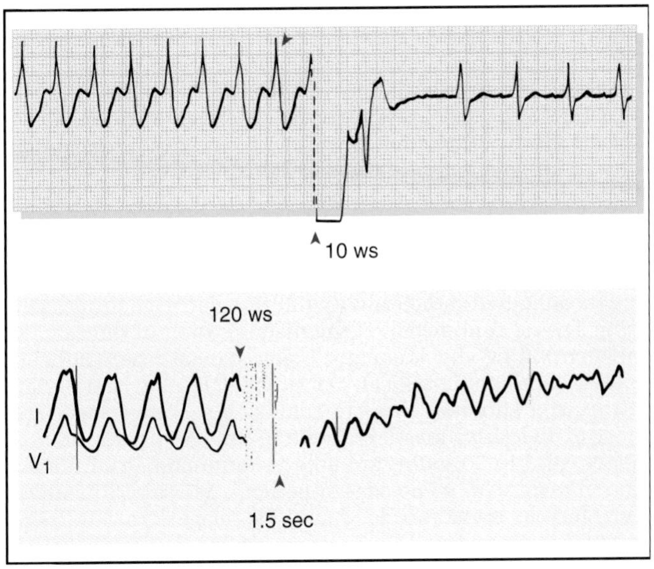

FIGURE 30–2 **Top,** A synchronized shock (note synchronization marks in the apex of the QRS complex [arrow]) during ventricular tachycardia is followed by a single repetitive ventricular response and then normal sinus rhythm. **Bottom,** A shock synchronized to the terminal portion of the QRS complex (arrow) in a patient with atrial fibrillation and conduction to the ventricle over an accessory pathway (Wolff-Parkinson-White syndrome) resulted in ventricular fibrillation that was promptly terminated by a 400-joule shock. Recording was lost for 1.5 seconds (arrow) owing to baseline drift after the shock. ws = watt seconds.

During elective cardioversion, a short-acting barbiturate such as methohexital, a sedative such as propofol, or an amnesic such as diazepam or midazolam can be used. A physician skilled in airway management should be in attendance, an IV route should be established, and pulse oximetry, the electrocardiogram, and blood pressure should be monitored. All equipment necessary for emergency resuscitation should be immediately accessible. Before cardioversion, 100 percent oxygen may be administered for 5 to 15 minutes by nasal cannula or face mask and is continued throughout the procedure. Manual ventilation of the patient may be necessary to avoid hypoxia during periods of deepest sedation. Adequate sedation of the patient undergoing even urgent cardioversion is essential; some patients who have needlessly been shocked while awake (because of uneasiness of the physician with the arrhythmia) have declined further medical care for their arrhythmias because of concern that they would again undergo cardioversion without appropriate sedation.

In up to 5 percent of patients with atrial fibrillation, sinus rhythm cannot be restored by external countershock despite all the preceding measures including ibutilide pretreatment and biphasic shocks. It is important to distinguish between inability to attain sinus rhythm, indicating inadequate energy delivery to the atria, and inability to maintain sinus rhythm following transient termination of fibrillation; the latter condition (early reinitiation of atrial fibrillation) does not respond to higher energy shocks because fibrillation has already been terminated (but quickly recurs). Pretreatment with an antiarrhythmic drug may help maintain sinus rhythm after subsequent shocks. Patients in whom atrial fibrillation simply cannot be terminated with external shock tend to be very obese or have severe obstructive lung disease. In such cases, internal cardioversion can be performed using specially configured catheters with multiple large electrodes covering several centimeters of the distal portion of the catheter for distributing shock energy. Using standard percutaneous access, these catheters can be situated in the lateral right atrium and coronary sinus to achieve a shock vector across most of the atrial mass. With such configurations, internal shocks of 2 to 15 joules are able to terminate atrial fibrillation in more than 90 percent of patients whose arrhythmia is refractory to transthoracic shock. Esophageal cardioversion has also been reported.

INDICATIONS. As a rule, any tachycardia that produces hypotension, congestive heart failure, or angina and does not respond promptly to medical management should be terminated electrically. Very rapid ventricular rates in patients with atrial fibrillation and Wolff-Parkinson-White syndrome are often best treated by electrical cardioversion. In almost all instances, the patient's hemodynamic status improves after cardioversion. An occasional patient may experience hypotension, reduced cardiac output, or congestive heart failure after the shock. This problem may be related to complications of the cardioversion, such as embolic events, myocardial depression resulting from the anesthetic agent or the shock itself, hypoxia, lack of restoration of left atrial contraction despite return of electrical atrial systole, or postshock arrhythmias. Direct-current countershock of digitalis-induced tachyarrhythmias is contraindicated.

Favorable candidates for electrical cardioversion of atrial fibrillation include patients who (1) have symptomatic atrial fibrillation of less than 12 months' duration and derive significant hemodynamic benefits from sinus rhythm, (2) continue to have atrial fibrillation after the precipitating cause has been removed (e.g., after treatment of thyrotoxicosis), and (3) have a rapid ventricular rate that is difficult to slow. In patients who have indications for chronic warfarin therapy to prevent stroke, the hope of avoiding anticoagulation by restoring sinus rhythm is not a reason to attempt cardioversion because these patients are still at increased risk for thromboembolic events. Several large trials[54] have shown that maintenance of sinus rhythm confers no survival advantage over rate control and anticoagulation; thus, not all patients with newly discovered atrial fibrillation warrant an attempt at restoring sinus rhythm. Treatment must be determined individually.

Unfavorable candidates include patients with (1) digitalis toxicity, (2) no symptoms and a well-controlled ventricular rate without therapy, (3) sinus node dysfunction and various unstable supraventricular tachyarrhythmias or bradyarrhythmias (often the bradycardia-tachycardia syndrome) who finally develop and maintain atrial fibrillation (which in essence represents a "cure" for the sick sinus syndrome), (4) little or no symptomatic improvement with normal sinus rhythm who promptly revert to atrial fibrillation after cardioversion despite drug therapy, (5) a large left atrium and longstanding atrial fibrillation, (6) infrequent episodes of atrial fibrillation that revert spontaneously to sinus rhythm, (7) no mechanical atrial systole after the return of electrical atrial systole, (8) atrial fibrillation and advanced heart block, (9) cardiac surgery planned in the near future, and (10) antiarrhythmic drug intolerance. Atrial fibrillation is likely to recur after cardioversion in patients who have significant chronic obstructive lung disease, congestive heart failure, mitral valve disease (particularly mitral regurgitation), atrial fibrillation longer than 1 year, and an enlarged left atrium (>4.5 cm by echocardiography).

In patients with atrial flutter, slowing the ventricular rate by administering digitalis or terminating the flutter with an antiarrhythmic agent may be difficult, and electrical cardioversion is often the initial treatment of choice. For the patient with other types of SVT, electrical cardioversion may be employed when (1) vagal maneuvers or simple medical management (e.g., IV adenosine and verapamil) has failed to terminate the tachycardia and (2) the clinical setting indicates that fairly prompt restoration of sinus rhythm is desirable because of hemodynamic decompensation or electrophysiological consequences of the tachycardia. Similarly, in patients with VT, the hemodynamic and electrophysiological consequences of the arrhythmias determine the need for and urgency of direct-current cardioversion. Electrical countershock is the initial treatment of choice for ventricular flutter or VF. Speed is essential.

If, after the first shock, reversion of the arrhythmia to sinus rhythm does not occur, a higher energy level should be tried. When transient ventricular arrhythmias result after an unsuccessful shock, a bolus of lidocaine can be given before delivering a shock at the next energy level. If sinus rhythm returns only transiently and is promptly supplanted by the tachycardia, a repeated shock can be tried, depending on the tachyarrhythmia being treated and its consequences. Administration of an antiarrhythmic agent intravenously may be useful before delivering the next cardioversion shock (such as ibutilide in resistant atrial fibrillation). After cardioversion, the patient should be monitored at least until full consciousness has been restored and preferably for several hours thereafter, depending on the duration of recovery from the particular form of sedation or anesthesia used. If ibutilide has been given, the electrocardiogram should be monitored for up to 8 hours because torsades de pointes can develop in the first few hours after administration.

RESULTS. Cardioversion restores sinus rhythm in 70 to 95 percent of patients, depending on the type of tachyarrhythmia. However, sinus rhythm remains after 12 months in less than one third to one half of the patients with chronic atrial fibrillation. Thus, maintenance of sinus rhythm, once established, is the difficult problem, not the immediate termination of the tachycardia. The likelihood of maintaining sinus rhythm depends on the particular arrhythmia, the presence of underlying heart disease, and the response to antiarrhythmic drug therapy. Atrial size decreases after termination of atrial fibrillation and restoration of sinus rhythm, and functional capacity improves.

COMPLICATIONS. Arrhythmias induced by electrical cardioversion are generally caused by inadequate synchronization, with the shock occurring during the ST segment or T wave. Occasionally, a properly synchronized shock can produce VF (see Fig. 30–2). Postshock arrhythmias are usually transient and do not require therapy. Embolic episodes are reported to occur in 1 to 3 percent of the patients converted from atrial fibrillation to sinus rhythm. Prior therapeutic anticoagulation (international normalized ratio, 2.0 to 3.0) consistently for at least 3 weeks should be employed for patients who have no contraindication to such therapy and have had atrial fibrillation present for longer than 2 to 3 days or of indeterminate duration. This approach is particularly true for those who are at high risk for emboli, such as those with mitral stenosis and atrial fibrillation of recent onset, a history of recent or recurrent emboli, a prosthetic mitral valve, an enlarged heart (including left atrial enlargement), or congestive heart failure. (It is important to note that 3 weeks of therapeutic anticoagulation is not the same as simply administering warfarin for 3 weeks.) Anticoagulation with warfarin for at least 4 weeks afterward is recommended because restoration of atrial mechanical function lags behind that of electrical systolic function, and thrombi can still form in largely akinetic atria, although they are electrocardiographically in sinus rhythm. Exclusion of left atrial thrombus by transesophageal echocardiography may not always preclude embolism after cardioversion of atrial fibrillation. Atrial thrombi may be present in patients with nonfibrillation atrial tachyarrhythmias such as atrial flutter and AT in patients with congenital heart disease.[55] The same precardioversion and postcardioversion anticoagulation recommendations apply to these patients as well as to those with atrial fibrillation. Although direct-current shock has been demonstrated in animals to cause myocardial injury, studies in humans indicate that elevations of myocardial enzymes after cardioversion are not common. ST segment elevation (sometimes dramatic) can occur immediately after elective direct-current cardioversion and last for 1 to 2 minutes, although cardiac enzymes and myocardial scintigraphy may be unremarkable. ST elevation lasting longer than 2 minutes usually indicates myocardial injury unrelated to the shock. A decrease in serum K^+ and Mg^{2+} can occur after cardioversion of VT.

Cardioversion of VT can also be achieved by a chest thump. Its mechanism of termination is probably related to a mechanically induced PVC that interrupts a tachycardia and may be related to commotio cordis (see Chap. 75). The thump cannot be timed very well and is probably effective only when delivered during a nonrefractory part of the cardiac cycle. The thump can alter a VT and possibly induce ventricular flutter or VF if it occurs during the vulnerable period of the T wave. Because there may be a slightly greater likelihood of converting a stable VT to VF than of terminating VT to sinus rhythm, the thump version should not be attempted unless a defibrillator is simply unavailable.

Implantable Electrical Devices for Treatment of Cardiac Arrhythmias

Implantable devices that monitor the cardiac rhythm and can deliver competing pacing stimuli and low- and high-energy shocks have been used effectively in selected patients and are discussed fully in Chapter 31.

Ablation Therapy for Cardiac Arrhythmias

The purpose of catheter ablation is to destroy myocardial tissue by delivering electrical energy over electrodes on a catheter placed next to an area of the endocardium integrally related to the onset or maintenance of the arrhythmia, or both. The first catheter ablation procedures were performed using direct-current shocks, but this energy source has been almost wholly supplanted by radiofrequency (RF) energy, which is delivered from an external generator and destroys tissue by controlled heat production.[56] Lasers and microwave energy sources have been used, but not commonly; cryothermal catheter ablation has been approved for use in humans.[57] When a target tissue has been identified at EPS, the tip of the ablation catheter is maneuvered into apposition with this tissue. After stable catheter position and recordings have been ensured, RF energy is delivered between the catheter tip and an indifferent electrode, usually an electrocautery-type grounding pad on the skin of the patient's thigh. Because energies in the RF portion of the electromagnetic spectrum are poorly conducted by cardiac tissue, RF energy instead causes resistive heating in the cells in close proximity to the catheter tip (i.e., these cells transduce the electrical energy into thermal energy). When the tissue temperature exceeds 50°C, irreversible cellular damage and tissue death occur. An expanding front of conducted heat emanates from the region of resistive heating while RF delivery continues, resulting in production of a homogenous hemispheric lesion of coagulative necrosis 3 to 5 mm in radius (Fig. 30–3). RF-induced heating of tissue that has inherent automaticity (His bundle, foci of automatic tachycardias) results in acceleration of a rhythm, whereas RF delivery during a reentrant arrhythmia typically causes slowing and termination of the arrhythmia. In most cases, RF delivery is painless, although ablation of atrial or RV tissue can be uncomfortable for some patients.

COOLED-TIP RADIOFREQUENCY ABLATION. There are situations in which the catheter can be delivered to the correct location but conventional RF energy delivery is unable to eliminate the tachycardia. In some such cases, the amount of damage (either depth or breadth) caused by standard RF is inadequate. Using standard RF, power delivery is usually regulated to maintain a preset catheter tip temperature (typically 55° to 70°C). Tip temperatures greater than 90°C are associated with coagulation of blood elements on the electrode that preclude further energy delivery and could also become detached and embolize. Cooling the catheter tip, by either internal circulation of liquid or continuous fluid infusion through the tip electrode, can prevent excessive heating of the tip and allow greater power delivery, thus effecting a larger lesion size and potentially enhancing efficacy. Cooled-tip ablation has been used to good advantage in cases in which standard (4-mm tip) catheter ablation has failed as well as for primary therapy in atrial flutter and some cases of VT associated with structural heart disease, in which additional damage to already diseased areas is not harmful and may be required to achieve the desired result.[58]

Catheter-delivered cryoablation causes tissue damage by freezing cellular structures. Nitrous oxide is delivered to the catheter tip, where it is allowed to boil, cooling the tip electrode, after which the gas is circulated back to the delivery console. Catheter tip temperature can be regulated, cooling to as low as –70°C. Cooling to 0°C causes reversible loss of function and can be used as a diagnostic test (i.e., termination of a tachycardia when the catheter is in contact with a group of cells critical to its perpetuation). The catheter tip can then be cooled more deeply to effect permanent damage and thus cure of the arrhythmia. Cryoablation appears to cause less endocardial damage and may thus engender less risk of thromboemboli following ablation.[59]

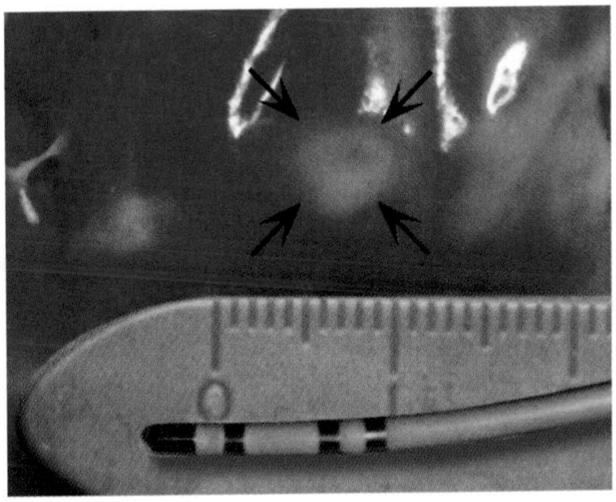

FIGURE 30–3 Radiofrequency lesion in human ventricular myocardium (explanted heart at the time of transplantation). A 30-second application of energy was made at the location denoted by arrows using the tip of the catheter shown. The lesion is 5 mm in diameter and has a clear border. A central depression in the lesion results from partial desiccation of tissue.

RADIOFREQUENCY CATHETER ABLATION OF ACCESSORY PATHWAYS

LOCATION OF PATHWAYS. The safety, efficacy, and cost-effectiveness of RF catheter ablation of an accessory AV pathway have made ablation the treatment of choice in most adult and many pediatric patients who have AV reentrant tachycardia (AVRT) or atrial flutter or fibrillation associated with a rapid ventricular response over the accessory pathway. However, the fact that the lesion size, when RF energy is delivered to an immature heart, can increase as the heart grows makes the long-term outlook for ablation less certain in the very young. RF energy has replaced direct-current shock as the optimal energy source.

An EPS is performed initially to determine that the accessory pathway is part of the tachycardia circuit or capable of rapid AV conduction during atrial fibrillation and to localize the accessory pathway (the optimal site for ablation). Pathways can exist in the right or left free wall or septum of the heart (Fig. 30-4). Septal accessory pathways are further classified as anteroseptal, midseptal, and posteroseptal. Rare parahisian pathways can be distinguished from anteroseptal pathways. Midseptal locations are true septal pathways, whereas those classified as anteroseptal generally have no septal connection but are located anteriorly along the central fibrous body or the right fibrous trigone at the right anterior free wall. Pathways classified as posteroseptal are located posterior to the central fibrous body within the so-called pyramidal space, which is bounded by the posterior superior process of the left ventricle and the inferomedial aspects of both atria. Anteroseptal pathways are found near the His bundle, and accessory pathway activation potential as well as His bundle potential can be recorded simultaneously from a catheter placed at the His bundle region. Midseptal pathways are classified as right midseptal if an accessory pathway potential is recorded through a catheter located in an area bounded anteriorly by the tip electrode of the His bundle catheter and posteriorly by the coronary sinus ostium. Pathways that are located in a similar region but can be ablated only from a left-sided approach are called left midseptal pathways. Right posteroseptal pathways insert along the tricuspid ring in the immediate vicinity of the coronary sinus ostium, whereas left posteroseptal pathways are close to the terminal portion of the coronary sinus and may be located at a subepicardial site around the proximal coronary sinus, within a middle cardiac vein or coronary sinus diverticulum, or subendocardially along the ventricular aspect of the mitral annulus. Pathways at all locations and in all age groups can be ablated successfully. Multiple pathways are present in about 5 percent of patients. Occasional epicardial locations may be more easily approached from within the coronary sinus. Rarely, pathways may connect an atrial appendage with adjacent ventricular epicardium, 2 cm or more from the AV groove (see Chap. 32).

ABLATION SITE. The optimal ablation site can be found by direct recordings of the accessory pathway (Fig. 30-5), although deflections that mimic accessory pathway potentials can be recorded at other sites. The ventricular insertion site can be determined by finding the site of the earliest onset of the ventricular electrogram in relation to the onset of the delta wave. Other helpful guidelines are unfiltered unipolar recordings that register a QS wave and the shortest AV conduction time during maximal preexcitation. A major ventricular potential synchronous with the onset of the delta wave can be a target site in left-sided preexcitation, whereas earlier ventricular excitation in relation to the delta wave can be found for right-sided preexcitation. The atrial insertion site of manifest or concealed pathways (i.e., delta wave present or absent, respectively) can be found by locating the site showing the shortest ventriculoatrial interval during retrograde conduction over the pathway. Reproducible mechanical inhibition of accessory pathway conduction during catheter manipulation and subthreshold stimulation have also been used to determine the optimal site. Accidental catheter trauma should be avoided, however, because it can "hide" the target for prolonged periods. Intracardiac echocardiography can be helpful at times in

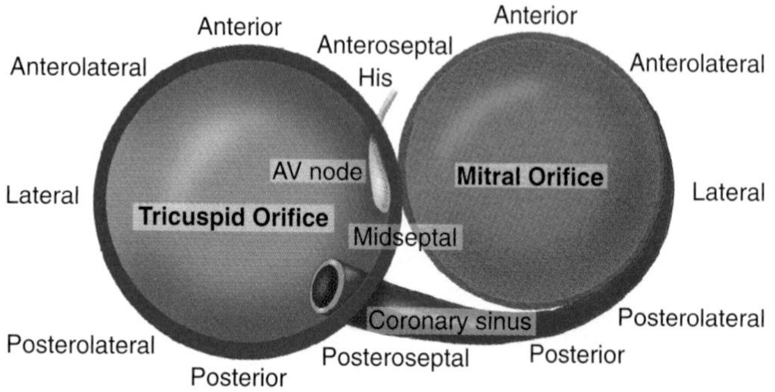

FIGURE 30–4 Locations of accessory pathways by anatomical region. Tricuspid and mitral valve annuli are depicted in a left anterior oblique view. Locations of coronary sinus, atrioventricular node, and bundle of His are shown. Accessory pathways may connect atrial to ventricular myocardium in any of the regions shown. AV = atrioventricular.

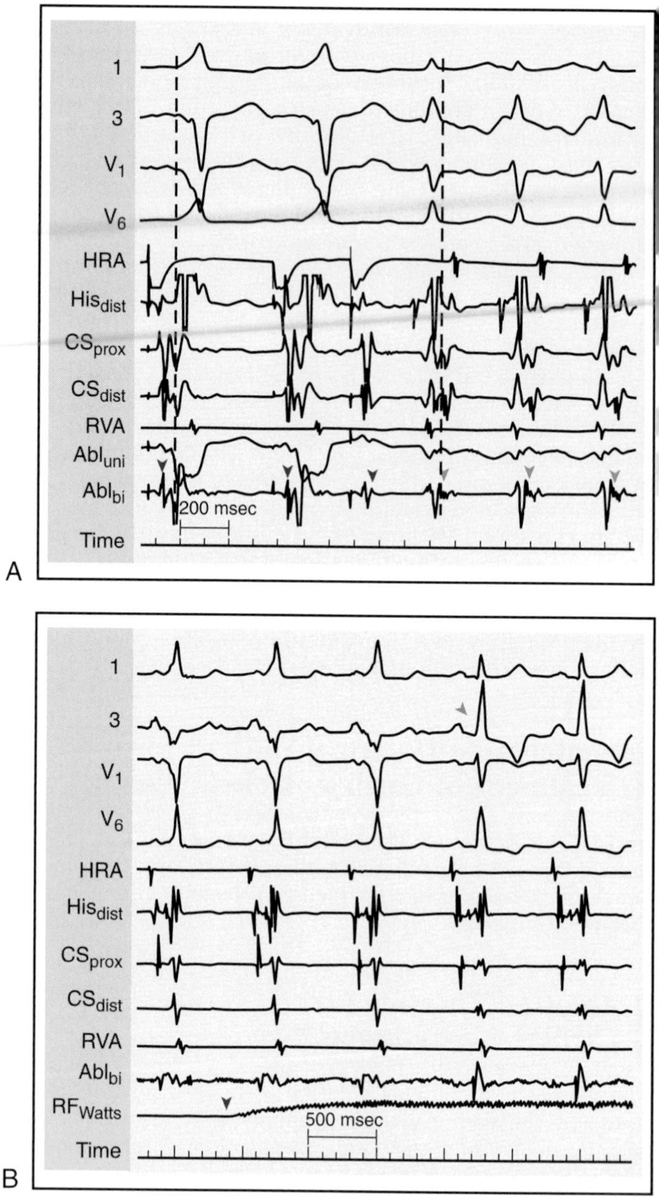

FIGURE 30–5 Wolff-Parkinson-White syndrome. Surface ECG leads 1, 3, V_1, and V_6 are shown with intracardiac recordings from high right atrium (HRA), distal His (His_{dist}) bundle region, proximal (CS_{prox}) and distal (CS_{dist}) coronary sinus, right ventricular apex (RVA), and unipolar (Abl_{uni}) and bipolar (Abl_{bi}) tip electrodes of ablation catheter. Radiofrequency powers in watts (RF_{Watts}) is also shown. **A,** Two beats of atrial pacing are conducted over the accessory pathway (blue arrows in Abl_{bi} recording, from the site of the accessory pathway) resulting in a delta wave on the electrocardiogram; a premature atrial stimulus (center) encounters accessory pathway refractoriness (red arrow) instead conducting over the atrioventricular (AV) node and bundle of His, resulting in a narrow QRS complex and starting an episode of AV reentrant tachycardia. After each narrow QRS complex is an atrial deflection, the earliest portion of which is recorded at the ablation site (green arrows). **B,** Ablation of this pathway is accomplished by delivery of radiofrequency (RF) energy from the ablation catheter tip. Blue arrow denotes onset of radiofrequency energy delivery; two QRS complexes later, the delta wave is abruptly lost (green arrow in lead 3) owing to elimination of conduction over the accessory pathway. T wave inversion in lead 3 is due to "memory" (see Chap. 32).

delineating unusual anatomy, guiding atrial septal puncture for left-sided access, and determining adequacy of catheter contact at ablation sites.

Left-sided accessory pathways often cross the mitral annulus obliquely. Consequently, the earliest site of retrograde atrial activation and the earliest site of anterograde ventricular activation are not directly across the AV groove from each other. Identification of the earliest site of atrial activation is usually performed during orthodromic AVRT or during relatively rapid ventricular pacing, so that retrograde conduction using the AV node does not confuse assessment of the location of the earliest atrial activation.

Successful ablation sites should exhibit stable fluoroscopic and electrical characteristics. During sinus rhythm, the local ventricular activation at the successful ablation site precedes the onset of the ECG delta wave by 10 to 35 milliseconds; during orthodromic AVRT, the interval between the onset of ventricular activation in any lead and local atrial activation is usually 70 to 90 milliseconds (see Fig. 30–5). When thermocouple- or thermistor-tipped ablation catheters are used, a stable rise in catheter tip temperature is a helpful indicator of catheter stability and adequate contact between the catheter and tissue.[60] In such an instance, the tip temperature generally exceeds 50°C. The retrograde transaortic and transseptal approaches have been used with equal success to ablate accessory pathways located along the mitral annulus. Routine EPS performed weeks after the ablation procedure is generally not indicated but should be considered in patients who have recurrent delta wave or symptoms of tachycardia. Catheter-delivered cryoablation may be useful in patients with septal accessory pathways (located near the AV conduction system). Using this system, the catheter tip and adjacent tissue can be reversibly cooled to test a potential site. If the accessory pathway conduction fails while normal AV conduction is preserved, deeper cooling can be performed at the site to complete the ablation. If, however, normal AV conduction is damaged, allowing the catheter to rewarm results in no permanent damage.

Patients with atriofascicular accessory pathways have connections consisting of a proximal portion responsible for conduction delay and decremental conduction properties and a long distal segment located along the endocardial surface of the right ventricular free wall that has electrophysiological properties similar to those of the right bundle branch. The distal end of the right atriofascicular accessory pathway can insert into the apical region of the right ventricular free wall close to the distal right bundle branch or can actually fuse with the latter. Right atriofascicular accessory pathways may actually represent a duplication of the AV conduction system and can be localized for ablation by recording potentials from the rapidly conducting distal component crossing the tricuspid annulus (analogous to the His bundle) and extending to the apical region of the right ventricular free wall. Ablation attempts should be performed more proximally to avoid inadvertently ablating the distal right bundle branch, which could actually be proarrhythmic and create incessant tachycardia by lengthening the reentrant circuit.

Indications. Ablation of accessory pathways is indicated in patients with symptomatic AVRT that is drug resistant or when the patient is drug intolerant or does not desire long-term drug therapy. It is also indicated in patients with atrial fibrillation (or other atrial tachyarrhythmias) and a rapid ventricular response by means of an accessory pathway when the tachycardia is drug resistant or when the patient is drug intolerant or does not desire long-term drug therapy. Other potential candidates include patients with AVRT or atrial fibrillation with rapid ventricular rates identified during EPS of another arrhythmia; asymptomatic patients with ventricular preexcitation whose livelihood, profession, important activities, insurability, mental well-being, or the public safety would be affected by spontaneous tachyarrhythmias or by the presence of the ECG abnormality; patients with atrial fibrillation and a controlled ventricular response by means of the accessory pathway; and patients with a family history of sudden cardiac death. Not all patients with accessory pathways need treatment; however, ablation has such a high success rate and low complication rate that in many centers patients who need any form of therapy are referred for catheter ablation.

Results. From the results of an early survey conducted by the North American Society of Pacing and Electrophysiology (NASPE),[61] successful ablation of left free wall accessory pathways was achieved in 2312 of 2527 (91 percent) patients; of septal accessory pathways, in 1115 of 1279 (87 percent); and of right free wall accessory pathways, in 585 of 715 (82 percent). Significant complications were reported in 94 of 4521 patients (2.1 percent), and there were 13 procedure-related deaths in 4521 studies of patients (0.2 percent). An update of this survey tallied only 651 accessory pathway ablation cases, among which successful ablation was achieved in 94 percent with a 2 percent complication rate and no deaths.[62] In Europe, the complication rate was 4.4 percent, with 3 deaths in 2222 patients.[49] A large study of patients using a temperature-controlled ablation system had similar success rates (overall success, 398 of 465 [93 percent] with an 8 percent recurrence rate).[60]

RADIOFREQUENCY CATHETER MODIFICATION OF THE AV NODE FOR AV NODAL REENTRANT TACHYCARDIAS. AV node reentry is a common cause of SVT episodes. Although controversy still exists about the exact nature of the tachycardia circuit, abundant evidence indicates that two pathways in the region of the AV node participate, one with relatively fast conduction but long refractoriness and the other with shorter refractoriness but slower conduction.[64] PACs can encounter refractoriness in the fast pathway, conduct down the slow pathway, and reenter the fast pathway retrogradely, initiating AV nodal reentrant SVT (Fig. 30–6). Although this is the most common presentation of AV node reentry, some patients have what appears to be propagation in the opposite direction in this circuit (anterograde fast, retrograde slow) as well as a "slow-slow" variant. Two or more of these variants can exist in the same patient (Fig. 30–7).

FAST-PATHWAY ABLATION. Ablation can be performed to eliminate conduction in the fast pathway or the slow pathway. In ablating the fast pathway, the electrode tip is positioned along the AV node–His bundle axis in the anterosuperior portion of the tricuspid annulus. The catheter is gradually withdrawn until the atrial electrogram amplitude equals or exceeds that of the ventricular electrogram and the His bundle recording is either absent or extremely small (0.05 mV). During energy delivery, the electrocardiogram is monitored for PR prolongation or the occurrence of AV block, or both. If accelerated junctional rhythm is noted during delivery of RF energy, the atrium can be paced at a faster rate to ensure integrity of AV conduction. The initial RF pulse is delivered at 15 to 20 watts for 10 to 15 seconds and gradually increased. Endpoints are PR prolongation, elimination of retrograde fast-pathway conduction, and noninducibility of AVNRT. An alternative approach is to apply RF current at the site of earliest retrograde atrial activation during tachycardia. RF current should be discontinued if the PR interval is prolonged by more than 50 percent or if AV block results. At present, fast-pathway ablation is rarely performed because it is associated with a prolonged PR interval, a higher recurrence rate (10 to 15 percent). and a slightly higher risk of complete AV block (2 to 5 percent) compared with slow-pathway ablation. One uncommon situation in which fast-pathway ablation may be preferred is in patients who have a markedly prolonged PR interval at rest and no evidence of anterograde fast-pathway conduction. In such cases, ablation of the anterograde slow pathway may produce complete AV block, whereas retrograde fast-pathway ablation can eliminate SVT without altering AV conduction.

SLOW-PATHWAY ABLATION. The slow pathway can be located by mapping along the posteromedial tricuspid annulus close to the coronary sinus os. Electrogram recordings are obtained with an atrial-to-ventricular electrogram ratio of less than 0.5 and either a multicomponent atrial electrogram or a recording of possible slow-pathway potential.[65] In the anatomical approach, target sites are selected fluoroscopically. A single RF application suffices in many cases, but in others serial RF lesions may be needed, starting at the most posterior site (near the coronary sinus os) and progressing to the more anterior locus (closer to the His bundle recording site). An accelerated junctional rhythm (Fig. 30–8) usually occurs when RF energy is applied at a site that will result in successful elimination of SVT. The success rate with the anatomical or electrogram mapping approach is equivalent, and, most often, combinations of both are used, yielding success rates approaching 100 percent with less than a 1 percent chance of complete heart block. Catheter-delivered cryoablation has been used for treatment of AVNRT with

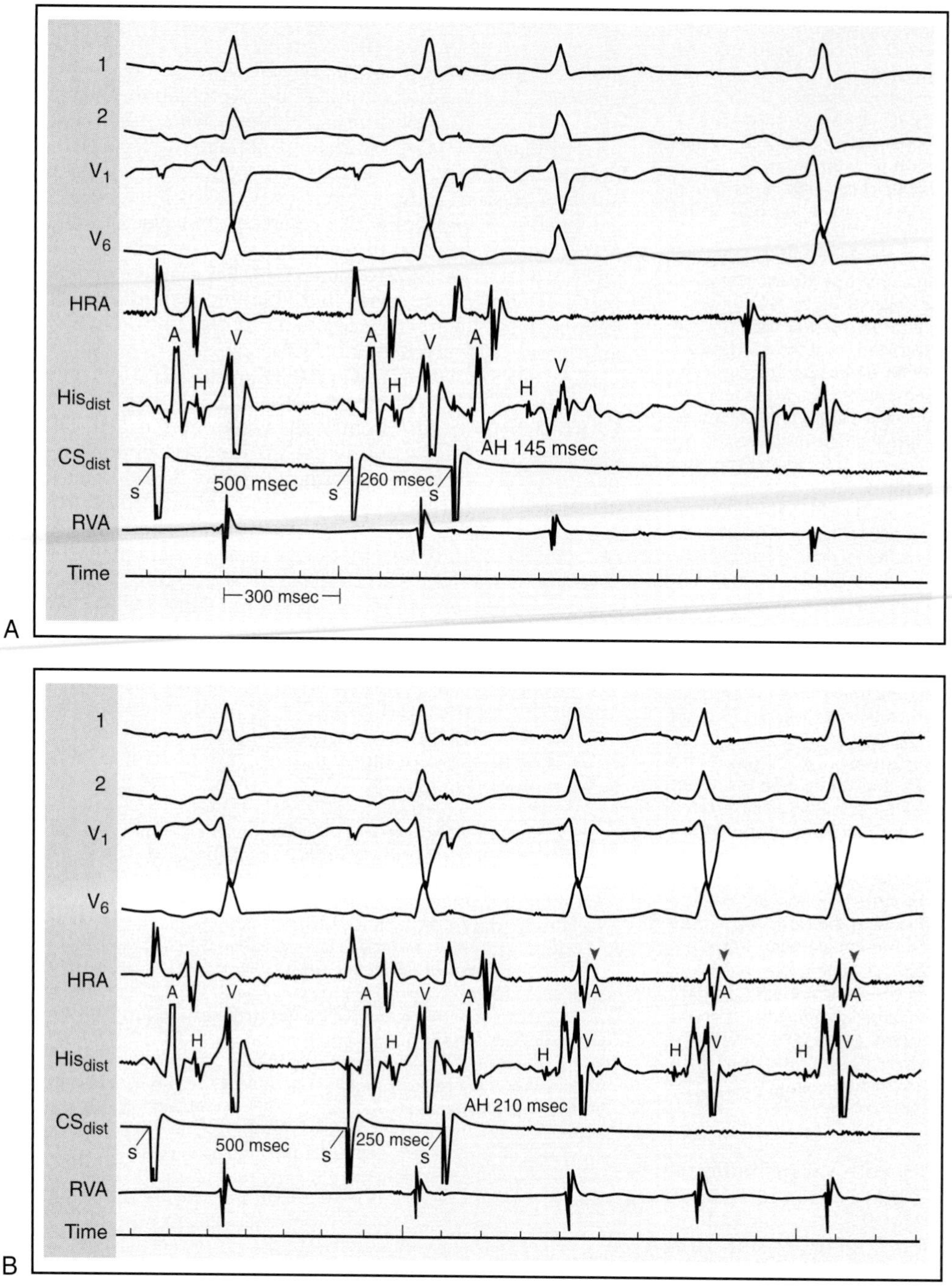

FIGURE 30–6 Atrioventricular (AV) node reentry. **A,** Two atrial paced complexes from the coronary sinus (CS) are followed by an atrial premature stimulus at coupling interval 260 milliseconds, resulting in an AH interval of 145 milliseconds. **B,** The same atrial drive train is followed by an atrial extrastimulus 10 milliseconds earlier than before (250 milliseconds). This results in a marked increase in the AH interval to 210 milliseconds, after which AV nodal reentrant tachycardia ensues because the extrastimulus encounters block in a "fast" AV node pathway, conducts down a "slow" pathway, and then conducts back up the fast pathway in a repeating fashion. Red arrows denote atrial electrograms coincident with QRS complexes, characteristic of the most common type of AV node reentry. Recording as in prior figures.

excellent results.[66] In theory, the ability to "cryomap" (test potential sites for slow-pathway block with moderate, reversible cooling) should almost entirely eliminate the risk of AV block with ablation.

Slow-pathway ablation results in an increase in the anterograde AV block cycle length and AV node ERP without a change in the AH interval or retrograde conduction properties of the AV node. Patients in whom slow-pathway conduction is completely eliminated almost never have recurrent SVT episodes; approximately 40 percent of patients can have evidence of residual slow-pathway function after successful elimination of sustained AVNRT (usually manifested as persistent dual AV node physiology and single AV node echoes during atrial extrastimulation). The surest endpoint for slow-pathway ablation is the elimination of sustained AVNRT both with and without an infusion of isoproterenol.

AVNRT recurs in about 5 percent of patients after slow-pathway ablation. In some patients, the ERP of the fast pathway decreases after slow-pathway ablation, possibly because of electrotonic interaction between the two pathways. Atypical forms of reentry can result after ablation, as can apparent parasympathetic denervation, resulting in inappropriate sinus tachycardia.

At present, the slow-pathway approach is the preferred method for ablation of typical AVNRT. Ablation of the slow pathway is also a safe and effective means for treating atypical AVNRT. In patients with AVNRT undergoing slow-pathway ablation, junctional ectopy during application of RF energy is a sensitive but nonspecific marker of successful ablation, occurring in longer bursts at effective target sites than at ineffective sites. Ventriculoatrial conduction should be expected during the junctional ectopy, and poor ventriculoatrial conduction or actual block may herald subsequent anterograde AV block in patients undergoing RF ablation of the slow pathway. Junctional ectopic rhythm is due to heating of the AV node and does not occur with cryoablation.

Indications. RF catheter ablation for AVNRT can be considered in patients with recurrent, symptomatic, sustained AVNRT that is drug resistant or when the patient is drug intolerant or does not desire long-term drug treatment. The procedure can also be considered in patients with sustained AVNRT identified during EPS or catheter ablation of another arrhythmia or when there is a finding of dual AV node pathway physiology and atrial echoes but without AVNRT during EPS in a patient suspected of having AVNRT clinically.

Results. Results of the NASPE survey indicate that 3052 patients had slow-pathway ablation with a 96 percent reported success rate, whereas 255 had fast-pathway ablation that was successful in 229 (90 percent). Significant complications occurred in 0.96 percent, but no procedure-related deaths were reported.[61] In Europe, the complication rate was 8.0 percent, mostly related to AV block after fast-pathway ablation, and there were no deaths in 815 patients.[61] Most centers currently employ slow-pathway ablation, resulting in a procedural success rate of 98 percent, recurrence rate of less than 2 percent, and incidence of heart block requiring permanent pacing of less than 1 percent.

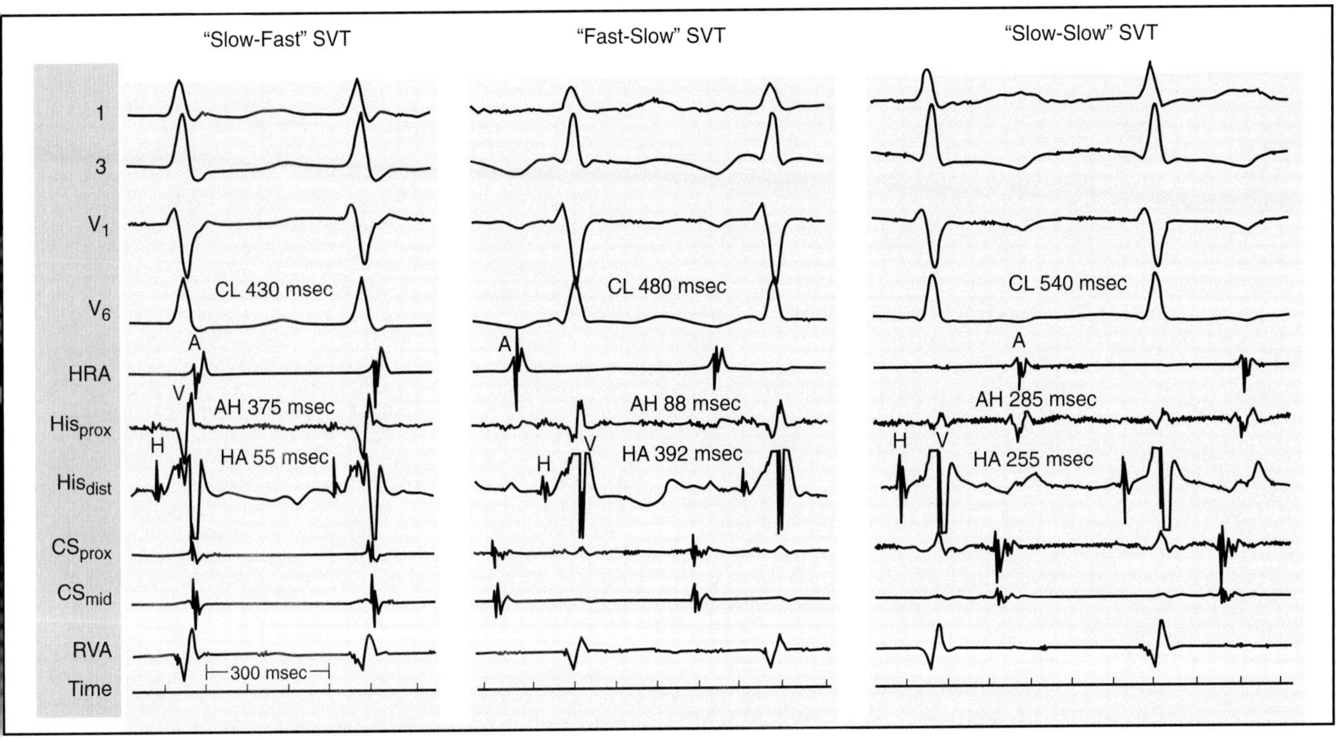

FIGURE 30–7 Three variants of atrioventricular (AV) node reentrant supraventricular tachycardia (SVT) in the same patient. Recordings as in other figures. The left panel shows the most common type of AV node SVT (anterograde slow pathway, retrograde fast); atrial activation is coincident with ventricular activation. The center panel shows "atypical" AV node reentry, with anterograde fast-pathway conduction and retrograde conduction over a slow pathway. A rare variety is shown in the right panel, with anterograde conduction over a slow pathway and retrograde conduction over a second slow pathway. Note the similar atrial activation sequences in the latter two (coronary sinus before right atrium), as distinct from that of slow-fast AV node reentry (coronary sinus and right atrial activation nearly simultaneous). Note also the different P-QRS relationships, from simultaneous activation (left, short RP interval) to P in front of the QRS (middle, long RP interval) and P midway in the cardiac cycle (right). CL = cycle length.

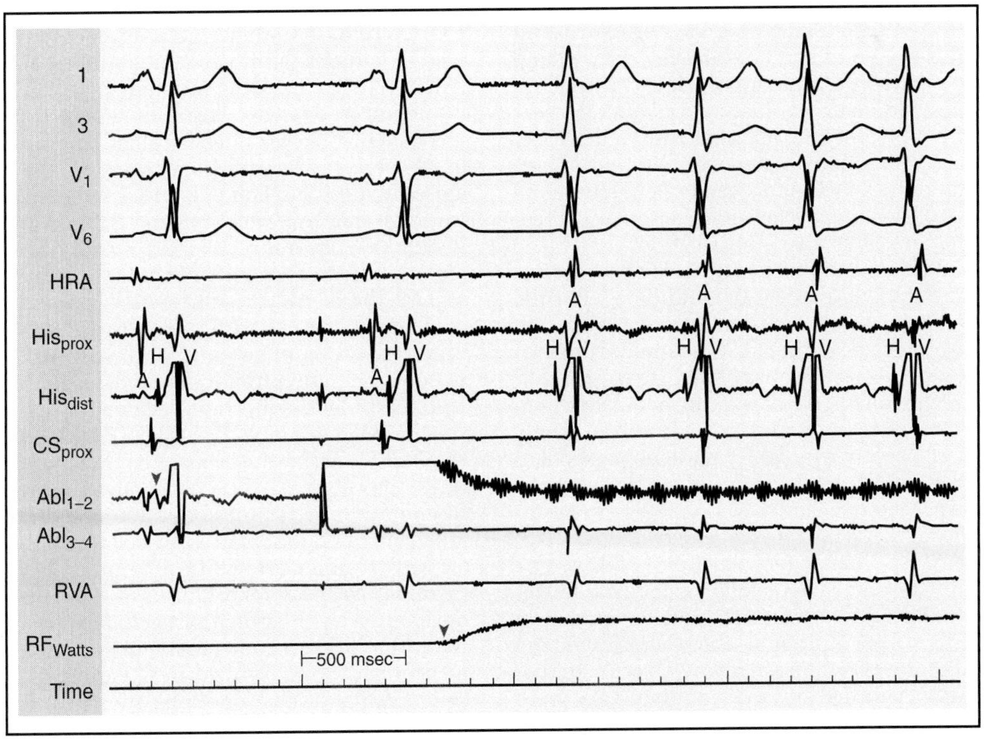

FIGURE 30–8 Atrioventricular (AV) node slow-pathway modification for cure of AV node reentrant supraventricular tachycardia. Recordings as in prior figures. The ablation recording (arrow in $Abl_{1\text{-}2}$) shows a slurred deflection between atrial and ventricular electrogram components; this may represent the AV node slow-pathway deflection (but it is not the bundle of His deflection, which is instead recorded from a separate catheter 15 mm away). Shortly after the onset of radiofrequency delivery (arrow in RF_{Watts}), an accelerated junctional rhythm begins and gradually speeds up further. Retrograde conduction is present during the junctional rhythm. $Abl_{3\text{-}4}$ = proximal electrode recording from ablation catheter.

ECTOPIC JUNCTIONAL TACHYCARDIA. Ectopic junctional tachycardia is a rare form of SVT in which the electrocardiogram resembles that in AVNRT but is distinct in that (1) the mechanism is automatic, not reentrant, and (2) the atrium is clearly not involved in the tachycardia. This disorder is most commonly observed in young healthy individuals, women more often than men, and is usually very catecholamine dependent. Ablation must be carried out very near the His bundle, and the risk of heart block requiring pacemaker insertion exceeds 5 percent.[67]

RADIOFREQUENCY CATHETER ABLATION OF ARRHYTHMIAS RELATED TO THE SINOATRIAL NODE. Reentry in or around the sinus node is an uncommon arrhythmia, characterized by episodes of tachycardia with a P wave identical to the sinus P wave, usually with a PR interval longer than in sinus (in physiological sinus tachycardia, the PR interval remains normal or shortens because of catecholamine effects on the AV node as well as on the sinus node). RF applications are placed around the region of the sinus node at sites of early activation (prior to P wave onset) until tachycardia terminates.

Inappropriate sinus tachycardia is a syndrome characterized by high sinus rates with exercise and at rest. Patients complain of palpitations at all times of day that correlate with inappropriately high sinus rates. They may not respond well to beta blocker therapy because of either lack of desired effect or occurrence of side effects. When the sinus node area is to be ablated, it can be identified anatomically as well as electrophysiologically, and ablation lesions are usually placed between the superior vena cava and crista terminalis at sites of early atrial activation. Isoproterenol may be helpful in "forcing" the site of impulse formation to cells with the most rapid discharge rate. Care must be taken to apply RF energy at the most cephalad sites first; initial ablation performed farther down the crista terminalis does not alter the atrial rate at the time but can damage subsidiary pacemaker regions that may be needed after the sinus node is eventually ablated.

Indications. Catheter ablation for sinus node reentrant tachycardia can be performed in patients with recurrent symptomatic episodes of sustained SVT that is drug resistant or when the patient is drug intolerant or does not desire long-term drug treatment. Patients with inappropriate sinus tachycardia should be considered for ablation only after clear failure of medical therapy because ablation results are often less than completely satisfactory. Whenever ablation is performed in the region of the sinus node, the patient should be apprised of the risk of needing a pacemaker after the procedure. Phrenic nerve damage is also a possibility.

Results. Sinus node reentrant tachycardia can be successfully ablated in more than 90 percent of candidates. Results are not as good for inappropriate sinus tachycardia; although a good technical result may be obtained at the time of the procedure, symptoms often persist because of recurrence of rapid sinus rates (at or near preablation rates) or for nonarrhythmic reasons. Multiple ablation sessions are needed in some patients, and about 20 percent eventually undergo pacemaker implantation (not all of whom have relief of palpitations despite a normal heart rate).

RADIOFREQUENCY CATHETER ABLATION OF ATRIAL TACHYCARDIA. ATs are a heterogeneous group of disorders with causes including rapid discharge of a focus (focal tachycardia) and reentry. The former can occur in anyone, irrespective of the presence of structural abnormalities of the atria, whereas reentrant ATs almost always occur in the setting of structurally damaged atria. Symptoms vary from none (in relatively infrequent or slow ATs in patients without heart disease) to syncope (rapid AT with compromised cardiac function) or heart failure (incessant AT over a period of weeks or months). All forms of AT are amenable to catheter ablation.

FOCAL ATRIAL TACHYCARDIA. In focal ATs (automatic or triggered foci or micro-reentry), activation mapping is used to determine the site of the AT by recording the earliest onset of local activation.[68] These tachycardias can behave capriciously and be practically noninducible at EPS despite the patient's complaining of multiple daily episodes for the week prior to EPS. Ten to 15 percent of patients can have multiple atrial foci. Sites tend to cluster near the pulmonary veins in the left atrium and the mouths of the atrial appendages and along the crista terminalis on the right (Fig. 30-9A; see Fig. 29-14). Activation times of these sites typically occur only 15 to 40 milliseconds prior to the onset of the P wave on the electrocardiogram. Care must be taken to avoid inadvertent damage to the phrenic nerve; its location can be determined by pacing at high current at a potential site of ablation, observing for diaphragmatic contraction. Ablation should not be performed at a site at which this is seen, if at all possible.

REENTRANT ATRIAL TACHYCARDIA. As noted, these ATs occur more commonly in the setting of structural heart disease, especially after prior atrial surgery. The region of slow conduction is typically related to an end of an atriotomy scar; this is, however, not in a constant anatomical location but varies from patient to patient depending on the operation performed. Therefore, preprocedure review of operative reports and careful electrophysiological mapping are essential. Because reentry within a complete circuit is occurring, activation can be recorded throughout the entire cardiac cycle. The ablation strategy is to identify regions with mid-diastolic atrial activation during tachycardia that can be proved by pacing techniques to be integral to the tachycardia (see Figs. 29-15 and 30-9B). Such sites are attractive ablation targets because they are composed of relatively few cells (hence electrical silence on the surface electrocardiogram in diastole) and are thus more easily ablated by a typical application of RF energy than other areas. Focal ablation of these sites can then be performed, but in many cases tachycardia can still be initiated (often at a slower rate) or recurs after the procedure. Because these sites are typically located at a relatively narrow zone between the ends of prior scars or surgical incisions and another nonconducting barrier (such as another scar, caval orifice, or valve annulus), another technique is to make a line of ablation lesions from the end of the scar to the nearest electrical barrier. Reentry can thus be prevented. This technique is analogous to that used in curing atrial flutter (see later). Because these patients often have extensive atrial disease with islands of scar that could serve as barriers for additional ATs, specialized mapping techniques may be needed to locate these regions and preemptively connect them with ablation lesions to prevent future AT episodes.

Indications. Catheter ablation for ATs should be considered in patients with recurrent episodes of symptomatic, sustained ATs that are drug resistant, or when the patient is drug intolerant or does not desire long-term drug treatment.

Results. Success rates for ablation of focal AT are from 80 to 95 percent, largely depending on the ability to induce episodes at EPS; when episodes can be initiated with pacing, isoproterenol, or other means, AT can usually be ablated. Reentrant ATs, although more readily induced at EPS, are often harder to eliminate completely; initial success rates are high (90 percent) but recurrences are seen in up to 20 percent of patients, necessitating drug therapy or another ablation procedure. Complications, occurring in 1 to 2 percent of patients, include phrenic nerve damage, cardiac tamponade, and heart block (with rare perinodal ATs).

RADIOFREQUENCY CATHETER ABLATION OF ATRIAL FLUTTER. Atrial flutter may be defined electrocardiographically (most typically, negative sawtooth waves in leads II and III and aVF at a rate of about 300 beats/min) or electrophysiologically (a rapid, organized macro-reentrant AT, the circuit for which is anatomically determined). Understanding the reentrant pathway for all forms of atrial flutter is essential for developing an ablation approach. Reentry in the right atrium, with the left atrium passively activated, constitutes the mechanism of the typical ECG variety of atrial flutter, with caudocranial activation along the right atrial septum and a craniocaudal activation of the right atrial free wall (Fig. 30–10A). In some cases, a zone of slow conduction exists in the low right atrium, which is typically bounded by the tricuspid annulus, the inferior vena cava, and the coronary sinus. In other cases, conduction velocity is more uniform

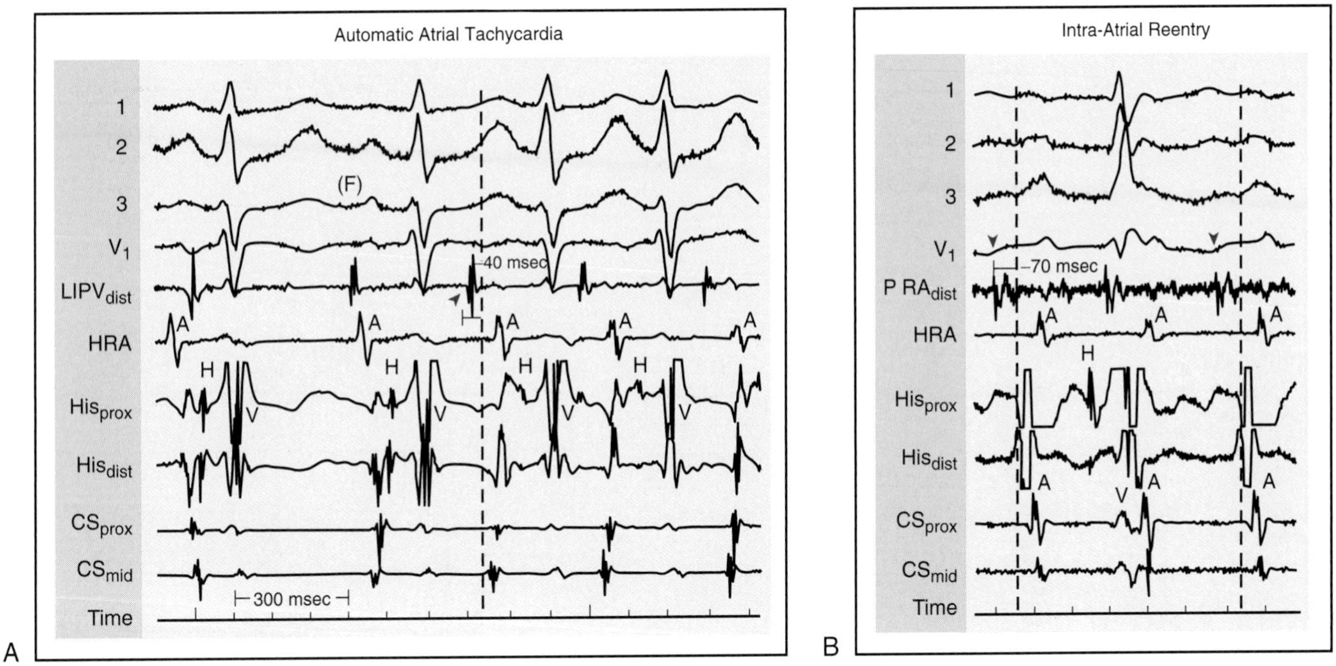

FIGURE 30–9 Atrial tachycardias. **A,** Automatic atrial tachycardia arising in the left inferior pulmonary vein (LIPV). A sinus beat is shown at left, followed by a fusion beat (F) of sinus and tachycardia activation. The last three beats in the panel are atrial tachycardia. The ablation catheter was within the LIPV and recorded a sharp potential (arrow) 40 milliseconds before the P wave onset (dashed line). Ablation at this site terminated the tachycardia. **B,** Intraatrial reentrant tachycardia in a patient who had undergone atrial septal defect repair years earlier. The ablation catheter is in the posterior right atrium (PRA), where a fragmented signal is recorded. A portion of this electrogram (arrows) precedes the P wave onset during tachycardia (dashed line) by 70 milliseconds. Ablation at this site terminated the tachycardia. Recordings as in prior figures.

throughout the large circuit. Placing an ablative lesion between any two anatomical barriers that transects a portion of the circuit necessary for perpetuation of reentry can be curative. Typically, this is across the isthmus of atrial tissue between the inferior vena caval orifice and tricuspid annulus (the cavotricuspid isthmus), a relatively narrow point in the circuit. Successful ablation can be accomplished where the advancing flutter wave front enters this zone in the low inferolateral right atrium, near the exit of this zone at the inferomedial right atrium, or in between these sites. Locations for RF delivery can be guided anatomically or electrophysiologically. Less commonly, the direction of wave front propagation in this large right atrial circuit is reversed ("clockwise" flutter proceeding cephalad up the right atrial free wall and caudad down the septum, with upright flutter waves in the inferior leads [see Fig. 30–10A]). This arrhythmia, which has been called "atypical atrial flutter," may also be ablated using the same techniques as with more typical atrial flutter. These two arrhythmias constitute "cavotricuspid isthmus–dependent" flutter and are distinct from other rapid atrial arrhythmias that may have a similar ECG appearance but utilize different (and often multiple) circuits in other parts of the right or left atrium. Ablation can be more difficult in these cases, which often occur in the setting of advanced lung disease or prior cardiac surgery. A common theme in these complex reentrant arrhythmias is the presence of an anatomically determined zone of inexcitability around which an electrical wave front can circulate. Specialized mapping tools and skills are necessary to effect successful ablation in such cases.

In patients with atrial fibrillation, an antiarrhythmic drug can slow intraatrial conduction to such a degree that atrial flutter results and fibrillation is no longer observed. In some of these, ablation of atrial flutter and having the patient continue to take the antiarrhythmic drug can prevent recurrences of these atrial arrhythmias.

The endpoint of atrial flutter ablation procedures was initially termination of atrial flutter with RF application accompanied by noninducibility of the arrhythmia. However, using these criteria, up to 30 percent of patients had recurrent flutter because of lack of complete and permanent conduction block in the cavotricuspid isthmus. In the last several years, the endpoint of ablation has changed to ensuring a line of bidirectional block in this region by pacing from opposite sides of the isthmus (see Fig. 30–10B) or other techniques.[69] Using these criteria, recurrence rates have fallen to less than 5 percent.

Indications. Candidates for RF catheter ablation include patients with recurrent episodes of atrial flutter that are drug resistant, those who are drug intolerant, or those who do not desire long-term drug therapy.

Results. Regardless of circuit location, atrial flutter can be successfully ablated in more than 90 percent of cases, although patients with complex right or left atrial flutters require more extensive and complex procedures. Recurrence rates are less than 5 percent except in patients with extensive atrial disease, in whom new circuits can develop over time as new areas of conduction delay and block form. Complications are rare, including inadvertent heart block and phrenic nerve paralysis.

ABLATION AND MODIFICATION OF ATRIOVENTRICULAR CONDUCTION FOR ATRIAL TACHYARRHYTHMIAS. In some patients with atrial tachyarrhythmias who have rapid ventricular rates despite optimal drug therapy, RF ablation can be used to eliminate or modify AV conduction to control the ventricular rates. To achieve RF catheter ablation of AV conduction, a catheter is placed across the tricuspid valve and positioned to record the largest His bundle electrogram associated with the largest atrial electrogram. RF energy is applied until complete AV block is achieved and is continued for an additional 30 to 60 seconds. If no change in AV conduction is observed after 15 seconds of RF ablation, the catheter is repositioned and the attempt is repeated. In occasional patients, attempts at RF ablation using this right-sided heart approach fail to achieve heart block. These patients can undergo an attempt from the left ventricle with

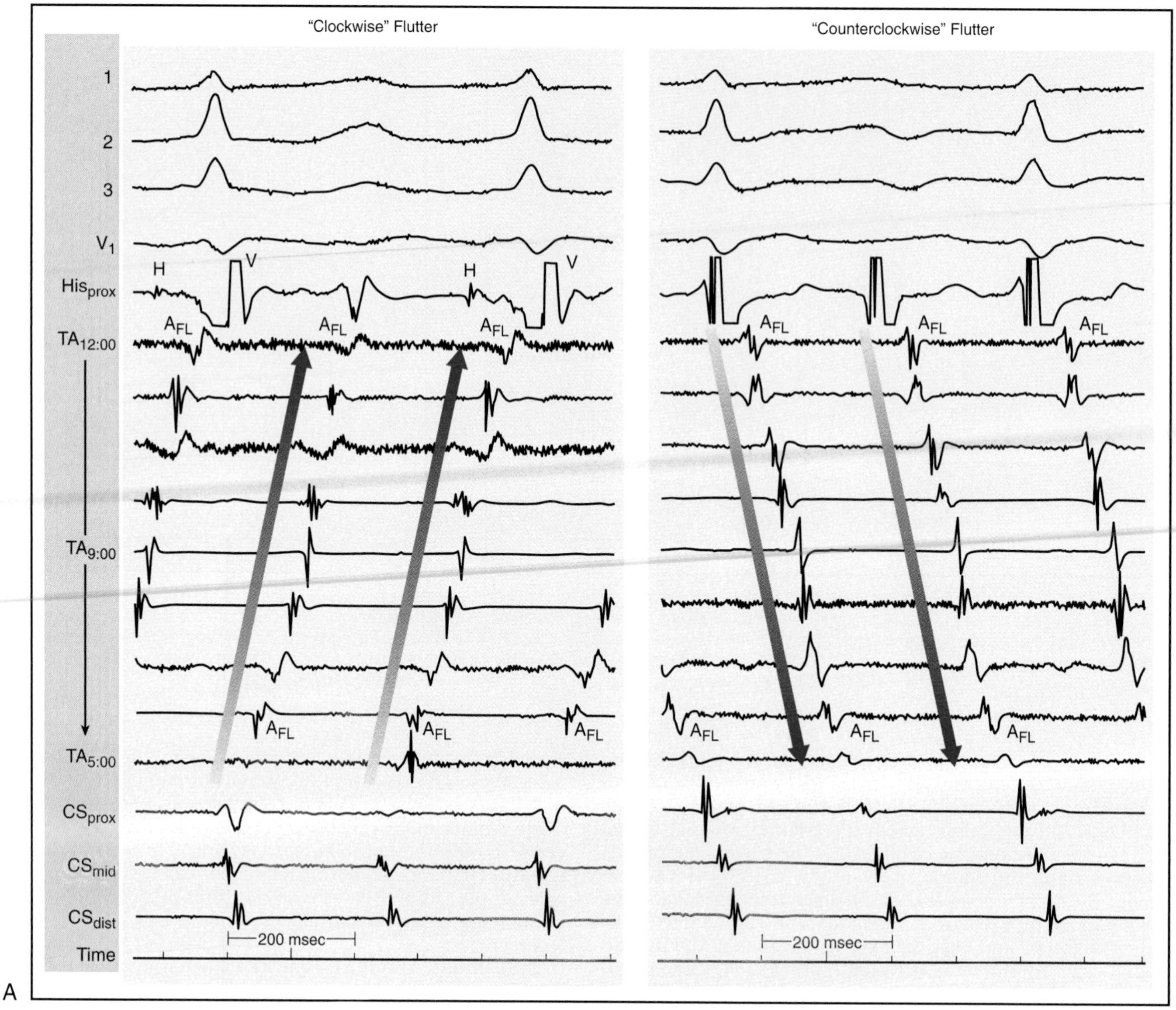

FIGURE 30–10 **A,** Two forms of atrial flutter in the same patient are shown. A "halo" catheter with 10 electrode pairs is situated on the atrial side of the tricuspid annulus (TA), with recording sites displayed from the top of the annulus ("12:00") to the inferomedial aspect ("5:00"), as shown in fluoroscopic views in **B**. On the left, the wave front of atrial activation proceeds in a "clockwise" fashion (arrows) along the annulus, whereas at the right the direction of propagation is the reverse.

a catheter positioned along the posterior interventricular septum just beneath the aortic valve to record a large His bundle electrogram. Energy is applied between the catheter electrode and the skin patch or between catheters in the left and right ventricles. Success rates currently approach 100 percent, with recurrence of AV conduction in less than 5 percent. Improved left ventricular function can result from both control of ventricular rate during atrial fibrillation and withdrawal of rate-controlling medications with negative inotropic action. Permanent ventricular or AV pacing is required after ablation.

In some cases, the AV junction can be modified to slow the ventricular rate without producing complete AV block by ablation in the region of the slow pathway, as described in connection with AV node modification for AV node reentry. Initial success rates for slowing the ventricular response are quite good; however, long-term results are less consistent.[70] Some patients have a gradual increase in ventricular rate to nearly preablation levels, whereas late complete heart block may occur in others. Nonetheless, this procedure can be tried before producing complete AV block.

Indications. Ablation and modification of AV conduction can be considered in (1) patients with symptomatic atrial tachyarrhythmias who have inadequately controlled ventricular rates unless primary ablation of the atrial tachyarrhythmia is possible; (2) similar patients when drugs are not tolerated or the patient does not wish to take them, even though the ventricular rate can be controlled; (3) patients with symptomatic, nonparoxysmal, junctional tachycardia that is drug resistant or in whom drugs are not tolerated or are not desired; (4) patients resuscitated from sudden cardiac death related to atrial flutter or atrial fibrillation with a rapid ventricular response in the absence of an accessory pathway; and (5) patients with a dual-chamber pacemaker and a pacemaker-mediated tachycardia that cannot be treated effectively by drugs or by reprogramming the pacemaker. The last three situations are rarely encountered.

Results. Results from the U.S. survey indicated that the procedure was successful in producing complete AV block in 95 percent of 1600 patients, with significant complications occurring in 21 (1.3 percent) and two procedure-related deaths (0.1 percent).[61] In Europe, the complication rate was

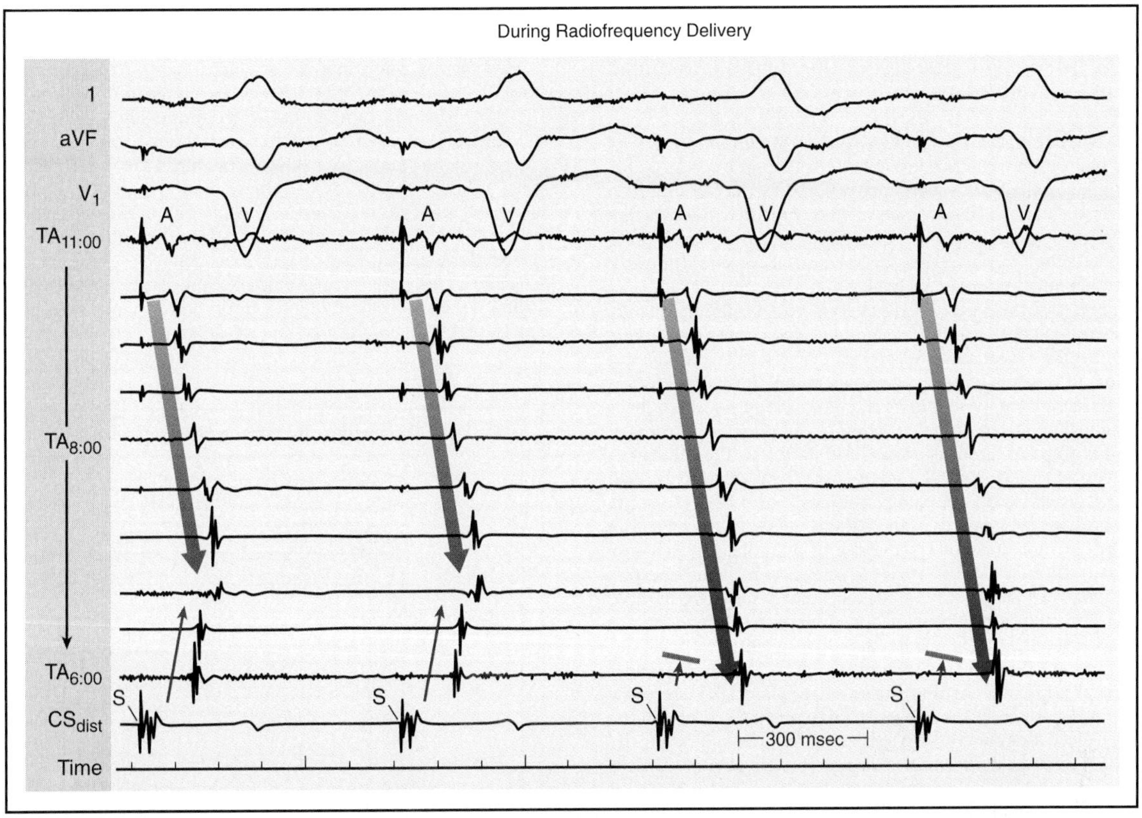

B

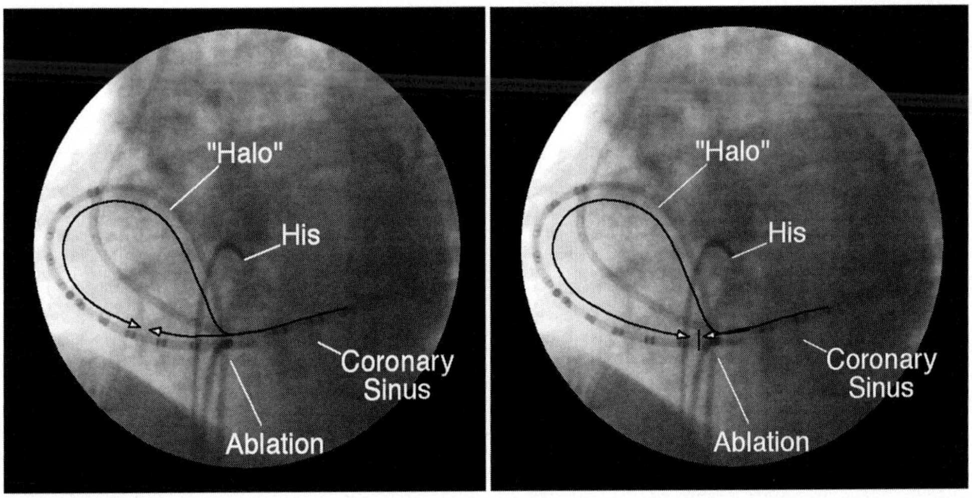

FIGURE 30–10, cont'd **B,** Ablation of the isthmus of atrial tissue between the tricuspid annulus and inferior vena caval orifice for cure of atrial flutter. Recordings are displayed from the multipolar catheter around much of the circumference of the tricuspid annulus (see left anterior oblique fluoroscopy images). Ablation of this isthmus is performed during coronary sinus pacing. In the two beats on the left, atrial conduction proceeds in two directions around the tricuspid annulus, as indicated by arrows and recorded along the halo catheter. In the two beats on the right, ablation has interrupted conduction in the floor of the right atrium, eliminating one path for transmission along the tricuspid annulus. The halo catheter now records conduction proceeding all the way around the annulus. This finding demonstrates unidirectional block in the isthmus; block in the other direction may be demonstrated by pacing from one of the halo electrodes and observing a similar lack of isthmus conduction. (The bundle of His recording in the right panel is lost owing to catheter movement.)

3.2 percent, and there was one death in 900 patients.[63] In early studies, up to 4 percent of patients had an episode of sudden death after AV junction ablation despite adequate pacemaker function, presumably because of relative bradycardia after long periods of rapid ventricular rates.[71] In one study, 6 of 100 patients died suddenly when the initial pacing rate was set to 60 beats/min, but none of 135 died suddenly when the rate was set to 90 beats/min for 1 to 3 months after ablation. Improvements in quality of life indices as well as cost-effectiveness have been demonstrated for this procedure.

RADIOFREQUENCY CATHETER ABLATION OF ATRIAL FIBRILLATION. Considerable progress has been made in understanding the pathophysiology of atrial fibrillation. The use of this information has translated directly into therapeutic advances. For example, it is now recognized that a significant proportion of patients with paroxysmal atrial fibrillation in the absence of structural heart disease have a focal origin of the arrhythmia; that is, rapid discharges from a focal source (often in a pulmonary vein) drive the atrium more rapidly than it can uniformly conduct, leading to the ECG appearance of atrial fibrillation. In other cases, a focal source can serve as a "trigger" that initiates episodes of fibrillation (see Chap. 32). In either scenario, if this focus can be located and ablated or its spread to the rest of the atrium eliminated, recurrences of atrial fibrillation are prevented.

LOCATION AND ABLATION OF FOCAL SOURCES. A variety of methods have been used to locate and ablate focal sources of atrial fibrillation. When first applied, PACs were mapped and the site from which they originated was ablated. This technique was limited by the fact that few patients have adequate frequency of PACs or short bursts of fibrillation to serve as either a good target for ablation or a useful indicator of success (i.e.,, elimination of PACs). In addition, the source of PACs or fibrillation in many cases was up to 3 cm deep within a pulmonary vein; ablation at these sites could result in pulmonary vein stenosis. As experience grew, it became clear that the majority of cases of paroxysmal atrial fibrillation originated within pulmonary veins; muscular sleeves extend from the left atrium for several centimeters along the pulmonary vein. Efforts then shifted to electrical isolation of the pulmonary veins to prevent spread of impulses from the sites of initiation to the remainder of the atrium. The advantages of this strategy over focal ablation are that (1) there is a greater likelihood of eliminating fibrillation because multiple veins may be arrhythmogenic, (2) the patient need not have PACs in order to perform the ablation, and (3) the risk of pulmonary vein stenosis may be lower. Although strands of atrial muscle enshroud the pulmonary veins, actual electrical connections may exist at only two or three discrete points. The pulmonary vein isolation strategy can be carried out either with mapping of the pulmonary veins to locate and ablate the discrete points of electrical connection between vein and atrium or with a purely anatomical approach. Mapping uses either a circular electrode catheter (Fig. 30–11) or a multipolar "basket" catheter situated within the ostium of the vein.[72] Pulmonary vein potentials, which might be the origin of fibrillation, appear as either sharp potentials (Fig. 30–12) or complex, fragmented signals following the nearby left atrial recording (Fig. 30–13).

Ablation is performed on the atrial side of the venoatrial junction until the pulmonary vein potentials are eliminated ("entrance block" into the vein). Ablation can be performed during sinus rhythm, atrial pacing, or even during atrial fibrillation (which often terminates during RF application).[73] Some advocate pacing from within the vein to demonstrate the more relevant "exit block" from vein to atrium. Using the anatomical approach, continuous lines of ablation are made that surround venous orifices. This method requires sophisticated mapping tools to be able to record the sites that have already been ablated and the areas that remain. In some cases, gaps in a line of ablation can be proarrhythmic by providing a path for macro-reentry in the left atrium. Some electrophysiologists make an additional line of ablation between the left inferior

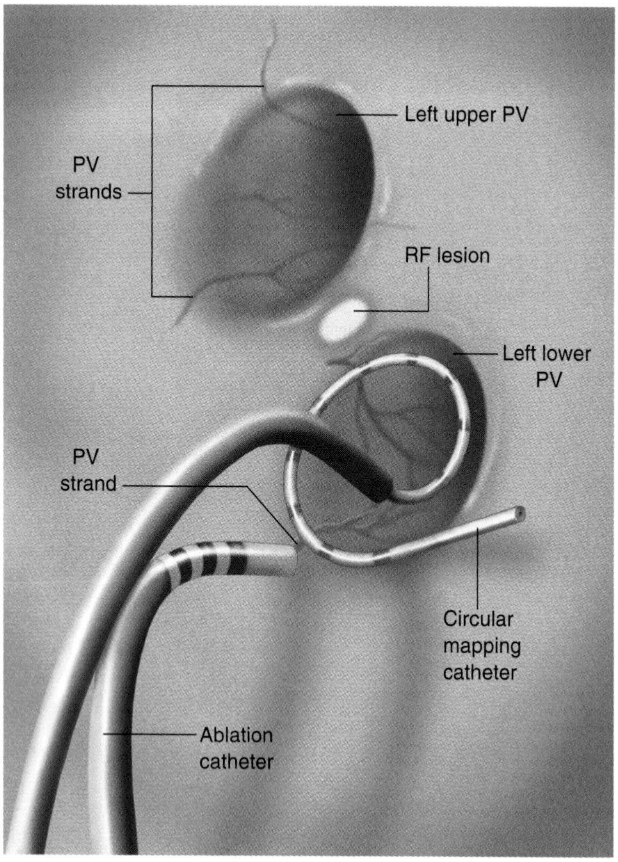

FIGURE 30–11 Depiction of catheters for pulmonary vein (PV) isolation. Both left PVs are illustrated with strands of atrial muscle connecting PV to left atrium at discrete points. A circular mapping catheter is shown resting in the ostium of the left lower PV and an ablation catheter with a large-tip electrode is shown adjacent to electrodes of the circular catheter that are recording a PV potential from the nearby strand. A radiofrequency (RF) lesion (between the two venous ostia) is at the site of a previously ablated strand.

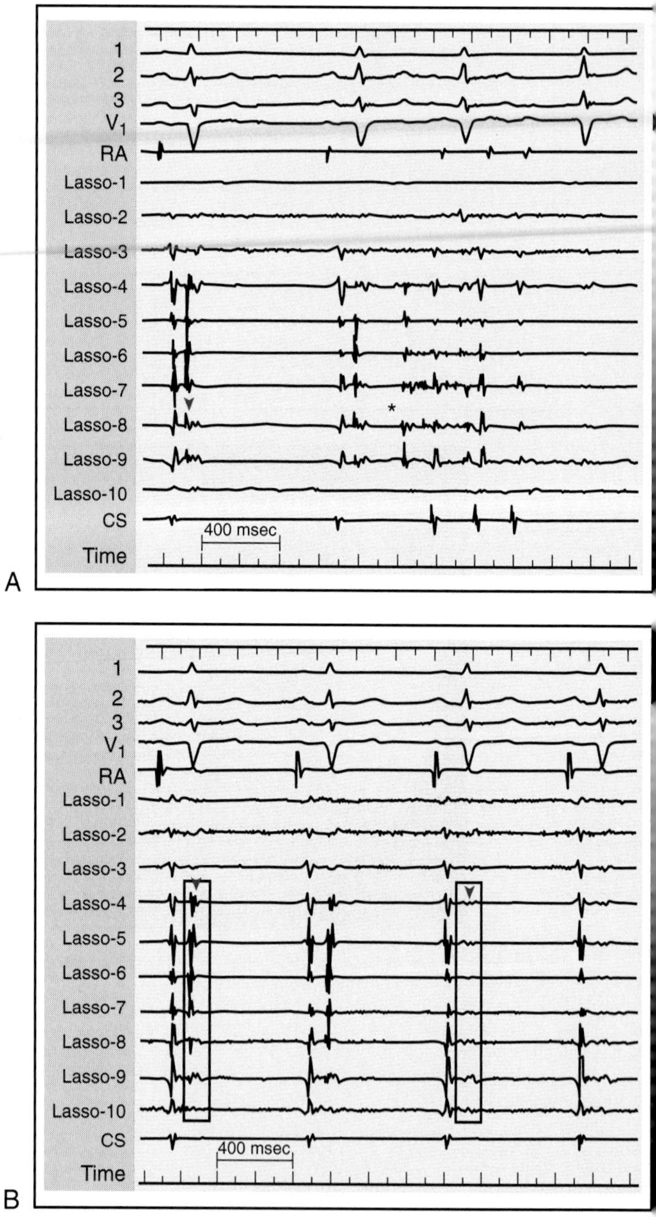

FIGURE 30–12 Sharp pulmonary vein potentials (PVPs). Surface electrocardiographic leads and intracardiac recordings from right atrium (RA), coronary sinus (CS), and a 10-electrode circular catheter (Lasso) situated in the ostium of a pulmonary vein. **A,** Lasso recordings show left atrial electrograms followed by sharp PV potentials in recordings Lasso-4 through Lasso-10 during a sinus beat (arrow points to earliest PVP at Lasso-8 as wave front enters vein); an asterisk marks an ectopic beat from this vein that initiates a very short episode of atrial fibrillation. **B,** Recorded during radiofrequency ablation near Lasso-8 recording site; the same sharp PVPs are seen in the first two beats (left arrow) but are absent during the last two beats (right arrow), leaving only the left atrial recordings. This vein has thus been electrically isolated from the left atrium.

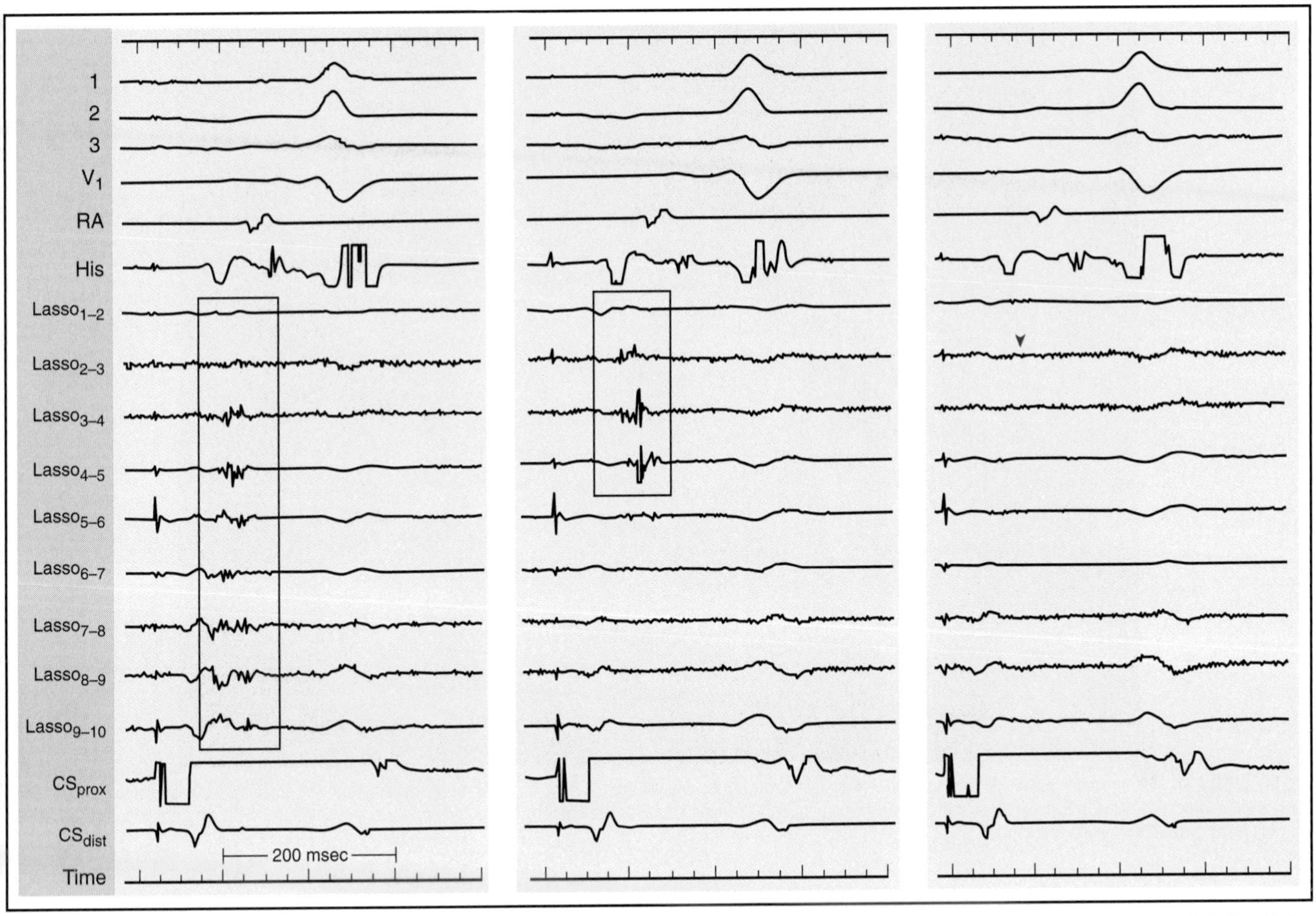

FIGURE 30–13 Low-amplitude, fragmented pulmonary vein potentials (PVPs). Recordings during coronary sinus pacing are similar to those in Figure 30–12. **Left,** Preablation recordings from PV; note fragmented recordings in Lasso-3 through Lasso-9 (within rectangle). **Middle,** Recordings partway through ablation; PVPs are no longer evident in Lasso-5 through Lasso-9. **Right,** Continued ablation eliminates all PVPs (arrow). This vein is now electrically isolated from the left atrium.

pulmonary vein and the mitral annulus to forestall this possibility. In many cases, a "flutter lesion" in the floor of the right atrium is also made because many patients undergoing a purely left atrial procedure have subsequent episodes of flutter. Each method of isolation requires left atrial access using a patent foramen ovale or the septal puncture technique, with full anticoagulation. This approach increases the risk of bleeding complications and still has not entirely prevented thromboemboli related to the procedure. The pulmonary vein isolation approach has been used primarily in younger patients with paroxysmal atrial fibrillation in the absence of structural heart disease; although experience with this technique in patients with chronic atrial fibrillation or those with structural heart disease is limited, preliminary results suggest nearly equivalent success rates. Before the ablation procedure, it is useful to obtain some type of noninvasive study to better define pulmonary venous anatomy, such as a high-resolution computed tomography or magnetic resonance imaging study (Fig. 30-14). This study aids the operator in planning the procedure so that anomalous venous anatomy does not interfere with successful ablation.

As noted earlier, some patients with atrial fibrillation show a transformation to stable atrial flutter when given antiarrhythmic drugs, particularly sodium channel blocking agents. In these patients, performing a flutter ablation and having the patient continue to take the same drug may prevent arrhythmia recurrence.[74]

The maze surgical procedure has become established as a successful technique for permanently restoring sinus rhythm. In 1994, the first reports appeared of replicating the surgically induced lines of block in the atria using catheter ablation in humans. The intent of the procedure is to compartmentalize the atrial muscle into segments too small to support fibrillation wave fronts yet have the segments connected enough to participate in contraction. Several techniques have been used, including creation of long, linear RF lesions limited to either the right or left atrium or both. This technique has been largely supplanted by pulmonary vein isolation, although it has been helpful in some patients who have had recurrent fibrillation after an apparently successful isolation procedure. These may be very long procedures, lasting 5 to 8 hours, and fluoroscopy times over 90 minutes are not uncommon.

Indications. Candidates for focal atrial fibrillation ablation have paroxysmal atrial fibrillation in the absence of structural heart disease and include those whose atrial fibrillation is either refractory to medications or who prefer not to take medications. Patients in whom linear ablation for atrial fibrillation might be considered are those with some degree of structural heart disease and persistent or chronic atrial fibrillation for whom maintenance of sinus rhythm is important and in whom atrial fibrillation recurs despite standard antiarrhythmic drugs or in whom drug therapy is not tolerated or preferred.

Results. Success rates of ablation for atrial fibrillation range from 70 to 85 percent. At present, there does not seem to be a preferred technique (mapping-guided segmental isolation of pulmonary venous ostia versus purely anatomically based ablation). Reasons for failure of ablation include (1) incomplete isolation of an arrhythmogenic vein, (2) restitution of conduction after apparently successful isolation, and (3) nonpulmonary venous sources of fibrillation. The risk of stroke related to extensive left atrial ablation is approximately 2 percent even with rigorous anticoagulation regimens. Pulmonary vein stenosis, more likely if ablation is performed within the vein itself rather than at the ostium, can cause dyspnea and pulmonary arterial hypertension. In some cases, angioplasty and stenting have been necessary.

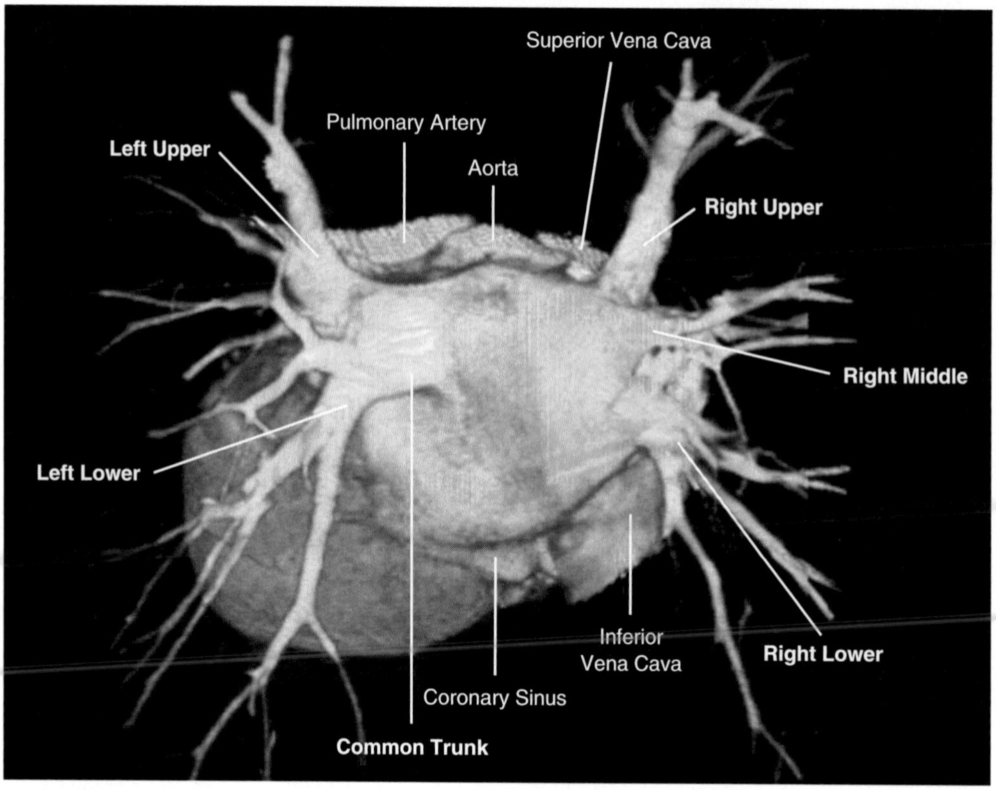

FIGURE 30–14 High-resolution computed tomographic view of the left atrium, viewed from behind to illustrate pulmonary vein (PV) anatomy. Instead of two veins entering the left atrium from each lung, this patient had both left veins emptying into a common trunk before entering the atrium and three veins from the right lung. This information helped plan the pulmonary vein isolation procedure.

Other nonpharmacological modalities for the treatment of atrial fibrillation, such as preventive pacing and implantable atrial defibrillators or atrial rhythm management devices, are discussed in Chapter 31.

RADIOFREQUENCY CATHETER ABLATION OF VENTRICULAR TACHYCARDIA. In general, the success rate for ablation of VTs is lower than that for AV node reentry or AV reentry. This lower success rate may be related to the fact that this procedure is often a last resort in patients with drug-resistant VTs, but it is also related to more difficult mapping in the ventricles. Furthermore, the VT induction must ideally be reproducible, uniform in QRS morphology from beat to beat, sustained, and hemodynamically stable so that the patient can tolerate the VT long enough during the procedure to undergo the extensive mapping necessary to localize optimal ablation target sites. (Patients with several electrocardiographically distinct, uniform morphologies of VT can still be candidates for ablation because in many instances a common reentrant pathway is shared by two or more VT morphologies.) Also, the origin of the VT must be fairly circumscribed and endocardially situated (rare cases of successful ablation only from the epicardial aspect have been reported[75]). Very rapid VT, polymorphic VT, and infrequent, nonsustained episodes are generally not amenable to this form of therapy at this time (see later).

LOCATION AND ABLATION. RF catheter ablation of VT can be divided into idiopathic VT that occurs in patients with essentially normal hearts, VT that occurs in a variety of disease settings but without coronary artery disease, and VT in patients with coronary artery disease and prior myocardial infarction. In the first group, VTs can arise in either ventricle. Right ventricular tachycardias most commonly originate in the outflow tract and have a characteristic left bundle branch block–like, inferior axis morphology; less often, VTs arise in the inflow tract or free wall. Initiation of tachycardia can often be facilitated by catecholamines. The majority of left ventricular VTs are septal in origin and have a characteristic QRS configuration (right bundle branch block, superior axis); other VTs occur less commonly and arise from other areas of the left ventricle, including the left ventricular outflow tract, and are similar in ECG appearance and clinical behavior to those arising in the right ventricular outflow tract (see Fig. 29–13). Abnormal patterns of sympathetic innervation may be present in some. VTs in abnormal hearts without coronary artery disease can be due to bundle branch reentry, most typically observed in patients with dilated cardiomyopathies. In these patients, ablation of the right bundle branch eliminates the tachycardia. VT can occur in right ventricular dysplasia, sarcoidosis, Chagas disease, hypertrophic cardiomyopathy, and a host of other noncoronary disease states (see Chap. 32).

Activation mapping and pace mapping are effective in patients with idiopathic VTs to locate the site of origin of the VT. In activation mapping, the timing of endocardial electrograms sampled by the mapping catheter is compared with the onset of the surface QRS complex. Sites that are activated before the surface QRS onset are near the origin of the VT (Fig. 30–15; see Fig. 29–13). In idiopathic VT, ablation at a site at which the unipolar electrogram shows a "QS" complex may yield greater success than if an "rS" potential is observed (Fig. 30–16). Pace mapping involves stimulation of various ventricular sites to initiate a QRS contour that duplicates the QRS contour of the spontaneous VT, thus establishing the apparent site of origin of the arrhythmia (see Fig. 30–15). This technique is limited by several methodological problems but may be useful when the tachycardia cannot be initiated and when a 12-lead electrocardiogram has been obtained during the spontaneous VT. Presystolic Purkinje potentials as well as very low-amplitude mid-diastolic signals can be recorded during VT from sites at which ablation cures VT in most patients with left ventricular VTs that have a right bundle branch block superior axis. Localization of optimal ablation sites for VT in patients with coronary artery disease and prior infarction is more difficult than in patients with structurally normal hearts because of the altered anatomy and electrophysiology. Pace mapping has lower sensitivity and specificity than it does for idiopathic VT. Furthermore, reentry circuits can sometimes be large and resistant to the relatively small lesions produced by RF catheter ablation in scarred endocardium.

Finding a protected region of diastolic activation used as a critical part of the reentrant circuit is desirable because ablation at this site has a good chance of eliminating the tachycardia (Fig. 30–17). Because of the extensive derangement in electrophysiology caused by the infarction, many areas of the ventricle may have diastolic activation but not be relevant to the perpetuation of the VT. These "bystander sites" make activation mapping more difficult. Pacing techniques such as entrainment can be used to test whether a site is truly part of a circuit or a bystander. Entrainment involves pacing for several seconds during a tachycardia at a rate slightly faster than the VT rate; after pacing ceases and the same tachycardia resumes, the timing of the first complex relative to the last paced beat is an indicator of how close the pacing site is to a part of the VT circuit. During entrainment, part of the ventricle is activated by the paced wave front and part by the VT wave front being forced to exit earlier than it ordinarily would, resulting in a fusion complex on the electrocardiogram. Pacing from within a critical portion of the circuit itself produces an exact QRS match with the VT; fusion occurs only within the circuit and is "concealed" on the surface electrocardiogram. Sites with a low-amplitude, isolated mid-diastolic potential that cannot be dissociated from the tachycardia by pacing perturbations, at which entrainment with concealed fusion can be demonstrated, are highly likely to be successful ablation sites.

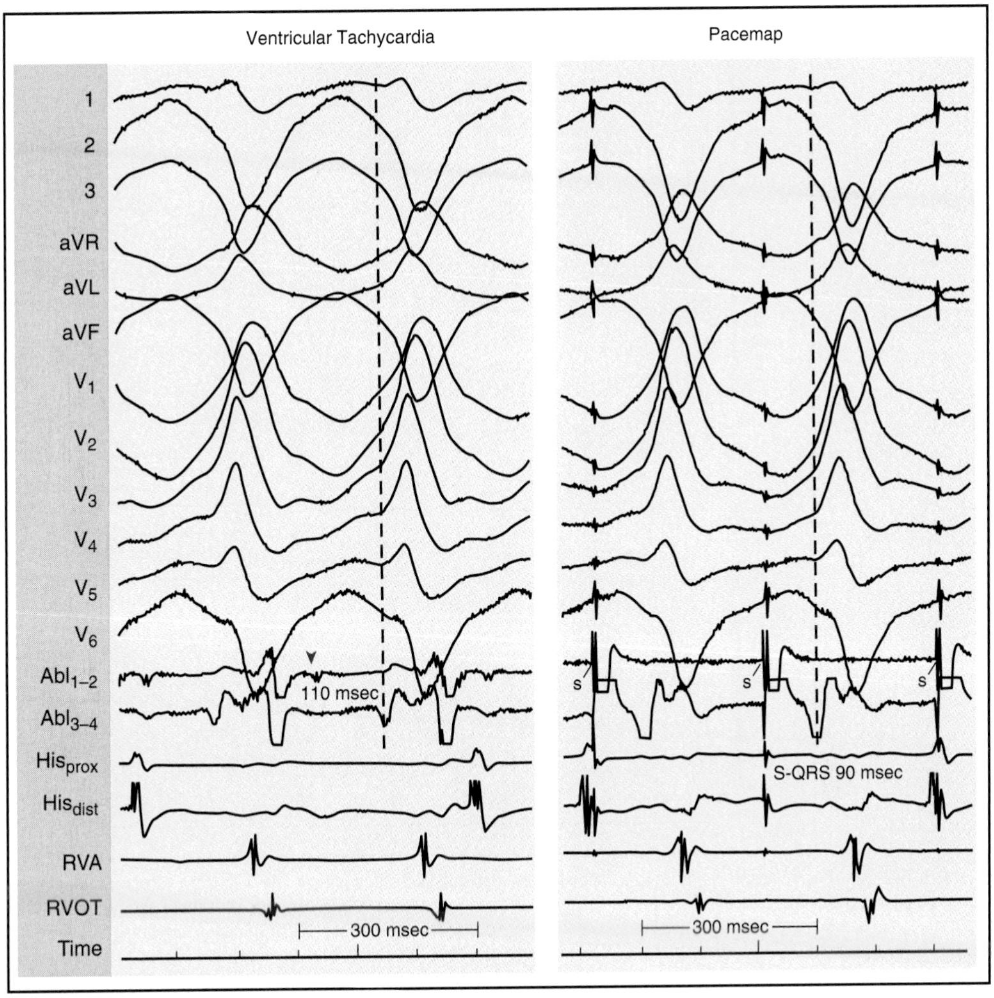

FIGURE 30–15 Ventricular tachycardia and pace mapping. All 12 surface electrocardiographic leads are shown along with intracardiac recordings during ventricular tachycardia (VT). The Abl_{1-2} recording shows a small deflection occurring early in electrical diastole (arrow) 110 milliseconds before the onset of the QRS (dashed line). In the right panel, pacing is performed from this site. This produces an identical QRS complex in each lead, with a stimulus–QRS onset interval similar to the electrogram–QRS onset interval during VT. Ablation at this site eliminated VT in 2 seconds. RVOT = right ventricular outflow tract.

In a significant proportion of patients with VT in the presence of structural heart disease, activation mapping and entrainment cannot be performed because of poor hemodynamic tolerance of the arrhythmia or inability to initiate sustained tachycardia at EPS. Some investigators have devised techniques to ascertain the location of myocardial regions at which ablation would decrease or eliminate VT recurrences. Such methods generally fall into a category of substrate mapping, in which areas of low electrical voltage or those from which very delayed potentials are recorded during sinus rhythm or at which pacing closely replicates a known VT 12-lead ECG morphology (pace mapping) are targeted for ablation without performing any mapping during VT.[76] Experience with these methods is limited, but results in decreasing the number of VT recurrences are thus far promising.

In patients without structural heart disease, only a single VT is usually present, and catheter ablation of that VT is curative. In patients with extensive structural heart disease, especially those with prior myocardial infarction, multiple VTs are usually present. Catheter ablation of a single VT in such patients may be only palliative and may not eliminate the need for further antiarrhythmic therapy. The genesis of multiple tachycardia morphologies is not clear, although in some cases they are merely different manifestations of one circuit (e.g., different directions of wave front propagation or exit to the ventricle as a whole), and ablation of one may prevent recurrence of others. The presence of multiple VT morphologies contributes to the difficulties in mapping and ablation of VT in these patients because pacing techniques employed to validate recordings at potential sites of ablation may result in a change in morphology to another VT that does not arise in the same region.

After ablation of VT, repeated ventricular stimulation is performed to assess efficacy. In some cases, rapid polymorphic VT or fibrillation is initiated. The clinical significance of these arrhythmias is unclear, but some evidence suggests that they have a low likelihood of spontaneous occurrence during follow-up.

As noted previously, most cases of polymorphic VT and VF are not currently amenable to ablation because of hemodynamic instability and beat-to-beat changes in activation sequence. However, rare reports of successful ablation of these arrhythmias in patients with apparent focal initiation have shown that at least some cases can be managed with ablation. In such cases, repeated episodes of arrhythmia have constant ECG features of the initiating beat or beats suggesting a consistent source, which may be in either ventricle. The electrogram at sites of successful ablation often has very sharp presystolic potentials reminiscent of Purkinje potentials.[77]

Indications. Patients considered for RF catheter ablation of VT in the absence of structural heart disease are those with symptomatic, sustained, monomorphic VT when the tachycardia is drug resistant, when the patient is drug intolerant, or when the patient does not desire long-term drug therapy. Patients with structural heart disease who are candidates for ablation include those with bundle branch reentrant VT and patients with sustained monomorphic VT and an ICD who are receiving multiple shocks not manageable by reprogramming or concomitant drug therapy. Occasionally, nonsustained VT or even severely symptomatic PVCs require RF catheter ablation.

Results. In the U.S. NASPE survey, 429 patients underwent ablation, with an overall success rate of 71 percent. In 224 patients with structurally normal hearts, the success rate

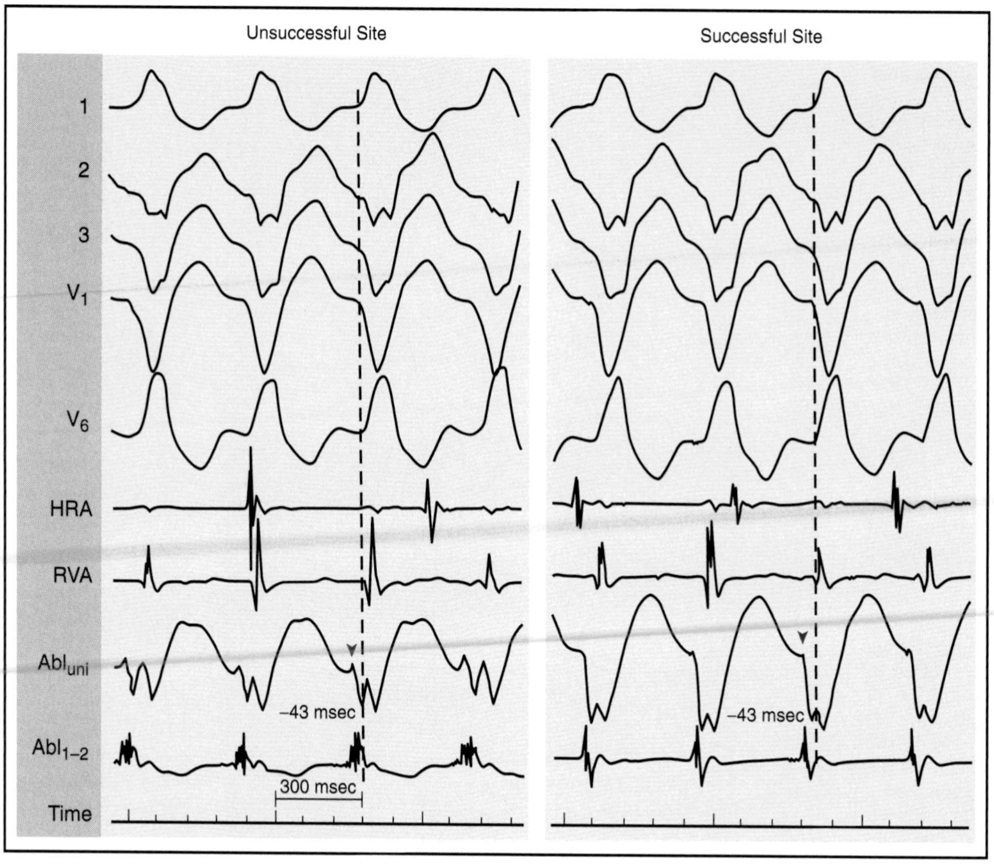

FIGURE 30–16 Recordings from unsuccessful and successful ablation sites in a patient with idiopathic ventricular tachycardia arising in the inferior right ventricular wall. In the recordings from the unsuccessful ablation site, the unipolar signal (arrow) has a small r wave, indicating that a portion of the wave front from the focus of tachycardia was approaching the site from elsewhere. At the successful site, the unipolar recording has a QS configuration, indicating that all depolarization was emanating from this site. In each site, the bipolar recording ($Abl_{1\text{-}2}$) occurs an identical 43 milliseconds before QRS onset (dashed lines).

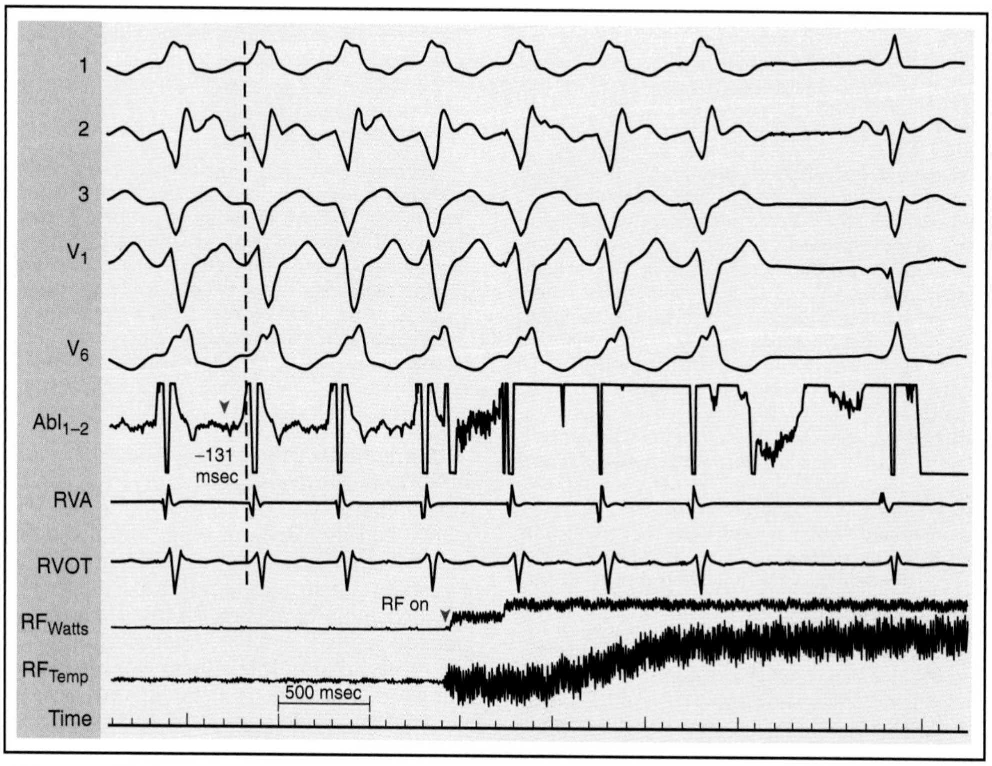

FIGURE 30–17 Radiofrequency (RF) ablation of postinfarct ventricular tachycardia (VT). Recordings are as in previous figures. The electrogram in the ablation recording ($Abl_{1\text{-}2}$, arrow) precedes the QRS onset (dashed line) by 131 milliseconds. Ablation here (RF on) results in slight deceleration of VT before termination in 1.3 seconds. Temperature monitored from the catheter tip had just peaked (approximately 70°C) at the time VT terminated.

was 85 percent. The success rate was 54 percent in 115 patients with VT related to ischemic heart disease and 61 percent in 90 patients with idiopathic cardiomyopathy. There were 13 significant complications (3.0 percent) and, interestingly, considering the nature of the disease, no procedure-related deaths.[61] The complication rate was 7.5 percent in the European survey, and there was one death in 320 patients.[63] Later series suggest a 30 percent "cure" rate for patients (no inducible ventricular arrhythmia of any type, no recurrences), whereas more than 70 percent of patients no longer have recurrences of VT after the procedure, despite inducibility of rapid VT or VF.

NEW MAPPING AND ABLATION TECHNOLOGIES

Multielectrode Mapping Systems. As noted earlier, many of the limitations of ablation are related to inadequate mapping. These problems include only isolated premature complexes during the EPS as opposed to sustained tachycardias (in idiopathic atrial and ventricular tachycardias), nonsustained episodes of VT, poor hemodynamic tolerance of VT, and multiple VT morphologies. Standard mapping techniques sample single sites sequentially and are poorly suited to these situations. New mapping systems are available that enable sampling of many sites simultaneously and incorporate sophisticated computer algorithms for analysis and display of global maps. These mapping systems use a variety of technologies, ranging from multiple electrodes situated on each of several splines of a basket catheter, to the use of low-intensity electrical or magnetic fields to localize the catheter tip in the heart and record and plot activation times on a contour map of the chamber, to the use of complex mathematics to compute "virtual" electrograms recorded from a mesh electrode situated in the middle of a chamber cavity.[78] Some of these systems are capable of generating activation maps of an entire chamber using only one complex, an obvious advantage in patients with only premature complexes, nonsustained arrhythmias, or poor hemodynamic tolerance. Although these mapping systems offer great assistance in selected cases, they are complex and expensive.

EPICARDIAL CATHETER MAPPING. Although the majority of VTs can be ablated from the endocardium, occasional cases are resistant to this therapy. In some of these cases, epicardial ablation may be successful.[75] Much of the work in this area has been performed in patients with VT related to Chagas disease, in whom a majority appear to require epicardial mapping and ablation; it is less frequently necessary in postinfarct or cardiomyopathy patients and those without structural heart disease. The technique for gaining access to the epicardium differs slightly from that for pericardiocentesis. A long spinal anesthesia needle is introduced from a subxiphoid approach under fluoroscopic guidance. As the pericardial surface is approached, a small amount of a radiocontrast agent is injected. If the needle tip is still outside the pericardium, the dye stays where injected; when the pericardial space has been entered, the dye disperses, outlining the heart. A guidewire can then be introduced through the needle and a standard vascular introducer sheath exchanged over the wire. The pericardial space is then accessible for a standard mapping ablation catheter. Standard mapping techniques can then be applied. When a site is selected for possible ablation, coronary arteriography may be warranted to avoid delivery of RF energy near a coronary artery. This is less important in postinfarct VT because the VT substrate is typically in a region of prior transmural infarction. The technique can be applied in patients who have had prior cardiac surgery, although adhesions may obliterate portions of the pericardial space.

CHEMICAL ABLATION. Chemical ablation with alcohol or phenol of an area of myocardium involved in a tachycardia has been used to create AV block in patients not responding to catheter ablation and to eliminate atrial and ventricular tachycardias. Recurrences of tachycardia several days after apparently successful ablation are common. Excessive myocardial necrosis is the major complication, and alcohol ablation should be considered only when other ablative approaches fail or cannot be done.

Surgical Therapy for Tachyarrhythmias

The objectives of a surgical approach to treating a tachycardia are to excise, isolate, or interrupt tissue in the heart critical for the initiation, maintenance, or propagation of the tachycardia while preserving or even improving myocardial function. In addition to a direct surgical approach to the arrhythmia, indirect approaches such as aneurysmectomy, coronary artery bypass grafting, and relief of valvular regurgitation or stenosis can be useful in selected patients by improving cardiac hemodynamics and myocardial blood flow. Cardiac sympathectomy alters adrenergic influences on the heart and has been effective in some patients, particularly those who have recurrent VT with the long QT syndrome.

Supraventricular Tachycardias

Surgical procedures exist for patients (adults and children) with ATs, atrial flutter, AV node reentry, and AV reentry (Fig. 30–18). RF catheter ablation adequately treats the vast majority of these patients and has thus replaced direct surgical intervention except for the occasional patient in whom RF catheter ablation fails or who is having concomitant cardiovascular surgery. In some instances, a prior attempt at RF catheter ablation complicates surgery by obliterating the normal tissue planes that exist in the AV groove of the heart or by rendering tissues too friable. Occasionally, patients with ATs have multiple foci that require surgical intervention.

The maze procedure, developed to treat patients with atrial fibrillation, eliminates the arrhythmia by reducing atrial tissue mass to a size at any instant in time too small to perpetuate the reentrant circuits responsible for atrial fibrillation.[79] It forces atrial activation to proceed along a surgically determined pathway, thus maintaining sinus rhythm with AV nodal conduction. The maze procedure permits organized electrical depolarization of the atria, restores atrial transport function, and in so doing decreases the risk of thromboembolism. Maintenance of sinus rhythm more than 3 months after the procedure approaches 100 percent, although up to 10 percent of patients require pacemakers because of chronotropic incompetence of the sinus node (related to either the surgery or the preexisting atrial pathology). The advent of minimally invasive endoscopic and endovascular techniques may make it possible to perform an equivalent of the maze procedure without thoracotomy in the future. The maze procedure or a variation of it is currently most commonly performed concomitantly with mitral valve surgery rather than as a primary indication. In many centers, intraoperative RF ablation has replaced surgical incisions for performing the maze procedure, although significant complications (such as esophageal erosion) have been reported.[80]

Ventricular Tachycardia

In contrast to patients with supraventricular arrhythmias, candidates for surgical therapy for ventricular arrhythmias often have severe left ventricular dysfunction, which is generally caused by coronary artery disease. The cause of the underlying heart disease influences the type of surgery performed. Candidates are patients with drug-resistant, symptomatic, recurrent ventricular tachyarrhythmias who ideally have a segmental wall motion abnormality (scar or aneurysm) with preserved residual left ventricular function, have not benefited from prior attempts at catheter ablation, or are not candidates for catheter ablation because of hemodynamic

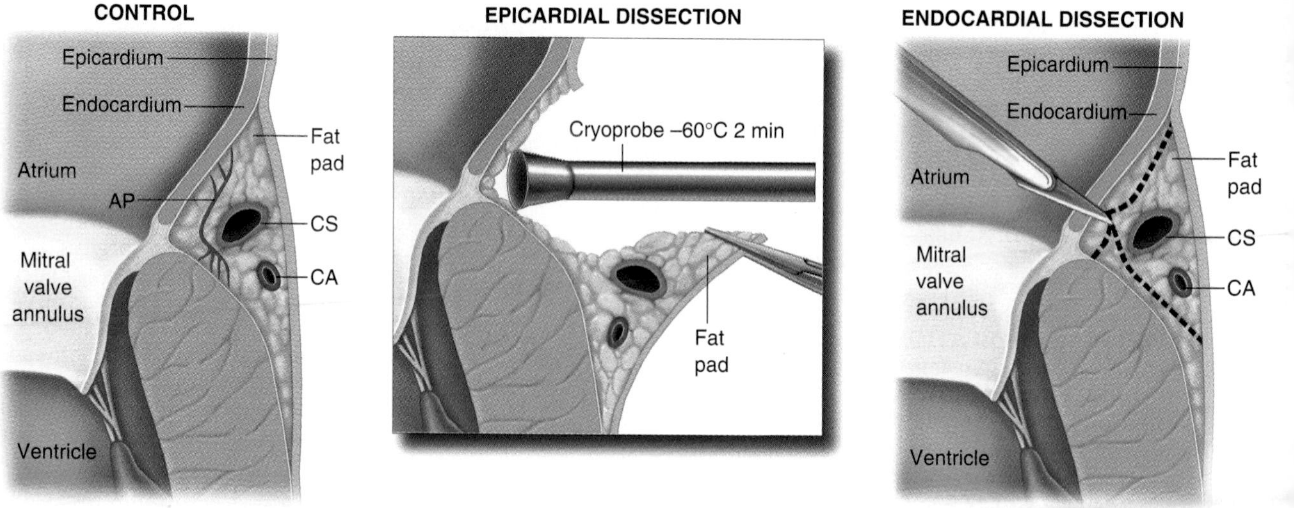

FIGURE 30–18 Schematic diagram showing the two approaches for surgical interruption of an accessory pathway. The left panel depicts the left atrioventricular groove and its vascular contents, the coronary sinus (CS) and circumflex coronary artery (CA). Multiple accessory pathways (APs) course through the fat pad. The middle panel shows the epicardial dissection approach, and the right panel exhibits the endocardial dissection. Both approaches clear out the fat pad and interrupt any accessory pathways. WPW = Wolff-Parkinson-White. (From Zipes DP: Cardiac electrophysiology: Promises and contributions. J Am Coll Cardiol 13:1329, 1989. Reprinted by permission of the American College of Cardiology.)

instability during VT or the presence of left ventricular thrombus. Poorer surgical results are obtained in patients with nonischemic cardiomyopathy.

ISCHEMIC HEART DISEASE. In almost all patients who have VT associated with ischemic heart disease, the arrhythmia, regardless of its configuration on the surface electrocardiogram, arises in the left ventricle or on the left ventricular side of the interventricular septum. The ECG contour of the VT can change from a right bundle branch block to a left bundle branch block pattern without a change in the site of earliest diastolic activation, suggesting that the site of the circuit within the left ventricle remains the same, often near the septum, but its exit pathway is altered.

Indirect surgical approaches, including cardiothoracic sympathectomy, coronary artery bypass grafting, and ventricular aneurysm or infarct resection with or without coronary artery bypass grafting, have been successful in 20 to 30 percent of reported cases. Coronary artery bypass grafting as a primary therapeutic approach has generally been successful only in patients who experience VT during ischemia as well as patients with ischemia-related VF but can sometimes be useful in patients with coronary disease resuscitated from sudden death who have no inducible arrhythmias at EPS. These patients generally have a clear relationship between episodes of ventricular arrhythmia and immediately antecedent severe ischemia and have either no evidence of infarction or minimal wall motion abnormalities with preserved overall left ventricular function. Patients with sustained monomorphic VT or only polymorphic VT rarely have their arrhythmias affected by coronary bypass surgery, although the latter can reduce the frequency of the arrhythmic episodes in some patients and prevent new ischemic events.

Surgical Techniques

Generally, two types of direct surgical procedures are used: resection and ablation (Fig. 30–19).[81] The first direct surgical approach to VT was encircling endocardial ventriculotomy, using a transmural ventriculotomy to isolate areas of endocardial fibrosis that were recognized visually; this procedure is rarely employed now. The rationale for subendocardial resection is based on animal and clinical data indicating that arrhythmias after myocardial infarction arise mostly at the subendocardial borders between normal and infarcted tissues. Subendocardial resection involves peeling off a 1- to 3-mm-thick layer of endocardium, often near the rim of an aneurysm, that has been demonstrated by means of mapping procedures to be the site of earliest activation recorded during the VT. Some VTs can arise from the epicardium. Tachycardias arising from near the base of the papillary muscles are treated using a cryoprobe cooled to −70°C. Cryoablation can also be used to isolate areas of the ventricle that cannot be resected and is often combined with resection. The neodymium:yttrium-aluminum-garnet laser approaches have been used as well with good success, but the equipment is expensive and difficult to work with.

RESULTS. For ventricular tachyarrhythmias, operative mortality ranges from 6 to 23 percent, with success rates defined as absence of recurrence of spontaneous ventricular arrhythmias ranging from 59 to 98 percent. In experienced centers, operative mortality can be as low as 5 percent in stable patients undergoing elective procedures, with 85 to 95 percent of survivors free of inducible or spontaneous ventricular tachyarrhythmias. Long-term recurrence rates range from 2 to 38 percent and correlate with results of the patient's postoperative electrophysiological stimulation study. Operative survival is strongly influenced by the degree of left ventricular dysfunction.

Operative mortality for nonthoracotomy ICD implantation is less than 1 percent, with an annual sudden cardiac death mortality rate of less than 1 percent. Because of the difference in operative survival and shorter hospital stay with ICD therapy compared with direct surgery for VT and the success rates for catheter ablation in patients who have an ICD but experience frequent episodes of VT, few curative surgical procedures are now performed.

Electrophysiological Studies

PREOPERATIVE ELECTROPHYSIOLOGICAL STUDY. In patients for whom direct surgical therapy for VT is planned, a preoperative EPS is usually warranted. This study involves initiation of the VT and electrophysiological mapping to localize the area to be resected, as is done with catheter ablation. A resolution of 4 to 8 cm^2 of ventricular endocardium is thereby achieved, although more accurate anatomical localization of the mapping electrode tip in the ventricle may be possible. Tachycardias that are too rapid, short in duration, or polymorphic cannot be mapped accurately unless multiple catheters or a multielectrode array is used. Administering a drug such as procainamide may slow the VT and transform a nonsustained polymorphic VT into a sustained VT of uniform contour that can be mapped. Preoperative catheter mapping is contraindicated in patients who have known left ventricular thrombus that might be dislodged by the mapping catheter.

INTRAOPERATIVE VENTRICULAR MAPPING. Electrophysiological mapping is also performed at the time of surgery, with the surgeon using a hand-held probe or an electrode array coupled with computer techniques that instantaneously provide an overall activation map cycle by cycle. The sequence of activation during VT can be plotted and the area of earliest activation determined. Resection or cryoablation of tissue from which these recordings are made usually cures the VT, indicating that they represent a critical portion of the reentrant circuit. However, it is quite clear that such electrical activity can be late following the preceding cycle or early in advance of the next cycle. When the earliest recordable endocardial electrical activity occurs less than 30 milliseconds before the onset of the QRS complex, the critical portions of the circuit may be in the interventricular septum or near the epicardium of the free wall.

The area of earliest recorded electrical activity during VT may not actually represent a critical portion of the tachycardia circuit because the latter may be several centimeters away (e.g., in a small, scarred area). The impulse may then be conducted slowly until it reaches more normally excitable tissue, where it exits and spreads rapidly to the rest of the endocardium to generate a QRS complex. However, this area of early activation is probably closely related to the origin of the tachycardia that, on the basis of the present state of knowledge and results from surgery, warrants surgical intervention at that site. Finding an area from which "continuous electrical activity" is recorded rarely, if ever, indicates that the entire circuit is being recorded. However, it is likely that a critical portion of the tachycardia circuit is close to the area of continuous electrical activity. In some patients, intramural mapping using a plunge needle electrode can be useful, particularly if the origin of the tachycardia is not in the subendocardium. Most centers now employ a strategy of "sequential" subendocardial resection, in which VT is initiated, mapped, and ablated (resected or cryoablated) and stimulation is immediately repeated. If VT can still be initiated, mapping and resection are also repeated until VT can no longer be initiated.

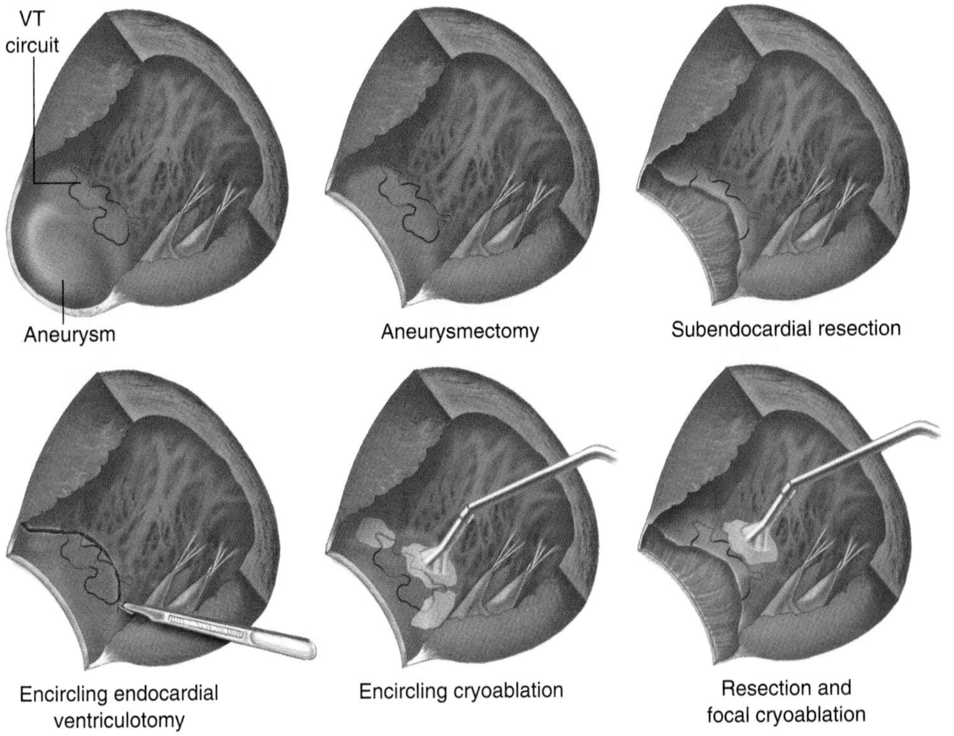

FIGURE 30–19 Schematic diagram showing surgical procedures for treatment of postinfarct ventricular tachycardia (VT) with left ventricular aneurysm. A damaged left ventricle is depicted as opened along the lateral wall and viewing the septum and papillary muscles. The tachycardia circuit (upper left) takes a meandering course near where the aneurysm meets normal myocardium and at times is superficial and at other times coursing deeper (green lines). Simple aneurysmectomy that leaves a portion of the aneurysm for suturing often misses the circuit and thus does not cure the arrhythmia. Using subendocardial resection, a layer of endocardium and subjacent tissue is removed, including at least some of the tachycardia circuit. This resection results in elimination of tachycardia. Encircling endocardial ventriculotomy attempts to isolate the circuit electrically without removing tissue, but it probably actually works by incising portions of the circuit. Cryoablation can be used to encircle the infarct zone or in combination with resection to damaged tissue too deep in the wall to be safely resected.

REFERENCES

1. Murgatroyd FD: "Pills and pulses": Hybrid therapy for atrial fiibrillation. J ardiovasc Electrophysiol 13:S40, 2002.

Pharmacological Therapy

2. Vaughan Williams EM: The relevance of cellular to clinical electrophysiology in classifying antiarrhythmic actions. J Cardiovasc Pharmacol 20:S1, 1992.
3. Members of the Sicilian Gambit: Antiarrhythmic Therapy: A Pathophysiologic Approach. Armonk, NY, Futura Publishing Company, 1994.
4. Kowey PR, Marinchak RA, Rials SJ, Bharucha DB: Classifiication and pharmacology o antiarrhythmic drugs. Am Heart J 140:12, 2000.
5. Napolitano C, Schwartz PJ, Brown AM, et al: Evidence for a cardiac ion channel mutation underlying drug-induced QT prolongation and life-threatening arrhythmias. J Cardiovasc Electrophysiol 11:691, 2000.
6. Naccarelli GV, Wolbrette DL, Khan M, et al: Old and new antiarrhythmic drugs for converting and maintaining sinus rhythm in atrial fiibrillation: Comparative effiicacy a results of trials. Am J Cardiol 91:15D, 2003.
7. Sarkozy A, Dorian P: Advances in the acute pharmacologic management of cardiac arrhythmias. Curr Cardiol Rep 5:387, 2003.
8. Choudhury L, Grais IM, Passman RS: Torsades de pointes due to drug interaction between disopyramide and clarithromycin. Heart Dis 1:206, 1999.
9. Somberg JC, Bailin SJ, Haffajee CI, et al: Intravenous lidocaine vs intravenous amiodarone (in a new aqueous formulation) for incessant ventricular tachycardia. Am J Cardiol 90:853, 2002.
10. Aliot E, De Roy L, Capucci A, et al: Safety of a controlled-release fllecainide acetate formulation in the prevention of paroxysmal atrial fiibrillation in outpatients. Ann Cardio Angeiol (Paris) 52:34, 2003.
11. Kowey PR, Yan GX, Winkel E, et al: Pharmacologic and nonpharmacologic options to maintain sinus rhythm: Guideline-based and new approaches. Am J Cardiol 91:33D, 2003.
12. Naccarelli GV, Wolbrette DL, Luck JC: Proarrhythmia. Med Clin North Am 85:503, 2001.
13. Flaker GC, Blackshear JL, McBride R, et al: Antiarrhythmic drug therapy and cardiac mortality in atrial fiibrillation. The Stroke Prevention in Atrial Fibrillation Investigators J Am Coll Cardiol 20:527, 1992.
14. The Cardiac Arrhythmia Suppression Trial Investigators: Preliminary report: Effect of encainide and fllecainide on mrtality in a randomized trial of arrhythmia suppression after myocardial infarction. N Engl J Med 321:406, 1989.

15. Wyse KR, Ye V, Campbell TJ: Action potential prolongation exhibits simple dose-dependence for sotalol, but reverse dose-dependence for quinidine and disopyramide: Implications for proarrhythmia due to triggered activity. J Cardiovasc Pharmacol 21:316, 1993.
16. Darbar D, Fromm MF, Dellorto S, Roden DM: Sympathetic activation enhances QT prolongation by quinidine. J Cardiovasc Electrophysiol 12:9, 2001.
17. Benton RE, Sale M, Flockhart DA, Woosley RL: Greater quinidine-induced QTc interval prolongation in women. Clin Pharmacol Ther 67:413, 2000.
18. Brembilla-Perrot B, Houriez P, Beurrier D, et al: Predictors of atrial fllutter with 1:1 coduction in patients treated with class I antiarrhythmic drugs for atrial tachyarrhythmias. Int J Cardiol 80:7, 2001.
19. Morita N, Kobayashi Y, Iwasaki YK, et al: Pronounced effect of procainamide on clockwise right atrial isthmus conduction compared with counterclockwise conduction: Possible mechanism of the greater incidence of common atrial fllutter during antiarrhythmi therapy. J Cardiovasc Electrophysiol 13:212, 2002.
20. Rials SJ, Britchkow D, Marinchak RA, Kowey PR: Electropharmacologic effect of a standard dose of intravenous procainamide in patients with sustained ventricular tachycardia. Clin Cardiol 23:171, 2000.

Class IB Antiarrhythmic Agents

CH 30

21. Ye VZ, Wyse KR, Campbell TJ: Lidocaine shows greater selective depression of depolarized and acidotic myocardium than propafenone: Possible implications for proarrhythmia. J Cardiovasc Pharmacol 21:47, 1993.
22. Dorian P, Cass D, Schwartz B, et al: Amiodarone as compared with lidocaine for shock-resistant ventricular fiibrillatio. N Engl J Med 346:884, 2002.
23. Yonezawa E, Matsumoto K, Ueno K, et al: Lack of interaction between amiodarone and mexiletine in cardiac arrhythmia patients. J Clin Pharmacol 42:342, 2002.
24. Azarbayjani F, Danielsson BR: Phenytoin-induced cleft palate: Evidence for embryonic cardiac bradyarrhythmia due to inhibition of delayed rectifiier $^{+}$ channels resulting in hypoxia-reoxygenation damage. Teratology 63:152, 2001.

Class IC Antiarrhythmic Agents

25. Ebenroth ES, Cordes TM, Darragh RK: Second-line treatment of fetal supraventricular tachycardia using fllecainide acetate. Pediatr Cardiol 22:483, 2001.
26. Arias C, Gonzalez T, Moreno I, et al: Effects of propafenone and its main metabolite, 5-hydroxypropafenone, on HERG channels. Cardiovasc Res 57:660, 2003.
27. Boriani G, Martignani C, Biffii M, et al: Oral loading with propafenone for conversion o recent-onset atrial fiibrillation: A review on in-hospital treatment. Drugs 62:415, 2002.
28. Geller JC, Geller M, Carlson MD, Waldo AL: Effiicacy and safety of moicizine in the maintenance of sinus rhythm in patients with recurrent atrial fiibrillation. Am J Cardio 87:172, 2001.
29. The Cardiac Arrhythmia Suppression Trial II Investigators: Effect of the antiarrhythmic agent moricizine on survival after myocardial infarction. N Engl J Med 327:227, 1992.

Class II Antiarrhythmic Agents

30. Singh BN, Sarma JSM: Beta-blockers and calcium channel blockers as antiarrhythmic drugs. *In* Zipes DP, Jalife J (eds): Cardiac Electrophysiology: From Cell to Bedside. 3rd ed. Philadelphia, WB Saunders, 1999, pp 903-920.
31. Connolly SJ, Cybulsky I, Lamy A, et al: Double-blind, placebo-controlled, randomized trial of prophylactic metoprolol for reduction of hospital length of stay after heart surgery: The beta-Blocker Length Of Stay (BLOS) study. Am Heart J 145:226, 2003.
32. Sun W, Sarma JS, Singh BN: Chronic and acute effects of dronedarone on the action potential of rabbit atrial muscle preparations: Comparison with amiodarone. J Cardiovasc Pharmacol 39:677, 2002
33. Aimond F, Beck L, Gautier P, et al: Cellular and in vivo electrophysiological effects of dronedarone in normal and postmyocardial infarcted rats. J Pharmacol Exp Ther 292:415, 2000.
34. Camm AJ, Yap YG: What should we expect from the next generation of antiarrhythmic drugs? J Cardiovasc Electrophysiol 10:307, 1999.

Class III Antiarrhythmic Agents

35. Doval HC, Nul DR, Grancelli HO, et al: Randomised trial of low-dose amiodarone in severe congestive heart failure. Grupo de Estudio de la Sobrevida en la Insufiicienci Cardiaca en Argentina (GESICA). Lancet 344:493, 1994.
36. Daoud EG, Strickberger SA, Man KC, et al: Preoperative amiodarone as prophylaxis against atrial fiibrillation after heart surgery. N Engl J Med 337:1785, 1997.
37. Dorian P, Mangat I: Role of amiodarone in the era of the implantable cardioverter defiirillator. J Cardiovasc Electrophysiol 14(Suppl 9):S78, 2003.
38. The AVID Investigators: Antiarrhythmics Versus Implantable Defiibrillators (AVID) Rationale, design, and methods. Am J Cardiol 75:470, 1995.
39. Ott MC, Khoor A, Leventhal JP, et al: Pulmonary toxicity in patients receiving low-dose amiodarone. Chest 123:646, 2003.
40. van Opstal JM, Schoenmakers M, Verduyn SC, et al: Chronic amiodarone evokes no torsades de pointes arrhythmias despite QT lengthening in an animal model of acquired long-QT syndrome. Circulation 104:2722, 2001.
41. Cardenas GA, Cabral JM, Leslie CA: Amiodarone induced thyrotoxicosis: Diagnostic and therapeutic strategies. Cleve Clin J Med 70:624, 628, 2003.
42. Sreih AG, Schoenfeld MH, Marieb MA: Optic neuropathy following amiodarone therapy. Pacing Clin Electrophysiol 22:1108, 1999.
43. Hohnloser SH, Woosley RL: Sotalol. N Engl J Med 331:31, 1994.
44. Pacifiico A, Hohnloser SH, Williams JH, et al: Prevention of implantable-defiibrillar shocks by treatment with sotalol. *d,l*-Sotalol Implantable Cardioverter-Defiibrillato Study Group. N Engl J Med 340:1855, 1999.
45. Eversole A, Hancock W, Johns T, et al: Ibutilide: Effiicacy and safety in atrial fiibrillati and atrial fllutter in a generl cardiology practice. Clin Cardiol 24:521, 2001.
46. Oral H, Souza JJ, Michaud GF, et al: Facilitating transthoracic cardioversion of atrial fiirillation with ibutilide pretreatment. N Engl J Med 340:1849, 1999.
47. Kalus JS, Mauro VF: Dofetilide: A class III–specifiic antiarrhythmic agent. Ann Pharmcother 34:44, 2000.
48. Pedersen OD, Bagger H, Keller N, et al: Effiicacy of dofetilide in the treatment of atria fiibrillation-fllutter in patients with reduced left ventricular function: A Danish investigations of arrhythmia and mortality on dofetilide (diamond) substudy. Circulation 104:292, 2001.
49. Clemett D, Markham A: Azimilide. Drugs 59:271, discussion, 278, 2000.
50. Abrol R, Page RL: Azimilide dihydrochloride: A new class III anti-arrhythmic agent. Expert Opin Investig Drugs 9:2705, 2000.

Class IV Antiarrhythmic Agents

51. De Simone A, De Pasquale M, De Matteis C, et al: Verapamil plus antiarrhythmic drugs reduce atrial fiibrillation recurrences after an electrical cardioversion (VEPARAF Study) Eur Heart J 24:1425, 2003.

Other Antiarrhythmic Agents

52. Strickberger SA, Man KC, Daoud EG, et al: Adenosine-induced atrial arrhythmia: A prospective analysis. Ann Intern Med 127:417, 1997.

Electrotherapy of Cardiac Arrhythmias

53. Mittal S, Ayati S, Stein KM, et al: Transthoracic cardioversion of atrial fiibrillation: Coparison of rectilinear biphasic versus damped sine wave monophasic shocks. Circulation 101:1282, 2000.
54. Wyse DG, Waldo AL, DiMarco JP, et al: Atrial Fibrillation Follow-up Investigation of Rhythm Management (AFFIRM) Investigators: A comparison of rate control and rhythm control in patients with atrial fiibrillation. N Enl J Med 347:1825, 2002.
55. Klein AL, Grimm RA, Murray RD, et al: Use of transesophageal echocardiography to guide cardioversion in patients with atrial fiibrillation. N Engl J Med 344:1411, 2001.
56. Morady F: Radio-frequency ablation as treatment for cardiac arrhythmias. N Engl J Med 340:534, 1999.
57. Kimman GJ, Szili-Torok T, Theuns DA, Jordaens LJ: Transvenous cryothermal catheter ablation of a right anteroseptal accessory pathway. J Cardiovasc Electrophysiol 12:1415, 2001.
58. Nabar A, Rodriguez LM, Timmermans C, Wellens HJ: Use of a saline-irrigated tip catheter for ablation of ventricular tachycardia resistant to conventional radiofrequency ablation: Early experience. J Cardiovasc Electrophysiol 12:153, 2001.
59. Rodriguez LM, Geller JC, Tse HF, et al: Acute results of transvenous cryoablation of supraventricular tachycardia (atrial fiibrillation, atrial flutter, Wolff-Parkins-White syndrome, atrioventricular nodal reentry tachycardia). J Cardiovasc Electrophysiol 13:1082, 2002.
60. Calkins H, Yong P, Miller JM, et al: Catheter ablation of accessory pathways, atrioventricular nodal reentrant tachycardia, and the atrioventricular junction: Final results of a prospective, multicenter clinical trial. The Atakr Multicenter Investigators Group. Circulation 99:262, 1999.
61. Scheinman MM: Patterns of catheter ablation practice in the United States: Results of the 1992 NASPE survey. North American Society of Pacing and Electrophysiology. Pacing Clin Electrophysiol 17:873, 1994.
62. Scheinman MM, Huang S: The 1998 NASPE prospective catheter ablation registry. Pacing Clin Electrophysiol 23:1020, 2000.
63. Hindricks G: The Multicentre European Radiofrequency Survey (MERFS): Complications of radiofrequency catheter ablation of arrhythmias. The Multicentre European Radiofrequency Survey (MERFS) investigators of the Working Group on Arrhythmias of the European Society of Cardiology. Eur Heart J 14:1644, 1993.
64. Wu J, Wu J, Olgin J, et al: Mechanisms underlying the reentrant circuit of atrioventricular nodal reentrant tachycardia in isolated canine atrioventricular nodal preparation using optical mapping. Circ Res 88:1189, 2001.
65. McGuire MA, de Bakker JM, Vermeulen JT, et al: Origin and signifiicance of doubl potentials near the atrioventricular node. Correlation of extracellular potentials, intracellular potentials, and histology. Circulation 89:2351, 1994.
66. Skanes AC, Dubuc M, Klein GJ, et al: Cryothermal ablation of the slow pathway for the elimination of atrioventricular nodal reentrant tachycardia. Circulation 102:2856, 2000.
67. Scheinman MM, Gonzalez RP, Cooper MW, et al: Clinical and electrophysiologic features and role of catheter ablation techniques in adult patients with automatic atrioventricular junctional tachycardia. Am J Cardiol 74:565, 1994.
68. Chen SA, Tai CT, Chiang CE, et al: Focal atrial tachycardia: Reanalysis of the clinical and electrophysiologic characteristics and prediction of successful radiofrequency ablation. J Cardiovasc Electrophysiol 9:355, 1998.
69. Tada H, Oral H, Sticherling C, et al: Double potentials along the ablation line as a guide to radiofrequency ablation of typical atrial flutter. J Am Coll Cariol 38:750, 2001.
70. Narasimhan C, Blanck Z, Akhtar M: Atrioventricular nodal modifiication and atrioventricular junctional ablation for control of ventricular rate in atrial fiibrillation. J Cardivasc Electrophysiol 9:S146, 1998.
71. Ozcan C, Jahangir A, Friedman PA, et al: Long-term survival after ablation of the atrioventricular node and implantation of a permanent pacemaker in patients with atrial fiibrillation. N Engl J Med 344:1043, 2001.
72. Marrouche NF, Martin DO, Wazni O, et al: Phased-array intracardiac echocardiography monitoring during pulmonary vein isolation in patients with atrial fiibrillation: Impac on outcome and complications. Circulation 107:2710, 2003.
73. Oral H, Knight BP, Ozaydin M, et al: Segmental ostial ablation to isolate the pulmonary veins during atrial fiibrillation: Feasibility and mechanistic insights. Circulatio 106:1256, 2002.
74. Nabar A, Rodriguez LM, Timmermans C, et al: Effect of right atrial isthmus ablation on the occurrence of atrial fiibrillation: Observations in fou patient groups having type I atrial fllutter with or without associated atrial fiibrillation. Circulation 99:1441, 1999

75. Sosa E, Scanavacca M, d'Avila A: Transthoracic epicardial catheter ablation to treat recurrent ventricular tachycardia. Curr Cardiol Rep 3:451, 2001.
76. Marchlinski FE, Callans DJ, Gottlieb CD, Zado E: Linear ablation lesions for control of unmappable ventricular tachycardia in patients with ischemic and nonischemic cardiomyopathy. Circulation 101:1288, 2000.
77. Haïssaguerre M, Shoda M, Jaïs P, et al: Mapping and ablation of idiopathic ventricular fibrillation. Circulation 106:962, 2002.
78. Strickberger SA, Knight BP, Michaud GF, et al: Mapping and ablation of ventricular tachycardia guided by virtual electrograms using a noncontact, computerized mapping system. J Am Coll Cardiol 35:414, 2000.

79. Gillinov AM, McCarthy PM, Marrouche N, Natale A: Contemporary surgical treatment for atrial fibrillation. Pacing Clin Electrophysiol 26:1641, 2003.
80. Melo J, Adragao PR, Neves J, et al: Electrosurgical treatment of atrial fibrillation with new intraoperative radiofrequency ablation catheter. Thorac Cardiovasc Surg 47(Suppl 3):370, 1999.
81. Miller JM, Rothman SA, Addonizio VP: Surgical techniques for ventricular tachycardia ablation. *In* Singer I (ed): Interventional Electrophysiology. New York, Williams & Wilkins, 1996, pp 641-684.

GUIDELINES *Thomas H. Lee*

Ambulatory Electrocardiography and Electrophysiological Testing

Guidelines for appropriate use of ambulatory electrocardiography (ECG) were first published by the American College of Cardiology/American Heart Association (ACC/AHA) in 1989[1] and updated in 1999.[2] In conjunction with other professional societies, the ACC/AHA issued a statement of requirements for clinical competence in ambulatory ECG in 2001.[3] Guidelines for performance of electrophysiology testing were first published in 1989[4] and updated in 1995[5]; a clinical competence statement was issued by the ACC/AHA for electrophysiology studies and catheter ablation in 2000.[6] The AHA and the North American Society of Pacing and Electrophysiology (NASPE) made recommendations on safety-related issues, such as restrictions on driving, for patients with arrhythmia in 1996.[7] Since then, efforts to update guidelines have focused on appropriateness of use of pacemakers and implantable defibrillators,[8] reflecting rapid advances in knowledge about the ability of implantable defibrillators to improve survival for patients with arrhythmia with or without electrophysiology testing.[9-11] Guidelines on the latter topic are addressed in the appendix to Chapter 31.

Ambulatory Electrocardiography

The evolution of guidelines for use of ambulatory ECG from 1989 to 1999[2] reflected important progress in several areas, including:

- Understanding of the limited usefulness of suppression of ventricular ectopy with drug therapy
- Solid-state digital technology that facilitates transtelephonic transmission of electrocardiographic data
- Technical advances in long-term event recorders
- Improved signal quality and interpretation
- Improved computer arrhythmia interpretation
- Increasingly sophisticated monitoring capacity of pacemakers and implantable defibrillators

As a result of progress in these areas, with increased knowledge about arrhythmias, ambulatory ECG is now considered to be of uncertain appropriateness for many indications for which it was once an accepted strategy.

As with other ACC/AHA guidelines, the indications for use of ambulatory ECG are classified into one of four classes:

- Class I: Conditions for which there is evidence and/or general agreement that the test is useful and effective.
- Class II: Conditions for which there is conflicting evidence and/or a divergence of opinion about the usefulness/efficacy of performing the test.
- Class IIa: Weight of evidence/opinion is in favor of usefulness/efficacy.
- Class IIb: Usefulness/efficacy is less well established by evidence/opinion.
- Class III: Conditions for which there is evidence and/or general agreement that the test is not useful/effective and in some cases may be harmful.

Diagnosis

In the assessment of symptoms that may be due to arrhythmias, ambulatory ECG is quite clearly established for evaluation of syncope (Table 30G–1). When continuous ambulatory ECG is not diagnostic, intermittent recorders may be useful. Ambulatory ECG is also supported for evaluation of recurrent palpitations, particularly if the frequency of these symptoms makes it reasonably likely that they can be correlated with the tracings obtained during a 24-hour monitoring period. The guidelines comment that data on the use of ambulatory ECG for near syncope or dizziness are insufficient to describe the diagnostic performance of this technology for patients with such symptoms.

The ACC/AHA guidelines explicitly discourage ambulatory ECG for patients with syncope or palpitations if other causes have been identified during the clinical evaluation and for patients with cerebrovascular accidents and no other evidence of arrhythmia. The guidelines seek to reduce performance of ambulatory ECG "for completeness" in such cases. Little support is provided for use of ambulatory ECG in cases in which the etiology of the patient's symptoms is unclear but in which the likelihood of detecting an unsuspected arrhythmia is low (class IIb indications).

Assessment of Risk

The ACC/AHA guidelines discouraged the use of ambulatory ECG for either arrhythmia detection or analysis of heart rhythm variability for the purpose of risk assessment among patients without symptoms of arrhythmia, even if they had cardiovascular conditions such as myocardial contusions, left ventricular hypertrophy, or valvular heart disease (see Table 30G–1). Routine use for patients in whom arrhythmia is a common cause of death (left ventricular dysfunction, hypertrophic cardiomyopathy) was considered a class IIb indication. These recommendations preceded data demonstrating the beneficial impact of implantable cardioverter-defibrillators (ICDs) in patients with left ventricular dysfunction after acute myocardial infarction even without symptoms of arrhythmia.[9] These more recent findings may lead to an expanded role for ambulatory ECG in determining which such asymptomatic patients most need these expensive devices.

Efficacy of Antiarrhythmic Therapy

In the absence of data demonstrating that oral antiarrhythmic therapy can improve survival through control of ventricular arrhythmias, ambulatory ECG has a diminished role as a test for evaluation of the efficacy of treatment (see Table 30G–1). Oral antiarrhythmic agents are important for control of supraventricular arrhythmias, but most patients with such arrhythmias do not have episodes every day. Event recorders can be useful for documenting the relationship between symptoms and recurrent arrhythmia and the interval between episodes, which can help guide therapy.

The guidelines provide some support for use of ambulatory ECG for detection of proarrhythmia during initiation of drug therapy, but patients at high risk for such complications tend to have initiation of these medications as inpatients.

TABLE 30G–1 ACC/AHA Guidelines for Ambulatory Electrocardiography for Assessment of Symptoms and Arrhythmias

Indication	Class I (Indicated)	Class IIa (Good Supportive Evidence)	Class IIb (Weak Supportive Evidence)	Class III (Not Indicated)
Assessment of symptoms possibly related to rhythm disturbances	Patients with unexplained syncope, near syncope, or episodic dizziness in whom the cause is not obvious Patients with unexplained recurrent palpitation		Patients with episodic shortness of breath, chest pain, or fatigue that is not otherwise explained Patients with neurological events when transient atrial fibrillation or flutter is suspected Patients with symptoms such as syncope, near syncope, episodic dizziness, or palpitation in whom a probable cause other than an arrhythmia has been identified but in whom symptoms persist despite treatment of this other cause	Patients with symptoms such as syncope, near syncope, episodic dizziness, or palpitation in whom other causes have been identified by history, physical examination, or laboratory tests Patients with cerebrovascular accidents, without other evidence of arrhythmia
Arrhythmia detection to assess risk for future cardiac events in patients without symptoms from arrhythmia			Post-MI patients with LV dysfunction (ejection fraction <40%) Patients with CHF Patients with idiopathic hypertrophic cardiomyopathy	Patients who have sustained myocardial contusion Systemic hypertensive patients with LV hypertrophy Post-MI patients with normal LV function Preoperative arrhythmia evaluation of patients for noncardiac surgery Patients with sleep apnea Patients with valvular heart disease
Measurement of heart rate variability to assess risk for future cardiac events in patients without symptoms from arrhythmia			Post-MI patients with LV dysfunction Patients with CHF Patients with idiopathic hypertrophic cardiomyopathy	Post-MI patients with normal LV function Diabetic subjects to evaluate for diabetic neuropathy Patients with rhythm disturbances that preclude HRV analysis (i.e., atrial fibrillation)
Assessment of antiarrhythmic therapy	To assess antiarrhythmic drug response in individuals in whom baseline frequency of arrhythmia has been characterized as reproducible and of sufficient frequency to permit analysis	To detect proarrhythmic responses to antiarrhythmic therapy in patients at high risk	To assess rate control during atrial fibrillation To document recurrent or asymptomatic nonsustained arrhythmias during therapy in the outpatient setting	

ACC/AHA = American College of Cardiology/American Heart Association; CHF = congestive heart failure; HRV = heart rhythm variability; LV = left ventricular; MI = myocardial infarction.

Assessment of Pacemaker and Implantable Cardioverter-Defibrillator Function

Ambulatory ECG was considered to be appropriate for evaluation of function of pacemakers and ICDs, but the role of ambulatory ECG is being eroded by increasing diagnostic and monitoring functions being built into these devices. Ambulatory ECG can provide useful information by correlating symptoms with device activity and by detecting abnormalities in sensing and capture during chronic follow-up (Table 30G–2). However, the ACC/AHA guidelines emphasize that ambulatory ECG should not be used when data available from device interrogation are sufficient to guide clinical management.

Monitoring for Myocardial Ischemia

The 1999 ACC/AHA guidelines do not provide strong support for any indications for routine clinical use of ambulatory ECG monitoring for myocardial ischemia (Table 30G–3). The only indication for which the task force felt there was good supportive evidence was in patients with suspected variant angina. This technology was not considered a first-choice alternative to exercise testing for patients who are unable to exercise.

TABLE 30G–2 ACC/AHA Guidelines for Ambulatory Electrocardiography for Assessment of Pacemaker and Implantable Cardioverter-Defibrillator Function

Class	Indication
Class I (indicated)	Evaluation of frequent symptoms of palpitations, syncope, or near syncope to assess device function to exclude myopotential inhibition and pacemaker-mediated tachycardia and to assist in the programming of enhanced features such as rate responsivity and automatic mode switching Evaluation of suspected component failure or malfunction when device interrogation is not definitive in establishing a diagnosis To assess the response to adjunctive pharmacological therapy in patients receiving frequent ICD therapy
Class IIa (good supportive evidence)	
Class IIb (weak supportive evidence)	Evaluation of immediate postoperative pacemaker function after pacemaker or ICD implantation as an alternative or adjunct to continuous telemetric monitoring Evaluation of the rate of supraventricular arrhythmias in patients with implanted defibrillators
Class III (not indicated)	Assessment of ICD or pacemaker malfunction when device interrogation, ECG, or other available data (chest radiograph and so forth) are sufficient to establish an underlying cause or diagnosis Routine follow-up in asymptomatic patients

ACC/AHA = American College of Cardiology/American Heart Association; ECG = electrocardiographic; ICD = implantable cardioverter-defibrillator.

TABLE 30G–3 ACC/AHA Guidelines for Ischemia Monitoring

Class	Indication
Class I (indicated)	
Class IIa (good supportive evidence)	Patients with suspected variant angina
Class IIb (weak supportive evidence)	Evaluation of patients with chest pain who cannot exercise Preoperative evaluation for vascular surgery of patients who cannot exercise Patients with known CAD and atypical chest pain syndrome
Class III (not indicated)	Initial evaluation of patients with chest pain who are able to exercise Routine screening of asymptomatic subjects

ACC/AHA = American College of Cardiology/American Heart Association; CAD = coronary artery disease.

Clinical Competence

The ACC/AHA statement on clinical competence recommended that trainees interpret at least 150 ambulatory electrocardiograms under supervision to acquire minimal competence with this technology.[3] A minimum of 25 test interpretations per year was recommended to maintain competence.

Electrophysiological Procedures for Diagnosis

The ACC/AHA guidelines for use of intracardiac electrophysiological procedures from 1989[4] and 1995[6] reflect the emerging role of catheter ablation as a therapeutic strategy but do not fully reflect the reduced importance of antiarrhythmic medications and growing role of ICDs that have occurred. Nevertheless, most of the basic themes of these guidelines remain valid today.

These guidelines, which are older than most of the ACC/AHA guidelines, use a simpler, three-category system for assessment of appropriateness, in which class II indications are not subdivided into indications with more and less support.

Evaluation of Sinus Node Function

Clinical evaluation of sinus node dysfunction is often difficult because of the episodic nature of symptomatic abnormalities and the wide variability in sinus node function among asymptomatic people. Invasive tests of sinus function can test the ability of the sinus node to recover from overdrive suppression and assess sinoatrial conduction by introducing atrial extrastimuli or by atrial pacing.

The ACC/AHA guidelines consider electrophysiological studies of sinus node function most appropriate for patients in whom dysfunction is suspected but not proved after a noninvasive evaluation (Table 30G–4). In contrast, the guidelines consider such studies inappropriate when a documented bradyarrhythmia has been found to be correlated with the patient's symptoms and management is unlikely to be influenced by an electrophysiological study. Studies are also considered inappropriate in asymptomatic patients and those who have sinus pauses only during sleep. When bradyarrhythmias were recognized as the cause of the patient's symptoms, electrophysiological studies were considered to have possible but uncertain appropriateness (class II) if such data might refine treatment choices.

Acquired Atrioventricular Block

The ACC/AHA guidelines emphasized that electrophysiological studies are inappropriate (class III) when ECG findings correlate with symptoms and the findings from electrophysiological studies are unlikely to alter management (e.g., documentation of His bundle conduction rarely improves management for a patient whose other clinical data indicate that placement of a permanent pacemaker is warranted because of symptomatic advanced atrioventricular [AV] block). Similarly, electrophysiological studies are not appropriate for asymptomatic patients with mild degrees of AV block who are not likely to warrant pacemaker implantation. According to these guidelines, electrophysiological studies of AV conduction should be performed when a relationship between symptoms and AV block has not been proved; in such patients, another arrhythmia could be the cause of symptoms.

Chronic Intraventricular Delay

According to ACC/AHA guidelines, the main role of electrophysiological testing in patients with prolonged H-V intervals is not to predict future complications but to determine whether the symptoms of arrhythmia are due to conduction delay or block versus some other arrhythmia. The only class I (clearly appropriate) indication for electrophysiological testing is in symptomatic patients in whom the cause of symptoms is not known. The guidelines specifically discourage such testing of asymptomatic patients and provide only equivocal support for asymptomatic patients with bundle branch block in whom treatment with drugs that might increase conduction delay is being considered.

Narrow and Wide Complex QRS Tachycardia. The ACC/AHA guidelines define different roles for electrophysiological testing in patients with narrow and wide complex tachycardias. In narrow QRS tachycardia, the site of abnormal impulse formation or the reentry circuit can often be determined from information from the 12-lead

TABLE 30G–4 ACC/AHA Guidelines for Clinical Intracardiac Electrophysiological Studies for Evaluation of Specific Electrocardiographic Abnormalities

Indication	Class I (Appropriate)	Class II (Equivocal)	Class III (Inappropriate)
Evaluation of sinus node function	Symptomatic patients in whom sinus node dysfunction is suspected as the cause of symptoms but a causal relation between an arrhythmia and the symptoms has not been established after appropriate evaluation	Patients with documented sinus node dysfunction in whom evaluation of atrioventricular (AV) or ventriculoatrial (VA) conduction or susceptibility to arrhythmias may aid in selection of the most appropriate pacing modality Patients with electrocardiographically documented sinus bradyarrhythmias to determine whether abnormalities are due to intrinsic disease, autonomic nervous system dysfunction, or the effects of drugs so as to help select therapeutic options Symptomatic patients with known sinus bradyarrhythmias to evaluate potential for other arrhythmias as the cause of symptoms	Symptomatic patients in whom an association between symptoms and a documented bradyarrhythmia has been established and choice of therapy would not be affected by results of an electrophysiological study Asymptomatic patients with sinus bradyarrhythmias or sinus pauses observed only during sleep, including sleep apnea
Acquired AV block	Symptomatic patients in whom His-Purkinje block, suspected as a cause of symptoms, has not been established Patients with second- or third-degree AV block treated with a pacemaker who remain symptomatic and in whom another arrhythmia is suspected as a cause of symptoms	Patients with second- or third-degree AV block in whom knowledge of the site of block or its mechanism or response to pharmacological or other temporary intervention may help direct therapy or assess prognosis Patients with premature, concealed junctional depolarizations suspected as a cause of second- or third-degree AV block pattern (i.e., pseudo AV block)	Symptomatic patients in whom the symptoms and presence of AV block are correlated by ECG findings Asymptomatic patients with transient AV block associated with sinus slowing (e.g., nocturnal type I second-degree AV block)
Chronic intraventricular conduction delay	Symptomatic patients in whom the cause of symptoms is not known	Asymptomatic patients with bundle branch block in whom pharmacological therapy that could increase conduction delay or produce heart block is contemplated	Asymptomatic patients with intraventricular conduction delay Symptomatic patients whose symptoms can be correlated with or excluded by ECG events
Narrow QRS tachycardia (QRS complex <0.12 sec)	Patients with frequent or poorly tolerated episodes of tachycardia that do not adequately respond to drug therapy and for whom information about site of origin, mechanism, and electrophysiological properties of the pathways of the tachycardia is essential for choosing appropriate therapy (drugs, catheter ablation, pacing, or surgery) Patients who prefer ablative therapy to pharmacological treatment	Patients with frequent episodes of tachycardia requiring drug treatment for whom there is concern about proarrhythmia or the effects of the antiarrhythmic drug on the sinus node or AV conduction	Patients with tachycardias easily controlled by vagal maneuvers and/or well-tolerated drug therapy who are not candidates for nonpharmacological therapy
Wide complex tachycardias	Patients with wide QRS complex tachycardia in whom correct diagnosis is unclear after analysis of available ECG tracings and for whom knowledge of the correct diagnosis is necessary for care	None	Patients with VT or supraventricular tachycardia with aberrant conduction or preexcitation syndromes diagnosed with certainty by ECG criteria and for whom invasive electrophysiological data would not influence therapy. However, data obtained at baseline electrophysiological study in these patients might be appropriate as a guide for subsequent therapy

TABLE 30G–4 ACC/AHA Guidelines for Clinical Intracardiac Electrophysiological Studies for Evaluation of Specific Electrocardiographic Abnormalities—cont'd

Indication	Class I (Appropriate)	Class II (Equivocal)	Class III (Inappropriate)
Prolonged QT interval syndrome	None	Identification of a proarrhythmic effect of a drug in patients experiencing sustained VT or cardiac arrest while receiving the drug Patients who have equivocal abnormalities of QT interval duration or TU wave configuration, with syncope or symptomatic arrhythmias, in whom catecholamine effects may unmask a distinct QT abnormality	Patients with clinically manifest congenital QT prolongation, with or without symptomatic arrhythmias Patients with acquired prolonged QT syndrome with symptoms closely related to an identifiable cause or mechanism
Wolff-Parkinson-White syndrome	Patients being evaluated for catheter ablation or surgical ablation of an accessory pathway Patients with ventricular preexcitation who have survived cardiac arrest or who have unexplained syncope Symptomatic patients in whom determination of the mechanism of arrhythmia or knowledge of the electrophysiological properties of the accessory pathway and normal conduction system would help in determining appropriate therapy	Asymptomatic patients with a family history of sudden cardiac death or with ventricular preexcitation but no spontaneous arrhythmia who engage in high-risk occupations or activities and in whom knowledge of the electrophysiological properties of the accessory pathway or inducible tachycardia may help determine recommendations for further activities or therapy Patients with ventricular preexcitation who are undergoing cardiac surgery for other reasons	Asymptomatic patients with ventricular preexcitation, except those in class II
Ventricular premature complexes, couplets, and nonsustained ventricular tachycardia	None	Patients with other risk factors for future arrhythmic events, such as a low ejection fraction, positive signal-averaged ECG, and nonsustained VT on ambulatory ECG recordings in whom electrophysiological studies will be used for further risk assessment and for guiding therapy in patients with inducible VT Patients with highly symptomatic, uniform morphology premature ventricular complexes, couplets, and nonsustained VT who are considered potential candidates for catheter ablation	Asymptomatic or mildly symptomatic patients with premature ventricular complexes, couplets, and nonsustained VT without other risk factors for sustained arrhythmias

ACC/AHA = American College of Cardiology/American Heart Association; ECG = electrocardiographic.

electrocardiogram. Thus, electrophysiological testing was considered more appropriate as a guide to therapy in this setting than as a tool for diagnosis. Class I indications for electrophysiological testing include patients with recurrent tachycardia for whom data from testing may help clinicians choose among drug therapy, catheter ablation, pacing, or surgery. However, testing was not considered useful for patients whose tachycardias were controlled by vagal maneuvers or medications and who are not candidates for nonpharmacological therapy.

In wide complex tachycardias, identification of the site of origin is frequently impossible from ECG tracings alone. However, electrophysiological testing permits accurate diagnosis in virtually all patients. Because knowledge of the mechanism of the arrhythmia is essential for selection of optimal therapy, electrophysiological testing was considered appropriate (class I) for the diagnosis of wide complex tachycardias in these guidelines. However, when the diagnosis is clear from other data and electrophysiological testing is not likely to influence therapy, the guidelines considered it inappropriate.

Prolonged QT Intervals. The ACC/AHA guidelines did not consider electrophysiological testing for any indications for routine use in patients with prolonged QT intervals. Whether catecholamine infusion during testing is useful for revealing patients who are at high risk for complications or whether electrophysiological testing can be used to evaluate proarrhythmic effects in this population was considered uncertain.

Wolff-Parkinson-White Syndrome. Electrophysiological testing is useful for patients with this syndrome for both diagnosis and planning of therapy. The ACC/AHA guidelines considered electrophysiological testing appropriate for patients who were candidates for catheter or surgical ablation, for those who had had cardiac arrests or unexplained syncope, or for patients whose management might be altered by knowledge of the electrophysiological properties of the accessory pathway and normal conduction system. For asymptomatic patients, however, electrophysiological studies were deemed inappropriate except in special situations, such as patients with high-risk occupations or those with a family history of sudden cardiac death.

More recently recognized entities such as Brugada syndrome, catecholaminergic tachycardia, and right ventricular cardiomyopathy were not considered.

Nonsustained Ventricular Tachycardia. For patients with ventricular premature complexes, couplets, and nonsustained ventricular tachycardia, the usefulness of electrophysiological testing is compromised by the lack of therapeutic strategies that have been shown to improve outcomes. There were no clearly appropriate indications for electrophysiological studies in these patients, and the guidelines discouraged testing in patients without other risk factors for sustained arrhythmias. Research published since these guidelines suggests that exceptions would include patients who fit the Multicenter Automatic Defibrillator Implantation Trial (MADIT) or Multicenter Unsustained Tachycardia Trial (MUSTT) criteria. For certain patients with other data suggesting an adverse prognosis, electrophysiological testing was believed to have possible but unproven appropriateness (class II).

Unexplained Syncope

The ACC/AHA guidelines recommend a low threshold for use of electrophysiological testing for patients with unexplained syncope if they also have structural heart disease (Table 30G–5). However, in patients without structural heart disease, the yield of electrophysiological testing is low. Thus, the ACC/AHA guidelines recommend a higher threshold for use of electrophysiological studies in such patients and suggest that head-up tilt testing may be a more useful test.

Survivors of Cardiac Arrest

The ACC/AHA guidelines considered electrophysiological testing appropriate for patients who were survivors of cardiac arrest other than in the earliest phase of acute myocardial infarction (see Table 30G–5). Since publication of these guidelines, acceptance of the usefulness of ICDs has become more widespread, and many of these patients receive such a device without electrophysiological testing or receive limited electrophysiological testing at device implantation. The guidelines considered electrophysiological studies inappropriate when cardiac arrest had occurred within the first 48 hours of myocardial infarction or when the cardiac arrest resulted from clearly definable specific causes.

Unexplained Palpitations

The procedure of choice to determine the cause of palpitations is ambulatory ECG, according to the ACC/AHA guidelines. The guidelines suggest that electrophysiological testing should be reserved for patients with palpitations that are associated with syncope or those in whom electrocardiograms have failed to capture a cause of the palpitations but who have been noted to have a rapid pulse rate by medical personnel (see Table 30G–5). Electrophysiological testing was considered of equivocal value in patients with symptoms so sporadic that they cannot be documented while ambulatory ECGs are performed.

Electrophysiological Studies for Therapeutic Intervention

The 1995 ACC/AHA guidelines for appropriateness of electrophysiological studies for guidance of drug therapy and implantable electrical devices do not fully reflect the decline in role of oral antiarrhythmic therapy and the rise in use of ICDs for treatment of patients who have had cardiac arrests (Table 30G–6). However, the guideline recommendations for the role of catheter ablation are still largely valid. The characteristics that are common among appropriate indications include supraventricular arrhythmias that are symptomatic; that cannot be controlled with medications because of either limited effectiveness, side effects, or inconvenience; or that have caused sudden cardiac death. Catheter ablation is also useful for some patients with ventricular tachycardia, although patients with extensive structural heart disease tend to have multiple sites of origin of their arrhythmia and may therefore be poor candidates for this procedure. Ablation is sometimes useful as an adjunct to ICD implantation to limit the episodes of ventricular tachycardia requiring ICD treatment.

TABLE 30G–5 ACC/AHA Guidelines for Clinical Intracardiac Electrophysiological Studies for Evaluation of Clinical Syndromes

Indication	Class I (Appropriate)	Class II (Equivocal)	Class III (Inappropriate)
Unexplained syncope	Patients with suspected structural heart disease and syncope that remain unexplained after appropriate evaluation	Patients with recurrent unexplained syncope without structural heart disease and a negative head-up tilt test	Patients with a known cause of syncope for whom treatment will not be guided by electrophysiological testing
Survivors of cardiac arrest	Patients surviving cardiac arrest without evidence of an acute Q wave MI Patients surviving cardiac arrest occurring more than 48 hr after the acute phase of MI in the absence of a recurrent ischemic event	Patients surviving cardiac arrest caused by bradyarrhythmia Patients surviving cardiac arrest thought to be associated with a congenital repolarization abnormality (long QT syndrome) in whom the results of noninvasive diagnostic testing are equivocal	Patients surviving a cardiac arrest that occurred during the acute phase (<48 hr) of MI Patients with cardiac arrest resulting from clearly definable specific causes such as reversible ischemia, severe valvular aortic stenosis, or noninvasively defined congenital or acquired long QT syndrome
Unexplained palpitations	Patients with palpitations who have a pulse rate documented by medical personnel as inappropriately rapid and in whom ECG recordings fail to document the cause of the palpitations Patients with palpitations preceding a syncopal episode	Patients with clinically significant palpitations, suspected to be of cardiac origin, in whom symptoms are sporadic and cannot be documented. Studies are performed to determine the mechanisms of arrhythmias, direct or provide therapy, or assess prognosis	Patients with palpitations documented to be due to extracardiac causes (e.g., hyperthyroidism)

ACC/AHA = American College of Cardiology/American Heart Association; ECG = electrocardiographic; MI = myocardial infarction.

TABLE 30G–6 ACC/AHA Guidelines for Clinical Intracardiac Electrophysiological Studies for Therapeutic Intervention

Indication	Class I (Appropriate)	Class II (Equivocal)	Class III (Inappropriate)
Guidance of drug therapy	Patients with sustained VT or cardiac arrest, especially those with prior MI Patients with AVNRT, AV reentrant tachycardia using an accessory pathway, or atrial fibrillation associated with an accessory pathway, for whom chronic drug therapy is planned	Patients with sinus node reentrant tachycardia, atrial tachycardia, atrial fibrillation, or atrial flutter without ventricular preexcitation syndrome, for whom chronic drug therapy is planned Patients with arrhythmias not inducible during control electrophysiological study for whom drug therapy is planned	Patients with isolated atrial or ventricular premature complexes Patients with ventricular fibrillation with a clearly identified reversible cause
Patients who are candidates for or who have implantable electrical devices	Patients with tachyarrhythmias, before and during implantation, and final (predischarge) programming of an electrical device to confirm its ability to perform as anticipated Patients with an implanted electrical antitachyarrhythmia device in whom changes in status or therapy may have influenced the continued safety and efficacy of the device Patients who have a pacemaker to treat a bradyarrhythmia and receive a cardioverter-defibrillator, to test for device interactions	Patients with previously documented indications for pacemaker implantation to test for the most appropriate long-term pacing mode and sites to optimize symptomatic improvement and hemodynamics	Patients who are not candidates for device therapy
Indications for catheter ablation procedures	Patients with symptomatic atrial tachyarrhythmias who have inadequately controlled ventricular rates unless primary ablation of the atrial tachyarrhythmia is possible Patients with symptomatic atrial tachyarrhythmias such as those above but when drugs are not tolerated or the patient does not wish to take them, even though the ventricular rate can be controlled Patients with symptomatic nonparoxysmal junctional tachycardia that is drug resistant or the patient is drug intolerant or does not wish to take it Patients resuscitated from sudden cardiac death caused by atrial flutter or atrial fibrillation with a rapid ventricular response in the absence of an accessory pathway	Patients with a dual-chamber pacemaker and pacemaker-mediated tachycardia that cannot be treated effectively by drugs or by reprogramming the pacemaker	Patients with atrial tachyarrhythmias responsive to drug therapy acceptable to the patient
Radiofrequency catheter ablation for AVNRT	Patients with symptomatic sustained AVNRT that is drug resistant or the patient is drug intolerant or does not desire long-term drug therapy	Patients with sustained AVNRT identified during electrophysiological study or catheter ablation of another arrhythmia The finding of dual AV nodal pathway physiology and atrial echoes but without AVNRT during electrophysiological study in patients suspected of having AVNRT clinically	Patients with AVNRT responsive to drug therapy that is well tolerated and preferred by the patient to ablation The finding of dual AV nodal pathway physiology (with or without echo complexes) during electrophysiological study in patients in whom AVNRT is not suspected clinically

Continued

TABLE 30G–6 ACC/AHA Guidelines for Clinical Intracardiac Electrophysiological Studies for Therapeutic Intervention—cont'd

Indication	Class I (Appropriate)	Class II (Equivocal)	Class III (Inappropriate)
Ablation of atrial tachycardia, flutter, and fibrillation: atrium/atrial sites	Patients with atrial tachycardia that is drug resistant or the patient is drug intolerant or does not desire long-term drug therapy Patients with atrial flutter that is drug resistant or the patient is drug intolerant or does not desire long-term drug therapy	Atrial flutter or atrial tachycardia associated with paroxysmal atrial fibrillation when the tachycardia is drug resistant or the patient is drug intolerant or does not desire long-term drug therapy Patients with atrial fibrillation and evidence of a localized site(s) of origin when the tachycardia is drug resistant or the patient is drug intolerant or does not desire long-term drug therapy	Patients with atrial arrhythmia that is responsive to drug therapy, well tolerated, and preferred by the patient to ablation Patients with multiform atrial tachycardia
Ablation of atrial tachycardia, flutter, and fibrillation: accessory pathways	Patients with symptomatic AV reentrant tachycardia that is drug resistant or the patient is drug intolerant or does not desire long-term drug therapy Patients with atrial fibrillation (or other atrial tachyarrhythmia) and a rapid ventricular response through the accessory pathway when the tachycardia is drug resistant or the patient is drug intolerant or does not desire long-term drug therapy	Patients with AV reentrant tachycardia or atrial fibrillation with rapid ventricular rates identified during electrophysiological study of another arrhythmia Asymptomatic patients with ventricular preexcitation whose livelihood or profession, important activities, insurability, or mental well-being or the public safety would be affected by spontaneous tachyarrhythmias or the presence of the ECG abnormality Patients with atrial fibrillation and a controlled ventricular response through the accessory pathway Patients with a family history of sudden cardiac death	Patients who have accessory pathway–related arrhythmias that are responsive to drug therapy, well tolerated, and preferred by the patient to ablation
Ablation of VT	Patients with symptomatic sustained monomorphic VT when the tachycardia is drug resistant or the patient is drug intolerant or does not desire long-term drug therapy Patients with bundle branch reentrant ventricular tachycardia Patients with sustained monomorphic VT and an ICD who are receiving multiple shocks not manageable by reprogramming or concomitant drug therapy	Nonsustained VT that is symptomatic when the tachycardia is drug resistant or the patient is drug intolerant or does not desire long-term drug therapy	Patients with VT that is responsive to drug, ICD, or surgical therapy and that therapy is well tolerated and preferred by the patient to ablation Unstable, rapid, multiple, or polymorphic VT that cannot be adequately localized by current mapping techniques Asymptomatic and clinically benign nonsustained VT

ACC/AHA = American College of Cardiology/American Heart Association; AV = atrioventricular; AVNRT = AV nodal reentrant tachycardia; ECG = electrocardiographic; ICD = implantable cardioverter-defibrillator; MI = myocardial infarction; VT = ventricular tachycardia.

Clinical Competence

The ACC/AHA statement on clinical competence from 2000[6] recommends that physicians specializing in electrophysiology undergo a minimum of 1 year of specialized training in electrophysiological studies, during which the physician should be the primary operator and analyze 100 to 150 initial diagnostic studies. At least 50 of these studies should involve patients with supraventricular arrhythmias. Because antiarrhythmic devices constitute a major part of current electrophysiology practice, the guidelines suggest that trainees should be the primary operators during at least 25 electrophysiological evaluations of implantable antiarrhythmic devices. For maintenance of competence, a minimum of 100 diagnostic electrophysiological studies per year is recommended. The statement also recommends that specialists in electrophysiology attend at least 30 hours of formal continuing medical education every 2 years to remain abreast of changes in knowledge and technology.

For physicians who perform catheter ablation, the NASPE Ad Hoc Committee on Catheter Ablation recommended that training should include at least 30 ablations, of which at least 15 are accessory pathway ablations.[12] The ACC/AHA statement recommended that physicians who perform ablations maintain a volume of at least 20 to 50 ablations per year.

Personal and Public Safety Issues

The AHA and the NASPE published a medical-scientific statement in 1996 that addressed many of the common issues regarding personal and public safety that arise in the care of patients with arrhythmias.[7] This publication summarized guidelines from other organizations, such as the U.S. Federal Aviation Administration, and the limited data available to estimate the risk of injury to the patient and others related to arrhythmias and provided recommendations about acceptable activities for patients with arrhythmias that may impair consciousness.

The AHA/NASPE guidelines divide patients into three classes. Class A patients should have no restrictions. Class B patients are restricted for a defined time without arrhythmia recurrence, usually after a therapeutic intervention (Table 30G–7). This time period is usually expressed as a subscript indicating the number of months of restriction (e.g., B_3). Patients in class C should have total restriction of potentially hazardous activities. Restrictions were divided into two categories: personal or noncommercial driving and commercial driving or flying. Except where stated otherwise, recommendations for flying were the same as those for commercial drivers. The guidelines noted that recommendations for restriction for commercial drivers might also be relevant to people in other potentially hazardous occupations, such as operators of heavy equipment.

The restrictions imposed by the guidelines vary depending on the severity of the arrhythmia and accompanying symptoms (see Table 30G–7). The duration of the restriction is shorter for patients who did not have impairment of symptoms with their arrhythmias but increases for patients who did have such symptoms and who had ventricular fibrillation or sustained ventricular tachycardia. Patients who had either of these arrhythmias should be totally restricted from commercial driving or flying according to these guidelines.

TABLE 30G–7 AHA/NASPE Guidelines for Safe Resumption of Activities (Classes of Restriction)

Arrhythmia	Private	Commercial
Nonsustained ventricular tachycardia	B_3 if symptoms of impaired consciousness with arrhythmia before treatment A if no impairment of consciousness with arrhythmia	B_6 if symptoms of impaired consciousness with arrhythmia before treatment A if no impairment of consciousness with arrhythmia
Sustained ventricular tachycardia	B_6 B_3 if idiopathic ventricular tachycardia (normal coronary arteries, normal ventricular function) and no impairment of consciousness	C B_6 if idiopathic ventricular tachycardia (normal coronary arteries, normal ventricular function) and no impairment of consciousness
Ventricular fibrillation	B_6	C
Asymptomatic or minimally symptomatic SVT (including WPW syndrome)	A	A
Symptomatic (evidence of hemodynamic compromise) SVT	B until after initiation of therapy that eliminates symptoms	B until after initiation of therapy that eliminates symptoms
Atrial fibrillation treated by catheter ablation of AV node	B	B
SVT with uncontrolled symptoms	C	C
Bradycardia without a pacemaker—no symptoms	A	A
Bradycardia without a pacemaker—syncope or near syncope	C	C
Bradycardia with a pacemaker—not pacemaker dependent*	A	A
Bradycardia with a pacemaker—pacemaker dependent*	B—1 wk	B—4 wk
Vasovagal syncope—mild	A	B_1
Vasovagal syncope—severe		
Treated vasovagal syncope	B_3	B_6
Untreated vasovagal syncope	C	C
Carotid sinus syncope—mild	A	A
Carotid sinus syncope—severe, treated with control	B_1	B_1
Carotid sinus syncope—severe, treated with uncertain control	B_3	B_6
Untreated	C	C

AHA/NASPE = American Heart Association/North American Society of Pacing and Electrophysiology; AV = atrioventricular; SVT = supraventricular tachycardia; WPW = Wolff-Parkinson-White.

Class A = no restriction; class B = restricted for months (in subscript); class C = total restriction.

*Patients who are pacemaker dependent are defined as those who have lost consciousness in the past because of bradyarrhythmias. This group may also include patients immediately after atrioventricular junction ablation or any other patient in whom sudden pacemaker failure would be likely to result in alteration of consciousness.

From Epstein AE, Miles WM, Benditt DG, et al: Personal and public safety issues related to arrhythmias that may affect consciousness: Implications for regulation and physician recommendations. Circulation 94:1147, 1996.

These recommendations were for patients who were treated with either antiarrhythmic drugs or ICDs. The guidelines recommended that noncommercial drivers should be prohibited from all driving for the first 6 months after ICD implantation; after this period, driving can be resumed if ICD discharge has not occurred. The guidelines recommend that all commercial driving be prohibited permanently after ICD implantation.

Special mention was made of patients with long QT syndromes. When the QT prolongation is acquired and due either wholly or in part to reversible factors such as electrolyte abnormalities, most patients can be allowed to drive after correction of these factors. Patients who have symptomatic long QT syndromes should not have driving privileges; those who are asymptomatic with or without treatment can receive driving privileges after a 6-month symptom-free interval.

For patients with supraventricular tachycardias, the guidelines did not impose harsher restrictions on commercial than on private drivers. No restrictions were recommended for patients with minimal or no symptoms with supraventricular tachycardia (see Table 30G–7). For patients who had symptoms suggestive of hemodynamic compromise (e.g., syncope, presyncope, chest pain, or dyspnea), the guidelines recommended restrictions until after initiation of therapy that eliminates symptoms. Patients with supraventricular tachycardia that appears to be successfully ablated can drive after recovery from the procedure. Patients treated with drug therapy should as a minimum have a 1-month symptom-free period before resuming driving, depending on the pretherapy frequency of tachycardia. If symptoms cannot be controlled, permanent full restrictions were recommended.

No restrictions were recommended for patients with bradyarrhythmias who were asymptomatic or who had a pacemaker but were not pacemaker dependent, i.e., patients who lost consciousness in the past because of bradyarrhythmias. "Pacemaker dependent" also included patients immediately after AV junction ablation or any other patient in whom sudden pacemaker failure would be likely to result in alteration of consciousness. Patients who were pacemaker dependent and had received a pacemaker should be restricted for 1 to 4 weeks, depending on whether they were private or commercial drivers. Patients who had had syncope or presyncope related to bradyarrhythmias who had not received a pacemaker should have full permanent restrictions.

No or only mild restrictions were recommended for patients with mild vasovagal syncope or carotid sinus syncope. The guidelines as written (see Table 30G–7) allow the clinician considerable leeway in determining the duration of restriction.

References

1. Knoebel SB, Crawford MH, Dunn MI, et al: Guidelines for ambulatory electrocardiography. A report of the American College of Cardiology/American Heart Association Task Force on Assessment of Diagnostic and Therapeutic Cardiovascular Procedures (Subcommittee on Ambulatory Electrocardiography). J Am Coll Cardiol 12:249, 1989.
2. Crawford MH, Bernstein SJ, Deedwania PC, et al: ACC/AHA guidelines for ambulatory electrocardiography. A report of the American College of Cardiology/American Heart Association Task Force on Practice Guidelines (Committee to Revise the Guidelines for Ambulatory Electrocardiography) J Am Coll Cardiol 34:866, 1999.
3. Kadish AH, Buxton AE, Kennedy HL, et al: ACC/AHA clinical competence statement on electrocardiography and ambulatory electrocardiography. A report of the ACC/AHA/ACP-ASIM Task Force on Clinical Competence (ACC/AHA Committee to Develop a Clinical Competence Statement on Electrocardiography and Ambulatory Electrocardiography). Circulation 104:3169, 2001.
4. Zipes DP, Akhtar M, Denes P, et al: Guidelines for clinical intracardiac electrophysiology studies. A report of the American College of Cardiology/American Heart Association Task Force on Assessment of Diagnostic and Therapeutic Cardiovascular Procedures (Subcommittee to Assess Clinical Intracardiac Electrophysiologic Studies). J Am Coll Cardiol 14:1827, 1989.
5. Zipes DP, DiMarco JP, Gillette PC, et al: Guidelines for clinical intracardiac electrophysiology studies and catheter ablation procedures. A report of the American College of Cardiology/American Heart Association Task Force on Practice Guidelines (Subcommittee on Clinical Intracardiac Electrophysiologic and Catheter Ablation Procedures). J Am Coll Cardiol 26:555, 1995.
6. Tracy CM, Akhtar M, DiMarco JP, et al: American College of Cardiology/American Heart Association Clinical Competence Statement on invasive electrophysiology studies, catheter ablation, and cardioversion. A report of the American College of Cardiology/American Heart Association/American College of Physicians-American Society of Internal Medicine Task Force on Clinical Competence. Circulation 102:2309, 2000.
7. Epstein AE, Miles WM, Benditt DG, et al: Personal and public safety issues related to arrhythmias that may affect consciousness: Implications for regulation and physician recommendations. Circulation 94:1147, 1996.
8. Gregoratos G, Abrams J, Epstein AE, et al: ACC/AHA/NASPE 2002 Guideline Update for Implantation of Cardiac Pacemakers and Antiarrhythmia Devices—summary article: A report of the American College of Cardiology/American Heart Association Task Force on Practice Guidelines (ACC/AHA/NASPE Committee to Update the 1998 Pacemaker Guidelines). J Am Coll Cardiol 40:1703, 2002.
9. Moss AJ, Zareba W, Hall WJ, et al: Prophylactic implantation of a defibrillator in patients with myocardial infarction and reduced ejection fraction. N Engl J Med 346:877, 2002.
10. Bansch D, Antz M, Boczor S, et al: Primary prevention of sudden death in idiopathic dilated cardiomyopathy: The Cardiomyopathy Trial (CAT). Circulation 105:1453, 2002.
11. Ezekowitz JA, Armstrong PW, McAlister FA: Implantable cardioverter defibrillators in primary and secondary prevention: A systematic review of randomized, controlled trials. Ann Intern Med 138:445, 2003.
12. Scheinman MM: Catheter ablation for cardiac arrhythmias, personnel, and facilities. North American Society of Pacing and Electrophysiology Ad Hoc Committee on Catheter Ablation. Pacing Clin Electrophysiol 15:715, 1992.

CHAPTER 31

Cardiac Pacemakers and Cardioverter-Defibrillators

David L. Hayes • Douglas P. Zipes

Implantable devices for the management of cardiac arrhythmias have evolved rapidly since the inception of cardiac pacing in the late 1950s. The collective intelligence of creative biomedical engineers and clinicians, coupled with the advent and increasing sophistication of the microprocessor, has made this possible. What began with asynchronous ventricular pacing as a therapy for patients with Stokes-Adams attacks has made momentous strides every decade. Device therapy is now rapidly expanding with implantable devices for hemodynamic monitoring and heart failure therapy. The rapid technological advancements in cardiac pacemakers have, at least to some degree, served as a catalyst for an even faster evolution in implantable cardioverter-defibrillators (ICDs) and cardiac resynchronization therapy (CRT) devices. The evolution of ICD and CRT technology has been staggering. As the technology for both pacemakers—ICDs and CRT—has evolved, clinical trials have been crucial to prove efficacy. Clinical trials are an integral part of the discipline of implantable device therapy and will remain so as we see further innovative improvements in the years to come.

Pacemaker Nomenclature

Pacemaker nomenclature was established in 1974, and it is necessary to know the nomenclature to understand the discipline of cardiac pacing (Table 31–1).[1] The code was updated in 2002 to include a "generic code" for the expanding field of multisite pacing therapy. The following is a brief description of the elements of the code that are shown in Table 31–1:

- The first position (I) refers to the chamber or chambers in which stimulation occurs: A = atrium; V = ventricle; and D = dual chamber, or both A and V.
- The second position (II) refers to the chamber or chambers in which sensing occurs. The letters are the same as those for the first position. (Manufacturers also use "S" in both the first and the second position to indicate that the device is capable of pacing only a single cardiac chamber.)
- The third position (III) refers to the mode of sensing, or how the pacemaker responds to a sensed event. An "I" indicates that a sensed event inhibits the output pulse and causes the pacemaker to recycle for one or more timing cycles. "T" means that an output pulse is triggered in response to a sensed event. "D" means that both "T" and "I" responses can occur. This designation is restricted to dual-chamber systems. An event sensed in the atrium inhibits the atrial output but triggers a ventricular output. Unlike a single-chamber triggered mode (VVT or AAT), in which an output pulse is triggered immediately on sensing, a dual-chamber mode has a delay between the sensed atrial event and the triggered ventricular output to mimic the normal PR interval. If a native ventricular signal or R wave is sensed, the ventricular output and possibly even the atrial output are inhibited, depending on where sensing occurs.
- The fourth position (IV) of the code indicates both programmability and rate modulation. An "R" in the fourth position indicates that the pacemaker incorporates a sensor to modulate the rate independently of intrinsic cardiac activity, such as with motion or respiration. From a practical standpoint, "R" is the only indicator commonly used in the fourth position.
- The fifth position (V) of the code is now used to indicate whether multisite pacing is present in (0) none of the cardiac chambers, (A) one or both atria, (V) one or both ventricles, or (D) any combination of atria and ventricles. To describe a patient with a DDDR (dual-chamber rate-adaptive) pacemaker with biventricular stimulation, the code would be DDDRV.

Indications for Cardiac Pacing

A joint committee of the American College of Cardiology (ACC), the American Heart

TABLE 31–1 Revised NASPE/BPEG Generic Code for Antibradycardia Pacing

Position	I	II	III	IV	V
Category	**Chamber(s) paced** O = None A = Atrium V = Ventricle D = Dual (A + V)	**Chamber(s) sensed** O = None A = Atrium V = Ventricle D = Dual (A + V)	**Response to sensing** O = None T = Triggered I = Inhibited D = Dual (T + I)	**Rate modulation** O = None R = Rate modulation	**Multisite pacing** O = None A = Atrium V = Ventricle D = Dual (A + V)
Manufacturers' designation only	S = Single (A or V)	S = Single (A or V)			

See text for explanation of use of the code.
BPEG = British Pacing and Electrophysiology Group; NASPE = North American Society of Pacing and Electrophysiology.
From Bernstein AD, Daubert JC, Fletcher RD, et al, and North American Society of Pacing and Electrophysiology/British Pacing and Electrophysiology Group: The revised NASPE/BPEG generic code for antibradycardia, adaptive-rate, and multisite pacing. Pacing Clin Electrophysiol 25:260-264, 2002.

Association (AHA), and the North American Society of Pacing and Electrophysiology (NASPE) has established indications for pacing into categories of "generally indicated," "may be indicated," and "not indicated."[2] Although some indications for permanent pacing are relatively certain or unambiguous, others require considerable expertise and judgment. The clinician prescribing permanent pacing systems should be aware of the published indications and controversies regarding indications.

The clinical need for pacing and appropriate objective data, such as electrocardiographic (ECG) tracings, must be documented clearly in the patient's medical record to ensure reimbursement by Medicare or third-party payers.

Indications are considered in categories of acquired atrioventricular (AV) block, congenital AV block, chronic bifascicular and trifascicular block, sinus node dysfunction, and neurocardiogenic syndromes. Currently, sinus node dysfunction is the most frequent indication for pacing, followed by AV node dysfunction. Pacing for tachyarrhythmias and miscellaneous indications comprises a relatively small percentage. Potential hemodynamic indications for permanent pacing are discussed separately.

Acquired AV Block

AV block is classified traditionally into first-, second-, and third-degree (or complete) heart block (see Chap. 32). Alternatively, it can be defined anatomically as supra-Hisian, intra-Hisian, or infra-Hisian. If the QRS complex is prolonged more than 0.12 second, there is a greater probability that the conduction disturbance is infra-Hisian. Acquired AV block is most commonly idiopathic and related to aging, but it has many potential causes. Indications for permanent pacing in acquired AV block are listed in Table 31–2.

Indications for permanent pacing for AV block that occurs with an acute myocardial infarction (see Chaps. 46 and 47) are more controversial. A pacemaker is generally considered indicated if complete AV block, Mobitz type II block, or bilateral or alternating bundle branch block persists for more than 72 hours after the acute event. Some clinicians consider new and persistent bifascicular block an indication for pacing, and others consider pacing for a new left anterior or left posterior hemiblock alone.

Congenital Complete Heart Block

Although some controversy remains about when to pace patients with congenital complete heart block, there is now a tendency to pace in all these patients and to do so earlier, even if they are asymptomatic. There is a high incidence of unpredictable syncope with significant mortality from initial attacks, a gradual decrease in heart rate, and a high incidence of acquired mitral regurgition.[3] In pediatric patients with congenital complete heart block, pacemaker implantation is recommended for congestive heart failure, average heart rate of less than 50 beats/min in the awake infant, history of

TABLE 31–2 Indications for Permanent Pacing in Atrioventricular Block

Type of AV Block	Pacemaker Necessary	Pacemaker Probably Necessary	Pacemaker not Necessary
Third	Symptomatic congenital CHB Acquired symptomatic AV block Atrial fibrillation with CHB Acquired asymptomatic CHB Neuromuscular diseases with AV block, with or without symptoms		AV block of any degree that is expected to resolve and unlikely to recur, e.g., drug toxicity, Lyme disease, sleep apnea, without treatment
Second	Symptomatic second-degree AV block regardless of type Asymptomatic advanced second-degree AV block with asystole ≥ 3.0 sec or escape rate < 40 beats/min in awake patients	Asymptomatic, type I, at intra-His or infra-His level* Hemodynamically symptomatic due to loss of AV synchrony Neuromuscular diseases with AV block, with or without symptoms	Asymptomatic, type I, at supra-His (AV node) level
First		Hemodynamically symptomatic due to loss of AV synchrony with markedly prolonged PR interval, e.g., > 300 msec	Asymptomatic

AV = atrioventricular; CHB = complete heart block.
*Shaw DB, Gowers JI, Kekwick CA, et al: Is Mobitz type I atrioventricular block benign in adults? Heart 90:169, 2004.

syncope or presyncope, significant ventricular ectopy, or exercise intolerance.

Chronic Bifascicular and Trifascicular Block

If bifascicular or trifascicular block is associated with transient complete heart block, whether symptomatic or not, pacing is indicated. Pacing in the patient with bifascicular or trifascicular block and syncope that cannot be attributed to any other cause is a class II ACC/AHA indication. If only fascicular block is noted in the asymptomatic patient, pacing is not indicated.

Sinus Node Dysfunction

Tachycardia-bradycardia syndrome, sick sinus syndrome, symptomatic sinus bradycardia, sinus arrest and sinus pauses, and chronotropic incompetence all are variants of sinus node dysfunction, and often the terms are used synonymously. The degree of bradycardia at which to consider pacing is controversial but is generally accepted to be rates of less than 40 beats/min during waking hours. There is disagreement about the absolute cycle length at which pacing should be considered. Although every patient needs to be considered individually, sinus pauses exceeding 3 seconds during waking hours are often considered abnormal and may warrant pacing if the patient has symptoms consistent with bradycardia. Pauses that occur during sleep are more difficult to categorize. Because of vagal influences, many normal persons display pauses significantly longer than 3 seconds during sleep. Permanent pacing should be considered for any patient who has symptomatic bradyarrhythmias if the cause of the bradyarrhythmia is not reversible or they require a drug, for example, a beta blocker, that produces symptomatic bradycardia. Examples of reversible conditions would include transient AV block secondary to an infectious disease that will respond to appropriate treatment, such as Lyme disease, untreated sleep disorder with secondary conduction abnormalities, and other hypervagal states.

Permanent pacing for patients with sinus node dysfunction after myocardial infarction is reserved for those who have symptoms during bradycardia. If drug therapy results in symptomatic bradycardia, criteria for permanent pacing should follow the guidelines given for sinus node dysfunction in Table 31–3.

Neurocardiogenic Syncope

Permanent pacing may be indicated for some of the several types of neurally mediated syncope.[4] Neurally mediated syncope includes carotid sinus hypersensitivity and vasovagal syncope (see Chap. 34).

The carotid sinus reflex is the physiological response to pressure applied to the carotid sinus. Although this reflex is physiological, some persons have an exaggerated or even pathological response. This reflex has two components: cardioinhibitory and vasodepressor. A cardioinhibitory response results predominantly from increased parasympathetic tone and may be manifested by sinus bradycardia, PR prolongation, or advanced AV block. The vasodepressor response is predominantly due to sympathetic withdrawal and secondary hypotension. Although a pure cardioinhibitory or pure vasodepressor response can occur, a mixed response is most common. Tilt-table testing can provide the physiological environment to reproduce vasovagal syncope. It is important to document whether the predominant cause of symptoms is cardioinhibitory or vasodepressor because therapy differs. Tilt-table testing is often helpful in determining the predominant cause.

Drugs such as beta blockers are commonly used as first-line therapy despite an absence of convincing efficacy data. Although significant controversy persists, vasovagal syncope can be aborted or blunted by dual-chamber pacing, and even if syncope does occur, pacing can prolong consciousness to avoid injury. In the North American Vasovagal Pacemaker Study I (VPS-I),[5] 46 patients with recurrent syncope and a positive tilt test were randomized to dual-chamber pacemaker with a special feature known as "rate drop" or to no pacemaker therapy. (The rate-drop algorithm allows the pacemaker to pace at a faster rate if bradycardia suddenly occurs.) Stopped prematurely because of the benefit observed with pacemaker therapy, the study revealed that only 17 percent of paced patients had recurrent syncope compared with 59 percent of patients without pacing.

The Vasovagal Syncope International Study (VASIS)[6] demonstrated a reduction in syncopal episodes, similar to VPS-I. This group of patients had experienced multiple episodes of vasovagal syncope as part of the inclusion criteria.

In the North American Vasovagal Pacemaker Study II (VPS-II),[7] all patients received a pacemaker implant and were then programmed to no pacing (ODO mode) or DDD with rate-drop response. In contrast to the initial trial,[5] there was no statistically significant improvement in the group of patients programmed to active pacing with rate-drop response.

Syncope and Falls in the Elderly Pacing and Carotid Sinus Evaluation 2 (SAFE PACE-2)[8] study is under way to assess pacing therapy in carotid sinus hypersensitivity (Table 31–4). In the precursor to this study, SAFE PACE-1,[11] there was a strong association between nonaccidental falls and cardioinhibitory carotid sinus hypersensitivity, and these patients should be referred for cardiovascular assessment.

Selection of the Appropriate Pacing Mode

When an indication for pacing has been identified, consideration should be given to selecting the most appropriate

TABLE 31–3 Indications for Permanent Pacing in Sinus Node Dysfunction (SND)

Pacemaker Necessary	Pacemaker Probably Necessary	Pacemaker not Necessary
Symptomatic sinus bradycardia	Symptomatic patients with SND who have documented rates of < 40 beats/min without a clear-cut association between significant symptoms and bradycardia	Asymptomatic SND
Symptomatic sinus bradycardia due to long-term drug therapy of a type and at a dose for which there is no accepted alternative	Syncope of unexplained origin when major abnormalities of sinus node function are discovered or provoked in electrophysiologic studies	

TABLE 31–4 Trials of Pacing Therapy in Neurocardiogenic Syncope

Study	Patient Inclusion Criteria	Endpoint(s)	Treatment Arms	Key Results
VPS-I[5]	≥Six lifetime episodes of syncope *and* Positive HUT test with syncope or presyncope Relative bradycardia	Time to recurrent syncope	Standard drug therapy *vs.* Pacemaker	85% risk reduction for recurrent syncope with pacing
VPS-II[7]	History strongly suggests vasovagal syncope ≥Six lifetime episodes of syncope *or* ≥Three in past 2 yr *or* One episode in past 6 mo *and* Positive HUT test with syncope or presyncope	Time to recurrent syncope Efficacy of RDR	Randomized to DDD or no pacing for 6 mo or until first episode of syncope Rerandomized to DDD pacing with or without RDR	No significant difference between pacing and no pacing
VASIS[6]	≥Three syncopal episodes in prior 2 yr Duration of symptoms > 6 mo	Recurrence of syncope Recurrence of presyncope Need for secondary pacemaker implant or drug therapy	Dual-chamber pacing with hysteresis *vs.* No pacing (no specific therapy)	5% incidence of syncope in paced group vs. 61% without pacing
SAFE PACE-2[8]	Age ≥ 50 yr ≥Two unexplained falls ± one syncopal episode in prior 12 mo >3-sec asystole on CSM No other cause of falls	Recurrent falls Time to first fall Frequency of dizziness or presyncope Health care utilization Quality of life	Pacemaker *vs.* Conventional therapy	In progress
SYDIT[9]	No cardiac disease Age > 35 yr ≥Three syncopal spells in preceding 2 yr Positive HUT test with HR ↓ ≥ 30% and bradycardia ≤ 50 beats/min	Recurrence of syncope	Atenolol vs. DDD pacing with RDR	Significant effect in favor of permanent pacing with recurrent syncope in 4.3% of patients with pacemaker and 25.5% of patients on atenolol
SYNPACE[10]	Symptomatic vasovagal syncope	Recurrence of syncope	Dual-chamber pacemaker with RDR on *vs.* Pacemaker implanted but programmed off	Active pacing not superior in preventing syncopal recurrence

CSM = carotid sinus massage; HR = heart rate; HUT = head-up tilt; RDR = rate drop response; SAFE PACE = Syncope and Falls in the Elderly Pacing and Carotid Sinus Evaluation; SYDIT = Syncope Diagnosis and Treatment Study; SYNPACE = Vasovagal Syncope and Pacing; VASIS = Vasovagal Syncope International Study; VPS = North American Vasovagal Pacemaker Study.

pacing mode for the patient. Factors to consider when choosing the pacing mode include the following:

- Underlying rhythm disturbance
- Overall physical condition
- Associated medical problems
- Exercise capacity
- Chronotropic response to exercise
- Effect of pacing mode on long-term morbidity and mortality

The effect of pacing mode on morbidity and mortality has been the basis of multiple randomized clinical trials.

Many investigators performed retrospective reviews to assess the effect of pacing mode on mortality. Despite the inherent weaknesses of retrospective analyses, it is difficult to dismiss the similar finding among all the studies of a significantly lower mortality with DDD or atrial inhibited (AAI) pacing than with ventricular inhibited (VVI) pacing and significantly lower incidences of atrial fibrillation.

Several prospective trials have been completed (Table 31-5). Andersen and colleagues[12] performed one of the first prospective studies on pacing mode and survival. In patients with sinus node dysfunction randomized to AAI or VVI pacing, the authors demonstrated a higher incidence of atrial fibrillation in the VVI group (14 percent of the AAI group vs. 23 percent of the VVI group; $p = 0.12$) and a higher incidence of thromboembolism in the VVI group than in the AAI group ($p = 0.0083$). Although no difference in mortality could be detected at the initial analysis at 3.3 years, subsequent analysis at 5.5 years showed improved survival and less heart failure in the AAI group.[12] In addition, there was a persistent reduction in the incidences of atrial fibrillation and thromboembolic events.

The Pacemaker Selection in the Elderly (PASE) trial, a prospective, randomized, single-blind trial, compared DDDR and VVIR pacing modes.[13] There was no statistically significant difference in quality of life between DDDR and VVIR pacing modes, but there was a trend toward improved quality of life in patients with sinus node dysfunction randomized to dual-chamber pacing. Perhaps more significant was a crossover of 26 percent of patients from ventricular pacing to dual-chamber pacing because of pacemaker syndrome.

TABLE 31–5 Trials Assessing the Effect of Pacing Mode on Morbidity and Mortality

Study	Patient Inclusion Criteria	Endpoint(s)	Treatment Arms	Key Results
Danish study[12]	Sick sinus syndrome requiring pacing	Mortality Cardiovascular death AF TE events Heart failure AV block	AAI pacing ($n = 110$) *vs.* VVI pacing ($n = 115$)	Cumulative incidence of CV death, PAF, chronic AF, and TE events lower with AAI pacing Less severe heart failure with AAI Multivariate analysis: AAI associated with freedom from TE events, survival from CV death
PASE[13]	Age ≥ 65 yr Need for PPM for prevention or treatment of bradycardia	QOL All-cause mortality First nonfatal CVA or death First hospitalization for CHF AF PM syndrome	Single-blind, randomized, controlled comparison; VVIR pacing *vs.* DDDR pacing	QOL improved significantly, but no difference between pacing modes 26% of patients with VVIR crossover to DDDR due to PM syndrome Trends of borderline statistical significance in endpoints favoring DDDR in patients with SND
CTOPP[14]	Initial PM Life expectancy > 1 yr Not in chronic AF	Cardiovascular mortality or stroke Paroxysmal or chronic AF Hospitalization for CHF QOL 6-min walk	DDDR or AAIR pacing *vs.* VVIR pacing	No difference in QOL, VVI vs. DDD/AAI No statistically significant difference in mortality or stroke No difference in hospitalizations 24% ↓ incidence of chronic or paroxysmal AF with DDD/AAI
MOST[15]	SND requiring PM NSR or atrial standstill at time of implantation	Stroke Health status Cost-effectiveness Total mortality CV mortality AF Heart failure score PM syndrome	DDDR *vs.* VVIR	Lower incidence of AF with DDDR No difference in any other endpoint
UKPACE[16]	AV block requiring PM Age > 70 yr	All-cause mortality Composite endpoint of CV deaths HF hospitalization AF CVA or events Reoperation	DDDR *vs.* VVI or VVIR	No difference in any endpoint
DANPACE[17]	Tachycardia-bradycardia syndrome with normal AV conduction	All-cause mortality CV mortality Incidence of AF and TE events QOL Cost-effectiveness	AAIR *vs.* DDDR	In progress

AF = atrial fibrillation; AV = atrioventricular; CHF = congestive heart failure; CTOPP = Canadian Trial of Physiologic Pacing; CV = cardiovascular; CVA = cardiovascular accident; DANPACE = Danish Pacing Trial; HF = heart failure; MOST = Mode Selection Trial; NSR = normal sinus rhythm; PAF = paroxysmal atrial fibrillation; PASE = Pacemaker Selection in the Elderly; PM = pacemaker; PPM = permanent pacemaker; QOL = quality of life; SND = sinus node dysfunction; TE = thromboembolic; UKPACE = United Kingdom Pacing and Cardiovascular Events.

The Canadian Trial of Physiologic Pacing (CTOPP)[14] compared VVIR with DDDR or AAIR and had primary endpoints of overall mortality and cerebrovascular accidents and secondary endpoints of atrial fibrillation, hospitalizations for congestive heart failure, and death due to a cardiac cause. CTOPP demonstrated that physiological pacing (DDD/AAI) was associated with a reduced incidence of chronic atrial fibrillation but no difference in quality of life or mortality.

The Mode Selection Trial (MOST) also randomized patients with sinus node dysfunction to either VVI or DDD pacing, with primary endpoints of all causes of mortality and cerebrovascular accidents.[15] MOST failed to demonstrate any difference in mortality but did demonstrate a lower incidence of atrial fibrillation with physiological pacing and also reduced the signs and symptoms of heart failure and slightly improved quality of life. The study concluded that, overall, dual-chamber pacing offers significant improvement compared with ventricular pacing.

The United Kingdom Pacing and Cardiovascular Events (UKPACE) trial compared DDD with VVI pacing modes in patients 70 years and older requiring permanent pacing for second- or third-degree AV block.[16] Results of this trial, presented (ACC March 2003) but not yet published, showed no significant difference between pacing modes in the primary endpoint of all-cause mortality or in the composite secondary endpoint of cardiovascular deaths, atrial fibrillation, heart failure hospitalizations, cerebrovascular accidents or thromboembolic events, and reoperation.

With the exception of PASE and UKPACE, the major trials discussed have demonstrated a lower incidence of atrial fibrillation with AAI or dual-chamber pacing.

Only one of the trials discussed demonstrated a lower mortality with physiological pacing. The difference in this trial design that may explain the mortality outcome merits discussion because of the larger implications for cardiac pacing. In the Andersen trial patients, the physiological pacing mode implemented was AAI mode. With AAI pacing, the patient maintains intrinsic AV conduction; perhaps more important, this avoids the abnormal depolarization pattern of right ventricular pacing that would occur with VVI or DDD pacing. There is growing sentiment, and data to support it, that the adverse effects of right ventricular apical pacing can lead to significant left ventricular dysfunction. This knowledge would support an effort to maintain intrinsic ventricular depolarization or pacing from some site that would enable more normal ventricular depolarization.[17]

Modes and Timing Cycles

The advantages and disadvantages of each pacing mode cannot be completely comprehended unless the timing cycle of each is understood.

Single-Chamber Triggered Pacing

Single-chamber triggered pacing (AAT and VVT) releases an output pulse every time a native event is sensed. This feature increases the current drain on the battery, accelerating its rate of depletion, and deforms the inscription of the intrinsic spontaneous complex on the ECG. However, it can serve as an excellent marker for the site of sensing within an intrinsic complex and can prevent inappropriate inhibition from oversensing when the patient does not have a stable escape rhythm. Triggered pacing is used infrequently.

Ventricular-Inhibited Pacing

VVI is a pacing mode that incorporates sensing on the ventricular channel, enabling a sensed ventricular event to inhibit pacemaker output (Fig. 31–1). VVI pacemakers are refractory for an interval after a paced or sensed ventricular event, the ventricular refractory period (VRP). Any ventricular event occurring within the VRP is not sensed and does not reset the ventricular timer.

VVI pacing is the most commonly used pacing mode worldwide. Although VVI pacing protects the patient from lethal bradycardias, it is significantly limited because it does not restore or maintain AV synchrony and does not provide rate responsiveness in the chronotropically incompetent patient, that is, the patient in whom the spontaneous sinus heart rate does not increase in response to a physiological demand. In addition, some patients with VVI pacing experience symptomatic hemodynamic deterioration during ventricular pacing. Adverse hemodynamics associated with a normally functioning pacing system that cause overt symptoms or limit the patient's ability to achieve optimal functional status are referred to as *pacemaker syndrome* (Fig. 31–2). Pacemaker syndrome was initially recognized with VVI pacing but can occur with any pacing mode if there is AV dissociation. The incidence of pacemaker syndrome is difficult to determine and depends on how the syndrome is defined. If the definition is restricted to patients with clinical limitations during any pacing mode that results in AV dissociation, the incidence is probably in the range of 7 to 10 percent of patients with VVI pacing. In a study of patients with DDD pacemakers who were randomized to DDD or VVI pacing mode, some degree of pacemaker syndrome was thought to be present in 83 percent. The most common symptoms reported were shortness of breath, dizziness, fatigue, pulsations in the neck or abdomen, cough, and apprehension. It can be concluded from this study that if patients with VVI pacing have some basis for comparison, they may be more aware of symptoms with VVI pacing.

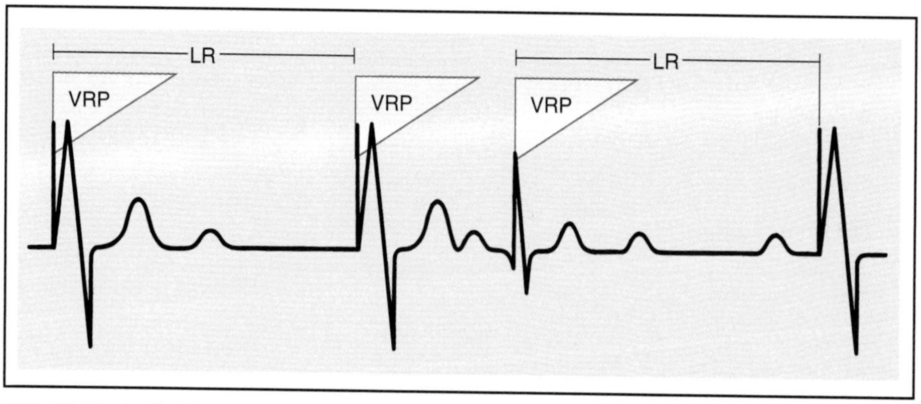

FIGURE 31–1 The VVI timing cycle consists of a defined lower rate limit (LR) and a ventricular refractory period (VRP, represented by triangle). When the LR timer is complete, a pacing artifact is delivered in the absence of a sensed intrinsic ventricular event. If an intrinsic QRS occurs, the LR timer is started from that point. A VRP begins with any sensed or paced ventricular activity.

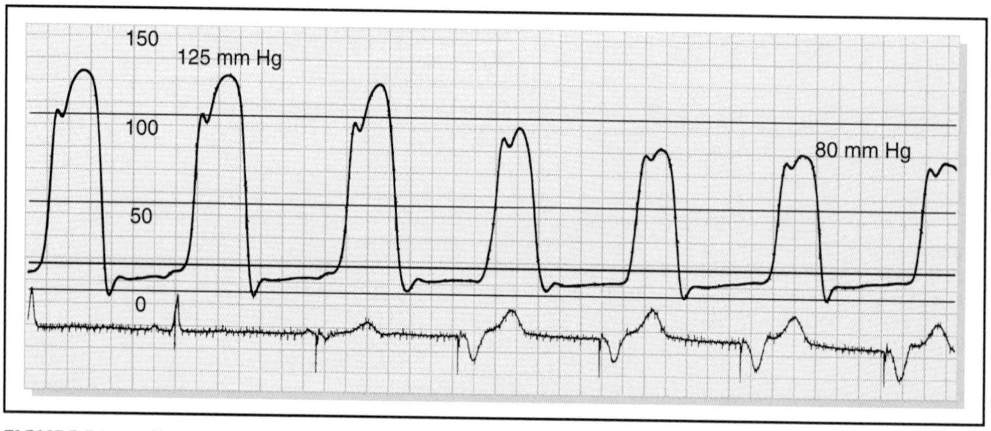

FIGURE 31–2 Hemodynamic tracing from a patient with pacemaker syndrome. In the initial portion of the tracing there is sinus rhythm with intrinsic atrioventricular node conduction with a systolic arterial pressure of approximately 125 mm Hg. This is followed by fusion beats and a progressive decrease in systolic pressure. When the ventricle is completely depolarized by the pacemaker, the systolic pressure decreases to approximately 80 mm Hg. This hemodynamic response is compatible with pacemaker syndrome.

Atrial-Inhibited Pacing

AAI pacing mode incorporates the same timing cycles, with the obvious difference that pacing and sensing occur from the atrium and pacemaker output is inhibited by a sensed atrial event (Fig. 31–3). An atrial paced or sensed event initiates a refractory period during which no spontaneous event is sensed by the pacemaker. When the atrial timing cycle ends, the atrial pacing artifact is delivered regardless of ventricular events because an AAI pacemaker should not sense ventricular events. The single exception to this rule is far-field sensing; that is, the ventricular signal is large enough to be inappropriately sensed by the atrial lead. In this situation, the atrial timing cycle is reset by events sensed in the ventricle. Sometimes this abnormality can be corrected by making the atrial channel less sensitive or by lengthening the refractory period.

AAI pacing is appropriate for patients with sinus node dysfunction and normal AV conduction. The obvious disadvantage of atrial pacing is lack of ventricular support should AV block occur. If the patient with sinus node dysfunction is assessed carefully for AV node disease at the time of pacemaker implantation, the occurrence of clinically significant AV node disease is very low (<2 percent per year). Assessment before use of an AAI system should include incremental atrial pacing at the time of pacemaker implantation. Although criteria vary among institutions and implanting physicians, the adult patient should be capable of 1:1 AV node conduction to rates of 120 to 140 beats/min.

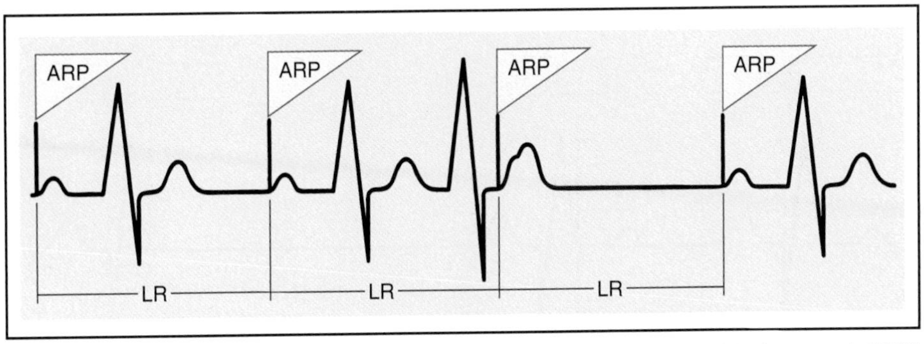

FIGURE 31–3 The AAI timing cycle consists of a defined lower rate (LR) limit and an atrial refractory period (ARP). When the LR cycle is complete, a pacing artifact is delivered in the atrium in the absence of a sensed atrial event. If an intrinsic P wave occurs, the LR timer is started from that point. An ARP begins with any sensed or paced atrial activity. The AAI timing cycle should not be affected by events in the ventricle. In this schematic example, a premature ventricular contraction (PVC) occurs. Appropriately, it is not sensed by the AAI pacemaker, and the atrial pacing artifact occurs in the T wave of the PVC. Even though atrial capture presumably would occur, there is no ventricular event after the paced atrial event because the ventricle is still refractory. However, the timing cycle will be reset by anything that is sensed on the atrial sensing circuit. In this schematic example, a PVC occurs. It is appropriately not sensed, and the pacing artifact is delivered after the PVC. Even though there appears to be atrial depolarization, no intrinsic ventricular depolarization occurs because the ventricle is refractory.

Dual-Chamber Pacing

AV Sequential, Non-P-Synchronous Pacing

AV sequential, non-P-synchronous pacing (DDI) is a pacing mode with dual-chamber sensing that incorporates atrial sensing as well as ventricular sensing, which prevents competitive atrial pacing (Fig. 31–4). The DDI mode of response is inhibition only; that is, no tracking of P waves can occur. Therefore, the programmed rate, which by definition is the lower rate, because only a single rate exists, is the fastest paced rate that can be seen. DDI is rarely the preimplantation mode of choice but remains a programmable option in most dual-chamber pacemakers. The DDI pacing mode could be considered for patients with intermittent atrial tachyarrhythmias, but DDD or DDDR pacing with mode switching is preferable.

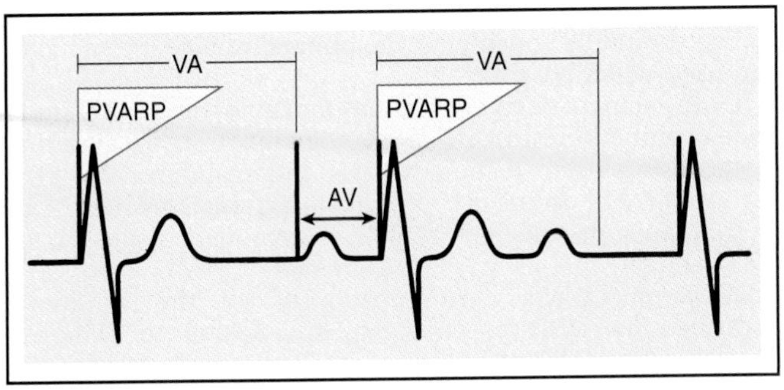

FIGURE 31–4 The timing cycle in DDI pacing consists of a lower rate limit, an atrioventricular (AV) interval, a ventricular refractory period (VRP), and an atrial refractory period (ARP). The VRP is initiated by any sensed or paced ventricular activity, and the ARP is initiated by any sensed or paced atrial activity. The lower rate limit cannot be violated even if the sinus rate is occurring at a faster rate. PVARP = postventricular atrial refractory period; VA = ventriculoatrial.

Atrial Synchronous Pacing

Atrial synchronous (VDD) pacemakers pace only in the ventricle, sense in both chambers, and respond both by inhibition of ventricular output due to intrinsic ventricular activity and by ventricular tracking of P waves. The VDD mode has become increasingly available as a single-lead pacing system. In this system, a single lead is capable of pacing in the ventricle in response to sensing atrial activity by way of a remote electrode situated on the intraatrial portion of the ventricular pacing lead.

In the VDD mode, sensed atrial events initiate the AV interval (AVI). If an intrinsic ventricular event occurs before the termination of the AVI, ventricular output is inhibited and the lower rate timing cycle is reset (Fig. 31–5). If a paced ventricular beat occurs at the end of the AVI, this beat resets the lower rate. If no atrial event occurs, the pacemaker escapes with a paced ventricular event at the lower rate limit; that is, the pacemaker displays VVI activity in the absence of a sensed atrial event. VDD pacing may be appropriate for the patient with normal sinus node function and conduction disease of the AV node.

Dual-Chamber Pacing and Sensing with Inhibition and Tracking

In the dual-chamber pacing and sensing with inhibition and tracking (DDD) mode, the basic timing circuit associated with lower rate pacing is divided into two sections: the ventriculoatrial (VA) interval and the AVI. The AVI may be defined by AV sequential pacing initiated by pacing with subsequent intrinsic ventricular conduction or initiated by a native P wave with subsequent ventricular pacing (Fig. 31–6).

The postventricular atrial refractory period (PVARP) is the period after a sensed or paced ventricular event during which the atrial sensing circuit is refractory. Any atrial event occurring during the PVARP is not sensed by the atrial sensing circuit. If a P wave occurs after the PVARP and is sensed, no atrial pacing artifact is delivered at the end of the VA interval (see Fig. 31–6). Because the maximum tracking rate of the pacemaker is determined by the total atrial refractory period (TARP), the PVARP is a significant determinant

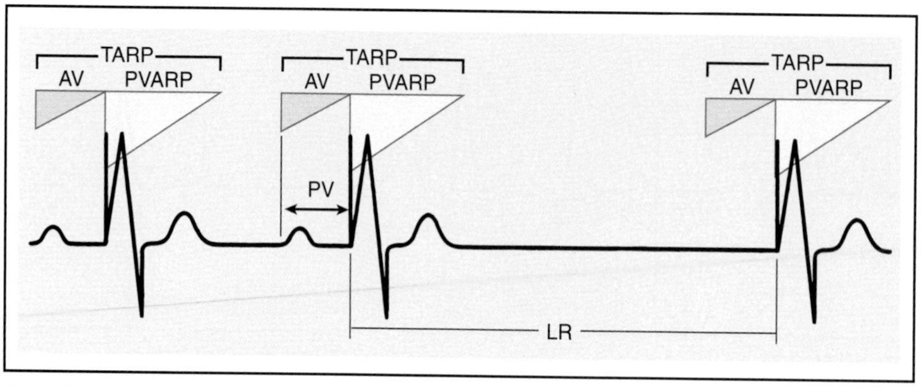

FIGURE 31–5 The timing cycle of VDD consists of a lower rate (LR) limit, an atrioventricular interval (AVI), a ventricular refractory period, a postventricular atrial refractory period (PVARP), and an upper rate limit. A sensed P wave initiates the AVI (during the AVI the atrial sensing channel is refractory). At the end of the AVI a ventricular pacing artifact is delivered if no intrinsic ventricular activity has been sensed; this represents P wave tracking pacing. Ventricular activity, paced or sensed, initiates the PVARP and the ventriculoatrial interval (the LR limit interval minus the AVI). If no P wave activity occurs, the pacemaker escapes with a ventricular pacing artifact at the LR limit. AV = atrioventricular; PV = interval from intrinsic atrial event to paced ventricular event; TARP = total atrial refractory period.

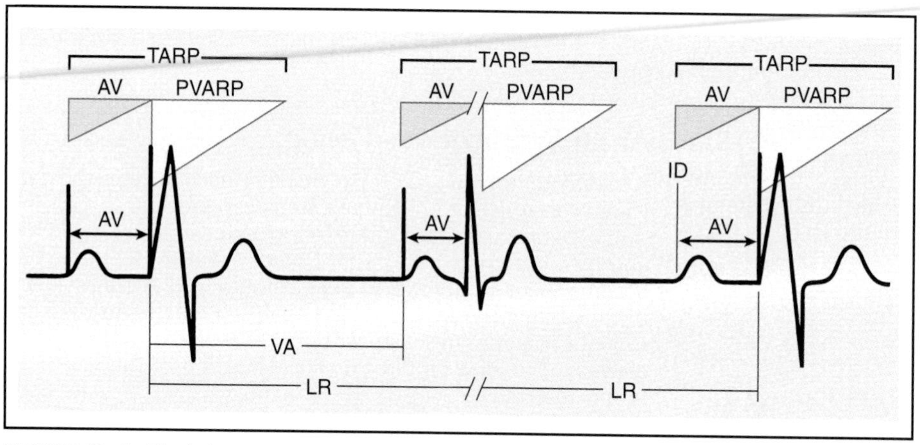

FIGURE 31–6 The timing cycle in DDD consists of a lower rate (LR) limit, an atrioventricular interval (AVI), a postventricular atrial refractory period (PVARP), and an upper rate limit. The AVI and PVARP together comprise the total atrial refractory period (TARP). If intrinsic atrial and ventricular activity occur before the LR times out, both channels are inhibited and no pacing occurs. If no intrinsic atrial or ventricular activity occurs, there is atrioventricular (AV) sequential pacing (first sequence). If no atrial activity is sensed before the ventriculoatrial (VA) interval is completed, an atrial pacing artifact is delivered, which initiates the AVI. If intrinsic ventricular activity occurs before the termination of the AVI, the ventricular output from the pacemaker is inhibited, that is, atrial pacing (second sequence). If a P wave is sensed before the VA interval is completed, output from the atrial channel is inhibited. The AVI is initiated, and if no ventricular activity is sensed before the AVI terminates, a ventricular pacing artifact is delivered, that is, P-synchronous pacing (third sequence). ID = intrinsic deflection.

of the upper rate limit. *The PVARP is especially important for the prevention of endless-loop, or pacemaker-mediated, tachycardia.*

Normal DDD function can appear electrocardiographically as (1) normal sinus rhythm, (2) atrial pacing only, (3) AV sequential pacing, or (4) P-synchronous pacing.

DDD pacing mode is most appropriate for patients with normal sinus node function and AV block. DDD pacing is often considered the mode of choice in neurocardiogenic syndromes with symptomatic cardioinhibition.

DDD pacing has limitations in the patient with sinus node dysfunction, because P-synchronous pacing is not possible in chronic atrial fibrillation or in patients with a paralyzed or nonexcitable atrium. Also, DDD pacing does not restore rate response in the chronotropically incompetent patient.

In any pacemaker capable of P-synchronous pacing, endless-loop tachycardia, also called *pacemaker reentrant tachycardia* or *pacemaker-mediated tachycardia*, can result. If AV synchrony is dissociated by any event, most commonly a premature ventricular complex (PVC), retrograde VA conduction can result in a retrograde P wave (Fig. 31–7). If the retrograde P wave is sensed by the atrial sensing circuit of the pacemaker, the AVI is initiated, resulting in a paced ventricular complex at a cycle length approximately equal to the maximum tracking rate. The paced ventricular event can again result in retrograde VA conduction, perpetuating this rapid reentrant circuit. Endless-loop tachycardia can be prevented by a PVARP that is long enough to prevent sensing of the retrograde P wave. Most pacemakers also have specific algorithms that attempt to recognize and abort endless-loop tachycardia.

Indications for Rate-Adaptive Pacing

Rate-adaptive pacemakers have the ability to increase the pacing rate through sensors that monitor physiological processes such as activity and minute ventilation. Single-chamber rate-adaptive pacing (AAIR, VVIR) has timing cycles that are not significantly different from those of its non–rate-adaptive counterparts. The difference lies in the potential variability of the paced rate. Depending on the sensor incorporated and the level of exertion of the patient, the basic interval shortens from the programmed lower rate limit to an upper rate limit programmed to define the absolute shortest cycle length allowable.

VVIR pacing, like VVI, is generally contraindicated if ventricular pacing results in retrograde (VA) conduction or a decrease in blood pressure. Also, if the sinus node is normal, P-synchronous pacing should be considered the optimal rate-adaptive mode and used when possible.

AAIR pacing can be considered for the patient with sinus node dysfunction and normal AV node function, because this mode restores rate responsiveness and maintains AV synchrony. If AAIR pacing is contemplated, normal AV node conduction must first be determined, as previously discussed for AAI pacing.

DDDR pacemakers are capable of all the variations described for DDD pacemakers. In addition to using P-synchronous pacing as a method for increasing heart rate, the sensor incorporated in the pacemaker can also drive the increase in heart rate. The resulting rhythm can be sinus driven or sensor driven. The ideal patient for DDDR pacing is one with combined sinus node and AV node dysfunction, because this mode allows restoration of rate responsiveness and AV synchrony.

Algorithms for determining the appropriate pacing mode for patients with sinus node disease and AV node disease are shown in Figure 31–8. In Figure 31-8A, a more complex algorithm, most of the available pacing modes are considered. The second algorithm is simpler and assumes that a pacemaker capable of rate adaptation is used (Fig. 31–8B).

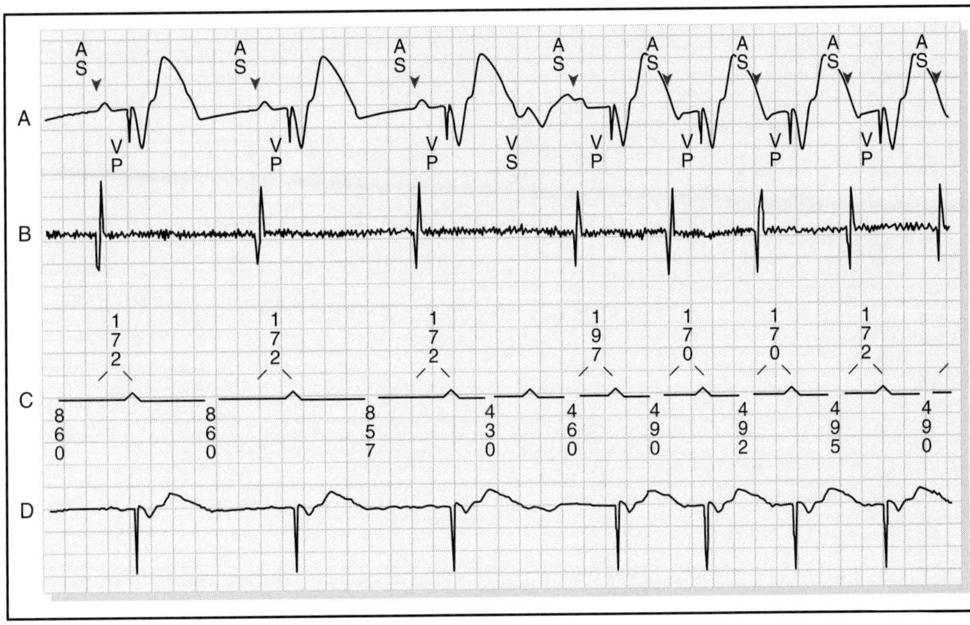

FIGURE 31–7 Electrocardiographic (ECG) example of pacemaker-mediated tachycardia (PMT) in a patient whose device is programmed to the DDD pacing mode. The ECG tracing **(A)** demonstrates P-synchronous pacing. The third paced QRS complex is followed by a ventricular sensed event that is followed by retrograde atrial sensing and subsequent ventricular pacing at a rate of approximately 115 beats/min. This appearance is consistent with PMT, or endless-loop tachycardia. **(B),** Atrial electrogram. **(C),** Marker channel. **(D),** Ventricular electrogram. VP = ventricular paced event; VS = ventricular sensed event; AS = atrial sensed event. Arrows indicate sensed or paced events. Numbers above the line indicate milliseconds between events. Numbers below the line indicate MS between ventricular events.

Selecting the Appropriate Sensor for Rate-Adaptive Pacing

Several varieties of sensors appropriate for rate-adaptive pacing have been developed and are displayed in Figure 31–9 as endpoints of some physiological response.[18] Although a number of sensors have been used clinically (some with clinical potential), only activity sensors, minute-ventilation sensors, and stimulus-T (QT interval) sensors have achieved clinical acceptance.

Activity Sensors

Activity sensing with vibration detection (piezoelectric crystal or accelerometer) has been the most widely used form of rate adaptation because it is simple, easy to apply clinically, and rapid in onset of rate response. The main difference between the piezoelectric crystal sensor and the accelerometer is that the former senses vibration from "up and down" motion and the latter in addition senses anterior and posterior motion. Accelerometers have become the activity sensor of choice, having been shown to have a slightly more physiological response than piezoelectric crystal sensors and, specifically, to have a more appropriate rate response to stair walking.[19]

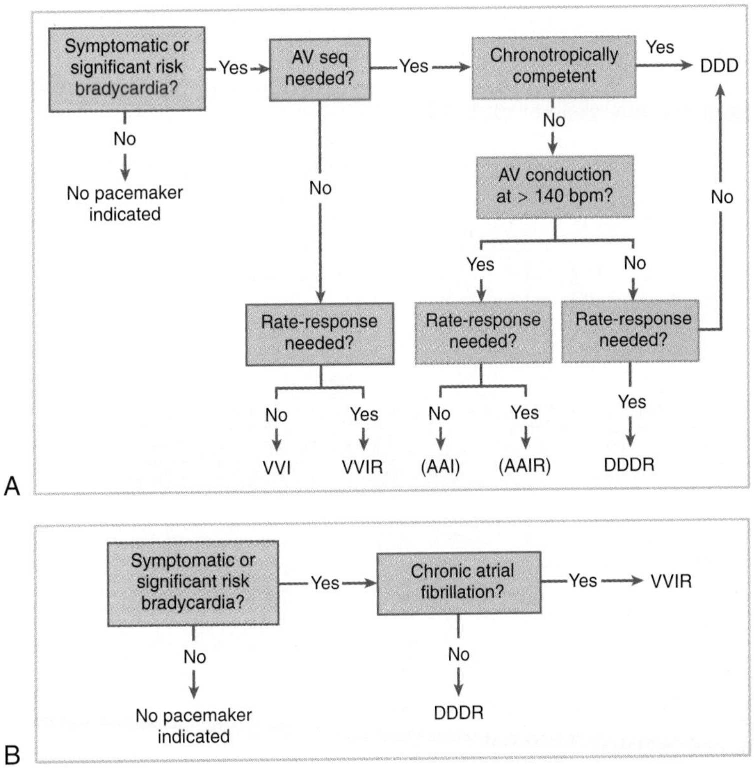

FIGURE 31–8 Algorithms for pacemaker mode selection. **A,** Choice of VVI, VVIR, AAI, AAIR, DDD, or DDDR is allowed. **B,** Only VVIR or DDDR is selected. AV = atrioventricular.

Minute-Ventilation Sensors

The minute-ventilation (respiratory rate × tidal volume) sensor has an excellent correlation with metabolic demand. In a rate-adaptive pacing system, minute volume is determined by emission of a small charge of known current from the pacemaker and measurement of the resulting voltage at the lead tip. When both current and voltage are known, transthoracic impedance can be measured between the ring electrode and the pacemaker. Because transthoracic impedance varies with respiration and its amplitude varies with tidal volume, the impedance measurement can be used to determine respiratory rate and tidal volume. A pacing algorithm uses the minute-volume measurements to alter pacing rate. Long-term reliability of the minute-ventilation sensor has been excellent.

Stimulus-T or QT-Sensing Pacemaker

The interval from the onset of a paced QRS complex to the end of the T wave has been used successfully for rate adaptation for many years. Autonomic activity and heart rate affect the stimulus-T interval, and the relationship allows

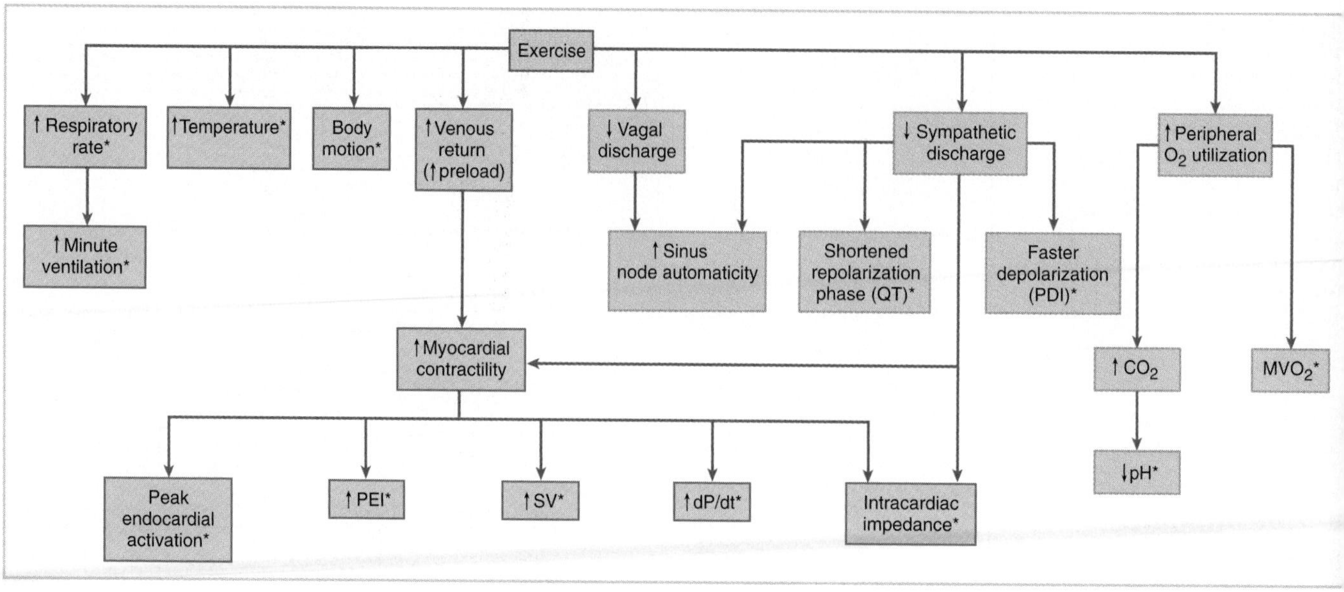

FIGURE 31–9 Physiological responses that have been investigated or clinically used for rate adaptation of permanent pacemakers. *Endpoints used for rate adaptation. PDI = paced depolarization integral; PEI = preejection interval; SV = stroke volume.

measurement of the stimulus-T interval to be used for rate adaptation.

Dual-Sensor Combinations

The overall performance of market-approved single-sensor rate-adaptive systems has been excellent. However, sensors have been combined in an effort to more closely mimic the normal sinus node at all levels of activity and during emotional stress.

The perfect sensor would be resistant to nonphysiological stimuli. A multisensor rate-adaptive pacing system could improve specificity by having one sensor verify or cross-check the other. For example, if one sensor indicated a rate increase and the other did not, a rate increase would not occur. Both sensors would have to indicate a rate increase before it would be allowed.

Pacing for Hemodynamic Improvement

In addition to hemodynamic improvements from pacing when a bradyarrhythmia is corrected, there are also nonbradyarrhythmic indications for permanent pacing for hemodynamic improvement.

Hypertrophic Obstructive Cardiomyopathy

Dual-chamber pacing has been used as a therapeutic modality for some patients with severe, symptomatic, medically refractory hypertrophic obstructive cardiomyopathy (HCM) (see Chap. 59).[20,21] The therapy is based on the concept that the altered septal activation caused by right ventricular apical pacing results in less narrowing of the left ventricular outflow tract and a subsequent decrease in the Venturi effect responsible for systolic anterior motion of the mitral valve.[20]

CLINICAL TRIALS

Pacing in HCM has been the subject of several randomized single-center and multicenter trials (Table 31–6). A single-center randomized crossover trial demonstrated symptomatic improvement in 63 percent of patients with pacing in the DDD mode.[22] However, 42 percent of patients had improvement when the pacemaker was programmed to a low pacing rate in the AAI mode, that is, effectively no pacing, suggesting a significant placebo effect.

In the Pacing in Cardiomyopathy (PIC) study, a multicenter, randomized, crossover study,[23] dual-chamber pacing resulted in a 50 percent reduction of the left ventricular outflow tract gradient, a 21 percent increase in exercise duration, and improvement in New York Heart Association (NYHA) functional class compared with baseline status. When clinical parameters, including chest pain, dyspnea, and subjective health status, were compared between DDD and back-up AAI pacing, there was no significant difference, again suggesting a significant placebo effect.

In the Multicenter Study of Pacing Therapy for Hypertrophic Cardiomyopathy (M-PATHY) trial, no significant differences were evident with randomization between pacing and no pacing, either subjectively or objectively, when exercise capacity, quality of life score, treadmill exercise time, and peak oxygen consumption were compared.[24] The investigators concluded that pacing should not be regarded as a primary treatment for HCM and that subjective benefit without objective evidence of improvement should be interpreted cautiously.

Pacing for the treatment of medically refractory HCM is currently a class IIb indication for pacing by the ACC/AHA guidelines.[2]

When pacing is applied in the patient with HCM, AVI programming is crucial to achieve optimal hemodynamic improvement. Ventricular depolarization must occur as a result of pacing. Therefore, the AVI must be short enough to result in depolarization by the paced event (Fig. 31–10). However, the shortest AVI is not necessarily the best.[22] Some experts have advocated AV node ablation to ensure paced ventricular depolarization if rapid intrinsic AV node conduction prevents total ventricular depolarization by means of the pacing stimulus.

Cardiac Resynchronization Therapy

Cardiac resynchronization therapy is the term applied to reestablishing synchronous contraction between the left ventricular free wall and the ventricular septum in an attempt

TABLE 31–6 Clinical Trials in Pacing for Hypertrophic Obstructive Cardiomyopathy

Study	Patient Inclusion Criteria	Endpoint(s)	Treatment Arms	Key Results
Mayo: Pacing in HCM[22]	Symptomatic HCM despite maximal medical regimen	LVOT gradient Quality of life Exercise duration Oxygen consumption	Blinded crossover of DDD pacing *vs.* No pacing (AAI)	Subjective improvement in ~60% of patients Significant placebo effect from pacing LVOT gradient reduced by mean of 33 ± 29 mm Hg
PIC[23]	Refractory symptoms from HCM despite stable drug regimen NYHA Class II or III Angina or dyspnea LVOT > 30 mm Hg	Exercise tolerance Dyspnea-angina symptom score NYHA Class Quality of life	Blinded crossover of DDD pacing *vs.* No pacing (AAI)	50% ↓ in LVOT gradient 21% ↑ in exercise duration 0.7 ↓ in NYHA Class
M-PATHY[24]	Symptomatic HCM despite maximal medical regimen LVOT ≥ 50 mm Hg	Quality of life Treadmill exercise duration Peak O_2 consumption ΔLVOT gradient ΔLV wall thickness	Blinded crossover of DDD pacing *vs.* No pacing (AAI at 30 beats/min)	No significant subjective or objective improvement with randomization Significant placebo effect

HCM = hypertrophic obstructive cardiomyopathy; LV = left ventricular; LVOT = left ventricular outflow tract; M-PATHY = Multicenter Study of Pacing Therapy for Hypertrophic Cardiomyopathy; NYHA = New York Heart Association; PIC = Pacing in Cardiomyopathy.

Data from Maron BJ, Nishimura RA, McKenna WJ, et al: Assessment of permanent dual-chamber pacing as a treatment for drug-refractory symptomatic patients with obstructive hypertrophic cardiomyopathy: A randomized, double-blind, crossover study (M-PATHY). Circulation 99:2927, 1999.

to improve left ventricular efficiency and, subsequently, to improve functional class. Generally, CRT has been used to describe biventricular or multisite ventricular pacing (Fig. 31–11), but cardiac resynchronization can be achieved by left ventricular pacing only in some patients.

Several randomized clinical trials have now been completed and have demonstrated the safety and efficacy of CRT. These trials are summarized in Table 31–7. In the most recent ACC/AHA/NASPE guidelines[2] for pacing, biventricular pacing in medically refractory, symptomatic NYHA Class III/IV patients with idiopathic dilated or ischemic cardiomyopathy, prolonged QRS interval (≥130 milliseconds), left ventricular end-diastolic diameter of 55 mm or more, and left ventricular ejection fraction of 0.35 or less is included as a class IIa indication. Similarly, the U.S. Food and Drug Administration labeling criteria for CRT are the following:

- NYHA functional Class III or IV
- QRS longer than 130 milliseconds
- Left ventricular ejection fraction of no more than 0.35
- Optimized medical therapy
- Normal sinus rhythm

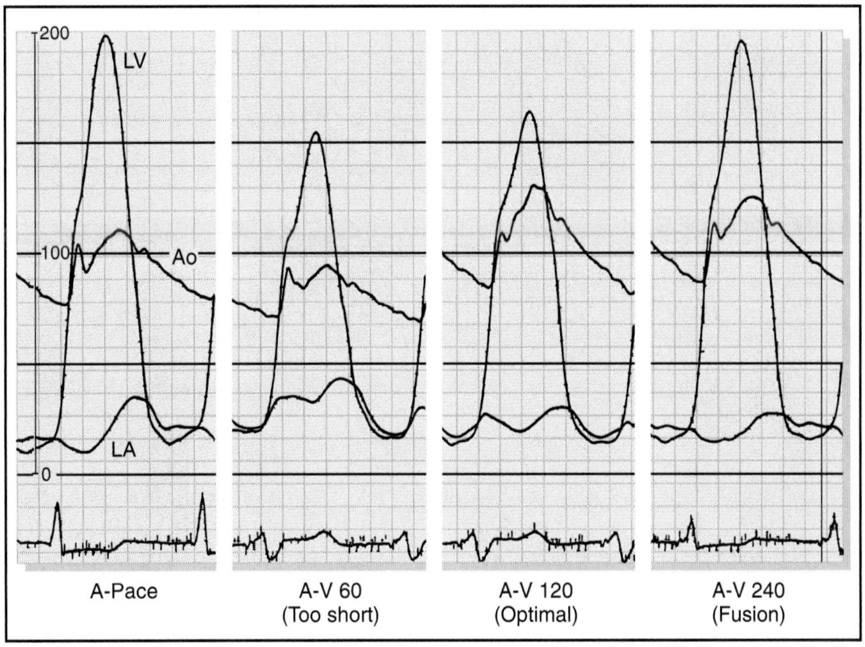

FIGURE 31–10 Pressure tracings at different atrioventricular (AV) intervals in a patient with hypertrophic obstructive cardiomyopathy. In this example, the outflow gradient was minimized at an AV interval of 120 milliseconds. LA = left atrium; LV = left ventricle; Ao = aorta.

CRT is rapidly gaining acceptance. Devices combining CRT and ICD capabilities are also available. The indications for such a device, often designated as *high-voltage CRT*, are discussed in the subsequent ICD section.

Pacing to Prevent Atrial Fibrillation

Multisite and alternate site atrial pacing have been used to prevent recurrent atrial tachyarrhythmias (see Chap. 32), presumably by decreasing the dispersion of refractoriness in the atrium.[25] Various techniques have been used to reduce or prevent atrial tachyarrhythmias (Table 31–8). Biatrial synchronous pacing with leads in the right atrial appendage and coronary sinus allows sensing from the lead in the right atrial appendage to be followed by immediate pacing at the coronary sinus site. The designation of *dual-site atrial pacing* has generally been used to describe one lead in a standard right atrial position and the other lead in the coronary sinus or near the coronary sinus ostium (Fig. 31–12). With both leads connected to the same port, there is simultaneous pacing at both sites. Dual-site pacing has been shown in a randomized clinical trial to decrease the number of episodes of paroxysmal atrial fibrillation and flutter and to increase the interval to

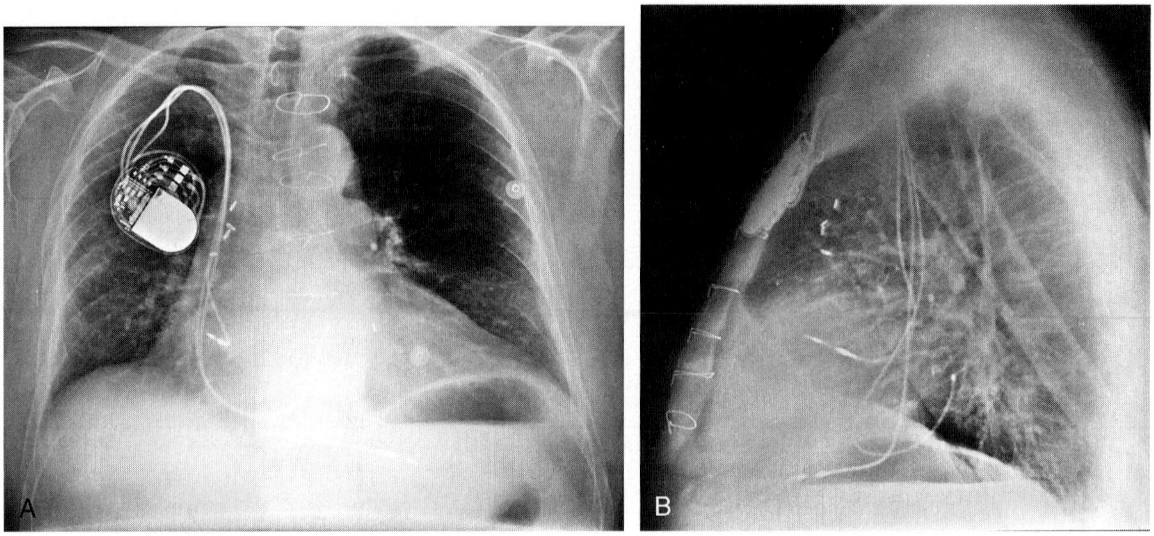

FIGURE 31–11 Posteroanterior **(A)** and lateral **(B)** chest radiographs demonstrating a biventricular pacing system. There are three leads: the first is positioned in the right atrium, a second is positioned in the right ventricular apex, and the third courses posteriorly in the coronary sinus and into the posterolateral cardiac vein.

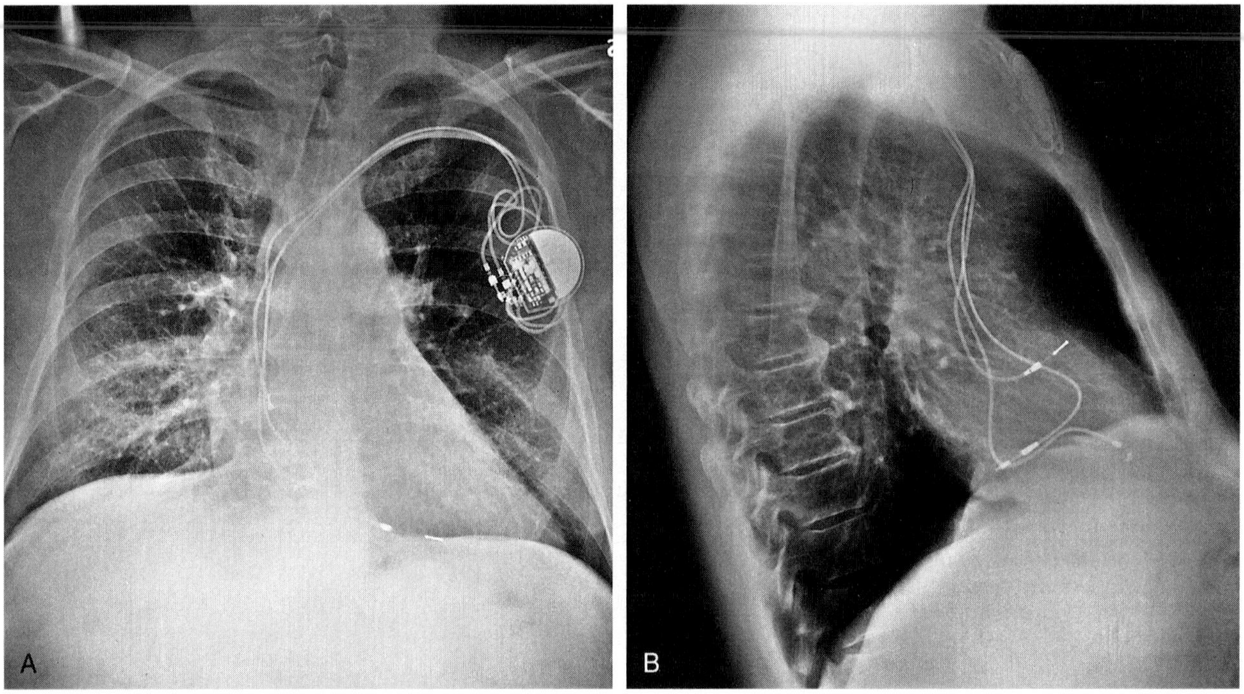

FIGURE 31–12 Posteroanterior **(A)** and lateral **(B)** chest radiographs in a patient with a dual-site atrial pacing system for the prevention of paroxysmal atrial fibrillation. Leads are positioned in the right atrium, near the coronary sinus ostium, and in the right ventricular apex.

recurrent atrial arrhythmias.[30] When "no pacing" was compared with dual-site or single-site atrial pacing, dual-site pacing was better, but single-site atrial pacing also resulted in a significant improvement over no pacing. Single-site atrial septal pacing[31] and Bachmann bundle pacing[32] have also been tested.

In addition to these alternate-pacing techniques, pacing algorithms have been incorporated in contemporary pacemakers in an effort to decrease the number of premature atrial complexes and maintain consistent atrial pacing (see Table 31–8). Multiple algorithms have been developed, and some pacemakers include as many as four different algorithms. A schematic representation of an algorithm that alters atrial pacing rate as a result of an atrial sensed event is shown in Figure 31–13.

Several clinical trials have been completed to assess these atrial pacing algorithms. A reduction in atrial fibrillation burden was demonstrated in two trials: the Atrial Dynamic Overdrive Pacing Trial (ADOPT)[33] (NASPE, 2002) and Atrial Fibrillation Therapy (AFT) trial (results not yet published) (European Society of Cardiology, 2002). Multiple additional trials are under way, but it is likely that atrial pacing algorithms will be included in the majority of future dual-chamber pacemakers.

Pacing in Long-QT Syndrome

The long-QT syndrome is characterized by abnormally prolonged ventricular repolarization and a risk of development

TABLE 31–7 Clinical Trials in Pacing for Congestive Heart Failure

Study	Patient Inclusion Criteria	Endpoint(s)	Treatment Arms	Key Results
InSync	NYHA Class III or IV on stable drug regimen LVEDD > 60 mm, LVEF ≤ 0.35 QRS width ≥ 150 msec	QOL NYHA Class 6-min hall walk	Nonrandomized	Sustained improvement in all three endpoints
MIRACLE	NYHA Class III or IV on stable drug regimen LVEDD ≥ 55 mm, LVEF ≤ 0.35 QRS width ≥ 130 msec	QOL NYHA Class 6-min hall walk	Randomized to pacing or no pacing for 6 mo and then to pacing	Sustained improvement in all three endpoints
PATH-CHF	DCM of any cause NYHA Class III or IV on stable drug regimen QRS ≥ 120 msec PR ≥ 150 msec	Acute maximum LV pressure derivative Aortic pulse pressure Chronic oxygen uptake Anaerobic threshold 6-min walk	Acute hemodynamic and chronic assessment of RV pacing *vs.* LV pacing *vs.* BiV pacing	Acute BiV and LV: ↑ LV pressure derivative and aortic pulse pressure more than RV pacing Sustained chronic improvement in all endpoints
MUSTIC-NSR	NYHA Class III Refractory symptoms on stable drug therapy LVEF < 0.35 LVEDD > 60 mm 6-min walk < 450 m NSR with QRS > 150 msec	Functional capacity QOL Metabolic exercise performance Mortality or need for transplant or LVAD Hospital admission for CHF	BiV pacing *vs.* No pacing with crossover	Sustained improvement in all endpoints Fewer hospital admissions with CRT
MUSTIC-AF	NYHA Class III Refractory symptoms on stable drug therapy LVEF < 0.35 LVEDD > 60 mm 6-min walk < 450 m AF with paced QRS > 200 msec	Functional capacity QOL Metabolic exercise performance Mortality or need for transplant or LVAD Hospital admission for CHF	BiV pacing *vs.* No pacing with crossover	Sustained improvement in all endpoints Fewer hospital admissions with CRT
InSync-III	NYHA Class III or IV on stable drug regimen LVEDD ≥ 60 mm, LVEF ≤ 0.35 QRS width ≥ 130 msec	QOL NYHA Class 6-min hall walk	BiV pacing with optimized AV and VV intervals *vs.* No pacing with crossover	Sustained improvement in all endpoints
CARE-HF	NYHA Class III or IV on stable drug regimen LVEDD ≥ 60 mm, LVEF ≤ 0.35 QRS width ≥ 150 msec or > 120 msec with echo study	Mortality QOL Economic outcomes Echo parameters Neurohormonal measurements	BiV pacing *vs.* No pacing with crossover	Enrollment completed (3/03)
PACMAN	Functional NYHA Class III CHF LVEF < 0.35 DCM of any etiology QRS > 150 msec Optimal medical management Hospitalization at least once in past 12 mo	Functional capacity by 6-min walk Secondary endpoints of QOL, adverse events, ventricular arrhythmias, hospitalizations	Observation over 1 yr with randomization of patients to CRT *vs.* No CRT (1:1 randomization)	Enrollment completed; in follow-up phase
VecToR	NYHA Class III or IV LVEF ≤ 0.35 QRS ≥ 140 msec LVEDD > 54 mm	QOL Mortality Echo parameters	BiV pacing *vs.* No pacing with crossover	In progress
ReLeVent	NYHA Class III or IV LVEF < 0.35 QRS > 140 msec LVEDD > 55 mm	6-min walk LVEDD LVESD Mortality QOL	BiV pacing *vs.* No pacing with crossover	In progress
PAVE	NYHA Class II or III Status post AV nodal ablation Able to complete 6-min hall walk 3 mo stable medical therapy	Exercise tolerance QOL	BiV pacing *vs.* RV pacing	In progress

Continued

TABLE 31–7 Clinical Trials in Pacing for Congestive Heart Failure—cont'd

Study	Patient Inclusion Criteria	Endpoint(s)	Treatment Arms	Key Results
MUSTIC-II	NYHA Class III or IV AF after ablation and paced for > 3 mo LVEDD > 60 mm QRS > 200 msec 6-min walk < 450 m LVEF < 0.35	Exercise tolerance QOL Hospitalization rates Modification of drug therapy	BiV pacing *vs.* No pacing with crossover	In progress

AF = atrial fibrillation; BiV = biventricular; CARE-HF = Cardiac Resynchronization in Heart Failure; CHF = congestive heart failure; CRT = cardiac resynchronization therapy; DCM = dilated cardiomyopathy; echo = echocardiographic; LV = left ventricular; LVAD = left ventricular assist device; LVEDD = left ventricular end-diastolic dimension; LVEF = left ventricular ejection fraction; LVESD = left ventricular end-systolic dimension; MIRACLE = Multicenter InSync Randomized Clinical Evaluation; MUSTIC = Multisite Stimulation in Cardiomyopathy; NSR = normal sinus rhythm; NYHA = New York Heart Association; PACMAN = Pacing for Cardiomyopathy: a European Study; PATH-CHF = Pacing Therapy in Congestive Heart Failure; PAVE = Left Ventricular Post-AV Nodal Ablation Evaluation; QOL = quality of life; ReLeVent = Remodeling of Cardiac Cavities by Long-Term Ventricular-Based Stimulation; RV = right ventricular; VecToR = Ventricular Resynchronization Therapy Randomized.

TABLE 31–8 Clinical Trials in Pacing for Prevention of Atrial Fibrillation

Study	Patient Inclusion Criteria	Endpoint(s)	Treatment Arms	Key Results
SYNBIAPACE	≥1-yr history of recurrent and drug-refractory AA P wave duration ≥ 120 msec and IACT ≥ 100 msec	Time to first AA recurrence	BASP at 70 beats/min *vs.* Single-site HRA at 70 beats/min *or* Single-site HRA at 40 beats/min	Trend to a ↓ in incidence of AA with BASP, but no real benefit of BASP
DAPPAF*	Bradycardia requiring pacing Two documented episodes of AF in prior 3 mo	Time to first recurrence of symptoms of AF Quality of life Safety of DAP	Dual-site right atrial pacing *or* Single-site atrial pacing *vs.* Support pacing mode (control arm)	Dual-site right atrial pacing prolonged or tended to prolong time to recurrent AF in presence of AAD Support pacing poorly tolerated and associated with highest recurrence rates of symptomatic AF
STOP-AF[26]	—	Time to recurrence of PAF	Physiological pacing *vs.* VVI pacing	In progress
PA3[27]	History of PAF with three or more episodes within year before Most recent PAF within 3 mo of entry At least one episode of PAF documented by ECG	Time to recurrence of PAF ≥ 5 min occurring ≥ 2 wk after entry Intervals between successive episodes of PAF Frequency of PAF Proportion of patients who chose to defer ablation	DDDR pacemaker implanted and randomized to atrial pacing or no pacing	Atrial RAP did not prevent PAF over short term in patients with drug-resistant PAF
PIPAF[28,29]	Indication for pacing Documented paroxysmal AAs for at least 1 yr, three episodes Stable drug therapy Fewer than two cardioversions in past year	Time to first recurrence of AA Cumulative arrhythmia duration	Comparison of six different lead and algorithm combinations	In progress

AA = atrial arrhythmia; AAD = antiarrhythmic drug; BASP = biatrial synchronous pacing; DAP = dual-site atrial pacing; DAPPAF = Dual-Site Atrial Pacing to Prevent Atrial Fibrillation; ECG = electrocardiography; HRA = high right atrium; IACT = interatrial conduction time; PA3 = Atrial Pacing Periablation for Prevention of Paroxysmal Atrial Fibrillation; PAF = paroxysmal atrial fibrillation; PIPAF = Pacing in Prevention of Atrial Fibrillation; RAP = rate-adaptive pacing; STOP-AF = Systematic Trial of Pacing for Atrial Fibrillation; SYNBIAPACE = Synchronous Biatrial Pacing.

*Data from Fitts SM, Hill MR, Mehra R, et al: DAPPAF Phase I Investigators: Design and implementation of the Dual Site Atrial Pacing to Prevent Atrial Fibrillation (DAPPAF) clinical trial. J Interv Card Electrophysiol 2:139, 1998.

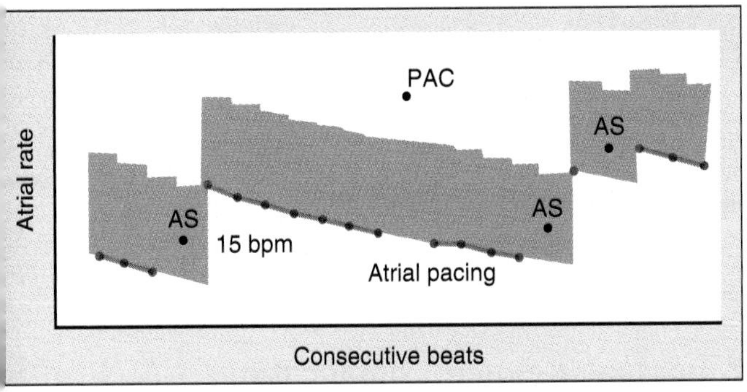

FIGURE 31–13 Schematic representation of an atrial pacing algorithm that increments the atrial pacing rate when a sensed atrial beat (AS) is detected to consistently overdrive the intrinsic atrial rhythm. The pacing rate would decrement after a specified period if no additional ASs were detected. PAC = premature atrial complex.

of life-threatening ventricular tachyarrhythmias (see Chaps. 28 and 32). Therapy must be individualized depending on the clinical situation. Therapeutic options include beta-blocker therapy, permanent pacing, and the ICD (see later).

Pulse Generator Implantation

Only qualified physicians should undertake pacemaker or ICD implantation. The recommended training requirements for pacemaker implantation[34] are as follows: a base of core knowledge for pacemaker follow-up, participation in at least 100 pacemaker follow-up visits, participation in at least 50 initial transvenous pacemaker implantations as the primary operator (recommended that at least one-half of these be dual-chamber), participation in at least 20 revisions of pacing systems, exposure to lead extraction techniques (suggested), and thorough knowledge of recognition and treatment of pacemaker and surgical complications and emergencies. A detailed description of pacemaker and ICD implantation technique can be found in texts devoted to these disciplines.[35] However, certain information related to the implantation technique is important for the referring physician to know.

Almost all pacemakers and defibrillators are now implanted transvenously, with the pulse generator placed in the upper anterior portion of the chest, just anterior to the pectoralis major muscle. Epicardial pacing is usually considered only in persons without reasonable venous access, that is, no access to the right ventricle because of an associated congenital anomaly, a prosthetic tricuspid valve, or an intracardiac right-to-left shunt.

Although multiple venous routes have been used for lead placement, the subclavian and cephalic veins are most commonly used. The subclavian approach involves a subclavian puncture and the use of one or more peel-away introducers. A lateral approach to the subclavian vein, often lateral enough to be the axillary vein, is preferred to minimize the risk of pneumothorax and to avoid subclavian crush injury to the lead, which is more common when a medial approach is used. The cephalic vein is often large enough to accept one or two pacing leads, and this approach avoids the risks associated with blind subclavian puncture. Potential complications of subclavian puncture include pneumothorax, hemopneumothorax, subclavian artery puncture, brachial nerve plexus injury, and thoracic duct injury.

Specific measurements must be obtained at the time of pacemaker or ICD implantation (Table 31–9).

After placement of the pulse generator, posteroanterior and lateral chest radiographs must be obtained to exclude pneumothorax and also to ensure adequate lead positioning. Before hospital dismissal, the pulse generator should be programmed to determine pacing and sensing thresholds for final programming with adequate safety margins. If the pulse generator is being programmed to a rate-adaptive pacing mode, adequate rate response should be assessed by formal or informal stress testing.

TABLE 31–9 Measurements During Implantation of Pacemaker or Cardioverter-Defibrillator

Threshold of stimulation
  Atrium*
  Ventricle

Measurement of electrogram†
  Atrium*
  Ventricle

Measurement of antegrade conduction‡   Wenckebach block point
Defibrillation threshold§

*Necessary only when an atrial lead is being placed.
†Electrogram measurement implies measurement of intrinsic amplitude of P wave (atrium) or QRS (ventricle); actual electrogram can easily be recorded by pacing system analyzer.
‡Necessary only when an AAI or AAIR system is implanted.
§Should be measured during all cardioverter-defibrillator implants.

Pacemaker Programming

All contemporary pacemakers have many programmable parameters that can be altered to optimize and troubleshoot pacemaker function. A detailed description of pacemaker programming is beyond the scope of this text. A few of the most critical parameters merit mention here, but any caregiver taking responsibility for pacemaker follow-up should have a thorough knowledge of all programming options.

Programming Pulse Width and Voltage Amplitude

Output programming is probably the most important aspect of programming that should be performed routinely. The output must be high enough to allow an adequate pacing margin of safety but should also be programmed with the intent of maximizing pacemaker longevity. A strength-duration curve plots voltage and pulse width thresholds and allows determination of appropriate values to ensure an adequate safety margin. There is no consensus of the best way to program output parameters, but options include doubling the voltage amplitude at threshold, tripling the pulse width at threshold, determining the threshold, or programming output parameters to achieve triple the threshold determined in microjoules. Some pacemakers automatically determine output parameters and others continually do surveillance of the capture threshold and automatically adjust output parameters.

AVI

In dual-chamber pacemakers, the interval corresponding to the intrinsic PR interval, that is, the interval between paced or sensed atrial event and paced ventricular event, must be programmed. Optimization of this interval is critical in some patients to obtain optimal hemodynamic benefit from the pacemaker. As mentioned earlier, there is currently a preference to maintain intrinsic ventricular activation, that is, program a longer AVI, when possible, to avoid the potential adverse effects of right ventricular apical pacing.

Mode Switching

Mode switching is the ability of the pacemaker to automatically change from one mode to another in response to an inappropriately rapid atrial rhythm (Fig. 31–14).[36] Mode switching is particularly useful for patients with paroxysmal supraventricular rhythm disturbances. In the DDD or DDDR pacing modes, if a supraventricular rhythm disturbance occurs and the pacemaker senses the pathological atrial rhythm, rapid ventricular pacing can occur. Any pacing mode that eliminates tracking of the pathological rhythm, that is, DDI, DDIR, DVI, or DVIR, also eliminates the ability to track normal sinus rhythm, which is usually the predominant rhythm. Mode switching avoids this limitation by switching from DDD or DDDR during sinus rhythm to a nontracking mode, such as DDIR, during the pathological atrial rhythm.

Rate-Adaptive Parameters

The goal of programming rate-adaptive pacemakers is to optimize the patient's chronotropic response. Some form of exercise is necessary to optimize rate-adaptive parameters. For patients who are limited to activities of daily living, informal exercise testing, such as walking at casual and brisk paces in the hospital corridor or in the outpatient facility, is often adequate. In determining the appropriate heart rate response, the patient's age and "usual activities" must be taken into consideration. If formal exercise testing is performed, a low-intensity exercise protocol that allows for a gradual increase may be preferable to a standard Bruce protocol. The chronotropic exercise assessment protocol allows for a gradual increase in speed and grade and thus mimics levels of exercise that are likely to occur during activities of daily living.

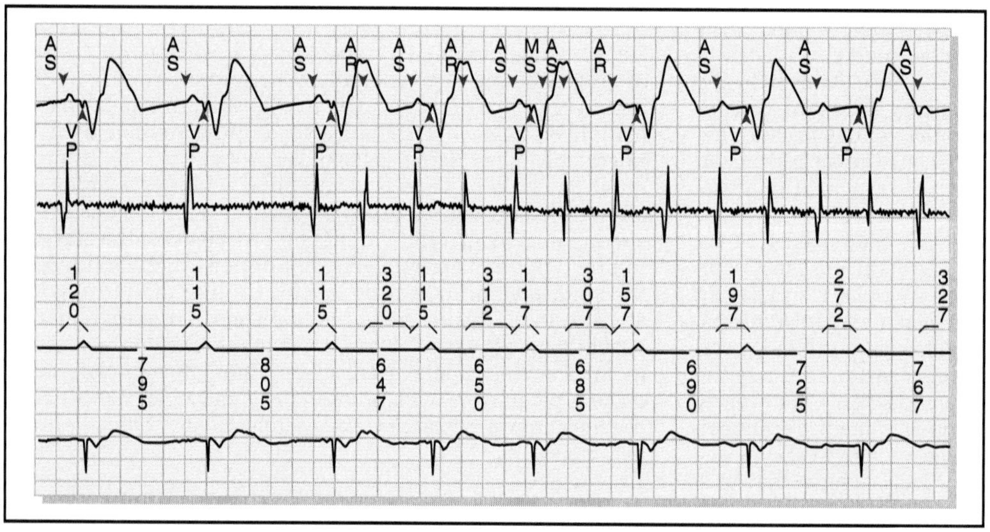

FIGURE 31–14 Electrocardiographic tracing from a patient with a DDD pacemaker. In the initial portion of the tracing, the pacing is in sinus rhythm. This is followed by the onset of an atrial tachyarrhythmia with initial tracking, but mode switching causes reversion to a DDI pacing mode. (The top tracing is the marker channel, the second tracing represents the atrial electrogram, and the third is the timing channel. The lower tracing represents the surface electrocardiogram.) Arrows indicate paced or sensed events or change in operation (mode switch [MS]). AR = atrial event in refractory period; AS = atrial sensed event; VP = ventricular paced event. Numbers above the line indicate milliseconds from one event to another (e.g., AS to VP). Numbers below the line indicate MS between ventricular events.

Pacemaker Complications

Complications can be divided into those related to implantation and those related to failure of a component of the pacing system. There are also problems encountered during follow-up that are actually pseudoabnormalities, that is, a normal response that appears abnormal because of unusual timing or because of idiosyncrasies of the device. Many complications are directly related to the experience of the implanter.

Implant-Related Complications

Most patients undergoing pacemaker implantation have some discomfort at the site of the incision in the early postoperative period. Mild analgesics may be required. Mild ecchymoses around the incision are not uncommon. As previously noted, if subclavian puncture is used for lead placement, several potential complications of this "blind" technique can occur, including the possibility of traumatic pneumothorax and hemopneumothorax, inadvertent arterial puncture, air embolism, arteriovenous fistula, thoracic duct injury, subcutaneous emphysema, and brachial plexus injury.

Hematoma formation at the pulse generator site occurs most commonly when anticoagulant therapy is initiated or reinstituted prematurely. A hematoma must be dealt with on the basis of its secondary consequences. Aspiration is generally not advised, and evacuation of the hematoma should be considered only if there is continued bleeding, potential compromise of the suture line or skin integrity, or pain from the hematoma that cannot be managed with analgesics.

Introduction of the lead or leads into the subclavian artery, the aorta, and the left ventricle usually is readily recognized because of the pulsatile flow of saturated blood. A pacing lead may also be placed in the left ventricle by passing it across an unsuspected atrial or ventricular septal defect (Fig. 31–15). Once the lead is within the subclavian artery, passage into the left ventricle is as easy as passage into the right ventricle via the venous system. Left ventricular lead placement should be recognized if lateral fluoroscopy is used or a lateral chest radiograph is obtained, because the lead is in the posterior aspect of the heart. The ECG during right ventricular pacing usually has a left bundle branch block (LBBB) pattern, and during left ventricular pacing, a right bundle branch block (RBBB) pattern is most common.

Although thresholds may be adequate, lead placement in the arterial circulation is associated with thrombus formation, embolization, and, consequently, stroke. The management of inadvertent left ventricular lead placement is dependent on the time it is discovered after implantation and individual patient needs and associated comorbid conditions.

Patients undergoing device implantation should be made aware of the potential for lead perforation. Although cardiac tamponade is the most dramatic outcome from perforation, lack of symptoms after ventricular perforation by a lead is not uncommon. The only sign may be a rising stimulation threshold. In other patients, the signs can include an RBBB pattern from a lead placed in the right ventricle, intercostal muscle, or diaphragmatic contraction; friction rub after implantation; and pericarditis, pericardial effusion, or cardiac tamponade. (Depending on lead

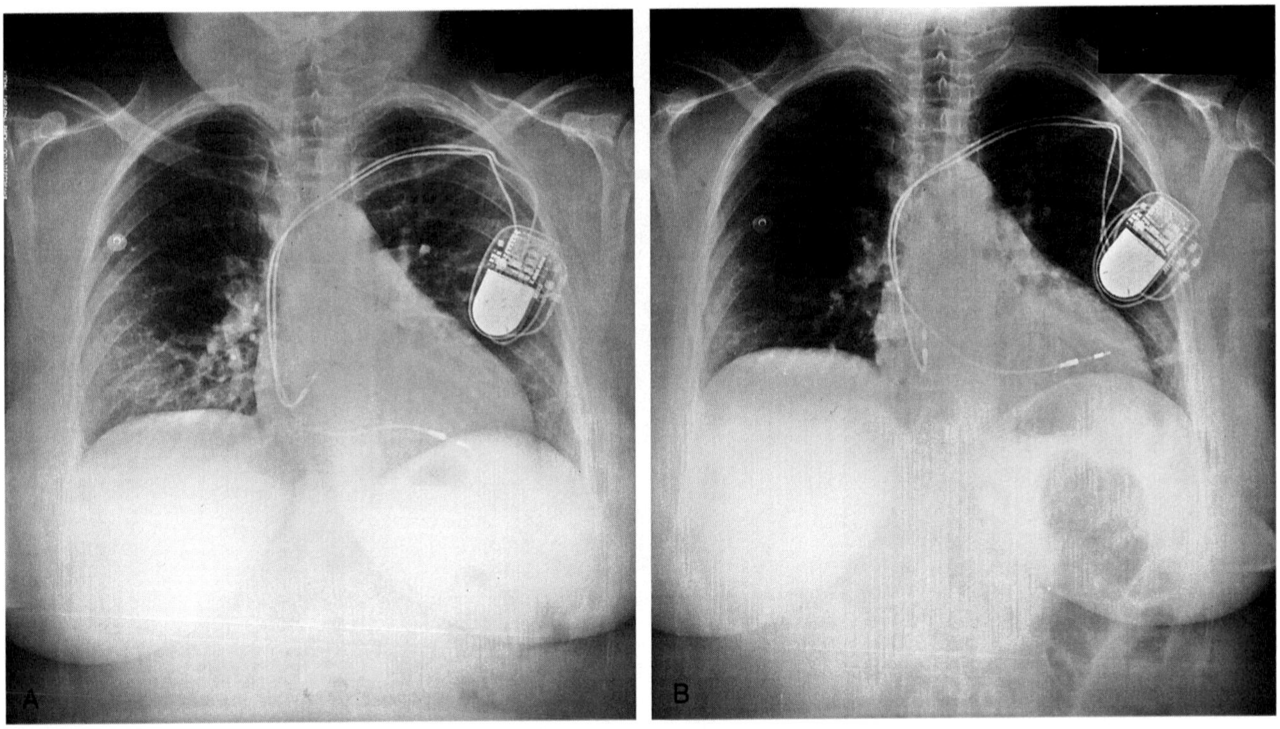

FIGURE 31–15 Posteroanterior chest radiographs of a dual-chamber pacemaker. **A,** Ventricular lead is passing through an atrial septal defect into the left ventricle. **B,** Lead is repositioned in the right ventricular apex.

position, an RBBB pattern is also possible when the lead is within the right ventricular cavity.)

Ventricular perforation may be suggested by radiography, ECG, and echocardiography. Once perforation is identified, lead withdrawal and repositioning are usually uncomplicated, although pericardial bleeding or tamponade results rarely.

Partial or silent inconsequential venous thrombosis of the subclavian vein is not uncommon after transvenous lead placement and is usually clinically insignificant. Such partial or silent thrombosis may limit venous access at the time of pacing system revision. Symptomatic thrombosis of the subclavian vein, with an edematous, painful upper extremity, is a relatively rare but recognized complication. Once again, management must be individualized. Anticoagulation will be necessary in some patients.

Lead-Related Complications

Several lead-related complications deserve attention, including lead dislodgment (Fig. 31–16), loose connector pin (Fig. 31–17), conductor coil (lead) fracture (Fig. 31–18), and insulation break.

Acceptable dislodgment rates should probably be less than 1 percent for ventricular leads and no more than 2 to 3 percent for atrial leads. Dislodgment may be radiographically evident (macrodislodgment) or not radiographically detectable (microdislodgment). Adequate lead position is assessed by posteroanterior and lateral chest radiographs and comparison with any previous chest radiographs.

Intermittent or complete failure of output can occur because of a loose connection at the interface of the lead and connector block (see Fig. 31-17), usually because the lead was inadequately secured at the time of pacemaker implantation. When a connection is loose, manipulating the pulse generator or pocket may reproduce the problem. The poor connection may be evident radiographically.

Loss of integrity of the insulating material is also uncommon and clinically can present as sensing or pacing abnormalities (or both). Both insulation defects and conductor fractures (see Fig. 31-18) can be caused by crush injury, specifically at the costoclavicular space when placement is by the subclavian puncture technique.

Supraventricular and ventricular arrhythmias, often encountered during pacemaker implantation, are usually inconsequential.

Extrasystoles can be seen in the early postimplantation period and are usually morphologically similar to the paced beats because they

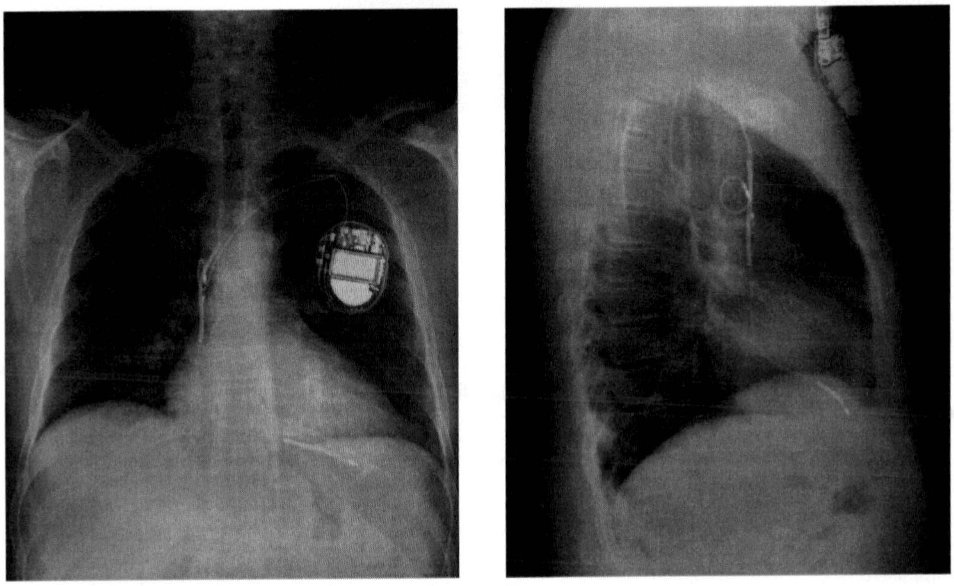

FIGURE 31–16 Posteroanterior chest radiographs of a dual-chamber pacemaker. **A,** The atrial lead, originally positioned in a right atrial appendage position, is clearly no longer apically positioned. **B,** Lateral view also demonstrates definite dislodgment of the ventricular lead.

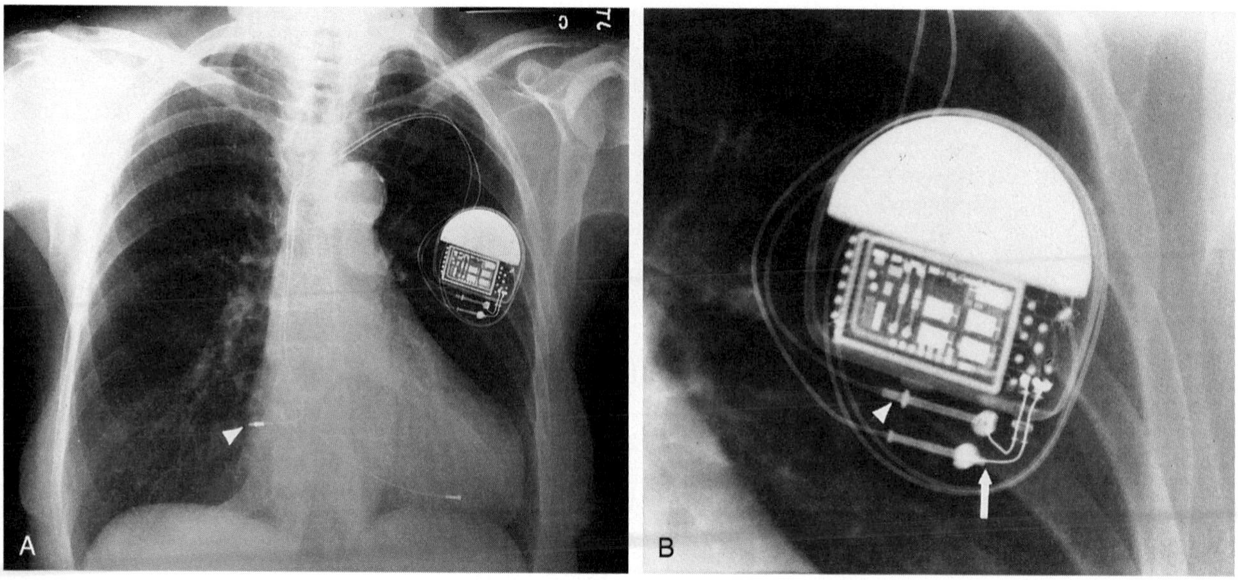

FIGURE 31–17 **A,** Posteroanterior chest radiograph in a patient with a VVI pacemaker and a bifurcated bipolar ventricular lead. The patient presented with recurrent near-syncope and intermittent failure to output. **B,** Close-up of the pacemaker shows that the lower connector pin is not securely in the connector block (arrow). (For comparison, the arrowhead indicates an appropriately engaged connector pin.) (**A** and **B,** From Hayes DL: Pacemaker radiography. *In* Furman S, Hayes DL, Holmes DR Jr [eds]: A Practice of Cardiac Pacing. 3rd ed. Mount Kisco, NY, Futura, 1993, p 361, By permission of Mayo Foundation.)

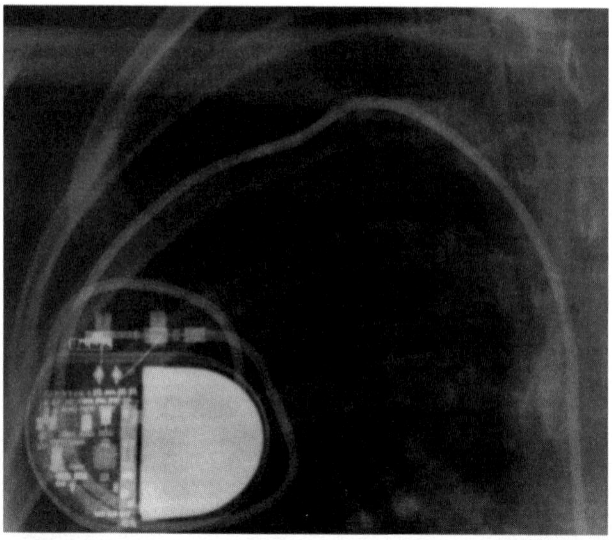

FIGURE 31–18 Close-up view of a portion of the posteroanterior chest radiograph in a patient with a single-chamber pacemaker. The lead has fractured where it passes below the clavicle. The patient presented with intermittent ventricular failure to capture and intermittent failure to output on the ventricular lead. Impedance was intermittently measured at more than 9999 Ω.

originate at the same site as the paced beats but are not preceded by a pacemaker stimulus. Such extrasystoles most often occur during the first 24 to 48 hours after implantation, usually resolve spontaneously, and almost never require pharmacological suppression. Extracardiac stimulation usually involves the diaphragm or pectoral muscle. Diaphragmatic stimulation may be due to direct stimulation of the diaphragm (usually stimulation of the left hemidiaphragm) or stimulation of the phrenic nerve (usually stimulation of the right hemidiaphragm). Diaphragmatic stimulation occurring during the early postimplantation period may be due to either microdislodgment or macrodislodgment of the pacing lead. Stimulation can be minimized or alleviated by decreasing the voltage output or pulse width (or both), but an adequate pacing margin of safety must be maintained after the output parameters are decreased. If the problem cannot be resolved by reprogramming the pacemaker output, lead repositioning will be required.

Pacemaker System Infection

Erosion is an uncommon complication that most commonly occurs because of an indolent infection, although it may also be the result of a pacemaker pocket that is too "tight."

If the patient seeks medical attention before the pacemaker has eroded through the skin, it may be possible to revise the pocket and reimplant the pacemaker. Impending erosion should be dealt with as an emergency because once any portion of the pacemaker has eroded through the skin, the only choice is removal of the pacemaker system and placement of a new system in another site.

Infection may be present even without purulent material; therefore, a specimen for culture should be obtained and proven negative before pocket revision. Adherence of the pacemaker to the skin strongly suggests an infection, and salvage of the site may not be possible.

The incidence of infection after pacemaker implantation should certainly be less than 2 percent and in most series has been less than 1 percent. Careful attention to surgical details and sterile procedures is of paramount importance in avoiding pacemaker site infection. Prophylactic use of antibiotics before implantation and in the immediate postoperative period remains controversial. Most studies do not show any significant difference in the rate of infection between patients who have had prophylactic administration of antibiotics and those who have not. Irrigation of the pacemaker pocket with an antibiotic solution at the time of pacemaker implantation is probably more important in the prevention of infection.

Pacemaker infection may appear as local inflammation or abscess formation in the pacemaker pocket, erosion of part of the pacing system with secondary infection, or sepsis with positive blood culture findings with or without a focus of infection elsewhere.

The most common clinical presentation is localized pocket infection; septicemia is uncommon. Many infectious agents can be responsible, but early infections are most commonly caused by *Staphylococcus aureus*, are aggressive, and are often associated with fever and systemic symptoms. Late infections commonly are caused by *Staphylococcus epidermidis* and are more indolent, usually without fever or systemic manifestation. Treatment for both organisms requires removal of the entire infected pacing system, pacemaker, and leads.

Troubleshooting Electrocardiographic Abnormalities

ECG abnormalities in the paced patient can be broadly grouped into failure to capture, failure to output, sensing abnormalities (undersensing or oversensing), and inappropriate rate change.

FAILURE TO CAPTURE

Failure to capture indicates that a pacing artifact is present without subsequent cardiac depolarization (Fig. 31-19). The possible causes of failure to capture are high thresholds with an inadequately programmed output, partial conductor coil fracture, insulation defect, lead dislodgment or perforation, impending total battery depletion, functional noncapture, poor or incompatible connection at the connector block, circuit failure, air in the pulse generator pocket (unipolar pacemaker), and elevated thresholds due to drugs or metabolic abnormality.

FAILURE TO PACE

Failure to pace, or failure to output, that is, failure to deliver an appropriate pacing stimulus, is often due to oversensing and inhibition of output but could also be due to true failure to output from the pacemaker or circuit interruption that prevents the electrical signal from reaching the heart (Fig. 31-20). The reasons for failure to output are circuit failure, complete or intermittent conductor coil fracture, intermittent or permanently loose set screw, incompatible lead or header, total battery depletion, internal insulation failure (bipolar lead), oversensing of any noncardiac activity, crosstalk (Fig. 31-21), and lack of anodal connector contact (e.g., unipolar lead in bipolar generator, bipolar lead in pacemaker programmed in unipolar mode, air in the pocket of a unipolar device, and unipolar pacemaker not in the pocket).

The differential diagnoses of failure to capture and failure to pace obviously overlap somewhat. For example, ECG manifestations of a conductor coil fracture may include failure to capture because of significant leakage of current at the incomplete fracture site and not enough current remaining to result in stimulation. Nonetheless, the pacemaker stimuli can appear. Alternatively, escaping current can be sensed by the pacemaker and inhibit pacemaker output. If the conductor coil is completely fractured, rendering the circuit incomplete, no pacemaker output will be detected on the ECG. Insulation defects can also be signaled by oversensing and failure to pace or by failure to capture, although the most common consequences of insulation failure are sensing abnormalities.

As the pacemaker battery reaches end stages of depletion, either failure to capture because of decreasing voltage output or failure to pace

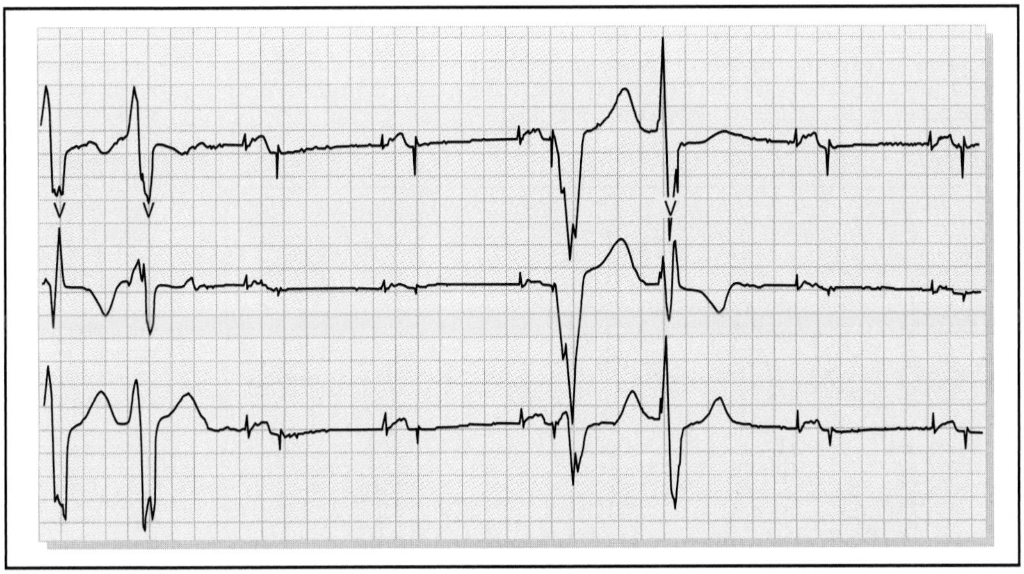

FIGURE 31–19 Electrocardiographic tracing from a patient with a DDDR pacemaker. All but one ventricular pacing artifact fail to result in ventricular depolarization, that is, failure to capture. In this patient, intermittent ventricular failure to capture was due to lead dislodgment.

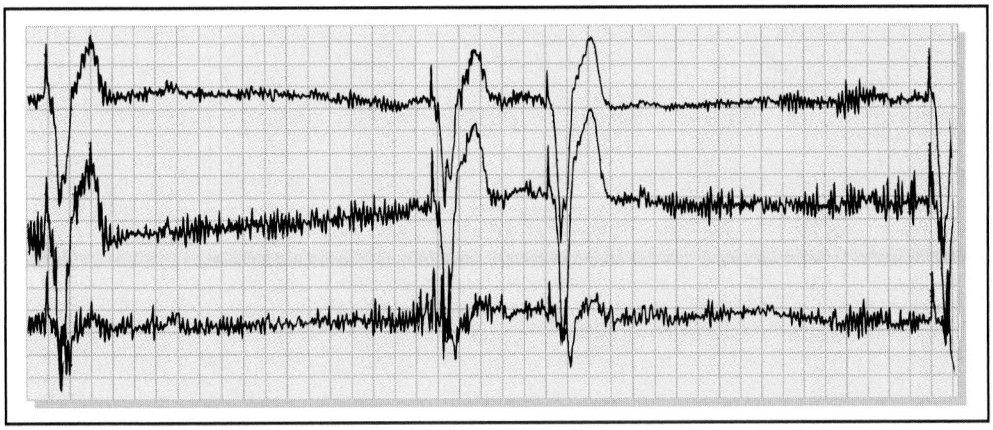

FIGURE 31–20 Electrocardiographic tracings. Patient with a VVIR pacemaker with a lower rate of 70 beats/min. After an initial paced ventricular beat, there is a pause of approximately 2.8 seconds with significant baseline artifact. After two additional paced beats, another pause of approximately 2.8 seconds occurs. This patient had a pacemaker programmed to a unipolar sensing configuration. Sensing of myopotentials led to symptomatic pauses, and reprogramming the pacemaker to a bipolar sensing configuration prevented subsequent myopotential oversensing.

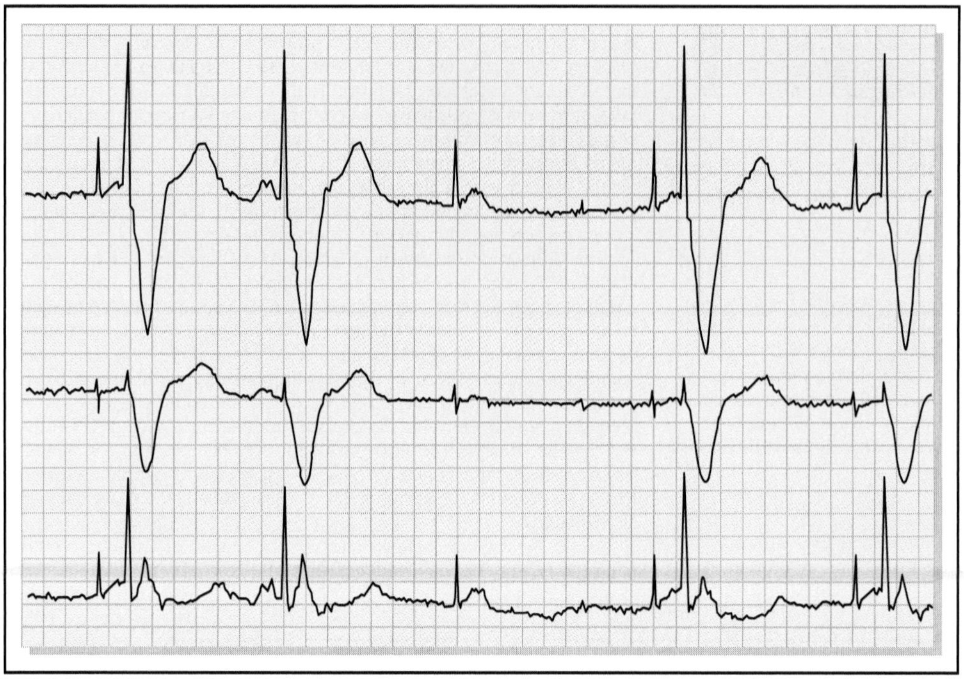

FIGURE 31–21 Patient with a DDD pacemaker. After the third atrial pacing artifact, there is evidence of atrial depolarization, but there is no ventricular pacing output. Failure to deliver the ventricular pacing artifact is due to crosstalk; that is, the atrial pacing output is sensed by the ventricular sensing circuit, with subsequent inhibition.

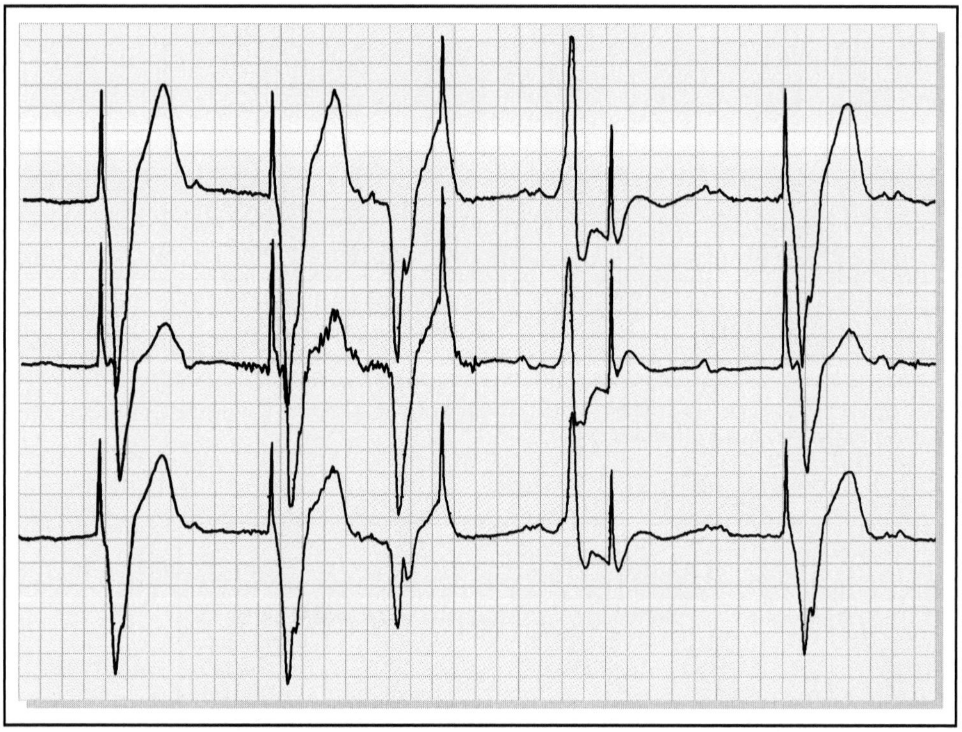

FIGURE 31–22 Electrocardiographic tracing from a patient with a VVI pacemaker with a programmed rate of 70 beats/min. After two paced ventricular complexes, a premature ventricular complex occurs. In approximately 260 milliseconds, a ventricular pacing artifact occurs. This is followed by a P wave with intrinsic atrioventricular nodal conduction and native QRS complex. A pacemaker artifact follows in approximately 220 milliseconds. This represents ventricular undersensing. In this patient, the abnormality occurred because of an insulation failure of the ventricular pacing lead.

because of total battery depletion can occur. This degree of battery depletion should be avoided by appropriate pacemaker follow-up.

Apparent failure to capture is noted if a pacemaker stimulus occurs during the refractory period of a spontaneous beat. This is referred to as *functional noncapture*.

FAILURE TO SENSE

Sensing abnormalities can be divided into *true abnormalities*, including undersensing (a failure to recognize normal intrinsic cardiac activity [Fig. 31-22] and oversensing (unexpected sensing of an intrinsic or extrinsic electrical signal [see Fig. 31-20]), and *functional sensing abnormalities*. The possible causes of sensing abnormalities are lead dislodgment or poor lead positioning, lead insulation failure, circuit failure, magnet application, malfunction of reed switch, electromagnetic interference (EMI), and battery depletion. The morphology of the intrinsic event is different from that measured at implantation.

True undersensing is most commonly due to lead dislodgment or inadequate initial lead placement. Sensing abnormalities can commonly be seen secondary to insulation defects and to intermittent "make-or-break" conductor fracture. A normally functioning pacing system at times fails to detect atrial or ventricular extrasystoles. The intrinsic events measured at the time of implantation generate an electrogram at the electrode tip. If an extrasystole is occurring elsewhere in the heart, the sensing vector is different from that of the normal intrinsic beat, and the resulting voltage generated may not be great enough to be sensed by the pacemaker. This anomaly cannot be anticipated unless extrasystoles of the same morphology occur during implantation and can be measured. It is reasonable to attempt reprogramming the sensitivity to allow the extrasystoles to be sensed, but if this is unsuccessful, it is rarely, if ever, necessary to reposition the lead for this abnormality.

Functional undersensing is present when an intrinsic cardiac event is not sensed because it falls within a programmed refractory period. For example, if an intrinsic atrial event occurs within the PVARP, the event is not, and should not be, sensed. However, without a thorough understanding of the timing cycle, it may appear as though there is true undersensing.

Fusion and pseudofusion beats occur as a result of superimposition of an ineffective pacemaker stimulus on a spontaneously occurring P wave or QRS complex (Fig. 31-23). ("Fusion" is present when the morphology of the cardiac event is a hybrid of the intrinsic morphology and the paced morphology. "Pseudofusion" is present when the pacemaker artifact occurs late enough that the intrinsic morphology is not deformed, but it may appear so because of distortion on the ECG by the superimposed pacing artifact.) Pseudofusion is usually the consequence of pacemaker discharge during the refractory period of intrinsic P or QRS before sufficient intracardiac voltage is generated to activate the sensing circuit. This is most likely to occur when the pacing rate and the intrinsic rate are similar. Also, pseudofusion beats can be the result of a delayed activation due to intraventricular conduction abnormalities.

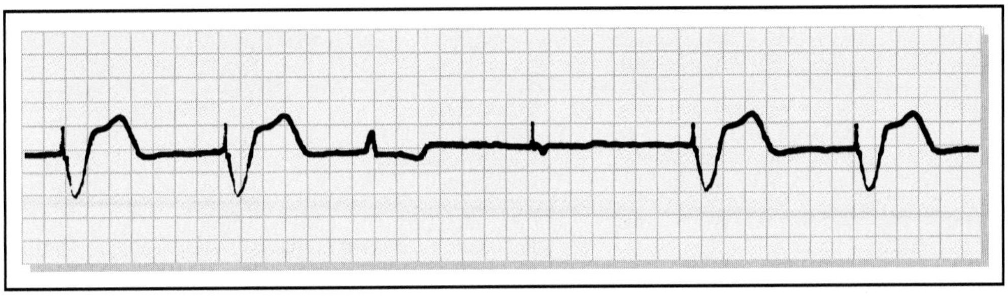

FIGURE 31–23 Electrocardiographic tracing from a patient with a VVI pacemaker. The first two complexes represent fully paced ventricular depolarizations. The third ventricular event is an intrinsic QRS complex, and the fourth event represents a fusion beat. This is followed by two paced ventricular complexes.

Implantable Cardioverter-Defibrillator Therapy

Indications for ICD Therapy

As previously noted, the ACC/AHA/NASPE guidelines for pacemakers and ICDs were updated in 2002.[2] These indications are summarized in Table 31–10, and significant changes from the previous guidelines are discussed in the following sections.

RANDOMIZED CLINICAL TRIALS OF ICD THERAPY

Clinical trials have been designed to determine the effect of ICD therapy (1) in secondary prevention of sudden cardiac death (Table 31-11), that is, in patients who have already experienced a life-threatening ventricular rhythm disturbance, and (2) in primary prevention, that is, in those who have not yet experienced a life-threatening ventricular tachyarrhythmia but are at high risk for sudden cardiac death (Table 31-12). The Antiarrhythmics Versus Implantable Defibrillators (AVID)[45] trial (secondary prevention), Multicenter Automatic Defibrillator Implantation Trial (MADIT)[46] (primary prevention), Cardiac Arrest Study Hamburg (CASH)[37] (secondary prevention), and Multicenter Unsustained Tachycardia Trial (MUSTT)[47] (primary prevention) all have demonstrated significant improvement in overall survival with ICD therapy compared with conventional or pharmacological treatment. No significant difference in overall survival was seen with ICD therapy in the Canadian Implantable Defibrillator Study (CIDS) trial (secondary prevention, probably underpowered) or the Coronary Artery Bypass Graft—Implantable Cardioverter-Defibrillator (CABG-PATCH)[48] study (primary prevention). CABG-PATCH should probably be considered separately because it randomized patients who were to undergo coronary artery bypass grafting to either ICD implantation at the time of bypass surgery or postoperative antiarrhythmic treatment. The study was terminated prematurely when the interim analysis failed to show a survival difference between the two study groups. The deaths in both groups were perioperative and, therefore, could not have been prevented by antiarrhythmic therapy. Analysis of subgroups showed the benefits of the ICD in patients at risk

TABLE 31–10 Implantable Cardioverter-Defibrillator Indications

Class I	Class II	Class III
Cardiac arrest due to VF or VT not due to a transient or reversible cause Spontaneous sustained VT associated with structural heart disease Syncope of undetermined origin with clinically relevant, hemodynamically significant sustained VT or VF induced at EP study when drug therapy is ineffective, not tolerated, or not preferred Nonsustained VT in patients with coronary disease, prior MI, LV dysfunction, and inducible VF or sustained VT at EP study not suppressible by an NYHA Class I antiarrhythmic drug Spontaneous sustained VT in patients without structural heart disease not amenable to other treatments	Patients with LVEF ≤ 30% at least 1 mo post MI and 3 mo post coronary artery revascularization surgery Cardiac arrest presumed due to VF when EP testing is precluded by other medical conditions Severe symptoms (e.g., syncope) attributable to sustained ventricular tachyarrhythmias while awaiting cardiac transplantation Familial or inherited conditions with a high risk for life-threatening ventricular tachyarrhythmias such as long-QT syndrome or hypertrophic cardiomyopathy Nonsustained VT with coronary artery disease, prior MI, and LV dysfunction, and inducible sustained VT or VF at EP study Recurrent syncope of undetermined cause in presence of ventricular dysfunction and inducible ventricular arrhythmias at EP study, when other causes of syncope have been excluded Syncope of unexplained origin or family history of unexplained sudden cardiac death associated with typical or atypical right bundle branch block and ST segment elevation (Brugada syndrome) Syncope in patients with advanced structural heart disease in whom thorough invasive and noninvasive investigations have failed to define a cause	Syncope of undetermined cause in a patient without inducible ventricular tachyarrhythmias and without structural heart disease Incessant VT or VF VF or VT resulting from arrhythmias amenable to surgical or catheter ablation, e.g., atrial arrhythmias associated with WPW, RVOT VT, idiopathic LV tachycardia, or fascicular VT Ventricular tachyarrhythmias due to transient or reversible disorder (e.g., AMI, electrolyte imbalance, drugs, or trauma) when correction of the disorder is considered feasible and likely to substantially reduce the risk of recurrent arrhythmia Significant psychiatric illnesses that may be aggravated by device implantation or may preclude systematic follow-up Terminal illnesses with projected life expectancy < 6 mo Patients with coronary artery disease with LV dysfunction and prolonged QRS duration in absence of spontaneous or inducible sustained or nonsustained VT who are undergoing coronary bypass surgery NYHA Class IV drug-refractory congestive heart failure in patients who are not candidates for cardiac transplantation

AMI = acute myocardial infarction; EP = electrophysiologic; LV = left ventricular; LVEF = left ventricular ejection fraction; MI = myocardial infarction; NYHA = New York Heart Association; RVOT = right ventricular outflow tract; VF = ventricular fibrillation; VT = ventricular tachycardia; WPW = Wolfe-Parkinson-White syndrome.

TABLE 31–11 Secondary Prevention of Sudden Cardiac Death

Study	Patient Inclusion Criteria	Endpoint(s)	Treatment Arms	Key Results
AVID	Survivor of cardiac arrest VT with syncope Symptomatic sustained VT with LVEF ≤ 0.40	Total mortality Mode of death Quality of life Cost benefit	Amiodarone or sotalol	Significant improvement in overall survival with ICD
CASH[37]	Survivor of cardiac arrest	Total mortality Recurrences of arrhythmias requiring CPR Recurrence of unstable VT	ICD Amiodarone, propafenone, or metoprolol	Significant improvement in overall survival with ICD
CIDS	Survivor of cardiac arrest Syncope with symptomatic sustained VT with LVEF ≤ 0.35 or syncope with inducible VT	Total mortality	Amiodarone	No significant improvement in survival with ICD
MAVERIC[38]	Resuscitated VT/VF, SCD Sustained nonsyncopal VT Dilated nonischemic cardiomyopathy with EF ≤ 0.35, syncope, and NSVT or positive SAECG	All-cause mortality Event-free survival Costs Quality of life Cost-effectiveness	Empirical amiodarone EP-guided therapy (drug or nondrug) Immediate ICD implantation	In progress
ASTRID	Patients with Ventak AV 1810 implanted for current indication DFT < 600 V and minimum 1 mV atrial, 5 mV ventricular EGM amplitudes at implantation	Time to first occurrence of inappropriate therapy Health care utilization Quality of life	Standard-features programming Enhanced-features programming	Completed; results not published

ASTRID = Atrial Sensing Trial to Prevent Inappropriate Detections; AVID = Antiarrhythmics Versus Implantable Defibrillators; CASH = Cardiac Arrest Study Hamburg; CIDS = Canadian Implantable Defibrillator Study; CPR = cardiopulmonary resuscitation; DFT = defibrillation threshold; EF = ejection fraction; EGM = electrogram; EP = electrophysiologic; ICD = implantable cardioverter-defibrillator; LVEF = left ventricular ejection fraction; MAVERIC = Midlands Trial of Empirical Amiodarone Versus Electrophysiologically Guided Intervention and Cardioverter Implant in Ventricular Arrhythmias; NSVT = nonsustained ventricular tachycardia; SAECG = signal-averaged electrocardiography; SCD = sudden cardiac death; VF = ventricular fibrillation; VT = ventricular tachycardia.

CH 31

for life-threatening ventricular tachyarrhythmia.[49] The role of ICD therapy for patients with asymptomatic sustained monomorphic ventricular tachycardia and structural heart disease but with an ejection fraction greater than 0.40 is less clear.[50]

Impact of Left Ventricular Function

Patients with coronary artery disease and reduced left ventricular function appear to experience greater benefit with ICD therapy than with drug therapy.[46] In the AVID trial, patients with an ejection fraction greater than 0.35 who received an ICD did not have a significant mortality benefit over those who received amiodarone therapy. Similarly, in post hoc analyses of MADIT-I, patients with a lower left ventricular ejection demonstrated the greatest mortality benefit.[46]

The MADIT-II trial evaluated ICD therapy as primary prevention in 1352 patients with a left ventricular ejection fraction no greater than 0.30 and a previous myocardial infarction.[9] Patients were randomized to ICD or conventional medical therapy. Patients who received an ICD had a 31 percent reduction in mortality (see Fig. 24–7). Based largely on this trial, the most recent ACC/AHA/NASPE guidelines include patients who meet MADIT-II criteria as a class IIa indication for ICD implantation. This significantly expands the patient population eligible for ICD therapy. MADIT-II criteria—previous myocardial infarction and left ventricular ejection fraction of 0.30 or less—have been approved as a reimbursable indication for ICD therapy but with the added criterion of QRS duration longer than 120 milliseconds.

Although MADIT-II addressed patients with reduced left ventricular function secondary to an ischemic event, it did not address patients with symptomatic congestive heart failure or those with an idiopathic dilated cardiomyopathy. In patients with idiopathic dilated cardiomyopathy (see Chap. 59), the combination of poor left ventricular function and nonsustained ventricular tachycardia is associated with an increased risk of sudden death (see Chap. 30).[45] A few trials evaluating ICD therapy as primary prevention in patients with dilated cardiomyopathy have been completed and several are under way (Table 31-13).

Trials evaluating combined CRT and ICD therapy have also been performed, with others in progress. The InSync ICD trial and CONTAK-CD studies included patients who met criteria for CRT and a clinical requirement for ICD therapy, that is, secondary prevention. Both trials demonstrated the safety and efficacy of a combined CRT and ICD device but were not designed as mortality trials.

The Comparison of Medical Therapy, Pacing, and Defibrillation (COMPANION) trial, presented but not published (ACC, 2003), was the first CRT and CRT with cardioverter-defibrillator capability (CRT/ICD) trial designed to assess all-cause mortality. In this trial, 1634 patients with left ventricular dysfunction of either idiopathic or ischemic etiology were randomized to optimized medical therapy, optimized medical therapy and CRT, or optimized medical therapy and CRT with ICD therapy. The study, terminated early by the data safety monitoring board, demonstrated a 43 percent decrease in mortality among patients who received CRT with ICD therapy when compared with the patients receiving only optimized medical therapy ($p = 0.02$). CRT therapy alone insignificantly reduced mortality by approximately 24 percent when compared with medical therapy ($p = 0.12$). Initial reports suggested that there was no difference in response or mortality outcomes between ischemic and nonischemic causes. Both CRT and CRT/ICD therapy decreased hospitalizations by approximately 19 percent over medical therapy alone.

The impact of CRT and CRT/ICD on mortality will be further defined by ongoing studies. The Cardiac Resynchronization in Heart Failure study has completed enrollment and will assess the effect of CRT on all-cause mortality and unplanned cardiovascular hospitalization as the primary endpoints.[51]

TABLE 31–12 Primary Prevention of Sudden Cardiac Death

Study	Patient Inclusion Criteria	Endpoint(s)	Treatment Arms	Key Results
MADIT	Q wave MI ≥ 3 wk Asymptomatic NSVT LVEF ≤ 0.35 Inducible and nonsuppressible VT on EPS with procainamide NYHA Classes I-III	Overall mortality Costs and cost-effectiveness	ICD ($n = 95$) Conventional therapy ($n = 101$)	ICDs reduced overall mortality by 54% ICDs cost $16,900 per life-year saved *vs.* Conventional therapy
CABG-PATCH	Scheduled for elective CABG surgery LVEF < 0.36 Abnormal SAECG	Overall mortality	ICD ($n = 446$) Standard treatment ($n = 454$)	Survival not improved by prophylactic implantation of ICD at time of elective CABG
MUSTT	CAD EF ≤ 0.40 NSVT Inducible VT or VF	Sudden arrhythmic death or spontaneous sustained VT	ICD in nonsuppressible group AAD therapy in suppressible group No therapy	Patients receiving ICD had > 70% risk reduction in arrhythmic death or cardiac arrest and > 50% reduction in total mortality
CAT[39]	Nonischemic DCM LVEF ≤ 0.30 NYHA Class II or III	Total mortality Sudden death Serious arrhythmia	ICD Standard treatment	Cumulative survival was not significantly different between the two groups at 2- and 4-yr follow-up
BEST-ICD[40]	Acute MI EF ≤ 0.40 SDRR < 70 msec or ≥ 109 PVCs/hr or abnormal SAECG	All-cause mortality Cost-effectiveness	Conventional + BB therapy EPS: if inducible, ICD and BB; if noninducible, BB	No significant survival improvement with ICD (concern that too few patients enrolled to draw firm conclusion)
DINAMIT	Acute MI (6-21 d) LVEF ≤ 0.35 HR ≥ 80 beats/min or SDRR < 70 msec	All-cause mortality Quality of life Cost-effectiveness	Conventional therapy ICD	Optimal medical therapy (OMT) *vs.* OMT + ICD Death from any cause NS, $p = 0.66$ Arrhythmic death lower with ICD, $p = 0.009$ Non-arrhythmic death. Risk lower in OMT group, $p = 0.016$
MADIT-II[41]	Prior MI EF ≤ 0.30	All-cause mortality Cost-effectiveness	Conventional therapy ICD	With ICD, 31% reduction in mortality
SCD-HeFT[42]	Ischemic or nonischemic cardiomyopathy EF ≤ 0.35 NYHA Class II or III Appropriate ACE inhibitor No history of sustained VT/VF	All-cause mortality Quality of life Cost-effectiveness Morbidity Incidence of arrhythmias	Placebo and standard therapy *vs.* Amiodarone and standard therapy *vs.* ICD and standard therapy	In progress; enrollment completed Mortality by intention to treat: Amiodarone *vs.* Placebo, NS, $p = 0.529$ ICD *vs.* Placebo, ICD lowers mortality by 23%, $p = 0.007$
DEBUT (SUDS)[43]	Survivor of sudden cardiac arrest from resuscitated VT/VF Probable sudden cardiac arrest with RBBB and ST elevation	All-cause mortality Rhythms via stored EGMs that triggered ICD shocks	ICD *vs.* BB	Study terminated early after no deaths in ICD group vs. four deaths in BB group
PRIDE	VT, VF, or nonischemic cardiomyopathy with EF < 0.35 and NSVT or positive SAECG	All-cause mortality Hospitalization due to CHF	ICD *vs.* EPS and randomization to ICD *vs.* Amiodarone or sotalol Negative EPS: therapy at physician discretion	In progress; follow-up to be completed in 2004

Continued

TABLE 31–12 Primary Prevention of Sudden Cardiac Death—cont'd

Study	Patient Inclusion Criteria	Endpoint(s)	Treatment Arms	Key Results
AMIOVIRT[44]	Patients with nonischemic dilated cardiomyopathy and nonsustained VT and EF ≤ 0.35	Primary Total mortality Secondary Arrhythmia-free survival Quality of life Costs	Amiodarone *vs.* ICD	Mortality and quality of life not significantly different between the two arms
SEDET	Acute MI (1-3 wk) Ineligible for thrombolysis EF ≥ 0.15 to ≤ 0.40 NSVT or ≥ 10 PVCs/hr between 6 and 21 d after MI	All-cause mortality Quality of life Incidence of VT Sudden and nonsudden death Cardiac death Predictive value of BRS and HRV	ICD *vs.* Conventional therapy	In progress
IRIS	Acute MI Fast NSVT > 150 beats/min HR > 100 beats/min at admission	All-cause mortality	ICD *vs.* Conventional therapy	In progress

AAD = antiarrhythmia drug; ACE = angiotensin-converting enzyme; AMIOVIRT = Amiodarone Versus Implantable Cardioverter-Defibrillator Trial; BB = beta blocker; BEST-ICD = Beta-Blocker Strategy Plus Implantable Cardioverter-Defibrillator; BRS = baroreceptor sensitivity; CABG = coronary artery bypass graft; CABG-PATCH = Coronary Artery Bypass Graft Patch Trial; CAD = coronary artery disease; CAT = Cardiomyopathy Trial; CHF = congestive heart failure; DCM = dilated cardiomyopathy; DEBUT (SUDS) = Defibrillator Versus Beta Blockers for Unexplained Death in Thailand (Sudden Unexplained Death Syndrome); DINAMIT = Defibrillator in Acute Myocardial Infarction Trial; EF = ejection fraction; EGM = electrogram; EPS = electrophysiologic study; HR = heart rate; HRV = heart rate variability; ICD = implantable cardioverter-defibrillator; IRIS = Immediate Risk Stratification Improves Survival; LVEF = left ventricular ejection fraction; MADIT = Multicenter Automatic Defibrillator Implantation Trial; MI = myocardial infarction; MUSTT = Multicenter Unsustained Tachycardia Trial; NSVT = nonsustained ventricular tachycardia; NYHA = New York Heart Association; PRIDE = Primary Implantation of Cardioverter-Defibrillator in High-Risk Ventricular Arrhythmias; PVC = premature ventricular contraction; RBBB = right bundle branch block; SAECG = signal-averaged electrocardiography; SCD-HeFT = Sudden Cardiac Death in Heart Failure Trial; SDRR = standard deviation of RR interval; SEDET = South European Defibrillator Trial; VF = ventricular fibrillation; VT = ventricular tachycardia.

There are a number of inherited arrhythmia conditions such as long-QT syndrome,[52] Brugada syndrome, right ventricular arrhythmogenic dysplasia (see Chap. 32), hypertrophic cardiomyopathy (see Chap. 59),[53] and others for which an ICD is often recommended.

The patient with idiopathic ventricular fibrillation should receive an ICD. Some patients with idiopathic ventricular tachycardia and no structural heart disease should probably be considered for catheter ablation before consideration of ICD therapy (see Chap. 32).

ICD Design

The basic components of the ICD are electronic circuitry, power source, and memory, with a microprocessor coordinating the various parts of the system.[54] High-voltage capacitors transform the battery-provided voltage into discharges ranging from less than 1 V for pacing to 750 V for defibrillation. ICDs incorporate a different sensing circuit than most pacemakers. Because of the need to reliably sense low-amplitude signals during ventricular fibrillation and to avoid sensing extracardiac noise and cardiac signals other than ventricular tachycardia or fibrillation, the sensing circuit is designed to automatically adjust either the gain or the sensing threshold.[54]

Virtually all ICD systems are implanted transvenously and include antitachycardia pacing (ATP) and ventricular bradycardia pacing, dual-chamber pacing with rate-adaptive options.[55] In addition, atrial defibrillation capabilities, as well as CRT features, are available in some devices. The longevity of ICDs depends on the frequency of shock delivery, the degree of pacemaker dependency, and other programmable options, but most are expected to last from 5 to 9 years. All currently available ICDs use biphasic shock waveforms, but the specifics of the waveform differ among various manufacturers.

The ICD functions by continuously monitoring the patient's cardiac rate and delivering therapy when the rate exceeds the programmed rate "cutoff." For example, if the ICD is programmed to treat ventricular tachyarrhythmias at a rate cutoff of 175 beats/min, once the ICD detects a rate greater than 175 beats/min it delivers ATP or charges and delivers a shock, depending on the programmed therapy.

ATP has the advantage of terminating a rhythm disturbance without delivery of a shock. ICDs capable of ATP have significant programming flexibility to adjust many aspects of tachycardia detection and therapy, thereby customizing therapy for the individual patient. Different "zones" or "tiers" of therapy can be programmed to detect ventricular tachyarrhythmias to allow slower arrhythmias to be treated with ATP before a shock is delivered but to still allow faster tachycardias to be treated more aggressively. The programming for a hypothetical patient is outlined in Table 31–14. In this patient, slower ventricular tachycardia in the range of 126 to 190 beats/min is treated with ATP therapies in zone 1. If initial ATP therapy (ATP-1) is unsuccessful, a second and different ATP therapy (ATP-2) is automatically delivered. If this is unsuccessful, lower energy shocks are attempted before high-energy shocks are delivered. Shocks are synchronized during ventricular tachycardia (cardioversion) or are asynchronous during ventricular fibrillation (defibrillation). A second zone of therapy is determined for a faster ventricular tachycardia, and still faster ventricular tachycardia or ventricular fibrillation is treated aggressively with a high-energy shock. In addition, current ICDs provide bradycardia support, as single- or dual-chamber devices.

The zones, detection rates of the different zones, specifics of the different therapies, and bradycardia pacing options all are programmable, and programming flexibility varies significantly from device to device.

TABLE 31–13 ICD Trials in Patients with Congestive Heart Failure and ICD/CRT Trials

Study	Patient Inclusion Criteria	Endpoint(s)	Treatment Arms	Key Results
VENTAK-CHF/ CONTAK CD	Indication for ICD Symptomatic CHF on stable drugs, including ACE inhibitors EF ≤ 0.35 QRS > 120 msec	Primary composite endpoint of mortality, HF, hospitalizations, and episodes of ventricular tachycardia or ventricular fibrillation	BiV pacing or no pacing and then crossover (ICD therapy was in both arms)	Composite endpoint insignificant trend favoring CRT Peak VO_2, 6-min hall walk, quality of life, NYHA Class all improved significantly with CRT
DEFINITE	Symptomatic nonischemic cardiomyopathy NSVT Low EF	All-cause mortality	ICD, standard drug therapy, and BB *vs.* Standard drug therapy and BB only	2-year mortality: no ICD, 13.8%; ICD, 8.1%; relative risk reduction (RR), 34%; arrhythmia deaths decrease (RR = 74%); $p = 0.01$).
Defibrillat	Patient with CHF awaiting heart transplant	Total mortality Serious arrhythmias	ICD Standard treatment	In progress
COMPANION	NYHA Classes II-IV EF ≤ 0.35 QRS ≥ 120 msec PR interval > 150 msec No conventional device indications	All-cause mortality and hospitalization Cardiac morbidity Long-term survival Functional capacity in HF patients (substudy)	Optimized medical therapy *vs.* CRT *vs.* CRT/ICD	43% mortality reduction with CRT/ICD 24% mortality reduction with CRT 19% reduction in hospitalization with CRT/ICD and CRT
BELIEVE	NYHA Classes II-IV QRS > 130 msec EF ≤ 0.35 LBBB LVEDD ≥ 55 mm ICD indications	LV-only pacing safe and effective BiV ATP safe and effective	LV CRT + RV ATP vs. BiV CRT + BiV ATP	In progress
MIRACLE-ICD	NYHA Classes II-IV QRS > 130 msec EF < 0.35 LVEDD > 55 mm Indication for ICD	Device safety and efficacy Quality of life 6-min walk		

ACE = angiotensin-converting enzyme; ATP = antitachycardia pacing; BB = beta blocker; BELIEVE = Biventricular Versus Left Ventricular Pacing in Italian Evaluation on Heart Failure Patients with Ventricular Arrhythmias; BiV = biventricular; CHF = congestive heart failure; COMPANION = Comparison of Medical Therapy, Pacing, and Defibrillation in Heart Failure; CRT = cardiac resynchronization therapy; CRT/ICD = CRT with cardioverter-defibrillator capability; Defibrillat = Defibrillator Implantation as a Bridge to Transplantation; DEFINITE = Defibrillators in Nonischemic Cardiomyopathy Treatment Evaluation; EF = ejection fraction; HF, heart failure; ICD = implantable cardioverter-defibrillator; LBBB = left bundle branch block; LV = left ventricular; LVEDD = left ventricular end-diastolic dimension; MIRACLE-ICD = Multicenter InSync Randomized Clinical Evaluation—Implantable Cardioverter-Defibrillator; NSVT = nonsustained ventricular tachycardia; NYHA = New York Heart Association; RV = right ventricular; VENTAK-CHF/CONTAK CD = Ventak-Congestive Heart Failure/Contak Cardioverter-Defibrillator.

TABLE 31–14 Implantable Cardioverter-Defibrillator Therapy

Zone	Tachycardia Rate (beats/min)	Sequence of Therapy Delivered
1	126-160	ATP-1, ATP-2, 1 J, 5 J, 34 J
2	161-200	ATP, 10 J, 34 J
3	>200	34 J

ATP = antitachycardia pacing therapy; ATP-1 = first ATP; ATP-2 = second (and different) ATP.

Device Selection

Considerations about the type of ICD to select for a given patient include whether the patient has bradycardia requiring pacing support, has associated atrial tachyarrhythmias, or would benefit from CRT (or a combination of these). The need for bradycardia support requires a choice between single- and dual-chamber ICD based on the mode selection algorithm already described.

The recent trend in the United States has been to implant more dual-chamber ICDs. However, data from the recent Dual-chamber and VVIT Implantable Defibrillator (DAVID) trial suggest that single-chamber ICD therapy may be advantageous if the patient does not have associated bradyarrhythmias.[56] In 506 patients with a left ventricular ejection fraction of 0.40 or less and no indication for cardiac pacing, dual-chamber pacing offered no clinical advantage over ventricular back-up pacing. Patients whose device was programmed to the DDD pacing at 70 beats/min experienced 1-year survival free of the composite endpoint (time to death or first hospitalization for congestive heart failure) of 73.3 percent compared with 83.9 percent for the VVI (40 beats/min) back-up pacing group (relative hazard, 1.61; 95 percent confidence interval [CI], 1.06 to 2.44). Mortality was also slightly higher (10.1 percent) for the dual-chamber patients than for the patients programmed to VVI at 40 beats/min (6.5 percent; relative hazard, 1.61; 95 percent CI, 0.84 to 3.09). The investigators suggested that the adverse effects of right ventricular apical pacing may account for the differences seen in the study.

If the patient has associated atrial tachyarrhythmias, a dual-chamber ICD capable of detecting and treating atrial tachyarrhythmias should be considered. Some devices also provide the ability to cardiovert atrial tachyarrhythmias.

As previously noted, devices that combine CRT and ICD therapy can be considered for patients who meet CRT criteria.

Issues Unique to ICD Implantation

When the ICD is placed transvenously with the pulse generator in the prepectoral position, the implantation technique and related complications are the same as those for pacemaker implantation, with the exception that complications can arise as a result of determining the defibrillation threshold (DFT). (*DFT* can be defined as the minimal energy that terminates ventricular fibrillation.[54]) Most ICD implantations are performed with conscious sedation and local anesthesia, with mask-supported ventilation. When DFT determination is completed, the patient can be allowed to recover from deeper anesthesia as the pocket is closed.

An acceptable DFT is a value that ensures an adequate safety margin for defibrillation, usually being at least 10 J less than the maximum output of the ICD, which ranges from 30 to 41 J of stored energy. It is difficult to state an "ideal" DFT because ideally it is the lowest achievable DFT with an adequate safety margin.

Generally, the preference is to implant the ICD in the left pectoral region because of a more favorable vector for delivery of the shock. Although successful defibrillation can usually be accomplished with a right-sided implant, the shocking vector is less optimal and may have an effect on achievable DFT.[57] Regardless of whether the ICD is placed on the right or the left side, in a small percentage of patients adequate DFT cannot be achieved with standard lead placement. In this situation, options include repositioning the ventricular lead to an alternative site or adding another lead in a subcutaneous position or within the superior vena cava.

Complications

Frequent ICD discharges may represent a clinical emergency. These discharges may be appropriate or inappropriate (Table 31–15). Appropriate discharges represent frequently occurring ventricular tachycardia or fibrillation or an electrical storm (see Chap. 32). If the device is discharging frequently because the defibrillation is unsuccessful, the device may have been programmed to an inappropriately low shock output or the DFT may have increased, for example, in response to a drug such as amiodarone (see Chap. 30).

Inappropriate discharges are usually the result of detection of a supraventricular tachyarrhythmia, most commonly atrial fibrillation. Inappropriate discharge can also be the result of device failure, for example, lead fracture with generation of make-or-break signals.

TABLE 31–15 Differential Diagnosis and Management of Multiple Implantable Cardioverter-Defibrillator (ICD) Shocks

Clinical Finding	Management
Frequent ventricular tachycardia or ventricular fibrillation (electrical storm)	Reassess antiarrhythmic therapy and programmed ICD therapy
Unsuccessful ICD therapy due to inappropriately low-output shock or elevation of defibrillation threshold	Reprogram ICD Assess potential causes of defibrillation threshold increase (e.g., drugs)
Lead fracture Lead dislodgment	Replace fractured lead Reposition lead
Sensing supraventricular rhythms	Reassess antiarrhythmic therapy Reprogram ICD parameters Ablate supraventricular arrhythmic focus
Oversensing separate pacing system	Reprogram pacemaker or ICD (or both) Reposition pacemaker or ICD leads (or both) Remove pacemaker and replace ICD with another ICD with more sophisticated bradycardia support
Oversensing electromagnetic interference	Avoid source Reprogram ICD
Oversensing intracardiac signals	Reprogram ICD Reposition sensing lead

Modified from Pinsky SL, Fahy GJ: Implantable cardioverter-defibrillators. Am J Med 106:446-458, 1999. Reprinted by permission of Excerpta Medica.

Electromagnetic Interference

EMI is defined as any signal—biological or nonbiological—that is within a frequency spectrum detectable by the sensing circuitry of the pacemaker or ICD. EMI can result in rate alteration, sensing abnormalities, asynchronous pacing, noise reversion, or reprogramming.[58] EMI can also cause failure to deliver antibradycardia pacing, inappropriate delivery of antitachycardia therapy, resetting of programmed parameters, and damage to the pulse generator or myocardial interface.

Other cardiac and extracardiac signals that can be falsely interpreted as a P wave or QRS complex and result in oversensing include T waves (Fig. 31–24), myopotential interference, afterpotential delay, and P waves.

Sources of EMI can be within and outside the hospital. Although multiple sources of EMI in the nonhospital environment can potentially result in single-beat inhibition, few, if any, of these are clinically significant and truly represent a threat to the paced patient.

Several potential sources of EMI require specific mention either because of their real potential for causing significant EMI or because of existing confusion or controversy. Industrial-strength welding equipment, certain degaussing equipment, and induction ovens are identified sources of EMI that can cause significant pacemaker or ICD interference. Most welding equipment used for "hobby" welding should not cause any significant problems. For the pacemaker-dependent patient who does hobby welding or any other activity that raises the clinician's concerns about EMI, the environment should be determined safe for the patient before the activity is condoned.

Currently, there is much interest in the potential EMI that may emanate from cellular telephones[59,60] and antitheft devices.[61] Available information suggests that commercially available cellular phones are safe for the device patient as long as some simple guidelines are followed. The patient should avoid having the "activated" cellular phone directly over the pacemaker or ICD, either from random motion of the phone or by carrying the activated phone in a breast pocket over the device.

Antitheft devices also have potential for pacemaker interference.[61] Practical suggestions are for patients with pacemakers or ICDs to be aware of electronic equipment for surveillance of articles and to avoid leaning on or lingering near such devices. If the patient passes through the equipment at a normal pace, adverse effects are quite unlikely. Any patient who feels unusual in any way when near electronic surveillance equipment should move away.

Hospital sources of potentially significant EMI are electrocautery, cardioversion, defibrillation, magnetic resonance imaging (MRI), lithotripsy,[62] radiofrequency ablation, electroshock therapy, and diathermy. The most important aspect of pacemaker or ICD care after exposure to any of these sources of EMI is to reassess the device to be certain that programmed parameters have not been changed.

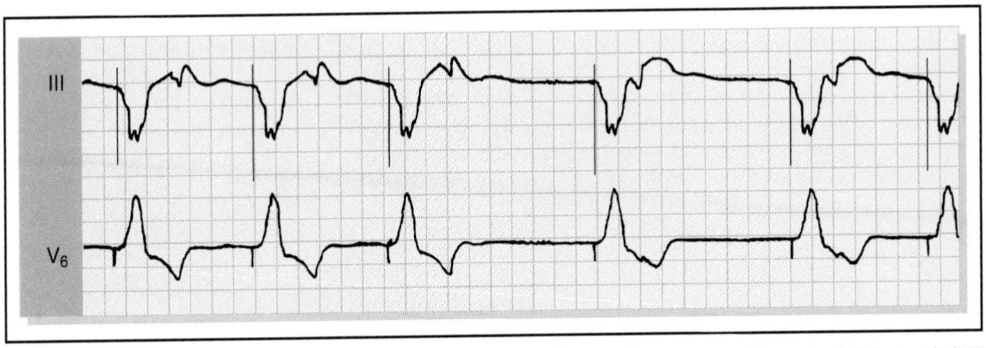

FIGURE 31–24 Electrocardiographic tracing from a patient with a VVI pacemaker programmed to a rate of 70 beats/min (857 milliseconds). The third and fourth VV cycles are longer than the programmed lower rate. Measuring 857 milliseconds backward from the ventricular pacing artifact at the end of the longer cycles locates the point at which there was oversensing. In this case, probably the T wave is sensed. Definite retrograde P waves can be recognized by deformation of the T wave. Although it is possible that the retrograde P wave is being oversensed, the relationship of the P waves does not appear to consistently coincide with the point of oversensing.

One of the most frequent questions asked is how to manage the patient with a pacemaker or ICD during an operative procedure, given the potential effects of electrocautery and guidelines for cardioversion and defibrillation. Routine interrogation of the device and deactivation of ICD therapy should be accomplished before the operation. After the procedure, the device should be reinterrogated and ICD therapy reinitiated. (During the time ICD therapy is "off," the patient must be monitored.) For pacemaker-dependent patients, it is reasonable to program the pacemaker to an asynchronous pacing mode, VOO or DOO, or to achieve the same effect by placing a magnet over the pacemaker throughout the procedure. The potential effects of electrocautery are reprogramming; permanent damage to the pulse generator; pacemaker inhibition; reversion to a fall-back mode, noise reversion mode,[63] or electrical reset; and myocardial thermal damage. The guidelines for cardioversion and defibrillation in the patient with a pacemaker or ICD are as follows: ideally, place paddles in the anteroposterior position, try to keep the paddles at least 4 inches from the pulse generator, have the appropriate pacemaker programmer available, and interrogate the pacemaker after the procedure.

Given the increasing utilization of MRI, potential interference with implantable devices merits mention. MRI is still considered a relative contraindication in patients with a pacemaker or ICD given the potential for induction of rapid hemodynamically unstable ventricular rhythms and the theoretical possibility of heating of the conductor coil and thermal damage at the electrode-myocardial interface. Although there are reports of MRI being performed safely in non–pacemaker-dependent patients, there are also reports of deaths resulting from MRI-induced rhythm disturbances.

Interference from Drugs and Metabolic Abnormalities

Drugs can affect sensing thresholds, pacing thresholds, and DFTs and result in ECG abnormalities.[58,64] Although many drugs have been reported to affect pacing thresholds, class 1C agents are the only drugs that commonly cause a problem. Flecainide and propafenone have the potential to increase pacing thresholds and sensing thresholds. If these drugs are administered to the patient with a pacemaker, especially a pacemaker-dependent patient, thresholds should be monitored for change. Amiodarone does not consistently affect pacing thresholds. Changes in drug therapy must also be monitored closely in the patient with an ICD.[64] In addition to altering pacing thresholds and increasing DFTs, certain drugs have the potential for interaction by altering the detection of ventricular tachycardia and producing proarrhythmic effects. Drug-induced slowing of the rate of ventricular tachycardia can result in inadequate detection of the arrhythmia. The DFT can increase from the administration of amiodarone.[65] Other drugs can theoretically increase the DFT or have been reported to do so in single case reports, but a clinically significant change does not often result.[64]

Electrolyte and metabolic abnormalities can also affect pacing and sensing thresholds. Hyperkalemia is the most common electrolyte abnormality to cause clinically significant problems, but severe acidosis or alkalosis, hypercapnia, severe hyperglycemia, hypoxemia, and hypothyroidism can also alter thresholds.

Device Follow-Up

Patients with pacemakers and ICDs must be followed on a regular schedule. There are different follow-up methods depending on clinician preference. For pacemaker follow-up, some caregivers prefer regular office assessment, others prefer transtelephonic follow-up, and still others prefer a combination of the two techniques. Transtelephonic assessment should include collection of a nonmagnet ECG strip, an ECG strip with magnet applied to the pacemaker, and measurement of magnet rate and pulse duration (pulse duration on both atrial and ventricular channels should be measured for a dual-chamber pacemaker). During an office visit, the same information should be collected. In addition, on some periodic basis, for example, once a year, patients whose device is programmed to a rate-adaptive pacing mode should be assessed to determine whether rate-response is appropriate.

Internet-based device follow-up has been introduced recently and marks the first major change in device follow-up in many years.[66,67]

Follow-up of the patient with an ICD must include periodic visits during which specific information is collected and assessed. In addition, patients may require interim assessment if there are concerns about the appropriateness of delivered therapy or other changes in the patient's medical status or drug regimen that could affect ICD therapy.

The electrophysiologist or an allied professional with ICD expertise and immediate access to the electrophysiologist should perform follow-up procedures. Aspects of follow-up include history with specific emphasis on awareness of delivered therapy and any tachyarrhythmic events, device interrogation, assessment of battery status and charge time, retrieval and assessment of stored diagnostic data, periodic radiographic assessment, and periodic arrhythmic induction in the electrophysiology laboratory to assess DFTs and efficacy.

Diagnostic information that can be retrieved varies with different ICDs. ICDs provide information about the cycle length or rate of the detected tachyarrhythmias (Fig. 31–25), and stored electrograms of detected arrhythmias (Fig. 31–26).

Follow-up protocols for patients with ICDs vary. Many caregivers are comfortable with follow-up every 3 to 6 months for the first 3 to 4 years, after which follow-up frequency increases. Currently, Internet-based retrieval is available but not widely used.

Frequency of DFT testing may depend on the type of ICD system and DFT at implant or change in medications.

COUNTER DATA REPORT -- Page 1 of 2

Date Interrogated: Jun 18, 1999 12:29:28
Counters Last Cleared: Jan 08, 1999 15:49:29

TACHYCARDIA COUNTERS:		BRADYCARDIA PACING COUNTERS:	
VF:	3	Total Brady Pulses:	8653351
FVT:	0	Runs of > 3 Consecutive Pulses:	65535
VT:	0		
ONSET CRITERION MET:	0	PREMATURE EVENT COUNTERS:	
		Isolated Premature Events:	0
		Runs of 2–4 Premature Beats:	0

VF THERAPY	Rx1	Rx2	Rx3	Rx4
INITIATED:	3	0	0	0
SUCCESSFUL:	3	0	0	0
ABORTED:	0	0	0	0
INEFFECTIVE:	0	0	0	0
CONVERTED TO VT:	0	0	0	0
CONVERTED TO FVT:	0	0	0	0
UNDETERMINED:	0	0	0	0

SN PCB200253R Rev 9891A221 Jun 18, 1999 12:29

A

EPISODE DATA REPORT -- Episode 1 of 3

19:53:54 VF detected VF Rx 1 Successful

INTERVAL (ms): VF = 260 VT = 350
STABILITY: OFF
ONSET: OFF

THERAPY SEQUENCE:
VF 1

PRE-DETECTION INTERVALS (ms):

−29.	740 VS	−14.	870 VS
−28.	130 FS	−13.	200 FS
−27.	270 TS	−12.	1200 VP
−26.	120 FS	−11.	330 TS
−25.	240 FS	−10.	150 FS
−24.	1180 VS	−9.	130 FS
−23.	130 FS	−8.	190 FS
−22.	240 FS	−7.	130 FS
−21.	1160 VS	−6.	120 FS
−20.	130 FS	−5.	130 FS
−19.	190 FS	−4.	740 VS
−18.	1010 VS	−3.	160 FS
−17.	210 FS	−2.	120 FS
−16.	190 FS	−1.	140 FS
−15.	120 FS	0.	120 FD

INTERVALS (ms): AFTER LAST Rx START:

1.	440 VS	11.	720 VS
2.	1210 CD	12.	770 VS
3.	530 VS	13.	860 VS
4.	680 VS	14.	1060 VS
5.	710 VS	15.	1080 VS
6.	640 VS	16.	1200 VP
7.	670 VS	17.	1000 VS
8.	670 VS	18.	1040 VS
9.	650 VS	19.	970 VS
10.	710 VS	20.	970 VS

SN PCB200253R Rev 9891A221 Jun 18, 1999 12:29

B

FIGURE 31–25 **A** and **B,** Printouts from an implantable cardioverter-defibrillator (ICD) programmer of a specific episode detected by the ICD. The text includes 29 VV interval lengths before therapy for ventricular fibrillation and 20 VV cycle lengths after therapy, documenting return to a nonpathological ventricular rhythm. FD = fibrillation detected; FS = fibrillation sensed; TS = tachycardia sensed; VS = ventricular sensed event.

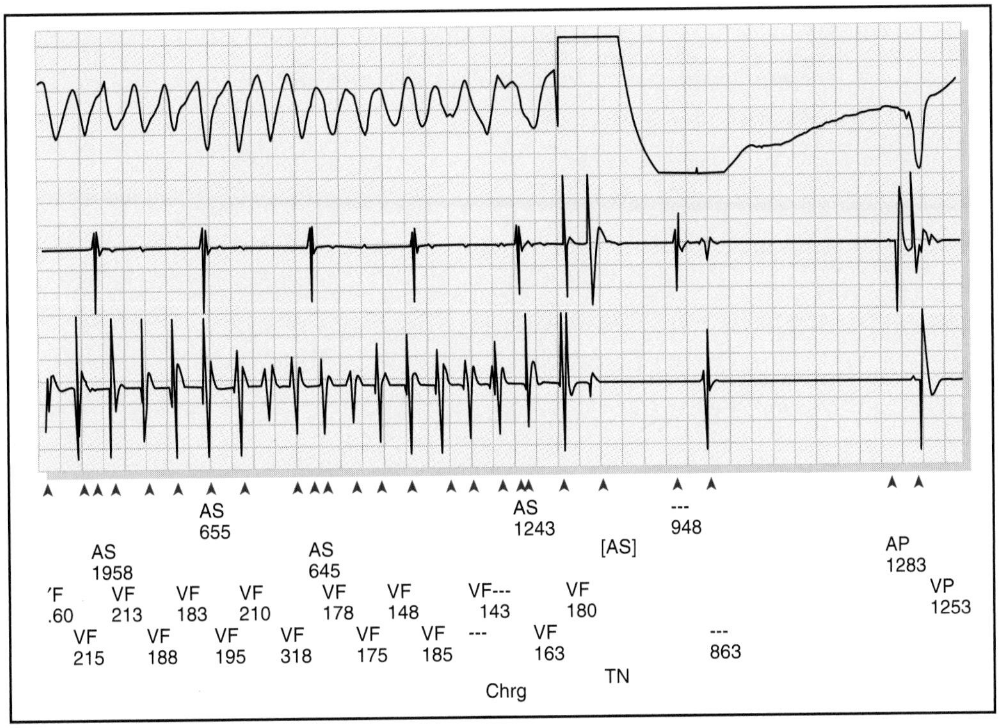

FIGURE 31–26 Stored electrogram from a patient with an episode of ventricular fibrillation and a dual-chamber pacemaker and implantable cardioverter-defibrillator. The **middle** tracing is the atrial electrogram, the **bottom** tracing is the ventricular electrogram, and the **upper** tracing is the surface electrocardiogram. AP = atrial paced event; AS = atrial sensed event; TN = telemetry noise; VF = ventricular fibrillation; VP = ventricular paced event. Chrg = charging. Numbers indicate milliseconds between events.

REFERENCES

Pacing Nomenclature

1. Bernstein AD, Daubert JC, Fletcher RD, et al, North American Society of Pacing and Electrophysiology/British Pacing and Electrophysiology Group: The revised NASPE/BPEG generic code for antibradycardia, adaptive-rate, and multisite pacing. Pacing Clin Electrophysiol 25:260, 2002.

Indications for Cardiac Pacing

2. Gregoratos G, Abrams J, Epstein AE, et al: ACC/AHA/NASPE 2002 guideline update for implantation of cardiac pacemakers and antiarrhythmia devices. Summary article: A report of the American College of Cardiology/American Heart Association Task Force on Practice Guidelines (ACC/AHA/NASPE Committee to Update the 1998 Pacemaker Guidelines). Circulation 106:2145, 2002.
3. Michaelsson M, Jonzon A, Riesenfeld T: Isolated congenital complete atrioventricular block in adult life: A prospective study. Circulation 92:442, 1995.
4. Sheldon R: Pacing to prevent vasovagal syncope. Cardiol Clin 18:81, 2000.
5. Connolly SJ, Sheldon R, Roberts RS, et al: The North American Vasovagal Pacemaker Study (VPS): A randomized trial of permanent cardiac pacing for the prevention of vasovagal syncope. J Am Coll Cardiol 33:16, 1999.
6. Vasovagal Syncope International Study: Is dual-chamber pacing efficacious in treatment of neurally mediated tilt-positive cardioinhibitory syncope? Pacemaker versus no therapy: A multicenter randomised study. Eur J Card Pacing Electrophysiol 3:169, 1993.
7. Connolly SJ, Sheldon R, Thorpe KE, et al, for the VPS-II Investigators: Pacemaker therapy for prevention of syncope in patients with recurrent severe vasovagal syncope. Second Vasovagal Pacemaker Study (VPS-II): A randomized trial. JAMA 289:2224, 2003.
8. Kenny RA, Seifer C: Brief report—SAFE PACE-2 Syncope and Falls in the Elderly Pacing and Carotid Sinus Evaluation: A randomized control trial of cardiac pacing in older patients with falls and carotid sinus hypersensitivity. Am J Geriatr Cardiol 8:87, 1999.
9. Ammirati F, Colivicchi F, Santini M, for the Syncope Diagnosis and Treatment Study Investigators: Permanent cardiac pacing versus medical treatment for the prevention of recurrent vasovagal syncope: A multicenter, randomized, controlled trial. Circulation 104:52, 2001.
10. Raviele A, Giada F, Sutton R, et al: The Vasovagal Syncope and Pacing (SYNPACE) trial: Rationale and study design. Europace 3:336, 2001.
11. Kenny RA, Richardson DA, Steen N, et al: Carotid sinus syndrome: A modifiable risk factor for nonaccidental falls in older adults (SAFE PACE). J Am Coll Cardiol 38:1491, 2001.

Selection of the Appropriate Pacing Mode

12. Andersen HR, Nielsen JC, Thomsen PE, et al: Long-term follow-up of patients from a randomised trial of atrial versus ventricular pacing for sick-sinus syndrome. Lancet 350:1210, 1997.
13. Lamas GA, Orav EJ, Stambler BS, et al, Pacemaker Selection in the Elderly Investigators: Quality of life and clinical outcomes in elderly patients treated with ventricular pacing as compared with dual-chamber pacing. N Engl J Med 338:1097, 1998.
14. Connolly SJ, Kerr CR, Gent M, et al, Canadian Trial of Physiologic Pacing Investigators: Effects of physiologic pacing versus ventricular pacing on the risk of stroke and death due to cardiovascular causes. N Engl J Med 342:1385, 2000.
15. Lamas GA, Lee KL, Sweeney MO, et al: Ventricular pacing or dual-chamber pacing for sinus node dysfunction. N Engl J Med 346:1854, 2002.
16. Toff WD, Skehan JD, De Bono DP, et al: The United Kingdom Pacing and Cardiovascular Events (UKPACE) trial: United Kingdom Pacing and Cardiovascular Events. Heart 78:221, 1997.
17. Andersen HR, Svendsen JH, on behalf of the DANPACE Investigators: The Danish multicenter randomized study on atrial-inhibited versus dual-chamber pacing in sick sinus syndrome (the DANPACE study): Purpose and design of the study. Heart Drug 1:67, 2001.

Indications for Rate-Adaptive Pacing

18. Leung SK, Lau CP: Developments in sensor-driven pacing. Cardiol Clin 18:113, 2000.
19. Alt E, Combs W, Willhaus R, et al: A comparative study of activity and dual sensor: Activity and minute ventilation pacing responses to ascending and descending stairs. Pacing Clin Electrophysiol 21:1862, 1998.

Pacing for Hemodynamic Improvement

20. Sorajja P, Elliott PM, McKenna WJ: Pacing in hypertrophic cardiomyopathy. Cardiol Clin 18:67, 2000.
21. Erwin JP III, Nishimura RA, Lloyd MA, et al: Dual-chamber pacing for patients with hypertrophic obstructive cardiomyopathy: A clinical perspective in 2000. Mayo Clin Proc 75:173, 2000.
22. Nishimura RA, Hayes DL, Ilstrup DM, et al: Effect of dual-chamber pacing on systolic and diastolic function in patients with hypertrophic cardiomyopathy: Acute Doppler echocardiographic and catheterization hemodynamic study. J Am Coll Cardiol 27:421, 1996.
23. Kappenberger L, Linde C, Daubert C, et al, PIC Study Group: Pacing in hypertrophic obstructive cardiomyopathy: A randomized crossover study. Eur Heart J 18:1249, 1997.
24. Maron BJ, Nishimura RA, McKenna WJ, et al: Assessment of permanent dual-chamber pacing as a treatment for drug-refractory symptomatic patients with obstructive hypertrophic cardiomyopathy: A randomized, double-blind, crossover study (M-PATHY). Circulation 99:2927, 1999.
25. Gillis AM: Pacing to prevent atrial fibrillation. Cardiol Clin 18:25, 2000.
26. Charles RG, McComb JM: Systematic Trial of Pacing to Prevent Atrial Fibrillation (STOP-AF). Heart 78:224, 1997
27. Gillis AM, Connolly SJ, Dubuc M, et al, for the PA3 Investigators: Circadian variation of paroxysmal atrial fibrillation. Am J Cardiol 87:794, 2001.
28. Djiane P: The best of cardiac pacing in 2002 [French]. Arch Mal Coeur Vaiss 96(Spec No. 1):35, 2003.

29. Anselme F, Saoudi N, Cribier A: Pacing in Prevention of Atrial Fibrillation—the PIPAF studies. J Interv Card Electrophysiol 4(Suppl 1):177, 2000.
30. Saksena S, Prakash A, Ziegler P, et al: Improved suppression of recurrent atrial fibrillation with dual-site right atrial pacing and antiarrhythmic drug therapy. J Am Coll Cardiol 40:1140, 2002.
31. Padeletti L, Pieragnoli P, Ciapetti C, et al: Randomized crossover comparison of right atrial appendage pacing versus interatrial septum pacing for prevention of paroxysmal atrial fibrillation in patients with sinus bradycardia. Am Heart J 142:1047, 2001.
32. Bailin SJ, Adler S, Giudici M: Prevention of chronic atrial fibrillation by pacing in the region of Bachmann's bundle: Results of a multicenter randomized trial. J Cardiovasc Electrophysiol 12:912, 2001.
33. Carlson MD, Ip J, Messenger J, et al: A new pacemaker algorithm for the treatment of atrial fibrillation: Results of the Atrial Dynamic Overdrive Pacing Trial (ADOPT). J Am Coll Cardiol 42:627, 2003.

Pulse Generator Implantation

34. Hayes DL, Naccarelli GV, Furman S, et al: NASPE policy statement: NASPE training requirements for cardiac implantable electronic devices: Selection, implantation, and follow-up. Pacing Clin Electrophysiol 26:1556-1562. 2003.
35. Ellenbogen KA, Kay GN, Wilkoff BL: Clinical Cardiac Pacing and Defibrillation. 2nd ed. Philadelphia, WB Saunders, 2000.

Pacemaker Programming

36. Fu EY, Ellenbogen KA: Management of atrial tachyarrhythmias in patients with implantable devices. Cardiol Clin 18:37, 2000.

Implantable Cardioverter-Defibrillator Therapy

37. Siebels J, Cappato R, Ruppel R, et al, CASH Investigators: Preliminary results of the Cardiac Arrest Study Hamburg (CASH). Am J Cardiol 72:109F, 1993.
38. Pathmanathan RK, Lau EW, Cooper J, et al: Potential impact of antiarrhythmic drugs versus implantable defibrillators on the management of ventricular arrhythmias: The Midlands trial of empirical amiodarone versus electrophysiologically guided intervention and cardioverter implant registry data. Heart 80:68, 1998.
39. Bansch D, Antz M, Boczor S, et al: Primary prevention of sudden cardiac death in idiopathic dilated cardiomyopathy: The Cardiomyopathy Trial (CAT). Circulation 105:1453, 2002.
40. Raviele A, Bongiorni MG, Brignole M, et al: Which strategy is "best" after myocardial infarction? The Beta-Blocker Strategy plus Implantable Cardioverter Defibrillator Trial: Rationale and study design. Am J Cardiol 83:104D, 1999.
41. Moss AJ, Zareba W, Hall WJ, et al: Prophylactic implantation of a defibrillator in patients with myocardial infarction and reduced ejection fraction. N Engl J Med 346:877, 2002.
42. Bardy GH, Lee KL, Mark DB, et al, and the SCD-HeFT Pilot Investigators: Sudden Cardiac Death in Heart Failure Trial: Pilot study [abstract]. Pacing Clin Electrophysiol 20:1148, 1997.
43. Nademanee K, Veerakul G, Mower M, et al: Defibrillator Versus β-Blockers for Unexplained Death in Thailand (DEBUT): A randomized clinical trial. Circulation 107:E9038, 2003.
44. Strickberger SA, Hummel JD, Bartlett TG, et al: Amiodarone versus implantable cardioverter-defibrillator: Randomized trial in patients with nonischemic dilated cardiomyopathy and asymptomatic nonsustained ventricular tachycardia—AMIOVIRT. J Am Coll Cardiol 41:1707, 2003.
45. The Antiarrhythmics Versus Implantable Defibrillators (AVID) Investigators: A comparison of antiarrhythmic drug therapy with implantable defibrillators in patients resuscitated from near-fatal ventricular arrhythmias. N Engl J Med 337:1576, 1997.
46. Moss AJ, Hall WJ, Cannom DS, et al, Multicenter Automatic Defibrillator Implantation Trial Investigators: Improved survival with an implanted defibrillator in patients with coronary disease at high risk for ventricular arrhythmia. N Engl J Med 335:1933, 1996.
47. Buxton AE, Fisher JD, Josephson ME, et al: Prevention of sudden death in patients wit coronary artery disease: The Multicenter Unsustained Tachycardia Trial (MUSTT). Pro Cardiovasc Dis 36:215, 1993.
48. Bigger JT Jr, Coronary Artery Bypass Graft (CABG) Patch Trial Investigators: Prophy lactic use of implanted cardiac defibrillators in patients at high risk for ventricula arrhythmias after coronary artery bypass graft surgery. N Engl J Med 337:1569, 1997.
49. Bigger JT Jr, Whang W, Rottman JN, et al: Mechanisms of death in the CABG-PATCH trial: A randomized trial of implantable cardiac defibrillator prophylaxis in patients a high risk of death after coronary artery bypass graft surgery. Circulation 99:1416, 1999.
50. Caruso AC, Marcus FI, Hahn EA, et al: Predictors of arrhythmic death and cardiac arres in the ESVEM trial: Electrophysiologic Study Versus Electromagnetic Monitoring. Circulation 96:1888, 1997.
51. Cleland JG, Daubert JC, Erdmann E, et al: The CARE-HF study (CArdiac REsynchronisation in Heart Failure study): Rationale, design, and end-points. Eur J Heart Fail 3:481 2001.
52. Groh WJ, Silka MJ, Oliver RP, et al: Use of implantable cardioverter-defibrillators in the congenital long-QT syndrome. Am J Cardiol 78:703, 1996.
53. Maron BJ, Shen WK, Link MS, et al: Efficacy of implantable cardioverter-defibrillators for the prevention of sudden death in patients with hypertrophic cardiomyopathy. N Engl J Med 342:365, 2000.
54. Pinski SL, Fahy GJ: Implantable cardioverter-defibrillators. Am J Med 106:446, 1999.
55. Higgins SL, Pak JP, Barone J, et al: The first-year experience with the dual-chamber ICD. Pacing Clin Electrophysiol 23:18, 2000.
56. Wilkoff BL, Cook JR, Epstein AE, et al: Dual-chamber pacing or ventricular backup pacing in patients with an implantable defibrillator: The Dual Chamber and VVI Implantable Defibrillator (DAVID) Trial. JAMA 288:3115, 2002.
57. Friedman PA, Rasmussen MJ, Grice S, et al: Defibrillation thresholds are increased by right-sided implantation of totally transvenous implantable cardioverter-defibrillators. Pacing Clin Electrophysiol 22:1186, 1999.

Electromagnetic Interference

58. Pinski SL, Trohman RG: Interference with cardiac pacing. Cardiol Clin 18:219, 2000.
59. Hayes DL, Wang PJ, Reynolds DW, et al: Interference with cardiac pacemakers by cellular telephones. N Engl J Med 336:1473, 1997.
60. Fetter JG, Ivans V, Benditt DG, et al: Digital cellular telephone interaction with implantable cardioverter-defibrillators. J Am Coll Cardiol 31:623, 1998.
61. Groh WJ, Boschee SA, Engelstein ED, et al: Interactions between electronic article surveillance systems and implantable cardioverter-defibrillators. Circulation 100:387, 1999.
62. Chung MK, Streem SB, Ching E, et al: Effects of extracorporeal shock wave lithotripsy on tiered therapy implantable cardioverter-defibrillators. Pacing Clin Electrophysiol 22:738, 1999.
63. Glikson M, Trusty JM, Grice SK, et al: Importance of pacemaker noise reversion as a potential mechanism of pacemaker-ICD interactions. Pacing Clin Electrophysiol 21:1111, 1998.

Interference from Drugs and Metabolic Abnormalities

64. Carnes CA, Mehdirad AA, Nelson SD: Drug and defibrillator interactions. Pharmacotherapy 18:516, 1998.
65. Kopp D, Kall J, Kinder C, et al: Effect of amiodarone and left ventricular mass on defibrillation energy requirements: Monophasic versus biphasic shocks. Pacing Clin Electrophysiol 18:872, 1995.

Device Follow-Up

66. Theuns DAMJ, Res JCJ, Jordaens LJ: Home monitoring in ICD therapy: Future perspectives. Europace 5:139, 2003.
67. Chun SH, Friday KJ, Chan A, et al: Clinical benefit and technical accuracy evaluation of wireless home monitoring pacemaker system: Multicenter clinical trial data. J Am Coll Cardiol 41(Suppl A):139A, 2003.

GUIDELINES *Thomas H. Lee*

Cardiac Pacemakers and Cardioverter-Defibrillators

Guidelines for implantation of cardiac pacemakers and antiarrhythmia devices were published by the American College of Cardiology/American Heart Association (ACC/AHA) and the North American Society for Pacing and Electrophysiology (NASPE) in 1998[1] and updated in 2002.[2] These guidelines continue to use the ACC/AHA classification system for the indications (class I for generally accepted indications; class IIa when indications are controversial, but the weight of evidence is supportive; class IIb when usefulness or efficacy is less well established; and class III when there is consensus against the usefulness of the intervention). The updated guidelines adopted a convention for rating levels of evidence on which recommendations have been based: *Level A* recommendations were derived from data from multiple randomized clinical trials; *level B* recommendations were derived from a single randomized trial or nonrandomized studies; and *level C* recommendations were based on the consensus opinion of experts.

Indications for Permanent Pacing (Tables 31G–1 to 31G–10)

Acquired AV Block. For patients with complete or second-degree atrioventricular (AV) block, the ACC/AHA guidelines consider permanent pacing to be appropriate when the abnormality causes complications and is not precipitated by a drug that can be discontinued (see Table 31G–1). Examples of complications include symptomatic bradycardia, congestive heart failure, and confusional states. For asymptomatic patients with complete or advanced second-degree AV block, permanent pacing was considered appropriate for patients with a high risk for development of complications, such as those with periods of asystole of 3 seconds or longer or an escape rate less than 40 beats/min, or patients who have had interventions or neuromuscular diseases that have damaged the AV node.

TABLE 31G–1 ACC/AHA Guidelines for Permanent Pacing in Acquired Atrioventricular Block in Adults

Class	Indication	Level of Evidence (see text)
I (indicated)	1. Third-degree and advanced second-degree AV block at any anatomic level, associated with any one of the following conditions:	
	a. Bradycardia with symptoms (including heart failure) presumed to be due to AV block	C
	b. Arrhythmias and other medical conditions requiring drugs that result in symptomatic bradycardia	C
	c. Documented periods of asystole ≥3.0 sec or any escape rate <40 beats/min in awake, symptom-free patients	B, C
	d. After catheter ablation of the AV junction; there are no trials to assess outcome without pacing, and pacing is virtually always planned in this situation unless the operative procedure is AV junction modification	B, C
	e. Postoperative AV block that is not expected to resolve after cardiac surgery	C
	f. Neuromuscular diseases with AV block, such as myotonic muscular dystrophy, Kearns-Sayre syndrome, Erb dystrophy (limb-girdle), and peroneal muscular atrophy, with or without symptoms, because there may be unpredictable progression of AV conduction disease	B
	2. Second-degree AV block regardless of type or site of block, with associated symptomatic bradycardia	B
IIa (good supportive evidence)	1. Asymptomatic third-degree AV block at any anatomic site with average awake ventricular rates of ≥40 beats/min, especially if cardiomegaly or LV dysfunction is present	B, C
	2. Asymptomatic type II second-degree AV block with a narrow QRS; when type II second-degree AV block occurs with a wide QRS, pacing becomes a class I recommendation	B
	3. Asymptomatic type I second-degree AV block at intra-His or infra-His levels found at electrophysiological study performed for other indications	B
	4. First- or second-degree AV block with symptoms similar to those of pacemaker syndrome	B
IIb (weak supportive evidence)	1. Marked first-degree AV block (>0.30 sec) in patients with LV dysfunction and symptoms of congestive heart failure in whom a shorter AV interval results in hemodynamic improvement, presumably by decreasing left atrial filling pressure	C
	2. Neuromuscular diseases such as myotonic muscular dystrophy, Kearns-Sayre syndrome, Erb dystrophy (limb-girdle), and peroneal muscular atrophy with any degree of AV block (including first-degree AV block), with or without symptoms, because there may be unpredictable progression of AV conduction disease	B
III (not indicated)	1. Asymptomatic first-degree AV block	B
	2. Asymptomatic type I second-degree AV block at the supra-His (AV node) level or not known to be intra-Hisian or infra-Hisian	B, C
	3. AV block expected to resolve and/or unlikely to recur (e.g., drug toxicity, Lyme disease, or during hypoxia in sleep apnea syndrome in absence of symptoms)	B

ACC = American College of Cardiology; AHA = American Heart Association; AV = atrioventricular; LV = left ventricular.

TABLE 31G–2 ACC/AHA Guidelines for Permanent Pacing in Chronic Bifascicular and Trifascicular Block

Class	Indication	Level of Evidence
I (indicated)	1. Intermittent third-degree AV block	B
	2. Type II second-degree AV block	B
	3. Alternating bundle branch block	C
IIa (good supportive evidence)	1. Syncope not demonstrated to be due to AV block when other likely causes have been excluded, specifically VT	B
	2. Incidental finding at electrophysiological study of markedly prolonged HV interval (≥100 msec) in asymptomatic patients	B
	3. Incidental finding at electrophysiological study of pacing-induced infra-His block that is not physiological	B
IIb (weak supportive evidence)	Neuromuscular diseases such as myotonic muscular dystrophy, Kearns-Sayre syndrome, Erb dystrophy (limb-girdle), and peroneal muscular atrophy with any degree of fascicular block, without symptoms, because there may be unpredictable progression of AV conduction disease	C
III (not indicated)	1. Fascicular block without AV block or symptoms	B
	2. Fascicular block with first-degree AV block without symptoms	B

ACC = American College of Cardiology; AHA = American Heart Association; AV = atrioventricular; VT = ventricular tachycardia.

CH 31

TABLE 31G–9 ACC/AHA Guidelines for Choice of Pacemaker

Type of Pacemaker	Sinus Node Dysfunction	AV Block	Neurally Mediated Syncope or Carotid Sinus Hypersensitivity
Single-chamber atrial	No suspected abnormality of AV conduction and not at increased risk for future AV block Maintenance of AV synchrony during pacing desired Rate response available if desired	Not appropriate	Not appropriate
Single-chamber ventricular	Maintenance of AV synchrony during pacing not necessary Rate response available if desired	Chronic atrial fibrillation or other atrial tachyarrhythmia or maintenance of AV synchrony during pacing not necessary Rate response available if desired	Chronic atrial fibrillation or other atrial tachyarrhythmia Rate response available if desired
Dual-chamber	AV synchrony during pacing desired Suspected abnormality of AV conduction or increased risk for future AV block Rate response available if desired	Rate response available if desired AV synchrony during pacing desired Atrial pacing desired	Sinus mechanism present Rate response available if desired
Single-lead, atrial-sensing ventricular	Not appropriate	Normal sinus node function and no need for atrial pacing Desire to limit the number of pacemaker leads	Not appropriate

ACC = American College of Cardiology; AHA = American Heart Association; AV = atrioventricular.

These recommendations differed from those in the prior ACC/AHA guidelines by supporting a lower threshold for use of pacemakers in patients with asymptomatic advanced second-degree heart block and by emphasizing the prognostic importance of the site of origin of the escape rhythm in cases of advanced AV block. For example, when type II second-degree AV block occurs with a wide QRS, pacing now becomes a class I recommendation, whereas this was a class IIa recommendation in the prior guidelines.

In addition, heart failure is now considered a complication of AV block that justifies a lower threshold for use of permanent pacing. This theme is also apparent in the class IIa recommendations, which consider evidence to be generally supportive for use of pacing in asymptomatic patients with third-degree AV block and ventricular rates or escape rates of 40 beats/min or more, especially if they have cardiomegaly or left ventricular dysfunction.

The guidelines do not support pacing for patients with asymptomatic first-degree or type I second-degree AV block, and they do not support the use of pacing for patients with hypoxia and sleep apnea syndrome in the absence of symptoms. The guidelines were written with awareness of a small study suggesting benefit from atrial pacing for patients with sleep apnea syndrome,[3] but the guideline authors considered support for routine use of pacing in this setting to be premature.

Chronic Bifascicular and Trifascicular Block. Syncope is common among patients with slowing of conduction below the AV node in the fascicles of the right and left bundles, but the risk of sudden death or progression to complete heart block varies among patient subsets. The ACC/AHA guidelines for pacing in these settings (see Table 31G–2) now include alternating bundle branch block as a class I indication for pacing, because this finding is recognized as a reflection of abnormal conduction in all three fascicles. The guidelines also provide some support for pacing in patients with findings of markedly abnormal conduction at electrophysiological studies, even if patients are asymptomatic (class IIa). Pacing is not supported for fascicular block without greater than first-degree AV block or symptoms.

Acute Myocardial Infarction. Symptoms do not play a role in appropriateness for pacing in patients with acute myocardial infarction because of the high risk for sudden death in postinfarction patients with conduction system disturbances (see Table 31G–3). The guidelines emphasize that the requirement for temporary pacing after acute myocardial infarction does not automatically indicate a need for permanent pacing (see Guidelines to Chap. 47). However, permanent pacemakers were supported for use in patients with persistent advanced-degree AV block or transient infranodal AV block and associated bundle branch block. The usefulness of permanent pacemakers for patients with advanced AV block at the AV node level was less clear (class IIb). Permanent pacing was discouraged if the only indication was transient AV conduction disturbances or left anterior hemiblock.

Sinus Node Dysfunction. As noted in the recommendations for pacing for patients with acquired AV block, the ACC/AHA guidelines support pacing for patients with symptoms due to bradycardia that is not due to a drug that can be discontinued. This theme is apparent in the indications for pacing in patients with sinus node dysfunction (see Table 31G–4). Pacing is discouraged in asymptomatic patients, even when resting heart rates are lower than 40 beats/min, and in symptomatic patients when symptoms cannot be proven to be due to bradycardia. A new class IIa recommendation is included in the 2002 guidelines that supports pacing in patients with syncope of unexplained origin when major abnormalities of sinus node function are demonstrated at electrophysiological testing.

Prevention and Termination of Tachyarrhythmias. In some patients with long-QT syndrome, continuous pacing can prevent recurrent tachyarrhythmias. In addition, paroxysmal reentrant tachyarrhythmias can be terminated in some patients through programmed stimulation and short bursts of rapid pacing. However, the ACC/AHA guidelines do not provide support for the routine use of antitachycardia pacemakers without extensive testing before implantation (see Table 31G–5). The 2002 guidelines actually raise the threshold for use of antitachycardia pacemakers by "downgrading" its class I indication for pacing in patients whose recurrent supraventricular tachycardia is unresponsive to antiarrhythmic drugs. This change reflects the Committee consensus that either drugs and/or ablation therapy should be first-line therapies for most patients. The guidelines continue to consider pacing appropriate (class I indication) for patients with sustained pause-dependent ventricular tachycardia, with or without prolonged QT, if the efficacy of pacing has been demonstrated (see Table 31G–6).

Carotid Sinus Syndrome and Neurocardiogenic Syncope. The only class I indication for permanent pacing in the ACC/AHA guidelines in patients with hypersensitive carotid sinus syndrome is

TABLE 31G–10 ACC/AHA Recommendations for ICD Therapy

Class	Indication	Level of Evidence
I (indicated)	1. Cardiac arrest due to VF or VT not due to a transient or reversible cause	A
	2. Spontaneous sustained VT in association with structural heart disease	B
	3. Syncope of undetermined origin with clinically relevant, hemodynamically significant sustained VT or VF induced at electrophysiological study when drug therapy is ineffective, not tolerated, or not preferred	B
	4. Nonsustained VT in patients with coronary disease, prior MI, LV dysfunction, and inducible VF or sustained VT at electrophysiological study not suppressible by a class I antiarrhythmic drug	A
	5. Spontaneous sustained VT in patients without structural heart disease not amenable to other treatments	C
IIa (good supportive evidence)	Patients with ejection fraction ≤30% at least 1 mo post MI and 3 mo post coronary artery revascularization surgery	B
IIb (weak supportive evidence)	1. Cardiac arrest presumed to be due to VF when electrophysiological testing is precluded by other medical conditions	C
	2. Severe symptoms (e.g., syncope) attributable to ventricular tachyarrhythmias in patients awaiting cardiac transplantation	C
	3. Familial or inherited conditions with a high risk for life-threatening ventricular tachyarrhythmias such as long-QT syndrome or hypertrophic cardiomyopathy	B
	4. Nonsustained VT with coronary artery disease, prior MI, LV dysfunction, and inducible sustained VT or VF at electrophysiological study	B
	5. Recurrent syncope of undetermined origin in the presence of ventricular dysfunction and inducible ventricular arrhythmias at electrophysiological study when other causes of syncope have been excluded	C
	6. Syncope of unexplained origin or family history of unexplained sudden cardiac death in association with typical or atypical right bundle branch block and ST segment elevations (Brugada syndrome)	C
	7. Syncope in patients with advanced structural heart disease in whom thorough invasive and noninvasive investigations have failed to define a cause	C
III (not indicated)	1. Syncope of undetermined cause in a patient without inducible ventricular tachyarrhythmias and without structural heart disease	C
	2. Incessant VT or VF	C
	3. VF or VT resulting from arrhythmias amenable to surgical or catheter ablation; e.g., atrial arrhythmias associated with Wolff-Parkinson-White syndrome, RV outflow tract VT, idiopathic LV tachycardia, or fascicular VT	C
	4. Ventricular tachyarrhythmias due to a transient or reversible disorder (e.g., acute MI, electrolyte imbalance, drugs, or trauma) when correction of the disorder is considered feasible and likely to substantially reduce the risk of recurrent arrhythmia	B
	5. Significant psychiatric illnesses that may be aggravated by device implantation or may preclude systematic follow-up	C
	6. Terminal illnesses with projected life expectancy <6 mo	C
	7. Patients with coronary artery disease with LV dysfunction and prolonged QRS duration in the absence of spontaneous or inducible sustained or nonsustained VT who are undergoing coronary bypass surgery	B
	8. NYHA Class IV drug-refractory congestive heart failure in patients who are not candidates for cardiac transplantation	C

ACC = American College of Cardiology; AHA = American Heart Association; ICD = implanted cardioverter-defibrillator; LV = left ventricular; MI = myocardial infarction; NYHA = New York Heart Association; RV = right ventricular; VF = ventricular fibrillation; VT = ventricular tachycardia.

recurrent syncope caused by carotid sinus stimulation in the absence of any drug that depresses the sinus node or AV conduction (see Table 31G–7). However, the guidelines added a new class IIa indication with support for pacing in patients with recurrent neurocardiogenic syncope associated with bradycardia, reflecting recent clinical trials showing the benefit of pacing in this setting. Pacing is discouraged in patients without symptoms or who have syncope without bradycardia.

Cardiomyopathy and after Cardiac Transplantation. For patients with hypertrophic or dilated cardiomyopathy or who have cardiac transplantation, class I indications for permanent pacing are similar to those in other patient populations (see Table 31G–8). The guidelines do not provide much support for the routine use of pacing in patients with hypertrophic cardiomyopathy for the purpose of reducing left ventricular outflow obstruction (class IIb indication). However, the 2002 guidelines add a new class IIa indication of biventricular pacing for patients with dilated cardiomyopathy and prolonged QRS intervals, reflecting multiple trials that have shown clinical and structural benefits from this intervention.

Selection of Pacemakers

The ACC/AHA guidelines provide recommendations (see Table 31G–9) and decision trees to help physicians choose the most appropriate type of pacemaker. These guidelines are aimed at helping physicians match patients' needs to the technology implanted and to anticipate future needs of the patient. Elderly patients should receive devices according to the same indications as younger patients, according to the guidelines.

Follow-Up of Patients with Pacemakers

The ACC/AHA guidelines do not directly address follow-up of patients with pacemakers but instead refer physicians to guidelines from other organizations.[4-8] Examples of reasonable follow-up schedules included twice in the first 6 months after implant of single-chamber pacemakers and then once every 12 months; and, for dual-chamber pacemakers, twice in the first 6 months, then once every 6 months.

 Guidelines for transtelephonic monitoring focus on content, not frequency.

Implantable Cardioverter-Defibrillator Therapy

The 2002 ACC/AHA guidelines reflect the continuing expansion of the role of implantable cardioverter-defibrillators (ICDs),[9-11] which are considered clearly appropriate for patients with cardiac arrests not due to transient or reversible causes and for patients with spontaneous sustained ventricular tachycardia associated with structural heart disease (see Table 31G–10). The guidelines note that ICD therapy is most efficacious in patients with sustained ventricular tachycardia and impaired left ventricular performance, whereas VT arising in structurally normal hearts can usually be treated pharmacologically or with catheter ablation.

The guidelines add a new class IIa indication for ICDs for patients with left ventricular ejection fraction less than 0.30 at least 1 month after myocardial infarction and 3 months after coronary artery revascularization surgery, reflecting recent data supporting the use of ICDs for primary prevention of cardiac arrest.[9,11] The Committee agreed that further risk stratification might help define the benefit of an ICD in such patients, and it identified this area as important for future research.

Only limited support (class IIb) was provided for the use of ICDs in patients with syncope of unexplained etiology or family history of unexplained sudden cardiac death in association with electrocardiographic abnormalities typical of Brugada syndrome. ICDs were considered contraindicated in patients in whom a triggering factor for ventricular tachycardia or ventricular fibrillation can be definitely identified, such as ventricular tachyarrhythmias in evolving acute myocardial infarction or electrolyte abnormalities.

See Guidelines in Chapter 30 for recommendations regarding resumption of driving or flying for patients who have received ICDs.

References

1. Gregoratos G, Cheitlin M, Conill A, et al: ACC/AHA guidelines for implantation of cardiac pacemakers and antiarrhythmia devices: A report of the American College of Cardiology/American Heart Association Task Force on Practice Guidelines (Committee on Pacemaker Implantation). J Am Coll Cardiol 31:1175, 1998.
2. Gregoratos G, Abrams J, Epstein AE, et al: ACC/AHA/NASPE 2002 Guideline Update for Implantation of Cardiac Pacemakers and Antiarrhythmia Devices—Summary Article: A Report of the American College of Cardiology/American Heart Association Task Force on Practice Guidelines (ACC/AHA/NASPE Committee to Update the 1998 Pacemaker Guidelines). J Am Coll Cardiol 40:1703-1719, 2002.
3. Garrigue S, Bordier P, Jais P, et al: Benefit of atrial pacing in sleep apnea syndrome. N Engl J Med 346:404-412, 2002.
4. Bernstein AD, Irwin ME, Parsonnet V, et al: Report of the NASPE Policy Conference on Antibradycardia Pacemaker Follow-Up: Effectiveness, needs, and resources. Pacing Clin Electrophysiol 17:1714-1729, 1994.
5. Levine PA, Belott PH, Bilitch M, et al: Recommendations of the NASPE policy conference on pacemaker programmability and follow-up programs. Pacing Clin Electrophysiol 6:1222-1223, 1983.
6. Levine PA: Proceedings of the Policy Conference of the North American Society of Pacing and Electrophysiology on Programmability and Pacemaker Follow-Up Programs. Clin Prog Pacing Electrophysiol 2:145-191, 1984.
7. Medicare Coverage Issues Manual. HCFA Publication No. 6, Thur Rev. 42. Baltimore, U.S. Department of Health and Human Services, Health Care Financing Administration, 1990.
8. Fraser JD, Gillis AM, Irwin ME, et al: Guidelines for pacemaker follow-up in Canada: A consensus statement of the Canadian Working Group on Cardiac Pacing. Can J Cardiol 16:355-376, 2000.
9. Moss AJ, Zareba W, Hall WJ, et al: Prophylactic implantation of a defibrillator in patients with myocardial infarction and reduced ejection fraction. N Engl J Med 346:877-883, 2002.
10. Bansch D, Antz M, Boczor S, et al: Primary prevention of sudden death in idiopathic dilated cardiomyopathy: The Cardiomyopathy Trial (CAT). Circulation 105:1453-1458, 2002.
11. Ezekowitz JA, Armstrong PW, McAlister FA: Implantable cardioverter defibrillators in primary and secondary prevention: A systematic review of randomized, controlled trials. Ann Intern Med 138:445-452, 2003.

CHAPTER 32

Specific Arrhythmias: Diagnosis and Treatment

Jeffrey E. Olgin • Douglas P. Zipes

Sinus Nodal Disturbances

Normal Sinus Rhythm

Normal sinus rhythm is arbitrarily limited to impulse formation beginning in the sinus node at frequencies between 60 and 100 beats/min. A range of 50 to 90 beats/min has been suggested. Infants and children generally have faster heart rates than adults do, both at rest and during exercise. The P wave is upright in electrocardiograph (ECG) leads I, II, and aV_f and negative in lead aV, with a vector in the frontal plane between 0 and +90 degrees. In the horizontal plane, the P vector is directed anteriorly and slightly leftward and can therefore be negative in leads V_1 and V_2 but positive in V_3 to V_6. The PR interval exceeds 120 milliseconds and can vary slightly with the rate. If the pacemaker site shifts, a change in morphology of the P wave can occur. The rate of sinus rhythm varies significantly and depends on many factors, including age, sex, and physical activity (Table 32–1).

The sinus nodal discharge rate responds readily to autonomic stimuli and depends on the effect of the two opposing autonomic influences. Steady vagal stimulation decreases the spontaneous sinus nodal discharge rate and predominates over steady sympathetic stimulation, which increases the spontaneous sinus nodal discharge rate. Single or brief bursts of vagal stimulation can speed, slow, or entrain sinus nodal discharge. A given vagal stimulus produces a greater absolute reduction in heart rate when the basal heart rate has been increased by sympathetic stimulation, a phenomenon known as *accentuated antagonism*.

Sinus Tachycardia

ECG RECOGNITION. *Tachycardia* (Fig. 32–1A) in an adult is defined as a rate faster than 100 beats/min. During sinus tachycardia, the sinus node exhibits a discharge frequency between 100 and 180 beats/min, but it may be higher with extreme exertion. The maximum heart rate achieved during strenuous physical activity decreases with age from near 200 beats/min to less than 140 beats/min. Sinus tachycardia generally has a gradual onset and termination. The P-P interval can vary slightly from cycle to cycle. P waves have a normal contour, but a larger amplitude can develop and the wave can become peaked. They appear before each QRS complex with a stable PR interval unless concomitant atrioventricular (AV) block ensues.

Accelerated phase 4 diastolic depolarization of sinus nodal cells is generally responsible for sinus tachycardia and is usually due to elevated adrenergic tone and/or withdrawal of parasympathetic tone. Carotid sinus massage and the Valsalva or other vagal maneuvers gradually slow sinus tachycardia, which then accelerates to its previous rate on cessation of enhanced vagal tone. More rapid sinus rates can fail to slow in response to a vagal maneuver, particularly those driven by high adrenergic tone.

CLINICAL FEATURES. Sinus tachycardia is common in infancy and early childhood and is the normal reaction to a variety of physiological or pathophysiological stresses such as fever, hypotension, thyrotoxicosis, anemia, anxiety, exertion, hypovolemia, pulmonary emboli, myocardial ischemia, congestive heart failure, or shock. Drugs such as atropine, catecholamines, and thyroid medications, as well as alcohol, nicotine, caffeine, and inflammation, can produce sinus tachycardia. Persistent sinus tachycardia can be a manifestation of heart failure.

In patients with structural heart disease, sinus tachycardia can result in reduced cardiac output or angina or can precipitate another arrhythmia, in part related to the abbreviated ventricular filling time and compromised coronary blood flow. Sinus tachycardia can be a cause of inappropriate defibrillator discharge in patients with an implantable automatic defibrillator. *Chronic inappropriate sinus tachycardia* has been described in otherwise healthy persons, possibly secondary to increased automaticity of the sinus node or an automatic atrial focus located near the sinus node.[1] The abnormality can result from a defect in either sympathetic or vagal nerve control of sinoatrial (SA) automaticity, or an abnormality of the intrinsic heart rate can be present.

MANAGEMENT. Management should focus on the *cause* of the sinus tachycardia. In the hospital inpatient setting, this is

TABLE 32–1 Arrhythmia Characteristics*

Type of Arrhythmia	P Waves Rate (beats/min)	P Waves Rhythm	P Waves Contour	QRS Complexes Rate (beats/min)	QRS Complexes Rhythm	QRS Complexes Contour
Sinus rhythm	60-100	Regular[†]	Normal	60-100	Regular	Normal
Sinus bradycardia	<60	Regular	Normal	<60	Regular	Normal
Sinus tachycardia	100-180	Regular	May be peaked	100-180	Regular	Normal
AV nodal reentry	150-250	Very regular except at onset and termination	Retrograde; difficult to see; lost in QRS complex	150-250	Very regular except at onset and termination	Normal
Atrial flutter	250-350	Regular	Sawtooth	75-175	Generally regular in absence of drugs or disease	Normal
Atrial fibrillation	400-600	Grossly irregular	Baseline undulation, no P waves	100-160	Grossly irregular	Normal
Atrial tachycardia with block	150-250	Regular; may be irregular	Abnormal	75-200	Generally regular in absence of drugs or disease	Normal
AV junctional rhythm	40-100[§]	Regular	Normal	40-60	Fairly regular	Normal
Reciprocating tachycardias using an accessory (WPW) pathway	150-250	Very regular except at onset and termination	Retrograde; difficult to see; monitor the QRS complex	150-250	Very regular except at onset and termination	Normal
Nonparoxysinal AV junctional tachycardia	60-100[¶]	Regular	Normal	70-130	Fairly regular	Normal
Ventricular tachycardia	60-100[¶]	Regular	Normal	110-250	Fairly regular; may be irregular	Abnormal, >0.12 sec
Accelerated idioventricular rhythm	60-100[¶]	Regular	Normal	50-110	Fairly regular; may be irregular	Abnormal, >0.12 sec
Ventricular flutter	60-100[¶]	Regular	Normal; difficult to see	150-300	Regular	Sine wave
Ventricular fibrillation	60-100[¶]	Regular	Normal; difficult to see	400-600	Grossly irregular	Baseline undulations; no QRS complexes
First-degree AV block	60-100**	Regular	Normal	60-100	Regular	Normal
Type I second-degree AV block	60-100**	Regular	Normal	30-100	Irregular[††]	Normal
Type II second-degree AV block	60-100**	Regular	Normal	30-100	Irregular[††]	Abnormal, >0.12 sec
Complete AV block	60-100[¶]	Regular	Normal	<40	Fairly regular	Abnormal, 0.12 sec
Right bundle branch block	60-100	Regular	Normal	60-100	Regular	Abnormal, 0.12 sec
Left bundle branch block	60-100	Regular	Normal	60-100	Regular	Abnormal, >0.12 sec

AV = atrioventricular; WPW = Wolff-Parkinson-White.

Modified from Zipes DP: Arrhythmias. *In* Andreoli K, Zipes DP, Wallace AG, et al (eds): Comprehensive Cardiac Care. 6th ed. St Louis, CV Mosby, 1987.

*In an effort to summarize these arrhythmias in tabular form, generalizations have to be made. For example, the response to carotid sinus massage may be slightly different from what is listed. Acute therapy to terminate a tachycardia may be different from chronic therapy to prevent recurrence. Some of the exceptions are indicated in the footnotes; the reader is referred to the text for a complete discussion.

[†]P waves initiated by sinus node discharge may not be precisely regular because of sinus arrhythmia.

[‡]Often, carotid sinus massage fails to slow a sinus tachycardia.

[§]Any independent atrial arrhythmia may exist or the atria may be captured retrogradely.

	P Waves		QRS Complexes	
		Physical Examination		
Ventricular Response to Carotid Sinus Massage	***Intensity of S_1***	***Splitting of S_2***	***a Waves***	***Treatment***
Gradual slowing and return to former rate	Constant	Normal	Normal	None
Gradual slowing and return to former rate	Constant	Normal	Normal	None, unless symptomatic; atropine
Gradual slowing[‡] and return to former rate	Constant	Normal	Normal	None, unless symptomatic; treat underlying disease
Abrupt slowing caused by termination of tachycardia, or no effect	Constant	Normal	Constant cannon *a* waves	Vagal stimulation, adenosine, verapamil, digitalis, propranolol, DC shock, pacing
Abrupt slowing and return to former rate; flutter remains	Constant; variable if AV block changing	Normal	Flutter waves	DC shock, digitalis, quinidine, propranolol, verapamil, adenosine
Slowing; gross irregularity remains	Variable	Normal	No *a* waves	Digitalis, quinidine, DC shock, verapamil, adenosine
Abrupt slowing and return to normal rate; tachycardia remains	Constant; variable if AV block changing	Normal	More *a* waves than *c-v* waves	Stop digitalis if toxic; digitalis if not toxic; possibly verapamil
None; may be slight slowing	Variables[¶]	Normal	Intermittent cannon waves	None, unless symptomatic; atropine
Abrupt slowing caused by termination of tachycardia, or no effect	Constant but decreased	Normal	Constant cannon waves	See AV nodal reentry above
None, may be slight slowing	Variable[¶]	Normal	Intermittent cannon waves[¶]	None, unless symptomatic: stop digitalis if toxic
None	Variable[¶]	Abnormal	Intermittent cannon waves[¶]	Lidocaine, procainamide, DC shock, quinidine, amiodarone
None	Variable[¶]	Abnormal	Intermittent cannon waves[¶]	None, unless symptomatic: lidocaine, atropine
None	Soft or absent	Soft or absent	Cannon waves	DC shock
None	None	None	Cannon waves	DC shock
Gradual slowing caused by sinus	Constant, diminished	Normal	Normal	None
Slowing caused by sinus slowing and an increase in AV black	Cyclic decrease, then increase after pause	Normal	Normal; increasing *a-c* interval; *a* waves without *c* waves	None, unless symptomatic: atropine
Gradual slowing caused by sinus slowing	Constant	Abnormal	Normal; constant *a-c* interval; *a* waves without *c* waves	Pacemaker
None	Variable**	Abnormal	Intermittent cannon waves**	Pacemaker
Gradual slowing and return to former rate	Constant	Wide	Normal	None
Gradual slowing and return to former rate	Constant	Paradoxical	Normal	None

¶Constant if the atria are captured retrogradely.
**Atrial rhythm and rate may vary, depending on whether sinus bradycardia, sinus tachycardia, or another abnormality is the atrial mechanism.
††Regular or constant if block is unchanging.

usually obvious (e.g., hemorrhage, sepsis, agitation). In the outpatient setting, the cause may be more elusive. The most common reversible causes include hyperthyroidism, anemia, diabetes, and hypovolemia . Elimination of tobacco, alcohol, coffee, tea, or other stimulants, such as the sympathomimetic agents in nose drops, may be helpful. Drugs such as propranolol or verapamil or fluid replacement in a hypovolemic patient or fever reduction in a febrile patient can be used to help slow the sinus nodal discharge rate. Treatment of inappropriate sinus tachycardia requires beta blockers, calcium-channel blockers, or digitalis, alone or in combination. In severe cases, sinus node radiofrequency or surgical ablation may be indicated.

Sinus Bradycardia

ECG RECOGNITION. Sinus bradycardia (Fig. 32–1B) exists in an adult when the sinus node discharges at a rate slower than 60 beats/min. P waves have a normal contour and occur before each QRS complex, usually with a constant PR interval greater than 120 milliseconds. Sinus arrhythmia often coexists.

CLINICAL FEATURES. Sinus bradycardia can result from excessive vagal and/or decreased sympathetic tone, as an effect of medications, or from anatomical changes in the sinus node. In most cases, symptomatic sinus bradycardia is due to the effects of medication. Asymptomatic sinus bradycardia frequently occurs in healthy young adults, particularly well-trained athletes, and decreases in prevalence with advancing age. During sleep, the normal heart rate can fall to 35 to 40 beats/min, especially in adolescents and young adults, with marked sinus arrhythmia sometimes producing pauses of 2 seconds or longer. Eye surgery, coronary arteriography, meningitis, intracranial tumors, increased intracranial pressure, cervical and mediastinal tumors, and certain disease states such as severe hypoxia, Chagas disease, myxedema, hypothermia, fibrodegenerative changes, convalescence from some infections, gram-negative sepsis, and mental depression can produce sinus bradycardia. Sinus bradycardia also occurs during vomiting or vasovagal syncope (see Chap. 34) and can be produced by carotid sinus stimulation or by the administration of parasympathomimetic drugs, lithium, amiodarone beta-adrenoceptor blocking drugs, clonidine, propafenone, or calcium antagonists. Conjunctival instillation of beta blockers for glaucoma can produce sinus or AV nodal abnormalities, especially in the elderly.

In most instances, sinus bradycardia is a benign arrhythmia and can actually be beneficial by producing a longer period of diastole and increasing the ventricular filling time It can be associated with syncope caused by an abnormal autonomic reflex (cardioinhibitory) (see Chap. 34). Sinus bradycardia occurs in 10 to 15 percent of patients with acute myocardial infarction and may be even more prevalent when patients are seen in the early hours of infarction. Unless accompanied by hemodynamic decompensation or arrhythmias, sinus bradycardia is generally associated with a more favorable outcome following myocardial infarction than is the presence of sinus tachycardia. It is usually transient and occurs more commonly during inferior than anterior myocardial infarction; it has also been noted during reperfusion with thrombolytic agents (see Chap. 48). Bradycardia following resuscitation from cardiac arrest is associated with a poor prognosis.

MANAGEMENT. Treatment of sinus bradycardia per se is not usually necessary. For example, if a patient with acute myocardial infarction is asymptomatic, it is probably best to not speed up the sinus rate. If cardiac output is inadequate or if arrhythmias are associated with the slow rate, atropine (0.5 mg intravenously [IV] as an initial dose, repeated if necessary) is usually effective. Lower doses of atropine, particularly when given subcutaneously or intramuscularly, can exert an initial parasympathomimetic effect, possibly via a central action. For symptomatic episodes of sinus bradycardia that are more than momentary or are recurrent (e.g., as during a myocardial infarction) temporary electrical pacing via a transveneous electrode is usually preferable to repeated or prolonged drug therapy. In some patients who experience congestive heart failure or symptoms of low cardiac output as a result of chronic sinus bradycardia, permanent electrical pacing may be needed (see Chap. 31). Atrial pacing is usually preferable to ventricular pacing to preserve sequential AV contraction and is preferable to drug therapy for long-term management of sinus bradycardia. As a general rule, no available drugs increase the heart rate reliably and safely over long periods without important side effects.

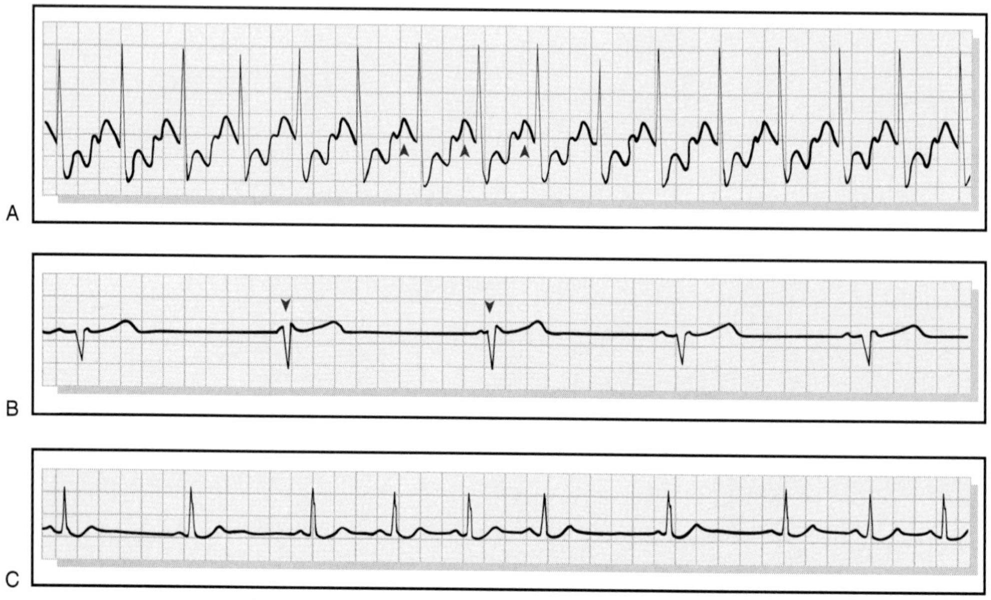

FIGURE 32–1 **A,** Sinus tachycardia (150 beats/min) in a patient during acute myocardial ischemia; note the ST segment depression. P waves are indicated by arrowheads. **B,** Sinus bradycardia at a rate of 40 to 48 beats/min. The second and third QRS complexes (arrowheads) represent junctional escape beats. Note the P waves at the onset of the QRS complex. **C,** Nonrespiratory sinus arrhythmia occurring as a consequence of digitalis toxicity. Monitor leads.

SINUS ARRHYTHMIA

Sinus arrhythmia (Fig. 32-1C) is characterized by a phasic variation in sinus cycle length during which the maximum sinus cycle length minus the minimum sinus cycle length exceeds 120 milliseconds or the maximum sinus cycle length minus the minimum sinus cycle length divided by the minimum sinus cycle length exceeds 10 percent. It is the most frequent form of arrhythmia and is considered to be a normal event. P wave morphology does not usually vary, and the PR interval exceeds 120 milliseconds and remains unchanged since the focus of discharge remains relatively fixed within the sinus node. Occasionally, the pacemaker focus can wander within the sinus node, or its exit to the atrium may change and produce P waves of a slightly different contour (but not retrograde) and a slightly changing PR interval that exceeds 120 milliseconds.

Sinus arrhythmia commonly occurs in the young, especially those with slower heart rates or following enhanced vagal tone, such as after the administration of digitalis or morphine, and decreases with age or with autonomic dysfunction, such as diabetic neuropathy. Sinus arrhythmia appears in two basic forms. In the *respiratory* form, the P-P interval cyclically shortens during inspiration, primarily as a result of reflex inhibition of vagal tone, and slows during expiration; breath-holding eliminates the cycle length variation (see Heart Rate Variability, Chap. 29). Efferent vagal effects alone have been suggested as being responsible for respiratory sinus arrhythmias. *Nonrespiratory* sinus arrhythmia is characterized by a phasic variation in the P-P interval unrelated to the respiratory cycle and may be the result of digitalis intoxication. Loss of sinus rhythm variability is a risk factor for sudden cardiac death (see Chap. 23).

Symptoms produced by sinus arrhythmia are uncommon, but on occasion, if the pauses between beats are excessively long, palpitations or dizziness may result. Marked sinus arrhythmia can produce a sinus pause sufficiently long to produce syncope if not accompanied by an escape rhythm.

Treatment is usually unnecessary. Increasing the heart rate by exercise or drugs generally abolishes sinus arrhythmia. Symptomatic individuals may experience relief from palpitations with sedatives, tranquilizers, atropine, ephedrine, or isoproterenol administration, as in the treatment of sinus bradycardia.

VENTRICULOPHASIC SINUS ARRHYTHMIA. The most common example occurs during complete AV block and a slow ventricular rate, when P-P cycles that contain a QRS complex are shorter than P-P cycles without a QRS complex. Similar lengthening can be present in the P-P cycle that follows a premature ventricular complex (PVC) with a compensatory pause. Alterations in the P-P interval are probably due to the influence of the autonomic nervous system responding to changes in ventricular stroke volume.

SINUS PAUSE OR SINUS ARREST

Sinus pause or sinus arrest (Fig. 32-2) is recognized by a pause in the sinus rhythm. The P-P interval delimiting the pause does not equal a multiple of the basic P-P interval. Differentiation of sinus arrest, which is thought to be due to slowing or cessation of spontaneous sinus nodal automaticity and therefore a disorder of impulse formation from SA exit block (see below) in patients with sinus arrhythmia, can be quite difficult without direct recordings of sinus node discharge.

Failure of sinus nodal discharge results in the absence of atrial depolarization and in periods of ventricular asystole if escape beats initiated by latent pacemakers do not occur (see Fig. 32-2). Involvement of the sinus node by acute myocardial infarction, degenerative fibrotic changes, effects of digitalis toxicity, stroke, or excessive vagal tone all can produce sinus arrest. Transient sinus arrest may have no clinical significance by itself if latent pacemakers promptly escape to prevent ventricular asystole or the genesis of other arrhythmias precipitated by the slow rates. Sinus arrest and AV block have been demonstrated in as many as 30 percent of patients with sleep apnea (see Chap. 68).

Treatment is as outlined earlier for sinus bradycardia. In patients who have a chronic form of sinus node disease characterized by marked sinus bradycardia or sinus arrest, permanent pacing is often necessary. However, as a general rule, chronic pacing for sinus bradycardia is indicated only in symptomatic patients or those with a sinus pause exceeding 3 seconds.[2]

SINOATRIAL EXIT BLOCK

This arrhythmia is recognized electrocardiographically by a pause resulting from absence of the normally expected P wave (Fig. 32-3). The duration of the pause is a multiple of the basic P-P interval. SA exit block is due to a conduction disturbance during which an impulse formed within the sinus node fails to depolarize the atria or does so with delay (Fig. 32-4). An interval without P waves that equals approximately two, three, or four times the normal P-P cycle characterizes type II second-degree SA exit block. During type I (Wenckebach) second-degree SA exit block, the P-P interval progressively shortens prior to the pause, and the duration of the pause is less than two P-P cycles. (See Chap. 27 for further discussion of Wenckebach intervals.) First-degree SA exit block cannot be recognized by ECG because SA nodal discharge is not recorded. Third-degree SA exit block can be manifested as a complete absence of P waves and is difficult to diagnose with certainty without sinus node electrograms.

Excessive vagal stimulation, acute myocarditis, infarction, or fibrosis involving the atrium, as well as drugs such as quinidine, procainamide, or digitalis, can produce SA exit block. SA exit block is usually transient. It may be of no clinical importance except to prompt a search for the underlying cause. Occasionally, syncope can result if the SA block is prolonged and unaccompanied by an escape rhythm. SA exit block can occur in well-trained athletes.

Therapy for patients who have symptomatic SA exit block is as outlined for sinus bradycardia.

WANDERING PACEMAKER

This variant of sinus arrhythmia involves passive transfer of the dominant pacemaker focus from the sinus node to latent pacemakers that have the next highest degree of automaticity located in other atrial sites (usually lower in the crista terminalis) or in AV junctional tissue. The change occurs in a gradual fashion over the duration of several beats; thus, only one pacemaker at a time controls the rhythm, in sharp contrast with AV dissociation. The ECG (Fig. 32-5) displays a cyclical increase in the R-R interval: a PR interval that gradually shortens and can become less than 120 milliseconds; and a change in the P wave contour, which becomes negative in lead I or II (depending on the site of discharge) or is lost within the QRS complex. Generally, these changes

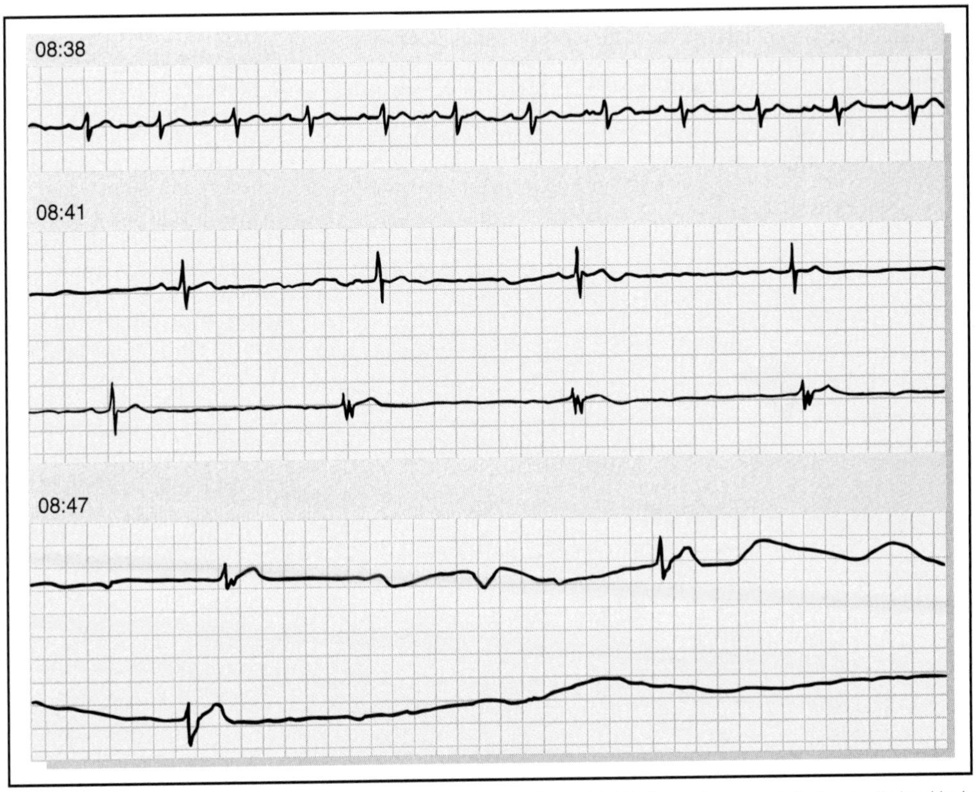

FIGURE 32-2 Sinus arrest. The patient had a long-term electrocardiographic (ECG) recorder connected when he died suddenly of cardiac standstill. The rhythms demonstrate progressive sinus bradycardia and sinus arrest at 8:41 A.M. The rhythm then becomes a ventricular escape rhythm, which progressively slows and finally ceases at 8:47 A.M. Monitor lead. The double ECG strips are continuous recordings.

occur in reverse as the pacemaker shifts back to the sinus node. Wandering pacemaker is a normal phenomenon that often occurs in the very young and particularly in athletes, presumably because of augmented vagal tone. Persistence of an AV junctional rhythm for long periods, however, may indicate underlying heart disease. *Treatment* is not usually indicated but, if necessary, is the same as that for sinus bradycardia (see earlier).

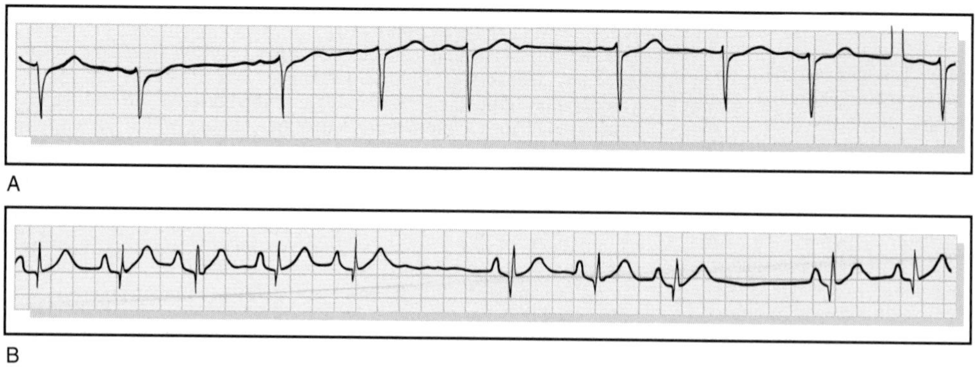

FIGURE 32–3 Sinus nodal exit block. **A,** A type I sinoatrial (SA) nodal exit block has the following features: The P-P interval shortens from the first to the second cycle in each grouping, followed by a pause. The duration of the pause is less than twice the shortest cycle length, and the cycle after the pause exceeds the cycle before the pause. The PR interval is normal and constant. Lead V_1. **B,** The P-P interval varies slightly because of sinus arrhythmia. The two pauses in sinus nodal activity equal twice the basic P-P interval and are consistent with a type II 2:1 SA nodal exit block. The PR interval is normal and constant. Lead III.

Hypersensitive Carotid Sinus Syndrome

(see also Chap. 34)

ECG RECOGNITION. Hypersensitive carotid sinus syndrome (Fig. 32–6) is characterized most frequently by ventricular asystole caused by cessation of atrial activity from sinus arrest or SA exit block. AV block is observed less frequently, probably in part because the absence of atrial activity from sinus arrest precludes the manifestations of AV block. However, if an atrial pacemaker maintained an atrial rhythm during the episodes, a higher prevalence of AV block would probably be noted. In symptomatic patients, AV junctional or ventricular escapes generally do not occur or are present at very slow rates, thus suggesting that heightened vagal tone and sympathetic withdrawal can suppress subsidiary pacemakers located in the ventricles, as well as supraventricular structures.

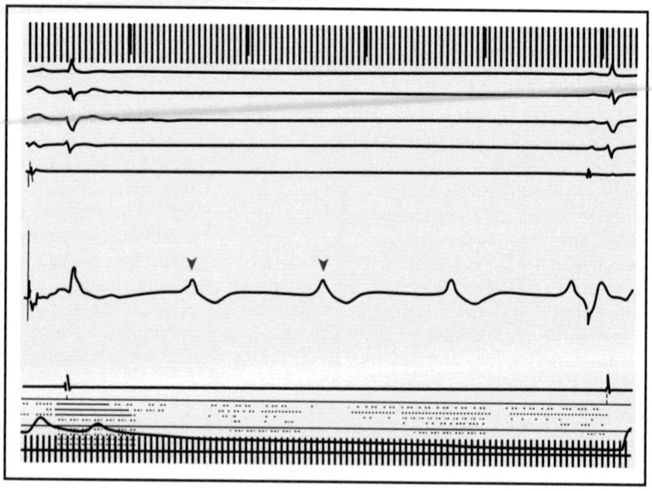

FIGURE 32–4 Sinus node exit block. After a period of atrial pacing (only the last paced cycle is shown), sinus node exit block developed. The tracing demonstrates sinus node potentials (arrowheads), recorded with a catheter electrode, not conducting to the atrium until the last complex. Recordings are leads I, II, III, and V_1, right atrial recording, sinus node recording, and right ventricular apical recording. The bottom tracing is femoral artery blood pressure.

CLINICAL FEATURES. Two types of hypersensitive carotid sinus responses are noted. *Cardioinhibitory* carotid sinus hypersensitivity is generally defined as ventricular asystole exceeding 3 seconds during carotid sinus stimulation, although normal limits have not been carefully established. In fact, asystole exceeding 3 seconds during carotid sinus massage is not common but can occur in asymptomatic subjects (see Fig. 32–6). *Vasodepressor* carotid sinus hypersensitivity is generally defined as a decrease in systolic blood pressure of 50 mm Hg or more without associated cardiac slowing or a decrease in systolic blood pressure exceeding 30 mm Hg when the patient's symptoms are reproduced.

Even if a hyperactive carotid sinus reflex is elicited in patients, particularly in older patients who complain of syncope or presyncope, the hyperactive reflex elicited with carotid sinus massage may not necessarily be responsible for these symptoms. Direct pressure or extension on the carotid sinus from head turning, neck tension, and tight collars can also be a source of syncope by reducing blood flow through the cerebral arteries. Hypersensitive carotid sinus reflex is most commonly associated with coronary artery disease. The mechanism responsible for hypersensitive carotid sinus reflex is not known.

MANAGEMENT. Atropine abolishes cardioinhibitory carotid sinus hypersensitivity. However, most symptomatic patients require pacemaker implantation.

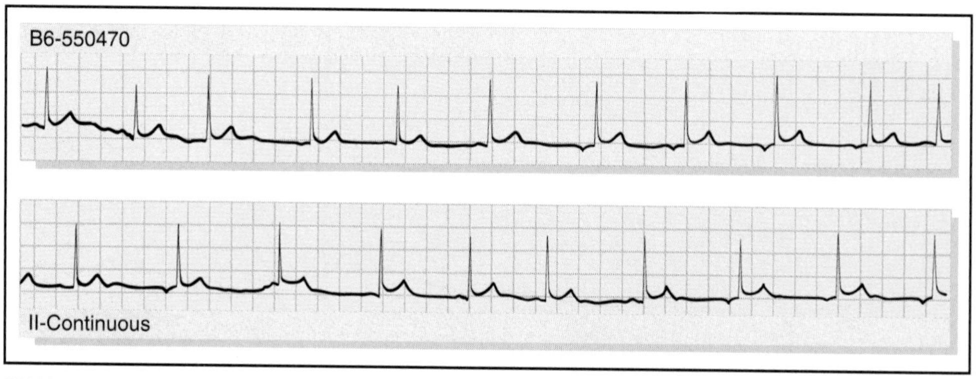

FIGURE 32–5 Wandering atrial pacemaker. As the heart rate slows, the P waves become inverted and then gradually revert toward normal when the heart rate speeds up again. The PR interval shortens to 0.14 second with the inverted P wave and is 0.16 second with the upright P wave. This phasic variation in cycle length with varying P wave contour suggests a shift in pacemaker site and is characteristic of wandering atrial pacemaker.

Because AV block can occur during periods of hypersensitive carotid reflex, some form of *ventricular* pacing, with or without atrial pacing, is generally required. Atropine and pacing do not prevent the decrease in systemic blood pressure in the vasodepressor form of carotid sinus hypersensitivity, which may result from inhibition of sympathetic vasoconstrictor nerves and possibly from activation of cholinergic sympathetic vasodilator fibers. Combinations of vasodepressor and cardioinhibitory types can occur, and vasodepression can account for continued syncope after pacemaker implantation in some patients. Patients who have a hyperactive carotid sinus reflex that does not cause symptoms require no treatment. Drugs such as digitalis, alpha-methyldopa, clonidine, and propranolol can enhance the response to carotid sinus massage and be responsible for symptoms in some patients. Elastic support hose and sodium-retaining drugs may be helpful in patients with vasodepressor responses.

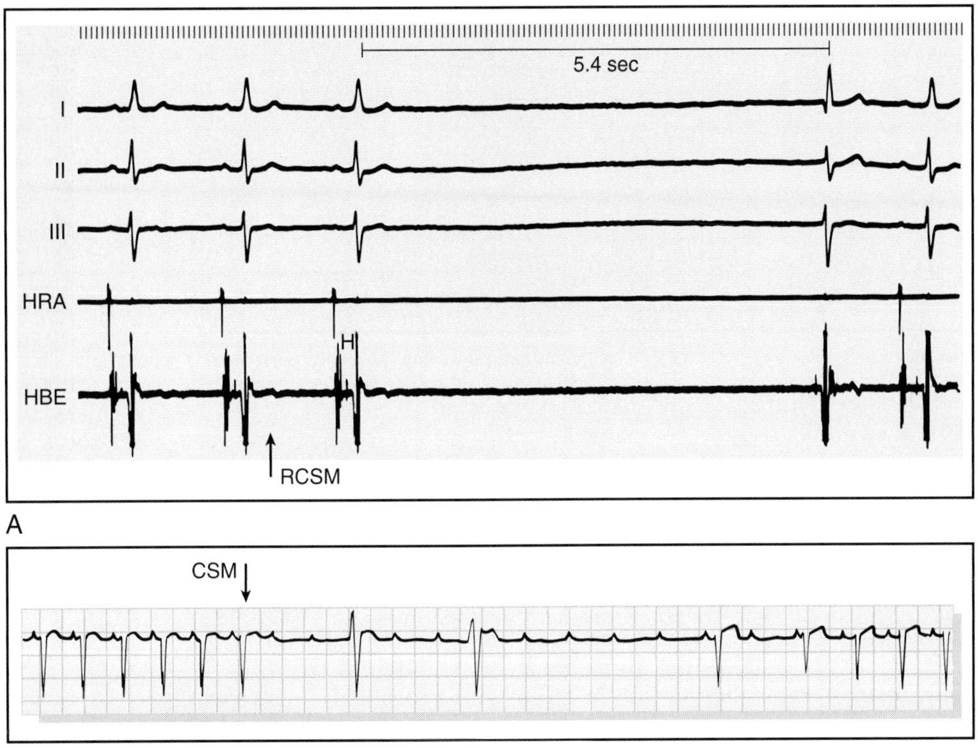

FIGURE 32–6 **A,** Right carotid sinus massage (RCSM) (arrow) results in sinus arrest and a ventricular escape beat (probably fascicular) 5.4 seconds later. Sinus discharge then resumes. **B,** Carotid sinus massage (CSM) (arrow; monitor lead) results in slight sinus slowing but, more important, advanced atrioventricular block. Obviously, an atrial pacemaker without ventricular pacing would be inappropriate for this patient.

Sick Sinus Syndrome

ECG RECOGNITION. *Sick sinus syndrome* is a term that is applied to a syndrome encompassing a number of sinus nodal abnormalities, including (1) persistent spontaneous sinus bradycardia not caused by drugs and inappropriate for the physiological circumstance; (2) sinus arrest or exit block (Fig. 32–7); (3) combinations of SA and AV conduction disturbances; or (4) alternation of paroxysms of rapid regular or irregular atrial tachyarrhythmias and periods of slow atrial and ventricular rates (bradycardia-tachycardia syndrome [Fig. 32–8]). More than one of these conditions can be recorded in the same patient on different occasions, and often their mechanisms can be shown to be causally interrelated and combined with an abnormal state of AV conduction or automaticity. Rapid atrial rates can "remodel" the sinus node and depress its automaticity, so the sinus bradycardia may be functional in part and reversible.[3]

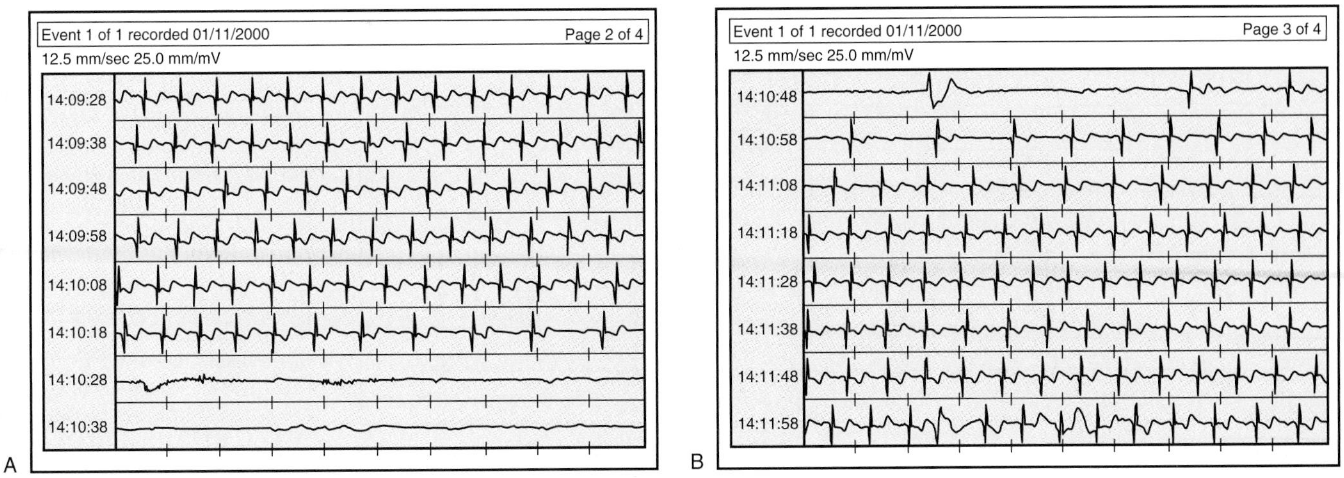

FIGURE 32–7 Continuous recording from an implanted loop recorder in a patient with syncope. The tracing shows paroxysmal sinus node arrest and a sinus pause of nearly 30 seconds. The preceding sinus cycle length appears to lengthen just prior to the pause, suggesting an autonomic component to the pause. There is also a single ventricular escape complex at 14:10:48.

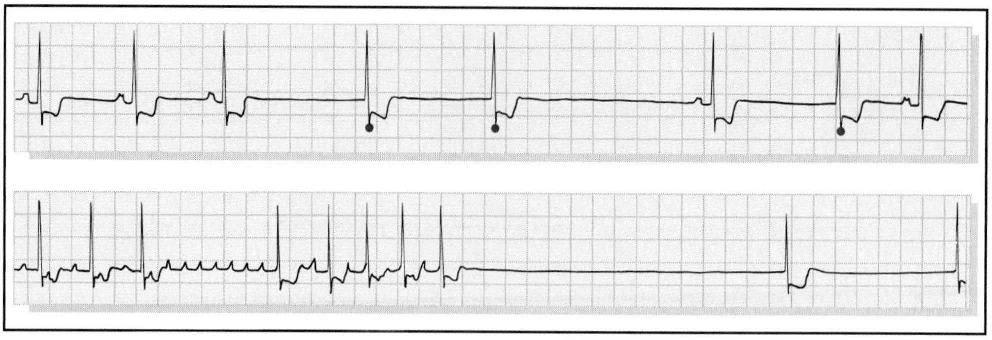

FIGURE 32–8 Sick sinus syndrome with bradycardia-tachycardia. **Top,** Intermittent sinus arrest is apparent with junctional escape beats at irregular intervals (red circles, top). **Bottom,** In this continuous monitor lead recording, a short episode of atrial flutter is followed by almost 5 seconds of asystole before a junctional escape rhythm resumes. The patient became presyncopal at this point.

Patients who have sinus node disease can be categorized as having intrinsic sinus node disease unrelated to autonomic abnormalities or combinations of intrinsic and autonomic abnormalities. Symptomatic patients with sinus pauses and/or SA exit block frequently show abnormal responses on electrophysiological testing and can have a relatively high incidence of atrial fibrillation. In children, sinus node dysfunction most commonly occurs in those with congenital or acquired heart disease, particularly following corrective cardiac surgery. Sick sinus syndrome can occur in the absence of other cardiac abnormalities. The course of the disease is frequently intermittent and unpredictable because it is influenced by the severity of the underlying heart disease. Excessive physical training can heighten vagal tone and produce syncope related to sinus bradycardia or AV conduction abnormalities in otherwise normal individuals.

The anatomical basis of sick sinus syndrome can involve total or subtotal destruction of the sinus node, areas of nodal-atrial discontinuity, inflammatory or degenerative changes in the nerves and ganglia surrounding the node, and pathological changes in the atrial wall. Fibrosis and fatty infiltration occur, and the sclerodegenerative processes generally involve the sinus node and the AV node or the bundle of His and its branches or distal subdivisions.[4] Occlusion of the sinus node artery may be important.

MANAGEMENT. For patients with sick sinus syndrome, treatment depends on the basic rhythm problem but generally involves permanent pacemaker implantation when symptoms are manifested (see Chap. 31). Pacing for the bradycardia, combined with drug therapy to treat the tachycardia, is required in those with bradycardia-tachycardia syndrome.

SINUS NODAL REENTRY TACHYCARDIA

ECG RECOGNITION. The rate of sinus nodal reentrant tachycardia varies from 80 to 200 beats/min but is generally slower than the other forms of supraventricular tachycardia, with an average rate of 130 to 140 beats/min (Fig. 32-9). Electrocardiographically, P waves are identical or very similar to the sinus P wave; the PR interval is related to the tachycardia rate, but generally the RP interval is long, with a shorter PR interval (Fig. 32-10D). AV block can occur without affecting the tachycardia, and vagal maneuvers can slow and then abruptly terminate the tachycardia. Electrophysiologically, the tachycardia can be initiated and terminated by premature atrial and, uncommonly, premature ventricular stimulation (see Fig. 32-9). Initiation of sinus nodal reentry does not depend on a critical degree of intraatrial or AV nodal conduction delay, and the atrial activation sequence is the same as during sinus rhythm. An AV nodal Wenckebach block during the tachycardia is common. The development of a bundle branch block does not affect the cycle length or PR interval during tachycardia.

Sinus nodal reentry may account for 5 to 10 percent of cases of supraventricular tachycardia. It occurs in all age groups without sex predilection. Patients may be slightly older and have a higher incidence of heart disease than do patients with supraventricular tachycardia resulting from other mechanisms. Many may not seek medical attention because the relatively slow rate of the tachycardia does not result in serious symptoms. On the other hand, sinus nodal reentry may be responsible for apparent "anxiety-related sinus tachycardia" in some patients. Drugs such as beta blockers, calcium-channel blockers, and digitalis may be effective in terminating and preventing recurrences of sinus node reentrant tachycardia. Catheter ablation is highly effective in treating this arrhythmia and does not produce sinus node dysfunction.

Disturbances of Atrial Rhythm

Premature Atrial Complexes

Premature complexes are among the most common causes of an irregular pulse. They can originate from any area in the heart—most frequently from the ventricles, less often from the atria and the AV junctional area, and rarely from the sinus node. Although premature complexes arise commonly in normal hearts, they are more often associated with structural heart disease and increase in frequency with age.

ECG RECOGNITION. The diagnosis of premature atrial complexes (Fig. 32–11) is indicated on the ECG by a premature P wave with a PR

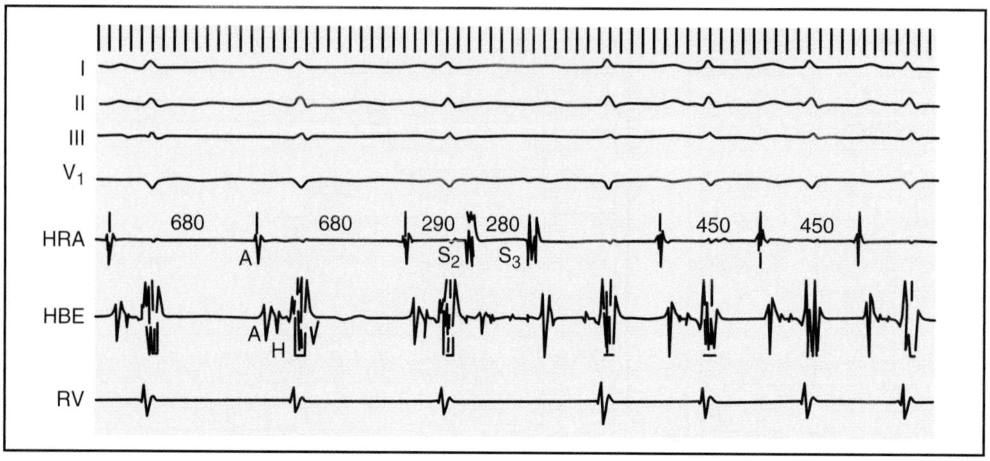

FIGURE 32–9 Sinus node reentry. After three spontaneous sinus-initiated beats, premature stimulation of the high right atrium (S_2, S_3) initiates a sustained tachycardia at a cycle length of 450 milliseconds that has the identical high-low atrial activation sequence characteristic of sinus node discharge. This is sinus node reentry. Leads I, II, III, and V_1 are scalar leads. A = atrial electrogram; H = His electrogram; HBE = His bundle electrogram; HRA = high right atrial electrogram; RV = right ventricular electrogram; V = ventricular electrogram. Numbers are milliseconds.

nterval exceeding 120 milliseconds (except in Wolff-Parkinson-White [WPW] syndrome, in which case the PR interval is usually less than 120 milliseconds). Although the contour of a premature P wave can resemble that of a normal sinus P wave, it generally differs. While variations in the basic sinus rate can at times make the diagnosis of prematurity difficult, differences in the contour of the P waves are usually apparent and indicate a different focus of origin. When a premature atrial complex occurs early in diastole, conduction may not be completely normal. The AV junction may still be refractory from the preceding beat and prevent propagation of the impulse (blocked or nonconducted premature atrial complex [Fig. 32–11A]) or cause conduction to be slowed (premature atrial complex with a prolonged PR interval). As a general rule, the RP interval is inversely related to the PR interval; thus, a short RP interval produced by an early premature atrial complex occurring close to the preceding QRS complex is followed by a long PR interval. When premature atrial complexes occur early in the cardiac cycle, the premature P waves can be difficult to discern because they are superimposed on T waves. Careful examination of tracings from several leads may be necessary before the premature atrial complex is recognized as a slight deformity of the T wave. Often, such premature atrial complexes are blocked before reaching the ventricle and can be misinterpreted as a sinus pause or sinus exit block (Fig. 32–11A).

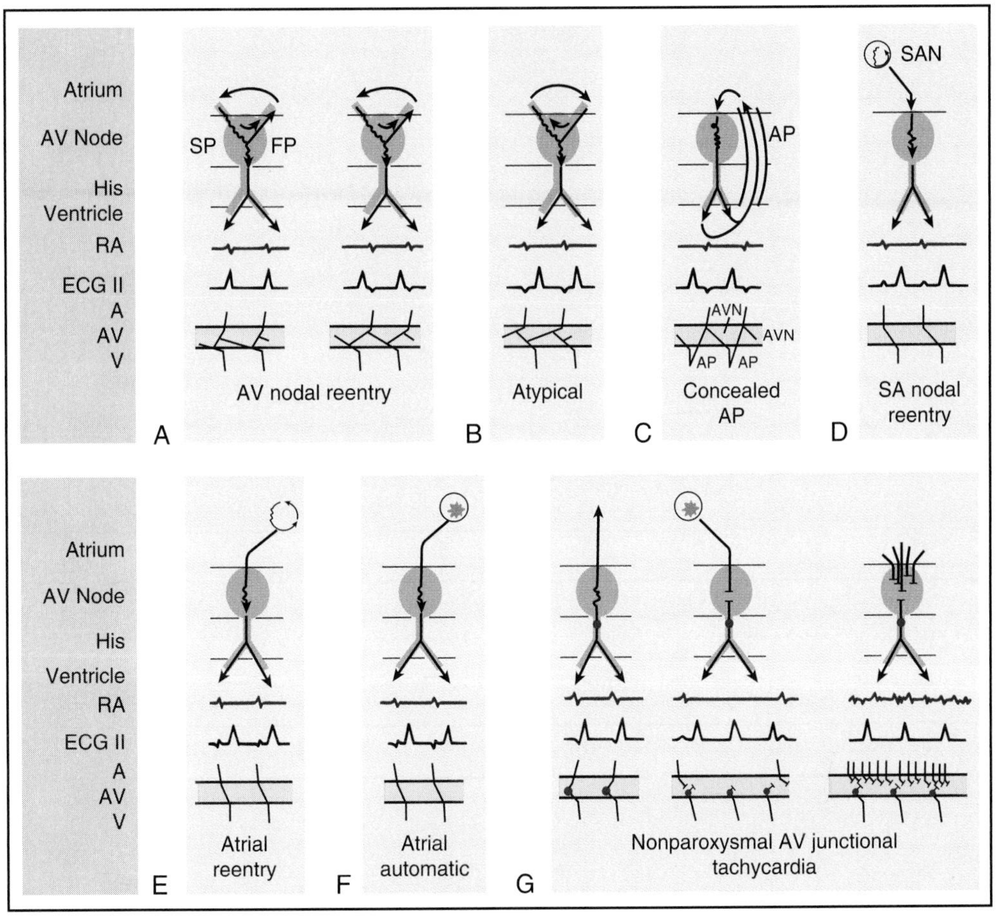

FIGURE 32–10 Diagrammatic representation of various tachycardias. In the upper portion of each example, a schematic of the presumed anatomical pathways is drawn; in the lower half, the electrocardiographic (ECG) appearance and the explanatory ladder diagram are depicted. **A,** Atrioventricular (AV) nodal reentry. In the left example, reentrant excitation is drawn with retrograde atrial activity occurring simultaneously with ventricular activity as a result of anterograde conduction over the slow AV nodal pathway (SP) and retrograde conduction over the fast AV nodal pathway (FP). In the right example, atrial activity occurs slightly later than ventricular activity because of retrograde conduction delay. **B,** Atypical AV nodal reentry caused by anterograde conduction over a fast AV nodal pathway and retrograde conduction over a slow AV nodal pathway. **C,** Concealed accessory pathway (AP). Reciprocating tachycardia is due to anterograde conduction over the AV node (AVN) and retrograde conduction over the accessory pathway. Retrograde P waves occur after the QRS complex. **D,** Sinus nodal reentry. The tachycardia is due to reentry within the sinus node, which then conducts the impulse to the rest of the heart. SA = sinoatrial; SAN = sinoatrial node. **E,** Atrial reentry. Tachycardia is due to reentry within the atrium, which then conducts the impulse to the rest of the heart. **F,** Automatic atrial tachycardia (star indicates origin). Tachycardia is due to automatic discharge in the atrium, which then conducts the impulse to the rest of the heart; it is difficult to distinguish from atrial reentry. **G,** Nonparoxysmal AV junctional tachycardia. Various manifestations of this tachycardia are depicted with retrograde atrial capture, AV dissociation with the sinus node in control of the atria, and AV dissociation with atrial fibrillation. Star indicates sinus node discharge. Red circles indicate site of junctional discharge.

The length of the pause following any premature complex or series of premature complexes is determined by the interaction of several factors. If the premature atrial complex occurs when the sinus node and perinodal tissue are not refractory, the impulse can be conducted into the sinus node, discharge it prematurely, and cause the next sinus cycle to begin from that time. The interval between the two normal P waves flanking a premature atrial complex that has reset the timing of the basic sinus rhythm is less than twice the normal P-P interval, and the pause after the premature atrial complex is said to be "noncompensatory." Referring to Figure 32-11E and F, reset (noncompensatory pause) occurs when the A_1-A_2 interval plus the A_2-A_3 interval is less than two times the A_1-A_1 interval and the A_2-A_3 interval is greater than the A_1-A_1 interval. The interval between the premature atrial complex (A_2) and the following sinus-initiated P wave (A_3) exceeds one sinus cycle but is less than "fully compensatory" (see later) because the A_2-A_3 interval is lengthened by the time that it takes the ectopic atrial impulse to conduct to the sinus node and depolarize it and then for the sinus impulse to return to the atrium. These factors lengthen the return cycle, that is, the interval between the premature atrial complex (A_2) and the following sinus-initiated P wave (A_3) (Fig. 32-11E and F). Premature discharge of the sinus node by an early premature atrial complex can temporarily depress sinus nodal automatic activity and cause the sinus node to beat more slowly initially (Fig. 32-11D). Often when this happens, the interval between the A_3 and the next sinus-initiated P wave exceeds the A_1-A_1 interval.

Less commonly, the premature atrial complex encounters a refractory sinus node or perinodal tissue (Fig. 32–11F), in which case the timing of the basic sinus rhythm is not altered since the sinus node is not reset by the premature atrial complex, and the interval between the two normal, sinus-initiated P waves flanking the premature atrial complex is twice the normal P-P interval. The interval following this premature atrial discharge is said to be a "full compensatory pause," that is, of sufficient duration so that the P-P interval bounding the premature atrial complex is twice the normal P-P interval. However, sinus arrhythmia can lengthen or shorten this pause. Rarely, an *interpolated premature atrial* complex

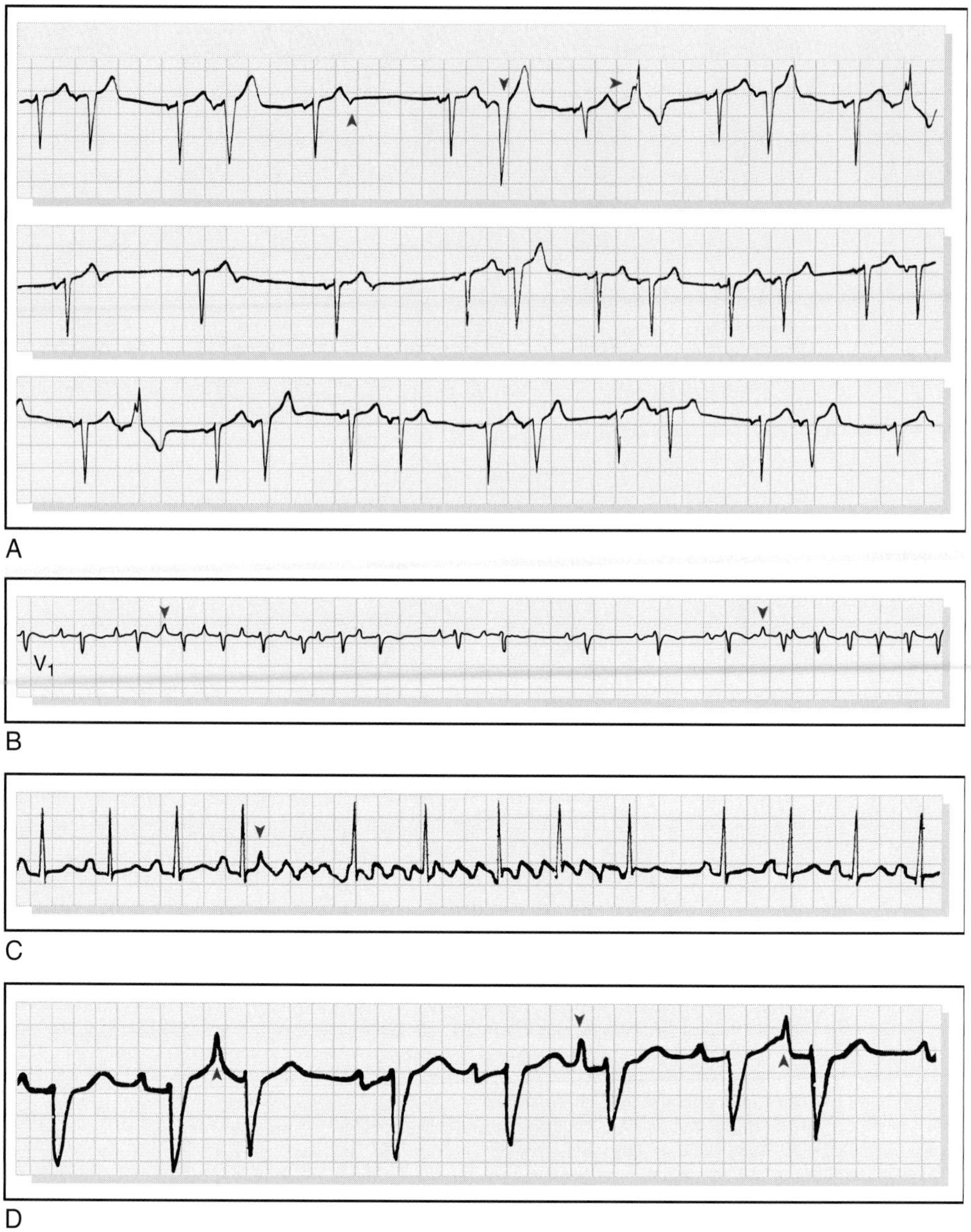

FIGURE 32–11 **A,** Premature atrial complexes (PACs) that block conduction entirely or conduct with a functional right or functional left bundle branch block. Depending on the preceding cycle length and coupling interval of the PAC, the latter blocks conduction entirely in the atrioventricular (AV) node (arrowhead ↑) or conducts with a functional left bundle branch block (arrowhead ↓) or functional right bundle branch block (arrowhead →). **B,** A PAC on the left (arrowhead) initiates AV nodal reentry that is due to reentry anterogradely and retrogradely over two slow AV nodal pathways, with a retrograde P wave produced midway in the cardiac cycle. On the right, a PAC (arrowhead) initiates AV nodal reentry as a result of anterograde conduction over the slow pathway and retrograde conduction over the fast pathway (see Fig. 32–10A), which produces a retrograde P wave in the terminal portion of the QRS complex that simulates an r′ wave. **C** and **D,** A PAC (arrowhead ↓) initiating a short run of atrial flutter **(C)** and a PAC (arrowhead ↑) depressing return of the next sinus nodal discharge **(D)**. A slightly later PAC (arrowhead ↓) in **D** does not depress sinus nodal automaticity. **B** to **D,** Monitor leads.

Continued

may occur. In this case, the pause after the premature atrial complex is very short, and the interval bounded by the normal sinus–initiated P waves on each side of the premature atrial complex is only slightly longer than or equals one normal P-P cycle length. The interpolated premature atrial complex fails to affect the sinus nodal pacemaker, and the sinus impulse following the premature atrial complex is conducted to the ventricles, often with a slightly lengthened PR interval. An interpolated atrial or ventricular premature complex of any type represents the only type of premature systole that does not actually replace the normally conducted beat. Premature atrial complexes can originate in the sinus node and are identified by premature P waves that have a contour identical to that of the normal sinus P wave.

On occasion, when the AV node has had sufficient time to repolarize and conduct without delay, the supraventricular QRS complex initiated by the premature atrial complex can be aberrant in configuration because the His-Purkinje system or ventricular muscle has *not* completely repolarized and conducts with a functional delay or block (Fig. 32–11A). The refractory period of cardiac fibers is directly related to cycle length. (In an adult, the AV nodal effective refractory period is prolonged at shorter cycle lengths.) A slow heart rate (long cycle length) produces a longer His-Purkinje refractory period than does a faster heart rate. As a consequence, a premature atrial complex that follows a long R-R interval (long refractory period) can result in a functional bundle branch block (aberrant ventricular conduction). Since the right bundle branch at long cycles has a longer refractory period than the left bundle branch does, aberration with a right bundle branch block pattern at slow rates occurs more commonly than aberration with a left bundle branch block pattern. At shorter cycles, the refractory period of the left bundle branch exceeds that of the right bundle branch, and a left bundle branch block pattern may be more likely to occur.

CLINICAL FEATURES. Premature atrial complexes can occur in a variety of situations, such as during infection, inflammation, or myocardial ischemia, or they can be provoked by a variety of medications, by tension states, or by tobacco, alcohol, or caffeine. Premature atrial complexes can precipitate or presage the occurrence of sustained supraventricular (Fig. 32–11B and C) and, rarely, ventricular tachyarrhythmias.

MANAGEMENT. Premature atrial complexes generally do not require therapy.[5] In symptomatic patients or when the premature atrial complexes precipitate tachycardias, treatment with digitalis, a beta blocker, or a calcium antagonist can be tried.

Atrial Flutter (see also Chap. 30)

Atrial flutter is now recognized as a macro-reentrant atrial rhythm. Typical atrial flutter (sometimes called *type I*) is a reentrant rhythm in the right atrium constrained anteriorly by the tricuspid annulus[6] and posteriorly by the crista terminalis and eustachian ridge. The flutter can circulate in a counterclockwise direction around the tricuspid annulus in the frontal plane (typical flutter, counterclockwise flutter) or in a clockwise direction (atypical, clockwise, or reverse flutter).[7,8] Since both of these forms of atrial flutter are constrained by anatomical structures, their rates and flutter wave morphology on surface ECG are consistent and predictable (see later).[7] Other forms of atrial flutter are now recognized as distinct types and include atrial macro-reentry caused by incisional scars from prior atrial surgery,[9] idiopathic fibrosis in areas of the atrium, or other anatomical or functional conduction barriers in the atria.[7,8,10] Because the barriers that constrain these atrial flutters are variable, the ECG pattern of these so-called atypical atrial flutters can be varied. Oftentimes, flutter wave morphology changes during the same episode of flutter, which indicates multiple circuits and/or nonfixed conduction barriers.

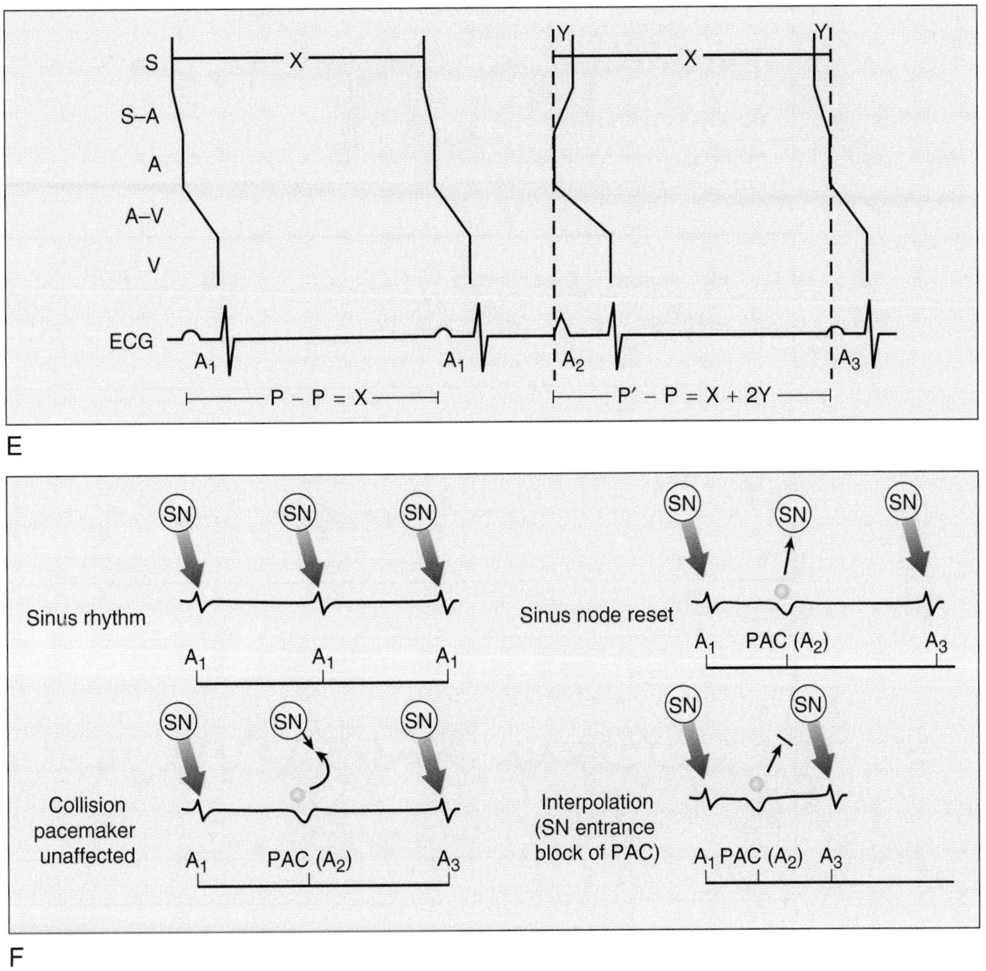

FIGURE 32–11, cont'd **E,** Diagrammatic example of the effects of a PAC. The sinus interval (A_1-A_1) equals X. The third P wave represents a PAC (A_2) that reaches and discharges the sinoatrial (SA) node, which causes the next sinus cycle to begin at that time. Therefore, the P-P (A_2-A_3) interval equals X + 2Y milliseconds, assuming no depression of SA nodal automaticity. **F,** Diagram of interactions of a PAC (yellow circles indicate origin; QRS complexes omitted) with the sinus node (SN) depending on the degree of prematurity. The top represents spontaneous sinus rhythm. The bottom is a late coupled PAC that collides with the exiting sinus impulse and therefore does not affect (or reset) the sinus pacemaker. The next sinus impulse (S_3) occurs at exactly twice the sinus interval. An early coupled PAC in the next diagram is able to penetrate the sinus node and thus resets the pacemaker, thereby resulting in resetting of the sinus node (as depicted in **E**). An even earlier coupled PAC in the lower figure reaches refractory tissue around the sinus node and is thus unable to penetrate the sinus node (SN entrance block); therefore, it does not affect sinus node discharge. The next spontaneous sinus beat (S_3) arrives exactly at the sinus interval. (**E,** Modified from Zipes DP, Fisch C: Premature atrial contraction. Arch Intern Med 128:453, 1971.)

ECG RECOGNITION. The atrial rate during typical atrial flutter is usually 250 to 350 beats/min, although it is occasionally slower, particularly when the patient is treated with antiarrhythmic drugs, which can reduce the rate to the range of 200 beats/min. If such slowing occurs, the ventricles can respond in a 1:1 fashion to the slower atrial rate. Ordinarily, the atrial rate is about 300 beats/min, and in untreated patients the ventricular rate is half the atrial rate, that is, 150 beats/min (Fig. 32–12A and F). A significantly slower ventricular rate (in the absence of drugs) suggests abnormal AV conduction. In children, in patients with the preexcitation syndrome (see Chap. 30), occasionally in patients with hyperthyroidism, and in those whose AV nodes conduct rapidly, atrial flutter can conduct to the ventricle in a 1:1 fashion and produce a ventricular rate of 300 beats/min.

In typical atrial flutter, the ECG reveals identically recurring regular sawtooth flutter waves (see Figs. 32–11C and 32–12B and F) and evidence of continual electrical activity (lack of an isoelectric interval between flutter waves), often best visualized in leads II, III, aV_f, or V_1 (Fig. 32–13). In some instances, transient slowing of the ventricular response, either with carotid sinus massage (see Fig. 32–12B) or with adenosine (see Fig. 32–12F), is necessary to visualize the flutter waves. The flutter waves for (type I) typical atrial flutter are inverted (negative) in these leads because of a counterclockwise reentrant pathway, and sometimes they are upright (positive) when the reentrant loop is clockwise (see Fig. 32–13). When the flutter waves are upright from clockwise rotation, they are often notched. If the AV conduction ratio remains constant, the ventricular rhythm will be regular; if the ratio of conducted beats varies (usually the result of a Wenckebach AV block), the ventricular rhythm will be irregular. Alternation between 2:1 and 4:1 AV conduction often occurs and can be due to two levels of block—2:1 high in the AV node and 3:2 lower down. The irregular ventricular response is frequently due to Wenckebach periodicity. Recurrent alternation of short and long ventricular intervals can be due to concealed conduction. Various degrees of penetration into the AV junction by flutter impulses can also influence AV conduction. The ratio of flutter waves to conducted ventricular complexes is most often an even number (e.g., 2:1, 4:1, and so on).

CLINICAL FEATURES. Atrial flutter is less common than atrial fibrillation. It can occur as a result of atrial dilation from septal defects, pulmonary emboli, mitral or tricuspid valve stenosis or regurgitation, or chronic ventricular failure but can also (rarely) occur without underlying heart disease. Toxic and metabolic conditions that affect the heart, such as thyrotoxicosis, alcoholism, and pericarditis, can cause atrial flutter. Occasionally, it can be congenital, follow surgery for congenital heart disease, or even occur in utero. When it

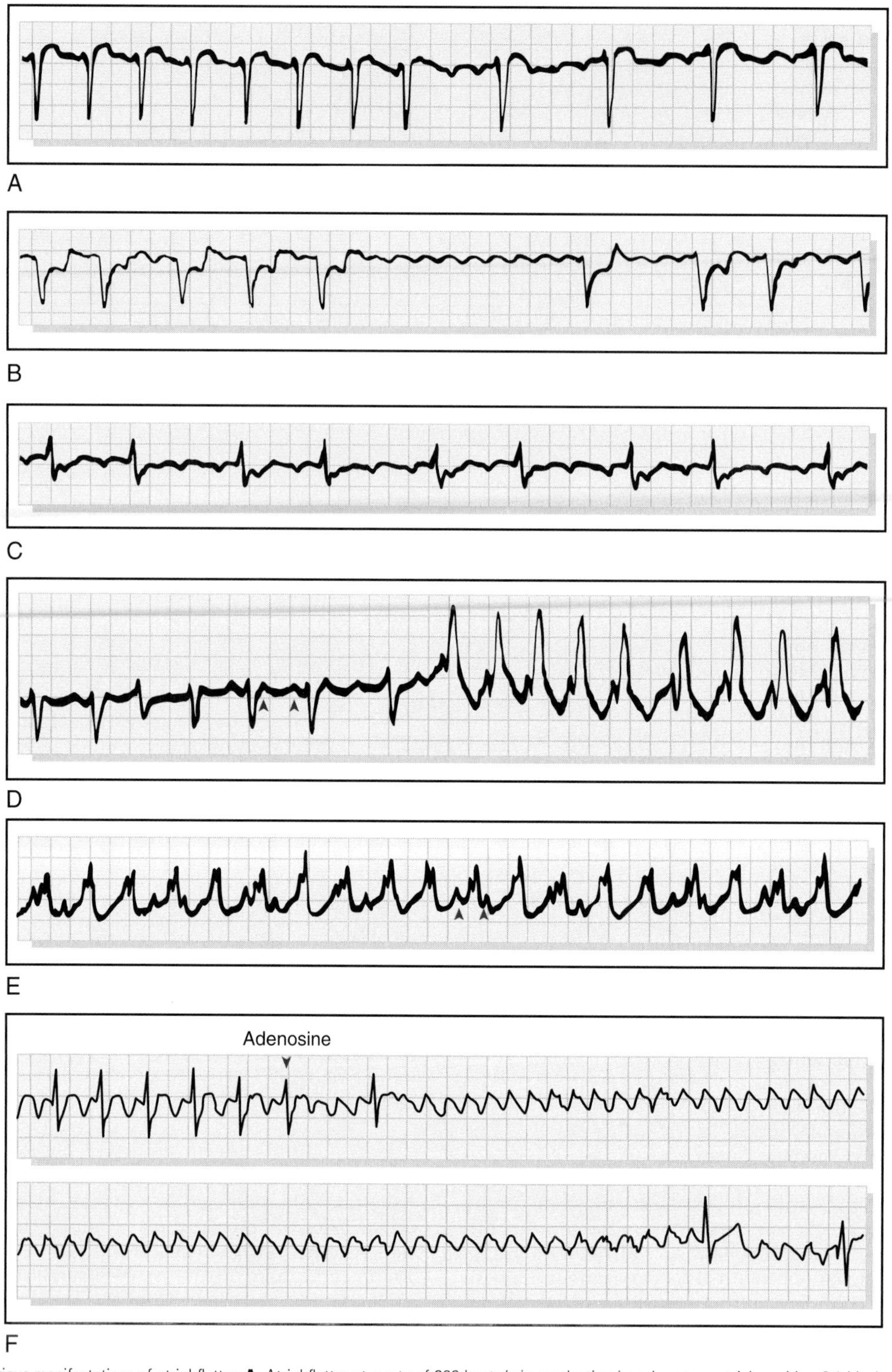

FIGURE 32–12 Various manifestations of atrial flutter. **A,** Atrial flutter at a rate of 300 beats/min conducting impulses to ventricles with a 2:1 block. In the midportion of the tracing, carotid sinus massage converts the block to 4:1, and the ventricular rate slows to 75 beats/min. **B,** Carotid sinus massage produces a transient period of atrioventricular (AV) block clearly revealing the flutter waves. **C,** Quinidine has slowed the atrial flutter rate to approximately 188 beats/min. The block is variable. **D,** Wide QRS complexes with an rSR′ configuration in V_1 begin after a short cycle that follows a long cycle in the midportion of the electrocardiogram strip. This pattern represents a functional right bundle branch block. Arrowheads indicate flutter waves. **E,** The QRS complexes are 0.12 second in duration and have a regular interval at a rate of 200 beats/min. Atrial activity is also regular at a rate of 300 beats/min and independent of ventricular activity (arrows). Thus, atrial flutter is present with a probable ventricular tachycardia, an example of complete AV dissociation. **F,** Adenosine injection given to a patient with a supraventricular tachycardia (SVT) at a rate of 150 beats/min reveals underlying atrial flutter, thus diagnosing the SVT as atrial flutter with 2:1 AV conduction and the flutter waves obscured within the T waves. Monitor leads in **A, B, C, E,** and **F**.

follows reparative surgery of congenital heart disease it usually involves an atriotomy and often occurs years after the surgery. In children, continued episodes of atrial flutter are associated with an increased possibility of sudden death.

Atrial flutter usually responds to carotid sinus massage with a decrease in the ventricular rate in stepwise multiples and returns in reverse manner to the former ventricular rate at the termination of carotid massage (see Fig. 32–12A). *Physical examination* may reveal rapid flutter waves in the jugular venous pulse. If the relationship of flutter waves to conducted QRS complexes remains constant, the first heart sound will have a constant intensity. Occasionally, sounds caused by atrial contraction can be auscultated.

MANAGEMENT. Cardioversion (see Chap. 30) is commonly the initial treatment of choice for atrial flutter since it promptly and effectively restores sinus rhythm. Cardioversion can be accomplished with synchronous direct current (DC), which often requires relatively low energies (<50 J). If the electrical shock results in atrial fibrillation, a second shock at a higher energy level is used to restore sinus rhythm or, depending on clinical circumstances, the atrial fibrillation can be left untreated. The latter can revert to atrial flutter or sinus rhythm. The short-acting antiarrhythmic medication ibutilide can also be given IV to convert atrial flutter. Ibutilide appears to successfully cardiovert about 60 to 90 percent of episodes of atrial flutter.[11,12] However, because this medication prolongs the QT interval, torsades de pointes is a potential complication during and shortly after the infusion. Other medications such as procainamide can be given to chemically convert atrial flutter. *Rapid atrial pacing* with a catheter in the esophagus or the right atrium can effectively terminate type I (counterclockwise and clockwise) and some forms of atypical atrial flutter in most patients and produce sinus rhythm or atrial fibrillation with a slowing of the ventricular rate and concomitant clinical improvement. Although the risk of thromboembolism is lower than that for atrial fibrillation, patients with atrial flutter do appear to have a risk of thromboembolism immediately after conversion to sinus rhythm.[13-15]

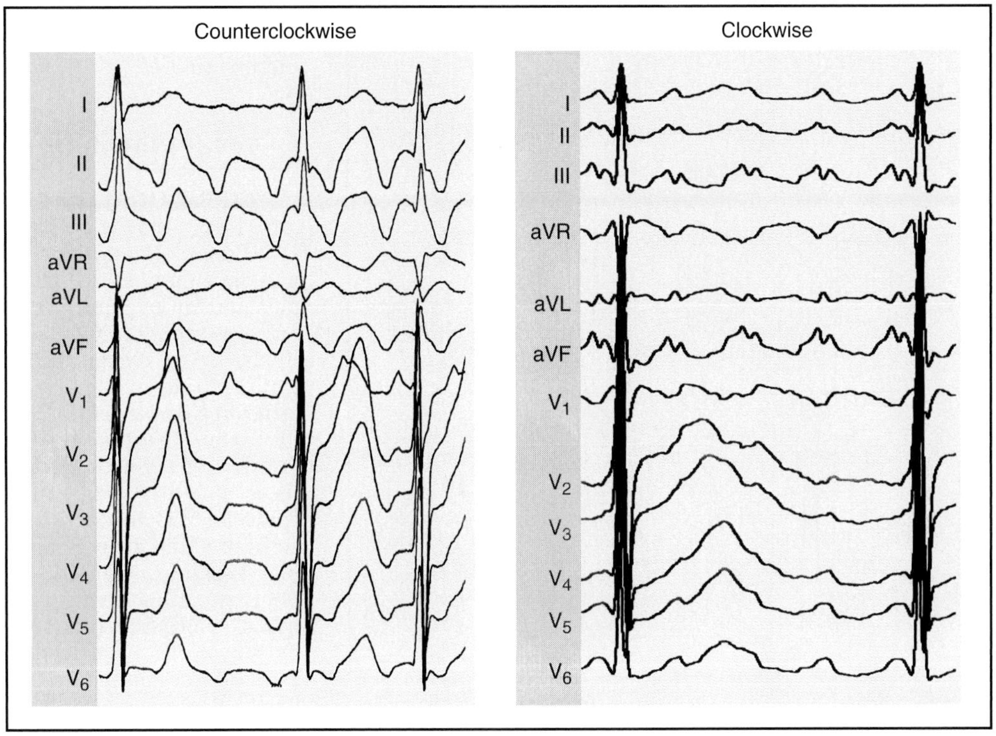

FIGURE 32–13 Twelve-lead electrocardiogram of counterclockwise and clockwise atrial flutter. In counterclockwise atrial flutter, the flutter waves are negative in leads II, III, aVL, and V_6 and upright in V_1. In counterclockwise atrial flutter, the flutter waves are upright in leads II, III, and aVF and often notched.

Verapamil (see Chap. 30) given as an initial bolus of 5 to 10 mg IV, followed by a constant infusion at a rate of 5 mg/kg/min, or *diltiazem* 0.25 mg/kg to slow the ventricular response, can be tried. *Adenosine* produces a transient AV block and can be used to reveal flutter waves if diagnosis of the arrhythmias is in doubt. It will not generally terminate the atrial flutter and can provoke atrial fibrillation. Esmolol, a beta-adrenergic blocker with a 9-minute elimination half-life, can be used to slow the ventricular rate.

If the flutter cannot be electrically cardioverted, terminated by pacing, or slowed by the aforementioned drugs, a *short-acting digitalis preparation* (such as digoxin or deslanoside) can be tried alone or with a calcium antagonist or beta blocker. The dose of digitalis necessary to slow the ventricular response varies and at times can result in toxic levels because it is often difficult to slow the ventricular rate during atrial flutter. Frequently, atrial fibrillation develops after digitalis administration and can revert to normal sinus rhythm on withdrawal of digitalis treatment; occasionally, normal sinus rhythm may occur without intervening atrial fibrillation. IV amiodarone has been shown to slow the ventricular rate as effectively as digoxin.

If the atrial flutter persists, class IA or IC drugs (see Chap. 30) can be tried in an attempt to restore sinus rhythm and prevent recurrence of atrial flutter. Amiodarone, especially in low doses of 200 mg/day, can also prevent recurrences. Side effects of these drugs, especially proarrhythmic responses, must be carefully considered and are dealt with at length in Chapter 30. Sometimes, treatment of the underlying disorder, such as thyrotoxicosis, is necessary to effect conversion to sinus rhythm. In certain instances, atrial flutter can continue, and if the ventricular rate can be controlled with drugs, conversion to sinus rhythm may not be indicated. Therapy with classes I and III drugs should be discontinued if flutter remains.

It is important to reemphasize that class I or III drugs should *not* be used unless the ventricular rate during atrial flutter has been *slowed* with digitalis or with a calcium antagonist or beta-blocking drug. Because of the vagolytic action of quinidine, procainamide, and disopyramide (see Chap. 30), but primarily because of the ability of class I drugs to slow the flutter rate, AV conduction can be *facilitated* sufficiently to result in a 1:1 ventricular response to the atrial flutter (Fig. 32–14).

Prevention of recurrent atrial flutter is often difficult to achieve medically but should be approached as outlined for the prevention of paroxysmal supraventricular tachycardia resulting from AV nodal reentry (see also Chap. 30). If recurrences cannot be prevented, therapy is directed toward controlling the ventricular rate when the flutter does recur with digitalis alone or combined with beta blockers or calcium antagonists. Mounting evidence indicates that the risk of emboli in atrial flutter may be more significant[13-15] than once thought. Because of this and since many patients with atrial flutter also have atrial fibrillation, anticoagulation is usually warranted. However, carefully controlled studies to determine the degree of embolic risk in patients with only atrial flutter are lacking. Long-term anticoagulation, as in atrial fibrillation, should probably be considered until more definitive data are available. Radiofrequency catheter ablation of typical flutter (counterclockwise and clockwise) is highly effective at curing atrial fibrillation and has a long-term success rate of 90 to 100 percent.[16] Because ablation of atrial flutter is highly effective with little risk, it can be offered as an alternative to

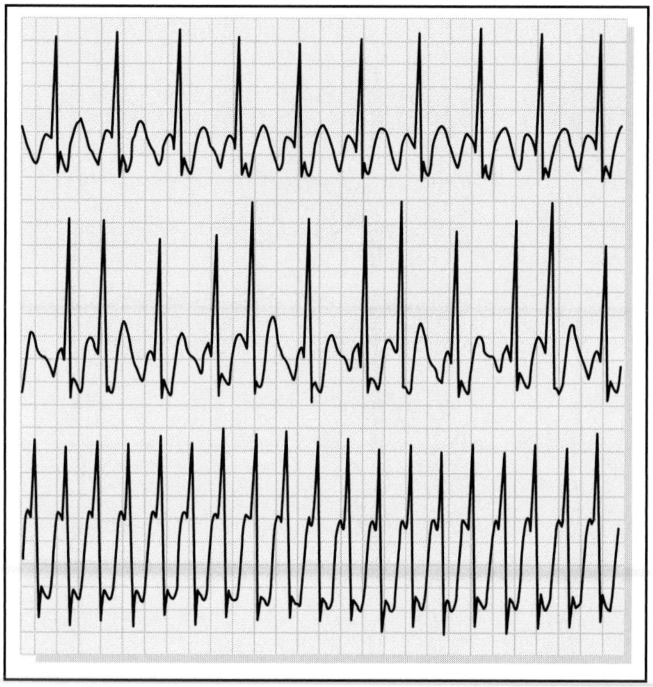

FIGURE 32–14 Atrial flutter with 1:1 conduction caused by flecainide. **Top,** Atrial flutter occurs with 2:1 conduction. **Middle,** 2:1 conduction alternates with 3:2 conduction. **Bottom,** Flecainide administration has been started, and the atrial flutter rate slows, with subsequent 1:1 conduction.

drug therapy. Ablation of other forms of atrial flutter is also effective, although success rates are somewhat lower and more variable.[9,10,17]

Atrial Fibrillation (see also Chap. 30)

ECG RECOGNITION. Atrial fibrillation (Fig. 32–15) is an arrhythmia that is characterized by seemingly disorganized atrial depolarizations without effective atrial contraction. It was once thought that all atrial fibrillation was due to a single mechanism of multiple wavelets propagating in random fashion throughout the atria. It is now apparent that there are likely several mechanisms and that there may be some organization to atrial fibrillation. For example, in many patients atrial fibrillation is due a focal discharge at rapid rates and fibrillatory conduction (heterogeneous conduction due to rapidity of activation) through the atria. Nonetheless, all of these potential mechanisms of atrial fibrillation have a common ECG appearance. During atrial fibrillation, electrical activity of the atrium can be detected on ECG as small, irregular baseline undulations of variable amplitude and morphology, called *f waves*, at a rate of 350 to 600 beats/min. At times, small, fine, rapid f waves can occur and are detectable only by right atrial leads or by intracavitary or esophageal electrodes. The ventricular response is grossly irregular ("irregularly irregular") and, in an untreated patient with normal AV conduction, is usually between 100 and 160 beats/min. In patients with WPW syndrome, the ventricular rate during atrial fibrillation can at times exceed 300 beats/min and lead to ventricular fibrillation. Atrial fibrillation should be suspected when the ECG shows supraventricular complexes at an irregular rhythm and no obvious P waves. The recognizable f waves probably do not represent total atrial activity but depict only the larger vectors generated by the multiple wavelets of depolarization that occur at any given moment.

Each recorded f wave is not conducted through the AV junction, so a rapid ventricular response comparable to the atrial rate does not occur. Many atrial impulses are concealed because of a collision of wavefronts, or they are blocked in the AV junction without reaching the ventricles (i.e., concealed conduction, which accounts for the irregular ventricular rhythm). The refractory period and conductivity of the AV node are determinants of the ventricular rate. When the ventricular rate is very rapid or very slow, it may appear to be more regular. Even though conversion of atrial fibrillation to atrial flutter is accompanied by slowing of the atrial rate, an increase in the ventricular response can result since more atrial impulses are transmitted to the ventricle

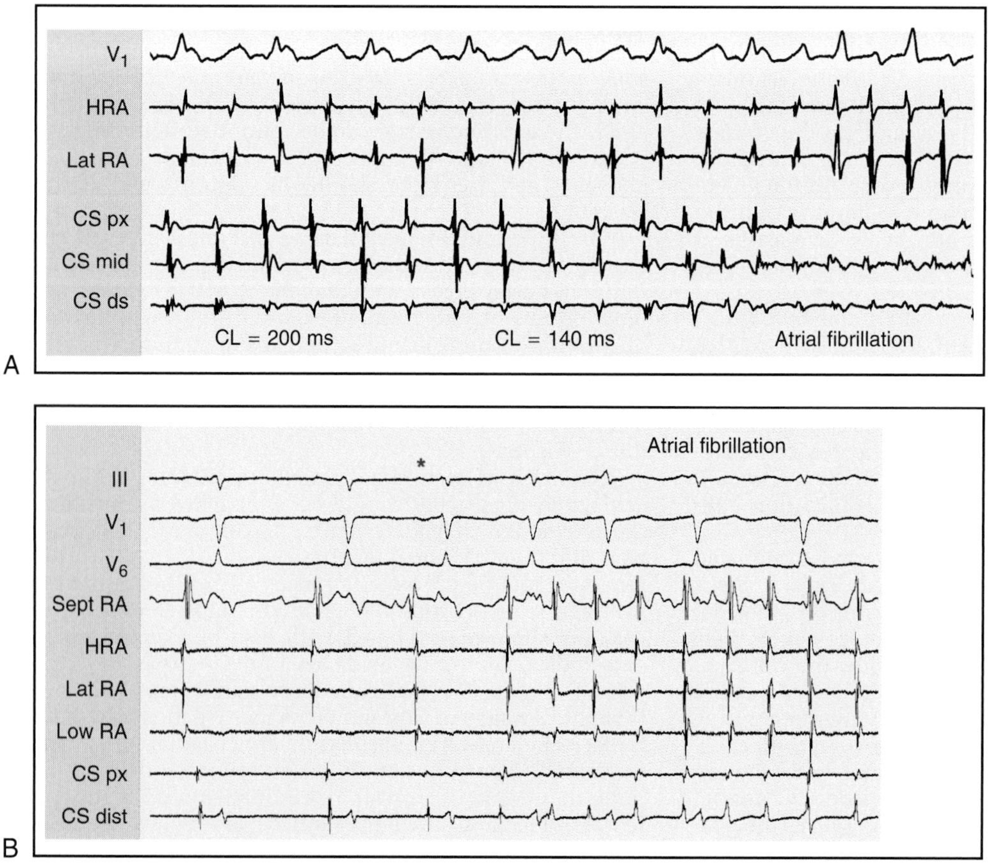

FIGURE 32–15 Atrial fibrillation produced by "focal" mechanisms. **A,** A rapid, regular atrial tachycardia (left side of figure) at a cycle length (CL) of 200 milliseconds degenerates into atrial fibrillation (right side of figure) characterized by rapid, irregular atrial depolarizations. **B,** A premature atrial complex (marked by the asterisk) induces atrial fibrillation (right side of figure). Elimination of these focal triggers for atrial fibrillation can eliminate the atrial fibrillation.

because of less concealed conduction. Also, it is easier to slow the ventricular rate during atrial fibrillation than during atrial flutter with drugs such as digitalis, calcium antagonists, and beta blockers because the increased concealed conduction makes it easier to produce an AV block.

CLINICAL FEATURES. Atrial fibrillation is a common arrhythmia that is found in 1 percent of persons older than 60 years to more than 5 percent of patients older than 69 years. The overall chance of atrial fibrillation developing over a period of two decades in patients older than 30 years, according to Framingham data, is 2 percent. Estimates are that 2.2 million Americans have atrial fibrillation, which occurs more commonly in men than in women.[18] A history of congestive heart failure, valvular heart disease and stroke, left atrial enlargement, abnormal mitral or aortic valve function, treated systemic hypertension, and advanced age are independently associated with the prevalence of atrial fibrillation. Four important aspects of atrial fibrillation are etiology, control of the ventricular rate, prevention of recurrences, and prevention of thromboembolic episodes. Occult or manifested thyrotoxicosis should be considered in patients with recent-onset atrial fibrillation. Atrial fibrillation can be intermittent or chronic and may be influenced by autonomic activity. Atrial fibrillation, whether it is persistent or intermittent, predisposes to stroke. Symptoms as a result of atrial fibrillation are determined by multiple factors, including the underlying cardiac status, the rapid ventricular rate, and loss of atrial contraction.

Physical findings include a slight variation in intensity of the first heart sound, absence of *a* waves in the jugular venous pulse, and an irregularly irregular ventricular rhythm. Often, with fast ventricular rates a significant pulse deficit appears, during which the auscultated or palpated apical rate is faster than the rate palpated at the wrist (pulse deficit) because each contraction is not sufficiently strong to open the aortic valve or transmit an arterial pressure wave through the peripheral artery. If the ventricular rhythm becomes regular in patients with atrial fibrillation, conversion to sinus rhythm, atrial tachycardia, or atrial flutter with a constant ratio of conducted beats or the development of junctional tachycardia or ventricular tachycardia (VT) should be suspected.

EMBOLIZATION AND ANTICOAGULATION. In addition to hemodynamic alterations, the risk of systemic emboli, probably arising in the left atrial cavity or appendage as a result of circulatory stasis, is an important consideration (see Chap. 80). Nonvalvular atrial fibrillation is the most common cardiac disease associated with cerebral embolism. In fact, almost half of cardiogenic emboli in the United States occur in patients with nonvalvular atrial fibrillation. The risk of stroke in patients with nonvalvular atrial fibrillation is five to seven times greater than that in controls without atrial fibrillation. Overall, 20 to 25 percent of ischemic strokes are due to cardiogenic emboli.

Many studies have evaluated the risk of stroke in patients with atrial fibrillation and the benefits of anticoagulation and antiplatelet therapy.[19-25] Patients with mitral stenosis and atrial fibrillation have a 4 to 6 percent incidence of embolism per year. Risk factors that predict stroke in patients with nonvalvular atrial fibrillation include a history of previous stroke or transient ischemic attack (relative risk 2.5), diabetes (relative risk 1.7), history of hypertension (relative risk 1.6), and increasing age (relative risk 1.4 for each decade). Patients with any of these risk factors have an annual stroke risk of at least 4 percent if untreated. Patients whose only stroke risk factor is congestive heart failure or coronary artery disease have stroke rates approximately three times higher than do patients without any risk factors. Left ventricular (LV) dysfunction and a left atrial size greater than 2.5 cm/m^2 on echocardiographic examination are associated with thromboembolism. Patients younger than 60 to 65 years of age who have a normal echocardiogram and no risk factors have an extremely low risk for stroke (1 percent per year). Therefore, the risk of stroke in patients with *lone atrial fibrillation,* that is, idiopathic atrial fibrillation in the absence of any structural heart disease or any of the risk factors discussed previously, is quite low.

The annual rate of stroke for the unanticoagulated control group in five large anticoagulation trials was 4.5 percent but was reduced to 1.4 percent (68 percent risk reduction) for the warfarin-treated group (60 percent risk reduction in men; 84 percent risk reduction in women). Aspirin, 325 mg/d, produced a risk reduction of 44 percent. The annual rate of major hemorrhage was 1 percent for the control group, 1 percent for the aspirin group, and 1.3 percent for the warfarin group. No difference in stroke risk occurs between paroxysmal (intermittent) atrial fibrillation and constant (chronic) atrial fibrillation. Anticoagulation therapy is approximately 50 percent more effective than aspirin therapy for the prevention of ischemic stroke in patients with atrial fibrillation. Risk factors for anticoagulant-associated intracranial hemorrhage include excessive anticoagulation and poorly controlled hypertension. Elderly individuals are at increased risk for anticoagulant-associated brain hemorrhage, especially if overanticoagulated.

From these and other data, it appears that individuals younger than 60 years of age without any clinical risk factors or structural heart disease (lone atrial fibrillation) do not require antithrombotic therapy for stroke prevention because of their low risk. The stroke rate is also low (~2 percent per year) in patients between the ages of 60 and 75 years with lone atrial fibrillation. These patients may be adequately protected from stroke by aspirin therapy. In very elderly (older than 75 years) patients with atrial fibrillation, anticoagulation should be used with caution and carefully monitored because of the potential increased risk of intracranial hemorrhage. Nevertheless, elderly patients with atrial fibrillation are still likely to benefit from anticoagulation because they are at particularly high stroke risk. Food and drugs such as antibiotics and antiarrhythmics (e.g., amiodarone) can influence the effects of warfarin (see Chap. 80).

The following recommendations for antithrombotic therapy can be made: Any patient with atrial fibrillation who has risk factors for stroke (prior stroke or transient ischemic attack, significant valvular heart disease, hypertension, diabetes, age older than 65 years, left atrial enlargement, coronary artery disease, or congestive heart failure) should be treated with warfarin anticoagulation to achieve an international normalized ratio (INR) of 2.0 to 3.0 for stroke prevention if the individual is a good candidate for oral anticoagulation. Patients with contraindications to anticoagulation and unreliable individuals should be considered for aspirin treatment. Patients with atrial fibrillation who do not have any of the preceding risk factors have a low stroke risk (2 percent per year or less) and can be protected from stroke with aspirin. In patients older than 75 years, anticoagulation should be used with caution and monitored carefully to keep the INR less than 3.0 because of the risk of intracranial hemorrhage.

The risk of embolism following cardioversion to sinus rhythm in patients with atrial fibrillation varies from 0 to 7 percent, depending on the underlying risk factors. This risk is independent of the mode of cardioversion, either by chemical (drug) or DC shock. Patients at high risk are those with prior embolism, a mechanical valve prosthesis, or mitral stenosis. Low-risk patients are those younger than 60 years without underlying heart disease. The high-risk group should receive chronic anticoagulation (see later), regardless of whether they will undergo cardioversion. Patients not in the low-risk group who have atrial fibrillation longer than 2 days should receive warfarin to achieve an INR of 2.0 to 3.0 for 3 weeks before elective cardioversion and for 3 to 4 weeks after reversion to sinus rhythm. An alternative strategy is to obtain a transesophageal echocardiogram to exclude the presence of an atrial thrombus. It appears that this technique predicts a group at low risk for the development of thromboembolism following cardioversion, provided that the patients are immediately treated with heparin followed by therapeutic doses of warfarin.[26] Anticoagulation with heparin has been recommended for emergency cardioversion when 3 weeks of anticoagulation or a transesophageal echocardiogram cannot be obtained. No matter which strategy is used, anticoagulation should be continued for at least 4 weeks following cardioversion since atrial contractile function may not fully return until then.[27,28]

These suggestions must be individualized for a given patient. For example, patients at risk of trauma by virtue of occupation, participation in sports, and episodes of dizziness or syncope are at increased risk of bleeding if given anticoagulants and should probably not receive warfarin. Patients should be warned about taking any new drugs, such as nonsteroidal antiinflammatory agents, if they are receiving warfarin.

There are no data to suggest that conversion to sinus rhythm eliminates the risk of thromboembolism and thus that should not be for the sole purpose of doing so. In fact, data from the Atrial Fibrillation Follow-Up Investigation of Rhythm Management (AFFIRM) trial suggest that the strategy of maintaining sinus rhythm is insufficient alone to prevent thromboembolism, and patients who are treated with a strategy of maintaining sinus rhythm should be continued on anticoagulation unless there is a contraindication.[29] Many patients can have asymptomatic recurrences of atrial fibrillation.

Newer strategies for stroke prevention are being developed. Oral thrombin inhibitors (e.g., ximelagatran and Melagatran)[30] have been shown to be effective in preventing postoperative deep vein thrombosis and have just been evaluated in a randomized trial for stroke prevention in atrial fibrillation (Stroke Prevention Using Oral Thrombin Inhibitor in Atrial Fibrillation [SPORTIF V]). Although the results of this study are not currently known, the potential advantage of these agents is their wider therapeutic window, not requiring monitoring like warfarin. Left atrial occlusion, either surgically[31] or with a catheter-based system,[32] is also in the early stages of evaluation as a method for stroke prevention.

MANAGEMENT. The goals of management of the patient with atrial fibrillation are to reduce the risk of thromboembolism (described earlier) and to control symptoms. The latter is accomplished by controlling the ventricular rate during atrial fibrillation and/or restoring and maintaining sinus rhythm. Currently, no clear benefit has been ascribed to one treatment strategy over the other (rate control vs. rhythm control), particularly since antiarrhythmic drugs are only 50 to 70 percent effective and carry risks of proarrhythmia (see later). Data from large clinical studies (e.g., AFFIRM, Pharmacologic Intervention in Atrial Fibrillation [PIAF], and Rate Control versus Electrical Cardioversion [RACE]) all demonstrate that both treatment strategies are reasonable.[29,33,34] In the largest of these studies, AFFIRM, 4060 patients with atrial fibrillation and risk factors for thromboembolism were randomized to either rhythm control or rate control treatment strategy, using standard pharmacological approaches. The study found no differences in mortality or quality of life between the two groups.[29] In both groups, thromboembolic events occurred in those patients in whom anticoagulation was stopped. These studies compared treatment strategies and did not compare sinus rhythm to atrial fibrillation with rate control. In the AFFIRM trial, only 60 percent of the patients in the rhythm control arm were in sinus rhythm at follow-up, and patients were not rigorously monitored for atrial fibrillation recurrences between visits.

The overall treatment strategy (i.e., ventricular rate control or restoration and maintenance of sinus rhythm) should be individualized for each patient and based on whether patients are symptomatic from uncontrolled ventricular rates or from atrial fibrillation itself (i.e., loss of AV synchrony and atrial contraction) and risk for side effects from drugs. It can sometimes be difficult to determine whether a patient's symptoms are due to rapid ventricular rates or the loss of atrial contraction. As a general rule, asymptomatic patients found to be in atrial fibrillation on routine ECG are not likely to require rhythm control, and rate control is usually sufficient. Ambulatory monitoring (see Chap. 30) correlating the patients' ventricular response and rhythm to symptoms and exercise testing can be useful to this end. Trials of aggressive rate control or, conversely, cardioversion and maintenance of sinus rhythm are sometimes necessary to make this determination. Intolerance to medications or excessive risk in one strategy may necessitate switching strategies. Again, a rhythm control strategy should not be an alternative to anticoagulation therapy to reduce stroke risk.

Many elderly patients tolerate atrial fibrillation well without therapy because the ventricular rate is slow as a result of concomitant AV nodal disease. These patients often have associated sick sinus syndrome, and the development of atrial fibrillation represents a cure of sorts. Such patients may demonstrate serious supraventricular and ventricular arrhythmias or asystole after cardioversion, so the likelihood of establishing and maintaining sinus rhythm should be weighed against the risks of cardioversion or other forms of therapy.

Acute Management. A patient with atrial fibrillation discovered for the first time should be evaluated for a precipitating cause, such as thyrotoxicosis, mitral stenosis, pulmonary emboli, or pericarditis. The patient's clinical status determines initial therapy, the objectives being to slow the ventricular rate and restore atrial systole. If sudden onset of atrial fibrillation with a rapid ventricular rate results in acute cardiovascular decompensation, electrical cardioversion is the initial treatment of choice. For other patients, the decision to cardiovert is largely based on the individual clinical situation. The need to restore sinus rhythm must be weighed against the likelihood of successful cardioversion and long-term maintenance of sinus rhythm.

Maintenance of sinus rhythm after cardioversion is influenced by the duration of atrial fibrillation and, in some adults, atrial dilation. Animal studies indicate that atrial fibrillation begets atrial fibrillation: The longer the patient has atrial fibrillation, the greater the likelihood that it will remain because of a process called *electrophysiological remodeling.* Similar electrophysiological abnormalities can be demonstrated in patients following short episodes of atrial fibrillation, but the mechanism(s) and clinical significance are currently unknown.[35-39] Although parameters such as atrial size and duration of atrial fibrillation predict the success of cardioversion in population studies, enlarged atria and atrial fibrillation of long duration are not absolute contraindications to attempted cardioversion. Internal cardioversion via intracavitary catheters can be effective when transthoracic shocks fail, particularly in obese patients or those with significant pulmonary disease.[40,41] However, with the advent of biphasic external defibrillators, the success rates and the energy requirement for cardioversion have improved and the need to perform internal cardioversions has decreased.[43-45] Alternatively, antiarrhythmic drugs that lower defibrillation thresholds such as ibutilide can be used to pretreat the patient and increase the success of DC cardioversion.[42] Atrial contraction may not return immediately after restoration of electrical systole, and clinical improvement may be delayed. DC cardioversion establishes normal sinus rhythm in more than 90 percent of patients, but sinus rhythm remains for 12 months in only 30 to 50 percent. Patients with atrial fibrillation of less than 12 months' duration have a greater chance of maintaining sinus rhythm after cardioversion. For patients who do not require emergent cardioversion, chemical cardioversion with IV antiarrhythmic drugs is effective in 35 to 75 percent of patients, depending on the population studied.[11,46] Although procainamide has been used extensively for years, no well-controlled studies have been performed to determine its efficacy. Outside the United States, IV flecainide has been used with good results.[46] IV amiodarone appears to be less effective, with no difference in conversion rates from placebo. IV ibulitide is also effective in about 35 to 75 percent of patients, depending on the population studied.[11,12,47] In the absence of decompensation, the patient can be treated with drugs such as digitalis, beta blockers, or calcium antagonists to maintain a resting apical rate of 60 to 80 beats/min that does not exceed 100 beats/min after slight exercise. The combined use of digitalis and a beta blocker or calcium antagonist can be helpful in slowing the ventricular rate. Digitalis may be more effective if associated LV dysfunction is present; without such dysfunction, a beta blocker may be preferable to control the ventricular rate.

Long-Term Management. For the *rate control strategy*, digitalis, calcium-channel blockers (diltiazem and verapamil) and beta blockers can be used alone or in combination. For chronic management, digitalis is usually insufficient for adequate rate control during periods of exertion. One should not rely on a resting heart rate during an office visit as the sole evaluation of the adequacy of rate control. Ambulatory monitoring and/or exercise testing can be useful to confirm adequate rate control during activity. In some patients with frequent recurrence and rapid ventricular rates not controlled by drugs or in patients intolerant to drugs, modification or elimination of AV nodal conduction by radiofrequency catheter ablation and implantation of a rate-adaptive VVI (VVIR) pacemaker is acceptable rate control therapy (see Chap. 31). Whenever possible, atrial or dual-chamber pacing is preferable since the incidence of atrial fibrillation and stroke appears to be reduced compared with VVI pacing.

If a decision to *maintain sinus rhythm* has been made, class IA, IC, and III (amiodarone, sotalol) agents can be used to terminate acute-onset atrial fibrillation and prevent recurrences of atrial fibrillation. No one drug, with the possible exception of amiodarone, appears clearly superior, and selection is often based on the side effect profile and risk of proarrhythmia.[46,48] This appears to be true for newer drugs, such as azimilide and dofetilide, as well, although comparative trials have not yet been done.[49,50] Most antiarrhythmic drugs increase the likelihood of maintaining sinus rhythm from about 30 to 50 percent to 50 to 70 percent of patients per year after cardioversion. Before electrical cardioversion, an antiarrhythmic agent is often administered for a few days to help prevent relapse of atrial fibrillation, as well as to convert some patients to sinus rhythm. For those patients who fail drug therapy, new catheter ablation approaches have been applied successfully. Ablation of a focus within the pulmonary vein (Fig. 32–16) or electrical isolation of the pulmonary veins is 70 to 85 percent effective in patients with paroxysmal atrial fibrillation in short-term follow-up studies.[51,52] The surgical Maze procedure has been used to eliminate atrial fibrillation, particularly in combination with valve surgery, with a high success rate (see Chap 30).[53]

Atrial Tachycardias

ECG RECOGNITION. Atrial tachycardia (Fig. 32–17) has an atrial rate of generally 150 to 200 beats/min with a P wave contour different from that of the sinus P wave. At onset, there may be some "warming up" of the rate, resulting in a slight increase in heart rate over the initial several complexes. Frequently, atrial tachycardias occur in short, recurrent bursts with spontaneous terminations. P waves are usually found in the second half of the tachycardia cycle (long RP/short PR tachycardia). If the atrial rate is not excessive and AV conduction is not depressed, each P wave can conduct to the ventricles. If the atrial rate increases and AV conduction becomes impaired, a Wenckebach (Mobitz type I) second-degree AV block can ensue. This aberration is sometimes called *atrial tachycardia with block.* When caused by digitalis, other manifestations of digitalis excess are present, such as PVCs. In nearly half the cases of atrial tachycardia with block, the atrial rate is irregular. Characteristic isoelectric intervals between P waves, in contrast to atrial flutter, are usually present in all leads. However, at rapid atrial rates, the distinction between atrial tachycardia with block and atrial flutter can be difficult. Analysis of P wave configuration during tachycardia indicates that a positive or biphasic P wave in V_1 predicts a right atrial focus, whereas a positive P wave in V_1 predicts a left atrial focus.

CLINICAL FEATURES. Although atrial tachycardia occurs commonly in patients with significant structural heart disease such as coronary artery disease, with or without myocardial infarction, cor pulmonale, or digitalis intoxication, it is also seen in patients without structural heart

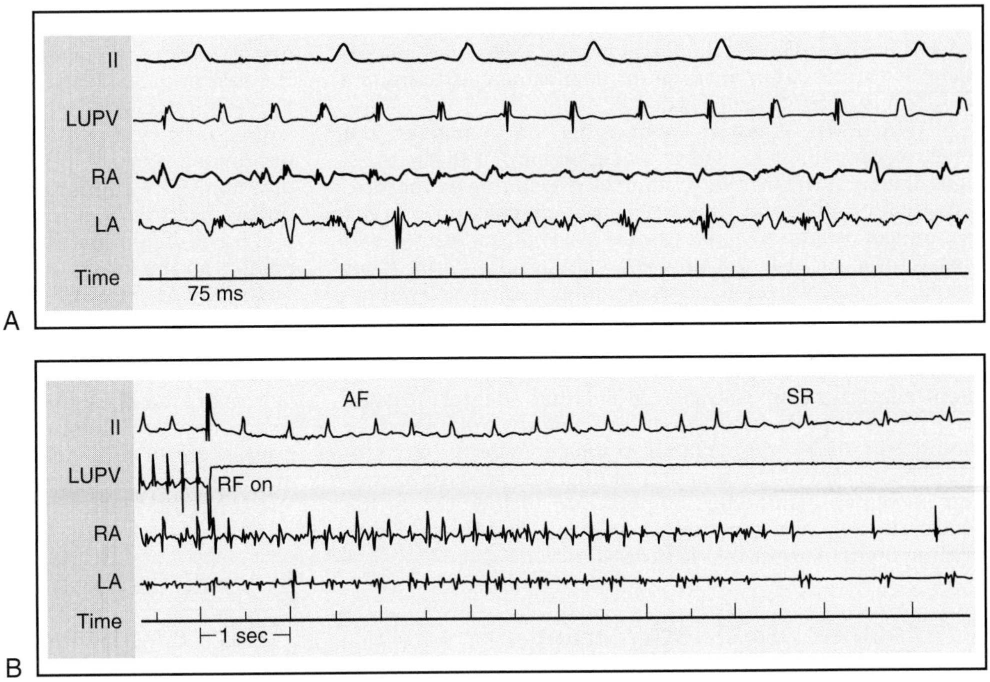

FIGURE 32–16 Focal atrial fibrillation arising from the left upper pulmonary vein (LUPV) **A,** During atrial fibrillation, irregular activity is recorded in the left atrium (LA) and the right atrium (RA). However, with a catheter at the focus in the LUPV, a regular sharp electrogram is recorded. **B,** During radiofrequency (RF) ablation at the site in **A,** the atrial fibrillation terminates within 7 seconds and sinus rhythm ensues.

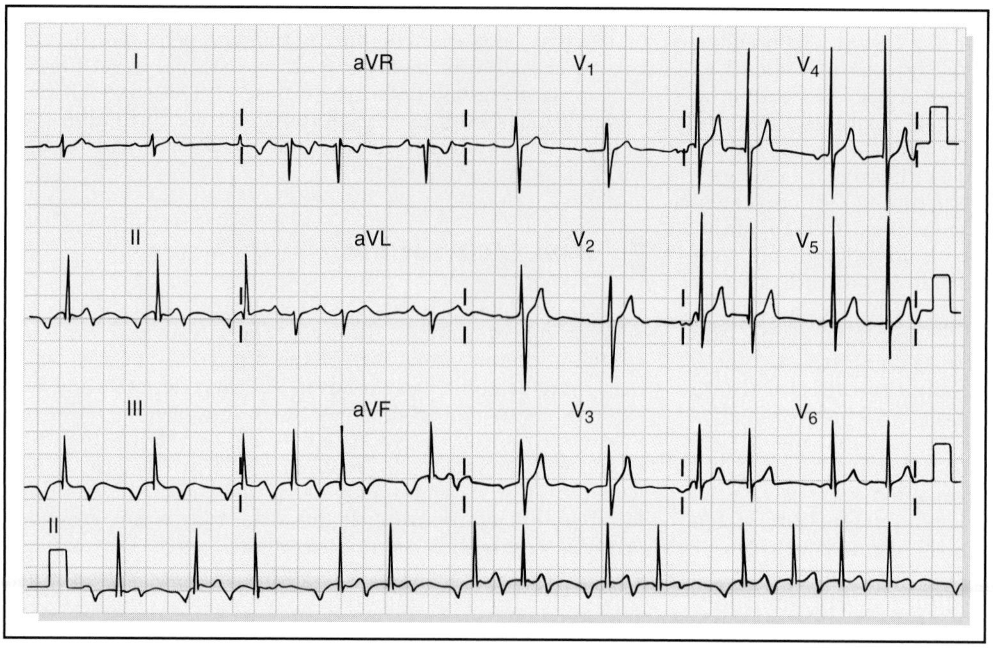

FIGURE 32–17 Atrial tachycardia. This 12-lead electrocardiogram and rhythm strip (bottom) demonstrate an atrial tachycardia at a cycle length of approximately 520 milliseconds. Conduction varies between 3:2 and 2:1. Note the negative P waves in leads II, III, and aVF and, when consecutive P waves are conducted, that the RP interval exceeds the PR interval. Note also that the tachycardia persists despite the development of atrioventricular (AV) block, an important finding that excludes the participation of an AV accessory pathway and sharply differentiates this tachycardia from the one shown in Figure 32–35.

disease. Potassium depletion can precipitate the arrhythmia in patients taking digitalis. The signs, symptoms, and prognosis are usually related to the underlying cardiovascular status and the rate of the tachycardia.

Physical findings during a variable rhythm include variable intensity of the first heart sound as a result of the varying AV block and PR interval. An excessive number of *a* waves can be seen in the jugular venous pulse. Carotid sinus massage or administration of adenosine increases the degree of AV block by slowing the ventricular rate in stepwise fashion without terminating the tachycardia, as in atrial flutter. It should be performed cautiously in patients with digitalis toxicity because serious ventricular arrhythmias can result. Occasionally, carotid sinus massage or adenosine can terminate some forms of atrial tachycardia.

MANAGEMENT. Atrial tachycardia in a patient not receiving digitalis is treated in a manner similar to the treatment of other atrial tachyarrhythmias. Depending on the clinical situation, digitalis, a beta blocker, or a calcium-channel blocker can be administered to slow the ventricular rate, and then if atrial tachycardia remains, class IA, IC, or III drugs can be added. Catheter ablation procedures are usually effective at eliminating the atrial tachycardia, depending on the mechanism and underlying heart disease (see Chap. 30).[9,17] However, atrial tachycardias can occasionally recur at a different site following a successful ablation attempt. If atrial tachycardia appears in a patient receiving digitalis, the drug should initially be assumed to be responsible for the arrhythmia. Therapy includes cessation of digitalis and administration of digitalis antibodies or potassium if low. Often, the ventricular response is not excessively fast, and simply withholding digitalis is all that is necessary.

Automatic Atrial Tachycardia

Three types of atrial tachycardias have been distinguished experimentally: automatic, triggered, and reentrant. The characteristics of automatic and reentrant tachycardias are discussed separately. Entrainment,[63] resetting curve patterns in response to overdrive pacing, the patient's response to adenosine, and recording of monophasic action potentials can be used to help distinguish one mechanism from the other. However, in most cases no clear identification of mechanism can be made clinically.

ECG FEATURES. Automatic atrial tachycardia (see Fig. 32–10F) is characterized electrocardiographically by a supraventricular tachycardia that generally accelerates after its initiation, with heart rates slower than 200 beats/min. The P wave contour differs from the sinus P wave, the PR interval is influenced directly by the tachycardia rate, and AV block can exist without affecting the tachycardia; that is, it continues uninterrupted. Vagal maneuvers do not generally terminate the tachycardia, even though they can produce AV nodal block. Thus, pharmacological or physiological maneuvers that selectively result in AV block do not affect the automatic focus, nor does the development of bundle branch block alter the PR or RP interval unless it is associated with prolongation of the H-V interval.

Initiation of tachycardia with premature atrial stimulation is not generally possible but is independent of intraatrial or AV nodal conduction delay when it occurs. The atrial activation sequence usually differs from a sinus-initiated P wave, and the A-H interval is related to the tachycardia rate. The first P wave of the tachycardia is the same as the subsequent P waves of the tachycardia, in contrast to most forms of reentrant supraventricular tachycardia, in which the initial and subsequent P waves differ. Usually, the tachycardia cannot be terminated by pacing, although it can exhibit overdrive suppression. The introduction of premature atrial complexes during tachycardia merely resets the timing of the tachycardia. It is difficult to differentiate this mechanism from microreentry by the leading-circle concept (see Chap. 27).

CLINICAL FEATURES. Many supraventricular tachycardias associated with AV block are probably due to automatic atrial tachycardia, including atrial tachycardia from digitalis intoxication (see Fig. 32–17). Automatic atrial tachycardia occurs in all age groups and is seen in settings of myocardial infarction, chronic lung disease (especially with acute infection), acute alcohol ingestion, a variety of metabolic derangements, or without any concomitant disease.

MANAGEMENT. Management is as discussed earlier.

Atrial Tachycardia Caused by Reentry

ECG RECOGNITION. Atrial tachycardia caused by reentry (Fig. 32–18; see also Fig. 32–10E). This arrhythmia is electrocardiographically manifest by a P wave that has a contour different from that of the sinus P wave, a PR interval

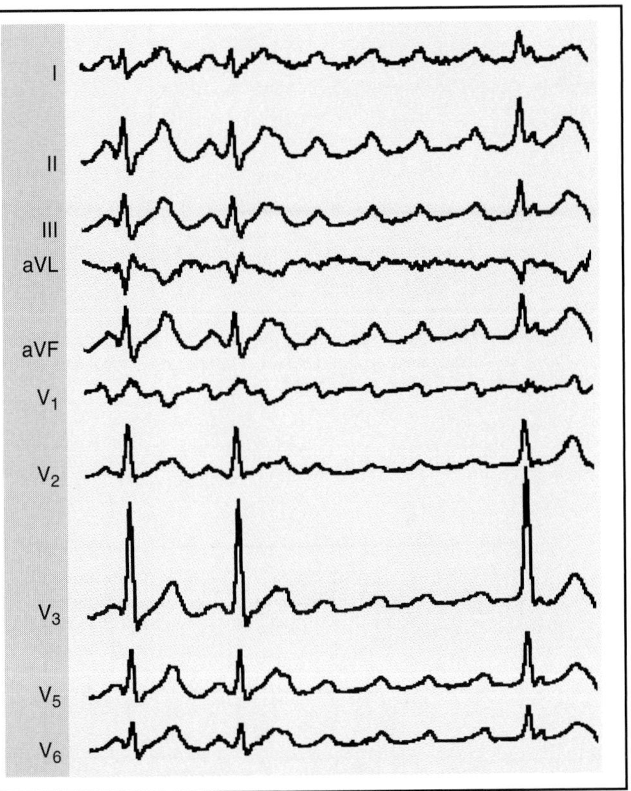

FIGURE 32–18 Macro-reentrant atrial tachycardia in a patient who underwent atrial septal defect repair 10 years earlier. This tachycardia uses a reentrant circuit established by the atriotomy on the lateral atrial wall. Ablation to extend the scar to the tricuspid annulus eliminated this tachycardia.

directly influenced by the tachycardia rate, and the capability to develop an AV block without interrupting the tachycardia. Atrial flutter (described earlier) is the prototypic atrial arrhythmia caused by reentry. Reentry can exist around a surgical scar, anatomical structure, or atriotomy incision.[9] Electrophysiologically, initiation of the tachycardia occurs with premature stimulation during the atrial relative refractory period, which results in a critical degree of intraatrial conduction delay, an atrial activation sequence different from what occurs during sinus rhythm, and an AV nodal conduction time related to the tachycardia rate. Occasionally, more aggressive stimulation is required to initiate some forms of reentrant atrial tachycardias. Vagal maneuvers generally do not terminate the tachycardia and can produce AV block.

CLINICAL FEATURES. Forms of atrial reentry producing atrial tachycardias include those that occur with atrial fibrosis (with pulmonary disease) or surgical atriotomy scars (see Fig. 32–18). The tachycardia can be started and stopped by an atrial extrastimulus. Spontaneous termination can be either sudden, with progressive slowing, or with alternating long-short cycle lengths.

CHAOTIC ATRIAL TACHYCARDIA

Chaotic (sometimes called *multifocal*) atrial tachycardia is characterized by atrial rates between 100 and 130 beats/min, with marked variation in P wave morphology and totally irregular P-P intervals (Fig. 32–19). Generally, at least three P wave contours are noted, with most P waves conducted to the ventricles, although often with variable PR intervals. This tachycardia occurs commonly in older patients with chronic obstructive pulmonary disease and congestive heart failure and may eventually develop into atrial fibrillation. Digitalis appears to be an unusual cause, and theophylline administration has been implicated. Chaotic atrial tachycardia can occur in childhood.

MANAGEMENT. Management is primarily directed toward the underlying disease. Antiarrhythmic agents are often ineffective in slowing either the rate of the atrial tachycardia or the ventricular response. Beta-adrenoreceptor blockers should be avoided in patients with bronchospastic pulmonary disease but can be effective if tolerated. Verapamil and amiodarone have been useful. Potassium and magnesium replacement may suppress the tachycardia.

AV Junctional Rhythm Disturbances

AV JUNCTIONAL ESCAPE COMPLEX

MECHANISM. Automatic fibers that are prevented from initiating depolarization by a pacemaker such as the sinus node, which possesses a more rapid rate of firing, are called *latent pacemakers.* Such latent pacemakers are found in some parts of the atrium, in the AV node–His bundle area, in the right and left bundle branches, in the Purkinje system and in the ventricular outflow tracts. A latent pacemaker can become the dominant pacemaker by default or usurpation, that is, by passive or active mechanisms. A decrease in the number of impulses arriving at a latent pacemaker site, the result of slowing of the sinus node or interruption of propagation of the normal impulse anywhere along its course, allows the latent pacemaker to escape and initiate depolarization passively, by default. An increase in the discharge rate of a latent pacemaker can capture pacemaker control actively, by usurpation. The implication of the two different mechanisms of ectopic impulse formation is important therapeutically.

ECG RECOGNITION. An AV junctional escape beat occurs when the rate of impulse formation of the primary pacemaker, generally the sinus node, becomes less than that of the AV junctional region or when impulses from the primary pacemaker do not penetrate to the region of the escape focus and allow the AV junctional focus to reach threshold and discharge. The interval from the last normally conducted beat to the AV junctional escape beat is a measure of the initial discharge rate of the AV junctional focus and generally corresponds to a rate of 35 to 60

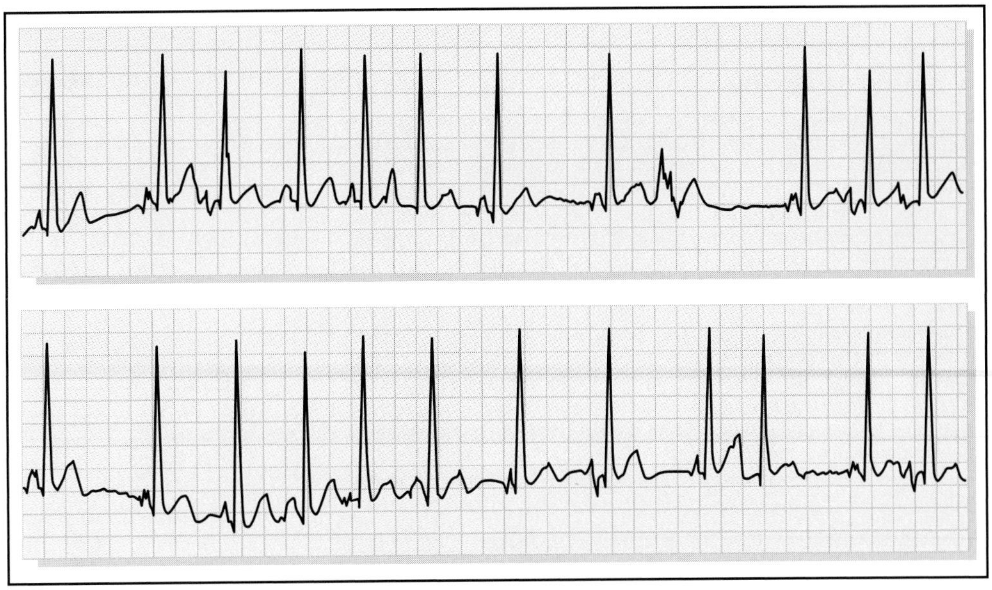

FIGURE 32–19 Chaotic (multifocal) atrial tachycardia. Premature atrial complexes occur at varying cycle lengths and with differing contours.

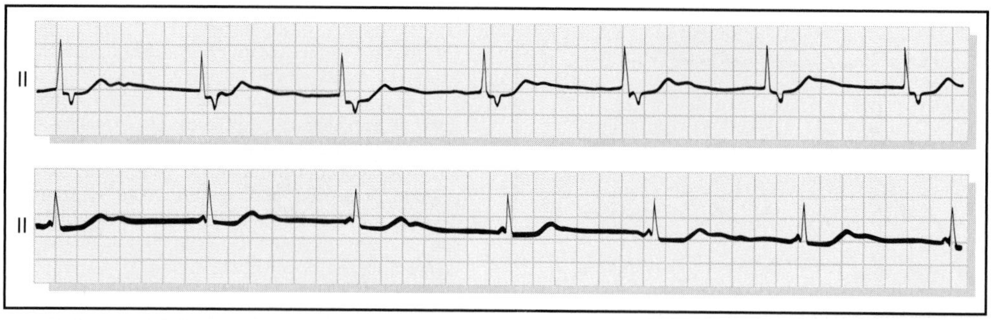

FIGURE 32–20 Atrioventricular (AV) junctional rhythm. **Top,** AV junctional discharge occurs fairly regularly at a rate of approximately 50 beats/min. Retrograde atrial activit follows each junctional discharge. **Bottom,** Recording made on a different day in the same patient. The AV junctional rate is slightly more variable, and retrograde P waves preced onset of the QRS complex. The positive terminal portion of the P wave gives the appearance of AV dissociation, which was not present.

beats/min (see Fig. 32-1B). Although an AV junctional escape rhythm is usually fairly regular, intervals between subsequent escape beats after the initial escape beat can gradually shorten as the rate of discharge of the escape focus increases, the so-called rhythm of development or warm-up phenomenon.

The ECG displays pauses longer than the normal P-P interval, interrupted by a QRS complex of supraventricular configuration with absent, retrograde, fusion, or sinus P waves that do not conduct to the ventricle. If P waves precede the QRS, they have a PR interval generally less than 0.12 second. The exact site of impulse formation (i.e., AN, N, or NH regions; low atrium; or His bundle) is not known and may differ from patient to patient and be influenced by the cause of the arrhythmia.

Treatment, if any, lies in increasing the discharge rate of the higher pacemakers and improving AV conduction and can require pacing. Frequently, no treatment is necessary.

PREMATURE AV JUNCTIONAL COMPLEXES

Premature AV junctional complexes are characterized by an impulse that arises prematurely in the AV junction (the exact site—i.e., AN, N, or NH regions; low atrium; or His bundle—is not known and may vary from patient to patient) and that attempts conduction in anterograde and retrograde directions. If unimpeded in its course, the impulse discharges the atrium to produce a premature retrograde P wave and a premature QRS complex with a supraventricular contour. The retrograde P wave can occur before, during, or after the QRS complex. Alterations in conduction time can influence the PR or RP relationships without a change in the site of origin of the impulse. Premature AV junctional complexes that conduct aberrantly are difficult to distinguish from PVCs observed on scalar ECG.

Treatment of premature AV junctional complexes is not generally necessary. However, since they may arise distal to the AV node, they can occur early in the cardiac cycle and can initiate a ventricular tachyarrhythmia in some instances. Under these circumstances, therapy is approached as for PVCs (see Chap. 30).

AV JUNCTIONAL RHYTHM

If the AV junctional escape complexes continue for a period, the rhythm is called an *AV junctional rhythm* (Fig. 32-20). Since the inherent rate of the AV junctional tissue is 35 to 60 beats/min, the AV junctional tissue can assume the role of the dominant pacemaker at this rate only by passive default of the sinus pacemaker. The ECG displays a normally conducted QRS complex, which can conduct retrogradely to the atrium or can occur independently of atrial discharge and produce AV dissociation.

An AV junctional escape rhythm can be a normal phenomenon in response to the effects of vagal tone, or it can occur during pathological sinus bradycardia or heart block. The escape complex or rhythm serves as a safety mechanism to prevent the occurrence of ventricular asystole. *Physical findings* vary depending on the P-QRS relationship. Large *a* waves in the jugular venous pulse and a loud, soft, or changing intensity of the first heart sound can be present if atrial contraction occurs when the tricuspid valve is shut.

Therapy is discussed under AV junctional escape complexes (see earlier).

NONPAROXYSMAL AV JUNCTIONAL TACHYCARDIA

ECG RECOGNITION. To usurp dominant pacemaker status, AV junctional tissue must exhibit an enhanced discharge rate such as during nonparoxysmal AV junctional tachycardia (Figs. 32-21 and 32-22). The

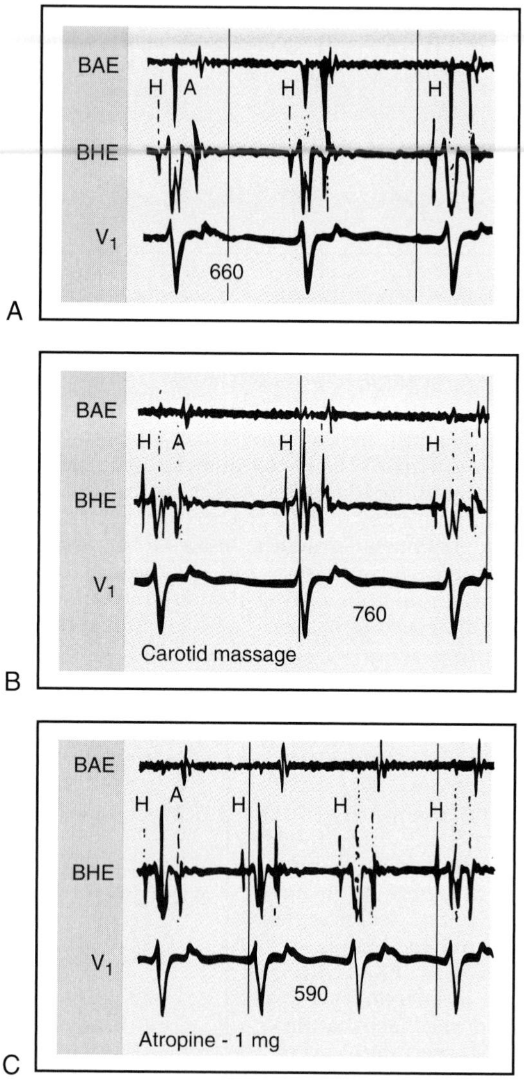

FIGURE 32–21 Nonparoxysmal atrioventricular (AV) junctional tachycardia. **A,** Control. **B,** Response to carotid sinus massage. **C,** Response to atropine 1 mg intravenously. Note that His bundle depolarization is the earliest recordable electrical activity in each cycle. The atria are depolarized retrogradely (low right atrial activity recorded in the BHE precedes high right atrial activity recorded in the BAE). Note also that carotid sinus massage slows the junctional discharge rate while atropine speeds it up. From these tracings alone one could not distinguish the rhythm from some other types of supraventricular tachycardia. However, the onset and termination of this tachycardia were typical of nonparoxysmal AV junctional tachycardia. BAE, bipolar atrial electrogram; BHE, bipolar His electrogram.

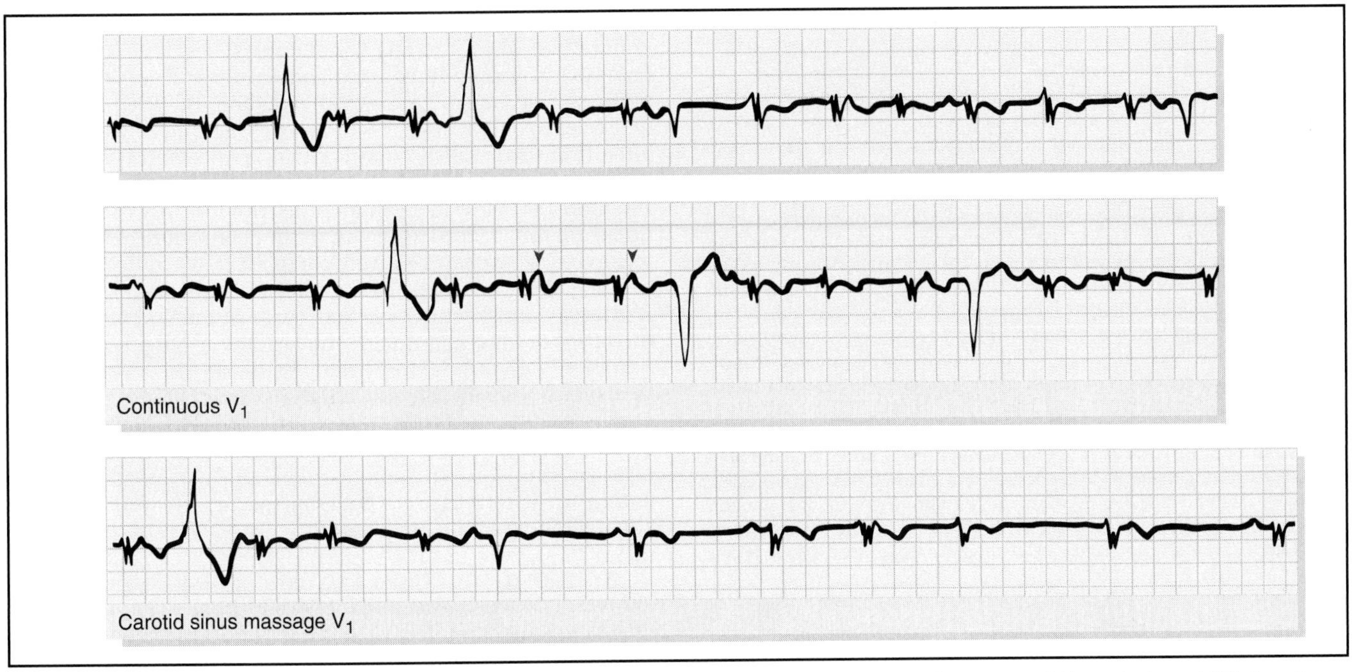

FIGURE 32–22 Nonparoxysmal atrioventricular junctional tachycardia in a healthy young adult. **Top,** This tachycardia occurs at a fairly regular interval ("W-shaped" complexes) and is interrupted intermittently with sinus captures that produce functional right and left bundle branch blocks. **Middle,** Two P waves are indicated by arrowheads. The junctional discharge rate is approximately 120 beats/min (cycle length = 500 milliseconds) and the rhythm irregular, sometimes shortened by sinus captures or delayed by concealed conduction that resets and displaces the junctional focus. **Bottom,** Carotid sinus massage slows the junctional as well as the sinus discharge rates.

tachycardia is usually of gradual onset and termination, hence the modifier *nonparoxysmal.* On occasion, nonparoxysmal AV junctional tachycardia can become manifest abruptly because slowing of the dominant pacemaker may then allow sudden capture and control of the rhythm by the AV junctional focus.

Nonparoxysmal AV junctional tachycardia is recognized by a QRS of supraventricular configuration at a fairly regular rate of 70 to 130 beats/min, but it can be faster. Accepted terminology assigns the label of tachycardia to rates exceeding 100 beats/min. The term *nonparoxysmal AV junctional tachycardia,* although not entirely correct when the rate is 70 to 100 beats/min, has generally been accepted since rates exceeding 60 beats/min in effect represent tachycardia for the AV junctional tissue. Enhanced vagal tone can slow while vagolytic agents can speed up the discharge rate. Although retrograde activation of the atria can occur, the atria are commonly controlled by an independent sinus, atrial, or on occasion, a second AV junctional focus resulting in AV dissociation (see Fig. 32-10G). The ECG diagnosis can be complicated by the presence of entrance and exit blocks at the AV junctional tissue level and incomplete forms of AV dissociation.

The cause of this arrhythmia is probably *accelerated automatic discharge* in or near the His bundle. It is possible that nonparoxysmal AV junctional tachycardia originates in atrial fibers without recognition of the latter's role from analysis of the scalar ECG or on intracardiac electrograms unless a careful search is made. Wenckebach periods can occur, but the presence of exit block has not yet been demonstrated by His bundle recording in humans, and the block can be in the AV node with the origin of the nonparoxysmal AV junctional tachycardia proximal to the site of the His bundle recording.

CLINICAL FEATURES. Nonparoxysmal AV junctional tachycardia occurs most commonly in patients with underlying heart disease, such as inferior infarction or myocarditis (often the result of acute rheumatic fever), or after open-heart surgery. An important cause is excessive digitalis, which can also produce the ECG manifestations of varying degrees of exit block (usually the Wenckebach type) from the accelerated AV junctional focus. Junctional tachycardia occurs commonly during radiofrequency catheter ablation of the slow pathway (see Chap. 30). Nonparoxysmal AV junctional tachycardia can occur in otherwise healthy individuals without symptoms (see Fig. 32-22) or can be a serious and difficult-to-control tachycardia, occasionally chronic, rapid, and long lasting. It can occur congenitally in infants or children and is associated with relatively high mortality.

The clinical features vary depending on the rate of the arrhythmia and the underlying etiology and severity of heart disease. As in most arrhythmias, the physical signs are determined by the relationship of the P wave to the QRS complex and the rate of atrial and ventricular discharge. The first heart sound can therefore be constant or varying, and cannon *a* waves may or may not occur in the jugular venous pulse.

The ventricular rhythm can be regular or irregular, often in a constant fashion. It is especially important to recognize slowing and regularization of the ventricular rhythm in a patient with atrial fibrillation as being caused by nonparoxysmal AV junctional tachycardia and as a possible early sign of *digitalis intoxication* (see Chap. 30). Initially, during atrial fibrillation, the regular ventricular rhythm can result from an AV junctional escape rhythm because the depressed AV conduction caused by digitalis blocks the passage of impulses from the fibrillating atria (see Fig. 32-10G). As digitalis administration is continued, the ventricular rate can then accelerate because of increased discharge of the AV junctional pacemaker but can still be regular. Further digitalis administration can produce a rate that is slow and irregular because of varying degrees of AV junctional exit block. The rhythm can be misdiagnosed as resumption of conduction from the fibrillating atria. The rate can then increase further because of development of VT.

MANAGEMENT. Therapy is directed toward the underlying etiological factor and functional support of the cardiovascular system. If the rhythm is regular, cardiovascular status is not compromised, and the patient is not taking digitalis, digitalis administration could be considered. If the patient tolerates the arrhythmia well, careful monitoring and attention to the underlying heart disease are usually all that are required in an adult. The arrhythmia generally abates spontaneously. If digitalis toxicity is the cause, treatment with the drug must be stopped and digitalis antibody given or potassium, if it is low. If digitalis is not involved, initial drug therapy with digitalis, calcium-channel blockers, or beta blockers can be tried. Other drug therapy can include agents from classes IA, IC, and III. Catheter ablation of the junctional site can be effective but carries a risk of complete heart block.

Tachycardias Involving the AV Junction

Much confusion exists regarding the nomenclature of tachycardias characterized by a supraventricular QRS complex, a regular R-R interval, and no evidence of ventricular preexcitation. Because it is now apparent that a variety of electrophysiological mechanisms can account for these tachycardias (see Fig. 32-10), the nonspecific term *paroxysmal supraventricular tachycardia* has been proposed to encompass the entire group. This term may be inappropriate because some tachycardias in patients with accessory pathways (see later) are no more supraventricular than they are ventricular in origin in that they may require participation of both the atria and the ventricles in the reentrant pathway and they exhibit a QRS complex of normal contour and duration only because anterograde conduction occurs over the normal AV node–His bundle pathways (see Fig. 32-10C). If conduction over the reentrant pathway reverses direction and travels in an "antidromic" direction (i.e., to the ventricles over the accessory pathway and to the atria over the AV node–His bundle), the QRS complex exhibits a prolonged duration, although the tachycardia is basically the same. The term *reciprocating tachycardia* has been offered as a substitute for paroxysmal supraventricular tachycardia, but use of such a term presumes the mechanism of the tachycardia to be reentrant (which is probably the case for many supraventricular tachycardias). Reciprocating tachycardia is probably the mechanism of many VTs as well. Thus, no universally acceptable nomenclature exists for these tachycardias. In this chapter, descriptive titles, although cumbersome, are used for the sake of clarity. In addition, the mechanism of reentry is assumed to be operative when the weight of evidence supports its presence even though unequivocal proof is not always available.

AV Nodal Reentrant Tachycardia

ECG RECOGNITION. Reentrant tachycardia in the AV node is characterized by a tachycardia with a QRS complex of supraventricular origin, with sudden onset and termination generally at rates between 150 and 250 beats/min (commonly 180 to 200 beats/min in adults) and with a regular rhythm. Uncommonly, the rate may be as low as 110 beats/min and occasionally, especially in children, may exceed 250 beats/min. Unless functional aberrant ventricular conduction or a previous conduction defect exists, the QRS complex is normal in contour and duration. P waves are generally buried in the QRS complex. Often, the P wave is seen just prior to or just after the end of the QRS and causes a subtle alteration in the QRS complex that results in a pseudo-S or pseudo-r′, which may be recognized only on comparison to the QRS complex in normal sinus rhythm (Fig. 32–23). AV nodal reentry recorded at the onset begins abruptly, usually following a premature atrial complex that conducts with a prolonged PR interval (see Figs. 32–10A and 32–11B). The R-R interval can shorten over the course of the first few beats at the onset or lengthen during the last few beats preceding termination of the tachycardia. Variation in cycle length is usually caused by variation in anterograde AV nodal conduction time. Cycle length and/or QRS alternans can occur, usually when the rate is very fast. Carotid sinus massage can slow the tachycardia slightly prior to its termination or, if termination does not occur, can produce only slight slowing of the tachycardia.

ELECTROPHYSIOLOGICAL FEATURES. An atrial complex that conducts with a critical prolongation of AV nodal conduction time generally precipitates AV nodal reentry (Figs. 32-24 to 32-26). Premature ventricular stimulation can also induce AV nodal reentry in about one third of patients. Data from radiofrequency catheter ablation results and mapping support the presence of differential atrial inputs into the AV node, the fast and slow pathways, to explain this tachycardia (see Chaps. 27 and 29). In Figure 32-30, as well as Figure 32-10A and B, the atria are shown as a necessary link between the fast and slow pathways. Whether these pathways are discrete pathways (perhaps due to anisotropy) or functional in nature is not known. In most examples, the retrograde P wave occurs at the onset of the QRS complex, clearly excluding the possibility of an accessory pathway. If an accessory pathway in the ventricle were part of the tachycardia circuit, the ventricles would have to be activated anterogradely before the accessory pathway could be activated retrogradely and depolarize the atria, thus placing the retrograde P wave no earlier than during the ST segment (see Preexcitation Syndrome, Chap. 30).

In approximately 30 percent of instances, atrial activation begins at the end of or just after the QRS complex and gives rise to a discrete P wave on the surface ECG (often appearing as a nubbin of an R in V_1) (see Fig. 32-10A), whereas in most patients, P waves are not seen since they are buried within the inscription of the QRS complex. In the most common variety of AV nodal reentrant tachycardia, the ventriculoatrial (VA) interval (i.e., the interval between the onset of QRS and the onset of atrial activity) is less than 50 percent of the R-R interval, and the ratio of the AV to the VA interval exceeds 1.0. These VA intervals are longer in patients with tachycardia related to accessory pathways, as well as in atypical forms of AV nodal reentry (see Fig. 32-10B).

Slow and Fast Pathways. In most patients, anterograde conduction to the ventricle occurs over the slow (alpha) pathway and retrograde conduction occurs over the fast (beta) pathway (see Chap. 27 and Fig. 32-10A and B). To initiate tachycardia, an atrial complex blocks conduction in the fast pathway anterogradely, travels to the ventricle over the slow

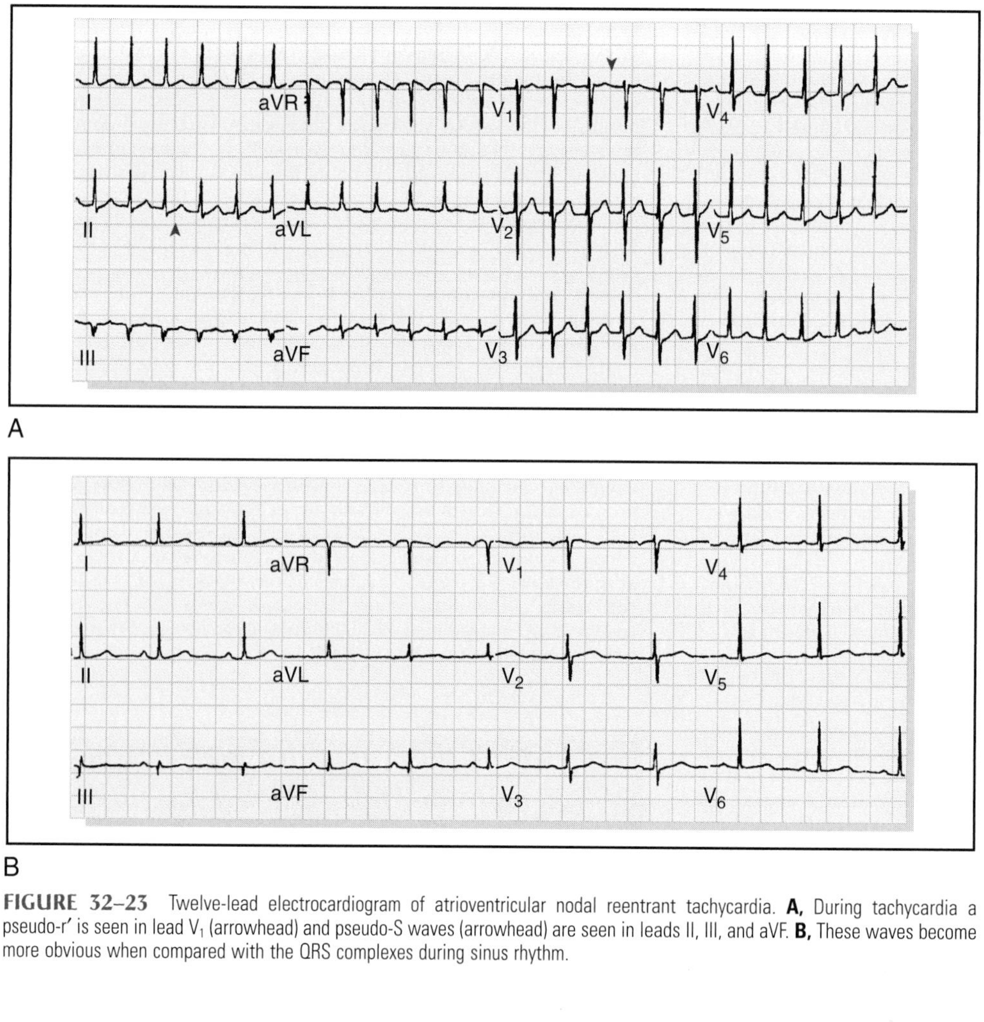

FIGURE 32–23 Twelve-lead electrocardiogram of atrioventricular nodal reentrant tachycardia. **A,** During tachycardia a pseudo-r′ is seen in lead V_1 (arrowhead) and pseudo-S waves (arrowhead) are seen in leads II, III, and aVF. **B,** These waves become more obvious when compared with the QRS complexes during sinus rhythm.

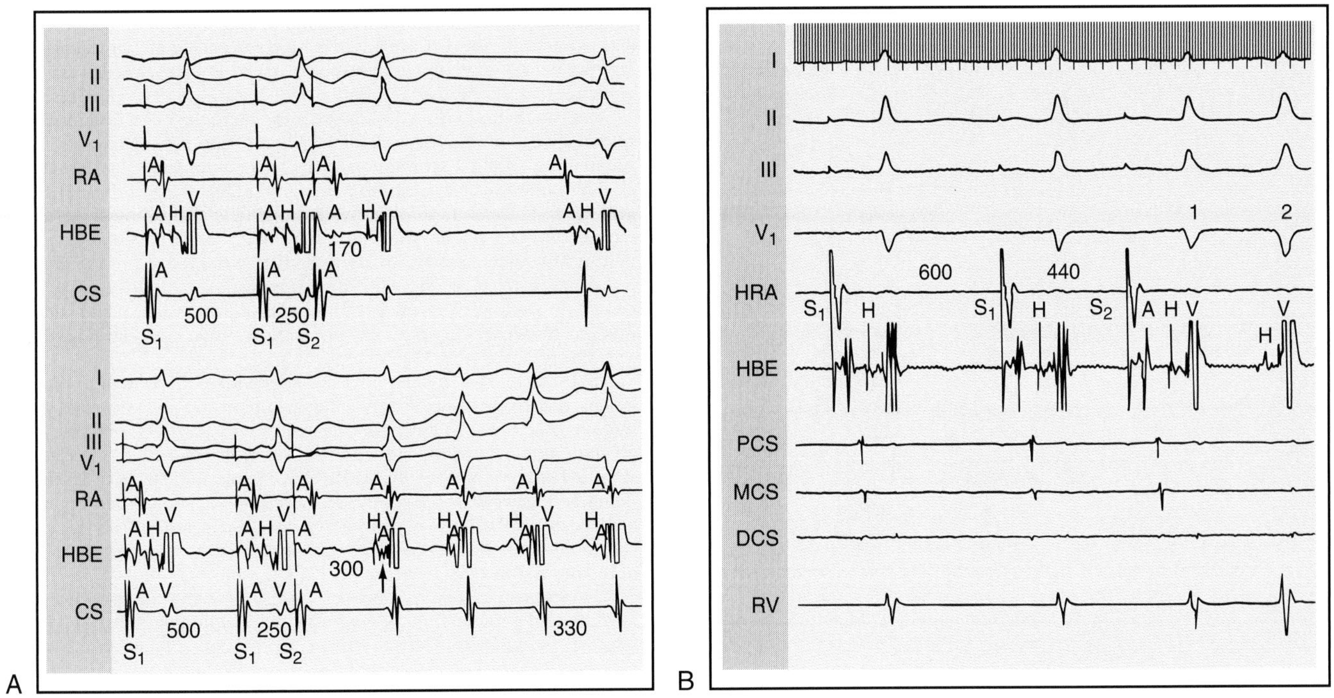

FIGURE 32–24 **A,** Initiation of atrioventricular (AV) nodal reentrant tachycardia in a patient with dual AV nodal pathways. **Upper** and **lower** panels show the last two paced beats of a train of stimuli delivered to the coronary sinus at a pacing cycle length of 500 milliseconds. The results of premature atrial stimulation at an S_1-S_2 interval of 250 milliseconds on two occasions are shown. In the **upper** panel, S_2 was conducted to the ventricle with an A-H interval of 170 milliseconds and was then followed by a sinus beat. In the **lower** panel, S_2 was conducted with an A-H interval of 300 milliseconds and initiated AV nodal reentry. Note that the retrograde atrial activity occurs (arrow) prior to the onset of ventricular septal depolarization and is superimposed on the QRS complex. Retrograde atrial activity begins first in the low right atrium (HBE lead) and then progresses to the high right atrium (RA) and coronary sinus (CS) recordings. **B,** Two QRS complexes in response to a single atrial premature complex. After a basic train of S_1 stimuli at 600 milliseconds, an S_2 at 440 milliseconds is introduced. The first QRS complex in response to S_2 occurs after a short (95 milliseconds) A-H interval caused by anterograde conduction over the fast AV nodal pathway. The first QRS complex is labeled number 1 (in lead V_1). The second QRS complex in response to the S_2 stimulus (labeled number 2) follows a long A-H interval (430 milliseconds) caused by anterograde conduction over the slow AV nodal pathway.

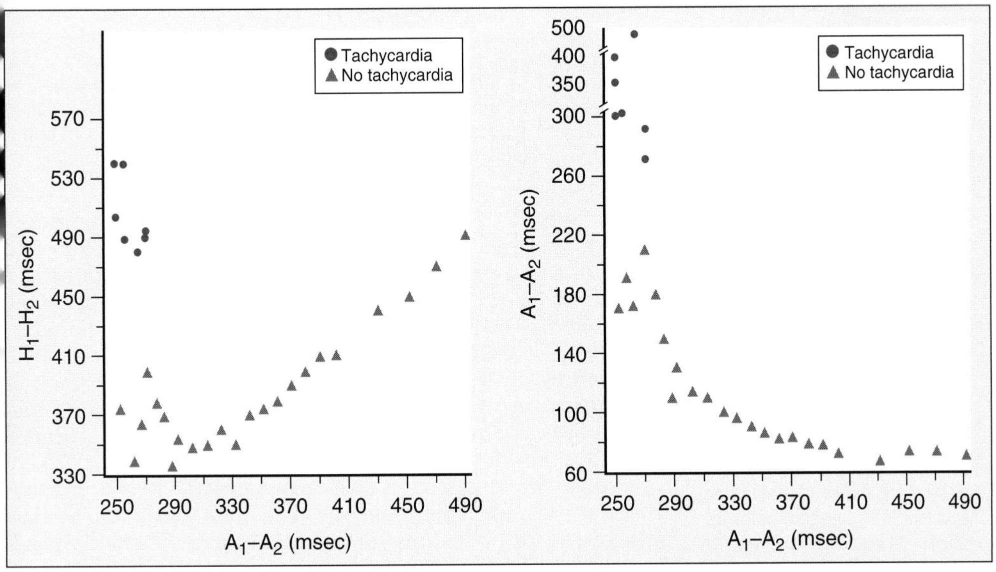

FIGURE 32–25 H_1-H_2 intervals **(left)** and A_2-H_2 intervals **(right)** at various A_1-A_2 intervals with a discontinuous atrioventricular (AV) nodal curve. At a critical A_1-A_2 interval the H_1-H_2 and the A_1-H_2 intervals increase markedly. At the break in the curves, AV nodal reentrant tachycardia is initiated.

pathway, and returns to the atrium over the previously blocked fast pathway ("slow-fast" form). The proximal and distal final pathways for this circus movement appear to be located within the AV node, so as currently conceived, the circus movement occurs over the two atrial approaches and the AV node (see Fig. 32–10A and B). The reentrant loop for typical AV nodal reentry is the anterograde slow AV nodal pathway to the final distal common pathway (probably the distal AV node), to the retrograde fast AV nodal pathway, and then to atrial myocardium. In atypical AV node reentry, the reentry occurs in the opposite direction. In some patients, the His bundle may be incorporated in the reentrant circuit. Less commonly, the reentry pathway can be over two slow pathways, the so-called slow-slow AV node reentry (see Fig. 32–11B). Some data are consistent with intranodal activity.

The cycle length of the tachycardia generally depends on how well the slow pathway conducts because the fast pathway usually exhibits excellent capability for retrograde conduction and has the shorter refractory period in the retrograde direction. Therefore, conduction time in the anterograde slow pathway is a major determinant of the cycle length of the tachycardia.

The Dual-Pathway Concept. Evidence supporting the dual-pathway concept derives from several observations, the most compelling of which is that radiofrequency catheter ablation of *either* the slow pathway or the fast pathway eliminates AV nodal reentry without eliminating AV nodal conduction. Other observations provide supporting proof. For example, in these patients a plot of the A_1-A_2 versus the A_2-H_2 or the A_1-A_2 versus the H_1-H_2 interval shows a discontinuous curve (see Fig. 32–25). The explanation is that at a crucial A_1-A_2 interval the impulse is suddenly blocked in the fast pathway and is conducted with delay over the slow pathway, with sudden prolongation of the A_2-H_2 (or H_1-H_2) interval. Generally, the A-H interval increases at least 50 milliseconds, with only a 10- to 20-millisecond decrease in the coupling interval of the premature atrial complex. Less commonly, dual pathways may be manifest by different PR

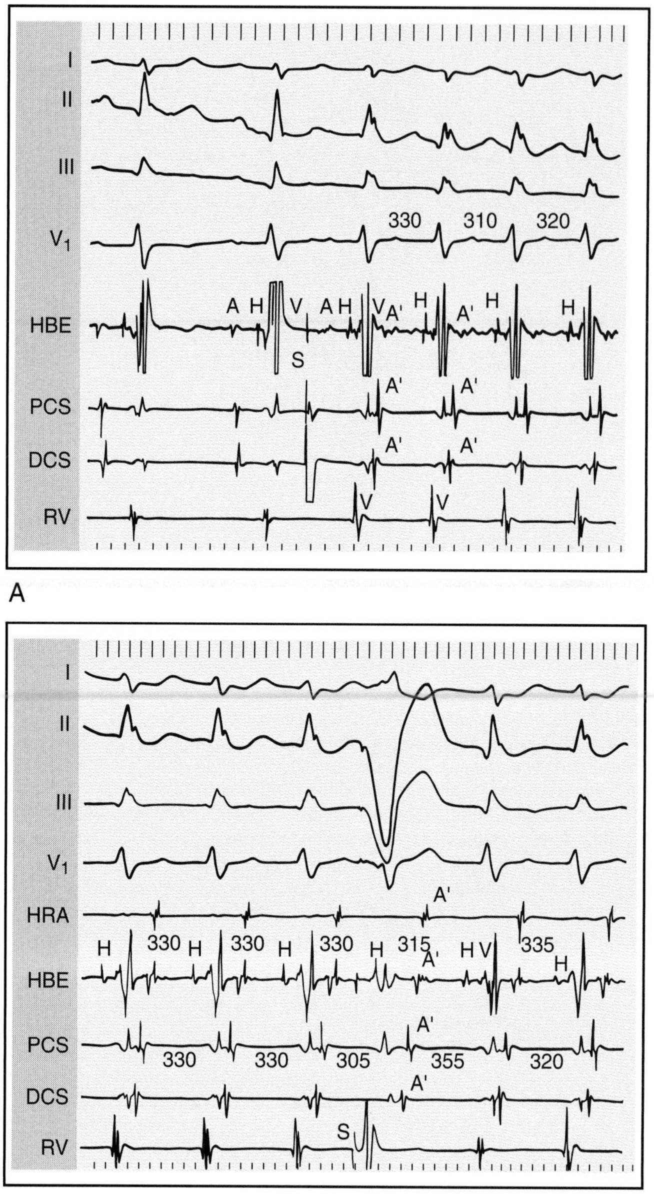

FIGURE 32–26 Atrial preexcitation during atrioventricular (AV) reciprocating tachycardia in a patient with a concealed accessory pathway. No evidence of accessory pathway conduction is present in the two sinus-initiated beats shown in **A.** A premature stimulus in the coronary sinus (S) precipitates a supraventricular tachycardia at a cycle length of approximately 330 milliseconds. The retrograde atrial activation sequence begins first in the distal coronary sinus (A′, DCS), followed by activation recorded in the proximal coronary sinus (PCS), low right atrium (HBE), and then the high right atrium (not shown). The QRS complex is normal and identical to the sinus-initiated QRS complex. (The terminal portion is slightly deformed by superimposition of the retrograde atrial recording.) Note that the RP interval is short and the PR interval is long. The shortest VA interval exceeds 65 milliseconds, consistent with conduction over a retrogradely conducting AV pathway. **B,** Premature ventricular stimulation at a time when the His bundle is still refractory from anterograde activation during tachycardia shortens the A-A interval from 330 to 305 milliseconds without a change in the retrograde atrial activation sequence. (Note that no change occurs in the H-H interval when the right ventricular stimulus, S, is delivered. H-H intervals are in milliseconds in the HBE lead.) Thus the ventricular stimulus, despite His bundle refractoriness, still reaches the atrium and produces an identical retrograde atrial activation sequence. The only way that this finding can be explained is via conduction over a retrogradely conducting accessory pathway. Therefore, the patient has a concealed accessory pathway with the Wolff-Parkinson-White syndrome.

or A-H intervals during sinus rhythm or at identical paced rates or by a sudden jump in the A-H interval during atrial pacing at a constant cycle length. Two QRS complexes in response to one P wave provide additional evidence (see Fig. 32–24B).

Some patients with AV nodal reentry may not have discontinuous refractory period curves, and some patients who do not have AV nodal reentry can exhibit discontinuous refractory curves. In the latter patients, dual AV nodal pathways can be a benign finding. Many of these patients also exhibit discontinuous curves retrogradely. Similar mechanisms of tachycardia can occur in children. Triple AV nodal pathways can be demonstrated in occasional patients. Virtually irrefutable proof of dual AV nodal pathways is the simultaneous propagation in opposite directions of two AV nodal wavefronts without collision (see Chap. 27) or the production of two QRS complexes from one P wave (see Fig. 32–24B) or two P waves from one QRS complex.

In less than 5 to 10 percent of patients with AV nodal reentry, anterograde conduction proceeds over the fast pathway and retrograde conduction over the slow pathway (termed the *unusual form* of "fast-slow" AV node reentry), with production of a long VA interval and a relatively short AV interval (generally AV/VA < 0.75; see Fig. 32–10B). The least common form ("slow-slow") exhibits a retrograde P wave midway in the cardiac cycle. Finally, it is possible to have tachycardias that use either the anterograde slow or fast pathways and conduct retrogradely over an accessory pathway (see later).

The ventricles are not needed to maintain AV nodal reentry in humans, and spontaneous AV block has been noted on occasion, particularly at the onset of the arrhythmia. Such block can take place in the AV node distal to the reentry circuit, between the AV node and bundle of His, within the bundle of His, or distal to it (see Chap. 27). Rarely, the block can be located between the reentry circuit in the AV node and the atrium. Most commonly, when block appears, it is below the bundle of His. Termination of the tachycardia generally results from a block in the anterogradely conducting slow pathway ("weak link"), so a retrograde atrial response is not followed by a His or ventricular response. Functional bundle branch block during AV nodal reentrant tachycardia does not modify the tachycardia significantly.

Retrograde Atrial Activation. The sequence of retrograde atrial activation is normal during AV nodal reentrant supraventricular tachycardia, which means that the earliest site of atrial activation during retrograde conduction over the fast pathway is recorded in the His bundle electrogram, followed by electrograms recorded from the os of the coronary sinus and then spreading to depolarize the rest of the right and left atria. During retrograde conduction over the slow pathway in the atypical type of AV nodal reentry, atrial activation recorded in the proximal coronary sinus precedes atrial activation recorded in the low right atrium, which suggests that the slow and fast pathways can enter the atria at slightly different positions.

CLINICAL FEATURES. AV nodal reentry commonly occurs in patients who have no structural heart disease and in the adult population frequently presents in the third and fourth decade of life. Symptoms frequently accompany the tachycardia and range from feelings of palpitations, nervousness, and anxiety to angina, heart failure, syncope, or shock, depending on the duration and rate of the tachycardia and the presence of structural heart disease. Tachycardia can cause syncope because of the rapid ventricular rate, reduced cardiac output, and cerebral circulation or because of asystole when the tachycardia terminates as a result of tachycardia-induced depression of sinus node automaticity. The prognosis for patients without heart disease is usually good.

MANAGEMENT

The Acute Attack. Management of AV nodal reentrant tachycardia depends on the underlying heart disease, how well the tachycardia is tolerated, and the natural history of previous attacks in the individual patient. For some patients, rest, reassurance, and sedation may be all that are required to abort an attack. Vagal maneuvers, including carotid sinus massage, the Valsalva and Mueller maneuvers, gagging, and occasionally exposure of the face to ice water, serve as the first line of therapy. These maneuvers may slightly slow the tachycardia rate, which then can speed up to the original rate following cessation of the attempt, or can terminate it. If vagal maneuvers fail, adenosine is the initial drug of choice. Digitalis, calcium antagonists, beta-adrenoceptor blockers, and adenosine normally depress conduction in the anterogradely conducting slow AV nodal pathway, whereas class IA and IC drugs depress conduction in the retrogradely conducting fast pathway (Table 32–2).

ADENOSINE. Adenosine (see Chap. 30) 6 to 12 mg given rapidly IV is the initial drug of choice and is successful at terminating the tachycardia in about 90 percent of cases.[64] *Verapamil* (see Chap. 30) 5 to 10 mg IV or diltiazem 0.25 to 0.35 mg/kg IV terminates AV nodal reentry successfully in about 2 minutes in approximately 90 percent of instances and is given when simple vagal maneuvers and adenosine fail.

DIGITALIS. Although it may be effective for longer-term management, digitalis has a slower onset of action than the agents described earlier and thus is not as useful in the acute management. If digitalis is used, digoxin can be given, 0.5 to 1 mg IV over a period of 10 to 15 minutes, followed by 0.25 mg every 2 to 4 hours, with a total dose less than 1.5 mg within any 24-hour period. *Oral digitalis* administration to terminate an acute attack is not generally indicated. Vagal maneuvers that were previously ineffective can terminate the tachycardia following digitalis administration and should therefore be repeated.

BETA-ADRENOCEPTOR BLOCKERS. Beta-adrenoceptor blockers must be used cautiously, if at all in patients with heart failure, chronic lung disease, or a history of asthma because their beta-adrenoceptor blocking action depresses myocardial contractility and can produce bronchospasm. Digitalis, calcium antagonists, beta blockers, and adenosine normally depress conduction in the anterogradely conducting slow pathway, whereas classes IA and IC drugs depress conduction in the retrogradely conducting fast pathway.

DC CARDIOVERSION. Before digitalis or a beta blocker is administered, it is advisable to reassess the clinical status of the patient and consider whether DC cardioversion may be advisable. DC shock administered to patients who have received excessive amounts of digitalis can be dangerous and result in serious postshock ventricular arrhythmias (see Chap. 30). Particularly if signs or symptoms of cardiac decompensation occur, DC electrical shock should be considered early. DC shock, synchronized to the QRS complex to avoid precipitating ventricular fibrillation, successfully terminates AV nodal reentry with energies in the range of 10 to 50 J; higher energies may be required in some instances.

PACING. If DC shock is contraindicated or if pacing wires are already in place (either postoperatively or if the patient has a permanent pacemaker), competitive *atrial* or *ventricular pacing* can restore sinus rhythm. In some instances, esophageal pacing can be useful (see Chap. 31).

Classes IA, IC, and III drugs are not usually required to terminate AV nodal reentry. Unless contraindicated, DC cardioversion should generally be attempted before using these agents, which are more often administered to prevent recurrence.

TABLE 32–2 Drugs that Slow Conduction in, and Prolong Refractoriness of, the Accessory Pathway and AV Node

Affected Tissue	Drugs
Accessory pathway AV node	Class IA Class II Class IV Adenosine Digitalis
Both	Class IC Class III (amiodarone)

AV = atrioventricular.

Pressor drugs can terminate AV nodal reentry by inducing reflex vagal stimulation mediated by baroreceptors in the carotid sinus and aorta when systolic blood pressure is acutely elevated to levels of about 180 mm Hg, but they are rarely needed unless the patient is also hypotensive.

Prevention of Recurrences. Initially, one must decide whether the frequency and severity of the attacks warrant long-term therapy. If the attacks of paroxysmal tachycardia are infrequent, well tolerated, and short lasting and either terminate spontaneously or are easily terminated by the patient, no prophylactic therapy may be necessary. If the attacks are sufficiently frequent and/or long lasting to necessitate therapy, the patient can be treated with drugs empirically or on the basis of serial electrophysiological testing. If empirical testing is desirable, digitalis, a long-acting calcium antagonist, or a long-acting beta-adrenoceptor blocker is a reasonable initial choice. The clinical situation and potential contraindications, such as beta blockers in an asthmatic, usually dictate the selection. If digitalis is used, rapid oral digitalization can be accomplished in 24 to 36 hours with digoxin at an initial dose of 1 to 1.5 mg, followed by 0.25 to 0.5 mg every 6 hours for a total dose of 2 to 3 mg. A less rapid oral regimen induces digitalization in 2 to 3 days with an initial dose of 0.75 to 1 mg, followed by 0.25 to 0.5 mg every 12 hours for a total dose of 2 to 3 mg. Alternatively, digoxin administered as a maintenance dose of 0.125 to 0.5 mg achieves digitalization in about 1 week. If any of these drugs are ineffective when taken singly, combinations can be tested.

RADIOFREQUENCY ABLATION. Radiofrequency ablation is more than 95 percent effective at curing patients long term, with a low incidence of complications. Because it is preferable to *cure* the patient of the tachycardia rather than use potentially toxic drugs to suppress it or to implant an antitachycardia device that terminates the tachycardia only after its onset (see Chap. 30), radiofrequency catheter ablation should be considered early in the management of patients with symptomatic recurrent episodes of AV node reentry. The procedure can be offered as an alternative to drug therapy in patients with frequent, symptomatic episodes. For patients who do not wish to take drugs, patients who are drug intolerant, or those in whom drugs are ineffective, radiofrequency catheter ablation is the treatment of choice. It should be considered before long-term therapy with class IA, IC, or III antiarrhythmic drugs. Ablation has replaced surgery in virtually all instances and may be considered the initial treatment of choice in many symptomatic patients.

Reentry over a Concealed (Retrograde-Only) Accessory Pathway

ECG RECOGNITION. The presence of an accessory pathway that conducts unidirectionally from the ventricle to the atrium but not in the reverse direction is not apparent by analysis of the scalar ECG during sinus rhythm because the ventricle is not preexcited (see Fig. 32–26).[65] Therefore, ECG manifestations of WPW syndrome are absent, and the accessory pathway is said to be "concealed." Since the mechanism responsible for most tachycardias in patients who have WPW syndrome is macro-reentry caused by anterograde conduction over the AV node–His bundle pathway and retrograde conduction over an accessory pathway, the latter, even if it only conducts retrogradely, can still participate in the reentrant circuit to cause an *AV reciprocating* tachycardia. Electrocardiographically, a tachycardia resulting from this mechanism can be *suspected* when the QRS complex is normal and the retrograde P wave occurs *after* completion of the QRS complex, in the ST segment, or early in the T wave (see Fig. 32–10C).

MECHANISMS. The cause of unidirectional propagation is not clear and can relate to multiple factors. During sinus rhythm, the atrial impulse probably enters the accessory pathway but is blocked near the ventricular insertion site with both right- and left-sided concealed accessory pathways. During functional block in patients with anterograde conduction over accessory pathways, block occurs near the ventricular insertion site most commonly with left-sided pathways but more often near the atrial insertion site with right-sided accessory pathways.

The P wave follows the QRS complex during tachycardia because the ventricle must be activated before the propagating impulse can enter the accessory pathway and excite the atria retrogradely. Therefore, the retrograde P wave must occur after ventricular excitation, in contrast to AV nodal reentry, in which the atria are usually excited during ventricular activation (see Fig. 32-10A). Also, the contour of the retrograde P wave can differ from that of the usual retrograde P wave since the atria may be activated eccentrically, that is, in a manner other than the normal retrograde activation sequence, which starts at the low right atrial septum as in AV nodal reentry. This eccentric activation occurs because the concealed accessory pathway in most instances is left sided, that is, inserts into the left atrium, which makes the left atrium the first site of retrograde atrial activation and causes the retrograde P wave to be negative in lead I (see Fig. 32-26).

Finally, since the tachycardia circuit involves the ventricles, if a functional bundle branch block occurs in the same ventricle in which the accessory pathway is located, the VA interval and cycle length of the tachycardia can become longer (see Fig. 32-31). This important change ensues because the bundle branch block lengthens the reentrant circuit (see Preexcitation Syndrome). For example, the normal activation sequence for a reciprocating tachycardia circuit with a left-sided accessory pathway but without a functional bundle branch block progresses from the atrium to the AV node–His bundle, to the right and left ventricles, to the accessory pathway, and then to the atrium. However, during a functional left bundle branch block, for example, the tachycardia circuit travels from the atrium to the AV node–His bundle, to the right ventricle, to the septum, to the left ventricle, to the accessory pathway, and then back to the atrium. This increase in the VA interval provides definitive proof that the ventricle and accessory pathway are part of the reentry circuit. The additional time required for the impulse to travel across the septum from the right to the left ventricle before reaching the accessory pathway and atrium lengthens the VA interval, which lengthens the cycle length of the tachycardia by an equal amount, assuming that no other changes in conduction times occur within the circuit. Thus, lengthening of the tachycardia cycle length by more than 35 milliseconds during an ipsilateral functional bundle branch block is diagnostic of a free wall accessory pathway if the lengthening can be shown to be due to VA prolongation only and not to prolongation of the H-V interval (which can develop with the appearance of a bundle branch block). In an occasional patient, the increase in cycle length because of prolongation of VA conduction can be nullified by a simultaneous decrease in the PR (A-H) interval.

The presence of an ipsilateral bundle branch block can facilitate reentry and cause an incessant AV reentrant tachycardia. A functional bundle branch block in the ventricle contralateral to the accessory pathway does not lengthen the tachycardia cycle if the H-V interval does not lengthen.

Septal Accessory Pathway. An exception to these observations occurs in a patient with a concealed septal accessory pathway. First, retrograde atrial activation is normal because it occurs retrogradely up the septum. Second, the VA interval and the cycle length of the tachycardia increase 25 milliseconds or less with the development of an ipsilateral functional bundle branch block.

Vagal maneuvers, by acting predominantly on the AV node, produce a response on AV reentry similar to AV nodal reentry, and the tachycardia can transiently slow and sometimes terminate. Generally, termination occurs in the anterograde direction, so the last retrograde P wave fails to conduct to the ventricle.

ELECTROPHYSIOLOGICAL FEATURES. Electrophysiological criteria supporting the diagnosis of tachycardia involving reentry over a concealed accessory pathway include the fact that initiation of tachycardia depends on a critical degree of AV delay (necessary to allow time for the accessory pathway to recover excitability so that it can conduct retrogradely), but the delay can be in the AV node or His-Purkinje system; that is, a critical degree of A-H delay is not necessary. Occasionally, a tachycardia can start with little or no measurable lengthening of AV nodal or His-Purkinje conduction time. The AV nodal refractory period curve is smooth, in contrast to the discontinuous curve found in many patients with AV nodal reentry. Dual AV nodal pathways can occasionally be noted as a concomitant, but unrelated finding.

Diagnosis of Accessory Pathways. Diagnosis can be accomplished by demonstrating that during ventricular pacing, premature ventricular stimulation activates the atria before retrograde depolarization of the His bundle, thus indicating that the impulse reached the atria before it depolarized the His bundle and must have traveled a different pathway to do so. Also, if the ventricles can be stimulated prematurely during tachycardia at a time when the His bundle is refractory and the impulse still conducts to the atrium, retrograde propagation traveled to the atrium over a pathway other than the bundle of His (see Fig. 32-26B). If the PVC depolarizes the atria without lengthening of the VA interval and with the same retrograde atrial activation sequence, one assumes that the stimulation site (i.e., ventricle) is within the reentrant circuit without intervening His-Purkinje or AV nodal tissue that might increase the VA interval and therefore the A-A interval. In addition, if a PVC delivered at a time when the His bundle is refractory terminates the tachycardia without activating the atria retrogradely, it most likely invaded and blocked conduction in an accessory pathway.

The VA interval (a measurement of conduction over the accessory pathway) is generally constant over a wide range of ventricular paced rates and coupling intervals of PVCs, as well as during the tachycardia in the absence of aberration. Similar short VA intervals can be observed in some patients during AV nodal reentry, but if the VA conduction time or RP interval is the same during tachycardia *and* ventricular pacing at comparable rates, an accessory pathway is almost certainly present. The VA interval is usually less than 50 percent of the R-R interval. The tachycardia can be easily initiated following premature ventricular stimulation that conducts retrogradely in the accessory pathway but blocks conduction in the AV node or His bundle. Atria and ventricles are required components of the macro-reentrant circuit; therefore, continuation of the tachycardia in the presence of AV or VA block excludes an accessory AV pathway as part of the reentrant circuit.

CLINICAL FEATURES. The presence of concealed accessory pathways is estimated to account for about 30 percent of patients with apparent supraventricular tachycardia referred for electrophysiological evaluation. The great majority of these accessory pathways are located between the left ventricle and left atrium and in the posteroseptal area, less commonly between the right ventricle and right atrium. It is important to be aware of a concealed accessory pathway as a possible cause of apparently "routine" supraventricular tachycardia since the therapeutic response may at times not follow the usual guidelines. Tachycardia rates tend to be somewhat faster than those occurring in AV nodal reentry (200 beats/min), but a great deal of overlap exists between the two groups.

Syncope can occur because the rapid ventricular rate fails to provide adequate cerebral circulation or because the tachyarrhythmia depresses the sinus pacemaker and causes a period of asystole when the tachyarrhythmia terminates. Physical examination reveals an unvarying, regular ventricular rhythm with constant intensity of the first heart sound. Jugular venous pressure can be elevated, but the waveform generally remains constant.

MANAGEMENT. The therapeutic approach to terminate this form of tachycardia acutely is as outlined for AV nodal reentry. It is necessary to achieve block of a single impulse from atrium to ventricle or ventricle to atrium. Generally, the most successful method is to produce a transient AV nodal block; therefore, vagal maneuvers, IV adenosine, verapamil or diltiazem, digitalis, and beta blockers are acceptable choices. Radiofrequency catheter ablation and conventional antiarrhythmic agents that prolong the activation time or refractory period in the accessory pathway need to be considered for chronic prophylactic therapy, similar to that discussed for reciprocating tachycardias associated with the preexcitation syndrome. Radiofrequency catheter ablation is curative, has low risk, and should be considered early for symptomatic patients (see Chap. 30).[65] The presence of atrial fibrillation in patients with a *concealed accessory pathway* should not be a greater therapeutic challenge than in patients who do not have such a pathway because anterograde AV conduction occurs only over the AV node and not over an accessory pathway. IV verapamil and digitalis are not contraindicated. However, under some circumstances, such as catecholamine stimulation, anterograde conduction can occur in the apparently concealed accessory pathway.

Preexcitation Syndrome

ECG RECOGNITION. Preexcitation, or the WPW ECG abnormality, occurs when the atrial impulse activates the whole or some part of the ventricle or the ventricular impulse activates the whole or some part of the atrium earlier than would be expected if the impulse traveled by way of the normal specialized conduction system only (Fig. 32–27).[65] This premature activation is caused by muscular connections composed of working myocardial fibers that exist outside the specialized conducting tissue and connect the atrium and ventricle while bypassing AV nodal conduction delay. They are named *accessory AV pathways* or connections and are responsible for the most common variety of preexcitation (incidentally noted in other species such as monkeys, dogs, and cats). The term *syndrome* is attached to this disorder when tachyarrhythmias occur as a result of the accessory pathway. Three basic features typify the ECG abnormalities of patients with the usual form of WPW conduction caused by an AV connection: (1) PR interval less than 120 milliseconds during sinus rhythm; (2) QRS complex duration exceeding 120 milliseconds with a slurred, slowly rising onset of the QRS in some leads (delta wave) and usually a normal terminal QRS portion; and (3) secondary ST-T wave changes that are generally directed in an opposite direction to the major delta and QRS vectors. Analysis of the scalar ECG can be used to localize the accessory pathway (Fig. 32–27D).[66]

In the *WPW syndrome,* the most common tachycardia is characterized by a normal QRS, a regular rhythm, ventricular rates of 150 to 250 beats/min (generally faster than AV nodal reentry), and sudden onset and termination, in most respects behaving like the tachycardia described for conduction over a concealed pathway (see Chap. 27). The major difference between the two is the capacity for anterograde conduction over the accessory pathway during atrial flutter or atrial fibrillation (see later).

Variants

A variety of other anatomical substrates exist and provide the basis for different ECG manifestations of several variations of the preexcitation syndrome (Fig. 32-28).[65] Fibers from the atrium to the His bundle bypassing the physiological delay of the AV node are called *atriohisian tracts* (Fig. 32-28B) and are associated with a short PR interval and a normal QRS complex. Although demonstrated anatomically (see later), the electrophysiological significance of these tracts in the genesis of tachycardias with a short PR interval and a normal QRS complex (Lown-Ganong-Levine [LGL] syndrome) remains to be established. Indeed, evidence does *not* support the presence of a specific LGL syndrome consisting of a short PR interval, normal QRS complex, and tachycardias related to an atriohisian bypass tract.

Another variant of accessory pathway conduction is that due to *atriofascicular* or *nodofascicular* accessory pathways. These fibers result in a unique AV conduction pattern (sometimes referred to as *Mahaim conduction*) characterized by the development of ventricular preexcitation (widened QRS and short H-V interval) with a progressive increase in the AV interval in response to atrial overdrive pacing, as opposed to the behavior of the usual accessory pathway in which preexcitation occurs with short AV intervals (Fig. 32-29). Because the accessory pathways responsible for this conduction pattern usually insert into the right bundle branch, preexcitation generally results in a left bundle branch block pattern. This phenomenon can be due to fibers passing from the AV node to the ventricle, called *nodoventricular fibers* (or nodofascicular if the insertion is into the right bundle branch rather than ventricular muscle) (see Fig. 32-28C). For nodoventricular connections, the PR interval may be normal or short, and the QRS complex is a fusion beat. This pattern of preexcitation can also result from *atriofascicular* accessory pathways. These fibers almost always represent a duplication of the AV node and the distal conducting system and are located in the right ventricular free wall. The apical end lies close to the lateral tricuspid annulus and conducts slowly, with AV node–like properties. After a long course, the distal portion of these fibers, which conducts rapidly, inserts into the distal right bundle branch or the apical region of the right ventricle.[65] No preexcitation is generally apparent during sinus rhythm but can be exposed by premature right atrial stimulation. The absence of retrograde conduction in these pathways produces only an antidromic AV reentry tachycardia ("preexcited" tachycardia) characterized by anterograde conduction over the accessory pathway and retrograde conduction over the right bundle branch–His bundle–AV node, thus making the atrium a necessary part of the circuit. The preexcited tachycardia has a left bundle branch block pattern, long AV interval (because of the long conduction time over the accessory pathway), and short VA interval. A right bundle branch block can be proarrhythmic by increasing the length of the tachycardia circuit (the VA interval is prolonged because of a delay in retrograde activation of the His bundle), and the tachycardia can become incessant.[65]

In patients who have an atriohisian tract, theoretically, the QRS complex would remain normal and the short A-H interval fixed or show very little increase during atrial pacing at more rapid rates. This response is uncommon. Rapid atrial pacing in patients who have nodoventricular or nodofascicular connections shortens the H-V interval and widens the QRS complex, with production of a left bundle branch block contour, but in contrast to the situation in patients who have an AV connection (Fig. 32-30), the AV interval also lengthens. In patients who have fasciculoventricular connections, the H-V interval remains short and the QRS complex unchanged and anomalous during rapid atrial pacing.

ELECTROPHYSIOLOGICAL FEATURES OF PREEXCITATION. If the accessory pathway is capable of anterograde conduction, two parallel routes of AV conduction are possible, one subject to physiological delay over the AV node and the other passing directly without delay from the atrium to the ventricle (Figs. 32-31 to 32-37; see also Figs. 32-28 to 32-30). This direct route of conduction produces the typical QRS complex that is a fusion beat as a result of depolarization of the ventricle in part by the wavefront traveling over the accessory pathway and in part by the wavefront traveling over the normal AV node–His bundle route. The delta wave represents ventricular activation from input over the accessory pathway. The extent of the contribution to ventricular deplorization by the wavefront over each route depends on their relative activation times. If AV nodal conduction delay occurs because of a rapid atrial pacing rate or premature atrial complex, for example, more of the ventricle becomes activated over the accessory pathway and the QRS complex becomes more anomalous in contour. Total activation of the ventricle over the accessory pathway can occur if the AV nodal conduction delay is sufficiently long. In contrast, if the accessory pathway is relatively far from the sinus node, for example, a left lateral accessory pathway, or if the AV nodal conduction time is relatively short, more of the ventricle may be activated by conduction over the normal pathway (see Fig. 32-30). The normal fusion beat during sinus rhythm has a short H-V interval, or His bundle activation actually begins after the onset of ventricular depolarization because part of the atrial impulse bypasses the AV node and activates the ventricle early, at a time when the atrial impulse traveling the normal route just reaches the His bundle. This finding of a short or negative H-V interval occurs *only* during conduction over an accessory pathway or from retrograde His activation during a complex originating in the ventricle, such as a VT.

Pacing the atrium at rapid rates, at premature intervals, or from a site close to the atrial insertion of the accessory pathway accentuates the anomalous activation of the ventricles and shortens the H-V interval even more (His activation may become buried in the ventricular electrogram, as in Fig. 32-30B). The position of the accessory pathway can be determined by careful analysis of the spatial direction of the delta wave in the 12-lead ECG in maximally preexcited beats (see Fig. 32-27).[66] T wave abnormalities can occur after the disappearance of preexcitation with orientation of the T wave according to the site of preexcitation (T wave

Text continued on p. 836

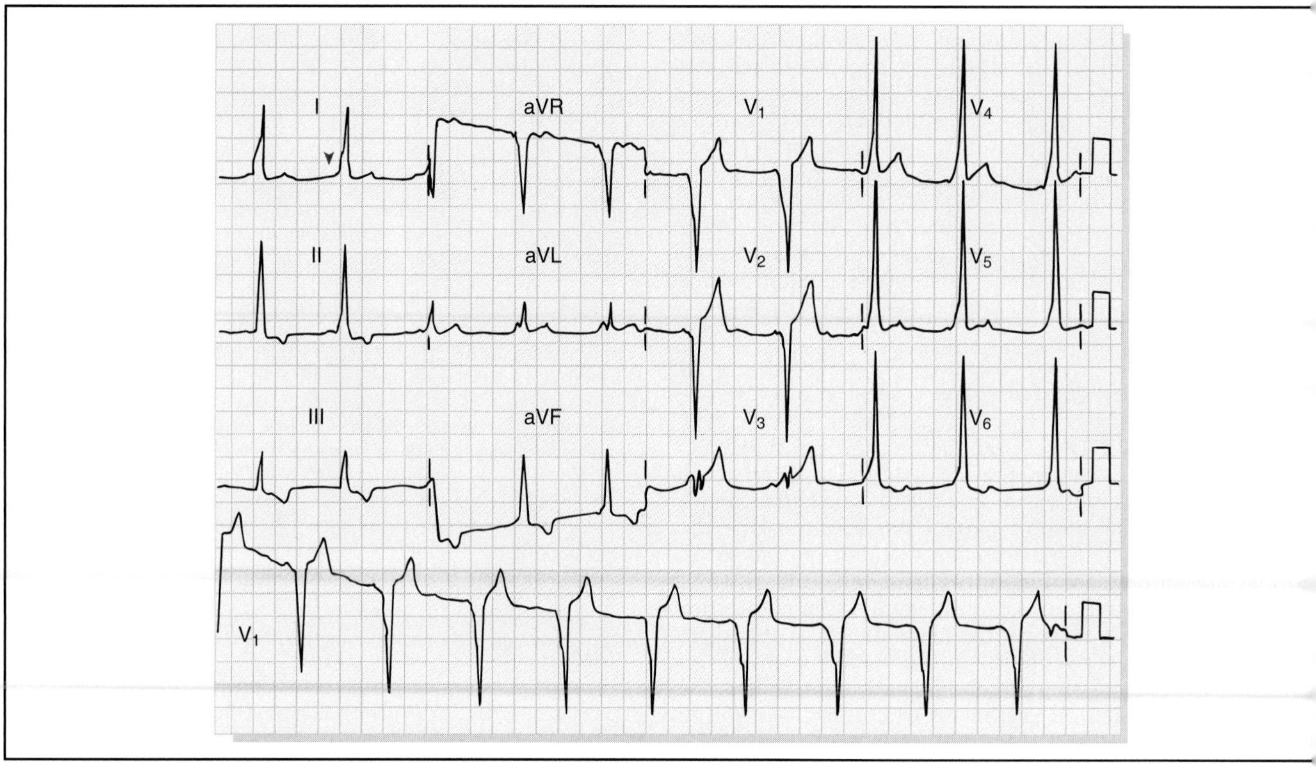

A

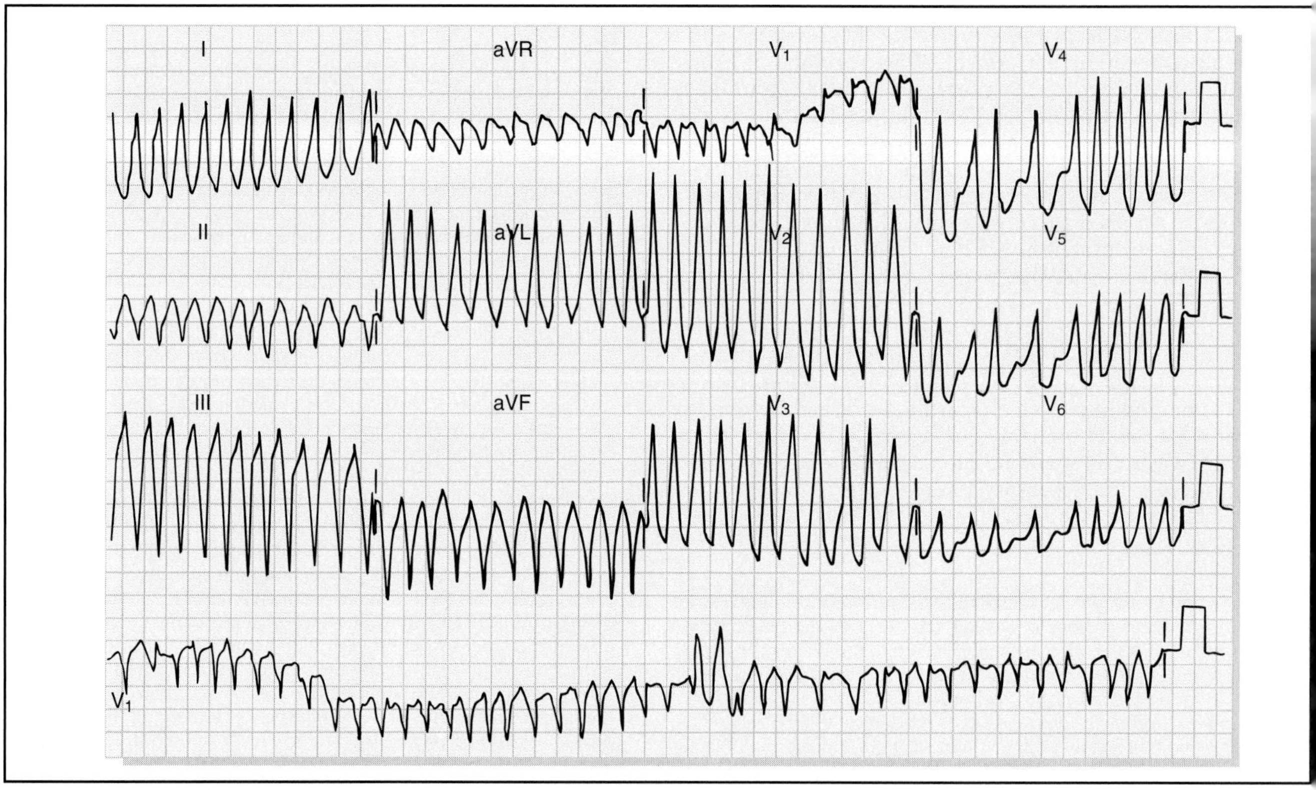

B

FIGURE 32–27 **A,** Right anteroseptal accessory pathway. The 12-lead electrocardiogram characteristically exhibits a normal to inferior axis. The delta wave is negative in V_1 and V_2, upright in leads I, II, aVL, and aVF, isoelectric in lead III, and negative in aVR. Location was verified at surgery. The arrowhead indicates a delta wave (lead I). **B,** Right posteroseptal accessory pathway. Negative delta waves in leads II, III, and aVF, upright in I and aVL, localize this pathway to the posteroseptal region. The negative delta wave in V_1 with sharp transition to an upright delta wave in V_2 pinpoints it to the right posteroseptal area. Atrial fibrillation is present. Location was verified at surgery. **C,** Left lateral accessory pathway. A positive delta wave in the anterior precordial leads and in leads II, III, and aVF, positive or isoelectric in leads I and aVL, and isoelectric or negative in V_5 and V_6 is typical of a left lateral accessory pathway. Rapid coronary sinus pacing (450-millisecond cycle length) was used to enhance preexcitation (negative P wave in leads I, II, III, aVF, and V_3 through V_6). Location was verified at surgery. **D,** Right free wall accessory pathway. The predominantly negative delta wave in V_1 and the axis more leftward than in **A** indicate the presence of a right free wall accessory pathway. **E,** Logic diagram to determine the location of accessory pathways. Begin with analysis of V_1 to determine whether the delta wave and the QRS complex are negative or positive. That establishes the ventricle in which the accessory pathway is located. Next, determine whether the delta wave and QRS complex are negative in leads II, III, and aVF. If so, the accessory pathway is located in a posteroseptal position. If the accessory pathway is located in the right ventricle, an inferior axis indicates an anteroseptal location, whereas a left axis indicates a right free wall location. If the accessory pathway is located in the left ventricle, an isoelectric or negative delta wave and QRS complex in leads I, aVL, V_5, and V_6 indicate a left lateral (free wall) location.

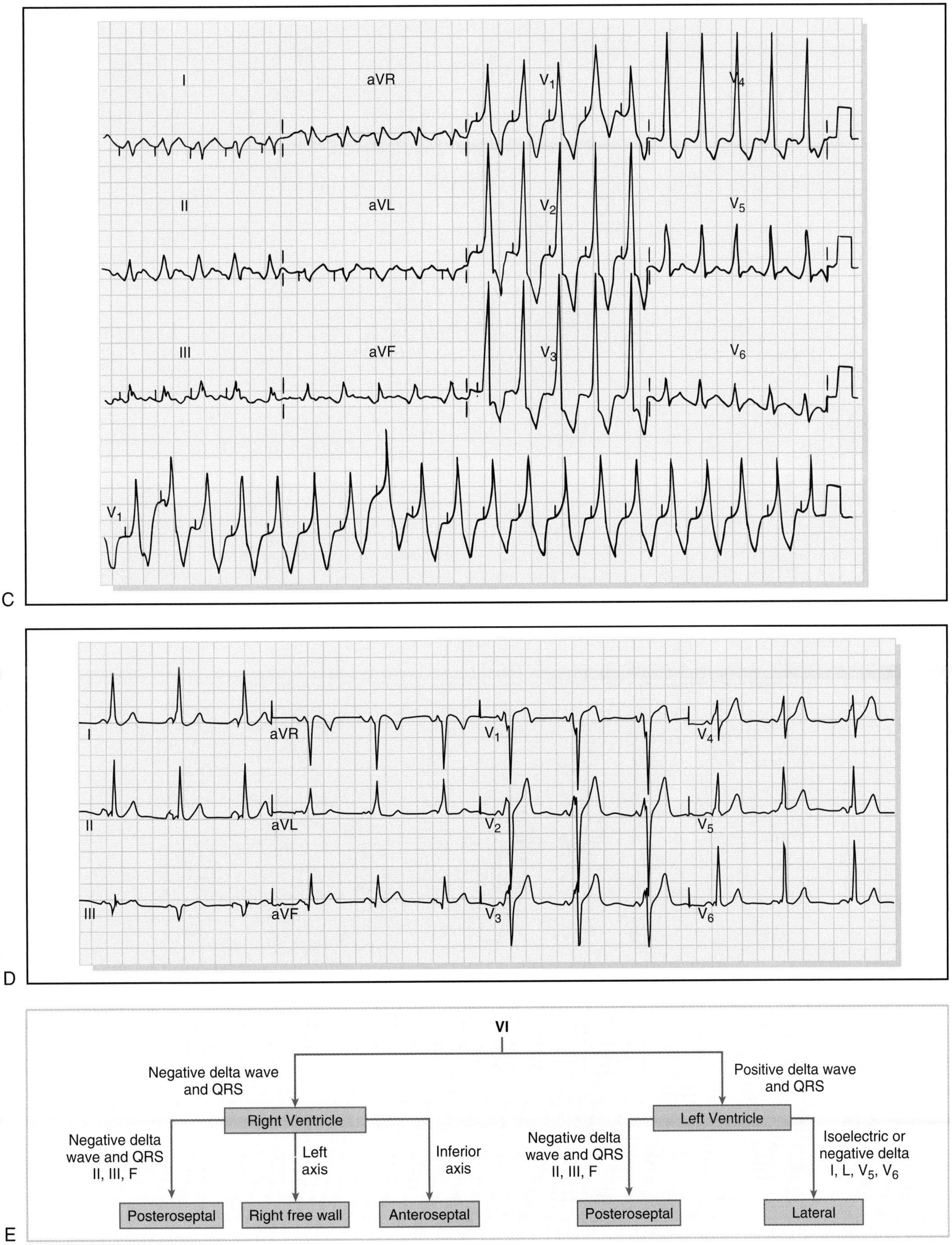

FIGURE 32–27 cont'd.

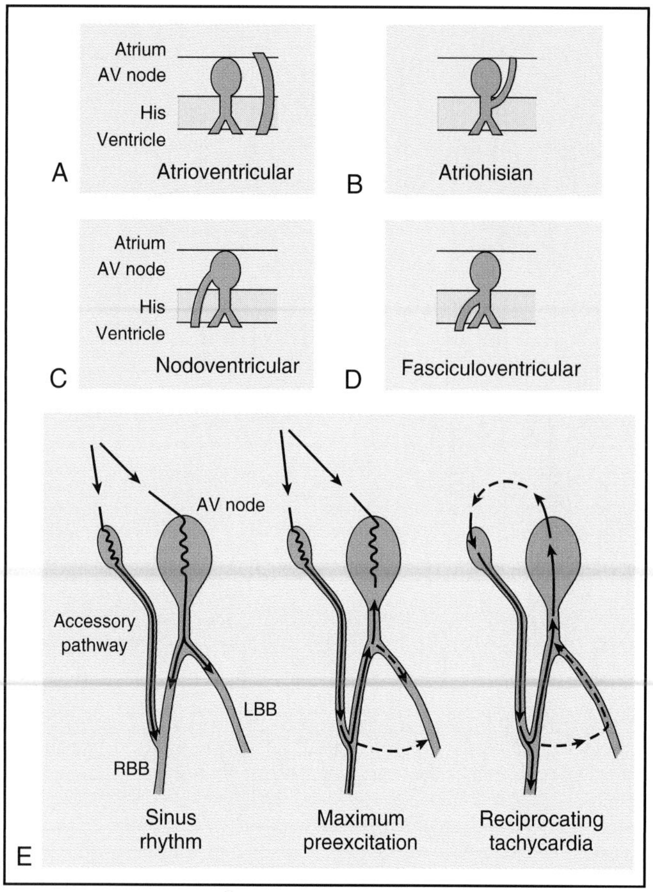

FIGURE 32–28 Schematic representation of accessory pathways. **A,** The "usual" atrioventricular (AV) accessory pathway giving rise to most clinical manifestations of tachycardia associated with Wolff-Parkinson-White (WPW) syndrome. **B,** The very uncommon atriohisian accessory pathway. If Lown-Ganong-Levine syndrome exists, it would have this type of anatomy, which has been demonstrated on occasion histopathologically. **C,** Nodoventricular pathways, original concept, in which anterograde conduction travels down the accessory pathway with retrograde conduction in the bundle branch–His bundle–AV node (see below). **D,** Fasciculoventricular connections, which are not thought to play an important role in the genesis of tachycardias. **E,** The current concept of nodofascicular accessory pathway in which the accessory pathway is an AV communication with AV nodal-like properties. Sinus rhythm results in a fusion QRS complex, as in the usual form of WPW syndrome shown in **A.** Maximum preexcitation results in ventricular activation over the accessory pathway, and the His bundle is activated retrogradely. During reciprocating tachycardia, anterograde conduction occurs over the accessory pathway with retrograde conduction over the normal pathway. LBBB = left bundle branch block; RBBB = right bundle branch block. (**E** from Benditt DG, Milstein S: Nodoventricular accessory connection: A misnomer or a structural/functional spectrum. J Cardiovasc Electrophysiol 1:231, 1990.)

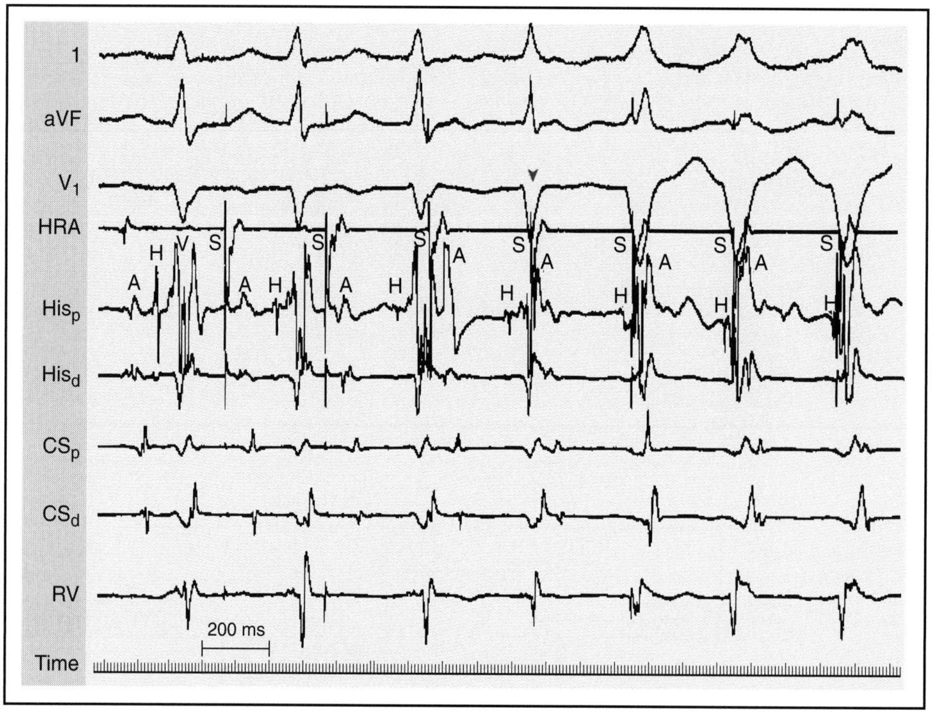

FIGURE 32–29 Development of preexcitation over an atriofascicular accessory pathway. During atrial pacing (S), on the left side of the figure, conduction occurs down the atrioventricular node as evidenced by a normal-appearing QRS complex and a normal H-V interval. The stimulus marked by the arrowhead conducts the impulse down an atriofascicular fiber, which results in a preexcited QRS, as evidenced by a widened QRS and short H-V interval.

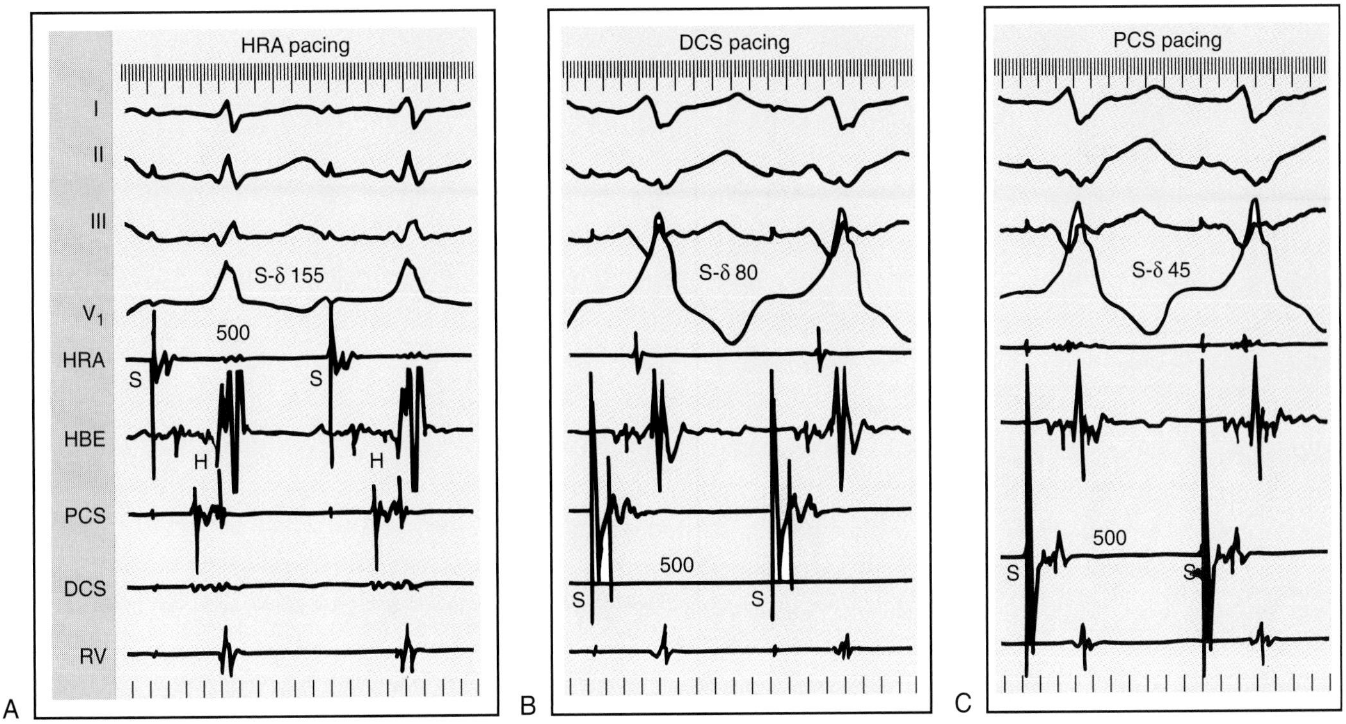

FIGURE 32–30 Atrial pacing at different atrial sites illustrating different conduction over the accessory pathway. **A,** High right atrial pacing at a cycle length of 500 milliseconds produces anomalous activation of the ventricle (note the upright QRS complex in V_1) and a stimulus-delta interval of 155 milliseconds (S-δ 155). This interval indicates that the time from the onset of the stimulus to the beginning of the QRS complex is relatively long because the stimulus is delivered at a fairly large distance from the accessory pathway. Note that His bundle activation (H) occurs at about the onset of the QRS complex. **B,** Atrial pacing occurs through the distal coronary sinus electrode (DCS). At the same pacing cycle length, DCS pacing results in more anomalous ventricular activation and a shorter stimulus-delta interval (80 milliseconds). His bundle activation is now buried within the inscription of the ventricular electrogram in the HBE lead. **C,** Pacing from the proximal coronary sinus electrode (PCS) results in the shortest stimulus-delta interval (45 milliseconds); such an interval indicates that the pacing stimulus is being delivered very close to the atrial insertion of the accessory pathway, which is located in the left posteroseptal region of the atrioventricular groove.

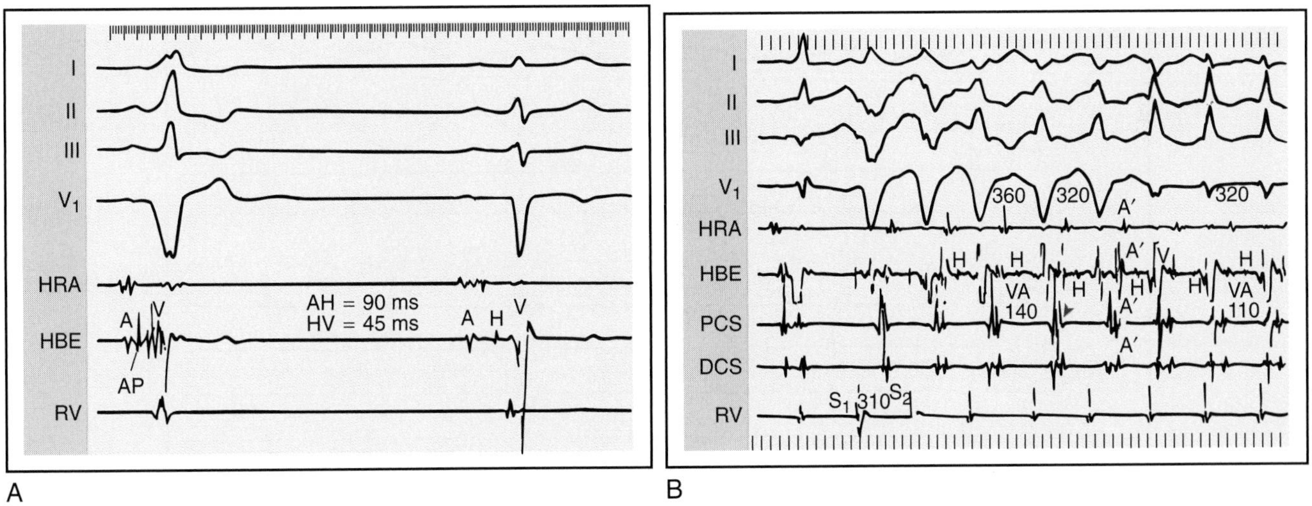

FIGURE 32–31 **A,** Recording of depolarization of an accessory pathway (AP) with a catheter electrode. The first QRS complex illustrates conduction over the AP. In the scalar ECG, a short P-R interval and delta wave (best seen in leads I and V_1) are apparent. His bundle activation is buried within the ventricular complex. In the following complex, conduction has blocked over the AP and a normal QRS complex results. His bundle activation clearly precedes the onset of ventricular depolarization by 45 milliseconds. The A-H interval for this complex is 90 milliseconds. **B,** Influence of functional ipsilateral bundle branch block on the VA interval during an atrioventricular reciprocating tachycardia. Partial preexcitation can be noted in the sinus-initiated complex (first complex). Two premature ventricular stimuli (S_1, S_2) initiate a sustained supraventricular tachycardia that persists with a left bundle branch block for several complexes before finally reverting to normal. The retrograde atrial activation sequence is recorded first in the proximal coronary sinus lead (arrowhead, PCS), then in the distal coronary sinus lead (DCS) and low right atrium (HBE), and then high in the right atrium (HRA). During the functional bundle branch block, the ventriculoatrial interval in the PCS lead is 140 milliseconds, which shortens to 110 milliseconds when the QRS complex reverts to normal. Such behavior is characteristic of a left-sided accessory pathway with prolongation of the reentrant pathway by the functional left bundle branch block. (**A,** From Prystowsky EN, Browne KF, Zipes DP: Intracardiac recording by catheter electrode of accessory pathway depolarization. J Am Coll Cardiol 1:468, 1983.)

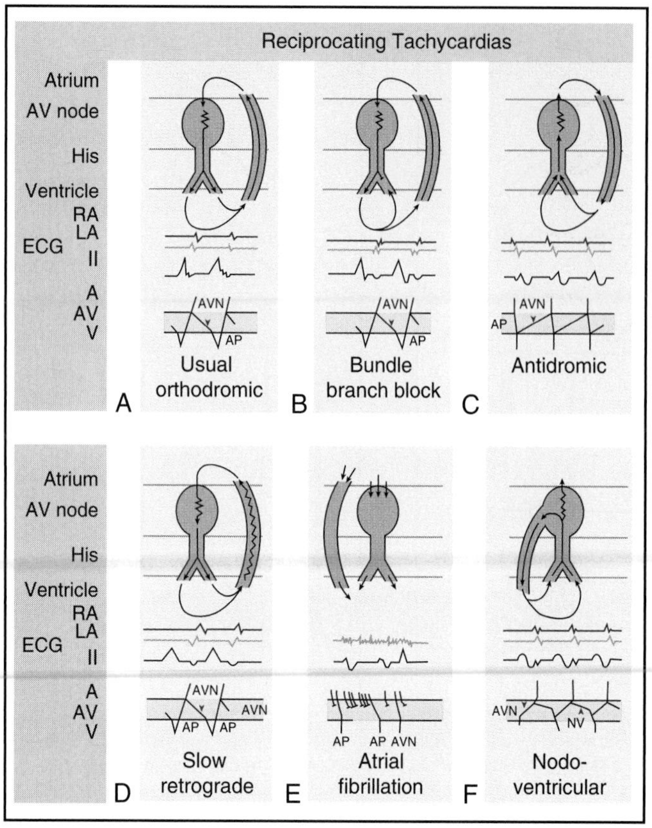

FIGURE 32–32 Schematic diagram of tachycardias associated with accessory pathways. **A,** Orthodromic tachycardia with anterograde conduction (arrow) over the atrioventricular (AV) node–His bundle route and retrograde conduction over the accessory pathway (left sided for this example, as depicted by left atrial activation preceding right atrial activation). **B,** Orthodromic tachycardia and ipsilateral functional bundle branch block. **C,** Antidromic tachycardia with anterograde conduction over the accessory pathway and retrograde conduction (arrow) over the AV node–His bundle. **D,** Orthodromic tachycardia with a slowly conducting accessory pathway (arrow). **E,** Atrial fibrillation with the accessory pathway as a bystander. **F,** Anterograde conduction over a portion of the AV node and a nodoventricular pathway and retrograde conduction over the AV node (arrows).

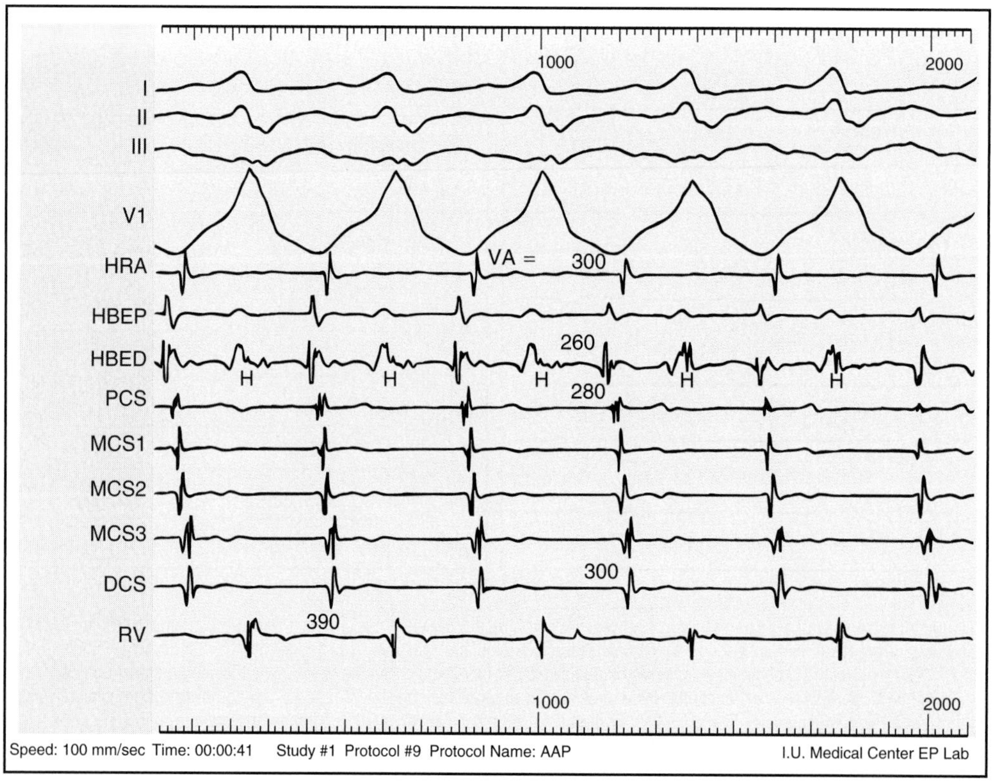

FIGURE 32–33 Antidromic atrioventricular (AV) reciprocating tachycardia. Tachycardia in this example is due to anterograde conduction over the accessory pathway (note the abnormal QRS complex of a left posterior accessory pathway) and a normal retrograde atrial activation sequence (beginning first in the HBED lead), which is due to retrograde conduction over the AV node. Tachycardia cycle length is 390 milliseconds, with a ventriculoatrial (VA) interval of 300 milliseconds measured in the high right atrial lead, 260 milliseconds in the distal His lead, and 280 milliseconds in the proximal coronary sinus lead. I, II, III, and V_1 are scalar leads. DCS = distal coronary sinus lead; HBEP and HBED leads = His bundle electrogram, proximal and distal; HRA = high right atrial electrogram; MCS1-3 = midcoronary sinus leads; PCS = proximal coronary sinus; RV = right ventricular electrogram.

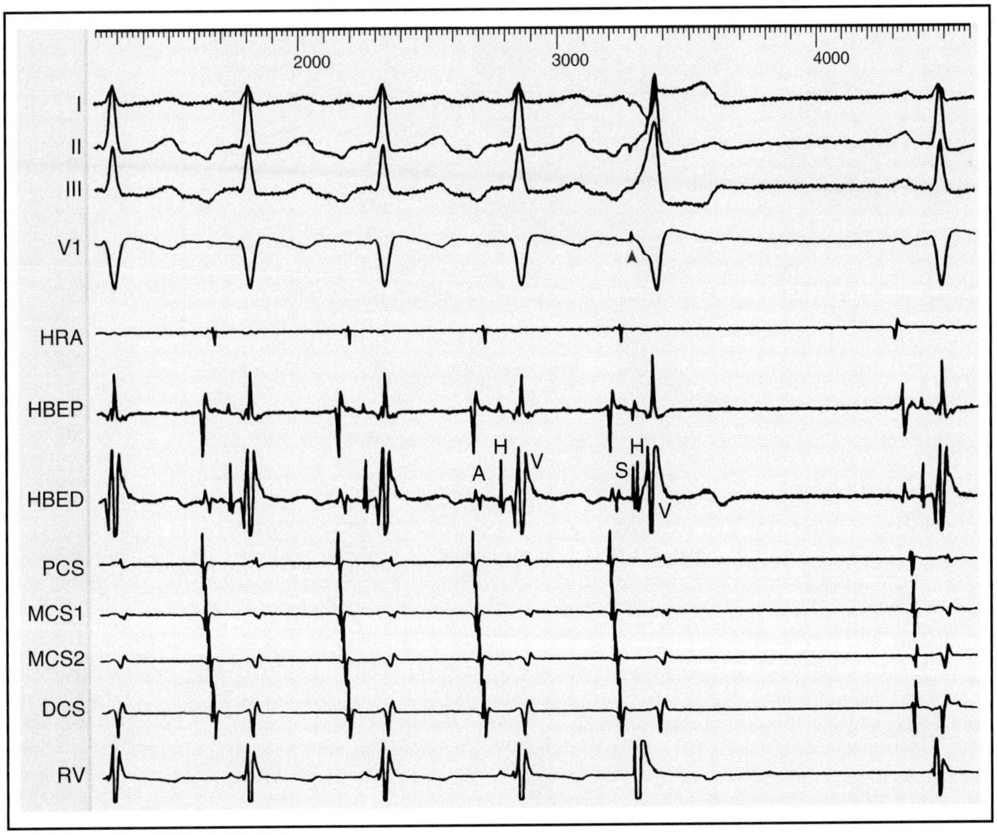

FIGURE 32–34 Termination of the permanent form of atrioventricular (AV) junctional reciprocating tachycardia (PJRT). In the left portion of this example, PJRT is present. The atrial activation sequence is indistinguishable from atypical AV nodal reentry and atrial tachycardia originating in the low right atrium. The response to premature stimulation identifies the tachycardia as PJRT. Premature ventricular stimulation (arrowhead) occurs at a time when the His bundle is refractory from depolarization during the tachycardia (second labeled H). Therefore, premature ventricular stimulation cannot enter the AV node. Furthermore, premature ventricular stimulation does not reach the atrium. Yet premature ventricular stimulation terminates the tachycardia. This detail can be explained only by the PVC invading and blocking in a retrogradely conducting accessory pathway. I, II, III, and V_1 are scalar electrocardiographic leads. DCS = distal coronary sinus electrograms; HBEP, HBED = His bundle electrogram, proximal and distal; HRA = high right atrial electrogram; MCS1, MCS2 = midcoronary sinus electrograms; PCS = proximal coronary sinus electrogram; RV = right ventricular electrogram.

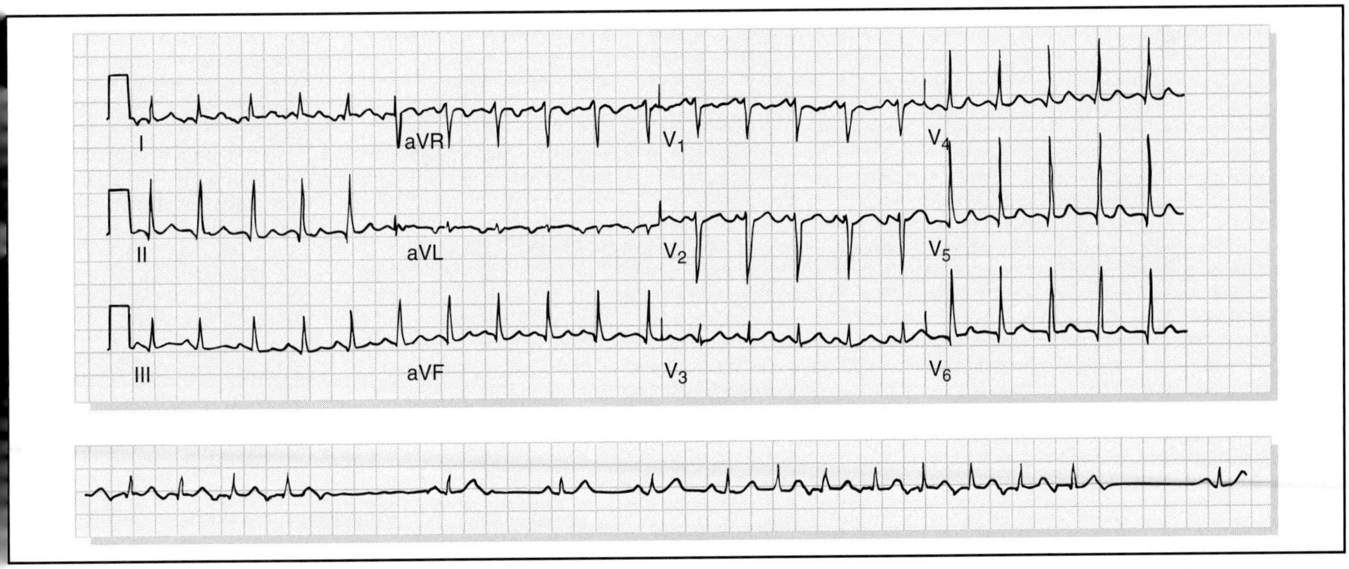

FIGURE 32–35 Permanent form of junctional reciprocating tachycardia (PJRT) in a patient with a left-sided accessory pathway. The 12-lead electrocardiogram demonstrates a long RP interval-short PR interval tachycardia, which in contrast to the usual form of PJRT, exhibits negative P waves in leads I and aVL. The rhythm strips below (lead I) indicate that whenever a nonconducted P wave occurs, the tachycardia always terminates, only to begin again after several sinus beats. This pattern is in marked contrast to that in Figure 32–12, in which the tachycardia continues despite nonconducted P waves.

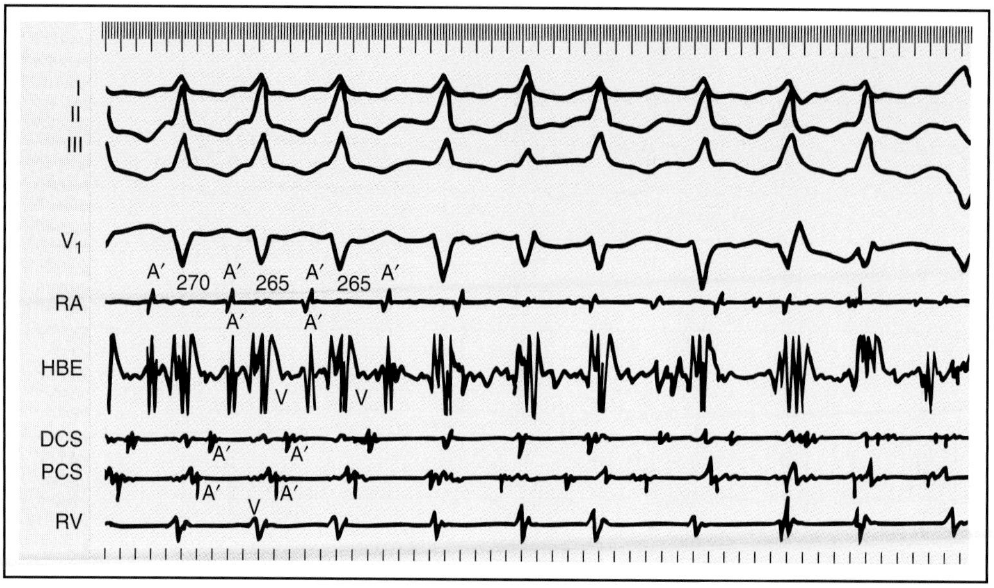

FIGURE 32–36 Atrioventricular (AV) reciprocating tachycardia disorganizing into atrial fibrillation. During sustained AV reciprocating tachycardia at a cycle length of approximately 265 milliseconds, the retrograde atrial activation sequence began first in the right paraseptal region (not shown in this example; location proved at surgery) and was then recorded in the proximal coronary sinus electrogram, followed by atrial activity in the distal coronary sinus, in the low right atrium recorded in the His bundle lead, and then in the high right atrium. Spontaneously, the atrial activation sequence becomes irregular (after the last A′) and atrial fibrillation begins. Note that the last QRS complex reflects conduction over the accessory pathway. Such a transformation occurred repeatedly in this patient and was associated with quickening of the ventricular rate. Atrial fibrillation did not recur following surgical interruption of the accessory pathway.

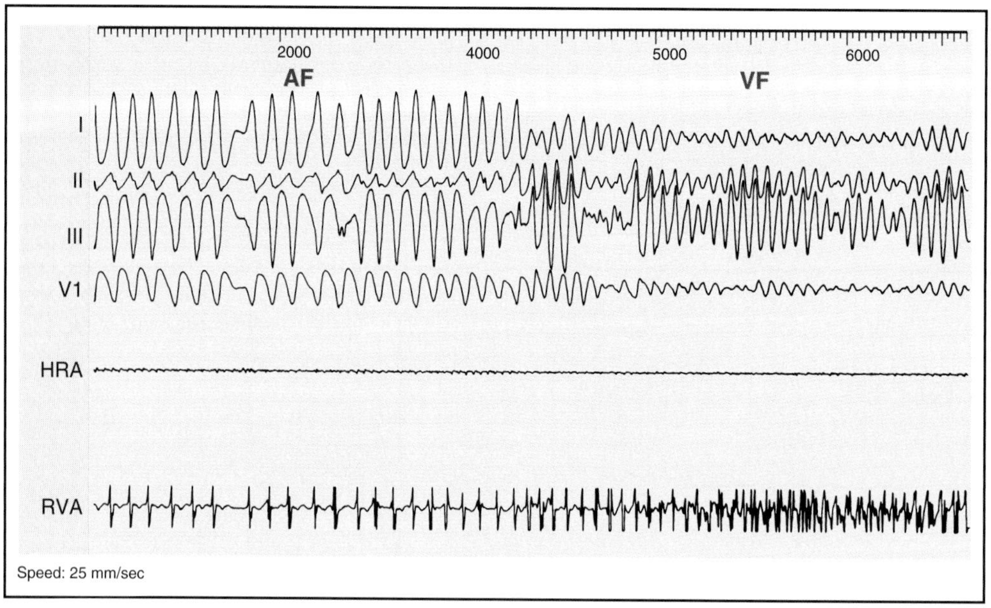

FIGURE 32–37 Atrial fibrillation (AF) becoming ventricular fibrillation (VF). In the left portion of this panel, the electrocardiogram (ECG) demonstrates AF with conduction over an accessory pathway producing a rapid ventricular response, at times in excess of 350 beats/min. In the midportion of the tracing VF can be seen to develop. I, II, III, and V_1 are scalar ECG leads. HRA = high right atrial electrogram; RVA = right ventricular apex electrogram.

memory). A variety of electrical, radionuclide, and echocardiographic techniques can be used to localize the insertion site of the accessory pathway (see Chap. 29).

ACCESSORY PATHWAY CONDUCTION. Even though the accessory pathway conducts more rapidly than the AV node (conduction velocity is faster in the accessory pathway), the accessory pathway usually has a longer refractory period during long cycle lengths (e.g., sinus rhythm); that is, it takes longer for the accessory pathway to recover excitability than it does for the AV node. Consequently, a premature atrial complex can occur sufficiently early to block conduction anterogradely in the accessory pathway and conduct to the ventricle only over the normal AV node–His bundle (see Fig. 32–32A and B). The resultant H-V interval and the QRS complex become normal. Such an event can initiate the most common type of reciprocating tachycardia, one characterized by anterograde conduction over the normal pathway and retrograde conduction over the accessory pathway (*orthodromic AV reciprocating tachycardia*) (see Fig. 32–32). The accessory pathway, which blocks conduction in an anterograde direction, recovers excitability in time to be activated after the QRS complex in a retrograde direction, thereby completing the reentrant loop.

Much less commonly, patients can have tachycardias called *antidromic* tachycardias during which anterograde conduction occurs over the accessory pathway and retrograde conduction over the AV node. The resultant QRS complex is abnormal because of total ventricular activation over the accessory pathway (see Figs. 32–32C and 32–33). In both tachycardias, the accessory pathway is an obligatory part of the reentrant circuit. In patients with bidirectional conduction over the accessory pathway, different fibers can be used anterogradely and retrogradely.

A small percentage of patients have multiple accessory pathways often suggested by various ECG clues, and on occasion, tachycardia can be due to a reentrant loop conducting anterogradely over one accessory pathway and retrogradely over the other. Fifteen to 20 percent of patients may exhibit AV nodal echoes or AV nodal reentry after interruption of the accessory pathway.

PERMANENT FORM OF AV JUNCTIONAL RECIPROCATING TACHYCARDIA. An incessant form of supraventricular tachycardia has been recognized that generally occurs with a long RP interval that exceeds the PR interval (see Figs. 32–34 and 32–35). Usually, a posteroseptal accessory pathway (most often the right ventricular but other locations as well) that conducts very slowly, possibly because of a long and tortuous route, appears responsible. Tachycardia is maintained by anterograde AV nodal conduction and retrograde conduction over the accessory pathway (see Fig. 32–32D). Although anterograde conduction over this pathway has been demonstrated, the long anterograde conduction time over the accessory pathway ordinarily prevents ECG manifestations of accessory pathway conduction during sinus rhythm. Therefore, during sinus rhythm, the QRS duration is prolonged from conduction over this accessory pathway only when conduction times through the AV node–His bundle exceed those in the accessory pathway.[65]

RECOGNITION OF ACCESSORY PATHWAYS. When retrograde atrial activation during tachycardia occurs over an accessory pathway that connects the left atrium to the left ventricle, the earliest retrograde activity is recorded from a left atrial electrode usually positioned in the coronary sinus (see Fig. 32-26). When retrograde atrial activation during tachycardia occurs over an accessory pathway that connects the right ventricle to the right atrium, the earliest retrograde atrial activity is generally recorded from a lateral right atrial electrode. Participation of a septal accessory pathway creates the earliest retrograde atrial activation in the low right portion of the atrium situated near the septum, anterior or posterior, depending on the insertion site. These mapping techniques provide an accurate assessment of the position of the accessory pathway, which can be anywhere in the AV groove except in the intervalvular trigone between the mitral valve and the aortic valve annuli. Recording electrical activity directly from the accessory pathway obviously provides precise localization.

It may be difficult to distinguish AV nodal reentry from participation of a septal accessory connection using the retrograde sequence of atrial activation because activation sequences during both tachycardias are similar. Other approaches to demonstrate retrograde atrial activation over the accessory pathway must be tried and can be accomplished by inducing PVCs during tachycardia to determine whether retrograde atrial excitation can occur from the ventricle at a time when the His bundle is refractory (see Fig. 32-26B). Since VA conduction cannot occur over the normal conduction system because the His bundle is refractory, an accessory pathway must be present for the atria to become excited. No patient with a reciprocating tachycardia from an accessory AV pathway has a VA interval of less than 70 milliseconds measured from the onset of ventricular depolarization to the onset of the earliest atrial activity recorded on an esophageal lead or a VA interval of less than 95 milliseconds when measured to the high right part of the atrium. In contrast, in most patients with reentry in the AV node, intervals from the onset of ventricular activity to the earliest onset of atrial activity recorded in the esophageal lead are less than 70 milliseconds.

Other Forms of Tachycardia in Patients with Wolff-Parkinson-White Syndrome

Patients can have other types of tachycardia during which the accessory pathway is a "bystander," that is, uninvolved in the mechanism responsible for the tachycardia, such as AV nodal reentry or an atrial tachycardia that conducts to the ventricle over the accessory pathway. In patients with atrial flutter or atrial fibrillation, the accessory pathway is not a requisite part of the mechanism responsible for tachycardia, and the flutter or fibrillation occurs in the atrium unrelated to the accessory pathway (see Fig. 32-32E). Propagation to the ventricle during atrial flutter or atrial fibrillation can therefore occur over the normal AV node–His bundle or accessory pathway. Patients with WPW syndrome who have atrial fibrillation almost always have inducible reciprocating tachycardias as well, which can develop into atrial fibrillation (see Fig. 32-36). In fact, interruption of the accessory pathway and elimination of AV reciprocating tachycardia usually prevent recurrence of the atrial fibrillation. Atrial fibrillation presents a potentially serious risk because of the possibility for very rapid conduction over the accessory pathway. At more rapid rates, the refractory period of the accessory pathway can shorten significantly and permit an extremely rapid ventricular response during atrial flutter or atrial fibrillation (see Fig. 32-27B). The rapid ventricular response can exceed the ability of the ventricle to follow in an organized manner; it can result in fragmented, disorganized ventricular activation and hypotension and lead to ventricular fibrillation (see Fig. 32-37). Alternatively, a supraventricular discharge bypassing AV nodal delay can activate the ventricle during the vulnerable period of the antecedent T wave and precipitate ventricular fibrillation. Patients who have had ventricular fibrillation have ventricular cycle lengths during atrial fibrillation in the range of 200 milliseconds or less.

Patients with preexcitation syndrome can have other causes of tachycardia such as AV nodal reentry, sometimes with dual AV nodal curves, sinus nodal reentry, or even VT unrelated to the accessory pathway. Some accessory pathways can conduct anterogradely only; more commonly, pathways conduct retrogradely only. If the pathway conducts only anterogradely, it cannot participate in the usual form of reciprocating tachycardia (see Fig. 32-32A). It can, however, participate in antidromic tachycardia (Fig. 32-32C), as well as conduct to the ventricle during atrial flutter or atrial fibrillation (Fig. 32-32E). Some data suggest that the accessory pathway demonstrates automatic activity, which could conceivably be responsible for some instances of tachycardia.

"WIDE-QRS" TACHYCARDIAS. In patients with preexcitation syndrome, so-called wide-QRS tachycardias can be due to multiple mechanisms, including sinus or atrial tachycardias, AV nodal reentry, and atrial flutter or fibrillation with anterograde conduction over the accessory pathway; orthodromic reciprocating tachycardia with functional or preexisting bundle branch block; antidromic reciprocating tachycardia; reciprocating tachycardia with anterograde conduction over one accessory pathway and retrograde conduction over a second one; tachycardias using nodofascicular or atriofascicular fibers; or VT.

CLINICAL FEATURES. The reported incidence of preexcitation syndrome depends in large measure on the population studied and varies from 0.1 to 3 per 1000 in apparently healthy subjects, with an average of about 1.5 per 1000. The incidence of the ECG pattern of WPW conduction in 22,500 healthy aviation personnel was 0.25 percent with a prevalence of documented tachyarrhythmias of 1.8 percent. Left free wall accessory pathways are most common, followed in frequency by posteroseptal, right free wall, and anteroseptal locations. WPW syndrome is found in all age groups from the fetal and neonatal periods to the elderly, as well as in identical twins. The prevalence is higher in men and decreases with age, apparently because of loss of preexcitation. Most adults with preexcitation syndrome have normal hearts, although a variety of acquired and congenital cardiac defects have been reported, including Ebstein anomaly, mitral valve prolapse, and cardiomyopathies. Patients with Ebstein anomaly (see Chap. 56) often have multiple accessory pathways, right sided either in the posterior septum or in the posterolateral wall, with preexcitation localized to the atrialized ventricle. They often have reciprocating tachycardia with a long VA interval and a right bundle branch block morphology.

The frequency of paroxysmal tachycardia apparently increases with age, from 10 per 100 patients with WPW syndrome in a 20- to 39-year-old age group to 36 per 100 in patients older than 60 years. Approximately 80 percent of patients with tachycardia have a reciprocating tachycardia, 15 to 30 percent have atrial fibrillation, and 5 percent have atrial flutter. VT occurs uncommonly. The anomalous complexes can mask or mimic myocardial infarction (see Chap. 46), bundle branch block, or ventricular hypertrophy, and the presence of the preexcitation syndrome can call attention to an associated cardiac defect. The prognosis is excellent in patients without tachycardia or an associated cardiac anomaly. For most patients with recurrent tachycardia, the prognosis is good, but sudden death occurs rarely, with an estimated frequency of 0.1 percent.

It is highly likely that an accessory pathway is congenital, although its manifestations can be detected in later years and appear to be "acquired." Relatives of patients with preexcitation, particularly those with multiple pathways, have an increased prevalence of preexcitation, thus suggesting a hereditary mode of acquisition. Some children and adults can lose their tendency for the development of tachyarrhythmias as they grow older, possibly as a result of fibrotic or other changes at the site of the accessory pathway insertion. Pathways can lose their ability to conduct anterogradely. Tachycardia beginning in infancy can disappear but frequently recurs. Tachycardia still present after 5 years of age persists in 75 percent of patients regardless of accessory pathway location. Intermittent preexcitation during sinus rhythm and abrupt loss of conduction over the accessory pathway after intravenous ajmaline or procainamide and with exercise suggest that the refractory period of the accessory pathway is long and that the patient is not at risk for a rapid ventricular rate should atrial flutter or fibrillation develop. These approaches are relatively specific, but not very sensitive, with a low positive predictive accuracy. Exceptions to these safeguards can occur.

TREATMENT. Patients with ventricular preexcitation who have only the ECG abnormality, without tachyarrhythmias, do not require electrophysiological evaluation or therapy. However, for patients with frequent episodes of symptomatic tachyarrhythmia, therapy should be initiated.

Three therapeutic options exist: electrical or surgical (see Chap. 30) ablation and pharmacological therapy. Drugs are chosen to prolong conduction time and/or refractoriness in the AV node, the accessory pathway, or both to prevent rapid rates from occurring. If successful, this therapy prevents maintenance of an AV reciprocating tachycardia or a rapid ventricular response to atrial flutter or atrial fibrillation. Some drugs can suppress premature complexes that precipitate the arrhythmias.

Adenosine, verapamil, propranolol, and digitalis all prolong conduction time and refractoriness in the AV node. Verapamil and propranolol do not directly affect conduction in the accessory pathway, and digitalis has had variable effects. Because digitalis has been reported to shorten refractoriness in the accessory pathway and speed the ventricular response in some patients with atrial fibrillation, it is advisable to *not* use digitalis as a single drug in patients with WPW syndrome who have or may have atrial flutter or atrial fibrillation. Since atrial fibrillation can develop *during* the reciprocating tachycardia in many patients (see Fig. 32–36), this caveat probably applies to *all* patients who have tachycardia and WPW syndrome. Rather, drugs that prolong the refractory period in the accessory pathway should be used, such as classes IA and IC drugs (see Chap. 30).

Class IC drugs, amiodarone, and sotalol can affect both the AV node and the accessory pathway. Lidocaine does not generally prolong refractoriness of the accessory pathway. Verapamil and IV lidocaine can *increase* the ventricular rate during atrial fibrillation in patients with WPW syndrome. IV verapamil can precipitate *ventricular fibrillation* when given to a patient with WPW syndrome who has a rapid ventricular rate during atrial fibrillation. This effect does not appear to happen with *oral* verapamil. Catecholamines can expose WPW syndromes, shorten the refractory period of the accessory pathway, and reverse the effects of some antiarrhythmic drugs.

Termination of an Acute Episode. Termination of an acute episode of reciprocating tachycardia, suspected electrocardiographically from a normal QRS complex, regular R-R intervals, a rate of about 200 beats/min, and a retrograde P wave in the ST segment, should be approached similar to AV nodal reentry. After vagal maneuvers, adenosine followed by IV verapamil or diltiazem is the initial treatment of choice. Atrial fibrillation can occur after drug administration, particularly adenosine, with a rapid ventricular response. An external cardioverter-defibrillator should be immediately available if necessary. For atrial flutter or fibrillation, the latter suspected from an anomalous QRS complex and grossly irregular R-R intervals (see Figs. 32–27B and 32–36), drugs must be used that prolong refractoriness in the accessory pathway, often coupled with drugs that prolong AV nodal refractoriness (e.g., procainamide and propranolol). In many patients, particularly those with a very rapid ventricular response and any signs of hemodynamic impairment, electrical cardioversion is the *initial* treatment of choice.

Prevention. For long-term therapy to prevent recurrence, it is not always possible to predict which drugs may be most effective for an individual patient. Some drugs can actually increase the frequency of episodes of reciprocating tachycardia by prolonging the duration of anterograde and not retrograde refractory periods of the accessory pathway, thereby making it easier for a premature atrial complex to block conduction anterogradely in the accessory pathway and initiate tachycardia. Oral administration of two drugs, such as flecainide and propranolol, to decrease conduction capability in both limbs of the reentrant circuit can be beneficial. Class IC drugs, amiodarone, or sotalol, which prolong refractoriness in both the accessory pathway and the AV node, can be effective. Depending on the clinical situation, empirical drug trials or serial electrophysiological drug testing can be used to determine optimal drug therapy for patients with reciprocating tachycardia. For patients who have atrial fibrillation with a rapid ventricular response, induction of atrial fibrillation while the patient is receiving therapy is essential to be certain that the ventricular rate is controlled. Exercise or isoproterenol can be superimposed to be certain that the rate is controlled. Patients who have accessory pathways with very short refractory periods may be poor candidates for drug therapy since the refractory periods may be insignificantly prolonged in response to the standard agents.

Electrical or Surgical Ablation (see Chap. 30). Radiofrequency catheter ablation of the accessory pathway is advisable for patients with frequent symptomatic arrhythmias that are not fully controlled by drugs, in patients who are drug intolerant, or in those who do not wish to take drugs. This option should be considered early in the course of treatment of a symptomatic patient because of its high success rate, low frequency of complications, and potential cost-effectiveness.[68] Rarely, surgical interruption of the accessory pathway may be necessary.

Summary of Electrocardiographic Diagnosis of Supraventricular Tachycardias

ECG clues that permit differentiation among the various supraventricular tachycardias are often present. P waves during tachycardia that are identical to sinus P waves and occur with a long RP interval and a short PR interval are most likely due to sinus nodal reentry, sinus tachycardia, or an atrial tachycardia arising from the right atrium near the sinus node. Retrograde (inverted in leads II, III, and aV_f) P waves generally represent reentry involving the AV junction, either AV nodal reentry or reciprocating tachycardia using a paraseptal accessory pathway. Tachycardia without manifest P waves is probably due to AV nodal reentry (P waves buried in QRS), whereas a tachycardia with an RP interval exceeding 90 milliseconds may be due to an accessory pathway. AV dissociation or AV block during tachycardia excludes the participation of an AV accessory pathway and makes AV nodal reentry less likely. Multiple tachycardias can occur at different times in the same patient. QRS alternans, thought to be a feature of AV reciprocating tachycardia, is more likely a rapid rate–related phenomenon independent of the tachycardia mechanism. RP-PR relationships (Table 32–3) help differentiate supraventricular tachycardias. QRS voltage can increase during supraventricular tachycardia.[69]

TABLE 32–3 Supraventricular Tachycardias

Short RP/Long PR Internal	Long RP/Short PR Internal
AV node reentry	Atrial tachycardia
AV reentry	Sinus node reentry Atypical AV node reentry AVRT with a slowly conducting accessory pathway (e.g., PJRT)

AV = atrioventricular; AVRT = AV reciprocating tachycardia; PJRT = paroxysmal junctional reciprocating tachycardia.

Ventricular Rhythm Disturbances

Premature Ventricular Complexes

ECG RECOGNITION. A PVC is characterized by the premature occurrence of a QRS complex that is abnormal in shape and has a duration usually exceeding the dominant QRS complex, generally greater than 120 milliseconds. The

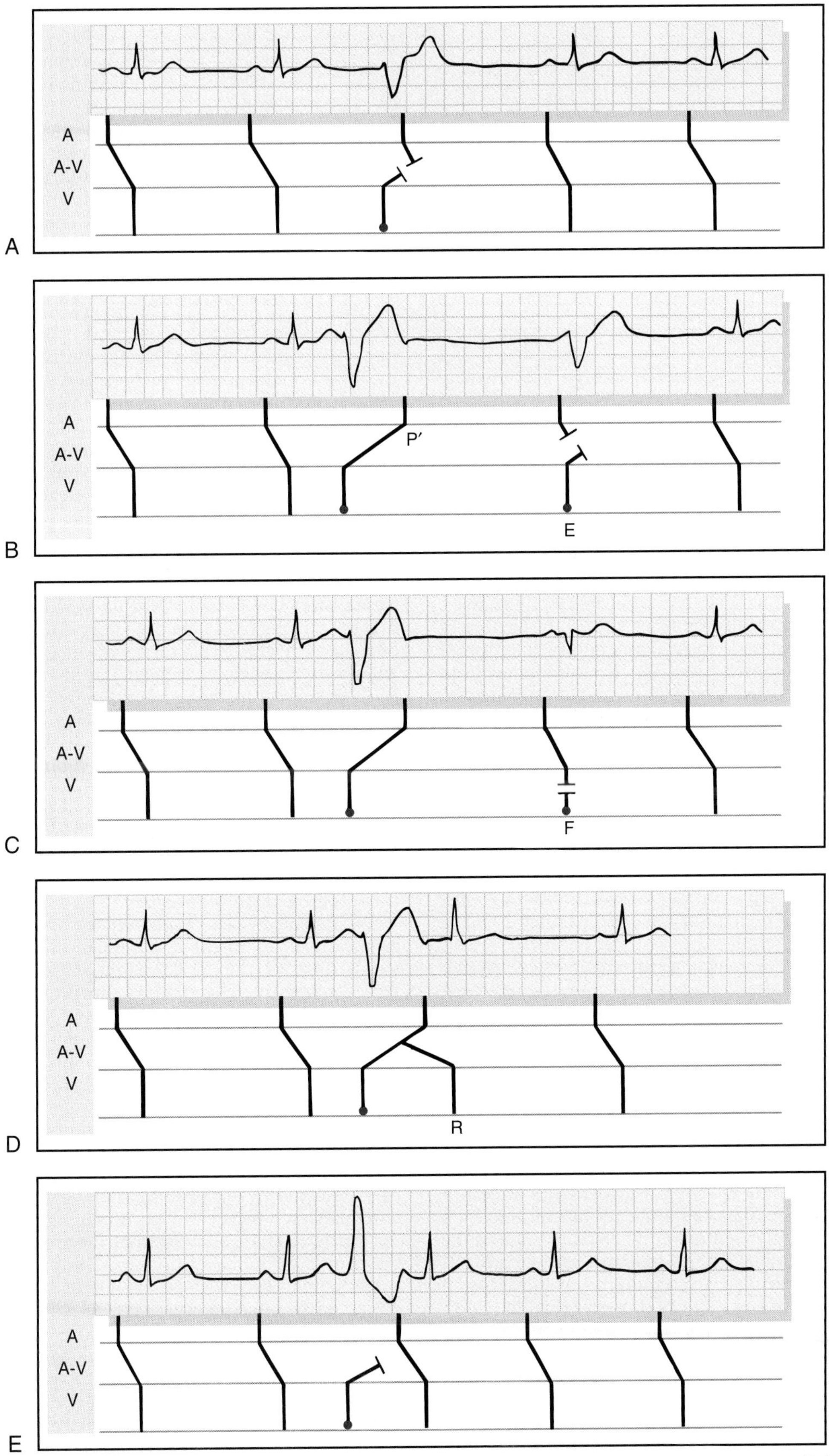

FIGURE 32–38 Premature ventricular complexes (PVCs). **A** to **D** were recorded in the same patient. **A,** A late results in a compensatory pause. **B,** A slower sinus rate and a slightly earlier premature ventricular complex result in retrograde atrial excitation (P). The sinus node is reset, followed by a noncompensatory pause. Before the sinus-initiated P wave that follows the retrograde P wave can conduct the impulse to the ventricle, ventricular escape (E) occurs. **C,** Events are similar to those in **B** except that a ventricular fusion beat (F) results after the PVC because of a slightly faster sinus rate. **D,** The impulse propagating retrogradely to the atrium reverses its direction after a delay and returns to reexcite the ventricles (R) to produce a ventricular echo. **E,** An interpolated PVC is followed by a slightly prolonged PR interval of the sinus-initiated beat. Lead II. Red circles indicate origin of PVCs.

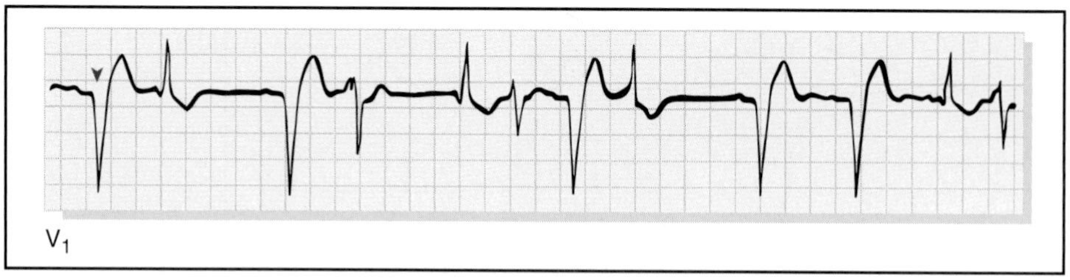

FIGURE 32–39 Multiform premature ventricular complexes (PVCs). The normally conducted QRS complexes exhibit a left bundle branch block contour (arrowhead) and are followed by PVCs with three different morphologies.

T wave is commonly large and opposite in direction to the major deflection of the QRS. The QRS complex is not preceded by a premature P wave but can be preceded by a nonconducted sinus P wave occurring at its expected time. The diagnosis of a PVC can never be made with unequivocal certainty from the scalar ECG since a supraventricular beat or rhythm can mimic the manifestations of ventricular arrhythmia (Fig. 32–38). Retrograde transmission to the atria from the PVC occurs fairly frequently but is often obscured by the distorted QRS complex and T wave. If the retrograde impulse discharges and resets the sinus node prematurely, it produces a pause that is not fully compensatory. More commonly, the sinus node and atria are not discharged prematurely by the retrograde impulse since interference of impulses frequently occurs at the AV junction in the form of collision between the anterograde impulse conducted from the sinus node and the retrograde impulse conducted from the PVC. Therefore, a fully compensatory pause usually follows a PVC: The R-R interval produced by the two sinus-initiated QRS complexes on either side of the premature complex equals twice the normally conducted R-R interval. The PVC may not produce any pause and may therefore be interpolated (Fig. 32–38E), or it may produce a postponed compensatory pause when an interpolated premature complex causes PR prolongation of the first postextrasystolic beat to such a degree that the P wave of the second postextrasystolic beat occurs at a very short RP interval and is therefore blocked.

Interference within the ventricle can result in *ventricular fusion beats* caused by simultaneous activation of the ventricle by two foci—one from the supraventricular impulse and the other from the PVC. On occasion, a fusion beat can be narrower than the dominant sinus beat when a right bundle branch block pattern of a PVC arising in the left ventricle fuses with the sinus-initiated complex conducting through the AV junction (see Fig. 32–32) or when a ventricle with a left bundle branch block pattern is paced artificially and a narrow ventricular fusion beat is produced between the paced and the sinus-conducted beats. Narrow PVCs have also been explained as originating at a point equidistant from each ventricle in the ventricular septum and by arising high in the fascicular system. Whether a compensatory or noncompensatory pause, retrograde atrial excitation, or an interpolated complex, fusion complex, or echo beat occurs (Fig. 32–38D), it is merely a function of how the AV junction conducts and the timing of the events taking place.

The term *bigeminy* refers to pairs of complexes and indicates a normal and premature complex, *trigeminy* indicates a premature complex following two normal beats, a premature complex following three normal beats is called *quadrigeminy,* and so on. Two successive PVCs are termed a *pair* or a *couplet,* whereas three successive PVCs are termed a *triplet.* Arbitrarily, three or more successive PVCs are termed *ventricular tachycardia.* PVCs can have different contours and are often called *multifocal* (Fig. 32–39). More properly they should be called *multiform, polymorphic,* or *pleomorphic* since it is not known whether multiple foci are discharging or whether conduction of the impulse originating from one site is merely changing.

PVCs can exhibit fixed or variable coupling; that is, the interval between the normal QRS complex and the PVC can be relatively stable or variable. Fixed coupling can be due to reentry, triggered activity (see Chap. 27), or other mechanisms. Variable coupling can be due to parasystole, to changing conduction in a reentrant circuit, or to changing discharge rates of triggered activity. Usually, it is difficult to determine the precise mechanism responsible for the PVC based on either constant or variable coupling intervals.

CLINICAL FEATURES. The prevalence of premature complexes increases with age, and they are associated with male sex and a reduced serum potassium concentration. PVCs are more frequent in the morning in patients after myocardial infarction, but this circadian variation is absent in patients with severe LV dysfunction. Symptoms of palpitations or discomfort in the neck or chest can result because of the greater than normal contractile force of the postextrasystolic beat or the feeling that the heart has stopped during the long pause after the premature complex. Long runs of frequent PVCs in patients with heart disease can produce angina, hypotension, or heart failure. Frequent interpolated PVCs actually represent a doubling of the heart rate and can compromise the patient's hemodynamic status. Activity that increases the heart rate can decrease the patient's awareness of the premature systole or reduce their number. Exercise can increase the number of premature complexes in some patients. Premature systoles can be quite uncomfortable in patients who have aortic regurgitation because of the large stroke volume. Sleep is usually associated with a decrease in the frequency of ventricular arrhythmias, but some patients can experience an increase.

PVCs occur in association with a variety of stimuli and can be produced by direct mechanical, electrical, and chemical stimulation of the myocardium. Often they are noted in patients with LV false tendons, during infection, in ischemic or inflamed myocardium, and during hypoxia, anesthesia, or surgery. They can be provoked by a variety of medications, by electrolyte imbalance, by tension states, by myocardial stretch, and by excessive use of tobacco, caffeine, or alcohol. Both central and peripheral autonomic stimulation have profound effects on the heart rate and can produce or suppress premature complexes.

Physical examination reveals the presence of a premature beat followed by a pause that is longer than normal. A fully compensatory pause can be distinguished from one that is not fully compensatory in that the former does not change the timing of the basic rhythm. The premature beat is often accompanied by a decrease in intensity of the heart sounds, often with auscultation of just the first heart sound, which can be sharp and snapping, and a decreased or absent peripheral (e.g., radial) pulse. The relationship of atrial to ventricular systole determines the presence of normal *a* waves or giant *a* waves in the jugular venous pulse, and the length of the PR interval determines the intensity of the first heart sound. The second heart sound can be abnormally split, depending on the origin of the ventricular complex.

The importance of PVCs depends on the clinical setting. In the absence of underlying heart disease, the presence of PVCs usually has no impact on longevity or limitation of activity; antiarrhythmic drugs are not indicated.[71] Patients should be reassured if they are symptomatic (see Chaps. 29 and 30). In men without apparent coronary disease, the incidental detection of ventricular arrhythmias is associated with a twofold increased risk for all-cause mortality and myocardial infarction or death from coronary disease. However, it has not been demonstrated that premature ventricular systoles or complex ventricular arrhythmias play a *precipitating* role in the genesis of sudden death in these patients, and the arrhythmias may simply be a marker of heart disease. Results from electrophysiological testing suggest that patients with PVCs who do not have VT induced at electrophysiological study have a low incidence of subsequent sudden death. Antiarrhythmic therapy given to suppress the premature ventricular systoles or complex ventricular arrhythmias has not been shown to reduce the incidence of sudden death in such apparently healthy men.

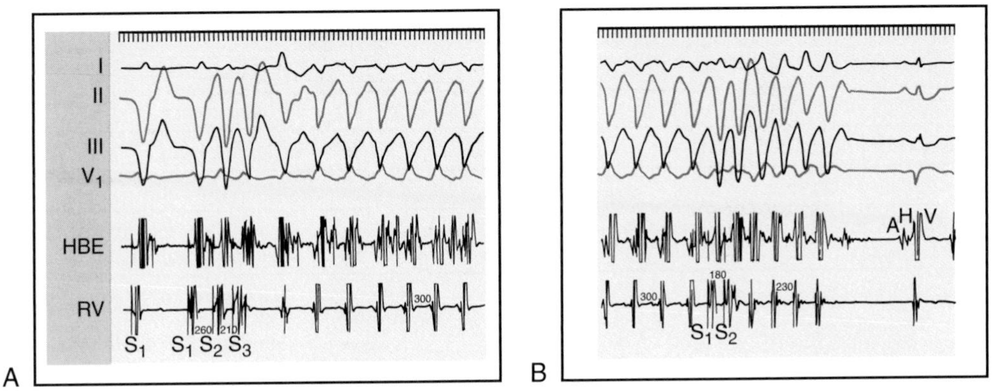

FIGURE 32–40 Initiation and termination of ventricular tachycardia by means of programmed ventricular stimulation. The last two ventricular-paced beats at a cycle length of 600 milliseconds are shown in **A.** A premature stimulus (S_2) at an S_1-S_2 interval of 260 milliseconds and another premature stimulus (S_3) at a cycle length of 210 milliseconds initiate a sustained monomorphic ventricular tachycardia at a cycle length of 300 milliseconds. Two premature ventricular stimuli (S_1-S_2) in **B** create an unstable ventricular tachycardia that persists for several beats at a shorter cycle length (230 milliseconds) and then terminates, followed by sinus rhythm.

In patients suffering from acute myocardial infarction, PVCs once considered to presage the onset of ventricular fibrillation, such as those occurring close to the preceding T wave, more than five or six per minute, bigeminal or multiform complexes, or those occurring in salvoes of two, three, or more, do not occur in about half the patients in whom ventricular fibrillation develops, and ventricular fibrillation does not develop in about half of the patients who have these PVCs. Thus these PVCs are not particularly helpful prognostically. The presence of 1 to more than 10 ventricular extrasystoles per hour can identify patients at increased risk for VT or sudden cardiac death after myocardial infarction but is likewise nonspecific.

MANAGEMENT. In most patients, PVCs (occurring as single PVCs, bigeminy, or trigeminy but excluding nonsustained VT [see later]) do not need to be treated, particularly if the patient does not have an acute coronary syndrome, and treatment is usually dictated by the presence of symptoms attributable to the PVCs. Both fast and slow heart rates can provoke the development of PVCs. PVCs accompanying slow ventricular rates can be abolished by increasing the basic rate with atropine or isoproterenol or by pacing, whereas slowing the heart rate in some patients with sinus tachycardia can eradicate PVCs. In hospitalized patients, IV lidocaine (see Chap. 30) is generally the initial treatment of choice to suppress PVCs. If maximum dosages of lidocaine are unsuccessful, procainamide given IV can be tried. Propranolol can be tried if the other drugs have been unsuccessful. IV magnesium can be useful. For long-term oral maintenance, a variety of classes I,[67] II,[72] and III drugs can be useful to prevent VT. Class IC drugs seem particularly successful in suppressing PVCs, but flecainide and moricizine have been shown to increase mortality in patients treated after myocardial infarction. Amiodarone can be quite effective. Athletes with structural heart disease and ventricular extrasystoles who are in high-risk groups can participate in low-intensity sports only.[5] Thrombolysis therapy does not influence the frequency of ventricular extrasystoles, which are related to residual LV pump performance after myocardial infarction. Low levels of serum potassium and magnesium are associated with higher prevalence rates of ventricular arrhythmias.

Ventricular Tachycardia

ECG RECOGNITION. VT arises distal to the bifurcation of the His bundle in the specialized conduction system, in ventricular muscle, or in combinations of both tissue types. Mechanisms include disorders of impulse formation and conduction considered earlier (see Chap. 27). Autonomic modulation can be important. The ECG diagnosis of VT is suggested by the occurrence of a series of three or more consecutive, abnormally shaped PVCs whose duration exceeds 120 milliseconds, with the ST-T vector pointing opposite the major QRS deflection. The R-R interval can be exceedingly regular or can vary. Patients can have VTs with multiple morphologies originating at the same or closely adjacent sites, probably with different exit paths. Others have multiple sites of origin. Atrial activity can be independent of ventricular activity, or the atria can be depolarized by the ventricles retrogradely (VA association). Depending on the particular type of VT, rates range from 70 to 250 beats/min, and the onset can be paroxysmal (sudden) or nonparoxysmal. QRS contours during the VT can be unchanging (uniform, monomorphic), can vary randomly (multiform, polymorphic, or pleomorphic), can vary in a more or less repetitive manner (torsades de pointes), can vary in alternate complexes (bidirectional VT), or can vary in a stable but changing contour (i.e., right bundle branch contour changing to a left bundle branch contour). VT can be sustained, defined arbitrarily as lasting longer than 30 seconds or requiring termination because of hemodynamic collapse, or nonsustained, when it stops spontaneously in less than 30 seconds. Most commonly, very premature stimulation is required to initiate VT electrically, whereas late coupled ventricular complexes usually initiate its spontaneous onset (Fig. 32–40).

Making the ECG distinction between supraventricular tachycardia with aberration and VT can be difficult at times since features of both arrhythmias overlap and under certain circumstances a supraventricular tachycardia can mimic the criteria established for VT.[73] Ventricular complexes with an abnormal and prolonged configuration indicate only that conduction through the ventricle is abnormal, and such complexes can occur in supraventricular rhythms as a result of preexisting bundle branch block, aberrant conduction during incomplete recovery of repolarization, conduction over accessory pathways, and several other conditions. These complexes do not necessarily indicate the origin of impulse formation or the reason for the abnormal conduction. Conversely, ectopic beats originating in the ventricle can

TABLE 32–4 Major Features in the Differential Diagnosis of Wide QRS Beats Versus Tachycardia

Supports SVT	Supports VT
Slowing or termination by vagal tone	Fusion beats
Onset with premature P wave	Capture beats
RP interval ≤ 100 msec	AV dissociation
P and QRS rate and rhythm linked to suggest that ventricular activation depends on atrial discharge, e.g., 2:1 AV block rSR′ V_1	P and QRS rate and rhythm linked to suggest that atrial activation depends on ventricular discharge, e.g., 2:1 VA block
Long-short cycle sequence	"Compensatory" pause Left axis deviation; QRS duration >140 msec Specific QRS contours (see text)

SVT = supraventricular tachycardia; VT = ventricular tachycardia.

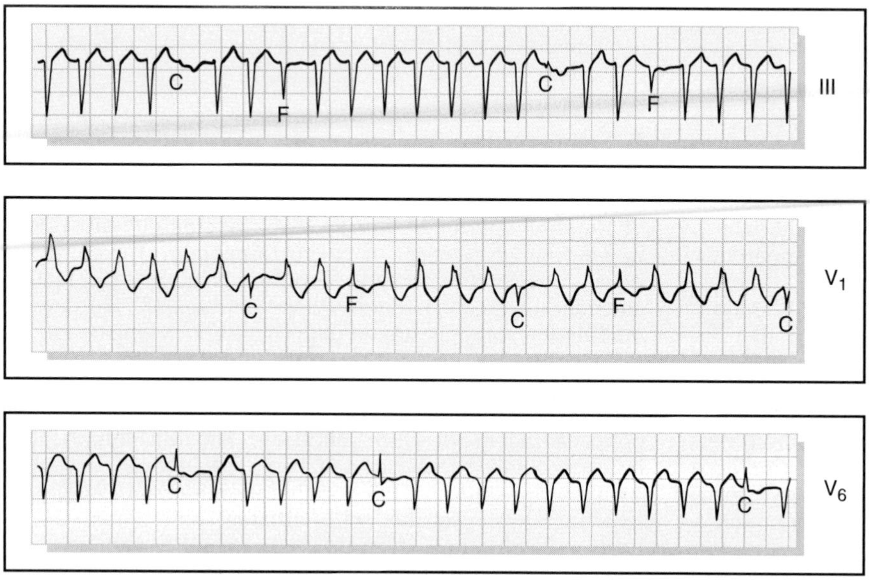

FIGURE 32–41 Fusion and capture beats during ventricular tachycardia. The QRS complex is prolonged, and the R-R interval is regular except for occasional capture beats (C) that have a normal contour and are slightly premature. Complexes intermediate in contour represent fusion beats (F). Thus, even though atrial activity is not clearly apparent, atrioventricular dissociation is present during ventricular tachycardia and produces intermittent capture and fusion beats.

uncommonly have a fairly normal duration and shape. However, VT is the most common cause of tachycardia with a wide QRS complex. A past history of myocardial infarction makes the diagnosis even more likely.

During the course of a tachycardia characterized by wide, abnormal QRS complexes, the presence of fusion beats and capture beats provides maximum support for the diagnosis of VT (Fig. 32–41 and Table 32–4). *Fusion beats* indicate activation of the ventricle from two different foci, with the implication that one of the foci had a ventricular origin. *Capture* of the ventricle by the supraventricular rhythm with a normal configuration of the captured QRS complex at an interval shorter than the tachycardia in question indicates that the impulse has a supraventricular origin. AV dissociation has long been considered a hallmark of VT. However, retrograde VA conduction to the atria from ventricular beats occurs in at least 25 percent of patients, and therefore, VT may not exhibit AV dissociation. AV dissociation can occur uncommonly during supraventricular tachycardias. Even if a P wave appears to be related to each QRS complex, it is at times difficult to determine whether the P wave is conducted anterogradely to the next QRS complex (i.e., supraventricular tachycardia with aberrancy and a long PR interval) or retrogradely from the preceding QRS complex (i.e., a VT). As a general rule, however, AV dissociation during tachycardia with a wide QRS is strong presumptive evidence that the tachycardia is of ventricular origin.

Differentiation Between Ventricular and Supraventricular Tachycardia. While fusion and capture beats and AV dissociation provide the strongest ECG evidence for differentiating VT from supraventricular tachycardia with aberrant conduction, these features are not always present. Therefore, other clues from the ECG may be required to help with this differentiation. Some ECG features characterizing supraventricular arrhythmia with aberrancy are (1) consistent onset of the tachycardia with a premature P wave; (2) a very short RP interval (0.1 second) often requiring an esophageal recording to visualize the P waves; (3) a QRS configuration the same as that occurring from known supraventricular conduction at similar rates; (4) P wave and QRS rate and rhythm linked to suggest that ventricular activation depends on atrial discharge (e.g., an AV Wenckebach block); and (5) slowing or termination of the tachycardia by vagal maneuvers.

Analysis of specific QRS contours can also be helpful in diagnosing VT and localizing its site of origin. For example, QRS contours suggesting VT include left-axis deviation in the frontal plane and a QRS duration exceeding 140 milliseconds with a QRS of normal duration during sinus rhythm. During VT with a right bundle branch block appearance, (1) the QRS complex is monophasic or biphasic in V_1 with an initial deflection different from that of the sinus-initiated QRS complex, (2) the amplitude of the R wave in V_1 exceeds the R′, and (3) a small R and large S wave or a QS pattern in V_6 may be present. With a VT having a left bundle branch block contour, (1) the axis can be rightward with negative deflections deeper in V_1 than in V_6, (2) a broad prolonged (>40 milliseconds) R wave can be noted in V_1, and (3) a small Q–large R wave or QS pattern in V_6 can exist. A QRS complex that is similar in V_1 through V_6, either all negative or all positive, favors a ventricular origin, as does the presence of a 2:1 VA block. (An upright QRS complex in V_1 through V_6 can also occur from conduction over a left-sided accessory pathway.) Supraventricular beats with aberration often have a triphasic pattern in V_1, an initial vector of the abnormal complex similar to that of the normally conducted beats, and a wide QRS complex that terminates a short cycle length following a long cycle (long-short cycle sequence). During atrial fibrillation, fixed coupling, short coupling intervals, a long pause after the abnormal beat, and runs of bigeminy rather than a consecutive series of abnormal complexes all favor a ventricular origin of the premature complex rather than a supraventricular origin with aberration. A grossly irregular, wide QRS tachycardia with ventricular rates exceeding 200 beats/min should raise the question of atrial fibrillation with conduction over an accessory pathway (see Fig. 32–4B). In the presence of a preexisting bundle branch block, a wide QRS tachycardia with a contour different from the contour during sinus rhythm is most likely a VT. Several algorithms, based on these criteria, for distinguishing VT from supraventricular tachycardia with aberrancy have been suggested. Exceptions exist to all the aforementioned criteria, especially in patients who have preexisting conduction disturbances or preexcitation syndrome; when in doubt, one must rely on sound clinical judgment and consider the ECG only one of several helpful ancillary tests.

Termination of a tachycardia by triggering vagal reflexes is considered diagnostic of supraventricular tachycardias. However, VT (especially if originating in the right ventricular outflow tract) can be stopped in a similar manner.

ELECTROPHYSIOLOGICAL FEATURES. Electrophysiologically, VT can be distinguished by a short or negative H-V interval (i.e., H begins after the onset of ventricular depolarization) because of retrograde activation from the ventricles (see Chap. 29). His bundle deflections are not usually apparent during VT because they are obscured by simultaneous ventricular septal depolarization or inadequate catheter position. The latter must be determined during supraventricular rhythm before the onset or after the termination of VT (see Fig. 32–40). His bundle deflections dissociated from ventricular activation are diagnostic, with rare exception. VT can produce QRS complexes of narrow duration and short H-V interval, most likely when the site of origin is close to the His bundle in the fascicles.

Successful electrical induction of VT by premature stimulation of the ventricle (see Fig. 32–40) depends on the characteristics of the VT and the anatomical substrate. Patients with sustained, hemodynamically stable VT and VT secondary to chronic coronary artery disease have monomorphic VT induced (90 percent) more frequently than do patients with nonsustained VT, VT from non–coronary-related causes or acute ischemia, and cardiac arrest (40 to 75 percent).[74] In general, it is more difficult to induce VT with late premature ventricular stimuli than with early premature stimuli, during sinus rhythm than during ventricular pacing, and with one premature stimulus than with two or three. The specificity of VT induction using more than two premature ventricular stimuli begins to decrease (while the sensitivity increases), and nonsustained polymorphic VT or ventricular fibrillation can be induced in patients who have no history of VT. Of patients with stable VT who have inducible sustained monomorphic VT, the latter is induced in about 25 percent with single extrastimuli, in 50 percent with double extrastimuli, and in 25 percent with triple extrastimuli. Occasionally, VT can be initiated only from the left ventricle or from specific sites in the right ventricle. Multiple premature stimuli reduce the need for LV stimulation. Drugs such as isoproterenol, various antiarrhythmic agents, and alcohol can facilitate the induction of VT. Coughing during VT that causes hypotension can help maintain blood pressure.

Termination by pacing depends significantly on the rate of the VT and the site of pacing. Slower VTs are terminated more easily and with fewer stimuli than are more rapid ones. An increasing number of stimuli are required to terminate more rapid VTs, which increases the risks of pacing-induced acceleration of the VT. Subthreshold stimulation and transthoracic stimulation can terminate VT. Atrial pacing, at times, can also induce and terminate VT (see Chap. 29).

CLINICAL FEATURES. Symptoms occurring during VT depend on the ventricular rate, duration of tachycardia, and the presence and extent of the underlying heart disease and peripheral vascular disease. VT can be in the form of short, asymptomatic, nonsustained episodes; sustained, hemodynamically stable events, generally occurring at slower rates or in otherwise normal hearts; or unstable runs, often degenerating into ventricular fibrillation. In some patients who have nonsustained VTs initially, sustained episodes or ventricular fibrillation later develops. The location of impulse formation and therefore the way in which the depolarization wave spreads across the myocardium can also be important. Physical findings depend in part on the P-to-QRS relationship. If atrial activity is dissociated from the ventricular contractions, the findings of AV dissociation are present. If the atria are captured retrogradely, regularly occurring cannon *a* waves appear when atrial and ventricular contractions occur simultaneously and signs of AV dissociation are absent.

More than half the patients treated for symptomatic recurrent VT have ischemic heart disease. The next biggest group has cardiomyopathy (both congestive and hypertrophic), with lesser percentages divided among those with primary electrical disease, mitral valve prolapse, valvular heart disease, congenital heart disease, and miscellaneous causes. LV hypertrophy can lead to ventricular arrhythmias. Coronary artery spasm can cause transient myocardial ischemia with severe ventricular arrhythmias in some patients (during ischemia as well as during the apparent reperfusion period).[74] Complex ventricular arrhythmias can occur *after* coronary artery bypass grafting. In patients resuscitated from sudden cardiac death (see Chap. 33), the majority (75 percent) have severe coronary artery disease, and ventricular tachyarrhythmias can be induced by premature ventricular stimulation in approximately 75 percent. When VT occurs in an ambulatory patient, it is uncommonly induced by R-on-T PVCs. Patients who have sustained VT are more likely to have a reduced ejection fraction (EF), slowed ventricular conduction and electrogram abnormalities, LV aneurysm, and previous myocardial infarction than are patients who have ventricular fibrillation, thus indicating different electrophysiological and anatomical substances. Young patients can also suffer cardiac arrest from VT or ventricular fibrillation, and persistent electrical inducibility of arrhythmias in these patients connotes a poor prognosis. In patients with coronary artery disease, sustained VT displays a circadian variation, with peak frequency in the morning.

Many approaches have been used to assess prognosis in patients with ventricular arrhythmias. Reduced baroreceptor sensitivity and heart period variability apparently caused by reduced vagal activity may indicate an increased risk of VT or sudden cardiac death. The presence of nonsustained VT after myocardial infarction often presages sudden cardiac death. Findings of reduced LV function, spontaneous ventricular arrhythmias, late potentials on signal-averaged ECG, QT interval dispersion, T wave alternans,[75,76] QRS duration, heart rate turbulence, and inducible sustained VTs at electrophysiological study all carry increased risk, further exaggerated when two or more of these features are present in the same patient. However, currently, no noninvasive technique reliably predicts outcome better than does assessment of LV function. LV function and inducibility of VT during electrophysiological study are the two strongest predictors of poor outcome. Early data suggest that T wave alternans may be as good as programmed stimulation.[77] Currently, T wave alternans is being evaluated in a prospective study to determine its value in risk stratification for implantable cardioverter-defibrillator (ICD) implantation. New risk factors such as elevated C-reactive protein, various cytokines, and genotypes may provide useful information in the future. In general, the prognosis for patients with idiopathic VT (see later), in the absence of structural heart disease or a prolonged QT interval, is good and warrants less aggressive treatment than in patients with structural heart disease.

MANAGEMENT. The dramatic changes in the management of VT and aborted sudden death over the past several years have been fueled by several large clinical trials (Table 32–5) and development of the ICD. Management decisions can be stratified into those involved in the acute management (or termination) and those involved in long-term therapy (or prevention of recurrence or sudden death) (see Chap. 33).

Acute Management of Sustained Ventricular Tachycardia. VT that does not cause hemodynamic decompensation can be treated medically to achieve acute termination by administering IV amiodarone, lidocaine, or procainamide, followed by an infusion of the successful drug. Lidocaine is often ineffective; amiodarone,[78] sotalol, and procainamide appear to be superior. In patients in whom procainamide is ineffective or in whom procainamide may be problematic

TABLE 32–5 Clinical Trials in the Treatment of Ventricular Tachycardia and Prevention of Cardiac Arrest

Study	Patient Inclusion	Endpoints	Treatment Arms	Key Results
Primary Prevention Studies				
BHAT[79]	*Post-MI*	Total mortality Sudden cardiac death	Propranolol Placebo	Total mortality and sudden cardiac death reduced in treatment arm
CAST[80]	*Post-MI* ≥6 PVCs/hr LVEF ≤40%	Arrhythmic death	Flecainide Encainide Moricizine Placebo	Arrhythmic death increased with all treatment arms
SWORD[81]	*Post-MI* LVEF <40% or Remote MI NYHA II, III	Total mortality	*d*-Sotalol Placebo	Increased mortality in treatment arm
EMIAT[82]	*Post-MI* LVEF <40%	Total mortality Arrhythmic death	Amiodarone Placebo	Amiodarone reduced arrhythmic death but not total mortality
CAMIAT[83]	*Post-MI* ≥10 PVCs/hr or NSVT	Arrhythmic death Total mortality	Amiodarone Placebo	Amiodarone reduced arrhythmic death but not total mortality
GESICA[84]	*CHF* LVEF ≤35%	Total mortality	Amiodarone Best therapy	Amiodarone reduced mortality. Patients with NSVT had higher mortality
CHF-STAT[85]	*CHF* LVEF ≤40% ≥10% PVCs/hr (asymptomatic)	Total mortality	Amiodarone Placebo	No effect in ischemic cardiomyopathy but trend toward reduced mortality in nonischemic cardiomyopathy
SCD-HeFT[87]	*CHF* LVEF ≤35% NYHA II, III	Total mortality Arrhythmic mortality Cost Quality of life	ICD Amiodarone Placebo	Ongoing
CABG Patch[88]	*CAD undergoing CABG* LVEF <36% Positive SAECG	Total mortality	CABG CABG + ICD	No difference in total mortality
MADIT[89]	*Post-MI* NSVT sustained LVEF ≤35% NYHA I-III Inducible VT not suppressed by procainamide	Total mortality	ICD Antiarrhythmic drug (80% amiodarone)	ICD reduced mortality
MADIT II[100]	*Post-MI* EF ≤30% >10 PVCs/hr or couplets	Total mortality	ICD No ICD	ICD reduced mortality
MUSTT[99]	*Post-MI* LVEF <40% NSVT sustained	Arrhythmic death or cardiac arrest	ICD in nonsuppressible group Antiarrhythmic drug in suppressible group No therapy	ICD reduced mortality
Secondary Prevention Studies				
ESVEM[91,92]	*Cardiac arrest, sustained VT or syncope* ≥10 PVCs/hr Inducible VT	Recurrence of arrhythmia	EP-guided antiarrhythmics (imipramine, mexiletine, procainamide, quinidine, sotalol, pirmenol, propafenone) Holter-guided antiarrhythmics	No difference between Holter- and EP-guided groups. Sotalol group had lowest recurrence rate of VT, arrhythmic death, and total death
CASCADE[93]	*Cardiac arrest* Not associated with acute MI	Cardiac mortality Aborted cardiac arrest	EP- or Holter-guided conventional drug therapy Empirical amiodarone	Amiodarone survival better than conventional drug therapy
CASH[94]	*Cardiac arrest* Not associated with acute MI	Total mortality	Empirical amiodarone Metoprolol Propafenone ICD	Sudden cardiac death mortality lowest in ICD arm. Increased mortality in propafenone arm
AVID[95]	*Cardiac arrest or sustained VT*	Total mortality Cost Quality of life	ICD Drug therapy (empirical amiodarone or EP/Holter-guided sotalol)	Survival better in ICD group, with most of benefit occurring in the first 9 m. Benefit most pronounced in patients with EF <35%
CIDS[96,97]	*Cardiac arrest or sustained VT*	Total mortality	ICD Amiodarone	Survival trended better in ICD group

CABG = coronary artery bypass grafting; CAD = coronary artery disease; CHF = congestive heart failure; EF = ejection fraction; EP = electrophysiology; ICD = implanted cardioverter-defibrillator; LVEF = left ventricular ejection fraction; MI = myocardial infarction; NSVT = nonsustained ventricular tachycardia; NYHA = New York Heart Association; PVC = premature ventricular complex; SAECG = signal-averaged electrocardiogram; VT = ventricular tachycardia.

(severe heart failure, renal failure), IV amiodarone is often effective. In general, an initial amiodarone loading dose of 15 mg/min is given over a 10-minute period. This dose is followed by an infusion of 1 mg/min for 6 hours and then a maintenance dose of 0.5 mg/min for the remaining 18 hours and for the next several days, as necessary. If VT does not terminate or if it recurs, a repeat loading dose can be given. Rarely, sinus bradycardia or AV block can be seen with IV amiodarone. The hypotension associated with IV amiodarone, caused largely by the diluent used in earlier formulations, does not seem to be as frequent a problem and is usually related to the rate of infusion. Bretylium is rarely used in this setting because of the frequently associated hypotension and because amiodarone appears to be more effective.

If the arrhythmia does not respond to medical therapy, electrical DC cardioversion can be used. VT that precipitates hypotension, shock, angina, congestive heart failure, or symptoms of cerebral hypoperfusion should be treated *promptly* with DC cardioversion (see Chaps. 30 and 33). Very low energies can terminate VT, beginning with a synchronized shock of 10 to 50 J. Digitalis-induced VT is best treated pharmacologically. After conversion of the arrhythmia to a normal rhythm, it is essential to institute measures to prevent recurrence.

Striking the patient's chest, sometimes called "thumpversion," can terminate VT by mechanically inducing a PVC that presumably interrupts the reentrant pathway necessary to support it. Chest stimulation at the time of the vulnerable period during the arrhythmia can accelerate the VT or possibly provoke ventricular fibrillation.

In some instances, such as VT associated with a remote myocardial infarction (which is due to reentry), ventricular pacing via a pacing catheter inserted into the right ventricle or transcutaneously at rates faster than the tachycardia can terminate the tachycardia. This procedure incurs the risk of accelerating the VT to ventricular flutter or ventricular fibrillation. In patients with recurrent VT, competitive ventricular pacing can be used to prevent recurrence. Intermittent VT, interrupted by several supraventricular beats, is generally best treated pharmacologically.

A search for reversible conditions contributing to the initiation and maintenance of VT should be made and the conditions corrected if possible. For example, VT related to ischemia, hypotension, or hypokalemia can at times be terminated by antianginal treatment, vasopressors, or potassium, respectively. Correction of heart failure can reduce the frequency of ventricular arrhythmias. Slow ventricular rates that are caused by sinus bradycardia or AV block can permit the occurrence of PVCs and ventricular tachyarrhythmias, which can be corrected by administering atropine, by temporary isoproterenol administration, or by transvenous pacing. Supraventricular tachycardia can initiate ventricular tachyarrhythmias and should be prevented if possible.

Long-Term Therapy for Prevention of Recurrences. The goal of long-term therapy is to prevent sudden cardiac death and recurrence of symptomatic VT. Asymptomatic nonsustained ventricular arrhythmias in low-risk populations (i.e., preserved LV function) often need not be treated. In patients with symptomatic nonsustained tachycardia, beta blockers are frequently effective in preventing recurrences. In patients refractory to beta blockers, class IC agents, sotalol, or amiodarone can be effective. However, class IC agents should be avoided in patients with structural heart disease, especially those with coronary artery disease because of the increased mortality associated with these drugs because of proarrhythmia. Sotalol should be used cautiously because of its potential for prolonging the QT interval and producing torsades des pointes. Patients with nonsustained VT after myocardial infarction and poor LV function are at significant risk for sudden death. The Multicenter Automatic Defibrillator Trial[98] (MADIT) found that patients with prior myocardial infarction and an EF of 0.35 or less who had inducible VT that was not suppressed with drugs[98] had better survival if treated with an ICD, with a hazard ratio of 0.46. In the Multicenter Unsustained Tachycardia Trial (MUSTT),[99] patients with an EF of 0.40 or less with coronary disease and asymptomatic nonsustained VT who had inducible sustained VT at electrophysiological study had a significant reduction in mortality if treated with an ICD. These studies suggest that patients with nonsustained VT and an EF of 0.35 to 0.40 or less should undergo electrophysiological study and, if they have inducible VT (i.e., not suppressed with procainamide), should have an ICD.[89] More recently, the MADIT-II study[100] found that patients with ischemic cardiomyopathy (prior myocardial infarction) with an EF of 0.30 or less and no requirement for ventricular arrhythmia had improved survival if treated with an ICD (hazard ratio of 0.69). This study suggests that patients with prior myocardial infarction and an EF of 0.30 or less ought to have a prophylactic ICD placed, regardless of the results of an electrophysiology study. Each of these trials demonstrated the superiority of the ICD over drugs as primary prevention of sudden cardiac death in patients at risk for a life-threatening ventricular arrhythmia. The Sudden Cardiac Death Heart Failure Trial (SCD-HeFT) is still ongoing and will investigate the role of ICDs in patients with classes II to III heart failure regardless of the presence of nonsustained VT or prior myocardial infarction. Whether additional risk stratifiers (such as T wave alternans) are beneficial is being investigated.

For secondary prevention of sustained VT or cardiac arrest (see Table 32–5 and Chaps. 30 and 33) in patients with structural heart disease, it is now clear from several clinical trials that (1) class I antiarrhythmic drugs produce a worse outcome than do class III antiarrhythmic drugs,[91,92,94] (2) empirical amiodarone results in better survival than does electrophysiology-guided antiarrhythmic drugs,[93] and (3) implantable defibrillators provide better survival than amiodarone does, particularly in patients with a left ventricular ejection fraction (LVEF) less than 0.35.[94-96] Therefore, in patients who have survived a cardiac arrest or who have sustained VT resulting in hemodynamic compromise and poor LV function (EF $<$ 0.35), an ICD is the treatment of choice.[95] For those with higher EFs, amiodarone may produce outcomes similar to those of implanted defibrillators. In patients who refuse a cardioverter-defibrillator, empirical amiodarone is the next best therapy.[93,94] The optimal therapy for patients with coronary disease who have preserved LV function with sustained VT is not currently known. Empirical amiodarone appears to be the safest therapy,[82-84] although Holter-guided sotalol has been advocated.[91,92] Some patients who receive ICDs have frequent shocks because of recurrent VT. In these patients, concomitant therapy with amiodarone may be required to reduce the frequency of VT or slow the rate of the VT to allow it to be pace terminated. Other drugs such as sotalol, procainamide, mexiletine, or flecainide may be required if amiodarone is not effective. Occasionally, a combination of drugs may be effective when a single drug is not. Although radiofrequency ablation (see Chap. 30) of certain types of idiopathic VT (see later) is very effective, ablation for postinfarct VT or that associated with dilated cardiomyopathy is somewhat less effective. In addition, because of the significant mortality associated with these arrhythmias in patients with structural heart disease and depressed LV function, ablation is generally used as an adjunct to ICD placement to reduce the frequency of VT and ICD shocks.[101-103] However, in patients with well-tolerated postinfarct VT and well-preserved LV function or in patients refractory to drugs, it may be used as first-line therapy.[101,103]

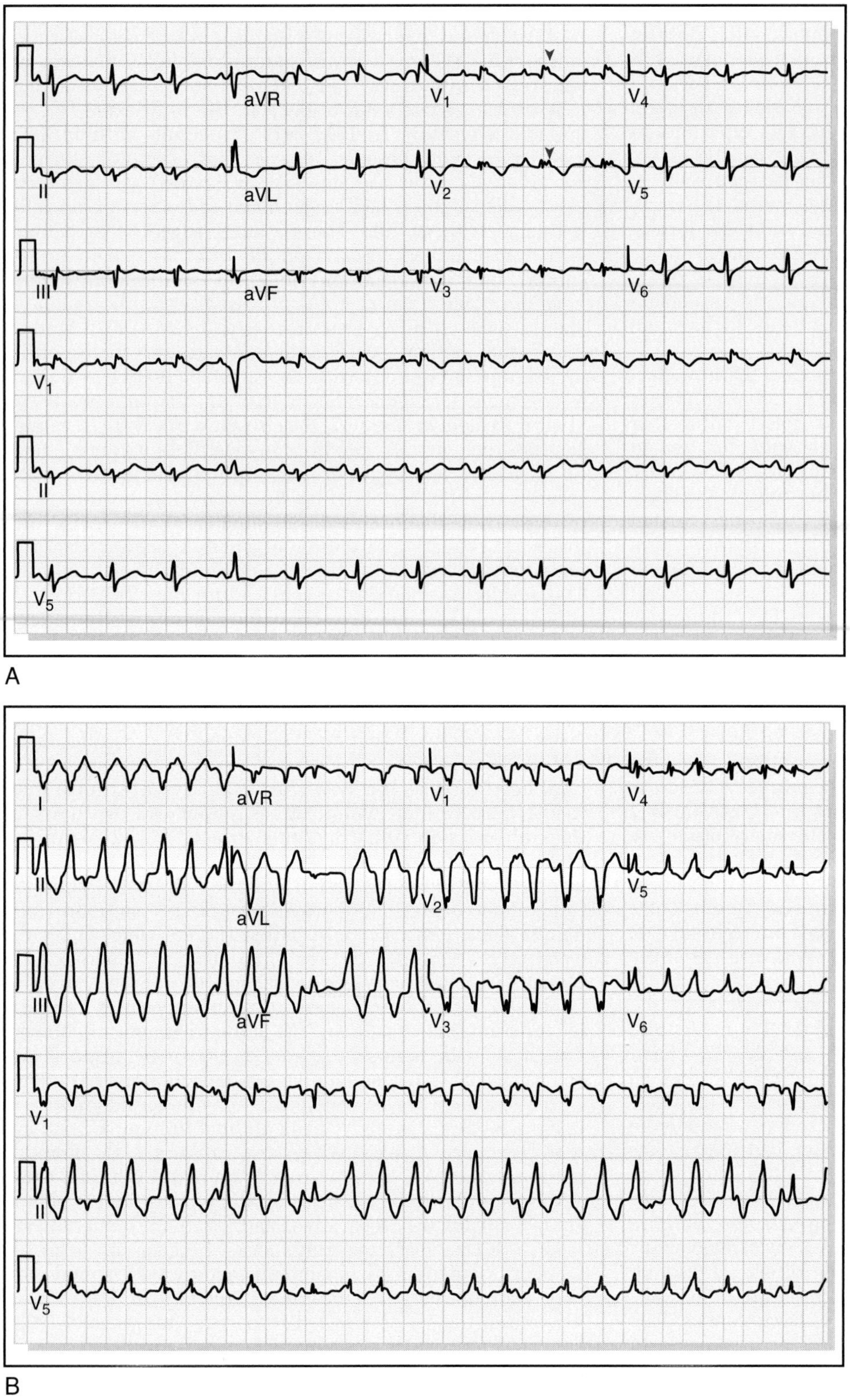

FIGURE 32–42 **A,** Normal sinus rhythm in a patient with arrhythmogenic right ventricular dysplasia. The arrowheads in V_1 and V_2 point to late right ventricular activation called an *epsilon wave.* **B,** Ventricular tachycardia in the same patient with right ventricular dysplasia.

Specific Types of Ventricular Tachycardia

A number of fairly specific types of VT have been identified, and distinction is based on either a constellation of distinctive ECG and electrophysiological features or a specific set of clinical events. Although our understanding of the electrophysiological mechanisms responsible for clinically occurring VTs is still naive, being able to identify different kinds of VTs is the first step toward understanding their mechanisms. These different kinds of VT often carry different prognoses and responses to different therapy. They are distinct from VTs associated with remote myocardial infarction or dilated cardiomyopathies.

Arrhythmogenic Right Ventricular Dysplasia

Patients with arrhythmogenic right ventricular dysplasia have VT that generally has a left bundle branch block contour (since the tachycardia arises in the right ventricle) often with right-axis deviation and T waves inverted over the right precordial leads (Fig. 32–42A). The VT may be due to reentry. Supraventricular arrhythmias can also occur, and exercise can induce the VT in some patients.

Arrhythmogenic right ventricular dysplasia is due to a type of cardiomyopathy, possibly familial in some patients, with hypokinetic areas involving the wall of the right ventricle. In the familial form, the genetic abnormality has been mapped to chromosomes 1 and 14q23-q24[104,105] and, most recently, chromosome 10, which has been implicated in apoptosis.[106,107] Mutations in the gene encoding the ryanodine receptor have also been identified in patients with arrhythmogenic right ventricular dysplasia (see Chap. 28).[108] Arrhythmogenic right ventricular dysplasia can be an important cause of ventricular arrhythmia in children and young adults with apparently normal hearts, as well as in older patients. Initial findings can be subtle and often mimic those of outflow tract VT (see later), that is, manifested only by tachycardia and no symptoms of right-sided heart failure. Right-sided heart failure or asymptomatic right ventricular enlargement can be present with normal pulmonary vasculature. Males predominate, and most patients usually show an abnormal right ventricle by echocardiography, computed tomography, right ventricular angiography, or magnetic resonance imaging, although this abnormality may not be apparent on initial evaluation. Two pathological patterns have been identified: fatty and fibrofatty infiltration. In the latter, myocardial atrophy appears to be the result of injury and myocyte death (perhaps from apoptosis) and culminates in fibrofatty replacement mediated by patchy myocarditis. The fatty degeneration preferentially occurs in the right ventricular inflow and outflow tracts and the apex. The left ventricle can be involved in advanced forms of the disease in up to 60 percent of patients.[104] Sympathetic innervation appears to be abnormal. The ECG during sinus rhythm can exhibit complete or incomplete right bundle branch block and T wave inversions in V_1 to V_3. A terminal notch in the QRS (called an *epsilon wave*) can be present as a result of slowed intraventricular conduction.[104] The signal-averaged ECG can be abnormal. Although there is no clinical trial at this point, ICDs are generally preferable to pharmacological approaches because of the progressive nature of the disease and poor prognosis, particularly if the patients have poorly tolerated VT (resulting in syncope or sudden cardiac death). Radiofrequency catheter ablation can be tried but is often not successful because of the multiple morphologies of VT and the progressive nature of the disease.

Tetralogy of Fallot

Chronic serious ventricular arrhythmias can occur in patients some years after repair of the *tetralogy of Fallot* (see Chap. 56). Sustained VT after repair can be caused by reentry at the site of previous surgery in the right ventricular outflow tract and can be cured by resection or catheter ablation of this area. The signal-averaged ECG can be abnormal. Decreased cardiac output can occur during VT and residual right ventricular outflow obstruction and lead to ventricular fibrillation.

Cardiomyopathies (see also Chap. 59)

Dilated Cardiomyopathy

Both dilated and hypertrophic cardiomyopathies can be associated with VTs and an increased risk of sudden cardiac death. Induction of VT by programmed stimulation does not reliably identify high-risk patients, whereas T wave alternans may be a useful means of risk stratifying patients with dilated cardiomyopathy.[109,110] Because it is difficult to predict patients at risk of sudden death or those who might respond favorably to an antiarrhythmic drug, ICDs have been advocated for patients with life-threatening ventricular arrhythmias and dilated cardiomyopathy. This recommendation has been supported by a large multicenter randomized trial (see Table 32–5) comparing amiodarone with implantable defibrillators in patients with poor ventricular function and symptomatic sustained VT; the study found improved survival in patients who received a defibrillator.[95] Bundle branch reentry may be the basis of some VTs in this population and can be treated by ablating the right bundle branch. Asymptomatic ventricular arrhythmias are common. The role of antiarrhythmic drugs and implantable defibrillators in the primary prevention of sudden cardiac death in patients with dilated cardiomyopathy may be warranted in certain high-risk patients, as discussed earlier. However, ongoing clinical trials will further clarify which patient population will benefit the most and which modality is most effective.

Hypertrophic Cardiomyopathy

The risk of sudden death in patients with hypertrophic cardiomyopathy (see Chap. 59) is increased by the presence of syncope, a family history of sudden death in first-degree relatives, septal thickness greater than 3 cm, or the presence of nonsustained VT on 24-hour ECG recordings. Asymptomatic or mildly symptomatic patients with brief and infrequent episodes of nonsustained VT have a low mortality. The use of electrophysiological testing to identify patients at increased risk of ventricular arrhythmias and sudden death is controversial. Amiodarone has been useful in some patients with mildly symptomatic, nonsustained VT but not in improving survival in patients without arrhythmias. QT dispersion is increased in those with ventricular arrhythmias and sudden death, as is T wave alternans.[111] DDD pacing has been useful in reducing the outflow gradient, but its role in affecting ventricular arrhythmia has not been established. Currently, no totally acceptable way to risk-stratify patients with hypertrophic cardiomyopathy in terms of VT has been identified. In patients believed to be at high risk of sudden death or those with sustained VT or frequent nonsustained VT, an implantable defibrillator may be indicated.[112] Alcohol ablation of the septum via direct injection into the septal branches of the coronary circulation has been used to improve outflow gradients, but its effect on ventricular arrhythmias and sudden cardiac death is not known.

Mitral Valve Prolapse

Patients with mitral valve prolapse (see Chap. 57) frequently have ventricular arrhythmias, although a causal relationship has not been clearly established between the arrhythmia and the mitral valve prolapse. The prognosis for most patients appears good, although sudden death can occur.

Idiopathic Ventricular Fibrillation

Idiopathic ventricular fibrillation can occur in about 1 to 8 percent of cases of out-of-hospital ventricular fibrillation and affects mostly men and those in middle age. Cardiovascular evaluation is normal except for the arrhythmia. Monomorphic VT is rarely induced at electrophysiological study. The natural history is incompletely known, but recurrences are not uncommon. It is important in this entity, as well as in patients with idiopathic VTs (see later), to remember that the arrhythmia may at times be an early manifestation of a developing cardiomyopathy, at least in some patients. Implantable defibrillators are useful therapeutic choices.

Catecholaminergic Polymorphic Ventricular Tachycardia

Catecholaminergic polymorphic ventricular tachycardia is an uncommon form of inherited VT that occurs in children and adolescents without any overt structural heart disease.[113] Patients typically present with syncope or aborted sudden death with highly reproducible, stress-induced VT that is often bidirectional. These patients have no structural heart disease and normal QT intervals. A family history of sudden death or stress-induced syncope is present in about 30 percent of the cases. During exercise, typical responses include initial sinus tachycardia and ventricular extrasystoles followed by salvos of monomorphic or bidirectional VT, which eventually leads to polymorphic VT as exercise continues. Recently, a genetic abnormality resulting in a mutation of the ryanodine receptor gene has been identified in many of these patients; those patients with this mutation appear to have a higher risk and earlier symptom (see Chap. 28).[114] The treatment of choice is beta blockers and ICDs.

Brugada Syndrome

Brugada syndrome is a distinct form of idiopathic ventricular fibrillation in which patients have right bundle branch block and ST segment elevation in the anterior precordial leads without evidence of structural heart disease (Fig. 32–43).[115-118] Mutations in a gene responsible for the sodium channel (*SCN5A*) have been identified in many families with Brugada syndrome.[119-121] Although the mutations are on the same gene as that responsible for one form of long-QT syndrome (long-QT-3) (see later), the site of mutation is different and does not result in a prolonged QT interval.[122] Mutations in the Brugada syndrome result either in acceleration of sodium-channel recovery or in nonfunctional sodium channels. This syndrome, common in apparently healthy young Southeast Asians, probably accounts for approxi-

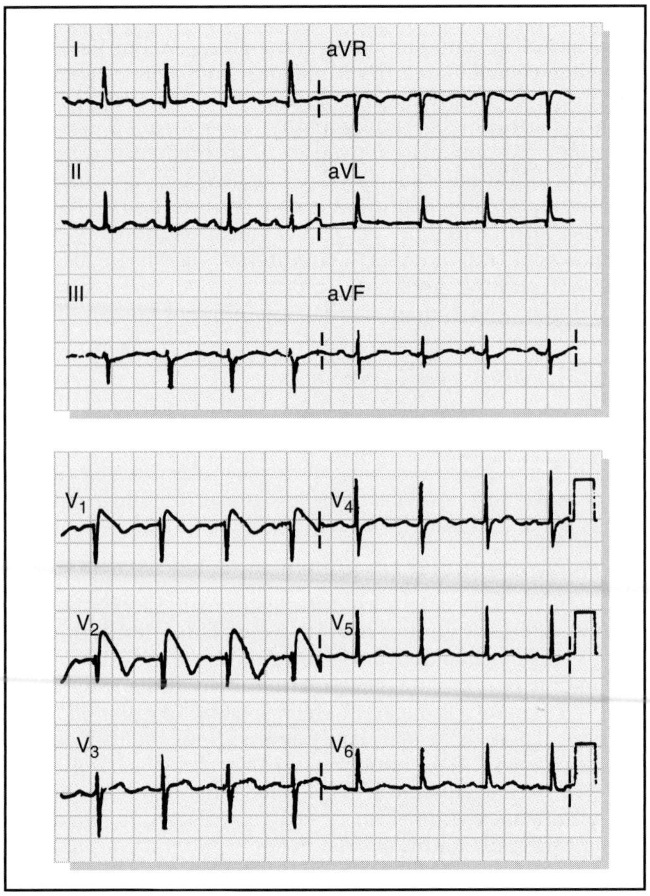

FIGURE 32–43 Twelve-lead electrocardiogram (ECG) of a patient with Brugada syndrome. The ECG is characterized by a right bundle branch block pattern and persistent ST elevation in V_1 through V_3. (From Brugada J, Brugada R, Brugada P: Right bundle branch block and ST segment elevation in leads V_1 through V_3: A marker for sudden death in patients without demonstrable structural heart disease. Circulation 97:457-460, 1998.)

mately 40 to 60 percent of all cases of idiopathic ventricular fibrillation.[119] The precise mechanism of the ECG changes and the development of ventricular fibrillation is not known. It is thought that loss of the action potential dome in the right ventricular epicardium, but not in the endocardium, results in the persistent ST segment elevation.[115] Heterogeneous loss of the action potential dome in the right ventricular epicardium leads to propagation of the dome from sites at which its presence is maintained to sites at which it is lost (phase 2 reentry), resulting in ventricular arrhythmias. Among several agents that can reproduce this ECG phenomenon are sodium-channel blockers. They can expose latent ECG forms of the syndrome and have been proposed as a provocative test. Currently, no pharmacological treatment can reliably prevent ventricular fibrillation in these patients. ICDs are the only effective treatment for preventing sudden death.

Idiopathic Ventricular Tachycardias

Idiopathic VTs with monomorphic contours can be divided into at least three types. Two types, paroxysmal VT and repetitive monomorphic VT, appear to originate from the region of the right ventricular outflow tract (Figs. 32–44 and 32–45). Right ventricular outflow tract VTs have a characteristic ECG appearance of a left bundle branch block contour in V_1 and an inferior axis in the frontal plane. Vagal maneuvers, including adenosine, terminate the VT, whereas exercise, stress, isoproterenol infusion, and rapid or premature stimulation can initiate or perpetuate the tachycardia. Beta blockers and verapamil can suppress this tachycardia as well. The mechanism responsible may be cyclic adenosine monophosphate–triggered activity[123,124] resulting from early or delayed afterdepolarizations. The paroxysmal form is exercise or stress induced, whereas the repetitive monomorphic type occurs at rest with sinus beats interposed between runs of nonsustained VT that may be precipitated by transient increases in sympathetic activity unrelated to exertion. The prognosis for most patients is quite good. Radiofrequency catheter ablation effectively eliminates this focal tachycardia in symptomatic patients. In others, antiarrhythmic drugs can be effective. An anatomical abnormality in the outflow tract of the right ventricle has been recognized in some patients.[123] In a small number of patients, the tachycardia seems to arise in the inflow tract or apex of the right ventricle. A similar tachycardia has been identified in the left ventricle and may mimic that of right ventricular outflow tract tachycardia.[125]

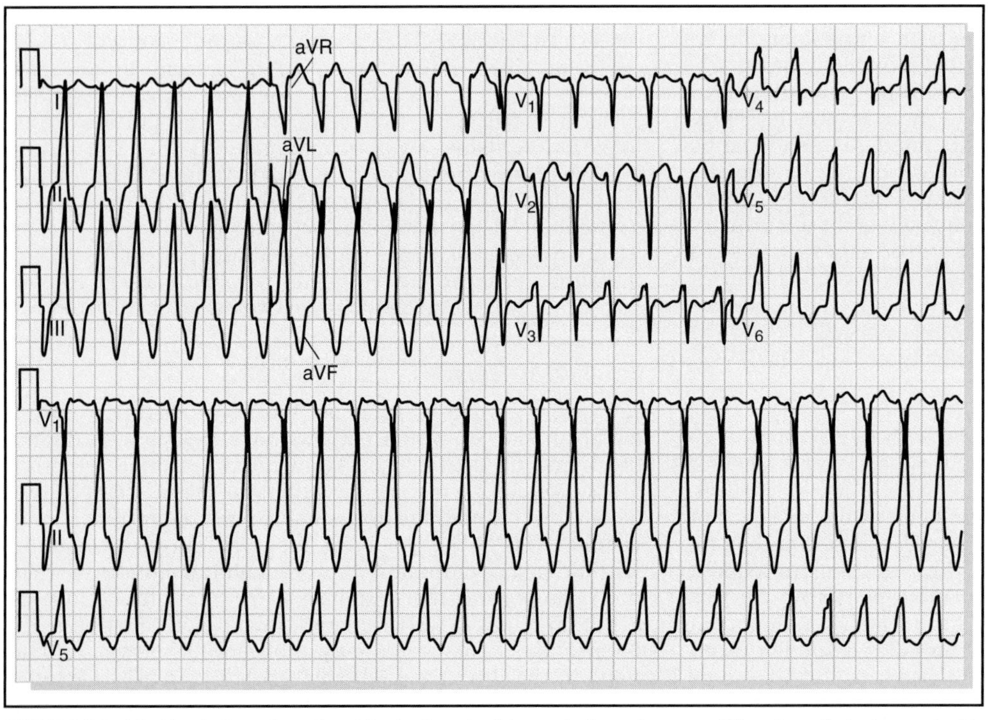

FIGURE 32–44 Ventricular tachycardia originating from the right ventricular outflow tract. This tachycardia is characterized by a left bundle branch block contour in V_1 and an inferior axis.

Left Septal Ventricular Tachycardia

A *left septal VT* has been described as arising in the left posterior septum, often preceded by a fascicular potential, and is sometimes called a *fascicular tachycardia* (Fig. 32–46). Entrainment has been demonstrated, which suggests reentry as a cause of some of the tachycardias. Verapamil or diltiazem suppresses this tachycardia, whereas adenosine does so only rarely. The response to verapamil suggests that the slow inward

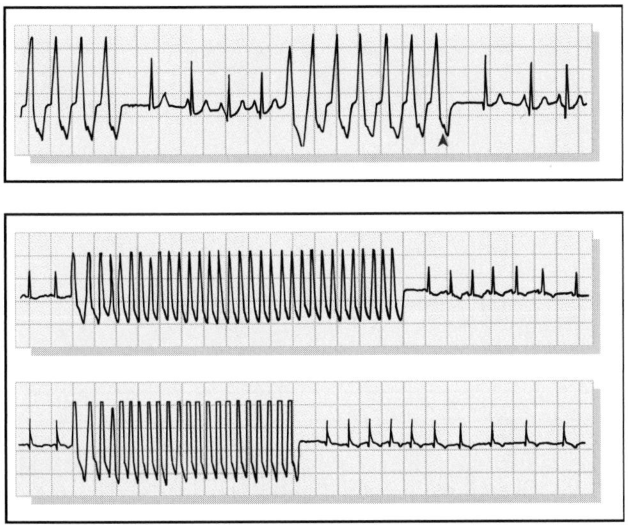

FIGURE 32–45 **A,** Repetitive monomorphic ventricular tachycardia. Short episodes of a monomorphic ventricular tachycardia at a rate of 160 beats/min repeatedly interrupt the normal sinus rhythm. Retrograde atrial capture probably occurs (the arrowhead points to the deflection in the ST segment), and the retrograde P wave of the last complex of the repetitive monomorphic ventricular tachycardia conducts over the normal pathway to produce a QRS complex with a normal contour. **B,** Short runs of a very rapid (260 beats/min) ventricular tachycardia of uniform contour. They probably provoke a compensatory sympathetic response because each is followed by a brief period of sinus tachycardia. The sinus pacemaker appears unstable as changes in P wave morphology result.

current may be important, possibly in a reentrant circuit or via delayed afterdepolarizations. Several mechanisms may be operative, and the group may not be homogeneous. Oral verapamil is not as effective as IV verapamil. Once initiated, the tachycardia is paroxysmal and sustained. It can be started by rapid atrial or ventricular pacing and sometimes by exercise or isoproterenol. Generally, the prognosis is good. Radiofrequency catheter ablation is effective in symptomatic patients. Late potentials have been reported in one-third of patients.

Sudden infant death syndrome is a syndrome of unexplained death that occurs in infancy. The precise cause is not known and is probably due to a variety of etiologies, both cardiac and noncardiac. It is not known what percentage, if any, is due to arrhythmias. Some have suggested that the long-QT (see later) and Brugada syndromes may be responsible in some cases (see Chap. 33).[126,127]

ACCELERATED IDIOVENTRICULAR RHYTHM

ECG RECOGNITION. The ventricular rate, commonly between 60 and 110 beats/min, usually hovers within 10 beats of the sinus rate, so control of the cardiac rhythm shifts between these two competing pacemaker sites. Consequently, fusion beats often occur at the onset and termination of the arrhythmia as the pacemakers vie for control of ventricular depolarization (Fig. 32-47). Because of the slow rate, capture beats are common. The onset of this arrhythmia is generally gradual (nonparoxysmal) and occurs when the rate of the VT exceeds the sinus rate because of sinus slowing or SA or AV block. The ectopic mechanism can also begin after a PVC, or the ectopic ventricular focus can simply accelerate sufficiently to overtake the sinus rhythm. The slow rate and nonparoxysmal onset avoid the problems initiated by excitation during the vulnerable period, and consequently, precipitation of more rapid ventricular arrhythmias is rarely seen. Termination of the rhythm generally occurs gradually as the dominant sinus rhythm accelerates or as the ectopic ventricular rhythm decelerates. The ventricular rhythm can be regular or irregular and can occasionally show sudden doubling, which suggests the presence of exit block. Many characteristics incriminate enhanced automaticity as the responsible mechanism.

The arrhythmia occurs as a rule in patients who have heart disease, such as those with acute myocardial infarction or with digitalis toxicity. It is transient and intermittent, with episodes lasting a few seconds to a minute, and does not appear to seriously affect the patient's clinical course or the prognosis. It commonly occurs at the moment of reperfusion of a previously occluded coronary artery, and it can be found during resuscitation.

MANAGEMENT

Suppressive therapy is rarely necessary because the ventricular rate is generally less than 100 beats/min, but such therapy may be considered when AV dissociation results in loss of sequential AV contraction, when an accelerated idioventricular rhythm occurs together with a more rapid VT, when an accelerated idioventricular rhythm begins with a PVC and causes discharges in the vulnerable period of the preceding T wave, when the ventricular rate is too rapid and produces symptoms, and if ventricular fibrillation develops as a result of the accelerated idioventricular rhythm. This last event appears to be fairly rare. Therapy, when indicated, should be as already noted for VT. Often, simply increasing the sinus rate with atropine or atrial pacing suppresses the accelerated idioventricular rhythm.

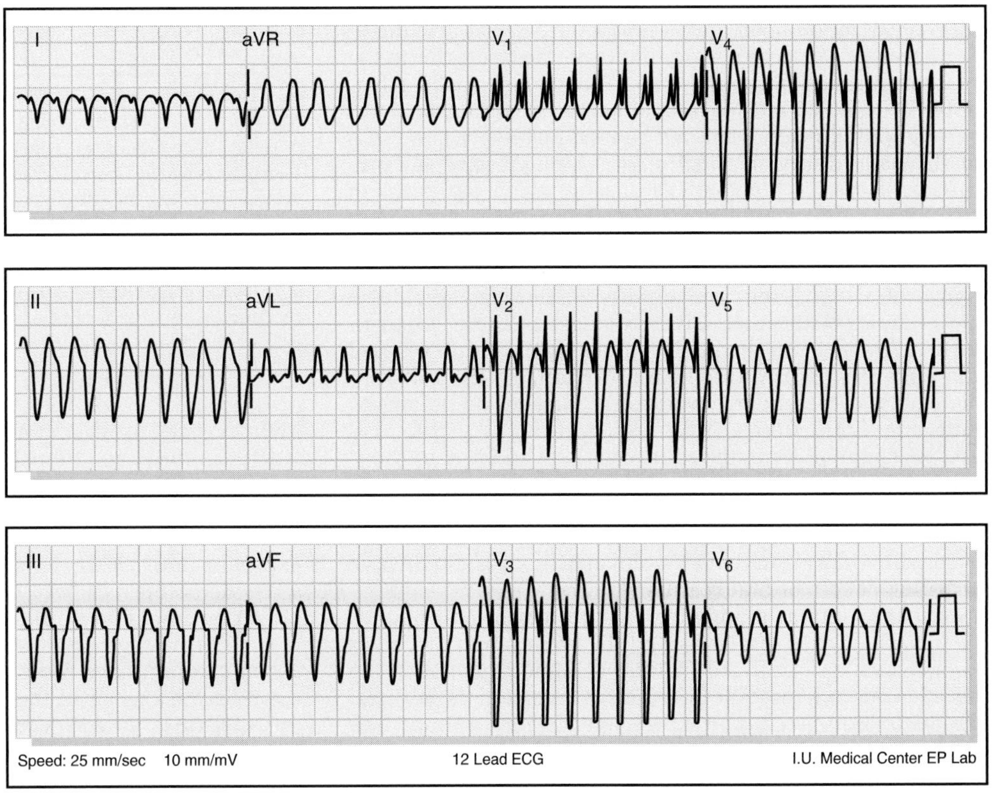

FIGURE 32–46 Left septal ventricular tachycardia. This tachycardia is characterized by a right bundle branch block contour. In this instance, the axis was rightward. The site of the ventricular tachycardia was established to be in the left posterior septum by electrophysiological mapping and ablation.

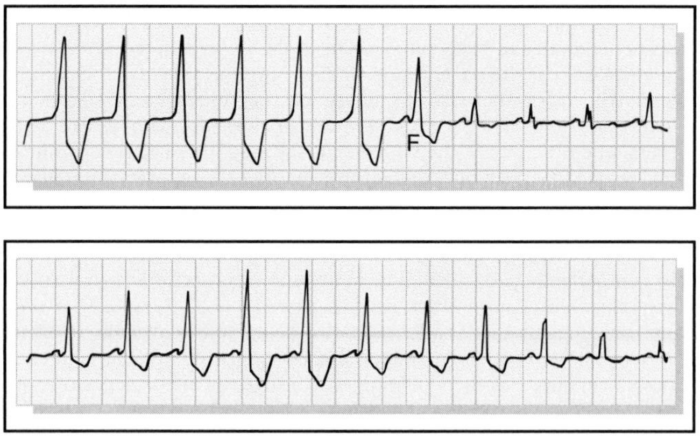

FIGURE 32–47 Accelerated idioventricular rhythm. In this continuous monitor lead recording, an accelerated idioventricular rhythm competes with the sinus rhythm. Wide QRS complexes at a rate of 90 beats/min fuse (F) with the sinus rhythm, which takes control briefly, generates the narrow QRS complexes, and then yields once again to the accelerated idioventricular rhythm as the P waves move "in and out" of the QRS complex. This example of isorhythmic atrioventricular dissociation may be due to hemodynamic modulation of the sinus rate via the autonomic nervous system.

Torsades de Pointes

ECG RECOGNITION. The term *torsades de pointes* refers to a VT characterized by QRS complexes of changing amplitude that appear to twist around the isoelectric line and occur at rates of 200 to 250/min (Fig. 32–48A).[128] Originally described in the setting of bradycardia caused by complete heart block, the term *torsades de pointes* is usually used to connote a *syndrome,* not simply an ECG description of the QRS complex of the tachycardia, characterized by prolonged ventricular repolarization with QT intervals generally exceeding 500 milliseconds. The U wave can also become prominent and merge with the T wave, but its role in this syndrome and in long-QT syndrome is not clear. The abnormal repolarization need not be present or at least prominent on all beats but may be apparent only on the beat prior to the onset of torsades de pointes (i.e., following a PVC). Long-short R-R cycle sequences commonly precede the onset of torsades de pointes from acquired causes. Relatively late PVCs can discharge during termination of the long T wave and precipitate successive bursts of VT during which the peaks of the QRS complexes appear successively on one side and then on the other side of the isoelectric baseline and give the typical twisting appearance with continuous and progressive changes in QRS contour and amplitude. Torsades de pointes can terminate with progressive prolongation in cycle length and larger and more distinctly formed QRS complexes and culminate in a return to the basal rhythm, a period of ventricular standstill, and a new attack of torsades de pointes or ventricular fibrillation.

A less common form, the short-coupled variant of torsades de pointes, is a malignant disease with a high mortality rate and shares several characteristics with idiopathic ventricular fibrillation. The ventricular arrhythmia in this setting is initiated with a close-coupled PVC and usually does not involve preceding pauses or bradycardia.[129]

VT that is similar morphologically to torsades de pointes and occurs in patients *without* QT prolongation, whether spontaneous or electrically induced, should generally be classified as polymorphic VT, not as torsades de pointes. The distinction has important therapeutic implications (see later).

ELECTROPHYSIOLOGICAL FEATURES. The electrophysiological mechanisms responsible for torsades de pointes are not completely understood. Most data suggest that early afterdepolarizations (see Chap. 27) are responsible for both long-QT syndrome and the torsades de pointes, or at least its initiation. Perpetuation may be due to triggered activity, reentry resulting from dispersion of repolarization produced by the early afterdepolarizations, or abnormal automaticity. Two out-of-phase discharging foci have been experimentally shown to produce a tachycardia similar to torsades de pointes, as have drifting rotors. Dispersion of repolarization from endocardium to epicardium may also play a role. A distinct group of cells, called *M cells,* located in the subepicardium have prolonged repolarization and may play a role in the genesis of torsades de pointes.[130]

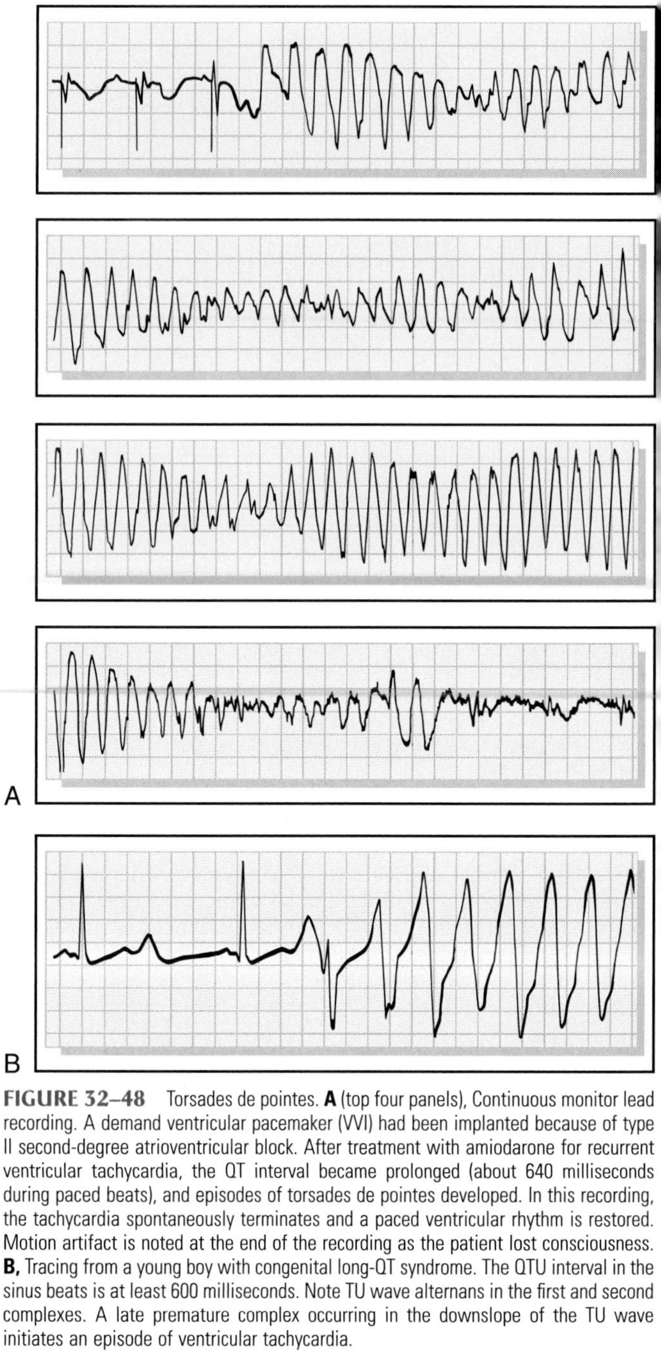

FIGURE 32–48 Torsades de pointes. **A** (top four panels), Continuous monitor lead recording. A demand ventricular pacemaker (VVI) had been implanted because of type II second-degree atrioventricular block. After treatment with amiodarone for recurrent ventricular tachycardia, the QT interval became prolonged (about 640 milliseconds during paced beats), and episodes of torsades de pointes developed. In this recording, the tachycardia spontaneously terminates and a paced ventricular rhythm is restored. Motion artifact is noted at the end of the recording as the patient lost consciousness. **B,** Tracing from a young boy with congenital long-QT syndrome. The QTU interval in the sinus beats is at least 600 milliseconds. Note TU wave alternans in the first and second complexes. A late premature complex occurring in the downslope of the TU wave initiates an episode of ventricular tachycardia.

CLINICAL FEATURES. Although many predisposing factors have been cited, the most common causes are congenital, severe bradycardia, potassium depletion, and use of medications (such as class IA, IC or III antiarrhythmic drugs). More than 50 drugs have been noted to prolong the QT interval (see Long-QT Syndrome). Clinical features depend on whether the torsades de pointes is due to the acquired or congenital (idiopathic) long-QT syndrome (see later). Symptoms from the tachycardia depend on its rate and duration, as with other VTs, and range from palpitations to syncope and death. Women, perhaps because of a longer QT interval, are at greater risk for torsades de pointes than are men.

MANAGEMENT. The approach to VT with a polymorphic pattern depends on whether it occurs in the setting of a prolonged QT interval. For this practical reason and because the mechanism of the tachycardia can differ depending on whether a long-QT interval is present, it is important to restrict the definition of torsades de pointes to the typical polymorphic VT in the setting of a long QT and/or U wave in the basal complexes. In all patients with torsades de pointes, administration of class IA, possibly some class IC, and class III antiarrhythmic agents (amiodarone and sotalol) can increase the abnormal QT interval and worsen the arrhythmia. IV magnesium is the initial treatment of choice for torsades de pointes from an acquired cause, followed by temporary ventricular or atrial pacing. Isoproterenol, given cautiously because it can exacerbate the arrhythmia, can be used to increase the rate until pacing is instituted. Lidocaine, mexiletine, or phenytoin can be tried. Potassium-channel openers may be useful. The cause of the long QT should be determined and corrected if possible. When the QT interval is normal, polymorphic VT *resembling* torsades de pointes is diagnosed, and standard antiarrhythmic drugs can be given. In borderline cases, the clinical context may help determine whether treatment should be initiated with antiarrhythmic drugs. Torsades de pointes resulting from congenital long-QT syndrome is treated with beta blockade, surgical sympathetic interruption, pacing, and implantable defibrillators (see later). ECGs taken on close relatives can help secure the diagnosis of long-QT syndrome in borderline cases.

Long-QT Syndrome

ECG RECOGNITION. The upper limit for duration of the normal QT interval *corrected* for heart rate (QTc) is often given as 0.44 seconds (Fig. 32–48B). However, the normal corrected QT interval may actually be longer (0.46 seconds for men and 0.47 seconds for women), with a normal range of plus or minus 15 percent of the mean value. Data from Holter recordings are consistent with a normal QTc less than 440 milliseconds.[131] The nature of the U wave abnormality and its relationship to long-QT syndrome is not clear. M cells may be responsible for the U wave (see Chap. 27). The probable risk of life-threatening ventricular arrhythmias developing in patients with idiopathic long-QT syndrome is exponentially related to the length of the QTc interval. T wave "humps" in the ECG suggest the presence of long-QT syndrome and may be caused by early afterdepolarizations. A point score system has been suggested to aid in the diagnosis. Unique T wave contours have been ascribed to specific genotypes causing long-QT syndrome.

CLINICAL FEATURES. Long-QT syndrome can be divided into idiopathic (congenital) and acquired forms.[128] The idiopathic form is a familial disorder that can be associated with sensorineural deafness (Jervell and Lange-Nielsen syndromes, autosomal recessive) or normal hearing (Romano-Ward syndrome, autosomal dominant). A nonfamilial form with normal hearing has been called the *sporadic form*.

The hypothesis that the idiopathic long-QT syndrome results from a preponderance of left sympathetic tone has been replaced by genetic information linking the disorder in different families to sites in several different chromosomes (see Table 28–1). The gene products from several of these mutations have been identified as potassium and sodium channels (see Table 38–1).[133-135] A detailed discussion of the genetics of long-QT syndrome is presented in Chapter 28.

The acquired form has a long-QT interval caused by various drugs (see Table 72–3) such as quinidine, procainamide, *N*-acetylprocainamide, sotalol, amiodarone, disopyramide, phenothiazines, or tricyclic antidepressants; cisapride; nonsedating antihistamines such as astemizole and terfenedine, whose actions can be exacerbated by drugs affecting their metabolism such as ketoconazoles; drugs such as erythromycin, pentamidine, and some antimalarials; electrolyte abnormalities such as hypokalemia and hypomagnesemia; the results of a liquid protein diet and starvation; central nervous system lesions; significant bradyarrhythmias; cardiac ganglionitis; mitral valve prolapse; and probucol. The acquired long-QT syndrome may be a forme fruste of the inherited form.[136,136a]

Patients with congenital long-QT syndrome can initially have syncope, at times misdiagnosed as epilepsy, from VTs that are often caused by torsades de pointes. Sudden death can occur in this group of patients, and it occurs in about 10 percent of pediatric patients without preceding symptoms. It is obvious that in some patients the ventricular arrhythmia becomes sustained and probably results in ventricular fibrillation. Patients with idiopathic long-QT syndrome who are at increased risk for sudden death include those with family members who died suddenly at an early age and those who have experienced syncope. It also appears that the specific mutations carry different risks, with long-QT-1 and long-QT-2 carrying the highest risk for arrhythmias. Although patients with the long-QT-3 mutation tend to have fewer cardiac events, they tend to be more lethal ones. Thus, the cumulative mortality appears to be the same for long-QT-1, long-QT-2, and long-QT-3.[137] Ventricular tachyarrhythmias commonly develop during periods of adrenergic stimulation, such as fright or exertion. However, some phenotypic variation is noted, such that patients with long-QT-1 and long-QT-2 mutations tend be more sympathetically driven, whereas long-QT-3 patients tend to have more events during sleep.[137] Syndactyly has recently been described in some patients with the idiopathic form.

Stress testing can prolong the QT interval and produce T wave alternans, the latter indicative of electrical instability. ECGs should be obtained for all family members when the propositus has symptoms. Patients should undergo prolonged ECG recording with various stresses designed to evoke ventricular arrhythmias, such as auditory stimuli, psychological stress, cold pressor stimulation, and exercise. The Valsalva maneuver can lengthen the QT interval and cause T wave alternans and VT in patients who have prolonged QT syndromes. Catecholamines can be infused in some patients, but this challenge must be performed cautiously, with resuscitative equipment along with alpha and beta antagonists close at hand. Stellate ganglion stimulation and blockade have been useful to provoke or abolish arrhythmias. Premature ventricular stimulation electrically does not generally induce arrhythmias in this syndrome and electrophysiology studies are usually not helpful in the diagnosis. Torsades de pointes commonly develops in patients with the acquired form during periods of bradycardia or after a long pause in the R-R interval, whereas those with the idiopathic form can have a sinus tachycardia preceding the ventricular arrhythmia. Competitive sports are contraindicated for patients with the congenital long-QT syndrome.[5]

MANAGEMENT. For patients who have idiopathic long-QT syndrome but do not have syncope, complex ventricular arrhythmias, or a family history of sudden cardiac death, generally no therapy or treatment with a beta blocker is recommended. In asymptomatic patients with complex ventricular arrhythmias or a family history of early sudden cardiac death, beta-adrenoceptor blockers at maximally tolerated doses are recommended. Implantation of a permanent pacemaker to prevent the bradycardia and/or pauses that may predispose to the development of torsades de pointes may be indicated.[2,138,139] In patients with syncope due to ventricular arrhythmias or aborted sudden death, an ICD is warranted. These patients should also be treated with concomitant beta blockers and perhaps overdrive atrial pacing (via the ICD) to minimize the frequency of ICD discharges. ICD is beneficial in these patient not simply because of the shocking capabilities but because of the ability to continually pace to prevent bradycardia-induced torsades and because of algorithms to prevent post-PVC pauses. The use of ICD in patients without syncope but with a long-QT interval and a strong family history of sudden death is still controversial but may be warranted in these high-risk patients. For patients who continue to have syncope despite maximum drug therapy, left-sided cervicothoracic sympathetic ganglionectomy that interrupts the stellate ganglion and the first three or four thoracic ganglia may be helpful. For patients with the acquired form and torsades de pointes, IV magnesium and atrial or ventricular pacing are initial choices. Class IB antiarrhythmic drugs or isoproterenol (cautiously) to increase the heart rate can be tried. Avoidance of precipitating drugs is mandatory. Potassium-channel–activating drugs such as pinacidil and cromakalim may be useful in both forms of long-QT syndrome.

Bidirectional Ventricular Tachycardia

Bidirectional VT is an uncommon type of VT that is characterized by QRS complexes with a right bundle branch block pattern, alternating polarity in the frontal plane from −60 to −90 degrees to +120 to +130 degrees, and a regular rhythm. The ventricular rate is between 140 and 200 beats/min. Although the mechanism and site of origin of this tachycardia have remained somewhat controversial, most evidence supports a ventricular origin.

Bidirectional VT can be a manifestation of digitalis excess, typically in older patients and in those with severe myocardial disease. When the tachycardia is due to digitalis, the extent of toxicity is often advanced, with a poor prognosis. Catecholaminergic polymorphic VT can present as bidirectional VT.

In addition to digoxin-binding antibodies (Digibind), drugs useful to treat digitalis toxicity such as lidocaine, potassium, phenytoin, and propranolol should be considered if excessive digitalis administration is suspected. Otherwise, the usual therapeutic approach to VT is recommended.

Bundle Branch Reentrant Ventricular Tachycardia

VT secondary to bundle branch reentry is characterized by a QRS morphology determined by the circuit established over the bundle branches or fascicles. Retrograde conduction over the left bundle branch system and anterograde conduction over the right bundle branch create a QRS complex with a left bundle branch block contour and constitute the most common form. The frontal plane axis may be about +30 degrees. Conduction in the opposite direction produces a right bundle branch block contour. Reentry can also occur over the anterior and posterior fascicles. Electrophysiologically, bundle branch reentrant complexes are started after a critical S_2-H_2 or S_3-H_3 delay. The H-V interval of the bundle branch reentrant complex equals or exceeds the H-V interval of the spontaneous normally conducted QRS complex.

Bundle branch reentry is a form of monomorphic sustained VT that is usually seen in patients with structural heart disease such as dilated cardiomyopathy. During follow-up, congestive heart failure is the most common cause of death in this population. Myocardial VTs can also be present. Uncommonly, bundle branch reentry can occur in the absence of myocardial disease.

The therapeutic approach is as for other types of VT. In the acute setting, pace termination is frequently effective. Long-term, catheter ablation effectively eliminates this form of VT.

Ventricular Flutter and Fibrillation (see also Chap. 33)

ECG RECOGNITION. These arrhythmias represent severe derangements of the heartbeat that usually terminate fatally within 3 to 5 minutes unless corrective measures are undertaken promptly. Ventricular flutter is manifested as a sine wave in appearance: regular large oscillations occurring at a rate of 150 to 300/min (usually about 200) (Fig. 32–49A). The distinction between rapid VT and ventricular flutter can be difficult and is usually of academic interest only. Hemodynamic collapse is present with both. Ventricular fibrillation is recognized by the presence of irregular undulations of varying contour and amplitude (Fig. 32–49B). Distinct QRS complexes, ST segments, and T waves are absent. Fine-amplitude fibrillatory waves (0.2 mV) are present with prolonged ventricular fibrillation. These fine waves identify patients with worse survival rates and are sometimes confused with asystole.[140]

MECHANISMS. Ventricular fibrillation occurs in a variety of clinical situations but is most commonly associated with coronary artery disease and as a terminal event (see Chap. 27).[141] Thrombolytic agents reduce the incidence of ventricular arrhythmias and inducible VT after myocardial infarction. Cardiovascular events, including sudden cardiac death from ventricular fibrillation, but not asystole, occur most frequently in the morning and may be related to increased platelet aggregability. Aspirin reduces this mortality. An excess in sudden deaths appears to occur during the winter months.[142] Ventricular fibrillation can occur during antiarrhythmic drug administration, hypoxia, ischemia, atrial fibrillation, and very rapid ventricular rates in the preexcitation syndrome; after electrical shock administered during cardioversion (see Chaps. 30 and 31) or accidentally by improperly grounded equipment; and during competitive ventricular pacing to terminate VT.

CLINICAL FEATURES. Ventricular flutter or ventricular fibrillation results in faintness, followed by loss of consciousness, seizures, apnea, and eventually, if the rhythm continues untreated, death. The blood pressure is unobtainable, and heart sounds are usually absent. The atria can continue to beat at an independent rhythm for a time or in response to impulses from the fibrillating ventricles. Eventually, electrical activity of the heart ceases.

In patients resuscitated from out-of-hospital cardiac

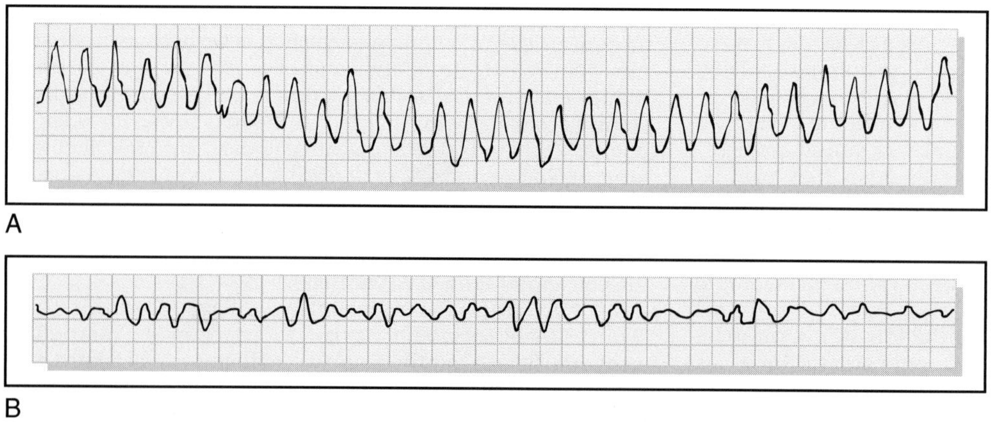

FIGURE 32–49 Ventricular flutter and ventricular fibrillation. **A,** The sine wave appearance of the complexes occurring at a rate of 300 beats/min is characteristic of ventricular flutter. **B,** The irregular undulating baseline typifies ventricular fibrillation.

arrest, 75 percent have ventricular fibrillation. Bradycardia or asystole, which can occur in 15 to 25 percent of these patients, is associated with a worse prognosis than is ventricular fibrillation and is usually associated with more advanced LV dysfunction. VT commonly precedes the onset of ventricular fibrillation, although frequently no consistent premonitory patterns emerge. Heart rate variability may be decreased.

Although 75 percent of resuscitated patients exhibit significant coronary artery disease, acute transmural myocardial infarction develops in only 20 to 30 percent. In one study, 73 percent had recent coronary artery thrombosis. Those in whom myocardial infarction does *not* develop have an increased recurrence rate for sudden cardiac death or ventricular fibrillation. Patients who have ventricular fibrillation and acute myocardial infarction have a recurrence rate at 1 year of 2 percent. In the past 20 years, there appears to have been an overall decrease in the incidence of sudden cardiac death, parallel to the decrease in death from coronary heart disease.

Predictors of death for resuscitated patients include a reduced EF, abnormal wall motion, history of congestive heart failure, history of myocardial infarction but no acute event, and the presence of ventricular arrhythmias. Patients discharged after an anterior myocardial infarction complicated by ventricular fibrillation appear to represent a subgroup at high risk of sudden death. Ventricular fibrillation can occur in infants, young people, athletes, and persons without known structural heart disease and in unexplained syndromes.

MANAGEMENT. Management should follow basic life support and advanced cardiac life support guidelines (see Chap. 33).[143] *Immediate* nonsynchronized DC electrical shock using 200 to 400 J is mandatory therapy for ventricular fibrillation and for ventricular flutter that has caused loss of consciousness. Automatic external defibrillators have facilitated the ability to defib-rillate early. Cardiopulmonary resuscitation is used only until the defibrillation equipment is readied. Time should not be wasted with cardiopulmonary resuscitation maneuvers if electrical defibrillation can be done promptly. Defibrillation requires fewer joules if done early. If the circulation is markedly inadequate despite return to sinus rhythm, closed-chest massage with artificial ventilation as needed should be instituted. The use of anesthesia during electrical shock is obviously dictated by the patient's condition and is not generally required. After conversion of the arrhythmia to a normal rhythm, it is essential to monitor the rhythm continuously and institute measures to prevent recurrence. Metabolic acidosis quickly follows cardiovascular collapse. If the arrhythmia is terminated within 30 to 60 seconds, significant acidosis does not occur. Judicious use of sodium bicarbonate to reverse the acidosis may be necessary, but its use should not delay administration of epinephrine or defibrillation shocks (see Chap. 33).

If the resuscitation time is short, artificial ventilation by means of a tightly fitting rubber face mask and an AMBU bag is quite satisfactory and eliminates the delay attending intubation by inexperienced personnel. If such a mask and bag are not available, mouth-to-mouth or mouth-to-nose resuscitation is indicated. It is important to reemphasize that there should be *no delay in instituting electrical shock.* If the patient is not monitored and it cannot be established whether asystole or ventricular fibrillation caused the cardiovascular collapse, the electrical shock should be administered *without* wasting precious seconds attempting to obtain an ECG. The DC shock may cause the asystolic heart to begin discharging and also terminate ventricular fibrillation, if the latter is present.

A search for conditions contributing to the initiation of ventricular flutter or fibrillation should be made and the conditions corrected, if possible. Initial medical approaches to prevent recurrence of ventricular fibrillation include IV administration of amiodarone, lidocaine, bretylium, or procainamide. Amiodarone tends to be the most effective and does not produce the ventricular dysfunction and hypotension often seen with bretylium or procainamide. Ventricular fibrillation rarely terminates spontaneously, and death results unless countermeasures are instituted immediately. Subsequent therapy is necessary to prevent recurrence. Implantable defibrillators have become the mainstay of chronic therapy in patients at continued risk for ventricular fibrillation or VT from nonreversible causes (see Chap. 31).

Heart Block

Heart block is a disturbance of impulse conduction that can be permanent or transient depending on the anatomical or functional impairment. It must be distinguished from *interference,* a normal phenomenon that is a disturbance of impulse conduction caused by physiological refractoriness resulting from inexcitability from a preceding impulse. Either interference or block can occur at any site where impulses are conducted, but they are recognized most commonly between the sinus node and atrium (SA block), between the atria and ventricles (AV block), within the atria (intraatrial block), or within the ventricles (intraventricular block). During AV block, the block can occur in the AV node, His bundle, or bundle branches. In some instances of bundle branch block the impulse may only be delayed and not completely blocked in the bundle branch, yet the resulting QRS complex may be indistinguishable from a QRS complex generated by a complete bundle branch block.

The conduction disturbance is classified by severity into three categories. During *first-degree heart block,* conduction time is prolonged but all impulses are conducted. *Second-degree heart block* occurs in two forms: Mobitz types I (Wenckebach) and II. Type I heart block is characterized by a progressive lengthening of the conduction time until an impulse is not conducted. Type II heart block denotes occasional or repetitive sudden block of conduction of an impulse without prior measurable lengthening of conduction time. When no impulses are conducted, *complete* or *third-degree block* is present. The degree of block may depend in part on the direction of impulse propagation. For unknown reasons, normal retrograde conduction can occur in the presence of advanced anterograde AV block. The reverse can also occur. Some electrocardiographers use the term *advanced heart block* to indicate blockage of two or more consecutive impulses.[144]

Certain features of type I second-degree block deserve special emphasis because when actual conduction times are not apparent in the ECG, for example, during SA, junctional, or ventricular exit block (Fig. 32–50), a type I conduction disturbance can be difficult to recognize. During a typical type I block, the increment in conduction time is greatest in the second beat of the Wenckebach group, and the absolute *increase* in conduction time *decreases* progressively over subsequent beats. These two features serve to establish the characteristics of classic Wenckebach group beating: (1) The interval between successive beats progressively decreases, although the conduction time increases (but by a decreasing function); (2) the duration of the pause produced by the nonconducted impulse is less than twice the interval preceding the blocked impulse (which is usually the shortest interval); and (3) the cycle following the nonconducted beat (beginning the Wenckebach group) is longer than the cycle preceding the blocked impulse. Although much emphasis has been placed on this characteristic grouping of cycles, primarily to be able

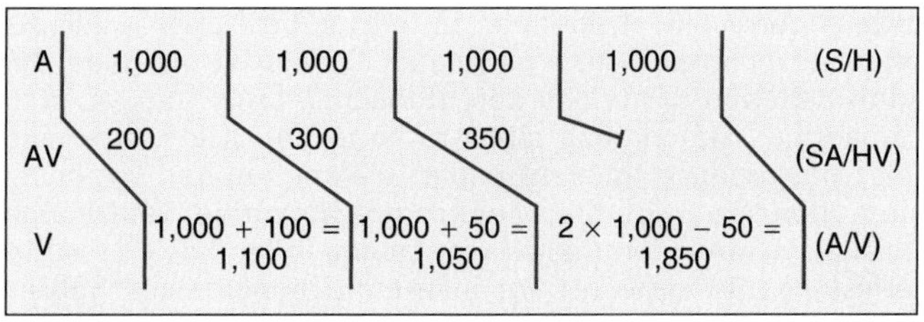

FIGURE 32–50 Typical 4:3 Wenckebach cycle. P waves ("A" tier) occur at a cycle length of 1000 milliseconds. The PR interval ("AV" tier) is 200 milliseconds for the first beat and generates a ventricular response ("V" tier). The PR interval increases by 100 milliseconds in the next complex, which results in an R-R interval of 1100 milliseconds (1000 + 100). The increment in the PR interval is only 50 milliseconds for the third cycle, and the PR interval becomes 350 milliseconds. The R-R interval shortens to 1050 milliseconds (1000 + 50). The next P wave is blocked, and an R-R interval is created that is less than twice the P-P interval by an amount equal to the increments in the PR interval. Thus, the Wenckebach features explained in the text can be found in this diagram. If the increment in the PR interval of the last conducted complex increased rather than decreased (e.g., 150 milliseconds rather than 50 milliseconds), the last R-R interval before the block would increase (1150 milliseconds) rather than decrease and thus become an example of an atypical Wenckebach cycle (see Fig. 32–44). If this were a Wenckebach exit block from the sinus node to the atrium, the sinus node cycle length (S) would be 1000 milliseconds, and the sinoatrial interval would increase from 200 to 300 to 350 milliseconds and culminate in a block. These events would be inapparent in the scalar electrocardiogram (ECG). However, the P-P interval in the ECG would shorten from 1100 to 1050 milliseconds, and finally, there would be a pause of 1850 milliseconds (A). If this rhythm were a junctional rhythm arising from the His bundle and conducting to the ventricle, the junctional rhythm cycle length would be 1000 milliseconds (H), and the H-V interval would progressively lengthen from 200 to 300 to 350 milliseconds, whereas the R-R interval would decrease from 1100 to 1050 milliseconds and then increase to 1850 milliseconds (V). The only clue to the Wenckebach exit block would be the cycle length changes in the ventricular rhythm.

to diagnose a Wenckebach exit block, this typical grouping occurs in fewer than 50 percent of patients who have a type I Wenckebach AV nodal block.

Differences in these cycle length patterns can result from changes in pacemaker rate (e.g., sinus arrhythmia), in neurogenic control of conduction, and in the increment of conduction delay. For example, if the PR increment in the last cycle *increases,* the R-R cycle of the last conducted beat can lengthen rather than shorten. In addition, since the last conducted beat is often at a critical state of conduction, it can become blocked and produce a 5:3 or 3:1 conduction ratio instead of a 5:4 or 3:2 ratio. During a 3:2 Wenckebach structure, the duration of the cycle following the nonconducted beat will be the same as the duration of the cycle preceding the nonconducted beat.

AV Block

An AV block exists when the atrial impulse is conducted with delay or is not conducted at all to the ventricle at a time when the AV junction is not physiologically refractory.

FIRST-DEGREE AV BLOCK. During first-degree AV block, every atrial impulse conducts to the ventricles and a regular ventricular rate is produced, but the PR interval exceeds 0.20 second in adults. PR intervals as long as 1.0 second have been noted and can at times exceed the P-P interval, a phenomenon known as "skipped" P waves. Clinically important PR interval prolongation can result from a conduction delay in the AV node (A-H interval), in the His-Purkinje system (H-V interval), or at both sites. Equally delayed conduction over both bundle branches can uncommonly produce PR prolongation without significant QRS complex aberration. Occasionally, an intraatrial conduction delay can result in PR prolongation. If the QRS complex in the scalar ECG is normal in contour and duration, the AV delay almost always resides in the AV node, rarely within the His bundle itself. If the QRS complex shows a bundle branch block pattern, the conduction delay may be within the AV node and/or His-Purkinje system (Fig. 32–51). In this latter instance, His bundle ECG is necessary to localize the site of conduction delay. Acceleration of the atrial rate or enhancement of vagal tone by carotid massage can cause first-degree AV nodal block to progress to type I second-degree AV block. Conversely, type I second-degree AV nodal block can revert to first-degree block with deceleration of the sinus rate.

SECOND-DEGREE AV BLOCK. Blocking of some atrial impulses conducted to the ventricle at a time when physiological interference is not involved constitutes second-degree AV block (Figs. 32–52 and 32–53; see also Fig. 32–50). The nonconducted P wave can be intermittent or frequent, at regular or irregular intervals, and can be preceded by fixed or lengthening PR intervals. A distinguishing feature is that conducted P waves relate to the QRS complex with recurring PR intervals; that is, the association of P with QRS is not random. Electrocardiographically, typical type I second-degree AV block is characterized by progressive PR prolongation culminating in a nonconducted P wave (see Fig. 32–52), whereas in type II second-degree AV block, the PR interval remains constant prior to the blocked P wave (Fig. 32–54A). In both instances the AV block is intermittent and

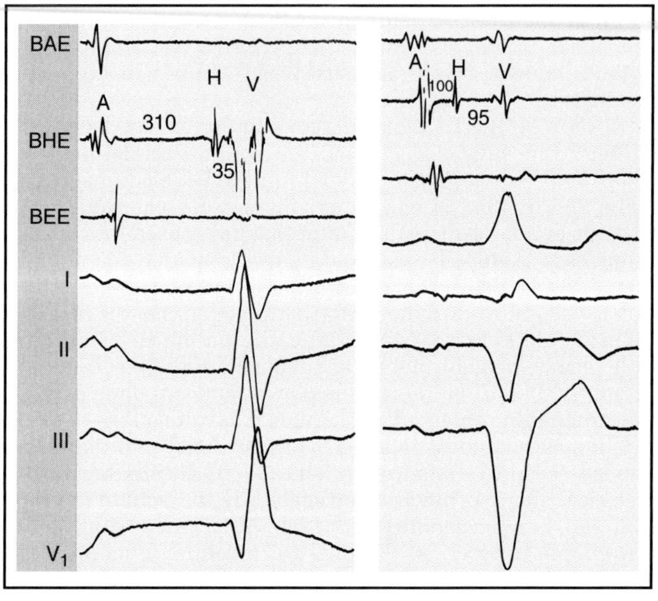

FIGURE 32–51 First-degree atrioventricular (AV) block. One complex during sinus rhythm is shown. **Left panel,** The PR interval measured 370 milliseconds (PA = 25 milliseconds; A-H = 310 milliseconds; H-V = 35 milliseconds) during a right bundle branch block. Conduction delay in the AV node causes the first-degree AV block. **Right panel,** The PR interval is 230 milliseconds (PA = 35 milliseconds; A-H = 100 milliseconds; H-V = 95 milliseconds) during a left bundle branch block. The conduction delay in the His-Purkinje system causes the first-degree AV block.

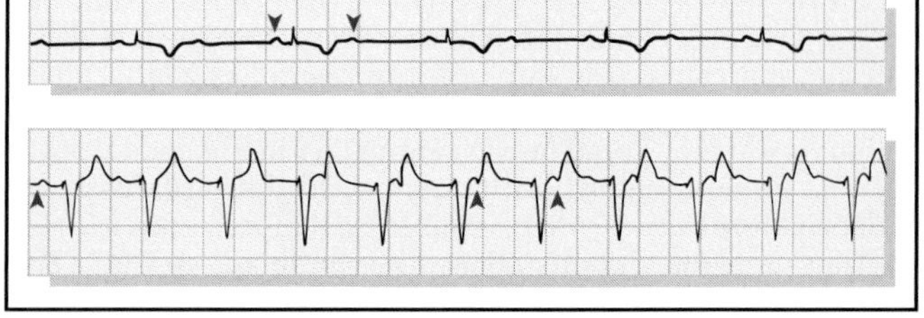

FIGURE 32–52 Unidirectional block. **Top,** During spontaneous sinus rhythm at a rate of 68 beats/min, 2:1 anterograde atrioventricular conduction occurs. In the **bottom** electrocardiogram, 1:1 retrograde conduction is seen during ventricular pacing at a rate of 70 beats/min. P waves are indicated by arrowheads.

generally repetitive and can block several P waves in a row. Often, the eponyms *Mobitz type I* and *Mobitz type II* are applied to the two types of block, whereas the term *Wenckebach block* refers to type I block only. A Wenckebach block in the His-Purkinje system in a patient with a bundle branch block can resemble an AV nodal Wenckebach block very closely (Fig. 32–54B).

Although it has been suggested that type I and type II AV blocks are different manifestations of the same electrophysiological mechanism that differ only quantitatively in the size of the increments, clinically separating second-degree AV block into type I and type II serves a useful function, and in most instances, the differentiation can be made easily and reliably from the surface ECG. Type II AV block often antedates the development of Adams-Stokes syncope and complete AV block, whereas type I AV block with a normal QRS complex is generally more benign and does not progress to more advanced forms of AV conduction disturbance. In older people, type I AV block with or without bundle branch block has been associated with a clinical picture similar to that in type II AV block.

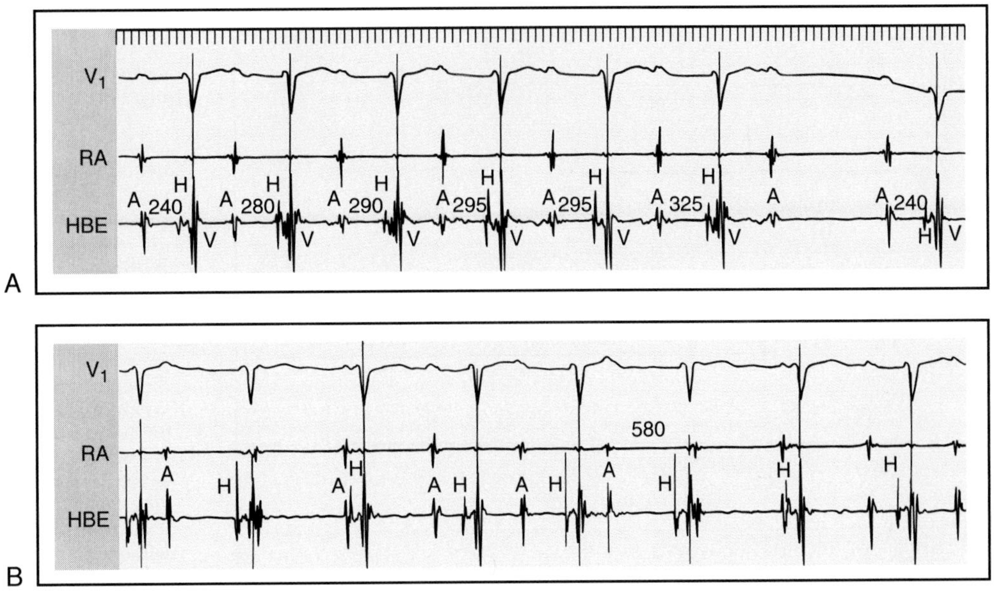

FIGURE 32–53 Type I (Wenckebach) atrioventricular (AV) nodal block **(A)**. During spontaneous sinus rhythm, progressive PR prolongation occurs and culminates in a nonconducted P wave. From the His bundle recording (HBE) it is apparent that the conduction delay and subsequent block occur within the AV node. Since the increment in conduction delay does not consistently decrease, the R-R intervals do not reflect the classic Wenckebach structure. **B** was recorded 5 minutes after the administration of 0.6 mg atropine intravenously. Atropine has had its predominant effect on sinus and junctional automaticity by this time, with little improvement in AV conduction. Consequently, more P waves are blocked and AV dissociation, caused by a combination of AV block and an enhanced junctional discharge rate, is present. At 8 minutes (not shown), when atropine finally improved AV conduction, 1:1 AV conduction occurred.

In a patient with an acute myocardial infarction, type I AV block usually accompanies inferior infarction (perhaps more often if a right ventricular infarction also occurs), is transient, and does not require temporary pacing, whereas type II AV block occurs in the setting of an acute anterior myocardial infarction, can require temporary or permanent pacing, and is associated with a high rate of mortality, generally from pump failure. A high degree of AV block can occur in patients with acute inferior myocardial infarction and is associated with more myocardial damage and a higher mortality rate than in those without AV block.

Although type I conduction disturbance is ubiquitous and can occur in any cardiac tissue in vivo, as well as in vitro, the site of block for the usual forms of second-degree AV block can be judged from the surface ECG with sufficient reliability to permit clinical decisions without requiring invasive electrophysiological studies in most instances. Type I AV block with a normal QRS complex almost always takes place at the level of the AV node, proximal to the His bundle. An exception is the uncommon patient with type I intrahisian block. Type II AV block, particularly in association with a bundle branch block, is localized to the His-Purkinje system. Type I AV block in a patient with a bundle branch block can be due to block in the AV node or in the His-Purkinje system. Type II AV block in a patient with a normal QRS complex can be due to an intrahisian AV block, but the block is likely to be a type I AV nodal block, which exhibits small increments in AV conduction time.

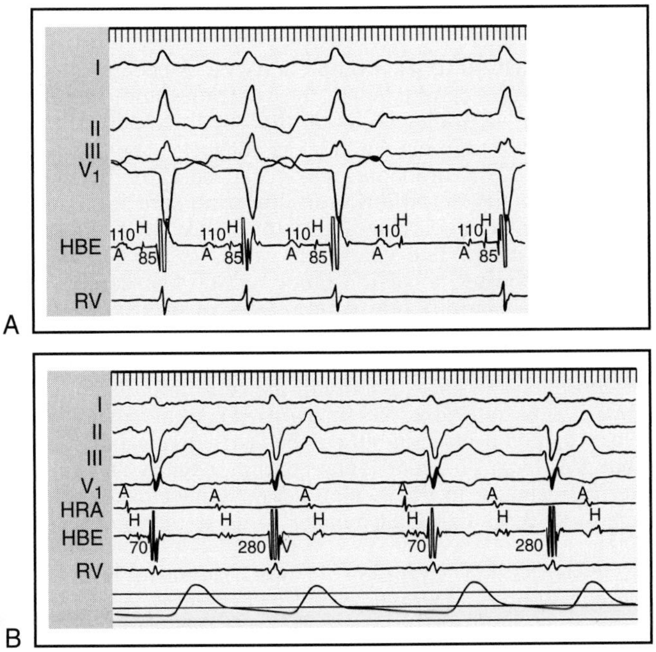

FIGURE 32–54 Type II atrioventricular (AV) block. **A,** The sudden development of a His-Purkinje block is apparent. The A-H and H-V intervals remain constant, as does the PR interval. Left bundle branch block is present. **B,** Wenckebach AV block in the His-Purkinje system. The QRS complex exhibits a right bundle branch block morphology. However, note that the second QRS complex in the 3:2 conduction exhibits a slightly different contour from the first QRS complex, particularly in V_1. This finding is the clue that the Wenckebach AV block might be in the His-Purkinje system. The H-V interval increases from 70 milliseconds to 280 milliseconds, and then block distal to the His bundle results.

DIFFERENTIATING TYPE I FROM TYPE II AV BLOCK. The preceding generalizations encompass the vast majority of patients with second-degree AV block. However, certain caveats must be heeded to avoid misdiagnosis because of subtle ECG changes or exceptions:

1. The 2:1 AV block can be a form of type I or type II AV block (Fig. 32-55). If the QRS complex is normal, the block is more likely to be type I and located in the AV node, and one should search for

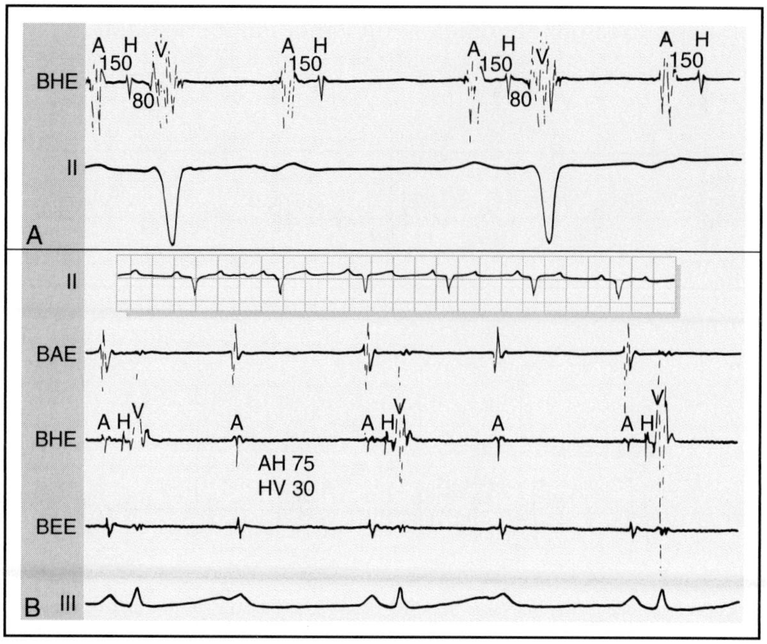

FIGURE 32–55 A 2:1 atrioventricular (AV) block proximal and distal to the His bundle deflection in two different patients. **A,** A 2:1 AV block seen in the scalar electrocardiogram occurs distal to the His bundle recording site in a patient with right bundle branch block and anterior hemiblock. The A-H interval (150 milliseconds) and H-V interval (80 milliseconds) are both prolonged. **B,** A 2:1 AV block proximal to the bundle of His in a patient with a normal QRS complex. The A-H interval (75 milliseconds) and the H-V interval (30 milliseconds) remain constant and normal.

transition of the 2:1 block to a 3:2 block, during which the PR interval lengthens in the second cardiac cycle. If a bundle branch block is present, the block can be located either in the AV node or in the His-Purkinje system.

2. AV block can occur simultaneously at two or more levels and can cause difficulty in distinguishing between types I and II.

3. If the atrial rate varies, it can alter conduction times and cause a type I AV block to stimulate a type II block or change a type II AV block into type I. For example, if the shortest atrial cycle length that just achieved 1:1 AV nodal conduction at a constant PR interval is decreased by as little as 10 or 20 milliseconds, the P wave of the shortened cycle can block conduction at the level of the AV node without an apparent increase in the antecedent PR interval. An apparent type II AV block in the His-Purkinje system can be converted to type I in the His-Purkinje system in some patients by increasing the atrial rate.

4. Concealed premature His depolarizations can create ECG patterns that simulate type I or type II AV block.

5. Abrupt, transient alterations in autonomic tone can cause sudden block of one or more P waves without altering the PR interval of the conducted P wave before or after the block. Thus, an apparent type II AV block would be produced at the AV node. Clinically, a burst of vagal tone usually lengthens the P-P interval, as well as producing an AV block.

6. The response of the AV block to autonomic changes either spontaneous or induced to distinguish type I from type II AV block can be misleading. Although vagal stimulation generally increases and vagolytic agents decrease the extent of type I AV block, such conclusions are based on the assumption that the intervention acts primarily on the AV node and fail to consider rate changes. For example, atropine can minimally improve conduction in the AV node and markedly increase the sinus rate, which results in an *increase* in AV nodal conduction time and the degree of AV block as a result of the faster atrial rate (see Fig. 32–53B). Conversely, if an increase in vagal tone minimally prolongs AV conduction time but greatly slows the heart rate, the net effect on type I AV block may be to improve conduction. In general, however, carotid sinus massage improves and atropine worsens AV conduction in patients with His-Purkinje block, whereas the opposite results are to be expected in patients who have AV nodal block. These two interventions can help differentiate the site of block without invasive study, although damaged His-Purkinje tissue may be influenced by changes in autonomic tone.

7. During type I AV block with high ratios of conducted beats, the increment in PR interval can be quite small and suggest a type II AV block if only the last few PR intervals before the blocked P wave are measured. By comparing the PR interval of the first beat in the long Wenckebach cycle with that of the beats immediately preceding the blocked P wave, the increment in AV conduction becomes readily apparent.

8. The classic AV Wenckebach structure depends on a stable atrial rate and a maximal increment in AV conduction time for the second PR interval of the Wenckebach cycle, with a progressive decrease in subsequent beats. Unstable or unusual alterations in the increment of AV conduction time or in the atrial rate, often seen with long Wenckebach cycles, result in atypical forms of type I AV block in which the last R-R interval can lengthen because the PR increment *increases;* these alterations are common.

9. Finally, it is important to remember that the PR interval in the scalar ECG is made up of conduction through the atrium, the AV node, and the His-Purkinje system. An increment in H-V conduction, for example, can be masked in the scalar ECG by a reduction in the A-H interval, and the resulting PR interval will not reflect the entire increment in His-Purkinje conduction time. Very long PR intervals (200 milliseconds) are more likely to result from AV nodal conduction delay (and block), with or without concomitant His-Purkinje conduction delay, although an H-V interval of 350 milliseconds is quite possible.

First-degree and type I second-degree AV block can occur in normal healthy children, and a Wenckebach AV block can be a normal phenomenon in well-trained athletes, probably related to an increase in resting vagal tone. Occasionally, progressive worsening of the Wenckebach AV conduction disorder can result and the athlete becomes symptomatic and has to decondition. In patients who have chronic second-degree AV nodal block (proximal to the His bundle) without structural heart disease, the course is relatively benign (except in older age groups), whereas in those who have structural heart disease the prognosis is poor and related to the underlying heart disease. *Advanced AV block* indicates a block of two or more consecutive P waves.

Complete AV Block

ECG RECOGNITION. Complete AV block occurs when no atrial activity is conducted to the ventricles and, therefore, the atria and ventricles are controlled by independent pacemakers. Thus, complete AV block is one type of complete AV dissociation. The atrial pacemaker can be sinus or ectopic (tachycardia, flutter, or fibrillation) or can result from an AV junctional focus occurring above the block with retrograde atrial conduction. The ventricular focus is usually located just below the region of the block, which can be above or below the His bundle bifurcation. Sites of ventricular pacemaker activity that are in or closer to the His bundle appear to be more stable and can produce a faster escape rate than can those located more distally in the ventricular conduction system. The ventricular rate in acquired complete heart block is less than 40 beats/min but can be faster in congenital complete AV block. The ventricular rhythm, usually regular, can vary in response to PVCs, a shift in the pacemaker site, an irregularly discharging pacemaker focus, or autonomic influences.

MECHANISMS. Complete AV block can result from block at the level of the AV node (usually congenital) (Fig. 32–56), within the bundle of His, or distal to it in the Purkinje system (usually acquired) (Fig. 32–57). Block proximal to the His bundle generally exhibits normal QRS complexes and rates of 40 to 60 beats/min because the escape focus that controls the ventricle arises in or near the His bundle. In complete AV nodal block, the P wave is not followed by a His deflection, but each ventricular complex is preceded by a His deflection (see Fig. 32–56). His bundle ECG can be useful to differentiate AV nodal from intrahisian block since the latter may carry a more serious prognosis than the former. Intrahisian block is recognized infrequently without invasive studies. In

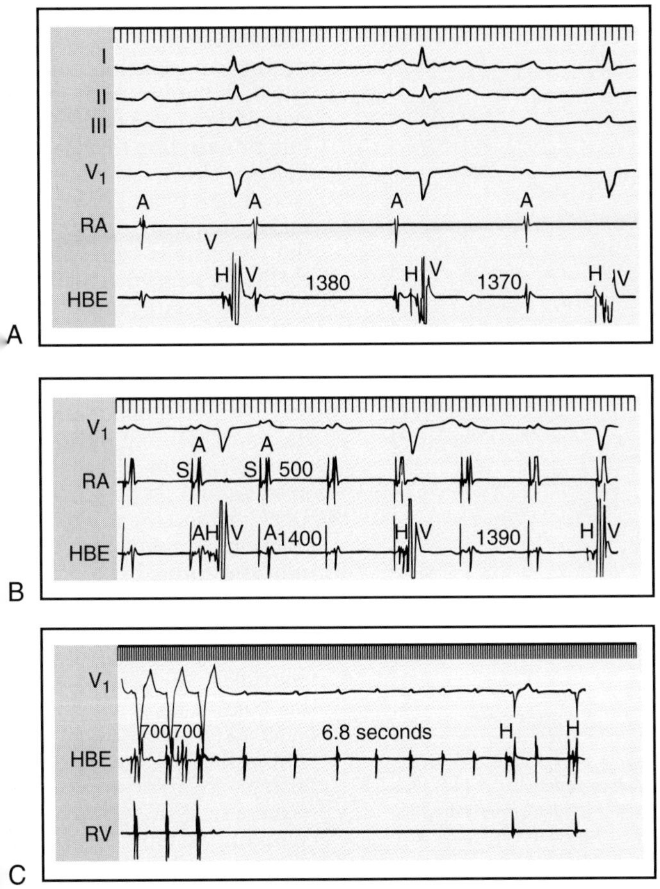

FIGURE 32–56 Congenital third-degree atrioventricular (AV) block. **A,** Complete AV nodal block is apparent. No P wave is followed by a His bundle potential, whereas each ventricular depolarization is preceded by a His bundle potential. **B,** Atrial pacing (cycle length of 500 milliseconds) fails to alter the cycle length of the functional rhythm. Still, no P wave is followed by a His bundle potential. **C,** After 30 seconds of ventricular pacing (cycle length of 700 milliseconds), suppression of the junctional focus results for almost 7 seconds (overdrive suppression of automaticity).

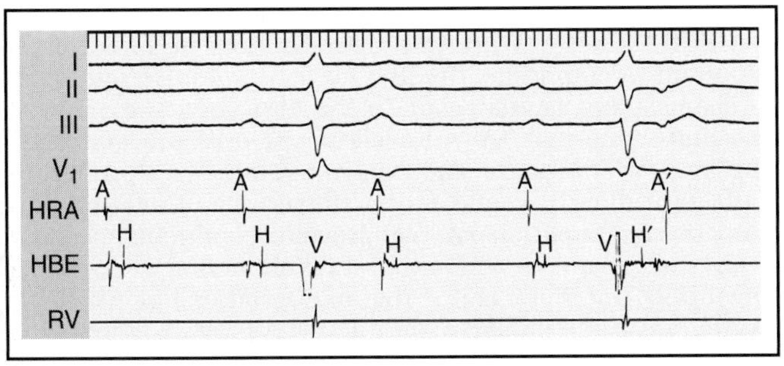

FIGURE 32–57 Complete anterograde atrioventricular (AV) block with retrograde ventriculoatrial conduction. All the sinus P waves are blocked distal to the His bundle, consistent with acquired complete AV block. The ventricles escape at a cycle length of approximately 1800 milliseconds (33 beats/min) and are not preceded by His bundle activation. The ventricular escape rhythm produces a QRS contour with left-axis deviation and right bundle branch block, possibly caused by impulse origin in the posterior fascicle of the left bundle branch. Of interest is the fact that the second ventricular escape beat conducts retrogradely through His (H) and to the atrium (note the low-high atrial activation sequence and the negative P wave in leads II and III). The first ventricular complex does not conduct retrogradely, probably because the His bundle is still refractory from the immediately preceding atrial impulse.

patients with AV nodal block, atropine usually speeds both the atrial and the ventricular rates. Exercise can reduce the extent of AV nodal block. Acquired complete AV block occurs most commonly distal to the bundle of His because of trifascicular conduction disturbance. Each P wave is followed by a His deflection, and the ventricular escape complexes are not preceded by a His deflection (see Fig. 32–57). The QRS complex is abnormal, and the ventricular rate is usually less than 40 beats/min. A hereditary form due to degeneration of the His bundle and bundle branches has been linked to the *SCN5A* gene that is also responsible for long-QT-3.[145]

Paroxysmal AV block in some instances can be due to hyperresponsiveness of the AV node to vagotonic reflexes. Surgery, electrolyte disturbances, myoendocarditis, tumors, Chagas disease, rheumatoid nodules, calcific aortic stenosis, myxedema, polymyositis, infiltrative processes (such as amyloid, sarcoid, or scleroderma), and an almost endless assortment of common and unusual conditions can produce AV block. In adults, rapid rates can sometimes be followed by block, an event known as *overdrive suppression* of conduction. This form of block may be important as a cause of paroxysmal AV block after cessation of a tachycardia.

AV Block in Children. In children, the most common cause of AV block is congenital (see Chap. 56). Under such circumstances, the AV block can be an isolated finding or be associated with other lesions. Connective tissue disease and the presence of anti-Rh_0-negative antibodies in the maternal sera of patients with congenital complete AV block raise the possibility that placentally transmitted antibodies play a role in some instances. Anatomical disruption between the atrial musculature and peripheral parts of the conduction system and nodoventricular discontinuity are two common histological findings. Children are most often asymptomatic; however, in some children symptoms develop that require pacemaker implantation. Mortality from congenital AV block is highest in the neonatal period, is much lower during childhood and adolescence, and increases slowly later in life. Adams-Stokes attacks can occur in patients with congenital heart block at any age. It is difficult to predict the prognosis in an individual patient. A persistent heart rate at rest of 50 beats/min or less correlates with the incidence of syncope, and extreme bradycardia can contribute to the frequency of Adams-Stokes attacks in children with congenital complete AV block. The site of block may not distinguish symptomatic children who have congenital or surgically induced complete heart block from those without symptoms. Prolonged recovery times of escape foci following rapid pacing (see Fig. 32–56C), slow heart rates on 24-hour ECG recordings, and the occurrence of paroxysmal tachycardias may be predisposing factors to the development of symptoms.

CLINICAL FEATURES. Many of the signs of AV block are evidenced at the bedside. First-degree AV block can be recognized by a long *a-c* wave interval in the jugular venous pulse and by diminished intensity of the first heart sound as the PR interval lengthens. In type I second-degree AV block, the heart rate may increase imperceptibly with gradually diminishing intensity of the first heart sound, widening of the *a-c* interval, terminated by a pause, and an *a* wave not followed by a *v* wave. Intermittent ventricular pauses and *a* waves in the neck not followed by *v* waves characterize type II AV block. The first heart sound maintains a constant intensity. In complete AV block, the findings are the same as those in AV dissociation (see later).

Significant clinical manifestations of first- and second-degree AV block usually consist of palpitations or subjective feelings of the heart "missing a beat." Persistent 2:1 AV block can produce symptoms of chronic bradycardia. Complete AV block can be accompanied by signs and symptoms of reduced cardiac output, syncope or presyncope, angina, or palpitations from ventricular tachyarrhythmias. It can occur in twins.

MANAGEMENT. For patients with transient or paroxysmal AV block who present with presyncope or syncope, the diagnosis can be elusive. Ambulatory monitoring (Holter or external loop recorders) can be useful, but on occasion monitoring for longer periods may be necessary and thus an

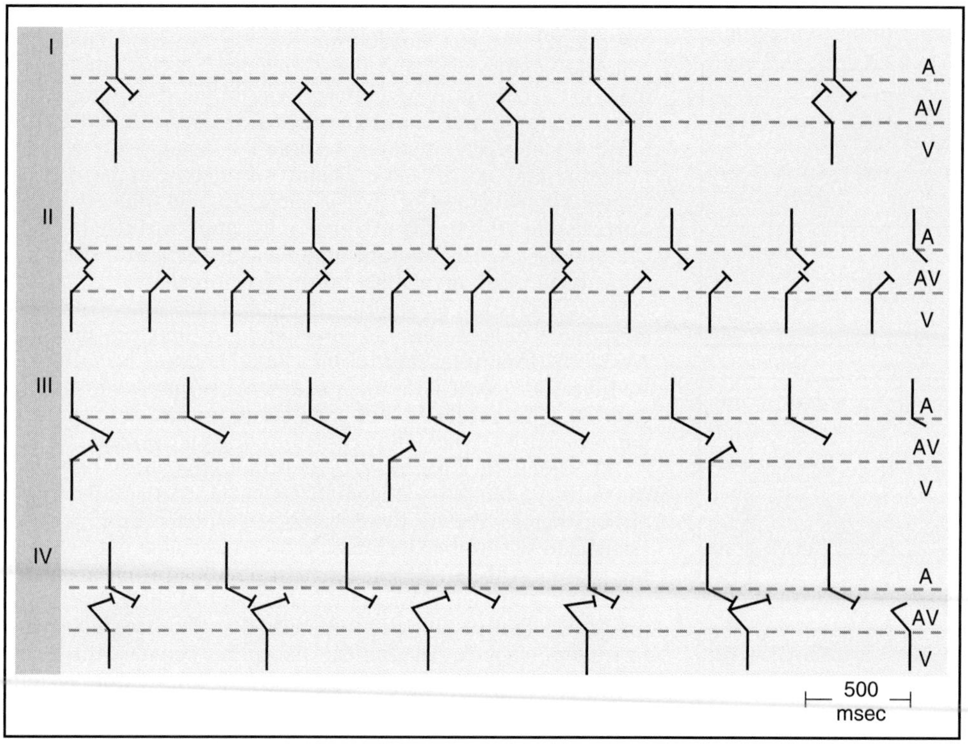

FIGURE 32–58 Diagrammatic illustration of the causes of atrioventricular (AV) dissociation. A sinus bradycardia allowing escape of an AV junctional rhythm that does not capture the atria retrogradely illustrates cause I **(top panel).** Intermittent sinus captures occur (third P wave) and produce incomplete AV dissociation. For cause II, ventricular tachycardia without retrograde atrial capture produces complete AV dissociation (see Figs. 32–22 and 32–41). As the third cause, complete AV block with a ventricular escape rhythm is diagrammed (see Figs. 32–56 and 32–57). The combination of causes II and III is shown in panel IV, which represents a nonparoxysmal AV junctional tachycardia and some degree of AV block.

implantable loop recorder may be needed to establish the diagnosis (see Chap. 29). Drugs cannot be relied on to increase the heart rate for more than several hours to several days in patients with symptomatic heart block without producing significant side effects. Therefore, temporary or permanent pacemaker insertion is indicated in patients with symptomatic bradyarrhythmias. Long-term right ventricular apical pacing can reduce cardiac function. For short-term therapy when the block is likely to be evanescent but still requires treatment or until adequate pacing therapy can be established, vagolytic agents such as atropine are useful for patients who have AV nodal disturbances, whereas catecholamines such as isoproterenol can be used transiently to treat patients who have heart block at any site (see Sinus Bradycardia). Isoproterenol should be used with extreme caution or not at all in patients who have acute myocardial infarction. The use of transcutaneous pacing is preferable.

AV Dissociation

CLASSIFICATION. As the term AV dissociation indicates, dissociated or independent beating of the atria and ventricles defines AV dissociation. AV dissociation is never a *primary* disturbance of rhythm but is a "symptom" of an underlying rhythm disturbance produced by one of three causes or a combination of causes (Fig. 32–58) that prevent the normal transmission of impulses from atrium to ventricle, as follows:

1. Slowing of the dominant pacemaker of the heart (usually the sinus node), which allows escape of a subsidiary or latent pacemaker. AV dissociation by *default* of the primary pacemaker to a subsidiary one in this manner is often a normal phenomenon. It may occur during sinus arrhythmia or sinus bradycardia and permit an independent AV junction rhythm to arise (see Fig. 32–1B).
2. Acceleration of a latent pacemaker that *usurps* control of the ventricles. An abnormally enhanced discharge rate of a usually slower subsidiary pacemaker is pathological and commonly occurs during nonparoxysmal AV junctional tachycardia or VT without retrograde atrial capture (see Figs. 32–22 and 32–41).
3. Block, generally at the AV junction, that prevents impulses formed at a normal rate in a dominant pacemaker from reaching the ventricles and allows the ventricles to beat under the control of a subsidiary pacemaker. Junctional or ventricular escape rhythm during AV block, without retrograde atrial capture, is a common example in which block gives rise to AV dissociation. Complete AV block is *not* synonymous with complete AV dissociation: Patients who have complete AV block have complete AV dissociation, but patients who have complete AV dissociation may or may not have complete AV block (see Figs. 32–56 and 32–57).
4. A combination of causes, for example, when digitalis excess results in the production of nonparoxysmal AV junctional tachycardia associated with SA or AV block.

MECHANISMS. With this classification in mind, it is important to emphasize that the term *AV dissociation* is *not* a diagnosis and is analogous to the term *jaundice* or *fever.* One must state that "AV dissociation is present *due to* . . ." and then give the cause. An accelerated rate of a slower, normally subsidiary pacemaker or a slower rate of a faster, normally dominant pacemaker that prevents conduction because of physiological collision and mutual extinction of opposing wavefronts (interference) or the manifestations of AV block are the basic disturbances producing AV dissociation. The atria in all these cases beat independently from the ventricles, under control of the sinus node or ectopic atrial or AV junctional pacemakers, and can exhibit any type of supraventricular rhythm. If a single pacemaker establishes control of both atria and ventricles for one beat (capture) or a series of beats (sinus rhythm, AV junctional rhythm with retrograde atrial capture, VT with retrograde atrial capture, and so forth), AV dissociation is abolished for that period. Conversely, as stated earlier, whenever the atria and ventricles fail to respond to a single impulse for one beat (PVC without retrograde capture of the atrium) or a series of beats (VT without retrograde atrial capture), AV dissociation exists for that period. The interruption of AV dissociation by one or a series of beats under the control of one pacemaker, either anterogradely or retrogradely, indicates that the AV dissociation is incomplete. Complete or incomplete dissociation can also occur in association with all forms of AV block. Commonly, when AV dissociation occurs as a result of AV block, the atrial rate exceeds the ventricular rate. For example, a subsidiary pacemaker with a rate of 40 beats/min can escape in the presence of a 2:1 AV block when the atrial rate is 78. If the AV block is bidirectional, AV dissociation results.

ECG AND CLINICAL FEATURES. The ECG demonstrates the independence of P waves and QRS complexes. The P wave morphology depends on the rhythm controlling the atria (sinus, atrial tachycardia, junctional, flutter, or fibrillation). During complete AV dissociation, both the QRS complex and the P waves appear regularly spaced without a fixed temporal relationship to each other. When the dissociation is incomplete, a QRS complex of supraventricular contour occurs early and is preceded by a P wave at a PR interval exceeding 0.12 second and within a conductable range. This combination indicates ventricular capture by the supraventricular focus. Similarly, a premature P wave with retrograde morphology and a conductable RP interval may indicate retrograde atrial capture by the subsidiary focus.

Physical findings include a variable intensity of the first heart sound as the PR interval changes, atrial sounds, and *a* waves in the jugular venous pulse lacking a consistent relationship to ventricular contraction. Intermittent large (cannon) *a* waves may be seen in the jugular venous pulse when atrial and ventricular contractions occur simultaneously. The second heart sound can split normally or paradoxically, depending on the manner of ventricular activation. A premature beat representing ventricular capture can interrupt a regular heart rhythm. When the ventricular rate exceeds the atrial rate, a cyclical increase in intensity of the first heart sound is produced as the PR interval shortens, climaxed by a very loud sound (bruit de canon). This intense sound is followed by a sudden reduction in intensity of the first heart sound and the appearance of giant *a* waves as the PR interval shortens and P waves "march through" the cardiac cycle.

MANAGEMENT. Management is directed toward the underlying heart disease and precipitating cause. The individual components *producing the AV dissociation*—not the AV dissociation per se—determine the specific type of antiarrhythmic approach. Therapy ranges from pacemaker insertion in a patient who has AV dissociation resulting from complete AV block to antiarrhythmic drug administration in a patient who has AV dissociation caused by VT.

A

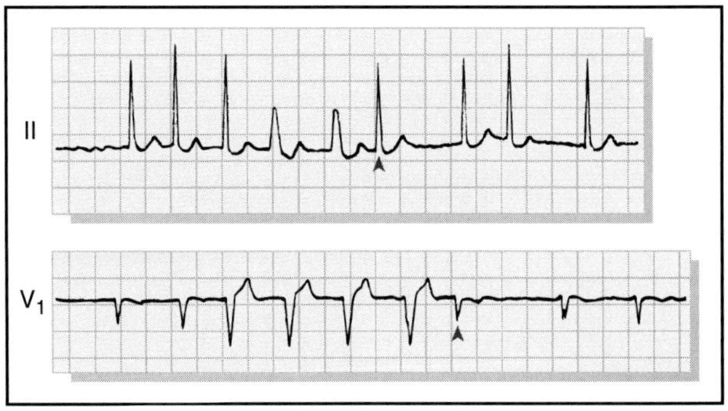

B

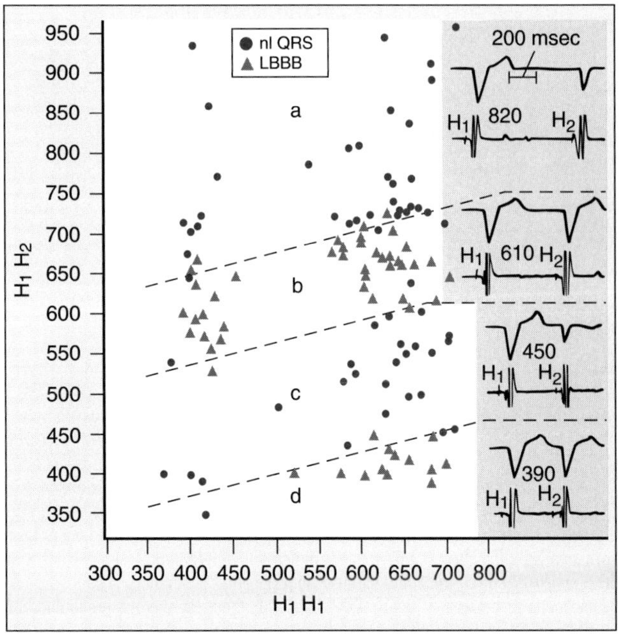

FIGURE 32–59 Supernormal conduction. **A,** Atrial fibrillation with long-short R-R cycle sequences giving rise to QRS complexes conducted with a functional left bundle branch block. In each example, however, a shorter R-R cycle length is terminated by a normal QRS complex (arrowhead), an example of supernormal conduction. **B,** Graph of the intervals and illustrative recordings during an electrophysiological study of the patient whose electrocardiogram is shown in **A**. The H-V interval of the complexes conducted with a left bundle branch block (LBBB) morphology is 45 milliseconds, whereas the H-V interval of those conducted with normal morphology is 35 milliseconds. The graph indicates the premature interval (H_1-H_2, ordinate) plotted against the preceding cycle length (H_1-H_1, abscissa). All H_1-H_1 intervals were taken from complexes with a left bundle branch block morphology. Normal complexes are represented by magenta circles and left bundle branch block contours by blue triangles. Four zones of conduction are identified and illustrated by the four examples to the right. The longest H_1-H_2 intervals are followed by normal intraventricular conduction (zone a), whereas at shorter intervals, left bundle branch block occurs (zone b). When the H_1-H_2 interval shortens further, normal intraventricular conduction returns and the H-V intervals shorten to 35 milliseconds (zone c, supernormal conduction). At the shortest H_1-H_2 interval, left bundle branch block again appears (zone d). (**B,** From Miles WM, Prystowsky EN, Heger JJ, Zipes DP: Evaluation of the patient with wide QRS tachycardia. Med Clin North Am 68:1015, 1984.)

Other Electrophysiological Abnormalities Leading to Cardiac Arrhythmias

SUPERNORMAL CONDUCTION

Supernormal conduction is the term applied to situations characterized by conduction that is better than expected but generally not as good as normal. The phenomenon almost always occurs when conduction is depressed but can be present in normal cardiac tissues as well. It generally occurs when conduction takes place during the relative refractory period of the preceding complex (Fig. 32-59). The electrophysiological basis can relate, in some examples, to supernormal excitability (see later) but probably to other mechanisms as well. Supernormal conduction has commonly been invoked to explain AV (most probably His-Purkinje rather than AV nodal) conduction that is more rapid than expected or AV conduction that results when AV block is expected.

SUPERNORMAL EXCITATION

Supernormal excitation results when a stimulus, normally subthreshold, occurs during the supernormal period of recovery of the preceding complex and produces a propagated response. Stimuli occurring earlier or later fail to produce a propagated response. Demonstrated in vitro in Purkinje fibers but not ventricular muscle, supernormal excitation occurs during phase 3 of the cardiac action potential, when the membrane potential, closer to threshold at the end of repolarization, requires less current to produce a propagated response. A similar phenomenon occurs during phase 4 diastolic depolarization or during afterdepolarizations that reduce the membrane potential closer to threshold. The phenomenon is most easily recognized when a nonsensing pacemaker, failing because of battery exhaustion and reduced output, produces a propagated response only when discharge falls during a specific period in a cardiac cycle (Fig. 32-60). Similar phenomena probably occur spontaneously with "weak" automatic foci, but recognition of these events clinically is difficult and often speculative.

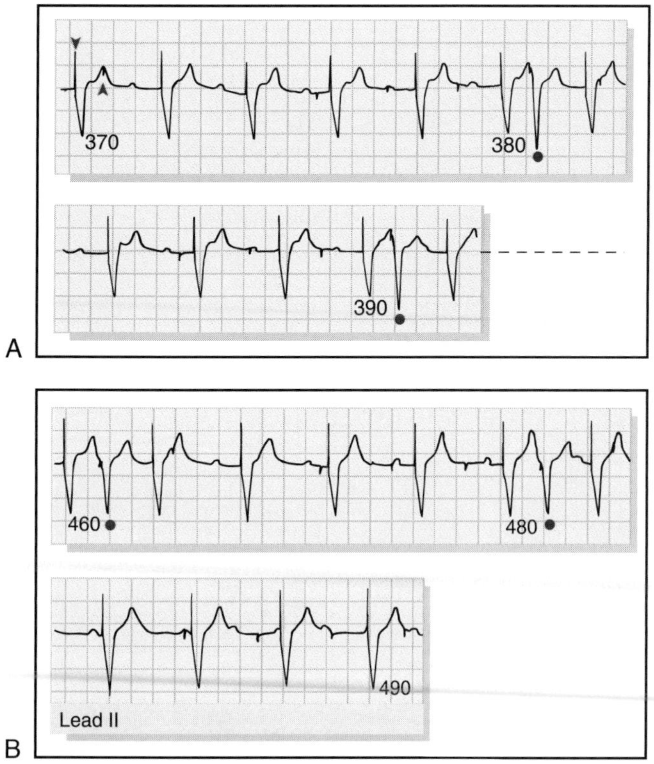

FIGURE 32–60 Supernormal excitation. **A** and **B,** Noncontiguous portions of a continuous electrocardiogram recording with a middle segment removed (dashed line). The patient had a bipolar pacemaker that had exceeded end-of-life status and was no longer consistently producing ventricular depolarization (small negative deflections indicated by the upright arrowhead). A temporary pacemaker was implanted and set at a fixed rate (asynchronous, VOO). These large deflections are indicated by the inverted arrowhead. The numbers in milliseconds indicate the interval between the onset of the QRS complex and the following subthreshold pacemaker stimulus. At intervals of 370 milliseconds (beginning, **A**) and 490 milliseconds (end, **B**), the subthreshold stimulus fails to produce a propagated ventricular response. However, at intervals between 380 and 480 milliseconds, ventricular depolarizations result (red circles). Thus, the period of supernormal excitation is 100 milliseconds in duration, from 380 to 480 milliseconds after the onset of the QRS complex.

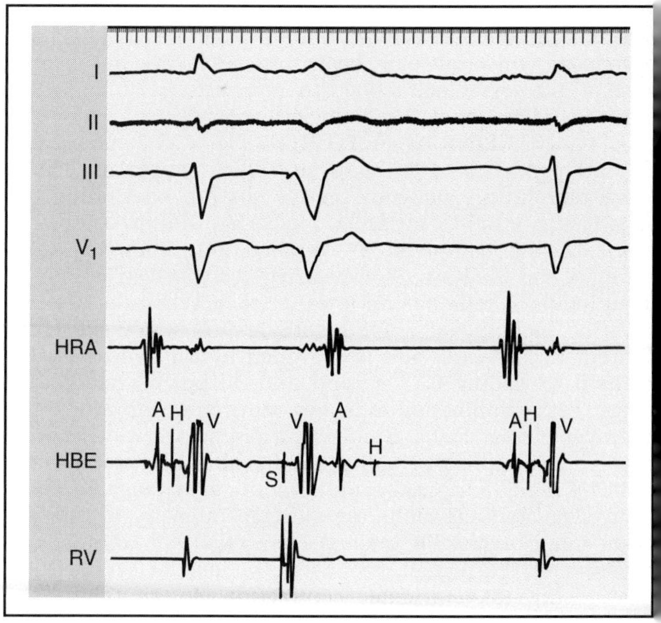

FIGURE 32–61 Concealed conduction. Following the first normally conducted sinus-initiated complex, a premature ventricular complex is stimulated (S). The next spontaneous sinus-initiated P wave is blocked and a fully compensatory pause is produced. The third sinus-initiated P wave is conducted normally. From the His bundle recording it is obvious that the nonconducted sinus beat is blocked distal to the His bundle recording site. Note that the A-H interval of the nonconducted sinus P wave beat is prolonged, which suggests that the retrogradely activated His and invaded the AV node, thereby making it partially refractory to the next sinus beat. Since retrograde conduction into the atrioventricular (AV) node is not recorded and can be surmised only on the basis of the increase in the following A-H interval, it is an example of concealed conduction. Furthermore, since retrograde His and AV node activation by the PVC would not be apparent in the scalar electrocardiogram but is responsible for the compensatory pause, the blocked P wave is an example of concealed conduction.

CONCEALED CONDUCTION

Concealed conduction describes the phenomenon during which impulses penetrate an area of the conduction tissue, the AV node commonly but other areas as well, without emerging. Since transmission of the impulse is concealed, that is, electrically silent in the standard ECG, concealed conduction becomes manifested only by its *effects* on the conduction and/or formation of subsequent impulses.[146] The most common example follows a PVC. Partial retrograde penetration of the AV node by the PVC is *deduced* because the following sinus-initiated P wave blocks conduction to produce a compensatory pause (Fig. 32-61) or conducts with a longer PR interval if the PVC is interpolated. The slower ventricular response when the atrial rate increases from atrial flutter to atrial fibrillation is due to a greater number of atrial impulses being blocked (conducting into, without emerging) in the AV node and is a manifestation of concealed conduction. Concealed conduction occurs in WPW syndrome and can be manifested by unidirectional block anterogradely or retrogradely in an accessory pathway. Concealed junctional extrasystoles can create ECG manifestations of apparent AV block. Strict confirmation of concealed conduction should be the demonstration of conduction, such as in the form of conducted junctional extrasystoles.

PARASYSTOLE

Parasystole (Fig. 32-62) refers to a cardiac arrhythmia characterized electrocardiographically by (1) a varying coupling interval between the ectopic (parasystolic) complex and the dominant (generally, sinus-initiated) complex; (2) a common minimal time interval between interectopic intervals, with the longer interectopic intervals being multiples of this minimal interval; (3) fusion complexes; and (4) presence of the

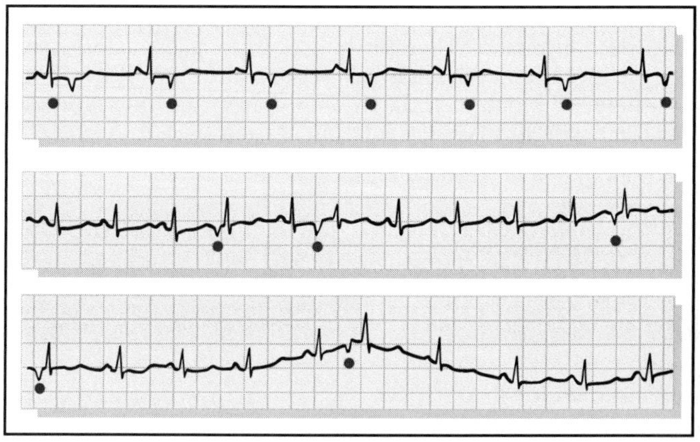

FIGURE 32–62 Atrial parasystole. **Top,** Atrial parasystolic impulses (red circles under the negative P waves) are present at a fixed coupling interval to the dominant sinus rhythm. The reason for the fixed coupling is as follows: Each time that the parasystolic impulse depolarizes the atrium, it also discharges the sinus node. Diastolic depolarization in the sinus node begins at that point (reset) and results in the following sinus P wave (positive P wave). Thus, the constant parasystolic discharge rate (interectopic interval approximately 960 milliseconds), resetting of the sinus node, and constant phase 4 diastolic depolarization in the sinus node combine to result in fixed coupling. **Middle** and **Bottom,** The sinus discharge rate is slightly faster. It is no longer discharged by the parasystolic impulse, which is still occurring at approximately 960 milliseconds (slightly longer interval in the bottom tracing). Variable coupling, the usual manifestation of parasystole, results. Lead II.

parasystolic impulse whenever the cardiac chamber is excitable. Parasystole with exit block is suspected when the parasystolic discharge focus fails to appear even though cardiac tissue is excitable. The analogy commonly invoked to represent parasystole is the behavior of a fixed-rate nonsensing (VOO) pacemaker (see Chap. 31). Parasystole can occur in the sinus and AV nodes, atrium and ventricle, and AV junction. The parasystolic mechanism presumably results from the regular discharge of an automatic focus that is independent of and protected from discharge by the dominant cardiac rhythm. A number of mechanisms have been postulated to explain the apparent protection enjoyed by the parasystolic rhythm.

These classic definitions of parasystole need to be modified because it has been well established that the dominant sinus beats can modulate the discharge rate of the parasystolic rhythm despite entrance block. Thus, wide variations in the modulated parasystolic cycle may occur. The "true," or unmodulated, parasystolic cycle length can be determined by finding two consecutive parasystolic complexes without intervening beats. Phase response curves can be generated. Fixed coupling between the dominant and parasystolic rhythms can occur through a variety of mechanisms, including entrainment. It is possible that modulated parasystole in the presence of supernormal excitability can trigger ventricular fibrillation.

REFERENCES

Individual Cardiac Arrhythmias and Sinus Nodal Disturbances

1. Olgin JE: Inappropriate sinus tachycardia and sinus node reentry. *In* Zipes D, Jalife J (eds): Cardiac Electrophysiology: From Cell to Bedside. 3rd ed. Philadelphia, WB Saunders, 2000, pp 459-468.
2. Gregoratos G, Cheitlin MD, Conill A, et al: ACC/AHA guidelines for implantation of cardiac pacemakers and antiarrhythmia devices: A report of the American College of Cardiology/American Heart Association Task Force on Practice Guidelines (Committee on Pacemaker Implantation). J Am Coll Cardiol 31:1175-1209, 1998.
3. Elvan A, Wylie K, Zipes DP: Pacing-induced chronic atrial fibrillation impairs sinus node function in dogs: Electrophysiological remodeling. Circulation 94:2953-2960, 1996.
4. Bharati S, Lev M: The pathologic changes in the conduction system beyond the age of ninety. Am Heart J 124:486-496, 1992.

Disturbances of Atrial Rhythm

5. Zipes DP, Garson A Jr: 26th Bethesda Conference: Recommendations for determining eligibility for competition in athletes with cardiovascular abnormalities. Task Force 6: Arrhythmias. Med Sci Sports Exerc 26(Suppl):276-283, 1994.
6. Kalman JM, Olgin JE, Saxon LA, et al: Activation and entrainment mapping defines the tricuspid annulus as the anterior barrier in typical atrial flutter. Circulation 94:398-406, 1996.
7. Olgin JE, Kalman JM, Fitzpatrick AP, Lesh MD: Role of right atrial endocardial structures as barriers to conduction during human type I atrial flutter: Activation and entrainment mapping guided by intracardiac echocardiography. Circulation 92:1839-1848, 1995.
8. Kalman JM, Olgin JE, Saxon LA, et al: Electrocardiographic and electrophysiologic characterization of atypical atrial flutter in man: Use of activation and entrainment mapping and implications for catheter ablation. J Cardiovasc Electrophysiol 8:121-144, 1997.
9. Kalman JM, VanHare GF, Olgin JE, et al: Ablation of "incisional" reentrant atrial tachycardia complicating surgery for congenital heart disease: Use of entrainment to define a critical isthmus of conduction. Circulation 93:502-512, 1996.
10. Olgin JE, Jayachandran JV, Engelstein E, et al: Atrial macroreentry involving the myocardium of the coronary sinus—a unique mechanism for atypical flutter. J Cardiovasc Electrophysiol 9:1094-1099, 1998.
11. Stambler BS, Wood MA, Ellenbogen KA, et al: Efficacy and safety of repeated intravenous doses of ibutilide for rapid conversion of atrial flutter or fibrillation. Ibutilide Repeat Dose Study Investigators. Circulation 94:1613-1621, 1996.
12. Abi-Mansour P, Carberry PA, McCowan RJ, et al: Conversion efficacy and safety of repeated doses of ibutilide in patients with atrial flutter and atrial fibrillation. Study Investigators. Am Heart J 136:632–642, 1998.
13. Weiss R, Marcovitz P, Knight BP, et al: Acute changes in spontaneous echo contrast and atrial function after cardioversion of persistent atrial flutter. Am J Cardiol 82:1052-1055, 1998.
14. Kontos MC, Paulsen WH: Impairment of left atrial appendage function after spontaneous conversion of atrial flutter. Clin Cardiol 21:769-771, 1998.
15. Sparks PB, Jayaprakash S, Vohra JK, et al: Left atrial "stunning" following radiofrequency catheter ablation of chronic atrial flutter. J Am Coll Cardiol 32:468-475, 1998.
16. Olgin JE, Lesh MD: The laboratory evaluation and role of catheter ablation for patients with atrial flutter. Cardiol Clin 15:677-688, 1997.
17. Olgin JE, Miles W: Ablation of atrial tachycardias. *In* Singor I, Barold S, Camm A (eds): Nonpharmacological Therapy of Arrhythmias for the 21st Century: The State of the Art. Mount Kisco, NY, Futura, 1998, pp 197-217.
18. Feinberg WM, Cornell ES, Nightingale SD, et al: Relationship between prothrombin activation fragment F1.2 and international normalized ratio in patients with atrial fibrillation. Stroke Prevention in Atrial Fibrillation Investigators. Stroke 28:1101-1106, 1997.
19. Warfarin versus aspirin for prevention of thromboembolism in atrial fibrillation: Stroke Prevention in Atrial Fibrillation II Study. Lancet 343:687-691, 1994.
20. Secondary prevention in non-rheumatic atrial fibrillation after transient ischaemic attack or minor stroke. EAFT (European Atrial Fibrillation Trial) Study Group. Lancet 342:1255-1262, 1993.
21. Ezekowitz MD, Bridgers SL, James KE, et al: Warfarin in the prevention of stroke associated with nonrheumatic atrial fibrillation. Veterans Affairs Stroke Prevention in Nonrheumatic Atrial Fibrillation Investigators. N Engl J Med 327:1406-1412, 1992.
22. Connolly SJ, Laupacis A, Gent M, et al: Canadian Atrial Fibrillation Anticoagulation (CAFA) Study. J Am Coll Cardiol 18:349-355, 1991.
23. The effect of low-dose warfarin on the risk of stroke in patients with nonrheumatic atrial fibrillation. The Boston Area Anticoagulation Trial for Atrial Fibrillation Investigators. N Engl J Med 323:1505-1511, 1990.
24. Petersen P, Boysen G, Godtfredsen J, et al: Placebo-controlled, randomised trial of warfarin and aspirin for prevention of thromboembolic complications in chronic atrial fibrillation. The Copenhagen AFASAK study. Lancet 1:175-179, 1989.
25. Stroke Prevention in Atrial Fibrillation Study. Final results. Circulation 84:527-539, 1991.
26. Klein AL, Grimm RA, Black IW, et al: Cardioversion guided by transesophageal echocardiography: The ACUTE Pilot Study. A randomized, controlled trial. Assessment of Cardioversion Using Transesophageal Echocardiography. Ann Intern Med 126:200-209, 1997.
27. Escudero EM, San Mauro M, Laugle C: Bilateral atrial function after chemical cardioversion of atrial fibrillation with amiodarone: An echo-Doppler study. J Am Soc Echocardiogr 11:365-371, 1998.
28. Omran H, Jung W, Luderitz B: Left atrial appendage function after internal atrial defibrillation. J Cardiovasc Electrophysiol 9(Suppl):97-103, 1998.
29. Wyse DG, Waldo AL, DiMarco JP, et al: A comparison of rate control and rhythm control in patients with atrial fibrillation. N Engl J Med 347:1825-1833, 2002.
30. Hopfner R: Ximelagatran (AstraZeneca). Curr Opin Investig Drugs 3:246-251, 2002.
31. Crystal E, Lamy A, Connolly SJ, et al: Left Atrial Appendage Occlusion Study (LAAOS): A randomized clinical trial of left atrial appendage occlusion during routine coronary artery bypass graft surgery for long-term stroke prevention. Am Heart J 145:174-178, 2003.
32. Sievert H, Lesh MD, Trepels T, et al: Percutaneous left atrial appendage transcatheter occlusion to prevent stroke in high-risk patients with atrial fibrillation: Early clinical experience. Circulation 105:1887-1889, 2002.
33. Hohnloser SH, Kuck KH, Lilienthal J: Rhythm or rate control in atrial fibrillation—Pharmacological Intervention in Atrial Fibrillation (PIAF): A randomised trial. Lancet 356:1789-1794, 2000.
34. Saxonhouse SJ, Curtis AB: Risks and benefits of rate control versus maintenance of sinus rhythm. Am J Cardiol 91:27-32, 2003.
35. Tieleman RG, Van Gelder IC, Crijns HJ, et al: Early recurrences of atrial fibrillation after electrical cardioversion: A result of fibrillation-induced electrical remodeling of the atria? J Am Coll Cardiol 31:167-173, 1998.
36. Franz MR, Karasik PL, Li C, et al: Electrical remodeling of the human atrium: Similar effects in patients with chronic atrial fibrillation and atrial flutter. J Am Coll Cardiol 30:1785-1792, 1997.
37. Daoud EG, Knight BP, Weiss R, et al: Effect of verapamil and procainamide on atrial fibrillation-induced electrical remodeling in humans. Circulation 96:1542-1550, 1997.
38. Olgin JE, Rubart M: Remodeling of the atria and ventricle due to rate. *In* Zipes D, Jalife J (eds): Cardiac Electrophysiology: From Cell to Bedside. 3rd ed. Philadelphia, WB Saunders, 2000, pp 364-378.
39. Sopher SM, Camm AJ: New trials in atrial fibrillation. J Cardiovasc Electrophysiol 9(Suppl):211-215, 1998.
40. Alt E, Ammer R, Schmitt C, et al: A comparison of treatment of atrial fibrillation with low-energy intracardiac cardioversion and conventional external cardioversion. Eur Heart J 18:1796-1804, 1997.
41. Levy S, Ricard P, Lau CP, et al: Multicenter low-energy transvenous atrial defibrillation (XAD) trial results in different subsets of atrial fibrillation. J Am Coll Cardiol 29:750-755, 1997.
42. Oral H, Souza JJ, Michaud GF, et al: Facilitating transthoracic cardioversion of atrial fibrillation with ibutilide pretreatment. N Engl J Med 340:1849-1854, 1999.
43. Mittal S, Ayati S, Stein KM, et al: Transthoracic cardioversion of atrial fibrillation: Comparison of rectilinear biphasic versus damped sine wave monophasic shocks. Circulation. 101:1282-1287, 2000.
44. Page RL, Kerber RE, Russell JK, et al: Biphasic versus monophasic shock waveform for conversion of atrial fibrillation: The results of an international randomized, double-blind multicenter trial. J Am Coll Cardiol 39:1956-1963, 2002.
45. Benditt DG, Samniah N, Iskos D, et al: Biphasic waveform cardioversion as an alternative to internal cardioversion for atrial fibrillation refractory to conventional monophasic waveform transthoracic shock. Am J Cardiol 88:1426-1428, 2001.
46. Viskin S, Barron H, Olgin JE, et al: The treatment of atrial fibrillation: Pharmacologic and non-pharmacological strategies. Curr Probl Cardiol 22:44-108, 1997.
47. Volgman AS, Carberry PA, Stambler B, et al: Conversion efficacy and safety of intravenous ibutilide compared with intravenous procainamide in patients with atrial flutter or fibrillation. J Am Coll Cardiol 31:1414-1419, 1998.
48. Olgin JE, Viskin S: Management of intermittent atrial fibrillation: Drugs to maintain sinus rhythm. J Cardiovasc Electrophysiol 10:433-441, 1999.
49. Lindeboom J, Kingma JH, Crijns HJ, Dunselman PH: Efficacy and safety of intravenous dofetilide for rapid termination of atrial fibrillation and atrial flutter. Am J Cardiol 85:1031-1033, 2000.
50. Sager PT: New advances in class III antiarrhythmic drug therapy. Curr Opin Cardiol 15:41-53, 2000.
51. Pappone C, Oreto G, Rosanio S, et al: Atrial electroanatomic remodeling after circumferential radiofrequency pulmonary vein ablation: Efficacy of an anatomic approach in a large cohort of patients with atrial fibrillation. Circulation 104:2539-2544, 2001.

52. Oral H, Knight BP, Tada H, et al: Pulmonary vein isolation for paroxysmal and persistent atrial fibrillation. Circulation 105:1077-1081, 2002.
53. Jessurun ER, Van Hemel NM, Defauw JJ, et al: A randomized study of combining maze surgery for atrial fibrillation with mitral valve surgery. J Cardiovasc Surg (Torino) 44:9-18, 2003.
54. Jais P, Haissaguerre M, Shah DC, et al: A focal source of atrial fibrillation treated by discrete radiofrequency ablation. Circulation 95:572-576, 1997.
55. Haissaguerre M, Jais P, Shah DC, et al: Spontaneous initiation of atrial fibrillation by ectopic beats originating in the pulmonary veins. N Engl J Med 339:659-666, 1998.
56. Haissaguerre M, Jais P, Shah DC, et al: Catheter ablation of chronic atrial fibrillation targeting the reinitiating triggers. J Cardiovasc Electrophysiol 11:2-10, 2000.
57. Wellens HJ, Lau CP, Luderitz B, et al: Atrioverter: An implantable device for the treatment of atrial fibrillation. Circulation 98:1651-1656, 1998.
58. Bailin SJ, Sulke N, Swerdlow CD: Clinical experience with a dual chamber implantable cardioverter defibrillator in patients with atrial fibrillation and flutter [abstract]. PACE 22:871, 1999.
59. Jung W, Wolpert C, Esmailzadeh B, et al: Clinical experience with implantable atrial and combined atrioventricular defibrillators. J Interv Cardiol Electrophysiol 4(Suppl 1):185-195, 2000.
60. Pollak A, Falk RH: Pacemaker therapy in patients with atrial fibrillation. Am Heart J 125:824-830, 1993.
61. Delfaut P, Saksena S, Prakash A, Krol RB: Long-term outcome of patients with drug-refractory atrial flutter and fibrillation after single- and dual-site right atrial pacing for arrhythmia prevention. J Am Coll Cardiol 32:1900-1908, 1998.
63. Waldo AL: Atrial flutter: Entrainment characteristics. J Cardiovasc Electrophysiol 8:337-352, 1997.

AV Junctional Rhythm Disturbances

64. Glatter KA, Cheng J, Dorostkar P, et al: Electrophysiologic effects of adenosine in patients with supraventricular tachycardia. Circulation 99:1034-1040, 1999.
65. Miles WM, Zipes DP: Atrioventricular reentry and variants: Mechanisms, clinical features, and management. *In* Zipes DP, Jalife J (eds): Cardiac Electrophysiology: From Cell to Bedside. 3rd ed. Philadelphia, WB Saunders, 2000, pp 638-655.
66. Arruda MS, McClelland JH, Wang X, et al: Development and validation of an ECG algorithm for identifying accessory pathway ablation site in Wolff-Parkinson-White syndrome. J Cardiovasc Electrophysiol 9:2-12, 1998.
68. Morady F: Radio-frequency ablation as treatment for cardiac arrhythmias. N Engl J Med 340:534-544, 1999.

Ventricular Rhythm Disturbances

69. Oreto G, Luzza F, Badessa F, et al: QRS complex voltage changes associated with supraventricular tachycardia. J Cardiovasc Electrophysiol 12:1358-1362, 2001.
71. Kennedy HL: Use of long-term (Holter) electrocardiographic recordings. *In* Zipes DP, Jalife J (eds): Cardiac Electrophysiology: From Cell to Bedside. 3rd ed. Philadelphia, WB Saunders, 2000, pp 716-730.
72. Singh BN: Beta-blockers and calcium channel blockers as anti-arrhythmic drugs. *In* Zipes DP, Jalife J (eds): Cardiac Electrophysiology: From Cell to Bedside. 3rd ed. Philadelphia, WB Saunders, 2000, pp 903-921.
73. Miller JM, Hsia HH, Rothman SA, Buxton AE: Ventricular tachycardia versus supraventricular tachycardia with aberration: Electrocardiographic distinctions. *In* Zipes DP, Jalife J (eds): Cardiac Electrophysiology: From Cell to Bedside. 3rd ed. Philadelphia, WB Saunders, 2000, pp 696-705.
74. Myerburg RJ, Kessler KM, Kimura S: Life-threatening ventricular arrhythmias: The link between epidemiology and pathophysiology. *In* Zipes DP, Jalife J (eds): Cardiac Electrophysiology: From Cell to Bedside. 3rd ed. Philadelphia, WB Saunders, 2000, pp 521 530.
75. Armoundas AA, Rosenbaum DS, Ruskin JN, et al: Prognostic significance of electrical alternans versus signal averaged electrocardiography in predicting the outcome of electrophysiological testing and arrhythmia-free survival. Heart 80:251-256, 1998.
76. Hohnloser SH, Klingenheben T, Li YG, et al: T wave alternans as a predictor of recurrent ventricular tachyarrhythmias in ICD recipients: Prospective comparison with conventional risk markers. J Cardiovasc Electrophysiol 9:1258-1268, 1998.
77. Gold MR, Bloomfield DM, Anderson KP, et al: A comparison of T-wave alternans, signal averaged electrocardiography, and programmed ventricular stimulation for arrhythmia risk stratification. J Am Coll Cardiol 36:2247-2253, 2000.
78. Somberg JC, Bailin SJ, Haffajee CI, et al: Intravenous lidocaine versus intravenous amiodarone (in a new aqueous formulation) for incessant ventricular tachycardia. Am J Cardiol 90:853-859, 2002.
79. A randomized trial of propranolol in patients with acute myocardial infarction: I. Mortality results. JAMA 247:1707-1714, 1982.
80. Echt DS, Liebson PR, Mitchell LB, et al: Mortality and morbidity in patients receiving encainide, flecainide, or placebo. The Cardiac Arrhythmia Suppression Trial. N Engl J Med 324:781-788, 1991.
81. Waldo AL, Camm AJ, deRuyter H, et al: Effect of *d*-sotalol on mortality in patients with left ventricular dysfunction after recent and remote myocardial infarction. The SWORD Investigators. Survival with Oral *d*-Sotalol. Lancet 348:7-12, 1996.
82. Julian DG, Camm AJ, Frangin G, et al: Randomised trial of effect of amiodarone on mortality in patients with left-ventricular dysfunction after recent myocardial infarction: EMIAT. European Myocardial Infarct Amiodarone Trial Investigators. Lancet 349:667-674, 1997.
83. Cairns JA, Connolly SJ, Roberts R, Gent M: Randomised trial of outcome after myocardial infarction in patients with frequent or repetitive ventricular premature depolarisations: CAMIAT. Canadian Amiodarone Myocardial Infarction Arrhythmia Trial Investigators. Lancet 349:675-682, 1997.
84. Doval HC, Nul DR, Grancelli HO, et al: Nonsustained ventricular tachycardia in severe heart failure: Independent marker of increased mortality due to sudden death. GESICA-GEMA Investigators. Circulation 94:3198-3203, 1996.
85. Singh SN, Fletcher RD, Fisher SG, et al: Amiodarone in patients with congestive heart failure and asymptomatic ventricular arrhythmia. Survival Trial of Antiarrhythmic Therapy in Congestive Heart Failure. N Engl J Med 333:77-82, 1995.
87. Klein H, Auricchio A, Reek S, Geller C: New primary prevention trials of sudden cardiac death in patients with left ventricular dysfunction: SCD-HEFT and MADIT-II. Am J Cardiol 83:91D-97D, 1999.
88. Bigger JT Jr, Whang W, Rottman JN, et al: Mechanisms of death in the CABG Patch trial: A randomized trial of implantable cardiac defibrillator prophylaxis in patients at high risk of death after coronary artery bypass graft surgery. Circulation 99:1416-1421, 1999.
89. Moss AJ, Hall WJ, Cannom DS, et al: Improved survival with an implanted defibrillator in patients with coronary disease at high risk for ventricular arrhythmia. Multicenter Automatic Defibrillator Implantation Trial Investigators. N Engl J Med 335:1933-1940, 1996.
90. Buxton AE, Lee KL, Fisher JD, et al: A randomized study of the prevention of sudden death in patients with coronary artery disease. Multicenter Unsustained Tachycardia Trial Investigators. N Engl J Med 341:1882-1890, 1999.
91. Mason JW: A comparison of electrophysiologic testing with Holter monitoring to predict antiarrhythmic-drug efficacy for ventricular tachyarrhythmias. Electrophysiologic Study versus Electrocardiographic Monitoring Investigators. N Engl J Med 329:445-451, 1993.
92. Mason JW: A comparison of seven antiarrhythmic drugs in patients with ventricular tachyarrhythmias. Electrophysiologic Study versus Electrocardiographic Monitoring Investigators. N Engl J Med 329:452-458, 1993.
93. Greene HL: The CASCADE Study: Randomized antiarrhythmic drug therapy in survivors of cardiac arrest in Seattle. CASCADE Investigators. Am J Cardiol 72:70F-74F, 1993.
94. Siebels J, Cappato R, Ruppel R, et al: Preliminary results of the Cardiac Arrest Study Hamburg (CASH). CASH Investigators. Am J Cardiol 72:109F-113F, 1993.
95. A comparison of antiarrhythmic-drug therapy with implantable defibrillators in patients resuscitated from near-fatal ventricular arrhythmias. The Antiarrhythmics versus Implantable Defibrillators (AVID) Investigators. N Engl J Med 337:1576-1583, 1997.
96. Cappato R: Secondary prevention of sudden death: The Dutch Study, the Antiarrhythmics Versus Implantable Defibrillator Trial, the Cardiac Arrest Study Hamburg, and the Canadian Implantable Defibrillator Study. Am J Cardiol 83:68D-73D, 1999.
97. Connolly SJ, Gent M, Roberts RS, et al: Canadian Implantable Defibrillator Study (CIDS): Study design and organization. CIDS Co-Investigators. Am J Cardiol 72:103F-108F, 1993.
98. Moss AJ, Hall WJ, Cannom DS, et al: Improved survival with an implanted defibrillator in patients with coronary disease at high risk for ventricular arrhythmia. Multicenter Automatic Defibrillator Implantation Trial Investigators. N Engl J Med 335:1933-1940, 1996.
99. Buxton AE, Lee KL, Fisher JD, et al: A randomized study of the prevention of sudden death in patients with coronary artery disease. Multicenter Unsustained Tachycardia Trial Investigators. N Engl J Med 341:1882-1890, 1999.
100. Moss AJ, Zareba W, Hall WJ, et al: Prophylactic implantation of a defibrillator in patients with myocardial infarction and reduced ejection fraction. N Engl J Med 346:877-883, 2002.
101. Rothman SA, Hsia HH, Cossu SF, et al: Radiofrequency catheter ablation of postinfarction ventricular tachycardia: Long-term success and the significance of inducible nonclinical arrhythmias. Circulation 96:3499-3508, 1997.
102. Strickberger SA, Man KC, Daoud EG, et al: A prospective evaluation of catheter ablation of ventricular tachycardia as adjuvant therapy in patients with coronary artery disease and an implantable cardioverter-defibrillator. Circulation 96:1525-1531, 1997.
103. Miller JM, Engelstein ED, Groh WJ, et al: Radiofrequency catheter ablation for postinfarct ventricular tachycardia. Curr Opin Cardiol 14:30-35, 1999.
104. Corrado D, Basso C, Thiene G, et al: Spectrum of clinicopathologic manifestations of arrhythmogenic right ventricular cardiomyopathy/dysplasia: A multicenter study. J Am Coll Cardiol 30:1512-1520, 1997.
105. Corrado D, Basso C, Schiavon M, Thiene G: Screening for hypertrophic cardiomyopathy in young athletes. N Engl J Med 339:364-369, 1998.
106. Li D, Ahmad F, Gardner MJ, et al: The locus of a novel gene responsible for arrhythmogenic right-ventricular dysplasia characterized by early onset and high penetrance maps to chromosome 10p12-p14. Am J Hum Genet 66:148-156, 2000.
107. Li D, Bachinski LL, Roberts R: Genomic organization and isoform-specific tissue expression of human NAPOR (CUGBP2) as a candidate gene for familial arrhythmogenic right ventricular dysplasia. Genomics 74:396-401, 2001.
108. Tiso N, Stephan DA, Nava A, et al: Identification of mutations in the cardiac ryanodine receptor gene in families affected with arrhythmogenic right ventricular cardiomyopathy type 2 (*ARVD2*). Hum Mol Genet 10:189-194, 2001.
109. Sakabe K, Ikeda T, Sakata T, et al: Comparison of T-wave alternans and QT interval dispersion to predict ventricular tachyarrhythmia in patients with dilated cardiomyopathy and without antiarrhythmic drugs: A prospective study. Jpn Heart J 42:451-457, 2001.
110. Sakabe K, Ikeda T, Sakata T, et al: Predicting the recurrence of ventricular tachyarrhythmias from T-wave alternans assessed on antiarrhythmic pharmacotherapy: A prospective study in patients with dilated cardiomyopathy. Ann Noninvasive Electrocardiol 6:203-208, 2001.
111. Kuroda N, Ohnishi Y, Yoshida A, et al: Clinical significance of T-wave alternans in hypertrophic cardiomyopathy. Circ J 66:457-462, 2002.
112. Primo J, Geelen P, Brugada J, et al: Hypertrophic cardiomyopathy: Role of the implantable cardioverter-defibrillator. J Am Coll Cardiol 31:1081-1085, 1998.
113. Leenhardt A, Lucet V, Denjoy I, et al: Catecholaminergic polymorphic ventricular tachycardia in children: A 7-year follow-up of 21 patients. Circulation 91:1512-1519, 1995.
114. Priori SG, Napolitano C, Memmi M, et al: Clinical and molecular characterization of patients with catecholaminergic polymorphic ventricular tachycardia. Circulation 106:69-74, 2002.

115. Gussak I, Antzelevitch C, Bjerregaard P, et al: The Brugada syndrome: Clinical, electrophysiologic, and genetic aspects. J Am Coll Cardiol 33:5-15, 1999.
116. Alings M, Wilde A: "Brugada" syndrome: Clinical data and suggested pathophysiological mechanism. Circulation 99:666-673, 1999.
117. Brugada P, Geelen P: Some electrocardiographic patterns predicting sudden cardiac death that every doctor should recognize. Acta Cardiol 52:473-484, 1997.
118. Brugada J, Brugada R, Brugada P: Right bundle-branch block and ST-segment elevation in leads V_1 through V_3: A marker for sudden death in patients without demonstrable structural heart disease. Circulation 97:457-460, 1998.
119. Chen Q, Kirsch GE, Zhang D, et al: Genetic basis and molecular mechanism for idiopathic ventricular fibrillation. Nature 392:293-296, 1998.
120. Potet F, Mabo P, Le Coq G, et al: Novel Brugada *SCN5A* mutation leading to ST segment elevation in the inferior or the right precordial leads. J Cardiovasc Electrophysiol 14:200-203, 2003.
121. Viswanathan PC, Benson DW, Balser JR: A common *SCN5A* polymorphism modulates the biophysical effects of an *SCN5A* mutation. J Clin Invest 111:341-346, 2003.
122. Veldkamp MW, Viswanathan PC, Bezzina C, et al: Two distinct congenital arrhythmias evoked by a multidysfunctional Na^+ channel. Circ Res 86:E91-E97, 2000.
123. Lerman BB, Dong B, Stein KM, et al: Right ventricular outflow tract tachycardia due to a somatic cell mutation in G protein subunit alpha 2. J Clin Invest 101:2862-2868, 1998.
124. Markowitz SM, Litvak BL, Ramirez de Arellano EA, et al: Adenosine-sensitive ventricular tachycardia: Right ventricular abnormalities delineated by magnetic resonance imaging. Circulation 96:1192-1200, 1997.
125. Callans DJ, Menz V, Schwartzman D, et al: Repetitive monomorphic tachycardia from the left ventricular outflow tract: Electrocardiographic patterns consistent with a left ventricular site of origin. J Am Coll Cardiol 29:1023-1027, 1997.
126. Schwartz PJ, Stramba-Badiale M, Segantini A, et al: Prolongation of the QT interval and the sudden infant death syndrome. N Engl J Med 338:1709-1714, 1998.
127. Priori SG, Napolitano C, Giordano U, et al: Brugada syndrome and sudden cardiac death in children. Lancet 355:808-809, 2000.
128. Schwartz PJ, Locati EH, Napolitano C: The long QT syndrome. *In* Zipes DP, Jalife J (eds): Cardiac Electrophysiology: From Cell to Bedside. 3rd ed. Philadelphia, WB Saunders, 2000, 788-811.
129. Viskin S, Belhassen B: Polymorphic ventricular tachyarrhythmias in the absence of organic heart disease: Classification, differential diagnosis, and implications for therapy. Prog Cardiovasc Dis 41:17-34, 1998.
130. Shimizu W, Antzelevitch C: Cellular basis for the ECG features of the LQT1 form of the long-QT syndrome: Effects of beta-adrenergic agonists and antagonists and sodium channel blockers on transmural dispersion of repolarization and torsades de pointes. Circulation 98:2314-2322, 1998.
131. Molnar J, Zhang F, Weiss J, et al: Diurnal pattern of QTc interval: how long is prolonged? Possible relation to circadian triggers of cardiovascular events. J Am Coll Cardiol 27:76-83, 1996.
133. Wang Q, Chen Q, Towbin JA: Genetics, molecular mechanisms and management of long QT syndrome. Ann Med 30:58-65, 1998.
134. Priori SG, Barhanin J, Hauer RN, et al: Genetic and molecular basis of cardiac arrhythmias: Impact on clinical management, parts I and II. Circulation 99:518-528, 1999.
135. Wang Q, Chen Q, Li H, Towbin JA: Molecular genetics of long QT syndrome from genes to patients. Curr Opin Cardiol 12:310-320, 1997.
136. Priori SG, Napolitano C, Schwartz PJ: Low penetrance in the long-QT syndrome: Clinical impact. Circulation 99:529-533, 1999.
136a. Roden DM: Drug-induced prolongations of the QT interval. N Engl J Med 350:1013–1022, 2004.
137. Zareba W, Moss AJ, Schwartz PJ, et al: Influence of genotype on the clinical course of the long-QT syndrome. International Long-QT Syndrome Registry Research Group. N Engl J Med 339:960-965, 1998.
138. Viskin S, Fish R, Roth A, Copperman Y: Prevention of torsades de pointes in the congenital long QT syndrome: Use of a pause prevention pacing algorithm. Heart 79:417-419, 1998.
139. Moss AJ: Clinical management of patients with the long QT syndrome: Drugs, devices, and gene-specific therapy. Pacing Clin Electrophysiol 20:2058-2060, 1997.
140. Epstein AE, Ideker RE: Ventricular fibrillation. *In* Zipes DP, Jalife J (eds): Cardiac Electrophysiology: From Cell to Bedside. 3rd ed. Philadelphia, WB Saunders, 2000, pp 927-933.
141. Zipes DP: Warning: The short days of winter may be hazardous to your health. Circulation 100:1590-1592, 1999.
143. Guidelines 2000 for Cardiopulmonary Resuscitation and Emergency Cardiovascular Care. Part 6: Advanced Cardiovascular Life Support: 7C: A Guide to the International ACLS algorithms. The American Heart Association in collaboration with the International Liaison Committee on Resuscitation. Circulation 102:I142-I157, 2000.

Heart Block

144. Rardon DP, Miles WM, Zipes DP: Atrioventricular block and AV dissociation. *In* Zipes DP, Jalife J (eds): Cardiac Electrophysiology: From Cell to Bedside. 3rd ed. Philadelphia, WB Saunders, 2000, pp 935-942.

Other Electyrophysiological Abnormalities Leading to Arrhythmias

145. Probst V, Kyndt F, Potet F, et al: Haploinsufficiency in combination with aging causes *SCN5A*-linked hereditary Lenegre disease. J Am Coll Cardiol 41:643-652, 2003.
146. Fisch C: Electrocardiographic manifestations of exit block, concealed conduction and "supernormal" conduction. *In* Zipes DP, Jalife J (eds): Cardiac Electrophysiology: From Cell to Bedside. 3rd ed. Philadelphia, WB Saunders, 2000, pp 955-976.

CHAPTER 33

Cardiac Arrest and Sudden Cardiac Death

Robert J. Myerburg • Agustin Castellanos

Definitions

Sudden cardiac death (SCD) is natural death from cardiac causes, heralded by abrupt loss of consciousness within 1 hour of the onset of acute symptoms. Preexisting heart disease may or may not have been known to be present, but the time and mode of death are unexpected. This definition incorporates the key elements of "natural," "rapid," and "unexpected." It consolidates previous definitions that have conflicted, largely because the most useful operational definition of SCD in the past differed for the clinician, the cardiovascular epidemiologist, the pathologist, and the scientist attempting to define pathophysiological mechanisms. As causes and mechanisms began to be understood, these differences faded.[1]

Four time elements must be considered in the construction of a definition of SCD to satisfy clinical, scientific, legal, and social considerations: (1) prodromes, (2) onset, (3) cardiac arrest, and (4) biological death (Fig. 33–1). Because the proximate cause of SCD is an abrupt disturbance of cardiovascular function, which is incompatible with maintaining consciousness because of abrupt loss of cerebral blood flow, any definition must recognize the brief time interval between the onset of the mechanism directly responsible for cardiac arrest and the consequent loss of consciousness (Fig. 33–1C). The 1-hour definition, however, refers to the duration of the "terminal event" (Fig. 33–1B), which defines the interval between the onset of symptoms signaling the pathophysiological disturbance leading to cardiac arrest and the onset of the cardiac arrest itself (Fig. 33–1B and C).

Premonitory signs and symptoms are often absent,[2] but nonspecific symptoms can occur during the days or weeks before a cardiac arrest. Prodromes (Fig. 33–1A) are poor predictors of an impending event because of low sensitivity but may be more specific for an imminent cardiac arrest when they begin abruptly. Sudden onset of chest pain, dyspnea, or palpitations and other symptoms of arrhythmias often precede the onset of cardiac arrest. The fourth element, *biological death* (Fig. 33–1D), was an immediate consequence of the clinical cardiac arrest in the past, usually occurring within minutes. However, since the development of community-based interventions and life support systems, patients may now remain biologically alive for a long period of time after the onset of a pathophysiological process that has caused irreversible damage and will ultimately lead to death. In this circumstance, the causative pathophysiological and clinical event is the cardiac arrest itself rather than the factors responsible for the delayed biological death. However, because of legal, forensic, and certain social considerations, biological death must continue to be used as the absolute definition of death. Finally, the forensic pathologist studying *unwitnessed deaths* may use the definition of sudden death for a person known to be alive and functioning normally 24 hours before, and this remains appropriate within obvious limits. The generally accepted clinical-pathophysiological definition of up to 1 hour between onset of the terminal event and biological death requires qualifications for specific circumstances.

The development of community-based intervention systems has also led to inconsistencies in the use of terms considered absolute. *Death* is defined biologically, legally, and literally as an absolute and irreversible event. Thus, SCD can be aborted, or a patient can survive cardiac arrest or cardiovascular collapse; however, survival after (sudden) death is a contradiction in terms. Table 33–1 provides definitions for events and terms related to the concept of SCD—death, cardiac arrest, and cardiovascular collapse.

Epidemiology

Epidemiological Overview

The worldwide incidence of SCD is difficult to estimate because it varies largely as a function of coronary heart disease prevalence in different countries (see Chap. 1).[3] Estimates for the United States, largely based upon retrospective death certificate

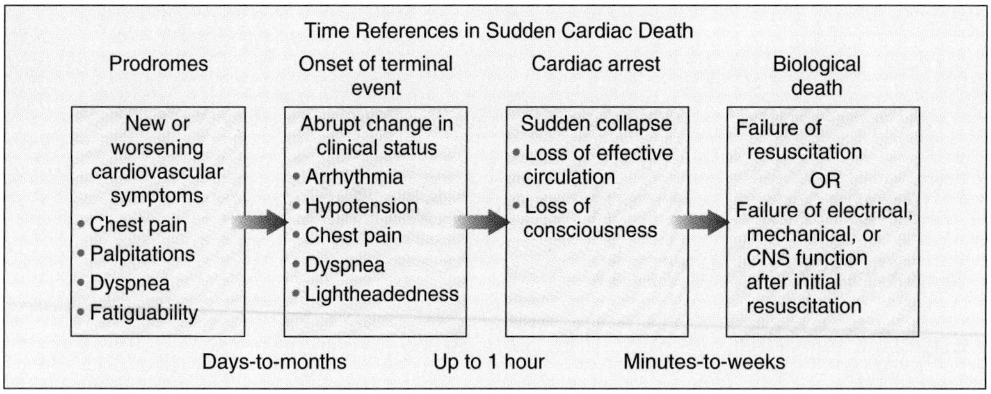

FIGURE 33–1 Sudden cardiac death viewed from four temporal perspectives: (1) prodromes, (2) onset of the terminal event, (3) cardiac arrest, and (4) progression to biological death. Individual variability of the components influences clinical expression. Some victims experience no prodromes, with onset leading almost instantaneously to cardiac arrest; others may have an onset that lasts up to 1 hour before clinical arrest. Some patients may live days to weeks after the cardiac arrest before biological death, often because of irreversible brain damage and dependence upon life support. These factors influence interpretation of the 1-hour definition. The two most relevant clinical factors are onset of the terminal event (2) and the clinical cardiac arrest itself (3); legal and social considerations focus on the time of biological death (4). CNS = central nervous system.

analyses[4-7] and an emergency rescue data base in one study,[8] range from less than 200,000 to more than 450,000 SCDs annually, with the most widely used estimates in the range of 300,000 to 350,000 SCDs annually.[9] The variation is based in part on the definition of sudden death and inclusion criteria used in individual studies, and the correct number can be found only from a carefully designed prospective epidemiological study.

The temporal definition of sudden death strongly influences epidemiological data. Retrospective death certificate studies have demonstrated that a temporal definition of death less than 2 hours after the onset of symptoms results in 12 to 15 percent of all natural deaths being defined as "sudden" and nearly 90 percent of all natural sudden deaths being due to cardiac causes. In contrast, the application of a 24-hour definition of sudden death increases the fraction of all natural deaths falling into the sudden category to more than 30 percent but reduces the proportion of all sudden natural deaths that are due to cardiac causes to 75 percent.

Prospective studies demonstrate that about 50 percent of all coronary heart disease deaths are sudden and unexpected, occurring shortly (instantaneous to 1 hour) after the onset of symptoms. Because coronary heart disease is the dominant cause of both sudden and nonsudden cardiac deaths in the United States, the fraction of total cardiac deaths that are sudden is similar to the fraction of deaths from coronary heart disease that are sudden, although there does appear to be a geographical variation in the fraction of coronary deaths that are sudden.[10] It is also of interest that the age-adjusted decline in coronary heart disease mortality in the United States during the past half-century[11] has not changed the fraction of coronary deaths that are sudden and unexpected,[12] even though there may be a decline in out-of-hospital deaths compared with emergency department deaths.[4] Furthermore, the decreasing age-adjusted mortality does not imply a decrease in absolute numbers of cardiac or sudden deaths because of the growth and aging of the U.S. population and the increasing prevalence of chronic heart disease.[13,14]

TABLE 33–1 Definition of Terms Related to Sudden Cardiac Death

Term	Definition	Qualifiers or Exceptions
Death	Irreversible cessation of all biological functions	None
Cardiac arrest	Abrupt cessation of cardiac pump function, which may be reversible but will lead to death in the absence of prompt intervention	Rare spontaneous reversions, likelihood of successful intervention relates to mechanism of arrest, clinical setting, and time to intervention
Cardiovascular collapse	A (sudden) loss of effective blood flow due to cardiac and/or peripheral vascular factors that may revert spontaneously (e.g., vasodepressor or cardioinhibitory syncope) or only with interventions (e.g., cardiac arrest)	Nonspecific term that includes cardiac arrest and its consequences and also events that characteristically revert spontaneously

FIGURE 33–2 Impact of population subgroups and time from events on the clinical epidemiology of sudden cardiac death (SCD). **A,** Estimates of incidence (percent per year) and the total number of events per year for the general adult population in the United States and for increasingly high risk subgroups. The overall adult population has an estimated sudden death incidence of 0.1 to 0.2 percent per year, accounting for a total of more than 300,000 events per year. With the identification of increasingly powerful risk factors, the incidence *increases* progressively, but it is accomplished by a progressive *decrease* in the total number of events represented by each group. The inverse relationship between incidence and total number of events occurs because of the progressively smaller denominator pool in the highest subgroup categories. Successful interventions among larger population subgroups require identification of specific markers to increase the ability to identify specific patients who are at particularly high risk for a future event. (Note: The horizontal axis for the incidence figures is not linear and should be interpreted accordingly. **B,** The distribution of clinical status of victims at the time of SCD. Nearly two-thirds of cardiac arrests occur as the first clinically manifest event or in the clinical setting of known disease in the absence of strong risk predictors. Less than 25 percent of the victims have high-risk markers based on arrhythmic or hemodynamic parameters. **C,** Idealized curves of SCD risk for a population of patients with known cardiovascular disease but at low risk because of freedom from major cardiovascular events (top curve) and for populations of patients who have survived a major cardiovascular event (bottom curve). Attrition over time is accelerated in both absolute and relative terms for the initial 6 to 18 months after the major cardiovascular event. After the initial attrition, the slopes of the curves for the high-risk and low-risk populations parallel each other, highlighting both the early attrition and the attenuation of risk after 18 to 24 months. These relations have been observed in diverse high-risk subgroups (cardiac arrest survivors, post-myocardial infarction patients with high-risk markers, recent onset of heart failure). AP = angina pectoris; EF = ejection fraction; M.I. = myocardial infarction. (**A,** From Myerburg et al, reference 14; reproduced with permission of the American Heart Association; **B,** modified from Myerburg RJ: Sudden cardiac death: Exploring the limits of our knowledge. J Cardiovasc Electrophysiol 12:369, 2001; **C,** modified from Myerburg RJ, Kessler KM, Castellanos A: Sudden cardiac death: Structure, function, and time-dependence of risk. Circulation 85[Suppl I]:I-2, 1992. Copyright 1992 American Heart Association.)

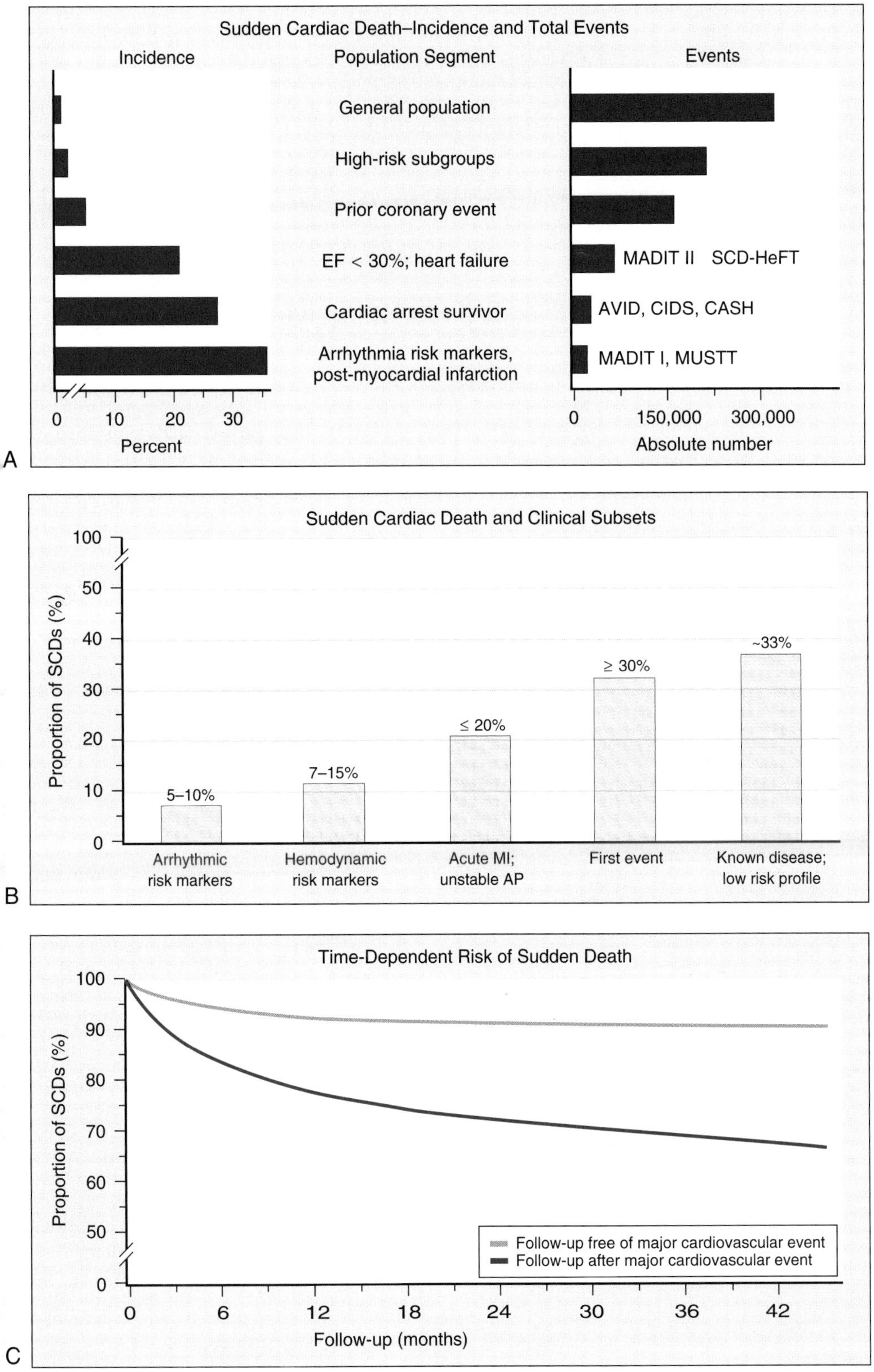

Population Pools and Time Dependence of Risk

Three factors are of primary importance for identifying populations at risk and consideration of strategies for prevention of SCD: (1) the absolute numbers and event rates (incidence) among population subgroups (Fig. 33–2A), (2) the clinical subgroups in which SCDs occur (Fig. 33–2B), and (3) the time dependence of risk (Fig. 33–2C).

POPULATION SUBGROUPS AND SUDDEN CARDIAC DEATH. When the more than 300,000 adult SCDs that occur annually in the United States are viewed as a global incidence in an unselected adult population, the overall incidence is 1 to 2 per 1000 population (0.1 to 0.2 percent) per year (see Fig. 33–2A). This large population base includes victims whose SCDs occur as a first cardiac event as well as those whose SCDs can be predicted with greater accuracy because they are included in higher risk subgroups (see Fig. 33–2B). Any intervention designed for the general population must, therefore, be applied to the 999 per 1000 who do not have an event in order to reach and possibly influence the 1 per 1000 who does. The cost and risk-to-benefit uncertainties limit the nature of such broad-based interventions and demand a higher resolution of risk identification. Figure 33–2A highlights this problem by expressing the incidence (percent per year) of SCD among various subgroups and comparing the incidence figures with the total number of events that occur annually in each subgroup. On moving from the total adult population to a subgroup at higher risk because of the presence of selected coronary risk factors, there may be a 10-fold or greater increase in the incidence of events annually, with the magnitude of increase dependent on the number of risk factors operating in the subgroup. The size of the denominator pool, however, remains very large, and implementation of interventions remains problematic, even at this heightened level of risk. Higher resolution is desirable and can be achieved by identification of more specific subgroups. However, the corresponding absolute number of deaths becomes progressively smaller as the subgroups become more focused (see Fig. 33–2A), limiting the potential benefit of interventions to a much smaller fraction of the total number of patients at risk. Various estimates suggest that at least one-third of all SCDs related to coronary heart disease occur as a first clinical event.

In addition, another one-third occur among subgroups of patients with known coronary heart disease profiled at relatively low risk for SCD (see Fig. 33–2B).[11]

BIOLOGICAL AND CLINICAL TIME-DEPENDENT RISK. Temporal elements in risk of SCD have been analyzed in the context of both biological and clinical chronology. In the former, epidemiological analyses of SCD risk among populations have identified three patterns: diurnal, weekly, and seasonal. General patterns of heightened risk during the morning hours, on Mondays, and during the winter months have been described.[15] In the clinical paradigm, risk of SCD is not linear as a function of time after changes in cardiovascular status.[9,14,16] Survival curves after major cardiovascular events, which identify risk for both sudden and total cardiac death, usually demonstrate that the most rapid rate of attrition occurs during the first 6 to 18 months after the index event (see Fig. 33–2C). Thus, there is a time dependence of risk that focuses the opportunity for maximum efficacy of an intervention during the early period after a conditioning event. Curves that have these characteristics have been generated from among survivors of out-of-hospital cardiac arrest, new onset of heart failure, and unstable angina and from high-risk subgroups of patients having recent myocardial infarction. Even though attrition rates decrease over time, an effective intervention can still cause late diversion of treated versus control risk curves, indicating continuing benefit. *The addition of time as a dimension for measuring risk may increase the resolution within subgroups.*

Age, Heredity, Gender, and Race

AGE. There are two ages of peak incidence of sudden death: between birth and 6 months of age (the sudden infant death syndrome) (see Chap 56) and between 45 and 75 years of age. Among the adult population, the *incidence* of sudden death caused by coronary heart disease increases as a function of advancing age,[17] in parallel with the age-related increase in incidence of total coronary heart disease deaths. The incidence is 100-fold less in adolescents and adults younger than 30 years (1 in 100,000 per year)[18-20] than it is in adults older than 35 years (1 in 1000 per year) (Fig. 33–3A).[11] In contrast to incidence, however, the *proportion* of deaths caused by coronary heart diseases that are sudden and unexpected decreases with advancing age. In the 20- to 39-year age group, approximately 75 percent of coronary heart disease deaths in men are sudden and unexpected, with the proportion falling to approximately 60 percent in the 45- to 54-year age group and hovering close to 50 percent thereafter. Age also influences the proportion of all cardiovascular causes among all causes of natural sudden death in that the proportion of coronary deaths and of all cardiac causes of death that are sudden is highest in the younger age groups, whereas the fraction of total sudden natural deaths that are due to any cardiovascular cause is higher in the older age groups. At the other end of the age range, only 19 percent of sudden natural deaths among children between 1 and 13 years of age are due to cardiac causes; the proportion increases to 30 percent in the 14- to 21-year-old age group.[21]

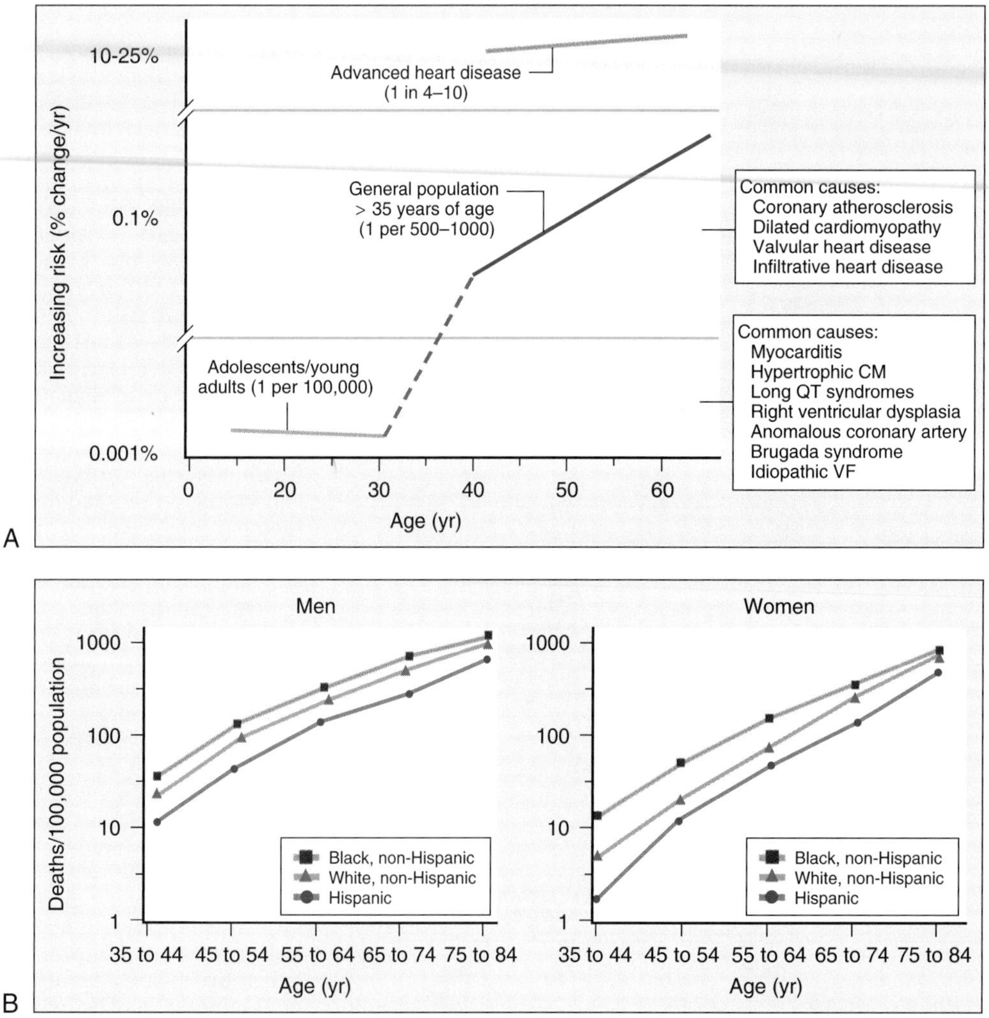

FIGURE 33–3 Age-, gender-, and race-specific risks of sudden cardiac death (SCD). **A,** Age-related and disease-specific risk for SCD. For the general population 35 years of age and older, SCD risk is 0.1 to 0.2 percent per year (1 per 500 to 1000 population). Among the general population of adolescents and adults younger than 30 years, the overall risk of SCD is 1 per 100,000 population or 0.001 percent per year. The risk of SCD increases dramatically beyond the age of 35 years and continues to increase past the age of 70 years. The greatest rate of increase is between 40 and 65 years (vertical axis is discontinuous). Among patients older than 30 years, with advanced structural heart disease and markers of high risk for cardiac arrest, the event rate may exceed 25 percent per year, and age-related risk attenuates. Among adolescents and young adults at risk for SCD because of specific identified causes, it is difficult to ascertain risk for individual patients because of variable expression of the disease state. The major risk is electrical, and the competing risk of mechanical heart dysfunction, as in advanced ischemic heart disease or dilated cardiomyopathy, does not contribute significantly to risk in many of these disorders. Therefore, effective electrical interventions are expected to have a better total mortality benefit (see text for details). **B,** SCD risk as a function of age, gender, and race or culture (white, black, and Hispanic). CM = cardiomyopathy; VF = ventricular fibrillation. (**B,** Modified from Gillum RF: Sudden cardiac death in Hispanic Americans and African Americans. Am J Public Health 87:1461, 1997.)

HEREDITY. Among the less common causes of SCD, hereditary patterns have been reported for specific syndromes[22] such as the congenital long QT interval syndromes,[23] hypertrophic cardiomyopathy,[24] right ventricular dysplasia,[25] the Brugada syndrome,[26] "idiopathic" ventricular tachycardia or fibrillation,[27,28] and yet-to-be-defined patterns of familial SCD in children and young adults (see Chap. 32). Mutations and functioning polymorphisms are being mapped to genes located on many chromosomes as the molecular bases for the entities are being defined. Although patients with stable congenital conducting system abnormalities have a good prognosis, progressive familial conducting system disease, which appears to have a hereditary pattern, carries an increased risk of SCD.[29] Familial sudden death associated with cardiac ganglionitis has been reported, but an inheritance pattern has not been demonstrated in the reports to date.

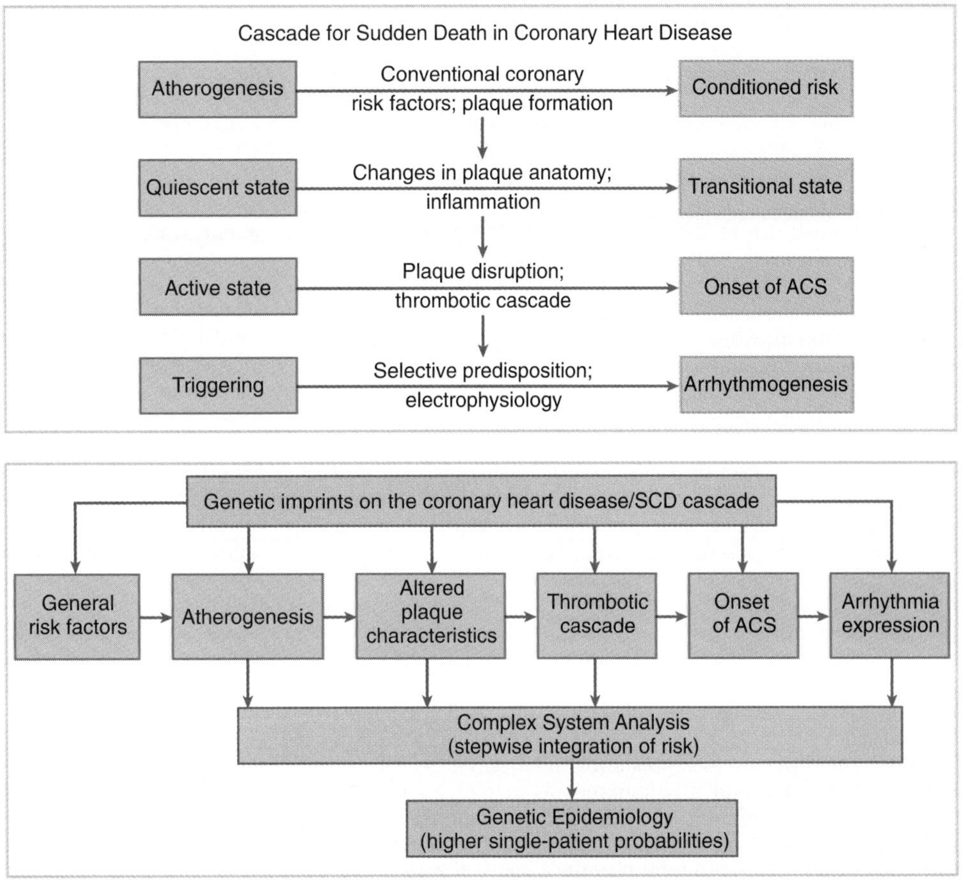

FIGURE 33–4 The coronary atherosclerosis heart disease cascade and genetic imprints on the progression to sudden cardiac death (SCD). **A,** The cascade from conventional risk factors for coronary atherosclerosis to arrhythmogenesis in SCD related to coronary heart disease. The cascade identifies four levels of risk, beginning with lesion initiation and development, progressing to the transition to an active state, then to acute coronary syndromes (ACS), and finally to the specific expression of life-threatening arrhythmias. Multiple factors enter at each level, including specific risk based upon genetic profiles of individual patients. **B,** Positions along multiple sites in the cascade from general risk factors for atherosclerosis to arrhythmic expression leading to SCD. Individual risk based on genetic profiles has been identified for atherogenesis, plaque evolution, the thrombotic cascade, and arrhythmia expression. Stepwise integration of these characteristics for individuals through complex analytical methods offers the hope of a field of genetic epidemiology that may lead to higher single-patient probabilities for SCD risk prediction. By integrating the risk associated with each step in the cascade, profiles become more highly specific for individual risk (see text for details). (Modified from Myerburg RJ: Scientific gaps in the prediction and prevention of sudden cardiac death. J Cardiovasc Electrophysiol 13:709, 2002.)

The multiple specific mutations at gene loci encoding ion channel proteins associated with the various inherited arrhythmia syndromes (see Chap. 28) provide a major advance in the understanding of a genetic and pathophysiological basis for these causes of sudden death. In addition, these observations may provide screening tools for individuals at risk as well as the potential for devising specific therapeutic strategies. These gene loci also serve as candidates for investigation of the role of low-penetrance mutations or polymorphisms in SCD related to more common causes, such as coronary heart disease. An example is a genetic variant in the cardiac sodium channel gene (*SCN5A*) observed among the African-American population (carrier rate = 13.2 percent) that appears to predispose to arrhythmias, even though it is not expressed as a prototypic long QT syndrome under control conditions.[30] Its role in predicting risk of SCD awaits clarification.

To the extent that SCD is an expression of underlying coronary heart disease, hereditary factors that contribute to coronary heart disease risk have been thought to operate nonspecifically for the SCD syndrome. However, studies have identified mutations and relevant polymorphisms along multiple steps of the cascade from atherogenesis to plaque destabilization, thrombosis, and arrhythmogenesis, each of which is associated with increased risk of a coronary event (Fig. 33–4).[31-34] Integration of these individual markers may provide more powerful individual risk prediction in the future. In addition, two population studies suggest that SCD, as an expression of coronary heart disease, clusters in specific families.[35,36] Whether this familial pattern is genetically or environmentally determined, or both, awaits further clarification.

GENDER. The SCD syndrome has a large preponderance in males compared with females during the young adult and early middle-age years because of the protection females enjoy from coronary atherosclerosis before menopause (see Fig. 33–3B).[37-39] Various population studies have demonstrated four- to sevenfold excesses of SCD among males compared with females prior to the 65-year-old and beyond age groups, in which the differences decrease to 2:1 or less. As coronary event risk increases in postmenopausal women, SCD risk increases proportionately.[37-39] Even though the overall risk is much lower in younger women, the classic coronary risk factors are still predictive of events among women,[37,40] including cigarette smoking, diabetes, use of oral contraceptives, and hyperlipidemia.

RACE. A number of studies comparing racial differences in relative risk of SCD in whites and blacks with coronary heart disease in the United States had yielded conflicting and inconclusive data. However, later studies have demonstrated excess risk of cardiac arrest and SCD among blacks compared with whites (see Fig. 33–3D).[39,41] SCD rates among Hispanic populations were smaller.[39] The differences were observed across all age groups.

Risk Factors for Sudden Cardiac Death

General Profile of Sudden Cardiac Death Risk

Risk profiling for coronary artery disease, by means of the conventional risk factors for coronary *atherogenesis*, is useful for identifying levels of population risk and individual risk[42] but cannot be used to distinguish individual patients at risk for SCD from those at risk for other manifestations of coronary heart disease. Multivariate analyses of selected risk factors (i.e., age, systolic blood pressure, heart rate, electrocardiographic abnormalities, vital capacity, relative weight, cigarette consumption, and serum cholesterol) have determined that approximately one-half of all SCDs occur among the 10 percent of the population in the highest risk decile, based upon multiple risk factors (Fig. 33–5). Thus, the cumulative risk derived from multiple risk factors exceeds the simple arithmetic sum of the individual risks.[42] The comparison of risk factors in the victims of SCD with those in people who developed any manifestations of coronary artery disease does not provide useful patterns, by either univariate or multivariate analysis, to distinguish victims of SCD from the overall pool. In addition, angiographic and hemodynamic patterns discriminate SCD risk from non-SCD risk only under limited conditions.[43] In contrast, familial clustering of SCD as a specific manifestation of the disease may lead to identification of specific genetic abnormalities that predispose to SCD.[35,36]

Hypertension is a clearly established risk factor for coronary heart disease and also emerges as a highly significant risk factor for incidence of SCD.[44,45] However, there is no influence of increasing systolic blood pressure levels on the ratio of sudden deaths to total coronary heart disease deaths. No relationship has been observed between cholesterol concentration and the proportion of coronary deaths that were sudden. Neither the electrocardiographic pattern of left ventricular hypertrophy nor nonspecific ST-T wave abnormalities influence the proportion of total coronary deaths that are sudden and unexpected; *only intraventricular conduction abnormalities are suggestive of a disproportionate number of SCDs.*[31] The latter is an old observation that is reinforced by data from device trials that suggests the importance of QRS duration as a risk marker.[46] A low vital capacity also suggests a disproportionate risk for sudden versus total coronary deaths. This is of interest because such a relationship was particularly striking in the Framingham Study in the analysis of data on women who had died suddenly.[37,38]

The conventional risk factors used in early studies of SCD are the risk factors for evolution of coronary artery disease. The rationale is based on two facts: (1) coronary disease is the structural basis for 80 percent of SCDs in the United States, and (2) the coronary risk factors are easy to identify because they tend to be present continuously over time (see Fig. 33–4A). However, risk factors specific for fatal arrhythmias are dynamic pathophysiological events and occur transiently.[47,48] Transient pathophysiological events are being modeled epidemiologically[49] in an attempt to express and use them as clinical risk factors for both profiling and intervention.[50]

FUNCTIONAL CAPACITY AND SUDDEN DEATH. The Framingham Study demonstrated a striking relationship between functional classification and death during a 2-year follow-up period. However, the proportion of deaths that were sudden did not vary with functional classification, ranging from 50 to 57 percent in all groups and from those free of clinical heart disease to those in functional class IV.[51] Other studies also suggest that patients with heart failure with better functional capacity are at lower risk of dying, as expected, but a higher proportion of those deaths are sudden.[12]

Life Style and Psychosocial Factors

LIFE STYLE. There is a strong association between *cigarette smoking* and all manifestations of coronary heart disease. The Framingham Study demonstrated that cigarette smokers have a twofold to threefold increase in sudden death risk in each decade of life at entry between 30 and 59 years and that this is one of the few risk factors in which the proportion of coronary heart disease deaths that are sudden increases in association with the risk factor.[51] In addition, in a study of 310 survivors of out-of-hospital cardiac arrest, the recurrent cardiac arrest rate was 27 percent at 3 years of follow-up among those who continued to smoke after their index event compared with 19 percent in those who stopped ($p < 0.04$).[52] Obesity is a second factor that appears to influence the proportion of coronary deaths that occur suddenly.[38,51] With increasing relative weight, the percentage of coronary heart disease deaths that were sudden in the Framingham Study increased linearly from a low of 39 percent to a high of 70 percent. Total coronary heart disease deaths increased with increasing relative weight as well.

Associations between levels of physical activity and SCD have been studied with variable results. Epidemiological observations have suggested a relationship between *low levels of physical activity* and increased coronary heart disease death risk. The Framingham Study, however, showed an *insignif-*

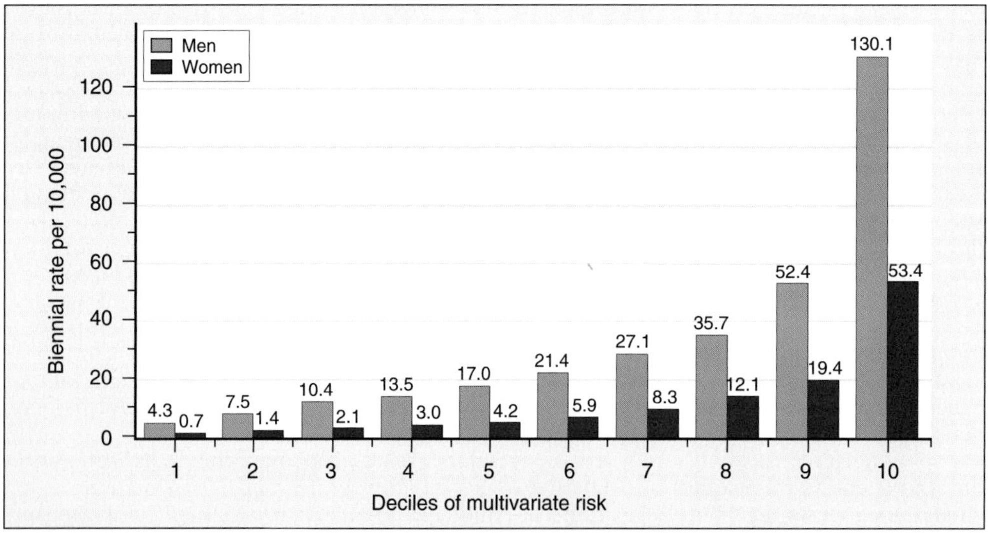

FIGURE 33–5 Risk of sudden death by decile of multivariant risk: 26-year follow-up, the Framingham Study. The variables included are age, systolic blood pressure, left ventricular hypertrophy, intraventricular block on the electrocardiogram, nonspecific electrocardiographic abnormalities, serum cholesterol, heart rate, vital capacity, cigarettes consumed per day, and relative weight. (Modified from Kannel WB, Shatzkin A: Sudden death: Lessons from subsets in population studies. Reprinted by permission of the American College of Cardiology. J Am Coll Cardiol 5[Suppl 6]:141B, 1985.)

cant relationship between low levels of physical activity and incidence of sudden death but a high proportion of sudden to total cardiac deaths at higher levels of physical activity.[51] An association between acute physical exertion and the onset of myocardial infarction has been suggested, particularly among individuals who are habitually physically inactive.[50] A subsequent case-crossover cohort study confirmed this observation for SCD, demonstrating a 17-fold relative increase in SCD associated with vigorous exercise compared with lower level activity or inactive states.[53] However, the absolute risk for events was very low (1 event per 1.5 million exercise sessions). Habitual vigorous exercise markedly attenuated risk. In contrast, SCD among young athletes has a higher incidence than among young nonathletic individuals in the same age range (see Chap. 75).[54] Information about physical activity relationships in various clinical settings, such as overt and silent disease states, is still lacking.

PSYCHOSOCIAL FACTORS. The magnitude of recent life changes in the realms of health, work, home and family, and personal and social factors has been related to myocardial infarction and SCD.[55-59] There is an association with significant elevations of life-change scores during the 6 months before a coronary event, and the association is particularly striking in victims of SCD. Among women, those who die suddenly are less often married, had fewer children, and had greater educational discrepancies with their spouses than did age-related control subjects living in the same neighborhood as the victims of sudden death. A history of psychiatric treatment, cigarette smoking, and greater quantities of alcohol consumption than the control subjects also characterized the sudden death group. Controlling for other major prognostic factors, risk of sudden and total deaths, and other coronary events is affected by social and economic stresses.[60] Alteration of modifiable life-style factors has been proposed as a strategy for reducing risk of SCD in patients with coronary heart disease,[61] although a study of treatment of depression following myocardial infarction failed to demonstrate an effect on event rates.[62] Acute psychosocial stressors have been associated with risk of cardiovascular events, including SCD.[63,64] The risk appears to cluster around the time of the stress and appears to occur among victims at preexisting risk, with the stressor simply advancing the time of an impending event.[63] In contrast, the possibility of physical stress–induced coronary plaque disruption has been suggested.[65]

Sudden Death and Previous Coronary Heart Disease

Although SCD is the first clinical manifestation of coronary heart disease in 20 to 25 percent or more of all coronary heart disease patients[1,9,11] and is the first clinical manifestation in more than 30 percent of coronary heart disease–related SCDs (see Fig. 33–2),[11,66] a previous myocardial infarction can be identified in as many as 75 percent of patients who die suddenly. The high incidence of both recognized and unrecognized prior myocardial infarction in victims of SCD has led to a search for predictors of SCD in survivors of myocardial infarction as well as in patients with other clinical manifestations of coronary heart disease and those with clinically silent disease.

LEFT VENTRICULAR EJECTION FRACTION IN CHRONIC ISCHEMIC HEART DISEASE. A marked reduction of the left ventricular ejection fraction is the most powerful predictor of SCD in patients with chronic ischemic heart disease as well as those at risk for SCD from other causes (see later). Increased risk, independent of other risk factors, is measurable at ejection fractions greater than 40 percent, but the greatest rate of change of risk is between 30 and 40 percent.[67] An ejection fraction equal to or less than 30 percent is the single most powerful independent predictor for SCD, but it has low specificity.

VENTRICULAR ARRHYTHMIAS IN CHRONIC ISCHEMIC HEART DISEASE. Most forms of ambient ventricular ectopic activity (premature ventricular complexes [PVCs] and short runs of nonsustained ventricular tachycardia [VT]) have a benign prognosis in the absence of structural heart disease.[68] An exception is polymorphic forms of nonsustained VT that occur in patients without structural heart disease but can have molecular, functional or drug- or electrolyte-related bases for high-risk arrhythmias.[69] When present in subjects in the coronary-prone age groups, however, PVCs select a subgroup with a higher probability of coronary artery disease and of SCD. Exercise-induced PVCs and short runs of nonsustained VT indicate some level of SCD risk,[70] even in the absence of recognizable structural heart disease. However, the data available to support this hypothesis are conflicting, with the possible exception of polymorphic runs of nonsustained VT.[69] Additional data suggest that PVCs and nonsustained VT during both the exercise and recovery phases of a stress test are predictive of increased risk.[71] Arrhythmias in the recovery phase, previously thought to be benign, appear to predict higher risk than arrhythmias in the exercise phase, and there is a gradient of risk with increasing severity of arrhythmias.

The occurrence of PVCs in survivors of myocardial infarction, particularly if frequent and of complex forms such as repetitive PVCs,[67] predicts an increased risk of SCD and total mortality during long-term follow-up. There are conflicting data on the role of measures of *frequency* and *forms* of ventricular ectopic activity as discriminators of risk, but most studies cite a frequency cutoff of 10 PVCs per hour as a threshold level for increased risk. Several investigators have emphasized that the most powerful predictors among the various forms of PVCs are runs of nonsustained VT, although this relationship is now questioned. Many of the reported studies have been based on a single ambulatory monitor sample recorded 1 week to several months after the onset of acute myocardial infarction, and the duration of the samples has ranged from 1 to 48 hours. Other studies have suggested that ambulatory ventricular arrhythmias in patients with heart failure do not specifically predict an increased risk of death.[72]

The results of the Cardiac Arrhythmia Suppression Trial (CAST) (see Chap. 30), designed to test the hypothesis that PVC suppression by antiarrhythmic drugs alters the risk of SCD after myocardial infarction, were surprising for two reasons.[73] First, the death rate in the randomized placebo group was lower than expected, and second, the death rate among patients in the encainide and flecainide arms exceeded control rates by more than three times. Subgroup analysis demonstrated increased risk in the placebo group for patients with nonsustained VT and with an ejection fraction of 30 percent or less, but excess risk in the treated group was still observed. The excess death rates may be accounted for by the occurrence of ischemic events in the presence of drug. No adverse effect (other than short-term proarrhythmic risk at initiation of therapy) was observed with the other drug in the study (moricizine), but no long-term benefit emerged either.[73] The Survival with Oral *d*-Sotalol (SWORD) study, a comparison of *d*-sotalol with placebo in a post-myocardial infarction population with a low death rate, also demonstrated excess risk in the drug-treated group.[74] Whether the conclusions from CAST, CAST II, and SWORD extend beyond the drugs studied, or to other diseases, remains to be learned.

Left ventricular dysfunction is the major modulator of risk implied by chronic PVCs after myocardial infarction.[67] The risk of death predicted by post-myocardial infarction PVCs is enhanced by the presence of left ventricular dysfunction

(Fig. 33–6); the latter appears to exert its influence most strongly in the first 6 months after infarction. Finally, there are data suggesting that the risk associated with postinfarction ventricular arrhythmias is higher in patients who have non-Q-wave infarctions than in those with transmural infarctions.[75]

Causes of Sudden Cardiac Death

Coronary heart disease and its consequences account for at least 80 percent of SCDs in Western cultures, and the cardiomyopathies cause another 10 to 15 percent (Table 33–2). Coronary heart disease is also the most common cause in many areas of the world in which its prevalence is lower. Despite the established relation between coronary heart disease and SCD, a complete understanding of SCD requires recognition of other causes that, although less common and often quite rare (see Table 33–2), may be recognizable before death, have therapeutic implications, and provide broad insight into the sudden death problem.[76,77] Many of these entities emerge as common causes of SCD in adolescents and young adults, among whom the prevalence of coronary atherosclerosis is much lower (see Fig. 33–3A).

Coronary Artery Abnormalities

Although structural abnormalities of coronary arteries other than coronary atherosclerosis are infrequent causes of SCD, the relative risk of SCD may be quite high for specific abnormalities. Nonatherosclerotic coronary artery abnormalities include congenital lesions, coronary artery embolism, coronary arteritis, and mechanical abnormalities of the coronary arteries. Among the congenital lesions, *anomalous origin of a left coronary artery from the pulmonary artery* (see Chaps. 56 and 75) is relatively common and associated with a high death rate in infancy and early childhood without surgical treatment. The early risk for SCD is not excessively high but patients who survive to adulthood without surgical intervention are at risk for SCD. Other forms of coronary arterial-venous fistulas are much less frequent and associated with a low incidence of SCD.

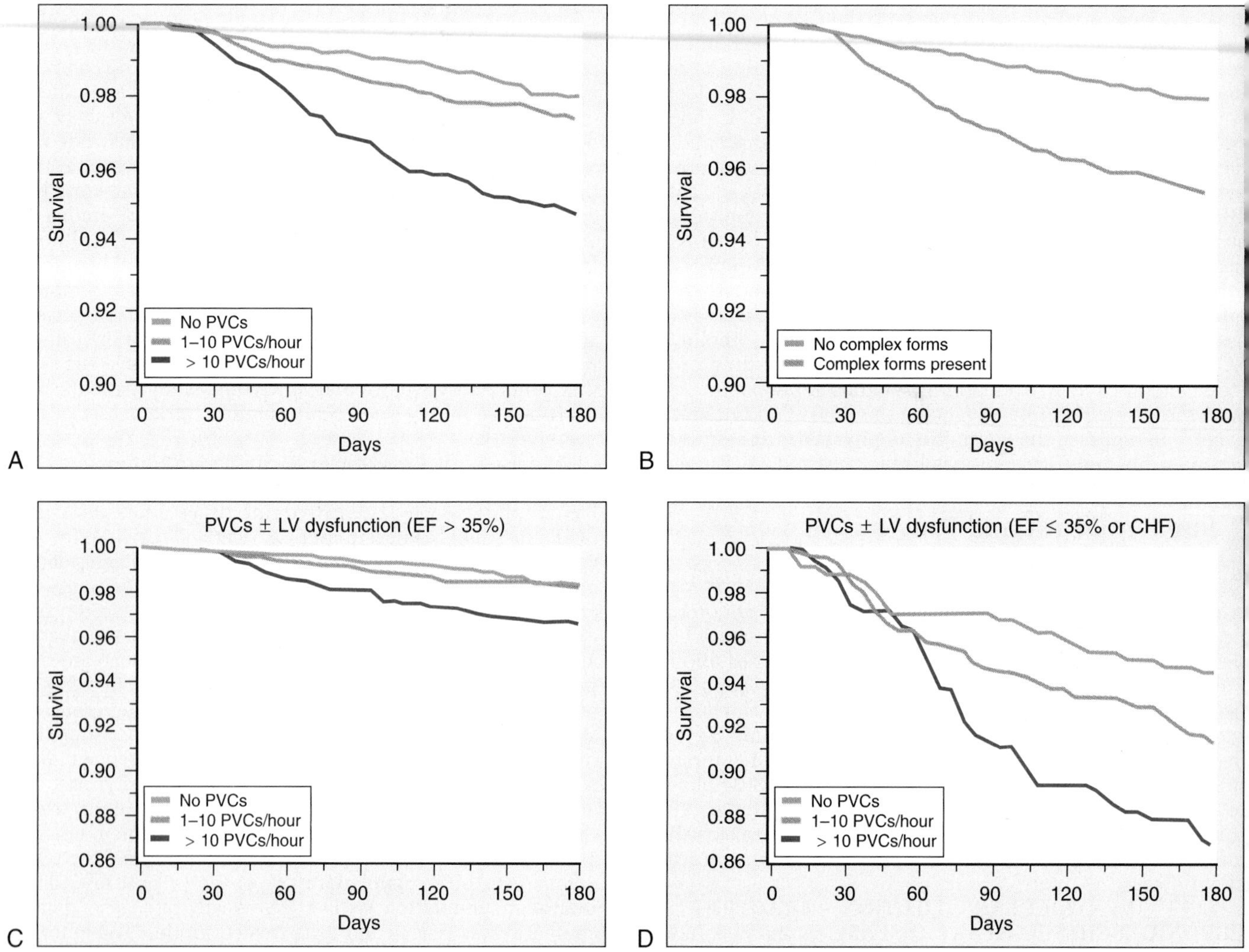

FIGURE 33–6 Prognostic significance of ventricular arrhythmias after myocardial infarction. The Gruppo Italiano per lo Studio della Sopravvivenza nell'Infarto Miocardico (GISSI)-2 data demonstrate that, in the thrombolytic era, frequent premature ventricular complexes (PVCs) carry prognostic information for mortality in the 6 months after an acute myocardial infarction, as previously reported in earlier studies. PVCs occurring at a frequency of greater than 10 per hour **(A)** and the presence of complex forms **(B)** both have an adverse effect on survival, although the latter did not hold up as an independent predictor on multivariate analysis. **C,** When PVCs occurred in the absence of left ventricular (LV) dysfunction (defined as ejection fraction [EF] less than 35 percent or the occurrence of congestive heart failure [CHF] during the event), the predictive power of frequent PVCs was reduced, and in the presence of LV dysfunction **(D)** it was enhanced. (From Maggioni AP, Zuanetti G, Franzosi MG, et al: Prevalence and prognostic significance of ventricular arrhythmias after acute myocardial infarction in the fibrinolytic era: GISSI-2 results. Circulation 87:312, 1993.)

TABLE 33–2 Causes and Contributing Factors in Sudden Cardiac Death

I. Coronary artery abnormalities
- A. Coronary atherosclerosis
  - 1. Chronic ischemic heart disease with transient supply-demand imbalance—thrombosis, spasm, physical stress
  - 2. Acute myocardial infarction
  - 3. Chronic atherosclerosis with change in myocardial substrate
- B. Congenital abnormalities of coronary arteries
  - 1. Anomalous origin from pulmonary artery
  - 2. Other coronary arteriovenous fistula
  - 3. Origin of a left coronary branch from right or noncoronary sinus of Valsalva
  - 4. Origin of right coronary artery from left sinus of Valsalva
  - 5. Hypoplastic or aplastic coronary arteries
  - 6. Coronary-intracardiac shunt
- C. Coronary artery embolism
  - 1. Aortic or mitral endocarditis
  - 2. Prosthetic aortic or mitral valves
  - 3. Abnormal native valves or left ventricular mural thrombus
  - 4. Platelet embolism
- D. Coronary arteritis
  - 1. Polyarteritis nodosa, progressive systemic sclerosis, giant cell arteritis
  - 2. Mucocutaneous lymph node syndrome (Kawasaki disease)
  - 3. Syphilitic coronary ostial stenosis
- E. Miscellaneous mechanical obstruction of coronary arteries
  - 1. Coronary artery dissection in Marfan syndrome
  - 2. Coronary artery dissection in pregnancy
  - 3. Prolapse of aortic valve myxomatous polyps into coronary ostia
  - 4. Dissection or rupture of sinus of Valsalva
- F. Functional obstruction of coronary arteries
  - 1. Coronary artery spasm with or without atherosclerosis
  - 2. Myocardial bridges

II. Hypertrophy of ventricular myocardium
- A. Left ventricular hypertrophy associated with coronary heart disease
- B. Hypertensive heart disease without significant coronary atherosclerosis
- C. Hypertrophic myocardium secondary to valvular heart disease
- D. Hypertrophic cardiomyopathy
  - 1. Obstructive
  - 2. Nonobstructive
- E. Primary or secondary pulmonary hypertension
  - 1. Advanced chronic right ventricular overload
  - 2. Pulmonary hypertension in pregnancy (highest risk peripartum)

III. Myocardial diseases and heart failure
- A. Chronic congestive heart failure
  - 1. Ischemic cardiomyopathy
  - 2. Idiopathic dilated cardiomyopathy
    - (a) Acquired
    - (b) Hereditary
  - 3. Alcoholic cardiomyopathy
  - 4. Hypertensive cardiomyopathy
  - 5. Postmyocarditis cardiomyopathy
  - 6. Peripartum cardiomyopathy
- B. Acute cardiac failure
  - 1. Massive acute myocardial infarction
  - 2. Acute myocarditis
  - 3. Acute alcoholic cardiac dysfunction
  - 4. Ball-valve embolism in aortic stenosis or prosthesis
  - 5. Mechanical disruptions of cardiac structures
    - (a) Rupture of ventricular free wall
    - (b) Disruption of mitral apparatus
      - (1) Papillary muscle
      - (2) Chordae tendineae
      - (3) Leaflet
    - (c) Rupture of interventricular septum
  - 6. Acute pulmonary edema in noncompliant ventricles

IV. Inflammatory, infiltrative, neoplastic, and degenerative processes
- A. Viral myocarditis, with or without ventricular dysfunction
  - 1. Acute phase
  - 2. Postmyocarditis interstitial fibrosis
- B. Myocarditis associated with the vasculitides
- C. Sarcoidosis
- D. Progressive systemic sclerosis
- E. Amyloidosis
- F. Hemochromatosis
- G. Idiopathic giant cell myocarditis
- H. Chagas disease

TABLE 33–2 Causes and Contributing Factors in Sudden Cardiac Death—cont'd

- I. Cardiac ganglionitis
- J. Arrhythmogenic right ventricular dysplasia; right ventricular cardiomyopathy
- K. Neuromuscular diseases (e.g., muscular dystrophy, Friedreich ataxia, myotonic dystrophy)
- L. Intramural tumors
  1. Primary
  2. Metastatic
- M. Obstructive intracavitary tumors
  1. Neoplastic
  2. Thrombotic

V. Diseases of the cardiac valves
- A. Valvular aortic stenosis/insufficiency
- B. Mitral valve disruption
- C. Mitral valve prolapse
- D. Endocarditis
- E. Prosthetic valve dysfunction

VI. Congenital heart disease
- A. Congenital aortic or pulmonic valve stenosis
- B. Right-to-left shunts with Eisenmenger physiology
  1. Advanced disease
  2. During labor and delivery
- C. Late after surgical repair of congenital lesions (e.g., tetralogy of Fallot)

VII. Electrophysiological abnormalities
- A. Abnormalities of the conducting system
  1. Fibrosis of the His-Purkinje system
     - (a) Primary degeneration (Lenegre disease)
     - (b) Secondary to fibrosis and calcification of the "cardiac skeleton" (Lev disease)
     - (c) Postviral conducting system fibrosis
     - (d) Hereditary conducting system disease
  2. Anomalous pathways of conduction (Wolff-Parkinson-White syndrome, short refractory period bypass)
- B. Abnormalities of repolarization
  1. Congenital long QT interval syndromes
     - (a) Romano-Ward syndrome (without deafness)
     - (b) Jervell and Lange-Nielsen syndrome (with deafness)
  2. Acquired (or provoked) long QT interval syndromes
     - (a) Drug effect (with genetic predisposition?)
       - (1) Cardiac, antiarrhythmic
       - (2) Noncardiac
       - (3) Drug interactions
     - (b) Electrolyte abnormality (response modified by genetic predisposition?)
     - (c) Toxic substances
     - (d) Hypothermia
     - (e) Central nervous system injury
  3. Brugada syndrome—right bundle branch block and ST segment elevations in the absence of ischemia
- C. Ventricular fibrillation of unknown or uncertain cause
  1. Absence of identifiable structural or functional causes
     - (a) "Idiopathic" ventricular fibrillation
     - (b) Short-coupled torsades de pointes, polymorphic ventricular tachycardia
     - (c) Nonspecific fibrofatty infiltration in previously healthy victim (variation of right ventricular dysplasia?)
  2. Sleep-death in Southeast Asians (see VII.B.3, Brugada syndrome)
     - (a) Bangungut
     - (b) Pokkuri
     - (c) Lai-tai

VIII. Electrical instability related to neurohumoral and central nervous system influences
- A. Catecholamine-dependent lethal arrhythmias
- B. Central nervous system related
  1. Psychic stress, emotional extremes
  2. Auditory related
  3. "Voodoo" death in primitive cultures
  4. Diseases of the cardiac nerves
  5. Congenital QT interval prolongation

IX. Sudden infant death syndrome and sudden death in children
- A. Sudden infant death syndrome
  1. Immature respiratory control functions
  2. Susceptibility to lethal arrhythmias (e.g., long QT syndrome)
  3. Congenital heart disease
  4. Myocarditis
- B. Sudden death in children
  1. Eisenmenger syndrome, aortic stenosis, hypertrophic cardiomyopathy, pulmonary atresia
  2. After corrective surgery for congenital heart disease
  3. Myocarditis
  4. Genetic disorders of electrical function (e.g., long QT syndrome)
  5. No identified structural or functional cause

TABLE 33–2 Causes and Contributing Factors in Sudden Cardiac Death—cont'd

X. Miscellaneous
   A. Sudden death during extreme physical activity (seek predisposing causes)
   B. Commotio cordis—blunt chest trauma
   C. Mechanical interference with venous return
      1. Acute cardiac tamponade
      2. Massive pulmonary embolism
      3. Acute intracardiac thrombosis
   D. Dissecting aneurysm of the aorta
   E. Toxic/metabolic disturbances
      1. Electrolyte disturbances
      2. Metabolic disturbances
      3. Proarrhythmic effects of antiarrhythmic drugs
      4. Proarrhythmic effects of noncardiac drugs
   F. Mimics sudden cardiac death
      1. "Cafe coronary"
      2. Acute alcoholic states ("holiday heart")
      3. Acute asthmatic attacks
      4. Air or amniotic fluid embolism

ANOMALOUS ORIGIN OF CORONARY ARTERIES FROM THE INAPPROPRIATE SINUS OF VALSALVA (see Chap. 75). These anatomical variants are associated with increased risk of SCD,[78] particularly during exercise. When the anomalous artery passes between the aortic and the pulmonary artery root, the takeoff angle of the anomalous ostium creates a slit-like opening of the vessel, reducing the effective cross-sectional area for blood flow. Congenitally hypoplastic, stenotic, or atretic left coronary arteries are uncommon abnormalities associated with a high risk of myocardial infarction but not of SCD.

EMBOLISM TO THE CORONARY ARTERIES. Coronary artery emboli occur most commonly in aortic valve endocarditis and from thrombotic material on diseased or prosthetic aortic or mitral valves. Emboli can also originate from left ventricular mural thrombi or as a consequence of surgery or cardiac catheterization. Symptoms and signs of myocardial ischemia or infarction are the most common manifestations. In each of these categories, SCD is a risk resulting from the electrophysiological consequences of the embolic ischemic event.

MUCOCUTANEOUS LYMPH NODE SYNDROME (KAWASAKI DISEASE) (see Chap. 82). This syndrome carries a risk of SCD in association with coronary arteritis. Polyarteritis nodosa and related vesiculitis syndromes can cause SCD presumably because of coronary arteritis, as can coronary ostial stenosis in syphilitic aortitis. The latter has become a rare manifestation of syphilis.

MECHANICAL OBSTRUCTION TO CORONARY ARTERIES. Several types of mechanical abnormalities are listed among causes of SCD. Coronary dissection, with or without dissection of the aorta, occurs in Marfan syndrome (see Chap. 56) and has also been reported after trauma and in the peripartum period of pregnancy. Among the rare mechanical causes of SCD is prolapse of myxomatous polyps from the aortic valve into coronary ostia, as well as dissection or rupture of a sinus of Valsalva aneurysm, with involvement of the coronary ostia and proximal coronary arteries. Finally, deep myocardial bridges over coronary arteries (see Chap. 75) have been reported in association with SCD occurring during strenuous exercise, possibly caused by dynamic mechanical obstruction. However, most myocardial bridges are inconsequential and SCD associated with this anatomy is uncommon.

CORONARY ARTERY SPASM (see Chap. 46). Coronary vasospasm may cause serious arrhythmias and SCD.[79] It is usually associated with some degree of concomitant coronary atherosclerotic disease. Painless myocardial ischemia, associated with either spasm or fixed lesions, is now recognized as a mechanism of previously unexplained sudden death.[79] Different patterns of silent ischemia (e.g., totally asymptomatic, post-myocardial infarction, and mixed silent-anginal pattern) may have different prognostic implications.[80]

VENTRICULAR HYPERTROPHY AND HYPERTROPHIC CARDIOMYOPATHY (see Chaps. 59 and 75). Left ventricular hypertrophy is an independent risk factor for SCD, accompanies many causes of SCD, and may be a physiological contributor to mechanisms of potentially lethal arrhythmias.[44,45] The underlying states resulting in hypertrophy include hypertensive heart disease with or without atherosclerosis, valvular heart disease, obstructive and nonobstructive hypertrophic cardiomyopathy, primary pulmonary hypertension with right ventricular hypertrophy, and advanced right ventricular overload secondary to congenital heart disease. Each of these conditions is associated with risk of SCD, and it has been suggested that patients with severely hypertrophic ventricles are particularly susceptible to arrhythmic death.[81]

Risk of SCD in obstructive and nonobstructive hypertrophic cardiomyopathy was identified in the early clinical and hemodynamic descriptions of this entity.[82] Among patients who have the obstructive form, up to 70 percent of all deaths are sudden. However, survivors of cardiac arrest in this group may have a better long-term outcome than survivors with other causes, and reports have suggested that the risk of *primary* cardiac arrest and SCD in hypertrophic cardiomyopathy is lower than previously thought.[83,84]

A substantial proportion of patients with obstructive and nonobstructive cardiomyopathy have a family history of affected relatives or premature SCDs of unknown cause. Genetic studies have confirmed autosomal dominant inheritance patterns, with a great deal of allele and phenotypic heterogeneity. Most of the mutations are at loci that encode elements in the contractile protein complex, the most common being beta-myosin heavy chain and cardiac troponin T, which together account for more than half of identified abnormalities.[24] In the beta-myosin heavy chain form, there is a relationship between severity of left ventricular hypertrophy and risk of SCD; in the troponin T form, left ventricular hypertrophy is less severe despite SCD risk. Thus, the specific defect, rather than the locus, is more relevant and may be independent of the severity of structural hypertrophy among different loci.[24]

Specific clinical markers have not been especially predictive of SCD in individual patients, although young age at onset, strong family history, magnitude of left ventricular mass, ventricular arrhythmias, and worsening symptoms (especially syncope) appear to indicate higher risk.[82-87] Early studies suggested that a low resting outflow gradient, with a substantial provocable gradient, identified high risk of SCD.[82] A more recent study supports the predictive power of a high resting gradient.[87] The mechanism of SCD in patients with hypertrophic obstructive cardiomyopathy was initially thought to involve outflow tract obstruction, possibly as a consequence of catecholamine stimulation, but later data have focused on lethal arrhythmias as the common mechanism of sudden death in this disease. Risk is also thought to be suggested by PVCs and nonsustained VT on ambulatory recording or the inducibility of potentially lethal arrhythmias during programmed electrical stimulation. However, stable and asymptomatic nonsustained VT has limited predictive power for SCD in these patients. Rapid or polymorphic symptomatic nonsustained tachycardias, or both, have better predictive power.

The question of whether the pathogenesis of the arrhythmias represents an interaction between electrophysiological and hemodynamic abnormalities or is a consequence of electrophysiological derangement of hypertrophied muscle[81] is unanswered. The observation that patients with nonobstructive hypertrophic cardiomyopathy have high-risk arrhythmias and are at increased risk for SCD suggests that an electrophysiological mechanism secondary to the hypertrophied muscle itself plays some role. In athletes younger than 35 years, hypertrophic cardiomyopathy is the most common cause of SCD, in contrast to athletes over the age of 35, among whom ischemic heart disease is the most common cause.[88]

DILATED CARDIOMYOPATHY AND HEART FAILURE. The advent of therapeutic interventions that provide better long-term control of congestive heart failure has improved long-term survival of such patients (see Chaps. 22 and 23). However, the proportion of patients with heart failure who die suddenly is substantial, especially among those who appear clinically stable (i.e., functional class I or II).[89] The mechanism of SCD (VT or ventricular fibrillation [VF] versus bradyarrhythmia or asystole) appears to be related to cause (i.e., ischemic versus nonischemic).[90] The absolute risk of SCD increases with deteriorating left ventricular function, but the ratio of sudden to nonsudden deaths is related inversely to the extent of functional impairment.[89] Among patients with cardiomyopathy who have good functional capacity (class I and II), total mortality risk is considerably lower than it is for those with poor functional capacity (class III and IV)(Fig. 33–7). Unexplained syncope has been observed to be a powerful predictor of SCD in patients who have functional class III or IV disease related to any cause of cardiomyopathy, although ambulatory ventricular arrhythmias do not appear to indicate specific SCD risk in such patients.[72,91,92]

The interaction between post-myocardial infarction ventricular arrhythmia and depressed ejection fraction in determining risk for SCD has been described.[67] The majority of studies addressing the relation between chronic congestive heart failure and SCD focused on patients with ischemic, idiopathic, alcoholic, and postmyocarditis congestive cardiomyopathy. Peripartum cardiomyopathy (see Chap. 74) may also cause SCD.

ACUTE HEART FAILURE. All causes of acute cardiac failure (see Chap. 21), in the absence of prompt interventions, can result in SCD caused by either the circulatory failure itself or secondary arrhythmias. The electrophysiological mechanisms involved have been proposed to be caused by acute stretching of myocardial fibers or the His-Purkinje system, on the basis of its experimentally demonstrated arrhythmogenic effects. However, the roles of neurohumoral mechanisms and acute electrolyte shifts have not been fully evaluated. Among the causes of acute cardiac failure that are associated with SCD are massive acute myocardial infarction, acute myocarditis, acute alcoholic cardiac dysfunction, acute pulmonary edema in any form of advanced heart disease, and a number of mechanical causes of heart failure, such as massive pulmonary embolism, mechanical disruption of intracardiac structures secondary to infarction or infection, and ball-valve embolism in aortic or mitral stenosis (see Table 33–2).

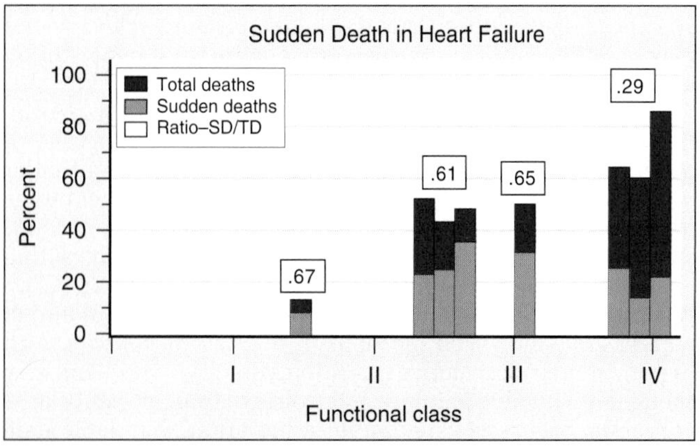

FIGURE 33–7 Risk of sudden cardiac death related to functional classification in heart failure. The relative probability of death being sudden is higher in the patients with better functional capacity who are at lower total mortality risk. SD = sudden death; TD = total death. (Modified from Kjekshus J: Arrhythmia and mortality in congestive heart failure. Am J Cardiol 65:42, 1990.)

INFLAMMATORY, INFILTRATIVE, NEOPLASTIC, AND DEGENERATIVE DISEASES OF THE HEART. Almost all diseases in this category have been associated with SCD, with or without concomitant cardiac failure. Acute viral myocarditis with left ventricular dysfunction (see Chap. 60) is commonly associated with cardiac arrhythmias, including potentially lethal arrhythmias. It is now recognized that serious ventricular arrhythmias or SCD can occur in myocarditis in the absence of clinical evidence of left ventricular dysfunction.[93,94] In a report of 19 SCDs among 1,606,167 previously screened U.S.Air Force recruits, 8 of the 19 (42 percent) had evidence of myocarditis (5 nonrheumatic, 3 rheumatic) at postmortem examination, and 15 (79 percent) suffered their cardiac arrests during strenuous exertion.[95] Viral carditis can also cause damage isolated to the specialized conducting system and result in a propensity to arrhythmias; the rare association of this process with SCD has been reported. Varicella in adults is a rare cause of striking conduction system disorders, but left ventricular function is usually preserved; its relationship to SCD is unclear.

Myocardial involvement in collagen-vascular disorders, tumors, chronic granulomatous diseases, infiltrative disorders, and protozoan infestations varies widely, but in all instances SCD can be the initial or terminal manifestation of the disease process. Among the granulomatous diseases, *sarcoidosis* (see Chap. 59) stands out because of the frequency of SCD associated with it. Roberts and coworkers[96] reported that SCD was the terminal event in 67 percent of sarcoid heart disease deaths; the occurrence of SCD has been related to the extent of cardiac involvement. In a report on the pathological findings in nine patients who died of *progressive systemic sclerosis* (see Chap. 59), eight who died suddenly had evidence of transient ischemia and reperfusion histologically, suggesting that this might represent Raynaud-like involvement of coronary vessels. *Amyloidosis* of the heart (see Chap. 59) may also cause sudden death. An incidence of 30 percent has been reported, and diffuse involvement of ventricular muscle or of the specialized conducting system may be associated with SCD.

ARRHYTHMOGENIC RIGHT VENTRICULAR DYSPLASIA OR RIGHT VENTRICULAR CARDIOMYOPATHY (see Chap. 32). This condition is associated with a high incidence of ventricular arrhythmias, including polymorphic nonsustained VT and VF as well as recurrent sustained monomorphic VT.[97] Although symptomatic monomorphic VT has been well recognized in the syndrome for many years, the risk of SCD was unclear and thought to be relatively low. However, the features of the disease and risks associated with it have now been clarified by a number of studies.[98-100] In a high proportion of victims, perhaps as many as 80 percent, the first manifestation of the disease is "unexplained" syncope or SCD.[98] SCD is often exercise related, and in some areas of the world where screening for hypertrophic cardiomyopathy has excluded the affected athletes from competition, right ventricular dysplasia has emerged as the most common cause of sport-related SCD.[101]

A genetic basis for right ventricular dysplasia is also being explored. A large proportion of the cases (up to an estimated 30 to 50 percent currently) appear to have a familial distribution.[22,99,100] The inheritance pattern is autosomal dominant except in one geographically isolated cluster in which it is autosomal recessive (Naxos disease—plakoglobin locus on chromosome 17).[22] To date, autosomal dominant mutations in two gene loci have been characterized (the ryanodine receptor locus on chromosome 1 [1q42][102] and the desmoplakin domain locus on chromosome 6 [6p24][103]), even though linkage analyses have implicated a heterogeneous distribution of multiple potential loci that may contribute to inheritance patterns (see Chap. 28).[22,25]

VALVULAR HEART DISEASE (see Chap. 57). Before the advent of surgery for valvular heart disease, severe *aortic stenosis* was associated with a high mortality risk. Approximately 70 percent of deaths were sudden, accounting for an absolute SCD mortality rate of 15 to 20 percent among all affected patients.[104] The advent of safe and effective procedures for aortic valve replacement has reduced the incidence of this cause of sudden death, but patients with prosthetic or heterograft aortic valve replacements remain at some risk for SCD caused by arrhythmias, prosthetic valve dysfunction, or coexistent coronary heart disease.[105] The incidence peaks 3 weeks after operation and then levels off after 8 months. Nonetheless, the risk is still appreciably lower than the historical risk among patients before the advent of valve surgery. A high incidence of ventricular arrhythmia has been observed during follow-up of patients with valve replacement, especially those who had aortic stenosis, multiple valve surgery, or cardiomegaly.[106] Sudden death during follow-up was associated with ventricular arrhythmias and thromboembolism. Hemodynamic variables were less predictive. Stenotic lesions of other valves imply a much lower risk of SCD. Regurgitant lesions, particularly chronic aortic regurgitation and acute mitral regurgitation, may cause SCD, but the risk is also lower than with aortic stenosis.

MITRAL VALVE PROLAPSE (see Chap. 57). This entity is prevalent, but probably less than previously thought,[107] and associated with a high incidence of annoying cardiac arrhythmias. However, a risk of SCD, although apparent, is quite low.[108] This uncommon complication appears to correlate with nonspecific ST-T wave changes in the inferior leads on the electrocardiogram (ECG). An association with redundancy of mitral leaflets on the echocardiogram has also been suggested. Reported associations between QT interval prolongation or preexcitation and SCD in mitral prolapse syndrome are less consistent.

ENDOCARDITIS OF THE AORTIC AND MITRAL VALVES (see Chap. 58). This may be associated with rapid death resulting from acute disruption of the valvular apparatus, coronary embolism, or abscesses of valvular rings or the septum; however, such deaths are rarely true sudden deaths as conventionally defined and tachyarrhythmic mechanisms are uncommon. Coronary embolism from valvular vegetations can trigger fatal ischemic arrhythmia on rare occasions.

CONGENITAL HEART DISEASE. The congenital lesions most commonly associated with SCD are aortic stenosis (see Chap. 56) and communications between the left and right sides of the heart with the Eisenmenger physiology. In the latter, the risk of SCD is a function of the severity of pulmonary vascular disease; also, there is an extraordinarily high risk of maternal mortality during labor and delivery in the pregnant patient with Eisenmenger syndrome (see Chap. 74).[109] Potentially lethal arrhythmias and SCD have been described as late complications after surgical repair of complex congenital lesions, particularly tetralogy of Fallot, transposition of the great arteries, and atrioventricular (AV) canal.[110] These patients should be observed closely and treated aggressively when cardiac arrhythmias are identified, although the late risk of SCD may not be as high as previously thought.

ELECTROPHYSIOLOGICAL ABNORMALITIES. Acquired disease of the AV node and His-Purkinje system and the presence of accessory pathways of conduction (see Chap. 32) are two groups of structural abnormalities of specialized conduction that may be associated with SCD. Epidemiological studies have suggested that intraventricular conduction disturbances in coronary heart disease are one of the few factors that can increase the proportion of SCD in coronary heart disease.[51] Several studies from the late 1970s and 1980s had demonstrated increased total mortality and SCD risk during the late in-hospital course and first few months after hospital discharge among patients with anterior myocardial infarctions and right bundle branch block or bifascicular block. In one study, 47 percent of patients who had late hospital VF had had the combination of anteroseptal infarction and bundle branch block. This finding corresponded to a VF incidence of 35 percent among a subgroup that represented only 4.1 percent of a total of 966 myocardial infarctions. In a later study, evaluating the impact of thrombolytic therapy on the prethrombolytic data, the incidence of pure right bundle branch block was actually higher but that of bifascicular block was lower, as were late complications and mortality.[111] These observations suggest a benefit of thrombolytic therapy, but the principle of increased risk among those who develop advanced conduction abnormalities (probably related to infarct size) is not attenuated by the therapy and the condition still requires aggressive management.

Primary fibrosis (Lenegre disease) or secondary mechanical injury (Lev disease) of the His-Purkinje system is commonly associated with intraventricular conduction abnormalities and symptomatic AV block and less commonly with SCD. The identification of people at risk and the efficacy of pacemakers for preventing SCD, rather than only ameliorating symptoms, have been subjects of debate. However, survival appears to depend more on the nature and extent of the underlying disease than on the conduction disturbance itself.

Patients with congenital AV block (see Chap. 32) or nonprogressive congenital intraventricular block, in the absence of structural cardiac abnormalities and with stable heart rate and rhythm, have been characterized as being at low risk for SCD in the past. In contrast, progressive congenital intraventricular blocks and the coexistence of structural congenital defects predicted a high risk and were considered pacemaker indications. Later data suggest that patients with the patterns of congenital AV block previously thought to be benign are at risk for a dilated cardiomyopathy,[112] and routine pacemaker implantation in patients older than 15 years, if not indicated sooner, has been suggested by at least one group.[113] Whether there is mortality benefit from pacemakers or a reduction in the incidence of dilated cardiomyopathy is not yet clear. A hereditary form of AV heart block has also been reported in association with a familial propensity to SCD.[29]

The anomalous pathways of conduction, bundles of Kent in the Wolff-Parkinson-White syndrome and Mahaim fibers, are commonly associated with nonlethal arrhythmias. However, when the anomalous pathways of conduction have short refractory periods, the occurrence of atrial fibrillation may allow the induction of VF during very rapid conduction across the bypass tract (see Chap. 32). The incidence of SCD in patients with short refractory period bypass tracts is unknown because an accurate estimate of its incidence among the population is not available. Patients who have multiple pathways appear to be at higher risk for SCD, as do patients with a familial pattern of anomalous pathways and premature SCD.[114] Family history is relevant because a genetic predisposition to Wolff-Parkinson-White syndrome has been suggested.[115]

THE LONG QT INTERVAL SYNDROMES (see also Chaps. 27 and 32). The *congenital* long QT interval syndrome is a functional abnormality caused by hereditary defects of molecular structure in ion channel proteins and is apparently associated with environmental or neurogenic triggers that can initiate lethal arrhythmias.[116-118] Two hereditary patterns have been described: the much more common autosomal dominant pattern known as the Romano-Ward syndrome and the rare autosomal recessive inheritance pattern, which is associated with deafness, the Jervell and Lange-Nielsen syndrome. There is a broad range of phenotypical expression. Some patients have prolonged QT intervals throughout life without any manifest arrhythmias, whereas others are highly susceptible to symptomatic and potentially fatal ventricular arrhythmias, particularly the torsades de pointes form of VT.[117,119] Moreover, genetic studies have demonstrated that penetrance may be low or variable in some families,[22] making electrocardiographic identification of affected members difficult. The relationship between low penetrance and risk of SCD remains undefined, but such patients are likely to be susceptible to QT-lengthening effects of drugs or serum electrolyte variations, expressed clinically as acquired long QT syndrome (see later).

Higher levels of risk are associated with female gender, greater degrees of QT prolongation or QT alternans, unexplained syncope, family history of premature SCD, and documented torsades de pointes or prior VF. Patients with the syndrome require avoidance of drugs that are associated with QT lengthening and careful medical management, which may include implantable defibrillators.[118,120] Moreover, efforts to identify and manage medically relatives who carry the mutation is an important preventive measure, given the familial pattern of expression of the entity (see Chaps. 27 and 32 for details). Mutations associated with the Romano-Ward inheritance pattern have been identified at loci on chromosomes 3, 4, 7, 11, and 21.[11] The Jervell and Lange-Nielsen form, in which the cardiac manifestations are associated with congenital deafness, has an autosomal recessive inheritance pattern. It is caused by inherited abnormalities of *KvLQT1* (chromosome 11) and *minK* (chromosome 21) or homozygous *KvLQT1* mutations.[22] It is likely that most of the mutations are not true recessives but rather variants with limited penetrance when heterozygous (see Chap. 27).

The *acquired form* of prolonged QT interval syndrome refers to excessive lengthening of the QT interval and the potential for developing torsades de pointes in response to environmental influences. As with congenital long QT, it is more common in women. The syndrome may be due to drug effects or individual patients' idiosyncrasies (particularly related to class IA or class III antiarrhythmic drugs and psychotropic drugs [see Chap. 72]), electrolyte abnormalities, hypothermia, toxic substances, bradyarrhythmia-induced QT adjustments, and central nervous system injury.[121] It has also been reported in intensive weight reduction programs that involve the use of liquid protein diets and in anorexia nervosa. Lithium carbonate can prolong the QT interval and has been reported to be associated with an increased incidence of SCD in cancer patients with preexisting heart disease. Drug interactions have been recognized as a mechanism of prolongation of the QT interval and torsades de pointes.[122] A growing body of evidence is suggesting that inherited polymorphisms or mutations with low penetrance, involving the same gene loci associated with phenotypically expressed long QT syndrome, underlie the susceptibility to the acquired form in many (if not most) instances.[30,123-125] In acquired prolonged QT syndrome, as in the congenital form, torsades de pointes is commonly the specific arrhythmia that triggers or degenerates into VF.

THE BRUGADA SYNDROME (see Chaps. 27 and 32). This disorder is characterized by right bundle branch block and an unusual form of nonischemic ST-T wave elevations in the anterior precordial leads (Fig. 33–8), associated with risk of SCD.[126] It is a familial disorder and occurs most commonly in young and middle-aged males. A mutation involving the cardiac Na^+ channel gene (*SCN5A*) has been observed in a minority of cases,[26] and there are compelling data suggesting that other ion channel defects may be a cause.[127] The right bundle branch block and ST-T wave changes may be intermittent and evoked or exaggerated by Na^+ channel blockers (e.g., flecainide). Risk of SCD is high and appears to be best predicted by the combination of persistent baseline ECG changes, syncope, life-threatening arrhythmias, a strong family history of SCD, and inducibility of ventricular tachyarrhythmias during electrophysiological testing.[128,129]

ELECTRICAL INSTABILITY RESULTING FROM NEUROHUMORAL AND CENTRAL NERVOUS SYSTEM INFLUENCES. Catecholamine-dependent lethal arrhythmias in the absence of QT interval prolongation, with control by beta adrenoceptor blocking agents, have been described.[130] In younger patients, more commonly males, bidirectional or polymorphic VT associated with SCD risk is related to a genetic disorder involving the ryanodine receptor locus, whereas the syndrome not associated with that genotype appears more likely to be in older patients, more commonly women.[131] Several central nervous system–related interactions with cardiac electrical stability have been suggested (see Chap. 85).[132] Epidemiological data also suggest an association between behavioral abnormalities and the risk of SCD. Psychic stress and emotional extremes have been suggested as triggering mechanisms for advanced arrhythmias and SCD for many years,[133,134] but there are only limited, largely observational, data supporting such associations. Stress-induced arrhythmias are better supported than stress-induced mortality risk, the latter requiring more study. Data from the 1994 Los Angeles earthquake identified an increased rate of fatal cardiac events on that day, but the event rate was reduced over the ensuing 2 weeks, suggesting a triggering of events about to happen rather than independent causation.[135] Associations between auditory stimulation and auditory auras and SCD have been reported. The auditory abnormalities in some forms of congenital QT prolongation have also been observed.

A variant of torsades de pointes, characterized by short coupling intervals between a normal impulse and the initiating impulse, has been described (Fig. 33–9).[136] It appears to have familial trends and to be related to alterations in autonomic nervous system activity. The 12-lead ECG demonstrates normal QT intervals, but VF and sudden death are common (see Chaps. 28 and 32).

The phenomenon of "voodoo death" has been studied in developing countries.[137] There appears to be an association between isolation from the tribe, a sense of hopelessness, severe bradyarrhythmias, and sudden death. With cultural changes in many of these areas, the syndrome has become less amenable to observation and study; however, there remain pockets of cultural isolation in which the syndrome may still exist.

SUDDEN INFANT DEATH SYNDROME AND SUDDEN CARDIAC DEATH IN CHILDREN. The sudden infant death syndrome (SIDS) occurs between birth and 6 months of age, is more common in males, and had an incidence of 0.1 to 0.3 percent of live births prior to widespread publication of appropriate sleep positions in at-risk infants.[138] Because of its abrupt nature, a cardiac mechanism has been suspected for many years, but a variety of causes, with central respiratory dysfunction playing a major role, are considered likely. Many cases of SIDS are believed to represent a form of "sleep apnea" that, if prolonged, can lead to hypoxia, cyanosis, and cardiac arrhythmias. Experience with "near misses" and the results of respiratory monitoring, in conjunction with the propensity of the syndrome to occur in premature infants, all suggest impaired central nervous system respiratory control reflexes, possibly owing to immaturity. There has been interest, however, in the possibility of obstructive apnea as another mechanism. Identification of individual infants at risk is difficult, but the risk does not persist beyond the first 6 months of life. Having infants sleep on their backs was anticipated to reduce the incidence of SIDS and appears to have achieved this goal in some studies,[139] but not all studies have demonstrated this improvement.

Primary cardiac causes have been considered the basis of this syndrome in some victims, and a large study of ECGs of infants suggested an association of risk of SIDS with prolonged QT interval as a potential cause.[140] Subsequently, a near-miss survivor was shown to have a de novo mutation of the Na^+ channel gene (*SCN5A*; chromosome 3), validating the concept that long QT may be one of the mechanisms of SIDS.[141] The combination of the relative incidence of SIDS among victims with the longer QT intervals and documentation of long QT–related arrhythmias in near misses supports the notion that a significant fraction of SIDS deaths occur by this mechanism. It does not, however, exclude the respiratory hypothesis as the mechanism for the majority of cases. Other cardiac causes have also been reported. Accessory pathways (two cases) and dispersed or immature AV nodal or bundle branch cells in the annulus fibrosus (four cases) were described among a group of seven SIDS victims studied by detailed histopathology.[142]

Sudden death in children beyond the age group at risk for SIDS is often associated with identifiable heart disease.[20,143] Although one earlier study identified cardiac causes in only 25 percent of victims of sudden natural death between the ages of 1 and 21 years,[21] a later report identified cardiac causes in 65 percent, with cardiac causes attributed in 80 percent of older children and adolescents.[20] About 25 percent of SCDs in children occur in those who have undergone previous surgery for congenital cardiac disease. Of the remaining 75 percent, more than one-half occur in children who have one of four lesions: congenital aortic stenosis, Eisenmenger syndrome, pulmonary stenosis or atresia, or obstructive hypertrophic cardiomyopathy. Neuspiel and Kuller[21] observed 14 cases of myocarditis among 51 SCDs in children (27 percent).

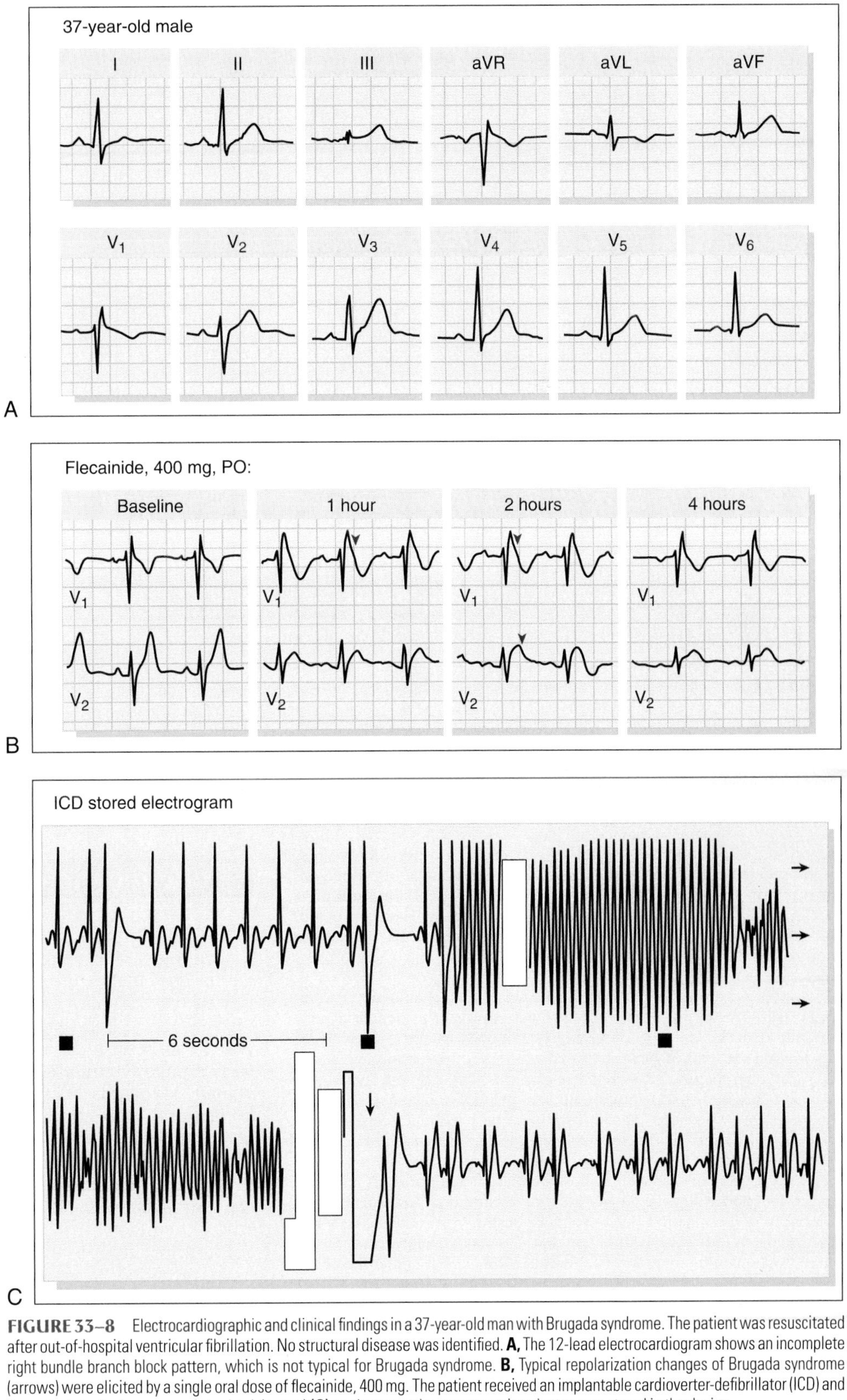

FIGURE 33–8 Electrocardiographic and clinical findings in a 37-year-old man with Brugada syndrome. The patient was resuscitated after out-of-hospital ventricular fibrillation. No structural disease was identified. **A,** The 12-lead electrocardiogram shows an incomplete right bundle branch block pattern, which is not typical for Brugada syndrome. **B,** Typical repolarization changes of Brugada syndrome (arrows) were elicited by a single oral dose of flecainide, 400 mg. The patient received an implantable cardioverter-defibrillator (ICD) and 6 months later had an appropriate shock (arrow) **(C)** as shown on the accompanying electrogram stored in the device.

OTHER CAUSES AND CIRCUMSTANCES ASSOCIATED WITH SUDDEN DEATH. SCD can occur during or after extreme physical activity in competing athletes or under special circumstances within the general population, examples of the latter being intense exercise and basic military training. Among adolescent and young adult competitive athletes, the incidence estimate is in the range of 1 per 75,000 annually in Italy,[144] compared with less than 1 per 125,000 for the general nonathlete population in the same age group.[54] However, Maron (see Chap. 75) reported the frequency of sudden unexpected death related to cardiovascular disease during competitive sports to be 1 in 200,000 individual student-athletes per academic year and in 1 in 70,000 over a 3-year high school career. Exercise-related incidence figures are more difficult to ascertain among other populations, but one study reported an incidence of one SCD per 1.5 million exercise sessions in health clubs.[53] The majority of both athletes and nonathletes have a previously known or unrecognized cardiac abnormality. In middle-aged and older adults, in whom coronary disease dominates as the cause of SCD, exercise-related deaths appear to be associated with acute plaque disruptions.[65] Whether exercise contributed to the initiation of plaque disruption or preexisting disruption simply set the stage for the fatal response during exercise remains unclear. Among athletes, hypertrophic cardiomyopathy with or without obstruction, occult congenital or acquired coronary artery disease, and valvular aortic stenosis are the

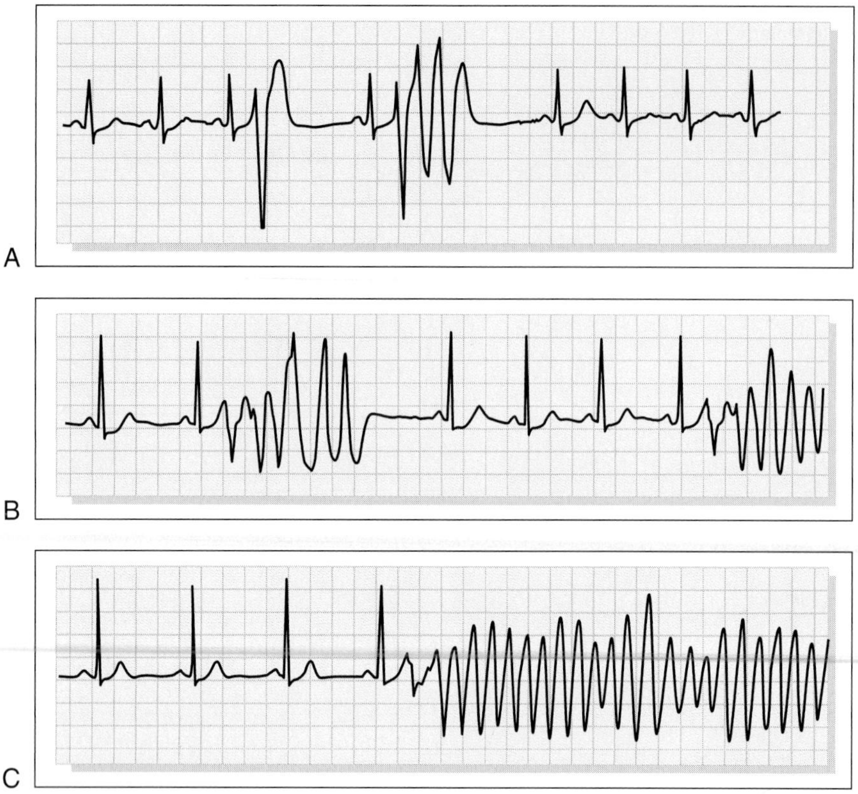

FIGURE 33–9 Short-coupled variant of torsades de pointes. This variant has been observed in people without structural heart disease and normal QT intervals. They are subject to spontaneous episodes of polymorphic ventricular tachycardia (torsades de pointes), which may degenerate into ventricular fibrillation. There is a high risk of sudden death in this uncommon syndrome.

most common causes identified after death (see Chap. 75).[88,144-149] In a report of a large cohort of U.S. Air Force recruits,[95] a surprisingly large fraction of people who died suddenly during exertion had unsuspected myocarditis. Diseases attributed to molecular structural abnormalities, such as long QT syndrome and right ventricular dysplasia, are being increasingly recognized as causes of SCD among athletes and exercising nonathletes.[88,146,147] Cardiac trauma (commotio cordis [see Chap. 59]) is the cause in some.[149]

Sudden death from true cardiac causes in athletes should not be confused with precipitous death related to heat stroke or malignant hyperthermia.[150] In the latter, excessive exercise in hot weather, sometimes in association with use of substances that cause heat production, and vasoconstriction impairing heat exchange can cause collapse with markedly elevated core body temperatures and irreversible organ system damage. Ingestion of exogenous dietary supplements, particularly ephedrine-related preparations in excess quantities, is being investigated for a role in precipitating SCD related to arrhythmia.

A small group of such victims, however, have neither previously determined functional abnormality nor identifiable structural abnormalities at postmortem examination. Such events or deaths, when associated with documented VF, are classified as idiopathic.[151] Although long-term survival after an idiopathic potentially fatal event is still unclear, some degree of risk appears to remain.[152] The idiopathic category is decreasing as the subtle molecular causes become better defined, including recognition by postmortem genetic studies. One pattern of so-called idiopathic VT has been associated with an inherited abnormality in calcium handling related to a ryanodine receptor mutation.[27] Limited data suggest that higher risk persists primarily in patients with subtle cardiac structural abnormalities, in contrast to patients who are truly normal. In addition, these events tend to occur in young, otherwise healthy people.

Long before Brugada's description of right bundle branch block, anterior nonischemic ST segment alterations, and sudden death predominantly in young males,[126] a specific pattern of SCD in young males had been observed in Southeast Asia. Syndromes referred to as *bangungut* in the Philippines, *pokkuri* in Japan, and *lai-tai* in Laos were reported. In each there was a tendency for death to occur unexpectedly during sleep, and at one time a toxic cause was suspected. Documented cases were reported in Laotians who came to the United States after the Vietnam War. The mechanism was identified as VF in some of these cases. The fact that these cases continue to occur in a new cultural setting suggested that there might be a hereditary predisposition. It is now accepted that many, if not all, of the subjects have Brugada syndrome.[153]

There also are a number of noncardiac conditions that *mimic* SCD. These include the so-called *cafe coronary* in which food, usually an unchewed piece of meat, lodges in the oropharynx and causes an abrupt obstruction at the glottis. The classic description of a cafe coronary is sudden cyanosis and collapse in a restaurant during a meal accompanied by lively conversation. The *holiday heart syndrome* is characterized by cardiac arrhythmias, most commonly atrial, and other cardiac abnormalities associated with acute alcoholic states. It has not been determined whether potentially lethal arrhythmias occurring in such settings account for reported sudden deaths associated with acute alcoholic states. *Massive pulmonary embolism* (see Chap. 66) can cause acute cardiovascular collapse and sudden death; sudden death in severe acute asthmatic attacks, without prolonged deterioration of the patient's condition, is well recognized. Air or amniotic fluid embolism at the time of labor and delivery may cause sudden death on rare occasions, with the clinical picture mimicking SCD. Peripartum air embolism caused by unusual sexual practices has been reported as a cause of such sudden deaths.

Finally, a number of abnormalities that do not directly involve the heart may cause SCD or mimic it. These include aortic dissection (see Chap. 53), acute cardiac tamponade (see Chap. 64), and rapid exsanguination.

Pathology and Pathophysiology

Pathological studies in SCD victims[154] reflect the epidemiological and clinical observations that coronary atherosclerosis is the major predisposing etiology.[76] Liberthson and coworkers[155] reported that 81 percent of 220 autopsied victims of SCD had significant coronary heart disease. At least one vessel with more than 75 percent stenosis was found in 94 percent of victims, acute coronary occlusion in 58 percent, healed myocardial infarction in 44 percent, and acute myocardial infarction in 27 percent. These observations are consistent with subsequent studies of the frequency of coronary disease in SCD victims, but the focus had evolved from the simple anatomical presence of coronary lesions to the specific associations with unstable plaques (see later).[65,156,157] All of the other causes of SCD (see Table 33–2) collectively account for no more than 15 to 20 percent of cases, but they have provided a large base of enlightening pathological data.[154]

The Pathology of Sudden Death Caused by Coronary Heart Disease

CORONARY ARTERIES. Extensive atherosclerosis has long been recognized as the most common pathological finding in the coronary arteries of victims of SCD. The combined results of a number of studies suggest a general pattern of at least two coronary arteries with 75 percent or greater narrowing among more than 75 percent of the victims. Several studies have demonstrated no specific pattern of distribution of coronary artery lesions that preselect for SCD. In a quantitative analysis comparing coronary artery narrowing at postmortem examination in SCD victims and control subjects, 36 percent of the 5-mm segments of the coronary arteries from the SCD group had 76 to 100 percent cross-sectional area reductions compared with 3 percent in the control group.[158] An additional 34 percent of the sections from the SCD group had 51 to 75 percent reductions in cross-sectional areas. Only 7 percent of the sections from the SCD patients had 0 to 25 percent reductions in cross-sectional areas.

The role of *active coronary artery* lesions, characterized by plaque fissuring, platelet aggregation, and thrombosis, as a major pathophysiological mechanism of the onset of cardiac arrest leading to SCD has become clarified.[65,156,157,159] Among 100 consecutive victims of sudden coronary death, 44 percent had major (more than 50 percent luminal occlusion) recent coronary thrombi, 30 percent had minor occlusive thrombi, and 21 percent had plaque fissuring. Only 5 percent had no acute coronary artery changes; 65 percent of the thrombi occurred at sites of preexisting high-grade stenoses, and an additional 19 percent were found at sites of more than 50 percent stenosis. In a subsequent study by the same investigators, 50 of 168 victims (30 percent) had occlusive intraluminal coronary thrombi, and 73 (44 percent) had mural intraluminal thrombi. Single-vessel disease, acute infarction at postmortem examination, and prodromal symptoms were associated with the presence of thrombi. In a later study, plaque rupture or erosion was observed in 66 percent of culprit vessel lesions among victims of SCD related to coronary heart disease.[48] Disruption, platelet aggregation, and thrombosis associate with markers of inflammation and various conventional risk factors for coronary atherosclerosis, such as cigarette smoking and hyperlipidemia.[160] *Coronary artery spasm,* an established cause of acute ischemia, can also cause SCD[79] and is recognizable in rare instances at postmortem examination.

MYOCARDIUM. Myocardial pathology in SCD caused by coronary heart disease reflects the extensive atherosclerosis usually present. Studies of victims of out-of-hospital SCD and from epidemiological sources indicate that healed myocardial infarction is a common finding in SCD victims, with most investigators reporting frequencies ranging from 40 to more than 70 percent.[155] In one study, 72 percent of men in the 25- to 44-year age group who died suddenly (24 or fewer hours) with no previous clinical history of coronary heart disease had scars of large (63 percent) or small (less than 1 cm cross-sectional area, 9 percent) areas of healed myocardial necrosis. The incidence of acute myocardial infarction is considerably less, with cytopathological evidence of recent myocardial infarction averaging about 20 percent. This estimate corresponds well with results of studies of out-of-hospital cardiac arrest survivors, who have an incidence of new myocardial infarction in the range of 20 to 30 percent. These pathological observations do not provide insight into the likely possibility that many SCDs occur by acute coronary syndrome mechanisms and progress from ischemia to fatal arrhythmias without time for structural markers to become visible. Even though there is an association of troponin elevations during chest pain syndromes with risk of cardiac death subsequently,[161] and troponin elevations occur in a substantial proportion of cardiac arrest survivors,[162] the question of whether the myocardial injury preceded or followed the cardiac arrest is difficult to resolve.

VENTRICULAR HYPERTROPHY. Myocardial hypertrophy can coexist and interact with acute or chronic ischemia but appears to confer an independent mortality risk.[44,45] There is not a close correlation between increased heart weight and severity of coronary heart disease in SCD victims; heart weights are higher in SCD victims than in those whose death is not sudden despite similar prevalences of history of hypertension before death. Hypertrophy-associated mortality risk is also independent of left ventricular function and extent of coronary artery disease.[163] Anderson[81] suggested that left ventricular hypertrophy itself may predispose to SCD. Experimental data also suggest increased susceptibility to potentially lethal ventricular arrhythmias in left ventricular hypertrophy with ischemia and reperfusion.[164] A study of massively enlarged hearts (i.e., weighing more than 1000 gm), however, did not indicate an excess incidence of SCD, but the underlying pathology in that study was dominated by lesions that produce volume overload.

SPECIALIZED CONDUCTING SYSTEM IN SUDDEN CARDIAC DEATH

Fibrosis of the specialized conducting system is a common but nonspecific endpoint of multiple causes. Although this process is associated with AV block or intraventricular conduction abnormalities, its role in SCD is uncertain. Lev and Lenegre diseases, ischemic injury caused by small-vessel disease, and numerous infiltrative or inflammatory processes all can result in such changes. In addition, active inflammatory processes such as myocarditis and infiltrative processes such as amyloidosis, scleroderma, hemochromatosis, and morbid obesity all may damage or destroy the AV node or bundle of His, or both, and result in AV block.[165]

Focal diseases such as sarcoidosis, Whipple disease, and rheumatoid arthritis and fibrotic or fatty infiltration of the AV node or His-Purkinje system with apparent discontinuities[93] can also involve the conducting system (see Chap. 32). These various categories of conducting system disease have been considered as possible pathological substrates for SCD that may be overlooked because of the difficulty in doing careful postmortem examinations of the conducting system routinely. Focal involvement of conducting tissue by tumors (especially mesothelioma of the AV node but also lymphoma, carcinoma, rhabdomyoma, and fibroma) has also been reported, and rare cases of SCD have been associated with these lesions. It has been suggested that abnormal postnatal morphogenesis of the specialized conducting system may be a significant factor in some SCDs in infants and children.

CARDIAC NERVES AND SUDDEN CARDIAC DEATH

Diseases of cardiac nerves have been postulated to have a role in SCD. Neural involvement may be the result of random damage to neural elements within the myocardium (i.e., "secondary" cardioneuropathy) or may be "primary," as in a selective cardiac viral neuropathy. Secondary involvement can be a consequence of ischemic neural injury in coronary heart disease and has been postulated to result in autonomic destabilization, enhancing the propensity to arrhythmias. Nerve sprouting may be important.[166] Some experimental data support this hypothesis, and a clinical technique for imaging cardiac neural fibers suggests a changing pattern over time after myocardial infarction. Viral, neurotoxic, and hereditary causes (e.g., progressive muscular dystrophy and Friedreich ataxia) have been emphasized.

Mechanisms and Pathophysiology

Electrical mechanisms of cardiac arrest are divided into tachyarrhythmic and bradyarrhythmia-asystolic events. The tachyarrhythmias include VF and sustained VT in which adequate blood flow cannot be maintained and perfusion is inadequate to meet the body's needs. Bradyarrhythmia-asystolic events include severe bradyarrhythmias—heart rates slow enough to impede adequate tissue perfusion and inability to generate a mechanical event because of either complete absence of electrical activity (asystole) or dissociation between abnormal spontaneous electrical activity and mechanical function (pulseless electrical activity). It is likely that VF, or VT deteriorating to VF, is the initiating event in the majority of cardiac arrests. After a variable period of time fibrillation may cease, and asystole or pulseless electrical activity emerges. In a significant minority of cases, however, the documented initial recording is asystole or pulseless electrical activity, which can continue as such or transform into VF.[167] More commonly, asystolic events or pulseless electrical activity follows an initial tachyarrhythmic event.

The occurrence of potentially lethal tachyarrhythmias, or of severe bradyarrhythmia or asystole, is the end of a cascade of pathophysiological abnormalities that result from complex interactions between coronary vascular events, myocardial injury, variations in autonomic tone, or the metabolic and electrolyte state of the myocardium (see Fig. 33–4).[12,168,169] There is no uniform hypothesis regarding mechanisms by which these elements interact to lead to the final pathway of lethal arrhythmias. However, Figure 33–10 shows a model of the pathophysiology of SCD in which the central event is the initiation of a potentially fatal arrhythmia. The risk of this event is conditioned by the presence of *structural abnormalities* and modulated by *functional variations*.[170]

Pathophysiological Mechanisms of Lethal Tachyarrhythmias

CORONARY ARTERY STRUCTURE AND FUNCTION. Among the 80 percent of SCDs associated with coronary atherosclerosis, the extent and distribution of chronic arterial narrowing have been well defined by pathological studies. However, the specific mechanisms by which these lesions lead to potentially lethal disturbances of electrical stability are no longer viewed as simply the consequence of steady-state reductions in regional myocardial blood flow in association with variable demands (see Chap. 35).[11,12,168] A simple increase in myocardial oxygen demand, in the presence of a fixed supply, may be a mechanism of exercise-induced arrhythmias and sudden death during intense physical activity or in others whose heart disease had not previously become clinically manifest. However, the dynamic nature of the pathophysiology of coronary events has led to the recognition that superimposed acute lesions create a setting in which alterations in the metabolic or electrolyte state of the myocardium are the common circumstance leading to disturbed electrical stability. Active vascular events, leading to acute or transient reduction in regional myocardial blood flow in the presence of a normal or previously compromised circulation, constitute a common mechanism of ischemia, angina pectoris, arrhythmias, and SCD.[11,79,168,169] Coronary artery spasm or modulation of coronary collateral flow, predisposed to by local endothelial dysfunction, exposes the myocardium to the double hazard of transient ischemia and reperfusion (Fig. 33–11).[151,168] Neurogenic influences may play a role but do not appear to be a sine qua non for the production of spasm. Vessel susceptibility and humoral factors, particularly those related to platelet activation and aggregation, also appear to be important mechanisms.

Transition of stable atherosclerotic plaques to an "active" state because of endothelial damage, with plaque fissuring leading to platelet activation and aggregation followed by thrombosis, is a mechanism that appears to be present in the majority of SCDs related to coronary heart disease (see Chap. 46).[156] Inflammatory responses in atherosclerotic plaques are now viewed as the condition leading to lesion progression, including erosion, disruption, platelet activation, and thrombosis. In addition to causing subacute or acute critical reduction in regional blood flow, these mechanisms produce a series of biochemical alterations that may enhance or retard susceptibility to VF by means of vasomotor modulation.

The final step in the role of coronary artery pathophysiology leading to ischemia-induced arrhythmias is platelet aggregation and thrombosis (see Fig. 33–4; see Chap. 35). Davies and Thomas[159] pointed out that 95 of 100 subjects who died suddenly (less than 6 hours after the onset of symptoms) had acute coronary thrombi, plaque fissuring, or both. This incidence was considerably higher than in many previous reports, but it is noteworthy that only 44 percent of the patients had the largest thrombus occluding 51 percent or more of the cross-sectional area of the involved vessel and only 18 percent of the patients had more than 75 percent occlusion. These findings raise questions about whether mechanical obstruction to flow was dominant or whether the high incidence of nonoccluding thrombi simply reflected the state of activation of the platelets. The discrepancy between the relatively high incidence of acute thrombi in postmortem studies and the low incidence of evolution of new myocardial infarction among survivors of out-of-hospital VF[155,171] highlights this question. Spontaneous thrombolysis, a dominant role of spasm induced by platelet products, or a combination may explain this discrepancy.

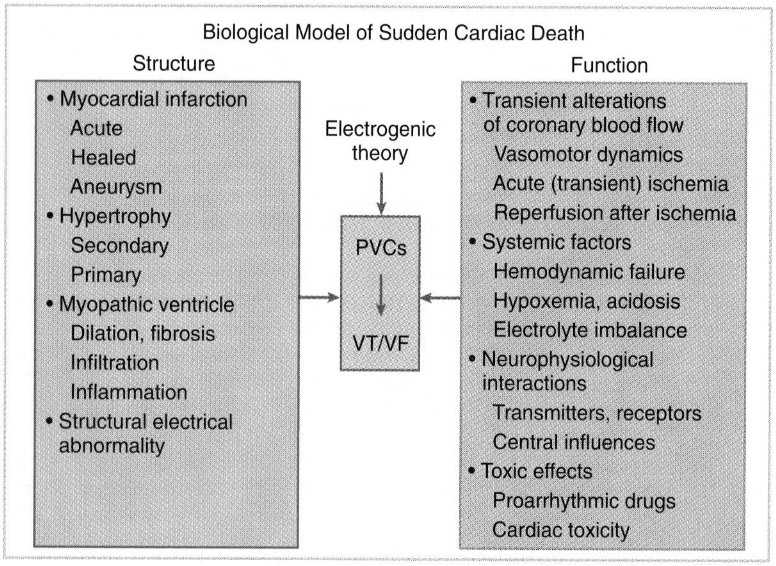

FIGURE 33–10 Biological model of sudden cardiac death (SCD). Structural cardiac abnormalities are commonly defined as the causative basis for SCD. However, functional alterations of the abnormal anatomical substrate are usually required to alter stability of the myocardium, permitting a potentially fatal arrhythmia to be initiated. In this conceptual model, short- or long-term structural abnormalities interact with functional modulations to influence the probability that premature ventricular contractions (PVCs) initiate ventricular tachycardia or fibrillation (VT/VF). (From Myerburg RJ, Kessler KM, Bassett AL, Castellanos A: A biological approach to sudden cardiac death: Structure, function, and cause. Am J Cardiol 63:1512, 1989.)

ACUTE ISCHEMIA AND INITIATION OF LETHAL ARRHYTHMIAS. The onset of acute ischemia produces immediate electrical, mechanical, and biochemical dysfunction of cardiac muscle (see Figs. 33–10 and 33–11). The specialized conducting tissue is more resistant to acute ischemia than working myocardium, and therefore the electrophysiological consequences are less intense and delayed in onset in specialized conduction tissue. Experimental studies have also provided data on the long-term consequences of left ventricular hypertrophy and healed experimental myocardial infarction. Tissue exposed to chronic stress produced by long-term left ventricular pressure overload and tissue that has healed after ischemic injury both show lasting cellular electrophysiological abnormalities, including regional changes in transmembrane action potentials and refractory periods.[169] Moreover, acute ischemic injury or acute myocardial infarction in the presence of healed myocardial infarction is more arrhythmogenic than the same extent of acute ischemia in previously normal tissue.[172] In addition to the direct effect of ischemia on normal or previously abnormal tissue, reperfusion after transient ischemia can cause lethal arrhythmias (see Fig. 33–11).[79,169] Reperfusion of ischemic areas can occur by three mechanisms: (1) spontaneous thrombolysis, (2) collateral flow from other coronary vascular beds to the ischemic bed, and (3) reversal of vasospasm. Some mechanisms of reperfusion-induced arrhythmogenesis appear to be related to the duration of ischemia before reperfusion. Experimentally, there is a window of vulnerability beginning 5 to 10 minutes after the onset of ischemia and lasting up to 20 to 30 minutes.

ELECTROPHYSIOLOGICAL EFFECTS OF ACUTE ISCHEMIA. Within the first minutes after experimental coronary ligation there is a propensity to ventricular arrhythmias that abates after 30 minutes and reappears after several hours. The initial 30 minutes of arrhythmias is divided into two periods, the first of which lasts for about 10 minutes and is presumably directly related to the initial ischemic injury. The second period (20 to 30 minutes) may be related either to reperfusion of ischemic areas or to the evolution of different injury patterns in the epicardial and endocardial muscle. Multiple mechanisms of reperfusion arrhythmias have been observed experimentally, including slow conduction and reentry[173] and afterdepolarizations and triggered activity.[164]

At the level of the myocyte, the immediate consequences of ischemia, which include alteration of cell membrane physiology with efflux of K^+, influx of Ca^{2+}, acidosis, reduction of transmembrane resting potentials,[174] and enhanced automaticity in some tissues, are followed by a separate series of changes during reperfusion. Those of particular interest are the possible continued influx of Ca^{2+}, which may produce electrical instability; responses to alpha or beta adrenoceptor stimulation, or both; and afterdepolarizations as triggering responses for Ca^{2+}-dependent arrhythmias. Other possible mechanisms studied experimentally include formation of superoxide radicals in reperfusion arrhythmias and differential responses of endocardial and epicardial muscle activation times and refractory periods during ischemia or reperfusion. The adenosine triphosphate-dependent K^+ current ($I_{K\text{-}ATP}$), which is inactive during normal conditions, is activated during ischemia.[175] Its activation results in a strong efflux of K^+ ions from myocytes, markedly shortening the time course of repolarization and leading to slow conduction and ultimately to inexcitability.[176] The fact that this response is more marked in epicardium than in endocardium leads to a prominent dispersion of repolarization across the myocardium during transmural ischemia. At an intercellular level, ischemia alters the distribution of connexin43, the primary gap junction protein between myocytes.[177] This alteration results in uncoupling of myocytes, a factor that is arrhythmogenic because of altered patterns of excitation and regional changes in conduction velocity.[178]

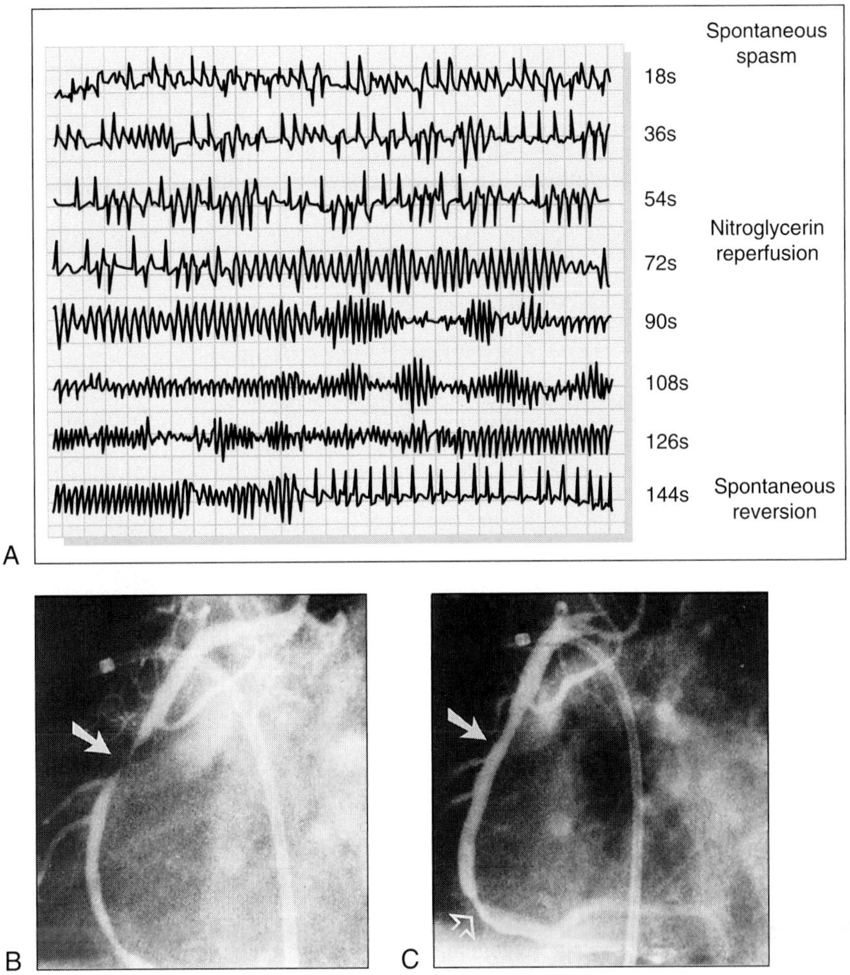

FIGURE 33–11 Life-threatening ventricular arrhythmias associated with acute myocardial ischemia related to coronary artery spasm and with reperfusion. **A,** Continuous lead II electrocardiographic monitor recording during ischemia (time 0 to 55 seconds) caused by spasm of the right coronary artery **(B)**. There is an abrupt transition (time 56 to 72 seconds) from repetitive ventricular ectopy to a rapid polymorphic, prefibrillatory tachyarrhythmia (time 80 to 130 seconds) associated with nitroglycerin-induced reversal of the spasm **(C)**. Closed arrows, site of spasm before and after nitroglycerin; open arrow, lower grade distal lesion.

The importance of the myocardial response to the onset of ischemia has been emphasized on the basis of the demonstration of dramatic cellular electrophysiological changes during the early period after coronary occlusion. However, the state of the myocardium at the time of onset of ischemia is a critical additional factor. Tissue healed after previous injury appears to be more susceptible to the electrical destabilizing effects of acute ischemia, as is chronically hypertrophied muscle. There are data suggesting that remodeling-induced local stretch, regional hypertrophy, or intrinsic cellular alteration may contribute to this vulnerability. Of more direct clinical relevance is the suggestion that K^+ depletion by diuretics and clinical hypokalemia may make ventricular myocardium more susceptible to potentially lethal arrhythmias.

The association of metabolic and electrolyte abnormalities, and neurophysiological and neurohumoral changes,[179] with lethal arrhythmias emphasizes the importance of integrating changes in the myocardial substrate with systemic influences. Most direct among myocardial metabolic changes in response to ischemia are local acute increase in interstitial K^+ levels to values exceeding 15 mM, a fall in tissue pH to below 6.0, changes in adrenoceptor activity, and alterations in autonomic nerve traffic, all of which tend to create and maintain electrical instability, especially if regional in distribution. Other metabolic changes such as cyclic adenosine monophosphate elevation, accumulation of free fatty acids and their metabolites, formation of lysophosphoglycerides, and impaired myocardial glycolysis have also been suggested as myocardial destabilizing influences.[180] These local myocardial changes integrate with systemic patterns of autonomic fluctuation that can be observed as patterns of altered heart rate variability and fractal dynamics,[181] potentially identifying subsets of patients predetermined to be at higher risk for SCD during an ischemic event.

TRANSITION FROM MYOCARDIAL INSTABILITY TO LETHAL ARRHYTHMIAS. Tshe combination of a triggering event and a susceptible myocardium is a fundamental electrophysiological concept for the mechanism of initiation of potentially lethal arrhythmias (see Figs. 33–4 and 33–10). The triggering event may be electrophysiological, ischemic, metabolic, or hemodynamic.[170] The endpoint of their interaction is disorganization of patterns of myocardial activation into multiple uncoordinated reentrant pathways (i.e., VF). Clinical, experimental, and pharmacological data all suggest that triggering events in the absence of myocardial instability are unlikely to initiate lethal arrhythmias. Therefore, in the absence of myocardial vulnerability, many triggering events, such as frequent and complex PVCs, may be innocuous.[170]

The onset of ischemia is accompanied by abrupt reductions in transmembrane resting potential and amplitude and in duration of the action potentials in the affected area with little change in remote areas. When ischemic cells depolarize to resting potentials less than −60 mV, they may become inexcitable and of little electrophysiological importance (see Chap. 27). As they are depolarizing to that range, however, or repolarizing as a consequence of reperfusion, the membranes pass through ranges of reduced excitability, upstroke velocity, and time courses of repolarization. These characteristics result in slow conduction and electrophysiological heterogeneity. When this occurs in ischemic myocardium that is adjacent to nonischemic tissue, it creates a setting for the key elements of reentry—slow conduction and unidirectional block—which makes the myocardium vulnerable to reentrant arrhythmias. When premature impulses are generated in this environment, regardless of their electrical mechanism (i.e., reentrant, triggered activity, automaticity), they may further alter the dispersion of recovery between ischemic tissue, chronically abnormal tissue, and normal cells, ultimately leading to complete disorganization and VF.

The dispersion of refractory periods produced by acute ischemia, which provides the substrate for reentrant tachycardias and VF, may be further enhanced by a healed ischemic injury. The time course of repolarization is lengthened after healing of ischemic injury and shortened by acute ischemia. The coexistence of the two appears to make the ventricle more susceptible to sustained arrhythmias in some experimental models.[172]

Bradyarrhythmias and Asystolic Arrest

The basic electrophysiological mechanism in this form of arrest is failure of normal subordinate automatic activity to assume the pacemaking function of the heart in the absence of normal function of the sinus node or AV junction, or both. Bradyarrhythmic and asystolic arrests are more common in severely diseased hearts and with cardiac arrest in patients with a number of end-stage disorders, both cardiac and noncardiac. These mechanisms may result, in part, from diffuse involvement of subendocardial Purkinje fibers in advanced heart disease. Systemic influences that increase extracellular K^+ concentration, such as anoxia, acidosis, shock, renal failure, trauma, and hypothermia, can result in partial depolarization of normal or already diseased pacemaker cells in the His-Purkinje system, with a decrease in the slope of spontaneous phase 4 depolarization and ultimate loss of automaticity. These processes can produce global dysfunction of automatic cell activity, in contrast to the regional dysfunction more common in acute ischemia. Functionally depressed automatic cells (e.g., owing to increased extracellular K^+ concentration) are more susceptible to overdrive suppression. Under these conditions, brief bursts of tachycardia may be followed by prolonged asystolic periods, with further depression of automaticity by the consequent acidosis and increased local K^+ concentration or by changes in adrenergic tone. The ultimate consequence may be degeneration into VF or persistent asystole.

Pulseless Electrical Activity

Pulseless electrical activity, formerly called electromechanical dissociation, is separated into *primary* and *secondary forms*. The common denominator in both is continued electrical rhythmicity of the heart in the absence of effective mechanical function. The secondary form includes the causes that result from an abrupt cessation of cardiac venous return, such as massive pulmonary embolism, acute malfunction of prosthetic valves, exsanguination, and cardiac tamponade from hemopericardium. The primary form is the more familiar; in it, none of these obvious mechanical factors are present but ventricular muscle fails to produce an effective contraction despite continued electrical activity (i.e., *failure of electromechanical coupling*). It usually occurs as an end-stage event in advanced heart disease, but it can occur in patients with acute ischemic events or, more commonly, after electrical resuscitation from a prolonged cardiac arrest. Although it is not thoroughly understood, it appears that diffuse disease, metabolic abnormalities, or global ischemia provides the pathophysiological substrate. The proximate mechanism for failure of electromechanical coupling may be abnormal intracellular Ca^{2+} metabolism, intracellular acidosis, or perhaps adenosine triphosphate depletion.

Clinical Characteristics of the Patient with Cardiac Arrest

Although the pathological anatomy associated with SCD related to coronary artery disease reflects the presence of the changes associated with acute coronary syndromes in the majority of cases, only a minority of survivors of out-of-hospital VF have clinical evidence of a new transmural myocardial infarction.[171,182,183] In the Seattle study, only one of five survivors had new transmural infarctions.[182] Nonetheless, many have enzyme elevations, with nonspecific ECG changes suggesting myocardial damage, which may be due to transient ischemia as a triggering event or a consequence of the loss of myocardial perfusion during the cardiac arrest.[162] The former supports the concept of transient pathophysiological changes associated with acute coronary syndromes as the trigger for cardiac arrest. The recurrence rate in survivors of out-of-hospital cardiac arrest was low in the subgroup of patients who had documentation of a new transmural myocardial infarction. In contrast, it was found to be 30 percent at 1 year and 45 percent at 2 years in the survivors who did not have a new transmural myocardial infarction.[182,183] Recurrence rates decreased subsequently,[171] possibly owing in part to long-term interventions. However, it is not known whether the decrease resulted from a change in the natural history, changes in preventive strategies for underlying disease, or long-term interventions for controlling arrhythmic risk.

Clinical cardiac arrest and SCD can be described in the framework of the same four phases of the event used to establish temporal definitions (see Fig. 33–1): prodromes, onset of the terminal event, the cardiac arrest, and progression to biological death or survival.

Prodromal Symptoms

Patients at risk for SCD can have prodromes such as chest pain, dyspnea, weakness or fatigue, palpitations, syncope, and a number of nonspecific complaints. Several epidemiological and clinical studies demonstrated that such symptoms can presage coronary events, particularly myocardial infarction and SCD, and result in contact with the medical system weeks to months before SCD. Among a group of patients successfully resuscitated after out-of-hospital cardiac arrest, 28 percent reported retrospectively that they had had new or changing angina pectoris or dyspnea in the 4 weeks before arrest and 31 percent had seen a physician during this time, but only 12 percent because of these symptoms.[182]

Attempts to identify early prodromal symptoms that are specific for the patient at risk for SCD have not been successful. Although several studies reported that 12 to 46 percent of fatalities occurred in patients who had seen a physician 1 to 6 months before death, such visits were more likely to presage myocardial infarction or nonsudden deaths, and the majority of complaints responsible for those visits were not heart related. However, patients who have chest pain as a prodrome to SCD appear to have a higher probability of intraluminal coronary thrombosis at postmortem examination.[184] Fatigue has been a particularly common symptom in the days or weeks before SCD in a number of studies, but this symptom is nonspecific. The symptoms that occur within the last hours or minutes before cardiac arrest are more specific for heart disease and may include symptoms of arrhythmias, ischemia, or heart failure. Liberthson and associates[155] reported specific cardiac symptoms at a mean interval of about 3.8 hours before collapse in 24 percent of victims of SCD. However, most studies have reported such symptoms even less commonly, particularly when victims whose deaths were instantaneous were included.

Onset of the Terminal Event

The period of 1 hour or less between acute changes in cardiovascular status and the cardiac arrest itself is defined as the "onset of the terminal event." A report on ambulatory recordings fortuitously obtained during the onset of an unexpected cardiac arrest indicated dynamic changes in cardiac electrical activity during the minutes or hours before the event.[185] This report suggested that increasing heart rate and advancing grades of ventricular ectopy are common antecedents of VF. Alterations in autonomic nervous system activity may also contribute to the onset of the event. Studies of short-term variations of heart rate variability, or related measures, have identified changes that correlate with the occurrence of ventricular arrhythmias.[186] Although these recordings suggest transient electrophysiological destabilization of the myocardium, the extent to which these objective observations are paralleled by clinical symptoms or events is less well documented.[187] SCDs caused by either arrhythmias or acute circulatory failure mechanisms correlate with a high incidence of acute myocardial disorders at the onset of the terminal event; such disorders are more likely to be ischemic when the death is due to arrhythmias and to be associated with low-output states or myocardial anoxia when the deaths are due to circulatory failure.

Abrupt, unexpected loss of effective circulation can be caused by cardiac arrhythmias or mechanical disturbances, but the majority of such events that terminate in SCD are arrhythmic. Hinkle and Thaler[188] classified cardiac deaths among 142 subjects who died during a follow-up of 5 to 10 years. Class I was labeled arrhythmic death and class II was death caused by circulatory failure. The distinction between the two classes was based on whether circulatory failure preceded (class II) or followed (class I) the disappearance of the pulse. Among deaths that occurred less than 1 hour after the onset of the terminal illness, 93 percent were due to arrhythmias; in addition, 90 percent of deaths caused by heart disease were initiated by arrhythmic events rather than circulatory failure. Deaths caused by circulatory failure occurred predominantly among patients who could be identified as having terminal illnesses (95 percent were comatose), were associated more frequently with bradyarrhythmias than with VF as the terminal arrhythmias, and were dominated by noncardiac events as the terminal illness. In contrast, 98 percent of the arrhythmic deaths were associated primarily with cardiac disorders.

Clinical Features of Cardiac Arrest

The cardiac arrest itself is characterized by abrupt loss of consciousness caused by lack of adequate cerebral blood flow. It is an event that uniformly leads to death in the absence of an active intervention, although spontaneous reversions occur rarely. The most common cardiac mechanism is VF, followed by asystole–pulseless electrical activity or severe bradyarrhythmias and sustained VT. Other mechanisms include rupture of the ventricle, cardiac tamponade, acute mechanical obstruction to flow, and acute disruption of a major blood vessel.

The potential for successful resuscitation is a function of the setting in which cardiac arrest occurs, the mechanism of the arrest, and the underlying clinical status of the victim. Closely related to the potential for successful resuscitation is the decision of whether to attempt to resuscitate.[189]

At present, there are fewer low-risk patients with otherwise uncomplicated myocardial infarctions weighting in-hospital cardiac arrest statistics than previously. Bedell and coworkers[190] reported that only 14 percent of patients receiving in-hospital cardiopulmonary resuscitation (CPR) were discharged from the hospital alive and that 20 percent of these patients died within the ensuing 6 months. Although 41 percent of the patients had suffered an acute myocardial infarction, 73 percent had a history of congestive heart failure and 20 percent had had prior cardiac arrests. The mean age of 70 years may have influenced the outcome statistics, but patients with high-risk complicated myocardial infarction and those with other high-risk markers heavily influenced the population of patients at risk for in-hospital cardiac arrest. Noncardiac clinical diagnoses were dominated by renal failure, pneumonia, sepsis, diabetes, and a history of cancer. The strong male preponderance consistently reported in out-of-hospital cardiac arrest studies is not present in in-hospital patients, but the better prognosis of VT or VF mechanisms, compared with bradyarrhythmic or asystolic mechanisms, persists (27 percent survival versus 8 percent survival). However, the proportion of arrests that are due to in-hospital VT or VF is considerably less (33 percent), with the combination of respiratory arrest, asystole, and electromechanical dissociation dominating the statistics (61 percent). In a more recent report, de Vos and colleagues[191] observed 22 percent survival to hospital discharge. Adverse risks were age older than 70 years, prior stroke or renal failure, or heart failure on admission. Better outcomes were predicted by prior angina pectoris or admission because of ventricular arrhythmias.

The important risk factors for death after CPR are listed in Table 33–3. The facts that the fraction of out-of-hospital cardiac arrest survivors who are discharged from the hospital alive may now equal or exceed the fraction of in-hospital cardiac arrest victims who are discharged alive and that the postdischarge mortality rate for in-hospital cardiac arrest survivors is higher than that for out-of-hospital cardiac arrest survivors[190] are telling clinical statistics. Not only do they emphasize the success of preventive measures for cardiac arrest in low-risk in-hospital patients, causing those statistics to be dominated by higher risk patients, but also they suggest the need for newer strategies for rapid in-hospital responses[192] in addition to emphasizing the need for improvement in prehospital and in-hospital care of out-of-hospital cardiac arrest victims.

Among elderly persons, the outcomes after community-based responses to out-of-hospital cardiac arrest are not as good as for younger victims. In one study comparing persons younger than 80 years (mean age = 64 years) with those in their 80s and 90s, survival to hospital discharge among the younger group was 19.4 percent compared with 9.4 percent for octogenarians and 4.4 percent for nonagenerians.[193]

TABLE 33–3 Predictors of Mortality after In-Hospital Cardiopulmonary Resuscitation

Before Arrest
Hypotension (systolic BP <100 mm Hg)
Pneumonia
Renal failure (BUN >50 mg/dl)
Cancer
Homebound life style
During Arrest
Arrest duration >15 min
Intubation
Hypotension (systolic BP <100 mm Hg)
Pneumonia
Homebound life style
After Resuscitation
Coma
Need for pressors
Arrest duration >15 min

BP = blood pressure; BUN = blood urea nitrogen.

Modified from Bedell SE, Delbanco TL, Cook EF, Epstein FH: Survival after cardiopulmonary resuscitation in the hospital. N Engl J Med 309:569, 1983. Copyright Massachusetts Medical Society.

However, when the groups were analyzed according to markers favoring survival (e.g., VF, pulseless VT), the incremental benefit was even better for the elderly than the younger patients (36, 24, and 17 percent, respectively). This finding suggests that age is only a weak predictor of an adverse outcome and should not be used in isolation as a reason not to resuscitate. Unfortunately, the frequency of ventricular tachyarrhythmias compared to nonshockable rhythms is lower among elderly persons.[193,194] Long-term neurological status and length of hospitalization were similar among older and younger surviving patients.

Progression to Biological Death

The time course for progression from cardiac arrest to biological death is related to the mechanism of the cardiac arrest, the nature of the underlying disease process, and the delay between onset and resuscitative efforts. The onset of irreversible brain damage usually begins within 4 to 6 minutes after loss of cerebral circulation related to unattended cardiac arrest, and biological death follows quickly. In large series, however, it has been demonstrated that a limited number of victims can remain biologically alive for longer periods and may be resuscitated after delays in excess of 8 minutes before beginning basic life support and in excess of 16 minutes before advanced life support. Despite these exceptions, it is clear that the probability of a favorable outcome deteriorates rapidly as a function of time after unattended cardiac arrest. Younger patients with less severe cardiac disease and the absence of coexistent multisystem disease appear to have a higher probability of a favorable outcome after such delays.

Irreversible injury of the central nervous system usually occurs before biological death, and the interval may extend to a period of weeks in patients who are resuscitated during the temporal gap between brain damage and biological death. In-hospital cardiac arrest caused by VF is less likely to have a protracted course between the arrest and biological death, with patients either surviving after a prompt intervention or succumbing rapidly because of inability to stabilize cardiac rhythm or hemodynamics.

The patients whose cardiac arrest is due to sustained VT with cardiac output inadequate to maintain consciousness can remain in VT for considerably longer periods, with blood flow that is marginally sufficient to maintain viability. Thus, there is a longer interval between the onset of cardiac arrest and the end of the period that allows successful resuscitation. The lives of such patients usually end in VF or an asystolic arrest if the VT is not actively or spontaneously reverted. Once the transition from VT to VF or to a bradyarrhythmia occurs, the subsequent course to biological death is similar to that in patients in whom VF or bradyarrhythmias are the initiating event.

The progression in patients with asystole or bradyarrhythmias as the initiating event is more rapid. Such patients, whether in an in-hospital or out-of-hospital environment, have a poor prognosis because of advanced heart disease or coexistent multisystem disease. They tend to respond poorly to interventions, even if the heart is successfully paced. Although a small subgroup of patients with bradyarrhythmias associated with electrolyte or pharmacological abnormalities may respond well to interventions, the majority progress rapidly to biological death. The infrequent cardiac arrests caused by mechanical factors such as tamponade, structural disruption, and impedance to flow by major thromboembolic obstructions to right or left ventricular outflow are reversible only in the instances in which the mechanism is recognized and an intervention is feasible. The vast majority of these events lead to rapid biological death, although prompt relief of tamponade may save some lives.

Hospital Course of Survivors of Cardiac Arrest

The conditions of patients who are resuscitated immediately from *primary* VF associated with acute myocardial infarction usually stabilize promptly, and they require no special management after the early phase of the infarction (see Chap. 47). The management after *secondary cardiac arrest in myocardial infarction* is dominated by the hemodynamic status of the patient. Among survivors of *out-of-hospital cardiac arrest,* the initial 24 to 48 hours of hospitalization are characterized by a tendency to ventricular arrhythmias, which usually respond well to antiarrhythmic therapy. The overall rate of recurrent cardiac arrest is low, 10 to 20 percent, but the mortality rate in patients who have recurrent cardiac arrests is about 50 percent. Only 5 to 10 percent of in-hospital deaths after out-of-hospital resuscitation are due to recurrent cardiac arrhythmias.[182,183] Patients who have recurrent cardiac arrest have a high incidence of either new or preexisting AV or intraventricular conduction abnormalities.[171]

The most common causes of death in hospitalized survivors of out-of-hospital cardiac arrest are noncardiac events related to central nervous system injury.[171,195] These include anoxic encephalopathy and sepsis related to prolonged intubation and hemodynamic monitoring lines. Fifty-nine percent of deaths during index hospitalization after prehospital resuscitation have been reported to be due to such causes. Approximately 40 percent of those who arrive in hospital in coma never awaken after admission to the hospital and die after a median survival of 3.5 days. Two-thirds of those who regain consciousness have no gross deficits, and an additional 20 percent have persisting cognitive deficits only. Of the patients who do awaken, 25 percent do so by admission, 71 percent by the first hospital day, and 92 percent by the third day. A small number of patients awakened after prolonged hospitalization. Among those who die in hospital, 80 percent do not awaken before death. Two studies suggest a potential benefit of therapeutic hypothermia for patients with post-cardiac arrest coma (see Post-Cardiac Arrest Care in Survivors of Out-of-Hospital Cardiac Arrest).[196,197]

Cardiac causes of delayed death during hospitalization after out-of-hospital cardiac arrest are most commonly related to hemodynamic deterioration, which accounts for about one-third of deaths in hospitals. Among all deaths, those that occurred within the first 48 hours of hospitalization were usually due to hemodynamic deterioration or arrhythmias regardless of the neurological status; later deaths were related to neurological complications. Admission characteristics most predictive of subsequent awakening included motor response, pupillary light response, spontaneous eye movement, and blood glucose level below 300 mg/dl.

Clinical Profile of Survivors of Out-of-Hospital Cardiac Arrest

The clinical features of survivors of out-of-hospital cardiac arrest are heavily influenced by the type and extent of the underlying disease associated with the event. Causation is dominated by coronary heart disease, which accounts for approximately 80 percent of out-of-hospital cardiac arrest in the United States[9] and is commonly extensive. The cardiomyopathies collectively account for another 10 to 15 percent, with all other structural heart diseases plus functional abnormalities and toxic or environmental causes accounting for the remainder (see Table 33–2).[76,198]

Ambient ventricular arrhythmias have been reported in the majority of survivors of prehospital cardiac arrest who had serial ambulatory monitor recordings. These arrhythmias show trends to higher grades of ventricular ectopy in victims of recurrent cardiac arrest compared with long-term survivors. Repetitive PVCs were strongly associated with a history of congestive heart failure or previous myocardial infarction.

LEFT VENTRICULAR FUNCTION. Left ventricular function is abnormal in the majority of survivors of out-of-hospital cardiac arrest, often severely so, but there is a wide variation, ranging from severe dysfunction to normal or near-normal measurements (Fig. 33–12).[199] The severity of myocardial dysfunction estimated shortly after cardiac arrest commonly improves within the first 24 hours of hospitalization.[200] Failure to begin improvement within that time frame is an adverse short-term prognostic sign. In a study of resuscitated out-of-hospital cardiac arrest victims admitted to hospital and subsequently discharged alive and neurologically intact, 47 percent had acute coronary syndromes identified during work-up and had a mean ejection fraction of 42 percent, compared with 32 percent among nonsurvivors.[201] Among survivors to hospital discharge, a reduced ejection fraction is an adverse long-term prognostic sign.

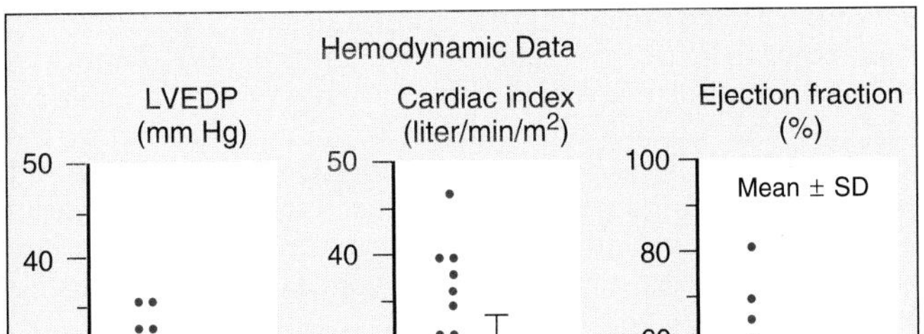

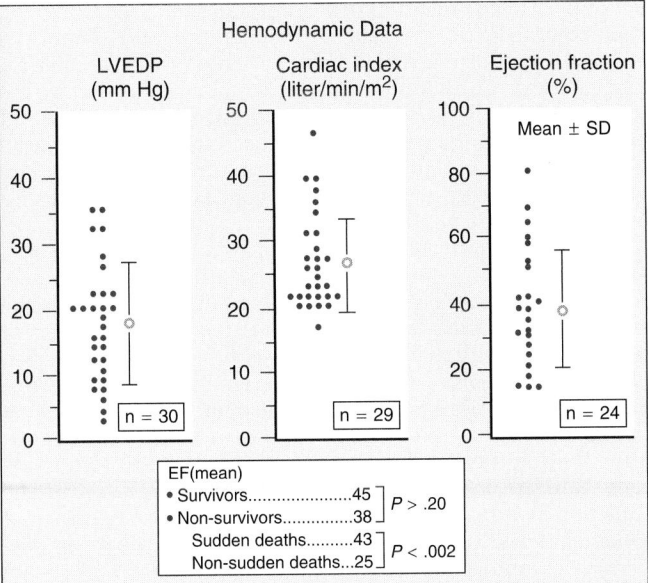

FIGURE 33–12 Hemodynamic data from victims of prehospital cardiac arrest studied during initial postarrest hospitalization. These data indicate a broad range of cardiac function and a statistically insignificant difference between ejection fraction at entry in long-term survivors and in victims of recurrent cardiac arrest. However, patients who died suddenly had significantly higher ejection fraction than those who died of non-sudden cardiac causes. LVEDP = left ventricular end-diastolic pressure. (From Myerburg RJ, Conde CA, Sung RJ, et al: Clinical, electrophysiologic and hemodynamic profile of patients resuscitated from prehospital cardiac arrest. Am J Med 68:568, 1980.)

CORONARY ANGIOGRAPHY. Studies of survivors of out-of-hospital cardiac arrest have shown that as a group this population tends to have extensive disease but no specific pattern of abnormalities. Acute coronary lesions, usually multifocal, are present in a majority of survivors.[168] Significant lesions in two or more vessels are present in at least 70 percent of patients who have any coronary lesion. Among patients who have recurrent cardiac arrests, the incidence of triple-vessel disease is higher than among those who do not. However, the frequency of moderate to severe stenosis of the left main coronary artery does not differ between cardiac arrest survivors and the overall population of patients with symptomatic coronary heart disease.

EXERCISE TESTING. Exercise testing is no longer commonly used to evaluate the need for, and response to, antiischemic therapy in survivors of out-of-hospital cardiac arrest, except when there is a question of transient ischemia as a mechanism for onset. The probability of a positive test related to ischemia is relatively low, although termination of testing because of fatigue is common.[171] Mortality during follow-up is greater in patients who have angina or failure of a normal rise in systolic blood pressure occurring during exercise.

ELECTROCARDIOGRAPHIC OBSERVATIONS. Among survivors of out-of-hospital cardiac arrest, the 12-lead ECG (see Chap. 9) has proved of value only for discriminating risk of recurrence among those whose cardiac arrest was associated with new transmural myocardial infarction. Patients who develop documented new Q waves in association with a clinical picture suggesting that an acute myocardial infarction began before the cardiac arrest itself are at lower risk for recurrence.[171] In contrast, nonspecific ECG markers of ischemia, associated with elevations of troponin or creatine kinase MB, indicate higher risk of recurrence.[162] A higher incidence of repolarization abnormalities (ST segment depression, flat T waves, prolonged QT) occurs in out-of-hospital cardiac arrest survivors than in post-myocardial infarction patients, and these might be markers for increased risk. Prolonged QRS duration is associated with increased mortality risk in patients with heart failure,[202] although it is not clear that this observation applies to sudden death specifically or to post-cardiac arrest victims in particular.

BLOOD CHEMISTRY. Lower serum K^+ levels are observed in survivors of cardiac arrest than in patients with acute myocardial infarction or stable coronary heart disease. This finding is probably a consequence of resuscitation interventions rather than a preexisting hypokalemic state owing to chronic diuretic use or other causes. Low ionized Ca^{2+} levels, with normal total calcium levels, were also observed during resuscitation from out-of-hospital cardiac arrest. Higher resting lactate levels have been reported in out-of-hospital cardiac arrest survivors than in normal subjects. Lactate levels correlated inversely with ejection fractions and directly with PVC frequency and complexity.

LONG-TERM PROGNOSIS. Studies from the early 1970s in both Miami[182] and Seattle[183] indicated that the risk of recurrent cardiac arrest in the first year after surviving an initial VT-VF event was about 30 percent and at 2 years was 45 percent. Total mortality at 2 years was about 60 percent in both studies. More recent total mortality data from the control groups of the secondary prevention implantable cardioverter-defibrillator (ICD) trials demonstrated a 2-year mortality rate between 20 and 25 percent.[203-205] The apparent improved outcomes, independent of the benefit provided by ICD therapy, are probably attributable to the current interventions used among survivors, such as beta adrenoceptor blockers, antiischemic procedures, amiodarone, and other therapies that were not available or in general use at the earlier time. Risk of recurrent cardiac arrest and all-cause mortality is higher during the first 12 to 24 months after the index event and relates best to ejection fraction during the first 6 months (Fig. 33–13).

Management of Cardiac Arrest

Community-Based Interventions

The initial systems responding to out-of-hospital cardiac arrests as developed in the United States were integrated into fire departments as primary emergency rescue systems. They employed paramedical personnel trained in CPR and the use of CPR monitoring equipment, defibrillators, and specific intravenous drug therapy. Although the initial out-of-hospital intervention experience in Miami and Seattle[182,183] reported in the mid-1970s yielded only 14 and 11 percent survivals to discharge, respectively, later improvements in the systems saved more lives (Fig. 33–14A).[206] By the early 1980s both had increased survival rates to about 25 percent[171,206] and by the late 1980s to 30 percent or more. Improvements correlated with the addition of emergency medical technicians as another tier of responders to provide CPR and earlier defibrillation. Survival rates have decreased since then, presumably because of the extension of rescue systems into less densely populated regions,[207] in addition to increased traffic congestion and verticalization of buildings

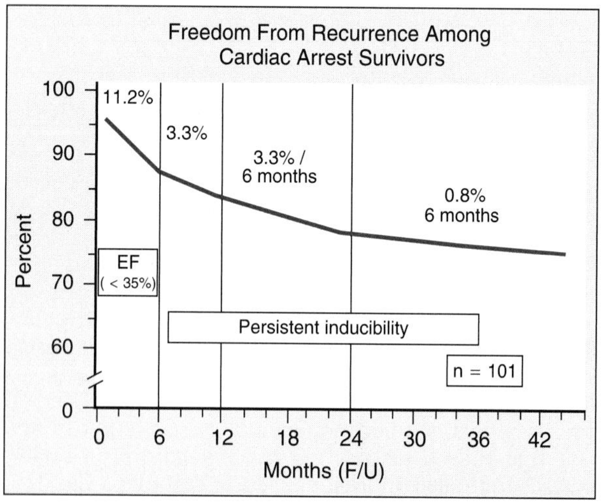

FIGURE 33–13 Time dependence of recurrences among survivors of cardiac arrest. Actuarial analysis of occurrences among a population of 101 cardiac arrest survivors with coronary artery disease is demonstrated. The risk was highest in the first 6 months (11.2 percent) and then fell to 3.3 percent per 6 months for the next three 6-month blocks. After 24 months, the rate fell to 0.8 percent per 6 months. A low ejection fraction (EF) was the most powerful predictor of death during the first 6 months; subsequently, persistent inducibility during programmed stimulation, despite drug therapy or surgery, was the most powerful predictor. F/U = follow-up. (Modified from Furukawa T, Rozanski JJ, Nogami A, et al: Time-dependent risk of and predictors for cardiac arrest recurrence in survivors of out-of-hospital cardiac arrest with chronic coronary artery disease. Circulation 80:599, 1989. The figure is reproduced from Myerburg RJ, Kessler KM, Castellanos A: Sudden cardiac death: Structure, function, and time-dependence of risk. Circulation 85[Suppl I]:I-2, 1992. Copyright 1992 American Heart Association.)

in urban areas (see Fig. 33–14A). Generally, rural areas have lower success rates,[208,209] and the national success rate for the United States is probably 5 percent or less.

Reports from very densely populated areas (i.e., Chicago and New York City) have also provided disturbing outcome data. The Chicago study reported that only 9 percent of out-of-hospital cardiac arrest victims survived to be hospitalized and that only 2 percent were discharged alive.[41] Moreover, outcomes in blacks were far worse than in whites (0.8 percent versus 2.6 percent). The fact that a large majority had bradyarrhythmias, asystole, or pulseless electrical activity on initial contact with emergency medical services suggests prolonged times between collapse and emergency medical service arrival or absent or ineffective bystander interventions, or both. The New York City report indicated a survival-to-hospital discharge rate of only 1.4 percent.[210] Among those who had bystander CPR, the rate increased to 2.9 percent, and bystander CPR plus VF as the initial rhythm yielded a further increase to 5.3 percent. Finally, for those whose arrests occurred after the arrival of emergency medical services, the success rate increased further to 8.5 percent. These trends suggest that delays and breaks in the "chain of survival"[211] have a major negative impact on results of emergency medical services in densely populated areas.

IMPORTANCE OF ELECTRICAL MECHANISMS. Several sources have identified a disturbing trend in initial rhythms recorded by emergency rescue personnel.[7,212,213] Compared with data from the 1970s and 1980s, there has been a decrease in the number of events in which ventricular tachyarrhythmias are the initial rhythm recorded, with a consequent reduction in the proportion of victims who have rhythms amenable to cardioversion-defibrillation (Fig. 33–15). Some studies now suggest that less than one-half of victims are in shockable rhythms at initial contact. This fact is associated with a reduction in cumulative survival probabilities from community-based interventions,[7] even though data from studies employing nonconventional automated external defibrillator (AED) strategies suggest improvement for outcomes in VT or VF victims.[212,213] Because this finding does not appear to be related to time from 911 summons to arrival, it is likely that pre-911 delays in recognition and reaction to an event may be playing a role, which suggests a need for more extensive public education programs. Thus "response times" may not be as close to true "down times" as one would hope, impairing the potential for success. The 4- to 6-minute time for a desirable response is not optimal. By 4 minutes significant circulatory and ischemic changes have occurred, and beyond that time conditions worsen rapidly.[214]

The electrical mechanism of out-of-hospital cardiac arrest, as defined by the initial rhythm recorded by emergency rescue personnel, has a powerful impact on outcome. The subgroup of patients who are in sustained VT at the time of first contact, although small, has the best outcome (Fig. 33–16). Eighty-eight percent of patients in cardiac arrest related to VT were successfully resuscitated and admitted to the hospital alive, and 67 percent were ultimately discharged alive.[171] However, this relatively low-risk group represents only 7 to 10 percent of all cardiac arrests. Because of the inherent time lag between collapse and initial recordings, it is likely that many more cardiac arrests begin as rapid sustained VT and degenerate into VF before arrival of rescue personnel.

Patients who have a bradyarrhythmia or asystole at initial contact have the worst prognosis; only 9 percent of such patients in the Miami study were admitted to the hospital alive and none was discharged.[171] In a later experience there was some improvement in outcome, although the improvement was limited to patients in whom the initial bradyarrhythmia recorded was an idioventricular rhythm that responded promptly to chronotropic agents in the field. Bradyarrhythmias also have adverse prognostic implications after defibrillation from VF in the field. Patients who developed a heart rate less than 60 beats/min after defibrillation regardless of the specific bradyarrhythmic mechanism had a poor prognosis, with 95 percent of such patients dying either before hospitalization or in the hospital.[182]

The outcome in the group of patients in whom VF is the initial rhythm recorded is intermediate between the outcomes associated with sustained VT and bradyarrhythmia and asystole. Figure 33–16 demonstrates that 40 percent of such patients were successfully resuscitated and admitted to the hospital alive and 23 percent were ultimately discharged alive.[171] Later data indicate improvement in outcome. The proportion of each of the electrophysiological mechanisms responsible for cardiac arrest varied among the earlier reports, with VF ranging from 65 to more than 90 percent of the study populations and bradyarrhythmia and asystole ranging from 10 to 30 percent. However, in reports from densely populated metropolitan areas, the ratios of tachyarrhythmic to bradyarrhythmic or pulseless activity events were reversed, and outcomes were far worse.[41,210]

A

History of Community-Based EMS Systems		
1971–1974	Initial Miami/Seattle outcomes	14%, 11%
1978–1985	Peak Miami/Seattle outcomes	25–35%
1984	Rural outcomes: Standard basic life support Ambulance-based expanded access	 3% 19%
1991	Estimated cumulative U.S. survival	1–3%
1992–1994	Major metropolitan population centers	≤ 2%
1996	Dade County, Florida, outcomes	9%
1996–1998	Current U.S. EMS outcomes, cumulative	< 5%
1999	"Optimized" systems (OPALS)	5%

B

AED Deployment Strategies				
Deployment	**Examples**	**Rescuers**	**Advantages**	**Limitations**
Emergency vehicles	Police cars Fire engines Ambulances	Trained emergency personnel	Experienced users Broad deployment Objectivity	Deployment time Arrival delays Community variations
Public access sites	Public buildings Stadiums, malls Airports Airliners	Security personnel Designated rescuers Random lay persons	Population density Shorter delays Lay and emergency personnel access	Low event rates Inexperienced users Panic and confusion
Multi-family dwellings	Apartments Condominiums Hotels	Security personnel Designated rescuers Family members	Familiar locations Defined personnel Shorter delays	Infrequent use Low event rates Geographic factors
Single-family dwellings	Private homes Apartments Neighborhood "Heart Watch"	Family members Security personnel Designated rescuers	Immediate access Familiar setting	Acceptance Victim may be alone One-time user; panic

FIGURE 33–14 Out-of-hospital cardiac arrest survival and deployment strategies for automated external defibrillators (AEDs). **A,** The history of out-of-hospital cardiac arrest survival statistics demonstrates that standard emergency rescue systems are not sufficient to have a meaningful impact on sudden cardiac death in the community. **B,** Various deployment strategies for nonconventional responders with access to AEDs. For each example, the type of rescuer and the advantages and limitations of each strategy are provided. It is unlikely that any single strategy will dominate; rather, there will be a cumulative benefit from the additive effect of multiple approaches. EMS = emergency medical service; OPALS = Ontario Prehospital Advanced Life Support. (From Myerburg RJ: Sudden cardiac death: Exploring the limits of our knowledge. J Cardiovasc Electrophysiol 12:369, 2001.)

Both improved prehospital care and improvements in in-hospital technology and practices can contribute to better outcomes, as described in the chain of survival concept.[211] Of these two general factors, the influence of prehospital care has been studied in more detail. The importance of early defibrillation for improving outcome is supported by a number of studies (Fig. 33–17).[214-218] In rural communities, earlier defibrillation by ambulance technicians yielded a 19 percent survival compared with only 3 percent for standard CPR. In another report, an analysis of the relationship between response delay and survival to hospital discharge revealed a 48 percent survival for response times of 2 minutes or less compared with less than 10 percent survival when responses were longer than 10 minutes (Fig. 33–18A).[215] Mean response time was approximately 13 minutes, and overall survival was 5 percent. It was 9.5 percent for those in VT or VF on first contact. These observations have motivated the search for strategies that shorten response times, such as deploying automatic external defibrillators in public places[218] and for use by nonconventional responders.[212,216,217] Preliminary data suggest that this strategy may improve outcome by substantial increments based upon the rationale of shortening response times (see later and Fig. 33–18B).

A second element in prehospital care that appears to contribute to outcome is the role of bystander CPR by laypeople awaiting the arrival of emergency rescue personnel.[219,220] It has been reported that although there was no significant difference in the percentage of patients successfully resuscitated and admitted to the hospital alive with (67 percent) or without (61 percent) bystander intervention, almost twice as many prehospital cardiac arrest victims were ultimately discharged alive when they had had bystander CPR (43 percent) than when such support was not provided (22 percent). Central nervous system protection, expressed as early regaining of consciousness, is the major protective element of bystander CPR. The rationale for bystander intervention is further highlighted by the relation between time to defibrillation and survival when analyzed as a function of time to initiation of basic CPR. It has been reported that more than 40 percent of victims whose defibrillation and other advanced life support activities were instituted more than 8

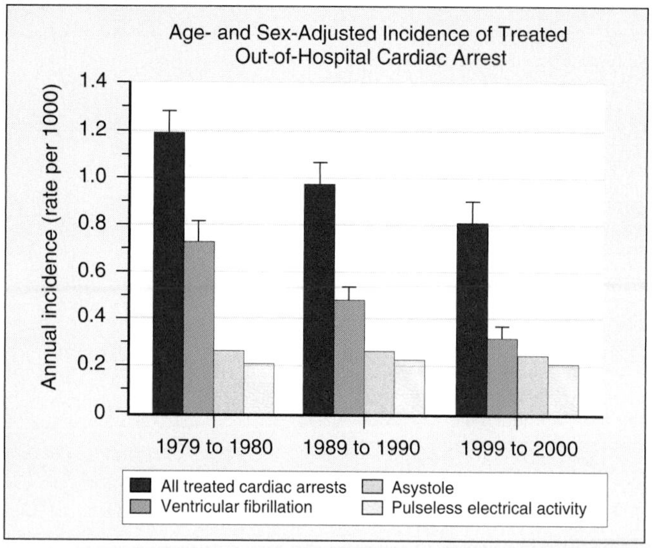

FIGURE 33–15 Changing incidence of ventricular fibrillation in the community. Between 1980 and 2000, there was a progressive decrease in the ventricular fibrillation event rate in the Seattle, Washington, community for unexplained reasons. Of note is the fact that there was not a concomitant increase in nonshockable rhythms. The proportion of events with ventricular fibrillation at initial contact is decreasing, as observed in several other studies. (Modified from Cobb LA, Fahrenbruch CE, Olsufka M, Copass MK: Changing incidence of out-of-hospital ventricular fibrillation, 1980-2000. JAMA 288:3008, 2002.)

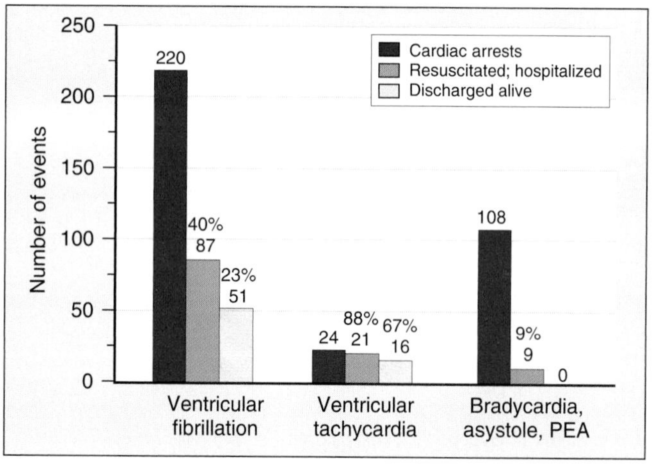

FIGURE 33–16 Survival after out-of-hospital cardiac arrest as function of the initial electrophysiological mechanism recorded by emergency rescue personnel. The mechanisms among 352 out-of-hospital cardiac arrest victims are separated into three categories: ventricular fibrillation (n = 220; 62 percent); ventricular tachycardia (n = 24; 7 percent); and bradycardia, asystole, and pulseless electrical activity (PEA) (n = 108; 31 percent). The purple bars illustrate the total number of events in each category. The blue bars illustrate the number and percentage of patients who were initially resuscitated in the field and reached the hospital alive in each category, and the yellow illustrate the percentage of total events in which patients were discharged from the hospital alive for each category. The data are derived from the Miami, Florida, experience.[211]

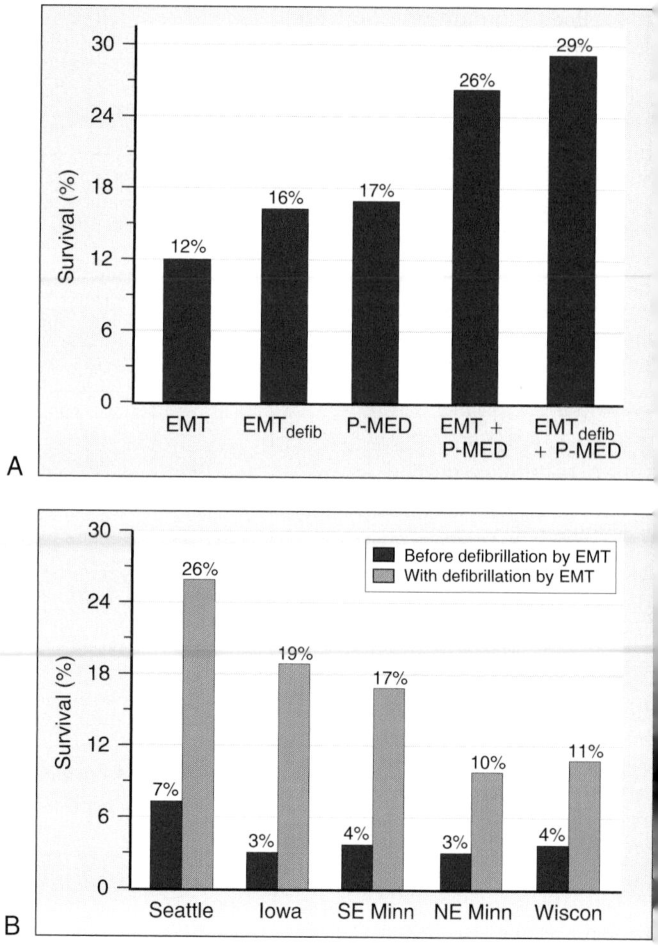

FIGURE 33–17 Impact of emergency rescue system design and immediate defibrillation on out-of-hospital cardiac arrest survival. **A,** Percent survival to hospital discharge with rescue activities by standard emergency medical technician (EMT) trained in cardiopulmonary resuscitation (CPR), EMTs allowed to defibrillate immediately (EMT_{defib}), initial response by paramedics (P-MED), two-tiered system with EMT and P-MED, and two-tiered system with EMTs allowed to defibrillate if they are the first responders plus P-MED. Training of first-responders (EMT_{defib}) and a two-tiered system have the best outcome. **B,** Comparison of outcomes observed in five geographic areas with EMTs providing only CPR (purple) versus EMTs trained to defibrillate as first responders (blue). In each group, there was a marked improvement in outcome when EMT personnel were trained and permitted to defibrillate. (Modified from Ornato JP, Om A: Community experience in treating out-of-hospital cardiac arrest. *In* Akhtar M, Myerburg RJ, Ruskin JN [eds]: Sudden Cardiac Death: Prevalence, Mechanisms and Approach to Diagnosis and Management. Baltimore, Williams & Wilkins, 1994, p 450.)

minutes after collapse survived if basic CPR had been initiated less than 2 minutes after onset of the arrest.[206] A period of CPR before defibrillation may also be helpful,[219] particularly if the time to defibrillation exceeds 4 minutes from onset of arrest.[214,221]

The time from onset of cardiac arrest to advanced life support influences outcome statistics. Improvement in both early neurological status and survival occurs in patients defibrillated by first responders, even if they are minimally trained emergency technicians allowed to carry out defibrillation as part of basic life support, compared with outcomes associated with awaiting more highly trained paramedics. Thus, the time to defibrillation plays a central role in determining outcome in cardiac arrest caused by VF. The development and deployment of AEDs (see Chap. 31) in the community hold promise for progress in the future.[218] This technology is potentially applicable with a number of different strategic models, each with its own benefits and limitations (see Fig. 33–14B).

Among the strategies that have yielded identifiable benefit to date are deployment in police vehicles,[212,213,217] airliners and airports,[224,225] casinos,[226] and more general community-based sites.[213,218] Police AED deployment data have been inconsistent among various studies,[209,212,213,217] possibly because of appropriateness for various types of communities and specific deployment strategies used, but data suggest that in large metropolitan areas there is benefit (Fig. 33–19).[212] Initial airline data were similarly uncertain, but a report on data from a large airline with a well-organized system sug-

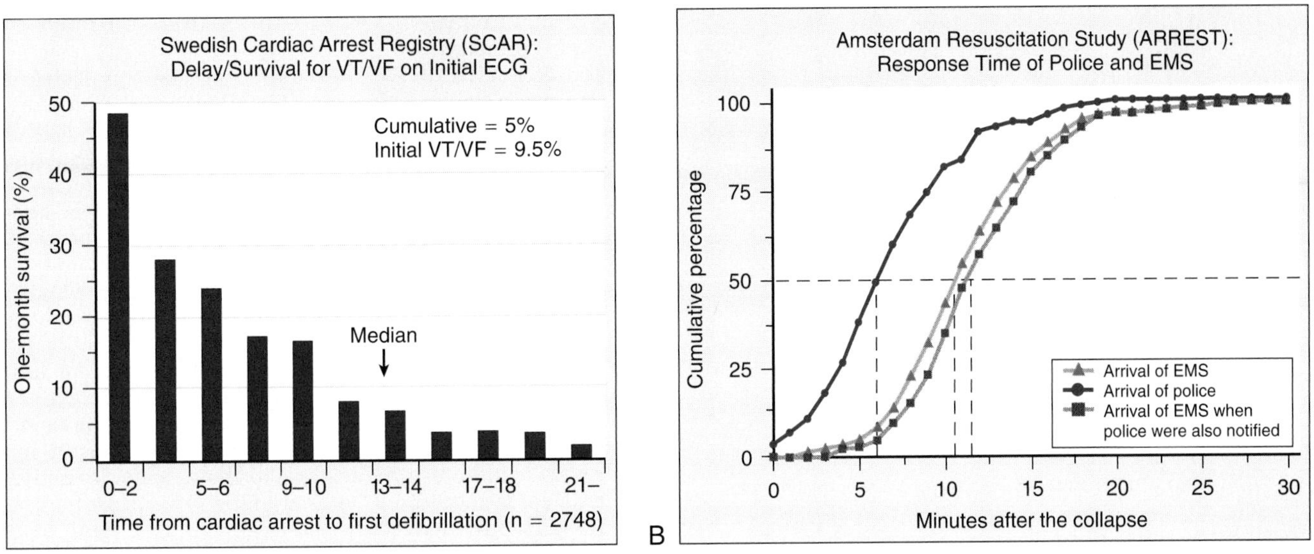

FIGURE 33–18 Influence of response time on survival from out-of-hospital cardiac arrest. **A,** The time from onset of cardiac arrest to initial defibrillation attempt is related to 1-month survival on the basis of data from the Swedish Cardiac Arrest Registry.[214] The cumulative survival rate was 5 percent, and the survival rate for victims whose initial rhythm was ventricular tachycardia (VT) or ventricular fibrillation (VF) was 9.5 percent. The median response time was nearly 13 minutes. Thirty-day survival ranged from a maximum of 48 percent with responses of less than 2 minutes to less than 5 percent with response time greater than 15 minutes. **B,** The potential for faster response systems, based on the Amsterdam Resuscitation Study, is demonstrated, comparing response times of police vehicles with those of conventional emergency medical systems (EMS). At the 50th percentile of response times, police vehicles provided a nearly 5-minute improvement in arrival time (approximately 6 minutes).[215]

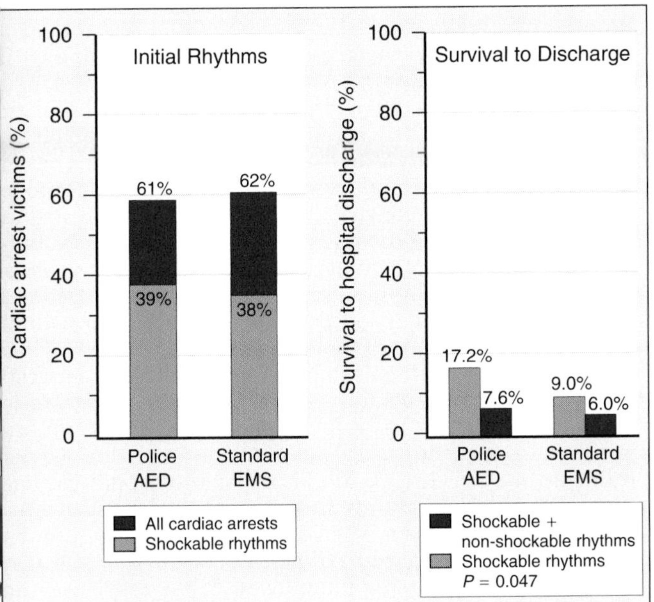

FIGURE 33–19 Rhythms at initial contact and survival statistics from the Miami–Dade County, Florida, police automated external defibrillator (AED) project. Shockable rhythms were observed in just under 40 percent in both the police AED program and the standard emergency medical system (EMS) historical control data. Those with shockable rhythms had improved survival to hospital discharge, with only a small improvement when both shockable and nonshockable rhythms were included in the analyzed data. (Modified from Myerburg RJ, Fenster J, Velez M, et al: Impact of community-wide police car deployment of automated external defibrillators on out-of-hospital cardiac arrest. Circulation 106:1058, 2002. Reproduced with permission of the American Heart Association).

gested benefit (Fig. 33–20A).[222] Similar encouraging results have been reported from deployment of AEDs in the Chicago airport system.[223] Finally, the special circumstance of casinos, in which continuous television monitoring alerts security officers to medical problems immediately, yielded impressive survival rates (Fig. 33–20B).[224] For more general community sites, defined as true public access including single-family dwellings, data are not yet available to determine benefit. However, there appears to be a great deal of variability of efficiency on the basis of expected event rates at different types of community sites.[218]

Management of Cardiac Arrest and Post-Cardiac Arrest Care

Management of the cardiac arrest victim is divided into five elements: (1) initial assessment, (2) basic life support, (3) advanced life support and definitive resuscitative efforts, (4) post-cardiac arrest care, and (5) long-term management. The first of these can be applied by a broad population base, which includes physicians and nurses as well as paramedical personnel, emergency rescue technicians, and laypeople educated in bystander intervention. The requirements for specialized knowledge and skills become progressively more focused as the patient moves through post-cardiac arrest management and into long-term follow-up care.[189]

Initial Assessment and Basic Life Support

This activity includes both diagnostic maneuvers and elementary interventions. The first action of the persons or persons in attendance when an individual collapses unexpectedly must be *confirmation that collapse is due to (or suspected to be due to) a cardiac arrest.* A few seconds of evaluation for response to voice, observation for respiratory movements and skin color, and simultaneous palpation of major arteries for the presence or absence of a pulse yield sufficient information to determine whether a life-threatening incident is in progress. Once a life-threatening incident is suspected or confirmed, contact with an available emergency medical rescue system (911) should be an immediate priority.[189]

The absence of a carotid or femoral pulse, particularly if confirmed by the absence of an audible heartbeat, is a primary diagnostic criterion. For lay responders, the pulse check is no longer recommended.[189] Skin color may be pale or intensely cyanotic. Absence of respiratory efforts or the presence of

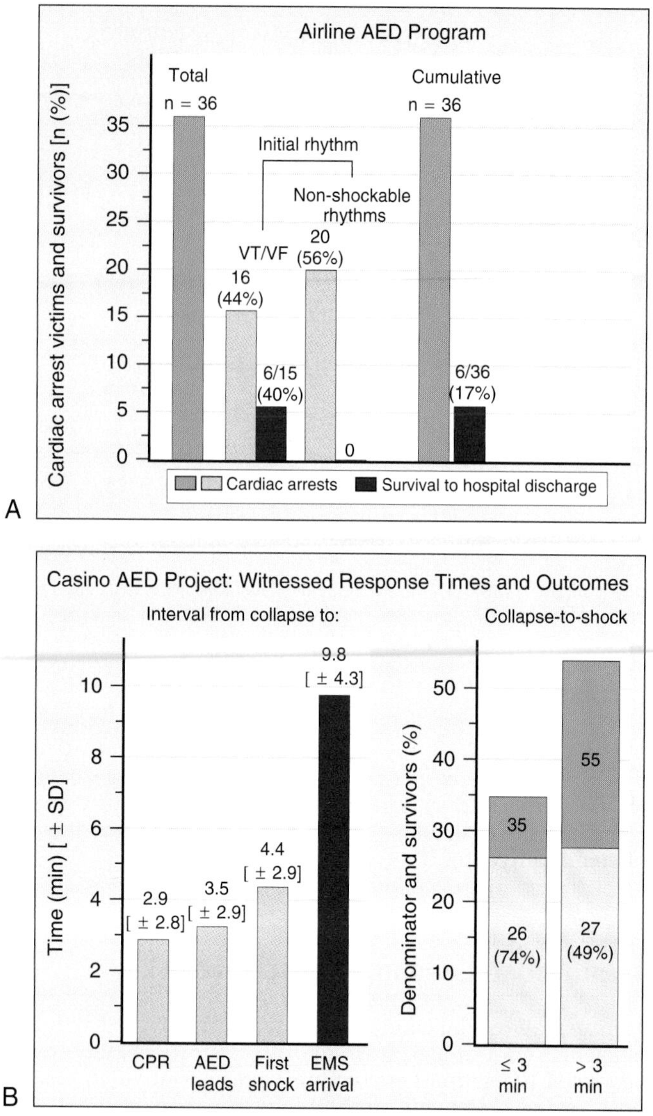

FIGURE 33–20 Outcomes of automated external defibrillator (AED) deployment programs at specific public sites. **A,** The data on outcomes after deployment of AEDs on a major airline demonstrated that approximately 44 percent of the cardiac arrests were associated with a documented ventricular tachycardia or fibrillation (VT/VF) mechanism and 40 percent of those victims survived. There were no survivors among the 56 percent of the victims who had nonshockable rhythms. Cumulative survival for the program was 17 percent. **B,** The results of AED deployment in the controlled environment of casinos. Because the onset of cardiac arrest can frequently be witnessed, short intervals from onset of collapse to cardiopulmonary resuscitation (CPR) and AED shocks were achieved. Response times were reduced by more than 50 percent compared with the standard emergency medical system (EMS). For those found in VT/VF, survival was better than expected from other community-based systems and approached 60 percent for VT/VF with a witnessed onset. When response time was less than 3 minutes, survival for VT/VF was more than 70 percent. (**A,** Modified from Page RL, Joglar JA, Kowal RC, et al. Use of automated external defibrillators by a U.S. airline. N Engl J Med 343:1210, 2000; **B,** modified from Valenzuela TD, Roe DJ, Nichol G, et al. Outcomes of rapid defibrillation by security officers after cardiac arrest in casinos. N Engl J Med 343:1206, 2000.)

only agonal respiratory efforts, in conjunction with an absent pulse, is diagnostic of cardiac arrest; however, respiratory efforts can persist for a minute or more after the onset of the arrest. In contrast, absence of respiratory efforts or severe stridor with persistence of a pulse suggests a primary respiratory arrest that will lead to a cardiac arrest in a short time. In the latter circumstance, initial efforts should include exploration of the oropharynx in search of a foreign body and the Heimlich maneuver, particularly if the incident occurs in a setting in which aspiration is likely (e.g., restaurant death or cafe coronary).

CHEST THUMP. When the diagnosis of a pulseless collapse (presumed cardiac arrest) is established, a blow to the chest (precordial thump, "thump-version") may be attempted by a properly trained rescuer. It has been recommended to be reserved as an advanced life support activity.[189] Caldwell and coworkers[225] supported its use on the basis of a prospective study in 5000 patients. Precordial thumps successfully reverted VF in 5 events, VT in 11, asystole in 2, and undefined cardiovascular collapse in 2 others in which the electrical mechanism was unknown. In no instance was conversion of VT to VF observed. Because the latter is the only major concern about the precordial thump technique and electrical activity can be initiated by mechanical stimulation in the asystolic heart, the technique is considered optional for responding to a *pulseless* cardiac arrest in the absence of monitoring when a defibrillator is not immediately available. It should not be used unmonitored for the patient with a rapid tachycardia without complete loss of consciousness. For attempted thump-version in cardiac arrest, one or two blows should be delivered firmly to the junction of the middle and lower thirds of the sternum from a height of 8 to 10 inches, but the effort should be abandoned if the patient does not immediately develop a spontaneous pulse and begin breathing. Another mechanical method, which requires that the patient is still conscious, is so-called cough-induced cardiac compression or cough-version. It is a conscious act of forceful coughing by the patient that may support forward flow by cyclic increases in intrathoracic pressure during VF or may cause conversion of sustained VT. Data supporting its successful use exist but are limited, and it is not considered an alternative to conventional techniques.

THE ABCS OF CARDIOPULMONARY RESUSCITATION. The goal of this activity is to maintain viability of the central nervous system, heart, and other vital organs until definitive intervention can be achieved. The activities included within basic life support encompass both the initial responses outlined earlier and their natural flow into establishing ventilation and perfusion. This range of activities can be carried out not only by professional and paraprofessional personnel but also by trained emergency technicians and laypeople. Time is the key issue, and there should be minimal delay between the diagnosis and preparatory efforts in the initial response and the institution of basic life support. This principle has measurable impact for both out-of-hospital and in-hospital cardiac arrest. Survival to discharge for in-hospital cardiac arrests, considering all etiologies and mechanisms, was reported to be 33 percent when CPR was initiated within the first minute compared with 14 percent when the time was more than 1 minute (odds ratio, 3.06).[192] When VF was the initial rhythm, the corresponding figures were 50 and 32 percent. In the out-of-hospital setting if only one witness is present, notification of emergency personnel (telephone 911) is the only activity that should precede basic life support.

AIRWAY. Clearing the airway is a critical step in preparing for successful resuscitation. This process includes tilting the head backward and lifting the chin in addition to exploring the airway for foreign bodies—including dentures—and removing them. The Heimlich maneuver should be performed if there is reason to suspect a foreign body lodged in the oropharynx. This maneuver entails wrapping the arms around the victim from the back and delivering a sharp thrust to the upper abdomen with a closed fist. If it is not possible for the person in attendance to carry out the maneuver because of insufficient physical strength, mechanical dislodgment of the foreign body can sometimes be achieved by abdominal thrusts with the unconscious patient in a supine position. The Heimlich maneuver is not entirely benign; ruptured abdominal viscera in the victim have been reported, as was an instance in which the rescuer disrupted his own aortic root and died. If there is strong suspicion that respiratory arrest precipitated cardiac arrest, particularly in the presence of a mechanical airway obstruction, a second precordial thump should be delivered after the airway is cleared.

BREATHING. With the head properly placed and the oropharynx clear, mouth-to-mouth respiration can be initiated if no specific rescue equipment is available. To a large extent, the procedure used for establishing ventilation depends on the site at which the cardiac arrest occurs. A variety of devices are available, including plastic oropharyngeal airways, esophageal obturators, the masked Ambu bag, and endotracheal tubes. Intubation is the preferred procedure, but time should not be sacrificed even in the in-hospital setting while awaiting an endotracheal tube or a person trained to insert it quickly and properly. Thus, in the in-hospital setting, temporary support with Ambu bag ventilation is the usual method until endotracheal intubation can be carried out, and in the out-of-hospital setting mouth-to-mouth resuscitation is used while awaiting emergency rescue personnel. The effect of the acquired immunodeficiency syndrome and hepatitis B transmission on attitudes toward mouth-to-mouth resuscitation by bystanders and even professional personnel in hospitals is an area of concern, but currently available data assessing risk of infection suggest that it is minimal.[189] The impact of this concern on attitudes toward, and outcomes of, resuscitative efforts has not been assessed.

Conventional CPR ventilatory techniques require that the lungs be inflated twice in succession after every 15 chest compressions.[189] Techniques of CPR based on the hypothesis that increased intrathoracic pressure is the prime mover of blood, rather than cardiac compression itself, have been evaluated; the cyclic ventilatory techniques are altered in these procedures (see later). However, clinical applicability is still not clarified.[226]

CIRCULATION (Fig. 33–21). This element of basic life support is intended to maintain blood flow (i.e., circulation) until definitive steps can be taken. The rationale is based on the hypothesis that chest compression allows the heart to maintain an externally driven pump function by sequential emptying and filling of its chambers, with competent valves favoring the forward direction of flow. In fact, the application of this technique has proved successful when used as recommended.[189] The palm of one hand is placed over the lower sternum and the heel of the other rests on the dorsum of the lower hand. The sternum is then depressed with the resuscitator's arms straight at the elbows to provide a less tiring and more forceful fulcrum at the junction of the shoulders and back (see Fig. 33–21). By using this technique, sufficient force is applied to depress the sternum about 4 to 5 cm, with abrupt relaxation, and the cycle is carried out at a rate of about 100 compressions per minute. Despite the fact that this conventional technique produces measurable carotid artery flow and a record of successful resuscitations, the absence of a pressure gradient across the heart in the presence of an extrathoracic arterial-venous pressure gradient has led to a concept that it is not cardiac compression per se but rather a pumping action produced by pressure changes in the entire thoracic cavity that optimizes systemic blood flow during resuscitation. Experimental work in which the chest is compressed during ventilations rather than between them (simultaneous compression-ventilation) had demonstrated better extrathoracic arterial flow. However, increased carotid artery flow does not necessarily equate with improved cerebral perfusion, and the reduction in coronary blood flow caused by elevated intrathoracic pressures by certain techniques may be too high a price for the improved peripheral flow. In addition, a high thoracoabdominal gradient has been demonstrated during experimental simultaneous compression-ventilation, which could divert flow from the brain in the absence of concomitant abdominal binding. On the basis of these observations, new mechanically assisted techniques, including an active decompression phase (i.e., active compression-decompression), have been evaluated for improved circulation during CPR.[226,227] More clinical studies are needed before establishing their general clinical applications.

Advanced Life Support and Definitive Resuscitation

This next step in the resuscitative sequence is designed to achieve definitive stabilization of the patient.[189] The implementation of advanced life support is not intended to suggest an abrupt cessation of basic life support activities but rather a merging and transition from one level of activity to the next. In the past, advanced life support required judgments and technical skills that removed it from the realm of activity of lay bystanders and even emergency medical technicians, limiting these activities to specifically trained paramedical

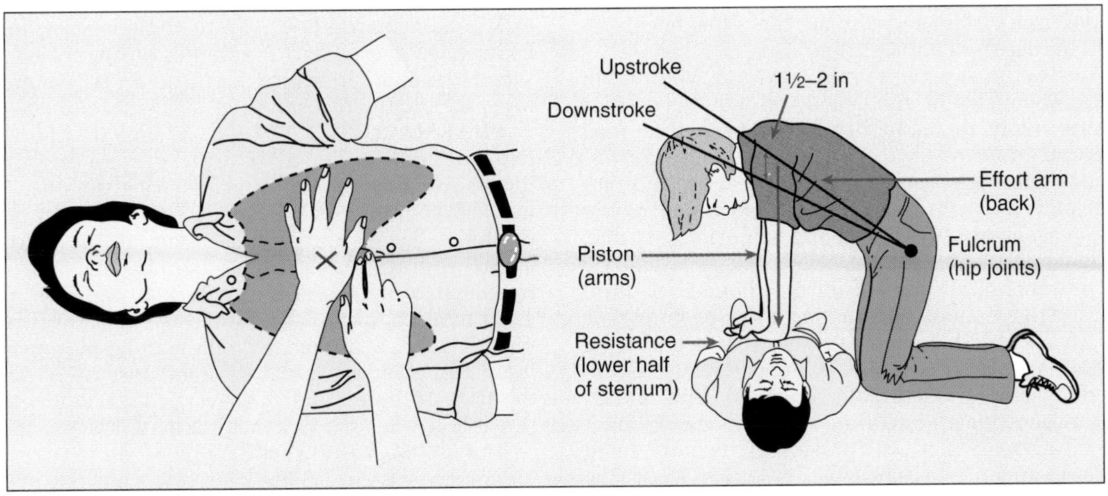

FIGURE 33–21 External chest compression. **Left,** Locating the correct hand position on the lower half of the sternum. **Right,** Proper position of the rescuer, with shoulders directly over the victim's sternum and elbows locked. (From Standards and guidelines for Cardiopulmonary Resuscitation [CPR] and Emergency Cardiac care [ECC]. National Academy of Sciences-National Research Council. JAMA 255:2906, 1986. Copyright 1986, the American Medical Association.)

personnel, nurses, and physicians. With further education of emergency technicians, most community-based CPR programs now permit them to carry out advanced life support activities. In addition, the development and testing of automatic external defibrillators that have the ability to sense and analyze cardiac electrical activity and prompt the user to deliver definitive electrical intervention[228] provides a role for less highly trained rescue personnel (i.e., police, ambulance drivers) and even untrained lay bystanders[218,223] for rapid defibrillation.

The general goals of advanced life support are to revert the cardiac rhythm to one that is hemodynamically effective, optimize ventilation, and maintain and support the restored circulation. Thus, during advanced life support, the patient's cardiac rhythm is promptly cardioverted or defibrillated as the first priority if appropriate equipment is immediately available. There is increasing evidence that a short period of closed-chest cardiac compression immediately before defibrillation enhances the probability of survival.[214,219,221] After the initial attempt to restore a hemodynamically effective rhythm, the patient is intubated and oxygenated, if needed, and the heart is paced if a bradyarrhythmia or asystole occurs. An intravenous line is established to deliver medications. After intubation, the goal of ventilation is to reverse hypoxemia and not merely achieve a high alveolar oxygen pressure (PO_2). Thus, oxygen rather than room air should be used to ventilate the patient; if possible, the arterial PO_2 should be monitored. Respirator support in hospital and an Ambu bag by means of an endotracheal tube, or facemasks in the out-of-hospital setting, are usually used.

DEFIBRILLATION-CARDIOVERSION (Fig. 33–22). Rapid conversion to an effective cardiac electrical mechanism is a key step for successful resuscitation. Delay should be minimal, even when conditions for CPR are optimal. When VF or a rapid VT is recognized on a monitor or by telemetry, defibrillation should be carried out immediately with a shock of 200 joules. From data based on monophasic waveforms, up to 90 percent of VF victims weighing up to 90 kg can be successfully resuscitated with a 200-joule shock, and a 300- or 360-joule shock may be used if this is not successful.[189] Failure of the initial shocks to cardiovert to an effective rhythm is a poor prognostic sign. After failure of three shocks up to a maximum of 360 joules of energy, CPR should be continued while the patient is intubated and intravenous access achieved. Epinephrine, 1 mg intravenously (IV), is administered and followed by repeated defibrillation attempts at 360 joules. Epinephrine may be repeated at 3- to 5-minute intervals with defibrillator shocks in between,[189] but high-dose epinephrine does not appear to provide added benefit.[229] Vasopressin, 40 units intravenously one time, has been suggested as an alternative to epinephrine.[230]

Simultaneously, the rescuer should focus on ventilation to correct the chemistry of the blood, efforts that render the heart more likely to reestablish a stable rhythm (i.e., improved oxygenation, reversal of acidosis, and improvement of the underlying electrophysiological condition). Although adequate oxygenation of the blood is crucial in the immediate management of the metabolic acidosis of cardiac arrest, additional correction can be achieved if necessary by intravenous administration of sodium bicarbonate. Sodium bicarbonate is recommended for circumstances of known or suspected preexisting bicarbonate-responsive causes of acidosis, certain drug overdoses, and prolonged resuscitation runs.[189] The more general role for bicarbonate during cardiac arrest has been questioned, but in any circumstance, much less sodium bicarbonate than was previously recommended is adequate for treatment of acidosis in this setting. Excessive quantities can be deleterious. Although some investigators have questioned the use of sodium bicarbonate at all because risks of alkalosis, hypernatremia, and hyperosmolality may outweigh its benefits, the circumstances cited may benefit from administration of 1 mEq/kg sodium bicarbonate while CPR is being carried out. Up to 50 percent of this dose may be repeated every 10 to 15 minutes during the course of CPR. When possible, arterial pH, PO_2, and PCO_2 should be monitored during the resuscitation.

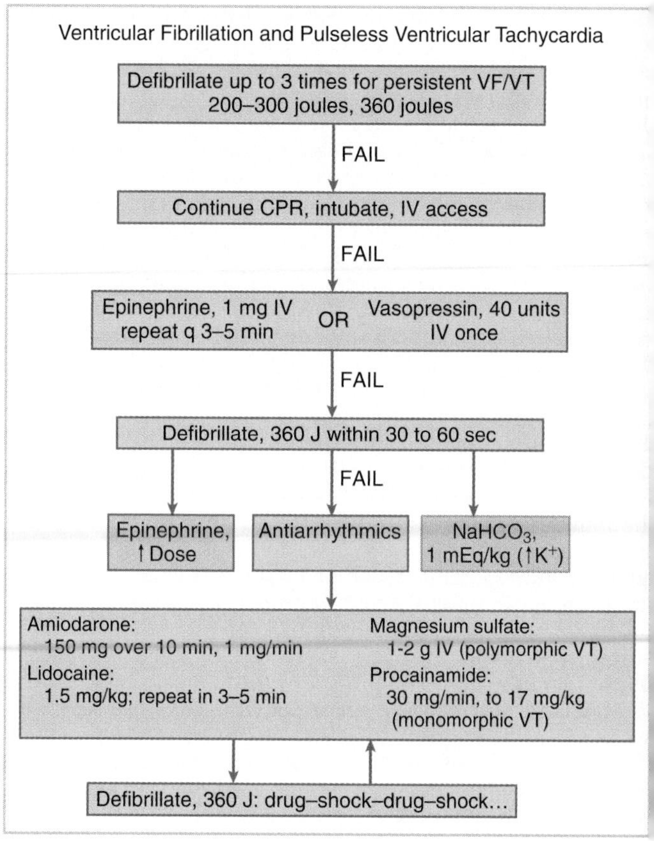

FIGURE 33–22 Advanced life support for ventricular fibrillation (VF) and pulseless ventricular tachycardia (VT). If initial defibrillation fails, the patient should be intubated and intravenous (I.V.) access immediately established while cardiopulmonary resuscitation (CPR) is continued. Epinephrine, 1 mg intravenously, should be administered and may be repeated several times with additional attempts to defibrillate with 360-joule shocks. If the conversion is still unsuccessful, epinephrine may be administered again, although it is unlikely that higher doses would provide any further benefit. Sodium bicarbonate should be administered at this time only if the patient is known to be hyperkalemic, but intravenous antiarrhythmic drugs should be tried (see text). Additional attempts to defibrillate should follow the administration of each drug attempted. (Modified from Emergency Cardiac Care Committee and Subcommittees, American Heart Association: Guidelines for cardiopulmonary resuscitation and emergency cardiac care. JAMA 268:2172, 1992. American Medical Association. See original reference for further details.)

PHARMACOTHERAPY (see Chap. 30). For the patient who continues to have VT or VF despite direct-current cardioversion after epinephrine, electrical stability of the heart may be achieved by intravenous administration of antiarrhythmic agents during continued resuscitation (see Fig. 33–22). Intravenous amiodarone has emerged as the initial treatment of choice (150 mg over 10 minutes, followed by 1 mg/min for up to 6 hours and 0.5 mg/min thereafter) (see Fig. 33–22).[167] Another regimen is 1 mg/min over the next 3 hours, followed by a maintenance dose of 0.5 mg/min over the next 18 hours and for several days as necessary. Additional bolus dosing, to a maximum of 500 mg, can be tried if the initial bolus is unsuccessful.

A bolus of 1.0 to 1.5 mg/kg of lidocaine may be given intravenously and the dose repeated in 2 minutes for patients in whom amiodarone is unsuccessful and possibly for those who have an acute transmural myocardial infarction as the triggering mechanism for the cardiac arrest. Intravenous procainamide (loading infusion of 100 mg per 5 minutes to a total dose of 500 to 800 mg, followed by continuous infusion at 2 to 5 mg/min) is rarely used in this setting any longer, but may be tried for persisting, hemodynamically stable arrhythmias.

For patients in whom acute hyperkalemia is the triggering event for resistant VF or who have hypocalcemia or are toxic from Ca^{2+} entry blocking drugs, 10 percent calcium gluconate, 5 to 20 ml infused at a rate of 2 to 4 ml/min, may be helpful.[189] Calcium should not be used routinely during resuscitation, even though ionized Ca^{2+} levels may be low during resuscitation from cardiac arrest. Some resistant forms of polymorphic VT or torsades de pointes, rapid monomorphic VT or ventricular flutter (rate ≥ 260/min), or resistant VF may respond to intravenous beta blocker therapy (propranolol, 1 mg IV boluses to a total dose of up to 15 to 20 mg; metoprolol, 5 mg IV, up to 20 mg) or intravenous $MgSO_4$ (1 to 2 gm IV given over 1 to 2 minutes).

BRADYARRHYTHMIC AND ASYSTOLIC ARREST; PULSELESS ELECTRICAL ACTIVITY (Fig. 33–23). The approach to the patient with bradyarrhythmic or asystolic arrest or pulseless electrical activity differs from the approach to patients with tachyarrhythmic events (VT or VF).[189] When this form of cardiac arrest is recognized, efforts should focus first on establishing control of the cardiorespiratory status (i.e., continue CPR, intubate, and establish intravenous access), then reconfirming the rhythm (in two leads if possible), and finally taking actions that favor the emergence of a stable spontaneous rhythm or attempt to pace the heart. Possible reversible causes, particularly for bradyarrhythmia and asystole, should be considered and excluded (or treated) promptly. These include hypovolemia, hypoxia, cardiac tamponade, tension pneumothorax, preexisting acidosis, drug overdose, hypothermia, and hyperkalemia. Epinephrine (1.0 mg IV every 3 to 5 minutes) and atropine (1.0 to 2.0 mg intravenously) are commonly used in an attempt to elicit spontaneous electrical activity or increase the rate of a bradycardia. These have had only limited success, as have intravenous isoproterenol infusions in doses up to 15 to 20 μg/min. In the absence of an intravenous line, epinephrine (1 mg [i.e., 10 ml of a 1:10,000 solution]) may be given by the intracardiac route, but there is danger of coronary or myocardial laceration. Sodium bicarbonate, 1 mEq/kg, may be tried for known or strongly suspected preexisting hyperkalemia or bicarbonate-responsive acidosis.

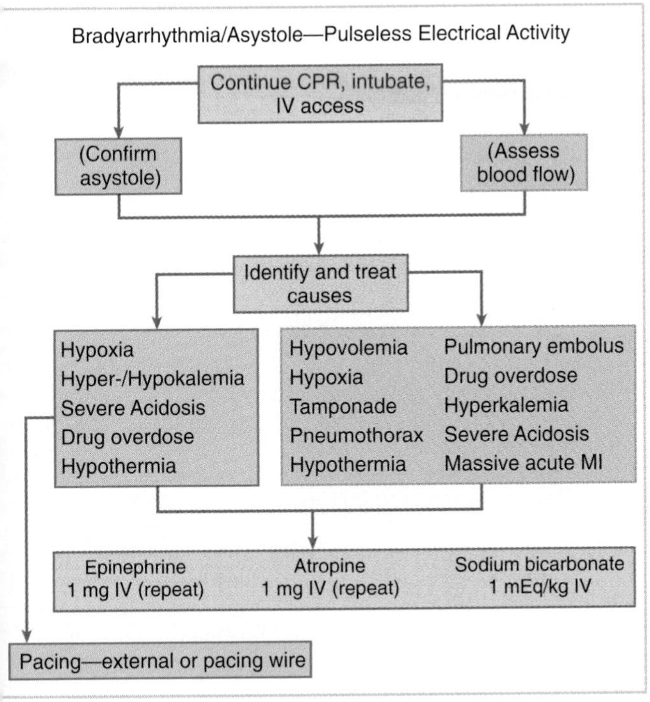

FIGURE 33–23 Advanced cardiac life support for patients with severe bradyarrhythmia, asystole, and pulseless electrical activity. The patient in any of these states should have continued cardiopulmonary resuscitation (CPR) and be intubated, with intravenous (I.V.) access established, before pharmacological treatment. The initial activity is to confirm persisting asystole or attempt to assess blood flow in patients thought to have pulseless electrical activity. An immediate attempt should be made to identify and treat reversible or treatable causes of these forms of cardiac arrest. Epinephrine is generally administered first, and atropine or bicarbonate, or both, may be administered subsequently. An attempt to pace the heart with an external device or an intracardiac pacing catheter is advisable, although usually not successful, except for certain reversible bradyarrhythmias. M.I. = myocardial infarction. (Modified from Emergency Cardiac Care Committee and Subcommittees, American Heart Association: Guidelines for cardiopulmonary resuscitation and emergency cardiac care. JAMA 268:2172, 1992. Copyright 1992, American Medical Association. See original reference for further details.)

Pacing of the bradyarrhythmic or asystolic heart has been limited in the past by the unavailability of personnel capable of carrying out such procedures at the scene of cardiac arrests. With the development of more effective external pacing systems, the role of pacing and its influence on outcome must now be reevaluated. Unfortunately, all data to date suggest that the *asystolic* patient continues to have a very poor prognosis despite new techniques.[231]

The published standards for CPR and emergency cardiac care[189] include a series of teaching algorithms to be used as guides to appropriate care. Figures 33–22 and 33–23 provide the algorithms for VF and pulseless VT, asystole (or cardiac standstill), and pulseless electrical activity. These general guides are not to be interpreted as inclusive of all possible approaches or contingencies. The special circumstance of CPR in pregnant women requires additional attention to effects of drugs on the gravid uterus and the fetus, mechanical and physiological influences of pregnancy on the efficacy of CPR, and risk of complications such as ruptured uterus and lacerated liver.

STABILIZATION. As soon as electrical resuscitation from VT, VF, bradycardia, asystole, or pulseless electrical activity is achieved, the focus of attention shifts to maintaining a stable electrical, hemodynamic, and central nervous system status. For electrical stability, a continuous infusion of an effective drug, based on observation during the cardiac arrest run, is commonly used. This drug may be lidocaine, 1 to 4 mg/min depending on size and clinical factors; intravenous amiodarone, 10 mg/kg/d (if this drug was required in the initial resuscitation); or procainamide, 2 to 4 mg/min. Occasionally, a continuous infusion of propranolol or esmolol is used. Catecholamines are used in cardiac arrest not only in an attempt to achieve better electrical stability (e.g., conversion from fine to coarse VF, or increasing the rate of spontaneous contraction during bradyarrhythmias) but also for their inotropic and peripheral vascular effects. Epinephrine is the first choice among the catecholamines for use in cardiac arrest because it increases myocardial contractility, elevates perfusion pressure, may convert electromechanical dissociation to electromechanical coupling, and improves chances for defibrillation. Because of its adverse effects on renal and mesenteric flow, norepinephrine is a less desirable agent despite its inotropic effects. When the chronotropic effect of epinephrine is undesirable, dopamine or dobutamine is preferable to norepinephrine for inotropic effect. Isoproterenol may be used for the treatment of primary or postdefibrillation bradycardia when heart rate control is the primary goal of therapy intended to improve cardiac output. Calcium chloride, 2 to 4 mg/kg, is sometimes used in patients with pulseless electrical activity that persists after administration of catecholamines. The efficacy of this intervention is uncertain. Stimulation of alpha adrenoceptors may be important during definitive resuscitative efforts. For instance, the alpha adrenoceptor–stimulating effects of epinephrine and higher dosages of dopamine, producing elevation of aortic diastolic pressures by peripheral vasoconstriction with increased cerebral and myocardial flow, have been reemphasized.

Post-Cardiac Arrest Care

For successfully resuscitated cardiac arrest victims, whether the event occurred in or out of hospital, post-cardiac arrest care includes admission to an intensive care unit and continuous monitoring for a minimum of 48 to 72 hours. Some elements of postarrest management are common to all resuscitated patients, but prognosis and certain details of management are specific for the clinical setting in which the cardiac arrest occurred. The major management categories include (1) primary cardiac arrest in acute myocardial infarction, (2) secondary cardiac arrest in acute myocardial infarction, (3) cardiac arrest associated with noncardiac disorders, and (4) survival after out-of-hospital cardiac arrest.

Primary Cardiac Arrest in Acute Myocardial Infarction

VF in patients with acute myocardial infarction free of concomitant hemodynamic complications (i.e., primary VF) (see also Chap. 47) is now less common in hospitalized patients than the 15 to 20 percent incidence before the availability of cardiac care units. The events that do occur are almost always successfully reverted by prompt interventions in properly equipped emergency departments or cardiac care units. After successful resuscitation, patients are often maintained with a lidocaine infusion at 2 to 4 mg/min. Antiarrhythmic support is usually discontinued after 24 hours if arrhythmias do not recur (see Chap. 30). The occurrence of VF during the early phase of acute myocardial infarction (i.e., first 24 to 48 hours) is not an indication for subsequent electrophysiological testing or long-term antiarrhythmic or device therapy. Rapid sustained VT producing the clinical picture of cardiac arrest in acute myocardial infarction is treated similarly; its intermediate- and long-term implications are the same as those of VF. Cardiac arrest caused by bradyarrhythmias or asystole in acute inferior wall myocardial infarction, in the absence of primary hemodynamic consequences, is uncommon and may respond to either atropine or pacing. The prognosis is good, with no special long-term care required in most instances. Rarely, symptomatic bradyarrhythmias that require permanent pacemakers persist in survivors. In contrast to inferior myocardial infarction, bradyarrhythmic cardiac arrest associated with large anterior wall infarctions (and AV or intraventricular block) has a poor prognosis.

Secondary Cardiac Arrest in Acute Myocardial Infarction

This condition is defined as cardiac arrest occurring in association with, or as a result of, hemodynamic or mechanical dysfunction. The immediate mortality among patients in this setting ranges from 59 to 89 percent, depending on the severity of the hemodynamic abnormalities and size of the myocardial infarction. Resuscitative efforts commonly fail in such patients, and when they are successful, the post-cardiac arrest management is often difficult. When secondary cardiac arrest occurs by the mechanisms of VT or VF, aggressive hemodynamic or antiischemic measures may help achieve rhythm stability. If recurrences of the arrhythmia continue, intravenous amiodarone has emerged as the antiarrhythmic therapy of choice.[167] Lidocaine may also be tried if the mechanism appears to be ischemic but is less likely to be successful in this setting than in primary VF. The success of interventions and prevention of recurrent cardiac arrest are related closely to the outcome of managing the hemodynamic status. The incidence of cardiac arrest caused by bradyarrhythmias or asystole, or by electromechanical dissociation, is higher in the secondary form of cardiac arrest in acute myocardial infarction. Such patients usually have large myocardial infarctions and major hemodynamic abnormalities and may be acidotic and hypoxemic. Even with aggressive therapy, the prognosis after a bradyarrhythmic or asystolic arrest in such patients is poor, and patients are resuscitated only rarely from electromechanical dissociation. All patients in circulatory failure at the onset of arrest are in a high-risk category, with only a 2 percent survival rate among hypotensive patients in one study.[190]

CARDIAC ARREST AMONG IN-HOSPITAL PATIENTS WITH NONCARDIAC ABNORMALITIES. These patients fall into two major categories: (1) those with life-limiting diseases such as malignancies, sepsis, organ failure, end-stage pulmonary disease, and advanced central nervous system disease and (2) those with acute toxic or proarrhythmic states that are potentially reversible. In the former category, the ratio of tachyarrhythmic to bradyarrhythmic cardiac arrest is low[190] and the prognosis for surviving cardiac arrest is poor. Although the data may be somewhat skewed by the practice of assigning "do not resuscitate" orders to patients with end-stage disease, available data for attempted resuscitations show a poor outcome. Only 7 percent of cancer patients, 3 percent of renal failure patients, and no patients with sepsis or acute central nervous system disease were successfully resuscitated and discharged from the hospital. For the few successfully resuscitated patients in these categories, postarrest management is dictated by the underlying precipitating factors.

Most antiarrhythmic drugs (see Chap. 30), a number of drugs used for noncardiac purposes, and electrolyte disturbances can precipitate potentially lethal arrhythmias and cardiac arrest. The class IA and class III antiarrhythmic drugs can cause proarrhythmic responses by lengthening the QT interval and generating torsades de pointes. The class IC drugs rarely cause torsades de pointes but cause excess SCD risk in patients with recent myocardial infarction, possibly by interacting with ischemia or other transient risk factors. Among other categories of drugs, the phenothiazines, tricyclic antidepressants, lithium, terfenadine interacting with ketoconazole (or other blockers of enzymes in the hepatic P450 system), pentamidine, cocaine, erythromycin, and cardiovascular drugs that are not antiarrhythmics—such as lidoflazine—are recognized causes. Beyond these, a broad array of pharmacological and pathophysiological-metabolic causes have been reported. Hypokalemia, hypomagnesemia, and perhaps hypocalcemia are the electrolyte disturbances most closely associated with cardiac arrest. Acidosis and hypoxia can potentiate the vulnerability associated with electrolyte disturbances. Proarrhythmic effects are often prewarned by prolongation of the QT interval, although this electrocardiographic change is not always present.[121]

Cardiac arrest caused by torsades de pointes is managed by intravenous administration of magnesium, pacing, or treatment with isoproterenol and removal of the offending agent. Class IC drugs may cause a rapid, sinusoidal VT pattern, especially among patients with poor left ventricular function. This VT has a tendency to recur repetitively after cardioversion until the drug has begun to clear and has been controlled by propranolol in some patients. When the patient's condition can be stabilized until the offending factor is removed (e.g., proarrhythmic drugs) or corrected (e.g., electrolyte imbalances, hypothermia), the prognosis is excellent. The recognition of torsades de pointes (see Chap. 32) and the identification of its risk by prolongation of the QT interval in association with the offending agent are helpful in managing these patients.

POST–CARDIAC ARREST CARE IN SURVIVORS OF OUT-OF-HOSPITAL CARDIAC ARREST. The initial management of survivors of out-of-hospital cardiac arrest centers on stabilizing the cardiac electrical status, supporting hemodynamics, and providing supportive care for reversal of organ damage that has occurred as a consequence of the cardiac arrest. The in-hospital risk of recurrent cardiac arrest is relatively low, and arrhythmias account for only 10 percent of in-hospital deaths after successful prehospital resuscitation.[232] However, the mortality rate during the index hospitalization is 50 percent, indicating that nonarrhythmic mortality dominates the mechanisms of early postresuscitation deaths (30 percent hemodynamic, 60 percent central nervous system related). Antiarrhythmic therapy, usually intravenous amiodarone, is used in an attempt to prevent recurrent cardiac arrest among patients who demonstrate residual electrophysiological instability and recurrent arrhythmia during the first 48 hours of postarrest hospitalization. Patients who have either preexisting or new AV or intraventricular conduction disturbances are at particularly high risk for recurrent cardiac arrest.[232] The routine use of temporary pacemakers has been evaluated in such patients but was not found to be helpful for preventing early recurrent cardiac arrest. Invasive techniques for hemodynamic monitoring are used in a patient whose condition is unstable but not routinely for those whose condition is stable on admission.

Anoxic encephalopathy is a strong predictor of in-hospital death. A suggested addition to the management of this condition is the use of induced mild hypothermia to reduce metabolic demands and cerebral edema.[196,197] When this strategy is applied promptly to the postarrest survivor who remains unconscious upon hospital admission, there is a modest but measurable survival benefit. During the later convalescent period, continued attention to central nervous system status, including physical rehabilitation, is of primary importance for an optimal outcome. Respiratory support by conventional methods is used as necessary. Management of other organ system injury (e.g., renal, hepatic), as well as early recognition and treatment of infectious complications, also contributes to ultimate survival.

Long-Term Management of Survivors of Out-of-Hospital Cardiac Arrest

When the survivor of an out-of-hospital cardiac arrest has awakened and achieved electrical and hemodynamic stability, usually between 1 and 7 days after the event, decisions must be made regarding the nature and extent of the work-up required to establish a long-term management strategy. The goals of the work-up are to identify the specific etiological and triggering cause of the cardiac arrest, clarify the functional status of the patient's cardiovascular system, and establish long-term therapeutic strategies. The extent of the work-up is largely dictated by the degree of central nervous system recovery and the factors already known to have contributed to the cardiac arrest. For instance, patients who have limited return of central nervous system function usually do not undergo extensive work-ups, and patients whose cardiac arrests were triggered by an acute transmural myocardial infarction have work-ups similar to those for other patients with acute myocardial infarction (see Chap. 47).

Survivors of out-of-hospital cardiac arrest not associated with acute myocardial infarction who have good return of neurological function appear to have a long-term survival probability commensurate with their age, gender, and extent of disease when treated according to existing guidelines.[201] These patients should undergo diagnostic work-ups to define the cause of cardiac arrest and tailor long-term therapy, the latter targeted to both the underlying disease and strategies for prevention of recurrent cardiac arrests or SCD. The work-up includes cardiac catheterization with coronary angiography if coronary atherosclerosis is known or considered to be the possible cause of the event,[233] an evaluation of the functional significance of coronary lesions by stress-imaging techniques if indicated, determination of functional and hemodynamic status, and estimation of baseline susceptibility to recurrent life-threatening arrhythmias and of the expected response to long-term therapy.

GENERAL CARE. The general management of survivors of cardiac arrest is determined by the specific cause and the pathophysiology of the underlying process. For patients with ischemic heart disease (see Chaps. 49 and 50), who constitute approximately 80 percent of cardiac arrest victims, interventions to prevent myocardial ischemia, optimization of therapy for left ventricular dysfunction, and attention to general medical status are all addressed. Although there are limited data suggesting that revascularization procedures may improve the recurrence rate and total mortality rates after survival from out-of-hospital cardiac arrest,[234] no properly controlled prospective studies have validated this impression for either bypass surgery or percutaneous interventions. Moreover, a randomized trial of prophylactic implantable defibrillators versus usual therapy in patients with low ejection fractions undergoing coronary bypass surgery in the absence of a history of cardiac arrest or other life-threatening arrhythmia or arrhythmia markers (the Coronary Artery Bypass Graft Patch Trial [CABG-Patch]) revealed no mortality benefit of implantable defibrillators after revascularization.[235] The indications for revascularization after a cardiac arrest are limited to those who have a generally accepted indication for angioplasty or surgery,[171] including (but not limited to) a documented ischemic mechanism for the cardiac arrest.

Although no data from placebo-controlled trials are available to define a benefit of various antiischemic strategies (including beta blockers or other medical antiischemic therapy) for long-term management after out-of-hospital cardiac arrest, medical, catheter interventional, or surgical antiischemic therapy, rather than antiarrhythmic drug therapy, is generally considered the primary approach to long-term management of the subgroup of prehospital cardiac arrest survivors in whom transient myocardial ischemia was the inciting factor. Moreover, in an uncontrolled observation comparing cardiac arrest survivors who had ever received beta blockers after the index event with those who had not received the drug, a significant improvement in long-term outcome was observed among those who had received beta blockers.[236] Further evaluation of the specific role of revascularization procedures and antiischemic medical therapy after out-of-hospital cardiac arrest is needed.

The long-term management of the consequences of left ventricular dysfunction by conventional means such as digitalis preparations and chronic diuretic use has been evaluated in several studies. Data from the Multiple Risk Factor Intervention Trial (MRFIT) suggested a higher mortality rate in the special intervention group, presumably related to diuretic use and K^+ depletion, and other data regarding the relation between K^+ depletion and arrhythmias have focused attention on routine use of such drugs. Although the facts are currently far from conclusive, it is advisable that diuretic use should be accompanied by careful monitoring of electrolytes. The use of digoxin in survivors of out-of-hospital cardiac arrest should be tailored to specific indications for left ventricular dysfunction.

The various pharmacological strategies (such as angiotensin-converting enzyme inhibitors, carvedilol and other beta-adrenergic blocking agents, and spironolactone) that have been shown to provide a clinical and mortality benefit in patients with left ventricular dysfunction, with or without heart failure, provide an SCD benefit in conjunction with total mortality benefit. The extent to which there is a specific SCD benefit for cardiac arrest survivors is uncertain, although some primary prevention trials suggest that such benefit occurs.

Prevention of Cardiac Arrest and Sudden Cardiac Death

Therapeutic strategies to prevent SCD can be classified into five categories: (1) prevention of recurrent events in survivors of cardiac arrest or hemodynamically compromising VT (secondary prevention); (2) prevention of an initial event among patients at high risk because of advanced heart disease with ejection fractions less than or equal to 35 percent (primary prevention); (3) primary prevention in patients with less advanced common or uncommon structural heart diseases and ejection fractions greater than 35 percent; (4) primary prevention in patients with structurally normal hearts, subtle or minor structural abnormalities, or molecular disorders associated with electrophysiological properties that establish risk for ventricular arrhythmias; and (5) primary prevention among the general population (Table 33–4). The last category includes the substantial proportion of SCDs that occur as a first cardiac event among victims previously free of known disease (see earlier).[169]

Four modes of antiarrhythmic therapy, which are not mutually exclusive, may be considered for patients at risk for cardiac arrest: antiarrhythmic drug therapy, surgery, catheter ablation, and implantable defibrillator therapy. The choice of therapy is based on estimation of the potential benefit determined by evaluation of the individual patient and available efficacy and safety data.

Antiarrhythmic Drug Strategies

The earliest approach, historically, to the management of risk of out-of-hospital cardiac arrest and VT with hemodynamic compromise was the use of pharmacological agents. This approach was based initially on the assumption that the high frequency of ambient ventricular arrhythmias constituted a triggering mechanism for potentially lethal arrhythmias and that the electrophysiological pathophysiology or instability of the myocardium that predisposed to potentially lethal arrhythmias could be modified by antiarrhythmic drugs. The therapeutic strategy for the former was the suppression of ambient ventricular arrhythmias by antiarrhythmic drugs and the strategy for the latter was the suppression of inducibility of VT or VF during programmed electrical stimulation studies. Observational data suggested that suppression of ambient arrhythmias, identified on ambulatory recorders, could be achieved by the empirical use of amiodarone, beta-adrenergic blocking agents, or membrane-active antiarrhythmic drugs. On the basis of historical expectations it was suggested, but not proved, that such suppressive techniques would improve mortality risk. For the membrane-active drugs, the observations that post-cardiac arrest survivors who had been treated with class I antiarrhythmic drugs had a worse outcome than those who were not treated challenged the concept of benefit,[236] and that skepticism was definitively reinforced by the results of CAST,[73] which demonstrated that certain class I antiarrhythmic drugs were neutral or did harm. In contrast, beta blocker therapy might have some benefit in such patients,[236,237] and amiodarone might also be effective for some patients.[238]

Another study, the Electrophysiologic Study Versus Electrocardiographic Monitoring (ESVEM) trial, designed to compare the value of ambulatory monitoring with programmed electrical stimulation techniques for predicting therapeutic outcome,[239] suggested that the class III antiarrhythmic drug sotalol was superior to class I membrane-active antiarrhythmic agents for patients with life-threatening ventricular tachyarrhythmias but provided no comparison with amiodarone or beta blockers. In summary, ambient arrhythmia suppression as a technique for reduction of risk enjoyed a short period of popularity for VT-VF survivors but in time yielded to the apparent greater benefits of amiodarone, and perhaps beta blockers,[240] prescribed empirically. The combination of amiodarone and beta blocker therapy in the post-myocardial infarction patient has been suggested as a strategy that provides greater benefit than either drug alone from subgroup analysis of the European Myocardial Infarct Amiodarone Trial (EMIAT) and Canadian Amiodarone Myocardial Infarction Trial (CAMIAT),[241] and another study reinforced the benefit of beta blockers for specific prevention of SCD in unselected post-myocardial infarction patients.[242]

TABLE 33–4 Categories of Therapeutic Strategies for Prevention of Recurrent Cardiac Arrest and Sudden Cardiac Death (SCD)

Prevention Targets	Clinical Examples	Estimate of Risk	Data Sources
Secondary*	Survivors of cardiac arrest; VF/VT	High	Observational; RCT: (+) control
Primary			
Advanced structural cardiac disease	CAD/DCM, EF < 35%	High	Observational; RCT: (+) control RCT: (−) control
Lower grade structural disease	CAD/DCM, EF > 35% RVD, sarcoidosis, HCM	Variable	Observational; RCT: Subgroup analyses
Functional cardiac disorders†	Long QT syndrome, Brugada syndrome	Variable	Observational
SCD as primary event in CAD†	Family history of SCD, risk factors for CAD	Low	Epidemiological; genetic (?)

Much of the data for secondary prevention, identified as a high-risk population because of the occurrence of a prior cardiac arrest, has derived from observational data and, more recently, from randomized controlled trials (RCTs), all of which have employed an active-therapy control group [(+) control], comparing outcomes between groups treated with implantable cardioverter-defibrillators (ICDs) and antiarrhythmic drugs (see Table 33–5).

RCTs are not feasible for primary prevention in patients with these lower risk conditions. However, some information can be acquired from subgroup analysis of larger studies: Decisions for ICD implantation in these patients must be judgment based rather than evidence based. Suggestions of familial clustering of sudden death, as a specific expression of coronary artery disease (CAD), raise the question of primary prevention in patients at risk for SCD using epidemiological and perhaps genetic markers in the future.

DCM = dilated cardiomyopathy; EF = ejection fraction; HCM = hypertrophic cardiomyopathy; RVD = right ventricular dysplasia; VF = ventricular fibrillation; VT = ventricular tachycardia.

Ambulatory Electrocardiographic Recording and Empirical Therapy

The development of reliable methods of analysis of ambulatory recordings led some investigators to study the usefulness of such recordings for profiling risk of sustained tachyarrhythmic events and to measure suppressibility of ambient arrhythmias as a specific and individualized means of evaluating drug therapy for prevention of SCD. This strategy is now obsolete as a primary approach in the cardiac arrest survivor, but ambulatory monitoring is still used for profiling the risk of developing life-threatening sustained arrhythmias in individuals with certain forms of structural or electrophysiological disease who are considered at high risk. For example, the strategies used in the Multicenter Automatic Defibrillator Implantation Trial (MADIT)[243] and the Multicenter Unsustained Tachycardia Trial (MUSTT)[244] employed identification of nonsustained VT in post-myocardial infarction patients with other risk markers for early mortality. Although the ambient arrhythmias were not a target for therapy in the design of the studies, they have established the usefulness of this technique for identifying risk. Similarly, ambulatory recordings, particularly among patients with symptoms, are used as an aid to risk profiling in disorders such as hypertrophic cardiomyopathy, long QT interval syndrome, and right ventricular dysplasia and in patients with dilated cardiomyopathy or heart failure.

Other investigators provided data suggesting the possibility that ambient arrhythmia suppression might be equivalent to suppression of inducible arrhythmias by programmed electrical stimulation for predicting outcome.[239] Moreover, analysis of the CAST data base also suggested an association between the ease of suppression of ambient ventricular arrhythmias and survival,[245] supporting the concept of a meaningful relationship between *suppressibility* of ambient arrhythmias and survival. Under circumstances in which amiodarone or beta-adrenergic blocking agents, or both, are used for primary prevention of cardiac arrest (and secondary prevention if ICDs are not available), baseline and follow-up ambulatory monitors are still used as a possible indicator of drug efficacy. This approach appears to have a rational basis for evaluating ambient arrhythmia responses, but there is still a level of uncertainty regarding its translation to actual cardiac arrest events.

Finally, empirical antiarrhythmic therapy, predominantly amiodarone, for prevention of recurrent cardiac arrest or other life-threatening arrhythmias has been observed to have a relative benefit in several studies. Whether it has an absolute mortality benefit can be determined only with data from placebo-controlled trials, which are not available. Moreover, several controlled trials have now suggested that empirical amiodarone is less effective than implantable defibrillators in reducing risk of death among survivors of life-threatening arrhythmic events (Antiarrhythmics Versus Implantable Defibrillators [AVID], Canadian Implantable Defibrillator Study [CIDS], and the Cardiac Arrest Study Hamburg [CASH]), particularly when the ejection fraction is less than 35 percent (see Chap. 31).[203-205]

PROGRAMMED ELECTRICAL STIMULATION

The second major antiarrhythmic strategy was based on suppression of inducibility of sustained ventricular arrhythmias, considered to be a marker of risk during electrophysiological testing. The use of programmed electrical stimulation to identify benefit on the basis of suppression of inducibility by an antiarrhythmic drug gained popularity for evaluating long-term therapy among survivors of out-of-hospital cardiac arrest. It evolved as the preferred method of management despite concerns about the sensitivity and specificity of the various pacing protocols and the extent to which the myocardial status at the time of the programmed electrical stimulation study reflected that present at the time of the clinical cardiac arrest. Nonetheless, most studies demonstrated limitations based on observations that a relatively small fraction of cardiac arrest survivors (an average of less than 50 percent on the basis of multiple studies) had inducible arrhythmias.

Drug suppression of inducibility during electrophysiological testing as an endpoint for either secondary prevention of SCD or primary prevention in high-risk post-myocardial infarction patients has yielded to the benefits of ICD therapy in most subgroups, with a few exceptions among primary prevention categories. It still has use, however, for risk profiling in a number of clinical circumstances.[243,244,246,247] Despite a large, albeit somewhat conflicting, data base on the role of electrophysiological testing for risk profiling, results of the secondary prevention trials among cardiac arrest survivors suggest that routine electrophysiological testing among such individuals is no longer necessary, particularly if ICD therapy is available to the patient. All of the secondary prevention trials demonstrated a benefit of the ICD over antiarrhythmic therapy, usually using amiodarone, without a determination that risk profiling by electrophysiological testing offered any benefit.[203-205] Under conditions in which a potentially reversible trigger for cardiac arrest can be identified, and perhaps among some cardiac arrest survivors in whom transient ischemia was the initiating mechanism and the ejection fraction is greater than 40 percent, there might be a persistent limited role for such testing as a guide to therapy. In contrast, several primary prevention trials such as MADIT[243] and MUSTT[244] used electrophysiological testing to profile risk and demonstrated large benefits. MADIT II,[248] which enrolled patients with lower ejection fractions than MADIT or MUSTT and did not employ arrhythmia markers, also demonstrated a survival benefit of ICD therapy. The extent to which MADIT II differs from MADIT and MUSTT and the question of whether the electrophysiological testing criteria in the latter are necessary have yet to be resolved. Until then, electrophysiological testing is used as the indicator leading to ICD use among candidates defined by MADIT and MUSTT criteria.

The implications of induced nonsustained forms of VT are more controversial. Although it has been suggested that induction of nonsustained ventricular rhythms may indicate risk, it is generally considered nonspecific in the absence of structural heart disease or when an aggressive protocol is used. The use of the suppression of nonsustained arrhythmias as an endpoint of therapy is not considered valid.

The significance of *non*inducibility at baseline electrophysiological stimulation testing in relation to risk and long-term management is also controversial. In the past, opinions ranged from the conclusion that potentially high-risk patients free of inducible ventricular arrhythmias were electrophysiologically stable and required no long-term antiarrhythmic therapy to the other extreme that such patients remained at risk but did not have an objective endpoint of therapy by this method and therefore must be treated by other techniques. Despite these conflicting opinions, it is generally accepted now that survivors of cardiac arrest without clearly identifiable transient and treatable causes remain at high risk regardless of inducibility status. Some out-of-hospital cardiac arrests can be clearly demonstrated to result from transient ischemia, and this subgroup appears to achieve benefit from antiischemic therapy.[201]

SURGICAL INTERVENTION STRATEGIES

The previously popular antiarrhythmic surgical techniques now have limited applications. Intraoperative map-guided cryoablation techniques may be used for patients who have inducible, hemodynamically stable sustained monomorphic VT during electrophysiological testing and have suitable ventricular and coronary artery anatomy, amenable to catheter ablation. However, they have little applicability to survivors of out-of-hospital cardiac arrest because the type of arrhythmia favoring this surgical approach is infrequently observed among cardiac arrest survivors. It can be used for patients whose arrhythmia frequency requires frequent ICD shocks as adjustive therapy to the device. In contrast, coronary revascularization procedures have a clearly defined role for cardiac arrest survivors in whom an ischemic mechanism was responsible for the event and suitable surgical anatomy is present.[234]

CATHETER ABLATION THERAPY

The use of catheter ablation techniques to treat ventricular tachyarrhythmias has been most successful for the benign focal tachycardias that originate in the right ventricle or left side of the interventricular septum (see Chap. 30) and for some reentrant VTs. With rare exceptions, catheter ablation techniques are not used for the treatment of higher risk ventricular tachyarrhythmias or for definitive therapy in patients at risk for progression of the arrhythmic substrate. For VT caused by bundle branch reentrant mechanisms, which occur in cardiomyopathies as well as other structural cardiac disorders, ablation of the right bundle branch to interrupt the reentrant cycle has been successful.[249] However, this has limited applicability to the large number of patients with structural heart disease at risk for SCD or those who have survived a cardiac arrest. On the other hand, the use of catheter ablation techniques for patients with ICDs who are having multiple tachyarrhythmic events is an appropriate and helpful adjunctive treatment strategy[250] rather than a preferred primary therapy for prevention of SCD.

Implantable Defibrillators

The development of the ICD added a new dimension to the management of patients at high risk for cardiac arrest (see Chap. 31). After the early reports by Mirowski and coworkers[251] and Echt and colleagues,[252] multiple observational studies confirmed that ICDs could achieve rates of sudden death consistently less than 5 percent at 1 year and total death rates in the 10 to 20 percent range among populations who have high mortality risks, as predicted by mortality surrogates such as historical controls or time to first appropriate shock.[253-256] Yet, determination of the mortality benefit of ICDs remained uncertain and they were debated for many years.[257] More than 16 years elapsed between the first clinical use of an implanted defibrillator[258] and publication of the first major randomized clinical trial comparing implantable defibrillator therapy with antiarrhythmic drug therapy.[243] Through that period of time, reports had documented the ability of implantable devices to revert potentially fatal arrhythmias but could not identify a valid relative or absolute mortality benefit because of confounding factors such as competing risks for sudden and nonsudden death and determination of whether appropriate shocks represented the interruption of an event that would have been fatal. Despite these limitations, ICD therapy continued to increase its relative position among other forms of therapy for survivors of out-of-hospital cardiac arrest and, to a lesser extent, for those considered to be at high risk for a primary cardiac arrest on the basis of specific clinical markers.

With publication of the results of MADIT,[243] information on the relative benefit of defibrillators over antiarrhythmic drug therapy (largely amiodarone) for primary prevention of SCD in a very high-risk population became available (Table 33–5; see also Fig. 33–24). The outcome demonstrated a 59 percent reduction in relative risk of total mortality at 2 years of follow-up (54 percent cumulative) and a 19 percent reduction in absolute risk of dying at 2 years of follow-up. One year later, the first adequately powered secondary prevention trial of ICDs versus antiarrhythmic drugs was published. This study, the AVID trial, demonstrated a 27 percent reduction in relative risk of total mortality at 2 years of follow-up with an absolute risk reduction of 7 percent.[203] The AVID trial was followed shortly by reports of two other studies—CIDS[204] and CASH[205]—both limited by the power of the enrollment numbers but suggesting trends toward similar benefits (see Table 33–5). As a consequence of the secondary prevention trials, ICDs have emerged as the preferred therapy for survivors of out-of-hospital cardiac arrest or hemodynamically important VT. A subgroup analysis of AVID suggested that the benefit is limited to patients with ejection fractions less than 35 percent; above that value, the outcome with either amiodarone or an ICD might be equivalent.[238]

Whereas the studies cited documented the ability of implantable devices to revert potentially fatal arrhythmias and subsequently showed a relative benefit over amiodarone in some groups of patients, the absence of placebo-controlled trials still prevents quantitation of the true magnitude of any mortality benefit because of the inability of positive

TABLE 33–5 Summary of Major Implantable Cardioverter-Defibrillator Trials for Prevention of Sudden Cardiac Deaths

		2-Year Outcomes (%)			
Trial	**Study Group**	***Control***	***ICDs***	***Rel RR***	***Abs RR***
Secondary prevention*					
AVID[202] (n = 1061)	VF, VT-syncope, VT: EF ≤ 40%	25	18	−27	−7
CIDS[203] (n = 659)	VF, VT-syncope, VT: EF ≤ 35% and CL < 400 ms	21	15	−30	−6
CASH[204] (n = 346)	Cardiac arrest survivors (VF, VT)	20 (combined)	12	−37	−8
		2-Year (MADIT, CABG-Patch, MADIT-2) and 5-Year (MUSTT, SCD-HeFT) Outcomes (%)			
		Control	***ICDs***	***Rel RR***	***Abs RR***
Primary prevention†					
MADIT[242] (n = 196)	Prior MI, EF ≤ 35%, NS VT, inducible VT, failed IV PA	32	13	−59	−19
MUSTT[243] (n = 704)	Prior MI, EF ≤ 40%, NS VT, inducible VT	55	24	−58	−31
CABG-Patch[234] (n = 900)	Coronary bypass surgery, EF < 36%, SAECG (+)	18	18	0	0
MADIT-2[248] (n = 1232)	Prior MI (>1 month), EF ≤ 30%	22	16	−28	−6
SCD-HeFT (n = 2521)‡	Class II-III CHF, EF ≤ 35%	36	29	−23	−7

Abs RR = absolute risk reduction; CHF = congestive heart failure; CL = cycle length; EF = ejection fraction; EP = electrophysiological; ICD = implantable cardioverter-defibrillator; IV PA = intravenous procainamide; MI = myocardial infarction; NS = nonsustained; Rel RR = relative risk reduction; SAECG = signal-averaged electrocardiogram; VF = ventricular fibrillation.

*Three major randomized trials for secondary prevention among survivors of out-of-hospital cardiac arrest, or high-risk ventricular tachycardia (VT), have been completed: the Antiarrhythmics Versus Implantable Defibrillators (AVID) trial, the Canadian Implantable Defibrillator Study (CIDS), and the Cardiac Arrest Study of Hamburg (CASH). Each used an active control, randomized design, comparing ICDs with antiarrhythmic drug (AAD) therapy, primarily amiodarone. The cumulative data, as well as the individual data from the larger studies, support the idea that the ICD is preferable to drug therapy for this high-risk population. However, the large relative benefits translated to more modest absolute benefits, with a large residual risk among the ICD-treated groups in each study.

†Four primary prevention trials among patients presumed to be at high risk but who have not had spontaneous life-threatening ventricular arrhythmias have been completed: the Multicenter Automatic Defibrillator Implantation Trial (MADIT), the Multicenter Unsustained Tachycardia Trial (MUSTT), the coronary artery bypass surgery/implantable defibrillator trial (CABG-Patch), and the Multicenter Automatic Defibrillator Implantation Trial-2 (MADIT-2). MADIT showed an advantage of ICD therapy over AAD therapy, MUSTT showed superiority of electrophysiologically (EP) guided evaluation leading to ICD therapy compared with that leading to drug therapy, and CABG-Patch showed no benefit to ICDs for patients undergoing routine coronary bypass surgery. MADIT-2 showed a benefit of ICD therapy compared with usual therapy for post-myocardial infarction patients with an EF ≤ 30%. The other large primary prevention trial, the Sudden Cardiac Death in Heart Failure Trail (SCD-HeFT), was in progress (along with a number of smaller trials) at time of writing.

‡Presented as a late-breaking trial at the Annual Scientific Sessions of the American College of Cardiology, March 8, 2004. No difference shown between amidiarone and control.

controlled trials to identify the absolute benefit of an intervention.[259] Despite these limitations, implantable defibrillator therapy is now the preferred therapy for survivors of cardiac arrest at risk for recurrences and for primary prevention in patients in a number of high-risk categories. Major questions still unanswered include the relative benefit of amiodarone versus defibrillators among lower risk subgroups of survivors of out-of-hospital cardiac arrest, the role of beta blockers, and the role of antiischemic surgical and medical therapy as definitive approaches.

A much larger issue, and one that has not yet been defined, is the use of implantable defibrillators among patients thought to be at intermediate levels of risk for cardiac arrest but who have not yet had an event. Several trials are in progress to determine whether preventive defibrillator therapy is an effective means of preventing the first cardiac arrest. Many of the trials are studying cost efficacy in addition to medical efficacy. One of the more important strategies being tested involves a comparison of defibrillator therapy and empirical amiodarone therapy with placebo in patients with heart failure without symptomatic arrhythmias or a history of cardiac arrest (see Chaps. 30 and 31).

Application of Therapeutic Strategies to Specific Groups of Patients

SECONDARY PREVENTION AFTER SURVIVING CARDIAC ARREST. As populations of cardiac arrest survivors began to accumulate from community-based emergency rescue activities, long-term therapeutic strategies intended to reduce recurrent cardiac arrest rates and total mortality risks emerged as a mandate for clinical investigators. The problem that affects all long-term strategies for cardiac arrest survivors, however, is the lack of a reliable concurrent natural history denominator against which to compare the results of interventions. This lack is a consequence of ethical concerns about withholding therapy in a placebo-controlled study model for patients at such high risk for dying[259] in conjunction with the likelihood that general therapies used in such patients may also improve total mortality risk. Earlier approaches to long-term therapy centered on the use of antiarrhythmic drug therapy, largely guided by the results of electrophysiological testing or the empirical use of antiarrhythmic drugs, particularly amiodarone. During the evolution of therapeutic strategies, various observational and positive-controlled studies suggested first that suppression of inducible ventricular arrhythmias yielded a better outcome than failure of suppression, then that amiodarone was better than class I antiarrhythmic drugs, and finally that ICDs were better than amiodarone. Therefore, ICD therapy has emerged as preferred therapy, absent absolute benefit data. Electrophysiological testing for secondary prevention—once routine—is now considered of questionable necessity and is commonly not performed.

Anatomically based antiarrhythmic surgery enjoyed a short period of popularity for secondary prevention, limited by the observation that surgical antiarrhythmic procedures appeared to provide benefit to only a small subset of such patients.[260] As the implantable defibrillator came into wider use, it also began to supplant pharmacological antiarrhythmic approaches, with the possible exception of amiodarone, even before the randomized clinical trials demonstrated relative ICD benefit. In the late 1990s, information from randomized clinical trials—AVID, CIDS, and CASH—provided compelling support for the use of ICDs as preferred therapy for secondary prevention of cardiac arrest related to ventricular tachyarrhythmias (Fig. 33–24).

PRIMARY PREVENTION OF OUT-OF-HOSPITAL CARDIAC ARREST WITH ADVANCED HEART DISEASE.

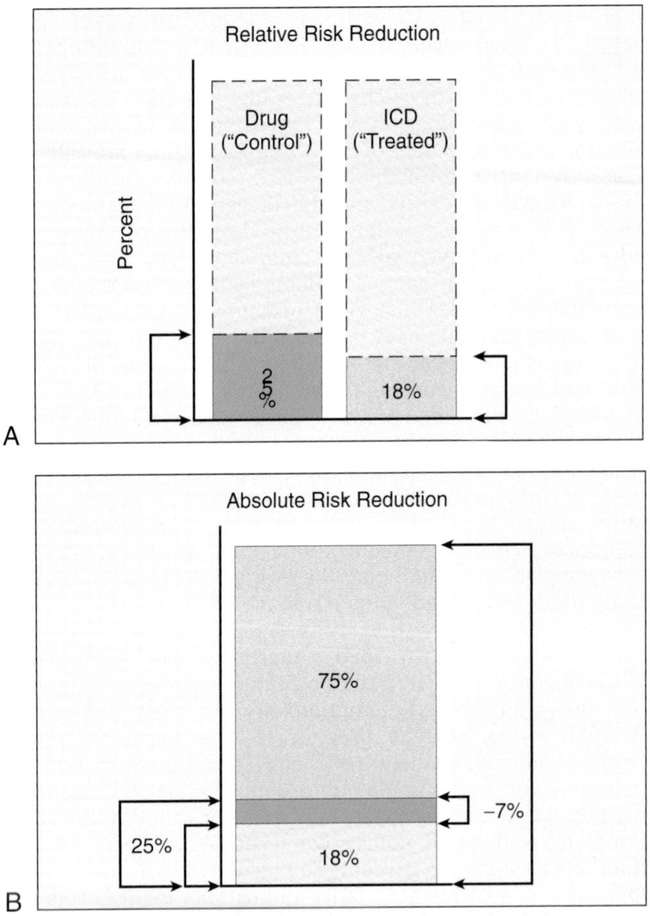

FIGURE 33–24 Relative and absolute benefit of implantable cardioverter-defibrillators (ICDs) in the Antiarrhythmics Versus Implantable Defibrillators (AVID) study. **A,** The ICD-treated subgroup had 18 percent mortality at 2 years versus 25 percent in the drug-treated group, a 27 percent *relative* reduction in the population having events. **B,** When relative reduction is extrapolated to the total target population, the *absolute* reduction of fatal events in the total population is 7 percent. (From Myerburg RJ, Mitrani R, Interian A Jr, Castellanos A: Interpretation of outcomes of antiarrhythmic clinical trials: Design features and population impact. Circulation 97:1514, 1998. Copyright 1998, American Heart Association.)

Because SCD is frequently the initial clinical expression of underlying structural heart disease or occurs in identified patients profiled to be at low risk (see Fig. 33–2), there has been a longstanding interest in therapeutic strategies targeted to primary prevention. After the disappointing outcome of CAST[73] and the disturbing suggestions of lack of efficacy or adverse effects of the class I antiarrhythmic drugs generally when used for primary or secondary prevention of SCD,[73,236] interest shifted to the use of amiodarone and implantable defibrillators. Two major trials of amiodarone in post-myocardial infarction patients,[261,262] one of which required ejection fractions less than 40 percent, demonstrated no total mortality benefit even though both trials demonstrated antiarrhythmic benefit, expressed as a reduction in arrhythmic deaths or resuscitated VF. Subgroup analyses suggested that the concomitant use of beta blockers did confer a mortality benefit.[241]

In parallel with the amiodarone trials, the randomized controlled trial comparing antiarrhythmic therapy (primarily amiodarone) with ICD therapy (MADIT) was carried out (see Table 33–5).[243] This trial randomly assigned patients with ejection fractions less than 35 percent, nonsustained VT during ambulatory recording, and inducible VT that was not suppressible by procainamide. This very high-risk group demonstrated a 54 percent reduction in total mortality with

ICD therapy compared with drug therapy, primarily amiodarone as noted earlier. At the same time, a trial comparing ICD implantation with no specific therapies for arrhythmias among patients with ejection fractions less than 36 percent who were undergoing coronary bypass surgery (CABG-Patch) demonstrated no benefit of defibrillators for total mortality.[235] The only marker for arrhythmic risk required for entry into the study was a positive signal-averaged ECG. A third trial, MUSTT,[244] was a complex study designed to determine whether electrophysiologically guided therapy provides an improved outcome among patients with nonsustained VT, inducible VT, and a history of prior myocardial infarction. The results demonstrated that although a statistically significant beneficial effect on total mortality was achieved by guiding therapy according to the results of electrophysiological testing, compared with patients with inducible tachycardia who did not receive therapy, the subgroup patients who received ICDs because they failed to respond to drug therapy did significantly better. There was 24 percent mortality among ICD-treated patients at 5 years of follow-up compared with 55 percent among those receiving electrophysiologically guided drug therapy and 48 percent among those randomly assigned to no therapy. MADIT II is the latest of the primary prevention trials reported to date.[248] In this study, ICD therapy provided a mortality benefit compared with conventional therapy among patients with prior myocardial infarction and ejection fractions less than 30 percent. Another study, still in progress, is the Sudden Cardiac Death–Heart Failure Trial (SCD-HeFT), designed to test the potential benefit of implantable defibrillators versus amiodarone, compared with placebo, among patients with functional class II or III congestive heart failure and ejection fractions less than 35 percent. The results of this study, when reported, should further clarify indications for ICD therapy for primary prevention in high-risk subgroups.

PRIMARY PREVENTION IN PATIENTS WITH LESS ADVANCED COMMON HEART DISEASES OR UNCOMMON DISEASES. Primary prevention trials have been designed to enroll populations of patients with advanced heart disease that were estimated to be at very high risk for SCD and total mortality as a consequence of the severity of the underlying disease. Most of the clinical trials testing the question of relative efficacy of antiarrhythmic versus ICD therapy have used the ejection fraction as the marker for advanced disease, with the qualifying criteria in the range of 30 to 40 percent or less. Moreover, in the secondary prevention trial AVID, a subgroup analysis suggested that there was no relative benefit of ICD therapy over amiodarone for patients with ejection fractions between 36 and 40 percent; all of the benefits accrued to those with ejection fractions of 35 percent or less.[238] This observation is important because it raises a question about therapeutic options—for both primary and secondary prevention strategies—when ejection fractions are greater than 35 percent. However, as a retrospective analysis, the observation calls for confirmation in a controlled trial.

Whereas the risk for SCD and total mortality is highest among patients with advanced structural heart disease and low ejection fractions or limited functional capacity, or both, a substantial portion of the total SCD burden occurs among patients with coronary heart disease or the various nonischemic cardiomyopathies with ejection fractions between 35 and 40 percent and higher. In addition, among patients with heart failure related to various forms of cardiomyopathy, whereas the total mortality risk is considerably lower among patients in functional class I or early class II than among those with late class III or class IV status, the probability of a death being sudden is higher in the former group.[263] Despite this observation, there are no data available to guide therapy for primary prevention of cardiac arrest in such patients.[12,169,264] This limitation is confounded by the fact that the patients in these categories generally have low event rates but cumulatively account for large numbers of SCDs (see Fig. 33–2A). In addition, certain other structural entities that are associated with some elevation of risk of sudden death in the absence of a severely reduced ejection fraction, such as some patterns of viral myocarditis, hypertrophic cardiomyopathy, right ventricular dysplasia, and sarcoidosis, are managed without the benefit of clinical trials to guide therapeutic decisions (see Table 33–4). Patients with symptomatic ventricular arrhythmias related to structural disorders such as right ventricular dysplasia, in which most of the mortality risk is arrhythmic, are often advised to have ICDs even in the absence of a prior cardiac arrest or hemodynamically significant VT. Whether antiarrhythmic therapy would be just as effective remains unknown, but the judgment of using defibrillators in patients with a disorder whose fatal expression is primarily arrhythmic carries the strength of logic, often supported by risk profiling based on observational data on clinical markers. Among the entities in which family history is helpful for defining risk, clinical judgment is made easier when there is a strong family history of SCD. Specific support for this approach derives from genetic studies in hypertrophic cardiomyopathy, in which a limited number of the known mutations appear to be associated with specific risk of SCD.[24] In addition, clinical observational data support the use of ICDs in high-risk subsets of patients with hypertrophic cardiomyopathy.[265]

PRIMARY PREVENTION IN PATIENTS WITH STRUCTURALLY NORMAL HEARTS OR MOLECULAR DISORDERS OF CARDIAC ELECTRICAL ACTIVITY. A new category of interest in primary preventive therapy has emerged. Clinically subtle or inapparent structural disorders or entities with pure electrophysiological expression, such as the congenital long QT interval syndromes, the Brugada syndrome, and idiopathic VF, have received increasing attention. The decision-making process for secondary prevention strategies for patients with the long QT interval syndrome is relatively easy. Individuals who have survived a cardiac arrest or potentially fatal arrhythmic event, especially when there is a family history of SCD, are generally treated with ICDs. Beta blockers are still considered useful for affected family members who have not had an event and perhaps for some subgroups with patients with syncope of undocumented mechanism.[119,120] In contrast, individuals who express the electrocardiographic phenotype of long QT interval syndrome without a family history of SCD or the absence of symptomatic arrhythmias, or both, are generally treated with beta blocker therapy at this time. Between these extremes are the asymptomatic affected family members of patients with symptomatic long QT syndrome. Given the complexity of the pathophysiology of potentially fatal arrhythmias among such patients, the threshold for considering ICD therapy is decreasing.[119] Genetic screening may ultimately prove useful for identifying specific risk, particularly if individual arrhythmic risk is demonstrated to be determined by one or more modifier genes interacting with the defect responsible for an ion channel pore defect (Fig. 33–25).[77] For the present, many such clinical therapeutic decisions remain judgment based rather than data driven. In this context, a family history of premature SCD in affected relatives appears to be useful for the decision-making process for preventive therapy in this general category of patients (see Chap. 28).

Among the other molecular arrhythmia syndromes, the Brugada syndrome is one in which management strategies remain problematic and debated.[266,267] The ICD is accepted as the preferred secondary prevention strategy among cardiac arrest survivors and symptomatic affected individuals even though it is based solely on observational data. However, primary prevention approaches for affected relatives, especially if asymptomatic, are unclear. Studies suggest that syncope associated with ECG changes suggestive of the disorder at baseline is a marker of risk sufficient to warrant ICD

Interactions Between Gene Products	
Direct ion channel modifiers:	
α-subunits	β-subunits
KvLQT1	minK
HERG	MiRP1
SCN5A	SCN1B
Related modifiers:	
Ion channel constructs	Ca^{2+}-handling
KvLQT1 + minK	RyR2
HERG + MiRP1	
SCN5A + SCN1B	
Integrated physiological functions:	
Arrhythmogenic constructs	Autonomic function
I_{K^+}, I_{Na^+}, $I_{Ca^{2+}}$ variants	β_1-AR functional polymorphisms

Gene/Non-Gene Interactions	
Molecular structure	Functional triggers
Inherited ion channel variants	β-adrenergic function (non-gene)
Reactive polymorphisms	Transient pathophysiological states;
Acquired (induced) DNA alterations	Pharmacological/metabolic factors

FIGURE 33–25 Gene-gene and gene-nongene interactions and risk profiling for sudden cardiac death. Genetic characteristics contribute to risk prediction at multiple points in the clinical-epidemiological cascade from the onset of atherogenesis to sudden cardiac death. Genetically determined influences on electrophysiology appear to play a complex role in the final step of the cascade—the onset of a fatal arrhythmia during an acute coronary syndrome. Multiple genes influencing inherent characteristics of ion channel structure and function, their integration with calcium handling and arrhythmogenesis, and individual variations in beta-adrenergic responses to stimulation all appear to play a role in this limited part of the overall cascade. Analysis of the interactions between direct modification of ion channel structure and function, other factors in arrhythmogenesis, and other activities that can be predicted by genetic profiling may provide greater power of prediction for individual risk of arrhythmias in the acutely ischemic setting. Genetically controlled variations, including polymorphisms that are expressed only in pathophysiological states ("reactive" polymorphisms) and acquired DNA alterations, may also play a role. Genetic factors then integrate with nongenetic factors as indicated. The chromosomes containing gene loci currently known to participate in control of several molecular characteristics are indicated. β_1-AR = beta$_1$-adrenergic receptor. (From Myerburg RJ: Scientific gaps in the prediction and prevention of sudden cardiac death. J Cardiovasc Electrophysiol 13:709, 2002.)

therapy[267] and that baseline ECG changes associated with inducibility of ventricular tachyarrhythmias during electrophysiological testing are also a marker of risk.[266] Conversely, the absence of right bundle branch block and ST-T wave changes without provocation suggested lower risk. However, a family history of SCD remains an important factor in judgment-based decisions. Similar arguments, but supported by even less data, apply to affected family members of patients with right ventricular dysplasia.

PRIMARY PREVENTION AMONG THE GENERAL POPULATION, INCLUDING ADOLESCENTS AND YOUNG ADULTS. To have a major impact on the problem of SCD among the general population, we need to move beyond the identification of high-risk patients who have specific clinical entities, advanced or subtle, that predict a high risk of SCD. Rather, it is necessary to find among the general population small subgroups of patients at specific risk for SCD as a manifestation of underlying heart disease, if and when that disease becomes manifest. As an example, the studies that have demonstrated familial clustering of SCD as the first expression of underlying coronary artery disease, suggesting genetic or behavioral predisposition, may provide some help for the future.[35,36] The report of a common genetic "variant" in the cardiac Na^+ channel gene (*SCN5A* on chromosome 3) among blacks with apparent susceptibility to arrhythmias and proarrhythmic responses to antiarrhythmic drugs[30] supports this concept. With a population frequency of affected individuals in the range of 13 percent, a valuable marker of risk may be offered if additional genetic epidemiological studies support the possibility that this is a marker of specific SCD risk during pathophysiological events. If highly specific markers can be found, either related to electrophysiological properties or along multiple points in the cascade of coronary events (see Fig. 33–4), preventive therapy before the first expression of an underlying disease may lead to a major impact on the population problem of SCD. Short of that, successes will be limited to community-based intervention and to the subgroups that are easier to identify and in whom it is more justifiable to use prophylactic interventional therapy on the basis of population size and magnitude of risk.[9,12,169,268]

Adolescents and young adults, including athletes (see Chap. 75), constitute a group for special consideration. The SCD risk among these groups is an order of magnitude of 1 percent of that of the general adult population older than 35 years (see Fig. 33–3A).[88,147,198,269] However, most of the causes of SCD among these populations are not characterized by advanced life-limiting structural heart disease, and therefore surviving cardiac arrest victims can, with appropriate long-term therapy, be expected to have significant extensions of life. Because the majority of deaths are arrhythmic, the ability to identify individuals at risk in advance of a life-threatening arrhythmic event offers more long-term impact than in the case of older populations. Among both the general young population and athletes, identification of individuals at risk may lead to prevention of events that are triggered by physical activity.[270,271] Strategies for screening adolescents, young adults, and athletes to identify the entities that create a risk have met with limited acceptance despite some data indicating both feasibility[146,272] and suggestions of cost-effectiveness.[271] ECG screening of the general adolescent population, including athletes, can identify many of those at potential risk because of congenital long QT syndrome, hypertrophic cardiomyopathy, right ventricular dysplasia, and Brugada syndrome. Although ECG screening in the adolescent and athletic subgroups is imperfect and commonly accompanied by depolarization and repolarization patterns that may be difficult to interpret, this strategy can lead to further testing in appropriate individuals. Echocardiography has also been suggested as a screening method, but it is more expensive and less cost efficient and does not recognize conditions such as long QT syndrome and Brugada syndrome. One study has demonstrated a reduction in SCDs among athletes with the use of widespread screening.[144]

Sudden Death and Public Safety

The unexpectedness of SCD has raised questions concerning secondary risk to the public created by people in the throes of a cardiac arrest. There are no data from controlled studies available to guide public policy regarding people at high risk for potentially lethal arrhythmias and for abrupt incapacitation. In a report of observations on 1348 sudden deaths caused by coronary heart disease in people 65 years of age or younger during a 7-year period in Dade County, Florida, 101 (7.5 percent) of the deaths occurred in people who were engaged in activities at the time of death that were potentially hazardous to the public (e.g., driving motor vehicles, working at altitude, piloting aircraft), and 122 (9.1 percent) of the victims had occupations that could create potential hazards to others if an abrupt loss of consciousness had occurred while they were at work.[273] There were no catastrophic events as a result of these cardiac arrests, only minor property damage in 19 and minor injuries in 5.

Other studies have also led to the conclusion that risk to the public is small. In specific reference to private automobile drivers, most of the data show that sudden death at the wheel usually involves enough of a prodrome to allow the driver to get to the roadside before losing consciousness.[274,275] An analysis of recurrent VT-VF events among cardiac arrest survivors suggested limitation of driving privileges for the first 8 months after the index event on the basis of the clustering of recurrent event rates early after the index event.[16,276] Therefore, although there are likely to be isolated instances in which cardiac arrest causes public hazards in the future, the risk appears to be small; and because it is difficult to identify specific individuals at risk, sweeping restrictions to avoid such risks appear unwarranted. The exceptions are people with multisystem disease, particularly senility, and individual circumstances that require specific consideration, such as high-risk patients who have special responsibilities—school bus drivers, aircraft pilots, train operators, and truck drivers.[16,273,276]

REFERENCES

Definitions

1. Torp-Pedersen C, Kober L, Elming H, Burchart H: Classification of sudden and arrhythmic death. Pacing Clin Electrophysiol 20:245, 1997.
2. Deedwania P: Global risk assessment in the presymptomatic patient. Am J Cardiol 88:17J, 2001.

Epidemiology

3. Priori SG, Aliot E, Blomstrom-Lundqvist C, et al: Task Force on Sudden Cardiac Death of the European Society of Cardiology. Eur Heart J 22:1374, 2001.
4. Gillum RF: Sudden coronary death in the United States: 1980-1985. Circulation 79:756, 1989.
5. Escobedo LG, Zack MM: Comparison of sudden and nonsudden coronary deaths in the United States. Circulation 93:2033, 1996.
6. American Heart Association. 2001 Heart and Stroke Statistical Update. Dallas, American Heart Association, 2000.
7. Zheng ZJ, Croft JB, Giles WH, Mensah GA: Sudden cardiac death in the United States, 1989 to 1998. Circulation 104:2158, 2001.
8. Cobb LA, Fahrenbruch CE, Olsufka M, Copass MK: Changing incidence of out-of-hospital ventricular fibrillation, 1980-2000. JAMA 288:3008, 2002.
9. Myerburg RJ, Kessler KM, Castellanos A: Sudden cardiac death: Epidemiology, transient risk, and intervention assessment. Ann Intern Med 119:1187, 1993.
10. Gillum RF: Geographic variations in sudden coronary death. Am Heart J 119:380, 1990.
11. Myerburg RJ: Sudden cardiac death: Exploring the limits of our knowledge. J Cardiovasc Electrophysiol 12:369, 2001.
12. Huikuri H, Castellanos A, Myerburg RJ: Sudden death due to cardiac arrhythmias. N Engl J Med 345:1473, 2001.
13. Braunwald E: Cardiovascular medicine at the turn of the millennium: Triumphs, concerns, and opportunities. N Engl J Med 337:1360, 1997.
14. Myerburg RJ, Kessler KM, Castellanos A: Sudden cardiac death: Structure, function, and time-dependence of risk. Circulation 85(Suppl I):I-2, 1992.
15. Arntz HR, Willich SN, Schreiber C, et al: Diurnal, weekly and seasonal variation of sudden death. Population-based analysis of 24,061 consecutive cases. Eur Heart J 21:315, 2000.
16. Larsen GC, Stupey MR, Wallace CG, et al: Recurrent cardiac events in survivors of ventricular fibrillation or tachycardia: Implications for driving restrictions. JAMA 271:1335, 1994.
17. Holmberg M, Holmberg S, Herlitz J: Incidence, duration and survival of ventricular fibrillation in out-of-hospital cardiac arrest patients in Sweden. Resuscitation 44:7, 2000.
18. Wren C, O'Sullivan JJ, Wright C: Sudden death in children and adolescents. Heart 83:410, 2000.
19. Kuisma M, Souminen P, Korpela R: Paediatric out-of-hospital cardiac arrests: Epidemiology and outcome. Resuscitation 30:141, 1995.
20. Steinberger J, Lucas RV Jr, Edwards JE, Titus JL: Causes of sudden, unexpected cardiac death in the first two decades of life. Am J Cardiol 77:992, 1996.
21. Neuspiel DR, Kuller LH: Sudden and unexpected natural death in childhood and adolescence. JAMA 254:1321, 1985.
22. Priori SG, Barhanin J, Hauer RNW, et al: Genetic and molecular basis of cardiac arrhythmias: Impact on clinical management. Circulation 99:518, 1999.
23. Schwartz PJ, Priori SG, Spazzolini C, et al: Genotype-phenotype correlation in the long-QT syndrome: Gene-specific triggers for life-threatening arrhythmias. Circulation 103:89, 2001.
24. Marian AJ, Roberts R: Molecular genetic basis of hypertrophic cardiomyopathy: Genetic markers for sudden cardiac death. J Cardiovasc Electrophysiol 9:88, 1998.
25. Danieli GA, Rampazzo A: Genetics of arrhythmogenic right ventricular cardiomyop thy. Curr Opin Cardiol 17:218, 2002.
26. Chen Q, Kirsch GE, Zhang D, et al: Genetic basis and molecular mechanism for idi pathic ventricular fibrillation. Nature 392:293, 1998.
27. Priori SG, Napolitano C, Memmi M, et al: Clinical and molecular characterization patients with catecholaminergic polymorphic ventricular tachycardia. Circulatic 106:69, 2002.
28. Lahat H, Pras E, Olender T, et al: A missense mutation in a highly conserved regio of *CASQ2* is associated with autosomal recessive catecholamine-induced polymorphi ventricular tachycardia in Bedouin families from Israel. Am J Hum Genet 69:137 2001.
29. Brookfield L, Bharati S, Denes P, et al: Familial sudden death: Report of a case an review of the literature. Chest 94:989, 1988.
30. Splawski I, Timothy KW, Tateyama M, et al: Variant of SCN5A sodium channel impl cated in risk of cardiac arrhythmia. Science 297:1333, 2002.
31. Boerwinkle E, Ellsworth DL, Hallman DM, Biddinger A: Genetic analysis of atherc sclerosis: A research paradigm for the common chronic diseases. Hum Mol Gene 5:1405, 1996.
32. Faber BC, Cleutjens KB, Niessen RL, et al: Identification of genes potentially involve in rupture of human atherosclerotic plaques. Circ Res 89:547, 2001.
33. Topol EJ, McCarthy J, Gabriel S, et al: Single nucleotide polymorphisms in multip novel thrombospondin genes may be associated with familial premature myocardia infarction. Circulation 104:2641, 2001.
34. Spooner PM, Albert C, Benjamin EJ, et al: Sudden cardiac death, genes, and arrhyth mogenesis: Consideration of new population and mechanistic approaches from National Heart, Lung, and Blood Institute Workshop. Part I: Circulation 103:2361; Pa II: Circulation 103:2447, 2001.
35. Friedlander Y, Siscovick DS, Weinmann S, et al: Family history as a risk factor fc primary cardiac arrest. Circulation 97:155, 1998.
36. Jouven X, Desnos M, Guerot C, Ducimetiere P: Predicting sudden death in the popu lation: The Paris Prospective Study I. Circulation 99:1978, 1999.
37. Schatzkin A, Cupples LA, Heeren T, et al: The epidemiology of sudden unexpecte death: Risk factors for men and women in the Framingham Heart Study. Am Heart 107:1300, 1984.
38. Schatzkin A, Cupples LA, Heeren T, et al: Sudden death in the Framingham Hea Study: Differences in incidence and risk factors by sex and coronary disease statu Am J Epidemiol 120:888, 1984.
39. Gillum RF: Sudden cardiac death in Hispanic Americans and African Americans. Ar J Public Health 87:1461, 1997.
40. Albert CM, Chae CU, Grodstein F, et al: Prospective study of sudden cardiac deat among women in the United States. Circulation 107:2096, 2003.
41. Becker LB, Han BH, Mayer PM, et al: Racial differences in the inci-dence of cardia arrest and subsequent survival. N Engl J Med 329:600, 1993.
42. Grundy SM, Balady GJ, Criqui MH, et al: Primary prevention of coronary heart disease Guidance from Framingham: A statement for healthcare professionals from the AH Task Force on Risk Reduction. Circulation 97:1876, 1998.
43. Holmes DR, Davis K, Gersh BJ, et al: Risk factor profiles of patients with sudden cardia death and death from other cardiac causes: A report from the Coronary Artery Surger Study (CASS). J Am Coll Cardiol 13:524, 1989.
44. Verdecchia P, Schillaci G, Borgioni C, et al: Prognostic significance of serial change in left ventricular mass in essential hypertension. Circulation 97:48, 1998.
45. Haider AW, Larson MG, Benjamin EJ, Levy D: Increased left ventricular mass an hypertrophy are associated with increased risk for sudden death. J Am Coll Cardic 32:1454, 1998.
46. Essebag V, Eisenberg MJ: Expanding indications for defibrillators after myocardia infarction: Risk stratification and cost effectiveness. Card Electrophysiol Rev 7:4 2003.
47. Myerburg RJ, Kessler KM, Kimura S, et al: Life-threatening ventricular arrhythmias The link between epidemiology and pathophysiology. *In* Zipes DP, Jalife J (eds): Cardia Electrophysiology. 2nd ed. Philadelphia, WB Saunders, 1995, p 723.
48. Taylor AJ, Burke AP, O'Malley PG, et al: A comparison of the Framingham risk index coronary artery calcification, and culprit plaque morphology in sudden cardiac death Circulation 101:1243, 2000.
49. Maclure M: The case-crossover design: A method for studying transient effects on th risk of acute events. Am J Epidemiol 33:144, 1991.
50. Mittleman MA, Maclure M, Tofler GH, et al: Triggering of acute myocardial infarctio by heavy physical exertion: Protection against triggering by regular exertion. N Engl Med 329:1677, 1993.
51. Kannel WB, Thomas HE: Sudden coronary death: The Framingham study. Ann N Acad Sci 382:3, 1982.
52. Hallstrom AP, Cobb LA, Ray R: Smoking as a risk factor for recurrence of sudde cardiac arrest. N Engl J Med 314:271, 1986.
53. Albert CM, Mittleman MA, Chae CU, et al: Triggering of sudden death from cardia causes by vigorous exertion. N Engl J Med 343:1355, 2000.
54. Thiene G, Basso C, Corrado D: Is prevention of sudden death in young athletes feasi ble? Cardiologia 44:497, 1999.
55. Rozanski A, Blumenthal JA, Kaplan J: Impact of psychological factors on the pathc genesis of cardiovascular disease and implications for therapy. Circulation 99:2192 1999.
56. Krantz DS, Sheps DS, Carney RM, Natelson BH: Effects of mental stress in patients wit coronary artery disease: Evidence and clinical implications. JAMA 283:1800, 2000.
57. Hemingway H, Malik M, Marmot M: Social and psychosocial influences on sudde cardiac death, ventricular arrhythmia and cardiac autonomic function. Eur Heart 22:1082, 2001.
58. Thomas SA, Friedmann E, Wimbush F, Schron E: Psychological factors and surviva in the cardiac arrhythmia suppression trial (CAST): A reexamination. Am J Crit Car 6:116, 1997.

59. Irvine J, Basinski A, Baker B, et al: Depression and risk of sudden cardiac death after acute myocardial infarction: Testing for the confounding effects of fatigue. Psychosom Med 61:729, 1999.
60. Williams RB, Barefoot JC, Califf RM, et al: Prognostic importance of social and economic resources among medically treated patients with angiographically documented coronary artery disease. JAMA 267:520, 1992.
61. de Vreede-Swagemakers JJ, Gorgels AP, Weijenberg MP, et al: Risk indicators for out-of-hospital cardiac arrest in patients with coronary artery disease. J Clin Epidemiol 52:601, 1999.
62. The Enhancing Recovery in Coronary Heart Disease Patients (ENRICHD) Randomized Trial Writing Committee: Effects of treating depression and low perceived social support on clinical events after myocardial infarction. JAMA 289:3106, 2003.
63. Leor J, Poole WK, Kloner RA: Sudden cardiac death triggered by an earthquake. N Engl J Med 334:413, 1996.
64. Lampert R, Joska T, Burg MM, et al: Emotional and physical precipitants of ventricular arrhythmia. Circulation 106:1800, 2002.
65. Burke AP, Farb A, Malcom GT, et al: Plaque rupture and sudden death related to exertion in men with coronary artery disease. JAMA 281:921, 1999.
66. de Vreede-Swagemakers JJ, Gorgels AP, Dubois-Arbouw WI, et al: Out-of-hospital cardiac arrest in the 1990's: A population-based study in the Maastricht area on incidence, characteristics and survival. J Am Coll Cardiol 30:1500, 1997.
67. Bigger JT, Fleiss JL, Kleiger R, et al: The relationships among ventricular arrhythmias, left ventricular dysfunction, and mortality in the 2 years after myocardial infarction. Circulation 69:250, 1984.
68. Kennedy HL, Whitlock JA, Sprague MK, et al: Long-term follow-up of asymptomatic healthy subjects with frequent and complex ventricular ectopy. N Engl J Med 312:193, 1985.
69. Viskin S, Belhassen B: Polymorphic ventricular tachyarrhythmias in the absence of organic heart disease: Classification, differential diagnosis, and implications for therapy. Prog Cardiovasc Dis 41:17, 1998.
70. Jouven X, Zureik M, Desnos M, et al: Long-term outcome in asymptomatic men with exercise-induced premature ventricular depolarizations. N Engl J Med 343:826, 2000.
71. Frolkis JP, Pothier CE, Blackstone EH, Lauer MS: Frequent ventricular ectopy after exercise as a predictor of death. N Engl J Med 348:781, 2003.
72. Teerlink JR, Jalaluddin M, Anderson S, et al: Ambulatory ventricular arrhythmias in patients with heart failure do not specifically predict an increased risk of sudden death. PROMISE (Prospective Randomized Milrinone Survival Evaluation) Investigators. Circulation 101:40, 2000.
73. Echt DS, Liebson PR, Mitchell LB, et al: Mortality and morbidity in patients receiving encainide, flecainide, or placebo: The Cardiac Arrhythmia Suppression Trial. N Engl J Med 324:781, 1991.
74. Waldo AL, Camm AJ, deRuyter H, et al, for the SWORD Investigators: Effect of d-sotalol on mortality in patients with left ventricular dysfunction after recent and remote myocardial infarction. Lancet 348:7, 1996.
75. Maisel AS, Scott N, Gilpin E, et al: Complex ventricular arrhythmias in patients with Q wave versus non-Q wave myocardial infarction. Circulation 72:963, 1985.

Causes of Sudden Cardiac Death

76. Myerburg RJ, Interian A Jr, Mitrani RM, et al: Frequency of sudden cardiac death and profiles of risk. Am J Cardiol 80:10F, 1997.
77. Myerburg RJ: Scientific gaps in the prediction and prevention of sudden cardiac death. J Cardiovasc Electrophysiol 13:709, 2002.
78. Frescura C, Basso C, Thiene G, et al: Anomalous origin of coronary arteries and risk of sudden death: A study based on an autopsy population of congenital heart disease. Hum Pathol 29:689, 1998.
79. Myerburg RJ, Kessler KM, Mallon SM, et al: Life-threatening ventricular arrhythmias in patients with silent myocardial ischemia due to coronary artery spasm. N Engl J Med 326:1451, 1992.
80. Sheps DS, Heiss G: Sudden death and silent myocardial ischemia. Am Heart J 117:177, 1989.
81. Anderson KP: Sudden death, hypertension, and hypertrophy. J Cardiovasc Pharmacol 6(Suppl 3):S498, 1984.
82. Braunwald E, Morrow AG, Cornell WP, et al: Idiopathic hypertrophic subaortic stenosis: Clinical, hemodynamic, and angiography manifestations. Am J Med 29:924, 1960.
83. Maron BJ, Spirito P: Impact of patient selection biases on the perception of hypertrophic cardiomyopathy and its natural history. Am J Cardiol 72:970, 1993.
84. Maron BJ, Casey SA, Poliac LC, et al: Clinical course of hypertrophic cardiomyopathy in a regional United States cohort. JAMA 281:650, 1999.
85. McKenna WJ, Behr ER: Hypertrophic cardiomyopathy: Management, risk stratification, and prevention of sudden death. Heart 87:169, 2002.
86. Elliott PM, Gimeno Blanes JR, Mahon NG, et al: Relation between severity of left-ventricular hypertrophy and prognosis in patients with hypertrophic cardiomyopathy. Lancet 357:420, 2001.
87. Maron MS, Olivotto I, Betocchi S, et al: Effect of left ventricular outflow tract obstruction on clinical outcome in hypertrophic cardiomyopathy. N Engl J Med 348:295, 2003.
88. Maron BJ, Shirani J, Poliac LC, et al: Sudden death in young competitive athletes. Clinical, demographic, and pathological profiles. JAMA 276:199, 1996.
89. Cleland JG, Chattopadhyay S, Khand A, et al: Prevalence and incidence of arrhythmias and sudden death in heart failure. Heart Fail Rev 7:229, 2002.
90. Stevenson WE, Stevenson LW, Middlekauff HR, et al: Sudden death prevention in patients with advanced ventricular dysfunction. Circulation 88:2953, 1993.
91. Middlekauff HR, Stevenson WG, Stevenson LW, et al: Syncope in advanced heart failure: High sudden death risk regardless of syncope etiology. J Am Coll Cardiol 21:110, 1993.
92. Knight BP, Goyal R, Pelosi F, et al: Outcome of patients with nonischemic dilated cardiomyopathy and unexplained syncope treated with an implantable defibrillator. J Am Coll Cardiol 33:1964, 1999.
93. Corrado D, Basso C, Thiene G: Sudden cardiac death in young people with apparently normal heart. Cardiovasc Res 50:399, 2001.
94. Theleman KP, Kuiper JJ, Roberts WC: Acute myocarditis (predominately lymphocytic) causing sudden death without heart failure. Am J Cardiol 88:1078, 2001.
95. Phillips M, Rabinowitz M, Higgins JR, et al: Sudden cardiac death in Air Force recruits. JAMA 256:2696, 1986.
96. Roberts WC, McAllister HA, Ferrans VJ: Sarcoidosis of the heart: A clinicopathologic study of 35 necropsy patients (group 1) and review of 78 previously described necropsy patients (group 11). Am J Med 63:86, 1977.
97. Corrado D, Basso C, Nava A, Thiene G: Arrhythmogenic right ventricular cardiomyopathy: Current diagnostic and management strategies. Cardiol Rev 9:259, 2001.
98. Thiene G, Nava A, Corrado D, et al: Right ventricular cardiomyopathy and sudden death in young people. N Engl J Med 318:129, 1988.
99. Fontaine G, Fontaliran F, Hebert JL, et al: Arrhythmogenic right ventricular dysplasia. Annu Rev Med 50:17, 1999.
100. Corrado D, Basso C, Thiene G, et al: Spectrum of clinicopathologic manifestations of arrhythmogenic right ventricular cardiomyopathy/dysplasia: A multicenter study. J Am Coll Cardiol 30:1512, 1997.
101. Furlanello F, Bertoldi A, Dallago M, et al: Cardiac arrest and sudden death in competitive athletes with arrhythmogenic right ventricular dysplasia. Pacing Clin Electrophysiol 21:331, 1998.
102. Tiso N, Stephan DA, Nava A, et al: Identification of mutations in the cardiac ryanodine receptor gene in families affected with arrhythmogenic right ventricular cardiomyopathy type 2 (ARVD2). Hum Mol Genet 10:189, 2001.
103. Rampazzo A, Nava A, Malacrida S, et al: Mutation in human desmoplakin domain binding to plakoglobin causes a dominant form of arrhythmogenic right ventricular cardiomyopathy. Am J Hum Genet 71:1200, 2002.
104. Sorgato A, Faggiano P, Aurigemma GP, et al: Ventricular arrhythmias in adult aortic stenosis: Prevalence, mechanisms, and clinical relevance. Chest 113:482, 1998.
105. McGiffin DC, O'Brien MF, Galbraith AJ, et al: An analysis of risk factors for death and mode-specific death after aortic valve replacement with allograft, xenograft, and mechanical valves. J Thorac Cardiovasc Surg 106:895, 1993.
106. Konishi Y, Matsuda K, Nishiwaki N, et al: Ventricular arrhythmias late after aortic and/or mitral valve replacement. Jpn Circ J 49:576, 1985.
107. Freed LA, Levy D, Levine RA, et al: Prevalence and clinical outcome of mitral valve prolapse. N Engl J Med 341:1, 1999.
108. Chugh SS, Kelly KL, Titus JL: Sudden cardiac death with apparently normal heart. Circulation 102:649, 2000.
109. Weiss BM, Hess OM: Pulmonary vascular disease and pregnancy: Current controversies, management strategies, and perspectives. Eur Heart J 21:104, 2000.
110. Gatzoulis MA, Balaji S, Webber SA, et al: Risk factors for arrhythmia and sudden cardiac death late after repair of tetralogy of Fallot: A multicentre study. Lancet 356:975, 2000.
111. Melgarejo-Moreno A, Galcera-Tomas J, Garcia-Alberola A, et al: Incidence, clinical characteristics, and prognostic significance of right bundle-branch block in acute myocardial infarction: A study in the thrombolytic era. Circulation 96:1139, 1997.
112. Udink ten Cate FE, Breur JM, Cohen MI, et al: Dilated cardiomyopathy in isolated congenital complete atrioventricular block: Early and long-term risk in children. J Am Coll Cardiol 37:1129, 2001.
113. Balmer C, Fasnacht M, Rahn M, et al: Long-term follow up of children with congenital complete atrioventricular block and the impact of pacemaker therapy. Europace 4:345, 2002.
114. Vidaillet HJ, Pressley JC, Henke E, et al: Familial occurrence of accessory atrioventricular pathways (preexcitation syndrome). N Engl J Med 317:65, 1987.
115. Gollob MH, Green MS, Tang AS, et al: Identification of a gene responsible for familial Wolff-Parkinson-White syndrome. N Engl J Med 344:1823, 2001.
116. Priori SG, Bloise R, Crotti L: The long QT syndrome. Europace 3:16, 2001.
117. Priori SG, Schwartz PJ, Napolitano C, et al: Risk stratification in the long-QT syndrome. N Engl J Med 348:1866, 2003.
118. Locati EH, Zareba W, Moss AJ, et al: Age- and sex-related differences in clinical manifestations in patients with congenital long-QT syndrome: Findings from the International LQTS Registry. Circulation 97:2237, 1998.
119. Moss AJ, Zareba W, Hall WJ, et al: Effectiveness and limitations of beta-blocker therapy in congenital long-QT syndrome. Circulation 101:616, 2000.
120. Zareba W, Moss AJ, Schwartz PJ, et al: Influence of genotype on the clinical course of the long-QT syndrome. N Engl J Med 339:960, 1998.
121. Fu EY, Clemo HF, Ellenbogen KA: Acquired QT prolongation: Mechanisms and implications. Cardiol Rev 6:319, 1998.
122. Woosley RL, Chen Y, Freiman JP, Gillis RA: Mechanism of cardiotoxic actions of terfenadine. JAMA 269:1532, 1993.
123. Sesti F, Abbott GW, Wei J, et al: A common polymorphism associated with antibiotic-induced cardiac arrhythmia. Proc Natl Acad Sci USA 97:10613, 2000.
124. Napolitano C, Schwartz PJ, Brown AM, et al: Evidence for a cardiac ion channel mutation underlying drug-induced QT prolongation and life-threatening arrhythmias. J Cardiovasc Electrophysiol 11:691, 2000.
125. Makita N, Horie M, Nakamura T, et al: Drug-induced long-QT syndrome associated with a subclinical SCN5A mutation. Circulation 106:1269, 2002.
126. Brugada J, Brugada R, Brugada P: Right bundle-branch block and ST-segment elevation in leads V1 through V3: A marker for sudden death in patients without demonstrable structural heart disease. Circulation 97:457, 1998.
127. Alings M, Wilde A: "Brugada" syndrome: Clinical data and suggested pathophysiological mechanism. Circulation 99:666, 1999.
128. Priori SG, Napolitano C, Gasparini M, et al: Natural history of Brugada syndrome: Insights for risk stratification and management. Circulation 105:1342, 2002.
129. Brugada J, Brugada R, Antzelevitch C, et al: Long-term follow-up of individuals with the electrocardiographic pattern of right bundle-branch block and ST-segment elevation in precordial leads V1 to V3. Circulation 105:73, 2002.

130. Coumel P, Rosengarten MD, Leclercq JF, Attuel P: Role of sympathetic nervous system in non-ischaemic ventricular arrhythmias. Br Heart J 47:137, 1982.
131. Priori SG, Napolitano C, Memmi M, et al: Clinical and molecular characterization of patients with catecholaminergic polymorphic ventricular tachycardia. Circulation 106:69, 2002.
132. Skinner JE: Neurocardiology. Brain mechanisms underlying fatal cardiac arrhythmias. Neurol Clin 11:325, 1993.
133. Krantz DS, Sheps DS, Carney RM, Natelson BH: Effects of mental stress in patients with coronary artery disease: Evidence and clinical implications. JAMA 283:1800, 2000.
134. Lampert R, Joska T, Burg MM, et al: Emotional and physical precipitants of ventricular arrhythmia. Circulation 106:1800, 2002.
135. Leor J, Poole WK, Kloner RA: Sudden cardiac death triggered by an earthquake. N Engl J Med 334:413, 1996.
136. Leenardt A, Glaser E, Burguera M, et al: Short-coupled variant of torsades de pointes: A new electrocardiographic entity in the spectrum of idiopathic ventricular tachyarrhythmias. Circulation 89:206, 1994.
137. Burrell RJW: The possible bearing of curse death and other factors in Bantu culture in the etiology of myocardial infarction. *In* James TN, Keyes JW (eds): The Etiology of Myocardial Infarction. Boston, Little, Brown, 1963, pp 95-100.
138. Hauck FR, Hunt CE: Sudden infant death syndrome in 2000. Curr Probl Pediatr 30:237, 2000.
139. Gibson E, Fleming N, Fleming D, et al: Sudden infant death syndrome rates subsequent to the American Academy of Pediatrics supine sleep position. Med Care 36:938, 1998.

140. Schwartz PJ, Stramba-Badiale M, Segantini A, et al: Prolongation of the QT interval and the sudden infant death syndrome. N Engl J Med 338:1709, 1998.
141. Schwartz P, Priori S, Dumaine R, et al: A molecular link between the sudden infant death syndrome and the long-QT syndrome. N Engl J Med 343:262, 2000.
142. Marino TA, Kane BM: Cardiac atrioventricular junctional tissues in hearts from infants who died suddenly. J Am Coll Cardiol 5:1178, 1985.
143. Topaz O, Edwards JE: Pathologic features of sudden death in children, adolescents, and young adults. Chest 87:476, 1985.
144. Corrado D, Basso C, Schiavon M, Thiene G: Screening for hypertrophic cardiomyopathy in young athletes. N Engl J Med 339:364, 1998.
145. Virmani R, Burke AP, Farb A, Kark JA: Causes of sudden death in young and middle-aged competitive athletes. Cardiol Clin 15:439, 1997.
146. Maron BJ, Thompson PD, Puffer JC, et al: Cardiovascular preparticipation screening of competitive athletes. A statement for health professionals from the Sudden Death Committee (clinical cardiology) and Congenital Cardiac Defects Committee (cardiovascular disease in the young), American Heart Association. Circulation 94:850, 1996.
147. Myerburg RJ, Mitrani R, Interian A Jr, Castellanos A: Identification of risk of cardiac arrest and sudden cardiac death in athletes. *In* Estes NAM, Salem DN, Wang PJ (eds): Sudden Cardiac Death in the Athlete. Armonk, NY, Futura, 1998, p 25.
148. Basso C, Maron BJ, Corrado D, Thiene G: Clinical profile of congenital coronary artery anomalies with origin from the wrong aortic sinus leading to sudden death in young competitive athletes. J Am Coll Cardiol 35:1493, 2000.
149. Maron BJ, Link MS, Wang PJ, Estes NA 3rd: Clinical profile of commotio cordis: An under appreciated cause of sudden death in the young during sports and other activities. J Cardiovasc Electrophysiol 10:114, 1999.
150. Armstrong LE, Maresh CM: Effects of training, environment, and host factors on the sweating response to exercise. Int J Sports Med 19(Suppl 2):S103, 1998.
151. Joint Steering Committees of the Unexplained Cardiac Arrest Registry of Europe and of the Idiopathic Ventricular Fibrillation Registry of the United States: Survivors of out-of-hospital cardiac arrest with apparently normal heart: Need for definition and standardized clinical evaluation. Circulation 95:265, 1997.
152. Meissner MD, Lehmann MH, Steinman RT: Ventricular fibrillation in patients without significant structural heart disease: A multicenter experience with implantable cardioverter-defibrillator therapy. J Am Coll Cardiol 21:1406, 1993.
153. Nademanee K, Veerakul G, Nimmannit S, et al: Arrhythmogenic marker for the sudden unexplained death syndrome in Thai men. Circulation 96:2595, 1997.

Pathology and Pathophysiology

154. Virmani R, Burke AP, Farb A: Sudden cardiac death. Cardiovasc Pathol 10:211, 2001.
155. Liberthson RR, Nagel EL, Hirschman JC, et al: Pathophysiologic observations in prehospital ventricular fibrillation and sudden cardiac death. Circulation 49:790, 1974.
156. Farb A, Tang AL, Burke AP, et al: Sudden coronary death: Frequency of active coronary lesions, inactive coronary lesions, and myocardial infarction. Circulation 92:1701, 1995.
157. Farb A, Burke AP, Tang AL, et al: Coronary plaque erosion without rupture into a lipid core: A frequent cause of coronary thrombosis in sudden coronary death. Circulation 93:1354, 1996.
158. Warnes CA, Roberts WC: Sudden coronary death: Relation of amount and distribution of coronary narrowing at necropsy to previous symptoms of myocardial ischemia, left ventricular scarring, and heart weight. Am J Cardiol 54:65, 1984.
159. Davies MJ, Thomas A: Thrombosis and acute coronary artery lesions in sudden cardiac ischemic death. N Engl J Med 310:1137, 1984.
160. Burke AP, Farb A, Malcom GT, et al: Coronary risk factors and plaque morphology in men with coronary disease who died suddenly. N Engl J Med 336:1276, 1997.
161. Antman EM, Tanasijevic MJ, Thompson B, et al: Cardiac-specific troponin I levels to predict the risk of mortality in patients with acute coronary syndromes. N Engl J Med 335:1342, 1996.
162. Mullner M, Hirschl MM, Herkner H, et al: Creatine kinase-MB fraction and cardiac troponin T to diagnose acute myocardial infarction after cardiopulmonary resuscitation. J Am Coll Cardiol 28:1220, 1996.
163. Cooper RS, Simmons BE, Castaner A, et al: Left ventricular hypertrophy is associated with worse survival independent of ventricular function and number of coronary arteries severely narrowed. Am J Cardiol 65:441, 1990.
164. Furukawa T, Bassett AL, Furukawa N, et al: The ionic mechanism of reperfusion-induced early afterdepolarizations in the feline left ventricular hypertrophy. J Clin Invest 91:1521, 1993.
165. Cohle SD, Suarez-Mier MP, Aguilera B: Sudden death resulting from lesions of the cardiac conduction system. Am J Forensic Med Pathol 23:83, 2002.
166. Liu YB, Wu CC, Lu LS, et al: Sympathetic nerve sprouting, electrical remodeling, and increased vulnerability to ventricular fibrillation in hypercholesterolemic rabbits. Circ Res 92:1145, 2003.
167. Dorian P, Cass D, Schwartz B, et al: Amiodarone as compared with lidocaine for shock-resistant ventricular fibrillation. N Engl J Med 347:368, 2002.
168. Mehta D, Curwin J, Gomes JA, Fuster V: Sudden death in coronary artery disease: Acute ischemia versus myocardial substrate. Circulation 96:3215, 1997.
169. Myerburg RJ, Kessler KM, Kimura S, Castellanos A: Sudden cardiac death: Future approaches based on identification and control of transient risk factors. J Cardiovasc Electrophysiol 3:626, 1992.
170. Myerburg RJ, Kessler KM, Bassett AL, Castellanos A: A biological approach to sudden cardiac death: Structure, function, and cause. Am J Cardiol 63:1512, 1989.
171. Myerburg RJ, Kessler KM, Zaman L, et al: Survivors of prehospital cardiac arrest. JAMA 247:1485, 1982.
172. Furukawa T, Moroe K, Mayrovitz HN, et al: Arrhythmogenic effects of graded coronary blood flow reductions superimposed on prior myocardial infarction in dogs. Circulation 84:368, 1991.
173. Coronel R, Wilms-Schopman FJG, Opthof T, et al: Reperfusion arrhythmias in isolated perfused pig hearts: Inhomogeneities in extra-cellular potassium, ST and QT potentials, and transmembrane action potentials. Circ Res 71:1131, 1992.
174. Vermeulen JT, Tan HL, Rademaker H, et al: Electrophysiologic and extracellular ionic changes during acute ischemia in failing and normal rabbit myocardium. J Mol Cell Cardiol 28:123, 1996.
175. Remme CA, Schumacher CA, de Jong JW, et al: K(ATP) channel opening during ischemia: Effects on myocardial noradrenaline release and ventricular arrhythmias. Cardiovasc Pharmacol 38:406, 2001.
176. Furukawa T, Kimura S, Furukawa N, et al: Role of cardiac ATP-regulated potassium channels in differential responses of endocardial and epicardial cells to ischemia. Circ Res 68:1693, 1991.
177. Beardslee MA, Lerner DL, Tadros PN, et al: Dephosphorylation and intracellular redistribution of ventricular connexin43 during electrical uncoupling induced by ischemia. Circ Res 87:656, 2000.
178. Yao JA, Hussain W, Patel P, et al: Remodeling of gap junctional channel function in epicardial border zone of healing canine infarcts. Circ Res 92:437, 2003.
179. Schwartz PJ: The autonomic nervous system and sudden death. Eur Heart J 19(Suppl F):F-72, 1998.
180. McLennan PL: Myocardial membrane fatty acids and the antiarrhythmic actions of dietary fish oil in animal models. Lipids 36(Suppl):S-111, 2001.
181. Makikallio TH, Koistinen J, Jordaens L, et al: Heart rate dynamics before spontaneous onset of ventricular fibrillation in patients with healed myocardial infarcts. Am J Cardiol 83:880, 1999.

Clinical Characteristics of the Patient with Cardiac Arrest

182. Liberthson RR, Nagel EL, Hirschman JC, Nussenfeld SR: Prehospital ventricular fibrillation: Prognosis and follow-up course. N Engl J Med 291:317, 1974.
183. Baum RS, Alvarez H, Cobb LA: Survival after resuscitation from out-of-hospital ventricular fibrillation. Circulation 50:1231, 1974.
184. Davies MJ, Bland JM, Hangartner JRW, et al: Factors influencing the presence or absence of acute coronary artery thrombi in sudden ischaemic death. Eur Heart J 10:203, 1989.
185. Bayes de Luna A, Coumel P, Leclercq JF: Ambulatory sudden death: Mechanisms of production of fatal arrhythmia on the basis of data from 157 cases. Am Heart J 117:151 1989.
186. Huikuri HV, Seppanen T, Koistinen MJ, et al: Abnormalities in beat-to-beat dynamics of heart rate before the spontaneous onset of life-threatening ventricular tachyarrhythmias in patients with prior myocardial infarction. Circulation 93:1836, 1996.
187. Huikuri HV, Makikallio TH, Raatikainen MJ, et al: Prediction of sudden cardiac death: Appraisal of the studies and methods assessing the risk of sudden arrhythmic death. Circulation 108:110, 2003
188. Hinkle LE, Thaler HT: Clinical classification of cardiac deaths. Circulation 65:457, 1982.
189. American Heart Association: International Guidelines 2000 for CPR and ECC. Circulation 102(Suppl I):I-1, 2000.
190. Bedell SE, Delbanco TL, Cook EF, Epstein FH: Survival after cardiopulmonary resuscitation in the hospital. N Engl J Med 309:569, 1983.
191. de Vos R, Koster RW, De Haan RJ, et al: In-hospital cardiopulmonary resuscitation: Prearrest morbidity and outcome. Arch Intern Med 159:845, 1999.
192. Herlitz J, Bang A, Alsen B, Aune S: Characteristics and outcome among patients suffering from in hospital cardiac arrest in relation to the interval between collapse and start of CPR. Resuscitation 53:21, 2002.
193. Kim C, Becker L, Eisenberg MS: Out-of-hospital cardiac arrest in octogenarians and nonagenarians. Arch Intern Med 160:3439, 2000.
194. Tresch DD, Thakur RK, Hoffmann RG, et al: Should the elderly be resuscitated following out-of-hospital cardiac arrest? Am J Med 86:145, 1989.
195. Kette F, Sbrojavacca R, Rellini G, et al: Epidemiology and survival rate of out-of-hospital cardiac arrest in northeast Italy: The F.A.C.S. study. Friuli Venezia Giulia Cardiac Arrest Cooperative Study. Resuscitation 36:153, 1998.
196. The Hypothermia after Cardiac Arrest Study Group: Mild therapeutic hypothermia to improve the neurologic outcome after cardiac arrest. N Engl J Med 346:549, 2002.
197. Bernard SA, Gray TW, Buist MD, et al: Treatment of comatose survivors of out-of-hospital cardiac arrest with induced hypothermia. N Engl J Med 346:557, 2002.

198. Myerburg RJ: Sudden cardiac death in persons with normal (or near normal) hearts. Am J Cardiol 79(Suppl 6A):3, 1997.
199. Gorgels AP, Gijsbers C, de Vreede-Swagemakers J, et al: Out-of-hospital cardiac arrest—The relevance of heart failure. The Maastricht Circulatory Arrest Registry. Eur Heart J 24:1204, 2003.
200. Laurent I, Monchi M, Chiche JD, et al: Reversible myocardial dysfunction in survivors of out-of-hospital cardiac arrest. J Am Coll Cardiol 40:2110, 2002.
201. Bunch TJ, White RD, Gersh BJ, et al: Long-term outcomes of out-of-hospital cardiac arrest after successful early defibrillation. N Engl J Med 348:2626, 2003.
202. Iuliano S, Fisher SG, Karasik PE, et al: QRS duration and mortality in patients with congestive heart failure. Am Heart J 143:1085, 2002.
203. The Antiarrhythmics versus Implantable Defibrillators (AVID) Investigators: A comparison of antiarrhythmic-drug therapy with implantable defibrillators in patients resuscitated from near-fatal ventricular arrhythmias. N Engl J Med 337:1576, 1997.
204. Connolly SJ, Gent M, Roberts RS, et al, on behalf of the CIDS Investigators: Canadian Implantable Defibrillator Study (CIDS): A randomized trial of the implantable cardioverter defibrillator against amiodarone. Circulation 101:1297, 2000.
205. Kuck KH, Cappato R, Siebels J, Ruppel R: Randomized comparison of antiarrhythmic drug therapy with implantable defibrillators in patients resuscitated from cardiac arrest: The Cardiac Arrest Study Hamburg (CASH). Circulation 102:748, 2000.

Management of Cardiac Arrest

206. Cobb LA, Weaver WD, Fahrenbrush CE: Community-based interventions for sudden cardiac death: Impact, limitations, and charges. Circulation 85(Suppl I): I-98, 1992.
207. Stults KR, Brown DD, Schug VL, Bean JA: Prehospital defibrillation performed by emergency medical technicians in rural communities. N Engl J Med 310:219, 1984.
208. Stapczynski JS, Svenson JE, Stone CK: Population density, automated external defibrillator use, and survival in rural cardiac arrest. Acad Emerg Med 4:552, 1997.
209. Groh WJ, Newman MM, Beal PE, et al: Limited response to cardiac arrest by police equipped with automated external defibrillators: Lack of survival benefit in suburban and rural Indiana—The police as responder automated defibrillation evaluation (PARADE). Acad Emerg Med 8:324, 2001.
210. Lombardi G, Gallagher J, Gennis P: Outcome of out-of-hospital cardiac arrest in New York City: The Pre-Hospital Arrest Survival Evaluation (PHASE) Study. JAMA 271:678, 1994.
211. Cummins RO, Ornato JP, Thies WH, Pepe PE: Improving survival from sudden cardiac arrest: The "chain of survival" concept: A statement for heart professionals from the Advanced Cardiac Life Support Subcommittee and the Emergency Cardiac Care Committee, American Heart Association. Circulation 83:1832, 1991.
212. Myerburg RJ, Fenster J, Velez M, et al: Impact of community-wide police car deployment of automated external defibrillators on out-of-hospital cardiac arrest. Circulation 106:1058, 2002.
213. Capucci A, Aschieri D, Piepoli MF, et al: Tripling survival from sudden cardiac arrest via early defibrillation without traditional education in cardiopulmonary resuscitation. Circulation 106:1065, 2002.
214. Weisfeldt ML, Becker LB: Resuscitation after cardiac arrest: A 3-phase time-sensitive model. JAMA 288:3035, 2002.
215. Holmberg M, Holmberg S, Herlitz J: The problem of out-of-hospital cardiac arrest: Prevalence of sudden death in Europe today. Am J Cardiol 83:88D, 1999.
216. Waalewijn RA, de Vos R, Koster RW: Out-of-hospital cardiac arrests in Amsterdam and its surrounding areas: Results from the Amsterdam resuscitation study (ARREST) in "Utstein" style. Resuscitation 38:157, 1998.
217. White RD, Hankins DG, Bugliosi TF: Seven years' experience with early defibrillation by police and paramedics in an emergency medical services system. Resuscitation 39:145, 1998.
218. Becker L, Eisenberg M, Fahrenbruch C, Cobb L: Public locations of cardiac arrest: Implications for public access defibrillation. Circulation 97:2106, 1998.
219. Cobb LA, Fahrenbruch CE, Walsh TR, et al: Influence of cardiopulmonary resuscitation prior to defibrillation in patients with out-of-hospital ventricular fibrillation. JAMA 281:1182, 1999.
220. Dowie R, Campbell H, Donohoe R, Clarke P: "Event tree" analysis of out-of-hospital cardiac arrest data: Confirming the importance of bystander CPR. Resuscitation 56:173, 2003.
221. Wik L, Hansen TB, Fylling F, et al: Delaying defibrillation to give basic cardiopulmonary resuscitation to patients with out-of-hospital ventricular fibrillation: A randomized trial. JAMA 289:1389, 2003.
222. Page RL, Joglar JA, Kowal RC, et al. Use of automated external defibrillators by a U.S. airline. N Engl J Med 343:1210, 2000.
223. Caffrey SL, Willoughby PJ, Pepe PE, Becker LB: Public use of automated external defibrillators. N Engl J Med 347:1242, 2002.
224. Valenzuela TD, Roe DJ, Nichol G, et al. Outcomes of rapid defibrillation by security officers after cardiac arrest in casinos. N Engl J Med 343:1206, 2000.
225. Caldwell G, Miller G, Quinn E, et al: Simple mechanical methods for cardioversion: Defense of the precordial thump and cough version. Br Med J (Clin Res Ed) 291:627, 1985.
226. Plaisance P, Lurie KG, Payen D: Inspiratory impedance during active compression-decompression cardiopulmonary resuscitation: A randomized evaluation in patients in cardiac arrest. Circulation 101:989, 2000.
227. Mauer D, Wolcke B, Dick W: Alternative methods of mechanical cardiopulmonary resuscitation. Resuscitation 44:81, 2000.
228. Kerber RE, Becker LB, Bourland JD, et al: Automatic external defibrillators for public access defibrillation: Recommendations for specifying and reporting arrhythmia analysis algorithm performance, incorporating new waveforms, and enhancing safety: A statement for health professionals from the American Heart Association Task Force on Automatic External Defibrillation, Subcommittee on AED Safety and Efficacy. Circulation 95:1677, 1997.
229. Gueugniaud PY, Mols P, Goldstein P, et al: A comparison of repeated high doses and repeated standard doses of epinephrine for cardiac arrest outside the hospital: European Epinephrine Study Group. N Engl J Med 339:1595, 1998.
230. Wenzel V, Lindner KH: Arginine vasopressin during cardiopulmonary resuscitation: Laboratory evidence, clinical experience and recommendations, and a view to the future. Crit Care Med 30(4 Suppl):S157, 2002.
231. Cummins RO, Graves JR, Larsen MP, et al: Out-of-hospital transcutaneous pacing by emergency medical technicians in patients with asystolic cardiac arrest. N Engl J Med 328:1377, 1993.
232. Myerburg RJ, Conde CA, Sung RJ, et al: Clinical, electrophysiologic and hemodynamic profile of patients resuscitated from prehospital cardiac arrest. Am J Med 68:568, 1980.
233. Spaulding CM, Joly LM, Rosenberg A, et al: Immediate coronary angiography in survivors of out-of-hospital cardiac arrest. N Engl J Med 336:1629, 1997.
234. Kelly P, Ruskin JN, Vlahakes GJ, et al: Surgical coronary revascularization in survivors of prehospital cardiac arrest. J Am Coll Cardiol 15:267, 1990.
235. Bigger JT Jr, for the Coronary Artery Bypass Graft (CABG) Patch Trial Investigators: Prophylactic use of implanted cardiac defibrillators in patients at high risk for ventricular arrhythmias after coronary-artery bypass graft surgery. N Engl J Med 337:1569, 1997.
236. Hallstrom AP, Cobb LA, Yu BH, et al: An antiarrhythmic drug experience in 941 patients resuscitated from an initial cardiac arrest between 1970 and 1985. Am J Cardiol 68:1025, 1991.

Prevention of Cardiac Arrest and Sudden Cardiac Death

237. Steinbeck G, Andresen S, Bach P, et al: A comparison of electrophysiologically guided antiarrhythmic drug therapy with beta-blocker therapy in patients with symptomatic sustained ventricular tachyarrhythmias. N Engl J Med 327:987, 1992.
238. Domanski MJ, Sakseena S, Epstein AE, et al, for the AVID Investigators: Relative effectiveness of the implantable cardioverter-defibrillator and antiarrhythmic drugs in patients with varying degrees of left ventricular dysfunction who have survived malignant ventricular arrhythmias. J Am Coll Cardiol 34:1090, 1999.
239. Mason JW, for The Electrophysiologic Study versus Electrocardiographic Monitoring Investigators: A comparison of electrophysiologic testing with Holter monitoring to predict antiarrhythmic-drug efficacy for ventricular tachyarrhythmias. N Engl J Med 329:445, 1993.
240. Reiter MJ, Reiffel JA: Importance of beta blockade in the therapy of serious ventricular arrhythmias. Am J Cardiol 82:9-I, 1998.
241. Boutitie F, Boissel JP, Connolly SJ, et al, for the EMIAT and CAMIAT Investigators: Amiodarone interaction with beta-blockers: Analysis of the merged EMIAT (European Myocardial Infarct Amiodarone Trial) and CAMIAT (Canadian Amiodarone Myocardial Infarction Trial) databases. The EMIAT and CAMIAT Investigators. Circulation 99:2268, 1999.
242. Huikuri HV, Tapanainen JM, Lindgran K, et al: Prediction of sudden cardiac death after myocardial infarction in the beta-blocking era. J Am Coll Cardiol 42:652, 2003.
243. Moss AJ, Hall WJ, Cannom DS, et al, for the Multicenter Automatic Defibrillator Implantation Trial Investigators: Improved survival with an implanted defibrillator in patients with coronary disease at high risk for ventricular arrhythmia. N Engl J Med 335:1933, 1996.
244. Buxton AE, Lee KL, Fisher JD, et al: A randomized study of the prevention of sudden death in patients with coronary artery disease. Multicenter Unsustained Tachycardia Trial Investigators. N Engl J Med 341:1882, 1999.
245. Goldstein S, Brooks MM, Ledingham R, et al: The association between ease of suppression of ventricular arrhythmias and survival. Circulation 91:79, 1995.
246. Priori SG, Aliot E, Blomstrom-Lundqvist C, et al: Task force report: Task Force on Sudden Cardiac Death of the European Society of Cardiology. Eur Heart J 22:1374, 2001.
247. Priori SG, Aliot E, Blomstrom-Lundqvist C, et al: Update of the guidelines on sudden cardiac death of the European Society of Cardiology. Eur Heart J 24:13, 2003.
248. Moss AJ, Zareba W, Hall WJ, et al: Prophylactic implantation of a defibrillator in patients with myocardial infarction and reduced ejection fraction. N Engl J Med 346:877, 2002.
249. Blanck Z, Dhala A, Deshpande S, et al: Bundle branch reentrant ventricular tachycardia. J Cardiovasc Electrophysiol 4:253, 1993.
250. Strickberger SA, Man KC, Daoud EG: A prospective evaluation of catheter ablation of ventricular tachycardia as adjuvant therapy in patients with coronary artery disease and an implantable cardioverter-defibrillator. Circulation 96:1525, 1997.
251. Mirowski M, Reid PR, Winkle RA, et al: Mortality in patients with implanted automatic defibrillators. Ann Intern Med 98:585, 1983.
252. Echt DS, Armstrong K, Schmidt P, et al: Clinical experience, complications, and survival in 70 patients with the automatic implantable cardioverter/defibrillator. Circulation 71:289, 1985.
253. Kelly PA, Cannom DS, Garan H, et al: The automatic implantable defibrillator (AICD): Efficacy, complications and survival in patients with malignant ventricular arrhythmias. J Am Coll Cardiol 11:1278, 1988.
254. Tchou PJ, Kadri N, Anderson J, et al: Automatic implantable cardioverter-defibrillators and survival of patients with left ventricular dysfunction and malignant ventricular arrhythmias. Ann Intern Med 109:529, 1988.
255. Myerburg RJ, Luceri RM, Thurer R, et al: Time to first shock and clinical outcome in patients receiving automatic implantable cardioverter-defibrillators. J Am Coll Cardiol 14:508, 1989.
256. Newman D, Sauve MJ, Herre J, et al: Survival after implantation of the cardioverter defibrillator. Am J Cardiol 69:699, 1992.
257. Myerburg RJ, Castellanos A: Clinical trials of implantable defibrillators. N Engl J Med 337:1621, 1997.
258. Mirowski M, Reid PR, Mower MM, et al: Termination of malignant ventricular arrhythmias with an implanted automatic defibrillator in human beings. N Engl J Med 303:322, 1980.

259. Myerburg RJ, Mitrani R, Interian A Jr, Castellanos A: Interpretation of outcomes of antiarrhythmic clinical trials: Design features and population impact. Circulation 97:1514, 1998.
260. Morris JJ, Rastogi A, Stanton MS, et al: Operation for ventricular tachyarrhythmias: Refining current treatment strategies. Ann Thorac Surg 58:1490, 1994.
261. Julian DG, Camm AJ, Frangin G, et al, for the European Myocardial Infarct Amiodarone Trial Investigators: Randomised trial of effect of amiodarone on mortality in patients with left-ventricular dysfunction after recent myocardial infarction: EMIAT. Lancet 349:667, 1997.
262. Cairns JA, Connolly SJ, Roberts R, Gent M, for the Canadian Amiodarone Myocardial Infarction Arrhythmia Trial Investigators: Randomised trial of outcome after myocardial infarction in patients with frequent or repetitive ventricular premature depolarisations: CAMIAT. Lancet 349:675, 1997.
263. MERIT-HF Study Group: Effect of metoprolol CR/XL in chronic heart failure: Metoprolol CR/XL Randomised Intervention Trial in Congestive Heart Failure (MERIT-HF). Lancet 353:2001, 1999.
264. Zipes DP, Wellens HJ: Sudden cardiac death. Circulation 98:2334, 1998.
265. Maron BJ, Shen WK, Link MS, et al: Efficacy of implantable cardioverter-defibrillators for the prevention of sudden death in patients with hypertrophic cardiomyopathy. N Engl J Med 342:365, 2000.
266. Brugada J, Brugada R, Antzelevitch C, et al: Long-term follow-up of individuals with the electrocardiographic pattern of right bundle-branch block and ST-segment elevation in precordial leads V_1 to V_3. Circulation 105:73, 2002.
267. Priori SG, Napolitano C, Gasparini M, et al: Natural history of Brugada syndrome: Insights for risk stratification and management. Circulation 105:1342, 2002.
268. Yusuf S, Sleight P, Pogue J, et al: Effects of an angiotensin-converting enzyme inhibitor, ramipril, on cardiovascular events in high-risk patients. The Heart Outcomes Prevention Evaluation Study Investigators. N Engl J Med 342:748, 2000.
269. Van Camp SP, Bloor CM, Mueller FO, et al: Nontraumatic sports death in high school and college athletes. Med Sci Sports Exerc 27:641, 1995.
270. Basilico FC: Cardiovascular disease in athletes. Am J Sports Med 27:108, 1999.
271. Fuller CM: Cost effectiveness analysis of screening of high school athletes for risk of sudden cardiac death. Med Sci Sports Exerc 32:887, 2000.
272. Maron BJ, Thompson PD, Puffer JC, et al: Cardiovascular preparticipation screening of competitive athletes: Addendum: An addendum to a statement for health professionals from the Sudden Death Committee (Council on Clinical Cardiology) and the Congenital Cardiac Defects Committee (Council on Cardiovascular Disease in the Young), American Heart Association. Circulation 97:2294, 1998.

Sudden Death and Public Safety

273. Myerburg RJ, Davis JH: The medical ecology of public safety: I. Sudden death due to coronary heart disease. Am Heart J 68:586, 1964.
274. Christian MS: Incidence and implications of natural deaths of road users. BMJ 297:1021, 1988.
275. Halinen MO, Jaussi A: Fatal road accidents caused by sudden death of the driver in Finland and Vaud, Switzerland. Eur Heart J 15:888, 1994.
276. Epstein AE, Miles WM, Benditt DG, et al: Personal and public safety issues related to arrhythmias that may affect consciousness: Implications for regulation and physician recommendations. A medical/scientific statement from the American Heart Association and the North American Society of Pacing and Electrophysiology. Circulation 94:1147, 1996.

CHAPTER 34

Hypotension and Syncope

Hugh Calkins • Douglas P. Zipes

Definition

Syncope is a sudden transient loss of consciousness and postural tone with spontaneous recovery. Loss of consciousness results from a reduction of blood flow to the reticular activating system located in the brain stem and does not require electrical or chemical therapy for reversal. The metabolism of the brain, in contrast to that of many other organs, is exquisitely dependent on perfusion. Consequently, cessation of cerebral blood flow leads to loss of consciousness within approximately 10 seconds. Restoration of appropriate behavior and orientation after a syncopal episode is usually immediate. Retrograde amnesia is uncommon. Syncope is an important clinical problem because it is common, is costly, is often disabling, may cause injury, and may be the only warning sign before sudden cardiac death.[1] Patients with syncope account for 1 percent of hospital admissions and 3 percent of emergency department visits. Elderly persons have a 6 percent annual incidence of syncope. Surveys of young adults have revealed that up to 50 percent report a prior episode of loss of consciousness; most of these episodes are isolated events that never come to medical attention. The Framingham Study, in which biennial examinations were performed on 7814 individuals, reported the incidence of a first report of syncope to be 6.2 per 1000 person-years follow-up.[2] The annual cost of evaluating and treating patients with syncope has been estimated to be $800 million.[3] Patients who experience syncope also report a markedly reduced quality of life.[4] The prognosis of patients with syncope varies greatly with the diagnosis. In the Framingham Study, for example, participants with syncope, including those with syncope of unknown origin, had increased mortality compared with participants without syncope. The highest mortality was observed among those with a cardiac cause of syncope. In contrast, the subgroup of participants with neurally mediated syncope (including orthostatic hypotension and medication-related syncope) did not experience increased mortality.[2]

Classification

The causes of syncope can be classified into six primary groups: vascular, cardiac, neurologic-cerebrovascular, psychogenic, metabolic-miscellaneous, and syncope of unknown origin (Table 34–1). A similar subclassification of the causes of syncope can be applied to the other diagnostic groups. Table 34–1 shows the types and relative frequencies with which various etiologies of syncope were established in three prospective clinical trials.[5-7] Vascular causes of syncope are most common, followed by cardiac causes of syncope. Psychogenic causes of syncope are now being recognized with increased frequency.[5-9] Some of the causes of syncope shown in Table 34–1 are not causes of "true syncope," which results from sudden transient global cerebral hypoperfusion. These "nonsyncopal" conditions (shown by an asterisk) include conditions in which consciousness is lost as a result of metabolic disorders, epilepsy, or alcohol as well as conditions in which consciousness is only apparently lost (i.e., conversion reaction).

Although knowledge of the common conditions that can cause syncope is essential and allows the clinician to arrive at a probable cause of syncope in the majority of patients, it is equally important for the clinician to be aware of several of the less common but potentially lethal causes of syncope, such as the long QT syndrome, arrhythmogenic right ventricular dysplasia, Brugada syndrome, hypertrophic cardiomyopathy, and pulmonary emboli.[10-12] It is also important to recognize that the distribution of the causes of syncope varies with age. In young individuals, neurally mediated syncope is by far most common, but neurally mediated syncope is an unusual type of syncope in elderly persons. Common causes of syncope in elderly persons include orthostatic hypotension, postprandial hypotension, medication, aortic stenosis, carotid sinus hypersensitivity, and bradyarrhythmias (i.e., sick sinus syndrome, heart block).

Vascular Causes of Syncope

Vascular causes of syncope, particularly reflex-mediated syncope and orthostatic hypotension, are by far the most common causes, accounting for at least one-third of all syncopal episodes.[13] In contrast, subclavian steal syndrome is an exceedingly uncommon cause of syncope, accounting for less than 0.1 percent of syncopal episodes.

ORTHOSTATIC HYPOTENSION. When a person stands, 500 to 800 ml of blood is displaced to the abdomen and lower extremities, resulting in an abrupt drop in venous return to the heart. This drop leads to a decrease in cardiac output and stimulation of aortic, carotid, and cardiopulmonary baroreceptors that trigger a reflex increase in sympathetic outflow. As a result, heart rate, cardiac contractility, and vascular resistance increase to maintain a stable systemic blood pressure on standing. Orthostatic hypotension, which is defined as a 20 mm Hg drop in systolic blood pressure or a 10 mm Hg drop in diastolic blood pressure within 3 minutes of standing, results from a defect in any portion of this blood pressure control system. Orthostatic hypotension can be asymptomatic or

TABLE 34–1 Causes of Syncope

Causes	Relative Frequency (%) Sarasin et al[7] (n = 611)	Ammirati et al[5] (n = 195)	Alboni et al[6] (n = 356)
Vascular	**62**	**42**	**58**
Anatomic			
Subclavian steal			
Orthostatic	24	6	2
Autonomic insufficiency			
Idiopathic			
Hypovolemia			
Drug-induced			
Reflex mediated			
Carotid sinus hypersensitivity	1	2	14
Neurally mediated syncope	37	30	33
Glossopharyngeal syncope			
Situational (cough, swallow, micturition)		4	7
Adenosine sensitive			2
Cardiac	**10**	**21**	**23**
Anatomic	4	3	3
Aortic stenosis			
Aortic dissection			
Atrial myxoma			
Cardiac tamponade			
Hypertrophic obstructive cardiomyopathy			
Mitral stenosis			
Myocardial ischemia/infarction			
Pulmonary embolus			
Pulmonary hypertension			
Arrhythmias			
Bradyarrhythmias	5	11	15
Sinus node dysfunction/bradycardia			
Atrioventricular block			
Tachycarrhythmias	2	7	5
Supraventricular arrhythmias			
Ventricular arrhythmias (including long QT syndrome)			
Neurologic / Cerebrovascular*	**5**	**14**	**0.70**
Arnold-Chiari malformation			
Migraine			
Seizure (partial complex, temporal lobe)		3	0.20
Vertebral-basilar insufficiency/transient ischemic attack		11	0.50
Metabolic / Miscellaneous	**2**	**1**	**0**
Metabolic*			
Drugs/alcohol			
Hyperventilation (hypocapnea)			
Hypoglycemia			
Hypoxemia			
Miscellaneous			
Cerebral syncope			
Hemorrhage			
Psychogenic syncope*	**1.50**	**6**	**0.20**
Hysterical			
Anxiety/panic disorder			
Somatization disorders			
Syncope of unknown origin	**14**	**18**	**18**

*Disorders resembling syncope.

associated with symptoms such as lightheadedness, dizziness, blurred vision, weakness, palpitations, tremulousness, and syncope. These symptoms are often worse immediately on arising in the morning or after meals or exercise. Syncope that occurs after meals, particularly in elderly people, can result from a redistribution of blood to the gut. A decline in systolic blood pressure of about 20 mm Hg approximately 1 hour after eating has been reported in up to one third of elderly nursing home residents. Although usually asymptomatic, it can result in lightheadedness or syncope.

Drugs that either cause volume depletion or result in vasodilation are the most common cause of orthostatic hypotension (Table 34–2). Elderly patients are particularly susceptible to the hypotensive effects of drugs because of reduced baroreceptor sensitivity, decreased cerebral blood flow, renal sodium wasting, and an impaired thirst mechanism that develops with aging. Orthostatic hypotension can also result from neurogenic causes, which can be subclassified into primary and secondary autonomic failure.[13,14] Primary causes are generally idiopathic, whereas secondary causes are associated with a known biochemical or structural anomaly or are seen as part of a particular disease or syndrome. There are three types of primary autonomic failure. Pure autonomic failure (Bradbury-Eggleston syn-

TABLE 34–2 Causes of Orthostatic Hypotension

Drugs
Diuretics
Alpha-adrenergic blocking drugs
Terazosin (Hytrin), labetalol
Adrenergic neuron blocking drugs
Guanethidine
Angiotensin-converting enzyme inhibitors
Antidepressants
Monoamine oxidase inhibitors
Alcohol
Diuretics
Ganglion-blocking drugs
Hexamethonium, mecamylamine
Tranquilizers
Phenothiazines, barbiturates
Vasodilators
Prazosin, hydralazine, calcium channel blockers
Centrally acting hypotensive drugs
Methyldopa, clonidine
Primary Disorders of Autonomic Failures
Pure autonomic failure (Bradbury-Eggleston syndrome)
Multiple system atrophy (Shy-Drager syndrome)
Parkinson disease with autonomic failure
Secondary Neurogenic
Aging
Autoimmune disease
Guillain-Barré syndrome, mixed connective tissue disease, rheumatoid arthritis
Eaton-Lambert syndrome, systemic lupus erythematosus
Carcinomatosis autonomic neuropathy
Central brain lesions
Multiple sclerosis, Wernicke encephalopathy
Vascular lesions or tumors involving the hypothalamus and midbrain
Dopamine beta-hydroxylase deficiency
Familial hyperbradykinism
General medical disorders
Diabetes, amyloid, alcoholism, renal failure
Hereditary sensory neuropathies, dominant or recessive
Infections of the nervous system
Human immunodeficiency virus infection, Chagas disease, botulism, syphilis
Metabolic disease
Vitamin B_{12} deficiency, porphyria, Fabry disease. Tangier disease
Spinal cord lesions

Adapted from Bannister SR (ed): Autonomic Failure, 2nd ed. Oxford, Oxford University Press, 1988, p 8.

drome) is an idiopathic sporadic disorder characterized by orthostatic hypotension, usually in conjunction with evidence of more widespread autonomic failure such as disturbances in bowel, bladder, thermoregulatory, and sexual function. Patients with pure autonomic failure have reduced supine plasma norepinephrine levels. Multiple system atrophy (Shy-Drager syndrome) is a sporadic, progressive, adult-onset disorder characterized by autonomic dysfunction, parkinsonism, and ataxia in any combination. The third type of primary autonomic failure is Parkinson disease with autonomic failure. A small subset of patients with Parkinson disease may also experience autonomic failure, including orthostatic hypotension. In addition to these forms of chronic autonomic failure is a rare acute panautonomic neuropathy. This neuropathy generally occurs in young people and results in widespread severe sympathetic and parasympathetic failure with orthostatic hypotension, loss of sweating, disruption of bladder and bowel function, fixed heart rate, and fixed dilated pupils.

Postural orthostatic tachycardia syndrome (POTS) is a milder form of chronic autonomic failure and orthostatic intolerance characterized by the presence of symptoms of orthostatic intolerance, an increase of 28 beats/min or more in heart rate, and absence of a significant change in blood pressure within 5 minutes of standing or upright tilt.[13] POTS appears to result from a failure of the peripheral vasculature to vasoconstrict appropriately under orthostatic stress. POTS can also be associated with syncope related to neurally mediated hypotension (see later).

REFLEX-MEDIATED SYNCOPE. There are many reflex-mediated syncopal syndromes (see Table 34–1). In each case, the reflex is composed of a trigger (the afferent limb) and a response (the efferent limb). This group of reflex-mediated syncopal syndromes has in common the response limb of the reflex, which consists of increased vagal tone and a withdrawal of peripheral sympathetic tone and leads to bradycardia, vasodilation, and, ultimately, hypotension, presyncope, or syncope. What distinguishes these causes of syncope are the specific triggers. For example, micturition syncope results from activation of mechanoreceptors in the bladder; defecation syncope results from neural inputs from gut wall tension receptors; and swallowing syncope results from afferent neural impulses arising from the upper gastrointestinal tract. The two most common types of reflex-mediated syncope, carotid sinus hypersensitivity and neurally mediated hypotension, are discussed later.

Neurally Mediated Hypotension or Syncope. The term *neurally mediated hypotension* or *syncope* (also known as neurocardiogenic, vasodepressor, and vasovagal syncope and as "fainting") has been used to describe a common abnormality of blood pressure regulation characterized by the abrupt onset of hypotension with or without bradycardia. Triggers associated with the development of neurally mediated syncope are those that either reduce ventricular filling or increase catecholamine secretion.[13-15] They include the sight of blood, pain, prolonged standing, a warm environment or hot shower, and stressful situations. In these types of situations, patients with this condition experience severe lightheadedness or syncope, or both. It has been proposed that these clinical phenomena result from a paradoxical reflex that is initiated when ventricular preload is reduced by venous pooling. This reduction leads to a reduction in cardiac output and blood pressure, which is sensed by arterial baroreceptors. The resultant increased catecholamine levels, combined with reduced venous filling, lead to a vigorously contracting volume-depleted ventricle. The heart itself is involved in this reflex by virtue of the presence of mechanoreceptors, or C-fibers, consisting of nonmyelinated fibers found in the atria, ventricles, and pulmonary artery. It has been proposed that vigorous contraction of a volume-depleted ventricle leads to activation of these receptors in susceptible individuals. These afferent C-fibers project centrally to the dorsal vagal nucleus of the medulla, leading to a "paradoxical" withdrawal of peripheral sympathetic tone and an increase in vagal tone, which, in turn, causes vasodilation and bradycardia. The ultimate clinical consequence is syncope or presyncope. Not all neurally mediated syncope results from activation of mechanoreceptors. In humans, it is well known that the sight of blood or extreme emotion can trigger syncope. These observations suggest that higher neural centers can also participate in the pathophysiology of vasovagal syncope. In addition, central mechanisms can contribute to the production of neurally mediated syncope.

Carotid Sinus Hypersensitivity. Syncope caused by *carotid sinus hypersensitivity* results from stimulation of carotid sinus baroreceptors, which are located in the internal carotid artery above the bifurcation of the common carotid artery. Carotid sinus hypersensitivity is diagnosed by applying gentle pressure over the carotid pulsation just below the angle of the jaw, where the carotid bifurcation is located. Pressure should be applied for 5 to 10 seconds. Studies have highlighted the importance of performing carotid sinus massage in both the supine and upright positions.[16,17] The main complications associated with performing carotid sinus massage are neurological. One study reported that persistent neurological complications are uncommon, occurring in 1 per 1000 patients.[18] Because of this complication, carotid sinus massage should be avoided in patients with prior transient ischemic attacks, strokes within the past 3 months, and carotid bruits.

A normal response to carotid sinus massage is a transient decrease in the sinus rate or slowing of atrioventricular (AV) conduction, or both. Carotid sinus hypersensitivity is defined as a sinus pause of more than 3 seconds duration and a fall in systolic blood pressure of 50 mm Hg or more. The response to carotid sinus massage can be classified as cardioinhibitory (asystole), vasodepressive (fall in systolic blood pressure), or mixed. Carotid sinus hypersensitivity is detected in approximately one third of elderly patients with syncope. Carotid sinus hypersensitivity is also commonly detected in elderly patients presenting after falls, with one study reporting the presence of carotid sinus hypersensitivity in approximately one fourth of patients presenting to an emergency room after falls.[19] It is important to recognize, however, that carotid sinus hypersensitivity is also commonly observed in asymptomatic elderly patients. Thus, the diagnosis of carotid sinus hypersensitivity should be approached cautiously after excluding alternative causes of syncope. Carotid sinus hypersensitivity is suggested in patients older than 40 years with syncope of unexplained cause following the initial history, physical examination, and electrocardiogram (ECG).[1] Once it is diagnosed, dual-chamber pacemaker implantation is recommended for patients with recurrent syncope resulting from carotid sinus hypersensitivity.[20]

Cardiac Causes of Syncope

Cardiac causes of syncope, particularly tachyarrhythmias and bradyarrhythmias (see Chap. 32), are the second most common causes, accounting for 10 to 20 percent of syncopal episodes. Ventricular tachycardia (VT) is the most common tachyarrhythmia that can cause syncope. Supraventricular tachycardia can also cause syncope, although the great majority of patients with supraventricular arrhythmias present with less severe symptoms such as palpitations, dyspnea, and lightheadedness. Bradyarrhythmias that can result in syncope include sick sinus syndrome as well as AV block. Anatomical causes of syncope include obstruction to blood flow, such as a massive pulmonary embolus, an atrial myxoma, or aortic stenosis.

Neurological Causes of Syncope

Neurological causes of syncope, including migraines, seizures, Arnold-Chiari malformations, and transient ischemic attacks, are surprisingly uncommon, accounting for less than 10 percent of all cases of syncope. The majority of patients in whom a "neurological" cause of syncope is established are found in fact to have had a seizure rather than true syncope.

Metabolic-Miscellaneous Causes of Syncope

Metabolic causes of syncope are rare, accounting for less than 5 percent of syncopal episodes. The most common metabolic causes of syncope are hypoglycemia, hypoxia, and hyperventilation. Establishing hypoglycemia as the cause of syncope requires demonstration of hypoglycemia during the syncopal episode. Although hyperventilation-induced syncope has been generally considered to be due to a reduction in cerebral blood flow, one study demonstrated that hyperventilation alone was not sufficient to cause syncope. This observation suggests that hyperventilation-induced syncope may also have a psychological component. Psychiatric disorders may also cause syncope. It has been reported that up to 25 percent of patients with syncope of unknown origin may have psychiatric disorders for which syncope is one of the presenting symptoms.[8,9] Cerebral syncope is a rare type of syncope resulting from cerebral vasoconstriction induced by orthostatic stress.[21]

RELATIONSHIP BETWEEN PROGNOSES AND THE CAUSE OF SYNCOPE. The prognosis for patients with syncope varies greatly with the diagnosis. Syncope of unknown origin or syncope with a noncardiac etiology (including reflex-mediated syncope) is generally associated with a benign prognosis. In contrast, syncope with a cardiac cause is associated with up to 30 percent mortality at 1 year.[1]

Diagnostic Tests

Identification of the precise cause of syncope is often challenging. Because syncope usually occurs sporadically and infrequently, it is extremely difficult to either examine a patient or obtain an ECG during an episode of syncope. For this reason, the primary goal in the evaluation of a patient with syncope is to arrive at a presumptive determination of the cause of syncope.

History and Physical Examination

The history and physical examination are by far the most important components of the evaluation of a patient with syncope (see Chap. 7). Several studies have reported that the probable cause of syncope can be identified on the basis of the history and physical examination alone in more than 25 percent of patients.[5-7] Maximal information can be obtained from the clinical history when it is approached in a systematic and detailed fashion. Initial evaluation should begin by determining whether the patient did, in fact, experience a syncopal episode. Every effort should be made to differentiate true syncope from alterations in consciousness resulting from nonsyncopal conditions such as metabolic and psychiatric disorders. Although falls can be differentiated from syncope by the absence of loss of consciousness, an overlap between symptoms of falls and syncope has been reported.[16,22] This overlap may reflect the fact that elderly individuals may experience amnesia for the episode of loss of consciousness. When evaluating a patient with syncope, particular attention should then be focused on (1) determining whether the patient has a history of cardiac disease or a family history of cardiac disease, syncope, or sudden death; (2) identifying medications that may have played a role in syncope; (3) quantifying the number and chronicity of prior syncopal and presyncopal episodes; (4) identifying precipitating factors including body position; and (5) quantifying the type and duration of prodromal and recovery symptoms. It is also useful to obtain careful accounts from witnesses who may have been present. The features of the clinical history most helpful in determining whether syncope resulted from neurally mediated hypotension, an arrhythmia, or a seizure are summarized in Table 34–3.

The clinical histories obtained from patients with syncope related to AV block and VT are similar. In each case, syncope

TABLE 34–3 Differentiating Syncope Caused by Neurally Mediated Hypotension, Arrhythmias, and Seizures

	Neurally Mediated Hypotension	Arrhythmias	Seizure
Demographics/clinical setting	Female > male gender Younger age (<55 yr) More episodes (>2) Standing, warm room, emotional upset	Male > female gender Older age (>54 yr) Fewer episodes (<3) Any setting	Younger age (<45 yr) Any setting
Premonitory symptoms	Longer duration (>5 sec) Palpitations Blurred vision Nausea Warmth Diaphoresis Lightheadedness	Shorter duration (<6 sec) Palpitations less common	Sudden onset or brief aura (déjà vu, olfactory, gustatory, visual)
Observations during the event	Pallor Diaphoretic Dilated pupils Slow pulse, low blood pressure Incontinence may occur. Brief clonic movements may occur.	Blue, not pale Incontinence can occur. Brief clonic movements can occur.	Blue face, no pallor Frothing at the mouth Prolonged syncope (duration >5 minutes) Tongue biting Horizontal eye deviation Elevated pulse and blood pressure Incontinence more likely* Tonic clonic movements if grand mal
Residual symptoms	Residual symptoms common Prolonged fatigue common (>90%) Oriented	Residual symptoms uncommon (unless prolonged unconsciousness) Oriented	Residual symptoms common Aching muscles Disoriented Fatigue Headache Slow recovery

*May be observed with any of these causes of syncope but more common with seizures.

typically occurs with less than 5 seconds of warning and few if any prodromal and recovery symptoms. Demographic features suggesting that syncope results from an arrhythmia such as VT or AV block include male gender, less than three prior episodes of syncope, and increased age. Features of the clinical history that point toward a vasovagal cause of syncope include palpitations, blurred vision, nausea, warmth, diaphoresis, or lightheadedness before syncope and the presence of nausea, warmth, diaphoresis, or fatigue after syncope.

The historical features of syncope were evaluated in 341 consecutive patients who were interviewed with a standard questionnaire.[6] A vascular cause of syncope was identified in 58 percent, a cardiac cause in 23 percent, a neurological or psychiatric cause in 1 percent, and syncope of unknown origin was diagnosed in 18 percent. This study initially evaluated the predictive ability of variables that are not part of the presentation of syncope: age, gender, and the presence of suspected cardiac disease (based on the initial evaluation that comprised the clinical history and ECG). Multivariate analysis revealed that the presence of suspected cardiac disease was the only independent predictor of a cardiac cause of syncope (odds ratio 16). The historical variables of syncope were then examined separately among the 191 patients with suspected cardiac disease and the 146 patients without suspected cardiac disease . The absence of suspected cardiac disease on the basis of the initial evaluation allowed a cardiac cause of syncope to be excluded in 142 of the 146 patients without suspected cardiac disease (97 percent). Among patients with suspected cardiac disease, variables that were predictive of a cardiac cause of syncope on multivariate analysis included duration of symptoms less than 4 years, history of presyncope, and blurred vision prior to syncope. Variables predictive of vascular syncope included duration of symptoms greater than 4 years, history of presyncope, and nausea. Among patients without suspected cardiac disease, the only variable predictive of a cardiac cause of syncope was palpitations before loss of consciousness. The only variable predictive of vascular syncope among patients without suspected cardiac disease was a duration of prodromal symptoms greater than 10 seconds. The authors concluded that the absence of suspected cardiac disease on initial evaluation together with the absence of palpitations prior to syncope allows exclusion of a cardiac cause of syncope. Although the presence of suspected cardiac disease is a strong predictor of a cardiac cause of syncope, its specificity is low.

The clinical history is also valuable in distinguishing seizures from syncope. Features of the clinical history that are useful in distinguishing seizures from syncope include orientation following an event, a blue face or not becoming pale during the event, frothing at the mouth, aching muscles, feeling sleepy after the event, and a duration of unconsciousness of more than 5 minutes. Tongue biting strongly points toward a seizure rather than syncope as the cause of loss of consciousness. Other findings suggestive of a seizure as a cause of the syncopal episode include (1) an aura before the episode, (2) horizontal eye deviation during the episode, (3) an elevated blood pressure and pulse during the episode, and (4) a headache following the event. Urinary or fecal incontinence can be observed in association with either a seizure or a syncopal episode but occurs more commonly in association with a seizure. Grand mal seizures are usually associated with tonic-clonic movements. It is important to note that syncope caused by cerebral ischemia can result in decorticate rigidity with clonic movements of the arms. Akinetic or petit mal seizures can be recognized by the patient's lack of responsiveness in the absence of a loss of postural tone. Temporal lobe seizures can also be confused with syncope. These seizures last several minutes and are characterized by confusion, changes in the level of consciousness, and autonomic signs such as flushing. Vertebral basilar insufficiency should be considered as the cause of syncope if syncope occurs in association with other symptoms of brain stem ischemia (i.e., diplopia, tinnitus, focal weakness or sensory loss, vertigo, or dysarthria). Migraine-mediated syncope is often associated with a throbbing unilateral headache, scintillating scotomata, and nausea.

In one study, a standardized questionnaire was administered to 102 patients with seizure and 569 patients with syncope.[23] The clinical symptoms reported by patients with syncope were compared with those reported by patients with seizure. Patients with seizure were more likely to have had a cut tongue, bedwetting, prodromal déjà vu, preoccupation, mood changes, hallucinations or trembling before loss of consciousness, postictal confusion, muscle pain, headaches, observed convulsive movements, head turning, unresponsiveness during loss of consciousness, and blue skin observed by a bystander. Patients with syncope were more likely to experience presyncope, have syncope associated with prolonged sitting or standing, or have presyncope with prolonged sitting or standing, warm environments, and exercise. Patients with syncope were also more likely to experience diaphoresis, dyspnea, chest pain, palpitations, warmth, nausea, and vertigo. The authors then developed a simple point score of diagnostic criteria that distinguishes seizures from syncope with 85 percent accuracy.

PHYSICAL EXAMINATION. After obtaining a careful history, evaluation should continue with a physical examination. In addition to a complete cardiac examination, particular attention should be focused on determining whether structural heart disease is present, defining the patient's level of hydration, and detecting the presence of significant neurological abnormalities suggestive of a dysautonomia or a cerebrovascular accident. Orthostatic vital signs are a critical component of the evaluation. The patient's blood pressure and heart rate should be obtained while he or she is supine and should then be obtained each minute for approximately 3 minutes. The three abnormalities that should be searched for are (1) early orthostatic hypotension, defined as a 20 mm Hg drop in systolic blood pressure or a 10 mm Hg drop in diastolic blood pressure within 3 minutes of standing; (2) POTS, which is defined as an increase of 28 beats/min or more within 5 minutes of standing with symptoms of orthostatic intolerance. The significance of POTS lies in its close overlap with neurally mediated syncope.[13]

Laboratory Tests

BLOOD TESTS. The routine use of blood tests, such as serum electrolytes, cardiac enzymes, glucose, and hematocrit levels, is of low diagnostic value.[24-26] As a result, the routine use of laboratory tests is not recommended for patients with syncope. Under rare circumstances, aspects of the patient's clinical presentation may suggest the diagnostic value of this type of testing.

CAROTID SINUS MASSAGE. Carotid sinus hypersensitivity is diagnosed by carotid massage, as outlined earlier.

TILT-TABLE TESTING. The tilt-table test (see Chap. 29) is a standard and widely accepted diagnostic test for evaluating patients with syncope.[1,27] To the extent that upright tilt testing provides diagnostic evidence indicating susceptibility to neurally mediated syncope, it is considered the "gold standard" for establishing this diagnosis. The American College of Cardiology published an expert consensus document that contains specific recommendations for performing and interpreting the results of this test.[27] Upright tilt testing is generally performed for 30 to 45 minutes at an angle between 60 and 80 degrees (with 70 degrees the most common). The sensitivity of the test can be increased, with an associated fall in specificity, by the use of longer tilt durations, steeper tilt angles, and provocative agents such as isoproterenol or nitroglycerin.[28-30] When isoproterenol is employed as a provocative agent, it is recommended that the infusion rate be increased incrementally from 1 to 3 μg/min in order to increase the heart rate to 25 percent greater than baseline. When nitroglycerin is employed, a fixed does of 400 μg nitroglycerine spray should be administered sublingually with the patient in the upright position. These two provocative approaches are equivalent in diagnostic accuracy. In the absence of pharmacological provocation, the specificity of the test has been estimated to be 90 percent.

There is general agreement that upright tilt testing is indicated in patients with recurrent syncope, in high-risk patients with a single syncopal episode for whom there is no evidence of structural heart disease or other causes of syncope have been excluded, and in the evaluation of patients for whom the cause of syncope has been determined (i.e., asystole) but the presence of neurally mediated syncope on upright tilt would influence treatment.[27] There is also general agreement that upright tilt-table testing is not necessary for patients who have experienced only a single syncopal episode that was highly typical for neurally mediated syncope and during which no injury occurred. Tilt-table testing is not useful in establishing a diagnosis of situation syncope (i.e., postmicturition syncope).[31]

ECHOCARDIOGRAPHY. Although echocardiograms are commonly used in the evaluation of patients with syncope, little objective evidence exists to support their use in patients with a normal physical examination and a normal ECG. The rationale for obtaining an echocardiogram in patients with syncope is to stratify the patient's risk by excluding the possibility of occult cardiac disease not apparent after the history, physical examination, and electrocardiography. The only situations in which an echocardiogram would be considered diagnostic of the cause of syncope are severe left ventricular outflow obstruction (see Chaps. 57 and 59) and atrial myxoma (see Chap. 11). Current guidelines recommend that an echocardiogram should not be obtained routinely for all patients with syncope but should be obtained when cardiac disease is suspected.[1]

STRESS TESTS, CARDIAC CATHETERIZATIONS. Myocardial ischemia is an unlikely cause of syncope and, when present, is usually accompanied by angina (see Chap. 49). Exercise stress testing and cardiac catheterization are unlikely to establish a diagnosis in patients presenting with syncope unless the clinical suspicion of ischemia is high.[32] The use of stress tests in the evaluation of patients with syncope is best reserved for those in whom syncope or presyncope occurred during or immediately after exertion or in association with chest pain. It should be noted that even among patients with syncope during exertion, exercise stress testing is highly unlikely to trigger another event. Patients suspected of having severe aortic stenosis or obstructive hypertrophic cardiomyopathy should not undergo exercise stress testing because it may precipitate a cardiac arrest. Current guidelines suggest that exercise stress testing be performed in patients who experience syncope during or shortly after exercise.[1] Exercise stress testing is not recommended for patients with non-exercise-related syncope.[32] Coronary angiography is recommended in patients with syncope suspected to be due, directly or indirectly, to myocardial ischemia.

ELECTROCARDIOGRAPHY. The 12-lead ECG is another important component in the work-up of a patient with syncope. The initial ECG results in establishment of a diagnosis in approximately 5 percent of patients and suggests a diagnosis in another 5 percent of patients.[24] Specific findings that can identify the probable cause of syncope include QT prolongation (long QT syndrome), the presence of a short PR interval and a delta wave (Wolff-Parkinson-White syndrome), the presence of a right bundle branch block pattern with ST segment elevation (Brugada syndrome), evidence of an acute myocardial infarction, high-grade AV block, or T wave inversion in the right precordial leads (arrhythmogenic right ventricular dysplasia) (see Chap. 32). Any abnormality of the baseline ECG is an independent predictor of cardiac syncope or increased mortality and suggests the need to pursue an evaluation of cardiac causes of syncope.[1] Most patients with syncope have a normal ECG. This finding is useful as it suggests a low likelihood of a cardiac cause of syncope and is associated with an excellent prognosis, particularly when observed in a young patient with syncope. Despite the low diagnostic yield of electrocardiography, the test is inexpensive and risk free. For these reasons, an ECG is considered a standard part of the evaluation of virtually all patients with syncope.[1,24]

SIGNAL-AVERAGED ELECTROCARDIOGRAPHY. Signal-averaged electrocardiography (SAECG) is a noninvasive technique used for the detection of low-amplitude signals in the terminal portion of the QRS complex (late potentials), which are a substrate for ventricular arrhythmias (see Chap. 29). In contrast to a standard ECG, the role of SAECG in the evaluation of patients with syncope is not well established. Studies in selected populations of patients have reported that SAECG has a sensitivity of 73 to 89 percent and a specificity of 89 to 100 percent for the prediction of inducible VT in patients with syncope.[24] Despite these encouraging results, no studies have evaluated the role of SAECG in unselected populations of patients. Furthermore, it is unknown whether SAECG can replace an electrophysiology (EP) study in the evaluation of patients with syncope in the setting of significant structural heart disease. These facts, combined with the inability of SAECG to provide the additional information routinely obtained during EP testing regarding sinus node function, AV conduction, and the presence of inducible supraventricular arrhythmias, limit the role of SAECG as a diagnostic tool in syncope. Another limitation of this technique is that criteria for the use of SAECG as a diagnostic tool in patients with a bundle branch block or nonspecific intraventricular conduction delay have not been developed. At present, SAECG testing is not recommended as a standard part of the evaluation of patients with syncope.[1,24] Perhaps one of the best uses of SAECG testing at present is to evaluate patients with possible arrhythmogenic right ventricular dysplasia.[10,33]

HOLTER RECORDING. Continuous ECG monitoring using telemetry or Holter monitoring, or both, is commonly performed in patients with syncope but is unlikely to identify the cause of syncope (see Chap. 29). The information provided by ECG monitoring at the time of syncope is extremely valuable because it allows an arrhythmic cause of syncope to be established or excluded. However, because of the infrequent and sporadic nature of syncope, the diagnostic yield of Holter monitoring in the evaluation of patients with syncope and presyncope is approximately 4 percent.[24] Another clinically useful finding is the detection of symptoms in the absence of an arrhythmia. This finding is observed in up to 15 percent of patients undergoing continuous ECG monitoring.[24] It is important to emphasize that the absence of an arrhythmia and symptoms during continuous ECG monitoring may not exclude an arrhythmia as the cause of syncope. In patients suspected of having an arrhythmia as the cause of syncope, additional evaluation such as EP testing or event monitoring should be considered. Holter or inpatient telemetric monitoring is indicated in patients with syncope suspected to result from an arrhythmia on the basis of features of the clinical history, an abnormal ECG, or the presence of structural heart disease.[1,24] Holter monitoring is most likely to be diagnostic when it is used in the occasional patient with frequent (i.e., daily) episodes of syncope or presyncope.

EVENT RECORDERS. Transtelephonic event monitors are small, portable ECG recording devices that are carried or worn continuously by the patient and can be activated by the patient to record a rhythm strip (see Chap. 29). The tracings can be stored and transmitted over telephone lines at a later time. Some event monitors, referred to as continuous-loop event monitors, are worn continuously and allow capture of both retrospective and prospective ECG recordings, whereas other types of event monitors record only when they are activated by the patient. Continuous-loop event monitors are preferred when used in the evaluation of a patient with syncope. These devices are often programmed with 4 minutes of retrospective memory and 1 minute of prospective memory on activation. Event monitors are indicated in the evaluation of patients with infrequent but recurrent episodes of presyncope or syncope, particularly when potentially malignant causes of syncope have been excluded.[1,24,34,35] When they are used in selected populations of patients, a diagnostic yield as high has 25 percent may be observed. However, a much lower diagnostic yield can be expected in less selected populations. One study, for example, reported that among 172 patients with syncope, no patient experienced frank syncope during the monitoring period.[35] A significant arrhythmia was detected in 6 percent of patients in association with less severe symptoms.

IMPLANTABLE EVENT RECORDERS. In some patients, episodes of syncope are extremely infrequent, occurring once or twice a year. In this population of patients, a traditional event monitor is unlikely to be diagnostic because of the prolonged length of recording that would be needed to record an event successfully. To address this problem, an implantable event monitor has been developed (Medtronic Reveal, Minneapolis, MN) (see Chap. 29). This lightweight and small device (61 × 19 × 8 mm), with a projected longevity of 18 to 24 months, incorporates two electrodes within its can and is implanted in the subcutaneous tissue of the chest. If necessary, the incision can be extended later to allow insertion of a pacemaker or implantable cardioverter-defibrillator. The ECG signal is stored in a circular buffer capable of recording up to 42 minutes of rhythm. The device can be configured to trigger automatically on the basis of programmed detection criteria as well as with a handheld activator.

In one series, a symptom-ECG correlation was reported in 50 of 85 patients (59 percent) during 10 ± 4 months of follow-up.[36] An arrhythmia was detected in 21 of the patients and sinus rhythm was detected in 29. Complications included two infections, one erosion, and one painful pocket requiring device reinsertion. The authors of the study subsequently performed a randomized trial to evaluate the diagnostic utility of the Reveal device compared with conventional testing.[37] Sixty patients with unexplained syncope after an initial evaluation consisting of a history, physical examination, and echocardiogram were enrolled. Patients with an ejection fraction less than 35 percent were excluded. Patients were randomly assigned to initial implantation of the Reveal monitor versus a standard evaluation consisting of an external event monitor, a tilt test, and an EP study. A diagnosis was established in 14 of 27 patients assigned to prolonged monitoring compared with 6 of 30 patients undergoing conventional testing. Although this implantable monitor provides a new tool for use in evaluating patients with syncope, a limitation of this diagnostic strategy is that it is expensive and requires that the patient experience another episode of syncope to establish a diagnosis. Current guidelines suggest that implantable event monitors be used in selected patients with recurrent and infrequent episodes of syncope when it is thought that there is a high probability of an arrhythmic cause of syncope.[1]

ELECTROPHYSIOLOGY TESTING. EP testing can provide important diagnostic and prognostic information in patients presenting with syncope (see Chaps. 29 and 30). The results of EP testing can be useful in establishing a diagnosis of sick sinus syndrome, carotid sinus hypersensitivity, heart block, supraventricular tachycardia, or VT. The indications for EP testing in the evaluation of patients with syncope have been established on the basis of an American College of Cardiology/American Heart Association Task Force Report.[20] There is general agreement that EP testing should be performed in patients with suspected structural heart disease and unexplained syncope (class 1 indication) and that EP testing should not be performed in patients with a known cause of syncope for whom treatment would not be influenced by the findings of the test (class 3 indication). The role of EP testing in evaluating patients with recurrent unexplained syncope who do not have structural heart disease and have had a negative tilt-table test remains controversial.

Sinus node function is evaluated during EP testing primarily by determining the sinus node recovery time (SNRT). The SNRT is determined by pacing the right atrium at cycle lengths between 600 and 350 milliseconds for 30 to 60 seconds. The SNRT is defined as the interval between the last paced atrial depolarization and the first spontaneous atrial depolarization resulting from activation of the sinus node. The SNRT is corrected for the underlying sinus cycle length (SCL) and expressed as the corrected SNRT (CSNRT = SNRT − SCL). A corrected SNRT greater than 525 milliseconds is generally considered abnormal. A secondary pause is defined as an inappropriately long pause among the beats that follow the first sinus recovery beat after atrial overdrive pacing. Evaluation of secondary pauses increases the sensitivity of the SNRT in the detection of sinus node dysfunction. Other, less widely used assays for evaluating sinus node function include the sinoatrial conduction time and the sinus node refractory period. Although the sinoatrial conduction time is a sensitive indicator of sinus node dysfunction, it lacks a high degree of specificity and has been of limited value in evaluating the need for a permanent pacemaker. Determination of sinus node refractoriness is another technique that has been reported to be useful in identifying patients with sinus node dysfunction. However, the usefulness of this parameter in selecting patients with syncope for pacemaker implantation has not been determined. Identification of sinus node dysfunction as the cause of syncope is uncommon during EP tests (<5 percent). It is also important to note that the absence of evidence of sinus node dysfunction during EP testing does not exclude a bradyarrhythmia as the cause of syncope.

During EP testing, AV conduction is assessed by measuring the AV nodal to His bundle conduction time (A-H interval) and the His bundle to ventricular conduction time (H-V interval) and also by determining the response of AV conduction to incremental atrial pacing and atrial premature stimuli. The findings obtained during EP testing that allow AV block to be established as the probable cause of syncope include an H-V interval of 100 milliseconds or more or infra-His block. Among studies that have reported the results of EP testing in evaluating patients with syncope, AV block was identified as the probable cause of syncope in approximately 10 to 15 percent of patients. Donateo and colleagues reported the results of a systematic evaluation of patients with syncope in the setting of a bundle branch block on their baseline ECG.[38] Of 347 patients referred for evaluation of syncope, 55 had a baseline bundle branch block pattern. Systematic evaluation of these patients, including EP testing, resulted in a diagnosis of cardiac syncope in 25 patients (45 percent): AV block in 20, sick sinus syndrome in 2, VT in 1, and aortic stenosis in 2. Neurally mediated syncope was diagnosed in 22 patients (40 percent) and syncope remained unexplained in 8 (15 percent).

It is uncommon for a supraventricular tachycardia to cause syncope unless the patient has underlying heart disease, the rate is extremely rapid, or the patient has a propensity for the development of neurally mediated syncope. The typical pattern that is observed is the development of syncope or near syncope at the onset of the supraventricular arrhythmia because of an initial drop in blood pressure. The patient often regains consciousness despite the continuation of the arrhythmia owing to the activation of a compensatory mechanism. Completion of a standard EP test allows accurate identification of most types of supraventricular arrhythmias that may have caused syncope. The study should be repeated during an isoproterenol infusion to increase the sensitivity of the study, particularly for detecting idiopathic VT or AV nodal reentrant tachycardia (see Chap. 32). A supraventricular arrhythmia is diagnosed as the probable cause of syncope in less than 5 percent of patients who undergo EP testing for evaluation of syncope of unknown origin.

VT is the most common abnormality that is uncovered during EP testing in patients with syncope. Among studies that have reported the results of EP testing in evaluating patients with syncope, VT was identified as the probable cause of syncope in approximately 20 percent of patients. An approximately 50 percent incidence of appropriate implantable defibrillator discharges has been reported in both patients with syncope who have inducible VT on EP testing and patients who present with a sustained ventricular arrhythmia and undergo cardiac defibrillator implantation.[39] In the past, an EP test was interpreted as positive for VT when sustained monomorphic VT was induced. The induction of polymorphic VT and ventricular fibrillation were considered to represent nonspecific responses to EP testing. More recent data suggest that the induction of polymorphic VT and ventricular fibrillation should also be considered abnormal findings during EP testing performed in a patient with syncope.[40,41] An analysis of data obtained as part of the Antiarrhythmics Versus Implantable Defibrillators (AVID) registry and an AVID syncope substudy showed no difference in the incidence of arrhythmic events among patients with syncope with inducible VT (<200 beats/min), inducible rapid VT (>200 beats/min), and inducible polymorphic VT or ventricular fibrillation.[40] In contrast, ejection fraction was highly predictive of arrhythmic events. At 1 year of follow-up, 15 percent of patients with an ejection fraction greater than 30 percent had an arrhythmic event compared with 38 percent of patients with syncope with an ejection fraction less than 30 percent.

Approximately 30 percent of patients with syncope referred for EP testing to evaluate syncope of unknown origin have a presumptive diagnosis established. Clinical factors identified as predictors of a positive response to EP testing include impaired ventricular function, male sex, prior myocardial infarction, bundle branch block, injury, and nonsustained VT.

Approximately 70 percent of patients referred for evaluation of syncope demonstrate a normal response to EP testing. A negative EP test has generally been considered predictive of a low risk of sudden death. However, studies have suggested that EP testing may have less predictive value in patients with markedly impaired ventricular function. One study reported that 7 of 14 patients with an idiopathic dilated cardiomyopathy who presented with syncope, had a negative EP test, and underwent placement of an implantable defibrillator received appropriate shocks for ventricular arrhythmias during 24 months of follow-up.[42] A similar study involving 46 patients with a nonischemic cardiomyopathy and a negative EP test reported that 33 percent of these patients received appropriate defibrillator therapy during follow-up.[43] Fonarow and colleagues reported the outcome of 147 patients referred for cardiac transplantation who had a nonischemic cardiomyopathy and syncope.[44] Management of patients, including whether to use an implantable defibrillator, was determined by their cardiologist. EP testing was not performed. The outcomes of the 25 patients who received an implantable defibrillator were compared with those of the 122 patients managed with conventional therapy alone. During a mean follow-up of 22 months, there were 31 deaths,

18 sudden, in patients treated with conventional therapy, whereas there were 2 deaths, neither sudden, in patients treated with an implantable defibrillator. An appropriate shock was received by 40 percent of defibrillator patients. The findings of these studies suggest that more sensitive diagnostic tests to evaluate patients' risk for sudden death or greater use of implantable cardioverter-defibrillators, or both, may be needed in this group of patients.

TEST TO SCREEN FOR NEUROLOGICAL CAUSES OF SYNCOPE. Syncope as an isolated symptom rarely has a neurological cause. Neurological causes of syncope are established in less than 5 percent of patients with syncope.[5-7] As a result, widespread use of tests to screen for neurological conditions is rarely diagnostic. In many institutions, computed tomography (CT) scans (see Chap. 15), electroencephalograms (EEGs), and carotid duplex scans are overused, being obtained for more than 50 percent of patients with syncope. A diagnosis is almost never uncovered that was not first suspected on the basis of a careful history and neurological examination. Transient ischemic attacks that result from carotid disease are not accompanied by loss of consciousness. No studies have suggested that carotid Doppler ultrasonography is beneficial in patients with syncope. Current guidelines for the evaluation of syncope suggest that EEGs be obtained only when there is a relatively high likelihood of epilepsy.[1] CT and magnetic resonance imaging should be avoided in patients with uncomplicated syncope.

Approach to the Evaluation of Patients with Syncope

Figure 34–1 outlines the approach to the diagnostic evaluation of a patient presenting with syncope proposed by the European Society of Cardiology Task Force on Syncope.[1] The initial evaluation begins with a careful history, physical examination, and 12-lead ECG. Various clinical features can help suggest a specific cause of the syncope (Table 34–4). On the basis of this initial evaluation performed in either an emergency department or outpatient setting, the probable cause of syncope can be identified in approximately 25 percent of patients. Common causes or types of syncope that can be identified at this initial stage include orthostatic hypotension, situational syncope, and neurally mediated syncope. This initial evaluation should also allow identification of patients who probably had a seizure rather than syncope. In another large group of patients the probable cause of syncope can be suspected and later confirmed with directed diagnostic testing. Causes or types of syncope that fall into this category include left ventricular outflow tract obstruction, neurally mediated syncope with a suggestive but not diagnostic clinical presentation, arrhythmias related to the long QT syndrome, Wolff-Parkinson-White syndrome, the Brugada syndrome, or arrhythmogenic right ventricular dysplasia as well as neurological causes of syncope. Among the remaining patients, the next step in the evaluation depends on the presence of structural heart disease as well as the physician's clinical suspicion that an arrhythmia may have been the cause of syncope. An echocardiogram is often obtained at this point to help determine whether structural heart disease is present. If the patient has significant structural heart disease or a clinical history suggestive of an arrhythmia, an EP test would be an appropriate next step. On the other hand, if structural heart disease is absent and the clinical history is not suggestive of an arrhythmia, the evaluation can be continued with a tilt test, event monitor, or clinical follow-up, depending on the severity and chronicity of the patient's symptoms. With this approach, a probable cause of syncope can be determined in 75 percent of patients.[5]

Management of Patients

The approach to treatment of a patient with syncope depends largely on the diagnosis that is established. For example, the appropriate treatment of a patient with syncope related to AV

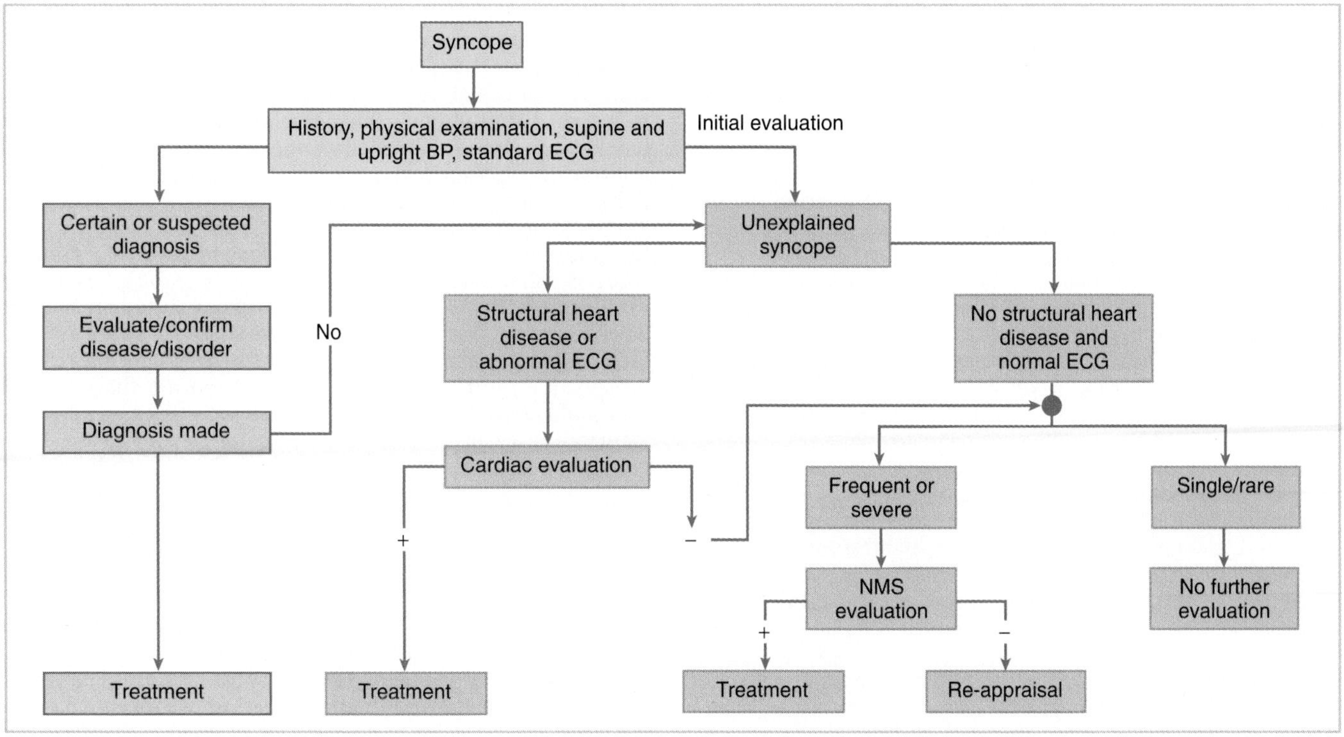

FIGURE 34–1 Diagnostic evaluation of syncope. BP = blood pressure; ECG = electrocardiogram; NMS = neurally mediated syncope.

TABLE 34–4 Clinical Features Suggestive of Specific Causes

Symptom or Finding	Diagnostic Consideration
After sudden unexpected pain, unpleasant sight, sound, or smell	Vasovagal syncope
During or immediately after micturition, cough, swallow, or defecation	Situational syncope
With neuralgia (glossopharyngeal or trigeminal)	Bradycardia or vasodepressor reaction
On standing	Orthostatic hypotension
Prolonged standing at attention	Vasovagal syncope
Well-trained athlete after exertion	Neurally mediated
Changing position (from sitting to lying, bending, turning over in bed)	Atrial myxoma, thrombus
Syncope with exertion	Aortic stenosis, pulmonary hypertension, pulmonary embolus, mitral stenosis, idiopathic hypertrophic subaortic stenosis, coronary artery disease, neurally mediated
With head rotation, pressure on carotid sinus (as in tumors, shaving, tight collars)	Carotid sinus syncope
Associated with vertigo, dysarthria, diplopia, and other motor and sensory symptoms of brain stem ischemia	Transient ischemic attack, subclavian steal, basilar artery migraine
With arm exercise	Subclavian steal
Confusion after episode	Seizure

block or sick sinus syndrome would probably involve placement of a permanent pacemaker (see Chap. 31), treatment of a patient with syncope related to the Wolff-Parkinson White syndrome would probably involve catheter ablation (see Chap. 30), and treatment of a patient with syncope related to VT would probably involve placement of an implantable defibrillator (see Chap. 31). For other types of syncope, optimal management may involve discontinuation of an offending pharmacological agent, an increase in salt intake, or education of the patient.

Other issues that need to be considered include the indication for hospitalization of a patient with syncope and duration of driving restrictions. Generally, hospital admission is indicated when there is concern regarding a potentially life-threatening cause of syncope or when significant injury has occurred. It would therefore be prudent to hospitalize a 65-year-old man with a prior history of a myocardial infarction and heart failure who presents with an initial episode of syncope that occurs without warning or residual symptoms. In this type of patient, the probability of VT as the cause of syncope is high. On the other hand, the evaluation of a young patient who presents with a clinical history suggestive of neurally mediated syncope and no clinical evidence of cardiac disease could be performed on an outpatient basis.

Physicians who care for patients with syncope are often asked to address the issue of driving risk. Patients who experience syncope while driving pose a risk both to themselves and to others. Although some would argue that all patients with syncope should never drive again because of the theoretical possibility of a recurrence, this is an impractical solution that would be ignored by many patients. Factors that should be considered when making a recommendation for a particular patient include (1) the potential for recurrent syncope, (2) the presence and duration of warning symptoms, (3) whether syncope occurs while seated or only when standing, (4) how often and in what capacity the patient drives, and (5) whether any state laws may be applicable. When considering these issues, physicians should note that acute illnesses, including syncope, are unlikely to cause a motor vehicle accident. The American Heart Association and the Canadian Cardiovascular Society have published guidelines concerning this issue. For noncommercial drivers, it is generally recommended that driving be restricted for several months. If the patient remains asymptomatic for several months, driving can then be resumed.

Neurally Mediated Syncope

Because neurally mediated syncope is so common, therapy is outlined in detail. Treatment begins with a careful history with particular attention focused on identifying precipitating factors, quantifying the degree of salt intake and current medication use, and determining whether the patient has a prior history of peripheral edema, hypertension, asthma, or other conditions that may alter the approach used to treat neurally mediated syncope. For many patients, particularly those with infrequent episodes associated with an identifiable precipitant, education about avoidance of predisposing factors and a moderate increase in salt intake are effective treatment. Patients can also be instructed to lie down at the beginning of symptoms or to cross their legs (if sitting) and squeeze them together. For others, treatment involves removal or avoidance of drugs that predispose to orthostatic hypotension or volume depletion, such as vasodilators and diuretics. One study reported that the actuarial probabilities of remaining syncope free 1 and 2 years after a positive tilt test were 72 and 60 percent, respectively.[45] The most powerful predictor of recurrence of syncope was the logarithm of the number of preceding syncopal spells.

Treatment with pharmacological agents is usually targeted at patients in whom syncope is recurrent or has been associated with physical injury. The medications that are generally relied on to treat neurally mediated syncope include beta blockers, fludrocortisone, serotonin reuptake inhibitors, and midodrine.[46] Despite the widespread use of these agents, none of these pharmacological agents have been demonstrated to be effective by the results of multiple large prospective randomized clinical trials. Perhaps the most carefully studied pharmacological agents are serotonin reuptake inhibitors such as paroxetine.[47] Several very small studies have reported that midodrine is effective.[48,49] Although beta blockers are considered by many as first-line therapy, a prospective randomized clinical trial reported that atenolol was ineffective.[50] Another study reported that a placebo was as effective as propranolol and nadolol in the treatment of neurally mediated syncope.[51]

Although pacemakers have also been found to be valuable in the treatment of some patients with neurally mediated syncope in several clinical trials, the Second Vasovagal Pacemaker Study, in which all subjects received pacemakers but pacing was activated in 50 percent of patients, showed no benefit of pacing.[52,53] Because of the variable results of these clinical trials and the profound implications of pacemaker implantation, considerable restraint should be exercised when considering the implantation of a pacemaker for treatment of neurally mediated syncope. The development of asystole during tilt-table testing is not considered to be an absolute indication for pacemaker implantation. Over the past several years, a number of studies have reported the efficacy of "orthostatic training" in the treatment of neurally mediated syncope.[54] This simple, inexpensive, and widely available approach deserves further study.

REFERENCES

Definition

1. Brignole M, Alboni P, Benditt D, et al, Task Force on Syncope, European Society of Cardiology: Guidelines on management (diagnosis and treatment) of syncope. Eur Heart J 22:1256, 2001.
2. Soteriades ES, Evand JC, Larson MG, et al: Incidence and prognosis of syncope. N Engl J Med 347:878, 2002.
3. Nyman JA, Krahn AD, Bland PC, et al: The costs of recurrent syncope of unknown origin in elderly patients. Pacing Clin Electrophysiol 22:1386, 1999.
4. Rose MS, Koshman ML, Spreng S, Sheldon R: The relationship between health-related quality of life and frequency of spells in patients with syncope. J Clin Epidemiol 53:1209, 2000.

Classification

5. Ammirati F, Colivicchi F, Santini M: Diagnosing syncope in clinical practice. Implementation of a simplified diagnostic algorithm in a multicentre prospective trial—The OESIL 2 study (Osservatorio Epidemiologico della Sincope nel Lazio). Eur Heart J 21:935, 2000.
6. Alboni P, Brignole M, Menozzi C, et al: Diagnostic value of history in patients with syncope with or without heart disease. J Am Coll Cardiol 37:1921, 2001.
7. Sarasin FP, Louis-Simonet M, Carballo D, et al: Prospective evaluation of patients with syncope: A population-based study. Am J Med 111:177, 2001.
8. Kapoor WN, Fortunato M, Hanusa BH, Schulberg HC: Psychiatric illnesses in patients with syncope. Am J Med 99:505, 1995.
9. Ventura R, Maas R, Rüppel R, et al: Psychiatric conditions in patients with recurrent unexplained syncope. Europace 3:311, 2001.
10. Nava A, Bauce B, Basso C, et al: Clinical profile and long-term follow-up of 37 families with arrhythmogenic right ventricular cardiomyopathy. J Am Coll Cardiol 36:226, 2000.
11. Elliott PM, Poloniecki J, Dickie S, et al: Sudden death in hypertrophic cardiomyopathy: Identification of high risk patients. J Am Coll Cardiol 36:2212, 2000.
12. Wilde A, Antzelevitch C, Borggrefe M, et al: Proposed diagnostic criteria for Brugada syndrome: Consensus report. Circulation 106:2514, 2002.
13. Grubb BP, Karas B: Clinical disorders of the autonomic nervous system associated with orthostatic intolerance: An overview of classification, clinical evaluation, and management. Pacing Clin Electrophysiol 22:798, 1999.
14. The Consensus Committee of the American Autonomic Society and the American Academy of Neurology: Consensus statement on the definition of orthostatic hypotension, pure autonomic failure, and multiple system atrophy. Neurology 46:1470, 1996.
15. Goldstein DS, Holmes C, Frank SM, et al: Sympathoadrenal imbalance before neurocardiogenic syncope. Am J Cardiol 91:53, 2003.
16. Kenny RAM, Richardson DA, Steen N, et al: Carotid sinus syndrome: A modifiable risk factor for nonaccidental falls in older adults (SAFE PACE). J Am Coll Cardiol 38:1491, 2001.
17. Morillo CA, Camacho ME, Wood MA, et al: Diagnostic utility of mechanical, pharmacological and orthostatic stimulation of the carotid sinus in patients with unexplained syncope. J Am Coll Cardiol 34:1587, 1999.
18. Richardson DA, Bexton R, Shaw RE, et al: Complications of carotid sinus massage—A prospective series of older patients. Age Ageing 29:413, 2000.
19. Richardson DA, Bexton RS, Shaw FE, Kenny RA: Prevalence of cardioinhibitory carotid sinus hypersensitivity in patients 50 years or over presenting to the accident and emergency department with "unexplained" or "recurrent" falls. Pacing Clin Electrophysiol 20:820, 1997.
20. Gregoratos G, Abrams J, Epstein A, et al: ACC/AHA/NASPE 2002 guideline update for implantation of cardiac pacemakers and antiarrhythmia devices: Summary article. A report of the American College of Cardiology/American Heart Association Task Force on practice guidelines (ACC/AHA/NASPE Committee to Update the 1998 Pacemaker Guidelines). Circulation 106:2145, 2002.
21. Grubb, BP, Samoil D, Kosinski D, et al: Cerebral syncope: Loss of consciousness associated with cerebral vasoconstriction in the absence of systemic hypotension. Pacing Clin Electrophysiol 21:652, 1998.

Diagnostic Tests

22. Close J, Ellis M, Hooper R, et al: Prevention of falls in the elderly trial (PROFET), a randomized controlled trial. Lancet 353:93, 1999.
23. Sheldon R, Rose S, Ritchie D, et al: Historical criteria that distinguish syncope from seizures. J Am Coll Cardiol 40:142, 2002.
24. Linzer M, Yang EH, Estes M, et al, for the Clinical Efficacy Assessment Project of the American College of Physicians: Clinical guideline. Diagnosing syncope. Part 1: Value of history, physical examination, and electrocardiography. Ann Intern Med 126:989, 1997.
25. Linzer M, Yang EH, Estes M III, et al, for the Clinical Efficacy Assessment Project of the American College of Physicians: Clinical guideline. Diagnosing syncope. Part 2: Unexplained syncope. Ann Intern Med 127:76, 1997.
26. Link MS, Lauer EP, Homoud MK, et al: Low yield of rule-out myocardial infarction protocol in patients presenting with syncope. Am J Cardiol 88:706, 2001.
27. Benditt DG, Ferguson DW, Grubb BP, et al: Tilt table testing for assessing syncope. J Am Coll Cardiol 28:263, 1996.
28. Takase B, Uehata A, Nishioka TI, et al: Different mechanisms of isoproterenol-induced and nitroglycerin-induced syncope during head-up tilt in patients with unexplained syncope: Important role of epinephrine in nitroglycerin-induced syncope. J Cardiovasc Electrophysiol 12:791, 2001.
29. Calkins H. Isoproterenol-provoked versus nitroglycerin-provoked tilt tests: Do they differ? J Cardiovasc Electrophysiol 12:797, 2001.
30. Raviele A, Giada F, Brignole M, et al: Comparison of diagnostic accuracy of sublingual nitroglycerin test and low-dose isoproterenol test in patients with unexplained syncope. Am J Cardiol 85:1194, 2000.
31. Sumiyoshi M, Nakata Y, Mineda Y, et al: Response to head-up tilt testing in patients with situational syncope. Am J Cardiol 82:1117, 1998.
32. Doi A, Tsuchihashi K, Kyuma M, et al: Diagnostic implications of modified treadmill and head-up tilt tests in exercise-related syncope: Comparative studies with situational and/or vasovagal syncope. Can J Cardiol 18:960, 2002.
33. Nasir K, Rutgerg J, Tandri H, et al: Utility of SAECG in arrhythmogenic right ventricle dysplasia. Ann Noninvasive Electrocardiol 8:112, 2003.
34. Fogel RI, Evans JJ, Prystowsky EN: Utility and cost of event recorders in the diagnosis of palpitations, presyncope, and syncope. Am J Cardiol 79:207, 1997.
35. Zimetbaum P, Kim KY, Ho KKL, et al: Utility of patient-activated cardiac event recorders in general clinical practice. Am J Cardiol 79:371, 1997.
36. Krahn AD, Klein GJ, Yee R, et al: Use of an extended monitoring strategy in patients with problematic syncope. Reveal Investigators. Circulation 99:406, 1999.
37. Krahn AD, Klein GJ, Yee R, Skanes AC: Randomized assessment of syncope trial. Conventional diagnostic testing versus a prolonged monitoring strategy. Circulation 104:46, 2001.
38. Donateo P, Brignole M, Alboni P, et al: A standardized conventional evaluation of the mechanism of syncope in patients with bundle branch block. Europace 4:357, 2002.
39. Andrews NP, Fogel RI, Pelargonio G, et al: Implantable defibrillator event rates in patients with unexplained syncope and inducible sustained ventricular tachyarrhythmias. J Am Coll Cardiol 34:2023, 1999.
40. Steinberg JS, Beckman K, Greene HL, et al: Follow-up of patients with unexplained syncope and inducible ventricular tachyarrhythmias: Analysis of the AVID registry and an AVID substudy. J Cardiovasc Electrophysiol 12:996, 2001.
41. Link MS, Costeas XF, Griffith JL, et al: High incidence of appropriate implantable cardioverter-defibrillator therapy in patients with syncope of unknown etiology and inducible ventricular arrhythmias. J Am Coll Cardiol 29:370, 1997.
42. Knight BP, Goyal R, Pelosi F, et al: Outcome of patients with nonischemic dilated cardiomyopathy and unexplained syncope treated with an implantable defibrillator. J Am Coll Cardiol 33:1964, 1999.
43. Russo AM, Verdino R, Schorr C, et al: Occurrence of implantable defibrillator events in patients with syncope and nonischemic dilated cardiomyopathy. Am J Cardiol 88:1444, 2001.
44. Fonarow GC, Feliciano Z, Boyle NG, et al: Improved survival in patients with nonischemic advanced heart failure and syncope treated with an implantable cardioverter-defibrillator. Am J Cardiol 85:981, 2000.

Approach to the Evaluation of Patients with Syncope and Management of Patients

45. Sheldon R, Rose S, Flanagan P, et al: Risk factors for syncope recurrence after a positive tilt table test in patients with syncope. Circulation 93:973, 1996.
46. Atiga W, Rowe P, Calkins H: Management of vasovagal syncope. J Cardiovasc Electrophysiol 10:874, 1999.
47. Girolamo ED, Iorio CD, Sabatini P, et al: Effects of paroxetine hydrochloride, a selective serotonin reuptake inhibitor, on refractory vasovagal syncope: A randomized, double-blind, placebo-controlled study. J Am Coll Cardiol 33:1227, 1999.
48. Ward CR, Gray JC, Gilroy JJ, et al: Midodrine: A role in the management of neurocardiogenic syncope. Heart 79:45, 1998.
49. Kaufmann H, Saadia D, Voustianiouk A: Midodrine in neurally mediated syncope: A double-blind, randomized, crossover study. Ann Neurol 52:342, 2002.
50. Madrid AH, Ortega J, Rebollo JG, et al: Lack of efficacy of atenolol for the prevention of neurally mediated syncope. J Am Coll Cardiol 37:554, 2001.
51. Flevari P, Livanis EG, Theodorakis GN, et al: Vasovagal syncope: A prospective, randomized, crossover evaluation of the effect of propranolol, nadolol and placebo on syncope recurrence and patients' well-being. J Am Coll Cardiol 40:499, 2002.
52. Connolly SJ, Sheldon R, Roberts RS, Gent M: The North American Vasovagal Pacemaker Study: A randomized trial of permanent cardiac pacing for the prevention of vasovagal syncope. J Am Coll Cardiol 33:16, 1999.
53. Connolly SJ, Sheldon R, Thorpe K, et al, for the VPS II Investigators: Pacemaker therapy for prevention of syncope in patients with recurrent severe vasovagal syncope. Second Vasovagal Pacemaker Study (VPS II): A randomized trial. JAMA 289:2224, 2003.
54. Girolamo ED, Iorio CD, Leonzio L, et al: Usefulness of a tilt training program for the prevention of refractory neurocardiogenic syncope in adolescents: A controlled study. Circulation 100:1798, 1999.

PART V

Preventive Cardiology

CHAPTER 35

The Vascular Biology of Atherosclerosis

Peter Libby

The 20th century witnessed a remarkable evolution in concepts concerning the pathogenesis of atherosclerosis. This disease has a venerable history, having left traces in the arteries of Egyptian mummies. Apparently uncommon in antiquity, atherosclerosis became epidemic as populations increasingly survived early mortality caused by infectious diseases. Also, many societies adopted dietary habits that may promote atherosclerosis, such as a surfeit of saturated fats, and curtailed physical activity (see Chaps. 1, 36, and 39).

Until very recently, most physicians viewed arteries as inanimate tubes rather than living, dynamic tissue. More than 100 years ago, Virchow recognized the participation of cells in atherogenesis. A controversy raged between Virchow, who viewed atherosclerosis as a proliferative disease, and Rokitansky, who believed that atheromata derived from healing and resorption of thrombi.[1] Experiments performed in the early part of the 20th century used dietary modulation to produce fatty lesions in the arteries of rabbits and ultimately identified cholesterol as the culprit. These observations, followed by the characterization of human lipoprotein particles at mid-century, promoted the concept of insudation of lipids as a cause for atherosclerosis.[1] We now recognize that elements of all these pathogenic theories participate in atherogenesis. This chapter summarizes evidence from human studies, animal experimentation, and in vitro work and highlights a synoptic view of atherogenesis, taking into account advances in vascular biology that have deepened our understanding of the process.

Acquaintance with the vascular biology of atherosclerosis should prove useful to the practitioner. Our daily contact with this common disease lulls us into a complacent belief that we understand it better than we actually do. For example, we are just beginning to learn why atherosclerosis affects certain regions of the arterial tree preferentially, and why its clinical manifestations occur only at certain times. Atherosclerosis can involve both large and mid-size arteries diffusely. Postmortem and intravascular ultrasonography studies have revealed widespread intimal thickening in patients with atherosclerosis. Many asymptomatic individuals have intimal lesions in their coronary or carotid arteries even in the early decades of life. At the same time, atherosclerosis is a focal disease that constricts areas of affected vessels much more than others. Understanding of the biological basis of the predilection of certain sites to develop atheroma is just beginning to emerge.[2]

Atherosclerosis also displays heterogeneity in time, being a disease with both chronic and acute manifestations. Few human diseases have a longer "incubation" period than atherosclerosis, which begins to affect arteries of many North Americans in the second and third decades of life (Fig. 35–1).[3] Indeed, one in six American teenagers have abnormal thickening of the coronary arteries.[4] Yet typically, symptoms of atherosclerosis do not occur until several decades later, characteristically occurring even later in women. Despite this indolent time course and prolonged period of clinical inactivity, the dreaded complications of atheroma such as myocardial infarction, unstable angina, or stroke typically occur suddenly.

Another poorly understood issue regarding atherogenesis is its role in causing narrowing, or stenosis, of some vessels and ectasia of others. Typically, we fear stenoses

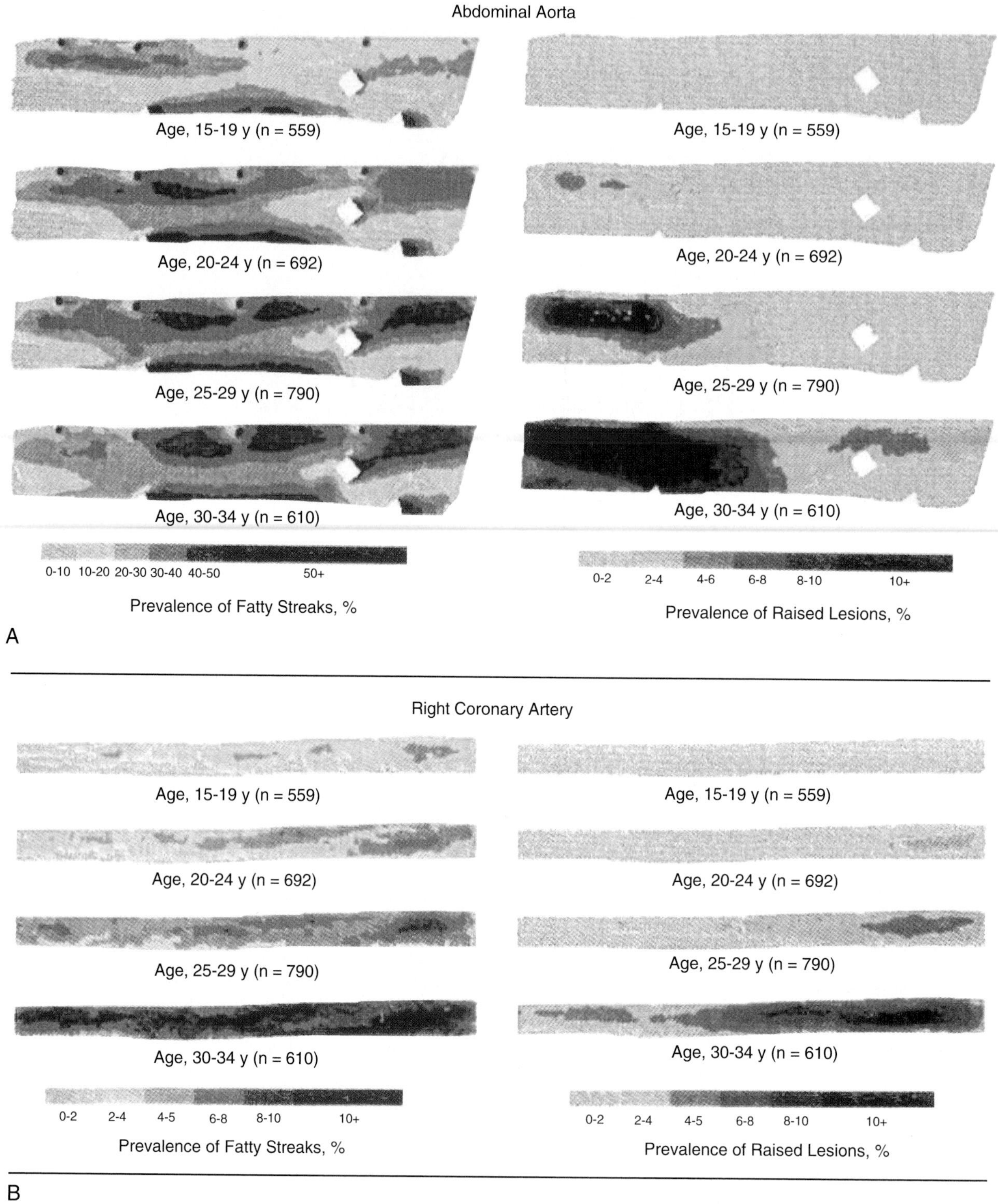

FIGURE 35–1 Prevalence maps of fatty streaks and raised lesions in the abdominal aorta. Composite data from the Pathobiological Determinants of Atherosclerosis In Youth (PDAY) Study show pseudocolored representation of morphometric analysis of more than 2800 aortas from Americans younger than 35 years of age who succumbed for noncardiac reasons. **A,** Note the early involvement of the dorsal surface of the infrarenal abdominal aorta by fatty streaks followed by raised lesions. **B,** A similar but slightly slower progression of lesions affects the right coronary artery. The scales at the bottoms of the panels show the coding of the pseudocoloring. (From Strong JP, Malcolm GT, McMahan CA, et al: Prevalence and extent of atherosclerosis in adolescents and young adults. JAMA 281:727, 1999.)

in coronary atherosclerosis. However, aneurysm is a common manifestation of this disease in other vessels, including the aorta. Even in the life history of a single atherosclerotic lesion, a phase of ectasia known as positive remodeling, or compensatory enlargement, precedes the formation of stenotic lesions.[5] Contemporary vascular biology is beginning to shed light on some of these apparent contradictions, or paradoxes, in understanding atherosclerosis.

Structure of the Normal Artery

Intima

Understanding the pathogenesis of atherosclerosis first requires knowledge of the structure and biology of the normal artery and its indigenous cell types. Normal arteries have a well-developed trilaminar structure (Fig. 35–2). The innermost layer, the tunica intima, is thin at birth in humans and many nonhuman species. Although often depicted as a monolayer of endothelial cells abutting directly on a basal lamina, the structure of the adult human intima is actually much more complex and heterogeneous. The endothelial cell of the arterial intima constitutes the crucial contact surface with blood. Arterial endothelial cells possess many highly regulated mechanisms of capital importance in vascular homeostasis that often go awry during the pathogenesis of arterial diseases.

For example, the endothelial cell provides one of the only surfaces, either natural or synthetic, that can maintain blood in a liquid state during protracted contact (Fig. 35–3). This remarkable blood compatibility derives in part from the expression of heparan sulfate proteoglycan molecules on the surface of the endothelial cell. These molecules, like heparin, serve as a cofactor for antithrombin III, causing a conformational change that allows this inhibitor to bind to and inactivate thrombin. The surface of the endothelial cell also contains thrombomodulin, which binds thrombin molecules and can exert antithrombotic properties by activating proteins S and C. Should a thrombus begin to form, the normal endothelial cell possesses potent fibrinolytic mechanisms associated with its surface. In this regard, the endothelial cell can produce both tissue- and urokinase-type plasminogen activators. These enzymes catalyze the activation of plasminogens to form plasmin, a fibrinolytic enzyme. (For a complete discussion of the role of endothelium in hemostasis and fibrinolysis, see Chapter 80.)

The endothelial monolayer rests on a basement membrane containing nonfibrillar collagen types, such as type IV collagen, laminin, fibronectin, and other extracellular matrix molecules. With aging, human arteries develop a more complex intima containing arterial smooth muscle cells and fibrillar forms of interstitial collagen (types I and III). The smooth muscle cell produces these extracellular matrix constituents of the arterial intima. The presence of a more complex intima, known by pathologists as *diffuse intimal thickening*, characterizes most adult human arteries. Some locales in the arterial tree tend to develop thicker intimas than other regions, even in the absence of atherosclerosis. For example, the proximal left anterior descending coronary artery often contains an intimal cushion of smooth muscle

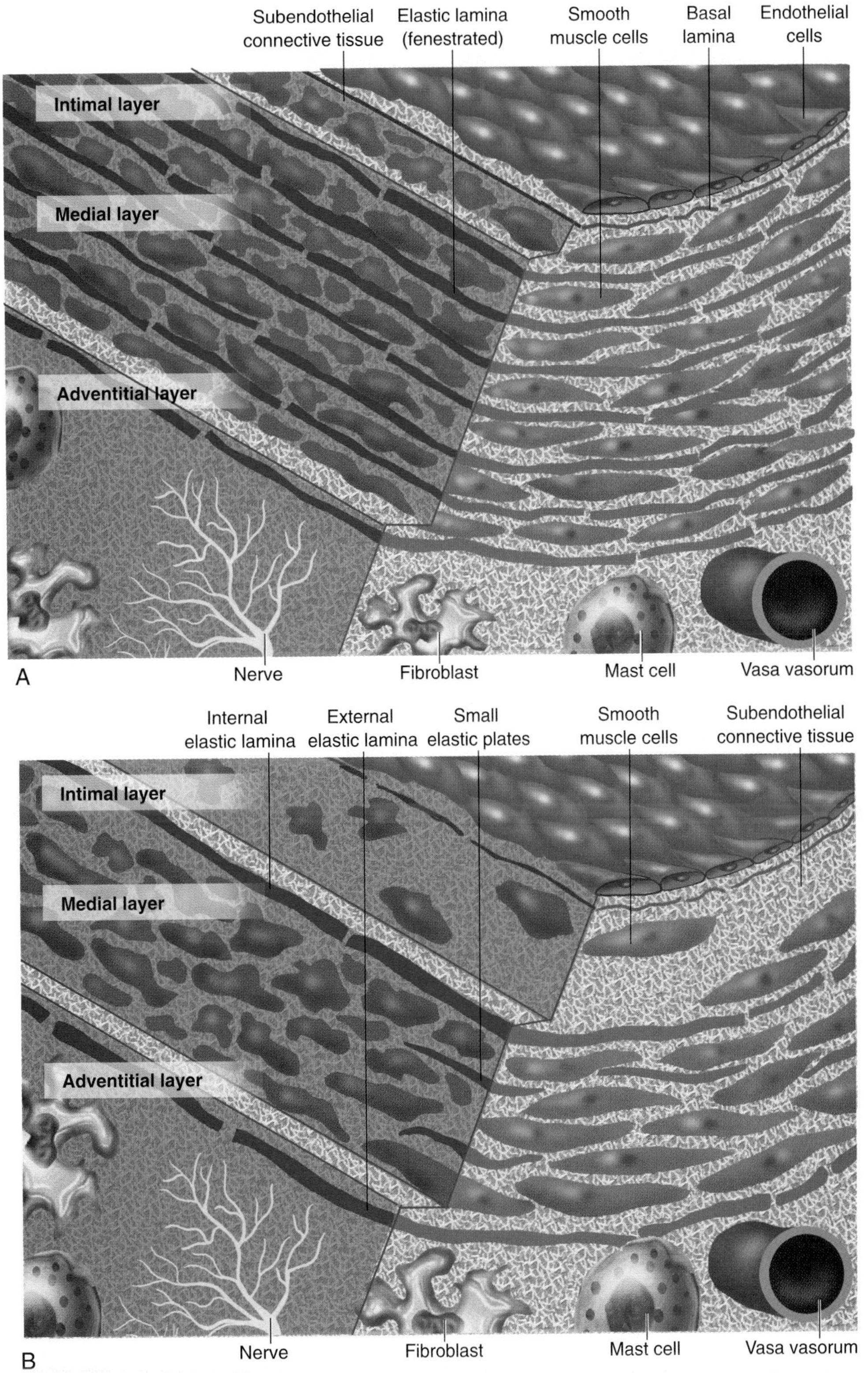

FIGURE 35–2 The structure of normal arteries. **A,** Elastic artery. Note the concentric laminae of elastic tissue that form “sandwiches” with successive layers of smooth muscle cells. Each level of the elastic arterial tree has a characteristic number of elastic laminae. **B,** Muscular artery. The smooth muscle cells are surrounded by a collagenous matrix but lack the concentric rings of well organized elastic tissue characteristic of the larger arteries.

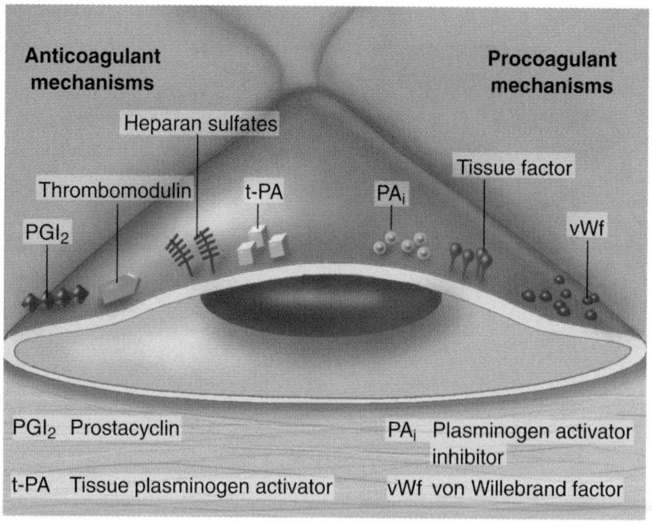

FIGURE 35–3 The endothelial thrombotic balance. This diagram depicts the anticoagulant profibrinolytic functions of the endothelial cell **(left)** and certain procoagulant and antifibrinolytic functions **(right)**. PA_i = plasminogen activator inhibitor; PGI_2 = prostacyclin; t-PA = tissue type plasminogen activator; vWf = von Willebrand factor.

cells more fully developed than that in typical arteries (see Chap. 54). The diffuse intimal thickening process does not necessarily go hand in hand with lipid accumulation and may occur in individuals without substantial burdens of atheroma. The internal elastic membrane bounds the tunica intima abluminally and serves as the border between the intimal layer and the underlying tunica media.

Tunica Media

The tunica media lies under the media and internal elastic lamina. The media of elastic arteries such as the aorta have well developed concentric layers of smooth muscle cells, interleaved with layers of elastin-rich extracellular matrix (see Fig. 35–2A). This structure appears well adapted to the storage of the kinetic energy of left ventricle systole by the walls of great arteries. The lamellar structure also doubtless contributes to the structural integrity of the arterial trunks. The media of smaller muscular arteries usually have a less stereotyped organization (see Fig. 35–2B). Smooth muscle cells in these smaller arteries generally embed in the surrounding matrix in a more continuous than lamellar array. The smooth muscle cells in normal arteries seldom proliferate. Indeed, rates of both cell division and cell death are quite low under usual circumstances. In the normal artery, a state of homeostasis of extracellular matrix also typically prevails. Because extracellular matrix neither accumulates nor atrophies, rates of arterial matrix synthesis and dissolution usually balance each other. The external elastic lamina bounds the tunica media abluminally, forming the border with the adventitial layer.

Adventitia

The adventitia of arteries has typically received little attention, although appreciation of its potential roles in arterial homeostasis and pathology has recently increased. The adventitia contains collagen fibrils in a looser array than usually encountered in the intima. Vasa vasorum and nerve endings localize in this outermost layer of the arterial wall. The adventitia has a sparser cellular population than do other arterial layers. Cells encountered in this layer include fibroblasts and mast cells (see Fig. 35–2).

Atherosclerosis Initiation

Extracellular Lipid Accumulation

The first steps in atherogenesis in humans remain largely conjectural. However, integration of observations of tissue obtained from young humans with the results of experimental studies of atherogenesis in animals provides hints in this regard. Upon initiation of an atherogenic diet, one typically rich in cholesterol and saturated fat, small lipoprotein particles accumulate in the intima (Fig. 35–4, 1&2).[6] These lipoprotein particles appear to decorate the proteoglycan of the arterial intima and tend to coalesce into aggregates (Fig. 35–5).[7] Detailed kinetic studies of labeled lipoprotein particles indicate that a prolonged residence time characterizes sites of early lesion formation in rabbits. The binding of lipoproteins to proteoglycan in the intima captures and retains these particles, accounting for their prolonged residence time.[7,8] Lipoprotein particles bound to proteoglycan have increased susceptibility to oxidative or other chemical modifications, considered by many investigators to be an important component of the pathogenesis of early atherosclerosis (see Fig. 35–4, 2).[7,9-11] Other studies suggest that permeability of the endothelial monolayer increases at sites of lesion predilection to low-density lipoprotein (LDL). Contributors to oxidative stress in the nascent atheroma could include NADH/NADPH oxidases expressed by vascular cells,[12] lipoxygenases expressed by infiltrating leukocytes,[13] or the enzyme myeloperoxidase.[14]

Leukocyte Recruitment

Another hallmark of atherogenesis, leukocyte recruitment and accumulation, also occurs early in lesion generation (Fig. 35–6; see also Fig. 35–4, 3). The normal endothelial cell generally resists adhesive interactions with leukocytes. Even in inflamed tissues, most recruitment and trafficking of leukocytes occurs in postcapillary venules, not in arteries. However, very early after initiation of hypercholesterolemia, leukocytes adhere to the endothelium and diapedese between endothelial cell junctions to enter the intima, where they begin to accumulate lipids and become foam cells (see Fig. 35–4, 5&6). In addition to the monocyte, T lymphocytes also tend to accumulate in early human and animal atherosclerotic lesions. The expression of certain leukocyte adhesion molecules on the surface of the endothelial cell regulates the adherence of monocytes and T cells to the endothelium. Two broad categories of leukocyte adhesion molecules exist. Members of the immunoglobulin superfamily include structures such as vascular cell adhesion molecule-1 (VCAM-1).[15,16] This adhesion molecule holds particular interest in the context of early atherogenesis because it interacts with an integrin (very late antigen-4 [VLA-4]) characteristically expressed by only those classes of leukocytes that accumulate in nascent atheroma, monocytes, and T cells. Moreover, studies in rabbits and mice have shown expression of VCAM-1 on endothelial cells overlying very early atheromatous lesions. Other members of the immunoglobulin superfamily of leukocyte adhesion molecules include intercellular adhesion molecule-1 (ICAM-1). This molecule is more promiscuous, both in the types of leukocytes it binds and because of its wide and constitutive expression at low levels by endothelial cells in many parts of the circulation.

Selectins constitute the other broad category of leukocyte adhesion molecules. The prototypical selectin, E-selectin (E for "endothelial," the cell type that selectively expresses this particular family member), probably has little to do with early atherogenesis. E-selectin preferentially recruits polymorphonuclear leukocytes, a cell type seldom if ever found in early atheroma (but an essential protagonist in acute

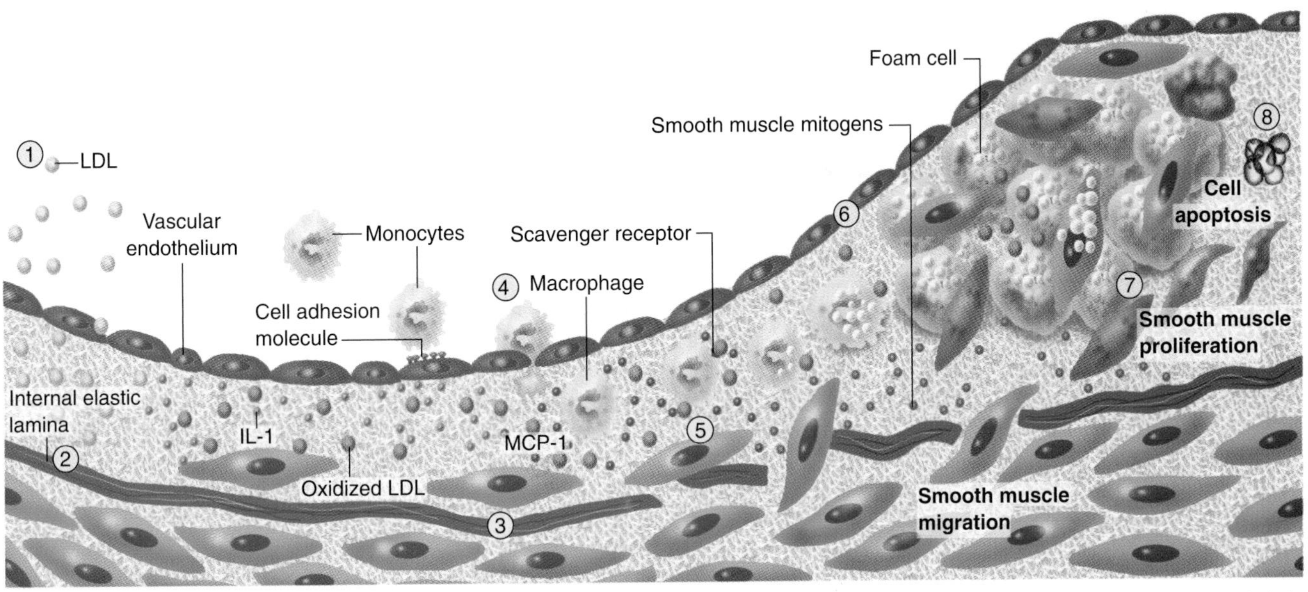

FIGURE 35–4 Schematic of the evolution of the atherosclerotic plaque. **1:** Accumulation of lipoprotein particles in the intima. The modification of these lipoproteins is depicted by the darker color. Modifications include oxidation and glycation. **2:** Oxidative stress, including products found in modified lipoproteins, can induce local cytokine elaboration. **3:** The cytokines thus induced increase expression of adhesion molecules for leukocytes that cause their attachment and chemoattractant molecules that direct their migration into the intima. **4:** Blood monocytes, upon entering the artery wall in response to chemoattractant cytokines such as monocyte chemoattractant protein 1 (MCP-1), encounter stimuli such as macrophage colony stimulating factor (M-CSF) that can augment their expression of scavenger receptors. **5:** Scavenger receptors mediate the uptake of modified lipoprotein particles and promote the development of foam cells. Macrophage foam cells are a source of mediators such as further cytokines and effector molecules such as hypochlorous acid, superoxide anion (O_2^-), and matrix metalloproteinases. **6:** Smooth muscle cells in the intima divide other smooth muscle cells that migrate into the intima from the media. **7:** Smooth muscle cells can then divide and elaborate extracellular matrix, promoting extracellular matrix accumulation in the growing atherosclerotic plaque. In this manner, the fatty streak can evolve into a fibrofatty lesion. **8:** In later stages, calcification can occur (not depicted) and fibrosis continues, sometimes accompanied by smooth muscle cell death (including programmed cell death, or apoptosis) yielding a relatively acellular fibrous capsule surrounding a lipid-rich core that may also contain dying or dead cells and their detritus. IL-1 = interleukin-1; LDL = low-density lipoprotein.

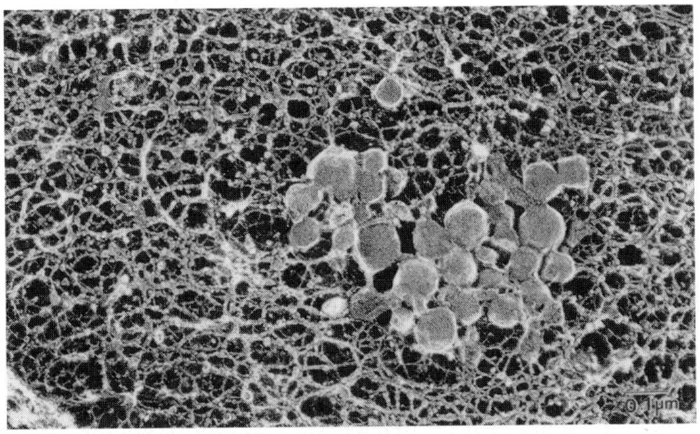

FIGURE 35–5 Scanning electron micrograph of a freeze etch preparation of rabbit aorta following an intravenous injection of human low-density lipoprotein (LDL). Round LDL particles decorate the strands of proteoglycan found in the subendothelial region of the intima. By binding LDL particles, proteoglycan molecules can retard their traversal of the intima and promote their accumulation. Proteoglycan-associated LDL appears particularly susceptible to oxidative modification. Accumulation of extracellular lipoprotein particles is one of the first morphological changes noted after initiation of an atherogenic diet in experimental animals. (From Nievelstein PF, Fogelman AM, Mottino G, Frank JS: Lipid accumulation in rabbit aortic intima 2 hours after bolus infusion of low density lipoprotein: A deep-etch and immunolocalization study of ultrarapidly frozen tissue. Arterioscler Thromb 11:1795, 1991.)

inflammation and host defenses against bacterial pathogens).[17] Moreover, endothelial cells overlying atheroma do not express high levels of this adhesion molecule. Other members of this family, including P-selectin (P for "platelet," the original source of this adhesion molecule), may play a greater role in leukocyte recruitment in atheroma, because endothelial cells overlying human atheroma do express this adhesion molecule.[18,19] Selectins tend to promote saltatory or rolling locomotion of leukocytes over the endothelium. Adhesion molecules belonging to the immunoglobulin superfamily tend to promote tighter adhesive interactions and immobilization of leukocytes. Studies in genetically altered mice have proven roles for VCAM-1 and P-selectin (including both platelet- and endothelial-derived P-selectin) in experimental atherosclerosis.[20-22]

Once adherent to the endothelium, leukocytes must receive a signal to penetrate the endothelial and enter the arterial wall (see Fig. 35–4, 4). The current concept of directed migration of leukocytes involves the action of protein molecules known as chemoattractant cytokines, or chemokines.[23] Two groups of chemokines have particular interest in recruiting the mononuclear cells characteristic of the early atheroma. One such molecule, known as monocyte chemoattractant protein-1 (MCP-1), is produced by the endothelium in response to oxidized lipoprotein and other stimuli. Cells intrinsic to the normal artery, including endothelium and smooth muscle, can produce this chemokine when stimulated by inflammatory mediators, as do many other cell types. MCP-1 selectively promotes the directed migration, or chemotaxis, of monocytes. Studies conducted with genetically modified mice lacking MCP-1 or its receptor CCR-2 have delayed and attenuated atheroma formation when placed on an atherosclerosis-prone hyperlipidemic genetic background.[24,25] Human atherosclerotic lesions express increased levels of MCP-1 compared with uninvolved vessels. Thus, several chemokines appear causally to contribute to monocyte recruitment during atherogenesis in vivo. Interleukin-8, a chemokine that binds to CXCR2 on leukocytes, also participates in experimental atherosclerosis.[26] Another unique cell-surface-bound chemokine, fractalkine, also appears to contribute to atherogenesis.[27] Another group of chemoattractant cytokines may heighten lymphocyte accumulation in

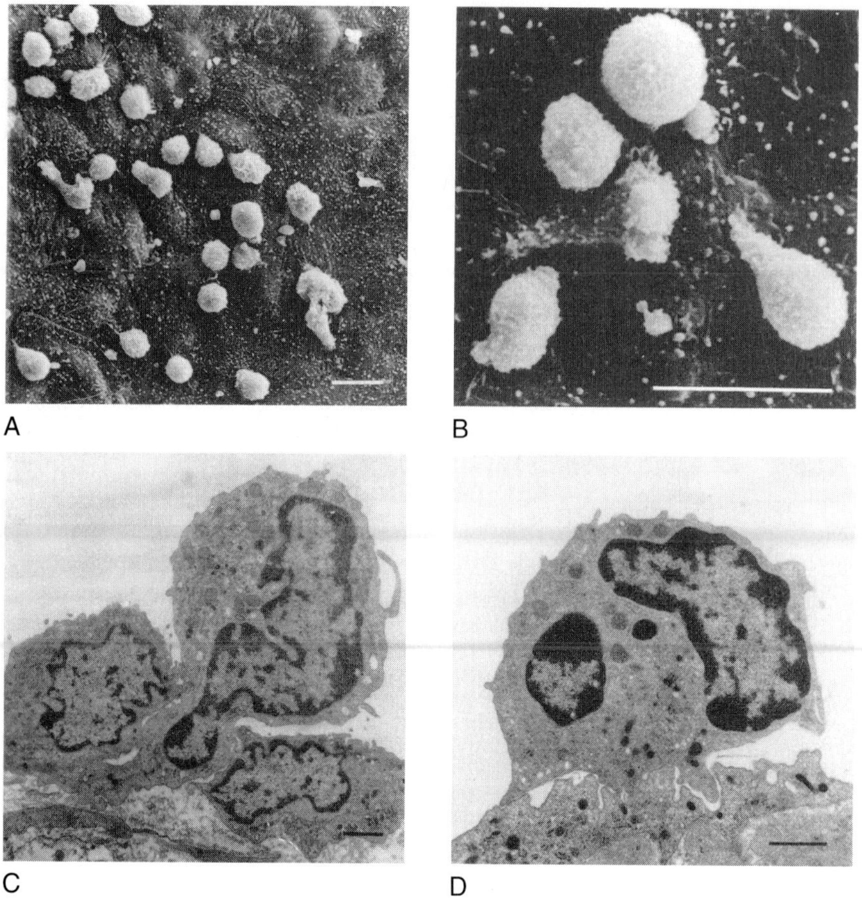

FIGURE 35–6 Electron microscopic examination of leukocyte interactions with the artery wall in hypercholesterolemic nonhuman primates. **A** and **B,** Scanning electron micrographs that demonstrate the adhesion of mononuclear phagocytes to the intact endothelium 12 days after initiating a hypercholesterolemic diet. **C** and **D,** Transmission electron micrographs. Note the abundant interdigitations and intimate association of the monocyte with the endothelium in part C. In part D, a monocyte appears to diapedese between two endothelial cells to enter the intima. (From Faggiotto A, Ross R, Harker L: Studies of hypercholesterolemia in the nonhuman primate. I. Changes that lead to fatty streak formation. Arteriosclerosis 4:323, 1984.)

plaques as well. Atheroma express a trio of lymphocyte-selective chemokines (IP-10, I-TAC, and MIG).[28] Gamma interferon, a cytokine known to be present in atheromatous plaques, induces the genes encoding this family of T-cell chemoattractants.

Focality of Lesion Formation

The spatial heterogeneity of atherosclerosis has proved challenging to explain in mechanistic terms. Equal concentrations of blood-borne risk factors such as lipoproteins bathe the endothelium throughout the vasculature. It is difficult to envisage how injury due to inhaling cigarette smoke could produce any local rather than global effect on arteries. Yet, atheromata typically form focally, as revealed by studies of morphology, lipid accumulation, and adhesion molecule expression. Some have invoked a multicentric origin hypothesis of atherogenesis, positing that atheroma arise as benign leiomyomata of the artery wall. The monotypia of various molecular markers such as glucose-6-phosphate dehydrogenase isoforms in individual atheroma supports this "monoclonal hypothesis" of atherogenesis.[29] However, the location of sites of lesion predilection at proximal portions of arteries after branch points or bifurcations at flow dividers suggests a hydrodynamic basis for early lesion development. Arteries without many branches (e.g., the internal mammary or radial arteries) tend not to develop atherosclerosis.

Two concepts can help one understand how local flow disturbances might render certain foci sites of lesion predilection. Locally disturbed flow could induce alterations that promote the steps of early atherogenesis. Alternatively, the laminar flow that usually prevails at sites that do *not* tend to develop early lesions may elicit antiatherogenic homeostatic mechanisms (atheroprotective functions).[30] The endothelial cell experiences the laminar shear stress of normal flow and the disturbed flow (usually yielding decreased shear stress) at predilected sites. In vitro data suggest that laminar shear stress can augment the expression of genes that may protect against atherosclerosis, including forms of the enzymes superoxide dismutase, or nitric oxide synthase. Superoxide dismutase can reduce oxidative stress by catabolizing the reactive and injurious superoxide anion. Endothelial nitric oxide synthase produces the well known endogenous vasodilator nitric oxide (•NO). However, beyond its vasodilating actions, •NO can resist inflammatory activation of endothelial functions such as expression of the adhesion molecule VCAM-1. Nitric oxide appears to exert this antiinflammatory action at the level of gene expression by interfering with the transcriptional regulator nuclear factor kappa B (NFκB). Nitric oxide actually increases the production of an intracellular inhibitor (IκBα) of this important transcription factor. The NFκB system regulates numerous genes involved in inflammatory responses in general and in atherogenesis in particular.[31] These examples show how basic vascular biology has yielded insights into previously obscure yet important aspects of atherogenesis. Future study of the molecular regulation of vascular cell function by mechanical stimuli should clarify the mechanisms of lesion formation at particular sites in the circulation.

Likewise, study of vascular developmental biology may aid understanding of the tendency of certain arteries to develop atherosclerosis at different rates and in different ways (see Chap. 54). Smooth muscle cells vary in embryological origin in different regions.[32] For example, upper body arteries can recruit smooth muscle from neurectoderm, whereas in the lower body smooth muscle cells derive principally from mesoderm. Coronary artery smooth muscle cells arise from an anlage known as the pro-epicardial organ.[33] After injury or transplantation, arteries can repopulate with smooth muscle cells derived from bone marrow.[34,35] How this heterogeneity in the origin of smooth muscle cells might affect human atherosclerosis and help explain some of the poorly understood issues regarding dispersion of atheroma in time and space remains intriguing yet speculative. (See Chapter 54 for further discussion of the cellular and molecular heterogeneity of blood vessels.)

Intracellular Lipid Accumulation: Foam Cell Formation

The monocyte, once recruited to the arterial intima, can there imbibe lipid and become a foam cell, or lipid-laden macrophage (see Fig. 35–4, 5). Most cells can express the classic cell surface receptor for LDL, but that receptor does not mediate foam cell accumulation (see Chap. 39). This is evident clinically, as patients lacking functional LDL receptors (familial hypercholesterolemia homozygotes) still develop tendinous xanthomata filled with foamy macrophages. The LDL receptor does not mediate foam cell formation because of its exquisite regulation by cholesterol. As soon as a cell collects enough cholesterol from low-density lipoprotein capture for its metabolic needs, an elegant transcriptional control mechanism quenches expression of the receptor (see Chap. 39).

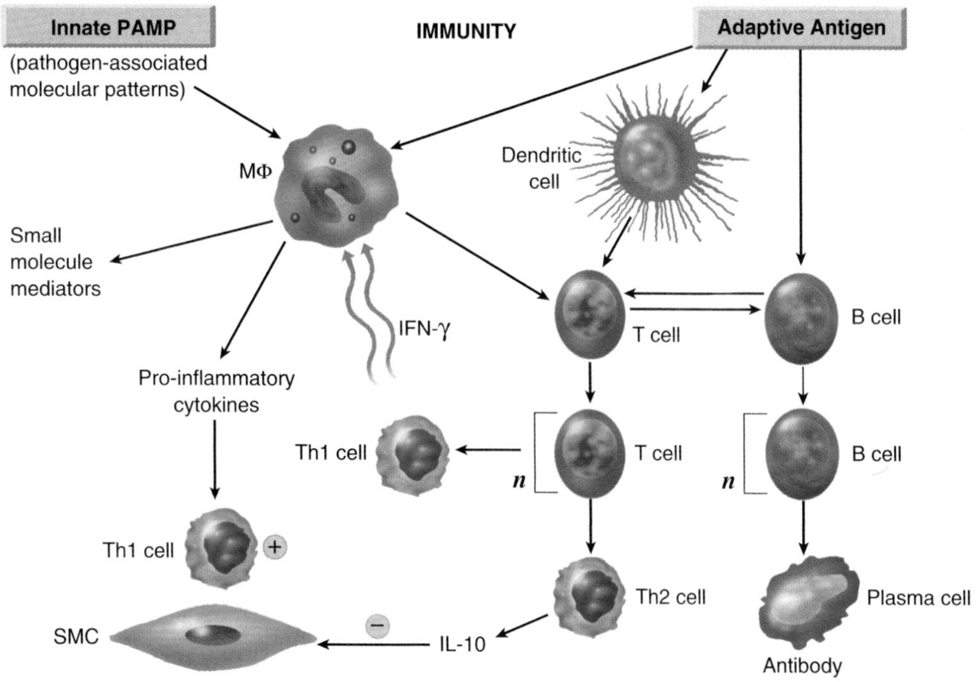

FIGURE 35–7 Innate and adaptive immunity in atherosclerosis. A diagram of the pathways of innate **(left)** and adaptive **(right)** immunity operating during atherogenesis. IFN-γ = interferon gamma; IL = interleukin; MΦ = macrophage; SMC = smooth muscle cell; Th = T helper cell. (Adapted from Hansson G, Libby P, Schoenbeck U, Yan Z-Q: Innate and adaptive immunity in the pathogenesis of atherosclerosis. Circ Res 91:281, 2002.)

Instead of the classic LDL receptor, various molecules known as *scavenger receptors* appear to mediate the excessive lipid uptake characteristic of foam cell formation.[36] The longest studied of these receptors belong to the scavenger receptor-A family. These surface molecules bind modified rather than native lipoproteins and apparently participate in their internalization. Atherosclerosis-prone mice with mutations that delete functional scavenger receptor-A have less exuberant fatty lesion formation than those with functional scavenger receptor-A molecules.[37] Other receptors that bind modified lipoprotein and that may participate in foam cell formation include CD36 and macrosialin, the latter exhibiting preferential binding specificity for oxidized forms of LDL. (See Chap. 39 for a table of scavenger receptors.)

Once macrophages have taken up residence in the intima and become foam cells, they not infrequently replicate. The factors that trigger macrophage cell division in the atherosclerotic plaque likely include macrophage-colony stimulating factor. This co-mitogen and survival factor for mononuclear phagocytes exists in human and experimental atheromatous lesions. Again, atherosclerosis-prone mice lacking functional macrophage-colony stimulating factor have retarded fatty lesion development as well.[38] Other candidates for macrophage mitogens or co-mitogens include interleukin-3 and granulocyte-macrophage colony stimulatory factor.

Up to this point in the development of the nascent atheroma, the lesion consists primarily of lipid-engorged macrophages. Complex features such as fibrosis, thrombosis, and calcification do not characterize the fatty streak, the precursor lesion of the complex atheroma (see Fig. 35–1). Several lines of evidence suggest that such fatty streaks may be reversible, at least to some extent.

Evolution of Atheroma

Innate and Adaptive Immunity: Mechanisms of Inflammation in Atherogenesis

Over the last decade, basic and clinical evidence have converged to demonstrate a fundamental role for inflammation in atherogenesis (see Chap. 36).[39,40] The macrophage foam cells recruited to the artery wall early in this process serve not only as a reservoir for excess lipid. In the established atherosclerotic lesion, these cells also provide a rich source of proinflammatory mediators, both proteins such as cytokines and chemokines and various eicosanoids and lipids such as platelet-activating factor. These phagocytic cells also can elaborate large quantities of oxidant species such as superoxide anion in the milieu of the atherosclerotic plaque.[41] This ensemble of inflammatory mediators can promote inflammation in the plaque and thus contribute to the progression of lesions. The term *innate immunity* describes this type of amplification of the inflammatory response that does not depend on antigenic stimulation (Fig. 35–7).

In addition to innate immunity, mounting evidence supports a prominent role for antigen-specific or adaptive immunity in plaque progression.[39,40] In addition to the mononuclear phagocytes, dendritic cells in atherosclerotic lesion can present antigens to the T cells that constitute an important minority of the leukocytes in the atherosclerotic lesion. Candidate antigens for stimulating this adaptive immune response include modified lipoproteins, heat shock proteins, beta-2 glycoprotein 1b, and infectious agents. The antigen-presenting cells (macrophages, dendritic cells, or endothelial cells) allow the antigen to interact with T cells in a manner that triggers their activation. The activated T cells then can secrete copious quantities of cytokines that can modulate atherogenesis.

The helper T cells (bearing CD4) fall into two general categories. The T helper 1 subtype elaborates proinflammatory cytokines such as interferon gamma, lymphotoxin, CD40 ligand, and tumor necrosis factor-alpha. This panel of Th1 cytokines can in turn activate vascular wall cells and orchestrate alterations in plaque biology that can lead to plaque destabilization and heightened thrombogenicity. On the other hand, helper T cells slanted toward the production of Th2 cytokines such as interleukin-10 may serve as inhibitors of inflammation in the context of atherogenesis.[42] Cytolytic T cells (bearing CD8) can express fas ligand and other cytotoxic factors that can promote cytolysis and apoptosis of target cells, including smooth muscle and endothelial cells, and macrophages.[43,44] The death of all three of these cell types can occur in the atherosclerotic lesion and may contribute to plaque progression and complications (see Fig. 35–4, 8). The role of B cells and antibody in atherosclerosis remains incompletely explored. Humoral immunity may have either atheroprotective or atherogenic properties, depending on the circumstances.

Smooth Muscle Cell Migration and Proliferation

While the early events in atheroma initiation involve primarily altered endothelial function and recruitment and accumulation of leukocytes, the subsequent evolution of atheroma into more complex plaques involves smooth muscle cells as well (see Fig. 35–4, 6&7). Smooth muscle cells in the normal arterial tunica media differ considerably from those in the intima of an evolving atheroma.[45,46] Whereas some smooth muscle cells likely arrive in the arterial intima early in life, others that accumulate in advancing atheroma likely arise from cells that have migrated from the underlying media into the intima. The chemoattractants for smooth muscle cells likely include molecules such as platelet-derived growth factor (PDGF), a potent smooth muscle cell chemoattractant secreted by activated macrophages and overexpressed in human atherosclerosis. These smooth muscle cells in the atherosclerotic intima can also multiply by cell division. Estimated rates of division of smooth muscle cells in the human atherosclerotic lesion are on the order of less than 1 percent. However, even such indolent replication might yield considerable smooth muscle cell accumulation over the decades of lesion evolution.

Smooth muscle cells in the atherosclerotic intima appear to exhibit a less mature phenotype than the quiescent smooth muscle cells in the normal arterial medial layer. Instead of expressing primarily isoforms of smooth muscle myosin characteristic of adult smooth muscle cells, those in the intima have higher levels of the embryonic isoform of smooth muscle myosin.[46] Thus, smooth muscle cells in the intima appear to recapitulate an embryonic phenotype. These intimal smooth muscle cells in atheroma appear morphologically distinct as well. They contain more rough endoplasmic reticulum and fewer contractile fibers than do normal medial smooth muscle cells.

Although replication of smooth muscle cells in the steady state appears infrequent in mature human atheroma, bursts of smooth muscle cell replication may occur during the life history of a given atheromatous lesion. For example, and as will be discussed in considerable detail later, episodes of plaque disruption with thrombosis may expose smooth muscle cells to potent mitogens, including the coagulation factor thrombin itself. Thus, accumulation of smooth muscle cells during atherosclerosis and growth of the intima may not occur in a continuous and linear fashion. Rather, "crises" may punctuate the history of an atheroma, during which bursts of smooth muscle replication and/or migration may occur (Fig. 35–8).

Smooth Muscle Cell Death During Atherogenesis

In addition to smooth muscle cell replication, death of these cells can also participate in the complication of the atherosclerotic plaque (see Fig. 35–4, 8). At least some smooth muscle cells in advanced human atheroma exhibit fragmentation of their nuclear DNA characteristic of programmed cell death, or apoptosis.[43,44] Apoptosis can occur in response to inflammatory cytokines known to be present in the evolving atheroma. In addition to soluble cytokines that can trigger programmed cell death, the T cells in atheroma can participate in eliminating some smooth muscle cells. In particular, certain T cell populations known to accumulate in plaques can express *fas* ligand on their surface. *Fas* ligand can engage *fas* on the surface of smooth muscle cells and, in conjunction with soluble proinflammatory cytokines, lead to death of the smooth muscle cell.[43,47]

Thus, smooth muscle cell accumulation in the growing atherosclerotic plaque probably results from a tug-of-war between cell replication and cell death.[43] Contemporary cell and molecular biological research has identified candidates for mediating both the replication and the attrition of smooth muscle cells, a concept that originated from the careful morphological observations of Virchow almost a century and a half ago. Referring to the smooth muscle cells in the intima, Virchow noted that early atherogenesis involves a "multiplication of their nuclei." However, he recognized that cells in lesions can "hurry on to their own destruction" because of death of smooth muscle cells.

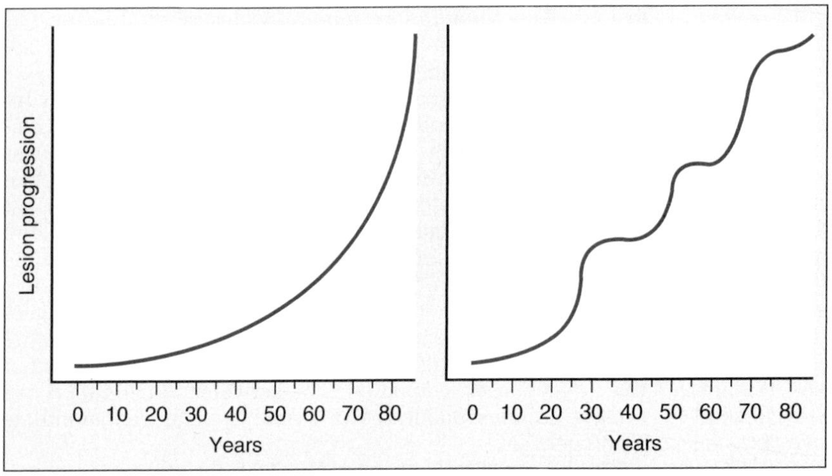

FIGURE 35–8 The time course of atherosclerosis. Traditional teaching held that atheroma formation followed an inexorably progressive course with age, depicted in the left-hand curve. Current thinking suggests an alternative model, a step function rather than a monotonically upward course of lesion evolution in time (right-hand curve). According to this latter model, "crises" can punctuate periods of relative quiescence during the life history of a lesion. Such crises might follow an episode of plaque disruption, with mural thrombosis, and healing, yielding a spurt in smooth muscle proliferation and matrix deposition. Intraplaque hemorrhage due to rupture of a friable microvessel might produce a similar scenario. Such episodes might usually be clinically inapparent. Extravascular events such as an intercurrent infection with systemic cytokinemia or endotoxemia could elicit an "echo" at the level of the artery wall, evoking a round of local cytokine gene expression by "professional" inflammatory leukocytes resident in the lesion. The episodic model of plaque progression shown on the right fits human angiographic data better than the continuous function, depicted on the left.

Arterial Extracellular Matrix

Extracellular matrix rather than cells themselves makes up much of the volume of an advanced atherosclerotic plaque. Thus, extracellular constituents of plaque also require consideration. The major extracellular matrix macromolecules that accumulate in atheroma include interstitial collagens (types I and III) and proteoglycans such as versican, biglycan, aggrecan, and decorin.[48,49] Elastin fibers can also accumulate in atherosclerotic plaques. The vascular smooth muscle cell produces these matrix molecules in disease, just as it does during development and maintenance of the normal artery (see Fig. 35–4, 7). Stimuli for excessive collagen production by smooth muscle cells include PDGF and transforming growth factor-beta (TGF-β), a constituent of platelet granules and a product of many cell types found in lesions.

Much like the accumulation of smooth muscle cells, extracellular matrix secretion also depends on a balance. In this case, the biosynthesis of the extracellular matrix molecules is balanced by breakdown catalyzed in part by catabolic enzymes known as matrix metalloproteinases (MMPs). Dissolution of extracellular matrix macromolecules undoubtedly plays a role in the migration of smooth muscle cells as they penetrate into the intima from the media through a dense extracellular matrix, traversing the elastin-rich internal elastic lamina. In injured arteries, overexpression of such proteinase inhibitors (known as tissue inhibitors of metalloproteinases) can delay smooth muscle accumulation in the intima of injured arteries.[50]

Extracellular matrix dissolution also likely plays a role in the arterial remodeling that accompanies lesion growth. During the first part of the life history of an atheromatous lesion, growth of the plaque is outward, in an abluminal direction, rather than inward in a way that would lead to luminal stenosis. This outward growth of the intima leads to an increase in the caliber of the entire artery. This so-called "positive" remodeling or "compensatory enlargement" must involve turnover of extracellular matrix molecules to accommodate the circumferential growth of the artery. Luminal stenosis tends to occur only after the plaque burden exceeds some 40 percent of the cross-sectional area of the artery.[5]

Angiogenesis in Plaques

The smooth muscle cell is not alone in its proliferation and migration within the evolving atherosclerotic plaque. Endothelial migration and replication also occur as plaques develop in microcirculation, characterized by plexi of newly formed vessels. Such plaque neovessels usually require special stains for visualization. However, histological examination with appropriate markers for endothelial cells reveals a rich neovascularization in evolving plaques. These microvessels likely form in response to angiogenic peptides overexpressed in atheroma. These angiogenesis factors include acidic and basic fibroblast growth factors, vascular endothelial growth factor,[51,52] placental growth factor,[53] and oncostatin M.[54]

These microvessels within plaques probably have considerable functional significance.[55] For example, the abundant microvessels in plaques provide a relatively large surface area for the trafficking of leukocytes, which could include both entry and exit of leukocytes. Indeed, in the advanced human atherosclerotic plaque, microvascular endothelium displays the mononuclear-selective adhesion molecules such as VCAM-1 much more prominently than does the macrovascular endothelium overlying the plaque. The microvascularization of plaques may also allow growth of the plaque overcoming diffusion limitations on oxygen and nutrient supply, analogous with the concept of tumor angiogenic factors and growth of malignant lesions. Consistent with this view, administration of inhibitors of angiogenesis to mice with experimentally induced atherosclerosis limits lesion expansion.[56] Finally, the plaque microvessels may be friable and prone to rupture like the neovessels in the diabetic retina.[57] Hemorrhage and thrombosis in situ could promote a local round of smooth muscle cell proliferation and matrix accumulation in the area immediately adjacent to the microvascular disruption (Fig. 35–9). This scenario illustrates a special case of one of the "crises" described earlier in the evolution of the atheromatous plaque (see Fig. 35–8). Attempts to augment myocardial perfusion by enhancing new vessel growth by transfer of angiogenic proteins or their genes might have adverse effects on lesion growth or clinical complications of atheroma by these mechanisms.

Plaque Mineralization

Plaques often develop areas of calcification as they evolve. Indeed, both Virchow and Rokitansky recognized morphological features of bone formation in atherosclerotic plaques in early microscopic descriptions of atherosclerosis. In recent years, understanding of the mechanism of mineralization during evolution of atherosclerotic plaques has advanced. Some subpopulations of smooth muscle cells may foster calcification by enhanced secretion of cytokines such as bone morphogenetic proteins, homologues of transforming growth factor-beta.[58] Atheromatous plaques can also contain proteins with gamma carboxylated glutamic acid residues specialized in sequestering calcium and thus promoting mineralization.[59]

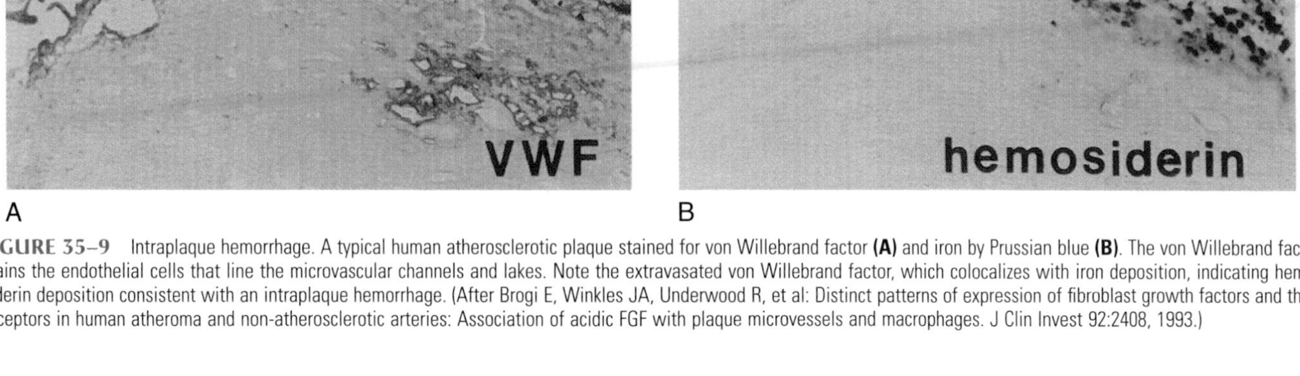

A B

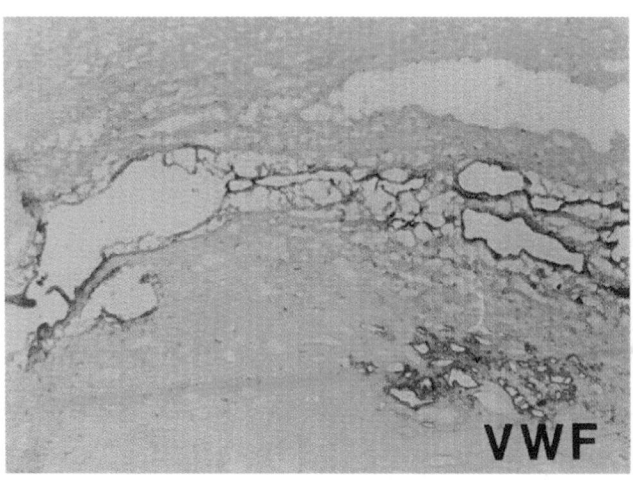

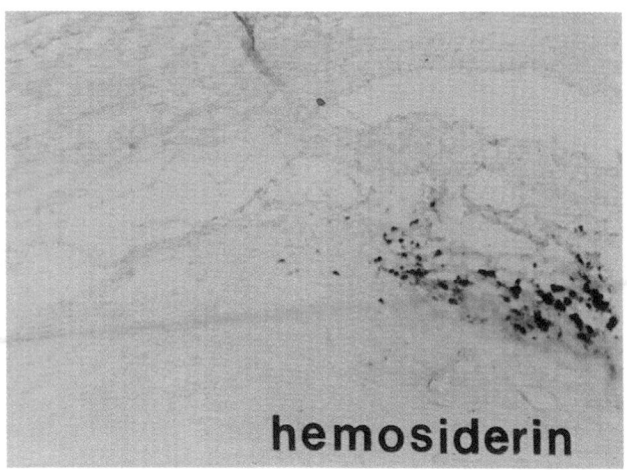

FIGURE 35–9 Intraplaque hemorrhage. A typical human atherosclerotic plaque stained for von Willebrand factor **(A)** and iron by Prussian blue **(B)**. The von Willebrand factor stains the endothelial cells that line the microvascular channels and lakes. Note the extravasated von Willebrand factor, which colocalizes with iron deposition, indicating hemosiderin deposition consistent with an intraplaque hemorrhage. (After Brogi E, Winkles JA, Underwood R, et al: Distinct patterns of expression of fibroblast growth factors and their receptors in human atheroma and non-atherosclerotic arteries: Association of acidic FGF with plaque microvessels and macrophages. J Clin Invest 92:2408, 1993.)

Arterial Stenoses and Their Clinical Implications

The previous sections have discussed the initiation and evolution of the atherosclerotic plaque. These phases of the atherosclerotic process generally last many years, during which time the affected individual often has no symptoms. After the plaque burden exceeds the capacity of the artery to remodel outward, encroachment on the arterial lumen begins. During the chronic asymptomatic or stable phase of lesion evolution, growth probably occurs discontinuously, with periods of relative quiescence punctuated by episodes of rapid progression (see Fig. 35–8). Human angiographic studies support this discontinuous growth of coronary artery stenoses.[60] Eventually, the stenoses can progress to a degree that impedes blood flow through the artery. Lesions that produce stenoses of greater than 60 percent can cause flow limitations under conditions of increased demand. This type of athero-occlusive disease commonly produces chronic stable angina pectoris or intermittent claudication upon increased demand. Thus, the symptomatic phase of atherosclerosis usually occurs many decades after lesion initiation.

In many cases of myocardial infarction, however, no history of prior stable angina heralds the acute event. Several kinds of clinical observation suggest that many myocardial infarctions result not from high-grade stenoses but from lesions that do not limit flow.[61,62] For example, in individuals who have undergone coronary arteriography in the months preceding myocardial infarction, the culprit lesion most often shows less than 50 percent stenosis. In a compilation of four such serial angiographic studies, only approximately 15 percent of acute myocardial infarctions arise from lesions with degrees of stenosis greater than 60 percent on an antecedent angiogram.

Instead of progressive growth of the intimal lesion to a critical stenosis, we now recognize that thrombosis, complicating a not necessarily occlusive plaque, most often causes episodes of unstable angina or acute myocardial infarction. Angiographic studies performed in individuals undergoing thrombolysis support this view. In one such study, almost half of patients undergoing thrombolysis for a first myocardial infarction had an underlying stenosis of less than 50 percent once the acute thrombus was lysed.

These findings do not imply that small atheromata cause most myocardial infarctions. Indeed, culprit lesions of acute myocardial infarction may actually be sizeable.[63] However, they may not produce a critical luminal narrowing because of the phenomenon of compensatory enlargement.[5,64,65] Of course, critical stenoses do cause myocardial infarctions. In fact, the high-grade stenoses are more likely to cause acute myocardial infarction than nonocclusive lesions. However, because the noncritical stenoses by far outnumber the tight focal lesions in a given coronary tree, the lesser stenoses cause more infarctions even though high-grade stenoses have a greater individual probability of causing myocardial infarction.

Thrombosis and Atheroma Complication

This evolution in our view of the pathogenesis of the acute coronary syndromes places new emphasis on thrombosis as the critical mechanism of transition from chronic to acute atherosclerosis. Understanding of the mechanisms of coronary thrombosis has advanced considerably. We now appreciate that a physical disruption of the atherosclerotic plaque commonly causes acute thrombosis. Several major modes of plaque disruption provoke most coronary thrombi. The first mechanism, accounting for some two thirds of acute myocardial infarctions, involves a fracture of the plaque's fibrous cap (Fig. 35–10). Another mode involves a superficial erosion of the intima (Fig. 35–11), accounting for up to one-quarter of acute myocardial infarctions in highly selected referral cases from medical examiners on individuals who have succumbed to sudden cardiac death. Superficial erosion appears more frequently in women than in men as a mechanism of coronary sudden death.[66]

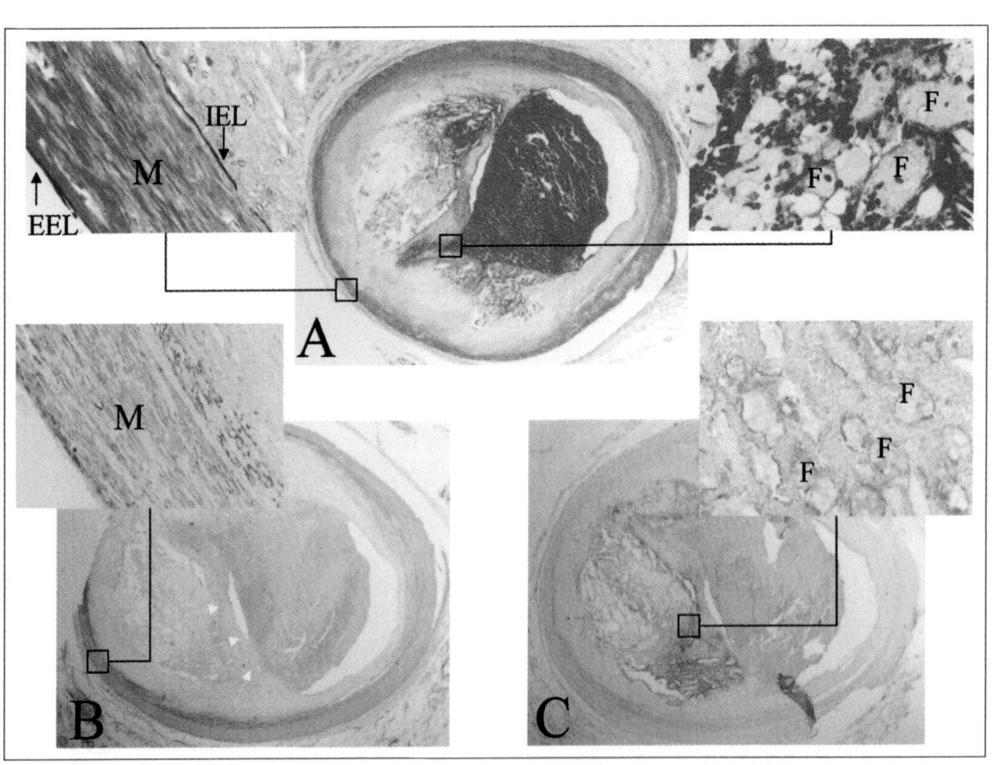

FIGURE 35–10 An example of a ruptured plaque that caused a fatal thrombosis. **A,** Movat stain. **B,** Immunostaining with HHF-35 discloses smooth muscle cells. Note the paucity of smooth muscle cells in the fibrous cap (white arrowheads), in contrast with the abundant smooth muscle cells in the medial layer (inset, M denotes the tunica media). **C,** Macrophage staining (CD-68) shows accumulation of the inflammatory cells near the fibrous cap (inset, F denotes foam cell). EEL = external elastic lamina; IEL = internal elastic lamina. (From Bezerra HG, Higuchi ML, Gutierrez PS, et al: Atheromas that cause fatal thrombosis are usually large and frequently accompanied by vessel enlargement. Cardiovasc Pathol 10:189, 2001.)

Plaque Rupture and Thrombosis

The rupture of the plaque's fibrous cap probably reflects an imbalance between the forces that impinge on the plaque's cap and the mechanical strength of the fibrous cap.[67] Interstitial forms of collagen provide most of the biomechanical resistance to disruption to the fibrous cap. Hence, the

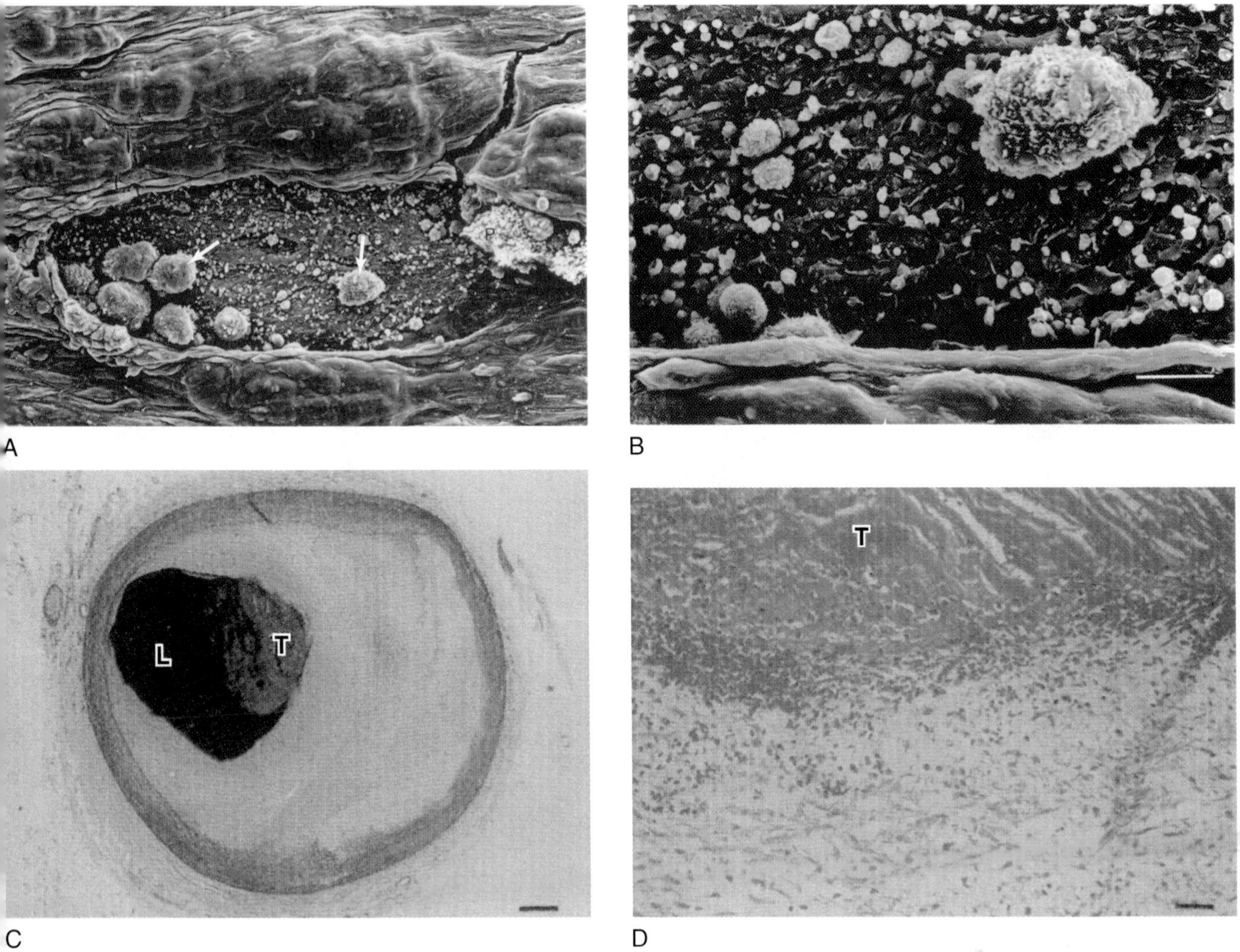

FIGURE 35–11 Superficial erosion of experimental atherosclerotic lesions shown by scanning electron microscopy. Advanced atherosclerotic plaques can promote thrombosis by superficial erosion of the endothelial layer, exposing the blood and platelets to the subendothelial basement membrane containing collagen platelet activation and thrombosis. **A,** In the low-power view, the rent in the endothelium is evident. Leukocytes have adhered to the subendothelium, which is beginning to be covered with a carpet of platelets (arrows). **B,** The high-power view shows a field selected from the center of part A that shows the leukocytes and platelets adherent to the subendothelium. **C,** A low-power histological section through a coronary artery thrombosed due to superficial erosion. **D,** A higher power histological section through a coronary artery thrombosed due to superficial erosion. L = lumen; T = thrombus. (**A** & **B,** from Faggiotto A, Ross R: Studies of hypercholesterolemia in the nonhuman primate. II. Fatty streak conversion to fibrous plaque. Arteriosclerosis 4: 341, 1984. **C** & **D,** from Farb A, Burke AP, Tang AL, et al: Coronary plaque erosion without rupture into a lipid core: A frequent cause of coronary thrombosis in sudden coronary death. Circulation 93:1354, 1996.)

metabolism of collagen probably participates in regulating the propensity of a plaque to rupture (Fig. 35–12). Factors that decrease collagen synthesis by smooth muscle cells can impair their ability to repair and maintain the plaque's fibrous cap. For example, the T-cell–derived cytokine interferon gamma potently inhibits smooth muscle cell collagen synthesis. On the other hand, as already noted, certain mediators released from platelet granules during activation can increase smooth muscle cell collagen synthesis, tending to reinforce the plaque's fibrous structure. Such mediators include TGF-β and PDGF.

In addition to reduced de novo collagen synthesis by smooth muscle cells, increased catabolism of the extracellular matrix macromolecules that comprise the fibrous cap can also contribute to weakening of this structure and rendering it susceptible to rupture and hence thrombosis. The same matrix-degrading enzymes thought to contribute to smooth muscle migration and arterial remodeling can also contribute to weakening of the fibrous cap (see Fig. 35–12). Macrophages in cases of advanced human atheroma overexpress matrix metalloproteinases and elastolytic cathepsins that can break down the collagen and elastin of the arterial extracellular matrix.[68,69] Thus, the strength of the plaque's fibrous cap is under dynamic regulation, linking the inflammatory response in the intima with the molecular determinants of plaque stability and hence thrombotic complications of atheroma. The thinning of the plaque's fibrous cap, a result of reduced collagen synthesis and increased degradation, probably explains why pathological studies have shown that thin fibrous cap characterizes atherosclerotic plaques that have ruptured and caused fatal myocardial infarction.[70]

Another feature of the so-called "vulnerable" atherosclerotic plaque defined by pathological analysis is a relative lack of smooth muscle cells (see Fig. 35–10B). As explained earlier, inflammatory mediators both soluble and associated with the surface of T-lymphocytes can provoke programmed cell death of smooth muscle cells. "Dropout" of smooth muscle cells from regions of local inflammation within plaques probably contributes to the relative lack of smooth muscle cells at places where plaques rupture. Since these cells are the source of the newly synthesized collagen needed to repair and maintain the matrix of the fibrous cap, the lack

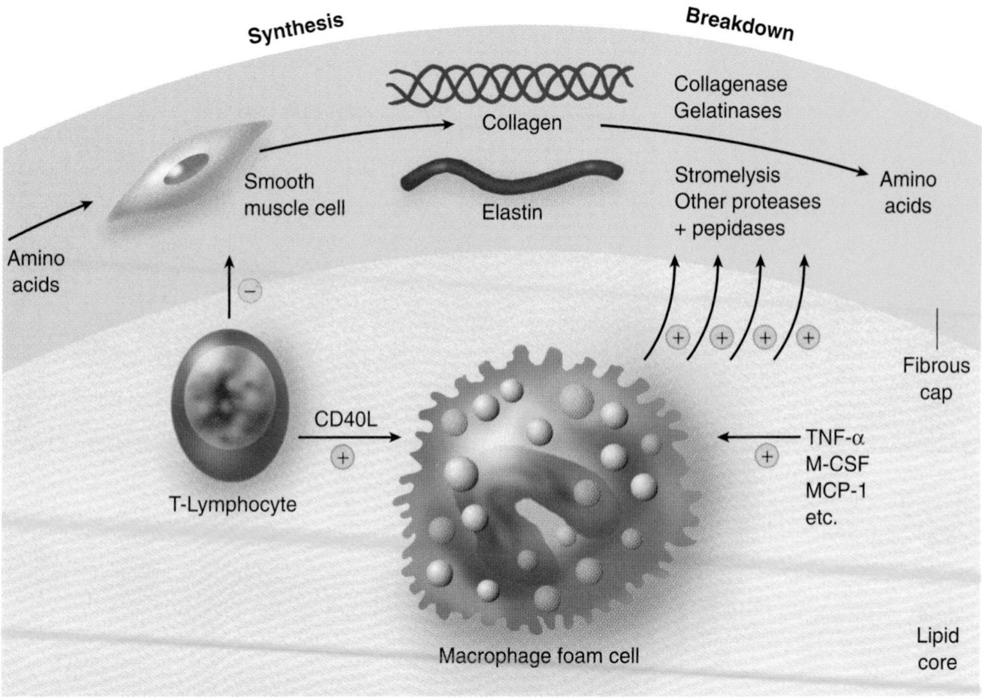

FIGURE 35–12 A schematic relating extracellular matrix metabolism to intimal inflammation during atherogenesis. The lymphocyte can elaborate gamma interferon (γ-IFN) that inhibits smooth muscle cell collagen production. The lymphocyte can also signal either by elaboration of soluble mediators or by contact activation of macrophages. Other cytokines produced in response to products of oxidized lipoproteins, among other stimuli, can further activate the macrophage. The activated phagocyte can release collagen degrading matrix metalloproteinases, and elastolytic enzymes including certain nonmetalloenzymes, such as cathepsins S and K. These enzymes promote matrix catabolism. Thus, in states characterized by heightened intimal inflammation, the extracellular matrix that confers biomechanical strength to the plaque's fibrous cap is under double attack: decreased synthesis and increased degradation. This results in a weakening and thinning of the fibrous cap, features associated in pathological studies with fatal atheromatous plaque disruptions and thrombosis. (From Libby P: The molecular bases of the acute coronary syndromes. Circulation 91:2844, 1995.)

of smooth muscle cells may contribute to weakening of the fibrous cap and hence the propensity of that plaque to rupture.[63]

A prominent accumulation of macrophages and a large lipid pool is a third microanatomical feature of the so-called "vulnerable" atherosclerotic plaque. From a strictly biomechanical viewpoint, a large lipid pool can serve to concentrate biomechanical forces on the shoulder regions of plaques, common sites of rupture of the fibrous cap. From a metabolic standpoint, the activated macrophage characteristic of the plaque's core region produces the cytokines and the matrix-degrading enzymes thought to regulate aspects of matrix catabolism and smooth muscle cell apoptosis in turn. Apoptotic macrophages as well as smooth muscle cells can generate particulate tissue factor, a potential instigator of microvascular thrombosis after spontaneous or iatrogenic plaque disruption. The success of lipid-lowering therapy in reducing the incidence of acute myocardial infarction or unstable angina in patients at risk may result from a reduced accumulation of lipid and decrease in inflammation and plaque thrombogenicity. Recent animal studies and monitoring of peripheral markers of inflammation in humans support this concept.[71-76]

Thrombosis due to Superficial Erosion of Plaques

The foregoing section discusses the pathophysiology of rupture of the plaque's fibrous cap. The pathobiology of superficial erosion is much less well understood. In experimental atherosclerosis in the nonhuman primate, areas of endothelial loss and platelet deposition occur in the more advanced plaques (see Fig. 35–11). In humans, superficial erosion appears more likely to cause fatal acute myocardial infarction in women and in individuals with hypertriglyceridemia and diabetes mellitus.[77,78] However, the underlying molecular mechanisms remain obscure. Apoptosis of endothelial cells could contribute to desquamation of endothelial cells in areas of superficial erosion. Likewise, matrix metalloproteinases such as certain gelatinases specialized in degrading the nonfibrillar collagen found in the basement membrane, such as collagen type IV, might also sever the tetherings of the endothelial cell to the subjacent basal lamina and promote their desquamation.[79]

Most plaque disruptions do not give rise to clinically apparent coronary events. Careful pathoanatomical examination of hearts obtained from individuals who have succumbed to noncardiac death have shown a surprisingly high incidence of focal plaque disruptions with limited mural thrombi. Moreover, hearts fixed immediately after explantation from individuals with severe but chronic stable coronary atherosclerosis and who had undergone transplantation for ischemic cardiomyopathy show similar evidence for ongoing but asymptomatic plaque disruption. Experimentally, in atherosclerotic nonhuman primates, mural platelet thrombi can complicate plaque erosions without causing arterial occlusion. Therefore, repetitive cycles of plaque disruption, thrombosis in situ, and healing probably contribute to lesion evolution and plaque growth. Such episodes of thrombosis and healing constitute one type of "crisis" in the history of a plaque that may cause a burst of smooth muscle cell proliferation, migration, and matrix synthesis. The TGF-β and PDGF released from platelet granules stimulate collagen synthesis by smooth muscle cells, as noted earlier. Thrombin, generated at sites of mural thrombosis, potently stimulates smooth muscle cell proliferation. The late-stage or "burned out" fibrous and calcific atheroma may represent a late stage of a plaque previously lipid-rich and vulnerable but now rendered fibrous and hypocellular due to a wound healing response mediated by the products of thrombosis.

Diffuse and Systemic Nature of Plaque Vulnerability and Inflammation in Atherogenesis

Studies at autopsy of atherosclerotic plaques that caused fatal thrombosis brought the notion of the vulnerability of high-risk plaque to the fore. This stimulated many investigators to seek ways of identifying and treating such high-risk atherosclerotic lesions.[80-84] However, current evidence suggests that such high-risk plaques are indeed numerous in a given coronary tree. Moreover, the inflammation thought to characterize the so-called vulnerable plaque appears widespread. Studies using various imaging modalities have underscored the multiplicity of such high-risk plaques. Careful analysis of angiograms of individuals with acute coronary syndromes has demonstrated evidence for plaque ulceration or thrombosis in more than one lesion in many cases.[85] Individuals with multiple unstable lesions by angiographic criteria tend to have worse outcomes during follow-up. Angioscopic studies have also shown multiple sites of intracoronary thrombosis in patients with acute coronary syndromes.[86] Systematic studies by intravascular ultrasonography of the coronary arterial system in individuals with acute coronary syndromes have revealed that more than 80 percent of such individuals have more than one disrupted atherosclerotic plaque.[87]

Several concordant lines of evidence support the systemic and diffuse nature of inflammation in individuals with acute coronary syndromes. Maseri's group demonstrated a transmyocardial gradient in the inflammatory marker myeloperoxidase when sampling from the great cardiac vein (draining the left coronary territory) in individuals with both left and right coronary artery culprit lesions.[88] Moreover, several studies have shown that various systemic markers of inflammation such as C-reactive protein increase in patients at risk for acute coronary syndromes. This is so even in the absence of biochemical evidence of myocardial injury (e.g., elevated troponin levels) that might elicit a secondary acute phase response.[89] Thus, a combination of imaging studies and investigations using inflammatory markers support the diffuse and systemic nature of instability of atheromata in individuals with or at risk for acute coronary syndromes. This recognition has important therapeutic implications. In addition to revascularization strategies, such individuals should have systemic therapy aimed at stabilizing the usually multiple high-risk lesions that may cause recurrent events.

Special Cases of Arteriosclerosis

Restenosis after Arterial Intervention

(see Chap. 52)

The problem of restenosis after percutaneous arterial intervention represents a special case of arteriosclerosis. After balloon angioplasty, luminal narrowing recurs in approximately one-third of cases within 6 months (see Chap. 52). Initially, work on the pathophysiology of restenosis after angioplasty focused on smooth muscle proliferation. A good deal of the thinking regarding the pathobiology of restenosis depended on extension to the human situation of the results of withdrawal of an overinflated balloon in a previously normal rat carotid artery. Study of this very well standardized preparation promoted precise understanding of the kinetics of intimal thickening after this type of injury. However, the attempts to transfer this information to cases of human restenosis met with considerable frustration. This disparity between the balloon withdrawal injury of animal arteries and human restenosis is not surprising. The substrate of animal studies was usually a normal rather than an atherosclerotic artery, with all the attendant cellular and molecular differences highlighted earlier. Moreover, a high-pressure inflation of an angioplasty balloon only vaguely resembles the overinflated balloon withdrawal injury commonly practiced in rats.

Although smooth muscle cell proliferation appears prominent in the simple experimental models of intimal thickening, observations on human specimens showed relatively low rates of smooth muscle cell proliferation and called into question therapeutic targeting of this process. Moreover, intravascular ultrasonographic studies in humans and considerable evidence from animal experimentation suggested that a substantial proportion of the loss of luminal caliber after balloon angioplasty resulted from a constriction of the vessel from the adventitial side ("negative remodeling").[5,90] These observations renewed interest in adventitial inflammation with scar formation and wound contraction as a mechanism of arterial constriction following balloon angioplasty.[91]

The widespread introduction of stents has changed the face of the restenosis problem. The process of in-stent stenosis, in contrast with restenosis after balloon angioplasty, depends uniquely on intimal thickening, as opposed to "negative remodeling." The stent provides a firm scaffold that prevents constriction from the adventitia. Histological analyses reveal that a great deal of the volume of the in-stent restenotic lesion is made up of "myxomatous" tissue, comprising occasional stellate smooth muscle cells embedded in a loose and highly hydrated extracellular matrix.[92]

The introduction of stents has reduced the clinical impact of restenosis because of the very effective increase in luminal diameter achieved by this technique. Even if a considerable degree of lumen loss occurs due to intimal thickening, the luminal caliber remains sufficient to alleviate the patient's symptoms because of the excellent dilation achieved. Radiation treatment, presumably targeting smooth muscle proliferation and matrix synthesis, proved useful as a therapeutic approach to limiting in-stent restenosis. Currently, stents that elaborate antiproliferative and antiinflammatory substances have shown great benefit in terms of preventing in-stent stenosis (see Chap. 52).[93-95]

Accelerated Arteriosclerosis after Transplantation

Since the advent of effective immunosuppressive therapy such as cyclosporin, the major limitation to long-term survival of cardiac allografts is the development of an accelerated form of arterial hyperplastic disease (see Chap. 26). We favor the term *arteriosclerosis* ("hardening of the arteries") rather than *atherosclerosis* ("gruel-hardening") to describe this process because of the inconstant association with lipids (the "gruel" in atherosclerosis).[96] This form of arterial disease often presents a diagnostic challenge. The patient may not experience typical anginal symptoms because of the interruption of cardiac denervation after transplantation. In addition, graft coronary disease is concentric and diffuse, not only affecting the proximal epicardial coronary vessels but also penetrating smaller intramyocardial branches (Fig. 35–13). For this reason, the angiogram, well suited to visualizing focal and eccentric stenoses, consistently underestimates the degree of transplantation arteriosclerosis.

In most centers, a majority of patients undergoing transplantation have atherosclerotic disease and ischemic cardiomyopathy. However, a sizeable minority of patients undergo heart transplantation for idiopathic dilated cardiomyopathy and may have few if any risk factors for atherosclerosis. Even in the absence of traditional risk factors, this latter group of individuals shares the risk of developing accelerated arteriosclerosis. This observation suggests that the pathophysiology of this form of accelerated arteriosclerosis differs from that of usual atherosclerosis.

The selective involvement of the engrafted vessels with sparing of the host's native arteries suggests that accelerated arteriopathy does not merely result from the immunosuppressive therapy or other systemic factors in the transplantation recipient. Rather, these observations suggest that the immunological differences between the host and the recipient vessels might contribute to the pathogenesis of this

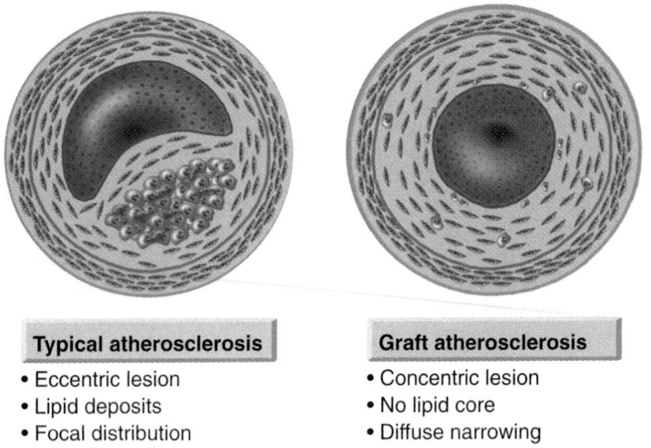

FIGURE 35–13 Comparison of usual atherosclerosis and transplantation arteriosclerosis. Usual atherosclerosis **(left panel)** characteristically forms an eccentric lesion with a lipid core and fibrous capsule. In contrast, the lesion of transplantation-associated accelerated arteriosclerosis **(right panel)** characteristically has a concentric intimal expansion without a clear central lipid core.

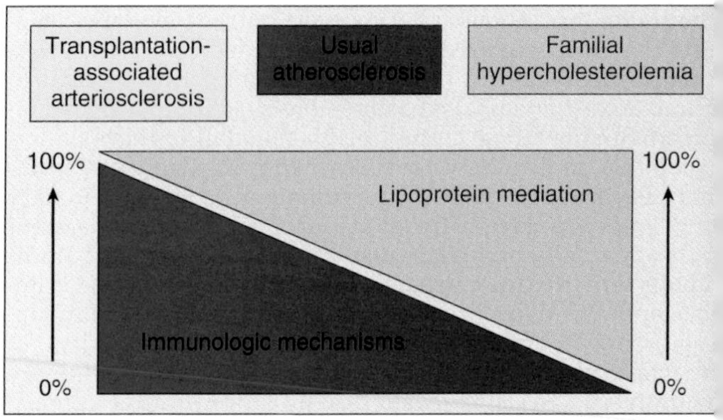

FIGURE 35–14 A multifactorial view of the pathogenesis of atherosclerosis. This diagram depicts two extreme cases of atherosclerosis. One **(far left)** represents accelerated arteriosclerosis that can occur in the transplanted heart in the absence of traditional coronary risk factors. This disease likely represents primarily immune-mediated arterial intimal disease. The other extreme **(far right)** depicts the case of a child who may succumb to rampant atherosclerosis in the first decade of life due solely to an elevated low-density lipoprotein (LDL) level caused by a mutation in the LDL receptor (homozygous familial hypercholesterolemia). Between these two extremes lie the vast majority of patients with atherosclerosis, probably involving various mixtures of immune and inflammatory and/or lipoprotein-mediated disease. One can further consider that this diagram extends to a third dimension that would involve other candidate risk factors such as homocysteine, lipoprotein (a), infection, tobacco abuse, and so on.

disease. Considerable evidence from both human and experimental studies currently supports this viewpoint. Endothelial cells in the transplanted coronary arteries express histocompatibility antigens that can engender an allogeneic immune response from host T cells. The activated T cells can secrete cytokines (e.g., interferon-gamma) that can augment histocompatibility gene expression, recruit leukocytes by induction of adhesion molecules, and activate macrophages to produce smooth muscle cell chemoattractants and growth factors. Interruption of interferon-gamma signaling can prevent experimental graft coronary disease in mice.[97] This disease appears to occur despite cyclosporin therapy, because this immunosuppressant is relatively ineffective as a suppressor of the endothelial allogeneic response. Indeed, immunosuppressive agents that more effectively suppress the endothelial allogeneic response appear effective in retarding graft arteriosclerosis.

The data summarized suggest that graft arteriosclerosis represents an extreme case of the immunologically driven arterial hyperplasia (Fig. 35–14) that can occur in the absence of other risk factors. On the other extreme, patients with homozygous familial hypercholesterolemia can develop fatal atherosclerosis in the first decade of life due solely to an elevation in LDL cholesterol. The vast majority of patients with atherosclerosis fall somewhere between these two extremes. Analysis of usual atherosclerotic lesions shows evidence for a chronic immune response and lipid accumulation. Therefore, by studying the extreme cases, such as transplantation arteriopathy and familial hypercholesterolemia, one can gain insight into elements of the pathophysiology that contribute to the multifactorial form of atherosclerosis that affects the majority of patients.

Aneurysmal Disease

Atherosclerosis produces not only stenoses but also aneurysmal disease (see Chap. 53). Why does a single disease process manifest itself in directionally opposite manner, for example, most commonly producing stenoses in the coronary arteries but causing ectasia of the abdominal aorta? In particular, aneurysmal disease characteristically affects the infrarenal abdominal aorta. This region is highly prone to the development of atherosclerosis. Data from the Pathobiological Determinants of Atherosclerosis In Youth Study (PDAY) show that the dorsal surface of the infrarenal abdominal aorta has a particular predilection for development of fatty streaks and raised lesions in Americans younger than 35 years of age who succumbed for noncardiac reasons (see Fig. 35–1).[3] Due to the absence of vasa vasorum, the relative lack of blood supply to the tunica media in this portion of the abdominal aorta might explain the regional susceptibility of this portion of the arterial tree to aneurysm formation. In addition, the lumbar lordosis of the biped human may alter the hydrodynamics of blood flow in the distal aorta, yielding flow disturbances that may promote lesion formation.

Histological examination shows considerable distinction between occlusive atherosclerotic disease and aneurysmal disease. In typical cases of coronary artery atherosclerosis, expansion of the intimal lesion produces stenotic lesions. The tunica media underlying the expanded intima is often thinned, but its general structure remains relatively well preserved. In contrast, transmural destruction of the arterial architecture occurs in patients with aneurysmal disease. In particular, the usually well defined laminar structure of the normal tunica media disappears with obliteration of the elastic laminae. The medial smooth muscle cells, usually well preserved in typical stenotic lesions, are notable for their paucity in the media of advanced aortic aneurysms.

Study of the pathophysiology that underlies these anatomical pathological findings has proved frustrating. Informative animal models are not available. The human specimens obtainable for analysis generally represent the late stages of this disease. Nonetheless, recent work has identified several mechanisms that may underlie the peculiar pathological features of aneurysmal disease. Widespread destruction of the elastic laminae suggests a role for degradation of elastin, collagen, and other constituents of the arterial extracellular matrix.[98] Many studies have documented overexpression of matrix-degrading proteinases, including matrix metalloproteinases in human aortic aneurysm specimens. Indeed, current clinical trials are testing the hypothesis that matrix metalloproteinase inhibitors can reduce the expansion of aneurysms.[99] Recent experimental work has implicated angiotensin II as a potentiator of aneurysm formation in atherosclerotic mice.[100]

Thus, heightened elastolysis may explain the breakdown of the usually ordered structure of the tunica media in cases of this disease. A slant toward T helper cell Th2 populations in cases of aneurysmal as opposed to occlusive disease may contribute to the overexpression of certain elastolytic enzymes.[101] In addition, aortic aneurysms show evidence for considerable inflammation, particularly in the adventitia.[102] The lymphocytes that characteristically abound on the adventitial side of aneurysmal tissue suggest that apoptosis of smooth muscle cells triggered by inflammatory mediators including soluble cytokines and *fas* ligand, elaborated by these inflammatory cells, may contribute to smooth muscle cell destruction and promote aneurysm formation.[103] Although extracellular matrix degradation and smooth muscle cell death also occur in sites where atherosclerosis causes stenosis, they appear to predominate in regions of aneurysm formation and to affect the tunica media much more extensively, for reasons that remain obscure.

Infection and Atherosclerosis

Recently, interest has increased in the possibility that infections may cause atherosclerosis. A considerable body of seroepidemiological evidence supports a role for certain bacteria, notably *Chlamydia pneumoniae*, and certain viruses, notably cytomegalovirus, in the origin of atherosclerosis.[104–106] The seroepidemiological studies have spurred a number of in vivo and in vitro experiments that lend varying degrees of support to this concept. In evaluation of the seroepidemiological evidence, several caveats apply. First, confounding factors should be carefully considered.[107] For example, smokers may have a higher incidence of bronchitis due to *C. pneumoniae*. Therefore, evidence of infection with *C. pneumoniae* may merely serve as a marker for tobacco use, a known risk factor for atherosclerotic events. Additionally, a strong bias favors publication of studies with positive findings over studies with negative findings. Thus, meta-analyses of seroepidemiological studies may be slanted toward the positive merely because of underreporting of negative findings. Finally, atherosclerosis is a common and virtually ubiquitous disease in developed countries. In most societies, many adults have serological evidence of prior infections with Herpes viridae such as cytomegalovirus and respiratory pathogens such as *C. pneumoniae*. It is difficult to sort out coincidence from causality when the majority of the population studied has evidence of both infection and atherosclerosis.

Although proof that bacteria or viruses can cause atherosclerosis remains elusive, it is quite plausible that infections can potentiate the action of traditional risk factors, such as hypercholesterolemia. Based on the vascular biology of atherosclerosis discussed in this chapter, a number of scenarios might apply. First, cells within the atheroma itself can be a site for infection. For example, macrophages existing in an established atherosclerotic lesion might become infected with *C. pneumoniae*, which could spur their activation and accelerate the inflammatory pathways that we currently believe operate within the atherosclerotic intima. Specific microbial products, such as lipopolysaccharides, heat shock proteins, or other virulence factors might act locally at the level of the artery wall to potentiate atherosclerosis in infected lesions.[108-114]

Extravascular infection might also influence the development of atheromatous lesions and provoke their complication. For example, circulating endotoxin or cytokines produced in response to a remote infection can act locally at the level of the artery wall to promote the activation of vascular cells and of leukocytes in preexisting lesions, producing an "echo" at the level of the artery wall of a remote infection.[105] Also, the acute phase response to an infection in a nonvascular site might affect the incidence of thrombotic complications of atherosclerosis by increasing fibrinogen or plasminogen activator inhibitor or otherwise altering the balance between coagulation and fibrinolysis. Such disturbance in the prevailing prothrombotic, fibrinolytic balance could critically influence whether a given plaque disruption will produce a clinically inapparent transient or nonocclusive thrombus, or sustained and occlusive thrombi that could cause an acute coronary event.

Acute infections might also produce hemodynamic alterations that could trigger coronary events. For example, the tachycardia and increased metabolic demands of fever could augment the oxygen requirements of the heart, precipitating ischemia in an otherwise compensated individual. These various scenarios illustrate how infectious processes, either local in the atheroma or extravascular, might aggravate atherogenesis, particularly in preexisting lesions or in concert with traditional risk factors. However, recent clinical trials have not shown that treatment with azithromycin for 12 weeks can reduce recurrent coronary events in survivors of myocardial infarction.[115] Even if the findings of ongoing studies with more prolonged antibiotic treatment were positive, they would not establish a role for a particular infectious agent, nor could they prove that the antibiotic effect of the agents tested, rather than some other action not related to their antimicrobial effect, produces benefit.[116,117]

REFERENCES

1. Libby P, Aikawa M, Schonbeck U: Cholesterol and atherosclerosis. Biochim Biophys Acta 1529:299, 2000.
2. Gimbrone MA Jr, Nagel T, Topper JN: Biomechanical activation: An emerging paradigm in endothelial adhesion biology. J Clin Invest 100:S61, 1997.
3. Strong JP, Malcom GT, McMahan CA, et al: Prevalence and extent of atherosclerosis in adolescents and young adults: Implications for prevention from the Pathobiological Determinants of Atherosclerosis in Youth Study. JAMA 281:727, 1999.
4. Tuzcu EM, Kapadia SR, Tutar E, et al: High prevalence of coronary atherosclerosis in asymptomatic teenagers and young adults: Evidence from intravascular ultrasound. Circulation 103:2705, 2001.
5. Pasterkamp G, de Kleijn DP, Borst C: Arterial remodeling in atherosclerosis, restenosis and after alteration of blood flow: Potential mechanisms and clinical implications. Cardiovasc Res 45:843, 2000.
6. Kruth HS: The fate of lipoprotein cholesterol entering the arterial wall. Curr Opin Lipidol 8:246, 1997.
7. Camejo G, Hurt-Camejo E, Wiklund O, et al: Association of apo B lipoproteins with arterial proteoglycans: Pathological significance and molecular basis. Atherosclerosis 139:205, 1998.
8. Williams KJ, Tabas I: The response-to-retention hypothesis of atherogenesis reinforced. Curr Opin Lipidol 9:471, 1998.
9. Witztum JL, Berliner JA: Oxidized phospholipids and isoprostanes in atherosclerosis. Curr Opin Lipidol 9:441, 1998.
10. Rong JX, Rangaswamy S, Shen L, et al: Arterial injury by cholesterol oxidation products causes endothelial dysfunction and arterial wall cholesterol accumulation. Arterioscler Thromb Vasc Biol 18:1885, 1998.
11. Tabas I: Nonoxidative modifications of lipoproteins in atherogenesis. Ann Rev Nutr 19:123, 1999.
12. Ushio-Fukai M, Alexander RW, Akers M, et al: p38 Mitogen-activated protein kinase is a critical component of the redox-sensitive signaling pathways activated by angiotensin II: Role in vascular smooth muscle cell hypertrophy. J Biol Chem 273:15022, 1998.
13. Cyrus T, Witztum JL, Rader DJ, et al: Disruption of the 12/15-lipoxygenase gene diminishes atherosclerosis in apo E-deficient mice. J Clin Invest 103:1597, 1999.
14. Sugiyama S, Okada Y, Sukhova GK, et al: Macrophage myeloperoxidase regulation by granulocyte macrophage colony-stimulating factor in human atherosclerosis and implications in acute coronary syndromes. Am J Pathol 158:879, 2001.
15. Nakashima Y, Raines EW, Plump AS, et al: Upregulation of VCAM-1 and ICAM-1 at atherosclerosis-prone sites on the endothelium in the apoE-deficient mouse. Arterioscler Thromb Vasc Biol 18:842, 1998.
16. Iiyama K, Hajra L, Iiyama M, et al: Patterns of vascular cell adhesion molecule-1 and intercellular adhesion molecule-1 expression in rabbit and mouse atherosclerotic lesions and at sites predisposed to lesion formation. Circ Res 85:199, 1999.
17. Ley K: The role of selectins in inflammation and disease. Trends Mol Med 9:263, 2003.
18. Vora DK, Fang ZT, Liva SM, et al: Induction of P-selectin by oxidized lipoproteins: Separate effects on synthesis and surface expression. Circ Res 80:810, 1997.
19. Dong ZM, Brown AA, Wagner DD: Prominent role of P-selectin in the development of advanced atherosclerosis in ApoE-deficient mice. Circulation 101:2290, 2000.
20. Ley K, Huo Y: VCAM-1 is critical in atherosclerosis. J Clin Invest 107:1209, 2001.
21. Cybulsky MI, Iiyama K, Li H, et al: A major role for VCAM-1, but not ICAM-1, in early atherosclerosis. J Clin Invest 107:1255, 2001.
22. Dong ZM, Chapman SM, Brown AA, et al: The combined role of P- and E-selectins in atherosclerosis. J Clin Invest 102:145, 1998.
23. Luster AD: Chemokines: Chemotactic cytokines that mediate inflammation. N Engl J Med 338:436, 1998.

24. Gu L, Okada Y, Clinton S, et al: Absence of monocyte chemoattractant protein-1 reduces atherosclerosis in low-density lipoprotein-deficient mice. Mol Cell 2:275, 1998.
25. Boring L, Gosling J, Cleary M, et al: Decreased lesion formation in CCR2-/- mice reveals a role for chemokines in the initiation of atherosclerosis. Nature 394:894, 1998.
26. Boisvert WA, Curtiss LK, Terkeltaub RA: Interleukin-8 and its receptor CXCR2 in atherosclerosis. Immunol Res 21:129, 2000.
27. Lesnik P, Haskell CA, Charo IF: Decreased atherosclerosis in CX3CR1-/- mice reveals a role for fractalkine in atherogenesis. J Clin Invest 111:333, 2003.
28. Mach F, Sauty A, Iarossi AS, et al: Differential expression of three T lymphocyte-activating CXC chemokines by human atheroma-associated cells. J Clin Invest 104:1041, 1999.
29. Murry CE, Gipaya CT, Bartosek T, et al: Monoclonality of smooth muscle cells in human atherosclerosis. Am J Pathol 151:697, 1997.
30. Gimbrone MA Jr, Resnick N, Nagel T, et al: Hemodynamics, endothelial gene expression, and atherogenesis. Ann N Y Acad Sci 811:1, 1997.
31. Collins T, Cybulsky MI: NF-kappaB: Pivotal mediator or innocent bystander in atherogenesis? J Clin Invest 107:255, 2001.
32. Majesky MW: Vascular smooth muscle diversity: Insights from developmental biology. Curr Atheroscler Rep 5:208, 2003.
33. Landerholm TE, Dong XR, Lu J, et al: A role for serum response factor in coronary smooth muscle differentiation from proepicardial cells. Development 126:2053, 1999.
34. Shimizu K, Mitchell RN: Stem cell origins of intimal cells in graft arterial disease. Curr Atheroscler Rep 5:230, 2003.
35. Saiura A, Sata M, Hirata Y, et al: Circulating smooth muscle progenitor cells contribute to atherosclerosis. Nat Med 7:382, 2001.
36. Miller YI, Chang MK, Binder CJ, et al: Oxidized low density lipoprotein and innate immune receptors. Curr Opin Lipidol 14:437, 2003.
37. Sakaguchi H, Takeya M, Suzuki H, et al: Role of macrophage scavenger receptors in diet-induced atherosclerosis in mice. Lab Invest 78:423, 1998.
38. Rajavashisth T, Qiao JH, Tripathi S, et al: Heterozygous osteopetrotic (op) mutation reduces atherosclerosis in LDL receptor-deficient mice. J Clin Invest 101:2702, 1998.
39. Hansson GK, Libby P, Schonbeck U, et al: Innate and adaptive immunity in the pathogenesis of atherosclerosis. Circ Res 91:281, 2002.
40. Binder CJ, Chang MK, Shaw PX, et al: Innate and acquired immunity in atherogenesis. Nat Med 8:1218, 2002.
41. Griendling KK, Harrison DG: Out, damned dot: Studies of the NADPH oxidase in atherosclerosis. J Clin Invest 108:1423, 2001.
42. Pinderski LJ, Fischbein MP, Subbanagounder G, et al: Overexpression of interleukin-10 by activated T lymphocytes inhibits atherosclerosis in LDL receptor-deficient mice by altering lymphocyte and macrophage phenotypes. Circ Res 90:1064, 2002.
43. Geng YJ, Libby P: Progression of atheroma: A struggle between death and procreation. Arterioscler Thromb Vasc Biol 22:1370, 2002.
44. Littlewood TD, Bennett MR: Apoptotic cell death in atherosclerosis. Curr Opin Lipidol 14:469, 2003.
45. Nagai R, Suzuki T, Aizawa K, et al: Phenotypic modulation of vascular smooth muscle cells: Dissection of transcriptional regulatory mechanisms. Ann N Y Acad Sci 947:56, 2001.
46. Manabe I, Nagai R: Regulation of smooth muscle phenotype. Curr Atheroscler Rep 5:214, 2003.
47. Boyle JJ, Weissberg PL, Bennett MR: Tumor necrosis factor-{alpha} promotes macrophage-induced vascular smooth muscle cell apoptosis by direct and autocrine mechanisms. Arterioscler Thromb Vasc Biol 23:1553, 2003.
48. Wight TN: Versican: A versatile extracellular matrix proteoglycan in cell biology. Curr Opin Cell Biol 14:617, 2002.
49. Williams KJ: Arterial wall chondroitin sulfate proteoglycans: Diverse molecules with distinct roles in lipoprotein retention and atherogenesis. Curr Opin Lipidol 12:477, 2001.
50. Dollery CM, Humphries SE, McClelland A, et al: In vivo adenoviral gene transfer of TIMP-1 after vascular injury reduces neointimal formation. Ann N Y Acad Sci 878:742, 1999.
51. Couffinhal T, Kearney M, Witzenbichler B, et al: Vascular endothelial growth factor/vascular permeability factor (VEGF/VPF) in normal and atherosclerotic human arteries. Am J Pathol 150:1673, 1997.
52. Ramos MA, Kuzuya M, Esaki T, et al: Induction of macrophage VEGF in response to oxidized LDL and VEGF accumulation in human atherosclerotic lesions. Arterioscler Thromb Vasc Biol 18:1188, 1998.
53. Pipp F, Heil M, Issbrucker K, et al: VEGFR-1-selective VEGF homologue P1GF is arteriogenic: Evidence for a monocyte-mediated mechanism. Circ Res 92:378, 2003.
54. Vasse M, Pourtau J, Trochon V, et al: Oncostatin M induces angiogenesis in vitro and in vivo. Arterioscler Thromb Vasc Biol 19:1835, 1999.
55. Libby P: Current concepts of the pathogenesis of the acute coronary syndromes. Circulation 104:365, 2001.
56. Moulton KS, Heller E, Konerding MA, et al: Angiogenesis inhibitors endostatin or TNP-470 reduce intimal neovascularization and plaque growth in apolipoprotein E-deficient mice. Circulation 99:1726, 1999.
57. Kolodgie FD, Gold HK, Burke AP, et al: Intraplaque hemorrhage and progression of coronary atheroma. N Engl J Med 349:2316, 2003.
58. Doherty TM, Asotra K, Fitzpatrick LA, et al: Calcification in atherosclerosis: Bone biology and chronic inflammation at the arterial crossroads. Proc Natl Acad Sci U S A 100:11201, 2003.
59. Bini A, Mann KG, Kudryk BJ, et al: Noncollagenous bone matrix proteins, calcification, and thrombosis in carotid artery atherosclerosis. Arterioscler Thromb Vasc Biol 19:1852, 1999.
60. Yokoya K, Takatsu H, Suzuki T, et al: Process of progression of coronary artery lesions from mild or moderate stenosis to moderate or severe stenosis: A study based on four serial coronary arteriograms per year. Circulation 100:903, 1999.
61. Naghavi M, Libby P, Falk E, et al: From vulnerable plaque to vulnerable patient: A cal for new definitions and risk assessment strategies: Part I. Circulation 108:1664, 2003
62. Naghavi M, Libby P, Falk E, et al: From vulnerable plaque to vulnerable patient: A cal for new definitions and risk assessment strategies: Part II. Circulation 108:1772, 2003
63. Bezerra HG, Higuchi ML, Gutierrez PS, et al: Atheromas that cause fatal thrombosi are usually large and frequently accompanied by vessel enlargement. Cardiovas Pathol 10:189, 2001.
64. Schoenhagen P, Ziada KM, Kapadia SR, et al: Extent and direction of arterial remodeling in stable versus unstable coronary syndromes: An intravascular ultrasound study Circulation 101:598, 2000.
65. Schoenhagen P, Stone GW, Nissen SE, et al: Coronary plaque morphology an frequency of ulceration distant from culprit lesions in patients with unstable and stabl presentation. Arterioscler Thromb Vasc Biol 23:1895, 2003.
66. Virmani R, Burke AP, Farb A, et al: Pathology of the unstable plaque. Prog Cardiovas Dis 44:349, 2002.
67. Lee R, Libby P: The unstable atheroma. Arterioscler Thromb Vasc Biol 17:1859, 1997
68. Sukhova GK, Shi GP, Simon DI, et al: Expression of the elastolytic cathepsins S and K in human atheroma and regulation of their production in smooth muscle cells. J Clir Invest 102:576, 1998.
69. Sukhova GK, Schonbeck U, Rabkin E, et al: Evidence for increased collagenolysis by interstitial collagenases-1 and -3 in vulnerable human atheromatous plaques. Circula tion 99:2503, 1999.
70. Kolodgie FD, Burke AP, Farb A, et al: The thin-cap fibroatheroma: A type of vulnera ble plaque: The major precursor lesion to acute coronary syndromes. Curr Opin Cardio 16:285, 2001.
71. Aikawa M, Rabkin E, Okada Y, et al: Lipid lowering by diet reduces matrix metallo proteinase activity and increases collagen content of rabbit atheroma: A potentia mechanism of lesion stabilization. Circulation 97:2433, 1998.
72. Aikawa M, Sugiyama S, Hill C, et al: Lipid lowering reduces oxidative stress anc endothelial cell activation in rabbit atheroma. Circulation 106:1390, 2002.
73. Aikawa M, Voglic SJ, Sugiyama S, et al: Dietary lipid lowering reduces tissue facto expression in rabbit atheroma. Circulation 100:1215, 1999.
74. Fukumoto Y, Libby P, Rabkin E, et al: Statins alter smooth muscle cell accumulatior and collagen content in established atheroma of Watanabe heritable hyperlipidemic rabbits. Circulation 103:993, 2001.
75. Ridker PM, Rifai N, Pfeffer MA, et al: Long-term effects of pravastatin on plasma concentration of C-reactive protein. The Cholesterol and Recurrent Events (CARE Investigators. Circulation 100:230, 1999.
76. Libby P, Aikawa M: Stabilization of atherosclerotic plaques: New mechanisms and clinical targets. Nat Med 8:1257, 2002.
77. Burke A, Farb A, Malcom G, et al: Coronary risk factors and plaque morphology in men with coronary disease who died suddenly. N Engl J Med 336:1276, 1997.
78. Burke AP, Farb A, Malcom GT, et al: Effect of risk factors on the mechanism of acute thrombosis and sudden coronary death in women. Circulation 97:2110, 1998.
79. Rajavashisth TB, Liao JK, Galis ZS, et al: Inflammatory cytokines and oxidized low density lipoproteins increase endothelial cell expression of membrane type 1-matrix metalloproteinase. J Biol Chem 274:11924, 1999.
80. Madjid M, Naghavi M, Malik BA, et al: Thermal detection of vulnerable plaque. Am J Cardiol 90:36L, 2002.
81. Stefanadis C, Vavuranakis M, Toutouzas P: Vulnerable plaque: The challenge to identify and treat it. J Interv Cardiol 16:273, 2003.
82. Schaar JA, De Korte CL, Mastik F, et al: Characterizing vulnerable plaque features with intravascular elastography. Circulation 108:2636, 2003.
83. Tearney GJ, Yabushita H, Houser SL, et al: Quantification of macrophage content in atherosclerotic plaques by optical coherence tomography. Circulation 107:113, 2003.
84. MacNeill BD, Lowe HC, Takano M, et al: Intravascular modalities for detection of vulnerable plaque: Current status. Arterioscler Thromb Vasc Biol 23:1333, 2003.
85. Goldstein JA, Demetriou D, Grines CL, et al: Multiple complex coronary plaques in patients with acute myocardial infarction. N Engl J Med 343:915, 2000.
86. Asakura M, Ueda Y, Yamaguchi O, et al: Extensive development of vulnerable plaques as a pan-coronary process in patients with myocardial infarction: An angioscopic study. J Am Coll Cardiol 37:1284, 2001.
87. Rioufol G, Finet G, Ginon I, et al: Multiple atherosclerotic plaque rupture in acute coronary syndrome: A three-vessel intravascular ultrasound study. Circulation 106:804, 2002.
88. Buffon A, Biasucci LM, Liuzzo G, et al: Widespread coronary inflammation in unstable angina. N Engl J Med 347:5, 2002.
89. Libby P, Ridker PM, Maseri A: Inflammation and atherosclerosis. Circulation 105:1135, 2002.
90. Mintz GS, Kent KM, Pichard AD, et al: Contribution of inadequate arterial remodeling to the development of focal coronary artery stenoses: An intravascular ultrasound study. Circulation 95:1791, 1997.
91. Libby P, Simon DI, Rogers C: Inflammation and arterial injury. *In* Topol EJ (ed): Textbook of Interventional Cardiology. 4th ed. Philadelphia, Elsevier Science, 2003, p 381.
92. Orford JL, Selwyn AP, Ganz P, et al: The comparative pathobiology of atherosclerosis and restenosis. Am J Cardiol 86:6H, 2000.
93. Moses JW, Leon MB, Popma JJ, et al: Sirolimus-eluting stents versus standard stents in patients with stenosis in a native coronary artery. N Engl J Med 349:1315, 2003.
94. Marks AR: Sirolimus for the prevention of in-stent restenosis in a coronary artery. N Engl J Med 349:1307, 2003.
95. Bennett MR: In-stent stenosis: Pathology and implications for the development of drug eluting stents. Heart 89:218, 2003.
96. Libby P, Zhao DX: Allograft arteriosclerosis and immune-driven angiogenesis. Circulation 107:1237, 2003.
97. Nagano H, Mitchell RN, Taylor MK, et al: Interferon-gamma deficiency prevents coronary arteriosclerosis but not myocardial rejection in transplanted mouse hearts. J Clin Invest 100:550, 1997.

98. Thompson RW: Reflections on the pathogenesis of abdominal aortic aneurysms. Cardiovasc Surg 10:389, 2002.
99. Thompson RW, Baxter BT: MMP inhibition in abdominal aortic aneurysms: Rationale for a prospective randomized clinical trial. Ann N Y Acad Sci 878:159, 1999.
100. Manning MW, Cassi LA, Huang J, et al: Abdominal aortic aneurysms: Fresh insights from a novel animal model of the disease. Vasc Med 7:45, 2002.
101. Schonbeck U, Sukhova GK, Gerdes N, et al: T(H)2 predominant immune responses prevail in human abdominal aortic aneurysm. Am J Pathol 161:499, 2002.
102. McMillan WD, Pearce WH: Inflammation and cytokine signaling in aneurysms. Ann Vasc Surg 11:540, 1997.
103. Henderson EL, Geng YJ, Sukhova GK, et al: Death of smooth muscle cells and expression of mediators of apoptosis by T lymphocytes in human abdominal aortic aneurysms. Circulation 99:96, 1999.
104. Danesh J: Coronary heart disease, *Helicobacter pylori*, dental disease, *Chlamydia pneumoniae*, and cytomegalovirus: Meta-analyses of prospective studies. Am Heart J 138:S434, 1999.
105. Libby P, Egan D, Skarlatos S: Roles of infectious agents in atherosclerosis and restenosis: An assessment of the evidence and need for future research [review]. Circulation 96:4095, 1997.
106. O'Connor S, Taylor C, Campbell LA, et al: Potential infectious etiologies of atherosclerosis: A multifactorial perspective. Emerg Infect Dis 7:780, 2001.
107. Ridker PM: Are associations between infection and coronary disease causal or due to confounding? [editorial; comment]. Am J Med 106:376, 1999.
108. Kol A, Sukhova GK, Lichtman AH, et al: Chlamydial heat shock protein 60 localizes in human atheroma and regulates macrophage TNF-alpha and matrix metalloproteinase expression. Circulation 98:300, 1998.
109. Kol A, Bourcier T, Lichtman AH, et al: Chlamydial and human heat shock protein 60s activate human vascular endothelium, smooth muscle cells, and macrophages. J Clin Invest 103:571, 1999.
110. Kalayoglu MV, Byrne GI: Induction of macrophage foam cell formation by *Chlamydia pneumoniae*. J Infect Dis 177:725, 1998.
111. Kalayoglu MV, Byrne GI: A *Chlamydia pneumoniae* component that induces macrophage foam cell formation is chlamydial lipopolysaccharide. Infect Immun 66:5067, 1998.
112. Kalayoglu MV, Hoerneman B, LaVerda D, et al: Cellular oxidation of low-density lipoprotein by *Chlamydia pneumoniae*. J Infect Dis 180:780, 1999.
113. Kol A, Lichtman AH, Finberg RW, et al: Heat shock protein (HSP) 60 activates the innate immune response: CD14 is an essential receptor for HSP60 activation of mononuclear cells. J Immunol 164:13, 2000.
114. Kalayoglu MV, Libby P, Byrne GI: *Chlamydia pneumoniae* as an emerging risk factor in cardiovascular disease. JAMA 288:2724, 2002.
115. O'Connor CM, Dunne MW, Pfeffer MA, et al: Azithromycin for the secondary prevention of coronary heart disease events: The WIZARD study: A randomized controlled trial. JAMA 290:1459, 2003.
116. Cannon CP, McCabe CH, Belder R, et al: Design of the Pravastatin or Atorvastatin Evaluation and Infection Therapy (PROVE IT)-TIMI 22 trial. Am J Cardiol 89:860, 2002.
117. Grayston JT: Secondary prevention antibiotic treatment trials for coronary artery disease. Circulation 102:1742, 2000.

CHAPTER 36

Risk Factors for Atherothrombotic Disease

Paul M. Ridker • Peter Libby

Cardiovascular disease is the single most common cause of death in the developed world and accounts for almost 1 million fatalities each year in the United States alone. Of these cardiovascular deaths, nearly half result directly from coronary artery disease and another 20 percent from stroke. Given our current understanding of atherothrombosis, it is historically surprising that the conceptual basis for considering specific "cardiovascular risk factors" did not formally exist until the initial findings of the Framingham Heart Study began to appear in the early 1960s.

From an epidemiological perspective, a "risk factor" is a characteristic or feature of an individual or population that is present early in life and is associated with an increased risk of developing future disease. The risk factor of interest may be an acquired behavior (such as smoking), an inherited trait (such as familial hyperlipidemia), or a laboratory measure (such as cholesterol or C-reactive protein). For a risk factor to be causal, the marker of interest must predate the onset of disease and must have biological plausibility. Most risk factors used in daily practice have demonstrated a consistent graded-response effect and are substantiated by a large series of consistent prospective epidemiological studies in broad populations. Several risk factors, such as hyperlipidemia and hypertension, are modifiable, and trials have demonstrated that lowering these factors reduces vascular risk.

This chapter reviews in two parts the epidemiological evidence underlying risk factors for atherothrombosis. The first section describes the conventional risk factors of smoking, hypertension, hyperlipidemia, insulin resistance and diabetes, physical activity, and obesity as well as general strategies for reducing risk related to these disorders. This section also briefly reviews evidence relating mental stress, depression, and vascular risk.

Not all coronary events occur in individuals with multiple traditional risk factors, however, and in some individuals isolated abnormalities of inflammation, hemostasis, and/or thrombosis appear to play critical roles. In particular, nearly half of all myocardial infarctions and strokes occur among individuals without hyperlipidemia. Thus, the second section of the chapter reviews in detail a series of novel atherothrombotic risk factors, including high sensitivity C-reactive protein (hsCRP) and other markers of inflammation, homocysteine, and lipoprotein(a). This chapter also reviews data regarding hemostatic and thrombotic markers of risk, including fibrinogen, D-dimer, and abnormalities of intrinsic fibrinolysis. In each case, we present the evidence that describes whether these novel risk indicators add to risk prediction over and above conventional factors.

Conventional Risk Factors

Smoking

Cigarette consumption remains the single most important modifiable risk factor for coronary artery disease and the leading preventable cause of death in the United States, where it accounts for more than 400,000 deaths annually.[1] Of these, ischemic heart disease causes 35 to 40 percent of all smoking-related deaths, with an additional 8 percent attributable to second-hand smoke exposure. Despite the relative stability (25 percent) in prevalence of current smokers in the United States, rates of tobacco use are increasing among adolescents, young adults, and women.[2,3] Close to 1 million young Americans begin smoking each year.[4] Although increased recognition of the hazards of smoking might be hoped to slow these trends, nearly 1 billion individuals now smoke worldwide. Smoking has a particularly large impact in the Third World. Almost one-half billion individuals worldwide will eventually die of smoking-related complications.[5] Even among nonsmokers, we now recognize that inhaled smoke, whether from passive exposure or from cigar and pipe consumption, also increases coronary risk.[6,7] Passive smoking exposure can cause endothelial dysfunction in the coronary circulation even among otherwise healthy young nonsmokers.[8] The impact of passive smoking is complex, as this exposure also results in increased bronchial responsiveness and concomitant pulmonary dysfunction.[9]

Landmark studies in the early 1950s first reported strong positive associations between cigarette smoke exposure and coronary heart disease. Over the next 50 years, an exceptionally consistent series of prospective studies have documented clearly the effects of smoking on coronary risk. These studies suggest that, compared with nonsmokers, persons who consume 20 or more cigarettes daily have a two- to threefold increase in total coronary heart disease. Moreover, these effects depend on dose; consumption of as few as one to four cigarettes daily increases coronary artery disease risk. Such "light" levels of smoking have a major impact on myocardial infarction and all-cause mortality even among smokers who do not report inhalation.[10] Smoking acts synergistically with oral contraceptive agents, placing younger women taking oral contraceptives at even higher relative risk. In addition to myocardial infarction, cigarette consumption directly relates to increased rates of sudden death, aortic aneurysm formation, symptomatic peripheral vascular disease, and ischemic stroke. As for coronary disease, the risk of ischemic stroke directly increases with the number of cigarettes consumed. Recent prospective evidence also has linked cigarette consumption to elevated risk of hemorrhagic stroke, including both intracranial hemorrhage and subarachnoid hemorrhage, again in a dose-response manner.[11] Not surprisingly, continued smoking is also a major risk factor for recurrent myocardial infarction.[12]

Historically, cigarette consumption was prevalent among men before women and, at least in the United States, smoking prevalence remains lower among women than men. However, this gender gap has markedly narrowed, with overall consumption rates among women now in excess of 20 percent. Native Americans and those with less education have higher rates, whereas black and Hispanic women appear to consume less than white women (Fig. 36–1). Due to adverse synergy with oral contraceptives, young female smokers who take oral contraceptives have particularly elevated risks of premature coronary disease and stroke. Smoking is especially hazardous among women with diabetes.[13]

Beyond acute unfavorable effects on blood pressure, sympathetic tone, and a reduction in myocardial oxygen supply, smoking affects atherothrombosis by several other mechanisms. In addition to accelerating atherosclerotic progression,[14] long-term smoking may enhance oxidation of low-density lipoprotein (LDL) cholesterol and impairs endothelium-dependent coronary artery vasodilation. This latter effect has now been linked directly to dysfunctional endothelial nitric oxide biosynthesis following chronic as well as acute cigarette consumption.[15-17] In addition, smoking has adverse hemostatic and inflammatory effects, including increased levels of hsCRP, soluble intercellular adhesion molecule-1 (ICAM-1), fibrinogen, and homocysteine.[18-20] Additionally, smoking is associated with spontaneous platelet aggregation,[21] increased monocyte adhesion to endothelial cells,[22] and adverse alterations in endothelial derived fibrinolytic and antithrombotic factors, including tissue-type plasminogen activator and tissue pathway factor inhibitor.[23-25] Compared with nonsmokers, smokers have an increased prevalence of coronary spasm and may have reduced thresholds for ventricular arrhythmia. Accruing evidence suggests that insulin resistance represents an additional mechanistic link between smoking and premature atherosclerosis.[26]

Cessation of cigarette consumption constitutes the single most important intervention in preventive cardiology. In a recent major overview, smoking cessation reduced coronary heart disease mortality by 36 percent as compared with mortality in subjects who continued smoking, an effect that did not vary by age, gender, or country of origin.[27] In this analysis, the reduction in nonfatal myocardial reinfarction among those who stopped smoking (relative risk, 0.68; 95 percent confidence interval, 0.57-0.82) was almost identical to the overall reduction in total cardiovascular mortality (RR, 0.64 95 percent CI, 0.58-0.71). These 35 to 40 percent risk reductions are at least as great as other secondary prevention interventions that have received far more attention from physicians, including the use of aspirin, statins, beta-blockade, and angiotensin-converting enzyme inhibitors. Similar benefits are present among persons with severe as well as mild systemic atherosclerosis.[28] Consistent data show that smoking cessation has immediate economic benefit across the health care system.[29]

In broad-based population studies, reductions in smoking from any mechanism improve health outcomes, particularly when linked to life-style changes, including exercise and dietary control.[30] Trials of nicotine replacement therapy using either transdermal nicotine or nicotine chewing gum have proven to greatly increase abstention rates after cessation. Such pharmacological programs, as well as physician-guided counseling, are cost-effective and should be provided as a standard prevention service.[31] Patients need to recognize that "low yield" cigarettes do not appear to reduce risks of myocardial infarction. Unfortunately, although the elevated cardiovascular risks associated with smoking decrease significantly after cessation, the risks of cancer of the lungs, pancreas, and stomach persist for more than a decade, as do the risks of developing chronic obstructive pulmonary disease. While smoking cessation has clear benefit, smoking reduction alone appears to have only marginal effect.[32]

Poor patient and physician understanding of the importance of smoking cessation continue. The observation that smoking predicts better outcome following various reperfusion strategies (the so-called "smoker's paradox") is not due to any benefit of smoking but simply to the fact that smokers are likely to undergo such procedures at a much younger age and hence have on average lower comorbidity. Despite public health legislation, the tobacco industry continues its aggressive targeting of young adults, who are most susceptible to new addiction.[33,34] Thus, primary prevention remains the most important population-based component of any smoking reduction strategy.

Hypertension (see Chaps. 37 and 38)

In contrast to cigarette consumption, hypertension is often a silent cardiovascular risk factor, and its prevalence is steadily increasing. Of the estimated 50 million Americans with high blood pressure, almost one-third evade diagnosis and only one-fourth receive effective treatment.[35] In the most recent National Health and Nutrition Examination Survey, 28.7 percent of subjects evaluated had a measured blood pressure greater than 140/90 mm Hg or reported use of antihypertensive medications, an increase of almost 4 percent from similar survey data a decade earlier.[36] Hypertension prevalence was highest in non-Hispanic blacks (33.5 percent), increased with age (reaching more than 65 percent after the age of 60 years), and tended to be more prevalent in women than men. Although 68 percent of

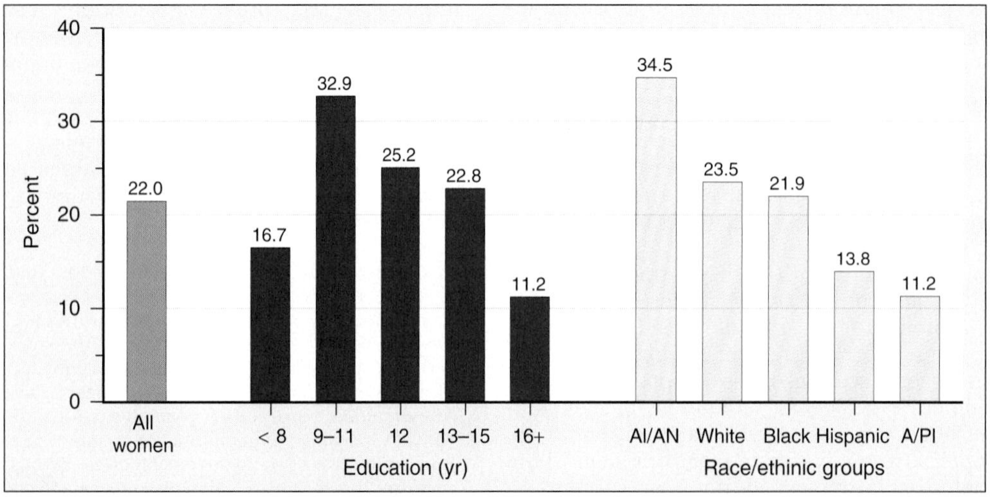

FIGURE 36–1 Prevalence of current smoking among American women aged 18 and older by education and by race/ethnicity. (From the National Health Interview Survey, US Department of Health and Human Services, Centers for Disease Control and Prevention.) AI/AN = American Indian/Alaska Native; A/PI = Asian/Pacific Islander.

he study participants were aware of their hypertension, only 58 percent were under therapy and 31 percent had their hypertension controlled (Fig. 36–2). Thus, in contrast to hyperlipidemia, hypertension prevalence is increasing and treatment rates remain poor, highlighting the need for programs targeting prevention. These trends are even more worrisome in Europe, where the prevalence of hypertension is 60 percent higher than in the United States and Canada. In sample surveys from nine nations, an average blood pressure observed in the European centers was 136/83 mm Hg, compared with an average blood pressure of 122/77 mm Hg in U.S. and Canadian centers.[37]

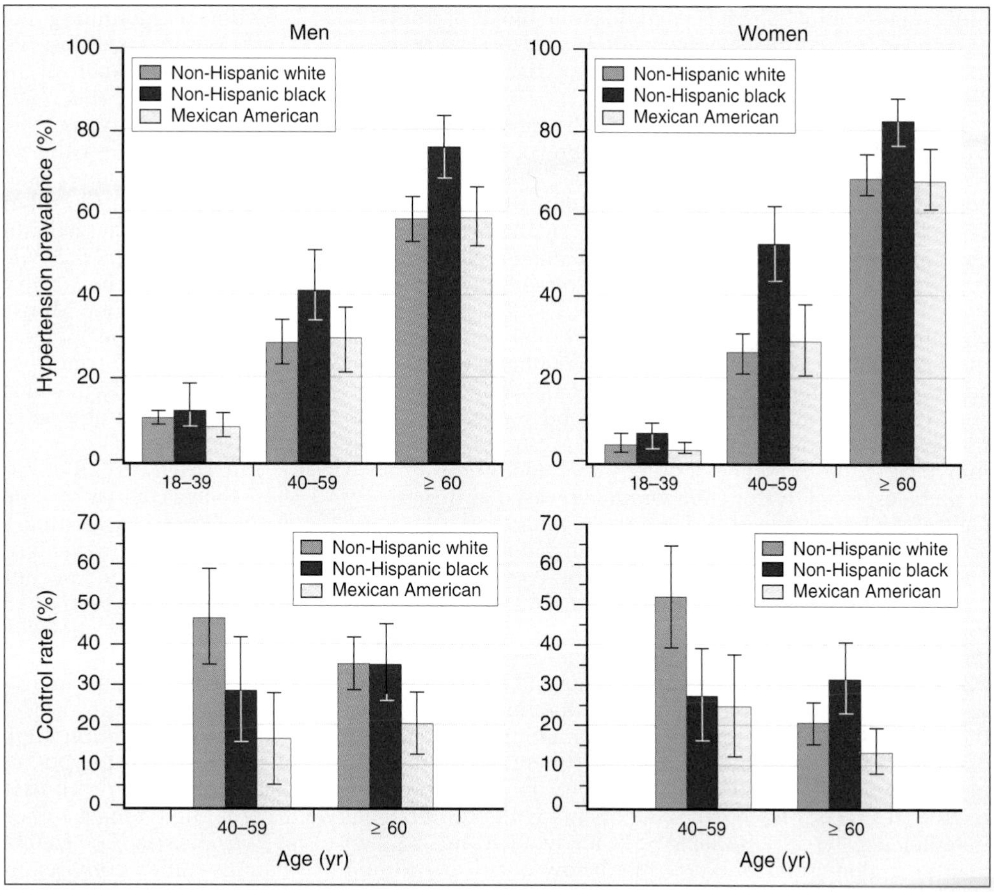

FIGURE 36–2 Hypertension prevalence **(top)** and hypertension control rates **(bottom)** by age and ethnicity among American men and women. (From Hajjar I, Kotchen TA: Trends in prevalence, awareness, treatment, and control of hypertension in the United States, 1988-2000. JAMA 290:199, 2003.)

Part of the complexity of hypertension as a risk factor relates to changing definitions of risk and an understanding that systolic blood pressure and pulse pressure may be of greater importance than diastolic blood pressure, contrary to decades of clinical teaching. Most epidemiological studies now recognize the joint contributions of systolic *and* diastolic blood pressure to the development of cardiovascular risk, an issue that has markedly changed strategies for risk detection.[38,39] Isolated systolic hypertension, in particular, is at least as important as diastolic blood pressure for the outcomes of total cardiovascular mortality and stroke.[40,41] These effects are greatest among older individuals and among those with known cardiovascular disease. Isolated systolic hypertension thus appears to represent a distinct pathophysiological state in which elevated blood pressure reflects reduced arterial elasticity not necessarily associated with increased peripheral resistance or an elevation in mean arterial pressure. In the Framingham Heart Study, even high-normal blood pressure (systolic blood pressure 130 to 139 mm Hg, diastolic blood pressure 85 to 89 mm Hg, or both) augments risk of cardiovascular disease twofold compared with lower levels.[42]

Pulse pressure, a potential surrogate for vascular wall stiffness, also potently predicts both first and recurrent myocardial infarction.[43] Defined as the difference between systolic and diastolic blood pressure, pulse pressure appears to predict independently cardiovascular events, particularly heart failure.[44-46] These data also stress the importance of arterial compliance and stiffness in atherogenesis as well as in the development of left ventricular hypertrophy. Several studies suggest that 24-hour ambulatory monitoring of blood pressure may provide a stronger predictor of cardiovascular morbidity and mortality when compared to office-based measures.[47] While ambulatory blood pressure monitoring has the advantage of correctly classifying as normal patients with "white-coat hypertension," recent data indicate that isolated ambulatory hypertension (in the setting of normal office blood pressure) also strongly correlates with cardiovascular morbidity.[48]

The importance of these changing definitions of hypertension is reflected by intervention trials that specifically target isolated systolic hypertension, all of which have shown benefit.[49-51] At the same time, major overviews continue to demonstrate that blood pressure reductions as small as 4 to 5 mm Hg result in large and clinically significant reductions in risk for stroke, vascular mortality, congestive heart failure, and total coronary heart disease in middle age, among the elderly, and in high-risk groups such as those with diabetes and peripheral arterial disease.[52] Among compliant patients, sodium reduction and weight loss can be effective.[53] However, not all patients respond to such measures, and the long-term success of nonpharmacological approaches to hypertension control has often proven disappointing. By contrast, relatively simple therapies such as low-dose diuretics can have major public health benefit. In an overview of 42 clinical trials that included 192,000 patients, low-dose diuretics compared to placebo yielded reductions of 21 percent in total coronary heart disease, 49 percent in congestive heat failure, 29 percent in stroke, and 19 percent in cardiovascular mortality.[54] Although combined therapy was often superior, none of the other first-line therapies for hypertension, including beta blockers, angiotensin-converting enzyme inhibitors, angiotensin receptor blockers, or calcium channel blockers, were significantly better than low-dose diuretics. Combined low-dose therapies, however, have considerable efficacy in terms of both blood pressure reduction and event prevention. In a comprehensive analysis of 354 randomized trials, regimens of multiple drugs given at low doses were estimated capable of reducing systolic blood pressure by 20 mm Hg and diastolic blood pressure by 11 mm Hg, effects that could result in stroke reductions of 63 percent and coronary heart disease risk reductions of 46 percent.[55]

In response to these observations, the most recent report from the Joint National Committee on Prevention, Detection, Evaluation, and Treatment of High Blood Pressure (JNC VII) continues to stress weight control, adoption of the DASH diet with sodium restriction and increased intake of potassium- and calcium-rich foods, moderation of alcohol consumption to fewer than two drinks daily, and increased physical activity (see Chap. 41).[35] However, the JNC VII also suggests a new classification of blood pressure, with normal defined as less than 120 mm Hg systolic and less than 80 mm Hg diastolic for adults and "pre-hypertension" defined as systolic blood pressure 120 to 139 mm Hg or diastolic blood pressure 80 to 89 mm Hg. In this latter category, pharmacological therapy is indicated in the presence of other major comorbidities such as diabetes, renal dysfunction, or known vascular disease. By contrast, pharmacological therapy is mandated for those with either stage 1 hypertension (systolic blood pressure 140-159 mm Hg or diastolic blood pressure 90-99 mm Hg) or stage 2 hypertension (systolic blood pressure >160 mm Hg or diastolic blood pressure >100 mm Hg). The treatment of hypertension is discussed at length in Chapter 38; a thiazide-type diuretic should be the first drug in almost all patients except those with hyponatremia or gout, and the diuretic should be the cornerstone of any multidrug combination. The majority of patients with overt hypertension will require two or more medications to achieve JNC VII target goal for blood pressure reduction. According to JNC VII, patients with chronic renal insufficiency (creatinine level >1.3 for women and >1.5 in men or a glomerular filtration rate below 60 ml/m^2) should also be targeted for blood pressure reduction, both for the prevention of cardiovascular disease and to slow progression to end-stage renal disease. Finally, as described later, patients with obesity, the metabolic syndrome, and frank diabetes represent high-risk groups. For all of these patients, target blood pressure should be in the "optimal" range of lower than 120/80 mm Hg.

Hyperlipidemia (see Chap. 39)

THE CHOLESTEROL HYPOTHESIS. The relationship between cholesterol and atherosclerosis currently enjoys wide acceptance.[56] In the 1850s, the German pathologist Virchow recognized in human atheromata "numerous plates of cholesterine . . . which display themselves even to the naked eye as glistening lamellae . . . which lie together in large numbers . . . and altogether produce a glittering reflection." In 1913, the Russian experimentalists Anitchkow and Chalatow observed that rabbits fed an egg-rich diet developed lipid-laden arterial lesions reminiscent of human atheromata. Later experiments identified cholesterol as the constituent of eggs that produced arterial lesions.

The biochemistry of cholesterol metabolism advanced throughout the 20th century. The advent of the ultracentrifuge enabled the characterization of the lipoprotein fractions in blood and furnished the foundation for detailed study of lipid metabolism. Armed with the ability to assay lipoproteins and cholesterol, translational investigators began to make clinical correlations. Cross-sectional studies of geographically dispersed populations revealed a relationship between serum cholesterol levels and coronary heart disease (CHD) death. Comparative study of ethnic Japanese living in Japan, the Hawaiian Islands, and the continental United States showed that in this relatively genetically homogeneous population, CHD death rates tracked with the environmentally induced augmentation in total serum cholesterol levels.

Various confounding factors can limit the validity of such cross-sectional studies. Thus, the emergence of data from cohort studies, such as that begun in Framingham in the 1950s, bolstered the relationship between cholesterol and CHD.[56] This study, as well as others performed in different populations around the world, established more firmly the concept of cholesterol as a culprit in coronary heart disease. Substantiation of the relationship between total cholesterol and CHD risk emerged from the Multiple Risk Factor Intervention (MRFIT) Trial, studies in the United Kingdom and Europe such as the Northwick Park Study and the Prospective Cardiovascular Munster (PROCAM) Cohort, and more recently the Atherosclerosis Risk in Communities (ARIC) study. The ARIC cohort has particular relevance to current clinical practice in the United States because it included substantial numbers of women and members of racial minority groups.

THE CHOLESTEROL CONTROVERSY. Although built on more than a century of experimental and clinical observation, doubt lingered regarding the role of cholesterol in atherosclerosis until surprisingly recently. Through the beginning of the 1990s, a cloud of controversy enveloped the role of cholesterol-lowering therapy in CHD risk reduction.[56] Despite the evidence that high cholesterol levels correlated with coronary death, the proposition that cholesterol-lowering therapy could reduce CHD morbidity remained unproven. Critics pointed to the apparently "J-shaped curve" describing the relationship of serum cholesterol with mortality. Advocates of the cholesterol hypothesis countered that the heightened risk for all-cause death in individuals with low levels of cholesterol might reflect comorbidities such as cancer, inanition, or liver disease. The goal of reducing CHD mortality by drug therapy eluded convincing proof for decades. Indeed, some cholesterol-lowering medications appeared to cause an increase in the incidence of some events, including noncoronary death. In the pioneering coronary drug project, estrogen treatment led to excess mortality in the cohort of men studied. The World Health Organization study of clofibrate showed increased noncoronary death. Dietary interventions to lower cholesterol often proved ineffective. Such results challenged the validity of cholesterol as a therapeutic target.

CLINICAL TRIALS SUBSTANTIATE THE CHOLESTEROL HYPOTHESIS (see Chap. 39). In the 1980s, clinical trial evidence first established a protective effect of pharmacological cholesterol reduction on coronary morbidity. The Lipid Research Clinic study showed that bile acid–binding resins could lower cholesterol levels in individuals with high baseline levels. A decrease in coronary morbidity accompanied the drop in serum cholesterol. However, total mortality did not change significantly. This finding fueled the fire of the skeptics.

Vindication of the cholesterol hypothesis awaited clinical trials of cholesterol lowering using the hydroxymethylglutaryl coenzyme A (HMG-CoA) reductase inhibitors. These drugs lowered LDL cholesterol more effectively than previously available agents. We now possess unassailable clinical trial evidence that lowering of LDL cholesterol can reduce coronary events in broad swaths of the population (see Chap. 39). First shown in survivors of myocardial infarction with relatively high cholesterol levels, recent clinical trials have extended the benefits of HMG-CoA reductase inhibitors to individuals without known atherosclerotic disease and with average levels of cholesterol. The ensemble of large clinical trials of HMG-CoA reductase inhibitors have substantiated a decrease in total mortality in the study populations. The HMG-CoA reductase inhibitors lowered LDL cholesterol levels 20 to 60 percent and reduced coronary events by up to one-third over a 5-year period. This result has vitiated previous concerns regarding increased noncardiac mortality due to cholesterol lowering. In addition, two very recent studies, the REVERSAL trial, which monitored intravascular coronary ultrasound, and the PROVE-IT trial of clinical endpoints, both demonstrate the benefit of aggressive as compared to moderate LDL cholesterol reduction.[56a,56b]

LOW-DENSITY LIPOPROTEIN CHOLESTEROL FULFILLS KOCH'S POSTULATES. The case for LDL cholesterol as a coronary heart disease risk factor meets most of the criteria established by Koch in the 19th century to inculpate an etiological agent in a disease. Although Koch's postulates deal with an infectious organism, the degree of rigor required to prove causality can apply to other agents of disease. High cholesterol levels consistently predict risk of future cardiovascular events in human populations. Animal studies in multiple species show a causal relationship between hypercholesterolemia and atherosclerosis. Knowledge of the LDL receptor pathway (see Chap. 39) plus emerging understanding of the vascular biology of atherosclerosis (see Chap. 35) provide biological plausibility for the involvement of LDL in atherogenesis. The human mutations in the LDL receptor produce hypercholesterolemia on a monogenic basis that causes rampant atherosclerosis as early as the first decade of life in individuals with homozygous familial hypercholesterolemia. Finally, intervention in large clinical trials to lower LDL cholesterol by a variety of pathways (bile acid–binding resins, intestinal bypass surgery, HMG-CoA reductase inhibitors) shows a reduction in cardiovascular events. Thus, LDL cholesterol fulfills these modified Koch's postulates as one etiological agent in atherosclerosis.

"AVERAGE" IS NOT NECESSARILY "NORMAL." The clinical chemistry laboratory establishes normal values based on the distribution of the variable in question in the general population. Several independent lines of evidence suggest that what we regard as "normal" cholesterol levels in Western society by these criteria exceed levels that good health requires, or that our species might normally have under different societal circumstances. The first line of evidence comes from comparing levels of cholesterol across different populations. Certain rural, agrarian societies have total cholesterol levels well below those accepted as normal in Western societies. Another line of evidence derives from phylogeny. Contemporary human beings have much higher total cholesterol levels than those of many other species of higher organisms that thrive nonetheless. While the current Adult Treatment Panel III defines "optimal" LDL cholesterol as below 100, the true optimum for our species may be considerably lower based on transcultural and phylogenetic considerations. Current clinical trials may inform further revisions of the guidelines and our concepts of "normal" in this regard.

THE RISK OF HYPERCHOLESTEROLEMIA BEGINS EARLY. Our current national guidelines use the Framingham Risk Equation. This instrument weights age heavily. However, for many patients and doctors, the relevant horizon of cardiovascular risk extends over a lifetime rather than 10 years, as predicated by the National Cholesterol Education Program Adult Treatment Panel III (NCEP ATP III) guidelines. For this reason, it is practically important to know whether cholesterol levels measured early in life influence long-term cardiovascular risk. Several data sets speak to this question. First, in the Bogalusa Heart Study, the burden of risk factors for atherosclerosis including hypercholesterolemia correlate with autopsy-proven fatty streak and raised lesion formation in the arterial tree. Studies performed on Johns Hopkins medical students upon matriculation with long-term follow-up suggested that cholesterol levels in the third decade correlate with long-term risk of myocardial infarction. A recent compilation of three major observational studies underscored the importance of cholesterol levels in young adulthood to long-term cardiovascular risk.[57] Thus, substantial evidence suggests that the burden of risk for cardiovascular disease begins in young adulthood. Well-known autopsy studies from the Korean and Vietnam conflicts, and recent explorations of coronary anatomy by intravascular ultrasonography, in conjunction with the Bogalusa Heart Study mentioned earlier, suggest that atherosclerosis can affect adolescents in our society. Because drug therapy will almost certainly prove neither cost-effective nor medically appropriate in primary prevention in younger populations, intensive life-style modification to reduce coronary risk due to lipid disorders should become a societal priority.

HIGH-DENSITY LIPOPROTEIN CHOLESTEROL. Several studies have found that CHD risk correlates inversely with high-density lipoprotein (HDL) cholesterol levels. Indeed, patients with angiographically proven coronary artery disease more often have low levels of HDL than high levels of LDL, as defined by current criteria. The process of reverse cholesterol transport may explain in part the apparent protective role of HDL against coronary death. According to this concept, HDL could ferry cholesterol from the vessel wall, augmenting peripheral catabolism of cholesterol. HDL can also carry antioxidant enzymes that may reduce the levels of oxidized phospholipids in atheromatous lesions that may enhance atherogenesis (see Chaps. 35 and 39). We lack a consistent body of clinical trial data on intervention to raise HDL cholesterol, in contrast to the case of LDL discussed previously. Yet, the consistency of the observational data, both cross-sectional and prospective, strongly support the HDL level as a "negative" risk factor, as incorporated in the ATP III guidelines.

TRIGLYCERIDE-RICH LIPOPROTEINS IN CARDIOVASCULAR RISK. In contrast to the compelling evidence favoring a causal role for LDL in atherogenesis, the role of triglycerides still engenders controversy. A number of issues foster this confusion. First, as triglyceride levels tend to vary inversely with HDL levels, demonstration of an unequivocal effect of triglycerides on cardiovascular events and mortality independent of HDL levels has proven elusive. Secondly, the level of triglycerides in the blood depends exquisitely on diet. Sampling serum for triglyceride levels in the fasting state avoids some of the variability in this measurement. However, most humans are in the postprandial state much of the day. The actual exposure of the artery wall to triglyceride-rich lipoprotein particles such as very-low-density lipoproteins (see Chap. 39) may indeed constitute a factor that promotes atherosclerosis that would be missed by the fasting lipid profile. For these reasons among others, current guidelines do not establish a target value of triglycerides. In view of the tight link of triglyceride levels with known risk factors for atherosclerosis (low HDL cholesterol level, uncontrolled diabetes, hypothyroidism), however, elevated triglyceride levels should enter into the overall risk assessment for an individual and stimulate consideration of the reason for triglyceride elevation (see Chap. 39).

Metabolic Syndrome, Insulin Resistance, and Diabetes (see Chap. 40)

Almost 35 million Americans have some degree of abnormal glucose tolerance, a condition along with obesity that markedly increases risk for type 2 diabetes and premature atherothrombosis.[58] Patients with diabetes have two- to eightfold higher rates of future cardiovascular events as compared with age- and ethnically matched nondiabetic individuals,[59] and three-fourths of all deaths among diabetic patients result from coronary heart disease.[60] Compared to unaffected individuals, diabetic patients have a greater atherosclerotic burden both in the major arteries and in the microvascular circulation. Not surprisingly, diabetic patients have substantially increased rates of atherosclerotic complications both in

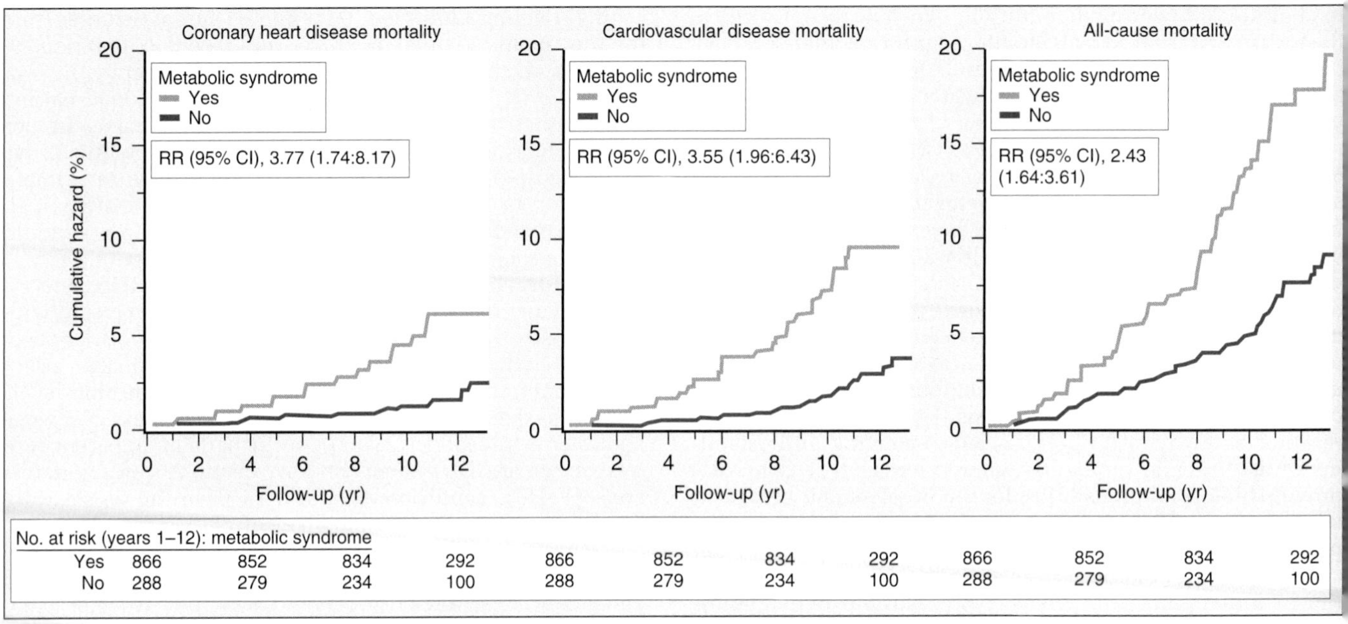

FIGURE 36–3 Cumulative hazard (unadjusted Kaplan-Meier hazard curves) for coronary heart disease, cardiovascular disease, and all-cause mortality among individuals with and without metabolic syndrome. (From Lakka H, Laaksonen DE, Lakka TA, et al: The metabolic syndrome and total and cardiovascular disease mortality in middle-aged men. JAMA 288:2709, 2002.)

the settings of primary prevention and after coronary interventional procedures. Moreover, the risk of cardiovascular disease starts to increase long before the onset of clinical diabetes, suggesting a "ticking clock" phenomenon. In an analysis of data from the Nurses Health Study of women who eventually developed type 2 diabetes, the relative risk of myocardial infarction was elevated threefold *before* the diagnosis of diabetes, a cardiovascular event rate almost as high as the rate in patients with frank diabetes at study entry.[61] These effects are amplified in ethnic minority populations[62] and in patients with other concomitant risk factors[63,64] and reflect subclinical disease in both the diabetic and the nondiabetic patient.[65] Thus, insulin resistance and diabetes rank among the major cardiovascular risk factors.

Although hyperglycemia is associated with microvascular disease, insulin resistance itself promotes atherosclerosis even before it produces frank diabetes, and available data corroborate the role of insulin resistance as an independent risk factor for atherothrombosis. This finding has prompted recommendations for increased surveillance for the metabolic syndrome, a cluster of glucose intolerance and hyperinsulinemia accompanied by hypertriglyceridemia, low HDL levels, hypofibrinolysis, hypertension, microalbuminuria, a predominance of small, dense LDL particles, and central obesity. Although several formal definitions of the metabolic syndrome have been proposed, the definition adopted by the National Cholesterol Education Program Adult Treatment Panel[66] requires at least three of the following five criteria: waist circumference greater than 102 cm in men and 88 cm in women; serum triglyceride levels of at least 150 mg/dl, HDL cholesterol less than 40 mg/dl in men and less than 50 mg/dl in women; blood pressure of at least 130/85 mm Hg; and serum glucose concentration of at least 110 mg/dl. Using these criteria, the prevalence of metabolic syndrome in the United States is almost 25 percent, or nearly 50 million (see Table 40–2).[67]

Several studies document that individuals with the metabolic syndrome have elevated vascular event rates. In the Kuopio Ischaemic Heart Disease Risk Factor Study, patients with metabolic syndrome showed markedly increased rates of coronary, cardiovascular, and all-cause mortality (Fig. 36–3).[68] However, not all individuals with metabolic syndrome have similar risk and, indeed, other markers may help to stratify clinical risk.[69] In particular, data from the Women's Health Study indicate that an hsCRP level greater than 3 mg/liter adds important prognostic information on cardiovascular risk at all levels of the metabolic syndrome (Fig. 36–4).[70] This observation is important, because levels of C-reactive protein measured with a high-sensitivity assay (hsCRP) also predict incident type 2 diabetes.[71-74a] Almost identical data regarding the additive value of hsCRP to the metabolic syndrome in terms of future vascular risk prediction derives from the West of Scotland Coronary Prevention Study.[75] As hsCRP levels correlate with systemic hypofibrinolysis and with basal insulin levels,[76] hsCRP evaluation may well become a routine part of the definition of metabolic syndrome.[77] As reviewed later in this chapter in sections

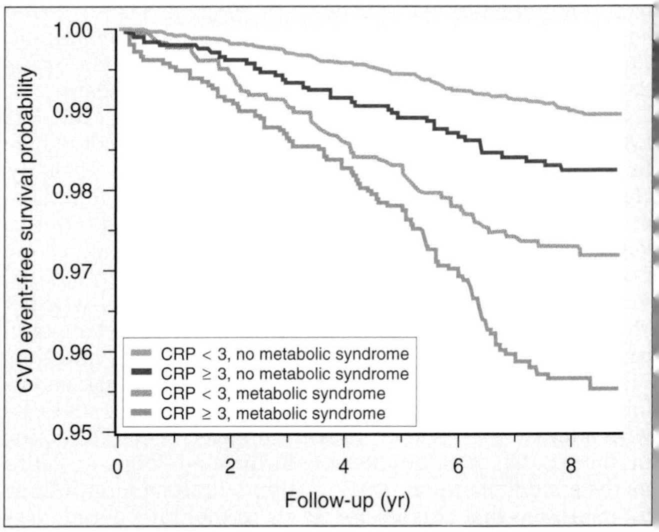

FIGURE 36–4 High-sensitivity C-reactive protein (CRP) adds prognostic information on risk among individuals with and without the metabolic syndrome. CVD = cardiovascular disease. (From Ridker PM, Buring JE, Cook NR, Rifai N: C-reactive protein, the metabolic syndrome, and risk of incident cardiovascular events: An 8-year follow-up of 14,719 initially healthy American women. Circulation 107:391, 2003.)

describing inflammatory markers, this conclusion is emerging in part from observations that atherosclerosis and type 2 diabetes share a common inflammatory basis.[78]

In addition to systemic metabolic abnormalities, hyperglycemia causes accumulation of advanced glycation end products associated with vascular damage.[79,80] Diabetic patients have markedly impaired endothelial and smooth muscle function and appear to have increased leukocyte adhesion to vascular endothelium, a critical early step in atherogenesis.[81] Diabetic nephropathy, detected by microalbuminuria, accelerates these adverse processes. Among individuals with non-insulin-dependent diabetes, microalbuminuria predicts both cardiovascular and all-cause mortality.[82] Abnormalities of endogenous fibrinolysis are also prevalent among diabetic and prediabetic patients, and therapies targeting plasminogen activator inhibitor have been proposed as a novel pathway for disease prevention in this setting.[83] The proinflammatory atherogenic mediator soluble CD40 ligand is elevated among diabetic patients and declines during thiazolidinedione therapy.[84] These effects, in concert with the impaired endothelium-dependent (nitric oxide–mediated) vasodilation common among diabetic patients, contribute to endothelial cell dysfunction and accelerated atherogenesis.[85] Chapters 40, 42, and 51 review the data about therapeutic interventions in patients with diabetes or the metabolic syndrome.

Exercise, Weight Loss, and Obesity

Regular physical exercise reduces myocardial oxygen demand and increases exercise capacity, both of which correlate with lower levels of coronary risk. The cardioprotective effects of exercise include adiposity, diabetes incidence, lowered blood pressure, and improvement of dyslipidemia, plasma rheology, and vascular inflammation. Exercise also enhances endothelial dysfunction, insulin sensitivity, and endogenous fibrinolysis.[86] It is thus not surprising that prospective epidemiological studies almost universally demonstrate strong graded associations between levels of physical activity and reduced rates of cardiovascular morbidity and all-cause mortality.

Recent observational studies cast doubt on the long-held belief that exercise must be vigorous to be beneficial. Exercise levels achieved with as little as 30 minutes of walking daily provide major coronary benefits. In the Women's Health Initiative, walking briskly for 30 minutes five times per week was associated with a 30 percent reduction in vascular events over a 3.5-year follow-up, an effect that persisted after adjustment for body mass index, age, and ethnicity (Fig. 36–5).[87] The Nurses Health Study yielded similar data: 3 hours of brisk walking per week conferred as much protection as did 1.5 hours of vigorous exercise per week.[88] In men participating in the Health Professional Follow-Up Study, 30 minutes of daily walking was associated with an 18 percent reduction in coronary risk. In that study, contrary to commonly given medical advice, resistance exercise and weight training were also found to have cardiovascular benefit.[89] Accumulated episodes of exercise, even if brief, have further demonstrated benefit, suggesting that prolonged vigorous work is not needed for risk reduction.[90] Smaller but consistent benefits of modest exercise have been observed for incident stroke, independent of hypertension.[91] Thus, a "no pain, no gain" approach to the prescription of physical activity to reduce vascular risk now appears passé.[92]

On the basis of these data, a joint statement from the Centers for Disease Control and the American College of Sports Medicine recommends that every American should accumulate at least 30 minutes of moderate-intensity physical activity daily.[93] Unfortunately, 7 of 10 American adults fail to meet this very modest level of activity, and one in three reports no leisure time activity at all.[94] Even though a

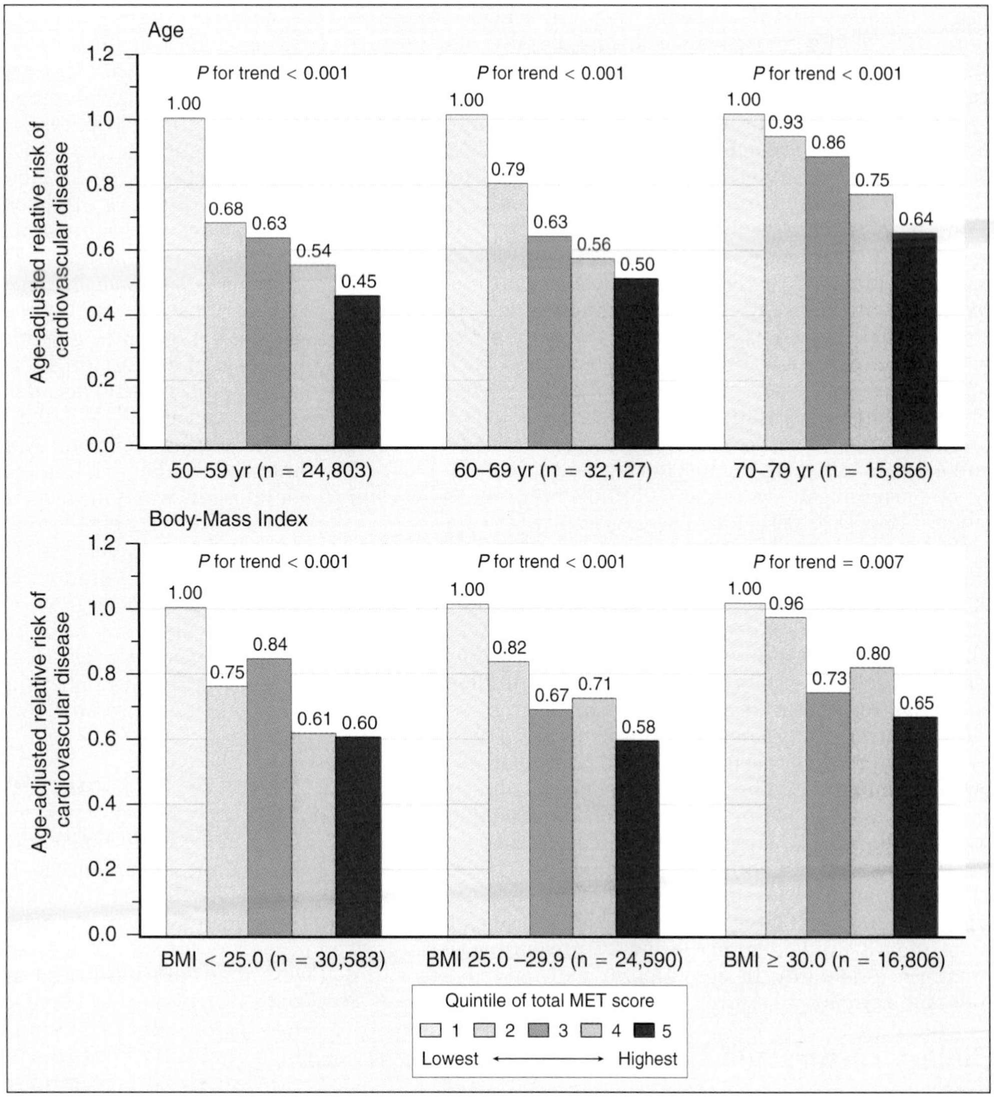

FIGURE 36–5 Relative risks of cardiovascular disease according to quintile of energy expenditure (MET Score) from recreational activities stratified by age **(top)** and body mass index **(bottom)**. (From Manson JE, Greenland P, LaCroix AZ, et al: Walking compared with vigorous exercise for the prevention of cardiovascular events in women. N Engl J Med 347:716, 2002.)

dose-response relationship is widely recognized between level of exercise and coronary risk, many experts worry that motivation to exercise might be undercut by even the slightly more aggressive recommendations from the Institute of Medicine to increase leisure time activity from 30 to 60 minutes daily.[95]

A recognized problem with the "30 minutes of walking per day" approach to vascular risk reduction is that this modest amount of exercise may not be adequate to reduce weight or maintain a healthy body mass index. In descriptive studies, long-term weight reduction requires more aggressive approaches among formerly obese patients, although one randomized trial showed short-term benefits of a less aggressive approach.[96]

Regular exercise affects multiple risk factors for atherosclerosis. In a recent meta-analysis of intervention trials, aerobic exercise was associated with a mean reduction of systolic blood pressure of 5 mm Hg among hypertensive participants, a level comparable to many drug interventions.[97] The degree of blood pressure reduction did not vary by frequency or intensity of exercise, and other studies show that walking alone has comparable effects.[98] Although exercise has been seen traditionally as having only modest effects on total and LDL cholesterol levels, improvements in HDL cholesterol level and reductions in triglycerides occur consistently, and more recent data indicate an increase in the average size of LDL particles without a change in plasma LDL concentration.[99] These effects occur even in the absence of clinically significant weight loss and were related more strongly with amount than intensity of exercise.

Exercise further improves insulin sensitivity and glycemic control with major benefits for diabetic patients. An analysis of 14 intervention trials of at least 8 weeks' duration showed clinically important reductions in glycated hemoglobin, along with reduced requirements for therapy.[100] These data agree with prospective epidemiological observations that moderate-intensity activity is associated with a reduced incidence of diabetes[101] and with randomized intervention studies such as the U.S. Diabetes Prevention Program, in which a 58 percent reduction in diabetes risk was observed with modest levels of exercise and a 5 to 7 percent reduction in body weight.[102] Finally, regular exercise lowers C-reactive protein levels,[103] improves coronary endothelial function,[104] and appears to benefit hemostatic variables, including tissue-type plasminogen activator, fibrinogen, von Willebrand factor, fibrin D-dimer, and plasma viscosity.[105]

Controversy remains as to whether obesity itself is a true risk factor for cardiovascular disease or whether its impact on vascular risk is mediated solely through interrelations with glucose intolerance, insulin resistance, hypertension, physical inactivity, and dyslipidemia. From an epidemiological perspective, obesity alone associates with elevated vascular risk regardless of activity levels, and the waist-to-hip ratio, a surrogate for centripetal or abdominal obesity, independently predicts vascular risk both in women and in older men.[106] Among U.S. adults, the prevalence of obesity (defined as a body mass index of 30 or greater) has doubled over the past decade and now reaches 30 percent across the population.[107] Even among children, particularly girls, obesity is a major problem, with rates in excess of 10 percent for white girls and 20 percent for black girls.[108] Thus, weight control must play a fundamental role in all preventive cardiology practices, preferably in conjunction with advice regarding diet and exercise.

Dietary Factors and Cardiovascular Risk (see Chaps. 41 and 42)

The fundamental role of diet, nutrition, and obesity in cardiovascular risk is discussed in detail in Chapter 41.

Mental Stress, Depression, and Cardiovascular Risk

Mental stress and depression both predispose to increased vascular risk and from a clinician's perspective should be considered as modifiable risk factors. The adrenergic stimulation of mental stress can augment myocardial oxygen requirements and aggravate myocardial ischemia. Mental stress can cause coronary vasoconstriction, particularly in atherosclerotic coronary arteries, and hence can influence myocardial oxygen supply as well. Recent studies have further linked mental stress to platelet and endothelial dysfunction,[109] the metabolic syndrome,[110,111] and the induction of ventricular arrhythmias.[112,113]

Acute stress such as that associated with natural disasters has long been recognized as a risk factor for coronary events.[114,115] More recently, work-related stress has gained recognition as a source of vascular risk. Work stress has two components: job strain (which combines high work demands and low job control) and effort-reward imbalance (which more closely reflects economic factors in the workplace). Both components are associated with an approximate doubling of risk for myocardial infarction and stroke in European[116] and Japanese populations.[117] Other psychological metrics, including anger and hostility scales, have also been associated with elevated vascular risk.

Clinical depression strongly predicts coronary heart disease. In a meta-analysis of 11 studies involving initially healthy individuals, those with depression had a significantly higher risk of developing coronary disease during follow-up, with clinical depression (RR, 2.7) being more important than depressive mood (RR, 1.5).[118] While depression is also associated with an increased prevalence of hypertension, smoking, and lack of physical activity, the effects of depression on overall risk remain after adjusting for these and other traditional risk factors.[119] Thus, findings that depressed individuals also have increased platelet activation, elevated levels of hsCRP, and decreased heart rate variability support depression as an independent predictor of events.

Onset of depression after myocardial infarction is common and predicts cardiovascular mortality independent of cardiac disease severity.[120] Whether therapy for postinfarction depression reduces recurrent event rates remains controversial. In the SADHART trial, a substantial proportion of cardiac depression was found to remit spontaneously, emphasizing the need for placebo-controlled studies.[121] By contrast, in the Enhancing Recovery in Coronary Heart Disease Patients (ENRICHD) trial, random allocation between usual care and formal psychosocial intervention resulted in modest improvements in measures of clinical depression but no significant improvement in event-free survival.[122] Ongoing studies will thus be critical to determine whether more aggressive interventions for depression can improve vascular outcomes.[123]

Novel Atherosclerotic Risk Factors

Despite the importance of blood lipids, half of all myocardial infarctions occur among individuals without overt hyperlipidemia. In fact, in a major prospective study of healthy American women, 77 percent of all future cardiovascular events occurred among patients with LDL cholesterol levels less than 160 mg/dl and 46 percent occurred among those with LDL cholesterol levels less than 130 mg/dl.[124] While the use of global prediction models like those developed in Framingham greatly improves the detection of heart disease risk, as many as 20 percent of all events occur in the absence of any of the major classic vascular risk factors.

This fact challenges several basic issues related to national screening programs for risk detection and disease prevention.

However, clinical data continue to accrue demonstrating the hazard of relying solely on classic risk factors. In one recent analysis of more than 120,000 patients with coronary heart disease, 15 percent of the men and 19 percent of the women had no evidence of hyperlipidemia, hypertension, diabetes, or smoking and more than half had only one of these general risk factors.[125] In another large analysis, between 85 and 95 percent of participants with coronary disease had at least one conventional risk factor, but so too did those participants without coronary disease despite follow-up for as long as 30 years.[126] Thus, because of the considerable need to improve vascular risk detection, much research over the past decade has focused on the identification and evaluation of novel atherosclerotic risk factors.[127,128]

When evaluating any novel risk factor as a potential new screening tool, clinicians need to consider (1) whether there is a standardized and reproducible assay for the marker of interest; (2) whether there is a consistent series of prospective studies demonstrating that a given parameter predicts future risk; (3) whether the novel marker adds to the predictive value of lipid screening; and (4) whether there is evidence that the novel marker adds to global risk prediction scores such as that in the Framingham Heart Study. The following section applies these basic epidemiological requirements to a series of novel risk factors, including hsCRP and other markers of inflammation, lipoprotein(a), homocysteine, and markers of fibrinolytic and hemostatic function such as fibrinogen, D-dimer, tissue plasminogen activator (t-PA), and plasminogen activator inhibitor (PAI-1) antigens (Table 36–1). Physicians should also consider the relative magnitude of novel markers in terms of risk prediction, particularly in comparison to lipid screening. Figure 36–6 shows data describing the relative efficacy of several variables measured at baseline in two large cohorts of initially healthy middle-aged men and women.

C-Reactive Protein (CRP)

Inflammation characterizes all phases of atherothrombosis and provides a critical pathophysiological link between plaque formation and acute rupture, leading to occlusion and infarction.[129] Formation of the fatty streak, the earliest phase of atherogenesis, involves recruitment of leukocytes due to the expression of adhesion molecules on endothelial cells in turn triggered by inflammatory cytokines such as interleukin-1 and tumor necrosis factor-alpha. Subsequent migration of inflammatory cells into the subendothelial space requires chemotaxis controlled by chemokines induced by the primary cytokines. Mononuclear cells within this initial infiltrate as well as intrinsic vascular cells subsequently release growth factors that stimulate proliferation of the smooth muscle cells and lead to plaque progression. The thrombotic complications of plaques often involve physical disruption, usually associated with signs of both local and systemic inflammation.[130] Other proinflammatory cytokines such as CD40 ligand can in turn induce tissue factor expression and promote thrombus formation. Moreover, the primary proinflammatory cytokines result in the expression of messenger cytokines such as interleukin-6, which can travel from local sites of inflammation to the liver, where it triggers a change in the program of protein synthesis characteristic of the acute phase response. The acute phase reactant, CRP, a simple downstream marker of inflammation, has now emerged as a major cardiovascular risk factor.[131]

Composed of five 23 kD subunits, CRP is a circulating member of the pentraxin family that plays a major role in the human innate immune response. Although it is primarily derived from the liver, recent data indicate that cells within human coronary arteries, particularly in the atherosclerotic intima, can elaborate CRP.[132,133] More than simply a marker of inflammation, CRP may influence directly vascular vulnerability through several mechanisms, including enhanced expression of local adhesion molecules, increased expression of endothelial PAI-1, reduced endothelial nitric oxide bioactivity, altered LDL uptake by macrophages, and colocalization with complement within atherosclerotic lesions.[134-137] Moreover, the expression of human CRP in CRP-

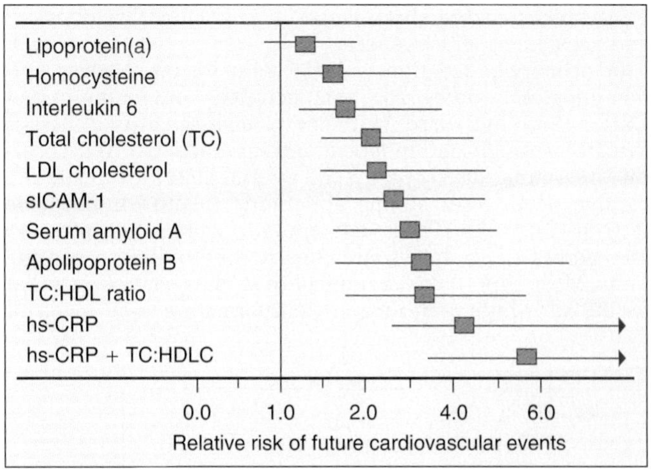

FIGURE 36–6 Relative risks of future myocardial infarction among apparently healthy women according to baseline levels of lipoprotein(a), homocysteine, interleukin-6, total cholesterol, low-density lipoprotein (LDL) cholesterol, soluble intercellular adhesion molecule-1 (sICAM-1), serum amyloid A, apolipoprotein B, the ratio of total cholesterol to high-density lipoprotein cholesterol (TC:HDLC), high-sensitivity C-reactive protein (hsCRP), and the combination of hsCRP with the TC:HDLC. (From Ridker PM: Clinical application of C-reactive protein for cardiovascular disease detection and prevention. Circulation 107:363, 2003.)

TABLE 36–1 Assessment of the Clinical Utility of Novel Markers of Cardiovascular Risk

Marker	Assay Conditions Standardized?	Prospective Studies Consistent?	Additive to Total Cholesterol and High-Density Lipoprotein Cholesterol?	Additive to Framingham Risk?
Lipoprotein(a)	–	+/–	+/–	–
Homocysteine	+	+	+/–	–
Tissue plasminogen activator and plasminogen activator inhibitor-1	+/–	+	+/–	–
Lipoprotein density	–	+/–	–	–
Fibrinogen	–	+	+	–
High-sensitivity C-reactive protein	+	+	+	+

transgenic mice directly enhances intravascular thrombosis[138] and accelerates atherogenesis.[138a]

In primary prevention, a large series of prospective epidemiological studies has demonstrated convincingly that CRP, when measured with new high-sensitivity assays (hsCRP), strongly and independently predicts risk of myocardial infarction, stroke, peripheral arterial disease, and sudden cardiac death even among apparently healthy individuals (Fig. 36–7).[124,139-143] These data apply to women as well as to men across all age levels and consistently to diverse populations. Most importantly, a number of studies have shown that hsCRP adds important prognostic information at all levels of LDL cholesterol and at all levels of risk as determined by the Framingham Risk Score (Fig. 36–8).[124,144] In the largest study to date, hsCRP levels predicted subsequent risk better than LDL cholesterol level. However, because hsCRP levels reflect a component of vascular risk quite different from that of cholesterol, the addition of hsCRP to lipid evaluation provides a major opportunity to improve global risk prediction. In clinical terms, absolute vascular risk is higher among individuals with elevated hsCRP and low levels of LDL cholesterol than among individuals with elevated levels of LDL cholesterol but low levels of hsCRP, yet current guidelines consider only the latter group at high risk (Fig. 36–9).

Additional data corroborating the ability of hsCRP to predict vascular risk after adjustment for traditional risk factors have been provided by several large cohorts in both the United States and Europe.[144a,b,c] These confirmatory studies include data from the Reykjavik Heart Study in which a 50 percent increase in risk associated with hsCRP was observed not only after control for Framingham covariates but also after additional control for diabetes, triglycerides, body mass index, and indices of pulmonary function.[144c] In that study, the odds ratio for hsCRP was identical to that of hypertension and statistically similar to that of smoking—data that demonstrate the clinical importance of inflammation in a population with much higher baseline cholesterol levels than those observed in contemporary U.S. cohorts.

Largely on the basis of these data, the American

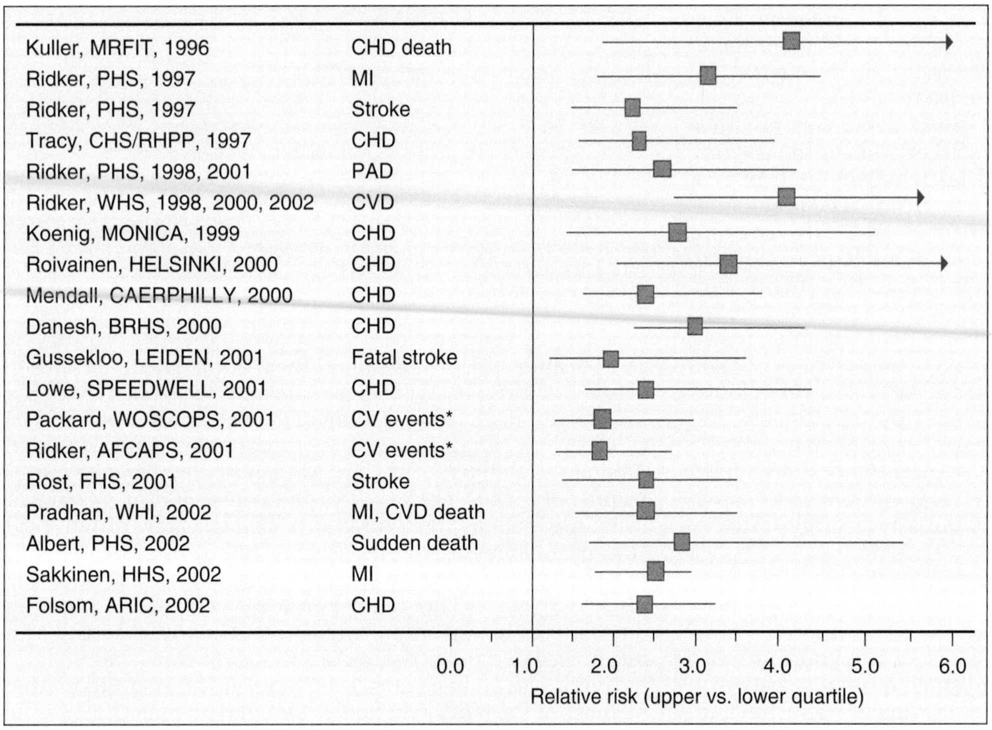

FIGURE 36–7 Prospective studies relating baseline high-sensitivity C-reactive protein levels to the risk of first cardiovascular events. CHD = coronary heart disease; CV = cardiovascular; CVD = cardiovascular disease; MI = myocardial infarction; PAD = pulmonary artery disease. (From Ridker PM: Clinical application of C-reactive protein for cardiovascular disease detection and prevention. Circulation 107:363, 2003.)

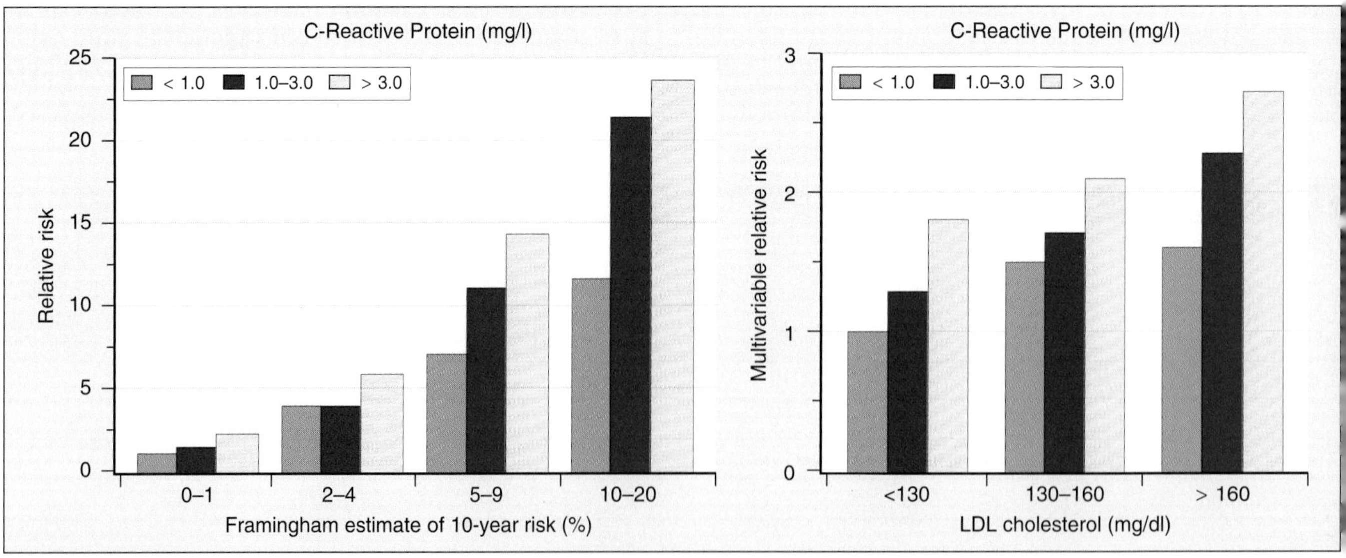

FIGURE 36–8 High-sensitivity C-reactive protein adds prognostic information at all levels of low-density lipoprotein (LDL) cholesterol after multivariate adjustment for traditional risk factors **(right)** and at all levels of the Framingham risk score **(left)**. (From Ridker PM, Rifai N, Rose L, et al: Comparison of C-reactive protein and low-density lipoprotein cholesterol levels in the prediction of first cardiovascular events. N Engl J Med 347:1557, 2002.)

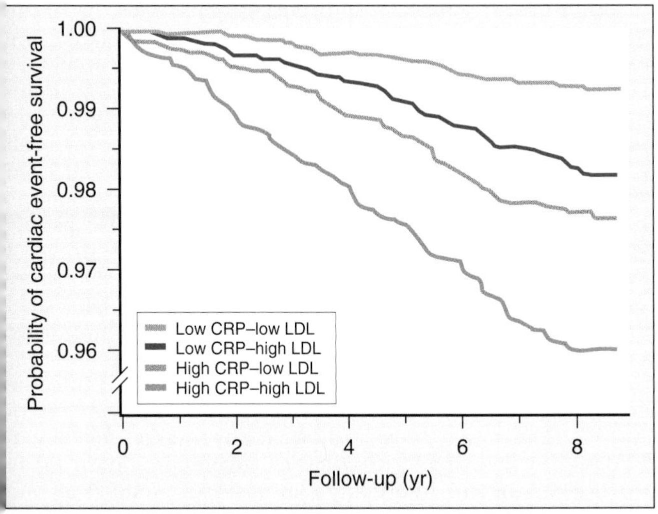

FIGURE 36–9 Cardiovascular event-free survival among apparently healthy individuals according to baseline levels of high-sensitivity C-reactive protein (CRP) and low-density lipoprotein (LDL) cholesterol. (From Ridker PM, Rifai N, Rose L, et al: Comparison of C-reactive protein and low-density lipoprotein cholesterol levels in the prediction of first cardiovascular events. N Engl J Med 347:1557, 2002.)

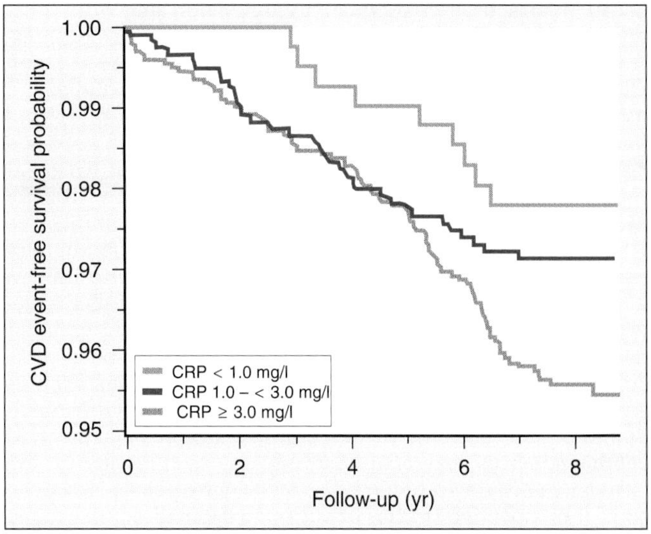

FIGURE 36–10 Cardiovascular disease (CVD) event-free survival among individuals with the metabolic syndrome, stratified by high-sensitivity C-reactive protein (CRP) levels at baseline. (From Ridker PM: Clinical application of C-reactive protein for cardiovascular disease detection and prevention. Circulation 107:363, 2003.)

Heart Association and the Centers for Disease Control and Prevention recently issued the first guidelines for the use of hsCRP in clinical practice.[145] In brief, hsCRP levels of less than 1, 1 to 3, and greater than 3 mg/liter should be interpreted as low, moderate, and high vascular risk, respectively. Screening for hsCRP should be done at the discretion of the physician as a part of global risk evaluation, not as a replacement for LDL and HDL testing. Although hsCRP predicts risk across the full population spectrum, its greatest utility is likely to be among those at "intermediate risk"; that is, individuals with anticipated 10-year event rates between 5 and 20 percent. Values of hsCRP in excess of 10 mg/liter may represent an acute-phase response due to an underlying inflammatory disease or intercurrent infection and should lead to repeat testing in approximately 2 to 3 weeks; consistently high values, however, represent very high risk of future cardiovascular disease because risk appears linear across the full range of hsCRP.[145a] Because hsCRP levels are stable over long periods of time, have no circadian variation, and are not affected by food intake, screening can easily be done on an outpatient basis at the time of cholesterol evaluation.

Levels of hsCRP greater than 3 mg/liter also appear to predict recurrent coronary events, thrombotic complications after angioplasty, poor outcome in the setting of unstable angina, and vascular complications after bypass surgery.[146-150] All of these data support the concept that inflammation plays a critical role throughout the atherothrombotic process. Additionally, hsCRP has prognostic utility in cases of acute ischemia even without troponin elevation, data suggesting that an enhanced inflammatory response at the time of hospital admission can determine subsequent plaque rupture.[151] These findings help explain why individuals with elevated hsCRP levels are also more likely to benefit from aggressive interventions compared to those with low levels.[152,153]

Elevated levels of hsCRP predict not only cardiovascular events but also the onset of type 2 diabetes mellitus,[71,72] perhaps because hsCRP levels correlate with several components of the metabolic syndrome, including those not easily measured in clinical practice such as insulin sensitivity, endothelial dysfunction, and hypofibrinolysis. Thus, hsCRP assessment also adds prognostic information at all levels of the metabolic syndrome.[70,75] Even among individuals with the ATP-III definition of metabolic syndrome, knowledge of hsCRP levels less than 1, 1 to 3, and greater than 3 mg/liter further defines low-, moderate-, and high-risk groups for future vascular events (Fig. 36–10).

Of commercially available novel risk factors, hsCRP has the greatest magnitude of predictive value. Further, unlike homocysteine, fibrinogen, and lipoprotein(a), hsCRP adds important prognostic information to global risk prediction. It is important to recognize, however, that no direct evidence to date shows that lowering hsCRP per se will reduce vascular risk. Nonetheless, smoking cessation, weight loss, diet, and exercise all reduce hsCRP levels and all lower cardiac risk. Thus the primary use of hsCRP at this time should be for improved targeting of primary prevention efforts directed at these modifiable risk factors.

Statins lower hsCRP levels in a manner largely unrelated to the magnitude of LDL cholesterol reduction.[154,155] Data in both primary and secondary prevention indicate that the relative benefit of statin therapy in terms of event reduction may be greater in the presence of elevated hsCRP levels. In the AFCAPS/TexCAPS trial, for example, lovastatin appeared to lower cardiovascular event rates even for those with below-median levels of LDL cholesterol but above-median levels of hsCRP.[156] By contrast, lovastatin did not reduce events among those with neither hyperlipidemia nor inflammation. These observations have led to the hypothesis that statin therapy prevents first vascular events not only among patients with elevated LDL cholesterol levels, but also among those with elevated levels of hsCRP. This critical hypothesis is now under direct investigation.[157]

In addition to statins, treatment with fibrates and niacin may also lower hsCRP levels, as does the use of thiazolidinediones. By contrast, oral preparations of hormone replacement therapy tend to increase hsCRP levels. While aspirin does not directly lower hsCRP levels, the utility of aspirin in preventing first vascular events appears to be greatest among patients with elevated hsCRP levels.

The hsCRP levels correlate only modestly with underlying atherosclerotic disease as measured by carotid intimal medial thickness or by coronary calcification. This observation suggests that hsCRP does not simply reflect the presence of subclinical disease but rather indicates an increased propensity for plaque disruption and/or thrombosis. Autopsy data support this hypothesis: elevated hsCRP levels occur more often among patients with frankly ruptured plaques than among those with erosive disease or among those who died of nonvascular causes.[158] Two recent studies showed that hsCRP levels predict incident hypertension and add prognostic information on vascular risk at all levels of blood pressure.[159,160] In patients with other conditions such as allograft atherosclerosis[161] and chronic renal failure and dialysis,[162] hsCRP levels have proven to predict strongly poor short- and long-term cardiovascular outcome.

Although inflammation clearly participates in vascular injury and hsCRP provides an inexpensive and clinically useful measure of this process, it remains uncertain as to what stimulus initiates the underlying proinflammatory response (see also Chap. 35). Patients with chronic inflammatory diseases such as rheumatoid arthritis tend to have elevated hsCRP levels and on average somewhat higher vascular risk, but a causal relationship in this setting has been difficult to establish. Patients with low-grade infections such as gingivitis or those who chronically carry *Chlamydia pneumoniae, Helicobacter pylori,* herpes simplex virus, and cytomegalovirus may also have higher vascular risk on the basis of a chronic systemic inflammatory response. However, careful prospective studies of antibody titers directed against these agents have not consistently found evidence of association, and a large antibiotic trial did not show reduced recurrent events in myocardial infarction survivors.[163] Whether novel targeted antiinflammatory therapies, including specific cytokine inhibitors, can improve coronary outcomes is an active area of research.

Given the robustness of laboratory and epidemiological data and the low cost of testing, we believe hsCRP evaluation will likely become a routine part of coronary risk prediction. In outpatient settings, hsCRP should be evaluated at the time of cholesterol screening if the practitioner wishes to use it as an adjunct to global risk prediction. For individuals with an LDL cholesterol level greater than 160 mg/dl, a finding of elevated hsCRP should provide an additional impetus for the physician to institute aggressive primary prevention and may help motivate some patients to comply with life-style modifications and, when indicated, pharmacotherapy.

For individuals with LDL cholesterol levels between 130 and 160 mg/dl, the finding of an elevated hsCRP level indicates substantial risk and should again lead to better adherence to preventive efforts and perhaps to earlier use of pharmacological approaches to risk reduction. For individuals with LDL cholesterol levels below 130 mg/dl, it is also clear that an elevated hsCRP value confers elevated risk. However, while post hoc analyses suggest that such patients may benefit from statin therapy, clinical trials testing this issue have only recently begun. Such individuals should thus aggressively undergo exercise, weight loss, and smoking cessation programs. In this setting, an elevated hsCRP level should provide considerable motivation to improve life-style, particularly for those previously told they were not at risk because of an absence of hyperlipidemia. Simple clinical algorithms for the use of hsCRP in primary care have recently become available.[164]

Approaches to hsCRP evaluation in secondary prevention and in acute coronary ischemia are evolving. A major area of concern is in the emergency room evaluation of patients with troponin-negative acute coronary ischemia. Because elevations in several inflammatory markers including hsCRP and myeloperoxidase occur in this setting and predict poor short-term outcomes, some form of inflammatory biomarker may aid the evaluation of chest pain (see also Chap. 45).

Other Markers of Inflammation

While hsCRP is by far the best-characterized inflammatory biomarker for clinical use, several other markers of inflammation have shown promise in terms of predicting vascular risk. These include cytokines such as interleukin-6,[152,165] soluble forms of certain cell adhesion molecules such as intercellular adhesion molecule (sICAM-1), P-selectin, or the mediator CD40 ligand,[166-170] as well as markers of leukocyte activation such as myeloperoxidase.[171] Other inflammatory markers associated with lipid oxidation such as lipoprotein-associated phospholipase A2[172,173] and pregnancy-associated plasma protein A have also shown promise.[174] However, each of these emerging biomarkers has analytical issues that need careful evaluation before routine clinical use. For example, the half-life of some is too short for clinical diagnostic testing, whereas the ability of others to predict risk in settings of broad populations has proved marginal thus far.[175] Nonetheless, several of these inflammatory biomarkers can shed critical pathophysiological light on the atherothrombotic process, particularly at the time of plaque rupture. For example, soluble CD40 ligand may provide insight into the efficacy of specific antithrombotic agents independent of CRP[176] and also may have a role as a novel target for thiazolidinedione therapy.[84] Similarly, myeloperoxidase may provide prognostic information in cases of acute ischemia over and above that associated with troponin or CRP.[130,177,178] Thus, continued evaluation of other inflammatory biomarkers may well provide novel targets for or monitors of therapy, particularly in the setting of acute coronary ischemia.

Homocysteine

Homocysteine is a sulfhydryl-containing amino acid derived from the demethylation of dietary methionine. Patients with rare inherited defects of methionine metabolism can develop severe hyperhomocysteinemia (plasma levels >100 μmol/liter) and have markedly elevated risk of premature atherothrombosis as well as venous thromboembolism. The mechanisms that account for these effects remain uncertain but include endothelial dysfunction, accelerated oxidation of LDL cholesterol, impairment of flow-mediated endothelial-derived relaxing factor with subsequent reduction in arterial vasodilation, platelet activation, increased expression of monocyte chemoattractant protein (MCP-1), and interleukin-8 leading to a proinflammatory response, and oxidative stress.[179-183]

In contrast to severe hyperhomocysteinemia, mild to moderate elevations of homocysteine (plasma levels >15 μmol/liter) are more common in the general population, primarily due to insufficient dietary intake of folic acid.[184] Other patient groups who tend to have elevated levels of homocysteine include those receiving folate antagonists such as methotrexate and carbamazepine, and those with impaired homocysteine metabolism due to hypothyroidism or to renal insufficiency.

A common polymorphism in the methylene tetrahydrofolate reductase (*MTHFR*) gene that encodes a thermolabile protein has also been linked to elevated homocysteine levels and to increased vascular risk, at least among individuals homozygous for the variant. Familial association studies report higher homocysteine levels among offspring of parents with premature coronary artery disease.[185] However, the clinical importance of the *MTHFR* polymorphism appears modest, and heterozygous individuals display little evidence of elevated homocysteine levels even among those with low folate intake. In a recent meta-analysis of 40 observational studies, individuals homozygous for the *MTHFR* 677 TT variant had only a 16 percent increase in relative risk (OR, 1.16; 95 percent CI, 1.05-1.28), and this observation was evident only in studies originating in Europe.[186] Thus, in populations in whom folate fortification exists, such as those in North America, no compelling evidence supports genetic evaluation of *MTHFR* to predict vascular risk.[187,188]

Until recently, total plasma homocysteine (the combination of free homocysteine, bound homocysteine, and mixed disulfides) was measured predominantly by high-performance liquid chromatography, which is accurate but requires a sophisticated analytic setting. Reliable and less expensive immunoassays have become available, however, that have made wider screening of homocysteine possible. Although a nonfasting evaluation of total plasma homocysteine suffices for most clinical purposes, measurement of homocysteine levels 2 to 6 hours after ingestion of an oral methionine load (0.1 gm/kg body mass) can identify individuals with impaired homocysteine metabolism despite normal fasting levels.

Despite availability of newer assays, measurement of homocysteine remains controversial and recent guidelines do not advocate their use. Several reasons suggest that this conservative approach is warranted for most patients. First, although early cross-sectional and retrospective studies reported strong positive associations between plasma homocysteine levels and risk, such study designs are subject to epidemiological bias and cannot establish a causal relationship, as homocysteine levels increase after myocardial infarction and stroke. This overestimation of effect appears to have been borne out now that a large series of prospective studies are available. In several recent meta-analyses, the magnitude and strength of association between baseline homocysteine levels and risk of subsequent disease has proven substantially smaller than previously reported.[189-192] Although there is some heterogeneity between the prospective studies, on average these meta-analyses report a 25 percent lower homocysteine level being associated with an approximate 11 percent lower risk of coronary heart disease, an estimate far smaller than hypothesized. Some of this reduction may reflect the introduction of folate fortification in 1998 to reduce the incidence of neural tube defects (see Chap. 41). However, many of the prospective studies began well before fortification and others have shown predictive value even among individuals taking and those not taking multivitamin supplements.[193] Fortification of the food supply has greatly reduced the frequency of low folate and elevated homocysteine levels, particularly for persons initially in the moderately elevated range.[194] Thus, the number of individuals potentially identifiable by general screening for homocysteine has decreased considerably.

Enthusiasm for population-based homocysteine evaluation has also been limited by a lack of evidence demonstrating that screening adds to standard lipid evaluation or to the Framingham risk score. Unlike inflammatory markers such as hsCRP, there is no evidence that homocysteine evaluation can identify high-risk populations who might benefit differentially from non-vitamin interventions such as statin therapy.[195] The cost of screening compared to the cost of folate supplementation has also been an issue. Folic acid, given in doses of up to 400 μg/day, can reduce homocysteine levels approximately 25 percent, and the addition of vitamin B12 will likely reduce levels another 7 percent.[196,197] Because this therapy is inexpensive and has low toxicity in the absence of vitamin B12 deficiency, vitamin supplementation may be a more cost-effective approach for high-risk groups than screening.[198] Finally, although several randomized trials are underway to evaluate the efficacy of folate and vitamin B supplementation to reduce vascular risk in general populations and in the setting of renal failure,[199-201] few have been reported to date, and concern has been raised that fortification may reduce the power of these trials to detect true differences.[202,203] For example, in the recent Vitamin Intervention for Stroke Prevention trial, moderate reduction in homocysteine with folic acid had no effect on vascular outcomes during two years follow-up.[203a]

There remain specific patient populations for whom homocysteine evaluation may prove appropriate, including those lacking traditional risk factors, in the setting of renal failure, or among those with premature atherosclerosis or a family history of myocardial infarction and stroke at a young age. In secondary prevention, persuasive data show that elevated homocysteine levels predict worse mortality, although no specific intervention has yet proven effective in this regard.[204,205] In the Swiss Heart Study, participants undergoing angioplasty appeared to have lower rates of restenosis, target lesion revascularization, and coronary events when given folate, vitamin B6, and vitamin B12,[206,207] although these data have not been reproduced elsewhere and predate widespread use of coronary stenting.

Current investigations are testing the potential input of homocysteine on nonthrombotic disease. Following observations in hyperhomocysteinemic hypertensive rats[208] and upon associations between homocysteine levels and extent of ventricular hypertrophy in renal failure patients,[209] investigators in the Framingham Study recently found plasma homocysteine levels to be associated with an increase in risk for congestive heart failure among adults without prior myocardial infarction.[210]

Fibrinogen and Fibrin D-Dimer

Plasma fibrinogen influences platelet aggregation and blood viscosity, interacts with plasminogen binding, and, in combination with thrombin, mediates the final step in clot formation and the response to vascular injury. In addition, fibrinogen associates positively with age, obesity, smoking, diabetes, and LDL cholesterol level, and inversely with HDL cholesterol level, alcohol use, physical activity, and exercise level.[211] Fibrinogen, like CRP, an acute phase reactant, increases during inflammatory responses.

Given these relationships, it is not surprising that fibrinogen was among the first "novel" risk factors evaluated. Early reports from the Gothenburg,[212] Northwick Park, and Framingham heart studies all found significant positive associations between fibrinogen levels and future risk of cardiovascular events. Since then, multiple other prospective studies have confirmed these findings[213,214] and in two recent meta-analyses, individuals with levels in the upper third had significantly elevated relative risks compared to those with the lowest levels (RR, 1.8; 95 percent CI, 1.6 to 2.0).[215,216] Fibrinogen levels also indicate increased risk of stroke and peripheral arterial disease.[217] In most studies, these effects were independent of other traditional risk factors, although in other settings fibrinogen was predictive only among those with concomitant elevation of lipoprotein(a)[218] or homocysteine.[219]

Despite the consistency of these data, fibrinogen evaluation has found limited use in clinical practice for several reasons. First, assay standardization for fibrinogen has been inadequate, and analytic consistency across reference laboratories remains poor. Second, at least in comparison to CRP, the predictive value of fibrinogen is modest. This likely results from a wider variation within individuals for fibrinogen levels than CRP and poorer assay characteristics for fibrinogen. Moreover, in several studies that evaluated both CRP and fibrinogen, only CRP independently predicted future vascular events.[143] Third, fibrinogen levels are elevated in certain groups, including women, persons taking estrogen, and smokers, thus complicating the interpretation of study results. Last, despite two decades of evaluation, we still lack data demonstrating additive value in risk assessment in primary prevention over Framingham scoring.

Fibrates and niacin lower fibrinogen levels but statin therapy does not, an effect different than that observed for CRP. To date, three clinical trials have evaluated the potential benefits of fibrinogen reduction, and all have found disappointing results. In the Bezafibrate Infarction Prevention Trial,[220] there was no reduction in event rates with active therapy despite a significant reduction in fibrinogen levels and despite evidence that within the study population baseline fibrinogen levels predicted vascular risk.[221] In a second trial of more than 1500 patients with peripheral vascular disease, bezafibrate reduced fibrinogen levels 13 percent but again had no significant effect on clinical outcomes.[222]

Finally, in the HERS trial and within the Women's Health Initiative, hormone replacement therapy lowered fibrinogen levels but had no benefit on outcome.[223]

Fibrin D-dimer reflects the extent of fibrin turnover in the circulation, and epidemiological evidence has found D-dimer levels to have modest predictive value for future vascular events.[224-226] As with fibrinogen, these studies, when taken together, suggest an approximate relative risk of 1.7 to 1.8 comparing those in the top to bottom thirds of the D-dimer distribution.[227] Following myocardial infarction, D-dimer levels also predict recurrent events[228] and like CRP, D-dimer predicts poor outcome in troponin-negative ischemia.[229] These studies have pathophysiological interest, and evidence has accumulated that genetic determinants of fibrinogen and D-dimer may lead to altered fibrin clot structure in susceptible individuals.[230] As with fibrinogen, however, the utility of D-dimer assessment for arterial thrombosis prediction appears limited in clinical settings. This finding contrasts markedly with the strong clinical utility of D-dimer evaluation in the setting of suspected venous thromboembolism.[231]

Markers of Fibrinolytic Function (Plasminogen Activator Inhibitor-1, Tissue Plasminogen Activator, Clot Lysis)

Impaired fibrinolysis can result from an imbalance between the clot-dissolving enzymes t-PA or urokinase-type plasminogen activator and their endogenous inhibitors, primarily PAI-1. Plasma levels of PAI-1 peak in the morning, whereas concentrations of t-PA demonstrate a less prominent circadian variation. On this basis, a relative hypofibrinolytic state may prevail in the morning that, along with increased platelet reactivity, may contribute to the increased risk of myocardial infarction seen in this time period. Visceral obesity yields enhanced PAI-1 production from adipocytes, and thus impaired fibrinolysis may help explain how weight gain and obesity influence atherothrombosis. Individuals with the insulin resistance syndrome commonly have impaired fibrinolysis, and, in the setting of metabolic syndrome, PAI-1 levels as well as CRP predict adverse vascular outcomes in addition to the onset of type 2 diabetes.[232]

Clinically, patients with isolated PAI-1 deficiencies have excess rates of hemorrhage, whereas genetically mediated PAI-1 excess may lead to spontaneous thrombosis. A consistent series of prospective studies has linked abnormalities of fibrinolysis to increased risk of arterial thrombosis. For example, prospective associations exist between PAI-1 antigen and activity levels and the risk of first and recurrent myocardial infarction. Perhaps paradoxically, individuals at risk for future coronary as well as cerebral thrombosis consistently also have elevated levels of circulating t-PA antigen.[233] These latter effects may represent evidence of underlying endothelial dysfunction among individuals at risk or a direct relationship between t-PA and PAI-1, or they may represent a biological response to impaired fibrinolysis. In this regard, reduced clot lysis time, an overall indicator of net fibrinolytic function, also predicts coronary risk. As reviewed earlier, several studies indicate that levels of D-dimer, a peptide released by plasmin's action on fibrin, also predicts myocardial infarction, peripheral atherosclerosis, and recurrent coronary events. These observations have recently been confirmed in women both taking and not taking hormone replacement therapy, an important issue because conjugated estrogens decrease PAI-1 antigen concentrations.[234,235]

Despite these data, the clinical use of fibrinolytic markers to determine coronary risk may offer marginal value, and no data available suggest that measures of fibrinolysis adds to traditional risk scores. Direct measurement of PAI-1 activity is difficult in clinical settings and requires special anticoagulants and precise phlebotomy techniques to avoid degranulation of platelets, a rich source of PAI-1. In addition, markers of fibrinolytic function such as PAI-1 have a wide circadian variation limiting use in outpatient settings as a risk determinant. Nonetheless, the recognition that fibrinolytic function contributes to atherothrombosis has yielded several practical applications. For example, PAI-1-resistant thrombolytic agents may provide a means to increase the efficacy of thrombolytic therapy for acute myocardial infarction. Further, the renin-angiotensin system plays an important role in the regulation of fibrinolysis, and angiotensin-converting enzyme inhibitors may favorably affect fibrinolytic balance.[236-238] Finally, well-described polymorphisms in the PAI-1 promoter and other components of the fibrinolytic system may contribute to interindividual differences in fibrinolytic function.[239,240]

Lipoprotein(a) (see Chap. 39)

Lipoprotein(a) consists of an LDL particle with its apo B-100 component linked by a disulfide bridge to apo(a), a variable-length protein that has sequence homology to plasminogen. The apo(a) component of lipoprotein(a) is a complex molecule composed in part of varying numbers of cysteine-rich kringle IV repeats that result in great heterogeneity. As such, plasma lipoprotein(a) concentrations vary inversely with apo(a) isoform size but also may vary even within isoform size based on differential levels of production. Underlying its molecular complexity, more than 25 heritable forms of lipoprotein(a) exist, demonstrating the importance of the genome in determining plasma levels, an important issue for risk prediction across different population groups.[241]

Although the biological function of lipoprotein(a) remains uncertain, the close homology between lipoprotein(a) and plasminogen has raised the possibility that this lipoprotein may inhibit endogenous fibrinolysis by competing with plasminogen binding on the endothelium. More recent data suggest that lipoprotein(a) binds and inactivates tissue factor pathway inhibitor and may upregulate the expression of plasminogen activator inhibitor, further linking lipoproteins and thrombosis.[242,243] Lipoprotein(a) also colocalizes within atherosclerotic lesions and may have local actions. Thus, several mechanisms may contribute to a role of lipoprotein(a) in atherothrombosis.

Although many retrospective and cross-sectional studies suggest a positive association between lipoprotein(a) and vascular risk, lipoprotein(a) levels rise after ischemia and with the acute phase response, and thus these studies cannot determine a causal relationship. A series of prospective studies that avoid this bias generally support this association, however. A recent meta-analysis of 27 prospective studies with a mean follow-up period of 10 years found that individuals with lipoprotein(a) levels in the top third of the distribution had a risk 1.6 times higher than those with lipoprotein(a) levels in the bottom third.[244] Adjustment for classic cardiovascular risk factors only modestly attenuated these effects, in part because there is little correlation between lipoprotein(a) and other markers of risk.

Whether the assessment of lipoprotein(a) truly adds prognostic information to overall risk in primary prevention remains uncertain, because in most studies lipoprotein(a) has been predictive only among those already known to be at high risk. For example, recent data from the Italian Longitudinal Study on Aging, the Prospective Cardiovascular Munster study, the Bruneck Heart Study, and the PRIME study suggest that high serum lipoprotein(a) level is an important risk factor primarily among individuals with type 2 diabetes[245,246] or overt hyperlipidemia.[247-249] Other investigators have found that lipoprotein(a) signifies elevated risk in limited situations such as the presence of hyperfibrinogenemia or elevated homocysteine level.[250,251] Several prospective evaluations have shown that lipoprotein(a) predicts risk in a nonlinear manner such that risk increases are very small until lipoprotein(a) levels within the top 5 to 10 percent are reached.[252,253] Large-scale prospective studies confirm these relationships but also find that lipoprotein(a) has modest predictive value in comparison with other novel risk factors.[142,154] Finally, some investigators have advocated lipoprotein(a) assessment in certain patient groups, such as those with established coronary disease[254] or renal failure, although data remain controversial.[255,256] Thus, in terms of general population screening, lipoprotein(a) evaluation appears to have limited utility.

Beyond these epidemiological considerations, several practical issues hamper lipoprotein(a) evaluation in clinical settings. Most importantly, standardization of commercial lipoprotein(a) assays remains problematic. A recent working group of the International Federation of Clinical Chemistry has reported that much of the inaccuracy of commercial lipoprotein(a) determination results from the use of techniques sensitive to apo(a) size.[257] Recognition of this issue, wider use of assays unaffected by apo(a) heterogeneity, and the establishment of reference standards should improve these limitations. We also have only limited data on risk prediction in non-white groups, although lipoprotein(a) levels vary widely on an ethnic basis. Finally, except for high-dose niacin, few interventions lower lipoprotein(a) level. This limitation, as well as the observation that LDL cholesterol reduction markedly reduces any hazard associated with lipoprotein(a), has also dampened enthusiasm for screening. Ongoing genetic investigation is yielding important insights into lipoprotein(a) regulation,[258] and the development of peptides that inhibit lipoprotein(a) assembly raise novel pathways for risk reduction that will require direct testing in clinical trials.[259] Evidence that children with recurrent ischemic stroke have elevated lipoprotein(a) levels also supports the potential use of this biomarker in unusual high-risk settings.[260]

Lipoprotein Subclasses, Particle Size, and Particle Concentration (see Chap. 39)

Although standard chemical measures for total and LDL cholesterol form the basis for current lipid screening and reduction guidelines, the amount of cholesterol carried by individual lipoprotein particles may influence their function and vary widely between individuals. Therefore, measures of core lipid composition and lipoprotein particle size and concentration might provide a better measure of risk prediction.[261] Several lines of evidence indicate that small LDL particles may be more atherogenic than large LDL particles and contribute to the dyslipidemia of diabetes.[262] Currently, a number of technologies are available for evaluation of LDL subclasses and particle size. Studies using density gradient ultracentrifugation and gradient gel electrophoresis have generally found that lipoprotein subclass identifies individuals at higher risk for coronary disease[263] and have successfully shown a preferential benefit of lipid-lowering therapy among patients with small, dense LDL particles as compared to large LDL particles.[264]

Recent studies have also found LDL particle concentration as measured by nuclear magnetic resonance to correlate well with coronary arterial lumen diameter after statin therapy[265] and to have predictive value for future vascular events. For example, in both the Women's Health Study[266] and the Cardiovascular Health Study,[267] LDL particle concentration measured by nuclear magnetic resonance predicted incident vascular events better than standard measurement of LDL cholesterol. These relationships remain complex, however, and have not always been consistent.[268] In addition, standardization across technologies available for lipoprotein subclassification has remained problematic. Thus, although intriguing pathophysiological information regarding lipid reduction with statins has come from studies of nuclear magnetic resonance spectroscopy as well as density gradient studies,[269] it remains unclear whether these novel methods of lipid evaluation greatly add to standard lipid screening. To date, no studies have tested whether such methods add to traditional scoring systems such as the Framingham Heart Study.

Future Directions in Cardiovascular Risk Assessment

Some 40 percent of the U.S. adult population is at "intermediate risk" but do not currently qualify for intensive risk factor intervention despite the presence of one or more traditional risk factors.[270] In the immediate future, the most important novel tool to improve risk stratification among these individuals will be the inflammatory biomarker hsCRP as an adjunct to global risk prediction. As reviewed earlier, strong evidence shows that hsCRP adds prognostic information at all levels of LDL cholesterol, at all levels of the Framingham risk score, and at all levels of the metabolic syndrome. Thus, hsCRP evaluation, along with standard lipid screening, will likely become common practice in the near future. Ongoing trials based on hsCRP evaluation will also probably have an impact on clinical practice guidelines.[157] The pathophysiological implications that follow from the inflammatory hypothesis of atherothrombosis should lead to novel interventions for primary prevention as well as the treatment of acute ischemia.

Direct Plaque Imaging

Aside from the use of inflammatory markers such as hsCRP, future strategies to detect vascular disease will likely take several forms. Most prominent may be the noninvasive detection of atherosclerotic plaque. At this time, a number of studies indicate that coronary calcification as detected by computed tomography can detect high-risk individuals and perhaps permit monitoring of lipid-lowering therapy.[271,272] It remains highly controversial, however, as to whether this approach is cost-effective or has an acceptable false-negative rate.[273] Enrollment in many such studies may be biased by referral patterns or self-selection by patients. Part of the difficulty with coronary calcification as a clinical surrogate is that CT imaging probably detects the very plaques least likely to rupture and does not detect the noncalcified, thin-walled lesions that appear to cause most clinical events. Thus, while coronary calcium provides a noninvasive measure of atherosclerotic burden, patients with low calcium scores cannot be dismissed as being at low risk. Further, the clinical determinants of calcification are largely unknown and may not reflect propensity to plaque rupture. Recent data demonstrating that hsCRP elevation corresponds to an approximate doubling of risk of plaque rupture at all levels of coronary calcium demonstrates the complexity of this approach.[274] Considerable public health concern has also been raised regarding the consequences of false-positive findings from imaging techniques such as coronary calcium scores. For example, in one recent study of currently asymptomatic individuals, 41 percent of all future vascular events occurred among those with coronary artery calcium scores (CACS) less than 100 and 17 percent occurred among those with CACS of zero.[274a] Thus, absence of CACS does not preclude risk of coronary events. Current guidelines do not support the routine use of coronary computed tomographic imaging.

A recent study showed that provision of calcium scores did not effectively motivate patients' adherence to risk reduction regimens.[275] Several other modalities for the noninvasive assessment of atherosclerosis are also available, ranging from those that are well documented and inexpensive (such as the ankle-brachial index) to those that are exploratory (such as thermography and magnetic resonance scanning). Perhaps the best studied noninvasive approach is the ultrasonic measurement of carotid intimal medial thickness. While somewhat operator dependent, this technique has proved to have strong predictive value in general population studies,[276,277] and no additional expense is required because most centers already have the required sonographic tools in place. Although carotid intimal medial thickness undoubtedly provides a valid research tool, its practical applicability in practice remains unproven. Whether any imaging technique will prove cost-effective as a screening tool is currently under study in the Multiethnic Study of Atherosclerosis (MESA) being funded by the National Heart, Lung, and Blood Institute.[278]

Genomic and Proteomic Approaches

The availability of a wide array of genetic data should also change coronary risk prediction in the future, and many large-scale evaluations of polymorphism and haplotype patterns designed to understand better the atherothrombotic process are well underway. For venous thrombosis, genetic detection of factor V Leiden and of a common promoter polymorphism in the prothrombin gene have already entered wide clinical practice. Proteomic studies that go a step further and evaluate all the products of these genes (and their post-transcriptional changes) have also already had an impact in our understanding of venous thromboembolism. By contrast, although family history contributes importantly to determining risk of myocardial infarction or stroke, studies of single nucleotide polymorphisms in arterial thrombosis have largely been disappointing to date. Continued methodological concerns about the reproducibility of published results and generalizability to usual populations suggest that the use of genetic data to predict arterial risk will take several more years of research to come to fruition. However, there is little doubt that major gene-environment and gene-gene interactions exist that, when carefully uncovered, will lead to novel methods of detection and prevention.

REFERENCES

1. Annual smoking-attributable mortality, years of potential life lost, and economic costs—United States, 1995-1999. MMWR Morb Mortal Wkly Rep 51:300, 2002.
2. U.S. Department of Health and Human Services: Women and Smoking. A Report of the Surgeon General. Rockville, Md, U.S. Department of Health and Human Services, Public Health Service, Office of the Surgeon General, 2001.
3. Cigarette smoking among adults—United States, 2000. MMWR Morb Mortal Wkly Rep 51:642, 2002.
4. Incidence of initiation of cigarette smoking—United States, 1965-1996. MMWR Morb Mortal Wkly Rep 47:837, 1998.
5. Peto R, Lopez AD, Boreham J, et al: Mortality from smoking worldwide. Br Med Bull 52:12, 1996.
6. Kawachi I, Colditz GA, Speizer FE, et al: A prospective study of passive smoking and coronary heart disease. Circulation 95:2374, 1997.
7. He J, Vupputuri S, Allen K, et al: Passive smoking and the risk of coronary heart disease: A meta-analysis of epidemiologic studies. N Engl J Med 340:920, 1999.
8. Otsuka R, Watanabe H, Hirata K, et al: Acute effects of passive smoking on the coronary circulation in healthy young adults. JAMA 286:436, 2001.
9. Janson C, Chinn S, Jarvis D, et al: Effect of passive smoking on respiratory symptoms, bronchial responsiveness, lung function, and total serum IgE in the European Community Respiratory Health Survey: A cross-sectional study. Lancet 358:2103, 2001.
10. Prescott E, Scharling H, Osler M, Schnohr P: Importance of light smoking and inhalation habits on risk of myocardial infarction and all cause mortality: A 22 year follow up of 12,149 men and women in The Copenhagen City Heart Study. J Epidemiol Community Health 56:702, 2002.
11. Kurth T, Kase CS, Berger K, et al: Smoking and the risk of hemorrhagic stroke in men. Stroke 34:1151, 2003.
12. Rea TD, Heckbert SR, Kaplan RC, et al: Smoking status and risk for recurrent coronary events after myocardial infarction. Ann Intern Med 137:494, 2002.
13. Al-Delaimy WK, Manson JE, Solomon CG, et al: Smoking and risk of coronary heart disease among women with type 2 diabetes mellitus. Arch Intern Med 162:273, 2002.
14. Howard G, Wagenknecht LE, Burke GL, et al: Cigarette smoking and progression of atherosclerosis: The Atherosclerosis Risk in Communities (ARIC) Study. JAMA 279:119, 1998.
15. Barua RS, Ambrose JA, Srivastava S, et al: Reactive oxygen species are involved in smoking-induced dysfunction of nitric oxide biosynthesis and upregulation of endothelial nitric oxide synthase: An in vitro demonstration in human coronary artery endothelial cells. Circulation 107:2342, 2003.
16. Barua RS, Ambrose JA, Eales-Reynolds LJ, et al: Dysfunctional endothelial nitric oxide biosynthesis in healthy smokers with impaired endothelium-dependent vasodilatation. Circulation 104:1905, 2001.
17. Tsuchiya M, Asada A, Kasahara E, et al: Smoking a single cigarette rapidly reduces combined concentrations of nitrate and nitrite and concentrations of antioxidants in plasma. Circulation 105:1155, 2002.
18. Tracy RP, Psaty BM, Macy E, et al: Lifetime smoking exposure affects the association of C-reactive protein with cardiovascular disease risk factors and subclinical disease in healthy elderly subjects. Arterioscler Thromb Vasc Biol 17:2167, 1997.
19. Blann AD, Steele C, McCollum CN: The influence of smoking on soluble adhesion molecules and endothelial cell markers. Thromb Res 85:433, 1997.
20. Bazzano LA, He J, Muntner P, et al: Relationship between cigarette smoking and novel risk factors for cardiovascular disease in the United States. Ann Intern Med 138:891, 2003.
21. Fusegawa Y, Goto S, Handa S, et al: Platelet spontaneous aggregation in platelet-rich plasma is increased in habitual smokers. Thromb Res 93:271, 1999.
22. Adams MR, Jessup W, Celermajer DS: Cigarette smoking is associated with increased human monocyte adhesion to endothelial cells: Reversibility with oral L-arginine but not vitamin C. J Am Coll Cardiol 29:491, 1997.
23. Newby DE, McLeod AL, Uren NG, et al: Impaired coronary tissue plasminogen activator release is associated with coronary atherosclerosis and cigarette smoking: Direct link between endothelial dysfunction and atherothrombosis. Circulation 103:1936, 2001.
24. Matetzky S, Tani S, Kangavari S, et al: Smoking increases tissue factor expression in atherosclerotic plaques: Implications for plaque thrombogenicity. Circulation 102:602, 2000.
25. Barua RS, Ambrose JA, Saha DC, Eales-Reynolds LJ: Smoking is associated with altered endothelial-derived fibrinolytic and antithrombotic factors: An in vitro demonstration. Circulation 106:905, 2002.
26. Reaven G, Tsao PS: Insulin resistance and compensatory hyperinsulinemia: The key player between cigarette smoking and cardiovascular disease? J Am Coll Cardiol 41:1044, 2003.
27. Critchley JA, Capewell S: Mortality risk reduction associated with smoking cessation in patients with coronary heart disease: A systematic review. JAMA 290:86, 2003.
28. van Domburg RT, Meeter K, van Berkel DF, et al: Smoking cessation reduces mortality after coronary artery bypass surgery: A 20-year follow-up study. J Am Coll Cardiol 36:878, 2000.
29. Lightwood JM, Glantz SA: Short-term economic and health benefits of smoking cessation: Myocardial infarction and stroke. Circulation 96:1089, 1997.
30. Hu FB, Stampfer MJ, Manson JE, et al: Trends in the incidence of coronary heart disease and changes in diet and lifestyle in women. N Engl J Med 343:530, 2000.
31. The Tobacco Use and Dependence Clinical Practice Guideline Panel, Staff, and Consortium Representatives: A clinical practice guideline for treating tobacco use and dependence: A U.S. Public Health Service report. JAMA 283:3244, 2000.
32. Godtfredsen NS, Holst C, Prescott E, et al: Smoking reduction, smoking cessation, and mortality: A 16-year follow-up of 19,732 men and women from The Copenhagen Centre for Prospective Population Studies. Am J Epidemiol 156:994, 2002.
33. Landman A, Ling PM, Glantz SA: Tobacco industry youth smoking prevention programs: Protecting the industry and hurting tobacco control. Am J Public Health 92:917, 2002.
34. Neuman M, Bitton A, Glantz S: Tobacco industry strategies for influencing European Community tobacco advertising legislation. Lancet 359:1323, 2002.
35. Chobanian AV, Bakris GL, Black HR, et al: The Seventh Report of the Joint National Committee on Prevention, Detection, Evaluation, and Treatment of High Blood Pressure: The JNC 7 report. JAMA 289:2560, 2003.
36. Hajjar I, Kotchen TA: Trends in prevalence, awareness, treatment, and control of hypertension in the United States, 1988-2000. JAMA 290:199, 2003.
37. Wolf-Maier K, Cooper RS, Banegas JR, et al: Hypertension prevalence and blood pressure levels in 6 European countries, Canada, and the United States. JAMA 289:2363, 2003.
38. Glynn RJ, L'Italien GJ, Sesso HD, et al: Development of predictive models for long-term cardiovascular risk associated with systolic and diastolic blood pressure. Hypertension 39:105, 2002.
39. Domanski M, Mitchell G, Pfeffer M, et al: Pulse pressure and cardiovascular disease-related mortality: Follow-up study of the Multiple Risk Factor Intervention Trial (MRFIT). JAMA 287:2677, 2002.
40. Staessen JA, Gasowski J, Wang JG, et al: Risks of untreated and treated isolated systolic hypertension in the elderly: Meta-analysis of outcome trials. Lancet 355:865, 2000.
41. O'Donnell CJ, Ridker PM, Glynn RJ, et al: Hypertension and borderline isolated systolic hypertension increase risks of cardiovascular disease and mortality in male physicians. Circulation 95:1132, 1997.
42. Vasan RS, Larson MG, Leip EP, et al: Impact of high-normal blood pressure on the risk of cardiovascular disease. N Engl J Med 345:1291, 2001.
43. Mitchell GF, Moye LA, Braunwald E, et al: Sphygmomanometrically determined pulse pressure is a powerful independent predictor of recurrent events after myocardial infarction in patients with impaired left ventricular function. SAVE investigators. Survival and Ventricular Enlargement. Circulation 96:4254, 1997.
44. Chae CU, Pfeffer MA, Glynn RJ, et al: Increased pulse pressure and risk of heart failure in the elderly. JAMA 281:634, 1999.
45. Vaccarino V, Holford TR, Krumholz HM: Pulse pressure and risk for myocardial infarction and heart failure in the elderly. J Am Coll Cardiol 36:130, 2000.
46. Haider AW, Larson MG, Franklin SS, Levy D: Systolic blood pressure, diastolic blood pressure, and pulse pressure as predictors of risk for congestive heart failure in the Framingham Heart Study. Ann Intern Med 138:10, 2003.
47. Staessen JA, Thijs L, Fagard R, et al: Predicting cardiovascular risk using conventional vs ambulatory blood pressure in older patients with systolic hypertension. Systolic Hypertension in Europe Trial Investigators. JAMA 282:539, 1999.
48. Bjorklund K, Lind L, Zethelius B, et al: Isolated ambulatory hypertension predicts cardiovascular morbidity in elderly men. Circulation 107:1297, 2003.
49. Liu L, Wang JG, Gong L, et al: Comparison of active treatment and placebo in older Chinese patients with isolated systolic hypertension. Systolic Hypertension in China (Syst-China) Collaborative Group. J Hypertens 16:1823, 1998.
50. SHEP Cooperative Research Group: Prevention of stroke by antihypertensive drug treatment in older persons with isolated systolic hypertension: Final results of the Systolic Hypertension in the Elderly Program (SHEP). JAMA 265:3255, 1991.
51. Staessen JA, Fagard R, Thijs L, et al: Randomised double-blind comparison of placebo and active treatment for older patients with isolated systolic hypertension. The Systolic Hypertension in Europe (Syst-Eur) Trial Investigators. Lancet 350:757, 1997.
52. Mehler PS, Coll JR, Estacio R, et al: Intensive blood pressure control reduces the risk of cardiovascular events in patients with peripheral arterial disease and type 2 diabetes. Circulation 107:753, 2003.

53. Whelton PK, Appel LJ, Espeland MA, et al: Sodium reduction and weight loss in the treatment of hypertension in older persons: A randomized controlled trial of nonpharmacologic interventions in the elderly (TONE). TONE Collaborative Research Group. JAMA 279:839, 1998.
54. Psaty BM, Lumley T, Furberg CD, et al: Health outcomes associated with various antihypertensive therapies used as first-line agents: A network meta-analysis. JAMA 289:2534, 2003.
55. Law MR, Wald NJ, Morris JK, Jordan RE: Value of low dose combination treatment with blood pressure lowering drugs: Analysis of 354 randomised trials. BMJ 326:1427, 2003.
56. Libby P, Aikawa M, Schonbeck U: Cholesterol and atherosclerosis. Biochim Biophys Acta 1529:299, 2000.
56a. Nissen SE, Tuzcu EM, Schoenhagen P, et al: Effect of intensive compared with moderate lipid-lowering therapy on progression of coronary atherosclerosis. JAMA 291:1071, 2004.
56b. Cannon CP, Braunwald E, McCabe CH, et al: Intensive versus moderate lipid lowering with statins after acute coronary syndromes. N Engl J Med 350:1495, 2004.
57. Stamler J, Daviglus ML, Garside DB, et al: Relationship of baseline serum cholesterol levels in 3 large cohorts of younger men to long-term coronary, cardiovascular, and all-cause mortality and to longevity. JAMA 284:311, 2000.
58. Grundy SM, Howard B, Smith S Jr, et al: Prevention Conference VI: Diabetes and Cardiovascular Disease: Executive summary: Conference proceeding for healthcare professionals from a special writing group of the American Heart Association. Circulation 105:2231, 2002.
59. Howard BV, Rodriguez BL, Bennett PH, et al: Prevention Conference VI: Diabetes and Cardiovascular disease: Writing Group I: Epidemiology. Circulation 105:e132, 2002.
60. Gu K, Cowie CC, Harris MI: Mortality in adults with and without diabetes in a national cohort of the U.S. population, 1971-1993. Diabetes Care 21:1138, 1998.
61. Hu FB, Stampfer MJ, Haffner SM, et al: Elevated risk of cardiovascular disease prior to clinical diagnosis of type 2 diabetes. Diabetes Care 25:1129, 2002.
62. Gillum RF, Mussolino ME, Madans JH: Diabetes mellitus, coronary heart disease incidence, and death from all causes in African American and European American women: The NHANES I epidemiologic follow-up study. J Clin Epidemiol 53:511, 2000.
63. Garber AJ: Attenuating CV risk factors in patients with diabetes: Clinical evidence to clinical practice. Diabetes Obes Metab 4(Suppl 1):S5, 2002.
64. Henry P, Thomas F, Benetos A, Guize L: Impaired fasting glucose, blood pressure and cardiovascular disease mortality. Hypertension 40:458, 2002.
65. Kuller LH, Velentgas P, Barzilay J, et al: Diabetes mellitus: Subclinical cardiovascular disease and risk of incident cardiovascular disease and all-cause mortality. Arterioscler Thromb Vasc Biol 20:823, 2000.
66. Executive Summary of the Third Report of the National Cholesterol Education Program (NCEP) Expert Panel on Detection, Evaluation, and Treatment of High Blood Cholesterol in Adults (Adult Treatment Panel III). JAMA 285:2486, 2001.
67. Ford ES, Giles WH, Dietz WH: Prevalence of the metabolic syndrome among U.S. adults: Findings from the third National Health and Nutrition Examination Survey. JAMA 287:356, 2002.
68. Lakka HM, Laaksonen DE, Lakka TA, et al: The metabolic syndrome and total and cardiovascular disease mortality in middle-aged men. JAMA 288:2709, 2002.
69. Isomaa B, Almgren P, Tuomi T, et al: Cardiovascular morbidity and mortality associated with the metabolic syndrome. Diabetes Care 24:683, 2001.
70. Ridker PM, Buring JE, Cook NR, Rifai N: C-reactive protein, the metabolic syndrome, and risk of incident cardiovascular events: An 8-year follow-up of 14,719 initially healthy American women. Circulation 107:391, 2003.
71. Pradhan AD, Manson JE, Rifai N, et al: C-reactive protein, interleukin 6, and risk of developing type 2 diabetes mellitus. JAMA 286:327, 2001.
72. Freeman DJ, Norrie J, Caslake MJ, et al: C-reactive protein is an independent predictor of risk for the development of diabetes in the West of Scotland Coronary Prevention Study. Diabetes 51:1596, 2002.
73. Albert CM, Campos H, Stampfer MJ, et al: Blood levels of long-chain n-3 fatty acids and the risk of sudden death. N Engl J Med 346:1113, 2002.
74. Barzilay JI, Abraham L, Heckbert SR, et al: The relation of markers of inflammation to the development of glucose disorders in the elderly: The Cardiovascular Health Study. Diabetes 50:2384, 2001.
74a. Hu FB, Meiss JB, Li TY, et al: Inflammatory markers and risk of developing type 2 diabetes in women. Diabetes 53:693, 2004.
75. Sattar N, Gaw A, Scherbakova O, et al: Metabolic syndrome with and without C-reactive protein as a predictor of coronary heart disease and diabetes in the West of Scotland Coronary Prevention Study. Circulation 108:414, 2003.
76. Pradhan AD, Cook NR, Buring JE, et al: C-reactive protein is independently associated with fasting insulin in nondiabetic women. Arterioscler Thromb Vasc Biol 23:650, 2003.
77. Festa A, D'Agostino R Jr, Howard G, et al: Chronic subclinical inflammation as part of the insulin resistance syndrome: The Insulin Resistance Atherosclerosis Study (IRAS). Circulation 102:42, 2000.
78. Pradhan AD, Ridker PM: Do atherosclerosis and type 2 diabetes share a common inflammatory basis? Eur Heart J 23:831, 2002.
79. Bierhaus A, Hofmann MA, Ziegler R, Nawroth PP: AGEs and their interaction with AGE-receptors in vascular disease and diabetes mellitus. I. The AGE concept. Cardiovasc Res 37:586, 1998.
80. Wautier JL, Guillausseau PJ: Diabetes, advanced glycation endproducts and vascular disease. Vasc Med 3:131, 1998.
81. Eckel RH, Wassef M, Chait A, et al: Prevention Conference VI: Diabetes and Cardiovascular Disease: Writing Group II: Pathogenesis of atherosclerosis in diabetes. Circulation 105:e138, 2002.
82. Valmadrid CT, Klein R, Moss SE, Klein BE: The risk of cardiovascular disease mortality associated with microalbuminuria and gross proteinuria in persons with older-onset diabetes mellitus. Arch Intern Med 160:1093, 2000.
83. Sobel BE: Effects of glycemic control and other determinants on vascular disease in type 2 diabetes. Am J Med 113(Suppl 6A):12S, 2002.
84. Varo N, Vicent D, Libby P, et al: Elevated plasma levels of the atherogenic mediator soluble CD40 ligand in diabetic patients: A novel target of thiazolidinediones. Circulation 107:2664, 2003.
85. Beckman JA, Creager MA, Libby P: Diabetes and atherosclerosis: Epidemiology, pathophysiology, and management. JAMA 287:2570, 2002.
86. Thompson PD, Buchner D, Pina IL, et al: Exercise and physical activity in the prevention and treatment of atherosclerotic cardiovascular disease: A statement from the Council on Clinical Cardiology (Subcommittee on Exercise, Rehabilitation, and Prevention) and the Council on Nutrition, Physical Activity, and Metabolism (Subcommittee on Physical Activity). Circulation 107:3109, 2003.
87. Manson JE, Greenland P, LaCroix AZ, et al: Walking compared with vigorous exercise for the prevention of cardiovascular events in women. N Engl J Med 347:716, 2002.
88. Manson JE, Hu FB, Rich-Edwards JW, et al: A prospective study of walking as compared with vigorous exercise in the prevention of coronary heart disease in women. N Engl J Med 341:650, 1999.
89. Tanasescu M, Leitzmann MF, Rimm EB, et al: Exercise type and intensity in relation to coronary heart disease in men. JAMA 288:1994, 2002.
90. Lee IM, Sesso HD, Paffenbarger RS Jr: Physical activity and coronary heart disease risk in men: Does the duration of exercise episodes predict risk? Circulation 102:981, 2000.
91. Hu FB, Stampfer MJ, Colditz GA, et al: Physical activity and risk of stroke in women. JAMA 283:2961, 2000.
92. Lee IM, Rexrode KM, Cook NR, et al: Physical activity and coronary heart disease in women: Is "no pain, no gain" passe? JAMA 285:1447, 2001.
93. Pate RR, Pratt M, Blair SN, et al: Physical activity and public health: A recommendation from the Centers for Disease Control and Prevention and the American College of Sports Medicine. JAMA 273:402, 1995.
94. Schoenborn CA, Barnes PM: Leisure-time physical activity among adults: United States, 1997-98. Advanced data from vital and health statistics; no.325. Hyattsville, Md, National Center for Health Statistics, 2002.
95. Institute of Medicine: Dietary reference intakes for energy, carbohydrates, fiber, fat, protein, and amino acids. Washington, DC, The National Academies Press, 2002.
96. Irwin ML, Yasui Y, Ulrich CM, et al: Effect of exercise on total and intra-abdominal body fat in postmenopausal women: A randomized controlled trial. JAMA 289:323, 2003.
97. Whelton SP, Chin A, Xin X, He J: Effect of aerobic exercise on blood pressure: A meta-analysis of randomized, controlled trials. Ann Intern Med 136:493, 2002.
98. Kelley GA, Kelley KS, Tran ZV: Walking and resting blood pressure in adults: A meta-analysis. Prev Med 33:120, 2001.
99. Kraus WE, Houmard JA, Duscha BD, et al: Effects of the amount and intensity of exercise on plasma lipoproteins. N Engl J Med 347:1483, 2002.
100. Boule NG, Haddad E, Kenny GP, et al: Effects of exercise on glycemic control and body mass in type 2 diabetes mellitus: A meta-analysis of controlled clinical trials. JAMA 286:1218, 2001.
101. Hu FB, Sigal RJ, Rich-Edwards JW, et al: Walking compared with vigorous physical activity and risk of type 2 diabetes in women: A prospective study. JAMA 282:1433, 1999.
102. Knowler WC, Barrett-Connor E, Fowler SE, et al: Reduction in the incidence of type 2 diabetes with lifestyle intervention or metformin. N Engl J Med 346:393, 2002.
103. Ford ES: Does exercise reduce inflammation? Physical activity and C-reactive protein among U.S. adults. Epidemiology 13:561, 2002.
104. Hambrecht R, Wolf A, Gielen S, et al: Effect of exercise on coronary endothelial function in patients with coronary artery disease. N Engl J Med 342:454, 2000.
105. Wannamethee SG, Lowe GD, Whincup PH, et al: Physical activity and hemostatic and inflammatory variables in elderly men. Circulation 105:1785, 2002.
106. Rexrode KM, Carey VJ, Hennekens CH, et al: Abdominal adiposity and coronary heart disease in women. JAMA 280:1843, 1998.
107. Flegal KM, Carroll MD, Ogden CL, Johnson CL: Prevalence and trends in obesity among U.S. adults, 1999-2000. JAMA 288:1723, 2002.
108. Ogden CL, Flegal KM, Carroll MD, Johnson CL: Prevalence and trends in overweight among U.S. children and adolescents, 1999-2000. JAMA 288:1728, 2002.
109. Ghiadoni L, Donald AE, Cropley M, et al: Mental stress induces transient endothelial dysfunction in humans. Circulation 102:2473, 2000.
110. Brunner EJ, Hemingway H, Walker BR, et al: Adrenocortical, autonomic, and inflammatory causes of the metabolic syndrome: Nested case-control study. Circulation 106:2659, 2002.
111. Hjemdahl P: Stress and the metabolic syndrome: An interesting but enigmatic association. Circulation 106:2634, 2002.
112. Lampert R, Jain D, Burg MM, et al: Destabilizing effects of mental stress on ventricular arrhythmias in patients with implantable cardioverter-defibrillators. Circulation 101:158, 2000.
113. Lampert R, Joska T, Burg MM, et al: Emotional and physical precipitants of ventricular arrhythmia. Circulation 106:1800, 2002.
114. Krantz DS, Santiago HT, Kop WJ, et al: Prognostic value of mental stress testing in coronary artery disease. Am J Cardiol 84:1292, 1999.
115. Krantz DS, Sheps DS, Carney RM, Natelson BH: Effects of mental stress in patients with coronary artery disease: Evidence and clinical implications. JAMA 283:1800, 2000.
116. Kivimaki M, Leino-Arjas P, Luukkonen R, et al: Work stress and risk of cardiovascular mortality: Prospective cohort study of industrial employees. BMJ 325:857, 2002.
117. Iso H, Date C, Yamamoto A, et al: Perceived mental stress and mortality from cardiovascular disease among Japanese men and women: The Japan Collaborative Cohort Study for Evaluation of Cancer Risk Sponsored by Monbusho (JACC Study). Circulation 106:1229, 2002.
118. Rugulies R: Depression as a predictor for coronary heart disease: A review and meta-analysis. Am J Prev Med 23:51, 2002.
119. Wulsin LR, Singal BM: Do depressive symptoms increase the risk for the onset of coronary disease? A systematic quantitative review. Psychosom Med 65:201, 2003.

120. Bush DE, Ziegelstein RC, Tayback M, et al: Even minimal symptoms of depression increase mortality risk after acute myocardial infarction. Am J Cardiol 88:337, 2001.
121. Glassman AH, O'Connor CM, Califf RM, et al: Sertraline treatment of major depression in patients with acute MI or unstable angina. JAMA 288:701, 2002.
122. Berkman LF, Blumenthal J, Burg M, et al: Effects of treating depression and low perceived social support on clinical events after myocardial infarction: The Enhancing Recovery in Coronary Heart Disease Patients (ENRICHD) Randomized Trial. JAMA 289:3106, 2003.
123. Frasure-Smith N, Lesperance F: Depression: A cardiac risk factor in search of a treatment. JAMA 289:3171, 2003.
124. Ridker PM, Rifai N, Rose L, et al: Comparison of C-reactive protein and low-density lipoprotein cholesterol levels in the prediction of first cardiovascular events. N Engl J Med 347:1557, 2002.
125. Khot UN, Khot MB, Bajzer CT, et al: Prevalence of conventional risk factors in patients with coronary heart disease. JAMA 290:898, 2003.
126. Greenland P, Knoll MD, Stamler J, et al: Major risk factors as antecedents of fatal and nonfatal coronary heart disease events. JAMA 290:891, 2003.
127. Ridker PM: Evaluating novel cardiovascular risk factors: Can we better predict heart attacks? Ann Intern Med 130:933, 1999.
128. Hackam DG, Anand SS: Emerging risk factors for atherosclerotic vascular disease: A critical review of the evidence. JAMA 290:932, 2003.
129. Libby P, Ridker PM, Maseri A: Inflammation and atherosclerosis. Circulation 105:1135, 2002.
130. Buffon A, Biasucci LM, Liuzzo G, et al: Widespread coronary inflammation in unstable angina. N Engl J Med 347:5, 2002.
131. Ridker PM: Clinical application of C-reactive protein for cardiovascular disease detection and prevention. Circulation 107:363, 2003.
132. Calabro P, Willerson JT, Yeh ET: Inflammatory cytokines stimulated C-reactive protein production by human coronary artery smooth muscle cells. Circulation 108:1930, 2003.
133. Jabs WJ, Theissing E, Nitschke M, et al: Local generation of C-reactive protein in diseased coronary artery venous bypass grafts and normal vascular tissue. Circulation 108:1428, 2003.
134. Pasceri V, Willerson JT, Yeh ET: Direct proinflammatory effect of C-reactive protein on human endothelial cells. Circulation 102:2165, 2000.
135. Zwaka TP, Hombach V, Torzewski J: C-reactive protein-mediated low density lipoprotein uptake by macrophages: Implications for atherosclerosis. Circulation 103:1194, 2001.
136. Venugopal SK, Devaraj S, Yuhanna I, et al: Demonstration that C-reactive protein decreases eNOS expression and bioactivity in human aortic endothelial cells. Circulation 106:1439, 2002.
137. Devaraj S, Xu DY, Jialal I: C-reactive protein increases plasminogen activator inhibitor-1 expression and activity in human aortic endothelial cells: Implications for the metabolic syndrome and atherothrombosis. Circulation 107:398, 2003.
138. Danenberg HD, Szalai AJ, Swaminathan RV, et al: Increased thrombosis after arterial injury in human C-reactive protein-transgenic mice. Circulation 108:512, 2003.
138a. Paul A, Ko KW, Yechoor V, et al: C-reactive protein accelerates the progression of atherosclerosis in apolipoprotein E-deficient mice. Circulation 109:647, 2004.
139. Pradhan AD, Manson JE, Rossouw JE, et al: Inflammatory biomarkers, hormone replacement therapy, and incident coronary heart disease: Prospective analysis from the Women's Health Initiative observational study. JAMA 288:980, 2002.
140. Albert CM, Ma J, Rifai N, et al: Prospective study of C-reactive protein, homocysteine, and plasma lipid levels as predictors of sudden cardiac death. Circulation 105:2595, 2002.
141. Ridker PM, Cushman M, Stampfer MJ, et al: Inflammation, aspirin, and the risk of cardiovascular disease in apparently healthy men. N Engl J Med 336:973, 1997.
142. Ridker PM, Hennekens CH, Buring JE, Rifai N: C-reactive protein and other markers of inflammation in the prediction of cardiovascular disease in women. N Engl J Med 342:836, 2000.
143. Ridker PM, Stampfer MJ, Rifai N: Novel risk factors for systemic atherosclerosis: A comparison of C-reactive protein, fibrinogen, homocysteine, lipoprotein(a), and standard cholesterol screening as predictors of peripheral arterial disease. JAMA 285:2481, 2001.
144. Albert MA, Glynn RJ, Ridker PM: Plasma concentration of C-reactive protein and the calculated Framingham Coronary Heart Disease Risk Score. Circulation 108:161, 2003.
144a. Ballantyne CM, Hoogeveen RC, Bang H, et al: Lipoprotein-associated phospholipase A2, high-sensitivity C-reactive protein, and risk for incident coronary heart disease in middle-aged men and women in the Atherosclerosis Risk In Communities (ARIC) Study. Circulation 109:837, 2004.
144b. Koenig W, Löwel H, Baumert J, Meisinger C: C-reactive protein modulates risk prediction based on the Framingham Score: Implications for future risk assessment. Circulation 109:1349, 2004.
144c. Danesh J, Wheeler JG, Hirschfield GM, et al: C-reactive protein and other circulating markers of inflammation in the prediction of coronary heart disease. N Engl J Med 350:1387, 2004.
145. Pearson TA, Mensah GA, Alexander RW, et al: Markers of inflammation and cardiovascular disease: Application to clinical and public health practice: A statement for healthcare professionals from the Centers for Disease Control and Prevention and the American Heart Association. Circulation 107:499, 2003.
145a. Ridker PM, Cook N. Clinical usefulness of very high and very low levels of C-reactive protein across the full range of Framingham risk scores. Circulation 109:1955, 2004.
146. Ridker PM, Rifai N, Pfeffer MA, et al: Inflammation, pravastatin, and the risk of coronary events after myocardial infarction in patients with average cholesterol levels. Cholesterol and Recurrent Events (CARE) Investigators. Circulation 98:839, 1998.
147. Liuzzo G, Biasucci LM, Gallimore JR, et al: The prognostic value of C-reactive protein and serum amyloid a protein in severe unstable angina. N Engl J Med 331:417, 1994.
148. Mueller C, Buettner HJ, Hodgson JM, et al: Inflammation and long-term mortality afte non-ST elevation acute coronary syndrome treated with a very early invasive strateg in 1042 consecutive patients. Circulation 105:1412, 2002.
149. Milazzo D, Biasucci LM, Luciani N, et al: Elevated levels of C-reactive protein befor coronary artery bypass grafting predict recurrence of ischemic events. Am J Cardic 84:459, A9, 1999.
150. Chew DP, Bhatt DL, Robbins MA, et al: Incremental prognostic value of elevated base line C-reactive protein among established markers of risk in percutaneous coronar intervention. Circulation 104:992, 2001.
151. Lindahl B, Toss H, Siegbahn A, et al: Markers of myocardial damage and inflamma tion in relation to long-term mortality in unstable coronary artery disease. FRISC Stud Group. Fragmin during Instability in Coronary Artery Disease. N Engl J Med 343:1139 2000.
152. Lindmark E, Diderholm E, Wallentin L, Siegbahn A: Relationship between interleuki 6 and mortality in patients with unstable coronary artery disease: Effects of an earl invasive or noninvasive strategy. JAMA 286:2107, 2001.
153. Dibra A, Mehilli J, Braun S, et al: Association between C-reactive protein levels anc subsequent cardiac events among patients with stable angina treated with coronary artery stenting. Am J Med 114:715, 2003.
154. Albert MA, Danielson E, Rifai N, Ridker PM: Effect of statin therapy on C-reactive protein levels: The pravastatin inflammation/CRP evaluation (PRINCE): A randomizec trial and cohort study. JAMA 286:64, 2001.
155. Ridker PM, Rifai N, Pfeffer MA, et al: Long-term effects of pravastatin on plasma con centration of C-reactive protein. The Cholesterol and Recurrent Events (CARE) Inves tigators. Circulation 100:230, 1999.
156. Ridker PM, Rifai N, Clearfield M, et al: Measurement of C-reactive protein for the tar geting of statin therapy in the primary prevention of acute coronary events. N Engl Med 344:1959, 2001.
157. Ridker PM: Rosuvastatin in the primary prevention of cardiovascular disease among patients with low LDL cholesterol and elevated high sensitivity C-reactive proteir (hsCRP): Rationale and design of the JUPITER trial. Circulation 108:2292, 2003.
158. Burke AP, Tracy RP, Kolodgie F, et al: Elevated C-reactive protein values and atherosclerosis in sudden coronary death: Association with different pathologies. Circulation 105:2019, 2002.
159. Sesso HD, Buring JE, Rifai N, et al: C-reactive protein and the risk of developing hypertension: Is hypertension an inflammatory disease? JAMA 290:2945, 2003.
160. Blake GJ, Rifai N, Buring JE, Ridker PM: Blood pressure, C-reactive protein, and risk of future cardiovascular events. Circulation 108:2993, 2003.
161. Labarrere CA, Lee JB, Nelson DR, et al: C-reactive protein, arterial endothelial activation, and development of transplant coronary artery disease: A prospective study. Lancet 360:1462, 2002.
162. Wanner C, Zimmermann J, Schwedler S, Metzger T: Inflammation and cardiovascular risk in dialysis patients. Kidney Int Suppl 80:99, May 2002.
163. O'Connor CM, Dunne MW, Pfeffer MA, et al: Azithromycin for the secondary prevention of coronary heart disease events: The WIZARD study: A randomized controlled trial. JAMA 290:1459, 2003.
164. Ridker PM: Cardiology Patient Page. C-reactive protein: A simple test to help predict risk of heart attack and stroke. Circulation 108:e81, 2003.
165. Ridker PM, Rifai N, Stampfer MJ, Hennekens CH: Plasma concentration of interleukin-6 and the risk of future myocardial infarction among apparently healthy men. Circulation 101:1767, 2000.
166. Ridker PM, Hennekens CH, Roitman-Johnson B, et al: Plasma concentration of soluble intercellular adhesion molecule 1 and risks of future myocardial infarction in apparently healthy men. Lancet 351:88, 1998.
167. Ridker PM, Buring JE, Rifai N: Soluble P-selectin and the risk of future cardiovascular events. Circulation 103:491, 2001.
168. Malik I, Danesh J, Whincup P, et al: Soluble adhesion molecules and prediction of coronary heart disease: A prospective study and meta-analysis. Lancet 358:971, 2001.
169. Pradhan AD, Rifai N, Ridker PM: Soluble intercellular adhesion molecule-1, soluble vascular adhesion molecule-1, and the development of symptomatic peripheral arterial disease in men. Circulation 106:820, 2002.
170. Schonbeck U, Varo N, Libby P, et al: Soluble CD40L and cardiovascular risk in women. Circulation 104:2266, 2001.
171. Zhang R, Brennan ML, Fu X, et al: Association between myeloperoxidase levels and risk of coronary artery disease. JAMA 286:2136, 2001.
172. Packard CJ, O'Reilly DS, Caslake MJ, et al: Lipoprotein-associated phospholipase A2 as an independent predictor of coronary heart disease. West of Scotland Coronary Prevention Study Group. N Engl J Med 343:1148, 2000.
173. Ballantyne CM, Houri J, Notarbartolo A, et al: Effect of ezetimibe coadministered with atorvastatin in 628 patients with primary hypercholesterolemia: A prospective, randomized, double-blind trial. Circulation 107:2409, 2003.
174. Bayes-Genis A, Conover CA, Overgaard MT, et al: Pregnancy-associated plasma protein A as a marker of acute coronary syndromes. N Engl J Med 345:1022, 2001.
175. Blake GJ, Dada N, Fox JC, et al: A prospective evaluation of lipoprotein-associated phospholipase A(2) levels and the risk of future cardiovascular events in women. J Am Coll Cardiol 38:1302, 2001.
176. Heeschen C, Dimmeler S, Hamm CW, et al: Soluble CD40 ligand in acute coronary syndromes. N Engl J Med 348:1104, 2003.
177. Baldus S, Heeschen C, Meinertz T, et al: Myeloperoxidase serum levels predict risk in patients with acute coronary syndromes. Circulation 108:1440, 2003.
178. Brennan ML, Penn MS, Van Lente F, et al: Prognostic value of myeloperoxidase in patients with chest pain. N Engl J Med 349:1595, 2003.
179. Welch GN, Loscalzo J: Homocysteine and atherothrombosis. N Engl J Med 338:1042, 1998.
180. Chambers JC, Ueland PM, Obeid OA, et al: Improved vascular endothelial function after oral B vitamins: An effect mediated through reduced concentrations of free plasma homocysteine. Circulation 102:2479, 2000.

181. Bellamy MF, McDowell IF, Ramsey MW, et al: Hyperhomocysteinemia after an oral methionine load acutely impairs endothelial function in healthy adults. Circulation 98:1848, 1998.
182. Poddar R, Sivasubramanian N, DiBello PM, et al: Homocysteine induces expression and secretion of monocyte chemoattractant protein-1 and interleukin-8 in human aortic endothelial cells: Implications for vascular disease. Circulation 103:2717, 2001.
183. Werstuck GH, Lentz SR, Dayal S, et al: Homocysteine-induced endoplasmic reticulum stress causes dysregulation of the cholesterol and triglyceride biosynthetic pathways. J Clin Invest 107:1263, 2001.
184. Jacques PF, Bostom AG, Wilson PW, et al: Determinants of plasma total homocysteine concentration in the Framingham Offspring cohort. Am J Clin Nutr 73:613, 2001.
185. Kark JD, Sinnreich R, Rosenberg IH, et al: Plasma homocysteine and parental myocardial infarction in young adults in Jerusalem. Circulation 105:2725, 2002.
186. Klerk M, Verhoef P, Clarke R, et al: MTHFR 677C→T polymorphism and risk of coronary heart disease: A meta-analysis. JAMA 288:2023, 2002.
187. Wilson PW: Homocysteine and coronary heart disease: How great is the hazard? JAMA 288:2042, 2002.
188. Malinow MR, Bostom AG, Krauss RM: Homocyst(e)ine, diet, and cardiovascular diseases: A statement for healthcare professionals from the Nutrition Committee, American Heart Association. Circulation 99:178, 1999.
189. Wald DS, Law M, Morris JK: Homocysteine and cardiovascular disease: Evidence on causality from a meta-analysis. BMJ 325:1202, 2002.
190. Homocysteine and risk of ischemic heart disease and stroke: A meta-analysis. JAMA 288:2015, 2002.
191. Kelly PJ, Rosand J, Kistler JP, et al: Homocysteine, MTHFR 677C→T polymorphism, and risk of ischemic stroke: Results of a meta-analysis. Neurology 59:529, 2002.
192. Ford ES, Smith SJ, Stroup DF, et al: Homocyst(e)ine and cardiovascular disease: A systematic review of the evidence with special emphasis on case-control studies and nested case-control studies. Int J Epidemiol 31:59, 2002.
193. Ridker PM, Manson JE, Buring JE, et al: Homocysteine and risk of cardiovascular disease among postmenopausal women. JAMA 281:1817, 1999.
194. Jacques PF, Selhub J, Bostom AG, et al: The effect of folic acid fortification on plasma folate and total homocysteine concentrations. N Engl J Med 340:1449, 1999.
195. Ridker PM, Shih J, Cook TJ, et al: Plasma homocysteine concentration, statin therapy, and the risk of first acute coronary events. Circulation 105:1776, 2002.
196. Lowering blood homocysteine with folic acid based supplements: Meta-analysis of randomised trials. Homocysteine Lowering Trialists' Collaboration. BMJ 316:894, 1998.
197. Wald DS, Bishop L, Wald NJ, et al: Randomized trial of folic acid supplementation and serum homocysteine levels. Arch Intern Med 161:695, 2001.
198. Tice JA, Ross E, Coxson PG, et al: Cost-effectiveness of vitamin therapy to lower plasma homocysteine levels for the prevention of coronary heart disease: Effect of grain fortification and beyond. JAMA 286:936, 2001.
199. Spence JD, Howard VJ, Chambless LE, et al: Vitamin Intervention for Stroke Prevention (VISP) trial: Rationale and design. Neuroepidemiology 20:16, 2001.
200. The VITATOPS (Vitamins to Prevent Stroke) Trial: Rationale and design of an international, large, simple, randomised trial of homocysteine-lowering multivitamin therapy in patients with recent transient ischaemic attack or stroke. Cerebrovasc Dis 13:120, 2002.
201. MacMahon M, Kirkpatrick C, Cummings CE, et al: A pilot study with simvastatin and folic acid/vitamin B12 in preparation for the Study of the Effectiveness of Additional Reductions in Cholesterol and Homocysteine (SEARCH). Nutr Metab Cardiovasc Dis 10:195, 2000.
202. Bostom AG, Selhub J, Jacques PF, Rosenberg IH: Power Shortage: Clinical trials testing the "homocysteine hypothesis" against a background of folic acid-fortified cereal grain flour. Ann Intern Med 135:133, 2001
203. Shemin D, Bostom AG, Selhub J: Treatment of hyperhomocysteinemia in end-stage renal disease. Am J Kidney Dis 38:S91, 2001.
203a. Toole JF, Malinow MR, Chambless LE, et al: Lowering homocysteine in patients with ischemic stroke to prevent recurrent stroke, myocardial infarction, and death. JAMA 291:565, 2004.
204. Nygard O, Nordrehaug JE, Refsum H, et al: Plasma homocysteine levels and mortality in patients with coronary artery disease. N Engl J Med 337:230, 1997.
205. Al-Obaidi MK, Stubbs PJ, Collinson P, et al: Elevated homocysteine levels are associated with increased ischemic myocardial injury in acute coronary syndromes. J Am Coll Cardiol 36:1217, 2000.
206. Schnyder G, Roffi M, Pin R, et al: Decreased rate of coronary restenosis after lowering of plasma homocysteine levels. N Engl J Med 345:1593, 2001.
207. Schnyder G, Roffi M, Flammer Y, et al: Effect of homocysteine-lowering therapy with folic acid, vitamin B12, and vitamin B6 on clinical outcome after percutaneous coronary intervention: The Swiss Heart study: A randomized controlled trial. JAMA 288:973, 2002.
208. Miller A, Mujumdar V, Palmer L, et al: Reversal of endocardial endothelial dysfunction by folic acid in homocysteinemic hypertensive rats. Am J Hypertens 15:157, 2002.
209. Blacher J, Demuth K, Guerin AP, et al: Association between plasma homocysteine concentrations and cardiac hypertrophy in end-stage renal disease. J Nephrol 12:248, 1999.
210. Vasan RS, Beiser A, D'Agostino RB, et al: Plasma homocysteine and risk for congestive heart failure in adults without prior myocardial infarction. JAMA 289:1251, 2003.
211. Margaglione M, Cappucci G, Colaizzo D, et al: Fibrinogen plasma levels in an apparently healthy general population: Relation to environmental and genetic determinants. Thromb Haemost 80:805, 1998.
212. Wilhelmsen L, Svardsudd K, Korsan-Bengtsen K, et al: Fibrinogen as a risk factor for stroke and myocardial infarction. N Engl J Med 311:501, 1984.
213. Folsom AR, Rosamond WD, Shahar E, et al: Prospective study of markers of hemostatic function with risk of ischemic stroke. The Atherosclerosis Risk in Communities (ARIC) Study Investigators. Circulation 100:736, 1999.
214. Ma J, Hennekens CH, Ridker PM, Stampfer MJ: A prospective study of fibrinogen and risk of myocardial infarction in the Physicians' Health Study. J Am Coll Cardiol 33:1347, 1999.
215. Danesh J, Collins R, Appleby P, Peto R: Association of fibrinogen, C-reactive protein, albumin, or leukocyte count with coronary heart disease: Meta-analyses of prospective studies. JAMA 279:1477, 1998.
216. Maresca G, Di Blasio A, Marchioli R, Di Minno G: Measuring plasma fibrinogen to predict stroke and myocardial infarction: An update. Arterioscler Thromb Vasc Biol 19:1368, 1999.
217. Lee AJ, Fowkes FG, Lowe GD, et al: Fibrinogen, factor VII and PAI-1 genotypes and the risk of coronary and peripheral atherosclerosis: Edinburgh Artery Study. Thromb Haemost 81:553, 1999.
218. Cantin B, Gagnon F, Moorjani S, et al: Is lipoprotein(a) an independent risk factor for ischemic heart disease in men? The Quebec Cardiovascular Study. J Am Coll Cardiol 31:519, 1998.
219. Acevedo M, Pearce GL, Kottke-Marchant K, Sprecher DL: Elevated fibrinogen and homocysteine levels enhance the risk of mortality in patients from a high-risk preventive cardiology clinic. Arterioscler Thromb Vasc Biol 22:1042, 2002.
220. Secondary prevention by raising HDL cholesterol and reducing triglycerides in patients with coronary artery disease: The Bezafibrate Infarction Prevention (BIP) study. Circulation 102:21, 2000.
221. Tanne D, Benderly M, Goldbourt U, et al: A prospective study of plasma fibrinogen levels and the risk of stroke among participants in the bezafibrate infarction prevention study. Am J Med 111:457, 2001.
222. Meade T, Zuhrie R, Cook C, Cooper J: Bezafibrate in men with lower extremity arterial disease: Randomised controlled trial. BMJ 325:1139, 2002.
223. Hulley S, Grady D, Bush T, et al: Randomized trial of estrogen plus progestin for secondary prevention of coronary heart disease in postmenopausal women. Heart and Estrogen/progestin Replacement Study (HERS) Research Group. JAMA 280:605, 1998.
224. Cushman M, Lemaitre RN, Kuller LH, et al: Fibrinolytic activation markers predict myocardial infarction in the elderly. The Cardiovascular Health Study. Arterioscler Thromb Vasc Biol 19:493, 1999.
225. Smith FB, Lee AJ, Fowkes FG, et al: Hemostatic factors as predictors of ischemic heart disease and stroke in the Edinburgh Artery Study. Arterioscler Thromb Vasc Biol 17:3321, 1997.
226. Lowe GD, Yarnell JW, Sweetnam PM, et al: Fibrin D-dimer, tissue plasminogen activator, plasminogen activator inhibitor, and the risk of major ischaemic heart disease in the Caerphilly Study. Thromb Haemost 79:129, 1998.
227. Danesh J, Whincup P, Walker M, et al: Fibrin D-dimer and coronary heart disease: Prospective study and meta-analysis. Circulation 103:2323, 1998.
228. Moss AJ, Goldstein RE, Marder VJ, et al: Thrombogenic factors and recurrent coronary events. Circulation 99:2517, 1999.
229. Menown IB, Mathew TP, Gracey HM, et al: Prediction of Recurrent Events by D-Dimer and Inflammatory Markers in Patients with Normal Cardiac Troponin I (PREDICT) Study. Am Heart J 145:986, 2003.
230. Mills JD, Ariens RA, Mansfield MW, Grant PJ: Altered fibrin clot structure in the healthy relatives of patients with premature coronary artery disease. Circulation 106:1938, 2002.
231. Wells PS, Anderson DR, Rodger M, et al: Evaluation of D-dimer in the diagnosis of suspected deep-vein thrombosis. N Engl J Med 349:1227, 2003.
232. Festa A, D'Agostino R Jr, Tracy RP, Haffner SM: Elevated levels of acute-phase proteins and plasminogen activator inhibitor-1 predict the development of type 2 diabetes: The insulin resistance atherosclerosis study. Diabetes 51:1131, 2002.
233. Thogersen AM, Jansson JH, Boman K, et al: High plasminogen activator inhibitor and tissue plasminogen activator levels in plasma precede a first acute myocardial infarction in both men and women: Evidence for the fibrinolytic system as an independent primary risk factor. Circulation 98:2241, 1998.
234. Brown NJ, Abbas A, Byrne D, et al: Comparative effects of estrogen and angiotensin-converting enzyme inhibition on plasminogen activator inhibitor-1 in healthy postmenopausal women. Circulation 105:304, 2002.
235. Pradhan AD, LaCroix AZ, Trevisan M, et al: Tissue plasminogen activator antigen and D-dimer as markers for atherothrombotic risk among healthy post-menopausal women: A report from the women's health initiative observational study. Circulation 2004, in press.
236. Vaughan DE, Rouleau JL, Ridker PM, et al: Effects of ramipril on plasma fibrinolytic balance in patients with acute anterior myocardial infarction. HEART Study Investigators. Circulation 96:442, 1997.
237. Brown NJ, Agirbasli MA, Williams GH, et al: Effect of activation and inhibition of the renin-angiotensin system on plasma PAI-1. Hypertension 32:965, 1998.
238. Pretorius M, Rosenbaum D, Vaughan DE, Brown NJ: Angiotensin-converting enzyme inhibition increases human vascular tissue-type plasminogen activator release through endogenous bradykinin. Circulation 107:579, 2003.
239. Festa A, D'Agostino R Jr, Rich SS, et al: Promoter (4G/5G) plasminogen activator inhibitor-1 genotype and plasminogen activator inhibitor-1 levels in blacks, Hispanics, and non-Hispanic whites: The Insulin Resistance Atherosclerosis Study. Circulation 107:2422, 2003.
240. Boekholdt SM, Bijsterveld NR, Moons AH, et al: Genetic variation in coagulation and fibrinolytic proteins and their relation with acute myocardial infarction: A systematic review. Circulation 104:3063, 2001.
241. Hobbs HH, White AL: Lipoprotein(a): Intrigues and insights. Curr Opin Lipidol 10:225, 1999.
242. Caplice NM, Panetta C, Peterson TE, et al: Lipoprotein(a) binds and inactivates tissue factor pathway inhibitor: A novel link between lipoproteins and thrombosis. Blood 98:2980, 2001.
243. Buechler C, Ullrich H, Ritter M, et al: Lipoprotein(a) up-regulates the expression of the plasminogen activator inhibitor 2 in human blood monocytes. Blood 97:981, 2001.

244. Danesh J, Collins R, Peto R: Lipoprotein(a) and coronary heart disease: Meta-analysis of prospective studies. Circulation 102:1082, 2000.
245. Solfrizzi V, Panza F, Colacicco AM, et al: Relation of lipoprotein(a) as coronary risk factor to type 2 diabetes mellitus and low-density lipoprotein cholesterol in patients > or = 65 years of age (The Italian Longitudinal Study on Aging). Am J Cardiol 89:825, 2002.
246. Koschinsky ML, Marcovina SM: The relationship between lipoprotein(a) and the complications of diabetes mellitus. Acta Diabetol 40:65, 2003.
247. von Eckardstein A, Schulte H, Cullen P, Assmann G: Lipoprotein(a) further increases the risk of coronary events in men with high global cardiovascular risk. J Am Coll Cardiol 37:434, 2001.
248. Kronenberg F, Kronenberg MF, Kiechl S, et al: Role of lipoprotein(a) and apolipoprotein(a) phenotype in atherogenesis: Prospective results from the Bruneck study. Circulation 100:1154, 1999.
249. Luc G, Bard JM, Arveiler D, et al: Lipoprotein(a) as a predictor of coronary heart disease: The PRIME Study. Atherosclerosis 163:377, 2002.
250. Foody JM, Milberg JA, Robinson K, et al: Homocysteine and lipoprotein(a) interact to increase CAD risk in young men and women. Arterioscler Thromb Vasc Biol 20:493, 2000.
251. Cantin B, Despres JP, Lamarche B, et al: Association of fibrinogen and lipoprotein(a) as a coronary heart disease risk factor in men (The Quebec Cardiovascular Study). Am J Cardiol 89:662, 2002.
252. Sweetnam PM, Bolton CH, Downs LG, et al: Apolipoproteins A-I, A-II and B, lipoprotein(a) and the risk of ischaemic heart disease: The Caerphilly study. Eur J Clin Invest 30:947, 2000.
253. Sharrett AR, Ballantyne CM, Coady SA, et al: Coronary heart disease prediction from lipoprotein cholesterol levels, triglycerides, lipoprotein(a), apolipoproteins A-I and B, and HDL density subfractions: The Atherosclerosis Risk in Communities (ARIC) Study. Circulation 104:1108, 2001.
254. Glader CA, Birgander LS, Stenlund H, Dahlen GH: Is lipoprotein(a) a predictor for survival in patients with established coronary artery disease? Results from a prospective patient cohort study in northern Sweden. J Intern Med 252:27, 2002.
255. Longenecker JC, Klag MJ, Marcovina SM, et al: Small apolipoprotein(a) size predicts mortality in end-stage renal disease: The CHOICE study. Circulation 106:2812, 2002.
256. Longenecker JC, Coresh J, Marcovina SM, et al: Lipoprotein(a) and prevalent cardiovascular disease in a dialysis population: The choices for healthy outcomes in caring for ESRD (CHOICE) study. Am J Kidney Dis 42:108, 2003.
257. Marcovina SM, Albers JJ, Scanu AM, et al: Use of a reference material proposed by the International Federation of Clinical Chemistry and Laboratory Medicine to evaluate analytical methods for the determination of plasma lipoprotein(a). Clin Chem 46:1956, 2000.
258. Holmer SR, Hengstenberg C, Kraft HG, et al: Association of polymorphisms of the apolipoprotein(a) gene with lipoprotein(a) levels and myocardial infarction. Circulation 107:696, 2003.
259. Sharp RJ, Perugini MA, Marcovina SM, McCormick SP: A synthetic peptide that inhibits lipoprotein(a) assembly. Arterioscler Thromb Vasc Biol 23:502, 2003.
260. Strater R, Becker S, von Eckardstein A, et al: Prospective assessment of risk factors for recurrent stroke during childhood: A 5-year follow-up study. Lancet 360:1540, 2002.
261. Otvos JD, Jeyarajah EJ, Cromwell WC: Measurement issues related to lipoprotein heterogeneity. Am J Cardiol 90:22i, 2002.
262. Sniderman AD, Scantlebury T, Cianflone K: Hypertriglyceridemic hyperapoB: The unappreciated atherogenic dyslipoproteinemia in type 2 diabetes mellitus. Ann Intern Med 135:447, 2001.
263. Lamarche B, Tchernof A, Moorjani S, et al: Small, dense low-density lipoprotein particles as a predictor of the risk of ischemic heart disease in men. Prospective results from the Quebec Cardiovascular Study. Circulation 95:69, 1997.
264. Zambon A, Hokanson JE, Brown BG, Brunzell JD: Evidence for a new pathophysiological mechanism for coronary artery disease regression: Hepatic lipase-mediated changes in LDL density. Circulation 99:1959, 1999.
265. Rosenson RS, Otvos JD, Freedman DS: Relations of lipoprotein subclass levels and low density lipoprotein size to progression of coronary artery disease in the Pravastatin Limitation of Atherosclerosis in the Coronary Arteries (PLAC-I) trial. Am J Cardiol 90:89, 2002.
266. Blake GJ, Otvos JD, Rifai N, Ridker PM: Low-density lipoprotein particle concentration and size as determined by nuclear magnetic resonance spectroscopy as predictors of cardiovascular disease in women. Circulation 106:1930, 2002.
267. Kuller L, Arnold A, Tracy R, et al: Nuclear magnetic resonance spectroscopy of lipoproteins and risk of coronary heart disease in the cardiovascular health study. Arterioscler Thromb Vasc Biol 22:1175, 2002.
268. Campos H, Moye LA, Glasser SP, et al: Low-density lipoprotein size, pravastatin treatment, and coronary events. JAMA 286:1468, 2001.
269. Otvos JD, Shalaurova I, Freedman DS, Rosenson RS: Effects of pravastatin treatment on lipoprotein subclass profiles and particle size in the PLAC-I trial. Atherosclerosis 160:41, 2002.
270. Greenland P, Smith SC Jr, Grundy SM: Improving coronary heart disease risk assessment in asymptomatic people: Role of traditional risk factors and noninvasive cardiovascular tests. Circulation 104:1863, 2001.
271. Keelan PC, Bielak LF, Ashai K, et al: Long-term prognostic value of coronary calcification detected by electron-beam computed tomography in patients undergoing coronary angiography. Circulation 104:412, 2001.
272. Achenbach S, Ropers D, Pohle K, et al: Influence of lipid-lowering therapy on the progression of coronary artery calcification: A prospective evaluation. Circulation 106:1077, 2002.
273. Detrano RC, Wong ND, Doherty TM, et al: Coronary calcium does not accurately predict near-term future coronary events in high-risk adults. Circulation 99:2633, 1999.
274. Park R, Detrano R, Xiang M, et al: Combined use of computed tomography coronary calcium scores and C-reactive protein levels in predicting cardiovascular events in nondiabetic individuals. Circulation 106:2073, 2002.
274a. Greenland P, LaBree L, Azen SP, et al: Coronary artery calcium score combined with Framingham score for risk prediction in asymptomatic individuals. JAMA 291:210, 2004.
275. O'Malley PG, Feuerstein IM, Taylor AJ: Impact of electron beam tomography, with or without case management, on motivation, behavioral change, and cardiovascular risk profile: A randomized controlled trial. JAMA 289:2215, 2003.
276. Hodis HN, Mack WJ, LaBree L, et al: The role of carotid arterial intima-media thickness in predicting clinical coronary events. Ann Intern Med 128:262, 1998.
277. O'Leary DH, Polak JF, Kronmal RA, et al: Carotid-artery intima and media thickness as a risk factor for myocardial infarction and stroke in older adults. Cardiovascular Health Study Collaborative Research Group. N Engl J Med 340:14, 1999.
278. Bild DE, Bluemke DA, Burke GL, et al: Multi-ethnic study of atherosclerosis: Objectives and design. Am J Epidemiol 156:871, 2002.

CHAPTER 37

Systemic Hypertension: Mechanisms and Diagnosis

Norman M. Kaplan

Recognition, Definitions, Prevalence, and Consequences of Hypertension

As the population grows older and more obese, the incidence of hypertension continues to increase, not only in the United States but in all developed and developing societies (Fig. 37–1).[1] At the same time, despite the widely recognized dangers of uncontrolled hypertension, the disease remains inadequately treated in the majority of patients.[2] Such inadequate management has been noted not only in closely observed communities[2] but also in carefully monitored antihypertensive drug trials.[3] As a consequence, cardiovascular risk remains high among the majority of hypertensive persons, whether treated or not.

Despite these disturbing figures, management of hypertension is now the leading indication for both visits to physicians and the use of prescription drugs in the United States.[4] Clearly, more attention is being directed toward hypertension, but adequate hypertension control remains elusive, in large part because of the asymptomatic nature of the disease for the first 15 to 20 years, even as it progressively damages the cardiovascular system. Asymptomatic patients are often unwilling to alter life style or take medication to forestall some far-off, poorly perceived danger, particularly when they are made uncomfortable in the process.

In view of these built-in barriers to effective control of the individual patient, population-wide application of preventive measures becomes inherently more attractive. Although the specific mechanisms for most hypertension remain unknown, it is highly likely that the process could be slowed, if not prevented, by the prevention of obesity, moderate reduction in sodium intake, higher levels of physical activity, and avoidance of excessive alcohol consumption.[5] Since hypertension will eventually develop in most people during their lifetime (Table 37–1),[6] the need for more widespread adoption of potentially effective and totally safe preventive measures is obvious. In the meantime, better management of those already afflicted must be practiced, starting with careful documentation of the diagnosis.

Measurement of Blood Pressure

Blood pressure typically changes considerably through the day and night. Such variability is seldom recognized by the relatively few office readings taken by most practitioners but can easily be identified by automatically recorded measurements taken throughout the day and night (Fig. 37–2). This variability can often be attributed to physical activity or emotional stress but is frequently without obvious cause. In a few patients, markedly elevated levels clearly indicate serious disease requiring immediate treatment. In most cases, however, initial readings are not high enough to indicate immediate danger, and the diagnosis of hypertension should be substantiated by repeated readings. The reason for such caution is obvious: The diagnosis of hypertension imposes psychological and socioeconomic burdens on an individual and usually implies the need for commitment to lifelong therapy.

Both transient and persistent elevations in blood pressure are common when the reading is taken in the physician's office or hospital. To identify the patient's usual range of blood pressure, more widespread use of out-of-the-office readings, either with semiautomatic inexpensive devices or with automatic ambulatory recorders, is encouraged both to establish the diagnosis and to monitor the patient's response to therapy.[7,8] A large body of data provides normal ranges for both home self-recorded and automatic ambulatory measurements.[9] Both average about 10/5 mm Hg lower than the average of multiple office readings. A closer correlation between the presence of various types of target organ damage, specifically, left ventricular hypertrophy (LVH), carotid wall thickness, proteinuria, and retinopathy, has been noted with ambulatory levels than with office levels. More importantly, increasing evidence supports a closer relation to future cardiovascular events with readings from ambulatory monitoring than with office readings (Fig. 37–3).[10] However, in the absence of adequate long-term follow-up, evidence of the risks associated with home monitoring, and the limited availability of ambulatory monitoring, office readings will continue to be the basis for the diagnosis and management of hypertension for most patients.

OUT-OF-THE-OFFICE MEASUREMENTS. A "white-coat effect," that is, a higher blood pressure on readings taken in the office than out of the office, is present in most patients. Therefore, whenever possible, office readings should be supplemented by out-of-the-office measurements, particularly when there is an apparent discrepancy between the level of blood pressure and the degree of target organ damage, in which case white coat hypertension should be suspected. In as many as one third of patients with office readings that remain elevated despite the use of three or more drugs, hypertension is found to be well controlled by out-of-the-office readings.[11] Purely white coat hypertension, that is, persistently elevated office readings at or above 140/90 mm Hg but persistently normal out-of-the-office

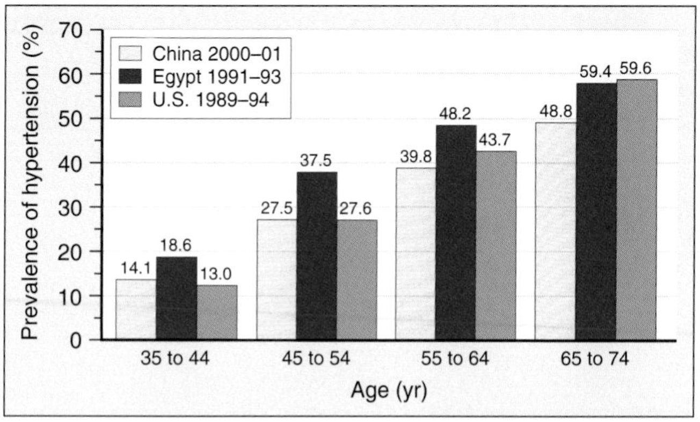

FIGURE 37–1 International Society of Hypertension prevalence of hypertension among three populations, ages 35 to 74 years: InterASIA (2000-2001), the Egyptian National Hypertension Project (1991-1993), and the Third National Health and Nutrition Examination Survey (1989-1994). (From Gu D, Reynolds K, Wu X, et al: Prevalence, awareness, treatment, and control of hypertension in China. Hypertension 40:925, 2002.)

TABLE 37–1 Residual Lifetime Risk of Hypertension According to Baseline Age*

	Women (%)		Men (%)	
Time, yrs	*55 yrs old* (*n* = 709)	*65 yrs old* (*n* = 549)	*55 yrs old* (*n* = 589)	*65 yrs old* (*n* = 438)
10	52	64	56	72
15	72	81	78	85
20	83	89	88	90
25	91	N/A	93	N/A

N/A = not applicable.
Modified from Vasan RS et al: JAMA 2002;287:1003-1010.
*For 55-year-old subjects, the risk for developing hypertension over 25 years represents their lifetime risk. For 65-year-old subjects, the risk for developing hypertension over 20 years indicates their lifetime risk.

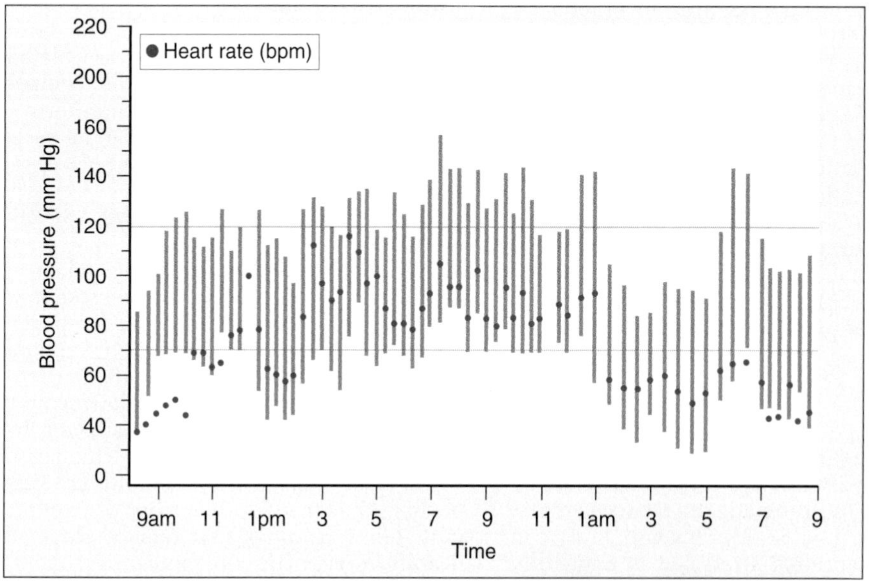

FIGURE 37–2 Computer printout of blood pressure readings obtained by ambulatory blood pressure monitoring over a 24-hour period beginning at 9 AM in a 50-year-old man with hypertension receiving no therapy. The patient slept from midnight until 6 AM. Solid circles indicate heart rate. (From Zachariah PK, Sheps SG, Smith RL: Defining the roles of home and ambulatory monitoring. Diagnosis 10:39, 1988. Copyright 1988, Medical Economics Publishing Company, Pradell, NJ. All rights reserved.)

readings at or below 135/85, is found in 20 to 30 percent of patients. The possibility of white-coat hypertension is increased in patients with these characteristics: (1) office blood pressure between 140 and 159 systolic or 90 and 99 diastolic; (2) female gender; (3) nonsmoking; (4) recent onset of hypertension; and (5) small left ventricular mass by echocardiography.[12] Obviously, the likelihood is also greater if only a few office readings have been taken.

Most such patients are free of the target organ damage and metabolic abnormalities (dyslipidemia, hyperinsulinemia) that are often found in patients with sustained hypertension, and follow-up for up to 10 years has found no increase in cardiovascular events.[12] Therefore, close observation and lifestyle modifications but not antihypertensive drug therapy seem appropriate management for such patients. On the other hand, a smaller portion of patients, particularly elderly subjects on treatment, may have "reverse white-coat" or "masked" hypertension, that is, normal office but elevated ambulatory readings.[13]

In addition to their role in the recognition of white coat and masked hypertension, out-of-the-office readings are essential for the recognition of persistently elevated pressures soon after arising, when the largest proportion of sudden deaths, myocardial infarctions, and strokes occur. The morning surge is dependent on physical activity after awakening and is related to increased sympathetic nervous activity.[14] The best way to blunt the early morning surge in pressure is to use antihypertensive drug formulations that provide full 24-hour coverage and to take them as early in the morning as possible. In view of the usual nocturnal fall in pressure (see Fig. 37–2), addition of the maximal antihypertensive effect of medication taken before bedtime could incite myocardial and cerebral ischemia during sleep.

Although a nocturnal fall or dipping in pressure is usual, little or no fall has been more frequently noted in various groups of hypertensive patients who have a more serious degree of target organ damage or subsequent major cardiovascular events. These groups include patients with LVH, diabetes, or renal damage and black patients. A smaller proportion of patients, mostly elderly, have excessive dipping, beyond 20 percent of the average daytime systolic level, and that too is associated with increased risk of cardiovascular morbidity.[15] Recognition of such abnormal nocturnal patterns of blood pressure then is another indication for more widespread use of automatic recordings.

BLOOD PRESSURE RESPONSE TO EXERCISE. Another source of potentially useful prognostic information is the blood pressure response to exercise, usually ascertained by treadmill testing. An exaggerated response in normotensive adults has been associated with a threefold greater likelihood of hypertension developing over the next 5 to 15 years[16] and a twofold greater cardiovascular mortality over a 21-year follow-up[17] compared to those without an exaggerated response during exercise. Since most normotensive subjects with an exaggerated response do not develop hypertension, exercise tests should not be done for predictive purposes. If, however, a supernormal response is noted, the subject should be advised to start a slowly progressive aerobic exercise program to moderate the response and, perhaps, delay the onset of hypertension.

DOCUMENTATION OF HYPERTENSION. For most patients who are in no immediate danger from markedly elevated pressure, that is, below approximately 170/110 mm Hg, the following guidelines are offered:

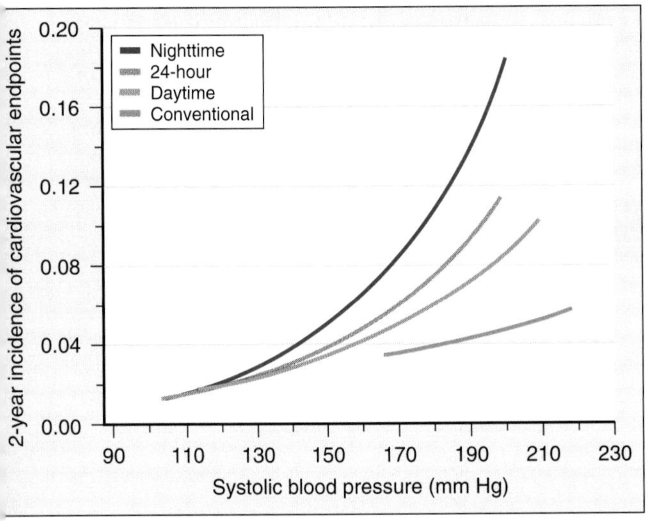

IGURE 37–3 The relation of systolic blood pressure by conventional (office) or 4-hour daytime and nighttime ambulatory measurements at entry as predictors of the -year incidence of cardiovascular endpoints in the placebo-treated older patients with ystolic hypertension. Incidence is given as a fraction (i.e., 0.02 is an incidence of 2 vents per 100 people). Using multiple Cox regression, the event rate was standardized o female gender, mean age of 69.6 years, no previous cardiovascular complications, onsmoking status, and residence in western Europe. (Modified from Staessen JA, Thijs , Fagard R, et al: Predicting cardiovascular risk using conventional vs. ambulatory blood ressure in older patients with systolic hypertension. JAMA 282:539, 1999.)

1. Multiple readings should be obtained with appropriate technique (Table 37–2). If possible, the readings should be taken under varying conditions and at various times for at least 4 to 6 weeks with a semiautomatic home device. If the diagnosis must be established more rapidly, a set of readings obtained by an automatic monitor over a single 24-hour period will be adequate.
2. Although the logical approach would be to calculate the average values from multiple readings when deciding whether hypertension is present, even a single high measurement should not be disregarded. In large populations, antecedent office measurements have been found to predict a greater likelihood of subsequent cardiovascular disease above and beyond current blood pressure levels.[18]
3. Elderly patients may have markedly sclerotic brachial arteries that are not occluded until very high pressures are exerted by the balloon; therefore, cuff levels may be considerably higher than those measured intraarterially. In patients with high cuff readings but little or no hypertensive retinopathy, cardiac hypertrophy, or other evidence of longstanding hypertension, "pseudohypertension" should be suspected and ruled out before treatment is begun.
4. Elderly persons with elevated systolic pressure should be monitored carefully for significant falls in pressure either with sudden upright posture or after meals. These changes reflect a progressive loss of autonomic responsiveness with age.

Definition of Hypertension

Blood pressure is distributed in a typical bell-shaped curve within the overall population. As seen in the 22-year follow-

TABLE 37–2 Guidelines in Measuring Blood Pressure

Conditions for the patient	*Posture:* For patients who are older than 65 years, diabetic, or receiving antihypertensive therapy, check for postural changes by taking readings after 5 min supine and immediately and 2 min after patient stands. Sitting pressures are usually adequate for routine follow-up. Patient should sit quietly with back supported for 5 min and arm supported at level of heart. *Circumstances:* No caffeine for preceding hour. No smoking for preceding 30 min. No exogenous adrenergic stimulants, e.g., phenylephrine in nasal decongestants. Quiet, warm setting. Home readings should be taken under varying circumstances throughout the day; for monitoring of therapy, an occasional reading taken soon after arising is usually adequate.
Equipment	Cuff size: The bladder should encircle and cover two-thirds of the length of the arm; if not, place the bladder over the brachial artery; if bladder is too small, spuriously high readings may result. Manometer: Aneroid gauges and electronic devices should be calibrated every 6 mo against a mercury manometer. For infants, use Doppler ultrasound equipment.
Technique	*Number of readings:* On each occasion, take at least two readings separated by as much time as practical. If readings vary by more than 5 mm Hg, take additional readings until two are close. For diagnosis, obtain at least three sets of readings at least 1 week apart; with home measurements, obtain multiple readings over 3-4 weeks. Initially, take pressure in both arms; if pressure differs, use arm with higher pressure. If arm pressure is elevated, take pressure in one leg, particularly in patients younger than 30 yr. *Performance:* Inflate the bladder quickly to a pressure 20 mm Hg above the systolic, as recognized by disappearance of the radial pulse. Deflate the bladder 3 mm Hg every second. Record the Korotkoff phase V (disappearance) except in children (<10 yrs), in whom use of phase IV (muffling) may be preferable. If Korotkoff sounds are weak, have the patient raise the arm and open and close the hand five to 10 times, after which the bladder should be inflated quickly. *Recordings:* Note the pressure, patient position, which arm, and cuff size (e.g., 140/90, seated, right arm, large adult cuff).

up of the almost 350,000 men screened for the Multiple Risk Factor Intervention Trial (MRFIT), the long-term risks for cardiovascular mortality associated with various levels of pressure rise progressively over the entire range of blood pressure, with no threshold that clearly identifies potential danger (Fig. 37–4).[19] Therefore, the definition of hypertension is somewhat arbitrary and usually taken as that level of pressure associated with a doubling of long-term risk. Perhaps the best operational definition is "the level at which the benefits (minus the risks and costs) of action exceed the risks and costs (minus the benefits) of inaction."

For the individual patient, hypertension should be diagnosed when most readings are at a level known to be associated with a significantly higher cardiovascular risk without treatment. The recommendations of the Sixth Joint National Committee (JNC-6) are shown in Table 37–3.[7] Note that systolic levels of 130 to 139 mm Hg and diastolic levels of 85 to 89 mm Hg are classified as high normal blood pressure, a classification associated with a significant increase in the risk of cardiovascular events over time (Fig. 37–5).[20] In view of this heightened risk, the JNC-7 report[8] defines levels above 120/80 to as high as 140/90 as "prehypertension." Therefore, persons with above-normal systolic or diastolic pressures should be advised that they may be at increased risk and counseled to follow better health habits in the hope of slowing the progression toward definite hypertension.

The criteria shown in Table 37–3 are based on at least three sets of measurements taken over at least a 3-month interval. Even more readings may be needed to establish a patient's usual level. Even though they are diagnosed as hypertensive, not all persons with usual levels above 140/90 mm Hg need be treated with drugs, although all should be advised to us the various life-style modifications described in Chapter 3ε The threshold for institution of drug therapy should be base on the overall cardiovascular risk profile.

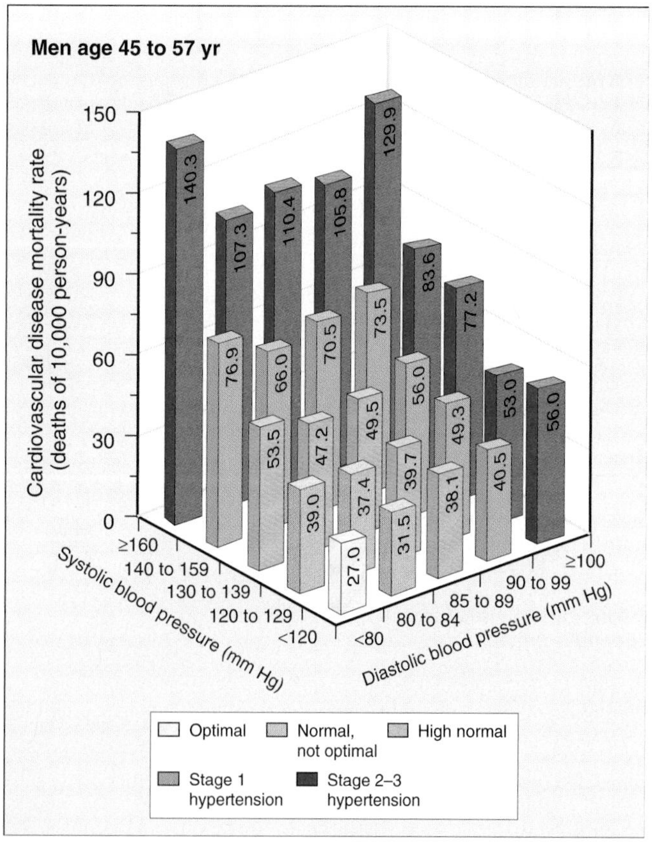

FIGURE 37–4 Age-adjusted cardiovascular disease mortality rate by systolic and diastolic blood pressure level used to define each JNC-VI stratum among the men aged 45 to 57 years enrolled in the Multiple Risk Factor Intervention Trial from 1973 to 1975 and followed through 1996. (Modified from Domanski M, Mitchell G, Pfeffer M, et al: Pulse pressure and cardiovascular disease-related mortality. JAMA 287:268, 2002.)

HYPERTENSION IN CHILDREN AND ADOLESCENTS Upper limits of normal in children of various ages wer

TABLE 37–3 JNC-6 Classification of Blood Pressure for Adults Aged 18 Years and Older*

Category	Blood Pressure (mm Hg)		
	Systolic		*Diastolic*
Optimal[†]	<120	*and*	<80
Normal	<130	*and*	<85
High-normal	130-139	*or*	85-89
Hypertension[‡]			
Stage 1	140-159	*or*	90-99
Stage 2	160-179	*or*	100-109
Stage 3	≥180	*or*	N ≥ 110

Adapted from The Sixth Report of the Joint National Committee on Preven tion, Detection, Evaluation and Treatment of High Blood Pressure. Arc Intern Med 157:2413, 1997. Copyright 1997, American Medical Association

*Not taking antihypertensive drugs and not acutely ill. When systolic and dias tolic blood pressure levels fall into different categories, the higher categor should be selected to classify the individual's blood pressure status. Fo example, 160/92 mm Hg should be classified as stage 2 hypertension, an 174/120 mm Hg should be classified as stage 3 hypertension. Isolated sys tolic hypertension is defined as systolic blood pressure 140 mm Hg or greate and diastolic blood pressure less than 90 mm Hg and staged approximatel (e.g., 170/82 mm Hg is defined as stage 2 isolated systolic hypertension). I addition to classifying stages of hypertension on the basis of average bloo pressure levels, clinicians should specify the presence or absence of targe organ disease and additional risk factors. This specificity is important fo risk classification and treatment (see Table 37–5).

[†]Optimal blood pressure with respect to cardiovascular risk is less than 120/8 mm Hg. However, unusually low readings should be evaluated for clinica significance.

[‡]Based on the average of two or more readings taken at each of two or mor visits after an initial screening.

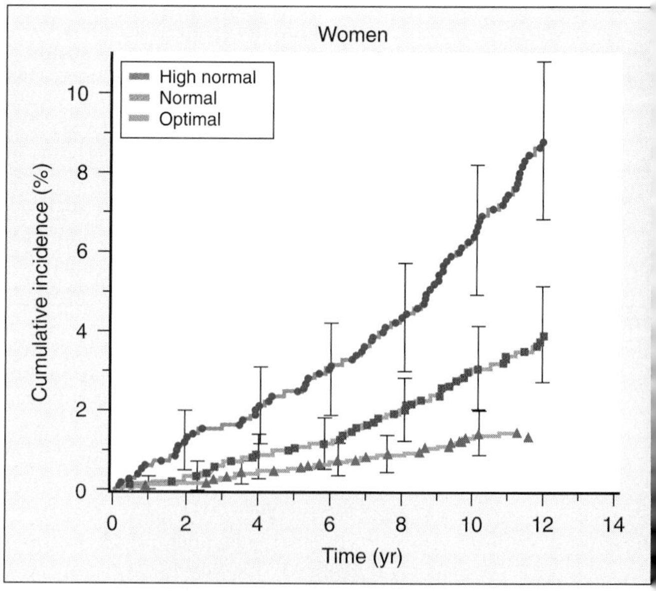

FIGURE 37–5 Cumulative incidence of cardiovascular events in women without hypertension, according to blood-pressure category at the baseline examination. Vertical bars indicate 95 percent confidence intervals. Optimal blood pressure is a systolic pressure of less than 120 mm Hg and a diastolic pressure of less than 80 mm Hg. High-normal blood pressure is a systolic pressure of 130 to 139 mm Hg or a diastolic pressure of 85 to 89. If the systolic and diastolic pressure readings for a subject were in different categories, the higher of the two categories was used. (Modified from Vasan RS, Larson MG, Leip EP, et al: Impact of high-normal blood pressure on the risk of cardiovascular disease. N Engl J Med 345:1295, 2001.)

proposed in the JNC-6 report (Table 37–4).[7] Increasing evidence documents a tracking of blood pressure during childhood with an association between levels at 6 months through adolescence.[21] Appropriate management for asymptomatic post-pubertal children with sustained elevations in blood pressure remains uncertain. Such patients should be monitored carefully, with particular emphasis placed on regular exercise and weight reduction for those who are overweight in the hope of preventing progression of the disease. If lifestyle modifications are not successful, antihypertensive agents should probably be prescribed for patients with sustained levels of blood pressure above the 95th percentile for age and height.

Prevalence of Hypertension

The prevalence of hypertension in the United States rises progressively with age in both men and women (Fig. 37–6).[22] The prevalence of hypertension among blacks is greater at every age beyond adolescence, and hypertension acts as an even stronger risk factor for coronary artery disease among blacks than among whites.[23] The prevalence of hypertension in Mexican Americans is lower than in non-Hispanic whites despite their greater obesity.[24]

After age 50, isolated systolic hypertension increasingly becomes the more common pattern. In the NHANES III survey of a representative sample of the U.S. population, among those not being adequately treated, isolated systolic hypertension was present in 54 percent of hypertensive subjects between the ages of 50 and 59 years and in 87 percent of hypertensive subjects older than 60 years of age.[25] As a consequence of arterial stiffness, systolic levels continue to rise with age, whereas diastolic levels tend to plateau during the fifth decade and to fall thereafter.[26]

SECONDARY HYPERTENSION. Once hypertension has been recognized, it is helpful to know whether some identifiable or secondary process—perhaps curable by surgery or more easily controlled by a specific drug—may be present (Table 37-5).

Most surveys to determine the relative proportion of various identifiable forms of hypertension are biased as a result of the selection process, with only the increasingly suspect population "funneled" to an investigator interested in a particular disease. Thus, estimates as high as 20 percent for certain secondary forms of hypertension have been reported, particularly among those resistant to usual therapy. However, these figures do not reflect the incidence in the population at large. Estimates more likely to be indicative of the situation in usual clinical practice almost all find about 90 percent of hypertensive patients to have primary (essential or idiopathic) disease, with renal parenchymal disease the most common secondary cause, followed by renovascular disease and various adrenal disorders.

SCREENING FOR SECONDARY HYPERTENSION. Because of the relatively low frequency of the various secondary diseases, the clinician should be selective in carrying out various screening and diagnostic tests. The presence of features inappropriate for the usual case of uncomplicated primary hypertension is an indication for additional tests (Table 37-6). However, for the 9 in 10 hypertensive patients without these features, a hematocrit, urine analysis, automated blood biochemical profile (including plasma glucose, potassium, creatinine, and total and high-density lipoprotein cholesterol), and an electrocardiogram are all

TABLE 37–4 Ninety-Fifth Percentile of Blood Pressure by Selected Ages in Girls and Boys in the 50th and 75th Height Percentiles

	Girls' SBP/DBP		Boys' SBP/DBP	
Age (yr)	*50th Percentile for Height*	*75th Percentile for Height*	*50th Percentile for Height*	*75th Percentile for Height*
1	104/58	105/59	102/57	104/58
6	111/73	112/73	114/74	115/75
12	123/80	124/81	123/81	125/82
17	129/84	130/85	136/87	138/88

DBP = diastolic blood pressure; SBP = systolic blood pressure.
Adapted from The Sixth Report of the Joint National Committee on Prevention, Detection, Evaluation and Treatment of High Blood Pressure. Arch Intern Med 157:2413, 1997. Copyright 1997, American Medical Association.

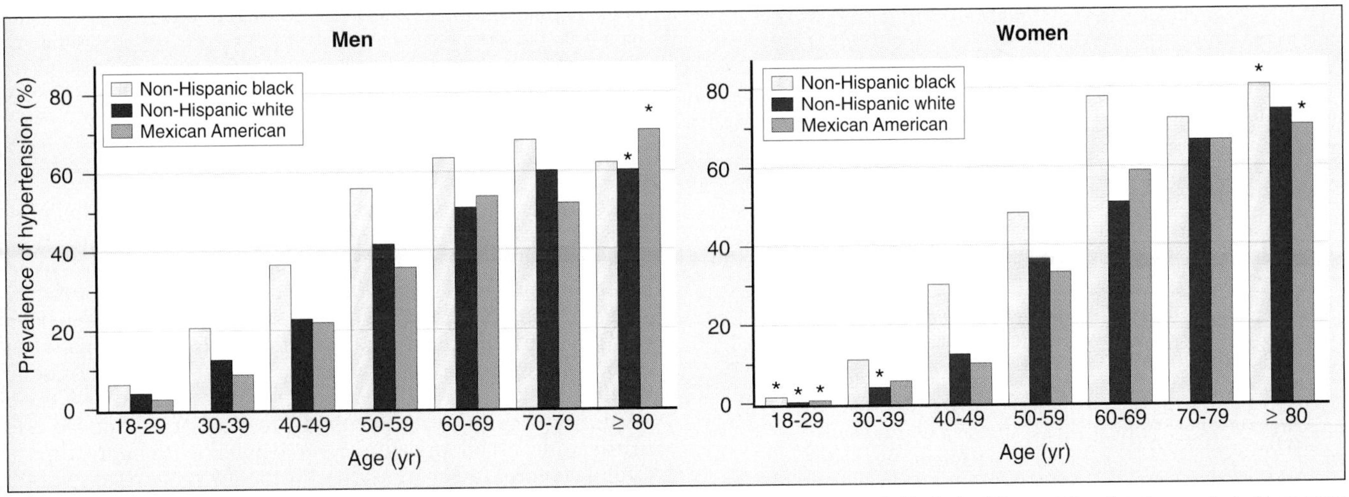

FIGURE 37–6 Prevalence of high blood pressure by age and race or ethnicity for men and women 18 years and older in the U.S. population. Data bars marked with an asterisk are based on a sample size that did not meet the minimum requirements of the National Health and Nutrition Examination Survey (NHANES) III design or relative SEM greater than 30 percent. (Data from Burt VL, Whelton P, Roccella EJ, et al: Prevalence of hypertension in the US adult population: Results from the Third National Health and Nutrition Examination Survey 1988-91. Hypertension 25:305, 1995.)

TABLE 37–5 Types of Hypertension

Systolic and Diastolic Hypertension	Primary, essential or idiopathic
	Identifiable (secondary)
	Renal
	Renal parenchymal disease
	Acute glomerulonephritis
	Chronic nephritis
	Polycystic disease
	Diabetic nephropathy
	Hydronephrosis
	Renovascular
	Renal artery stenosis
	Intrarenal vasculitis
	Renin-producing tumors
	Renoprival
	Primary sodium retention (Liddle syndrome, Gordon syndrome)
	Endocrine
	Acromegaly
	Hypothyroidism
	Hyperthyroidism
	Hypercalcemia (hyperparathyroidism)
	Adrenal
	Cortical
	Cushing syndrome
	Primary aldosteronism
	Congenital adrenal hyperplasia
	Medullary: pheochromocytoma
	Extraadrenal chromaffin tumors
	Apparent mineralocorticoid excess (licorice)
	Carcinoid
	Exogenous hormones
	Estrogen
	Glucocorticoids
	Mineralocorticoids
	Sympathomimetics
	Erythropoietin
	Tyramine-containing foods and monoamine oxidase inhibitors
	Coarctation of the aorta
	Pregnancy-induced hypertension
	Neurological disorders
	Increased intracranial pressure
	Sleep apnea (usually obstructive)
	Quadriplegia
	Acute porphyria
	Familial dysautonomia
	Guillain-Barré syndrome
	Acute stress, including surgery
	Psychogenic hyperventilation
	Hypoglycemia
	Burns
	Alcohol withdrawal
	Sickle cell crisis
	Postresuscitation
	Perioperative
	Increased intravascular volume
	Exogenous causes
	Alcohol abuse
	Nicotine
	Immunosuppressive drugs
	Heavy metal toxicity
Systolic Hypertension	Increased cardiac output
	Aortic valvular insufficiency
	Arteriovenous fistula, patent ductus
	Thyrotoxicosis
	Paget disease of bone
	Beriberi
	Rigidity of the aorta

TABLE 37–6 Features of "Inappropriate" Hypertension

Onset before 20 or after 50 years of age
Level of blood pressure >180/110 mm Hg
Organ damage Funduscopic findings of grade 2 or higher Serum creatinine >1.5 mg/100 ml Cardiomegaly or left ventricular hypertrophy
Features indicative of secondary causes Unprovoked hypokalemia Abdominal bruit Variable pressures with tachycardia, sweating, tremor Family history of renal disease
Poor response to therapy that is usually effective

that is required. Although some practitioners would include other tests, an inordinate number of screening tests for relatively rare diseases will increase the likelihood of a false-positive result. For example, according to Bayes' theorem, at a prevalence rate of 2 percent for renovascular hypertension, which is probably higher than seen in the overall hypertensive population, the predictive value of an abnormal renogram suggestive of this diagnosis is only 10 percent, and an abnormal renogram is more likely to be a false-positive finding than be true-positive.

If a secondary cause for hypertension is suspected from the initial evaluation, additional diagnostic studies should be obtained in a sequential manner (Table 37–7). More about these and other identifiable causes will be provided at the end of this chapter.

Natural History of Untreated Hypertension

The changing pattern of blood pressure with age—rising systolic and falling diastolic levels—primarily reflects atherosclerotic rigidity of large capacitance arteries and a faster reflection of the pulse wave from arteriosclerotic stiffness of smaller peripheral arteries.[26] Both the rising systolic and falling diastolic levels logically are associated with an increased risk for atherosclerotic vascular diseases. The resultant widening pulse pressure has been widely reported to be the best prognostic indicator of cardiovascular risk. However, an analysis of data from almost one million adults in 61 prospective studies found that, for predicting mortality from both stroke and coronary disease, the systolic blood pressure is slightly more informative than the diastolic blood pressure and that pulse pressure is much less informative.[27]

SYMPTOMS AND SIGNS. Uncomplicated hypertension is almost always asymptomatic, so that patients may be unaware of the consequent progressive cardiovascular damage for as long as 10 to 20 years. Only if blood pressure is measured frequently and people are made aware that hypertension may be harmful even if asymptomatic will the majority of people with unrecognized or inadequately treated hypertension be managed effectively. Symptoms often attributed to hypertension—headache, tinnitus, dizziness, and fainting—may be observed just as commonly in the normotensive population. Moreover, many symptoms attributed to the elevated blood pressure are psychogenic in origin, often reflecting hyperventilation induced by anxiety over the diagnosis of a lifelong, insidious disease that threatens well-being and survival.[28] Even headache, long considered a frequent symptom of hypertension, is poorly related to the level of blood pressure.

COURSE OF UNTREATED HYPERTENSION. The relationship between increasing blood pressure and cardiovascular mortality is direct, continuous, and independent of other risk factors. The findings in the long follow-up of subjects screened for the MRFIT study (see Fig. 37–4)[19] have been confirmed by the meta-analysis of the relationship between blood pressure and cardiovascular mortality in almost one million adults in 61 prospective observational studies.[27] Each 20 mm Hg rise in systolic blood pressure or 10 mm Hg rise in diastolic blood pressure is associated with more than a twofold increase in mortality from stroke and a twofold increase in mortality from coronary disease.

As noted in Figure 37–5, even minimal hypertension is accompanied by significant increases in cardiovascular mortality. These figures may be misleading, however, since they

TABLE 37–7 Overall Guide to Work-up for Identifiable Causes of Hypertension

Diagnosis	Diagnostic Procedure: *Initial*	*Additional*
Chronic renal disease	Urinalysis, serum creatinine, renal sonography	Isotopic renogram, renal biopsy
Renovascular disease	Captopril-enhanced isotopic renogram, duplex sonography	Magnetic resonance or CT angiogram, aortogram
Coarctation	Blood pressure in legs	Echocardiogram, aortogram
Primary aldosteronism	Plasma and urinary potassium, plasma renin and aldosterone	Plasma or urinary aldosterone after saline load, adrenal CT and venous sampling
Cushing syndrome	Morning plasma cortisol after 1 mg dexamethasone at bedtime	Urinary cortisol after variable doses of dexamethasone, adrenal CT, and scintiscans
Pheochromocytoma	Plasma metanephrine Spot urine for metanephrine	Urinary catechols; plasma catechols (basal and after 0.3 mg clonidine) Adrenal CT and scintiscans

CT = computed tomography.

seem to imply that most hypertensive subjects, including those with minimally elevated pressure, will experience adverse consequences of hypertension, and rather quickly. In fact, the usual presentation of data as *relative* risk suggests a much greater danger than is shown when data are presented as *absolute* risk. The issue is well identified in the data from the Pooling Project,[29] which includes many prospective follow-up studies, including the Framingham cohort. These data indicate that white men with diastolic pressures of 80 to 87 mm Hg had a 52 percent greater relative risk of having a major coronary event over an 8.6-year period than did those with diastolic pressures below 80. However, this large increased relative risk translates to an absolute excess risk of only 3.5 men per 100 over the 8.6-year interval. Obviously, the majority of those with even higher diastolic pressures did not suffer a major coronary event.

Nonetheless, because so many persons have hypertension, the fact that even a minority of them will suffer a premature cardiovascular event in the course of their disease makes hypertension a major societal problem. In fact, when the cardiovascular death rates for various levels of systolic or diastolic blood pressure are multiplied by the proportion of people in the population who have these various levels, the majority of excess deaths attributable to hypertension are found to occur among those with minimally elevated pressure (Fig. 37–7).

As the public and the medical profession have become aware of the overall societal consequences of even mild hypertension, enthusiasm for early recognition and aggressive treatment of hypertension has continued to mount. A closer look at the issue of deciding on the need for therapy is provided in Chapter 38. However, further consideration of the natural course of hypertension, as it applies to the individual patient, is needed to answer a basic question: Are the blood pressure and the consequent risk high enough to justify medical intervention? Unless the risk is high enough to mandate some form of intervention, there seems to be no need to identify and label the person as hypertensive, since psychological and socioeconomic burdens accompany this label; unless risks clearly outweigh these burdens, caution is obviously advised.

We are thus left with a dilemma: For hypertensive subjects as a group, even among those with the least elevated pressures, risk is increased; for the individual hypertensive subject, the risk may not justify the labeling or treatment of the condition.

Assessment of Individual Risk

Guidelines are available to help practitioners resolve this dilemma in dealing with the individual patient. These guidelines are based on the overall assessment of cardiovascular

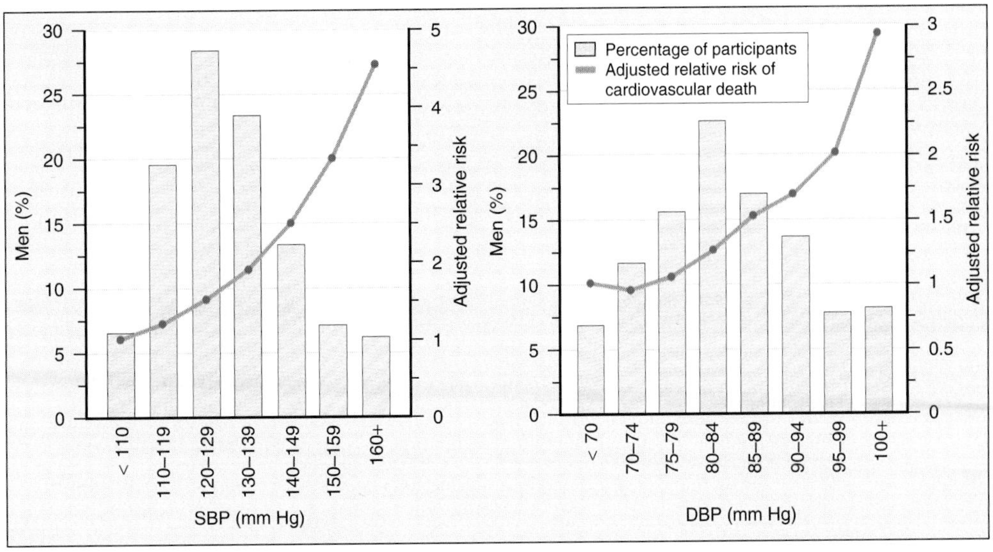

FIGURE 37–7 **Left,** Percentage distribution of systolic blood pressure (SBP) for men screened for the Multiple Risk Factor Intervention Trial who were 35 to 57 years old and had no history of myocardial infarction ($n = 347{,}978$) (shaded bars) and corresponding 12-year rates of cardiovascular mortality by SBP level adjusted for age, race, total serum cholesterol level, cigarettes smoked per day, reported use of medications for diabetes mellitus, and estimated household income (using census tract of residence). **Right,** Percentage distribution of diastolic blood pressure (DBP) in the same group ($n = 356{,}222$). (From National High Blood Pressure Education Program Working Group: National High Blood Pressure Education Program Working Group report on primary prevention of hypertension. Arch Intern Med 153:186, 1993. Copyright 1993, American Medical Association.)

risk and the biological aggressiveness of the hypertension. They are intended to apply only to those with stage 1 (formerly referred to as mild) hypertension, that is, systolic pressure between 140 and 159 mm Hg or diastolic pressure between 90 and 99 mm Hg; those with higher levels have been shown to be at high enough risk from the hypertension per se to justify immediate intervention. Recall, however, that most hypertensive persons are in the range between 140 and 159 mm Hg systolic or 90 and 99 mm Hg diastolic (Fig. 37–7). On the other hand, patients at high overall cardiovascular risk, even with high normal blood pressure, are deemed to be in need of active drug therapy.[7]

OVERALL CARDIOVASCULAR RISK. The Framingham Study and other epidemiological surveys have clearly defined certain risk factors for premature cardiovascular disease in addition to hypertension (see Chap. 36). For varying levels of blood pressure, the Framingham data show the increasing likelihood of a vascular event over the next 10 years for both men and women at various ages as more and more risk factors are added (Fig. 37–8). For example, a 55-year-old man with a systolic blood pressure of 160 mm Hg who is otherwise at low risk would have a 13.7 percent chance of a vascular event in the next 10 years. A man of the same age with the same pressure but with all the additional risk factors (elevated serum total cholesterol, low high-density lipoprotein cholesterol, cigarette smoking, glucose intolerance, and LVH on the electrocardiogram) has a 59.5 percent chance. Obviously, the higher the overall risk, the more intensive the interventions should be.

Several approaches have been taken to apply the Framingham risk data to individual patients. As perhaps first and best articulated by a group of New Zealand physicians,[30] the degree of risk from hypertension can be categorized with reasonable accuracy by taking into account (1) the level of blood pressure, (2) the biological nature of the hypertension based on the degree of target organ damage, and (3) the coexistence of other risks. The JNC-6 report provides a stratification of risk into three groups based on known components of risk (Table 37–8) and levels of blood pressure, which are, in turn, used as the basis for deciding upon initial treatment (Table 37–9). According to this stratification, active drug

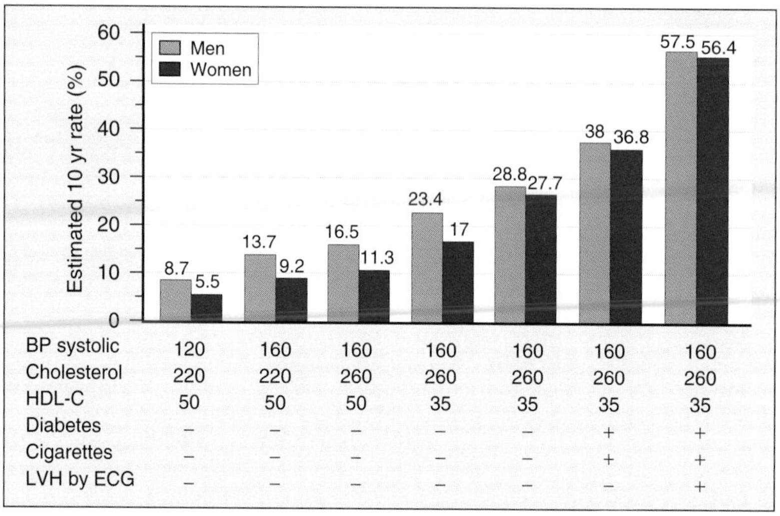

FIGURE 37–8 Estimated 10-year risk of coronary artery disease in hypothetical 55-year-old men and women according to levels of various risk factors. Lipid units are milligrams per deciliter. BP = blood pressure; ECG = electrocardiogram; HDL-C = high-density lipoprotein cholesterol; LVH = left ventricular hypertrophy. (From O'Donnell CJ, Kannel WB: Cardiovascular risks of hypertension: Lessons from observational studies. J Hypertens 16(Suppl 6):3, 1998.)

CH 37

TABLE 37–8 Components of Cardiovascular Risk Stratification in Patients with Hypertension

Major Risk Factors	Target Organ Damage/Clinical Cardiovascular Disease
Smoking	Heart diseases
Dyslipidemia	Left ventricular hypertrophy
Diabetes mellitus	Angina or prior myocardial infarction
Age >60 yr	Prior coronary revascularization
Sex (men and postmenopausal women)	Heart failure
Family history of cardiovascular disease	Stroke or transient ischemic attack
Women >65 yr or men >55 yr	Nephropathy
	Peripheral arterial disease
	Retinopathy

From The Sixth Report of the Joint National Committee on Prevention, Detection, Evaluation and Treatment of High Blood Pressure. Arch Intern Med 157:2413 1997. Copyright 1997, American Medical Association.

TABLE 37–9 Risk Stratification and Treatment*

Blood Pressure Stages (mm Hg)	Risk Group A (No risk factors: no TOD/CCD)	Risk Group B (At least 1 risk factor, not including diabetes: no TOD/CCD)	Risk Group C (TOD/CCD and/or diabetes, with or without other risk factors)
High-normal (130-139/85-89)	Life-style modification	Life-style modification	Drug therapy
Stage 1 (140-159/90-99)	Life-style modification (up to 12 months)	Life-style modification (up to 6 months)	Drug therapy
Stages 2 and 3 (>160/>100)	Drug therapy	Drug therapy	Drug therapy

CCD = clinical cardiovascular disease; TOD = target organ disease.

From The Sixth Report of the Joint National Committee on Prevention, Detection, Evaluation and Treatment of High Blood Pressure. Arch Intern Med 157:2413, 1997. Copyright 1997, American Medical Association.

*Note: For example, a patient with diabetes and a blood pressure of 142/94 mm Hg plus left ventricular hypertrophy should be classified as having stage 1 hypertension with target organ disease (left ventricular hypertrophy) and with another major risk factor (diabetes). This patient would be categorized as "stage 1, risk group C," and recommended for immediate initiation of pharmacological treatment. Life-style modification should be adjunctive therapy for all patients recommended for pharmacological therapy.

herapy is recommended for high-risk patients even if blood pressure is only high normal, whereas life-style modifications are recommended for low-risk patients even if blood pressure is as high as 159/99 mm Hg. In the 2003 JNC-7 report, drug therapy is recommended for the majority of patients with blood pressure above 140/90 mm Hg.[8]

Both the 1997 JNC-6 and the 1999 WHO-ISH[31] guidelines identify a large number of patients in whom risk is considered high enough to warrant drug therapy who would not be so identified by other risk estimates.[32] Although there is an increasing acceptance of using an overall coronary risk of 15 percent or higher over 10 years as an appropriate criterion for antihypertensive drug therapy, risk evaluation remains an inexact science. The addition of echocardiography and carotid ultrasonography markedly elevates the estimate of risk in patients who are considered low-risk by JNC-6 or WHO-ISH criteria.[33] Those procedures have not been advocated, however, largely on the basis of cost-benefit analysis.

It is obvious that since the course of the blood pressure cannot be predicted with certainty, even hypertensive subjects who are not treated should be monitored, and recognition of their hypertension should motivate them to follow good health habits. In this way, no harm should be done, and the potential benefit may be considerable if progression of the disease can be slowed by life-style modifications.

Complications of Hypertension

The purpose of risk assessment is to assist clinicians in determining the appropriate treatment of individual patients to best protect against the various complications associated with hypertension. The higher the degree of risk, the more likely that various cardiovascular diseases will develop prematurely through acceleration of atherosclerosis, the pathological hallmark of uncontrolled hypertension. If untreated, about 50 percent of hypertensive patients die of coronary heart disease or congestive failure, about 33 percent of stroke, and 10 to 15 percent of renal failure. Those with rapidly accelerating hypertension die more frequently of renal failure, as do those who are diabetic once proteinuria or other evidence of nephropathy develops. It is easy to underestimate the role of hypertension in producing the underlying vascular damage that leads to these cardiovascular catastrophes. Death is usually attributed to stroke or myocardial infarction instead of to the hypertension that was largely responsible. Moreover, hypertension may not persist after a myocardial infarction or stroke.

The biological aggressiveness of a given level of hypertension varies among individuals. This inherent propensity to induce vascular damage can best be ascertained by examination of the eyes, heart, and kidney.

FUNDUSCOPIC EXAMINATION (see also Chap. 8). Vascular changes in the fundus reflect both hypertensive retinopathy and arteriosclerotic retinopathy. The two processes first induce narrowing of the arteriolar lumen (grade 1) and then sclerosis of the adventitia and/or thickening of the arteriolar wall, visible as arteriovenous nicking (grade 2). Progressive hypertension induces rupture of small vessels, seen as hemorrhage and exudate (grade 3) and eventually papilledema (grade 4). The grade 3 and 4 changes are clearly indicative of an accelerated-malignant form of hypertension, whereas the lesser changes have been correlated with the risk of coronary disease.[34]

CARDIAC INVOLVEMENT. Hypertension places increased tension on the left ventricular myocardium that is manifested as stiffness and hypertrophy, which accelerates the development of atherosclerosis within the coronary vessels. The combination of increased demand and lessened supply increases the likelihood of myocardial ischemia and thereby leads to a higher incidence of myocardial infarction, arrhythmias, and congestive failure in hypertensive patients.

Abnormalities in Left Ventricular Function. Even before LVH develops, changes in both systolic and diastolic function can be seen. Those patients with minimally increased left ventricular muscle mass may have supernormal contractility as reflected by an increased inotropic state with a high percentage of fractional shortening and increased wall stress.[35] The earliest functional cardiac changes in hypertension are in left ventricular diastolic function, with lower E/A ratio and longer isovolemic relaxation time (see Chap. 11).[36]

With increasing hemodynamic load, either systolic or diastolic dysfunction may evolve and progress to different forms of congestive heart failure (Fig. 37–9).[37] In addition, impaired coronary flow reserve and thallium perfusion defects may be observed in hypertensive patients without obstructive coronary disease.[38] Hypertensive black patients are at a higher risk for progression to heart failure and death from left ventricular dysfunction than are similarly treated white patients.[39]

Left Ventricular Hypertrophy. Hypertrophy as a response to the increased afterload associated with elevated systemic vascular resistance can be viewed as necessary and protective up to a certain point. Beyond that point, a variety of dysfunctions accompany LVH, including lower coronary vasodilatory capacity, depressed left ventricular wall mechanics, and abnormal left ventricular diastolic filling pattern.[40]

Whereas LVH is identified by electrocardiography in only 5 to 10 percent of hypertensive patients, LVH is found by echocardiography in nearly 30 percent of unselected hypertensive adults and up to 90 percent of persons with severe hypertension.[41] The patterns of LVH differ by the type of hemodynamic load: volume overload leads to eccentric hypertrophy, whereas pure blood pressure overload leads to an increase in LV wall thickness without concomitant increase in cavity volume (i.e., concentric hypertrophy). The pattern of LVH can also be modified by increased arterial stiffness, increased pulse wave velocity, and blood viscosity.

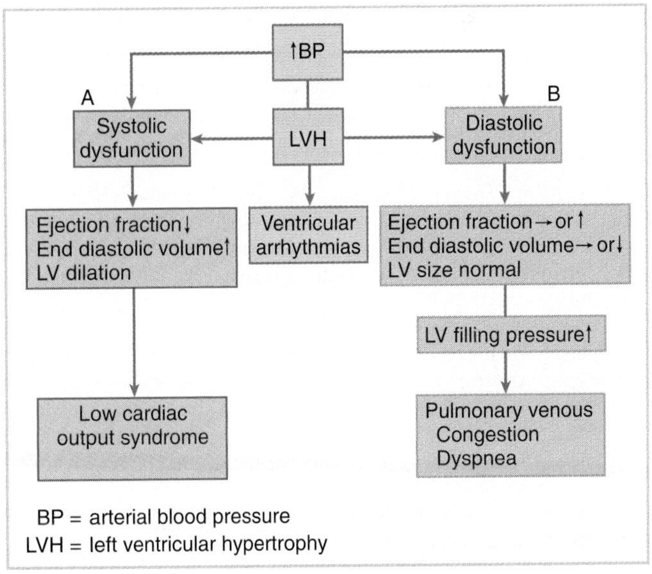

FIGURE 37–9 Consequences of systolic and diastolic dysfunction related to hypertension. **A,** Systolic dysfunction and congestive heart failure caused by impaired ventricular contraction may occur late in the evolution of hypertensive heart disease. **B,** Diastolic dysfunction is the most common manifestation of the effect of hypertension on cardiac function and can also lead to congestive heart failure from increased filling pressures. BP = blood pressure; LV = left ventricular; LVH = left ventricular hypertrophy. (From Shepherd RFJ, Zachariah PK, Shub C: Hypertension and left ventricular diastolic function. Mayo Clin Proc 64:1521, 1989. By permission of the Mayo Foundation.)

In one series of 913 patients with varying stages of hypertension, these percentages of various patterns were found by echocardiography: normal geometry, 19 percent; concentric remodeling, 11 percent; eccentric hypertrophy, 47 percent; and concentric hypertrophy, 23 percent.[42] The presence of LVH is consistently and strongly related to subsequent cardiovascular morbidity and mortality.

Since the presence of LVH may connote a number of deleterious effects of hypertension on cardiac function, a great deal of effort has been expended in showing that treatment of hypertension will cause LVH to regress. Treatment with all antihypertensive drugs except those that further activate sympathetic nervous system activity, for example, direct vasodilators such as hydralazine when used alone, has been shown to cause LVH regression. With regression, left ventricular function usually improves and cardiovascular morbidity decreases.[43]

Congestive Heart Failure (see Chap. 22). The various alterations of systolic and diastolic function seen with LVH obviously can progress into congestive heart failure (CHF). A 20 mm Hg increment in systolic blood pressure conferred a 56 percent increased risk for CHF in the Framingham cohort.[44] Hypertension remains the major preventable factor in the disease that is now the leading cause of hospitalization in the United States for adults older than 65 years of age. It is likely that antihypertensive treatment does not completely prevent CHF but postpones its development by several decades.

Most episodes of CHF in hypertensive patients are associated with systolic dysfunction as reflected in a reduced ejection fraction. However, about 40 percent of episodes of CHF are associated with diastolic dysfunction and preserved left ventricular systolic function. For example, in a series of patients with acute pulmonary edema and systolic blood pressure above 160 mm Hg, an exacerbation of diastolic dysfunction was responsible rather than systolic dysfunction in almost half the cases.[37] Vasan and Benjamin[45] explain the susceptibility of hypertensive patients, particularly those with LVH, to diastolic heart failure:

> When hemodynamically challenged by stress (such as exercise, tachycardia, increased afterload, or excessive preload), persons with hypertension are unable to increase their end-diastolic volume (i.e., they have limited preload reserve), because of decreased left ventricular relaxation and compliance. Consequently, a cascade begins, in which the left ventricular end-diastolic blood pressure rises, left atrial pressure increases, and pulmonary edema develops.

Coronary Heart Disease. As detailed elsewhere (see Chap. 36), hypertension is a major risk factor for myocardial infarction (MI), and ischemia. Moreover, the prevalence of silent MI is significantly increased in hypertensive subjects,[46] and they have a greater risk for mortality after an initial MI.[47] Hypertension may play an even greater role in the pathogenesis of coronary heart disease than is commonly realized, since preexisting hypertension may go unrecognized in patients first seen after an MI. Although acute rises in blood pressure may follow the onset of ischemic pain, the blood pressure often falls immediately after the infarct if pump function is impaired.

Once an MI occurs, the prognosis is affected by both the preexisting and the subsequent blood pressure. The 28-day case fatality rate among 635 men who had an acute MI was 24.5 percent in those with prior systolic blood pressure below 140 mm Hg, 35.6 percent with prior systolic blood pressure of 140 to 159 mm Hg, and 48.2 percent with prior systolic blood pressure of 160 mm Hg or higher.[48] On the other hand, an increase in post-MI mortality has been noted among those whose blood pressure fell significantly, presumably a reflection of poor pump function.[49] If the blood pressure of these subjects remained elevated, the prognosis was even worse, likely representing a severe load on a damaged myocardium, so that care must be taken with patients who have either lower or higher blood pressure after an infarction.

RENAL FUNCTION. Renal dysfunction too subtle to be recognized may be responsible for the development of most cases of primary (essential) hypertension. As discussed later (see Renal Retention of Sodium), increased renal retention of salt and water may be a mechanism initiating primary hypertension, but the retention is so small that it escapes detection. With detailed study, both structural damage and functional derangements reflecting intraglomerular hypertension often reflected by microalbuminuria can be found in most hypertensive persons. Microalbuminuria in hypertensive patients has been correlated with left ventricular hypertrophy and carotid artery thickness.[50] As hypertension-induced nephrosclerosis proceeds, the plasma creatinine level begins to rise and eventually, renal insufficiency may develop. However, despite the epidemiological evidence for an association between hypertension and renal disease, some investigators question the relationship, postulating that the renal damage seen in hypertensive patients is usually secondary to underlying renal diseases that may, in turn, be aggravated by the presence of hypertension.

CEREBRAL INVOLVEMENT. Hypertension may accelerate cognitive decline with age.[51] Hypertension, particularly systolic, is a major risk factor for both ischemic stroke and intracerebral hemorrhage. Cerebral white matter lesions are a common finding by brain magnetic resonance imaging (MRI) seen in 41 percent of asymptomatic, middle-aged hypertensive patients[52] and brain atrophy is more common past the age 67 years in hypertensive than in normotensive subjects.[53] Blood pressure usually rises further during the acute phases of a stroke, and caution is advised in lowering blood pressure during this crucial period.

Mechanisms of Primary (Essential) Hypertension

No single or specific cause is known for most cases of hypertension, and the condition is referred to as *primary* in preference to *essential.* Since persistent hypertension can develop only in response to an increase in cardiac output or a rise in peripheral resistance, defects may be present in one or more of the multiple factors that affect these two forces (Fig. 37–10). The interplay of various derangements in factors affecting cardiac output and peripheral resistance may precipitate the disease, and these abnormalities may differ in both type and degree in different patients.

Hemodynamic Patterns

Before describing specific abnormalities in the various factors shown in Figure 37–10 to affect the following basic equation

$$\text{blood pressure} = \text{cardiac output} \times \text{peripheral resistance}$$
$$(BP = CO \times PR)$$

the hemodynamic patterns that have been measured in patients with hypertension will be considered. One cautionary factor should be kept in mind: Development of the disease is slow and gradual. By the time that blood pressure becomes elevated, the initiating factors may no longer be apparent because they may have been "normalized" by multiple compensatory interactions. Nonetheless, when a group of untreated young hypertensive patients was studied initially, cardiac output was normal or slightly increased and peripheral resistance was normal.[54] Over the next 20 years, cardiac output fell progressively while peripheral resistance rose. In

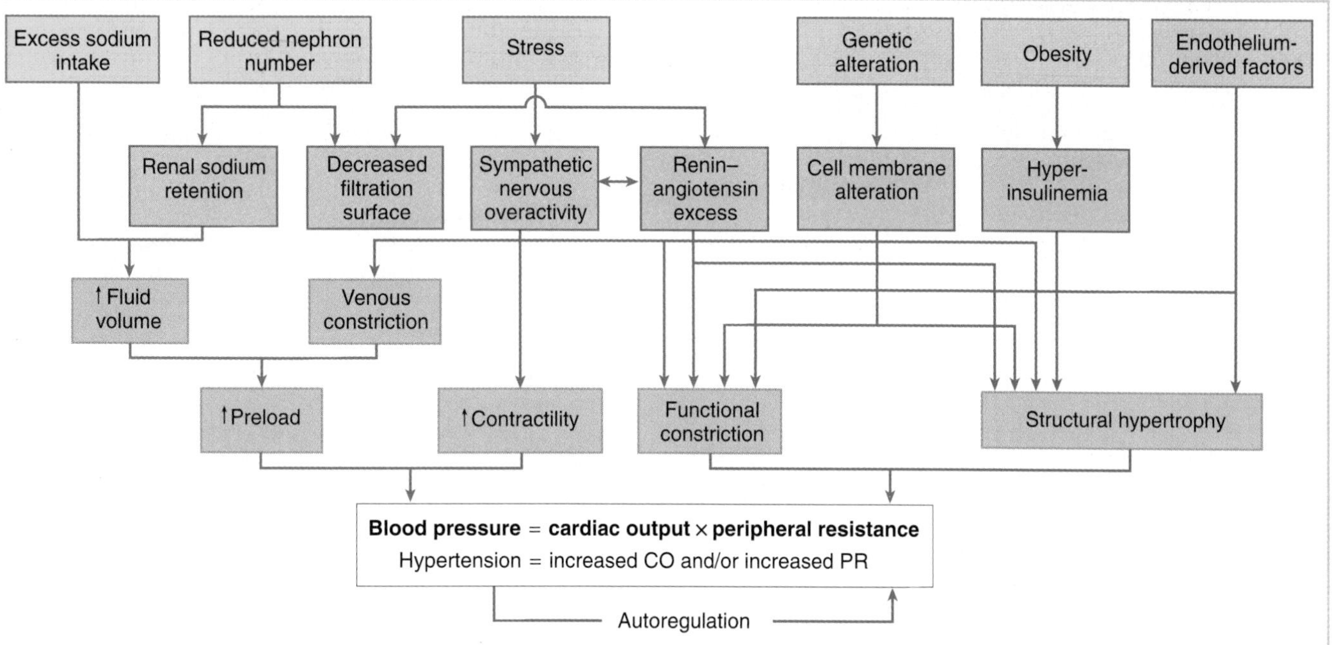

FIGURE 37–10 Some of the factors involved in the control of blood pressure that affect the basic equation blood pressure = cardiac output (CO) × peripheral resistance (PR). (From Kaplan NM: Clinical Hypertension. 8th ed. Baltimore, Lippincott Williams & Wilkins, 2002, p 63.)

a much larger study involving more than 2600 subjects in Framingham who were monitored for 4 years by echocardiography, an increased cardiac index and end-systolic wall stress were related to the development of hypertension,[55] and in a 10-year follow-up of 4700 young people, an increased heart rate, presumably associated with a reflection of increased cardiac output, has been found to be a predictor of future hypertension.[56]

Regardless of how hypertension begins, eventually increased peripheral resistance becomes the primary hemodynamic fault of sustained hypertension.

Genetic Predisposition

As discussed in Chapter 70 and shown in Figure 37–10, genetic alterations may initiate the cascade to permanent hypertension. In studies of twins and family members in which the degree of familial aggregation of blood pressure levels is compared with the closeness of genetic sharing, the genetic contributions have been estimated to range from 30 to 60 percent.[57] Unquestionably, multiple environmental factors play a role, interacting with multiple genes to skew the distribution of blood pressure to higher levels (Fig. 37–11).[58] Essential hypertension is almost certainly a polygenic disorder, involving multiple genes, each having small effects on blood pressure.[59] Linkage genome scans on more than 6000 relatives of hypertensive patients have failed to find regions with large effects.[60]

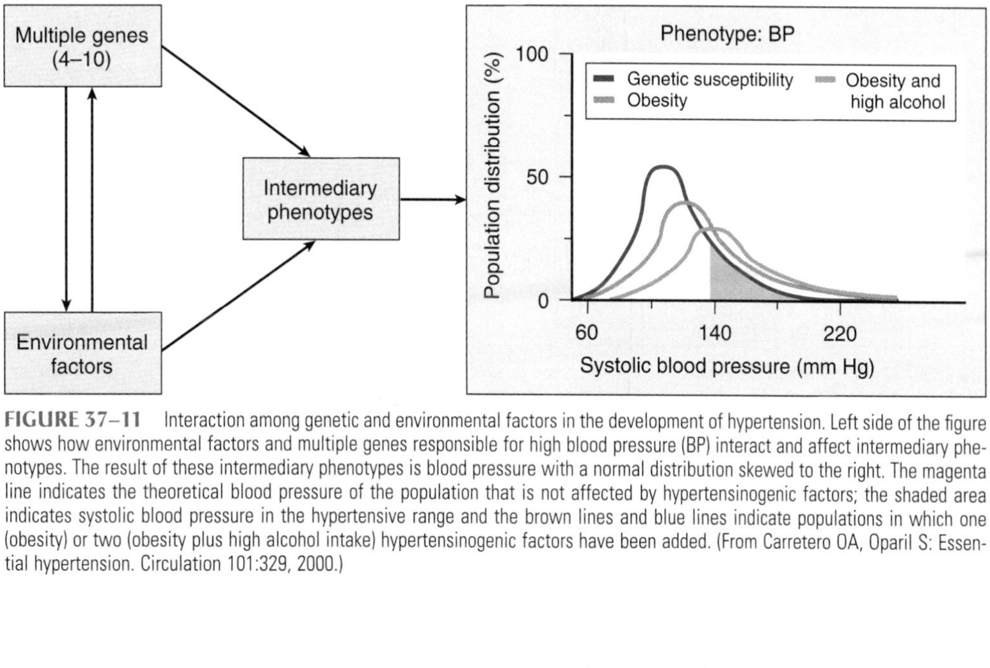

FIGURE 37–11 Interaction among genetic and environmental factors in the development of hypertension. Left side of the figure shows how environmental factors and multiple genes responsible for high blood pressure (BP) interact and affect intermediary phenotypes. The result of these intermediary phenotypes is blood pressure with a normal distribution skewed to the right. The magenta line indicates the theoretical blood pressure of the population that is not affected by hypertensinogenic factors; the shaded area indicates systolic blood pressure in the hypertensive range and the brown lines and blue lines indicate populations in which one (obesity) or two (obesity plus high alcohol intake) hypertensinogenic factors have been added. (From Carretero OA, Oparil S: Essential hypertension. Circulation 101:329, 2000.)

A number of rare forms of hypertension have been found to be caused by a monogenic abnormality, including glucocorticoid-remediable aldosteronism, Liddle syndrome, and apparent mineralocorticoid excess.[61] Virtually all of these involve renal sodium transport in some manner. A monogenic form should be suspected with a strong family history of early onset of hypertension.

In addition to the search for specific causes of hypertension, genetic profiling may make it possible to direct antihypertensive therapy more precisely. For now, children and siblings of hypertensive patients should be more carefully screened. They should be vigorously advised to avoid environmental factors known to aggravate hypertension and increase cardiovascular risk (e.g., smoking, inactivity, and excess sodium).

The Fetal Environment

Environmental factors may come into play very early. Low birth weight as a consequence of fetal undernutrition has been repeatedly found to be followed by an increased incidence of high blood pressure later in life with an overall estimate that a 1 kg lower birth weight is associated with a 2 to 4 mm Hg higher systolic blood pressure in adulthood.[62] However, an analysis of 55 studies that reported regression coefficients of systolic blood pressure on birth weight found progressively weaker associations with increased numbers of participants in the studies and a common inappropriate adjustment for current weight and other confounding factors, leading to the conclusion that "birth weight is of little relevance to blood pressure levels in later life."[63] Moreover, increasing weight gain during childhood has been found to have an even greater impact on adult blood pressure.[62]

Despite these objections to the role of the "low birth weight" hypothesis originally proposed by Professor David Barker, increasing evidence for an effect of intrauterine growth retardation on nephrogenesis provides support for the hypothesis of Brenner and colleagues that a reduced number of nephrons eventuates in hypertension (Fig. 37–12).[64] In addition to experimental evidence,[65] even stronger support comes from a postmortem study of patients with primary hypertension who were found to have half the total number of glomeruli per kidney than matched normotensive control subjects.[66] This lower nephron number presumably was congenital and not acquired after development of hypertension, since there were very few obsolescent glomeruli in the hypertensive subjects' kidneys.

These data fit nicely with Brenner's explanation for the inexorable progression of renal damage once it begins and the concept that hypertension may begin by renal sodium retention induced by the decreased filtration surface area. Other subtle acquired renal injuries induced by vasoconstriction may also contribute to the development of sodium-sensitive hypertension.[67]

Renal Retention of Sodium

A considerable amount of circumstantial evidence supports a role for sodium in the genesis of hypertension (Table 37–10). To induce hypertension, some of that excess sodium must be retained by the kidneys. Such retention could arise in a number of ways, including the following:

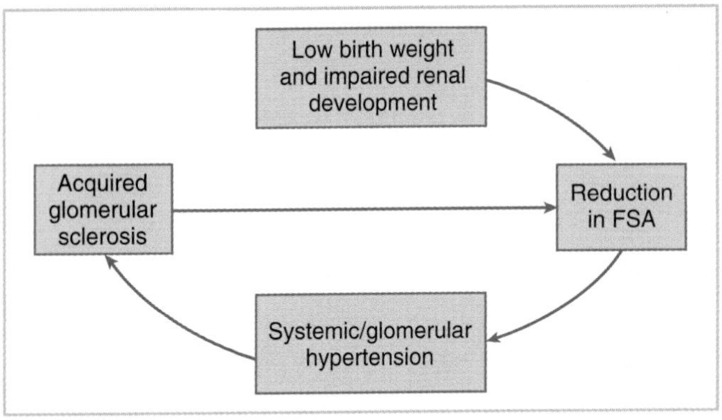

FIGURE 37–12 The risk of essential hypertension and progressive renal injury developing in adult life is increased as a result of congenital oligonephropathy, an inborn deficit of filtration surface area (FSA) caused by impaired renal development. Low birth weight resulting from intrauterine growth retardation or prematurity contributes to this oligonephropathy. Systemic and glomerular hypertension in later life results in progressive glomerular sclerosis, further reducing FSA and thereby perpetuating a vicious cycle that leads, in the extreme, to end-stage renal failure. (From Brenner BM, Chertow GM: Congenital oligonephropathy: An inborn cause of adult hypertension and progressive renal injury? Curr Opin Nephrol Hypertens 2:691, 1993.)

- A decrease in filtration surface by a congenital or acquired deficiency in nephron number or function.
- A resetting of the normal pressure-natriuresis relationship wherein a rise in pressure invokes an immediate increase in renal sodium excretion, thereby shrinking fluid volume and returning the pressure to normal—the Guyton hypothesis.
- Nephron heterogeneity, described as the presence of "a subpopulation of nephrons that is ischemic either from afferent arteriolar vasoconstriction or from an intrinsic narrowing of the lumen. Renin secretion from this subgroup of nephrons is tonically elevated. This increased renin secretion then interferes with the compensatory capacity of intermingled normal nephrons to adaptively excrete sodium and, consequently, perturbs overall blood pressure homeostasis."[68]
- An acquired inhibitor of the sodium pump or other abnormalities in sodium transport.[69]

Thus, more than enough ways are available to incite renal retention of even a very small bit of the excess sodium typically ingested that could eventually expand body fluid volume. Individuals who are more sodium sensitive have been found to have more markers of endothelial damage, nondipping of nocturnal blood pressure, and increased mortality[70] than do those who are less sodium sensitive.

Vascular Hypertrophy

Both excess sodium intake and renal sodium retention would presumably work primarily on increasing fluid volume and cardiac output. A number of other factors may work primarily on the second part of the equation $BP = CO \times PR$ (see Fig. 37–10). Most of these factors can cause both functional contraction and structural remodeling and hypertrophy. These pressor-growth promoters may result in both vascular contraction and hypertrophy simultaneously, but perpetuation of hypertension involves hypertrophy. Various hormonal mediators, such as angiotensin II and endothelin, may serve as the initiator of what eventuates as increased peripheral resistance. To explain this process, Lever and Harrap[71] have postulated that

> Most forms of secondary hypertension have two pressor mechanisms: a primary cause, e.g., renal clip, and a second process, which is slow to develop, capable of maintaining hypertension after removal of the primary cause, and probably self-perpetuating in nature. We suggest that essential hypertension also has two mechanisms, both based upon cardiovascular hypertrophy: (1) a growth-promoting process in children (equivalent to the primary cause in secondary hypertension) and (2) a self-perpetuating mechanism in adults.

TABLE 37–10 Evidence for Role of Sodium in Primary (Essential) Hypertension

In multiple populations, the rise in blood pressure with age is directly correlated with increasing levels of sodium intake.
Multiple, scattered groups who consume little sodium (<50 mmol/d) have little or no hypertension. When they consume more sodium, hypertension appears.
Hypertension develops in animals given sodium loads, if genetically predisposed.
In some people, large sodium loads given over short periods cause an increase in vascular resistance and blood pressure.
An increased concentration of sodium is present in the vascular tissue and blood cells of most hypertensives.
Sodium restriction to a level below 100 mmol/d will lower blood pressure in most people. The antihypertensive action of diuretics requires an initial natriuresis.

These investigators have built on the original proposal of Folkow[72] of a "positive feedback interaction" wherein even mild functional pressor influences, if repeatedly exerted, may lead to structural hypertrophy, which in turn reinforces and perpetuates the elevated pressure (Fig. 37–13).

This scheme to explain an immediate pressor action and a slow hypertrophic effect is thought to be common to the action of pressor-growth promoters. When present in high concentrations over long periods, as with angiotensin II in renal artery stenosis, each of these pressor-growth promoters causes hypertension. No marked excess of any known pressor hormone is identifiable in the majority of hypertensive patients. Nonetheless, a lesser excess of one or more may have been responsible for initiation of the process sustained by positive feedback. If this double process is fundamental to the pathogenesis of primary hypertension, the difficulty in recognizing the initiating causal factor is easily explained. As formulated by Lever,[73]

> The primary cause of hypertension will be most apparent in the early stages; in the later stages, the cause will be concealed by an increasing contribution from hypertrophy . . . A particular form of hypertension may wrongly be judged to have 'no known cause' because each mechanism considered is insufficiently abnormal by itself to have produced the hypertension. The cause of essential hypertension may have been considered already but rejected for this reason.

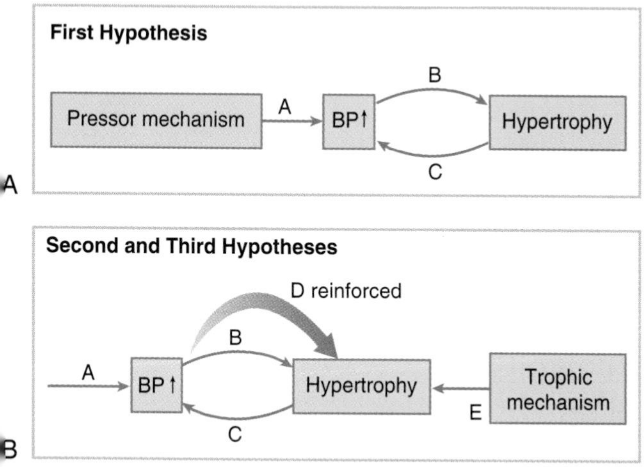

FIGURE 37–13 Hypotheses for the initiation and maintenance of hypertension. **A,** Folkow's first proposal that minor overactivity of a pressor mechanism (A) raises blood pressure (BP) slightly, which initiates positive feedback (B-C-B) and a progressive rise in blood pressure. **B,** As in part **A,** with two additional signals: D, an abnormal or "reinforced" hypertrophic response to pressure; and E, increase in a humoral agent causing hypertrophy directly. (From Lever AF, Harrap SB: Essential hypertension: A disorder of growth with origins in childhood? J Hypertens 10:101, 1992.)

Endothelial Cell Dysfunction

These pressor-growth promoters have traditionally been assumed to be circulating and passing through an inert endothelium. Over the past decade, the endothelial cell has been recognized to be an active participant, the source of multiple relaxing and constricting substances, most having a local, paracrine influence on underlying smooth muscle cells (Fig. 37–14).[74]

NITRIC OXIDE (see Chap. 44). Hypertensive patients have been shown to have a reduced vasodilatory response to various stimuli of nitric oxide release that appears to be independent of the origin of the hypertension and the degree of gross vascular structural alteration. Impaired nitric oxide–mediated vasodilation may promote abnormal vascular remodeling and serves as a marker of future cardiovascular events. Nitric oxide–mediated forearm responsiveness has been restored by normalization of blood pressure by antihypertensive drugs with different modes of action.

ENDOTHELIN. A number of endothelium-derived constricting factors are shown in Figure 37–14. Of these,

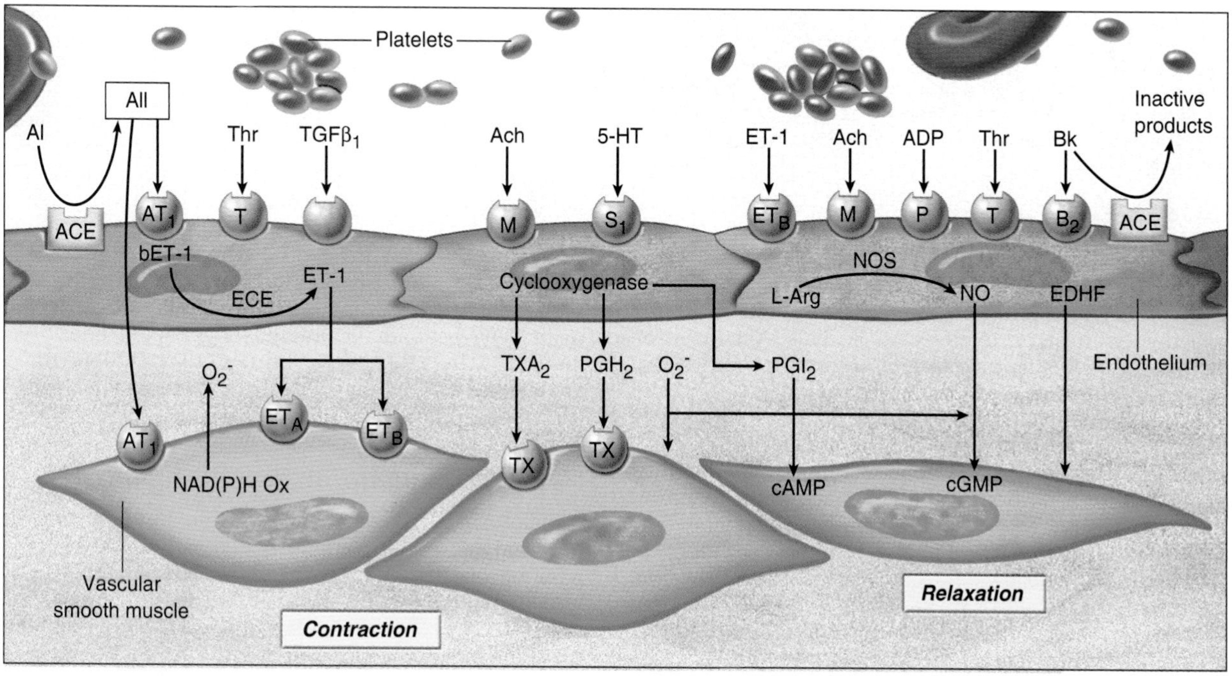

FIGURE 37–14 Endothelium-derived vasoactive substances. Various blood- and platelet-derived substances can activate specific receptors (orange circles) on the endothelial membrane to release relaxing factors such as nitric oxide (NO), prostacyclin (PGI_2), and an endothelium-derived hyperpolarizing factor (EDHF). Other contracting factors are released, such as endothelin-1 (ET-1), angiotensin (A), and thromboxane A_2 (TXA_2), as well as prostaglandin H_2 (PGH_2). ACE = angiotensin-converting enzyme; Ach = acetylcholine; 5-HT = 5-hydroxytryptamine, or serotonin; BK = bradykinin; ECE = endothelin-converting enzyme; L-Arg = L-arginine; NOS = nitric oxide synthase; O_2^- = superoxide; TGF-β_1 = transforming growth factor-beta$_1$; Thr = thrombin. (From Ruschitzka F, Corti R, Noll G, Lüscher TF, et al: A rationale for treatment of endothelial dysfunction in hypertension. J Hyperten 17(Suppl 1):25, 1999.)

endothelin-1 appears to be of particular importance because it causes pronounced and prolonged vasoconstriction and because blockade of its receptors improves endothelium-dependent vasodilation in hypertensive patients.[75] Its role in human hypertension, however, remains uncertain.

A large number of circulating hormones and locally acting substances may be involved in the development of hypertension. Support exists for each of those shown as potential instigators in Figure 37–10.

Sympathetic Nervous Hyperactivity

Young hypertensive patients tend to have increased levels of circulating catecholamines, augmented sympathetic nerve traffic in muscles, faster heart rate, and heightened vascular reactivity to alpha-adrenergic agonists.[76] These changes could raise blood pressure in a number of ways—either alone or in concert with stimulation of renin release by catecholamines—by causing arteriolar and venous constriction, by increasing cardiac output, or by altering the normal renal pressure-volume relationship.

Repetitive stress or an accentuated, exaggerated response to stress is the logical means by which sympathetic activation would arise. Among middle-aged men in Framingham, the development of hypertension over an 18- to 20-year period was associated with heightened anxiety and anger intensity and suppressed expression of anger at baseline.[77] Similarly, among middle-aged men, the systolic pressure reaction to mental stress was positively correlated with higher systolic blood pressures 10 years later.[78] Moreover, the association between progressively lower socioeconomic status and the incidence of hypertension could obviously involve increased levels of stress.

Sympathetic nervous activity could be activated from the brain without the mediation of stress or emotional distress. Hypertension has been induced in animals by various neurogenic defects. An intriguing association has been reported but not well documented between hypertension, increased central sympathetic outflow, and compression of the ventrolateral medulla by loops of the posterior inferior cerebellar artery seen by magnetic resonance tomography.[79]

Whatever the specific role of sympathetic activity in the pathogenesis of hypertension, it appears to be involved in the increased cardiovascular morbidity and mortality that affect hypertensive patients during the early morning hours as noted earlier in this chapter.[14] Increased alpha-sympathetic activity occurs in the early morning in association with the assumption of upright posture after overnight recumbency, raising blood pressure abruptly and markedly. This rise must be at least partly responsible for the increase in cardiovascular catastrophes in the early morning hours.

Renin-Angiotensin System

Both as a direct pressor and as a growth promoter, the renin-angiotensin mechanism is likely involved in the pathogenesis of hypertension. All functions of renin are mediated through the synthesis of angiotensin II. This system is the primary stimulus for the secretion of aldosterone and hence mediates mineralocorticoid responses to varying sodium intake and volume load. When sodium intake is reduced or effective plasma volume shrinks, the increase in renin-angiotensin II stimulates aldosterone secretion, which in turn is responsible for a portion of the enhanced renal retention of sodium and water (Fig. 37–15). As noted elsewhere (see Chap. 79), aldosterone may have additional pathological roles, including a contribution to myocardial fibrosis.

According to the feedback shown in Figure 37–15, any rise in blood pressure inhibits release of renin from the renal juxtaglomerular cells. Therefore, primary (essential) hypertension would be expected to be accompanied by low, suppressed levels of plasma renin activity (PRA). However, when large populations of hypertensive subjects are surveyed, only about 30 percent have low PRA levels, whereas 50 percent have normal levels and the remaining 20 percent have high levels.

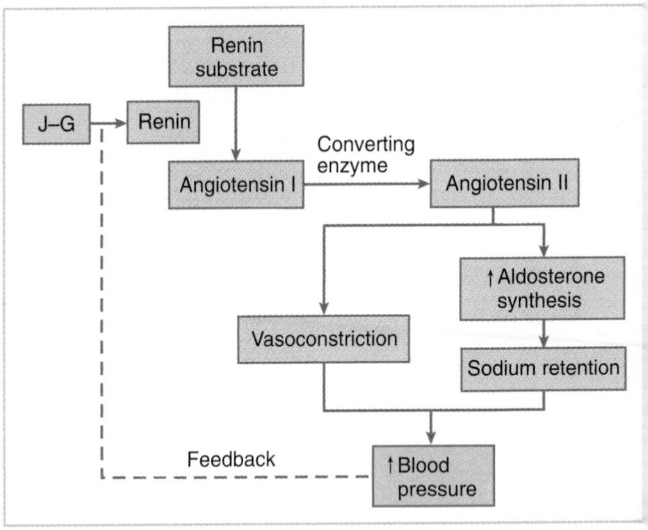

FIGURE 37–15 Overall scheme of the renin-angiotensin mechanism. J-G = juxtaglomerular.

NORMAL- AND HIGH-RENIN HYPERTENSION. A number of explanations have been offered for these "inappropriately normal" or high levels, beyond the proportion expected in a normal gaussian distribution curve. One of the more attractive explanations is the concept of "nephron heterogeneity,"[68] which assumes a mixture of normal and ischemic nephrons caused by afferent arteriolar narrowing. Excess renin from the ischemic nephrons could raise the total blood renin level to varying degrees and cause normal or high renin levels in patients with primary hypertension.

Williams and coworkers[80] have found that about half of normal-renin hypertensive subjects are nonmodulators; that is, they do not normally increase aldosterone secretion in response to sodium restriction and do not normally increase renal blood flow in response to sodium loading. Such nonmodulation in the presence of usual high sodium intake would help explain the pathogenesis of both sodium-sensitive hypertension and the continued secretion of renin due to a defective feedback mechanism.

The renin-angiotensin system is active in multiple organs, either from in situ synthesis of various components or by transport from renal juxtaglomerular cells through the circulation. Most of the important pathophysiological effects are mediated through the angiotensin II type I receptor, but some effects may involve the type II receptor. The presence of the complete system in endothelial cells, the brain, the heart, and the adrenal cortex broadens the potential role of this mechanism even beyond its previously accepted boundaries. As described in Chapter 38, drugs that inhibit the renin-angiotensin mechanism have assumed a major role in the treatment of hypertension.

Hyperinsulinemia/Insulin Resistance

An association between hypertension and hyperinsulinemia has been recognized for many years, particularly with accompanying obesity but also in about 20 percent of nonobese hypertensive patients. Virtually all obese people are hyperinsulinemic secondary to insulin resistance and even more so if the obesity is predominantly visceral—abdominal or upper body—wherein decreased hepatic uptake of insulin contributes to the hyperinsulinemia. The hyperinsulinemia of hypertension also arises as a consequence of resistance to the effects of insulin on peripheral glucose utilization.

The cause of the insulin resistance in nonobese hypertensive persons is unknown. It could reflect a simple reduced ability of insulin to reach skeletal muscle cells, wherein its major peripheral actions on glucose metabolism occur. This impairment may in turn result from a defect in the usual vasodilatory effect of insulin mediated through increased synthesis of nitric oxide, which normally counters the multiple pressor effects of insulin. These pressor effects include activation of sympathetic activity, a trophic action on vascular hypertrophy, and increased renal sodium reabsorption (Fig. 37–16).

The failure of vasodilation to antagonize the multiple pressor effects of insulin presumably eventuates in a rise in blood pressure that may be either a primary cause of hypertension or, at least, a secondary potentiator. In addition, the underlying insulin resistance is often associated with the metabolic syndrome, including dyslipidemia and diabetes along with hypertension, which combine to be a major risk factor for premature coronary disease.

Other Possible Mechanisms

The preceding description of the possible roles of the various mechanisms portrayed in Figure 37–10 does not exhaust the list of putative contributors to the pathogenesis of primary hypertension. Defects in ion transport across cell membranes and deficiencies of various vasodepressor hormones may also be involved. Moreover, a number of associations between hypertension and other conditions have been noted and may offer additional insight into the potential causes and possible prevention of the disease.

ASSOCIATION OF HYPERTENSION WITH OTHER CONDITIONS

Obesity

Hypertension is more common among obese individuals and adds to their increased risk for ischemic heart disease, particularly if it is abdominal or visceral in location as part of the metabolic syndrome. In the Framingham study, the incidence of hypertension was increased 46 percent in men and 75 percent in women who were overweight, defined as a body mass index of 25.0 to 29.9, compared to normal-weight persons.[81] Even small amounts of weight gain are associated with a marked increase in the incidence of hypertension and coronary events. Unfortunately, there is a worldwide epidemic of obesity, perhaps most widespread in the United States, where the prevalence of obesity, defined as a body mass index above 30, increased by 50 percent from 1980 to 1995.[82] Obesity is rapidly increasing among U.S. children, and children seem particularly vulnerable to the hypertensive effects of weight gain.[83] Therefore, avoidance of childhood obesity in the hope of avoiding subsequent hypertension is important. The evidence that weight reduction will lower established hypertension is discussed later.

Sleep Apnea

One of the contributors to hypertension in obese persons is obstructive sleep apnea. Snoring and sleep apnea are often associated with hypertension, which may in turn be induced by increased sympathetic activity and endothelin release in response to hypoxemia during apnea.[84] Relief of sleep apnea may alleviate hypertension.

Physical Inactivity

Physical fitness can help prevent hypertension, and persons who are already hypertensive can lower their blood pressure by means of regular aerobic exercise. The relationship may involve a restoration of age-related declines in endothelium-dependent vasodilation.[85]

Alcohol Intake

Alcohol in small amounts (less than one or two usual portions a day) provides protection from coronary disease, congestive heart failure, stroke, and dementia[86] and, at least in women, reduces the incidence of hypertension.[87] In larger amounts (more than two portions a day and even more so when drunk in binges), alcohol increases blood pressure and arterial stiffness. The reduction in coronary disease in persons who ingest small amounts of alcohol may reflect an improvement in lipid profile, a reduction in factors that encourage thrombosis, and an improvement in insulin sensitivity.

The pressor effect of larger amounts of alcohol primarily reflects an increase in cardiac output and heart rate, possibly a consequence of increased sympathetic nerve activity. Alcohol also alters cell membranes and allows more calcium to enter, perhaps by inhibition of sodium transport.

Smoking (see Chap. 36)

Cigarette smoking raises blood pressure, probably through the nicotine-induced release of norepinephrine from adrenergic nerve endings. In addition, smoking causes an acute and marked reduction in radial artery compliance independent of the increase in blood pressure. When smokers quit, a rise in blood pressure may occur, probably reflecting a gain in weight.

Hematological Findings

Higher hematocrits are found in hypertensive persons and are associated with abnormal left ventricular filling on echocardiography.[88] Whole-blood viscosity is increased by about 10 percent in persons with untreated mild hypertension, comparable to the increase in their peripheral resistance.[89]

Hyperuricemia

Hyperuricemia is present in 25 to 50 percent of individuals with untreated primary hypertension, about five times the frequency found in normotensive persons. Hyperuricemia probably reflects decreased renal blood flow, presumably a reflection of nephrosclerosis.

Hypercholesterolemia

Hypercholesterolemia frequently coexists with hypertension, at least in part because it impairs endothelium-dependent vasodilation. Lipid-lowering therapy restores the bioavailability of nitric oxide, reduces arterial stiffness, and lowers blood pressure.[90] In addition to these conditions often associated with hypertension, distinctive features of hypertension may be important in various special groups of people.

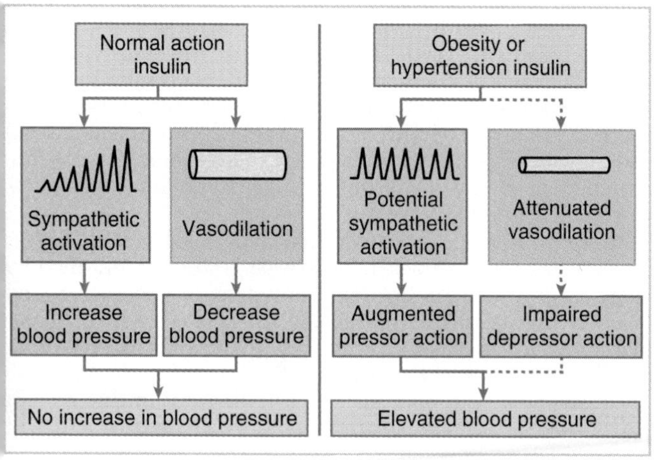

FIGURE 37–16 **Left,** Insulin's actions in normal humans. Although insulin causes a marked increase in sympathetic neural outflow, which would be expected to increase blood pressure, it also causes vasodilation, which would decrease blood pressure. The net effect of these two opposing influences is no change or a slight decrease in blood pressure. There may be an imbalance between the sympathetic and vascular actions of insulin in conditions such as obesity or hypertension. **Right,** Insulin may cause potentiated sympathetic activation or attenuated vasodilation. An imbalance between these pressor and depressor actions of insulin may result in elevated blood pressure. (From Anderson EA, Mark AL: Cardiovascular and sympathetic actions of insulin: The insulin hypothesis of hypertension revisited. Cardiovasc Risk Factors 3:159, 1993.)

Hypertension in Special Groups

Blacks

Although, on average, blood pressure in black persons is not higher than in white persons during adolescence, adult blacks have hypertension more frequently, with higher rates of morbidity and mortality. These higher rates may reflect a higher incidence of low birth weight from intrauterine growth retardation, a lesser tendency for the pressure to fall during sleep, hyperresponsivity to stress, and impaired nitric oxide–induced vasodilation,[91] but the lower socioeconomic status and lesser access to adequate health care of black persons as a group are probably more important. In particular, blacks suffer more renal damage, even with apparently effective blood pressure control, which leads to a significantly greater prevalence of end-stage disease.[92] When given a high-sodium diet, most blacks but not whites tend to have renal vasoconstriction and an increase in the glomerular filtration rate, thus providing a possible mechanism for increased glomerular sclerosis. Hypertension in blacks has been characterized as having a relatively greater component of fluid volume excess, including a higher prevalence of low PRA and greater responsiveness to diuretic therapy.

Perhaps black persons as a group evolved the physiological machinery that would offer protection in their ancestral habitat, hot, arid climates in which avid sodium conservation was necessary for survival because the diet was relatively low in sodium. When they migrate to areas where sodium intake is excessive, they are then more susceptible to "sodium overload." In addition, blacks may also be more susceptible to hypertension because as a group they tend to ingest less potassium.[93]

TABLE 37–11 Most Common Causes for Chronic Hypertension in Childhood

Newborn	
	Renal artery stenosis or thrombosis
	Congenital renal structural abnormalities
	Coarctation of the aorta
	Bronchopulmonary dysplasia
Infancy to 6 yr	
	Renal structural and inflammatory diseases
	Coarctation of the aorta
	Renal artery stenosis
	Wilms tumor
6-10 yr	
	Renal structural and inflammatory diseases
	Renal artery stenosis
	Essential (primary) hypertension
	Renal parenchymal diseases
Adolescence	
	Primary hypertension
	Renal parenchymal diseases

From Loggie JMH: Hypertension in children. Heart Dis Stroke 3:147, 1994.

Women

In general, women suffer less cardiovascular morbidity and mortality than men do for any degree of hypertension.[94] Moreover, before menopause, hypertension is less common in women than in men, perhaps reflecting the lower blood volume afforded women by menses. Eventually, however, more women than men have a hypertension-related cardiovascular complication because there are more elderly women than elderly men and hypertension is both more common and more dangerous in the elderly.

Children and Adolescents

As in adults, care is needed in establishing the presence of persistently elevated blood pressure in children when using the upper limits of normal shown in Table 37–4. Surveillance of blood pressure as children grow older shows an overall tracking of systolic levels,[21] but the positive predictive value of a blood pressure reading above the 95th percentile in a 10-year-old boy being at a hypertensive level at age 20 is only 0.44.[95] Nonetheless, most authorities[96] agree that children with "significant" hypertension (levels above the 95th percentile) should be given a limited work-up for target organ damage and secondary causes (perhaps including an echocardiogram and probably including a renal isotopic scan); if results of these tests are negative, the children should be carefully monitored and given nonpharmacological therapy. Those with "severe" hypertension (levels above the 99th percentile) should be more rapidly and completely evaluated and given appropriate pharmacological therapy.

EPIDEMIOLOGY. The older the child is, the more likely it is that the hypertension is of unknown cause, that is, primary or essential. In prepubertal children, chronic hypertension is more likely caused by congenital or acquired renal parenchymal or vascular disease (Table 37–11). In adolescents, primary hypertension is the most likely diagnosis. Factors that increase the likelihood for early onset of hypertension include a positive family history of hypertension, obesity, poor physical fitness, and an increase in thickness of the interventricular septum during systole on echocardiography.

MANAGEMENT. Once persistently elevated blood pressure is identified in children and adolescents and an appropriate work-up has been performed, weight reduction if the patient is overweight, regular dynamic exercise, and moderate restriction of dietary sodium should be encouraged. Those children deemed to be in need of drug therapy are usually treated in the way adults are managed, as described in Chapter 38.

The Elderly

As more people live longer, more hypertension, particularly systolic, will be seen. By the usual criteria of the average of three blood pressure measurements on one occasion at or above 140 mm Hg systolic and/or 90 mm Hg diastolic or the taking of antihypertensive medication, 54 percent of men and women aged 65 to 74 years have hypertension; among blacks, the prevalence is 72 percent.[22] Most of this hypertension is isolated systolic hypertension (>140/<90 mm Hg). Partly because systolic levels are more resistant to therapy and partly because practitioners are often hesitant to treat older patients, the rate of control among the elderly is much lower than among persons younger than 65 years of age.[97] The risks of both pure systolic and combined systolic and diastolic hypertension at every level are greater in the elderly, at least to age 80, than in younger patients as a result of the adverse effects of age-related atherosclerosis and concomitant conditions. It comes as no surprise that elderly subjects achieved even greater reductions in coronary disease and heart failure by effective therapy than did younger hypertensive subjects in multiple clinical trials.[98]

There is evidence, however, that hypertension is no longer a risk factor for cardiovascular disease in those older than 80 years of age.[99] The limited data from seven placebo-controlled trials involving 1670 hypertensive subjects 80 years of age or older reveal significant reductions in major cardiovascular events—strokes by 34 percent, heart failure by 39 percent—in those given antihypertensive drug therapy, but no benefit for mortality.[100] Obviously, more evidence is needed and will be provided by ongoing trials in very old subjects.

As noted before, elderly patients may display three features that reflect age-related cardiovascular changes. The first is pseudohypertension from markedly sclerotic arteries that do not collapse under the blood pressure cuff and therefore cause much higher cuff pressures than present within the vessels. The second feature, seen in 20 to 30 percent of the elderly population, is postural and postprandial hypotension, which usually reflects a progressive loss of baroreceptor responsiveness with age. A standing blood pressure reading should always be taken in patients older than 65 years, particularly if seated or supine hypertension is noted; if postural hypotension is present, maneuvers to overcome the precipitous falls in pressure should be attempted before the seated and supine hypertension is cautiously treated. More about the special therapeutic challenges often found in the elderly is provided in Chapter 38.

The third, increasing arterial stiffness, is largely responsible for the progressively higher levels of systolic pressure (and lower levels of diastolic pressure) with age. Current measures of arterial stiffness have many limitations, but considerable effort is being expended to make them clinically useful.[101] They may prove to be valuable in managing the elderly hypertensive patient.

Patients with Diabetes Mellitus (see Chap. 51)

Hypertension and diabetes coexist more commonly than predicted by chance. They act in a synergistic manner to markedly accelerate cardiovascular damage, which is in turn largely responsible for the premature disabilities and higher rates of mortality that afflict diabetic patients.[102] Among some 1500 diabetic subjects included in the NHANES III survey, 71 percent were hypertensive but only 12 percent had good control—that is, blood pressure below 130/80 mm Hg—whereas 55 percent had blood pressure above 140/90 mm Hg.[103] Not only is hypertension more common in diabetic patients, but it also tends to be more persistent, with less of the usual nocturnal fall in pressure. The absence of a nocturnal fall in pressure may reflect autonomic neuropathy or incipient diabetic nephropathy. Since ambulatory monitoring is not generally available, home measurements of early morning blood pressure should be used. Patients with readings above 130/85 mm Hg are more likely to develop nephropathy and other complications.[104]

When hypertensive, patients with diabetes mellitus may confront some unusual problems. With progressive renal insufficiency, they may have few functional juxtaglomerular cells, and as a result, the syndrome of hyporeninemic hypoaldosteronism may appear, usually manifested by hyperkalemia. If hypoglycemia develops because of too much insulin or other drugs, severe hypertension may occur as a result of stimulated sympathetic nervous activity. Diabetic neuropathy may add to the postural hypotension that is commonly seen in elderly hypertensive individuals. As will be noted in Chapter 38, diabetic patients are also susceptible to special problems associated with antihypertensive therapy. On the other hand, successful control of blood pressure has clearly been shown to protect such patients from the otherwise inexorable progress of diabetic nephropathy. Even more encouraging are the results of large trials documenting the ability of life-style modifications to prevent the onset of diabetes.

Identifiable (Secondary) Forms of Hypertension (see Tables 37–5 and 37–7)

Oral Contraceptive and Postmenopausal Estrogen Use

The use of estrogen-containing oral contraceptive pills is probably the most common cause of secondary hypertension in young women. Most women who take them experience a slight rise in blood pressure. In a prospective cohort study of almost 70,000 nurses, over the 4 years between 1989 and 1993, those who were current users of oral contraceptives had an overall risk for hypertension 50 percent higher than never-users and 10 percent higher than former users.[105] The 50 percent increase in relative risk translated to 41 cases per 10,000 person-years of oral contraceptive use. The incidence of hypertension is likely even less with present-day lower dose formulations.

The dangers of oral contraceptives should be kept in proper perspective. While it is true that use of these drugs is associated with increased morbidity and mortality, the absolute numbers are quite small, as noted in the nurses study.[105] Most adverse effects, including hypertension, occur in women older than 35 years of age who smoke and have other cardiovascular risk factors.[106]

CLINICAL FEATURES. In most women, the hypertension is mild; however, in some, it may accelerate rapidly and cause severe renal damage. When use of the pill is discontinued, blood pressure falls to normal within 3 to 6 months in about half the patients. Whether the pill caused permanent hypertension in the other half or just uncovered primary hypertension at an earlier time is not clear.

MECHANISMS OF HYPERTENSION. Oral contraceptive use probably causes hypertension by volume expansion, since both estrogens and the synthetic progestogens used in oral contraceptive pills cause sodium retention. Although plasma renin levels rise in response to increased levels of angiotensinogen, angiotensin-converting enzyme (ACE) inhibition did not alter blood pressure any more in women with oral contraceptive–induced hypertension than in women with essential hypertension.[107]

MANAGEMENT. The use of estrogen-containing oral contraceptives should be restricted in women older than 35 years, particularly if they also smoke or are hypertensive or obese. Women given the pill should be properly monitored as follows: (1) The initial supply should be limited; (2) they should be asked to return for a blood pressure check before an additional supply is provided; and (3) if blood pressure has risen, an alternative contraceptive method should be offered. If the pill remains the only acceptable contraceptive method, the elevated blood pressure can be reduced with appropriate therapy. In view of the possible role of aldosterone, use of a diuretic-spironolactone combination seems appropriate. In women who stop taking oral contraceptives, evaluation for secondary hypertensive diseases should be postponed for at least 3 months to allow changes in the renin-angiotensin-aldosterone system to remit. If the hypertension does not recede, additional work-up and therapy may be needed.

POSTMENOPAUSAL ESTROGEN USE. Millions of women take estrogen replacement therapy after menopause. Estrogen replacement therapy does not appear to induce hypertension, even though it does induce the various changes in the renin-angiotensin-aldosterone system seen with oral contraceptive use. In fact, most controlled trials find a decrease in daytime ambulatory blood pressure and a greater dipping of nocturnal blood pressure in estrogen replacement therapy users[108] and most hypertensive women have a fall in blood pressure with transdermal estradiol.[109] Such lower blood pressures may reflect a number of effects, including improved endothelium-dependent vasodilation and reduced muscle sympathetic nerve activity.

Renal Parenchymal Disease (see Chap. 86)

Subtle renal dysfunction has been previously described as a likely initiator of primary hypertension, and renal parenchymal disease is the most common cause of secondary hypertension, responsible for 2 to 5 percent of cases. As chronic glomerulonephritis has become less common, hypertensive nephrosclerosis and, to an even greater degree, diabetic nephropathy have become the most common causes of chronic renal disease.[110] The prevalence of chronic renal disease, defined by a reduction in glomerular filtration rate to less than 60 ml/min/1.73 m^2 or persistent albuminuria of more than 300 mg/day, is estimated to be 11 percent (19.2 million) of the adult U.S. population.[111] The higher prevalence of hypertension among U.S. blacks is probably responsible for their significantly higher rate of end-stage renal disease with hypertension as the underlying cause in as many as half of these patients.

As previously noted, even microalbuminuria, 30 to 300 mg/day, is closely related to target organ damage in hypertensive persons,[50] and it likely should be looked for routinely in the evaluation of every new hypertensive patient in a "spot" urine collection. Measurement of serum creatinine is routine but by itself is an inadequate screening test for significant renal damage, particularly in elderly patients.[112] Therefore, a creatinine clearance should be calculated with either the Cockcroft-Gault formula or the Modification of Diet in Renal Disease (MDRD) equation, taking age, gender, and body weight into account.

Once it begins, renal disease is usually progressive, following the concept that a loss of filtration surface leads to both glomerular and systemic hypertension, which engenders more glomerular sclerosis, setting up a cycle of progressive disease (see Fig. 37–12). Therefore, it is critical to identify renal damage early, since removal of causal or aggravating factors can prevent the otherwise inexorable progress of renal damage. These factors include obstruction of the urinary tract, depletion of effective circulating volume, nephrotoxic agents, and, most importantly, uncontrolled hypertension.

In addition to these and other factors involved in chronic renal disease, a number of acute conditions may be responsible for renal damage and hypertension.

ACUTE RENAL DISEASES. Hypertension may appear with any sudden, severe insult to the kidneys that either markedly impairs excretion of salt and water, which leads to volume expansion, or reduces renal blood flow, which sets off the renin-angiotension-aldosterone mechanism. Bilateral ureteral obstruction is an example of the former; sudden bilateral renal artery occlusion, as by cholesterol emboli, is an example of the latter. Relief of either may dramatically reverse severe hypertension. Such reversal of hypertension has been particularly striking in men with high-pressure chronic retention of urine, who may manifest both renal failure and severe hypertension, both of which may be ameliorated by relief of the obstruction.[113] Some collagen diseases may also produce rapidly progressive vasculitis and renal damage.

Two commonly used classes of drugs—nonsteroidal antiinflammatory drugs and inhibitors of the renin-angiotensin system—may suddenly worsen renal function in patients with preexisting renal diseases. Nonsteroidal antiinflammatory drugs, by blocking synthesis of prostaglandins, which act as vasodilators within the kidney, may cause an abrupt loss of renal function. Renin-angiotensin inhibitors, both ACE inhibitors and angiotensin II receptor blockers (ARBs), may precipitate acute renal failure in patients with bilateral renovascular disease whose renal profusion is dependent on high levels of renin-angiotensin.[114]

CHRONIC RENAL DISEASES. All chronic renal diseases are associated with a higher prevalence of hypertension, and the presence of hypertension accelerates the progression of renal damage. Although it is uncertain that hypertension by itself can lead to renal failure in persons who are not black, there is no doubt that hypertension can accelerate the progress of all underlying renal diseases.

The control of hypertension can slow or stop the progression of renal diseases and of cardiovascular sequelae (Fig. 37-17).[115] As noted in the Heart Outcomes Prevention Evaluation (HOPE) trial,[116] the presence of microalbuminuria was associated with an increase in cardiovascular morbidity and mortality in subjects with microalbuminuria (26.4 percent) compared with those without microalbuminuria (15.4 percent). With the further lowering of blood pressure by the addition of the ACE inhibitor ramipril, individuals with microalbuminuria had even greater reduction in their risk. This protection may reflect special advantages of ACE inhibition, but the lowering of blood pressure must also be a factor.

Uncertainty remains as to the goal of antihypertensive therapy in patients with chronic renal disease. In two large trials of nondiabetic patients with chronic renal disease, more intensive therapy to reach a goal of 125/75 mm Hg did not slow the rate of fall of glomerular filtration rate more than did less intensive therapy to a level of 140/85 mm Hg, except in patients with more than 1 g of proteinuria per day.[117,118]

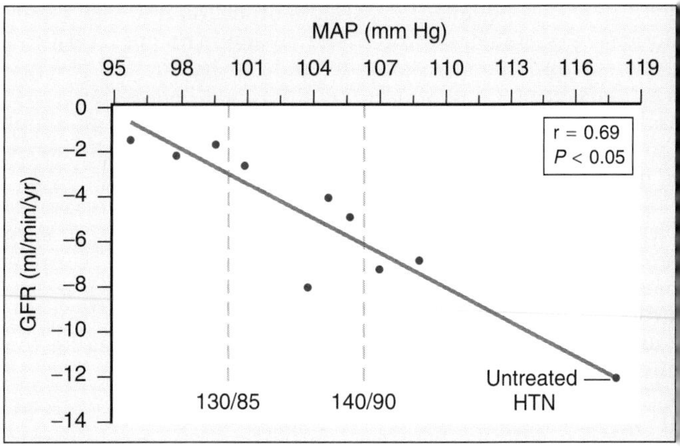

FIGURE 37–17 Relationship between achieved blood pressure control and declines in glomerular filtration rate (GFR) in six clinical trials of patients with diabetic renal disease and three trials of patients with nondiabetic renal disease. HTN = hypertension; MAP = mean arterial pressure. (From Bakris GL, Williams M, Dworkin L, et al: Preserving renal function in adults with hypertension and diabetes: A consensus approach. Am J Kidney Dis 36:646, 2000.)

Issues as to the preferred choices of antihypertensive agents in patients with chronic renal disease are addressed in Chapter 38. Suffice it to note that an ACE inhibitor or an ARB is always indicated as the initial choice, almost always in combination with a diuretic. With whatever drugs chosen, but particularly with ACE inhibitors and ARBs, caution is needed in lowering blood pressure in the presence of previously unrecognized bilateral renovascular disease, which has been found in as many as 20 percent of patients with progressive renal damage.[114] However, a modest increase in serum creatinine, averaging 30 percent above baseline, has been found to predict a better preservation of renal function, presumably reflecting a successful reduction in intraglomerular pressure.[119]

DIABETIC NEPHROPATHY (see Chaps. 51 and 86)**.** The most impressive protection against progressive renal damage by reduction of elevated blood pressure has been seen in patients with diabetic nephropathy.[110] Such protection has been observed to extend to diabetic retinopathy and neuropathy, both in normotensive[120] and hypertensive[121] type 2 diabetic patients with proteinuria. The consensus advice is to start antihypertensive therapy in diabetic patients with or without nephropathy at a blood pressure of 140/90 mm Hg or higher and to reach a level of 130/80 mm Hg or lower.[115] Such intensive control of hypertension has been shown to be much more cost-effective than either intensive glycemic control or reduction in hypercholesterolemia.[122]

Hypertension During Chronic Dialysis and after Renal Transplantation

In patients with end-stage renal disease who are on dialysis, hypertension is a significant risk factor for mortality. Beyond the primary influence of excess fluid volume, hypertension can be accentuated by the accumulation of endogenous inhibitors of nitric oxide synthase. With neither the vasoconstrictor effects of renal renin nor the vasodepressor actions of various renal hormones, blood pressure may be particularly labile and sensitive to changes in fluid volume. Among patients receiving maintenance hemodialysis every 48 hours, elevated blood pressures tend to fall progressively after dialysis is completed, remain depressed during the remainder of the first 24 hours, and rise again during the second day as a consequence of excessive fluid retention. By increasing the time of dialysis treatment and thereby reducing dry weight, blood pressure can be better controlled.[123] As with other forms of renal disease, ACE inhibitors may provide special benefits to hemodialysis patients.[124]

Although successful renal transplantation may cure primary hypertension, various problems can result, with about half of the recipients becoming hypertensive within 1 year. These problems include stenosis of the renal artery at the site of anastomosis, rejection reactions, high doses of adrenal steroids and cyclosporine or tacrolimus, and excess renin derived from the retained diseased kidneys. ACE inhibitor therapy may obviate the need to remove the native diseased kidneys to relieve hypertension caused by their persistent secretion of renin. The source of the donor kidney may also play a role in the subsequent development of hypertension in the recipient. More hypertension has been observed when donors had a family history of hypertension or when the donors had died of subarachnoid hemorrhage and had probably been hypertensive.

Renovascular Hypertension

Renovascular hypertension is among the most common secondary forms of hypertension and is not easily recognizable. The prevalence of proven renovascular hypertension in the overall hypertensive population is unknown, but significant renal artery disease (defined as a 60 percent or greater reduction of diameter on duplex sonography) has been found in 6.8 percent of 824 elderly people in North Carolina[125] and in 7 percent of hypertensive patients undergoing coronary angiography (defined as a 70 percent or greater stenosis on renal angiography).[126]

It has long been known that the presence of renovascular disease does not, in itself, prove that the renovascular lesion is responsible for renovascular hypertension. Therefore, screening should focus on those hypertensive patients who have multiple features known to be associated with renovascular hypertension. The greater the number of clues, the more extensive the search (Table 37–12). The search likely should start with renal arteriography in those who are at high likelihood, since no other screening study can rule out the presence of the disease.

Classification

In adults, the two major types of renovascular disease tend to appear at different times and affect the sexes differently (Table 37–13). Atherosclerotic disease affecting mainly the proximal third of the main renal artery is seen mostly in older men. Fibroplastic disease involving mainly the distal two-thirds and branches of the renal arteries appears most commonly in younger women. As the population grows older, 80 percent of cases are caused by atherosclerotic disease and fewer than 20 percent by fibroplastic disease. Although the nonatherosclerotic stenoses may involve all layers of the renal artery, the most common is medial fibroplasia.

A number of other intrinsic and extrinsic causes of renovascular hypertension are known, including cholesterol emboli within the renal artery or compression of this vessel by nearby tumors. Most renovascular hypertension develops from partial obstruction of one main renal artery, but only a branch need be involved; segmental disease has been found in about 10 percent of cases. On the other hand, if apparent complete occlusion of the renal artery is slow in developing, enough collateral flow will become available to preserve the viability of the kidney. In this way, the seemingly nonfunctioning kidney may be responsible for continued renin secretion and hypertension. If recognized, such totally occluded vessels can sometimes be repaired, with return of renal function and relief of hypertension.[127]

Renovascular stenosis is often bilateral, although usually one side is clearly predominant. The possibility of bilateral disease should be suspected in those with renal insufficiency, particularly if rapidly progressive oliguric renal failure develops without evidence of obstructive uropathy and even more so if it develops after the start of ACE inhibitor or ARB therapy.[114]

Mechanisms

The sequence of changes in patients with renovascular hypertension starts with the release of increased amounts of renin when sufficient ischemia is induced to diminish pulse pressure against the juxtaglomerular cells in the renal afferent arterioles. A reduction in renal perfusion pressure by 50 percent leads to an immediate and persistent increase in renin secretion from the ischemic kidney, along with

TABLE 37–12 Clinical Clues for Renovascular Hypertension

History
Onset of hypertension before 30 or after 50 years of age
Abrupt onset of hypertension
Severe or resistant hypertension
Symptoms of atherosclerotic disease elsewhere
Negative family history of hypertension
Smoker
Worsening renal function with angiotensin-converting enzyme inhibition
Recurrent flash pulmonary edema
Examination
Abdominal bruits
Other bruits
Advanced fundal changes
Laboratory
Secondary aldosteronism
Higher plasma renin
Low serum potassium
Low serum sodium
Proteinuria, usually moderate
Elevated serum creatinine
>1.5 cm difference in kidney size on sonography

Adapted from McLaughlin K, Jardine AG, Moss JG. Renal artery stenosis. Br Med J 320:1124, 2000.

TABLE 37–13 Features of the Two Major Forms of Renal Artery Disease

Cause	Incidence (%)	Age (yr)	Location of Lesion in Renal Artery	Natural History
Atherosclerosis	80-90	>50	Proximal 2 cm; branch disease rare	Progression in 50%, often to total occlusion
Fibromuscular dysplasias				
Intimal	1-2	Birth-25	Midportion of main renal artery and/or branches	Progression in most cases; dissection and/or thrombosis common
Medial	10-20	25-50	Distal segment of main renal artery and/or branches	Progression in 33%; dissection and/or thrombosis rare
Periarterial	1-2	15-30	Middle to distal segments of main renal artery or branches	Progression in most cases; dissection and/or thrombosis common

From Kaplan NM: Kaplan's Clinical Hypertension. 8th ed. Baltimore, Lippincott Williams & Wilkins, 2002, p 385.

suppression of secretion from the contralateral one. With time, renin levels fall (but not to the low level expected from the elevated blood pressure), accompanied by an expanded body fluid volume and increased cardiac output.

Diagnosis

The presence of the clinical features listed in Table 37–12, found in perhaps 5 to 10 percent of all hypertensive persons, indicates the need for a screening test for renovascular hypertension. A positive screening test result, or very strong clinical features, calls for more definitive confirmatory tests. Recurrent flash pulmonary edema has been associated with renovascular hypertension, so this clinical manifestation has been added to the indication for diagnostic work-up.[128] The initial diagnostic study in most patients should be noninvasive and, if abnormal, followed by a study of renal perfusion to ensure that any renovascular lesion is pathogenic, to decide whether revascularization is indicated (Fig. 37–18).[129]

There are problems with all screening studies. Considerable asymmetry of renal blood flow, 25 percent or more, was found in 148 hypertensive patients with patent renal arteries on prior angiography.[130] Such normal asymmetry likely is responsible for the low sensitivity and specificity of captopril-enhanced renal scans. On the other hand, the sensitivity of renal duplex sonography for the detection of hemodynamically significant renovascular disease has been reported to be only 50 percent.[131] The accuracy of ultrasonography is very much operator-dependent, often requiring scanning times of 1 hour or longer, so its use has been limited. However, a strong association with the outcome of revascularization has been reported with the use of a resistance index to assess flow in segmental arteries.[132] Patients with high resistance-index values above 80, reflecting marked intrarenal vascular disease, had generally poor outcomes. Those with lower values had generally good outcomes.

Over the past few years, both contrast-enhanced computed tomography and magnetic resonance angiography have been increasingly used to screen for renovascular hypertension. Magnetic resonance angiography will likely be more widely used, since it avoids the possibility of dye-induced nephrotoxicity and ionizing radiation as well as its greater potential for an assessment of renal function.

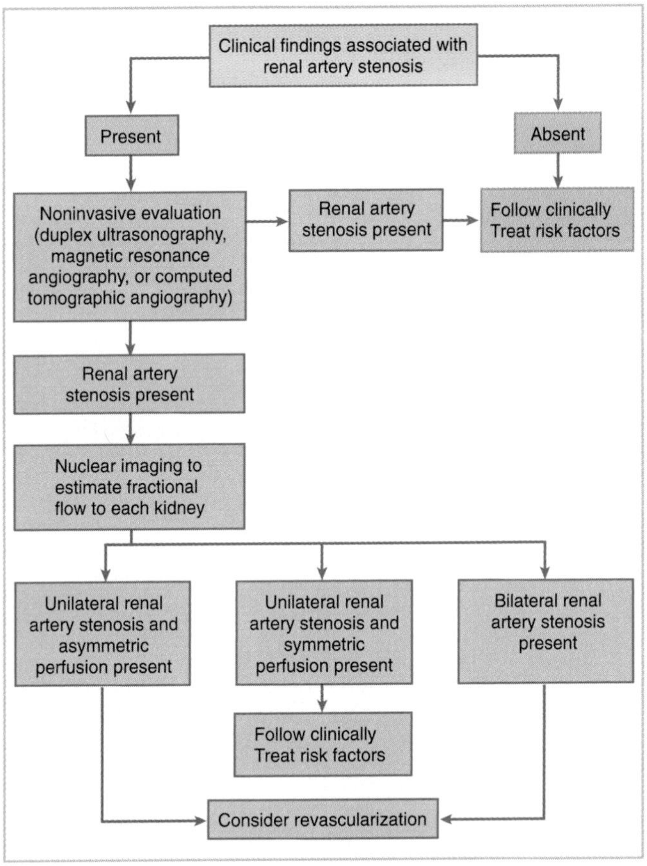

FIGURE 37–18 Algorithm for evaluating patients in whom renal artery stenosis is suspected. Clinical follow-up includes periodic reassessment with duplex ultrasonography, magnetic resonance angiography, and nuclear imaging to estimate fractional blood flow to each kidney. The treatment of risk factors includes smoking cessation and the use of aspirin, lipid-lowering agents, and antihypertensive therapy. (Modified from Safian RD, Textor SC: Renal-artery stenosis. N Engl J Med 344:431, 2001.)

Management

MEDICAL. The availability of ACE inhibitors can be considered a two-edged sword; one edge provides better control of renovascular hypertension than may be possible with other antihypertensive medications, while the other edge exposes the already ischemic kidney to further loss of blood flow by removing the high level of angiotensin II that was supporting its circulation. Other antihypertensive drugs may be almost as effective as ACE inhibitors and perhaps safer, but there are no comparative data.

ANGIOPLASTY (see Chap. 55). Angioplasty has been shown to improve blood pressure (at least transiently) in 60 to 70 percent of patients, more with fibromuscular disease than with atherosclerosis, as is also the case for surgery. In three small but controlled trials, balloon angioplasty was shown to provide a modest but significantly greater reduction in blood pressure than medical therapy.[133] Placement of an arterial stent reduced the likelihood of restenosis and is increasingly performed as the initial procedure to preserve renal function.[134]

SURGERY. Revascularization by surgery is indicated in patients whose hypertension is not well controlled or whose renal function deteriorates with medical therapy and in those with only a transient response to angioplasty or in whom lesions are not amenable to that procedure. Surgery is recommended more to preserve renal function than to relieve hypertension and should be undertaken before serum creatinine level rises above 3 mg/dl.[129]

Renin-Secreting Tumors

Made up of juxtaglomerular cells or hemangiopericytomas, renin-secreting tumors have been found mostly in young patients with severe hypertension, very high renin levels in both peripheral blood and the kidney harboring the tumor, and secondary aldosteronism manifested by hypokalemia.[135] The tumor can generally be recognized by selective renal angiography, usually performed for suspected renovascular hypertension, although a few are extrarenal. More commonly, children with Wilms tumors (nephroblastoma) may have hypertension and high plasma renin and prorenin levels that revert to normal after nephrectomy.[136]

Adrenal Causes of Hypertension

Adrenal causes of hypertension include primary excesses of aldosterone, cortisol, and catecholamines; more rarely, excess deoxycorticosterone is present along with congenital adrenal hyperplasia. Together, these conditions cause less than 1 percent of all hypertensive diseases, although, as will be noted, primary aldosteronism may be more common than previously thought. Each can usually be recognized with relative ease, and patients suspected of having these disorders can be screened by readily available tests.

More of a problem than the diagnosis of these adrenal disorders is the need to exclude their presence because of the increasing identification of incidental adrenal masses when abdominal computed tomography (CT) is done to diagnose intraabdominal pathological conditions. Unsuspected adrenal tumors have been found on about 1 percent of abdominal CT scans obtained for reasons unrelated to the adrenal gland. As delineated in Table 37–7, screening for hormonal excess should be performed if an adrenal tumor is found. Most of these "incidentalomas" appear to be nonfunctional on the basis of normal basal adrenal hormone levels. When more detailed studies are done, however, a significant number show incomplete suppression of cortisol by dexamethasone, that is, subclinical Cushing disease that does not appear to progress to overt hypercortisolism but may be associated with insulin resistance and osteopenia.[137]

The benign nature of smaller tumors can usually be assured by appropriate imaging studies. The threat of malignancy can probably be best excluded by adrenal scintigraphy with NP-59, a radioiodinated derivative of cholesterol. Benign lesions almost always take up the isotope, whereas malignant ones almost always do not. Most tumors larger than 4 cm are resected, since a significant number of them are malignant.

Primary Aldosteronism

This disease has been considered to be relatively rare in unselected populations, but it has been recognized in considerably more patients screened by a plasma aldosterone/renin activity ratio.[138]

PATHOPHYSIOLOGY OF MINERALOCORTICOID EXCESS. A number of syndromes with mineralocorticoid excess have been recognized (Table 37-14), with primary aldosteronism being by far the most common. Until recently, the most frequently found source of hyperaldosteronism was a solitary aldosterone-producing adenoma. Recently, as milder forms of hyperaldosteronism have been recognized by measurements of plasma renin and aldosterone, bilateral adrenal hyperplasia (BAH) has become far more common.

Aldosterone excess from any source causes hypertension and renal potassium wastage, which should induce hypokalemia (Fig. 37-19). However, the majority of patients with aldosteronism caused by BAH are normokalemic.[138] The lack of overt hypokalemia could be explained in numerous ways: (1) potassium wastage has lowered the serum potassium level, but not yet to hypokalemic levels; (2) with milder degrees of aldosteronism, as are typical with BAH, the excess of aldosterone induces hypertension without causing potassium wastage, a scenario that has never been experimentally or clinically recognized; or (3) the BAH is related to the typical progressive increase in adrenal nodular hyperplasia with age that has no relationship to hypertension.[139] The third explanation would fit with the long-held belief that BAH is simply a form of low-renin hypertension, that is, primary (essential) hypertension with plasma renin levels that are known to fall progressively with age while plasma aldosterone levels remain stable.[140]

TABLE 37–14 Syndromes of Mineralocorticoid Excess

Adrenal origin
Aldosterone excess (primary)
Aldosterone-producing adenoma
Bilateral hyperplasia
Primary unilateral adrenal hyperplasia
Glucocorticoid-remediable aldosteronism (familial hyperaldosteronism, type I)
Adrenal carcinoma
Extraadrenal tumors
Deoxycorticosterone excess
Deoxycorticosterone-secreting tumors
Congenital adrenal hyperplasia
11β-hydroxylase deficiency
17α-hydroxylase deficiency
Cortisol excess
Cushing syndrome from ACTH-producing tumor
Glucocorticoid receptor resistance
Renal origin
Activating mutation of mineralocorticoid receptor
Pseudohypoaldosteronism, type II (Gordon)
11β-hydroxysteroid dehydrogenase deficiency
Congenital: apparent mineralocorticoid excess
Acquired: licorice, carbenoxolone

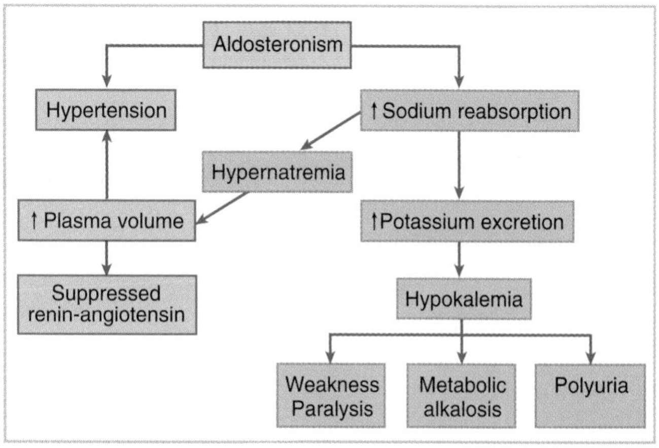

FIGURE 37–19 Pathophysiology of primary aldosteronism.

This third explanation could account for the common finding of an increased aldosterone/renin ratio, due not to increased aldosterone but to decreased renin as well as the presence of BAH in the majority of normokalemic hypertensive patients reported in recent series.[138] In an analysis of the aldosterone/renin ratio in 505 patients with essential hypertension, an elevated ratio was found to be a measure of low renin alone without increased aldosterone in 36 percent and the positive predictive value of the ratio to identify patients with increased aldosterone and low renin was only 34 percent.[141]

This examination of the pathophysiology of hyperaldosteronism does not deny the existence of autonomous hypersecretive from hyperplastic glands. However, most patients with an elevated aldosterone/renin ratio and BAH do not have autonomous hyperaldosteronism.[142]

DIAGNOSIS. Despite the enthusiasm to screen virtually all hypertensive patients with an aldosterone/renin ratio measurement,[138] there are good reasons to limit use of the test and, rather than using a ratio that could be high entirely because of a low renin level, to simply confirm an elevated plasma aldosterone level, above 15 ng/dl, and a low renin level. This more conservative view is based on the strong likelihood that only a very few normokalemic patients harbor an adenoma that should be resected and that there is no need to identify the presence of bilateral hyperplasia in normokalemic patients, mainly because identification of BAH usually requires an expensive, difficult, and occasionally harmful study, bilateral adrenal venous sampling.[143]

Therefore, screening is recommended only for hypertensive subjects who have a higher likelihood of primary aldosteronism, including those with (1) unprovoked, unexplainable hypokalemia; (2) hypokalemia induced by diuretics but resistant to correction; (3) family history of aldosteronism; or (4) hypertension resistant to appropriate therapy wherein the resistance cannot be explained. Hyperaldosteronism has been found in as many as 20 percent of resistant hypertensive patients, but BAH is the usual finding and therapy with the aldosterone blocker spironolactone significantly reduced blood pressure,[144] alleviating the need for extensive evaluation for aldosteronism in most such patients.

If the screening plasma aldosterone and renin levels are suggestive, a saline suppression study, either oral or intravenous, should be done to document autonomy of hyperaldosteronism (Fig. 37-20). If the aldosteronism persists, either a CT or an MRI scan should look for adrenal pathological lesions. If a solitary adenoma larger than 1 cm is present, the diagnosis of an aldosterone-producing adenoma can be reasonably ensured and consideration given to adrenalectomy. Because some nodularity is common even with a single hypersecreting adenoma, however, most experts suggest adrenal venous sampling before surgery is recommended.[145]

OTHER FORMS OF MINERALOCORTICOID EXCESS. Table 37-14 lists a number of other causes for real or apparent mineralocorticoid excess. One, familial glucocorticoid-remediable aldosteronism, is caused by a mutation in the genes involved in coding for the aldosterone synthase enzyme normally found only in the outer zona glomerulosa and the 11-beta-hydroxylase enzyme in the zona fasciculata. The chimeric

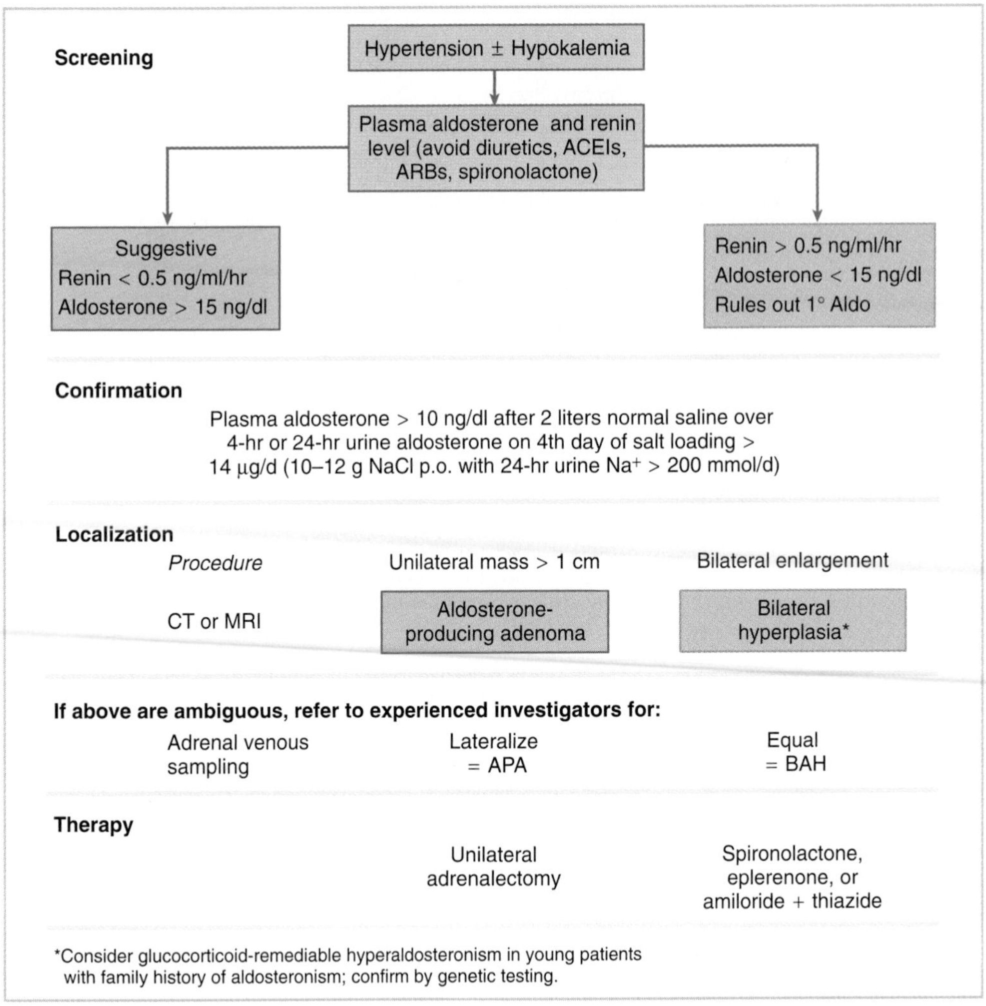

FIGURE 37–20 A diagnostic flow chart for evaluating and treating patients with primary aldosteronism. 1° Aldo = primary aldosteronism; ACEI = angiotensin-converting enzyme inhibitor; APA = aldosterone-producing adenoma; ARB = angiotensin II receptor blocker; BAH = bilateral adrenal hyperplasia; CT = computed tomography; MRI = magnetic resonance imaging; 18-OH-B, 18-hydroxycorticosterone. (Modified from Kaplan NM: Kaplan's Clinical Hypertension. 8th ed. Baltimore, Lippincott Williams & Wilkins, 2002, p 464.)

gene induces an enzyme that catalyzes the synthesis of 18-hydroxylated cortisol in the zona fasciculata. Since this zone is under the control of adrenocorticotropic hormone (ACTH), the glucocorticoid suppressibility of the syndrome is explained. The diagnosis should be made by genetic testing for the chimeric gene and treatment provided with glucocorticoid suppression.[146]

Another rare form is apparent mineralocorticoid excess caused by deficiency of the enzyme 11-beta-hydroxysteroid dehydrogenase type 2 (11β-OHSD2) in the renal tubule, where it normally converts cortisol (which has the ability to act on the mineralocorticoid receptor) to cortisone (which does not). Persistence of high levels of cortisol induces all the features of mineralocorticoid excess. The 11β-OHSD enzyme may be congenitally absent (the syndrome of apparent mineralocorticoid excess) or inhibited by the glycyrrhetenic acid contained in licorice.[147] Another unusual syndrome with hypertension and hypokalemia but suppressed mineralocorticoid secretion is Liddle syndrome, wherein the kidney reabsorbs excess sodium and wastes potassium because of a mutation in the beta or gamma subunits of the epithelial sodium channel.[148]

THERAPY. Once the diagnosis of primary aldosteronism is made and the type of adrenal disorder has been established, the choice of therapy is easy: Patients with a solitary adenoma should have the tumor resected, now more and more frequently done by laparoscopic surgery, and those with bilateral hyperplasia should be treated with an aldosterone blocker, either spironolactone or eplerenone and, if necessary, a thiazide diuretic or other antihypertensive drugs.[149] When an adenoma is resected, about half the patients will become normotensive, whereas the others, although improved, remain hypertensive, either from preexisting primary hypertension or from renal damage caused by prolonged secondary hypertension.

Cushing Syndrome
(see Chap. 79)

Hypertension occurs in about 80 percent of patients with Cushing syndrome. If left untreated, it can cause marked LVH and CHF. As with hypertension of other endocrine causes, the longer it is present, the less likely it is to disappear when the underlying cause is relieved.

MECHANISM OF HYPERTENSION. Blood pressure can increase for a number of reasons.[150] Secretion of mineralocorticoids can also be increased along with cortisol. The excess cortisol can overwhelm the ability of renal 11β-OHSD2 to convert it to the inactive cortisone, and renal mineralocorticoid receptors are activated by the excess cortisol to retain sodium and expand fluid volume. Cortisol stimulates the synthesis of renin substrate and the expression of angiotensin II receptors, which may be responsible for enhanced pressor effects.

DIAGNOSIS. The syndrome should be suspected in patients with truncal obesity, thin skin, muscle weakness, and osteoporosis. If clinical features are suggestive, the diagnosis can be either ruled out or virtually ensured by the measurement of free cortisol in a 24-hour urine sample or the simple overnight dexamethasone suppression test.[151] In normal subjects, the level of plasma cortisol in a sample drawn at 8 AM after a bedtime dose of 1 mg of dexamethasone should be lower than 2 μg/100 ml. If the level is higher, additional work-up is in order to establish both the diagnosis of cortisol excess and the pathological type. A lack of suppression may be noted in patients who are depressed or are alcohol abusers.

When an abnormal screening test result is present, most authorities continue to recommend an additional high-dose dexamethasone suppression test at 2.0 mg every 6 hours for 2 days, with measurement of urinary free cortisol excretion and plasma cortisol levels. If Cushing syndrome is caused by excess pituitary ACTH drive with bilateral adrenal hyperplasia, urinary free cortisol will be suppressed to below 40 percent of the control value with the 2.0 mg dose. Plasma ACTH assays provide an additional means of differentiating pituitary and ectopic ACTH excess from adrenal tumors with ACTH suppression. The response to corticotropin-releasing hormone and inferior petrosal sinus sampling may be needed to identify a pituitary cause of the syndrome.

THERAPY. In about two-thirds of patients with Cushing syndrome, the process begins with overproduction of ACTH by the pituitary, which leads to bilateral adrenal hyperplasia. Although pituitary hyperfunction may reflect a hypothalamic disorder, the majority of patients have discrete pituitary adenomas that can usually be resected by selective transsphenoidal microsurgery.

If an adrenal tumor is present, it should be removed surgically. With earlier diagnosis and more selective surgical therapy, it is hoped that more patients with Cushing syndrome will be cured without a need for lifelong glucocorticoid replacement therapy and with permanent relief of their hypertension. Temporarily, and rarely permanently, therapy may require one of a number of drugs.[152]

Congenital Adrenal Hyperplasia

Enzymatic defects may induce hypertension by interfering with cortisol biosynthesis. Low levels of cortisol lead to increased ACTH, which increases the accumulation of precursors proximal to the enzymatic block, specifically deoxycorticosterone, which induces mineralocorticoid hypertension. The more common of these is 11-hydroxylase deficiency, which has been attributed to various mutations in the gene[153] and leads to virilization (from excessive androgens) and hypertension with hypokalemia (from excessive deoxycorticosterone). The other is 17-hydroxylase deficiency, which also causes hypertension from excess deoxycorticosterone but, in addition, causes failure of secondary sexual development because sex hormones are also deficient.[154] Affected children are hypertensive, but the defect in sex hormone synthesis may not become obvious until after puberty. Thereafter, affected males display ambiguity of sexual development and fail to mature.

Pheochromocytoma (see Chap. 79)

The wild fluctuations in blood pressure and dramatic symptoms of pheochromocytoma usually alert both the patient and the physician to the possibility of this diagnosis. However, such fluctuations may be missed, or, as occurs in half the patients, the hypertension may be persistent, with headache, sweating, and palpitations. On one hand, the spells that are typical of a pheochromocytoma may be incorrectly attributed to migraine, menopause, or panic attacks. On the other, some patients with severe paroxysmal hypertension do not have a pheochromocytoma but rather marked anxiety.[155] Unfortunately, if the diagnosis of pheochromocytoma is missed, severe complications can arise from exceedingly high blood pressure and damage to the heart by catecholamines. Stroke and hypertensive crises with encephalopathy and retinal hemorrhage may occur, probably because blood pressure levels soar in vessels unprepared by a chronic hypertensive condition. Fortunately, a single blood test will detect the disease with virtual certainty,[156] so diagnostic indecision should be minimized.

PATHOPHYSIOLOGY. Tumors arising from chromaffin cells, that is, pheochromocytomas, occur at all ages anywhere along the sympathetic chain and rarely in aberrant sites. About 15 percent of pheochromocytomas are extraadrenal, that is, paragangliomas. Paragangliomas below the head and neck are often functional; those in the head and neck usually present with a mass effect.

Of the 85 percent of pheochromocytomas that arise in the adrenal medulla, 10 percent are bilateral and another 10 percent are malignant. Familial pheochromocytomas are inherited as an autosomal dominant trait alone or in one of four syndromes with recognized genetic mutations: in about half of patients with multiple endocrine neoplasia types 2A or 2B, in 25 percent of those with von Hippel-Lindau disease, and rarely in those with neurofibromatosis type 1. Such germ-line mutations have been found in 25 percent of 271 patients with sporadic, nonsyndromic, nonfamilial pheochromocytoma, a much higher prevalence than the generally reported 10 percent of pheochromocytomas.[157] Therefore, a higher index of suspicion for familial syndromes is needed, particularly in young patients or those with multiple extraadrenal tumors, prompting a thorough family history and a careful search for other components of a hereditary syndrome. Genetic testing should become more readily available.

Secretion from nonfamilial pheochromocytomas varies considerably, with small tumors tending to secrete larger proportions of active catecholamines. If the predominant secretion is epinephrine, which is formed primarily in the adrenal medulla, the symptoms reflect its effects, mainly systolic hypertension caused by increased cardiac output, tachycardia, sweating, flushing, and apprehension. If norepinephrine is predominantly secreted, as from some of the adrenal tumors and from almost all extraadrenal tumors, the symptoms include both systolic and diastolic hypertension from peripheral vasoconstriction but less tachycardia, palpitations, and anxiety.

DIAGNOSIS. Many more hypertensive patients have variable blood pressure and "spells" than the 0.1 percent or so who harbor a pheochromocytoma. Spells with paroxysmal hypertension may occur with a number of stresses, and a large number of conditions may involve transient catecholamine release. A pheochromocytoma should be suspected in patients with hypertension that is either paroxysmal or persistent and accompanied by the symptoms and signs listed in Table 37–15. In addition, children and patients with rapidly accelerating hypertension should be screened. Those whose tumors secrete predominantly epinephrine are prone to postural hypotension from a contracted blood volume and blunted sympathetic reflex tone. Suspicion should be heightened if activities such as bending over, exercise, palpation of the abdomen, smoking, or dipping snuff cause repetitive spells that begin abruptly, advance rapidly, and subside within minutes.

High levels of catecholamines can induce myocarditis (see Chap. 60), which can progress to cardiomyopathy and left ventricular failure. Electrocardiographic changes of ischemia can also be seen. Beta blockers given to such patients can raise the pressure and induce coronary spasm through blockade of beta-mediated vasodilation.

LABORATORY CONFIRMATION. The easiest and best procedure is a plasma free metanephrine assay,[156] which provides better sensitivity and specificity than other blood or urine catecholamine assays. The test has been found to be equally sensitive for detection of pheochromocytomas in children as part of one of the autosomal dominant familial disorders.[158]

At the Mayo Clinic, measures of urinary metanephrine and catecholamine excretion provided equal sensitivity and better specificity than plasma free metanephrine assays, so the urinary assays are recommended for testing low-risk patients to avoid false-positive results.[159]

If basal levels are equivocal, a clonidine suppression test can be performed, using the plasma free metanephrine assay.[160]

LOCALIZATION OF THE TUMOR. Once the diagnosis has been made, medical therapy should be started and the tumor localized by CT or MRI, which usually demonstrates these typically large tumors with ease. In the few patients in whom localization is not possible by CT or MRI, radioisotopes that localize in chromaffin tissue are available for imaging.

THERAPY. Once diagnosed and localized, pheochromocytomas should be resected. Although preoperative alpha-adrenergic blockade has been recommended, fewer operative and postoperative problems were encountered in one series of patients who had been treated with a calcium channel blocker.[161] If the tumor is unresectable, chronic medical therapy with the alpha blocker phenoxybenzamine (Dibenzyline) or the inhibitor of catechol synthesis alpha-methyltyrosine (Demser) can be used.

Other Causes of Hypertension

A host of other causes of hypertension are known (see Table 37–5). One that is probably becoming more common is ingestion of various drugs, prescribed (e.g., cyclosporine,

TABLE 37–15 Features Suggestive of Pheochromocytoma

Hypertension: Persistent or Paroxysmal
Markedly variable blood pressures (± orthostatic hypotension)
Sudden paroxysms (± subsequent hypertension) in relation to
Stress: anesthesia, angiography, parturition
Pharmacological provocation: histamine, nicotine, caffeine, beta blockers, glucocorticoids, tricyclic antidepressants
Manipulation of tumors: abdominal palpation, urination
Rare patients persistently normotensive
Unusual settings
Childhood, pregnancy, familial
Multiple endocrine adenomas: medullary carcinoma of the thyroid (MEN-2), mucosal neuromas (MEN-2B)
von Hippel-Lindau syndrome
Neurocutaneous lesions: neurofibromatosis
Associated Symptoms
Sudden spells with headache, sweating, palpitations, nervousness, nausea, and vomiting
Pain in chest or abdomen
Associated Signs
Sweating, tachycardia, arrhythmia, pallor, weight loss

MEN = multiple endocrine neoplasia.

tacrolimus, and erythropoietin), over-the-counter (e.g., ephedra), and illicit (e.g., cocaine). As previously noted, obstructive sleep apnea has been well characterized as a cause of significant, and reversible, hypertension.

Coarctation of the Aorta (see Chap. 56)

Congenital narrowing of the aorta can occur at any level of the thoracic or abdominal aorta. It is usually found just beyond the origin of the left subclavian artery or distal to the insertion of the ligamentum arteriosum. With less severe postductal lesions, symptoms may not appear until the teenage years or later, particularly during pregnancy.

Hypertension in the arms, weak or absent femoral pulses, and a loud murmur heard over the back are the classic features of coarctation. The pathogenesis of the hypertension can be more complicated than simple mechanical obstruction; a generalized vasoconstrictor mechanism is likely involved. The lesion can be detected by two-dimensional echocardiography, and aortography proves the diagnosis. Once repaired, patients may continue to have hypertension that should be carefully monitored[162] and treated.

Hormonal Disturbances

Hypertension is seen in as many as half of patients with a variety of hormonal disturbances, including acromegaly,[163] hypothyroidism,[164] and hyperparathyroidism.[165] Diagnosis of the latter two conditions has been made easier by readily available blood tests, and affected hypertensive patients can be relieved of their high blood pressure by correction of the hormonal disturbance. Such relief happens more frequently in patients with hypothyroidism than in those with hyperparathyroidism.

Perioperative Hypertension

If at all possible, preexisting hypertension should be well controlled before elective surgery, with particular attention to correction of diuretic-induced hypokalemia. Caution is advised in abruptly discontinuing antihypertensive agents preoperatively, in particular beta-blockers or clonidine. Fortunately, intravenous formulations of most classes are available if oral intake is not possible. A skin patch of clonidine can treat the patient through surgery.

Hypertension may appear or worsen in the perioperative period, perhaps more commonly with cardiac than noncardiac surgery (Table 37–16).[166] Patients at high risk for cardiac events have been found to be protected by the use of beta-blockers prior to either cardiac or noncardiac surgery.[167]

Hypertension is of particular concern after heart transplantation, appearing for a number of reasons but in particular because the denervation of cardiac volume receptors prevents the normal suppression of the renin-angiotensin mechanism with volume expansion.[168] Reduction of dietary sodium intake and ACE inhibitor or ARB therapy should be especially beneficial.

TABLE 37–16 Hypertension Associated with Cardiac Surgery

Preoperative
- Anxiety, angina, etc.
- Discontinuation of antihypertensive therapy
- Rebound from beta blockers in patients with coronary artery disease

Intraoperative
- Induction of anesthesia: tracheal intubation; nasopharyngeal, urethral, or rectal manipulation
- Precardiopulmonary bypass (during sternotomy and chest retraction)
- Cardiopulmonary bypass
- Postcardiopulmonary bypass (during surgery)

Postoperative
- Early (within 2 h)
  - Obvious cause: hypoxia, hypercarbia, ventilatory difficulties, hypothermia, shivering, arousal from anesthesia
  - With no obvious cause: after myocardial revascularization; less frequently after valve replacement; after resection of aortic coarctation
- Late (weeks to months)
  - After aortic valve replacement by homografts

Data from Estafanous FG, Tarazi RC: Systemic arterial hypertension associated with cardiac surgery. Am J Cardiol 46:685, 1980.

Hypertension During Pregnancy (see Chap. 74)

In about 12 percent of first pregnancies in previously normotensive women, hypertension appears after 20 weeks (gestational hypertension) and in about half this hypertension will progress to preeclampsia when complicated by proteinuria, edema, or hematological or hepatic abnormalities, which, in turn, increase the risk of progress to eclampsia, defined by the occurrence of convulsions. Women with hypertension predating pregnancy have an even higher incidence of preeclampsia and a greater likelihood of early delivery of small-for-gestational-age babies.

Preeclampsia is of unknown cause but occurs more frequently in primigravid women and in pregnancies involving either men or women who were the product of a pregnancy complicated by preeclampsia,[169] supporting a genetic role. Additional predisposing factors include increased age, black race, multiple gestations, concomitant heart or renal disease, and chronic hypertension.

The diagnosis is usually based on a rise in pressure of 30/15 mm Hg or more to a level above 140/90 mm Hg. As with other forms of hypertension, the diagnosis is most precisely made by ambulatory blood pressure monitoring.[170]

Clinical Features

The features shown in Table 37–17 should help distinguish gestational hypertension and preeclampsia from chronic,

TABLE 37–17 Differences Between Preeclampsia and Chronic Hypertension

Feature	Preeclampsia	Chronic Hypertension
Age (yr)	Young (<20)	Older (>30)
Parity	Primigravida	Multigravida
Onset	After 20 wk of pregnancy	Before 20 wk of pregnancy
Weight gain and edema	Sudden	Gradual
Systolic blood pressure	<160 mm Hg	>160 mm Hg
Funduscopic findings	Spasm, edema	Arteriovenous nicking, exudates
Left ventricular hypertrophy	Rare	More common
Proteinuria	Present	Absent
Plasma uric acid	Increased	Normal
Blood pressure after delivery	Normal	Elevated

primary hypertension. The distinction should be made because management and prognosis are different: Gestational hypertension is self-limited and less commonly recurs in subsequent pregnancies, whereas chronic hypertension progresses and usually complicates subsequent pregnancies. Separation may be difficult because of a lack of knowledge of prepregnancy blood pressure and because of the usual tendency for high pressure to fall considerably during the middle trimester so that hypertension present before pregnancy may not be recognized.

Mechanisms

The hemodynamic features of gestational hypertension are a further rise in cardiac output than usually seen in normal pregnancy, accompanied by profound vasoconstriction that reduces intravascular capacity even more than blood volume that may reflect increased central and peripheral sympathetic activity.[171] The mother may be particularly vulnerable to encephalopathy because of her previously normal blood pressure. As is described in more detail under Hypertensive Crisis, cerebral blood flow is normally maintained constant over a fairly narrow range of mean arterial pressure, roughly between 60 and 100 mm Hg in normotensive individuals. In a previously normotensive young woman, an acute rise in blood pressure to 150/100 mm Hg can exceed the upper limit of autoregulation and result in a "breakthrough" of cerebral blood flow (acute dilation) that leads to cerebral edema and convulsions.

Increasingly strong evidence indicates that preeclampsia starts from deficient trophoblast invasion that, in some manner, sets off a systemic maternal inflammatory response. A variety of triggers have been proposed,[172] but the specific mechanisms remain unknown.

Prevention

Beyond delay of pregnancy until after the teens and better prenatal care, the only other maneuver that has been shown to prevent preeclampsia is the use of low doses of aspirin.[173]

Treatment

The only cure for preeclampsia is delivery, which removes the diseased placenta. To achieve this apparently simple end, the clinician must detect the symptomless prodromal condition by screening all pregnant women, admit to hospital those with advanced preeclampsia so as to keep track of an unpredictable situation, and time preemptive delivery to maximize the safety of mother and baby.

Caution is advised in the use of drugs for gestational hypertension, traditionally limited to methyldopa. Drug treatment of maternal blood pressure does not improve perinatal outcome and may be associated with fetal growth retardation. Most authorities recommend antihypertensive drugs only if diastolic pressures remain above 100 mm Hg.[174] The only drugs that are contraindicated are ACE inhibitors and ARB because of their propensity to induce neonatal renal failure.

Chronic Hypertension

If pregnancy begins while a woman is receiving antihypertensive drug therapy, the medications, including diuretics but excluding ACE inhibitors and ARBs, are usually continued in the belief that the mother should be protected and that the fetus will not suffer from any sudden hemodynamic shifts such as occur when therapy is first begun. However, despite modern treatment, the incidence of perinatal mortality and fetal growth retardation remains higher in patients with chronic hypertension.

Management of Eclampsia

With appropriate care of gestational hypertension, eclampsia hardly ever supervenes; when it does, however, maternal and fetal mortality increase markedly. Excellent results have been reported with the use of magnesium sulfate to prevent and treat convulsions.[175] Caution is needed to avoid volume overload, since pulmonary edema is the most common cause of maternal mortality. When compared with women who were normotensive, the overall prognosis for women who had hypertension during pregnancy is not as good, probably because of causes other than preeclampsia, including unrecognized chronic primary hypertension.

After delivery, transient or persistent hypertension can develop in the mother. In many, early primary hypertension may have been masked by the hemodynamic changes of pregnancy. Peripartum cardiomyopathy is a rare form of left ventricular systolic dysfunction appearing during the last month of pregnancy or within a few months after delivery in the absence of known causes.[176]

Hypertensive Crisis

Definitions

A number of clinical circumstances require rapid reduction of blood pressure (Table 37–18). These circumstances can be separated into *emergencies,* which require immediate reduction of blood pressure (within 1 hour), and *urgencies,* which can be treated more slowly. A persistent diastolic pressure exceeding 130 mm Hg is often associated with acute vascular damage; some patients may suffer vascular damage from lower levels of pressure, whereas others are able to withstand even higher levels without apparent harm. As discussed subsequently, the rapidity of the rise may be more important than the absolute level in producing acute vascular damage. Therefore, in practice, all patients with diastolic blood pressure above 130 mm Hg should be treated, some more rapidly with parenteral drugs and others more slowly with oral agents.

When the rise in pressure causes retinal hemorrhages, exudates, or papilledema, the term *accelerated-malignant hypertension* is used. *Hypertensive encephalopathy* is characterized by headache, irritability, alterations in consciousness, and other manifestations of central nervous dysfunction with sudden and marked elevations in blood pressure.

Incidence

Fewer than 1 percent of patients with primary hypertension progress to an accelerated-malignant phase. The incidence is probably falling as a consequence of more widespread

TABLE 37–18 Circumstances Requiring Rapid Treatment of Hypertension

Accelerated-malignant hypertension with papilledema
Cerebrovascular Hypertensive encephalopathy Atherothrombotic brain infarction with severe hypertension Intracerebral hemorrhage Subarachnoid hemorrhage
Cardiac Acute aortic dissection Acute left ventricular failure Acute or impending myocardial infarction After coronary bypass surgery
Renal Acute glomerulonephritis Renal crises from collagen-vascular diseases Severe hypertension after kidney transplantation
Excessive circulating catecholamines Pheochromocytoma crisis Food or drug interactions with monoamine oxidase inhibitors Sympathomimetic drug use (cocaine) Rebound hypertension after sudden cessation of antihypertensive drugs
Eclampsia
Surgical Severe hypertension in patients requiring immediate surgery Postoperative hypertension Postoperative bleeding from vascular suture lines
Severe body burns
Severe epistaxis
Thrombotic thrombocytopenic purpura

From Kaplan NM: Kaplan's Clinical Hypertension. 8th ed. Baltimore, Lippincott Williams & Wilkins, 2002, p 340.

treatment of hypertension. Any hypertensive disease can initiate a crisis. Some, including pheochromocytoma and renovascular hypertension, do so at a higher rate than seen with primary hypertension. However, since hypertension is of unknown cause in more than 90 percent of all patients, most hypertensive crises appear in the setting of preexisting primary hypertension.

PATHOPHYSIOLOGY. Whenever blood pressure rises and remains above a critical level, various processes set off a series of local and systemic effects that cause further rises in pressure and vascular damage eventuating in accelerated-malignant hypertension.

Studies in animals and humans by Strandgaard and Paulson have elucidated the mechanism of hypertensive encephalopathy.[177] First, they directly measured the caliber of pial arterioles over the cerebral cortex in cats whose blood pressure was varied over a wide range of infusion by vasodilators or angiotensin II. As the pressure fell, the arterioles became dilated; as the pressure rose, they become constricted. Thus, constant cerebral blood flow was maintained by means of autoregulation, which is dependent on the cerebral sympathetic nerves. However, when mean arterial pressure rose above 180 mm Hg, the tightly constricted vessels could no longer withstand the pressure and suddenly dilated. This dilation began in an irregular manner, first in areas with less muscle tone and then diffusely with production of generalized vasodilation. This "breakthrough" of cerebral blood flow hyperperfuses the brain under high pressure and thereby causes leakage of fluid into the perivascular tissue and results in cerebral edema and the syndrome of hypertensive encephalopathy.

In human subjects, cerebral blood flow was measured repetitively by an isotopic technique while blood pressure was lowered or raised with vasodilators or vasoconstrictors in a manner similar to that used in the animal studies.[177] Curves depicting cerebral blood flow as a function of arterial pressure demonstrated autoregulation with a constancy of flow over mean pressures in normotensive persons from about 60 to 120 mm Hg and in hypertensive patients from about 110 to 180 mm Hg (Fig. 37-21). This "shift to the right" in hypertensive patients is the result of structural thickening of the arterioles as an adaptation to the chronically elevated pressure. When pressure was raised beyond the upper limit of autoregulation, the same "breakthrough" with hyperperfusion occurred as was seen in the animal studies. In previously normotensive persons whose vessels have not been altered by prior exposure to high pressure, breakthrough occurred at a mean arterial pressure of about 120 mm Hg; in hypertensive patients, the breakthrough occurred at about 180 mm Hg.

These studies confirm clinical observations. In previously normotensive persons, severe encephalopathy occurs with relatively little hypertension. In children with acute glomerulonephritis and in women with eclampsia, convulsions can occur as a result of hypertensive encephalopathy, with blood pressure readings as low as 150/100 mm Hg. Obviously, chronically hypertensive patients withstand such pressures without difficulty; however, when pressure increases significantly, encephalopathy can develop even in these patients.

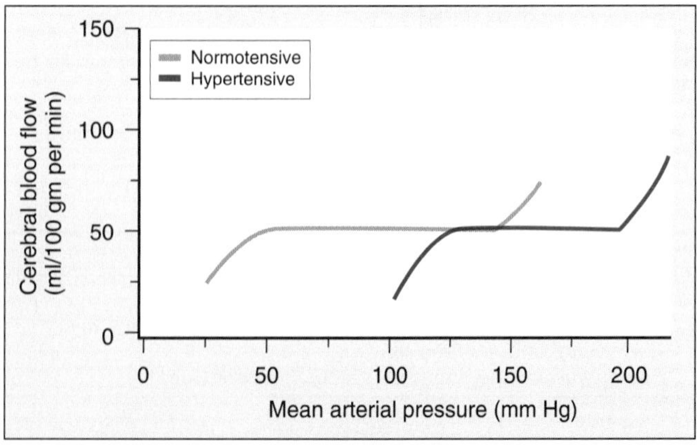

FIGURE 37–21 Idealized curves of cerebral blood flow at varying levels of systemic blood pressure in normotensive and hypertensive subjects. Rightward shift in autoregulation is shown with chronic hypertension. (Adapted from Strandgaard S, Olesen J, Skinhtoi E, Lassen NA: Autoregulation of brain circulation in severe arterial hypertension. Br Med J 1:507, 1973.)

Manifestations and Course

The symptoms and signs of hypertensive crises are usually dramatic (Table 37–19), likely reflecting acute damage to endothelium and platelet activation.[178] However, some patients may be relatively asymptomatic despite markedly elevated pressure and extensive organ damage. Young black men are particularly prone to hypertensive crisis with severe renal insufficiency but little obvious prior distress. Even in elderly persons, however, hypertension can initially present in an accelerated-malignant phase.

If left untreated, patients die quickly of brain damage or more gradually of renal damage. Before effective therapy was available, fewer than 25 percent of patients with malignant hypertension survived 1 year and only 1 percent survived 5 years. With therapy, including renal dialysis, more than 90 percent survive 1 year and about 80 percent survive 5 years.

Differential Diagnosis

The presence of hypertensive encephalopathy or accelerated-malignant hypertension demands immediate, aggressive therapy to lower blood pressure effectively, often before the specific cause is known. However, certain serious diseases, as well as psychogenic problems, can mimic a hypertensive crisis (Table 37–20) and management of these conditions usually requires different diagnostic and therapeutic approaches. In particular, blood pressure should not be lowered too abruptly in a patient with a stroke.[179] Specific therapy for hypertensive crises is described in Chapter 38.

TABLE 37–19 Clinical Characteristics of Hypertensive Crisis

Blood pressure: usually >140 mm Hg diastolic
Funduscopic findings: hemorrhages, exudates, papilledema
Neurological status: headache, confusion, somnolence, stupor, visual loss, focal deficits, seizures, coma
Cardiac findings: prominent apical impulse, cardiac enlargement, congestive failure
Renal: oliguria, azotemia
Gastrointestinal: nausea, vomiting

From Kaplan NM: Kaplan's Clinical Hypertension. 8th ed. Baltimore, Lippincott Williams & Wilkins, 2002, p 341.

TABLE 37–20 Conditions That Can Mimic a Hypertensive Crisis

Acute left ventricular failure
Uremia from any cause, particularly with volume overload
Cerebrovascular accident
Subarachnoid hemorrhage
Brain tumor
Head injury
Epilepsy (postictal)
Collagen diseases, particularly lupus, with cerebral vasculitis
Encephalitis
Sympathomimetics: cocaine, amphetamines, etc.
Hypercalcemia
Acute anxiety with hyperventilation syndrome

REFERENCES

Recognition, Definitions, and Prevalence

1. Gu D, Reynolds K, Wu X, et al: Prevalence, awareness, treatment, and control of hypertension in China. Hypertension 40:920, 2002.
2. Lloyd-Jones DM, Evans JC, Larson MG, Levy D: Treatment and control of hypertension in the community: A prospective analysis. Hypertension 40:640, 2002.
3. Mancia G, Grassi G: Systolic and diastolic blood pressure control in antihypertensive drug trials. J Hypertens 20:1461, 2002.
4. Cherry DK, Woodwell DA: National Ambulatory Medical Care Survey: 2002 summary. Advance data from vital and health statistics; No. 328. Hyattsville, MD, National Center for Health Statistics, 2002.
5. Whelton PK, He J, Appel LJ, et al: Primary prevention of hypertension: Clinical and public health advisory from the National Blood Pressure Education Program. JAMA 288:1882, 2002.
6. Vasan RS, Beiser A, Seshadri S, et al: Residual lifetime risk for developing hypertension in middle-aged women and men. The Framingham Heart Study. JAMA 287:1003, 2002.
7. Joint National Committee: The sixth report of the Joint National Committee on detection, evaluation, and treatment of high blood pressure (JNC VI). Arch Intern Med 157:2413, 1997.
8. Joint National Committee: The seventh report of the Joint Committee on Prevention, Detection, Evaluation, and Treatment of High Blood Pressure (JNC-7 Express). JAMA 289:2560, 2003.
9. Appel L, Robinson K, Guallar E: Utility of blood pressure monitoring outside of the clinic setting. Evidence Report/Technology Assessment No. 63. AHRQ Publication No. 03-E004. Rockville, MD: Agency for Healthcare Research and Quality, 2002.
10. Staessen JA, Thijs L, Fagard R, et al: Predicting cardiovascular risk using conventional vs ambulatory blood pressure in older patients with systolic hypertension. JAMA 282:539, 1999.
11. Brown MA, Buddle ML, Martin A: Is resistant hypertension really resistant? Am J Hypertens 14:1263, 2001.
12. Verdecchia P, O'Brien E, Pickering T, et al: When can the practicing physician suspect white coat hypertension? Statement from the Working Group on Blood Pressure Monitoring of the European Society of Hypertension. Am J Hypertens 16:87, 2003.
13. Wing LMH, Brown MA, Beilin LJ, et al: 'Reverse white-coat hypertension' in older hypertensives. J Hypertens 20:639, 2002.
14. Marfella R, Gualdiero P, Siniscalchi M, et al: Morning blood pressure peak, QT intervals, and sympathetic activity in hypertensive patients. Hypertension 41:237, 2003.
15. Kario K, Pickering TG, Matsuo T, et al: Stroke prognosis and abnormal nocturnal blood pressure falls in older hypertensives. Hypertension 38:852, 2001.
16. Matthews CE, Pate RP, Jackson KL, et al: Exaggerated blood pressure response to dynamic exercise and risk of future hypertension. J Clin Epidemiol 51:29, 1998.
17. Kjeldsen SE, Mundal R, Sandvik L, et al: Supine and exercise systolic blood pressure predict cardiovascular death in middle-aged men. J Hypertens 19:1343, 2001.
18. Vasan RS, Massaro JM, Wilson PWF, et al: Antecedent blood pressure and risk of cardiovascular disease. The Framingham Heart Study. Circulation 105:48, 2002.
19. Domanski M, Mitchell G, Pfeffer M, et al: Pulse pressure and cardiovascular disease-related mortality: Follow-up study of the Multiple Risk Factor Intervention Trial (MRFIT). JAMA 287:2677, 2002.
20. Vasan RS, Larson MG, Leip EP, et al: Impact of high-normal blood pressure on the risk of cardiovascular disease. N Engl J Med 345:18:1291, 2001.
21. Fuentes RM, Notkola I-L, Shemeikka S, et al: Tracking of systolic blood pressure during childhood: A 15-year follow-up population-based family study in eastern Finland. J Hypertens 20:195, 2002.
22. Burt VL, Whelton P, Roccella EJ, et al: Prevalence of hypertension in the US adult population. Results from the Third National Health and Nutrition Examination Survey, 1988-1991. Hypertension 25:3050, 1995.
23. Jones DW, Chambless LE, Folsom AR, et al: Risk factors for coronary heart disease in African Americans. Arch Intern Med 162:2565, 2002.
24. Lorenzo C, Serrano-Rios M, Martinez-Larrad MT, et al: Prevalence of hypertension in Hispanic and non-Hispanic white populations. Hypertension 39:203, 2002.
25. Franklin SS, Jacobs MJ, Wong ND, et al: Predominance of isolated systolic hypertension among middle-aged and elderly US hypertensives. Analysis based on National Health and Nutrition Examination Survey (NHANES) III. Hypertension 37:869, 2001.
26. Lakatta EG, Levy D: Arterial and cardiac aging: Major shareholders in cardiovascular disease enterprises. Part I: Aging arteries: A "set up" for vascular disease. Circulation 103:139, 2003.
27. Prospective Studies Collaboration: Age-specific relevance of usual blood pressure to vascular mortality: A meta-analysis of individual data for one million adults in 61 prospective studies. Lancet 360:1903, 2002.
28. Kaplan NM: Anxiety-induced hyperventilation: A common cause of symptoms in patients with hypertension. Arch Intern Med 157:945, 1997.
29. The Pooling Project Research Group: Relationship of blood pressure, serum cholesterol, smoking habit, relative weight and ECG abnormalities to incidence of major coronary events. Final report of the pooling project. J Chronic Dis 31:201, 1978.
30. Baker S, Priest P, Jackson R: Using thresholds based on risk of cardiovascular disease to target treatment for hypertension: Modelling events averted and number treated. Br Med J 320:680, 2000.
31. Guidelines Subcommittee 1999 World Health Organization: International Society of Hypertension guidelines for the management of hypertension. J Hypertens 17:151, 1999.
32. Yikona JI, Wallis EJ, Ramsay LE, Jackson PR: Coronary and cardiovascular risk estimation in uncomplicated mild hypertension: A comparison of risk assessment methods. J Hypertens 20:2173, 2002.
33. Cuspidi C, Ambrosioni E, Mancia G, et al: Role of echocardiography and carotid ultrasonography in stratifying risk in patients with essential hypertension: The Assessment of Prognostic Risk Observational Survey. J Hypertens 20:1307, 2002.
34. Wong TY, Klein R, Sharrett AR, et al: Retinal arteriolar narrowing and risk of coronary heart disease in men and women: The Atherosclerosis Risk in Communities Study. JAMA 287:1153, 2002.
35. Schussheim AE, Devereux RB, de Simone G: Usefulness of subnormal midwall fractional shortening in predicting left ventricular exercise dysfunction in asymptomatic patients with systemic hypertension. Am J Cardiol 79:1070, 1997.
36. Aeschbacher BC, Hutter D, Fuhrer J, et al: Diastolic dysfunction precedes myocardial hypertrophy in the development of hypertension. Am J Hypertens 14:106, 2001.
37. Gandhi SK, Powers JC, Nomeir A-M, et al: The pathogenesis of acute pulmonary edema associated with hypertension. N Engl J Med 344:17, 2001.
38. Gimelli A, Schneider-Eicke J, Neglia D, et al: Homogeneously reduced versus regionally impaired myocardial blood flow in hypertensive patients: Two different patterns of myocardial perfusion associated with degree of hypertrophy. J Am Coll Cardiol 31:366, 1998.
39. Dries DL, Exner DV, Gersh BJ, et al: Racial differences in the outcome of left ventricular dysfunction. N Engl J Med 340:609, 1999.
40. Kozàkovà M, de Simone G, Morizzo C, Palombo C: Coronary vasodilator capacity and hypertension-induced increase in left ventricular mass. Hypertension 41:224, 2003.
41. Schmieder RE, Messerli FH: Hypertension and the heart. J Hum Hypertens 14:597, 2000.
42. Wachtell K, Rokkedal J, Bella JN, et al: Effect of electrocardiographic left ventricular hypertrophy on left ventricular systolic function in systemic hypertension. Am J Cardiol 87:54, 2001.
43. Verdecchia P, Schillaci G, Borgioni C, et al: Prognostic significance of serial changes in left ventricular mass in essential hypertension. Circulation 97:48, 1998.
44. Haider AW, Larson MG, Franklin SS, Levy D: Systolic blood pressure, diastolic blood pressure, and pulse pressure as predictors of risk for congestive heart failure in the Framingham Heart Study. Ann Intern Med 138:10, 2003.
45. Vasan RS, Benjamin EJ: Diastolic heart failure. N Engl J Med 344:56, 2001.
46. Boon D, Piek JJ, van Montfrans GA: Silent ischaemia and hypertension. J Hypertens 18:1355, 2000.
47. Haider AW, Chen L, Larson MG, et al: Antecedent hypertension confers increased risk for adverse outcomes after initial myocardial infarction. Hypertension 30:1020, 1997.
48. Njølstad I, Arnesen E: Preinfarction blood pressure and smoking are determinants for a fatal outcome of myocardial infarction. Arch Intern Med 158:1326, 1998.
49. Flack JM, Neaton J, Grimm R Jr, et al: Blood pressure and mortality among men with prior myocardial infarction. Circulation 92:2437, 1995.
50. Leoncini G, Sacchi G, Ravera M, et al: Microalbuminuria is an integrated marker of subclinical organ damage in primary hypertension. J Hum Hypertens 16:399, 2002.
51. Reinprecht F, Elmståhl S, Janzon L, André-Petersson L: Hypertension and changes of cognitive function in 81-year-old men: A 13-year follow-up of the population study 'Men Born in 1914', Sweden. J Hypertens 21:57, 2003.
52. Sierra C, de la Sierra A, Mercader J, et al: Silent cerebral white matter lesions in middle-aged essential hypertensive patients. J Hypertens 20:519, 2002.
53. Goldstein IB, Bartzokis G, Guthrie D, Shapiro D: Ambulatory blood pressure and brain atrophy in the healthy elderly. Neurology 59:713, 2002.

Mechanisms of Primary (Essential) Hypertension

54. Lund-Johnson P: Central haemodynamics in essential hypertension at rest and during exercise: A 20-year follow-up study. J Hypertens 7(Suppl):52, 1989.
55. Post WS, Larson MG, Levy D: Hemodynamic predictors of incident hypertension. Hypertension 24:585, 1994.
56. Kim J-R, Kiefe CI, Liu K, et al: Heart rate and subsequent blood pressure in young adults: The CARDIA study. Hypertension 33:640, 1999.
57. Iliadou A, Lichtenstein P, Morgenstern R, et al: Repeated blood pressure measurements in a sample of Swedish twins: Heritabilities and associations with polymorphisms in the renin-angiotensin-aldosterone system. J Hypertens 20:1543, 2002.
58. Carretero OA, Oparil S: Essential hypertension. Circulation 101:329, 2000.
59. Luft FC: Hypertension as a complex genetic trait. Semin Nephrol 22:115, 2002.
60. Province MA, Kardia SLR, Ranade K, et al: A meta-analysis of genome-wide linkage scans for hypertension: The National Heart, Lung and Blood Institute Family Blood Pressure Program. Am J Hypertens 16:144, 2003.
61. Lifton RP, Gharavi AG, Geller DS: Molecular mechanisms of human hypertension [review]. Cell 104:545, 2001.
62. Law CM, Shiell AW, Newsome CA, et al: Fetal, infant, and childhood growth and adult blood pressure: A longitudinal study from birth to 22 years of age. Circulation 105:1088, 2002.
63. Huxley R, Neil A, Collins R: Unravelling the fetal origins hypothesis: Is there really an inverse association between birthweight and subsequent blood pressure? Lancet 360:659, 2002.
64. Brenner BM, Chertow GM: Congenital oligonephropathy: An inborn cause of adult hypertension and progressive renal injury? Curr Opin Nephrol Hypertens 2:691, 1993.
65. Moritz KM, Wintour EM, Dodic M: Fetal uninephrectomy leads to postnatal hypertension and compromised renal function. Hypertension 39:1071, 2002.
66. Keller G, Zimmer G, Mall G, et al: Nephron number in patients with primary hypertension. N Engl J Med 348:101, 2003.
67. Johnson RJ, Herrera-Acosta J, Schreiner GF, Rodríguez-Iturbe B: Subtle acquired renal injury as a mechanism of salt-sensitive hypertension. N Engl J Med 346:913, 2002.
68. Sealey JE, Blumenfeld JD, Bell GM, et al: On the renal basis for essential hypertension: Nephron heterogeneity with discordant renin secretion and sodium excretion causing a hypertensive vasoconstriction-volume relationship. J Hypertens 6:763, 1988.
69. Aperia A: Regulation of sodium/potassium ATPase activity. Curr Hypertens Rep 3:165, 2001.

70. Weinberger MH, Fineberg NS, Fineberg SE, Weinberger M: Salt sensitivity, pulse pressure and death in normal and hypertensive humans. Hypertension 37:429, 2001.
71. Lever AF, Harrap SB: Essential hypertension: A disorder of growth with origins in childhood? J Hypertens 10:101, 1992.
72. Folkow B: "Structural factor" in primary and secondary hypertension. Hypertension 16:89, 1990.
73. Lever AF: Slow pressor mechanisms in hypertension: A role for hypertrophy of resistance vessels? J Hypertens 4:515, 1986.
74. Cosentino F, Lüscher TF: Effects of blood pressure and glucose on endothelial function. Curr Hypertens Rep 3:79, 2001.
75. Cardillo C, Campia U, Kilcoyne CM, et al: Improved endothelium-dependent vasodilation after blockade of endothelin receptors in patients with essential hypertension. Circulation 105:452, 2002.
76. Esler M, Rumantir M, Lambert G, Kaye D: The sympathetic neurobiology of essential hypertension. Am J Hypertens 14(Suppl):139S, S2001.
77. Markovitz JH, Matthews KA, Kannel WB, et al: Psychological predictors of hypertension in the Framingham Study: Is there tension in hypertension? JAMA 270:2439, 1993.
78. Carroll D, Smith GD, Shipley MJ, et al: Blood pressure reactions to acute psychological stress and future blood pressure status: A 10-year follow-up of men in the Whitehall II study. Psychosomatic Med;63:737, 2001.
79. Schobel HP, Frank H, Naraghi R, et al: Hypertension in patients with neurovascular compression is associated with increased central sympathetic outflow. J Am Soc Nephrol 13:35, 2002.
80. Williams GH, Fisher NDL, Hunt SC, et al: Effects of gender and genotype on the phenotypic expression of nonmodulating essential hypertension. Kidney Int 57:1404, 2000.
81. Wilson PWF, D'Agostino R, Sullivan L, et al: Overweight and obesity as determinants of cardiovascular risk. The Framingham experience. Arch Intern Med 162:1867, 2002.
82. Flegal KM, Carroll MD, Ogden CL, Johnson CL: Prevalence and trends in obesity among US adults, 1999-2000. JAMA 288:1723, 2002.
83. Ogden CL, Flegal KM, Carroll MD, Johnson CL: Prevalence and trends in overweight among US children and adolescents, 1999-2000. JAMA 288:1728, 2002.
84. Malhotra A, White DP: Obstructive sleep apnea. Lancet 360:237, 2002.
85. DeSouza CA, Shapiro LF, Clevenger CM, et al: Regular aerobic exercise prevents and restores age-related declines in endothelium-dependent vasodilation in healthy men. Circulation 102:1351, 2000.
86. Mukamal KJ, Kuller LH, Fitzpatrick AL, et al: Prospective study of alcohol consumption and risk of dementia in older adults. JAMA 289:1405, 2003.
87. Thadhani R, Camargo CA Jr, Stampfer MJ, et al: Prospective study of moderate alcohol consumption and risk of hypertension in young women. Arch Intern Med 162:569, 2002.
88. Schunkert H, Koenig W, Bröckel U, et al: Haematocrit profoundly affects left ventricular diastolic filling as assessed by Doppler echocardiography. J Hypertens 18:1483, 2000.
89. Devereux RB, Case DB, Alderman MH, et al: Possible role of increased blood viscosity in the hemodynamics of systemic hypertension. Am J Cardiol 85:1265, 2000.
90. Ferrier KE, Muhlmann MH, Baguet J-P, et al: Intensive cholesterol reduction lowers blood pressure and large artery stiffness in isolated systolic hypertension. J Am Coll Cardiol 39:1020, 2002.

Hypertension in Special Groups

91. Kahn DF, Duffy SJ, Tomasian D, et al: Effects of black race on forearm resistance vessel function. Hypertension 40:195, 2002.
92. Marcantoni C, Ma L-J, Federspiel C, Fogo AB: Hypertensive nephrosclerosis in African Americans versus Caucasians. Kidney Int 62:172, 2002.
93. Morris RC Jr, Sebastian A, Forman A, et al: Normotensive salt sensitivity. Hypertension 33:18, 1999.
94. O'Donnell CJ, Kannel WB: Cardiovascular risks of hypertension: Lessons from observational studies. J Hypertens 16(Suppl 6):S3, 1998.
95. Gillman MW, Cook N, Rosner B, et al: Identifying children at high risk for the development of essential hypertension. J Pediatr 122:837, 1993.
96. Lieberman E: Hypertension in childhood and adolescence. *In* Kaplan N (ed): Kaplan's Clinical Hypertension, 8th ed. Philadelphia, Lippincott Williams & Wilkins, 2002.
97. Hyman DJ, Pavlik VN: Characteristics of patients with uncontrolled hypertension in the United States. N Engl J Med 345:479, 2001.
98. Staessen JA, Gasowski J, Wang JG, et al: Risks of untreated and treated isolated systolic hypertension in the elderly. Lancet 355:865, 2000.
99. Arima H, Tanizaki Y, Kiyohara Y, et al: Validity of the JNC VI recommendations for the management of hypertension in a general population of Japanese elderly. The Hisayama study. Arch Intern Med 163:361, 2003.
100. Gueyffier F, Bulpitt C, Boissel J-P, et al: Antihypertensive drugs in very old people. Lancet 353:793, 1999.
101. O'Rourke MF, Staessen JA, Vlachopoulos C, et al: Clinical applications of arterial stiffness: Definitions and reference values. Am J Hypertens 15:426, 2002.
102. Mooradian AD: Cardiovascular disease in type 2 diabetes mellitus: Current management guidelines. Arch Intern Med 163:33, 2003.
103. Geiss LS, Rolka DB, Engelgau MM: Elevated blood pressure among U.S. adults with diabetes, 1988-1994. Am J Prev Med 22:42, 2002.
104. Kamoi K, Mihakoshi M, Soda S, et al: Usefulness of home blood pressure measurement in the morning in type 2 diabetic patients. Diabetes Care 25:2218, 2002.

Identifiable (Secondary) Forms of Hypertension

105. Chasan-Taber L, Willett WC, Manson JE, et al: Prospective study of oral contraceptives and hypertension among women in the United States. Circulation 94:483, 1996.
106. Seibert C, Barbouche E, Fagan J, et al: Prescribing oral contraceptives for women older than 35 years of age. Ann Intern Med 138:54, 2000.
107. Ribstein J, Halimi J-M, du Cailar G, Mimran A: Renal characteristics and effect of angiotensin suppression in oral contraceptive users. Hypertension 33:90, 1999.
108. Butkevich A, Abraham C, Phillips RA: Hormone replacement therapy and 24-hour blood pressure profile on postmenopausal women. Am J Hypertens 13:1039, 2000.
109. Modena MG, Molinari R, Muia N Jr, et al: Double-blind randomized placebo-controlled study of transdermal estrogen replacement therapy on hypertensive postmenopausal women. Am J Hypertens 12:1000, 1999.
110. Remuzzi G, Schieppati A, Ruggenenti P: Nephropathy in patients with type 2 diabetes. N Engl J Med 346:1145, 2002.
111. Coresh J, Astor BC, Greene T, et al: Prevalence of chronic kidney disease and decreased kidney function in the adult US population: Third National Health and Nutrition Examination Survey. Am J Kidney Dis 41:1, 2003.
112. Swedko PJ, Clark HD, Paramsothy K, Akbari A: Serum creatinine is an inadequate screening test for renal failure in elderly patients. Arch Intern Med 163:356, 2003.
113. Ghose RR, Harinda V: Unrecognized high pressure chronic retention of urine presenting with systemic arterial hypertension. Br Med J 298:1626, 1989.
114. Textor SC, Wilcox CS: Ischemic nephropathy/azotemic renovascular disease. Semin Nephrol 20:489, 2000.
115. Bakris GL, Williams M, Dworkin L, et al: Preserving renal function in adults with hypertension and diabetes: A consensus approach. Am J Kidney Dis 36:646, 2000.
116. The Heart Outcomes Prevention Evaluation Study Investigators: Effects of an angiotensin-converting-enzyme inhibitor, ramipril, on cardiovascular events in high-risk patients. N Engl J Med 342:145, 2000.
117. Lazarus JM, Bourgoignie JJ, Buckalew VM, et al: Achievement and safety of a low blood pressure goal in chronic renal disease: The modification of diet in renal disease study group. Hypertension 29:641, 1997.
118. Wright JT Jr, Bakris G, Greene T, et al: Effect of blood pressure lowering and antihypertensive drug class on progression of hypertensive kidney disease: Results from the AASK trial. JAMA 288:2421, 2002.
119. Palmer BF: Renal dysfunction complicating the treatment of hypertension. N Engl Med 347:1256, 2002.
120. Schrier RW, Estacio RO, Esler A, Mehler P: Effects of aggressive blood pressure control in normotensive type 2 diabetic patients on albuminuria, retinopathy and strokes. Kidney Int 61:1086, 2002.
121. Gæde P, Vedel P, Larsen N, et al: Multifactorial intervention and cardiovascular disease in patients with type 2 diabetes. N Engl J Med 348:383, 2003.
122. The CDC Diabetes Cost-effectiveness Group: Cost-effectiveness of intensive glycemic control, intensified hypertension control, and serum cholesterol level reduction for type 2 diabetes. JAMA 287:2542, 2002.
123. Rahman M, Dixit A, Donley V, et al: Factors associated with inadequate blood pressure control in hypertensive hemodialysis patients. Am J Kidney Dis 33:498, 1999.
124. Efrati S, Zaidenstein R, Dishy V, et al: ACE inhibitors and survival of hemodialysis patients. Am J Kidney Dis 40:1023, 2002.
125. Hansen KJ, Edwards MS, Craven TE, et al: Prevalence of renovascular disease in the elderly: A population-based study. J Vasc Surg 36:443, 2002.
126. Rihal CS, Textor SC, Breen JF, et al: Incidental renal artery stenosis among a prospective cohort of hypertensive patients undergoing coronary angiography. Mayo Clin Proc 77:309, 2002.
127. Oskin TC, Hansen KJ, Deitch JS, et al: Chronic renal artery occlusion: Nephrectomy versus revascularization. J Vasc Surg 29:140, 1999.
128. Block MJ, Trost DW, Pickering TG, et al: Prevention of recurrent pulmonary edema in patients with bilateral renovascular disease through renal artery stent placement. Am J Hypertens 12:1, 1999.
129. Safian RD, Textor SC: Renal-artery stenosis. N Engl J Med 344:431, 2001.
130. van Onna M, Houben AJHM, Kroon AA, et al: Asymmetry of renal blood flow in patients with moderate to severe hypertension. Hypertension 41:108, 2003.
131. de Haan MW, Kroon AA, Flobbe K, et al: Renovascular disease in patients with hypertension: Detection with duplex ultrasound. J Human Hypertens 16:501, 2002.
132. Radermacher J, Chavan A, Bleck J, et al: Use of Doppler ultrasonography to predict the outcome of therapy for renal-artery stenosis. N Engl J Med 344:410, 2001.
133. Nordmann AJ, Woo K, Parkes R, Logan AG: Balloon angioplasty or medical therapy for hypertensive patients with atherosclerotic renal artery stenosis? A meta-analysis of randomized controlled trials. Am J Med 114:44, 2003.
134. Leertouwer TC, Derkx FHM, Pattynama PMT, et al: Functional effects of renal artery stent placement on treated and contralateral kidneys. Kidney Int 62:574, 2002.
135. Haab F, Duclos JM, Guyenne T, et al: Renin secreting tumors: Diagnosis, conservative surgical approach and long term results. J Urol 153:1781, 1995.
136. Leckie BJ, Birnie G, Carachi R: Renin in Wilms' tumor: Prorenin as an indicator. J Clin Endocrinol Metab 79:1742, 1994.
137. Hadjidakis D, Tsagarakis S, Roboti C, et al: Does subclinical hypercortisolism adversely affect the bone mineral density in patients with adrenal incidentalomas? Clin Endocrinol 58:72, 2003.
138. Gordon RD, Stowasser M, Rutherford JC: Primary aldosteronism: Are we diagnosing and operating on too few patients? World J Surg 25:941, 2001.
139. Tracy RE, White S: A method for qualifying adrenocortical nodular hyperplasia at autopsy: Some use of the methods in illuminating hypertension and atherosclerosis. Ann Diagn Pathol 6:20, 2002.
140. Padfield PL: Primary aldosteronism, a common entity? The myth persists. J Hum Hypertens 16:159, 2002.
141. Schwartz GL, Chapman AB, Boerwinkle E, et al: Screening for primary aldosteronism: Implications of an increased plasma aldosterone/renin ratio. Clin Chem 48:1919, 2002.
142. Rossi E, Regolisti G, Negro A, et al: High prevalence of primary aldosteronism using postcaptopril plasma aldosterone to renin ratio as a screening test among Italian hypertensives. Am J Hypertens 15:896, 2002.
143. Magill SB, Raff H, Shaker JL, et al: Comparison of adrenal vein sampling and computed tomography in the differentiation of primary aldosteronism. J Clin Endocrinol Metab 86:1066, 2001.

144. Lim PO, Jung RT, MacDonald TM: Is aldosterone the missing link in refractory hypertension? Aldosterone-to-renin ratio as a marker of inappropriate aldosterone activity. J Human Hypertens 16:153, 2002.
145. Rossi GP, Sacchetto A, Chiesura-Corona M, et al: Identification of the etiology of primary aldosteronism with adrenal vein sampling in patients with equivocal computed tomography and magnetic resonance findings: Results in 104 consecutive cases. J Clin Endocrinol Metab 86:1083, 2001.
146. Dluhy RG, Lifton RP: Glucocorticoid-remediable aldosteronism. J Clin Endocrinol Metab 84:4341, 1999.
147. Cooper M, Stewart PM: The syndrome of apparent mineralocorticoid excess. Q J Med 91:453, 1998.
148. Yamashita Y, Koga M, Takeda Y, et al: Two sporadic cases of Liddle's syndrome caused by de novo ENaC mutations. Am J Kidney Dis 37:499, 2001.
149. Lim PO, Young WF, MacDonald TM: A review of the medical treatment of primary aldosteronism. J Hypertens 19:353, 2001.
150. Whitworth JA, Mangos GJ, Kelly JJ: Cushing, cortisol, and cardiovascular disease. Hypertension 36:912, 2000.
151. Boscaro M, Barzon L, Fallo F, Sonino N: Cushing's syndrome. Lancet 357:783, 2001.
152. Chu JW, Matthias DF, Belanoff J, et al: Successful long-term treatment of refractory Cushing's disease with high-dose mifepristone (RU 486). J Clin Endocrinol Metab 86:3568, 2001.
153. Chabre O, Portrat-Doyen S, Chaffanjon P, et al: Bilateral laparoscopic adrenalectomy for congenital adrenal hyperplasia with severe hypertension, resulting from two novel mutations in splice donor sites of CYP11B1. J Clin Endocrinol Metab 85:4060, 2000.
154. Hermans C, de Plaen J-F, de Nayer P, Maiter D: Case report: 17 α-Hydroxylase/17,20-lase deficiency: A rare cause of endocrine hypertension. Am J Med 312:126, 1996.
155. Mann SJ: Severe paroxysmal hypertension (pseudopheochromocytoma). Arch Intern Med 159:670, 1999.
156. Lenders JWM, Pacak K, Walther MM, et al: Biochemical diagnosis of pheochromocytoma: Which test is best? JAMA 287:1427, 2002.
157. Neumann HPH, Bausch B, McWhinney SR, et al: Germ-line mutations in nonsyndromic pheochromocytoma. N Engl J Med 346:1459, 2002.
158. Weise M, Merke DP, Pacak K, et al: Utility of plasma free metanephrines for detecting childhood pheochromocytoma. J Clin Endocrinol Metab 87:1955, 2002.
159. Sawka AM, Jaeschke R, Singh RJ, Young WF Jr: A comparison of biochemical tests for pheochromocytoma: Measurement of fractionated plasma metanephrines compared with the combination of 24-hour urinary metanephrines and catecholamines. J Clin Endocrinol Metab 88:553, 2003.
160. Eisenhofer G: Biochemical diagnosis of pheochromocytoma. Ann Intern Med 134:317, 2001.
161. Ulchaker JC, Goldfarb DA, Bravo EL, Novick AC: Successful outcomes in pheochromocytoma surgery in the modern era. J Urol 161:764, 1999.
162. Swan L, Goyal S, Hsia C, et al: Exercise systolic blood pressures are of questionable value in the assessment of the adult with a previous coarctation repair. Heart 89:189, 2003.
163. Colao A, Baldelli R, Marzullo P, et al: Systemic hypertension and impaired glucose tolerance are independently correlated to the severity of the acromegalic cardiomyopathy. J Clin Endocrinol Metab 85:193, 2000.
164. Fommei E, Iervasi G: The role of thyroid hormone in blood pressure homeostasis: Evidence from short-term hypothyroidism in humans. J Clin Endocrinol Metab 87:1996, 2002.
165. Silverberg SJ: Cardiovascular disease in primary hyperparathyroidism. J Clin Endocrinol Metab 85:3513, 2000.
166. Vuylsteke A, Feneck RO, Jolin-Mellgård Å, et al: Perioperative blood pressure control: A prospective study of patient management in cardiac surgery. J Cardiothor Vasc Anesth 14:269, 2000.
167. Auerbach AD, Goldman L: β-blockers and reduction of cardiac events in noncardiac surgery: Scientific review. JAMA 287:1435, 2002.
168. Eisen HJ: Hypertension in heart transplant recipients: More than just cyclosporine. J Am Coll Cardiol 41:433, 2003.
169. Esplin MS, Fausett MB, Fraser A, et al: Paternal and maternal components of the predisposition to preeclampsia. N Engl J Med 344:867, 2001.
170. Hermida RC, Ayala DE, Mojón A, et al: Differences in circadian blood pressure variability during gestation between healthy and complicated pregnancies. Am J Hypertens 16:200, 2003.
171. Greenwood JP, Scott EM, Walker JJ, et al: The magnitude of sympathetic hyperactivity in pregnancy-induced hypertension and preeclampsia. Am J Hypertens 16:194, 2003.
172. Leach RE, Romero R, Kim YM, et al: Pre-eclampsia and expression of heparin-binding EGF-like growth factor. Lancet 360:1215, 2002.
173. Duley L, Henderson-Smart D, Knight M, King J: Antiplatelet drugs for prevention of pre-eclampsia and its consequences: Systematic review. Br Med J 322:329, 2001.
174. National High Blood Pressure Education Program Working Group on High Blood Pressure in Pregnancy: Report of the National High Blood Pressure Education Program Working Group on High Blood Pressure in Pregnancy. Am J Obstet Gynecol 183:S1, 2000.
175. The Magpie Trial Collaborative Group: Do women with pre-eclampsia, and their babies, benefit from magnesium sulphate? The Magpie Trial: A randomized placebo-controlled trial. Lancet 359:1877, 2002.
176. Pearson GD, Veille J-C, Rahimtoola, et al: Peripartum cardiomyopathy. JAMA 283:1183, 2000.
177. Strandgaard S, Paulson OB: Cerebral blood flow and its pathophysiology in hypertension. Am J Hypertens 2:486, 1989.
178. Preston RA, Jy W, Jinenez JJ, et al: Effects of severe hypertension on endothelial and platelet microparticles. Hypertension 41:211, 2003.
179. Chalmers J, Beilin L, Mancia G, et al: International Society of Hypertension (ISH): Statements on blood pressure and stroke. J Hypertens 21:649, 2003.

CHAPTER 38

Systemic Hypertension: Therapy

Norman M. Kaplan

As noted at the beginning of Chapter 37, the number of patients being treated for hypertension has expanded markedly during the past 30 years so that hypertension is now the leading reason for visits by nonpregnant adults to physicians' offices. Nonetheless, in various developed countries—from the United Kingdom and Canada, which have national health schemes that cover everyone, to the United States, with its sporadic coverage—only a third or less of hypertensive patients have their disease under good control.[1] This apparent paradox of expanded coverage but continued poor control is the consequence of multiple factors, including (1) worsening life-style habits, particularly weight gain and physical inactivity, which engender hypertension; (2) poor adherence to long-term prescribed medications; (3) lack of appreciation of the risks associated with even small degrees of elevated blood pressure; and (4) physicians' unwillingness to prescribe the therapy needed to lower the often recalcitrant systolic hypertension so common in elderly patients. Nonetheless, when therapy is pushed to reach appropriate goals, at least two thirds of patients can achieve control.[2] Relatively few patients are truly resistant to therapy.

Fundamental to the difficulty of controlling hypertension is the inherent nature of the disease: induced by common but unhealthy life styles, asymptomatic, and persistent, with overt consequences delayed by 10 to 30 years so that the costs of therapy, both in money and in adverse effects, seem on the surface to outweigh benefits to be derived from adherence to the regimen. Furthermore, behind the inherent nature of the disease lurks yet another disquieting feature of the therapy of most hypertension: it may not benefit the majority of patients who adhere faithfully to their treatment. Even among such elderly patients as enrolled in the Systolic Hypertension in the Elderly Program (SHEP) trial, 111 would need to be treated for 5 years to prevent one cardiovascular death and 19 treated to prevent one cardiovascular event.[3] Because of the costs and side effects of therapy, the use of medication as a preventive measure has not been deemed appropriate.

Yet another element, the issue of cost-effectiveness, has been introduced into the debate about the value of treating all patients with any degree of hypertension. As the escalating costs of health care consume a greater share of society's resources, two opposing forces have risen: one, the need for less expensive illness care, and the other, the relatively large cost of prevention when indiscriminately applied to low-risk subjects. Therefore, it is likely that antihypertensive therapy will be more selective and targeted in the future.

Benefits of Therapy

The treatment of hypertension is aimed not at simple reduction of blood pressure but at prevention of the cardiovascular complications that are known to accompany the high pressure. During the past 35 years, many randomized controlled trials (RCTs) have tested the ability of antihypertensive drugs to prevent strokes and heart attacks.[4] Few other aspects of clinical practice have as strong an evidence base as does the treatment of hypertension.

A meta-analysis of 27 large RCTs wherein systolic blood pressures were provided portrays the effects of therapy in 136,124 patients (Fig. 38–1).[4] Beyond the progressive reduction in cardiovascular mortality that is directly correlated with the degree of systolic blood pressure lowering, reduction in morbidity from stroke and, to a larger degree, from myocardial infarction has also been clearly documented. Over the 35 years encompassed by these trials, benefits of treatment were first documented for patients with severe hypertension, then for those with moderate disease, and only later for those with lesser degrees of hypertension.[3]

The protection against stroke has been shown to apply even to a limited number of patients older than 80 years.[5] In the six trials that included 1670 patients older than 80 years, the half who were treated with either diuretics or dihydropyridine (DHP) calcium antagonists had a 36 percent reduction in stroke, a 39 percent reduction in heart failure, and a statistically significant 22 percent reduction in major coronary events.[5] Moreover, in the one RCT in which dementia was carefully ascertained, treatment of elderly patients with isolated systolic hypertension based on a DHP–calcium channel blocker (CCB) reduced the incidence of dementia by 55 percent over an 8-year follow-up.[6]

The difficulty in showing clear benefits of treatment in the larger part of the hypertensive population, those with stage 1 or blood pressures from 140/90 to 160/100 mm Hg, must be reconciled with the fact that even though their individual risk is relatively low, their sheer number causes them to make the major contribution to the overall population risk from hypertension, as shown in Figure 37–7. This fact has given rise to two important guidelines for clinical practice: first, the critical need for prevention of hypertension by population-wide life-style modifications[7]; and second, the rationale for considering blood pressure in the larger context of overall cardiovascular risk.[8]

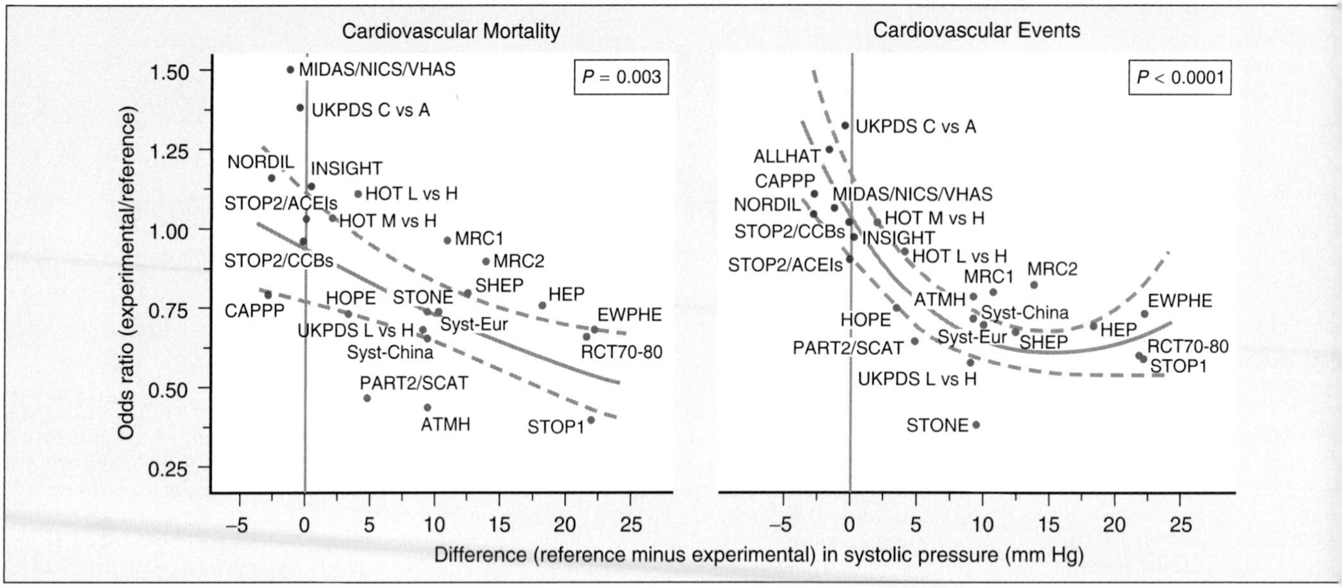

FIGURE 38–1 Relation between the odds ratio for cardiovascular mortality and all cardiovascular events and corresponding differences in systolic blood pressure minus the effect of placebo in 27 published randomized controlled trials of the treatment of hypertension. Magenta dots denote trials that compared new with old drugs. (Modified from Staessen JA, Wang J-G, Thijs L: Cardiovascular protection and blood pressure reduction. Lancet 358:1309, 2001.)

Threshold for Therapy

The value of life-style modifications is documented in the next section of this chapter. The rationale for a broader look at risk beyond blood pressure that was first formalized by a group of investigators from New Zealand[8] has now been incorporated into virtually all guidelines from expert committees.[9,10] The threshold for institution of active drug therapy has generally been taken as an absolute risk of cardiovascular disease of 15 percent or higher in 10 years. The World Health Organization–International Society of Hypertension report provides additional data on the absolute effects of treatment on patients at various levels of cardiovascular risk (Table 38–1).[10] As shown, relatively small benefits have been seen in RCTs of about 5 years' duration in low-risk patients, although with more intensive therapy to lower blood pressure by 20/10 mm Hg, they too can achieve more impressive protection.

As noted in the previous chapter, these relatively crude risk estimates may mark many more patients for antihypertensive

TABLE 38–1 Absolute Effects of Treatment on Cardiovascular Risk

- From the results of randomized, controlled trials, it appears that each reduction of 10 to 14 mm Hg in systolic blood pressure and 5 to 6 mm Hg in diastolic blood pressure confers about two fifths less stroke, one sixth less coronary heart disease, and, in Western populations, one third fewer major cardiovascular events overall.
- In patients with grade I hypertension, monotherapy with most agents produces reductions in blood pressure of about 10/5 mm Hg. In patients with higher grades of hypertension, it is possible to achieve sustained blood pressure reductions of 20/10 mm Hg or more, particularly if combination drug therapy is used.
- The estimated absolute effects of such blood pressure reductions on cardiovascular disease (CVD) risk (fatal plus nonfatal stroke or myocardial infarction) are as follows:

Group of Patients	Absolute Risk (CVD Events over 10 Years) (%)	Absolute Treatment Effects (CVD Events Prevented per 1000 Patient-Years)	
		10/5 mm Hg	*20/10 mm Hg*
Low risk	<15	<5	<8
Medium risk	15-20	5-7	8-11
High risk	20-30	7-10	11-17
Very high risk	>30	>10	>17

- Between these strata, the estimated absolute treatment benefits range from less than 5 events prevented per thousand patient-years of treatment (low risk) to more than 17 events prevented per thousand patient-years of treatment (very high risk).
- The absolute benefits for stroke and coronary artery disease will be augmented by smaller absolute benefits for congestive heart failure and renal disease.
- These estimates of benefit are based on relative risk reductions observed in trials of about 5 years' duration. Longer term treatment over decades could produce larger risk reductions.

From Guidelines Subcommittee: 1999 World Health Organization–International Society of Hypertension guidelines for the management of hypertension. J Hypertens 17:151, 1999.

drug therapy than provided by more careful assessments. On the other hand, the argument has been made that drug therapy should be considered in more presumably low-risk patients even in the absence of evidence that they benefit, largely because there have been no adequate outcome trials in low-risk patients with blood pressure below 140/90 mm Hg. Recall the evidence from the Framingham Study showing that presumably low-risk subjects with high-normal blood pressure—that is, 130 to 139 systolic and 85 to 89 diastolice—had three to four times more cardiovascular events over a 12-year follow-up than occurred among those with lower blood pressure (see Fig. 37–5).[11] On the basis of such evidence, a more liberal approach has been advocated in the 2003 Joint National Committee (JNC)-7 Express report[1]: all patients with sustained blood pressure greater than140/90 are recommended for antihypertensive drug therapy along with appropriate life-style modifications.

These recommendations have placed the decision to treat individual patients with different levels of blood pressure and degrees of overall cardiovascular risk into a much more rational framework. If drug therapy is *not* given, close surveillance must still be provided because from 10 to 17 percent of the placebo-treated patients in various RCTs had progression of their blood pressure to a level above that considered an indication for active treatment. Moreover, all patients should be strongly advised to use the appropriate life-style modifications (see Life-Style Modifications).

Systolic Pressure in Elderly Patients

Current guidelines recommend that therapy be given to elderly patients with isolated systolic hypertension (ISH) because they generally have a higher absolute risk of cardiovascular disease and therefore derive greater benefit from treatment. As previously noted, in the data from eight RCTs involving elderly patients with ISH, those given drugs achieved impressive reductions in cardiovascular morbidity compared with those given placebo,[12] and in the one trial in which cognitive function was specifically monitored, those given drug therapy had a 55 percent reduction in onset of dementia over an 8-year follow-up.[6]

It should be noted that the diagnosis of ISH in these trials was based on a systolic level of 160 mm Hg or higher. A large percentage of elderly persons have systolic pressures above 140 but below 160 with diastolic pressures below 90. As yet there are no data to document benefit in this population, but because many of them are inherently at high risk, the JNC-7 report recommends active drug therapy for those with systolic levels above 140 mm Hg.[1]

USE OF SURROGATE ENDPOINTS. All of the preceding discussion of the benefits of therapy and the threshold for treatment has involved "hard" endpoints: morbidity and mortality. Some argue that softer endpoints should also be taken into account, using as surrogates one or another sign of cardiovascular damage that may be easier to assess and quicker to appear. These include regression of left ventricular hypertrophy (LVH) or carotid artery stenosis and reduction of proteinuria. Most, however, hold to the need for the hard endpoints for large outcome trials.

Goal of Therapy

When the decision has been made to treat, the clinician must consider the goal of therapy. In the past, most physicians assumed that the effects of reduction of blood pressure on cardiovascular risk would fit a straight line downward (line A in Fig. 38–2), justifying the opinion "the lower, the better." However, data from multiple large trials indicated a more

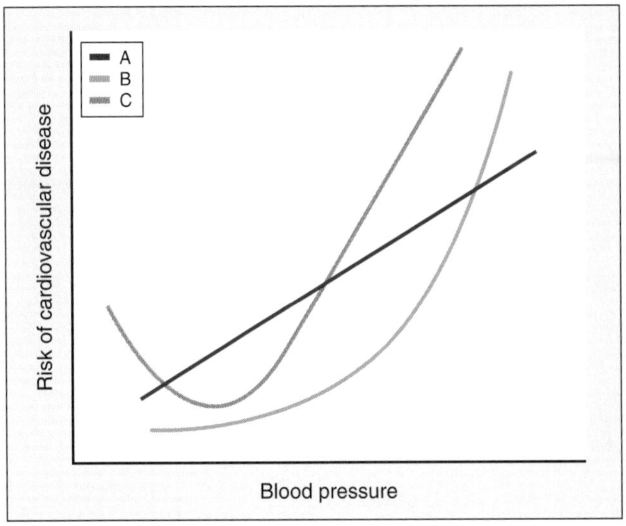

FIGURE 38–2 Three models representing hypothetical relationships between levels of blood pressure and risk of cardiovascular disease. (See text.)

gradual decline in risk when pressures were reduced to moderate levels (line B in Fig. 38–2). Subsequently, evidence has been presented suggesting a J curve, i.e., a fall in risk until some critical level of pressure below which the risk goes back up (line C in Fig. 38–2).[13] The J curve has been claimed for coronary events with falls in diastolic pressure below 85 in patients with diastolic hypertension and for strokes with falls below 65 mm Hg in patients with ISH.

In an attempt to ascertain the presence of a J curve, the Hypertension Optimal Treatment (HOT) trial was performed.[14] Almost 19,000 patients with an initial mean blood pressure of 170/105 mm Hg were randomly allocated to one of three target diastolic pressures: 90, 85, or 80 mm Hg. Diastolic pressures were significantly reduced in all three groups, but at the end, only 4 mm Hg separated them, and it was not possible to prove or disprove a J curve. The least cardiovascular mortality was seen at a blood pressure of 139/86 mm Hg; the least morbidity at 138/83 mm Hg. In the absence of a placebo group, the absolute degree of protection could not be ascertained, but most of the benefit was noted in the 1500 diabetic patients who had a 51 percent reduction in major cardiovascular events in those in the below 80 mm Hg target group compared with the below 90 mm Hg target group.

Another analysis of evidence for a J curve was based on data for individual patients from seven RCTs involving over 40,000 patients given either placebo or drug therapy.[15] A J curve between both systolic and diastolic pressures and cardiovascular mortality was seen, but it occurred in both the treated and the nontreated groups, with the nadir being 5 mm Hg lower in the treated patients (Fig. 38–3). The authors concluded that "The increased risk of events observed with low blood pressure was not related to antihypertensive treatment. . . . Poor health conditions leading to low blood pressure and an increased risk for death probably explain the J-shaped curve."[15]

Certainly, poor general health may cause low blood pressure and increase the risk for death. Nonetheless, excessive antihypertensive treatment may increase cardiovascular morbidity and mortality. The problem may be even more ominous in elderly patients with ISH, whose diastolic pressures are often low before therapy is started. In the SHEP trial, an increased risk for death and stroke was seen with a fall in diastolic pressure below 65 mm Hg.[16]

Nevertheless, the major clinical problem is not overtreatment but undertreatment. Even in carefully conducted clinical trials in which good control should be at a maximum, systolic blood pressures usually remain above 140 mm Hg even though diastolic levels can usually be brought down to below 90 mm Hg. Moreover, even with presumably adequate control, target organ damage may not be reversed. Hypertensives who were treated down to an average level of 128/80 mm Hg maintained a greater left ventricular mass than that seen in normotensive persons, although less than that seen in untreated patients.[17]

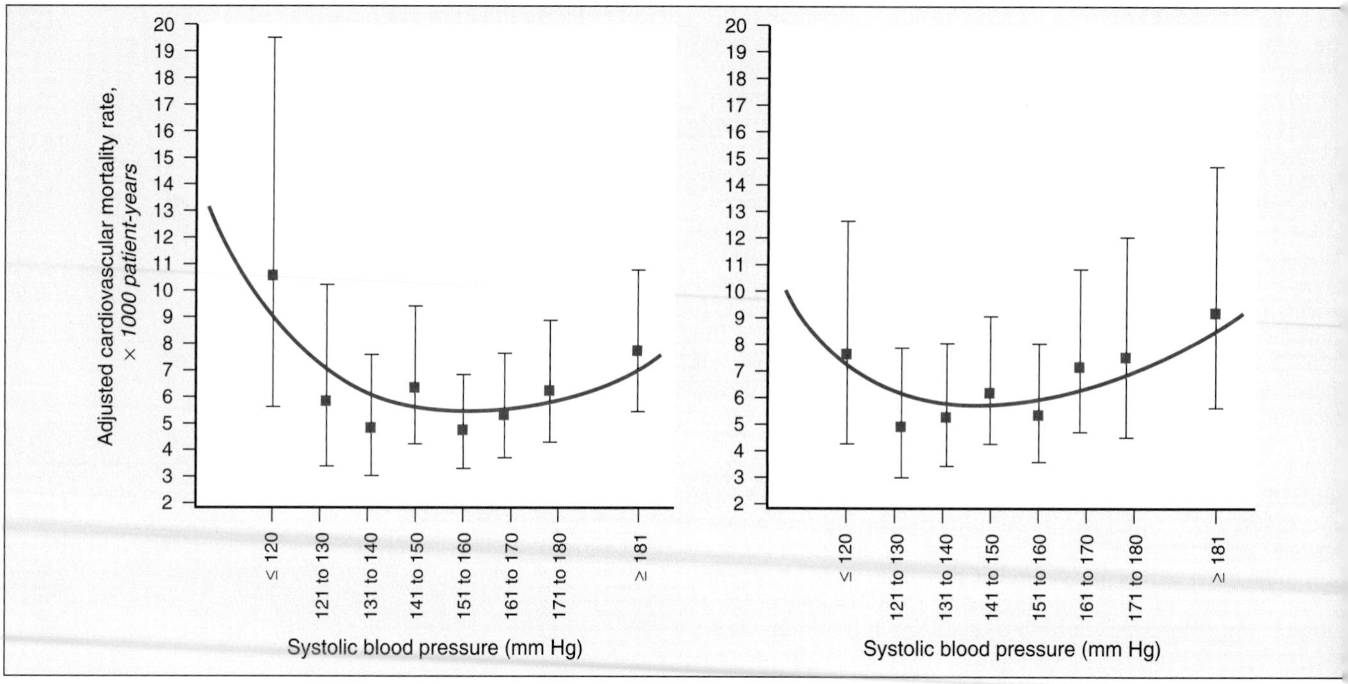

FIGURE 38–3 Age- and sex-adjusted rates of events in eight categories of achieved systolic blood pressure and predicted continuous relationship in active control **(left)** and treatment **(right)** groups from seven randomized controlled trials. (Modified from Boutitie F, Gueyffier F, Pocock S, et al: J-shaped relationship between blood pressure and mortality in hypertensive patients: New insights from a meta-analysis of individual-patient data. Ann Intern Med 136:443, 2002.)

In conclusion, the optimal goal of antihypertensive therapy in most patients with combined systolic and diastolic hypertension who were not at high risk is a blood pressure of less than 140/90 mm Hg. The greatest benefit is probably derived from lowering the diastolic pressure to 80 to 85 mm Hg. Not only is there no proven benefit with more intensive control, but also added cost and probable increased side effects are associated with more aggressive antihypertensive therapy.

In elderly patients with ISH, the goal should be a systolic blood pressure of 140 to 145 mm Hg, as that was the level reached in the RCTs wherein benefit was shown. Caution is advised if, inadvertently, diastolic pressures fall below 65 mm Hg. In such an event, less than ideal reductions in systolic levels need to be balanced against the potential for harm if diastolic levels fall below that level.[13]

More intensive therapy to attain a diastolic pressure of 80 mm Hg or lower may be desirable in some groups, including the following:

- Black patients, who are at greater risk for hypertensive complications and who may continue to have progressive renal damage despite a diastolic pressure of 85 to 90 mm Hg.
- Patients with diabetes mellitus, in whom a blood pressure of less than 130/85 mm Hg reduces the incidence of cardiovascular events.[14] In the United Kingdom Prospective Diabetes Study population of 3642 type 2 diabetic hypertensives, no threshold of risk for systolic pressure was noted: the lower the systolic blood pressure down to 110 mm Hg, the lower was the risk of both micro- and macrovascular complications related to diabetes.[18] (No data on diastolic pressures were provided.)
- Patients with slowly progressive chronic renal disease excreting more than 1 to 2 gm of protein per day, in whom reducing the blood pressure to 125/75 mm Hg may slow the rate of loss of renal function.[19] However, in the African American Study of Kidney Disease (AASK) trial involving 1094 blacks with nondiabetic hypertensive renal disease, those given more therapy to reach a level of 128/78 mm Hg had no better preservation of renal function than those treated to a higher level of 141/85 mm Hg.[19]

Despite the difficulties in achieving the appropriate goal of therapy, good control can be achieved in most patients if they are given enough antihypertensive medication in a progressive manner. Control is enhanced when access to health care is readily available and frequent contact with the same physician is maintained. In addition, the use of life-style modifications markedly improves the chances of adequate control.[1]

Life-Style Modifications

Life-style modifications are indicated for virtually all hypertensives (Table 38–2). Adverse life-style habits are ubiquitous in those with hypertension and may play a major role in the development of the disease. Multiple modifications of life style can lower blood pressure, and their use has been highly correlated with the control of hypertension in the Third National Health and Nutrition Examination Survey (NHANES III) population.[1] Life-style changes are the only maneuvers that have been found to delay, if not stop, the development of hypertension.[7]

Observational and trial data support the importance of multiple simultaneous modifications of life style to accomplish the greatest benefit. Although success in modifying life style may be as difficult or even more difficult to achieve than having patients continue long-term antihypertensive drug therapy, even a small persistent reduction in blood pressure can have a major protective effect on cardiovascular diseases. Moreover, even modest improvements in life style have been shown to reduce the incidence of type 2 diabetes, a common contributor to hypertension.[20]

AVOIDANCE OF TOBACCO. Even though smoking cigarettes has long been known to be a major risk factor for cardiovascular disease, almost 25 percent of U.S. adults now smoke. Part of their risk comes from the major pressor effect of tobacco, which is easily missed because patients are not

TABLE 38–2 Life-Style Modifications to Manage Hypertension

Modification	Recommendation	Approximate Systolic Blood Pressure Reduction (range)
Weight reduction	Maintain normal body weight (body mass index 18.5-24.9 kg/m²)	50-20 mm Hg/10 kg
Adopt DASH eating plan	Consume a diet rich in fruits, vegetables, and low-fat dairy products with a reduced content of saturated and total fat	8-14 mm Hg
Dietary sodium reduction	Reduce dietary sodium intake to no more than 100 mmol/d (2.4 gm sodium or 6 gm sodium chloride)	2-8 mm Hg
Physical activity	Engage in regular aerobic physical activity such as brisk walking (at least 30 min/d, most days of the week)	4-9 mm Hg
Moderation of alcohol consumption	Limit consumption to no more than two drinks (1 oz or 30 ml ethanol; 24 oz beer, 10 oz wine, or 3 oz 80-proof whiskey) per day in most men and to no more than one drink per day in women and lighter weight persons	2.5-4 mm Hg

DASH = Dietary Approaches to Stop Hypertension.
From Joint National Committee: The seventh report of the Joint National Committee on Prevention, Detection, Evaluation, and Treatment of High Blood Pressure (JNC-7 Express). JAMA 289:2560, 2003.

allowed to smoke in places where blood pressures are recorded. With automatic monitoring, the effect is easy to demonstrate, and blood pressure usually falls immediately when smokers quit.

Tolerance does not develop to the pressor effect of nicotine and sympathetic outflow increases with each cigarette, leading to an increase in arterial stiffness. The noxious effects of smoking include an increase in insulin resistance, visceral obesity, and a particularly detrimental effect on progression of nephropathy. Those who smoke must be told to stop on every contact with a health practitioner. Nicotine replacement therapies are effective and have minimal pressor effects, probably because they provide a lesser and slower rise in plasma nicotine.

WEIGHT REDUCTION. Obesity is growing rapidly in the United States and in all developed and developing societies. The consequences of even small amounts of increased weight are impressive. Over 18 years, women with an initial body mass index (BMI) of 24 were five times more likely to have diabetes and twice as likely to have hypertension as women with a BMI of 21 or lower.[21] In many people, most of this increased weight is deposited in the upper body, constituting a major component of the metabolic syndrome (see Chap. 40), which is now present in almost half of U.S. men and women older than 60. Such upper body obesity is a risk factor for hypertension independent of BMI. Upper body obesity is also more commonly associated with obstructive sleep apnea (see Chap. 68), which is much more common than now recognized, found in more than 10 percent of hypertensives.[22] Obstructive sleep apnea can lead to sustained hypertension, and relief of apnea can lower blood pressure.

In virtually every study of weight reduction, systolic blood pressure is reduced, even if the degree of weight loss is small; each 1.0-kg decrease in body weight is associated with an average blood pressure reduction of 1.6/1.3 mm Hg.

PHYSICAL ACTIVITY. An increase in physical activity is almost always essential for weight reduction. Even without weight loss, however, physical activity can lower the incidence of hypertension and diabetes and protect against cardiovascular disease.[20] The blood pressure falls during aerobic exercise and remains lower for the remainder of the day. The overall antihypertensive effect is greater with longer duration but not with more intensive aerobic exercise.[23]

DIETARY CHANGES

Dietary Sodium Restriction. Evidence incriminating the typically high sodium content of the diet of persons living in developed, industrialized societies was presented earlier as a cause of hypertension. When hypertension is present, modest salt restriction may help lower the blood pressure. In an analysis by He and MacGregor of 28 well-controlled intervention studies that lasted at least 4 weeks in which daily intake (based on urinary sodium excretion) was reduced by a median of 78 mmol per 24 hours, blood pressures fell an average of 5.0/2.7 mm Hg in 734 hypertensive subjects and 2.0/1.0 mm Hg in 2220 normotensive subjects (Fig. 38–4).[24] There was a dose-response relationship—the more sodium reduction, the greater the blood pressure decline. However, the maintenance of dietary sodium restriction over 6 months or longer in 11 controlled trials averaged only 33 mmol per 24 hours and was associated with only a 1.1/0.6 mm Hg reduction in blood pressure.[25]

Not all hypertensive persons respond to a moderate degree of sodium restriction to the recommended level of 100 mmol

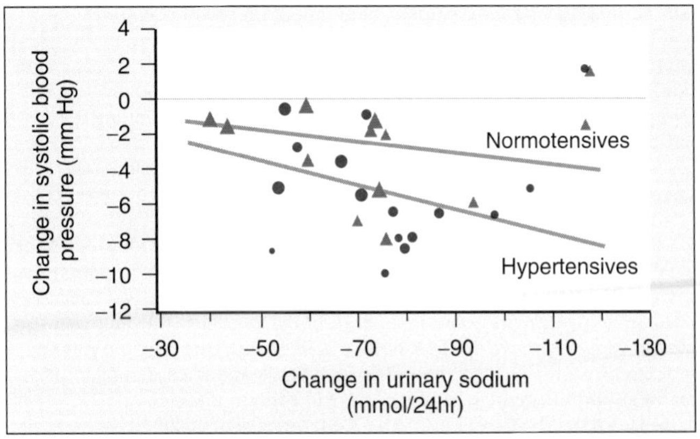

FIGURE 38–4 Relationship between the net change in urinary sodium excretion and systolic blood pressure. The blue triangles represent normotensive and the magenta circles represent hypertensive subjects. The slope is weighted by the inverse of the variance of the net change in systolic blood pressure. The size of the circle is in proportion to the weight of the trial. (Modified from He FJ, MacGregor GA: Effect of modest salt reduction on blood pressure: A meta-analysis of randomized trials. Implications for public health. J Hum Hypertens 16:766, 2002.)

sodium or 2.4 gm/d. Blacks and elderly patients may be more responsive to sodium restriction, perhaps because of their lower renin responsiveness. Nevertheless, even if the blood pressure does not fall with moderate degrees of sodium restriction, patients may still benefit. Multiple cardiovascular and noncardiovascular ill effects have been noted with high sodium intake. In a prospective follow-up of 2400 Finnish men and women, a 100 mmol per 24 hours higher sodium excretion was accompanied by a 45 percent increase in the hazard ratio for cardiovascular disease and a 26 percent increase in all-cause mortality.[26]

However, rigid degrees of sodium restriction not only are difficult for patients to achieve but also may be counterproductive. The marked stimulation of renin-aldosterone and sympathetic nervous activity that accompanies rigid sodium restriction may prevent the blood pressure from falling and increase the amount of potassium wastage if diuretics are used concomitantly.

Therefore, I consider sodium restriction to be useful for all persons, as a preventive measure in those who are normotensive and, more certainly, as partial therapy in those who are hypertensive. The easiest way to accomplish moderate sodium restriction is to substitute natural foods for processed foods because natural foods are low in sodium and high in potassium whereas most processed foods have had sodium added and potassium removed. It is hoped that food processors will gradually reduce the large amounts of salt they often add to processed foods, but in the meantime, patients should be asked to avoid foods whose label indicates more than 300 mg of sodium per portion. Additional guidelines include the following:

- Add no sodium chloride to food during cooking or at the table.
- If a salty taste is desired, use a half sodium and half potassium chloride preparation (such as Lite-Salt) or a pure potassium chloride substitute.
- Avoid or minimize the use of "fast foods," many of which have high sodium content.
- Recognize the sodium content of some antacids and proprietary medications. (For example, Alka-Seltzer contains more than 500 mg of sodium; Rolaids are virtually sodium free.)

POTASSIUM SUPPLEMENTATION. Some of the advantages of a lower sodium intake may be related to its tendency to increase body potassium content, both by a coincidental increase in dietary potassium intake and by a decrease in potassium wastage if diuretics are being used. Low dietary potassium intake is associated with an increased risk of stroke that may be independent of an effect on blood pressure.[27]

Potassium supplements have been shown to reduce the blood pressure an average of 3.1/2.0 mm Hg in 33 RCTs, with the effect being greater in blacks and in the presence of higher dietary sodium intake.[28] Nonetheless, potassium supplements are too costly and potentially hazardous for routine use in normokalemic hypertensive persons. Patients should be protected from potassium depletion and encouraged to increase dietary potassium intake, which may be enough to lower blood pressure.

CALCIUM SUPPLEMENTS. In 42 mostly short-term studies of either calcium supplements (in 33) or dietary intervention (in 9) in 4560 nonpregnant adults, the blood pressure fell 1.44/0.84 mm Hg.[29] Because calcium supplements sometimes raise blood pressure and increase the risk of kidney stones, the best course is to ensure that calcium intake is not inadvertently reduced by reduction of milk and cheese consumption in an attempt to reduce saturated fat and sodium intake.

MAGNESIUM SUPPLEMENTS. A meta-analysis of 20 RCTs of magnesium supplements, averaging 15.4 mmol per 24 hours, found a statistically insignificant fall in blood pressure of 0.6/0.8 mm Hg.[30]

OTHER DIETARY CONSTITUENTS. Significant reductions in blood pressure were observed in a controlled trial of 690 normotensive persons, half of whom ate a diet rich in fruits and vegetables.[31] This fall in blood pressure could reflect increases in fiber, potassium, or other ingredients. Some lowering of the blood pressure has been noted in studies of high fiber intake and high doses of omega-3 fatty acids from fish oil. Supplements of vitamin C have had various effects on blood pressure.

In 11 carefully controlled trials involving 522 subjects who consumed an average of five cups of caffeine-containing coffee, the mean blood pressure rose 2.4/1.2 mm Hg.[32] A pressor response has been noted with decaffeinated coffee as well. Even though consumption of tea has been found to be associated with a lower risk of myocardial infarction, it too may raise blood pressure.

MODERATION OF ALCOHOL. Alcohol is a two-edged sword. Too much, particularly in a binge, raises blood pressure and can have lethal effects; too little can deny multiple cardiovascular benefits (see Chap. 36). The "safe" level of regular alcohol consumption with regard to hypertension in men is less than two portions per 24 hours, although even less was found to increase the incidence in black men.[33] A portion is defined as about 12 ml of alcohol—the equivalent of 12 oz of beer, 4 oz of wine, or 1.5 oz of liquor. Among women, the incidence of hypertension was reduced by 14 percent in those who consumed an average of one half-portion per 24 hours and was increased by 31 percent in those who drank more than two portions per 24 hours.[34] On the other hand, regular consumption of moderate amounts of alcohol reduces the risk of coronary disease, heart failure, ischemic stroke, diabetes, and dementia, perhaps at least in part through an antiinflammatory mechanism.[35]

RELAXATION TECHNIQUES. Most studies of various cognitive-behavioral therapies have shown transient but not sustained lowering of blood pressure. However, more impressive effects were found in 45 hypertensives who received 10 hours of individualized stress management; after 6 months, ambulatory blood pressure levels were reduced by 6.1/4.3 mm Hg.[36] Perhaps acting in ways beyond relaxation, slow breathing guided by a device has also been found to lower blood pressure.[37]

COMBINED THERAPIES. When several life-style modifications are combined, additional antihypertensive effects may accrue. Perhaps the best study is the placebo arm of the Treatment of Mild Hypertension Study (TOMHS),[38] in which 234 mildly hypertensive persons followed a 48-month regimen of moderate sodium restriction, weight loss, regular exercise, and moderation of alcohol use. Despite relatively small changes in weight (average loss of 6.6 pounds), sodium intake (reduction of 10 percent), exercise level, and alcohol consumption, these patients had an 8.6/8.6 mm Hg decline in blood pressure at the end of the 4-year program. Moreover, they experienced improvements in lipid profile and reduction in left ventricular mass.

Nonetheless, despite the need to rely on life-style modifications in the hope of preventing hypertension and in managing the disease once it has developed, the limited success of achieving significant life-style changes in clinical practice must be recognized. Therefore, although life-style changes should be pursued, patients must not be denied the proven benefits of antihypertensive drug therapy.

Antihypertensive Drug Therapy

If the life-style modifications just described are not adequate to bring the blood pressure to goal (<140/90 mm Hg for most, <130/80 mm Hg for those with diabetes or renal insufficiency) or if the level of hypertension at the onset is so high that immediate drug therapy is deemed necessary (>160/100 mm Hg), the JNC-7 report provides an overall algorithm for treatment (Fig. 38–5).[1]

General Guidelines

When drug therapy is decided upon, the guidelines listed in Table 38–3 should be followed in order to provide effective 24-hour control of hypertension in a manner that encourages adherence to the regimen. The approach is based on known pharmacological principles and proven ways to improve adherence.[39]

For the majority of patients who do not require more intensive immediate therapy, once the selection of the most appropriate agent for initial therapy has been made (by a process that is discussed further in the next section), a relatively low dose of a single drug should be started, aiming for a reduction of 5 to 10 mm Hg in blood pressure at each step. Many physicians, by nature and training, wish to control a patient's

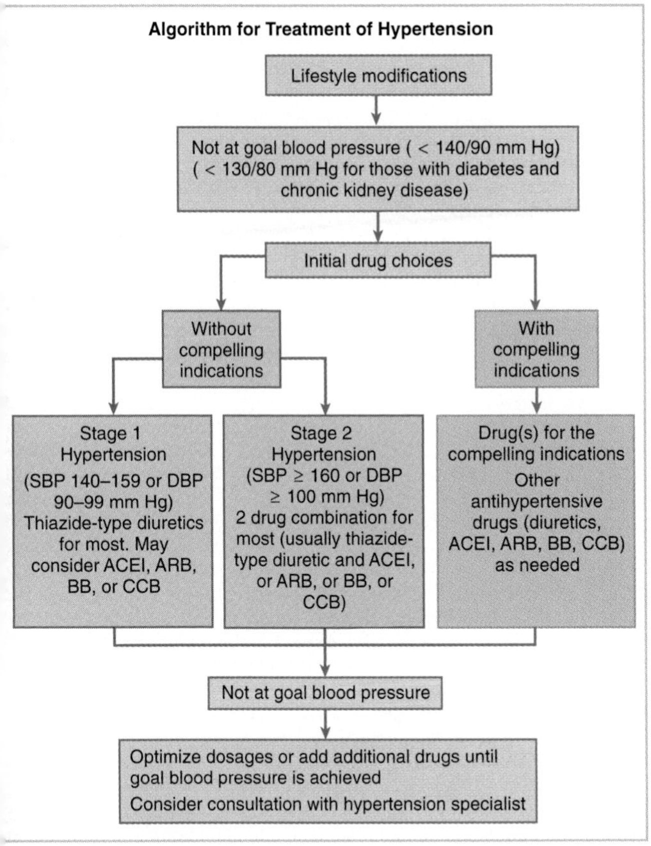
Algorithm for Treatment of Hypertension
Lifestyle modifications
Not at goal blood pressure (< 140/90 mm Hg) (< 130/80 mm Hg for those with diabetes and chronic kidney disease)
Initial drug choices
Without compelling indications
With compelling indications
Stage 1 Hypertension (SBP 140–159 or DBP 90–99 mm Hg) Thiazide-type diuretics for most. May consider ACEI, ARB, BB, or CCB
Stage 2 Hypertension (SBP ≥ 160 or DBP ≥ 100 mm Hg) 2 drug combination for most (usually thiazide-type diuretic and ACEI, or ARB, or BB, or CCB)
Drug(s) for the compelling indications Other antihypertensive drugs (diuretics, ACEI, ARB, BB, CCB) as needed
Not at goal blood pressure
Optimize dosages or add additional drugs until goal blood pressure is achieved
Consider consultation with hypertension specialist

FIGURE 38–5 Treatment of hypertension according to the level of blood pressure and cardiovascular risk as recommended by Joint National Committee (JNC)-7. ACEI = angiotensin-converting enzyme inhibitor; ARB = angiotensin II receptor blocker; BB = beta blocker; CCB = calcium channel blocker; DBP = diastolic blood pressure; SBP = systolic blood pressure. (Modified from Joint National Committee: The seventh report of the Joint Committee on Prevention, Detection, Evaluation, and Treatment of High Blood Pressure (JNC-7 Express). JAMA 289:2560, 2003.)

hypertension rapidly and completely. Regardless of which drugs are used, this approach often leads to undue fatigue, weakness, and postural dizziness, which many patients find intolerable, particularly when they felt well before therapy was begun. Although hypokalemia and other electrolyte abnormalities may be responsible for some of these symptoms, a more likely explanation has been provided by the studies of Strandgaard and Haunsø.[40] As shown in Figure 38–6, they demonstrated the constancy of cerebral blood flow by autoregulation over a range of mean arterial pressures from about 60 to 120 mm Hg in normal subjects and from 110 to 180 mm Hg in patients with hypertension. This shift to the right protects hypertensive patients from a surge of blood flow, which could cause cerebral edema. However, the shift also predisposes hypertensive patients to cerebral ischemia when blood pressure is lowered.

The lower limit of autoregulation necessary to preserve a constant cerebral blood flow in hypertensive patients is a mean of about 110 mm Hg. Thus, acutely lowering the pressure from 160/110 mm Hg (mean = 127) to 140/85 mm Hg (mean = 102) may induce cerebral hypoperfusion, although hypotension in the accepted sense has not been produced. This observation provides a probable explanation for what many patients experience at the start of antihypertensive therapy (i.e., fatigue, lethargy, and dizziness), even though blood pressure levels do not seem inordinately low.

Thus, the approach to antihypertensive therapy should be gradual in order to avoid symptoms related to overly intensive blood pressure reduction. Fortunately, as shown in the middle of Figure 38–6, if therapy is continued for a period, the curve of cerebral autoregulation shifts back toward normal, allowing patients to tolerate greater reductions in blood pressure without experiencing symptoms.

TABLE 38–3 Guidelines to Improve Maintenance of Antihypertensive Therapy

Be aware of the problem and be alert to signs of inadequate intake of medications Recognize and manage depression
Articulate the goal of therapy: to reduce blood pressure to near normotension with few or no side effects
Educate the patient about the disease and its treatment Provide individual assessments of current risks and potential benefits of control Involve the patient in decision-making Provide written instructions Encourage family support
Maintain contact with the patient Encourage visits and calls to allied health personnel Allow the pharmacist to monitor therapy Give feedback to the patient through home blood pressure readings Make contact with patients who do not return
Keep care inexpensive and simple Do the least work-up needed to rule out secondary causes Obtain follow-up laboratory data only yearly unless indicated more often Use home blood pressure readings Use nondrug, low-cost therapies Use once-daily doses of long-acting drugs Use generic drugs and break larger doses of tablets in half If appropriate, use combination tablets Use calendar blister packs (if and when they are marketed) Tailor medication to daily routines Use detailed clinical protocols monitored by nurses and assistants
Prescribe according to pharmacological principles Add one drug at a time Start with small doses, aiming for reductions of 5 to 10 mm Hg at each step Have medication taken immediately on awakening in the morning or after 4 AM if patient awakens to void
Be willing to stop unsuccessful therapy and try a different approach
Anticipate and address side effects Adjust therapy to ameliorate side effects that do not disappear spontaneously
Continue to add effective and tolerated drugs, stepwise, in sufficient doses to achieve the goal of therapy
Provide feedback and validation of success

STARTING DOSAGES. The need to start with a fairly small dose also reflects a greater responsiveness of some patients to doses of medication that may be appropriate for the majority. All drugs exert increasing effect with increasing doses, portrayed by a log-linear dose-response curve (Fig. 38-7).[41] However, different patients require different absolute amounts of drug for their own dose response.

As a hypothetical example, for the majority of patients, 50 mg of the beta blocker atenolol would provide a moderate response, shown as point A on the therapeutic effect curve, whereas a dose of 25 mg would provide only a minimal response. At dose A, providing the significant albeit partial response, the side effects would be minimal, as shown by point A′ on the curve of toxic effect. If a starting dose of 100 mg were used, the therapeutic effect would be near maximal (point B) but the side effects would be much greater as well (point B′). Therefore, a lower starting dose is preferable for most patients.

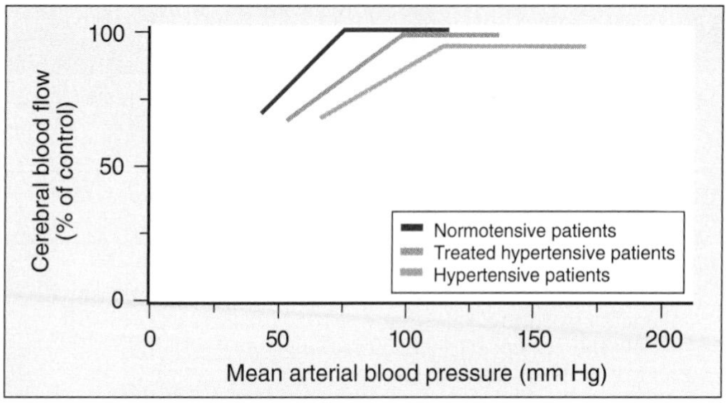

FIGURE 38–6 Mean cerebral blood flow autoregulation curves from normotensive, severely hypertensive, and effectively treated hypertensive patients are shown. (Modified from Strandgaard S: Autoregulation of cerebral blood flow in hypertensive patients. The modifying influence of prolonged antihypertensive treatment on the tolerance to acute, drug-induced hypotension. Circulation 53:720, 1976; and Strandgaard S, Haunsø S: Why does antihypertensive treatment prevent stroke but not myocardial infarction? Lancet 2:658, 1987.)

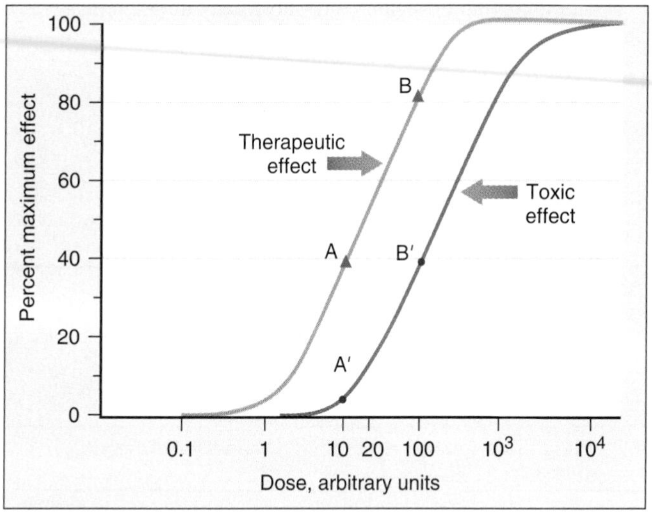

FIGURE 38–7 Theoretical therapeutic and toxic logarithmic-linear dose-response curves. The horizontal axis is the logarithmic scale with arbitrary dose units. The vertical axis is a linear scale showing percentage of maximum possible response. (Modified from Fagan TC: Remembering the lessons of basic pharmacology. Arch Intern Med 154:1430, 1994. Copyright 1994 American Medical Association.)

However, the response to a given dose is not the same for all patients but rather assumes a bell-shaped curve; some patients are very sensitive to that dose and some very resistant, with the majority having a moderate response. Therefore, a significant minority of patients—the very sensitive ones—would have a near-maximal response to the 25-mg dose and would better be started on 12.5 mg in order to achieve a moderate therapeutic effect (point A) with minimal side effects (point A′). Without knowing how individual patients will respond, the safest and easiest approach is to start at a dose that probably is not enough for most patients.

To allow autoregulation of blood flow to maintain perfusion to vital organs when perfusion pressure is lowered, the decline in pressure should be relatively small and gradual. More precipitous reductions in pressure, as frequently occur with larger starting doses, may induce considerable hypoperfusion that results in symptoms that are at least bothersome (fatigue, impotence) and that may be potentially hazardous (postural hypotension, coronary ischemia). It is far better to start low and go slow.

CHOICE OF INITIAL DRUG. In the past, the choice of initial drug was largely based on perceived differences in the efficacy of lowering blood pressure and the likelihood of side effects. Although comparative trials did show some differences, largely determined by age and race,[42] most found that moderate doses of all classes of drugs provided similar efficacy.[3] This conclusion is hardly surprising because the formulations of virtually all antihypertensive drugs are designed to do the same thing: lower the blood pressure at least 10 percent in the majority of hypertensive patients. More than that would probably be unacceptable to patients; less than that would be unacceptable to practitioners.

Recommendations for the choice of initial therapy have been increasingly based on the "compelling" indications of other conditions that frequently coexist with hypertension (Table 38–4).[9,10] In the last 10 years, large trials have examined the ability of different classes to reduce morbidity and mortality, and the results of these outcome trials should now direct the choice of therapy.

The first clear documentation of superiority of one class was a meta-analysis of 19 RCTs comparing outcomes with high and low doses of diuretics and beta blockers, all against placebo (Table 38–5).[43] Low doses of diuretic were seen to protect better against coronary disease than high doses of diuretic or beta blockers.

From 1995 to 2000, eight trials involving 37,872 patients compared different regimens against one other (Table 38–6).[44] The relative risk for stroke was lower for CCB-based therapy than for therapy based on diuretics with or without beta blockers, but the risks for coronary disease and heart failure were lower for therapy based on angiotensin-converting enzyme inhibitors (ACEIs) than for CCB-based therapy. Two points need to be considered in interpreting the data in Table 38–6: (1) in all trials, the primary drug was often admixed with other drugs in order to reach the goal of therapy, and (2) the data comparing ACEI versus CCB came from one large trial that found no significant differences between the two[45] and a much smaller trial that found a highly significant difference.[46] The authors of the meta-analysis concluded that "the evidence suggestive of greater benefits of stroke and lesser benefits for coronary heart disease with calcium-antagonist-based regimens is not sufficiently reliable to allow precise assessments."[45]

THREE RANDOMIZED CLINICAL TRIALS. Since 2000, the results of two larger RCTs comparing different agents in predominantly[2] or exclusively[47] elderly patients have been published. In addition, another large RCT compared an angiotensin II (AII) receptor blocker (ARB) against a beta blocker in the ability to protect hypertensives with LVH.[48]

In brief, the Antihypertensive and Lipid-Lowering Treatment to Prevent Heart Attack Trial (ALLHAT), the largest RCT now available, compared regimens based on a diuretic (chlorthalidone) against either an ACEI (lisinopril) or a CCB (amlodipine) in high-risk hypertensive patients older than 55 years (mean age of 67).[2] Diuretic-based therapy was as effective as ACEI- or CCB-based therapy in preventing the primary endpoint, major coronary events; superior to both in preventing heart failure; and superior to the ACEI in preventing stroke. A large part of the differences in the secondary outcomes may reflect the greater reduction in blood pressure achieved with the diuretic. Moreover, only 35 percent of the patients were treated with their primary drug alone. As with virtually all trials, most patients required more than one drug to achieve the goal of therapy.

A second large outcome trial compared a diuretic-based regimen (hydrochlorothiazide) against an ACEI-based regimen (enalapril) in 6083 hypertensive patients aged 65 to 84.[47] Despite similar reductions in blood pressure, averaging 26/12 mm Hg, those in the ACEI group had an 11 percent greater reduction than the diuretic group in the primary endpoints of cardiovascular events or death. This difference was almost entirely related to a decrease in myocardial infarction in the men, whereas women showed no differences in outcomes, and there was no difference in stroke in either men or women.

In the Losartan Intervention For Endpoint reduction (LIFE) trial, 9193 hypertensive subjects with LVH ascertained by electrocardiography were assigned to either a beta blocker (atenolol) or an ARB (losartan).[48] With equal degrees of blood pressure reduction, those receiving the ARB had a 13 percent lower relative risk of the primary endpoints (death, myocardial infarction, or stroke). This difference was entirely composed of a 25 percent lower risk of stroke; myocardial infarctions were slightly *more* common in those given the ARB, even though more regression of LVH was seen with the ARB. In the LIFE trial, only 11 percent of the patients took only their primary drug and more than 80 percent of both groups also received hydrochlorothiazide.

AN OVERALL ALGORITHM. On the basis of these data and more and in agreement with the JNC-7 algorithm (see Fig. 38–5), the algorithm shown in Figure 38–8 seems to be an appropriate approach to the treatment of stage 1 hypertension. A low-dose thiazide diuretic should be the foundation but is likely to be adequate by itself in only about 30

TABLE 38–4 Indications and Contraindications for the Use of Antihypertensive Drugs

Class of Drug	Indications	Contraindications
Diuretics	Heart failure Advanced age Systolic hypertension	Gout
Beta blockers	Angina or previous myocardial infarction Heart failure Tachyarrhythmias Migraine	Asthma or chronic obstructive pulmonary disease Heart block
Alpha blockers	Prostatic hypertrophy	Incipient heart failure
Calcium channel blockers	Advanced age Systolic hypertension Cyclosporine-induced hypertension	Heart block (verapamil, diltiazem)
ACE inhibitors	Heart failure or left ventricular dysfunction Previous myocardial infarction Diabetic or other nephropathy or proteinuria	Pregnancy Bilateral renal artery stenosis Hyperkalemia
Angiotensin receptor blockers	ACE inhibitor–associated cough Diabetic or other nephropathy Congestive heart failure	Pregnancy Bilateral renal artery stenosis Hyperkalemia

ACE = angiotensin-converting enzyme.

TABLE 38–5 Randomized Controlled Trials in Hypertension: First Drug Therapy

	Relative Risk Versus Placebo			
Agent	*Stroke*	*Coronary Heart Disease*	*Congestive Heart Failure*	*Cardiovascular Mortality*
High-dose thiazide diuretic (50-100 mg)*	0.49	0.99	0.17	0.78
Low-dose thiazide diuretic (12.5-25 mg)*	0.66	0.72	0.58	0.76
Beta blocker	0.71	0.93	0.58	0.89

*Doses are for hydrochlorothiazide or its equivalent.

Modified from Psaty BM, Smith NL, Siscovick DS, et al: Health outcomes associated with antihypertensive therapies used as first-line agents, JAMA 277:739, 1997.

TABLE 38–6 Prospective Overview of Randomized Trials for Hypertension

	Relative Risks (Confidence Interval)					
Therapy	*Stroke*	*CHD*	*CHF*	*Major CV Events*	*CV Death*	*Total Mortality*
ACEI versus placebo (4 trials; 12,124 patients)	0.70 (0.57-0.85)	0.80 (0.72-0.89)	0.84 (0.68-1.04)	0.79 (0.73-0.86)	0.74 (0.64-0.85)	0.84 (0.76-0.94)
CCB versus placebo (2 trials; 5220 patients)	0.61 (0.44-0.85)	0.79 (0.59-1.06)	0.72 (0.48-1.07)	0.72 (0.59-0.87)	0.72 (0.52-0.98)	0.87 (0.70-1.09)
ACEI versus D/βB (3 trials; 16,161 patients)	1.05 (0.92-1.19)	1.00 (0.88-1.14)	0.92 (0.77-1.09)	1.00 (0.93-1.08)	1.00 (0.87-1.15)	1.03 (0.93-1.14)
CCB versus D/βB (5 trials; 23,454 patients)	0.87 (0.77-0.98)	1.12 (1.0-1.26)	1.12 (0.95-1.33)	1.02 (0.95-1.10)	1.05 (0.92-1.2)	1.01 (0.92-1.11)
ACEI versus CCB (2 trials; 4871 patients)	1.02 (0.85-1.21)	0.81 (0.68-0.97)	0.82 (0.67-1.0)	0.92 (0.83-1.01)	1.04 (0.87-1.24)	1.03 (0.91-1.18)

ACEI = angiotensin-converting enzyme inhibitor; CCB = calcium channel blocker; D/βB = diuretic/beta-blacker; CHD = coronary heart disease; CHF = congestive heart failure; CV = cardiovascular.

From Neal B, MacMahon S, Chapman N—Blood Pressure Lowering Treatment Trialists' Collaboration: Effects of ACE inhibitors, calcium antagonists, and other blood-pressure-lowering drugs: Results of prospectively designed overviews of randomised trials. Blood Pressure Lowering Treatment Trialists' Collaboration. Lancet 356:1955, 2000.

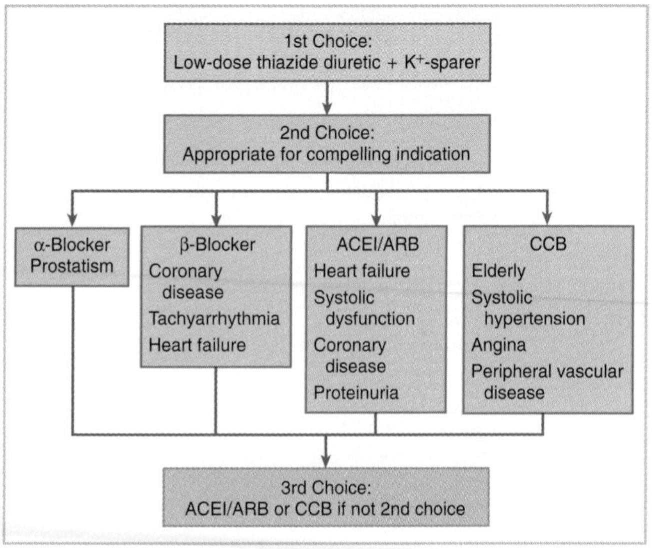

FIGURE 38–8 An algorithm for therapy of hypertension. ACEI = angiotensin-converting enzyme inhibitor; ARB = angiotensin II receptor blocker; CCB = calcium channel blocker.

percent of patients. The remainder should then be given whatever choice seems appropriate for their coexisting conditions (see Table 38–4). On the basis of these short-term efficacy trials, those with only hypertension could logically be given an ACEI if they are younger or nonblack or a CCB if they are older or black. In fact, because the differential responses in blood pressure reduction are largely removed when a diuretic is also given, there seems little reason to favor any drug class in the absence of a specific indication or contraindication.

COMBINATION THERAPY. Because a low dose of a thiazide diuretic potentiates the effect of all other drug classes and because most patients, particularly those with diabetes, renal disease, or levels of blood pressure above 160/100, require two or more drugs for adequate control, a combination of a low-dose diuretic and the appropriate second choice may logically be used at the onset of therapy as recommended by JNC-7. Other combinations are also available and may improve control of hypertension by lowering the cost and improving adherence to therapy.

COMPLETE COVERAGE WITH ONCE-DAILY DOSING. A number of choices within each of the six major classes of antihypertensive drugs now available provide full 24-hour efficacy. Therefore, single daily dosing should be feasible for virtually all patients, resulting in improved adherence to therapy. The use of longer acting agents avoids the potential for inducing too great a peak effect in order to provide an adequate effect at the end of the dosing interval (the trough). Moreover, because many patients occasionally skip a dose of their drugs, there is an additional value in using agents with an inherently long duration of action that covers the skipped dose as well.

Long-acting choices are available within each class. However, because patients differ not only in terms of degree of response but also in terms of the duration of effect, the prudent course is to document the patient's response at the end of the dosing interval by home or ambulatory monitoring. With this approach, the abrupt surge in blood pressure that occurs on awakening is blunted, and, it is hoped, patients can be better protected from the increased incidence of cardiovascular catastrophes at this critical time.

If short-acting medications are taken at bedtime to ensure coverage in the early morning, ischemia to vital organs might be induced by the combination of the maximal effect of the drug within the first 3 to 6 hours after intake and the usual nocturnal decline in pressure. Therefore, the safest course is to take medications with a 24-hour duration of action as early in the morning as possible.

With the general principles of therapy in mind, particulars about the various classes of drugs available are now covered.

Diuretics (see also Chap. 23)

Diuretics may be divided into four major groups by their primary site of action within the tubule, starting in the proximal portion and moving to the collecting duct: (1) agents acting on the proximal tubule, such as carbonic anhydrase inhibitors, which have limited antihypertensive efficacy; (2) loop diuretics; (3) thiazides and related sulfonamide compounds; and (4) potassium-sparing agents (Table 38–7). A thiazide is the usual choice, often in combination with a potassium-sparing agent. Loop diuretics should be reserved for patients with renal insufficiency or resistant hypertension. The availability of a more specific aldosterone blocker, eplerenone, may considerably broaden the use of this class of drug beyond that of spironolactone.

MECHANISM OF ACTION. All diuretics initially lower the blood pressure by increasing urinary sodium excretion and by reducing plasma volume, extracellular fluid volume, and cardiac output. Within 6 to 8 weeks, the lowered plasma, extracellular fluid volume, and cardiac output return toward normal. At this point and beyond, the lower blood pressure is related to a decline in peripheral resistance, thereby improving the underlying hemodynamic defect of hypertension. The mechanism responsible for the lowered peripheral resistance may involve a vasorelaxant effect, but initial diuresis is needed because diuretics fail to lower the blood pressure when the excreted sodium is returned or when given to patients who have nonfunctioning kidneys and are undergoing long-term dialysis. With the shrinkage in blood volume and lower blood pressure, increased secretion of renin and

TABLE 38–7 Representative Diuretics and Potassium-Sparing Agents

Agent	Daily Dose (mg)	Duration of Action (hr)
Thiazides		
Bendroflumethiazide (Naturetin)	1.25-5.0	>18
Cyclothiazide (Anhydron)	0.125-1	18-24
Hydrochlorothiazide (Esidrix, HydroDIURIL, Oretic)	6.25-50	12-18
Methyclothiazide (Enduron)	2.5-5.0	>24
Trichlormethiazide (Metahydrin, Naqua)	1-4	>34
Related Sulfonamide Compounds		
Chlorthalidone (Hygroton)	12.5-50	24-72
Indapamide (Lozol)	1.25-2.5	24
Metolazone (Mykrox, Zaroxolyn)	0.5-10	24
Loop Diuretics		
Bumetanide (Bumex)	0.5-5	4-6
Ethacrynic acid (Edecrin)*	25-100*	12*
Furosemide (Lasix)	40-480	4-6
Torsemide (Demadex)	5-40	12
Potassium-Sparing Agents		
Amiloride (Midamor)	5-10	24
Eplerenone (Inspra)	50-200	24
Spironolactone (Aldactone)	25-100	8-12
Triamterene (Dyrenium)	50-100	12

*No longer available in the United States.

ldosterone retards the continued sodium diuresis. Both enin-induced vasoconstriction and aldosterone-induced odium retention prevent continued diminution of body uids and progressive reduction in blood pressure while iuretic therapy is continued.

CLINICAL EFFECTS. With daily diuretic therapy, systolic ressure usually falls about 10 mm Hg, although the degree epends on various factors, including the initial height of ne pressure, the quantity of sodium ingested, the adequacy f renal function, and the intensity of the counterregulatory enin-aldosterone response. Those with initially lower renin r aldosterone levels, including many elderly or black hyper- ensives, tend to have a greater antihypertensive effect.[49] The ntihypertensive effect of the diuretic persists indefinitely, lthough it may be overwhelmed by excessive dietary sodium ntake.

If other antihypertensive drugs are used, a diuretic may lso be needed. Without a concomitant diuretic, antihyper- ensive drugs that do not block the renin-aldosterone mech- nism may cause sodium retention. This mechanism robably reflects the success of the drugs in lowering the lood pressure and may involve the abnormal renal pressure- atriuresis relationship that is presumably present in primary ypertension. Just as more pressure is needed to excrete a iven load of sodium in a hypertensive individual, so does a owering of pressure toward normal lead to sodium retention.

The critical need for adequate diuretic therapy to keep ntravascular volume slightly diminished has been repeat- dly documented. Drugs that inhibit the renin-aldosterone nechanism, such as ACEIs, or drugs that induce some natri- resis themselves, such as calcium antagonists, may continue o work without the need for concomitant diuretics. However, diuretic enhances the effectiveness of all other types of lrugs, including calcium antagonists. Moreover, the results f multiple comparative trials including ALLHAT[2] and those hown in Tables 38–5 and 8–6 reconfirm the cardio- ascular protective effects of liuretic-based therapy.

The benefits of diuretics nay be even greater in atients who are more odium sensitive, perhaps as consequence of genetic ariants. In a case-controlled tudy, the hypertensives who arried the alpha-adducin ene variant were found to ave an even lower risk for oronary and stroke events vhen given a diuretic than vith other agents.[50]

DOSAGE AND CHOICE OF AGENT. Most patients vith mild to moderate hyper- ension and serum creatinine oncentrations less than .5 mg/dl respond to the ower doses of the various liuretics (thiazides and elated compounds) listed n Table 38–7. An amount quivalent to 12.5 mg of ydrochlorothiazide is usually adequate. For ncomplicated hyperten- sion, a single morning dose of hydrochlorothiazide pro- vides a 24-hour antihyper- ensive effect. The non- thiazide agent indapamide has special properties that make it an attractive choice. With renal damage, manifested by a serum creatinine level exceeding 1.5 mg/dl or creatinine clearance less than 30 ml/min, thiazides are usually not effective, and repeated daily doses of furosemide, one or two doses of torsemide, or a single dose of metolazone is usually needed. The combination of a thiazide with a loop diuretic may provide even better efficacy by countering the distal nephron hypertrophy seen with loop diuretics alone.

SIDE EFFECTS. A number of biochemical changes often accompany successful diuresis, including a decrease in plasma potassium level and increases in glucose, insulin, and cholesterol levels (Fig. 38–9). Most of these are minimized or absent with low doses of diuretic.

HYPOKALEMIA. The degree of potassium wastage and hypokalemia is directly related to the dose of diuretic; serum potassium level falls an average of 0.7 mmol/liter with 50 mg of hydrochlorothiazide, 0.4 with 25, and little if any with 12.5.[3] Hypokalemia related to high doses of diuretic may precipitate potentially hazardous ventricular ectopic activity and increase the risk of primary cardiac arrest, even in patients not known to be susceptible because of concomitant digitalis therapy or myocardial irritability.

The following maneuvers should help prevent diuretic-induced hypokalemia:

- Use the smallest dose of diuretic needed.
- Use a moderately long-acting (12- to 18-hour) diuretic, such as hydrochlorothiazide, because longer acting drugs (e.g., chlorthalidone) may increase potassium loss.
- Restrict sodium intake to less than 100 mmol/d.
- Increase dietary potassium intake.
- Use a combination of a thiazide with a potassium-sparing agent except in patients with renal insufficiency or in association with an ACEI or ARB.
- Use a concomitant beta blocker, an ACEI, or an ARB, which diminishes potassium loss by blunting the diuretic-induced rise in renin and aldosterone.

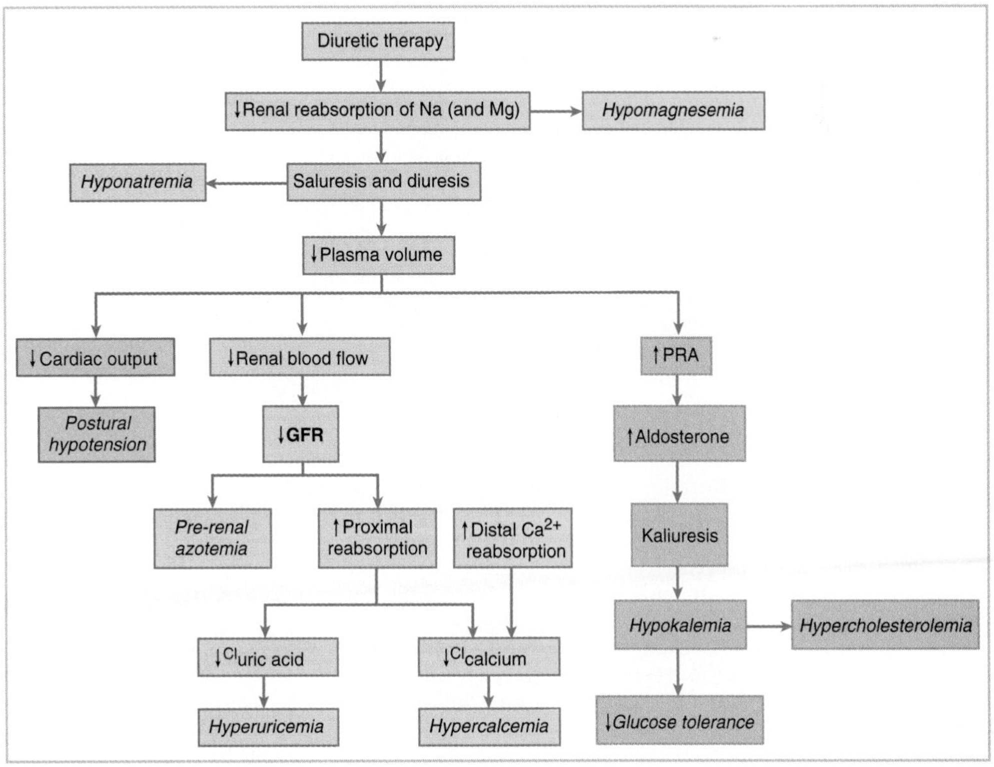

FIGURE 38–9 The mechanisms by which chronic diuretic therapy may lead to various complications. The mechanism for hypercholesterolemia remains in question, although it is shown as arising through hypokalemia. Cl = clearance; GFR = glomerular filtration rate; PRA = plasma renin activity. (Modified from Kaplan NM: Kaplan's Clinical Hypertension. 8th ed. Baltimore, Lippincott Williams & Wilkins, 2002, p 246.)

HYPOMAGNESEMIA. In some patients, concomitant diuretic-induced magnesium deficiency prevents restoration of intracellular deficits of potassium, so that hypomagnesemia should be corrected. Magnesium deficiency may also be responsible for some of the arrhythmias ascribed to hypokalemia.

HYPERURICEMIA. The serum uric acid level is elevated in as many as one third of untreated hypertensive patients. With long-term high-dose diuretic therapy, hyperuricemia appears in another third of patients as a consequence of increased proximal tubule reabsorption accompanying volume contraction and may precipitate acute gout. Because asymptomatic hyperuricemia does not cause urate deposition, most investigators agree that it need not be treated.

HYPERGLYCEMIA AND INSULIN RESISTANCE. High doses of diuretics may impair glucose tolerance and precipitate diabetes mellitus, probably because they increase insulin resistance and hyperinsulinemia.

HYPERCALCEMIA. A slight rise in serum calcium levels, less than 0.5 mg/dl, is frequently seen with thiazide diuretic therapy and is accompanied by a 40 to 50 percent decrease in urinary calcium excretion. Thiazide therapy thereby protects against renal stones and osteoporosis.

HYPONATREMIA. Thiazides may cause insidious hyponatremia, usually in elderly women.

ERECTILE DYSFUNCTION. An increase in the incidence of impotence was noted among men who took 15 mg of chlorthalidone, with the diuretic being the only one of five classes of agents attended by this effect.[51]

RENAL CELL CARCINOMA. A significant but numerically small increase in renal cell carcinoma among diuretic users has been documented.[52]

SULFA SENSITIVITY. Ethacrynic acid, the only diuretic that does not have a sulfonamide structure, is no longer available. A slow rechallenge with a sulfonamide diuretic may be successful in overcoming sulfa sensitivity.

LOOP DIURETICS. Loop diuretics are usually needed in the treatment of hypertensive patients with renal insufficiency, defined here as a serum creatinine level exceeding 1.5 mg/dl. Furosemide has been most widely used, although metolazone may be as effective and requires only a single daily dose. Many physicians use furosemide in the management of uncomplicated hypertension, but this drug provides less antihypertensive action when given once or twice a day than do longer acting diuretics, which maintain the slight volume contraction that is needed for the antihypertensive effect of diuretics.

POTASSIUM-SPARING AGENTS. These drugs are normally used in combination with a thiazide diuretic. Of the four currently available, two (eplerenone and spironolactone) are aldosterone antagonists; the other two (triamterene and amiloride) are direct inhibitors of potassium secretion. In combination with a thiazide diuretic, they diminish the amount of potassium wasting. Although they are more expensive than thiazides alone, they may decrease the total cost of therapy by reducing the need to monitor and treat potassium depletion. Moreover, low doses of spironolactone have been found to prevent myocardial fibrosis and reduce mortality in patients with heart failure.[53]

Eplerenone is a more selective aldosterone antagonist than spironolactone and exerts an impressive antihypertensive effect without the gynecomastia and menstrual irregularities sometimes seen with spironolactone.[54] In view of the increasing evidence that even normal levels of aldosterone induce fibrosis in various tissues,[55] such a selective aldosterone blocker may find much wider use as a potassium sparer.

An Overview of Diuretics in Hypertension

A low dose of a thiazide diuretic should almost always be the initial choice of drug therapy for most hypertensives. If not the first choice, a diuretic should certainly be the second drug used. In those with more severe hypertension or renal damage, larger doses of a thiazide or a loop-acting agent are needed. The potential for multiple adverse effects that can be associated with diuretics requires appropriate surveillance but, overall, they remain the least expensive choice and one that may provide other benefits, e.g., protection against osteoporosis, as well.

Adrenergic Inhibitors

A number of drugs that inhibit the adrenergic nervous system are available, including some that act centrally on vasomotor center activity, peripherally on neuronal catecholamine discharge, or by blocking alpha- or beta-adrenergic receptors, or both (Table 38–8); some act at numerous sites. Figure 38–10, a schematic view of the ending of an adrenergic nerve and the effector cell with its receptors, depicts how some of these drugs act.

An important aspect of sympathetic activity involves the feedback of norepinephrine to alpha- and beta-adrenergic receptors located on the neuronal surface, i.e., presynaptic receptors. Presynaptic alpha-adrenergic receptor activation inhibits release, whereas presynaptic beta activation stimulates further norepinephrine release. The presynaptic receptors have a role in the action of some of the drugs to be discussed.

Drugs That Act Within the Neuron

Reserpine, guanethidine, and related compounds act differently to inhibit the release of norepinephrine from peripheral adrenergic neurons.

RESERPINE. Reserpine, the most active and widely used of the derivatives of the rauwolfia alkaloids, depletes the postganglionic adrenergic neurons of norepinephrine by inhibiting its uptake into storage vesicles, exposing it to degradation by cytoplasmic monoamine oxidase. The peripheral effect is predominant, although the drug enters the brain and depletes central catecholamine stores as well. This effect probably accounts for the sedation and depression accompanying reserpine use. The drug has certain advantages: only one dose a day is needed; in combination with a diuretic, the antihypertensive effect is significant; little postural hypotension is noted; and many patients experience no side effects. The drug has a relatively flat dose-response curve, so that a dose of only 0.05 mg/d gives almost as much antihypertensive effect as 0.125

TABLE 38–8 Adrenergic Inhibitors Used in Treatment of Hypertension

Peripheral Neuronal Inhibitors
Reserpine
Guanethidine (Ismelin)
Guanadrel (Hylorel)
Bethanidine (Tenathan)
Central Adrenergic Inhibitors
Methyldopa (Aldomet)
Clonidine (Catapres)
Guanabenz (Wytensin)
Guanfacine (Tenex)
Alpha Receptor Blockers
$Alpha_1$ and $alpha_2$ receptor
Phenoxybenzamine (Dibenzyline)
Phentolamine (Regitine)
$Alpha_1$ receptor
Doxazosin (Cardura)
Prazosin (Minipress)
Terazosin (Hytrin)
Beta Receptor Blockers
Acebutolol (Sectral)
Atenolol (Tenormin)
Betaxolol (Kerlone)
Bisoprolol (Zebeta)
Carteolol (Cartrol)
Metoprolol (Lopressor, Toprol)
Nadolol (Corgard)
Penbutolol (Levatol)
Pindolol (Visken)
Propranolol (Inderal)
Timolol (Blocadren)
Alpha and Beta Receptor Blockers
Labetalol (Normodyne, Trandate)
Carvedilol (Coreg)

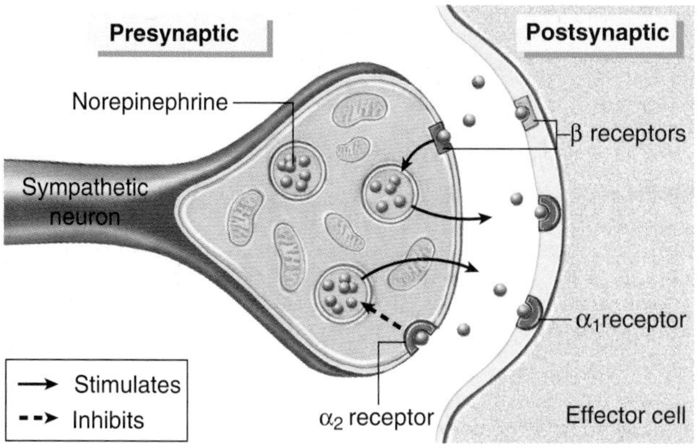

FIGURE 38–10 Simplified schematic view of the adrenergic nerve ending showing that norepinephrine (NE) is released from its storage granules when the nerve is stimulated and enters the synaptic cleft to bind to alpha$_1$ and beta receptors on the effector cell (postsynaptic). In addition, a short feedback loop exists in which NE binds to alpha$_2$ and beta receptors on the neuron (presynaptic) to inhibit or to stimulate further release, respectively.

or 0.25 mg/d but with fewer side effects. Although it remains popular in some places and is recommended as an inexpensive choice where resources are limited, use of reserpine has progressively declined because it has no commercial sponsor.

GUANETHIDINE. This agent and a series of related guanidine compounds, including guanadrel, bethanidine, and debrisoquine, act by inhibiting the release of norepinephrine from the adrenergic neurons. Blood pressure is reduced mainly when the patient is upright, owing to gravitational pooling of blood in the legs, because compensatory sympathetic nervous system–mediated vasoconstriction is blocked. This effect results in the most common side effect, postural hypotension. Unlike reserpine, guanethidine has a steep dose-response curve, so that it can be successfully used in treating hypertension of any degree in daily doses of 10 to 300 mg. As other drugs have become available, guanethidine and related compounds have been relegated mainly to the treatment of severe hypertension unresponsive to all other agents.

Drugs That Act on Receptors

Predominantly Central Alpha-Agonists

Of these, only clonidine has much current use, although methyldopa remains one of the few drugs approved for treatment of pregnancy-induced hypertension (see also Chap. 74).

METHYLDOPA. The primary site of action of methyldopa is within the central nervous system, where alpha-methylnorepinephrine, derived from methyldopa, is released from adrenergic neurons and stimulates central alpha-adrenergic receptors, reducing the sympathetic outflow from the central nervous system. The blood pressure falls mainly as a result of a decrease in peripheral resistance with little effect on cardiac output. Renal blood flow is well maintained, and significant postural hypotension is unusual.

Methyldopa need be given no more than twice daily, in doses ranging from 250 to 3000 mg/d.

Side effects include some that are common to centrally acting drugs that reduce sympathetic outflow: sedation, dry mouth, impotence, and galactorrhea. However, methyldopa causes some unique side effects that are probably of an autoimmune nature because a positive antinuclear antibody test result is obtained in about 10 percent of patients who take the drug, and red cell autoantibodies occur in about 20 percent. Inflammatory disorders in various organs have been reported, most commonly involving the liver (with diffuse parenchymal injury similar to that in viral hepatitis).

CLONIDINE. Although of different structure, clonidine shares many features with methyldopa. It acts at the same central sites, has similar antihypertensive efficacy, and causes many of the same bothersome but less serious side effects (e.g., sedation, dry mouth). It does not, however, induce the autoimmune and inflammatory side effects.

The drug has a fairly short biological half-life, so that when it is discontinued, the inhibition of norepinephrine release disappears within about 12 to 18 hours and plasma catecholamine levels rise. This effect is responsible for the rapid rebound of the blood pressure to pretreatment levels and the occasional appearance of withdrawal symptoms, including tachycardia, restlessness, and sweating. If the rebound requires treatment, clonidine may be reintroduced or alpha-adrenergic receptor antagonists given.

Clonidine is available in a *transdermal* preparation, which may provide smoother blood pressure control for as long as 7 days with fewer side effects. Bothersome skin rashes preclude its use in perhaps one fourth of patients, however.

GUANABENZ. This drug differs in structure from but shares many characteristics with both methyldopa and clonidine, acting primarily as a central alpha-agonist.

GUANFACINE. This drug is also similar to clonidine but is longer acting, which enables once-daily dosing and minimizes rebound hypertension. This agent, although used less than clonidine, is the preferred choice of a central alpha-agonist.

Alpha-Adrenergic Receptor Antagonists

These agents may have many attractive features but their use has been limited, initially because of the potential for postural hypotension, more recently because of a greater likelihood of fluid retention that may provoke congestive heart failure.[56] The first of this class was prazosin but the two now used, doxazosin and terazosin, have slower onset and longer duration of action so that they may be given once daily with less propensity for first-dose hypotension.

Selective alpha blockers are as effective as other antihypertensives.[38] When given to patients whose condition is poorly controlled by two or more agents, they may reduce blood pressure even more than anticipated. The favorable hemodynamic changes—a fall in peripheral resistance with maintenance of cardiac output—make them an attractive choice for patients who wish to remain physically active. In addition, blood lipids and insulin sensitivity are not adversely altered and may actually improve with alpha blockers, unlike the adverse effects observed with diuretics and beta blockers.[57]

Despite these attractive features, alpha blockers have not been widely used for hypertension. Their use is likely to diminish further because of the ALLHAT trial data.[56] In this large, double-blind, randomized trial involving older patients with hypertension, the alpha-adrenergic blocker doxazosin, when compared with the diuretic chlorthalidone, was associated with significantly higher risks for stroke and congestive heart failure but no increase in mortality.

The higher risk of stroke could be due to the lesser reduction of blood pressure with the alpha blocker than the diuretic. The design of the study may be largely responsible for the increased risk of congestive heart failure. Many of the enrollees were at high risk for heart failure and had to stop abruptly whatever drugs they had been taking, including diuretics or ACEIs, that were effectively keeping them out of failure, and switched to 1 mg of doxazosin. The resultant fluid retention may have precipitated congestive heart failure.

Nonetheless, the ALLHAT data clearly indicate the need to use a diuretic with the alpha blocker, particularly in those with LVH or other risk factors for congestive heart failure. Meanwhile, alpha blockers are now being used primarily for relief of prostatism. By decreasing the tone of the smooth muscle at the bladder neck and prostate, they relieve the obstructive symptoms of prostatic hypertrophy.

Beta-Adrenergic Receptor Antagonists (see also Chaps. 23 and 50)

In the 1980s, beta-adrenergic receptor blockers became the most popular form of antihypertensive therapy after diuretics, reflecting their relative effectiveness and freedom from many bothersome side effects. Because beta blockers have been found to reduce mortality if taken either before or after acute myocardial infarction (i.e., secondary prevention), it was assumed that they might offer special protection against initial coronary events (i.e., primary prevention). However, in large clinical trials, a beta blocker provided less protection than did a low-dose diuretic (see Table 38–5).[43] Nevertheless, their efficacy in treatment of congestive heart failure has stimulated their use.

THE VARIOUS BETA BLOCKERS. Beta blockers now available in the United States are shown in Figure 38–11. Pharmacologically, those now available differ considerably from one another with respect to degree of absorption, protein binding, and bioavailability. However, the three most important differences affecting their clinical use are cardioselectivity, intrinsic sympathomimetic activity, and lipid solubility. Despite these differences, they all seem to be about equally effective as antihypertensives.

Cardioselectivity. Cardioselectivity refers to the relative blocking effect on the $beta_1$-adrenergic receptors in the heart compared with that on the $beta_2$ receptors in the bronchi, peripheral blood vessels, and elsewhere. Such cardioselectivity can easily be shown using small doses in acute studies; with the rather high doses used to treat hypertension, much of this selectivity is lost. However, more cardioprotective drugs may be better tolerated in patients with reactive airway disease or peripheral vascular disease.[58]

Intrinsic Sympathomimetic Activity. Some of these drugs have intrinsic sympathomimetic activity, interacting with beta receptors to cause a measurable agonist response but at the same time blocking the greater agonist effects of endogenous catecholamines. As a result, although in usual doses they lower the blood pressure about the same degree as do other beta blockers, they cause a smaller decline in heart rate, cardiac output, and renin levels.

Lipid Solubility. Atenolol and nadolol are among the least lipid soluble of the beta blockers so that they escape hepatic metabolism and are excreted unchanged. Lipid-soluble agents, e.g., metoprolol and propranolol, are taken up and metabolized in the liver and so are more bioavailable after intravenous than oral administration.

Mechanism of Action. Despite these and other differences, the various beta blockers now available are approximately equipotent as antihypertensive agents. A number of possible mechanisms are likely to be involved in their antihypertensive action. For those without intrinsic sympathomimetic activity, cardiac output falls 15 to 20 percent and renin release is reduced about 60 percent. Central nervous system beta-adrenergic receptor blockade may reduce sympathetic discharge.

At the same time that beta blockers lower blood pressure through various means, their blockade of peripheral beta-adrenergic receptors inhibits vasodilation, leaving alpha receptors open to catecholamine-mediated vasoconstriction. Over time, however, vascular resistance tends to return to normal, which presumably preserves the antihypertensive effect of a reduced cardiac output.

Clinical Effects. Even in small doses, beta blockers begin to lower the blood pressure within a few hours. Although progressively higher doses have usually been given, careful study has shown a near-maximal effect from smaller doses. Beta blockers are particularly well suited for younger and middle-aged hypertensive patients, especially nonblacks, and for patients with tachyarrhythmias, myocardial ischemia, and high levels of stress. Because the hemodynamic responses to physical stress are reduced, however, they may interfere with the ability to exercise.

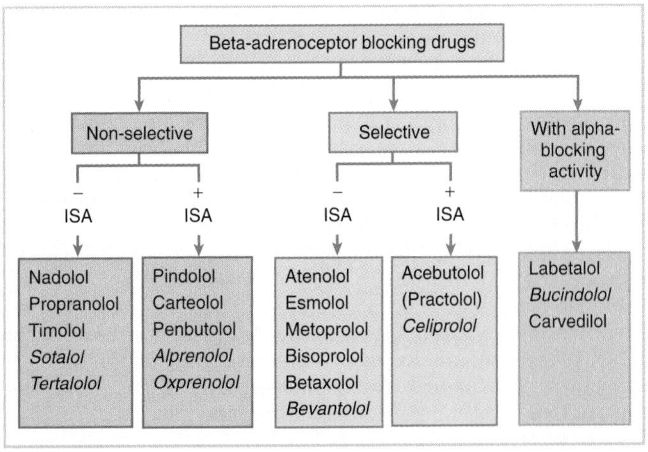

FIGURE 38–11 Classification of beta-adrenoreceptor blockers on the basis of cardioselectivity and intrinsic sympathomimetic activity. Drugs not approved for use in the United States for treatment of hypertension are in italics. ISA = intrinsic sympathomimetic activity. (Modified from Kaplan NM: Kaplan's Clinical Hypertension. 8th ed. Baltimore, Lippincott Williams & Wilkins, 2002, p 262.)

SPECIAL USES FOR BETA BLOCKERS

COEXISTING ISCHEMIC HEART DISEASE. Even without evidence that beta blockers protect patients from initial coronary events, the antiarrhythmic and antianginal effects of these drugs make them especially valuable in hypertensive patients with coexisting coronary disease.

COEXISTING HEART FAILURE. As described elsewhere (see Chap. 23), beta blockers have been found to reduce mortality in patients with congestive heart failure.

HYPERKINETIC HYPERTENSION. Some hypertensive patients have increased cardiac output that may persist for many years. Beta blockers should be particularly effective in such patients but may reduce their ability to exercise.

MARKED ANXIETY. The somatic manifestations of anxiety—tremor, sweating, and tachycardia—can be helped without the undesirable effects of methods commonly used to control anxiety, such as alcohol and tranquilizers.

PERIOPERATIVE STRESS. Beta blockers have been found to reduce cardiovascular events in high-risk patients who have noncardiac surgery.[59]

SIDE EFFECTS. Most of the side effects of beta blockers are related to their major pharmacological action, the blockade of beta-adrenergic receptors. Certain concomitant problems may worsen when beta-adrenergic receptors are blocked, including peripheral vascular disease and bronchospasm. However, in a meta-analysis of 29 studies, cardioselective beta blockers did not have clinically significant adverse respiratory effects in patients with mild to moderate reactive airway disease or chronic obstructive pulmonary disease, leading the authors to conclude that these drugs should not be withheld from such patients who have an indication for their use.[58]

The most common side effect is fatigue, probably a consequence of decreased cardiac output and peripheral and cerebral blood flow. Sexual dysfunction was also increased by use of beta blockers in RCTs involving patients with myocardial infarction, congestive heart failure, or hypertension, but depression was not.[60] However, the effect on depression remains uncertain and others have reported an increase in suicide among users of beta blockers compared with ACEIs or CCBs.[61]

The use of beta blockers increases the incidence of diabetes,[62] presumably through a decrease in insulin sensitivity. Diabetic patients may have additional problems with beta blockers, more so with nonselective ones. The responses to hypoglycemia, both the symptoms (except sweating) and the counterregulatory hormonal changes that raise blood glucose levels, are partially dependent on sympathetic nervous activty. Diabetic patients who are susceptible to hypoglycemia nay not be aware of the usual warning signals and may not ebound as quickly.

Perturbations of lipoprotein metabolism accompany the ise of beta blockers. Nonselective agents cause greater rises n triglycerides and reductions in cardioprotective high-lensity lipoprotein cholesterol levels. When a beta blocker is uddenly discontinued, angina pectoris and myocardial nfarction may occur. Because patients with hypertension are nore susceptible to coronary disease, they should be weaned radually and given appropriate coronary vasodilator herapy.

Caution is advised in the use of beta blockers in patients suspected of harboring a pheochromocytoma (see Chaps. 37 and 79) because unopposed alpha-adrenergic agonist action nay precipitate a serious hypertensive crisis if this disease s present. The use of beta blockers during pregnancy has een clouded by scattered case reports of various fetal roblems.

AN OVERVIEW OF BETA BLOCKERS IN HYPERTENSION. Beta blockers are specifically recommended for hypertensive patients with concomitant coronary disease, particularly after a myocardial infarction, congestive heart ailure, or tachyarrhythmias (see Table 38–4). If a beta blocker s chosen, the agents that are more cardioselective offer the ikelihood of fewer perturbations of lipid and carbohydrate netabolism and greater adherence of patients to therapy; nly one dose a day is needed, and side effects are probably ninimized.

Alpha- and Beta-Adrenergic Receptor Antagonists

The combination of an alpha and a beta blocker in a single nolecule is available in the forms of labetalol and carvedilol, vith the latter agent approved for treatment of heart failure s well. The fall in pressure results mainly from a decrease n peripheral resistance, with little or no decline in cardiac output. The most bothersome side effects are related to postural hypotension; the most serious side effect is hepatoxicity. Intravenous labetalol is used to treat hypertensive emergencies.

Vasodilators

n the past, direct-acting arteriolar vasodilators were used nainly as third drugs, when combinations of a diuretic and adrenergic blocker failed to control blood pressure. However, vith the availability of vasodilators of different types, i.e., ACEIs, ARBs, and CCBs, which can be easily tolerated when used as first or second drugs, wider and earlier application of vasodilators in therapy of hypertension has evolved.

Direct Vasodilators

Hydralazine is the most widely used agent of this type. Minoxidil is more potent but is usually reserved for patients vith severe, refractory hypertension associated with enal failure. Nitroprusside and nitroglycerin are given ntravenously for hypertensive crises and are discussed later see Therapy for Hypertensive Crises).

HYDRALAZINE. Hydralazine, in combination with a diuretic and a beta blocker, has been used frequently to treat severe hypertension. The drug acts directly to relax the smooth muscle in precapillary resistance vessels, with little or no effect on postcapillary venous capacitance vessels. As a result, blood pressure falls by a reduction in peripheral resistance, but in the process a number of compensatory processes, which are activated by the arterial baroreceptor arc, blunt the decrease in pressure and cause side effects. With concomitant use of a diuretic to overcome the tendency for fluid retention and an adrenergic inhibitor to prevent the reflex increase in sympathetic activity and rise in renin, the vasodilator is more effective and causes few, if any, side effects.

The drug need be given only twice a day. Its daily dose should be kept below 400 mg to prevent the lupus-like syndrome that appears in 10 to 20 percent of patients who receive more. This reaction, although uncomfortable to the patient, is almost always reversible. The reaction is uncommon with daily doses of 200 mg or less and is more common in slow acetylators of the drug.

MINOXIDIL. This drug vasodilates by opening potassium channels in vascular smooth muscle. Its hemodynamic effects are similar to those of hydralazine, but minoxidil is even more effective and may be used once a day. It is particularly useful in patients with severe hypertension and renal failure. Even more than with hydralazine, diuretics and adrenergic receptor blockers must be used with minoxidil to prevent the reflex increase in cardiac output and fluid retention. Pericardial effusions have appeared in about 3 percent of those given minoxidil, in some without renal or cardiac failure. The drug also causes hair to grow profusely, and the facial hirsutism precludes use of the drug in most women.

Calcium Channel Blockers (see also Chap. 50)

These drugs are among the most popular classes of agents used in the treatment of hypertension. Claims of multiple serious side effects of their use, mostly based on biased observational studies, have been repudiated by data from multiple RCTs including ALLHAT, wherein coronary events were the same for the CCB as for the diuretic or ACEI and mortality from noncardiovascular causes was significantly lower in the CCB group than the diuretic or ACEI group.[2]

MECHANISMS OF ACTION. All currently available CCBs interact with the same L-type voltage-gated plasma membrane channel but at different sites and with different consequences. DHPs have the greatest peripheral vasodilatory action with little effect on cardiac automaticity, conduction, or contractility. However, comparative trials have shown that verapamil and diltiazem, which do affect these properties, are also effective antihypertensives, and they may cause fewer side effects related to vasodilation, such as flushing and ankle edema.

CLINICAL USE. CCBs are effective in hypertensive patients of all ages and races.[42] Against placebo in RCTs, DHP-CCBs reduced cardiovascular events and deaths (see Table 38–6).[44] Compared with other classes of drugs, they may protect better against stroke but less well against heart failure.[2,44]

CCBs have been found to be particularly effective in prevention of stroke in elderly hypertensives, perhaps because they tend to have a greater antihypertensive effect than seen in younger patients.[63] They also appear to lower blood pressure in blacks better than other classes,[64] but with equal degrees of blood pressure reduction as among the blacks in the ALLHAT trial,[2] they are no better in cardioprotection than a diuretic or an ACEI.

Calcium antagonists may cause at least an initial natriuresis, probably by producing renal vasodilation, which may lessen the need for concurrent diuretic therapy. In fact, unlike all other antihypertensive agents, they may have their effectiveness reduced rather than enhanced by concomitant dietary sodium restriction, whereas most careful studies show an enhancement of their effect by concomitant diuretic therapy.[65]

The use of CCBs has been contentious in two important groups of hypertensives: those with diabetes and those with nephropathy. Concerning the use of CCBs in patients with type 2 diabetes, a DHP-CCB, nitrendipine, provided excellent protection in those enrolled in the Systolic Hypertension in Europe (Syst-Eur) trial, even better than that provided by a diuretic in the SHEP trial.[66] Therapy based on the DHP-CCB felodipine provided a 51 percent reduction in major cardiovascular events in the 1501 patients with diabetes enrolled in the HOT trial.[14] Among the almost 12,000 diabetics in the ALLHAT trial, the CCB amlodipine was as protective as the ACEI or diuretic.[2]

Concerning the use of CCBs in patients with nephropathy, experts agree that an ACEI or ARB should be the first drug used.[67] However, in order to provide the degree of blood pressure reduction required to protect such patients maximally, additional drugs are almost always required. A CCB is an appropriate choice as the third drug, with a diuretic as the second. Clearly, a CCB is not as renoprotective as an ACEI[19] or an ARB[68] when used as the initial drug, but, if needed to achieve the goal of therapy, a CCB is just as clearly an appropriate addition.[69]

On the basis of a greater reduction in proteinuria seen with non–DHP-CCBs than with DHP-CCBs, some believe a non–DHP-CCB should be used.[67] However, the addition of a DHP-CCB does not interfere with the renoprotective effect of ACEIs or ARBs.[70] Moreover, renal function, assessed by estimated glomerular filtration rate, was better preserved by the DHP-CCB than by either the diuretic or the ACEI in ALLHAT.[2]

SIDE EFFECTS. Side effects preclude the use of these drugs in perhaps 10 percent of patients. Most side effects—headaches, flushing, local ankle edema—are related to the vasodilation for which the drugs are given. With slow-release and longer acting formulations, vasodilative side effects are reduced. It should be no surprise that, in a few patients, the antihypertensive effect of the short-acting agents, particularly liquid nifedipine, may be so marked as to reduce blood flow and induce ischemia of vital organs, calling for a moratorium on their use.[71]

A potentially serious adverse effect of the use of calcium antagonists to treat hypertension was described in a case-control study in which more hypertensive patients who had a myocardial infarction were taking short-acting calcium antagonists than hypertensive patients who had not had an infarct.[72] The most likely explanation for the finding is exclusion bias, which is an inherent problem with case-control studies in which the cases are at greater risk for the complication than the controls; i.e., higher risk patients are excluded from the control group but not from the case group.[73] The decrease in coronary events in large RCTs with *long-acting* DHPs is the best proof of the safety of these agents. Similar claims based on case-control studies that calcium antagonists increase cancer and gastrointestinal bleeding have also been refuted.[2]

Calcium antagonists may be unique in not having their antihypertensive efficacy blunted by nonsteroidal anti-inflammatory drugs (NSAIDs).[74]

AN OVERVIEW OF CALCIUM CHANNEL BLOCKERS. CCBs have been found to reduce stroke more but heart attacks less than other therapies while having similar effects on overall mortality.[44] They work well and are usually well tolerated across the entire spectrum of hypertensives. They have some particular niches: coexisting angina and cyclosporine or NSAID use. If chosen, an inherently long-acting, second-generation DHP seems the best choice because it maintains better blood pressure control in the critical early morning hours and on throughout the next day if the patient misses a dose.[75] Rate-slowing CCBs, e.g., verapamil or diltiazem, may be preferable in certain circumstances.

Angiotensin-Converting Enzyme Inhibitors

Activity of the renin-angiotensin system may be inhibited in four ways, three of which can be applied clinically. The first, use of beta-adrenergic receptor blockers to inhibit the release of renin, was discussed earlier. The second, direct inhibition of renin activity by specific renin inhibitors, is being investigated.[76] The third, inhibition of the enzyme that converts the inactive decapeptide angiotensin I to the active octapeptide AII, is being widely used with orally effective ACEIs. The fourth, blockade of angiotensin's actions by a competitive receptor blocker, is the basis for the fastest growing class of antihypertensive agents—the ARBs. ARBs may offer additional benefits, but their immediate advantage is the absence of cough that often accompanies ACEIs as well as less angioedema. The ARBs are considered after the ACEIs.

MECHANISM OF ACTION. The first of the ACEIs, captopril, was synthesized as a specific inhibitor of the converting enzyme that, in the classic pathway shown in Figure 86–1, breaks the peptidyl dipeptide bond in angiotensin I, preventing the enzyme from attaching to and splitting the angiotensin I structure. Because AII cannot be formed and angiotensin I is inactive, the ACEI paralyzes the classic renin-angiotensin system, thereby removing the effects of most endogenous AII as both a vasoconstrictor and a stimulant to aldosterone synthesis.

Interestingly, with long-term use of ACEIs, the plasma AII levels actually return to previous values while the blood pressure remains lowered,[77] which suggests that the antihypertensive effect may involve other mechanisms. Because the same enzyme that converts angiotensin I to AII is also responsible for inactivation of the vasodilating hormone bradykinin, by inhibiting the breakdown of bradykinin, ACEIs increase the concentration of a vasodilating hormone while they decrease the concentration of a vasoconstrictor hormone. The increased plasma kinin levels may contribute to the vasodilation and other beneficial effects of ACEIs,[78] but they are also probably responsible for the most common and bothersome side effects of their use, a dry, hacking cough and, less frequently, angioedema.[79]

Regardless of their mechanism of action, ACEIs lower blood pressure mainly by reducing peripheral resistance with little, if any, effect on heart rate, cardiac output, or body fluid volumes, probably reflecting preservation of baroreceptor reflexes.[80] As they restore endothelium-dependent relaxation, resistance arteries become less thickened and more responsive.[81]

CLINICAL USE. In patients with uncomplicated primary hypertension, ACEIs as monotherapy provide antihypertensive effects that are equal to those with other classes, but they are somewhat less effective in blacks and elderly people because of their lower renin levels.[42] Addition of a diuretic, even as little as 6.25 mg of hydrochlorothiazide, enhances the efficacy of an ACEI.[82] More important, ACEI-based therapy has provided significant protection against cardiovascular disease and death when compared against placebo and comparable if not better protection than other classes of drugs (see Table 38–6).[44] In the ALLHAT trial involving predominantly elderly, high-risk hypertensives, ACEI-based therapy was equal to diuretic- or CCB-based therapies in most regards except against strokes in the black enrollees,[2] probably because of less antihypertensive efficacy. In the Australian National Blood Pressure Study involving elderly but lower risk hypertensives, ACEI-based therapy provided better protection against cardiovascular events than diuretic-based therapy for the men but not for the women.[47]

ACEIs have been impressively effective in treatment of hypertensives (and nonhypertensives) with coronary disease or congestive heart failure as detailed in Chapters 23 and 50. Another area in which they have become the drug of choice is chronic renal disease, whether diabetic[67] or nondiabetic[8] in origin. The high levels of renin, arising in the JG cells within the renal afferent arterioles, flood the glomeruli and renal efferent arterioles, providing ACEIs (and ARBs) the opportunity to dilate these vessels selectively and lower intraglomerular pressure more effectively than other classes of drugs. These hemodynamic effects may lower renal perfusion and glomerular filtration. However, because acute increases of serum creatinine of up to 30 percent that stabilize within the first 2 months of ACEI therapy are associated with *better* long-term renoprotection,[84] such rises should not prompt withdrawal of the drug.

Whether ACEIs (and ARBs) provide renal (and cardiac) protection beyond their antihypertensive effects remains in question. The issue has been most intensively studied in patients with proteinuria because it is so easy to measure. Controlled trials suggest that the antiproteinuric effect of an ACEI is directly related to its antihypertensive effect,[85] but there are inadequate data to be sure. As noted later (see Angiotensin II Receptor Blockers, Clinical Use), the potential for an additional antihypertensive effect of an ARB added to an ACEI also remains uncertain.

These drugs have been a mixed blessing for patients with renovascular hypertension. On the one hand, they usually control the blood pressure effectively.[86] On the other hand, the removal of the high levels of AII that they produce may deprive the stenotic kidney of the hormonal drive to its blood flow, thereby causing a marked decline in renal perfusion so that patients with solitary kidneys or bilateral disease may develop acute and sometimes persistent renal failure.

Another potential special indication for ACEI therapy may be in protection against recurrent stroke. In a study of 6105 patients who had a history of prior stroke or transient ischemic attack, the ACEI perindopril plus a diuretic provided a 43 percent relative reduction in recurrent stroke.[87] By itself, the ACEI had an inconsequential effect.

SIDE EFFECTS. Most patients who take an ACEI experience neither the side effects nor the biochemical changes often accompanying other drugs that may be of even more concern even though they are not as obvious; neither rises in lipids, glucose, or uric acid nor reductions in potassium levels are noted. To be sure, ACEIs may have both specific and nonspecific adverse effects. Among the specific ones are rare rashes, loss of taste, and leukopenia. In addition, they may cause a hypersensitivity reaction with angioneurotic edema[79] or a cough that, although often persistent, is infrequently associated with pulmonary dysfunction.[88] The cough, affecting more than 10 percent of women and about half as many men, may not disappear for 3 weeks after the ACEI is discontinued. If a cough appears in a patient who needs an ACEI, an ARB should be substituted.

The antihypertensive efficacy of ACEIs may be blunted by large (300 mg) doses of aspirin and most NSAIDs, with the apparent exception of celecoxib.[89] Finally, patients with renal insufficiency or those taking potassium supplements or potassium-sparing agents may not be able to excrete potassium loads and therefore may develop hyperkalemia.[90]

AN OVERVIEW OF ANGIOTENSIN-CONVERTING ENZYME INHIBITORS. The rationale for the use of ACEIs in the treatment of hypertension has steadily expanded beyond their proven efficacy as antihypertensive agents. In particular, they have been shown to provide special advantages in three large groups of patients: those with heart failure, coronary ischemia, or nephropathy. As seen in Table 38–4, they are clearly the drugs of choice for such patients. Moreover, the evidence from the Heart Outcomes Prevention Evaluation (HOPE) trial[91] has led to the recommendation that an ACEI be given to all patients at high risk for coronary disease, whether hypertensive or not. Although an ACEI-based therapy did not outperform a diuretic or a CCB in the ALLHAT trial,[2] their proven special benefits ensure their continued growth.

Even as ACEIs have become increasingly popular, their position has been threatened by the introduction of ARBs, agents acting at a more distal site of the renin-angiotensin system.

Angiotensin II Receptor Blockers

MECHANISMS OF ACTION. ARBs displace AII from its specific AT_1 receptor, antagonizing all of its known effects and resulting in a dose-dependent fall in peripheral resistance and little change in heart rate or cardiac output.[92] As a consequence of the competitive displacement, circulating levels of AII increase and at the same time the blockade of the renin-angiotensin mechanism is more complete, including any AII that is generated through pathways that do not involve ACEI. No obvious good or bad effects of the increased AII levels have been noted (along with the higher renin levels, as seen with ACEIs).

The major obvious difference between ARBs and ACEIs is the absence of an increase in kinin levels that may be responsible for some of the beneficial effects of ACEIs and probably even more of their side effects. Direct comparisons between the two types of drugs show little difference in antihypertensive efficacy, but cough is not provoked by the ARB[93] although angioedema has been reported.[94] Losartan has a uricosuric effect that is not seen with other ARBs.[95] As seen with ACEIs, ARBs have been found to improve endothelial dysfunction[96] and correct the altered structure of resistance arteries in patients with hypertension.[97]

CLINICAL USE. In the recommended doses, all six currently available ARBs have comparable antihypertensive efficacy and all are potentiated by addition of a diuretic. The dose-response curve is fairly flat for all, although increasing doses of candesartan have an increasing effect.[98] Moreover, in this study, the effect of candesartan persisted for 36 hours after a purposely missed dose whereas the effect of losartan was largely dissipated after 12 hours.

The addition of ARB to a presumed maximal dose of an ACEI was not shown to increase the antihypertensive effect[99] but did reduce the progression of nondiabetic nephropathy.[100] ARB-based therapy has been shown to reduce the progress of renal damage in patients with type 2 diabetes with nephropathy.[68,70,101] Their use in heart failure is described in Chapter 23. Therapy based on the ARB losartan caused LVH to regress and reduced the number of cardiovascular events more than therapy based on the beta blocker atenolol in the LIFE trial of hypertensives with LVH.[48]

SIDE EFFECTS. Whether or not they are more effective than ACEIs, ARBs are easier to take. In various clinical trials, side effects were generally no greater than with placebo, and the agent was better tolerated than other antihypertensive agents. Fetal toxicity, hyperkalemia, hypotension, and renal impairment are almost certain to be noted occasionally because they are expected consequences of blockade of the renin-angiotensin mechanism, but, as yet, no major surprises have surfaced.

OVERVIEW OF ANGIOTENSIN II RECEPTOR BLOCKERS. As reflected in the fast growth of the use of ARBs, they are surely being prescribed for many more patients than the 10 percent or so who are intolerant of an ACEI. With the intensely competitive market for the six (or more) of these agents now being heavily promoted, their use will surely continue to grow. However, caution is advised; additional outcome data are needed to know whether they are as good as the proven ACEIs. All current expert guidelines recommend ARBs only for those who should receive an ACEI but are intolerant, usually because of cough. Many outcome trials now in progress should provide proof of their value beyond that found in type II diabetic nephropathy.[102]

Other Agents

The first of the most promising new class of drugs, neutral endopeptidase inhibitors, was waylaid by a high incidence of angioedema. An old vasodilator now used extensively for coronary ischemia, the nitrate isosorbide, has been shown to be an attractive agent[103] but is not likely to be tested properly because of the lack of a commercial sponsor. Meanwhile, glitazones, which are now used for the treatment of diabetes, have been shown to lower blood pressure in nondiabetic hypertensives, logically as a consequence of improved insulin sensitivity.[104]

Special Considerations in Therapy

WITHDRAWAL OF DRUGS. As many as 20 percent of treated patients with well-controlled hypertension are able to maintain normotension for as long as 1 year after withdrawal of their drugs.[105] Considering how difficult it may be to achieve adequate control, withdrawal seems inappropriate if the therapy is causing no adverse effects.

RESISTANT HYPERTENSION. There are numerous causes of resistance to therapy, usually defined as the failure of diastolic blood pressure to fall below 90 mm Hg despite the use of three or more drugs (Table 38–9). Patients often do not respond well because they do not take their medications. On the other hand, what appears to be a poor response on the basis of office readings of blood pressure may be disclosed to be an adequate response when ambulatory or home readings are obtained.[106] A number of factors may be responsible for a poor response even if the appropriate medication is taken regularly. Most common is volume overload owing either to inadequate diuretic or to excessive dietary sodium intake. Larger doses or more potent diuretics often bring resistant hypertension under control.

TABLE 38–9 Causes of Inadequate Responsiveness to Therapy

Pseudoresistance	
"White coat" or office elevations	
Pseudohypertension in the elderly	
Nonadherence to Therapy	
Side effects of medication	
Cost of medication	
Lack of consistent and continuous primary care	
Inconvenient and chaotic dosing schedules	
Instructions not understood	
Inadequate education of patients	
Organic brain syndrome (e.g., memory deficit)	
Drug-Related Causes	
Doses too low	
Inappropriate combinations (e.g., two centrally acting adrenergic inhibitors)	
Rapid inactivation (e.g., hydralazine)	
Drug interactions	
Nonsteroidal antiinflammatory drugs	Oral contraceptives
Sympathomimetics	Adrenal steroids
Nasal decongestants	Licorice (chewing tobacco)
Appetite suppressants	Cyclosporine
Cocaine	Erythropoietin
Caffeine	Cholestyramine
Antidepressants (monoamine oxidase inhibitors, tricyclics)	
Excessive volume contraction with stimulation of renin and aldosterone	
Hypokalemia (usually diuretic induced)	
Rebound after clonidine withdrawal	
Associated Conditions	
Smoking	
Increasing obesity	
Sleep apnea	
Insulin resistance or hyperinsulinemia	
Ethanol intake more than 1 oz/d (>three portions)	
Anxiety-induced hyperventilation or panic attacks	
Chronic pain	
Intense vasoconstriction (Raynaud, arteritis)	
Secondary Hypertension	
Renal insufficiency	
Renovascular hypertension	
Pheochromocytoma	
Primary aldosteronism	
Volume Overload	
Excess sodium intake	
Progressive renal damage (nephrosclerosis)	
Fluid retention related to reduction of blood pressure	
Indequate diuretic therapy	

Modified from The sixth report of the Joint National Committee on Prevention, Detection, Evaluation and Treatment of High Blood Pressure. Arch Intern Med 157:2413, 1997. Copyright 1997, American Medical Association.

ANESTHESIA IN HYPERTENSIVE PATIENTS. In the absence of significant cardiac dysfunction, hypertension adds little to the cardiovascular risks of surgery. If possible, however, hypertension should be well controlled by means of medications before anesthesia and surgery to reduce the risk of myocardial ischemia. Therefore, patients taking antihypertensive medications should continue these drugs, if necessary using dermal or intravenous formulations, as long as the anesthesiologist is aware of their use and takes reasonable precautions to prevent wide swings in pressure. The very short-acting beta blocker esmolol has been successful in preventing surges in blood pressure during intubation, and the use of the beta blocker bisoprolol reduced cardiac events in high-risk patients undergoing vascular surgery.[107]

Hypertension is often observed during and immediately after coronary bypass surgery (see Chap. 50). Various intravenous agents have been used successfully to lower the pressure. Nitroprusside has been the usual choice during the postoperative period, but esmolol, labetalol, or nicardipine may be better choices.

HYPERTENSIVE CHILDREN. Almost nothing is known about the effects of various antihypertensive medications given to children over long periods. In the absence of adequate data, an approach similar to that advocated for adults is advised.[108] Emphasis should be placed on weight reduction in hypertensive children who are obese in the hope of attempting to control hypertension without the need for drug therapy.

HYPERTENSION DURING PREGNANCY. This topic is discussed in Chapters 37 and 74.

HYPERTENSION IN ELDERLY PERSONS. Some elderly persons may have high blood pressure as measured by the sphygmomanometer but may have less or no hypertension when direct intraarterial readings are made, i.e., pseudohypertension related to rigid arteries that do not collapse under the cuff.

If either the systolic pressure alone or both systolic and diastolic levels are elevated, careful lowering of blood pressure with either diuretics or DHP calcium antagonists has been unequivocally documented to reduce cardiovascular morbidity in older hypertensive patients,[12] extending to those older than 80 years.[5] Care is needed because they may have a number of problems with the medications (Table 38–10). In view of the reduced effectiveness of the baroceptor reflex and the failure of peripheral resistance to rise appropriately with

TABLE 38–10 Factors That Might Contribute to Increased Risk of Pharmacological Treatment of Hypertension in Elderly Persons

Factors	Potential Complications
Diminished baroreceptor activity	Orthostatic hypotension
Decreased intravascular volume	Orthostatic hypotension, dehydration
Sensitivity to hypokalemia	Arrhythmia, muscle weakness
Decreased renal and hepatic function	Drug accumulation
Polypharmacy	Drug interaction
Central nervous system changes	Depression, confusion

standing, postural hypotension should be carefully looked for and, if present, addressed before starting antihypertensive therapy. All drugs should be given in slowly increasing doses to prevent excessive lowering of the pressure.

For those who start with systolic pressures exceeding 160 mm Hg, the goal of therapy should be a level around 140 mm Hg with caution about further reductions in already low diastolic levels.[16]

PATIENTS WITH HYPERTENSION AND DIABETES. Special attention should be given to diabetic patients with hypertension. The two commonly coexist and multiply the cardiovascular risks of each alone. Fortunately, evidence from several trials now documents the protection provided by *intensive* control of hypertension, in concert with management of the diabetes and the dyslipidemia that commonly accompanies the two. Most diabetic hypertensive patients need two or more antihypertensive drugs to bring their pressure to below 130/80 mm Hg, which is probably the highest level that should be tolerated. The benefits of such intensive management were clearly documented in a 7.8-year follow-up of 160 patients with type 2 diabetes and hypertension with microalbuminuria.[109] In the half given more intensive management, the risks of having a cardiovascular event, nephropathy, retinopathy, or autonomic neuropathy were all reduced by 50 percent or more.

An ACEI or ARB should be included if proteinuria is present. A diuretic and a beta blocker are appropriate, and a long-acting DHP is likely to be required.

HYPERTENSIVE PATIENTS WITH IMPOTENCE. Erectile dysfunction is common in hypertensive patients, even more so in those who are also diabetic. The problem may be exacerbated by diuretic therapy, even in appropriately low doses.[51] Fortunately, sildenafil usually returns erectile ability even in the presence of various antihypertensive drugs with no greater likelihood of adverse events than in those not receiving antihypertensive therapy.[110]

HYPERTENSION WITH CONGESTIVE HEART FAILURE. Cardiac output may fall so markedly in hypertensive patients who are in heart failure with systolic dysfunction that their blood pressure is reduced, obscuring the degree of hypertension; often, however, the diastolic blood pressure is raised by intense vasoconstriction while the systolic pressure falls as a result of the reduced stroke volume. Lowering the blood pressure may, by itself, relieve the heart failure. Chronic unloading has been most efficiently accomplished with ACEIs, and beta blockers have been shown to reduce morbidity and mortality further in ACEI-treated patients in heart failure.

As noted in Chapter 37, LVH is frequently found by echocardiography, even in patients with mild hypertension. All antihypertensive drugs except direct vasodilators have been shown to cause LVH to regress, and regression may continue for as long as 5 years of treatment.

HYPERTENSION WITH ISCHEMIC HEART DISEASE. The coexistence of ischemic heart disease makes antihypertensive therapy even more essential because relief of the hypertension may ameliorate the coronary disease. Beta blockers and calcium antagonists are particularly useful if angina or arrhythmias are present. Caution is needed to avoid decreased coronary perfusion that may be responsible for the J curve seen in several trials (see Goal of Therapy).[14]

The often markedly high levels of blood pressure during the early phase of an acute myocardial infarction may reflect sympathetic nervous hyperreactivity to pain. Antihypertensive drugs that do not decrease cardiac output may be utilized cautiously in the immediate postinfarction period, whereas beta blockers and ACEIs have been shown to provide long-term benefit.

Therapy for Hypertensive Crises

When diastolic blood pressure exceeds 140 mm Hg, rapidly progressive damage to the arterial vasculature is demonstrable experimentally, and a surge of cerebral blood flow may rapidly lead to encephalopathy (see Chap. 37). If such high pressures persist or if there are any signs of encephalopathy, the pressures should be lowered using parenteral agents in patients considered to be in immediate danger or oral agents in those who are alert and in no other acute distress.[111]

A number of drugs for this purpose are currently available (Table 38–11). If diastolic pressure exceeds 140 mm Hg and the patient has any complications, such as an aortic dissection, a constant infusion of nitroprusside is most effective and almost always lowers the pressure to the desired level. Constant monitoring with an intraarterial line is mandatory because a slightly excessive dose may lower the pressure abruptly to levels that induce shock. The potency and rapidity of action of nitroprusside have made it the treatment of choice for life-threatening hypertension. However, because nitroprusside acts as a venous and arteriolar dilator, venous return and cardiac output are lowered and intracranial pressures may increase. Therefore, other parenteral agents are being more widely used. These include labetalol and the calcium antagonist nicardipine.

With any of these agents, intravenous furosemide is often needed to lower the blood pressure further and prevent retention of salt and water. Diuretics should not be given if volume depletion is initially present. For patients in less immediate danger, oral therapy may be used. Almost every drug has been used and most, with repeated doses, reduce high pressures. The prior preference for liquid nifedipine by mouth or sublingually has been diminished because of occasional ischemic complications resulting from too rapid reduction in blood pressure.[71] Oral doses of other short-acting formulations may be used, including furosemide, propranolol, captopril, or felodipine. A safer course for any patients, particularly if their current high pressures are simply a reflection of stopping previously effective oral medication and they are asymptomatic, is simply to restart the previous medication and monitor their response closely. If their nonadherence to therapy was caused by side effects, appropriate changes should be made.

Most centers are seeing fewer patients in hypertensive crisis, presumably because more patients are diagnosed and treated before the disease enters this malignant course. The continued successful treatment of many more hypertensive persons will prevent the more frequent long-range cardiovascular complications of hypertension.

TABLE 38–11 Parenteral Drugs for Treatment of Hypertensive Emergency

Drug*	Dose	Onset of Action	Adverse Effects†
Diuretics			
Furosemide	20-40 mg in 1-2 min, repeated and higher doses with renal insufficiency	5-15 min	Volume depletion, hypokalemia
Vasodilators			
Nitroprusside (Nipride, Nitropress)	0.25-10 μg/kg/min as IV infusion	Immediate	Nausea, vomiting, muscle twitching, sweating, thiocyanate and cyanide intoxication
Nitroglycerin (Nitro-Bid IV)	5-100 μg/min as IV infusion	2-5 min	Headache, vomiting, methemoglobinemia, tolerance with prolonged use
Fenoldopam (Corlopam)	0.1-0.6 μg/kg/min as IV infusion	4-5 min	Reflex tachycardia, increased intraocular pressure, headache
Nicardipine‡ (Cardene I.V.)	5-15 mg/h IV	5-10 min	Headache, nausea, flushing, tachycardia, local phlebitis
Hydralazine (Apresoline)	10-20 mg IV 10-50 mg IM	10-20 min 20-30 min	Tachycardia, flushing, headache, vomiting, worsening of angina
Enalaprilat (Vasotec I.V.)	1.25-5 mg every 6 hr	15 min	Precipitous fall in pressure in high-renin states; response variable
Adrenergic Inhibitors			
Phentolamine	5-15 mg IV	1-2 min	Tachycardia, flushing, headache
Esmolol (Brevibloc)	200-500 μg/kg/min for 4 min, then 50-300 μg/kg/min IV	1-2 min	Hypotension, nausea
Labetalol (Normodyne, Trandate)	20-80 mg IV bolus every 10 min 2 mg/min IV infusion	5-10 min	Vomiting, scalp tingling, burning in throat, dizziness, nausea, heart block, orthostatic hypotension

From Kaplan NM: Kaplan's Clinical Hypertension. 8th ed. Baltimore, Lippincott Williams & Wilkins, 2002, p 348.
*In order of rapidity of action.
†Hypotension may occur with any.
‡Intravenous formulations of other calcium channel blockers are also available.

REFERENCES

1. Joint National Committee: The seventh report of the Joint Committee on Prevention, Detection, Evaluation, and Treatment of High Blood Pressure (JNC-7 Express). JAMA 289:2560, 2003.
2. ALLHAT Officers and Coordinators for the ALLHAT Collaborative Research Group: Major outcomes in high-risk hypertensive patients randomized to angiotensin-converting enzyme inhibitor or calcium channel blocker vs diuretic. JAMA 288:2981, 2002.
3. Kaplan NM: Treatment of hypertension: Drug therapy. *In* Kaplan NM: Kaplan's Clinical Hypertension. 8th ed. Philadelphia, Lippincott Williams & Wilkins, 2002, pp 237-338.
4. Staessen JA, Wang J-G, Thijs L: Cardiovascular protection and blood pressure reduction. Lancet 358:1305, 2001.
5. Gueyffier F, Bulpitt C, Boissel J-P, et al: Antihypertensive drugs in very old people: A subgroup meta-analysis of randomised controlled trials. Lancet 353:793, 1999.
6. Forette F, Seux M-L, Staessen JA, et al: The prevention of dementia with antihypertensive treatment: New evidence from the Systolic Hypertension in Europe (Syst-Eur) study. Arch Intern Med 162:2046, 2002.
7. Whelton PK, He J, Appel LJ, et al: Primary prevention of hypertension: Clinical and public health advisory from the National High Blood Pressure Education Program. JAMA 288:1882, 2002.
8. Jackson R: Updated New Zealand cardiovascular disease risk-benefit prediction guide. BMJ 320:709. 2000.

Threshold for and Goal of Therapy

9. European Society of Hypertension-European Society of Cardiology Guidelines Committee: 2003 European Society of Hypertension-European Society of Cardiology guidelines for the management of arterial hypertension. J Hypertens 21:1011, 2003.
10. Guidelines Subcommittee: 1999 World Health Organization–International Society of Hypertension guidelines for the management of hypertension. J Hypertens 17:151, 1999.
11. Vasan RS, Larson MG, Leip EP, et al: Impact of high-normal blood pressure on the risk of cardiovascular disease. N Engl J Med 345: 1291, 2001.
12. Staessen JA, Gasowski J, Wang JG, et al: Risks of untreated and treated isolated systolic hypertension in the elderly. Lancet 355:865, 2000.
13. Kaplan NM: What is goal blood pressure for the treatment of hypertension? Arch Intern Med 161:1480, 2001.
14. Hansson L, Zanchetti A, Carruthers SG, et al: Effects of intensive blood-pressure lowering and low-dose aspirin in patients with hypertension: Principal results of the Hypertension Optimal Treatment (HOT) randomised trial. Lancet 351:1755, 1998.
15. Boutitie F, Gueyffier F, Pocock S, et al: J-shaped relationship between blood pressure and mortality in hypertensive patients: New insights from a meta-analysis of individual-patient data. Ann Intern Med 136:438, 2002.
16. Somes GW, Pahor M, Shorr RI, et al: The role of diastolic blood pressure when treating isolated systolic hypertension. Arch Intern Med 159:2004, 1999.
17. Mancia G, Carugo S, Grassi G, et al: Prevalence of left ventricular hypertrophy in hypertensive patients without and with blood pressure control: Data from the PAMELA population. Hypertension 39:744, 2002.
18. Adler AI, Stratton IM, Neil HAW, et al: Association of systolic blood pressure with macrovascular and microvascular complications of type 2 diabetes (UKPDS 36). BMJ 321:412, 2000.
19. Wright JT Jr, Bakris G, Greene T, et al: Effect of blood pressure lowering and antihypertensive drug class on progression of hypertensive kidney disease. Results from the AASK trial. JAMA 288:2421, 2002.

Life-Style Modifications

20. Diabetes Prevention Program Research Group: Reduction in the incidence of type 2 diabetes with lifestyle intervention or metformin. N Engl J Med 346:393, 2002.
21. Willett WC, Dietz WH, Colditz GA: Guidelines for healthy weight. N Engl J Med 341:427, 1999.
22. Sjöström C, Lindberg E, Elmasry A, et al: Prevalence of sleep apnoea and snoring in hypertensive men: A population based study. Thorax 57:602, 2002.
23. Whelton SP, Chin A, Xin X, He J: Effect of aerobic exercise on blood pressure: A meta-analysis of randomized, controlled trials. Ann Intern Med 136:493, 2002.
24. He FJ, MacGregor GA: Effect of modest salt reduction on blood pressure: A meta-analysis of randomized trials. Implications for public health. J Hum Hypertens 16:761, 2002.
25. Hooper L, Bartlett C, Smith GD, Ebrahim S: Systematic review of long term effects of advice to reduce dietary salt in adults. BMJ 325:628, 2002.
26. Tuomilehto J, Jousilahti P, Rastenyte D, et al: Urinary sodium excretion and cardiovascular mortality in Finland: A prospective study. Lancet 357:848, 2001.
27. Bazzano LA, He J, Ogden LG, et al: Dietary potassium intake and risk of stroke in US men and women: National Health Nutrition Examination Survey I Epidemiologic Follow-up Study. Stroke 32:1473, 2001.
28. He J, Whelton PK: What is the role of dietary sodium and potassium in hypertension and target organ injury? Am J Med Sci 317:152, 1999.
29. Griffith LE, Guyatt GH, Cook RJ, et al: The influence of dietary and nondietary calcium supplementation on blood pressure. Am J Hypertens 12:84, 1999.
30. Jee SH, Miller ER, Guallar E, et al: The effect of magnesium supplementation on blood pressure: A meta-analysis of randomized clinical trials. Am J Hypertens 15:691, 2002.
31. John JH, Ziebland S, Yudkin P, et al: Effects of fruit and vegetable consumption on plasma antioxidant concentrations and blood pressure: A randomised controlled trial. Lancet 359:1969, 2002.
32. Jee SH, He J, Whelton PK, et al: The effect of chronic coffee drinking on blood pressure. Hypertension 33:647, 1999.
33. Fuchs FD, Chambless LE, Whelton PK, et al: Alcohol consumption and the incidence of hypertension: The Atherosclerosis Risk in Communities Study. Hypertension 37:1242, 2001.

34. Thadhani R, Camargo CA Jr, Stampfer MJ, et al: Prospective study of moderate alcohol consumption and risk of hypertension in young women. Arch Intern Med 162:569, 2002.
35. Albert MA, Glynn RJ, Ridker PM: Alcohol consumption and plasma concentration of C-reactive protein. Circulation 107:443, 2003.
36. Linden W, Lenz JW, Con AH: Individualized stress management for primary hypertension: A randomized trial. Arch Intern Med 161:1071, 2001.
37. Rosenthal T, Alter A, Peleg E, Gavish B: Device-guided breathing exercises reduce blood pressure: Ambulatory and home measurements. Am J Hypertens 14:74, 2001.
38. Neaton JD, Grimm RH Jr, Prineas RJ, et al: Treatment of mild hypertension study (TOMHS). JAMA 270:713, 1993.

Antihypertensive Drug Therapy

39. Haynes RB, McDonald HP, Garg AX: Helping patients follow prescribed treatment: Clinical applications. JAMA 288:2880, 2002.
40. Strandgaard S, Haunsø S: Why does antihypertensive treatment prevent stroke but not myocardial infarction? Lancet 2:658, 2987.
41. Fagan TC: Remembering the lessons of basic pharmacology. Arch Intern Med 154:1430, 1994.
42. Materson BJ, Reda DJ, Cushman WC, et al: Single-drug therapy for hypertension in men. N Engl J Med 328:914, 1993.
43. Psaty BM, Smith NL, Siscovick DS, et al: Health outcomes associated with antihypertensive therapies used as first-line agents. JAMA 277:739, 1997.
44. Blood Pressure Lowering Treatment Trialists' Collaboration: Effects of ACE inhibitors, calcium antagonists, and other blood-pressure-lowering drugs. Lancet 355:1955, 2000.
45. Hansson L, Lindholm LH, Ekbom T, et al: Randomised trial of old and new antihypertensive drugs in elderly patients. Lancet 354:1751, 1999.
46. Schrier RW, Estacio RO: Additional follow-up from the ABCD trial in patients with type 2 diabetes and hypertension. N Engl J Med 343:1969, 2000.
47. Wing LMH, Reid CM, Ryan P, et al: A comparison of outcomes with angiotensin-converting-enzyme inhibitors and diuretics for hypertension in the elderly. N Engl J Med 348:583, 2003.
48. Dalhöf B, Devereux RB, Kjeldsen SE, et al: Cardiovascular morbidity and mortality in the Losartan Intervention For Endpoint reduction in hypertension study (LIFE): A randomized trial against atenolol. Lancet 359:995, 2002.

Diuretics

49. Chapman AB, Schwartz GL, Boerwinkle E, Turner ST: Predictors of antihypertensive response to a standard doze of hydrochlorothiazide for essential hypertension. Kidney Int 61:1047, 2002.
50. Psaty BM, Smith NL, Heckbert SR, et al: Diuretic therapy, the α-adducin gene variant, and the risk of myocardial infarction or stroke in persons with treated hypertension. JAMA 287:1680, 2002.
51. Grimm RH Jr, Grandits GA, Prineas RJ, et al: Long-term effects on sexual function of five antihypertensive drugs and nutritional hygienic treatment of hypertensive men and women. Hypertension 29:8, 1997.
52. Grossman E, Messerli FH, Goldbourt U: Antihypertensive therapy and the risk of malignancies. Eur Heart J 22:1343, 2001.
53. Pitt B, Zannad F, Remme WJ, et al: The effect of spironolactone of morbidity and mortality in patients with severe heart failure. N Engl J Med 341:709, 1999.
54. Weinberger MH, Roniker B, Krause SL, Weiss RJ: Eplerenone, a selective aldosterone blocker, in mild-to-moderate hypertension. Am J Hypertens 15:709, 2002.
55. Young MJ, Funder JW: Mineralocorticoid receptors and pathophysiological roles for aldosterone in the cardiovascular system. J Hypertens 20:1465, 2002.

Adrenergic Inhibitors

56. ALLHAT Officers and Coordinators for the ALLHAT Collaborative Research Group: Major cardiovascular events in hypertensive patients randomized to doxazosin vs chlorthalidone. JAMA 283:1967, 2000.
57. Levy D, Walmsley P, Levenstein M: Principal results of the hypertension and lipid trial (HALT): A multicenter study of doxazosin in patients with hypertension. Am Heart J 131:966, 1996.
58. Salpeter SR, Ormiston TM, Salpeter EE: Cardioselective β-blockers in patients with reactive airway disease: A meta-analysis. Ann Intern Med 137:715, 2002.
59. Auerbach AD, Goldman L: β-Blockers and reduction of cardiac events in noncardiac surgery. Scientific review. JAMA 287:1435, 2002.
60. Ko DT, Hebert PR, Coffey CS, et al: β-Blocker therapy and symptoms of depression, fatigue, and sexual dysfunction. JAMA 288:351, 2002.
61. Sørensen HT, Mellemkjaer L, Olsen JH: Risk of suicide in users of β-adrenoceptor blockers, calcium channel blockers and angiotensin converting enzyme inhibitors. Br J Clin Pharmacol 52:313, 2001.
62. Gress TW, Nieto FJ, Shahar E, et al: Hypertension and antihypertensive therapy as risk factors for type 2 diabetes mellitus. N Engl J Med 342:905, 2000.

Vasodilators

63. Lernfelt B, Landahl S, Johansson P, et al: Haemodynamic and renal effects of felodipine in young and elderly patients. Eur J Clin Pharmacol 54:595, 1998.
64. Sareli P, Radevski IV, Valtchanova ZP, et al: Efficacy of different drug classes used to initiate antihypertensive treatment in black subjects: Results of a randomized trial in Johannesburg, South Africa. Arch Intern Med 161:965, 2001.
65. Stergiou GS, Malakos JS, Achimastos AD, Mountokalakis TD: Additive hypotensive effect of a dihydropyridine calcium antagonist to that produced by a thiazide diuretic. J Cardiovasc Pharmacol 29:412, 1997.
66. Tuomilehto J, Rastenyte D, Birkenhäger WH, et al: Effects of calcium-channel blockade in older patients with diabetes and systolic hypertension. N Engl J Med 340:677, 1999.
67. Remuzzi G, Schieppati A, Ruggenenti P: Nephropathy in patients with type 2 diabetes. N Engl J Med 346:1145, 2002.
68. Lewis EJ, Hunsicker LG, Clarke WR, et al: Renoprotective effect of the angiotensin-receptor antagonist irbesartan in patients with nephropathy due to type 2 diabetes. N Engl J Med 345:851, 2001.
69. Zanchetti A, Ruilope LM: Antihypertensive treatment in patients with type-2 diabetes mellitus: What guidance from recent controlled randomized trials? J Hypertens 20:2099, 2002.
70. Brenner BM, Cooper ME, de Zeeuw D, et al: Effects of losartan on renal and cardiovascular outcomes in patients with type 2 diabetes and nephropathy. N Engl J Med 345:861, 2001.
71. Grossman E, Messerli FH, Grodzicki T, Kowey P: Should a moratorium be placed on sublingual nifedipine capsules given for hypertensive emergencies and pseudoemergencies? JAMA 276:1328, 1996.
72. Psaty BM, Heckbert SR, Koepsell TD, et al: The risk of myocardial infarction associated with antihypertensive drug therapies. JAMA 274:620, 1995.
73. Leader S, Mallick R, Roht L: Using medication history to measure confounding by indication in assessing calcium channel blockers and other antihypertensive therapy. J Hum Hypertens 15:153, 2001.
74. Celis H, Thijs L, Staessen JA, et al: Interaction between nonsteroidal anti-inflammatory drug intake and calcium-channel blocker-based antihypertensive treatment in the Syst-Eur trial. J Hum Hypertens 15:613, 2001.
75. Elliott HL, Elawad M, Wilkinson R, Singh SP: Persistence of antihypertensive efficacy after missed doses: Comparison of amlodipine and nifedipine gastrointestinal therapeutic system. J Hypertens 20:333, 2002.
76. van Paassen P, de Zeeuw D, Navis G, de Jong PE: Renal and systemic effects of continued treatment with renin inhibitor remikiren in hypertensive patients with normal and impaired renal function. Nephrol Dial Transplant 15:637, 2000.
77. Forclaz A, Maillard M, Nussberger J, et al: Angiotensin II receptor blockade: Is there truly a benefit of adding an ACE inhibitor? Hypertension 41:31, 2003.
78. Pretorius M, Rosenbaum D, Vaughan DE, Brown NJ: Angiotensin-converting enzyme inhibition increases human vascular tissue-type plasminogen activator release through endogenous bradykinin. Circulation 103:579, 2003.
79. Nussberger J, Cugno M, Cicardi M: Bradykinin-mediated angioedema. N Engl J Med 347:621, 2002.
80. Grassi G, Turri C, Dell'Oro R, et al: Effect of chronic angiotensin converting enzyme inhibition on sympathetic nerve traffic and baroreflex control of the circulation in essential hypertension. J Hypertens 16:1789, 1998.
81. Taddei S, Virdis A, Ghiadoni L, et al: Restoration of nitric oxide availability after calcium antagonist treatment in essential hypertension. Hypertension 37:943, 2001.
82. Cheng A, Frishman WH: Use of angiotensin-converting enzyme inhibitors as monotherapy and in combination with diuretics and calcium channel blockers. J Clin Pharmacol 38:477, 1998.
83. Levey AS: Nondiabetic kidney disease. N Engl J Med 347:1505, 2002.
84. Bakris GL, Weir MR: Angiotensin-converting enzyme inhibitor-associated elevations in serum creatinine. Arch Intern Med 160:685, 2000.
85. Haas M, Leko-Mohr Z, Erler C, Mayer G: Antiproteinuric versus antihypertensive effects of high-dose ACE inhibitor therapy. Am J Kidney Dis 40:458, 2002.
86. Losito A, Gaburri M, Errico R, et al: Survival in patients with renovascular disease and ACE inhibition. Clin Nephrol 52:339, 1999.
87. PROGRESS Collaborative Group: Randomised trial of a perindopril-based blood-pressure-lowering regimen among 6105 individuals with previous stroke or transient ischaemic attack. Lancet 358:1033, 2001.
88. Wood R: Bronchospasm and cough as adverse reactions to the ACE inhibitors captopril, enalapril, lisinopril. Br J Clin Pharmacol 39:265, 1995.
89. White WB, Kent J, Taylor A, et al: Effects of celecoxib on ambulatory blood pressure in hypertensive patients on ACE inhibitors. Hypertension 39:929, 2002.
90. Schepkens H, Vanholder R, Billiouw J-M, Lameire N: Life-threatening hyperkalemia during combined therapy with angiotensin-converting enzyme inhibitors and spironolactone: An analysis of 25 cases. Am J Med 110:438, 2001.
91. Heart Outcomes Prevention Evaluation (HOPE) Study Investigators: Effects of an angiotensin-converting-enzyme inhibitor, ramipril, on cardiovascular events in high-risk patients. N Engl J Med 342:145, 2000.
92. Burnier M, Brunner HR: Angiotensin II receptor antagonists. Lancet 355:637, 2000.
93. Tanser PH, Campbell LM, Carranza J, et al: Candesartan cilexetil is not associated with cough in hypertensive patients with enalapril-induced cough. Am J Hypertens 13:214, 2000.
94. Warner KK, Visconti JA, Tschampel MM: Angiotensin II receptor blockers in patients with ACE inhibitor–induced angioedema. Ann Pharmacother 34:526, 2000.
95. Würzner G, Gerster J-C, Chiolero A, et al: Comparative effects of losartan and irbesartan on serum uric acid in hypertensive patients with hyperuricaemia and gout. J Hypertens 19:1855, 2001.
96. Klingbeil AU, John S, Schneider MP, et al: Effect of AT_1 receptor blockade on endothelial function in essential hypertension. Am J Hypertens 16:123, 2003.
97. Schiffrin EL, Park JB, Intengan HD, Touyz RM: Correction of arterial structure and endothelial dysfunction in human essential hypertension by the angiotensin receptor antagonist losartan. Circulation 101:1653, 2000.
98. Lacourcière Y, Asmar R: A comparison of the efficacy and duration of action of candesartan cilexetil and losartan as assessed by clinic and ambulatory blood pressure after a missed dose, in truly hypertensive patients. Am J Hypertens 12:1181, 1999.
99. Agarwal R: Add-on angiotensin receptor blockade with maximized ACE inhibition. Kidney Int 59:2282, 2001.
100. Nakao N, Yoshimura A, Morita H, et al: Combination treatment of angiotensin-II receptor blocker and angiotensin-converting-enzyme inhibitor in non-diabetic renal disease (COOPERATE): A randomized controlled trial. Lancet 361:117, 2003.

101. Parving H-H, Lehnert H, Bröchner-Mortensen J, et al: The effect of irbesartan on the development of diabetic nephropathy in patients with type 2 diabetes. N Engl J Med 345:870, 2001.
102. Brunner HR, Gavras H: Angiotensin blockade for hypertension: A promise fulfilled. Lancet 359:990, 2002.
103. Stokes GS, Barin ES, Gilfillan KL: Effects of isosorbide mononitrate and AII inhibition on pulse wave reflection in hypertension. Hypertension 41:297, 2003.
104. Raji A, Seely EW, Bekins SA, et al: Rosiglitazone improves insulin sensitivity and lowers blood pressure in hypertensive patients. Diabetes Care 26:172, 2003.

Special Considerations in Therapy

105. Nelson MR, Reid CM, Krum H, et al: Short-term predictors of maintenance of normotension after withdrawal of antihypertensive drugs in the Second Australian National Blood Pressure Study (ANBP2). Am J Hypertens 16:39, 2003.
106. Redon J, Campos C, Narciso ML, et al: Prognostic value of ambulatory blood pressur monitoring in refractory hypertension. Hypertension 31:712, 1998.
107. Poldermans D, Boersma E, Bax JJ, et al: The effect of bisoprolol on perioperative mortality and myocardial infarction in high-risk patients undergoing vascular surgery. N Engl J Med 341:1789, 1999.
108. Flynn JT: Pharmacologic management of childhood hypertension: Current status future challenges. Am J Hypertens 15(Suppl):30S, 2002.
109. Gæde P, Vedel P, Larsen N, et al: Multifactorial intervention and cardiovascular disease in patients with type 2 diabetes. N Engl J Med 348:383, 2003.
110. Kloner RA, Brown M, Prisant LM, Collins M, for the Sildenafil Study Group: Effect of sildenafil in patients with erectile dysfunction taking antihypertensive therapy. Am J Hypertens 14:70, 2001.
111. Mansoor GA, Frishman WH: Comprehensive management of hypertensive emergencies and urgencies. Heart Dis 4:358, 2002.

GUIDELINES *Thomas H. Lee*

Treatment of Hypertension

The major U.S. guidelines for management of hypertension are issued by the Joint National Committee on Prevention, Detection, Evaluation, and Treatment of High Blood Pressure, a group coordinated by the National Heart Lung and Blood Institute (NHLBI). Their seventh and most recent guidelines were published in 2003, and are known as JNC-7.[1] Other recent recommendations have been published in other countries, such as guidelines from the British Hypertension Society.[2] In 2003, recommendations regarding blood pressure control in patients with diabetes were issued by the American College of Physicians,[3] and for African Americans by the International Society on Hypertension in Blacks.[4]

Initial Evaluation

JNC-7 updated NHLBI recommendations from prior guidelines issued in 1997[5] in several important ways. First, JNC-7 introduced the concept of "prehypertension," which is systolic blood pressures of 120 to 139 mm Hg or a diastolic blood pressure of 80 to 89 mm Hg. JNC-7 recommended a more aggressive approach to patients with blood pressures in this range, with an emphasis on lifestyle modifications to prevent cardiovascular disease. JNC-7 describes "normal" blood pressure as systolic pressures below 120 mm Hg and diastolic blood pressures below 80 mm Hg. Stage 1 hypertension is systolic blood pressure 140 to 159 mm Hg or diastolic blood pressure 90 to 99 mm Hg. Patients with higher blood pressures have Stage 2 hypertension.

JNC-6 gives recommendations for follow-up of patients after initial measurement of blood pressure (Table 38G–1). These recommendations should be guided by the blood pressure and other clinical data, including past blood pressure measurements, other cardiovascular risk factors, or target organ disease. JNC-7 recommends routine laboratory tests before initiation of therapy that include 12-lead electrocardiogram; urinalysis; blood glucose and hematocrit; serum potassium, creatinine, and calcium; and lipid profile. More extensive testing for identifiable causes of hypertension is not indicated routinely.

Initial Management Strategy

The goal of treatment according to JNC-7 is to reduce blood pressure to below 140 mm Hg systolic and 90 mm Hg diastolic; in patients with concomitant diabetes or renal disease, the goal is blood pressure below 130/80 mm Hg.

These guidelines recommend that initial management be based upon the patient's blood pressure stage and other medical issues (Table 38G–2). Life-style modifications should be encouraged for all patients, including those with normal blood pressures, and should be used as the sole therapy for patients with prehypertension unless they have clinical evidence of "compelling indications." These indications include heart failure, postmyocardial infarction, high coronary artery disease risk, diabetes, chronic kidney disease, and need for recurrent stroke prevention.

Recommended life-style modifications include:

- Weight reduction to maintain normal body weight (body mass index 18.5 to 24.9 kg/m^2)
- Adoption of the Dietary Approaches to Stop Hypertension (DASH) eating plan[6]
- Dietary sodium reduction to no more than 100 mmol per day (2.4 g sodium or 6 g sodium chloride)
- Physical activity—at least 30 minutes per day, most days of the week
- Limit alcohol intake to no more than 2 drinks (1 oz or 30 m ethanol; e.g., 24 oz beer, 10 oz wine, or 3 oz 80-proof whiskey) per day in most men and to no more than 1 drink per day in women and lighter weight persons.

Drug Therapy

JNC-7 guidelines recommend thiazide-type diuretics as the initial therapy for most patients with hypertension, either alone or in combination with one of the other classes. Table 38G–3 describes JNC-7's list of "compelling indications" and recommended therapies. The guidelines note that most patients who are hypertensive will require two or more antihypertensive agents to achieve their blood pressure goals. When blood pressure is more than 20/10 mm Hg above goal the guidelines recommend that clinicians consider initiating therapy with two drugs.

Guidelines from other organizations vary slightly in thresholds for initiating therapy. For example, the British Hypertension Society's guidelines support initiation of drug therapy for all patients with systolic blood pressure ≥ 160 mm Hg or sustained diastolic blood pressure ≥ 100 mm Hg despite nonpharmacological measures. Drug treatment is also indicated in patients with sustained systolic blood pressures of 140 to 159 mm Hg or diastolic blood pressures of 90 to 99 mm Hg if target organ damage is present, or there is evidence of established cardiovascular disease, or diabetes, or the 10-year coronary heart disease risk is greater than 15%. For most patients, these guidelines recommend a target of reducing systolic pressure below 140 mm Hg and diastolic pressure below 85 mm Hg. For patients with diabetes a lower target is recommended. These guidelines recommend initiation of therapy with a diuretic unless there is a contraindication or a compelling indication for another drug class.

For patients with hypertension and diabetes, the 2003 recommendations from the American College of Physicians include a target blood pressure of no more than 135/80 mm Hg.[3] These guidelines recommend thiazide diuretics or ACE inhibitors as first-line agents for blood pressure control in most patients.

TABLE 38G–1 Joint National Committee (JNC)-6 Guidelines for Follow-Up Based on Initial Blood Pressure Measurements for Adults

Initial Blood Pressure* (mm Hg)		
Systolic	*Diastolic*	*Follow-Up Recommended*
<130	<85	Recheck in 2 yr
130-139	85-89	Recheck in 1 yr (provide information about life-style modifications)
140-159	90-99	Confirm within 2 mo (provide information about life-style modifications)
160-179	100-109	Evaluate or refer to source of care within 1 mo
≧180	≧110	Evaluate or refer to source of care immediately or within 1 wk depending on clinical situation

*If systolic and diastolic categories are different, follow recommendations for shorter time follow-up.

TABLE 38G–2 Joint National Committee (JNC)-7 Guidelines for Classification and Management of Hypertension in Adults

				Initial Drug Therapy	
Blood Pressure Classification	**Systolic Blood Pressure (mm Hg)**	**Diastolic Blood Pressure (mm Hg)**	**Life-style Modification**	***Without Compelling Indications***	***With Compelling Indications****
Normal	<120	And <80	Encourage	No antihypertensive drug indicated	Drug(s) for compelling indications[†]
Prehypertension	120-139	Or 80-89	Yes		
Stage 1 hypertension	140-159	Or 90-99	Yes	Thiazide-type diuretics for most	Drug(s) for compelling indications.[†] Other antihypertensive drugs (diuretics, ACEI, ARB, BB, CCB) as needed
Stage 2 hypertension	≧160	Or ≧100	Yes	Two-drug combination for most (usually thiazide-type diuretic and ACEI or ARB or BB or CCB)	

ACEI, angiotensin-converting enzyme inhibitor; ARB, angiotensin receptor blocker; BB, beta blocker; CCB, calcium channel blocker.
*Heart failure, postmyocardial infarction, high coronary artery disease risk, diabetes, chronic kidney disease, recurrent stroke prevention.
[†]Treat patients with chronic kidney disease or diabetes to blood pressure goal of <130/80 mm Hg.

TABLE 38G–3 Joint National Committee (JNC)-7 Guidelines for Recommended Drugs for Patients with Compelling Indications

	Recommended Drugs					
Compelling Indication	***Diuretic***	***Beta Blocker***	***ACE Inhibitor***	***Angiotensin Receptor Blocker***	***Calcium Channel Blocker***	***Aldosterone Antagonist***
Heart failure	+	+	+	+		+
Postmyocardial infarction		+	+			+
High coronary disease risk	+	+	+		+	
Diabetes	+	+	+	+	+	
Chronic kidney disease			+	+		
Recurrent stroke prevention	+		+			

ACE = angiotensin-converting enzyme.

Guidelines developed for treatment of African Americans recommend lower thresholds for drug therapy and more aggressive treatment strategies.[4] These guidelines recommend a lower blood pressure target (130/80 mm Hg) for African Americans with hypertension who also have conditions such as heart disease, kidney disease, or diabetes. This statement notes that physicians should have a low threshold for using more than one drug for treatment of hypertension in blacks.

Follow-Up and Referral to Specialists

In follow-up, the JNC-7 guidelines recommend that most patients should be seen at approximately monthly intervals until the blood pressure goal is reached. More frequent visits are recommended for patients with Stage 2 hypertension or with complicating comorbid conditions. Serum potassium and creatinine should be monitored at least 1 to 2 times per year. After blood pressure is at goal and stable, follow-up visits can be scheduled at 3- to 6-month intervals. Low-dose aspirin therapy should be considered only after blood pressure is controlled due to risk of hemorrhagic stroke in patients with uncontrolled hypertension.

References

1. Chobanian AV, et al: The Seventh Report of the Joint National Committee on Prevention, Detection, Evaluation, and Treatment of High Blood Pressure. NIH Publication No. 03-5233, 2003.
2. Ramsay LE, Williams B, Johnston GD, et al: Guidelines for management of hypertension: Report of the third working party of the British Hypertension Society. J Hum Hypertens 13:569, 1999.
3. Snow V, Weiss KB, Mottur-Pilson C, for the Clinical Efficacy Assessment Subcommittee of the American College of Physicians: The evidence base for tight blood pressure control in the management of type 2 diabetes mellitus. Ann Intern Med 138:587, 2003.
4. Douglas JG, Bakris GL, Epstein M, et al: Management of high blood pressure in African Americans: Consensus Statement of the Hypertension in African Americans Working Group of the International Society of Hypertension in Blacks. Arch Intern Med 163:525, 2003.
5. Sheps SG, et al: The Sixth Report of the Joint National Committee on Prevention, Detection, Evaluation, and Treatment of High Blood Pressure. NIH Publication No. 98-4080, 1997.
6. Sacks FM, Svetkey LP, Vollmer WM, et al: Effects on blood pressure of reduced dietary sodium and the Dietary Approaches to Stop Hypertension (DASH) diet. DASH-Sodium Collaborative Research Group. N Engl J Med 344:3, 2001.

CHAPTER 39

Lipoprotein Disorders and Cardiovascular Disease

Jacques Genest • Peter Libby • Antonio M. Gotto, Jr.

The lipid fractions of blood have proved to be among the most potent and best substantiated risk factors for atherosclerosis in general and coronary heart disease (CHD) in particular. Chapter 35 discusses the biological basis of atherosclerosis. Chapter 36 presents the observational data on lipids as a key component of the palette of cardiovascular risk factors. This chapter deals with the fundamentals of lipid metabolism, the therapeutic approaches to treatment of lipid disorders, and the evidence base regarding their clinical use.

Although the term *hyperlipidemia* has long been used in clinical practice, the term *dyslipoproteinemia* more appropriately reflects the disorders of the lipid and lipoprotein transport pathways associated with arterial diseases. *Dyslipidemia* encompasses disorders often encountered in clinical practice such as low high-density lipoprotein (HDL) cholesterol level and elevated triglyceride level but an average total plasma cholesterol level. Certain rare lipoprotein disorders can cause overt clinical manifestations, but most common dyslipoproteinemias themselves only rarely cause symptoms or produce clinical signs that are evident on physical examination. Rather, they require laboratory tests for detection. Dyslipoproteinemias constitute a major risk factor for atherosclerosis and coronary artery disease, and their proper recognition and management can reduce cardiovascular and total mortality rates. Thus the fundamentals of lipidology presented here have importance for the daily practice of cardiovascular medicine.

Lipoprotein Transport System

Biochemistry of Lipids

The lipid transport system has evolved to carry hydrophobic molecules (fat) from sites of origin to sites of utilization through the aqueous environment of plasma. The proteins (apolipoproteins) that mediate this process are conserved throughout evolution in organisms with a circulatory system. Most apolipoproteins derive from an ancestral gene and contain both hydrophilic and hydrophobic domains. This amphipathic structure enables these proteins to bridge the interface between the aqueous environment of plasma and the phospholipid constituents of the lipoprotein.[1] The major types of lipids that circulate in plasma include cholesterol and cholesteryl esters, phospholipids, and triglycerides (Fig. 39–1).

Cholesterol is an essential component of mammalian cell membranes and furnishes the substrate for steroid hormones and bile acids. Many cell functions depend critically upon membrane cholesterol, and cells tightly regulate cholesterol content. Most of the cholesterol in plasma circulates in the form of cholesteryl esters, in the core of lipoprotein particles. The enzyme lecithin:cholesterol acyltransferase (LCAT) forms cholesteryl esters by transferring a fatty acyl chain from phosphatidyl choline to cholesterol.

Triglycerides consist of a three-carbon glycerol backbone covalently linked to three fatty acids. The fatty acid composition varies in terms of chain length and presence of double bonds (degree of saturation). Triglyceride molecules are nonpolar and hydrophobic. Hydrolysis of triglycerides by lipases generates free fatty acids used for storage or energy utilization.

Phospholipids are constituents of all cellular membranes and consist of a glycerol molecule linked to two fatty acids. The fatty acids differ in length and in the presence of a single (monounsaturated) or multiple (polyunsaturated) double bonds. The third carbon of the glycerol moiety carries a phosphate group to which one of four molecules is linked: choline (forming phosphatidyl choline—or lecithin), ethanolamine (forming phosphatidylethanolamine), serine (forming phosphatidyl serine), or inositol (forming phosphatidylinositol). A related phospholipid, sphingomyelin, has special functions in the plasma membrane in the formation of membrane microdomains, such as rafts and caveolae. The structure of sphingomyelin resembles that of phosphatidylcholine. The backbone of sphingolipids uses serine rather than glycerol. Phospholipids are polar molecules, more soluble than triglycerides or cholesterol or its esters. Phospholipids participate in signal transduction pathways: hydrolysis by membrane-associated phospholipases generates second messengers such as diacyl

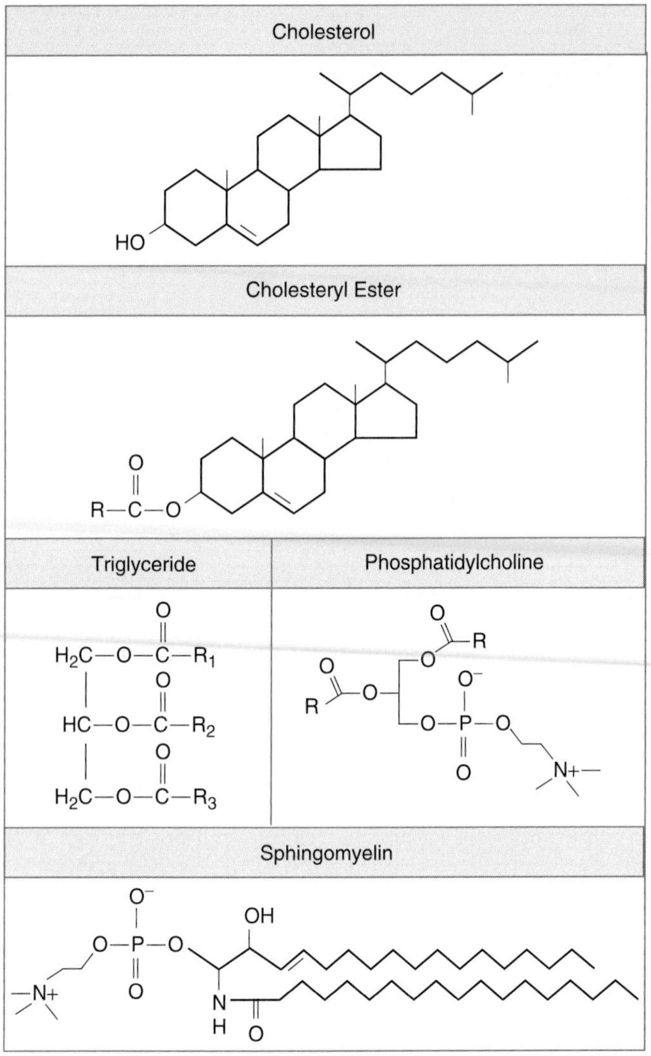

FIGURE 39–1 Biochemical structure of the major lipid molecules: cholesterol, cholesteryl esters, triglycerides, and phospholipids (phosphatidylcholine and sphingomyelin).

glycerols, lysophospholipids, phosphatidic acids, and free fatty acids such as arachidonate that can regulate many cell functions.

Lipoproteins, Apolipoproteins, Receptors, and Processing Enzymes

The apolipoprotein coating packages the hydrophobic cholesteryl esters and triglycerides in the core of spherical lipoprotein particles, enabling their transport in blood (Fig. 39–2). Lipoproteins vary in size, density in the aqueous environment of plasma, and lipid and apolipoprotein content (Fig. 39–3, Table 39–1). The classification of lipoproteins reflects their density in plasma (1.006 gm/ml) as gauged by flotation in the ultracentrifuge. The triglyceride-rich lipoproteins consisting of chylomicrons and very-low-density lipoprotein (VLDL) have a density less than 1.006 gm/ml. The rest of the ultracentrifuged plasma consists of low-density lipoprotein (LDL), HDL, and lipoprotein(a).

APOLIPOPROTEINS, RECEPTORS, AND PROCESSING PROTEINS. Apolipoproteins have four major roles: (1) assembly and secretion of the lipoprotein (apo B_{100} and B_{48}); (2) structural integrity of the lipoprotein (apo B, apo E, apo AI, apo AII); (3) coactivators or inhibitors of enzymes (apo AI, CI, CII, CIII); and (4) binding or docking to specific receptors and proteins for cellular uptake of the entire particle or selective uptake of a lipid component (apo AI, B_{100}, E) (Table 39–2). The role of several apolipoproteins (AIV, AV, D, and J) remain incompletely understood.

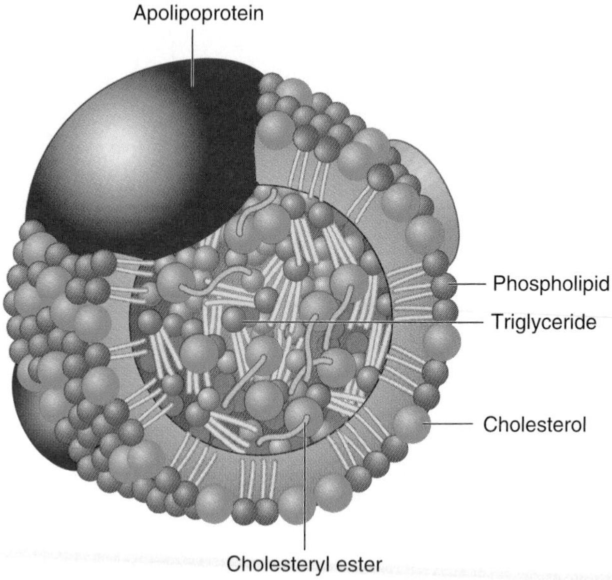

FIGURE 39–2 Structure of lipoproteins. Phospholipids are oriented with their polar head toward the aqueous environment of plasma. Free cholesterol is inserted within the phospholipid layer. The core of the lipoprotein is made up of cholesteryl esters and triglycerides. Apolipoproteins are involved in the secretion of the lipoprotein, provide structural integrity, and act as cofactors for enzymes or as ligands for various receptors.

Many proteins regulate the synthesis, secretion, and metabolic fate of lipoproteins; their characterization has provided insight in molecular cellular physiology and provided targets for drug development (Table 39-3). The discovery of the LDL receptor furnished a landmark in understanding cholesterol metabolism and receptor-mediated endocytosis. The LDL receptor regulates the entry of cholesterol into cells, as tight control mechanisms alter its expression on the cell surface, depending on need. Other receptors for lipoproteins include several that bind VLDL but not LDL. The LDL receptor-related peptide, which mediates the uptake of chylomicron remnants and VLDL, preferentially recognizes apolipoprotein E (apo E).[2] The LDL receptor–related peptide interacts with hepatic lipase. A specific VLDL receptor has also been isolated.[3] The interaction between hepatocytes and the various lipoproteins containing apo E is complex and involves cell surface proteoglycans that provide a scaffolding for lipolytic enzymes (lipoprotein lipase and hepatic lipase) involved in remnant lipoprotein recognition.[4-6] Macrophages express receptors that bind modified (especially oxidized) lipoproteins. These scavenger lipoprotein receptors mediate the uptake of oxidized LDL into macrophages. In contrast to the exquisitely regulated LDL receptor, high cellular cholesterol content does not suppress scavenger receptors, enabling the intimal macrophages to accumulate abundant cholesterol, become foam cells, and form fatty streaks. Endothelial cells can also take up modified lipoproteins through a specific receptor, such as Lox-1.[7]

At least two physiologically relevant receptors bind HDL particles: the scavenger receptor class B (SR-B1; also named CLA-1 in humans)[8] and the adenosine triphosphate–binding cassette transporter A1 (ABCA1). SR-B1 is a ligand for HDL (also for LDL and VLDL, but with less affinity). SR-B1 mediates the selective uptake of HDL cholesteryl esters in steroidogenic tissues, hepatocytes, and endothelium. The ABCA1 mediates cellular phospholipid (and possibly cholesterol) efflux and contributes importantly to the formation of HDL particles.

Lipoprotein Metabolism and Transport

The lipoprotein transport system has two major roles: the efficient transport of triglycerides from the intestine and the liver to sites of utilization (fat tissue or muscle) and the transport of cholesterol to peripheral tissues, for membrane synthesis and for steroid hormone production or to the liver for bile acid synthesis.

TABLE 39–1 Plasma Lipoprotein Composition

	Origin	Density (gm/ml)	Size (nm)	% Protein	[Cholesterol] in plasma†	[Triglyceride] in fasting plasma‡	Major apo	Other apo
Chylomicrons	Intestine	<0.95	100-1000	1-2	0.0	0	B48	AI, C's
VLDL	Liver	<1.006	40-50	10	0.1-0.4	0.2-1.2	B100	AI, C's
IDL	VLDL	1.006-1.019	25-30	18	0.1-0.3	0.1-0.3	B100, E	
LDL	IDL	1.019-1.063	20-25	25	1.5-3.5	0.2-0.4	B100	
HDL	Tissues	1.063-1.210	6-10	40-55	0.9-1.6	0.1-0.2	AI	AII, AIV
Lipoprotein (a)	Liver	1.051-1.082	25	30-50			B100, (a)	

apo = apolipoproteins; HDL = high-density lipoprotein; IDL = intermediate-density lipoprotein; LDL = low-density lipoprotein; VLDL = very-low-density lipoprotein.
†In mmol/L; for mg/dl, multiply by 38.67.
‡In mmol/L; for mg/dl, multiply by 88.5.

INTESTINAL PATHWAY (CHYLOMICRONS TO CHYLOMICRON REMNANTS). Life requires fats. The human body derives essential fatty acids that it cannot make from the diet. Fat typically furnishes 20 to 40 percent of daily calories. The major portion of fats ingested is in the form of triglycerides. For an individual consuming 2000 kcal/day, with 30 percent in the form of fat, this represents approximately 66 gm of triglycerides per day and approximately 250 mg (0.250 gm) of cholesterol.

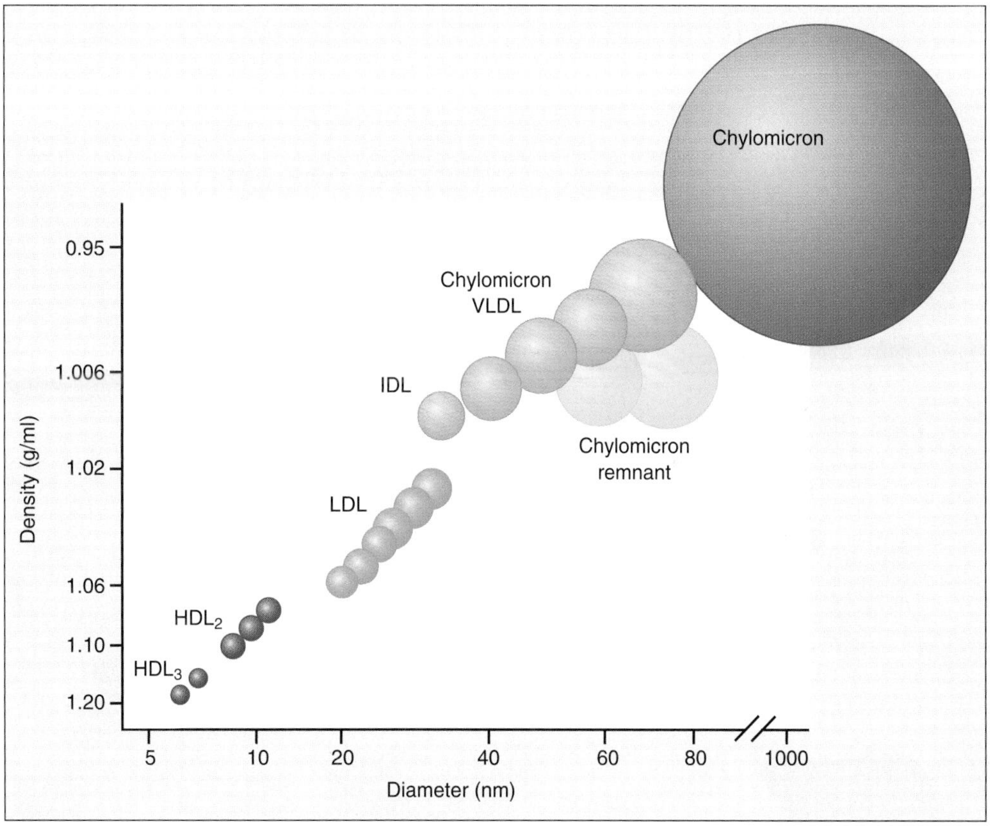

FIGURE 39–3 Relative size of plasma lipoproteins according to their hydrated density. HDL = high-density lipoprotein; IDL = intermediate-density lipoprotein; LDL = low-density lipoprotein.

Upon ingestion, pancreatic lipases hydrolyze triglycerides into free fatty acids and mono- or diglycerides. Emulsification by bile salts leads to the formation of intestinal micelles. Micelles resemble lipoproteins in that they consist of phospholipids, free cholesterol, bile acids, di- and monoglycerides, free fatty acids, and glycerol. The mechanism of micelle uptake by the intestinal brush border cells still engenders debate. Recent work has identified Niemann-Pick C1-like 1 protein as an intestinal cholesterol transporter, and potential target for the cholesterol absorption inhibitor ezetimibe[8a] (see below). The advent of selective inhibitors of cholesterol uptake (ezetimibe; see later) has rekindled interest in the mechanisms of intestinal fat absorption. After uptake into intestinal cells, fatty acids re-esterified to form triglycerides and packaged into chylomicrons inside the intestinal cell enter the portal circulation (Fig. 39–4, part 1). Chylomicrons contain apo B48, the amino-terminal component of apo B100. In the intestine, the apo B gene is modified during transcription into mRNA with a substitution of a uracil for a cytosine by an apo B48 editing enzyme complex (ApoBec). This mechanism involves a cytosine deaminase and leads to a termination codon at residue 2153 and a truncated form of apo B. Only intestinal cells express ApoBec.

Chylomicrons rapidly enter the plasma compartment after meals. In capillaries of adipose tissue or muscle cells in the peripheral circulation, chylomicrons encounter lipoprotein lipase (LPL), an enzyme attached to heparin sulfate and present on the luminal side of endothelial cells (Fig. 39–4, part 2). LPL activity is modulated by apo CII (an activator) and by apo CIII (an inhibitor).[9] Lipoprotein lipase has broad specificity for triglycerides; it cleaves all fatty acyl residues attached to glycerol, generating three molecules of free fatty acid for each molecule of glycerol. Muscle cells rapidly take up fatty acids. Adipose cells can store triglycerides made from fatty acids for energy utilization, a process that requires insulin. Fatty acids can also bind to fatty acid–binding proteins and travel to the liver, where they are repackaged in VLDL. Peripheral resistance to insulin can thus increase the delivery of free fatty acids to the liver with a consequent increase in VLDL secretion and increased apo B particles in plasma. As discussed later, this is one of the consequences of the metabolic syndrome (see Chap. 40). The remnant particles, derived from chylomicron following LPL action, contain apo E and enter the liver for degradation and reutilization of its core constituents (Fig. 39–4, part 3).

TABLE 39–2 Apolipoproteins

	Predominant Lipoprotein	Molecular Weight (kDa)	Plasma Concentration (mg/dl)	Chromosome	Role	Human Disease
Apo AI	HDL	28.3	90-160	11q23	ACAT activation, structural	HDL deficiency
Apo AII	HDL	17	25-45	1q21-23	Structural	
Apo AIV	HDL	45	10-20	11q23	Structural, absorption	
Apo AV	VLDL, HDL			11q23	TRL metabolism[72]	
Apo B100	LDL, VLDL	512	50-150	2q23-24	Structural, LDL-R binding	Hypobetalipoproteinemia
Apo B48	Chylomicrons	241	0-100	2q23-24	Structural	
Apo CI	Chylomicrons	6.63	5-6	19q13.2	TRL metabolism	
Apo CII	Chylomicrons, VLDL	8.84	3-5	19q13.2	LPL activation	Hyperchylomicronemia
Apo CIII	Chylomicrons, VLDL	8.76	10-14	11q23	LPL inhibition	Hypertriglyceridemia
Apo D	HDL	33	4-7	3q26.2	LCAT	
Apo E	Chylomicrons remnant, IDL	34	2-8	19q13.2	LDL-R, ApoE-R binding	Type III
Apo J	HDL	70	10	18p21	Complement system	
Apo(a)	Lipoprotein(a)	250-800	0-200	6q27	Tissue injury?	

Apo = apolipoprotein; ApoE-R = Apo E receptor; HDL = high-density lipoprotein; IDL = intermediate-density lipoprotein; LCAT = lecithin:cholesterol acyltransferase; LDL = low-density lipoprotein; LDL-R = LDL receptor; TRL = triglyceride-rich lipoprotein; VLDL = very-low-density lipoprotein.

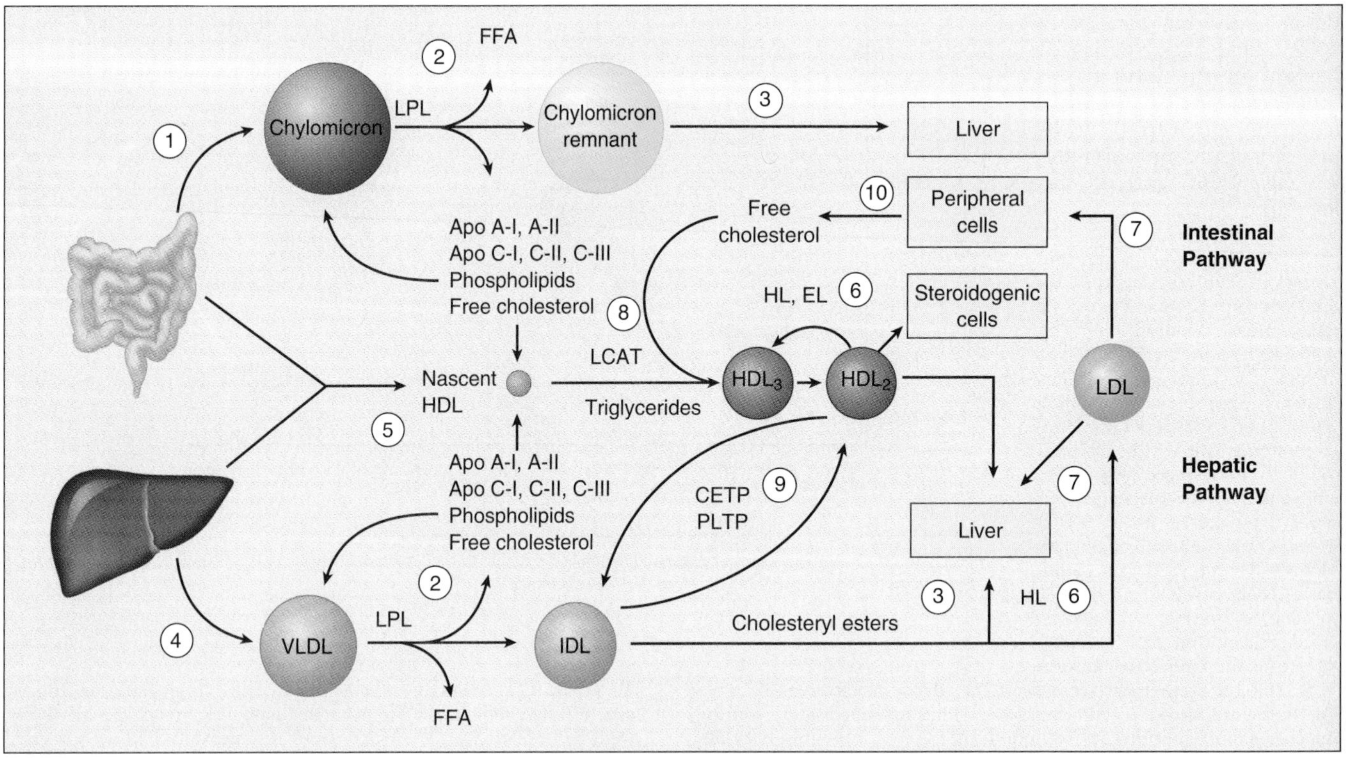

FIGURE 39–4 Schematic diagram of the lipid transport system. Numbers in circles refer to explanation in text. Apo = apolipoprotein; CETP = cholesteryl ester transfer protein; EL = endothelial lipase; FFA = free fatty acids; HL = hepatic lipase; HDL = high-density lipoprotein; IDL = intermediate-density lipoprotein; LCAT = lecithin cholesterol acyltransferase; LDL = low-density lipoprotein; LPL = lipoprotein lipase; PLTP = phospholipid transfer protein; VLDL = very-low-density lipoprotein.

TABLE 39–3 Lipoprotein Processing Enzymes, Receptors, Modulating Proteins

Abreviation	Name	Role	Chromosome	Human Disease
ABCA1	ATP binding cassette AI	Cellular phospholipid efflux	9q31	Tangier disease
ABCG5/G8	ATP binding cassette G5 and G8	Intestinal sitosterol transporter	21	Sitosterolemia
ACAT1	Acyl:CoA cholesterol acyl-transferase 1	Cholesterol esterification	1q22.3	Cellular cholesterol esterification
ACAT2	Acyl:CoA cholesterol acyl-transferase 2	Cholesterol esterification	6q25.3	Cellular cholesterol esterification
ApoE-R	ApoE containing lipoprotein	TRL uptake	1p34	
CD36	Fatty acid translocase	Fatty acid transport	7q11.2	See ref. 73
CETP	Cholesteryl ester transfer protein	Lipid exchange in plasma	16q21	Elevated HDL cholesterol
EL	Endothelial lipase	Tg hydrolysis	18q21.1	See ref. 79
HL	Hepatic lipase	Tg hydrolysis	15q21	Remnant accumulation[75,76]
HSL (LIPE)	Hormone-sensitive lipase	Fatty acid release from adipocytes	19q13.2	
LCAT	Lecithin:cholesterol acyltransferase	Cholesterol esterification	16q22.1	LCAT deficiency, low HDL
LDL-R	Low-density lipoprotein receptor	LDL uptake	19p13	Familial hypercholesterolemia
Lox1	Scavenger receptor	OxLDL uptake, endothelium	12p12-13	Oxidized lipoprotein uptake
LPL	Lipoprotein lipase	Tg hydrolysis	8p22	Hyperchylomicronemia
LRP1	LDL-R–related protein	Protease uptake, many ligands	19q12	
LRP2	LDL-R–related protein 2 (megalin)	Protease uptake, apo J	2q24-31	See ref. 74
MTP	Microsomal triglyceride transfer	Apo B assembly	4q22-24	Abetalipoproteinemia
NPC1	Niemann-Pick C gene product	Cellular cholesterol transport	18q11-12	Niemann-Pick type C
NPC1L1	Niemann-Pick C1-like 1 protein	Intestinal cholesterol absorption	7p13	See ref. 8a
PLTP	Phospholipid transfer protein	Lipid exchange in plasma	20q12	See ref. 77
PCSK9	Proprotein convertase, subtilisin/kexin type 9	Protein cleavage	1p34.1	Hypercholesterolemia
SRA	Scavenger receptor A	OxLDL uptake, macrophages	8p21	
SR-B1	Scavenger receptor B1	HDL CE uptake	12	See ref. 78
VLDL-R	Very-low-density lipoprotein receptor	VLDL uptake	9q24	

CE = cholesterol esters; HDL = high-density lipoprotein; LDL = low-density lipoprotein; OxLDL = oxidized low-density lipoprotein; Tg = triglyceride; TRL = triglyceride-rich lipoprotein; VLDL = very-low-density lipoprotein.

HEPATIC PATHWAY (VERY-LOW-DENSITY LIPOPROTEIN TO INTERMEDIATE-DENSITY LIPOPROTEIN). Food is not always available, and dietary fat content is not always constant. The body must ensure readily available triglyceride molecules for energy demands. Hepatic secretion of VLDL particles serves this function (Fig. 39–4, part 4). VLDLs are triglyceride-rich lipoproteins smaller than chylomicrons (see Table 39–1 and Fig. 39–3). They contain apo B100 as their main lipoprotein. As opposed to apo B48, apo B100 contains a domain recognized by the LDL receptor (the apo B/E receptor). VLDL particles follow the same catabolic pathway through lipoprotein lipase as chylomicrons (Fig. 39–4, part 2). During hydrolysis of triglyceride-rich lipoproteins by LPL, an exchange of proteins and lipids takes place: VLDL particles (and chylomicrons) acquire apo Cs and apo E, in part from HDL particles. VLDLs also exchange triglycerides for cholesteryl esters from HDL (mediated by cholesteryl ester transfer protein [CETP]) (Fig. 39–4, parts 5 and 9). Such bidirectional transfer of constituents between lipoproteins serves several purposes, allowing lipoproteins to acquire specific apolipoproteins that will dictate their metabolic fate; transfer of phospholipids onto nascent HDL particles mediated by phospholipid transfer protein (PLTP)[10] (during the loss of core triglycerides, the phospholipid envelope becomes redundant and is shed off to apo AI to form new HDL particles); and transfer of cholesterol from HDL to VLDL remnants so it can be metabolized in the liver. This exchange constitutes a major part of the reverse cholesterol transport pathway.

After hydrolysis of triglycerides partly depletes VLDL of triglycerides, VLDL particles have relatively more cholesterol, shed several apolipoproteins (especially the C apolipoproteins), and acquire apo E. The VLDL remnant lipoprotein, called *intermediate-density lipoprotein*, is taken up by the liver via its apo E moiety (Fig. 39–4, part 3) or further delipidated by hepatic lipase to form an LDL particle (Fig. 39–4, part 6). There are at least four receptors for triglyceride-rich lipoprotein (TRL), TRL remnants, and apo B–containing lipoproteins: the VLDL receptor, the remnant receptor, the LDL receptor (also called the apo B/E receptor), and the LDL receptor–related peptide. A common feature of most hepatic receptors is their recognition of apo E, which mediates uptake of several classes of lipoproteins, including VLDL and intermediate-density lipoprotein. The interaction between apo E and its ligand is complex and involves the "docking" of TRL on heparan sulfate proteoglycans before presentation of the ligand to its receptor.

LOW-DENSITY LIPOPROTEINS. LDL particles contain predominantly cholesteryl esters packaged with the protein moiety apo B100. Normally, triglycerides constitute only 4 to 8 percent of the LDL mass. In the presence of elevated plasma triglyceride levels, LDL particles can become enriched in triglycerides and depleted in core cholesteryl esters. LDL particle size variation results from changes in core constituents, with an increase in triglycerides and a relative decrease in cholesteryl esters leading to smaller, denser LDL particles.

The LDL particles in most higher mammals, including humans and nonhuman primates, serve as the main carriers of cholesterol. In other mammals, such as rodents or rabbits, VLDL and HDL particles transport most of the cholesterol. The cholesterol molecule is required for membrane biosynthesis, steroid hormone production, or bile acid synthesis in the liver. Cells can either make cholesterol from acetate through enzymatic reactions requiring at least 33 steps or obtain it as cholesteryl esters from LDL particles. Cells internalize LDL via the LDL receptor (LDL-R) (Fig. 39–5A). LDL particles contain one molecule of apo B. While several domains of apo B are highly lipophilic and associate with phospholipids, a region surrounding residue 3500 binds with high affinity and saturability to the LDL-R. The LDL-R localizes in a region of the plasma membrane rich in the protein clathrin (Figs. 39–4, part 7 and 39–5A). Once bound to the receptor, clathrin polymerizes and forms an endosome that contains LDL bound to its receptor, a portion of the plasma membrane, and clathrin. This internalized particle then fuses with a lysosome that will release its catalytic enzymes (cholesteryl ester hydrolase, cathepsins), which in turn will release free cholesterol and degrade apo B. The LDL-R will detach itself from its ligand and recycle to the plasma membrane.

Cells tightly regulate cholesterol content by (1) cholesterol synthesis in the smooth endoplasmic reticulum (via the rate-limiting step hydroxymethylglutaryl coenzyme A [HMG-CoA] reductase); (2) receptor-mediated endocytosis of LDL (two mechanisms under the control of the steroid-responsive element binding protein [SREBP]); (3) cholesterol efflux from plasma membrane to cholesterol acceptor particles (predominantly HDL); and (4) intracellular cholesterol esterification via the enzyme acyl-CoA: cholesteryl acyltransferase (ACAT) (see Fig. 39–5A, B). The SREBP coordinately regulates the first two pathways at the level of gene transcription. Cellular cholesterol binds to a protein called SCAP (SREPB cholesterol-activated protein), which is located on the endoplasmic reticulum. Cholesterol inhibits the interaction of SCAP with SREPB. In the absence of cholesterol, SCAP will mediate the cleavage of SREBP at two sites by specific proteases and release an amino (NH_2) fragment of SREBP. The SREBP NH_2 fragment will migrate to the nucleus and increase the transcriptional activity of genes involved in cellular cholesterol and fatty acid homeostasis. Cleavage of SREBP depends on a proprotein convertase related to the subtilisin/kexin family of convertases.[11] The ACAT pathway is regulated at the level of protein regulation by cholesterol content in membranes.[12] Humans express two separate forms of ACAT. ACAT1 and ACAT2 derive from different genes and mediate cholesterol esterification in cytoplasm and in the endoplasmic reticulum lumen for lipoprotein assembly and secretion.[13]

Regulation of cholesterol efflux depends in part on the ABCA1 pathway, controlled in turn by hydroxysterols (especially 22-OH cholesterol, which acts as a ligand for the liver-specific receptor [LXR] family of transcriptional regulatory factors). In conditions of cellular cholesterol excess, the cell can decrease its input of cholesterol by decreasing the de novo synthesis of cholesterol. The cell can also decrease the amount of cholesterol that enters the cell via the LDL-R, increase the amount stored as cholesteryl esters, and promote the removal of cholesterol by increasing its movement to the plasma membrane for efflux.

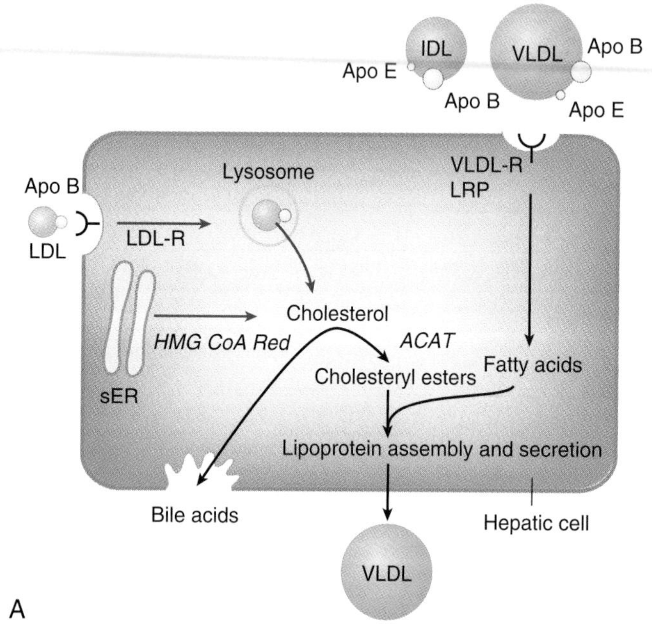

A

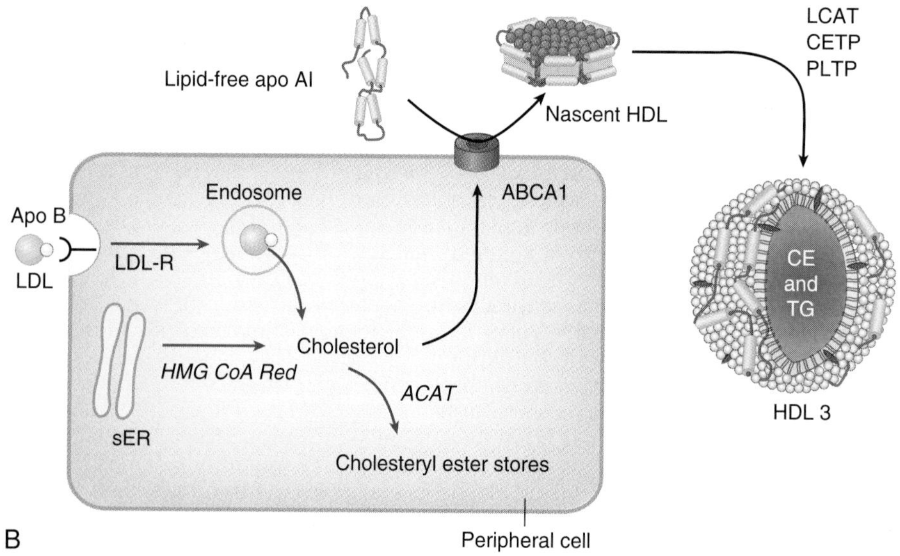

B

FIGURE 39–5 Cellular cholesterol homeostasis in various tissues. **A,** Cholesterol homeostasis (hepatocytes). **B,** Cellular cholesterol efflux (peripheral cells). *See opposite page for definitions and parts C and D.*

HIGH-DENSITY LIPOPROTEIN AND REVERSE CHOLESTEROL TRANSPORT. Epidemiological studies consistently have shown an inverse relationship between plasma levels of HDL cholesterol and the presence of coronary artery disease. HDL promotes reverse cholesterol transport and can prevent lipoprotein oxidation and exert antiinflammatory actions in vitro. In a process called *selective uptake of cholesterol*, HDL also provides cholesterol to steroid hormone–producing tissues and the liver through the scavenger SR-B1 receptor (see Fig. 39–5C).[14,15]

The metabolism of HDL is complex and only partly understood. The complexity arises from the consideration that HDL particles acquire their components from several sources while these components also are metabolized at different sites. Apolipoprotein AI, the main protein of HDL, is synthesized in the intestine and the

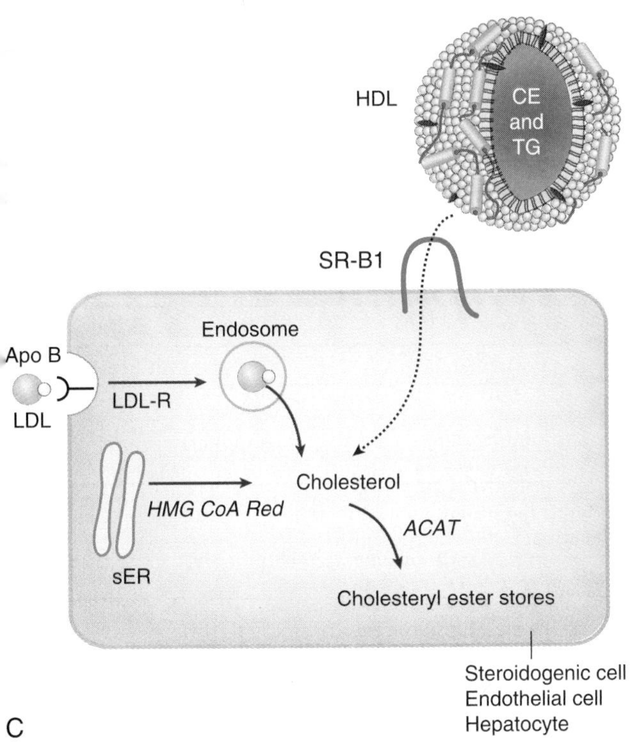

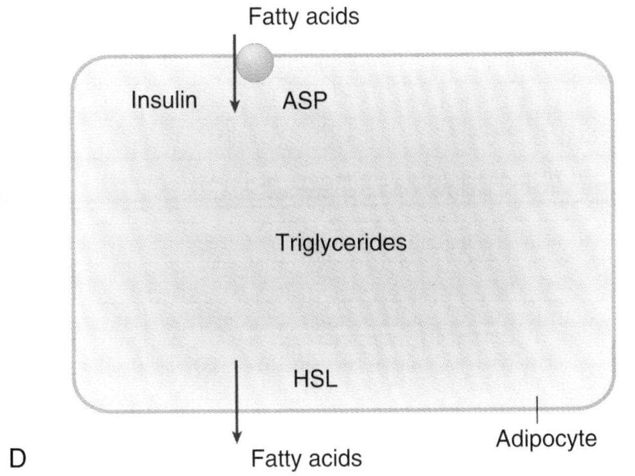

FIGURE 39–5—cont'd **C,** Selective uptake of cholesterol (adrenal cells, hepatocytes, endothelial cells). **D,** Adipocytes. ABCA1 = ATP-binding cassette transporter A1; ACAT = acyl–coenzyme A:cholesterol acyltransferase; Apo = apolipoprotein; ASP = acylation-stimulating protein; CE = cholesterol esters; CETP = cholesteryl ester transfer protein; HDL = high-density lipoprotein; HMG CoA Red = hydroxymethylglutaryl coenzyme A reductase; HSL = hormone-sensitive lipase; IDL = intermediate-density lipoprotein; LCAT = lecithin cholesterol acyltransferase; LDL = low-density lipoprotein; LDL-R = low-density lipoprotein receptor; LRP = low-density lipoprotein receptor–related peptide; PLTP = phospholipid transfer protein; sER = smooth endoplasmic reticulum; SR-B1 = scavenger receptor B1; TG = triglycerides; VLDL = very-low-density lipoprotein; VLDL-R = very-low-density lipoprotein receptor.

liver. Lipid-free apo AI acquires phospholipids from cell membranes and from redundant phospholipids shed during hydrolysis of triglyceride-rich lipoproteins. Lipid-free apo AI binds to ABCA1 and promotes its phosphorylation via cyclic adenosine monophosphate, which increases the net efflux of phospholipids and cholesterol onto apo AI to form a nascent HDL particle (Fig. 39–4, part 10).[16,17] This particle, containing apo AI and phospholipids (and little cholesterol) resembles a flattened disk in which the phospholipids form a bilayer surrounded by two molecules of apo AI arranged in a circular fashion at the periphery of the disk (see Fig. 39–5B). These nascent HDL particles will mediate further cellular

cholesterol efflux. Currently, standard laboratory tests do not measure these HDL precursors because they contain little or no cholesterol. Upon reaching a cell membrane, the nascent HDL particles will capture membrane-associated cholesterol and promote the efflux of free cholesterol onto other HDL particles (see Fig. 39–4, part 10). Conceptually, the formation of HDL particles appears to be a two-step phenomenon, the first step being ABCA1-mediated and the second probably not dependent on ABCA1.[18] The plasma enzyme LCAT, an enzyme activated by apo AI, then esterifies the free cholesterol (see Figs. 39–4, part 8, and 39–5B). LCAT transfers an acyl chain (a fatty acid) from the R2 position of a phospholipid to the 3′OH residue of cholesterol, resulting in the formation of a cholesteryl ester (see Fig. 39–1).

Because cholesteryl esters are hydrophobic, they move to the core of the lipoprotein and the HDL particle now assumes a spherical configuration (a particle denoted HDL_3). With further cholesterol esterification, the HDL particle increases in size to become the more buoyant HDL_2. Cholesterol within HDL particles can exchange with triglyceride-rich lipoproteins via cholesteryl ester transfer protein (CETP), which mediates an equimolar exchange of cholesterol from HDL to triglyceride-rich lipoprotein and triglyceride movement from triglyceride-rich lipoprotein onto HDL (Fig. 39–4, part 9). Phospholipid transfer protein (PLTP) mediates the transfer of phospholipids between triglyceride-rich lipoprotein and HDL particles. Triglyceride-enriched HDL are denoted HDL_{2b}. Hepatic lipase can hydrolyze triglycerides within these particles, converting them back to HDL_3 particles.

One mechanism of reverse cholesterol transport includes the uptake of cellular cholesterol and its esterification by LCAT, transport by large HDL particles, and exchange for one triglyceride molecule by CETP. Originally on an HDL particle, the cholesterol molecule can now be taken up by hepatic receptors on a triglyceride-rich lipoprotein or LDL particle. HDL particles, therefore, act as shuttles between tissue cholesterol, triglyceride-rich lipoprotein, and the liver.

The catabolism of HDL particles has been a matter of debate among lipoprotein researchers. The protein component of HDL particles is exchangeable with lipoproteins of other classes. The kidneys appear to be a route of elimination of apolipoprotein AI and other HDL apolipoproteins.[19] The lipid component of HDL particles also follow a different metabolic route (see Fig. 39–5A, B, and C).

Lipoprotein Disorders

Definitions

Time and new knowledge have brought necessary changes to the classification of lipoprotein disorders. The original classification of lipoprotein disorders by Fredrickson, Lees, and Levy was based on the measurement of total plasma cholesterol and triglycerides and analyzed lipoproteins patterns after separation by electrophoresis. This classification recognized elevations of chylomicrons (type I), VLDL or pre-beta lipoproteins (type IV), "broad beta" disease (or type III hyperlipoproteinemia), beta lipoproteins (LDL) (type II), and elevations of both chylomicrons and VLDL (type V). In addition, the combined elevations of pre-beta (VLDL) and beta (LDL) lipoproteins was recognized as type IIb hyperlipoproteinemia. Though providing a useful conceptual framework, this classification has some drawbacks: it does not include HDL cholesterol, and it does not differentiate severe monogenic lipoprotein disorders from the more common polygenic disorders. Subsequently, the World Health Organization, the European Atherosclerosis Society and, more recently, the National Cholesterol Education Program have classified lipoprotein disorders on the basis of arbitrary cut-points.

A practical approach describes the lipoprotein disorder by the absolute plasma levels of lipids (cholesterol and triglycerides) and lipoprotein cholesterol levels (LDL and HDL cholesterol) and considers clinical manifestations of hyperlipoproteinemia in the context of biochemical characterization. For example, a young patient presenting with eruptive xanthomas and a plasma triglyceride level of 11.3 mmol/liter (1000 mg/dl) is likely to have familial hyperchylomicronemia. An obese, hypertensive middle-aged man with a cholesterol level of 6.4 mmol/liter (247 mg/dl), a triglyceride level of 3.1 mmol/liter (274 mg/dl), a HDL cholesterol level of 0.8 mmol/liter (31 mg/ml), and a calculated LDL cholesterol level of 4.2 mmol/liter (162 mg/dl) likely has the metabolic syndrome, the concomitant conditions of which, such as hypertension, hyperglycemia, and hyperuricemia, should be sought.

The clinical usefulness of apolipoprotein levels has stirred debate. Although a useful research tool in general, the measurement of apolipoproteins AI and B practically may add little substantial information to that provided by the conventional lipid profile. Taken as a single measurement, the apo B level provides information on the number of potentially atherogenic particles and can be used as a goal of lipid-lowering therapy.[20] Similarly, LDL particle size correlates highly with plasma HDL cholesterol and triglyceride levels, and most studies do not show it to be an independent cardiovascular risk factor. The presence of small, dense LDL particles can be related to features of the metabolic syndrome, which is characterized by the presence of abdominal obesity, peripheral insulin resistance, high blood pressure, and dyslipoproteinemia with elevated plasma triglycerides and reduced HDL cholesterol levels. In some studies, improvement in LDL particle size correlated with angiographic improvement of coronary artery disease. Other studies showed that large LDL particles correlate with recurrent coronary events in survivors of myocardial infarction.[21] It remains uncertain whether in addition to LDL particle number reduction, a change in LDL particle size will bring further clinical benefit.[22]

Genetic Lipoprotein Disorders

Understanding of the genetics of lipoprotein metabolism has expanded rapidly. Classification of genetic lipoprotein disorders usually requires a biochemical phenotype in addition to a clinical phenotype. With the exception of familial hypercholesterolemia, monogenic disorders tend to be infrequent or very rare. Disorders considered heritable on careful family study may be difficult to characterize unambiguously because of age, gender, penetrance, and gene-gene and environmental interactions. Most common lipoprotein disorders encountered clinically result from the interaction of increasing age, lack of physical exercise, weight gain, and a suboptimal diet with individual genetic make-up.

Genetic lipoprotein disorders can affect LDL, lipoprotein(a), remnant lipoproteins, triglyceride-rich lipoproteins (chylomicrons and VLDL), or HDL (Table 39–4). Within each of these, genetic disorders can cause an excess or a deficiency of a specific class of lipoprotein.

TABLE 39–4 Genetic Lipoprotein Disorders

Disorder	Gene	Figure 4
LDL Particles		
Familial hypercholesterolemia	LDL-R	7
Familial defective apo B-100	Apo B	7
Autosomal dominant hypercholesterolemia	PCSK9	
Abetalipoproteinemia	MTP	
Hypobetalipoproteinemia	Apo B	
Familial sitosterolemia	ABCG5/ABCG8	
Lipoprotein(a)		
Familial lipoprotein(a) hyperlipoproteinemia	Apo (a)	
Remnant Lipoproteins		
Dysbetalipoproteinemia type III	Apo E	3
Hepatic lipase deficiency	HL	6
Triglyceride-rich Lipoproteins		
Lipoprotein lipase deficiency	LPL	2
Apo CII deficiency	Apo CII	2
Familial hypertriglyceridemia	Polygenic	
Chylomicron retention disease	?	
Familial combined hyperlipidemia	Polygenic	
HDL Particles		
Apo AI deficiency	Apo AI	
Familial HDL deficiency/Tangier disease	ABCA1	10
Familial LCAT deficiency syndromes	LCAT	8
CETP deficiency	CETP	9
Niemann-Pick disease types A and B	SMPD1	

CETP = cholesteryl ester transfer protein; HDL = high-density lipoprotein; LCAT = lecithin cholesterol acyltransferase.

Low-Density Lipoproteins (Type II Hyperlipidemia)

FAMILIAL HYPERCHOLESTEROLEMIA. Familial hypercholesterolemia is the most thoroughly studied lipoprotein disorder. The elucidation of the pathway by which complex molecules enter the cell by receptor-mediated endocytosis and the discovery of the LDL receptor represent landmarks in cell biology and clinical medicine. Affected subjects have an elevated LDL cholesterol level greater than the 95th percentile for age and gender. In adulthood, clinical manifestations include corneal arcus, tendinous xanthomas over the extensor tendons (metacarpophalangeal joints, Achilles tendons), and xanthelasmas. Transmission is autosomal codominant. The prevalence of familial hypercholesterolemia is estimated at approximately 1:500, although this prevalence is higher in populations with founder effects. Patients with familial hypercholesterolemia are at high risk of developing coronary artery disease (CAD) by the third to fourth decade in men and approximately 8 to 10 years later in women. Diagnosis is based on elevated plasma LDL cholesterol level, family history of premature CAD, and the presence of xanthomas. A molecular diagnosis is sometimes required. Defects of the *LDL-R* gene cause an accumulation of LDL particles in plasma and thus alter the function of the LDL-R protein and cause familial hypercholesterolemia (Fig. 39–4, part 7). To date, there are well over 600 identified mutations of the *LDL-R* gene (see http://www.umd.necker.fr).[23]

FAMILIAL DEFECTIVE APO B. Mutations within the apo B gene that lead to an abnormal ligand-receptor interaction can cause a form of familial hypercholesterolemia clinically indistinguishable from the primary form. This disorder, familial defective apo B 100, is caused by several mutations at the postulated binding site to the LDL-R (Fig. 39–4, part 7). These consist of apo $B_{Arg3500Gln}$, apo $B_{Arg3500Trp}$, and apo $B_{Arg3531Cys}$.[24] The apo $B_{Arg3500Gln}$ results from a G→A substitution at nucleotide 3500 within exon

26 of the apo B gene. The defective apo B has a reduced affinity (20 to 30 percent of control) for the LDL-R. LDL particles with defective apo B have a plasma half-life three- to fourfold greater than the half-life of normal LDL. Because of their increased half-life, these LDL particles can more readily undergo oxidative modifications that can enhance their atherogenicity. Affected subjects usually have elevated LDL cholesterol levels up to 400 mg/dl (10.4 mmol/liter) but may also have normal levels. Familial defective apo B 100 has a prevalence similar to that of familial hypercholesterolemia (1/500). In subjects with the classic presentation of familial hypercholesterolemia, the prevalence of familial defective apo B 100 is reported to be 1 in 50 to 1 in 20. The reasons for the variability of plasma LDL cholesterol levels remain unexplained.

Mutations within the apo B gene can lead to truncations of the mature apo B_{100} peptide. Many such mutations cause a syndrome characterized by reduced LDL and VLDL cholesterol but little or no clinical manifestations and no known risk of cardiovascular disease. Apo B truncated close to its amino terminus loses the ability to bind lipids, producing a syndrome similar to abetalipoproteinemia, a rare recessive lipoprotein disorder of infancy that causes mental retardation and growth abnormalities. Abetalipoproteinemia is caused by a mutation in gene coding for the microsomal triglyceride transfer protein (MTP) required for assembly of apo B-containing lipoproteins in the liver and the intestine.[25] The resulting lack of apo B-containing lipoproteins in plasma causes a marked deficiency of fat-soluble vitamins (A, D, E, and K) that circulate in lipoproteins.

An autosomal dominant form of hypercholesterolemia has been mapped to chromosome 1p34.1. The genetic basis for this condition is mutation within the proprotein convertase, subtilisin/kexin type 9 gene (*PCSK9*). *PCSK9* codes for a protein identified as neural apoptosis-regulated convertase 1 (NARC1), a novel proprotein convertase belonging to the subtilase family of convertases. It is related to subtilisin/kexin isoenzyme-1 (site-1 protease) required for cleavage of SREBP.[11]

SITOSTEROLEMIA. A rare condition of increased intestinal absorption and decreased excretion of plant sterols (sitosterol and campesterol) can mimic severe familial hypercholesterolemia, with extensive xanthoma formation. Premature atherosclerosis, often apparent clinically before adulthood, occurs frequently in patients with sitosterolemia. Diagnosis requires specialized analysis of plasma sterols demonstrating an elevation in sitosterol, campesterol, cholestanol, sitostanol, and campestanol. Interestingly, plasma cholesterol is normal or reduced, and triglycerides are normal. Positional cloning techniques have localized the defect to chromosome 2p21. Mutations in the adenosine triphosphate binding cassette G5 and G8 genes (*ABCG5* and *ABCG8*) have been found in patients with sitosterolemia. The gene products of *ABCG5* and *ABCG8* are half ABC transporters and are thought to form a heterodimer characteristic of the full ABC transporters. The complex is located in the villous border of intestinal cells and actively pumps plant sterols back into the intestinal lumen. A defect in either of the genes renders the complex inactive, and absorption of plant sterols (rather than their elimination) ensues. *ABCG5* and *ABCG8* mutations leading to sitosterolemia are very rare.[26]

LIPOPROTEIN(A) (see Chap. 36). Lipoprotein(a) consists of an LDL particle linked covalently with one molecule of apo (a). The apo (a) moiety consists of a protein with a high degree of homology with plasminogen. The apo (a) gene appears to have arisen from the plasminogen gene by nonhomologous recombination. The apo (a) gene has multiple repeats of one of the kringle motifs (kringle IV), varying in number from 12 to more than 40 in each individual. Plasma lipoprotein(a) levels depend almost entirely on genetics and correlate inversely with the number of kringle repeats and, therefore, with the molecular weight of apo (a).[27] Few environmental factors or medications modulate plasma lipoprotein(a) levels. The pathogenesis of lipoprotein(a) may result from an antifibrinolytic potential and/or ability to bind oxidized lipoproteins. Some prospective epidemiological studies have shown a positive (albeit weak) association between lipoprotein(a) and coronary artery disease (see Chap. 36).[28]

Triglyceride-Rich Lipoproteins

In subjects with the metabolic syndrome and in diabetic patients, elevation of plasma triglyceride level occurs most often in the presence of visceral (abdominal) obesity and a diet rich in calories, carbohydrates, and saturated fats. Severe elevation of plasma triglycerides can result from genetic disorders of the processing enzymes or apolipoproteins and poorly controlled diabetes.

FAMILIAL HYPERTRIGLYCERIDEMIA (TYPE IV HYPERLIPOPROTEINEMIA). Familial hypertriglyceridemia is not associated with clinical signs such as corneal arcus, xanthoma, and xanthelasmas. Plasma triglycerides, VLDL cholesterol, and VLDL triglycerides are moderately to markedly elevated; LDL cholesterol level is usually low, and HDL cholesterol level is also reduced. Total cholesterol is normal or elevated, depending on VLDL cholesterol levels. Fasting plasma concentrations of triglycerides are in the range of 2.3 to 5.7 mmol/liter (200 to 500 mg/dl). After a meal, plasma triglycerides may exceed 11.3 mmol/liter (1000 mg/dl). The disorder is found in first-degree relatives, but phenotypic variability is related to gender, age, hormone use (especially estrogens), and diet. Alcohol intake potently stimulates hypertriglyceridemia in these subjects, as does caloric or carbohydrate intake. The relationship with coronary artery disease is not as strong as with familial combined hyperlipidemia and has not been found consistently. Depending on criteria used, the prevalence of familial hypertriglyceridemia ranges from 1 in 100 to 1 in 50. The disorder is highly heterogeneous and likely results from several genes, with a strong environmental influence. An unrelated disorder, familial glycerolemia, a chromosome X-linked genetic disorder, may mimic familial hypertriglyceridemia because most measurement techniques for triglycerides use the measurement of glycerol after enzymatic hydrolysis of triglycerides.[29] The diagnosis of familial hyperglycerolemia requires ultracentrifugation of plasma and analysis of glycerol.

The metabolic defect in familial hypertriglyceridemia is hepatic overproduction of VLDL (Fig. 39-4, part 4); the catabolism (uptake) of VLDL particles can be normal or reduced. Lipolysis by LPL appears not to be a limiting factor, although the triglyceride load, especially in the postprandial state, may limit processing of VLDL particles. The genetic basis of familial hypertriglyceridemia is unknown, and the candidate approach to find the gene or genes involved (apo B, LDL, apo CIII) has not yielded fruit thus far. Treatment is based first on lifestyle modifications, including withdrawal of hormones (estrogens and progesterone), limiting alcohol intake, reducing caloric intake, and increasing exercise. The decision to treat this disorder with medications depends on global cardiovascular risk.

An infrequent disorder characterized by severe elevation in plasma triglyceride levels (both VLDL and chylomicrons) is associated with a fat-rich diet, obesity, and poorly controlled diabetes. Recognized as type V hyperlipidemia, the pathogenesis is multifactorial and results from overproduction of both VLDL and chylomicrons and decreased catabolism of these particles.

FAMILIAL HYPERCHYLOMICRONEMIA (TYPE I HYPERLIPIDEMIA). This is a rare disorder of severe hypertriglyceridemia associated with elevations in fasting plasma triglycerides greater than 11.3 mmol/liter (>1000 mg/dl). These patients have recurrent bouts of pancreatitis and eruptive xanthomas. Interestingly, severe hypertriglyceridemia can also be associated with xerostomia, xerophthalmia, and behavioral abnormalities. The hypertriglyceridemia results from a markedly reduced or absent LPL activity or, more rarely, the absence of its activator, apo CII (Fig. 39–4, part 2).[30] These defects lead to a lack of hydrolysis of chylomicrons and VLDL and their accumulation in plasma, especially after meals. Extreme elevations of plasma triglycerides (>113 mmol/liter; >10 000 mg/dl) can result.

Plasma from a patient with very high triglycerides is milky white, and a clear band of chylomicrons can be seen on top of the plasma after it stands overnight in a refrigerator. Populations with a founder effect can have high prevalence of LPL mutations. At least 60 LPL mutations can cause LPL deficiency. LPL_{188}, $LPL_{asn291ser}$, and LPL_{207} are frequently associated hyperchylomicronemia. Heterozygotes for the disorder tend to have an increase in fasting plasma triglycerides and smaller, denser LDL particles. Many patients with complete LPL deficiency present in childhood fail to thrive and have recurrent bouts of pancreatitis. To underscore the importance of LPL's role, the LPL knockout mouse leads to a perinatal lethal phenotype.[31] The treatment of acute pancreatitis includes intravenous hydration and avoidance of fat in the diet (including in parenteral nutrition). Plasma filtration is required only rarely. Chronic treatment includes avoidance of alcohol and dietary fats. To make the diet more palatable, short-chain fatty acids (which are not incorporated in chylomicrons) can be used to supplement the diet.

TYPE III HYPERLIPOPROTEINEMIA. Type III hyperlipoproteinemia, also referred to as *dysbetalipoproteinemia* or *broad beta disease*, is a rare genetic lipoprotein disorder characterized by an accumulation in plasma of remnant lipoprotein particles. On lipoprotein agarose gel electrophoresis, a typical pattern of a broad band between the pre-beta (VLDL) and beta (LDL) lipoproteins is observed, hence the name "broad beta disease." Patients with this disease clearly have increased cardiovascular risk. The clinical presentation consists of pathognomonic tuberous xanthomas and palmar striated xanthomas. The lipoprotein profile shows increased cholesterol and triglyceride levels and reduced HDL cholesterol. Remnant lipoproteins (partly catabolized chylomicrons and VLDL) accumulate in plasma and accumulate cholesterol esters. The defect is due to abnormal apo E, which does not bind to hepatic receptors using apo E as a ligand (Fig. 39–4, part 3).[32] The ratio of VLDL cholesterol to triglycerides, normally less than 0.7 mmol/liter (<0.30 mg/dl), is elevated in patients with type III hyperlipoproteinemia, owing to cholesteryl ester enrichment of remnant particles. The diagnosis includes plasma ultracentrifugation for lipoprotein separation, lipoprotein electrophoresis, and apo E phenotyping or genotyping. Patients with type III hyperlipoproteinemia have the apo E2/2 phenotype or genotype. There are three common alleles for apo E: apo E2, E3, and E4. The apo E2 allele has markedly decreased binding to the apo B/E receptor.

In a normal population, the prevalence of the apo E2/2 phenotype is approximately 0.7 to 1.0 percent. Type III hyperlipoproteinemia occurs in approximately 1 percent of subjects bearing the apo E2/2 phenotype. The reasons for the relative rarity of type III dyslipoproteinemia are not fully understood. As discussed previously, a second "hit" is thought to impart the full expression of the disorder. Other rare mutations of the apo E gene can cause type III hyperlipoproteinemia.[32] Apo E-deficient mice currently serve as a model for the study of atherosclerosis.[13] In general, type III dyslipoproteinemia responds well to dietary therapy, correction of other metabolic abnormalities (diabetes, obesity), and, in cases requiring drug therapy, fibric acid derivatives or statins.

FAMILIAL COMBINED HYPERLIPIDEMIA. One of the most common familial lipoprotein disorders is familial combined hyperlipoproteinemia. Described initially in survivors of myocardial infarction, the definition of familial combined hyperlipoproteinemia has undergone several refinements. It is characterized by the presence of elevated total cholesterol and/or triglyceride levels based on arbitrary cut-points in several members of the same family. Advances in analytical techniques have added the measurement of LDL cholesterol and, in some cases, apo B levels. Because of the lack of a clear-cut clinical or biochemical marker, considerable overlap exists between familial combined hyperlipoproteinemia, familial dyslipidemic hypertension, the metabolic syndrome, and hyperapobetalipoproteinemia. Genetic heterogeneity probably underlies familial combined hyperlipoproteinemia, which has a prevalence of approximately 1 in 50 and accounts for 10 to 20 percent of patients with premature CAD.[33] The condition has few clinical signs; corneal arcus, xanthomas, and xanthelasmas occur infrequently. The biochemical abnormalities include elevation of plasma total and LDL cholesterol levels (>90th to 95th percentile) and/or an elevation of plasma triglycerides (>90th to 95th percentile)—a type IIb lipoprotein phenotype, often in correlation with low HDL cholesterol and elevated apo B levels; small, dense LDL particles are seen frequently. For a diagnosis of familial combined hyperlipoproteinemia, the disorder must be identified in at least one first-degree relative. The underlying metabolic disorder appears to be hepatic overproduction of apo B–containing lipoproteins, delayed postprandial triglyceride-rich lipoprotein clearance, and increased flux of free fatty acids (FFA) to the liver.

Experimental data have shown that hepatic apo B secretion is substrate driven, the most important substrates being FFA and cholesteryl esters. Increased delivery of FFA to the liver, as occurs in states of insulin resistance, leads to increased hepatic apo B secretion (see Chap. 40). Familial combined hyperlipoproteinemia has complex genetics. It was initially considered an autosomal codominant trait; modifying factors include gender, age of onset, and comorbid states such as obesity, lack of exercise, and diet. Initial reports of linkage with the apo AI-CIII-AIV and LPL genes remain unsubstantiated. A novel locus on chromosome 1 in Finnish families currently appears to be a promising candidate gene related to familial combined hyperlipoproteinemia.[34]

Recent reports of the acylation-stimulating protein (ASP), also known as complement C3desARG pathway, suggests that abnormal peripheral uptake of FFA may underlie some cases of familial combined hyperlipoproteinemia and the insulin-resistance metabolic syndrome.[35] A putative receptor for ASP has been identified recently as the orphan receptor C2L5, the complement C5 receptor that also binds complement C3desARG.[36] Abnormal binding of ASP to peripheral cells has been reported in subjects with familial combined hyperlipoproteinemia. Abnormal ASP binding causes decreased uptake of FFAs into adipocytes and subsequent increased flux of FFAs to the liver (see Fig. 39–5D). FFAs are a major substrate for hepatic apo B-containing lipoprotein assembly and secretion.

High-Density Lipoproteins

Reduced plasma levels of HDL cholesterol consistently correlate with the development or presence of CAD (see Chap. 36). Most cases of reduced HDL cholesterol are secondary to elevated plasma triglycerides or apo B levels and often keep company with other features of the metabolic syndrome. Primary forms of reduced HDL cholesterol have been identified in cases of premature CAD and helped shed light on the complex metabolism of HDL particles. Genetic disorders of HDL can result from decreased production or abnormal maturation and increased catabolism. Genetic lipoprotein disorders leading to moderate to severe elevations in plasma triglycerides cause a reduction in HDL cholesterol levels. Familial hyperchylomicronemia, familial hypertriglyceridemia, and familial combined hyperlipoproteinemia are all associated with reduced HDL cholesterol levels. In complex disorders of lipoprotein metabolism such as familial combined hyperlipidemia, the metabolic syndrome, and common forms of hypertriglyceridemia, several factors most likely correlate to low HDL cholesterol level. Plasma triglycerides and HDL cholesterol levels vary inversely. For several reasons, patients with elevated apo B levels also have reduced HDL cholesterol levels. First, decreased lipolysis of triglyceride-rich lipoproteins (each VLDL contains one molecule of apo B) decrease the substrate (phospholipids) available for HDL maturation. Second, triglyceride enrichment of HDL increases their catabolic rate and hence reduces their plasma concentration. Third, exchange of lipids between HDL and triglyceride-rich lipoprotein is reduced, leading to a more rapid disappearance of HDL from plasma.[37] The inverse relationship between HDL cholesterol levels and plasma triglycerides reflects the interdependency of the metabolism of triglyceride-rich lipoproteins and HDL particles.

APO AI GENE DEFECTS. Primary defects affecting production of HDL particles consist predominantly of apo AI-CIII-AIV gene defects. More than 46 mutations affect the structure of apo AI,[38] leading to a marked reduction in HDL cholesterol levels. Not all of these defects are associated with premature cardiovascular disease. Clinical presentations can vary from extensive atypical xanthomatosis and corneal infiltration of lipids to no manifestations at all. Treatment of these apo AI gene defects generally fails to raise HDL cholesterol levels. Other mutations of apo AI lead to increased catabolic rate of apo AI and may not be associated with cardiovascular disease. One such mutation, apo AI_{Milano} (apo $AI_{Arg173Cys}$), may be associated with longevity despite very low HDL levels.[38]

LCAT, CETP DEFICIENCY. Genetic defects in the HDL-processing enzymes give rise to interesting phenotypes. Deficiencies of LCAT, the enzyme that catalyzes the formation of cholesteryl esters in plasma, cause corneal infiltration of neutral lipids and hematological abnormalities due to abnormal constitution of red blood cell membranes. LCAT deficiency can lead to an entity called "fish eye disease" because of the characteristic pattern of corneal infiltration observed in affected individuals.[39]

Patients without CETP have very elevated HDL cholesterol levels, enriched in cholesteryl esters. Because CETP facilitates the transfer of HDL cholesteryl esters into triglyceride-rich lipoproteins, a deficiency of this enzyme causes accumulation of cholesteryl esters within HDL particles. CETP deficiency is not associated with premature CAD but may not afford protection against CAD.[40,41]

TANGIER DISEASE AND FAMILIAL HIGH-DENSITY LIPOPROTEIN DEFICIENCY. A rare disorder of HDL deficiency was identified in a proband from the Chesapeake Bay island of Tangier in the United States. The proband, whose sister was also affected, had markedly enlarged yellow tonsils and nearly absent HDL cholesterol levels, an entity now called *Tangier disease*. The cellular defect in Tangier disease consists of a reduced cellular cholesterol efflux in skin fibroblasts and macrophages from affected subjects.[42] A more common entity, familial HDL deficiency, was also found to result from decreased cellular cholesterol. The genetic defect in Tangier disease and in familial HDL deficiency results from mutations at the ATP binding cassette A1 gene (*ABCA1*) that encodes the ABCA1 transporter (see Fig. 39–5B).[43-45] At least 50 mutations have been reported within ABCA1, causing Tangier disease (homozygous or compound heterozygous mutations) or familial HDL deficiency (heterozygous mutations). Although subjects with Tangier disease and familial HDL deficiency are at increased risk for CAD, their very low levels of LDL cholesterol appear to have a protective effect. ABCA1 appears to shuttle from the late endosomal compartment to the plasma membrane and act as a membrane-bound transporter of phospholipids (and possibly cholesterol) onto acceptor proteins such as apo AI and apo E. Hydroxysterols regulate ABCA1 via the LXR/RXR nuclear receptor pathway. ABCA1 undergoes phosphorylation via protein kinase A and acts as a receptor for apo AI.

OTHER CHOLESTEROL TRANSPORT DEFECTS. Niemann-Pick type C disease is a disorder of lysosomal cholesterol transport. In patients with Niemann-Pick type C disease, mental retardation and neurological manifestations occur frequently. The cellular phenotype involves markedly decreased cholesterol esterification and cellular cholesterol transport defect to the Golgi apparatus. Unlike Tangier disease/familial HDL deficiency, the cellular defect in Niemann-Pick type C disease appears proximal to the transport of cholesterol to the plasma membrane. The gene for Niemann-Pick type C disease (*NPC1*) has been mapped to 18q21 and the gene codes for a 1278–amino acid protein, the role of which appears to be involved in cholesterol shuttling between the late endosomal pathway and the plasma membrane. The NPC1 gene product shares homology with the morphogen receptor *patched* and the SREBP cleavage activating protein (SCAP).[46] Niemann-Pick type I disease (subtypes A and B), caused by mutations at the sphingomyelin phosphodiesterase-1 (*SMPD-1*) gene, is associated with a low HDL cholesterol level. The *SMPD-1* gene codes for a lysosomal (acidic) and secretory sphingomyelinase. The cause of the low HDL cholesterol level in Niemann-Pick A and B patients appears to be due to a decrease in LCAT reaction because of abnormal HDL constituents.[47]

Secondary Causes of Hyperlipidemia and the Metabolic Syndrome

Several clinical disorders lead to alterations in lipoprotein status (Table 39–5).

HORMONAL CAUSES. Hypothyroidism, a not infrequent cause of secondary lipoprotein disorders, often manifests with elevated LDL cholesterol, triglycerides, or both. An elevated level of thyroid-stimulating hormone is key to the diagnosis, and the lipoprotein abnormalities often revert to normal after correction of thyroid status. Rarely, hypothyroidism may uncover a genetic lipoprotein disorder such as type III hyperlipidemia. Estrogens can elevate plasma triglycerides and HDL cholesterol levels, probably because of increases in both hepatic VLDL and apo AI production. In postmenopausal women, estrogens may reduce LDL cholesterol by 0 to 15 percent. The use of estrogens for the treatment of lipoprotein disorders is no longer recommended because of the slight increase in cardiovascular risk with prolonged use of estrogens in the postmenopausal period (see Chaps. 42 and 73).[48a] Rarely, pregnancy is associated with severe increases in plasma triglycerides, on a background of lipoprotein lipase deficiency. Such cases present a serious threat to mother and child and must be referred to specialized centers. Male sex hormones and anabolic steroids can increase hepatic lipase activity and have been used in the treatment of hypertriglyceridemia in men. Growth hormone can reduce LDL cholesterol and augment HDL cholesterol but is not recommended in the treatment of lipoprotein disorders.

METABOLIC CAUSES. The most frequent secondary cause of dyslipoproteinemia is probably the constellation of metabolic abnormalities seen in patients with the metabolic syndrome (see Chaps. 40 and 42). The finding of increased visceral fat (abdominal obesity), elevated blood pressure, and peripheral insulin resistance often clusters with increased plasma triglycerides and a reduced HDL cholesterol level. Overt diabetes, especially type 2 diabetes, frequently elevates plasma triglycerides and reduces HDL cholesterol. These abnormalities have prognostic implications in patients with type 2 diabetes. Poor control of diabetes, obesity, and moderate to severe hyperglycemia can yield severe hypertriglyceridemia with chylomicronemia and increased VLDL cholesterol levels. Subjects with juvenile diabetes can also have severe hypertriglyceridemia when the diabetes is poorly controlled. Familial lipodystrophy (complete or partial) may be associated with increased VLDL secretion. Dunnigan

TABLE 39–5 Secondary Causes of Dyslipoproteinemias

Metabolic	Diabetes Lipodystrophy Glycogen storage disorders
Renal	Chronic renal failure Glomerulonephritis
Hepatic	Obstructive liver disease Cirrhosis
Hormonal	Estrogens Progesterones Growth hormone Thyroid disorders (hypothyroidism) Corticosteroids
Lifestyle	Physical inactivity Obesity Diet rich in fats, saturated fats Alcohol intake
Medications	Retinoic acid derivatives Glucocorticoids Exogenous estrogens Thiazide diuretics Beta-adrenergic blockers (selective) Testosterone Immunosuppresive medications (cyclosporine) Antiviral medications (human immunodeficiency virus protease inhibitors)

lipodystrophy, a genetic disorder with features of the metabolic syndrome, is caused by mutations within the Lamin A/C gene and is associated with limb-girdle fat atrophy. Excess plasma triglycerides often accompany glycogen storage disorders.

RENAL DISORDERS. In subjects with glomerulonephritis and protein-losing nephropathies, a marked increase in secretion of hepatic lipoproteins can raise LDL cholesterol levels, which may approach the levels seen in subjects with familial hypercholesterolemia. By contrast, patients with chronic renal failure have a pattern of hypertriglyceridemia with reduced HDL cholesterol. Patients with end-stage renal disease, including those on hemodialysis or chronic ambulatory peritoneal dialysis, have a poor prognosis and accelerated atherosclerosis and should undergo aggressive treatment of lipoprotein disorders. After organ transplantation, the immunosuppressive regimen (glucocorticoids and cyclosporine) typically elevates triglycerides and reduces HDL cholesterol levels. Because transplant patients generally have an increase in cardiovascular risk, a secondary hyperlipidemia may warrant treatment. Patients receiving the combination of statin plus cyclosporine merit careful dose titrations and monitoring for myopathy.

LIVER DISEASE. Obstructive liver disease, especially primary biliary cirrhosis may lead to the formation of an abnormal lipoprotein termed *lipoprotein-x*. This type of lipoprotein is found in cases of LCAT deficiency and consists of an LDL-like particle but with a marked reduction in cholesteryl esters. Extensive xanthoma formation on the face and palmar areas can result from accumulation of lipoprotein-x.

LIFESTYLE. Factors contributing to obesity, such as an imbalance between caloric intake and energy expenditure, lack of physical activity, and a diet rich in saturated fats and refined sugars, contribute in large part to the lipid and lipoprotein lipid levels within a population (see Chaps. 36 and 41).

MEDICATION. Several medications can alter lipoproteins. Thiazide diuretics can increase plasma triglyceride levels. Beta blockers, especially non-beta-1 selective, increase triglycerides and lower HDL cholesterol levels. Retinoic acid and estrogens can increase triglyceride levels, sometimes dramatically. Corticosteroids and immunosuppressive agents can increase plasma triglyceride levels and lower HDL cholesterol levels. Estrogens can increase plasma HDL cholesterol significantly and may also increase triglyceride concentrations.

In clinical practice, many dyslipoproteinemias, other than the genetic forms mentioned earlier, share an important environmental cause. Lifestyle changes (diet, exercise, reduction of abdominal obesity) should be the cornerstone of the treatment of most dyslipidemias. The effects of marked alterations in lifestyle, reduction in dietary fats, especially saturated fats, and exercise can lead to an improved cardiovascular prognosis. Translating these findings into practice, however, has been more difficult. For example, dietary manipulations as performed in a physician's office lead to relatively small reductions in plasma lipid and lipoprotein cholesterol levels (see Chaps. 36, 41, and 42).

Drugs that Affect Lipid Metabolism (Table 39–6)

Resins

The bile acid–binding resins interrupt the enterohepatic circulation of bile acids by inhibiting their reabsorption in the intestine (bile acids, which contain cholesterol, are more than 90 percent reabsorbed via this pathway). Currently, their main use is adjunctive therapy in patients with severe hypercholesterolemia due to increased LDL cholesterol. Since bile acid–binding resins are not absorbed systemically (they remain in the intestine and are eliminated in the stool), they are considered safe in children. Cholestyramine (Questran) is used in 4-gm unit doses as powder, and colestipol (Colestid) is used in 5-gm unit doses; a 1-gm tablet of colestipol is available. Effective doses range from 2 to 6 unit doses/day, always taken with meals. The most important side effects are predominantly gastrointestinal, with constipation, a sensation of fullness, and gastrointestinal discomfort. Hypertriglyceridemia can result from the use of these drugs. Decreased drug absorption dictates careful scheduling of medications 1 hour before or 3 hours after the patient takes bile acid–binding resins. Bile acid–binding resins can be used in combination with statins and/or cholesterol absorption inhibitors in cases of severe hypercholesterolemia.

TABLE 39–6 Current Lipid-Lowering Medications

Generic Name	Trade Name	Recommended Dose Range
Statins		
Atorvastatin	Lipitor	10-80 mg
Fluvastatin	Lescol	20-80 mg
Lovastatin	Mevacor	20-80 mg
Pravastatin	Pravachol	10-40 mg
Rosuvastatin	Crestor	10-40 mg
Simvastatin	Zocor	10-80 mg
Bile Acid Absorption Inhibitors		
Cholestyramine	Questran	2-24 gm
Colestipol	Colestid	5-30 gm
Colesevelam	WelChol	3.8-4.5 gm
Cholesterol Absorption Inhibitors		
Ezetimibe	Zetia (Ezetrol)	10 mg
Fibrates*		
Bezafibrate	Bezalip	400 mg
Fenofibrate	Tricor (Lipidil Micro)	67-200 mg
Gemfibrozil†	Lopid	600-1200 mg
Niacin‡		
Nicotinic acid		1-3 gm

*Avoid in patients with renal insufficiency.
†Not recommended in combination with statins.
‡Use with caution in patients with diabetes or glucose intolerance.

Hydroxymethylglutaryl–Coenzyme A Reductase Inhibitors (Statins)

Statins inhibit HMG-CoA reductase and prevent the formation of mevalonate, the rate-limiting step of sterol synthesis. To maintain cellular cholesterol homeostasis, expression of the LDL-R increases and the rate of cholesteryl ester formation declines. These homeostatic adjustments to HMG-CoA reductase inhibition increase LDL cholesterol clearance from plasma and decrease hepatic production of VLDL and LDL. In addition to blocking the synthesis of cholesterol, statins also interfere with the synthesis of lipid intermediates with important biological effects. In the cholesterol synthetic pathway, intermediate molecules of dimethylallyl pyrophosphate are metabolized by prenyl transferase into geranyl pyrophosphate and subsequently into farnesyl pyrophosphate. This step occurs before the formation of squalenes.[49] These intermediates, geranylgeranyl and farnesyl, are used for protein prenylation, a mechanism by which a lipid moiety attaches covalently to a protein, allowing anchoring into cell membranes and enhancing its biological activity. This is the case for the GTP-binding proteins Rho A, Rac, and Ras. Indeed, statins may increase HDL cholesterol in part by preventing the geranylgeranylation of Rho A and phosphorylation of perisome proliferator–activated receptor alpha (PPARα), a factor that regulates apo AI transcription.[49] Altered protein prenylation may also mediate some of the putative effects of statins not related to a reduction in LDL cholesterol levels.

Atherosclerosis is an inflammatory disease.[50] Statins decrease C-reactive protein, induce apoptosis in smooth muscle cells, alter collagen content of atherosclerotic plaques, alter endothelial function, and decrease the inflammatory component of plaques.[51,52] Some investigators argue that statins possess effects independent of their inhibition of HMG CoA reductase. In clinical practice, the role of these possible LDL-independent actions is difficult to assess. It remains speculative that clinically important differences exist in efficacy between statins for a given percentage reduction in LDL cholesterol.

Statins are generally well tolerated; side effects include reversible elevation in transaminases and myositis, which causes discontinuation of the drug in less than 1 percent of patients. The currently available drugs are fluvastatin (Lescol), 20 to 80 mg/day; lovastatin (Mevacor), 20 to 80 mg/day; pravastatin (Pravachol), 20 to 40 mg/day; simvastatin (Zocor), 10 to 80 mg/day; atorvastatin (Lipitor), 10 to 80 mg/day; and rosuvastatin (Crestor), 10 to 40 mg/day. Concomitant drugs that interfere with the metabolism of statins by inhibiting the cytochrome P450 3A4 and 2C9 systems can increase plasma concentrations of statins. These include antibiotics, antifungal medications, certain antiviral drugs, grapefruit juice, cyclosporine, amiodarone, and several others.

Cholesterol Absorption Inhibitors

The development of selective inhibitors of intestinal sterol absorption has significantly advanced the treatment of lipoprotein disorders. Ezetimibe is the first such compound. Ezetimibe appears to limit selective uptake of cholesterol and other sterols by intestinal epithelial cells, perhaps by interfering with the Niemann-Pick C1-like 1 protein 1.[8a] It is particularly indicated for patients with LDL cholesterol levels above target on maximally tolerated statin dose. Ezetimibe lowers LDL cholesterol by about 18 percent and is additive to the effect of statins.[53] Because ezetimibe also prevents the intestinal absorption of sitosterol, it might be the drug of choice in cases of sitosterolemia. The current dose of ezitimibe is 10 mg/day.

Fibric Acid Derivatives (Fibrates)

Three derivatives of fibric acid are currently available in the United States and two more are available in Canada and Europe. Gemfibrozil (Lopid) is used at a dose of 600 mg twice a day and is indicated in cases of hypertriglyceridemia and in the secondary prevention of cardiovascular diseases in patients with a low HDL cholesterol levels. These latter recommendations are based on the Veterans Administration HDL Intervention Trial (VA-HIT). Fenofibrate (Tricor, Lipidil Micro) is used to treat hypertriglyceridemia and combined hyperlipoproteinemia. The dose is 200 mg/day and a new formulation is available to vary the dose from 67 mg (especially in cases of renal failure) to 267 mg/day. Clofibrate (Atromid) is still available in some centers, although its use has declined since the introduction of newer molecules. Ciprofibrate (Lypanthyl, Lipanor) and bezafibrate (Bezalip) are more widely used in Europe. The main indications for the use of fibrates is hypertriglyceridemia when diet and lifestyle changes are not sufficient. Another indication is in the prevention of cardiovascular diseases in patients with elevated plasma triglycerides and low HDL cholesterol. The mechanism of action of fibrates involves interaction with the nuclear transcription factor PPARα that regulates the transcription of the LPL, apo CII, and apo AI genes. The side effects of fibrates include cutaneous manifestations, gastrointestinal effects (abdominal discomfort, increased bile lithogenicity), erectile dysfunction, elevated transaminases, interaction with oral anticoagulants, and elevated plasma homocysteine, especially with fenofibrate and, to a lesser extent, with bezafibrate.[54] Because fibrates augment LPL activity, LDL cholesterol levels may rise in patients with hypertriglyceridemia treated with this class of medications. Fibrates, especially gemfibrozil, can inhibit the glucuronidation of statins, and thus retard their elimination. For this reason, combination of gemfibrozil with statins may increase the risk of myotoxicity.

Nicotinic Acid (Niacin)

Niacin has been used for decades for the treatment of dyslipidemias and is particularly effective in increasing HDL cholesterol and lowering triglyceride levels. The effect of niacin on LDL cholesterol is more modest. Effective doses of niacin are in the range of 3000 mg/day, in three separate doses. It is preferable to use an escalating dose schedule to reach the full dose in 2 to 3 weeks rather than starting with the full dose. Slow-release forms of niacin decrease the side effect profile of the drug. Skin flushing can be attenuated by taking a daily aspirin. Niacin decreases the hepatic secretion of VLDL from the liver and decreased FFA mobilization for the periphery. Although niacin has been shown in the long-term follow-up of the Coronary Drug Project to decrease mortality at 15 years, its use has been hampered by significant and sometimes common minor side effects and much less frequent serious adverse actions, and by the development of statins. Side effects of niacin include flushing, hyperuricemia, hyperglycemia, hepatotoxicity, acanthosis nigricans, and gastritis. Close laboratory monitoring of side effects is warranted. Long-acting niacin has the advantage of a once- or twice-daily dosing schedule, but older preparations of slow-release niacin were potentially more hepatotoxic. Niacin effectively raises HDL cholesterol levels and, in combination with low-dose statin, can retard the angiographic progression of CAD and decrease adverse cardiac events.[55] Recent work has identified cell surface receptors for nicotinic acid that belong to the G-protein–coupled heptahelical superfamily. This discovery may speed the elucidation of the molecular mechanism of nicotinic acid's effects on lipid metabolism.[56,57]

Fish Oils

Fish oils are rich in polyunsaturated fatty acids such as eicosapentaenoic acid or docosahexaenoic acid, with the first double in the omega-3 position. These fatty acids lower plasma triglyceride levels and have antithrombotic properties. Although employed in the treatment of hypertriglyceridemia, their use is reserved in cases of severe hypertriglyceridemia refractory to conventional therapy. Fish oils decrease VLDL synthesis and decrease VLDL apo B. The response to fish oils depends on dose, requiring a daily intake of 10 to 15 gm of eicosapentaenoic acid or docosahexaenoic acid for a significant benefit on plasma triglyceride levels.

Phytosterols

Phytosterols are derivatives of cholesterol from plants and trees. They interfere with the formation of micelles in the intestine and prevent intestinal cholesterol absorption. They can be obtained as "neutraceuticals" or can be incorporated in soft margarines. The sterols may prove useful for the adjunctive management of lipoprotein disorders and are part of the therapeutic lifestyle change regimen in the current guidelines (see later).

Other Medications

Probucol was used as an antioxidant and had modest effects on plasma lipoprotein levels. The lack of conclusive evidence that probucol has beneficial effects and profound reduction in HDL levels and prolongation of QT interval led to its withdrawal. A recent study indicates that it may have a role in the prevention of restenosis after coronary angioplasty if used before the procedure.[58] Thyroxine is no longer used as a lipid modulator unless hypothyroidism has been documented.

Monitoring of Lipid Therapy

After initiation of medical therapy, the response should be checked within the first 3 months, along with transaminases and creatinine kinase. Thereafter, clinical judgment should dictate the interval between follow-up visits. Although frequent visits are probably not useful in the detection of serious side effects, they serve to encourage compliance and adherence to diet and lifestyle changes.

Clinical Trials of Drugs Affecting Lipid Metabolism

Numerous pathological, epidemiological, genetic, and interventional trials have validated the central tenet of the "lipid hypothesis," which proposes a causal relationship between dyslipidemia and atherogenesis and identifies lipid modification as a risk-reducing strategy for CHD (see Chap. 36). A number of small trials using dietary or drug therapies have demonstrated the angiographic benefit of managing elevated total cholesterol and LDL cholesterol. Early clinical trials using bile-acid sequestrants, fibrates, or nicotinic acid reported modest reductions in coronary risk with modest reductions in LDL cholesterol. We refer readers interested in these earlier trials to previous editions of this textbook.

The advent of the HMG-CoA reductase inhibitors, or statins, in the mid-1980s made possible more aggressive reduction of LDL cholesterol. By the late 1990s, several large-scale, prospective randomized trials with these drugs had reported robust reductions in relative cardiovascular risks, compared with placebo (Tables 39–7 and 39–8, Fig. 39–6).[59-63] This section discusses the more recently representative or in-progress trials in this area, in the context of some of the unanswered questions about the effects of cholesterol treatment. The focus on statin trials reflects the widespread contemporary interest and clinical success of this category of drugs. Ample reviews have considered the results of the older trials.

Treating High-Risk Patients

As the interaction of multiple coronary risk factors has received greater clinical importance, recommendations for clinical practice have increasingly embraced the concept of global risk management. In the 2001 U.S. Adult Treatment Panel (ATP III) guidelines, the patient's overall risk for developing CHD in the next 10 years determines the intensity of lipid intervention.[64] This global risk is calculated using an algorithm that considers not only total cholesterol but also HDL cholesterol, smoking, age, hypertension, and gender (see Chap. 36).

Because global risk assessment shifts emphasis away from abnormal lipids alone to the patient's overall risk profile, it raises an important issue for the future of lipid management. That is, should the decision to initiate lipid modification for cardiovascular risk reduction be based on high risk or high cholesterol? Recent trials have evaluated this question (Table 39–9).

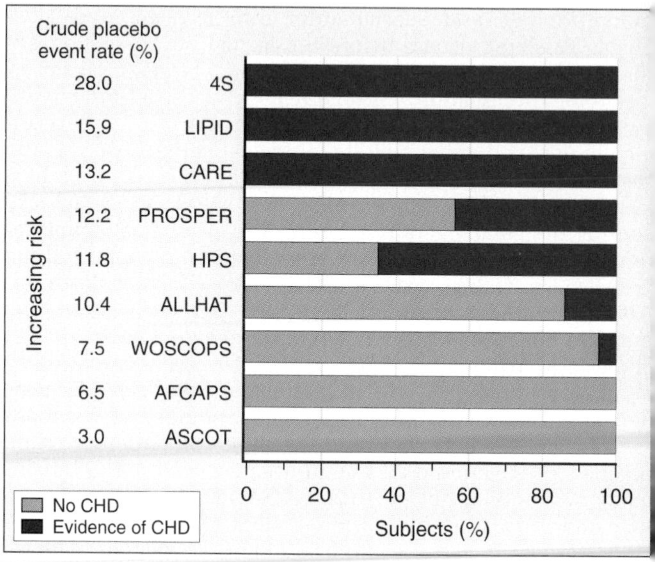

FIGURE 39–6 Clinical trials of statin therapy have demonstrated benefits in patients across the spectrum of coronary disease.

TABLE 39–7 Primary Prevention Trials of Statin Therapy

	WOSCOPS	AFCAPS/TexCAPS
N (% women)	6596 (0)	6605 (15)
Duration (yrs)	4.9	5.2
Intervention	Pravastatin, 40 mg/day	Lovastatin, 20-40 mg/day
Baseline lipids (mg/dl)		
Total cholesterol	272	221
LDL cholesterol	192	150
HDL cholesterol	44	36 men; 40 women
Triglycerides	164	158
% Lipid changes, treatment vs. placebo		
Total cholesterol	−20	−19
LDL cholesterol	−26	−26
HDL cholesterol	+5	+5
Triglycerides	−12	−13
Endpoints (% changes in risk), treatment vs. placebo		
Nonfatal MI/CHD death	**−31**	−25
Fatal/nonfatal MI	—	−40
Acute major coronary events	—	**−37**
Total mortality	−22	+3 (NS)
CHD mortality	−28	too few
Revascularizations	−37	−33
Stroke	−11 (NS)	—

AFCAPS/TexCAPS = Air Force/Texas Coronary Atherosclerosis Prevention Study; CHD = coronary heart disease; HDL = high-density lipoprotein; LDL = low-density lipoprotein; MI = myocardial infarction; NS = nonsignificant; WOSCOPS = West of Scotland Coronary Prevention Study; **bold** = study's primary endpoint; — = not reported.

TABLE 39–8 Secondary Prevention Trials of Statin Therapy

	4S	CARE	LIPID
N (% women)	4444 (19)	4159 (14)	9014 (17)
Duration (yrs)	5.4	5	6.1
Intervention	Simvastatin, 10-40 mg/day	Pravastatin, 40 mg/day	Pravastatin, 40 mg/day
Baseline lipids (mg/dl)			
Total cholesterol	261	209	218
LDL cholesterol	188	139	150
HDL cholesterol	46	39	36
Triglycerides	135	155	138
% Lipid changes, treatment vs. placebo			
Total cholesterol	−26	−20	−18
LDL cholesterol	−36	−28	−25
HDL cholesterol	+7	+5	+5
Triglycerides	−17	−14	−11
Endpoints (% changes in risk), treatment vs. placebo			
Nonfatal MI/CHD death	−34	**−24**	−24
Fatal/nonfatal MI	−42	−25	−24
Acute major coronary events	—	—	−29
Total mortality	**−30**	−9 (NS)	−22
CHD mortality	−42	−20	**−24**
Revascularizations	−37	−27	−20
Stroke	−30	−31	−19

CARE = Cholesterol and Recurrent Events; CHD = coronary heart disease; HDL = high-density lipoprotein; LDL = low-density lipoprotein; LIPID = Long-term Intervention with Pravastatin in Ischemic Disease; MI = myocardial infarction; NS = nonsignificant; 4S = Scandinavian Simvastatin Survival Study; **bold** = study's primary endpoint; — = not reported.

THE HEART PROTECTION STUDY. The Medical Research Council/British Heart Foundation Heart Protection Study (HPS) evaluated the role of statin therapy in at-risk patients for whom guidelines at the time would not have recommended drug intervention.[65] Participants in the HPS had increased risk for vascular disease, but many did not meet existing criteria for hypolipidemic therapy. The two-by-two factorial design of the HPS intended to analyze the effect of simvastatin, 40 mg/day, versus placebo with or without a combination of antioxidant vitamins (600 mg alpha tocopherol, 250 mg ascorbic acid, 20 mg beta carotene) on the risk of major vascular events.

Patients were selected on the basis of being at increased risk for CHD because of either the presence of documented coronary atherosclerosis or having risk factors considered to confer a level of risk equivalent to having CHD. The trial thus enrolled not only individuals with prior myocardial infarction, unstable or stable angina, coronary artery bypass grafting, or angioplasty eligible for randomization, but also patients with occlusive disease of noncoronary arteries, diabetes, or treated hypertension. The study included patients from 40 to 80 years of age and with total serum cholesterol concentrations of at least 135 mg/dl (3.5 mmol/liter).

The combination of antioxidant vitamins did not affect morbidity or mortality. Simvastatin treatment, on the other hand, reduced the risk for any major vascular event by 24 percent ($p < 0.0001$), with an absolute risk reduction of 5.4 percent (25.2 percent in the placebo group minus 19.8 percent in the simvastatin group). The all-cause mortality rate fell by 13 percent ($p = 0.0003$), with a significant 17 percent reduction ($p < 0.0001$) in deaths attributed to any vascular cause. There was no increase in noncardiac causes of mortality, such as neoplasia, respiratory disease, or other nonvascular deaths.

The HPS population included individuals who would qualify as traditional candidates for primary prevention because of their history of no previous coronary event. A substantial number of individuals without known CHD (n = 7150) had a CHD-equivalent risk profile: diabetes (n = 3982), peripheral vascular disease (n = 2701), or cerebrovascular disease

TABLE 39–9 Trials of Statin Therapy in High-Risk Patients

	HPS	ALL-HAT LLT	ASCOT LLA	PROSPER
N (% women)	20536 (24.7)	10355 (48.8)	10305 (18.8)	5804 (51.7)
Duration (yrs)	5	4.8	3.3	3.2
Percent with Hx of CVD or CHD	65%	14%	14%	44%
Statin crossover rate	17%	26.1%	9%	10%
Intervention	Simvastatin, 40 mg/day vs. placebo	Pravastatin, 20-40 mg/day vs. usual care	Atorvastatin, 10 mg/day vs. placebo	Pravastatin, 40 mg/day vs. placebo
Baseline lipids, mg/dL (mmol/liter)				
Total cholesterol	228 (5.9)	224 (5.8)	213 (5.5)	221 (5.7)
LDL cholesterol	132 (3.4)	146 (3.8)	132 (3.4)	147 (3.8)
HDL cholesterol	41 (1.06)	48 (1.2)	50 (1.3)	50 (1.3)
Triglycerides	124 (1.4)	152 (1.7)	152 (1.7)	58 (1.5)
% Lipid changes, treatment vs. placebo				
Total cholesterol	−20	−10	−24	NR
LDL cholesterol	−29	−17	−35	−34
HDL cholesterol	+3	+1	0	+5
Triglycerides	−21	—	−17	−13
Endpoints (% changes in risk), treatment vs. placebo				
Major cardiovascular events	**−24**	—	—	**+15**
Nonfatal MI/CHD death	−27	NS	**+36**	−19
Fatal/nonfatal MI	—	—	—	—
Total mortality	−13	**NS**	NS	NS
CHD mortality	−17	NS	NS	−24
Revascularizations	−24	—	—	NS
Stroke	−25	NS	−27	NS

HPS = Heart Protection Study; ALL-HAT LLT = Antihypertensive and Lipid-Lowering Treatment to Prevent Heart Attack Trial; ASCOT LLA = Anglo-Scandinavian Cardiac Outcomes Trial Lipid Lowering Arm; PROSPER = Prospective Study of Pravastatin in the Elderly at Risk; LDL = low-density lipoprotein; HDL = high-density lipoprotein; MI = myocardial infarction; CHD = coronary heart disease; NS = nonsignificant; **bold** = study's primary endpoint; — = not reported.

(n = 1820). Statin treatment exhibited clinical benefit regardless of the presence of known vascular disease, baseline LDL cholesterol level, age, or sex.

PROSPER. Coronary and cerebrovascular atherosclerosis in the elderly is a growing clinical problem because of the population's increasing longevity. Older chronological age in and of itself should not exclude patients from receiving therapy, especially if an otherwise healthy older patient's remaining years of life could benefit from prevention of the morbidity associated with a coronary event. Indeed, age is one of the most potent cardiovascular risk factors.

The Prospective Evaluation of Pravastatin in the Elderly (PROSPER) assessed the impact of treatment with pravastatin 40 mg/day versus placebo in 5804 men and women aged 70 to 82 years of age with a history of vascular disease (coronary, cerebrovascular, or peripheral vascular) or a risk factor profile consistent with high risk (smoking, hypertension, or diabetes).[66] Participants in this study had plasma total cholesterol levels between 155 and 350 mg/dl (4.0 to 9.0 mmol/liter) and triglyceride concentrations less than 530 mg/dl (6.0 mmol/liter). Women accounted for more than half of the individuals in PROSPER.

The mean follow-up was 3.2 years and the composite primary endpoint included coronary death, nonfatal myocardial infarction, and fatal or nonfatal stroke. Pravastatin treatment reduced the relative risk for this endpoint significantly by 15 percent ($p = 0.014$) and for CHD death by 24 percent ($p = 0.043$). The treatment showed similar benefit across many subgroups: those with versus those without prior vascular disease; men versus women; tertiles of baseline LDL cholesterol; current smokers versus nonsmokers; and those with and those without a history of hypertension. Participants in the lowest tertile of baseline HDL cholesterol (<1.11 mmol/liter) experienced greater benefit than those in the higher tertiles.

Lipid-modifying treatment had no effect on the risk for stroke or on cognitive function, both of which are important endpoints in an older population. There were no safety differences between pravastatin and placebo, except for a greater number of new cancer diagnoses in pravastatin patients that is inconsistent with the overall clinical experience with this drug and may have arisen from recruitment of patients with occult disease. Despite these concerns, as a whole, the results of PROSPER favor treatment of the elderly to reduce CHD risk and affirm the findings of subgroup analyses from earlier statin trials.

ALLHAT (LIPID-LOWERING ARM). The large Antihypertensive and Lipid-Lowering Treatment to Prevent Heart Attack Trial (ALLHAT) sought to determine whether cholesterol lowering with open-label pravastatin 20 to 40 mg/day (plus resin, if needed) would reduce total mortality in 10,355 moderately hypercholesterolemic, hypertensive men and women, aged 55 years or older, with at least one other CHD risk factor, as compared with usual care.[67] The ALLHAT patients met lipid criteria of a LDL cholesterol level of 120 to 189 mg/dl (3.1 to 5 mmol/liter) (or 100 to 129 mg/dl [2.6 to 3.3 mmol/liter] in those with CHD) and triglycerides less than 350 mg/dl (<3.9 mmol/liter).

In contrast with other studies in this section, ALLHAT reported no benefit and no harm of treatment compared with usual care on any study endpoint. Several aspects of this trial may help explain this null finding.[68] The study may have been underpowered because of difficulties related to patient recruitment. The trial was open-labeled, and there was declining adherence in the pravastatin group and a high crossover rate to statin therapy in the usual-care group (by 6 years, more than 25 percent of these patients were receiving a statin). Indeed, the absolute difference in total cholesterol between the pravastatin and the usual-care group by the end of the trial was only 9.6 percent, which was approximately half of the reduction achieved in other statin trials.

ASCOT. The lipid-lowering arm of the Anglo-Scandinavian Cardiac Outcomes Trial (ASCOT) assessed the clinical effect of atorvastatin, 10 mg/day, versus placebo in 10,305 hypertensive patients with a total cholesterol level of less than 250 mg/dl (6.5 mmol/liter) and a high-risk profile.[6] Although the trial excluded individuals with previous myocardial infarction, current angina, or cerebrovascular disease within 3 months before randomization, the randomized patients had evidence of other vascular disease or CHD risk equivalents (left ventricular hypertrophy, other electrocardiographic abnormalities, peripheral arterial disease, previous cerebrovascular disease, diabetes), or several other CHD risk factors.

Originally planned to have a follow-up period of 5 years the ASCOT ended early after a median follow-up of 3.3 years after 100 primary endpoint events had occurred in the atorvastatin group compared with 154 in the placebo group. The relative risk reduction was 36 percent ($p = 0.0005$), and the benefit became apparent within a year of the study's initiation. Benefit was similar across prespecified subgroups. Atorvastatin reduced the relative risk for stroke by 27 percent ($p = 0.024$) and for total cardiovascular events by 21 percent ($p = 0.0005$). Total mortality and adverse events did not differ between the treatment groups.

The ASCOT and ALLHAT are the only two published lipid-lowering clinical trials performed in hypertensive patients. The statin crossover rate in the placebo group was only 9 percent in ASCOT compared with approximately 26 percent in the usual-care group of ALLHAT. Adherence to the study drug was also better in ASCOT than in ALLHAT.

CARDS. Because of their high risk for developing CHD, diabetic patients warrant aggressive lipid modification, according to U.S. guidelines (see Chap. 40). However, few trials have evaluated the effects of lipid modification on clinical endpoints in this population, and the evidence of benefit derives largely from subgroup analyses. The Collaborative Atorvastatin Diabetes Study (CARDS) is a multicenter, randomized, placebo-controlled, primary-prevention study in patients with type 2 diabetes.[70] Entry criteria included not only diabetes but also at least one other CHD risk factor: current smoking, hypertension, retinopathy, or micro- or macroalbuminuria. The trial enrolled individuals with LDL cholesterol levels less than 160 mg/dl (4.14 mmol/liter) and triglycerides less than 600 mg/dl (6.78 mmol/liter). The study included 2838 men and women, 40 to 75 years of age. The trial utilized a fixed dosage of atorvastatin of 10 mg/day compared with placebo. The primary efficacy parameter is the time from randomization to the occurrence of a first primary endpoint event, which may include major coronary events, revascularizations, stroke, unstable angina, or resuscitated cardiac arrest. The study was stopped prematurely for benefit.[71]

Does Lipid Lowering Benefit Patients with Acute Coronary Syndromes?

Earlier secondary prevention statin studies generally selected patients who were at least 3 to 6 months postcoronary event and stabilized. Substantial interest has turned to the question of statin treatment in the period immediately following an acute coronary syndrome. Conflicting observational data, however, have reported either a beneficial or a null effect of early statin treatment on subsequent coronary risk.[72,73]

The Myocardial Ischemia Reduction and Aggressive Cholesterol Lowering (MIRACL) trial examined the premise that early and intensive treatment with high-dose atorvastatin therapy begun immediately after the onset of an acute coronary event might produce beneficial clinical effects in a much larger cohort (n = 3086).[74] The composite primary endpoint of MIRACL included nonfatal acute myocardial infarction, cardiac arrest, or symptomatic myocardial ischemia. Atorvastatin resulted in a modest albeit statistically significant 16 percent improvement in relative risk for the primary endpoint ($p = 0.048$). The major effect of early atorvastatin was a reduction in recurrent myocardial ischemia, which was decreased by 26 percent ($p = 0.02$). While statistically significant, the clinical benefits observed in MIRACL were not as robust as those seen in the larger and longer 4S and LIPID trials. However, MIRACL does provide reassurance regarding the safety of aggressive lipid lowering with a statin in the immediate aftermath of an acute coronary event.

Several other trials in this emerging area have been completed or are in progress. The Aggrastat-to-Zocor (A-2-Z) study will first randomize postacute coronary event patients to treatment with tirofiban and unfractionated versus low-molecular-weight heparin, then re-randomize them to receive either simvastatin, 40 to 80 mg/day, versus diet plus simvastatin, 20 mg/day.[75] Its results are expected in 2004. The Pravastatin or Atorvastatin Evaluation and Infection Therapy (PROVE-IT) trial compared pravastatin, 40 mg/day, with atorvastatin, 80 mg/day, in 4162 postacute coronary event patients.[76] This study also has an antibiotic treatment arm. The lipid-lowering arm of PROVE-IT showed that in patients who have recently survived an acute coronary syndrome, an intensive statin regimen that yielded a median LDL cholesterol of 62 mg/dl (1.60 mmol/liter) provided greater protection against death or major cardiovascular events than less aggressive therapy that lowered LDL cholesterol to a median of 95 mg/dl (2.46 mmol/liter), a level below the upper limit recommended by ATP-III as a target for this category of patients. Thus, PROVE-IT suggests that ACS survivors benefit from early statin treatment to levels of LDL cholesterol considerably below current target levels.[76a]

Medical Therapy Versus Revascularization

The Atorvastatin versus Revascularization Treatment (AVERT) trial evaluated the potential benefits of aggressive lipid lowering with open-label atorvastatin, 80 mg/day, versus usual care on ischemic events in a cohort of 341 patients with stable atherosclerosis who were scheduled to undergo an elective percutaneous revascularization procedure.[77] Follow-up was 18 months. Qualification requirements included at least one native coronary vessel with 50 percent or greater stenosis and an LDL cholesterol level in excess of 115 mg/dl. Exclusion criteria included triglycerides in excess of 500 mg/dl, ejection fraction less than 40 percent, inability to complete 4 minutes of exercise on a standard Bruce protocol, left main or triple vessel coronary atherosclerosis, or recent unstable angina or myocardial infarction (<14 days).

The composite primary endpoint in the AVERT trial encompassed the incidence of ischemic events, defined as cardiac death, resuscitation after cardiac arrest, nonfatal myocardial infarction, stroke, worsening angina, or revascularization (coronary artery bypass graft or repeat angioplasty). The patients randomized to usual care received percutaneous coronary interventions, and approximately one-third of the patients with treated lesions underwent placement of a coronary stent. The patients treated with angioplasty could receive hypolipidemic therapy as part of usual care. Lipid-lowering drugs were administered in 73 percent of patients in this group at some time during the follow-up (71 percent of the total group received statins). Despite this crossover, the atorvastatin group had lower total cholesterol, LDL cholesterol, and triglycerides relative to usual care.

A total of 22 ischemic events occurred in the group randomized to receive aggressive lipid-lowering therapy, compared with 37 events in the usual-care group (36 percent reduction; $p = 0.048$). The difference in the treatment arms tended toward statistical significance, since the significance level was adjusted to 0.045 because of the performance of two interim analyses. Atorvastatin treatment significantly delayed the time to the first event ($p = 0.027$) compared with usual care, but 54 percent of angioplasty patients compared with 41 percent of atorvastatin patients had improvement of Canadian Cardiovascular Society (CCS) classification of angina symptoms ($p = 0.009$). Seventeen serious adverse events were reported in the atorvastatin group, although none were attributed to atorvastatin. Twenty-eight of the patients in the angioplasty group had serious adverse events; six of these patients had events attributable to the angioplasty.

These results support a strategy of aggressive lipid-lowering therapy to complement revascularization in patients with stable angina. The multicenter, randomized Clinical Outcomes Utilizing Revascularization and Aggressive Drug Evaluation (COURAGE) trial may elucidate the issue further through its investigation of whether combining percutaneous coronary intervention with maximal statin intervention will provide greater benefits than statin intervention alone in more than 3000 patients.[78] The COURAGE protocol targets global risk reduction, emphasizing (1) lifestyle modification; (2) maximal use of drugs to lower blood pressure to Joint National Committee on Prevention, Detection, Evaluation, and Treatment of High Blood Pressure (JNC) VI goals; (3) maximal use of simvastatin, 80 mg/day, to lower cholesterol to below current US goals for secondary prevention; and (4) maximal use of drug to alleviate anginal symptoms with or without the best interventional devices to conduct percutaneous coronary intervention. Patients will be treated to a target LDL cholesterol level of 60 to 85 mg/dl and will be followed for a minimum of 3 years. The main outcome will be all-cause mortality or nonfatal myocardial infarction.

What Are the Optimal Limits of Therapy?

No statin clinical trial has rigorously identified a threshold below which LDL cholesterol reduction was not beneficial. Therefore, the optimal LDL cholesterol goal for therapy remains unclear. The Reversal of Atherosclerosis with Lipitor (REVERSAL) trial used intravascular ultrasonography to examine the effect of differing degrees of lipid-lowering on plaque volume. Over 18 months, patients treated with pravastatin (40 mg/day) had a 25 percent drop in LDL cholesterol, and those randomized to atorvastatin (80 mg/day) had a 46 percent decrease, to an average LDL cholesterol level of 79 mg/dl. The more aggressive lipid-lowering regimen reduced lesion volume.[78a] Trials that are tracking clinical events in patients treated to different levels of LDL cholesterol are currently underway. The Study of the Effectiveness of Additional Reductions in Cholesterol and Homocysteine (SEARCH) will examine the effect of high-dosage (80 mg/day) versus low-dosage simvastatin (20 mg/day), with or without folic acid, on clinical endpoints in approximately 12,000 CHD patients. Participants had total cholesterol greater than 135 mg/dl, or greater than 174 mg/dl if no previous statin use, and the high-dosage group will have an LDL cholesterol goal of 70 mg/dl compared with a goal of 100 mg/dl in the low-dosage patients. Will a greater reduction in LDL cholesterol using high-dose therapy translate into greater clinical benefit? The primary efficacy endpoint will be the effect of such treatment on the incidence of CHD death and nonfatal myocardial infarction. The secondary objective will be to assess the effect of high-dose compared with low-dose therapy on stroke, other mortality, and conditions requiring hospitalization. The use of folic acid supplementation will test the hypothesis that reducing homocysteine will reduce CHD risk.[79]

Similarly, the Treating to New Targets (TNT) trial will assess whether lowering LDL cholesterol levels beyond current recommendations with high-dosage versus low-dosage atorvastatin in patients with clinically evident CHD will lower clinical coronary event rates.[80] Patients aged 35 to 75 years with prior myocardial infarction, prior or present angina with objective evidence of atherosclerotic CHD, or prior coronary revascularization procedures and LDL cholesterol and triglyceride levels of 130 to 250 mg/dl (3.36 to 6.46 mmol/liter) and less than 600 mg/dl (6.77 mmol/liter), respectively, will undergo an 8-week open-label treatment phase with atorvastatin. Those patients attaining LDL cholesterol levels less than 130 mg/dl (3.36 mmol/liter) will be randomized to double-blind treatment with atorvastatin 10 mg/d or 80 mg/d; the anticipated LDL cholesterol goals at these dosages are 100 mg/dl (2.58 mmol/liter) and 75 mg/dl (1.93 mmol/liter), respectively. A projected total of 8600 patients will receive randomized treatment for an average of 5 years or until the number of primary coronary events reaches 750. The main efficacy measure is the occurrence of CHD death or nonfatal myocardial infarction. Secondary outcome measures include the incidence of any coronary event (primary event, coronary artery bypass grafting or other coronary revascularization, documented angina), cerebrovascular events, peripheral vascular disease, hospitalization with a primary diagnosis of CHD, any cardiovascular event, and all-cause mortality.

Fibrate Trials

VA-HIT. Of recent fibrate trials, perhaps the most necessary to mention is the Veteran's Affairs Cooperative Studies Program High Density Lipoprotein Cholesterol Intervention Trial (VA-HIT), a multicenter, randomized study that assessed the effects of gemfibrozil at a dose of 1200 mg/day versus dietary therapy on the incidence of cardiovascular events in 2531 men with known CHD and low baseline HDL cholesterol levels.[81] Enrollment criteria for VA-HIT required a HDL cholesterol level of 40 mg/dl (1.03 mmol/liter) or less or LDL cholesterol level of less than 140 mg/dl (3.6 mmol/liter) and triglycerides at 300 mg/dl (3.39 mmol/liter) or less.

The mean age of subjects in the VA-HIT was 64 years, with more than 75 percent of the patients older than 60 years of age. The participants in the VA-HIT had a mean body mass index of 29, a waist-hip ratio of 0.96, and a 25 percent prevalence of diabetes mellitus. Approximately 57 percent of the population was hypertensive and 20 percent were smokers. Baseline lipids in the VA-HIT revealed a total cholesterol level of 175 mg/dl, HDL cholesterol of 32 mg/dl, LDL cholesterol of 111 mg/dl, and triglycerides of 161 mg/dl. Gemfibrozil therapy resulted in essentially minimal alterations in total cholesterol and LDL levels. Total cholesterol was decreased by 4 percent as compared with placebo, and no significant change was demonstrable with LDL cholesterol concentrations. Triglycerides, on the other hand, fell by 31 percent and HDL cholesterol increased by 6 percent. The primary endpoint of the VA HIT was the combination of CHD death and nonfatal myocardial infarction. Patients randomized to receive placebo accounted for 275 events, compared with 219 events in the gemfibrozil group. The decline in coronary events represented a 22 percent risk reduction that was statistically significant ($p = 0.006$). The event curves began to diverge at approximately 2 years after the beginning of the trial.

A number of safety analyses were performed and found no differences in death from malignancies or violent deaths, and the only adverse event observed more frequently in the gemfibrozil group was dyspepsia. The VA-HIT reinforces the importance of targeting low HDL cholesterol as a major coronary risk factor.

BIP. The Bezafibrate Infarction Prevention (BIP) study reported no reduction in fatal and nonfatal myocardial infarction and CHD death in a cohort of 3090 men and women with CHD, total cholesterol of 180 to 250 mg/dl, HDL cholesterol less than 45 mg/dl (1.2 mmol/liter), triglycerides less than 300 mg/dl (3.4 mmol/liter), and LDL cholesterol less than 180 mg/dl (4.7 mmol/liter), who were treated with either bezafibrate, 400 mg/day, or placebo.[19] Despite producing an increase in HDL cholesterol of 14 percent and reduction in triglycerides of 25 percent compared with placebo, fibrate treatment did not reduce CHD risk. After 6.2 years, the reduction in the cumulative probability of the primary endpoint was 7.3 percent ($p = 0.24$). However, a substantial risk reduction with bezafibrate (39.5 percent; $p = 0.02$) was observed post hoc in the small subgroup of patients with elevated triglycerides at baseline (>200 mg/dl [2.3 mmol/liter]).

The lack of effect in BIP can be in part explained by the use of adjuvant open-label lipid-modifying drugs in the placebo group: 15 percent of patients in the placebo group were receiving this additional treatment before the end of the study, compared with 11 percent in the bezafibrate group. Also, compared with the VA-HIT, the BIP cohort had a lower placebo event rate, fewer diabetic participants, higher baseline HDL and LDL cholesterol levels, and lower baseline triglycerides.

ACCORD. The Action to Control Cardiovascular Risk in Diabetes (ACCORD) study, sponsored by the US National Heart, Lung, and Blood Institute, anticipates enrolling 10,000 patients with type 2 diabetes mellitus (from www.accordtrial.org, accessed April 14, 2004). The trial will compare effects on cardiovascular disease events of three strategies: intensive glycemic control; increasing HDL cholesterol and lowering triglycerides (with good LDL cholesterol and glycemic control); and intensive blood pressure control (in the context of good glycemic control). The lipid-modification arm of ACCORD will evaluate a fibrate intended to lower triglycerides and increase HDL cholesterol, combined with a statin to lower the LDL cholesterol level. The ACCORD study, therefore, will assess the effect of multiple risk factor intervention in diabetic patients and will also provide valuable information about the use of the statin-fibrate combination in preventing clinical events. In January 2003, the ACCORD main trial began a 30-month recruiting period. Follow-up will continue until 2009.[82]

In recent years, our understanding of cardiovascular risk management has grown increasingly sophisticated largely because of the growing dominance of global risk assessment as the conceptual basis of treatment decisions. The clinical trial database has undergone a parallel evolution in which early clinical trials of lipid modification using strategies capable of only modest lipid changes yielded important, but less than robust, results. The arrival of statin therapy made possible substantially greater LDL cholesterol reductions, and the trials using these drugs in the middle to late 1990s provided the most compelling evidence of benefit seen to date (see Fig. 39–6). With the database thus expanded, the questions being asked in trials have by necessity become increasingly specific. We no longer wonder whether reducing cholesterol will yield coronary benefit—it does—and therefore clinical trialists must turn toward the next direction: identifying the optimal conditions for achieving benefit. What kinds of patients will most likely benefit? What are the optimal goals of therapy? What clinical presentations of atherosclerotic disease will treatment affect most? The answers to these questions will shape the future of cardiovascular guidelines.

Overall Approach to the Treatment of Lipoprotein Disorders

Patients with lipoprotein disorders should undergo comprehensive evaluation and management in the context of a global risk reduction program (see Chap. 42). Most patients with dyslipoproteinemias lack symptoms, except for those with severe hypertriglyceridemia who can present with acute pancreatitis and those with familial lipoprotein disorders who have cutaneous manifestations (xanthomas, xanthelasmas). In the evaluation of patients with dyslipidemia, secondary causes should be sought and treated. The clinical evaluation should include a thorough history, including a complete family history that may reveal clues as to the genetic cause but also to the genetic susceptibility to cardiovascular disease. The physician should seek and address other risk factors (cigarette smoking, diabetes) and institute a management plan to improve lifestyle, such as diet, physical activity, and alcohol intake. Such interventions should make use of nonphysician health professionals (e.g., those with training in diet and nutrition or smoking cessation). The ATP III Therapeutic Lifestyle Change program offers one such approach. Concomitant medication use in addition to lifestyle change will often be needed to achieve current guideline goals.

The physical examination should include a search for xanthomas (in extensor tendons, including hands, elbows, knees, Achilles tendons, and palmar xanthomas); the presence of xanthelasmas, corneal arcus, and corneal opacifications. The blood pressure, waist circumference, weight, and height should be recorded and signs of vascular compromise must be carefully examined. A complete cardiovascular examination must be performed. The evaluation of peripheral pulses

TABLE 39–10 Laboratory Tests for the Diagnosis of Lipoprotein Disorders

Lipid Profile	May Help in Diagnosis	Specialized Centers	Research Tools
Cholesterol	Lipoprotein separation by UTC†	LDL particle size	Molecular diagnosis
Triglycerides	Apo B	LPL assay	
HDL cholesterol	Apo AI	LCAT assay	
LDL cholesterol*	Apo E genotype/ phenotype	Apo E levels	
	Lipoprotein(a)	Apolipoprotein separation by PAGE	
		LDL-R assay	
		Apo CII, CIII	

Apo = apolipoprotein; HDL = high-density lipoprotein; LCAT = lecithin cholesterol acyltransferase; LDL = low-density lipoprotein; LDL-R = LDL receptor; LPL = lipoprotein lipase.

*Calculated as LDL cholesterol = cholesterol (triglycerides/2.2 + HDL cholesterol) in mmol/liter (or triglycerides divided by 5 in mg/dl); valid for triglycerides <4.5 mmol/liter (<400 mg/dl). LDL cholesterol can also be directly measured in plasma.

†Ultracentrifugation.

and the determination of the ankle-brachial index may reveal important clues for the presence of peripheral vascular disease (see Chap. 54).

The diagnosis of lipoprotein disorders depends on laboratory measurements (Table 39–10). The lipid profile generally suffices for most lipoprotein disorders, and specialized laboratories can refine the diagnosis and provide expertise for extreme cases. Additional tests often involve considerable expense and may not increase the predictive value beyond that of the lipid profile, although they can help in refining the diagnosis. To assess baseline risk in individuals on lipid-lowering therapy, the medication should be stopped for 1 month before a lipid profile is measured. Many tests are available in specialized centers (see Table 39–10) but should not be requested unless results of the test will alter clinical judgment and influence treatment.

After diagnosis of a lipid disorder (based on at least two lipid profiles), secondary causes should be evaluated by measurement of thyroid stimulating hormone and glucose. Patients who will receive medications should have measurement of baseline liver function (alanine aminotransferase [ALT]) and creatinine kinase. A decision to treat high-risk subjects (for example, patients with an acute coronary syndrome or post-myocardial infarction or coronary revascularization) should be implemented immediately and should commence concomitantly with lifestyle changes.[51]

Target Levels (see Chap. 42)

The National Cholesterol Education Program Adult Treatment Panel III (NCEP ATP III)[64] has made recommendations for the treatment of hypercholesterolemia. Target levels depend on overall risk of cardiovascular death or nonfatal myocardial infarction. Patients with CAD or atherosclerosis of other vascular beds (carotids or peripheral vascular disease), adults with diabetes, and those patients with an estimated 10-year risk of developing CAD of greater than 20 percent fall into a high-risk category and merit aggressive treatment, including medications along with lifestyle modifications, exercise, and diet to achieve a primary target of an LDL cholesterol level less than 2.6 mmol/liter (100 mg/dl). In subjects with triglycerides greater than 200 mg/dl, ATP III presents a secondary target of a non-HDL cholesterol level less than 3.4 mmol/liter (130 mg/dl). Many of these individuals have the metabolic syndrome.

Lifestyle Changes

TREATMENT. The therapeutic options consist of lifestyle modifications, treatment of secondary causes, and, if possible, diet and medications.

DIET (see Chap. 41). Individuals with dyslipoproteinemias should always adopt dietary therapy. High-risk subjects should have medications started concomitantly with a diet because in many cases, diet may not suffice to reach target levels. The diet should have three objectives. First, it should allow the patient to reach and maintain ideal body weight. Second, it should provide a well-balanced diet with fruits, vegetables, and whole grains and it should be restricted in saturated fats and refined carbohydrates. Dietary counseling should involve a professional dietitian. Often, the help of dietitians, weight loss programs, or diabetic outpatient centers can aid sustained weight loss. Currently, the ATP III and the American Heart Association[16] recommend a diet in which protein intake represents 15 to 20 percent of calories, fats represent less than 35 percent, with only 7 percent from saturated fats, and the remaining calories derive from carbohydrates. Cholesterol intake should be less than 300 mg/day.

Treatment of Combined Lipoprotein Disorders

Combined lipoprotein disorders, characterized by an increase in plasma total cholesterol and triglycerides, frequently occur in clinical practice and represent difficult challenges. Patients with combined lipoprotein disorders have an increase in LDL cholesterol and LDL particle number (as reflected by an increase in total or LDL apo B), small, dense LDL particles, increased VLDL cholesterol and VLDL triglycerides, and a reduced HDL cholesterol level. Patients with this pattern of combined dyslipidemia often have obesity and the metabolic syndrome. Treatment should begin with lifestyle modifications, with a diet reduced in total calories and saturated fats, weight reduction, and increased exercise. Drug treatment, when warranted, aims to correct the predominant lipoprotein abnormality. Statins can reduce plasma triglyceride levels, particularly in individuals with high baseline triglyceride levels. Fibrates reduce triglycerides and may change the composition of LDL particles to a larger and less dense phenotype. Although fibric acid derivatives have a role in the secondary prevention of cardiovascular diseases in subjects with low HDL cholesterol levels, they can paradoxically increase LDL cholesterol levels (because of increased lipoprotein lipase activity). Plasma total homocysteine levels may increase with fenofibrate and to a lesser extent with bezafibrate. In view of gemfibrozil's effects on glucuronidation of statins, we advise against its use in combination therapy. The combination of a statin with a fibrate has proven highly effective in correcting the combined dyslipoproteinemias. Patients taking a fibrate plus a statin merit close medical follow-up for evidence of hepatotoxicity or myositis within the first 6 weeks of therapy and every 6 months thereafter. Other combinations, including fibric acid derivatives with bile acid–binding resins and niacin with bile acid–binding resins, have also proved to be useful in specific cases. The combination of fibrates or statins with niacin requires experience and care because of the risk of hepatotoxicity and myositis. The search for correctable causes (e.g., uncontrolled diabetes, obesity, hypothyroidism, and alcohol use) of combined dyslipidemia and the benefit of lifestyle modifications require reemphasis. Often, the help of dietitians, weight loss programs, or diabetic outpatient centers is highly beneficial.

EXTRACORPOREAL LOW-DENSITY LIPOPROTEIN FILTRATION. Patients with severe hypercholesterolemia, especially those with homozygous familial hypercholesterolemia or severe heterozygous familial hypercholesterolemia may warrant treatment by extracorporeal LDL elimination. These techniques use selective filtration, adsorption, or precipitation of LDL (or apo B–containing particles) after plasma separation. Specialized centers have LDL-pheresis available. This approach can dramatically reduce the risk of developing cardiovascular disease and improve survival.[83]

Novel Approaches

The development of novel pharmaceutical agents for the treatment of lipoprotein disorders will likely continue because cardiovascular disease due to atherosclerosis represents the largest burden of disease for the near future. Better targeting of high-risk individuals will allow optimization of expensive therapies. The finding that subjects who were previously identified as being at relatively low risk of CAD on the basis of their LDL cholesterol levels but who have an elevated C-reactive protein level derive benefit from a statin in the primary prevention of CAD may radically alter the concept of cardiovascular risk stratification.[84,85] If cardiovascular risk can be better identified using markers of inflammation, in addition to conventional risk factors, physicians' attitudes should embrace these findings. This hypothesis is undergoing rigorous testing in a clinical trial.[85]

The burgeoning field of pharmacogenetics might, in the near future, allow treatment of patients on the basis of their genetic make-up. Genetic screening may become a useful clinical tool, as technology improves and rapid genotyping for diagnostic and prognostic purposes becomes available for clinicians. Other than cost issues, the ethics of screening for genetic predisposition to disease and access to information represent daunting challenges. The discovery that the apo E4 allele carries the risk of early-onset Alzheimer disease, one of the familial forms of the disorder, illustrates the ethical complexities of genetic testing in the realm of lipoprotein disorders.

Drug Development and Future Directions

Novel proteins that regulate the synthesis of lipids have become therapeutic targets for drug development. The development of competitive inhibitors of HMG-CoA reductase leading to statin drugs provides a good example. These drugs have an important impact on cardiovascular morbidity and mortality reduction in high-risk individuals. Inhibitors of pancreatic lipases are being used to treat obesity.[86] Future potential drug targets might include inhibition of apo B secretion by inhibiting the microsomal triglyceride transfer protein, which is crucial in the assembly of apo B–containing lipoproteins.[87] Hepatic steatosis may limit this therapeutic option in humans. Selective inhibition of ACAT may also provide a therapeutic target to inhibit cholesterol absorption through the intestinal wall, inhibit secretion from the liver of apo B–containing lipoproteins, and interfere with foam cell formation.[12] Drugs that increase cellular cholesterol efflux to increase HDL cholesterol levels may also prove useful in the treatment of dyslipoproteinemias.

Other therapeutic modalities in the treatment of atherosclerosis by modulating lipoprotein metabolism include the development of inhibitors of CETP to increase HDL cholesterol levels[87a] or modulation of LCAT, and inhibitors of bile acid transport to decrease intestinal cholesterol uptake. Clinical studies currently in progress are testing the effect of CETP inhibitors on human atherosclerosis. Pharmacological modulation of HDL cholesterol levels, other than by niacin, has not led to results proportional to those achieved for LDL cholesterol. Potential modulators of HDL cholesterol levels include SR-B1, ABCA1 pathways, apo A1, and its homologues and mimetics.[88]

Gene Therapy

Severe, homozygous, monogenic disorders may eventually b treated by gene therapy. The initial trials of gene therapy i cases of homozygous familial hypercholesterolemia have no led to a major improvement and have largely been aban doned. However, the lifelong burden of these rare disorder and the potential for cure makes this approach very appeal ing. Other diseases, such as abetalipoproteinemia, LPL defi ciency, Niemann-Pick type C disease, sitosterolemia, an Tangier disease may become therapeutic targets for gen therapy. If the approach to correct these disorders is suc cessful, the more widespread applications of gene-based ther apies for the purpose of reducing potential cardiovascula risk will become a daunting medical, social, and ethica problem.

REFERENCES

1. Sorci-Thomas MG, Curtiss L, Parks JS, et al: The hydrophobic face orientation c apolipoprotein A-I amphipathic helix domain 143-164 regulates lecithin:cholester acyltransferase activation. J Biol Chem 273:11776, 1998.
2. Hiltunen TP, Luoma JS, Nikkari T, Yla-Herttuala S: Expression of LDL receptor, VLD receptor, LDL receptor-related protein, and scavenger receptor in rabbit atheroscleroti lesions: Marked induction of scavenger receptor and VLDL receptor expression durin lesion development. Circulation 97:1079, 1998.
3. Nimpf J, Schneider WJ: The VLDL receptor: An LDL receptor relative with eight ligan binding repeats, LR8. Atherosclerosis 141:191, 1998.
4. Mahley RW, Ji ZS: Remnant lipoprotein metabolism: Key pathways involving cel surface heparan sulfate proteoglycans and apolipoprotein E. J Lipid Res 40:1, 1999.
5. Brown ML, Ramprasad MP, Umeda PK, et al: A macrophage receptor for apolipoprotei B48: Cloning, expression, and atherosclerosis. Proc Natl Acad Sci U S A 97:7488, 200
6. de Man FH, de Beer F, van der Laarse A, et al: Lipolysis of very low density lipopro teins by heparan sulfate proteoglycan-bound lipoprotein lipase. J Lipid Res 38:2465 1997.
7. Sawamura T, Kume N, Aoyama T, et al: An endothelial receptor for oxidized low-densit lipoprotein. Nature 386:73, 1997.
8. Acton S, Rigotti A, Landschulz KT, et al: Identification of scavenger receptor SR-BI a a high density lipoprotein receptor. Science 271:518, 1996.
8a. Altmann SW, Davis HR Jr, Zhu LJ, et al: Niemann-Pick C1 like 1 protein is critical fo intestinal cholesterol absorption. Science 303:1201, 2004.
9. Mann CJ, Troussard AA, Yen FT, et al: Inhibitory effects of specific apolipoprotein C-I isoforms on the binding of triglyceride-rich lipoproteins to the lipolysis-stimulate receptor. J Biol Chem 272:31348, 1997.
10. van Tol A: Phospholipid transfer protein. Curr Opin Lipidol 13:135, 2002.
11. Abifadel M, Varret M, Rabes JP, et al: Mutations in PCSK9 cause autosomal dominan hypercholesterolemia. Nat Genet 34:154, 2003.
12. Willner EL, Tow B, Buhman KK, et al: Deficiency of acyl CoA:cholesterol acyltransferas 2 prevents atherosclerosis in apolipoprotein E-deficient mice. Proc Natl Acad Sci U S A 100:1262, 2003.
13. Zhang SH, Reddick RL, Piedrahita JA, Maeda N: Spontaneous hypercholesterolemia an arterial lesions in mice lacking apolipoprotein E. Science 258:468, 1992.
14. O'Connell BJ, Genest J Jr: High-density lipoproteins and endothelial function. Circula tion 104:1978, 2001.
15. Li XA, Titlow WB, Jackson BA, et al: High density lipoprotein binding to scavenge receptor, class B, type I activates endothelial nitric-oxide synthase in a ceramide dependent manner. J Biol Chem 277:11058, 2002.
16. Oram JF: HDL apolipoproteins and ABCA1: Partners in the removal of excess cellula cholesterol. Arterioscler Thromb Vasc Biol 23:720, 2003.
17. Haidar B, Denis M, Krimbou L, et al: cAMP induces ABCA1 phosphorylation activit and promotes cholesterol efflux from fibroblasts. J Lipid Res 43:2087, 2002.
18. Fielding PE, Nagao K, Hakamata H, et al: A two-step mechanism for free cholesterol an phospholipid efflux from human vascular cells to apolipoprotein A-1. Biochemistry 39:14113, 2000.
19. Hammad SM, Stefansson S, Twal WO, et al: Cubilin, the endocytic receptor for intrinsic factor-vitamin B(12) complex, mediates high-density lipoprotein holoparticle endocytosis. Proc Natl Acad Sci U S A 96:10158, 1999.
20. Grundy SM: Low-density lipoprotein, non-high-density lipoprotein, and apolipoprotein B as targets of lipid-lowering therapy. Circulation 106:2526, 2002.
21. Campos H, Moye LA, Glasser SP, et al: Low-density lipoprotein size, pravastatin treatment, and coronary events. JAMA 286:1468, 2001.
22. Sacks FM, Campos H: Clinical review 163: Cardiovascular endocrinology: Low-density lipoprotein size and cardiovascular disease: A reappraisal. J Clin Endocrinol Metab 88:4525, 2003.
23. Wilson DJ, Gahan M, Haddad L, et al: A World Wide Web site for low-density lipoprotein receptor gene mutations in familial hypercholesterolemia: Sequence-based, tabular, and direct submission data handling. Am J Cardiol 81:1509, 1998.
24. Hansen PS, Defesche JC, Kastelein JJ, et al: Phenotypic variation in patients heterozygous for familial defective apolipoprotein B (FDB) in three European countries. Arterioscler Thromb Vasc Biol 17:741, 1997.
25. Wetterau JR, Aggerbeck LP, Bouma ME, et al: Absence of microsomal triglyceride transfer protein in individuals with abetalipoproteinemia. Science 258:999, 1992.

26. Berge KE, Tian H, Graf GA, et al: Accumulation of dietary cholesterol in sitosterolemia caused by mutations in adjacent ABC transporters. Science 290:1771, 2000.
27. Mooser V, Mancini FP, Bopp S, et al: Sequence polymorphisms in the apo(a) gene associated with specific levels of Lp(a) in plasma. Hum Mol Genet 4:173, 1995.
28. Danesh J, Collins R, Peto R: Lipoprotein(a) and coronary heart disease: Meta-analysis of prospective studies. Circulation 102:1082, 2000.
29. Sjarif DR, Sinke RJ, Duran M, et al: Clinical heterogeneity and novel mutations in the glycerol kinase gene in three families with isolated glycerol kinase deficiency. J Med Genet 35:650, 1998.
30. Santamarina-Fojo S: The familial chylomicronemia syndrome. Endocrinol Metab Clin North Am 27:551, viii, 1998.
31. Weinstock PH, Bisgaier CL, Aalto-Setala K, et al: Severe hypertriglyceridemia, reduced high density lipoprotein, and neonatal death in lipoprotein lipase knockout mice: Mild hypertriglyceridemia with impaired very low density lipoprotein clearance in heterozygotes. J Clin Invest 96:2555, 1995.
32. Mahley RW, Huang Y, Rall SC Jr: Pathogenesis of type III hyperlipoproteinemia (dysbetalipoproteinemia): Questions, quandaries, and paradoxes. J Lipid Res 40:1933, 1999.
33. Genest JJ Jr, Martin-Munley SS, McNamara JR, et al: Familial lipoprotein disorders in patients with premature coronary artery disease. Circulation 85:2025, 1992.
34. Pajukanta P, Nuotio I, Terwilliger JD, et al: Linkage of familial combined hyperlipidaemia to chromosome 1q21-q23. Nat Genet 18:369, 1998.
35. Murray I, Kohl J, Cianflone K: Acylation-stimulating protein (ASP): Structure-function determinants of cell surface binding and triacylglycerol synthetic activity. Biochem J 342:41, 1999.
36. Kalant D, Cain SA, Maslowska M, et al: The chemoattractant receptor-like protein C5L2 binds the C3a des-Arg77/acylation-stimulating protein. J Biol Chem 278:11123, 2003.
37. Lamarche B, Uffelman KD, Carpentier A, et al: Triglyceride enrichment of HDL enhances in vivo metabolic clearance of HDL apo A-I in healthy men. J Clin Invest 103:1191, 1999.
38. Sorci-Thomas MG, Thomas MJ: The effects of altered apolipoprotein A-I structure on plasma HDL concentration. Trends Cardiovasc Med 12:121, 2002.
39. Kuivenhoven JA, Jukema JW, Zwinderman AH, et al: The role of a common variant of the cholesteryl ester transfer protein gene in the progression of coronary atherosclerosis. The Regression Growth Evaluation Statin Study Group. N Engl J Med 338:86, 1998.
40. Kuivenhoven JA, Pritchard H, Hill J, et al: The molecular pathology of lecithin:cholesterol acyltransferase (LCAT) deficiency syndromes. J Lipid Res 38:191, 1997.
41. Zhong S, Sharp DS, Grove JS, et al: Increased coronary heart disease in Japanese-American men with mutation in the cholesteryl ester transfer protein gene despite increased HDL levels. J Clin Invest 97:2917, 1996.
42. Ma K, Cilingiroglu M, Otvos JD, et al: Endothelial lipase is a major genetic determinant for high-density lipoprotein concentration, structure, and metabolism. Proc Natl Acad Sci U S A 100:2748, 2003.
43. Marcil M, Brooks-Wilson A, Clee SM, et al: Mutations in the ABC1 gene in familial HDL deficiency with defective cholesterol efflux. Lancet 354:1341, 1999.
44. Rust S, Rosier M, Funke H, et al: Tangier disease is caused by mutations in the gene encoding ATP-binding cassette transporter 1. Nat Genet 22:352, 1999.
45. Bodzioch M, Orso E, Klucken J, et al: The gene encoding ATP-binding cassette transporter 1 is mutated in Tangier disease. Nat Genet 22:347, 1999.
46. Carstea ED, Morris JA, Coleman KG, et al: Niemann-Pick C1 disease gene: Homology to mediators of cholesterol homeostasis. Science 277:228, 1997.
47. Lee CY, Krimbou L, Vincent J, et al: Compound heterozygosity at the sphingomyelin phosphodiesterase-1 (SMPD1) gene is associated with low HDL cholesterol. Hum Genet 112:552, 2003.
48. Herrington DM, Vittinghoff E, Lin F, et al: Statin therapy, cardiovascular events, and total mortality in the Heart and Estrogen/Progestin Replacement Study (HERS). Circulation 105:2962, 2002.
48a. Anderson GL, Limacher M, Assaf AR: Effects of conjugated equine estrogen in postmenopausal women with hysterectomy: The Women's Health Initiative randomized controlled trial. JAMA 291:1701, 2004.
49. Martin G, Duez H, Blanquart C, et al: Statin-induced inhibition of the Rho-signaling pathway activates PPARalpha and induces HDL apoA-I. J Clin Invest 107:1423, 2001.
50. Libby P, Ridker PM, Maseri A: Inflammation and atherosclerosis. Circulation 105:1135, 2002.
51. Genest J, Pedersen TR: Prevention of cardiovascular ischemic events: High-risk and secondary prevention. Circulation 107:2059, 2003.
52. Libby P, Aikawa M: Stabilization of atherosclerotic plaques: New mechanisms and clinical targets. Nat Med 8:1257, 2002.
53. Gagne C, Bays HE, Weiss SR, et al: Efficacy and safety of ezetimibe added to ongoing statin therapy for treatment of patients with primary hypercholesterolemia. Am J Cardiol 90:1084, 2002.
54. Bissonnette R, Treacy E, Rozen R, et al: Fenofibrate raises plasma homocysteine levels in the fasted and fed states. Atherosclerosis 155:455, 2001.
55. Brown BG, Zhao XQ, Chait A, et al: Simvastatin and niacin, antioxidant vitamins, or the combination for the prevention of coronary disease. N Engl J Med 345:1583, 2001.
56. Wise A, Foord SM, Fraser NJ, et al: Molecular identification of high and low affinity receptors for nicotinic acid. J Biol Chem 278:9869, 2003.
57. Soga T, Kamohara M, Takasaki J, et al: Molecular identification of nicotinic acid receptor. Biochem Biophys Res Commun 303:364, 2003.
58. Cote G, Tardif JC, Lesperance J, et al: Effects of probucol on vascular remodeling after coronary angioplasty. Multivitamins and Protocol Study Group. Circulation 99:30, 1999.
59. Downs JR, Clearfield M, Weis S, et al: Primary prevention of acute coronary events with lovastatin in men and women with average cholesterol levels: Results of AFCAPS/TexCAPS. Air Force/Texas Coronary Atherosclerosis Prevention Study. JAMA 279:1615, 1998.
60. Shepherd J, Cobbe SM, Ford I, et al: Prevention of coronary heart disease with pravastatin in men with hypercholesterolemia. West of Scotland Coronary Prevention Study Group. N Engl J Med 333:1301, 1995.
61. Sacks FM, Pfeffer MA, Moye LA, et al: The effect of pravastatin on coronary events after myocardial infarction in patients with average cholesterol levels. Cholesterol and Recurrent Events Trial investigators. N Engl J Med 335:1001, 1996.
62. Prevention of cardiovascular events and death with pravastatin in patients with coronary heart disease and a broad range of initial cholesterol levels. The Long-Term Intervention with Pravastatin in Ischaemic Disease (LIPID) Study Group. N Engl J Med 339:1349, 1998.
63. Randomised trial of cholesterol lowering in 4444 patients with coronary heart disease: The Scandinavian Simvastatin Survival Study (4S). Lancet 344:1383, 1994.
64. Executive Summary of the Third Report of the National Cholesterol Education Program (NCEP) Expert Panel on Detection, Evaluation, And Treatment of High Blood Cholesterol In Adults (Adult Treatment Panel III). JAMA 285:2486, 2001.
65. MRC/BHF Heart Protection Study of cholesterol lowering with simvastatin in 20,536 high-risk individuals: A randomised placebo-controlled trial. Lancet 360:7, 2002.
66. Shepherd J, Blauw GJ, Murphy MB, et al: Pravastatin in elderly individuals at risk of vascular disease (PROSPER): A randomised controlled trial. Lancet 360:1623, 2002.
67. Major outcomes in moderately hypercholesterolemic, hypertensive patients randomized to pravastatin vs usual care: The Antihypertensive and Lipid-Lowering Treatment to Prevent Heart Attack Trial (ALLHAT-LLT). JAMA 288:2998, 2002.
68. Pasternak RC: The ALLHAT lipid lowering trial—less is less. JAMA 288:3042, 2002.
69. Sever PS, Dahlof B, Poulter NR, et al: Prevention of coronary and stroke events with atorvastatin in hypertensive patients who have average or lower-than-average cholesterol concentrations, in the Anglo-Scandinavian Cardiac Outcomes Trial—Lipid Lowering Arm (ASCOT-LLA): A multicentre randomised controlled trial. Lancet 361:1149, 2003.
70. Colhoun HM, Thomason MJ, Mackness MI, et al: Design of the Collaborative AtoRvastatin Diabetes Study (CARDS) in patients with type 2 diabetes. Diabet Med 19:201, 2002.
71. Colhoun HM, Thomason MJ, Mackness MI, et al: Design of the collaborative Ato Rvastatin Diabetes Study (CARDS) in patients with type 2 diabetes. Diabet Med 19:201, 2002.
72. Stenestrand U, Wallentin L: Early statin treatment following acute myocardial infarction and 1-year survival. JAMA 285:430, 2001.
73. Newby LK, Kristinsson A, Bhapkar MV, et al: Early statin initiation and outcomes in patients with acute coronary syndromes. JAMA 287:3087, 2002.
74. Schwartz GG, Olsson AG, Ezekowitz MD, et al: Effects of atorvastatin on early recurrent ischemic events in acute coronary syndromes: The MIRACL study: A randomized controlled trial. JAMA 285:1711, 2001.
75. Blazing MA, De Lemos JA, Dyke CK, et al: The A-to-Z Trial: Methods and rationale for a single trial investigating combined use of low-molecular-weight heparin with the glycoprotein IIb/IIIa inhibitor tirofiban and defining the efficacy of early aggressive simvastatin therapy. Am Heart J 142:211, 2001.
76. Cannon CP, McCabe CH, Belder R, et al: Design of the Pravastatin or Atorvastatin Evaluation and Infection Therapy (PROVE IT)-TIMI 22 trial. Am J Cardiol 89:860, 2002.
76a. Cannon CP, Braunwald E, McCabe CH, et al: Intensive versus moderate lipid lowering with statins after acute coronary syndromes. N Engl J Med 350:1495, 2004.
77. Pitt B, Waters D, Brown WV, et al: Aggressive lipid-lowering therapy compared with angioplasty in stable coronary artery disease. Atorvastatin versus Revascularization Treatment Investigators. N Engl J Med 341:70, 1999.
78. Chiquette E, Chilton R: Aggressive medical management of coronary artery disease versus mechanical revascularization. Curr Atheroscler Rep 5:118, 2003.
78a. Nissen SE, Tuzcu EM, Schoenhagen P, et al: Effect of intensive compared with moderate lipid-lowering therapy on progression of coronary atherosclerosis: A randomized controlled trial. JAMA 291:1071, 2004.
79. McMahon M, Kirkpatrick C, Cummings CE, et al: A pilot study with simvastatin and folic acid/vitamin B_{12} in preparation for the Study of the Effectiveness of Additional Reductions in Cholesterol and Homocysteine (SEARCH). Nutr Metab Cardiovasc Dis 10:195, 2000.
80. Waters DD, Guyton JR, Herrington DM, et al: Treating to New Targets (TNT): Does lowering low-density lipoprotein in cholesterol levels below currently recommended guidelines yield incremental clinical benefits. Am J Cardiol 193:154, 2004.
81. Rubins HB, Robins SJ, Collins D, et al: Gemfibrozil for the secondary prevention of coronary heart disease in men with low levels of high-density lipoprotein cholesterol. Veterans Affairs High-Density Lipoprotein Cholesterol Intervention Trial Study Group. N Engl J Med 341:410, 1999.
82. Secondary prevention by raising HDL cholesterol and reducing triglycerides in patients with coronary artery disease: The Bezafibrate Infarction Prevention (BIP) study. Circulation 102:21, 2000.
83. Nishimura S, Sekiguchi M, Kano T, et al: Effects of intensive lipid lowering by low-density lipoprotein apheresis on regression of coronary atherosclerosis in patients with familial hypercholesterolemia: Japan Low-density Lipoprotein Apheresis Coronary Atherosclerosis Prospective Study (L-CAPS). Atherosclerosis 144:409, 1999.
84. Ridker PM, Rifai N, Rose L, et al: Comparison of C-reactive protein and low-density lipoprotein cholesterol levels in the prediction of first cardiovascular events. N Engl J Med 347:1557, 2002.
85. Ridker PM: Rosuvastatin in the primary prevention of cardiovascular disease among patients with low levels of low-density lipoprotein cholesterol and elevated high-sensitivity C-reactive protein: Rationale and design of the JUPITER trial. Circulation 108:2292, 2003.
86. Hvizdos KM, Markham A: Orlistat: A review of its use in the management of obesity. Drugs 58:743, 1999.
87. Narcisi TM, Shoulders CC, Chester SA, et al: Mutations of the microsomal triglyceride-transfer-protein gene in abetalipoproteinemia. Am J Hum Genet 57:1298, 1995.
87a. Brousseau ME, Schaefer EJ, Wolfe ML, et al: Effects of an inhibitor of cholesteryl ester transfer protein on HDL cholesterol. N Engl J Med 350:1505, 2004.
88. Nissen SE, Tsunoda T, Tuzcu EM, et al: Effect of recombinant ApoA-I Milano on coronary atherosclerosis in patients with acute coronary syndromes: A randomized controlled trial. JAMA 290:2292, 2003.

CHAPTER 40

Diabetes Mellitus, the Metabolic Syndrome, and Atherosclerotic Vascular Disease

Joshua A. Beckman • Peter Libby • Mark A. Creager

Vascular diseases account for most morbidity and mortality in patients with diabetes mellitus.[1-3] Diabetes causes microvascular diseases, such as nephropathy, neuropathy, and retinopathy, and macrovascular disease, that is, atherosclerosis. Atherosclerosis of the coronary, cerebral, and peripheral arteries accounts for approximately 80 percent of mortality and 75 percent of hospitalizations in persons with diabetes.

Approximately 8 percent of the U.S. population has diabetes, undiagnosed in half the cases.[4] The prevalence of diabetes follows that of obesity, which affected approximately 18 percent of the U.S. population in 1998.[5,6] Hispanics, blacks, Native Americans, and Asian Indians bear a disproportionate burden of diabetic cardiovascular disease.[7] The predilection for these ethnic groups to develop obesity and glucose intolerance on a western diet may have a genetic basis, because the ability to store fat may have conferred a survival advantage in populations subject to famine. This selective pressure could enrich the population in genes that facilitate fat storage, the so-called "thrifty gene" hypothesis.[8,9]

The prevalence of diabetes is increasing within the U.S. population (Fig. 40–1) and has grown from approximately 2 million cases in the early 1960s to 15 million in 2000. Americans born in 2000 will have an estimated 36 percent chance of developing diabetes in their lifetime.[10] Current estimates project 22 million cases by 2025.[11] When viewed in the light of the rapidly expanding diabetic population, these data raise the specter of a reversal in the improvement in cardiovascular outcomes over the last two decades. The general population in the United States has enjoyed an impressive decline in the mortality associated with heart disease in the last decades. However, the drop in cardiovascular mortality in diabetic men and women has lagged well behind that of the general population.[12]

Cardiovascular disease in diabetes also impacts the economic resources of the health care system. Data from a managed care organization on the 1-year costs of treating more than 85,000 patients with diabetes compared with age- and sex-matched nondiabetic counterparts attributes the largest proportion (17 percent) of the excess costs associated with diabetes to coronary artery disease (CAD).[13] In comparison, end-stage renal disease accounted for only 11 percent of the excess costs of treatment.

Better implementation of therapies that reduce cardiovascular risk in diabetic patients will require moving beyond the traditional primary focus on glycemic control.[14] A working knowledge of the effects of diabetes mellitus on the heart and blood vessels will aid physicians caring for these patients.

Diagnostic Criteria for Diabetes Mellitus

In 1997, the American Diabetes Association (ADA) promulgated new criteria for the diagnosis of diabetes mellitus.[15] These criteria use a single blood glucose determination after an 8-hour fast (fasting plasma glucose [FPG]) as the major diagnostic criterion (Table 40–1). An FPG of less than 110 mg/dl is considered normal. A new diagnostic category known as impaired fasting glucose (IFG) encompasses FPGs higher than 110 but lower than 126 mg/dl. An FPG of higher than 126 mg/dl establishes the diagnosis of diabetes mellitus. Type 2 diabetes mellitus, previously known as non-insulin-dependent or adult-onset diabetes, represents 90 percent of the diabetic population. Type 1 diabetes, known previously as insulin-dependent or juvenile-onset diabetes, accounts for the remaining 10 percent. Both forms of diabetes confer independent risk for cardiovascular events, although patients with type 1 diabetes generally develop cardiovascular disease at a much younger age than those with type 2 diabetes.

Epidemiology of Cardiovascular Disease in Diabetes Mellitus

The clinical manifestations of diabetes-related atherosclerosis occur in every major vascular territory, notably the coronary, cerebral, and peripheral (limb) arteries.

Coronary Artery Disease

Patients with diabetes have a twofold to fourfold increase in the risk of CAD.[16] In the Multiple Risk Factor Intervention (MRFIT) study, more than 5000 men (of ~350,000 screened) who reported taking medications for diabetes were followed for an average of 12 years.[17] For every age stratum, ethnic background, and risk factor level, men with diabetes had an absolute risk of CAD death more than 3 times higher than that in the nondiabetic cohort, even after adjustment for established risk factors.[18] Another large cohort of 11,554 white men and 666 black men between 35 and 64 years of age, screened from 1967 to 1973 and followed prospectively for 22 years, showed similar findings.[18]

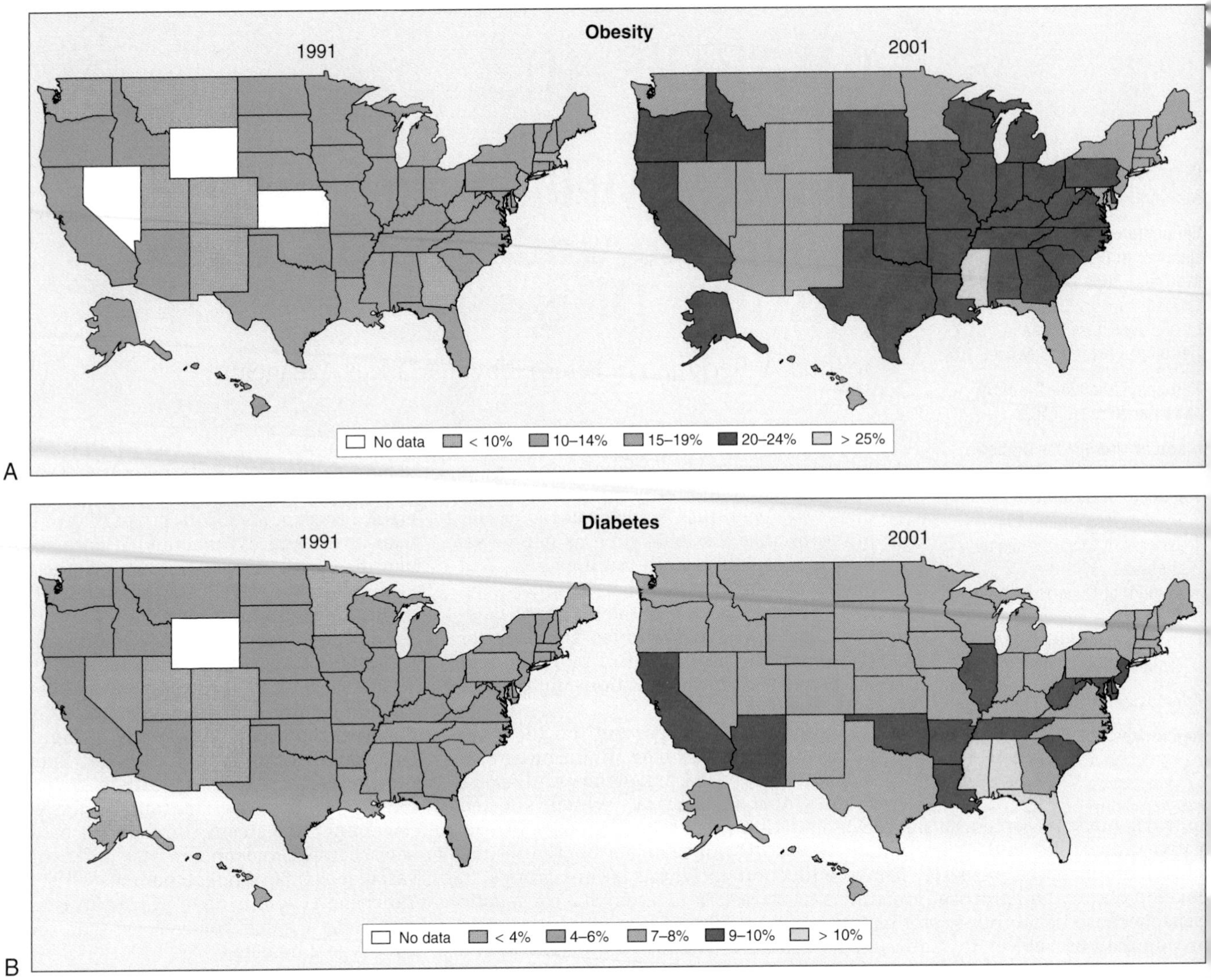

FIGURE 40–1 Obesity and diabetes mellitus in U.S. adults. Over the 10-year period of 1991 to 2001, the prevalence of obesity and diabetes among U.S. adults increased in every region of the nation. Obesity is associated with the development of type 2 diabetes mellitus and may serve as the root cause underlying the increased prevalence of type 2 diabetes. (From Mokdad AH, Ford ES, Bowman BA, et al: Prevalence of obesity, diabetes, and obesity-related health risk factors, 2001. JAMA 289:76-79, 2003.) (See also Chap. 41.)

TABLE 40–1 Criteria for the Diagnosis of Diabetes Mellitus*

Normal	Impaired Fasting Glucose	Diabetes Mellitus
FPG < 110 mg/dl	FPG ≥ 110 mg/dl and <126 mg/dl (IFG)	FPG ≥ 126 mg/dl
2-hr PG < 140 mg/dl	2-hr PG ≥ 140 mg/dl and <200 mg/dl (IGT)	2-hr PG ≥ 200 mg/dl Symptoms of diabetes mellitus and random plasma glucose concentration ≥200 mg/dl

FPG = fasting postload glucose; IFG = impaired fasting glucose; IGT = impaired glucose tolerance; PG = postload glucose.
Data from American Diabetes Association: Clinical practice recommendations. Diabetes Care 22(Suppl 1): S5-S19, 1999.
*Rather than employing the classic glucose tolerance curve with multiple time points sampled, the new criteria employ, in parallel to the FPG measurements, a 2-hr PG set of criteria. The plasma sample is obtained 2 hr following an oral administration of 75 gm of anhydrous glucose in aqueous solution.

In the general population, women experience relative protection from myocardial infarction and usually develop CAD approximately 10 years later than men. However, diabetes blunts the cardiovascular benefit of female gender.[19] Diabetic U.S. women of either European or African ancestry have this heightened risk.[20] Diabetes increases the risk of death after myocardial infarction in women more than men (see Chap. 51).[21] In the First National Health and Nutrition Examination Survey (NHANES) and the NHANES Epidemiologic Follow-Up Survey conducted 10 years apart, age-adjusted mortality decreased in nondiabetic men and women, less so in diabetic men, but increased by 23 percent in diabetic women.[12]

Multiple studies support the notion that acute and long-term adverse cardiovascular events have substantially increased in patients with diabetes. A Finnish epidemiological survey compared the rates of myocardial infarction in nondiabetic and diabetic populations (Fig. 40–2).[22] In this study, patients with diabetes but without prior myocardial infarction had the same level of risk for subsequent acute coronary

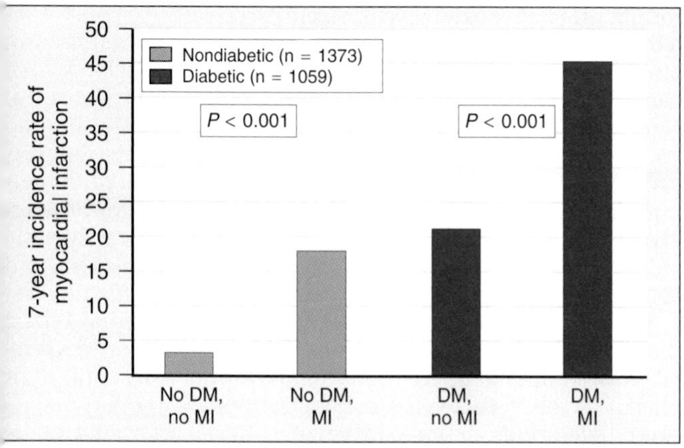

FIGURE 40–2 Marked increase in risk of coronary artery disease in patients with type 2 diabetes mellitus (DM). These data show a striking increase in the risk of first or recurrent myocardial infarction (MI) in diabetic patients compared with nondiabetic subjects in a population-based study in Finland over a 7-year follow-up period. These data also show that the diabetic patient without history of previous myocardial infarction has an approximately equal risk for first myocardial infarction as a nondiabetic subject who has already sustained myocardial infarction. These data support recent recommendations from the American Diabetes Association to treat diabetic subjects as if they already have established coronary artery disease. (From Haffner SM, Lehto S, Ronnemaa T, et al: Mortality from coronary heart disease in subjects with type 2 diabetes and in nondiabetic subjects with and without prior myocardial infraction. N Engl J Med 339:229-234, 1998.)

events as did nondiabetic persons with a history of previous myocardial infarction.

In the six-nation OASIS study, diabetic patients presenting with unstable angina or non-Q wave myocardial infarction had increased rates of stroke, congestive heart failure, and death during the index hospitalization compared with nondiabetic patients.[23] In the Gruppo Italiano per lo Studio della Sopravvivenza nell'Infarto Miocardico-2 (GISSI-2) study of thrombolytic therapy in patients with myocardial infarction, diabetes increased the rate of death in men by 40 percent and women by 90 percent.[24] In the Should We Emergently Revascularize Occluded Coronaries for Cardiogenic Shock (SHOCK) trial, which evaluated a strategy of early revascularization in patients with myocardial infarction complicated by cardiogenic shock, 31.1 percent of the patients had diabetes—a much greater percentage than in the population in general.[25] Moreover, the patients with diabetes experienced a 36 percent excess in mortality compared to patients without diabetes.[26] In the Finnish contribution to the WHO MONICA Project (World Health Organization Multinational Monitoring of Trends and Determinants of Cardiovascular Disease), 1-year mortality was 38 percent higher for diabetic men and 86 percent higher for diabetic women.[21] In a follow-up study of more than 5000 patients who presented to an emergency department with symptoms suggestive of myocardial infarction, diabetic patients had a 53.5 percent 5-year mortality rate compared with 23.3 percent among nondiabetic patients.[27] These trends toward an increasing risk of death among diabetic subjects are even greater in younger patients. In a statewide analysis of myocardial infarction, the risk of death in diabetic subjects was 87 percent greater than in nondiabetics aged 30 to 49 years but only 17 percent greater in the 70- to 89-year age group.[28]

Cerebrovascular Disease

Diabetes mellitus increases the frequency of cerebral atherosclerosis and the risk of stroke. Among patients presenting with a stroke, the prevalence of diabetes is thrice that of matched controls, and diabetes increases the risk of stroke up to fourfold.[29-31] In the MRFIT study, diabetic subjects who required medication for glucose control were threefold as likely to develop a stroke as nondiabetic subjects.[17] Similarly, in more than 12,000 male and female subjects followed for 6 to 8 years in the Atherosclerosis Risk in Communities Study, the relative risk of an ischemic stroke was increased nearly fourfold by the presence of diabetes.[32] Moreover, insulin resistance varies inversely with the risk of stroke.[29] Diabetic subjects have more severe carotid atherosclerosis as assessed by ultrasonography and a fivefold excess prevalence of calcified carotid atheroma as observed on dental panoramic radiographs.[33]

Diabetes puts younger patients at particular risk for stroke. Diabetes decreases the age at presentation for stroke compared to persons who do not have diabetes. One in 10 stroke victims is younger than 55 years of age, and diabetes increases the stroke risk more than 10-fold in this age group.[34] In the Baltimore-Washington Cooperative Young Stroke Study of 296 cases of incident ischemic stroke subjects aged 18 to 44 years, diabetes markedly increased the risk of stroke.[35] The age-adjusted odds ratio for stroke was 3.3 for black women, 4.2 for black men, 6.2 for white women, and 23.1 for white men (Fig. 40–3).

Most studies have shown that diabetes increases the risk of stroke more in women than men.[36,37] In the Renfrew/Paisley Study, a 20-year follow-up study in Scotland of 7052 men and 8354 women aged 45 to 64 years, diabetic women had a nearly threefold excess in stroke.[38] The 52 percent increase in diabetic men did not achieve statistical significance.[38] Further, diabetic women also had a higher risk of death from stroke. In another study of 16,600 patients, diabetes accounted for 16 percent of stroke-related mortality in men and 33 percent in women.[39] Diabetes augments the risk of stroke more among blacks and Caribbean Hispanics than whites. In the Northern Manhattan Stroke Study, the odds ratio for stroke risk was 1.8 for blacks and 2.1 for Caribbean Hispanics compared to whites.[40] Diabetes also increased the risk of stroke-related dementia more in blacks and Hispanics than in whites.[41]

Diabetes worsens stroke outcome as well. Diabetes doubles the risk of recurrent stroke,[42] more than trebles the risk of stroke-related dementia,[41] and markedly increases mortality, both total and stroke related.[37,39,43] In the Renfrew-Paisley

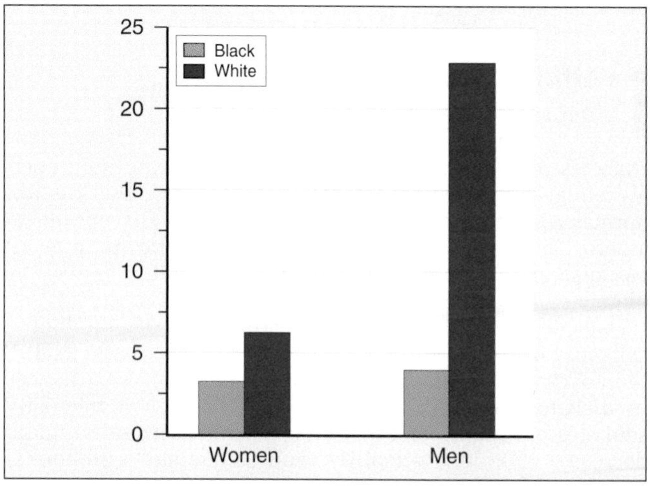

FIGURE 40–3 Odds ratio for stroke in diabetic patients aged 18 to 44 years. These data show a marked increase in the risk of stroke in diabetic persons compared to nondiabetic persons, highlighting a marked increase in risk among young adults. These data support recommendations to treat hypertension aggressively in patients with diabetes to reduce the risk of stroke and death. (From Rohr J, Kittner S, Feeser B, et al: Traditional risk factors and ischemic stroke in young adults: The Baltimore-Washington Cooperative Young Stroke Study. Arch Neurol 53:603-607, 1996.)

study, diabetes raised the relative risk of death after stroke by 290 percent in men and 400 percent in women over 20 years of follow-up.[44]

Peripheral Arterial Disease

Diabetes increases the incidence of peripheral arterial disease (PAD) twofold to fourfold.[2] Diabetic patients more often have femoral bruits and absent pedal pulses.[45] The prevalence of PAD in unselected persons with diabetes, based on decreased ankle-brachial indices (see Chap. 54) ranges from 12 to 16 percent.[46] In whites of European ancestry, the prevalence of PAD ranges from 7 percent in those with normal glucose tolerance to 20.9 percent in patients with diabetes requiring multiple medications.[47]

The duration of diabetes and the severity of hyperglycemia correlate with the prevalence and severity of PAD.[48,49] In addition to increasing the frequency of PAD, diabetes affects the distribution of atherosclerosis in the lower extremity. PAD in diabetic patients typically affects tibial and peroneal arteries, as well as femoral and popliteal arteries. Moreover, the atherosclerotic lesions in diabetic patients are more likely to manifest vascular calcification than those in nondiabetic cohorts.[49,50]

In addition to an increased frequency of lower extremity atherosclerosis, diabetes mellitus augments the likelihood of developing the symptomatic forms of PAD. In the Framingham study, diabetes mellitus increased the risk of claudication by 350 percent in men and 860 percent in women.[51] The duration of diabetes also increases the risk of developing claudication in most but not all studies.[48,52] Diabetes also increases the risk of developing critical limb ischemia and tissue loss and more than doubles the risk of critical limb ischemia in men with intermittent claudication and toe pressures of less than 40 mm Hg.[45] Diabetes is the most common cause of amputation in the United States.[53] The relative risk for amputation is increased 12.7-fold in diabetic compared with nondiabetic persons in the Medicare population in Minnesota. In the highest-risk age group, diabetic persons aged 65 to 74 years, the relative risk of amputation increases 23.5-fold. These trends extend beyond the United States. The Global Lower Extremity Amputation Study Group reports that the percentage of patients with diabetes may reach as high as 90 percent in patients undergoing their first ever amputations in populations studied in North America, Europe, and east Asia.[54]

Pathophysiology of Diabetic Vascular Disease

Diabetes involves metabolic abnormalities, including hyperglycemia, dyslipidemia, and insulin resistance, that disrupt normal arterial function and render arteries susceptible to atherosclerosis. Diabetes specifically alters the function of vascular endothelium and smooth muscle cells, as well as platelets, in ways that promote atherogenesis.

Diabetes impairs the vasodilator function of endothelial cells and decreases the bioavailability of nitric oxide (NO).[55] Moreover, each of the fundamental metabolic disturbances in diabetes, including hyperglycemia, increased free fatty acid concentrations, and insulin resistance, can individually decrease NO bioavailability and attenuate endothelial function.[56-58]

Hyperglycemia decreases NO production from endothelial NO synthase (eNOS) and increases its degradation via generation of reactive oxygen species. Hyperglycemia triggers the production of reactive oxygen species in vascular cells through enzymatic (protein kinase C [PKC] and NADPH oxidases) and nonenzymatic sources of oxidant stress (e.g., the formation of advanced glycation end products [AGEs]).[59,60] As oxidative stress increases, the eNOS cofactor tetrahydrobiopterin becomes oxidized and uncouples eNOS, which causes this enzyme to produce superoxide anion instead of NO.[61] Superoxide anion quenches NO in a diffusion-limited reaction to produce peroxynitrite.[62] Peroxynitrite inhibits prostacyclin synthase and endothelium-dependent hyperpolarizing factor activity.[63,64] Similar to the effects of hyperglycemia, free fatty acids activate intracellular enzymatic oxidant sources, including PKC, NADPH oxidases, and eNOS, yielding analogous increases in superoxide anion.[65]

The excess adipose tissue that usually accompanies type 2 diabetes mellitus releases excess fatty acids. Reduced skeletal muscle uptake of free fatty acids further augments their plasma levels.[66] Increased concentrations of free fatty acids exert deleterious actions in several areas. Free fatty acids independently activate intracellular enzymatic oxidant sources, including PKC, NADPH oxidases, and eNOS, yielding analogous increases in superoxide anion to hyperglycemia.[65] Indeed, free fatty acids likely represent an independent source of pathogenic oxygen-derived free radicals in insulin-resistant states prior to hyperglycemia—a state associated with impaired vascular function.[67] In healthy humans, free fatty acid infusion impairs endothelial function, and the coinfusion of an antioxidant restores it.[68] Moreover, free fatty acids interfere with intracellular signaling pathways to cause not only muscle and visceral insulin resistance but vascular insulin resistance as well.[69]

In diabetes, hyperglycemia and increased free fatty acids increase the concentration in the cell of the metabolite diacylglycerol.[70] Diacylglycerol, in turn, is a classic activator of a family of enzymes, known as PKC, that perform key regulatory functions by phosphorylating proteins important in metabolic control. Recent work has implicated activation of the PKC family in cardiovascular complications of diabetes.[71] Activation of PKC can inhibit the expression of eNOS, augment cytokine-induced tissue factor gene expression and procoagulant activity in human endothelial cells, and increase the production of proinflammatory cytokines, the proliferation of vascular wall cells, and the production of extracellular matrix macromolecules that accumulate during atherosclerotic lesion formation.[71,72] In vivo evidence supports a role of PKC activation in the pathogenesis of various aspects of vascular dysfunction in vivo. Administration of a selective inhibitor of PKC-β to diabetic rats improves retinal blood flow and prevents impaired endothelial function in healthy humans exposed to hyperglycemia (Fig. 40–4).[73,74]

Although typically associated with impairments in skeletal glucose muscle uptake, many tissues in the diabetic patient demonstrate insulin resistance, including adipose, liver, and endothelial cells.[75] Normal vascular function requires intact endothelial insulin signaling. For example, in genetically engineered mice that lack the endothelial cell insulin receptor, vascular eNOS concentration decreases 60 percent.[76] Endothelial insulin resistance alters the pattern of activation of intracellular signaling pathways, favoring stimulation of mitogen-activated protein (MAP) kinases over phosphatidylinositol kinase. Preferential activation of the MAP kinase pathway decreases NO production, increases endothelin production, stimulates the transcription of pro-inflammatory genes, and increases the tendency to coagulation.[77]

Recent work has identified a novel potential mechanism for mediating impaired endothelial-dependent vasodilator function. An endogenous competitive inhibitor of NO synthase, known as asymmetrical dimethylarginine (ADMA), increases directly with insulin resistance in nondiabetic subjects and glycemic control in diabetes[78,79] and improves with glycemic control.[80] The accumulation of ADMA may result from inhibition of its catabolism due to reduction in activity of the ɜnzyme dimethylarginine limethylaminohydrolase.[81] Recent evidence suggests hat dysregulation of this ɜnzyme may raise levels of ADMA in diabetics.[82] These new findings provide yet another potential molecular pathway of impaired vascu-ar function in diabetes.

Diabetes also disturbs vas-cular function through non-enzymatic glycation of macromolecules. In states of hyperglycemia and increased oxidative stress, many pro-eins and even lipids undergo nonenzymatic gly-cation. For example, hemo-globin A1c, the glycated form of hemoglobin, provides the clinician with an integrated gauge of hyperglycemia. Glycated proteins can form structures known as AGEs hat actually cause the macromolecule to take on a brown hue, similar to burnt sugar. Numerous chemical studies have characterized he structure of AGEs, which appear to contribute to the pathobiology of complica-ions of diabetes, notably the accelerated vascular disease characteristic of this condi-ion.[83-87] Recent studies have shown accumulation of AGE-modified proteins in diabetic subjects. The presence of gly-cated forms of low-density ipoprotein (LDL) can engen-der an immune response and contribute to macrovascular disease.[88] Phospholipids and apolipoproteins can form AGEs.[83] AGE-modified LDL apopro-ein and LDL lipid increase in diabetic subjects compared to nondiabetics.[85]

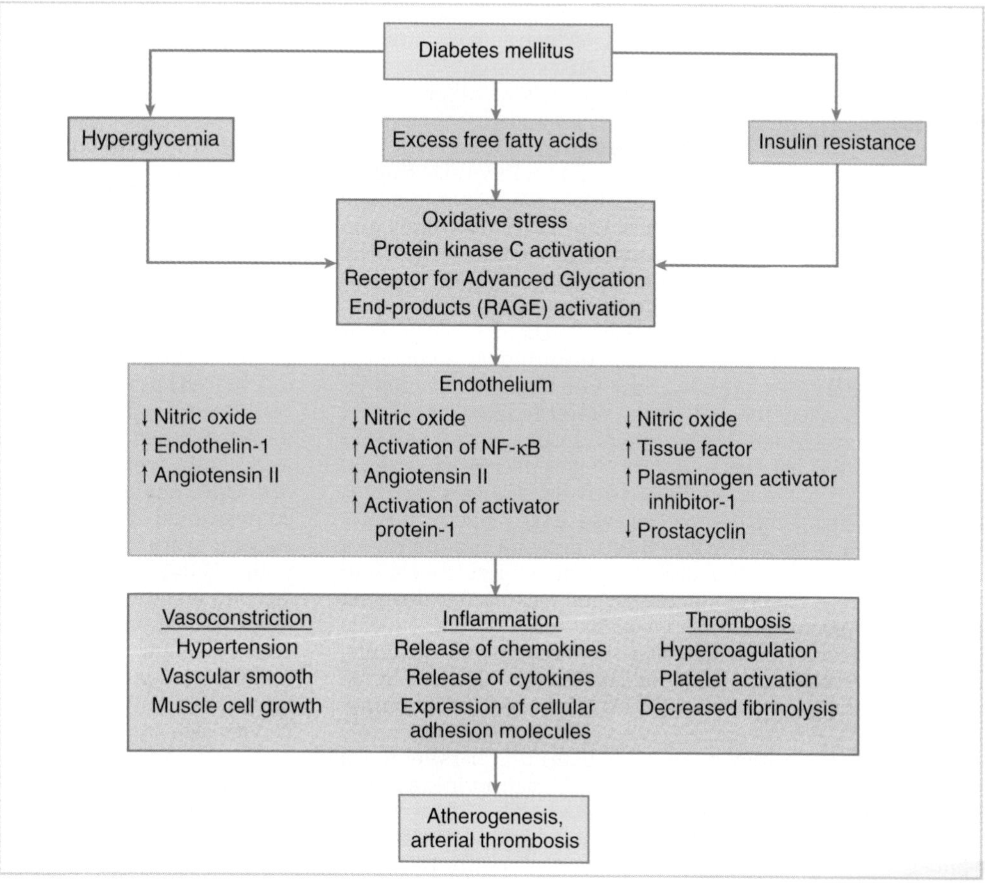

FIGURE 40–4 Endothelial dysfunction in diabetes. Normally, the endothelium maintains vascular homeostasis by promoting vasodilation, minimizing inflammation, and preventing thrombosis. In diabetes, hyperglycemia, excess free fatty acid release, dyslipidemia, and insulin resistance increase reactive oxygen species production, formation of advanced glycation end-products (AGE), and activation of protein kinase C, diminishing the bioavailability of nitric oxide and decreasing its potent vasodilatory, antiinflammatory, and antithrombotic effects. Diabetes impairs endothelial function and promotes vasoconstriction, inflammation, and thrombosis. Decreasing nitric oxide and increasing endothelin 1 and angiotensin II concentrations increases vascular tone and vascular smooth muscle cell growth and migration. Activation of inflammatory transcription factors nuclear factor-kappa B (NF-κB) and activator protein 1 induces liberation of leukocyte-attracting chemokines, production of inflammatory cytokines, and expression of cell adhesion molecules. Attenuated nitric oxide and prostacyclin activate platelets, whereas increases in plasmin activator inhibitor-1 and tissue factor create a prothrombotic milieu.

Cells have several surface receptors for AGEs that mediate heir biological effects. Exposure to AGE-modified proteins can elicit the production of inflammatory cytokines from vas-cular cells, cause impaired endothelial-dependent vasodila-or function, and augment endothelial expression of various eukocyte adhesion molecules implicated in atherogenesis in vivo.[85] One extensively characterized receptor for AGE is known as RAGE. Recent experiments support a functional role for RAGE in development of experimental atherosclero-sis. Mice lacking the apolipoprotein E gene are susceptible o atherosclerosis. Administration of an antibody fragment hat neutralizes RAGE attenuates atherosclerosis in these mutant mice. This beneficial effect on atherosclerotic lesion development does not depend on a change in blood sugar or lipoprotein profile,[90] supporting a role for AGE in atherogenesis.

Through decreases in NO, increases in oxidative stress, AGE production and activation of its receptor, and insulin resistance, diabetes increases vascular inflammation via the activation and nuclear translocation of intracellular trans-cription factors, nuclear factor (NF)-κB and activator protein 1 (AP-1).[91-93] These factors cause the expression of genes responsible for producing chemokines, cytokines, leukocyte adhesion molecules, and proinflammatory mediators, such as tumor necrosis factor-alpha.[94,95] Diabetes further aggravates plaque progression by causing endothelial cells to produce cytokines that decrease collagen production by vascular smooth muscle cells and to enhance endothelial cell production of matrix metalloproteinases and tissue factor.[96] These changes may decrease the stability of the atherosclerotic plaque's fibrous cap, increasing the likelihood and severity of plaque rupture and thrombosis (see also Chap. 35).

Numerous basic science and clinical studies indicate an increased level of oxidative stress in diabetes.[84] The reactive oxygen species in turn can augment the formation of reactive carbonyl species. Nonoxidative reactions can also increase the concentrations of reactive carbonyl compounds under hyperglycemic conditions. The reactive carbonyl species can derivatize proteins and lipids. Among the products of reactions of proteins with reactive oxygen and carbonyl species are the AGEs, discussed earlier. There is little doubt that products of glycoxidation accumulate in diabetic patients. However, they accumulate in nondiabetic elderly individuals as well.[84] Recent evidence suggests that overwhelming detoxifying mechanisms of the reactive carbonyl groups may account for the increase in oxidant and carbonyl stress in diabetics.

Diabetes impairs vascular smooth muscle function and augments the production of vasoconstrictor mediators including endothelin 1,[97] which causes vascular smooth muscle growth and inflammation.[98] Levels of other atherogenic mediators, including angiotensin II and vasoconstrictor prostanoids, increase in diabetes as well.[2] Patients with type 2 diabetes have impaired vasodilation, possibly reflecting an abnormality in NO signal transduction.[55] Moreover, diabetic patients have attenuated vasoconstriction to endothelin 1 and angiotensin.[99,100] The relative contribution of the sympathetic nervous system to vascular smooth muscle function remains unclear. Experimentally, norepinephrine re-uptake by sympathetic nerve neurons is reduced.[101] Diabetes may alter subcellular calcium distribution,[102] resulting in augmented vasoconstriction in response to norepinephrine and phenylephrine. However, most diabetic patients have peripheral autonomic impairment at the time of diagnosis, and vascular beds regulated by these nerves have decreased arterial resistance.[103,104] Akin to endothelial cells, diabetes activates atherogenic mechanisms within vascular smooth muscle cells, including PKC, RAGE, NF-κB, and the production of oxidative stress.[65,105] Diabetes heightens vascular smooth muscle cell migration in atherosclerotic lesions.[106] Advanced atherosclerotic lesions have fewer vascular smooth muscle cells in diabetic patients than in nondiabetic patients, possibly resulting in decreased resiliency of the fibrous cap and thereby increasing the risk of rupture and luminal thrombosis.[107]

Platelet abnormalities occur in diabetes that parallel those found in endothelial cells, including activation of PKC, decreased production of platelet-derived NO, and increased oxidative stress.[108-110] Diabetes impairs platelet calcium homeostasis,[111] which may contribute importantly to abnormal platelet activity since calcium regulates platelet shape change, secretion, aggregation, and thromboxane formation. Moreover, platelets from patients with diabetes have increased expression of the adhesive glycoproteins Ib and IIb/IIIa.[2] Type 2 diabetes and its associated metabolic abnormalities favor an imbalance in the coagulation/fibrinolytic systems that support clot formation and stability. Type 2 diabetes increases plasminogen activator inhibitor type 1 levels, impairing fibrinolytic capacity in atherosclerotic lesions.[112] Moreover, diabetes increases the expression of tissue factor and the levels of plasma coagulation factors, and it decreases levels of endogenous anticoagulants.[113,114] These various abnormalities may contribute to heightened susceptibility to the thrombotic complications of atherosclerosis.

Medical Therapy for Diabetic Vascular Disease

Over the last decade, treatment of diabetes has evolved from a focus on hyperglycemia to a broader view encompassing all of the metabolic disturbances associated with diabetes: insulin resistance, dyslipidemia, hypertension, and thrombosis (see Fig. 40–3). Each of these abnormalities plays an important role in cardiovascular disease development and progression.

Treatment of Hyperglycemia and Insulin Resistance

Hyperglycemia, a fundamental component of diabetes, adversely affects vascular function and directly correlates with cardiovascular events. In the United Kingdom Prospective Diabetes Study (UKPDS), hemoglobin A1c levels above 6.2 percent were associated with an increased risk of macrovascular disease.[115] For each 1 percent elevation in hemoglobin A1c, coronary heart disease (CHD) risk increased by 11 percent. A meta-analysis of nearly 100,000 diabetic patients found that increases in plasma glucose concentrations correlated with augmented cardiovascular risk, beginning with glucose concentrations below the diabetic threshold.[116] Data concerning the role of glucose intolerance are inconsistent. Large trials such as the Honolulu Heart Program demonstrated an increasing risk of CHD with greater glycemia, whereas the Paris Prospective Study did not.[117,118] However, in UKPDS, it appeared that the relative risk of CHD did not increase in association with hemoglobin A1c levels above 7 percent, suggesting a threshold.

Several clinical trials have sought to determine whether intensive treatment of blood glucose levels can reduce the risk of CHD associated with diabetes. In the Diabetes Control and Complications Trial (DCCT), 1441 patients with type 1 diabetes (mean age 27 years) without significant retinopathy at baseline were randomized to intensive glycemic control (external insulin pump or ≥3 insulin injections per day) or conventional therapy (1 or 2 insulin injections per day).[119] Patients were followed prospectively for a mean of 6.5 years, with regular assessments of microvascular and macrovascular outcomes. After 5 years, the cumulative incidence of retinopathy was approximately 50 percent less in the intensive-treatment group than in the conventional-treatment group ($p < 0.001$). Intensive therapy also reduced the risk of macrovascular disease (cardiovascular and peripheral vascular disease) by 41 percent, although the difference between groups lacked statistical significance. A second, smaller Veterans Affairs (VA) study that tested the feasibility of intensive blood glucose control in type 2 diabetics also showed no significant differences in cardiovascular endpoints between treatment arms.[120] These two trials had a number of important limitations. Both lacked adequate power to detect a difference in macrovascular events between treatment groups, given the small number of events in each group. In the DCCT, the low event rate probably resulted from the relative youth of the study population and, in the VA study, likely resulted from a small patient population and a short follow-up period.

Larger, adequately powered studies, such as UKPDS, showed a nonsignificant trend in favor of intensive blood glucose control in terms of reduction of myocardial infarction.[121] This trial randomized 3867 patients with newly diagnosed type 2 diabetes to intensive therapy (diet plus oral therapy or insulin) or to conventional therapy. Patients entered into the study had a low background prevalence of CHD and a low rate of CHD risk factors, and were followed for approximately 10 years. As in the DCCT, microvascular endpoints were improved in the intensive-therapy arm. There was also a trend for a reduced rate of myocardial infarction in the group receiving intensive blood glucose control ($p = 0.052$).[121]

More recent data support the notion that tight glycemic control may decrease the rate of cardiovascular morbidity and mortality. In the Epidemiology of Diabetes Interventions and Complications study, the long-term follow-up study of patients in the DCCT trial, type 1 subjects underwent carotid ultrasound 1 to 2 years after the end of DCCT and again 4 years later.[122] The subjects in the intensive glycemic control arm had significantly less progression of their carotid intima-media thickness (IMT) than the patients in the usual control arm. Recently, in the STOP-Noninsulin-Dependent Diabetes Mellitus (NIDDM) trial, patients with impaired glucose tolerance were randomized to acarbose, an alpha-glucosidase inhibitor, or matching placebo and followed for an average of 3.3 years.[123] Patients taking acarbose had significantly fewer cardiovascular events (including myocardial infarction, new angina, revascularization, cardiovascular death, congestive heart failure, cerebrovascular events, and PAD) than subjects taking placebo. Ongoing clinical trials with more aggressive glycemic control may enable a better evaluation of the hypothesis that glycemic control serves an important role in the prevention of cardiovascular disease.

Insulin resistance may provide the crucial link between hyperglycemia and cardiovascular disease (Table 40–2). This collective occurrence of multiple metabolic abnormalities in an individual patient has been termed variously, *syndrome X*, the *insulin resistance syndrome*, and *cardiovascular dysmetabolic syndrome*, or simply *metabolic syndrome*. Data from a number of studies indicate that insulin resistance independently predicts cardiovascular disease risk. In a large triethnic population comprising equal numbers of subjects with diabetes, hyperglycemia, and normal glucose tolerance, insulin resistance correlated positively with atherosclerosis as assessed by carotid intima-media thickness.[124] Since insulin resistance typically precedes the development of hyperglycemia, these findings may explain, in part, the elevated risk of CHD in individuals with newly diagnosed type 2 diabetes. Indeed, the severity of insulin resistance directly correlates with rates of myocardial infarction,[125] stroke,[29,32] and PAD.[126] In UKPDS, improving insulin resistance with metformin decreased macrovascular events. This result has engendered some controversy because the addition of metformin to sulfonylurea therapy seemed to increase cardiovascular risk.[53,127] The recent availability of the thiazolidinediones (TZDs) provides a second approach to improve insulin sensitivity and glycemic control.[128] TZDs bind and activate peroxisome proliferator-activated receptor-γ (PPAR-γ), a nuclear receptor that regulates functions of adipose, inflammatory, and vascular cells.[129] In addition to improving insulin sensitivity, PPAR-γ agonists may have antiinflammatory activity and directly retard atherogenesis.[130] TZDs also may decrease the concentration of small, dense LDL[131] and augment LDL resistance to oxidation.[132] However, total, LDL, and HDL cholesterol concentrations increase,[133,134] making the net effect on the lipid profile unclear. TZDs have complex effects as activation of PPAR-γ may theoretically promote foam cell formation.[135,136] Ongoing clinical trials will determine whether improvements in insulin resistance with TZDs or other drugs will decrease cardiovascular morbidity and mortality in patients with diabetes.

Treatment of Dyslipidemia in Diabetes

(see also Chap. 39)

Even though patients with diabetes typically have LDL cholesterol levels in the average range, these patients often have elevated triglycerides, decreased high-density lipoprotein (HDL) cholesterol, and more small, dense LDL. Increased delivery of free fatty acids to the liver due to excess adipose efflux and impaired skeletal muscle uptake increases hepatic production of very low density lipoprotein (VLDL) and cholesteryl ester synthesis (Fig. 40–5).[137] Overproduction of triglyceride-rich lipoproteins and impaired clearance by lipoprotein lipase lead to hypertriglyceridemia in diabetes.[138,139]

Triglyceride levels tend to vary inversely with HDL levels as cholesteryl ester transfer protein mediates exchanges of cholesterol from HDL to VLDL.[137] The combination of elevated triglycerides and low HDL is more common than elevated total and LDL cholesterol in diabetic patients with CAD.[140] In addition to abnormalities of concentration, functional defects in the HDL of diabetic subjects and a diminished capacity to prevent LDL oxidation also may promote atherogenesis.[141] Increased concentrations of small, dense LDL in diabetic person results from abnormal cholesterol and triglyceride transfer between VLDL and LDL and depends on increased levels of VLDL, particularly when triglyceride concentrations are higher than 130 mg/dl.[137] Small, dense LDL particles are proatherogenic. They bind readily to intimal proteoglycans, which enhances their retention in the intima, promoting their oxidative modification and hence take-up by macrophages and smooth muscle cells.[142]

Life-style modification should be the first prescription to improve the lipid profile. Indeed, each component of diabetic dysmetabolism improves with weight loss, exercise, and dietary modification. Strict glycemic control may lessen hepatic VLDL production.[138] Large clinical trials have demonstrated the benefits of pharmacological interventions. Lipid-lowering therapy, particularly with 3-hydroxy-3-methylglutaryl coenzyme A reductase inhibitors, or statins, results in a proportionally greater cardiovascular risk reduction in diabetic than in nondiabetic subjects (Table 40–3).[143,144] In the Scandinavian Simvastatin Survival Study

TABLE 40–2 Components of the Metabolic Syndrome

Variable	Parameter
Hyperglycemia	>110 mg/dl
Dyslipidemia	HDL cholesterol Men < 40 mg/dl Women < 50 mg/dl Triglycerides > 150 mg/dl
Obesity	Waist circumference Men > 40 in Women > 35 in
Hypertension	Blood pressure >130/85 mm Hg
Age	Men > 45 yr Women > 55 yr

HDL = high-density lipoprotein.

Adapted from Executive Summary of the Third Report of the National Cholesterol Education Program (NCEP) Expert Panel on Detection, Evaluation, and Treatment of High Blood Cholesterol in Adults (Adult Treatment Panel III). JAMA 285:2486, 2001.

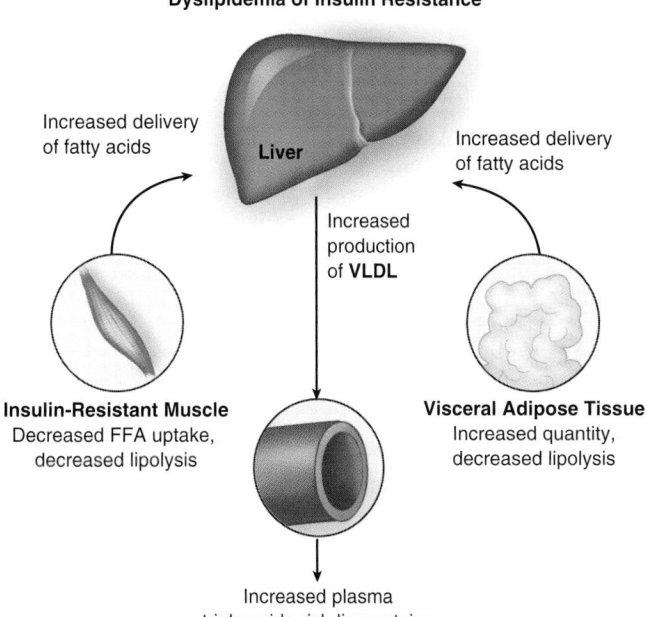

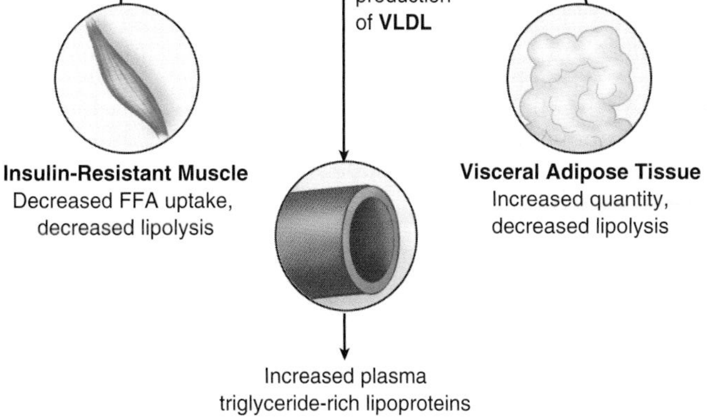

FIGURE 40–5 Pathogenesis of diabetic dyslipidemia. Increased production of very low density lipoprotein (VLDL) from the liver results from increased delivery of fatty acids because of decreased utilization by muscle and increased delivery of fatty acids from visceral abdominal fat to the liver via the portal circulation. Decreased catabolism of postprandial triglyceride-rich lipoprotein particles due to reduced lipoprotein lipase activity (lipolysis) accentuates diabetic dyslipidemia. FFA = free fatty acid.

TABLE 40–3 Statin Therapy in Diabetes

Trial*	No. of Patients	Indication	Drug	Duration (yr)	CV Outcome	Risk Reduction (%)
AFCAPS/ TexCAPS	155	PP, average TC Low HDL	Lovastatin	5.2	FMI, NFMI, SD	43
4S	202	Stable CAD Elevated TC	Simvastatin	5.3	Fatal CHD + NFMI	51
CARE	602	Stable CAD Average TC	Pravastatin	5	Fatal CHD + NFMI + CR	22
LIPID	782	Stable CAD Average TC	Pravastatin	6.1	Fatal CHD + NFMI	17
HPS	5983	Diabetes	Simvastatin	4.8	MI + CVA + CR + NCR	33

*The trials are identified as follows: AFCAPS = Air Force Coronary Artery Prevention Study; 4S = Scandinavian Simvastatin Survival Study; CARE = Cholesterol and Recurrent Events; CAD = coronary artery disease; CHD = coronary heart disease; CR = coronary revascularization; CV = cardiovascular; CVA = cerebrovascular accident; FMI = fatal myocardial infarction; HDL = high-density lipoprotein; HPS = heart protection study; LIPID = Long-term Intervention with Pravastatin in Ischemic Disease; MI = myocardial infarction; NCR = noncoronary revascularization; NFMI = nonfatal myocardial infarction; PP = Primary prevention; SD = sudden death; TC = total cholesterol.

(4S) trial, simvastatin reduced total mortality by 43 percent in diabetics compared with 29 percent in nondiabetics.[144] Similarly, myocardial infarction was reduced by 55 percent versus 32 percent in diabetic and nondiabetic cohorts, respectively.[144] In the Cholesterol and Recurrent Events (CARE) trial, which included subjects with average LDL levels and CAD, pravastatin reduced the absolute risk of coronary events for diabetic and nondiabetic patients by 8.1 percent and 5.2 percent, respectively.[143] In the Heart Protection Study (HPS), which included 5963 subjects with diabetes, simvastatin decreased the risk of coronary death, nonfatal myocardial infarction, stroke, or revascularization by 25 percent in the diabetic subgroup.[145] The reduction risk even extended to patients with pretreatment LDL cholesterol levels below 100 mg/dL.

Fibric acid derivatives address particularly the increased triglyceride and decreased HDL concentrations characteristic of diabetic dyslipidemia. In the VA High-Density Lipoprotein Cholesterol Intervention Trial (VA-HIT), treatment with gemfibrozil resulted in a 24 percent risk reduction for myocardial infarction in the diabetic subjects, who represented one fourth of enrolled subjects, an outcome similar to that observed in nondiabetic subjects.[146]

In the Diabetes Atherosclerosis Intervention Study (DAIS), fenofibrate limited angiographic progression of coronary artery lesions in a diabetic cohort, but the event reduction did not achieve statistical significance owing to the small sample size in this angiographic trial.[147] Akin to TZDs, fibrates may have antiatherogenic effects independent of lipid lowering. Fibrates bind to PPAR-α, which exerts anti-inflammatory effects that include the reduction of endothelial cell activation by pro-inflammatory cytokines and decreased tissue factor production by human macrophages.[148-150] Fibric acid derivatives may prove of value, typically as a second lipid agent in diabetic patients with persistently elevated triglycerides and low HDL. Combinations of statins and fibrates warrant careful monitoring for muscle injury. Despite concern over worsening glycemic control, nicotinic acid may be useful in diabetic persons to increase HDL.

Treatment of Hypertension in Diabetic Patients

Hypertension and insulin resistance frequently occur together as part of the metabolic syndrome.[151,152] The addition of hypertension to the clinical picture of diabetes amplifies the already high cardiovascular disease risk in these patients. Aggressive blood pressure control prevents further cardiovascular events more in diabetics than nondiabetics.[153] Indeed, the Appropriate Blood Pressure Control in Diabetes (ABCD) trial investigated the effect of aggressive blood pressure control in type 2 diabetic patients with PAD. The intensively treated group (128/75 mm Hg) had no increased risk of cardiovascular events over 4 years of follow-up.[154,155]

The role of specific classes of antihypertensive drugs in reducing cardiovascular morbidity and mortality in patients with diabetes has engendered controversy. Two trials compared the effects of calcium-channel blockers and angiotensin-converting enzyme (ACE) inhibitors in patients with type 2 diabetes.[156,157] In these trials, the ACE inhibitor reduced cardiovascular endpoints more effectively than the dihydropyridine calcium-channel blockers. The results of these two studies suggest that calcium-channel blockers do not benefit and might even harm diabetic patients at high risk for cardiovascular events. Neither the UKPDS nor the Systolic Hypertension in Europe Trial (Sys-Eur) has supported the findings of the two smaller trials noted earlier and, indeed, have shown beneficial effects for both ACE inhibitors and calcium-channel blockers in patients with diabetes (Table 40–4). Also, in UKPDS,[158] 1148 hypertensive patients with type 2 diabetes responded equally well to captopril or atenolol in terms of achieving blood pressure control and had similar reductions in the risk of macrovascular disease. Aggressive blood pressure reduction with either agent significantly reduced stroke and deaths due to diabetes. Myocardial infarction declined 21 percent in the group randomized to tight blood pressure control (p = NS). Although blood pressure in the UKPDS subgroup assigned to tight blood pressure control was good (averaging 144/82 mm Hg), data from the Syst-Eur trial[153,159] and the HOT trial[160] indicate that achieving even lower blood pressure with calcium-channel blockers further lowers the rate of cardiovascular complications compared with moderate blood pressure control. Achieving ADA target blood pressure (130/80 mm Hg) almost always requires more than one agent.[53,160,161]

Modulation of the renin-angiotensin system has particular importance in diabetic patients. ACE inhibitors reduce nephropathy and end-stage renal disease in patients with type 1 diabetes, and angiotensin receptor blockers reduce risk of these microvascualar disorders in patients with type 2 diabetes.[162-164] In the recent Heart Outcomes and Prevention Evaluation (HOPE) study, ramipril significantly decreased the rates of myocardial infarction, stroke, and death in patients with diabetes and a mean blood pressure of 140/80 mm Hg.[165] In the Losartan Intervention For Endpoint (LIFE) study,[166] 1195 diabetic subjects were enrolled as part of the cohort. All

TABLE 40–4 Treatment of Hypertension in Diabetes

Trial*	No. of Patients	Population	Drug	Duration (yr)	BP Control: *Tight (mm Hg)*	BP Control: *Less Tight*	CV Outcome	Risk Reduction (%)
Placebo Controlled Trials								
SHEP	583	Elderly T2	Chlorthalidone	5	143/68	155/72	CHD CV mortality	56 34
HOT	1501	T2, 50-80 yr	Felodipine	3	140/81	144/85	CV events MI	51 50
Syst-Eur	492	T2	Nitrendipine	2	153/76	182/81	CVA CV mortality	69 70
UKPDS	1148	T2	Captopril or atenolol	8.4	144/82	154/87	CVA Death	44 37
HOPE	3547	T2 + 1 RF	Ramipril	4.5	140/77	143/77	MI CVA Mortality	22 33 24
Drug Comparison Trials			**Initial Therapy**		**Drug 1**	**Drug 2**		
CAPP	572	DM	Captopril vs. diuretic or beta blocker	7	155/89	153/88	FMI/NFMI + CVA/CVD	41
LIFE	1195	DM + LVH	Losartan vs. atenolol	4.8	146/79	148/79	CV events Mortality	22 39

DM = diabetes mellitus; LVH = left ventricular hypertrophy; RF = Risk factor; T2 = Type 2 diabetic patients; for other abbreviations see Table 40–3.
*The trials are identified as follows: SHEP = Systolic Hypertension in the Elderly; HOT = Hypertension Optimal Treatment; Syst-Eur = Systolic Hypertension in Europe; UKPDS = United Kingdom Prospective Diabetes Study; HOPE = Heart Outcomes and Prevention Evaluation; CAPP = Captopril Prevention Project; LIFE = Losartan Intervention for Endpoint.

subjects were hypertensive and had evidence of left ventricular hypertrophy. Subjects were randomized to losartan or atenolol. Despite equivalent blood pressure lowering, the subjects randomized to losartan experienced a 39 percent reduction in all-cause mortality, a 37 percent reduction in cardiovascular mortality, and a 21 percent reduction in stroke.[166]

Comprehensive Risk Factor Modification

Aggressive modification of every risk factor may produce results with greater than additive benefit than expected from treatment of each individual risk factor. The Steno-2 trial randomized 160 subjects to intensive multifactorial risk factor modification including dietary modification (fat intake <30 percent of total consumption), light to moderate exercise three to five times per week, smoking cessation courses, ACE inhibitors, multivitamins, aspirin, intensive glucose control, and lipid modification or to conventional therapy.[167] This combination of interventions significantly and markedly reduced the rate of cardiovascular events from 85 events among 35 patients in the conventional arm to 33 events among 19 patients in the intensive risk factor modification group. Aggressive therapies to modify the risks of cardiovascular disease will diminish the clinical manifestations of vascular disease and should be implemented (Fig. 40–6).

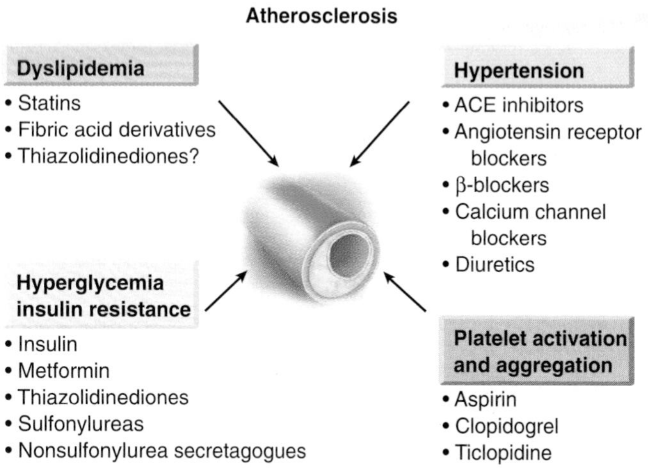

FIGURE 40–6 Antiatherosclerosis therapy in diabetes. To stem the onset and progression of atherosclerosis, patients with diabetes require therapy for each metabolic abnormality. Statins and fibric acid derivatives improve the lipid profile and decrease the risk of myocardial infarction and death. The clinical benefit of thiazolidinediones for cardiovascular outcomes therapy is under investigation. Treatment of hypertension decreases the rate of myocardial infarction and stroke in diabetes. Therapy should include angiotensin-converting enzyme (ACE) inhibitors for their proven microvascular and atherosclerotic benefits. The heightened thrombotic potential of the diabetic state supports the use of platelet antagonists such as aspirin and clopidogrel. Although strict treatment of hyperglycemia does not significantly reduce the incidence of myocardial infarction or death, the improvement in microvascular outcomes itself warrants vigorous pursuit of rigorous glycemic control in diabetes.

Conclusion

Atherosclerosis and its complications cause most deaths and much of the disability in patients with diabetes mellitus. Intensive treatment of the entire scope of metabolic abnormalities beyond hyperglycemia alone significantly reduces the rates of adverse cardiovascular events. As the prevalence of patients with diabetes increases, strategies to ensure the appropriate and aggressive use of medical therapy will help stem the tide of death and disability in this high-risk population.

REFERENCES

1. Resnick HE, Shorr RI, Kuller L, et al: Prevalence and clinical implications of American Diabetes Association–defined diabetes and other categories of glucose

dysregulation in older adults: The health, aging and body composition study. J Clin Epidemiol 54:869-876, 2001.
2. Beckman JA, Creager MA, Libby P: Diabetes and atherosclerosis: epidemiology, pathophysiology, and management. JAMA 287:2570-2581, 2002.
3. Grundy SM, Benjamin IJ, Burke GL, et al: Diabetes and cardiovascular disease: A statement for healthcare professionals from the American Heart Association. Circulation 100:1134-1146, 1999.
4. Mokdad AH, Ford ES, Bowman BA, et al: Prevalence of obesity, diabetes, and obesity-related health risk factors, 2001. JAMA 289:76-79, 2003.
5. Mokdad AH, Bowman BA, Engelgau MM, Vinicor F: Diabetes trends among American Indians and Alaska natives—1990–1998. Diabetes Care 24:1508-1509, 2001.
6. Wilson PW, Kannel WB, Silbershatz H, D'Agostino RB: Clustering of metabolic factors and coronary heart disease. Arch Intern Med 159:1104-1109, 1999.
7. Brancati FL, Kao WH, Folsom AR, et al: Incident type 2 diabetes mellitus in African American and white adults: The Atherosclerosis Risk in Communities Study. JAMA 283:2253-2259, 2000.
8. Carter JS, Pugh JA, Monterrosa A: Non-insulin-dependent diabetes mellitus in minorities in the United States. Ann Intern Med 125:221-232, 1996.
9. Lindeman RD, Romero LJ, Hundley R, et al: Prevalences of type 2 diabetes, the insulin resistance syndrome, and coronary heart disease in an elderly, biethnic population. Diabetes Care 21:959-966, 1998.
10. Narayan KMV, Boyle JP, Thompson TJ, et al: Lifetime risk for diabetes mellitus in the United States. JAMA 290:1884-1890, 2003.
11. Fujimoto WY: The importance of insulin resistance in the pathogenesis of type 2 diabetes mellitus. Am J Med 108(Suppl 6a):9S-14S, 2000.
12. Gu K, Cowie CC, Harris MI: Diabetes and decline in heart disease mortality in U.S. adults. JAMA 281:1291-1297, 1999.
13. Selby JV, Ray GT, Zhang D, Colby CJ: Excess costs of medical care for patients with diabetes in a managed care population. Diabetes Care 20:1396-1402, 1997.

14. Libby P, Plutzky J: Diabetic macrovascular disease: The glucose paradox? Circulation 106:2760-2763, 2002.
15. Report of the Expert Committee on the Diagnosis and Classification of Diabetes Mellitus. Diabetes Care 20:1183-1197, 1997.
16. Kris-Etherton PM: AHA Science Advisory. Monounsaturated fatty acids and risk of cardiovascular disease. American Heart Association. Nutrition Committee. Circulation 100:1253-1258, 1999.
17. Stamler J, Vaccaro O, Neaton JD, Wentworth D: Diabetes, other risk factors, and 12-year cardiovascular mortality for men screened in the Multiple Risk Factor Intervention Trial. Diabetes Care 16:434-444, 1993.
18. Lowe LP, Liu K, Greenland P, et al: Diabetes, asymptomatic hyperglycemia, and 22-year mortality in black and white men. The Chicago Heart Association Detection Project in Industry Study. Diabetes Care 20:163-169, 1997.
19. Hu FB, Stampfer MJ, Solomon CG, et al: The impact of diabetes mellitus on mortality from all causes and coronary heart disease in women: 20 years of follow-up. Arch Intern Med 161:1717-1723, 2001.
20. Gillum RF, Mussolino ME, Madans JH: Diabetes mellitus, coronary heart disease incidence, and death from all causes in African American and European American women: The NHANES I epidemiologic follow-up study. J Clin Epidemiol 53:511-518, 2000.
21. Miettinen H, Lehto S, Salomaa V, et al: Impact of diabetes on mortality after the first myocardial infarction. The FINMONICA Myocardial Infarction Register Study Group. Diabetes Care 21:69-75, 1998.
22. Haffner SM, Lehto S, Ronnemaa T, et al: Mortality from coronary heart disease in subjects with type 2 diabetes and in nondiabetic subjects with and without prior myocardial infarction. N Engl J Med 339:229-234, 1998.
23. Malmberg K, Yusuf S, Gerstein HC, et al: Impact of diabetes on long-term prognosis in patients with unstable angina and non-Q-wave myocardial infarction: Results of the OASIS (Organization to Assess Strategies for Ischemic Syndromes) Registry. Circulation 102:1014-1019, 2000.
24. Zuanetti G, Latini R, Maggioni AP, et al: Influence of diabetes on mortality in acute myocardial infarction: Data from the GISSI-2 study. J Am Coll Cardiol 22:1788-1794, 1993.
25. Hochman JS, Sleeper LA, Webb JG, et al: Early revascularization in acute myocardial infarction complicated by cardiogenic shock. SHOCK Investigators: Should We Emergently Revascularize Occluded Coronaries for Cardiogenic Shock. N Engl J Med 341:625-634, 1999.
26. Shindler DM, Palmeri ST, Antonelli TA, et al: Diabetes mellitus in cardiogenic shock complicating acute myocardial infarction: A report from the SHOCK Trial Registry. SHould we emergently revascularize Occluded Coronaries for cardiogenic shocK? J Am Coll Cardiol 36(3 Suppl A):1097-1103, 2000.
27. Herlitz J, Karlson BW, Lindqvist J, Sjolin M: Rate and mode of death during five years of follow-up among patients with acute chest pain with and without a history of diabetes mellitus. Diabet Med 15:308-314, 1998.
28. Abbud ZA, Shindler DM, Wilson AC, Kostis JB: Effect of diabetes mellitus on short- and long-term mortality rates of patients with acute myocardial infarction: A statewide study. Myocardial Infarction Data Acquisition System Study Group. Am Heart J 130:51-58, 1995.
29. Adachi H, Hirai Y, Tsuruta M, et al: Is insulin resistance or diabetes mellitus associated with stroke? An 18-year follow-up study. Diabetes Res Clin Pract 51:215-223, 2001.
30. Jamrozik K, Broadhurst RJ, Forbes S, et al: Predictors of death and vascular events in the elderly: The Perth Community Stroke Study. Stroke 31:863-868, 2000.
31. Wannamethee SG, Perry IJ, Shaper AG: Nonfasting serum glucose and insulin concentrations and the risk of stroke. Stroke 30:1780-1786, 1999.
32. Folsom AR, Rasmussen ML, Chambless LE, et al: Prospective associations of fasting insulin, body fat distribution, and diabetes with risk of ischemic stroke. The Atherosclerosis Risk in Communities (ARIC) Study Investigators. Diabetes Care 22:1077-1083, 1999.
33. Friedlander AH, Maeder LA: The prevalence of calcified carotid artery atheromas on the panoramic radiographs of patients with type 2 diabetes mellitus. Oral Surg Oral Med Oral Pathol Oral Radiol Endod 89:420-424, 2000.
34. You RX, McNeil JJ, O'Malley HM, et al: Risk factors for stroke due to cerebral infarction in young adults. Stroke 28:1913-1918, 1997.
35. Rohr J, Kittner S, Feeser B, et al: Traditional risk factors and ischemic stroke in young adults: The Baltimore-Washington Cooperative Young Stroke Study. Arch Neurol 53:603-607, 1996.
36. Kuusisto J, Mykkanen L, Pyorala K, Laakso M: Non-insulin-dependent diabetes and its metabolic control are important predictors of stroke in elderly subjects. Stroke 25:1157-1164, 1994.
37. Stegmayr B, Asplund K: Diabetes as a risk factor for stroke: A population perspective. Diabetologia 38:1061-1068, 1995.
38. Hart CL, Hole DJ, Smith GD: Risk factors and 20-year stroke mortality in men and women in the Renfrew/Paisley study in Scotland. Stroke 30:1999-2007, 1999.
39. Tuomilehto J, Rastenyte D, Jousilahti P, et al: Diabetes mellitus as a risk factor for death from stroke: Prospective study of the middle-aged Finnish population. Stroke 27:210-215, 1996.
40. Sacco RL, Boden-Albala B, Abel G, et al: Race-ethnic disparities in the impact of stroke risk factors: The Northern Manhattan Stroke Study. Stroke 32:1725-1731, 2001.
41. Luchsinger JA, Tang MX, Stern Y, et al: Diabetes mellitus and risk of Alzheimer's disease and dementia with stroke in a multiethnic cohort. Am J Epidemiol 154:635-641, 2001.
42. Hankey GJ, Jamrozik K, Broadhurst RJ, et al: Long-term risk of first recurrent stroke in the Perth Community Stroke Study. Stroke 29:2491-2500, 1998.
43. Jorgensen H, Nakayama H, Raaschou HO, Olsen TS: Stroke in patients with diabetes. The Copenhagen Stroke Study. Stroke 25:1977-1984, 1994.
44. Hart CL, Hole DJ, Smith GD: Comparison of risk factors for stroke incidence and stroke mortality in 20 years of follow-up in men and women in the Renfrew/Paisley Study in Scotland. Stroke 31:1893-1896, 2000.
45. Abbott RD, Brand FN, Kannel WB: Epidemiology of some peripheral arterial findings in diabetic men and women: Experiences from the Framingham Study. Am J Med 88:376-381, 1990.
46. Meijer WT, Hoes AW, Rutgers D, et al: Peripheral arterial disease in the elderly: The Rotterdam Study. Arterioscler Thromb Vasc Biol 18:185-192, 1998.
47. Beks PJ, Mackaay AJ, de Neeling JN, et al: Peripheral arterial disease in relation to glycaemic level in an elderly Caucasian population: The Hoorn study. Diabetologia 38:86-96, 1995.
48. Katsilambros NL, Tsapogas PC, Arvanitis MP, et al: Risk factors for lower extremity arterial disease in non-insulin-dependent diabetic persons. Diabet Med 13:243-246, 1996.
49. Jude EB, Oyibo SO, Chalmers N, Boulton AJ: Peripheral arterial disease in diabetic and nondiabetic patients: A comparison of severity and outcome. Diabetes Care 24:1433-1437, 2001.
50. Mozes G, Keresztury G, Kadar A, et al: Atherosclerosis in amputated legs of patients with and without diabetes mellitus. Int Angiol 17:282-286, 1998.
51. Kannel WB, McGee DL: Update on some epidemiologic features of intermittent claudication: The Framingham Study. J Am Geriatr Soc 33:13-18, 1985.
52. Fowkes FG, Housley E, Riemersma RA, et al: Smoking, lipids, glucose intolerance, and blood pressure as risk factors for peripheral atherosclerosis compared with ischemic heart disease in the Edinburgh Artery Study. Am J Epidemiol 135:331-340, 1992.
53. Diabetes-related amputations of lower extremities in the Medicare population—Minnesota, 1993-1995. MMWR Morb Mortal Wkly Rep 47:649-652, 1998.
54. Group TG: Epidemiology of lower extremity amputation in centres in Europe, North America, and East Asia: The Global Lower Extremity Amputation Study Group. Br J Surg 87:328-337, 2000.
55. Beckman JA, Goldfine AB, Gordon MB, et al: Oral antioxidant therapy improves endothelial function in type 1 but not type 2 diabetes mellitus. Am J Physiol Heart Circ Physiol 285:H2392-H2398, 2003.
56. Williams SB, Goldfine AB, Timimi FK, et al: Acute hyperglycemia attenuates endothelium-dependent vasodilation in humans in vivo. Circulation 97:1695-1701, 1998.
57. Steinberg HO, Tarshoby M, Monestel R, et al: Elevated circulating free fatty acid levels impair endothelium- dependent vasodilation. J Clin Invest 100:1230-1239, 1997.
58. Steinberg HO, Chaker H, Leaming R, et al: Obesity/insulin resistance is associated with endothelial dysfunction: Implications for the syndrome of insulin resistance. J Clin Invest 97:2601-2610, 1996.
59. Nishikawa T, Edelstein D, Du XL, et al: Normalizing mitochondrial superoxide production blocks three pathways of hyperglycaemic damage. Nature 404:787-790, 2000.
60. Brownlee M: Biochemistry and molecular cell biology of diabetic complications. Nature 414:813-820, 2001.
61. Shinozaki K, Kashiwagi A, Nishio Y, et al: Abnormal biopterin metabolism is a major cause of impaired endothelium-dependent relaxation through nitric oxide/O_2^- imbalance in insulin-resistant rat aorta. Diabetes 48:2437-2445, 1999.
62. Beckman JS, Koppenol WH: Nitric oxide, superoxide, and peroxynitrite: The good, the bad, and ugly. Am J Physiol 272:C1424-C1437, 1996.
63. Zou M, Yesilkaya A, Ullrich V: Peroxynitrite inactivates prostacyclin synthase by heme-thiolate-catalyzed tyrosine nitration. Drug Metab Rev 31:343-349, 1999.
64. Liu Y, Terata K, Chai Q, et al: Peroxynitrite inhibits Ca^{2+}-activated K^+ channel activity in smooth muscle of human coronary arterioles. Circ Res 91:1070-1076, 2002.
65. Inoguchi T, Li P, Umeda F, et al: High glucose level and free fatty acid stimulate reactive oxygen species production through protein kinase C–dependent activation of NAD(P)H oxidase in cultured vascular cells. Diabetes 49:1939-1945, 2000.
66. Goldstein BJ: Insulin resistance as the core defect in type 2 diabetes mellitus. Am J Cardiol 90:3G-10G, 2002.
67. Steinberg HO, Baron AD: Vascular function, insulin resistance, and fatty acids. Diabetologia 45:623-634, 2002.
68. Pleiner J, Schaller G, Mittermayer F, et al: FFA-induced endothelial dysfunction can be corrected by vitamin C. J Clin Endocrinol Metab 87:2913-2917, 2002.

69. Griffin ME, Marcucci MJ, Cline GW, et al: Free fatty acid–induced insulin resistance is associated with activation of protein kinase C theta and alterations in the insulin signaling cascade. Diabetes 48:1270-1274, 1999.
70. Itani SI, Ruderman NB, Schmieder F, Boden G: Lipid-induced insulin resistance in human muscle is associated with changes in diacylglycerol, protein kinase C, and I kappa B-alpha. Diabetes 2002;51(7):2005-11.
71. Koya D, King GL: Protein kinase C activation and the development of diabetic complications. Diabetes 47:859-866, 1998.
72. Terry CM, Callahan KS: Protein kinase C regulates cytokine-induced tissue factor transcription and procoagulant activity in human endothelial cells. J Lab Clin Med 127:81-93, 1996.
73. Ishii H, Jirousek MR, Koya D, et al: Amelioration of vascular dysfunctions in diabetic rats by an oral PKC beta inhibitor. Science 272:728-731, 1996.
74. Beckman JA, Goldfine AB, Gordon MB, et al: Inhibition of protein kinase C beta prevents impaired endothelium-dependent vasodilation caused by hyperglycemia in humans. Circ Res 90:107-111, 2002.
75. Kaburagi Y, Yamauchi T, Yamamoto-Honda R, et al: The mechanism of insulin-induced signal transduction mediated by the insulin receptor substrate family. Endocr J 46(Suppl):S25-S34, 1999.
76. Vicent D, Ilany J, Kondo T, et al: The role of endothelial insulin signaling in the regulation of vascular tone and insulin resistance. J Clin Invest 111:1373-1380, 2003.
77. Montagnani M, Golovchenko I, Kim I, et al: Inhibition of phosphatidylinositol 3-kinase enhances mitogenic actions of insulin in endothelial cells. J Biol Chem 277:1794-1799, 2002.
78. Stuhlinger MC, Abbasi F, Chu JW, et al: Relationship between insulin resistance and an endogenous nitric oxide synthase inhibitor. JAMA 287:1420-1426, 2002.
79. Paiva H, Lehtimaki T, Laakso J, et al: Plasma concentrations of asymmetric-dimethyl-arginine in type 2 diabetes associate with glycemic control and glomerular filtration rate but not with risk factors of vasculopathy. Metabolism 52:303-307, 2003.
80. Asagami T, Abbasi F, Stuelinger M, et al: Metformin treatment lowers asymmetric dimethylarginine concentrations in patients with type 2 diabetes. Metabolism 51:843-846, 2002.
81. Ito A, Tsao PS, Adimoolam S, et al: Novel mechanism for endothelial dysfunction: Dysregulation of dimethylarginine dimethylaminohydrolase. Circulation 99:3092-3095, 1999.
82. Lin KY, Ito A, Asagami T, et al: Impaired nitric oxide synthase pathway in diabetes mellitus: Role of asymmetric dimethylarginine and dimethylarginine dimethylaminohydrolase. Circulation 106:987-992, 2002.
83. Wendt T, Bucciarelli L, Qu W, et al: Receptor for advanced glycation endproducts (RAGE) and vascular inflammation: Insights into the pathogenesis of macrovascular complications in diabetes. Curr Atheroscler Rep 4:228-237, 2002.
84. Baynes JW, Thorpe SR: Role of oxidative stress in diabetic complications: A new perspective on an old paradigm. Diabetes 48:1-9, 1999.
85. Brownlee M: Negative consequences of glycation. Metabolism 49(2 Suppl 1):9-13, 2000.
86. Stitt AW, Bucala R, Vlassara H: Atherogenesis and advanced glycation: Promotion, progression, and prevention. Ann N Y Acad Sci 811:115-127, 1997; discussion, 127-129.
87. Wautier JL, Guillausseau PJ: Diabetes, advanced glycation end products, and vascular disease. Vasc Med 3:131-137, 1998.
88. Witztum JL: Role of modified lipoproteins in diabetic macroangiopathy. Diabetes 46(Suppl 2):S112-S114, 1997.
89. Schmidt AM, Yan SD, Wautier JL, Stern D: Activation of receptor for advanced glycation end products: A mechanism for chronic vascular dysfunction in diabetic vasculopathy and atherosclerosis. Circ Res 84:489-497, 1999.
90. Park L, Raman KG, Lee KJ, et al: Suppression of accelerated diabetic atherosclerosis by the soluble receptor for advanced glycation end products. Nat Med 4:1025-1031, 1998.
91. Morigi M, Angioletti S, Imberti B, et al: Leukocyte-endothelial interaction is augmented by high glucose concentrations and hyperglycemia in a NF-κB–dependent fashion. J Clin Invest 101:1905-1915, 1998.
92. El Bekay R, Alvarez M, Monteseirin J, et al: Oxidative stress is a critical mediator of the angiotensin II signal in human neutrophils: Involvement of mitogen-activated protein kinase, calcineurin, and the transcription factor NF-kappaB. Blood 102:662-671, 2003.
93. Pieper GM, Riaz ul-Haq: Activation of nuclear factor-kappaB in cultured endothelial cells by increased glucose concentration: Prevention by calphostin C. J Cardiovasc Pharmacol 30:528-532, 1997.
94. Rosen P, Nawroth PP, King G, et al: The role of oxidative stress in the onset and progression of diabetes and its complications: A summary of a Congress Series sponsored by UNESCO-MCBN, the American Diabetes Association, and the German Diabetes Society. Diabetes Metab Res Rev 17:189-212, 2001.
95. Schmidt AM, Stern D: Atherosclerosis and diabetes: The RAGE connection. Curr Atheroscler Rep 2:430-436, 2000.
96. Uemura S, Matsushita H, Li W, et al: Diabetes mellitus enhances vascular matrix metalloproteinase activity: Role of oxidative stress. Circ Res 88:1291-1298, 2001.
97. Park JY, Takahara N, Gabriele A, et al: Induction of endothelin-1 expression by glucose: An effect of protein kinase C activation. Diabetes 49:1239-1248, 2000.
98. Browatzki M, Schmidt J, Kubler W, Kranzhofer R: Endothelin-1 induces interleukin-6 release via activation of the transcription factor NF-kappaB in human vascular smooth muscle cells. Basic Res Cardiol 95:98-105, 2000.
99. Ang C, Hillier C, Cameron AD, et al: The effect of type 1 diabetes mellitus on vascular responses to endothelin-1 in pregnant women. J Clin Endocrinol Metab 86:4939-4942, 2001.
100. McAuley DF, McGurk C, Nugent AG, et al: Vasoconstriction to endothelin-1 is blunted in non-insulin-dependent diabetes: A dose-response study. J Cardiovasc Pharmacol 36:203-208, 2000.
101. Tesfamariam B, Cohen RA: Enhanced adrenergic neurotransmission in diabetic rabbit carotid artery. Cardiovasc Res 29:549-554, 1995.
102. Fleischhacker E, Esenabhalu VE, Spitaler M, et al: Human diabetes is associated with hyperreactivity of vascular smooth muscle cells due to altered subcellular Ca^{2+} distribution. Diabetes 48:1323-1330, 1999.
103. Stansberry KB, Hill MA, Shapiro SA, et al: Impairment of peripheral blood flow responses in diabetes resembles an enhanced aging effect. Diabetes Care 20:1711-1716, 1997.
104. Takahashi T, Nishizawa Y, Emoto M, et al: Sympathetic function test of vasoconstrictor changes in foot arteries in diabetic patients. Diabetes Care 21:1495-1501, 1998.
105. Hattori Y, Hattori S, Sato N, Kasai K: High-glucose-induced nuclear factor kappaB activation in vascular smooth muscle cells. Cardiovasc Res 46:188-197, 2000.
106. Suzuki LA, Poot M, Gerrity RG, Bornfeldt KE: Diabetes accelerates smooth muscle accumulation in lesions of atherosclerosis: Lack of direct growth-promoting effects of high glucose levels. Diabetes 50:851-860, 2001.
107. Fukumoto H, Naito Z, Asano G, Aramaki T: Immunohistochemical and morphometric evaluations of coronary atherosclerotic plaques associated with myocardial infarction and diabetes mellitus. J Atheroscler Thromb 5:29-35, 1998.
108. Assert R, Scherk G, Bumbure A, et al: Regulation of protein kinase C by short-term hyperglycaemia in human platelets in vivo and in vitro. Diabetologia 44:188-195, 2001.
109. Martina V, Bruno GA, Zumpano E, et al: Administration of glutathione in patients with type 2 diabetes mellitus increases the platelet constitutive nitric oxide synthase activity and reduces PAI-1. J Endocrinol Invest 24:37-41, 2001.
110. Schaeffer G, Wascher TC, Kostner GM, Graier WF: Alterations in platelet Ca^{2+} signalling in diabetic patients is due to increased formation of superoxide anions and reduced nitric oxide production. Diabetologia 42:167-176, 1999.
111. Li Y, Woo V, Bose R: Platelet hyperactivity and abnormal Ca^{2+} homeostasis in diabetes mellitus. Am J Physiol Heart Circ Physiol 280:H1480-H1489, 2001.
112. Pandolfi A, Cetrullo D, Polishuck R, et al: Plasminogen activator inhibitor type 1 is increased in the arterial wall of type 2 diabetic subjects. Arterioscler Thromb Vasc Biol 21:1378-1382, 2001.
113. Bruno G, Cavallo-Perin P, Bargero G, et al: Hyperfibrinogenemia and metabolic syndrome in type 2 diabetes: A population-based study. Diabetes Metab Res Rev 17:124-130, 2001.
114. Carr ME: Diabetes mellitus: A hypercoagulable state. J Diabetes Complications 15:44-54, 2001.
115. Turner RC: The U.K. Prospective Diabetes Study: A review. Diabetes Care 21(Suppl 3):C35-C38, 1998.
116. Coutinho M, Gerstein HC, Wang Y, Yusuf S: The relationship between glucose and incident cardiovascular events: A metaregression analysis of published data from 20 studies of 95,783 individuals followed for 12.4 years. Diabetes Care 22:233-240, 1999.
117. Rodriguez BL, Lau N, Burchfiel CM, et al: Glucose intolerance and 23-year risk of coronary heart disease and total mortality: The Honolulu Heart Program. Diabetes Care 22:1262-1265, 1999.
118. Fontbonne A, Charles MA, Thibult N, et al: Hyperinsulinaemia as a predictor of coronary heart disease mortality in a healthy population: The Paris Prospective Study, 15-year follow-up. Diabetologia 34:356-361, 1991.
119. The effect of intensive treatment of diabetes on the development and progression of long-term complications in insulin-dependent diabetes mellitus. The Diabetes Control and Complications Trial Research Group. N Engl J Med 329:977-986, 1993.
120. Abraira C, Colwell J, Nuttall F, et al: Cardiovascular events and correlates in the Veterans Affairs Diabetes Feasibility Trial. Veterans Affairs Cooperative Study on Glycemic Control and Complications in Type 2 Diabetes. Arch Intern Med 157:181-188, 1997.
121. Intensive blood-glucose control with sulphonylureas or insulin compared with conventional treatment and risk of complications in patients with type 2 diabetes (UKPDS 33). UK Prospective Diabetes Study (UKPDS) Group. Lancet 352:837-853, 1998.
122. Nathan DM, Lachin J, Cleary P, et al: Intensive diabetes therapy and carotid intima-media thickness in type 1 diabetes mellitus. N Engl J Med 348:2294-2303, 2003.
123. Chiasson JL, Josse RG, Gomis R, et al: Acarbose treatment and the risk of cardiovascular disease and hypertension in patients with impaired glucose tolerance: The STOP-NIDDM trial. JAMA 290:486-494, 2003.
124. Howard G, O'Leary DH, Zaccaro D, et al: Insulin sensitivity and atherosclerosis. The Insulin Resistance Atherosclerosis Study (IRAS) Investigators. Circulation 93:1809-1817, 1996.
125. Lempiainen P, Mykkanen L, Pyorala K, et al: Insulin resistance syndrome predicts coronary heart disease events in elderly nondiabetic men. Circulation 100:123-128, 1999.
126. Schaper NC, Nabuurs-Franssen MH, Huijberts MS: Peripheral vascular disease and type 2 diabetes mellitus. Diabetes Metab Res Rev 16(Suppl 1):S11-S15, 2000.
127. Effect of intensive blood-glucose control with metformin on complications in overweight patients with type 2 diabetes (UKPDS 34). UK Prospective Diabetes Study (UKPDS) Group. Lancet 352:854-865, 1998.
128. Aronoff S, Rosenblatt S, Braithwaite S, et al: Pioglitazone hydrochloride monotherapy improves glycemic control in the treatment of patients with type 2 diabetes: A 6-month randomized placebo-controlled dose-response study. The Pioglitazone 001 Study Group. Diabetes Care 23:1605-1611, 2000.
129. Plutzky J: Peroxisome proliferator-activated receptors in vascular biology and atherosclerosis: Emerging insights for evolving paradigms. Curr Atheroscler Rep 2:327-335, 2000.
130. Marx N, Sukhova G, Murphy C, et al: Macrophages in human atheroma contain PPARgamma: Differentiation-dependent peroxisomal proliferator-activated receptor gamma (PPARgamma) expression and reduction of MMP-9 activity through PPARgamma activation in mononuclear phagocytes in vitro. Am J Pathol 153:17-23, 1998.
131. Tack CJ, Smits P, Demacker PN, Stalenhoef AF: Troglitazone decreases the proportion of small, dense LDL and increases the resistance of LDL to oxidation in obese subjects. Diabetes Care 21:796-799, 1998.
132. Cominacini L, Young MM, Capriati A, et al: Troglitazone increases the resistance of low-density lipoprotein to oxidation in healthy volunteers. Diabetologia 40:1211-1218, 1997.

133. Parulkar AA, Pendergrass ML, Granda-Ayala R, et al: Nonhypoglycemic effects of thiazolidinediones. Ann Intern Med 134:61-71, 2001.
134. Ghazzi MN, Perez JE, Antonucci TK, et al: Cardiac and glycemic benefits of troglitazone treatment in NIDDM. The Troglitazone Study Group. Diabetes 46:433-439, 1997.
135. Nagy L, Tontonoz P, Alvarez JG, et al: Oxidized LDL regulates macrophage gene expression through ligand activation of PPARgamma. Cell 93:229-240, 1998.
136. Tontonoz P, Nagy L, Alvarez JG, et al: PPARgamma promotes monocyte/macrophage differentiation and uptake of oxidized LDL. Cell 93:241-252, 1998.
137. Sniderman AD, Scantlebury T, Cianflone K: Hypertriglyceridemic hyperapob: The unappreciated atherogenic dyslipoproteinemia in type 2 diabetes mellitus. Ann Intern Med 135:447-459, 2001.
138. Malmstrom R, Packard CJ, Caslake M, et al: Defective regulation of triglyceride metabolism by insulin in the liver in NIDDM. Diabetologia 40:454-462, 1997.
139. Nesto RW, Libby P: Diabetes mellitus and the cardiovascular system. *In* Braunwald E, Zipes DP, Libby P (eds): Heart Disease. 6th ed. Philadelphia, WB Saunders, 2001, pp 2133-2150.
140. Rubins HB, Robins SJ, Collins D, et al: Distribution of lipids in 8,500 men with coronary artery disease. Department of Veterans Affairs HDL Intervention Trial Study Group. Am J Cardiol 75:1196-1201, 1995.
141. Gowri MS, Van der Westhuyzen DR, Bridges SR, Anderson JW: Decreased protection by HDL from poorly controlled type 2 diabetic subjects against LDL oxidation may be due to the abnormal composition of HDL. Arterioscler Thromb Vasc Biol 19:2226-2233, 1999.
142. Williams KJ, Tabas I: The response-to-retention hypothesis of atherogenesis reinforced. Curr Opin Lipidol 9:471-474, 1998.
143. Goldberg RB, Mellies MJ, Sacks FM, et al: Cardiovascular events and their reduction with pravastatin in diabetic and glucose-intolerant myocardial infarction survivors with average cholesterol levels: Subgroup analyses in the cholesterol and recurrent events (CARE) trial. The Care Investigators. Circulation 98:2513-2519, 1998.

144. Pyörala K, Pedersen TR, Kjekshus J, et al: Cholesterol lowering with simvastatin improves prognosis of diabetic patients with coronary heart disease: A subgroup analysis of the Scandinavian Simvastatin Survival Study (4S). Diabetes Care 20:614-620, 1997.
145. Collins R, Armitage J, Parish S, et al: MRC/BHF Heart Protection Study of cholesterol-lowering with simvastatin in 5963 people with diabetes: A randomised placebo-controlled trial. Lancet 361:2005-2016, 2003.
146. Rubins HB, Robins SJ, Collins D, et al: Gemfibrozil for the secondary prevention of coronary heart disease in men with low levels of high-density lipoprotein cholesterol. Veterans Affairs High-Density Lipoprotein Cholesterol Intervention Trial Study Group. N Engl J Med 341:410-418, 1999.
147. Effect of fenofibrate on progression of coronary-artery disease in type 2 diabetes: The Diabetes Atherosclerosis Intervention Study, a randomised study. Lancet 357:905-910, 2001.
148. Marx N, Sukhova GK, Collins T, et al: PPARalpha activators inhibit cytokine-induced vascular cell adhesion molecule-1 expression in human endothelial cells. Circulation 99:3125-3131, 1999.
149. Marx N, Mackman N, Schonbeck U, et al: PPARalpha activators inhibit tissue factor expression and activity in human monocytes. Circulation 103:213-219, 2001.
150. Neve BP, Corseaux D, Chinetti G, et al: PPARalpha agonists inhibit tissue factor expression in human monocytes and macrophages. Circulation 103:207-212, 2001.
151. Sowers JR, Epstein M: Diabetes mellitus and associated hypertension, vascular disease, and nephropathy: An update. Hypertension 26:869-879, 1995.
152. Gress TW, Nieto FJ, Shahar E, et al: Hypertension and antihypertensive therapy as risk factors for type 2 diabetes mellitus. Atherosclerosis Risk in Communities Study. N Engl J Med 342:905-912, 2000.
153. Tuomilehto J, Rastenyte D, Birkenhager WH, et al: Effects of calcium-channel blockade in older patients with diabetes and systolic hypertension. Systolic Hypertension in Europe Trial Investigators. N Engl J Med 340:677-684, 1999.
154. Mehler PS, Jeffers BW, Estacio R, Schrier RW: Associations of hypertension and complications in non-insulin-dependent diabetes mellitus. Am J Hypertens 10:152-161, 1997.
155. Mehler PS, Coll JR, Estacio R, et al: Intensive blood pressure control reduces the risk of cardiovascular events in patients with peripheral arterial disease and type 2 diabetes. Circulation 107:753-756, 2003.
156. Tatti P, Pahor M, Byington RP, et al: Outcome results of the Fosinopril versus Amlodipine Cardiovascular Events Randomized Trial (FACET) in patients with hypertension and NIDDM. Diabetes Care 21:597-603, 1998.
157. Estacio RO, Schrier RW: Antihypertensive therapy in type 2 diabetes: Implications of the appropriate blood pressure control in diabetes (ABCD) trial. Am J Cardiol 82:9R-14R, 1998.
158. Efficacy of atenolol and captopril in reducing risk of macrovascular and microvascular complications in type 2 diabetes: UKPDS 39. UK Prospective Diabetes Study Group. BMJ 317:713-720, 1998.
159. Staessen JA, Fagard R, Thijs L, et al: Randomised double-blind comparison of placebo and active treatment for older patients with isolated systolic hypertension. The Systolic Hypertension in Europe (Syst-Eur) Trial Investigators. Lancet 350:757-764, 1997.
160. Hansson L, Zanchetti A, Carruthers SG, et al: Effects of intensive blood-pressure lowering and low-dose aspirin in patients with hypertension: Principal results of the Hypertension Optimal Treatment (HOT) randomised trial. HOT Study Group. Lancet 351:1755-1762, 1998.
161. Sowers JR, Epstein M, Frohlich ED: Diabetes, hypertension, and cardiovascular disease: An update. Hypertension 37:1053-1059, 2001.
162. Parving HH, Hommel E, Jensen BR, Hansen HP: Long-term beneficial effect of ACE inhibition on diabetic nephropathy in normotensive type 1 diabetic patients. Kidney Int 60:228-234, 2001.
163. Kvetny J, Gregersen G, Pedersen RS: Randomized placebo-controlled trial of perindopril in normotensive, normoalbuminuric patients with type 1 diabetes mellitus. QJM 94:89-94, 2001.
164. Lewis EJ, Hunsicker LG, Clarke WR, et al: Renoprotective effect of the angiotensin-receptor antagonist irbesartan in patients with nephropathy due to type 2 diabetes. N Engl J Med 345:851-860, 2001.
165. Effects of ramipril on cardiovascular and microvascular outcomes in people with diabetes mellitus: Results of the HOPE study and MICRO-HOPE substudy. Heart Outcomes Prevention Evaluation Study Investigators. Lancet 355:253-259, 2000.
166. Lindholm LH, Ibsen H, Dahlof B, et al: Cardiovascular morbidity and mortality in patients with diabetes in the Losartan Intervention For Endpoint reduction in hypertension study (LIFE): A randomised trial against atenolol. Lancet 359:1004-1010, 2002.
167. Gaede P, Vedel P, Larsen N, et al: Multifactorial intervention and cardiovascular disease in patients with type 2 diabetes. N Engl J Med 348:383-393, 2003.

CHAPTER 41

Nutrition and Cardiovascular Disease

Ronald M. Krauss

Appropriate nutritional practices are of central importance in managing risk for atherosclerotic cardiovascular disease. Indeed, many of the current dietary guidelines for the health of the general population aim to prevent cardiovascular disease. These recommendations are based on considerable evidence for nutritional influences on cardiovascular disease risk and a smaller but compelling number of studies indicating that certain dietary modifications can reduce that risk. Additional dietary interventions can benefit patients at higher risk because of specific conditions such as dyslipidemia, hypertension, and obesity. Because of the complexities of testing specific nutrient effects and the inherent difficulties of conducting randomized, controlled clinical endpoint trials for nutritional interventions, they generally cannot be subjected to the same evidence-based criteria that are used to assess drug treatments. Nevertheless, a body of information supports a number of dietary interventions for reducing cardiovascular disease risk and calls into question others that are promoted without an adequate scientific basis.

For dietary recommendations to be effective, they must be provided to patients in a manner that promotes implementation and long-term adherence. The involvement of dietitians and other trained members of a health care team can greatly aid this goal. Of critical importance is the commitment of the health care provider to nutritional guidance and the ability to convey this in terms that patients can accept and readily integrate into their daily lives. Ensuring the patient's understanding of the principles and the goals of the dietary recommendations is an essential element of this process.

The information in this chapter is consistent with dietary guidelines prepared in recent years by the American Heart Association (AHA),[1] the Adult Treatment Panel III of the National Cholesterol Education Program,[2] the National Heart, Lung, and Blood Institute (NHLBI) Joint National Committee on Prevention, Detection, Evaluation and Treatment of High Blood Pressure,[3] and the NHLBI Clinical Guidelines on the Identification, Evaluation, and Treatment of Overweight and Obesity in Adults.[4]

Effects of Overall Dietary Pattern and Specific Food Categories on Cardiovascular Disease

Observational Evidence

Numerous epidemiological studies have identified dietary patterns and food categories associated with reduced risk of cardiovascular disease.[5] Although the interpretation of these studies is limited by their observational nature, the imprecision of the dietary information collected, and the difficulty of correcting for confounding effects of other health behaviors, nevertheless they represent the only feasible approach for drawing conclusions regarding the overall impact of dietary pattern and intake of specific food categories on health outcomes. These analyses permit the general conclusion that lower risk for cardiovascular disease is promoted by emphasis on intake of fruits and vegetables, whole grains, nuts and legumes, fish (preferably fatty), poultry and lean meats, low fat and fat-free dairy products, and liquid vegetable oils. Major nutrient characteristics of these diets include high density of micronutrients and fiber, moderate amounts of unsaturated fats, including omega-3 fatty acids, and lower content of saturated and *trans* fatty acids, sugars, and starches with a high glycemic effect. The relation of these nutrients to cardiovascular disease risk are described further later in the chapter. Epidemiological studies have reported that adherence to such patterns is associated with reductions in cardiovascular disease risk of 30 percent or more.[6-9] However, it is important to recognize that the nutrient composition of these dietary patterns agrees with current recommended dietary intakes for overall health.

A large number of epidemiological studies have reported relationships of specific food categories within these dietary patterns to cardiovascular disease risk, and these studies have formed the basis for recommended intakes of these foods in current dietary guidelines.[1]

FRUITS AND VEGETABLES. Consumption of fruits and vegetables of three or more servings per day versus less than once per day was associated with a 27 percent reduction in cardiovascular disease risk,[10] consistent with results from other studies in which there was a graded risk reduction associated with higher intakes.[11-13] Data suggest that intake of green leafy vegetables and foods rich in carotenoids and vitamin C contribute particularly strongly to this relationship. Based on these data, together with evidence from the Dietary Approaches to Stop Hypertension (DASH) trial, described further later,[14,15] consumption of at least five portions per day of a variety of fruits and vegetables is generally recommended for maintaining cardiovascular health.[1]

WHOLE GRAINS AND FIBER. Consumption of whole grains has been associated with reduced cardiovascular disease risk in a number of studies.[16,17] While this effect may be related to fiber intake,[18,19] not all studies have indicated that the relationship with fiber intake is independent of other variables.[20] There is indeed reason to implicate effects of other nutrients in whole grains that are shared by other plant foods, particularly, vitamins, phytoestrogens, phenols, omega-3 fatty acids, resistant starch, and minerals.

Another issue surrounding intake of whole grains is the potential inverse relationship with consumption of sugars and starches with a high glycemic effect, which may have adverse effects on cardiovascular risk.[21] The magnitude of glycemia, namely the blood glucose elevation following consumption of a dietary carbohydrate, primarily reflects the rate of starch digestion and absorption from the intestine, and this in turn can lead to undesirable metabolic consequences, such as a greater rate of increase in postprandial insulin and an increase in plasma triglycerides.[22] A value ("glycemic index") can be assigned to a food based on the magnitude of blood glucose elevation following consumption of this food in relation to that following a standard food (white bread).[22] However, the reliability of this index as a measure of metabolic effects of meals, and the relation of glycemic load (the quantity of foods with high glycemic index) to disease risk has been challenged.[23]

This food category therefore illustrates the general difficulty of statistically dissociating the effects of a single food category from others that are part of an overall dietary pattern. Nevertheless, a recent meta-analysis indicated an average 27 percent reduction in coronary heart disease independently associated with whole grain consumption and suggested an intake of at least three servings per day for cardiovascular health.[24]

LEGUMES. Increased intake of legumes (e.g., peas, beans, soybeans, lentils) has been associated with reduced cardiovascular disease risk in some,[25,26] but not all[11] analyses. In the case of soy, beneficial effects may derive from cholesterol-lowering effects of soy protein as well as vascular effects of soy isoflavones,[27] but there is little direct evidence for reduced cardiovascular risk.

NUTS. Several large studies have indicated an association of nut consumption with reduced cardiovascular disease risk.[28-30] Women who consumed 5 oz. of nuts per week had a 35 percent lower risk of nonfatal myocardial infarction compared with those eating less than 1 oz. per month,[29] while men who consumed nuts twice per week or more had a 47 percent reduction in risk for sudden cardiac death and a 30 percent reduction in total coronary heart disease mortality compared with those who rarely or never consume nuts.[30] As with other complex plant foods, it is difficult to determine which components of nuts may be responsible for these beneficial associations. Nuts are good sources of monounsaturated fatty acids, fiber, minerals, and flavonoids. Walnuts are particularly rich in polyunsaturated fatty acids such as linoleic and alpha-linolenic acid. Recent studies of almond intake have indicated beneficial effects on plasma lipoproteins,[31] but comparisons with the effects of other nuts have not been reported.

FISH AND FISH OIL. There is strong evidence that consumption of fish, especially those species with high content of omega-3 fatty acids, confers protection from ischemic heart disease[32,33] and that this relationship is particularly strong for coronary heart disease mortality and sudden cardiac death, which has been reported to be on average 52 percent lower in men consuming fish at least once weekly versus men consuming less.[34] Although fish have a number of important nutritive qualities, it is likely that their major cardiovascular benefit is due to their content of the omega-3 fatty acids, eicosapentanoic acid (EPA) and docosahexanoic acid (DHA). Increased plasma levels of these fatty acids predicted a considerable reduction in sudden cardiac death,[35] a result consistent with that of a report indicating that intake of 5.5 gm per/mo of EPA plus DHA (equivalent to one portion of fatty fish per week) was associated with a 50 percent lower incidence of primary cardiac arrest compared with individuals consuming no fish.[36] This effect appears to be related to enrichment of membrane phospholipids with omega-3 fatty acids and a resulting reduction in risk for abnormal cardiac electrical conductivity.[36] Other properties of these fatty acids that may benefit risk for coronary heart disease include antiplatelet and antiinflammatory effects, as well as reduction in plasma triglycerides at higher doses.[33]

Based on these studies, as well as results of intervention trials with omega-3 fatty acids described later, the AHA has recommended consumption of two portions of fish per week,[1] particularly those fish rich in omega-3 fatty acids (e.g., salmon, mackerel, albacore tuna, swordfish, herring, sardines, lake trout). Because these fish (particularly predatory fish such as swordfish and some types of tuna) can contain significant quantities of contaminants including methylmercury, polychlorinated biphenyls, and dioxin, the U.S. Environmental Protection Agency and the U.S. Food and Drug Administration (FDA) have provided guidelines for maximal intakes, an issue of particular concern for children and women of childbearing age. In most cases, however, the recommendation of two portions per week falls within these guidelines.

Clinical trials have supported evidence from epidemiological studies[32] that higher intakes of fish may particularly benefit patients with coronary heart disease (Table 41–1).[33] In the Gruppo Italiano per lo Studio della Sopravvivenza nell'Infarto Miocardio (GISSI) secondary prevention trial,[37,38] a supplement containing a total of 0.85 gm/d of EPA and DHA resulted in reductions of 45 percent and 30 percent in sudden and cardiovascular death. Total mortality and sudden death were reduced after 3 and 4 months of treatment, respectively, consistent with reduction of arrhythmia by the treatment. Based on the overall evidence to date, the AHA has recommended that supplemental EPA plus DHA at doses of up to 1 gm/d may be considered for risk reduction in patients with coronary heart disease in consultation with their physician.[33] Supplements also could be a component of the medical management of hypertriglyceridemia, a setting in which even larger doses (2 to 4 gm/d) are required. The availability of high-quality omega-3 fatty acid supplements, free of contaminants, is an important prerequisite to their use.

ALCOHOL. Moderate alcohol consumption (one to three alcoholic beverages per day) is strongly and consistently associated with lower risk for coronary heart disease than either abstention or higher intakes.[39] Some data have suggested that wine, particularly red varieties, is of particular benefit, possibly due to its content of polyphenols such as resveratrol that may have direct benefits on vascular reactivity, thrombosis, and oxidative stress.[40] However, most studies have not documented such a differential benefit of red versus white wine, and it appears likely that the major benefit of alcohol consumption is related to an increase in high-density lipoprotein (HDL) cholesterol and perhaps to other effects such as reduced fibrinogen, platelet aggregation, and inflammation.[39,41,42] In a recent study, men who consumed alcohol three or four times per week had a 37 percent reduction in risk for myocardial infarction compared to men who drank less than once per week, and the risk reduction was no greater with more frequent consumption.[43] Current recommendations from the AHA[1] and the U.S. Dietary Guidelines Advisory Committee are that men who drink alcohol may consume up to two alcoholic beverages per day, and women no more than one per day, in part because of alcohol-related breast cancer risk. Because of the potential hazards associated with habituation to alcohol, the potential for adverse effects such as hepatoxicity and aggravation of hypertriglyceridemia, and the favorable benefit/risk ratio of other dietary practices and therapeutic interventions, individuals should not begin to consume alcohol as a means of reducing coronary disease risk.[44]

Clinical Trials (see Table 41–1)

Relatively few clinical trials have examined the effects of overall dietary patterns or specific food categories on

TABLE 41–1 Trials of Dietary Interventions and Coronary Events

Trial	Patients in Intervention Group	Dietary Intervention	Dietary Fat (Energy) in Treatment Group, %	Energy From P and S Fat in Treatment Group, %	Overall Trial Duration, y	Change in Serum Cholesterol Level, %[†]	Change in CHD, %[‡]
Low-Fat Approach							
MRC (low fat)	123 male MI patients	Reduce total fat	22	NR	3	−5	+5
DART	1015 male MI patients	Reduce total fat	32	NR	2	−4	−9
High-Polyunsaturated-Fat Approach							
Finnish Mental Hospital Study	676 men without CHD	Reduce saturated fat, increase polyunsaturated fat	35	P = 13; S = 9	6	−15	−44[§]
Los Angeles Veteran Study	424 men; most had no evidence of existing CHD	Reduce saturated fat, increase polyunsaturated fat	40	P = 16; S = 9	8	−13[§]	−20 in CHD, −31[§] in cardiovascular events
Oslo Diet-Heart Study	206 male MI patients	Reduce saturated fat, increase polyunsaturated fat	39	P = 21; S = 9	5	−14[§]	−25[§]
MRC (soy oil)	199 male MI patients	Reduce saturated fat, increase polyunsaturated fat	46	P:S ratio = 2	4	−15[§]	−12
Minnesota Coronary Survey	4393 men and 4664 women	Reduce saturated fat, increase polyunsaturated fat	38	P = 15; S = 9	1[‖]	−14[§]	0
Increase Omega-3 Fatty Acid							
DART	1015 male MI patients	Fish twice per week or fish oil (1.5 gm/d)	NR	NR	2	NR	−16 on CHD events, −29[§] in total mortality
GISSI-Prevenzione	5666 MI patients, primarily men	Fish oil (EPA + DHA, 1 gm/d)	NR	NR	3.5	0	−30[§] in cardiovascular death, −45[§] in sudden death
Indian Experiment of Infarct Survival 4	242 MI patients, primarily men	Fish oil (EPA, 1.08 gm/d) or mustard oil (ALA, 2.9 gm/d)	NR	NR	1	0	−30[‡] in fish oil group, −19 in mustard oil group
Whole-Diet Approach							
Lyon Diet Heart Study	302 MI patients, primarily men	High ALA intake and Mediterranean diet	31	P:S ratio = 0.7	3.8	0	−72[§]
Indian Experiment of Infarct Survival	204 MI patients, primarily men	High intake of fruits, vegetables, nuts, fish, and pulses	24	P:S ratio = 1.2	1	−9[§]	−40[§]

ALA = α-linolenic acid; CHD = coronary heart disease; DART = Diet and Reinfarction Trial; DHA = docosahexaenoic acid; EPA = eicosapentaenoic acid; GISSI = Gruppo Italiano per lo Studio della Sopravvivenza nell'Infarto Miocardico; MI = myocardial infarction; NR = not reported; MRC = Medical Research Council; P = polyunsaturated fat; S, saturated fat.

*From Hu FB, Willett WC: Optimal diets for prevention of coronary artery disease: JAMA 288:2569, 2002.

[†]Change in cholesterol level refers to the percentage change in serum cholesterol level in the treatment group compared with the change in the control group.

[‡]Change in CHD refers to the percentage difference in coronary event rates in the treatment group compared with the control group.

[§]$P < .05$

[‖]The total duration of the study was 4.5 years, but the mean duration of the intervention was only 1 year.

cardiovascular disease endpoints. Early randomized trials (Wadsworth Veterans Affairs Hospital, Oslo Diet-Heart, Finnish Mental Hospital Study) tested the effectiveness of cholesterol-lowering diets enriched in polyunsaturated fatty acids.[45] These trials showed a 25 to 50 percent reduction in cardiovascular disease endpoints over 5 to 12 years in conjunction with a 13 to 15 percent reduction in blood cholesterol levels. Notably, these diets were not low in total fat (30 to 40 percent of calories).

More recently, the Lyon Diet Heart Study tested the effects of a Mediterranean-style diet in 423 patients with documented coronary artery disease who were followed for a mean of 3.8 years.[46] Compared with the control diet, the experimental diet had increased amounts of fruits, vegetables, legumes, and fiber and reductions of meats, butter, and cream (but not cheese). In addition, the diet contained a margarine enriched in alpha-linolenic acid, an omega-3 fatty acid precursor of the longer chain EPA plus DHA found in fatty fish. Total fat was approximately 31 percent in both diets. Despite lower content of dietary saturated fat, there were no differences in plasma lipids, lipoproteins, or other major risk factors between the two diets. There were, however, significant reductions in all outcome measures, including all-cause mortality (56 percent), cardiac mortality (65 percent), and nonfatal myocardial infarction (70 percent) (Fig. 41–1).[45,46] Although many components of the dietary program may have contributed to these results, the authors suggested a particularly important role for increased omega-3 fatty acid intake.

The effects of a very low fat diet in the context of an intensive life-style intervention have been evaluated in the Life-Style Heart Trial[47] and a more recent multicenter extension of this program.[48] The regimen includes a vegetarian diet with 10 percent total fat, as well as aerobic exercise training, stress management, smoking cessation, and psychosocial support. In the Life-Style Heart Trial, 48 men with coronary artery disease were allocated to intervention and control groups, and 35 completed a 5-year follow-up. In the experimental group, the average percent diameter stenosis at baseline decreased 1.75 absolute percentage points after 1 year (a 4.5

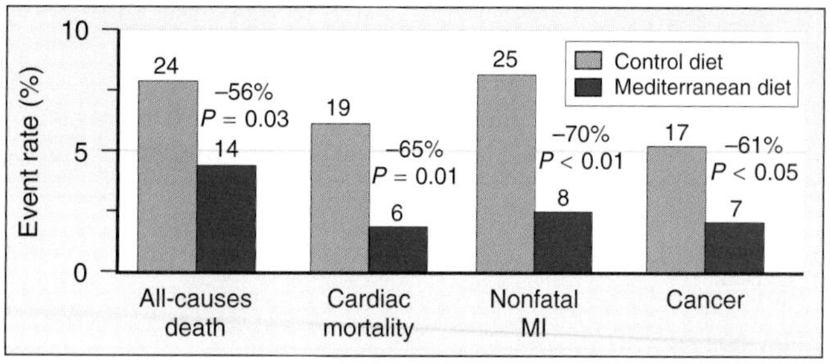

FIGURE 41–1 The effect of a Mediterranean diet on total mortality, coronary disease events, and cancer in men after acute myocardial infarction (MI): the Lyon Heart Study. (From Sacks FM, Katan M: Randomized clinical trials on the effects of dietary fat and carbohydrate on plasma lipoproteins and cardiovascular disease. Am J Med 113:13S, 2002.)

percent relative improvement) and by 3.1 absolute percentage points after 5 years (a 7.9 percent relative improvement). In contrast, the average percent diameter stenosis in the control group increased by 2.3 percentage points after 1 year (a 5.4 percent relative worsening) and by 11.8 percentage points after 5 years (a 27.7 percent relative worsening) (p = .001 between groups). Twenty-five cardiac events occurred in 28 experimental group patients versus 45 events in 20 control group patients during the 5-year follow-up (risk ratio for any event for the control group, 2.47 [95 percent confidence interval, 1.48 to 4.20]). Among major cardiovascular risk factors, the intervention program versus control resulted in a significant 40 percent versus 1 percent reduction of low-density lipoprotein (LDL) cholesterol and a 17 percent versus 4 percent reduction in body weight, with no significant changes in HDL, cholesterol, triglyceride, or blood pressure. Thus, this approach offers an effective means of coronary disease risk reduction, although the magnitude of the contribution of the very low fat diet per se, in the context of the overall program and in comparison with more moderate dietary regimens, has not been established.

Effects of Specific Dietary Components on Risk Factors for Cardiovascular Disease

The effects of dietary patterns and specific food categories on cardiovascular disease risk may operate in part through their effects on risk factors. The major diet-related risk factors are obesity, plasma lipids and lipoproteins, and blood pressure. Other factors for which dietary benefits are less well established include homocysteine, inflammation, and oxidative stress. Other than antiplatelet effects of omega-3 fatty acids, there is little indication of dietary effects on thrombosis.

Overweight and Obesity

Overweight and obesity, defined respectively as body mass index higher than 25 and more than 30 kg/m^2, respectively,[4] are progressively increasing in prevalence in the United States and globally.[49] These conditions are associated with numerous comorbidities affecting cardiovascular disease risk, notably dyslipidemia, hypertension, diabetes, and metabolic syndrome.[49,50] The underlying guidelines for prevention and treatment of excess body weight as articulated in the AHA Dietary Guidelines target both diet and physical activity[1]:

1. Match intake of energy (calories) to overall energy needs; limit consumption of foods with a high-caloric density and/or low nutritional quality, including those with a high content of sugars.
2. Maintain a level of physical activity that achieves fitness and balances energy expenditure with energy intake; for weight reduction, expenditure should exceed intake.

These principles, which agree with those of the NHLBI,[4] recognize that weight reduction requires achieving a negative energy balance. In this regard, carefully controlled metabolic studies have established that at a given level of physical activity, reduced energy intake will result in weight loss irrespective of the macronutrient (carbohydrate, fat, protein) composition of the diet over a rather wide range.[51,52] Nonetheless, considerable controversy persists as to whether diets with differing macronutrient composition differ in their effectiveness in achieving short-term or long-term weight loss. A detailed discussion of this controversy exceeds the scope of this chapter, but arguments based on observational data, or on intervention programs that incorporate dietary change with increases in physical activity and other behavioral changes, do not adequately address the question of diet composition per se as a factor that affects the efficacy of weight loss. In fact, studies of individuals who have achieved long-term weight loss indicate that these individuals employ a number of behavioral changes to control dietary fat intake, have higher levels of physical activity (especially strenuous activity), and maintain a greater frequency of self-weighing.[53]

However, even this information does not help to establish whether alternate dietary strategies, such as very-low-carbohydrate and/or high-protein diets may prove even more effective, based on either their metabolic effects or their influence on eating behavior. Only recently have studies specifically tested the efficacy of such dietary approaches.[54-56] Results to date suggest that at least over periods up to 6 months, average weight loss is higher for diets with very low carbohydrate content (e.g., <35 g/day) than with diets containing more conventional amounts of carbohydrate that are restricted in total fat (Table 41–2).[57] Possible explanations for this finding include the restricted food choices, and the possibility that higher dietary content of protein and/or lower content of carbohydrates, especially simple sugars and rapidly digested starches with lower glycemic effects, increase satiety. Differing effects of these diets on body fat or body composition have not been demonstrated. However, questions remain regarding the long-term safety and overall health effects of such diets, particularly since they lack many of the foods associated with maintaining cardiovascular and overall health, including fruits, vegetables, and whole grains. Additionally, they are high in saturated and *trans* fats and cholesterol, although as described later, the expected effects of these fats on LDL cholesterol levels appear to be attenuated. Another major concern is whether diets with extreme deviations from conventional food choices, i.e., very low in either carbohydrate or fat, can be effectively sustained over the long term (e.g., years). In the case of low-fat diets, this appears possible at least for highly motivated individuals,[48,53] and for population groups such as East Asians, but it remains undetermined for very-low-carbohydrate/high-protein/high-fat diets, regimens for which little long-term population experience exists. There are also specific concerns regarding long-term consequences of high protein intake, particularly in the setting of renal or hepatic impairment.[58]

Plasma Lipids

TOTAL AND LDL CHOLESTEROL. Dietary management of LDL cholesterol remains a major goal of coronary artery disease risk management.[2] Although diet-induced lowering of LDL cholesterol has not been firmly proved to reduce coronary disease risk, this conclusion is reasonable based both on the results of dietary trials designed to lower LDL described

TABLE 41–2 Comparison of Low-Carbohydrate and Reduced-Fat Diets

Variable	Low-Carbohydrate Diet*	Reduced-Fat Diet†
Caloric restriction	Not necessary; ketosis may help reduce intake	Necessary
Food choices	Highly restricted	Moderately restricted
Initial rate of weight loss	Rapid, with increased diuresis	Gradual, with some diuresis
Weight loss	Dependent on duration	Dependent on duration
Weight maintenance	Unproven over the long term	Unproven over the long term
Cholesterol		
LDL	No change	Decrease
HDL	Greater increase	Increase
Triglycerides	Greater decrease	Decrease
Potential long-term concerns	Calciuria (renal stones and decreased bone mass) Relatively high-protein content (patients with renal or hepatic disease) Atherogenicity (high saturated fat, trans fat, and cholesterol levels and relative absence of fruits, vegetables, and whole grains	None

*A low-carbohydrate diet is defined as one that provides <35 gm of carbohydrate per day. The Atkins diet begins with a stricter limitation (20 gm/day) for at least the first 2 weeks, with a gradual increase of 5 gm/week to achieve a rate of weight loss of approximately 2 lb (0.9 kg) per week until a weight within 5 to 10 lb (2.3 to 4.5 kg) of the goal is achieved. Carbohydrate intake is then further increased by 10 gm/week until weight loss ceases.

†A reduced-fat diet is defined as one in which fat constitutes <30% of the total caloric intake; under certain circumstances (e.g., in some patients with the metabolic syndrome), fat intake of ≤35% of the total caloric intake is recommended.

LDL = low-density lipoprotein; HLD = high-density lipoprotein.

From Bonow RO, Eckel RH: Diet, obesity, and cardiovascular risk. N Engl J Med 348:2057, 2003.

earlier and the relation of drug-induced reductions in LDL cholesterol to decreases in coronary disease morbidity and mortality. Nutritional factors known to increase LDL cholesterol levels include saturated and *trans* fatty acids, dietary cholesterol, and excess body weight. While total fat intake tends to correlate with that of saturated fat, there is no evidence that LDL levels rise due to increased dietary total fat intake per se. In fact, as mentioned earlier, trials employing high total and unsaturated fat consumption resulted in lower LDL cholesterol and reduced heart disease risk. Moreover, recent studies have indicated that at least over the short term, very low carbohydrate diets with high levels of total fat and protein blunt the expected increases in LDL cholesterol expected from high saturated fat intake.[54-56]

Substitution of carbohydrate and/or unsaturated fatty acids for saturated and *trans* fatty acids results in reduction of LDL cholesterol. Many studies have assessed the quantitative effects of these dietary changes on LDL and other lipids and lipoproteins, as recently summarized and reviewed (Fig. 41–2).[59,60] When substituted for carbohydrate, the greatest increases in LDL cholesterol result from C12 : 0 (lauric), C14 : 0 (myristic), and C16 : 0 (palmitic) fatty acids found in dairy fat, meat, and tropical oils, with equivalent changes induced by *trans* monounsaturated fatty acids found in baked goods, stick margarine, and in fried "fast foods" such as french fries. In contrast, 18 : 0 fatty acid (stearic), which is found in many of the same foods, generally does not raise LDL cholesterol levels. No increases in LDL cholesterol follow intake of monounsaturated fatty acids, principally 18 : 1 (oleic), a major component of olive and canola oils, and polyunsaturated fatty acids of the omega-6 series, principally 18 : 2 (linoleic), found in vegetable and seed oils such as corn, safflower, and sunflower oils. Current guidelines recommend consumption of less than 10 percent of calories as saturated fat for the general population and further limitation to 7 percent or less for those with a level of LDL cholesterol higher than that recommended for their overall risk status.[1,2] For *trans* fatty acids, it is recommended that intake be reduced to a minimum, a goal that will be easier to achieve once *trans* fatty acid content is indicated on food labels.

With the exception of egg yolk and shellfish, dietary cholesterol is found in foods of animal origin that are also high

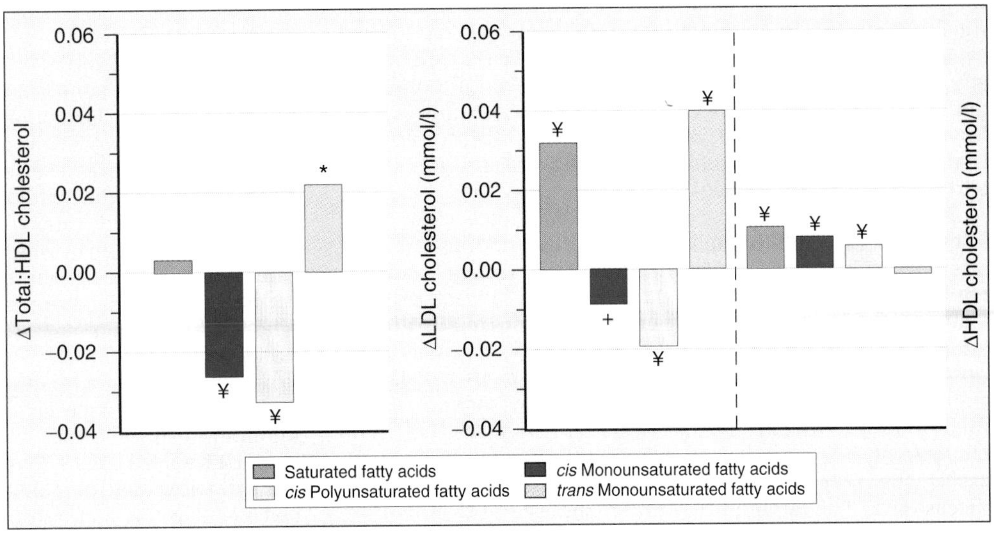

FIGURE 41–2 Predicted changes (Δ) in the ratio of serum total to HDL cholesterol and in LDL- and HDL-cholesterol concentrations when carbohydrates constituting 1 percent of energy are replaced isoenergetically with saturated, *cis* monosaturated, *cis* polyunsaturated, or *trans* monounsaturated fatty acids. *$p < 0.05$; +$p < 0.01$; ¥$p < 0.001$. (From Mensink RP, Zock PL, Kester AD, Katan MB: Effects of dietary fatty acids and carbohydrates on the ratio of serum total to HDL cholesterol and on serum lipids and apolipoproteins: A meta-analysis of 60 controlled trials. Am J Clin Nutr 77:1146, 2003.)

in saturated fat. On average, an increase of 100 mg/d of dietary cholesterol increases total serum cholesterol about 2 to 3 mg/dl, of which approximately 70 percent is in the LDL fraction. This effect of added cholesterol varies considerably among individuals and is attenuated at higher cholesterol intakes. The LDL cholesterol increase would predict approximately a 1 to 2 percent increase in coronary heart disease risk, with possibly offsetting effects of concomitantly increased HDL cholesterol. An effect of this magnitude is difficult to detect in epidemiological data and may contribute to the reported lack of association of egg yolk intake with coronary disease risk for amounts up to 1 or more eggs (~215 mg cholesterol) per day, except in patients with diabetes.[61] Based on available data, as well as the infeasibility of consuming diets with markedly restricted cholesterol content, current guidelines[1,2] recommend limiting intake to less than 300 mg/d for the general population and less than 200 mg/d for individuals at increased risk for heart disease by National Cholesterol Education Program criteria.

Although there is wide interindividual variation in response to these changes,[62,63] the reductions in LDL cholesterol that may be expected with adoption of diets low in saturated fat and cholesterol are generally in the range of 5 to 10 percent. Near-maximal response of LDL cholesterol to dietary change occurs as early as 3 to 4 weeks, and thereafter it can be determined whether additional therapeutic measures will be required to achieve the desired LDL cholesterol target.

Some epidemiological analyses have shown positive independent associations of saturated fat intake with coronary heart disease risk, but the relationships have been relatively weak and inconsistent.[64] This likely reflects several factors including the relatively small average effects of saturated fat on LDL cholesterol and the possible offsetting increases in HDL cholesterol as described later. On the other hand, *trans* fatty acid intake appears to have a stronger relationship with coronary heart disease risk,[64] perhaps reflecting the finding that HDL cholesterol levels are not increased by *trans* fat or perhaps the existence of other adverse effects of these fatty acids on disease mechanisms.

Other nutritional measures that can reduce LDL cholesterol include weight loss, which may be particularly effective in some cases, and addition of plant sterol and stanol esters,[65] viscous fiber (in particular, beta-glucan, a component of oat fiber),[66] soy protein,[27] and nuts.[31] LDL cholesterol has been found to fall by a mean of 28 percent on a diet that combines diet components in amounts (per 1000 kcal) that have been reported to be beneficial individually: plant sterols 1.0 gm, soy protein 21.4 gm, viscous fibers 9.8 gm, and almonds 14 gm.[67] This reduction was comparable to that achieved by lovastatin 10 mg/d (30.9 percent) and significantly greater than with a diet low in saturated fat (4.5 percent of energy) and cholesterol (8.0 percent).

HDL CHOLESTEROL. Although HDL cholesterol correlates inversely and independently with risk for coronary artery disease, it remains uncertain whether changes in HDL cholesterol, and in particular those induced by diet, predict changes in risk. There are two general categories of nutritional effect on HDL: those due to changes in dietary fatty acid composition and those due to factors that also affect plasma triglyceride levels, as described in the next section. Since dietary fatty acids have major effects on LDL as well as HDL cholesterol, it is necessary to examine these effects jointly to assess the potential impact of HDL change on coronary disease risk. The ratio of LDL or total cholesterol to HDL cholesterol permits assessment of these joint effects. A review of 60 dietary trials has indicated that the plasma cholesterol to HDL cholesterol ratio did not change if saturated fatty acids replaced an isocaloric amount of dietary carbohydrates. However, this ratio decreased if *cis* unsaturated fatty acids replaced saturated fatty acids (see Fig. 41–2).[59] The effect on total:HDL cholesterol of replacing *trans* fatty acids with a mix of carbohydrates and *cis* unsaturated fatty acids was almost twice as large as that of replacing saturated fatty acids. Lauric acid greatly increased total cholesterol, but much of its effect was on HDL cholesterol, resulting in a lower ratio of total:HDL cholesterol for oils rich in lauric acid, such as coconut oil. As discussed earlier, the tandem effects of dietary saturated fatty acids as well as dietary cholesterol on total and HDL cholesterol may contribute to the relatively weak relationship of these nutrients to coronary heart disease risk.

TRIGLYCERIDE AND THE ATHEROGENIC DYSLIPIDEMIA OF OBESITY, DIABETES, AND THE METABOLIC SYNDROME. Elevated plasma triglyceride independently but rather weakly predicts coronary heart disease risk. Its principal cardiovascular significance is as a component of, and a marker for, the atherogenic dyslipidemia commonly found in patients with excess adiposity, the metabolic syndrome, and type 2 diabetes mellitus (see Chaps. 39 and 40).[6] The triad of lipid abnormalities in these conditions consists of elevated plasma triglyceride (≥150 mg/dl), reduced HDL cholesterol, and a relative excess of small, dense LDL particles with total LDL cholesterol levels that are generally average.[69] Adiposity itself is the principal nutritionally related influence on atherogenic dyslipidemia. Among nutrients, the major determinant of this dyslipidemic triad is carbohydrate.[70] In general, simple sugars and rapidly hydrolyzed starches have a greater glyceridemic effect than more complex carbohydrates and those consumed in conjunction with higher intake of fiber. The glyceridemic effects of carbohydrates tend to correlate with their glycemic effects.[2] Dietary carbohydrate-induced increases in plasma triglyceride are often accompanied by decreases in HDL cholesterol and increases in levels of small, dense LDL particles.[7] Although there is no direct evidence that these diet-induced changes contribute to increased coronary heart disease risk, it has been reported that dietary glycemic load, a measure of the quantity of high glycemic foods related to high plasma triglyceride and low HDL cholesterol, strongly and independently predicts coronary heart disease risk.[21] Hence limitation of sugars and high glycemic/glyceridemic carbohydrates is advisable in patients with this form of dyslipidemia.

Blood Pressure

Current recommendations for nonpharmacological management of elevated blood pressure include weight reduction, moderation in alcohol consumption, limitation of sodium intake, and increased intake of certain other minerals (see Chap. 38).[1,3] Another important therapeutic modality for reducing blood pressure is the DASH combination diet.[14,15] Taken together, the evidence supporting these recommendations described later reinforces the roles of multiple components of an overall dietary pattern in promoting cardiovascular and general health.

BODY WEIGHT. Numerous clinical trials reviewed elsewhere[1,3] have documented a substantial and significant relation between change in weight and change in blood pressure. It has been estimated that a reduction of more than 1 mm Hg in systolic and diastolic blood pressure may occur for each kilogram of weight loss.

DIETARY SODIUM. Numerous observational studies and clinical trials have demonstrated that a high intake of sodium can result in an increase in blood pressure.[72] Meta-analyses of randomized trials have shown that on average, reducing sodium intake by about 80 mmol (1.8 gm)/d yields systolic and diastolic blood pressure reductions of about 4 and 2 mm Hg in hypertensive patients and smaller reductions in normotensive subjects.[73] Although the blood pressure response to change in salt intake varies among individuals, in part because of genetic factors and other variables such as age, classification of individuals as "responders" or "nonresponders" can be difficult.[74]

The Trials of Hypertension Prevention documented that sodium reduction, alone or combined with weight loss, can lower incidence of hypertension by about 20 percent (Fig. 41–3).[75] In the Trials of Nonpharmacologic Interventions in the Elderly, a reduced salt intake with or without weight loss significantly reduced blood pressure and the need for antihypertensive medication in older persons.[76] In both trials, the dietary interventions reduced total sodium intake to about 100 mmol/d. Although the DASH-sodium trial has shown that further blood pressure reduction can be achieved by lowering sodium intake to 50 mmol/d (see later), such a limitation is extremely difficult to implement because of the high sodium content of many prepared foods. Overall, the available data support the current AHA population guideline of limiting salt intake to 6 gm/d, the equivalent of 100 mmol of sodium (2400 mg) per day.[1] Careful selection of foods and limitation of added salt can substantially lower sodium intake, and these measures can be particularly beneficial in hypertensive patients.

ALCOHOL. Observational data have consistently demonstrated a relationship between heavy drinking (three or more standard drinks per day) and higher blood pressure.[77] Clinical trials of reducing alcohol consumption have yielded less conclusive findings.[78] As stated previously, the totality of the evidence supports a recommendation to limit alcohol intake to no more than two drinks per day for men and one drink per day for women.

POTASSIUM, MAGNESIUM, AND CALCIUM INTAKE. As reviewed elsewhere,[72,79] observational data have provided evidence that increased intakes of these minerals are associated with lower blood pressure. Clinical trials have also documented a beneficial impact of potassium supplements on blood pressure, but the evidence for calcium and magnesium is less consistent.[72,79] A meta-analysis of randomized trials of the effects of potassium supplementation[80] found that, on average, supplementation of diets with 60 to 120 mmol/d reduced systolic and diastolic blood pressure by 4.4 and 2.5 mm Hg in hypertensive patients and by 1.8 and 1.0 mm Hg in normotensive subjects. Because a high dietary intake of potassium, magnesium, and calcium can be achieved from food sources and because diets rich in these minerals provide a variety of other nutrients, the preferred strategy for increasing mineral intake is through foods rather than supplements.

DIETARY PATTERN. The DASH study[14,81] found that a diet rich in fruits and vegetables (five to nine servings per day) and low-fat dairy products (two to four servings a day), and with reduced saturated and total fat content, reduced systolic and diastolic blood pressure by 5.5 and 3.0 mm Hg more than did a control diet of equal sodium content that produced no differences in sodium or body weight. As with other interventions, reductions were substantially greater in hypertensive than normotensive subjects, and reductions were larger in black than nonblack subjects. In a second trial, the DASH-sodium study, progressive sodium restriction in the DASH diet (from a daily intake of 150 to 100 mmol and 50 mmol) further reduced blood pressure, such that the DASH diet with the lowest sodium intake led to a mean systolic blood pressure that was 7.1 mm Hg lower in participants without hypertension and 11.5 mm Hg lower in participants with hypertension.[15,82] However, particularly among normotensive and nonblack subjects, most of the blood pressure reduction could be accounted for by the DASH diet rather than additional sodium restriction.

Due to the multifactorial dietary intervention of DASH, its mechanisms of effectiveness cannot be determined. However, the diet was rich in potassium, calcium, and magnesium, and hence the findings are consistent with the possibility that these elements contributed to the observed reductions in blood pressure. A similar conclusion may be drawn from the Vanguard study, a trial that used a dietary regimen based on prepackaged foods.[83]

OTHER DIETARY EFFECTS ON BLOOD PRESSURE. Limited data support the possible beneficial effects of additional dietary measures on blood pressure. These include fish,[84] whole grains (in particular, oats),[85] and protein (in particular, soy).[86-88] The suggestion that soy isoflavone content may contribute to this benefit is consistent with a recent report that polyphenols in dark chocolate can also promote blood pressure reduction.[89]

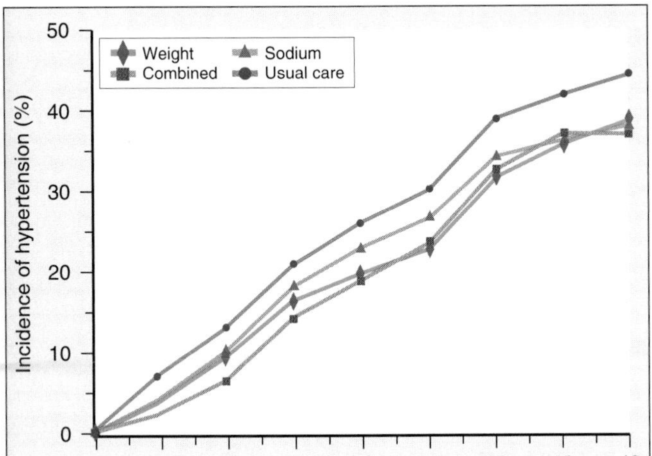

FIGURE 41–3 Plot of the incidence of hypertension for the respective randomized groups through 48 months of follow-up, from life-table analysis in the Trials of Hypertension Prevention, Phase II. (From The Trials of Hypertension Prevention Collaborative Research Group: Effects of weight loss and sodium reduction intervention on blood pressure and hypertension incidence in overweight people with high-normal blood pressure. The Trials of Hypertension Prevention, Phase II. Arch Intern Med 157:657, 1997.)

Other Cardiovascular Risk Factors Related to Diet (see also Chap. 36)

HOMOCYSTEINE. Recent meta-analyses have concluded that elevated plasma homocysteine levels modestly increase the risk for ischemic heart disease and stroke.[90,91] Folic acid, as well as pyridoxine and cyanocobalamin (vitamins B_6 and B_{12}), are the major dietary components influencing plasma homocysteine levels.[92] There is as yet little information regarding the potential benefit of plasma homocysteine reduction on cardiovascular disease risk. A placebo-controlled, randomized trial of a daily regimen of folic acid 1 mg, cyanocobalamin 400 μg, and pyridoxine 10 mg significantly reduced a composite endpoint for adverse cardiovascular outcomes in patients undergoing coronary angioplasty.[93] Although, as expected, plasma homocysteine levels were substantially reduced by treatment, it cannot be determined to what extent this contributed to the outcome. Nevertheless, if this finding is confirmed by other ongoing studies, this could provide a basis for future recommendations of supplemental vitamin therapy for high-risk patients. However, such studies may be difficult to carry out, since population levels of plasma homocysteine in the United States have decreased since fortification of cereal grain flour mandated by the FDA in 1998, and it has been shown that folic acid supplementation causes only modest further reductions in homocysteine in coronary artery disease patients who are exposed to cereal products.[94] Administration of folic acid supplements in the absence of adequate cyanocobalamin may lead to masking of pernicious anemia.[92]

DIETARY INFLUENCES ON C-REACTIVE PROTEIN. A number of nutritional factors influence C-reactive protein, a well-established coronary artery disease risk factor (see Chap. 36).[95] Chief among these is adiposity, which in turn appears to exert its effect by increasing insulin resistance.[96] Weight loss reduces C-reactive protein levels.[97] Glycemic load is positively associated with plasma C-reactive protein levels[98] and inversely with alcohol intake,[42] but prospective clinical studies of these effects have not been reported. Higher glycemic loads associate with elevated levels of C-reactive protein in both normal and overweight women (Fig. 41–4). The "portfolio" diet containing multiple supplements that lowered plasma LDL cholesterol also lowered C-reactive protein to a level similar to that obtained with low-dose statin therapy.[67]

ANTIOXIDANT VITAMINS. Despite the evidence supporting the role of oxidative stress in atherogenesis and observational data relating antioxidant intake to reduced risk of cardiovascular disease, there is insufficient evidence from clinical trials to support the use of antioxidant vitamins for the prevention of ischemic heart disease.[99,100] Notably, no benefit was observed with a supplement of 600 mg of vitamin E, 250 mg of vitamin C, and 20 mg of beta carotene daily in the randomized, placebo-controlled Heart Protection Study trial of 20,536 high-risk individuals. In a smaller study, the cardiovascular protective effects of statin plus niacin therapy in patients with coronary artery disease were attenuated by coadministration of a mixture of antioxidants that also resulted in reductions of large HDL particles.[101] It is possible that the observational studies reflect confounding effects of other dietary or lifestyle practices that correlate with antioxidant consumption either in foods or supplements or that longer-term consumption is necessary to achieve benefits.

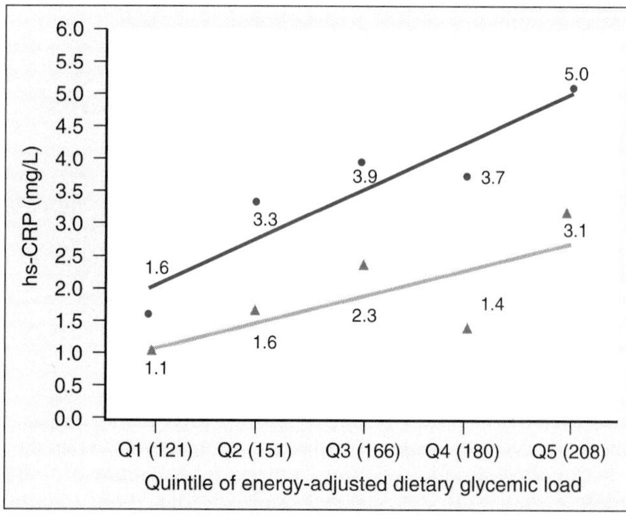

FIGURE 41–4 Adjusted geometric mean plasma concentrations of high-sensitivity C-reactive protein (hs-CRP) by quintiles (Q1 to Q5) of energy-adjusted dietary glycemic load in 244 women in two body mass index categories: BMI < 25 (▲ and blue regression line) and BMI ≥ 25 (• and magenta regression line). Multiple linear regression models were used to adjust for potential confounding factors, including age; randomized treatment status; smoking status; BMI; physical activity levels; alcohol intake; parental history of myocardial infarction before the age of 60 years; history of diabetes mellitus; history of hypertension; history of high cholesterol; postmenopausal hormone use; and intakes of dietary fiber, folate, protein, cholesterol, and total energy. $p = 0.01$ for the interaction between BMI and dietary glycemic load. Mean dietary glycemic load for each quintile is shown in parentheses. (From Liu S, Manson JE, Buring JE, et al: Relation between a diet with a high glycemic load and plasma concentrations of high-sensitivity C-reactive protein in middle-aged women. Am J Clin Nutr 75:492, 2002.)

However, given the available data, no recommendation can be made at this time for the use of antioxidant supplements to reduced cardiovascular disease risk.

Lp(a). This risk factor for cardiovascular disease and stroke is under strong genetic regulation, and dietary influences on plasma Lp(a) levels are modest and variable. Increased *trans* fatty acid intake can lead to variable but generally small increases in Lp(a) levels,[102] in contrast to the effects of saturated fatty acids, which reduce Lp(a).[103]

Conclusion

In conclusion, physicians caring for individuals with or at risk of cardiovascular diseases should emphasize the need for implementing "heart healthy" nutritional measures such as those outlined here. Often, nutritional counseling should use allied health professionals such as dietitians for therapeutic nutritional intervention. The epidemic of obesity and its attendant cardiovascular risks warrant heightened attention to nutrition by practitioners and public alike.

REFERENCES

General Dietary Guidelines

1. Krauss RM, Eckel RH, Howard B, et al: AHA Dietary Guidelines—revision 2000: A statement for healthcare professionals from the Nutrition Committee of the American Heart Association. Circulation 102:2284, 2000.
2. Expert Panel on Detection, Evaluation, and Treatment of High Blood Cholesterol in Adults. Executive Summary of the Third Report of The National Cholesterol Education Program (NCEP) Expert Panel on Detection, Evaluation, and Treatment of High Blood Cholesterol in Adults (Adult Treatment Panel III). JAMA 285:2486, 2001.
3. Chobanian AV, Bakris GL, Black HR, et al: The Seventh Report of the Joint National Committee on Prevention, Detection, Evaluation, and Treatment of High Blood Pressure: The JNC 7 report. JAMA 289:2560, 2003.
4. National Heart, Lung, and Blood Institute. Clinical Guidelines on the Identification, Evaluation, and Treatment of Overweight and Obesity in Adults: The Evidence Report. Rockville, MD, National Heart, Lung, and Blood Institute, 1998.

Diets and Nutrients to Prevent Cardiovascular Disease

5. Hu FB, Willett WC: Optimal diets for prevention of coronary heart disease. JAMA 288:2569, 2002.
6. Stampfer MJ, Hu FB, Manson JE, et al: Primary prevention of coronary heart disease in women through diet and lifestyle. N Engl J Med 343:16, 2000.
7. Hu FB, Rimm EB, Stampfer MJ, et al: Prospective study of major dietary patterns and risk of coronary heart disease in men. Am J Clin Nutr 72:912, 2000.
8. Trichopoulou A, Costacou T, Bamia C, Trichopoulos D: Adherence to a Mediterranean diet and survival in a Greek population. N Engl J Med 348:2599, 2003.
9. Barzi F, Woodward M, Marfisi RM, et al: Mediterranean diet and all-causes mortality after myocardial infarction: Results from the GISSI-Prevenzione trial. Eur J Clin Nutr 57:604, 2003.
10. Bazzano LA, He J, Ogden LG, et al: Fruit and vegetable intake and risk of cardiovascular disease in U.S. adults: The First National Health and Nutrition Examination Survey Epidemiologic Follow-up Study. Am J Clin Nutr 76:93, 2002.
11. Joshipura KJ, Hu FB, Manson JE, et al: The effect of fruit and vegetable intake on risk for coronary heart disease. Ann Intern Med 134:1106, 2001.
12. Liu S, Lee IM, Ajani U, et al: Intake of vegetables rich in carotenoids and risk of coronary heart disease in men: The Physicians' Health Study. Int J Epidemiol 30:130, 2001.
13. Liu S, Manson JE, Lee IM, et al: Fruit and vegetable intake and risk of cardiovascular disease: The Women's Health Study. Am J Clin Nutr 72:922, 2000.
14. Appel LJ, Moore TJ, Obarzanek E, et al: A clinical trial of the effects of dietary patterns on blood pressure. DASH Collaborative Research Group. N Engl J Med 336:1117, 1997.
15. Sacks FM, Svetkey LP, Vollmer WM, et al: Effects on blood pressure of reduced dietary sodium and the Dietary Approaches to Stop Hypertension (DASH) diet. DASH-Sodium Collaborative Research Group. N Engl J Med 344:3, 2001.
16. Liu S, Stampfer MJ, Hu FB, et al: Whole-grain consumption and risk of coronary heart disease: Results from the Nurses' Health Study. Am J Clin Nutr 70:412, 1999.
17. Jacobs DR Jr, Meyer KA, Kushi LH, Folsom AR: Whole-grain intake may reduce the risk of ischemic heart disease death in postmenopausal women: The Iowa Women's Health Study. Am J Clin Nutr 68:248, 1998.
18. Wolk A, Manson JE, Stampfer MJ, et al: Long-term intake of dietary fiber and decreased risk of coronary heart disease among women. JAMA 281:1998, 1999.
19. Bazzano LA, He J, Ogden LG, et al: Dietary fiber intake and reduced risk of coronary heart disease in U.S. men and women: The National Health and Nutrition Examination Survey I Epidemiologic Follow-up Study. Arch Intern Med 163:1897, 2003.
20. Liu S, Buring JE, Sesso HD, et al: A prospective study of dietary fiber intake and risk of cardiovascular disease among women. J Am Coll Cardiol 39:49, 2002.
21. Liu S, Willett WC, Stampfer MJ, et al: A prospective study of dietary glycemic load, carbohydrate intake, and risk of coronary heart disease in U.S. women. Am J Clin Nutr 71:1455, 2000.

22. Jenkins DJ, Kendall CW, Augustin LS, et al: Glycemic index: Overview of implications in health and disease. Am J Clin Nutr 76:266S, 2002.
23. Pi-Sunyer FX: Glycemic index and disease. Am J Clin Nutr 76:290S, 2002.
24. Anderson JW, Hanna TJ, Peng X, Kryscio RJ: Whole-grain foods and heart disease risk. J Am Coll Nutr 19:291S, 2000.
25. Bazzano LA, He J, Ogden LG, et al: Legume consumption and risk of coronary heart disease in U.S. men and women: NHANES I Epidemiologic Follow-up Study. Arch Intern Med 161:2573, 2001.
26. Kushi LH, Meyer KA, Jacobs DR Jr: Cereals, legumes, and chronic disease risk reduction: Evidence from epidemiologic studies. Am J Clin Nutr 70:451S, 1999.
27. Erdman JW Jr: AHA Science Advisory: Soy protein and cardiovascular disease: A statement for healthcare professionals from the Nutrition Committee of the AHA. Circulation 102:2555, 2000.
28. Sabate J: Nut consumption, vegetarian diets, ischemic heart disease risk, and all-cause mortality: Evidence from epidemiologic studies. Am J Clin Nutr 70:500S, 1999.
29. Hu FB, Stampfer MJ, Manson JE, et al: Frequent nut consumption and risk of coronary heart disease in women: Prospective cohort study. BMJ 317:1341, 1998.
30. Albert CM, Gaziano JM, Willett WC, Manson JE: Nut consumption and decreased risk of sudden cardiac death in the Physicians' Health Study. Arch Intern Med 162:1382, 2002.
31. Jenkins DJ, Kendall CW, Marchie A, et al: Dose response of almonds on coronary heart disease risk factors: Blood lipids, oxidized low-density lipoproteins, lipoprotein(a), homocysteine, and pulmonary nitric oxide: A randomized, controlled, crossover trial. Circulation 106:1327, 2002.
32. Marckmann P, Gronbaek M: Fish consumption and coronary heart disease mortality: A systematic review of prospective cohort studies. Eur J Clin Nutr 53:585, 1999.
33. Kris-Etherton PM, Harris WS, Appel LJ: Fish consumption, fish oil, omega-3 fatty acids, and cardiovascular disease. Circulation 106:2747, 2002.
34. Albert CM, Hennekens CH, O'Donnell CJ, et al: Fish consumption and risk of sudden cardiac death. JAMA 279:23, 1998.
35. Albert CM, Campos H, Stampfer MJ, et al: Blood levels of long-chain n-3 fatty acids and the risk of sudden death. N Engl J Med 346:1113, 2002.
36. Siscovick DS, Raghunathan T, King I, et al: Dietary intake of long-chain n-3 polyunsaturated fatty acids and the risk of primary cardiac arrest. Am J Clin Nutr 71:208S, 2000.
37. Gruppo Italiano per lo Studio della Sopravvivenza nell'Infarto Miocardico: Dietary supplementation with n-3 polyunsaturated fatty acids and vitamin E after myocardial infarction: results of the GISSI-Prevenzione trial. Lancet 354:447, 1999
38. Marchioli R, Barzi F, Bomba E, et al: Early protection against sudden death by n-3 polyunsaturated fatty acids after myocardial infarction: Time-course analysis of the results of the Gruppo Italiano per lo Studio della Sopravvivenza nell'Infarto Miocardico (GISSI)-Prevenzione. Circulation 105:1897, 2002.

Alcohol Consumption and Cardiovascular Disease

39. Vogel RA: Alcohol, heart disease, and mortality: A review. Rev Cardiovasc Med 3:7, 2002.
40. Goldberg IJ, Mosca L, Piano MR, Fisher EA: AHA Science Advisory: Wine and your heart: A science advisory for healthcare professionals from the Nutrition Committee, Council on Epidemiology and Prevention, and Council on Cardiovascular Nursing of the American Heart Association. Stroke 32:591, 2001.
41. Sierksma A, van der Gaag MS, Kluft C, Hendriks HF: Moderate alcohol consumption reduces plasma C-reactive protein and fibrinogen levels: A randomized, diet-controlled intervention study. Eur J Clin Nutr 56:1130, 2002.
42. Albert MA, Glynn RJ, Ridker PM: Alcohol consumption and plasma concentration of C-reactive protein. Circulation 107:443, 2003.
43. Mukamal KJ, Conigrave KM, Mittleman MA, et al: Roles of drinking pattern and type of alcohol consumed in coronary heart disease in men. N Engl J Med 348:109, 2003.
44. Pearson TA: AHA Science Advisory: Alcohol and heart disease. Nutrition Committee of the American Heart Association. Am J Clin Nutr 65:1567, 1997.

Diet, Lifestyle Modification, Obesity, and Cardiovascular Disease

45. Sacks FM, Katan M: Randomized clinical trials on the effects of dietary fat and carbohydrate on plasma lipoproteins and cardiovascular disease. Am J Med 113(Suppl 9B):13S, 2002.
46. de Lorgeril M, Salen P, Martin JL, et al: Mediterranean diet, traditional risk factors, and the rate of cardiovascular complications after myocardial infarction: Final report of the Lyon Diet Heart Study. Circulation 99:779, 1999.
47. Ornish D, Scherwitz LW, Billings JH, et al: Intensive lifestyle changes for reversal of coronary heart disease. JAMA 280:2001, 1998.
48. Koertge J, Weidner G, Elliott-Eller M, et al: Improvement in medical risk factors and quality of life in women and men with coronary artery disease in the Multicenter Lifestyle Demonstration Project. Am J Cardiol 91:1316, 2003.
49. Mokdad AH, Ford ES, Bowman BA, et al: Prevalence of obesity, diabetes, and obesity-related health risk factors. JAMA 289:76, 2001
50. Eckel RH: Obesity and heart disease: A statement for healthcare professionals from the Nutrition Committee, American Heart Association. Circulation 96:3248, 1997.
51. Lean ME, Han TS, Prvan T, et al: Weight loss with high and low carbohydrate 1200 kcal diets in free living women. Eur J Clin Nutr 51:243, 1997.
52. Hirsch J, Hudgins LC, Leibel RL, Rosenbaum M: Diet composition and energy balance in humans. Am J Clin Nutr 67:551S, 1998.
53. McGuire MT, Wing RR, Klem ML, Hill JO: Behavioral strategies of individuals who have maintained long-term weight losses. Obes Res 7:334, 1999.
54. Samaha FF, Iqbal N, Seshadri P, et al: A low-carbohydrate as compared with a low-fat diet in severe obesity. N Engl J Med 348:2074, 2003.
55. Foster GD, Wyatt HR, Hill JO, et al: A randomized trial of a low-carbohydrate diet for obesity. N Engl J Med 348:2082, 2003.
56. Westman EC, Yancy WS, Edman JS, et al: Effect of 6-month adherence to a very low carbohydrate diet program. Am J Med 113:30, 2002.
57. Bonow RO, Eckel RH: Diet, obesity, and cardiovascular risk. N Engl J Med 348:2057, 2003.
58. St Jeor ST, Howard BV, Prewitt TE, et al: Dietary protein and weight reduction: A statement for healthcare professionals from the Nutrition Committee of the Council on Nutrition, Physical Activity, and Metabolism of the American Heart Association. Circulation 104:1869, 2001.
59. Mensink RP, Zock PL, Kester AD, Katan MB: Effects of dietary fatty acids and carbohydrates on the ratio of serum total to HDL cholesterol and on serum lipids and apolipoproteins: A meta-analysis of 60 controlled trials. Am J Clin Nutr 77:1146, 2003.
60. National Academy of Sciences and Institute of Medicine: Dietary Reference Intakes: Energy, carbohydrate, fiber, fat, fatty acids, cholesterol, protein, and amino acids. Washington, DC, National Academies Press, 2002.
61. Hu FB, Stampfer MJ, Rimm EB, et al: A prospective study of egg consumption and risk of cardiovascular disease in men and women. JAMA 281:1387, 1999.
62. Dreon DM, Krauss RM: Diet-gene interactions in human lipoprotein metabolism. J Am Coll Nutr 16:313, 1997.
63. Schaefer EJ, Lamon-Fava S, Ausman LM, et al: Individual variability in lipoprotein cholesterol response to National Cholesterol Education Program Step 2 diets. Am J Clin Nutr 65:823, 1997.
64. Hu FB, Manson JE, Willett WC: Types of dietary fat and risk of coronary heart disease: A critical review. J Am Coll Nutr 20:5, 2001.
65. Lichtenstein AH, Deckelbaum RJ: AHA Science Advisory. Stanol/sterol ester-containing foods and blood cholesterol levels: A statement for healthcare professionals from the Nutrition Committee of the Council on Nutrition, Physical Activity, and Metabolism of the American Heart Association. Circulation 103:1177, 2001.
66. Van Horn L: Fiber, lipids, and coronary heart disease: A statement for healthcare professionals from the Nutrition Committee, American Heart Association. Circulation 95:2701, 1997.
67. Jenkins DJ, Kendall CW, Marchie A, et al: Effects of a dietary portfolio of cholesterol-lowering foods versus lovastatin on serum lipids and C-reactive protein. JAMA 290:502, 2003.
68. Grundy SM: Hypertriglyceridemia, atherogenic dyslipidemia, and the metabolic syndrome. Am J Cardiol 81:18B, 1998.
69. Berneis KK, Krauss RM: Metabolic origins and clinical significance of LDL heterogeneity. J Lipid Res 43:1363, 2002.
70. Parks EJ, Hellerstein MK: Carbohydrate-induced hypertriacylglycerolemia: Historical perspective and review of biological mechanisms. Am J Clin Nutr 71:412, 2000.
71. Krauss RM: Dietary and genetic effects on low-density lipoprotein heterogeneity. Annu Rev Nutr 21:283, 2001.

Dietary Factors and Blood Pressure Control

72. Kotchen TA, McCarron DA: Dietary electrolytes and blood pressure: A statement for healthcare professionals from the American Heart Association Nutrition Committee. Circulation 98:613, 1998.
73. Graudal NA, Galloe AM, Garred P: Effects of sodium restriction on blood pressure, renin, aldosterone, catecholamines, cholesterols, and triglyceride: A meta-analysis. JAMA 279:1383, 1998.
74. Obarzanek E, Proschan MA, Vollmer WM, et al: Individual blood pressure responses to changes in salt intake: Results from the DASH-Sodium Trial. Hypertension 42:459, 2003.
75. Trials of Hypertension Prevention Collaborative Research Group. Effects of weight loss and sodium reduction intervention on blood pressure and hypertension incidence in overweight people with high-normal blood pressure: The Trials of Hypertension Prevention, Phase II. Arch Intern Med 157:657, 1997.
76. Whelton PK, Appel LJ, Espeland MA, et al: Sodium reduction and weight loss in the treatment of hypertension in older persons: A randomized controlled trial of nonpharmacologic interventions in the elderly (TONE). TONE Collaborative Research Group. JAMA 279:839, 1998.
77. Klatsky AL: Alcohol and cardiovascular disease—more than one paradox to consider. Alcohol and hypertension: does it matter? Yes. J Cardiovasc Risk 10:21, 2003.
78. Cushman WC, Cutler JA, Hanna E, et al: Prevention and Treatment of Hypertension Study (PATHS): Effects of an alcohol treatment program on blood pressure. Arch Intern Med 158:1197, 1998.
79. Vaskonen T: Dietary minerals and modification of cardiovascular risk factors. J Nutr Biochem 14:492, 2003.
80. Whelton PK, He J, Cutler JA, et al: Effects of oral potassium on blood pressure: Meta-analysis of randomized controlled clinical trials. JAMA 277:1624, 1997.
81. Svetkey LP Simons-Morton D, Vollmer WM, et al: Effects of dietary patterns on blood pressure: Subgroup analysis of the Dietary Approaches to Stop Hypertension (DASH) randomized clinical trial. Arch Intern Med 159:285, 1999.
82. Vollmer WM, Sacks FM, Ard J, et al: Effects of diet and sodium intake on blood pressure: Subgroup analysis of the DASH-Sodium trial. Ann Intern Med 135:1019, 2001.
83. Resnick LM, Oparil S, Chait A, et al: Factors affecting blood pressure responses to diet: The Vanguard study. Am J Hypertens 13:956, 2000.
84. Bao DQ, Mori TA, Burke V, et al: Effects of dietary fish and weight reduction on ambulatory blood pressure in overweight hypertensives. Hypertension 32:710, 1998.
85. Saltzman E, Das SK, Lichtenstein AH, et al: An oat-containing hypocaloric diet reduces systolic blood pressure and improves lipid profile beyond effects of weight loss in men and women. J Nutr 131:1465, 2001.
86. Burke V, Hodgson JM, Beilin LJ, et al: Dietary protein and soluble fiber reduce ambulatory blood pressure in treated hypertensives. Hypertension 38:821, 2001.
87. Teede HJ, Dalais FS, Kotsopoulos D, et al: Dietary soy has both beneficial and potentially adverse cardiovascular effects: A placebo-controlled study in men and postmenopausal women. J Clin Endocrinol Metab 86:3053, 2001.
88. Rivas M, Garay RP, Escanero JF, et al: Soy milk lowers blood pressure in men and women with mild to moderate essential hypertension. J Nutr 132:1900, 2002.

89. Taubert D, Berkels R, Roesen R, Klaus W: Chocolate and blood pressure in elderly individuals with isolated systolic hypertension. JAMA 290:1029, 2003.
90. Bautista LE, Arenas IA, Penuela A, Martinez LX: Total plasma homocysteine level and risk of cardiovascular disease: A meta-analysis of prospective cohort studies. J Clin Epidemiol 55:882, 2002.
91. Homocysteine Cooperative Research Group. Homocysteine and risk of ischemic heart disease and stroke: A meta-analysis. JAMA 288:2015, 2002.
92. Malinow MR, Bostom AG, Krauss RM: Homocyst(e)ine, diet, and cardiovascular diseases: A statement for healthcare professionals from the Nutrition Committee, American Heart Association. Circulation 99:178, 1999.
93. Schnyder G, Roffi M, Flammer Y, et al: Effect of homocysteine-lowering therapy with folic acid, vitamin B_{12}, and vitamin B_6 on clinical outcome after percutaneous coronary intervention: The Swiss Heart study: A randomized controlled trial. JAMA 288:973, 2002.
94. Bostom AG, Jacques PF, Liaugaudas G, et al: Total homocysteine-lowering treatment among coronary artery disease patients in the era of folic acid–fortified cereal grain flour. Arterioscler Thromb Vasc Biol 22:488, 2002.

Other Dietary Factors and Cardiovascular Risk

95. Pearson TA, Mensah GA, Alexander RW, et al: Markers of inflammation and cardiovascular disease—application to clinical and public health practice: A statement for healthcare professionals from the Centers for Disease Control and Prevention and the American Heart Association. Circulation 107:499, 2003.
96. McLaughlin T, Abbasi F, Lamendola C, et al: Differentiation between obesity and insulin resistance in the association with C-reactive protein. Circulation 106:2908, 2002.
97. Esposito K, Pontillo A, Di Palo C, et al: Effect of weight loss and lifestyle changes on vascular inflammatory markers in obese women: A randomized trial. JAMA 289:1799, 2003.
98. Liu S, Manson JE, Buring JE, et al: Relation between a diet with a high glycemic load and plasma concentrations of high-sensitivity C-reactive protein in middle-aged women. Am J Clin Nutr 75:492, 2002.
99. Tribble DL: AHA Science Advisory. Antioxidant consumption and risk of coronary heart disease: Emphasis on vitamin C, vitamin E, and beta-carotene: A statement for healthcare professionals from the American Heart Association. Circulation 99:591, 1999.
100. Morris CD, Carson S: Routine vitamin supplementation to prevent cardiovascular disease: A summary of the evidence for the U.S. Preventive Services Task Force. Ann Intern Med 139:56, 2003.
101. Brown BG, Zhao XQ, Chait A, et al: Simvastatin and niacin, antioxidant vitamins, or the combination for the prevention of coronary disease. N Engl J Med 345:1583, 2001.
102. Lichtenstein AH: Dietary *trans* fatty acid. J Cardiopulm Rehabil 20:143, 2000.
103. Ginsberg HN, Kris-Etherton P, Dennis B, et al: Effects of reducing dietary saturated fatty acids on plasma lipids and lipoproteins in healthy subjects: The DELTA Study, protocol 1. Arterioscler Thromb Vasc Biol 18:441, 1998.

CHAPTER 42

Primary and Secondary Prevention of Coronary Heart Disease

J. Michael Gaziano • JoAnn E. Manson • Paul M. Ridker

Both primary and secondary prevention of coronary heart disease (CHD) have indisputable public health importance. Given the prevalence of CHD, preventing even a small proportion of cases would save thousands of lives, avoid inestimable suffering, and save billions of health care dollars. In addition, measures that prevent CHD may also mitigate other manifestations of atherosclerosis, such as stroke and peripheral artery disease, and may have an impact on hypertension, diabetes, cancer, cognitive function, depression, and other chronic conditions as well. Because cardiovascular diseases (CVDs) will soon become the number one killer worldwide,[1] widespread deployment of affordable preventive strategies should have high priority in both developed and developing countries.[2]

The great strides made over the last 50 years toward understanding the pathophysiology of atherosclerosis and identifying a large number of life-style, biochemical, and genetic factors potentially associated with CHD have contributed to significant declines in age-adjusted cardiovascular mortality (Fig. 42–1). The first step toward prevention entails using these factors to predict who is likely to experience atherosclerotic events. Several scores have been developed that use different risk factors to estimate an individual's risk of future cardiovascular events. Yet the process of disease prevention must push beyond using factors to predict future events and move toward establishing interventions that definitively reduce risk. Weighing the benefits of given interventions against their risks and costs has led to the establishment of guidelines for health providers and the general public. Implementing these guidelines, however, remains a difficult task. Lack of time is certainly one hurdle. Delivering only those cardiovascular-related preventive services recommended by the U.S. Preventive Services Task Force would take the representative clinician a minimum of 1.5 hours per day.[3] Lack of reimbursement also limits the delivery of preventive interventions.

This chapter defines risk factors in a novel way. First, we discuss the various types of risk factors and their utility in predicting risk. Then we present a scheme for prioritizing preventive interventions that divides these interventions into the following three categories:

- Class 1 interventions are those for risk factors with a clear causal relationship with heart disease where the benefits of intervention have been established.
- Class 2 interventions are those for risk factors that appear to have a causal relationship with heart disease and for which the data suggest that intervention will probably reduce coronary events, but for which there are limited data regarding the benefits, risks, and costs of the intervention.
- Class 3 interventions are those for which an independent causal relationship with heart disease is suspected but as yet unproved.

The chapter then examines 13 potentially modifiable risk factor domains and interventions, with information on prevalence, associated risk, benefit of treatment, cost efficacy, and recommendations/guidelines for each. It concludes with a discussion of multiple risk factor interventions.

About Risk Factors

In addition to detailed descriptions of the natural history and epidemiology of atherosclerosis and coronary disease, the Framingham Heart Study gave modern medicine the term *risk factor.* In a 1961 report, Kannel and colleagues described "factors of risk" associated with the development of CHD.[4] Since then, the term has become an integral part of the language of epidemiology, cardiology, and a host of other disciplines.

"Risk factor" generally applies to a parameter that can predict a future cardiovascular event. For the purposes of risk prediction, what matters is the predictive value of the risk factor, the feasibility of assessing it, and the cost of assessment. Age, for example, is a useful predictor, because it is strongly associated with cardiovascular risk and can be assessed easily and at no cost. However, when trying to identify potential targets for intervention, it is worth considering which factors can be modified to lower risk, such as smoking. Risk factors can be divided into four basic categories (Table 42–1): predisposing factors, risk-modifying behaviors, metabolic risk factors, and disease markers.

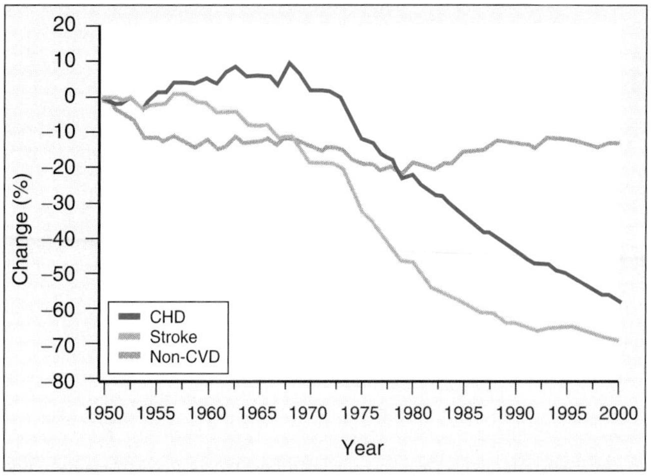

FIGURE 42–1 Change in age-adjusted mortality from coronary heart disease (CHD), stroke, and non-CVD in the United States, 1950 to 2000. CVD = cardiovascular disease. (From Morbidity and Mortality: 2002 Chart Book on Cardiovascular, Lung, and Blood Diseases. Bethesda, MD, National Heart, Lung, and Blood Institute, 2002, p 23.) (See also Chap. 36.)

TABLE 42–1 Four Basic Categories of Risk Factors

Category	Risk Factors
Predisposing factors	Age, sex, family history, genes
Risk-modifying behaviors	Smoking, atherogenic diet, alcohol intake, physical activity
Metabolic risk factors	Dyslipidemias, hypertension, obesity, diabetes, metabolic syndrome
Disease markers	Calcium score, catheterization results, stress test results, left ventricular hypertrophy on echocardiogram, personal history of vascular disease (prior myocardial infarction or stroke, angina, peripheral vascular disease), inflammatory state

These distinctions may be useful but are somewhat arbitrary. At times it may be difficult to classify a factor in a distinct category. For example, family history could represent an individual's genes *or* behaviors that are passed from one generation to the next. Is hypertension a metabolic risk factor that results in part from the influence of risk-modifying behaviors such as an atherosclerotic diet or physical inactivity, or is it a marker of endothelial dysfunction and atherosclerosis? Similarly, an inflammatory state as measured by high-sensitivity C-reactive protein (hs-CRP) could be considered as a metabolic intermediate, such as high cholesterol, or may be a marker of ongoing atherosclerosis. The four categories of risk factors described earlier are useful in considering potential targets for intervention but require evaluation in clinical trials to confirm any suspected modifiability.

In this framework, predisposing factors such as genes interact with behavioral factors and lead to metabolic abnormalities that may eventually lead to cardiovascular disease. For example, an atherogenic diet and lack of exercise in a genetically susceptible individual increase low-density lipoprotein (LDL) cholesterol, which leads to endothelial dysfunction, fatty streaks, atherosclerotic plaques, and eventually to cardiovascular events. Metabolic factors can interact in similar ways to accelerate this process.

For a factor to be useful in prediction, it must be easy and inexpensive to measure—a major potential limitation for expensive techniques such as screening with electron-beam computed tomography (CT). Further, the false-positive rate associated with screening must be low to avoid unnecessary and potentially hazardous consequences. Although predictive value is *necessary* to infer that modification of a risk factor will lead to reduced risk, it is not *sufficient.* The benefit of intervention must clearly exceed any risks and be worth the cost. Then it must be implemented in appropriate populations.

Figure 42–2 describes a way of classifying risk factors by their ability to predict disease and their proven utility for modifying the chance of future events. Although some risk factors that correctly predict disease may be targets for future interventions, we consider only those factors for which there is strong evidence that modification reduces cardiovascular risk. Several preventive medications, such as aspirin, and cardiovascular interventions have been added to the list of interventions that modify risk because of their ability to lower the risk of future events, and therefore they must be considered when addressing prevention for a patient. This chapter considers only those factors that modify intermediate or long-term risk. Interventions used acutely to modify short-term risk, such as aspirin in the setting of an acute myocardial infarction, are considered elsewhere in this text (see Chap. 47).

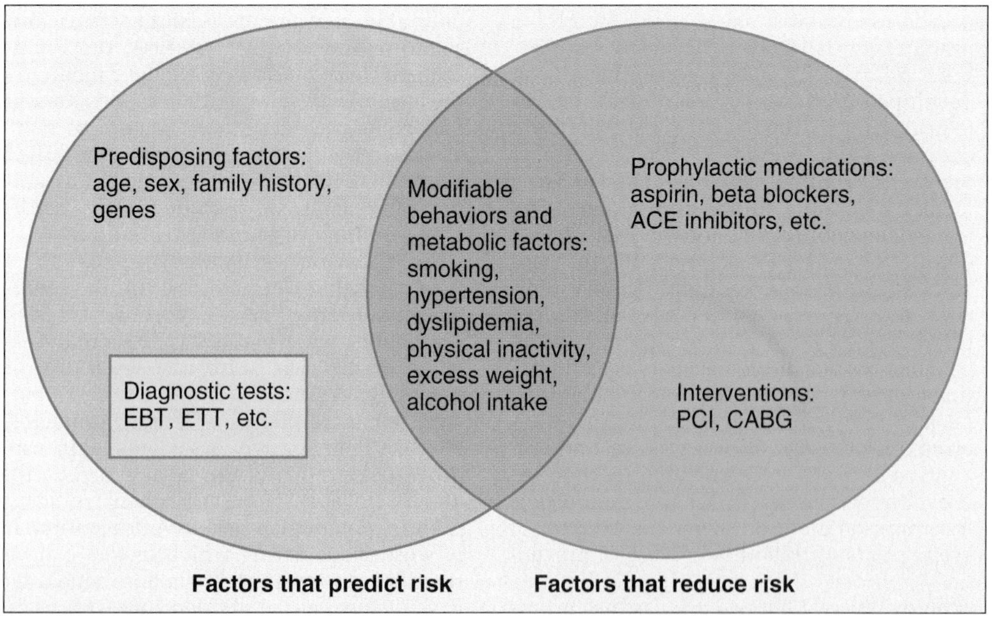

FIGURE 42–2 Classification of risk factors by their ability to predict disease and their proven utility for modifying the chance of future events. EBT = electron-beam tomography; ETT = exercise tolerance test; ACE = angiotensin-converting enzyme; PCI = percutaneous coronary intervention; CABG = coronary artery bypass graft. (See also Chap. 36.)

Predicting Risk

A fundamental step in establishing individual or population-wide preventive strategies involves assessing the risk of development of clinically relevant outcomes because the cost efficacy of any intervention varies according to global risk in a given individual or population. Since absolute risk among those with known disease is higher than among those at lower risk, fewer high-risk individuals require treatment to save one life or prevent one event in comparison to those at lower risk, even if relative risk reductions are identical in both groups. To illustrate this concept, assume that an intervention reduces mortality by 25 percent in both primary and secondary prevention. Furthermore, assume that a high-risk individual with CHD has a 20 percent chance of death from cardiovascular disease over the next 10 years while a low-risk individual has a 1 percent chance of death over the same period. To save a life among those at high risk, one would have to treat only 20 patients (4 of whom are destined to die) for 10 years so that a 25 percent relative risk reduction would result in 1 life saved (3 deaths instead of 4). On the other hand, one would have to treat 400 low-risk patients (4 of whom are also destined to die) so that the same 25 percent relative risk reduction would yield 3 deaths instead of 4. Thus, the total cost per lives saved is considerably lower ($\frac{1}{20}$ the cost) among individuals at higher absolute risk. Assessing an individual's absolute risk enables cost-effective targeting of interventions. Accordingly, the National Cholesterol Education Program (NCEP) Adult Treatment Panel (ATP) III[5] and the Seventh Joint National Committee on Prevention, Detection, Evaluation, and Treatment of High Blood Pressure (JNC-7)[6] now use absolute risk to gauge the intensity of intervention. The American Diabetes Association also recommends a tiered approach to management based on absolute risk.[7]

Assessing Individual Risk

A crude way to categorize individuals as being at higher or lower risk is by the presence or absence of cardiovascular disease. Those with known cardiovascular disease, including coronary, cerebrovascular, or peripheral artery disease, are on average at much higher risk than those without known disease. Approximately 80% of those with known cardiovascular disease will die of some form of cardiovascular disease, whereas those without known cardiovascular disease have approximately half that cardiovascular disease mortality rate. As discussed later in this chapter, those with cardiovascular disease generally warrant aggressive preventive interventions. Risk reduction in those with known cardiovascular disease is referred to as *secondary prevention*, as opposed to primary prevention among those without overt cardiovascular disease. Individuals with diabetes comprise a second high-risk group. Rates of cardiovascular disease events and mortality among diabetic patients considerably exceed those in the general population; thus, patients with diabetes warrant aggressive preventive interventions. Another group of patients that is at exceedingly high risk for cardiovascular disease events and death are those with chronic renal failure, many of whom have diabetes.

For those without overt cardiovascular disease or diabetes, other predictive risk factors should be used to assess overall risk. Several risk prediction strategies have been developed using some of the predictive risk factors outlined in Figure 42–2. Framingham Heart Study investigators have developed a useful tool to assess risk of a first cardiovascular event based on age, gender, total or LDL cholesterol, high-density lipoprotein (HDL) cholesterol, systolic and diastolic blood pressure, and history of diabetes and cigarette smoking (Fig. 42–3).[8] Point-based weights are assigned to the presence and/or level of each risk factor. Once the points have been assigned and summed, the total score can be translated to an estimated absolute risk of a CHD event occurring within the next 10 years. The National Heart, Lung, and Blood Institute has made available an online version of the 10-year risk calculator (hin.nhlbi.nih.gov/atpiii/calculator.asp), as well as versions that can be downloaded to a clinician's desktop computer (hin.nhlbi.nih.gov/atpiii/riskcalc.htm) or handheld device (hin.nhlbi.nih.gov/atpiii/atp3palm.htm).

Risk assessment scales are also available from the Framingham investigators for the secondary prevention of myocardial infarction and stroke. However, since all patients with prior evidence of cardiovascular disease have high risk for recurrent events and require aggressive preventive efforts, the utility of these tools is unclear.

The European Society of Cardiology (ESC) has also assembled recommendations for the prevention of heart disease that stratify preventive interventions according to whether a patient is at high, intermediate, or low risk.[9] Those with known CHD constitute the highest-risk category because most of these individuals have a greater than 20 percent chance of subsequent events over the next 10 years. Individuals without known CHD are assessed for risk with a modified Framingham assessment tool. This tool, presented in a series of easy-to-use charts, allows clinicians to assess risk over the next 10 years based on age, gender, smoking status, diabetes, level of cholesterol, and blood pressure (Fig. 42–4). Those for whom the risk of a primary event exceeds 20 percent over the next 10 years are recommended for aggressive management. Those for whom risk is lower are prescribed a less intense and less costly approach.

A third method of assessing absolute risk in men has emerged from the Prospective Cardiovascular Munster (PROCAM) Study, a long-term follow-up study of more than 5000 men aged 35 to 65 years recruited between 1979 and 1985. Risk factors included in the PROCAM algorithm include cigarette smoking, systolic blood pressure, LDL cholesterol, HDL cholesterol, fasting triglycerides, diabetes, family history of myocardial infarction, and age. Answers to questions regarding these factors is tallied into a point score, just as with the Framingham algorithm, and this point score is converted into a 10-year absolute risk of fatal or nonfatal myocardial infarction or sudden cardiac death.[10] Scores for women are not yet available.

These scores provide a good initial method for assessing risk at low cost. A number of diagnostic tests and novel biochemical markers have emerged as potential ways to augment these simple scores. Calcium scores determined by electron-beam CT and exercise tolerance tests represent two such diagnostic tests for which substantial data are available. Another is hs-CRP, a marker of inflammation that holds promise in providing incremental predictive value. As reviewed in Chapter 36, hs-CRP adds prognostic information at all levels of LDL cholesterol, at all levels of the metabolic syndrome, and at all levels of the Framingham Risk Score. However, these tests entail costs and potential consequences, and their utility in prevention remains controversial.

Although the various risk prediction scores tend to categorize individuals similarly, there are differences. Compared to the ESC score, the Framingham Heart Study score tends to predict slightly higher overall risk.[11] However, for the purposes of broad categorization of individuals, there is generally good agreement between the two scores.

Assessing Risk at a Population Level: Incidence, Prevalence, and Population-Attributable Risk

Sound public policy also requires evaluation of the impact of different factors on the *population*. Population risk depends not only on the strength of the risk factor–disease association and the benefit of intervention but also on how common the factor is in the general population. These concepts are captured in incidence, prevalence, and population-attributable risk. Although incidence rates reflect the frequency of new cases of disease or a risk factor over a given period, prevalence reflects the proportion of individuals with a given condition or factor at a single point. Population-attributable risk, or how much of the population's risk of disease is attributable to a

Step 1

Age		
Years	LDL Pts	Chol Pts
30–34	−1	[−1]
35–39	0	[0]
40–44	1	[1]
45–49	2	[2]
50–54	3	[3]
55–59	4	[4]
60–64	5	[5]
65–69	6	[6]
70–74	7	[7]

Step 2

LDL-C		
(mg/dl)	(mmol/L)	LDL Pts
< 100	< 2.59	−3
100–129	2.60–3.36	0
130–159	3.37–4.14	0
160–190	4.15–4.92	1
≥ 190	≥ 4.92	2

Cholesterol		
(mg/dl)	(mmol/L)	Chol Pts
< 160	< 4.14	[−3]
160–199	4.15–5.17	[0]
200–239	5.18–6.21	[1]
240–279	6.22–7.24	[2]
≥ 280	≥ 7.25	[3]

Step 3

HDL-C			
(mg/dl)	(mmol/L)	LDL Pts	Chol Pts
< 35	< 0.90	2	[2]
35–44	0.91–1.16	1	[1]
45–49	1.17–1.29	0	[0]
50–59	1.30–1.55	0	[0]
≥ 60	≥ 1.56	−1	[−2]

Step 4

Blood Pressure					
Systolic	Diastolic (mm Hg)				
(mm Hg)	< 80	80–84	85–89	90–99	≥ 100
< 120	0 [0] pts				
120–129		0 [0] pts			
130–139			1 [1] pt		
140–159				2 [2] pts	
≥ 160					3 [3] pts

Note: When systolic and diastolic pressures provide different estimates for point scores, use the higher number

Step 5

Diabetes		
	LDL Pts	Chol Pts
No	0	[0]
Yes	2	[2]

Step 6

Smoker		
	LDL Pts	Chol Pts
No	0	[0]
Yes	2	[2]

Step 7 (sum from steps 1-6)

Adding up the points	
Age	______
LDL-C or Chol	______
HDL-C	______
Blood Pressure	______
Diabetes	______
Smoker	______
Point Total	______

Step 8 (determine CHD risk from point total)

CHD Risk			
LDL Pts Total	10-Yr CHD Risk	Chol Pts Total	10-Yr CHD Risk
< −3	1%		
−2	2%		
−1	2%	[< −1]	[2%]
0	3%	[0]	[3%]
1	4%	[1]	[3%]
2	4%	[2]	[4%]
3	6%	[3]	[5%]
4	7%	[4]	[7%]
5	9%	[5]	[8%]
6	11%	[6]	[10%]
7	14%	[7]	[13%]
8	18%	[8]	[16%]
9	22%	[9]	[20%]
10	27%	[10]	[25%]
11	33%	[11]	[31%]
12	40%	[12]	[37%]
13	47%	[13]	[45%]
≥ 14	≥ 56%	[≥ 14]	[≥ 53%]

Step 9 (compare to average person your age)

Comparative Risk			
Age (years)	Average 10-Yr CHD Risk	Average 10-Yr Hard* CHD Risk	Low† 10-Yr CHD Risk
30–34	3%	1%	2%
35–39	5%	4%	3%
40–44	7%	4%	4%
45–49	11%	8%	4%
50–54	14%	10%	6%
55–59	16%	13%	7%
60–64	21%	20%	9%
65–69	25%	22%	11%
70–74	30%	25%	14%

Relative Risk
- Very low
- Low
- Moderate
- High
- Very high

* Hard CHD events exclude angina pectoris

† Low risk was calculated for a person the same age, optimal blood pressure, LDL-C 100–129 mg/dl or cholesterol 160–199 mg/dl, HDL-C 45 mg/dl for men or 55 mg/dl for women, nonsmoker, no diabetes

Risk estimates were derived from the experience of the Framingham Heart Study, a predominantly Caucasian population in Massachusetts, USA

A

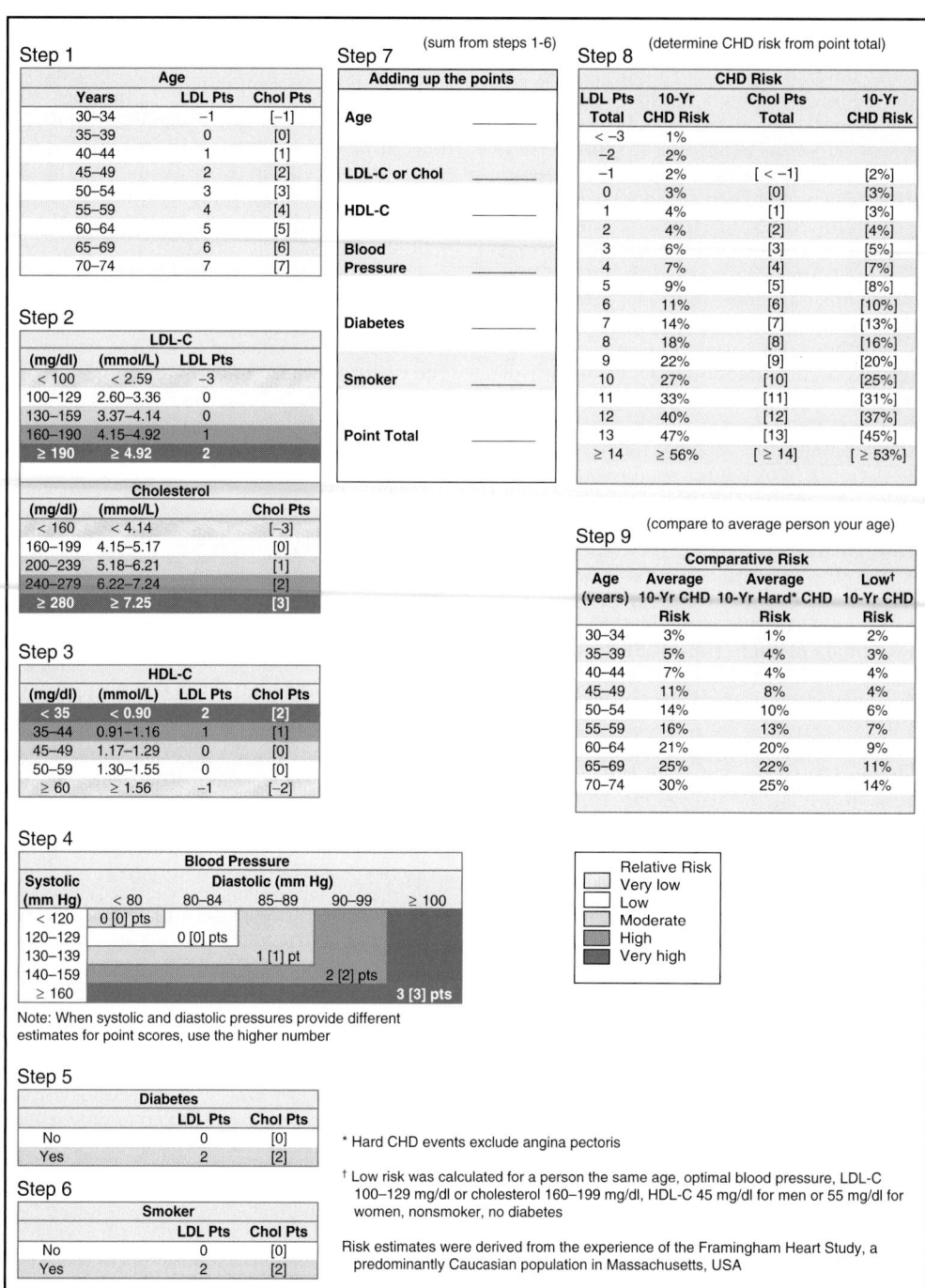

FIGURE 42–3 Coronary heart disease (CHD) score sheets for calculating 10-year CHD risk according to age, total cholesterol (TC) (or low-density lipoprotein cholesterol [LDL-C]), high-density lipoprotein cholesterol (HDL-C), blood pressure, diabetes, and smoking. **A,** Score sheet for men based on the Framingham experience in men 30 to 74 years of age at baseline. Average risk estimates are based on typical Framingham subjects, and estimates of idealized risk are based on optimal blood pressure, TC of 160 to 199 mg/dl (or LDL of 100 to 129 mg/dl), HDL-C of 45 mg/dl, no diabetes, and no smoking.

given factor, is driven by the proportion of the public with a given risk factor and the magnitude of the associated risk.

Population-attributable risk also reflects the shape of the relationship between the exposure and the disease. Many factors increase risk in a linear fashion, so population-attributable risk can be computed against an ideal standard or a low-risk individual. For example, the relationship between hypertension and heart disease and stroke is linear. Thus, lowering blood pressure at any level in the pathological range reduces risk. In contrast, the shape of the risk curve for obesity appears nonlinear, with risk increasing logarithmically (Fig. 42–5). Thus, each incremental pound gained is associated with much more risk in those who are already overweight. Population-attributable risk is an important concept for determining resource allocation between various preventive interventions.

Preventive Intervention Strategies for Modifiable Risk Factors

Some predictive risk factors are potential targets for intervention. A crucial step in developing preventive intervention

Step 1

Age		
Years	LDL Pts	Chol Pts
30–34	−9	[−9]
35–39	−4	[−4]
40–44	0	[0]
45–49	3	[3]
50–54	6	[6]
55–59	7	[7]
60–64	8	[8]
65–69	8	[8]
70–74	8	[8]

Step 2

LDL-C		
(mg/dl)	(mmol/L)	LDL Pts
< 100	< 2.59	−2
100–129	2.60–3.36	0
130–159	3.37–4.14	0
160–190	4.15–4.92	2
≥ 190	≥ 4.92	2

Cholesterol		
(mg/dl)	(mmol/L)	Chol Pts
< 160	< 4.14	[−2]
160–199	4.15–5.17	[0]
200–239	5.18–6.21	[1]
240–279	6.22–7.24	[1]
≥ 280	≥ 7.25	[3]

Step 3

HDL-C			
(mg/dl)	(mmol/L)	LDL Pts	Chol Pts
< 35	< 0.90	5	[5]
35–44	0.91–1.16	2	[2]
45–49	1.17–1.29	1	[1]
50–59	1.30–1.55	0	[0]
≥ 60	≥ 1.56	−2	[−3]

Step 4

Blood Pressure					
Systolic	Diastolic (mm Hg)				
(mm Hg)	< 80	80–84	85–89	90–99	≥ 100
< 120	−3 [−3] pts				
120–129		0 [0] pts			
130–139			0 [0] pts		
140–159				2 [2] pts	
≥ 160					3 [3] pts

Note: When systolic and diastolic pressures provide different estimates for point scores, use the higher number

Step 5

Diabetes		
	LDL Pts	Chol Pts
No	0	[0]
Yes	4	[4]

Step 6

Smoker		
	LDL Pts	Chol Pts
No	0	[0]
Yes	2	[2]

Step 7 (sum from steps 1-6)

Adding up the points	
Age	_______
LDL-C or Chol	_______
HDL-C	_______
Blood Pressure	_______
Diabetes	_______
Smoker	_______
Point Total	_______

Step 8 (determine CHD risk from point total)

CHD Risk			
LDL Pts Total	10-Yr CHD Risk	Chol Pts Total	10-Yr CHD Risk
≤ −2	1%	[≤ −2]	[1%]
−1	2%	[−1]	[2%]
0	2%	[0]	[2%]
1	2%	[1]	[2%]
2	3%	[2]	[3%]
3	3%	[3]	[3%]
4	4%	[4]	[4%]
5	5%	[5]	[4%]
6	6%	[6]	[5%]
7	7%	[7]	[6%]
8	8%	[8]	[7%]
9	9%	[9]	[8%]
10	11%	[10]	[10%]
11	13%	[11]	[11%]
12	15%	[12]	[13%]
13	17%	[13]	[15%]
14	20%	[14]	[18%]
15	24%	[15]	[20%]
16	27%	[16]	[24%]
≥ 17	≥ 32%	[≥ 17]	[≥ 27%]

Step 9 (compare to average person your age)

Comparative Risk			
Age (years)	Average 10-Yr CHD Risk	Average 10-Yr Hard* CHD Risk	Low† 10-Yr CHD Risk
30–34	< 1%	< 1%	< 1%
35–39	< 1%	< 1%	1%
40–44	2%	1%	2%
45–49	5%	2%	3%
50–54	8%	3%	5%
55–59	12%	7%	7%
60–64	12%	8%	8%
65–69	13%	8%	8%
70–74	14%	11%	8%

Relative Risk
- Very low
- Low
- Moderate
- High
- Very high

* Hard CHD events exclude angina pectoris

† Low risk was calculated for a person the same age, optimal blood pressure, LDL-C 100–129 mg/dl or cholesterol 160–199 mg/dl, HDL-C 45 mg/dl for men or 55 mg/dl for women, nonsmoker, no diabetes

Risk estimates were derived from the experience of the Framingham Heart Study, a predominantly Caucasian population in Massachusetts, USA

B

IGURE 42–3, cont'd **B,** Score sheet for women based on Framingham experience in women 30 to 74 years of age at baseline. Average risk estimates are based on typical ramingham subjects, and estimates of idealized risk are based on optimal blood pressure, TC of 160 to 199 mg/dl (or LDL of 100 to 129 mg/dl), HDL-C of 55 mg/dl, no diabetes, nd no smoking. Use of the LDL-C categories is appropriate when fasting LDL-C measurements are available. Pts = points. (From Wilson PW, D'Agostino RB, Levy D, et al: Prediction of coronary heart disease using risk factor categories. Circulation 97:1837-1847, 1998.)

s the establishment of cause and effect. Data from several types of research are needed to establish a causal relationship between exposure and disease (Table 42–2). Basic research provides insight into the mechanisms underlying atherogenesis and helps elucidate the biological plausibility of potential interventions to modify these effects. Basic research has proven particularly successful in drug discovery. The development of preventive strategies also depends heavily on a number of complementary methods of population research, including descriptive studies (cross-sectional surveys and cross-cultural analyses), analytical studies (case-control and prospective cohort studies), and intervention studies (randomized trials).

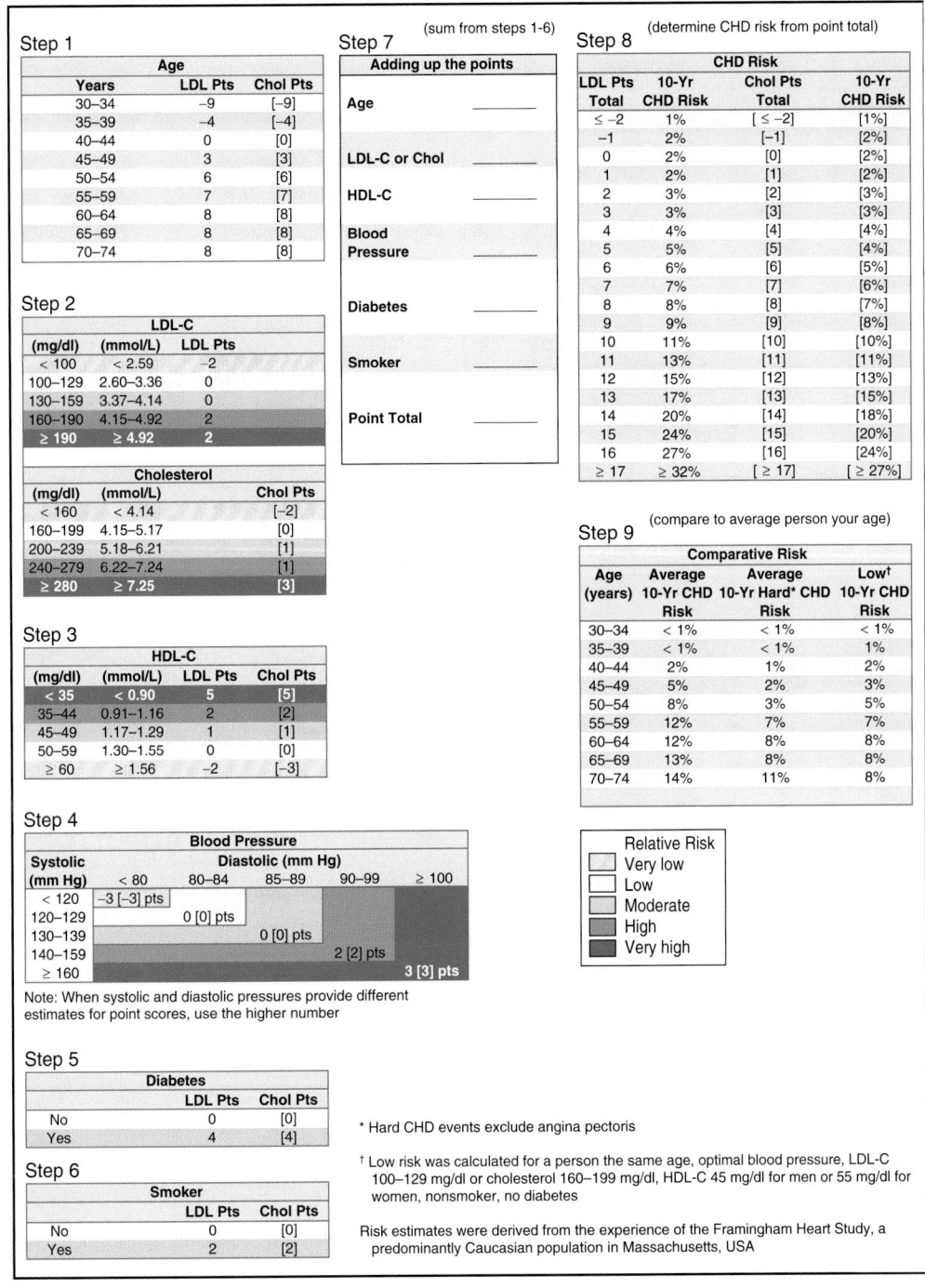

Each of these strategies has strengths and weaknesses. Descriptive studies (case reports, case series, cross-sectional surveys, cross-cultural studies, and studies of population-based temporal trends) have considerable value for their ability to generate hypotheses. However, their design prevents adequate control for potential factors that may confound apparent associations. Observational studies (case-

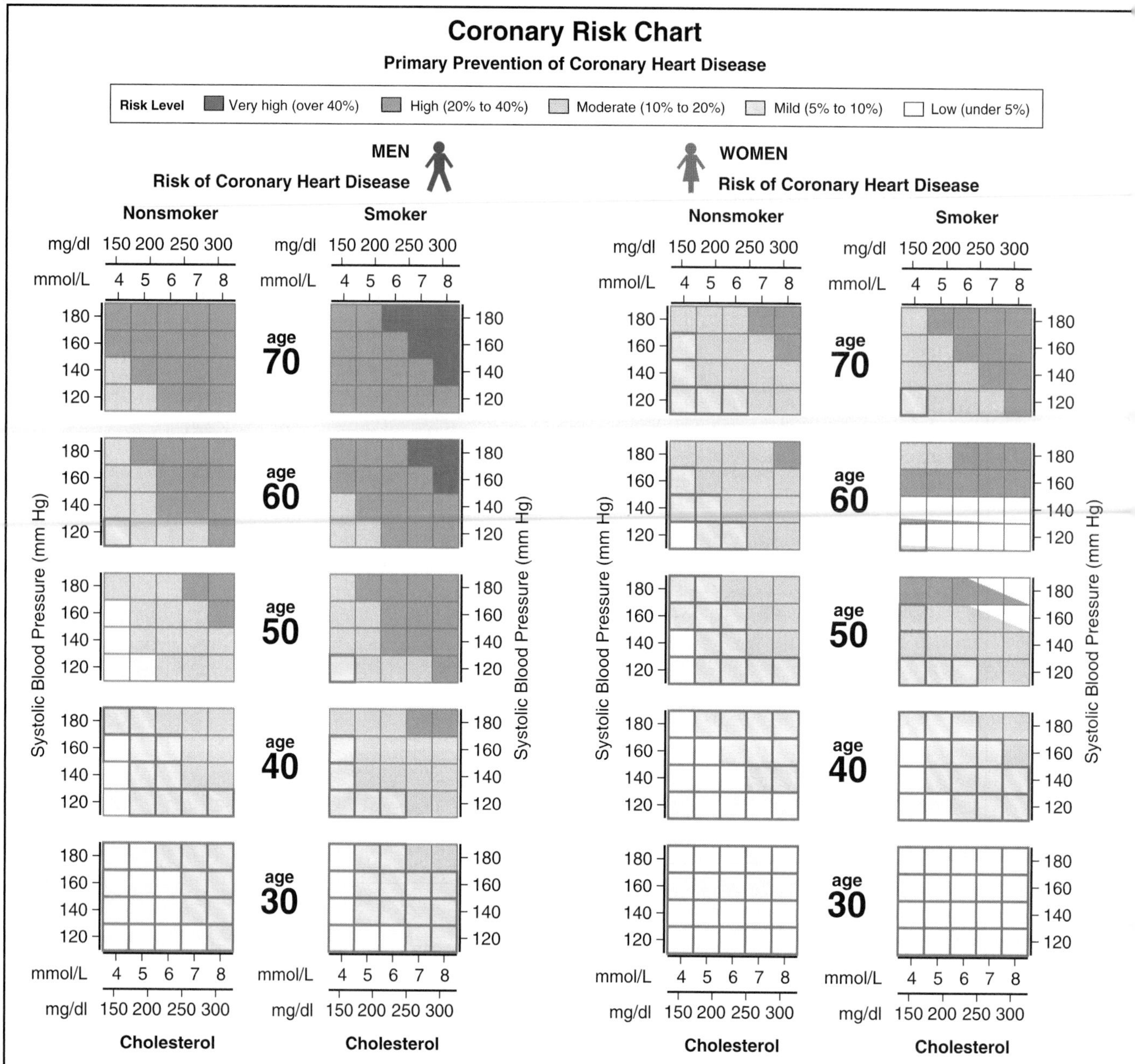

How to use the Coronary Risk Chart for Primary Prevention

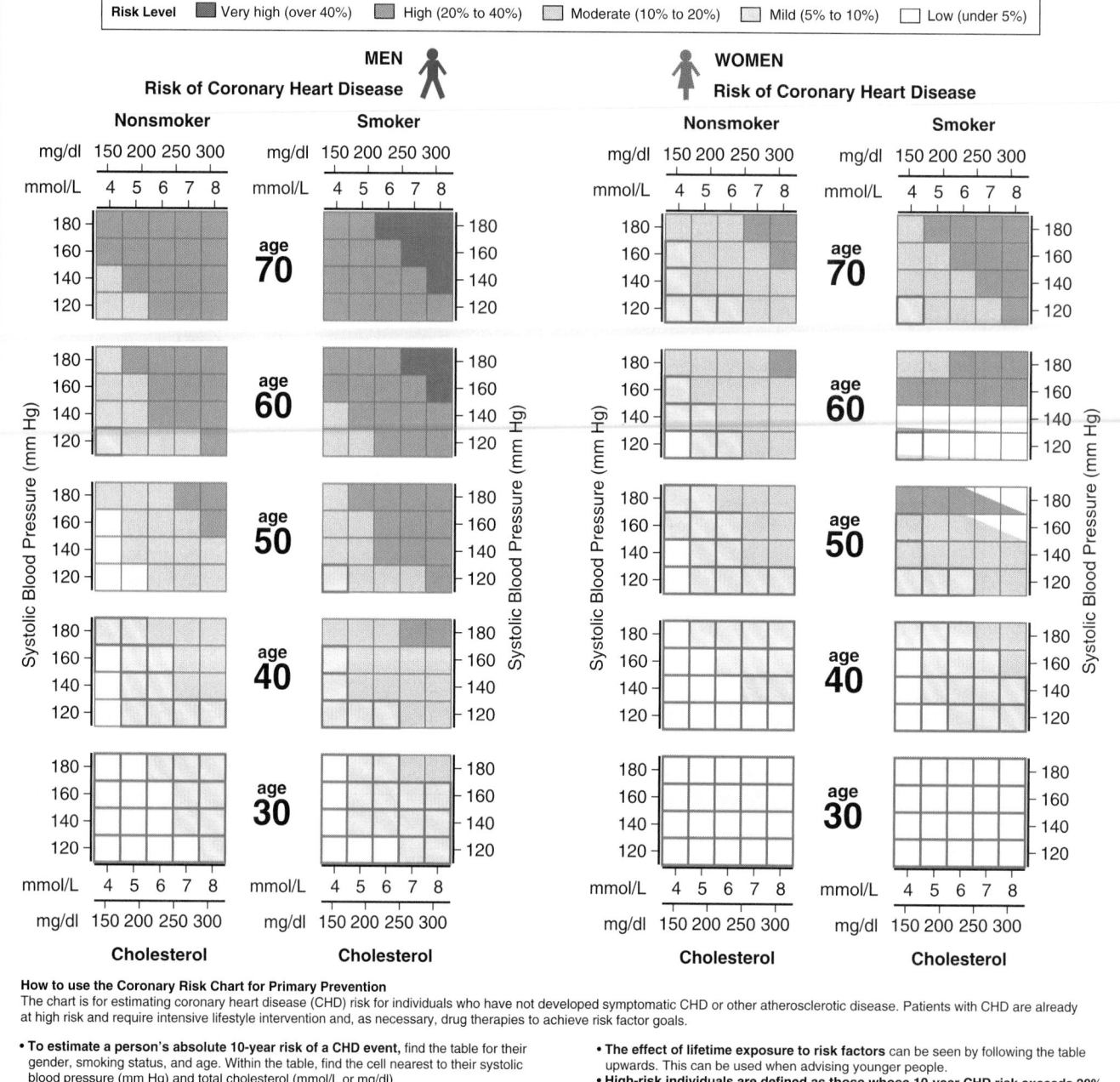

The chart is for estimating coronary heart disease (CHD) risk for individuals who have not developed symptomatic CHD or other atherosclerotic disease. Patients with CHD are already at high risk and require intensive lifestyle intervention and, as necessary, drug therapies to achieve risk factor goals.

- **To estimate a person's absolute 10-year risk of a CHD event,** find the table for their gender, smoking status, and age. Within the table, find the cell nearest to their systolic blood pressure (mm Hg) and total cholesterol (mmol/L or mg/dl).
- **CHD risk is higher than indicated** in the chart for those with:-
  Familial hyperlipidaemia
  Diabetes: risk is approximately doubled in men and more than doubled in women
  Those with a family history of premature cardiovascular disease
  Those with low HDL cholesterol. These tables assume HDL cholesterol to be 1.0 mmol/L (39 mg/dl) in men and 1.1 (43) in women
  Those with raised triglyceride levels > 2.0 mmol/L (> 180 mg/dl)
  As the person approaches the next age category.
- **The effect of lifetime exposure to risk factors** can be seen by following the table upwards. This can be used when advising younger people.
- **High-risk individuals are defined as those whose 10-year CHD risk exceeds 20% or will exceed 20% if projected to age 60.**
- **To find a person's relative risk,** compare their risk category with that for other people of the same age. The absolute risk shown here may not apply to all populations, especially those with a low CHD incidence. Relative risk is likely to apply to most populations.
- **The effect of changing** cholesterol, smoking status, or blood pressure can be read from the chart.

FIGURE 42–4 Risk assessment tool using cholesterol levels, blood pressure, and smoking status devised by a European task force on coronary prevention. (From Wood D, DeBacker G, Faergeman O, et al: Prevention of coronary heart disease in clinical practice: Recommendations of the Second Joint Task Force of European and other Societies on Coronary Prevention. Eur Heart J 19:1434-1503, 1998.)

control and prospective cohort studies) give researchers greater control over potential confounders. They are extremely useful in establishing risk attributable to a single factor, particularly when the effect of a given factor is large, as is the case for smoking and lung cancer. Yet when searching for small-to-moderate effects, the amount of uncontrolled confounding in observational studies may be as large as the probable risk reduction itself. In such cases, randomized trials are essential for confirming causation. Even when causality is not in question, trials help quantify the magni-

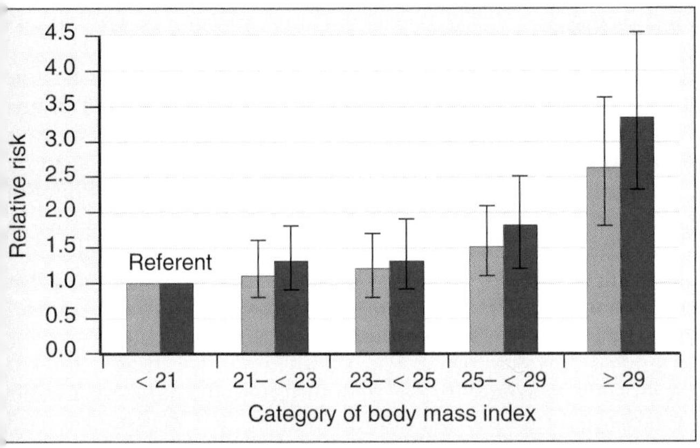

IGURE 42–5 Association between body mass index and relative risk of nonfatal nyocardial infarction and fatal coronary heart disease among women. Light bars show ne relative risks for age and smoking. The vertical lines represent 95 percent confidence intervals.

TABLE 42–2	Types of Studies Used in Establishing Preventive Strategies
Basic research	
In vitro studies	
Animal studies	
Clinical investigation	
Epidemiological studies	
Descriptive studies	
Case reports	
Cross-sectional surveys	
Cross-cultural comparison studies	
Temporal trend studies	
Analytical studies	
Observational	
Case-control studies	
Cohort studies	
Intervention (randomized trials)	
Cost-efficacy studies	
Meta-analyses	

tude of an intervention's effect. In addition, when the intervention is associated with competing risks and benefits, randomized trials are needed to determine the net clinical effect of the intervention.

Once a factor has been established as causally related to disease, interventions to modify the factor must be developed and tested. This is of critical importance because the magnitude of associated risk is not necessarily related to the magnitude of benefit derived from the intervention. Such lack of correlation may be due to the inability of the intervention to achieve the necessary change, or a change in the parameter may not result in the necessary change in risk in a proportional manner. An example is the difference between the observed risk associated with a 1-mm Hg rise in blood pressure and the lower-than-anticipated benefit on CHD derived from reducing blood pressure by this amount.[8,12] Similarly, even though elevated levels of homocysteine have been implicated as a risk factor for CHD and folic acid reduces homocysteine levels, evidence is not yet available from randomized trials indicating that reducing homocysteine levels with folic acid reduces vascular risk. In a similar manner, although hs-CRP is a strong independent predictor of vascular risk, data are not yet available demonstrating that reduction of hs-CRP per se will result in reduced risk.

In addition to providing information on the causal nature of an association, randomized trials generally provide the best data on the magnitude of benefit and risk from a given intervention. This information is essential for assessing cost efficacy and developing preventive strategies.

Cost Efficacy of Preventive Interventions

(see also Chap. 2)

Once reasonable estimates of benefit and risk have been established for a given factor, cost-effectiveness analyses can help establish guidelines for intervention. The common currency used to compare interventions is the quality-adjusted life-year (QALY) or disability-adjusted life-year (DALY). Estimates derived from cost- and risk-benefit analyses are dependent on the underlying assumptions made in a given analysis. In particular, because prevention measures have a long time horizon (decades or more), the consequences of initial assumptions can be much more significant than those of interventions with a short time horizon. Nonetheless, the cost-effectiveness of interventions to prevent heart disease is important because of the prevalence of CHD and the high cost of treatment.

Cost-effectiveness estimates are calculated as the ratio of net cost to gain in life expectancy. Interventions with an incremental cost-effectiveness ratio less than $40,000 per QALY are comparable to other chronic interventions such as hypertension management and hemodialysis. Those with a cost-effectiveness ratio under $20,000 per QALY are very favorable, whereas those exceeding $40,000 per QALY tend to be higher than generally accepted by most insurers.

Interventions at an Individual and Population Level

Three complementary approaches may be used to reduce the population burden of cardiovascular disease: (1) therapeutic interventions for secondary prevention in patients with known cardiovascular disease, (2) identification and targeting of high-risk individuals for primary prevention through mass screening or case finding, and (3) general recommendations disseminated throughout the population. Each of these approaches has merit in different situations. For example, targeted interventions such as specialized cardiac rehabilitation and life-style programs show the greatest efficacy among motivated individuals who hope to avoid a recurrent myocardial infarction, whereas mass screening programs for high blood pressure and hyperlipidemia are cost-effective. Population-wide campaigns against cigarette smoking offer an example of an effective public health approach. Implementation of the first two strategies requires risk assessment at the individual level, while the latter one requires knowledge of risk at the population level.

Classification of Interventions for Modifiable Risk Factors

Implementation of preventive strategies requires a practical, systematic approach to prioritizing interventions and allocating resources. The American College of Cardiology's Bethesda conferences placed risk factors into four categories according to the likelihood that modification of the factor will result in lower risk.[13] These categories include (1) factors for which interventions have been proved to reduce risk; (2) factors for which interventions are likely to lower the incidence of events; (3) factors clearly associated with CHD risk that, if modified, might lower the incidence of coronary events; and (4) factors associated with CHD risk that cannot be modified or, if modified, are not likely to decrease risk

(Table 42–3). Adapting this useful classification scheme to clinical practice requires consideration of cost efficacy. We present a modified classification scheme of interventions for major modifiable risk factors based not only on the strength of the association and evidence of benefit of intervention but also on cost efficacy (Table 42–4).

CLASS 1 INTERVENTIONS. Class 1 interventions have a clear causal relationship with heart disease (Table 42–5). Solid data, generally from randomized clinical trials, demonstrate the magnitude of the intervention's benefit, as well as its risks and cost. Cigarette smoking, hypertension, and dyslipidemias are causally related to CHD, and the corresponding interventions—smoking cessation, blood pressure management, and lipid profile management—all are cost-effective in both primary and secondary prevention. For management of hypertension and dyslipidemia, extensive trial and cost efficacy data enable a tiered approach based on absolute risk at baseline. Other pharmacological approaches proven to be beneficial and cost-effective include aspirin, beta blockers, and angiotensin-converting enzyme (ACE) inhibitors in secondary prevention and aspirin in primary prevention.

CLASS 2 INTERVENTIONS. Class 2 includes interventions for which the available data (largely basic research and human observational studies) strongly indicate a causal relationship and suggest that intervention will probably reduce the incidence of events but for which data on the benefits, risks, and costs of intervention are limited. Class 2 factors that clearly increase the risk of CHD include diabetes, obesity, and physical inactivity. Light-to-moderate alcohol consumption and the use of oral anticoagulants appear to reduce the risk of CHD. Trial data on interventions are forthcoming for several of these factors. It is unlikely, however, that there will ever be data from large-scale randomized trials on alcohol intake. Despite their limitations, class 2 interventions are useful in assessing global risk and have the potential to lower the risk of initial or recurrent CHD. Although it makes sense to invest more resources to modify these factors in individuals at highest risk, guidelines for class 2 factors do not generally distinguish between high- and low-risk individuals.

TABLE 42–3 Evidence Supporting the Association of Risk Factors with Cardiovascular Disease, the Usefulness of Measuring Them, and Their Responsiveness to Intervention

Risk Factor	Evidence for Association with CVD: *Epidemiological*	Evidence for Association with CVD: *Clinical Trials*	Clinical Measurement Useful?	Response to *Nonpharmacological Therapy*	Response to *Pharmacological Therapy*
Category I (Risk Factors for which Interventions Have Been Proved to Lower CVD Risk)					
Cigarette smoking	+++	++	+++	+++	++
LDL cholesterol	+++	+++	+++	+++	+++
High-fat/high-cholesterol diet	+++	++	++	++	–
Hypertension	+++	+++ (Stroke)	+++	+	+++
Left ventricular hypertrophy	+++	+	++	–	++
Category II (Risk Factors for which Interventions Are Likely to Lower CVD Risk)					
Diabetes mellitus	+++	+	+++	++	+++
Physical inactivity	+++	++	++	++	–
HDL cholesterol	+++	+	+++	++	+
Triglycerides; small, dense LDL	++	++	+++	++	+++
Obesity	+++	–	+++	++	+
Postmenopausal status (women)	+++	–	+++	–	+++
Category III (Factors Associated with Increased CVD Risk that, if Modified, Might Lower Risk)					
Psychosocial factors	++	+	+++	+	–
Lipoprotein (a)	+	–	+	–	+
Homocysteine	++	–	+	++	++
Oxidative stress	+	–	–	+	++
No alcohol consumption	+++	–	++	++	–
Category IV (Factors Associated with Increased CVD Risk but Cannot be Modified)					
Age	+++	–	+++	–	–
Male gender	+++	–	+++	–	–
Low socioeconomic status	+++	–	++	–	–
Family history of early-onset CVD	+++	–	+++	–	–

+ = weak, somewhat consistent evidence; ++ = moderately strong, rather consistent evidence; +++ = very strong, consistent evidence; – = poor or nonexistent evidence. CVD = cardiovascular disease; HDL = high-density lipoprotein; LDL = low-density lipoprotein.

Modified from Pearson TA. McBride PE, Miller NH, Smith SC: 27th Bethesda Conference: Matching the intensity of risk factor management with the hazard for coronary disease events. Task Force 8. Organization or preventive cardiology service. J Am Coll Cardiol 27:1039-1047, 1996.

TABLE 42–4 Classification Scheme for Modifiable Risk Factors	
Class	Definition
1	Basic research and human observational studies indicate a clear causal relationship Intervention data (typically from randomized trials) demonstrate the magnitude of the benefit and risk Interventions are cost-effective
2	Basic research and human observational studies indicate a causal relationship Intervention data from large-scale trials are limited Lack of adequate intervention data precludes determination of cost-effectiveness
3	Basic research and human observational studies demonstrate associations, but the independent nature of a causal relationship is not yet clear Interventions are not yet available or have not been adequately tested

TABLE 42–5 Cardiovascular Disease Risk Factors and Interventions

Risk Factor	Intervention	Secondary Prevention	Primary Prevention
Cigarette smoking	Smoking cessation	Class 1	Class 1
High blood pressure	Blood pressure management	Class 1	Class 1
High cholesterol	Cholesterol lowering	Class 1	Class 1
Low HDL	Increase HDL	Class 1, 2	Class 2
High triglycerides	Triglyceride lowering	Class 2	Class 2
Pharmacotherapy	Aspirin therapy Beta blockers ACE inhibitors Oral anticoagulants	Class 1 Class 1 Class 1 Class 1, 2	Class 2 — — —
Diabetes	Diabetes control	Class 2	Class 2
Obesity	Weight reduction	Class 2	Class 2
Physical inactivity	Increase activity	Class 2	Class 2
Dietary factors	Improved diet Moderate alcohol consumption	Class 3 Class 2, 3	Class 3 Class 2, 3
Menopause	Hormone replacement therapy	Class 2	Class 2

ACE = angiotensin-converting enzyme; HDL = high-density lipoprotein.

CLASS 3 INTERVENTIONS. Class 3 interventions are currently under active investigation. For many factors in this class, data are incomplete and an independent causal relationship with CHD cannot be inferred. For others where data are promising, such as homocysteine and C-reactive protein, interventions are not yet available or widely tested even though causal relationships are apparent. Thus, although these factors may have utility for risk assessment, their role in preventing CHD is uncertain. For these reasons, dietary practices such as the consumption of nutritional supplements, psychological factors, the use of hormone replacement therapy after menopause, and novel biochemical and genetic markers are currently considered class 3 factors. It is possible that the identification of high risk may in and of itself provide motivation for better compliance with life-style modifications. For example, individuals with elevated levels of hs-CRP may be more likely to comply with dietary advice and smoking cessation if they understand that they are, in fact, at elevated vascular risk. In several instances, an intervention has proven efficacy in secondary prevention but data are not yet available to support that intervention in primary prevention. For this reason, a factor may be a class 1 intervention for secondary prevention but a class 2 intervention with respect to primary prevention.

Class 1 Interventions

Cigarette Smoking/Cessation (see Chap. 36)

PREVALENCE. In the United States, per capita cigarette consumption rose dramatically in the first half of the 20th century. More than 65 percent of men born between 1911 and 1920 were smoking by 1945.[14] Annual per capita consumption of cigarettes hit an astonishing 4286 (more than 200 packs per year) in 1963, but has since declined to 1875.[15] The prevalence of smoking among men peaked at 55 percent in 1955 and, among women, 10 years later at 34 percent.[16] Since then, smoking rates have declined substantially, although the rate of decline differs by gender. Among men, smoking rates have declined by approximately half, whereas among women, rates have dropped by only one-third, primarily because of increasing smoking rates among women younger than 30 years. Currently, approximately 25 percent of men aged 18 and older are smokers, as compared with 21 percent of women.[17] Smoking rates among high school seniors rose from 30 percent in the mid-1980s to approximately 36.5 percent by 1997[18] but now appear to be on a gradual downward trend.[19] Smoking rates tend to be higher among blacks, those with lower socioeconomic status, and those with a high school education or less.[20]

ASSOCIATED RISK. Smoking increases the risk of CHD (see Chap. 36). By the middle of the 20th century, seminal studies linking smoking and heart disease had been published. The Surgeon General's report in 1964 reaffirmed the epidemiological relationship between the two, and by 1983 the Surgeon General firmly established cigarette smoking as the leading avoidable cause of cardiovascular disease. The Surgeon General's 1989 report presented definitive data from observational case-control and cohort studies, largely among men, that demonstrated that smoking doubles the incidence of CHD and increases CHD mortality by 50 percent, and that these risks increase with age and the number of cigarettes smoked. Similar increases in the relative risk for CHD have been observed among women.

In the United States, cigarette smoking is the leading preventable cause of death and accounts for an estimated 440,000 deaths each year—more than 40 percent of which result from cardiovascular disease—and almost 6 million years of potential life lost.[21] Worldwide, smoking rates continue to rise, with the greatest increases in the developing world[22]; 1 million more deaths were attributable to tobacco in 2000 than in 1990.[23]

BENEFIT OF INTERVENTION. Although data from large-scale, randomized trials concerning the risk reduction associated with smoking cessation are limited, observational studies demonstrate clear benefits of smoking cessation. Smokers who quit reduce their excess risk of a coronary event by 50 percent in the first year or two after cessation, with much of this gain in the first few months. This period is followed by a more gradual decline, with the risk of former smokers approaching that of never smokers after 5 to 15 years.

COST EFFICACY. Smoking cessation is highly cost-effective in both primary and secondary prevention. The intervention is usually short term and thus low cost. In fact, smoking cessation programs generally cost less than continued smoking. The gains in life expectancy are large, and the earlier in life an individual stops smoking, the larger the potential gain—a 35-year-old male smoker may add 3 years to his life expectancy on cessation. Costs vary, depending on the intensity of intervention and the use of pharmacological agents, from $1100 to $4500 (in 1995 dollars) for every QALY saved.[24]

GUIDELINES/RECOMMENDATIONS. Clinical practice guidelines from the U.S. Public Health Service recognize that tobacco dependence is a chronic condition that generally requires repeated intervention.[25] They recommend asking patients about tobacco use at every visit, a strategy supported by the U.S. Preventive Services Task Force.[26] The Public Health Service guidelines support a combination of counseling and pharmacological therapy, when necessary. Three types of counseling and behavioral therapies appear to be particularly effective: (1) provision of problem solving and skills training, (2) provision of social support in treatment, and (3) help securing social support outside of treatment. Six first-line pharmacotherapies that reliably increase long-term smoking abstinence were also identified. These are sustained-release bupropion hydrochloride, nicotine gum, nicotine patch, nicotine inhaler, nicotine nasal spray, and nicotine lozenge.

In view of the addictive nature of smoking and the tendency to increase smoking over time, smoking reduction—as opposed to smoking cessation—is not an acceptable strategy. The efficacy of smoking intervention programs ranges from a 6 percent 1-year success rate for physician counseling to 18 percent for self-help programs and 20 to 40 percent for cessation programs with pharmacological interventions with nicotine gum or patches.[27]

Although it is important to counsel patients at all stages about the hazards of smoking and the benefits of quitting, the period soon after a cardiac event is an opportune time to encourage a patient to make an effort to stop smoking.

FUTURE CHALLENGES. In the United States, the prevalence of smoking is increasing among young women, particularly minority women. Worldwide, intense public health efforts are needed to reverse the alarming rise in smoking rates occurring in many developing countries. The low rates of success in cessation efforts offer a challenge to clinicians and greater emphasis must be placed on preventing smoking in the first place.

Hypertension/Blood Pressure Control

(see also Chap. 38)

PREVALENCE. As defined by JNC-7,[6] an estimated 50 million Americans are hypertensive and another 45 million fall into a new category called *prehypertension* (Table 42–6). High blood pressure is more common among blacks than whites and among men than women. The prevalence of hypertension clearly increases with age, from 9 percent of those aged 19 to 24 years to 75 percent of those older than 75 years.[28] Data from the Framingham Heart Study suggest that normotensive individuals at age 55 have a 90 percent lifetime risk for developing hypertension.[29] In the United States, hypertension prevalence appears to be increasing, and control rates remain low (~30 percent).[30]

ASSOCIATED RISK. Elevated systolic or diastolic blood pressure is clearly associated with an increased risk of CHD (see Chaps. 36 and 37). The best estimate for the magnitude of associated risk derives from a meta-analysis of nine large prospective, observational studies with 420,000 participants who accrued more than 4850 CHD events during follow-up.[12] A 7-mm Hg increase in diastolic blood pressure over any baseline reading was associated with a 27 percent increase in CHD risk and a 42 percent increase in stroke risk. Hypertension is also associated with increased risk of heart failure, stroke, and kidney disease. The shape of the cardiovascular disease risk curve is linear. For individuals aged 40 to 70 years, each increment of 20 mm Hg in systolic blood pressure or 10 mm Hg in diastolic blood pressure doubles the risk of cardiovascular disease across a blood pressure range from 115/75 to 185/115 mm Hg.[31]

BENEFIT OF INTERVENTION. Beginning in the late 1960s, a number of randomized trials confirmed the protective effect of treating mild to moderate hypertension. These early trial data led to the establishment of treatment guidelines in the 1970s. The most precise estimates of risk reduction have come from meta-analyses reporting that lowering diastolic blood pressure by 5 to 6 mm Hg results in a 42 percent reduction in the risk of stroke and a 15 percent reduc-

TABLE 42–6 Classification and Management of Blood Pressure (BP) for Adults

			Management		
				Initial Drug Therapy	
BP classification	**Systolic BP (mm Hg)**	**Diastolic BP (mm Hg)**	**Lifestyle Modification**	***Without Compelling Indication***	***With Compelling Indication***
Normal	<120	*and* <80	Encourage		
Prehypertension	120-139	*or* 80-89	Yes	None indicated	Drugs for compelling indications* (treat to BP target <130/80)
Stage 1 hypertension	140-159	*or* 90-99	Yes	Thiazide-type diuretics for most. May consider ACEI, ARB, BB, CCB, or combination	Drug(s) for compelling indications* Other antihypertensive drugs (diuretics, ACEI, ARB, BB, CCB) as needed
Stage 2 hypertension	≥160	*or* ≥100	Yes	Two-drug combination for most (usually thiazide-type diuretic and ACEI or ARB or BB or CCB)	

ACEI = angiotensin-converting enzyme inhibitor; ARB = angiotensin-receptor blocker; BB = beta blocker; CCB = calcium channel blocker.

From Chobanian AV, Bakris GL, Black HR, et al: The Seventh Report of the Joint National Committee on Prevention, Detection, Evaluation, and Treatment of High Blood Pressure: The JNC 7 Report. JAMA 289:2560-2572, 2003.

*Patients with chronic kidney disease or diabetes.

ion in the risk of CHD events.[32] Ogden and colleagues ɪpplied the risk stratification system of JNC-6 to data from the National Health and Nutrition Examination Survey Epidemiologic Follow-up Study and found that the absolute benefits of antihypertensive therapy depended on baseline blood pressure as well as the presence or absence of additional cardiovascular disease risk factors, preexisting clinical cardiovascular disease, or target organ damage. Among individuals with stage 1 hypertension and additional cardiovascular risk factors, sustaining a 12-mm Hg decrease in systolic blood pressure for 10 years would prevent 1 death for every 11 patients treated. In the presence of cardiovascular disease or target-organ damage, such a reduction would prevent 1 death for every 9 patients treated.[33]

The Antihypertensive and Lipid-Lowering Treatment to Prevent Heart Attack Trial (ALLHAT) demonstrated the efficacy of thiazide diuretics compared with other antihypertensive agents.[34]

COST EFFICACY. Detection and management of hypertension are highly cost-effective in both primary and secondary prevention (see Chap. 2). However, more aggressive management in those at high risk based on the existence of cardiovascular disease or diabetes is warranted based on greater cost efficacy. In secondary prevention, for agents such as diuretics and beta blockers, the cost is below $10,000 per QALY for patients with established CHD, even when blood pressure is only mildly elevated.[35] In primary prevention, cost ranges between $10,000 and $20,000 per QALY among individuals with moderate to severe elevations in blood pressure. However, the cost approaches an unacceptable range of $100,000 per QALY for higher-priced medications. In contrast to some estimates for lipid lowering, cost efficacy decreases with increasing age. Given these issues, careful cost-efficacy evaluation is needed for newer recommendations from JNC-7 since this guideline suggests the use of multiple agents and favors intervention for a wider group of individuals, including those with minor elevations of blood pressure.

GUIDELINES/TREATMENT. The U.S. Preventive Services Task Force recommends routine blood pressure testing of all adults.[36] The JNC-7[6] defines four levels of blood pressure according to the risk imparted (see Table 42–6).

Recommendations for intervention from the JNC-7 are based on the level of blood pressure and the level of absolute risk. The absolute risk strata are defined according to the presence or absence of target-organ disease, clinical cardiovascular disease, diabetes, and cardiovascular risk factors such as smoking, hyperlipidemia, age older than 60 years, gender, and family history of early-onset cardiovascular disease. The JNC-7 sets a blood pressure goal of 140/90 mm Hg for lower-risk patients and 130/80 mm Hg for those with cardiovascular disease, diabetes, or chronic kidney disease. Since the relationship of blood pressure to risk of cardiovascular disease is linear, a significant portion of the population-attributable risk occurs among those with blood pressure in the JNC-7 category of prehypertension—a systolic blood pressure of 120 to 139 mm Hg or a diastolic pressure of 80 to 89 mm Hg.

For all individuals with blood pressure of 120/80 mm Hg or greater, JNC-7 recommends life-style modifications, including smoking cessation, weight reduction if needed, increased physical activity, limited alcohol intake, limited sodium intake, maintenance of adequate potassium and calcium intake, and adoption of the Dietary Approaches to Stop Hypertension (DASH) eating plan—a diet with a reduced content of saturated and total fat that is also rich in fruits, vegetables, and low-fat dairy products (see Chap. 41).[37,38]

Initiation of drug therapy depends on blood pressure and the absolute level of risk. For example, among individuals with stage 1 hypertension but no evidence of end-organ damage, vascular disease, or diabetes and one cardiovascular disease risk factor, life-style modification and drug therapy is recommended. Data from ALLHAT indicate that a thiazide-type diuretic should be the preferred agent for first-step antihypertensive therapy.[34] For individuals with stage 2 hypertension, combination therapy that usually includes a thiazide-type diuretic is the starting point for therapy. The guidelines also recommend initiating therapy with two drugs, one of which is a diuretic, when blood pressure is more than 20/10 mm Hg above the target level. The specific therapeutic agents recommended by JNC-7 are provided in Table 42–7 and discussed at length in Chapter 38. Most patients require more than one agent to achieve their blood pressure goal.

Guidelines from the ESC stratify initial therapy somewhat differently.[9] Drug therapy is recommended for individuals with less than 20 percent absolute risk and blood pressure in excess of 160/95 mm Hg only after at least 6 months of life-style modification; for individuals with greater than 20 percent absolute risk if their blood pressure exceeds 140/90 mm Hg after 3 months of life-style modification; and immediately for individuals whose blood pressure exceeds 180/100 mm Hg, regardless of absolute risk. As with the JNC-7 recommendations, life-style modifications should always be used as an adjunct to drug therapy.

FUTURE CHALLENGES. In the developed world, the prevalence of hypertension is increasing as populations age. In the United States, the proportion of patients with hypertension managed appropriately has decreased, thus reversing a two-decade trend.[39] Approximately 40 percent of those with hypertension do not know they have this condition and are not being treated for it, and only one-third of patients treated for hypertension have their blood pressure under control.[6] In

TABLE 42–7 Compelling Indications for Individual Antihypertensive Drug Classes

High-Risk Indications with Compelling Indication	Recommended Drugs					
	Diuretic	*Beta Blocker*	*ACE Inhibitor*	*ARB*	*CCB*	*Aldosterone Antagonist*
Heart failure	×	×	×	×	×	×
Prior myocardial infarction		×	×			×
High CHD risk	×	×	×		×	
Diabetes	×	×	×	×	×	
Chronic kidney disease				×	×	
Prior stroke	×		×			

ACE = angiotensin-converting enzyme; ARB = angiotensin-receptor blocker; CCB = calcium-channel blocker; CHD = coronary heart disease.
From Chobanian AV, Bakris GL, Black HR, et al: The Seventh Report of the Joint National Committee on Prevention, Detection, Evaluation, and Treatment of High Blood Pressure: The JNC 7 Report. JAMA 289:2560-2572, 2003.

developing countries, hypertension rates are rising rapidly with urbanization and changes in life-style habits. The attributable risk for hypertension tends to be greater in the developing world because the low rates of detection and treatment in such countries result in a proportionately higher rate of hypertensive heart disease and stroke.[40]

Hypercholesterolemia/Lipid Control

(see also Chap. 39)

PREVALENCE. Mean age-adjusted cholesterol levels have declined modestly in the United States since the early 1960s.[28] Even with this decline, half of all American adults have cholesterol levels greater than 200 mg/dl, and 18 percent have cholesterol levels higher than 240 mg.[28]

ASSOCIATED RISK. Elevated serum cholesterol is causally associated with increased risk of CHD. Specifically, a 10 percent increase in serum cholesterol is associated with a 20 to 30 percent increase in risk for CHD, and elevations earlier in life may be associated with higher increases in risk.[41,42]

BENEFIT OF INTERVENTION. Clear benefits have been demonstrated for dietary and pharmacological treatments that lower serum cholesterol (see Chap. 39).[43] A number of completed large-scale primary and secondary prevention trials using 3-hydroxy-3-methylglutaryl coenzyme A reductase inhibitors (statins), beginning with the Scandinavian Simvastatin Survival Study, have demonstrated significant reductions in fatal and nonfatal CHD in a variety of populations. These include patients with established CHD; those with coronary disease, other occlusive arterial disease, or diabetes but usual cholesterol levels; those without clinically evident atherosclerotic cardiovascular disease and average total and LDL cholesterol levels; elderly individuals at risk of vascular disease; and hypertensive patients with average or lower-than-average cholesterol levels. Some,[44] but not all,[45] trial data support the early initiation of statin therapy following myocardial infarction or coronary artery bypass grafting.

A meta-analysis of five primary and secondary trials (30,817 participants and >166,000 person-years of follow-up) demonstrated that statin therapy for an average duration of 5.4 years was associated with average reductions of 20 percent in total cholesterol, 28 percent in LDL, and 13 percent in triglycerides and a 5 percent increase in HDL. Compared with placebo, statin therapy in these trials reduced the risk of major coronary events by 31 percent and all-cause mortality by 21 percent, with similar reductions in men and women, as well as in those younger and older than 65 years.[46] Cholesterol-lowering trials also demonstrate reductions in stroke.[47] These data indicate that long-term compliance is important for successful intervention. Indeed, long-term daily compliance is far more important in determining outcome efficacy than any demonstrated differences between statins in terms of potency.

Several early trials raised concerns that cholesterol lowering might increase the risk of nonvascular mortality. However, data from the large statin trials provide reassuring data that cholesterol reduction does not increase the risk of nonvascular mortality.

COST EFFICACY. The cost efficacy of nonpharmacological interventions to lower LDL cholesterol is unclear (see Chap. 2). Pharmacological intervention, however, is clearly cost-effective under certain conditions, and available data permit tailoring recommendations to the level of baseline CHD risk. Early analyses of cholesterol reduction for secondary prevention (which used data from cholestyramine trials) resulted in very costly interventions, largely because the available drugs were relatively ineffective. In contrast, data for statin therapy are remarkably consistent.

For example, in the Scandinavian Simvastatin Survival Study, the direct cost per life-year saved was $5400 for men and $10,500 for women. As expected, cost decreased as the baseline cholesterol level increased. For example, the direct cost per life saved was $11,400 for a man with a baseline total cholesterol of 213 mg/dl (5.5 mmol/liter) and $6700 for a man with a cholesterol level of 309 mg/dl (8.0 mmol/liter). Furthermore, the direct cost tended to be lower with increasing age, a finding in stark contrast to early estimates based on the Coronary Heart Disease Policy Model.

To determine a more modern cost-effectiveness of statin therapy, Prosser and colleagues[48] applied data from several large-scale, long-term, randomized, controlled trials of statins to the Coronary Heart Disease Policy. They divided men and women aged 35 to 85 years with LDL levels higher than 160 mg/dl into 240 risk subgroups according to age, sex, and the presence of four major CHD risk factors (smoking status, blood pressure, LDL level, and HDL level).[48] In primary prevention, statins failed to reach a cost-effectiveness ratio of $50,000 per QALY in any of the risk subgroups and ranged as high as $1.4 million per QALY. In contrast, primary prevention with a Step I diet ranged from $1900 per QALY to $500,000. In secondary prevention, statin therapy was clearly cost-effective, ranging from $1800 per QALY for a man aged 45 to 54 years to $40,000 for a woman aged 35 to 44 years. Statin therapy is also effective and cost-effective for secondary prevention in patients 75 to 84 years of age.[48,49] All of these QALY evaluations are highly sensitive to drug cost and can be expected to decline substantially as statin agents transition into generic drugs.

GUIDELINES/TREATMENT. All patients with cardiovascular disease should be screened for serum cholesterol levels. In primary prevention, some controversy remains regarding screening. The NCEP recommends routine screening of all adults older than 20 years,[5] the American College of Physicians (ACP) recommends screening only men ages 35 to 65 and women ages 45 to 65,[50] and the U.S. Preventive Services Task Force recommends screening all men aged 35 and older and all women aged 45 and older.[26]

To reduce the prevalence of hyperlipidemia in the United States, the NCEP issued its first *Adult Treatment Panel* (ATP) report in 1988. The latest one was published in 2002.[5] Under the latest NCEP guidelines, the number of U.S. adults eligible for lipid modification has increased from 52 million to 65 million for therapeutic life-style changes, and from approximately 13 million to 36 million for drug therapy. The goals of intervention are based on the level of CHD risk for an individual (Fig. 42–6).

The ATP III guidelines recommend different therapeutic targets depending on a patients' overall risk, which includes calculation of his or her Framingham risk score (see Fig. 42–3). Patients with existing CHD (or a CHD risk equivalent such as diabetes or peripheral arterial disease) are at the highest risk for a cardiovascular event and thus have the lowest LDL target (<100 mg/dl) and receive the most intensive treatment (Table 42–8). Patients without CHD are treated depending on their overall risk. Those with two or more risk factors, or zero or one risk factor and a 10-year overall risk less than 20 percent, should be treated to an LDL target less than 130 mg/dl. Patients with lower risk should be treated to a target LDL less than 160 mg/dl.

As part of its first-line Therapeutic Life-style Changes, the NCEP recommends a diet that includes 25 to 35 percent of calories from fat, with saturated fat accounting for less than 7 percent of fat intake and cholesterol intake limited to less than 200 mg/d. Carbohydrates, predominantly from whole grains and other foods rich in complex carbohydrates, should account for 50 to 60 percent of calories, and protein for 15 percent. These guidelines also recommend including 20 to 30 gm/d of dietary fiber (especially soluble fiber), as well

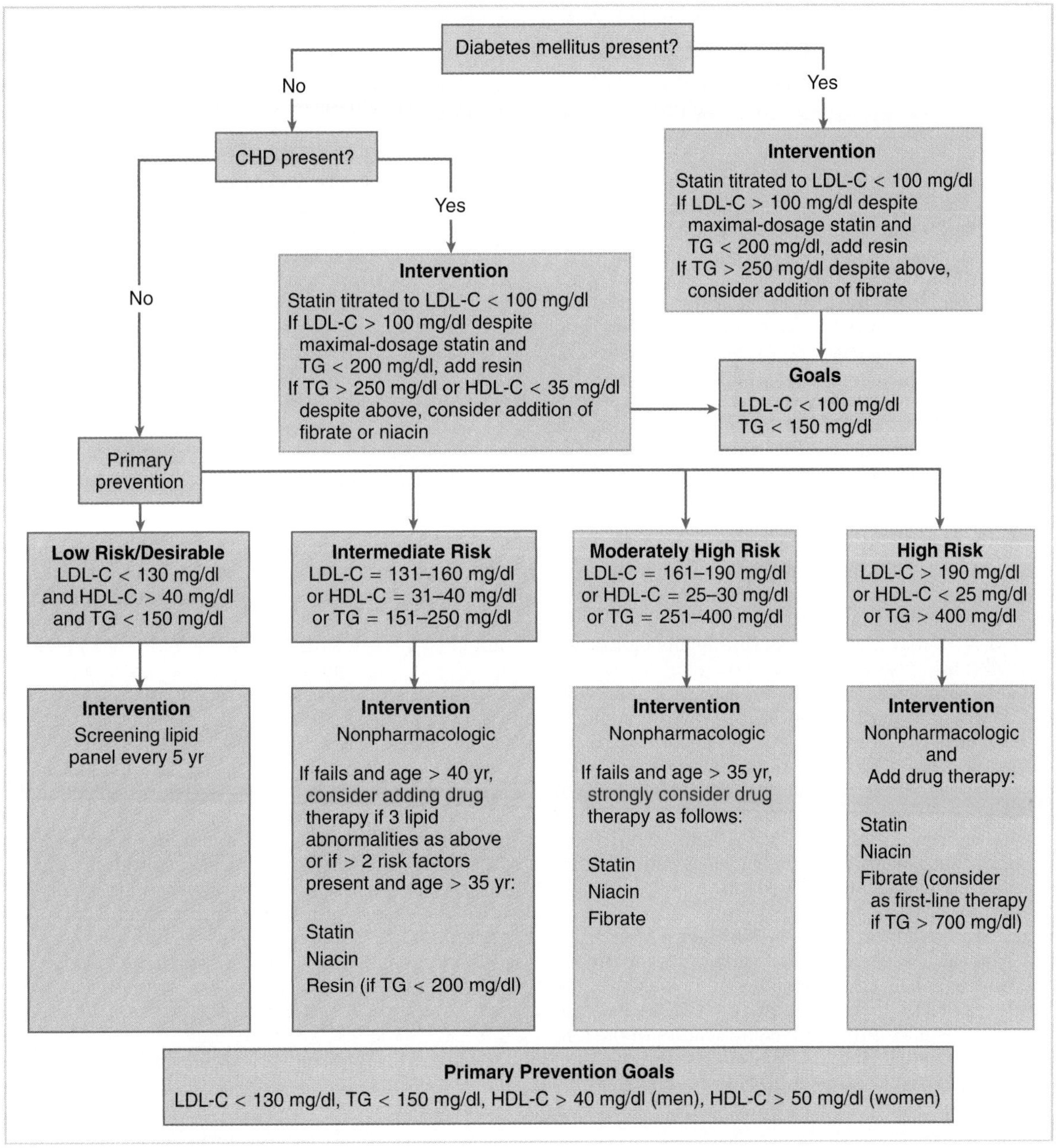

FIGURE 42–6 Algorithm for lipid-lowering therapy based on findings from intervention trials. CHD = coronary heart disease; HDL-C = high-density lipoprotein cholesterol; LDL-C = low-density lipoprotein cholesterol; TG = triglycerides. (From Third Report of the National Cholesterol Education Program [NCEP] Expert Panel on Detection, Evaluation, and Treatment of High Blood Cholesterol in Adults [Adult Treatment Panel III]: Final report. Circulation 106:3143-3421, 2002.) (See also Chap. 39.)

TABLE 42–8 Low-Density Lipoprotein (LDL) Goals for Three Risk Levels

Risk Level	LDL Goal (mg/dl)
CHD and CHD risk equivalent*	<100
Multiple (2+) risk factors	<130[†]
0-1 risk factor	<160

CHD = coronary heart disease.

From Third Report of the National Cholesterol Education Program (NCEP) Expert Panel on Detection, Evaluation, and Treatment of High Blood Cholesterol in Adults (Adult Treatment Panel III) final report. Circulation 106:3143-3421, 2002.

*Diabetes, chronic kidney disease.

†LDL goal for individuals with multiple risk factors and a 10-yr overall risk >20% is <100 mg/dl.

as 2 gm of plant stanols/sterols. Weight management and increased physical activity are also stressed.

Since patients may find it difficult to understand percent calories, translating these guidelines into grams of fat, protein, and other dietary constituents may be helpful. Such reporting is now mandated on labels of all food sold in the United States. Professional counseling with a dietitian may also be helpful. If dietary therapy does not achieve the target LDL level, drug therapy should be started (see Chap. 39). In all cases, drug therapy should be an adjunct to dietary therapy and increased physical activity.

A variety of drugs are available for lowering total and LDL cholesterol (see Chap. 39). The most commonly used are the statins. Others include niacin, fibrates, bile acid sequestrants, and cholesterol absorption inhibitors.

Guidelines from the ESC also have three tiers.[9] Although the target is identical for all patients (total cholesterol of

≤190 mg/dl [5 mmol/liter] and LDL cholesterol of ≤115 mg/dl [3 mmol/liter]) the timing and intensity of drug therapy are different. For individuals with CHD, diet and drug therapy are initiated simultaneously. In primary prevention, if either the absolute 10-year risk of a CHD event or the projected risk at age 60 is greater than 20 percent, life-style modifications are recommended and lipids are checked in 3 months. If at 3 months the total or LDL cholesterol level is above target, drug therapy may be instituted. For those with a current or projected risk less than 20 percent, life-style advice but not drug therapy is recommended.

FUTURE CHALLENGES. Additional randomized trial data are needed to clarify the role of cholesterol screening and the association between reducing serum cholesterol and stroke prevention. Ongoing trials comparing intensive LDL reduction to moderate LDL reduction will be important for determining appropriate targets for intervention across different risk levels. Although cholesterol levels are falling or stable in industrialized countries, they are rising in developing countries as "Western" diets are increasingly adopted.

HDL and Triglycerides (see also Chap. 39)

PREVALENCE. Low HDL and high triglyceride levels tend to coincide and often result from metabolic phenomena that are distinct from those leading to high levels of LDL cholesterol. Thus, low HDL and high triglyceride levels can occur alone or in combination with high LDL levels.

ASSOCIATED RISK. HDL cholesterol has emerged as an important independent predictor of CHD—every 1 mg/dl decrease in HDL cholesterol causes a 3 to 4 percent increase in coronary artery disease.[5] Furthermore, an emerging body of evidence indicates that the ratio of total or LDL cholesterol to HDL cholesterol may be a better predictor of CHD risk than LDL alone. Data from the Physicians' Health Study, for example, suggest that a 1-unit decrease in this ratio (which is easily achievable with statin drugs) reduces the risk of myocardial infarction by 53 percent.

Imprecision in triglyceride measurements, within-individual variability, and complex interactions between triglycerides and other lipid parameters may obscure the impact of triglycerides in the development of CHD. However, fasting triglyceride levels represent a useful marker of the risk for CHD, particularly when HDL levels are considered.[51] This independence suggests that some triglyceride-rich lipoproteins are atherogenic. Meta-analyses suggest that elevated triglycerides are an independent risk factor for CHD.[52,53]

BENEFIT OF INTERVENTION. Gemfibrozil, an agent that increases HDL and lowers triglyceride levels, reduces risk among those with high total and LDL cholesterol. In the Veterans Affairs High-Density Lipoprotein Cholesterol Intervention Trial (VA-HIT), a 22 percent reduction in cardiovascular events was observed with gemfibrozil treatment in a population with low HDL (<40 mg/dl [1 mmol/liter]).[54] This risk reduction occurred in the absence of any substantial change in LDL cholesterol, data that support the potential for agents targeted at HDL and triglyceride levels. It remains unclear, however, whether therapy targeted at increasing HDL will necessarily reduce vascular risk since diverse metabolic pathways lead to changes in HDL and may be differentially affected by different pharmacological strategies.

RECOMMENDATIONS. Screening of patients with cardiovascular disease should include a full fasting lipid profile, including total cholesterol, HDL, and triglycerides. For patients without cardiovascular disease, screening for HDL remains controversial, with the NCEP recommending for screening and the ACP recommending against it. Because HDL and the ratio of total cholesterol to HDL cholesterol powerfully predict risk and aid in the detection of individuals who have elevated LDL despite moderate levels of total cholesterol, it seems prudent to check HDL along with total cholesterol.

All patients with low HDL and/or high triglycerides should receive recommendations for life-style modifications that include a diet low in saturated fat and increased physical activity.[5] In secondary prevention, individuals with high LDL who also have low HDL or high triglycerides should be treated aggressively and consideration given to combination therapy (see Chap. 39). Further, for those with known disease who have low HDL and normal LDL, consideration can be given to pharmacological intervention based on the results of VA-HIT. In primary prevention, nonpharmacological interventions are warranted for individuals who have a normal LDL level but a low HDL and/or high triglycerides because trial data regarding drug therapy in such cases are insufficient. Intervention data regarding patients with isolated elevated triglyceride levels are needed.

Cardiac Protection with Aspirin, Beta Blockers, and ACE Inhibitors

Several pharmacological interventions have proved highly effective in the prevention of cardiovascular disease. Pharmacological reduction of risk during or immediately after the development of CHD has been demonstrated for aspirin, beta blockers, and ACE inhibitors. Each of these agents has proven efficacy in intermediate and longer-term secondary prevention among various subgroups of patients. Aspirin is also an effective primary prevention agent for some groups.

ASPIRIN IN SECONDARY PREVENTION. Aspirin therapy in patients with existing cardiovascular disease (see Chaps. 36 and 50) reduces the risk of subsequent events by 25 percent. Meta-analyses demonstrate clear reductions in mortality and nonfatal cardiovascular disease events among those with prior myocardial infarction, stroke, bypass surgery, angioplasty, peripheral vascular surgery, or angina.[55]

Unless contraindicated, aspirin should be used by most patients with known cardiovascular disease. Other antiplatelet agents with demonstrated efficacy such as ticlopidine and clopidogrel should be considered for patients with aspirin allergy or intolerance. However, the cost efficacy of these agents is less favorable than the cost efficacy of aspirin. Data from the Coronary Heart Disease Policy Model suggest that extending the use of aspirin therapy for secondary prevention from current levels to all eligible patients for 25 years would have an estimated cost-effectiveness ratio of about $11,000 per QALY gained. Clopidogrel alone in all patients or in routine combination with aspirin had an incremental cost of more than $130,000 per QALY gained.[56]

ASPIRIN IN PRIMARY PREVENTION. Five large-scale trials, performed primarily in men, have assessed the benefits of low-dose aspirin in the prevention of cardiovascular disease. Taken together, these studies suggest a benefit of prophylactic aspirin in primary prevention among men.[57] However, concerns over increased risk of hemorrhagic stroke have not been fully assessed, and data in women remain limited.

In 1997, the American Heart Association recommended against the use of aspirin for primary prevention, largely on the basis of the unknown benefit-risk ratio. Five years later, the U.S. Preventive Services Task Force concluded that there was sufficient evidence that aspirin decreases the incidence of CHD in adults at increased risk for heart disease.[58] Among individuals with a 10-year risk of CHD of 6 percent or greater, the Task Force determined that the benefits of taking aspirin outweighed the increased risk of gastrointestinal bleeding or hemorrhagic stroke. The ESC recommends low-dose aspirin (75 mg) in primary prevention only for men at particularly high risk of CHD.[9]

For women, the Women's Health Study, which is scheduled to end in 2005, is addressing the benefit-risk ratio of aspirin therapy for primary prevention of cardiovascular disease.

BETA BLOCKERS. A number of trials have demonstrated the long-term efficacy of beta blockade after myocardial infarction in reducing mortality, and meta-analyses suggest a 23 percent mortality reduction with long-term use.[59] Long-term use of beta blockers also lowers the risk of recurrent cardiovascular events. Cross-trial comparisons suggest that the higher the level of beta blockade, as measured by heart rate reduction relative to the control group, the greater the benefit. Beta blockade after myocardial infarction and in the setting of congestive heart failure is also extremely cost-effective. Data from the Coronary Heart Disease Policy Model suggest that implementing beta-blocker therapy in all first-myocardial infarction survivors annually over 20 years would prevent 62,000 myocardial infarctions and result in 72,000 fewer CHD deaths; the cost-effectiveness of beta-blocker therapy would be less than $11,000 per QALY gained, even under unfavorable assumptions.[60]

ACE INHIBITORS. The benefit of ACE inhibitors among individuals at high risk for CHD events is substantial. Following myocardial infarction, the use of an ACE inhibitor is associated with a 7 percent reduction in mortality at 30 days.[61,62] Among individuals with a low ejection fraction after myocardial infarction, total mortality is reduced by 26 percent (see Chap. 50). A meta-analysis of six randomized, controlled trials suggests that long-term ACE inhibitor therapy reduces the risk of major clinical outcomes by 22 percent.[63] Findings from the Heart Outcomes Prevention Evaluation (HOPE) Study suggest that the benefits of ACE inhibitors extend to those with clinical CHD (see Chap. 50) and diabetes, even in the absence of left ventricular dysfunction.[64] Results from the Candesartan in Heart Failure Assessment of Reduction in Mortality and Morbidity (CHARM) trials indicate that the use of an angiotensin-receptor blocker such as candesartan among patients with heart failure can prevent 1 death for every 63 patients treated, prevent 1 first hospitalization with heart failure for 23 patients treated, and prevent 1 new case of diabetes for every 71 patients treated.[65]

RECOMMENDATIONS. For secondary prevention, aspirin, beta blockers, and ACE inhibitors are cost-effective and should be considered standard therapy in appropriate patients—aspirin for any patient with cardiovascular disease, beta blockers after myocardial infarction, and ACE inhibitors in patients with a low ejection fraction, as well as in others with cardiovascular disease and diabetes. All three agents are recommended for secondary prevention by the American Heart Association, the American College of Cardiology, and the ESC. The U.S. Preventive Services Task Force recommends aspirin in primary prevention for those with 5-year cardiovascular disease risk of 3 percent or higher.

Class 2 Interventions

Class 2 interventions relate to risk factors that appear to have strong causal associations with CHD risk and for which intervention has the potential to reduce risk but for which intervention data are limited (see Table 42–4). Factors in this category include diabetes, obesity, physical inactivity, and alcohol intake. In general, cost efficacy data are not available because of a lack of adequate intervention data.

Diabetes/Diabetes Control, Prediabetes, and Metabolic Syndrome (see also Chap. 40)

PREVALENCE. In the United States, nearly 17 million people—6.2 percent of the U.S. population—have diabetes mellitus; approximately 90 percent of cases are type 2 diabetes.[66] Fully one-third of people with diabetes are not aware they have this disease. The prevalence of diabetes appears to have increased over the last decade, which may be a reflection of increasing body mass index (BMI).[67] Another alarming trend is the recent increase in type 2 diabetes (formerly called *adult-onset diabetes*) among children, who account for more than 30 percent of new cases in some parts of the U.S.[68,69]

ASSOCIATED RISK. Diabetes is a powerful risk factor for atherosclerotic disease, its complications, and cardiovascular-related mortality. By age 40 years, CHD is the leading cause of death in both diabetic men and women, with surveys showing CHD listed on 69 percent of death certificates in a representative national cohort of adults with diabetes.[70] Age-adjusted rates for CHD are two to three times higher among diabetic men and three to seven times higher among diabetic women than among their counterparts without diabetes.[71] During 10 years of follow-up in the Health Professionals Follow-Up Study, the multivariate relative risks for fatal CHD were 3.84 (95 percent confidence interval [CI], 3.12 to 4.71) for those with diabetes only, 7.88 (95 percent CI, 6.86 to 9.05) for those with myocardial infarction only, and 13.41 (95 percent CI, 10.49 to 17.16) for those with both diabetes and myocardial infarction compared with men without diabetes or prior myocardial infarction at baseline.[72] Similar, though not quite as pronounced, associations were observed among women in the Nurses' Health Study over a 20-year period.[73] Thus, individuals with diabetes must be considered at high risk for CHD, regardless of the presence or absence of other risk factors.

BENEFIT OF TREATMENT. Maintaining normoglycemia may reduce the risk of microvascular (renal and eye) disease. However, data demonstrating reduced risk of CHD with tight glycemic control are scant. In the Diabetes Complications and Control Trial (DCCT), an apparent reduction in CHD events among patients with type 1 diabetes assigned to intensive therapy did not achieve statistical significance, possibly because of the small number of events in this relatively young cohort. Although oral hypoglycemic agents and insulin can improve glycemic control, their role in the reduction of risk from macrovascular complications of type 2 diabetes mellitus remains unclear.[74,75] The recent HOPE trial showed that ACE inhibitor therapy reduced the onset of diabetes.[64,76]

Aggressive multifactorial intervention among diabetics does appear effective in reducing CHD events. In a recent trial of 160 patients with type 2 diabetes and microalbuminuria who were allocated to conventional care or intensive therapy (life-style and pharmacological interventions intended to maintain glycosylated hemoglobin below 6.5 percent, total cholesterol below 175 mg/dl, triglycerides below 150 mg/dl, and blood pressure below 130/80 mm Hg), rates of incident cardiovascular events were more than halved over an 8-year follow-up period (hazard ratio 0.47; 95 percent CI, 0.24 to 0.73).[77] Given beneficial results among diabetic patients enrolled in cardiovascular event reduction trials of statins, aspirin, and ACE inhibitors, these data regarding the continued importance of life-style management are important. Improved screening must also be undertaken if the diabetic population is to benefit from these advances; in a recent study of Medicare beneficiaries with diabetes, half had not undergone lipid evaluation.[78] Most important with regard to cardiovascular disease, subgroup analyses of large placebo-controlled trials of cholesterol- and triglyceride-lowering therapy indicate that individuals with diabetes benefit as much from these therapies as do nondiabetics.[5]

GUIDELINES/RECOMMENDATIONS. Diet and exercise are integral components of the treatment strategy for patients with diabetes. In many patients with type 2 diabetes, glycemic control can be achieved by modest weight loss through diet and exercise.[79]

In contrast with patients with type 1 diabetes, those with type 2 diabetes are much more likely to have multiple coronary risk factors than is the case in the general population. Thus, aggressive modification of associated risk factors—including treatment of hypertension, aggressive reduction of serum cholesterol, reduction of weight, and increased physical activity—is of paramount importance in reducing the risk of CHD among people with diabetes.

Guidelines from the American Diabetes Association call for treating patients with diabetes and hypertension to a target blood pressure lower than 130/80 mm Hg. Although initial drug therapy with any drug class may be indicated for hypertension, some drug classes (ACE inhibitors, beta blockers, and diuretics) have shown particular benefits in reducing cardiovascular disease events among diabetic patients.[80] Current guidelines from the NCEP consider diabetes to be a CHD equivalent.[5] Thus, even for diabetic patients without previous CHD, the LDL cholesterol goal is lower than 100 mg/dl.[7] Life-style changes should be attempted first and supplemented with a statin when necessary or if starting LDL levels are higher than 130 mg/dl. If the HDL level is less than 40 mg/dl, a fibrate may also be used. Initial therapy for hypertriglyceridemia is improved glycemic control. Additional triglyceride lowering can be achieved with high-dose statins (for subjects with both high LDL and triglyceride levels), a fibrate, or niacin. Administration of a drug that inhibits intestinal absorption of cholesterol, such as ezetimibe, also appears to raise HDL.[81] The American Diabetes Association also recommends daily low-dose aspirin therapy among diabetics with evidence of large-vessel disease (those with a history of myocardial infarction, vascular bypass procedure, stroke or transient ischemic attack, peripheral vascular disease, claudication, and/or angina), as well as among those without evidence of cardiovascular disease but who are at high risk for it based on cardiovascular risk factors such as smoking, hypercholesterolemia, hypertension, or obesity.[82]

Prediabetes and Metabolic Syndrome. The *metabolic syndrome* is a cluster of metabolic abnormalities that includes insulin resistance, dyslipidemia, hypertension, and excess weight, particularly around the waist (see Chaps. 36 and 40). The syndrome is quite common. In age-adjusted estimates from the National Health and Nutrition Examination Survey (NHANES) III, approximately 24 percent of U.S. adults met the criteria for metabolic syndrome.[83] Individuals with this syndrome are at increased risk for diabetes and cardiovascular disease and at increased risk of mortality from cardiovascular disease.[84]

Benefits of Treatment. Two recent randomized clinical trials demonstrate that patients with metabolic syndrome or impaired glucose tolerance benefit markedly from life-style interventions. In the Finnish Diabetes Prevention Study, 522 overweight individuals with impaired glucose tolerance received no intervention or individualized counseling with regard to reducing weight, total fat intake, and physical activity. Over a 3.2-year follow-up period, weight loss was significantly greater in the active intervention group, and the incidence of type 2 diabetes was reduced from 23 percent to 11 percent, a risk reduction of almost 60 percent ($p < 0.001$).[85] Using this simple intervention, 5 subjects with impaired glucose tolerance treated for 5 years would prevent one case of incident type 2 diabetes. In a critical test of this hypothesis, the Diabetes Prevention Program randomly assigned 3234 nondiabetic American patients with abnormal glucose metabolism to either placebo, metformin, or a life-style reduction program targeting weight loss and exercise.[86] In this trial, the life-style intervention reduced the incidence of type 2 diabetes by 58 percent as compared to placebo, whereas metformin reduced risk by 31 percent. Most important, the life-style-induced reduction was significantly greater than that achieved with pharmacological therapy.

Taken together, these two pivotal trials demonstrate that type 2 diabetes can be prevented or delayed, an effect that in turn will likely reduce atherosclerotic complications in this high-risk group. However, precise estimates for reduction in risk of cardiovascular disease events are unknown, and therefore cost efficacy data are not available.

The population impact of life-style intervention is likely to be large. In a prospective study of women, more than 90 percent of all incident cases of diabetes occurred among those who failed to exercise, had a BMI greater than 25, smoked, or had poor dietary habits.[87] The impact of exercise cannot be underestimated, because nearly one-third of all diabetic patients report a life-long pattern of minimal physical exertion.[88] Although a 2-hour postchallenge glucose measure provides improved sensitivity for risk detection in nondiabetic patients compared to fasting glucose levels, the clinical utility of this approach appears modest.[89]

Recommendations. Both the ATP III[5] and JNC-7[6] guidelines address the metabolic syndrome. Patients are classified as having it if they have three or more of the following: waist size > 40 inches for men or > 35 inches women; blood pressure > 135/85 mm Hg; HDL < 40 mg/dl for men or 50 mg/dl for women; triglycerides > 150 mg/dl; and fasting blood sugar > 100 mg/dl.

The main target of therapy is the underlying insulin resistant state. The safest and most effective strategies for reducing insulin resistance include weight reduction in overweight and obese patients and increased physical activity. Although drugs that can improve insulin resistance are available, there is no clear evidence that they reduce CHD risk in patients with metabolic syndrome. There is evidence that drug therapy to improve the lipid profile, lower blood pressure, and treat the prothrombotic state reduces cardiac risk in this population.[5]

Obesity/Weight Loss (see also Chap. 41)

PREVALENCE. Over the past four decades, the proportion of the U.S. population considered to be overweight (BMI ≥ 25.0) and obese (BMI ≥ 30.0) has risen steadily (Fig. 42–7). In the National Health Examination Survey (1960 to 1962), an estimated 31.6 percent of men and women met the definition for overweight (BMI of 25.0 to 29.9 kg/m^2), of whom 13.4

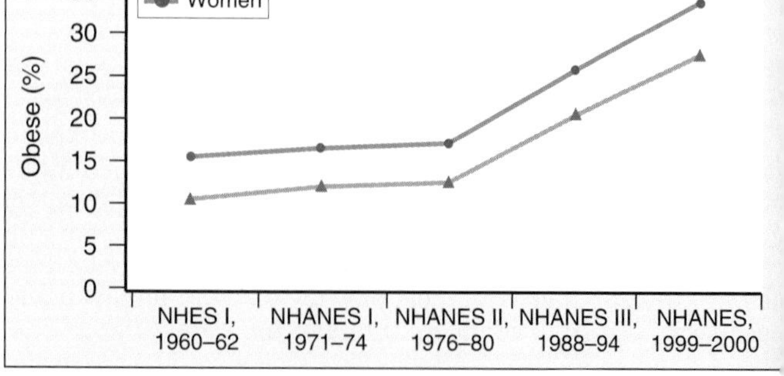

FIGURE 42-7 Percentage of U.S. adults classified as obese (body mass index > 30 kg/m^2) in health surveys from 1960 to 2000. NHES = National Health Examination Survey; NHANES = National Health and Nutrition Examination Survey. (Data from Flegal KM, Carroll MD, Ogden CL, Johnson CL: Prevalence and trends in obesity among U.S. adults, 1999-2000. JAMA 288:1723-1727, 2002.)

percent were obese (BMI > 30 kg/m^2).[90] Today, people who are overweight or obese make up a majority of the U.S. population, with the 1999 to 2000 NHANES showing 64.5 percent of men and women classified as overweight, of whom 30.5 percent were obese.[91]

The prevalence of overweight and obesity in children and adolescents is rising in parallel with that in adults. An estimated 15 percent of those aged 6 to 19 years and 10.4 percent of those aged 2 to 5 years are considered overweight or obese,[92] an alarming trend in view of the fact that early obesity is a strong predictor of later cardiovascular disease. Of considerable concern, excess weight may explain the surprising and dramatic increases in type 2 diabetes among children. In some parts of the United States, more than 30 percent of new cases of type 2 diabetes are in children, and most of these are attributable to obesity.[68,69]

ASSOCIATED RISK. Because various measures have been used to define overweight and obesity, reports on the magnitude of their association with CHD are not entirely consistent. Whether excess weight is an independent risk factor for CHD is disputed because its impact on CHD risk may be mediated, at least in part, by other coronary risk factors such as hypertension, dyslipidemia, glucose intolerance, and possibly hemostatic and inflammatory factors. However, obesity clearly associates with CHD and is thus an important and easily assessed marker of risk.

Data from numerous cohort and metabolic studies provide consistent evidence linking excess weight and inactivity with impaired health. Excess weight increases the risks of metabolic disorders such as hypertension, dyslipidemia, insulin resistance, and glucose intolerance. For example, in the Marks and Spencer Cardiovascular Risk Factor Study of 14,077 middle-aged women, highly significant age-adjusted differences were observed across seven categories of BMI (<20 to >30 kg/m^2) for systolic and diastolic blood pressure, serum total cholesterol, LDL cholesterol, HDL cholesterol, triglycerides, apolipoprotein A1, apolipoprotein B, and fasting blood glucose.[93] Excess weight is associated with increases in inflammatory markers such as C-reactive protein and fibrinogen in adults and children, increases that have been associated with elevated risks of cardiovascular disease.[94-96] Excess weight is also strongly linked to increased risk of CHD, ischemic stroke, type 2 diabetes mellitus, and a host of other chronic conditions.[97-101]

The distribution of body fat may also play a role in the development of CHD, with abdominal adiposity posing a substantially greater risk in both women[102] and men.[103] A waist circumference greater than 35 inches in women and greater than 40 inches in men is an easily measured marker of increased CHD risk.

The personal and economic burdens of excess weight are enormous. Recent estimates from six large prospective cohorts suggest that excess weight accounts for an estimated 280,000 to 320,000 deaths a year in the United States, more than 80 percent of which occur among individuals with BMI greater than 30 kg/m^2.[104] Data from a national survey of almost 10,000 U.S. adults suggest that obesity is associated with more chronic disorders and poorer health-related quality of life than smoking or problem drinking.[105] Medical spending for weight-related conditions accounted for an estimated 9 percent of the total annual U.S. medical expenses in 1998, or $78 billion,[106,107] an amount that rivals expenditures on smoking-related conditions.

BENEFIT OF INTERVENTION. No large-scale randomized trials of weight reduction as an isolated intervention are available on which to estimate the benefits of weight loss in lowering risk of CHD. However, sufficient information is available from numerous observational studies and small or short-term randomized clinical trials[97,108] to conclude that weight loss offers substantial health benefits (Table 42–9).

TABLE 42–9 Benefits of Weight Loss and Physical Activity among Overweight/obese Individuals or Those with Insufficient Daily Activity

Disease/Risk Factor	Weight Loss	Physical Activity
Hypertension	↓↓↓[97]	↓↓↓[109]
Type 2 diabetes mellitus	↓↓↓[85,86,110]	↓↓[85,86,110]
Lipid profile	Definite improvement[97]	Definite improvement[111]
Coronary heart disease	↓↓[108]	↓↓↓[108]
Stroke	↓[112]	↓↓[113]
Colorectal cancer	↓[114]	↓↓[114]
Breast cancer	↓[115]	↓[115]
Osteoarthritis	↓↓[116]	↓[117]
Osteoporosis	↔	↓↓↓[118,119]
Gallbladder disease	↓[120]	↓[121]
Sleep apnea	↓↓[122]	Unknown
Mental health	Probable improvement[123]	Probable improvement[123]

From Manson JE, Skerrett PJ, Greenland P, VanItallie TB: The escalating pandemics of obesity and sedentary lifestyle: A call to action for clinicians. Arch Intern Med 164:249-258, 2004.
↓↓↓: strong decrease in risk; ↓↓: moderate decrease in risk; ↓: slight decrease in risk; ↔: no benefit.

Modest weight loss, on the order of 5 percent to 10 percent, is associated with a significant improvement in blood pressure among individuals with and without hypertension.[97] Modest weight loss is also associated with improvements in the lipoprotein profile—lower levels of serum triglycerides, higher levels of HDL cholesterol, and small reductions in total and LDL cholesterol—as well as improvements in glucose tolerance and/or insulin resistance.[97] It is also associated with improvements in sleep apnea.[124]

There is little consensus, however, on the ideal approach to weight reduction.[125] Promoting life-style changes to encourage weight reduction has been universally disappointing. Although 25 percent of American men and 43 percent of American women may attempt to lose weight in any given year,[126] failure rates are exceedingly high. One reason may be that most individuals who are trying to lose weight are not following recommendations to reduce calorie intake and engage in at least 150 minutes of leisure time activity per week.[126] Effective treatment strategies generally involve a multifaceted approach, including dietary counseling, behavioral modification, increased physical activity, and psychosocial support. For some obese patients, pharmacotherapy or bariatric surgery may be necessary.[127]

COST EFFICACY. Without precise estimates of the benefit and with substantial variability in the intervention strategy, it is currently impossible to estimate the cost-benefit ratio of weight loss programs or interventions.

RECOMMENDATIONS/GUIDELINES. Numerous options are available for helping patients lose weight. Guidelines produced by the National Heart, Lung, and Blood Institute and the North American Association for the Study of Obesity[97] emphasize a three-part strategy for weight loss that includes caloric restriction, structured physical activity, and behavior therapy for all patients with a BMI greater than 30 kg/m^2 and those with a BMI of 25.0 to 29.9 kg/m^2 and a history of CHD or two or more disease risk factors.

Physical Inactivity/Exercise

(see also Chaps. 36 and 43)

PREVALENCE. Physical activity is an exceptionally common modifiable risk factor for CHD. Data from the Behavioral Risk Factor Surveillance System (BRFSS) suggest that 75 percent of adult Americans do not meet the current recommendation of 30 minutes of leisure-time physical activity on most, if not all, days of the week.[128] Nearly one-third do not engage in any leisure-time physical activity.[129] Lack of sufficient physical activity is also endemic among children. Only a minority of schoolchildren have daily physical education classes,[130,131] while walking and bicycling by children has declined.[132] In contrast, the time spent in sedentary activities such as watching television, playing video games, or using a computer has dramatically increased.[133] Older individuals, who are most at risk for cardiovascular disease, are less likely to be physically active than younger individuals, and women tend to be less active than men.

ASSOCIATED RISK. Data from more than 40 observational studies demonstrate clear evidence of an inverse linear dose-response relation between volume of physical activity and all-cause mortality rates in younger and older men and women. Minimal adherence to current physical activity guidelines, which yield an energy expenditure of about 1000 kcal/wk, is associated with a significant 20 to 30 percent reduction in risk of all-cause mortality.[134]

Data available in the mid-1950s showed that CHD rates were lower among bus conductors and mail carriers than sedentary bus drivers and postal supervisors. By incorporating estimates of leisure-time activity in their analyses, these investigators found that civil servants with sedentary jobs who engaged in vigorous sports were half as likely to suffer myocardial infarction as those who did not engage in leisure-time physical activity. Since then, a number of observational studies have reported similar inverse associations between activity level from work or play and CHD. In a 1990 meta-analysis of 27 observational cohort studies, Berlin and Colditz demonstrated that the risk of CHD in sedentary individuals was almost twice that of active individuals after controlling for other coronary risk factors. Long-term prospective studies of men and women consistently demonstrate that regular physical activity protects against death from CHD.[135-137] These benefits apply to activities as simple as brisk walking, which has been shown to reduce the risk of CHD in women[138] and men,[139,140] as well as the risk of type 2 diabetes.[110] Shifting even late in life from a sedentary life style to a more active one confers a reduction in mortality from CHD.[141,142] Physical activity is also associated with a decreased risk of stroke in men[143,144] and women,[145] primarily because of its beneficial effects on body weight, blood pressure, serum cholesterol, and glucose tolerance.

Although no large-scale, randomized trials of physical activity are available, numerous trials of moderate size and duration have been conducted among healthy individuals, those at high risk for cardiovascular disease, and those with existing cardiovascular disease. Despite differences in design, these trials generally demonstrate a benefit.[108] The ideal intensity, frequency, and duration of physical activity, however, have still not been determined.

BENEFIT OF INTERVENTION. While cessation of activity appears to result in increased risk of CHD, the lack of large-scale, randomized, primary prevention trials on the benefits of physical activity makes it difficult to determine the precise benefit of exercise in terms of CHD reduction. Physical activity does, however, have clearly demonstrated benefits on cardiovascular risk factors. Exercise increases HDL, reduces LDL[146] and triglycerides, increases insulin sensitivity,[147,148] and reduces blood pressure in both hypertensive and normotensive individuals.[149] Exercise also improves endothelial function.[150]

In secondary prevention, cardiac rehabilitation programs with an exercise component tend to report benefit in reducing subsequent events. Pooled data from many of these trials suggest reductions in total and cardiovascular mortality of about 25 percent.[151]

GUIDELINES/TREATMENT. For secondary prevention, guidelines from the American Heart Association/American College of Cardiology recommend encouraging patients to be physically active. An "exercise prescription" might include walking, jogging, cycling, swimming, or other aerobic activity for 30 to 60 minutes on at least most days of the week supplemented with an increase in daily life-style activities such as walking up stairs when possible.[152] Strength training may offer additional cardiovascular and other benefits.[153] Structured exercise programs may enhance long-term compliance. For primary prevention, the U.S. Surgeon General's recommendation is an excellent starting point—every adult should accumulate 30 minutes of moderately intense physical activity on most, if not all, days of the week.[154]

Moderate Alcohol Consumption

Alcohol consumption has complex effects on cardiovascular disease. Observational studies demonstrate that heavy alcohol intake increases total mortality and cardiovascular disease mortality. In contrast, more than 100 prospective studies show an inverse association between moderate drinking and risk of heart attack, ischemic stroke, peripheral vascular disease, sudden cardiac death, and death from all cardiovascular causes.[155] The effect is relatively consistent, corresponding to a 20 to 45 percent reduction in risk. An association between moderate alcohol consumption and decreased cardiovascular risk has been observed in both primary and secondary prevention and among men and women. Mechanisms underlying the effect of moderate alcohol consumption, defined as one or two drinks daily, include raising HDL levels, improving fibrinolytic capacity, and reducing platelet aggregation and hs-CRP.[156]

RECOMMENDATIONS. While the association of alcohol and CHD is likely to be causal, any individual or public health recommendation must consider the complexity of alcohol's metabolic, physiological, and psychological effects. With alcohol, the difference between daily intake of small-to-moderate quantities and large quantities may be the difference between preventing and causing disease. For appropriate patients, a discussion of alcohol intake can be a part of routine preventive counseling. In general, one or two drinks per day may be safe for men. For women, because of their generally smaller BMIs and potential differences in liver metabolism, lower levels may be more prudent. However, counseling must be individualized—other medical problems, including other coronary risk factors (particularly hypertension and diabetes), liver disease, tendency toward excess use, family history of alcoholism, and possibly a family history of breast and colon cancer, should be taken into account when discussing alcohol consumption.

Oral Anticoagulants (see also Chaps. 50 and 80)

Oral anticoagulants prevent embolic events in patients with prosthetic heart valves and atrial fibrillation. Less certain is their role, either alone or in combination with aspirin, in the secondary prevention of events in those with CHD. The results of randomized, controlled trials are inconsistent, a troubling issue because oral anticoagulants have significant bleeding as a side effect.

A meta-analysis provided a comprehensive summary of data on high-, moderate-, and low-intensity oral anticoagulants alone or in combination with aspirin versus placebo or aspirin alone among those with cardiovascular disease.[157] In this analysis, high- and moderate-intensity oral anticoagulation reduced myocardial infarction and stroke rates when compared with placebo but increased the risk of hemorrhage. The combination of low-intensity oral anticoagulation plus aspirin did not appear to confer any benefit over aspirin alone, whereas the combination of moderate- or high-intensity oral anticoagulation plus aspirin did appear to offer promising benefits. These findings require confirmation from ongoing clinical trials.

Class 3 Interventions

Class 3 interventions relate to risk factors that are currently under investigation (see Table 42–3). For some of them, a causal relationship with CHD cannot be determined because of limited data. For others, where causal relationships are apparent, interventions are not yet available or tested.

Postmenopausal Estrogen Therapy

(see also Chap. 73)

RISK ASSOCIATED WITH MENOPAUSE. Before age 45, cardiovascular disease afflicts relatively few women in the United States and other developed countries. By age 60, however, it is the leading cause of death among women.[158] Although men exhibit a higher incidence of CHD at every age, as well as higher mortality rates from it, the gap narrows substantially after both natural menopause and bilateral oophorectomy.

A wide range of factors may explain the increased risk of CHD after menopause. These include adverse changes in lipid and glucose metabolism that result in an increase in LDL cholesterol and a decrease in HDL cholesterol, an increase in glucose intolerance, and changes in hemostatic factors and vascular function. These changes have long been attributed to the decline in endogenous estrogen that accompanies menopause. Physiological effects of exogenous estrogen are consistent with a cardioprotective effect. Estrogen reduces LDL and increases HDL levels; reduces Lp(a) lipoprotein, plasminogen-activator inhibitor type 1, and insulin levels; inhibits oxidation of LDL; and improves endothelial vascular function.[159] The effects of estrogen on inflammation are complex, as levels of fibrinogen decrease while levels of hs-CRP increase. Many of these effects are minimal when estrogen is given transdermally, suggesting a first-pass effect. Estrogen may also play one or more roles in maintaining normal hemostasis and improving glucose tolerance.

Considerable evidence from observational studies had suggested that the use of postmenopausal hormone therapy reduced the risk of CHD. A meta-analysis of 40 cohort and case-control studies suggested a 50 percent reduction in the risk of CHD associated with current estrogen use.[160] In an early study from the Nurses' Health Study, the largest prospective cohort study to address this question, current users of estrogen had about half the risk of CHD (relative risk, 0.51; 95 percent CI, 0.37 to 0.70) as nonusers did. The association appeared even stronger among women with known CHD. Such data provided the foundation for widespread use of postmenopausal hormone therapy to prevent cardiovascular disease.

EFFECTS OF INTERVENTION. Data from seven recent randomized trials (five on secondary prevention and two on primary prevention) not only failed to support the possible benefit of hormone therapy on CHD but indicated that combined estrogen and progestin may actually *increase* CHD risk.[161] This abrupt about-face with regard to the possible benefits of hormone therapy illustrates the problem of confounding and the importance of randomized, controlled trials.

The first secondary prevention trial, the Heart and Estrogen/progestin Replacement Study (HERS), found no cardiovascular benefit of estrogen-progestin supplementation even with extended follow-up.[162] Subsequent trials found no beneficial effect of hormone therapy or an increased risk of CHD events.[163-166]

One arm of the large, ongoing Women's Health Initiative was designed to evaluate the relative benefits and risks of estrogen plus progestin among 16,608 postmenopausal women aged 50 to 79 years with an intact uterus at baseline over a planned 8.5-year period. However, after a mean of 5.2 years of follow-up, the trial's data and safety monitoring board recommended stopping the trial because the test statistic for invasive breast cancer exceeded the stopping boundary for this adverse effect, and the global index statistic supported risks exceeding benefits. At this time, the estimated hazard ratios were 1.29 (95 percent CI, 1.02 to 1.63) for CHD; 1.41 (95 percent CI, 1.07 to 1.85) for stroke; and 2.13 (95 percent CI, 1.39 to 3.25) for pulmonary embolism. The hazard ratio for total cardiovascular disease was 1.22 (95 percent CI, 1.09 to 1.36).[161] The absolute excess cardiovascular risks per 10,000 person-years attributable to estrogen plus progestin were seven more CHD events, eight more strokes, and eight more pulmonary emboli.

The use of unopposed estrogen, other forms of estrogen, selective estrogen receptor modulators, and phytoestrogens in cardiovascular risk prevention remains unproven (see Chap. 73).[167]

RECOMMENDATIONS. Hormone therapy is no longer recommended as an approach to the prevention of cardiovascular disease. The U.S. Preventive Services Task Force recommends against the routine use of estrogen and progestin for the prevention of chronic conditions, including cardiovascular disease, in postmenopausal women.[168] Guidelines from the North American Menopause Society state that estrogen/progestin therapy should not be used for primary or secondary prevention of CHD.[169] Furthermore, in 2003 the U.S. Food and Drug Administration revised the labeling for all postmenopausal hormone therapies containing estrogen alone or estrogen plus a progestogen to include a boxed warning that highlights the increased risk for heart disease, myocardial infarction, stroke, and breast cancer.[170]

Dietary Factors (see also Chap. 41)

Diet clearly has an impact on CHD risk. Cross-cultural studies suggest that diet plays a role in CHD as well as other chronic diseases. For example, the Ni-Hon-San study demonstrated that Japanese immigrants who moved to Hawaii and California developed CHD and ischemic stroke at rates comparable to lifetime residents of the United States. However, understanding the specific components of the Western diet that impart this risk has been challenging. Dietary research is hampered by the complexity and difficulty of measuring dietary components.

Observational Studies

Observational studies have suggested a number of dietary factors that may increase the risk of CHD. One of the key features of the Western life style is an excess of caloric intake relative to caloric expenditure. One of the most consistent findings in observational dietary research is that individuals who consume higher amounts of fresh fruits and vegetables have lower rates of heart disease[171] and stroke.[172] Other components of the Western diet that have been implicated in increasing the risk of CHD include saturated and *trans* fats, simple carbohydrates that represent a glycemic load, and lack of fiber.

Metabolic trials suggest that diet is an important component of any prevention program for several reasons. It can have a potentially profound effect on weight reduction, which can improve dyslipidemia, hypertension, and diabetes. Even without weight loss, a healthy diet can improve the lipid profile and deliver nutrients that have salutary effects on the cardiovascular system. In the DASH Trial, 459 adults with systolic blood pressure lower than 160 mm Hg and diastolic pressure lower than 80 to 95 mm Hg were randomized to (1) a control diet low in fruits, vegetables, and dairy products and with a fat content of 37 percent; (2) a diet rich in fruits and vegetables; or (3) a combination diet rich in fruits, vegetables, and low-fat dairy products. Both of the intervention diets substantially reduced systolic and diastolic blood pressure in individuals with and without hypertension.[37]

A review of data from 147 metabolic studies, prospective cohort studies, and clinical trials suggests that at least three dietary strategies are effective in preventing CHD. These include substituting nonhydrogenated unsaturated fats for saturated and *trans* fats; increasing consumption of omega-3 fatty acids from fish, fish oil supplements, or plant sources; and adhering to a diet high in fruits, vegetables, nuts, and whole grains and low in refined grain products.[173]

Diet Trials with CHD Endpoints

Trial data exploring the impact of dietary changes alone on CHD events are limited. The Lyon Diet Heart Study randomized 605 survivors of a first myocardial infarction to a Mediterranean-type diet or a "prudent Western-type diet." After a mean follow-up of 46 months, the risk of cardiac death or acute myocardial infarction was 65 percent lower for those consuming the Mediterranean diet.[174] In the Gruppo Italiano per lo Studio della Sopravvivenza nell'Infarto Miocardico (GISSI), 11,324 survivors of a recent myocardial infarction were randomized to daily supplements containing 1 gm of n-3 polyunsaturated fatty acids, 300 mg of vitamin E, both, or neither for 3.5 years. Treatment with the n-3 polyunsaturated fatty acids, but not vitamin E, lowered the relative risk of the primary endpoint, which included death, nonfatal myocardial infarction, and stroke, by 10 percent (95 percent CI, 1 to 18).[175] This benefit was primarily attributable to a decrease in the risk of death rather than nonfatal myocardial infarction or stroke.

Specific Foods and Nutrients

A host of foods and micronutrients are under investigation as agents for reducing the risk of cardiovascular disease (see Chap. 41). These include whole grains, fiber, fish and fish oils, soy protein, folate, vitamin B_6, and antioxidants such as vitamin E and ubiquinone (coenzyme Q_{10}). Observational studies tend to report lower rates of CHD events among those who take antioxidant vitamins and folate supplements; however, studies are inconsistent and the effects are modest.

The importance of randomized clinical trials with regard to "heart healthy" foods and nutrients is best illustrated by briefly describing the ups and downs of vitamin E. Basic research strongly suggests that oxidative stress plays an important role in the development of atherosclerotic disease and that vitamin E may delay or prevent various steps in atherosclerosis. By the mid-1990s, observational data strongly suggested that high doses of vitamin E reduced the risk of CHD, particularly with regard to secondary prevention.[176] Completed secondary prevention trials, however, have demonstrated that vitamin E supplementation has little impact on CHD risk.[175,177,178] Several large, ongoing trials will determine whether vitamin E supplementation is effective for the primary prevention of cardiovascular disease.

RECOMMENDATIONS. Given the limited trial data, it is difficult to answer the patient question, "What should I eat to prevent heart disease?" Elements of that answer should include the following:

- Total caloric intake must be balanced with energy expenditure.
- Minimize intake of saturated and *trans* fat as well as rapidly digested carbohydrates. Instead, select monounsaturated and polyunsaturated fats and whole grains.
- Maximize fruit and vegetable intake. The U.S. Department of Agriculture recommends at least two servings of fresh fruit and at least three servings of fresh vegetables per day.
- Adequate intake of omega-3 fatty acids also appears to reduce the incidence of cardiovascular disease and especially sudden cardiac death.[179] Inclusion of two or three servings of fish per week (particularly fatty fish) may help prevent cardiovascular events.

Psychosocial Factors/Counseling

(see also Chaps. 36 and 84)

Like diet, the study of psychosocial factors as potential risk factors for CHD is hampered by imprecision in definitions and widely accepted metrics. Psychosocial factors such as depression, chronic hostility, social isolation, and perceived lack of social support have been consistently linked with risk of CHD.[180] Further data are needed, however, to confirm these relationships and establish the efficacy of interventional strategies. Data are inconsistent regarding associations between vascular risk and other psychological factors such as work-related stress, type A behavior, and anxiety.

Studies of therapeutic interventions, although not blinded, suggest a role for improving psychosocial factors as part of prevention programs, particularly in secondary prevention. The strongest evidence comes from post–myocardial infarction patients.[181] Although abundant data suggest that stress and depression are prevalent and predict events after myocardial infarction, data on interventions are limited. A meta-analysis of 37 small studies of health education and stress-management programs for CHD patients suggested that such efforts might reduce cardiac mortality by 34 percent and recurrent myocardial infarction by 29 percent, quite possibly through favorable effects on blood pressure, cholesterol, body weight, smoking behavior, physical activity, and dietary habits.[181]

The Enhancing Recovery in Coronary Heart Disease Patients (ENRICHD) randomized trial recruited 2481 patients (26 percent with perceived low social support, 39 percent with clinical depression, and 34 percent with both low social support and depression) within 4 weeks of myocardial infarction.[182] Half were randomized to cognitive behavioral therapy and drug therapy, if needed, and half to usual medical care. The intervention did not increase event-free survival. It did improve depression and social isolation, although the relative improvement in the intervention group compared with the usual care group was less than expected due to substantial improvement in usual care patients.

Preliminary evidence suggests that pharmacotherapy for depression following myocardial infarction, revascularization, or the diagnosis of coronary disease may improve morbidity and mortality. The Sertraline Antidepressant Heart Attack Randomized Trial (SADHART) demonstrated the safety of this selective serotonin re-uptake inhibitor as a treatment for recurrent depression in cardiovascular patients. Sertraline had no more impact on left ventricular ejection fraction, treatment-emergent ventricular premature complex runs, or other cardiac measures than placebo.[183] Scores on depression and mood scales were better in the sertraline group, particularly among those who had been depressed before their heart attacks, a group in which postattack depression is especially likely. Of note, rates of second heart attacks, heart failure, episodes of chest pain, or heart-related deaths were lower in the sertraline group than the placebo group. In the ENRICHD trial, antidepressant use was also associated with significantly lower risks of nonfatal myocardial infarction or death.[182]

Novel Biochemical and Genetic Markers

(see also Chap. 36)

Hemostatic and inflammatory markers, novel lipid parameters, cellular adhesion molecules, indicators of prior infection, and markers of oxidative stress all have been linked to steps in atherogenesis, thrombosis, or cardiovascular disease events (reviewed in detail in Chap. 36). Of these novel risk factors, only hs-CRP has been shown to add prognostic information over and above that provided by global risk prediction models such as the Framingham Risk Score. Recent guidelines from the Centers for Disease Control and Prevention and the American Heart Association encourage the use of hs-CRP as an adjunct to risk prediction, particularly among those at "intermediate risk."[184] In part, this endorsement of hs-CRP reflects the low cost of evaluation, particularly in comparison to other screening approaches based on imaging techniques such as CT scans for coronary calcium.

Other novel risk factors such as Lp(a) lipoprotein and homocysteine have more limited use in general screening but are likely to be helpful in settings of premature disease and in families affected by atherosclerosis who lack clusters of traditional risk factors. Novel markers such as the cytokine interleukin-6, the adhesion molecule known as intercellular adhesion molecule 1, CD40 ligand, myeloperoxidase, and lipoprotein-associated phospholipase A_2 have shown efficacy in several settings but currently lack standardized commercial assays for evaluation. A common limitation to all these novel markers is that no data yet exist that lowering levels leads to reduced vascular risk, and thus their use is largely limited to risk identification and motivation for life-style change. For example, although statin therapy lowers hs-CRP levels and post hoc analyses of completed statin trials suggest survival benefits for those with elevated hs-CRP levels, prospective trials directly testing the use of hs-CRP to target statin therapy are only now being initiated. Similarly, although folate lowers homocysteine levels, evidence that this approach lowers vascular risk is lacking. The potential clinical utility of these markers[185] and current evidence regarding their modification are covered in Chapter 36.

A number of common genetic polymorphisms have been associated with coronary risk factors. For example, carriers of a common mutation in the *MTHFR* gene have elevated levels of homocysteine, and there are multiple inherited abnormalities of lipid metabolism linked both to hyperlipidemia and elevated vascular risk. Similarly, almost half of the variance in hs-CRP is heritable. However, as discussed in Chapter 36, there is no evidence that screening for any of these polymorphisms substantially adds to information more easily obtained from direct plasma measures of homocysteine, lipids, or hs-CRP. This finding for arterial thrombosis is in marked contrast to findings for venous thromboembolism, where evaluation for factor V Leiden and the prothrombin mutation has proven clinically useful. Thus, although genetic screening holds great promise for identifying individuals at risk for subsequent events, its role in primary or secondary prevention remains unproven for atherothrombotic disease at this time. However, one can envision a time when genetic assays will play a role in identifying at-risk individuals and targeting therapies to reduce their risk of subsequent events.[186]

Multiple Risk Factor Intervention Programs

Although most prevention studies focus on changing a single factor, several have attempted to measure the impact of simultaneously changing multiple risk factors. In theory, the potential for synergistic effects between risk factors could lead to substantial reductions in risk that are multiplicative and offer the possibility of meaningful reductions in the risk of cardiovascular disease.[187]

Although these multiple risk factor intervention trials (Table 42–10) have made major contributions to our understanding of cardiovascular risk, as well as our knowledge of what makes for effective—and ineffective—intervention strategies, their results have been mixed. It is clear that intervention on multiple levels can reduce risk factors and that this reduction can be sustained over time. In a Belgian study that was part of the World Health Organization (WHO) European Collaborative Trial in the Multifactorial Prevention of Coronary Heart Disease, an intervention program composed of face-to-face counseling about eating habits, smoking, and physical activity substantially reduced predictors of coronary risk when compared with a control program that offered no such advice. The effect was sustained for 5 years.

A common result from multiple risk factor intervention trials is a change in risk factor levels or composite scores among those receiving intervention. However, this change has not always translated into lower event rates. Explanations for this inconsistency include the possibility that the magnitude of intervention was too small or that control patients may also have improved their health habits over time. What is clear from these trials, however, is that multiple simultaneous interventions can reduce cardiovascular risk when the planned interventions are large enough and are adequately implemented.

In an analysis of seven multiple intervention trials, Kornitzer plotted change in the multiple logistic function of risk against the reduction in risk of CHD. The strong linear relationship (Fig. 42–8) suggests that as long as risk factors are truly modified, event rates will also be reduced.

Summary of Recommendations

In this section we outline a general approach to a patient. The appropriate strategy for any given patient begins with an assessment of the overall risk of a first or subsequent cardiovascular event. Patients can be classified into two broad groups: (1) those with overt cardiovascular disease, including previous myocardial infarction, stroke, peripheral vascular disease, angina, or prior vascular procedure and (2) those without overt cardiovascular disease. Those without cardiovascular disease can be further subdivided into three risk strata: diabetics, high-risk nondiabetics, and low-risk nondiabetics. Those with cardiovascular disease and diabetes are generally straightforward to identify. Stratifying the remaining group requires the use of an algorithm such as those developed by the Framingham Heart Study (see Fig. 42–3) or the ESC.

Table 42–11 summarizes the interventional approach for all three classes. Many of these activities can be undertaken by allied health professionals in a prevention program. Case management models of prevention have been demonstrated as useful among higher-risk groups following myocardial infarction or bypass surgery.[188]

Current data strongly support a role for risk factors in the prediction of future risk and in the modification of that risk in both primary and secondary prevention of CHD. For several risk factors—cigarette smoking, dyslipidemias, and hypertension—the strength and consistency of association with atherosclerotic disease indicate a causal relationship, and the benefits of intervention are well documented in both primary and secondary prevention. There is little doubt that diabetes, physical inactivity, and obesity increase the risk of CHD and that light-to-moderate alcohol consumption reduces the risk, but the precise magnitude of the effect attributable to intervention for these factors has been difficult to docu-

TABLE 42–10 Multiple Intervention Trials

Trial	Population	Intervention
Multiple Risk Factor Intervention Trial[189]	12,866 men aged 35-57 yr at high risk for CHD; average 7-yr follow-up	Stepped-care therapy for high BP, counseling for smoking cessation, and dietary advice for high cholesterol; *or* usual care
Oslo Trial[190]	1232 men aged 40-49 yr with coronary risk in upper quartile; 5-yr follow-up	Diet similar to AHA step 1, counseling to stop smoking; *or* usual care
WHO Multifactorial Trial[191]	60,881 men aged 40-59 yr from 80 factories in Belgium, Italy, Poland, and United Kingdom; average 6 yr of intervention and follow-up	Educational materials or individual counseling regarding diet, smoking cessation, physical activity, and BP; drug therapy as needed for BP control; *or* no intervention
North Karelia Project[192]	11,992 men and women aged 25-59 yr; 10-yr follow-up	Population-based prevention program with outreach for smoking cessation and for reducing BP, serum cholesterol and other CVD risk factors
Goteborg Primary Prevention Trial[193]	Random sample of 20,000 men aged 47–55 yr; average 10 yr of intervention and follow-up	Antihypertensive treatment in subjects with SBP > 175 mm Hg or DBP > 115 mm Hg, dietary advice for subjects with serum cholesterol levels > 260 mg/dl, and smoking cessation advice; *or* usual care
Minnesota Heart Health Program[194]	400,000 residents aged 30-74 yr from 6 (3 paired) Midwestern communities; 5- to 6-yr intervention program	Individual counseling and community outreach on decreasing BP and serum cholesterol, smoking cessation, and increasing physical activity; *or* no intervention
Pawtucket Heart Health Program[195]	140,000 residents aged 18-64 yr of Pawtucket, RI, and a reference community; 7-yr intervention program	Community-wide educational programs designed to help individuals lower cholesterol and BP, stop smoking, maintain healthy weight, and increase physical activity
Stanford Five-City Project[196]	320,300 residents of 5 California cities (2 intervention, 3 comparison); 5-yr intervention program	Individual counseling and community outreach regarding decreasing BP and serum cholesterol, smoking cessation, and increasing physical activity
Lifestyle Heart Trial[187]	48 men and women aged 35-75 yr with ischemic heart disease; 4-yr intervention and follow-up	Low-fat vegetarian diet, moderate aerobic exercise, stress management training, smoking cessation, and group support; *or* usual care
Heidelberg Trial[197]	113 men and women recruited after coronary angiography for stable angina pectoris; 6-yr intervention and follow-up	Intervention group: AHA step 3 diet, 30 min of exercise daily, and two 60-min group counseling sessions per week; *or* advice about the AHA step 1 diet and encouragement of moderate aerobic exercise
Stanford Coronary Risk Intervention Project[198]	300 men and women < age 75 yr without severe congestive heart failure, pulmonary disease, intermittent claudication, or noncardiac life-threatening illness	Low-fat diet (<20% of calories from fat and <75 mg of cholesterol/d), physical activity, and counseling for smoking cessation, with cholesterol-lowering medication as needed; *or* usual care with personal physician

AHA = American Heart Association; BMI = body mass index; BP = blood pressure; CAD = coronary artery disease; CHD = coronary heart disease; CVD = cardiovascular disease; DBP = diastolic BP; HDL-C = high-density lipoprotein cholesterol; LDL-C = low-density lipoprotein cholesterol; MI = myocardial infarction; SBP = systolic BP; WHO = World Health Organization.

ment. For these factors low-cost behavioral interventions appear warranted.

Future Challenges

Primary and secondary prevention have contributed substantially to the reduction in CHD mortality rates. Yet challenges remain. First, as the population ages, the number of individuals with factors that put them at risk for cardiovascular disease will increase even if age-adjusted risk factor rates decline. Similarly, the number of people living with cardiovascular disease will increase, thus necessitating greater secondary preventive efforts.

Second, trends of several modifiable risk factors are troubling. Obesity and physical inactivity are epidemic among all

Change in Risk Factor(s)	Impact on Endpoint(s)
Coronary risk factors declined in both groups, though to a greater degree in intervention group	Nonsignificant change in CHD death: 17.9/1000 in intervention group, 19.3/1000 in usual care group
LDL-C (13%), triglycerides (20%), tobacco consumption (45%), and weight were lower in intervention group than usual care group; in both groups, physical activity and BP unchanged vs. baseline	Significant reduction in fatal MI, nonfatal MI, sudden death, and cerebrovascular accidents in intervention vs. control; 55% decrease in CHD death and 32% decrease in total mortality
Coronary risk predictors were significantly lower in intervention group during first 5 yr of trial; by trial's end, differences were statistically significant only for high-risk subjects who received face-to-face counseling	Nonsignificant differences in all-cause mortality (−5.3%), total CHD (−10.2%; $p = 0.07$), fatal CHD (6.9%), and nonfatal MI (−14.8%; $p = 0.06$) for intervention group vs. nonintervention group
In intervention group, 28% decrease in smoking, 3% decrease in serum cholesterol, and 3% decrease in BP vs. reference group	Age-adjusted CHD mortality decreased 22% in intervention group, 12% in reference group, and 11% in all of Finland ($p < 0.05$)
BP, serum cholesterol, and smoking all decreased markedly in both intervention and control groups	No significant differences in total mortality, stroke, and CHD incidence
Generally favorable, though not statistically significant changes in intervention group vs. reference group	No significant difference in CAD death rate
Small, not statistically significant decreases in serum cholesterol and BP in Pawtucket; slightly less smoking in the reference community	Projected CVD rates significantly (16%) less in Pawtucket during education program, but dropped to 8% after education program
Statistically significant reductions in community averages of plasma cholesterol level (2%), BP (4%), resting pulse rate (3%), and smoking rate (13%) in intervention communities vs. reference communities	Decreased composite total mortality risk scores (15%) and CHD risk scores (16%) in intervention communities vs. reference communities
After 4 yr, participants in intervention group were exercising more, practicing more stress management, and consuming less cholesterol and fewer fat calories than those in usual care group	In intervention group after 4 yr, significant reductions in frequency, duration, and severity of angina; fewer revascularizations (21% vs. 60%); and regression of atherosclerotic lesions (vs. continued worsening in usual care group)
Nonsignificant reductions in total cholesterol and triglycerides, maintenance of BMI, and significant increase in physical work capacity among those in intervention group	As assessed by coronary arteriography, significantly slower progression of coronary artery stenosis in intervention group, combined with significant improvements in myocardial perfusion
Significant improvements in percent body fat, weight, BP, LDL-C, triglycerides, HDL-C, and exercise capacity in treatment group vs. controls	Although progression of coronary artery disease occurred in both groups, intervention group had a 47% lower rate of progression per individual and a 58% lower rate of progression in diseased vessel segments than reference group

sectors of the population, including children. These factors will tend to increase rates of diabetes and hypertension and slow the favorable trends in mean lipid levels.

Third, in addition to developing a better understanding of the mechanistic and epidemiological determinants of atherosclerotic disease, we must pay more attention to finding effective strategies for prioritizing factors in prevention programs, implementing existing guidelines for risk factor modification, and developing low-cost interventions for factors for which guidelines are not yet available. Many life-style changes are difficult to achieve and even harder to maintain over the long term. Such interventions need to involve not only the affected individuals but also families, workplaces, schools, and even whole communities.

Finally, for clinicians, identifying a successful strategy for each patient is of critical importance. Further research on cost-benefit and risk-benefit ratios will enable better targeting of interventions for maximal individual and societal benefit. More widespread use of multifaceted self-help and health professional–directed prevention programs should help sustain the decline in cardiovascular disease mortality rates in the United States.

TABLE 42–11 Modifiable Risk Factors for the Prevention of Cardiovascular Disease

Factor	Effect	Intervention	Comment
Class 1 Risk Factors and Interventions in the Prevention of Cardiovascular Disease			
Smoking	2-3-fold increased risk	Smoking cessation with behavior and pharmacological intervention	Smoking cessation results in a 60% reduction in CHD risk by 3 yr; about half of that benefit occurs in first 3-6 mo after quitting. Interventions are cost-effective in both primary and secondary prevention
Hypertension	7 mm Hg increase in BP over baseline increases risk of CVD by 27%	Life-style modifications, weight loss, limited alcohol intake, aerobic exercise, and medications	A 5- to 6-mm Hg reduction in BP results in 42% reduction in risk of stroke and 16% reduction in risk of CVD. Extensive trial and cost-efficacy data support a tiered approach based on underlying risk
Dyslipidemias			
Hypercholesterolemia	10% increase in serum cholesterol increases risk of CVD by 20-30%	Dietary changes, lipid-lowering medications	Reduction in serum cholesterol by 10% reduces CVD death by 10% and CVD events by 18%. Treatment for >5 yr reduces CVD events by 25%. Extensive trial and cost-efficacy data support a tiered approach based on underlying risk
Elevated fasting triglyceride levels and low HDL levels	Increases risk	Diet, exercise, and lipid-lowering therapy	HDL and triglyceride measures are useful markers of CHD risk, and limited trial data suggest that intervention reduces risk
Pharmacological Therapies			
Aspirin in secondary prevention	Reduces CVD events by 25%	Daily low-dose aspirin	Reduces risk among those with any form of CVD
Beta blockers following MI	Reduces CVD events by 18%	Daily beta blocker use	Trial data suggest that the benefit may increase with increasing dose
ACE inhibitors for patients with low EF and following MI	Reduces CVD events by 22% in those with low EF and by 7% following MI	Daily ACE inhibitor use	Trial data suggest that the benefit may increase with increasing dose
Class 2 Risk Factors and Interventions in the Prevention of Cardiovascular Disease			
Insulin-dependent diabetes	Increases risk 2-4-fold in men and 3-7-fold in women	Maintaining normoglycemia with diet, exercise, weight management, and insulin	Trial data strongly suggest that tight control with insulin reduces risk of microvascular disease and may reduce the risk of CVD events
NIDDM	Increases risk 2-4-fold in men and 3-7-fold in women	Maintaining normoglycemia with diet, exercise, weight management, oral agents, and insulin as needed	Tight control appears to reduce microvascular disease, but data on the risk of CHD are not available. Those with NIDDM are likely to have multiple coronary risk factors that should be aggressively modified
Obesity and physical inactivity	Increases risk	Diet, exercise, and weight management programs	In addition to improving other CVD risk factors, maintaining ideal body weight and a physically active life style may reduce risk of MI as much as 50%, but trial data are limited
Moderate alcohol intake (one drink per day)	Decreases risk of MI by 30-50%	Discussion of alcohol intake with all patients	Risk/benefit ratio for moderate alcohol consumption may vary widely by gender and is based on underlying risk of CHD; recommendations must be made individually with careful regard for conditions such as hypertension, diabetes, liver disease, history of alcohol abuse, risk of breast cancer
Pharmacological Therapies			
Aspirin in primary prevention	Pooled trial data in men suggest a 33% reduction in risk of first MI	Daily or alternate-day low-dose aspirin	Prophylactic aspirin use in older men, particularly with risk factors, may reduce risk of MI. Data among women are limited but forthcoming

TABLE 42–11 Modifiable Risk Factors for the Prevention of Cardiovascular Disease—cont'd

Category	Specific Factors	Comment
Class 3 Factors and Interventions in the Prevention of Cardiovascular Disease		
Menopause	Increases CVD risk. Evidence from large RCTs suggests that hormone replacement therapy may increase, not decrease, this risk, and long-term use is associated with increased risk of endometrial and breast cancer	The combination of estrogen and progestin is not recommended as a strategy for decreasing the risk of heart disease in postmenopausal women
Dietary factors	Fruit and vegetable intake, type and amount of fat, type and amount of carbohydrate, fiber, *trans*-fatty acids, dietary antioxidants, dietary bioflavonoids, dietary folate, fish and fish oils, garlic, etc.	USDA recommends 5 servings of fruit and vegetables per day. Reduction in saturated and *trans*-fatty acid intake appears to be warranted
Dietary supplements	Multivitamins, antioxidant supplements, folate, vitamins B_{12} and B_6, fish oils, etc.	Randomized trials of antioxidant supplements have been disappointing. Randomized trial data on antioxidants and folate are forthcoming
Psychological factors	Depression, lack of social support, stress, type A personality, etc.	Trials of antidepressants in secondary prevention are forthcoming
Novel biochemical markers	Fibrinogen, homocysteine, Lp(a), t-PA, von Willebrand factor, factor VII, C-reactive protein, soluble adhesion molecules (sICAM, sVCAM), antibodies to various infectious agents, measures of oxidative stress, etc.	Additional observational data are needed to clarify the role of these factors in clinical practice
Novel genetic markers	LDL receptor, factor V Leiden, ACE, etc.	Potential genetic markers and therapies are emerging at a rapid rate

ACE = angiotensin-converting enzyme; BP = blood pressure; CHD = coronary heart disease; CVD = cardiovascular disease; EF = ejection fraction; HDL = high-density lipoprotein; LDL = low-density lipoprotein; Lp(a) = lipoprotein little A antigen; MI = myocardial infarction; NIDDM = non-insulin-dependent diabetes mellitus; RCTs = randomized controlled trials; sICAM = soluble intercellular adhesion molecule; sVCAM = soluble vascular cell adhesion molecule; t-PA = tissue-type plasminogen activator; USDA = U.S. Department of Agriculture.

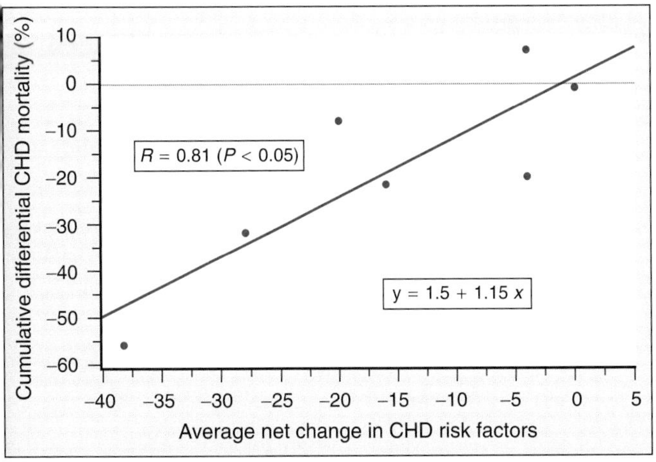

FIGURE 42–8 For seven trials, four of which made up the World Health Organization European Collaborative Trial in Multifactorial Prevention of Coronary Heart Disease, Kornitzer plotted the difference in a composite risk factor score between treated and untreated groups and showed a statistically significant correlation between the magnitude of risk factor improvement and coronary heart disease (CHD) mortality. (From Kornitzer M: Changing individual behavior. *In* Marmot M, Elliott P [eds]: Coronary Heart Disease Epidemiology: From Aetiology to Public Health. Oxford, Oxford University Press, 1992, p 492.)

REFERENCES

1. Murray CJL, Lopez AD: The Global Burden of Disease. Cambridge, MA, Harvard School of Public Health, 1996.
2. Howson CP, Reddy SK, Ryan TJ, Bale JR: Control of Cardiovascular Diseases in Developing Countries. Washington, DC, National Academy Press, 1998.
3. Yarnall KS, Pollak KI, Ostbye T, et al: Primary care: Is there enough time for prevention? Am J Public Health 93:635-641, 2003.
4. Kannel WB, Dawber TR, Kagan A, et al: Factors of risk in the development of coronary heart disease—six year follow-up experience: The Framingham Study. Ann Intern Med 55:33-50, 1961.
5. Third Report of the National Cholesterol Education Program (NCEP) Expert Panel on Detection, Evaluation, and Treatment of High Blood Cholesterol in Adults (Adult Treatment Panel III) final report. Circulation 106:3143-3421, 2002.
6. Chobanian AV, Bakris GL, Black HR, et al: The Seventh Report of the Joint National Committee on Prevention, Detection, Evaluation, and Treatment of High Blood Pressure: The JNC-7 Report. JAMA 289:2560-2572, 2003.
7. Haffner SM: Management of dyslipidemia in adults with diabetes. Diabetes Care 26(Suppl 1):S83-S86, 2003.
8. Wilson PW, D'Agostino RB, Levy D, et al: Prediction of coronary heart disease using risk factor categories. Circulation 97:1837-1847, 1998.
9. Wood D, De Backer G, Faergeman O, et al: Prevention of coronary heart disease in clinical practice: Recommendations of the Second Joint Task Force of European and other Societies on Coronary Prevention. Eur Heart J 19:1434-1503, 1998.
10. Assmann G, Cullen P, Schulte H: Simple scoring scheme for calculating the risk of acute coronary events based on the 10-year follow-up of the prospective cardiovascular Munster (PROCAM) study. Circulation 105:310-315, 2002.
11. Orford JL, Sesso HD, Stedman M, et al: A comparison of the Framingham and European Society of Cardiology coronary heart disease risk prediction models in the normative aging study. Am Heart J 144:95-100, 2002.
12. MacMahon S, Peto R, Cutler J, et al: Blood pressure, stroke, and coronary heart disease: I. Prolonged differences in blood pressure: Prospective observational studies corrected for the regression dilution bias. Lancet 335:765-774, 1990.
13. Pearson TA, McBride PE, Miller NH, Smith SC: 27th Bethesda Conference: Matching the intensity of risk factor management with the hazard for coronary disease events. Task Force 8. Organization of preventive cardiology service. J Am Coll Cardiol 27:1039-1047, 1996.

Cigarette Smoking

14. Strategies to control tobacco use in the United States: A blueprint for public health action in the 1990s. NIH Publication No. 92-3316. Bethesda, MD, U.S. Department of Health and Human Services, Public Health Service, National Institutes of Health, National Cancer Institute, 1991.
15. Cigarette report for 2001. Federal Trade Commission, 2003. (http://www.ftc.gov/os/2003/06/2001cigreport.pdf)
16. Office on Smoking and Health: Percentage of smoking prevalence among U.S. adults, 18 years of age and older, 1955-1994. National Center for Chronic Disease and Prevention, Centers for Disease Control and Prevention, 1996. (http://www.cdc.gov/tobacco/prevali.htm)
17. Cigarette smoking among adults—United States, 2000. MMWR Morb Mortal Wkly Rep 51:642-645, 2002.
18. Johnston LD, O'Malley PM, Bachman JG: National survey results on drug use from the Monitoring the Future study, 1975-1998. Vol I: secondary school students. NIH Publication No. 99-4660. Rockville, MD, National Institutes of Health, National Institute on Drug Abuse, 1999.
19. Trends in cigarette smoking among high school students—United States, 1991–2001. MMWR Morb Mortal Wkly Rep 51:409-412, 2002.

20. Cigarette smoking among adults—United States, 1997. MMWR Morb Mortal Wkly Rep 48:993-996, 1999.
21. Annual smoking—attributable mortality, years of potential life lost, and economic costs: United States, 1995-1999. MMWR Morb Mortal Wkly Rep 51:300-303, 2002.
22. Jha P, Chaloupka FJ: Curbing the epidemic: Governments and the economics of tobacco control. Washington, DC, World Bank, 1999.
23. Reducing risks, promoting healthy life: World Health Report 2002. Geneva, World Health Organization, 2002.
24. Cromwell J, Bartosch WJ, Fiore MC, et al: Cost-effectiveness of the clinical practice recommendations in the AHCPR guideline for smoking cessation. Agency for Health Care Policy and Research. JAMA 278:1759-1766, 1997.
25. A clinical practice guideline for treating tobacco use and dependence: A U.S. Public Health Service report. The Tobacco Use and Dependence Clinical Practice Guideline Panel, Staff, and Consortium Representatives. JAMA 283:3244-3254, 2000.
26. U.S. Preventive Services Task Force: Guide to Clinical Preventive Services. 3rd ed. Rockville, MD, Agency for Healthcare Research and Quality, 2000-2003.
27. Thomson CC, Rigotti NA: Hospital- and clinic-based smoking cessation interventions for smokers with cardiovascular disease. Prog Cardiovasc Dis 45:459-479, 2003.

Hypertension

28. National Center for Health Statistics: Health, United States, 2002. Hyattsville, MD, U.S. Department of Health and Human Services, Centers for Disease Control and Prevention, 2002.
29. Vasan RS, Beiser A, Seshadri S, et al: Residual lifetime risk for developing hypertension in middle-aged women and men: The Framingham Heart Study. JAMA 287:1003-1010, 2002.
30. Hajjar I, Kotchen TA: Trends in prevalence, awareness, treatment, and control of hypertension in the United States, 1988-2000. JAMA 290:199-206, 2003.
31. Lewington S, Clarke R, Qizilbash N, et al: Age-specific relevance of usual blood pressure to vascular mortality: A meta-analysis of individual data for one million adults in 61 prospective studies. Lancet 360:1903-1913, 2002.
32. Collins R, Peto R, MacMahon S, et al: Blood pressure, stroke, and coronary heart disease: II. Short-term reductions in blood pressure: Overview of randomised drug trials in their epidemiological context. Lancet 335:827-838, 1990.
33. Ogden LG, He J, Lydick E, Whelton PK: Long-term absolute benefit of lowering blood pressure in hypertensive patients according to the JNC-VI risk stratification. Hypertension 35:539-543, 2000.
34. Major outcomes in high-risk hypertensive patients randomized to angiotensin-converting enzyme inhibitor or calcium channel blocker versus diuretic: The Antihypertensive and Lipid-Lowering Treatment to Prevent Heart Attack Trial (ALLHAT). JAMA 288:2981-2997, 2002.
35. Pearce KA, Furberg CD, Psaty BM, Kirk J: Cost-minimization and the number needed to treat in uncomplicated hypertension. Am J Hypertens 11:618-629, 1998.
36. Guide to Clinical Preventive Services. 2nd ed. Baltimore, MD, Williams & Wilkins, 1996.
37. Appel LJ, Moore TJ, Obarzanek E, et al: A clinical trial of the effects of dietary patterns on blood pressure. DASH Collaborative Research Group. N Engl J Med 336:1117-1124, 1997.
38. Sacks FM, Svetkey LP, Vollmer WM, et al: Effects on blood pressure of reduced dietary sodium and the Dietary Approaches to Stop Hypertension (DASH) diet. DASH-Sodium Collaborative Research Group. N Engl J Med 344:3-10, 2001.
39. The sixth report of the Joint National Committee on Prevention, Detection, Evaluation, and Treatment of High Blood Pressure. Arch Intern Med 157:2413-2446, 1997.
40. Bertrand E: Cardiovascular disease in developing countries. *In* Dalla Volta S (ed): Cardiology. New York, McGraw-Hill, 1999, pp 825-834.

Dyslipidemia

41. Law MR, Wald NJ, Thompson SG: By how much and how quickly does reduction in serum cholesterol concentration lower risk of ischaemic heart disease? BMJ 308:367-372, 1994.
42. Law MR, Wald NJ, Wu T, et al: Systematic underestimation of association between serum cholesterol concentration and ischaemic heart disease in observational studies: Data from the BUPA study. BMJ 308:363-366, 1994.
43. Maron DJ, Fazio S, Linton MF: Current perspectives on statins. Circulation 101:207-213, 2000.
44. Schwartz GG, Olsson AG, Ezekowitz MD, et al: Effects of atorvastatin on early recurrent ischemic events in acute coronary syndromes. The MIRACL Study: A randomized controlled trial. JAMA 285:1711-1718, 2001.
45. Newby LK, Kristinsson A, Bhapkar MV, et al: Early statin initiation and outcomes in patients with acute coronary syndromes. JAMA 287:3087-3095, 2002.
46. LaRosa JC, He J, Vupputuri S: Effect of statins on risk of coronary disease: A meta-analysis of randomized controlled trials. JAMA 282:2340-2346, 1999.
47. Warshafsky S, Packard D, Marks SJ, et al: Efficacy of 3-hydroxy-3-methylglutaryl coenzyme A reductase inhibitors for prevention of stroke. J Gen Intern Med 14:763-774, 1999.
48. Prosser LA, Stinnett AA, Goldman PA, et al: Cost-effectiveness of cholesterol-lowering therapies according to selected patient characteristics. Ann Intern Med 132:769-779, 2000.
49. Ganz DA, Kuntz KM, Jacobson GA, Avorn J: Cost-effectiveness of 3-hydroxy-3-methylglutaryl coenzyme A reductase inhibitor therapy in older patients with myocardial infarction. Ann Intern Med 132:780-787, 2000.
50. Guidelines for using serum cholesterol, high-density lipoprotein cholesterol, and triglyceride levels as screening tests for preventing coronary heart disease in adults. American College of Physicians. Ann Intern Med 124:515-517, 1996.
51. Gaziano JM, Hennekens CH, O'Donnell CJ, et al: Fasting triglycerides, high-density lipoprotein, and risk of myocardial infarction. Circulation 96:2520-2525, 1997.
52. Austin MA, Hokanson JE, Edwards KL: Hypertriglyceridemia as a cardiovascular risk factor. Am J Cardiol 81:7B-12B, 1998.
53. Assmann G, Schulte H, Funke H, von Eckardstein A: The emergence of triglycerides as a significant independent risk factor in coronary artery disease. Eur Heart J 19(Suppl M):M8-M14, 1998.
54. Rubins HB, Robins SJ, Collins D, et al: Gemfibrozil for the secondary prevention of coronary heart disease in men with low levels of high-density lipoprotein cholesterol. Veterans Affairs High-Density Lipoprotein Cholesterol Intervention Trial Study Group. N Engl J Med 341:410-418, 1999.

Secondary Prevention

55. Collaborative meta-analysis of randomised trials of antiplatelet therapy for prevention of death, myocardial infarction, and stroke in high risk patients. BMJ 324:71-86, 2002.
56. Gaspoz JM, Coxson PG, Goldman PA, et al: Cost-effectiveness of aspirin, clopidogrel, or both for secondary prevention of coronary heart disease. N Engl J Med 346:1800-1806, 2002.
57. Eidelman RS, Hebert PR, Weisman SM, Hennekens CH: An update on aspirin in the primary prevention of cardiovascular disease. Arch Intern Med 163:2006-2010, 2003.
58. Aspirin for the primary prevention of cardiovascular events: Recommendation and rationale. Ann Intern Med 136:157-160, 2002.
59. Freemantle N, Cleland J, Young P, et al: Beta blockade after myocardial infarction: Systematic review and meta regression analysis. BMJ 318:1730-1737, 1999.
60. Phillips KA, Shlipak MG, Coxson P, et al: Health and economic benefits of increased beta-blocker use following myocardial infarction. JAMA 284:2748-2754, 2000.
61. Indications for ACE inhibitors in the early treatment of acute myocardial infarction: Systematic overview of individual data from 100,000 patients in randomized trials. ACE Inhibitor Myocardial Infarction Collaborative Group. Circulation 97:2202-2212, 1998.
62. Domanski MJ, Exner DV, Borkowf CB, et al: Effect of angiotensin-converting enzyme inhibition on sudden cardiac death in patients following acute myocardial infarction: A meta-analysis of randomized clinical trials. J Am Coll Cardiol 33:598-604, 1999.
63. Teo KK, Yusuf S, Pfeffer M, et al: Effects of long-term treatment with angiotensin-converting-enzyme inhibitors in the presence or absence of aspirin: A systematic review. Lancet 360:1037-1043, 2002.
64. Yusuf S, Sleight P, Pogue J, et al: Effects of an angiotensin-converting enzyme inhibitor, ramipril, on cardiovascular events in high-risk patients. The Heart Outcomes Prevention Evaluation Study Investigators. N Engl J Med 342:145-153, 2000.
65. Pfeffer MA, Swedberg K, Granger CB, et al: Effects of candesartan on mortality and morbidity in patients with chronic heart failure: The CHARM-Overall programme. Lancet 362:759-766, 2003.

Diabetes, Metabolic Syndrome, and Obesity

66. National Diabetes Fact Sheet: General Information and National Estimates on Diabetes in the United States, 2000. Atlanta, Centers for Disease Control and Prevention, 2002.
67. Harris MI, Flegal KM, Cowie CC, et al: Prevalence of diabetes, impaired fasting glucose, and impaired glucose tolerance in U.S. adults. The Third National Health and Nutrition Examination Survey, 1988–1994. Diabetes Care 21:518-524, 1998.
68. Type 2 diabetes in children and adolescents. American Diabetes Association. Diabetes Care 23:381-389, 2000.
69. Fagot-Campagna A, Pettitt DJ, Engelgau MM, et al: Type 2 diabetes among North American children and adolescents: An epidemiologic review and a public health perspective. J Pediatr 136:664-672, 2000.
70. Gu K, Cowie CC, Harris MI: Mortality in adults with and without diabetes in a national cohort of the U.S. population, 1971-1993. Diabetes Care 21:1138-1145, 1998.
71. Barrett-Connor EL, Cohn BA, Wingard DL, Edelstein SL: Why is diabetes mellitus a stronger risk factor for fatal ischemic heart disease in women than in men? The Rancho Bernardo Study. JAMA 265:627-631, 1991.
72. Hu FB, Stampfer MJ, Solomon CG, et al: The impact of diabetes mellitus on mortality from all causes and coronary heart disease in women: 20 years of follow-up. Arch Intern Med 161:1717-1723, 2001.
73. Cho E, Rimm EB, Stampfer MJ, et al: The impact of diabetes mellitus and prior myocardial infarction on mortality from all causes and from coronary heart disease in men. J Am Coll Cardiol 40:954-960, 2002.
74. Intensive blood glucose control with sulphonylureas or insulin compared with conventional treatment and risk of complications in patients with type 2 diabetes (UKPDS 33). UK Prospective Diabetes Study (UKPDS) Group. Lancet 352:837-853, 1998.
75. Abraira C, Colwell J, Nuttall F, et al: Cardiovascular events and correlates in the Veterans Affairs Diabetes Feasibility Trial. Veterans Affairs Cooperative Study on Glycemic Control and Complications in Type II Diabetes. Arch Intern Med 157:181-188, 1997.
76. Gerstein HC, Mann JF, Pogue J, et al: Prevalence and determinants of microalbuminuria in high-risk diabetic and nondiabetic patients in the Heart Outcomes Prevention Evaluation Study. The HOPE Study Investigators. Diabetes Care 23(Suppl 2):B35-B39, 2000.
77. Gaede P, Vedel P, Larsen N, et al: Multifactorial intervention and cardiovascular disease in patients with type 2 diabetes. N Engl J Med 348:383-393, 2003.
78. Arday DR, Fleming BB, Keller DK, et al: Variation in diabetes care among states: Do patient characteristics matter? Diabetes Care 25:2230-2237, 2002.
79. Markovic TP, Jenkins AB, Campbell LV, et al: The determinants of glycemic responses to diet restriction and weight loss in obesity and NIDDM. Diabetes Care 21:687-694, 1998.
80. Arauz-Pacheco C, Parrott MA, Raskin P: Treatment of hypertension in adults with diabetes. Diabetes Care 26(Suppl 1):S80-S82, 2003.
81. Ballantyne CM, Houri J, Notarbartolo A, et al: Effect of ezetimibe coadministered with atorvastatin in 628 patients with primary hypercholesterolemia: A prospective, randomized, double-blind trial. Circulation 107:2409-2415, 2003.
82. Colwell JA: Aspirin therapy in diabetes. Diabetes Care 26(Suppl 1):S87-S88, 2003.
83. Ford ES, Giles WH, Dietz WH: Prevalence of the metabolic syndrome among U.S. adults: Findings from the Third National Health and Nutrition Examination Survey. JAMA 287:356-359, 2002.

84. Wilson PW, Grundy SM: The metabolic syndrome: practical guide to origins and treatment: Parts I and II. Circulation 108:1422-1424 and 1537-1540, 2003.
85. Tuomilehto J, Lindstrom J, Eriksson JG, et al: Prevention of type 2 diabetes mellitus by changes in lifestyle among subjects with impaired glucose tolerance. N Engl J Med 344:1343-1350, 2001.
86. Knowler WC, Barrett-Connor E, Fowler SE, et al: Reduction in the incidence of type 2 diabetes with lifestyle intervention or metformin. N Engl J Med 346:393-403, 2002.
87. Hu FB, Manson JE, Stampfer MJ, et al: Diet, lifestyle, and the risk of type 2 diabetes mellitus in women. N Engl J Med 345:790-797, 2001.
88. Nelson KM, Reiber G, Boyko EJ: Diet and exercise among adults with type 2 diabetes: Findings from the Third National Health and Nutrition Examination Survey (NHANES III). Diabetes Care 25:1722-1728, 2002.
89. Smith NL, Barzilay JI, Shaffer D, et al: Fasting and 2-hour postchallenge serum glucose measures and risk of incident cardiovascular events in the elderly: The Cardiovascular Health Study. Arch Intern Med 162:209-216, 2002.
90. Flegal KM, Carroll MD, Kuczmarski RJ, Johnson CL: Overweight and obesity in the United States: Prevalence and trends, 1960-1994. Int J Obes Relat Metab Disord 22:39-47, 1998.
91. Flegal KM, Carroll MD, Ogden CL, Johnson CL: Prevalence and trends in obesity among U.S. adults, 1999-2000. JAMA 288:1723-1727, 2002.
92. Ogden CL, Flegal KM, Carroll MD, Johnson CL: Prevalence and trends in overweight among U.S. children and adolescents, 1999-2000. JAMA 288:1728-1732, 2002.
93. Ashton WD, Nanchahal K, Wood DA: Body mass index and metabolic risk factors for coronary heart disease in women. Eur Heart J 22:46-55, 2001.
94. Ford ES, Galuska DA, Gillespie C, et al: C-reactive protein and body mass index in children: Findings from the Third National Health and Nutrition Examination Survey, 1988-1994. J Pediatr 138:486-492, 2001.
95. Duncan BB, Schmidt MI, Chambless LE, et al: Fibrinogen, other putative markers of inflammation, and weight gain in middle-aged adults—the ARIC study. Atherosclerosis Risk in Communities. Obes Res 8:279-286, 2000.
96. Visser M, Bouter LM, McQuillan GM, et al: Elevated C-reactive protein levels in overweight and obese adults. JAMA 282:2131-2135, 1999.
97. Clinical Guidelines on the Identification, Evaluation, and Treatment of Overweight and Obesity in Adults. National Institutes of Health, National Heart, Lung, and Blood Institute, Obesity Education Initiative, 1998. (http://www.nhlbi.nih.gov/guidelines/obesity/ob_gdlns.htm)
98. Overweight, Obesity, and Health Risk: National Task Force on the Prevention and Treatment of Obesity. Arch Intern Med 160:898-904, 2000.
99. Thompson D, Edelsberg J, Colditz GA, et al: Lifetime health and economic consequences of obesity. Arch Intern Med 159:2177-2183, 1999.
100. Oster G, Thompson D, Edelsberg J, et al: Lifetime health and economic benefits of weight loss among obese persons. Am J Public Health 89:1536-1542, 1999.
101. Must A, Spadano J, Coakley EH, et al: The disease burden associated with overweight and obesity. JAMA 282:1523-1529, 1999.
102. Rexrode KM, Carey VJ, Hennekens CH, et al: Abdominal adiposity and coronary heart disease in women. JAMA 280:1843-1848, 1998.
103. Rexrode KM, Buring JE, Manson JE: Abdominal and total adiposity and risk of coronary heart disease in men. Int J Obes Relat Metab Disord 25:1047-1056, 2001.
104. Allison DB, Fontaine KR, Manson JE, et al: Annual deaths attributable to obesity in the United States. JAMA 282:1530-1538, 1999.
105. Sturm R, Wells KB: Does obesity contribute as much to morbidity as poverty or smoking? Public Health 115:229-235, 2001.
106. Finkelstein EA, Fiebelkorn IC, Wang G: National medical spending attributable to overweight and obesity: How much, and who's paying? Health Aff (Millwood) 22:Web supplement, 2003.
107. Finkelstein EA, Fiebelkorn IC, Wang G: National medical spending attributable to overweight and obesity. Health Affairs, 2003. (http://www.healthaffairs.org/WebExclusives/Finkelstein_Web_Excl_051403.htm)
108. Stefanick ML. Exercise and weight loss. *In* Hennekens CH (ed): Clinical Trials in Cardiovascular Disease: A Companion Guide to Braunwald's Heart Disease. Philadelphia, WB Saunders, 1999, pp 375-391.
109. Halbert JA, Silagy CA, Finucane P, et al: The effectiveness of exercise training in lowering blood pressure: A meta-analysis of randomised controlled trials of 4 weeks or longer. J Hum Hypertens 11:641-649, 1997.
110. Hu FB, Sigal RJ, Rich-Edwards JW, et al: Walking compared with vigorous physical activity and risk of type 2 diabetes in women: A prospective study. JAMA 282:1433-1439, 1999.
111. Hardman AE: Interaction of physical activity and diet: Implications for lipoprotein metabolism. Public Health Nutr 2:369-276, 1999.
112. Rexrode KM, Hennekens CH, Willett WC, et al: A prospective study of body mass index, weight change, and risk of stroke in women. JAMA 277:1539-1545, 1997.

Physical Activity

113. Fletcher GF: Exercise in the prevention of stroke. Health Rep 6:106-110, 1994.
114. Shike M: Diet and lifestyle in the prevention of colorectal cancer: An overview. Am J Med 106:11S-15S; discussion 50S-51S, 1999.
115. McTiernan A: Associations between energy balance and body mass index and risk of breast carcinoma in women from diverse racial and ethnic backgrounds in the U.S. Cancer 88:1248-1255, 2000.
116. Ettinger WH Jr, Burns R, Messier SP, et al: A randomized trial comparing aerobic exercise and resistance exercise with a health education program in older adults with knee osteoarthritis. The Fitness Arthritis and Seniors Trial (FAST). JAMA 277:25-31, 1997.
117. Messier SP, Loeser RF, Mitchell MN, et al: Exercise and weight loss in obese older adults with knee osteoarthritis: A preliminary study. J Am Geriatr Soc 48:1062-1072, 2000.
118. Berard A, Bravo G, Gauthier P: Meta-analysis of the effectiveness of physical activity for the prevention of bone loss in postmenopausal women. Osteoporos Int 7:331-337, 1997.
119. Bonaiuti D, Shea B, Iovine R, et al: Exercise for preventing and treating osteoporosis in postmenopausal women. Cochrane Database Syst Rev CD000333, 2002.
120. The Surgeon General's Call to Action to Prevent and Decrease Overweight and Obesity. Rockville, MD, U.S. Department of Health and Human Services, Public Health Service, Office of the Surgeon General, 2001.
121. Leitzmann MF, Rimm EB, Willett WC, et al: Recreational physical activity and the risk of cholecystectomy in women. N Engl J Med 341:777-784, 1999.
122. Peppard PE, Young T, Palta M, et al: Longitudinal study of moderate weight change and sleep-disordered breathing. JAMA 284:3015-3021, 2000.
123. Physical Activity and Health: A report of the Surgeon General. U.S. Department of Health and Human Services, Centers for Disease Control and Prevention, 1996. (http://www.cdc.gov/nccdphp/sgr/sgr.htm)
124. Peppard PE, Young T, Palta M: Longitudinal study of moderate weight change and sleep-disordered breathing. JAMA 284:3015-3021, 2000.
125. Schmitz MK, Jeffery RW: Public health interventions for the prevention and treatment of obesity. Med Clin North Am 84:491-512, viii, 2000.
126. Serdula MK, Mokdad AH, Williamson DF, et al: Prevalence of attempting weight loss and strategies for controlling weight. JAMA 282:1353-1358, 1999.
127. The Practical Guide: Identification, Evaluation, and Treatment of Overweight and Obesity in Adults. NIH Publication No. 00-4084. Washington DC, National Heart, Lung, and Blood Institute, North American Association for the Study of Obesity, 2000. (available online at<http://www.nhlbi.nih.gov/guidelines/obesity/practgde.htm>)
128. Physical activity trends—United States, 1990–1998. MMWR Morb Mortal Wkly Rep 50:166-169, 2001.
129. Healthy People 2010: Understanding and Improving Health. U.S. Department of Health and Human Services, 2000. (http://www.healthypeople.gov/Document/pdf/uih/2010uih.pdf)
130. Lowry R, Wechsler H, Kann L, Collins JL: Recent trends in participation in physical education among U.S. high school students. J Sch Health 71:145-152, 2001.
131. National Institute of Child Health and Human Development Study of Early Child Care and Youth Development Network: Frequency and intensity of physical activity of third grade children in physical education. Arch Pediatr Adolesc Med 157:185-190, 2003.
132. U.S. Department of Transportation: Nationwide Personal Transportation Survey. Washington DC, Federal Highway Administration, 1997.
133. Rideout VJ, Foehr UG, Roberts DF, Brodie M: Kids and media at the new millennium: A comprehensive national analysis of children's media use. Menlo Park, CA, Kaiser Family Foundation, 1999.
134. Lee IM, Skerrett PJ: Physical activity and all-cause mortality: What is the dose-response relation? Med Sci Sports Exerc 33:S459-S471; discussion S493-S494, 2001.
135. Folsom AR, Arnett DK, Hutchinson RG, et al: Physical activity and incidence of coronary heart disease in middle-aged women and men. Med Sci Sports Exerc 29:901-909, 1997.
136. Leon AS, Myers MJ, Connett J: Leisure time physical activity and the 16-year risks of mortality from coronary heart disease and all-causes in the Multiple Risk Factor Intervention Trial (MRFIT). Int J Sports Med 18(Suppl 3):S208-S215, 1997.
137. Rosengren A, Wilhelmsen L: Physical activity protects against coronary death and deaths from all causes in middle-aged men: Evidence from a 20-year follow-up of the primary prevention study in Goteborg. Ann Epidemiol 7:69-75, 1997.
138. Manson JE, Greenland P, LaCroix AZ, et al: Walking compared with vigorous exercise for the prevention of cardiovascular events in women. N Engl J Med 347:716-725, 2002.
139. Hakim AA, Curb JD, Petrovitch H, et al: Effects of walking on coronary heart disease in elderly men: The Honolulu Heart Program. Circulation 100:9-13, 1999.
140. Tanasescu M, Leitzmann MF, Rimm EB, et al: Exercise type and intensity in relation to coronary heart disease in men. JAMA 288:1994-2000, 2002.
141. Gregg EW, Cauley JA, Stone K, et al: Relationship of changes in physical activity and mortality among older women. JAMA 289:2379-2386, 2003.
142. Wannamethee SG, Shaper AG, Walker M: Changes in physical activity, mortality, and incidence of coronary heart disease in older men. Lancet 351:1603-1608, 1998.
143. Lee IM, Hennekens CH, Berger K, et al: Exercise and risk of stroke in male physicians. Stroke 30:1-6, 1999.
144. Lee IM, Paffenbarger RS Jr: Physical activity and stroke incidence: The Harvard Alumni Health Study. Stroke 29:2049-2054, 1998.
145. Hu FB, Stampfer MJ, Colditz GA, et al: Physical activity and risk of stroke in women. JAMA 283:2961-2967, 2000.
146. Stefanick ML, Mackey S, Sheehan M, et al: Effects of diet and exercise in men and postmenopausal women with low levels of HDL cholesterol and high levels of LDL cholesterol. N Engl J Med 339:12-20, 1998.
147. Henriksen EJ: Effects of acute exercise and exercise training on insulin resistance. J Appl Physiol 93:788-796, 2002.
148. Schmitz KH, Jacobs DR Jr, Hong CP, et al: Association of physical activity with insulin sensitivity in children. Int J Obes Relat Metab Disord 26:1310-1316, 2002.
149. Whelton SP, Chin A, Xin X, He J: Effect of aerobic exercise on blood pressure: A meta-analysis of randomized, controlled trials. Ann Intern Med 136:493-503, 2002.
150. Stewart KJ: Exercise training and the cardiovascular consequences of type 2 diabetes and hypertension: Plausible mechanisms for improving cardiovascular health. JAMA 288:1622-1631, 2002.
151. Jolliffe JA, Rees K, Taylor RS, et al: Exercise-based rehabilitation for coronary heart disease. Cochrane Database Syst Rev 3, 2003.
152. Smith SC Jr, Blair SN, Bonow RO, et al: AHA/ACC Guidelines for Preventing Heart Attack and Death in Patients with Atherosclerotic Cardiovascular Disease: 2001 Update. A statement for healthcare professionals from the American Heart Association and the American College of Cardiology. J Am Coll Cardiol 38:1581-1583, 2001.
153. Pollock ML, Franklin BA, Balady GJ, et al: Resistance exercise in individuals with and without cardiovascular disease: Benefits, rationale, safety, and prescription: An advisory from the Committee on Exercise, Rehabilitation, and Prevention, Council on Clinical Cardiology, American Heart Association. Position paper endorsed by the American College of Sports Medicine. Circulation 101:828-833, 2000.

154. Physical Activity and Health: A Report of the Surgeon General. Washington, DC, U.S. Department of Health and Human Services, Centers for Disease Control and Prevention, 1996.

Alcohol Intake

155. Goldberg IJ, Mosca L, Piano MR, Fisher EA: AHA Science Advisory: Wine and your heart: A science advisory for healthcare professionals from the Nutrition Committee, Council on Epidemiology and Prevention, and Council on Cardiovascular Nursing of the American Heart Association. Circulation 103:472-475, 2001.
156. Rimm EB, Williams P, Fosher K, et al: Moderate alcohol intake and lower risk of coronary heart disease: Meta-analysis of effects on lipids and haemostatic factors. BMJ 319:1523-1528, 1999.
157. Anand SS, Yusuf S: Oral anticoagulant therapy in patients with coronary artery disease: A meta-analysis. JAMA 282:2058-2067, 1999.

Hormone Therapy

158. Anderson R: Deaths: Leading Causes for 2000. National Vital Statistics Reports. Vol 50, No. 16. Hyattsville, MD, National Center for Health Statistics, 2002.
159. Manson JE, Martin KA: Clinical practice: Postmenopausal hormone-replacement therapy. N Engl J Med 345:34-40, 2001.
160. Grodstein F, Stampfer MJ: The epidemiology of postmenopausal hormone therapy and cardiovascular disease. *In* Goldhaber SZ, Ridker PM (eds): Thrombosis and Thromboembolism. New York, Marcel Dekker, 2002, pp 67-78.
161. Rossouw JE, Anderson GL, Prentice RL, et al: Risks and benefits of estrogen plus progestin in healthy postmenopausal women: Principal results From the Women's Health Initiative randomized controlled trial. JAMA 288:321-333, 2002.
162. Grady D, Herrington D, Bittner V, et al: Cardiovascular disease outcomes during 6.8 years of hormone therapy: Heart and Estrogen/progestin Replacement Study follow-up (HERS II). JAMA 288:49-57, 2002.

163. Herrington DM, Reboussin DM, Brosnihan KB, et al: Effects of estrogen replacement on the progression of coronary artery atherosclerosis. N Engl J Med 343:522-529, 2000.
164. Clarke SC, Kelleher J, Lloyd-Jones H, et al: A study of hormone replacement therapy in postmenopausal women with ischaemic heart disease: The Papworth HRT atherosclerosis study. Br J Obstet Gynaecol 109:1056-1062, 2002.
165. Waters DD, Alderman EL, Hsia J, et al: Effects of hormone replacement therapy and antioxidant vitamin supplements on coronary atherosclerosis in postmenopausal women: A randomized controlled trial. JAMA 288:2432-2440, 2002.
166. Cherry N, Gilmour K, Hannaford P, et al: Oestrogen therapy for prevention of reinfarction in postmenopausal women: A randomised placebo controlled trial. Lancet 360:2001-2008, 2002.
167. Lissin LW, Cooke JP: Phytoestrogens and cardiovascular health. J Am Coll Cardiol 35:1403-1410, 2000.
168. Postmenopausal hormone replacement therapy for the primary prevention of chronic condition: Recommendations and rationale. U.S. Preventive Services Task Force. Am Fam Physician 67:358-364, 2003.
169. Amended report from the NAMS Advisory Panel on Postmenopausal Hormone Therapy. Menopause 10:6-12, 2003.
170. FDA approves new labels for estrogen and estrogen with progestin therapies for postmenopausal women following review of Women's Health Initiative data. Washington, DC, U.S. Food and Drug Administration, 2003. (http://www.fda.gov/bbs/topics/NEWS/2003/NEW00863.html)

Diet

171. Ness AR, Powles JW: Fruit and vegetables, and cardiovascular disease: A review. Int J Epidemiol 26:1-13, 1997.
172. Joshipura KJ, Ascherio A, Manson JE, et al: Fruit and vegetable intake in relation to risk of ischemic stroke. JAMA 282:1233-1239, 1999.
173. Hu FB, Willett WC: Optimal diets for prevention of coronary heart disease. JAMA 288:2569-2578, 2002.
174. de Lorgeril M, Salen P, Martin JL, et al: Mediterranean diet, traditional risk factors, and the rate of cardiovascular complications after myocardial infarction: Final report of the Lyon Diet Heart Study. Circulation 99:779-785, 1999.
175. Dietary supplementation with n-3 polyunsaturated fatty acids and vitamin E after myocardial infarction: Results of the GISSI-Prevenzione trial. Gruppo Italiano per lo Studio della Sopravvivenza nell'Infarto miocardico. Lancet 354:447-455, 1999.
176. Tribble DL: AHA Science Advisory. Antioxidant consumption and risk of coronary heart disease: Emphasis on vitamin C, vitamin E, and beta-carotene: A statement for healthcare professionals from the American Heart Association. Circulation 99:591-595, 1999.
177. MRC/BHF Heart Protection Study of antioxidant vitamin supplementation in 20,536 high-risk individuals: A randomised placebo-controlled trial. Lancet 360:23-33, 2002.
178. Yusuf S, Dagenais G, Pogue J, et al: Vitamin E supplementation and cardiovascular events in high-risk patients. The Heart Outcomes Prevention Evaluation Study Investigators. N Engl J Med 342:154-160, 2000.
179. Kris-Etherton PM, Harris WS, Appel LJ: Fish consumption, fish oil, omega-3 fatty acids, and cardiovascular disease. Circulation 106:2747-2757, 2002.

Psychosocial Factors

180. Allan R, Scheidt S. Psychosocial factors. *In* Hennekens CH (ed): Clinical Trials in Cardiovascular Disease: A Companion Guide to Braunwald's Heart Disease. Philadelphia, WB Saunders, 1999, pp 315-323.
181. Dusseldorp E, van Elderen T, Maes S, et al: A meta-analysis of psychoeduational programs for coronary heart disease patients. Health Psychol 18:506-519, 1999.
182. Effects of treating depression and low perceived social support on clinical events after myocardial infarction: The Enhancing Recovery in Coronary Heart Disease Patients (ENRICHD) Randomized Trial. JAMA 289:3106-3116, 2003.
183. Glassman AH, O'Connor CM, Califf RM, et al: Sertraline treatment of major depression in patients with acute MI or unstable angina. JAMA 288:701-709, 2002.

Novel Risk Markers

184. Pearson TA, Mensah GA, Alexander RW, et al: Markers of inflammation and cardiovascular disease: Application to clinical and public health practice: A statement for healthcare professionals from the Centers for Disease Control and Prevention and the American Heart Association. Circulation 107:499-511, 2003.
185. Ridker PM: Evaluating novel cardiovascular risk factors: Can we better predict heart attacks? Ann Intern Med 130:933-937, 1999.
186. Libby P, Ridker PM: Novel inflammatory markers of coronary risk: Theory versus practice. Circulation 100:1148-1150, 1999.

Global Risk Modification

187. Ornish D, Hart JA: Multiple risk factor intervention trials. *In* Hennekens CH (ed): Clinical Trials in Cardiovascular Disease: A Companion Guide to Braunwald's Heart Disease. Philadelphia, WB Saunders, 1999, pp 432-446.
188. DeBusk RF, West JA, Miller NH, Taylor CB: Chronic disease management: Treating the patient with disease(s) versus treating disease(s) in the patient. Arch Intern Med 159:2739-2742, 1999.
189. Multiple Risk Factor Intervention Trial. Risk factor changes and mortality results. Multiple Risk Factor Intervention Trial Research Group. JAMA 248:1465-1477, 1982.
190. Hejermann I: A randomized primary preventive trial in coronary heart disease: The Oslo study. Prev Med 12:181-184, 1983.
191. European Collaborative Trial of Multifactorial Prevention of Coronary Heart Disease: Final report on the 6-year results. World Health Organization European Collaborative Group. Lancet 1:869-872,1986.
192. Puska P, Tuomilehto J, Nissinen A, Salonen J: Ten years of the North Karelia project. Acta Med Scand Suppl 701:66-71, 1985.
193. Wilhelmsen L, Berglund G, Elmfeldt D, et al: The Multifactor Primary Prevention Trial in Goteborg, Sweden. Eur Heart J 7:279-288, 1986.
194. Luepker RV, Rastam L, Hannan PJ, et al: Community education for cardiovascular disease prevention. Morbidity and mortality results from the Minnesota Heart Health Program. Am J Epidemiol 144:351-362, 1996.
195. Carelton RA, Lasater TM, Assaf AR et al: The Pawtucket Heart Health Program: Community changes in cardiovascular risk factors and projected disease risk. Am J Public Health 85:777-785, 1995.
196. Farquhar JW, Fortmann SP, Flora JA, et al: Effects of communitywide education on cardiovascular disease risk factors. The Stanford Five-City Project. JAMA 264:359-365, 1990.
197. Niebauer J, Hambrecht R, Velich T, et al: Attenuated progression of coronary artery disease after 6 years of multifactorial risk intervention: Role of physical exercise. Circulation 96:2534-2541, 1997.
198. Haskell WL, Alderman EL, Fair JM, et al: Effects of intensive multiple risk factor reduction on coronary atherosclerosis and clinical cardiac events in men and women with coronary artery disease. The Stanford Coronary Risk Intervention Project (SCRIP). Circulation 89:975-990, 1994.

CHAPTER 43

Comprehensive Rehabilitation of Patients with Cardiovascular Disease

Richard C. Pasternak

Fifty years ago, patients who survived a myocardial infarction were confined to bed for 2 months or longer and then urged to limit their activity indefinitely. Avoidance of physical activity was likewise advocated for those with angina. The realization that bed rest hindered recovery and contributed to complications radically altered the rehabilitation of cardiac patients. Early efforts aimed at progressive activity gradually coalesced into formal cardiac rehabilitation programs. Although such programs initially emphasized exercise training before and after hospital discharge, contemporary programs have evolved into comprehensive multidisciplinary efforts that, in addition to exercise training, include modification of other risk factors as well as personal and vocational adjustment and education.

In the United States alone, well more than 1 million individuals per year become candidates for cardiac rehabilitation.[1] Unfortunately, up to 90 percent of patients who could benefit from cardiac rehabilitation do not get it; of those who do, 25 to 50 percent drop out within weeks to months.[2] Women and older patients are less likely to participate in a program than are men and younger patients.[3]

Numerous factors contribute to this dismal participation rate, including transportation issues, motivation, comorbidities, misunderstanding of the value of these programs, reimbursement issues, and suboptimal referral rates. Of 100 consecutive patients undergoing coronary artery bypass grafting (CABG) at a major teaching hospital, 78 percent of those who did not participate in a cardiac rehabilitation program cited lack of physician referral.[4]

HISTORY OF CARDIAC REHABILITATION

Until fairly recently, the treatment of patients with heart disease generally followed this Hippocratic suggestion: "In every movement of the body, whenever one begins to endure pain, it will be relieved by rest."[5] By the time Herrick clinically described the link between coronary thrombosis and myocardial infarction in 1912,[6] absolute bed rest for 6 to 8 weeks was the standard first step in recovery and rehabilitation. Lewis, for example, recommended that during this period, "the patient is to be guarded by day and night nursing and helped in every way to avoid voluntary movement or effort."[7] The rationale for immobility was that exertion could lead to ventricular aneurysm formation and ventricular rupture, and the hypoxia associated with exertion could lead to arrhythmia, recurrent myocardial infarction, or sudden death. Following discharge from the hospital, even moderately stressful activity such as climbing stairs was discouraged for a year or more, and return to work or normal activity was the exception rather than the rule.[8]

Dramatic successes in medical rehabilitation achieved during the course of World War II[8] helped clinicians question the benefits of extended immobility. Vilifying extended bed rest as something that "saps morale, provokes desperation, unleashes anxiety, and ushers in hopelessness of the capacity of resuming a normal life,"[9] Levine advocated limited early activity after myocardial infarction. Early mobilization first took the form of "chair therapy," described by Levine and Lown in 1951. It encouraged patients to sit in a chair for 1 to 2 hours a day as soon as the first day following myocardial infarction.[10] Other attempts at early mobilization coupled with results from the Dallas Bed Rest Study[11] demonstrating that deconditioning was associated with greater immobility gradually began to convince clinicians that early mobilization was beneficial rather than harmful. By the early 1970s, clinical practice in the United States varied considerably—the duration of enforced bed rest varied from 1 day to 4 weeks after myocardial infarction and the duration of hospitalization varied from 2 to 6 weeks.[12]

Early mobilization came to be called phase I or inpatient cardiac rehabilitation.[13] Its goal was to condition the patient to carry out safely activities of daily living following discharge. Such programs entailed prescribing activity in rigid steps with successively higher metabolic equivalents (METs). Early phase I programs included up to 14 separate steps.[12] Comprehensive rehabilitation programs eventually grew to include four phases (Table 43-1).

Early rehabilitation programs focused almost exclusively on exercise. Over time they have evolved to encompass what the World Health Organization called the "sum of activity required to ensure cardiac patients the best possible physical, mental, and social conditions so that [patients] may, by their own efforts, regain as normal as possible a place in the community and lead an active life."[14]

Contemporary Cardiac Rehabilitation

Although exercise remains a central part of modern cardiac rehabilitation, it has broadened to include all relevant aspects of secondary prevention (Table 43–2). In addition to risk factor management, the goals of such a secondary prevention program include reduction in both symptoms and risk of premature death and improvement in quality of life. Strategies to improve adherence to all medical therapies and life-style changes are employed. An additional goal is to provide information to patients' family members and others.

TABLE 43–1 Traditional Terminology for the Phases of Cardiac Rehabilitation
Phase I Inpatient rehabilitation, usually lasting for the duration of hospitalization. It emphasizes a gradual, progressive approach to exercise and an education program that helps the patient understand the disease process, the rehabilitation process, and initial preventive efforts to slow the progression of disease.
Phase II Multifaceted outpatient rehabilitation, lasting 2 to 3 mo. Emphasizes safe physical activity to improve conditioning with continued behavior modification aimed at smoking cessation, weight loss, healthy eating, and other factors to reduce disease risk. Initiate an exercise prescription.
Phase III Supervised rehabilitation, lasting 6 to 12 mo. Establishes a prescription for safe exercise that can be performed at home or in a community service facility, such as a senior center or YMCA, and continues to emphasize risk factor reduction.
Phase IV Maintenance, indefinite

Modern rehabilitation programs generally include three stages: inpatient rehabilitation, outpatient rehabilitation, and maintenance (Fig. 43–1). Responsibilities may lie with different or overlapping groups, e.g., a physical therapy department for an inpatient program and a nurse-managed cardiac rehabilitation specialist for an outpatient program. Because hospital stays after uncomplicated acute myocardial infarction or cardiac procedures have decreased in the United States, comprehensive inpatient rehabilitation is not possible. It is still routine, however, in many other countries. Outpatient programs are traditionally conducted in hospital-based cardiac rehabilitation centers. Community-based centers or home-based programs can also provide a beneficial experience for selected and motivated patients.[15,16]

Inpatient Cardiac Rehabilitation

As soon as it is safe to do so when a patient has been stabilized after initial treatment of an acute coronary syndrome or CABG, he or she should be encouraged to sit in a chair and begin to take a few steps, even in intensive care units. Limited range-of-motion exercises are also advisable, except in unstable patients. When the patient has been transferred out of intensive care, assisted walking should be encouraged unless the patient remains symptomatic. Activity levels are gradually increased during hospitalization with encouragement to perform activities of daily living. Pharmacological therapies to improve the patient's risk factor profile and improve long-term event-free survival should be initiated in the hospital or at discharge.

Short stays make it difficult to do more than introduce patients to the disease process, the factors that maintain it, and strategies for reducing risk. Patients should, however, become familiar with the symptoms of recurrent ischemia, heart failure, and hypertension and should be instructed in the proper response to symptoms if they arise. They should also be provided with key telephone numbers of the responsible physician as well as other important contacts, including hospitals and cardiac rehabilitation programs.

Patients are often overwhelmed during the hospital stay by the volume of new information they must assimilate. Thus, an appropriate trend in inpatient programs is an emphasis on evaluation of risks and a focus on referral to and participation in an appropriate outpatient cardiac rehabilitation program.

Outpatient Cardiac Rehabilitation

The traditional outpatient cardiac rehabilitation model is a formal, institution-based program conducted by a team of rehabilitation professionals. Current programs include efforts that were once accomplished as part of phase II and phase III programs (see Fig. 43–1). Programs now offer the structure, support, and feedback that many individuals need in order to make important behavioral changes (see Table 43–2).

Alternatives to Hospital-Based Cardiac Rehabilitation

Because enrollment in traditional hospital-based cardiac rehabilitation programs is suboptimal, relatively costly, and, under some circumstances, not reimbursed by insurance, a number of alternative models have been devised and tested. These include modified protocols with early transition to community-based or independent programs; physician-supervised, nurse-managed programs; community-based programs supervised by exercise physiologists guided by a computerized management system based on national guidelines; and home-based programs. Small, randomized trials suggest that such alternatives may be as effective as a hospital-based rehabilitation program for some patients.[15-17]

Maintenance

Following more structured outpatient programs are long-term "maintenance" programs, often conducted in the same facilities as structured programs but with fewer staff. In the absence of formal guidelines or reimbursement for these programs, there is less consistency to what they offer. The model for many programs is a supervised health club, for which patients pay a monthly fee.

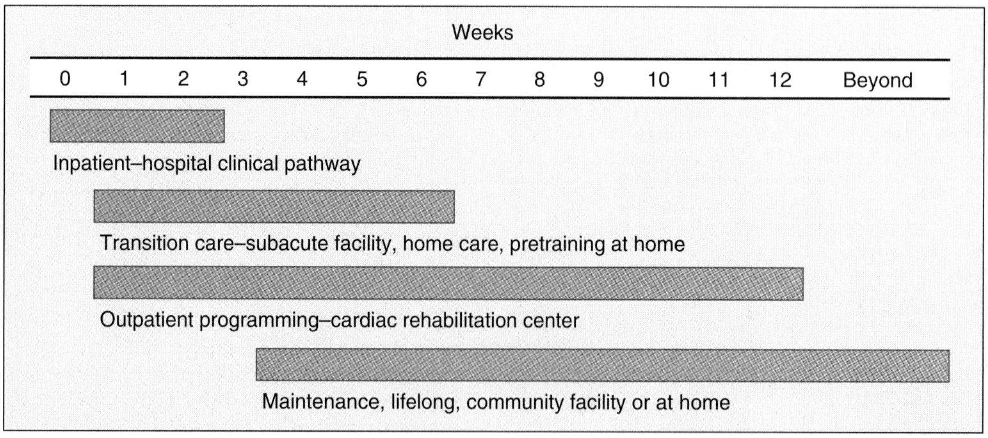

FIGURE 43–1 Recommended continuum of care for cardiac rehabilitative services.

Evidence Base for Cardiac Rehabilitation

Considerably less clinical research has been focused on cardiac rehabilitation than

TABLE 43–2 Components of Cardiac Rehabilitation and Associated Goals

Initial Evaluation
Take medical history and perform physical examination
Measure risk factors
Obtain electrocardiograms at rest and during exercise
Provide vocational counseling
Determine level of risk
Goal: formulation of preventive plan in collaboration with primary care physician
Management of Lipid Levels
Assess and modify diet, physical activity, and drug therapy
Primary goal: LDL cholesterol level < 100 mg/dl
Secondary goals: non-HDL cholesterol level < 130 mg/dl, HDL cholesterol level > 45 mg/dl, triglyceride level < 200 mg/dl
Management of Hypertension
Measure blood pressure frequently at rest and during exercise
If resting systolic pressure is 130 to 139 mm Hg or diastolic pressure is 85 to 89 mm Hg, recommend life-style modifications, including exercise, weight management, sodium restriction, and moderation of alcohol intake; if patient has diabetes or chronic renal or heart failure, consider drug therapy
If resting systolic pressure is ≥140 mm Hg or diastolic pressure is ≥90 mm Hg, recommend drug therapy
Monitor effects of intervention in collaboration with primary care physician
Goal: blood pressure < 140/90 mm Hg (or < 130/85 mm Hg if patient has diabetes or chronic heart or renal failure); optimal < 120/80 mm Hg
Cessation of Smoking
Document smoking status (never smoked, stopped smoking in remote past, stopped smoking recently, or currently smokes)
Determine patient's readiness to quit; if ready, pick a date for quitting
Offer nicotine replacement therapy, bupropion, or both
Offer behavioral advice and group or individual counseling
Goal: long-term abstinence
Weight Reduction
Consider for patients with BMI > 25 or waist circumference > 102 cm (in men) or > 88 cm (in women), particularly if associated with hypertension, hyperlipidemia, or insulin resistance or diabetes
Provide behavioral and nutritional counseling with follow-up to monitor progress in achieving goals
Goals: loss of 5 to 10% of body weight and modification of associated risk factors
Management of Diabetes
Identify candidates on the basis of the medical history and baseline glucose test
Develop a regimen of dietary modification, weight control, and exercise combined with oral hypoglycemic agents and insulin therapy
Monitor glucose control before and after exercise sessions and communicate results to primary care physician
For newly detected diabetes, refer patient to primary care physician for evaluation and treatment
Goals: normalization of fasting plasma glucose level (80 to 110 mg/dl) or glycosylated hemoglobin level (<7.0%) and control of associated obesity, hypertension, and hyperlipidemia
Psychosocial Management
Identify psychosocial problems such as depression, anxiety, social isolation, anger, and hostility by means of an interview, standardized questionnaires, or both
Provide individual or group counseling, or both, for patients with clinically significant psychosocial problems
Provide stress reduction classes for patients
Goal: absence of clinically significant psychosocial problems and acquisition of stress management skills
Physical Activity Counseling and Exercise Training
Assess current physical activity and exercise tolerance with monitored exercise stress test
Identify barriers to increased physical activity
Provide advice regarding increasing physical activity
Develop an individualized regimen of aerobic and resistance training, specifying frequency, intensity, duration, and types of exercise
Goals: increases in regular physical activity, strength, and physical functioning, expenditure of at least 1000 kcal/wk in physical activity

BMI = body mass index; HDL = high-density lipoprotein; LDL = low-density lipoprotein.

Adapted from Balady GJ, Ades PA, Comoss P, et al: Core components of cardiac rehabilitation/secondary prevention programs: A statement for healthcare professionals from the American Heart Association and the American Association of Cardiovascular and Pulmonary Rehabilitation Writing Group. Circulation 102:1069, 2000.

on many other areas of cardiology. Yet, we possess sufficient evidence upon which to base recommendations for rehabilitation following acute myocardial infarction, CABG, or percutaneous coronary intervention. In 1995, the federal Agency for Health Care Policy Research issued a clinical practice guideline with the Public Health Service and the National Heart, Lung, and Blood Institute.[2] Standards for exercise training relevant to cardiac rehabilitation have been issued and updated by the American Heart Association.[18]

Numerous randomized clinical trials of exercise-based cardiac rehabilitation have been conducted in North America and Europe. Although they have generally demonstrated a trend toward reduced mortality, virtually all of these trials had insufficient statistical power to demonstrate the efficacy of cardiac rehabilitation.

Two early meta-analyses that each included approximately 4500 patients concluded that exercise-based cardiac rehabilitation reduced both total and cardiac mortality by 20 to 25 percent but had little effect on nonfatal myocardial infarction or sudden death.[19,20] In a 19-year follow-up of one of the trials included in these meta-analyses, the U.S. National Exercise and Heart Disease Project, all-cause mortality risk estimates were nonsignificantly lower in the intervention group after 3 years (relative risk, 0.69; 95 percent confidence interval [CI], 0.39 to 1.25) but rose gradually with increased follow-up—0.84 after 5 years, 0.95 after 10 years, 1.02 after 15 years, and 1.09 after 19 years.[21] These results suggest either that protective mechanisms associated with cardiac rehabilitation operate in the short term or that patients stop performing the protective activities they engaged in as part of the program.

The latest meta-analysis of exercise-based cardiac rehabilitation, conducted for the Cochrane Collaboration (Fig. 43–2),[22] adds approximately 4000 patients to the prior meta-analyses. Using data from 36 trials and almost 8500 patients, the investigators were able to analyze separately exercise-only and comprehensive programs. The pooled effect estimate for total mortality demonstrated a 27 percent reduction in total mortality for the exercise-only programs (odds ratio [OR], 0.73; 95 percent CI, 0.54 to 0.98) and a 13 percent reduction for comprehensive interventions (OR, 0.87; 95 percent CI, 0.71 to 1.05). The exercise-only interventions appeared to reduce total cardiac mortality slightly more than comprehensive interventions (OR, 0.69; 95 percent CI, 0.51 to 0.94 for exercise only and OR, 0.74; 95 percent CI, 0.57 to 0.96 for comprehensive programs). Neither had an effect on nonfatal myocardial infarction. In addition to confirming the results of the prior meta-analyses that exercise-based cardiac rehabilitation reduces cardiac mortality without reducing the risk of recurrent infarction, the work by Jolliffe and colleagues supports the role of exercise as a critical component of rehabilitation.[22]

Most of the studies in the three meta-analyses preceded widespread use of acute thrombolytic therapy, primary angioplasty, and early revascularization as well as standard secondary prevention therapies including statins and angiotensin-converting enzyme (ACE) inhibitors. Thus, trials that include contemporary rehabilitation programs and emphasize adherence to comprehensive secondary prevention efforts might show greater effects on total and cardiovascular mortality and also affect recurrent myocardial infarction.

Exercise training can affect cardiovascular and overall health in numerous ways. Smoking cessation has an almost immediate effect on cardiovascular health. Even modest reductions in blood pressure result in a 15 percent reduction in the risk of coronary heart disease (CHD) events and a 42 percent reduction in risk of stroke.[23] Reducing serum cholesterol by 10 percent reduces the risk of a CHD event by 15 percent.[24] Among overweight individuals, modest weight loss corresponding to 5 to 10 percent of starting body weight is associated with significant improvements in blood pressure, serum lipids, and glucose tolerance or insulin resistance, or both.[25] (See Chaps. 41 and 42 for details of risk reduction for specific factors.)

A prospective, 1-year controlled study demonstrated the beneficial effects of early short-term intensive cardiac rehabilitation on traditional cardiac risk factors. Within 1 to 4 weeks of hospital discharge for acute myocardial infarction or CABG, 109 patients began a multidisciplinary ambulatory cardiac rehabilitation program. At the study's end, 9 to 10 months later, there was a high rate of aspirin intake, a low rate of smoking (14 percent of the patients), a 15 percent increase in physical capacity, a decrease in resting heart rate of 7 beats/min, and a 4 mg/dl increase in high-density lipoprotein (HDL) cholesterol.[26]

In summary, the aggregate evidence from randomized controlled trials demonstrates that exercise-based cardiac rehabilitation can prevent premature morbidity and mortality. Although there is insufficient evidence to determine whether interventions that include exercise and comprehensive risk factor reduction are the equivalent of exercise-only interventions, most studies were conducted before the current era of aggressive management of coronary disease and newer secondary prevention strategies. Given that the age of large prospective randomized trials for cardiac rehabilitation is probably over, cost, local access to available services, and national consensus guidelines are likely to drive clinicians' choices.

Components of a Cardiac Rehabilitation Program

It is now widely recognized that cardiac rehabilitation and comprehensive secondary rehabilitation programs are integral to the complete management of patients with cardiovascular disease. The most comprehensive statement addressing the core requirements came from the American Association of Cardiovascular and Pulmonary Rehabilitation[27] and has been reviewed and endorsed by the American College of Cardiology and the American Heart Association (see Table 43–2).

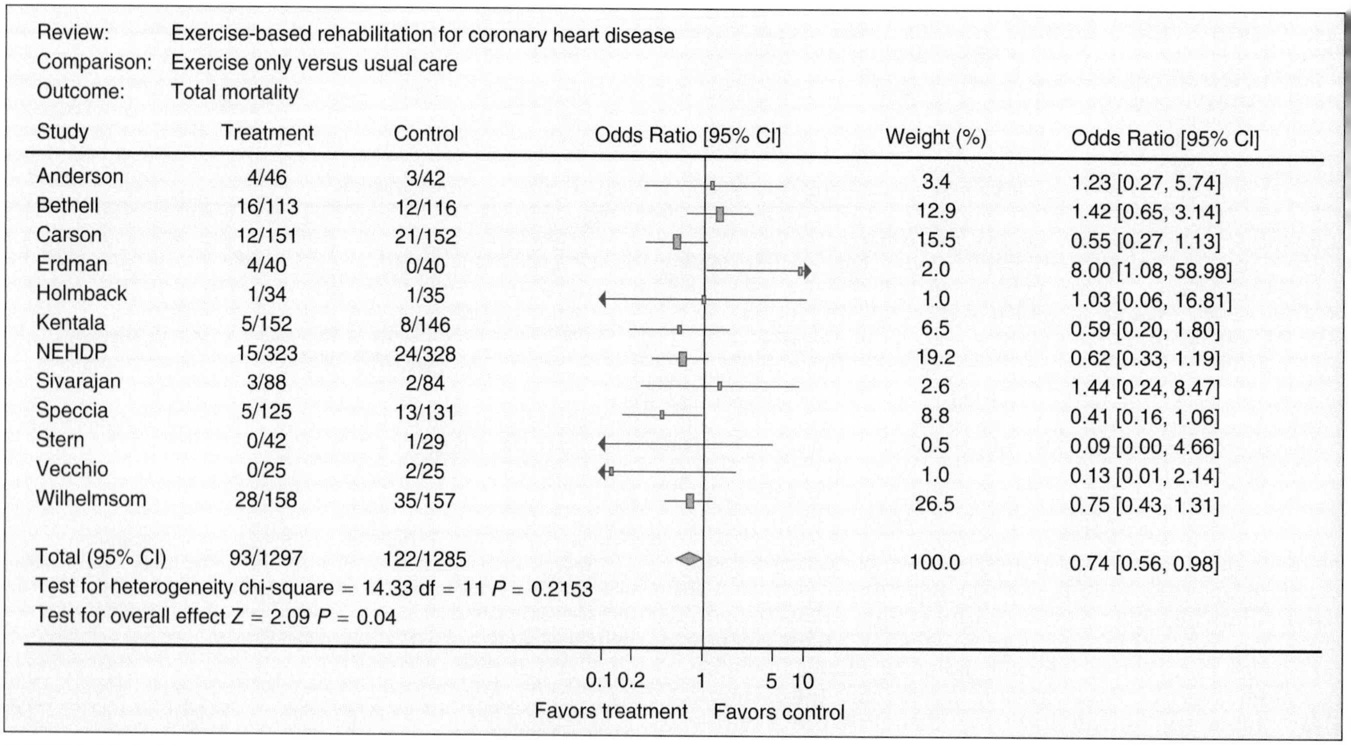
Review: Exercise-based rehabilitation for coronary heart disease
Comparison: Exercise only versus usual care
Outcome: Total mortality
Study | Treatment | Control | Odds Ratio [95% CI] | Weight (%) | Odds Ratio [95% CI]
Anderson 4/46 3/42 3.4 1.23 [0.27, 5.74]
Bethell 16/113 12/116 12.9 1.42 [0.65, 3.14]
Carson 12/151 21/152 15.5 0.55 [0.27, 1.13]
Erdman 4/40 0/40 2.0 8.00 [1.08, 58.98]
Holmback 1/34 1/35 1.0 1.03 [0.06, 16.81]
Kentala 5/152 8/146 6.5 0.59 [0.20, 1.80]
NEHDP 15/323 24/328 19.2 0.62 [0.33, 1.19]
Sivarajan 3/88 2/84 2.6 1.44 [0.24, 8.47]
Speccia 5/125 13/131 8.8 0.41 [0.16, 1.06]
Stern 0/42 1/29 0.5 0.09 [0.00, 4.66]
Vecchio 0/25 2/25 1.0 0.13 [0.01, 2.14]
Wilhelmsom 28/158 35/157 26.5 0.75 [0.43, 1.31]
Total (95% CI) 93/1297 122/1285 100.0 0.74 [0.56, 0.98]
Test for heterogeneity chi-square = 14.33 df = 11 P = 0.2153
Test for overall effect Z = 2.09 P = 0.04
0.1 0.2 1 5 10
Favors treatment
Favors control

FIGURE 43–2 Meta-analysis of the effect of exercise-based rehabilitation for coronary heart disease on mortality. For information on individual studies listed (left-hand column), see references. (From Jolliffe JA, Rees K, Taylor RS, et al: Exercise-based rehabilitation for coronary heart disease. Cochrane Database Syst Rev [1]:CD001800, 2001 [jajollif@exeter.ac.uk].)

Exercise

Definition of Terms

A variety of terms are used to describe exercise-related activity, often with overlapping definitions. The following are used in this chapter:

- *Physical activity.* Any body movement produced by skeletal muscles that results in energy expenditure beyond resting expenditure.
- *Exercise.* Physical activity that is planned, structured, repetitive, and purposeful, usually aimed at improving or maintaining physical fitness.
- *Physical fitness.* Attributes that people have or achieve related to the ability to perform physical activity, including cardiorespiratory fitness, muscle strength, body composition, and flexibility.
- *Dose.* The total amount of energy expended in physical activity.
- *Intensity.* The absolute or relative rate of energy expenditure during activity. Absolute intensity reflects the rate of energy expenditure during exercise and is usually expressed in metabolic equivalents (METs). Relative intensity refers to the percentage of aerobic power utilized during exercise and is usually expressed as percentage of maximal heart rate or percentage of maximum oxygen consumption ($\dot{V}O_{2max}$) (Table 43–3).
- *Metabolic equivalents.* One MET equals the resting metabolic rate of 3.5 ml O_2/kg/min (Table 43–4).
- *Moderate-intensity activity.* Activity performed at a relative intensity of 40 to 60 percent of $\dot{V}O_{2max}$ or an absolute intensity of 4 to 6 METs.
- *Vigorous-intensity activity.* Activity performed at a relative intensity of greater than 60 percent of $\dot{V}O_{2max}$ or an absolute intensity greater than 6 METs.

Exercise Physiology

Exercise induces a large increase in cardiac output that provides for the metabolic needs of exercising muscles, prevents hyperthermia, and ensures adequate blood flow to essential organs. This increase results from changes in both heart rate and stroke volume.

HEART RATE. Within seconds of increased physical activity, the heart rate begins to increase. During strenuous activity, heart rate can attain values of 160 to 180 beats/min. Rates as high as 240 beats/min have been observed during short periods of maximal exercise. Vagal withdrawal rather than an increase in sympathetic tone is the likely cause of the almost instantaneous acceleration in heart rate with exercise, whereas later increases stem from reflex activation of pulmonary stretch receptors and increased levels of circulating adrenal catecholamines. The increase in heart rate during exercise accounts for more of the increase in cardiac output than does the increase in stroke volume. Stroke volume normally reaches its maximum when cardiac output has increased by only half its maximum, and further increases in cardiac output occur by increasing the heart rate alone.

STROKE VOLUME. Exercise affects both physiological mechanisms that influence stroke volume—increased venous return (increased preload) and more forceful contractions (increased inotropy). In the upright position at rest, the diminished venous return to the heart (compared with the supine position) results in smaller stroke volume and cardiac output. During upright exercise, however, stroke volume can approach the maximum stroke volume observed in the recumbent position, achieved in part by increased venous tone and skeletal muscle compression. Exercise also increases inotropy because of catecholamine release.

DISTRIBUTION OF CARDIAC OUTPUT. Sympathetic activity dominates during exercise. Increases in plasma norepinephrine and epinephrine levels constrict the majority of vascular beds, except those in the exercising muscles and the coronary and cerebral circulations. During light and moderate exercise, cutaneous blood flow increases to facilitate body cooling, whereas more vigorous exercise causes a progressive decrease in skin flow. The kidneys and splanchnic tissue can tolerate considerable reductions in blood flow through increased extraction of oxygen from the available blood supply. The heart's limited reserve—it extracts approximately 75 percent of the oxygen in the coronary blood flow at rest—requires that it meet increased oxygen demands during exercise by an increase in coronary blood flow. Cerebral blood flow also increases during exercise.

The cessation of exercise rapidly decreases heart rate and cardiac output because of a decrease in sympathetic drive and the reactivation of vagal activity, while systemic vascular resistance remains lower for some time. As a result, arterial pressure often falls to below preexercise levels for several hours after exercise and then returns to normal levels.

CARDIOVASCULAR RESPONSE TO DIFFERENT TYPES OF EXERCISE. Contraction of large muscle groups that results in movement (*isotonic exercise*) places a volume load on the heart reflected by significant increases in both cardiac output and oxygen consumption and a fall in systemic vascular resistance. Constant muscular contraction of smaller

TABLE 43–3 Classification of Physical Activity Intensity

	Relative Intensity			Endurance-Type Activity, Absolute Intensity in Healthy Adults (age), METS					Strength-Type Exercise/Relative Intensity*
Intensity	$\dot{V}O_{2max}$† (%)	Maximum Heart Rate‡ (%)	RPE§	Young (20-39)	Middle-Aged (40-64)	Old (65-79)	Very Old (80+)	RPE§	Maximum Voluntary Contraction
Very light	<20	<35	<10	<2.4	<2.0	<1.6	<1.0	<10	<30
Light	20-39	35-54	10-11	2.4-4.7	2.0-3.9	1.6-3.1	1.1-1.9	10-11	30-49
Moderate	40-59	55-69	12-13	4.8-7.1	4.0-5.9	3.2-4.7	2.0-2.9	12-13	50-69
Hard	60-84	70-89	14-16	7.2-10.1	6.0-8.4	4.8-6.7	3.0-4.25	14-16	70-84
Very hard	≥85	≥90	17-19	≥10.2	≥8.5	≥6.8	≥4.25	17-19	≥85
Maximum‖	100	100	20	12.0	10.0	8.0	5.0	20	100

MET = metabolic equivalent.

From Fletcher GF, Balady GJ, Amsterdam EA, et al: Exercise standards for testing and training: A statement for healthcare professionals from the American Heart Association. Circulation 104:1694, 2001.

*Based on 8 to 12 repetitions for persons younger than 50 to 60 years and 10 to 15 repetitions for persons older than 50 to 60 years.

†$\dot{V}O_2$, measured oxygen intake.

‡Maximum heart rate indicates 220 minus age or peak heart rate on exercise test.

§Borg rating of relative perceived exertion (RPE), scale of 6 to 20.

‖Maximum values are mean values achieved during maximum exercise by healthy adults. Absolute intensity values are approximate mean values for men. Mean values for women are approximately 1 to 2 METs lower than those for men.

TABLE 43–4 Energy Requirements of Common Daily Activities*

Activities	METs
Leisure activities	
Mild	
Playing the piano	2.3
Canoeing (leisurely)	2.5
Golf (with cart)	2.5
Walking (2 mph)	2.5
Dancing (ballroom)	2.9
Moderate	
Walking (3 mph)	3.3
Cycling (leisurely)	3.5
Calisthenics (no weight)	4.0
Golf (without cart)	4.4
Swimming (slow)	4.5
Walking (4 mph)	4.5
Vigorous	
Chopping wood	4.9
Tennis (doubles)	5.0
Ballroom (fast) or square dancing	5.5
Cycling (moderately)	5.7
Skiing (water or downhill)	6.8
Climbing hills (no load)	6.9
Swimming	7.0
Walking (5 mph)	8.0
Jogging (10-min mile)	10.2
Rope skipping	12.0
Squash	12.1
Activities of daily living	
Lying quietly	1.0
Sitting; light activity	1.5
Walking from house to car or bus	2.5
Watering plants	2.5
Loading and unloading car	3.0
Taking out trash	3.0
Walking the dog	3.0
Household tasks, moderate effort	3.5
Vacuuming	3.5
Lifting items continuously	4.0
Raking lawn	4.0
Gardening (no lifting)	4.4
Mowing lawn (power mower)	4.5

MET = metabolic equivalent or a unit of sitting, resting oxygen uptake.
*These activities can often be done at variable intensities, assuming that the intensity is not excessive and that the courses are flat (no hills) unless so specified. Categories are based on experience or tolerance; if an activity is perceived to be more than indicated, it should be judged accordingly.

muscle groups without movement (*isometric exercise*) tends to exert a pressure load rather than a volume load on the heart that is characterized by increases in systemic vascular resistance and blood pressure with minimal changes in cardiac output and oxygen consumption. *Resistance exercises* such as weight lifting produce muscular contraction with movement and thus, depending on intensity, can produce both volume and pressure loads. Most activities usually combine all three types of exercise.

CHRONIC ADAPTATIONS TO EXERCISE. Over time, regular exercise increases the ability of the cardiovascular system to deliver oxygen to the tissues while at the same time improving the ability of muscles to use oxygen. The combination of increased cardiac output and peripheral adaptations that improve oxygen extraction associated with regular exercise can increase maximum oxygen consumption twofold to threefold. Regular exercise also reduces resting heart rate and blood pressure. By improving functional work capacity, it also reduces the metabolic and circulatory demands of activities of daily living.

Possible Biological Mechanisms for the Benefits of Exercise (Table 43–5)

Physical activity appears to lower cardiovascular disease risk by effects on traditional coronary risk factors, as discussed

TABLE 43–5 Possible Mechanisms for Exercise-Induced Reductions in Morbidity and Mortality

Cardiovascular influences
Reduction of resting and exercise heart rates
Reduction of resting and exercise blood pressures
Reduction of myocardial oxygen demand at submaximal levels of physical activity
Expansion of plasma volume
Increase in myocardial contractility
Increase in peripheral venous tone
Favorable changes in fibrinolytic system
Increased endothelium-dependent vasodilation
Increased gene expression for nitric oxide synthase
Enhanced parasympathetic tone
Possible increases in coronary blood flow, coronary collateral vessels, and myocardial capillary density
Metabolic influences
Reduction of obesity
Enhanced glucose tolerance
Improved lipid profile
Life-style influences
Decreased likelihood of smoking
Possible reduction of stress, depression
Short-term reduction of appetite

From Shephard RJ, Balady GJ: Exercise as cardiovascular therapy. Circulation 99:963, 1999.

subsequently. Regular exercise may also improve fibrinolytic and endothelial vasodilator function.

WEIGHT. Exercise by itself yields modest weight loss, with exercise randomized clinical trials showing losses of 2 to 3 kg in the exercise group. However, exercise appears to complement dietary approaches to weight loss—the combination achieves an average weight loss of 8.5 kg.[28] Exercise may play an even more important role in maintenance of weight loss. A meta-analysis of studies of long-term weight loss maintenance found that groups who exercised more had significantly greater weight loss maintenance than those who exercised less.[29] Exercise also improves body composition and fat distribution, both of which are linked to cardiovascular mortality.[30]

BLOOD PRESSURE. Cohort and clinical studies indicate that exercise reduces blood pressure independent of weight loss. A meta-analysis of 54 randomized, controlled trials that included 2419 participants whose intervention and control groups differed only in aerobic exercise demonstrated a clear association between exercise and blood pressure. Aerobic exercise was associated with a 3.84 mm Hg (95 percent CI, 4.97 to 2.72 mm Hg) reduction in mean systolic blood pressure and a 2.58 mm Hg (95 percent CI, 3.35 to 1.81 mm Hg) reduction in diastolic blood pressure. Reductions occurred in men and women, hypertensive and normotensive participants, and overweight and normal-weight participants.[31] The reduction in blood pressure related to aerobic exercise did not differ significantly according to frequency or intensity of aerobic exercise.

DIABETES MELLITUS. Physical activity has beneficial effects on both glucose metabolism and insulin sensitivity.[32] Even moderate-intensity activities such as walking are associated with both prevention of diabetes[33] and reductions in cardiovascular disease and mortality among individuals with diabetes.[34,35] The Diabetes Prevention Program demonstrated the powerful effect that physical activity and weight loss can exert in preventing the onset of type 2 diabetes in individuals at high risk for this disease. Compared with usual care, there was a 58 percent reduction in the onset of type 2 diabetes over 2.8 years among individuals randomly assigned to a life-style intervention that produced an average

4-kg decrease in body weight and an 8-MET-hr/wk increase in physical activity.[36]

LIPIDS. Despite the extensive research focused on the effects of exercise on lipid levels, the benefits of exercise are not precisely known owing to the heterogeneity of study methods, populations, and exercise interventions. A meta-analysis of 52 exercise training trials lasting more than 12 weeks that included 4700 subjects demonstrated an average 4.6 percent increase in HDL levels and reductions in triglyceride and low-density lipoprotein (LDL) concentrations of 3.7 and 5.0 percent, respectively.[37] In the largest and most carefully controlled of these trials, the *HE*alth, *RI*sk factors, Exercise *T*raining, *A*nd *GE*netics (HERITAGE) study, 5 months of exercise training among 675 normolipidemic subjects induced a 1.1-mg/dl increase in HDL among men along with a 5.9-mg/dl decrease in triglycerides and a 0.9-mg/dl decrease in LDL. Among women, HDL increased 1.4 mg/dl, triglycerides decreased 0.6 mg/dl, and LDL decreased 4.4 mg/dl.[38] It is possible that larger exercise-related increases in HDL may occur in individuals with baseline hypertriglyceridemia or in studies of longer duration, but few studies have addressed the effect of exercise in subjects with lipid disorders.

Exercise may also alter the distribution of lipid fractions. Among 111 sedentary, overweight men and women with mild to moderate dyslipidemia randomly assigned to 8 months of exercise or a nonexercise control group, exercising at a caloric equivalent of 17 to 18 miles per week at an intensity equivalent to that of jogging at a moderate pace significantly decreased the concentrations of both small LDL and total LDL particles and increased the average size of LDL particles without changing the plasma LDL cholesterol concentration. The total HDL concentration, concentration of large HDL particles, and average size of HDL particles were also increased, whereas the concentrations of triglycerides and total very low-density lipoprotein triglycerides decreased.[39] The dose of exercise appeared to contribute more to plasma lipoprotein concentrations than the intensity of exercise.

A patient's genotype may influence the impact of exercise duration or intensity on cardiovascular risk factors. Exerting a larger fraction of the total energy expenditure in high-intensity activities, for example, may lead to greater improvements in HDL and triglycerides among individuals with the ApoE4 allele.[40]

THROMBOSIS. Exercise training favorably affects the fibrinolytic system by reducing plasma fibrinogen and plasminogen activator inhibitor-1 levels and increasing tissue plasminogen activator (t-PA) levels. Among 3810 British men observed for 20 years after an initial screening, physical activity showed an inverse dose-response relationship with fibrinogen, plasma and blood viscosity, platelet count, coagulation factors VIII and IX, von Willebrand factor, fibrin D-dimer, tissue plasminogen activator antigen, C-reactive protein, and white cell count.[41] Among sedentary older men, 3 months of aerobic exercise increased endothelial capacity to release t-PA by 55 percent to levels similar to those of young adults and older endurance-trained men.[42] Acute exercise may increase platelet activation and reactivity, especially in sedentary individuals, and thus increase the risk of myocardial infarction or unstable angina. Regular exercise, in comparison, appears to reduce platelet aggregability.

ENDOTHELIAL FUNCTION. Arterial tone and platelet aggregation depend in part on release of nitric oxide from the vascular endothelium. Patients with atherosclerosis or coronary risk factors have impaired endothelium-dependent dilation. Exercise can limit or reverse this dysfunction among patients with coronary disease,[43,44] peripheral arterial disease,[45] heart failure,[46] and diabetes.[47]

AUTONOMIC FUNCTION. Heart rate is modulated by the interplay between sympathetic and parasympathetic activity. Chronic activation of the sympathetic nervous system or neutralization of parasympathetic (vagal) tone, or both, increases the risk of adverse cardiovascular events as well as mortality, especially among patients with heart disease.[48] One measure of autonomic function is heart rate variability. Low heart rate variability has been associated with increased risk of CHD and mortality.[49] Among healthy older adults[50] and those with coronary disease, exercise training significantly improves heart rate variability.[51]

Benefits of Exercise

Data from more than 40 observational studies demonstrate clear evidence of an inverse linear dose-response relation between volume of physical activity and all-cause mortality rates in younger and older men and women. Minimal adherence to current physical activity guidelines, which yield an energy expenditure of about 1000 kcal/wk, is associated with a significant 20 to 30 percent reduction in risk of all-cause mortality.[52]

Exercise capacity is an important prognostic factor in patients with cardiovascular disease. It also predicts mortality among individuals with symptoms that suggested CHD. Among 6213 consecutive men referred for treadmill exercise testing for clinical reasons and observed for a mean of 6.2 years, peak exercise capacity measured in METs was the strongest predictor of the risk of death among both normal subjects and those with cardiovascular disease. Each 1-MET increase in exercise capacity conferred a 12 percent improvement in survival.[53]

Exercise training is useful for patients with angina pectoris who are not candidates for revascularization or who choose not to have it. The symptomatic improvement in exercise tolerance after exercise training results primarily from a reduction in the heart rate and systolic blood pressure or rate-pressure product at submaximal workloads. It is also possible that exercise training improves myocardial oxygen delivery by altering the coronary vasomotor response to exercise.[43]

Although no large studies have directly addressed the benefits of exercise training following coronary revascularization, it is likely to be beneficial in this population as well. The Exercise Training Intervention after Coronary Angioplasty (ETICA) trial randomly assigned 118 consecutive patients to 6 months of exercise training or a control group. Trained patients demonstrated a significant 26 percent increase in peak O_2 and improvement in quality of life.[54] Over almost 3 years of follow-up, the exercise-trained patients had fewer cardiac events (11.9 versus 32.2 percent) and hospital readmissions (18.6 versus 46 percent) than subjects assigned to usual care. In the trained subjects, residual coronary stenosis was reduced by 30 percent and recurrent cardiac events by 29 percent.

Exercise Testing

Exercise testing (see Chap. 10) offers important information regarding a patient's cardiovascular status. Determination of functional capacity in patients referred for cardiac rehabilitation is essential for developing an appropriate exercise prescription (Table 43–6). Thus, exercise testing may be performed as part of cardiac rehabilitation to provide necessary information for the development of the exercise prescription, to assess the impact of exercise training occurring as part of the cardiac rehabilitation program, and to provide feedback to the patient.[55]

Principles of Exercise Prescription

Exercise therapy must be individualized on the basis of the patient's specific characteristics, abilities, and comorbidities. In fact, much like pharmacological therapy, it requires a prescription with a careful consideration of both appropriate dosage and possible side effects (see Table 43–6).

TABLE 43–6 Exercise Prescription for Endurance and Resistance Training

Endurance Training	
Frequency	3-5 d/wk
Intensity	See Table 43–3 and text
Duration	20-60 min
Modality	
Lower extremity	Walking Jogging/running Stairclimber Cycling
Upper extremity	Arm ergometry
Combined	Rowing Cross-country ski machine Combined arm-leg cycle Swimming Aerobics
Resistance Training	
Frequency	2-3 d/wk
Intensity	1-3 sets of 8-15 RM for each muscle group
Modality	
Lower extremity	Legs extensions, curls, presses Adductors-abductors
Upper extremity	Biceps curls Triceps extensions Bench-overhead presses Lateral pulldowns-raises Benchovers–seated rowing

RM = maximum number of times a load can lifted before fatigue.

From Shephard RJ, Balady GJ: Exercise as cardiovascular therapy. Circulation 99:963, 1999.

AEROBIC EXERCISE PRESCRIPTION FOR PATIENTS WITH CARDIOVASCULAR DISEASE

Adequate exercise training is a function of variables that include type of exercise, intensity, frequency, duration, and total energy expenditure.

TYPE OF EXERCISE. Walking is the preferred initial mode of exercise because it requires no special training or equipment and can be performed at any time of day. Because the energy cost of walking varies little from person to person, it is relatively simple to specify the dose of exercise in terms of a distance to be covered within a specified time. However, depending on patients' preferences, other activities such as stationary cycling or rowing may be substituted.

INTENSITY (see also Table 43–3). It was once thought that aerobic training response required exercise at an intensity sufficient to achieve 60 to 80 percent of an individual's maximal Vo_2. For many individuals, however, the largest reduction in overall mortality over time occurs with moving from the lowest to the next lowest quintile of fitness.[56] Thus, for sedentary older adults—the most likely beneficiaries of cardiac rehabilitation programs—aerobic fitness can be enhanced by exercise intensities as low as 40 percent of Vo_{2max}.[57] For some individuals, effort insufficient to augment aerobic power may nevertheless confer some health benefits.

For most patients, exercise intensity should be prescribed at 50 to 80 percent of Vo_{2max} as determined by an exercise test or by the estimated numbers of METs achieved. A training heart rate is generally designated as 65 to 85 percent of the maximal measured heart rate from the exercise test.[58] If an exercise test is not initially performed, a target of 20 beats/min above the resting heart rate is adequate until test results are available. For patients who develop symptoms, ST depression, or arrhythmias, a target of approximately 10 beats/min below the rate at which these occurred should be used.

FREQUENCY. At the beginning of cardiac rehabilitation, as many as three sessions per week may be undertaken under medical supervision. These supervised sessions can be tapered off as home exercise becomes increasingly important. Eventually, aerobic exercise should be performed on most days of the week.[27,58,59]

DURATION. With increasing fitness, patients should be encouraged to achieve a minimum of 30 minutes of aerobic exercise per day.[27,59] This is best accomplished in a single bout of exercise but may be divided into two or three parts. However, divided exercise produce less cardiovascular fitness.

TOTAL ENERGY EXPENDITURE. Because many of the benefits of exercise depend upon the total dose of exercise, patients should be encouraged to engage in as many activities as is practical. They can, at least partially, make up for a "deficit" on one day with a greater dose on the next. In addition to duration, the exercise prescription should specify the pace of activities such as walking or jogging.

ADVANCING THE PRESCRIPTION. As patients become more conditioned, the exercise prescription should be advanced. The scale developed by Borg (see Table 43–3) is useful for this. In general, exercise should be performed at a rate of perceived exertion (RPE) of 13 to 15 on the Borg scale. For some individuals an RPE of 14 to 15 represents exercise too strenuous to sustain, as evidenced by heart rates over target. When this is the case, less aggressive targets should be used. As the RPE falls with improving fitness, the intensity of exercise may be increased, usually in increments of 5 to 10 percent of the maximal heart rate. Most asymptomatic patients should have as a goal the ability to exercise at 85 percent of their peak heart rate for the full exercise session. For symptomatic or high-risk patients or those who experience ischemia or arrhythmias with exercise, repeated exercise testing may be required before safely advancing the prescription.

RESISTANCE TRAINING PRESCRIPTION FOR PATIENTS WITH CARDIOVASCULAR DISEASE

Range-of-motion and resistance exercises are necessary to counter the muscle atrophy induced by aging, surgery, or bed rest. Following CABG, range-of-motion exercises are needed to prevent the development of adhesions and help avoid muscle weakness or loss. Although stretching or flexibility activities can begin as early as 24 hours after CABG or 2 days after myocardial infarction, low-level resistance training should not begin until 2 to 3 weeks after myocardial infarction.[60] In general, surgical patients should avoid strength-training exercises that pull on the sternum for 3 months after CABG surgery.

Otherwise, selected patients should begin the same type of strength-training program recommended for healthy older adults. Patients should start with a weight low enough to allow one set of 10 to 15 repetitions and increase weight slowly (2 to 5 pounds/wk for arms and 5 to 10 pounds/wk for legs). Given the slow course of muscle hypertrophy, current recommendations call for at least two sessions of resistance exercise per week. The prescription for resistance training may differ depending on comorbid conditions and other limitations. Pure isometric exercise is not recommended for cardiac rehabilitation.

Electrocardiographic Monitoring

Practice varies considerably regarding the number of electrocardiographically monitored exercise sessions. Guidelines recommend using as few monitored sessions as possible.[18] The decision should be based on the patient's risk (Table 43–7), available staff, and the exercise setting. Electrocardiographic (ECG) monitoring is generally performed with either hardwired or telemetric systems and should be continuous. Telephonic home ECG monitoring has been used and appears to be effective in selected circumstances.[61]

Safety of Exercise Training and Cardiac Rehabilitation

Among patients with coronary artery disease, the risk of an adverse event during exercise testing is up to 100-fold higher than during usual activity. Even so, exercise training as part of a cardiac rehabilitation program is quite safe, with exceedingly low rates of coronary events reported in the rehabilitation setting. In a survey of 167 supervised programs, the

TABLE 43–7 Criteria for Electrocardiographic Monitoring During Exercise

Severely depressed left ventricular function (ejection fraction < 30%)
Resting complex ventricular arrhythmia
Ventricular arrhythmias appearing or increasing with exercise
Decrease in systolic blood pressure with exercise
Survivors of sudden cardiac death
Survivors of myocardial infarction complicated by congestive heart failure, cardiogenic shock, serious ventricular arrhythmias, or some combination of the three
Severe coronary artery disease and marked exercise-induced ischemia (ST segment depression greater than or equal to 2 mm)
Inability to self-monitor heart rate because of physical or intellectual impairment

From Cardiac Rehabilitation: Clinical Practice Guideline No. 17. Bethesda, Md, Agency for Health Care Policy and Research, National Heart, Lung, and Blood Institute, 1995; and Fletcher GF, Balady GJ, Amsterdam EA, et al: Exercise standards for testing and training: A statement for healthcare professionals from the American Heart Association. Circulation 104:1694, 2001.

incidence rate of cardiac events was quite low: 8.9 per million patient-hours of exercise for cardiac arrest, 3.4 per million patient-hours for myocardial infarction, and 1.3 per million patient-hours for fatalities.[58] In a 16-year follow-up of medically supervised exercise in a single cardiac rehabilitation center, five major cardiovascular complications (three nonfatal myocardial infarctions and two cardiac arrests) were recorded during 292,254 patient exercise hours, yielding an incidence rate of 17.1 per million patient-hours of exercise.[62]

The rate of sudden cardiac arrests among exercising individuals with known cardiovascular disease appears to be considerably higher, approximately 1 per 60,000 person-hours,[18] supporting the concept that supervised exercise, even among higher risk individuals, is far safer in the setting of cardiac rehabilitation.

Strength training is also a safe mode of exercise for cardiac rehabilitation, even among deconditioned patients. A review of 12 studies of resistance training in cardiac rehabilitation in men demonstrated improvements in muscular strength and endurance as well as absence of anginal symptoms, ischemic ST segment depression, abnormal hemodynamics, complex ventricular dysrhythmias, and cardiovascular complications.[2] Unfortunately, similar data for women are lacking. Table 43–8 lists the clinical circumstances in which exercise as part of cardiac rehabilitation is potentially dangerous and thus contraindicated.

Nutrition (see also Chap. 41)

Nutrition has direct effects on weight, serum lipids, blood pressure, blood sugar and insulin sensitivity, cardiac rhythm, endothelial function, and oxidative stress, all factors associated with cardiovascular health and disease.[63] Poor nutrition can thus increase the risk of coronary events, and healthy eating can decrease the risk.

At least five randomized trials with clinical endpoints have demonstrated that different approaches to diet can provide significant reductions in cardiac events such as myocardial infarction and sudden cardiac death.[64-68] Although not all diet studies have demonstrated benefits, more recent ones have been strikingly positive, with reductions in coronary events from 40 to 72 percent and mortality reductions as high as 30 percent.[63] The choice of diet to be recommended as part of

TABLE 43–8 Clinical Contraindications for Inpatient and Outpatient Cardiac Rehabilitation Exercise

Unstable angina
Resting SBP ≥ 180 mm Hg or resting DBP ≥ 100 mm Hg (evaluate on case-by-case basis)
Orthostatic blood pressure drop > 20 mm Hg with symptoms
Critical aortic stenosis
Acute systemic illness or fever
Uncontrolled atrial or ventricular arrhythmia
Uncontrolled sinus tachycardia (>120 beats/min)
Uncompensated CHF
Third-degree AV block (without pacemaker)
Active pericarditis or myocarditis
Recent embolism
Thrombophlebitis
Resting ST displacement (≥2 mm); ≥3 mm if patient is taking digitalis)
Uncontrolled diabetes
Severe orthopedic problems that would prohibit exercise
Other metabolic problems such as acute thyroiditis, hypo- or hyperkalemia, hypovolemia

AV = atrioventricular; CHF = congestive heart failure; DBP = diastolic blood pressure; SBP = systolic blood pressure.

Adapted from American College of Sports Medicine: Guidelines for Graded Exercise Testing and Prescription. 5th ed. Baltimore, Williams & Wilkins, 1995, p 179.

comprehensive cardiac rehabilitation should be based on both existing evidence of a beneficial effect and the social and cultural needs of the patient.

Intervention

Nutritional evaluation, counseling, and tracking must occur as part of a comprehensive cardiac rehabilitation program. Assessment of dietary patterns must begin before active participation with specific goals determined and communicated to the patient. For patients who are overweight (body mass index > 25 kg/m^2), a healthy eating strategy must include a specific weight management component. Interventions to promote weight loss should focus on adjusting caloric intake and increasing caloric expenditure with increased daily physical activity and regular exercise. Referral for medical intervention in the form of pharmacotherapy or bariatric surgery may be considered for patients whose obesity is seriously detrimental to their health. A rate of weight loss of 1 to 2 pounds per week or 1 percent of body weight per week is considered safe.[25]

In spite of intense public debate regarding the relative merits of low-fat versus low-carbohydrate diets, the optimal eating strategy for losing weight is not likely to be resolved soon.[69] It is possible that the specific components of a diet are not as important as achieving continued caloric restriction. Data from the National Weight Control Registry, which has enrolled approximately 3000 women and men who lost more than 30 pounds and kept them off for at least a year, suggest three important strategies for successful weight loss: exercise (an average of 400 calories per day, or the equivalent of 1 hour of brisk walking), consumption of fewer calories (registry members consumed, on average, 1400 calories a day), and a lower fat diet rich in fruits and vegetables and low in sugars and sweets.[70]

Two useful basic plans have been developed. Each one can be easily adapted into cardiac rehabilitation programs.

- The dietary component of the National Cholesterol Education Program's *Therapeutic Lifestyle Changes*[71]: 25 to 35 percent of calories from fat, saturated fat less than 7 percent of caloric intake, and cholesterol intake less than 200 mg/d. Carbohydrates (from whole grains and other foods rich in complex carbohydrates) constitute 50 to 60 percent of calories, protein 15 percent, and 20 to 30 gm of dietary fiber (especially soluble fiber) per day.
- The *Dietary Approaches to Stop Hypertension* (DASH) eating plan[72]: this diet, which emerged from the randomized DASH trial, is low in saturated fat, cholesterol, and total fat, and emphasizes fruits, vegetables, low-fat dairy foods, whole-grain products, fish, poultry, and nuts.

Increased intake of omega-3 fatty acids from fish, fish oil supplements, or plant sources should also be encouraged. Omega-3 fatty acids may reduce the risk of cardiac events, in particular sudden cardiac death.[73]

Regardless of specific nutrition issues, long-term dietary adherence remains problematic. A successful cardiac rehabilitation program provides patients with not only specific dietary information but also critically important strategies to improve adherence based on sound principles from behavioral medicine (see Chap. 84).

Smoking

Cigarette smoking is the leading cause of preventable death,[74] more than 40 percent of which results from smoking-related cardiovascular disease. Tobacco smoke contains a multitude of cardiotoxic substances, of which nicotine is probably the most important.[75] The smoke of as little as one cigarette elevates blood pressure and heart rate, probably related to nicotine-induced release of catecholamines. Cigarette smoking increases platelet activation and impairs fibrinolysis,[76] adversely affects the lipoprotein profile by raising triglycerides and lowering HDL,[77] lowers the threshold for arrhythmia,[78] impairs endothelial function,[79,80] and promotes the progression of atherosclerosis.[81]

Cessation of smoking yields a 50 percent reduction in the risk of a coronary event in the first year or two after quitting, with the risk of former smokers approaching that of nonsmokers after 5 to 15 years. Patients who quit smoking have a 36 percent reduction in crude relative risk of mortality compared with those who continue smoking.[82] A 20-year follow-up of patients after CABG showed that those who continued smoking had a 1.75 relative risk of cardiac death compared with those who stopped smoking for at least 1 year after surgery.[83]

Smoking cessation efforts conducted during the course of a comprehensive cardiac rehabilitation program can have a significant impact on smoking rates. In a study of a combined educational and behavioral intervention, 17 to 26 percent of patients stopped smoking.[84] In a later example, among 109 patients referred to a 2- to 3-month multidisciplinary ambulatory cardiac rehabilitation program within 1 to 4 weeks after hospital discharge for acute myocardial infarction or CABG, smoking rates dropped to 14 percent at 12 months.[26]

Smoking Cessation Intervention

The period following an acute coronary event, revascularization procedure, or diagnosis of cardiovascular disease is an ideal time to encourage patients to stop smoking. Providing information about the link between smoking and cardiovascular disease at this vulnerable time may supply the motivation to stop smoking. This motivation must be carefully nurtured and supported with effective interventions. Guidelines from the U.S. Public Health Service[85] recommend a combination of behavioral counseling and pharmacological therapy for nicotine withdrawal. Social support and training in problem solving appear to be effective behavioral interventions. First-line pharmacotherapies include sustained-release bupropion hydrochloride and nicotine replacement (Table 43–9). These therapies have been demonstrated to be safe, even among patients with CHD.[86] However, current clinical guidelines recommend that these first-line therapies not be used in patients with unstable angina or a myocardial infarction in the previous 2 weeks because there are few data to support their use in this period.[87]

Exposure to passive smoke may explain why counseling the patient alone may not be sufficient for smoking cessation. In a survey of 103 consecutive patients attending a hospital-based 10-week multidisciplinary cardiac rehabilitation program, 40 percent reported living with someone else who smoked, most often a spouse.[88] Thus, interventions to modify the smoking behavior of other members of the cardiac patient's household may be needed to achieve optimum secondary prevention. Smokers who are depressed are more likely to relapse after hospitalization or during cardiac rehabilitation; thus, assessment and treatment of depression should proceed in concert with, or prior to, smoking cessation efforts.

Psychosocial Factors

A wide variety of psychosocial factors influence outcomes in CHD patients. Detection of and intervention for many of these can and should occur in connection with cardiac rehabilitation. Depression and perceived lack of social support are common among patients with CHD, affecting one third or more of this population.[89] Both are associated with increases in cardiac morbidity and mortality up to eightfold among patients with CHD.[90,91] Following myocardial infarction, depression is a risk factor for mortality independent of the severity of cardiac disease,[92] and there is some evidence that depression during admission for myocardial infarction is more closely linked to long-term survival than depression after the event.[93] Although major depression is clearly detrimental, even minimal symptoms of depression increase the risk of mortality after myocardial infarction.[94]

Depression and low social support may predispose a patient to be nonadherent to medications, exercise programs, and other secondary prevention efforts.[95] Depression and stress may also affect biological factors that increase risk of cardiac events, such as ventricular irritability, low heart rate variability, and increased platelet activation.[96,97] Other factors including anxiety, life stress, vital exhaustion (defined as a combination of fatigue, lack of energy, feelings of hopelessness, and loss of libido), and hostility[98] have been shown to influence CHD outcomes. Hostility has attracted attention as the possible "toxic" element of a type A personality. Studies have linked its presence to increased risk.

Two meta-analyses have assessed the impact of psychosocial interventions in cardiac rehabilitation. Linden and colleagues demonstrated that psychosocially treated patients showed greater reductions in psychological distress, systolic blood pressure, heart rate, and cholesterol level, whereas patients who did not receive psychosocial treatment showed significantly greater mortality and cardiac recurrence rates during the first 2 years of follow-up.[99] A meta-analysis by Dusseldorp and colleagues that included 37 studies suggested that psychosocial interventions were associated with a 34 percent reduction in cardiac mortality, a 29 percent reduction in recurrence of myocardial infarction, and significant beneficial effects on blood pressure, cholesterol, body weight, smoking, physical activity, and eating habits.[100]

TABLE 43–9 First-Line Medications to Treat Nicotine Addiction

Medication	Advantages	Side Effects	Considerations
Nicotine patch	Easy to use, steady-state blood levels	Skin reactions, disturbed sleep	Available over the counter, low liability for long-term use
Nicotine gum	Can be used ad libitum	Sore mouth, hiccups, dyspepsia, sore jaw	Compliance can be increased with careful instructions: chew slowly and intermittently, avoid acidic beverages. Available over the counter
Nicotine inhaler	Can be used ad libitum	Mouth-throat irritation, coughing,	Acidic beverages reduce nicotine absorption
Nicotine nasal spray	Can be used ad libitum; causes rapid rise in blood nicotine levels	Nasal irritation or congestion, rhinitis	More likely to be abused than other therapies
Nicotine lozenge	Can be used ad libitum; oral substitute for cigarettes	Sore mouth, dyspepsia, hiccups	Available over the counter
Sustained-release bupropion	Nonnicotine treatment; easy to use and well tolerated	Insomnia, dry mouth	Can be safely used with nicotine replacement therapy; avoid in patients with seizure disorder, history of alcoholism, or severe uncontrolled hypertension

Adapted from Thomson CC, Rigotti NA: Hospital- and clinic-based smoking cessation interventions for smokers with cardiovascular disease. Prog Cardiovasc Dis 45:459, 2003.

In the Enhancing Recovery in Coronary Heart Disease Patients (ENRICHD) trial, 2481 patients with recent myocardial infarction were randomly assigned to 6 months of cognitive behavioral therapy or usual care. In the treatment arm, an antidepressant was prescribed for patients who did not respond within 5 weeks to this therapy or with high scores on the Hamilton Rating Scale for Depression. Psychosocial outcomes were significantly better in the treatment group.[89] There were no significant differences, however, in survival or recurrent myocardial infarction. This null result may be attributed to frequent interventions in the control group—among patients with depression, 28 percent of those in the treatment arm and 20.6 percent of those in the control arm were taking an antidepressant. The interventions employed in the ENRICHD trial can be adjusted and adapted into cardiac rehabilitation programs.

Easing the stress and distress that follow myocardial infarction, revascularization, or a diagnosis of CHD may be one avenue by which comprehensive cardiac rehabilitation programs improve survival. A 3-month nonrandomized trial evaluated 150 men who received either standard medical care (n = 72) or an accelerated comprehensive rehabilitation program that included counseling sessions aimed at coping with stress. At the program's end, rehabilitation patients reported more improvement and less deterioration in mood than control patients. After 9 years of follow-up, the most significant predictors of mortality were left ventricular ejection fraction less than 50 percent (odds ratio, 3.2; 95 percent CI, 1.1 to 9.8) and rehabilitation (odds ratio, 0.2; 95 percent CI, 0.1 to 0.7).[101]

Pharmacotherapy may be an important adjunct to behavioral therapy in treating depression. In the Sertraline Antidepressant Heart Attack Randomized Trial (SADHART), sertraline therapy was judged to be safe following an acute coronary syndrome.[102] The incidence of severe adverse cardiovascular events was 14.5 percent in the sertraline group and 22.4 percent in the placebo group. In the ENRICHD trial, subgroup analysis of patients taking a selective serotonin reuptake inhibitor antidepressant showed significant improvements in cardiac outcomes. Use of a serotonin reuptake inhibitor was associated with a 43 percent lower risk of myocardial infarction and a 42 percent lower risk of death.[89]

Intervention

A rehabilitation program provides an excellent setting in which to identify patients who are significantly depressed, isolated, excessively stressed, or easily angered and to begin appropriate interventions that may act synergistically with other component of the program. Exercise, for example, may help improve depression, and the dynamics of a group setting may provide the seeds of a potentially helpful social support network.[103]

Some cardiac rehabilitation programs offer psychological interventions as a component of the program itself. These include group psychotherapy, individual psychotherapy, behavior counseling, and relaxation or stress management classes. All programs should include an assessment or screening for the presence of psychosocial problems and should provide an opportunity for referral to other experts if conditions merit.

Other Therapy (Aspirin, Statins, Angiotensin-Converting Enzyme Inhibitors, Beta Blockers)

Pharmacotherapy for secondary prevention is covered in detail in Chapters 39 and 42. Participation in cardiac rehabilitation should enhance adherence to recommended pharmacological interventions.[59]

Education

Education of patients is such an integral part of any cardiac rehabilitation program that it was included as a critical component of cardiac rehabilitation in the 1995 Agency for Health Care Policy and Research guideline[2] and is required for certification by the American Association of Cardiovascular and Pulmonary Rehabilitation. Structural aspects of the cardiac rehabilitation program, training expertise, and interests of the staff as well as the needs, abilities, and cultural differences among the patients all influence the important process of information delivery and behavior change that constitute education of patients. Timing of education is of critical importance, because the initial period in outpatient cardiac rehabilitation often represents a time when motivation is likely to be high, but also when there are major deficits in knowledge and important misconceptions. The experience of group cardiac rehabilitation is optimal for improving this situation in a supportive environment in which both experienced professionals and other patients experiencing similar conditions combine their communication efforts to build knowledge and assist with behavior change.

Several principles of behavior change are helpful in improving the participant's motivation as well as an individual's ability to comprehend and digest a broad array of information. None of these principles are mutually exclusive, and many are often combined in programs, depending on staff organization and patients' needs.[104]

LEARNING NEEDS. In many cases, learning depends on what the individual perceives as his or her need to learn. Thus, after a recent cardiovascular event or procedure, learning can be enhanced by structuring information around patient-specific events and findings (the use of anatomical models and diagrams), and such information can be blended with advice on behavior change and awareness of warning signs.

OUTCOME MODEL. Many individuals find it easier to change behavior when specific goals or targets are placed on the horizon. Such a process involves knowing not only what ideal goals should be from the professional standpoint, but also the optimal achievable goals from the patient's perspective. It is also essential to know what resources are available and what experience the individual has had with respect to specific goals. Specific and reasonable outcome goals can be elucidated. Some have found it useful to document these goals explicitly in the form of "contracts."

SELF-EFFICACY. A concept based on Bandura's social learning theory[105] has become important in understanding both barriers to behavior change and strategies to improve healthy behaviors. Self-efficacy concepts tested in the cardiac rehabilitation setting have been shown to improve learning and behavior change. There are two critical components of the self-efficacy concept. The first is an "outcome expectancy," which is an individual's belief that a particular behavior will lead to a specific outcome. The second is an "efficacy expectation" that he or she can be successful in modifying the behavior necessary to produce the outcome. Self-esteem appears to be a critical component of this concept; thus, individuals with low self-esteem are often both less motivated and less able to make behavior change. Strategies that improve self-esteem or self-efficacy, or both, have been shown to improve life-style risk factor change.

STAGES OF CHANGE. The stages of change model, also called the transtheoretical model, developed by Prochaska and DiClemente[106] has been widely applied to smoking cessation and is also being used to understand and improve behavior change efforts for other risk factors. This model generally defines four stages in the process of behavior change: precontemplation, contemplation, action, and maintenance. When an individual's current stage has been identified, educational interventions are targeted to that specific stage. Thus, for an individual who is not yet thinking of stopping smoking (precontemplation), efforts need to be directed at understanding why that patient smokes and what it might take for him or her to consider smoking cessation. Strategies for someone already in the process of planning to stop smoking are quite different—that patient not only needs specific information about why smoking is bad but also needs help with strategies to aid in smoking cessation, including preparation for withdrawal symptoms. Similar strategies could be applied to individuals beginning exercise.

PERFORMED LEARNING STYLE. People understand and remember new information in a variety of different ways. This model emphasizes assessment of which mode of learning suits an individual best (e.g., oral, pictorial, graphic).

Although it would be impractical to tailor all educational efforts to highly specific individual needs, clearly the option of independent learning modalities within a cardiac rehabilitation setting is optimal. Most successful programs include classes (some of which are optional), the opportunities for one-on-one learning, written materials, video materials, and now Internet-based materials.

In addition to imparting knowledge and assisting with behavior change, education of patients in the context of cardiac rehabilitation should optimally be responsive to other learning needs:

- Inclusion of family members and significant others in teaching
- Maintenance of change and prevention of relapse
- Provision of learning resources in different forms—written, video, computer (Internet based)
- Access to other community resources (e.g., local American Heart Association)

Sexual Activity after Myocardial Infarction

Issues of sexual activity must also be addressed. Because patients are often reluctant to discuss sexuality or sexual dysfunction, members of the cardiac rehabilitation team should address these issues, including the possible effect of medications on sexual function. The most common sexual problems encountered by cardiac patients are reduced or extinguished libido and avoidance of sexual activity. Men also commonly experience impotence or premature or delayed ejaculation. Factors contributing to sexual dysfunction include depression, fear of precipitating a cardiovascular event on the part of the individual or his or her partner, and medications particularly beta blockers and diuretics.

The hemodynamic response to usual sexual activity approximates the maximal heart rate attained with other customary activities, such as walking up one or two flights of stairs.[107] The response may be significantly higher with an unfamiliar partner, in unfamiliar circumstances, or after excessive eating or alcohol consumption. Low-risk patients (those with mild, stable angina, successful coronary revascularization, uncomplicated myocardial infarction, or mild valvular disease) can be safely encouraged to initiate or resume sexual activity or to receive treatment for sexual dysfunction. It is important to stress that sildenafil or other phosphodiesterase-5 inhibitors must not be used by patients taking nitrates in any form. Higher risk patients should receive further cardiological evaluation before recommendations are made regarding sexual activity.[108] Patients should be encouraged to report symptoms lasting more than 10 minutes after sexual activity.

Successful education of the patient in cardiac rehabilitation depends upon the educator's ability to communicate and knowledge of appropriate learning and behavior strategies. Opportunities to obtain competence in these areas are important, and ongoing assessment of abilities allows individual participants to benefit greatly from the cardiac rehabilitation experience and to continue to benefit when the formal program has been completed.

Adherence

To state the obvious, interventions proved to improve outcomes require implementation and adherence to have their desired effect. Patients often have difficulty adhering to even a single intervention such as taking a statin for high cholesterol.[109] Comprehensive cardiac rehabilitation entails more than a dozen separate interventions, making adherence quite complex. Indeed, up to half of individuals who begin a cardiac rehabilitation program fail to complete it.

A review of studies examining participation in and adherence to cardiac rehabilitation reveals several factors consistently associated with participation. These include referral by physicians, specific cardiac diagnoses, reimbursement issues, self-efficacy, perceived benefits of cardiac rehabilitation, distance and transportation, self-motivation, family composition, social support, self-esteem, and occupation. Factors associated with nonadherence include being older, being female, having fewer years of formal education, depression, and difficulty in perceiving the benefits of cardiac rehabilitation.[110]

Successful cardiac rehabilitation depends upon implementation and integration at the levels of the patient, provider, and system. Because these programs are multidisciplinary, often hospital based, and interact at all three levels when optimally designed and utilized, they represent an ideal opportunity to enhance adherence to all secondary prevention interventions. A number of interventions are available to improve adherence at all levels (Table 43–10). The most effective interventions—those with multiple components and a continued maintenance intervention—can be delivered through a model in which physicians provide advice and other members of the health care team provide more in-depth behavioral counseling and follow-up.

Adherence to smoking cessation, dietary change, and psychosocial interventions presents challenges specific to the problems themselves. For example, counseling designed to identify and deal with "triggers" to unhealthy behaviors improves adherence to both smoking cessation and caloric restriction. Uniquely, successful smoking cessation requires specific counseling regarding withdrawal symptoms. Group sessions help some patients with stress reduction and anger management techniques, but depression generally requires individual attention. Indeed, inadequate attention to depression often leads to poor adherence with other behavior changes and medical interventions as well.[95]

A case management system can provide an important framework for the delivery of care by integrating the patient, family, environment, life style, and community.[111] In this model, a single individual, usually a nurse or exercise physiologist, coordinates all aspects of care, engaging physicians and other specialists when necessary.

Rehabilitation for Other Populations

Cardiac rehabilitation is also beneficial for patients with a variety of other cardiovascular diseases. Medicare provides payments for cardiac rehabilitation only for the diagnoses of myocardial infarction, coronary artery bypass surgery, and stable angina. Unfortunately, reimbursement is not available for patients who have undergone percutaneous revascularization, heart transplantation, and heart valve surgery or for patients with heart failure. Insurance coverage by other third-party payers varies considerably throughout the United States.

TABLE 43–10 Interventions to Improve Adherence with Cardiac Rehabilitation

Focus on the Patient
Simplify medication regimens
Provide explicit instructions and teach the patient how to follow the prescribed treatment
Encourage the use of prompts to help patients remember treatment regimens
Use systems to reinforce adherence and maintain contact
Encourage the support of family and friends
Reinforce and reward adherence
Increase patients' visits for persons unable to achieve treatment goal
Increase the convenience and access to care
Involve patients in their care through self-monitoring
Focus on Provider and Medical Office
Implement prevention guidelines
Use reminders to prompt physicians to attend to prevention
Identify a patient advocate in the office
Develop a standardized treatment plan to structure care
Use feedback from past performance to foster change in future care
Remind patients of appointments and follow up missed appointments
Focus on the Health Delivery System
Use case management by nurses
Use telemedicine when possible
Collaborate with pharmacists
Develop and use critical care pathways

Adapted from National Cholesterol Education Program (NCEP) Expert Panel on Detection, Evaluation, and Treatment of High Blood Cholesterol in Adults (Adult Treatment Panel III): Third Report of the National Cholesterol Education Program (NCEP) Expert Panel on Detection, Evaluation, and Treatment of High Blood Cholesterol in Adults (Adult Treatment Panel III) final report. Circulation 106:3143, 2002.

HEART FAILURE (see also Chap. 24)

Exercise intolerance is a cardinal symptom of heart failure. In addition to myocardial dysfunction, other contributors to this syndrome include abnormalities in peripheral blood flow, skeletal muscle morphology, and metabolism. For many years, bed rest was a primary treatment for congestive heart failure. However, pioneering work from Duke in the late 1980s showed significant improvements in exercise capacity and associated physiological changes with progressive exercise. Since then, a profusion of mostly small, short-term trials has generally demonstrated benefits of exercise in a variety of aspects of heart failure domains. These include increased peak oxygen consumption, improvement in autonomic regulation of cardiovascular activity, improved endothelial function and skeletal muscle function, and favorable effects on ventilatory function as well as improvements in the ability to perform activities of daily living, anxiety, depression, and general well-being.[112] There is, however, no clear evidence yet that exercise therapy improves survival in patients with heart failure.

EXERCISE PRESCRIPTION FOR PATIENTS WITH HEART FAILURE. Guidelines from the Agency for Health Care Policy and Research[2] and from the American Heart Association[112] recommend exercise training for patients with stable heart failure. Because an exercise prescription specifically tailored for patients with heart failure has not yet been devised, it is prudent to use the American Heart Association's exercise standards for exercise testing and training for patients with cardiovascular disease[18] as a template for an individual prescription.

Among patients with advanced disease, exercise prescriptions based on heart rate may not be accurate, given their limited chronotropic reserve. Widespread use of beta blockers in this population also makes it impractical to use heart rate alone to measure exercise intensity. Instead, a peak Vo_2 of 70 to 80 percent may provide a better target for the intensity of exercise. For debilitated patients or those unused to aerobic activity, lower intensity activities (peak Vo_2 of 60 to 65 percent) with programmed periods of rest may be adequate. The duration of exercise should include an adequate warm-up period that may be longer (10 to 15 minutes) than for other cardiac rehabilitation patients. The warm-up period is followed by an exercise period of 20 to 30 minutes at the desired intensity and a cool-down period. Three to five times per week is the usual frequency for training. Resistance training can strengthen individual muscle groups. Guidelines from the American Association of Cardiovascular and Pulmonary Rehabilitation[27] call for direct monitoring and supervision at first, possibly followed by home training.

SAFETY OF REHABILITATION FOR PATIENTS WITH HEART FAILURE. No large-scale trials have focused specifically on the safety of exercise training for patients with heart failure. There is, however, little evidence that exercise worsens left ventricular function or increases the size of heart chambers. Data from the European Heart Failure Training Group confirm the beneficial effects of exercise rehabilitation on functional capacity.[113] In the randomized Exercise Rehabilitation Trial, 12 months of exercise training improved peak oxygen uptake and strength with no significant differences in total mortality, hospitalization for heart failure, or worsening of heart failure.[114] Contraindications for exercise among patients with heart failure are similar to those for patients with coronary artery disease (see Table 43–7).

REHABILITATION FOR CARDIAC TRANSPLANTATION PATIENTS

Candidates for heart transplantation are generally quite debilitated and deconditioned. Following transplantation, persistent heart failure, diminished aerobic capacity, muscle atrophy, and premature coronary atherosclerosis are common. Functional capacity during exercise testing is reduced to 50 percent in heart transplant recipients compared with age-matched healthy control subjects.[115] Case series and several small clinical studies[116-118] have demonstrated that exercise training has the potential for reversing or diminishing physiological abnormalities in heart transplant patients. Thus, training that includes both aerobic and resistance exercise is recommended before and after transplantation.[2,112,118]

Most studies of rehabilitation before or after heart transplantation have followed a standard cardiac rehabilitation model, with exercise sessions conducted three or four times per week from 8 to 12 weeks at moderate intensity. Improvements in aerobic capacity range from 20 to 50 percent. Resistance training offers an opportunity to increase lean muscle mass and bone density.[116]

Published studies to date do not address the progressive, diffuse atherosclerosis that tends to occur after heart transplantation, which is a common cause of late cardiac graft failure and patients' death (see Chaps. 26 and 35). Cardiac rehabilitation and secondary prevention interventions could delay or prevent progression of coronary artery disease in the transplanted heart. Coping with the ongoing medical consequences of heart transplantation presents a substantial challenge to patients. A multidisciplinary cardiac rehabilitation program that includes exercise, education, nutrition, and behavioral interventions is ideally suited to these patients.

REHABILITATION FOR PATIENTS WITH ARRHYTHMIAS

Patients with a variety of arrhythmias can benefit from cardiac rehabilitation. Indeed, exercise can potentially suppress some arrhythmias at rest, possibly because of exercise-induced vagal withdrawal and increased sympathetic stimulation.[18,119] However, exercise programs for these patients vary widely. At one end of the spectrum, those with nonsustained ventricular arrhythmias and normal myocardial function generally require only a few sessions of electrocardiogram-monitored exercise before graduating to a nonmonitored or home exercise program. At the other end, patients with an implantable cardioverter-defibrillator (ICD) related to prior ventricular fibrillation require a much longer period of electrocardiogram-monitored exercise. Unfortunately, exercise training for patients with arrhythmias has received little attention in the literature.

ATRIAL FIBRILLATION. Exercise improves exercise performance in patients with atrial fibrillation to the same extent that it does in those without it.[120] For patients with controlled ventricular rates during atrial fibrillation, the use of a target heart range during exercise is preferred to a specific heart rate. Uncontrolled ventricular rate during atrial fibrillation is a contraindication to exercise training because it can lead to hemodynamic instability.

PREMATURE VENTRICULAR COMPLEXES. Frequent premature ventricular complexes may decrease coronary perfusion, cardiac output, and blood pressure. These, in turn, can lead to ventricular arrhythmias. Thus, patients with frequent premature ventricular complexes should be closely monitored during exercise, and the appearance of exercise-induced arrhythmias should mandate reducing the intensity of exercise or stopping altogether.

PACEMAKER. For patients with pacemakers enrolled in a cardiac rehabilitation program, it is essential to identify the rhythm and conduction history for which the pacemaker has been implanted. Both the exercise prescription and its monitoring must be tailored to the characteristics of the device.

IMPLANTABLE CARDIOVERTER-DEFIBRILLATOR. Patients with an ICD are often physically or psychologically disabled by their disease or the possibility of a sudden ICD discharge, or both. Thus, an important part of cardiac rehabilitation involves allaying fears that activity or exercise will cause a discharge. Baseline exercise testing can help determine whether exercise provokes ventricular arrhythmias as well as establishes the upper limit of exercise (10 to 15 beats/min below the device trigger point). A slow progression from low to moderate exercise intensity may be necessary because of prior deconditioning and to avoid overshooting the target heart rate. Perceived exertion (the Borg scale; see Table 43-3) offers a good guide for increasing exercise intensity. Given these caveats, exercise-based cardiac rehabilitation can offer substantial benefits to patients with ICDs. In a 12-week study of comprehensive cardiac rehabilitation among 16 patients who had undergone implantation of an ICD, no ventricular arrhythmias or device discharges occurred during the exercise components of the program, exercise times increased by 16 percent, and anxiety and depression decreased significantly.[121]

Cardiac Rehabilitation for Elderly Patients (see also Chap. 72)

Given the high prevalence of CHD among those older than 65 years,[1] elderly persons represent a large proportion of potential candidates for cardiac rehabilitation. In addition to improving cardiovascular health and reducing risk factors for cardiovascular and other chronic diseases,[122] rehabilitation programs can enhance functional independence and overall well-being.[123] The benefits of cardiac rehabilitation do not appear to be age limited and are beneficial[124] and cost-effective[125] even in the ninth decade of life. As at other ages, a cardiac rehabilitation program under the direction of trained personnel is often the ideal setting for the provision of education, counseling, and behavioral and exercise interventions for elderly individuals.

In general, the exercise prescription described earlier is appropriate for older patients. However, because the exercise capacity of elderly people is usually lower than that of younger individuals (Table 43–11), activities that require lower levels of energy expenditure (40 to 50 percent of VO_{2max}) are generally necessary, especially during the first weeks of a rehabilitation program. For individuals who require lower intensity activity, lengthening the duration of activity per session can increase caloric expenditure. Individuals for whom physical or psychosocial problems limit exercise duration may require more frequent episodes of exercise. Guidelines for other comprehensive secondary prevention efforts in elderly persons have been elaborated by the American Heart Association.[126]

Cardiac Rehabilitation for Patients with Diabetes (see also Chaps. 40 and 51)

Of the rapidly growing population of patients with diabetes, more than half exhibit hypertension, an atherogenic lipid profile, abdominal obesity, and endothelial dysfunction. Diabetes increases the risk of cardiovascular disease two- to fourfold,[127] and cardiovascular disease contributes to approximately 70 percent of deaths among individuals with diabetes.[128] The well-established beneficial effects of weight loss and exercise on insulin resistance and the other metabolic disorders associated with diabetes make this population particularly well suited for a comprehensive cardiac rehabilitation program.

Data from cohort studies involving diabetic men[35] and women[129] have demonstrated 35 to 45 percent reductions in risk of cardiovascular disease and mortality with walking and other forms of physical activity. In the Steno-2 study, conducted among 160 patients with type 2 diabetes and microalbuminuria, random assignment to a targeted, multifactorial, risk factor reduction intervention reduced the risk of cardiovascular disease by 53 percent and the risk of microvascular complications such as nephropathy, retinopathy, and autonomic neuropathy by approximately 60 percent after 8 years compared with standard care.[130]

Exercise Prescription and Precautions

Although the balance of benefits and risks of exercise-based cardiac rehabilitation is quite favorable for most patients with diabetes, some precautions are warranted. Given the potential complications of poor glycemic control, peripheral and autonomic neuropathy, and diabetic retinopathy, exercise prescriptions must be individualized. Detailed guidelines for exercise testing and training are available from the American College of Sports Medicine[131] and the American Diabetes Association.[132] In general, the exercise prescription for individuals with uncomplicated diabetes calls for 30 to 45

TABLE 43–11 Age-Associated Changes in Physiological Response to Aerobic Exercise

Reduced aerobic capacity—a decline in maximum oxygen consumption of 8-10%/yr in nontrained populations
Reduced maximum heart rate of 1 beat/min/yr
More rapid increase in systolic blood pressure with exercise
Attenuated elevation in left ventricular ejection fraction

minutes of aerobic exercise three or four times per week and resistance training one or two times per week, with appropriate warm-up and cool-down periods. The intensity of aerobic exercise is generally set at 55 to 80 percent of maximum heart rate for patients with multiple risk factors, autonomic neuropathy, or no exercise testing and at 50 to 60 percent of maximum heart rate for patients with a low initial level of fitness.

Contraindications to exercise based on glycemic control exist for type 1 diabetes,[132] but guidelines for type 2 diabetes are less definitive. Among more than 550 individuals with type 2 diabetes not requiring insulin and with baseline glucose levels ranging from 60 to 400 mg/dl (3.3 to 22.2 mmol/liter) monitored for 24 hours after exercise, no episodes of ketosis or hypoglycemia were observed and the occurrence of hypoglycemia was 2 percent.[133] Thus, patients with type 2 diabetes who do not require insulin may not need routine blood glucose testing while exercising. Supplementary food is generally not necessary unless exercise is exceptionally vigorous or long. Recurrent episodes of hypoglycemia should lead to downward adjustment of preexercise medications or ingestion of carbohydrate before exercise. Evening exercise sessions can occasionally induce early morning hypoglycemia and thus necessitate a bedtime snack or a change in the timing of exercise sessions. Emergency equipment, including glucose tablets or gels and glucagon injection kits, should be readily available to treat hypoglycemic episodes.

Screening for sensory deficits, cutaneous lesions, ingrown toenails, or foot deformities is an important part of intake evaluation for exercise rehabilitation programs. Such patients should be encouraged to examine their feet before and after exercise and to wear proper footwear, with orthotics when necessary. Many patients with autonomic neuropathy have decreased maximum heart rates and resting tachycardia; thus, targets for exercise should be based on perceived exertion rather than heart rate. Swimming, bicycling, rowing, and arm or chair calisthenics may be appropriate for patients with severe neuropathy.[131,132]

Patients with active proliferative diabetic retinopathy, as well as those with moderate or severe nonproliferative diabetic retinopathy, should avoid exercise that involves straining because of concern about vitreous hemorrhage or traction retinal detachment retinopathy.[134] Patients with nonproliferative retinopathy can engage in most forms of exercise with minimal risk of progressive disease.[131,132,135]

Cardiac Rehabilitation for Obese Patients

Mirroring trends in the general population, the majority of candidates for cardiac rehabilitation are overweight or obese. In one survey of 449 consecutive cardiac rehabilitation patients, 88 percent were overweight or obese.[136]

Most controlled exercise training studies among overweight or obese patients show modest improvements in weight (2 to 3 kg), body mass index, and percentage of body fat.[137] Adding a behavioral intervention and increasing the caloric expenditure can significantly increase weight loss.[138,139]

The exercise prescription for most overweight or obese patients should be much like that for other cardiac rehabilitation patients (see Table 43–6). Low-impact exercises, such as brisk walking or cycle ergometry, may be performed with greater duration and frequency and less intensity.

Cardiac Rehabilitation for Patients with Chronic Obstructive Pulmonary Disease

Patients with chronic obstructive pulmonary disease who have suffered a cardiac event or have been diagnosed with cardiovascular disease can generally take part in and benefit from a standard cardiac rehabilitation program. Patients with resting or exercise-induced hypoxia (oxygen saturation < 88 percent) should receive continuous supplemental oxygen during exercise training. Close monitoring generally precludes the use of a home-based program.

CARDIAC REHABILITATION FOR PATIENTS WITH END-STAGE RENAL DISEASE (see also Chap. 86)

Cardiovascular disease is the leading cause of morbidity and mortality in patients with end-stage renal disease, accounting for more than half of deaths.[140] The benefits of exercise training among renal disease patients with cardiovascular disease should be similar to those derived by the cardiac rehabilitation population at large, but such programs are underused in this high-risk cohort. Because of possible limitations in exercise capacity, careful selection of rehabilitation candidates and appropriate medical supervision are important.

As a result of age, poor nutrition, deconditioning, and advanced cardiovascular disease, many patients with end-stage renal disease have reduced exercise capacity. Exercising to target heart rates 50 to 70 percent of those achieved on exercise tests may lead to improvements in exercise capacity and symptoms similar to those attained by individuals able to exercise at higher intensities.[2] Given that ventricular arrhythmias are common among patients with end-stage renal disease undergoing hemodialysis and last for several hours afterward,[141] it is prudent to schedule exercise training sessions and hemodialysis on alternate days.

Cost-Effectiveness of Cardiac Rehabilitation

In the current era of cost containment, cost-effectiveness has become an important element in determining which primary and secondary prevention therapies to pursue. Interventions are generally compared using the quality-adjusted life-year (QALY) or disability-adjusted life-year (DALY). Interventions with an incremental cost-effectiveness ratio under $20,000 per QALY are generally considered to be quite favorable (see Chap. 2).

A cost-effectiveness analysis suggests that cardiac rehabilitation improves life expectancy by 0.2 years at a cost below $5000 per life-year saved.[142] It is more cost effective than many other post-myocardial infarction treatment interventions (Table 43-12).

Modified protocols may be even more cost-effective. Carlson and colleagues randomly assigned 80 low- to moderate-risk cardiac patients to a traditional cardiac rehabilitation program or a modified program for 6 months. The traditional program included three supervised exercise sessions per week with an ECG monitor for the first 3 months as well as one-on-one education about risk factors. The modified program discontinued ECG monitoring after the first month and gradually moved patients to an off-site exercise regimen supplemented with educational support and telephone follow-up. Patients in the modified program had

TABLE 43–12 Comparative Cost-Effectiveness of Treatments for Coronary Heart Disease

Intervention	Cost-Effectiveness ($/LYS)
Cardiac rehabilitation versus usual care	$2130-4950
Smoking cessation	$220-728
Statin therapy	
Secondary prevention	$9630
Primary prevention	$17,000-38,000
Coronary artery bypass grafting versus medical care	$8500-114,000

LYS = life-year saved.
From Ades PA, Pashkow FJ, Nestor JR: Cost-effectiveness of cardiac rehabilitation after myocardial infarction. J Cardiopulm Rehabil 17:222, 1997.

higher rates of off-site exercise over 6 months and total exercise during the final 3 months; other measures, such as lipid levels and maximal oxygen uptake, were the same in both groups. The modified protocol cost $830 less per patient ($1519 versus $2349) and required 30 percent less staff (full-time equivalents) than the traditional protocol.[17]

The number needed to treat (NNT) is an estimate of the number of patients who must be treated to achieve an additional favorable outcome or prevent an additional adverse outcome. Oldridge and colleagues determined the NNT for mortality in three meta-analyses of cardiac rehabilitation trials as 32, 46, and 72.[143] The result compares favorably with the NNT for other common secondary prevention interventions such as aspirin (67)[144] and beta blockers (42).[145] Among patients with stable chronic heart failure, Georgiou and colleagues determined that long-term exercise therapy increased life expectancy by 1.82 years over a 15.5-year period at a cost of $1773 per life-year saved.[146]

Disease Management

As cardiac rehabilitation has evolved from specifically phased programs (I to IV) to more complex multidisciplinary programs that respond to patients' needs after a cardiac event or procedure (in hospital) or after the onset of angina, newer models for the delivery of comprehensive secondary prevention services have appeared.

Case management models for cardiac rehabilitation have been successfully utilized and have demonstrated improved risk factor[16,84] and clinical[147] outcomes. In these models, a case manager (usually a cardiac nurse or exercise physiologist) develops an individualized program that optimizes preventive management across the individual's spectrum of risk factors and behaviors. For those at lower risk, such programs can be carried out remotely, facilitated by telephone or computer-based systems. These programs also allow continued surveillance of prevention issues beyond the duration of customary cardiac rehabilitation programs, often at relatively low cost. Alternatively, many traditional cardiac rehabilitation programs have added a "maintenance" phase to allow patients to continue cardiac rehabilitation at a lower level of supervision following completion of a formal program. Unfortunately, reimbursement is not generally available for such programs.

Case management and newer cardiac rehabilitation models overlap with health care delivery strategies, commonly referred to as "disease management." Disease management programs have arisen from both academia and the largely for-profit disease management industry. Because the latter has often focused on programs that provide a clear and early return on investment, they tend to enroll higher risk individuals (e.g., patients with heart failure). Nevertheless, secondary prevention disease management programs are being tested and utilized. As the health care information technology infrastructure improves, such programs are likely to be integrated into the delivery of comprehensive cardiac rehabilitation. Unfortunately, reimbursement for cardiac rehabilitation remains one of the key barriers to more complete delivery of this crucial service.

Acknowledgment

The author gratefully acknowledges the superb and expert editorial collaboration by Patrick J. Skerrett.

REFERENCES

1. American Heart Association: Heart Disease and Stroke Statistics—2003 Update. Dallas, American Heart Association, 2003.
2. Agency for Health Care Policy and Research: Cardiac Rehabilitation: Clinical Practice Guideline No. 17 (AHCPR Publication No. 96-0672). Bethesda, Md, National Heart, Lung, and Blood Institute, 1995.
3. Evenson KR, Rosamond WD, Luepker RV: Predictors of outpatient cardiac rehabilitation utilization: The Minnesota Heart Surgery Registry. J Cardiopulm Rehabil 18:192, 1998.
4. Pasquali SK, Alexander KP, Lytle BL, et al: Testing an intervention to increase cardiac rehabilitation enrollment after coronary artery bypass grafting. Am J Cardiol 88:1415 A6, 2001.

History of Cardiac Rehabilitation

5. Hippocrates: The Genuine Works of Hippocrates. Huntington, NY, RE Krieger, 1972.
6. Herrick JB: Clinical features of sudden obstruction of the coronary arteries. JAMA 59:2015, 1912.
7. Lewis T: Diseases of the Heart. New York, Macmillan, 1933.
8. White PD, Rusk HA, Lee PR, Williams B: Rehabilitation of the Cardiovascular Patient New York, McGraw-Hill, 1958.
9. Levine SA: Some harmful effects of recumbency in the treatment of heart disease JAMA 126:80, 1944.
10. Levine SA, Lown B: The "chair" treatment of acute coronary thrombosis. Trans Assoc Am Physicians 64:316, 1951.
11. Saltin B, Blomqvist G, Mitchell JH, et al: Response to exercise after bed rest and after training. Circulation 38:VII1-78, 1968.
12. Wenger NK, Hellerstein HK, Blackburn H, Castranova SJ: Uncomplicated myocardial infarction. Current physician practice in patient management. JAMA 224:511, 1973.
13. Wenger NK, Gilbert C, Skoropa M: Cardiac conditioning after myocardial infarction An early intervention program. J Card Rehabil 2:17, 1971.
14. World Health Organization: Rehabilitation of Patients with Cardiovascular Disease (Technical Report Series No. 270). Geneva, World Health Organization, 1964.

Contemporary Cardiac Rehabilitation

15. Arthur HM, Smith KM, Kodis J, McKelvie R: A controlled trial of hospital versus home-based exercise in cardiac patients. Med Sci Sports Exerc 34:1544, 2002.
16. Gordon NF, English CD, Contractor AS, et al: Effectiveness of three models for comprehensive cardiovascular disease risk reduction. Am J Cardiol 89:1263, 2002.
17. Carlson JJ, Johnson JA, Franklin BA, VanderLaan RL: Program participation, exercise adherence, cardiovascular outcomes, and program cost of traditional versus modified cardiac rehabilitation. Am J Cardiol 86:17, 2000.

Evidence Base for Cardiac Rehabilitation

18. Fletcher GF, Balady GJ, Amsterdam EA, et al: Exercise standards for testing and training: A statement for healthcare professionals from the American Heart Association Circulation 104:1694, 2001.
19. Oldridge NB, Guyatt GH, Fischer ME, Rimm AA: Cardiac rehabilitation after myocardial infarction. Combined experience of randomized clinical trials. JAMA 260:945 1988.
20. O'Connor GT, Buring JE, Yusuf S, et al: An overview of randomized trials of rehabilitation with exercise after myocardial infarction. Circulation 80:234, 1989.
21. Dorn J, Naughton J, Imamura D, Trevisan M: Results of a multicenter randomized clinical trial of exercise and long-term survival in myocardial infarction patients: The National Exercise and Heart Disease Project (NEHDP). Circulation 100:1764, 1999.
22. Jolliffe JA, Rees K, Taylor RS, et al: Exercise-based rehabilitation for coronary heart disease. Cochrane Database Syst Rev, 2003.
23. Chobanian AV, Bakris GL, Black HR, et al: The Seventh Report of the Joint National Committee on Prevention, Detection, Evaluation, and Treatment of High Blood Pressure: The JNC 7 report. JAMA 289:2560, 2003.
24. Gould AL, Rossouw JE, Santanello NC, et al: Cholesterol reduction yields clinical benefit: Impact of statin trials. Circulation 97:946, 1998.
25. Obesity Education Initiative: Clinical guidelines on the identification, evaluation, and treatment of overweight and obesity in adults. National Institutes of Health, National Heart, Lung, and Blood Institute, 1998. (http://www.nhlbi.nih.gov/guidelines/obesity/ob_gdlns.htm)
26. Detry JR, Vierendeel IA, Vanbutsele RJ, Robert AR: Early short-term intensive cardiac rehabilitation induces positive results as long as one year after the acute coronary event: A prospective one-year controlled study. J Cardiovasc Risk 8:355, 2001.

Components of a Cardiac Rehabilitation Program

27. American Association of Cardiovascular and Pulmonary Rehabilitation: Guidelines for Cardiac Rehabilitation and Secondary Prevention Programs. 3rd ed. Champaign, Ill, Human Kinetics, 1999.
28. Blair SN: Evidence for success of exercise in weight loss and control. Ann Intern Med 119:702, 1993.
29. Anderson JW, Konz EC, Frederich RC, Wood CL: Long-term weight-loss maintenance: A meta-analysis of US studies. Am J Clin Nutr 74:579, 2001.
30. Brochu M, Poehlman ET, Ades PA: Obesity, body fat distribution, and coronary artery disease. J Cardiopulm Rehabil 20:96, 2000.
31. Whelton SP, Chin A, Xin X, He J: Effect of aerobic exercise on blood pressure: A meta-analysis of randomized, controlled trials. Ann Intern Med 136:493, 2002.
32. Henriksen EJ: Effects of acute exercise and exercise training on insulin resistance. J Appl Physiol 93:788, 2002.
33. Hu FB, Sigal RJ, Rich-Edwards JW, et al: Walking compared with vigorous physical activity and risk of type 2 diabetes in women: A prospective study. JAMA 282:1433, 1999.
34. Gregg EW, Gerzoff RB, Caspersen CJ, et al: Relationship of walking to mortality among US adults with diabetes. Arch Intern Med 163:1440, 2003.
35. Tanasescu M, Leitzmann MF, Rimm EB, Hu FB: Physical activity in relation to cardiovascular disease and total mortality among men with type 2 diabetes. Circulation 107:2435, 2003.
36. Knowler WC, Barrett-Connor E, Fowler SE, et al: Reduction in the incidence of type 2 diabetes with lifestyle intervention or metformin. N Engl J Med 346:393, 2002.
37. Leon AS, Sanchez OA: Response of blood lipids to exercise training alone or combined with dietary intervention. Med Sci Sports Exerc 33:S502; discussion S528, 2001.

38. Couillard C, Despres JP, Lamarche B, et al: Effects of endurance exercise training on plasma HDL cholesterol levels depend on levels of triglycerides: Evidence from men of the Health, Risk Factors, Exercise Training and Genetics (HERITAGE) Family Study. Arterioscler Thromb Vasc Biol 21:1226, 2001.
39. Kraus WE, Houmard JA, Duscha BD, et al: Effects of the amount and intensity of exercise on plasma lipoproteins. N Engl J Med 347:1483, 2002.
40. Bernstein MS, Costanza MC, James RW, et al: Physical activity may modulate effects of ApoE genotype on lipid profile. Arterioscler Thromb Vasc Biol 22:133, 2002.
41. Wannamethee SG, Lowe GD, Whincup PH, et al: Physical activity and hemostatic and inflammatory variables in elderly men. Circulation 105:1785, 2002.
42. Smith DT, Hoetzer GL, Greiner JJ, et al: Effects of ageing and regular aerobic exercise on endothelial fibrinolytic capacity in humans. J Physiol (Lond) 546:289, 2003.
43. Hambrecht R, Wolf A, Gielen S, et al: Effect of exercise on coronary endothelial function in patients with coronary artery disease. N Engl J Med 342:454, 2000.
44. Gokce N, Vita JA, Bader DS, et al: Effect of exercise on upper and lower extremity endothelial function in patients with coronary artery disease. Am J Cardiol 90:124, 2002.
45. Brendle DC, Joseph LJ, Corretti MC, et al: Effects of exercise rehabilitation on endothelial reactivity in older patients with peripheral arterial disease. Am J Cardiol 87:324, 2001.
46. Linke A, Schoene N, Gielen S, et al: Endothelial dysfunction in patients with chronic heart failure: Systemic effects of lower-limb exercise training. J Am Coll Cardiol 37:392, 2001.
47. Maiorana A, O'Driscoll G, Cheetham C, et al: The effect of combined aerobic and resistance exercise training on vascular function in type 2 diabetes. J Am Coll Cardiol 38:860, 2001.
48. Curtis BM, O'Keefe JH Jr: Autonomic tone as a cardiovascular risk factor: The dangers of chronic fight or flight. Mayo Clin Proc 77:45, 2002.
49. Dekker JM, Crow RS, Folsom AR, et al: Low heart rate variability in a 2-minute rhythm strip predicts risk of coronary heart disease and mortality from several causes: The ARIC Study. Atherosclerosis Risk In Communities. Circulation 102:1239, 2000.
50. Stein PK, Ehsani AA, Domitrovich PP, et al: Effect of exercise training on heart rate variability in healthy older adults. Am Heart J 138:567, 1999.
51. Iellamo F, Legramante JM, Massaro M, et al: Effects of a residential exercise training on baroreflex sensitivity and heart rate variability in patients with coronary artery disease: A randomized, controlled study. Circulation 102:2588, 2000.
52. Lee I-M, Skerrett PJ: Physical activity and all-cause mortality—What is the dose-response relation? Med Sci Sports Exerc 33(6 Suppl):S459, 2001.
53. Myers J, Prakash M, Froelicher V, et al: Exercise capacity and mortality among men referred for exercise testing. N Engl J Med 346:793, 2002.
54. Belardinelli R, Paolini I, Cianci G, et al: Exercise training intervention after coronary angioplasty: The ETICA trial. J Am Coll Cardiol 37:1891, 2001.
55. Rodgers GP, Ayanian JZ, Balady G, et al: American College of Cardiology/American Heart Association Clinical Competence Statement on Stress Testing. A Report of the American College of Cardiology/American Heart Association/American College of Physicians–American Society of Internal Medicine Task Force on Clinical Competence. Circulation 102:1726, 2000.
56. Blair SN, Kampert JB, Kohl HW 3rd, et al: Influences of cardiorespiratory fitness and other precursors on cardiovascular disease and all-cause mortality in men and women. JAMA 276:205, 1996.
57. American College of Sports Medicine Position Stand. The recommended quantity and quality of exercise for developing and maintaining cardiorespiratory and muscular fitness, and flexibility in healthy adults. Med Sci Sports Exerc 30:975, 1998.
58. Ades PA: Cardiac rehabilitation and secondary prevention of coronary heart disease. N Engl J Med 345:892, 2001.
59. Smith SC J., Blair SN, Bonow RO, et al: AHA/ACC guidelines for preventing heart attack and death in patients with atherosclerotic cardiovascular disease: 2001 update. J Am Coll Cardiol 38:1581, 2001.
60. Pollock ML, Franklin BA, Balady GJ, et al: AHA Science Advisory. Resistance exercise in individuals with and without cardiovascular disease: Benefits, rationale, safety, and prescription: An advisory from the Committee on Exercise, Rehabilitation, and Prevention, Council on Clinical Cardiology, American Heart Association; Position paper endorsed by the American College of Sports Medicine. Circulation 101:828, 2000.
61. Shaw DK, Sparks KE, Jennings HS 3rd: Transtelephonic exercise monitoring: A review. J Cardiopulm Rehabil 18:263, 1998.
62. Franklin BA, Bonzheim K, Gordon S, Timmis GC: Safety of medically supervised outpatient cardiac rehabilitation exercise therapy: A 16-year follow-up. Chest 114:902, 1998.
63. Hu FB, Willett WC: Optimal diets for prevention of coronary heart disease. JAMA 288:2569, 2002.
64. Burr ML, Fehily AM, Gilbert JF, et al: Effects of changes in fat, fish, and fibre intakes on death and myocardial reinfarction: Diet and reinfarction trial (DART). Lancet 2:757, 1989.
65. Singh RB, Rastogi SS, Verma R, et al: Randomised controlled trial of cardioprotective diet in patients with recent acute myocardial infarction: Results of one year follow up. BMJ 304:1015, 1992.
66. Singh RB, Dubnov G, Niaz MA, et al: Effect of an Indo-Mediterranean diet on progression of coronary artery disease in high risk patients (Indo-Mediterranean Diet Heart Study): A randomised single-blind trial. Lancet 360:1455, 2002.
67. Ornish D, Scherwitz LW, Billings JH, et al: Intensive lifestyle changes for reversal of coronary heart disease. JAMA 280:2001, 1998.
68. de Lorgeril M, Salen P, Martin JL, et al: Mediterranean diet, traditional risk factors, and the rate of cardiovascular complications after myocardial infarction: Final report of the Lyon Diet Heart Study. Circulation 99:779, 1999.
69. Ware JH: Interpreting incomplete data in studies of diet and weight loss. N Engl J Med 348:2136, 2003.
70. Wing RR, Hill JO: Successful weight loss maintenance. Annu Rev Nutr 21:323, 2001.
71. National Cholesterol Education Program (NCEP) Expert Panel on Detection, Evaluation, and Treatment of High Blood Cholesterol in Adults (Adult Treatment Panel III): Third Report of the National Cholesterol Education Program (NCEP) Expert Panel on Detection, Evaluation, and Treatment of High Blood Cholesterol in Adults (Adult Treatment Panel III) final report. Circulation 106:3143, 2002.
72. Sacks FM, Svetkey LP, Vollmer WM, et al: Effects on blood pressure of reduced dietary sodium and the Dietary Approaches to Stop Hypertension (DASH) diet. DASH-Sodium Collaborative Research Group. N Engl J Med 344:3, 2001.
73. Leaf A, Kang JX, Xiao YF, Billman GE: Clinical prevention of sudden cardiac death by n-3 polyunsaturated fatty acids and mechanism of prevention of arrhythmias by n-3 fish oils. Circulation 107:2646, 2003.
74. Annual smoking-attributable mortality, years of potential life lost, and economic costs—United States, 1995-1999. MMWR Morb Mortal Wkly Rep 51:300, 2002.
75. Benowitz NL, Gourlay SG: Cardiovascular toxicity of nicotine: Implications for nicotine replacement therapy. J Am Coll Cardiol 29:1422, 1997.
76. Fisher SD, Zareba W, Moss AJ, et al: Effect of smoking on lipid and thrombogenic factors two months after acute myocardial infarction. Am J Cardiol 86:813, 2000.
77. Craig WY, Palomaki GE, Haddow JE: Cigarette smoking and serum lipid and lipoprotein concentrations: An analysis of published data. BMJ 298:784, 1989.
78. Sheps DS, Herbst MC, Hinderliter AL, et al.: Production of arrhythmias by elevated carboxyhemoglobin in patients with coronary artery disease. Ann Intern Med 113:343, 1990.
79. Neunteufl T, Heher S, Kostner K, et al: Contribution of nicotine to acute endothelial dysfunction in long-term smokers. J Am Coll Cardiol 39:251, 2002.
80. Winkelmann BR, Boehm BO, Nauck M, et al: Cigarette smoking is independently associated with markers of endothelial dysfunction and hyperinsulinaemia in nondiabetic individuals with coronary artery disease. Curr Med Res Opin 17:132, 2001.
81. Howard G, Wagenknecht LE, Burke GL, et al: Cigarette smoking and progression of atherosclerosis: The Atherosclerosis Risk in Communities (ARIC) Study. JAMA 279:119, 1998.
82. Critchley JA, Capewell S: Mortality risk reduction associated with smoking cessation in patients with coronary heart disease: A systematic review. JAMA 290:86, 2003.
83. van Domburg RT, Meeter K, van Berkel DF, et al: Smoking cessation reduces mortality after coronary artery bypass surgery: A 20-year follow-up study. J Am Coll Cardiol 36:878, 2000.
84. DeBusk RF, Miller NH, Superko HR, et al.: A case-management system for coronary risk factor modification after acute myocardial infarction. Ann Intern Med 120:721, 1994.
85. A clinical practice guideline for treating tobacco use and dependence: A US Public Health Service report. The Tobacco Use and Dependence Clinical Practice Guideline Panel, Staff, and Consortium Representatives. JAMA 283:3244, 2000.
86. Joseph AM, Fu SS: Safety issues in pharmacotherapy for smoking in patients with cardiovascular disease. Prog Cardiovasc Dis 45:429, 2003.
87. Fiore MC, Bailey WC, Cohen SJ, et al: Treating tobacco use and dependence: Clinical practice guideline. Rockville, Md, U.S. Department of Health and Human Services, Public Health Service, 2000.
88. Hevey D, Slack K, Cahill A, et al: Rates of smoking in the households of cardiac patients. J Cardiovasc Risk 9:271, 2002.
89. Berkman LF, Blumenthal J, Burg M, et al, Enhancing Recovery in Coronary Heart Disease Patients Investigators (ENRICHD): Effects of treating depression and low perceived social support on clinical events after myocardial infarction: The Enhancing Recovery in Coronary Heart Disease Patients (ENRICHD) Randomized Trial. JAMA 289:3106, 2003.
90. Berkman LF, Leo-Summers L, Horwitz RI: Emotional support and survival after myocardial infarction. A prospective, population-based study of the elderly. Ann Intern Med 117:1003, 1992.
91. Frasure-Smith N, Lesperance F, Gravel G, et al: Social support, depression, and mortality during the first year after myocardial infarction. Circulation 101:1919, 2000.
92. Frasure-Smith N, Lesperance F: Depression and other psychological risks following myocardial infarction. Arch Gen Psychiatry 60:627, 2003.
93. Lesperance F, Frasure-Smith N, Talajic M, Bourassa MG: Five-year risk of cardiac mortality in relation to initial severity and one-year changes in depression symptoms after myocardial infarction. Circulation 105:1049, 2002.
94. Bush DE, Ziegelstein RC, Tayback M, et al: Even minimal symptoms of depression increase mortality risk after acute myocardial infarction. Am J Cardiol 88:337, 2001.
95. DiMatteo MR, Lepper HS, Croghan TW: Depression is a risk factor for noncompliance with medical treatment: Meta-analysis of the effects of anxiety and depression on patient adherence. Arch Intern Med 160:2101, 2000.
96. Stein PK, Carney RM, Freedland KE, et al: Severe depression is associated with markedly reduced heart rate variability in patients with stable coronary heart disease. J Psychosom Res 48:493, 2000.
97. Markovitz JH, Shuster JL, Chitwood WS, et al: Platelet activation in depression and effects of sertraline treatment: An open-label study. Am J Psychiatry 157:1006, 2000.
98. Rozanski A, Blumenthal JA, Kaplan J: Impact of psychological factors on the pathogenesis of cardiovascular disease and implications for therapy. Circulation 99:2192, 1999.
99. Linden W, Stossel C, Maurice J: Psychosocial interventions for patients with coronary artery disease: A meta-analysis. Arch Intern Med 156:745, 1996.
100. Dusseldorp E, van Elderen T, Maes S, et al: A meta-analysis of psychoeducational programs for coronary heart disease patients. Health Psychol 18:506, 1999.
101. Denollet J, Brutsaert DL: Reducing emotional distress improves prognosis in coronary heart disease: 9-year mortality in a clinical trial of rehabilitation. Circulation 104:2018, 2001.
102. Glassman AH, O'Connor CM, Califf RM, et al: Sertraline treatment of major depression in patients with acute MI or unstable angina. JAMA 288:701, 2002.
103. Burnett RE, Blumenthal JA: Biobehavioral aspects of coronary artery disease: Considerations for prognosis and treatment. *In* Pollock ML, Schmidt DH (eds): Heart Disease and Rehabilitation. 3rd ed. Champaign, Ill, Human Kinetics, 1995, pp 41-55.

104. Hansen M, Streff MM: Patient education: Practical guidelines. *In* Pollock ML, Schmidt DH (eds): Heart Disease and Rehabilitation. 3rd ed. Champaign, Ill, Human Kinetics, 1995, pp 277-286.
105. Bandura A: Social Learning Theory. Englewood Cliffs, NJ, Prentice Hall, 1977.
106. Prochaska JO, DiClemente CC: Stages of change in the modification of problem behaviors. Prog Behav Modif 28:183, 1992.
107. Falk RH: The cardiovascular response to sexual activity: Do we know enough? Clin Cardiol 24:271, 2001.
108. DeBusk R, Drory Y, Goldstein I, et al: Management of sexual dysfunction in patients with cardiovascular disease: Recommendations of The Princeton Consensus Panel. Am J Cardiol 86:175, 2000.
109. Jackevicius CA, Mamdani M, Tu JV: Adherence with statin therapy in elderly patients with and without acute coronary syndromes. JAMA 288:462, 2002.
110. Daly J, Sindone AP, Thompson DR, et al: Barriers to participation in and adherence to cardiac rehabilitation programs: A critical literature review. Prog Cardiovasc Nurs 17:8, 2002.
111. Ades PA, Balady GJ, Berra K: Transforming exercise-based cardiac rehabilitation programs into secondary prevention centers: A national imperative. J Cardiopulm Rehabil 21:263, 2001.

Rehabilitation for Other Populations

112. Pina IL, Apstein CS, Balady GJ, et al: Exercise and heart failure: A statement from the American Heart Association Committee on exercise, rehabilitation, and prevention. Circulation 107:1210, 2003.
113. Experience from controlled trials of physical training in chronic heart failure. Protocol and patient factors in effectiveness in the improvement in exercise tolerance. European Heart Failure Training Group. Eur Heart J 19:466, 1998.
114. McKelvie RS, Teo KK, Roberts R, et al: Effects of exercise training in patients with heart failure: The Exercise Rehabilitation Trial (EXERT). Am Heart J 144:23, 2002.

115. Keteyian S, Shepard R, Ehrman J, et al: Cardiovascular responses of heart transplant patients to exercise training. J Appl Physiol 70:2627, 1991.
116. Braith RW, Welsch MA, Mills RM Jr, et al: Resistance exercise prevents glucocorticoid-induced myopathy in heart transplant recipients. Med Sci Sports Exerc 30:483, 1998.
117. Kavanagh T, Mertens DJ, Shephard RJ, et al: Long-term cardiorespiratory results of exercise training following cardiac transplantation. Am J Cardiol 91:190, 2003.
118. Kobashigawa JA, Leaf DA, Lee N, et al: A controlled trial of exercise rehabilitation after heart transplantation. N Engl J Med 340:272, 1999.
119. Billman GE: Aerobic exercise conditioning: A nonpharmacological antiarrhythmic intervention. J Appl Physiol 92:446, 2002.
120. Vanhees L, Schepers D, Defoor J, et al: Exercise performance and training in cardiac patients with atrial fibrillation. J Cardiopulm Rehabil 20:346, 2000.
121. Fitchet A, Doherty PJ, Bundy C, et al: Comprehensive cardiac rehabilitation programme for implantable cardioverter-defibrillator patients: A randomised controlled trial. Heart 89:155, 2003.
122. Marchionni N, Fattirolli F, Fumagalli S, et al: Improved exercise tolerance and quality of life with cardiac rehabilitation of older patients after myocardial infarction: Results of a randomized, controlled trial. Circulation 107:2201, 2003.
123. Richardson LA, Buckenmeyer PJ, Bauman BD, et al: Contemporary cardiac rehabilitation: Patient characteristics and temporal trends over the past decade. J Cardiopulm Rehabil 20:57, 2000.
124. Vonder Muhll I, Daub B, Black B, et al: Benefits of cardiac rehabilitation in the ninth decade of life in patients with coronary heart disease. Am J Cardiol 90:645, 2002.
125. Paniagua D, Lopez-Jimenez F, Londono JC, et al: Outcome and cost-effectiveness of cardiopulmonary resuscitation after in-hospital cardiac arrest in octogenarians. Cardiology 97:6, 2002.
126. Williams MA, Fleg JL, Ades PA, et al: Secondary prevention of coronary heart disease in the elderly (with emphasis on patients > or = 75 years of age): An American Heart Association scientific statement from the Council on Clinical Cardiology Subcommittee on Exercise, Cardiac Rehabilitation, and Prevention. Circulation 105:1735, 2002.
127. Marks JB, Raskin P: Cardiovascular risk in diabetes: A brief review. J Diabetes Complications 14:108, 2000.
128. 1102Gu K, Cowie CC, Harris MI: Mortality in adults with and without diabetes in a national cohort of the U.S. population, 1971-1993. Diabetes Care 21:1138, 1998.
129. Hu FB, Stampfer MJ, Solomon C, et al: Physical activity and risk for cardiovascular events in diabetic women. Ann Intern Med 134:96, 2001.
130. Gaede P, Vedel P, Larsen N, et al: Multifactorial intervention and cardiovascular disease in patients with type 2 diabetes. N Engl J Med 348:383, 2003.
131. Albright A, Franz M, Hornsby G, et al: American College of Sports Medicine position stand. Exercise and type 2 diabetes. Med Sci Sports Exerc 32:1345, 2000.
132. Ruderman N, Devlin JT, Schneider S, Kriska A: Handbook of Exercise in Diabetes. 2nd ed. Alexandria, Va, American Diabetes Association, 2002.
133. Badenhop DT, Dunn CB, Eldridge S: Monitoring and management of cardiac rehabilitation patients with type 2 diabetes. Clin Exerc Physiol 3:71, 2001.
134. Aiello LP, Wong J, Cavallerano JD, et al: Retinopathy. *In* Ruderman N, Devlin JT, Schneider S, Kriska A (eds): Handbook of Exercise in Diabetes. 2nd ed. Alexandria, Va, American Diabetes Association, 2002, pp 401-413.
135. Rauramaa R, Salonen JT, Seppanen K, et al: Inhibition of platelet aggregability by moderate-intensity physical exercise: A randomized clinical trial in overweight men. Circulation 74:939, 1986.
136. Bader DS, Maguire TE, Spahn CM, et al: Clinical profile and outcomes of obese patients in cardiac rehabilitation stratified according to National Heart, Lung, and Blood Institute criteria. J Cardiopulm Rehabil 21:210, 2001.
137. Lavie CJ, Milani RV: Benefits of cardiac rehabilitation and exercise training. Chest 117:5, 2000.
138. Savage PD, Brochu M, Poehlman ET, Ades PA: Reduction in obesity and coronary risk factors after high caloric exercise training in overweight coronary patients. Am Heart J 146:317, 2003.
139. Savage PD, Lee M, Harvey-Berino J, et al: Weight reduction in the cardiac rehabilitation setting. J Cardiopulm Rehabil 22:154, 2002.
140. Collins AJ: Cardiovascular mortality in end-stage renal disease. Am J Med Sci 325:163 2003.
141. Meier P, Vogt P, Blanc E: Ventricular arrhythmias and sudden cardiac death in end-stage renal disease patients on chronic hemodialysis. Nephron 87:199, 2001.

Cost Effectiveness of Cardiac Rehabilitation

142. Ades PA, Pashkow FJ, Nestor JR: Cost-effectiveness of cardiac rehabilitation after myocardial infarction. J Cardiopulm Rehabil 17:222, 1997.
143. Oldridge N, Perkins A, Marchionni N, et al: Number needed to treat in cardiac rehabilitation. J Cardiopulm Rehabil 22:22, 2002.
144. Weisman SM, Graham DY: Evaluation of the benefits and risks of low-dose aspirin in the secondary prevention of cardiovascular and cerebrovascular events. Arch Intern Med 162:2197, 2002.
145. Freemantle N, Cleland J, Young P, et al: Beta blockade after myocardial infarction: Systematic review and meta regression analysis. BMJ 318:1730, 1999.
146. Georgiou D, Chen Y, Appadoo S, et al: Cost-effectiveness analysis of long-term moderate exercise training in chronic heart failure. Am J Cardiol 87:984, 2001.

Disease Management

147. Haskell WL, Alderman EL, Fair JM, et al.: Effects of intensive multiple risk factor reduction on coronary atherosclerosis and clinical cardiac events in men and women with coronary artery disease. The Stanford Coronary Risk Intervention Project (SCRIP). Circulation 89:975, 1994.

PART VI

Atherosclerotic Cardiovascular Disease

CHAPTER 44

Coronary Blood Flow and Myocardial Ischemia

Morton J. Kern*

The coronary circulation supplies the heart with oxygen and nutrients to maintain cardiac function and thus supply the remainder of the body with blood. The systemic metabolic needs may change rapidly and widely, thus requiring rapid adaptation of cardiac function and coronary blood flow. Imbalance in myocardial oxygen demand and supply can produce myocardial ischemia with contractile cardiac dysfunction, arrhythmias, infarction, and possibly death. Knowledge of the coronary anatomy and flow mechanics of different regions helps us understand the clinical presentations of myocardial ischemia.

The flow through the coronary arteries is pulsatile, with characteristic phasic systolic and diastolic flow components. Systolic compression of the intramural coronary vessels causes mean systolic arterial flow to be reduced relative to diastolic flow, despite having a higher systolic driving pressure. The systolic flow wave has rapid, brief retrograde responses corresponding to phasic myocardial compliance over the cardiac cycle. Diastolic flow occurs during the relaxation phase after myocardial contraction with an abrupt increase above systolic levels and a gradual decline parallel with that of aortic diastolic pressure.

Intramural coronary blood volume changes during each heartbeat, with the myocardium acting as a capacitance circuit to accommodate the volume change brought about by muscular contraction. Coronary venous flow is out of phase with coronary arterial flow, occurring predominantly in systole and nearly absent during diastole. The arterial and venous pulsatile flow characteristics describing the heart as a pump are dependent on intramyocardial compliance. The capacity of the pump as reservoir is controlled by resistance arterioles to coronary vascular inflow, whereas outlet resistance is related to intramural cardiac veins. The intramyocardial capillary resistance influences both arterial and venous responses but predominantly acts in concert with outlet resistance. The coronary blood flow not only is phasic but also varies with the type of vessel and location in the myocardium. The nonlinear and time-dependent behavior of coronary flow may not be negligible under specific experimental or clinical conditions.

Myocardial Oxygen Supply and Demand Relationship

The basic concept of the myocardial supply and demand relationship is that for any given oxygen need, the heart will be supplied with a sufficient quantity to prevent underperfusion leading to ischemia or infarction. Myocardial oxygen demand (MVO_2) has been indexed by the product of systolic aortic pressure and systolic duration. Myocardial oxygen supply (flow) can be indexed by the product of diastolic time and mean diastolic pressure. Figure 44–1 displays major factors of the supply-and-demand relationship.

The heart, an aerobic organ, relies almost exclusively on the oxidation of substrates for energy generation. It can develop only a small oxygen debt. In a steady state, MVO_2 provides an accurate measure of its total metabolism. MVO_2 correlates directly with the fraction of energy derived from the metabolism of fatty acids, which varies directly with the arterial concentration of fatty acids and inversely with that of glucose and insulin. The total metabolism of the arrested, quiescent heart is only a small fraction of that of the working organ. The MVO_2 of the beating canine heart ranges from 8 to 15 ml/min/100 gm, whereas the MVO_2 of the noncontracting heart is approximately 1.5 ml/min/100 gm, an amount required for those physiological processes

*Portions of this chapter have been taken and incorporated from Drs. Peter Ganz and William Ganz, coauthors of this chapter in the sixth edition of this book.

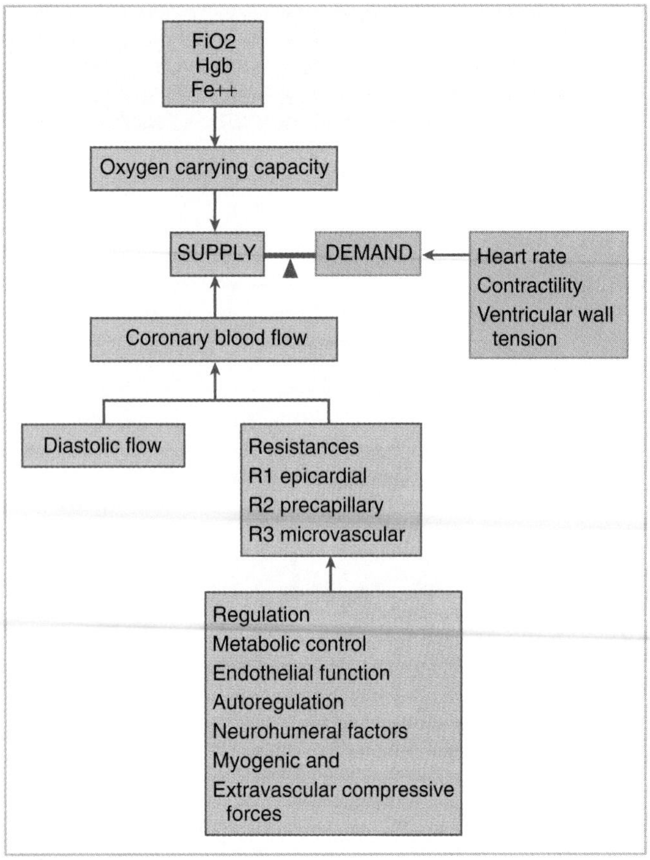

FIGURE 44–1 Factors influencing myocardial oxygen supply and demand. FiO_2 = fraction of inspired oxygen; Hgb = hemoglobin.

not directly associated with contraction. Increases in the frequency of depolarization of the noncontracting heart are accompanied by only small increases in MVO_2 (Table 44–1).

Determinants of Myocardial Oxygen Demand

The three major determinants of MVO_2 are heart rate, myocardial contractility, and myocardial wall tension or stress.[1] Additional factors are shown in Table 44–2.

TABLE 44–1 Myocardial O_2 Consumption Components*

Total 6-8 ml/min/100 gm
Distribution Basal, 20% Electrical, 1% Volume work, 15% Pressure work, 64%
Effects on MVo2 of 50% Increase In Wall stress, 25% Contractility, 45% Pressure work, 50% Heart rate, 50% Volume work, 4%

From Gould KL: Coronary Artery Stenosis. New York, Elsevier, 1991, p 8.
*The table demonstrates the dominant contribution to myocardial O_2 consumption (MVO_2) made by pressure work and prominent effects of increasing pressure work and heart rate on MVO_2.

TABLE 44–2 Determinants of Myocardial O_2 Consumption

Heart rate
Contractile state
Tension development
Activation
Depolarization
Direct metabolic effect of catecholamines
Family history of coronary artery disease
Fatty acid uptake
Maintenance of active state
Maintenance of cell viability in basal state
Shortening against a load (Fenn effect)

Heart Rate

Heart rate is the most important determinant of MVO_2. When heart rate doubles, myocardial oxygen uptake approximately doubles. Heart rate is a dominant factor in the supply-demand ratio for two reasons: (1) increases in heart rate also increase oxygen consumption and (2) increases in heart rate reduce subendocardial coronary flow due to diminution of the diastolic filling period. As demonstrated by Spaan,[2] subendocardial ischemia occurs during tachycardia because of a declining MVO_2–heart rate slope, whereas the relationship between increasing demand (tachycardia) and maximal flow for the subepicardium is relatively stable (Fig. 44–2).

Myocardial Contractility

MVO_2 is determined by the summed responses relating contractility and generated pressure on a per-beat basis. The net effect of positive inotropic stimuli (e.g., Ca^{2+} and catecholamines) on MVO_2 is the result of two major determinants that change in opposite directions in the intact heart. These are *wall tension*, which declines as a consequence of reduction in heart size, and *myocardial contractility*, which, by definition, is augmented by inotropic stimuli. In the failing, dilated ventricle, the increased contractility reduces the left ventricular pressure and volume. On the basis of the Laplace relation, the reduction in ventricular volume leads to a reduction in myocardial tension, which reduces MVO_2. However, the decrease in MVO_2 that might be expected to result from falling ventricular wall tension is opposed by the increase in

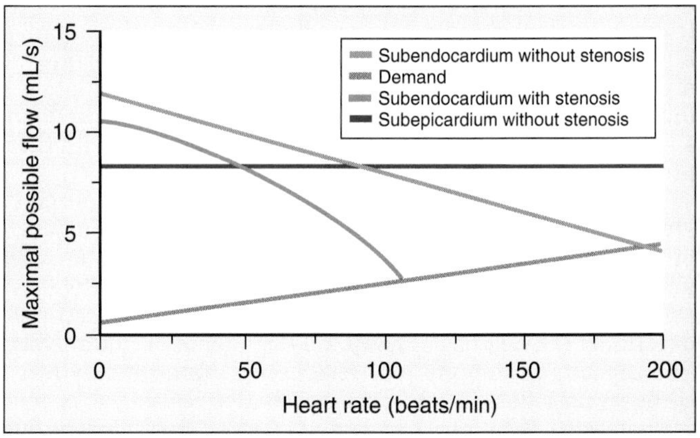

FIGURE 44–2 Schematic representation of the effect of heart rate on myocardial blood flow: The myocardial oxygen demand for unit weight of tissue is similar for the two layers in the heart, but the maximum flow at the subendocardium decreases with heart rate faster than the demand increases, especially in the presence of the stenosis. The maximum flow curve for the subepicardium in the presence of a stenosis has not been drawn. (Modified from Spaan JAE, Piek JJ, Siebes M: Coronary circulation and hemodynamics. *In* Kurachi Y, Terzic A, Cohen M, et al [eds]: Heart Physiology and Pathophysiology. 4th ed. Boston, Academic Press, 2001.)

contractility, which tends to augment MVO_2. Thus, the change in MVO_2 consequent to an inotropic stimulus depends on the extent to which intramyocardial tension is reduced in relation to the extent to which contractility is augmented. In the absence of heart failure, drugs that stimulate myocardial contractility elevate MVO_2 because heart size and therefore wall tension are not reduced substantially and do not offset the effect of the stimulation of contractility. The increase in MVO_2 produced by positive inotropic agents, such as Ca^{2+} and epinephrine, results from the energy costs of enhanced excitation-contraction coupling.

Myocardial Wall Tension

Myocardial tension developed during systole is proportionate to the aortic pressure, myocardial fibril length, and ventricular volume. MVO_2 doubles as mean aortic pressure increases from 75 to 175 mm Hg, at constant heart rate and stroke volume. The myocardial inotropic state determines ventricular performance independent of preload and afterload and increases 30% when the rate of pressure development in the left ventricle (dP/dt) is doubled, such as occurs following extrasystolic potentiation or by norepinephrine when heart rate, aortic pressure, and cardiac output are maintained constant. Comparing the relative effects of ventricular pressure, stroke volume, and heart rate on MVO_2, it was found that ventricular pressure development is a key determinant of MVO_2. MVO_2 per beat correlated well with the area under the left ventricular pressure curve (time × pressure), termed the *tension-time index*.[2,3] Subsequently, the myocardial wall tension–time integral was found to be a more accurate determinant of MVO_2 than is the developed pressure. An augmentation of *heart rate* elevates MVO_2 by increasing the frequency of tension development per unit time, as well as by increasing contractility.

MVO_2 is also influenced by the degree of myocardial shortening during stroke volume ejection, although less than by tension development. The systolic pressure-rate product (also known as the *double product*) can be used as an estimate of MVO_2 in a clinical setting, such as exercise or pacing tachycardia, recognizing the limited accuracy. MVO_2 closely correlates with the left ventricular systolic pressure-volume loop area (the external mechanical work) and the end-systolic elastic potential energy in the ventricular wall (the area enclosed by the systolic pressure-volume trajectory, and the E_{max} line) (Fig. 44–3).

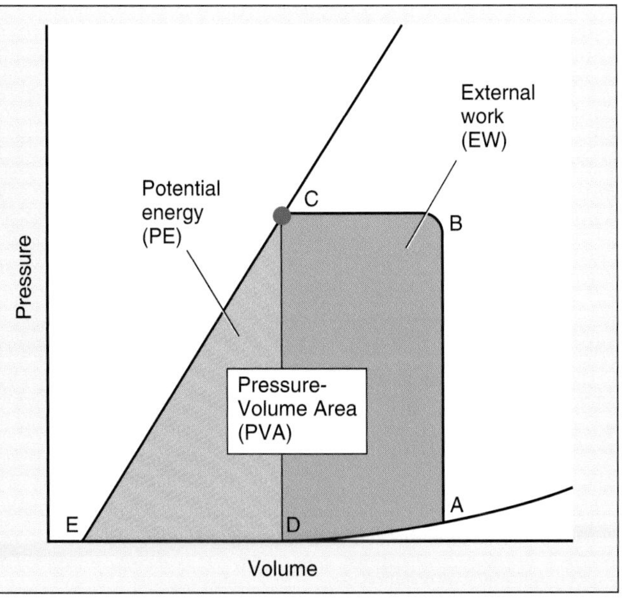

FIGURE 44–3 Myocardial oxygen consumption correlates with the left ventricular pressure-volume area (PVA). PVA is the area in the pressure-volume (PV) diagram that is circumscribed by the end-systolic PV line (E-C), the end-diastolic PV relation curve (D-A), and the systolic segment of the PV trajectory (E-A-B-C-E). PVA consists of the external work (EW) performed during systole and the end-systolic elastic potential energy (PE) stored in the ventricular wall at end-systole. EW is the area within the PV loop trajectory (A-B-C-D-A), and PE is the area between the end-systolic PV line and the end-diastolic PV relation curve to the left of EW (E-C-D-E). (From Kameyama T, Asanoi H, Ishizaka S, et al: Energy conversion efficiency in human left ventricle. Circulation 85:988, 1992.)

Determinants of Myocardial Oxygen Supply

Myocardial oxygen supply is provided by the coronary arterial and capillary inflow and a satisfactory capability of hemoglobin to transport and deliver oxygen to the myocardial cells. A breakdown in any link of this chain can result in an inadequate myocardial oxygen supply.

OXYGEN TRANSPORT AND DELIVERY. Satisfactory oxygen transport and delivery require an adequate inspired quantity of oxygen and red blood cells with normally functioning hemoglobins. Hypoxia from pneumonia or carbon monoxide overdose, anemia, or hemoglobinopathies can produce myocardial ischemia despite adequate coronary blood flow.

REGULATION OF CORONARY BLOOD FLOW AND RESISTANCE. Approximately 75 percent of total coronary resistance occurs in the arterial system, which comprises conductance (R1), prearteriolar (R2), and arteriolar and intramyocardial capillary vessels (R3).[4] Normal epicardial coronary arteries in humans are typically 0.3 to 5 mm in caliber and do not offer appreciable resistance to blood flow. Even at the highest level of blood flow, there is no detectable resistance that would manifest as a pressure drop along the length of human epicardial arteries.[5] Normally, large epicardial vessel resistance (R1) is trivial until atherosclerotic obstructions compromise the lumen. During systole, the blood volume increases approximately 25 percent as antegrade flow from the aorta enters and retrograde flow is squeezed from the myocardial vessels. Elastic energy of the vessel wall during systole is transformed into blood kinetic energy at the beginning of diastole. Since most of the vessel wall comprises a muscular media that responds to changes in aortic pressure and modulates coronary tone in response to flow-mediated endothelium-dependent vasodilators, circulating vasoactive substance, and neurostimuli, conductive activity is impaired when vascular wall disease is present. Large conduit arteries are unaffected by myocardial metabolites because of their extramural location.

Precapillary arterioles (R2) are resistive vessels connecting epicardial to myocardial capillaries and are the principal controllers of coronary blood flow.[4] Precapillary arterioles (100 to 500 μm in size) contribute approximately 25 to 35 percent of total coronary resistance (Fig. 44–4). The prearteriolar resistance function maintains driving pressure at the origin of the precapillary arterioles within a preset autoregulatory pressure range. This regulatory function is also mediated by myogenic autoregulation and flow-dependent vasodilation related to shear stress.

Distal precapillary arteriolar vessels are the main site of *metabolic* regulation of coronary blood flow. These vessels (<100 μm in diameter) are responsible for 40 to 50 percent of coronary flow resistance. The distal arteriolar tone is modulated by neurogenic stimuli and local vasoactive products. In some settings, the effects of vasoconstrictor stimuli are strong enough to induce myocardial ischemia unopposed by locally released myocardial vasodilatory metabolites.

The dense network of about 4000 capillaries per square millimeter ensures that each myocyte is adjacent to a capillary. Capillaries are not uniformly patent because precapillary sphincters regulate flow according to the needs of the myocardium. This capillary density is reduced in the presence of ventricular hypertrophy. Several conditions, such as left ventricular hypertrophy, myocardial ischemia, or diabetes can impair the microcirculatory resistance (R3), blunting the maximal absolute increase in coronary flow in times of increased oxygen demand. Increased R3 resistance may also be associated with elevated resting blood flow above that expected for the existing MVO_2, resulting in reduced coronary flow reserve.

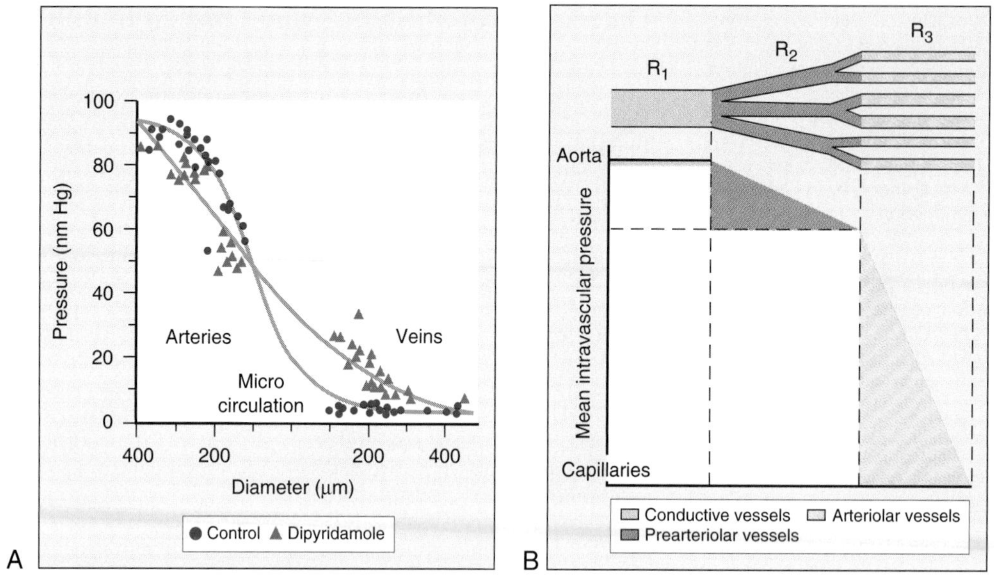

FIGURE 44–4 **A,** Pressure distribution as a function of vessel diameter in the cat. **B,** Schematic representation of the coronary arterial system and its subdivisions. Resistance to blood flow is highest in the arteriolar bed, in which vasodilator activity is under myocardial metabolic regulation. Prearteriolar vessels also contribute to coronary resistance but are not influenced by direct metabolic control. The prearteriolar vessels function to maintain pressure at the origin of the arterioles within a narrow range under varying aortic pressure and coronary flow. The conductive vessels provide negligible resistance to flow. (**A,** From Chilian WM, Layne SM, Klausner ED, et al: Redistribution of coronary microvascular resistance produced by dipyridamole. Am J Physiol 256:H383-390, 1989. **B,** From Maseri A: Ischemic Heart Disease. New York, Churchill Livingstone, 1995.)

Control heterogeneity of the coronary resistance vessels has been demonstrated with specialized resistance vessel function according to their size.[4] For example, in the smallest arterioles (<30 μm), metabolic vasodilation occurs predominantly, whereas intermediate arterioles (30 to 60 μm) are the principal site of myogenic regulation. The large arterioles (100 to 150 μm) appear to be the sites of flow-mediated dilation.[6] A system of multiple functional "valves" permits fine control of the coronary circulation. The smallest arterioles dilate during metabolic stress resulting in reduced microvascular resistance and increased myocardial perfusion. As the upstream arteriolar pressure decreases owing to a fall in distending pressure across a stenosis, myogenic dilation of slightly larger arterioles upstream occurs and causes an additional decrease in resistance. Increased flow in the largest arterioles augments shear stress and triggers flow-mediated dilation, further reducing the resistance of this network. Thus, coronary arterioles appear to have specialized regulatory elements along their length that operate "in series" in an integrated manner.

As in any vascular bed, blood flow to the myocardium depends on the coronary artery driving pressure and the resistance offered by the resistance components. Coronary vascular resistance, in turn, is regulated by several interrelated control mechanisms that include myocardial metabolism (metabolic control), endothelial (and other humoral) control, autoregulation, myogenic control, extravascular compressive forces, and neural control. These control mechanisms may be impaired in disease states, thereby contributing to the development of myocardial ischemia (Tables 44–3 and 44–4).

TABLE 44–3 Regulation of Coronary Circulation

Mechanism	Effector
Autoregulation	Intrinsic vasoconstrictor tone
Perfusion pressure	Aortic or poststenotic pressure
Metabolic activity	Exercise, ischemia
Myocardial compression and myogenic mechanisms	Systolic-diastolic interaction
Neural control	Sympathetic, parasympathetic, pain
Endothelium	EDRF, EDCF
Pharmacologic	Dipyridaimole, adenosine, acetylcholine, α, β, agonists and antagonists, and so forth

EDRF = endothelial-derived relaxing factor; EDCF = endothelial-derived constricting factor.

Modified from Gould L: Coronary Artery Stenosis and Reversing Atherosclerosis. 2nd ed. New York, Arnold and Oxford University Press, 1998.

TABLE 44–4 Mediators of Coronary Vasodilation*

Stimulus	Epicardial Arteries	Arterioles, Increased Flow
Acetylcholine	*Nitric oxide*	*Endothelial*
Flow shear	*Endothelial*	*Nitric oxide*
Exercise	*Nitric oxide*, neural	*Metabolic*, nitric oxide, neural
Pacing	*Nitric oxide*	*Nitric oxide*, metabolic
Ischemia or hypoxia	*Metabolic*, nitric oxide	*Metabolic*, nitric oxide
Perfusion pressure	*Myogenic*	*Myogenic*
Reactive hyperemia	*Myogenic*, flow shear	*Myogenic*, flow shear, metabolic, nitric oxide, prostacycline
Dipyridamole, adenosine	No direct effect	*Direct dilator*, nitric oxide
Nitroglycerine	*Direct dilator*	No direct effect
Collaterals	—	*Nitric oxide*, prostaglandin

From Gould L: Coronary Artery Stenosis and Reversing Atherosclerosis. 2nd ed. New York, Arnold and Oxford University Press, 1998.

*Italics, primary mechanism followed by secondary or contributing mechanisms; endothelial, unknown mediator, not oxide; metabolic, unknown mediators or mechanisms but in part mediated by adenosine.

Endothelial Function

The vascular endothelium performs an array of homeostatic functions within normal blood vessels. Located between the blood lumen and the vascular smooth muscle cells, the endothelium is a monolayer of cells capable of transducing blood-borne signals, sensing mechanical forces within the lumen, and regulating vascular tone through the production of a variety of vasoactive humoral factors (Table 44-5; see also Fig. 37-14).[7] Endothelium produces both potent vasodilators, such as endothelium-derived relaxing factor (EDRF), nitric oxide (NO), prostacyclin, and endothelium-derived hyperpolarizing factor (EDHF), and vasoconstrictors, such as endothelin 1 (ET-1). Normally, the endothelium promotes vasodilatory functions in response to a variety of systemic, neurohumoral, and mechanical stimuli. Inappropriate vasoconstriction characterizes the vascular response in patients with endothelial dysfunction.[8]

An imbalance among the endothelium-derived counteracting vasoactive factors occurs in vascular segments damaged early in the atherosclerotic process. Dysfunctional endothelium, common in patients with cardiovascular risk factors, leads to disturbances in coronary blood flow, promoting myocardial ischemia, and accelerating the evolution of atherosclerosis and thrombosis.[9]

Endothelium-dependent vasodilation not only operates in large (conductance) arteries, but is also an important mechanism that controls dilation in small (resistance) vessels. Although atherosclerosis does not directly involve resistance vessels, coronary risk factors markedly impair resistance vessel responses to endothelium-dependent vasodilator stimuli.[8] Endothelial dysfunction in resistance vessels may be an important factor in preventing increases in coronary blood flow during times of augmented metabolic stress. Impaired endothelium-dependent dilation of coronary resistance vessels also accounts for some of the cases of syndrome X (patients with normal coronary angiography, chest pain, and evidence of stress-induced myocardial ischemia).[10] For example, in normal subjects, exercise induces coronary vasodilation, whereas in patients with atherosclerotic coronary artery disease and stable angina, exercise produces paradoxical vasoconstriction typically at the site of coronary stenoses or mildly irregular arterial segments. Vasomotor changes during exercise parallel the responses observed to the endothelium-dependent agent, acetylcholine. Paradoxical constriction of atherosclerotic coronary arteries has also been observed with mental stress, the cold pressor test, and tachycardia,[11] conditions normally activating the sympathetic nervous system, increasing circulating catecholamines and coronary blood flow secondary to a rise in MVO_2. The loss of endothelium-dependent dilation occurs early in atherosclerosis, even prior to its detection by angiography, and is related to risk factors for atherosclerosis (Table 44-6).[12] Oxidized low-density lipoprotein (LDL) and small, dense LDL particles reduce NO synthase.[2] Degradation of chylomicrons and very low-density lipoprotein produce highly atherogenic remnant particles associated with endothelial dysfunction and reduced NO.[13]

ENDOTHELIUM-DERIVED RELAXING FACTORS. In healthy arteries, endothelium-dependent vasodilation predominates over direct smooth muscle vasoconstriction. EDRF is produced from an intact endothelium and mediates acetylcholine-induced vasodilation.[14] EDRF has been identified as the NO radical formed in endothelial cells from L-arginine by the action of NO synthase (Fig. 44-5).[15] The activity of the reaction is also controlled by calcium and calmodulin. NO diffuses into smooth muscle cells activating intracellular guanylate cyclase, increasing cyclic guanosine monophosphate (GMP), and consequently decreasing intracellular calcium. Once released from endothelial cells, NO has a very short half-life due to interaction with other free radicals in tissues, principally superoxide, and is destroyed after entering red blood cells to react with oxyhemoglobin. Endothelium-dependent vasodilation by NO secretion in healthy human epicardial arteries can be inhibited by specifically blocking NO synthesis with N^G-monomethyl-L-arginine (L-NMMA).[16]

TABLE 44-5 Autocrine and Paracrine Substances Released from the Endothelium

Type of Substance	Specific Substances
Vasodilators	NO, prostacyclin, endothelium-derived hyperpolarizing factor, bradykinin, adrenomedullin, C-natriuretic peptide
Vasoconstrictors	ET-1, angiotensin II, thromboxane A_2, oxidant radicals, prostaglandin H_2
Antiproliferative	NO, prostacyclin, transforming growth factor-β, heparin sulfate
Proproliferative	ET-1, angiotensin II, oxidant radicals, platelet-derived growth factor, basic fibroblast growth factor, insulin-like growth factor, interleukins
Antithrombotic	NO, prostacyclin, plasminogen activator, protein C, tissue factor inhibitor, von Willebrand factor
Prothrombotic	ET-1, oxidant radicals, plasminogen-activator inhibitor-1, thromboxane A_2, fibrinogen, tissue factor
Inflammatory markers	CAMs (P- and E-selectin, ICAM, VCAM) chemokines, nuclear factor κB
Permeability	Receptor for advanced glycosylation end-products
Angiogenesis	Vascular endothelial growth factor

CAM = cellular adhesion molecule; ET = endothelin 1; ICAM = intercellular adhesion molecule; NO = nitric oxide; VCAM = vascular cellular adhesion molecule.

Modified from Verma S, Anderson T: Fundamentals of endothelial function for the clinical cardiologist. Circulation 105:546-549, 2002.

TABLE 44-6 Risk Factors Associated with Impaired Endothelium-Dependent Vasodilation

Dyslipidemia
Hypertension
Diabetes mellitus
Cigarette smoking
Menopause
Hyperhomocysteinemia
Aging
Family history of coronary artery disease
Mutations in eNOS

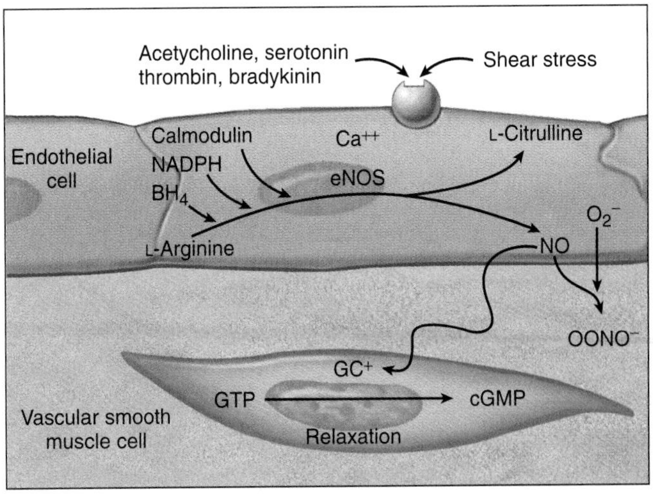

FIGURE 44-5 Endothelial cell production of nitric oxide (NO) by the action of nitric oxide synthase (eNOS) on L-arginine. This reaction requires a number of cofactors such as tetrahydrobiopterin (BH_4), calmodulin, and NADPH. eNOS stimulation by vasodilator agonists or shear stress is mediated by rise in intracellular calcium (Ca^{2+}). NO may be broken down by free radicals (O_2^-), producing peroxinitrite ($OONO^-$), which is vasoinactive. NO acts on vascular smooth muscle cells to cause relaxation by activating guanylate cyclase (GC^+), thereby increasing intracellular cyclic guanosine monophosphate (cGMP).

The release of NO is stimulated by products of thrombosis (thrombin), aggregating platelets (serotonin, adenosine diphosphate [ADP]), other chemical stimuli (histamine, bradykinin), and increased shear stress with flow-mediated vasodilation. In contrast to NO, the nitrovasodilators (e.g., nitroglycerin, nitroprusside) and prostacyclin act independently of the endothelium and directly on vascular smooth muscle.[7] Adenosine elicits both endothelium-independent and endothelium-dependent vasodilation; at high concentration of adenosine, endothelium-independent dilation dominates.

NO also inhibits the recruitment and differentiation of inflammatory cells by inhibiting the production of chemoattractant cytokines, leukocyte adhesion molecules, and factors encouraging the differentiation of monocytes into macrophages. Reductions in NO are associated with activation of potentially vulnerable atherosclerotic plaques and acute coronary syndromes.[17]

Endothelium-dependent vasodilation also occurs by hyperpolarizing the underlying smooth muscle through activation of Ca^{2+}-activated K^+ channels, a response attributed to a diffusible factor termed *EDHF* (also known as *11,12-epoxyeicosatrienoic acid*).[18] EDHF appears to be far more important in small arterioles than in larger conduit arteries.[19] It is released by many of the same stimuli that stimulate NO, including acetylcholine, bradykinin, substance P, and shear stress. Although there may be more than one EDHF molecule, cytochrome P450–dependent metabolites of arachidonic acid, especially the epoxide EDHF, also act as mediators of endothelium-dependent hyperpolarization and have antiinflammatory properties. NO inhibits the production of EDHF. A decrease in NO bioavailability maintains endothelial vasodilator function by upregulation of EDHF.[19]

ENDOTHELIUM-DERIVED CONSTRICTING FACTORS. The endothelium not only mediates vasodilation but also is a source of vasoconstrictor factors, the best characterized being the endothelins. ET-1 is a 21-amino-acid peptide that has a potent vasoconstrictor activity. Two other isoforms of ET have been discovered (ET-2 and ET-3), but endothelium produces only ET-1. Beginning with a large precursor molecule, preproendothelin is converted by the action of endothelin-converting enzyme to the fully active ET-1.[20]

Unlike NO, which can be released rapidly in response to vasodilator stimuli and then inactivated within seconds, ET-1–mediated constriction is slow in onset and lasts over minutes to hours. Agents that stimulate ET-1, such as thrombin, angiotensin II, epinephrine, or vasopressin, do so by de novo transcription of messenger RNA. ET-1 contributes to the regulation of vascular tone primarily by exerting a tonic vasoconstrictor influence and stimulates smooth muscle proliferation, vascular remodeling, and leukocyte adhesion and recruitment.[21] Plasma concentrations of ET-1 are elevated in a number of cardiovascular disorders including hypercholesterolemia, hypertension, atherosclerosis, acute myocardial infarction, and congestive heart failure.[21] Oxidized LDL associated with vulnerable plaque activators is a potent stimulus to ET-1 synthesis. ET-1 exerts its vascular effects by binding to two specific receptors named ET-A and ET-B. ET-A receptors are present on vascular smooth muscle cells and promote vasoconstriction and smooth muscle proliferation. ET-B receptors are located on endothelial cells, where they mediate endothelium-dependent dilation by releasing NO, and also on smooth muscle cells, where they mediate constriction.[22]

ENDOTHELIAL FUNCTION TESTING. Endothelial function can be tested by examining the angiographic vasodilatory responses to intracoronary infusions of endothelial-dependent and -independent vasodilators. The infusion of acetylcholine evokes an endothelium-dependent NO-mediated vasodilatory response. In patients with endothelial dysfunction the normal vasodilatory response is blunted or paradoxic vasoconstriction occurs. Endothelial function of microvascular reserve is assessed by intracoronary Doppler flow velocity measurements during intracoronary infusions of acetylcholine and adenosine for endothelial-dependent and -independent responses, respectively.

Noninvasive assessments of coronary endothelial function, evaluating coronary epicardial blood flow and microcirculatory responses, have been obtained by Doppler echocardiography, positron-emission tomography, and phase-contrast magnetic resonance imaging. The most widely used noninvasive method to assess endothelial function of the peripheral circulation is brachial artery reactive hyperemia obtained during upper arm arterial occlusion and release. Normal endothelial function produces flow-mediated vasodilation of the arterial diameter assessed by continuous ultrasound scanning. Peripheral vascular resistance using strain-gauge venous impedance plethysmography examines forearm blood flow in response to intraarterial administration of vascular agonist into the brachial artery. Brachial artery responses have been generally related to coronary endothelial function. (Fig. 44–6 illustrates changes in coronary diameter and flow during endothelial function testing.) Abnormal endothelial responses can be restored by treatment with angiotensin-converting enzyme inhibitors, antioxidants, and the oral administration of L-arginine.[23] Table 44–7 lists strategies to counter endothelial dysfunction.

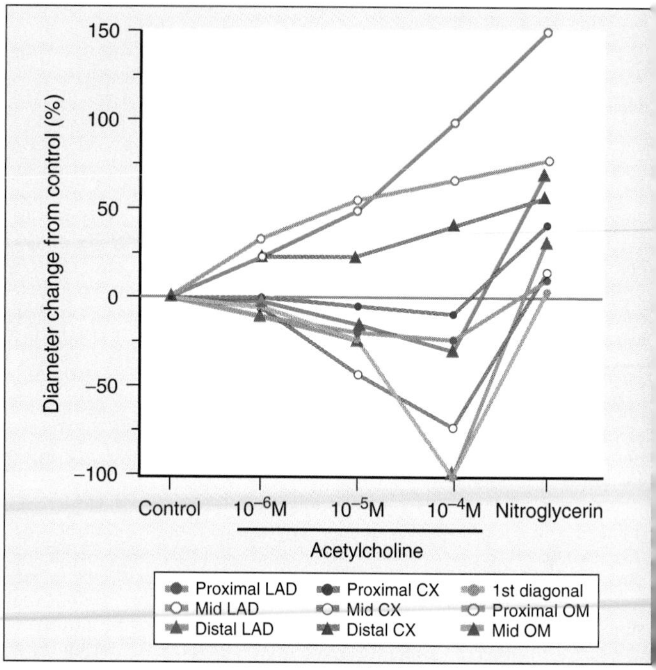

FIGURE 44–6 Heterogeneous responses of coronary artery diameter to the intracoronary acetylcholine in a patient with coronary artery disease. CX = circumflex artery LAD = left anterior descending [coronary artery]; OM = obtuse marginal artery. (From El-Tamini H, Mansour M, Wargovich TJ, et al: Constrictor and dilator responses to intracoronary acetylcholine in adjacent segments of the same coronary artery in patients with coronary artery disease. Circulation 89:45-51, 1994.)

Autoregulation

Foremost in the control of coronary blood flow is the fundamental relationship that myocardial oxygen supply rises and falls in response to the oxygen (energy) demands of the myocardium. Sudden alterations in systemic hemodynamics are matched with abrupt and transitory changes in blood flow, promptly returning to the resting steady state after activity has ceased. The ability to maintain myocardial perfusion at constant levels in the face of changing driving pressure is termed *autoregulation* (Fig. 44–7). Autoregulation maintains coronary perfusion at relatively constant levels over a wide range of mean aortic pressure from130 to 40 mm Hg in experimental animals and humans.[24] When aortic pressure exceeds its upper or lower limits, coronary blood flow precipitously declines or increases proportionately. Normally functioning autoregulation prevents myocardial ischemia at rest. When reduced perfusion pressure distal to stenoses is not compensated by autoregulatory dilation of the resistance vessels, ischemia occurs. Chronic hypertension and left ventricular hypertrophy narrow the range of autoregulation, especially in the subendocardium. In some patients, exhaustion of subendocardial autoregulation may lead to ischemia in the absence of a significant coronary stenosis.

Systemic hypotension can lower perfusion pressure below the critical lower limit of effective autoregulation, producing myocardial ischemia that increases left ventricular filling pressure, further reducing the coronary perfusion gradient. Hypotension begets a deteriorating, self-perpetuating ischemic spiral, especially deadly in patients with critical coronary stenoses, such as those with left main or with three-vessel coronary disease. Augmenting coronary (diastolic)

TABLE 44–7 Conditions Associated with Impaired Endothelial Function, Strategies to Counter Endothelial Dysfunction, and Surrogate Soluble Markers of Endothelial Dysfunction

Conditions associated with impaired endothelial function	Atherosclerosis, hypercholesterolemia, high LDL-C, low HDL-C, high lipoprotein (a), small dense LDL-C, oxidized LDL-C, hypertension, high homocysteine, aging, vasculitis, preeclampsia, metabolic syndrome, variant angina, diabetes, active smoking, passive smoking, ischemia-reperfusion, transplant atherosclerosis, cardiopulmonary bypass, postmenopause, Kawasaki disease, Chagas disease, family history CAD, infections, depression, inactivity, obesity, renal failure, increased CRP, congestive heart failure, left ventricular hypertrophy, postprandial state
Interventions to improve endothelial function	ACE inhibitors, angiotensin receptor blockers, endothelin blockers, statins, tetrahydrobiopterin, folates, exercise, improving insulin sensitivity, LDL reduction, HDL augmentation, antioxidants, estrogen, L-arginine, desferoxamine, glutathione, homocysteine reduction, lowering CRP, reducing free fatty acid flux
Soluble surrogate markers of endothelial dysfunction	CAMs, von Willbebrand factor, ET-1, nitrites, asymmetric dimethylarginine, CRP, tissue plasminogen activator, fibrinogen, amyloid A

Modified from Verma S, Anderson T: Fundamentals of endothelial function for the clinical cardiologist. Circulation 105:546-549, 2002.
ACE = angiotensin-converting enzyme; CAM = cellular adhesion molecule; CAD = coronary artery disease; CRP = C-reactive protein; ET = endothelin; HDL = high-density lipoprotein; LDL = low-density lipoprotein.

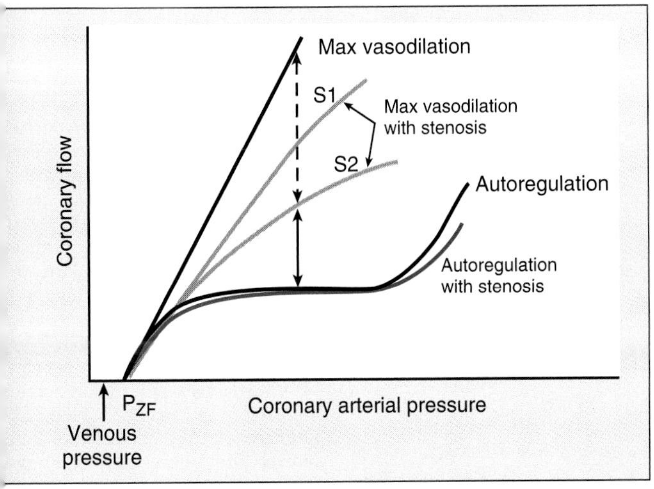

FIGURE 44–7 Coronary pressure-flow relations with and without stenosis. Autoregulation of flow at rest without stenosis and maximal vasodilation without stenosis are indicated in black lines. S1 has mild stenosis compared to S2. The solid arrow illustrates the reduced coronary flow reserve related to the presence of a severe stenosis. The dashed arrow indicates the dilatory reserve loss because of the stenosis. P_{ZF} is pressure at zero flow. (From Spaan JAE, Piek JJ, Siebes M: Coronary circulation and hemodynamics. *In* Kurachi Y, Terzic A, Cohen M, et al [eds]: Heart Physiology and Pathophysiology. 4th ed. Boston, Academic Press, 2001.)

perfusion pressure with intraaortic balloon pumping in this setting restores coronary pressure so that autoregulation is reestablished and the cycle of myocardial ischemia may be attenuated or terminated.

Metabolic Regulation

Coronary blood flow is closely coupled to MVO_2 in normal hearts because (1) the myocardium depends almost entirely on aerobic metabolism; (2) the myocardial oxygen extraction saturation is very high as evidenced by low coronary venous oxygen saturation (25 to 30 percent at rest); and (3) oxygen stores in the heart are meager. Potent vasodilator agents such as NO, adenosine, and dipyridamole can relax vascular smooth muscle in coronary arterioles and can attenuate autoregulation. Release of intrinsic vasodilators links myocardial oxygen supply to demand.

ADENOSINE. Adenosine, the principal mediator of coronary blood flow and local metabolic regulation, is formed by degradation of adenine nucleotides. Degradation occurs when adenosine triphosphate (ATP) utilization exceeds the capacity of myocardial cells to resynthesize high-energy phosphate compounds (a process dependent on mitochondrial oxidative phosphorylation). This results in the production of adenosine monophosphate (AMP). The enzyme 5′-nucleotidase is responsible for the formation of adenosine from AMP (Fig. 44–8). Accordingly, adenosine diffuses from myocytes into the interstitial fluid and the coronary venous effluent. Adenosine is a powerful coronary dilator, and its production increases during an imbalance in the oxygen supply-to-demand ratio. The rise in the interstitial concentration of adenosine parallels the increase in coronary blood flow. The inhibition of adenosine, either by its destruction by adenosine deaminase or by administration of adenosine receptor antagonists, does not always reduce the magnitude of the hyperemia in response to metabolic stimuli in animals or humans.[25] Adenosine is certainly not the *only* vasoactive factor involved in the metabolic regulation of coronary blood flow. NO, vasodilator prostaglandins, ATP-sensitive K^+ channels (K^+-ATP channels), and myocardial oxygen and carbon dioxide tensions also contribute to metabolic regulation.

NITRIC OXIDE AND OTHER METABOLIC MEDIATORS. NO increases blood flow in response to metabolic stimuli. Inhibition of NO reduces the magnitude of metabolic dilation in animals and in the peripheral and coronary circulation in humans.[25] Metabolic stimuli augment NO production by at least two mechanisms: (1) hypoxia-stimulated release of NO from the endothelium and (2) coronary flow–mediated vasodilation. Although hypoxia may initiate hyperemia, flow-mediated dilation sustains and amplifies it.

Prostaglandins and K^+-ATP channels also act in concert to regulate coronary flow in response to metabolic needs.[26] A loss or inhibition of one mediator is compensated for by upregulation of others. Although the inhibition of K^+-ATP channels, adenosine, and NO individually have, at most, a modest effect on the increase in coronary blood flow during exercise in dogs, inhibition of all three simultaneously nearly abolishes the flow increase.[27]

Neural and Neurohumeral Control

Neural control of the coronary circulation complements local metabolic, autoregulatory, and endothelial mechanisms.[28] Epicardial arteries and coronary arterioles are innervated by sympathetic and parasympathetic fibers, with extensive adrenergic and muscarinic receptor supply (Table 44-8). In addition to acetylcholine and norepinephrine, nonadrenergic and noncholinergic neurotransmitters have been identified modulating adrenergic and cholinergic output.[28,29] These substances include purines (ATP), amines (serotonin and dopamine), and peptides (neuropeptide Y, calcitonin-gene related peptide [CGRP], substance P, and vasoactive intestinal peptide). Neuropeptide Y released during sympathetic nerve stimulation causes ischemia by microvascular constriction. Intracoronary infusion of CGRP and substance P cause release of EDRF and dose-dependent vasodilation of epicardial vessels equivalent to that produced by nitrates.[30]

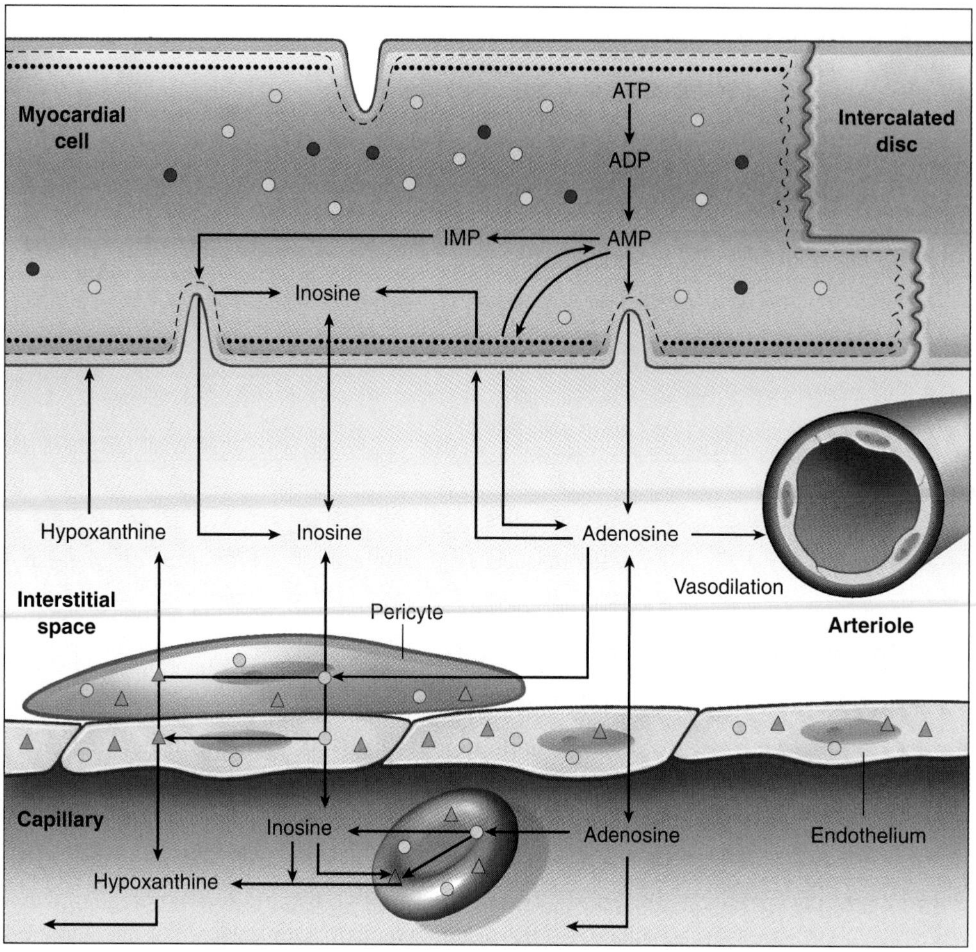

FIGURE 44–8 Schematic depiction of a myocardial interstitial space, an arteriole, and a capillary with the localization of enzymes involved in the formation and fate of adenosine. Adenosine formed by 5′-nucleotidase from adenosine monophosphate (AMP) (which in turn arises from adenosine triphosphate) can enter the interstitial space. There it can induce arteriolar dilation and reenter the myocardial cell, where it is either phosphorylated to AMP by adenosine kinase or deaminated to inosine monophosphate (IMP) by adenosine deaminase, or it can enter the capillaries and leave the tissue. A large fraction of adenosine that crosses the capillary wall is deaminated to inosine, which in turn is split to hypoxanthine and ribose-1-PO_4 by nucleoside phosphorylase located in the endothelial cells, pericytes, and erythrocytes. Most of the adenosine is taken up by the myocardial cells. Adenosine escaping into the circulation is largely in the form of inosine and hypoxanthine. Because adenylic acid deaminase (which deaminates AMP to IMP) is in low concentration in heart muscle, the major degradative pathway from AMP is by means of dephosphorylation to adenosine. Open circles = adenosine deaminase; closed circles = adenylic acid deaminase; triangles = nucleoside phosphorylase; dashed lines = 5′-nucleotidase; dotted lines = adenosine kinase. (From Berne RM, Rubio R: Coronary circulation. *In* Berne RM, Sperelakis N, Geiger SR [eds]: Handbook of Physiology, Section 2. The Cardiovascular System. Bethesda, MD, American Physiological Society, 1979, p 924.)

SYMPATHETIC CONTROL. The effect of stimulation of the adrenergic system depends on the net result of alpha- and beta-receptor activation, with alpha-mediated vasoconstriction normally balanced by beta$_1$-mediated vasodilation (Table 44–9). In the presence of beta-adrenoreceptor antagonists, electrical activation of sympathetic fibers results in coronary vasoconstriction mediated by alpha receptors and attenuated by alpha-adrenergic antagonists. Alpha-adrenergic vasoconstriction competes with metabolic regulation.[31]

Reflex alpha-adrenergic vasoconstriction occurs in response to hypotension mediated through the carotid baroreceptor reflex, which produces activation of sympathetic fibers and inhibition of vagal discharge. The resultant increase in MV_{O_2} and blood flow is countered by alpha-adrenergic–mediated vasoconstriction. This restraint imposed by the alpha-adrenergic system results in increased myocardial oxygen extraction. In humans, alpha-adrenergic coronary constriction can be demonstrated by activation of another reflex sympathetic pathway by the cold pressor test and its potentiation by pretreatment with beta-adrenergic blockade and attenuation by selective alpha$_1$-adrenergic antagonism. Selective alpha$_1$-adrenergic and alpha$_2$-adrenergic blockade improves coronary vasodilation and reserve after epicardial stenting by increasing both the epicardial vasodilation and flow velocity, suggesting that the adrenergic system may limit the vasodilatory capacity in patients with coronary artery disease.[32]

Alpha-adrenergic coronary vasoconstriction has also been observed during exercise in conscious dogs wherein myocardial oxygen delivery increased markedly but not maximally, because the increase in blood flow was blunted by alpha-adrenergic activation. The apparent

TABLE 44–8 Neural Control of Coronary Blood Flow

	Neural	Metabolic
Parasympathetic Vagal stimulation CSP vagotonic Bezold-Jarish reflex	Vasodilation flow ↑	HR, BP ↓, vasoconstrict, flow ↓
Sympathetic Alpha stimulation Beta stimulation Stellectomy relieves chronic alpha constrictor tone	Vasoconstriction flow ↓ Vasodilation flow ↑ (β_2)	BP ↑, vasodilation, flow ↑ HR, contractility ↑ dilation, flow (β_1)
Metabolic	Overrides neural control, but alpha constriction limits vasolation	

BP = blood pressure; CSP = carotid sinus pressure; HR = heart rate.
Modified from Gould L: coronary Artery Stenosis and Reversing Atherosclerosis, 2nd ed. Arnold and Oxford University Press, New York, 1998.

TABLE 44–9 Actions of the Sympathetic Neural Systems

Receptor	Site	Action
β_1	Myocardium SA, AV nodes	Increased contractility Increased heart rate and conduction
β_2	Coronary arterioles Peripheral arterioles Large coronary arteries Peripheral arterioles Lungs	Vasodilation Vasodilation Bronchodilation
α	Large coronary arteries Coronary arterioles Peripheral arterioles	Vasoconstriction Vasoconstriction Vasoconstriction

AV = atrioventricular; SA = sinoatrial.

paradox of sympathetic coronary constriction during exercise results in the favorable transmural distribution of blood in the left ventricular wall away from the endocardium. Recently, a genetic link to alpha-adrenergic coronary vasoconstriction has been demonstrated,[33] and a genetic predisposition to alpha$_2$-adrenergic coronary vasoconstriction has been identified as a risk factor for fatal myocardial infarction and sudden death.[34]

Beta-receptor activation leads to coronary vasodilation under experimental conditions during which adrenergic activation does not alter MVO_2. This vasodilation is mediated predominantly by a beta$_1$ receptor in conduit arteries and by beta$_2$ receptors in resistance arterioles.[28]

PARASYMPATHETIC CONTROL. When MVO_2 is held constant, stimulation of the parasympathetic nervous system releases acetylcholine, leading to vasodilation of the epicardial arteries. Although the small release of acetylcholine from nerve terminals occurs at the medial-adventitial junction, sufficient amount diffuses to stimulate the endothelium.

Myogenic Control and Extravascular Compressive Forces

Arteriolar smooth muscle reacts to increased intraluminal pressure by contracting. The consequent augmentation of resistance tends to return blood flow toward normal despite the higher perfusion pressure. This regulatory mechanism, referred to as *myogenic control*, is important in some vascular beds. Although myogenic responses are present in coronary resistance arteries, their contribution to autoregulation is relatively small.[35]

Because systolic ventricular wall contraction compresses intramyocardial vessels, most of the coronary blood flow to the left ventricle occurs during diastole. At peak systole, there is detectable retrograde flow in the coronary arteries, particularly in the intramural and small epicardial arteries.[36] The extravascular systolic compressive force has two components. The first is left ventricular systolic intracavitary pressure, which is transmitted fully to the subendocardium but declines to almost zero near the epicardial surface. The second, and perhaps even more important, component is the vascular narrowing caused by compression and bending of vascular arterioles coursing through the ventricular wall as the heart contracts. The effect of systole on reducing myocardial perfusion is particularly important when systolic intraventricular pressure exceeds coronary perfusion pressure, as may occur with valvular or subvalvular aortic stenosis, or with severe aortic regurgitation.[37] Extravascular compressive forces are magnified when coronary vascular tone is diminished after arteriolar vasodilation or during metabolic vasodilation associated with exercise.

Because compressive forces exerted by the right ventricle are far smaller than those of the left ventricle, right ventricular perfusion is reduced but not interrupted during systole. When the right ventricular systolic pressure is elevated by disease (e.g., pulmonic stenosis), the phasic blood flow pattern of the arteries perfusing the right ventricle resembles that of the left ventricle.

Transmural Distribution of Myocardial Blood Flow

Extravascular compressive forces are greater in the subendocardium than in the subepicardial layer (Fig. 44–9). Subendocardial arterioles are particularly susceptible to compression as they arborize from long, transmural vessels. Therefore, *systolic* flow is reduced more in the subendocardium than the subepicardium. Nevertheless, in conscious dogs under resting physiological conditions, the ratio of endocardial to epicardial flow averaged throughout the cardiac cycle is approximately 1.25:1 due to preferential dilation of the

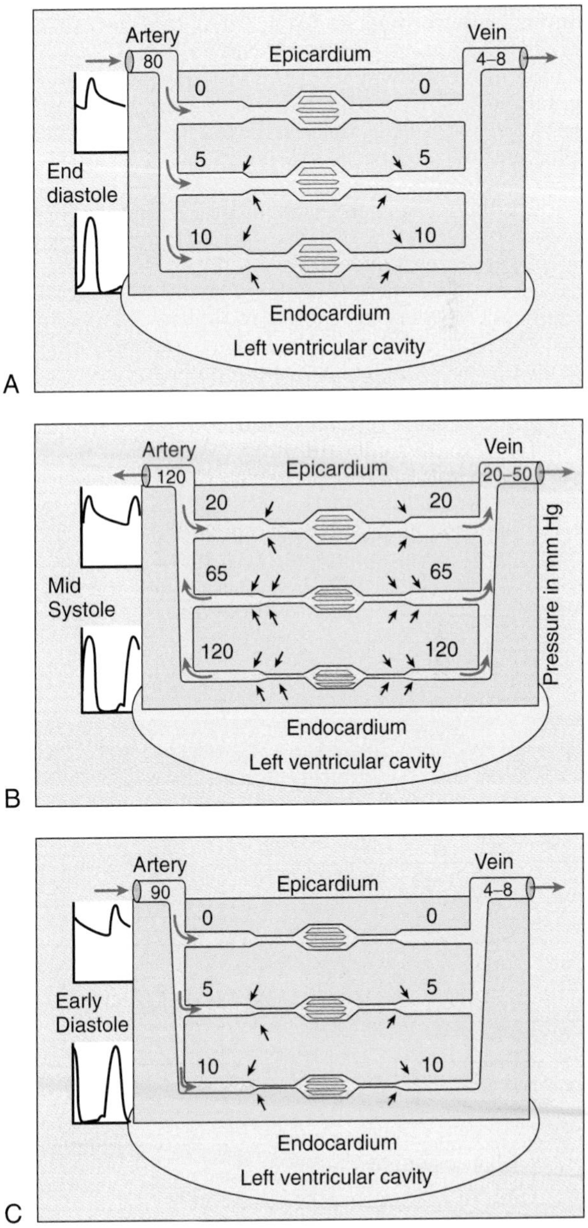

FIGURE 44–9 **A** to **C**, Changes in interstitial and intravascular pressure in vessel flow across left ventricular free wall during the cardiac cycle. During systole, interstitial tissue pressures are greater in subendocardium than in subepicardium. The subendocardial vessels are squeezed more than subepicardial vessels at the end of systole and take longer to resume full diastolic dimension. In the presence of low perfusion pressure, subendocardial flow is impaired by reduced diastolic time, especially with tachycardia and by elevated left ventricular diastolic pressure. (**A** to **C**, Modified from Hoffman JIE, Baer RW, Hanley FL, et al: Regulation of transmural myocardial blood flow. J Biochem Eng 107:2, 1985.)

subendocardial arterioles, causing a large increase in diastolic flow in the subendocardium. The greater subendocardial blood flow appears to be secondary to the wall stress (and therefore oxygen consumption per unit weight).[38]

The subendocardium is more vulnerable to ischemic damage than the mid-myocardium or subepicardium. Epicardial coronary stenoses are associated with reductions in the subendocardial-to-subepicardial flow ratio.[38] When coronary arteries were constricted sufficiently to reduce total coronary flow to approximately 40 percent of control, endocardial-to-epicardial flow ratio fell from 1.16 at baseline to 0.37. This pattern of redistribution of flow away from the endocardium is further exaggerated during exercise, mental stress, and pacing-induced tachycardia. Potent arteriolar vasodilators, such as dipyridamole or adenosine, also cause redistribution of blood flow from the endocardium to the epicardium. In the presence of epicardial stenoses, this transmural redistribution leads to a "coronary steal," or vertical diversion of blood away from the subendocardial layer with flow falling below resting values. Severe left ventricular hypertrophy, as well as heart failure with elevated left ventricular end-diastolic pressure, may also reduce the endocardial-to-epicardial flow ratio.

A low subendocardial-to-subepicardial flow ratio can be increased by elevation of aortic pressure, which preferentially increases perfusion of subendocardial region whose arterioles are maximally dilated and are, in this setting, pressure dependent. Overperfusion of the epicardial region is prevented by autoregulatory arteriolar constriction. Potent vasoconstrictors such as ET-1 and alpha-adrenergic agonists or inhibitors of adenosine-induced arteriolar dilation such as theophylline cause arteriolar constriction and redistribution of blood flow to the endocardium.[38,39] As long as the absolute blood flow is not reduced appreciably, these measures may lessen myocardial ischemia. Reduction of MV_{O_2}, for example by beta blockers, also decreases epicardial blood flow and increases perfusion pressure and flow to the ischemic subendocardial region. Table 44–10 compares characteristics of the subepicardial and subendocardial circulatory responses.

TABLE 44–10 Characteristics of Subendocardium and Subepicardium

Variable	Subendocardium	Subepicardium
Wall stress	++	+
V_{O_2}	++	+
Tissue P_{O_2}	+	++
Perfusion pressure	+	++
SV_{O_2}, ATP	+	++
Lactate	++	+
Flow reserve	+	++
Resistance	+	++
Capillaries open, systolic flow decrease	+++	+
Due to compression, diastolic flow increase	+	++
Due to resistance	++	+
Mean flow (equal)	++	++

Strength of effects: + = mild; ++ = moderate; +++ = prominent or large.
ATP = adenosine triphosphate.
Modified from Gould L: Coronary Artery Stenosis and Reversing Atherosclerosis. 2nd ed. New York, Arnold and Oxford University Press, 1998.

Influence of a Stenosis on Coronary Blood Flow

A stenosis produces resistance to blood flow related directly to the morphologic features of the stenosis. Resistance to flow changes exponentially with lumen cross-sectional area (the most commonly used measure of severity) and linearly with lesion length. Additional factors contributing to resistance include the shape of the entrance and exit orifices, vessel stiffness, and distensibility of the diseased segment (permitting active or passive vasomotion) and the variable lumen obstruction that may be superimposed by platelet aggregation and thrombosis compromising lumen area, a process active in acute coronary syndromes.

As blood traverses a stenosis, pressure (energy) is lost resulting in a pressure gradient (ΔP) across the stenosis. Using a simplified Bernoulli formula of fluid dynamics (Fig 44–10), pressure loss across a stenosis can be estimated as follows:

(1)
$$\Delta P = fQ + sQ^2$$

(2)
$$\Delta P = \frac{1.8 \bullet Q}{d_{sten}^4} + \frac{6.1 \bullet Q^2}{d_{sten}^4}$$

where ΔP is the pressure drop across a stenosis in millimeters of mercury, Q is the flow across the stenosis in milliliters per second, and d_{sten} is the minimal diameter of the stenosis lumen in millimeters. In equation 1, the first term (f) accounts energy losses due to viscous friction between laminar layers of fluid.

$$f = \frac{8\pi\mu L}{A_s^2}$$

where A_s is the stenotic segment cross-sectional area, μ is the blood viscosity, and L is the stenosis length.

In equation 1, the second term (s) reflects energy loss when normal arterial flow is transformed first to high-velocity flow in the stenosis and then to the turbulent nonlaminar distal flow eddies at the exit from the stenosis (inertia and expansion).

$$s = \frac{\rho}{2}\left[\frac{1}{A_s} - \frac{1}{A_n}\right]^2$$

where ρ is the blood density, and A_n represents the normal artery cross-sectional area. This results in energy loss due to flow separation and disturbed laminar flow.

As described by the Bernoulli formula (equation 1), the separation energy loss term (s) increases with the *square* of the

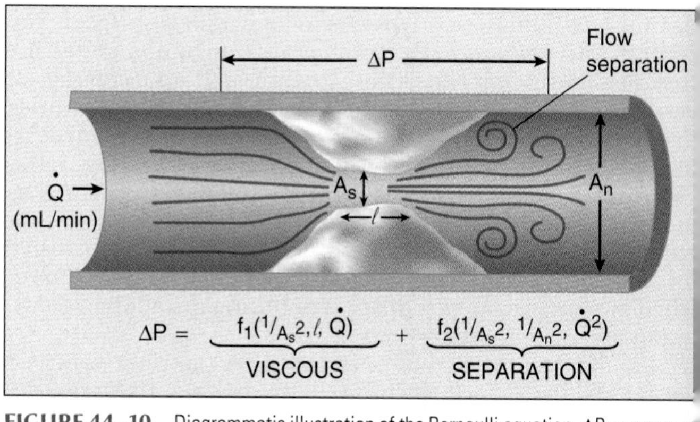

FIGURE 44–10 Diagrammatic illustration of the Bernoulli equation. ΔP = pressure gradient; A_s = area of the stenosis; A_n = area of the normal segment; L = stenosis length; $\dot{Q}$ = flow; f_1 = viscous factor; f_2 = separation factor. See text for details.

flow while viscous energy loss (f) becomes negligible. Thus, increases in coronary blood flow augment the associated pressure gradient in an exponential manner (Fig. 44–11). Despite augmentation of coronary blood flow, the increasing pressure loss across the stenosis reduces myocardial perfusion pressure and lowers the threshold for myocardial ischemia relative to demand.[40]

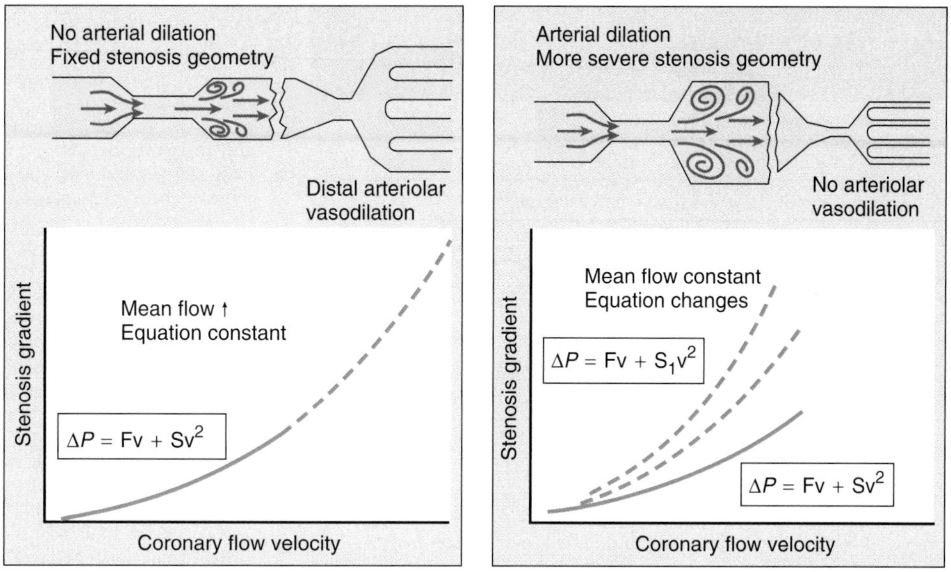

FIGURE 44–11 Conceptional diagrams of the effects of distal arteriolar vasodilation and proximal epicardial vasodilation on the geometry of the stenosis and pressure gradient (ΔP)–velocity relationship. With arteriolar vasodilation alone, stenosis geometry is constant and ΔP increases proportionally with velocity, V, according to the Bernoulli equation. With large epicardial artery vasodilation, the relative percent stenosis would become worse since the stenotic segment would remain fixed while the adjacent normal segment of the artery would become larger. The angle of divergence of flow exiting the lesion would become greater; consequently, greater pressure loss due to flow separation would occur, increasing the gradient-velocity curve. The separation coefficient would likewise increase from S to S_1. (From Gould L: Pressure-flow characteristics of coronary stenoses in unsedated dogs at rest and during coronary vasodilation. Circ Res 43:242-253, 1978.)

Factors Influencing Resistance Across a Stenosis

At any level of blood flow, the single most important determinant of stenosis resistance is the minimum diameter of the stenosis. The transstenotic pressure drop is inversely proportional to the *fourth* power of the lumen radius. As a consequence, in a severe stenosis, relatively small changes in luminal diameter (such as caused by active or passive vasomotion or transient obstruction by thrombus) can produce marked hemodynamic effects. For example, when the diameter stenosis is increased from 80 to 90 percent, the resistance of a stenosis rises nearly threefold. For most stenoses, the length of the narrowing has only a modest effect on its physiological significance. However, in very long, narrowed segments, significant turbulence occurs along the walls of the stenotic segment, and energy is dissipated as heat when eddies form and impact on the vessel wall. A preserved arc of vascular smooth muscle in some diseased arteries may be compliant and subject to dynamic changes that can alter luminal caliber and stenosis resistance. Dynamic changes in stenosis severity and resistance can also occur passively in response to changes in intraluminal distending pressure, or selective dilation of distal resistance vessels with agents such as dipyridamole. A single pressure-flow curve thus cannot be applied to a compliant or dynamic stenosis, because the pressure-flow relationship moves over a family of curves reflecting altered stenosis diameter and variable distending pressure. Despite the theoretical concerns, coronary artery pressures always remain positive, and collapse of distal segments is unlikely when intracoronary pressure is high due to microvascular compression.

The physiological effect of a coronary stenosis also depends on the degree to which the resistance to flow can be compensated by dilation of the microcirculation distal to the stenosis. *Resting* coronary flow is not impeded by mild or moderate stenoses and is maintained by normal vasodilatory regulation of the microcirculation. Resting coronary blood flow remains constant up to the point where an epicardial coronary constriction exceeds 85 to 90 percent of the normal segment diameter. However, unlike resting flow, *maximal* hyperemic coronary blood flow begins to decline when diameter stenosis exceeds 45 to 60 percent (Fig. 44–12). The capacity to increase coronary blood flow in response to a hyperemic stimulus, called *coronary flow reserve* (CFR), is abolished when diameter stenosis exceeds 90 percent. Factors responsible for reduced CFR in the absence of epicardial stenosis are shown in Table 44–11.

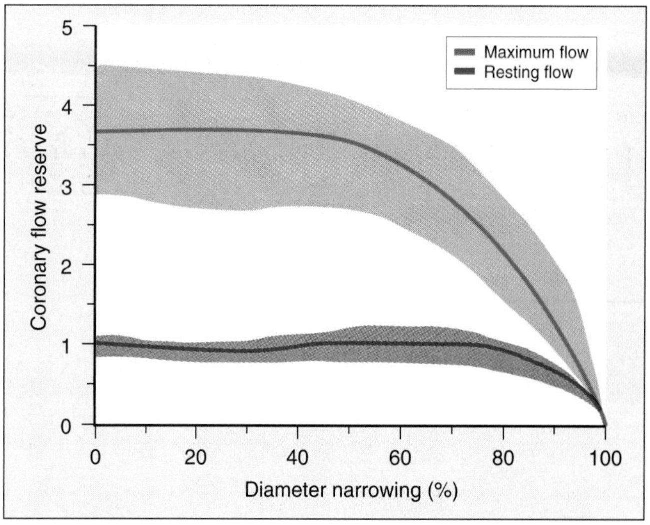

FIGURE 44–12 Coronary flow reserve expressed as the ratio of maximum to resting flow plotted as a function of percent diameter narrowing. With progressive narrowing, resting flow does not change (magenta line) whereas maximum potential increase in flow (blue line) and coronary flow reserve begin to be impaired at approximately 50 percent diameter narrowing. The shaded area represents the limits of variability of data about the mean. (From Gould KL, Lipscomb K, Hamilton GW: Physiologic basis for assessing critical coronary stenosis: Instantaneous flow response and regional distribution during coronary hyperemia as measures of coronary flow reserve. Am J Cardiol 33:87-94, 1974.)

CORONARY PRESSURE AND FLOW FOR THE PHYSIOLOGICAL ASSESSMENT OF A CORONARY STENOSIS

The limitations of angiography to determine the functional significance of an intermediate coronary stenosis can be overcome by measurements of coronary blood flow and pressure as estimates of coronary reserve. These measurements provide important information that complements the anatomical (most often angiographic) evaluation and facilitates clinical decision making. The hemodynamic significance of a given stenosis in humans can be measured by the pressure-flow relationship using sensor angioplasty guidewires.[41]

TABLE 44–11 Factors Responsible for Microvascular Disease and the Reduction of Coronary Flow Reserve
Abnormal vascular reactivity
Abnormal myocardial metabolism
Abnormal sensitivity toward vasoactive substances
Coronary vasospasm
Myocardial infarction
Hypertrophy
Vasculitis syndromes
Hypertension
Diabetes
Recurrent ischemia

From Baumgart D, Haude M, Liu F, et al: Current concepts of coronary flow reserve for clinical decision making during cardiac catheterization. Am Heart J 136:136-149, 1998.

Coronary Hyperemia

The myocardium can increase coronary flow from its basal level to a maximal flow in response to physiology or pharmacological stimuli. The most basic form of CFR is *reactive hyperemia* produced by transient severe myocardial ischemia, which produces maximal coronary dilation and a marked increase in coronary flow. Reactive hyperemia follows an occlusion as short as 200 milliseconds. *Maximal reactive hyperemia* follows coronary occlusion of 20 seconds. Longer occlusion increases the duration but not the amplitude of the hyperemic response. Reactive hyperemia is a response partly driven by metabolic regulation, fulfilling a requirement to repay oxygen debt. However, the hyperemic response is less pronounced when coronary arteries are perfused with deoxygenated blood for the same duration, suggesting that factors other than hypoxia, such as the local accumulation of adenosine, prostacyclin, and NO, stimulate the hyperemic response. At maximal hyperemia, autoregulation is also abolished and coronary blood flow is directly related to the driving pressure. Therefore, maximal hyperemic coronary blood flow is closely dependent on the coronary arterial pressure at the time of the measurement, a fact that is used in the derivation of pressure-derived fractional flow reserve of the myocardium (see later).

Three types of stimuli have been used to elicit maximal coronary blood flow in humans: (1) transient coronary occlusion during angioplasty (reactive hyperemia); (2) pharmacological vasodilators; and (3) metabolic stress. Adenosine, dipyridamole, and papaverine are the principal pharmacological vasodilators used to elicit coronary hyperemia. Adenosine, the most commonly used agent in the catheterization laboratory, can be administered by the intravenous or intracoronary route. Adenosine is benign in the appropriate dosages (20 to 30 μg in the right coronary artery or 30 to 50 μg in the left coronary artery or infused intravenously at 140 μg/kg/min) (Fig. 44–13). In a small (8 percent) percentage of patients, maximal coronary hyperemia may require higher (>50 μg) intracoronary adenosine doses.[42] Intravenous dobutamine (10 to 40 μg/kg/min) can also produce maximal hyperemia without modifying the angiographic area of the epicardial stenosis.[43]

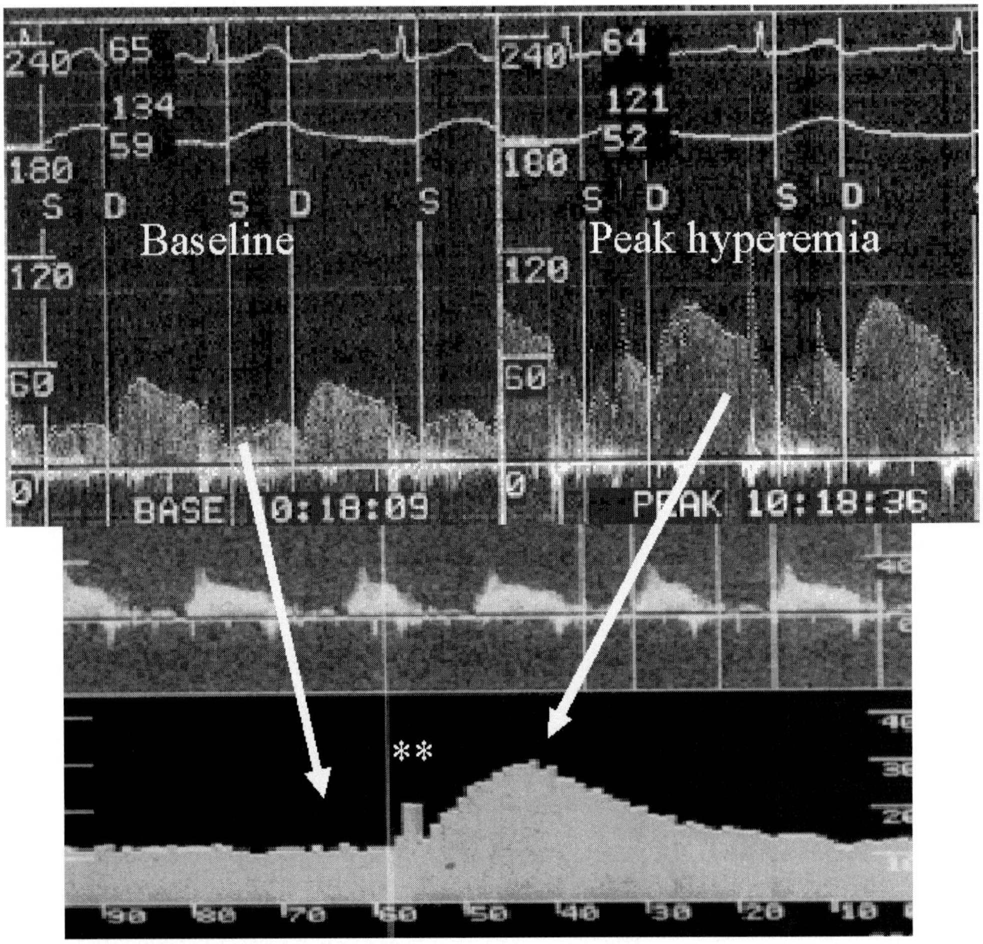

FIGURE 44–13 Coronary Doppler flow velocity signals used for the measurement of coronary flow velocity reserve in the cardiac catheterization laboratory. **Top panel,** Divided into the baseline (left) and the peak hyperemic velocity (right) signals, phasic flow-velocity tracing is demarcated by systolic (S) and diastolic (D) markers, corresponding to the electrocardiogram and aortic pressure at top of panels. Diastolic flow normally predominates over systolic flow. (Flow velocity scale is 0 to 240 cm/sec). **Bottom panel,** Continuous trend plot of average peak velocity (APV) showing the baseline and time course of peak hyperemia. The effect of an intracoronary bolus of adenosine (**) can be seen by the rapid increase in APV. The phasic peak hyperemic velocity signal was captured and displayed in the upper right panel. (The APV trend plot scale is from 0 to 60 cm/sec, with a time base of 0 to 90 seconds). In this example, baseline flow is 13 cm/sec and peak hyperemic flow is 30 cm/sec, for a coronary flow reserve of 2.3.

Measurement of Coronary Flow Reserve

CFR is defined as the ratio of maximal to basal coronary flow. CFR measures the ability of the two components of myocardial perfusion, namely the epicardial stenosis resistance and the microvascular resistance, to achieve maximal blood flow. There are two methods available to measure coronary blood flow in the catheterization laboratory: intracoronary Doppler flow velocity[41] and coronary thermodilution.[44]

Coronary Doppler measures the velocity of red blood cells moving past the ultrasound emitter/receiver on the end of a Doppler-tipped angioplasty guidewire. Velocity is determined from the frequency shift, defined by the Doppler equation (see Chap. 11). Volumetric flow is the product of vessel area (square centimeters) and flow velocity (centimeters per second) yielding a value in cubic centimeter per second. Absolute Doppler flow velocities represent changes in volumetric coronary flow when the vessel cross-sectional area remains constant over the measurement period. Compared to volumetric measurements, velocity may underestimate the volumetric CFR in some vessels that demonstrate intact endothelial-mediated vasodilation. The coronary thermodilution technique uses thermistors on a pressure-sensor angioplasty guidewire and measures the arrival time of room temperature saline bolus indicator injections through the guiding catheter into the coronary artery.[44] When combined with poststenotic pressure measurements, CFR measurements can provide a complete description of the pressure-flow relationship and the response of the microcirculation.

Normal CFR in young patients with normal arteries by intravascular ultrasound commonly exceeds 3.0.[45] In patients with chest pain undergoing cardiac catheterization with angiographically normal vessels, the CFR averages 2.7 ± 0.6[46] and is related, in part, to comorbid conditions such as hyperlipidemia, hypertension, or diabetes mellitus. Changes in heart rate, blood pressure, and contractility alter CFR by changing resting basal flow or maximal hyperemic flow or both. Tachycardia increases basal flow, reducing CFR. Increasing mean arterial pressure reduces maximal vasodilation, reducing hyperemic flow more than basal flow. CFR may be reduced in patients with normal coronary arteries who have essential hypertension or aortic stenosis. Diabetes mellitus also reduces CFR, especially in patients with diabetic retinopathy, due to reduced volumetric coronary blood flow (velocity × vessel cross-sectional area) during hyperemia and higher baseline flow compared to nondiabetic control subjects.[47]

RELATIVE CORONARY FLOW VELOCITY. Because CFR is the summed response of the major two coronary flow resistances, an abnormal value cannot distinguish between increased epicardial resistance or microvascular flow impairment (Fig. 44-14). To identify the resistance level, a relative CFR (rCFR) can be calculated as the ratio of maximal flow in the coronary with stenosis (Q^S) to flow in a normal coronary without stenosis (Q^N), assuming basal flows are the same. It was shown that rCFR is independent of the aortic pressure and heart rate pressure product and was well suited to assess the physiological significance of coronary stenoses. Using coronary flow velocity in the catheterization laboratory, rCFR is defined as the ratio of CFR_{target} to CFR in an angiographically normal reference vessel,

$$rCFR = (Q^S/Q_{base})/(Q^N/Q_{base}) = CFR_{target}/CFR_{reference}$$

and assumes both that basal flow in the two vessels is similar and that the microcirculatory response is uniform in the regions measured. A normal range for rCFR is 0.8 to 1.0. rCFR but cannot be used in patients with three-vessel coronary disease who have no suitable reference vessel. Because it relies on the assumption that the microvascular circulation is uniformly distributed, rCFR is of no value in patients with myocardial infarction, in patients with left ventricular regional dysfunction, or patients in whom the microcirculatory responses are heterogeneous. Because of the inherent difficulties and variability of both absolute and relative coronary flow velocity measurements, pressure-derived measurements are the preferred invasive method of physiological stenosis assessment.[48]

PRESSURE-DERIVED FRACTIONAL FLOW RESERVE OF THE MYOCARDIUM. Using coronary pressure distal to a stenosis measured at constant and minimal myocardial resistances (i.e., maximal hyperemia), Pijls and associates[49] derived an estimate of the percentage of normal coronary blood flow expected to go through a stenotic artery. This pressure-derived ratio is called the fractional flow reserve (FFR) and can be subdivided into three components describing the flow contributions by the coronary artery, the myocardium, and the collateral supply. FFR of the coronary artery (FFR_{cor}) is defined as the maximum coronary artery flow in the presence of a stenosis divided by the normal theoretical maximum flow of the artery (i.e., the maximum flow in that artery if no stenosis were present). Similarly, FFR of the myocardium (FFR_{myo}) is defined as maximum myocardial (artery and bed) blood flow distal to an epicardial stenosis divided by its value if no epicardial stenosis were present. Stated another way, FFR represents that fraction of normal maximum flow that remains despite the presence of an epicardial lesion (Fig. 44-15). The difference between FFR_{myo} and FFR_{cor} is FFR of the collateral flow (see later).

The FFR of a coronary artery and its dependent myocardium can be calculated by the following equations:

(1) $FFR_{cor} = (P_d - P_w)/(P_a - P_w)$
(2) $FFR_{myo} = (P_d - P_v)/(P_a - P_v)$
(3) $FFR_{collateral} = FFR_{myo} - FFR_{cor}$

where P_a, P_d, and P_w are pressures of the aorta, distal artery, and coronary wedge (during balloon occlusion), respectively, taken at maximum vasodilation, and P_v is venous or right atrial pressure. Because FFR_{cor} uses P_w, it can be calculated only during balloon coronary angioplasty. However, FFR_{myo} can be calculated during diagnostic procedures (Fig. 44-16). FFR reflects both antegrade and collateral myocardial perfusion rather than merely transstenotic pressure loss (i.e., a stenosis pressure gradient). Because it is calculated only at peak hyperemia, FFR is differentiated from CFR by being largely independent of basal flow, driving pressure, heart rate, systemic blood pressure, or status of the microcirculation.[50]

The FFR, but not the resting pressure or hyperemic pressure gradient, is strongly related to provocable myocardial ischemia demonstrated by comparisons to different clinical stress testing modalities in patients with stable angina. The nonischemic threshold value of FFR is greater than 0.75 (Fig. 44-17). In patients with an abnormal microcirculation, it can be argued that a normal FFR indicates the conduit resistance is not a major contributing factor to perfusion impairment and that focal conduit enlargement (e.g., stenting) would not restore normal perfusion.

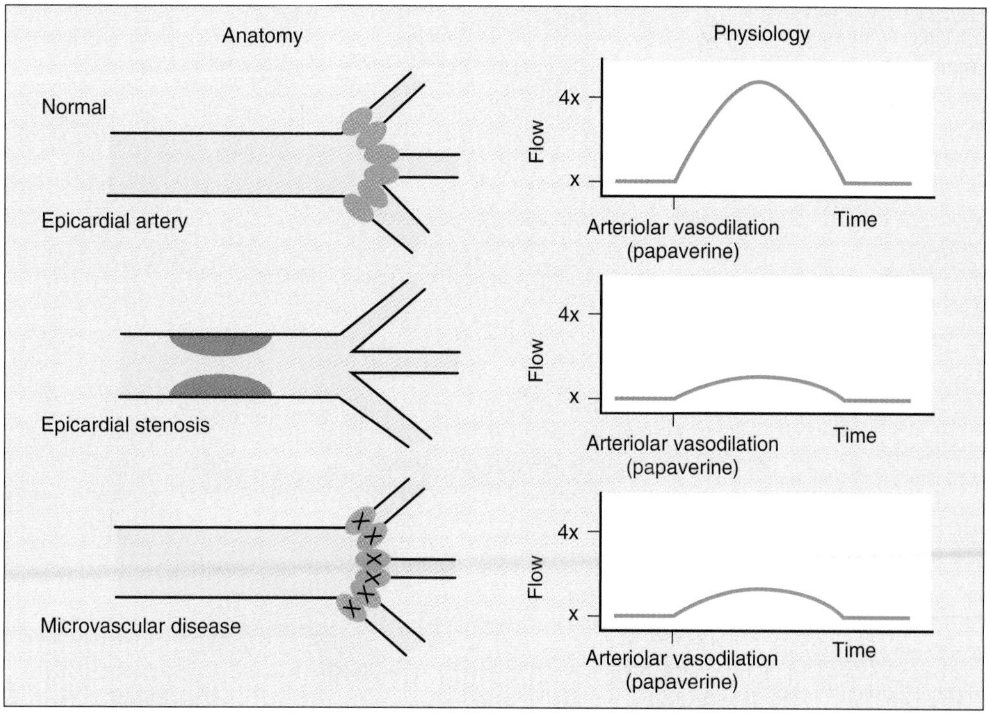

FIGURE 44–14 Interaction of the two major components of coronary flow reserve. **Top,** The two components—the epicardial artery and microcirculation—when both are normal, produce a normal coronary flow velocity reserve that is more than three times basal flow. **Middle,** With an epicardial stenosis and normal microcirculation, coronary flow reserve is impaired. **Bottom,** With microvascular disease and a normal epicardial, coronary artery flow reserve is also impaired. Coronary flow reserve alone thus cannot differentiate between an epicardial stenosis and an impaired microvascular disease. X = impaired microcirculation. (Modified from Wilson RF, Laxson DD: Caveat emptor: A clinician's guide to assessing the physiologic significance of arterial stenoses. Cathet Cardiovasc Diagn 29:93-98, 1993.)

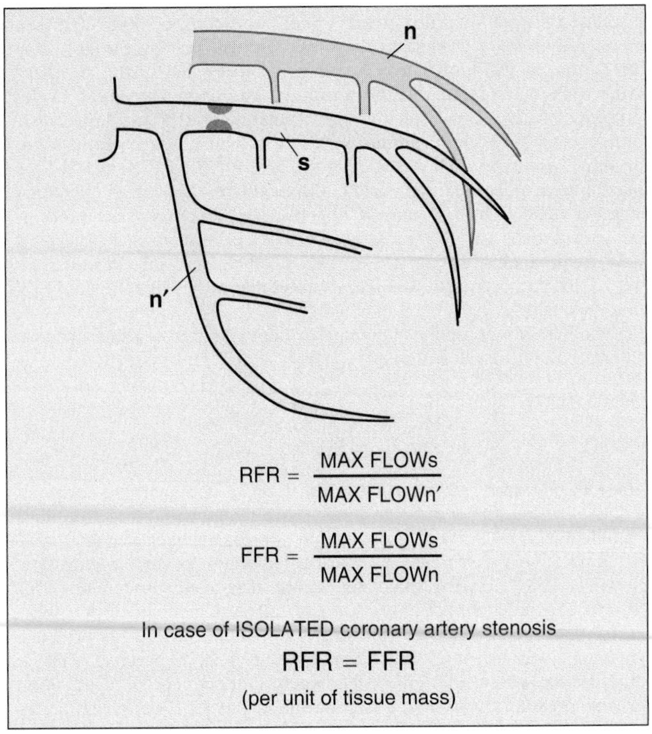

FIGURE 44–15 Diagram of an artery illustrating the rationale of comparing relative and fractional myocardial flow reserve. The relative flow reserve RFR) is the ratio of hyperemic flow in the anterior region (depending on the stenotic left anterior descending (LAD) coronary artery) to the hyperemic flow in the normal region (depending on the left circumflex coronary artery). The myocardial fractional flow reserve (FFR) is the ratio of hyperemic flow in the anterior region (depending on the stenotic LAD coronary artery) to hyperemic flow in that same region in the hypothetical case of a normal LAD coronary artery (faint lines). These measurements are derived from the mean pressure distal to the stenosis divided by the mean pressure proximal to the stenosis at maximal hyperemia. In the case of a similar decrease of myocardial resistance during hyperemia in the LAD area and the left circumflex area, the value of both the relative and the fractional myocardial flow reserves should be identical. n = the hypothetical normal left anterior descending coronary artery; n′ = normal left circumflex coronary artery; s = stenotic left anterior descending coronary artery. (From De Bruyne B, Banohuin T, Melin J, et al: Coronary flow reserve calculated from pressure measurements in humans: Validation with positron emission tomography. Circulation 89:1013-1022, 1994.)

FFR is thus specific for stenosis resistance and by design excludes the assessment and influence of the microcirculation.

SIMULTANEOUS PRESSURE-FLOW VELOCITY (P-V) RELATIONSHIPS. In a manner similar to that proposed by Gould and colleagues (see Fig. 44-16), Marques and coworkers[51] demonstrated the pressure-velocity flow (P-V) relationships characterizing mild, moderate, and severe human coronary stenoses.The P-V data also demonstrated that the variability of microvascular resistance possibly contributed to discrepancies between FFR and coronary blood flow velocity reserve in intermediate coronary lesions (Fig. 44-18)[52] with concordance between FFR and CFR occurring in 73 percent of patients. Minimum microvascular resistance (the ratio of mean distal pressure to average peak blood flow velocity during hyperemia) was significantly higher in patients with FFR greater than 0.75 and CFR less than 2.0.A hyperemic stenosis resistance index (defined as the ratio of hyperemic stenosis pressure gradient [mean aortic—mean distal pressure] divided by hyperemic average peak

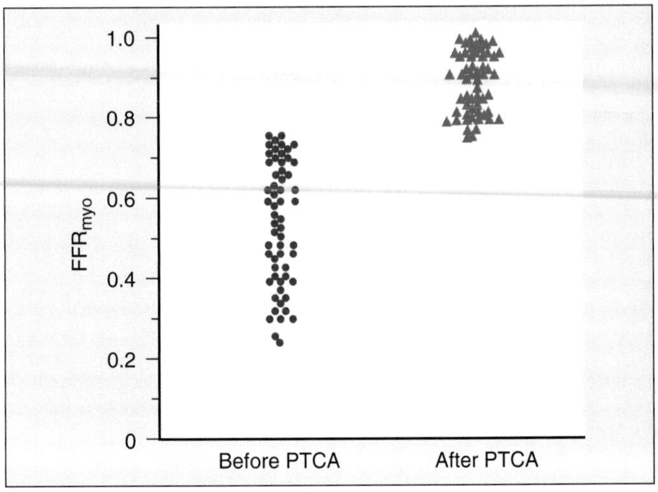

FIGURE 44–17 Values of fractional flow reserve of the myocardium (FFR_{myo}) before and after percutaneous transluminal coronary angioplasty (PTCA). Values associated with proven myocardial ischemia are indicated by magenta circles, and values definitely not associated with ischemia are indicated by blue triangles. The threshold of FFR below which exertional ischemia is observed and above which no ischemia occurs is 0.74. (From Pijls NH, De Bruyne B, Peels K, et al: Measurement of fractional flow reserve to assess the functional severity of coronary artery stenoses. N Engl J Med 334:1703-1708, 1996.)

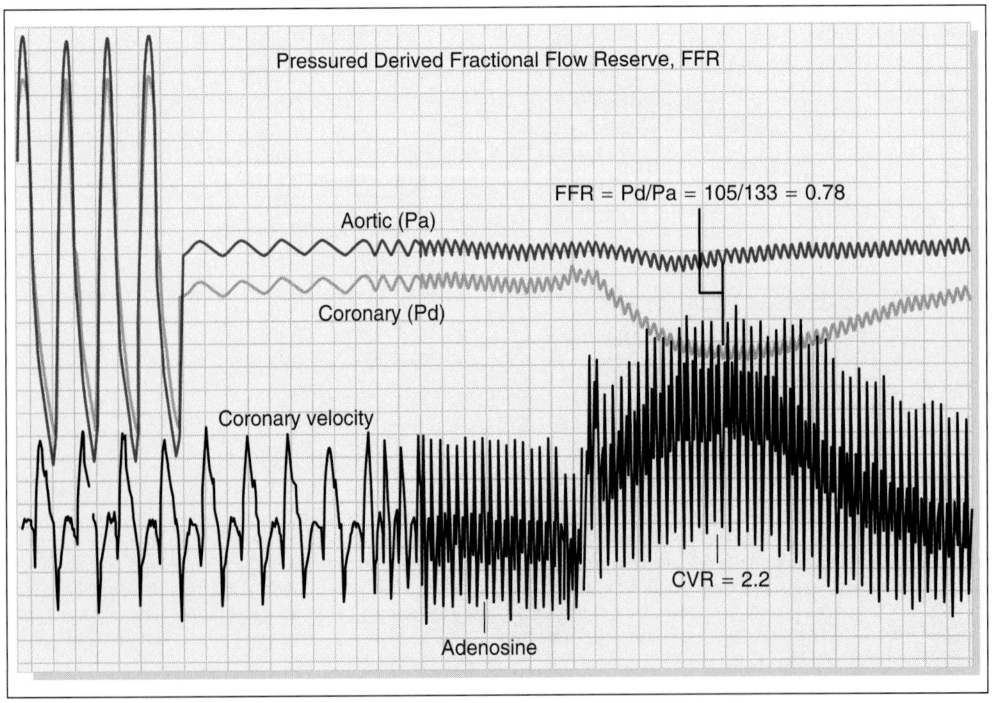

FIGURE 44–16 Pressure and flow velocity signals obtained in a patient with intermediate severity of coronary artery disease. A coronary flow velocity tracing is used to demonstrate timing of coronary hyperemia and coronary vasodilatory reserve (CVR). Mean aortic (P_a) and distal coronary pressures (P_d) during adenosine hyperemia are used to compute fractional flow reserve (FFR). FFR = 0.78 when CVR = 2.2. (Courtesy of B. DeBruyne.)

A

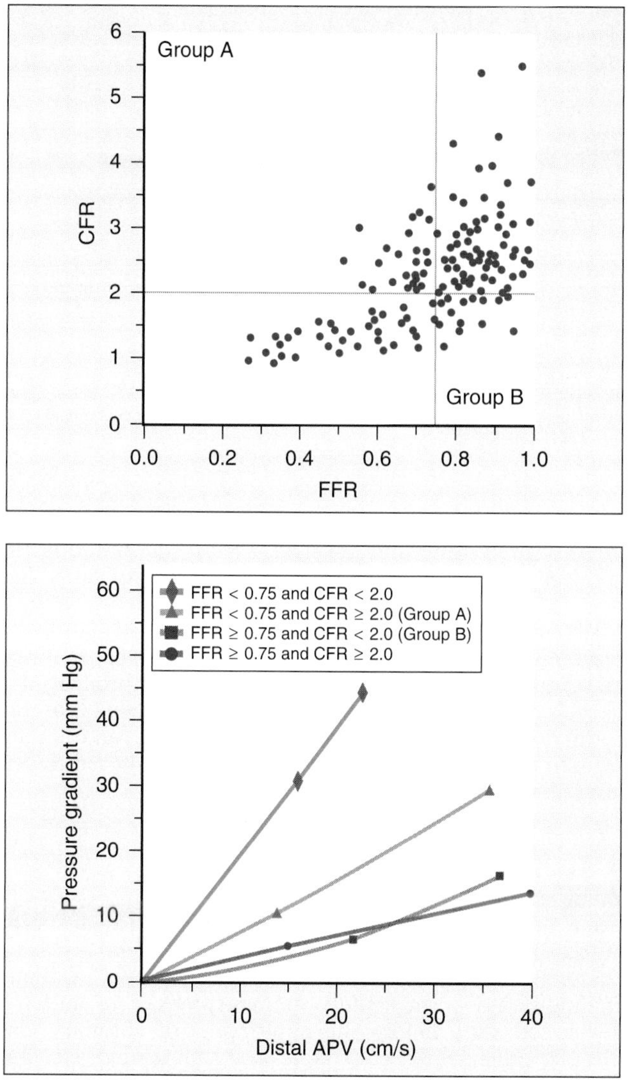

B

FIGURE 44–18 Comparison of fractional flow reserve (FFR) and coronary flow reserve (CFR) in 150 patients. Data are categorized on the basis of threshold values. **A,** Group A, FFR < 0.75 and CFR > 2.0, and Group B, FFR > 0.75 and CFR ≤ 2. **B,** Pressure gradient-flow velocity relation showing average data at baseline and hyperemia for all groups. APV = average peak velocity. (**A** and **B,** From Meuwissen M, Chamuleau S, Siebes M, et al: Role of variability in microvascular resistance on fractional flow reserve and coronary blood flow velocity reserve in intermediate coronary lesions. Circulation 103:184-187, 2001.)

velocity [APV]) was determined to be more specific for agreement with perfusion imaging by single-photon emission tomography in lesions with discordant FFR and CFR.[53] Thus, combined P-V measurements are needed to describe the contribution of both the epicardial and microvascular resistance to myocardial perfusion.

Clinical Outcomes of Coronary Blood Flow Measurements

Strong correlations exist between inducible myocardial ischemia by stress testing and FFR or CFR. An FFR less than 0.75 or abnormal CFR (<2.0) identified physiologically significant stenoses associated with inducible myocardial ischemia, with high (>90 percent) sensitivity, specificity, positive predictive value, and overall accuracy.[41,50,53-55] FFR or CFR values above the ischemic thresholds have been used safely to defer coronary interventions for intermediate stenoses, with clinical event rates of less than 10 percent over a 2-year follow-up period.[56-59]

Percutaneous intervention of lesions with normal FFR has a worse outcome than when such patients are treated medically. Bech and associates[59] studied 325 patients with intermediate coronary stenosis without documented myocardial ischemia. When FFR was greater than 0.75, patients were randomly assigned to a deferral group ($n = 91$) or a performance group ($n = 90$). If FFR was less than 0.75, percutaneous transluminal coronary angioplasty (PTCA) was performed as planned (reference group, $n = 144$). At clinical follow-up to 24 months, the event-free survival was higher in the deferral than in the performance group (89 percent vs. 83 percent) and significantly lower in the reference group (78 percent). FFR identified those patients in whom percutaneous coronary intervention (PCI) provides no additional clinical benefit (Fig. 44–19).

The AHA/ACC recommendations[60] for use of physiological measurements during invasive procedures are provided in Table 44–12.

DIFFUSE ATHEROSCLEROSIS. Coronary arteries without focal stenosis are generally considered non–flow limiting. A diffusely diseased atherosclerotic coronary artery can be viewed as a series of branching units diverting and gradually distributing flow and reducing pressure longitudinally along the conduit. In such a vessel, a reduced CFR is not associated with any single location of stenotic pressure loss. Diffuse atherosclerosis, rather than a focal narrowing, is characterized by a continuous and gradual pressure recovery from distal to proximal without a localized abrupt increase in pressure related to an isolated stenosis. De Bruyne and colleagues[5] examined FFR in normal arteries and in atherosclerotic nonstenotic arteries. FFR in the normal group was 0.97 ± 0.02 but was significantly lower, 0.89 ± 0.08, in the diffuse disease group indicating significant arterial resistance without focal obstruction. In 8 percent of arteries in the diffusely diseased group FFR was less than 0.75, well below the ischemic

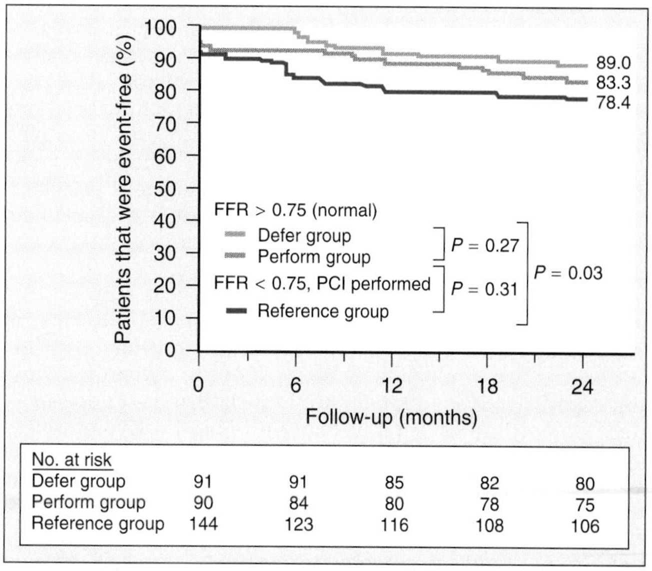

FIGURE 44–19 Clinical outcome of deferring or treating patients with intermediate stenosis and fractional flow reserve (FFR) > 0.75. Event-free Kaplan-Meier curves for three strategies are shown. The top curve are patients with intermediate coronary stenosis with FFR > 0.75 and in whom intervention was deferred (blue). The bottom curve is the reference group (magenta) in whom FFR was < 0.75 and percutaneous coronary intervention (PCI) was performed. The middle curve is the group of patients with FFR > 0.75 who had PCI performed (brown). In a follow-up over 2 years, events were higher in the FFR > 0.75 PCI-perform group than in the PCI-deferred group. PCI offered no advantage in terms of events or symptom relief to these patients. (From Bech GJW, De Bruyne B, Pijls NHJ, et al: Fractional flow reserve to determine the appropriateness of angioplasty in moderate coronary stenosis: A randomized trial. Circulation 103:2928-2934, 2001.)

TABLE 44–12 Recommendations for Intracoronary Physiologic Measurements (Doppler Ultrasound, FFR)

Class	Indication	Level of Evidence
IIa	1. Assessment of the physiological effects of intermediate coronary stenosis (33-70% luminal narrowing) in patients with anginal symptoms. Coronary pressure (FFR) of Doppler velocimetry may also be useful as an alternative to performing noninvasive functional testing (e.g., when the functional study is absent or ambiguous) to determine whether an intervention is warranted	B
IIb	1. Evaluation of the success of percutaneous coronary revascularization in restoring flow reserve and to predict the risk of restenosis	C
	2. Evaluation of patients with anginal symptoms without an apparent angiographic culprit lesion	C
III	1. Routine assessment of the severity of angiographic disease in patients with a positive, unequivocal noninvasive function study	C

FFR = fractional flow reserve.
From Smith SC Jr, Dove JT, Jacobs AK, et al: ACC/AHA guidelines for percutaneous coronary intervention (revision of the 1993 PTCA Guidelines)—executive summary. A report of the American College of Cardiology/American Heart Association Task Force on Practice Guidelines (committee to revise the 1993 guidelines for percutaneous transluminal coronary angioplasty. J Am Coll Cardiol 37:2215-2238, 2001).

threshold (Fig. 44–20). In this setting, mechanical therapy to treat a presumed focal flow limiting plaque would be futile. Diffuse atherosclerosis also explains persistently abnormal perfusion imaging studies in some patients despite unobstructed proximal coronary artery segments.

PERCUTANEOUS CORONARY INTERVENTIONS (see Chap. 52). Sequential flow velocity data have confirmed that the normalization of CFR occurring in only 50 percent of patients after PTCA alone was due to angiographically unapparent residual lumen obstruction. CFR may normalize in 80 percent of patients after stenting, corresponding to improved lumen area as the mechanism responsible for improved coronary blood flow. The remaining 20 percent of patients with widely patent stents had impaired CFR (<2.0) attributed to microvascular disease and/or transient emboli from PCI. A low postprocedural CFR has been associated with a worse periprocedural outcome.

FFR after *stenting* also predicts adverse cardiac events at follow-up. In a multicenter study, Pijls and coworkers[61] examined FFR and clinical outcomes in 750 patients 6 months after stent placement. FFR immediately after stenting was an independent variable related to all adverse cardiac events. The event rate was 5 percent in patients in whom FFR normalized, 6 percent in patients with poststent FFR between 0.90 and 0.95, and 20 percent in those with FFR less than 0.90. In patients with FFR less than 0.80, the event rate was 30 percent (Fig. 44–21). These data suggest that lack of normalization of FFR and diffuse disease are associated with worse long-term outcome independent of final stent diameter.

ACUTE MYOCARDIAL INFARCTION (see Chap. 46). Measurements of coronary blood flow or pressure during or immediately after acute myocardial infarction may not represent true lesion physiology because of the dynamic nature and recovery of the microcirculation. De Bruyne and associates[62] demonstrated that a normal FFR is indicative of reversal of myocardial perfusion defects in patients with acute myocardial infarction after 6 days. Excluding false-positive and -negative studies, the corresponding sensitivity, specificity, and predictive accuracy of FFR values were 87 percent, 100 percent, and 94 percent, respectively. An FFR greater than 0.75 distinguished patients after myocardial infarction with negative perfusion scintigraphic imaging (Fig. 44–22).

Postinfarction viability is associated with preservation of the microcirculation as reflected by phasic flow velocity characteristics (Fig. 44–23). Phasic coronary blood flow characteristics correlate with myocardial recovery after rescue PCI for acute myocardial infarction[63-65] and differentiated patients with Thrombolysis in Myocardial Infarction (TIMI)-2 versus TIMI-3 angiographic flow. Patients with reduced APV and prolonged diastolic deceleration time and small diastolic-to-systolic velocity ratio had better left ventricular recovery than those with systolic flow reversal, a rapid deceleration time, and negative diastolic-to-systolic flow velocity ratio. Similarly, after acute myocardial infarction, patients in whom APV increased after only a transient decline had significantly greater left ventricular systolic functional recovery than those in whom the APV progressively decreased throughout the next day.[66] These findings suggest that maneuvers that might maintain or augment coronary blood flow (e.g., an intraaortic balloon pumping or adenosine) could be monitored to determine the impact on myocardial salvage.

Coronary Collateral Circulation

After total or near-total occlusion of a coronary artery, myocardial perfusion occurs by way of collaterals—vascular channels that interconnect epicardial arteries.[67] Collateral channels may form acutely or may preexist in an underdeveloped state before the appearance of coronary artery disease. Preexisting collaterals are thin-walled structures ranging in diameter from 20 to 200 μm, with a variable density among different species. Preexisting collaterals are normally closed and nonfunctional because no pressure gradient exists to drive flow between the arteries they connect. After coronary occlusion, the distal pressure drops precipitously and preexisting collaterals open virtually instantly.

Collateral Growth and Function

The transformation of preexisting collaterals into mature collaterals, called *arteriogenesis,* occurs in three stages. The initial stage (first 24 hours) involves *passive widening* of the preexisting channels, facilitating increased flow. Endothelial cells become *activated* by increased blood flow velocity and shear stress and secrete proteolytic enzymes that fragment the basement membrane and dissolve extracellular matrix (an essential process in the upcoming migration of endothelial cells).[68] Shear stress induces widespread functional changes in the endothelium, many of which reflect new gene expression, including upregulation of leukocyte adhesion molecules and production of proinflammatory cytokines (monocyte chemoattractant protein-1, tumor necrosis factor-alpha, granulocyte-macrophage colony-stimulating factor).[68,69]

The second stage (1 day to 3 weeks) is characterized by *inflammation and cellular proliferation.* Monocytes migrate into the vascular wall and secrete cytokines and growth factors. Over several weeks, proliferating endothelial and smooth muscle cells arrange themselves into circular and longitudinal layers. During these first two phases, the luminal diameter of collateral channels increases nearly 10-fold. The third stage of collateral maturation (3 weeks to 6 months) involves thickening of the vessel wall due to *deposition of extracellular matrix* and further cellular proliferation in part stimulated by a variety of growth factors.[70] This is balanced by inhibitory factors such as angiostatin (a fragment of plasminogen), endostatin (a proteolytic fragment of collagen) and thrombospondin-1.[71] The mature collateral vessel may reach 1 mm in luminal

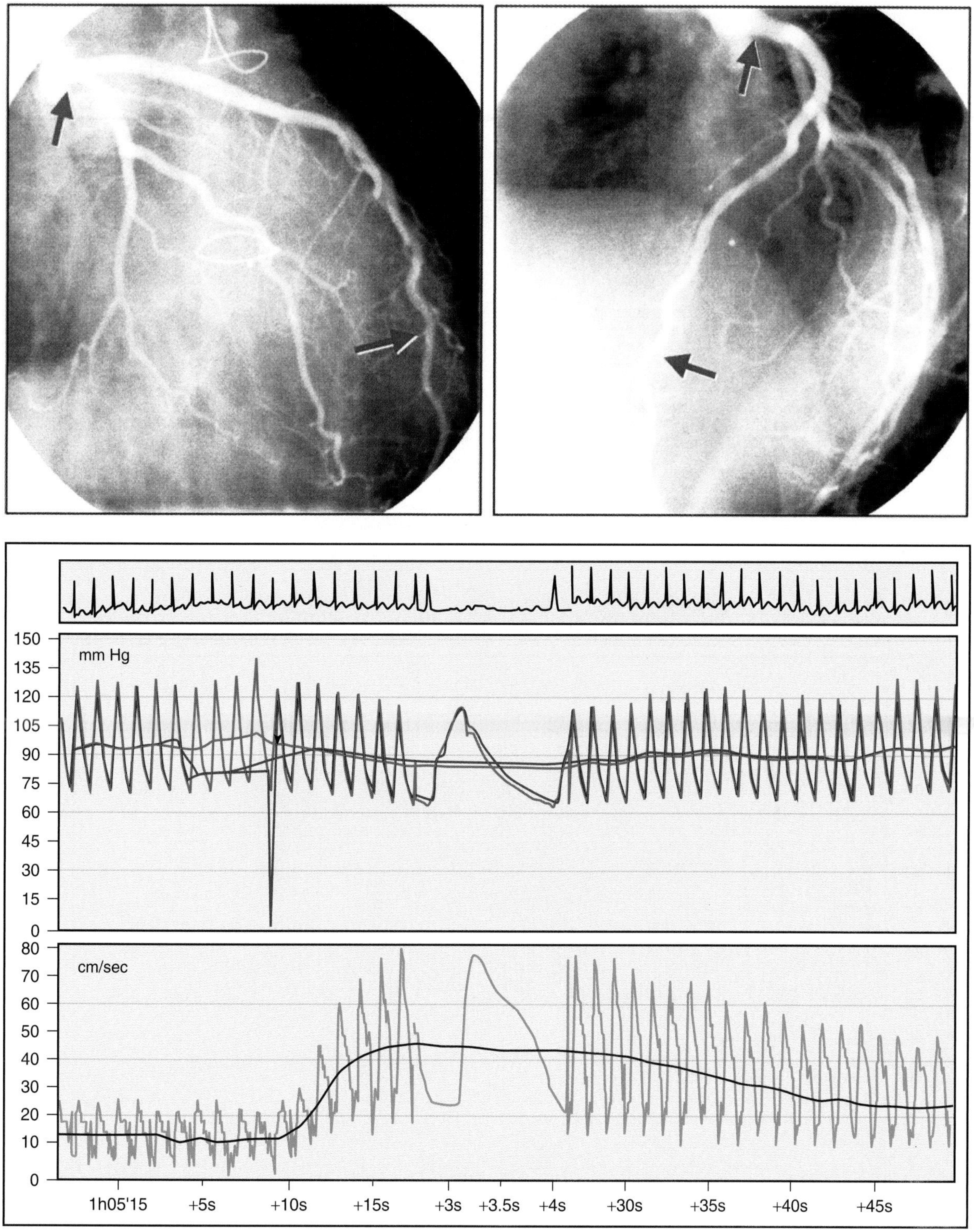

IGURE 44–20 **A,** Angiograms **(upper panels),** aortic and distal coronary pressures **(middle panel),** and coronary flow velocity data **(bottom panel)** in a normal coronary rtery. Coronary pressure (blue curve) and aortic pressure (magenta curve) remain identically matched during maximal hyperemia in arteries without evidence of atherosclerosis, ndicating normal fractional flow reserve (FFR). The black curve in the **bottom panel** is average peak velocity. Red and blue arrows in the angiograms indicate locations of the red nd blue pressure measurements, respectively.

Continued

diameter. Its three-layer structure is nearly indistinguishable from a normal coronary artery of the same size.[67,69]

The severity of coronary obstruction is a critical determinant of the development of coronary collateral channels. In patients, coronary collaterals do not develop until a coronary stenosis of at least 70 percent diameter narrowing is present. The same risk factors that predispose to atherosclerosis may limit the formation of collateral pathways. For example, patients with diabetes mellitus have an impaired ability to develop collateral blood vessels in the setting of obstructive coronary artery disease.[72]

The mature coronary collaterals can appreciably dilate or constrict in response to vasoactive stimuli. Conditions that reduce endothelium-derived NO, including coronary risk factors, may reduce the dilator reserve of coronary collaterals, a condition correctable by the administration of exogenous nitrates.[73] Coronary collaterals can mitigate the severity of myocardial ischemia and, in acute myocardial infarction,

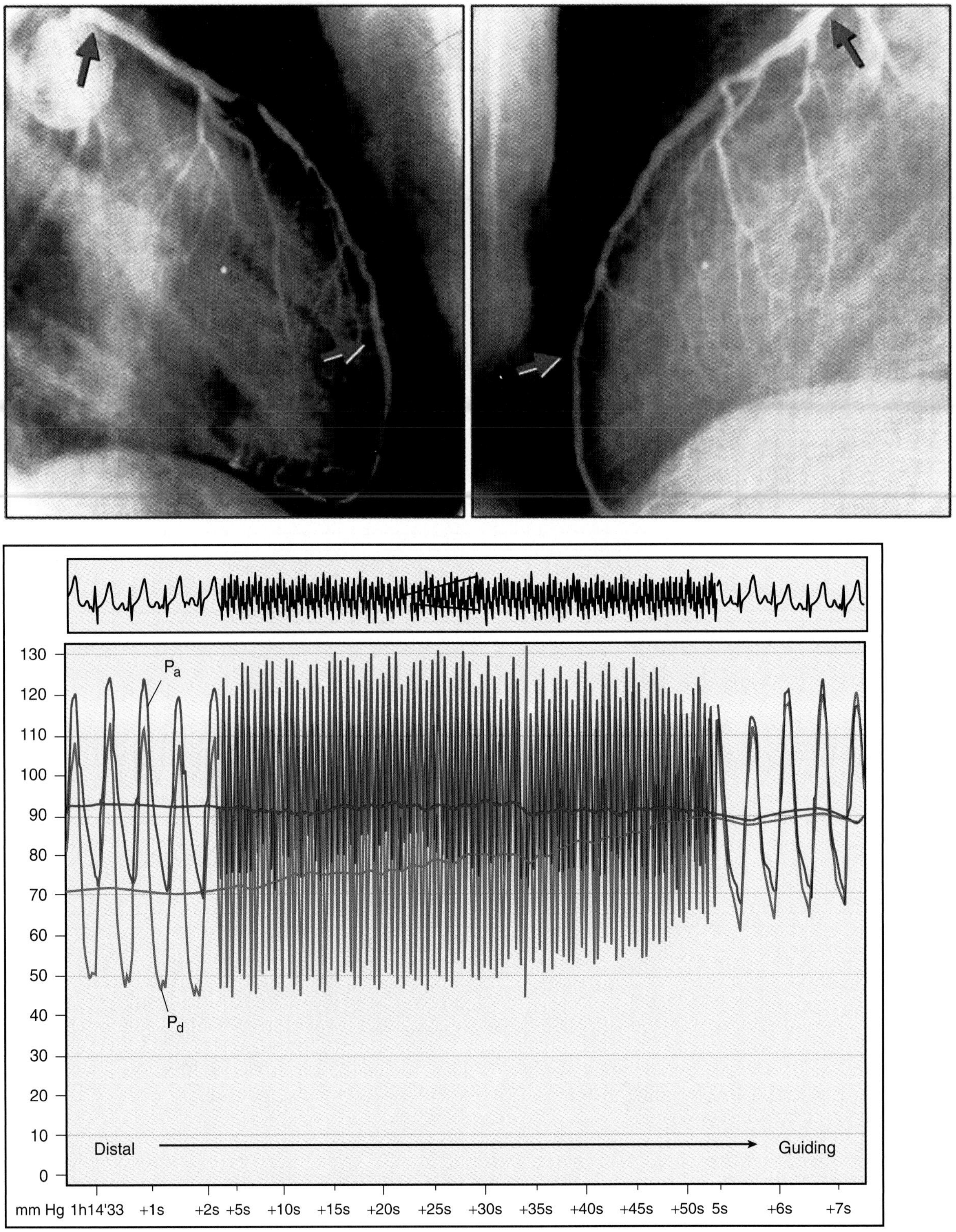

FIGURE 44–20, cont'd **B,** Example of a 44-year-old man with stable angina pectoris. A tight stenosis in the mid-right coronary artery was treated by angioplasty. The coronary angiogram of the left anterior descending coronary artery **(upper panels)** did not show any focal stenosis, but luminal irregularities suggested diffuse atherosclerosis. Aortic (Pa) and distal coronary (Pd) pressures recordings **(lower panel)** during adenosine-induced maximal hyperemia show a pressure gradient of 23 mm Hg (corresponding to an FFR of 0.76) when the pressure sensor is located in the distal left anterior descending coronary artery. This pressure gradient indicates that the diffusely atherosclerotic artery is responsible for approximately one-fourth of the total resistance to blood flow. When the sensor is slowly pulled back, a graded, continuous increase in distal coronary pressure is observed, which indicates diffuse atherosclerosis, not focal stenosis. The exact locations of aortic and distal coronary pressure measurements are indicated by the red and blue arrows, respectively.

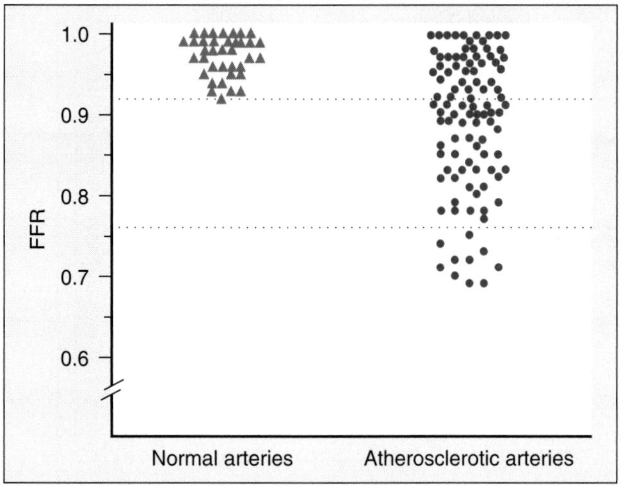

C

FIGURE 44–20, cont'd **C,** Graphs of individual values of FFR in normal arteries and in atherosclerotic coronary arteries without focal stenosis on arteriogram. The upper dotted line indicates the lowest value of FFR in normal coronary arteries. The lower dotted line indicates the threshold level of greater than 0.75. (From De Bruyne B, Hersbach F, Pijls NHJ, et al: Abnormal epicardial coronary resistance in patients with diffuse atherosclerosis but "normal" coronary angiography. Circulation 104:2401-2406, 2001.)

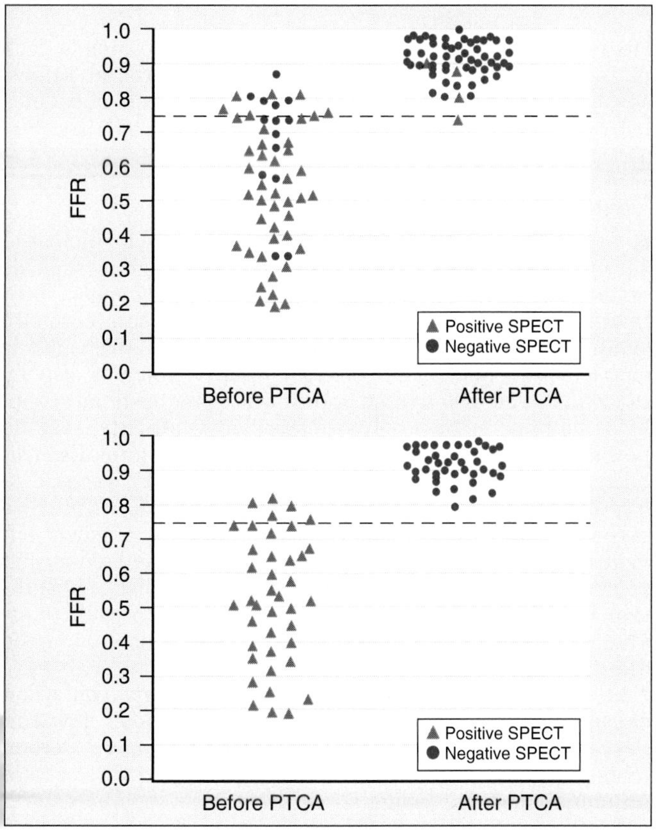

FIGURE 44–22 Fractional flow reserve (FFR) in patients after myocardial infarction. Values of FFR before and after percutaneous transluminal coronary angioplasty (PTCA) according to results of sestamibi single-photon emission computed tomography (SPECT) myocardial perfusion imaging in the patient population as a whole **(top)** and in patients with truly positive and negative SPECT imaging **(bottom)**. (From De Bruyne B, Pijls NHJ, Bartunek J, et al: Fractional flow reserve in patients with prior myocardial infarction. Circulation 104:157-162, 2001.)

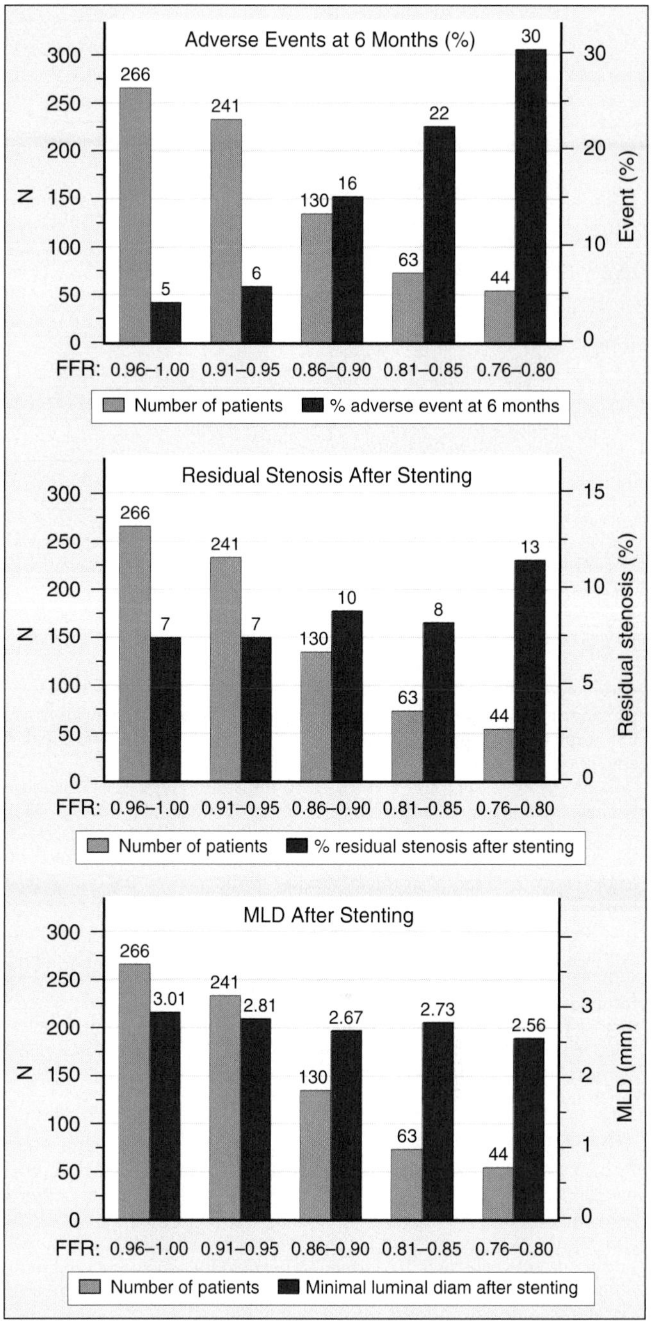

FIGURE 44–21 Clinical outcome of stenting and relationship to fractional flow reserve (FFR) in the FFR-post Stent Registry, involving 750 patients. **Top,** Distribution of the study population over the five FFR categories. A strong inverse correlation was present between FFR after stenting and event rate at 6-month follow-up. **Middle,** Distribution of percent residual stenosis in the five FFR categories. **Bottom,** Minimal luminal diameter (MLD) in the five FFR categories. (From Pijls NHJ, Klauss V, Siebert U, et al: Coronary pressure measurement after stenting predicts adverse events at follow-up: A multicenter registry. Circulation 105:2950-2954, 2002.)

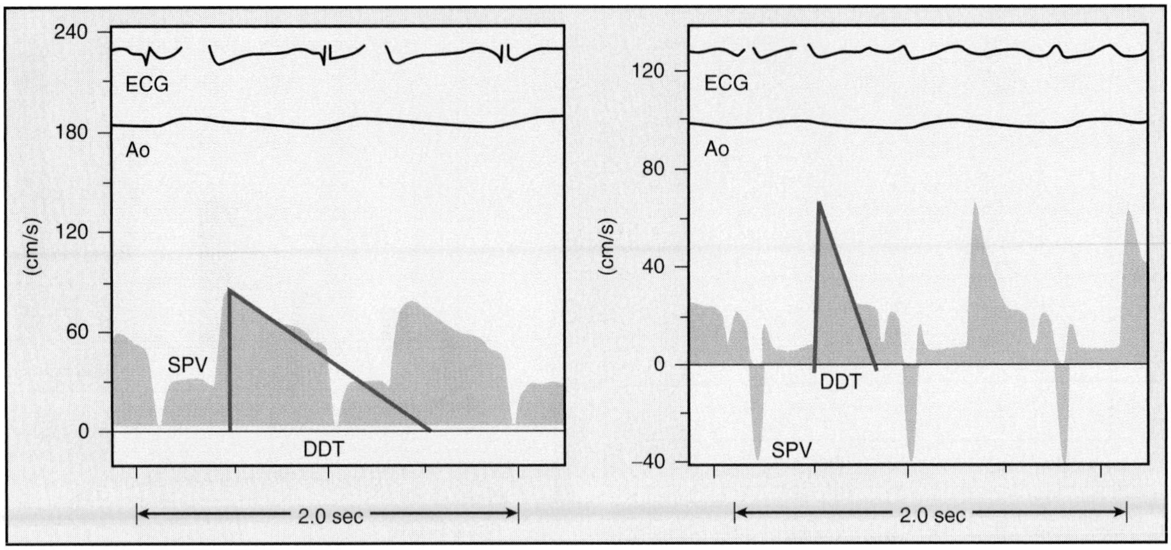

FIGURE 44–23 Phasic flow velocity signals in two patients with acute myocardial infarction demonstrating diastolic deceleration time (DDT) and systolic peak velocity (SPV). A rapid DDT and the presence of systolic flow reversal (negative SPV), as shown in the **right panel,** is associated with poor myocardial functional recovery after infarction. ECG = electrocardiogram; Ao = aorta. (From Yamamuro A, Akasaka T, Tamita K, et al: Coronary flow velocity pattern immediately after percutaneous coronary intervention as a predictor of complications and in-hospital survival after acute myocardial infarction. Circulation 106:3051-3056, 2002.)

provide significant myocardial blood flow, decrease infarct size, improve left ventricular function, reduce the likelihood of left ventricular aneurysm formation, and improve survival.

Coronary pressure and flow distal to the site of angioplasty balloon occlusion can be used to quantitate recruitable collateral perfusion (Fig. 44-24).[74,75] Patients in whom recruitable collateral blood flow exceeded 28 percent of normal maximal myocardial blood flow were free of ischemia at the time of coronary occlusion induced by balloon angioplasty.[76] This approach has also shown that collateral circulation rarely provides blood flow increases adequate to meet the MV_{O_2} of maximal physical exercise; it is typically limited to less than 50 percent of maximal CFR.[74] In addition, quantitatively determined collateral flow is related to future ischemic events.[75] In 403 patients with stable coronary artery disease followed over a 2-year period (Fig. 44-25), those with well-developed collateral supply, (collateral flow index > 0.25) had substantially significantly reduced events compared to those with collateral flow index less than 0.25 (2 percent vs 9 percent).

Arteriogenesis and Angiogenesis

In contrast to *arteriogenesis*, which refers to formation of mature collaterals by enlargement of preexisting rudimentary collaterals, *angiogenesis* refers to *sprouting of new vessels* from preexisting blood vessels and usually results in formation of smaller, capillary-like structures. Subendocardial collaterals may be formed in this manner. Angiogenic stimuli initiate activation of endothelial cells of capillaries or postcapillary venules. This results in local vasodilation, increased vascular permeability, and degradation of the basement membrane. Migration and proliferation of endothelial cells occur with formation of capillary sprouts. Further endothelial proliferation elongates the sprouts, and adjacent sprouts connect to form capillary loops that can carry blood flow. Maturation of the sprouts is associated with deposition of basement membrane.[68]

Angiogenic growth factors can promote formation of new collateral channels in animal models of peripheral and myocardial ischemia. The angiogenic growth factors used in these studies, administered as recombinant protein or by gene transfer, included vascular endothelial growth factor, fibroblast growth factors 1 and 2, hepatocyte growth factor, and hypoxia inducible factor 1. Each of these growth factors can stimulate the critical steps in angiogenesis, including endothelial activation and mitogenesis and upregulation of matrix proteins and matrix proteinases.[77]

In *therapeutic angiogenesis*, exogenous angiogenic growth factors (or genes encoding these growth factors) are administered to stimulate neovascularization of ischemic issues.[77] Therapeutic angiogenesis has since been carried out successfully in several animal species for the treatment of peripheral ischemia. Whether vessels formed in this manner arise from preexisting rudimentary collaterals by arteriogenesis or whether they are vessels newly formed by angiogenesis remains to be determined.

Myocardial Ischemia

Historically, ischemia has been defined as tissue anemia (lack of red blood cells) due to obstruction of arterial inflow. Myocardial ischemia is characterized by an imbalance between myocardial oxygen supply and demand (see Fig. 44–1).

Supply Ischemia

A reduction of arterial blood flow secondary to increased coronary vascular tone (vasospasm) or obstruction (stenosis or thrombus formation) results in *supply ischemia* or *low-flow ischemia* and is often associated with acute coronary syndromes or myocardial infarction. Low-flow ischemia is characterized not only by oxygen deprivation but also by inadequate removal of metabolites due to reduced perfusion. In patients with low-flow ischemia, left ventricular systolic performance is lower and left ventricular diastolic distensibility greater than when the same patients were exposed to high-flow ischemia or hypoxia. This response occurs because coronary flow and perfusion pressure normally augment left ventricular systolic performance (Gregg effect) and reduce left ventricular diastolic distensibility (Salisbury effect). In addition, buildup of tissue metabolites, especially inorganic phosphate, reduces calcium sensitivity of myofilaments, thereby diminishing contractility.

Myocardial ischemia may also be caused by *hypoxia*, when oxygen supply is reduced despite adequate blood flow and tissue perfusion. It may be present in asphyxiation, carbon monoxide poisoning, cyanotic congenital heart disease, cor pulmonale, severe anemia, or hemoglobinopathies with reduced oxygen-carrying capacity.

Demand Ischemia

In the presence of severe chronic coronary obstruction with relatively fixed coronary blood flow, an increase in MV_{O_2} due to exercise, tachycardia, or emotion with insufficient increases in coronary blood flow produces *demand ischemia* or *high-flow ischemia*. Demand ischemia is generally associated with episodes of chronic stable angina. In most clinical presentations, myocardial ischemia usually results from both an increase in oxygen demand and a reduction in myocardial oxygen supply. These mechanisms may act singly or in combination in the same patient at the same or during different episodes of ischemia.

Effects of Ischemia and the Ischemic Cascade

The heart has virtually no stores of oxygen and relies almost entirely on aerobic metabolism to provide for its high rate of energy expenditure. Within seconds of coronary occlusion, myocardial oxygen tension rapidly falls and left ventricular dysfunction occurs. Impairment of systolic and diastolic function are likely related to alterations in intracellular calcium handling. Ischemic regional asynergy may be so extensive that the uninvolved myocardium cannot sustain the normal hemodynamic function, resulting in systolic heart failure. Ischemia changes myocardial stiffness, shifting the diastolic pressure-volume relationship, adding to left ventricular diastolic failure, increasing the resistance to ventricular filling, elevating ventricular filling pressures, and ultimately causing symptoms of pulmonary congestion.

When an epicardial stenosis limits coronary blood flow, compensatory mechanisms are activated to preserve myocardial perfusion. Distal vessels dilate in response to reduced transmural perfusion pressure and release of metabolic vasodilators, and these newly released vasodilatory stimuli enhance flow from preexisting collateral connections. Subendocardial blood flow diminishes because of the higher intramyocardial forces acting on vessels in this region. The subendocardium has less vasodilatory reserve and is thus unable to compensate completely for the fall in coronary perfusion pressure. Subsequently, subendocardial ischemia reduces ventricular contractile force, ultimately stretching and paradoxically elongating the myocardium during ventricular systole. The depression of contractile force during moderate ischemia appears to be mediated by cardiac myocyte K^+-ATP channels. Adenosine stimulates opening of these channels. Although the energy balance may return to normal with recovery of phosphocreatine, contractile function usually remains depressed.

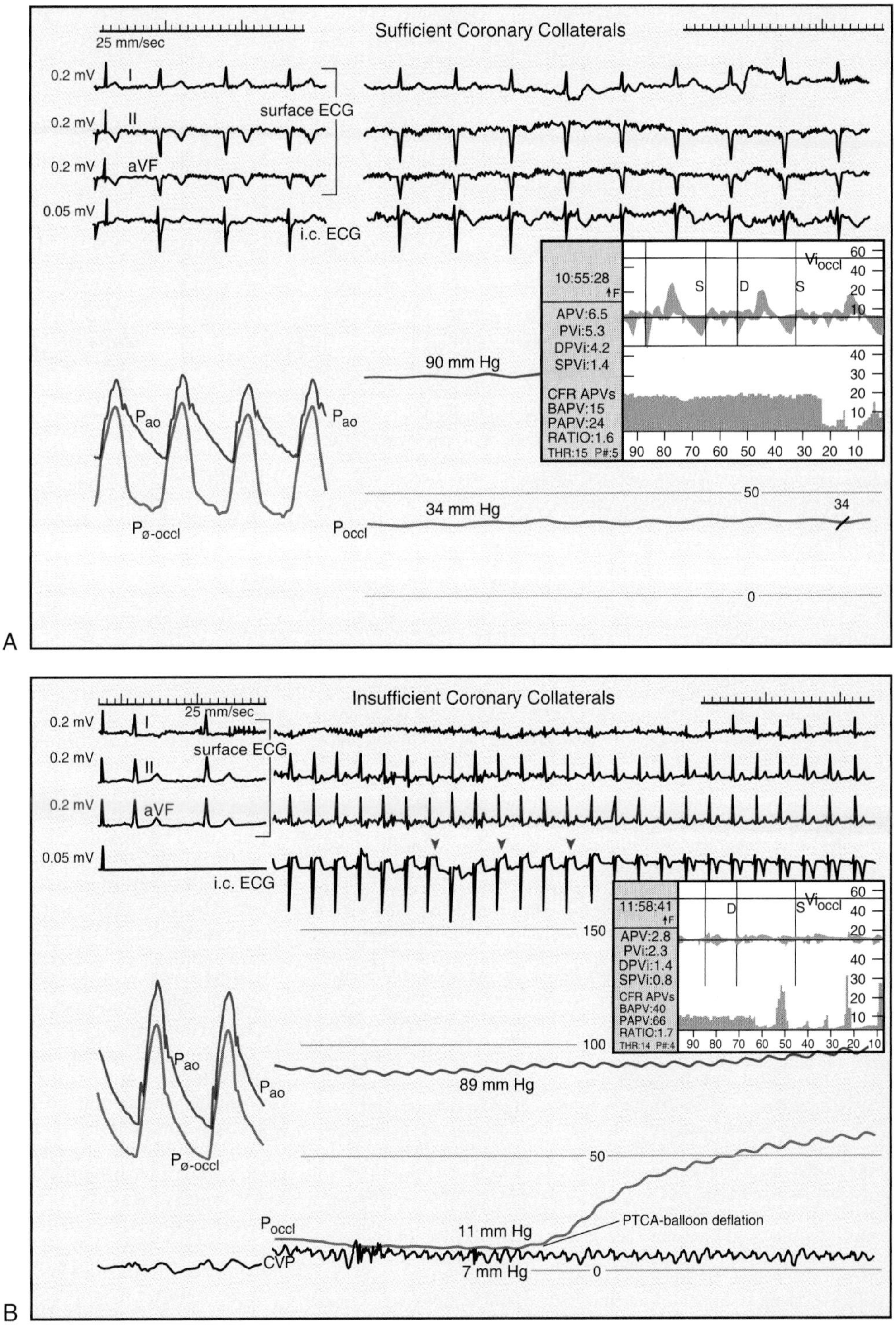

FIGURE 44–24 Pressure and flow tracings during balloon occlusion in two patients, one with sufficient collaterals **(A)** and one with insufficient collaterals **(B)**. Note that the coronary balloon occlusion pressure in the patient with sufficient collaterals is 34 mm Hg with maintained distal flow velocity. The patient with insufficient collaterals has an occlusion pressure of 11 mm Hg and reduced distal coronary occlusion pressure. P_{ao} = aortic guide catheter pressure; P_{occl} = distal coronary pressure during balloon occlusion; Vi_{occl} = distal flow velocity integral during balloon occlusion; CVP = central venous pressure; i.c. = intracoronary; ECG = electrocardiogram; PTCA = percutaneous transluminal coronary angioplasty; AVP = average peak velocity. (From Seiler C, Fleisch M, Billinger M, Meier B: Simultaneous intracoronary velocity- and pressure-derived assessment of adenosine-induced collateral hemodynamics in patients with one- to two-vessel coronary artery disease. J Am Coll Cardiol 34:1985-1994, 1999.)

The sudden cessation of myocardial blood flow due to occlusion of an epicardial artery is followed by predictable physiologic and metabolic changes within seconds following the occlusion. Myocardial energy metabolism immediately shifts from aerobic or mitochondrial metabolism to anaerobic glycolysis in a few seconds as underperfused tissue consumes oxygen from oxyhemoglobin and oxymyoglobin. Simultaneous with energy depletion, myocardial contraction diminishes and then stops. The myocardium elongates rather than shortens with each subsequent systole. The cellular membrane potential decreases and ischemic electrocardiographic abnormalities appear.[78,79]

Anaerobic glycolysis provides 80 percent of new high-energy phosphates in the ischemic zone. As this is insufficient to meet energy demands, high-energy phosphate stores decrease. Tissue ATP is metabo-

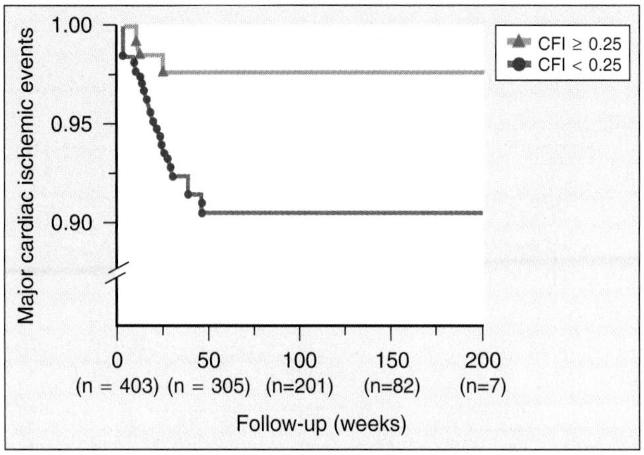

FIGURE 44–25 Clinical outcome in patients with sufficient collateral flow index (CFI): Cumulative event rate analysis and time to occurrence of major adverse cardiac events (death, myocardial infarction, and unstable angina) during follow-up of 200 weeks. Only 3 patients (2 percent) with good collaterals, but 24 patients (9 percent) with poor collaterals, had major adverse cardiac ischemic events during the first year after successful percutaneous coronary intervention. (From Billinger M, Kloos P, Eberli FR, et al: Physiologically assessed coronary collateral flow and adverse cardiac ischemic events: A follow-up study in 403 patients with coronary artery disease. J Am Coll Cardiol 40:1545-1550, 2002.)

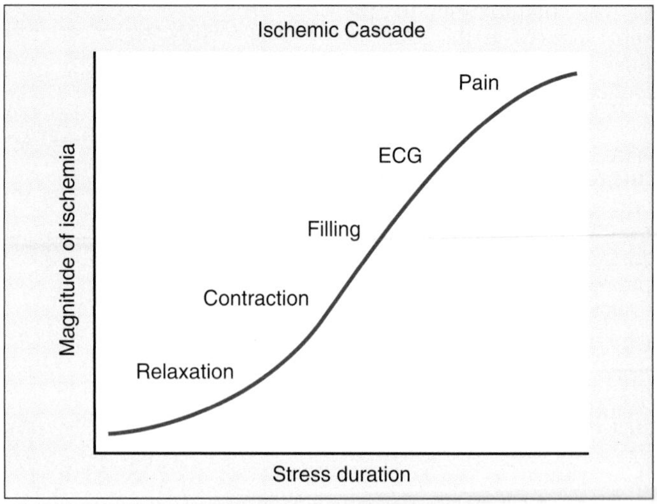

FIGURE 44–26 Schema of the ischemic cascade. The events (on the vertical) are related to the time course of occurrence on the horizontal. The first changes of ischemia are biochemical, followed by diastolic dysfunction, systolic dysfunction, electrocardiographic (ECG) changes, and ultimately angina.

lized and ADP accumulates. Creatinine phosphate, a source of high energy, decreases quickly, whereas ATP is more gradually metabolized. In reversible ischemia, 75 to 80 percent of ATP present at the initiation of the ischemic event is depleted. Because glucose trapped in the extracellular fluid is minimal, anaerobic glycolysis uses glucose-1-phosphate from glycogenolysis as its active substrate. Lactate and its associated hydrogen ion accumulate immediately during ischemia. Continued ischemia decreases tissue glycogen stores and increases anaerobic glycolysis, releasing glucose-1-phosphate, glucose-6-phosphate, alphaglycerophosphate, and lactate. ADP is rapidly generated, whereas rephosphorylation of the adenine nucleotide pool to ATP is retarded by acidosis and lactate. During ischemia, adenosine diffuses into the extracellular fluid and is removed from the adenine nucleotide pool. Adenosine is further degraded to inosine and hypoxanthine, which accumulate during ischemia, resulting in a reduction of the size of the adenosine pool to 30 to 40 percent of its initial levels. Additional metabolites such as bradykinin, opioids, norepinephrine, and angiotensin are also released and participate in receptor activation of myocytes, stimulating intracellular signaling systems. Intracellular ionic calcium rises during ischemia, and intracellular sodium competes to expel calcium via the sodium-calcium exchange system. During reperfusion after ischemia, many of these basic processes can be attenuated or reduced; however, ischemic reperfusion is associated with its own set of biochemical alterations and only partial restoration of function.[78,79]

Thus, ischemia produces a typical cascade of events beginning with metabolic and biochemical alternations leading to impaired ventricular relaxation and diastolic dysfunction, impaired systolic function, and electrocardiographic abnormalities with ST segment alterations, followed by increased end-diastolic pressure with left ventricular dyssynchrony, hypokinesis, akinesis, and dyskinesis and, lastly, painful symptoms of angina (Fig. 44–26). The sequence of hemodynamic and electrocardiographic events can be reproduced by transient epicardial coronary artery occlusion during angioplasty or during spontaneous coronary vasospasm.

Myocardial Stunning and Hibernation

A brief episode of severe ischemia may produce prolonged myocardial dysfunction with a gradual return of contractile activity, a condition termed *myocardial stunning.* Myocardial stunning is represented by persistent regional dysfunction at a time when chest pain, ST segment deviation, and regional perfusion have recovered.[75,79] In patients with a myocardial infarction (with and without thrombolytic therapy), stunned myocardium lies adjacent to infarcted myocardium. Improvement in ventricular function occurs gradually over the course of days to weeks. Myocardial stunning is also an important feature of unstable angina.[80]

There are three major mechanisms in the pathogenesis of myocardial stunning (Fig. 44–27): (1) generation of oxygen-derived free radicals, (2) calcium overload, and (3) reduced sensitivity of myofilaments to calcium and loss of myofilaments.[78] In the first minutes of reperfusion after transient ischemia, the increased production of superoxide and hydroxyl radicals inactivate enzymes and cause lipid peroxidation. The presumed targets of oxygen-derived free radicals include sarcolemmal Na^+,K^+-ATPase and calcium-stimulated adenosine triphosphatase (ATPase) and, in the sarcoplasmic reticulum, calcium-stimulated ATPase. The result is increased influx of calcium through the sarcolemma and diminished calcium reuptake by the sarcoplasmic reticulum, resulting in cellular calcium overload and, ultimately, in impaired excitation-contraction coupling. Calcium overload can also activate enzymes that further damage the sarcolemma and sarcoplasmic reticulum. Ischemia followed by reperfusion also results in decreased calcium sensitivity of myofilaments, at least in part due to oxidation of critical thiol groups and in part due to partial proteolysis of troponin.[81] Recent evidence suggests that calcium overload may activate calpains, resulting in selective proteolysis of myofibrils.[79] Although antioxidants are effective, they do not prevent stunning completely because of two postulated interrelated components of stunning: an ischemic component not responsive to antioxidants and a second, larger component related to reperfusion.[78]

Impaired resting left ventricular function due to chronically reduced coronary blood flow that can be restored by revascularization has been attributed to *myocardial hibernation.* Even some akinetic segments can occasionally regain systolic contraction after revascularization. Conceptually, hibernation represents a condition in which the myocardium reduces its contractility (and hence its MVO_2) to match reduced perfusion, thereby preserving cellular viability. Hibernating myocardium is present in approximately one-third of patients with coronary artery disease and impaired left ventricular function. The time course of recovery of hibernating myocardium after revascularization is quite variable, ranging from days to months. Slower recovery is typically associated with longer duration of hibernation. Revascularization can be effective whether achieved by coronary bypass grafting or by coronary angioplasty.[82]

Dysfunctional, hibernating myocardium can be identified by noninvasive methods such as echocardiography, nuclear perfusion imaging, and magnetic resonance imaging (see Chaps. 11, 13, and 14). This has significant practical importance because revascularization can improve left ventricular function, alleviate symptoms of heart failure, and, in the long term, forestall myocardial necrosis. Features of ischemia, stunning, and hibernation are summarized in Table 44–13.

Myocardial Necrosis

Unrelieved ischemia produces cell death. Because energy requirements, rates of metabolic activity, and oxygen extraction are greatest in the subendocardium, the subendocardium is the most susceptible region to ischemic injury and necrosis.[83] Severely ischemic myocardium undergoes necrosis first in the subendocardium, beginning as early as 15 to 20 minutes after coronary artery occlusion. Necrosis progresses toward the epicardium in a wavefront, gradually involving the less severely ischemic outer epicardial layers. The progression of the wavefront is slowed by the presence of residual blood flow when the coronary occlusion is incomplete or when mature collaterals are present at the time of occlusion. The wavefront conversely is accelerated when myocardial ischemia is unusually severe or when collateral blood flow is low, MVO_2 is high, or marked arterial hypotension is present (e.g., in patients in cardiogenic shock). In dogs with acute coronary occlusion, the subendocardial lateral boundaries of myocardial infarcts are established early in the first hour, whereas the myocardial infarct enlarges in the transmural direction over 4 to 6 hours, a finding similarly noted in humans. The recognition of the time-dependent progression of necrosis is the basis of timely interventions to salvage myocardium.[83,84]

The clinical presentations of myocardial ischemia are reflective of distinct pathogenic mechanisms. Clinical syndromes are often but not always associated with anginal pain and include chronic stable angina, unstable angina, variant (vasospastic) angina, and myocardial infarction (Fig. 44–28) (see Chaps. 46, 49, and 50). Atherosclerotic coronary stenosis is the most common cause of myocardial ischemia because of the high disease prevalence. Acute thrombosis superimposed on atherosclerotic plaque is associated with acute

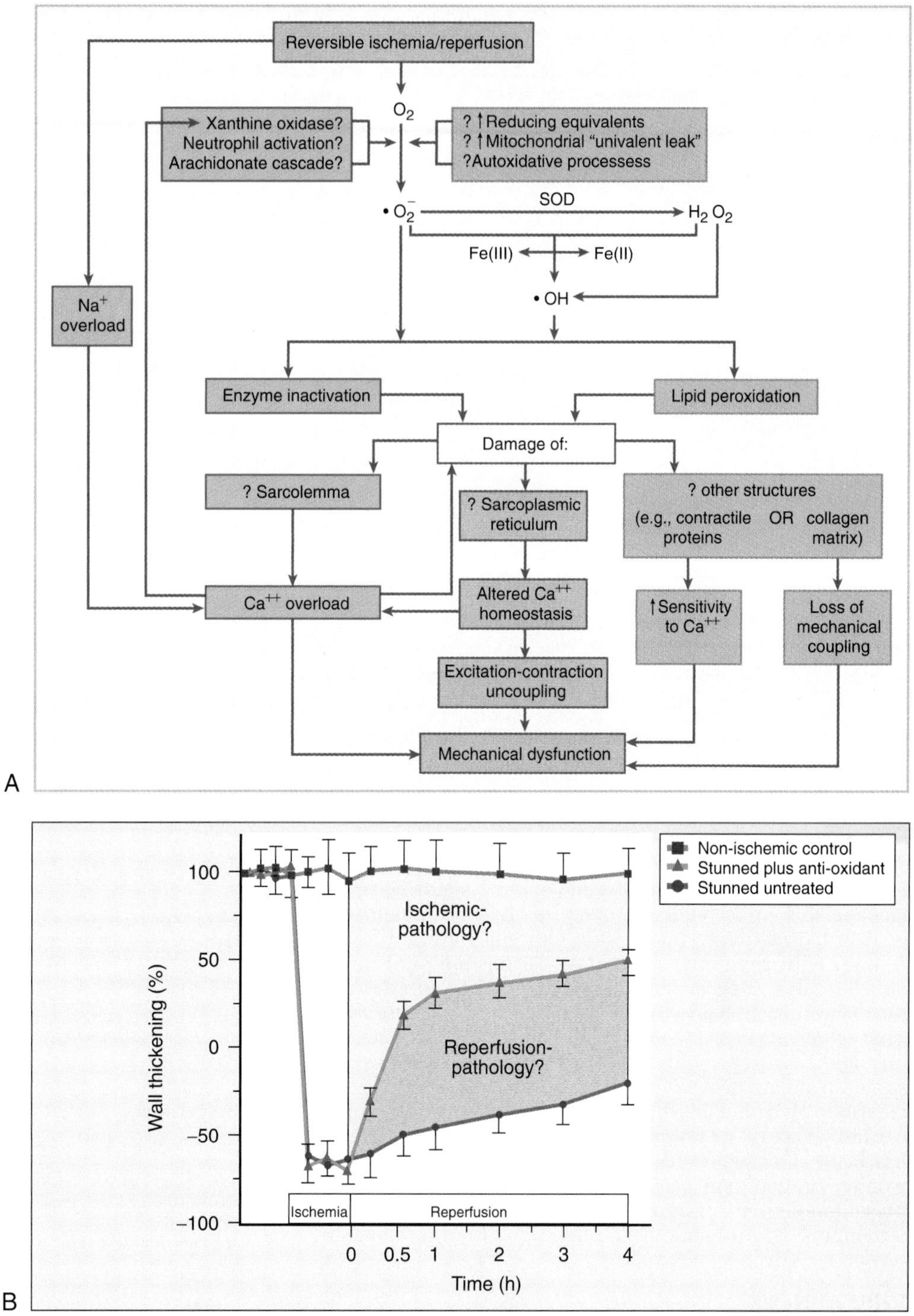

FIGURE 44–27 **A,** Illustration of proposed mechanisms of postischemic myocardial dysfunction integrating the mechanisms into three major hypotheses involving calcium overload, increased sensitivity to calcium, and loss of mechanical coupling. SOD = sodium oxide dismutase. **B,** Components of postischemic dysfunction: myocardial stunning probably arises from the additive effects of a reperfusion-induced pathology (magenta shading) of the contractile deficit, which can be restored through the use of antioxidant intervention transiently at the time of reperfusion. The second component (blue shading) incorporates pathology from which the heart is slowly recovering together with additional reperfusion-induced components not amenable to intervention. (Adapted from Hearse DJ: Stunning: A radical re-view. Cardiovasc Drugs Ther 5:853, 1991; Opie LH [ed]: Stunning, Hibernation, and Calcium in Myocardial Ischemia and Reperfusion Loss in Massachusetts. Dordrecht, Kluwer, 1992, pp 10-55; and Kloner RA, Bolli R, Marban E, et al: Medical and cellular implications of stunning, hibernation, and preconditioning: An NHLBI workshop. Circulation 97:1848-1867, 1998.)

TABLE 44–13 Features of Ischemia, Stunning, and Hibernation

Variable	Coronary Blood Flow	Lactate Production	Contractile Function
Ischemia/infarction	Markedly reduced/absent	Yes	Impaired transiently or permanently Recovers after relief of ischemia
Stunning	Preserved	No	Impaired, improved by inotropic with patent artery stimulation Recovers spontaneously
Hibernation	Reduced with abnormal myocardium	No	Impaired; recovery after revascularization

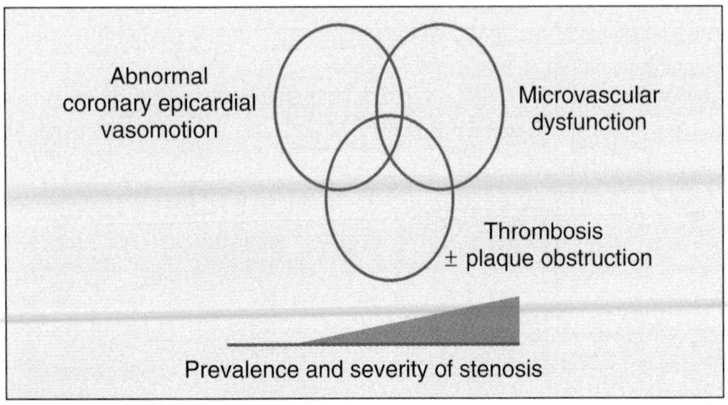

FIGURE 44–28 Pathophysiological components of myocardial ischemia. Different clinical ischemic syndromes result from fixed obstruction to coronary blood flow by atherosclerotic plaques, thrombosis, and/or coronary vasoconstriction of epicardial or microvascular vessels. These events may occur together or separately. (Modified from Maseri A, Crea F, Lanza GA, et al: Coronary vasoconstriction: Where do we stand in 1999? An important, multifaceted but elusive role. Cardiologia 44:115, 1999.)

myocardial infarction and unstable anginal syndromes. The mechanisms underlying the onset of unstable angina and myocardial infarction include not only plaque fissuring and rupture with superimposed platelet aggregation and thrombus but also coronary vasoconstriction. The products of platelet aggregation and thrombosis dilate normal arteries but can severely constrict the atherosclerotic artery. Patients with unstable coronary syndromes and complex plaques demonstrate augmented release of serotonin into the coronary circulation. Dynamic narrowing of coronary arteries due to coronary vasospasms or dynamic reduction in stenosis areas has been associated with cocaine use, cigarette smoking in women, or other nonspecific neurogenic stimuli. The clinical presentations and findings of the different myocardial ischemic syndromes are further described in other chapters.

REFERENCES

Myocardial Oxygen Supply and Demand Relationship

1. Braunwald E: Myocardial oxygen consumption: The quest for its determinants and some clinical fallout. J Am Coll Cardiol 35:45B, 2000.
2. Spaan JAE: Coronary Blood Flow: Mechanics, Distribution, and Control. Dordrecht, Netherlands, Kluwer, 1991.
3. Kal JE, Van Wezel HB, Vergroesen I: A critical appraisal of the rate pressure product as index of myocardial oxygen consumption for the study of metabolic coronary flow regulation. Int J Cardiol 71:141-148, 1999.
4. Chilian WM: Coronary microcirculation in health and disease: Summary of an NHLBI workshop. Circulation 95:522-528, 1997.
5. De Bruyne B, Hersbach F, Pijls NHJ, et al: Abnormal epicardial coronary resistance in patients with diffuse atherosclerosis but "normal" coronary angiography. Circulation 104:2401-2406, 2001.
6. Stepp DW, Nishikawa Y, Chilian WM: Regulation of shear stress in the canine coronary microcirculation. Circulation 100:1555-1561, 1999.

Endothelial Function

7. Mombouli JV, Vanhoutte PM: Endothelial dysfunction: From physiology to therapy. J Mol Cell Cardiol 31:61-74, 1999.
8. Verman S, Anderson TJ: Fundamentals of endothelial function for the clinical cardiologist. Circulation 105:546-549, 2002.
9. Selwyn AP, Kinlay S, Libby P, Ganz P: Atherogenic lipids, vascular dysfunction, and clinical signs of ischemic heart disease. Circulation 95:5-7, 1997.
10. Hasdai D, Gibbons RJ, Holmes DR Jr, et al: Coronary endothelial dysfunction in humans is associated with myocardial perfusion defects. Circulation 96:3390-3395, 1997.
11. Drexler H: Endothelial dysfunction: Clinical implications. Prog Cardiovasc Dis 39:287-324, 1997.
12. Thorne S, Mullen MJ, Clarkson P, et al: Early endothelial dysfunction in adults at risk from atherosclerosis: Different responses to L-arginine. J Am Coll Cardiol 32:110-116, 1998.
13. Inoue T, Saniabadi AR, Matsunaga R, et al: Impaired endothelium-dependent acetylcholine-induced coronary artery relaxation in patients with high serum remnant lipoprotein particles. Atherosclerosis 139:363-367, 1998.
14. Xu WM, Liu LZ: Nitric oxide: From a mysterious labile factor to the molecule of the Nobel Prize. Recent progress in nitric oxide research. Cell Res 8:251-258, 1998.
15. Moncada S: Nitric oxide: Discovery and impact on clinical medicine. J R Soc Med 92:164-169, 1999.
16. Ignarro LJ, Cirino G, Casini A, Napoli C: Nitric oxide as a signaling molecule in the vascular system: An overview. J Cardiovasc Pharmacol 34:879-886, 1999.
17. Lee RT, Libby P: The unstable atheroma. Arterioscler Thromb Vasc Biol 17:1859-1867, 1997.
18. Quilley J, Fulton D, McGiff JC: Hyperpolarizing factors. Biochem Pharmacol 54:1059-1070, 1997.
19. Bauersachs J, Popp R, Fleming I, Busse R: Nitric oxide and endothelium-derived hyperpolarizing factor: Formation and interactions. Prostaglandins Leukot Essent Fatty Acids 57:439-446, 1997.
20. Ortega Mateo A, de Artinano AA: Highlights on endothelins: A review. Pharmacol Res 36:339-351, 1997.
21. Kelly JJ, Whitworth JA: Endothelin-1 as a mediator in cardiovascular disease. Clin Exp Pharmacol Physiol 26:158-161, 1999.
22. Verhaar MC, Strachan FE, Newby DE, et al: Endothelin A receptor antagonist–mediated vasodilatation is attenuated by inhibition of nitric oxide synthesis and by endothelin-B receptor blockade. Circulation 97:752-756, 1998.
23. Heitzer T, Schlinzig T, Krohn K, et al: Endothelial dysfunction, oxidative stress, and risk of cardiovascular events in patients with coronary artery disease. Circulation 104:2673-2678, 2001.

Autoregulation

24. Pijls NHJ, De Bruyne B: Coronary Pressure. Dordrecht, Netherlands, Kluwer, 1997, pp 12-13.
25. Yada T, Richmond KN, Van Bibber R, et al: Role of adenosine in local metabolic coronary vasodilation. Am J Physiol 276:H1425-H1433, 1999.
26. Duffy SJ, Castle SF, Harper RW, Meredith IT: Contribution of vasodilator prostanoids and nitric oxide to resting flow, metabolic vasodilation, and flow-mediated dilation in human coronary circulation. Circulation 100:1951-1957, 1999.
27. Ishibashi Y, Duncker DJ, Zhang J, Bache RJ: ATP-sensitive K^+ channels, adenosine, and nitric oxide–mediated mechanisms account for coronary vasodilation during exercise. Circ Res 82:346-359, 1998.
28. Feigl EO: Neural control of coronary blood flow. J Vasc Res 35:85-92, 1998.
29. Saetrum OO, Gulbenkian S, Edvinsson L: Innervation and effects of vasoactive substances in the coronary circulation. Eur Heart J 18:1556, 1997.
30. Tanaka E, Mori H, Chujo M, et al: Coronary vasoconstrictive effects of neuropeptide Y and their modulation by the ATP-sensitive potassium channel in anesthetized dogs. J Am Coll Cardiol 29:1380, 1997.
31. Heusch G; Baumgart D, Camici P, et al: Alpha-adrenergic coronary vasoconstriction and myocardial ischemia in humans. Circulation 101:689, 2000.
32. Gregorini L, Marco J, Farah B, et al: Effects of selective α_1- and α_2-adrenergic blockade on coronary flow reserve after coronary stenting. Circulation 106:2901-2907, 2002.
33. Heusch G, Erbel R, Siffert W: Genetic determinants of coronary vasomotor in humans. Am J Physiol Heart Circ Physiol 281:H1465, 2001.
34. Snapir A, Mikkelsson J, Perola M, et al: Variation in the $alpha_2$-B adrenoceptor gene as a risk factor for pre-hospital fatal myocardial infarction and sudden death. J Am Coll Cardiol 41:190-194, 2003.
35. Rajagopalan S, Dube S, Canty JM Jr: Regulation of coronary diameter by myogenic mechanisms in arterial microvessels greater than 100 microns in diameter. Am J Physiol 268:H788-H793, 1995.
36. Morita K, Mori H, Tsujioka K, et al: Alpha-adrenergic vasoconstriction reduces systolic retrograde coronary blood flow. Am J Physiol 273:H2746-H2755, 1997.

37. Zhang J, Duncker DJ, Ya X, et al: Effect of left ventricular hypertrophy secondary to chronic pressure overload on transmural myocardial 2-deoxyglucose uptake: A ^{31}P NMR spectroscopic study. Circulation 92:1274-1283, 1995.
38. Duncker DJ, Traverse JH, Ishibashi Y, Bache RJ: Effect of NO on transmural distribution of blood flow in hypertrophied left ventricle during exercise. Am J Physiol 276:H1305-H1312, 1999.
39. Duncker DJ, Ishibashi Y, Bache RJ: Effect of treadmill exercise on transmural distribution of blood flow in hypertrophied left ventricle. Am J Physiol 275:H1274-H1282, 1998.

Influence of a Stenosis on Coronary Blood Flow

40. Siebes M, Campbell CS, D'Argenio DZ: Fluid dynamics of a partially collapsible stenosis in a flow model of the coronary circulation. ASME J Biomech Eng 118:489-497, 1996.
41. Kern M: Curriculum in interventional cardiology: Coronary pressure and flow measurements in the cardiac catheterization laboratory. Cathet Cardiovasc Intervent 54:378-400, 2002.
42. Jeremias A, Whitbourn RJ, Filardo SD, et al: Adequacy of intracoronary versus intravenous adenosine-induced maximal coronary hyperemia for fractional flow reserve measurements. Am Heart J 140:651-657, 2000.
43. Bartunek J, Winjs W, Heyndrickx GR, de Bruyne B: Effects of dobutamine on coronary stenosis: Physiology and morphology comparison with intracoronary adenosine. Circulation 100:243-249, 1999.
44. Pijls NH, De Bruyne B, Smith L, et al: Coronary thermodilution to assess flow reserve: Validation in humans. Circulation 105:2482-2486, 2002.
45. Baumgart D, Haude M, Liu F, et al: Current concepts of coronary flow reserve for clinical decision making during cardiac catheterization. Am Heart J 136:136-149, 1998.
46. Kern MJ, Bach RG, Mechem C, et al: Variations in normal coronary vasodilatory reserve stratified by artery, gender, heart transplantation and coronary artery disease. J Am Coll Cardiol 28:1154-1160, 1996.
47. Akasaka T, Yoshida K, Hozumi T, et al: Retinopathy identifies marked restriction of coronary flow reserve in patients with diabetes mellitus. J Am Coll Cardiol 30:935-941, 1997.

Measurement of Coronary Flow Reserve

48. Kern MJ: Coronary physiology revisited: Practical insights from the cardiac catheterization laboratory. Circulation 101:1344-1351, 2000.
49. Pijls NH, Van Gelder B, Van der Voort P, et al: Fractional flow reserve: A useful index to evaluate the influence of an epicardial coronary stenosis on myocardial blood flow. Circulation 92:3183-3193, 1995.
50. De Bruyne B, Bartunek J, Sys SU, et al: Simultaneous coronary pressure and flow velocity measurements in humans: Feasibility, reproducibility, and hemodynamic dependence of coronary flow velocity reserve, hyperemic flow versus pressure slope index, and fractional flow reserve. Circulation 94:1842-1849, 1996.
51. Marques KMJ, Spruijt HJ, Boer C, et al: The diastolic flow-pressure gradient relation in coronary stenoses in humans. J Am Coll Cardiol 39:1630-1636, 2002.
52. Meuwissen M, Chamuleau S, Siebes M, et al: Role of variability in microvascular resistance on fractional flow reserve and coronary blood flow velocity reserve in intermediate coronary lesions. Circulation 103:184-187, 2001.
53. Meuwissen M, Siebes M, Chamuleau SAJ, et al: Hyperemic stenosis resistance index for evaluation of functional coronary lesion severity. Circulation 106:441-446, 2002.
54. Pijls NH, De Bruyne B, Peels K, et al: Measurement of fractional flow reserve to assess the functional severity of coronary artery stenoses. N Engl J Med 334:1703-1708, 1996.
55. Chamuleau SAJ, Meuwissen M, van Eck-Smit BLF, et al: Fractional flow reserve, absolute and relative coronary blood flow velocity reserve in relation to the results of technetium-99m sestamibi single-photon emission computed tomography in patients with two-vessel coronary artery disease. J Am Coll Cardiol 37:1316-1322, 2001.
56. Kern MJ, Donohue TJ, Aguirre FV, et al: Clinical outcome of deferring angioplasty in patients with normal translesional pressure-flow velocity measurements. J Am Coll Cardiol 25:178-187, 1995.
57. Bech GJ, De Bruyne B, Bonnier HJRM, et al: Long-term follow-up after deferral of percutaneous transluminal coronary angioplasty of intermediate stenosis on the basis of coronary pressure measurement. J Am Coll Cardiol 31:841-847, 1998.
58. Bech GJW, Pijls NHJ, De Bruyne B, et al: Usefulness of fractional flow reserve to predict clinical outcome after balloon angioplasty. Circulation 99:883-888, 1999.
59. Bech GJW, De Bruyne B, Pijls NHJ, et al: Fractional flow reserve to determine the appropriateness of angioplasty in moderate coronary stenosis: A randomized trial. Circulation 103:2928-2934, 2001.
60. Smith SC Jr, Dove JT, Jacobs AK, et al: ACC/AHA guidelines for percutaneous coronary intervention (revision of the 1993 PTCA guidelines)—executive summary. A report of the American College of Cardiology/American Heart Association Task Force on Practice Guidelines (committee to revise the 1993 guidelines for percutaneous transluminal coronary angioplasty. J Am Coll Cardiol 37:2215-2238, 2001.
61. Pijls NHJ, Klauss V, Siebert U, et al: Coronary pressure measurement after stenting predicts adverse events at follow-up: A multicenter registry. Circulation 105:2950-2954, 2002.
62. De Bruyne B, Pijls NHJ, Bartunek J, et al: Fractional flow reserve in patients with prior myocardial infarction. Circulation 104:157-162, 2001.
63. Akasaka T, Yoshida K, Kawamoto T, et al: Relation of phasic coronary flow velocity characteristics with TIMI perfusion grade and myocardial recovery after primary percutaneous transluminal coronary angioplasty and rescue stenting. Circulation 101:2361-2367, 2000.
64. Yamamuro A, Akasaka T, Tamita K, et al: Coronary flow velocity pattern immediately after percutaneous coronary intervention as a predictor of complications and in-hospital survival after acute myocardial infarction. Circulation 106:3051-3056, 2002.
65. Kawamoto T, Yoshida K, Akasaka T, et al: Can coronary blood flow velocity pattern after primary percutaneous transluminal coronary angiography predict recovery of regional left ventricular function in patients with acute myocardial infarction? Circulation 100:339-345, 1999.
66. Tsunoda T, Nakamura M, Wakatsuki T, et al: The pattern of alteration in flow velocity in the recanalized artery is related to left ventricular recovery in patients with acute infarction and successful direct balloon angioplasty. J Am Coll Cardiol 32:338-344, 1998.

Coronary Collateral Circulation

67. Schaper W, Ito WD: Molecular mechanisms of coronary collateral vessel growth. Circ Res 79:911-919, 1996.
68. Pepper MS: Manipulating angiogenesis: From basic science to the bedside. Arterioscler Thromb Vasc Biol 17:605-619, 1997.
69. Wolf C, Cai WJ, Vosschulte R, et al: Vascular remodeling and altered protein expression during growth of coronary collateral arteries. J Mol Cell Cardiol 30:2291-2305, 1998.
70. Stetler-Stevenson WG: Matrix metalloproteinases in angiogenesis: A moving target for therapeutic intervention. J Clin Invest 103:1237-1241, 1999.
71. Majno G: Chronic inflammation: Links with angiogenesis and wound healing. Am J Pathol 153:1035-1039, 1998.
72. Schaper W, Buschmann I: Collateral circulation and diabetes. Circulation 99:2224-2226, 1999.
73. Klassen CL, Traverse JH, Bache RJ: Nitroglycerin dilates coronary collateral vessels during exercise after blockade of endogenous NO production. Am J Physiol 277:H918-H923, 1999.
74. Pijls NH, Bech GJ, el Gamal MI, et al: Quantification of recruitable coronary collateral blood flow in conscious humans and its potential to predict future ischemic events. J Am Coll Cardiol 25:1522-1528, 1995.
75. Billinger M, Kloos P, Eberli FR, et al: Physiologically assessed coronary collateral flow and adverse cardiac ischemic events: A follow-up study in 403 patients with coronary artery disease. J Am Coll Cardiol 40:1545-1550, 2002.
76. Seiler C, Fleisch M, Billinger M, Meier B: Simultaneous intracoronary velocity- and pressure-derived assessment of adenosine-induced collateral hemodynamics in patients with one- to two-vessel coronary artery disease. J Am Coll Cardiol 34:1985-1994, 1999.
77. Isner JM, Asahara T: Angiogenesis and vasculogenesis as therapeutic strategies for postnatal neovascularization. J Clin Invest 103:1231-1236, 1999.

Myocardial Ischemia

78. Kloner RA, Bolli R, Marban E, et al: Medical and cellular implications of stunning, hibernation, and preconditioning: An NHLBI workshop. Circulation 97:1848-1867, 1998.
79. Bolli R, Marban E: Molecular and cellular mechanisms of myocardial stunning. Physiol Rev 79:609-634, 1999.
80. Gerber BL, Wijns W, Vanoverschelde JL, et al: Myocardial perfusion and oxygen consumption in reperfused noninfarcted dysfunctional myocardium after unstable angina: Direct evidence for myocardial stunning in humans. J Am Coll Cardiol 34:1939-1946, 1999.
81. Perez NG, Marban E, Cingolani HE: Preservation of myofilament calcium responsiveness underlies protection against myocardial stunning by ischemic preconditioning. Cardiovasc Res 42:636-643, 1999.
82. Elsasser A, Schlepper M, Klovekorn WP, et al: Hibernating myocardium: An incomplete adaptation to ischemia. Circulation 96:2920-2931, 1997.
83. Bogaert J, Maes A, Van de Werf F, et al: Functional recovery of subepicardial myocardial tissue in transmural myocardial infarction after successful reperfusion: An important contribution to the improvement of regional and global left ventricular function. Circulation 99:36-43, 1999.
84. Jennings RB, Steenbergen C Jr, Reimer KA: Myocardial ischemia and reperfusion. Monogr Pathol 37:47-80, 1995.

CHAPTER 45

Approach to the Patient with Chest Pain

Thomas H. Lee • Christopher P. Cannon

Acute chest pain remains a difficult challenge for clinicians, and the percentage of patients who present to the emergency department with acute chest pain and are then admitted to the hospital may be increasing.[1-4] The reasons for caution include short-term mortality rates that are about twice as high for patients with acute myocardial infarction (MI) who are mistakenly discharged from the emergency department compared to what would be expected if they were admitted.[5,6] The legal costs that result from missed diagnoses of MI represent the largest category of losses from emergency medicine malpractice litigation.[7] For patients with low risks of complications, however, these concerns must be balanced against the costs and inconvenience that accompany admission to the hospital, and the risks of complications from tests and procedures with a low probability of improving patient outcomes.

Several advances in recent years have enhanced the accuracy and efficiency of the evaluation of patients with acute chest pain.[8] These advances include better serum markers for myocardial injury; decision aids to stratify patients according to their risks of complications; early and even immediate exercise testing and radionuclide scanning for lower risk patient subsets; and use of chest pain units and critical pathways for efficient and rapid evaluations of lower risk patients.

Causes of Acute Chest Pain

In a typical population of patients presenting for evaluation of acute chest pain in emergency departments, about 20 percent have acute MI or unstable angina.[5] A small percentage have other life-threatening problems, such as pulmonary embolism or acute aortic dissection, but most are discharged without a diagnosis or with a diagnosis of a noncardiac condition. These noncardiac conditions include musculoskeletal syndromes, disorders of abdominal viscera, and psychological conditions (Table 45–1).

MYOCARDIAL ISCHEMIA OR INFARCTION (see Chaps. 46 and 49). The most common serious cause of acute chest discomfort is myocardial ischemia or infarction, which occurs when the myocardial oxygen supply is inadequate compared to myocardial oxygen needs. Myocardial ischemia usually occurs in the setting of coronary atherosclerosis but also may reflect dynamic components of coronary vascular resistance. Coronary spasm can occur in normal coronary arteries, or, in patients with coronary disease, near atherosclerotic plaques and in smaller coronary arterioles (see Chap. 49). Other, less common causes of impaired coronary blood flow include syndromes that compromise the orifices of the coronary arteries or the arteries themselves, such as syphilitic aortitis, collagen-vascular diseases, aortic dissection, myocardial bridges, or congenital abnormalities of the coronary arteries.

Ischemic chest pain also can result from any disease process that causes occlusion of a coronary artery, such as thrombosis arising at the site of a ruptured atherosclerotic plaque. Other potential causes include coronary artery emboli such as may occur in patients with infectious or noninfectious endocarditis, or a clot in the left atrium or left ventricle.

Myocardial ischemia can be precipitated by conditions that cause a mismatch between the perfusion pressure within the coronary arteries and myocardial oxygen demand, such as aortic stenosis, aortic regurgitation, or hypertrophic cardiomyopathy. Increases in heart rate can markedly exacerbate ischemia in such patients because, even while oxygen demand is rising, myocardial perfusion falls due to a reduction in the proportion of time that the heart is in diastole, thereby decreasing the available time for coronary perfusion. Other clinical conditions can worsen oxygen delivery and/or raise oxygen need, although they generally cause myocardial ischemia and chest pain only when accompanied by coronary atherosclerosis. Such conditions include anemia, sepsis, and thyrotoxicosis.

The classic manifestation of ischemia is angina, which is usually described as a heavy chest pressure or squeezing, a "burning" feeling, or difficulty breathing. It is often associated with radiation to the left shoulder, neck, or arm. It typically builds in intensity over a period of a few minutes. The pain may begin with exercise or psychological stress, but acute coronary syndromes most commonly occur without obvious precipitating factors.

"Atypical" descriptions of chest pain reduce the likelihood that the symptoms represent myocardial ischemia or injury. The American College of Cardiology and the American Heart Association (ACC/AHA) guidelines list the following as pain descriptions that are *not* characteristic of myocardial ischemia[9]:

- Pleuritic pain (i.e., sharp or knife-like pain brought on by respiratory movements or cough)
- Primary or sole location of discomfort in the middle or lower abdominal region
- Pain that may be localized at the tip of one finger, particularly over the left ventricular (LV) apex
- Pain reproduced with movement or palpation of the chest wall or arms
- Constant pain that persists for many hours
- Very brief episodes of pain that last a few seconds or less
- Pain that radiates into the lower extremities

TABLE 45–1 Common Causes of Acute Chest Pain

System	Syndrome	Clinical description	Key Distinguishing Features
Cardiac	Angina	Retrosternal chest pressure, burning, or heaviness; radiating occasionally to neck, jaw, epigastrium, shoulders, or left arm	Precipitated by exercise, cold weather, or emotional stress; duration <2-10 minutes.
	Rest or unstable angina	Same as angina, but may be more severe	Usually <20 minutes; lower tolerance for exertion
	Acute myocardial infarction	Same as angina, but may be more severe	Sudden onset, usually lasting 30 minutes or longer. Often associated with shortness of breath, weakness, nausea, vomiting
	Pericarditis	Sharp, pleuritic pain aggravated by changes in position; highly variable duration	Pericardial friction rub
Vascular	Aortic dissection	Excruciating, ripping pain of sudden onset in anterior of chest, often radiating to back	Marked severity of unrelenting pain; usually occurs in setting of hypertension or underlying connective tissue disorder such as Marfan syndrome
	Pulmonary embolism	Sudden onset of dyspnea and pain, usually pleuritic with pulmonary infarction	Dyspnea, tachypnea, tachycardia, and signs of right heart failure
	Pulmonary hypertension	Substernal chest pressure, exacerbated by exertion	Pain associated with dyspnea and signs of pulmonary hypertension
Pulmonary	Pleuritis and/or pneumonia	Pleuritic pain, usually brief, over involved area	Pain pleuritic and lateral to midline, associated with dyspnea
	Tracheobronchitis	Burning discomfort in midline	Midline location, associated with coughing
	Spontaneous pneumothorax	Sudden onset of unilateral pleuritic pain, with dyspnea	Abrupt onset of dyspnea and pain
Gastrointestinal	Esophageal reflux	Burning substernal and epigastric discomfort, 10-60 minutes in duration	Aggravated by large meal and postprandial recumbency; relieved by antacid
	Peptic ulcer	Prolonged epigastric or substernal burning	Relieved by antacid or food
	Gallbladder disease	Prolonged epigastric, right upper quadrant pain	Unprovoked or following meal
	Pancreatitis	Prolonged, intense epigastric and substernal pain	Risk factors including alcohol, hypertriglyceridemia, and medications
Musculoskeletal	Costochondritis	Sudden onset of intense fleeting pain	May be reproduced by pressure over affected joint; occasional patients have swelling and inflammation over costochondral joint
	Cervical disc disease	Sudden onset of fleeting pain	May be reproduced with movement of neck
Infectious	Herpes zoster	Prolonged burning pain in dermatomal distribution	Vesicular rash, dermatomal distribution
Psychological	Panic disorder	Chest tightness or aching, often accompanied by dyspnea and lasting 30 minutes or more, unrelated to exertion or movement	Patient may have other evidence of emotional disorder

However, data from large populations of patients with acute chest pain indicate that acute coronary syndromes occur in patients with atypical symptoms with sufficient frequency that no single factor should be used to exclude the diagnosis of acute ischemia heart disease.[10]

PERICARDIAL DISEASE (see Chap. 64). The visceral surface of the pericardium is insensitive to pain, as is most of the parietal surface. Therefore, noninfectious causes of pericarditis (such as uremia) usually cause little or no pain. In contrast, infectious pericarditis nearly always involves surrounding pulmonary pleura, so that patients typically experience pleuritic pain with breathing, coughing, and changes in position. Swallowing may induce the pain because of the proximity of the esophagus to the posterior heart. Because the central diaphragm receives its sensory supply from the phrenic nerve, and the phrenic nerve arises from the third to fifth cervical segments of the spinal cord, pain from infectious pericarditis is frequently felt in the shoulders and neck. Involvement of the more lateral diaphragm can lead to symptoms in the upper abdomen and back, creating confusion with pancreatitis or cholecystitis. Pericarditis occasionally causes a steady, crushing substernal pain that is similar to that of acute myocardial infarction.[11]

VASCULAR DISEASE. Acute aortic dissection (see Chap. 53) usually is accompanied by sudden onset of excruciating, ripping pain, the location of which reflects the site and progression of the dissection.[12] Ascending aortic dissections tend to manifest with pain in the midline of the anterior chest, and posterior descending aortic dissections manifest with pain in the back of the chest. Aortic dissections usually occur in the presence of risk factors that include hypertension, pregnancy, atherosclerosis, and other conditions that lead to degeneration of the aortic media, such as Marfan and Ehlers-Danlos syndromes.

Pulmonary emboli (see Chap. 66) may be asymptomatic but often cause sudden onset of dyspnea and pleuritic chest pain.[13] Massive pulmonary emboli tend to cause severe and persistent substernal pain, which is believed to be due to distention of the pulmonary artery. Smaller emboli that lead to pulmonary infarction can cause lateral pleuritic chest pain. Hemodynamically significant pulmonary emboli may cause hypotension, syncope, and signs of right heart failure.

Pulmonary hypertension (see Chap. 67) can cause chest pain similar to angina pectoris, presumably because of right heart hypertrophy and ischemia.[14]

PULMONARY. Pulmonary conditions that cause chest pain usually produce dyspnea and pleuritic symptoms, the location of which reflect the site of pulmonary disease.[15] Tracheobronchitis tends to be associated with a burning midline pain,[16] whereas pneumonia can produce pain over the involved lung. The pain of a pneumothorax is sudden in onset and is usually accompanied by dyspnea.

GASTROINTESTINAL. Irritation of the esophagus by acid reflux can produce a burning discomfort that is exacerbated by alcohol, aspirin, and some foods. Symptoms often are worsened by a recumbent position and relieved by sitting upright and by acid-reducing therapies.[17] Esophageal spasm can produce a squeezing chest discomfort similar to that of angina.[18] Mallory-Weiss tears of the esophagus can occur in patients who have had prolonged vomiting episodes.

Chest pain due to ulcer disease usually occurs 60 to 90 minutes after meals and is typically relieved rapidly by acid-reducing therapies. This pain is usually epigastric in location but can radiate into the chest and shoulders.

Cholecystitis produces a wide range of pain syndromes and usually causes right upper quadrant abdominal pain. Chest and back pain due to cholecystitis is not unusual, however. The pain is often described as aching or colicky. Pancreatitis typically causes an intense aching epigastric pain that may radiate to the back. Relief through acid-reducing therapies is limited.

MUSCULOSKELETAL AND OTHER CAUSES. Chest pain can be caused by musculoskeletal disorders involving the chest wall, such as costochondritis, or by conditions affecting the nerves of the chest wall, such as cervical disc disease or herpes zoster. Musculoskeletal syndromes causing chest pain are often induced by direct pressure over the affected area or by movement of the patient's neck. The pain itself can be fleeting, or a dull ache that lasts for hours.

Panic syndrome is a major cause of chest discomfort among emergency department patients.[19] The symptoms typically include chest tightness, often accompanied by shortness of breath and a sense of anxiety, and generally lasting for 30 minutes or more.

CLINICAL EVALUATION. When evaluating patients with acute chest pain, the clinician must address a series of issues related to prognosis and immediate management. Even before trying to arrive at a definite diagnosis, high-priority questions include the following:

- *Clinical stability:* Is the patient in need of immediate treatment of circulatory collapse or respiratory insufficiency?
- *Immediate prognosis:* If the patient is currently clinically stable, what is the risk that the patient has a life-threatening condition, such as an acute coronary syndrome, pulmonary embolism, or aortic dissection?
- *Safety of triage options:* If the risks of life-threatening conditions are low, would it be safe to discharge the patient for outpatient management, or should the patient have further testing and/or observation to guide management?

Initial Assessment

The evaluation of the patient with acute chest pain actually begins before the physician sees the patient, and its effectiveness depends on the actions of office staff and other nonphysician personnel. Guidelines from the ACC/AHA[9] (see Guidelines section of Chap. 49) emphasize that patients with symptoms consistent with acute coronary syndromes should *not* be evaluated solely over the telephone but should be referred to facilities that allow evaluation by a physician and the recording of a 12-lead electrocardiogram.[19] These guidelines also recommend strong consideration of immediate referral to an emergency department or a specialized chest pain unit for patients with suspected acute coronary syndrome with chest discomfort at rest for more than 20 minutes, hemodynamic instability, or recent syncope or presyncope. Transport as a passenger in a private vehicle is considered an acceptable alternative to an emergency vehicle only if the wait would lead to a delay of greater than 20 to 30 minutes.

The National Heart Attack Alert Program guidelines recommend that patients with the following chief complaints should have immediate assessment by triage nurses and should be referred for further evaluation[20]:

- Chest pain, pressure, tightness, or heaviness; pain that radiates to neck, jaw, shoulders, back, or one or both arms
- Indigestion or "heartburn"; nausea and/or vomiting associated with chest discomfort
- Persistent shortness of breath
- Weakness, dizziness, lightheadedness, loss of consciousness

EXAMINATION. If the patient is not in immediate need of interventions because of circulatory collapse or respiratory insufficiency, the physician's assessment should begin with a clinical history that captures the characteristics of pain, the time of onset, and the duration of symptoms and an examination that emphasizes vital signs and cardiovascular status. This evaluation should be focused on screening for the most common life-threatening conditions: acute myocardial infarction, pulmonary embolism, and acute aortic dissection (see Table 45–1). Although information on coronary risk factors can help clinicians in the assessment of whether a patient has coronary artery disease, available data indicate that such information has limited ability to improve risk stratification of patients with acute chest pain, presumably because the probability of acute complications is dominated by other factors, such as the presence or absence of evidence of ischemia on the electrocardiogram.[3] Younger patients have a lower risk of acute coronary syndrome[21] but should be screened with greater care for histories of recent cocaine use (see Chap. 62).[22]

ELECTROCARDIOGRAM. The most important single source of data, the electrocardiogram, should be obtained within 10 minutes after presentation in patients with ongoing chest discomfort and as rapidly as possible in patients who have a history of chest discomfort consistent with acute coronary syndrome but whose discomfort has resolved by the time of evaluation,[19] to permit identification of patients who might benefit from primary angioplasty or thrombolytic therapy. When the electrocardiogram shows ST-segment changes or T-wave abnormalities that are consistent with the presence of ischemia and are not known to be old, discharging the patient home without further evaluation is hazardous both clinically and legally. The prevalence of acute MI is 80 percent among patients with 1 mm or more of new ST-segment elevation and 20 percent among patients with ST-segment depression or T-wave inversion not known to be old. However, if the electrocardiogram does not show changes consistent with ischemia, the risk of acute MI is about 4 percent among patients with a history of coronary artery disease and 2 percent among patients with no such history.[8] Failure to perform an electrocardiogram is one of the most important factors in malpractice losses related to patients with acute chest pain, followed by failure to interpret the electrocardiogram correctly.

For patients with a moderate or high probability of acute coronary syndromes, physicians usually perform assays of markers of myocardial injury such as the cardiac troponins T or I (cTnT or cTnI) or creatine kinase MB isoenzyme (CK-MB). Many hospital laboratories perform these tests on a "stat" basis, and point of care ("bedside") assays for these markers are now widely available; thus, results are often available to inform initial management decisions (see Chap. 46).

Studies of the diagnostic performance of cTnI or cTnT or CK-MB indicate that when any of these test findings are abnormal, the patient has a high likelihood of having an acute coronary syndrome (Fig. 45–1; Tables 45–2 and 45–3). The more challenging issues in the interpretation of these test findings during the initial evaluation of acute chest pain are (1) the frequency and causes of false-positive results; (2) the prognostic implications of abnormal test results; and (3) the interpretation of single values of these tests, such as are available during the initial evaluation of acute chest pain.

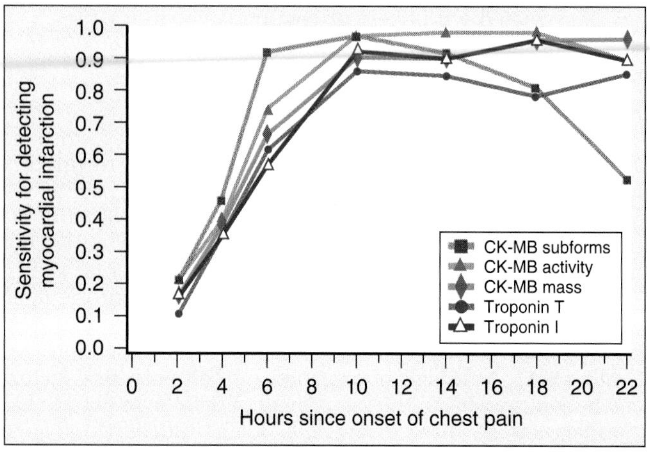

FIGURE 45–1 Diagnostic sensitivity of macromolecular markers of myocardial infarction according to the length of time from the onset of chest pain. CK-MB = creatine kinase MB isoenzyme. (Data from Zimmerman J, Fromm R, Meyer D, et al: Diagnostic marker cooperative study for the diagnosis of myocardial infarction. Circulation 99:1671, 1999.)

DIAGNOSTIC PERFORMANCE. Studies of the major assays used to evaluate patients with acute chest pain (CK-MB, cTnI, and cTnT) indicate that with serial sampling, these agents all have excellent sensitivity for detection of acute MI.[23-29] Cardiac troponin abnormalities persist for several days after myocardial injury; hence, after 24 hours from symptom onset, these assays are significantly more sensitive than CK-MB. The oldest of these three assays, CK-MB, provides the benchmark against which the other two are evaluated. Meta-analysis of published data indicate that CK-MB mass has a clinical sensitivity for acute myocardial infarction of 97 percent and specificity of 90 percent.[30]

Creatine Kinase MB Isoenzyme. The dissemination of the radioimmunoassay for CK-MB (versus the older activity assay and electrophoretic assays) have greatly reduced false-positive rates; measured CK-MB with the mass assay can be reliably assumed to represent true CK-MB. However, noncardiac muscle frequently has trace amounts of true CK-MB, and these amounts are increased in patients with conditions that cause chronic muscle destruction and regeneration, such as muscular dystrophy or high performance athletics (e.g., marathon running).[31] CK-MB elevations are particularly common in emergency department patients, who have higher rates of histories of alcohol abuse or trauma.

In addition to the problem of "false-positive" CK-MB results due to CK-MB from noncardiac sources, clinicians also struggle with uncertainty as to whether the amount of CK-MB measured represents a pathological elevation. Although there is no physiological basis for such an index, many clinicians calculate a "CK-MB mass index" dividing the CK-MB mass level by the total CK activity level. Ratios greater than 2.5 percent are considered suggestive of myocardial damage.[32] This ratio may be inaccurate when (1) high levels of total CK are present because of skeletal muscle injury, (2) chronic skeletal muscle injuries release greater amounts of CK-MB, and (3) total CK measurements are within normal reference range for the laboratory and while the CK-MB level is elevated.[33]

For several years, there has been investigative interest in CK-MB isoforms as a possible refinement to measurement of CK-MB. CK-MB exists in only one form in myocardial tissue (CK-MB2) but is modified in plasma so that another isoform (CK-MB1) also exists. An absolute level of CK-MB2 greater

TABLE 45–2 Likelihood that Signs and Symptoms Represent an Acute Coronary Syndrome

Feature	High Likelihood (any of the following)	Intermediate Likelihood (absence of high-likelihood features and presence of any of the following)	Low Likelihood (absence of high- or intermediate-likelihood features but may have any of the following)
History	• Chest or left arm pain or discomfort as chief symptom reproducing prior documented angina • Known history of coronary artery disease, including myocardial infarction	• Chest or left arm pain or discomfort as chief symptom • Age >70 years • Male sex • Diabetes mellitus	• Probable ischemic symptoms in absence of any of the intermediate likelihood characteristics • Recent cocaine use
Examination	• Transient mitral regurgitation, hypotension, diaphoresis, pulmonary edema, or rales	• Extracardiac vascular disease	• Chest discomfort reproduced by palpation
Electrocardiogram	• New, or presumably new, transient ST-segment deviation (≥0.05 mV) or T-wave inversion (≥0.2 mV) with symptoms	• Fixed Q waves • Abnormal ST segments or T waves not documented to be new	• T-wave flattening or inversion in leads with dominant R waves • Normal ECG
Cardiac markers	Elevated cardiac TnI, TnT, or CK-MB	Normal	Normal

From Fleet RP, Dupuis G, Marchand A, et al: ACC/AHA 2002 guideline update for the management of patients with unstable angina and non–ST-segment elevation myocardial infarction: Summary article. A report of the American College of Cardiology/American Heart Association Task Force on Practice Guidelines (Committee on the Management of Patients With Unstable Angina). Circulation 106:1893, 2002.

TABLE 45–3 Short-Term Risk of Death or Nonfatal Myocardial Ischemia in Patients with Unstable Angina			
Feature	**High Likelihood (any of the following)**	**Intermediate Likelihood (absence of high-likelihood features and presence of any of the following)**	**Low Likelihood (absence of high- or intermediate-likelihood features but may have any of the following)**
History	Accelerating tempo of ischemic symptoms in preceding 48 hours	Prior MI, peripheral or cerebrovascular disease, or CABG; prior aspirin use	
Character of pain	Prolonged ongoing (>20 minutes) rest pain	• Prolonged (>20 min) rest angina, now resolved, with moderate or high likelihood of coronary artery disease • Rest angina (<20 min) or relieved with rest or sublingual NTG	New-onset or progressive Canadian Cardiovascular System Class III or IV angina the past 2 weeks without prolonged (>20 min) rest pain but with moderate or high likelihood of coronary artery disease
Clinical findings	• Pulmonary edema, most likely due to ischemia • New or worsening mitral regurgitation murmur • S_3 or new/worsening rales • Hypotension, bradycardia, tachycardia • Age >75 years	Age >70 years	
Electrocardiogram	• Angina at rest with transient ST-segment changes >0.05 mV • Bundle-branch block, new or presumed new • Sustained ventricular tachycardia	• T-wave inversions >0.2 mV • Pathological Q waves	• Normal or unchanged ECG during an episode of chest discomfort
Cardiac markers	Elevated (e.g., TnT or TnI >0.1 ng/ml)	Slightly elevated (e.g., TnT >0.01 but <0.1 ng/ml)	Normal

CABG = coronary artery bypass grafting; ECG = electrocardiogram; MI = myocardial infarction; NTG = nitroglycerin.
From Fleet RP, Dupuis G, Marchand A, et al: ACC/AHA 2002 guideline update for the management of patients with unstable angina and non–ST-segment elevation myocardial infarction: Summary article. A report of the American College of Cardiology/American Heart Association Task Force on Practice Guidelines (Committee on the Management of Patients With Unstable Angina). Circulation 106:1893, 2002.

than 1 U/liter and a ratio of CK-MB2 to CK-MB1 greater than 1.5 indicates fresh release of CK-MB and, when measured within the first 6 hours of symptoms, has better sensitivity for MI than conventional CK-MB assays.[34] The CK-MB isoform assay is not widely available, however, and, as is true of the conventional CK-MB assay, suffers from lack of specificity of CK-MB to myocardial tissues.

Troponins. The troponins T and I are encoded by different genes in cardiac muscle, slow skeletal muscle, and fast skeletal muscle; hence, the assays that were developed for the cardiac troponins are more specific than CK-MB for myocardial injury. Assessment of the diagnostic performance of the cardiac troponin assays is complicated by the known limitations of the CK-MB assay, which, by necessity, is used to determine whether newer assays have provided a misleading result. Using combinations of clinical criteria including CK-MB data, cardiac troponins have had good but not perfect sensitivity (84 to 89 percent) for detecting acute MIs.[25,27] cTnI and cTnT have been described as having a lower specificity for MI than the traditional CK-MB assays, but these findings may be due to greater sensitivity for smaller degrees of myocardial damage than can be detected with CK-MB assays.

Because the cardiac troponins are highly specific to myocardial tissues, "false-positive" elevations usually represent myocardial damage from causes other than coronary artery disease. Such damage may occur with myopericarditis, trauma, congestive heart failure, pulmonary embolus, and sepsis. Elevated levels of cardiac troponins have been reported in patients with renal disease and connective tissue diseases.[35,36] In patients with acute coronary syndromes, even minor elevations of cTnI and cTnT have been shown to identify patients with an increased risk of complications who benefit from aggressive management strategies.[37]

Rapid bedside assays for cTnT and cTnI using whole blood samples yield results that are in close agreement with serum cTnT concentrations measured by the standard enzyme immunoassay.[28,38,39] For example, in one multicenter study, 95 percent of all samples with cTnT concentration below 0.3 ng/ml were negative on the bedside assay, and 99 percent of samples above 0.3 ng/ml were positive.[38] In this study, the "gray zone" in which the bedside assay was not perfect extended from 0.1 to 0.5 ng/ml. A bedside assay for cTnI has also been reported to have diagnostic efficacy comparable to the standard enzyme-linked immunosorbent assay (ELISA).[39] One of the few studies that assessed both rapid cardiac troponin assays found that 94 percent of patients with MI had a positive cTnT result at least within 6 hours from the onset of chest pain and all had a positive cTnI result; the specificities were 89 percent and 83 percent, respectively.[25] Hence, diagnostic performance with the two cardiac troponins appears essentially the same.

Myoglobin. Serum myoglobin has long interested clinicians as a potential aid to early detection of MI, because this smaller molecule diffuses through interstitial fluids more rapidly after cell death than the larger CK and troponin molecules. It therefore becomes abnormal as early as 30 minutes after myocardial injury. However, myoglobin is not specific to myocardial tissue, so false-positive rates in emergency department populations are high.

Prognostic Implications of Test Results. Abnormal levels of CK-MB, cTnI, and cTnT are predictors of increased risk of complications (see Tables 45–2 and 45–3).[25,40-44] Even if patients do not have CK-MB elevations, cTnI and cTnT are useful for early risk stratification in patients with acute chest pain, particularly those without ST-segment elevation.[40] For example, in the GUSTO-IIa troponin T substudy, which enrolled patients with acute ischemic syndromes, patients with elevated cTnT at baseline had a 30-day mortality rate of 10 percent, compared with 5 percent in patients with late positive cTnT levels (8-16 hours) and 0 percent in those with persistently normal cTnT results.[44] The prognostic value of cTnI seems to be comparable to that of cTnT in patients with unstable angina.[45]

Test Performance of Single Assays. Although high sensitivities and specificities for diagnosis of myocardial injury can be achieved for several assays through serial sampling, the diagnostic performance of a single value of any of these tests is not nearly as good. A single CK-MB value in emergency department patients with acute chest pain has a sensitivity for detecting acute MI of 34 percent and a specificity of 88 percent[46]; a single value of cTnI has a sensitivity of about 40 percent.[27]

The diagnostic performance of single values of these tests is influenced considerably by the time elapsed since the onset of symptoms. For example, a single CK-MB mass or troponin drawn within 4 hours of the onset of symptoms has a sensitivity of less than 25 percent.[27,46,47] However, single values of CK-MB mass and troponins that are drawn more than 12 hours after the onset of symptoms have sensitivities for myocardial infarction in the range of 70 to 90 percent.

INTERPRETATION OF TESTS: RELATIONSHIP BETWEEN PRETEST PROBABILITY AND POSTTEST PROBABILITY. As is true of most tests in medicine, results should be interpreted in the context of the patient's overall probability of having the diagnosis of interest. Thus, a normal result on a test or series of tests in a patient with a high clinical probability of acute coronary syndrome does not exclude this diagnosis, although it raises the question of whether any myocardial injury may have occurred several days previously. Similarly, an abnormal test result in a patient with a low probability of coronary disease does not necessarily mean that the patient has had myocardial injury, although it may suggest that a reassessment of the patient's clinical data is in order.

To formalize such analyses, cardiac markers can be interpreted in a bayesian framework in which pretest probabilities are modified by test results (Fig. 45–2). These calculations of posttest probabilities assume that the sensitivity and specificity of serial sampling of CK-MB mass values, for example, in patients presenting within 24 hours of the onset of symptoms are about 95 percent (see Fig. 45–2A). In contrast, the impact of single CK-MB mass results on patients' probabilities of coronary disease is quite modest (see Fig. 45–2B). These analyses assume a sensitivity of 56 percent and a specificity of 98 percent for single CK-MB mass values greater than 5 ng/ml at admission.[27]

TESTING STRATEGY. Guidelines from the ACC/AHA recommend measurement of biomarkers of cardiac injury in patients with symptoms that are consistent with acute coronary syndromes (Table 45–4).[19] Implicit is this recommendation is recognition that patients with very low probability of acute coronary syndrome should not undergo measurement of biomarkers, because of the possibility that false-positive results will lead to unnecessary hospitalizations, tests, procedures, and their complications. Because single values of these assays have limited sensitivity for detecting myocardial injury, a single negative biomarker does not really "rule out" myocardial injury for these low-risk patients.

The ACC/AHA guidelines recommend that cTnI or cTnT are the preferred first-line markers but note that CK-MB (by mass assay) is an acceptable alternative. The preference for cardiac troponins reflects the greater specificity of these markers compared with CK-MB and the prognostic value of troponin elevations in the presence of normal CK-MB levels. If the initial set of markers is negative in patients who have presented within the first 6 hours of the onset of pain, the guidelines recommend that another sample should be drawn in the 6- to 12-hour time frame.

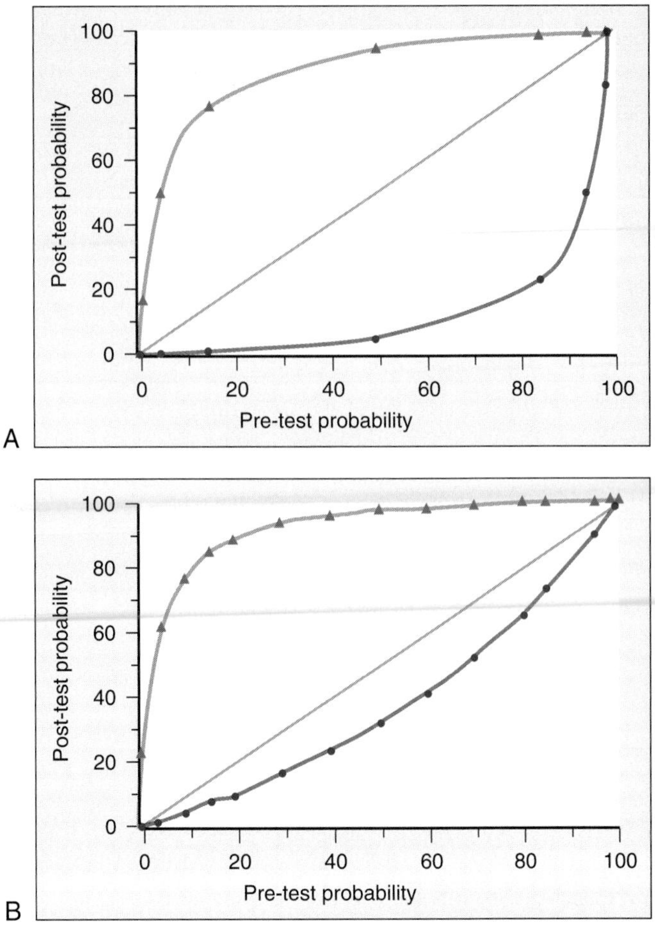

FIGURE 45–2 Effect of serial CK-MB results **(A)** and single CK-MB values **(B)** on the probability of acute myocardial infarction. The pretest probabilities, as marked along the *x* axis, can be derived through use of computerized algorithms, personal experience, or analysis of published data. Posttest probabilities are plotted on the *y* axis. The curves correspond to posttest probabilities of infarction with normal (magenta) or elevated (blue) creatine kinase MB isoenzyme (CK-MB) results, assuming a 95 percent sensitivity and 95 percent specificity for serial sampling of CK-MB levels.

Initial Risk Stratification

For patients with chest pain, the initial risk stratification focuses on the safety of various triage and testing options. These options include the following:

- Immediate treatment of acute coronary syndrome with invasive therapy or thrombolytic agents
- Admission to a coronary care or other intensive care unit
- Admission to an intermediate care facility with central electrocardiographic monitoring, such as chest pain units
- Further data collection, such as via immediate exercise testing or radionuclide imaging
- Discharge to home

The decision among these options is made on the basis of information from the history, physical examination, electrocardiogram, and, for patients with suspected acute coronary syndrome, one or more sets of biomarkers for myocardial injury. Key factors suggesting a high risk of acute coronary syndrome and its complications include prolonged or accelerating ischemic symptoms; evidence of congestive heart

TABLE 45–4 ACC/AHA Recommendations for Early Risk Stratification

	Indication	Level of Evidence
Class I (indicated)	1. A determination should be made in all patients with chest discomfort of the likelihood of acute ischemia caused by CAD as high, intermediate, or low.	C
	2. Patients who present with chest discomfort should undergo early risk stratification that focuses on anginal symptoms, physical findings, ECG findings, and biomarkers of cardiac injury.	B
	3. A 12-lead ECG should be obtained immediately (within 10 min) in patients with ongoing chest discomfort and as rapidly as possible in patients who have a history of chest discomfort consistent with ACS but whose discomfort has resolved by the time of evaluation.	C
	4. Biomarkers of cardiac injury should be measured in all patients who present with chest discomfort consistent with ACS. A cardiac-specific troponin is the preferred marker, and if available, it should be measured in all patients. CK-MB by mass assay is also acceptable. In patients with negative cardiac markers within 6 hr of the onset of pain, another sample should be drawn in the 6- to 12-hr time frame (e.g., at 9 hr after the onset of symptoms).	C
Class IIa (good supportive evidence)	For patients who present within 6 hr of the onset of symptoms, an early marker of cardiac injury (e.g., myoglobin or CK-MB subforms) should be considered in addition to a cardiac troponin.	C
Class IIb (weak supportive evidence)	C-reactive protein and other markers of inflammation should be measured.	B
Class III (not indicated)	Total CK (without MB), aspartate aminotransferase (AST, SGOT), beta-hydroxybutyric dehydrogenase, and/or lactate dehydrogenase should be the markers for the detection of myocardial injury in patients with chest discomfort suggestive of ACS.	C

ACS = acute coronary syndrome; CAD = coronary artery disease; CK-MB = creatine kinase MB isoenzyme; ECG = electrocardiogram.
From Braunwald E, Antman EM, Beasley JW, et al: ACC/AHA 2002 guideline update for the management of patients with unstable angina and non–ST-segment elevation myocardial infarction: Summary article. A report of the American College of Cardiology/American Heart Association Task Force on Practice Guidelines (Committee on the Management of Patients With Unstable Angina). Circulation 106:1893, 2002.

failure on physical examination; electrocardiographic abnormalities consistent with ischemia that are not known to be old, and elevated markers for myocardial injury (see Tables 45–2 and 45–3). The association of these findings with risks of complications is discussed in Chapters 46 and 49. This discussion focuses on the ability of various data to improve initial patient management.

Clinical History

Other factors from the history contribute to risk stratification in addition to the assessment of whether the patient's symptoms are consistent with myocardial ischemia, and whether the duration and pattern of symptoms suggest an elevated risk for complications (see Tables 45–2 and 45–3). A prior history of myocardial infarction is associated not only with a high risk of obstructive coronary disease but also with an increased risk of multivessel disease.[48] Women with suspected acute coronary syndrome are less likely to have coronary disease than are men with similar clinical presentations, and, when coronary disease is present, it tends to be less severe.[49,50] Older patients, particularly beyond 70 years of age, have a higher risk for coronary disease and higher risk for adverse outcomes.[51]

Information on traditional risk factors, especially diabetes, can help identify high-risk patients among those with acute coronary syndrome. However, risk factor data are of relatively little value in the diagnosis of patients with acute ischemia after consideration of other data from the history, electrocardiogram, and cardiac markers.[51] Thus, ACC/AHA guidelines recommend that these data should *not* be used to determine whether a patient should be admitted.[19] Similarly, the guidelines note that a family history of premature coronary disease is *not* a useful indicator of diagnosis or prognosis for patients with acute chest pain.

The Physical Examination

The initial examination of patients with acute chest pain is directed toward identifying potential precipitating causes of myocardial ischemia[52] (e.g., uncontrolled hypertension); important comorbid conditions (e.g., chronic obstructive pulmonary disease); and evidence of hemodynamic complications (e.g., congestive heart failure, new mitral regurgitation, or hypotension). The ACC/AHA guidelines recommend that every patient with suspected acute coronary syndrome have blood pressure measured in both arms, as well as documentation of heart rate and temperature and a thorough cardiovascular and chest examination. The examination of the peripheral vessels should include assessment of the presence of bruits or pulse deficits that might suggest extracardiac vascular disease.

For patients whose clinical presentations are not suggestive of myocardial ischemia, the search for noncoronary causes of chest pain should focus first on potentially life-threatening issues (aortic dissection, pulmonary embolism), and then turn to the possibility of other cardiac (e.g., pericarditis) and noncardiac (e.g., esophageal discomfort) diagnoses. Aortic dissection is suggested by pulse deficits or a new murmur of aortic regurgitation in the presence of back or midline anterior chest pain. Differences in breath sounds in the presence of acute dyspnea and pleuritic chest pain raises the possibility of pneumothorax. Tachycardia and tachypnea may be the major manifestations of pulmonary embolism on physical examination.

The Electrocardiogram

The electrocardiogram provides critical information for both diagnosis and prognosis (see Tables 45–2 and 45–3), particularly when a tracing is obtained during episodes of pain. New persistent or transient ST-segment changes (≥0.05 mV) that develop during a symptomatic episode at rest and resolve when the symptoms resolve strongly suggest acute ischemia and severe coronary disease. Nonspecific ST-segment and T-wave changes are usually defined as lesser amounts of ST-segment deviation or T-wave inversion of less than or equal to 0.2 mV and are less helpful in risk stratification. A completely normal electrocardiogram (ECG) does not exclude the possibility of acute coronary syndrome; about 1 to 6 percent of such patients with acute chest pain are subsequently found to have acute MI, although the prognosis of patients with a normal or near-normal ECG is better than that of patients with clearly abnormal ECGs at presentation.[53,54]

The availability of a prior ECG improves diagnostic accuracy and is associated with a reduced rate of admission for patients with abnormal baseline tracings.[55] Serial ECG tracings improve the clinician's ability to diagnose acute MI,[56] particularly if combined with serial measurement of cardiac markers.[57] Continuous ECG monitoring to detect ST-segment shifts is technically feasible, but the contribution to patient management is uncertain.[19,58]

Decision Aids

Multivariate algorithms have been developed and prospectively validated with the goal of improving the stratification of risk in patients with acute chest pain. These algorithms can be used to estimate the probability for individual patients of acute myocardial infarction,[2] acute ischemic heart disease,[1,4] or the risk of major cardiac complications.[3] These algorithms have been used mainly to identify patients who are at low risk for complications and who therefore do not require admission to the hospital or coronary care unit.

A prospectively validated algorithm for prediction of risk of complications requiring intensive care unit care[3] is presented as a flow chart in Figure 45–3. In this algorithm, patients with suspected myocardial infarction on ECG are immediately classified as having a high risk (>16 percent) of major complications within the next 72 hours. Patients whose ECGs are consistent with ischemia but not infarction are then classified as intermediate (approximately 8 percent) or high risk for complications depending on the presence or absence of clinical risk factors, including systolic blood pressure below 100 mm Hg; bilateral rales heard above the bases; and known unstable ischemic heart disease (defined as worsening of previously stable angina, a new onset of angina after infarction or after a coronary revascularization procedure, or pain that was the same as that associated with a prior MI). These same risk factors are used to stratify patients without ischemic changes on their ECGs.

Validated algorithms for prediction of acute ischemic heart disease and the risks and benefits of thrombolytic therapy have been incorporated into computerized reports of electrocardiograms to help clinicians make decisions about admission[4] and to help them assess the risks and benefits of using thrombolytic therapy in individual cases.[59] In a multicenter randomized trial, an intervention in which information about the expected impact of the use of thrombolytic therapy on the electrocardiogram led to an increase in the use of thrombolytic therapy for women (from 18 to 22 percent) and was associated with an improvement in timeliness of treatment.

Prospective trials indicate that these algorithms have little effect in the routine clinical practice of clinicians who have not received training in their use.[4,60,61] Among the reasons that practicing physicians do not use algorithms are that they are too busy, are unsure of their value, or are concerned about the legal and clinical consequences of inappropriately discharging patients who are subsequently found to have had MI.[61,62]

Immediate Management

The ACC/AHA guidelines suggest an approach to the immediate management of patients with possible acute coronary syndrome (ACS) that integrates information from the history, physical examination, 12-lead ECG, and initial cardiac marker tests to assign patients to four categories: noncardiac diagnosis, chronic stable angina, possible ACS, and definite ACS (Fig. 45–4). In this algorithm, patients with ST elevation are triaged immediately for reperfusion therapy, according to ACC/AHA guidelines for acute MI. For patients with acute coronary syndrome who have ST or T wave changes, ongoing pain, positive cardiac markers, or hemodynamic abnormalities, admission to hospital for management of acute ischemia is recommended. Cost-effectiveness analyses support triage of such patients to the coronary care unit for their initial care.[63] For patients with possible or definite acute coronary syndrome who do not have diagnostic electrocardiograms and whose initial serum cardiac markers are within normal limits, observation in a chest pain unit or other nonintensive care facility is appropriate.[19]

Chest Pain Protocols and Units

Until the 1980s, most patients with suspected acute coronary syndrome were triaged to coronary care units, where they underwent 2 to 3 days of "rule out MI" evaluations.[64] In the last two decades, however, economic pressures and advances in risk stratification have led many institutions to develop "critical pathways" to standardize management of lower risk patients with acute chest pain.[65] These critical pathways make explicit the timing and sequence of key tests and triage decisions.

The main elements of a typical chest pain critical pathway are included in the bottom part of Figure 45–4. According to the ACC/AHA recommendations,[19] patients with a low risk of acute coronary syndrome or associated complications can be observed for 4 to 8 hours while undergoing electrocardiographic monitoring and serial measurement of cardiac markers. Patients who develop evidence of ischemia or other indicators of increased risk should be admitted to the coronary care unit for further manage-

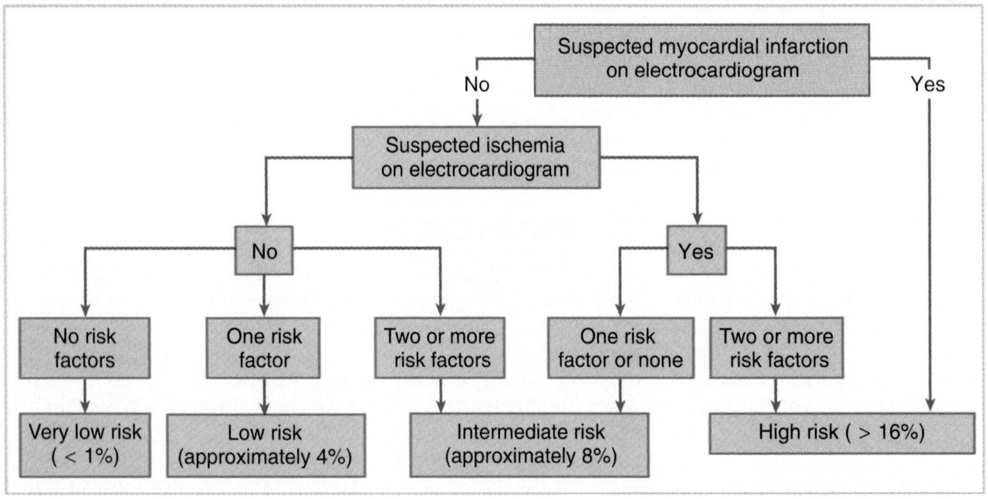

FIGURE 45–3 Derivation and validation of four groups into which patients can be categorized according to risk of major cardiac events within 72 hours after admission. (From Goldman L, Cook EF, Johnson PA, et al: Prediction of the need for intensive care in patients who come to emergency departments with acute chest pain. N Engl J Med 334:1498, 1966.)

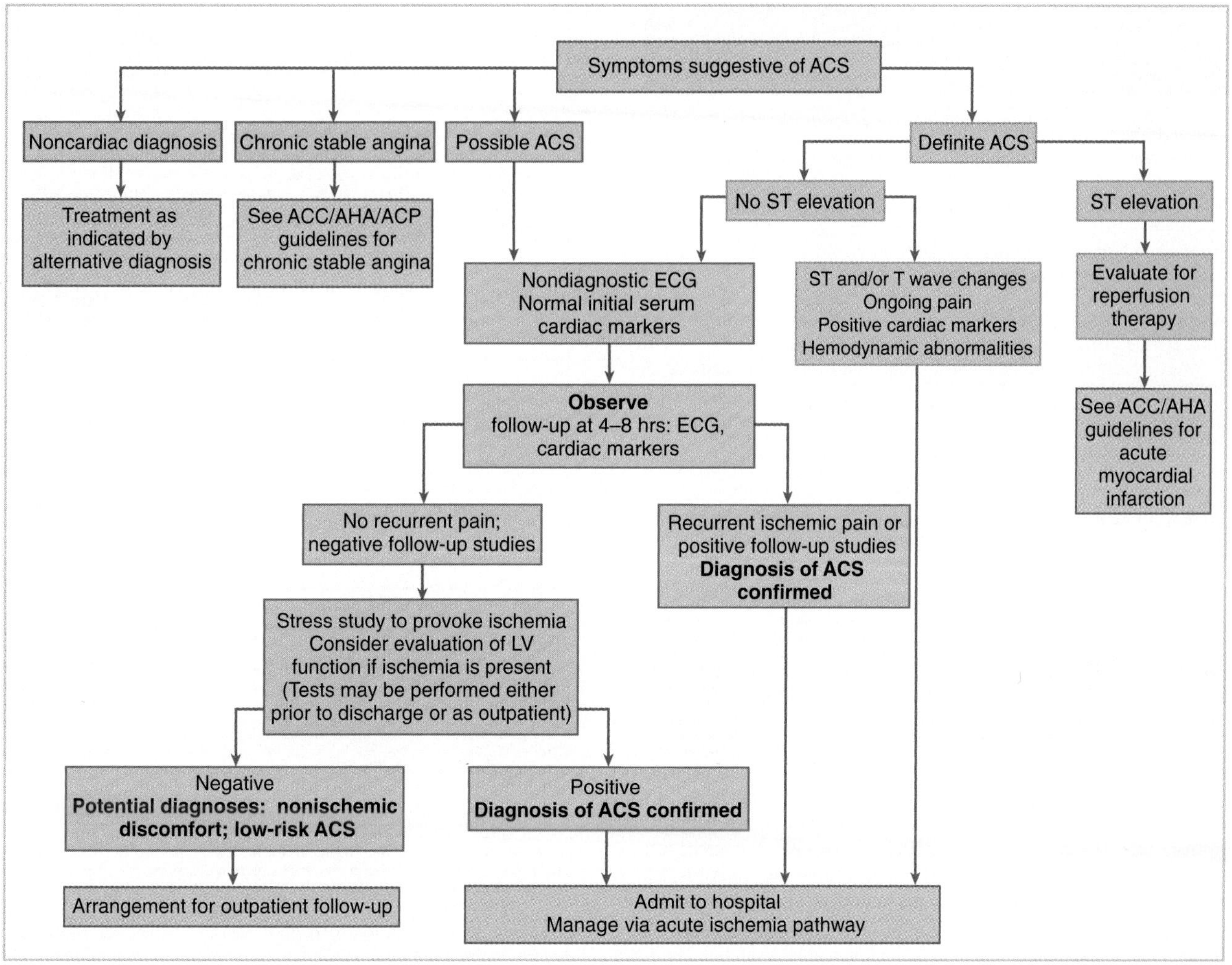

FIGURE 45–4 Algorithm for evaluation and management of patients suspected of having acute coronary syndrome (ACS). (From Braunwald E, Antman EM, Beasley JW, et al: ACC/AHA guideline update for the management of patients with unstable angina and non-ST-segment elevation myocardial infarction—Summary article 2002: A report of the American College of Cardiology/American Heart Association Task Force on Practice Guidelines [Committee on the Management of Patients With Unstable Angina]. Circulation 106:1893, 2002.)

ment. Patients who do not develop recurrent pain or other predictors of increased risk can be triaged for early noninvasive testing (see below) either before or after discharge.

To enhance the efficiency and reliability of implementation of such chest pain protocols, many hospitals triage low-risk patients with chest pain to special chest pain units.[66-69] These units are often adjacent to or in emergency departments but are sometimes located elsewhere in the hospital. In most such units, the rate of MI has been about 1 to 2 percent. These units have proved safe and cost-saving sites of care for low-risk patients[68,69] because fewer personnel are involved than in coronary-care units and there is an explicit emphasis on a protocol-driven approach.

Chest pain units are also sometimes used for intermediate-risk patients, such as patients with a prior history of coronary disease but no other high-risk predictors. In one community-based randomized trial, patients with unstable angina and an overall intermediate risk of complications had similar outcomes and lower costs if they were triaged to a chest pain unit versus conventional hospital management.

Early Noninvasive Testing

TREADMILL ELECTROCARDIOGRAPHY. A major goal of the initial short period of observation of low-risk patients in chest pain units is to determine whether performance of exercise testing or other noninvasive tests is safe. Treadmill exercise electrocardiography is an inexpensive test that is available at many hospitals 7 days per week and beyond traditional laboratory hours, and prospective data indicate that early exercise test results provide reliable prognostic information for low-risk patient populations. Most studies have used the Bruce or modified Bruce treadmill protocol. One study found that, among low-risk patients who had exercise testing within 48 hours of presentation for acute chest pain, the 6-month event rate among 195 patients with a negative test was 2 percent, in contrast to a rate of 15 percent among patients with a positive or equivocal test result.[70]

Studies have shown that patients who have a low clinical risk of complications can safely undergo exercise testing within 6 to 12 hours after presentation at the hospital[66-68] or even immediately.[71] In general, protocols for early or immediate exercise testing exclude patients with electrocardiographic changes consistent with ischemia not known to be old, ongoing chest pain, or evidence of congestive heart failure. Analyses of pooled data suggest that the prevalence of coronary disease in populations undergoing early exercise testing averages about 5 percent, and that the rate of adverse events is negligible.[66] Indications and contraindications for exercise ECG testing in the emergency department from an Advisory Statement from the American Heart Association are summarized in Table 45–5.[66]

TABLE 45–5 Indications and Contraindications for Exercise Electrocardiographic Testing in the Emergency Department

Requirements before exercise ECG testing that should be considered in the emergency department setting
- Two sets of cardiac enzymes at 4-hr intervals should be normal.
- ECG at the time of presentation, and preexercise 12-lead ECG shows no significant change.
- Absence of rest ECG abnormalities that would preclude accurate assessment of the exercise ECG.
- From admission to the time results are available from the second set of cardiac enzymes: patient asymptomatic, lessening chest pain symptoms, or persistent atypical symptoms.
- Absence of ischemic chest pain at the time of exercise testing.

Contraindications to exercise ECG testing in the emergency department setting
- New or evolving ECG abnormalities on the rest tracing.
- Abnormal cardiac enzymes.
- Inability to perform exercise.
- Worsening or persistent ischemic chest pain symptoms from admission to the time of exercise testing.
- Clinical risk profiling indicating imminent coronary angiography is likely.

IMAGING TESTS. Stress echocardiography or radionuclide scans are the preferred noninvasive testing modalities for patients who cannot undergo treadmill ECG testing due to physical disability or ECGs that do lend themselves to interpretation. Imaging technologies are less readily available and more expensive than exercise electrocardiography but have increased sensitivity for detection of coronary disease and the ability to quantify the extent of jeopardized myocardium. High-risk rest perfusion scans are associated with an increased risk of major cardiac complications, whereas patients with low-risk scans have low 30 day cardiac event rates (<2 percent).[72,73]

In addition to stress imaging studies to detect provokable ischemia, rest radionuclide scans also can help determine whether a patient's symptoms represent myocardial ischemia.[74] In a multicenter prospective randomized trial of 2475 adult emergency department patients with chest pain or other symptoms suggestive of acute cardiac ischemia and with normal or nondiagnostic initial ECG results, patients were randomly assigned to receive either the usual evaluation strategy or the usual strategy supplemented with results from acute resting myocardial perfusion imaging.[74] The availability of scan results did not influence management of patients with acute MI or unstable angina, but rates of hospitalization for patients without acute cardiac ischemia were reduced among patients who underwent scanning (52 to 42 percent).

Echocardiography can also be used with and without physical stress to detect wall-motion abnormalities consistent with myocardial ischemia.[75,76] The presence of induced or baseline regional wall motion abnormalities is associated with worse prognosis. Cost-effectiveness analyses indicated that radionuclide imaging, stress echocardiography, and prompt coronary angiography may all be appropriate for diagnosing coronary artery disease in some subgroups of patients,[77,78] but guidelines recommend exercise electrocardiography as the preferred first-line test.[15,66]

REFERENCES

Causes of Chest Pain

1. Pozen MW, D'Agostino RB, Selker HP, et al: A predictive instrument to improve coronary-care unit admission practices in acute ischemic heart disease: A prospective multicenter clinical trial. N Engl J Med 310:1273, 1984.
2. Goldman L, Cook EF, Brand DA, et al: A computer protocol to predict myocardial infarction in emergency department patients with chest pain. N Engl J Med 318:797, 1988.
3. Goldman L, Cook EF, Johnson PA, et al: Prediction of the need for intensive care in patients who come to emergency departments with acute chest pain. N Engl J Med 334:1498, 1996.
4. Selker HP, Beshansky JR, Griffith JL, et al: Use of the acute cardiac ischemic time-insensitive predictive instrument (ACI-TIPI) to assist with triage of patients with chest pain or other symptoms suggestive of acute cardiac ischemia: A multicenter, controlled clinical trial. Ann Intern Med 129:845, 1998.
5. Pope JH, Aufderheide TP, Ruthazer R, et al: Missed diagnoses of acute cardiac ischemia in the emergency department. N Engl J Med 342:1163, 2000.
6. Lee TH, Rouan GW, Weisberg MC, et al: Clinical characteristics and natural history of patients with acute myocardial infarction sent home from the emergency room. Am J Cardiol 60:219, 1987.
7. Rusnak RA, Stair TO, Hansen K, Fastow JS: Litigation against the emergency physician: Common features in cases of missed myocardial infarction. Ann Emerg Med 18:1029, 1989.
8. Lee TH, Goldman L: Evaluation of the patient with acute chest pain. N Engl J Med 342:1187, 2000.
9. Braunwald E, Antman EM, Beasley JW, et al: ACC/AHA guidelines for the management of patients with unstable angina and non-ST-segment elevation myocardial infarction. J Am Coll Cardiol 36:970, 2000.
10. Lee TH, Cook EF, Weisberg M, et al: Acute chest pain in the emergency room: Identification and examination of low risk patients. Arch Intern Med 145:65, 1985.
11. Spodick D: Acute pericarditis: Current concepts and practice. JAMA 289:1150, 2003.
12. Hagan PG, Nienaber CA, Isselbacher EM, et al: The International Registry of Acute Aortic Dissection (IRAD): New insights into an old disease. JAMA 283:897, 2000.
13. Goldhaber SZ: Medical progress: Pulmonary embolism. N Engl J Med 339:93, 1998.
14. Fedulla PF, Auger WR, Kerr KM, Rubin LJ: Chronic thromboembolic pulmonary hypertension. N Engl J Med 345:1465, 2001.
15. Halm EA, Tierstein AS: Management of community-acquired pneumonia. N Engl J Med 347:2039, 2002.
16. Long W, Tate RB, Neuman M, et al: Respiratory symptoms in a susceptible population due to burning of agricultural residue. Chest 113:351, 1998.
17. Pandak WM, Arezo S, Everett S, et al: Short course of omeprazole: A better first diagnostic approach to noncardiac chest pain than endoscopy, manometry, or 24-hour esophageal pH monitoring. J Clin Gastroenterol 35:307, 2002.
18. Spechler SJ, Castell DO: Classification of oesophageal motility abnormalities. Gut 49:145, 2001.
19. Fleet RP, Dupuis G, Marchand A, et al: ACC/AHA 2002 guideline update for the management of patients with unstable angina and non-ST-segment elevation myocardial infarction: Summary article: A report of the American College of Cardiology/American Heart Association Task Force on Practice Guidelines (Committee on the Management of Patients With Unstable Angina). Circulation 106:1893, 2002.
20. National Heart Attack Alert Program: Emergency department: Rapid identification and treatment of patients with acute myocardial infarction. US Department of Health and Human Services, US Public Health Service, National Institutes of Health, National Heart, Lung, and Blood Institute; September 1993; NIH Publication No. 93-3278.
21. Walker NJ, Sites FD, Shofer FS, Hollander JE: Characteristics and outcomes of young adults who present to the emergency department with chest pain. Acad Emerg Med 8:703, 2001.
22. Lange RA, Hillis LD: Cardiovascular complications of cocaine use. N Engl J Med 345:351, 2001.
23. Antman EM, Tanasijevic MJ, Thompson B, et al: Cardiac-specific troponin I levels to predict the risk of mortality in patients with acute coronary syndromes. N Engl J Med 335:1342, 1996.
24. Newby LK, Christenson RH, Ohman EM, et al: Value of serial troponin T measures for early and late risk stratification in patients with acute coronary syndromes. Circulation 98:1853, 1998.
25. Hamm CW, Goldmann BU, Heeschen C, et al: Emergency room triage of patients with acute chest pain by means of rapid testing for cardiac troponin T or troponin I. N Engl J Med 337:1648, 1997.
26. Zimmerman J, Fromm R, Meyer D, et al: Diagnostic marker cooperative study for the diagnosis of myocardial infarction. Circulation 99:1671, 1999.
27. Polanczyk CA, Lee TH, Cook EF, et al: Cardiac troponin I as a predictor of major cardiac events in emergency department patients with acute chest pain. J Am Coll Cardiol 32:8, 1998.
28. Antman EM, Grudzien C, Sacks DB: Evaluation of a rapid bedside assay for detection of serum cardiac troponin T. JAMA 273:1279, 1995.
29. Polanczyk CA, Johnson PA, Cook EF, Lee TH: A proposed strategy for utilization of creatine kinase-MB and troponin I in the evaluation of acute chest pain. Am J Cardiol 83:1175, 1999.
30. Christenson RH, Duh SH: Evidence based approach to practice guides and decision thresholds for cardiac markers. Scand J Clin Lab Invest Suppl 230:90, 1999.
31. Lee TH, Goldman L: Serum enzyme assays in the diagnosis of myocardial infarction. Recommendations based on a quantitative analysis. Ann Intern Med 105:221, 1986.
32. Pearson JR, Carrea F: Evaluation of the clinical usefulness of a chemiluminometric method for measuring creatine kinase MB. Clin Chem 36:1809, 1990.
33. Adams JE, Abendschein DR, Jaffe AS: Biochemical markers of myocardial injury: Is MB creatine kinase the choice for the 1990s? Circulation 88:750, 1993.
34. Puleo PR, Meyer D, Warthen C, et al: Use of a rapid assay of subforms of creatine kinase-MB to diagnose or rule out acute myocardial infarction. N Engl J Med 331:561, 1994.
35. Mockel M, Schindler R, Knorr L, et al: Prognostic value of cardiac troponin T and I elevations in renal disease patients without acute coronary syndromes: A 9-month outcome analysis. Nephrol Dial Transplant 14:1489, 1999.
36. Krahn J, Parry DM, Leroux M, Dalton J: High percentage of false positive cardiac troponin I results in patients with rheumatoid factor. Clin Biochem 32:477, 1999.

37. Morrow DA, Cannon CP, Rifai N, et al: Ability of minor elevations of troponins I and T to predict benefit from an early invasive strategy in patients with unstable angina and non-ST elevation myocardial infarction. JAMA 286:2405, 2001.
38. Collinson PO, Gerhardt W, Katus HA, et al: Multicentre evaluation of an immunological rapid test for the detection of troponin T in whole blood samples. Eur J Clin Chem Clin Biochem 34:591, 1996.
39. Heeschen C, Goldman BU, Moeller RH, Hamm CW: Analytical performance and clinical application of a new rapid bedside assay for the detection of serum cardiac troponin I. Clin Chem 44:1925, 1998.
40. Hoekstra JW, Hedges JR, Gibler WB, et al: Emergency department CK-MB: A predictor of ischemic complications. Acad Emerg Med 1:17, 1994.
41. Galvani M, Ottani F, Ferrini D, et al: Prognostic influence of elevated values of cardiac troponin I in patients with unstable angina. Circulation 95:2053, 1997.
42. Hillis GS, Taggart P, Dalsey WC, Mangione A: Utility of cardiac troponin I, creatine kinase-MB (mass), myosin light chain 1, and myoglobin in the early in-hospital triage of "high risk" patients with chest pain. Heart 82:614, 1999.
43. Ohman EM, Armstrong PW, Christenson RH, et al: Cardiac troponin T levels for risk stratification in acute myocardial ischemia. GUSTO IIA Investigators. N Engl J Med 335:1333, 1996.
44. Newby LK, Christenson RH, Ohman EM, et al: Value of serial troponin T measures for early and late risk stratification in patients with acute coronary syndromes. Circulation 1998:1853, 1998.
45. Luscher MS, Thygesen K, Ravkilde J, Heickendorff L: Applicability of cardiac troponin T and I for early risk stratification in unstable coronary artery disease. TRIM Study Group. Thrombin Inhibition in Myocardial ischemia. Circulation 96:2578, 1997.
46. Lee TH, Weisberg MC, Cook EF, et al: Evaluation of creatine kinase and creatine kinase-MB for diagnosing myocardial infarction: Clinical impact in the emergency room. Arch Intern Med 147:115, 1987.
47. Brogan GX Jr, Hollander JE, McCuskey CF, et al: Evaluation of a new assay for cardiac troponin I vs creatine kinase-MB for the diagnosis of acute myocardial infarction. Biochemical Markers for Acute Myocardial Ischemia (BAMI) Study Group. Acad Emerg Med 4:6, 1997.

Initial Risk Stratification

48. Brieger DB, Mak KH, White HD, et al: Benefit of early sustained reperfusion in patients with prior myocardial infarction (the GUSTO-I trial). Global Utilization of Streptokinase and TPA for Occluded Arteries. Am J Cardiol 81:282, 1998.
49. Hochman JS, Tamis JE, Thompson TD, et al, for the Global Use of Strategies to Open Occluded Coronary Arteries in Acute Coronary Syndromes IIb Investigators: Sex, clinical presentation, and outcome in patients with acute coronary syndromes. N Engl J Med 341:226, 1999.
50. Hochman JS, McCabe CH, Stone PH, et al, for the TIMI Investigators: Thrombolysis In Myocardial Infarction: Outcome and profile of women and men presenting with acute coronary syndromes: a report from TIMI IIIB. J Am Coll Cardiol 30:141, 1997.
51. White HD, Barbash GI, Califf RM, et al: Age and outcome with contemporary thrombolytic therapy: Results from the GUSTO-I trial. Global Utilization of Streptokinase and TPA for Occluded coronary arteries trial. Circulation 94:1826, 1996.
52. Jayes RLJ, Beshansky JR, D'Agostino RB, Selker HP: Do patients' coronary risk factor reports predict acute cardiac ischemia in the emergency department? A multicenter study. J Clin Epidemiol 45:621, 1992.
53. Rouan GW, Lee TH, Cook EF, et al: Clinical characteristics and outcome of acute myocardial infarction in patients with initially normal or nonspecific electrocardiograms (a report from the Multicenter Chest Pain Study). Am J Cardiol 64:1087, 1989.
54. Slater DK, Hlatky MA, Mark DB, et al: Outcome in suspected acute myocardial infarction with normal or minimally abnormal admission electrocardiographic findings. Am J Cardiol 60:766, 1987.
55. Lee TH, Cook EF, Weisberg MC, et al: Impact of the availability of a prior electrocardiogram on the triage of the patient with acute chest pain. J Gen Intern Med 5:381, 1990.
56. Kudenchuk PJ, Maynard C, Cobb LA, et al: Utility of the prehospital electrocardiogram in diagnosing acute coronary syndromes: The Myocardial Infarction Triage and Intervention (MITI) Project. J Am Coll Cardiol 32:17, 1998.
57. Hedges JR, Young GP, Henkel GF, et al: Serial ECGs are less accurate than serial CK-MB results for emergency department diagnosis of myocardial infarction. Ann Emerg Med 21:1445, 1992.
58. Patel DJ, Knight CJ, Holdright DR, et al: Long-term prognosis in unstable angina: The importance of early risk stratification using continuous ST segment monitoring. Eur Heart J 19:240, 1998.
59. Selker HP, Beshansky JR, Griffith JL, for the TPI Trial Investigators: Use of the electrocardiograph-based thrombolytic predictive instrument to assist thrombolytic and reperfusion therapy for acute myocardial infarction: A multicenter, randomized, controlled, clinical effectiveness trial. Ann Intern Med 137:87, 2002.
60. Corey GA, Merenstein JH: Applying the acute ischemic heart disease predictive instrument. J Fam Pract 25:127, 1987.
61. Pearson SD, Goldman L, Garcia TB, et al: Physician response to a prediction rule for the triage of emergency department patients with chest pain. J Gen Intern Med 9:241, 1994.
62. Lee TH, Pearson SD, Johnson PA, et al: Failure of information as an intervention to modify clinical management: A time-series trial in patients with acute chest pain. Ann Intern Med 122:434, 1995.

Immediate Management

63. Tosteson ANA, Goldman L, Udvarhelyi IS, Lee TH: Cost-effectiveness of a coronary care unit versus an intermediate care unit for emergency department patients with chest pain. Circulation 94:143, 1996.
64. Lee TH, Goldman L: The coronary care unit turns 25: Historical trends and future directions. Ann Intern Med 108:887, 1988.
65. Nichol G, Walls R, Goldman L, et al: A critical pathway for management of patients with acute chest pain who are at low risk for myocardial ischemia: Recommendations and potential impact. Ann Intern Med 127:996, 1997.
66. Stein RA, Chaitman BR, Balady GJ, et al: Safety and utility of exercise testing in emergency room chest pain centers: An advisory from the Committee on Exercise, Rehabilitation, and Prevention, Council on Clinical Cardiology, American Heart Association. Circulation 102:1463, 2000.
67. Farkouh ME, Smars PA, Reeder GS, et al: A clinical trial of a chest-pain observation unit for patients with unstable angina. N Engl J Med 339:1882, 1998.
68. Gibler WB, Runyon JP, Levy RC, et al: A rapid diagnostic and treatment center for patients with chest pain in the emergency department. Ann Emerg Med 25:1, 1995.
69. Gomez MA, Anderson JL, Karagounis LA, et al: An emergency department-based protocol for rapidly ruling out myocardial ischemia reduces hospital time and expense: Results of a randomized study (ROMIO). J Am Coll Cardiol 28:25, 1996.
70. Polanczyk CA, Johnson PA, Hartley LH, et al: Clinical correlates and prognostic significance of early negative exercise tolerance test in patients with acute chest pain seen in the hospital emergency department. Am J Cardiol 81:288, 1998.
71. Lewis WR, Amsterdam EA, Turnipseed S, Kirk JD: Immediate exercise testing of low risk patients with known coronary artery disease presenting to the emergency department with chest pain. J Am Coll Cardiol 33:1843, 1999.
72. Hilton TC, Fulmer H, Abuan T, et al: Ninety-day follow-up of patients in the emergency department with chest pain who undergo initial single-photon emission computed tomographic perfusion scintigraphy with technetium 99m-labeled sestamibi. J Nucl Cardiol 3:308, 1996.
73. Kontos MC, Jesse RL, Schmidt KL, et al: Value of acute rest sestamibi perfusion imaging for evaluation of patients admitted to the emergency department with chest pain. J Am Coll Cardiol 30:976, 1997.
74. Udelson JE, Beshansky JR, Ballin DS, et al: Myocardial perfusion imaging for evaluation and triage of patients with suspected acute cardiac ischemia: A randomized controlled trial. JAMA 288:2693, 2002.
75. Colon PJ III, Mobarek SK, Milani RV, et al: Prognostic value of stress echocardiography in the evaluation of atypical chest pain patients without known coronary artery disease. Am J Cardiol 81:545, 1998.
76. Fleischmann KE, Lee TH, Come PC, et al: Echocardiographic predictors of complications in patients with chest pain. Am J Cardiol 79:292, 1997.
77. Kuntz KM, Fleischmann KE, Hunink MG, Douglas PS: Cost-effectiveness of diagnostic strategies for patients with chest pain. Ann Intern Med 130:709, 1999.
78. Garber AM, Solomon NA: Cost-effectiveness of alternative test strategies for the diagnosis of coronary artery disease. Ann Intern Med 130:719, 1999.

CHAPTER 46

ST-Elevation Myocardial Infarction: Pathology, Pathophysiology, and Clinical Features

Elliott M. Antman • Eugene Braunwald

Definition

The *pathological* diagnosis of myocardial infarction (MI) requires evidence of myocyte cell death as a consequence of prolonged ischemia. Characteristic findings include coagulation necrosis and contraction band necrosis, often with patchy areas of myocytolysis at the periphery of the infarct. The *clinical* diagnosis of MI requires an integrated assessment of the history with some combination of indirect evidence of myocardial necrosis using biochemical, electrocardiographic, and imaging modalities (Table 46–1). The sensitivity and specificity of the various clinical tools for diagnosing MI vary considerably, and at varying times after the onset of the infarction.

Epidemiological reports from the World Heath Organization and American Heart Association beginning in the late 1950s required the presence of at least two of the following: characteristic symptoms, electrocardiographic changes, and a typical rise and fall in biochemical markers for the diagnosis of myocardial infarction.[1] This epidemiological approach was then generally adopted in routine clinical practice, although the rigor with which clinicians apply the electrocardiographic and biochemical criteria for infarction varies considerably.

Since the original epidemiological efforts, considerable advances have occurred in the electrocardiographic and biochemical aspects of the definition of infarction. The electrocardiographic criteria for MI were codified and scoring systems were developed for estimation of infarct size.[2] Biochemical assays became available for markers more specific for cardiac damage. Thus, assays for lactic dehydrogenase and creatine kinase activity (CK) have been superseded by mass assays for the MB fraction of CK and immunoassays for cardiac-specific troponins. The cardiac-specific troponin assays have nearly absolute myocardial tissue specificity and have become the preferred biomarker for diagnosing MI. Advances in the techniques for diagnosing MI, especially the introduction of assays for cardiac-specific troponins, were the impetus for a consensus document published jointly by the European Society of Cardiology and the American College of Cardiology.[2] The main features of the revised definition of MI are summarized in Table 46–2. The revised definition of MI has important implications not only for clinical care of patients but also for tracking epidemiological trends, public policy, and clinical trials.[3,4] The paradigm shift to cardiac-specific troponins as the markers of choice for the diagnosis of MI requires new cutoff values for cardiac injury. The term *normal range* has been replaced by *upper reference limit*, defined as the 99th percentile of a normal reference control group.[5]

As discussed later, the contemporary approach to patients presenting with ischemic discomfort is to consider that they are experiencing an acute coronary syndrome. The 12-lead electrocardiogram (ECG) is pivotal for segregating patients into those presenting with ST-segment elevation, the subject of Chapters 46 through 48, and those presenting without ST-segment elevation, the subject of Chapter 49.[6] Although the revised definition of MI has greater impact on the non-ST-segment elevation end of the acute coronary syndrome spectrum (i.e., distinction between unstable angina and non-ST-segment elevation MI), the issues are also pertinent to discussion of ST-segment elevation myocardial infarction (STEMI).

Changing Patterns in Clinical Care

Despite impressive advances in diagnosis and management over the last four decades, STEMI continues to be a major public health problem in the industrialized world and is becoming an increasingly important problem in developing countries (see Chap. 1).[7,8] In the United States, nearly 1.0 million patients annually suffer from an acute MI.[9] More than 1 million patients with suspected acute MI are admitted yearly to coronary care units in the United States.[9]

TABLE 46–1 Aspects of Diagnosis of Myocardial Infarction by Different Techniques

Pathology	Myocardial cell death
Biochemistry	Markers of myocardial cell death recovered from blood samples
Electrocardiography	Evidence of myocardial ischemia (ST and T wave abnormalities) Evidence of loss of electrically functioning cardiac tissue (Q waves)
Imaging	Reduction or loss of tissue perfusion Cardiac wall motion abnormalities

Adapted from Alpert JS, Thygesen K, Antman E, et al: Myocardial infarction redefined—A consensus document of The Joint European Society of Cardiology/American College of Cardiology Committee for the redefinition of myocardial infarction. J Am Coll Cardiol 36:959, 2000.

TABLE 46–2 Revised Definition of Myocardial Infarction (MI)

Criteria for acute, evolving, or recent MI
Either one of the following criteria satisfies the diagnosis for an acute, evolving, or recent MI:
1. Typical rise and gradual fall (troponin) or more rapid rise and fall (CK-MB) of biochemical markers of myocardial necrosis with at least one of the following: a. Ischemic symptoms b. Development of pathologic Q waves on the ECG reading c. ECG changes indicative of ischemia (ST-segment elevation or depression) d. Coronary artery intervention (e.g., coronary angioplasty)
2. Pathological findings of an acute MI
Criteria for established MI
Either of the following criteria satisfies the diagnosis for established MI:
1. Development of new pathological Q waves on serial ECG readings. The patient may or may not remember previous symptoms. Biochemical markers of myocardial necrosis may have normalized, depending on the length of time that has passed since the infarct developed.
2. Pathological findings of a healed or healing MI

CK = creatine kinase; ECG = electrocardiographic.

From Alpert JS, Thygesen K, Antman E, et al: Myocardial infarction redefined—A consensus document of The Joint European Society of Cardiology/American College of Cardiology Committee for the redefinition of myocardial infarction. J Am Coll Cardiol 36:959, 2000.

The development of STEMI is a fatal event in approximately one-third of patients, with about half of the deaths occurring within 1 hour of the event from ventricular tachyarrhythmias. Because STEMI can strike an individual during the most productive years, it can have profound deleterious psychosocial and economic ramifications.

Of particular concern from a global perspective are projections from the World Heart Federation that the burden of disease in developing countries will become similar to those now afflicting developed countries.[9] Given the wide disparity of available resources to treat STEMI in developing countries, major efforts are needed on an international level to strengthen primary prevention programs at the community level.[10]

IMPROVEMENTS IN OUTCOME

A steady decline in the mortality rate from STEMI has been observed across several population groups since 1960.[11] This drop in mortality appears to be caused by a fall in the incidence of STEMI (replaced in part by an increase in the rate of unstable angina/non-ST-segment elevation MI[12]) and a fall in the case fatality rate once STEMI has occurred.[13]

Several phases in the management of patients have contributed to the decline in mortality from STEMI.[14] The "clinical observation phase" of coronary care consumed the first half of the 20th century and focused on a detailed recording of physical and laboratory findings, whereas treatment consisted of strict bed rest and sedation. Subsequently, the "coronary care unit phase" began in the mid-1960s and was notable for detailed analysis and vigorous management of cardiac arrhythmias. The "high-technology phase" was ushered in by the introduction of the pulmonary artery balloon flotation catheter, setting the stage for bedside hemodynamic monitoring and more precise management of heart failure and cardiogenic shock associated with STEMI. A battery of tests, sometimes providing overlapping information, was developed during the high-technology phase. The modern "reperfusion era" of coronary care was introduced by intracoronary and then intravenous fibrinolysis, increased use of aspirin, and development of primary percutaneous coronary intervention (PCI).

Driven in large part by the need for cost-saving measures, contemporary care of patients with STEMI has entered the "evidence-based coronary care phase" and is becoming increasingly influenced by managed care systems and guidelines for clinical practice (see Chap. 47, Guidelines).[15] Coronary care practice is better equipped than other fields of cardiovascular medicine to face this transition from pathophysiologically based decision-making to evidence-based decision-making, given the rich data base of patients with suspected STEMI studied in clinical trials and registries and efforts at summarizing a vast amount of data using meta-analysis.[16] New therapies for STEMI are being evaluated not only for evidence of safety and efficacy but also for their cost-effectiveness in caring for patients and their impact on quality of life. However, despite an abundance of cost-effectiveness information using data from clinical trials, clinicians weighing the risk-benefit ratio of any given intervention at the bedside of an individual patient may have difficulty applying the findings for several reasons: uncertainty about whether the benefits observed in a strictly defined trial population are applicable to a wider selection of patients, limited data on specific subgroups, variations in the absolute level of baseline risk, and variations in patient preferences.[17]

LIMITATIONS OF CURRENT THERAPY. Despite the gratifying success of medical therapy for STEMI, several observations indicate that considerable room for improvement exists. The short-term mortality rate of patients with STEMI who receive aggressive pharmacological reperfusion therapy as part of a randomized trial is in the range of 6.5 to 7.0 percent,[18] whereas observational data bases suggest that the mortality rate in STEMI patients in the community is 15 to 20 percent.[19] In part, this difference relates to the selection of patients without serious comorbidities for clinical trials.

Although the survival of elderly patients (>65 years of age) after STEMI has improved significantly, advanced age consistently emerges as one of the principal determinants of mortality in patients with STEMI.[20] Despite reluctance to use potentially life-saving drug therapies in elderly patients, cardiac catheterization and other invasive procedures are being performed more commonly at some point during hospitalization in elderly patients with STEMI. Nevertheless, evidence suggests that the greatest reductions in mortality for elderly patients are derived from those strategies employed during the first 24 hours, a time frame in which prompt and appropriate use of life-saving pharmacotherapy is of paramount importance, emphasizing the need to extend advances in drug therapy for STEMI to the elderly.[16]

Despite trends toward greater use of mortality-reducing therapies such as fibrinolytics, aspirin, and beta-adrenoceptor blockers in patients with STEMI, these drugs still appear to be underutilized.[17] Considerable variation exists in practice patterns for management of patients with STEMI.[21] Mortality rates for STEMI are lower in hospitals with a high clinical volume, a high rate of invasive procedures, and a top ranking in quality reports (see Chap. 4).[22,23] Variation has also been observed in the treatment patterns of certain population subgroups with STEMI, notably women and blacks. Although the unadjusted rates of fibrinolytic use and referral for cardiac catheterization and angioplasty are lower and unadjusted mortality rates are higher in women with STEMI, gender differences are less apparent (but may not disappear entirely) once adjustment is made for baseline variables such as comorbidities and age (see Chap. 73).[19] Of interest, after STEMI, younger women but not older women have higher rates of in-hospital mortality than men of the same age.[24]

Pathology

Almost all MIs result from coronary atherosclerosis, generally with superimposed coronary thrombosis. Nonatherogenic forms of coronary artery disease are discussed later in this chapter and causes of STEMI without coronary atherosclerosis are shown in Table 46–3.

Prior to the fibrinolytic era, clinicians typically divided patients with MI into those suffering a Q-wave and those suffering a non-Q-wave infarct, based on the evolution of the pattern on the ECG over several days. The term *Q-wave infarction* was frequently considered to be virtually synonymous with *transmural infarction*, whereas *non-Q-wave infarctions* were often referred to as *subendocardial infarctions*. Phibbs summarized the arguments that previous distinctions between Q-wave infarction and non-Q-wave infarctions were based on erroneous interpretation of pathological data and should not serve as the basis for designing therapy.[25] A more suitable framework based on pathophysiology is referred to as the *acute coronary syndromes* (Fig. 46–1).

Plaque

Slowly accruing high-grade stenoses of epicardial coronary arteries can progress to complete occlusion but do not usually precipitate STEMI, probably because of the development of a

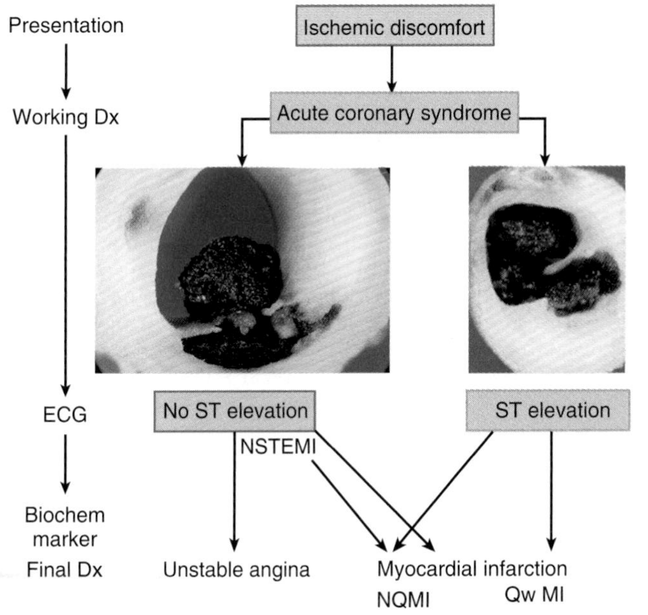

FIGURE 46–1 Nomenclature of acute coronary syndromes. Patients with ischemic discomfort present with or without ST-segment elevation on the electrocardiogram (ECG). The majority of patients with ST-segment elevation ultimately develop a Q wave acute myocardial infarction (QwMI), whereas a minority develop a non-Q-wave myocardial infarction (NQMI). Patients who present without ST-segment elevation are either experiencing unstable angina or a non-ST-segment elevation myocardial infarction (NSTEMI). The distinction between these two diagnoses is ultimately made based on the presence or absence of a cardiac biomarker detected in the blood. Most patients with NSTEMI do not evolve a Q wave on the 12-lead ECG and are subsequently referred to as having sustained an NQMI; only a minority of NSTEMI patients develop a Q wave MI and are later diagnosed as Q wave MI. The spectrum of clinical conditions ranging from unstable angina to non-Q wave MI constitutes the acute coronary syndromes. (From Braunwald E, Antman EM, Beasley JW, et al: ACC/AHA guidelines for the management of patients with unstable angina: A report of the American College of Cardiology/American Heart Association Task Force on Practice Guidelines [Committee on the Management of Patients With Unstable Angina]. J Am Coll Cardiol 36:970, 2000.)

TABLE 46–3 Causes of Myocardial Infarction without Coronary Atherosclerosis

Coronary Artery Disease Other than Atherosclerosis
Arteritis
Luetic
Granulomatous (Takayasu disease)
Polyarteritis nodosa
Mucocutaneous lymph node (Kawasaki) syndrome
Disseminated lupus erythematosus
Rheumatoid spondylitis
Ankylosing spondylitis
Trauma to coronary arteries
Laceration
Thrombosis
Iatrogenic
Radiation (radiation therapy for neoplasia)
Coronary mural thickening with metabolic disease or intimal proliferative disease
Mucopolysaccharidoses (Hurler disease)
Homocysteinuria
Fabry disease
Amyloidosis
Juvenile intimal sclerosis (idiopathic arterial calcification of infancy
Intimal hyperplasia associated with contraceptive steroids or with the postpartum period
Pseudoxanthoma elasticum
Coronary fibrosis caused by radiation therapy
Luminal narrowing by other mechanisms
Spasm of coronary arteries (Prinzmetal angina with normal coronary arteries)
Spasm after nitroglycerin withdrawal
Dissection of the aorta
Dissection of the coronary artery
Emboli to Coronary Arteries
Infective endocarditis
Nonbacterial thrombotic endocarditis
Prolapse of mitral valve
Mural thrombus from left atrium, left ventricle, or pulmonary veins
Prosthetic valve emboli
Cardiac myxoma
Associated with cardiopulmonary bypass surgery and coronary arteriography
Paradoxical emboli
Parpillary fibroelastoma of the aortic valve ("fixed embolus")
Thrombi from intracardiac catheters or guidewires
Congenital Coronary Artery Anomalies
Anomalous origin of left coronary from pulmonary artery
Left coronary artery from anterior sinus of Valsalva
Coronary arteriovenous and arteriocameral fistulas
Coronary artery aneurysms
Myocardial Oxygen Demand-Supply Disproportion
Aortic stenosis, all forms
Incomplete differentiation of the aortic valve
Aortic insufficiency
Carbon monoxide poisoning
Thyrotoxicosis
Prolonged hypotension
Hematological (in situ Thrombosis)
Polycythemia vera
Thrombocytosis
Disseminated intravascular coagulation
Hypercoagulability, thrombosis, thrombocytopenic purpura
Miscellaneous
Cocaine abuse
Myocardial contusion
Myocardial infarction with normal coronary arteries
Complication of cardiac catheterization

Modified from Cheitlin MD, McAllister HA, de Castro CM: Myocardial infarction without atherosclerosis. JAMA 231:951, 1975. Copyright 1975, American Medical Association.

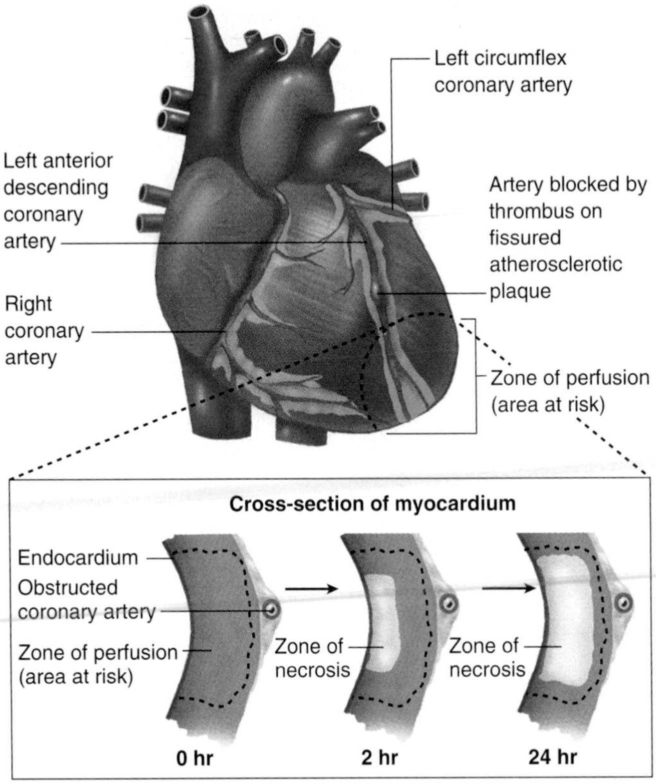

FIGURE 46–2 Schematic representation of the progression of myocardial necrosis after coronary artery occlusion. Necrosis begins in a small zone of the myocardium beneath the endocardial surface in the center of the ischemic zone. This entire region of myocardium (dashed outline) depends on the occluded vessel for perfusion and is the area at risk. Note that a very narrow zone of myocardium immediately beneath the endocardium is spared from necrosis because it can be oxygenated by diffusion from the ventricle. (From Schoen FJ: The heart. *In* Cotran RS, Kumar V, Collins T [eds]: Pathologic Basis of Disease. 6th ed. Philadelphia, WB Saunders, 1999, p 557.)

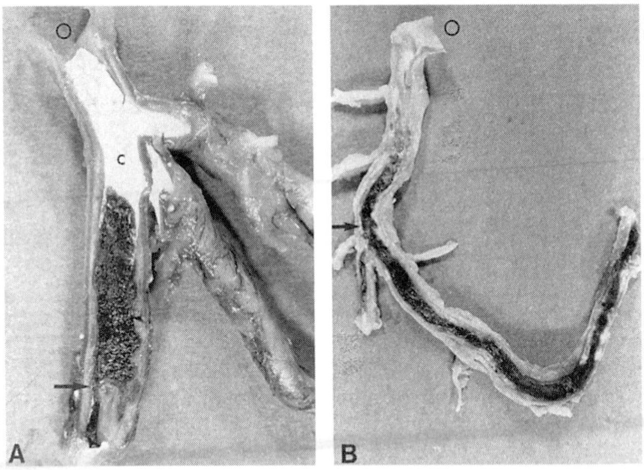

FIGURE 46–3 Thrombus propagation. **A,** Left anterior descending coronary artery cut open longitudinally, showing a dark (red) stagnation thrombosis propagating upstream from the initiating rupture/platelet-rich thrombus at the arrow. In this case, the thrombus has propagated proximally up to the nearest major side branch (the first diagonal branch). **B,** The right coronary artery cut open longitudinally, showing a huge stagnation thrombosis propagating downstream from the initiating rupture/platelet-rich thrombus at the arrow. Unlike upstream thrombus propagation, downstream propagation may, as in this case, occlude major side branches. c = contrast medium injected postmortem; O = coronary ostium. (From Falk E: Coronary thrombosis: Pathogenesis and clinical manifestations. Am J Cardiol 68:28B, 1991.)

rich collateral network over time. However, during the natural evolution of atherosclerotic plaques, especially those that are lipid-laden, an abrupt and catastrophic transition can occur, characterized by plaque disruption. Some patients have a systemic predisposition to plaque disruption that is independent of traditional risk factors.[16,26,27] After plaque disruption, there is exposure of substances that promote platelet activation and aggregation, thrombin generation, and ultimately thrombus formation.[28,29] The resultant thrombus that is formed interrupts blood flow and leads to an imbalance between oxygen supply and demand and, if this imbalance is severe and persistent, to myocardial necrosis (Fig. 46–2).

COMPOSITION OF PLAQUES. At autopsy, the atherosclerotic plaque of patients who died of STEMI is composed primarily of fibrous tissue of varying density and cellularity with superimposed thrombus. Calcium, lipid-laden foam cells, and extracellular lipid each constitutes 5 to 10 percent of the remaining area. The atherosclerotic plaques that are associated with thrombosis and a total occlusion, located in infarct-related vessels, are generally more complex and irregular than those in vessels not associated with STEMI. Histological studies of these lesions often reveal plaque rupture or erosion. Coronary arterial thrombi responsible for STEMI are approximately 1 cm in length in most cases, adhere to the luminal surface of an artery, and are composed of platelets, fibrin, erythrocytes, and leukocytes (Fig. 46–3). The composition of the thrombus may vary at different levels: a white thrombus is composed of platelets, fibrin, or both, and a red thrombus is composed of erythrocytes, fibrin, platelets, and leukocytes.[27] Early thrombi are usually small and nonocclusive and are composed predominantly of platelets.

PLAQUE FISSURING AND DISRUPTION. In atherosclerotic plaques prone to disruption, there is an increased rate of formation of metalloproteinase enzymes such as collagenase, gelatinase, and stromelysin that degrade components of the protective interstitial matrix.[26] These proteinases can be elaborated by activated macrophages and mast cells that have been shown to accumulate in high concentration at the site of atheromatous erosions and plaque disruption in patients who died of STEMI.[26] Examination of specimens from atherectomy reveals a much higher content of macrophages and tissue factor in patients with unstable angina or STEMI compared with patients with chronic stable angina.[30] In addition to these structural aspects of vulnerable or high-risk plaques, stresses induced by intraluminal pressure, coronary vasomotor tone, tachycardia (cyclic stretching and compression), and disruption of nutrient vessels combine to produce plaque disruption at the margin of the fibrous cap near an adjacent plaque-free segment of the coronary artery wall (shoulder region of plaque).[28] A number of key physiological parameters such as systolic blood pressure, heart rate, blood viscosity, endogenous tissue plasminogen activator (t-PA) activity, plasminogen activator inhibitor-1 (PAI-1) levels, plasma cortisol levels, and plasma epinephrine levels that exhibit circadian and seasonal variations are increased at times of stress. They act in concert to produce a heightened propensity to plaque disruption and coronary thrombosis, yielding the clustering of STEMI in the early morning hours, and especially in the winter and after natural disasters.[31]

Acute Coronary Syndromes

When plaque disruption occurs, a sufficient quantity of thrombogenic substances is exposed, and the coronary artery lumen may become obstructed by a combination of platelet aggregates, fibrin, and red blood cells (see Fig. 46–3). An adequate collateral network that prevents necrosis from occurring can result in clinically silent episodes of coronary occlusion. Disruption of plaques is now considered to be the common pathophysiological substrate of the acute coronary syndromes (ACS) (see Fig. 46–1).[16] Characteristically, such completely occlusive thrombi lead to a large zone of necrosis involving the full or nearly full thickness of the ventricular wall in the myocardial bed subtended by the affected coronary artery and typically produce ST elevation on the ECG (see Fig. 46–2). The infarction process alters the sequence of depolarization ultimately reflected as changes in the surface of QRS.[25] The most characteristic change in the QRS that develops in about 75 percent of patients initially presenting with ST elevation is the evolution of Q waves in the leads overlying the infarct zone—leading to the term *Q-wave infarction* (see Fig. 46–1). In about 25 percent of patients presenting with ST elevation, no Q waves develop,[32] but other abnormalities of the QRS complex are frequently seen such as diminution in R wave height and notching or splintering of the QRS. Patients presenting without ST elevation are initially diagnosed as suffering either from a non-ST-elevation MI (NSTEMI) or unstable angina (see Fig. 46–1 and Chap. 49).

The ACS spectrum concept, organized around a common pathophysiological substrate, is a useful framework for developing therapeutic strategies.[15] Patients presenting with persistent ST-segment elevation are candidates for reperfusion therapy (either pharmacological or catheter-based) to restore flow in the occluded epicardial infarct-related artery. ACS patients presenting without ST segment elevation are not candidates for pharmacological reperfusion but should receive antiischemic therapy, often followed by PCI. Antithrombin therapy and antiplatelet therapy should be administered to all patients with ACS regardless of the presence or absence of ST-segment elevation. Thus, the 12-lead ECG remains at the center of the decision pathway for management of patients with ACS to distinguish between presentations with ST elevation and without ST elevation (see Fig. 46–1).[12] The ECG lacks sufficient sensitivity and specificity to permit reliable distinction of transmural from subendocardial infarcts. Categorization of patients into those with Q-wave and those with non-Q-wave infarction pattern is best conceived of as only a crude guide to the extent of ventricular damage—prognostic considerations must take into account other important factors, such as whether the ECG abnormality is due to a first infarct versus subsequent infarct, the location of infarction (anterior versus inferior), infarct size, and demographic factors such as patient age.[25]

The Heart Muscle

Gross Pathology

On gross inspection, MI can be divided into two major types: transmural infarcts, in which myocardial necrosis involves the full thickness (or nearly full thickness) of the ventricular wall, and subendocardial (nontransmural) infarcts, in which the necrosis involves the subendocardium, the intramural myocardium, or both without extending all the way through the ventricular wall to the epicardium (Fig. 46–4).

An occlusive coronary thrombosis appears to be far more common when the infarction is transmural and localized to the distribution of a single coronary artery (see Fig. 46–3). Nontransmural infarctions, however, frequently occur in the presence of severely narrowed but still patent coronary arteries. Patchy nontransmural infarction may arise from thrombolysis or PCI of an originally occlusive thrombus with restoration of blood flow *before* the wavefront of necrosis has extended from the subendocardium across the full thickness of the ventricular wall (see Fig. 46–2). Paradoxically, before their infarction, patients with nontransmural infarcts have, on average, a more severe stenosis in the infarct-related coronary artery than do patients suffering from transmural infarcts. This finding suggests that a more severe obstruction occurring before coronary occlusion protects against the development of transmural infarction, perhaps by fostering the development of collateral circulation. It also accords with the concept that less severely stenotic but lipid-laden plaques with a fragile cap are responsible for the abrupt presentation of ST-segment elevation that may evolve to transmural infarctions.

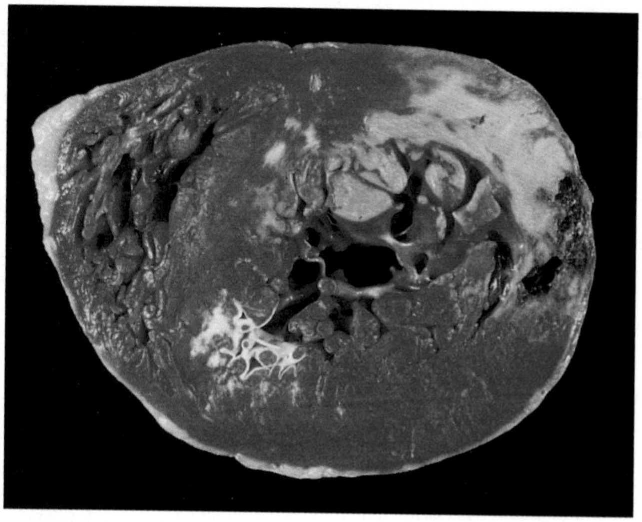

FIGURE 46–4 Acute myocardial infarction, predominantly of the posterolateral left ventricle, demonstrated histochemically by a lack of staining by the triphenyltetrazolium chloride (TTC) stain in areas of necrosis. The staining defect is due to the enzyme leakage that follows cell death. Note the myocardial hemorrhage at one edge of the infarct that was associated with cardiac rupture, and the anterior scar (lower left), indicative of old infarct. (Specimen oriented with posterior wall at top.) (From Schoen FJ: The heart. *In* Cotran RS, Kumar V, Collins T [eds]: Pathologic Basis of Disease. 6th ed. Philadelphia, WB Saunders, 1999, p 559.)

THE FIRST HOURS. Gross alterations of the myocardium are difficult to identify until at least 6 to 12 hours have elapsed following the onset of necrosis (Fig. 46–5). However, a variety of histochemical stains can be used to identify zones of necrosis that can be discerned after only 2 to 3 hours. Tissue slices of suspected infarct sites are immersed in a solution of triphenyltetrazolium chloride (TTC), which stains viable myocardium brick red (because of preserved dehydrogenase enzymes that form a red formazan precipitate) and leaves the infarcted region pale as a result of failure of uptake of the vital dye (see Fig. 46-4). The nitroblue tetrazolium (NBT) staining technique can similarly distinguish viable zones of myocardium, which stain dark blue, from necrotic areas of myocardium that therefore remain uncolored and identifiable. Other approaches include autofluorescence staining, immunohistochemical analysis, and, more recently, special DNA staining techniques to identify apoptotic bodies in myocardial sections.[33]

THE FIRST DAYS. Initially, the myocardium in the affected region may appear pale and slightly swollen. Eighteen to 36 hours after the onset of the infarct, the myocardium is tan or reddish purple (due to trapped erythrocytes), with a serofibrinous exudate evident on the epicardium in transmural infarcts. These changes persist for approximately 48 hours; the infarct then turns gray, and fine yellow lines, secondary to neutrophilic infiltration, appear at its periphery. This zone gradually widens and during the next few days extends throughout the infarct.

THE FIRST WEEKS. Eight to 10 days after infarction, the thickness of the cardiac wall in the area of the infarct is reduced as necrotic muscle is removed by mononuclear cells.

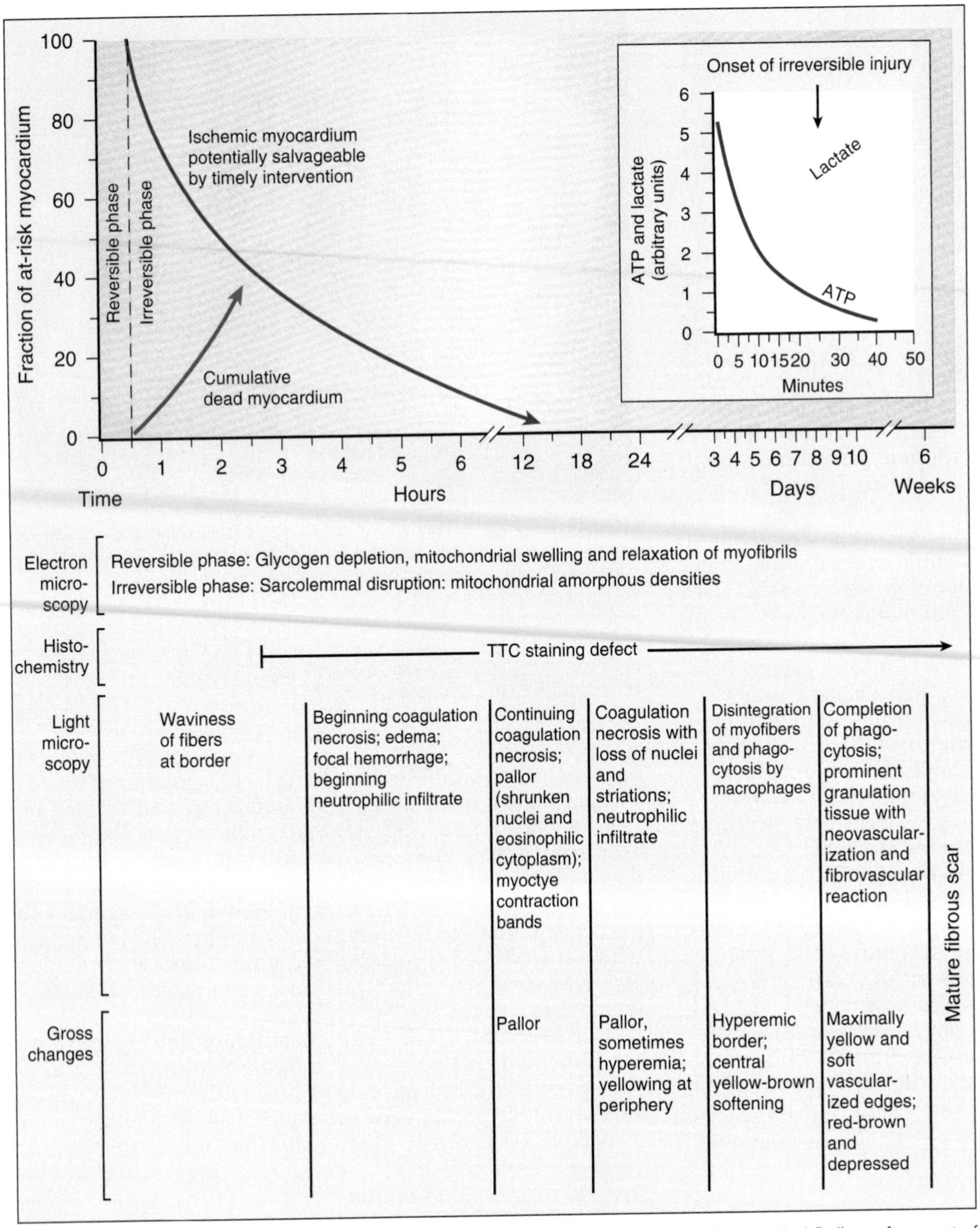
100
80
60
40
20
0
Fraction of at-risk myocardium
Reversible phase
Irreversible phase
Ischemic myocardium potentially salvageable by timely intervention
Cumulative dead myocardium
0 1 2 3 4 5 6 12 18 24
3 4 5 6 7 8 9 10
6
Time
Hours
Days
Weeks
Onset of irreversible injury
ATP and lactate (arbitrary units)
Lactate
ATP
0 5 10 15 20 30 40 50
Minutes
Electron microscopy
Reversible phase: Glycogen depletion, mitochondrial swelling and relaxation of myofibrils
Irreversible phase: Sarcolemmal disruption: mitochondrial amorphous densities
Histochemistry
TTC staining defect
Light microscopy
Waviness of fibers at border
Beginning coagulation necrosis; edema; focal hemorrhage; beginning neutrophilic infiltrate
Continuing coagulation necrosis; pallor (shrunken nuclei and eosinophilic cytoplasm); myoctye contraction bands
Coagulation necrosis with loss of nuclei and striations; neutrophilic infiltrate
Disintegration of myofibers and phagocytosis by macrophages
Completion of phagocytosis; prominent granulation tissue with neovascularization and fibrovascular reaction
Mature fibrous scar
Gross changes
Pallor
Pallor, sometimes hyperemia; yellowing at periphery
Hyperemic border; central yellow-brown softening
Maximally yellow and soft vascularized edges; red-brown and depressed

FIGURE 46–5 Temporal sequence of early biochemical, ultrastructural, histochemical, and histological findings after onset of myocardial infarction. At the top of the figure are schematically shown the time frames for early and late reperfusion of the myocardium supplied by an occluded coronary artery. For approximately $^1/_2$ hour after the onset of even the most severe ischemia, myocardial injury is potentially reversible; after that there is progressive loss of viability that is complete by 6 to 12 hours. The benefits of reperfusion (both early and late) are greatest when it is achieved early, with progressively smaller benefits occurring as reperfusion is delayed. ATP = adenosine triphosphate; TTC = triphenyltetrazolium chloride. (From Schoen FJ: Pathologic considerations of the surgery of adult heart disease. *In* Edmunds LH [ed]: Cardiac Surgery in the Adult. New York, McGraw Hill, 1997, p 85.)

The cut surface of an infarct of this age is yellow, surrounded by a reddish purple band of granulation tissue that extends through the necrotic tissue by 3 to 4 weeks. Commencing at this time and extending over the next 2 to 3 months, the infarcted area gradually acquires a gelatinous, ground-glass, gray appearance, eventually converting into a shrunken, thin, firm scar, which whitens and firms progressively with time (see Fig. 46–4).[34] This process begins at the periphery of the infarct and gradually moves centrally. The endocardium below the infarct increases in thickness and becomes gray and opaque.

Histological and Ultrastructural Changes

LIGHT MICROSCOPY

In some infarcts, a pattern of wavy myocardial fibers may be seen as early as 1 to 3 hours after onset, especially at the periphery of the infarct (Figs. 46–5 and 46–6). It is hypothesized that wavy fibers result from the stretching and buckling of noncontractile fibers as forces are transmitted to them from adjacent viable contractile fibers.[34] After 8 hours, edema of the interstitium becomes evident, as do increased fatty deposits in the muscle fibers, along with infiltration of neutrophilic polymorphonuclear leukocytes and red blood cells. Muscle cell nuclei become pyknotic and then undergo karyolysis, and small blood vessels undergo necrosis.

By 24 hours, there is clumping of the cytoplasm and loss of cross-striations, with appearance of focal hyalinization and irregular cross-bands in the involved myocardial fibers. The nuclei become pyknotic and sometimes even disappear. The myocardial capillaries in the involved region dilate, and polymorphonuclear leukocytes accumulate, first at the periphery and then in the center of the infarct. During the first 3 days, the interstitial tissue becomes edematous and red blood cells may extravasate (see Fig. 46–5). Generally, on about the fourth day after infarction, removal of necrotic fibers by macrophages begins, again commencing at the periphery (see Figs. 46–5 and 46–6). Later, lymphocytes, macrophages, and fibroblasts infiltrate between myocytes, which become fragmented. At 8 days, the necrotic muscle fibers have become dissolved; by about 10 days, the number of polymorphonuclear leukocytes is reduced, and granulation tissue first appears at the periphery (see Figs. 46–5 and 46–6). Ingrowth of blood vessels and fibroblasts continues, along with removal of necrotic muscle cells, until the fourth to sixth week after infarction, by which time much of the necrotic myocardium has been removed. This process continues along with increasing collagenization of the infarcted area. By the sixth week, the infarcted area has usually been converted into a firm connective tissue scar with interspersed intact muscle fibers (see Figs. 46–5 and 46–6).

PATTERNS OF MYOCARDIAL NECROSIS

COAGULATION NECROSIS. This results from severe, persistent ischemia and is usually present in the central region of infarcts, which results in the arrest of muscle cells in the relaxed state and the passive stretching of ischemic muscle cells. On light microscopy, the myofibrils are stretched, many with nuclear pyknosis, vascular congestion, and healing by phagocytosis of necrotic muscle cells (see Fig. 46–5). There is evidence of mitochondrial damage with prominent amorphous (flocculent) densities but no calcification.

NECROSIS WITH CONTRACTION BANDS. This form of myocardial necrosis, also termed *contraction band necrosis* or *coagulative myocytolysis*, results primarily from severe ischemia followed by reflow.[34] It is characterized by hypercontracted myofibrils with contraction bands and mitochondrial damage, frequently with calcification, marked vascular congestion, and healing by lysis of muscle cells. It is caused by increased Ca^{2+} influx into dying cells, resulting in the arrest of cells in the contracted state. It is seen in the periphery of large infarcts and is present to a greater extent in nontransmural than in transmural infarcts. The entire infarct may show this form of necrosis after reperfusion (Figs. 46-6 and 46-7).[35] The presence of contraction band necrosis in a large segment of the infarcts of patients who did not receive reperfusion therapy suggests that reperfusion through spontaneous fibrinolysis and/or the release of spasm have occurred.

MYOCYTOLYSIS. Ischemia without necrosis generally causes no acute changes that are visible by light microscopy. However, severe prolonged ischemia can cause myocyte vacuolization, often termed *myocytolysis*. Prolonged severe ischemia, which is potentially reversible, causes cloudy swelling, as well as hydropic, vascular, and fatty degeneration. Frequently seen at the borders of an infarct as well as in patchy areas of infarction in patients with chronic ischemic heart disease, myocytolysis is characterized by edema and cell swelling, lysis of myofibrils and nuclei, no neutrophilic response, and healing by lysis and phagocytosis of necrotic myocytes and ultimately scar formation.

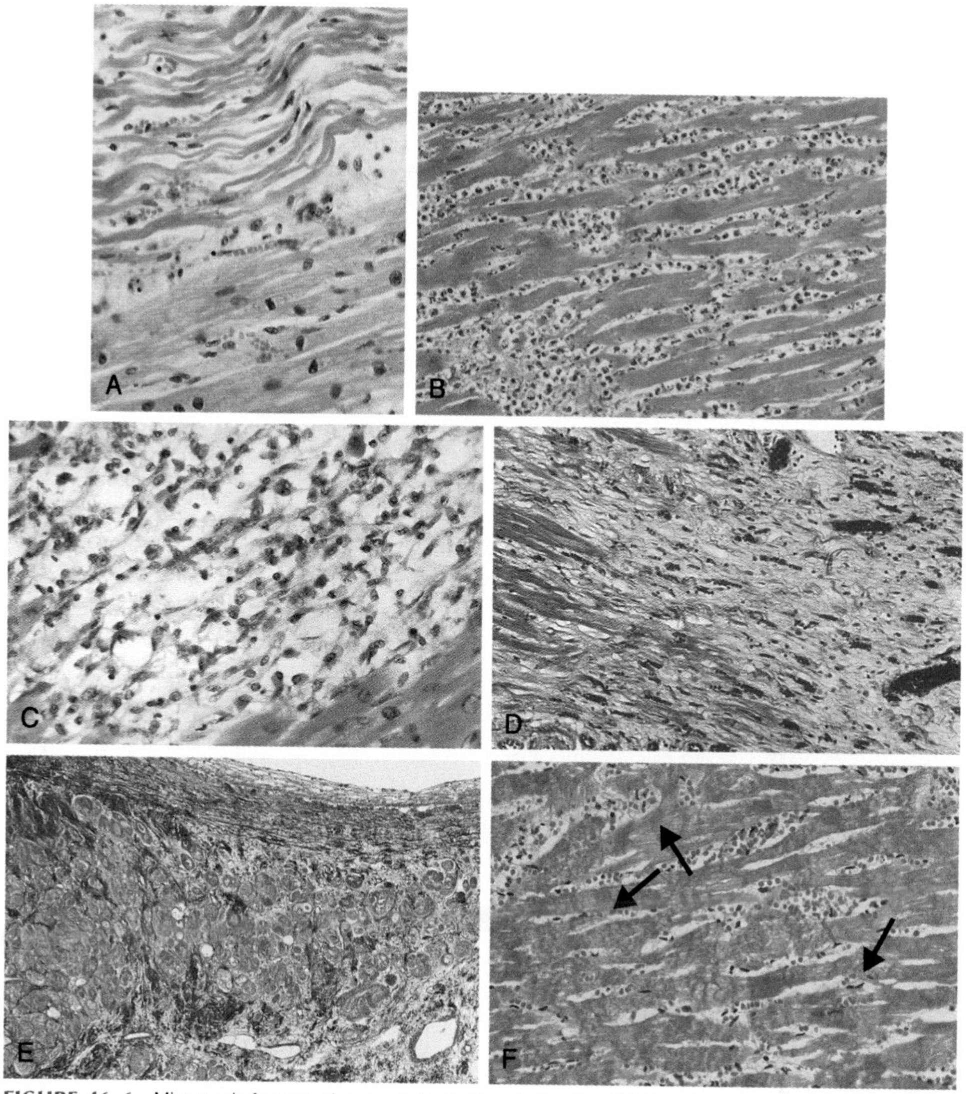

FIGURE 46–6 Microscopic features of myocardial infarction. **A,** One-day-old infarct showing coagulative necrosis, wavy fibers with elongation, and narrowing, compared with adjacent normal fibers (lower right). Widened spaces between the dead fibers contain edema fluid and scattered neutrophils. **B,** Dense polymorphonuclear leukocytic infiltrate in an area of acute myocardial infarction of 3 to 4 days' duration. **C,** Nearly complete removal of necrotic myocytes by phagocytosis (approximately 7 to 10 days). **D,** Granulation tissue with a rich vascular network and early collagen deposition, approximately 3 weeks after infarction. **E,** Well-healed myocardial infarct with replacement of the necrotic fibers by dense collagenous scar. A few residual cardiac muscle cells are present. (In **D** and **E,** collagen is highlighted as blue in this Masson trichrome stain). **F,** Myocardial necrosis with hemorrhage and contraction bands, visible as dark bands spanning some myofibers (arrows). This is the characteristic appearance of markedly ischemic myocardium that has been reperfused. (From Schoen FJ: The heart. *In* Cotran RS, Kumar V, Collins T [eds]: Pathologic Basis of Disease. 6th ed. Philadelphia, WB Saunders, 1999, pp 560-561.)

ELECTRON MICROSCOPY

In experimental infarction, the earliest ultrastructural changes in cardiac muscle following ligation of a coronary artery, noted within 20 minutes, consist of reduction in the size and number of glycogen granules, intracellular edema, and swelling and distortion of the transverse tubular system, the sarcoplasmic reticulum, and the mitochondria (see Fig. 46-5).[33] These early changes are reversible. Changes after 60 minutes of occlusion include myocardial cell swelling, swelling and internal disruption of mitochondria, and development of amorphous, flocculent aggregation and margination of nuclear chromatin, and relaxation of myofibrils. After 20 minutes to 2 hours of ischemia, changes in some cells become irreversible, and there is progression of these alterations; additional changes include indistinct tight junctions at the intercalated discs, swollen sacs of the sarcoplasmic reticulum at the level of the A band, greatly enlarged mitochondria with few cristae, thinning and fractionation of myofilaments, disappearance of the heterochromatin, rarefaction of the euchromatin and peripheral aggregation of chromatin in the nucleus, disorientation of myofibrils, and clumping of mitochondria. Cells irreversibly damaged by ischemia are usually swollen, with an enlarged sarcoplasmic space; the sarcolemma may peel off the cells, defects in the plasma membrane may appear, and the mitochondria are fragmented. The swollen mitochondria obtained from ischemic myocardium contain deposits of calcium phosphate and amorphous matrix densities. Many of these changes become more intense when blood flow is restored.[34]

MODIFICATION OF PATHOLOGICAL CHANGES BY REPERFUSION

When reperfusion of myocardium undergoing the evolutionary changes from ischemia to infarction occurs sufficiently early (i.e., within 15 to 20 minutes), it can successfully prevent necrosis from developing. Beyond this early stage, the number of salvaged myocytes and therefore the amount of salvaged myocardial tissue (area of necrosis/area at risk) is directly related to the length of time the coronary artery has been totally occluded, the level of myocardial oxygen consumption, and the collateral blood flow (see Fig. 46-7). Typical pathological findings of reperfused infarcts include a histological mixture of necrosis, hemorrhage within zones of irreversibly injured myocytes, coagulative necrosis with contraction bands, and distorted architecture of the cells in the reperfused zone (see Fig. 46-7).[33] After reperfusion, mitochondria in nonviable myocytes may develop deposits of calcium phosphate. Reperfusion of infarcted myocardium also accelerates the washout of intracellular proteins ("serum cardiac markers"), producing an exaggerated and early peak value of substances such as CK-MB and cardiac-specific troponin T and I (see Fig. 46-5).[36]

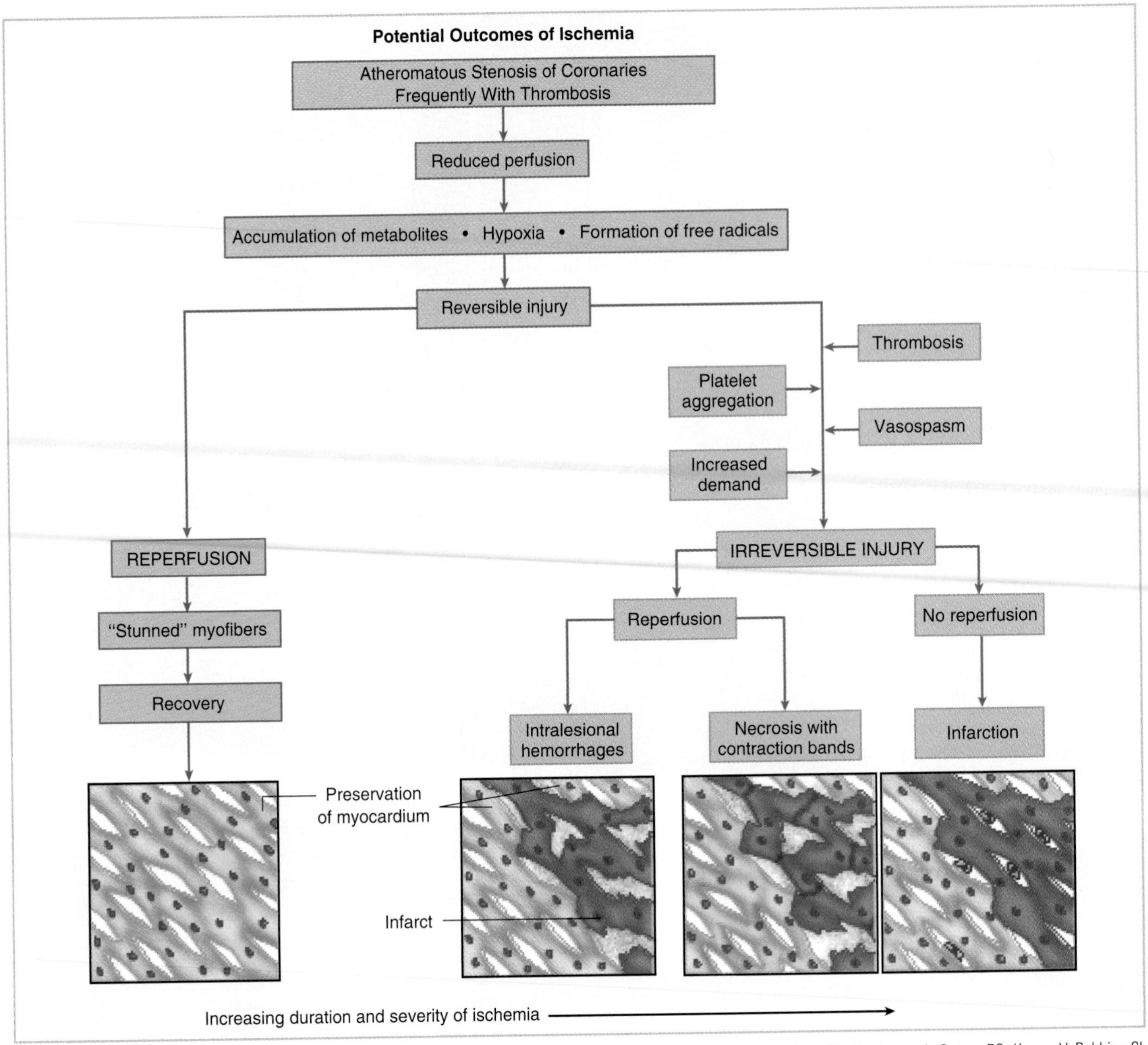

FIGURE 46–7 Several potential outcomes of reversible and irreversible ischemic injury to the myocardium. (From Schoen FJ: The heart. *In* Cotran RS, Kumar V, Robbins SL [eds]: Pathologic Basis of Disease. 5th ed. Philadelphia, WB Saunders, 1994, p 538.)

CORONARY ANATOMY AND LOCATION OF INFARCTION

In more than 75 percent of patients with STEMI who come to autopsy, more than one coronary artery is severely narrowed. Approximately one-half of patients with STEMI have critical obstruction (to less than 25 percent of luminal area) of all three coronary arteries, whereas the remainder are equally divided between those having one-vessel disease and those having two-vessel disease. Coronary arteriographic studies in surviving patients show that a higher percentage have one-vessel disease. Angiographic studies performed in the earliest hours of STEMI have revealed approximately a 90 percent incidence of total occlusion of the infarct-related vessel.[37] Recanalization from spontaneous thrombolysis as well as attrition due to some mortality among those patients with total occlusion results in a diminishing incidence of angiographically totally occluded vessels in the period following the onset of MI (Fig. 46–8). Pharmacological thrombolysis markedly increases the proportion of patients with a patent infarct-related artery early after STEMI (see Fig. 46–8).

A STEMI with transmural necrosis occurs distal to an acutely totally occluded coronary artery with thrombus superimposed on a ruptured plaque. The converse is not the case, however, in that chronic total occlusion of a coronary artery is not always associated with MI. Collateral blood flow and other factors—such as the level of myocardial metabolism, the presence and location of stenoses in other coronary arteries, the rate of development of the obstruction, and the quantity of myocardium supplied by the obstructed vessel—all influence the viability of myocardial cells distal to the occlusion. In many series of patients studied at necropsy or by coronary arteriography, a small number (5 percent) of patients with STEMI are found to have normal coronary vessels. In these patients, an embolus that has lysed, a transiently occlusive platelet aggregate, or a prolonged episode of severe coronary spasm may have been responsible for the reduction in coronary flow.

Studies of patients who ultimately develop STEMI after having undergone coronary angiography at some time before its occurrence have been helpful in clarifying coronary anatomy before infarction. Although high-grade stenoses, when present, more frequently lead to STEMI than do less severe lesions, the majority of occlusions actually occur in vessels with a previously identified stenosis of less than 50 percent on angiograms performed months to years earlier. This finding supports the

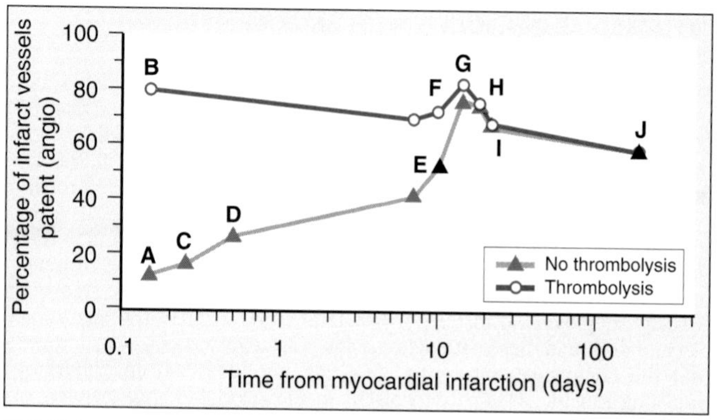

FIGURE 46–8 Comparison of angiographically documented infarct-related coronary artery patency rates in 10 separate clinical studies and time from myocardial infarction as modulated by early administration of a thrombolytic agent versus nonthrombolytic (conventional) therapy. The *x*-axis is a semilogarithmic scale of time in days from myocardial infarction. Note that the difference in patency rates becomes diminishingly small within the first 2 to 3 weeks after infarction. (From Rumberg JA, Gersh BJ: Coronary artery patency and left ventricular remodeling after myocardial infarction: Mechanisms and mechanics. *In* Califf RM, Mark DB, Wagner GS [eds]: Acute Coronary Care. St. Louis, Mosby-Year Book, 1995, p 122.)

concept that STEMI occurs as a result of sudden thrombotic occlusion at the site of rupture of previously nonobstructive but lipid-rich plaques.

When an area of the ventricle is perfused by collateral vessels, an infarct may occur at a distance from a coronary occlusion. For example, following the gradual obliteration of the lumen of the right coronary artery, the inferior wall of the left ventricle can be kept viable by collateral vessels arising from the left anterior descending coronary artery. Later, an occlusion of the left anterior descending artery may cause an infarct of the diaphragmatic wall.

RIGHT VENTRICULAR INFARCTION. Approximately 50 percent of patients with inferior infarction have some involvement of the right ventricle.[38] Among these patients, right ventricular infarction occurs exclusively in those with transmural infarction of the inferoposterior wall and the posterior portion of the septum. Right ventricular infarction almost invariably develops in association with infarction of the adjacent septum and left ventricular myocardium, but isolated infarction of the right ventricle is seen in 3 to 5 percent of autopsy-proven cases of MI (Fig. 46–9).

Regardless of whether it is combined with involvement of the left ventricle, right ventricular infarction is generally associated with obstructive lesions of the right coronary artery. However, right ventricular infarction occurs less commonly than would be anticipated from the frequency of atherosclerotic lesions involving the right coronary artery. This discrepancy probably can be explained by the lower oxygen demands of the right ventricle, because right ventricular infarcts occur more commonly in conditions associated with increased right ventricular oxygen needs such as pulmonary hypertension and right ventricular hypertrophy. Moreover, the intercoronary collateral system of the right ventricle is richer than that of the left, and the thinness of the right ventricular wall allows the chamber to derive some nutrition from the blood within the right ventricular cavity. Therefore, the right ventricle can sustain long periods of ischemia but still demonstrate excellent recovery of contractile function after reperfusion.[39]

ATRIAL INFARCTION. This can be seen in up to 10 percent of patients with STEMI if PR-segment displacement is used as the criterion for atrial infarction. Although isolated atrial infarction is observed in 3.5 percent of autopsies of patients with STEMI, it often occurs in conjunction with ventricular infarction and can cause rupture of the atrial wall.[40] This type of infarct is more common on the right side

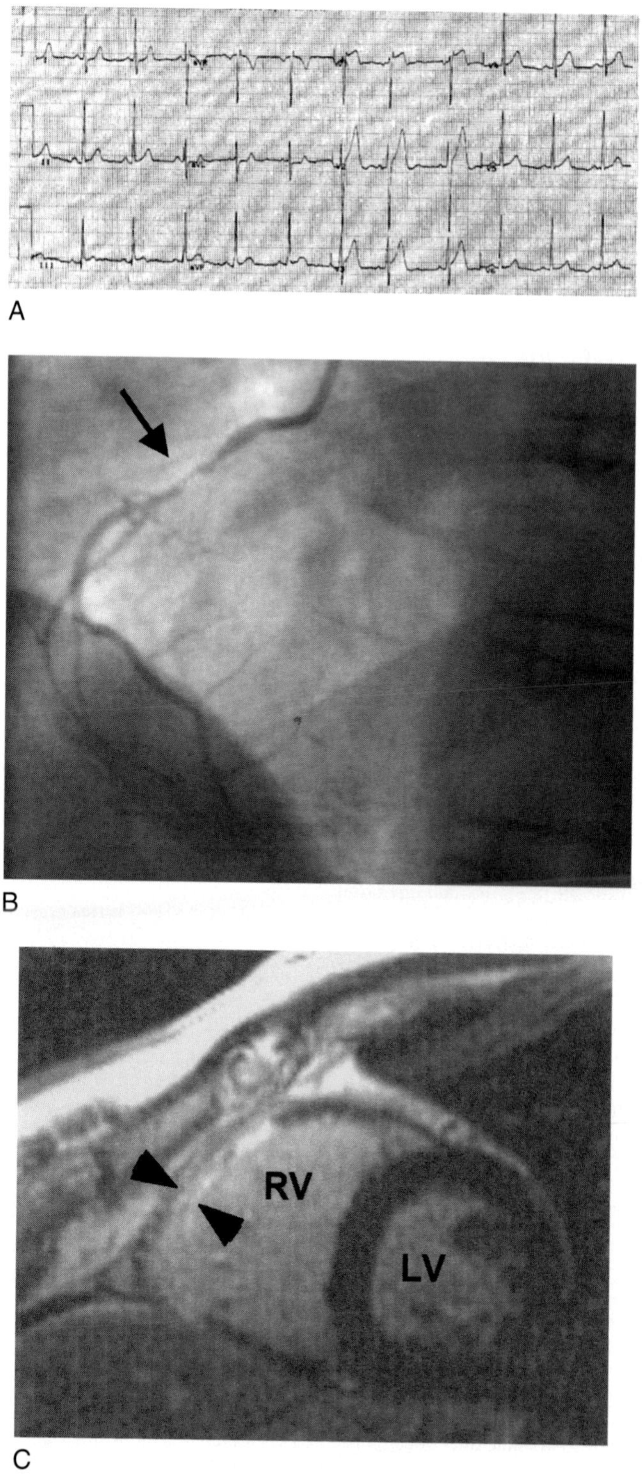

FIGURE 46–9 A 47-year-old man with no prior history of cardiac disease presented to an outside hospital describing "an awesome feeling that just sat in my chest" associated with bilateral arm weakness. The initial electrocardiogram **(A)** revealed ST-segment elevation in the right precordial leads and to a lesser extent in the inferior leads. The patient was treated with fibrinolytic therapy and transferred for catheterization. Angiography revealed a tight stenosis of a proximal nondominant right coronary artery (**B,** arrow) without significant disease in the left coronary artery. Contrast-enhanced cardiac magnetic resonance imaging **(C)** demonstrated delayed hyperenhancement consistent with injury of the right ventricle (RV) with distinct involvement of the right ventricular free wall (arrowhead), sparing the left ventricle (LV) as well as the right ventricular apex. The patient remained hemodynamically stable throughout his hospital course and was discharged home. (From Finn AV, Antman EM: Images in clinical medicine. Isolated right ventricular infarction. N Engl J Med, 349:1636, 2003.)

than on the left side, occurs more frequently in the atrial appendages than in the lateral or posterior walls of the atrium, and can result in thrombus formation. The difference in incidence between right and left atrial infarction might be explained by the considerably higher oxygen content of left atrial blood. Atrial infarction is frequently accompanied by atrial arrhythmias.[41] It has also been reported to be associated with reduced secretion of atrial natriuretic peptide and a low cardiac output syndrome when right ventricular infarction coexists.

COLLATERAL CIRCULATION IN ACUTE MYOCARDIAL INFARCTION (see Chap. 50)

The coronary collateral circulation is particularly well developed in patients with (1) coronary occlusive disease, especially when it is severe, with the reduction of the luminal cross-sectional area by more than 75 percent in one or more major vessels; (2) chronic hypoxia, as occurs in cases of severe anemia, chronic obstructive pulmonary disease, and cyanotic congenital heart disease; and (3) left ventricular hypertrophy, which intensifies coronary collaterals.

The magnitude of coronary collateral flow is one of the principal determinants of infarct size. Indeed, it is rather common for patients with abundant collaterals to have totally occluded coronary arteries without evidence of infarction in the distribution of that artery; thus, the survival of the myocardium distal to such occlusions must depend on collateral blood flow. Even if collateral perfusion existing at the time of coronary occlusion is not successful in preventing infarction, it may still exert a beneficial effect by preventing the formation of a left ventricular aneurysm. Some collaterals are seen in nearly 40 percent of patients with an acute total occlusion, and more begin to appear soon after the total occlusion occurs.[37] It is likely that the presence of a high-grade stenosis (90 percent), possibly with periods of intermittent total occlusion, permits the development of collaterals that remain only as potential conduits until a total occlusion occurs or recurs. Total occlusion then brings these channels into full operation.[42]

The incidence of collaterals 1 to 2 weeks after STEMI varies considerably and may be as high as 75 to 100 percent in patients with persistent occlusion of the infarct vessel, or as low as 17 to 42 percent in patients with subtotal occlusion.

NONATHEROSCLEROTIC CAUSES OF ACUTE MYOCARDIAL INFARCTION

Numerous pathological processes other than atherosclerosis can involve the coronary arteries and result in STEMI (see Table 46-3). For example, coronary arterial occlusions can result from embolization of a coronary artery. Emboli most frequently lodge in the distribution of the left anterior descending coronary artery, commonly in the distal epicardial and intramural branches. The causes of coronary embolism are numerous: infective endocarditis and nonbacterial thrombotic endocarditis (see Chap. 58), mural thrombi, prosthetic valves, neoplasms, air that is introduced at the time of cardiac surgery, and calcium deposits from manipulation of calcified valves at operation. In situ thrombosis of coronary arteries can occur secondary to chest wall trauma (see Chap. 65).

A variety of inflammatory processes can be responsible for coronary artery abnormalities, some of which mimic atherosclerotic disease and may predispose to true atherosclerosis. Epidemiological evidence suggests that viral infections, particularly with coxsackie B, may be an uncommon cause of MI. Viral illnesses precede MI occasionally in young persons who are later shown to have normal coronary arteries.

Syphilitic aortitis can produce marked narrowing or occlusion of one or both coronary ostia, whereas Takayasu arteritis can result in obstruction of the coronary arteries (see Chap. 53). Necrotizing arteritis, polyarteritis nodosa, mucocutaneous lymph node syndrome (Kawasaki disease), systemic lupus erythematosus (see Chap. 82), and giant cell arteritis can cause coronary occlusion. Therapeutic levels of mediastinal radiation can cause thickening and hyalinization of the walls of coronary arteries, with subsequent infarction. MI can also be the result of coronary arterial involvement in patients with amyloidosis (see Chap. 59), Hurler syndrome, pseudoxanthoma elasticum, and homocystinuria.

As cocaine abuse has become more common, reports of MI after the use of cocaine have appeared with increasing frequency (see Chap. 62). Cocaine can cause MI in patients with normal coronary arteries, preexisting MI, documented coronary artery disease, or coronary artery spasm.

MYOCARDIAL INFARCTION WITH ANGIOGRAPHICALLY NORMAL CORONARY VESSELS

Approximately 6 percent of all patients with STEMI and perhaps four times that percentage of patients with this diagnosis younger than 35 years of age do not have coronary atherosclerosis demonstrated by coronary arteriography or at autopsy.[37] Perhaps half of the patients of this group, in turn, have a variety of other lesions involving the coronary vessels or myocardium (see Table 46-3), whereas the others have no detectable coronary obstructive lesions. Patients with STEMI and normal coronary arteries tend to be young and to have relatively few coronary risk factors, except that they often have a history of cigarette smoking. Usually they have no history of angina pectoris prior to the infarction. The infarction in these patients is usually not preceded by any prodrome, but the clinical, laboratory, and ECG features of STEMI are otherwise indistinguishable from those present in the overwhelming majority of patients with STEMI who have classic obstructive atherosclerotic coronary artery disease. In patients who recover, areas of localized dyskinesis and hypokinesis can often be demonstrated by left ventricular angiography. Many of these cases are caused by coronary artery spasm and/or thrombosis, perhaps with underlying endothelial dysfunction or small plaques that are not apparent on coronary angiography.

Additional suggested causes include (1) coronary emboli (perhaps from a small mural thrombus, a prolapsed mitral valve, or a myxoma); (2) coronary artery disease in vessels too small to be visualized by coronary arteriography or coronary arterial thrombosis with subsequent recanalization; (3) a variety of hematological disorders causing in situ thrombosis in the presence of normal coronary arteries (polycythemia vera, cyanotic heart disease with polycythemia, sickle cell anemia, disseminated intravascular coagulation, thrombocytosis, and thrombotic thrombocytopenic purpura); augmented oxygen demand (thyrotoxicosis, amphetamine use); (5) hypotension secondary to sepsis, blood loss, or pharmacological agents; and (6) anatomical variations such as anomalous origin of a coronary artery (see Chap. 56), coronary arteriovenous fistula (see Chap. 56), or a myocardial bridge (see Chap. 18).

PROGNOSIS. The long-term outlook for patients who have survived a STEMI with angiographically normal coronary vessels on arteriography appears to be substantially better than for patients with STEMI and obstructive coronary artery disease. After recovery from the initial infarct, recurrent infarction, heart failure, and death are unusual in patients with normal coronary arteries. Indeed, most of these patients have normal exercise ECGs and only a minority develop angina pectoris.

Pathophysiology

Left Ventricular Function

Systolic Function

Upon interruption of antegrade flow in an epicardial coronary artery, the zone of myocardium supplied by that vessel immediately loses its ability to shorten and perform contractile work. Four abnormal contraction patterns develop in sequence: (1) dyssynchrony, that is, dissociation in the time course of contraction of adjacent segments; (2) hypokinesis, reduction in the extent of shortening; (3) akinesis, cessation of shortening; and (4) dyskinesis, paradoxical expansion, and systolic bulging.[43,44] Accompanying dysfunction of the infarcting segment initially is hyperkinesis of the remaining normal myocardium. The early hyperkinesis of the noninfarcted zones is thought to be the result of acute compensatory mechanisms, including increased activity of the sympathetic nervous system and the Frank-Starling mechanism. A portion of this compensatory hyperkinesis is ineffective work because contraction of the noninfarcted segments of myocardium causes dyskinesis of the infarct zone. Increased motion of the noninfarcted region subsides within 2 weeks of infarction, during which time some degree of recovery can be seen in the infarct region as well, particularly if reperfusion of the infarcted area occurs and myocardial stunning diminishes.

Patients with STEMI often also show reduced myocardial contractile function in noninfarcted zones. This may result from previous obstruction of the coronary artery supplying the noninfarcted region of the ventricle and loss of collaterals from the freshly occluded infarct-related vessel, a condition that has been termed *ischemia at a distance*.[45] Conversely, the presence of collaterals developing before STEMI may allow for greater preservation of regional systolic function in an area of distribution of the occluded artery and improvement in left ventricular ejection fraction early after infarction.

If a sufficient quantity of myocardium undergoes ischemic injury, left ventricular pump function becomes depressed; cardiac output, stroke volume, blood pressure, and peak dP/dt are reduced[44]; and end-systolic volume is increased. The degree to which end-systolic volume increases is perhaps the most powerful predictor of mortality following STEMI.[46] Paradoxical systolic expansion of an area of ventricular myocardium further decreases left ventricular stroke volume. As necrotic myocytes slip past each other, the infarct zone thins and elongates, especially in patients with large anterior infarcts, leading to infarct expansion. As the ventricle dilates during the first few hours to days after infarction, regional and global wall stress increase according to Laplace's law. In some patients, a vicious circle of dilation begetting further dilation is initiated.[47] The degree of ventricular dilation, which depends closely on infarct size, patency of the infarct-related artery,[48,49] and activation of the local renin-angiotensin system in the noninfarcted portion of the ventricle, can be favorably modified by angiotensin-converting enzyme (ACE) inhibition therapy, even in the absence of symptomatic left ventricular dysfunction.[50]

With the passage of time, edema and cellular infiltration and ultimately fibrosis increase the stiffness of the infarcted myocardium back to and beyond control values. Increasing stiffness in the infarcted zone of myocardium improves left ventricular function because it prevents paradoxical systolic wall motion (dyskinesia).

The likelihood of developing clinical symptoms such as dyspnea and ultimately a shock-like state correlate with specific parameters of left ventricular function. The earliest abnormality is a reduction in diastolic compliance (see later), which can be observed with infarcts that involve only 8 percent of the total left ventricle on angiographic examination. When the abnormally contracting segment exceeds 15 percent, the ejection fraction may be reduced and elevations of left ventricular end-diastolic pressure and volume occur. The risk of developing physical signs and symptoms of left ventricular failure also increase proportionally to increasing areas of abnormal left ventricular wall motion.[44] Clinical heart failure accompanies areas of abnormal contraction exceeding 25 percent, and cardiogenic shock, often fatal, accompanies loss of more than 40 percent of the left ventricular myocardium.

Unless infarct extension occurs, some improvement in wall motion takes place during the healing phase, as recovery of function occurs in initially reversibly injured (stunned) myocardium (Fig. 46–7). Regardless of the age of the infarct, patients who continue to demonstrate abnormal wall motion of 20 to 25 percent of the left ventricle are likely to manifest hemodynamic signs of left ventricular failure.

Diastolic Function

The diastolic properties of the left ventricle (see Chap. 21) are altered in infarcted and ischemic myocardium. These changes are associated with a decrease in the peak rate of decline in left ventricular pressure [peak (−)dP/dt], an increase in the time constant of the fall in left ventricular pressure, and an initial rise in left ventricular end-diastolic pressure. Over a period of several weeks, end-diastolic volume increases and diastolic pressure begins to fall toward normal. As with impairment of systolic function, the magnitude of the diastolic abnormality appears to be related to the size of the infarct.

Circulatory Regulation

The abnormality in circulatory regulation that is present in patients with STEMI is diagrammed in Figure 46–10. The process begins with an anatomical or functional obstruction in the coronary vascular bed, which results in regional myocardial ischemia and, if the ischemia persists, in infarction. If the infarct is of sufficient size, it depresses overall left

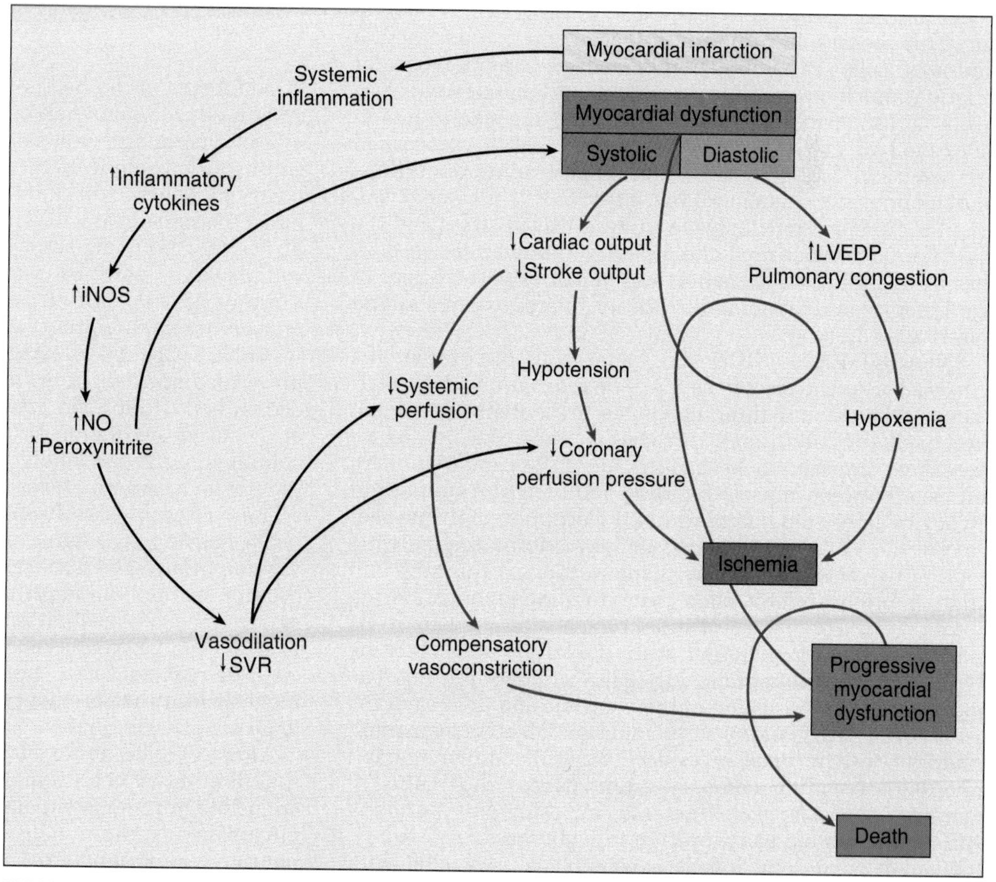

FIGURE 46–10 Classic shock paradigm is shown in black. The influence of the inflammatory response syndrome initiated by a large myocardial infarction is illustrated in red. LVEDP = left ventricular end-diastolic pressure. (From Hochman J: Cardiogenic shock complicating acute myocardial infarction: Expanding the paradigm. Circulation 107:2998, 2003.)

ventricular function so that left ventricular stroke volume falls and filling pressures rise. A marked depression of left ventricular stroke volume ultimately lowers aortic pressure and reduces coronary perfusion pressure; this condition may intensify myocardial ischemia and thereby initiate a vicious circle (see Fig. 46–10). Systemic inflammation leads to the release of cytokines that contribute to vasodilation and a fall in systemic vascular resistance.[51]

The inability of the left ventricle to empty normally also leads to an increased preload; that is, it dilates the well-perfused, normally functioning portion of the left ventricle. This compensatory mechanism tends to restore stroke volume to normal levels, but at the expense of a reduced ejection fraction. The dilation of the left ventricle also elevates ventricular afterload, however, because Laplace's law dictates that at any given arterial pressure, the dilated ventricle must develop a higher wall tension. This increased afterload not only depresses left ventricular stroke volume but also elevates myocardial oxygen consumption, which in turn intensifies myocardial ischemia. When regional myocardial dysfunction is limited and the function of the remainder of the left ventricle is normal, compensatory mechanisms sustain overall left ventricular function. If a large portion of the left ventricle becomes necrotic, pump failure occurs; that is, overall left ventricular function becomes so depressed that the circulation cannot be sustained despite the dilation of the remaining viable portion of the ventricle.

Ventricular Remodeling

As a consequence of STEMI, the changes in left ventricular size, shape, and thickness involving both the infarcted and the noninfarcted segments of the ventricle described earlier occur and are collectively referred to as *ventricular remodeling*. This process, in turn, can influence ventricular function and prognosis.[47] A combination of changes in left ventricular dilation and hypertrophy of residual noninfarcted myocardium is responsible for remodeling. After the size of infarction, the two most important factors driving the process of left ventricular dilation are ventricular loading conditions and infarct artery patency (Fig. 46–11).[47,49,52] Elevated ventricular pressure contributes to increased wall stress and the risk of infarct expansion, and a patent infarct artery accelerates myocardial scar formation and increases tissue turgor in the infarct zone, reducing the risk of infarct expansion and ventricular dilation.

INFARCT EXPANSION. An increase in the size of the infarcted segment, known as *infarct expansion*, is defined as "acute dilation and thinning of the area of infarction not explained by additional myocardial necrosis."[53] Infarct expansion appears to be caused by (1) a combination of slippage between muscle bundles, reducing the number of myocytes across the infarct wall; (2) disruption of the normal myocardial cells; and (3) tissue loss within the necrotic zone.[53] It is characterized by disproportionate thinning and dilation of the infarct zone prior to formation of a firm, fibrotic scar. The degree of infarct expansion appears to be related to the preinfarction wall thickness, with existing hypertrophy possibly protecting against infarct thinning. The apex is the thinnest region of the ventricle and an area of the heart that is particularly vulnerable to infarct expansion.[54] Infarction of the apex secondary to occlusion of the left anterior descending coronary artery causes the radius of curvature at the apex to increase, exposing this normally thin region to a marked elevation in wall stress.

When it is present, infarct expansion is associated with both a higher mortality and a higher incidence of nonfatal complications, such as heart failure and ventricular aneurysm. Infarct expansion has been noted in more than

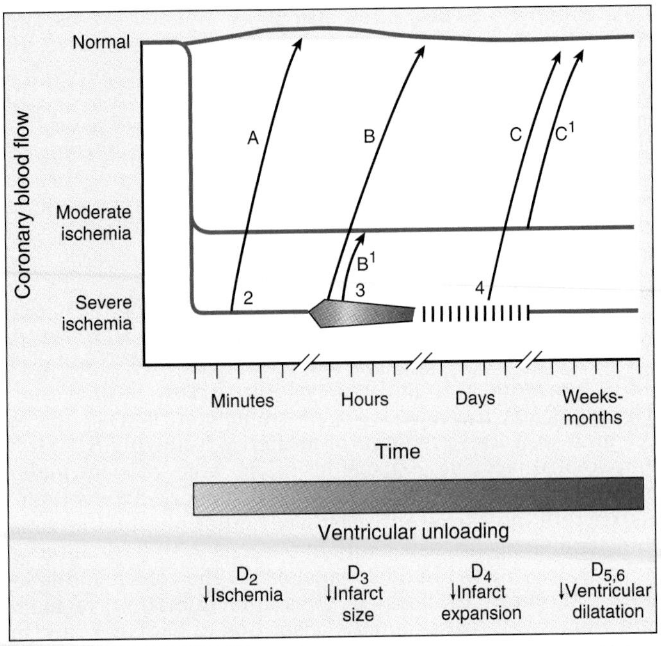

FIGURE 46–11 Therapeutic maneuvers in various stages of ischemia and infarction. Severely ischemic tissue (2) may be reperfused, thereby averting myocardial infarction (A). Infarcting tissue (3) may be reperfused, leading to sparing of myocardial tissue (B). If blood flow is restored only in part B, the myocardium may remain noncontractile although viable, that is, hibernating. After completion of the infarct (4), late reperfusion (C) may still be useful. Mechanical reperfusion of moderately ischemic myocardium (C) may restore contractility of hibernating myocardium to normal. Ventricular unloading may be useful throughout the preinfarct and postinfarct periods. Unloading may reduce ischemia (D_2), infarct size (D_3), infarct expansion (D_4), and ventricular dilatation ($D_{5,6}$). (From Braunwald E, Pfeffer MA: Ventricular enlargement and remodeling following acute myocardial infarction: Mechanisms and management. Am J Cardiol 68:4D, 1991.)

three-fourths of the hearts of patients succumbing to STEMI and one-third to one-half of all patients with anterior Q-wave infarctions. Infarct expansion is best recognized echocardiographically as elongation of the noncontractile region of the ventricle. When expansion is severe enough to cause symptoms, the most characteristic clinical finding is deterioration of systolic function associated with new or louder gallop sounds and new or worsening pulmonary congestion. Rupture of the ventricle may be considered to be a consequence of extreme infarct expansion.

VENTRICULAR DILATION. Although infarct expansion plays an important role in the ventricular remodeling that occurs early following myocardial infarction, remodeling is also caused by dilation of the viable portion of the ventricle, commencing immediately after STEMI and progressing for months or years thereafter (see Fig. 46–11). Dilation may be accompanied by a shift of the pressure-volume curve of the left ventricle to the right, resulting in a larger left ventricular volume at any given diastolic pressure (see Chap. 21). This dilation of the noninfarct zone can be viewed as a compensatory mechanism that maintains stroke volume in the face of a large infarction. However, ventricular dilation is also associated with nonuniform repolarization of the myocardium that predisposes the patient to life-threatening ventricular arrhythmias.

After STEMI, an extra load is placed on the residual functioning myocardium, a load that presumably is responsible for the compensatory hypertrophy of the uninfarcted myocardium. This hypertrophy could help to compensate for the functional impairment caused by the infarct and may be responsible for some of the hemodynamic improvement seen in the months after infarction in some patients.

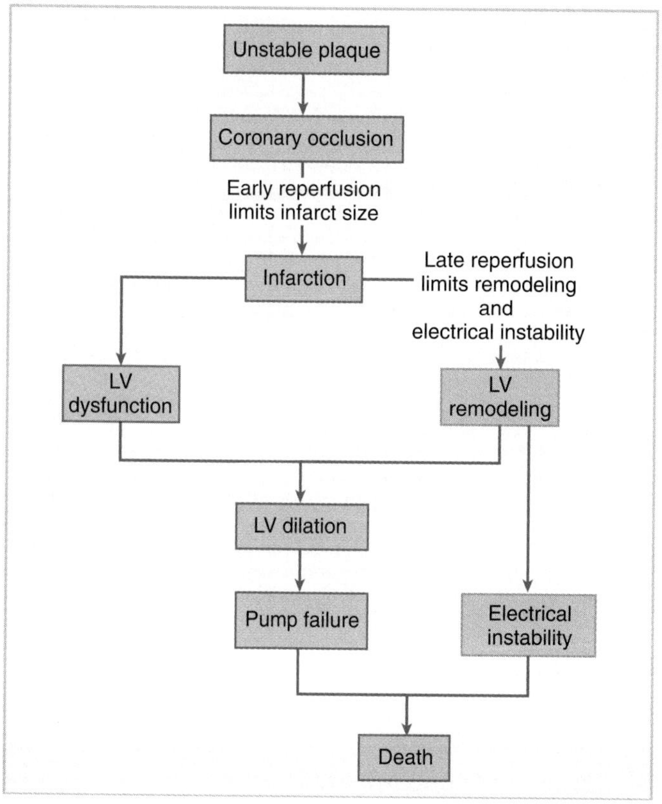

FIGURE 46–12 Flow chart showing postulated sequence of events from an unstable atherosclerotic plaque to death. The original paradigm emphasizing early reperfusion is shown at the left; the expanded paradigm illustrating the benefits of late reperfusion is shown at the right. LV = left ventricular. (Modified from Kim CB, Braunwald E: Potential benefits of late reperfusion of infarcted myocardium: The open artery hypothesis. Circulation 88:2426, 1993. Copyright 1993 American Heart Association.)

EFFECTS OF TREATMENT. Ventricular remodeling after STEMI can be affected by several factors, the first of which is infarct size (see Fig. 46–11). Acute reperfusion and other measures to restrict the extent of myocardial necrosis limit the increase in ventricular volume after STEMI, and evidence suggests that an open infarct artery per se, achieved even late after coronary occlusion, also attenuates ventricular enlargement (Fig. 46–12).[49] The second factor is scar formation in the infarct. Glucocorticosteroids and nonsteroidal antiinflammatory agents given early after MI can cause scar thinning and greater infarct expansion, whereas ACE inhibitors[47] attenuate ventricular enlargement (see Figs. 46–11 and 46–12). Additional beneficial consequences of inhibition of angiotensin II that may contribute to myocardial protection include attenuation of endothelial dysfunction and direct antiatherogenic effects.[55]

Pathophysiology of Other Organ Systems

PULMONARY FUNCTION

Changes in pulmonary gas exchange, ventilation, and distribution of perfusion occur with STEMI. There is an inverse relationship between arterial oxygen tension and pulmonary artery diastolic pressure. This suggests that increased pulmonary capillary hydrostatic pressure leads to interstitial edema, which results in arteriolar and bronchiolar compression that ultimately causes perfusion of poorly ventilated alveoli with resultant hypoxemia (see Chap. 22). In addition to hypoxemia, there is a fall in diffusing capacity. Hyperventilation often occurs in patients with STEMI and may cause hypocapnia and respiratory alkalosis, particularly in restless, anxious patients with pain. With reversal of heart failure, hypoxemia and intrapulmonary shunting diminish.

INCREASE IN INTERSTITIAL WATER. A positive correlation has been demonstrated between pulmonary extravascular (interstitial) water content, left ventricular filling pressure, and the clinical signs and symptoms of left ventricular failure. The increase in pulmonary extravascular water may be responsible for the alterations in pulmonary mechanics observed in patients with STEMI; that is, reduction of airway conductance, pulmonary compliance, forced expiratory volume and midexpiratory flow rate, and an increase in closing volume, the last presumably related to the widespread closure of small, dependent airways during the first 3 days after STEMI. Ultimately, severe increases in extravascular water may lead to pulmonary edema. Recovery of left ventricular function or diuresis reduces back to normal the abnormally elevated values for closing volumes, such as the lung volume at which airway closure commences.

The "closing volume" can encroach on and sometimes exceed functional residual volume. This can lead to arterial hypoxemia by the shunting of blood through alveoli that are not well ventilated.

REDUCTION OF VITAL CAPACITY. Virtually all lung volume indices—total lung capacity, functional residual capacity, and residual volume, as well as vital capacity—fall in the presence of STEMI.[56] These reductions correlate with the elevations of left-sided filling pressures and are most probably due to increases in pulmonary extravascular water. Lung volumes, oxygenation, and airway resistance all return toward normal by the time of hospital discharge for most patients. Increased pulmonary venous pressure also results in redistribution of pulmonary blood flow from the bases to the apices of the lung in patients with STEMI, altering the relationship between ventilation and perfusion. At follow-up examination 3 to 25 weeks after STEMI, however, the ventilation-perfusion relationship has usually returned to normal or almost so.

REDUCTION OF AFFINITY OF HEMOGLOBIN FOR OXYGEN. In patients with MI, particularly when complicated by left ventricular failure or cardiogenic shock, the affinity of hemoglobin for oxygen is reduced; that is, the P_{50} is increased. The increase in P_{50} results from increased levels of erythrocyte 2,3-diphosphoglycerate (2,3-DPG), which constitutes an important compensatory mechanism, responsible for an estimated 18 percent increase in oxygen release from oxyhemoglobin in patients with cardiogenic shock.

ENDOCRINE FUNCTION

PANCREAS. Hyperglycemia and impaired glucose tolerance are common in patients with STEMI. Although the absolute levels of blood insulin are often in the normal range, they are usually inappropriately low for the level of blood sugar, and there may be relative insulin resistance as well. Patients with cardiogenic shock often demonstrate marked hyperglycemia and depressed levels of circulating insulin, often with complete suppression of insulin secretion in response to tolbutamide. These abnormalities in insulin secretion and the resultant impaired glucose tolerance appear to be secondary to a reduction in pancreatic blood flow as a consequence of splanchnic vasoconstriction accompanying severe left ventricular failure. In addition, increased activity of the sympathetic nervous system with augmented circulating catecholamines inhibits insulin secretion and augments glycogenolysis, also contributing to the elevation of blood sugar.[57]

Glucose appears to be a more favorable energy source than free fatty acids for the ischemic myocardium by more efficiently replenishing the Krebs cycle and stimulating contractile performance.[58] Because hypoxic heart muscle derives a considerable portion of its energy from the metabolism of glucose (see Chap. 19) and because insulin is essential for the uptake of glucose by the myocardium as well as for myocardial protein synthesis and inhibition of lysosomal activity, the deleterious effects of insulin deficiency are clear. These metabolic considerations, combined with epidemiological observations that diabetic patients have a markedly worse prognosis, have served as the foundation for efforts to more aggressively administer insulin-glucose infusions to diabetic patients with STEMI.

ADRENAL MEDULLA. Excessive secretion of catecholamines produces many of the characteristic signs and symptoms of STEMI. The plasma and urinary catecholamine levels are highest during the first 24 hours after the onset of chest pain,[57] with the greatest rise in plasma catecholamine secretion occurring during the first hour after the onset of STEMI. These high levels of circulating catecholamines in patients with STEMI correlate with the occurrence of serious arrhythmias and result in an increase in myocardial oxygen consumption, both directly and indirectly, as a consequence of catecholamine-induced elevation of circulating free fatty acids. As might be anticipated, the concentration of circulating catecholamines correlates with the extent of myocardial damage and incidence of cardiogenic shock, as well as both early and late mortality rates.

Circulating catecholamines enhance platelet aggregation; when this occurs in the coronary microcirculation, the release of the potent local vasoconstrictor thromboxane A_2 may further impair cardiac perfusion. The marked increase in sympathetic activity associated with STEMI serves as the foundation for beta-adrenoceptor blocker regimens in the acute phase.

LOCAL MYOCARDIAL AND SYSTEMIC RENIN-ANGIOTENSIN SYSTEM. Noninfarcted regions of the myocardium appear to exhibit activation of the tissue renin-angiotensin system with increased angiotensin II production. Both locally and systemically generated angiotensin II can stimulate the production of various growth factors, such as platelet-derived growth factor and transforming growth factor, that promote compensatory hypertrophy in the noninfarcted myocardium as well as control the structure and tone of the infarct-related coronary and other myocardial vessels. Additional potential actions of angiotensin II that have a more negative impact on the infarction process include release of endothelin, PAI-1, and aldosterone, which may cause vasoconstriction, impaired fibrinolysis, and increased sodium retention, respectively. Inhibition of generation of circulating and tissue angiotensin II is one of the proposed mechanisms of benefit from ACE inhibitors in STEMI.

NATRIURETIC PEPTIDES. The peptides atrial natriuretic factor (ANF) and N-terminal pro-ANF are released from cardiac atria in response to elevation of atrial pressure. Brain natriuretic peptide (BNP), originally isolated from porcine brain, has been shown to be secreted by human ventricular myocardium (see Chap. 21). It appears to be released early after STEMI, peaking at about 16 hours. Patients with anterior infarction, lower cardiac index, and more significant congestive heart failure after STEMI have higher levels of BNP and also show a second peak of BNP release about 5 days after infarction. These intriguing observations suggest that BNP levels may be a marker of the degree of left ventricular dysfunction in patients with STEMI and that markedly elevated levels of BNP correlate with a worse prognosis.[59-61]

ADRENAL CORTEX. Plasma and urinary 17-hydroxycorticosteroids and ketosteroids, as well as aldosterone, are also markedly elevated in patients with STEMI.[57] Their concentrations correlate directly with the peak level of serum CK, implying that the stress imposed by larger infarcts is associated with greater secretion of adrenal steroids. The magnitude of the elevation of cortisol correlates with infarct size and mortality. Glucocorticosteroids also contribute to the impairment of glucose tolerance.

THYROID GLAND. Although patients with STEMI are generally euthyroid clinically, there is evidence of a transient decrease in serum triiodothyronine (T_3) levels, a fall that is most marked on about the third day after the infarct. This fall in T_3 is usually accompanied by a rise in reverse T_3, with variable changes or no change in thyroxine (T_4) and thyroid-stimulating hormone (TSH) levels. The alteration in peripheral T_4 metabolism appears to correlate with infarct size and may be mediated by the rise in endogenous levels of cortisol that accompanies STEMI.

RENAL FUNCTION

Both prerenal azotemia and acute renal failure can complicate the marked reduction of cardiac output that occurs in cardiogenic shock. On the other hand, an increase in circulating atrial natriuretic peptide occurs following STEMI, which is correlated with the severity of left ventricular failure. An increase in natriuretic peptide is also found when right ventricular infarction accompanies inferior wall infarction, suggesting that this hormone may play a role in the hypotension that accompanies right ventricular infarction.

HEMATOLOGICAL FUNCTION

PLATELETS. STEMI generally occurs in the presence of extensive coronary and systemic atherosclerotic plaques, which may serve as the site for the formation of platelet aggregates, a sequence that has been suggested as the initial step in the process of coronary thrombosis, coronary occlusion, and subsequent MI. Circulating platelets are hyperaggregable in patients with STEMI. Platelets from STEMI patients have an increased propensity for aggregation locally in the area of a disrupted plaque and also release vasoactive substances such as thromboxane A_2.[27]

HEMOSTATIC MARKERS. Elevated levels of serum fibrinogen degradation products, an end-product of thrombosis, as well as release of distinctive proteins when platelets are activated, such as platelet factor 4 and beta-thromboglobulin, have been reported in some patients with STEMI. Fibrinopeptide A, a protein released from fibrin by thrombin, is a marker of ongoing thrombosis and is increased during the early hours of STEMI. Marked elevation of hemostatic markers such as FPA, TAT, and F1&2 is associated with an increased risk of mortality in STEMI patients[62] (see Chap. 80). The interpretation of the coagulation tests in patients with STEMI may be complicated by elevated blood levels of catecholamines, concomitant shock, and/or pulmonary embolism, conditions that are all capable of altering various tests of platelet and coagulation function.

LEUKOCYTES. STEMI is usually accompanied by leukocytosis, which is related to the magnitude of the necrotic process, elevated glucocorticoid levels, and possibly inflammation in the coronary arteries. The magnitude of elevation of the leukocyte count is associated with in-hospital mortality after STEMI.[63] Activation of neutrophils may produce important intermediates, such as leukotriene B_4 and oxygen free radicals, which have important microcirculatory effects.

BLOOD VISCOSITY. Clinical and epidemiological studies suggest that several hemostatic and hemorheological factors (e.g., fibrinogen, factor VII, plasma viscosity, hematocrit, red blood cell aggregation, total white blood cell count) are involved in the pathophysiology of atherosclerosis and also play an integral role in acute thrombotic events. An increase in blood viscosity also occurs in patients with STEMI. During the first few days after infarction, this is mainly attributable to hemoconcentration, but later the increases in plasma viscosity and red blood cell aggregation correlate with elevated serum concentrations of alpha$_2$-globulin and fibrinogen, which are nonspecific reactions to tissue necrosis and are also responsible for the elevated sedimentation rate characteristic of STEMI. The high values of blood viscosity indices are observed most frequently in patients with complications such as left ventricular failure, cardiogenic shock, and thromboembolism.

Clinical Features

Predisposing Factors

The risk factors for atherosclerotic coronary artery disease are discussed in Chapter 36.

In as many as one-half of patients with STEMI, a precipitating factor or prodromal symptoms can be identified. Evidence suggests that unusually heavy exercise (particularly in fatigued or emotionally stressed, habitually inactive patients) may play a role in precipitating STEMI.[64] Such infarctions could be the result of marked increases in myocardial oxygen consumption in the presence of severe coronary arterial narrowing. Patients with known coronary disease who have been hospitalized for treatment of an acute coronary syndrome–related event and who subsequently report a high level of stress in their life have an increased risk of rehospitalization for cardiovascular reasons and also for "hard" events such as death and myocardial infarction.

Accelerating angina and rest angina, two patterns of unstable angina, may culminate in STEMI (see Fig. 46–1). Noncardiac surgical procedures have also been noted as precursors of STEMI. Perioperative risk stratification and the use of beta blockers may reduce the likelihood of STEMI and cardiac-related mortality (see Chap. 77).[65] Reduced myocardial perfusion secondary to hypotension (e.g., hemorrhagic or septic shock) and increased myocardial oxygen demands secondary to aortic stenosis, fever, tachycardia, and agitation can also be responsible for myocardial necrosis. Other factors reported as predisposing to STEMI include respiratory infections, hypoxemia of any cause, pulmonary embolism, hypoglycemia, administration of ergot preparations, use of cocaine, sympathomimetics, serum sickness, allergy, and, on rare occasion, wasp stings. In patients with Prinzmetal angina (see Chap. 49), STEMI may develop in the territory of the coronary artery that repeatedly undergoes spasm.[66] Rarely, munition workers exposed to high concentrations of nitroglycerin develop MI when they are withdrawn from this exposure, suggesting that it is caused by vasospasm.

CIRCADIAN PERIODICITY. An analysis of a large number of patients hospitalized with MI, studied as a part of the Multicenter Investigation of Limitation of Infarct Size (MILIS), revealed a pronounced circadian periodicity for the time of onset of STEMI, with peak incidence of events between 6 AM and 12 noon. This observation has been confirmed repeatedly.[64] Circadian rhythms affect many physiological and biochemical parameters; the early morning hours are associated with rises in plasma catecholamines and cortisol and increases in platelet aggregability.[67] Interestingly, the characteristic circadian peak was *absent* in patients receiving beta blocker or aspirin before their presentation with STEMI. The concept of "triggering" a STEMI is a complex one and likely involves the superimposition of multiple factors such as time of day, season, and the stress of natural disasters.[64]

History

PRODROMAL SYMPTOMS. Despite advances in the laboratory detection of STEMI, the patient's history remains of substantial value in establishing a diagnosis. The prodrome is usually characterized by chest discomfort, resembling classic angina pectoris, but it occurs at rest or with less activity than usual and can therefore be classified as unstable angina. However, it is often not disturbing enough to induce patients to seek medical attention, and if they do, they may not be hospitalized. A feeling of general malaise or frank exhaustion often accompanies other symptoms preceding STEMI.

NATURE OF THE PAIN (see Chap. 7). The pain of STEMI is variable in intensity; in most patients, it is severe and in some instances intolerable. The pain is prolonged, usually lasting for more than 30 minutes and frequently for a number of hours. The discomfort is described as constricting, crushing, oppressing, or compressing; often the patient complains of a sensation of a heavy weight or a squeezing in the chest. Although the discomfort is typically described as a choking, vise-like, or heavy pain, it can also be characterized as a stabbing, knife-like, boring, or burning discomfort. The pain is usually retrosternal in location, spreading frequently to both sides of the anterior chest, with predilection for the left side. Often the pain radiates down the ulnar aspect of the left arm, producing a tingling sensation in the left wrist, hand, and fingers. Some patients note only a dull ache or numbness of the wrists in association with severe substernal or precordial discomfort. In some instances, the pain of STEMI may begin in the epigastrium and simulate a variety of abdominal disorders, a fact that often causes STEMI to be misdiagnosed as "indigestion." In other patients, the discomfort of STEMI radiates to the shoulders, upper extremities, neck, jaw, and interscapular region, again usually favoring the left side. In patients with preexisting angina pectoris, the pain of infarction usually resembles that of angina with respect to location. However, it is generally much more severe, lasts longer, and is not relieved by rest and nitroglycerin.

The pain of STEMI may have disappeared by the time the physician first encounters the patient (or the patient reaches the hospital), or it may persist for many hours. Opiates, in particular morphine, usually relieve the pain. Both angina pectoris and the pain of STEMI are thought to arise from nerve endings in ischemic or injured, but not necrotic, myocardium. Thus, in cases of STEMI, stimulation of nerve fibers in an ischemic zone of myocardium surrounding the necrotic central area of infarction probably gives rise to the pain.

The pain often disappears suddenly and completely when blood flow to the infarct territory is restored. In patients in whom reocclusion occurs after thrombolysis, pain recurs if the initial reperfusion has left viable myocardium. Thus, what has previously been thought of as the "pain of infarction," sometimes lasting for many hours, probably represents pain caused by ongoing ischemia. The recognition that pain implies ischemia and not infarction heightens the importance of seeking ways to relieve the ischemia, for which the pain is a marker. This finding suggests that the clinician should not be complacent about ongoing cardiac pain under any circumstances. In some patients, particularly the elderly, STEMI is manifested clinically not by chest pain but rather by symptoms of acute left ventricular failure and chest tightness or by marked weakness or frank syncope. These symptoms may be accompanied by diaphoresis, nausea, and vomiting.

OTHER SYMPTOMS. Nausea and vomiting may occur, presumably owing to activation of the vagal reflex or to stimulation of left ventricular receptors as part of the Bezold-Jarisch reflex. These symptoms occur more commonly in patients with inferior STEMI than in those with anterior STEMI. Moreover, nausea and vomiting are common side effects of opiates. When the pain of STEMI is epigastric in location and is associated with nausea and vomiting, the clinical picture can easily be confused with that of acute cholecystitis, gastritis, or peptic ulcer. Occasionally, a patient complains of diarrhea or a violent urge to evacuate the bowels during the acute phase of STEMI. Other symptoms include feelings of profound weakness, dizziness, palpitations, cold perspiration, and a sense of impending doom. On occasion, symptoms arising from an episode of cerebral embolism or other systemic arterial embolism are the first signs of STEMI. The aforementioned symptoms may or may not be accompanied by chest pain.

Differential Diagnosis

The pain of STEMI may simulate the pain of acute pericarditis (see Chap. 64), which is usually associated with some pleuritic features: it is aggravated by respiratory movements and coughing and often involves the shoulder, ridge of the trapezius, and neck. An important feature that distinguishes pericardial pain from ischemic discomfort is that ischemic discomfort never radiates to the trapezius ridge, a characteristic site of radiation of pericardial pain.[68] Pleural pain is usually sharp, knife-like, and aggravated in a cyclical fashion by each breath, which distinguishes it from the deep, dull, steady pain of STEMI. Pulmonary embolism (see Chap. 66) generally produces pain laterally in the chest, is often pleuritic in nature, and may be associated with hemoptysis. The pain due to acute aortic dissection (see Chap. 53) is usually localized to the center of the chest, is extremely severe and described by the patient as a "ripping" or "tearing" sensation, is at its maximal intensity shortly after onset, persists for many hours, and often radiates to the back or the lower extremities. Often one or more major arterial pulses are absent. Pain arising from the costochondral and chondrosternal articulations may be associated with localized swelling and redness; it is usually sharp and "darting" and is characterized by marked localized tenderness. Episodes of retrosternal discomfort induced by peristalsis in patients with increased esophageal stiffness and also episodes of sustained esophageal contraction can mimic the pain of STEMI.[69]

SILENT STEMI AND ATYPICAL PRESENTATION. Nonfatal STEMI can be unrecognized by the patient and discovered only on subsequent routine electrocardiographic or postmortem examinations. Of these unrecognized infarctions, approximately half are truly silent, with the patients unable to recall any symptoms whatsoever. The other half of patients with so-called silent infarction can recall an event characterized by symptoms compatible with acute infarction when leading questions are posed after the electrocardiographic abnormalities are discovered. Unrecognized or silent infarction occurs more commonly in patients without antecedent angina pectoris and in patients with diabetes and hypertension.[70] Silent STEMI is often followed by silent ischemia (see Chap. 50). The prognoses of patients with silent and symptomatic presentations of STEMI appear to be similar.

Atypical presentations of STEMI include the following: (1) heart failure, that is, dyspnea without pain beginning de novo or worsening of established failure; (2) classic angina pectoris without a particularly severe or prolonged episode; (3) atypical location of the pain; (4) central nervous system manifestations, resembling those of stroke, secondary to a sharp reduction in cardiac output in a patient with cerebral arteriosclerosis; (5) apprehension and nervousness; (6) sudden mania or psychosis; (7) syncope; (8) overwhelming weakness; (9) acute indigestion; and (10) peripheral embolization.

Physical Examination

GENERAL APPEARANCE. Patients suffering STEMI often appear anxious and in considerable distress. An anguished facial expression is common, and—in contrast to patients with severe angina pectoris, who often lie, sit, or stand still, recognizing that all forms of activity increase the discomfort—some patients suffering STEMI may be restless and move about in an effort to find a comfortable position. They often massage or clutch their chests and frequently describe their pain with a clenched fist held against the sternum (the Levine sign, named after Dr. Samuel A. Levine). In patients with left ventricular failure and sympathetic stimulation, cold perspiration and skin pallor may be evident; they typically sit or are propped up in bed, gasping for breath. Between breaths, they may complain of chest discomfort or a feeling of suffocation. Cough productive of frothy, pink, or blood-streaked sputum is common.

Patients in cardiogenic shock often lie listlessly, making few if any spontaneous movements. The skin is cool and clammy, with a bluish or mottled color over the extremities, and there is marked facial pallor with severe cyanosis of the lips and nailbeds. Depending on the degree of cerebral perfusion, the patient in shock may converse normally or may evidence confusion and disorientation.

HEART RATE. The heart rate can vary from a marked bradycardia to a rapid regular or irregular tachycardia, depending on the underlying rhythm and the degree of left ventricular failure. Most commonly, the pulse is rapid and regular initially (sinus tachycardia at 100 to 110 beats/min), slowing as the patient's pain and anxiety are relieved; premature ventricular beats are common, occurring in more than 95 percent of patients evaluated within the first 4 hours after the onset of symptoms.

BLOOD PRESSURE. The majority of patients with uncomplicated STEMI are normotensive, although the reduced stroke volume accompanying the tachycardia can cause declines in systolic and pulse pressures and elevation of diastolic pressure. Among previously normotensive patients, a hypertensive response occasionally is seen during the first few hours, with the arterial pressure exceeding 160/90 mm Hg, presumably as a consequence of adrenergic discharge secondary to pain anxiety and agitation. It is common for previously hypertensive patients to become normotensive without treatment after STEMI, although many of these previously hypertensive patients eventually regain their elevated levels of blood pressure, generally 3 to 6 months after infarction. In patients with massive infarction, arterial pressure falls acutely, owing to left ventricular dysfunction and venous pooling secondary to administration of morphine or nitrates or both; as recovery occurs, the arterial pressure tends to return to preinfarction levels.

Patients in cardiogenic shock by definition have systolic pressures below 90 mm Hg and evidence of end-organ hypoperfusion. However, hypotension alone does not necessarily signify cardiogenic shock, because some patients with inferior infarction in whom the Bezold-Jarisch reflex is activated may also transiently have systolic blood pressure below 90 mm Hg. Their hypotension eventually resolves spontaneously, although the process can be accelerated by intravenous atropine (0.5-1.0 mg) and assumption of the Trendelenburg position. Other patients who are initially only slightly hypotensive may demonstrate gradually falling blood pressures with progressive reduction in cardiac output over several hours or days as they develop cardiogenic shock as a consequence of increasing ischemia and extension of infarction (see Fig. 46–10). Evidence of autonomic hyperactivity is common, varying in type with the location of the infarction. At some time in their initial presentation, more than half of patients with inferior STEMI have evidence of excess parasympathetic stimulation, with hypotension, bradycardia, or both, whereas about half of patients with anterior STEMI show signs of sympathetic excess, having hypertension, tachycardia, or both.[71]

TEMPERATURE AND RESPIRATION. Most patients with extensive STEMI develop fever, a nonspecific response to tissue necrosis, within 24 to 48 hours of the onset of infarction. Body temperature often begins to rise within 4 to 8 hours after the onset of infarction, and rectal temperature may reach 38.3° to 38.9° C (101°-102° F). Fever usually resolves by the fourth or fifth day after infarction.

The respiratory rate may be slightly elevated soon after the development of STEMI; in patients without heart failure, it results from anxiety and pain because it returns to normal with treatment of physical and psychological discomfort. In patients with left ventricular failure, the respiratory rate correlates with the severity of failure; patients with pulmonary edema may have respiratory rates exceeding 40 per minute. However, the respiratory rate is not necessarily elevated in patients with cardiogenic shock. Cheyne-Stokes (periodic) respiration (see Chap. 8) may occur in elderly individuals with cardiogenic shock and heart failure, particularly after opiate therapy and in the presence of cerebrovascular disease.

JUGULAR VENOUS PULSE. The height and contour of the jugular venous pulse reflect right atrial and right ventricular diastolic pressures (see Chap. 8). Because these pressures are usually normal or only slightly elevated in patients with STEMI (even in the presence of mild to moderate left ventricular failure), it is not surprising that usually the jugular venous pulse fails to show any abnormalities. The *a* wave may be prominent in patients with pulmonary hypertension secondary to left ventricular failure or reduced compliance. In contrast, right ventricular infarction (whether or not it accompanies left ventricular infarction) often results in marked jugular venous distention and, when it is complicated by necrosis or ischemia of right ventricular papillary muscles, tall *c-v* waves of tricuspid regurgitation are evident. In patients with STEMI and cardiogenic shock, the jugular venous pressure is usually elevated. In patients with STEMI, hypotension, and hypoperfusion (findings that may resemble those of patients with cardiogenic shock) but who have flat neck veins, it is likely that the depression of left ventricular performance may be related, at least in part, to hypovolemia. The differentiation can be made only by assessing left ventricular performance using echocardiography or by measuring left ventricular filling pressure with a pulmonary artery flotation catheter.

CAROTID PULSE. Palpation of the carotid arterial pulse provides a clue to the left ventricular stroke volume; a small pulse suggests a reduced stroke volume, whereas a sharp, brief upstroke is often observed in patients with mitral regurgitation or ruptured ventricular septum with a left-to-right shunt. Pulsus alternans reflects severe left ventricular dysfunction.

THE CHEST. Moist rales are audible in patients who develop left ventricular failure and/or a reduction of left ventricular compliance with STEMI. Diffuse wheezing can present in patients with severe left ventricular failure. Cough with hemoptysis, suggesting pulmonary embolism with infarction, can also occur. In 1967, Killip proposed a prognostic classification scheme based on the presence and severity of rales detected in patients presenting with STEMI.[72] Class I patients are free of rales and a third heart sound. Class II patients have rales but only to a mild to moderate degree (<50 percent of lung fields) and may or may not have an S_3. Patients in class III have rales in more than half of each lung field and frequently have pulmonary edema. Finally, class IV patients are in cardiogenic shock. Despite overall improvement in mortality rate in each class, compared with data observed during the original development of the classification scheme, the classification scheme remains useful today as evidenced by data from large MI trials of STEMI patients.[18,73]

Cardiac Examination

PALPATION. Despite severe symptoms and extensive myocardial damage, the findings on examination of the heart may be quite unremarkable in patients with STEMI. Palpation of the precordium may yield normal findings, but in patients with transmural STEMI, it more commonly reveals a presystolic pulsation, synchronous with an audible fourth heart sound, reflecting a vigorous left atrial contraction filling a ventricle with reduced compliance. In the presence of left ventricular systolic dysfunction, an outward movement of the left ventricle can be palpated in early diastole, coincident with a third heart sound.

AUSCULTATION (see Chap. 8). The heart sounds, particularly the first sound, are frequently muffled and occasionally inaudible immediately after the infarct, and their intensity increases during convalescence. A soft first heart sound may also reflect prolongation of the P-R interval. Patients with marked ventricular dysfunction and/or left bundle branch block may have paradoxical splitting of the second heart sound.

A fourth heart sound is almost universally present in patients in sinus rhythm with STEMI and is usually best heard between the left sternal border and the apex. This sound reflects the atrial contribution to ventricular filling and is particularly prominent in STEMI patients due to a reduction in left ventricular compliance and elevation of left ventricular end-diastolic pressure, even in the absence of left ventricular systolic dysfunction. This finding is of limited diagnostic value because it is commonly audible in most patients with chronic ischemic heart disease and is recordable, although not often audible, in many normal subjects older than 45 years.

A third heart sound in patients with STEMI usually reflects severe left ventricular dysfunction with elevated ventricular filling pressure. It is caused by rapid deceleration of transmitral blood flow during protodiastolic filling of the left ventricle with resultant oscillations of the cardiohemic system (i.e., myocardium and stream of blood flowing from left atrium to left ventricle) and is usually heard in patients with large infarctions. This sound is detected best at the apex, with the patient in the left lateral recumbent position, and is more common in patients with transmural anterior infarctions than in those with inferior or nontransmural infarctions. A third heart sound may be caused not only by left ventricular failure but also by increased inflow into the left ventricle, as occurs when mitral regurgitation or ventricular septal defect complicates STEMI (see Chap. 8). Third and fourth heart sounds emanating from the left ventricle are heard best at the apex; in patients with right ventricular infarcts, these sounds can be heard along the left sternal border and are intensified by inspiration.

Systolic murmurs, transient or persistent, are commonly audible in patients with STEMI and generally result from mitral regurgitation secondary to dysfunction of the mitral valve apparatus (papillary muscle dysfunction, left ventricular dilation). A new, prominent, apical holosystolic murmur, accompanied by a thrill, may represent rupture of a head of a papillary muscle. The findings in cases of rupture of the interventricular septum are similar, although the murmur and thrill are usually most prominent along the left sternal border and may be audible at the right sternal border as well. The systolic murmur of tricuspid regurgitation (caused by right ventricular failure due to pulmonary hypertension and/or right ventricular infarction or by infarction of a right ventricular papillary muscle) is also heard along the left sternal border. It is characteristically intensified by inspiration and is accompanied by a prominent *c-v* wave in the jugular venous pulse and a right ventricular fourth sound.

Pericardial friction rubs may be heard in patients with STEMI, especially those sustaining large transmural infarctions.[68] Rubs are notorious for their evanescence and hence are probably even more common than reported; frequent auscultation in patients with transmural infarction often results in the discovery of a rub that might otherwise have gone unnoticed. Although friction rubs can be heard within 24 hours or as late as 2 weeks after the onset of infarction, most commonly they are noted on the second or third day.[68] Occasionally, in patients with extensive infarction, a loud rub can be heard for many days. Patients with STEMI and a pericardial friction rub may have a pericardial effusion on echocardiographic study, but only rarely are the classic electrocardiographic changes of pericarditis seen.[68] Delayed onset of the rub and the associated discomfort of pericarditis (as late as 3 months post infarction) are characteristic of the now rare post-myocardial infarction (Dressler) syndrome.

Pericardial rubs are most readily audible along the left sternal border or just inside the point of maximal impulse. Loud rubs may be audible over the entire precordium and even over the back. Occasionally, only the systolic portion of a rub is heard; it can be confused with a systolic murmur, and the diagnosis of rupture of the ventricular septum or mitral regurgitation may be incorrectly considered.

OTHER FINDINGS

FUNDI. Hypertension, diabetes, and generalized atherosclerosis commonly accompany STEMI, and because these conditions can produce characteristic changes in the fundus, a funduscopic examination may provide information concerning the underlying vascular status; this is particularly useful in patients unable to provide a detailed history.

ABDOMEN. As already noted, in patients with STEMI, particularly in an inferior location with diaphragmatic irritation, the pain may be localized to the epigastrium or the right upper quadrant. Pain in the abdomen associated with nausea, vomiting, restlessness, and even abdominal distention is often interpreted by patients as a sign of "indigestion," resulting in self-medication with antacids, and it can suggest an acute abdominal process to the physician. Right heart failure, characterized by hepatomegaly and a positive abdominojugular reflux, is unusual in patients with acute left ventricular infarction but does occur in patients with severe and prolonged left ventricular failure or right ventricular infarction.

EXTREMITIES. Coronary atherosclerosis is often associated with systemic atherosclerosis, and therefore patients with STEMI commonly have a history of intermittent claudication and demonstrate physical findings of peripheral vascular disease. Thus, diminished peripheral arterial pulses, loss of hair, and atrophic skin in the lower extremities are noted frequently in patients with coronary artery disease. Peripheral edema is a manifestation of right ventricular failure and, like congestive hepatomegaly, is unusual in patients with acute left ventricular infarction. Cyanosis of the nailbeds is common in patients with severe left ventricular failure and is particularly striking in patients with cardiogenic shock.

NEUROPSYCHIATRIC FINDINGS. Except for the altered mental status that occurs in patients with STEMI who have a markedly reduced cardiac output and cerebral hypoperfusion, the neurological examination findings are normal unless the patient has suffered cerebral embolism secondary to a mural thrombus. The coincidence between these two conditions can be explained by systemic hypotension due to STEMI precipitating a cerebral infarction and the converse, as well as by mural emboli from the left ventricle causing cerebral emboli.

Patients with STEMI often exhibit alterations of the emotional state, including intense anxiety, denial, and depression. Medical staff caring for STEMI patients must be sensitive to changes in the patient's emotional state; a calm, professional atmosphere, with thorough explanations of equipment and prognosis, can help alleviate the distress associated with STEMI.

Laboratory Findings

Serum Markers of Cardiac Damage

The classic World Health Organization (WHO) criteria for the diagnosis of MI require that at least two of the following three elements be present: a history of ischemic-type chest discomfort, evolutionary changes on serially obtained ECG tracings, and a rise and fall in serum cardiac markers.[74] There is considerable variability in the pattern of presentation of MI with respect to these three elements, as exemplified by the following statistics. ST-segment elevation and Q waves on the ECG, two features that are highly indicative of MI, are seen in only about half of MI cases on presentation. Approximately one-fourth of patients with MI do not present with classic chest pain, and the event would go unrecognized unless an ECG were recorded fortuitously in temporal proximity to the infarction or permanent pathological Q waves are seen on later tracings. Nondiagnostic ECGs are recorded in approximately half of patients presenting to emergency departments with chest pain suspicious for MI who ultimately are shown to have an MI. Among patients admitted to the hospital with a chest pain syndrome, fewer than 20 percent are subsequently diagnosed as having had an MI. In the majority of patients, therefore, clinicians must obtain serum cardiac marker measurements at periodic intervals to either establish or exclude the diagnosis of MI; such measurements can also be useful for a rough quantitation of the size of infarction.

The availability of serum cardiac markers with markedly enhanced sensitivity for myocardial damage enables clinicians to diagnose MI in about an additional one-third of patients who would not have fulfilled criteria for MI in the past.[75] The increased use of more sensitive biomarkers of MI combined with more precise imaging techniques has necessitated establishment of new criteria for MI (see Table 46–2).

As myocytes become necrotic, the integrity of the sarcolemmal membrane is compromised and intracellular macromolecules (serum cardiac markers) begin to diffuse into the cardiac interstitium and ultimately into the microvasculature and lymphatics in the region of the infarct (Fig. 46–13 and Table 46–4).[76] The rate of appearance of these macromolecules in the peripheral circulation depends on several factors, including intracellular location, molecular weight, local blood and lymphatic flow, and the rate of elimination from the blood.[76]

Given the accelerated pace of decision-making in patients with acute coronary syndromes and emphasis on reduction of length of hospital stay, there is considerable interest in evaluating new serum cardiac markers, shortening assay time in the central chemistry laboratory, and designing rapid whole blood bedside assays.[77] For optimal specificity, a serum marker of MI should be present in high concentration in the myocardium and be absent from nonmyocardial tissue and serum. For optimal sensitivity, it should be rapidly released

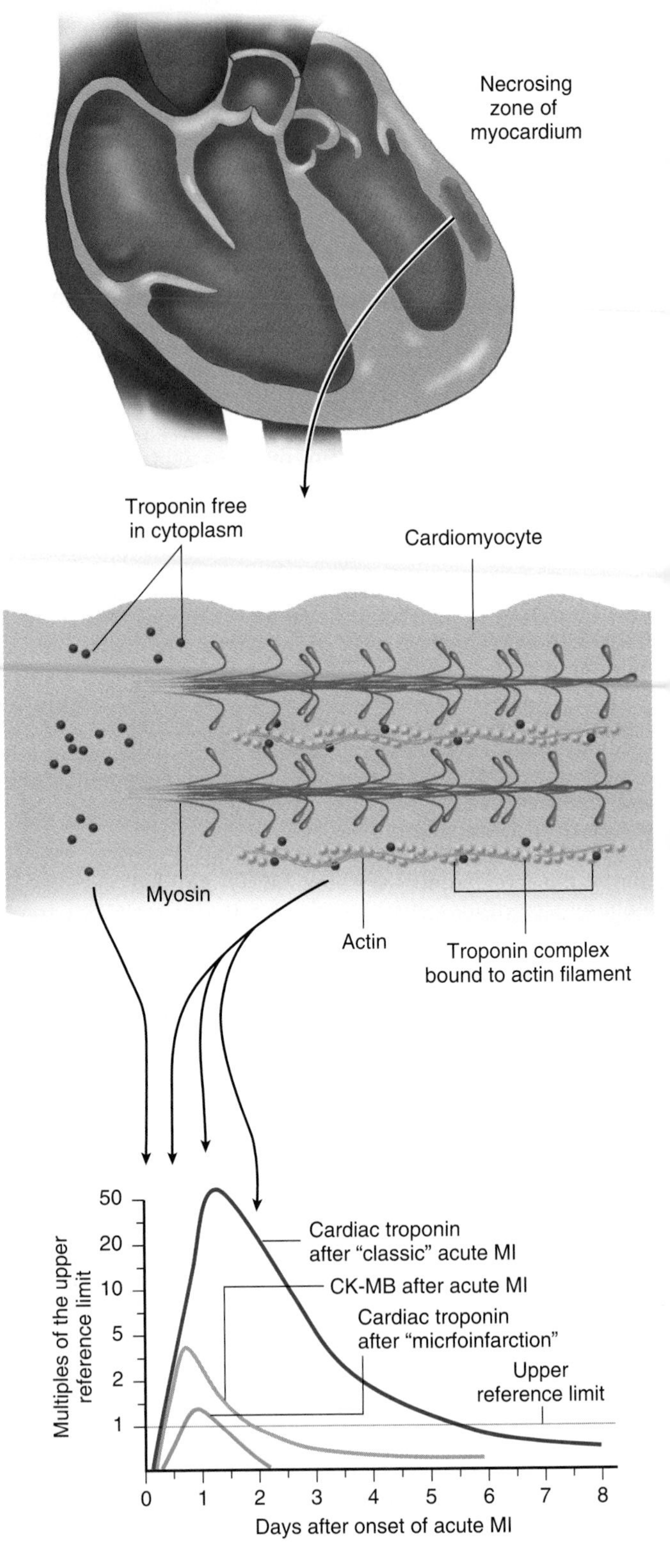

FIGURE 46–13 The zone of necrosing myocardium is shown at the top of the figure, followed in the middle portion of the figure by a diagram of a cardiomyocyte that is in the process of releasing biomarkers. Most troponin exists as a tripartite complex of C, I, and T components that are bound to actin filaments, although a small amount of troponin is free in the cytoplasm. After disruption of the sarcolemmal membrane of the cardiomyocyte, the cytoplasmic pool of troponin is released first (left-most arrow in bottom portion of figure), followed by a more protracted release from the disintegrating myofilaments that may continue for several days (three-headed arrow). Cardiac troponin levels rise to about 20 to 50 times the upper reference limit (the 99th percentile of values in a reference control group) in patients who have a "classic" acute myocardial infarction (MI) and sustain sufficient myocardial necrosis to result in abnormally elevated levels of the MB fraction of creatine kinase (CK-MB). Clinicians can now diagnose episodes of microinfarction by sensitive assays that detect cardiac troponin elevations above the upper reference limit, even though CK-MB levels may still be in the normal reference range (not shown). (From Antman EM: Decision making with cardiac troponin tests. N Engl J Med 346:2079, 2002.)

TABLE 46–4 Molecular Biomarkers for the Evaluation of Patients with ST-Elevation Myocardial Infarction

Biomarker	Molecular Weight (D)	Range of Times to Initial Elevation (h)	Mean Time to Peak Elevations (Nonreperfused)	Time to Return to Normal Range
Frequently used in clinical practice				
MB-CK	86,000	3-12	24 h	48-72 h
cTnI	23,500	3-12	24 h	5-10 d
cTnT	33,000	3-12	12 h-2 d	5-14 d
Infrequently used in clinical practice				
Myoglobin	17,800	1-4	6-7 h	24 h
MB-CK tissue isoform	86,000	2-6	18 h	Unknown
MM-CK tissue isoform	86,000	1-6	12 h	38 h

*Increased sensitivity can be achieved with sampling every 6 or 8 h.

CP = chest pain; cTnI = cardiac troponin I; cTnT = cardiac troponin T; MB-CK = MB isoenzyme of creatine kinase (CK); MM-CK = MM isoenzyme of CK.

Modified from Adams J III, Abendschein D, Jaffe A: Biochemical markers of myocardial injury. Is MB creatine kinase the choice for the 1990s? Circulation 1993;88: 750. Copyright 1993 American Heart Association.

into the blood after myocardial injury, and there should be a stoichiometric relationship between the plasma level of the marker and the extent of myocardial injury. For ease of clinical use, the marker should persist in blood for an appropriate length of time to provide a convenient diagnostic time window (see Table 46–4). Finally, the assay methodology should be inexpensive and easy to use.[78]

CREATINE KINASE. Serum CK activity exceeds the normal range within 4 to 8 hours after the onset of STEMI and declines to normal within 2 to 3 days (see Fig. 46–13). Although the peak CK occurs on average at about 24 hours, peak levels occur earlier in patients who have had reperfusion as a result of the administration of fibrinolytic therapy or mechanical recanalization (as well as in patients with early spontaneous fibrinolysis). Because the time-activity curve of serum CK is influenced by reperfusion, and because reperfusion itself influences infarct size, reperfusion interferes with estimation of infarct size by enzyme analysis (Fig. 46–14).[79]

Although elevation of the serum CK concentration is a sensitive enzymatic detector of STEMI that is routinely available in most hospitals,[80] important drawbacks include false-positive results in patients with muscle disease, alcohol intoxication, diabetes mellitus, skeletal muscle trauma, vigorous exercise, convulsions, intramuscular injections, thoracic outlet syndrome, and pulmonary embolism.[80]

CREATINE KINASE ISOENZYMES. Three isoenzymes of CK (MM, BB, and MB) have been identified by electrophoresis. Extracts of brain and kidney contain predominantly the BB isoenzyme; skeletal muscle contains principally MM but does contain some MB (1 to 3 percent); and both MM and MB isoenzymes are present in cardiac muscle. The MB isoenzymes of CK can also be present in minor quantities in the small intestine, tongue, diaphragm, uterus, and prostate. Strenuous exercise, particularly in trained long-distance runners or professional athletes, can cause elevation of both total CK and CK-MB.[81] Since CK-MB can be detected in the blood of healthy subjects, the cutoff value for abnormal elevation of CK-MB is usually set a few units above the upper reference limit for a given laboratory (see Fig. 46–13).[80] Despite the fact that small quantities of CK-MB isoenzyme are found in tissues other than the heart, elevated levels of CK-MB may be considered, for practical purposes, to be the result of MI (except in the case of trauma or surgery on the aforementioned organs).

Creatine kinase MB is analyzed in most laboratories by highly sensitive and specific enzyme immunoassays that utilize monoclonal antibodies directed against CK-MB.[80] Mass assays report results in nanograms per milliliter rather than units per milliliter and have been confirmed to be more accurate than CK-MB activity assays, especially in patients presenting within 4 hours of the onset of STEMI. It has been proposed that a ratio (relative index) of CK-MB mass to CK activity of about 2.5 is indicative of a myocardial rather than a skeletal source of the CK-MB elevation. Although this ratio may be satisfied by many patients with STEMI, it is inaccurate in several circumstances: (1) when high levels of total CK are present because of skeletal muscle injury (a large quantity of CK-MB must be released from the myocardium to satisfy criteria); (2) when chronic skeletal muscle injury releases large amounts of CK-MB; and (3) when total CK

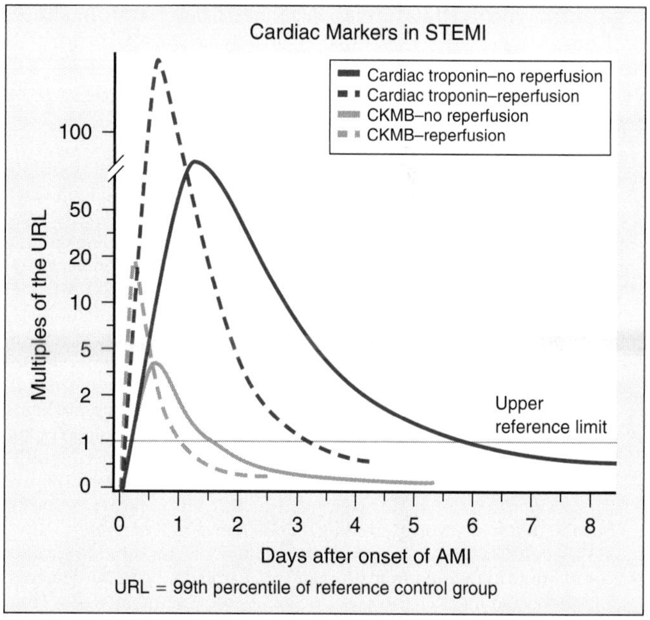

FIGURE 46–14 The kinetics of release of creatine kinase MB (CKMB) and cardiac troponin in patients who do not undergo reperfusion are shown in the solid green and red curves as multiples of the upper reference limit (URL). Note that when patients with ST-segment elevation myocardial infarction (STEMI) undergo reperfusion, as depicted in the dashed green and red curves, the cardiac biomarkers are detected sooner, rise to a higher peak value, but decline more rapidly, resulting in a smaller area under the curve and limitation of infarct size. AMI = acute myocardial infarction. (Adapted from Alpert JS, Thygesen K, Antman E, Bassand JP: Myocardial infarction redefined—A consensus document of The Joint European Society of Cardiology/American College of Cardiology Committee for the redefinition of myocardial infarction. J Am Coll Cardiol 36:959, 2000; and from Wu AH, Apple FS, Gibler WB, et al: National Academy of Clinical Biochemistry Standards of Laboratory Practice: Recommendations for the use of cardiac markers in coronary artery diseases. Clin Chem 45:1104, 1999.)

measurements are within the normal reference range for the laboratory and CK-MB is elevated (possibly indicating that a microinfarction has occurred). Patients with minimally elevated CK-MB and normal CK have a prognosis that is generally worse than that for patients with suspected MI but no CK-MB elevation. Elevation of CK-MB following PCI is associated with increased late (1-3 years) cardiac mortality.[82]

Clinicians should not rely on measurements of CK and CK-MB at a single point in time but instead should evaluate the temporal rise and fall of serially obtained values; skeletal muscle release of CK-MB generally remains elevated for a longer time than myocardial release of CK-MB and produces a "plateau" pattern of CK-MB values over several days, in contrast to the shorter time course of skeletal muscle CK-MB elevation, as depicted in Figure 46–13. Of note, since cardiac-specific troponins I and T (cTnI and cTnT) (see Fig. 46–13 and Tables 46–2 and 46–3) accurately distinguish skeletal from cardiac muscle damage, the troponins are now considered the preferred biomarker for diagnosing MI.[76]

In addition to STEMI secondary to coronary obstruction, other forms of injury to cardiac muscle, such as those resulting from myocarditis, trauma, cardiac catheterization, shock, and cardiac surgery, may also produce elevated serum CK-MB levels.[80] These latter causes of elevation of serum CK-MB values can usually be readily distinguished from STEMI by the clinical setting.

CREATINE KINASE ISOFORMS. Isoforms of the MM and MB isoenzymes have been identified.[83] These are subtypes of the individual isoenzymes and are formed in the circulation when the enzyme carboxypeptidase cleaves lysine residues from the carboxy terminus of the myocardial forms of the enzyme (CK-MM3 and CK-MB2), producing isoforms with a different electrophoretic mobility (CK-MM2, CK-MM1, and CK-MB1). Certain isoforms appear to be released into the blood quite rapidly, perhaps as soon as 1 hour, after the onset of infarction. An absolute level of CK-MB2 isoform greater than 1.0 U/liter or a ratio of CK-MB2 to CK-MB1 greater than 2.5 has a sensitivity for diagnosing MI of 46.4 percent at 4 hours and of 91.5 percent at 6 hours.[84] A rapid high-voltage electrophoretic assay for these isoforms is available, and results from experienced research laboratories suggest that it could permit early identification of patients with MI and early detection of successful reperfusion (peak CK-MB2/CK-MB1 > 3.8 at 2 hours), but controversy exists about the utility of CK isoforms in general clinical practice.[78]

MYOGLOBIN. This low-molecular-weight heme protein is released into the circulation from injured myocardial cells and can be detected within a few hours after the onset of infarction (see Table 46–3). Peak levels of serum myoglobin are reached considerably earlier (1 to 4 hours) than peak values of serum CK.[85] Because of its lack of cardiac specificity, an isolated measurement of myoglobin within the first 4 to 8 hours after the onset of chest discomfort in patients with a nondiagnostic ECG should not be relied upon to make the diagnosis of MI but should be supplemented by a more cardiac-specific marker such as cTnI or cTnT (see Table 46–3).[86]

In contrast to CK, myoglobin is readily excreted into the urine. A more rapid rise in serum myoglobin has been observed after reperfusion, and its measurement has been suggested as a useful index of successful reperfusion[79,87,88] and even infarct size. In patients presenting less than 6 hours from symptom onset and with ST elevation in whom the diagnosis of STEMI is not in doubt, an elevated myoglobin level is associated with an increased risk of mortality.[89] The adverse prognostic significance of an elevated myoglobin level at presentation is probably due to a combination of a large amount of myocardial damage and a delay of at least several hours from onset of symptoms to blood sampling.

CARDIAC-SPECIFIC TROPONINS. The troponin complex consists of three subunits that regulate the calcium-mediated contractile process of striated muscle. These include troponin C, which binds Ca^{2+}; troponin I (TnI), which binds to actin and inhibits actin-myosin interactions; and troponin T (TnT), which binds to tropomyosin, thereby attaching the troponin complex to the thin filament. Although the majority of TnT is incorporated in the troponin complex, approximately 6 percent is dissolved in the cytosol; about 2 to 3 percent of TnI is found in a cytosolic pool.

Although both TnT and TnI are present in cardiac and skeletal muscle, they are encoded by different genes and the amino acid sequence differs. This permits the production of antibodies that are specific for the cardiac form (cTnT and cTnI) and has led to the development of quantitative assays for cTnT and cTnI that have been approved by the Food and Drug Administration for clinical use[76] (see Fig. 46–13 and Table 46–4). Several studies have confirmed the reliability of these new quantitative assays for detecting myocardial injury, and measurement of cTnT or cTnI is now at the center of a new diagnostic criteria for STEMI.[90,91] Qualitative, rapid, bedside assays for cTnT and cTnI have also been approved for diagnosing MI.[92]

When interpreting the results of assays for cTnT or cTnI, clinicians must be cognizant of several analytical issues. The first-generation assay for cTnT exhibited some nonspecific binding to skeletal muscle troponin, but this was corrected in subsequent generations of assays.[93] The cTnT assays are produced by a single manufacturer, leading to relative uniformity of cutoffs, whereas several manufacturers produce cTnI assays. The majority of cTnI released into the bloodstream in patients with STEMI is complexed with cardiac troponin C.[94] Variations in the cutoff concentration for abnormal levels of cTnI in the clinically available immunoassays may be due in part to different specificities of the antibodies used for detecting free and complexed cTnI.[94] Thus, when using the measurement of cTnI for diagnosing STEMI, clinicians should apply the cutoff values for the particular assay used in their laboratory.[95] For both cTnT and cTnI, the definition of an abnormally increased level is a value exceeding that of 99 percent of a reference control group.[90]

Cutoff Values. Because cTnT or cTnI is not detected in the peripheral circulation under normal circumstances, the cutoff value for these analytes may be set only slightly above the "noise" level of the assay. Furthermore, whereas CK-MB usually increases 10- to 20-fold above the upper limit of the reference range, cTnT and cTnI typically increase more than 20 times above the reference range. These features of the cardiac-specific troponin assays provide an improved signal-to-noise ratio, enabling the detection of even minor degrees of myocardial necrosis.[96] In patients with MI, cTnT and cTnI first begin to rise above the upper reference limit by 3 hours from the onset of chest pain. Due to a continuous release from a degenerating contractile apparatus in necrotic myocytes, elevations of cTnI may persist for 7 to 10 days after MI; elevations of cTnT may persist for up to 10 to 14 days. The prolonged time course of elevation of cTnT and cTnI is advantageous for the late diagnosis of MI (see Fig. 46–13).

Patients with STEMI who undergo successful recanalization of the infarct-related artery have a rapid release of cardiac troponins that may be useful as an indicator of reperfusion, although myoglobin appears slightly more efficient in this regard (see Fig. 46–14).[79,97]

Troponin versus CK-MB. When comparing the diagnostic efficiency of the cardiac troponins versus CK-MB for MI, it is important to bear in mind that the troponin assays are probably capable of detecting episodes of myocardial necrosis that are below the detection limit of the current CK-MB assays, leading to a number of "false-positive" cases of troponin elevations if CK-MB is used as the gold standard. The somewhat vague terms *minor myocardial damage* and *microinfarction* have been used to describe the pathological process in patients who have a chest pain syndrome and elevated cardiac troponin but in whom CK-MB is in the normal range.[98] From a clinical perspective, it is desirable to have diagnostic tests for MI with increased sensitivity to increase the number of MI cases identified and increased specificity to reduce the number of cases incorrectly diagnosed and treated for MI. In addition, cardiac troponin measurements have been shown to have prognostic value for identifying patients with an acute coronary syndrome at risk for adverse clinical outcomes and who also exhibit enhanced responsiveness to new therapies such as glycoprotein IIb/IIIa inhibitors and low-molecular-weight heparins. The prognostic value of the troponins is independent of other risk factors such as age and ECG abnormalities, as well as the measurement of classic biomarkers such as CK-MB.[76]

Interpretation of Troponin Elevations. Balanced against the advantages of the troponins for improved detection of MI and prognostication of risk are the epidemiological, social, and health care delivery implications of assigning a diagnosis of MI to a larger cohort of patients than was the case in an earlier era (see Table 46–2).[99] Revised criteria for MI have an impact on our ability to monitor trends in the incidence of MI and draw comparisons with previous observations, on the psychological status of the patient, on patients' ability to obtain driving and pilot licenses, on disability applications, and on hospital reimbursement.[90] There is no clear solution to these issues.

Recommendations for Measurement of Serum Markers

It seems reasonable for clinicians to measure either cTnT or cTnI in patients with suspected MI. From a cost-effectiveness perspective, it is unnecessary to measure both a cardiac-specific troponin and CK-MB at all time points.[100] Routine diagnosis of MI can be accomplished within 12 hours using CK-MB, cTnT, or cTnI by obtaining measurements approximately every 8 to 12 hours (see Table 46–2). Retrospective diagnosis or diagnosis of MI in the presence of skeletal muscle injury is more readily accomplished with cTnT or cTnI.

Although serum cardiac markers have been used successfully to stratify patients for risk of cardiac events when the presenting ECG does not show ST elevation, bedside assays for troponin or myoglobin either alone or in combination with the ECG also are useful for stratifying risk in patients with STEMI.[89,101]

OTHER LABORATORY MEASUREMENTS

Numerous nonspecific manifestations can be recognized in patients with STEMI. Although they are not generally employed in establishing the diagnosis, awareness of their coexistence with infarction is important to avoid misinterpretation or erroneous diagnosis of other disorders.

SERUM LIPIDS. These are often determined in patients with STEMI. However, the results may be misleading because numerous factors that can alter the values are operating at the time of the patient's admission to the hospital. Serum triglycerides are affected by caloric intake, intravenous glucose, and recumbency.

During the first 24 to 48 hours after admission, total cholesterol and high-density lipoprotein (HDL) cholesterol remain at or near baseline values but generally fall precipitously after that. The fall in HDL cholesterol after STEMI is greater than the fall in total cholesterol; thus, the ratio of total cholesterol to HDL cholesterol is no longer useful for risk assessment early after MI. A lipid profile should be obtained on all STEMI patients who are admitted within 24 to 48 hours of symptoms. Based on the success of lipid-lowering therapy in primary and secondary prevention studies and evidence that hypolipidemic therapy improves endothelial function and inhibits thrombus formation,[102] it has been argued that early management of serum lipids in patients hospitalized for STEMI is advisable.[103,104] For patients admitted beyond 24 to 48 hours, more accurate determinations of serum lipid levels are obtained about 8 weeks after the infarction has occurred.

HEMATOLOGICAL FINDINGS. The elevation of the white blood cell count usually develops within 2 hours after the onset of chest pain, reaches a peak 2 to 4 days after infarction, and returns to normal in 1 week; the peak white blood cell count usually ranges between 12 and 15×10^3/ml but occasionally rises to as high as 20×10^3/ml in patients with large STEMI. Often there is an increase in the percentage of polymorphonuclear leukocytes and a shift of the differential count to band forms. An epidemiological association has been reported indicating a worse angiographic appearance of culprit lesions and increased risk of adverse clinical outcomes the higher the white blood cell count at presentation with an acute coronary syndrome.[63,105]

The erythrocyte sedimentation rate (ESR) is usually normal during the first day or two after infarction, even though fever and leukocytosis may be present. It then rises to a peak on the fourth or fifth day and may remain elevated for several weeks. The increase in the ESR is secondary to elevated plasma alpha$_2$-globulin fibrinogen, but the peak does not correlate well with the size of the infarction or with the prognosis. The hematocrit often increases during the first few days after infarction as a consequence of hemoconcentration. Although an elevated C-reactive protein (CRP) level appears to identify patients at increased risk of coronary heart disease, evidence also exists that in patients presenting with STEMI, an elevated CRP is associated with worse angiographic appearance of the infarct artery and a greater likelihood of developing heart failure.[106,107]

Electrocardiography (see Chap. 9)

In the majority of patients with STEMI, some change can be documented when serial ECGs are compared. However, many factors limit the ability of the ECG to diagnose and localize MI: the extent of myocardial injury, the age of the infarct, its location, the presence of conduction defects, the presence of previous infarcts or acute pericarditis, changes in electrolyte concentrations, and the administration of cardioactive drugs. Changes in the ST segment and T wave are quite nonspecific and may occur in a variety of conditions, including stable and unstable angina pectoris, ventricular hypertrophy, acute and chronic pericarditis, myocarditis, early repolarization, electrolyte imbalance, shock, and metabolic disorders and following the administration of digitalis. Serial ECGs may be of considerable aid in differentiating these conditions from STEMI. Transient changes favor angina or electrolyte disturbances, whereas persistent changes argue for infarction if other causes such as shock, administration of digitalis, and persistent metabolic disorders can be eliminated. Nevertheless, serial standard 12-lead ECGs remain a potent and extremely clinically useful method for the detection and localization of MI.[108] Analysis of the constellation of ECG leads showing ST elevation may also be useful for identifying the site of occlusion in the infarct artery.[108] The extent of ST deviation on the ECG, location of infarction, and QRS duration correlate with risk of adverse outcomes.[109] Even when left bundle branch block is present on the ECG, MI can be diagnosed when striking ST segment deviation is present beyond that which can be explained by the conduction defect.[108] In addition to the diagnostic and prognostic information contained within the 12-lead ECG, it also provides valuable noninvasive information about the success of reperfusion for STEMI (see Chap. 47).[108,110]

Although general agreement exists on electrocardiographic and vectorcardiographic criteria for the recognition of infarction of the anterior and inferior myocardial walls, less agreement is found on criteria for lateral and posterior infarcts[111]; in this area, even the terminology can be confusing. It has been reported that patients with an abnormal R wave in V_1 (0.04 sec in duration and/or R/S ratio ≥ 1 in the absence of preexcitation or right ventricular hypertrophy) with inferior or lateral Q waves have an increased incidence of isolated occlusion of a dominant left circumflex coronary artery without collateral circulation; such patients have a lower ejection fraction, increased end-systolic volume, and higher complication rate than patients with inferior infarction due to isolated occlusion of the right coronary artery.

More sophisticated forms of ECG recordings, including high-resolution electrocardiography, body surface potential mapping of ST segments, and continuous vectorcardiography, have all been reported in small series of patients to augment the 12-lead ECG in diagnosing MI, but the lack of ready availability of equipment and the special expertise required limits the use of these techniques.

Although most patients continue to demonstrate the ECG changes from an infarction for the rest of their lives, particularly if they evolve Q waves, in a substantial minority the typical changes disappear, Q waves can regress, and the ECG can even return to normal after a number of years. Under many circumstances, Q-wave patterns simulate MI. Conditions that may mimic the electrocardiographic features of MI by producing a pattern of "pseudoinfarction" include ventricular hypertrophy, conduction disturbances, preexcitation, primary myocardial disease, pneumothorax, pulmonary embolus, amyloid heart disease, primary and metastatic tumors of the heart, traumatic heart disease, intracranial hemorrhage, hyperkalemia, pericarditis, early repolarization, and cardiac involvement with sarcoidosis.

Q-WAVE AND NON-Q-WAVE INFARCTION. As noted earlier, the presence or absence of Q waves on the surface ECG does not reliably predict the distinction between transmural and nontransmural (subendocardial) MI.[25] Q waves on the ECG signify abnormal electrical activity but are not synonymous with irreversible myocardial damage. Also, the absence of Q waves may simply reflect the insensitivity of the standard 12-lead ECG, especially in the posterior zones of the left ventricle. True pathological subendocardial MI, as recognized at autopsy, is seen with ST-segment depression and/or T-wave changes only about 50 percent of the time.[112] Angiographic studies in MI patients without ST-segment elevation show a higher incidence of subtotal occlusion of the culprit coronary vessel and greater collateral flow to the infarct zone. Observational data suggest that MI without ST-segment elevation is seen more commonly in elderly patients and patients with a prior MI.

ISCHEMIA AT A DISTANCE. Patients with new Q waves and ST-segment elevation diagnostic for STEMI in one territory often have ST-segment depression in other territories. These additional ST-segment changes are caused either by ischemia in a territory other than the area of infarction, termed *ischemia at a distance*, or by reciprocal electrical phenomena. A good deal of attention has been directed to associated ST-segment depression in the anterior leads, when it occurs in patients with acute inferior STEMI. However, despite the clinical importance of differentiation among causes of anterior ST-segment depression in such patients, including anterior ischemia, posterior wall infarction, and true reciprocal changes, such a differentiation cannot be made reliably by electrocardiographic or even vectorcardiographic techniques. Although precordial ST-segment depression is more commonly associated with extensive infarction of the posterior, lateral, or inferior septal segments, rather than anterior wall subendocardial ischemia, imaging techniques such as two-dimensional echocardiography are necessary to ascertain whether an anterior wall motion abnormality is present.[113] Regardless of whether the anterior ST-segment changes reflect anterior wall ischemia or are reciprocal to changes elsewhere, this finding, as with ischemia at a distance, implies a poorer prognosis than if such changes were not present.[114]

RIGHT VENTRICULAR INFARCTION. ST-segment elevation in right precordial leads (V_1, V_3R-V_6R) is a relatively sensitive and specific sign of right ventricular infarction.[108,115] Occasionally, ST-segment elevation in leads V_2 and V_3 is due to acute right ventricular infarction; this appears to occur only when the injury to the left inferior wall is minimal.[116–118] Usually, the concurrent inferior wall injury suppresses this anterior ST-segment elevation resulting from right ventricular injury. Likewise, right ventricular infarction appears to reduce the anterior ST-segment depression often observed with inferior wall myocardial infarction. A QS or QR pattern in leads V_3R and/or V_4R also suggests right ventricular myocardial necrosis but has less predictive accuracy than ST-segment elevation in these leads.

ATRIAL INFARCTION. The most common electrocardiographic patterns are depression or elevation of the PR segment, alterations in the contour of the P wave, and abnormal atrial rhythms, including atrial flutter, atrial fibrillation, wandering atrial pacemaker, and atrioventricular nodal rhythm.[40]

Imaging

Roentgenography (see Chap. 12)

The initial chest roentgenogram in patients with STEMI is almost invariably a portable film obtained in the emergency room or the coronary care unit. When present, prominent pulmonary vascular markings on the roentgenogram reflect elevated left ventricular end-diastolic pressure, but significant temporal discrepancies can occur because of what have been termed *diagnostic lags* and *post-therapeutic lags*. Up to 12 hours can elapse before pulmonary edema accumulates after ventricular filling pressure has become elevated. The post-therapeutic phase lag represents a longer time interval; up to 2 days are required for pulmonary edema to resorb and the radiographic signs of pulmonary congestion to clear after ventricular filling pressure has returned toward normal. The degree of congestion and the size of the left side of the heart on the chest film are useful for defining groups of patients with STEMI who are at increased risk of dying after the acute event.[119]

Echocardiography (see Chap. 11)

TWO-DIMENSIONAL ECHOCARDIOGRAPHY. The relative portability of echocardiographic equipment makes this technique ideal for the assessment of patients with MI hospitalized in the coronary care unit or even in the emergency department before admission.[113] In patients with chest pain compatible with MI but with a nondiagnostic ECG, the finding on echocardiography of a distinct region of disordered contraction can be helpful diagnostically because it supports the diagnosis of myocardial ischemia. Echocardiography is also useful in evaluating patients with chest pain and a nondiagnostic ECG who are suspected of having an aortic dissection. The identification of an intimal flap consistent with an aortic dissection is a critical observation because it represents a major contraindication to fibrinolytic therapy (see Chap. 47).

Areas of abnormal regional wall motion are observed almost universally in patients with MI, and the degree of wall motion abnormality can be categorized with a semiquantitative wall motion score index. Of note, abnormal wall motion is less often noted echocardiographically when the infarction is small and the age of regional wall motion abnormality cannot always be determined. Left ventricular function estimated from two-dimensional echocardiograms correlates well with measurements from angiography and is useful in establishing prognosis after MI.[113] Furthermore, the early use of echocardiography can aid in the early detection of potentially viable but stunned myocardium (contractile reserve), residual provocable ischemia, patients at risk for the development of congestive heart failure after MI, and mechanical complications of MI.[113]

Although transthoracic imaging is adequate in most patients, occasional patients have poor echo windows, especially if they are undergoing mechanical ventilation. In such patients, transesophageal echocardiography can be safely performed and can be useful in evaluating ventricular septal defects and papillary muscle dysfunction.[120]

DOPPLER ECHOCARDIOGRAPHY. This technique (see Chap. 11) allows assessment of blood flow in the cardiac chambers and across cardiac valves. Used in conjunction with two-dimensional echocardiography, it is helpful in detecting and assessing the severity of mitral or tricuspid regurgitation after STEMI. Identification of the site of acute ventricular septal rupture, quantification of shunt flow across the resulting defect, and assessment of acute cardiac tamponade are also possible.[120,121]

Other Imaging Modalities

COMPUTED TOMOGRAPHY (see Chap. 15). This technique can provide useful cross-sectional information in patients with MI. In addition to the assessment of cavity dimensions and wall thickness, left ventricular aneurysms can be detected, and, of particular importance in patients with STEMI, intracardiac thrombi can be identified. Although cardiac computed tomography is a less convenient technique, it probably is more sensitive for thrombus detection than is echocardiography.

MAGNETIC RESONANCE IMAGING (see Chap. 14). In addition to localizing and sizing the area of infarction, magnetic resonance imaging techniques are capable of early recognition of MI and of providing an assessment of the severity of the ischemic insult. This modality is attractive because of its ability to assess perfusion of infarcted and noninfarcted tissue as well as of reperfused myocardium; to identify areas of jeopardized but not infarcted myocardium; to identify myocardial edema, fibrosis, wall thinning, and hypertrophy; to assess ventricular chamber size and segmental wall motion; and to identify the temporal transition between ischemia and infarction.[122] It has limited practical application, however, because of the need to transport patients with MI to the magnetic resonance imaging facility.

NUCLEAR IMAGING (see Chap. 13). Radionuclide angiography, perfusion imaging, infarct-avid scintigraphy, and positron emission tomography have been used to evaluate patients with STEMI.[123] Nuclear cardiac imaging techniques can be useful for detecting MI; assessing infarct size, collateral flow, and jeopardized myocardium; determining the effects of the infarct on ventricular function; and establishing prognosis of patients with STEMI.[123] However, the necessity of moving a critically ill patient from the coronary care unit (CCU) to the nuclear medicine department limits their practical application unless a portable gamma camera is available. Cardiac radionuclide imaging for the diagnosis of MI should be restricted to special limited situations in which the triad of clinical history, ECG findings, and serum marker measurements is unavailable or unreliable.

Estimation of Infarct Size

ELECTROCARDIOGRAPHY. Interest in limiting infarct size, in large part because of the recognition that the quantity of myocardium infarcted has important prognostic implications, has focused attention on the accurate determination of MI size. The sum of ST-segment elevations measured from multiple precordial leads correlates with the extent of myocardial injury in patients with anterior MI.[108] QRS scoring systems and planar or vectorcardiographic techniques to estimate infarct size have also been developed. Although they demonstrate good correlations with infarct size at autopsy and with enzymatic estimates, formal sizing of infarcts by ECG technique is not necessary in most patients. Of note, however, there is a relationship between the number of ECG leads showing ST-segment elevation and mortality rate: patients with 8 or 9 of 12 leads with ST-segment elevation have three to four times the mortality of those with only 2 or 3 leads with ST-segment elevation. The duration of ischemia time as estimated from continuous ST-segment monitoring is correlated with infarct size, the ratio of infarct size to area at risk, and the extent of regional wall motion abnormality observed subsequently.[124]

SERUM CARDIAC MARKERS. To estimate infarct size by analysis of serum cardiac markers, it is necessary to account for the quantity of the marker lost from the myocardium, its volume of distribution, and its release ratio.[125] Serial measurements of proteins released by necrotic myocardium are helpful in determining MI size. Clinically, the peak CK or CK-MB provides an approximate estimate of infarct size and is widely used prognostically. In the prethrombotic era, quantification of the cumulative release of CK or CK-MB correlated with other techniques for estimating infarct size in vivo as well as with the area of necrosis at autopsy. However, coronary artery reperfusion dramatically changes the wash-out kinetics of CK and other markers from myocardium, resulting in early and exaggerated peak levels and limiting the usefulness of such curves as a measure of infarct size.

NONINVASIVE IMAGING TECHNIQUES. Echocardiography (see Chap. 11), radionuclide scintigraphy (see Chap. 13),[123] computed tomography (see Chap. 15), and magnetic resonance imaging (see Chap. 14) have all been utilized for the clinical and experimental assessment of infarct size. Infarct-avid scintigraphy and myocardial perfusion imaging have been used to quantify infarct size. Estimation of infarct size by quantitative tomographic ^{99m}Tc-sestamibi imaging appears to be less limited by ventricular geometry and can distinguish small infarcts and ischemia from infarcted myocardium more readily than other noninvasive methods.[126] Tomography has improved on planar techniques employing technetium-99m pyrophosphate to image MI.[127] Contrast-enhanced magnetic resonance imaging has been helpful in demonstrating the regional heterogeneity of infarction patterns in patients with persistently occluded infarct arteries versus those with successfully reperfused vessels.[128]

REFERENCES

1. Luepker RV, Apple FS, Christenson RH, et al: Case definitions for acute coronary disease in epidemiology and clinical research studies. Circulation 108:2543, 2003.
2. Alpert JS, Thygesen K, Antman E, et al: Myocardial infarction redefined: A consensus document of The Joint European Society of Cardiology/American College of Cardiology Committee for the redefinition of myocardial infarction. J Am Coll Cardiol 36:959, 2000.
3. Newby LK, Alpert JS, Ohman EM, et al: Changing the diagnosis of acute myocardial infarction: Implications for practice and clinical investigators. Am Heart J 144:957, 2002.
4. White HD: Things ain't what they used to be: Impact of a new definition of myocardial infarction. Am Heart J 144:933, 2002.
5. Apple FS, Wu AHB, Jaffe AS: European Society of Cardiology and American College of Cardiology guidelines for the redefinition of myocardial infarction: How to use existing assays clinically and for clinical trials. Am Heart J 144:981, 2002.
6. Hamm CW, Bertrand M, Braunwald E: Acute coronary syndrome without ST elevation: Implementation of new guidelines. Lancet 358:1533, 2001.
7. Rogers WJ, Canto JG, Lambrew CT, et al: Temporal trends in the treatment of over 1.5 million patients with myocardial infarction in the US from 1990 through 1999: The National Registry of Myocardial Infarction 1, 2 and 3. J Am Coll Cardiol 36:2056, 2000.
8. Kesteloot H, Sans S, Kromhout D: Evolution of all-causes and cardiovascular mortality in the age-group 75-84 years in Europe during the period 1970-1996: A comparison with worldwide changes. Eur Heart J 23:384, 2002.
9. American Heart Association: Heart Disease and Stroke Statistics—2004 Update. Dallas, American Heart Association, 2003.
10. Ezzati M, Vander Hoorn S, Rodgers A, et al: Estimates of global and regional potential health gains from reducing multiple major risk factors. Lancet 362:271, 2003.
11. Tunstall-Pedoe H, Mahonen M, Tolonen H, et al: Contribution of trends in survival and coronary-event rates to changes in coronary heart disease mortality: 10-year results from 37 WHO MONICA Project populations. Lancet 353:1547, 1999.
12. Braunwald E, Antman EM, Beasley JW, et al: ACC/AHA 2002 guideline update for the management of patients with unstable angina and non-ST-segment elevation myocardial infarction—summary article: A report of the American College of Cardiology/American Heart Association task force on practice guidelines (Committee on the Management of Patients With Unstable Angina). J Am Coll Cardiol 40:1366, 2002.
13. Tunstall-Pedoe H, Vanuzzo D, Hobbs M, et al: Estimation of contribution of changes in coronary care to improving survival, event rates, and coronary heart disease mortality across the WHO MONICA Project populations. Lancet 355:688, 2000.
14. Braunwald E, Antman EM: Evidence-based coronary care. Ann Intern Med 126:551, 1997.
15. Antman EM, et al: ACC/AHA Guidelines for the Management of Patients with ST-Elevation Myocardial Infarction. 2004 (http://www.acc.org/clinical/guidelines/stemi/index.htm).

16. Boersma E, Mercado N, Poldermans D, et al: Acute myocardial infarction. Lancet 361:847, 2003.
17. Burwen DR, Galusha DH, Lewis JM, et al: National and state trends in quality of care for acute myocardial infarction between 1994-1995 and 1998-1999: The medicare health care quality improvement program. Arch Intern Med 163:1430, 2003.
18. Assessment of the Safety and Efficacy of a New Thrombolytic Regimen (ASSENT)-3 Investigators: Efficacy and safety of tenecteplase in combination with enoxaparin, abciximab, or unfractionated heparin: The ASSENT-3 randomised trial in acute myocardial infarction. Lancet 358:605, 2001.
19. Canto JG, Rogers WJ, Chandra NC, et al: The association of sex and payer status on management and subsequent survival in acute myocardial infarction. Arch Intern Med 162:587, 2002.
20. White HD: Thrombolytic therapy in the elderly. Lancet 356:2028, 2000.
21. Krumholz HM, Chen J, Rathore SS, et al: Regional variation in the treatment and outcomes of myocardial infarction: Investigating New England's advantage. Am Heart J 146:242, 2003.
22. Thiemann DR, Coresh J, Oetgen WJ, et al: The association between hospital volume and survival after acute myocardial infarction in elderly patients. N Engl J Med 340:1640, 1999.
23. Chen J, Radford MJ, Wang Y, et al: Do "America's Best Hospitals" perform better for acute myocardial infarction? N Engl J Med 340:286, 1999.
24. Vaccarino V, Parsons L, Every NR, et al: Sex-based differences in early mortality after myocardial infarction. National Registry of Myocardial Infarction 2 Participants. N Engl J Med 341:217, 1999.
25. Phibbs B, Marcus F, Marriott HJC, et al: Q-wave versus non-Q wave myocardial infarction: A meaningless distinction. J Am Coll Cardiol 33:576, 1999.

Pathology

26. Libby P: Current concepts of the pathogenesis of the acute coronary syndromes. Circulation 104:365, 2001.
27. Fuster V, Corti R, Fayad ZA, et al: Integration of vascular biology and magnetic resonance imaging in the understanding of atherothrombosis and acute coronary syndromes. J Thromb Haemost 1:1410, 2003.
28. Malek AM, Alper SL, Izumo S: Hemodynamic shear stress and its role in atherosclerosis. JAMA 282:2035, 1999.
29. Rosenberg RD, Aird WC: Vascular-bed-specific hemostasis and hypercoagulable states. N Engl J Med 340:1555, 1999.
30. Ardissino D, Merlini PA, Ariens R, et al: Tissue-factor antigen and activity in human coronary atherosclerotic plaques. Lancet 349:769, 1997.
31. Kloner RA, Leor J: Natural disaster plus wake-up time: A deadly combination of triggers. Am Heart J 137:779, 1999.
32. Goodman SG, Langer A, Ross AM, et al: Non-Q-wave versus Q-wave myocardial infarction after thrombolytic therapy: Angiographic and prognostic insights from the global utilization of streptokinase and tissue plasminogen activator for occluded coronary arteries-I angiographic substudy. GUSTO-I Angiographic Investigators. Circulation 97:444, 1998.
33. Vargas SO, Sampson BA, Schoen FJ: Pathologic detection of early myocardial infarction: A critical review of the evolution and usefulness of modern techniques. Mod Pathol 12:635, 1999.
34. Schoen FJ: The heart. *In* Cotran FS, Kumar V, Collins T (eds): Pathologic Basis of Disease. 7th ed. Philadephia, WB Saunders, 2004.
35. Kloner RA, Ellis SG, Lange R, et al: Studies of experimental coronary artery reperfusion: Effects on infarct size, myocardial function, biochemistry, ultrastructure and microvascular damage. Circulation 68:15, 1983.
36. Lehrke S, Giannitsis E, Steen H, et al: Cardiac troponin T in ST-segment elevation acute myocardial infarction revisited. Cardiovasc Toxicol 1:99, 2001.
37. DeWood MA, Spores J, Notske RN, et al: Prevalence of total coronary artery occlusion during the early hours of transmural myocardial infarction. N Engl J Med 303:897, 1980.
38. Ozdemir K, Altunkeser BB, Icli A, et al: New parameters in identification of right ventricular myocardial infarction and proximal right coronary artery lesion. Chest 124:219, 2003.
39. Bowers TR, O'Neill WW, Grines C, et al: Effect of reperfusion on biventricular function and survival after right ventricular infarction. N Engl J Med 338:933, 1998.
40. Neven K, Crijns H, Gorgels A: Atrial infarction: A neglected electrocardiographic sign with important clinical implications. J Cardiovasc Electrophysiol 14:306, 2003.
41. Kyriakidis M, Barbetseas J, Antonopoulos A, et al: Early atrial arrhythmias in acute myocardial infarction. Role of the sinus node artery. Chest 101:944, 1992.
42. Fujita M, Nakae I, Kihara Y, et al: Determinants of collateral development in patients with acute myocardial infarction. Clin Cardiol 22:595, 1999.

Pathophysiology

43. Swan HJC, Forrester JS, Diamond G, et al: Hemodynamic spectrum of myocardial infarction and cardiogenic shock. Circulation 45:1097, 1972.
44. Forrester JS, Wyatt HL, Daluz PL, et al: Functional significance of regional ischemic contraction abnormalities. Circulation 54:64, 1976.
45. Schuster EH, Bulkley BH: Ischemia at a distance after acute myocardial infarction: A cause of early postinfarction angina. Circulation 62:509, 1980.
46. White HD, Norris RM, Brown MA, et al: Left ventricular end-systolic volume as the major determinant of survival after recovery from myocardial infarction. Circulation 76:44, 1987.
47. Pfeffer MA, Braunwald E: Ventricular remodeling after myocardial infarction. Experimental observations and clinical implications. Circulation 81:1161, 1990.
48. Sadanandan S, Buller CE, Menon V, et al: The late open artery hypothesis—A decade later. Am Heart J 142:411, 2001.
49. Braunwald E, Kim CB: Late establishment of patency of the infarct-related artery. *In* Julian D, Braunwald E (eds): Acute Myocardial Infarction. London, WB Saunders, 1994, pp 147-162.
50. Pfeffer MA, Lamas GA, Vaughan DE, et al: Effect of captopril on progressive ventricular dilatation after anterior myocardial infarction. N Engl J Med 319:80, 1988.
51. Hochman JS: Cardiogenic shock complicating acute myocardial infarction: Expanding the paradigm. Circulation 107:2998, 2003.
52. Pfeffer JM, Pfeffer MA, Fletcher PJ, et al: Progressive ventricular remodeling in rat with myocardial infarction. Am J Physiol 260:H1406, 1991.
53. Weisman HF, Bush DE, Mannisi JA, et al: Cellular mechanisms of myocardial infarct expansion. Circulation 78:186, 1988.
54. Pfeffer MA: Left ventricular remodeling after acute myocardial infarction. Ann Rev Med 46:455, 1995.
55. Schmermund A, Lerman LO, Ritman EL, et al: Cardiac production of angiotensin II and its pharmacologic inhibition: Effects on the coronary circulation. Mayo Clin Proc 74:503, 1999.
56. Gray BA, Hyde RW, Hodges M, et al: Alterations in lung volume and pulmonary function in relation to hemodynamic changes in acute myocardial infarction. Circulation 59:551, 1979.
57. Ceremuzynski L: Hormonal and metabolic reactions evoked by acute myocardial infarction. Circulation Res 48:767, 1981.
58. Sack MN, Yellon DM: Insulin therapy as an adjunct to reperfusion after acute coronary ischemia: A proposed direct myocardial cell survival effect independent of metabolic modulation. J Am Coll Cardiol 41:1404, 2003.
59. Stein BC, Levin RI: Natriuretic peptides: Physiology, therapeutic potential, and risk stratification in ischemic heart disease. Am Heart J 135:914, 1998.
60. de Lemos JA, Morrow DA, Bentley JH, et al: The prognostic value of B-type natriuretic peptide in patients with acute coronary syndromes. N Engl J Med 345:1014, 2001.
61. Morrow DA, Braunwald E: Future of biomarkers in acute coronary syndromes: Moving toward a multimarker strategy. Circulation 108:250, 2003.
62. Li YH, Teng JK, Tsai WC, et al: Prognostic significance of elevated hemostatic markers in patients with acute myocardial infarction. J Am Coll Cardiol 33:1543, 1999.
63. Sabatine MS, Morrow DA, Cannon CP, et al: Relationship between baseline white blood cell count and degree of coronary artery disease and mortality in patients with acute coronary syndromes: A TACTICS-TIMI 18 (Treat Angina with Aggrastat and determine Cost of Therapy with an Invasive or Conservative Strategy-Thrombolysis in Myocardial Infarction 18 trial) substudy. J Am Coll Cardiol 40:1761, 2002.

Clinical Features

64. Singh JP, Muller JE: Triggers to acute coronary syndromes. *In* Theroux P (ed): Acute Coronary Syndromes: A Companion to Braunwald's Heart Disease. Philadelphia, WB Saunders, 2003, pp 108-118.
65. Eagle KA, Berger PB, Calkins H, et al: ACC/AHA guideline update for perioperative cardiovascular evaluation for noncardiac surgery—Executive summary: A report of the American College of Cardiology/American Heart Association Task Force on Practice Guidelines (Committee to Update the 1996 Guidelines on Perioperative Cardiovascular Evaluation for Noncardiac Surgery). J Am Coll Cardiol 39:542, 2002.
66. Maseri A, L`Abbate A, Baroldi G, et al: Coronary vasospasm as a possible cause of myocardial infarction. N Engl J Med 299:1271, 1978.
67. Muller JE, Abela GS, Nesto RW, et al: Triggers, acute risk factors and vulnerable plaques: The lexicon of a new frontier. J Am Coll Cardiol 23:809, 1994.
68. Spodick DH: Pericardial complications of myocardial infarction. *In* Francis GS, Alpert JS (eds): Coronary Care. 2nd ed. Boston, Little, Brown & Company, 1995, pp 333-341.
69. Balaban DH, Yamamoto Y, Liu J, et al: Sustained esophageal contraction: A marker of esophageal chest pain identified by intraluminal ultrasonography. Gastroenterology 116:29, 1999.
70. McGuire DK, Granger CB: Diabetes and ischemic heart disease. Am Heart J 138:366, 1999.
71. Webb SW, Adgey AA, Pantridge JF: Autonomic disturbance at onset of acute myocardial infarction. BMJ 818:89, 1982.
72. Killip T, Kimball JT: Treatment of myocardial infarction in a coronary care unit: A two year experience with 250 patients. Am J Cardiol 20:457, 1967.
73. Magnesium in Coronaries (MAGIC) Trial Investigators: Early administration of intravenous magnesium to high-risk patients with acute myocardial infarction in the Magnesium in Coronaries (MAGIC) Trial: A randomised controlled trial. Lancet 360:1189, 2002.
74. Pedoe-Tunstall H, Kuulasmaa K, Amouyel P, et al: Myocardial infarction and coronary deaths in the World Health Organization MONICA Project. Circulation 90:583, 1994.
75. Ravkilde J, Horder M, Gerhardt W, et al: Diagnostic performance and prognostic value of serum troponin T in suspected acute myocardial infarction. Scand J Clin Lab Invest 53:677, 1993.
76. Antman EM: Decision making with cardiac troponin tests. N Engl J Med 346:2079, 2002.
77. Hamm CW: Cardiac biomarkers for rapid evaluation of chest pain. Circulation 104:1454, 2001.
78. Penttila K, Koukkunen H, Halinen M, et al: Myoglobin, creatine kinase MB isoforms and creatine kinase MB mass in early diagnosis of myocardial infarction in patients with acute chest pain. Clin Biochem 35:647, 2002.
79. French JK, Ramanathan K, Stewart JT, et al: A score predicts failure of reperfusion after fibrinolytic therapy for acute myocardial infarction. Am Heart J 145:508, 2003.
80. Apple FS, Quist HE, Doyle PJ, et al: Plasma 99th percentile reference limits for cardiac troponin and creatine kinase MB mass for use with European Society of Cardiology/American College of Cardiology consensus recommendations. Clin Chem 49:1331, 2003.
81. Apple FS: Tissue specificity of cardiac troponin I, cardiac troponin T and creatine kinase-MB. Clin Chim Acta 284:151, 1999.

82. Gibson CM, Murphy SA, Marble SJ, et al: Relationship of creatine kinase-myocardial band release to thrombolysis in myocardial infarction perfusion grade after intracoronary stent placement: An ESPRIT substudy. Am Heart J 143:106, 2002.
83. Roberts R, Kleiman N: Earlier diagnosis and treatment of acute myocardial infarction necessitates the need for a "new diagnostic mind-set." Circulation 89:872, 1994.
84. Zimmerman J, Fromm R, Meyer D, et al: Diagnostic marker cooperative study for the diagnosis of myocardial infarction. Circulation 99:1671, 1999.
85. Apple FS: Creatine kinase isoforms and myoglobin: Early detection of myocardial infarction and reperfusion. Coron Artery Dis 10:75, 1999.
86. Wu AH, Apple FS, Gibler WB, et al: National Academy of Clinical Biochemistry Standards of Laboratory Practice: Recommendations for the use of cardiac markers in coronary artery diseases. Clin Chem 45:1104, 1999.
87. de Lemos JA, Morrow DA, Gibson CM, et al: Early noninvasive detection of failed epicardial reperfusion after fibrinolytic therapy. Am J Cardiol 88:353, 2001.
88. Srinivas VS, Cannon CP, Gibson CM, et al: Myoglobin levels at 12 hours identify patients at low risk for 30-day mortality after thrombolysis in acute myocardial infarction: A Thrombolysis in Myocardial Infarction 10B substudy. Am Heart J 142:29, 2001.
89. de Lemos JA, Antman EM, Giugliano RP, et al: Very early risk stratification after thrombolytic therapy with a bedside myoglobin assay and the 12-lead electrocardiogram. Am Heart J 140:373, 2000.
90. Alpert JS, Thygesen K, Antman E, Bassand JP: Myocardial infarction redefined—A consensus document of the Joint European Society of Cardiology/American College of Cardiology Committee for the redefinition of myocardial infarction. J Am Coll Cardiol 36:959, 2000.
91. Jaffe AS, Ravkilde J, Roberts R, et al: It's time for a change to a troponin standard. Circulation 102:1216, 2000.
92. Apple FS, Murakami MM, Jesse RL, et al: Near-bedside whole-blood cardiac troponin I assay for risk assessment of patients with acute coronary syndromes. Clin Chem 48:1784, 2002.
93. Aviles RJ, Askari AT, Lindahl B, et al: Troponin T levels in patients with acute coronary syndromes, with or without renal dysfunction. N Engl J Med 346:2047, 2002.
94. Katrukha AG, Bereznikova AV, Esakova TV, et al: Troponin I is released in bloodstream of patients with acute myocardial infarction not in free form but as complex. Clin Chem 43:1379, 1997.
95. Cheitlin MD, Khayam-Bashi H: Biomarkers of myocardial infarction: Finding the right cut-off point. Cardiol Rev 9:323, 2001.
96. Antman EM, Grudzien C, Sacks DB: Evaluation of a rapid bedside assay for detection of serum cardiac troponin T. JAMA 273:1279, 1995.
97. Tanasijevic MJ, Cannon CP, Antman EM, et al: Myoglobin, creatine-kinase-MB and cardiac troponin-I 60-minute ratios predict infarct-related artery patency after thrombolysis for acute myocardial infarction: Results from the Thrombolysis in Myocardial Infarction study (TIMI) 10B. J Am Coll Cardiol 34:739, 1999.
98. Panteghini M, Apple FS, Christenson RH, et al: Use of biochemical markers in acute coronary syndromes. IFCC Scientific Division, Committee on Standardization of Markers of Cardiac Damage. International Federation of Clinical Chemistry. Clin Chem Lab Med 37:687, 1999.
99. Apple FS, Wu AH: Myocardial infarction redefined: Role of cardiac troponin testing. Clin Chem 47:377, 2001.
100. Collinson PO, Stubbs PJ, Kessler AC: Multicentre evaluation of the diagnostic value of cardiac troponin T, CK-MB mass, and myoglobin for assessing patients with suspected acute coronary syndromes in routine clinical practice. Heart 89:280, 2003.
101. Ohman EM, Armstrong PW, White HD, et al: Risk stratification with a point-of-care cardiac troponin T test in acute myocardial infarction. Am J Cardiol 84:1281, 1999.
102. Wolfrum S, Jensen KS, Liao JK: Endothelium-dependent effects of statins. Arterioscler Thromb Vasc Biol 23:729, 2003.
103. Teo KK, Burton JR: Who should receive HMG CoA reductase inhibitors? Drugs 62:1707, 2002.
104. MRC/BHF Heart Protection Study of cholesterol lowering with simvastatin in 20,536 high-risk individuals: A randomised placebo-controlled trial. Lancet 360:7, 2002.
105. Barron HV, Cannon CP, Murphy SA, et al: Association between white blood cell count, epicardial blood flow, myocardial perfusion, and clinical outcomes in the setting of acute myocardial infarction: A thrombolysis in myocardial infarction 10 substudy. Circulation 102:2329, 2000.
106. Berton G, Cordiano R, Palmieri R, et al: C-reactive protein in acute myocardial infarction: Association with heart failure. Am Heart J 145:1094, 2003.
107. Sano T, Tanaka A, Namba M, et al: C-reactive protein and lesion morphology in patients with acute myocardial infarction. Circulation 108:282, 2003.

Electrocardiography

108. Zimetbaum PJ, Josephson ME: Use of the electrocardiogram in acute myocardial infarction. N Engl J Med 348:933, 2003.
109. Manes C, Pfeffer MA, Rutherford JD, et al: Value of the electrocardiogram in predicting left ventricular enlargement and dysfunction after myocardial infarction. Am J Med 114:99, 2003.
110. Feldman LJ, Coste P, Furber A, et al: Incomplete resolution of ST-segment elevation is a marker of transient microcirculatory dysfunction after stenting for acute myocardial infarction. Circulation 107:2684, 2003.
111. Cooksey JD, Dunn M, Massie E: Clinical Vectorcardiography and Electrocardiography. 2nd ed. Chicago, Year Book Medical Publishers, 1977.
112. Levine HD: Subendocardial infarction in retrospect: Pathologic, cardiographic, and ancillary features. Circulation 72:790, 1985.
113. Cheitlin MD, Armstrong WF, Aurigemma GP, et al: ACC/AHA/ASE 2003 guideline update for the clinical application of echocardiography: A report of the American College of Cardiology/American Heart Association Task Force on Practice Guidelines (ACC/AHA/ASE Committee to Update the 1997 Guidelines on the Clinical Application of Echocardiography). American College of Cardiology, 2003. (http://www.acc.org/clinical/guidelines/echocardiography/dirIndex.htm)
114. Mirvis DM: Physiologic bases for anterior ST segment depression in patients with acute inferior wall myocardial infarction. Am Heart J 116:1308, 1988.
115. Lopez-Sendon J, Coma-Canella I, Alcasena S, et al: Electrocardiographic findings in acute right ventricular infarction: Sensitivity and specificity of electrocardiographic alterations in right precordial leads V4R, V3R, V1, V2, and V3. J Am Coll Cardiol 6:1273, 1985.
116. Geft IL, Shah PK, Rodriguez L, et al: ST elevations in leads V1 to V5 may be caused by right coronary artery occlusion and acute right ventricular infarction. Am J Cardiol 53:991, 1984.
117. Acikel M, Yilmaz M, Bozkurt E, et al: ST segment elevation in leads V1 to V3 due to isolated right ventricular branch occlusion during primary right coronary angioplasty. Catheter Cardiovasc Interv 60:32, 2003.
118. Finn AV, Antman EM: Images in clinical medicine. Isolated right ventricular infarction. N Engl J Med 349:1636, 2003.

Imaging

119. Brattler A, Karliner JS, Higgins CB, et al: The initial chest x-ray in acute myocardial infarction: Prediction of early and late mortality and survival. Circulation 61:1004, 1980.
120. Reimold SC, Antman EM: Noninvasive cardiac imaging in chest pain syndromes. J Thrombosis Thrombolysis 6:239, 1998.
121. Spodick DH: Acute cardiac tamponade. N Engl J Med 349:684, 2003.
122. Pohost GM, Hung L, Doyle M: Clinical use of cardiovascular magnetic resonance. Circulation 108:647, 2003.
123. Klocke FJ, Baird MG, Bateman TM, et al: ACC/AHA/ASNC guidelines for the clinical use of cardiac radionuclide imaging: A report of the American College of Cardiology/American Heart Association Task Force on Practice Guidelines (ACC/AHA/ASNC Committee to Revise the 1995 Guidelines for the Clinical Use of Radionuclide Imaging). American College of Cardiology, 2003 (http://www.acc.org/clinical/guidelines/radio/dirIndex.htm).
124. Krucoff MW, Johanson P, Crater SW, et al: The clinical utility of serial and continuous ST-segment recovery in patients with acute ST elevation myocardial infarction: Assessing the dynamics of epicardial and myocardial reperfusion. Circulation 2004, in press.
125. Adams J III, Abendschein D, Jaffe A: Biochemical markers of myocardial injury. Is MB creatine kinase the choice for the 1990s? Circulation 88:750, 1993.
126. Gibbons RJ, Miller TD, Christian TF: Infarct size measured by single photon emission computed tomographic imaging with (99m)Tc-sestamibi : A measure of the efficacy of therapy in acute myocardial infarction. Circulation 101:101, 2000.
127. Kopecky SL, Aviles RJ, Bell MR, et al: A randomized, double-blinded, placebo -controlled, dose-ranging study measuring the effect of an adenosine agonist on infarct size reduction in patients undergoing primary percutaneous transluminal coronary angioplasty: The ADMIRE (AmP579 Delivery for Myocardial Infarction REduction) study. Am Heart J 146:146, 2003.
128. Kwong RY, Yucel EK: Computed tomography and magnetic resonance imaging. Circulation 108:e104, 2003.

CHAPTER 47

ST-Elevation Myocardial Infarction: Management

Elliott M. Antman

Although considerable advances have been made in the process of care for patients with ST-elevation myocardial infarction (STEMI), room for improvement exists, especially in special populations such as the very elderly and members of ethnic minority groups.[1-4] It is useful to organize a discussion of the phases of management of STEMI along the chronology of the interface of clinicians with the patient. Primary and secondary prevention of STEMI are discussed in Chapter 42. Treatment at the time of onset of STEMI (prehospital issues, initial recognition and management in the emergency department, reperfusion), hospital management (medications, arrhythmics, complications, preparation for discharge), and secondary prevention of STEMI are discussed in this chapter. The reader is referred to Chapter 48 for a discussion of percutaneous coronary intervention (PCI) in patients with STEMI.

PREHOSPITAL CARE. The prehospital care of patients with suspected STEMI is a crucial element bearing directly on the likelihood of survival. Most deaths associated with STEMI occur within the first hour of its onset and are usually due to ventricular fibrillation (see Chap. 32). Accordingly, the importance of the immediate implementation of definitive resuscitative efforts and of rapidly transporting the patient to a hospital cannot be overemphasized. Major components of the delay from the onset of symptoms consistent with acute myocardial infarction to reperfusion include the following[5]: (1) the time for the patient to recognize the seriousness of the problem and seek medical attention; (2) prehospital evaluation, treatment, and transportation; (3) the time for diagnostic measures and initiation of treatment in the hospital (e.g., "door-to-needle" time for patients receiving a thrombolytic agent and "door-to-balloon" time for patients undergoing a catheter-based reperfusion strategy); and (4) the time from initiation of treatment to restoration of flow (Fig. 47–1).

Patient-related factors that correlate with a longer time to the decision to seek medical attention include older age, female gender, African-American race, low socioeconomic status, low emotional or somatic awareness, history of angina, diabetes, or both, consulting a spouse or other relative, and consulting a physician.[5,6] Health care professionals should heighten the level of awareness of patients at risk for STEMI (e.g., those with hypertension, diabetes, history of angina pectoris).[5,7] They should review and reinforce with patients and their families the need to seek urgent medical attention for a pattern of symptoms including chest discomfort, extreme fatigue, and dyspnea, especially if accompanied by diaphoresis, lightheadedness, palpitations, or a sense of impending doom.[8,9] Although many patients shun such discussions and tend to minimize the likelihood of ever needing emergency cardiac treatment, emphasis should be placed on the prevention and treatment of potentially fatal arrhythmias as well as salvage of the jeopardized myocardium by reperfusion, for which time is crucial.[8] Patients should also be instructed in the proper use of sublingual nitroglycerin and to call 911 emergency services if the ischemic-type discomfort persists for more than 5 minutes.[10,11]

EMERGENCY MEDICAL SERVICES (EMS) SYSTEMS. These have three major components: emergency medical dispatch, first response, and EMS ambulance response. Ongoing efforts to shorten the time to treatment of patients with STEMI include improvement in the medical dispatch component by expanding 911 coverage, providing automated external defibrillators to first responders, placing automated external defibrillators in critical public locations, and greater coordination of EMS ambulance response.[12,13] Well-equipped ambulances and helicopters staffed by personnel trained in the acute care of the STEMI patient allow definitive therapy to commence while the patient is being transported to the hospital (Table 47–1). To be used effectively, they must be placed strategically within a community, and excellent radio communication systems must be available. These units should be equipped with battery-operated monitoring equipment, a DC defibrillator, oxygen, endotracheal tubes and suction apparatus, and commonly used cardiovascular drugs. Radiotelemetry systems that allow transmission of the electrocardiographic (ECG) signal to a medical control officer are highly desirable to facilitate triage of STEMI patients and are becoming increasingly available in many communities (Fig. 47–2). Observations of simple variables such as age, heart rate, and blood pressure permit initial classification of patients into high- or low-risk subgroups.[14]

In addition to prompt defibrillation, the efficacy of prehospital care appears to depend on several factors, including early relief of pain with its deleterious physiological sequelae, reduction of excessive activity of the autonomic nervous system, and abolition of prelethal arrhythmias, such as ventricular tachycardia. However, these efforts must not inhibit rapid transfer to the hospital (see Fig. 47–2).

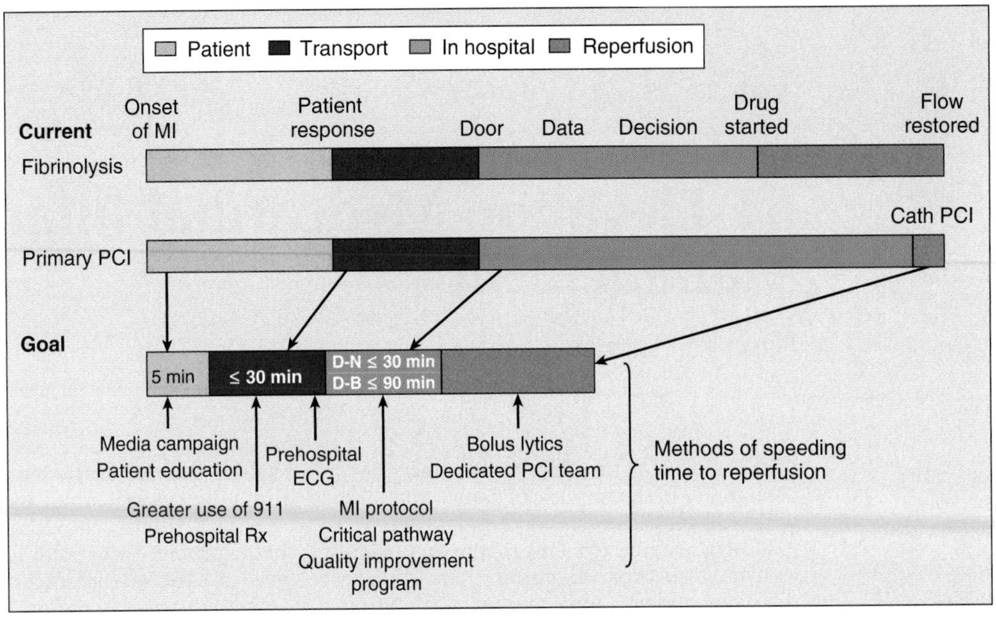

FIGURE 47–1 Major components of time delay between onset of infarction and restoration of flow in the infarct-related artery. Plotted sequentially from left to right are the time for patients to recognize symptoms and seek medical attention, transportation to the hospital, in-hospital decision-making and implementation of reperfusion strategy, and time for restoration of flow once the reperfusion strategy has been initiated. The time to initiate fibrinolytic therapy is the "door-to-needle" (D-N) time; this is followed by the period of time required for pharmacological restoration of flow. More time is required to move the patient to the catheterization laboratory for a percutaneous coronary interventional (PCI) procedure, referred to as the "door-to-balloon" (D-B) time, but restoration of flow in the epicardial infarct-related artery occurs promptly after PCI. At the bottom are shown a variety of methods for speeding the time to reperfusion along with the goals for the time intervals for the various components of the time delay. (Adapted from Cannon CP, Antman EM, Walls R, Braunwald E: Time as adjunctive agent to thrombolytic therapy. J Thromb Thrombolysis 1:27, 1994.)

TABLE 47–1 Reperfusion Checklist for Evaluation of the STEMI Patient

Step One: Has patient experienced chest discomfort for **greater than** 15 min and **less than** 12 hr?

YES → Step Two

NO → STOP

Step Two: Are there contraindications to fibrinolysis?
If ANY of the following are CHECKED, fibrinolysis ***MAY*** be contraindicated.

Systolic blood pressure greater than 180 mm Hg	■ **YES**	NO
Diastolic blood pressure greater than 110 mm Hg	■ **YES**	NO
Right vs. left arm systolic blood pressure difference greater than 15 mm Hg	■ **YES**	NO
History of structural central nervous system disease	■ **YES**	NO
Significant closed head/facial trauma within the previous 3 mo	■ **YES**	NO
Recent (within 6 wk) major trauma, surgery (including laser eye surgery), gastrointestinal or genitourinary bleed	■ **YES**	NO
Bleeding or clotting problem on blood thinners	■ **YES**	NO
CPR more than 10 min	■ **YES**	NO
Pregnant female	■ **YES**	NO
Serious systemic disease (e.g., advanced/terminal cancer, severe liver or kidney disease)	■ **YES**	NO

Step Three: Does the patient have severe heart failure or cardiogenic shock such that percutaneous coronary intervention is preferable?

Pulmonary edema (rales greater than halfway up)	■ YES	**NO**
Systemic hypoperfusion (cold, clammy)	■ YES	**NO**

From Antman EM, et al: ACC/AHA Guidelines for the Management of Patients with ST-Elevation Myocardial Infarction, 2004 (http://www.acc.org/clinical/guidelines/stemi/index.htm).

A
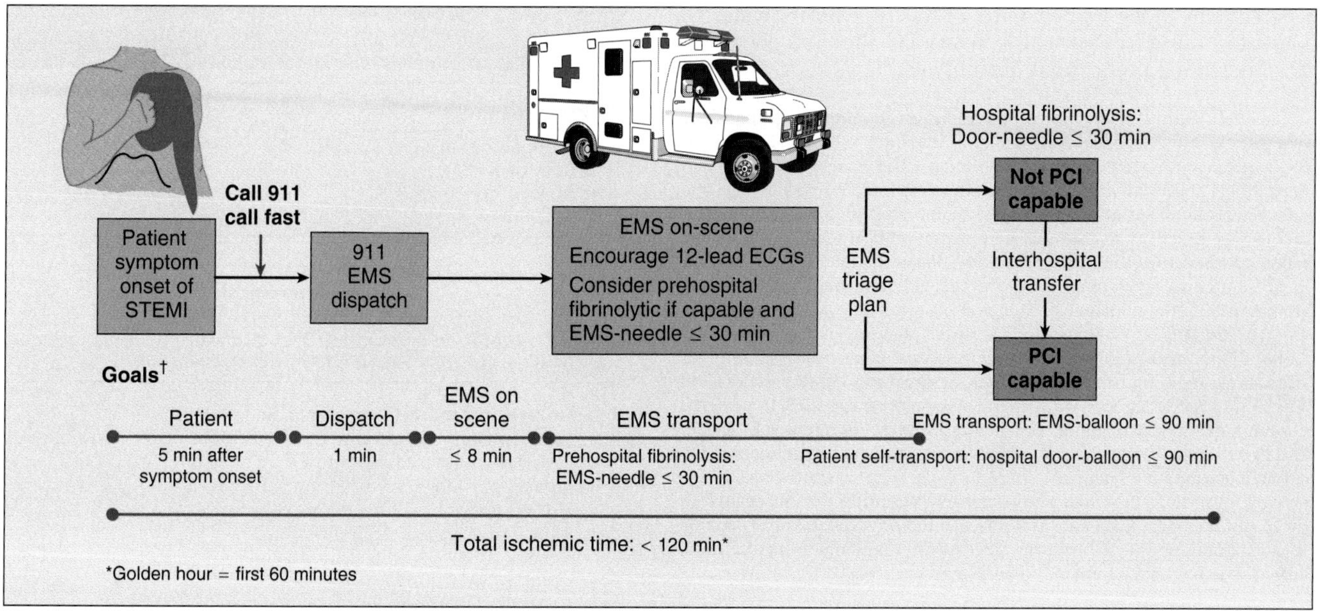

B
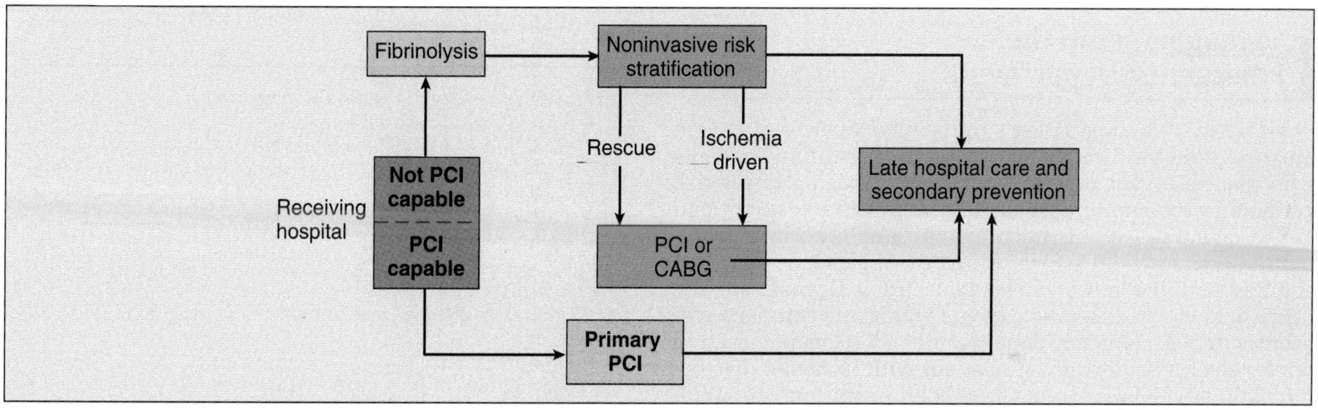

FIGURE 47–2 Options for transportation of STEMI patients and initial reperfusion treatment. Reperfusion in patients with STEMI can be accomplished by the pharmacological (fibrinolysis) or catheter-based (primary PCI) approaches. Implementation of these strategies varies based on the mode of transportation of the patient and capabilities at the receiving hospital. **A,** Patient transported by emergency medical services (EMS) after calling 911. Transport time to the hospital is variable from case to case, but the goal is to keep total ischemic time less than 120 minutes. There are three possibilities. (1) If EMS has fibrinolytic capability and the patient qualifies for therapy, prehospital fibrinolysis should be started within 30 minutes of EMS arrival on scene. (2) If EMS is not capable of administering prehospital fibrinolysis and the patient is transported to a non-PCI capable hospital, the hospital door-to-needle time should be less than or equal to 30 minutes for patients in whom fibrinolysis is indicated. (3) If EMS is not capable of administering prehospital fibrinolysis and the patient is transported to a PCI-capable hospital, the hospital door-to-balloon time should be less than or equal to 90 minutes.

Interhospital transfer. It is also appropriate to consider emergency interhospital transfer of the patient to a PCI-capable hospital for mechanical revascularization if (1) there is a contraindication to fibrinolysis; (2) PCI can be initiated promptly (≤90 min after the patient presented to the initial receiving hospital or ≤60 min compared to when fibrinolysis could be initiated at the initial receiving hospital; (3) fibrinolysis is administered and is unsuccessful (i.e., "rescue PCI"). Secondary nonemergency interhospital transfer can be considered for recurrent ischemia **(B)**.

Patient self-transport. Patient self-transportation is discouraged. If the patient arrives at a non-PCI-capable hospital, the door-to-needle time should be 30 minutes or less. If the patient arrives at a PCI-capable hospital, the door-to-balloon time should be 90 minutes or less. The treatment options and time recommendations after first hospital arrival are the same.

B, For patients who receive fibrinolysis, noninvasive risk stratification is recommended to identify the need for rescue PCI (failed fibrinolysis) or ischemia drive PCI. Regardless of the initial method of reperfusion treatment, all patients should receive late hospital care and secondary prevention of STEMI.

†The medical system goal is to facilitate rapid recognition and treatment of patients with STEMI such that door-to-needle (or EMS-to-needle) for initiation of fibrinolytic therapy can be achieved within 30 minutes or that door-to-balloon (or EMS-to-balloon) or PCI can be achieved within 90 minutes. These goals should not be understood as "ideal" times, but rather the longest times that should be considered acceptable for a given system. Systems that are able to achieve even more rapid times for treatment of patients with STEMI should be encouraged. (Adapted from Armstrong PW, Collen D, Antman E: Fibrinolysis for acute myocardial infarction: The future is here and now. Circulation 107:2533, 2003; and Antman EM, et al: ACC/AHA Guidelines for the Management of Patients with ST-Elevation Myocardial Infarction, 2004 [http://www.acc.org/clinical/guidelines/stemi/index.htm]).

PREHOSPITAL FIBRINOLYSIS. The potential benefits of prehospital versus in-hospital fibrinolysis have been evaluated in several randomized trials. Although none of the individual trials showed a significant reduction in mortality with prehospital-initiated thrombolytic therapy, there was a generally consistent observation of benefit from earlier treatment, and a meta-analysis of all the available trials demonstrated a 17 percent reduction in mortality.[15] The CAPTIM trial reported a trend toward a lower rate of mortality among STEMI patients receiving prehospital fibrinolysis as compared with primary PCI, especially if patients were treated within 2 hours of the onset of symptoms.[16,17] Additional support for the benefit of prehospital lysis is found in a report from a French registry of STEMI patients treated less than 12 hours from the onset of symptoms; the 1-month mortality rate was 14.7 percent in patients who did not receive reperfusion,

9 percent in those treated with in-hospital fibrinolysis, 7.9 percent in those treated with primary PCI, and 3.2 percent in those receiving prehospital fibrinolysis.[18]

Several factors must be weighed when communities consider whether their ambulances and emergency transport vehicles should have the capability to initiate fibrinolytic therapy. The greatest reduction in mortality is observed when reperfusion can be initiated within 60 to 90 minutes of the onset of symptoms.[19] Streamlining of emergency department triage practices so that treatment can be started within 30 minutes, when coupled with the 15- to 30-minute transport time that is common in most urban centers, may be more cost-effective than equipping all ambulances to administer prehospital fibrinolytic therapy (see Fig. 47-2).[7] The latter would require extensive training of personnel (see Table 47-1), installation of computer-assisted electrocardiography or systems for radio transmission of the ECG signal to a central station, and stocking of medicine kits with the necessary drug supplies. In selected communities where transport delays may be 60 to 90 minutes or longer and experienced personnel are available on ambulances, prehospital fibrinolytic therapy is beneficial.[20] Therefore, prehospital fibrinolysis is reasonable in settings in which physicians are present in the ambulance or there is a well-organized EMS system with full-time paramedics, capability for obtaining and transmitting 12-lead ECG readings from the field, and on-line medical command to authorize prehospital fibrinolysis.

Management in the Emergency Department

Physicians evaluating patients in the emergency department must confront the difficult task of rapidly identifying patients who require urgent reperfusion therapy, triaging lower risk patients to the appropriate facility within the hospital, and not discharging patients home inappropriately while avoiding unnecessary admissions. A history of ischemic-type discomfort and the initial 12-lead electrocardiogram are the primary tools for screening patients with acute coronary syndromes in the emergency department.[21] ST segment elevation on the electrocardiogram of a patient with ischemic discomfort is highly suggestive of thrombotic occlusion of an epicardial coronary artery, and its presence should serve as the trigger for a well-rehearsed sequence of rapid assessment of the patient for contraindications to fibrinolysis and initiation of a reperfusion strategy (Tables 47–2 and 47–3).[7] Since the 12-lead electrocardiogram is at the center of the decision pathway for initiation of reperfusion therapy, it should be obtained promptly (≤10 minutes) in patients presenting with ischemic discomfort.

Because lethal arrhythmias can occur suddenly in patients with STEMI, all patients should be attached to a bedside ECG monitor and intravenous access obtained for infusion of 5 percent dextrose in water. If the initial ECG reading shows ST segment elevation of 1 mm or more in at least two contiguous leads or a new or presumably new left bundle branch block, the patient should be evaluated immediately for a reperfusion strategy. Critical factors to be considered when selecting a reperfusion strategy include (1) the time elapsed since the onset of symptoms, (2) the risk associated with STEMI, (3) the risk of administering fibrinolysis, and (4) the time required to initiate an invasive strategy (see Table 47–2). There is controversy about which form of reperfusion therapy is superior. A detailed discussion of the issues is found later in this chapter.

Given the importance of time to reperfusion,[13] the concept of medical system goals has arisen. Benchmarks for medical systems to use when assessing the quality of their performance are a door-to-needle time of ≤30 minutes for initiation of fibrinolytic therapy and a door-to-balloon time of ≤90 minutes for PCI (see Fig. 47–2).[7] With increasing sophistication of EMS systems, it is possible to initiate the process of evaluation/implementation of a reperfusion strategy even before the patient arrives in the emergency department. For those patients transported by ambulance, the medical system goals can be restated as an EMS-to-needle time of ≤30 minutes for initiation of fibrinolysis and an EMS-to-balloon time of ≤90 minutes for initiation of PCI (see Fig. 47–2).[7,22] An intriguing proposal that may also facilitate care of patients with STEMI is the development of regionalized centers for care of patients with acute ischemic heart disease.[23] Implementation of such "centers of excellence" requires a coordinated commitment of multiple components of the health care system—a formidable challenge, but one that many authorities believe is a vital step toward improvement of care of patients with STEMI.[24]

Patients with an initial ECG reading that reveals new or presumably new ST segment depression and/or T wave inversion, while not considered candidates for thrombolytic therapy, should be treated as though they are suffering from myocardial infarction without ST elevation or unstable

TABLE 47–2 Assessment of Reperfusion Options for STEMI Patients

Step 1: Assess time and risk.

- Time since onset of symptoms
- Risk of STEMI
- Risk of fibrinolysis
- Time required for transport to a skilled PCI lab

Step 2: Determine if fibrinolysis or invasive strategy is preferred.

- *If presentation is less than 3 hr and there is no delay to an invasive strategy, there is no preference for either strategy.*

Fibrinolysis is generally preferred if:

- Early presentation (≤ 3hr from symptom onset and delay to invasive strategy) (see below)
- Invasive strategy is not an option
  - Catheterization lab occupied or not available
  - Vascular access difficulties
  - Lack of access to a skilled PCI lab†‡
- Delay to invasive strategy
  - Prolonged transport
  - (Door-to-Balloon)–(Door-to-Needle) more than 1 hr*§
  - Medical contact-to-balloon or door-to-balloon more than 90 min

An invasive strategy is generally preferred if:

- Skilled PCI lab available with surgical backup
  - Skilled PCI lab is available, defined by:†‡
  - Medical contact-to-balloon or door-to-balloon less than 90 min
  - (Door-to-Balloon)–(Door-to-Needle) less than 1 hr*
- High risk from STEMI
  - Cardiogenic shock
  - Killip class ≥ 3
- Contraindications to fibrinolysis including increased risk of bleeding and ICH
- Late presentation
  - Symptom onset was more than 3 hr ago
- Diagnosis of STEMI is in doubt

*Applies to fibrin-specific agents.
†Operator experience greater than a total of 75 primary PCI cases/yr.
‡Team experience greater than a total of 36 primary PCI cases/yr.
§This calculation implies that the estimated delay to the implementation of the invasive strategy is greater than 1 hr versus initiation of fibrinolytic therapy immediately.
ICH = intracranial hemorrhage; PCI = percutaneous coronary intervention; STEMI = ST-elevation myocardial infarction.
From Antman EM, et al: ACC/AHA Guidelines for the Management of Patients with ST-Elevation Myocardial Infarction. 2004 (http://www.acc.org/clinical/guidelines/stemi/index.htm).

TABLE 47–3 Contraindications and Cautions for Fibrinolytic Use in STEMI*

Absolute contraindications
- Any prior intracranial hemorrhage
- Known structural cerebral vascular lesion (e.g., arteriovenous malformation)
- Known malignant intracranial neoplasm (primary or metastatic)
- Ischemic stroke within 3 months EXCEPT acute ischemic stroke within 3 hours
- Suspected aortic dissection
- Active bleeding or bleeding diathesis (excluding menses)
- Significant closed head or facial trauma within 3 months

Relative contraindications
- History of chronic severe poorly controlled hypertension
- Severe uncontrolled hypertension on presentation (SBP greater than 180 or DBP greater than 110 Hg)†
- History of prior ischemic stroke greater than 3 months, dementia, or known intracranial pathology not covered in contraindications
- Traumatic or prolonged (more than 10 min) CPR or major surgery (less than 3 wk)
- Recent (within 2-4 weeks) internal bleeding
- Noncompressible vascular punctures
- For streptokinase/anistreplase: prior exposure (more than 5 days ago) or prior allergic reaction to these agents
- Pregnancy
- Active peptic ulcer
- Current use of anticoagulants: the higher the INR, the higher the risk of bleeding

CPR = cardiopulmonary resuscitation; DBP = diastolic blood pressure; INR = international normalized ratio; SBP = systolic blood pressure; STEMI = ST-elevation myocardial infarction.

From Antman EM, et al: ACC/AHA Guidelines for the Management of Patients with ST-Elevation Myocardial Infarction. 2004 (http://www.acc.org/clinical/guidelines/stemi/index.htm).

*Viewed as advisory for clinical decision-making and may not be all-inclusive or definitive.

†Could be an absolute contraindication in low-risk patients with myocardial infarction.

angina (a distinction to be made subsequently after scrutiny of serial electrocardiograms and serum cardiac marker measurements) (see Chaps. 46 and 49).

In patients with a clinical history suggestive of STEMI (see Chap. 46) and an initial nondiagnostic ECG reading (i.e., no ST segment deviation or T wave inversion), serial tracings should be obtained while the patients are being evaluated in the emergency department. Emergency department staff can be alerted to the sudden development of ST segment elevation by periodic visual inspection of the bedside ECG monitor, by continuous ST segment recording, or by auditory alarms when the ST segment deviation exceeds programmed limits. Decision aids such as computer-based diagnostic algorithms, identification of high-risk clinical indicators, rapid determination of cardiac serum markers, two-dimensional echocardiographic screening for regional wall motion abnormalities, and myocardial perfusion imaging are of greatest clinical utility when the ECG reading is nondiagnostic. In an effort to improve the cost-effectiveness of care of patients with a chest pain syndrome, nondiagnostic ECG reading, and low suspicion of myocardial infarction but in whom the diagnosis has not been entirely excluded, many medical centers have developed critical pathways that involve a coronary observation unit with a goal of ruling out myocardial infarction in less than 12 hours.[25]

General Treatment Measures

ASPIRIN. This agent not only is useful for the primary prevention of vascular events (see Chap. 42) but is also effective across the entire spectrum of acute coronary syndromes and forms part of the initial management strategy for patients with suspected STEMI. The pharmacology of aspirin is presented in Chapter 80. The goal of aspirin treatment is to quickly block formation of thromboxane A_2 in platelets by cyclooxygenase inhibition. Because low doses (40 to 80 mg) take several days to achieve full antiplatelet effect, at least 162 to 325 mg should be administered acutely in the emergency department.[7] To achieve therapeutic blood levels rapidly, the patient should chew the tablet, thus promoting buccal absorption rather than absorption through the gastric mucosa.

CONTROL OF CARDIAC PAIN. Analgesia is an important element of management of STEMI patients in the emergency department. Often there is a tendency to underdose the patient for fear of obscuring response to antiischemic or reperfusion therapy. This should be avoided, because pain contributes to the heightened sympathetic activity that is particularly prominent during the early phase of STEMI. Control of cardiac pain is typically accomplished with a combination of nitrates, analgesics (e.g., morphine), oxygen, and beta-adrenoceptor blockers. Similar pharmacological principles apply in the coronary care unit, where many of the therapies discussed herein are continued after initial dosing in the emergency department. Because the pain associated with STEMI is related to ongoing ischemia, many interventions that act to improve the oxygen supply-demand relationship (by either increasing supply or decreasing demand) have a functional analgesic effect.

Analgesics. Although a wide variety of analgesic agents has been used to treat the pain associated with STEMI, including meperidine, pentazocine, and morphine, morphine remains the drug of choice, except in patients with well-documented morphine hypersensitivity. Four to 8 mg should be administered intravenously and doses of 2 to 8 mg repeated at intervals of 5 to 15 minutes until the pain is relieved or evident toxicity—hypotension, depression of respiration, or severe vomiting—precludes further administration of the drug. In some patients, remarkably large cumulative doses of morphine (2-3 mg/kg) may be required and are usually tolerated.

The reduction of anxiety resulting from morphine diminishes the patient's restlessness and the activity of the autonomic nervous system, with a consequent reduction of the heart's metabolic demands. The beneficial effect of morphine in patients with pulmonary edema is unequivocal and may be related to several factors, including peripheral arterial and venous dilation (particularly among patients with excessive sympathoadrenal activity), reduction of the work of breathing, and slowing of heart rate secondary to combined withdrawal of sympathetic tone and augmentation of vagal tone.

Hypotension following the administration of nitroglycerin and morphine can be minimized by maintaining the patient in a supine position and elevating the lower extremities if systolic arterial pressure declines below 100 mm Hg. Such positioning is undesirable in the presence of pulmonary edema, but morphine rarely produces hypotension under these circumstances. The concomitant administration of atropine in doses of 0.5 to 1.5 mg intravenously may be helpful in reducing the excessive vagomimetic effects of morphine, particularly when hypotension and bradycardia are present before it is administered.[7] Respiratory depression is an unusual complication of morphine in the presence of severe pain or pulmonary edema, but as the patient's cardiovascular status improves, impairment of ventilation may supervene. It can be treated with naloxone, in doses of 0.1 to 0.2 mg intravenously initially, repeated after 15 minutes if necessary. Nausea and vomiting may be troublesome side effects of large doses of morphine and can be treated with a phenothiazine.

Nitrates. By virtue of their ability to enhance coronary blood flow by coronary vasodilation and to decrease ventricular preload by increasing venous capacitance, sublingual nitrates are indicated for most patients with an acute coronary syndrome. At present, the only groups of patients with STEMI in whom sublingual nitroglycerin should *not* be given are those with inferior myocardial infarction and suspected right ventricular infarction[26] or marked hypotension (systolic pressure < 90 mm Hg), especially if accompanied by bradycardia.

Once it is ascertained that hypotension is not present, a sublingual nitroglycerin tablet should be administered and the patient observed carefully for improvement in symptoms or change in hemodynamics. If an initial dose is well tolerated and appears to be of benefit, further nitrates should be administered, with monitoring of the vital signs. Even small doses can produce sudden hypotension and bradycardia, a reaction that can be life-threatening but can usually be easily reversed with intravenous atropine if it is recognized quickly. Long-acting oral nitrate preparations should be avoided in the very early course of STEMI because of the frequently changing hemodynamic status of the patient. In patients with a prolonged period of waxing and waning chest pain, intravenous nitroglycerin may be of benefit in controlling symptoms and correcting ischemia, but frequent monitoring of blood pressure is required.

Beta-Adrenoceptor Blockers. These drugs relieve pain, reduce the need for analgesics in many patients, and reduce infarct size. A popular and relatively safe protocol for the use of a beta blocker in this situation is as follows. (1) Patients with heart failure (rales > 10 cm up from diaphragm), hypotension (blood pressure < 90 mm Hg), bradycardia (heart rate < 60 beats/min), or heart block (PR interval > 0.24 sec) are first excluded. (2) Metoprolol is given in three 5-mg boluses. (3) Patients are observed for 2 to 5 minutes after each bolus, and if the heart rate falls below 60 beats/min or systolic blood pressure falls below 100 mm Hg, no further drug is given; a total of three intravenous doses (15 mg) is administered. (4) If hemodynamic stability continues, 15 minutes after the last intravenous dose, the patient is begun on oral metoprolol, 50 mg every 6 hours for 2 days, then switched to 100 mg twice daily. An infusion of an extremely short-acting beta blocker, esmolol (50 to 250 mg/kg/min), may be useful in patients with relative contraindications to beta blockade in whom heart rate slowing is considered highly desirable.

Oxygen. Hypoxemia can occur in patients with STEMI and is usually secondary to ventilation-perfusion abnormalities that are sequelae of left ventricular failure; pneumonia and intrinsic pulmonary disease are additional causes of hypoxemia. It is common practice to treat all patients hospitalized with STEMI with oxygen for at least 24 to 48 hours, based on the empirical assumption of hypoxia and evidence that increased oxygen in the inspired air may protect ischemic myocardium. However, this practice may not be cost-effective. Augmentation of the fraction of oxygen in the inspired air does not elevate oxygen delivery significantly in patients who are not hypoxemic. Furthermore, it may increase systemic vascular resistance and arterial pressure and thereby lower cardiac output slightly.

In view of these considerations, arterial oxygen saturation can be estimated by pulse oximetry (an increasingly available technology), and oxygen therapy can be omitted if it is normal. On the other hand, oxygen should be administered to patients with STEMI when arterial hypoxemia is clinically evident or can be documented by measurement (e.g., SaO_2 < 90 percent).[7] In these patients, serial arterial blood gas measurements can be employed to follow the efficacy of oxygen therapy. The delivery of 2 to 4 liters/min of 100 percent oxygen by mask or nasal prongs for 6 to 12 hours is satisfactory for most patients with mild hypoxemia. If arterial oxygenation is still depressed on this regimen, the flow rate may have to be increased, and other causes for hypoxemia should be sought. In patients with pulmonary edema, endotracheal intubation and positive-pressure controlled ventilation may be necessary.

Limitation of Infarct Size

Infarct size is an important determinant of prognosis in patients with STEMI. Patients who succumb from cardiogenic shock generally exhibit either a single massive infarct or a small to moderate-sized infarct superimposed on multiple prior infarctions.[27] Survivors with large infarcts frequently exhibit late impairment of ventricular function, and the long-term mortality rate is higher than for survivors with small infarcts, who tend not to develop cardiac decompensation.[27]

In view of the prognostic importance of infarct size, the concept that modification of infarct size is possible has attracted a great deal of experimental and clinical attention (see Fig. 46–12).[13,28] Efforts to limit the size of the infarct have been divided among several different (sometimes overlapping) approaches: (1) early reperfusion, (2) reduction of myocardial energy demands, (3) manipulation of sources of energy production in the myocardium, and (4) prevention of reperfusion injury. Although early reperfusion ("time-dependent effect of reperfusion") has been the major focus of modern management strategies for STEMI, it is important to note that in addition to the limitation of infarct size, late reperfusion of ischemic myocardium may convey several benefits that contribute to mortality reduction ("time-independent effect of reperfusion") (see Fig. 46–12).[29]

THE DYNAMIC NATURE OF INFARCTION. STEMI is a dynamic process that does not occur instantaneously but evolves over hours. The fate of jeopardized, ischemic tissue can be affected favorably by interventions that restore myocardial perfusion, reduce microvascular damage in

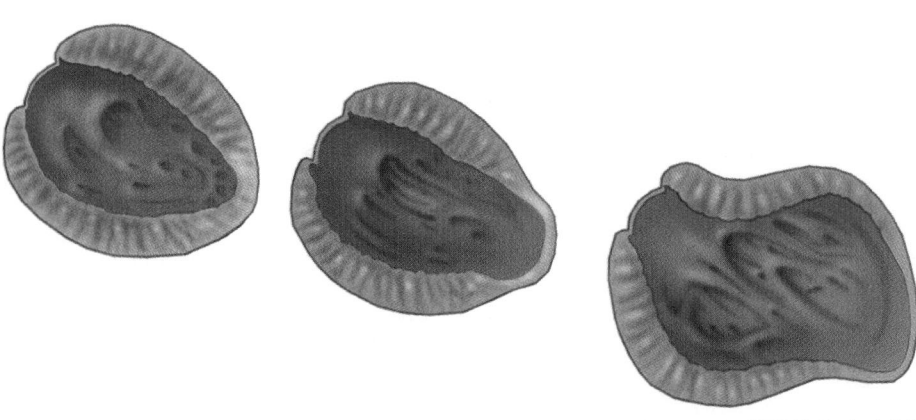

FIGURE 47–3 Remodeling of left ventricle after ST segment elevation myocardial infarction (STEMI). On the left is shown an apical STEMI (white zone of left ventricle). Over time, the infarct zone elongates and thins. Progressive remodeling of the left ventricle occurs (center and right images) ultimately converting the left ventricle from an oval shape to a spherical shape. Pharmacological and catheter-based reperfusion strategies for STEMI have a favorable impact on this process by minimizing the extent of myocardial necrosis (left) through prompt restoration of flow in the epicardial infarct vessel. (Adapted from McMurray JJV, Pfeffer MA (eds): Heart Failure Updates. London, Martin Dunitz, 2003.)

the infarct zone, reduce myocardial oxygen requirements, inhibit accumulation of or facilitate wash-out of noxious metabolites, augment the availability of substrate for anaerobic metabolism, or blunt the effects of mediators of injury that compromise the structure and function of intracellular organelles and constituents of cell membranes.[30-32] Strong evidence in experimental animals and suggestive evidence in patients indicate that ischemic preconditioning, a form of endogenous protection against STEMI (see Chap. 19), prior to sustained coronary occlusion decreases infarct size and is associated with a more favorable outcome, with decreased risk of extension of infarction and recurrent ischemic events. Brief episodes of ischemia in one coronary vascular bed may precondition myocardium in a remote zone, attenuating the size of infarction in the latter when sustained coronary occlusion occurs.[33]

The perfusion of the myocardium in the infarct zone appears to be reduced maximally immediately following coronary occlusion. Up to one-third of patients develop spontaneous recanalization of an occluded infarct-related artery beginning at 12 to 24 hours. This delayed spontaneous reperfusion has been associated with improvement of left ventricular function because it improves healing of infarcted tissue, prevents ventricular remodeling, and reperfuses hibernating myocardium. However, to *maximize* the amount of salvaged myocardium by *accelerating* the process of reperfusion and also implementing it in those patients who would otherwise have an occluded infarct-related artery, the strategies of pharmacologically induced and catheter-based reperfusion of the infarct vessel have been developed (Fig. 47-3) (see Chap. 48).

Additional factors that may contribute to limitation of infarct size in association with reperfusion include relief of coronary spasm, prevention of damage to the microvasculature, improved systemic hemodynamics (augmentation of coronary perfusion pressure and reduced left ventricular end-diastolic pressure), and development of collateral circulation. The prompt implementation of measures designed to protect ischemic myocardium and support myocardial perfusion may provide sufficient time for the development of anatomical and physiological compensatory mechanisms that limit the ultimate extent of infarction (see Fig. 46-3). It is possible that interventions designed to protect ischemic myocardium during the initial event may also reduce the incidence of extension of infarction or early reinfarction.

ROUTINE MEASURES FOR INFARCT SIZE LIMITATION. Although reperfusion of ischemic myocardium is the most important technique for limiting infarct size, several routine measures to accomplish this goal are applicable to all patients with STEMI, whether or not reperfusion therapy is prescribed. The treatment strategies discussed in this section can be initiated in the emergency department and then continued in the coronary care unit.

It is important to maintain an optimal balance between myocardial oxygen supply and demand so that as much as possible of the jeopardized zone of the myocardium surrounding the most profoundly ischemic zones of the infarct can be salvaged. During the period before irreversible injury has occurred, myocardial oxygen consumption should be minimized by maintaining the patient at rest, physically and emotionally, and by utilizing mild sedation and a quiet atmosphere that may lower heart rate, a major determinant of myocardial oxygen consumption. If the patient was receiving a beta-adrenoceptor blocking agent at the time the clinical manifestations of the infarction commenced, the drug should be continued unless a specific contraindication develops, such as left ventricular systolic failure or bradyarrhythmia. Marked sinus bradycardia (heart rate less than approximately 50 beats/min) and the frequently coexisting hypotension should be treated with postural maneuvers (the Trendelenburg position) to increase central blood volume and atropine and electrical pacing, but not with isoproterenol. On the other hand, the routine administration of atropine, with the resultant increase in heart rate, to patients without serious bradycardia is contraindicated. All forms of tachyarrhythmias require prompt treatment because they increase myocardial oxygen needs.[7]

Congestive heart failure should be treated promptly. Given their multiple beneficial actions in STEMI patients, inhibitors of the renin-angiotensin-aldosterone system are indicated in the treatment of congestive heart failure associated with STEMI unless the patient is hypotensive. Inotropic agents such as isoproterenol that increase myocardial oxygen consumption should be avoided.

As discussed earlier, arterial oxygenation should be restored to normal in patients with hypoxemia, such as occurs in patients with chronic pulmonary disease, pneumonia, or left ventricular failure. Oxygen-enriched air should be administered to patients with hypoxemia, and bronchodilators and expectorants should be used when indicated. Severe anemia, which can also extend the area of ischemic injury, should be corrected by the cautious administration of packed red blood cells, accompanied by a diuretic if there is any evidence of left ventricular failure. Associated conditions, particularly infections and the accompanying tachycardia, fever, and elevated myocardial oxygen needs, require immediate attention.

Systolic arterial pressure should not be allowed to deviate by more than approximately 25 to 30 mm Hg from the patient's usual level unless marked hypertension had been present before the onset of STEMI. It is likely that each patient has an optimal range of arterial pressure; as coronary perfusion pressure deviates from this level, the unfavorable balance between oxygen supply (which is related to coronary perfusion pressure) and myocardial oxygen demand (which is related to ventricular wall tension) that ensues increases the extent of ischemic injury.

Reperfusion Therapy

GENERAL CONCEPTS. Although late spontaneous reperfusion occurs in some patients, persistent thrombotic occlusion is present in the majority of patients with STEMI while the myocardium is undergoing necrosis.[34] Timely reperfusion of jeopardized myocardium represents the most effective way of restoring the balance between myocardial oxygen supply and demand. When fibrinolysis is administered, the extent of protection appears to be related directly to the rapidity with which reperfusion is implemented after the onset of coronary occlusion.[34] Evidence exists to suggest that the extent of myocardial salvage when reperfusion is achieved with PCI (including stent deployment) is less time dependent than that for fibrinolysis.[28] The mechanisms underlying the therapy-dependent influence of time-to-treatment on myocardial salvage are not clear but probably include restoration of full antegrade flow in the infarct artery with PCI and decreasing efficacy of fibrinolytic agents as coronary thrombi mature with the passage of time.[28] It should be noted, however, that analyses adjusting for baseline risk demonstrate a statistically significant increase in mortality with progressive delays between the onset of symptoms and PCI.[35] For every 30-minute delay from symptom onset to PCI, there is an 8 percent increase in the relative risk of 1-year mortality (Fig. 47–4).[36]

In some patients, particularly those with cardiogenic shock, tissue damage occurs in a "stuttering" manner rather than abruptly, a condition that might more properly be termed *subacute infarction*. This concept of the nature of the infarction process, as well as the observation that the incidence of complications of STEMI in both the early and late postinfarction periods is a function of infarct size, underscores the need for careful history-taking to ascertain whether the patient appears to have had repetitive cycles of sponta-

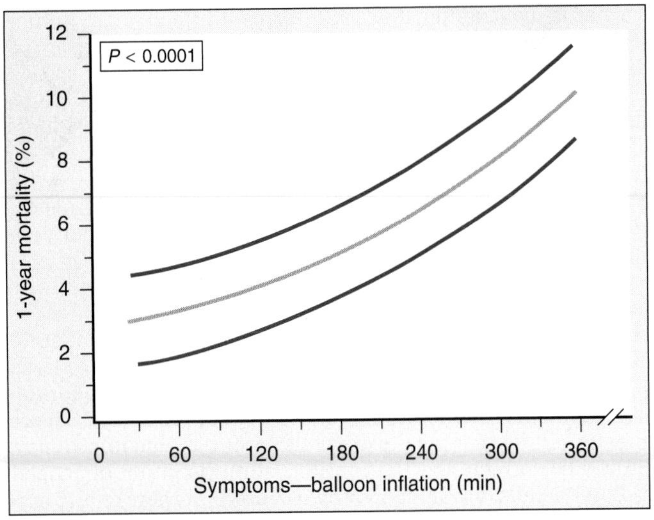

FIGURE 47–4 Importance of time to reperfusion in patients undergoing primary percutaneous coronary intervention (PCI) for ST segment elevation myocardial infarction (STEMI). This plot is based on the pooled data from 1791 patients undergoing primary PCI for STEMI. After adjusting for baseline risk, there is a curvilinear relationship between the time elapsed from the onset of symptoms to balloon inflation and the rate of mortality at 1 year. For every 30-minute delay from onset of symptoms to primary PCI, there is an 8 percent increase in the relative risk of 1-year mortality. (From De Luca G, Suryapranata H, Ottervanger JP, et al: Time-delay to treatment and mortality in primary angioplasty for acute myocardial infarction: Every minute counts. Circulation 109:1223, 2004.)

neous reperfusion and reocclusion. "Fixing" the time of onset of the infarction process in such patients can be difficult. In such patients with waxing and waning ischemic discomfort, a rigid time interval from the first episode of pain should not be used when determining whether a patient is "outside the window" for benefit from acute reperfusion therapy.

PATHOPHYSIOLOGY OF MYOCARDIAL REPERFUSION. Prevention of cell death by the restoration of blood flow depends on the severity and duration of preexisting ischemia. Substantial experimental and clinical evidence exists indicating that the earlier blood flow is restored, the more favorably influenced are recovery of left ventricular systolic function, improvement in diastolic function, and reduction in overall mortality.[19] Collateral coronary vessels also appear to play a role in the resultant left ventricular function following reperfusion.[37] They provide sufficient perfusion of myocardium to retard cell death and are probably of greater importance in patients having reperfusion later rather than 1 to 2 hours after coronary occlusion.

Even after successful reperfusion and despite the absence of irreversible myocardial damage, a period of postischemic contractile dysfunction can occur—a phenomenon referred to as *myocardial stunning*.[38] Periods of myocardial stunning are well described in experimental animals but have also been confirmed in STEMI patients using positron emission tomography (PET) scanning after percutaneous transluminal coronary angiography (PTCA) to measure myocardial blood flow and oxygen consumption.[39]

REPERFUSION INJURY

The process of reperfusion, although beneficial in terms of myocardial salvage, may come at a cost due to a process known as *reperfusion injury*. Kloner has summarized the data on the four types of reperfusion injury that have been observed in experimental animals. These consist of (1) lethal reperfusion injury—a term referring to reperfusion-induced death of cells that were still viable at the time of restoration of coronary blood flow; (2) vascular reperfusion injury—progressive damage to the microvasculature such that there is an expanding area of no reflow and loss of coronary vasodilatory reserve[40]; (3) stunned myocardium—salvaged myocytes display a prolonged period of contractile dysfunction following restoration of blood flow owing to abnormalities of intracellular biochemistry leading to reduced energy production; and (4) reperfusion arrhythmias—bursts of ventricular tachycardia and on occasion ventricular fibrillation that occur within seconds of reperfusion. The available evidence suggests that vascular reperfusion injury, stunning, and reperfusion arrhythmias can all occur in patients with acute myocardial infarction. The concept of lethal reperfusion injury of potentially salvageable myocardium remains controversial, both in experimental animals and in patients.[41]

Reperfusion increases the cell swelling that occurs with ischemia. Reperfusion of the myocardium in which the microvasculature is damaged leads to the creation of a hemorrhagic infarct (see Fig. 46-6). Fibrinolytic therapy appears more likely to produce hemorrhagic infarction than reperfusion by mechanical means. Although concern has been raised that this hemorrhage may lead to extension of the infarct, this does not appear to be the case. Histological study of patients not surviving in spite of successful reperfusion has revealed hemorrhagic infarcts, but this hemorrhage usually does not extend beyond the area of necrosis.[41]

PROTECTION AGAINST REPERFUSION INJURY. A variety of adjunctive approaches have been taken to protect the myocardium against injury that occurs after reperfusion: (1) preservation of microvascular integrity by using antiplatelet agents and antithrombins to minimize embolization of atheroembolic debris[42,43]; (2) prevention of inflammatory damage[31,44-47]; and (3) metabolic support of the ischemic myocardium.[48-50] The effectiveness of agents directed against reperfusion injury rapidly declines the later they are administered after reperfusion; eventually, no beneficial effect is detectable in animal models after 45 to 60 minutes of reperfusion has elapsed.[48]

REPERFUSION ARRHYTHMIAS

Transient sinus bradycardia occurs in many patients with inferior infarcts at the time of acute reperfusion; it is most often accompanied by some degree of hypotension. This combination of hypotension and bradycardia with a sudden increase in coronary flow has been ascribed to the activation of the Bezold-Jarisch reflex.[51] Premature ventricular contractions, accelerated idioventricular rhythm, and nonsustained ventricular tachycardia are also seen commonly following successful reperfusion. In experimental animals with STEMI, ventricular fibrillation occurs shortly after reperfusion, but this arrhythmia is not as frequent in patients as in the experimental setting. Although some investigators have postulated that early afterdepolarizations participate in the genesis of reperfusion ventricular arrhythmias, early afterdepolarizations are present both during ischemia and during reperfusion and are therefore unlikely to be involved in the development of reperfusion ventricular tachycardia or fibrillation.

When present, rhythm disturbances may actually be a marker of successful restoration of coronary flow. However, although reperfusion arrhythmias have a high sensitivity for detecting successful reperfusion, the high incidence of identical rhythm disturbances in patients without successful coronary artery reperfusion limits their specificity for detection of restoration of coronary blood flow. In general, clinical features are poor markers of reperfusion, with no single clinical finding or constellation of findings being reliably predictive of angiographically demonstrated coronary artery patency.[52]

Although reperfusion arrhythmias may show a temporal clustering at the time of restoration of coronary blood flow in patients with successful fibrinolysis, the overall incidence of such arrhythmias appears to be similar in patients not receiving a thrombolytic agent who may develop these arrhythmias as a consequence of spontaneous coronary artery reperfusion or the evolution of the infarct process itself. These considerations, as well as the fact that the brief "electrical storm" occurring at the time of reperfusion is generally innocuous, indicate that no prophylactic antiarrhythmic therapy is necessary when thrombolytics are prescribed.

LATE ESTABLISHMENT OF PATENCY OF THE INFARCT VESSEL

It has been suggested that improved survival and ventricular function after successful reperfusion are not due entirely to limitation of infarct size (see Fig. 46-12).[53] Both experimental and clinical evidence indicate that the benefits of a patent artery include a favorable effect on ventricular remodeling (improved healing of infarcted tissue and prevention of infarct expansion), enhancement of collateral flow, improvement in diastolic and systolic function, increased electrical stability, and reduced long-term mortality. Late reperfusion of the artery perfusing an infarction provides a vascular scaffolding in the infarct zone and increases the influx of inflammatory cells that participate in the formation of a mature fibrous scar. The vascular scaffold and firmer myocardial scar prevent infarct segment lengthening and decrease the tendency to infarct expansion and aneurysm formation.[29] Poorly contracting or noncontracting myocardium in a zone that is supplied by a stenosed infarct-related artery with slow antegrade perfusion may still contain viable myocytes. This situation is referred to as *hibernating myocardium*,[54] and its function can be improved by PCI to augment flow in the infarct-related artery. Late reperfusion of the infarct-related artery by thrombolysis or late restoration of flow via PCI enhances the electrical stability of the infarcted zone and is probably related to the reduced incidence of ventricular fibrillation and of automatic firing of implantable cardioverter-defibrillator devices.[53] The beneficial effect of late reperfusion of the infarct-related artery is independent of left ventricular function and other mortality-reducing therapies such as angiotensin-converting enzyme (ACE) inhibitors. Several clinical trials are testing the benefits of late reperfusion of an occluded infarct artery in asymptomatic patients (see Fig. 46-12).[29,55]

SUMMARY OF EFFECTS OF MYOCARDIAL REPERFUSION. Rupture of an unstable plaque in the culprit vessel produces complete occlusion of the infarct-related coronary artery. STEMI occurs with the ensuing development of left ventricular dilation and ultimate death through a combination of pump failure and electrical instability (Fig. 47–3; see also Fig. 46–12). Early reperfusion shortens the duration of coronary occlusion, minimizes the degree of ultimate left ventricular dysfunction and dilation, and reduces the probability that the STEMI patient will develop pump failure or malignant ventricular tachyarrhythmias.[34,56] Late reperfusion may favorably affect the process of infarct healing and minimize left ventricular remodeling and the ultimate development of pump dysfunction and electrical instability.[57]

Coronary Fibrinolysis

Many years elapsed between the first report of intracoronary clot lysis in an experimental animal and the widespread use of fibrinolytic agents in patients with STEMI. With publication of the first GISSI trial of more than 11,000 patients in 1986, in which intravenous streptokinase was shown to result in a significant reduction in the rate of mortality in patients treated within 6 hours of the onset of symptoms, the use of fibrinolytic therapy in cases of STEMI was established.[34] It is now clear that fibrinolysis recanalizes thrombotic occlusion associated with STEMI, and restoration of coronary flow reduces infarct size and improves myocardial function and survival over both the short and the long terms.[58] The majority of the mortality benefit seen at 10-year follow-up in the GISSI trial was obtained prior to hospital discharge, since no survival difference was seen in fibrinolysed and control patients discharged alive except for those treated within the first hour after onset of symptoms.[59]

INTRACORONARY THROMBOLYSIS. Clinical investigation of pharmacological reperfusion of ischemic myocardium initially focused on intracoronary thrombolysis in the early hours of STEMI. Because of the delay involved in catheterizing patients with STEMI, current consensus is that intracoronary administration of fibrinolytic therapy should be reserved for the rare situation in which a patient develops coronary thrombosis during the course of an angiographic procedure and in whom either a coronary catheter is already in place or such placement is easily and rapidly achieved. In contemporary practice, however, such patients are more likely to be treated by PCI (see Chap. 48).

INTRAVENOUS FIBRINOLYSIS

TIMI Flow Grade. To provide a level of standardization for comparison of the various regimens, most investigators describe the flow in the infarct vessel according to the Thrombolysis in Myocardial Infarction trial (TIMI) grading system: grade 0 is complete occlusion of the infarct related artery; grade 1, some penetration of the contrast material beyond the point of obstruction but without perfusion of the distal coronary bed; grade 2, perfusion of the entire infarct vessel into the distal bed but with delayed flow compared with a normal artery; and grade 3, full perfusion of the infarct vessel with normal flow.[60,61] When evaluating reports of angiographic studies of fibrinolytic agents, it must be kept in mind that only in studies in which a pretreatment coronary arteriogram documents occlusion of the culprit vessel can the term *recanalization* be applied if flow is restored. If the status of the culprit vessel is not known prior to treatment, the only fact that can be stated with certainty is the *patency rate* of the vessel at the moment the contrast material is injected. This snapshot in time does not reflect the fluctuating status of flow in the infarct vessel that characteristically undergoes repeated cycles of patency and reocclusion, as has been documented angiographically and by continuous ST segment monitoring.

Issues of the fluctuating nature of patency of the infarct-related artery notwithstanding, the majority of angiographic studies of reperfusion regimens for STEMI used an assessment of the TIMI flow grade at 90 or preferably 60 minutes after the start of fibrinolytic therapy.[62]

Initially, TIMI grade 2 and grade 3 flows were lumped into the favorable category of coronary patency that was compared with a combined TIMI grade 0 and grade 1 flow in an unfavorable category of persistent occlusion. It has been learned, however, that TIMI grade 2 flow should not be combined with grade 3 flow because it has been recognized that TIMI grade 3 flow is far superior to grade 2 in terms of infarct size reduction and both short-term and long-term mortality benefit.[30] Therefore, TIMI grade 3 flow should be considered to be the goal when assessing flow in the epicardial infarct artery (Fig. 47-5).[30]

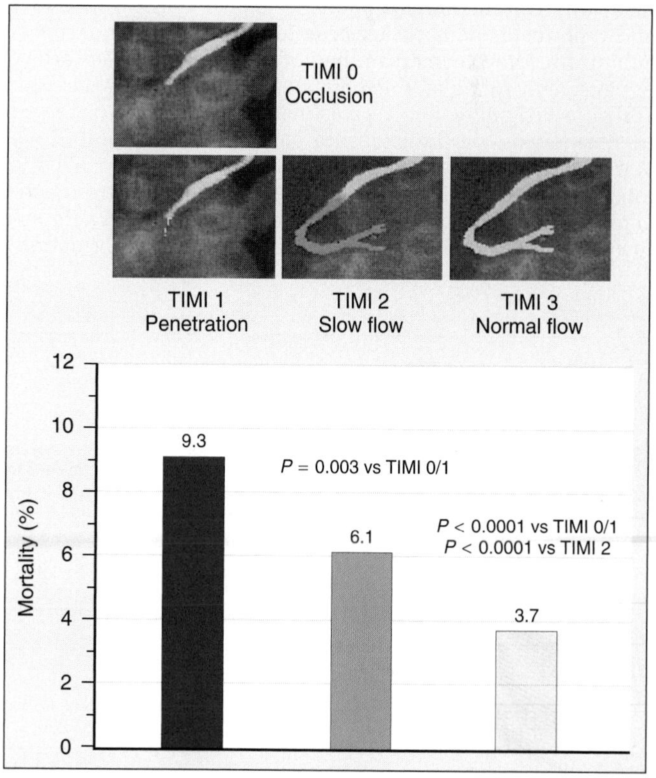

FIGURE 47–5 Correlation of TIMI flow grade and mortality. A pooled analysis of data from 5498 patients in several angiographic trials of reperfusion for ST elevation myocardial infarction showed a gradient of mortality when the angiographic findings were stratified by TIMI flow grade. Patients with TIMI 0 or TIMI 1 flow had the highest rate of mortality; TIMI 2 flow was associated with an intermediate rate of mortality; the lowest rate of mortality was observed in patients with TIMI 3 flow. (Dr. Michael Gibson, personal communication.)

THE TIMI FRAME COUNT. In an effort to provide a more quantitative statement of the briskness of coronary blood flow in the infarct artery and also to account for differences in the size and length of vessels (e.g., left anterior descending versus right coronary artery) and interobserver variability, Gibson and coworkers developed the *TIMI frame count*—a simple count of the number of angiographic frames elapsed until the contrast material arrives in the distal bed of the vessel of interest. This is an objective and quantitative index of coronary blood flow, is an independent predictor of in-hospital mortality from STEMI, and also discriminates patients with TIMI grade 3 flow into low- and high-risk groups.[63] Using the TIMI frame count, Gibson and coworkers determined that the following were univariate predictors of delayed coronary blood flow following fibrinolytic administration: a greater percentage diameter stenosis, a decreased minimum lumen diameter, a greater percentage of the culprit artery distal to stenosis, and the presence of delayed achievement of patency, a culprit artery location in the left coronary circulation, pulsatile flow (i.e., reversible flow in systole), or intraluminal thrombus.[64] The TIMI frame count can also be used to quantitate coronary blood flow (cc's per second) calculated at

$$21 \div (\text{observed TIMI frame count}) \times 1.7$$

(based on Doppler velocity wire data showing that normal flow equals 1.7 cm^3 per second, which is proportional to 21 frames). The relationship between calculated coronary perfusion and mortality for patients treated with fibrinolytics and primary PCI is illustrated in Figure 47–6.

MYOCARDIAL PERFUSION. Despite intense interest in the development of reperfusion regimens that normalize flow in the epicardial infarct-related artery, the real goal of reperfusion in patients with STEMI is to improve myocardial perfusion in the infarct zone. Of course, myocardial perfusion cannot be improved adequately without restoration of flow in the occluded infarct-related artery. However, even patients with TIMI grade 3 flow may not achieve adequate myocardial perfusion. The two major impediments to normalization of myocardial perfusion are microvascular damage (Fig. 47–7) and reperfusion injury.[30] Obstruction of the distal microvasculature in the downstream bed of the infarct-related artery is caused by platelet microemboli and thrombi. Microembolization of platelet aggregates may actually be exacerbated by fibrinolysis via the exposure of clot-bound thrombin, an extremely potent platelet agonist. Spasm can also occur in the microvasculature due to the release of substances from activated platelets such as serotonin and thromboxane A_2. Reperfusion injury results in cellular edema, free radical formation, and calcium overload. In addition, cytokine activation leads to neutrophil accumulation and inflammatory mediators that contribute to tissue injury.

Several techniques have been used to evaluate the adequacy of myocardial perfusion. Electrocardiographic ST segment resolution is a strong predictor of outcome in STEMI patients but is a better predictor of an occluded than of a patent infarct-related artery.[65,66] Absence of early ST segment resolution after angiographically successful primary PCI identifies patients with a higher risk of left ventricular dysfunction and mortality, presumably because of microvascular damage in the infarct zone. Thus, the 12-lead electrocardiogram is a marker of the biological integrity of myocytes in the infarct zone and can reflect inadequate myocardial perfusion even in the presence of TIMI 3 flow.[40,67] Given the dynamic nature of coronary occlusion, it has been proposed that continuous ST segment monitoring is more informative than static 12-lead ECG recordings, but practical limitations have prevented continuous ST monitoring from widespread clinical application.[66] Defects in perfusion patterns seen with myocardial contrast echocardiography correlate with regional wall motion abnormalities and lack of myocardial viability on dobutamine stress echocardiography. A practical limitation to myocardial contrast echocardiography is the need for intracoronary injection of echo contrast, although this can be circumvented by the availability of new echo contrast agents that can be injected intravenously. Doppler flow wire studies, magnetic resonance imaging, and nuclear imaging with positron emission tomography have also been used to define abnormalities of myocardial perfusion (Fig. 47–8).[30]

A new angiographic method for assessing myocardial perfusion has also been introduced by Gibson and colleagues: the TIMI myocardial perfusion grade (see Fig. 47–9). Abnormalities of increasing myocardial perfusion as assessed by the TIMI myocardial perfusion grade correlate with mortality risk even after adjusting for the presence of TIMI grade 3 flow or a normal TIMI frame count.[68]

Effect of Fibrinolytic Therapy on Mortality

There is no doubt that early intravenous fibrinolysis improve survival in patients with STEMI.[58] Mortality varies considerably depending on the patients included for study and the adjunctive therapies employed. The benefit of fibrinolytic therapy appears to be greatest when agents are administered as early as possible, with the most dramatic results when the drug is given less than 2 hours after symptoms begin.[69]

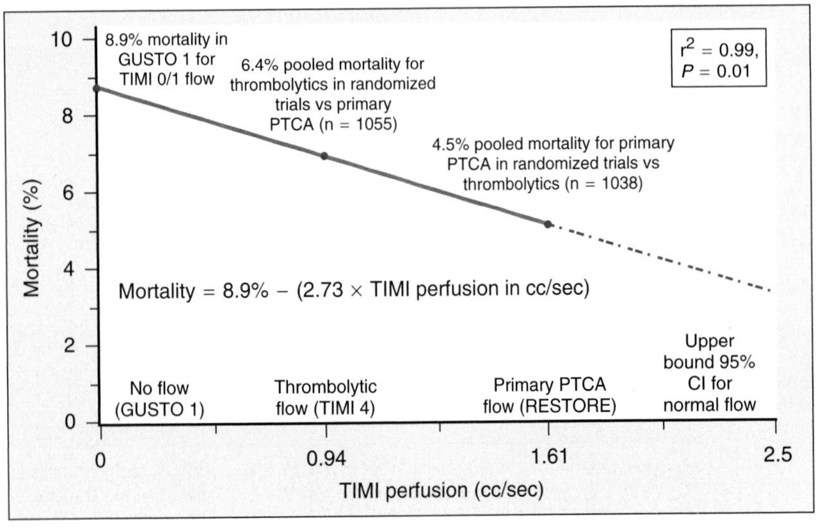

FIGURE 47–6 Relationship between coronary blood flow and mortality rate in patients with acute myocardial infarction. (From Gibson CM: Primary angioplasty, rescue angioplasty, and new devices. *In* Hennekens CH [ed]: Clinical Trials in Cardiovascular Disease: A Companion to Braunwald's Heart Disease. Philadelphia, WB Saunders, 1999, p 194.)

The Fibrinolytic Therapy Trialists' Collaborative Group (FTT) has performed a comprehensive overview of nine trials of thrombolytic therapy, each of which enrolled more than 1000 patients (Fig. 47–10).[19] The database for the FTT overview consisted of 58,600 patients, including 6177 (10.5 percent) who died, 564 (1.0 percent) who sustained a stroke, and 436 (0.7 percent) who sustained major noncerebral bleeds. The absolute mortality rates for the control and fibrinolytic groups stratified by presenting features are shown in Figure 47–10. The overall results indicated an 18 percent reduction in short-term mortality, but as much as a 25 percent reduction in mortality for the subset of 45,000 patients with ST segment elevation or bundle branch block. Two trials, LATE and EMERAS, viewed together provide evidence that a mortality reduction may still be observed in patients treated with thrombolytic agents between 6 and 12 hours from the onset of ischemic symptoms. The data from LATE and EMERAS and the FTT overview form the basis for extending the window of treatment with fibrinolytics up to 12 hours from the onset of symptoms. Boersma and

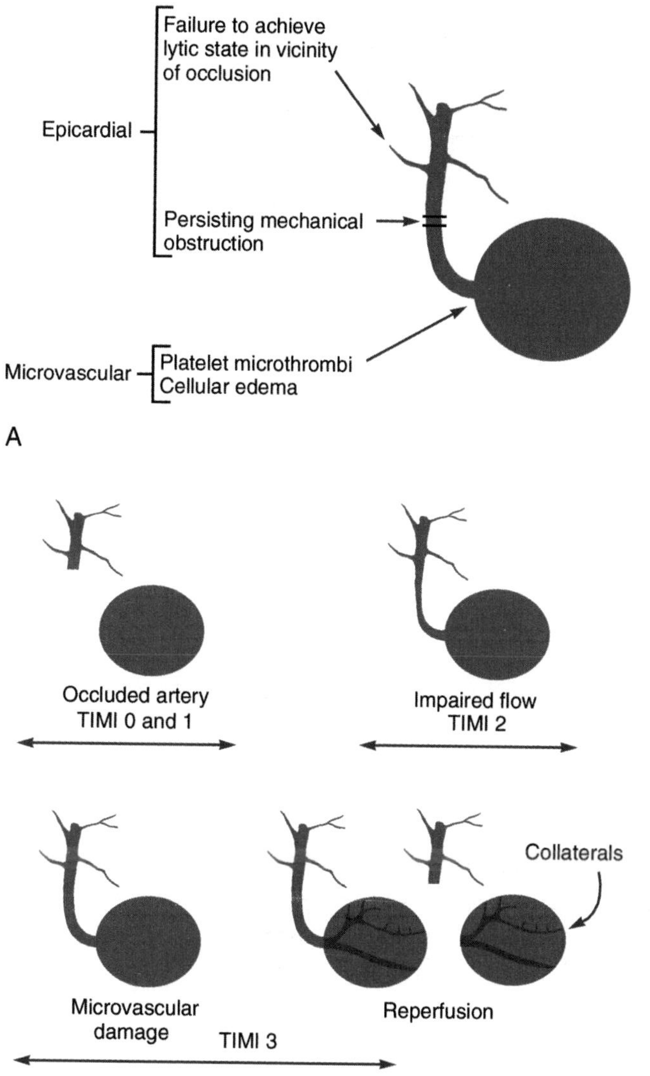

FIGURE 47–7 Patterns of response to fibrinolysis. **A,** Failure of epicardial reperfusion can occur due to failure to induce a lytic state or due to mechanical factors at the site of occlusion. Failure of microvascular reperfusion is due to a combination of platelet microthrombi followed by endothelial swelling and myocardial edema ("no reflow"). **B,** Fibrinolysis may fail due to persistent occlusion of the epicardial infarct-related artery (TIMI grades 0 and 1), patency of an epicardial artery in the presence of impaired (TIMI grade 2) flow, or microvascular occlusion in the presence of angiographically normal (TIMI grade 3) flow. Successful reperfusion requires a patent artery with an intact microvascular network. Conversely, reperfusion may occur despite an occluded epicardial artery due to the presence of collateral arteries. (From Davies CH, Ormerod OJ: Failed coronary thrombolysis. Lancet 351:1191, 1998.)

colleagues pooled the trials in the FTT overview, two smaller studies with data on time to randomization, and 11 additional trials of more than 100 patients. Patients were divided into six time categories from symptom onset to randomization. A nonlinear relationship of treatment benefit to time was observed, with the greatest benefit occurring in the first 1 to 2 hours from the onset of symptoms (Fig. 47–11).[69]

The mortality effect of fibrinolytic therapy in elderly patients is of considerable interest and controversy. Although patients older than 75 years of age were initially excluded from randomized trials of fibrinolytic therapy, they now constitute about 15 percent of the patients studied in contemporary megatrials of fibrinolysis and about 35 percent of patients analyzed in registries of STEMI patients.[70-72] Barriers to initiation of therapy in older patients with STEMI include a protracted period of delay in seeking medical care, a lower incidence of ischemic discomfort and greater incidence of atypical symptoms and concomitant illnesses, and an increased incidence of nondiagnostic ECG readings.[7] Younger patients with STEMI achieve a slightly greater relative reduction in mortality compared with elderly patients, but the higher absolute mortality in the elderly results in similar absolute mortality reductions. Thus, as seen in Figure 47–10, there was a 26 percent decrease in mortality in patients who were younger than 55 years of age (11 lives saved per 1000 with thrombolytic therapy) and a 4 percent reduction in mortality in patients older than 75 years of age (10 lives saved per 1000 treated).[73] Data from a Swedish national registry in patients 75 years of age or older with a first STEMI support the use of fibrinolysis in the elderly in that there was a 13 percent relative risk reduction ($p = 0.001$) in the composite of mortality and cerebral bleeding at 1 year compared to no fibrinolysis (Fig. 47–12).[72]

Other important baseline characteristics that have an impact on the mortality effect of fibrinolytic therapy include the vital signs at presentation and the presence of diabetes mellitus (see Fig. 47–10). For example, there was an 18 percent decrease in mortality for patients presenting with a systolic pressure less than 100 mm Hg (62 lives saved per 1000 treated), compared with a 12 percent reduction in mortality for patients with a systolic pressure of 175 mm Hg or more (10 lives saved per 1000 treated). Patients with a history of diabetes mellitus experienced a mortality reduction of 21 percent (37 lives saved per 1000 treated), compared with a mortality reduction of 15 percent (15 lives saved per 1000 treated) in patients without a history of diabetes.

A number of models have been developed to integrate the many clinical variables that affect a patient's mortality risk before administration of fibrinolytic therapy. A convenient, simple, bedside risk-scoring system for predicting 30-day mortality at presentation for fibrinolytic-eligible patients with STEMI was developed by Morrow and associates using the InTIME-II trial database (Fig. 47–13).[74,75] However, modeling of mortality risk cannot cover all clinical scenarios and should not substitute for clinical judgment in individual cases. For example, patients with inferior STEMI who might

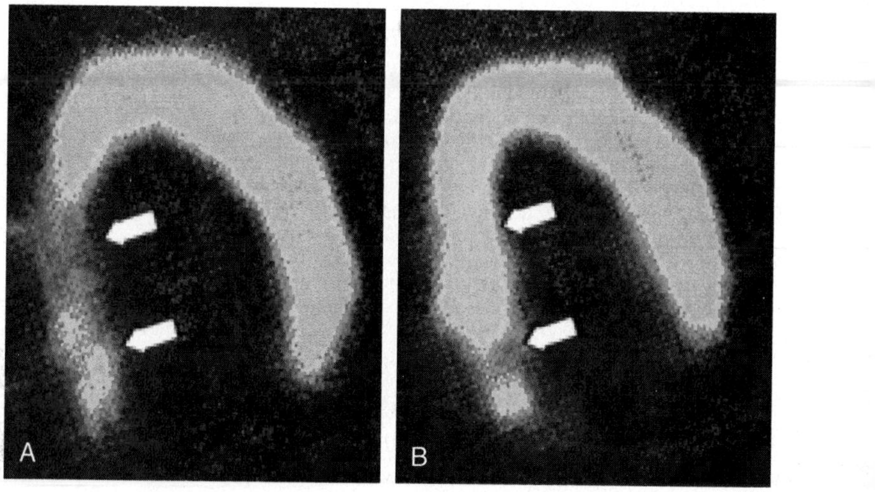

FIGURE 47–8 Myocardial perfusion in a case of acute myocardial infarction. **A,** ^{99m}Tc-sestamibi single-photon emission computed tomography (SPECT) before reperfusion; vertical long axis slice; reduced tracer uptake of basal inferior left ventricular myocardium (arrows). **B,** ^{99m}Tc-sestamibi SPECT 7 days after stenting of left circumflex coronary artery; nearly normal tracer uptake of basal inferior left ventricular myocardium. (From Horcher J, Blasini R, Martinoff S, et al: Myocardial perfusion in acute coronary syndrome. Circulation 99:e15, 1999.)

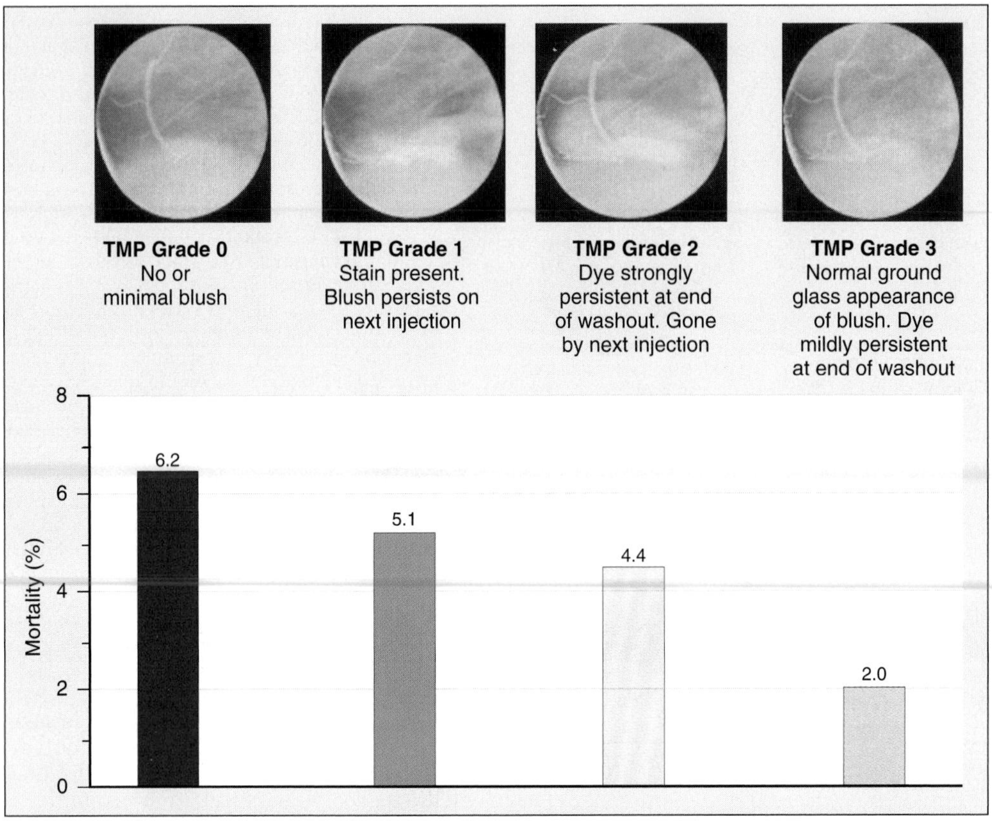

FIGURE 47–9 Relationship between TIMI myocardial perfusion grade and mortality. TIMI myocardial perfusion grade 0 or no perfusion of the myocardium is associated with the highest rate of mortality. If the stain of the myocardium is present (grade 1), mortality is also high. A reduction in mortality is seen if the dye enters the microvasculature but is still persistent at the end of the washout phase (grade 2). The lowest mortality rate is observed in those patients with normal perfusion (grade 3) where the dye is minimally persistent at the end of the washout phase. (From Gibson CM, Murphy SA, Rizzo MJ, et al: Relationship between TIMI frame count and clinical outcomes after thrombolytic administration. Thrombolysis In Myocardial Infarction [TIMI] Study Group. Circulation 99:1945, 1999.)

otherwise be considered to have a low risk of mortality and for whom many physicians have questioned the benefits of fibrinolytic therapy might be in a much higher mortality risk subgroup if their inferior infarction is associated with right ventricular infarction, precordial ST segment depression, or ST segment elevation in the lateral precordial leads.

The short-term survival benefit enjoyed by patients who receive fibrinolytic therapy is maintained over the 1- to 10-year follow-up.[59] Room for improvement remains, however, given reports of reocclusion rates of the infarct-related artery as high as 10 percent in hospital and up to 30 percent by 3 months,[76] and reinfarction rates as high as 9.5 percent within 6 weeks in fibrinolytic-treated patients.[77]

COMPARISON OF FIBRINOLYTIC AGENTS (see Chap. 80)

Some comparative features of the approved fibrinolytic agents for intravenous therapy are presented in Table 47–4.

The tissue plasminogen activator (t-PA) molecule contains the following five domains: finger, epidermal growth factor, kringle 1 and kringle 2, and serum protease (Fig. 47–14).[78] In the absence of fibrin, t-PA is a weak plasminogen activator; fibrin provides a scaffold on which t-PA and plasminogen are held in such a way that the catalytic efficiency for plasminogen activation of t-PA is increased many-fold. Plasma clearance of t-PA is mediated to a varying degree by residues in each of the domains except the serine protease domain, which is responsible for the enzymatic activity of t-PA. The accelerated dose regimen of t-PA over 90 minutes produces more rapid thrombolysis than the standard 3-hour infusion of t-PA. The recommended dosage regimen for t-PA is a 15 mg intravenous bolus followed by an infusion of 0.75 mg/kg (maximum 50 mg) over 30 minutes, and then an infusion of 0.5 mg/kg (maximum 35 mg) over 60 minutes.

Modifications of the basic t-PA structure have been made to yield a group of third-generation fibrinolytics (see Fig. 47–14 and Table 47–4). A common feature among the third-generation fibrinolytics is prolonged plasma clearance, allowing them to be administered as a bolus rather than the bolus and double-infusion technique by which accelerated-dose t-PA is administered.[78]

RETEPLASE. This is a recombinant deletion mutant form of t-PA lacking the finger, epidermal growth factor, and kringle 1 domains as well as the carbohydrate side chains (see Fig. 47–14 and Table 47–4).

The GUSTO III trial compared the 10 + 10 unit regimen of reteplase with accelerated t-PA in 15,059 patients.[79] The 30-day mortality rate was 7.47 percent in the reteplase group and 7.24 percent in the t-PA group corresponding to an absolute difference of 0.23 percent with a 95 percent confidence interval of −0.66 to +1.1 percent. The results of GUSTO III did not demonstrate superiority of reteplase over t-PA, and, using a 1 percent absolute difference as a boundary for equivalence, the mortality results also do not formally demonstrate equivalence.[80,81] The intracranial hemorrhage rate was 0.91 percent with reteplase and 0.87 percent with t-PA. The secondary composite endpoint of net clinical benefit (death or disabling stroke) was 7.89 percent with reteplase and 7.91 percent with accelerated t-PA. Although GUSTO III did not fulfill formal criteria for equivalence of reteplase and t-PA, many clinicians consider the two agents to be therapeutically similar and consider the double bolus method of administration of reteplase to be an advantage over t-PA.

TENECTEPLASE. Tenecteplase is a mutant of t-PA with specific amino acid substitutions in the kringle 1 domain and

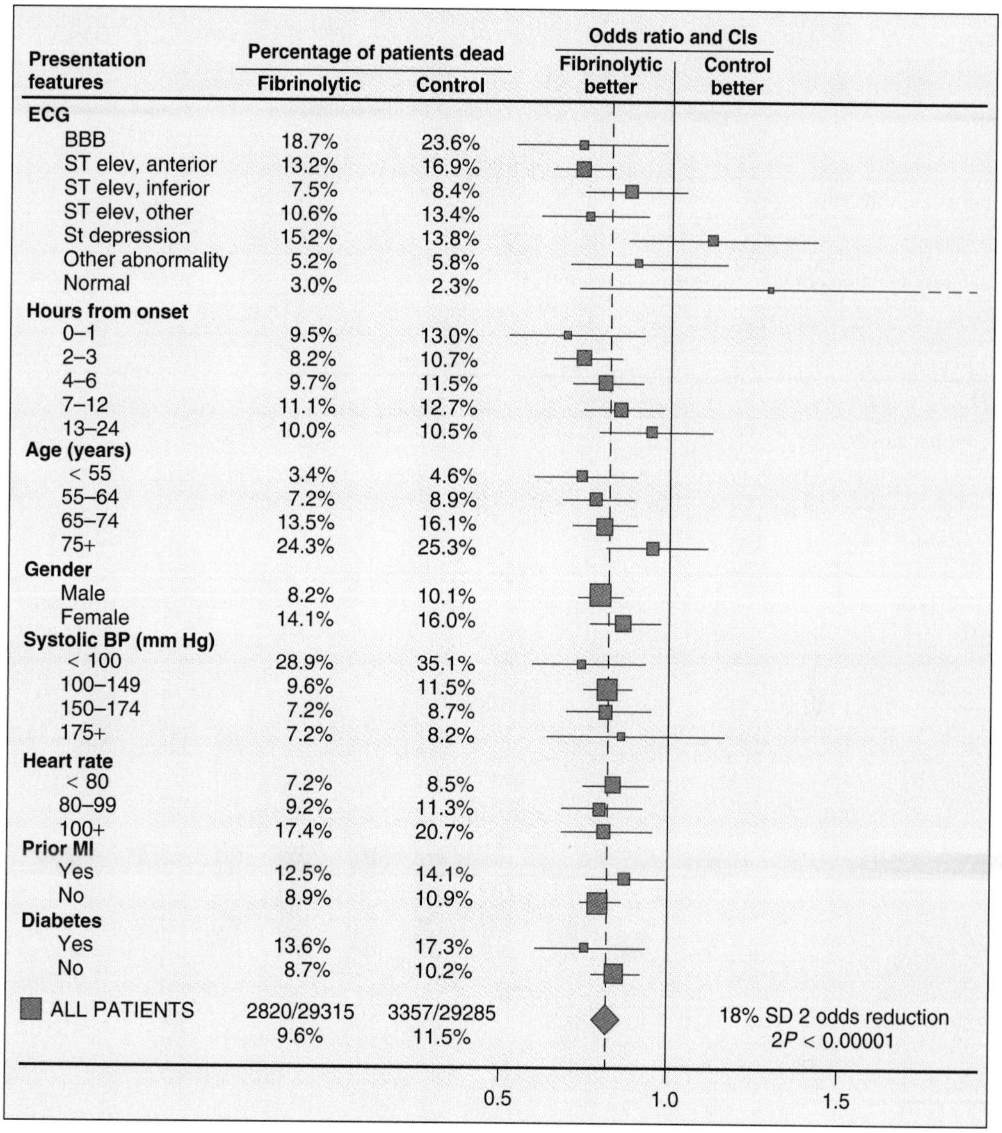
Odds ratio and CIs
Presentation features
Percentage of patients dead
Fibrinolytic
Control
Fibrinolytic better
Control better
ECG
BBB 18.7% 23.6%
ST elev, anterior 13.2% 16.9%
ST elev, inferior 7.5% 8.4%
ST elev, other 10.6% 13.4%
St depression 15.2% 13.8%
Other abnormality 5.2% 5.8%
Normal 3.0% 2.3%
Hours from onset
0–1 9.5% 13.0%
2–3 8.2% 10.7%
4–6 9.7% 11.5%
7–12 11.1% 12.7%
13–24 10.0% 10.5%
Age (years)
< 55 3.4% 4.6%
55–64 7.2% 8.9%
65–74 13.5% 16.1%
75+ 24.3% 25.3%
Gender
Male 8.2% 10.1%
Female 14.1% 16.0%
Systolic BP (mm Hg)
< 100 28.9% 35.1%
100–149 9.6% 11.5%
150–174 7.2% 8.7%
175+ 7.2% 8.2%
Heart rate
< 80 7.2% 8.5%
80–99 9.2% 11.3%
100+ 17.4% 20.7%
Prior MI
Yes 12.5% 14.1%
No 8.9% 10.9%
Diabetes
Yes 13.6% 17.3%
No 8.7% 10.2%
ALL PATIENTS 2820/29315 3357/29285
9.6% 11.5%
18% SD 2 odds reduction
2P < 0.00001
0.5
1.0
1.5

FIGURE 47–10 Mortality differences during days 0 to 35 subdivided by presentation features in a collaborative overview of results from nine trials of thrombolytic therapy. The absolute mortality rates are shown for fibrinolytic and control groups in the center portion of the figure for each of the clinical features at presentation listed on the left side of the figure. The ratio of the odds of death in the fibrinolytic group to that in the control group is shown for each subdivision (colored square), along with its 99 percent confidence interval (horizontal line). The summary odds ratio at the bottom of the figure corresponds to an 18 percent proportional reduction in 35-day mortality and is highly statistically significant. This translates to a reduction of 18 deaths per 1000 patients treated with thrombolytic agents. (From Fibrinolytic Therapy Trialists' [FTT] Collaborative Group: Indications for fibrinolytic therapy in suspected acute myocardial infarction: Collaborative overview of mortality and major morbidity results from all randomized trials of more than 1000 patients. Lancet 343:311, 1994. Copyright by The Lancet Ltd.)

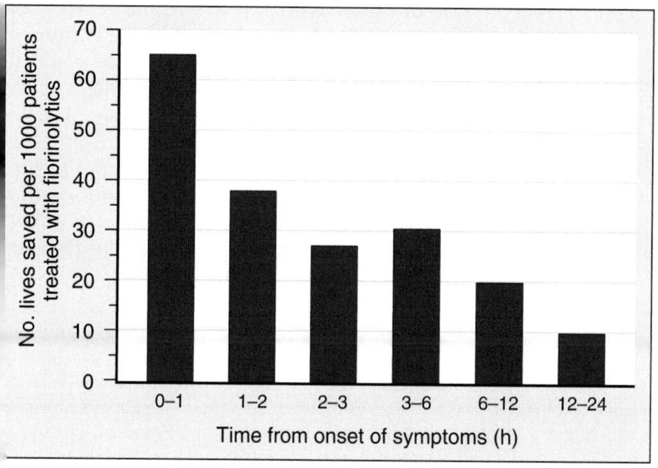

FIGURE 47–11 Importance of time to reperfusion in patients receiving fibrinolytic therapy for ST segment elevation myocardial infarction. The data from 22 trials of fibrinolytic therapy were pooled and the findings stratified by the six time categories shown in the figure. The number of lives saved per 1000 patients treated with fibrinolytics compared with placebo is greatest the earlier treatment is initiated after the onset of symptoms and this decreases in a nonlinear fashion with incremental time delays. Since the life-saving effect of fibrinolysis is maximal in the first hour from onset of symptoms, this has been referred to as the "golden hour" for pharmacological reperfusion. (From Boersma E, Maas AC, Deckers JW, et al: Early thrombolytic treatment in acute myocardial infarction: Reappraisal of the golden hour. Lancet 348:771, 1996.)

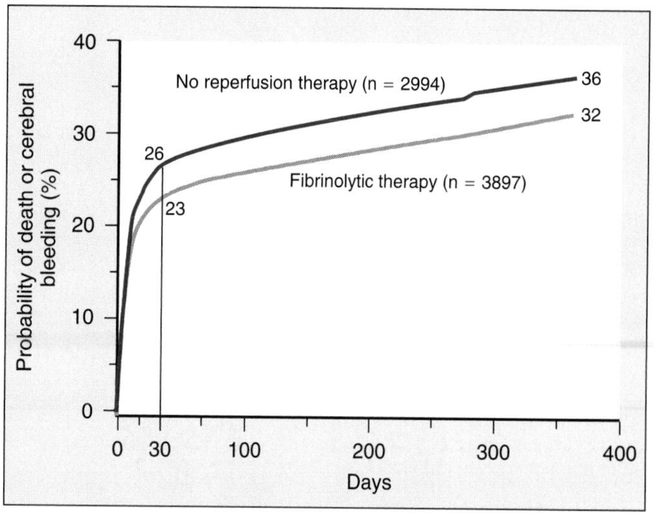

FIGURE 47–12 Probability of death or cerebral bleeding in elderly patients with ST segment elevation myocardial infarction. Patients older than 75 years of age entered in a Swedish national registry had significantly lower rates of death or cerebral bleeding if they received fibrinolytic therapy compared to no reperfusion therapy. The adjusted relative risk of death or cerebral bleeding through 1 year was 0.87 (0.80-0.94; $p = 0.001$). (From Stenestrand U, Wallentin L: Fibrinolytic therapy in patients 75 years and older with ST-segment-elevation myocardial infarction: One-year follow-up of a large prospective cohort. Arch Intern Med 163:965, 2003.)

TABLE 47–4 Comparison of Approved Fibrinolytic Agents

	Streptokinase	Alteplase	Reteplase	TNK-t-PA
Dose	1.5 MU in 30-60 min	Up to 100 mg in 90 min (based on weight)	10 U × 2 each over 2 min	30-50 mg based on weight*
Bolus administration	No	No	Yes	Yes
Antigenic	Yes	No	No	No
Allergic reactions (hypotension most common)	Yes	No	No	No
Systemic fibrinogen depletion	Marked	Mild	Moderate	Minimal
90-min patency rates (%)	Approximately 50	Approximately 75	Approximately 75	Approximately 75†
TIMI grade 3 flow (%)	32	54	60	63
Cost per dose (U.S. $)‡	568	2750	2750	2750 for 50 mg

Data from *Armstrong PW, Collen D: Circulation 103:2862, 2001; †Cannon CP, Gibson CM, McCabe CH, et al: Circulation 98:2805, 1998; and ‡Medical Economics Staff: 2001 Drug Topics Red Book. 105th ed. Montvale, NJ, Medical Economics Company, 2001.

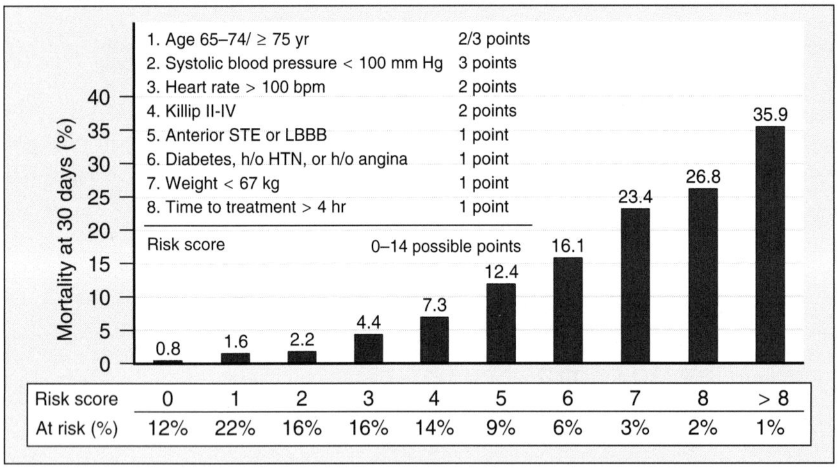

FIGURE 47–13 TIMI risk score for ST segment elevation myocardial infarction predicting 30-day mortality. h/o = history of; HTN = hypertension; LBBB = left bundle branch block; STE = ST segment elevation. (From Morrow DA, Antman EM, Charlesworth A, et al: The TIMI risk score for ST elevation myocardial infarction: A convenient, bedside, clinical score for risk assessment at presentation: An InTIME II substudy. Circulation 102:2031, 2000.)

protease domain introduced to decrease plasma clearance, increase fibrin specificity, and reduce sensitivity to plasminogen activator inhibitor-1 (see Fig. 47–14 and Table 47–4). The phase II angiographic dose-ranging studies TIMI 10A and TIMI 10B helped to define the optimum dose of tenecteplase with respect to efficacy.[82,83] An analysis comparing the weight-adjusted dose of tenecteplase compared with TIMI grade 3 flow indicated that a dose of 0.53 mg/kg was optimal for achieving high rates of TIMI grade 3 flow.[83] The safety of tenecteplase was evaluated in both TIMI 10B and another large phase II clinical trial called ASSENT 1.[84]

ASSENT 2 was a randomized, double-blind, phase III equivalence trial comparing single bolus tenecteplase with accelerated dose t-PA in 16,949 patients.[85] The 30-day mortality rate with tenecteplase was 6.179 percent and with t-PA it was 6.151 percent (p = 0.0059 for equivalence). The rate of intracranial hemorrhage was 0.93 percent with tenecteplase and 0.94 percent with t-PA. Major bleeding occurred in 4.66 percent of tenecteplase-treated patients compared with 5.94 percent of t-PA-treated patients (peak was 0.0002). There was no specific subgroup of patients in whom tenecteplase or t-PA was significantly better, with the exception of patients treated after 4 hours from the onset of symptoms, among whom the mortality rate was 7.0 percent with tenecteplase and 9.2 percent with t-PA ($p = 0.018$).

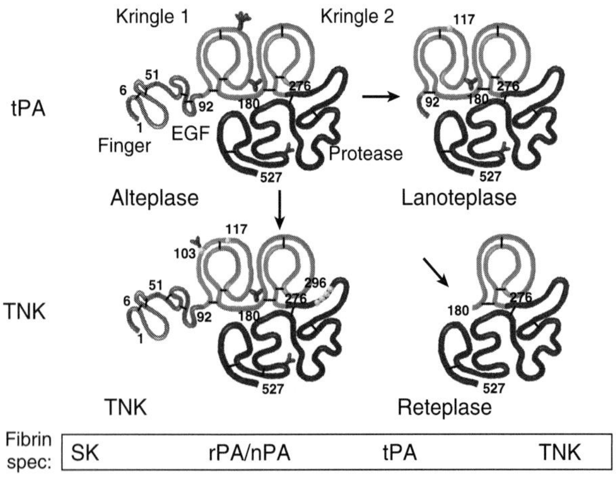

FIGURE 47–14 Molecular structure of alteplase (tPA), lanoteplase (nPA), reteplase (rPA), and tenecteplase (TNK). Streptokinase is the least fibrin-specific thrombolytic agent in clinical use; the progressive increase in relative fibrin specificity for the various thrombolytics is shown at the bottom. (Modified from Brener SJ, Topol EJ: Third-generation thrombolytic agents for acute myocardial infarction. *In* Topol EJ [ed.]: Acute Coronary Syndromes. New York, Marcel Dekker, 1998, p 169.)

OTHER FIBRINOLYTIC AGENTS. *Lanoteplase* is a novel plasminogen activator that is a mutant of t-PA lacking the finger and epidermal growth factor domains and also containing an amino acid substitution in the kringle 1 domain, leading to deletion of a glycosylation site (see Fig. 47-14). InTIME-II was a phase III double-blind equivalence trial in 15,078 patients comparing 120 kU/kg of lanoteplase with 100 mg of accelerated-dose t-PA. The 30-day mortality rate was 6.61 percent in the t-PA group and 6.75 percent in the lanoteplase group (RR, 1.02; p = 0.075 for equivalence).[86] The intracranial hemorrhage rate was 0.64 percent for t-PA and 1.12 percent for lanoteplase (p = 0.004). Because of the increased rate of intracranial hemorrhage with lanoteplase compared to t-PA in the dose studied, it is no longer being pursued for clinical development.

Urokinase is used on rare occasion as an intracoronary infusion (6000 IU/min) to an average cumulative dose of 5,000,000 IU to lyse intracoronary thrombi that are believed to be responsible for an evolving STEMI.

Anistreplase, usually administered in a dose of 30 mg over 2 to 5 minutes intravenously, has a side-effect profile similar to that of streptokinase, a patency profile similar to that of conventional-dose t-PA, and a mortality benefit similar to that of streptokinase or t-PA (double-chain form, duteplase). The lack of any compelling advantages (other than bolus administration) and costs higher than streptokinase have relegated anistreplase to an extremely infrequently prescribed drug for acute myocardial infarction in the United States.

Staphylokinase is a highly fibrin-specific plasminogen activator that requires priming on the surface of a clot. A pegylated, recombinant form of staphylokinase has been shown to yield TIMI grade 3 flow rates similar to those obtained with t-PA.[87]

Effect on Left Ventricular Function

Although precise measurements of infarct size would be an ideal endpoint for clinical reperfusion studies, such measures have been found to be impractical. Attempts to use left ventricular ejection fraction as a surrogate for infarct size have not been productive because little difference is seen in ejection fraction between treatment groups that show a significant difference in mortality. Methods of assessing left ventricular function, such as end-systolic volume or quantitative echocardiography, are more revealing because patients with smaller volumes and better preserved ventricular shape have an improved survival. The myocardial salvage index, defined as the difference between an initial perfusion defect (e.g., by sestamibi scintigraphy) and final perfusion defect, is a useful means for comparing the effectiveness of reperfusion therapies.[28]

As with survival, improvement in global left ventricular function is related to the time of fibrinolytic treatment, with greatest improvement occurring with earliest therapy.[28] Greater improvement in left ventricular function has been reported with anterior than with inferior infarcts. The angiographic substudy in GUSTO I reported detailed regional wall motion analyses stratified by thrombolytic regimen.[88] Patients who received the accelerated t-PA regimen had significantly less depression of regional wall motion in the ischemic zone, as evidenced by fewer abnormal chords when their ventricular silhouettes were subjected to segmental wall motion analysis. In addition, this patient group tended to have a slightly higher global ejection fraction and slightly reduced end-systolic volume index at 90 minutes following initiation of thrombolytic therapy. The totality of the data presented in the GUSTO I angiographic substudy[88] is consistent with the hypothesis that more rapid and complete restoration of normal coronary blood flow in the infarct-related artery with t-PA was associated with an improvement in regional and global left ventricular function (presumably through greater myocardial salvage in the ischemic zone) and that this difference in function compared with that obtained with streptokinase may have contributed to the mortality differences observed at 30 days and beyond.

Complications of Fibrinolytic Therapy

Recent (<1 year) exposure to streptococci or streptokinase produces some degree of antibody-mediated resistance to streptokinase (and anistreplase) in most patients. Although this is of clinical consequence only rarely, it is recommended that patients not receive streptokinase for STEMI if they have been treated with a streptokinase product within the last year. Bleeding complications are, of course, most common and potentially the most serious. Most bleeding is relatively minor with all agents, with more serious episodes occurring in patients requiring invasive procedures.[89] Intracranial hemorrhage is the most serious complication of fibrinolytic therapy; its frequency varies with the clinical characteristics of the patient and the fibrinolytic agent prescribed (Fig. 47–15).[7]

There have been reports of an "early hazard" with fibrinolytic therapy, that is, an excess of deaths in the first 24 hours in fibrinolytic-treated patients compared with control subjects (especially in elderly patients treated more than 12 hours).[19] However, this excess early mortality is more than offset by the deaths prevented beyond the first day, culminating in an 18 percent (range, 13 to 23 percent) reduction in mortality by 35 days.[19] The mechanisms responsible for this

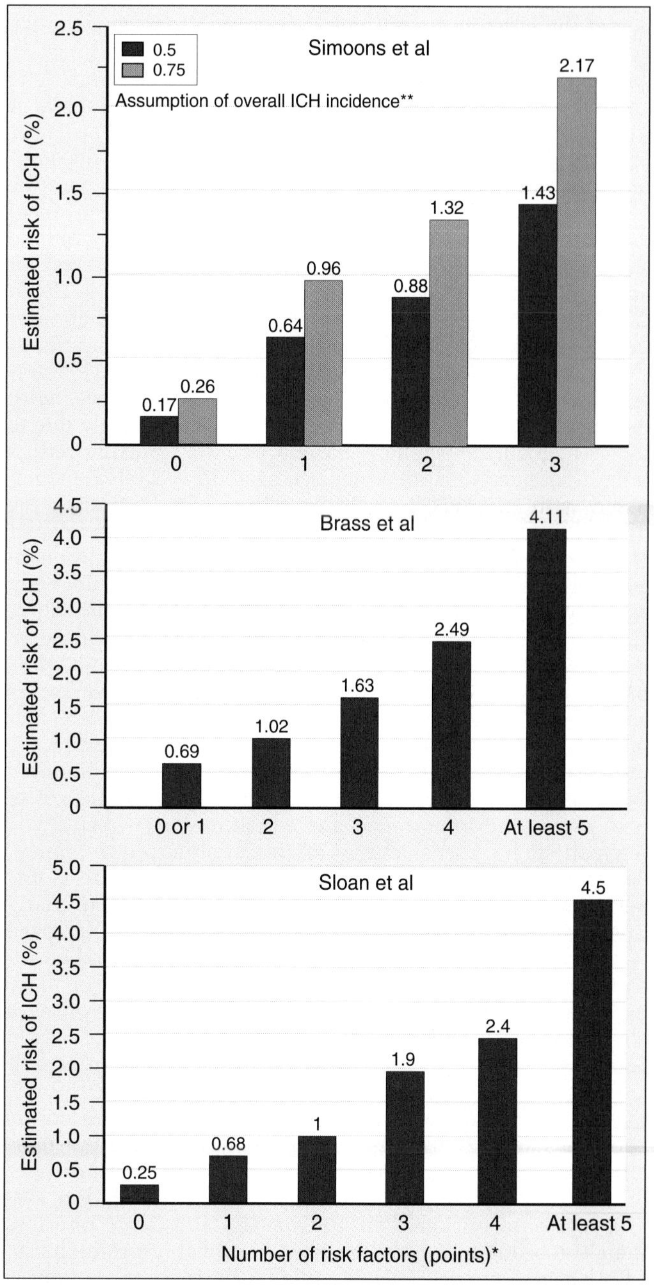

FIGURE 47–15 Estimation of risk of intracranial hemorrhage (ICH) with fibrinolysis. *The number of risk factors is the sum of the points based on criteria established in the studies shown. Although the exact risk factors varied among the studies, common risk factors across all the studies include increased age, low body weight, and hypertension on admission. **If the overall incidence of ICH is assumed to be 0.75 percent, patients without risk factors who receive streptokinase have a 0.26 percent probability of ICH. The risk is 0.96, 1.32, and 21.7 percent in patients with one, two, or three risk factors, respectively. See references for further discussion. (Data from Simoons et al: Lancet 342:1523, 1993; Brass et al: Stroke 31:1802, 2000; Sloan et al: J Am Coll Cardiol:37(Suppl A):372A, 2001.)

early hazard are not clear but probably are multiple, including an increased risk of myocardial rupture (particularly in the elderly), fatal intracranial hemorrhage,[90] inadequate myocardial reperfusion resulting in pump failure and cardiogenic shock,[91] and possible reperfusion injury of reperfused myocardium. Reports of more unusual complications such as splenic rupture, aortic dissection, and cholesterol embolization have also appeared.

Recommendations for Fibrinolytic Therapy

NET CLINICAL BENEFIT OF FIBRINOLYSIS. Perhaps one of the most important messages from all of the available evidence is that fibrinolytic therapy is underutilized in patients with STEMI.[92] Hesitancy in prescribing a fibrinolytic agent is often the result of uncertainty about the risk of bleeding. Patients with a higher baseline risk of mortality are more likely to benefit from fibrinolytic therapy. Against the mortality benefit associated with fibrinolytic therapy must be weighed the excess risk of stroke. Using the net clinical benefit composite endpoint of 30-day mortality or nonfatal stroke, a small but statistically significant benefit is seen for accelerated-dose t-PA compared with streptokinase. Given the data from the GUSTO 3 and ASSENT-2 trials, it appears that the net clinical benefit of accelerated-dose t-PA is similar to that obtained with reteplase or tenecteplase.[79,85] Of interest, the rate of noncerebral major bleeding was lower with tenecteplase than t-PA in the ASSENT-2 trial, possibly due to the greater fibrin specificity of tenecteplase.[85] Further reduction in noncerebral bleeding occurred in ASSENT-3 compared with ASSENT-2, probably due to a reduction in the dose of unfractionated heparin used in ASSENT-3.[93]

CHOICE OF AGENT. Analysis of the net clinical benefit and cost-effectiveness of t-PA versus streptokinase does not easily yield recommendations for treatment because clinicians must weigh the risk of mortality and the risk of intracranial hemorrhage when confronting a fibrinolytic-eligible patient with STEMI; additional considerations may be the constraints placed on physicians' therapeutic decision-making by the health care system in which they are practicing. In the subgroup of patients presenting within 4 hours of symptom onset, the speed of reperfusion of the infarct vessel is of paramount importance, and a high-intensity fibrinolytic regimen such as accelerated t-PA is the preferred treatment, except in those individuals in whom the risk of death is low (e.g., a young patient with a small inferior myocardial infarction) and the risk of intracranial hemorrhage is increased (e.g., acute hypertension), in whom streptokinase and accelerated t-PA are approximately equivalent choices. For those patients presenting between 4 and 12 hours after the onset of chest discomfort, the speed of reperfusion of the infarct vessel is of lesser importance, and therefore streptokinase and accelerated t-PA are generally equivalent options, given the difference in costs. Of note, for those patients presenting between 4 and 12 hours from symptom onset with a low mortality risk but an increased risk of intracranial hemorrhage (e.g., elderly patients with inferior myocardial infarction, systolic pressure greater than 100 mm Hg, and heart rate less than 100 beats/min), streptokinase is probably preferable to t-PA because of cost considerations if fibrinolytic therapy is prescribed at all in such patients.

In those patients considered appropriate candidates for fibrinolysis and in whom t-PA would have been selected as the agent of choice in the past, we believe clinicians should now consider using a bolus thrombolytic such as reteplase or tenecteplase. The rationale for this recommendation is that bolus fibrinolysis has the advantage of ease of administration, a lower chance of medication errors (and the associated increase in mortality when such medication errors occur), and less noncerebral bleeding and also offers the potential for prehospital treatment.[94,95]

LATE THERAPY. No mortality benefit was demonstrated in the LATE and EMERAS trials when fibrinolytics were routinely administered to patients between 12 and 24 hours, although we believe it is still reasonable to consider fibrinolytic therapy in appropriately selected patients with persistent symptoms and ST elevation on the electrocardiogram beyond 12 hours. Persistent chest pain late after the onset of symptoms correlates with a higher incidence of collateral or antegrade flow in the infarct zone and is therefore a marker for patients with viable myocardium that might be salvaged. Because elderly patients treated with fibrinolytic agents more than 12 hours after the onset of symptoms are at increased risk of cardiac rupture, it is our practice to restrict late fibrinolytic administration to younger patients (<65 years) with ongoing ischemia, especially those with large anterior infarctions. The elderly patient with ongoing ischemic symptoms but presenting late (>12 hours) is probably better managed with PCI (see Chap. 48) than with fibrinolytic therapy.

Before the institution of fibrinolytic therapy, consideration should be given to the patient's need for intravascular catheterization, as would be required for the placement of an arterial pressure monitoring line, a pulmonary artery catheter for hemodynamic monitoring, or a temporary transvenous pacemaker. If any of these are required, ideally they should be placed as expeditiously as possible *before* infusion of the fibrinolytic agent. If such procedures require an additional delay of more than 30 minutes, they should be deferred as long as possible after fibrinolytic therapy is begun. In the early hours after institution of fibrinolytic therapy, such catheterization should be performed only if crucial to the patient's survival, and then sites where excessive bleeding can be controlled should be chosen (e.g., subclavian vein catheterization should be avoided).

As noted earlier, all patients with suspected STEMI should receive aspirin (160-325 mg) regardless of the fibrinolytic agent prescribed. Aspirin should be continued indefinitely. The issues surrounding antithrombin therapy as an adjunct to thrombolysis are complex and are discussed in detail in a subsequent section.

Catheter-Based Reperfusion Strategies

Reperfusion of the infarct artery can also be achieved by a catheter-based strategy. This approach has evolved from passage of a balloon catheter over a guidewire to now include potent antiplatelet therapy (intravenous glycoprotein IIb/IIIa inhibitors, thienopyridines) and coronary stents.[56] When PCI is used in lieu of fibrinolytic therapy, it is referred to as direct or primary PCI. When fibrinolysis has failed to reperfuse the infarct vessel, or a severe stenosis is present in the infarct vessel, a rescue PCI can be performed. A more conservative approach of elective PCI can be used to manage STEMI patients only when spontaneous or exercise-provoked ischemia occurs, whether or not they have received a previous course of fibrinolytic therapy. Discussion of the use of PCI in STEMI patients and recommendations for catheter-based reperfusion strategies are found in Chapter 48.

SURGICAL REPERFUSION. Despite the extensive improvement in intraoperative preservation with cardioplegia and hypothermia and numerous surgical techniques (see Chap. 76), it is not logistically possible to provide surgical reperfusion in a timely fashion. Therefore, patients with STEMI who are candidates for reperfusion routinely receive either fibrinolysis or PCI. However, about 10 to 20 percent of STEMI patients are currently referred for coronary bypass grafting for one of the following indications: persistent or recurrent chest pain despite fibrinolysis or PCI, high-risk coronary anatomy (e.g., left main stenosis) discovered at catheterization, or a complication of STEMI such as ventricular septal rupture or severe mitral regurgitation due to papillary muscle dysfunction. Patients with STEMI with continued severe ischemic and hemodynamic instability are likely to benefit from emergency revascularization. PCI with stenting as needed is the preferable technique when revascularization is needed in the first 48 to 72 hours following STEMI; surgery should be reserved for patients in whom PCI has been unsuccessful or whose anatomy dictates the need for coronary artery bypass grafting, such as patients with left main or extensive multivessel coronary artery disease.

Patients undergoing successful fibrinolysis but with important residual stenoses, who on anatomical grounds are more suitable for surgical revascularization than for PCI, have undergone coronary artery bypass grafting with quite low rates of mortality (about 4 percent) and morbidity, *provided* that they are operated on more than 24 hours from STEMI; those patients requiring urgent or emergency coronary artery bypass grafting within 24 to 48 hours of acute myocardial infarction have mortality rates between 12 and 15 percent.[96] When surgery is performed under urgent conditions with active and ongoing ischemia or cardiogenic shock, the operative mortality rate rises steeply.

Selection of Reperfusion Strategy

Despite strong evidence in the literature that prompt use of reperfusion therapy improves survival of STEMI patients, room for improvement exists, since reperfusion therapy is underutilized and often not administered soon after presentation.[92,97] Considerable controversy exists about the optimum form of reperfusion therapy.[98] An important factor that continues to fuel this controversy is the dynamic and rapidly changing evidence base regarding the best approach to reperfusion for patients with STEMI. With respect to pharmacological reperfusion, new fibrinolytic agents, modified dosing regimens, and combinations of adjunctive treatments have produced a continuous process of refinement and improvement in medical measures to restore flow in the infarct artery (Fig. 47–16). From the perspective of PCI, improvements in catheterization laboratory facilities, new forms of stents, and distal embolization protection devices have dramatically improved the efficacy and safety of PCI for patients with STEMI (see Chap. 48). Improvements in pharmacological and PCI-based reperfusion strategies rapidly make prior studies less relevant to contemporary practice. In addition, progressive reductions in mortality from STEMI have made it increasingly difficult to conduct clinical trials of a practical size. Investigators frequently use composite endpoints that combine mortality with nonfatal events such as recurrent myocardial infarction, recurrent ischemia, or target vessel revascularization.

In a pooled analysis of 23 randomized trials comparing PCI versus fibrinolysis for STEMI over both the short and the long terms, PCI was superior to fibrinolysis for almost all of the endpoints analyzed (see Fig. 48–2).[99] However, the absolute risk difference between the two reperfusion strategies varied depending on the endpoint; this translates into a wide range of patients who need to be treated (or who are harmed) to prevent one event using PCI as compared with fibrinolysis as the reperfusion strategy for patients with STEMI.

Several issues should be considered in selecting the type of reperfusion therapy:

1. *Time from the onset of symptoms to initiation of fibrinolytic therapy*: This is an important predictor of infarct size and patient outcome.[66] Schomig and colleagues reported that the influence of time-to-treatment interval on myocardial salvage in patients with STEMI depends on the type of reper-

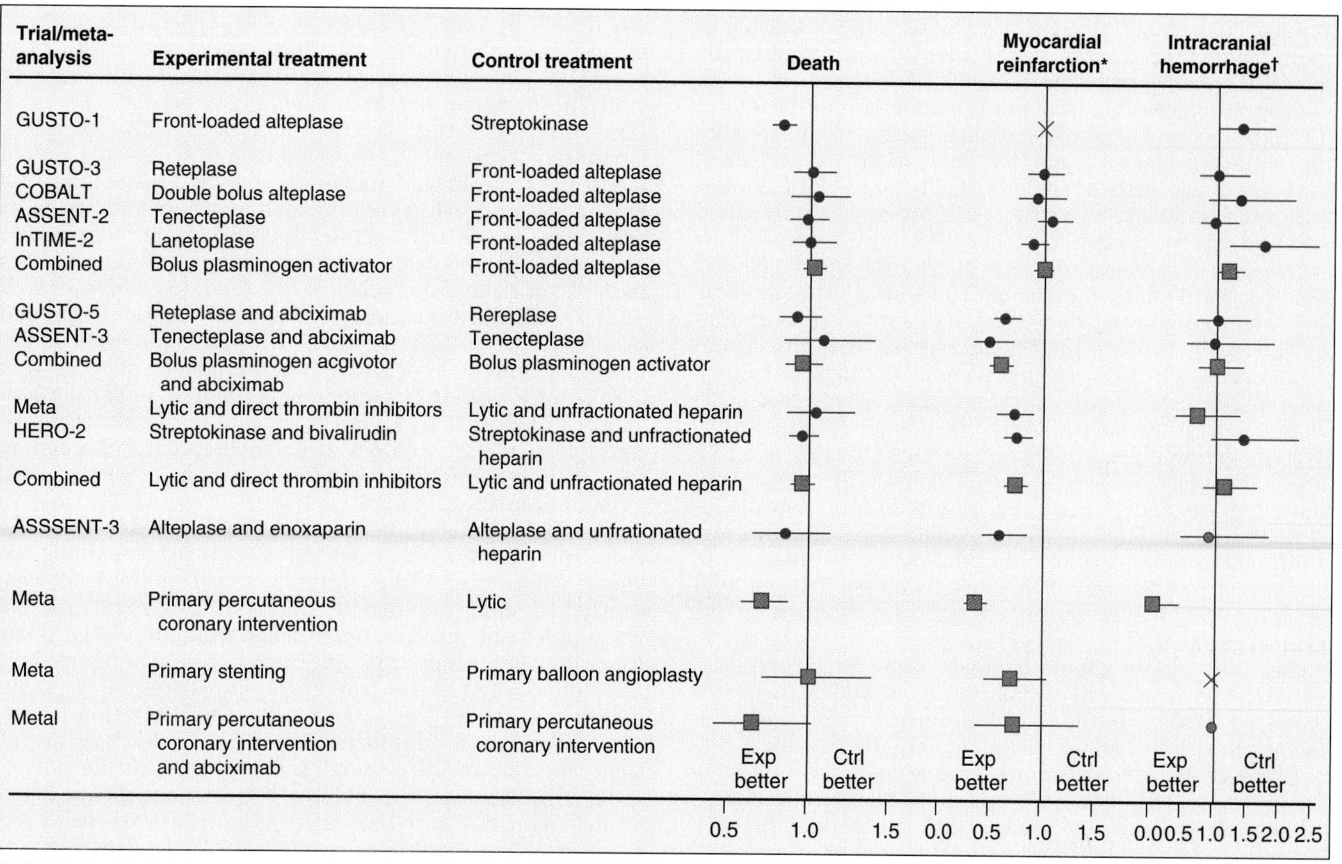

FIGURE 47–16 Relative treatment effect associated with several acute reperfusion modalities in patients presenting with ST segment elevation myocardial infarction (STEMI). Data are odds ratios and 95 percent confidence intervals. (Modified from Boersma E, Mercado N, Poldermans, et al: Acute myocardial infarction. Lancet 361:851, 2003.)

fusion therapy.[28] Patients who were treated with fibrinolysis less than 165 minutes, 165 to 280 minutes, and more than 280 minutes from the onset of symptoms had final infarct sizes of 13.6 percent, 20.2 percent, and 24.0 percent of the left ventricle; in patients treated with stenting, the final infarct sizes were 10.1 percent, 9.4 percent, and 11.1 percent, respectively, in the same time intervals. Despite the time-dependent increase in infarct size in patients treated with fibrinolysis and the more stable pattern of smaller infarcts in patients treated with PCI, no consistent time-dependent pattern was seen in clinical outcomes with either reperfusion strategy.[28] The lack of a consistent relationship between infarct size and clinical outcomes regardless of reperfusion strategy suggests that a complex interplay of multiple factors determines the likelihood of clinical events. While infarct size is one such factor, others include the coexistence of obstructions in noninfarct-related coronary arteries, the level of electrical stability of the myocardium, the extent of left ventricular remodeling, and the number of medications prescribed following STEMI as well as the patient's response to them. Thus, for patients treated by fibrinolysis or PCI, time from the onset of symptoms is an important predictor of mortality, underscoring the need for prompt reperfusion, whichever strategy is selected (see Figs. 47–1 and 47–2).[35–36,69]

2. *Risk of the STEMI*: Patients presenting with cardiogenic shock have an improved 1-year survival chance if they are treated with an early revascularization strategy (PCI and/or coronary artery bypass grafting as indicated).[100] Observational data from the Second National Registry of Myocardial Infarction also suggests the superiority of PCI compared with fibrinolysis for patients presenting with a condition of a Killip class ≥ II.[101] Kent and associates performed an analysis to test whether subgroups of patients with STEMI with a high risk of mortality might be especially likely to benefit from PCI and those at lower risk might be less likely to benefit.[102] Patients at highest risk of mortality from STEMI account for the majority of deaths from STEMI (see Fig. 47–13). Accordingly, the mortality benefit associated with PCI is largest in patients who are at highest risk of mortality; the mortality benefit of PCI decreases progressively as the patient's risk of mortality from STEMI decreases, such that the mortality advantage of PCI is no longer evident among patients whose 30-day mortality rate is estimated to be between 2 and 3 percent if treated with fibrinolytic therapy.[102]

3. *Risk of bleeding*: In patients with an increased risk of bleeding, particularly intracranial hemorrhage, therapeutic decision making strongly favors a PCI-based reperfusion strategy[103] (see Fig. 47–15). If PCI is unavailable, then the benefit of pharmacological reperfusion should be balanced against the risk of bleeding. A decision analysis suggests that when no PCI is available, fibrinolytic therapy should still be favored over no reperfusion treatment until the risk of a life-threatening bleed exceeds 4 percent. For patients who are not candidates for acute reperfusion because of lack of availability of PCI and contraindications to fibrinolysis, aspirin and antithrombin therapy with either unfractionated heparin or enoxaparin can be prescribed. There is no benefit to amplifying the antiplatelet regimen by adding tirofiban to the medical regimen.[104]

Thus, every effort should be made to provide reperfusion therapy even in clinical circumstances in which there is a perceived increase in the risk of bleeding. Arrangements for urgent primary PCI should be made for patients with a constellation of advanced age, low body weight, and hypertension on presentation because of the substantially increased risk of intracranial hemorrhage with fibrinolytic therapy. When the estimated delay to implementation of primary PCI is substantial (much greater than 90 minutes), fibrinolysis (with a fibrin-specific agent) may be preferable to no reperfusion therapy in such patients when the risk from the STEMI is high (e.g., anterior infarction with hemodynamic compromise). In the setting of absolute contraindications to fibrinolysis (see Table 47–3) and lack of access to PCI facilities, antithrombin therapy with unfractionated heparin or enoxaparin and antiplatelet therapy with aspirin should be prescribed because of the small but finite chance (10 percent) of restoration of TIMI grade 3 flow in the infarct vessel and decreasing the chance of thrombotic complications of STEMI.[88]

4. *Time required for transportation to a skilled PCI center*: The greatest operational impediment to routine implementation of a PCI reperfusion strategy is the delay required for transportation to a skilled PCI center (see Figs. 47–1 and 47–2).[98] Although several trials reported that referral to a PCI center was superior to fibrinolysis administered in a local hospital, such studies were conducted in dedicated health care systems with extremely short transportation and door-to-balloon times at the PCI centers.[105-107] Evidence exists to suggest that for every 10 minutes of delay to perform primary PCI versus administration of fibrinolytic therapy, there is a 1 percent absolute reduction in the mortality difference originally favoring primary PCI.[108] Thus, a 1-hour delay for initiation of primary PCI may equalize the mortality benefit of primary PCI versus administration of fibrin-specific fibrinolytic therapy.

Circumstances in which fibrinolysis or PCI is the preferred reperfusion strategy are summarized in Table 47–2. The assessment of reperfusion options for STEMI is a two-step process. Step one involves the integrated assessment of the time since onset of symptoms (see Figs. 47–4 and 47–11), risk of STEMI (see Fig. 47–13), risk of bleeding if fibrinolysis were to be administered (see Fig. 47–15), and time required for transportation to a skilled PCI center (see Fig. 47–4 and Chap. 48). The complexities of clinical medicine do not permit the decision-making to be reduced to a simple equation or "one size fits all" approach to selection of the reperfusion strategy. Instead, for step two, it is best to conceive of circumstances in which fibrinolysis is generally preferred and those in which an invasive strategy is generally preferred.

Fibrinolysis is the preferred reperfusion strategy under circumstances in which there is no ready access to a skilled PCI facility (prolonged transportation time, catheterization laboratory occupied, only inexperienced operator/team is available), PCI is not technically feasible (vascular access difficulties), or the decision-making favors initiation of lysis rather than risking the delay to PCI (door-to-balloon time is >90 minutes, the difference between door-to-balloon time and prompt initiation of lysis with a fibrin-specific agent [door-to-needle time] is >1 hour). When the patient presents very early after the onset of symptoms (<3 hours), either fibrinolysis or PCI is acceptable, but in most clinical circumstances fibrinolysis is preferred because of the anticipated delay to PCI, which would put the patient at risk of a substantial amount of myocardium.

An invasive strategy is generally preferred, the greater the risk. This risk may be from the STEMI itself (cardiogenic shock, Killip class ≥ II) or from bleeding if fibrinolysis were prescribed. When a skilled PCI operator/team is available and can implement an invasive strategy without undue delay (door-to-balloon time < 90 minutes or within 1 hour of the time a fibrinolytic agent could be administered), it is preferable to take the STEMI patient to the catheterization laboratory rather than administer fibrinolysis. Because of the increased risk of intracranial hemorrhage with fibrinolysis with advanced age, the elderly patient is probably better treated with PCI, provided there is no excessive delay. As coronary thrombi mature over time, they become increasingly resistant to fibrinolysis. Thus, PCI is the preferred reperfusion strategy if more than 3 hours have elapsed from the onset of symptoms, again assuming there is no significant delay in the anticipated time to balloon inflation (see Fig. 47–4). Finally, when the diagnosis is in doubt, an invasive strategy is clearly the preferred strategy, since it not only provides key diagnostic information regarding the patient's symptoms but does so without the risk of intracranial hemorrhage associated with fibrinolysis.

Antithrombin and Antiplatelet Therapy

Antithrombin Therapy

The rationale for administering antithrombin therapy acutely in STEMI patients includes prevention of deep venous thrombosis, pulmonary embolism, ventricular thrombus formation, and cerebral embolization. In addition, establishing and maintaining patency of the infarct-related artery, whether or not a patient receives fibrinolytic therapy, is another common rationale for antithrombin therapy in cases of STEMI (Fig. 47–17).

EFFECT ON MORTALITY. Randomized trials in STEMI patients conducted in the prefibrinolytic era showed that the risks of pulmonary embolism, stroke, and reinfarction were reduced in patients who received intravenous heparin, providing the support for prescription of heparin to STEMI patients not treated with fibrinolytic therapy. With the introduction of the fibrinolytic era and, importantly, after the publication of the ISIS-2 trial,[109] the situation became more complicated because of strong evidence of a substantial mortality reduction with aspirin alone and confusing and conflicting data regarding the risk-benefit ratio of heparin used as an adjunct to aspirin or in combination with aspirin and a fibrinolytic agent. For every 1000 patients treated with heparin compared with aspirin alone, there are 5 fewer deaths ($p = 0.03$) and 3 fewer recurrent infarctions ($p = 0.04$), at the expense of 3 more major bleeds ($p < 0.001$).[110] Nonrandomized subgroup analyses from the LATE trial of 2821 patients who received t-PA showed a 35-day mortality rate of 7.6 percent when intravenous heparin was administered, compared with 10.4 percent when no heparin was given. Heparin was administered as adjunctive therapy in randomized trials of reteplase and tenecteplase under the supposition that those agents were more fibrin-specific than streptokinase and required concomitant use of heparin.[84,111]

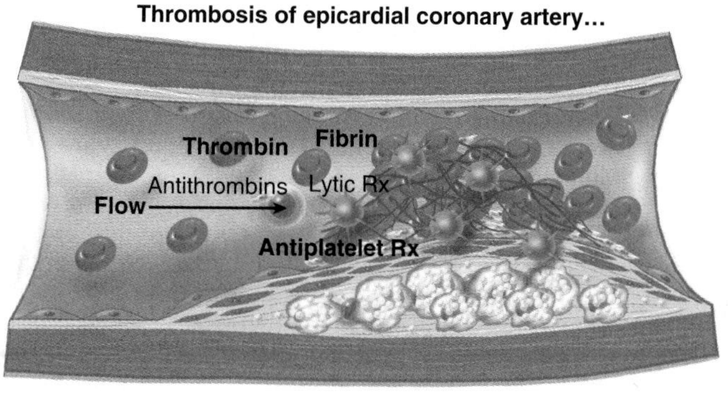

FIGURE 47–17 Pharmacological dissolution of thrombus in infarct-related artery. This figure shows a schematic view of a longitudinal section of an infarct-related artery at the level of the obstructive thrombus. Following rupture of a vulnerable plaque (bottom center), the coagulation cascade is activated, ultimately leading to the deposition of fibrin strands (blue curvilinear arcs); platelets are activated and begin to aggregate (transition from flat discs representing inactive platelets to green spiked ball elements representing activated and aggregating platelets). The mesh of fibrin strands and platelet aggregates obstructs flow (normally moving from left to right) in the infarct-related artery; this would correspond to TIMI grade 0 on angiography. Pharmacological reperfusion is a multipronged approach consisting of fibrinolytic agents that digest fibrin, antithrombins that prevent the formation of thrombin and inhibit the activity of thrombin that is formed, and antiplatelet therapy. (Courtesy of Luke Wells, The Exeter Group.)

OTHER EFFECTS. A number of angiographic studies have examined the role of heparin therapy in establishing and maintaining patency of the infarct-related artery in patients with STEMI. Comparison of these trials is difficult because of potentially important differences in study design, including whether aspirin was administered along with heparin, the fibrinolytic agent that was administered, and variations in the time of diagnostic coronary arteriography. Although the evidence favoring the use of heparin for enhancing patency of the infarct artery when a fibrin-specific fibrinolytic agent is prescribed is not conclusive, the suggestion of a mortality benefit and amelioration of the pattern of left ventricular thrombus (less protuberant) that develops after STEMI indicates it is prudent to use heparin for at least 48 hours after fibrinolysis and to maintain an activated partial thromboplastin time (aPTT) target of one-and-a-half to two times that of control.[7,112]

Although heparin may induce thrombocytopenia through an immunological mechanism, this is seen only rarely, probably occurring in only 2 to 3 percent of patients.[113] The most serious complication of antithrombotic therapy is bleeding, especially intracranial hemorrhage, when fibrinolytic agents are prescribed. Major hemorrhagic events occur more frequently in patients of low body weight, advanced age, female gender, marked prolongation of the aPTT (greater than 90 to 100 seconds), and the performance of invasive procedures.[112] Frequent monitoring of the aPTT (facilitated by use of a bedside testing device) reduces the risk of major hemorrhagic complications in patients treated with heparin. It should be noted, however, that during the first 12 hours following fibrinolytic therapy, the aPTT may be elevated from the fibrinolytic agent alone (particularly if streptokinase is administered), making it difficult to accurately interpret the effects of a heparin infusion on the patient's coagulation status.

NEW ANTITHROMBOTIC AGENTS

Potential disadvantages of unfractionated heparin include dependency on antithrombin III for inhibition of thrombin activity, sensitivity to platelet factor 4, inability to inhibit clot-bound thrombin, marked interpatient variability in therapeutic response, and the need for frequent aPTT monitoring. In an effort to circumvent these disadvantages of unfractionated heparin, there has been interest in the development of novel antithrombotic compounds.[114]

HIRUDIN AND BIVALIRUDIN. Direct thrombin inhibitors such as hirudin or bivalirudin have not been shown to reduce mortality compared with heparin when used as adjuncts to fibrinolysis.[115,116] While recurrent myocardial infarction is reduced by 25 to 30 percent compared with heparin, this benefit is primarily observed during the period of administration of the direct thrombin inhibitor and decreases in magnitude over time. In addition, both hirudin and bivalirudin have been associated with higher rates of major bleeding versus heparin when used with fibrinolytic agents.[115,116]

LOW-MOLECULAR-WEIGHT HEPARINS. These are formed by controlled enzymatic or chemical depolymerization, producing chains of glycosaminoglycans of varying length but with a mean molecular weight of approximately 5000.[114] Advantages of low-molecular-weight heparins include a stable, reliable anticoagulant effect, high bioavailability, permitting administration via the subcutaneous route, and a high antiXa:antiIIa ratio, producing blockade of the coagulation cascade in an upstream location, resulting in a marked decrement in thrombin generation. Compared with unfractionated heparin, the rate of early (60-90 minutes) reperfusion of the infarct artery, either assessed angiographically or by noninvasive means, is not enhanced by administration of a low-molecular-weight heparin.[117-119] However, the rates of reocclusion of the infarct artery, reinfarction, or recurrent ischemic events appear to be reduced by low-molecular-weight heparins.

The ASSENT-3 trial compared unfractionated heparin with enoxaparin (30 mg intravenous bolus followed by subcutaneous injections of 1 mg/kg every 12 hours until hospital discharge).[93] The composite endpoint of 30-day mortality, in-hospital reinfarction, or in-hospital refractory ischemia was reduced from 15.4 percent with unfractionated heparin to 11.4 percent with enoxaparin (RR, 0.74; 95 percent CI, 0.63-0.87). The rate of intracranial hemorrhage was similar with unfractionated heparin versus enoxaparin (0.93 percent versus 0.88 percent; $p = 0.98$).

The ASSENT-3 PLUS study compared the same unfractionated heparin and enoxaparin regimens but initiated therapy in the prehospital setting.[120] The composite endpoint of 30-day mortality, in-hospital reinfarction, or in-hospital refractory ischemia was reduced from 17.4 percent with unfractionated heparin to 14.2 percent with enoxaparin ($p = 0.08$). Of concern, however, was the increased rate of intracranial hemorrhage observed in ASSENT-3 PLUS: 1.0 percent with unfractionated heparin versus 2.2 percent with enoxaparin ($p = 0.05$). The increase in intracranial hemorrhage in ASSENT-3 PLUS was seen predominantly in patients older than 75 years of age: 0.8 percent with unfractionated heparin versus 6.7 percent with enoxaparin ($p = 0.01$). The ongoing ExTRACT-TIMI 25 trial is testing the hypothesis that enoxaparin is superior to unfractionated heparin when administered as an adjunct to fibrinolytic therapy with respect to the primary composite endpoint of death or nonfatal recurrent myocardial infarction through 30 days. Because of the observations noted earlier regarding the excess risk of intracranial hemorrhage in elderly patients receiving enoxaparin, a dose modification has been introduced so that elderly patients do not receive an initial 30 mg intravenous bolus and receive 0.75 mg/kg subcutaneously every 12 hours throughout the index hospitalization; this represents 75 percent of the maintenance dose administered to patients younger than 75 years of age.

Recommendations for Antithrombin Therapy

Given the pivotal role thrombin plays in the pathogenesis of STEMI, antithrombotic therapy remains an important intervention (see Fig. 47–17). Patients undergoing percutaneous or surgical revascularization should receive unfractionated heparin (see Chaps. 48 and 76). Patients undergoing reperfusion therapy with alteplase, reteplase, or tenecteplase should receive unfractionated heparin as a weight-based bolus of 60 U/kg (maximum 4000 U) followed by an initial infusion of 12 U/kg/hr (maximum 1000 U/hr) adjusted to maintain an aPTT at one and a half to two times control.[7] Unfractionated heparin should also be given intravenously to patients treated with nonselective fibrinolytic agents (e.g., streptokinase) who are at high risk for systemic emboli (large or anterior myocardial infarction, atrial fibrillation, previous embolus, or known left ventricular thrombus). It is not unreasonable to also consider administration of unfractionated heparin intravenously to all patients undergoing reperfusion therapy with streptokinase.

Low-molecular-weight-heparin can be considered an acceptable alternative to unfractionated heparin as ancillary therapy for patients younger than 75 years of age who are receiving fibrinolytic therapy if significant renal dysfunction (serum creatinine > 2.5 mg/dl in men or > 2.0 mg/dl in women) is not present. Enoxaparin (30-mg intravenous bolus followed by 1.0 mg/kg subcutaneously every 12 hours until hospital discharge) used in combination with full-dose tenecteplase is the most comprehensively studied regimen in patients younger than 75 years of age. Low-molecular-weight heparin should not be used as an alternative to unfractionated heparin as ancillary therapy in patients older than 75 years of age who are receiving fibrinolytic therapy until a safe dosing regimen for elderly patients is established from clinical trials.

In patients with known heparin-induced thrombocytopenia, it is reasonable to consider bivalirudin as a useful alternative to heparin to be used in conjunction with streptokinase. Dosing according to the HERO 2 regimen (a bolus of 0.25 mg/kg followed by an intravenous infusion of 0.5 mg/kg/hr for the first 12 hours and 0.25 mg/kg/hr for the subsequent 36 hours) is recommended but with a reduction in the infusion rate if the aPTT is greater than 75 seconds within the first 12 hours.[116] (Bivalirudin is currently indicated only for anticoagulation in patients with unstable angina who are undergoing percutaneous coronary angioplasty, but in view of the limited alternatives available to clinicians when treating patients with heparin-induced thrombocytopenia, the recommendation noted above should be considered.)

Antiplatelet Therapy

Platelets play a major role in the thrombotic response to disruption of a coronary artery plaque (see Fig. 46–1).[121] Platelets are activated in response to fibrinolysis, and platelet-rich thrombi are also more resistant to fibrinolysis than are fibrin and erythrocyte-rich thrombi (Fig. 47–17).[122] Thus, there is a sound scientific basis for inhibiting platelet aggregation in *all* STEMI patients, regardless of whether a thrombolytic agent is prescribed. Comprehensive overviews of randomized trials of antiplatelet therapy have summarized the overwhelming evidence of benefit of antiplatelet therapy for a wide range of vascular disorders.[123] In patients at risk for STEMI, patients with a documented prior STEMI, and patients in the acute phase of STEMI, there is a 22 percent reduction in the odds of the composite endpoint of death, nonfatal recurrent infarction, and nonfatal stroke with antiplatelet therapy (Fig. 47–18). Not unexpectedly, the absolute benefits are greatest in those patients at highest baseline risk. Although several antiplatelet regimens have been evaluated, the agent most extensively tested has been aspirin, and this also is the drug for which the most compelling evidence of benefit exists.

The ISIS-2 study was the largest trial of aspirin in STEMI patients; it provides the single strongest piece of evidence that aspirin reduces mortality in STEMI patients.[109] In contrast to the observations of a time-dependent mortality effect of fibrinolytic therapy, the mortality reduction with aspirin was similar in patients treated within 4 hours (25 percent reduction in mortality), between 5 and 12 hours (21 percent reduction), and between 13 and 24 hours (21 percent reduction). There was an overall 23 percent reduction in mortality from aspirin in ISIS-2 that was largely additive to the 25 percent reduction in mortality from streptokinase, so that patients receiving both therapies experienced a 42 percent reduction in mortality.[109] The mortality reduction was as high as 53 percent in those patients who received both aspirin and streptokinase within 6 hours of symptoms. Of particular interest was the finding that the combination of streptokinase and aspirin reduced mortality *without* increasing the risk of stroke or hemorrhage.

Obstructive arterial thrombi that are platelet rich are resistant to fibrinolysis and have an increased tendency to produce reocclusion after initial successful reperfusion in patients with STEMI.[124] Despite the inhibition of cyclooxygenase by aspirin, platelet activation continues to occur through thromboxane A_2-independent pathways, leading to platelet aggregation and increased thrombin formation. Activation of platelets by a variety of agonists results in the expression of functional receptors for fibrinogen and other ligands on the platelet surface—the glycoprotein (GP) IIb/IIIa receptor.[125] GP IIb/IIIa inhibition accelerates fibrinolysis and prevents reocclusion of successfully recanalized infarct arteries.[126] Potential mechanistic explanations for the beneficial of the effects of GP IIb/IIIa inhibition when combined with fibrinolytics center around important interactions between fibrinolytics and platelets (see Fig. 47–17). Platelets can be stimulated by fibrinolytics—for example, by the exposure of clot-bound thrombin. A narrowed lumen and a highly stenosed infarct-related artery generates high shear forces, a potent stimulus to platelet activation. Activated platelets may inhibit thrombolysis through the release of substances such as plasminogen activator inhibitor-1, alpha-2 plasminogen inhibitor, and factor XIII, which stabilize the clot and also

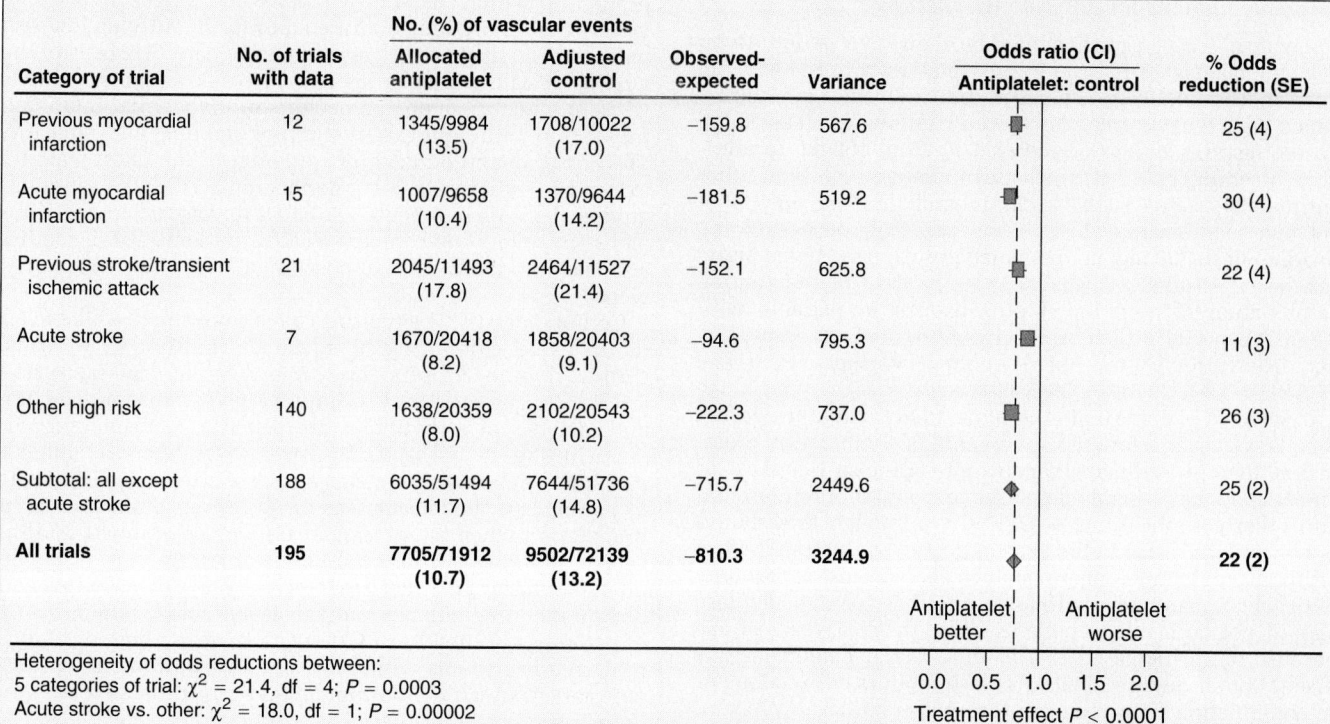

Category of trial	No. of trials with data	No. (%) of vascular events: Allocated antiplatelet	No. (%) of vascular events: Adjusted control	Observed-expected	Variance	Odds ratio (CI) Antiplatelet: control	% Odds reduction (SE)
Previous myocardial infarction	12	1345/9984 (13.5)	1708/10022 (17.0)	−159.8	567.6		25 (4)
Acute myocardial infarction	15	1007/9658 (10.4)	1370/9644 (14.2)	−181.5	519.2		30 (4)
Previous stroke/transient ischemic attack	21	2045/11493 (17.8)	2464/11527 (21.4)	−152.1	625.8		22 (4)
Acute stroke	7	1670/20418 (8.2)	1858/20403 (9.1)	−94.6	795.3		11 (3)
Other high risk	140	1638/20359 (8.0)	2102/20543 (10.2)	−222.3	737.0		26 (3)
Subtotal: all except acute stroke	188	6035/51494 (11.7)	7644/51736 (14.8)	−715.7	2449.6		25 (2)
All trials	**195**	**7705/71912 (10.7)**	**9502/72139 (13.2)**	**−810.3**	**3244.9**		**22 (2)**

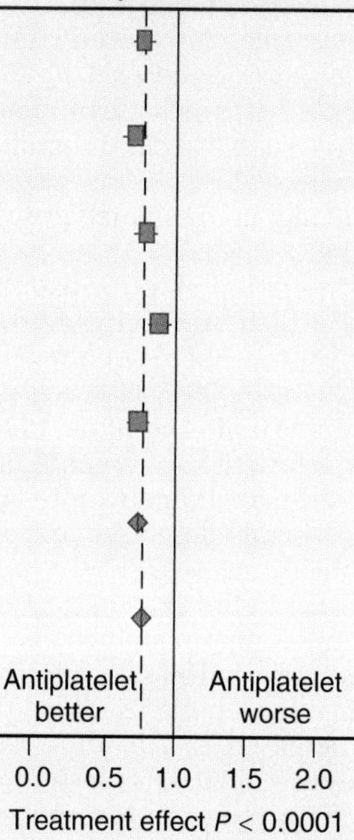

Heterogeneity of odds reductions between:
5 categories of trial: $\chi^2 = 21.4$, df = 4; $P = 0.0003$
Acute stroke vs. other: $\chi^2 = 18.0$, df = 1; $P = 0.00002$

FIGURE 47–18 Proportional effects of antiplatelet therapy on vascular events (myocardial infarction, stroke, or vascular death) in the main high-risk categories. Stratified ratio of odds of an event in treatment groups to that in control groups is plotted for each group of trials (square) along with its 99 percent confidence interval (horizontal line). Meta-analysis of results for all trials (and 95 percent confidence interval) is represented by a diamond. (From Antithromboitc Trialists' Collaboration: Collaborative meta-analysis of randomised trials of antiplatelet therapy for prevention of death, myocardial infarction, and stroke in high-risk patients. BMJ 324:71, 2002.)

enhance clot retraction—all features that make the clot more resistant to thrombolysis. Observations such as those noted earlier served as the foundation for testing the hypothesis that GP IIb/IIIa inhibition is a potent and safe addition to thrombolytic regimens and introduced the concept of *combination reperfusion* for patients with STEMI.

Aspirin only partially inhibits platelet aggregation by inhibiting the thromboxane A_2 pathway. Thienopyridines such as ticlopidine and clopidogrel inhibit binding to the adenosine diphosphate receptor and also block adenosine diphosphate-dependent pathways for platelet activation. Platelet inhibition by aspirin and the thienopyridines block only a limited number of the pathways of platelet activation. Irrespective of the stimulus for platelet activation, the final common pathway is expression of the GP IIb/IIIa receptor on the platelet surface. Therefore, direct inhibition of the GP IIb/IIIa receptor with intravenous agents such as abciximab, tirofiban, and eptifibatide has been studied in patients with STEMI.[34]

COMBINATION PHARMACOLOGICAL REPERFUSION. Several studies evaluated the combination of GP IIb/IIIa inhibitors and fibrinolytics.[127] The first series of trials combined full doses of thrombolytic agents with IIb/IIIa inhibitors.[128-131] Although these initial trials provided proof of the concept that the addition of an intravenous GP IIb/IIIa inhibitor enhanced the efficacy of a full dose of a fibrinolytic agent, unacceptably high rates of major bleeding were observed.

The combination of a reduced dose of a fibrinolytic agent and IIb/IIIa inhibitor was tested in a subsequent series of trials.[62,132-135] The rates of TIMI grade 3 flow at 60 and 90 minutes were only slightly higher with combination reperfusion compared with full-dose fibrinolytic monotherapy. A generally consistent observation across the trials was evidence of improved myocardial perfusion reflected in enhanced ST segment resolution and faster angiographic frame counts.[132,134-136]

GLYCOPROTEIN IIB/IIIA INHIBITION. The GUSTO V trial tested half-dose reteplase (5 U and 5 U) and full-dose abciximab compared with full-dose reteplase (10 U and 10 U) in 16,588 patients in the first 6 hours of STEMI.[137] Thirty-day mortality rates were similar in the two treatment groups (5.9 percent versus 5.6 percent). However, nonfatal reinfarction and other complications of myocardial infarction were reduced in the group receiving combination reperfusion therapy. Although the rates of intracranial hemorrhage were the same in the two treatment groups (0.6 percent), moderate to severe bleeding was significantly increased from 2.3 percent to 4.6 percent with combination reperfusion therapy ($p < 0.001$). This excess bleeding risk appeared to be limited to patients older than 75 years of age. The greatest mortality benefit was observed in those patients who presented with anterior myocardial infarction.

The ASSENT-3 trial randomized 6095 patients with STEMI to full-dose tenecteplase with unfractionated heparin versus full-dose tenecteplase with enoxaparin or half-dose tenecteplase plus abciximab (with weight-adjusted reduced-dose unfractionated heparin).[93] Similar to the GUSTO V trial, combination reperfusion therapy with half-dose tenecteplase and abciximab was not associated with a reduction in 30-day mortality; however, in-hospital reinfarction and refractory ischemia were reduced with combination reperfusion therapy. Of note, the major bleeding rate other than intracranial hemorrhage was increased from 2.2 percent to 4.3 percent with combination reperfusion therapy ($p < 0.0005$). The elderly were at greatest risk for excess bleeding, experiencing a threefold increase in the rate of that complication.

Nonenteric-coated aspirin should be chewed by patients who have not taken aspirin prior to presentation with STEMI. The dose should be 162 to 325 mg initially. During the maintenance phase of antiplatelet therapy following STEMI, the dose of aspirin should be reduced to 75 to 162 mg to minimize bleeding risk.[138] If true aspirin allergy is present, other antiplatelet agents such as clopidogrel (loading dose 300-600 mg; maintenance dose 75 mg per day) or ticlopidine (loading dose 500 mg; maintenance dose 250 mg twice daily) can be substituted. The efficacy and safety of the routine combination of clopidogrel plus aspirin in patients with STEMI, especially those receiving fibrinolytic therapy, has not been established but is being investigated in the CLARITY-TIMI 28 and COMMIT trials.

In selected patients (anterior myocardial infarction, age less than 75 years, and low risk for bleeding), combination reperfusion therapy with abciximab and half-dose reteplase or tenecteplase can be considered for prevention of reinfarction and other complications of STEMI,[137] although this should not be undertaken with the expectation of a reduction in mortality. Combination pharmacological reperfusion therapy with abciximab and half-dose reteplase or tenecteplase should not be given to patients older than 75 years of age because of an increased risk of intracranial hemorrhage. A discussion of the use of GP IIb/IIIa inhibitors either alone or in combination with reduced dose fibrinolytic as a preparatory regimen in patients for whom PCI is planned (i.e., facilitated PCI) is found in Chapter 48.

Hospital Management

Coronary Care Units

Deaths from primary ventricular fibrillation in patients with STEMI have been prevented because the coronary care unit (CCU) allows continuous monitoring of cardiac rhythm by highly trained nurses with the authority to initiate immediate treatment of arrhythmias in the absence of physicians, and because of the specialized equipment (defibrillators, pacemakers) and drugs available. Although all of these benefits can be achieved for patients scattered throughout the hospital, the clustering of patients with STEMI in the CCU has greatly improved the efficient use of the trained personnel, facilities, and equipment. With increasing emphasis on hemodynamic monitoring and treatment of the serious complications of STEMI with such modalities as pharmacological or catheter-based reperfusion therapy, afterload reduction, and intraaortic balloon counterpulsation, the presence of a CCU and experienced teams of physicians has assumed even greater importance. Improvements in the 30-day survival rate of elderly patients with STEMI can be traced to advances in therapy delivered in CCUs.[139] As reperfusion strategies including fibrinolytic therapy and PCI are used more routinely in STEMI patients, facilities in which patients can undergo diagnostic and therapeutic angiographic procedures are being integrated into an expanded structure of a coronary care team.[140]

At the same time, the value of CCUs for patients with uncomplicated STEMI has been questioned and restudied.[7] With increasing attention directed to the limitations of resources and to the economic impact of intensive care, efforts have been made to select patients likely to benefit from hospitalization in a CCU. The ECG reading, on presentation, particularly in conjunction with previous tracings and an immediate general clinical assessment, can be useful both for predicting which patients will have the diagnosis of acute myocardial infarction confirmed and for identifying low-risk patients who may require less intensive care. Analysis of the quality of pain can help identify low-risk patients. Patients without a history of angina pectoris or myocardial infarction presenting with pain that is sharp or stabbing and pleuritic, positional, or reproduced by palpation of the chest wall are extremely unlikely to be experiencing STEMI.[25] Computer-guided decision protocols are being developed to aid clinicians in identifying those STEMI patients who require admission to the CCU as opposed to a less intensive hospital ward.[141]

Contemporary CCUs typically have equipment available for noninvasive monitoring of single or multiple ECG leads, cardiac rhythm, ST segment deviation, arterial pressure, and arterial oxygen saturation. Computer algorithms for detection and analysis of arrhythmias are superior to visual surveillance by skilled CCU staff. However, even the most sophisticated ECG monitoring systems are susceptible to artifacts due to patient movement or noise on the signal from poor skin preparation when monitoring electrodes are applied. Noninvasive monitoring of arterial blood pressure using a sphygmomanometric cuff that undergoes cycles of inflation and deflation at programmed intervals is suitable for the majority of patients admitted to a CCU. Invasive arterial monitoring is preferred in patients with a low output syndrome under circumstances in which inotropic therapy is initiated for severe left ventricular failure.

The CCU remains the appropriate hospital unit for patients with complicated infarctions (e.g., hemodynamic instability, recurrent arrhythmias) and those patients requiring intensive nursing care for devices such as an intraaortic balloon pump. STEMI patients with an uncomplicated status, such as those without a history of previous infarction, persistent ischemic-type discomfort, congestive heart failure, hypotension, heart block, or hemodynamically compromising ventricular arrhythmias, can be safely transferred out of the CCU within 24 to 36 hours. In patients with a complicated STEMI, the duration of the CCU stay should be dictated by the need for "intensive" care; that is, hemodynamic monitoring, close nursing supervision, intravenous vasoactive drugs, and frequent changes in the medical regimen.

For patients with a low risk of mortality from STEMI, the clinician should consider admission to an intermediate care facility (see later) equipped with simple ECG monitoring and resuscitation equipment.[7] This strategy has been shown to be cost-effective and may reduce CCU use by one-third, shorten hospital stays, and have no deleterious effect on patients' recovery. Intermediate care units for low-risk STEMI patients can also be appealing to patients who stand to gain little benefit from the high staffing, intense activity, and elaborate technology available in current CCUs (with their attendant high costs) and who may be disturbed by that activity and equipment.

General Measures

The CCU staff must be sensitive to patient concerns about mortality, prognosis, and future productivity. A calm, quiet atmosphere and the "laying on of hands" with a gentle but confident touch help allay anxiety and reduce sympathetic tone, ultimately leading to a reduction in hypertension, tachycardia, and arrhythmias.[7] To reduce the risk of nausea and vomiting early after infarction and to reduce the risk of aspiration, during the first 4 to 12 hours after admission patients should receive either nothing by mouth or a clear liquid diet (see Table 47–5). Subsequently, a diet with 50 to 55 percent of calories from complex carbohydrates and up to 30 percent from mono- and unsaturated fats should be given. The diet should be enriched in foods that are high in

TABLE 47–5 Sample Admitting Orders for the STEMI patient

1. Condition: Serious
2. IV: NS on D_5W to keep vein open. Start a second IV if IV medication is being given. This may be a saline lock.
3. Vital signs: every 1.5 hours until stable, then every 4 hours and as needed. Notify physician if HR is less than 60 beats/min or greater than 100 beats/min, BP is less than 100 mm Hg systolic or greater than 150 mm Hg systolic, respiratory rate is less than 8 or greater than 22.
4. Monitor: Continuous ECG monitoring for dysrhythmia and ST segment deviation
5. Diet: NPO except for sips of water until stable. Then start 2 gm sodium/day, low saturated fat (less than 7% of total calories/day), low cholesterol (less than 200 mg/day) diet, such as Total Lifestyle Change (TLC) diet
6. Activity: Bedside commode and light activity when stable
7. Oxygen: Continuous oximetry monitoring. Nasal cannula at 2 liters/min when stable for 6 hr, reassess for oxygen need (i.e., O_2 saturation of less than 90%) and consider discontinuing oxygen.
8. Medications:
   a. Nitroglycerin (NTG)
      1. Use sublingual NTG 0.4 mg every 5 min as needed for chest discomfort.
      2. Intravenous NTG for CHF, hypertension, or persistent ischemia.
   b. ASA
      1. If ASA not given in the emergency department (ED), chew nonenteric-coated ASA* 162-325 mg.
      2. If ASA has been given, start daily maintenance of 75-162 mg daily; may use enteric coated for gastrointestinal protection.
   c. Beta blocker
      1. If not given in the ED, assess for contraindications, i.e., bradycardia and hypotension; continue daily assessment to ascertain eligibility for beta blocker.
      2. If given in the ED, continue daily dose and optimize as dictated by heart rate and blood pressure.
   d. ACE inhibitor
      1. Start ACE inhibitor orally in patients with pulmonary congestion or LVEF less than 40 percent if the following are absent: hypotension (SBP less than 100 mm Hg or less than 30 mm Hg below baseline) or known contraindications to this class of medications.
   e. Angiotensin receptor blocker (ARB)
      1. Start ARB orally in patients who are intolerant of ACE inhibitors and with either clinical or radiological signs of heart failure or LVEF less than 40 percent.
   f. Pain medications
      1. IV morphine sulfate 2-4 mg with increments of 2-8 mg IV at 5- to 15-min intervals as needed to control pain.
   g. Anxiolytics (based on a nursing assessment)
   h. Daily stool softener

Modified from Ryan TJ, Antman EM, Brooks NH, et al: 1999 update: ACC/AHA guidelines for the management of patients with acute myocardial infarction. A report of the American College of Cardiology/American Heart Association Task Force on Practice Guidelines (Committee on Management of Acute Myocardial Infarction). J Am Coll Cardiol 34:890, 1999.

*Although some trials have used enteric-coated ASA for initial dosing, more rapid buccal absorption occurs with nonenteric-coated formulations.

potassium, magnesium, and fiber but low in sodium (Table 47–5).

The results of laboratory tests obtained in the CCU should be scrutinized for any derangements potentially contributing to arrhythmias, such as hypoxemia, hypovolemia, disturbances of acid-base balance or of electrolytes, and drug toxicity. Oxazepam, 15 to 30 mg orally four times a day, is useful to allay the anxiety that is common in the first 24 to 48 hours (see Table 47–5). Delirium can be provoked by medications frequently used in the CCU, including antiarrhythmic drugs, H_2 blockers, narcotics, and beta blockers. Potentially offending agents should be discontinued in patients with an abnormal mental status. Haloperidol, a butyrophenone, can be used safely in patients with STEMI beginning with a dose of 2 mg intravenously for mildly agitated patients and 5 to 10 mg for progressively more agitated patients. Hypnotics, such as temazepam, 15 to 30 mg or an equivalent, should be provided as needed for sleep. Dioctyl sodium sulfosuccinate, 200 mg daily, or another stool softener should be used to prevent constipation and straining (see Table 47–5).

"Coronary precautions" that do *not* appear to be supported by evidence from clinical research include the avoidance of iced fluids, hot beverages, caffeinated beverages, rectal examinations, and back rubs.[7]

PHYSICAL ACTIVITY. In the absence of complications, patients with STEMI need not be confined to bed for more than 12 hours and, unless they are hemodynamically compromised, they may use a bedside commode shortly after admission (see Table 47–5). Progression of activity should be individualized depending on the patient's clinical status, age, and physical capacity.

In patients without hemodynamic compromise, early ambulation, including dangling the feet on the side of the bed, sitting in a chair, standing, and walking around the bed, does not cause important changes in heart rate, blood pressure, or pulmonary wedge pressure. Although heart rate increases slightly (usually by less than 10 percent), pulmonary wedge pressures fall slightly as the patient assumes the upright posture for activities. Early ambulatory activities are rarely associated with any symptoms, and when symptoms do occur, they generally are related to hypotension. Thus, when Levine and Lown proposed the "armchair" treatment of STEMI in the 1950s, they were undoubtedly correct that stress to the myocardium is less in the upright position. As long as blood pressure and heart rate are monitored, early ambulation offers considerable psychological and physical benefit without any clear medical risk.

The Intermediate Coronary Care Unit

Patients with STEMI are at risk for late in-hospital mortality from recurrent ischemia or infarction, hemodynamically significant ventricular arrhythmias, and severe congestive heart failure after discharge from the CCU. Therefore, continued surveillance in intermediate CCUs (also called step-down units) is justifiable. Risk factors for mortality in the hospital after discharge from the coronary care unit include significant congestive heart failure evidenced by persistent sinus tachycardia for more than 2 days and rales greater than one-third of the lung fields; recurrent ventricular tachycardia and ventricular fibrillation; atrial fibrillation or flutter while in the CCU; intraventricular conduction delays or heart block; anterior location of infarction; and recurrent episodes of angina with marked electrocardiographic ST-segment abnormalities at low activity levels.

The availability of intermediate care units may also be helpful in identifying those patients who remain free of complications and are suitable candidates for early discharge from the hospital. Aggressive reperfusion protocols with angioplasty or thrombolytics can reduce the length of hospital stay.[142] In patients who are believed to have undergone successful reperfusion, the *absence* of early sustained ventricular tachyarrhythmias, hypotension, or heart failure, coupled with a well-preserved left ventricular ejection fraction, predicts a low risk of late complications in-hospital.[143] Such patients are suitable candidates for discharge from the hospital in less than 5 days from the onset of symptoms.

Following STEMI, patients are often eager for information, in need of reassurance, confused by misinformation and prior impressions, capable of counterproductive denial, and simply frightened. Intermediate care facilities provide ideal settings and ample opportunities to begin the rehabilitation process.[144] The capacity for the early detection of problems following STEMI and the social and educational benefits of grouping such patients together strongly argue for continued utilization of intermediate CCUs. Furthermore, the economic advantage of grouping such patients together for sharing of skilled personnel and resources outweighs any questions raised by the lack of a clear consensus regarding reduced mortality. An additional potential advantage is the facilitation of patient education in a group setting with lectures and audiovisual programs.

Pharmacological Therapy

Beta Blockers (see Chaps. 49 and 50)

The effects of beta blockers in the treatment of patients with STEMI can be divided into those that are immediate (when the drug is given very early in the course of infarction) and those that are long-term (secondary prevention), when the drug is initiated sometime after infarction. The immediate intravenous administration of beta-adrenoceptor blockers reduces cardiac index, heart rate, and blood pressure.[50] The net effect is a reduction in myocardial oxygen consumption per minute and per beat. Favorable effects of acute intravenous administration of beta-adrenoceptor blockers on the balance of myocardial oxygen supply and demand are reflected in reductions in chest pain, in the proportion of patients with threatened infarction who actually evolve STEMI, and in the development of ventricular arrhythmias.[145] Because beta-adrenoceptor blockade diminishes circulating levels of free fatty acids by antagonizing the lipolytic effects of catecholamines and because elevated levels of fatty acids augment myocardial oxygen consumption and probably increase the incidence of arrhythmias, these metabolic actions of beta-blocking agents may also be beneficial to the ischemic heart.

Objective evidence of beneficial effects of beta blockers in acute myocardial ischemia has been reported using the precordial ST segment mapping technique. Acute beta blockade probably reduces infarct size in patients with STEMI. Reduction in release of serum cardiac biomarkers with beta blockade is suggestive of a smaller infarct, as is the preservation of R waves and reduction in the development of Q waves.

At least 30 randomized beta blocker trials involving more than 29,000 patients have been undertaken. Intravenous followed by oral beta blocker therapy is associated with about a 13 percent relative reduction in the risk of mortality (Fig. 47–19). Although antagonism of sympathetic stimulation to the heart might be expected to exacerbate pulmonary edema in patients with occult heart failure, usually only small changes in pulmonary capillary wedge pressure occur when the drug is used in patients with STEMI. Thus, in appropriately selected patients (Table 47–6), the benefits occur at a cost of about a 3 percent incidence of provocation of congestive heart failure or complete heart block and a 2 percent incidence of the development of cardiogenic shock.

Because reduction of infarct size in STEMI patients treated with beta blockers is likely to occur only with early treatment (<4 hours from the onset of pain), investigators have sought other explanations for the reduction in the mortality in the acute phase that has been observed. Intriguing observations from the ISIS-1 trial raise the possibility that a reduction in the development of cardiac rupture or electromechanical dissociation during the first day is achieved with early beta blockade.[146]

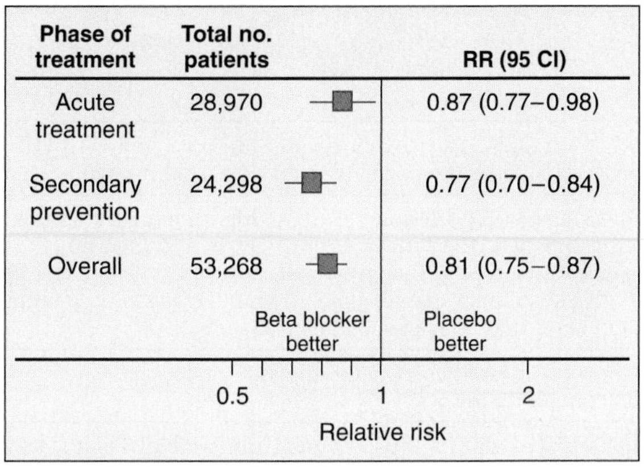

FIGURE 47–19 Effect of beta blockers on mortality rate in patients with myocardial infarction. The relative risk of mortality is reduced with beta blockers both during the acute phase of treatment and when prescribed as secondary prevention after acute myocardial infarction. (Data from Chae CU, Hennekens CH: Beta blockers. *In* Hennekens CH [ed]: Clinical Trials in Cardiovascular Disease: A Companion to Braunwald's Heart Disease. Philadelphia, WB Saunders, 1999, p 84.)

TABLE 47–6 Contraindications to Beta-Adrenoceptor Blocker Therapy in Acute Myocardial Infarction

Heart rate < 60 beats/min
Systolic arterial pressure < 100 mm Hg
Moderate or severe left ventricular failure
Signs of peripheral hypoperfusion
PR interval > 0.24 second
Second- or third-degree atrioventricular block
Severe chronic obstructive pulmonary disease
History of asthma
Severe peripheral vascular disease
Insulin-dependent diabetes mellitus

In the TIMI-II trial, the addition of a beta blocker (metoprolol) to fibrinolytic therapy was studied.[147] Although recurrent ischemia and reinfarction were reduced by immediate intravenous versus delayed use of metoprolol, mortality was not reduced, nor was ventricular function improved. Thus, immediate intravenous beta blockade, although clinically beneficial, may not enhance salvage of myocardium in the setting of early reperfusion but may confer clinical benefit by means of its antiischemic effect.[148]

Substantial proportions of elderly patients who are hospitalized with STEMI and are ideal candidates for early beta blocker therapy do not receive this treatment.[50] Compared with elderly patients who receive early beta blockade in STEMI, those who do not receive beta blockade are older, more likely to be women, and less likely to be white. Elderly patients who receive early beta blocker therapy have significantly lower in-hospital mortality rates than those who do not receive beta blockers.

RECOMMENDATIONS. Given the overwhelming evidence of benefits of early blockade in STEMI, patients without a contraindication who can be treated within 12 hours of the onset of infarction, irrespective of administration of concomitant thrombolytic therapy or performance of primary PCI, should receive beta blockers. A regimen that we like to use is metoprolol 5 mg intravenously every 2 to 5 minutes for three doses provided the heart rate does not fall below 60 beats/min and the systolic blood pressure does not drop below 100 mm Hg. Oral maintenance dosing is initiated with metoprolol 50 mg every 6 hours for 2 days and then 100 mg twice daily.

Beta blockers are especially helpful in patients in whom STEMI is complicated by persistent or recurrent ischemic pain, progressive or repetitive serum enzyme elevations suggestive of infarct extension, or tachyarrhythmias early after the onset of infarction. If adverse effects of beta blockers develop or if patients present with complications of infarction that are contraindications to beta blockade such as heart failure or heart block, the beta blocker should be withheld. Unless there are contraindications (Table 47–6), beta blockade probably should be continued in patients who develop STEMI.

Selection of Beta Blocker. Favorable effects have been reported with metoprolol, atenolol, timolol, and alprenolol; these benefits probably occur with propranolol and with esmolol, an ultra-short-acting agent, as well. In the absence of any favorable evidence supporting the benefit of agents with intrinsic sympathomimetic activity, such as pindolol and oxprenolol, and with some unfavorable evidence for these agents in secondary prevention, beta blockers with intrinsic sympathomimetic activity probably should not be chosen for treatment of STEMI. The CAPRICORN trial randomized 1959 patients with myocardial infarction and systolic dysfunction (ejection fraction < 40 percent) to carvedilol or placebo in addition to contemporary pharmacotherapy, including ACE inhibitors in 98 percent of patients.[149] All-cause mortality was reduced from 15.3 percent in the placebo group to 11.9 percent in the carvedilol group (23 percent relative risk reduction; $p = 0.031$). Thus, CAPRICORN confirms the benefit of beta blockade in addition to ACE inhibitor therapy in patients with transient or sustained left ventricular dysfunction after myocardial infarction. An algorithm for the use of beta blockers in the STEMI patients is shown in Figure 47–20.

Occasionally, the clinician may wish to proceed with beta blocker therapy even in the presence of relative contraindications, such as a history of mild asthma, mild bradycardia, mild heart failure, or first-degree heart block. In this situation, a trial of esmolol may help determine whether the patient can tolerate beta blockade. Because the hemodynamic effects of this drug, with a half-life of 9 minutes, disappear in less than 30 minutes, it offers considerable advantage over

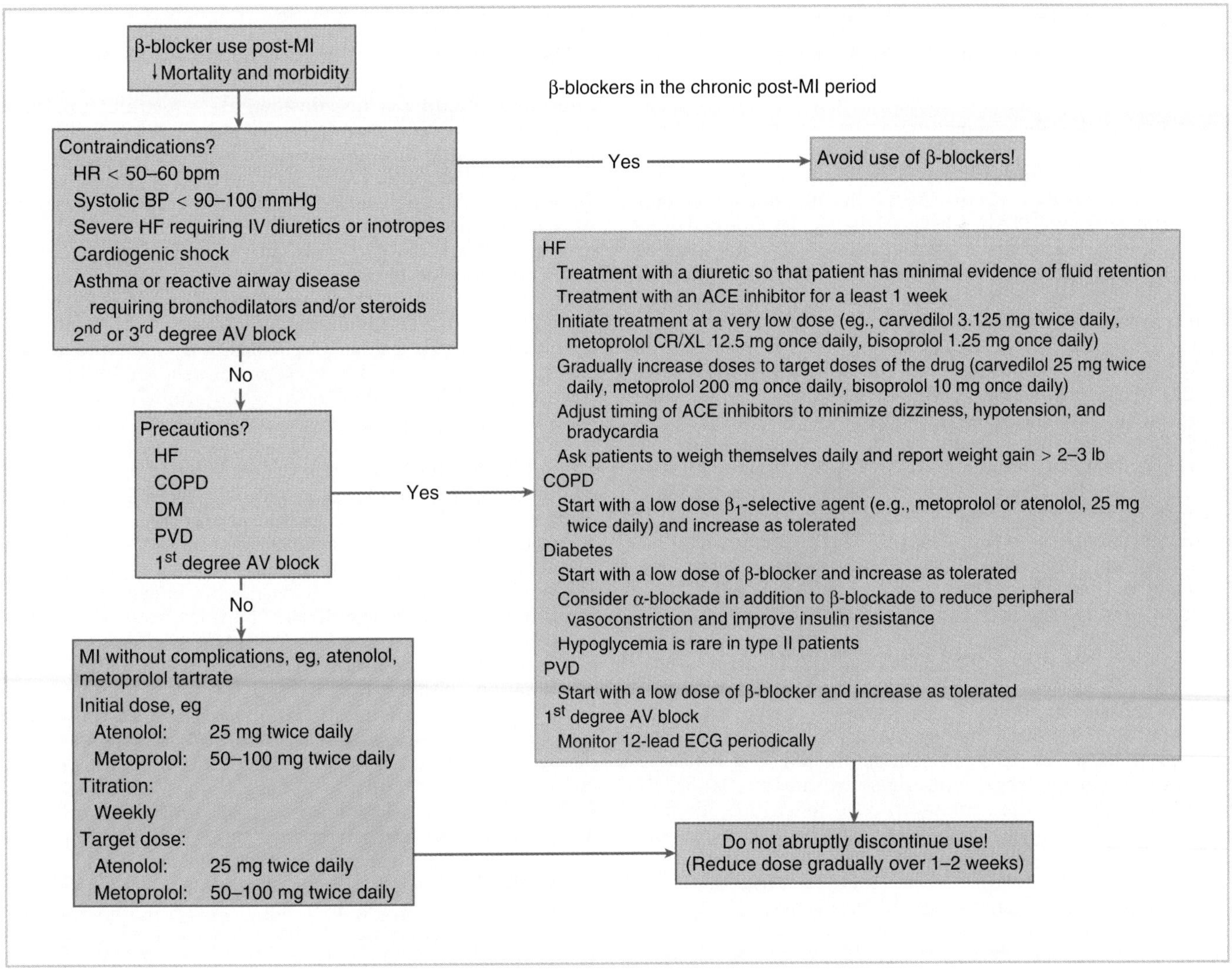

FIGURE 47–20 Algorithm for use of beta blockers in the treatment of patients with ST segment elevation myocardial infarction. COPD = chronic obstructive pulmonary disease; DM = diabetes mellitus; HF = heart failure; PVD = peripheral vascular disease. (From Gheorghiade M, Goldstein S: Beta-blockers in the post-myocardial infarction patient. Circulation 106:394, 2002.)

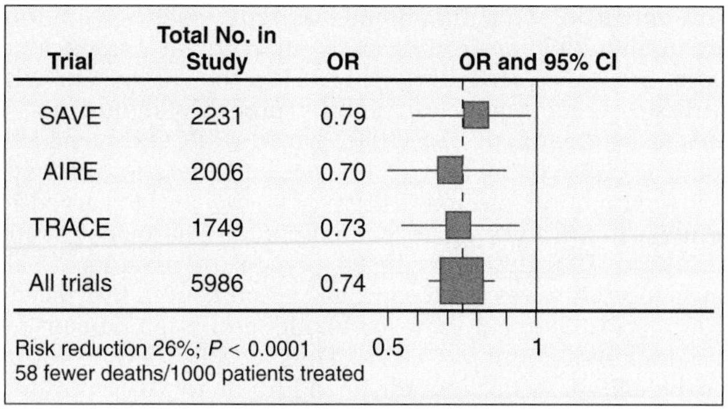

FIGURE 47–21 Effect of angiotensin-converting enzyme inhibitors on mortality after myocardial infarction: results from the long-term trials. (From Flather MD, Pfeffer MA: Angiotensin-converting enzyme inhibitors. *In* Hennekens CH [ed]: Clinical Trials in Cardiovascular Disease: A Companion to Braunwald's Heart Disease. Philadelphia, WB Saunders, 1999, p 97.)

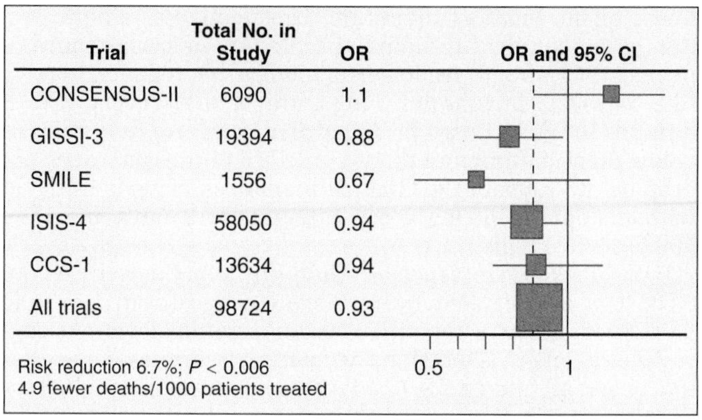

FIGURE 47–22 Effects of angiotensin-converting enzyme inhibitors on mortality after myocardial infarction: results from the short-term trials. (From Flather MD, Pfeffer MA: Angiotensin-converting enzyme inhibitors. *In* Hennekens CH [ed]: Clinical Trials in Cardiovascular Disease: A Companion to Braunwald's Heart Disease. Philadelphia, WB Saunders, 1999, p 101.)

longer acting agents when the risk of a beta blocker complication is relatively high.

Inhibition of the Renin-Angiotensin-Aldosterone System

In 1992, with the publication of the SAVE trial, ACE inhibitors were established as an important addition to the list of treatments for STEMI. The rationale for their use includes experimental and clinical evidence of a favorable impact on ventricular remodeling, improvement in hemodynamics, and reductions in congestive heart failure.[150] There is now unequivocal evidence from randomized, placebo-controlled mortality trials that ACE inhibitors reduce the rate of mortality from STEMI. These trials can be grouped into two categories. The first consisted of *selected* myocardial infarction patients for randomization, based on features indicative of increased mortality such as left ventricular ejection fraction less than 40 percent, clinical signs and symptoms of congestive heart failure,[151] anterior location of infarction,[152] and abnormal wall motion score index (Fig. 47–21).[153] The second group were *unselective* trials that randomized all patients with myocardial infarction provided they had a minimum systolic pressure of approximately 100 mm Hg (ISIS-4,[154] GISSI-3,[155] CONSENSUS II,[156] and Chinese Captopril Study) (Fig. 47–22). With the exception of the SMILE trial,[152] all of the selective trials initiated ACE inhibitor therapy between 3 and 16 days after myocardial infarction and maintained it for 1 to 4 years, whereas the unselective trials all initiated treatment within the first 24 to 36 hours and maintained it for only 4 to 6 weeks.

A consistent survival benefit was observed in all of the trials already noted, except for CONSENSUS II, the one study that utilized an intravenous preparation early in the course of myocardial infarction.[156] An estimate of the mortality benefit of ACE inhibitors in the unselective, short duration of therapy trials was 5 per 1000 patients treated.[157,158] Analysis of these unselective short-term trials indicates that approximately one-third of the lives saved occurred within the first 1 to 2 days. Certain subgroups, such as patients with anterior infarction, showed proportionately greater benefit from early administration (11 lives saved per 1000) of ACE inhibitors. Not unexpectedly, greater survival benefits of 42 to 76 lives saved per 1000 patients treated were obtained in the *selective*, long duration of therapy trials. Of note, there was generally a 20 percent reduction in the risk of death attributable to ACE inhibitor treatment in the selective trials. The mortality reduction with ACE inhibitors is accompanied by significant reductions in the development of congestive heart failure, supporting the underlying pathophysiological rationale for administering this class of drugs in patients with STEMI.[151,153,155] In addition, some data suggest that ischemic events, including recurrent infarction and the need for coronary revascularization, can also be reduced by chronic administration of ACE inhibitors after a STEMI.[159]

The mortality benefits of ACE inhibitors are additive to those achieved with aspirin and beta blockers.[155] Thus, ACE inhibitors should not be considered a substitute for these other therapies with proven benefit in STEMI patients. The benefits of ACE inhibition appear to be a class effect because mortality and morbidity have been reduced by several agents. To replicate these benefits in clinical practice, however, physicians should select a specific agent and prescribe the drug according to the protocols utilized in the successful clinical trials reported to date.

The major *contraindications* to the use of ACE inhibitors in patients with STEMI include hypotension in the setting of adequate preload, known hypersensitivity, and pregnancy. Adverse reactions include hypotension, especially after the first dose, and intolerable cough with chronic dosing; much less commonly, angioedema can occur (see Chap. 38).

An alternative method of pharmacological inhibition of the renin-angiotensin-aldosterone system is by administration of angiotensin-2 receptor blockers (ARBs). The OPTIMAAL trial evaluated the effects of the ARB losartan versus captopril on survival and other major cardiovascular outcomes in myocardial infarction patients with clinical evidence of heart failure. Although losartan was significantly better tolerated than captopril, there was a nonsignificant trend favoring captopril in terms of total mortality.[160] The VALIANT trial compared the effects of the ARB valsartan versus captopril alone and in combination with captopril on mortality in patients with acute myocardial infarction complicated by left ventricular systolic dysfunction and/or heart failure.[161] Patients were randomized within 10 days of myocardial infarction to valsartan (20 mg initially, titrated to 160 mg twice daily), valsartan added to captopril (20 mg and 6.25 mg initially, titrated to 80 mg twice daily and 50 mg three times daily), or captopril (6.25 mg initially, titrated to 50 mg three times daily), added to conventional therapy. Rates of mortality were similar in the three treatment groups: 19.9 percent in the valsartan group, 19.3 percent in the valsartan plus captopril group, and 19.5 percent in the captopril alone group (Fig. 47–23). Permanent discontinuation of study medication was more frequent in the groups receiving captopril (valsartan, 20.5 percent; valsartan plus captopril 23.4 percent; captopril alone

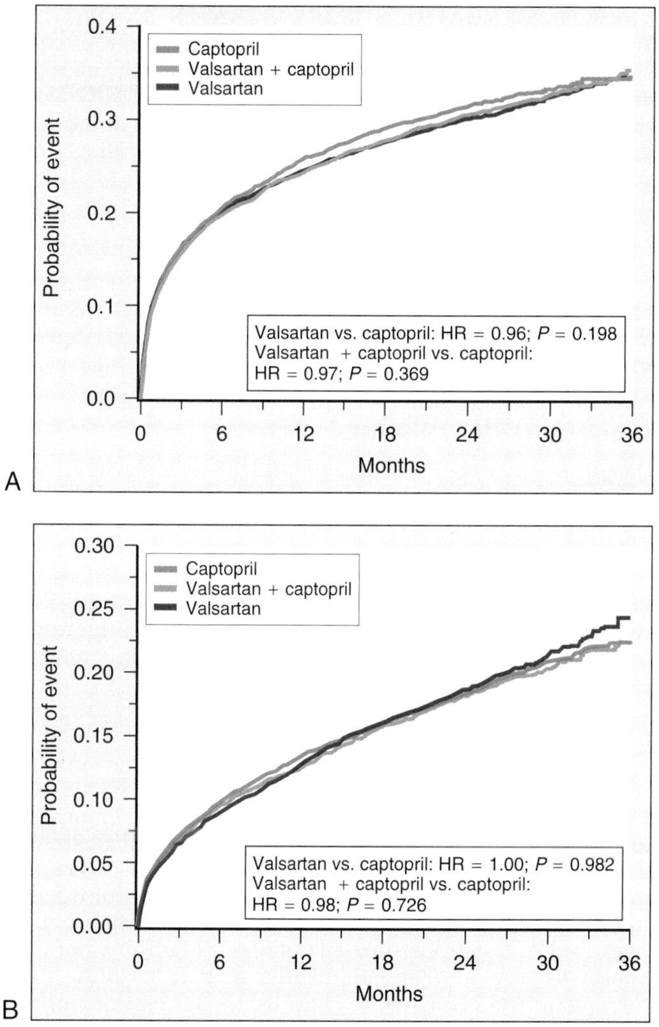

FIGURE 47–23 Effects of an angiotensin-converting enzyme inhibitor (captopril), angiotensin receptor blocker (valsartan), or the combination after myocardial infarction. The Kaplan-Meier estimates of **(A)** mortality and **(B)** cardiovascular death, reinfarction, or hospitalization for heart failure, by treatment in the VALIANT trial are depicted. (From Pfeffer M, McMurray JJ, Velasquez EJ, et al: Effects of valsartan relative to captopril in patients with myocardial infarction complicated by heart failure and or left ventricular dysfunction. N Engl J Med 349:1893, 2003.)

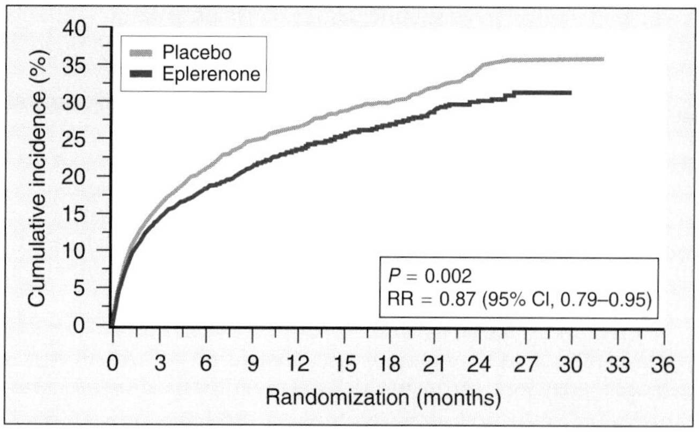

FIGURE 47–24 Effect of a selective aldosterone receptor blocker (eplerenone) after myocardial infarction. The Kaplan-Meier estimates of the rate of death from cardiovascular causes or hospitalization for cardiovascular events in the EPHESUS trial are depicted. (From Pitt B, Remme W, Zannad F, et al: Eplerenone, a selective aldosterone blocker, in patients with left ventricular dysfunction after myocardial infarction (abstract). N Engl J Med 348:14, 2003.)

21.6 percent; $p = 0.129$ for valsartan compared to captopril and $p = 0.021$ for valsartan plus captopril versus captopril alone).

Aldosterone blockade is the last pharmacological strategy for inhibition the renin-angiotensin-aldosterone system. The EPHESUS trial randomized 6642 patients with acute myocardial infarction complicated by left ventricular dysfunction and heart failure to the selective aldosterone blocker eplerenone or placebo in conjunction with contemporary postinfarction pharmacotherapy.[162] During a mean follow-up period of 16 months, there was a 15 percent reduction in the relative risk of mortality favoring eplerenone (Fig. 47–24). Cardiovascular mortality or hospitalization for cardiovascular events was also reduced by eplerenone. Serious hyperkalemia (serum potassium concentration ≥ 6.0 mmol/liter) occurred in 5.5 percent of patients in the eplerenone group compared with 3.9 percent of patients in the placebo group ($p = 0.002$).

RECOMMENDATIONS. After administration of aspirin and initiation of reperfusion strategies and, where appropriate, beta blockade, *all* STEMI patients should be considered for inhibition of the renin-angiotensin-aldosterone system. Although there is little disagreement that high-risk STEMI patients (elderly, anterior infarction, prior infarction, Killip class II or greater, and asymptomatic patients with evidence of depressed global ventricular function on an imaging study) should receive life-long treatment with ACE inhibitors,[163] short-term (4-6 weeks) therapy to a broader group of patients has also been proposed based on the pooled results of the unselective mortality trials.[154]

Considering all the available data, we favor a strategy of an initial trial of oral ACE inhibitors in all STEMI patients with congestive heart failure as well as in hemodynamically stable patients with ST segment elevation or left bundle branch block, commencing within the first 24 hours.[158,164] ACE inhibition therapy should be continued indefinitely in patients with congestive heart failure, evidence of a reduction in global function, or a large regional wall motion abnormality. In patients without these findings at discharge, ACE inhibitors can be discontinued.

The results of the VALIANT trial expand the range of options available to clinicians treating patients with STEMI. Since the ARB was at least as effective as the ACE inhibitor in reducing mortality and other adverse cardiovascular outcomes following myocardial infarction, it should be considered as a clinically effective alternative to captopril. The choice between ACE inhibition and angiotensin receptor blockade following STEMI should be based on physician experience with the agents, patient tolerability, safety, convenience, and cost. Finally, based on experience from the EPHESUS study, long-term aldosterone blockade with eplerenone 25 mg/day initially and then titrated to 50 mg/day for high-risk patients following STEMI (ejection fraction ≤ 40 percent, clinical heart failure, diabetes mellitus) should be considered. Given the small but definite increase in the risk of serious hypokalemia when aldosterone blockade is prescribed, particularly when other measures for inhibition of the renin-angiotensin-aldosterone system are used concurrently, periodic monitoring of the serum potassium level should be undertaken.[165]

Nitrates (see Chap. 50)

Sublingual nitroglycerin very rarely opens occluded coronary arteries. However, in patients with STEMI, the potential for reductions in ventricular filling pressures, wall tension, and cardiac work coupled with improvement in coronary blood flow, especially in ischemic zones, and antiplatelet effects make nitrates a logical and attractive pharmacological intervention.[7]

In patients with STEMI, the administration of nitrates reduces pulmonary capillary wedge pressure and systemic arterial pressure, left ventricular chamber volume, infarct size, and the incidence of mechanical complications. As with other interventions to spare ischemic myocardium in cases of STEMI, intravenous nitroglycerin appears to be of greatest benefit in patients treated earliest after the onset of symptoms.

CLINICAL TRIAL RESULTS. In the prefibrinolytic era, 10 randomized trials of acute administration of intravenous nitroglycerin (or nitroprusside, another nitric oxide donor) collectively enrolled 2042 patients. A meta-analysis of these trial results showed a reduction in mortality of 35 percent associated with nitrate therapy.

In the fibrinolytic era, two megatrials of nitrate therapy have been conducted: GISSI-3[155] and ISIS-4.[154] In GISSI-3, there was no independent effect of nitrates on short-term mortality.[155] Similarly, in ISIS-4, no effect of a mononitrate on 35-day mortality was observed. A pooled analysis of more than 80,000 patients treated with nitrate-like preparations intravenously or orally in 22 trials revealed a mortality rate of 7.7 per cent in the control group, which was reduced to 7.4 percent in the nitrate group. These data are consistent with a small treatment effect of nitrates on mortality such that 3 to 4 fewer deaths would occur for every 1000 patients treated.[154]

NITRATE PREPARATIONS AND MODE OF ADMINISTRATION. Intravenous nitroglycerin can be administered safely to patients with evolving STEMI as long as the dose is titrated to avoid induction of reflex tachycardia or systemic arterial hypotension. Patients with inferior wall infarction are particularly sensitive to an excessive fall in preload, particularly if concurrent right ventricular infarction is present.[166] In such cases, nitrate-induced venodilation could impair cardiac output and reduce coronary block flow, thus worsening myocardial oxygenation rather than improving it.

A useful regimen employs an initial infusion rate of 5 to 10 mg/min with increases of 5 to 20 mg/min until the mean arterial blood pressure is reduced by 10 percent of its baseline level in normotensive patients and by 30 percent for hypertensive patients, but in no case below a systolic pressure of 90 mm Hg. Alternatively, nitroglycerin can be administered as a sustained-release oral preparation (30-60 mg/day) or as an ointment (1 to 3 inches every 6 to 8 hours for patients with a systolic pressure greater than 120 mm Hg). Nitroglycerin can also be given sublingually at doses of 0.3 to 0.6 mg. This route can be more hazardous because the rate of absorption is difficult to control and arterial pressure may decline precipitously.

ADVERSE EFFECTS. Clinically significant methemoglobinemia has been reported to occur during administration of intravenous nitroglycerin. Although uncommon, this problem is seen when unusually large doses of nitrates are administered. It is important not only for its potential to cause symptoms of lethargy and headache but also because elevated methemoglobin levels can impair the oxygen-carrying capacity of blood, potentially exacerbating ischemia. Dilation of the pulmonary vasculature supplying poorly ventilated lung segments may produce a ventilation-perfusion mismatch.

Tolerance to intravenous nitroglycerin (as manifested by increasing nitrate requirements) develops in many patients, often as soon as 12 hours after the infusion is started. Despite the theoretical and demonstrated benefit of sulfhydryl agents in diminishing tolerance, their use has not become widespread.

RECOMMENDATIONS FOR NITRATES IN PATIENT WITH STEMI. Nitroglycerin is indicated for the relief of persistent pain and as a vasodilator in patients with infarction associated with left ventricular failure. In the absence of recurrent angina or congestive heart failure, we do not routinely prescribe them for STEMI patients. Higher risk patients such as those with large transmural infarctions, especially of the anterior wall, have the most to gain from nitrates in terms of reduction of ventricular remodeling, and we therefore routinely use intravenous nitrates for 24 to 48 hours in such patients. There is no clear benefit to empirical long-term cutaneous or oral nitrates in the asymptomatic patient, and we therefore do not prescribe nitrates beyond the first 48 hours unless angina or ventricular failure is present.

Calcium Antagonists (see Chap. 50)

Despite sound experimental and clinical evidence of an anti-ischemic effect, calcium antagonists have *not* been found to be helpful in the acute phase of STEMI, and concern has been raised in several systematic overviews about an increased risk of mortality when they are prescribed on a routine basis. A distinction should be made between the dihydropyridine type of calcium antagonists (e.g., nifedipine) and the nondihydropyridine calcium antagonists (e.g., verapamil and diltiazem).

NIFEDIPINE. In multiple trials involving more than 5000 patients, the immediate-release preparation of nifedipine has not resulted in any reduction in infarct size, prevention of progression to infarction, control of recurrent ischemia, or lowering of mortality rate. When trials of the immediate-release form of nifedipine are pooled in a meta-analysis, evidence suggests a dose-related increased risk of in-hospital mortality (especially at a dose higher than 80 mg of nifedipine), although posthospital mortality does not appear to be increased in nifedipine-treated patients. Nifedipine does not appear to be helpful in conjunction with either fibrinolytic therapy or beta blockade.[167] Thus, we do not recommend the use of immediate-release nifedipine early in the treatment of STEMI. No trials of the sustained-release preparations of nifedipine in patients with acute myocardial infarction have been reported to date.

VERAPAMIL AND DILTIAZEM. When administered during the acute phase of STEMI, these drugs have not had any demonstrated favorable effect on infarct size or other important endpoints in patients with STEMI, with the exception of control of supraventricular arrhythmias.[168] The INTERCEPT trial compared 300 mg of diltiazem with placebo in patients who received fibrinolytic therapy for STEMI.[169] Diltiazem did not reduce the cumulative occurrence of cardiac death, nonfatal reinfarction, or refractory ischemia during a 6-month follow-up.

Based on the available data, we do *not* recommend the routine use of either verapamil or diltiazem in patients with STEMI. Verapamil and diltiazem can be given for relief of ongoing ischemia or slowing of a rapid ventricular response in atrial fibrillation in patients for whom beta blockers are ineffective or contraindicated.[7] Their use should be avoided in patients with Killip class II or greater hemodynamic findings.

OTHER THERAPIES

MAGNESIUM. Patients with STEMI may have a total body deficit of magnesium because of a low dietary intake, advanced age, or prior diuretic use. They may also acquire a functional deficit of available magnesium due to trapping of free magnesium in adipocytes, as soaps are formed when free fatty acids are released by catecholamine-induced lipolysis with the onset of infarction.

The ISIS-4 investigators enrolled 58,050 patients, 29,011 to magnesium and 29,039 to control. The control group mortality was 7.2 percent in ISIS-4 compared with 7.6 percent in the magnesium group.[154] The MAGIC trial investigated the benefits of early administration of intravenous magnesium to high-risk patients with STEMI.[48] At 30 days, the mortality rate was 15.3 percent in the magnesium group and 15.2 percent in the placebo group (OR, 1.0; 95 percent CI, 0.9-1.2; $p = 0.96$).

RECOMMENDATIONS. Because of the risk of cardiac arrhythmias when electrolyte deficits are present in the early phase of infarction, all patients with STEMI should have a serum magnesium measurement on admission. We advocate repleting magnesium deficits to maintain a serum magnesium level of 2.0 mEq/liter or more. In the presence of hypokalemia (<4.0 mEq/liter) during the course of treatment of STEMI, the serum magnesium level should be rechecked and repleted if necessary because it is often difficult to correct a potassium deficit in the presence of a concurrent magnesium deficit. Episodes of torsades de pointes should be treated with 1 to 2 gm of magnesium delivered as a bolus over about 5 minutes. Between 1980 and 2002, 68,684 patients were studied in a series of 14 randomized trials. Based on the totality of available evidence and current coronary care practice, there is no indication for the routine administration of intravenous magnesium to patients with STEMI at any level of risk.

GLUCOSE-INSULIN-POTASSIUM. Administration of a solution of glucose-insulin-potassium (GIK) lowers the concentration of plasma free fatty acids and improves ventricular performance, as reflected in systolic arterial pressure, cardiac output, and stroke work at any level of left ventricular filling pressure; also, the frequency of ventricular premature beats decreases. Fath-Ordoubadi and colleagues reported in a meta-analysis of nine studies conducted between 1965 and 1987 enrolling a cumulative total of 1932 patients that the mortality rate was reduced from 21 percent in the placebo group to 16.1 percent in the GIK group (OR, 0.72; 95 percent CI, 0.57-0.90; $p = 0.004$).[170] Subsequently, the ECLA group performed a randomized trial of STEMI patients treated within 24 hours of the onset of symptoms.[171] The mortality rate was reduced from 15.2 percent in the control group to 5.2 percent in the GIK group for the subset of patients who received thrombolysis (OR, 0.34; 95 percent CI, 0.15-0.77; $p = 0.01$).

The DIGAMI (Diabetes Mellitus Insulin-Glucose Infusion in Acute Myocardial Infarction) Study reported a significant 30 percent relative decrease in mortality at 1 year in diabetic patients with myocardial infarction who received a strict regimen of an insulin-glucose infusion for 24 hours, followed by 3 months of subcutaneous injections of insulin four times daily as compared with standard therapy. Thus, infusions of GIK may provide necessary metabolic support for the ischemic myocardium; this could be particularly important in patients with large anterior infarcts and cardiogenic shock.

The most contemporary of the studies of GIK treatment in cases of STEMI was conducted by Dutch investigators who randomized 940 patients treated with PCI to either a GIK infusion (3 ml/kg/hr over 8 to 12 hours) or no infusion.[49] The 30-day mortality rate was 4.8 percent in patients receiving GIK compared with 5.8 percent in the control group (RR, 0.82; 95 percent CI, 0.46-1.46). Among the 91 percent of patients who presented without heart failure (Killip class I), the 30-day mortality rate was 1.2 percent in the GIK group versus 4.2 percent in the control group (RR, 0.28; 95 percent CI, 0.1-0.75). Among the 8.9 percent of patients with Killip class ≥ II, the 30-day mortality rate was 36 percent in the GIK group versus 26.5 percent in the control group (RR, 1.44; 95 percent CI, 0.65-3.22). As pointed out by Apstein, the rate of the GIK infusion in the Dutch study (3.8 ml/kg/hr) was twice as high as that used in the ECLA study (1.5 ml/kg/hr). For example, in the Dutch study, an 80 kg patient with heart failure received approximately 2 liters of fluid in the first 8 hours—a volume load that may have not been tolerated and was associated with an increased mortality risk.[172]

Thus, the benefits of routine administration of GIK to patients with STEMI, although intriguing, remain controversial. Additional studies are required to define the optimal dose and rate of infusion of GIK as well as the cohort of STEMI patients for whom GIK is efficacious and safe.

INTRAAORTIC BALLOON COUNTERPULSATION (see also Chap. 25). From a theoretical standpoint, intraaortic balloon counterpulsation might be expected to limit infarct size for several reasons. In experimental animals, intraaortic balloon counterpulsation decreases preload, increases coronary blood flow, and improves cardiac performance. No definitive information is available indicating that intraaortic balloon counterpulsation alters the prognosis in patients with relatively uncomplicated STEMI, especially in the context of other proven mortality-reducing therapies used in contemporary clinical practice. Intraaortic balloon pumping should be reserved for hemodynamically compromised patients and for those with refractory ischemia. Although noninvasive external forms of counterpulsation have been developed, these approaches have not been rigorously studied in patients with STEMI.

OTHER AGENTS. Several adjunctive pharmacotherapies have been investigated to prevent inflammatory damage in the infarct zone.[173] Trials with antibodies against the CD11/CD18 receptor on white blood cells failed to show a reduction in infarct size.[44,45]

Pexelizumab, a monoclonal antibody against the C5 component of complement had no effect on infarct size in STEMI patients treated either with fibrinolytics or PCI.[31,47] However, the rate of mortality was lower in the pexelizumab group compared with the placebo group in patients treated with PCI, prompting further clinical trials with this agent.

The AMISTAD II trial was a dose-ranging study of adenosine in patients with anterior STEMI.[174] Although high-dose adenosine (70 μg/kg/min infusion for 3 hours) was associated with a reduction in infarct size, neither high- nor low-dose adenosine reduced the primary composite clinical endpoint of death or the development of heart failure at 6 months compared with placebo.

Contrary to earlier beliefs that the heart is a terminally differentiated organ without the capacity to regenerate, evidence now exists that human cardiac myocytes divide after STEMI, and stem cells can promote regeneration of cardiac tissue.[175,176] These observations open up the possibility of myocardial replacement therapy after STEMI.[177]

Hemodynamic Disturbances

Hemodynamic Assessment

In patients with clinically uncomplicated STEMI, invasive hemodynamic monitoring is not necessary because the status of the circulation can be assessed by clinical evaluation. This ordinarily consists of monitoring of heart rate and rhythm, repeated measurement of systemic arterial pressure by cuff, obtaining chest radiographs to detect heart failure, repeated auscultation of the lung fields for pulmonary congestion, measurement of urine flow, examination of the skin and mucous membranes for evidence of the adequacy of perfusion, and arterial sampling for P_{O_2}, P_{CO_2}, and pH when hypoxemia or metabolic acidosis is suspected.

In contrast, in patients with STEMI whose ventricular contractile performance is not normal, as evidenced by clinical signs and symptoms of heart failure, it is important to assess the degree of hemodynamic compromise to initiate therapy with drugs such as vasodilators and diuretics. In the past, central venous or right atrial pressure was used to gauge the degree of left ventricular failure in patients with STEMI. However, this technique is fraught with error because central venous pressure actually reflects right rather than left ventricular function. Right ventricular function and therefore systemic venous pressure may be normal or nearly so in patients with significant left ventricular failure. Conversely, patients with right ventricular failure due to right ventricular infarction or pulmonary embolism may exhibit elevated right atrial and central venous pressures despite normal left ventricular function. Low values for right atrial and central venous pressures imply hypovolemia, whereas elevated right atrial pressures usually result from right ventricular failure secondary to left ventricular failure, pulmonary hypertension, or right ventricular infarction, or less commonly from tricuspid regurgitation or pericardial tamponade.

Major advances in the management of STEMI have resulted from the hemodynamic monitoring that has become widespread in CCUs (Table 47–7). This often consists of both an intraarterial catheter and a pulmonary artery catheter for measurement of pulmonary artery, pulmonary artery occlusive (equivalent to pulmonary wedge), and right atrial

TABLE 47–7 Indications for Hemodynamic Monitoring in Patients with STEMI

Management of complicated acute myocardial infarction Hypovolemia vs. cardiogenic shock Ventricular septal rupture vs. acute mitral regurgitation Severe left ventricular failure Right ventricular failure
Refractory ventricular tachycardia
Differentiating severe pulmonary disease from left ventricular failure
Assessment of cardiac tamponade
Assessment of therapy in *selected* individuals Afterload reduction in patients with severe left ventricular failure Inotropic agent therapy Beta blocker therapy Temporary pacing (ventricular vs. atrioventricular) Intraaortic balloon counterpulsation Mechanical ventilation

From Gore JM, Zwernet PL: Hemodynamic monitoring of acute myocardial infarction. *In* Francis GS, Alpert JS (eds): Modern Coronary Care, Boston, Little, Brown. 1990, p 138.

pressures, and cardiac output by thermodilution. In patients with hypotension, a Foley catheter provides accurate and continuous measurement of urine output.

NEED FOR INVASIVE MONITORING. The use of invasive hemodynamic monitoring is based on the following principal factors:

1. Difficulty in interpreting clinical and radiographic findings of pulmonary congestion because of phase lags, such as those occurring after diuretic therapy. Severe depression of cardiac index and/or elevation of left ventricular filling pressure may be unsuspected in as many as 15 percent of patients when estimates are based exclusively on clinical criteria.
2. Need for identifying noncardiac causes of arterial hypotension, particularly hypovolemia.
3. Possible contribution of reduced ventricular compliance to impaired hemodynamics, requiring judicious adjustment of intravascular volume to optimize left ventricular filling pressure.
4. Difficulty in assessing the severity and sometimes even determining the presence of lesions such as mitral regurgitation and ventricular septal defect when the cardiac output or the systemic pressures are depressed.
5. Establishing a baseline of hemodynamic measurements and guiding therapy in patients with clinically apparent pulmonary edema or cardiogenic shock.
6. Underestimation of systemic arterial pressure by the cuff method in patients with intense vasoconstriction.

The prognosis and the clinical status are related to both the cardiac output and the pulmonary artery wedge pressure. Patients with normal cardiac output after STEMI have an extremely low expected chance of mortality; prognosis worsens as cardiac output declines. Patients with intraventricular conduction defects, atrioventricular (AV) block, or both after anterior infarction have lower cardiac indices and higher pulmonary capillary wedge pressures than do patients without these conduction disturbances. On the other hand, patients with these conduction defects and inferior STEMI usually do not demonstrate such hemodynamic abnormalities.

PULMONARY ARTERY PRESSURE MONITORING. Patients most likely to benefit from pulmonary artery catheter monitoring include those whose STEMI is complicated by (1) hypotension that is not easily corrected by fluid administration; (2) hypotension in the presence of congestive heart failure; (3) hemodynamic compromise severe enough to require intravenous vasopressors or vasodilators or intraaortic balloon counterpulsation; (4) mechanical lesions (or suspected ones) such as cardiac tamponade, severe mitral regurgitation, and a ruptured ventricular septum; and (5) right ventricular infarction.[26] Other indications for hemodynamic monitoring include assessment of the effects of mechanical ventilation, differentiating pulmonary disease from left ventricular failure as the cause of hypoxemia, and management of septic shock (see Table 47–7).[7]

Before inserting a pulmonary artery catheter into a patient with STEMI, the physician must weigh that the potential benefit of the information to be obtained outweighs any potential risks. Major complications from pulmonary artery catheters are relatively rare (about 3 to 5 percent of cases), but severe problems can occur, including sepsis, pulmonary infarction, and pulmonary artery rupture. By minimizing the duration of catheterization and by strict adherence to aseptic techniques, risk can be diminished. Catheter-related bloodstream infections can also be reduced by using antiseptic-impregnated catheters.[178]

Accurate determination of hemodynamics by clinical assessment is difficult in critically ill patients. The use of a pulmonary artery catheter often leads to important changes in therapy that would not have occurred if the hemodynamic information had not been available. Of note, reports exist that rates of complications and mortality may be higher in patients who undergo pulmonary artery catheterization, although such patients are often at higher risk initially. These observations emphasize the importance of patient selection, meticulous technique, and correct interpretation of the data obtained.

Hemodynamic Abnormalities

In 1976, Swan, Forrester, and their associates measured the cardiac output and wedge pressure simultaneously in a large series of patients with acute myocardial infarction and identified four major hemodynamic subsets of patients (Table 47–8): (1) patients with normal perfusion and without pulmonary congestion (normal cardiac output and normal wedge pressure); (2) patients with normal perfusion and pulmonary congestion (normal cardiac output and elevated wedge pressure); (3) patients with decreased perfusion but without pulmonary congestion (reduced cardiac output and normal wedge pressure); and (4) patients with decreased perfusion and pulmonary congestion (reduced cardiac output and elevated wedge pressure). This classification, which overlaps with a crude clinical classification proposed earlier by Killip and Kimball (Table 47–9), has proved to be quite useful, but it should be noted that patients frequently pass from one category to another with therapy and sometimes apparently even spontaneously.

HEMODYNAMIC SUBSETS. These are usually reflected in the patient's clinical status. Hypoperfusion usually becomes evident clinically when the cardiac index falls below approximately 2.2 liters/min/m^2, whereas pulmonary congestion is noted when the wedge pressure exceeds approximately 20 mm Hg. However, approximately 25 percent of patients with cardiac indices less than 2.2 liters/min/m^2 and 15 percent of patients with elevated pulmonary capillary wedge pressures are not recognized clinically. Discrepancies in hemodynamic and clinical classification of patients with STEMI arise for a variety of reasons.

Patients may exhibit "phase lags" as clinical pulmonary congestion develops or resolves, symptoms secondary to chronic obstructive pulmonary disease may be confused with those resulting from pulmonary congestion, or longstanding left ventricular dysfunction may mask signs of hypoperfusion secondary to compensatory vasoconstriction.

The hemodynamic findings shown in Tables 47–8 and 47–9 allow for rational approaches to therapy. The goals of hemodynamic therapy are to maintain ventricular performance, support blood pressure, and protect jeopardized myocardium. Because these goals occasionally may be at cross purposes, recognition of the hemodynamic profile, as assessed clinically or as available from hemodynamic monitoring, is required before optimal therapeutic interventions can be designed along the lines discussed later.

HYPOTENSION IN THE PREHOSPITAL PHASE. During the prehospital phase of STEMI, invasive hemodynamic monitoring is not feasible, and during this period, therapy should be guided by frequent clinical assessment and measurement of arterial pressure by cuff, with the recognition that intense vasoconstriction can provide a falsely low pressure measured by this method. Hypotension associated with bradycardia often reflects excessive vagotonia. Relative or absolute hypovolemia is often present when hypotension occurs with a normal or rapid heart rate, particularly among patients receiving diuretics just prior to the occurrence of infarction. Marked diaphoresis, reduction of fluid intake, or vomiting during the period preceding and accompanying the onset of STEMI may all contribute to the development of hypovolemia. Even if the effective vascular volume is normal, relative hypovolemia may be present because ventricular compliance is reduced in cases of STEMI and a left ventricular filling pressure as high as 20 mm Hg may be needed to provide an optimal preload.

MANAGEMENT. In the absence of rales involving more than one-third of the lung fields, the patient should be put in the reverse Trendelenburg position, and in patients with sinus bradycardia and hypotension, atropine should be administered (0.3-0.6 mg IV repeated at 3- to 10-minute intervals up to 2.0 mg). If these measures do not correct the hypotension, normal saline should be administered intravenously, beginning with a bolus of 100 ml followed by 50 ml increments every 5 minutes. The patient should be observed and the infusion stopped when the systolic pressure returns to approximately 100 mm Hg, if the patient becomes dyspneic, or if pulmonary rales develop or increase. Because of the poor correlation between left ventricular filling pressure and mean right atrial pressure, assessment of systemic (even central) venous pressure is of limited value as a guide to fluid therapy.

Administration of cardiotonic agents is indicated during the prehospital phase if systemic hypotension persists despite correction of hypovolemia and excessive vagotonia. In the absence of invasive hemodynamic monitoring, assessment of peripheral vascular resistance must be based on clinical observations. If cutaneous vasoconstriction is present, therapy with dobutamine, which stimulates cardiac contractility without unduly accelerating heart rate and which does not increase the impedance to ventricular outflow, may be helpful. In hypotensive patients with STEMI with clinical evidence of vasodilation, an uncommon circumstance, phenylephrine hydrochloride is preferable, although this agent, which increases coronary as well as peripheral vascular tone, should be used with caution.

HYPOVOLEMIC HYPOTENSION. Recognition of hypovolemia is of particular importance in hypotensive patients with STEMI because of the hazard it poses and because of the improvement in circulatory dynamics that can be achieved so readily and safely by augmentation of vascular volume. Because hypovolemia is often occult, it is frequently over-

TABLE 47–8 Hemodynamic Classifications of Patients with Acute Myocardial Infarction

A. Based on Clinical Examination		B. Based on Invasive Monitoring	
Class	*Definition*	*Subset*	*Definition*
A	Rales and S_3 absent	I	Normal hemodynamics PCWP < 18, CI > 2.2
B	Rales over >50% of lung	II	Pulmonary congestion PCWP > 18, CI > 2.2
C	Rales over <50% of lung fields (pulmonary edema)	III	Peripheral hypoperfusion PCWP < 18, CI < 2.2
D	Shock	IV	Pulmonary congestion and peripheral hypoperfusion PCWP > 18, CI < 2.2

A, Modified from Killip T, Kimball J: Treatment of myocardial infarction in a coronary care unit. A two year experience with 250 patients. Am J Cardiol *20*:457, 1967; and B, From Forrester J, Diamond G, Chatterjee K, et al: Medical therapy of acute myocardial infarction by the application of hemodynamic subsets. N Engl J Med 295:1356, 1976.

PCWP = pulmonary capillary wedge pressure; CI = cardiac index.

TABLE 47–9 Hemodynamic Patterns for Common Clinical Conditions

	Chamber Pressure (mm Hg)				
Cardiac Condition	*RA*	*RV*	*PA*	*PCW*	*CI*
Normal	0-6	25/0-6	25/0-12	6-12	≥2.5
AMI without LVF	0-6	25/0-6	30/12-18	≤18	≥2.5
AMI with LVF	0-6	30-40/0-6	30-40/18-25	>18	>2.0
Biventricular failure	>6	50-60/>6	50-60/25	18-25	>2.0
RVMI	12-20	30/12-20	30/12	≤12	<2.0
Cardiac tamponade	12-16	25/12-16	25/12-16	12-16	<2.0
Pulmonary embolism	12-20	50-60/12-20	50-60/12	<12	<2.0

AMI = acute myocardial infarction; CI = cardiac index; LVF = left ventricular failure; PA = pulmonary artery; PCW = pulmonary capillary wedge; RA = right atrium; RV = right ventricle; RVMI = right ventricular myocardial infarction.

From Gore JM, Zwerner PL: Hemodynamic monitoring of acute myocardial infarction. *In* Francis GS, Alpert JS (eds): Modern Coronary Care, 1990, pp 139-164.

looked in the absence of invasive hemodynamic monitoring. Hypovolemia may be absolute, with low left ventricular filling pressure (8 mm Hg), or relative, with normal (8 to 12 mm Hg) or even modestly increased (13 to 18 mm Hg) left ventricular filling pressures. Because of the reduction of left ventricular compliance that occurs with acute ischemia and infarction, left ventricular filling pressures between 13 and 18 mm Hg, although above the upper limits of normal, may actually be suboptimal.

Exclusion of hypovolemia as the cause of hypotension requires the documentation of a reduced cardiac output despite left ventricular filling pressure exceeding 18 mm Hg. If, in a hypotensive patient, the pulmonary capillary wedge pressure (ordinarily measured as the pulmonary artery occlusive pressure) is below this level, fluid challenge should be carried out as described earlier. If hypovolemia is documented or suspected, the fluid replaced should resemble the fluid lost. Thus, when a low hematocrit complicates STEMI, infusion of packed red blood cells or whole blood is the treatment of choice.[179] On the other hand, crystalloid or colloid solutions should be administered when the hematocrit is normal or elevated.

Hypotension caused by right ventricular infarction may be confused with that caused by hypovolemia because both are associated with a low, normal, or minimally elevated left ventricular filling pressure. The findings and management of right ventricular infarction are discussed elsewhere in this chapter.

THE HYPERDYNAMIC STATE. When infarction is not complicated by hemodynamic impairment, no therapy other than general supportive measures and treatment of arrhythmias is necessary. However, if the hemodynamic profile is of the hyperdynamic state, that is, elevation of sinus rate, arterial pressure, and cardiac index, occurring singly or together in the presence of a normal or low left ventricular filling pressure, and if other causes of tachycardia such as fever, infection, and pericarditis can be excluded, treatment with beta-adrenoceptor blockers is indicated. Presumably, the increased heart rate and blood pressure are the result of inappropriate activation of the sympathetic nervous system, possibly secondary to augmented release of catecholamines, pain and anxiety, or some combination of these.

Left Ventricular Failure

Left ventricular dysfunction is the single most important predictor of mortality following STEMI (Fig. 47–25).[79,85] In patients with STEMI, heart failure is characterized either by systolic dysfunction alone or by both systolic and diastolic dysfunction. Left ventricular diastolic dysfunction leads to pulmonary venous hypertension and pulmonary congestion, whereas systolic dysfunction is principally responsible for a depression of cardiac output and of the ejection fraction. Clinical manifestations of left ventricular failure become more common as the extent of the injury to the left ventricle increases.[180] In addition to infarct size, other important predictors of the development of symptomatic left ventricular dysfunction include advanced age and diabetes.[180] Mortality increases in association with the severity of the hemodynamic deficit.

THERAPEUTIC IMPLICATIONS. Classification of patients with STEMI by hemodynamic subsets has therapeutic relevance. As already noted, patients with normal wedge pressures and hypoperfusion often benefit from infusion of fluids, because the peak value of stroke volume is usually not attained until left ventricular filling pressure reaches 18 to 24 mm Hg. However, a low level of left ventricular filling pressure does not imply that left ventricular damage is necessarily slight. Such patients may be relatively hypovolemic

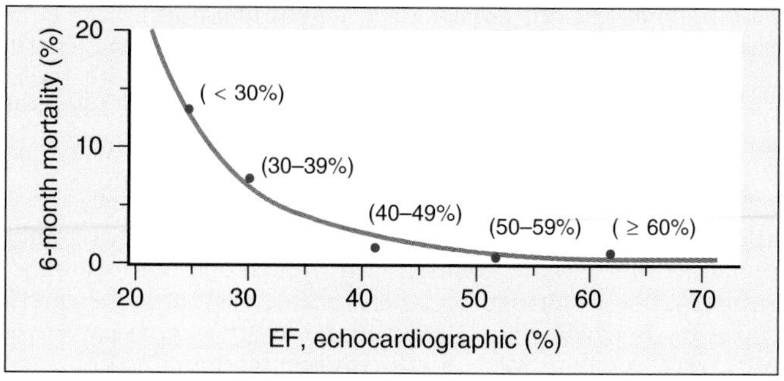

FIGURE 47–25 Impact of left ventricular function on survival following myocardial infarction. The curvilinear relationship between left ventricular ejection fraction (LVEF) for patients treated in the fibrinolytic era is shown. Among patients with an LVEF below 40 percent, the rate of mortality is markedly increased at 6 months. Thus, interventions such as thrombolysis, aspirin, and angiotensin-converting enzyme inhibitors should be of considerable benefit in patients with acute myocardial infarction to minimize the amount of left ventricular damage and interrupt the neurohumoral activation seen with congestive heart failure. (Adapted from Volpi A, De VC, Franzosi MG, et al: Determinants of 6-month mortality in survivors of myocardial infarction after thrombolysis. Results of the GISSI-2 data base. The Ad Hoc Working Group of the Gruppo Italiano per lo Studio della Sopravvivenza nell'Infarto Miocardico (GISSI)-2 Data Base. Circulation 88:416, 1993.)

and/or may have suffered a right ventricular infarct with or without severe left ventricular damage.

The relationship between ventricular filling pressure and cardiac index when preload is increased by an infusion of saline or dextran can provide valuable hemodynamic information, in addition to that obtained from baseline measurements. For example, the ventricular function curve rises steeply (marked increase in cardiac index, small increase in filling pressure) in patients with normal left ventricular function and hypovolemia, whereas the curve rises gradually or remains flat in those patients with a combination of hypovolemia and depressed cardiac function.

Invasive hemodynamic monitoring is essential to guide therapy of patients with severe left ventricular failure (pulmonary capillary wedge pressure > 18 mm Hg *and* cardiac index < 2.5 liters/min/m^2).

AVOIDANCE OF HYPOXEMIA. Patients whose STEMI is complicated by congestive heart failure characteristically develop hypoxemia due to a combination of pulmonary vascular engorgement (and in some cases pulmonary interstitial edema), diminished vital capacity, and respiratory depression from narcotic analgesics. Hypoxemia can impair the function of ischemic tissue at the margin of the infarct and thereby contribute to establishing or perpetuating the vicious circle (see Fig. 46–10). The ventilation-perfusion mismatch that results in hypoxemia requires careful attention to ventilatory support. Increasing fractions of inspired oxygen (FIO_2) via face mask should be used initially, but if the oxygen saturation of the patient's blood cannot be maintained above 85 to 90 percent on 100 percent FIO_2, strong consideration should be given to endotracheal intubation with positive-pressure ventilation. The improvement of arterial oxygenation and hence myocardial oxygen supply may help to restore ventricular performance. Positive end-expiratory pressure may diminish systemic venous return and reduce effective left ventricular filling pressure. This may require reduction in the amount of positive end-expiratory pressure, normal saline infusions to maintain left ventricular filling pressure, adjustment of the rate of infusion of vasodilators such as nitroglycerin, or some combination of these. Because myocardial ischemia frequently occurs during the return to unsupported spontaneous breathing, the weaning process should be accompanied by observation for signs of ischemia and is potentially facilitated by a period of intermittent mandatory ventilation or pressure support ventilation before extubation.

Although positive inotropic agents can be useful, they do not represent the initial therapy of choice in patients with STEMI. Instead, heart failure is managed most effectively first by reduction of ventricular preload, and then, if possible, by lowering of afterload. Arrhythmias can contribute to hemodynamic compromise and should be treated promptly in patients with left ventricular failure.

DIURETICS (see Chaps. 23 and 38). Mild heart failure in patients with STEMI frequently responds well to diuretics such as furosemide, administered intravenously in doses of 10 to 40 mg, repeated at 3- to 4-hour intervals if necessary. The resultant reduction of pulmonary capillary pressure reduces dyspnea, and the lowering of left ventricular wall tension that accompanies the reduction of left ventricular diastolic volume diminishes myocardial oxygen requirements and may lead to improvement of contractility and augmentation of the ejection fraction, stroke volume, and cardiac output. The reduction of elevated left ventricular filling pressure may also enhance myocardial oxygen delivery by diminishing the impedance to coronary perfusion attributable to elevated ventricular wall tension. It may also improve arterial oxygenation by reducing pulmonary vascular congestion.

The intravenous administration of furosemide reduces pulmonary vascular congestion and pulmonary venous pressure within 15 minutes, before renal excretion of sodium and water has occurred; presumably this action results from a direct dilating effect of this drug on the systemic arterial bed. It is important not to reduce left ventricular filling pressure much below 18 mm Hg, the lower range associated with optimal left ventricular performance in STEMI, because this may reduce cardiac output further and cause arterial hypotension. Excessive diuresis may also result in hypokalemia, with its attendant risk of digitalis intoxication.

AFTERLOAD REDUCTION. Myocardial oxygen requirements depend on left ventricular wall stress, which in turn is proportional to the product of peak developed left ventricular pressure, volume, and wall thickness. Vasodilator therapy is recommended in patients with STEMI complicated by (1) heart failure unresponsive to treatment with diuretics, (2) hypertension, (3) mitral regurgitation, or (4) ventricular septal defect. In these patients, treatment with vasodilator agents increases stroke volume and may reduce myocardial oxygen requirements and thereby lessen ischemia. Hemodynamic monitoring of systemic arterial and, in many cases, pulmonary capillary wedge (or at least pulmonary artery) pressure and cardiac output in patients treated with these agents is important. Improvement of cardiac performance and energetics requires three simultaneous effects: (1) reduction of left ventricular afterload, (2) avoidance of excessive systemic arterial hypotension to maintain effective coronary perfusion pressure, and (3) avoidance of excessive reduction of ventricular filling pressure with consequent diminution of cardiac output. In general, pulmonary capillary wedge pressure should be maintained at approximately 20 mm Hg and arterial pressure above 90/60 mm Hg in patients who were normotensive before developing the STEMI.

Vasodilator therapy is particularly useful when STEMI is complicated by mitral regurgitation or rupture of the ventricular septum. In such patients, vasodilators alone or in combination with intraaortic balloon counterpulsation can sometimes serve as a "holding maneuver" and provide hemodynamic stabilization to permit definitive catheterization and angiographic studies to be carried out and to prepare the patient for early surgical intervention. Because of the precarious state of patients with complicated infarction and the need for meticulous adjustment of dosage, therapy is best initiated with agents that can be administered intravenously and that have a short duration of action, such as nitroprusside, nitroglycerin, or isosorbide dinitrate. After initial stabilization, the medication of choice is generally an ACE inhibitor, but long-acting nitrates given by mouth, sublingually, or by ointment can also be useful.

Nitroglycerin. This drug has been shown in animal experiments to be less likely than nitroprusside to produce a "coronary steal"—that is, to divert blood flow from the ischemic to the nonischemic zone. Therefore, apart from consideration of its routine use in STEMI patients discussed earlier, it may be a particularly useful vasodilator in patients with STEMI complicated by left ventricular failure. Ten to 15 mg/min is infused and the dose is increased by 10 mg/min every 5 minutes until (1) the desired effect (improvement of hemodynamics or relief of ischemic chest pain) is achieved or (2) a decline in systolic arterial pressure to 90 mm Hg, or by more than 15 mm Hg, has occurred. Although both nitroglycerin and nitroprusside lower systemic arterial pressure, systemic vascular resistance, and the heart rate-systolic blood pressure product, the reduction of left ventricular filling pressure is more prominent with nitroglycerin because of its relatively greater effect than nitroprusside on venous capacitance vessels. Nevertheless, in patients with severe left ventricular failure, cardiac output often increases despite the reduction in left ventricular filling pressure produced by nitroglycerin.

Oral Vasodilators. The use of oral vasodilators in the treatment of chronic congestive heart failure is discussed in Chapter 23. In patients with STEMI and persistent heart failure, long-term inhibition of the renin-angiotensin-aldosterone system should be carried out. This reduced ventricular load decreases the remodeling of the left ventricle that occurs commonly in the period after STEMI and thereby reduces the development of heart failure and risk of death.[181]

DIGITALIS (see Chap. 23). Although digitalis increases the contractility and the oxygen consumption of normal hearts, when heart failure is present the diminution of heart size and wall tension frequently results in a net reduction of myocardial oxygen requirements. In animal experiments, it fails to improve ventricular performance immediately following experimental coronary occlusion, but salutary effects are elicited when it is administered several days later. The absence of early beneficial effects may be due to the inability of ischemic tissue to respond to digitalis or the already maximal stimulation of contractility of the normal heart by circulating and neuronally released catecholamines.

Although the issue is still controversial, arrhythmias can be increased by digitalis glycosides when they are given to patients in the first few hours after the onset of STEMI, particularly in the absence of hypokalemia. Also, undesirable peripheral systemic and coronary vasoconstriction can result from the rapid intravenous administration of rapidly acting glycosides such as ouabain.

Administration of digitalis to patients with STEMI in the hospital phase should generally be reserved for the management of supraventricular tachyarrhythmias such as atrial flutter and fibrillation and of heart failure that persists despite treatment with diuretics, vasodilators, and beta-adrenoceptor agonists. There is no indication for its use as an inotropic agent in patients without clinical evidence of left ventricular dysfunction, and it is too weak an inotropic agent to be relied upon as the principal cardiac stimulant in patients with overt pulmonary edema or cardiogenic shock. It may, however, be useful as a supplement to agents that inhibit the renin-angiotensin-aldosterone system and in the maintenance phase of treatment for persistent or recurrent left ventricular failure.[182]

BETA-ADRENOCEPTOR AGONISTS. When left ventricular failure is severe, as manifested by marked reduction of cardiac index (<2 liters/min/m^2), and pulmonary capillary wedge pressure is at optimal (18-24 mm Hg) or excessive (>24 mm Hg) levels despite therapy with diuretics, beta-adrenoceptor agonists are indicated. Although isoproterenol is a potent cardiac stimulant and improves ventricular performance, it should be avoided in STEMI patients. It also causes tachycardia and augments myocardial oxygen consumption and lactate production; in addition, it reduces coronary perfusion pressure by causing systemic vasodilation and in animal experiments it increases the extent of experimentally induced infarction. Norepinephrine also increases myocardial oxygen consumption because of its peripheral vasoconstrictor as well as positive inotropic actions.

Dopamine and dobutamine (see Chap. 23) can be particularly useful in patients with STEMI and reduced cardiac output, increased left ventricular filling pressure, pulmonary vascular congestion, and hypotension. Fortunately, the potentially deleterious alpha-adrenergic vasoconstrictor effects exerted by dopamine occur only at higher doses than those required to increase contractility. The vasodilating actions of dopamine on renal and splanchnic vessels and its positive inotropic effects generally improve hemodynamics and renal function. In patients with STEMI and severe left ventricular failure, this drug should be administered at a dose of 3 μg/kg/min while pulmonary capillary wedge and systemic arterial pressures as well as cardiac output are monitored. The dose can be increased stepwise to 20 μg/kg/min to reduce pulmonary capillary wedge pressure to approximately 20 mm Hg and elevate cardiac index to exceed 2 liters/min/m^2. It must be recognized, however, that doses exceeding 5 μg/kg/min activate peripheral alpha receptors and cause vasoconstriction.

Dobutamine has a positive inotropic action comparable to that of dopamine but a slightly less positive chronotropic effect and less vasoconstrictor activity. In patients with STEMI, dobutamine improves left ventricular performance without augmenting enzymatically estimated infarct size. It can be administered in a starting dose of 2.5 μg/kg/min and increased stepwise to a maximum of 30 μg/kg/min. Both dopamine and dobutamine must be given carefully and with constant monitoring of the electrocardiogram, systemic arterial pressure, and pulmonary artery or pulmonary artery occlusive pressure and, if possible, with frequent measurements of cardiac output. The dose must be reduced if the heart rate exceeds 100 to 110 beats/min, if supraventricular or ventricular tachyarrhythmias are precipitated, or if ST segment changes increase.

OTHER POSITIVE INOTROPIC AGENTS. Milrinone is a noncatecholamine, nonglycoside, phosphodiesterase inhibitor with inotropic and vasodilating actions. It is useful in selected patients whose heart failure persists despite treatment with diuretics, who are not hypotensive, and who are likely to benefit from both an enhancement in contractility and afterload reduction. Milrinone should be given as a loading dose of 0.5 μg/kg/min over 10 minutes, followed by a maintenance infusion of 0.375 to 0.75 μg/kg/min.

Cardiogenic Shock

Cardiogenic shock is the most severe clinical expression of left ventricular failure and is associated with extensive damage to the left ventricular myocardium in more than 80 percent of STEMI patients in whom it occurs; the remainder have a mechanical defect such as ventricular septal or papillary muscle rupture or predominant right ventricular infarction.[27] In the past, cardiogenic shock has been reported to occur in up to 20 percent of patients with STEMI, but estimates from recent large randomized trials of fibrinolytic therapy and observational databases report an incidence rate in the range of 7 percent.[27] About 10 percent of patients with cardiogenic shock present with this condition at the time of admission, whereas 90 percent develop it during hospitalization. This low-output state is characterized by elevated ventricular filling pressures, low cardiac output, systemic hypotension, and evidence of vital organ hypoperfusion (e.g., clouded sensorium, cool extremities, oliguria, acidosis). Patients with cardiogenic shock due to STEMI are more likely to be older, to have a history of a prior myocardial infarction or congestive heart failure, and to have sustained an anterior infarction at the time of development of shock. Of note, although the incidence of cardiogenic shock in patients with STEMI has been relatively stable since the mid-1970s, the short-term mortality rate has decreased from 70 to 80 percent in the 1970s to 50 to 60 percent in the 1990s.[183] Cardiogenic shock is the cause of death in about 60 percent of patients dying after fibrinolysis for STEMI.[27]

PATHOLOGICAL FINDINGS. At autopsy, more than two-thirds of patients with cardiogenic shock demonstrate stenosis of 75 percent or more of the luminal diameter of all three major coronary vessels, usually including the left anterior descending coronary artery.[184] Almost all patients with cardiogenic shock are found to have thrombotic occlusion of the artery supplying the major region of recent infarction, with loss of about 40 percent of the left ventricular mass.[27] In addition to culprit vessel location, correlates of 1-year survival in patients with shock complicating STEMI include age, the initial TIMI flow grade, and extent of left ventricular dysfunction.[185] Other causes of cardiogenic shock in patients with STEMI include mechanical defects such as rupture of the ventricular septum, a papillary muscle, or free wall with tamponade; right ventricular infarction; or marked reduction of preload due to conditions such as hypovolemia.[27]

Patients who die as a consequence of cardiogenic shock often have "piecemeal" necrosis, that is, progressive myocardial necrosis from marginal extension of their infarct into an ischemic zone bordering on the infarction. This is generally associated with persistent elevation of creatine kinase-MB (CK-MB). Early deterioration in left ventricular function secondary to apparent extension of infarction may, in some cases, result from expansion of the necrotic zone of myocardium without actual extension of the necrotic process. Shear forces that develop during ventricular systole can disrupt necrotic myocardial muscle bundles, with resultant expansion and thinning of the akinetic zone of myocardium, which in turn results in deterioration of overall left ventricular function.

At autopsy, patients with cardiogenic shock consistently demonstrate marginal extension of recent areas of infarction. Additionally, focal areas of necrosis are frequently found in regions of the left and right ventricles that are not adjacent to the major area of recent infarction. Such extensions and focal lesions are probably in part the result of the shock state itself, because they can also be found in the hearts of patients dying of noncardiogenic shock. Infarction of the ischemic periinfarction zone can be precipitated by a number of factors that adversely affect the supply of oxygen or the metabolic demand in this zone of myocardium. These include a reduction of coronary perfusion pressure causing impaired myocardial perfusion in the presence of atherosclerotic obstructions of the nonculprit artery. An augmentation of myocardial oxygen demand resulting from the local release of catecholamines from ischemic adrenergic nerve endings in the heart as well as from circulating endogenous or infused catecholamines may also play a role. Patients with shock due to a mechanical defect often have smaller infarcts than do those with cardiogenic shock secondary to ventricular failure without a mechanical lesion. The prognosis is better in such patients because the smaller infarct allows their left ventricle to support the circulation if the mechanical defect has been corrected surgically.

PATHOPHYSIOLOGY. The shock state in patients with STEMI appears to be the result of a vicious circle, demonstrated in Figure 46–10.

DIAGNOSIS. Cardiogenic shock is characterized by marked and persistent (>30 min) hypotension with systolic arterial pressure less than 80 mm Hg and a marked reduction of cardiac index (generally <1.8 liters/mm/m^2) in the face of elevated left ventricular filling pressure (pulmonary capillary wedge pressure > 18 mm Hg). Spurious estimates of left ventricular filling pressure based on measurements of the pulmonary artery wedge pressure can occur in the presence of marked mitral regurgitation, in which the tall *v* wave in the left atrial (and pulmonary artery wedge) pressure tracing elevates the mean pressure above left ventricular end-diastolic pressure. Accordingly, mitral regurgitation and other mechanical lesions such as ventricular septal defect, ventricular aneurysm, and pseudoaneurysm must be excluded before the diagnosis of cardiogenic shock due to impairment of left ventricular function can be established. Mechanical complications should be suspected in any patient with acute myocardial infarction in whom circulatory collapse occurs.[27] Immediate hemodynamic, angiographic, and echocardiographic evaluations are necessary in patients with cardiogenic shock. It is important to exclude mechanical complications, because primary therapy of such lesions usually requires immediate operative treatment with intervening support of the circulation by intraaortic balloon counterpulsation.

Medical Management

When the aforementioned mechanical complications are not present, cardiogenic shock is due to impairment of left ventricular function. Although dopamine or dobutamine usually improves the hemodynamics in these patients, unfortunately neither appears to improve hospital survival significantly. Similarly, vasodilators have been used in an effort to elevate cardiac output and to reduce left ventricular filling pressure. However, by lowering the already markedly reduced coronary perfusion pressure, myocardial perfusion can be compromised further, accelerating the vicious circle illustrated in Figure 46–10. Vasodilators may nonetheless be used in conjunction with intraaortic balloon counterpulsation and inotropic agents in an effort to increase cardiac output while sustaining or elevating coronary perfusion pressure.

The systemic vascular resistance is usually elevated in patients with cardiogenic shock, but occasionally resistance is normal and in a few cases vasodilation actually predominates.[186] When systemic vascular resistance is not elevated (i.e., <1800 dynes/sec/cm^5) in patients with cardiogenic shock, norepinephrine, which has both alpha- and beta-adrenoceptor agonist properties (in doses ranging from 2 to 10 μg/min), can be employed to increase diastolic arterial pressure, maintain coronary perfusion, and improve contractility. Norepinephrine should be used only when other means, including balloon counterpulsation, fail to maintain arterial diastolic pressure above 50 to 60 mm Hg in a previously normotensive patient. The use of alpha-adrenoceptor agents such as phenylephrine and methoxamine is contraindicated in patients with cardiogenic shock (unless systemic vascular resistance is inordinately low). Inspired by the observation that many patients with shock have a low systemic vascular resistance, Cotter and associates evaluated the benefit of the nitric oxide synthase inhibitor L-NMMA in patients in refractory shock.[187] The favorable impact of L-NMMA on the hemodynamics and clinical outcomes in this pilot study serves as the foundation for further investigation of nitric oxide synthase inhibition of cardiogenic shock.[186]

Intraaortic Balloon Counterpulsation (see Chap. 25)

Intraaortic balloon counterpulsation is used in the treatment of STEMI in three groups of patients: (1) those whose conditions are hemodynamically unstable and in whom support of the circulation is required for the performance of cardiac catheterization and angiography carried out to assess lesions that are potentially correctable surgically or by angioplasty; (2) those with cardiogenic shock that is unresponsive to medical management; and (3) rarely, those with persistent ischemic pain that is unresponsive to treatment with inhalation of 100 percent oxygen, beta-adrenoceptor blockade, and nitrates. Unfortunately, among patients with cardiogenic shock, improvement is often only temporary, and "balloon dependence" commonly develops. Patients with cardiogenic shock treated with this modality can be successfully weaned from the supporting system only occasionally. Counterpulsation alone does not improve overall survival in patients either with or without a surgically remediable mechanical lesion.

COMPLICATIONS. Complications occur infrequently but include damage to or perforation of the aortic wall, ischemia distal to the site of insertion of the balloon in the femoral artery, thrombocytopenia, hemolysis, renal emboli, and mechanical failure such as rupture of the balloon. Patients at highest risk include those with peripheral vascular disease, the elderly, and women, particularly if they are small. These factors should be taken into consideration before an attempt is made to institute intraaortic balloon counterpulsation. Because of the potential for vascular bleeding complications, there has been a reluctance to use intraaortic pumps in patients who have undergone fibrinolytic therapy. However, despite the increased bleeding risk, because of the poor outcome among patients with shock following thrombolysis (usually ineffective thrombolysis), this modality should be considered in selected patients who are candidates for an aggressive approach to revascularization.

Revascularization

Of the five therapies frequently used to treat patients with cardiogenic shock (vasopressors, intraaortic balloon counterpulsation, fibrinolysis, PCI, and coronary artery bypass surgery), the first two are useful temporizing maneuvers. Surgical treatment in patients with cardiogenic shock (aside from correcting mechanical abnormalities) may involve bypassing occluded as well as severely obstructed nonoccluded vessels. Occlusion of one major vessel can cause left ventricular dysfunction and hypotension, which can then lead to hypoperfusion and ischemia of myocardium subserved by the other diseased vessels. Left ventricular function can be improved by relief of this ischemia with revascularization.

The SHOCK study evaluated early revascularization for the treatment of patients with acute myocardial infarction complicated by cardiogenic shock. Patients with shock due to left ventricular failure complicating STEMI were randomized to emergency revascularization (n = 152), accomplished by either coronary artery bypass grafting or angioplasty, or initial medical stabilization (n = 150). In 86 percent of patients in both groups, intraaortic balloon counterpulsation was performed. The primary endpoint was all-cause mortality at 30 days; a secondary endpoint was mortality at 6 months. At 30 days, the overall mortality rate was 46.7 percent in the revascularization group, not significantly different from the 56.0 percent mortality rate observed in the medical therapy group ($p = 0.11$). Subgroups of patients in the SHOCK trial that showed particular benefit from the early revascularization strategy (i.e., reduced 6-month mortality) were those who were younger than 75 years of age, had a prior myocardial infarction, and were randomized less than 6 hours from onset of infarction.[188] The 1-year survival rate was significantly higher in the revascularization group than in the medical therapy group, with rates of 46.7 percent versus 33.6 percent, respectively ($p = 0.027$).

RECOMMENDATIONS. We recommend assessment of patients on an individualized basis to determine their desire for aggressive care and overall candidacy for further treatment (e.g., age, mental status, comorbidities). Patients who are potential candidates for revascularization should then rapidly receive intraaortic balloon counterpulsation and be referred for coronary arteriography. Those with suitable anatomy should be revascularized as completely as possible with PCI and/or coronary artery bypass surgery.[189] Encouraging initial experience has been reported with a percutaneous left ventricular assist device as a bridge to a revascularization procedure.[190] In appropriately selected patients, emergency cardiac transplantation has also been used successfully to manage cardiogenic shock.

Right Ventricular Infarction

A characteristic hemodynamic pattern (Table 47–10) has been observed in patients with right ventricular infarction, which frequently accompanies inferior left ventricular infarction or rarely occurs in isolated form. Right-heart filling pressures (central venous, right atrial, and right ventricular end-diastolic pressures) are elevated, whereas left ventricular filling pressure is normal or only slightly raised; right ventricular systolic and pulse pressures are decreased, and cardiac output is often markedly depressed. Rarely, this disproportionate elevation of right-sided filling pressure causes right-to-left shunting through a patent foramen ovale. This possibility should be considered in patients with right ventricular infarction who have unexplained systemic hypoxemia. The finding of an elevation in atrial natriuretic factor level in patients with this condition has led to the suggestion that abnormally high levels of this peptide might be in part responsible for the hypotension seen in patients with right ventricular infarction. Of note, the same protective effect of ischemic preconditioning that has been described in cases of infarction of the left ventricle has also been reported in patients with infarction of the right ventricle.[191]

TABLE 47–10 Features of Right Ventricular Myocardial Infarction
Clinical Findings
Normal or depressed right ventricular function
Shock
Tricuspid regurgitation
Ruptured ventricular septum
Hemodynamic Measurements
Abnormally elevated right atrial pressure
Normal right ventricular and pulmonary artery systolic pressures
Increased ratio of right ventricular to left ventricular filling presure
Depressed right ventricular function curve
Scintigraphy
Uptake in right ventricular free wall
Increased right ventricular dimensions and decreased wall motion
Echocardiography
Increased right ventricular dimension
Absence of pericardial effusion
Cardiac Biomarkers
Increased magnitude of biomarker values relative to degree of left ventricular dysfunction
Cardiac Catheterization
Involvement of right (usually) or left (rarely) circumflex coronary arteries
Right ventricular akinesis
Differential Diagnosis
Hypotension with acute myocardial infarction
Pericardial tamponade
Constrictive pericarditis
Pulmonary embolus

Modified from Rackley CE, Russell RO Jr, Mantle JA, et al: Right ventricular infarction and function. Am Heart J 101:215, 1981.

Diagnosis

Many patients with the combination of normal left ventricular filling pressure and depressed cardiac index have right ventricular infarcts (with accompanying inferior left ventricular infarcts). The hemodynamic picture may superficially resemble that seen in patients with pericardial disease (see Chap. 64). It includes elevated right ventricular filling pressure; steep, right atrial *y* descent; and an early diastolic drop and plateau (resembling the square root sign) in the right ventricular pressure tracing. Moreover, the Kussmaul sign (an increase in jugular venous pressure with inspiration) and pulsus paradoxus (a fall in systolic pressure of greater than 10 mm Hg with inspiration) may be present in patients with right ventricular infarction.[26] In fact, Kussmaul sign in the setting of inferior STEMI is highly predictive of right ventricular involvement.

The electrocardiogram can provide the first clue that right ventricular involvement is present in the patient with inferior STEMI. Most patients with right ventricular infarction have ST segment elevation in lead V_4R (right precordial lead in V_4 position).[192] Transient elevation of the ST segment in any of the right precordial leads can occur with right ventricular myocardial infarction, and the presence of ST segment elevation of 0.1 mV or more in any one or combination of leads V_4R, V_5R, and V_6R in patients with the clinical picture of acute myocardial infarction is highly sensitive and specific for the diagnosis of right ventricular myocardial infarction. Wellens has emphasized that in addition to noting the presence or absence of convex upward ST elevation in V_4R, clinicians should determine whether the T wave is positive or negative—such distinctions help distinguish proximal versus distal occlusion of the right coronary artery versus occlusion of the left circumflex artery.[193] Elevation of the ST segments in leads V_1 through V_4 due to right ventricular infarction can be confused with elevation due to anteroseptal infarction. Although the elevated ST segments are oriented anteriorly in both cases, it is the frontal plane that provides important clues—the ST segments are oriented to the right in right ventricular infarction (e.g., +120 degrees) whereas they are oriented to the left in anteroseptal infarction (e.g., −30 degrees).[194]

ECHOCARDIOGRAPHY AND RADIONUCLIDE ANGIOGRAPHY. Echocardiography is helpful in the differential diagnosis because in right ventricular infarction, in contrast to pericardial tamponade, no significant quantities of pericardial fluid are seen. On two-dimensional echocardiography, abnormal wall motion of the right ventricle as well as right ventricular dilation and depression of right ventricular ejection fraction are noted.[26] Gated equilibrium radionuclide angiography is also useful for recognizing right ventricular infarction. Serial studies have shown that some degree of recovery of an initially depressed right ventricular ejection fraction is the rule with right ventricular infarction, whereas this is less apparent in cases of left ventricular ejection fraction.[26]

HEMODYNAMICS. Loss of atrial transport in patients with right ventricular infarction can result in marked reductions in stroke volume and arterial blood pressure. As already noted, disproportionate elevation of the right-sided filling pressure is the hemodynamic hallmark of right ventricular infarction. Therefore, ventricular pacing may fail to increase cardiac output, and atrioventricular sequential pacing may be required.

Treatment

Because of their ability to reduce preload, medications routinely prescribed for left ventricular infarction may produce profound hypotension in patients with right ventricular infarction.[26] In patients with hypotension due to right ventricular myocardial infarction, hemodynamics can be improved by a combination of expanding plasma volume to augment right ventricular preload and cardiac output and, when left ventricular failure is present, arterial vasodilators. The initial therapy for hypotension in patients with right ventricular infarction should almost always be volume expansion. If hypotension has not been corrected after 1 or more liters of fluid have been administered briskly, however, consideration should be given to hemodynamic monitoring with a pulmonary artery catheter, because further volume infusion may be of little use and may produce pulmonary congestion. Vasodilators reduce the impedance to left ventricular outflow and in turn left ventricular diastolic, left atrial, and pulmonary (arterial) pressures, thereby lowering the impedance to right ventricular outflow and enhancing right ventricular output.

Right ventricular infarction is common among patients with inferior left ventricular infarction. Therefore, otherwise unexplained systemic arterial hypotension or diminished cardiac output, or marked hypotension in response to small doses of nitroglycerin in patients with inferior infarction, should lead to the prompt consideration of this diagnosis. In view of the importance of atrial transport, patients requiring pacing should have atrial or atrioventricular sequential pacing.[195] Successful reperfusion of the right coronary artery significantly improves right ventricular mechanical function and lowers in-hospital mortality in patients with right ventricular infarction. Replacement of the tricuspid valve and repair of the valve with annuloplasty rings have been carried out in the treatment of severe tricuspid regurgitation secondary to right ventricular infarction.

Mechanical Causes of Heart Failure

Free Wall Rupture

The most dramatic complications of STEMI are those that involve tearing or rupture of acutely infarcted tissue (Fig. 47–26).[7] The clinical characteristics of these lesions vary considerably and depend on the site of rupture, which may involve the papillary muscles, the interventricular septum, or the free wall of either ventricle. The overall incidence of these complications is hard to assess because clinical and autopsy series differ considerably.[196] The comparative clinical profile of these complications, as gathered from different studies, is shown in Table 47–11. The incidence of myocardial rupture has increased since the late 1960s. The prior use of corticosteroids or nonsteroidal antiinflammatory agents has been implicated as predisposing to rupture as a result of impaired healing. Controversy remains about the actual relationship between the use of such agents and the frequency of rupture, with several series suggesting a correlation of rupture with their use and others not. Conversely, the early use of fibrinolytic therapy appears to reduce the incidence of cardiac rupture, an effect that is responsible in part for improved survival with effective fibrinolysis. Late fibrinolytic therapy may actually *increase* the risk of cardiac rupture despite improving overall survival.

Rupture of the free wall of the infarcted ventricle (see Fig. 47–26) occurs in up to 10 percent of patients dying in the hospital of STEMI.[197] Thinness of the apical wall, marked intensity of necrosis at the terminal end of the blood supply, poor collateral flow, the shearing effect of muscular contraction against an inert and stiffened necrotic area, and aging of the myocardium with laceration of the myocardial microstructure have all been proposed as the local factors that lead to rupture (Fig. 47–27).[198]

CLINICAL CHARACTERISTICS. The following are some features that characterize this serious complication of STEMI[199]:

1. Occurs more frequently in elderly patients and possibly more frequently in women than in men with infarction.[197]
2. Appears to be more common in hypertensive than in normotensive patients.

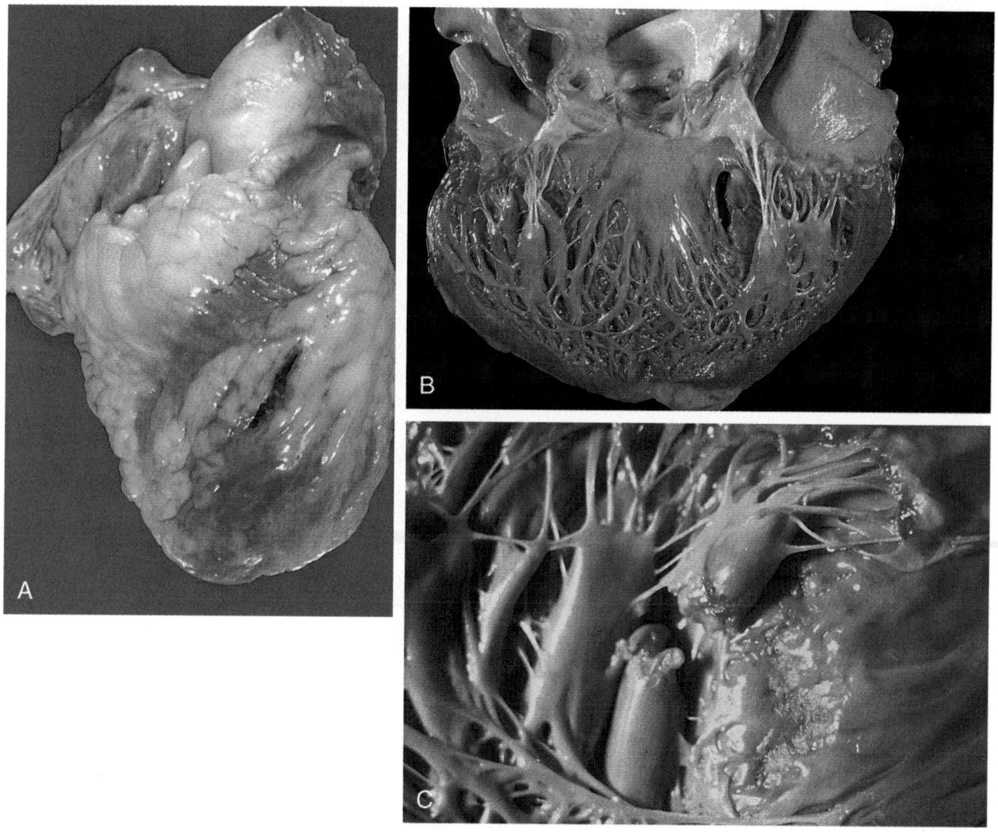

FIGURE 47–26 Cardiac rupture syndromes complicating STEMI. **A,** Anterior myocardial rupture in an acute infarct (arrow). **B,** Rupture of the ventricular septum (arrow). **C,** Complete rupture of a necrotic papillary muscle. (From Schoen FJ: The heart. *In* Cotran RS, Kumar V, Collins T [eds]: Pathologic Basis of Disease. 6th ed. Philadelphia, WB Saunders Company, 1999, p 562.)

TABLE 47–11 Clinical Profile of Mechanical Complications of Myocardial Infarction

Variable	Ventricular Septal Defect	Free Wall Rupture	Papillary Muscle Rupture
Age (mean, yr)	63	69	65
Days post-MI	3-5	3-6	3-5
Anterior MI	66%	50%	25%
New murmur	90%	25%	50%
Palpable thrill	Yes	No	Rare
Previous MI	25%	25%	30%
Echocardiographic findings			
Two-dimensional	Visualize defect	May have pericardial effusion	Flail or prolapsing leaflet
Doppler	Detect shunt		Regurgitant jet in LA
PA catheterization	Oxygen step-up in RV	Equalization of diastolic pressure	Prominent *c-v* wave in PCW tracing
Mortality			
Medical	90%	90%	90%
Surgical	50%	Case reports	40-90%

MI = myocardial infarction; LA = left atrium; PA = pulmonary artery; RV = right ventricle; PCW = pulmonary capillary wedge.
Modified from Labovitz AJ, et al: Mechanical complications of acute myocardial infarction. Cardiovasc Rev Rep 5:948, 1984.

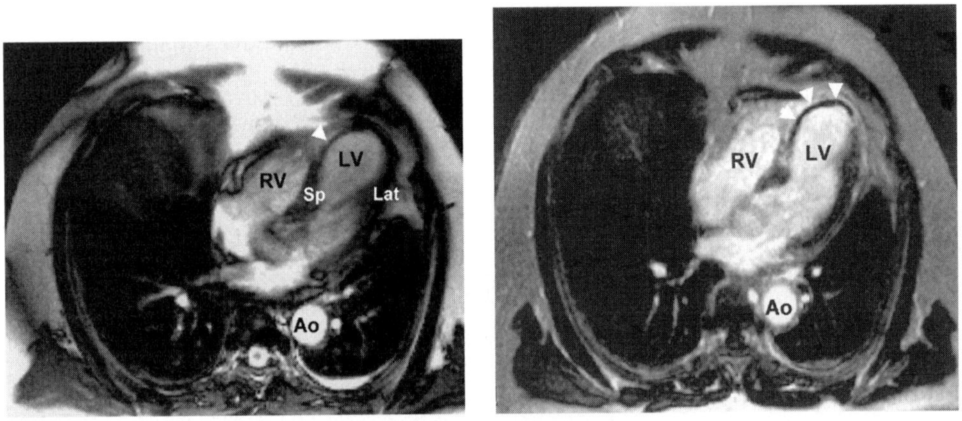

A B

FIGURE 47–27 **A,** Gadolinium-enhanced cardiac magnetic resonance horizontal long-axis image at end diastole. The white arrowhead indicates a very dark region in the mid- to distal septum and true apical regions. The lack of gadolinium perfusion represents microvascular obstruction. **B,** Cine images show dyskinetic systolic wall motion in the regions with microvascular obstruction (as in part A). Marked wall thinning is again visible. Ao = aorta; Lat = lateral left wall; LV = left ventricular cavity; RV = right ventricular cavity; Sp = interventricular septum. (From Lesser JR, Johnson K, Lindberg JL, et al: Myocardial rupture, microvascular obstruction, and infarct expansion: Elucidation by cardiac magnetic resonance. Circulation 108:116, 2003.

3. Occurs more frequently in the left than in the right ventricle and seldom occurs in the atria.
4. Usually involves the anterior or lateral walls[197] of the ventricle in the area of the terminal distribution of the left anterior descending coronary artery.
5. Is usually associated with a relatively large transmural infarction involving at least 20 percent of the left ventricle.
6. Occurs between 1 day and 3 weeks, but most commonly 1 to 4 days, after infarction.
7. Is usually preceded by infarct expansion, that is, thinning and a disproportionate dilation within the softened necrotic zone (see Fig. 47–27).
8. Most commonly results from a distinct tear in the myocardial wall or a dissecting hematoma that perforates a necrotic area of myocardium (see Fig. 47–26).
9. Usually occurs near the junction of the infarct and the normal muscle.
10. Occurs less frequently in the center of the infarct, but when rupture occurs here, it is usually during the second rather than the first week after the infarct.
11. Rarely occurs in a greatly thickened ventricle or in an area of extensive collateral vessels.
12. Most often occurs in patients *without* previous infarction.
13. There is no evidence that the intensity of anticoagulation influences the occurrence of rupture.[200]
14. Occurs more commonly in patients who received reperfusion therapy with a fibrinolytic versus PCI.[197]

Rupture of the free wall of the left ventricle usually leads to hemopericardium and death from cardiac tamponade. Occasionally, rupture of the free wall of the ventricle occurs as the first clinical manifestation in patients with undetected or silent myocardial infarction, and then it may be considered a form of "sudden cardiac death" (see Chap. 33).

The course of rupture varies from catastrophic, with an acute tear leading to immediate death, to subacute, with nausea, hypotension, and pericardial type of discomfort being the major clinical clues to its presence.[198] Survival depends on the recognition of this complication, hemodynamic stabilization of the patient—usually with inotropic agents and/or intraaortic balloon pump—and most importantly on prompt surgical repair.

PSEUDOANEURYSM. Incomplete rupture of the heart may occur when organizing thrombus and hematoma, together with pericardium, seal a rupture of the left ventricle and thus prevent the development of hemopericardium (Fig. 47–28). With time, this area of organized thrombus and pericardium can become a pseudoaneurysm (false aneurysm) that maintains communication with the cavity of the left

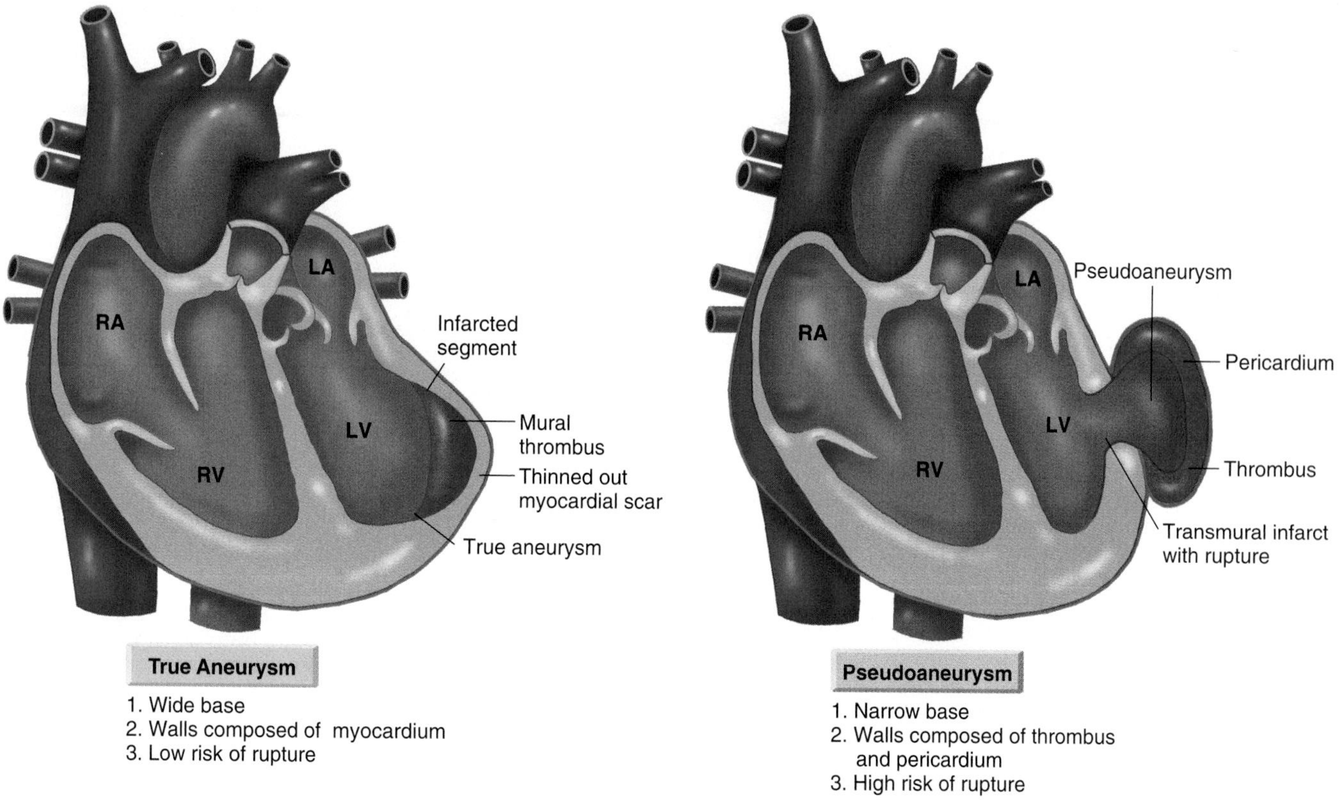

FIGURE 47–28 Differences between a pseudoaneurysm and a true aneurysm. (From Shah PK: Complications of acute myocardial infarction. *In* Parmley W, Chatterjee K [eds]: Cardiology. Philadelphia, JB Lippincott, 1987.)

ventricle. In contrast to true aneurysms, which always contain some myocardial elements in their walls, the walls of pseudoaneurysms are composed of organized hematoma and pericardium and lack any elements of the original myocardial wall. Pseudoaneurysms can become quite large, even equaling the true ventricular cavity in size, and they communicate with the left ventricular cavity through a narrow neck. Frequently, pseudoaneurysms contain significant quantities of old and recent thrombi, superficial portions of which can cause arterial emboli. Pseudoaneurysms can drain off a portion of each ventricular stroke volume exactly as do true aneurysms. The diagnosis of pseudoaneurysm can usually be made by two-dimensional echocardiography and contrast angiography, although at times differentiation between true aneurysm and pseudoaneurysm can be difficult by any imaging technique.[201]

DIAGNOSIS. The rupture usually is first suggested by the development of sudden profound shock, often rapidly leading to electromechanical dissociation due to pericardial tamponade. Immediate pericardiocentesis confirms the diagnosis and relieves the pericardial tamponade, at least momentarily. If the patient's condition is relatively stable, echocardiography may help in establishing the diagnosis of tamponade.[7] Under the most favorable conditions, cardiac catheterization can be carried out, not necessarily to confirm the diagnosis of rupture but to delineate the coronary anatomy. This is helpful so that, in addition to ventricular repair, coronary artery bypass surgery can be performed in patients in whom high-grade obstructive lesions are present. In patients in whom hemodynamics are critically compromised, establishment of the diagnosis should be followed immediately by surgical resection of the necrotic and ruptured myocardium with primary reconstruction (Fig. 47–29). When rupture is subacute and a pseudoaneurysm is suspected or present, prompt elective surgery is indicated

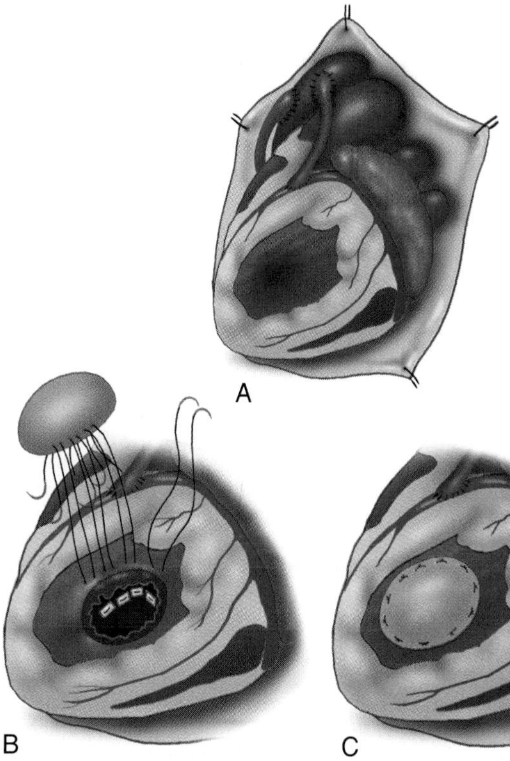

FIGURE 47–29 Management of free wall rupture. **A,** Typically, the rupture site is within a larger area of necrotic muscle. **B,** After debridement, pledgeted sutures are placed inside the ventricle and through a tailored prosthetic patch. **C,** The patch is then secured to the free wall. (Courtesy of Dr. David Adams, Mt. Sinai Hospital, New York.)

because rupture of the pseudoaneurysm occurs relatively frequently.

Rupture of the Interventricular Septum

Although rupture of the interventricular septum previously was reported in up to 11 percent of autopsied cases and 2 percent of acute myocardial infarction patients in the prefibrinolytic era, it occurs in only 0.2 percent of patients in contemporary fibrinolytic trials.[196] Clinical features associated with an increased risk of rupture of the interventricular septum include lack of development of a collateral network, advanced age, hypertension, anterior location of infarction, and possibly thrombolysis.[196] Patients who develop a rupture of the interventricular septum after STEMI have a much higher 30-day mortality rate (74 percent) than patients who do not develop this complication (7 percent).[202]

The perforation can range in length from one to several centimeters (see Fig. 47–26). It can be a direct through-and-through opening or more irregular and serpiginous. The size of the defect determines the magnitude of the left-to-right shunt and the extent of hemodynamic deterioration, which in turn affects the likelihood of survival.[196] As in rupture of the free wall of the ventricle, transmural infarction underlies rupture of the ventricular septum. Rupture of the septum with an anterior infarction tends to be apical in location, whereas inferior infarctions are associated with perforation of the basal septum and with a worse prognosis than those in an anterior location. In contrast with rupture of the free wall, rupture of the ventricular septum is more likely (20-30 percent of cases) to be associated with complete heart block, right bundle branch block, and atrial fibrillation.[203] Virtually all patients have multivessel coronary artery disease, with the majority exhibiting lesions in all of the major vessels. The likelihood of survival depends on the degree of impairment of ventricular function and the size of the defect.[196]

A ruptured interventricular septum is characterized by the appearance of a new harsh, loud holosystolic murmur that is heard best at the lower left sternal border and that is usually accompanied by a thrill.[7] Biventricular failure generally ensues within hours to days. The defect can also be recognized by two-dimensional echocardiography with color flow Doppler imaging or insertion of a pulmonary artery balloon catheter to document the left-to-right shunt. Catheter placement of an umbrella-shaped device within the ruptured septum has been reported to stabilize the conditions of critically ill patients with acute septal rupture after STEMI.

Rupture of a Papillary Muscle

Partial or total rupture of a papillary muscle is a rare but often fatal complication of transmural myocardial infarction (see Fig. 47–26).[204] Inferior wall infarction can lead to rupture of the posteromedial papillary muscle, which occurs more commonly than rupture of the anterolateral muscle, a consequence of anterolateral myocardial infarction. Rupture of a right ventricular papillary muscle is rare but can cause massive tricuspid regurgitation and right ventricular failure. Complete transection of a left ventricular papillary muscle is incompatible with life because the sudden massive mitral regurgitation that develops cannot be tolerated. Rupture of a portion of a papillary muscle, usually the tip or head of the muscle, resulting in severe, although not necessarily overwhelming, mitral regurgitation, is much more frequent and is not immediately fatal (Fig. 47–30). Unlike rupture of the ventricular septum, which occurs with large infarcts, papillary muscle rupture occurs with a relatively small infarction in approximately one-half of the cases seen. The extent of coronary artery disease in these patients sometimes is modest as well.

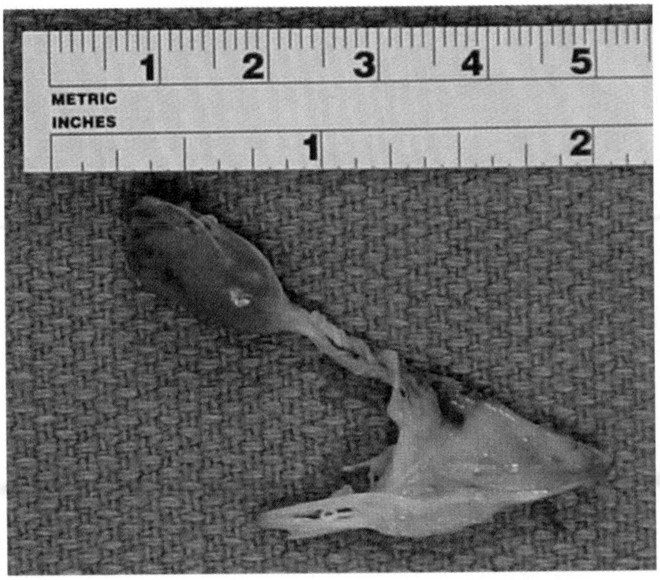

FIGURE 47–30 Surgical specimen showing papillary muscle (top left), chordae, and anterior mitral leaflet (bottom right) from a patient who had partial rupture of the papillary muscle and underwent mitral valve replacement for severe mitral regurgitation after ST elevation myocardial infarction. (Courtesy of John Byrne, MD, Brigham and Women's Hospital, Boston.)

In a small number of patients, rupture of more than one cardiac structure is noted clinically or at postmortem examination; all possible combinations of rupture of the free left ventricular wall, the interventricular septum, and papillary muscles have been described.[203]

As with patients who have a ruptured ventricular septal defect, those with papillary muscle rupture manifest a new holosystolic murmur and develop increasingly severe heart failure. In both conditions, the murmur may become softer or disappear as arterial pressure falls. Mitral regurgitation due to partial or complete rupture of a papillary muscle can be promptly recognized echocardiographically.[205] Color flow Doppler imaging is particularly helpful in distinguishing acute mitral regurgitation from a ventricular septal defect in the setting of STEMI (see Table 47–11).[7] Therefore, an echocardiogram should be obtained immediately on any patient in whom the diagnosis is suspected, because hemodynamic deterioration can ensue rapidly. Echocardiography also often permits differentiation of papillary muscle rupture from other, generally less severe forms of mitral regurgitation that occur with STEMI.

Differentiation Between Ventricular Septal Rupture and Mitral Regurgitation

It may be difficult, on clinical grounds, to distinguish between acute mitral regurgitation and rupture of the ventricular septum in patients with STEMI who suddenly develop a loud systolic murmur. This differentiation can be made most readily by color flow Doppler echocardiography. In addition, a right-heart catheterization with a balloon-tipped catheter can readily distinguish between these two complications. Patients with ventricular septal rupture demonstrate a "step-up" in oxygen saturation in blood samples from the right ventricle and pulmonary artery compared with those from the right atrium. Patients with acute mitral regurgitation lack this step-up; they may demonstrate tall *c-v* waves in both the pulmonary capillary and pulmonary arterial pressure tracings.

Invasive monitoring, which is essential in these patients, also allows for the critically important assessment of ventricular function.[7] Right and left ventricular filling pressures (right atrial pressure and pulmonary capillary wedge pressure) dictate fluid administration or the use of diuretics, whereas measurements of cardiac output and mean arterial pressure are obtained for calculation of systemic vascular resistance as a guide for vasodilator therapy. Unless systolic pressure is below 90 mm Hg, this therapy, generally using nitroglycerin or nitroprusside, should be instituted as soon as possible once hemodynamic monitoring is available. This may be critically important for stabilizing the patient's condition in preparation for further diagnostic studies and surgical repair. If vasodilator therapy is not tolerated or if it fails to achieve hemodynamic stability, intraaortic balloon counterpulsation should be rapidly instituted.

Surgical Treatment

Operative intervention is most successful in patients with STEMI and circulatory collapse when a surgically correctable mechanical lesion such as ventricular septal defect or mitral regurgitation can be identified and repaired. In such patients, the circulation should at first be supported by intraaortic balloon pulsation and a positive inotropic agent such as dopamine or dobutamine in combination with a vasodilator, unless the patient is hypotensive. Surgery should not be delayed in patients with a correctable lesion who agree to an aggressive management strategy and require pharmacological and/or mechanical (counterpulsation) support. Such patients frequently develop a serious complication—infection, adult respiratory distress syndrome, extension of the infarct, or renal failure—if surgery is delayed. Surgical survival is predicted by early operation, short duration of shock, and mild degrees of right and left ventricular impairment. When the hemodynamic status of a patient with one of these mechanical lesions complicating STEMI remains stable after the patient has been weaned from pharmacological and/or mechanical support, it may be possible to postpone the operation for 2 to 4 weeks to allow some healing of the infarct to occur. Surgical repair involves correction of mitral regurgitation, insertion of a prosthetic mitral valve repair, or closure of a ventricular septal defect, usually accompanied by coronary revascularization (Figs. 47–31 and 47–32).[7]

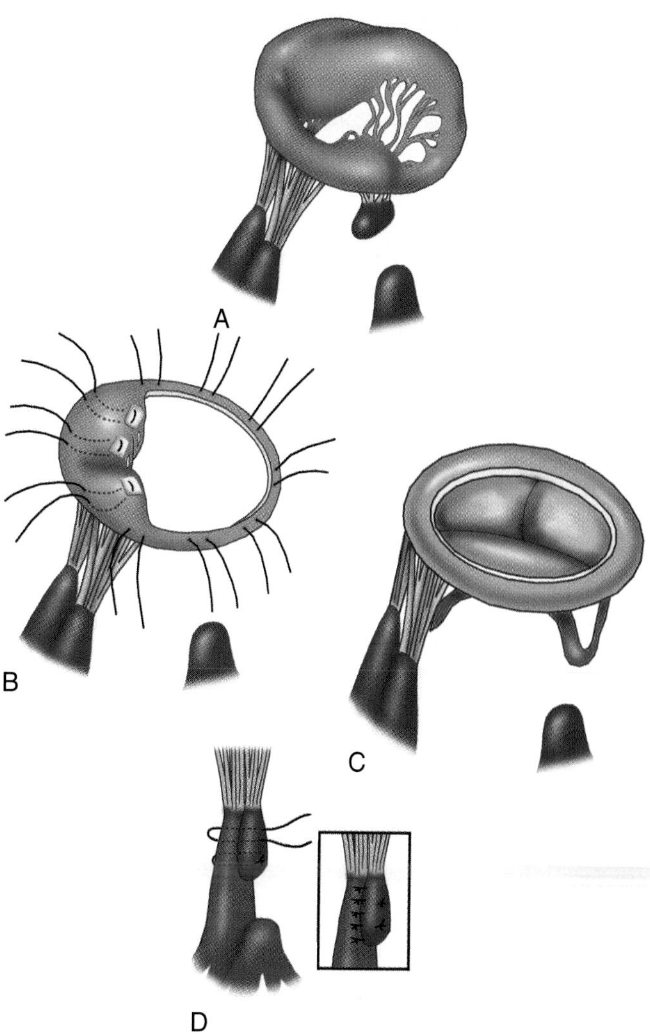

FIGURE 47–31 Surgical management of mitral regurgitation due to ruptured papillary muscle. **A,** Acute papillary muscle rupture results in severe mitral regurgitation due to leaflet and commissural prolapse. Mitral valve replacement is usually necessary. **B,** Mitral debridement with retention of the unruptured commissural and leaflet segment is performed to preserve partial annular papillary continuity. **C,** Mitral valve replacement is then performed. **D,** Occasionally, mitral valve repair can be performed by transfer of a papillary head to a nonrupture segment. (Courtesy of Dr. David Adams, Mt. Sinai Hospital, New York.)

Arrhythmias

The genesis and diagnosis of arrhythmias are presented in Chapters 27 and 29 and their treatment in Chapters 30 and 31. The role of arrhythmias in complicating the course of patients with STEMI and the prevention and treatment of these arrhythmias in this setting are discussed here and summarized in Table 47–12.

The incidence of arrhythmias is higher in patients the earlier they are seen after the onset of symptoms. Many serious arrhythmias develop before hospitalization, even before the patient is monitored. Some abnormality of cardiac rhythm also occurs in the majority of patients with STEMI treated in CCUs. When patients are seen very early during the course of STEMI, they almost invariably exhibit evidence of increased activity of the autonomic nervous system. Thus, sinus bradycardia, sometimes associated with AV block, and hypotension reflect augmented vagal activity.

MECHANISM OF ARRHYTHMIAS. A leading hypothesis for a major mechanism of arrhythmias in the acute phase of coronary occlusion is reentry due to inhomogeneity of the electrical characteristics of ischemic myocardium.[206] The cellular electrophysiological mechanisms for reperfusion arrhythmias appear to include washout of various ions such as lactate and potassium and toxic metabolic substances that have accumulated in the ischemic zone.

HEMODYNAMIC CONSEQUENCES. Patients with significant left ventricular dysfunction have a relatively fixed stroke volume and depend on changes in heart rate to alter cardiac output. However, there is a narrow range of heart rate over which the cardiac output is maximal, with significant reductions occurring at both faster and slower rates. Thus, all forms of bradycardia and tachycardia can depress the cardiac output in patients with STEMI. Although the optimal rate insofar as cardiac output is concerned may exceed 100 beats/min, it is important to consider that heart rate is one of the major determinants of myocardial oxygen consumption and that at more rapid heart rates, myocardial energy needs can be elevated to levels that adversely affect ischemic myocardium. Therefore, in patients with STEMI, the optimal rate is usually lower, in the range of 60 to 80 beats/min.

A second factor to consider in assessing the hemodynamic consequences of a particular arrhythmia is the loss of the atrial contribution to ventricular preload. Studies in patients without STEMI have demonstrated that loss of atrial transport decreases left ventricular output by 15 to 20 percent. In patients with reduced diastolic left ventricular compliance of any cause (including STEMI), however, atrial systole is of greater importance for left ventricular filling. In patients with STEMI, atrial systole boosts end-diastolic volume by 15 percent, end-diastolic pressure by 29 percent, and stroke volume by 35 percent.

TABLE 47–12 Cardiac Arrhythmias and Their Management During Acute Myocardial Infarction

Category	Arrhythmia	Objective of Treatment	Therapeutic Options
1. Electrical instability	Ventricular premature beats	Correction of electrolyte deficits and increased sympathetic tone	Potassium and magnesium solutions, beta blocker
	Ventricular tachycardia	Prophylaxis against ventricular fibrillation, restoration of hemodynamic stability	Antiarrhythmic agents; cardioversion/defibrillation
	Ventricular fibrillation	Urgent reversion to sinus rhythm	Defibrillation; bretylium tosylate
	Accelerated idioventricular rhythm	Observation unless hemodynamic function is compromised	Increase sinus rate (atropine, atrial pacing); antiarrhythmic agents
	Nonparoxysmal atrioventricular junctional tachycardia	Search for precipitating causes (e.g., digitalis intoxication); suppress arrhythmia only if hemodynamic function is compromised	Atrial overdrive pacing; antiarrhythmic agents; cardioversion relatively contraindicated if digitalis intoxication present
2. Pump failure/excessive sympathetic stimulation	Sinus tachycardia	Reduce heart rate to diminish myocardial oxygen demands	Antipyretics; analgesics; consider beta blocker unless congestive heart failure present; treat latter if present with anticongestive measures (diuretics, afterload reduction)
	Atrial fibrillation and/or atrial flutter	Reduce ventricular rate; restore sinus rhythm	Verapamil, digitalis glycosides; anticongestive measures (diuretics, afterload reduction); cardioversion; rapid atrial pacing (for atrial flutter)
	Paroxysmal supraventricular tachycardia	Reduce ventricular rate; restore sinus rhythm	Vagal maneuvers; verapamil, cardiac glycosides, beta-adrenergic blockers; cardioversion; rapid atrial pacing
3. Bradyarrhythmias and conduction disturbances	Sinus bradycardia	Acceleration of heart rate only if hemodynamic function is compromised	Atropine; atrial pacing
	Junctional escape rhythm	Acceleration of sinus rate only if loss of atrial "kick" causes hemodynamic compromise	Atropine; atrial pacing
	Atrioventricular block and intraventricular block		Insertion of pacemaker

Modified from Antman EM, Rutherford JD (eds): Coronary Care Medicine: A Practical Approach. Boston, Martinus Nijhoff Publishing, 1986, p 78.

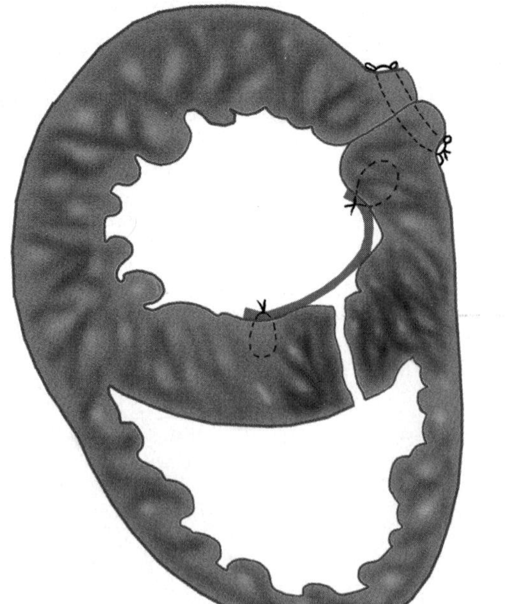

FIGURE 47–32 Repair of ischemic ventricular septal defect. The infarct typically involves a free wall and septum. Repair of the defect is performed through an incision in the ventricular wall infarct. The septal defect is closed with a prosthetic patch and a second patch is used to close the incision in the free wall. (Courtesy of Dr. David Adams, Mt. Sinai Hospital, New York.)

VENTRICULAR ARRHYTHMIAS (see Chap. 29)

Ventricular Premature Complexes

Prior to the widespread use of reperfusion therapy, aspirin, beta blockers, and intravenous nitrates in the management of STEMI, it was believed that frequent ventricular premature complexes (more than 5 per minute), ventricular premature complexes with multiform configuration, early coupling (the "R-on-T" phenomenon), and repetitive patterns in the form of couplets or salvos presaged ventricular fibrillation. It is now clear, however, that such "warning arrhythmias" are present in as many patients who do not develop fibrillation as those who do. Several reports have shown that primary ventricular fibrillation (see later) occurs without antecedent warning arrhythmias and may even develop in spite of suppression of warning arrhythmias.[207] Both primary ventricular fibrillation and ventricular premature complexes, especially R-on-T beats, occur during the early phase of STEMI, when considerable heterogeneity of electrical activity is present. Although R-on-T beats expose this heterogeneity and can precipitate ventricular fibrillation in a small minority of patients, the ubiquitous nature of VPCs in patients with STEMI and the extremely infrequent nature of ventricular fibrillation in the current era of STEMI management produces unacceptably low sensitivity and specificity of ECG patterns observed on monitoring systems for identifying patients at risk of ventricular fibrillation.

MANAGEMENT. Since the incidence of ventricular fibrillation in patients with STEMI seen in CCUs over the last three decades appears to be declining, the prior practice of prophylactic suppression of ventricular premature beats with antiarrhythmic drugs no longer is necessary and there is the possibility that its use may actually be associated with an increased risk of fatal bradycardic and asystolic events.[208] Therefore, we pursue a conservative course when ventricular premature complexes are observed in STEMI patients and do not routinely prescribe

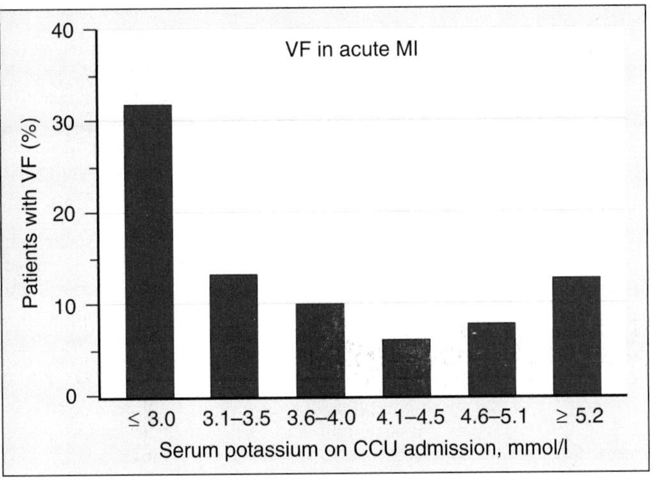

FIGURE 47–33 Importance of electrolyte deficits, as shown in this study in which the risk for ventricular fibrillation (VF) was strikingly increased in patients who presented to the critical care unit (CCU) with hypokalemia. MI = myocardial infarction. (From Nordrehaug JE, van der Lippe G: Hypokalemia and ventricular fibrillation in acute myocardial infarction. Br Heart J 50:525, 1983.)

antiarrhythmic drugs but instead determine whether recurrent ischemia or electrolyte (Fig. 47–33) or metabolic disturbances are present.[207,209]

When, at the very inception of an infarction, ventricular premature complexes are encountered in the presence of sinus tachycardia, augmented sympathoadrenal stimulation is often a contributing factor and can be treated by beta-adrenoceptor blockade. In fact, early administration of an intravenous beta blocker is effective in reducing the incidence of ventricular fibrillation in cases of evolving myocardial infarction.

ACCELERATED IDIOVENTRICULAR RHYTHM. This arrhythmia is seen in up to 20 percent of patients with STEMI. It occurs frequently during the first 2 days, with about equal frequency in anterior and inferior infarctions. Most episodes are of short duration. Accelerated idioventricular rhythm is often observed shortly after successful reperfusion has been established. However, the frequent occurrence of this rhythm in patients without reperfusion limits their reliability as markers of restoration of patency of the infarct-related coronary artery.[7] In contrast to rapid ventricular tachycardia, accelerated idioventricular rhythm is thought not to affect prognosis, and we do not routinely treat accelerated idioventricular rhythms.

Ventricular Tachycardia

Nonsustained runs of ventricular tachycardia do not appear to be associated with an increased mortality risk, either during hospitalization or over the first year. Ventricular tachycardia occurring late in the course of STEMI is more common in patients with transmural infarction and left ventricular dysfunction, is likely to be sustained, usually induces marked hemodynamic deterioration, and is associated with increased rates of both hospital mortality and long-term mortality.

MANAGEMENT. Since hypokalemia can increase the risk of developing ventricular tachycardia, low serum potassium levels should be identified quickly after a patient's admission for STEMI and should be treated promptly. We strive to maintain the serum potassium level above 4.5 mEq/liter and serum magnesium level above 2 mEq/liter. Rapid abolition of sustained ventricular tachycardia in patients with STEMI is mandatory because of its deleterious effect on pump function and because it frequently deteriorates into ventricular fibrillation. After reversion to sinus rhythm, every effort should be made to correct underlying abnormalities such as hypoxia, hypotension, acid-base or electrolyte disturbances, and digitalis excess. Although no definitive data are available, it is a common clinical practice to continue maintenance infusions of antiarrhythmic drugs for several days after an index episode of ventricular tachycardia and to discontinue the drug and either observe the patient for recurrence or perform a diagnostic electrophysiology study. Patients with recurrent or refractory ventricular tachycardia should be considered for specialized procedures such as implantation of antitachycardia devices or surgery. Occasionally, urgent attempts at revascularization with angioplasty or coronary artery bypass graft surgery help control refractory ventricular tachycardia.

Ventricular Fibrillation

Ventricular fibrillation can occur in three settings in hospitalized patients with STEMI. (Its occurrence as a mechanism of sudden death is discussed in Chapter 33.) *Primary* ventricular fibrillation occurs suddenly and unexpectedly in patients with no or few signs or symptoms of left ventricular failure. Although primary ventricular fibrillation occurred in up to 10 percent of patients hospitalized with STEMI several decades ago, analyses suggest that its incidence has declined. *Secondary* ventricular fibrillation is often the final event of a progressive downhill course with left ventricular failure and cardiogenic shock. So-called *late* ventricular fibrillation develops more than 48 hours after STEMI and frequently but not exclusively occurs in patients with large infarcts and ventricular dysfunction. Patients with intraventricular conduction defects and anterior wall infarction, patients with persistent sinus tachycardia, atrial flutter, or fibrillation early in the clinical course, and patients with right ventricular infarction who require ventricular pacing are at higher risk for suffering late in-hospital ventricular fibrillation than are patients without these features.

PROGNOSIS. The effect of primary ventricular fibrillation on prognosis continues to be debated.[208] The MILIS study, conducted in the prethrombolytic era, suggested that it does not have an adverse effect on hospital mortality, whereas the GISSI investigators reporting observations in large cohorts of thrombolytic-treated patients, suggested there was an excess mortality due to primary ventricular fibrillation during the hospital phase but not thereafter.[210] Now, with the availability of amiodarone and implantable cardioverter-defibrillators, the prognosis of late ventricular fibrillation is improving and is probably driven more by residual ventricular function and recurrent ischemia than by the arrhythmic risk per se.

PROPHYLAXIS. Lidocaine prophylaxis to prevent primary ventricular fibrillation is no longer advised. There is an association between hypokalemia and the risk of ventricular fibrillation in the CCU (see Fig. 47–33). Although it has not been conclusively shown that correction of hypokalemia to a level of 4.5 mEq/liter actually reduces the incidence of ventricular fibrillation, our experience suggests that this probably is protective and of little risk. Despite the fact that no consistent relationship between hypomagnesemia and ventricular fibrillation has been observed, magnesium deficits may still be involved in the risk of ventricular fibrillation because intracellular magnesium levels are reduced in patients with STEMI and are not adequately reflected by serum measurements. For these reasons, plus the fact that it is often difficult to repair a potassium deficit without administering supplemental magnesium, we routinely replete magnesium to a level of 2 mEq/liter.

The only situation in which we might consider prophylactic lidocaine (bolus of 1.5 mg/kg followed by 20-50 μg/kg/min) would be the unusual circumstance in which a patient within the first 12 hours of a STEMI must be managed in a facility where cardiac monitoring is not available and equipment for prompt defibrillation is not readily accessible.

MANAGEMENT (see Chaps. 32 and 33). Treatment for ventricular fibrillation consists of an unsynchronized electrical countershock with at least 200 to 300 joules, implemented as rapidly as possible.[7] When ventricular fibrillation occurs outside an intensive care unit, resuscitative efforts are much less likely to be successful, primarily because the time interval between the onset of the episode and institution of definitive therapy tends to be prolonged. Failure of electrical countershock to restore an effective cardiac rhythm is almost always due to rapidly recurrent ventricular tachycardia or ventricular fibrillation, to electromechanical dissociation, or, very rarely, to electrical asystole.

Successful interruption of ventricular fibrillation or prevention of refractory recurrent episodes can also be facilitated by administration of intravenous amiodarone. When synchronous cardiac electrical activity is restored by countershock but contraction is ineffective—that is, during electromechanical dissociation—the usual underlying cause is very extensive myocardial ischemia or necrosis or rupture of the ventricular free wall or septum. If rupture has not occurred, intracardiac administration of calcium gluconate or epinephrine may promote restoration of an effective heartbeat. We do *not* usually administer bicarbonate injections to correct acidosis because of the high osmotic load they impose and the fact that hyperventilation of the patient is probably a more suitable means of clearing the acidosis.

BRADYARRHYTHMIAS (see Chap. 29)

Sinus Bradycardia

Sinus bradycardia is a common arrhythmia occurring during the early phases of STEMI, and it is particularly frequent in patients with inferior and posterior infarction.[7,211] On the basis of data obtained in experimental infarction and from some clinical observations, it appears that the increased vagal tone that produces sinus bradycardia during the early phase of STEMI may actually be protective, perhaps because it reduces myocardial oxygen demands.[212] Thus, the acute mortality rate appears to be as low in patients with sinus bradycardia as in patients without this arrhythmia.

MANAGEMENT. Isolated sinus bradycardia, unaccompanied by hypotension or ventricular ectopy, should be observed rather than treated initially. In the first 4 to 6 hours after infarction, if the sinus rate is extremely slow (less than 40 to 50 beats/min) and associated with hypotension, intravenous atropine in aliquots of 0.3 to 0.6 mg every 3 to 10 minutes (with a total dose not exceeding 2 mg) can be administered to bring the heart rate up to approximately 60 beats/min.

Atrioventricular and Intraventricular Block

Ischemic injury can produce conduction block at any level of the AV or intraventricular conduction system. Such blocks can occur in the atrioventricular node and the bundle of His, producing various grades of AV block; in either main bundle branch, producing right or left bundle branch block; and in the anterior and posterior divisions of the left bundle, producing left anterior or left posterior (fascicular) divisional blocks. Disturbances of conduction can, of course, occur in various combinations. Clinical features of proximal and distal AV conduction disturbances in patients with STEMI are summarized in Table 47-13.

FIRST-DEGREE ATRIOVENTRICULAR BLOCK. First-degree AV block generally does not require specific treatment. Beta blockers and calcium antagonists (other than nifedipine) prolong AV conduction and may be responsible for first-degree AV block as well. However, discontinuation of these drugs in the setting of STEMI has the potential of increasing ischemia and ischemic injury. Therefore, it is our practice not to decrease the dosage of these drugs unless the PR interval is greater than 0.24 second. Only if higher degree block or hemodynamic impairment occurs should these agents be stopped. If the block is a manifestation of excessive vagotonia and is associated with sinus bradycardia and hypotension, administration of atropine, as already outlined, may be helpful. Continued electrocardiographic monitoring is important in such patients in view of the possibility of progression to higher degrees of block.

SECOND-DEGREE ATRIOVENTRICULAR BLOCK. First-degree and type I second-degree AV blocks do not appear to affect survival, are most commonly associated with occlusion of the right coronary artery, and are caused by ischemia of the AV node (see Table 47-13). Specific therapy is not required in patients with second-degree AV block of the type I variety when the ventricular rate exceeds 50 beats/min and premature ventricular contractions, heart failure, and bundle branch block are absent. However, if these complications develop or if the heart rate falls below approximately 50 beats/min and the patient is symptomatic, immediate treatment with atropine (0.3 to 0.6 mg) is indicated; temporary pacing systems are almost never needed in the management of this arrhythmia.

Type II second-degree block usually originates from a lesion in the conduction system below the bundle of His (see Table 47-13). Because of its potential for progression to complete heart block, type II second-degree AV block should be treated with a temporary external or transvenous demand pacemaker with the rate set at approximately 60 beats/min.[7]

COMPLETE (THIRD-DEGREE) ATRIOVENTRICULAR BLOCK. Complete AV block can occur in patients with either anterior or inferior

TABLE 47-13 Atrioventricular (AV) Conduction Disturbances in Acute Myocardial Infarction

	Location of AV Conduction Disturbance	
	Proximal	***Distal***
Site of block	Intranodal	Infranodal
Site of infarction	Inferoposterior	Anteroseptal
Compromised arterial supply	RCA (90%), LCX (10%)	Septal perforators of LAD
Pathogenesis	Ischemia, necrosis, hydropic cell swelling, excess parasympathetic activity	Ischemia, necrosis, hydropic cell swelling
Predominant type of AV nodal block	First-degree (PR > 200 msec) Mobitz type I second-degree	Mobitz type II second-degree Third-degree
Common premonitory features of third-degree AV block	(a) First–second-degree AV block (b) Mobitz I pattern	(a) Intraventricular conduction block (b) Mobitz II pattern
Features of escape rhythm following third-degree block (a) Location (b) QRS width (c) Rate (d) Stability of escape rhythm	 (a) Proximal conduction system (His bundle) (b) <0.12/sec* (c) 45-60/min but may be as low as 30/min (d) Rate usually stable; asystole uncommon	 (a) Distal conduction system (bundle branches) (b) >0.12/sec (c) Often <30/min (d) Rate often unstable with moderate to high risk of ventricular asystole
Duration of high-grade AV block	Usually transient (2-3 days)	Usually transient but some form of AV conduction disturbance and/or intraventricular defect may persist
Associated mortality rate	Low unless associated with hypotension and/or congestive heart failure	High because of extensive infarction associated with power failure or ventricular arrhythmias
Pacemaker therapy (a) Temporary (b) Permanent	 (a) Rarely required; may be considered for bradycardia associated with left ventricular power failure, syncope, or angina (b) Almost never indicated because conduction defect is usually transient	 (a) Should be considered in patients with anteroseptal infarction and acute bifascicular block (b) Indicated for patients with high-grade AV block with block in His-Purkinje system and those with transient advanced AV block and associated bundle branch block

LAD = left anterior descending coronary artery. LCX = left circumflex coronary artery; RCA = right coronary artery.

Modified from Antman EM, Rutherford JD: Coronary Care Medicine: A Practical Approach. Boston, Martinus Nijhoff, 1986; and Dreifus LS, et al: Guidelines for implantation of cardiac pacemakers and antiarrhythmia devices. J Am Coll Cardiol 18:1, 1991. Reprinted with permission from the American College of Cardiology.

*Some studies suggest that a wide QRS escape rhythm (>0.12 sec) following high-grade AV block in inferior infarction is associated with a worse prognosis.

infarction. Complete heart block in patients with inferior infarction usually results from an intranodal or supranodal lesion and develops gradually, often progressing from first-degree or type I second-degree block. The escape rhythm is usually stable without asystole and often junctional, with a rate exceeding 40 beats/min and a narrow QRS complex in 70 percent of cases and a slower rate and wide QRS in the others. This form of complete AV block is often transient, may be responsive to pharmacological antagonism of adenosine with methylxanthines,[213] and resolves in the majority of patients within a few days (see Table 47-13).

In patients with anterior infarction, third-degree AV block often occurs suddenly, 12 to 24 hours after the onset of infarction, although it is usually preceded by intraventricular block and often type II (not first-degree or type I) AV block. Such patients have unstable escape rhythms with wide QRS complexes and rates less than 40 beats/min; ventricular systole may occur quite suddenly. In patients with anterior infarction, AV block usually develops as a result of extensive septal necrosis that involves the bundle branches. The high rate of mortality in this group of patients with slow idioventricular rhythm and wide QRS complexes is the consequence of extensive myocardial necrosis resulting in severe left ventricular failure and often shock (see Table 47-13).

Patients with inferior infarction often have concomitant ischemia or infarction of the AV node secondary to hypoperfusion of the AV node artery. However, the His-Purkinje system usually escapes injury in such individuals. Patients with inferior STEMI who develop AV block usually have lesions in both right and left anterior descending coronary arteries. Likewise, patients with inferior STEMI and AV block have larger infarcts and more depressed right ventricular and left ventricular function than do patients with inferior infarct and no AV block. As already noted, junctional escape rhythms with narrow QRS complexes occur commonly in this setting.

Although data suggest that complete AV block is *not* an independent risk factor for mortality, whether temporary transvenous pacing per se improves survival of patients with anterior STEMI remains controversial. Some investigators contend that ventricular pacing is useless when employed to correct complete AV block in patients with anterior infarction in view of the poor prognosis in this group regardless of therapy. However, pacing may protect against transient hypotension with its attendant risks of extending infarction and precipitating malignant ventricular tachyarrhythmias. Also, pacing protects against asystole (see Chap. 31), a particular hazard in patients with anterior infarction and infranodal block. Improved survival with pacing probably occurs in only a small fraction of patients with complete AV block and anterior wall infarcts, because the extensive destruction of the myocardium that almost invariably accompanies this condition results in a very high mortality rate, even in paced patients. Given these considerations, an extremely large series of patients would be required to demonstrate the small reduction of mortality that might be achieved by pacing. The absence of data supporting such an effect, however, by no means excludes the possibility that it may be present.

Pacing is not usually needed in patients with inferior wall infarction and complete AV block that is often transient in nature, but it is indicated if the ventricular rate is very slow (<40 to 50 beats/min), if ventricular arrhythmias or hypotension is present, or if pump failure develops; atropine is only rarely of value in these patients. Only when complete heart block develops in less than 6 hours after the onset of symptoms is atropine likely to abolish the AV block or cause acceleration of the escape rhythm. In such cases, the AV block is more likely to be transient and related to increases in vagal tone, rather than the more persistent block seen later in the course of STEMI, which generally requires cardiac pacing.

Intraventricular Block

The right bundle branch and the left posterior division have a dual blood supply from the left anterior descending and right coronary arteries, whereas the left anterior division is supplied by septal perforators originating from the left anterior descending coronary artery. Not all conduction blocks observed in patients with STEMI can be considered to be complications of infarcts, because almost half are already present at the time the first electrocardiogram is recorded, and they may represent antecedent disease of the conduction system.[214] Compared with patients without conduction defects, STEMI patients with bundle branch blocks have more comorbid conditions, are less likely to receive therapies such as thrombolytics, aspirin, and beta blockers, and have an increased in-hospital mortality rate.[215] In the prefibrinolytic era, studies of intraventricular conduction disturbances—that is, block within one or more of the three subdivisions (fascicles) of the His-Purkinje system (the anterior and posterior divisions of the left bundle and the right bundle)—had been reported to occur in 5 to 10 percent of patients with STEMI. More recent series in the fibrinolytic era suggest that intraventricular blocks occur in about 2 to 5 percent of patients with myocardial infarction.[216]

ISOLATED FASCICULAR BLOCKS. Isolated left anterior divisional block is unlikely to progress to complete AV block. Mortality is increased in these patients, although not as much as in patients with other forms of conduction block. The posterior fascicle is larger than the anterior fascicle, and, in general, a larger infarct is required to block it. As a consequence, mortality is markedly increased. Complete AV block is not a frequent complication of either form of isolated divisional block.

RIGHT BUNDLE BRANCH BLOCK. This conduction defect alone can lead to AV block because it is often a new lesion, associated with anteroseptal infarction. Isolated right bundle branch block is associated with an increased mortality risk in patients with anterior STEMI even if complete AV block does not occur, but this appears to be the case only if it is accompanied by congestive heart failure.

BIFASCICULAR BLOCK. The combination of right bundle branch block with either left anterior or posterior divisional block or the combination of left anterior and posterior divisional blocks (i.e., left bundle branch block) is known as bidivisional or bifascicular block. If new block occurs in two of the three divisions of the conduction system, the risk of developing complete AV block is quite high. Mortality is also high because of the occurrence of severe pump failure secondary to the extensive myocardial necrosis required to produce such an extensive intraventricular block.[216] Patients with intraventricular conduction defects, particularly right bundle branch block, account for the majority of patients who develop ventricular fibrillation late in their hospital stay. However, the high rate of mortality in these patients occurs even in the absence of high-grade AV block and appears to be related to cardiac failure and massive infarction rather than to the conduction disturbance.[215]

Preexisting bundle branch block or divisional block is less often associated with the development of complete heart block in patients with STEMI than are conduction defects acquired during the course of the infarct. Bidivisional block in the presence of prolongation of the P-R interval (first-degree AV block) may indicate disease of the third subdivision rather than of the AV node and is associated with a greater risk of complete heart block than if first-degree AV block is absent.

Complete bundle branch block (either left or right), the combination of right bundle branch block and left anterior divisional (fascicular) block, and any of the various forms of trifascicular block are all more often associated with anterior than with inferoposterior infarction. All these forms are more frequent with large infarcts and in older patients and have a higher incidence of other accompanying arrhythmias than is seen in patients without bundle branch block.

Use of Pacemakers in Patients with Acute Myocardial Infarction (see Chap. 31)

TEMPORARY PACING. Just as is the case for complete AV block, transvenous ventricular pacing has not resulted in statistically demonstrable improvement in prognosis among patients with acute myocardial infarction who develop intraventricular conductions defects. However, temporary pacing is advisable in some of these patients because of the high risk of developing complete AV block. This includes patients with new bilateral (bifascicular) bundle branch block—that is, right bundle branch block with left anterior or posterior divisional block and alternating right and left bundle branch block; first-degree AV block adds to this risk. Isolated new block in only one of the three fascicles even with P-R prolongation and preexisting bifascicular block and normal P-R interval poses somewhat less risk; these patients should be monitored closely, with insertion of a temporary pacemaker deferred unless higher degree AV block occurs.

Noninvasive external temporary cardiac pacing is possible routinely in conscious patients and is acceptable to many but not all patients despite the discomfort. Used in a standby mode, it is virtually free of complications and contraindications and provides an important alternative to transvenous endocardial pacing.[7] Once it is clinically evident that continuous pacing is required, external pacing, which is generally not well tolerated for more than minutes to hours, should be replaced by a temporary transvenous pacemaker.

ASYSTOLE. The presence of apparent ventricular asystole on monitor displays of continuously recorded electrocardiograms may be misleading, because the mechanism may in fact be fine ventricular fibrillation. Because of the predominance of ventricular fibrillation as the cause of cardiac arrest in this setting, initial therapy should include electrical countershock, even if definitive electrocardiographic documentation of this arrhythmia is not available. In the rare instance in which asystole can be documented to be the responsible electrophysiological disturbance, immediate transcutaneous pacing (or stimulation with a transvenous pacemaker if one is already in place) is indicated.[7]

PERMANENT PACING. The question of the advisability of permanent pacemaker insertion is complicated by the fact that not all sudden deaths in STEMI patients with conduction defects are due to high-grade AV block. A high incidence of late ventricular fibrillation occurs in CCU survivors with anterior STEMI complicated by either right or left bundle branch block. Therefore, ventricular fibrillation rather than asystole due to failure of AV conduction and infranodal pacemakers could be responsible for late sudden death.

Long-term pacing is often helpful when complete heart block persists throughout the hospital phase in a patient with STEMI, when sinus node function is markedly impaired, or when type II second- or third-degree block occurs intermittently.[7] When high-grade AV block is associated with newly acquired bundle branch block or other criteria of impairment of conduction system function, prophylactic long-term pacing may be justified as well. Additional considerations that drive a decision to insert a permanent pacemaker include whether the patient is a candidate for an implantable cardioverter-defibrillator or has severe heart failure that might be improved with biventricular pacing (see Chap. 24).

SUPRAVENTRICULAR TACHYARRHYTHMIAS (see Chap. 29)

SINUS TACHYCARDIA. This arrhythmia is typically associated with augmented sympathetic activity and may provoke transient hypertension or hypotension. Common causes are anxiety, persistent pain, left ventricular failure, fever, pericarditis, hypovolemia, pulmonary embolism, and the administration of cardioaccelerator drugs such as atropine, epinephrine, or dopamine; rarely, it occurs in patients with atrial infarction. Sinus tachycardia is particularly common in patients with anterior infarction, especially if there is significant accompanying left ventricular dysfunction. It is an undesirable rhythm in patients with STEMI because it results in an augmentation of myocardial oxygen consumption, as well as a reduction in the time available for coronary perfusion, thereby intensifying myocardial ischemia and/or external myocardial necrosis. Persistent sinus tachycardia can signify persistent heart failure and under these circumstances is a poor prognostic sign associated with an excess mortality. An underlying cause should be sought and appropriate treatment instituted, such as analgesics for pain; diuretics for heart failure; oxygen, beta blockers, and nitroglycerin for ischemia; and aspirin for fever or pericarditis.

Administration of beta-adrenoceptor blocking agents, in the dosage and manner described elsewhere in this chapter, may be helpful in the treatment of sinus tachycardia, particularly when this arrhythmia is a manifestation of a hyperdynamic circulation, which is seen particularly in young patients with an initial STEMI without extensive cardiac damage. Beta blockade is contraindicated, however, in patients in whom the sinus tachycardia is a manifestation of hypovolemia or of pump failure, the latter reflected by a systolic arterial pressure below 100 mm Hg, rales involving more than one-third of the lung fields, a pulmonary capillary wedge pressure exceeding 20 to 25 mm Hg, or a cardiac index below approximately 2.2 liters/min/m^2. A possible exception to this is a patient in whom persistent ischemia is believed to be the cause or the result of tachycardia-cautious administration of an ultra-short-acting beta-adrenoceptor blocker such as esmolol (25 to 200 μg/kg/min) can be tried to ascertain the patient's response to slowing of the heart rate.

ATRIAL FLUTTER AND FIBRILLATION. Atrial flutter is usually transient, and in patients with STEMI it is typically a consequence of augmented sympathetic stimulation of the atria, often occurring in patients with left ventricular failure or pulmonary emboli in whom the arrhythmia intensifies hemodynamic deterioration (see Table 47-12).

As with atrial premature complexes and atrial flutter, fibrillation is usually transient and tends to occur in patients with left ventricular failure but is also observed in patients with pericarditis and ischemic injury to the atria and right ventricular infarction.[26] The increased ventricular rate and the loss of the atrial contribution to left ventricular filling result in a significant reduction in cardiac output. Atrial fibrillation during STEMI is associated with increased mortality and stroke, particularly in patients with anterior wall infarction.[217] However, because it is more common in patients with clinical and hemodynamic manifestations of extensive infarction and a poor prognosis, atrial fibrillation is probably a marker of poor prognosis, with only a small independent contribution to increased mortality.

Management. Atrial flutter and fibrillation in patients with STEMI are treated in a manner similar to these conditions in other settings (see Chap. 29). Patients with recurrent episodes of atrial fibrillation should be treated with oral anticoagulants (to reduce the risk of stroke), even if sinus rhythm is present at the time of hospital discharge, because no antiarrhythmic regimen can be relied upon to be completely effective in suppressing atrial fibrillation. In the absence of contraindications, patients should receive a beta blocker after STEMI; in addition to their several other beneficial effects, these agents are helpful in slowing the ventricular rate, should atrial fibrillation recur.

Other Complications

Recurrent Chest Discomfort

Evaluation of postinfarction chest discomfort is sometimes complicated by previous abnormalities on the electrocardiogram and a vague description of the discomfort by the patient, who either may be exquisitely sensitive to fleeting discomfort or may deny a potential recrudescence of symptoms. The critical task for clinicians is to distinguish recurrent angina or infarction from nonischemic causes of discomfort that might be caused by infarct expansion, pericarditis, pulmonary embolism, and noncardiac conditions. Important diagnostic maneuvers include a repeat physical examination, repeat ECG reading, and assessment of the response to sublingual nitroglycerin, 0.4 mg. (The use of noninvasive diagnostic evaluation for recurrent ischemia in patients whose symptoms appear only with moderate levels of exertion is discussed elsewhere in this chapter.)

RECURRENT ISCHEMIA AND INFARCTION. The incidence of postinfarction angina without reinfarction is 20 percent in patients treated with fibrinolytics and is significantly reduced to 6 percent in patients undergoing primary PCI for STEMI.[99] It does not appear to be reduced by the use of thrombolytic therapy as the management strategy during the acute phase[218] but has been reported to be lower in patients who undergo primary percutaneous transluminal coronary angioplasty for acute myocardial infarction, especially if stents are used.[219] When accompanied by ST and T wave changes in the same leads where Q waves have appeared, it may be due to occlusion of an initially patent vessel, reocclusion of an initially recanalized or stented vessel, or coronary spasm.

DIAGNOSIS. *Extension* of the original zone of necrosis or *reinfarction* in a separate myocardial zone can be a difficult diagnosis, especially within the first 24 hours after the index event. It is more convenient to refer to both extension and reinfarction collectively under the more general term *recurrent infarction.* Serum cardiac markers may still be elevated from the initial infarction, and it may not be possible to distinguish the ECG changes that are part of the normal evolution after the index infarction from those due to recurrent infarction. Because the levels of cardiac-specific troponins remain elevated for more than 1 week following the index event, they are of less value for diagnosing recurrent infarction than are more rapidly rising and falling markers, such as CK-MB. Within the first 18 to 24 hours following the initial infarction, when serum cardiac markers may not have returned to the normal range, recurrent infarction should be strongly considered when there is repeat ST segment elevation on the electrocardiogram. Although pericarditis remains a possibility in such patients, the two can usually be distinguished by the presence of a rub and lack of responsiveness to nitroglycerin in patients with pericardial discomfort.

Beyond the first 24 hours, when serum cardiac markers such as CK-MB have usually returned to the normal range, recurrent infarction can be diagnosed either by re-elevation of the CK-MB level above the upper limit of normal and increased by at least 50 percent of the previous value or the appearance of new Q waves on the ECG reading.[7] Because of variations in patient populations and definitions of recurrent infarction, estimates of the incidence of this complication vary; large fibrinolytic trials report 30-day reinfarction rates of about 5 to 6 percent as compared with about 20 percent in patients undergoing primary PCI.[79,85,99,220] Reinfarction is more common in patients with diabetes mellitus and those with a previous myocardial infarction. In patients treated with fibrinolytics, the rate of reinfarction is lower if a low-molecular-weight heparin or direct thrombin inhibitor is used instead of unfractionated heparin as adjunctive antithrombin therapy.[67] The predominant angiographic predictors of reinfarction in patients undergoing primary PCI include a final coronary stenosis greater than 30 percent, post-PCI coronary dissection, and post-PCI intracoronary thrombus.[220]

PROGNOSIS. Regardless of whether postinfarction angina is persistent or limited, its presence is important because the short-term morbidity rate is higher among such patients; mortality is increased if the recurrent ischemia is accompanied by ECG changes and hemodynamic compromise.[7] Recurrent infarction (due in many cases to reocclusion of the infarct-related coronary artery) carries serious adverse prognostic information because it is associated with two- to fourfold higher rates of in-hospital complications (congestive heart failure, heart block) and early and long-term mortality.[221] Presumably, the higher mortality rate is related to the larger mass of myocardium whose function becomes compromised.

Of the standard therapies that are routinely prescribed during the acute phase of STEMI, aspirin and beta blockers have been associated with a reduction in the incidence of recurrent infarction.[147,166]

Management. As with the acute phase of treatment of STEMI, algorithms for management of patients with recurrent ischemic discomfort at rest center on the 12-lead electrocardiogram (Fig. 47–34). Patients with ST segment re-elevation should be referred for urgent catheterization and PCI; repeat fibrinolysis can be considered if PCI is not available. Insertion of an intraaortic balloon pump may help stabilize the patient while other procedures are being arranged. For patients believed to have recurrent ischemia who do not have evidence of hemodynamic compromise, an attempt should be made to control symptoms with sublingual or intravenous nitroglycerin and intravenous beta blockade to slow the heart rate to 60 beats/min. When hypotension, congestive heart failure, or ventricular arrhythmias develop during recurrent ischemia, urgent catheterization and revascularization are indicated.

Prior studies failed to show any benefit of a strategy of *routine* referral for catheterization and revascularization, either early or after a delay of 1 or 2 days. It should be realized, however, that those studies were conducted in an era in which the catheterization equipment was less technologically advanced than it is today and glycoprotein IIb/IIIa inhibitors and stents were not part of the interventionist's armamentarium. The de facto practice in many centers currently is to pursue a routine invasive strategy after fibrinolysis for STEMI. Although no large-scale randomized trials have been conducted in the contemporary era to support such a practice, we find it quite persuasive. Investigators in Germany reported lower rates of the composite endpoint of death/recurrent myocardial infarction/target vessel revascularization/ischemic events in patients treated with routine PCI as compared to a conservative strategy of medical therapy with referral for PCI when symptoms recurred.[222,223] The expanded use of PCI beyond rescue PCI, referred to by Dauerman and Sobel as "pharmacoinvasive recanalization," is in need of more vigorous testing but holds considerable promise for reducing rates of mortality and morbidity after STEMI.[224-227]

Pericardial Effusion and Pericarditis (see Chap. 64)

PERICARDIAL EFFUSION. Effusions are generally detected echocardiographically, and their incidence varies with technique, criteria, and laboratory expertise.[228] Effusions are more common in patients with anterior STEMI and with larger infarcts and when congestive failure is present. The majority of pericardial effusions that are seen following STEMI do not cause hemodynamic compromise; when

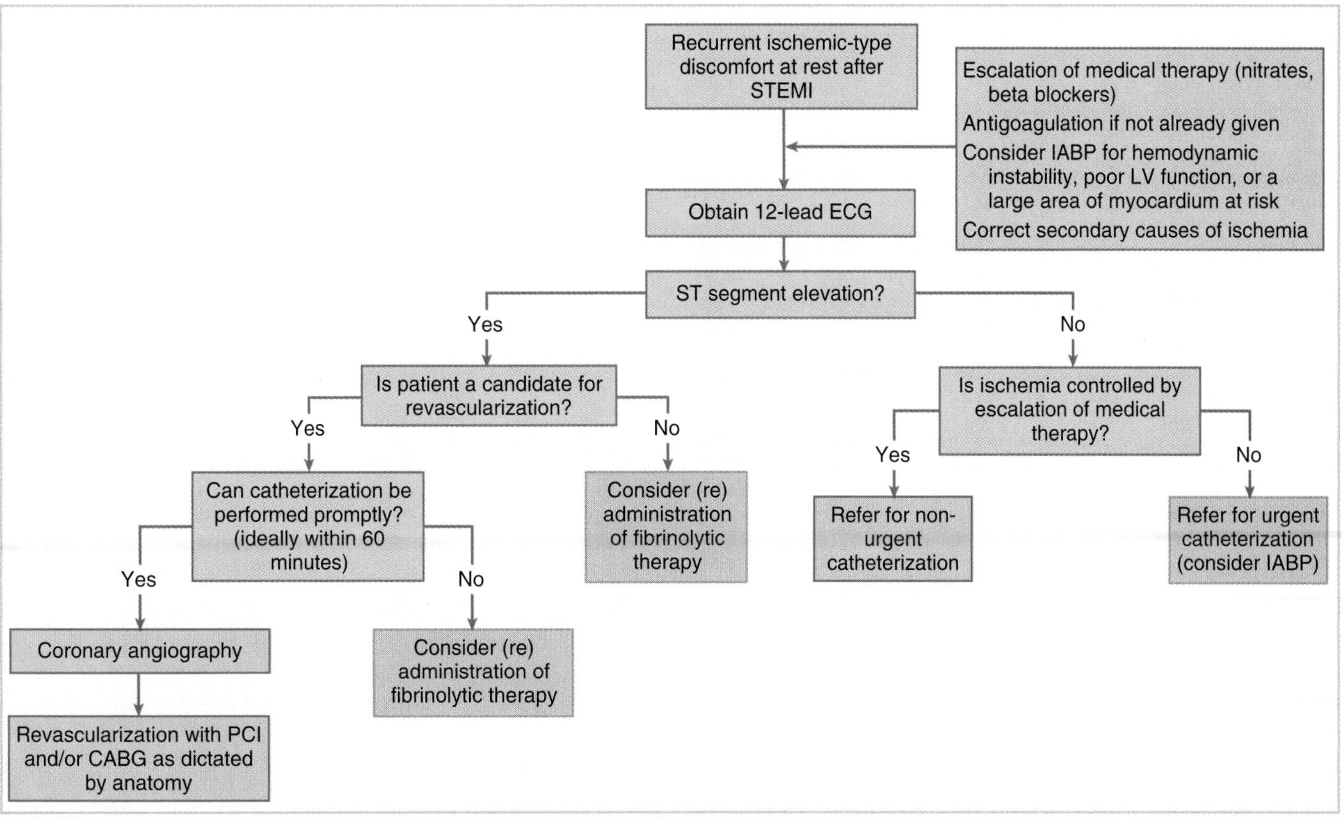

FIGURE 47–34 Algorithm for management of ischemia/infarction after ST segment elevation myocardial infarction (STEMI). CABG = coronary artery bypass grafting; ECG = electrocardiogram; IABP = intraaortic balloon pump; PCI = percutaneous coronary intervention. (Modified from Braunwald E, Zipes D, Libby P: Heart Disease: A Textbook of Cardiovascular Medicine. 6th ed. Philadelphia, WB Saunders, 2001, p 1195.)

tamponade occurs, it is usually due to ventricular rupture or hemorrhagic pericarditis.

The reabsorption rate of a postinfarction pericardial effusion is slow, with resolution often taking several months. The presence of an effusion does not indicate that pericarditis is present; although they may occur together, the majority of effusions occur without other evidence of pericarditis.

PERICARDITIS. Pericarditis can produce pain as early as the first day and as late as 6 weeks after STEMI. The pain of pericarditis may be confused with that resulting from postinfarction angina, recurrent infarction, or both. An important distinguishing feature is the radiation of the pain to either trapezius ridge, a finding that is nearly pathognomonic of pericarditis and rarely seen with ischemic discomfort. Transmural myocardial infarction, by definition, extends to the epicardial surface and is responsible for local pericardial inflammation. An acute fibrinous pericarditis (pericarditis epistenocardica) occurs commonly after transmural infarction, but the majority of patients do not report any symptoms from this process. Although transient pericardial friction rubs are relatively common among patients with transmural infarction within the first 48 hours, pain or electrocardiographic changes occur much less often. However, the development of a pericardial rub appears to be correlated with a larger infarct and greater hemodynamic compromise. The discomfort of pericarditis usually becomes worse during a deep inspiration, but it can be relieved or diminished when the patient sits up and leans forward.

Although anticoagulation clearly increases the risk for hemorrhagic pericarditis early after STEMI, this complication has not been reported with sufficient frequency during heparinization or following fibrinolytic therapy to warrant absolute prohibition of such agents when a rub is present. Nevertheless, the detection of a pericardial effusion on echocardiogram is usually an indication for discontinuation of anticoagulation. In patients in whom continuation or initiation of anticoagulant therapy is strongly indicated (such as during cardiac catheterization or following coronary angioplasty), heightened monitoring of clotting parameters and observation for clinical signs of possible tamponade are needed. Late pericardial constriction due to anticoagulant-induced hemopericardium has been reported.

Treatment of pericardial discomfort consists of aspirin, but usually in higher doses than prescribed routinely following infarction—doses of 650 mg orally every 4 to 6 hours may be needed. Nonsteroidal anti-inflammatory agents and steroids should be avoided because they may interfere with myocardial scar formation.[7]

DRESSLER SYNDROME. Also known as the *postmyocardial infarction syndrome*, Dressler syndrome usually occurs 1 to 8 weeks after infarction. Dressler cited an incidence of 3 to 4 percent of all myocardial infarction patients in 1957, but the incidence has decreased dramatically since that time. Clinically, patients with Dressler syndrome present with malaise, fever, pericardial discomfort, leukocytosis, an elevated sedimentation rate, and a pericardial effusion. At autopsy, patients with this syndrome usually demonstrate localized fibrinous pericarditis containing polymorphonuclear leukocytes. The cause of this syndrome is not clearly established, although the detection of antibodies to cardiac tissue has raised the notion of an immunopathological process. Treatment is with aspirin, 650 mg, as often as every 4 hours. Glucocorticosteroids and nonsteroidal antiinflammatory agents are best avoided in patients with Dressler syndrome within 4 weeks of STEMI because of their potential to impair infarct healing, to cause ventricular rupture,[229] and to increase coronary vascular resistance. Aspirin in large doses is effective.

Venous Thrombosis and Pulmonary Embolism

Almost all pulmonary emboli originate from thrombi in the veins of the lower extremities; much less commonly, they originate from mural thrombi overlying an area of right ventricular infarction. Bed rest and heart failure predispose to venous thrombosis and subsequent pulmonary embolism, and both of these factors occur commonly in patients with STEMI, particularly those with large infarcts. At a time when patients with STEMI were routinely subjected to prolonged periods of bed rest, significant pulmonary embolism was found in more than 20 percent of patients with STEMI coming to autopsy, and massive pulmonary embolism accounted for 10 percent of deaths from myocardial infarction. In contemporary practice, with early mobilization and the widespread use of low-dose anticoagulant prophylaxis especially using low-molecular-weight heparins, pulmonary embolism has become an uncommon cause of death in patients with STEMI. When pulmonary embolism does occur in patients with STEMI, management is generally along the lines described for noninfarction patients (see Chap. 66).

Left Ventricular Aneurysm

The term *left ventricular aneurysm* (often termed *true aneurysm*) is generally reserved for a discrete, dyskinetic area of the left ventricular wall with a broad neck (to differentiate it from pseudoaneurysm due to a contained myocardial rupture). Dyskinetic or akinetic areas of the left ventricle are far more common than true aneurysms after STEMI; such poorly contracting segments are referred to as *regional wall motion abnormalities*.[228] True left ventricular aneurysms probably develop in less than 5 percent of all patients with STEMI and perhaps somewhat more frequently in patients with transmural infarction (especially anterior).[41] The wall of the true aneurysm is thinner than the wall of the rest of the left ventricle (see Fig. 47–28), and it is usually composed of fibrous tissue as well as necrotic muscle, occasionally mixed with viable myocardium.

PATHOGENESIS. Aneurysm formation presumably occurs when intraventricular tension stretches the noncontracting infarcted heart muscle, thus producing infarct expansion, a relatively weak, thin layer of necrotic muscle, and fibrous tissue that bulges with each cardiac contraction. With the passage of time, the wall of the aneurysm becomes more densely fibrotic, but it continues to bulge with systole causing some of the left ventricular stroke volume during each systole to be ineffective.

When an aneurysm is present after anterior STEMI, there is generally a total occlusion of a poorly collateralized left anterior descending coronary artery. An aneurysm is rarely seen with multivessel disease when there are either extensive collaterals or a nonoccluded left anterior descending artery. Aneurysms usually range from 1 to 8 cm in diameter. They occur approximately four times more often at the apex and in the anterior wall than in the inferoposterior wall. The overlying pericardium is usually densely adherent to the wall of the aneurysm, which may even become partially calcified after several years. True left ventricular aneurysms (in contrast to pseudoaneurysms) rarely rupture soon after development. Late rupture, when the true aneurysm has become stabilized by the formation of dense fibrous tissue in its wall almost never occurs.

The rate of mortality in patients with a left ventricular aneurysm is up to six times higher than in patients without aneurysms, even when compared with that in patients with comparable left ventricular ejection fraction. Death in these patients is often sudden and presumably related to the high incidence of ventricular tachyarrhythmias that occur with aneurysms.[207]

DIAGNOSIS. The presence of persistent ST segment elevation in an electrocardiographic area of infarction, classically thought to suggest aneurysm formation, actually indicates a large infarct with a regional wall motion abnormality but does not necessarily imply an aneurysm. The diagnosis of aneurysm is best made noninvasively by an echocardiographic study by radionuclide ventriculography or at the time of cardiac catheterization by left ventriculography. With the loss of shortening from the area of the aneurysm, the remainder of the ventricle must be hyper-

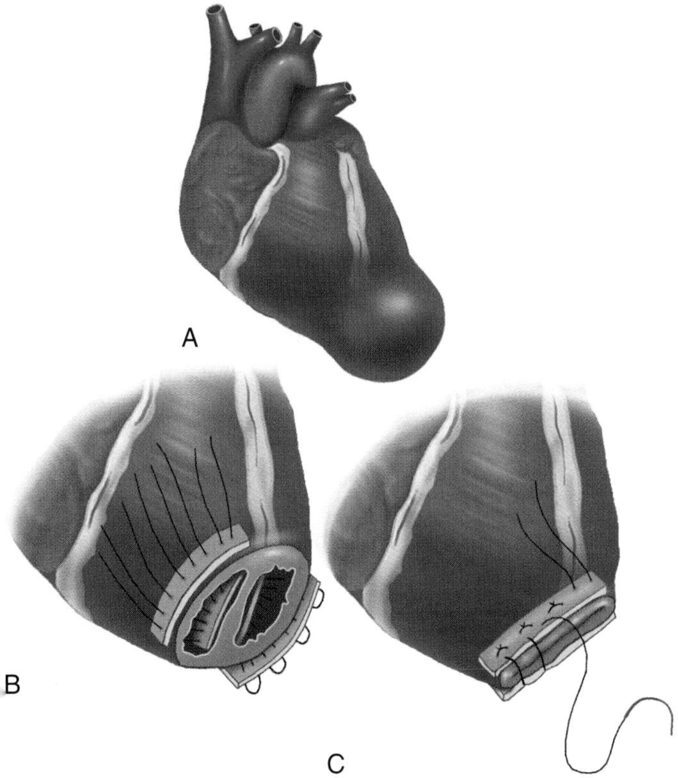

FIGURE 47–35 Surgical management of ventricular aneurysm. **A,** In this case, the aneurysm is located at the apex. **B,** The aneurysmal segment is resected and felt pledget strips are used to reinforce interrupted suture closure of the apex. **C,** Completed repair partially restores apical geometry. (Courtesy of Dr. David Adams, Division of Cardiac Surgery, Mt. Sinai Hospital, New York.)

kinetic in order to compensate. With relatively large aneurysms, complete compensation is impossible. The stroke volume falls, or, if it is maintained, it is at the expense of an increase in end-diastolic volume, which in turn leads to increased wall tension and myocardial oxygen demand. Heart failure may ensue, and angina may appear or worsen.

TREATMENT. Aggressive management of STEMI, including prompt reperfusion, may diminish the incidence of ventricular aneurysms. Surgical aneurysmectomy generally is successful only if there is relative preservation of contractile performance in the nonaneurysmal portion of the left ventricle (Fig. 47–35). In such circumstances, when the operation is performed for worsening heart failure or angina, operative mortality is relatively low and clinical improvement can be expected.[230] Aneurysmectomy and special procedures carried out to control ventricular tachyarrhythmias occurring with left ventricular aneurysms are described elsewhere in this chapter. Because of the risk of mural thrombosis and systemic embolization, we favor long-term oral anticoagulation with warfarin in patients with a left ventricular aneurysm after STEMI.

LEFT VENTRICULAR THROMBUS AND ARTERIAL EMBOLISM

The most convenient and accurate method for diagnosing left ventricular thrombosis is two-dimensional echocardiography.[228] It is hypothesized that endocardial inflammation during the acute phase of infarction provides a thrombogenic surface for clots to form in the left ventricle. With extensive transmural infarction of the septum, however, mural thrombi may overlie infarcted myocardium in both ventricles. Prospective studies have suggested that patients who develop a mural thrombus early (within 48 to 72 hours of infarction) have an extremely poor early prognosis,[231] with a high rate of mortality from the complications of a large infarction (shock, reinfarction, rupture, and ventricular tachyarrhythmia), rather than emboli from the left ventricular thrombus.

Although a mural thrombus adheres to the endocardium overlying the infarcted myocardium, superficial portions of it can become detached and produce systemic arterial emboli. Although estimates vary based on patient selection, about 10 percent of mural thrombi result in systemic embolization.[231] Echocardiographically detectable features that suggest that a given thrombus is more likely to embolize include increased mobility and protrusion into the ventricular chamber, visualization in multiple views, and contiguous zones of akinesis and hyperkinesis.

MANAGEMENT. Data from previous trials with limited sample size suggested that anticoagulation (intravenous heparin or high-dose subcutaneous heparin) reduced the development of left ventricular *thrombi* by 50 percent, but, because of the low event rate, it was not possible to demonstrate a reduction in the incidence of *systemic embolism.* Fibrinolysis reduces the rate of thrombus formation and the character of the thrombi so that they are less protuberant. Of note, however, the data from fibrinolytic trials are difficult to interpret because of the confounding effect of antithrombotic therapy with heparin. Recommendations for anticoagulation vary considerably, and fibrinolysis has precipitated fatal embolization. Nevertheless, anticoagulation for 3 to 6 months with warfarin is advocated for many patients with demonstrable mural thrombi.[7,232]

Based on the available data, it is our practice to recommend anticoagulation (intravenous heparin to elevate the aPTT to one and a half to two times that of control, followed by a minimum of 3 to 6 months of warfarin) in the following clinical situations: (1) an embolic event has already occurred, or (2) the patient has a large anterior infarction whether or not a thrombus is visualized echocardiographically. We are also inclined to follow the same anticoagulation practice in patients with infarctions other than in the anterior distribution if a thrombus or large wall motion abnormality is detected.

Aspirin, although probably not capable of affecting thrombus size in most patients, may prevent further platelet deposition on existing thrombi and also is protective against recurrent ischemic events. It should be prescribed in conjunction with warfarin to patients who are candidates for long-term anticoagulation therapy based on the indications discussed earlier.

Convalescence, Discharge, and Post-Myocardial Infarction Care

TIMING OF HOSPITAL DISCHARGE. The timing of discharge from the hospital is variable. As noted earlier, patients who have undergone aggressive reperfusion protocols and have no significant ventricular arrhythmias, recurrent ischemia, or congestive heart failure have been safely discharged in less than 5 days. More commonly, discharge occurs 5 or 6 days after admission for patients who experience no complications, who can be followed readily at home, and whose family setting is conducive to convalescence. Most complications that would preclude early discharge occur within the first day or two of admission; therefore, patients suitable for early discharge can be identified early during the hospitalization.[233] Several controlled trials and many uncontrolled trials of early discharge after STEMI have failed to show any increase in risk in patients appropriately selected for early discharge. The decision regarding timing of discharge in the patients with uncomplicated STEMI should take into account the patient's psychological state after STEMI, the adequacy of the dose titration for essential drugs such as beta blockers and inhibitors of the renin-angiotensin-aldosterone system, and the availability and timing of follow-up with visiting nurses and the patient's primary care physician.[144]

For patients who have experienced a complication, discharge is deferred until their condition has been stable for several days and it is clear that they are responding appropriately to necessary medications such as antiarrhythmic agents, vasodilators, or positive inotropic agents or that they have undergone the appropriate work-up for recurrent ischemia.

COUNSELING. Before discharge from the hospital, all patients should receive detailed instruction concerning physical activity. Initially, this should consist of ambulation at home but avoidance of isometric exercise such as lifting; several rest periods should be taken daily. In addition, the patient should be given fresh nitroglycerin tablets and instructed in their use and should receive careful instructions about the use of any other medications prescribed. As convalescence progresses, graded resumption of activity should be encouraged. Many approaches have been utilized, ranging from formal rigid guidelines to general advice advocating moderation and avoidance of any activity that evokes symptoms. Sexual counseling is often overlooked during recovery from STEMI and should also be included as part of the educational process. Such counseling should begin early after STEMI and should include the recommendation that sexual activity be resumed after successful completion of either early submaximal or later symptom-limited exercise stress testing.[7]

Some evidence indicates that behavioral alteration is possible after recovery from STEMI and that this may improve prognosis. A cardiac rehabilitation program with supervised physical exercise and an educational component has been recommended for most STEMI patients after discharge. Although the overall clinical benefit of such programs continues to be debated, there is little question that most people derive considerable knowledge and psychological security from such interventions, and they continue to be endorsed by experienced clinicians.[7] Meta-analyses of randomized trials of medically supervised rehabilitation programs versus usual care that were conducted in an era before widespread use of beta-adrenoceptor blockers and aggressive reperfusion strategies have shown a reduction in cardiovascular death but no change in the incidence of nonfatal reinfarction. Given the relationship between depression and STEMI, interest has arisen in psychosocial intervention programs in the convalescent phase of STEMI.[234] Psychosocial intervention programs have been shown to be helpful for decreasing symptoms of depression and are a useful adjunct to standard cardiac rehabilitation programs after STEMI; however, they do not have a significant impact on the risk of mortality or recurrent myocardial infarction after STEMI.[234] More detailed information on physical and psychological aspects of rehabilitation of patients convalescing from STEMI is given in Chapter 43.

Risk Stratification After STEMI

The process of risk stratification following STEMI occurs in several stages: initial presentation, in-hospital course (CCU, intermediate care unit), and at the time of hospital discharge. The tools used to form an integrated assessment of the patient consist of baseline demographic information, serial electrocardiograms and serum cardiac marker measurements, hemodynamic monitoring data, a variety of noninvasive tests, and, if performed, the findings at cardiac catheterization (Fig. 47–36).[7]

INITIAL PRESENTATION. Certain demographic and historical factors are associated with a poor prognosis in patients with STEMI, including female gender, age greater than 70 years, a history of diabetes mellitus, prior angina pectoris, and previous myocardial infarction (see Fig. 47-10).[143] Diabetes mellitus, in particular, appears to confer a three- to fourfold increase in risk. Whether this is due to accelerated atherosclerosis or some other characteristic induced by the diabetic state (such as a larger infarct size) is unclear. (Surviving diabetic patients also experience a more complicated post-myocardial infarction course, including a greater incidence of postinfarction angina, infarct extension, and heart failure.[7])

In addition to playing a central role in the decision pathway for management of patients with STEMI based on the presence or absence of ST segment elevation, the 12-lead electrocardiogram carries important prognostic information. Mortality is greater in patients experiencing anterior wall myocardial infarction than after inferior myocardial infarction, even when corrected for infarct size. Patients with right ventricular infarction complicating inferior infarction, as suggested by ST segment elevation in V_4R, have a greater mortality rate than patients sustaining an inferior infarction without right ventricular involvement.[26,235] Patients with multiple leads showing ST elevation and a high sum of ST segment elevation have an increased mortality rate, especially if their infarct is anterior in location.[235] Patients whose electrocardiogram demonstrates persistent advanced heart block (e.g., type II, second-degree, or third-degree AV block) or new intraventricular conduction abnormalities (bifascicular or trifascicular) in the course of a STEMI have a worse prognosis than do patients without these abnormalities. The influence of high degrees of heart block is particularly important in patients with right ventricular infarction, because such patients have a markedly increased mortality risk. Other electrocardiographic findings that augur poorly are persistent horizontal or downsloping ST segment depression, Q waves in multiple leads, evidence of right ventricular infarction accompanying inferior infarction,[26] ST segment depressions in anterior leads in patients with inferior infarction,[235] and atrial arrhythmias (especially atrial fibrillation).

HOSPITAL COURSE. Soon after CCUs were instituted, it became apparent that left ventricular function is an important early determinant of survival. Hospital mortality from acute myocardial infarction depends directly on the severity of left ventricular dysfunction.[143] Risk stratification via clinical findings, estimation of infarct size, and, in appropriate patients, invasive hemodynamic monitoring in the CCU provide an assessment of the likelihood of a complicated hospital course and may also identify important abnormalities, such as hemodynamically significant mitral regurgitation, that convey an adverse long-term prognosis (see Table 47-8).

Recurrent ischemia and infarction following STEMI, either in the same location as the index infarction or "at a distance," influence prognosis adversely.[221] Poor prognosis comes from the loss of viable myocardium, with the resulting larger area of infarction creating a greater compromise in ventricular function. Postinfarction angina generally connotes a less favorable prognosis because it indicates the presence of jeopardized myocardium. In the current era of aggressive revascularization, early postinfarction angina often leads to early interventions that tend to improve outcome, diminishing the long-term impact and significance of angina early after STEMI.[220]

Assessment at Hospital Discharge

Both short-term and long-term survival after STEMI depend on three factors: resting left ventricular function, residual potentially ischemic myocardium, and susceptibility to serious ventricular arrhythmias. The most important of these factors is the state of left ventricular function (see Fig. 47-25).[7] The second most important factor is how the severity and extent of the obstructive lesions in the coronary vascular bed perfusing residual viable myocardium affect the risk of recurrent infarction, additional myocardial damage, and serious ventricular arrhythmias.[7] Thus, survival relates to the quantity of myocardium that has become necrotic and the quantity at risk of becoming necrotic.

At one end of the spectrum, the prognosis is best for the patient with normal intrinsic coronary vessels whose completed infarction constitutes a small fraction (5 percent) of the left ventricle as a consequence of a coronary embolus and who has no jeopardized myocardium. At the other extreme is the patient with a massive infarct with left ventricular failure whose residual viable myocardium is perfused by markedly obstructed vessels. Progression of atherosclerosis or lowering of perfusion pressure in these vessels impairs the function and viability of the residual myocardium on which left ventricular function depends. The situation may not be hopeless even in such a patient, however, because revascularization may reduce the threat to the jeopardized myocardium. The third risk factor, the susceptibility to serious arrhythmias, is reflected in ventricular ectopic activ-

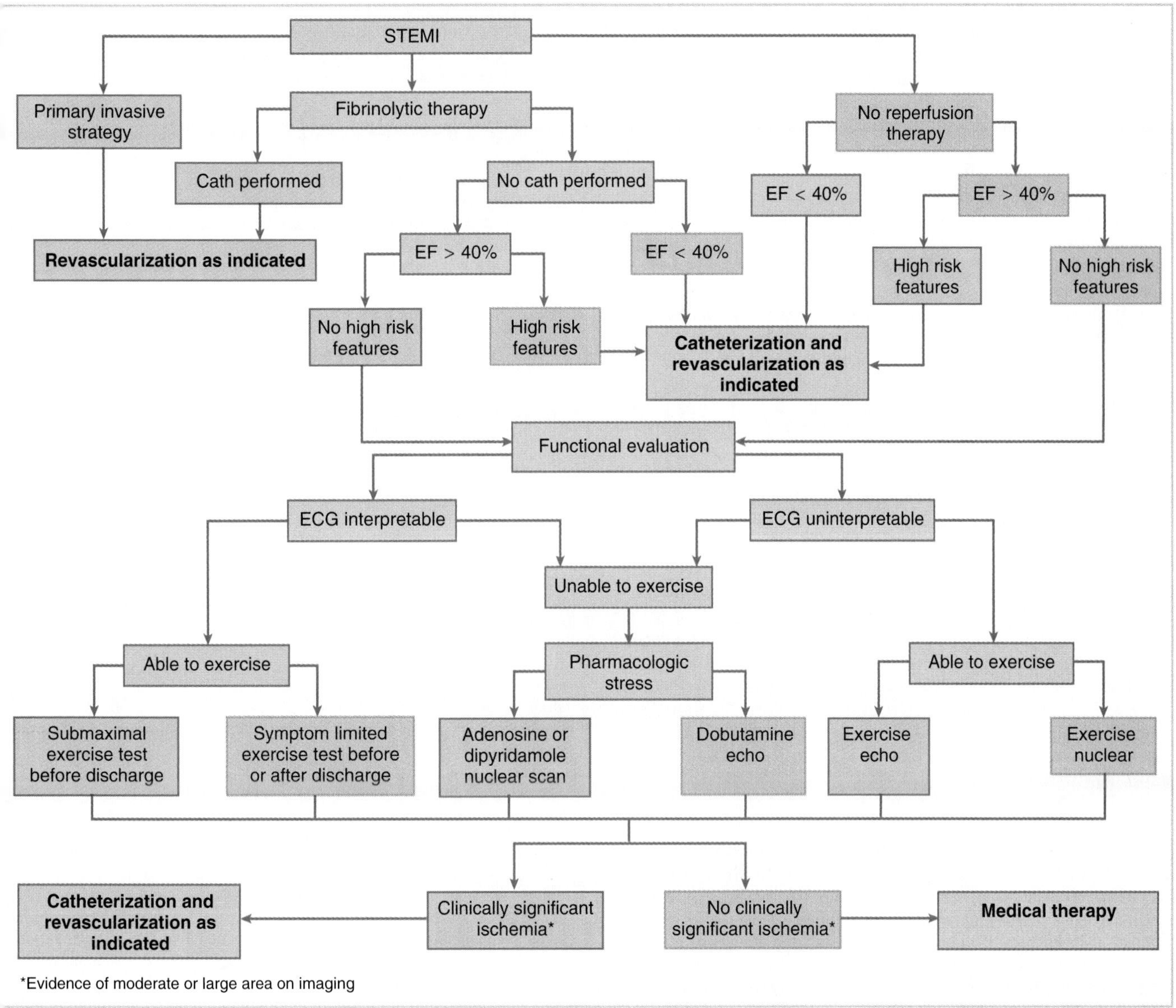

FIGURE 47–36 Algorithm for catheterization and revascularization after ST segment elevation myocardial infarction (STEMI). The algorithm shows the treatment paths for patients who initially undergo a primary invasive strategy, receive fibrinolytic therapy, or do not undergo reperfusion therapy for STEMI. Patients who have not undergone a primary invasive strategy and have no high-risk features should undergo functional evaluation using one of the noninvasive tests shown. When clinically significant ischemia (evidence of moderate or large area of ischemia by imaging) is detected, patients should undergo catheterization and revascularization as indicated; if no clinically significant ischemia is detected, medical therapy is prescribed post-STEMI. (From Antman EM, et al: ACC/AHA Guidelines for the Management of Patients with ST-Elevation Myocardial Infarction. 2004 [http://www.acc.org/clinical/guidelines/stemi/index.htm].)

ity and other indicators of electrical instability, such as reduced heart rate variability or baroreflex sensitivity and an abnormal signal-averaged electrocardiogram. All of these identify patients at increased risk of death.

In addition, patients with an occluded infarct-related artery late (e.g., 1 to 2 weeks) after STEMI have a higher long-term mortality rate.[29] Persistent occlusion of the culprit artery is associated with an increased incidence of abnormal late potentials on the electrocardiogram and appears to have an adverse prognostic effect independent of the level of ventricular function.

ASSESSMENT OF LEFT VENTRICULAR FUNCTION. Left ventricular ejection fraction may be the most easily assessed measurement of left ventricular function and is extremely useful for risk stratification (see Fig. 47–25). However, imaging of the left ventricle at rest may not distinguish adequately between infarcted, irreversibly damaged, and stunned or hibernating myocardium. To circumvent this difficulty, a variety of techniques has been investigated to assess the extent of residual viable myocardium, including exercise and pharmacological stress echocardiography, stress radionuclide ventricular angiography, perfusion imaging in conjunction with pharmacological stress, and positron emission tomography.[236] All of these techniques can be performed safely in postinfarction patients. Since no study has clearly shown one imaging modality to be superior to others, clinicians should be guided in their selection of ventricular imaging technique by the availability and level of expertise with a given modality at their local institution.[143,228,237]

In patients with low left ventricular ejection fraction, the measurement of exercise capacity is useful for further identifying those patients at particularly high risk and also for establishing safe exercise limits after discharge.[238] Patients with a good exercise capacity despite a reduced ejection fraction have a better long-term outcome than those who cannot perform more than modest exercise.

ASSESSMENT OF MYOCARDIAL ISCHEMIA. Because of the potent adverse consequences of recurrent myocardial infarction after STEMI, it is important to assess a patient's risk for future ischemia and infarction. Given the increasing array of pharmacological, interventional catheterization, and surgical options available to modify the likelihood of developing recurrent episodes of myocardial ischemia, most clinicians find it helpful to identify patients at risk for provocable myocardial ischemia prior to discharge. A predischarge evaluation for ischemia allows clinicians to select patients who might benefit from catheterization and revascularization following STEMI and to assess the adequacy of medical therapy for those patients who are suitable for a more conservative management strategy (see Fig. 47–36).

Exercise Testing. An exercise test also offers the clinician an opportunity to formulate a more precise exercise prescription and is helpful in boosting patients' confidence in their ability to conduct their daily activities after discharge. Patients who are unable to exercise can be evaluated by the use of a pharmacological stress protocol, such as an infusion of dobutamine or dipyridamole with echocardiography or perfusion imaging (see Fig. 47–36).

Treadmill exercise testing after STEMI has traditionally utilized a submaximal protocol that requires the patient to exercise until symptoms of angina appear, electrocardiographic evidence of ischemia is seen, or a target workload (approximately 5 metabolic equivalents) has been reached (see Chap. 10). It has been proposed that symptom-limited exercise tests can be safely performed before discharge in patients with an uncomplicated postinfarction course in-hospital.[238] Variables derived from exercise tests after STEMI that have been evaluated for their ability to predict the occurrence of death or recurrent nonfatal infarction include the development and magnitude of ST segment depression, the development of angina, exercise capacity, and the systolic blood pressure response during exercise.

The DANAMI (Danish Acute Myocardial Infarction) investigators reported that when patients with provocable ischemia after infarction were randomized to catheterization and revascularization versus conservative medical therapy, they experienced a lower requirement for antianginal medications, less unstable angina, and fewer nonfatal infarctions.[239] These observations, coupled with emerging data on the potential benefits of PCI after fibrinolysis, lend support for the increasingly common practice of routine referral for catheterization after lytic therapy.

ASSESSMENT FOR ELECTRICAL INSTABILITY. After STEMI, patients are at greatest risk for the development of sudden cardiac death due to malignant ventricular arrhythmias over the course of the first 1 to 2 years.[240] Several techniques have been devised to stratify patients into those who are at increased risk of sudden death following STEMI: measurement of Q-T dispersion (variability of Q-T intervals between ECG leads), ambulatory ECG recordings for detection of ventricular arrhythmias (Holter monitoring), invasive electrophysiological testing, recording a signal-averaged electrocardiogram (a measure of delayed, fragmented conduction in the infarct zone), and measuring heart rate variability (beat-to-beat variability in R-R intervals) or baroreflex sensitivity (slope of a line relating beat-to-beat change in sinus rate in response to alteration of blood pressure).[207]

Despite the increased risk of arrhythmic events following acute myocardial infarction in patients who are found to have abnormal results on one or more of the noninvasive tests described earlier, several points should be emphasized. The low positive predictive value (<30 percent) for the noninvasive screening tests limits their usefulness when viewed in isolation. Although the predictive value of screening tests can be improved by combining several of them together, the therapeutic implications of an increased risk profile for arrhythmic events have not been established. The mortality reductions achievable with the general use of beta blockers, ACE inhibitors, aspirin, and revascularization when appropriate after infarction, coupled with concerns about the efficacy and safety of antiarrhythmic drugs and the cost of implanted defibrillators, leave considerable uncertainty about the therapeutic implications of an abnormal noninvasive test for electrical instability in an asymptomatic patient. Additional data on patient outcomes when clinicians act on the results of an abnormal finding are required before definitive recommendations can be made for asymptomatic patients.[166] The management of patients with sustained, hemodynamically compromising arrhythmias is discussed in Chapters 30 and 31.

PROPHYLACTIC ANTIARRHYTHMIC THERAPY. Although it has been recognized for decades that antiarrhythmic therapy can control atrial and ventricular arrhythmias effectively in many patients, reviews of clinical trials following STEMI have reported an increased risk of mortality with type I drugs. The most notable postinfarction trial in this area was the Cardiac Arrhythmia Suppression Trial (CAST), which tested whether encainide, flecainide, or moricizine for suppression of ventricular arrhythmias detected on ambulatory electrocardiographic monitoring would reduce the risk of cardiac arrest and death over the long term. Both the first phase of the trial (encainide or flecainide versus placebo) and the second phase of the trial (moricizine versus placebo) were stopped prematurely because of increased mortality in the active treatment groups. The mechanism of the increased risk after STEMI remains a subject of investigation, but one hypothesis that has been put forth is an adverse interaction between recurrent ischemia and the presence of an antiarrhythmic drug because the risk of death or cardiac arrest was greater in patients with a non-Q-wave acute myocardial infarction than with Q-wave myocardial infarction. Sodium channel blockade by antiarrhythmics may exacerbate electrophysiological differences between subepicardial and subendocardial zones of myocardium, rendering the latter more susceptible to ischemic injury.

Subsequent to CAST, another postinfarction prophylactic antiarrhythmic drug trial was undertaken with oral D-sotalol (Survival With ORal D-sotalol, or SWORD). This trial was designed to test the hypothesis that prophylactic administration of D-sotalol to patients with depressed left ventricular function (ejection fraction < 40 percent) and either a recent (6 to 42 days) or remote (42 days) acute myocardial infarction would reduce total mortality. SWORD also was stopped prematurely after enrollment of only 3121 of a planned 6400 patients because statistical evidence of increased mortality emerged in the active treatment group.

The Canadian Amiodarone Myocardial Infarction Trial (CAMIAT) showed that amiodarone reduced the frequency of ventricular premature depolarization in patients with recent myocardial infarction; this correlated with a reduction in arrhythmic death or resuscitation from ventricular fibrillation.[241] However, 42 percent of patients discontinued amiodarone during maintenance therapy in CAMIAT because of intolerable side effects. The European Amiodarone Myocardial Infarction Trial (EMIAT) showed a reduction in arrhythmic death after myocardial infarction in patients with depressed left ventricular function, but there was no reduction in total mortality or other cardiovascular-related mortality.[242]

RECOMMENDATIONS. At this time, the *routine* use of antiarrhythmic agents (including amiodarone) cannot be recommended. Given the data cited earlier on the protective effects of beta-adrenoceptor blockers against sudden death and the ability of aspirin to reduce the risk of reinfarction, it is unclear that additional mortality reductions would be achieved by the empirical addition of amiodarone in the patient who is convalescing from a STEMI and is free of symptomatic sustained ventricular arrhythmias.

Several trials that included post-STEMI patients in the study population have shown significant mortality reductions in patients randomized to ICD implantation versus conventional medical therapy (see Chap. 31). At present, the selection of STEMI patients who are candidates for ICD implantation is based on the left ventricular ejection fraction and the time since the acute STEMI event. An algorithm incorporating these factors is given in Figure 47–37.

Secondary Prevention of Acute Myocardial Infarction (see Chap. 42)

The concept of secondary prevention of reinfarction and death after recovery from a STEMI has been investigated actively for several decades. Problems in proving the efficacy of various interventions have been related both to the ineffectiveness of certain strategies and to the difficulty in proving a benefit as mortality and morbidity have improved after STEMI. Nevertheless, patients who survive the initial course of STEMI are at increased risk because of coronary artery disease and its complications; therefore, it is imperative that efforts be made to reduce this risk. Although secondary prevention drug trials generally have tested one form of therapy against placebo in an attempt to demonstrate a benefit of that therapy, the physician must remember that disciplined clinical care of the individual patient is far more important than rote use of an agent found beneficial in the latest drug trial.

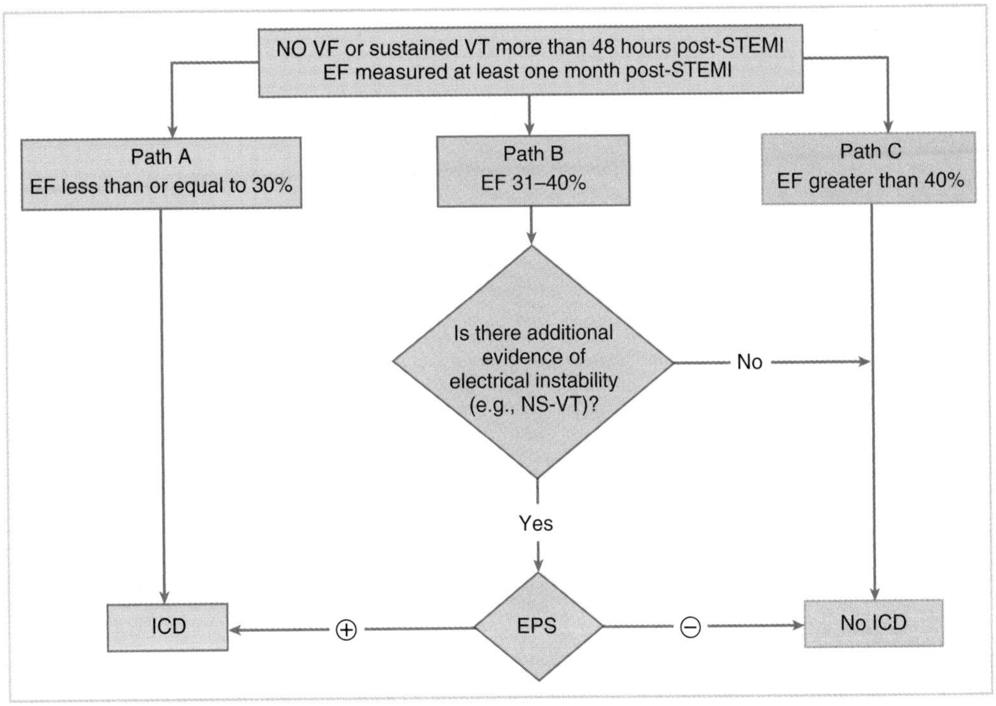

FIGURE 47–37 Algorithm for assessment of need for electrophysiological study and implantation of an implantable cardioverter-defibrillator (ICD) in ST segment elevation myocardial infarction (STEMI) patients without ventricular fibrillation (VF) or sustained ventricular tachycardia (VT) more than 72 hours after STEMI. The appropriate management path is selected based on the timing and measurement of left ventricular ejection fraction (EF) (see table at top of figure). EF measurements obtained 3 days or less after STEMI should be repeated before proceeding with the algorithm. In path A, patients with markedly depressed left ventricular function at least 1 month post-STEMI are referred for insertion of an ICD. Path B illustrates the management of patients in an intermediate-risk category who require further evaluation with an electrophysiology study (EPS). If the EPS reveals inducible ventricular tachycardia/ventricular fibrillation, an ICD is implanted; if the EPS is negative, no ICD is implanted and the patient receives medical therapy post-STEMI. Path C illustrates the management of patients with preserved left ventricular function who do not receive an ICD and are treated with medical therapy post-STEMI. LOE = level of evidence; NS-VT = nonsustained ventricular tachycardia. (From Antman EM, et al: ACC/AHA Guidelines for the Management of Patients with ST-Elevation Myocardial Infarction. 2004 [http://www.acc.org/clinical/guidelines/stemi/index.htm].)

LIFE-STYLE MODIFICATION. Efforts to improve survival and the quality of life after myocardial infarction that relate to life-style modification of known risk factors are considered in Chapter 42. Of these, cessation of smoking and control of hypertension are probably most important. It has been shown that within 2 years of quitting smoking, the risk of a nonfatal myocardial infarction in former smokers falls to a level similar to that in patients who never smoked. Being hospitalized for a STEMI is a powerful motivation for patients to cease cigarette smoking, and this is an ideal time to encourage that clearly beneficial and highly cost-effective life-style change. It is also an ideal time to begin to treat hypertension, to counsel patients to achieve optimal body weight, and to consider various strategies to improve the patient's lipid profile.[7]

DEPRESSION. Physicians caring for patients following a STEMI need to be sensitive to the fact that some patients experience major depression after infarction, and the development of this problem is an independent risk factor for mortality. In addition, lack of an emotionally supportive network in the patient's environment after discharge is associated with an increased risk of mortality and recurrent cardiac events.[7] The precise mechanisms relating depression and lack of social support to worse prognosis after STEMI are not clear, but one possibility is lack of adherence to prescribed treatments, a behavior that has been shown to be associated with increased risk of mortality after infarction.[7] Evidence exists that a comprehensive rehabilitation program utilizing primary health care personnel who counsel patients and make home visits favorably impacts the clinical course of patients after infarction and reduces the rate of rehospitalization for recurrent ischemia and infarction. A supportive physician attitude can also have a positive impact on the rate of return to work after STEMI.

MODIFICATION OF LIPID PROFILE. Compelling evidence now exists that an increased cholesterol level, and most importantly an increased low-density lipoprotein (LDL) cholesterol level, is associated with an increased risk of coronary heart disease (see Chap. 39). Based on this observation and the finding that lowering cholesterol reduces the risk of coronary heart disease, a target LDL cholesterol level of less than 100 mg/dl has been recommended in patients with clinically evident coronary heart disease.[243] This recommendation clearly applies to patients with STEMI, and it is therefore important to obtain a lipid profile on admission in all patients admitted with acute infarction. (It should be recalled that cholesterol levels may fall 24 to 48 hours after infarction.) In addition to lowering LDL cholesterol, therapy with statins reduces levels of C-reactive protein, suggesting an antiinflammatory effect.[244]

Surveys of physician practice in the past have revealed a disappointingly low rate of treatment of hypercholesterolemia in patients with proven coronary artery disease, indicating considerable room for improvement in this aspect of secondary prevention after STEMI.

Recommendations. The dietary prescription after STEMI should be low saturated fat (<7 percent of total calories) and low cholesterol (<200 mg/day). Patients with an LDL cholesterol level greater than 100 mg/dl should be discharged on statin therapy with the goal of reducing the LDL level to less than 70 mg/dl (see Chap. 49). It is also reasonable to prescribe statin therapy to patients recovering from STEMI whose LDL cholesterol level is either unknown or is less than 100 mg/dl.[7] For many patients recovering from an acute myocardial infarction, a low high-density lipoprotein cholesterol level is their primary lipid abnormality. Gemfibrozil (1200 mg/day) reduces the risk of death, reinfarction, and stroke in such patients.[7]

ANTIPLATELET AGENTS. On the basis of the compelling data from the Antiplatelet Trialists' Collaboration of a 22 percent reduction in the risk of recurrent infarction, stroke, or vascular death in high-risk vascular patients receiving prolonged antiplatelet therapy in the absence of a true aspirin allergy, all STEMI patients should receive 75 to 162 mg of aspirin daily indefinitely.[123,138] Additional benefits of long-term aspirin that can accrue in the STEMI patient are an increased likelihood of patency of the infarct artery and smaller infarcts if recurrent myocardial infarction does take place. Patients with true aspirin allergy can be treated with clopidogrel (75 mg once daily), based on experience from patients with unstable angina/non-ST segment elevation myocardial infarction (see Chap. 49).

INHIBITION OF THE RENIN-ANGIOTENSIN-ALDOSTERONE SYSTEM. The rationale for inhibition of this neurohormonal axis after STEMI was discussed earlier. To prevent late remodeling of the left ventricle and also to decrease the likelihood of recurrent ischemic events, we advocate indefinite therapy with an ACE inhibitor to all patients with clinically evident congestive heart failure, a moderate decrease in global ejection fraction, or a large regional wall-motion abnormality, even in the face of a normal global ejection fraction. Once the STEMI patient is discharged from the hospital, the evidence base on long-term management of patients with chronic coronary artery disease is the most relevant for long-term decision-making. Based on the results of the HOPE and EUROPA trials, we advocate indefinite treatment with an ACE inhibitor in all STEMI patients, provided no contraindications exist.[245,246] As discussed earlier, the VALIANT trial results suggest that valsartan may be used as an alternative to an ACE inhibitor for long-term management of patients with left ventricular dysfunction after STEMI.[161]

BETA-ADRENOCEPTOR BLOCKERS. Meta-analyses of trials from the prethrombolytic era involving more than 24,000 patients who received beta-adrenoceptor blockers in the convalescent phase of STEMI have shown a 23 percent reduction in long-term mortality (see Fig. 47-19). When beta blockade is initiated early (6 hours) in the acute phase of infarction and continued in the chronic phase of treatment, some of the benefit may result from a reduction in infarct size. In the majority of patients who have beta blockade initiated during the convalescent phase of STEMI, however, reduction in long-term mortality is probably due to a combination of an antiarrhythmic effect (prevention of sudden death) and prevention of reinfarction. Beta blockade over the long term is also effective for reducing the rate of mortality in patients who have undergone revascularization.[247]

Given the well-documented benefits of beta-adrenoceptor blockade, it is disturbing that this form of therapy continues to be underutilized, especially in high-risk groups such as the elderly.[7] Patients with a relative contraindication to beta blockade (moderate heart failure, bradyarrhythmias) should undergo a monitored trial of therapy in the hospital. The dosage should be sufficient to blunt the heart rate response to stress or exercise. Much of the impact of beta blockers in preventing mortality occurs in the first weeks; treatment should commence as soon as possible. Evidence exists that programs providing physician feedback improve adherence to guidelines such as those noted earlier for prescription of beta-adrenoceptor blockers after acute myocardial infarction.[1]

Some controversy exists as to how long patients should be treated. The collective data from five trials providing information on long-term follow-up of beta-adrenoceptor blockers after infarction suggest that therapy should be continued for at least 2 to 3 years (see Fig. 47-19). At that time, if the beta blocker is well tolerated and if there is no reason to discontinue therapy, such therapy probably should be continued in most patients.

Not all patients derive the same benefit from beta blocker therapy. The cost-effectiveness of treatment in medium- or high-risk persons compares very favorably with that of many other accepted interventions, such as coronary bypass surgery, angioplasty, and lipid-lowering therapy. In patients with an extremely good prognosis (first acute myocardial infarction, good ventricular function, no angina, negative stress test result, and no complex ventricular ectopy) among whom a mortality rate of

TABLE 47–14 Aspirin vs. Warfarin Therapy after ST-Elevation Myocardial Infarction (STEMI)

Study	Study Design	Drugs Used	ASA	Second Arm	Third Arm
STEMI-Specific Trials					
WARIS II*	Randomized Open label N = 3630 FU = Mean 4 yr	ASA monotherapy vs. warfarin monotherapy vs. warfarin + ASA	160 mg daily	Dosed to target INR 2.8-4.2	Dosed to target INR 2.0-2.5 + ASA 75 mg daily
APRICOT II†	Randomized Open label N = 308 FU = 3 mo	ASA monotherapy vs. warfarin + ASA	If TIMI grade 3 post 48 hr UFH then 160 mg initially and then 80 mg daily	Dosed to target INR 2-3 if TIMI 3 post 48 hr UFH + 160 mg initially and then 80 mg daily	N/A
Trials not Specific to STEMI					
ASPECT II‡	Randomized Open label N = 999 FU = 26 mo	ASA monotherapy vs. warfarin monotherapy vs.warfarin + ASA	80 mg daily	Dosed to target INR 3-4	Dosed to target INR 2-2.5 + ASA 80 mg daily
CHAMP§	Randomized Open label N = 5059 FU = median 2.7 yr	ASA monotherapy vs. warfarin +ASA	162 mg daily	Dosed to target INR 1.5-2.5 + 81 mg ASA daily	N/A
CARS¶	Randomized Blinded N = 8803 FU = 33 mo Median = 14 mo	ASA monotherapy vs. warfarin 1 mg + ASA	160 mg daily (avg INR @ wk 4 = 1.02	1 mg + 80 mg ASA (avg INR @ wk 4 = 1.05)	N/A

N/A = not applicable; ASA = acetylsalicylic acid (aspirin); FU = follow-up; INR = international normalized ratio; MI = myocardial infarction; STEMI = ST-elevation myocardial infarction; Tx = treatment; UA = unstable angina; UFH = unfractionated heparin.

*Hurlen M, et al: N Engl J Med 347:969, 2002.

†Brouwer MA, et al: Circulation 106:659, 2002.

‡Van Es RF, et al: Lancet 360:109, 2002.

approximately 1 percent per year can be anticipated, beta blockers would have a smaller impact on survival. However, it is our preference to prescribe beta blockers to such patients for whatever postinfarction benefit is achieved and also to have them as part of the patient's usual regimen should acute myocardial infarction recur at an unpredictable time in the future.

NITRATES. Although these agents are suitable for management of specific conditions after STEMI, such as recurrent angina or as part of a treatment regimen for congestive heart failure, little evidence indicates that they reduce mortality over the long term when prescribed on a routine basis to all patients with infarction.[7]

ANTICOAGULANTS. At least three theoretical reasons exist for anticipating that anticoagulants might be beneficial in the long-term management of patients after STEMI. (1) Because the coronary occlusion responsible for the STEMI is often due to a thrombus, anticoagulants might be expected to halt progression, slow progression, or prevent the development of new thrombi elsewhere in the coronary arterial tree. (2) Anticoagulants might be expected to diminish the formation of mural thrombi and resultant systemic embolization. (3) Anticoagulants might be expected to reduce the incidence of venous thrombosis and pulmonary embolization.

After several decades of evaluation, the weight of evidence now suggests that anticoagulants have a favorable effect on late mortality, stroke, and reinfarction among patients hospitalized with STEMI (Table 47-14). Given the complexities of combining long-term therapy with warfarin alone with antiplatelet therapy, clinicians must weigh the need for warfarin based on established indications for anticoagulation and the risk of bleeding. An algorithm to guide decision-making is given in Figure 47-38.

CALCIUM ANTAGONISTS. At present, we do not recommend the routine use of calcium antagonists for secondary prevention of infarction. A possible exception is a patient who cannot tolerate a beta-adrenoceptor blocker because of adverse effects on bronchospastic lung disease but who has well-preserved left ventricular function; such patients may be candidates for a rate-slowing calcium antagonist such as diltiazem or verapamil.

HORMONE THERAPY. The decision to prescribe hormone therapy is often a complex one that involves the desire to suppress postmenopausal symptoms versus the risks of breast and endometrial cancer and vascular events. Despite improvement in lipid profiles, hormone therapy with estrogen plus progestin to postmenopausal women with established coronary heart disease does not prevent recurrent coronary events and is associated with significantly increased risk of coronary heart disease and venous thromboembolic events.[7] At present, we recommend not starting hormone therapy with estrogen plus progestin after STEMI and discontinuing it in postmenopausal women after STEMI.

ANTIOXIDANTS. Dietary supplementation with omega-3 polyunsaturated fatty acids has been associated with a reduction in congestive heart disease death and nonfatal reinfarction in patients within 3 months of a myocardial infarction.[248] Vitamin E (300 mg/day) was not associated with any significant clinical benefit, however.[248]

		Results		
Patients	**Endpoints**	*ASA Alone*	*Warfarin Alone*	*ASA + Warfarin*
Age < 75 yr Hospitalized for acute MI **% STEMI = 71.8**	Death, nonfatal reinfarction, or thromboembolic stroke Major, nonfatal bleeding ($p < 0.001$)	20% 0.17%	16.7% ($p = 0.03$ vs. ASA) 0.68%	15% ($p = 0.001$ vs. ASA) 0.57%
Age ≤ 76 yr Acute ST MI ≤ 6 hr prior to thrombolytic Tx **% STEMI = 100**	Reooclusion (TIMI ≤ 2) ($p < 0.02$) Total occlusion (TIMI 0-1) ($p < 0.02$) Revascularization ($p < 0.01$) Reinfarction ($p < 0.05$) Event-free survival rate* ($p < 0.01$) Bleeding (TIMI major and minor ($p = NS$)	28% 20% 31% 8% 66% 3%	N/A	15% 9% 13% 2% 86% 5%
Acute MI or UA within preceding 8 wk	Death, MI, or stroke ($p = 0.0479$) Major bleeding Minor bleeding ($p < 0.0001$) Almost 20% of the warfarin and combined group discontinued therapy; 40% in therapeutic range	9% 1% 5%	5% 1% 8%	5% 2% 15%
Acute MI within preceding 14 days prior to enrollment	Death ($p = 0.76$) Recurrent MI ($p = 0.78$) Stroke ($p = 0.52$) Major bleeding ($p = 0.001$)	17.3% 13.1% 3.5% 0.72**	N/A	17.6% 13.3% 3.1% 1.2**
Age 21-85 yr (82% < 70 yr) MI 3-21 days (mean 9.6 days) prior to enrollment	Ischemic stroke ($p = 0.0534$)	0.6%	N/A	1.1%

§Fiore LD, et al: Circulation 105:557, 2002.
¶O'Connor CM, et al: Am J Cardiol 88:541, 2001.
**Reported as number of events per 100 person-years of follow-up.
Adapted from Antman EM, et al: ACC/AHA Guidelines for the Management of Patients with ST-Elevation Myocardial Infarction. 2004 (http://www.acc.org/clinical/guidelines/stemi/index.htm).

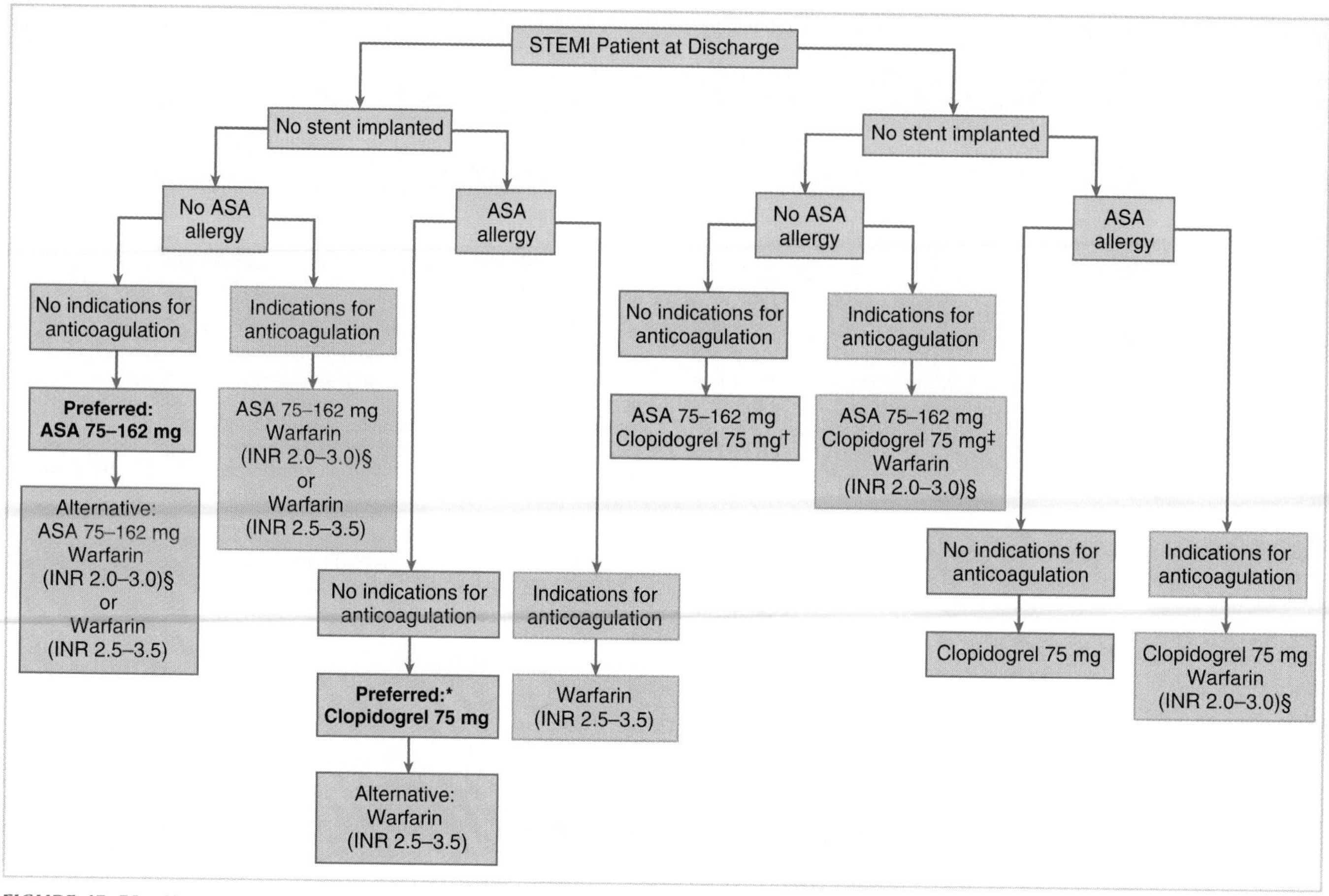

FIGURE 47–38 Algorithm for antithrombotic therapy at hospital discharge after ST segment elevation myocardial ischemia (STEMI). *Clopidogrel is preferred over warfarin due to increased risk of bleeding and low patient compliance in warfarin trials. †For 12 months. ‡Discontinue clopidogrel 1 month after implantation of a bare metal stent or several months after implantation of a drug-eluting stent (3 months after sirolimus and 6 months after paclitaxel) because of the potential increased risk of bleeding with warfarin and two antiplatelet agents. Continue ASA and warfarin long term if warfarin is indicated for other reasons such as atrial fibrillation, LV thrombus, cerebral emboli, or extensive regional wall motion abnormality. §An INR of 2.0–3.0 is acceptable with tight control, but the lower end of this range is preferable. The combination of antiplatelet therapy and warfarin may be considered in patients aged less than 75 years, with low bleeding risk, who can be monitored reliably. ASA = acetylsalicyclic acid; INR = international normalized ratio; LV = left ventricular. (From Antman EM, et al: ACC/AHA Guidelines for the Management of Patients with ST-Elevation Myocardial Infarction. 2004 [http://www.acc.org/clinical/guidelines/stemi/index.htm].)

REFERENCES

1. Mehta RH, Montoye CK, Gallogly M, et al: Improving quality of care for acute myocardial infarction: The Guidelines Applied in Practice (GAP) Initiative. JAMA 287:1269, 2002.
2. Jencks SF, Huff ED, Cuerdon T: Change in the quality of care delivered to Medicare beneficiaries, 1998-1999 to 2000-2001. JAMA 289:305, 2003.
3. National Committee for Quality Assurance: The State of Health Care Quality. Washington, DC, NCQA, 2003.
4. Schneider EC, Zaslavsky AM, Epstein AM: Racial disparities in the quality of care for enrollees in medicare managed care. JAMA 287:1288, 2002.
5. Faxon D, Lenfant C: Timing is everything: Motivating patients to call 9-1-1 at onset of acute myocardial infarction. Circulation 104:1210, 2001.

Prehospital Care

6. Luepker RV, Raczynski JM, Osganian S, et al: Effect of a community intervention on patient delay and emergency medical service use in acute coronary heart disease: The Rapid Early Action for Coronary Treatment (REACT) Trial. JAMA 284:60, 2000.
7. Antman EM, et al: ACC/AHA Guidelines for the Management of Patients with ST-Elevation Myocardial Infarction. 2004 (http://www.acc.org/clinical/guidelines/stemi/index.htm).
8. Ornato JP, Hand MM: Warning signs of a heart attack. Circulation 104:1212, 2001.
9. Canto JG, Zalenski RJ, Ornato JP, et al: Use of emergency medical services in acute myocardial infarction and subsequent quality of care: Observations from the National Registry of Myocardial Infarction 2. Circulation 106:3018, 2002.
10. National Heart Lung and Blood Institute: Act in time to heart attack signs. Accessed 10/6/03. (www.nhlbi.nih.gov/actintime)
11. American Heart Association. Accessed 10/6/03. (www.americanheart.org.)
12. Caffrey SL, Willoughby PJ, Pepe PE, et al: Public use of automated external defibrillators. N Engl J Med 347:1242, 2002.
13. Gibson CM: Time is myocardium and time is outcomes. Circulation 104:2632, 2001.
14. Morrow DA, Antman EM, Giugliano RP, et al: A simple risk index for rapid initial triage of patients with ST-elevation myocardial infarction: An InTIME II substudy. Lancet 358:1571, 2001.
15. Morrison LJ, Verbeek PR, McDonald AC, et al: Mortality and prehospital thrombolysis for acute myocardial infarction: A meta-analysis. JAMA 283:2686, 2000.
16. Bonnefoy E, Lapostolle F, Leizorovicz A, et al: Primary angioplasty versus prehospital fibrinolysis in acute myocardial infarction: A randomised study. Lancet 360:825, 2002.
17. Steg G, Bonnefoy E, Chabaud S, et al: Impact of time to treatment on mortality after prehospital fibrinolysis or primary angioplasty: Data from the CAPTIM randomized clinical trial. Circulation 108:2851, 2003.
18. Hanamia G, Sauval P, LaBlanche JM, et al: Impact of prehospital thrombolysis on 1-month outcome after ST-elevation myocardial infarction: Data from the nationwide French USIC 2000 survey. Abstract 2703. Vienna, European Society of Cardiology, 2003.
19. Fibrinolytic Therapy Trialists (FTT) Collaborative Group: Indications for fibrinolytic therapy in suspected acute myocardial infarction: Collaborative overview of early mortality and major morbidity results from all randomised trials of more than 1000 patients. Lancet 343:311, 1994.
20. Pedley DK, Bissett K, Connolly EM, et al: Prospective observational cohort study of time saved by prehospital thrombolysis for ST elevation myocardial infarction delivered by paramedics. BMJ 327:22, 2003.

Care in the Emergency Department

21. Hamm CW, Bertrand M, Braunwald E: Acute coronary syndrome without ST elevation: Implementation of new guidelines. Lancet 358:1533, 2001.
22. Van de Werf F, Ardissino D, Betriu A, et al: Management of acute myocardial infarction in patients presenting with ST-segment elevation. The Task Force on the Management of Acute Myocardial Infarction of the European Society of Cardiology. Eur Heart J 24:28, 2003.
23. Califf RM, Faxon DP: Need for centers to care for patients with acute coronary syndromes. Circulation 107:1467, 2003.
24. Willerson JT: Editor's commentary: Centers of excellence. Circulation 107:1471, 2003.
25. Braunwald E, Antman EM, Beasley JW, et al: ACC/AHA 2002 guideline update for the management of patients with unstable angina and non-ST-segment elevation myocardial infarction—Summary article: A report of the American College of Cardiology/

American Heart Association task force on practice guidelines (Committee on the Management of Patients With Unstable Angina). J Am Coll Cardiol 40:1366, 2002.
26. Pfisterer M: Right ventricular involvement in myocardial infarction and cardiogenic shock. Lancet 362:392, 2003.
27. Holmes DR Jr: Cardiogenic shock: A lethal complication of acute myocardial infarction. Rev Cardiovasc Med 4:131, 2003.
28. Schomig A, Ndrepepa G, Mehilli J, et al: Therapy-dependent influence of time-to-treatment interval on myocardial salvage in patients with acute myocardial infarction treated with coronary artery stenting or thrombolysis. Circulation 108:1084, 2003.
29. Sadanandan S, Buller CE, Menon V, et al: The late open artery hypothesis—A decade later. Am Heart J 142:411, 2001.
30. Gibson CM: Has my patient achieved adequate myocardial reperfusion? Circulation 108:504, 2003.
31. Granger CB, Mahaffey KW, Weaver WD, et al: Pexelizumab, an anti-C5 complement antibody, as adjunctive therapy to primary percutaneous coronary intervention in acute myocardial infarction: The COMplement inhibition in Myocardial infarction treated with Angioplasty (COMMA) trial. Circulation 108:1184, 2003.
32. Kopecky SL, Aviles RJ, Bell MR, et al: A randomized, double-blinded, placebo-controlled, dose-ranging study measuring the effect of an adenosine agonist on infarct size reduction in patients undergoing primary percutaneous transluminal coronary angioplasty: The ADMIRE (AmP579 Delivery for Myocardial Infarction REduction) study. Am Heart J 146:146, 2003.
33. Przyklenk K, Bauer B, Ovize M, et al: Regional ischemic 'preconditioning' protects remote virgin myocardium from subsequent sustained coronary occlusion. Circulation 87:893, 1993.
34. Katritsis D, Karvouni E, Webb-Peploe MM: Reperfusion in acute myocardial infarction: Current concepts. Prog Cardiovasc Dis 45:481, 2003.
35. De Luca G, Suryapranata H, Zijlstra F, et al: Symptom-onset-to-balloon time and mortality in patients with acute myocardial infarction treated by primary angioplasty. J Am Coll Cardiol 42:991, 2003.
36. De Luca G, Suryapranata H, Ottervanger JP, et al: Time-delay to treatment and mortality in primary angioplasty for acute myocardial infarction: every minute counts. Circulation 109:1223, 2004.
37. Fujita M, Nakae I, Kihara Y, et al: Determinants of collateral development in patients with acute myocardial infarction. Clin Cardiol 22:595, 1999.
38. Bolli R, Marban E: Molecular and cellular mechanisms of myocardial stunning. Physiol Rev 79:609, 1999.
39. Gerber BL, Wijns W, Vanoverschelde JL, et al: Myocardial perfusion and oxygen consumption in reperfused noninfarcted dysfunctional myocardium after unstable angina: Direct evidence for myocardial stunning in humans. J Am Coll Cardiol 34:1939, 1999.
40. Davies CH, Ormerod OJ: Failed coronary thrombolysis. Lancet 351:1191, 1998.
41. Vargas SO, Sampson BA, Schoen FJ: Pathologic detection of early myocardial infarction: A critical review of the evolution and usefulness of modern techniques. Mod Pathol 12:635, 1999.
42. de Lemos JA, Gibson CM, Antman EM, et al: Abciximab and early adjunctive percutaneous coronary intervention are associated with improved ST-segment resolution after thrombolysis: Observations from the TIMI 14 Trial. Am Heart J 141:592, 2001.
43. Antman EM, Cooper HA, Gibson CM, et al: Determinants of improvement in epicardial flow and myocardial perfusion for ST elevation myocardial infarction: Insights from TIMI 14 and InTIME-II. Eur Heart J 23:928, 2002.
44. Baran KW, Nguyen M, McKendall GR, et al: Double-blind, randomized trial of an anti-CD18 antibody in conjunction with recombinant tissue plasminogen activator for acute myocardial infarction: Limitation of myocardial infarction following thrombolysis in acute myocardial infarction (LIMIT AMI) study. Circulation 104:2778, 2001.
45. Faxon DP, Gibbons RJ, Chronos NA, et al: The effect of blockade of the CD11/CD18 integrin receptor on infarct size in patients with acute myocardial infarction treated with direct angioplasty: The results of the HALT-MI study. J Am Coll Cardiol 40:1199, 2002.
46. Wang K, Zhou X, Zhou Z, et al: Recombinant soluble P-selectin glycoprotein ligand-Ig (rPSGL-Ig) attenuates infarct size and myeloperoxidase activity in a canine model of ischemia-reperfusion. Thromb Haemost 88:149, 2002.
47. Mahaffey KW, Granger CB, Nicolau JC, et al: Effect of pexelizumab, an anti-C5 complement antibody, as adjunctive therapy to fibrinolysis in acute myocardial infarction: The COMPlement inhibition in myocardial infarction treated with thromboLYtics (COMPLY) trial. Circulation 108:1176, 2003.
48. Magnesium in Coronaries (MAGIC) Trial Investigators: Early administration of intravenous magnesium to high-risk patients with acute myocardial infarction in the Magnesium in Coronaries (MAGIC) Trial: A randomised controlled trial. Lancet 360:1189, 2002.
49. van der Horst IC, Zijlstra F, van't Hof AW, et al: Glucose-insulin-potassium infusion inpatients treated with primary angioplasty for acute myocardial infarction: The glucose-insulin-potassium study: A randomized trial. J Am Coll Cardiol 42:784, 2003.
50. Gheorghiade M, Goldstein S: Beta-blockers in the post-myocardial infarction patient. Circulation 106:394, 2002.
51. Chiladakis JA, Patsouras N, Manolis AS: The Bezold-Jarisch reflex in acute inferior myocardial infarction: Clinical and sympathovagal spectral correlates. Clin Cardiol 26:323, 2003.
52. Hochman JS, Califf RM: Acute myocardial infarction. *In* Antman E (ed): Cardiovascular Therapeutics: A Companion to Braunwald's Heart Disease. 2nd ed. Philadelphia, WB Saunders, 2002, pp 233-291.
53. Sadanandan S, Hochman JS: Early reperfusion, late reperfusion, and the open artery hypothesis: An overview. Prog Cardiovasc Dis 42:397, 2000.
54. Kloner RA, Jennings RB: Consequences of brief ischemia: Stunning, preconditioning, and their clinical implications: Part 2. Circulation 104:3158, 2001.
55. Yousef ZR, Redwood SR, Bucknall CA, et al: Late intervention after anterior myocardial infarction: Effects on left ventricular size, function, quality of life, and exercise tolerance: Results of the Open Artery Trial (TOAT Study). J Am Coll Cardiol 40:869, 2002.
56. Van De Werf F, Baim DS: Reperfusion for ST-segment elevation myocardial infarction: An overview of current treatment options. Circulation 105:2813, 2002.
57. Nakatani D, Sato H, Kinjo K, et al: Effect of successful late reperfusion by primary coronary angioplasty on mechanical complications of acute myocardial infarction. Am J Cardiol 92:785, 2003.

Coronary Fibrinolysis

58. Boersma E, Mercado N, Poldermans D, et al: Acute myocardial infarction. Lancet 361:847, 2003.
59. Franzosi MG, Santoro E, De Vita C, et al: Ten-year follow-up of the first megatrial testing thrombolytic therapy in patients with acute myocardial infarction: Results of the Gruppo Italiano per lo Studio della Sopravvivenza nell'Infarto-1 study. The GISSI Investigators. Circulation 98:2659, 1998.
60. TIMI Study Group: The Thrombolysis in Myocardial Infarction (TIMI) Trial; Phase I findings. N Engl J Med 312:932, 1985.
61. Chesebro JH, Knatterud G, Roberts R, et al: Thrombolysis in Myocardial Infarction (TIMI) Trial, Phase 1: A comparison between intravenous tissue plasminogen activator and intravenous streptokinase. Circulation 76:142, 1987.
62. Antman EM, Giugliano RP, Gibson CM, et al: Abciximab facilitates the rate and extent of thrombolysis: Results of the thrombolysis in myocardial infarction (TIMI) 14 trial. The TIMI 14 Investigators. Circulation 99:2720, 1999.
63. Gibson CM, Murphy SA, Rizzo JM, et al: Relationship between TIMI frame count and clinical outcomes after thrombolytic administration. Thrombolysis In Myocardial Infarction (TIMI) Study Group. Circulation 99:1945, 1999.
64. Gibson CM, Murphy S, Menown IB, et al: Determinants of coronary blood flow after thrombolytic administration. TIMI Study Group. Thrombolysis in Myocardial Infarction. J Am Coll Cardiol 34:1403, 1999.
65. Schroder R: ST segment resolution on 12-lead ECG. Circulation 2004, in press.
66. Krucoff MW, Johanson P, Crater SW, et al: The clinical utility of serial and continuous ST-segment recovery in patients with acute ST elevation myocardial infarction: Assessing the dynamics of epicardial and myocardial reperfusion. Circulation 2004, in press.
67. Armstrong PW, Collen D, Antman E: Fibrinolysis for acute myocardial infarction: The future is here and now. Circulation 107:2533, 2003.
68. Angeja BG, Gunda M, Murphy SA, et al: TIMI myocardial perfusion grade and ST segment resolution: Association with infarct size as assessed by single photon emission computed tomography imaging. Circulation 105:282, 2002.
69. Boersma E, Maas AC, Deckers JW, et al: Early thrombolytic treatment in acute myocardial infarction: Reappraisal of the golden hour. Lancet 348:771, 1996.
70. Thiemann DR, Coresh J, Schulman SP, et al: Lack of benefit for intravenous thrombolysis in patients with myocardial infarction who are older than 75 years. Circulation 101:2239, 2000.
71. Berger AK, Radford MJ, Wang Y, et al: Thrombolytic therapy in older patients. J Am Coll Cardiol 36:366, 2000.
72. Stenestrand U, Wallentin L: Fibrinolytic therapy in patients 75 years and older with ST-segment-elevation myocardial infarction: One-year follow-up of a large prospective cohort. Arch Intern Med 163:965, 2003.
73. White HD: Thrombolytic therapy in the elderly. Lancet 356:2028, 2000.
74. Morrow DA, Antman EM, Charlesworth A, et al: TIMI risk score for ST-elevation myocardial infarction: A convenient, bedside, clinical score for risk assessment at presentation: An intravenous nPA for treatment of infarcting myocardium early II trial substudy. Circulation 102:2031, 2000.
75. Morrow DA, Antman EM, Parsons L, et al: Application of the TIMI risk score for ST-elevation MI in the National Registry of Myocardial Infarction 3. JAMA 286:1356, 2001.
76. Brouwer MA, van den Bergh PJ, Aengevaeren WR, et al: Aspirin plus coumarin versus aspirin alone in the prevention of reocclusion after fibrinolysis for acute myocardial infarction: Results of the Antithrombotics in the Prevention of Reocclusion In Coronary Thrombolysis (APRICOT)-2 Trial. Circulation 106:659, 2002.
77. Aversano T, Aversano LT, Passamani E, et al: Thrombolytic therapy vs primary percutaneous coronary intervention for myocardial infarction in patients presenting to hospitals without on-site cardiac surgery: A randomized controlled trial. JAMA 287:1943, 2002.
78. Llevadot J, Giugliano RP, Antman EM: Bolus fibrinolytic therapy in acute myocardial infarction. JAMA 286:442, 2001.
79. The Global Use of Strategies to Open Occluded Coronary Arteries (GUSTO III) Investigators: A comparison of reteplase with alteplase for acute myocardial infarction. N Engl J Med 337:1118, 1997.
80. Ware JH, Antman EM: Equivalence trials. N Engl J Med 337:1159, 1997.
81. White HD: Thrombolytic therapy and equivalence trials. J Am Coll Cardiol 31:494, 1998.
82. Cannon CP, McCabe CH, Gibson CM, et al: TNK-tissue plasminogen activator in acute myocardial infarction. Results of the Thrombolysis in Myocardial Infarction (TIMI) 10A dose-ranging trial. Circulation 95:351, 1997.
83. Cannon CP, Gibson CM, McCabe CH, et al: TNK-tissue plasminogen activator compared with front-loaded alteplase in acute myocardial infarction: Results of the TIMI 10B trial. Thrombolysis in Myocardial Infarction (TIMI) 10B Investigators. Circulation 98:2805, 1998.
84. Van de Werf F, Cannon CP, Luyten A, et al: Safety assessment of single-bolus administration of TNK tissue-plasminogen activator in acute myocardial infarction: The ASSENT-1 trial. The ASSENT-1 Investigators. Am Heart J 137:786, 1999.
85. Assessment of the Safety and Efficacy of a New Thrombolytic (ASSENT-2) Investigators: Single-bolus tenecteplase compared with front-loaded alteplase in acute myocardial infarction: The ASSENT-2 double-blind randomised trial. Assessment of the Safety and Efficacy of a New Thrombolytic Investigators. Lancet 354:716, 1999.
86. The InTIME-II Investigators: Intravenous NPA for the treatment of infarcting myocardium early; InTIME-II, a double-blind comparison of single-bolus lanoteplase

vs accelerated alteplase for the treatment of patients with acute myocardial infarction. Eur Heart J 21:2005, 2000.
87. Armstrong PW, Burton J, Pakola S, et al: Collaborative Angiographic Patency Trial Of Recombinant Staphylokinase (CAPTORS II). Am Heart J 146:484, 2003.
88. The GUSTO Angiographic Investigators: The comparative effects of tissue plasminogen activator, streptokinase, or both on coronary artery patency, ventricular function and survival after acute myocardial infarction. N Engl J Med 329:1615, 1993.
89. Dubois CL, Belmans A, Granger CB, et al: Outcome of urgent and elective percutaneous coronary interventions after pharmacologic reperfusion with tenecteplase combined with unfractionated heparin, enoxaparin, or abciximab. J Am Coll Cardiol 42:1178, 2003.
90. Gore JM, Granger CB, Simoons ML, et al: Stroke after thrombolysis: Mortality and functional outcomes in the GUSTO-I Trial. Circulation 92:2811, 1995.
91. Kleiman NS, Terrin M, Mueller H, et al: Mechanisms of early death despite thrombolytic therapy: Experience from the Thrombolysis in Myocardial Infarction Investigation Phase II (TIMI II) Study. J Am Coll Cardiol 19:1129, 1992.
92. Eagle KA, Goodman SG, Avezum A, et al: Practice variation and missed opportunities for reperfusion in ST-segment-elevation myocardial infarction: Findings from the Global Registry of Acute Coronary Events (GRACE). Lancet 359:373, 2002.
93. Assessment of the Safety and Efficacy of a New Thrombolytic Regimen (ASSENT)-3 Investigators: Efficacy and safety of tenecteplase in combination with enoxaparin, abciximab, or unfractionated heparin: The ASSENT-3 randomised trial in acute myocardial infarction. Lancet 358:605, 2001.
94. Van de Werf F, Barron HV, Armstrong PW, et al: Incidence and predictors of bleeding events after fibrinolytic therapy with fibrin-specific agents: A comparison of TNK-tPA and rt-PA. Eur Heart J 22:2253, 2001.
95. Giugliano RP, Antman EM: Caeteris paribus—All things being equal. Eur Heart J 22:2221, 2001.
96. Lee DC, Oz MC, Weinberg AD, et al: Optimal timing of revascularization: Transmural versus nontransmural acute myocardial infarction. Ann Thorac Surg 71:1197, discussion 1202, 2001.
97. Hasdai D, Behar S, Wallentin L, et al: A prospective survey of the characteristics, treatments and outcomes of patients with acute coronary syndromes in Europe and the Mediterranean basin: The Euro Heart Survey of Acute Coronary Syndromes (Euro Heart Survey ACS). Eur Heart J 23:1190, 2002.
98. Weaver WD: All hospitals are not equal for treatment of patients with acute myocardial infarction. Circulation 108:1768, 2003.
99. Keeley EC, Boura JA, Grines CL: Primary angioplasty versus intravenous thrombolytic therapy for acute myocardial infarction: A quantitative review of 23 randomised trials. Lancet 361:13, 2003.
100. Hochman JS, Sleeper LA, White HD, et al: One-year survival following early revascularization for cardiogenic shock. JAMA 285:190, 2001.
101. Wu AH, Parsons L, Every NR, et al: Hospital outcomes in patients presenting with congestive heart failure complicating acute myocardial infarction: A report from the Second National Registry of Myocardial Infarction (NRMI-2). J Am Coll Cardiol 40:1389, 2002.
102. Kent DM, Schmid CH, Lau J, et al: Is primary angioplasty for some as good as primary angioplasty for all? J Gen Intern Med 17:887, 2002.
103. Grzybowski M, Clements EA, Parsons L, et al: Mortality benefit of immediate revascularization of acute ST-segment elevation myocardial infarction in patients with contraindications to thrombolytic therapy: A propensity analysis. JAMA 290:1891, 2003.
104. Herrmann HC: Optimizing outcomes in ST-segment elevation myocardial infarction. J Am Coll Cardiol 42:1357, 2003.
105. Widimsky P, Budesinsky T, Vorac D, et al: Long distance transport for primary angioplasty vs immediate thrombolysis in acute myocardial infarction: Final results of the randomized national multicentre trial—PRAGUE-2. Eur Heart J 24:94, 2003.
106. Andersen HR, Nielsen TT, Rasmussen K, et al: A comparison of coronary angioplasty with fibrinolytic therapy in acute myocardial infarction. N Engl J Med 349:733, 2003.
107. Dalby M, Lechat P, Montalescot G: Transfer for primary angioplasty versus immediate thrombolysis in acute myocardial infarction. Circulation 108:1809, 2003.
108. Nallamothu BK, Bates ER: Percutaneous coronary intervention versus fibrinolytic therapy in acute myocardial infarction: Is timing (almost) everything? Am J Cardiol 92:824, 2003.

Antithrombin and Antiplatelet Therapy

109. ISIS-2 (Second International Study of Infarct Survival) Collaborative Group: Randomised trial of intravenous streptokinase, oral aspirin, both, or neither among 17,187 cases of suspected acute myocardial infarction: ISIS-2. Lancet 2:349, 1988.
110. Baigent C, Collins R: Aspirin and heparin. *In* Hennekens CH (ed): Clinical Trials in Cardiovascular Disease: Companion to Braunwald's Health Disease. Philadelphia, WB Saunders, 1999, p 60.
111. The Global Use of Strategies to Open Occluded Coronary Arteries (GUSTO) IIb Investigators: A comparison of recombinant hirudin with heparin for the treatment of acute coronary syndromes. N Engl J Med 335:775, 1996.
112. Menon V, Berkowitz SD, Antman EM, et al: New heparin dosing recommendations for patients with acute coronary syndromes. Am J Med 110:641, 2001.
113. Hirsh J, Anand SS, Halperin JL, et al: Guide to anticoagulant therapy: Heparin: A statement for healthcare professionals from the American Heart Association. Circulation 103:2994, 2001.
114. Antman EM: The search for replacements for unfractionated heparin. Circulation 103:2310, 2001.
115. Direct Thrombin Inhibitor Trialists' Collaborative Group: Direct thrombin inhibitors in acute coronary syndromes: Principal results of a meta-analysis based on individual patients' data. Lancet 359:294, 2002.
116. White H: Thrombin-specific anticoagulation with bivalirudin versus heparin in patients receiving fibrinolytic therapy for acute myocardial infarction: The HERO-2 randomised trial. Lancet 358:1855, 2001.
117. Ross AM, Molhoek P, Lundergan C, et al: Randomized comparison of enoxaparin, a low-molecular-weight heparin, with unfractionated heparin adjunctive to recombinant tissue plasminogen activator thrombolysis and aspirin: Second trial of Heparin and Aspirin Reperfusion Therapy (HART II). Circulation 104:648, 2001.
118. Simoons M, Krzeminska-Pakula M, Alonso A, et al: Improved reperfusion and clinical outcome with enoxaparin as an adjunct to streptokinase thrombolysis in acute myocardial infarction. The AMI-SK study. Eur Heart J 23:1282, 2002.
119. Antman EM, Louwerenburg HW, Baars HF, et al: Enoxaparin as adjunctive antithrombin therapy for ST-elevation myocardial infarction: Results of the ENTIRE-Thrombolysis in Myocardial Infarction (TIMI) 23 Trial. Circulation 105:1642, 2002.
120. Wallentin L, Goldstein P, Armstrong PW, et al: Efficacy and safety of tenecteplase in combination with the low-molecular-weight heparin enoxaparin or unfractionated heparin in the prehospital setting: The Assessment of the Safety and Efficacy of a New Thrombolytic Regimen (ASSENT)-3 PLUS randomized trial in acute myocardial infarction. Circulation 108:135, 2003.
121. Naghavi M, Libby P, Falk E, et al: From vulnerable plaque to vulnerable patient: A call for new definitions and risk assessment strategies: Part I. Circulation 108:1664, 2003.
122. Serebruany VL, Malinin AI, Callahan KP, et al: Effect of tenecteplase versus alteplase on platelets during the first 3 hours of treatment for acute myocardial infarction: The Assessment of the Safety and Efficacy of a New Thrombolytic Agent (ASSENT-2) platelet substudy. Am Heart J 145:636, 2003.
123. Antithrombotic Trialists' Collaboration: Collaborative meta-analysis of randomised trials of antiplatelet therapy for prevention of death, myocardial infarction, and stroke in high risk patients. BMJ 324:71, 2002.
124. Gawaz M, Neumann FJ, Schomig A: Evaluation of platelet membrane glycoproteins in coronary artery disease: Consequences for diagnosis and therapy. Circulation 99:E1, 1999.
125. Moliterno DJ, Chan AW: Glycoprotein IIb/IIIa inhibition in early intent-to-stent treatment of acute coronary syndromes: EPISTENT, ADMIRAL, CADILLAC, and TARGET. J Am Coll Cardiol 41:49S, 2003.
126. Vivekananthan DP, Patel VB, Moliterno DJ: Glycoprotein IIb/IIIa antagonism and fibrinolytic therapy for acute myocardial infarction. J Interv Cardiol 15:131, 2002.
127. Eisenberg MJ, Jamal S: Glycoprotein IIb/IIIa inhibition in the setting of acute ST-segment elevation myocardial infarction. J Am Coll Cardiol 42:1, 2003.
128. Kleiman N, Ohman EM, Califf RM, et al: Profound inhibition of platelet aggregation with monoclonal antibody 7E3 Fab after thrombolytic therapy: Results of the Thrombolysis and Angioplasty in Myocardial Infarction (TAMI) 8 pilot study. J Am Coll Cardiol 22:381, 1993.
129. Ohman EM, Kleiman NS, Gacioch G, et al: Combined accelerated tissue-plasminogen activator and platelet glycoprotein IIb/IIIa integrin receptor blockade with Integrilin in acute myocardial infarction. Results of a randomized, placebo-controlled, dose-ranging trial. IMPACT-AMI Investigators. Circulation 95:846, 1997.
130. Ronner E, van Kesteren HA, Zijnen P, et al: Safety and efficacy of eptifibatide vs placebo in patients receiving thrombolytic therapy with streptokinase for acute myocardial infarction: A phase II dose escalation, randomized, double-blind study. Eur Heart J 21:1530, 2000.
131. The PARADIGM Investigators: Combining thrombolysis with the platelet glycoprotein IIb/IIIa inhibitor lamifiban: Results of the Platelet Aggregation Receptor Antagonist Dose Investigation and Reperfusion Gain in Myocardial Infarction (PARADIGM) trial. J Am Coll Cardiol 32:2003, 1998.
132. Strategies for Patency Enhancement in the Emergency Department (SPEED) Group: Trial of abciximab with and without low-dose reteplase for acute myocardial infarction. Circulation 101:2788, 2000.
133. Brener SJ, Zeymer U, Adgey AA, et al: Eptifibatide and low-dose tissue plasminogen activator in acute myocardial infarction: The integrilin and low-dose thrombolysis in acute myocardial infarction (INTRO AMI) trial. J Am Coll Cardiol 39:377, 2002.
134. Giugliano RP, Roe MT, Harrington RA, et al: Combination reperfusion therapy with eptifibatide and reduced-dose tenecteplase for ST-elevation myocardial infarction: Results of the integrilin and tenecteplase in acute myocardial infarction (INTEGRITI) Phase II Angiographic Trial. J Am Coll Cardiol 41:1251, 2003.
135. Ohman EM, Oliverio RM, Harrelson L: Results of the Fibrinolytics and Aggrastat in ST Elevation Resolution (FASTER, TIMI 24) randomized trial. 2004, in press.
136. de Lemos JA, Antman EM, Gibson CM, et al: Abciximab improves both epicardial flow and myocardial reperfusion in ST-elevation myocardial infarction: Observations from the TIMI 14 trial. Circulation 101:239, 2000.
137. Topol EJ: Reperfusion therapy for acute myocardial infarction with fibrinolytic therapy or combination reduced fibrinolytic therapy and platelet glycoprotein IIb/IIIa inhibition: The GUSTO V randomised trial. Lancet 357:1905, 2001.
138. Peters RJ, Mehta SR, Fox KA, et al: Effects of aspirin dose when used alone or in combination with clopidogrel in patients with acute coronary syndromes: Observations from the Clopidogrel in Unstable angina to prevent Recurrent Events (CURE) Study. Circulation 108:1682, 2003.
139. Reikvam A, Kvan E, Aursnes I: Use of cardiovascular drugs after acute myocardial infarction: A marked shift towards evidence-based drug therapy. Cardiovasc Drugs Ther 16:451, 2002.
140. Fonarow GC, Gawlinski A, Moughrabi S, et al: Improved treatment of coronary heart disease by implementation of a Cardiac Hospitalization Atherosclerosis Management Program (CHAMP). Am J Cardiol 87:819, 2001.
141. Pope JH, Selker HP: Diagnosis of acute cardiac ischemia. Emerg Med Clin North Am 21:27, 2003.
142. Bartholomew BA, Harjai KJ, Grines CL, et al: Variation in hospital length of stay in patients with acute myocardial infarction undergoing primary angioplasty and the need to change the diagnostic-related group system. Am J Cardiol 92:830, 2003.
143. Peterson ED, Shaw LJ, Califf RM: Risk stratification after myocardial infarction. Ann Intern Med 126:561, 1997.
144. Antman EM, Kuntz KM: The length of the hospital stay after myocardial infarction. N Engl J Med 342:808, 2000.

Pharmacological Therapy

145. Freemantle N, Cleland J, Young P, et al: Beta blockade after myocardial infarction: Systematic review and meta regression analysis. BMJ 318:1730, 1999.
146. ISIS-1 (First International Study of Infarct Survival) Collaborative Group: Mechanisms for the early mortality reduction produced by beta-blockade started early in acute myocardial infarction: ISIS-1. Lancet 1:921, 1988.
147. The TIMI Study Group: Comparison of invasive and conservative strategies after treatment with intravenous tissue plasminogen activator in acute myocardial infarction: Results of the Thrombolysis in Myocardial Infarction (TIMI) Phase II Trial. N Engl J Med 320:618, 1989.
148. Roberts R, Rogers WJ, Mueller HS, et al: Immediate versus deferred B-blockade following thrombolytic therapy in patients with acute myocardial infarction: Results of the Thrombolysis in Myocardial Infarction (TIMI) II-B Study. Circulation 83:422, 1991.
149. Dargie HJ: Effect of carvedilol on outcome after myocardial infarction in patients with left-ventricular dysfunction: The CAPRICORN randomised trial. Lancet 357:1385, 2001.
150. Pfeffer MA: Left ventricular remodeling after acute myocardial infarction. Ann Rev Med 46:455, 1995.
151. The Acute Infarction Ramipril Efficacy (AIRE) Study Investigators: Effect of ramipril on mortality and morbidity of survivors of acute myocardial infarction with clinical evidence of heart failure. Lancet 342:821, 1993.
152. Ambrosioni E, Borghi C, Magnani B, et al: Effects of the early administration of zofenopril on mortality and morbidity in patients with anterior myocardial infarction: Results of the Survival of Myocardial Infarction Long-Term Evaluation Trial. N Engl J Med 332:280, 1995.
153. Kobler L, Torp-Pedersen C, Carlsen JE, et al: A clinical trial of the angiotensin-converting-enzyme inhibitor trandolapril in patients with left ventricular dysfunction after myocardial infarction. N Engl J Med 333:1670, 1995.
154. ISIS-4 Collaborative Group: ISIS-4: A randomized factorial trial assessing early oral captopril, oral mononitrate, and intravenous magnesium sulphate in 58,050 patients with suspected acute myocardial infarction. Lancet 345:669, 1995.
155. Gruppo Italiano per lo Studio della Sopravvivenza nell'Infarto Miocardico: GISSI-3: Effects of lisinopril and transdermal glyceryl trinitrate singly and together on 6-week mortality and ventricular function after acute myocardial infarction. Lancet 343:1115, 1994.
156. Swedberg K, Held P, Kjekshus J, et al: Effects of early administration of enalapril on mortality in patients with acute myocardial infarction. Results of the Cooperative North Scandinavian Enalapril Survival Study II (CONSENSUS II). N Engl J Med 327:678, 1992.
157. ACE Inhibitor Myocardial Infarction Collaborative Group: Indications for ACE inhibitors in the early treatment of acute myocardial infarction: Systematic overview of individual data from 100,000 patients in randomized trials. Circulation 97:2202, 1998.
158. Pfeffer MA: ACE inhibitors in acute myocardial infarction: Patient selection and timing. Circulation 97:2192, 1998.
159. Rutherford JD, Pfeffer MA, Moye LA, et al: Effects of captopril on ischemic events after myocardial infarction. Results of the Survival and Ventricular Enlargement Trial. Circulation 90:1731, 1994.
160. Dickstein K, Kjekshus J: Effects of losartan and captopril on mortality and morbidity in high-risk patients after acute myocardial infarction: The OPTIMAAL randomised trial. Optimal Trial in Myocardial Infarction with Angiotensin II Antagonist Losartan. Lancet 360:752, 2002.
161. Pfeffer MA: Effects of valsartan relative to captopril in patients with myocardial infarction complicated by heart failure and/or left ventricular dysfunction. N Engl J Med 349:1843, 2003.
162. Pitt B, Remme W, Zannad F, et al: Eplerenone, a selective aldosterone blocker, in patients with left ventricular dysfunction after myocardial infarction. N Engl J Med 348:1309, 2003.
163. Lindsay HSJ, Zaman AG, Cowan JC: ACE inhibitors after myocardial infarction: Patient selection or treatment for all? Br Heart J 73:397, 1995.
164. Pfeffer MA, Greaves SC, Arnold JM, et al: Early versus delayed angiotensin-converting enzyme inhibition therapy in acute myocardial infarction: The healing and early afterload reducing therapy trial. Circulation 95:2643, 1997.
165. Pitt B: Aldosterone blockade in patients with systolic left ventricular dysfunction. Circulation 108:1790, 2003.
166. Ryan TJ, Antman EM, Brooks NH, et al: 1999 update: ACC/AHA Guidelines for the Management of Patients with Acute Myocardial Infarction: Executive Summary and Recommendations: A report of the American College of Cardiology/American Heart Association Task Force on Practice Guidelines (Committee on Management of Acute Myocardial Infarction). Circulation 100:1016, 1999.
167. Report of the Holland Interuniversity Nifedipine/Metoprolol Trial Research Group: Early treatment of unstable angina in the coronary care unit: A randomised, double-blind, placebo-controlled comparison of recurrent ischaemia and thrombolytic therapy in patients treated with nifedipine or metoprolol or both. Br Heart J 56:400, 1986.
168. The Danish Study Group on Verapamil in Myocardial Infarction: Verapamil in acute myocardial infarction. Eur Heart J 54:516, 1984.
169. Boden WE, van Gilst WH, Scheldewaert RG, et al: Diltiazem in acute myocardial infarction treated with thrombolytic agents: A randomised placebo-controlled trial. Incomplete Infarction Trial of European Research Collaborators Evaluating Prognosis post-Thrombolysis (INTERCEPT). Lancet 355:1751, 2000.
170. Fath-Ordoubadi F, Beatt KJ: Glucose-insulin-potassium therapy for treatment of acute myocardial infarction: An overview of randomized placebo-controlled trials. Circulation 96:1152, 1997.
171. Diaz R, Paolasso EA, Piegas LS, et al: Metabolic modulation of acute myocardial infarction. The ECLA (Estudios Cardiologicos Latinoamerica) Collaborative Group. Circulation 98:2227, 1998.
172. Apstein CS: The benefits of glucose-insulin-potassium for acute myocardial infarction (and some concerns). J Am Coll Cardiol 42:792, 2003.
173. Falati S, Liu Q, Gross P, et al: Accumulation of tissue factor into developing thrombi in vivo is dependent upon microparticle P-selectin glycoprotein ligand 1 and platelet P-selectin. J Exp Med 197:1585, 2003.
174. Ross A, Gibbons R, Kloner RA, et al: Acute Myocardial Infarction Study of Adenosine (AMISTAD II). J Am Coll Cardiol 39:883, 2002.
175. Beltrami AP, Urbanek K, Kajstura J, et al: Evidence that human cardiac myocytes divide after myocardial infarction. N Engl J Med 344:1750, 2001.
176. Quaini F, Urbanek K, Beltrami AP, et al: Chimerism of the transplanted heart. N Engl J Med 346:5, 2002.
177. Siminiak T, Kurpisz M: Myocardial replacement therapy. Circulation 108:1167, 2003.

Hemodynamic Disturbances

178. Veenstra DL, Saint S, Saha S, et al: Efficacy of antiseptic-impregnated central venous catheters in preventing catheter-related bloodstream infection: A meta-analysis. JAMA 281:261, 1999.
179. Wu WC, Rathore SS, Wang Y, et al: Blood transfusion in elderly patients with acute myocardial infarction. N Engl J Med 345:1230, 2001.
180. Lewis EF, Moye LA, Rouleau JL, et al: Predictors of late development of heart failure in stable survivors of myocardial infarction: The CARE study. J Am Coll Cardiol 42:1446, 2003.
181. Udelson JE, Patten RD, Konstam MA: New concepts in post-infarction ventricular remodeling. Rev Cardiovasc Med 4(Suppl 3):S3, 2003.
182. Eichhorn EJ, Gheorghiade M: Digoxin—New perspective on an old drug. N Engl J Med 347:1394, 2002.
183. Goldberg RJ, Samad NA, Yarzebski J, et al: Temporal trends in cardiogenic shock complicating acute myocardial infarction. N Engl J Med 340:1162, 1999.
184. Webb JG, Lowe AM, Sanborn TA, et al: Percutaneous shock intervention for cardiogenic shock in the SHOCK Trial. J Am Coll Cardiol 42:1380, 2003.
185. Sanborn TA, Sleeper LA, Webb JG, et al: Correlates of one-year survival in patients with cardiogenic shock complicating acute myocardial infarction: Angiographic findings from the SHOCK trial. J Am Coll Cardiol 42:1373, 2003.
186. Hochman JS: Cardiogenic shock complicating acute myocardial infarction: Expanding the paradigm. Circulation 107:2998, 2003.
187. Cotter G, Kaluski E, Milo O, et al: LINCS: L-NAME (a NO synthase inhibitor) in the treatment of refractory cardiogenic shock: A prospective randomized study. Eur Heart J 24:1287, 2003.
188. Hochman JS, Sleeper LA, Webb JG, et al: Early revascularization in acute myocardial infarction complicated by cardiogenic shock. SHOCK Investigators: Should we emergently revascularize occluded coronaries for cardiogenic shock? N Engl J Med 341:625, 1999.
189. Bertrand M, McFadden E: Cardiogenic shock: Is there light at the end of the tunnel? J Am Coll Cardiol 42:1387, 2003.
190. Lemos PA, Cummins P, Lee CH, et al: Usefulness of percutaneous left ventricular assistance to support high-risk percutaneous coronary interventions. Am J Cardiol 91:479, 2003.
191. Inoue K, Ito H, Kitakaze M, et al: Antecedent angina pectoris as a predictor of better functional and clinical outcomes in patients with an inferior wall acute myocardial infarction. Am J Cardiol 83:159, 1999.
192. Zimetbaum PJ, Josephson ME: Use of the electrocardiogram in acute myocardial infarction. N Engl J Med 348:933, 2003.
193. Wellens HJ: The value of the right precordial leads of the electrocardiogram. N Engl J Med 340:381, 1999.
194. Hurst JW: Comments about the electrocardiographic signs of right ventricular infarction. Clin Cardiol 21:289, 1998.
195. Jacobs AK, Leopold JA, Bates E, et al: Cardiogenic shock caused by right ventricular infarction: A report from the SHOCK registry. J Am Coll Cardiol 41:1273, 2003.
196. Birnbaum Y, Fishbein MC, Blanche C, et al: Ventricular septal rupture after acute myocardial infarction. N Engl J Med 347:1426, 2002.
197. Sugiura T, Nagahama Y, Nakamura S, et al: Left ventricular free wall rupture after reperfusion therapy for acute myocardial infarction. Am J Cardiol 92:282, 2003.
198. Birnbaum Y, Chamoun AJ, Anzuini A, et al: Ventricular free wall rupture following acute myocardial infarction. Coron Artery Dis 14:463, 2003.
199. Figueras J, Cortadellas J, Calvo F, et al: Relevance of delayed hospital admission on development of cardiac rupture during acute myocardial infarction: Study in 225 patients with free wall, septal or papillary muscle rupture. J Am Coll Cardiol 32:135, 1998.
200. Becker RC, Hochman JS, Cannon CP, et al: Fatal cardiac rupture among patients treated with thrombolytic agents and adjunctive thrombin antagonists: Observations from the Thrombolysis and Thrombin Inhibition in Myocardial Infarction 9 Study. J Am Coll Cardiol 33:479, 1999.
201. Reynen K, Strasser RH: Images in clinical medicine. Impending rupture of the myocardial wall. N Engl J Med 348:e3, 2003.
202. Crenshaw BS, Granger CB, Birnbaum Y, et al: Risk factors, angiographic patterns, and outcomes in patients with ventricular septal defect complicating acute myocardial infarction. Circulation 101:27, 2000.
203. Figueras J, Cortadellas J, Soler-Soler J: Comparison of ventricular septal and left ventricular free wall rupture in acute myocardial infarction. Am J Cardiol 81:495, 1998.
204. Birnbaum Y, Chamoun AJ, Conti VR, et al: Mitral regurgitation following acute myocardial infarction. Coron Artery Dis 13:337, 2002.
205. Dias B, Graba J, Siu S, et al: Papillary muscle rupture complicating an acute myocardial infarction. Can J Cardiol 17:722, 2001.

206. Carmeliet E: Cardiac ionic currents and acute ischemia: From channels to arrhythmias. Physiol Rev 79:917, 1999.
207. Cannom DS, Prystowsky EN: Management of ventricular arrhythmias: Detection, drugs, and devices. JAMA 281:172, 1999.
208. Tan HL, Lie KI: Prophylactic lidocaine use in acute myocardial infarction revisited in the thrombolytic era. Am Heart J 137:770, 1999.
209. Thompson CA, Yarzebski J, Goldberg RJ, et al: Changes over time in the incidence and case-fatality rates of primary ventricular fibrillation complicating acute myocardial infarction: Perspectives from the Worcester Heart Attack Study. Am Heart J 139:1014, 2000.
210. Volpi A, Cavalli A, Santoro L, et al: Incidence and prognosis of early primary ventricular fibrillation in acute myocardial infarction—Results of the Gruppo Italiano per lo Studio della Sopravvivenza nell'Infarto Miocardico (GISSI-2) database. Am J Cardiol 82:265, 1998.
211. Brady WJ Jr, Harrigan RA: Diagnosis and management of bradycardia and atrioventricular block associated with acute coronary ischemia. Emerg Med Clin North Am 19:371, xi, 2001.
212. Zuanetti G, Mantini L, Hernandez-Bernal F, et al: Relevance of heart rate as a prognostic factor in patients with acute myocardial infarction: Insights from the GISSI-2 study. Eur Heart J 19(Suppl F):F19, 1998.
213. Altun A, Kirdar C, Ozbay G: Effect of aminophylline in patients with atropine-resistant late advanced atrioventricular block during acute inferior myocardial infarction. Clin Cardiol 21:759, 1998.
214. Herlitz J, Karlson BW, Bang A, et al: Mortality and risk indicators for death during five years after acute myocardial infarction among patients with and without ST elevation on admission electrocardiogram. Cardiology 89:33, 1998.
215. Go AS, Barron HV, Rundle AC, et al: Bundle-branch block and in-hospital mortality in acute myocardial infarction. National Registry of Myocardial Infarction 2 Investigators. Ann Intern Med 129:690, 1998.
216. Sgarbossa EB, Pinski SL, Topol EJ, et al: Acute myocardial infarction and complete bundle branch block at hospital admission: Clinical characteristics and outcome in the thrombolytic era. GUSTO-I Investigators. Global Utilization of Streptokinase and t-PA [tissue-type plasminogen activator] for Occluded Coronary Arteries. J Am Coll Cardiol 31:105, 1998.
217. Pedersen OD, Bagger H, Kober L, et al: The occurrence and prognostic significance of atrial fibrillation/flutter following acute myocardial infarction. TRACE Study group. TRAndolapril Cardiac Evalution. Eur Heart J 20:748, 1999.
218. The GUSTO Investigators: An international randomized trial comparing four thrombolytic strategies for acute myocardial infarction. N Engl J Med 329:673, 1993.
219. Grines CL, Cox DA, Stone GW, et al: Coronary angioplasty with or without stent implantation for acute myocardial infarction. N Engl J Med 341:1949, 1999.
220. Kernis SJ, Harjai KJ, Stone GW, et al: The incidence, predictors, and outcomes of early reinfarction after primary angioplasty for acute myocardial infarction. J Am Coll Cardiol 42:1173, 2003.
221. Gibson CM, Karha J, Murphy SA, et al: Early and long-term clinical outcomes associated with reinfarction following fibrinolytic administration in the Thrombolysis in Myocardial Infarction trials. J Am Coll Cardiol 42:7, 2003.
222. Scheller B, Hennen B, Hammer B, et al: Beneficial effects of immediate stenting after thrombolysis in acute myocardial infarction. J Am Coll Cardiol 42:634, 2003.
223. Zeymer U, Uebis R, Vogt A, et al: Randomized comparison of percutaneous transluminal coronary angioplasty and medical therapy in stable survivors of acute myocardial infarction with single vessel disease: A study of the Arbeitsgemeinschaft Leitende Kardiologische Krankenhausarzte. Circulation 108:1324, 2003.
224. Dauerman HL, Sobel BE: Synergistic treatment of ST-segment elevation myocardial infarction with pharmacoinvasive recanalization. J Am Coll Cardiol 42:646, 2003.
225. O'Neill WW: "Watchful waiting" after thrombolysis: It's time for a re-evaluation. J Am Coll Cardiol 42:17, 2003.
226. Dauerman HL: The early days after ST-segment elevation acute myocardial infarction: Reconsidering the delayed invasive approach. J Am Coll Cardiol 42:420, 2003.
227. McKay RG: Evolving strategies in the treatment of acute myocardial infarction in the community hospital setting. J Am Coll Cardiol 42:642, 2003.
228. Cheitlin MD, Armstrong WF, Aurigemma GP, et al: ACC/AHA/ASE 2003 guideline update for the clinical application of echocardiography: A report of the American College of Cardiology/American Heart Association Task Force on Practice Guidelines (ACC/AHA/ASE Committee to Update the 1997 Guidelines on the Clinical Application of Echocardiography). American College of Cardiology, 2003 (http://www.acc.org/clinical/guidelines/echocardiography/dirIndex.htm. 2003).
229. Reinecke H, Wichter T, Weyand M: Left ventricular pseudoaneurysm in a patient with Dressler's syndrome after myocardial infarction. Heart 80:98, 1998.
230. Ohara K: Current surgical strategy for post-infarction left ventricular aneurysm—From linear aneurysmectomy to Dor's operation. Ann Thorac Cardiovasc Surg 6:289, 2000.
231. Barbera S, Hillis LD: Echocardiographic recognition of left ventricular mural thrombus. Echocardiography 16:289, 1999.
232. Hirsh J, Fuster V, Ansell J, et al: American Heart Association/American College of Cardiology Foundation guide to warfarin therapy. Circulation 107:1692, 2003.

Post-Myocardial Infarction Care

233. Newby LK, Califf RM, Guerci A, et al: Early discharge in the thrombolytic era: An analysis of criteria for uncomplicated infarction from the Global Utilization of Streptokinase and t-PA for Occluded Coronary Arteries (GUSTO) trial. J Am Coll Cardiol 27:625, 1996.
234. Berkman LF, Blumenthal J, Burg M, et al: Effects of treating depression and low perceived social support on clinical events after myocardial infarction: The Enhancing Recovery in Coronary Heart Disease Patients (ENRICHD) Randomized Trial. JAMA 289:3106, 2003.
235. Birnbaum Y, Drew BJ: The electrocardiogram in ST elevation acute myocardial infarction: Correlation with coronary anatomy and prognosis. Postgrad Med J 79:490, 2003.
236. Agati L, De Majo F, Madonna MP, et al: Assessment of myocardial viability in patients with postischemic left ventricular dysfunction: Role of myocardial contrast echocardiography. Echocardiography 20(Suppl 1):S19, 2003.
237. Klocke FJ, Baird MG, Bateman TM, et al: ACC/AHA/ASNC guidelines for the clinical use of cardiac radionuclide imaging: A report of the American College of Cardiology/American Heart Association Task Force on Practice Guidelines (ACC/AHA/ASNC Committee to Revise the 1995 Guidelines for the Clinical Use of Radionuclide Imaging). American College of Cardiology, 2003. (http://www.acc.org/clinical/guidelines/radio/dirIndex.htm. 2003).
238. Gibbons RJ, Balady GJ, Bridker JT, et al: ACC/AHA 2002 guideline update for exercise testing: A report of the American College of Cardiology/American Heart Association Task Force on Practice Guidelines (Committee on Exercise Testing). 2002. American College of Cardiology, 2002 (http://www.acc.org/clinical/guidelines/exercise/dirIndex.htm. 2002).
239. Madsen JK, Grande P, Saunamaki K, et al: Danish multicenter randomized study of invasive versus conservative treatment in patients with inducible ischemia after thrombolysis in acute myocardial infarction (DANAMI). DANish trial in Acute Myocardial Infarction. Circulation 96:748, 1997.
240. Moss AJ, Zareba W, Hall WJ, et al: Prophylactic implantation of a defibrillator in patients with myocardial infarction and reduced ejection fraction. N Engl J Med 346:877, 2002.
241. Cairns JA, Connolly SJ, Roberts R, et al: Randomised trial of outcome after myocardial infarction in patients with frequent or repetitive ventricular premature depolarisations: CAMIAT. Canadian Amiodarone Myocardial Infarction Arrhythmia Trial Investigators. Lancet 349:675, 1997.
242. Julian DG, Camm AJ, Frangin G, et al: Randomised trial of effect of amiodarone on mortality in patients with left-ventricular dysfunction after recent myocardial infarction: EMIAT. European Myocardial Infarct Amiodarone Trial Investigators. Lancet 349:667, 1997.
243. Expert Panel on Detection, Evaluation, and Treatment of High Blood Cholesterol in Adults: Executive Summary of The Third Report of The National Cholesterol Education Program (NCEP) Expert Panel on Detection, Evaluation, And Treatment of High Blood Cholesterol In Adults (Adult Treatment Panel III). JAMA 285:2486, 2001.
244. Libby P, Ridker PM, Maseri A: Inflammation and atherosclerosis. Circulation 105:1135, 2002.
245. Yusuf S, Sleight P, Pogue J, et al: Effects of an angiotensin-converting-enzyme inhibitor, ramipril, on cardiovascular events in high-risk patients. The Heart Outcomes Prevention Evaluation Study Investigators. N Engl J Med 342:145, 2000.
246. Fox KM: Efficacy of perindopril in reduction of cardiovascular events among patients with stable coronary artery disease: Randomised, double-blind, placebo-controlled, multicentre trial (the EUROPA study). Lancet 362:782, 2003.
247. Chen J, Radford MJ, Wang Y, et al: Are beta-blockers effective in elderly patients who undergo coronary revascularization after acute myocardial infarction? Arch Intern Med 160:947, 2000.
248. Gruppo Italiano per lo Studio della Sopravvivenza nell'Infarto Miocardico: Dietary supplementation with n-3 polyunsaturated fatty acids and vitamin E after myocardial infarction: Results of the GISSI-Prevenzione trial. Lancet 354:447, 1999.

CHAPTER 48

Primary Percutaneous Coronary Intervention in the Management of Acute Myocardial Infarction

Gary E. Lane • David R. Holmes, Jr.

The restoration of blood flow to ischemic myocardium is established as the preeminent objective for treatment of patients with acute myocardial infarction. Primary angioplasty or percutaneous coronary intervention (PCI) has evolved through continued innovation of the method and dissemination to an expanding proportion of patients. This chapter examines the evidence favoring a primary angioplasty (PCI) strategy, modern application of the technique, and emerging innovations in reperfusion science.

OBSERVATIONAL DATA

Multiple centers have described their experience with primary angioplasty over the past 20 years. These series have frequently included patients with contraindications to thrombolysis and cardiogenic shock. For example, O'Keefe and colleagues[1] reported a large consecutive series (1980 to 1993) of 1000 patients (7.9 percent with cardiogenic shock). The infarct artery was recanalized in 94 percent and the overall mortality was 7.8 percent (44 percent with cardiogenic shock). Historically, these reports may be compromised by selection bias, but they established primary angioplasty as an alternative reperfusion modality.

Several large registries have been reported comparing primary angioplasty with thrombolysis. Although these registries evaluate reperfusion treatment in contemporary practice, their importance is limited by significant drawbacks including nonuniform availability of primary angioplasty, unidentified imbalance of patients' characteristics, and the influence of clinical opinions concerning treatment. Nevertheless, they provide information regarding the applicability of lessons learned from randomized trials.

The Myocardial Infarction Triage and Intervention (MITI) registry ($n = 3145$) (1988 to 1994) did not identify differences in mortality (hospital or at 3 years) or reinfarction, although 26 percent of patients in the thrombolytic group underwent "rescue" revascularization.[2] In the Second National Registry of Myocardial Infarction (NRMI-2) ($n = 29{,}644$) (1994 to 1995) total strokes were less (0.7 percent versus 1.6 percent, $p < 0.0001$) with primary angioplasty but the combined endpoint of death and nonfatal stroke was equivalent (5.6 percent for angioplasty and 6.2 percent for thrombolysis).[3]

In contrast, logistic regression multivariate analysis of the combined German Maximal Individual Therapy in Acute Myocardial Infarction–Myocardial Infarction Registry (MITRA-MIR) registries ($n = 9906$) (1994 to 1998) found a significantly reduced risk of hospital mortality for patients undergoing primary angioplasty compared with thrombolysis (6.4 percent versus 11.3 percent; odds ratio [OR] 0.54, confidence interval [CI] 0.43 to 0.67).[4] This effect was persistent across almost all preidentified subgroups of patients analyzed, including those related to gender, age, and infarct location. Furthermore, as mortality in the groups of patients increased, presumably reflecting higher risk patients, there was an increase in the absolute benefit of primary angioplasty compared with thrombolysis. The advantage noted in this analysis may reflect the improving methodology of catheter-based reperfusion. A separate examination of this registry revealed an improving hospital mortality from 1994 to 1998 with primary angioplasty but not with thrombolytic therapy.[5] From registry data, it appears that interventional advances have led to continued separation in the relative benefits of the two reperfusion strategies.

Randomized Trials Comparing Primary Angioplasty with Thrombolysis

The foundation of evidence-based medicine rests on the data obtained from carefully conducted randomized trials. On the question of reperfusion strategy, significant information has accumulated, yet even randomized trials may have inherent limitations including the inability to "blind" treatment groups and the common crossover to revascularization in patients allocated to thrombolysis.

Three randomized trials published simultaneously in 1993 provided a stimulus for expanded application and investigation of the primary angioplasty strategy. The largest ($n = 395$) of these trials, the Primary Angioplasty in Myocardial Infarction (PAMI) trial, achieved reperfusion success in 97 percent (94 percent Thrombolysis in Myocardial Infarction [TIMI] 3 flow) within 60 minutes in the angioplasty group.[6] Although there was no significant improvement in left ventricular function during rest or exercise at 6-week follow-up, there was a trend for a reduction of in-hospital mortality (2.6 percent versus 6.5 percent, $p = 0.06$) in the angioplasty group in comparison with the group treated with tissue plasminogen activator (t-PA). There was a significant reduction in combined death or reinfarction (5.1 percent versus 12 percent, $p = 0.02$) and intracranial hemorrhage (0 percent versus 2.0 percent, $p = 0.05$) with angioplasty. Patients classified as "not low risk" (older than 70 years, anterior infarction or heart rate >100) had a lower mortality rate (2.0 percent versus 10.4 percent, $p = 0.01$) with angioplasty.

The Mayo Clinic trial ($n = 108$, primary angioplasty versus t-PA) assessed myocardial salvage by technetium-99m sestamibi tomographic imaging in 108 patients.[7] No significant difference in salvage was detected. The Netherlands (Zwolle) trial compared primary angioplasty with streptokinase in 142 patients and found a significant reduction in reinfarction with angioplasty (0 percent versus 13 percent, $p = 0.003$) and a higher predischarge left ventricular ejection fraction (0.51 versus 0.45, $p = 0.004$).[8]

The Global Use of Strategies to Open Occluded Coronary Arteries in Acute Coronary Syndromes (GUSTO-IIb) angioplasty substudy was the largest trial comparing primary balloon angioplasty with thrombolysis (t-PA).[9] Although the incidence of the primary endpoint (death, nonfatal reinfarction, or disabling stroke at 30 days) was significantly reduced in the angioplasty group (9.6 percent versus 13.7 percent, $p = 0.033$), there was no significant advantage evident at 6 months (14.1 percent versus 16.1 percent, p = not significant). In comparison of this trial with other trials, it has been noted that only 81 percent of patients assigned to angioplasty underwent the procedure and TIMI-3 flow was achieved in only 73 percent. This finding may reflect the number of relatively inexperienced centers in this trial.

Evidence favoring the primary angioplasty strategy was derived from the Primary Coronary Angioplasty Trialists (PCAT) meta-analysis of 10 randomized trials (conducted 1989 to 1996).[10] The details of these trials are highlighted in Table 48–1. Primary balloon angioplasty resulted in a significant reduction in 30-day mortality (4.4 percent versus 6.5 percent, $p = 0.02$; 34 percent risk reduction) and the combination of death plus reinfarction (7.2 percent versus 11.9 percent, $p < 0.001$; 40 percent risk reduction). These effects were not significantly affected by the thrombolytic regimen. Primary angioplasty was also associated with a reduction in total stroke (0.7 percent versus 2.0 percent, $p = 0.007$) and a marked decrease in hemorrhagic stroke (0.1 percent versus 1.1 percent, $p < 0.001$).

A follow-up study from the PCAT investigators revealed that 26 lives were saved per 1000 patients treated with a primary angioplasty strategy.[11] This beneficial effect persisted at 6 months (Fig. 48–1). A similar reduction in estimated relative risk of death or reinfarction was noted across each of the major clinical subgroups analyzed, but the absolute benefits were greater in proportion to baseline risk. A 5-year follow-up from the Zwolle investigators has demonstrated the durability of primary angioplasty results with a persistent attenuation of mortality (13 percent versus 24 percent, $p < 0.01$) and reinfarction (6 percent versus 22 percent, $p < 0.001$).[12]

These studies occurred before adoption of more advanced angioplasty techniques. More recent trials have compared thrombolysis with catheter-based reperfusion utilizing stents and glycoprotein (GP) IIb/IIIa receptor inhibitors. For example, the Stent versus Thrombolysis for Occluded Coronary Arteries in Patients with Acute Myocardial Infarction (STOPAMI) trial compared patients reperfused with a stent plus abciximab with patients receiving t-PA.[13] Scintigraphic infarct size was significantly reduced in the stent group because of a larger salvage index. In addition, the composite endpoint of death, reinfarction, and stroke was lower in the stent group (8.5 percent versus 23.2 percent at 6 months, $p = 0.02$). Conversely, primary angioplasty was compared with

TABLE 48–1 Randomized Trials Comparing Primary Angioplasty with Thrombolysis*

Reference	N	Population of Patients	Symptom Duration (hr)	Thrombolytic Regimen	Treatment Interval (min) PTCA	Treatment Interval (min) Thrombolysis	Primary Follow-Up Duration (d)	Trial Period	Stents	IIb/IIIa
Dewood[†25]	90	<75 yr; ↑ST	<12	Duteplase (4 hr)	126	84	30	—	No	No
PAMI-1[†6]	395	↑ST	<12	t-PA (3 hr)	60	32	D/C	90-92	No	No
Zijlstra[†8]	294	<75 yr; ↑ST	<6	Streptokinase	68	30	30	90-92	No	No
Mayo[†7]	103	<80 yr; ↑ST	<12	Duteplase (4 hr)	45	20	D/C	89-91	No	No
Zijlstra[†22]	95	Low risk; ↑ST	<6	Streptokinase	68	30	30	93-95	No	No
Ribeiro[†23]	100	<75 yr; ↑ST	<6	Streptokinase	238	179	D/C	89	No	No
Grinfeld[†24]	112	↑ST	<12	Streptokinase	63	18	30	96[‡]	No	No
Ribichini[†26]	83	<80 yr: IWMI	<6	t-PA (90 min)	40	43	D/C	93-96	Yes	No
Garcia[†27]	189	AWMI	5	t-PA (90 min)	84	69	30	91-96	No	No
GUSTO IIB[†9]	1138	↑ST, LBBB	<12	t-PA (90 min)	114	72	30	94-96	No	No
Akhras[28]	87	↑ST	<12	Streptokinase	—	—	240	97[‡]	No	No
de Boer[29]	87	>75 yr; ↑ST	<6	Streptokinase	59	31	30	96-99	Yes	No
STOPAMI[13]	140	↑ST	<12	t-PA (90 min)	65	30	180	97-99	Yes	Yes
STAT[30]	133	↑ST, LBBB	<12	t-PA (90 min)	77	15	180	97-99	Yes	Yes
Kastrati[31]	162	↑ST, LBBB	<12	t-PA (90 min)	75	35	180	99-01	Yes	Yes
PRAGUE-1[15]	200	↑ST, LBBB	<6	Streptokinase	93	10	30	97-99	Yes	No
PRAGUE-2[16]	850	↑ST	<12	Streptokinase	94	12	30	99-02	Yes	No
LIMI[32]	150	<80 yr; ↑ST	<6	t-PA (90 min)	100	45	42	95-97	Yes	No
Air-PAMI[17]	137	↑ST; high risk	<12	t-PA/streptokinase	155	155	55	—	Yes	Yes
DANAMI-2[18]	1129	↑ST	<12	t-PA (90 min)	100	40	30	—	Yes	NA
C-PORT[20]	451	↑ST	<12	t-PA (90 min)	101	46	42/180	96-99	Yes	Yes
CAPTIM[14]	840	↑ST	<6	t-PA (90 min)	190	130	30	97-00	Yes	Yes
SHOCK[§33]	302	Cardiogenic shock	<36	t-PA (90 min)	152	150	30	93-98	Yes	Yes

AW = anterior wall; D/C = hospital discharge; IW = inferior wall; LBBB = left bundle branch block; MI = myocardial infarction; NA = not available; t-PA = tissue plasminogen activator. Trials: Air-PAMI = Air Primary Angioplasty in Myocardial Infarction; CAPTIM = Comparison of Angioplasty and Prehospital Thrombolysis In acute Myocardial infarction; C-PORT = Atlantic Cardiovascular Patient Outcomes Research Team; DANAMI = DANish trial in Acute Myocardial Infarction; GUSTO = Global Use of Strategies to Open Occluded Coronary Arteries in Acute Coronary Syndromes; PAMI = Primary Angioplasty in Myocardial Infarction; PRAGUE = PRimary Angioplasty in patients transferred from General community hospitals to specialized PTCA Units without Emergency thrombolysis; SHOCK = SHould we emergently revascularize Occluded coronaries for Cardiogenic shocK; STAT = Stenting versus Thrombolysis in Acute myocardial infarction Trial; STOPAMI = Stent versus Thrombolysis for Occluded Coronary Arteries in Patients with Acute Myocardial Infarction.

*The first 10 trials (above the horizontal line) were included in the PCAT analysis conducted in 1989-1996. The other 13 trials (below the horizontal line) were conducted in 1997-2002.

†Initial PCAT analysis trials.

‡Publication date.

§In the SHOCK trial patients were randomly assigned to revascularization or medical treatment (see text).

Data from Keeley EC, Boura JA, Grines CL: Primary angioplasty versus intravenous thrombolytic therapy for acute myocardial infarction: A quantitative review of 23 randomised trials. Lancet 361:13-20, 2003.

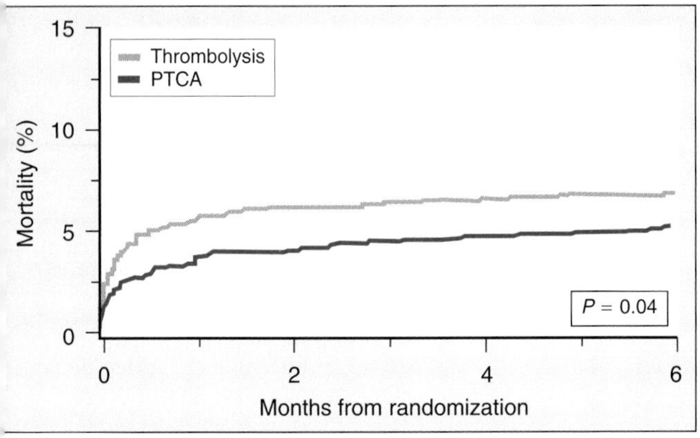

FIGURE 48–1 Mortality over 6 months from Primary Coronary Angioplasty Trialists analysis of 11 randomized trials.[11] PTCA = percutaneous transluminal coronary angioplasty.

prehospital thrombolysis in the Comparison of Angioplasty and Prehospital Thrombolysis In acute Myocardial infarction (CAPTIM) trial.[14] Although the trial was discontinued prematurely because of lack of funding, there was no significant difference in the primary endpoint of death, reinfarction, or stroke at 30 days. Rescue angioplasty was performed in 26 percent of the prehospital thrombolysis group, and a physician was part of the ambulance team. Notably, the incidence of cardiogenic shock on admission was significantly reduced in the thrombolysis group.

Additional data from randomized trials comparing primary angioplasty and thrombolysis have accumulated from trials examining logistical constraints to the application of catheter-based reperfusion. Several trials have compared a protocol of on-site thrombolysis with interhospital transport for primary angioplasty (Table 48–2). The PRimary Angioplasty in patients transferred from General community hospitals to specialized PTCA Units without Emergency thrombolysis (PRAGUE) 1 and 2,[15,16] Air Primary Angioplasty in Myocardial Infarction (Air PAMI),[17] and Danish multicenter randomized on thrombolytic treatment versus acute coronary angioplasty (DANAMI-2)[18] trials all demonstrated more favorable outcomes for patients treated with primary angioplasty despite the intrinsic transportation delay. Pooled analysis of comparative interhospital transportation trials ($n = 1242$) revealed a significant reduction in 30-day mortality (6.8 percent versus 9.6 percent, $p = 0.01$).[19] The Atlantic Cardiovascular Outcomes Research Team (C-PORT) trial compared thrombolysis (t-PA) with primary angioplasty at hospitals without on-site cardiac surgery.[20] The composite endpoint (death, reinfarction, stoke) was lower with primary angioplasty at 6 weeks (10.7 percent versus 17.7 percent, $p = 0.03$) and 6 months (12.4 percent versus 19.9 percent, $p = 0.03$).

A comprehensive review by Keeley and colleagues[21] combined the previous trials from the PCAT analysis[6-9,22-27] with 13 (conducted 1997 to 2002) more recent investigations[13-18,20,28-33] (see Table 48–1) in which stents were utilized in 12 of 13 and GP IIb/IIIa inhibitors in 7 of 13. The summary results (Fig. 48–2) ($n = 7437$) delineated a significant reduction in death, reinfarction, stroke, and hemorrhagic stroke.[21] Major hemorrhage (5 percent versus 7 percent, $p = 0.032$) was increased in the angioplasty patients. The benefit was similar irrespective of the thrombolytic regimen. Long-term (6 months) outcomes in several trials were persistently favorable for the angioplasty patients.

As with registry observations, the increasing advantage of catheter-based reperfusion strategies over thrombolysis in the more recently conducted (1996 to 2002) trials may represent increased institutional experience and advancing technology.

Advantages of the Primary Angioplasty (Percutaneous Coronary Intervention) Strategy

SUPERIOR RESTORATION OF FLOW. The GUSTO-I trial confirmed the critical link between early establishment of TIMI-3 flow and myocardial salvage and subsequent survival (Table 48–3).[34] A relationship between TIMI-3 flow and survival has also been verified for primary angioplasty.[35] Catheter-based reperfusion techniques attain TIMI-3 flow in 93 to 98 percent of patients.[6,7,36,37] In contrast, only 54 percent of patients achieve this reperfusion benchmark with accelerated t-PA.[34] This discrepancy provides a theoretical basis for

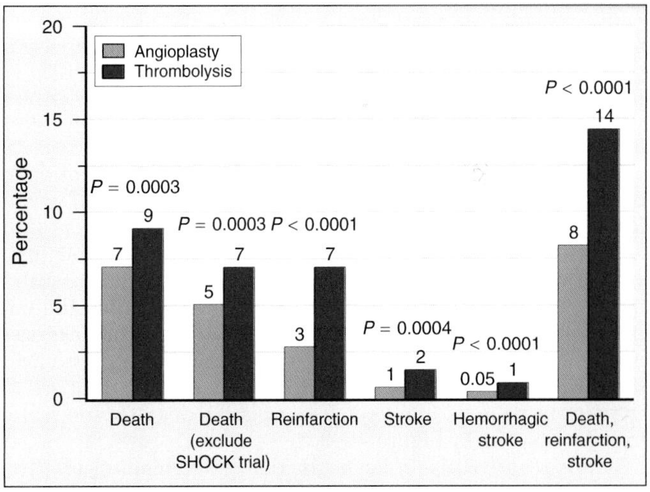

FIGURE 48–2 Short-term clinical outcomes of patients in 23 randomized trials of primary angioplasty versus thrombolysis.[21]

TABLE 48–2 Trials of Thrombolysis versus Transfer for Primary Angioplasty

			Treatment Interval (min)		% Death, Reinfarction, Stroke at 30 days		
Trial	*n*	Lytic Agent	*PTCA*	*Thrombolysis*	*PTCA*	*Thrombolysis*	*p*
PRAGUE-1[15]	200	SK	93	10	8	23	<0.02
PRAGUE-2[16]	850	SK	94	12	8.4	15.2	<0.003
Air-PAMI[17]	138	t-PA/SK	155	51	8.4	13.6	0.33
DANAMI-2[18]	1129	t-PA	100	40	8.5	14.2	0.002

Air-PAMI = Air Primary Angioplasty in Myocardial Infarction; DANAMI = DANish trial in Acute Myocardial Infarction; PRAGUE = PRimary Angioplasty in patients transferred from General community hospitals to specialized PTCA Units without Emergency thrombolysis; SK = streptokinase; t-PA = tissue plasminogen activator.

TABLE 48–3 TIMI Flow Grade Classification Scheme[42]

Flow Grade	Definition
Grade 0	No perfusion. No antegrade flow beyond the point of occlusion.
Grade 1	Penetration without perfusion. Contrast material passes beyond the area of obstruction but fails to opacify the entire coronary bed distal to the obstruction for the duration of the cineangiographic filming sequence.
Grade 2	Partial perfusion. Contrast material passes across the obstruction and opacifies the coronary distal to the obstruction. However, the rate of entry of contrast material into the vessel distal to the obstruction or its rate of clearance form the distal bed (or both) is perceptibly slower than its flow into or clearance from comparable areas not perfused by the previously occluded vessel.
Grade 3	Complete perfusion. Antegrade flow into the bed distal to the obstruction occurs as promptly as antegrade flow into the bed proximal to the obstruction, and clearance of contast material from the involved bed is as rapid as clearance from an uninvolved bed in the same vessel or the opposite artery.

TIMI: Thrombolysis In Myocardial Infarction.

the incremental improvement in outcomes with primary angioplasty.

Modification of pharmacological reperfusion utilizing a reduced-dose lytic agent and addition of a GP IIb/IIIa inhibitor resulted in TIMI-3 flow rates as high as 76 percent at 90 minutes.[38] This combination therapy was tested in the GUSTO-V and Assessment of the Safety and Efficacy of a New Thrombolytic Regimen (ASSENT)-3 trials.[39,40] Although a reduction in early ischemic events (including reinfarction) was seen, there was no reduction in 30-day[39,40] or 1-year mortality[40] compared with standard lytic therapy.

Despite restoration of epicardial flow, many patients exhibit suboptimal tissue level perfusion. This has been demonstrated by several techniques including myocardial contrast echocardiography, magnetic resonance imaging, scintigraphic methods, and Doppler flow wire measurements.[41] Epicardial flow has been more precisely quantitated utilizing the TIMI frame count,[42] and angiographic assessments of perfusion have been introduced including the TIMI myocardial perfusion grade (Table 48–4)[43] and blush score.[44] The implication of inadequate perfusion despite adequate flow is depicted in Figure 48–3.[43]

Blended into this concept is the phenomenon of "no reflow" indicating impaired function of the microvasculature within the distribution of the infarct.[45] The impaired perfusion is associated with adverse left ventricular remodeling, heart failure, and reduced survival.[41,45] A multitude of factors contribute to microvascular dysfunction including platelet embolization and obstruction, vasoconstriction, and reperfusion injury processes leading to neutrophil adhesion or infiltration, endothelial cell damage, and edema.[41,45,46]

Although a significant proportion of patients exhibit impaired perfusion (30 to 70 percent)[43,44,47] after successful restoration of infarct artery flow, there appears to be more preserved microvascular perfusion among patients undergoing primary angioplasty. In a study of patients with TIMI-3 flow, 72 percent of patients treated with t-PA exhibited persistent microvascular dysfunction (myocardial echo contrast defects) at 1 month compared with 31 percent of patients treated by primary angioplasty.[47] Analysis of ST segment resolution during infarction provides a simple surrogate for monitoring

TABLE 48–4 TIMI Myocardial Perfusion Grades[43]

Perfusion Grade	Definition
Grade 0	Minimal or no myocardial blush.
Grade 1	Dye stains the myocardium and this stain persists on the next injection.
Grade 2	Dye enters the myocardium but washes out slowly so that dye is strongly persistent at the end of the injection.
Grade 3	There is normal entrance and exit of dye in the myocardium so that dye is mildly persistent at the end of the injection.

TIMI = Thrombolysis In Myocardial Infarction.

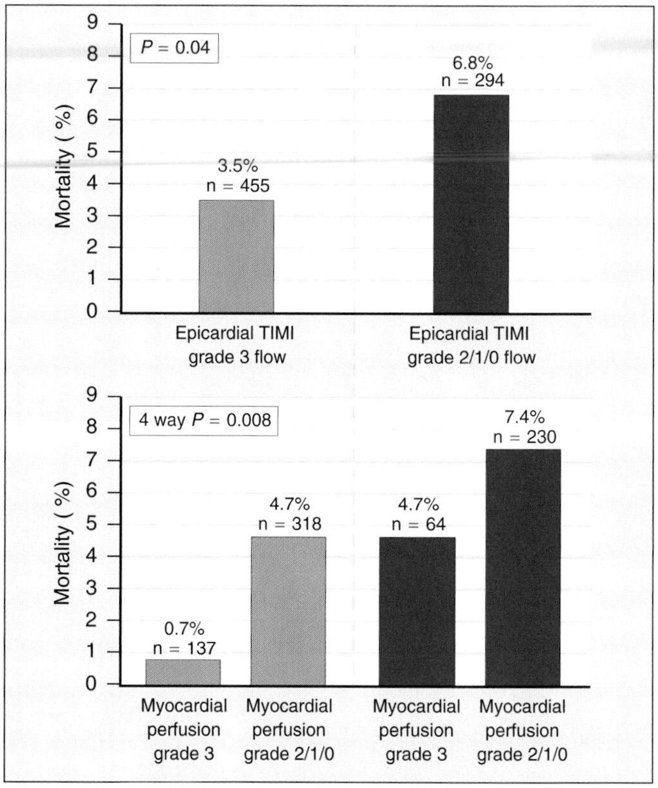

FIGURE 48–3 Relationship of both the Thrombolysis in Myocardial Infarction (TIMI) flow grade and TIMI myocardial perfusion grade at 90 minutes in the TIMI 10B trial (randomized comparison of TNK and tissue plasminogen activator). Even among patients with TIMI-3 flow, 30-day mortality was increased as myocardial perfusion decreased.[43]

myocardial perfusion. In a retrospective study of thrombolytic ($n = 851$) and primary angioplasty ($n = 528$) reperfusion, ST resolution was accelerated in the latter group and this correlated with an improved outcome.[48]

Modern objectives for reperfusion therapy should include the maintenance of microvascular integrity. Continued investigation into methods to prevent embolization, modify distal vascular tone, and enhance the microcirculatory environment may augment the results of reperfusion therapy.[41,45]

TREATMENT OF THE INCITING PATHOBIOLOGY IN ACUTE MYOCARDIAL INFARCTION. Although reperfusion therapy is based upon thrombotic coronary occlusion, thrombus may not play the predominant role in a significant proportion of acute myocardial infarctions. One study found that intracoronary aspiration thrombectomy successfully resolved coronary occlusion in 58 percent of patients, whereas thrombectomy alone or followed by primary angioplasty was successful in more than 90 percent.[49] The thrombectomy success is similar to that seen with optimal thrombolysis. Dynamic occlusive events apart from thrombus, including plaque rupture, intramural hemorrhage, dissection, and spasm, may explain at least part of the advantage of primary angioplasty over thrombolysis.

After successful thrombolysis, a significant residual stenosis remains in the majority of patients (Fig. 48–4).[50] Among patients in the TIMI trials the composite of death, reinfarction, and congestive heart failure was higher with a residual stenosis greater than 50 percent (7.8 percent versus 2.8 percent, $p = 0.03$). Treatment of the stenosis during primary angioplasty appears to lower the risk of recurrent ischemic events. In the meta-analysis of randomized trials, reinfarction was reduced to 3 percent with primary angioplasty compared with 7 percent for thrombolytic therapy ($p < 0.0001$).[21]

Late reocclusion rates (5 to 14 percent) compare favorably with those reported after thrombolysis (25 to 30 percent).[51,52] Restenosis after primary balloon angioplasty has been reported in 28 to 47 percent of patients.[51-53] Stenting further reduces the risk of reocclusion (5.1 percent versus 9.3 percent with percutaneous transluminal coronary angioplasty [PTCA], $p = 0.04$ in Stent Primary Angioplasty in Myocardial Infarction [Stent-PAMI]) and restenosis (20.3 percent versus 33.5 percent, $p < 0.001$).[36,53]

ANATOMICAL DEFINITION AND RISK STRATIFICATION. The angiographic and hemodynamic data obtained at the time of emergency catheterization impart valuable decision-facilitating information and more precise risk stratification. Definition of the coronary pathology is confirmed in patients with equivocal or uninterpretable electrocardiographic changes. After urgent coronary angiography, approximately 5 percent of patients require emergent coronary bypass surgery for severe multivessel or left main coronary artery disease.[54] Mechanical complications can also be identified during cardiac catheterization. An additional 5 percent of patients exhibit spontaneous reperfusion without a significant residual stenosis.

Stratification of patients into a low-risk group (age ≤ 70 years, left ventricular ejection fraction > 0.45, one- or two-vessel disease, successful angioplasty, no persistent arrhythmias) at the time of the procedure facilitates rapid safe recovery. It may allow omission of intensive care and noninvasive testing with early (day 3) hospital discharge.[55]

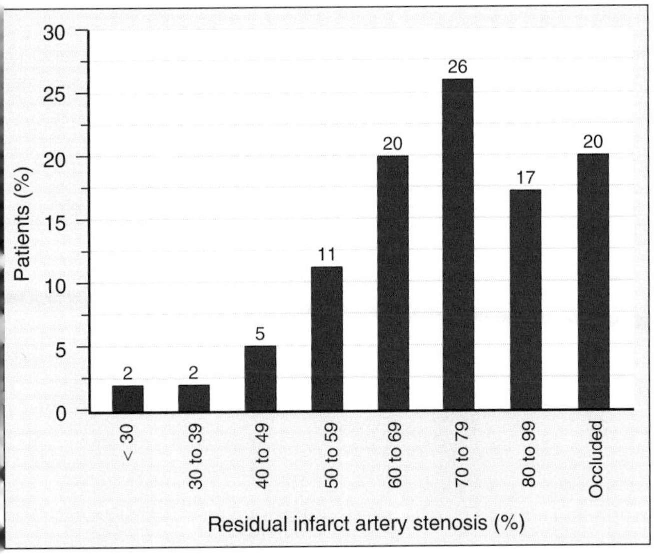

FIGURE 48–4 Distribution of residual stenosis in the infarct-related artery at 90 minutes after thrombolysis in 2119 patients in the TIMI 4, 10A, 10B, and 14 trials. (Modified from Llevadot J, Giugliano RP, McCabe CH, et al: Degree of residual stenosis in the culprit coronary artery after thrombolytic administration (Thrombolysis in Myocardial Infarction [TIMI] trials). Am J Cardiol 85:1409, 2000.)

REDUCTION IN COMPLICATIONS. Treatment with primary angioplasty appears to reduce the complications of myocardial infarct rupture. In a combined meta-analysis of the GUSTO-I and PAMI-I/II trials, primary angioplasty resulted in an 86 percent reduction in the risk of mechanical complications compared with that of patients undergoing thrombolysis.[56] There was a significant reduction in acute mitral regurgitation (0.31 percent versus 1.73 percent, $p < 0.001$) and ventricular septal defects (0.0 percent versus 0.47 percent, $p < 0.001$). In a multivariate analysis of 1375 patients, treatment with primary angioplasty was independently associated with a lower risk of free wall rupture.[57]

Intracranial hemorrhage remains a serious complication of thrombolysis. In the NRMI-2 registry the overall risk after t-PA therapy was 1.0 percent.[3] A primary angioplasty strategy nearly eliminated the peril of this complication.[21] One-third of the mortality reduction with primary angioplasty compared with thrombolysis has been attributed to curtailment of intracranial hemorrhage.[10]

Challenging Groups of Patients

ELDERLY PATIENTS. The population of elderly patients (older than 65 years) accounts for 85 percent of deaths from myocardial infarction.[58] Senescent transformation of the cardiovascular system limits cardiac reserve and complicates the management of myocardial injury.

Although the relative benefit of thrombolytic therapy is diminished in elderly patients, an analysis of the Fibrinolytic Trialists' data demonstrated a 15 percent reduction in mortality for eligible patients older than 75 years[59] compared with conservative therapy. Despite this evidence, reperfusion therapy is applied to less than half of eligible elderly patients.[60] Apprehension regarding the risk of intracranial hemorrhage significantly contributes to this diminished treatment.

Observations from the Cooperative Cardiovascular Project (CCP) Medicare data base identified a 38 percent statistically significant relative increase in mortality for thrombolysis-treated patients 76 to 84 years of age compared with conservative management.[61] The risk of intracranial hemorrhage was 2.5 percent among those older than 75 years in the NRMI-2 registry.[3] Trials of thrombolytic therapy including more aged patients have demonstrated a 2 to 3 percent risk of intracranial hemorrhage in this group. Attempts to enhance the results of thrombolysis with combination regimens in the ASSENT-3 and GUSTO-V trials did not improve overall efficacy and increased bleeding risk in patients older than 75 years.[39,40]

In contrast, the CCP patients undergoing primary angioplasty ($n = 2038$) exhibited lower 30-day (8.7 percent versus 11.9 percent, $p = 0.001$) and 1-year (14.4 percent versus 17.6 percent, $p = 0.001$) mortality compared with those undergoing thrombolysis ($n = 18{,}645$).[60] For patients older than 75 years in the NRMI-2 registry, the combined endpoint of death and nonfatal stroke was significantly higher in patients treated with t-PA compared with primary angioplasty (18.4 percent versus 14.6 percent, $p = 0.001$).[3]

Pooled analysis of the PAMI, Zwolle, and Mayo Clinic randomized trials revealed a significant mortality reduction for the elderly (older than 70 years) subgroup treated with angioplasty (3.5 percent versus 16 percent, $p = 0.02$) but not for younger patients.[62] A small randomized trial demonstrated no advantage for primary balloon angioplasty over conservative therapy in 120 patients older than 80 years.[63] However a trial ($n = 87$) comparing streptokinase (perhaps the preferred lytic agent in elderly patients) with angioplasty (stents in 51 percent) demonstrated a striking reduction (9 percent versus 29 percent, $p = 0.01$) in the primary endpoint (death, reinfarction, or stroke) and considerable reduction in 30-day (7 percent versus 22 percent, $p = 0.04$) and 1-year mortality (11 percent versus 29 percent, $p = 0.03$) with angioplasty in patients older than 75 years.[29]

Despite a shortage of randomized trial data, the advantage of primary angioplasty may be magnified in the elderly population. Clearly, further investigation is needed emphasizing the selection of patients who can safely benefit from reperfusion therapy.

PRIOR CORONARY BYPASS SURGERY. Mortality is increased in patients with prior coronary bypass surgery and acute myocardial infarction.[64,65] The increased risk of mortality and infarct complications may be attributed to more frequent coexistent factors such as advanced age, prior infarction, multivessel disease, diabetes, and impaired ventricular function. However, prior bypass surgery remains an independent risk factor for mortality.[66] No randomized controlled trials specifically address reperfusion therapy in this cohort.

In the NRMI-2 registry, 2544 patients with previous bypass surgery were treated with t-PA and 375 underwent primary angioplasty.[65] There was no significant difference in the mortality rate. The large thrombus burden often present in vein grafts may be more resistant to the action of lytic agents. In the GUSTO-I trial of thrombolysis, TIMI-3 flow in bypass grafts was achieved in only 32 percent compared with 49.2 percent without previous surgery.[64]

Primary balloon angioplasty of vein grafts has been associated with higher rates of TIMI-3 flow compared with thrombolysis (83 percent in the PAMI trials, $n = 93$) but reduced rates compared with native vessel reperfusion.[66,67] In addition to more extensive thrombus, vein graft angioplasty is often complicated by graft ectasia, limited runoff, atherosclerotic debris, and increased risk of distal embolization. Reperfusion of the infarct artery through the native circulation should be attempted if feasible.

In a retrospective series of 158 patients with acute vein graft occlusion, primary stenting ($n = 74$) resulted in more frequent TIMI-3 flow than balloon angioplasty ($n = 84$) (96 percent versus 72 percent, $p = 0.0001$) but without a difference in clinical outcome.[68] The role of GP IIb/IIIa inhibitors is unclear, although they appear to be of little value during vein graft intervention in other settings. Alternative methodology (thrombectomy, distal protection devices, ultrasound thrombolysis) requires investigation to optimize reperfusion within bypass grafts.

PATIENTS WITH THROMBOLYTIC CONTRAINDICATIONS. A significant proportion (25 to 30 percent) of patients presenting with ST elevation (or left bundle branch block) infarction who are eligible do not receive reperfusion therapy. In the Global Registry of Acute Coronary Events (GRACE) registry, 2084 patients presented within 12 hours of the onset of ST elevation infarction.[69] Thrombolytic contraindications were present in 15 percent, and overall 30 percent of eligible patients did not receive reperfusion therapy. Correlates of the latter group included prior bypass surgery, diabetes, history of congestive failure, and age older than 75 years. There remains a bias against thrombolysis particularly for elderly patients. Patients with clear-cut and relative contraindications to thrombolysis are at higher risk for death.

Patients with thrombolytic contraindications who underwent primary angioplasty in the MITRA registry had significantly lower mortality than conservatively managed patients (2.2 percent versus 24.7 percent, $p = 0.001$).[70] Juliard and colleagues[71] reported that reperfusion therapy with thrombolysis or angioplasty, or both, could be accomplished in 98 percent of 500 consecutive patients. Primary angioplasty can be applied in most higher risk patients who are not ideal candidates for thrombolytic therapy. The contraindications to primary angioplasty are limited to patients who cannot receive heparin or aspirin-thienopyridines, patients with documented life-threatening contrast allergy, or those with lack of vascular access.

CARDIOGENIC SHOCK. Infarct artery patency correlates with improved survival in cardiogenic shock secondary to left ventricular damage. Multiple observational series of patients undergoing angioplasty in cardiogenic shock have demonstrated an improved hemodynamic status and suggested enhanced survival.[72]

In contrast, thrombolysis appears to be less effective when administered to patients in shock. Limited trial data suggest an equivocal or marginal benefit in cardiogenic shock.[72] Intraaortic balloon counterpulsation may improve the results of thrombolytic therapy in cardiogenic shock.[73]

The SHould we emergently revascularize Occluded Coronaries for cardiogenic shocK (SHOCK) trial[33] verified a role for revascularization in cardiogenic shock. Patients ($n = 302$) were randomly assigned to an early (within 6 hours) revascularization strategy (angioplasty [55 percent] or bypass surgery [38 percent]) or medical stabilization (thrombolysis 63 percent) with delayed revascularization if appropriate. Intraaortic balloon support was recommended (86 percent in both groups). A significant survival advantage for revascularization was noted at 6 months and 1 year but not at the 30-day primary endpoint (Fig. 48–5).[74] The 30-day mortality was significantly lower with early revascularization for patients younger than 75 years (41 percent versus 57 percent, $p < 0.05$). These data strongly support the utilization of early revascularization in patients with shock younger than 75 years. The approach in elderly patients is less clear, although a survival advantage was seen for those older than 75 years who were clinically selected for early revascularization in the SHOCK registry.[75] Clearly, rapid reperfusion is critical to success in patients with cardiogenic shock (Fig. 48–6).[76]

Multivessel or left main disease is found in 60 to 90 percent of patients with cardiogenic shock.[72] In the SHOCK trial angioplasty was recommended for patients with one- or two-vessel disease and bypass surgery for those with left main or three-vessel disease. The role for multivessel angioplasty in cardiogenic shock remains to be defined, but stenting may allow safer application of this strategy.

THE LOGISTIC CHALLENGE OF EFFECTIVE REPERFUSION THERAPY

Rapid reperfusion of the infarct artery leading to myocardial salvage has remained the basis for the reperfusion paradigm. The survival benefit of

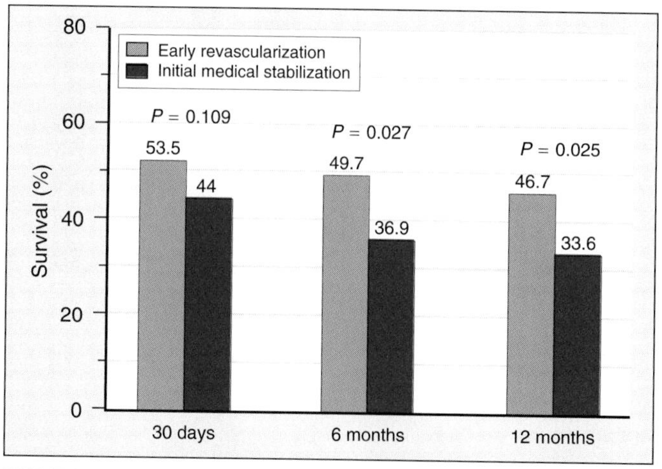

FIGURE 48–5 The temporal relation to survival for patients randomized in the SHould we emergently revascularize Occluded Coronaries for cardiogenic shocK (SHOCK) trial by treatment strategy.[74]

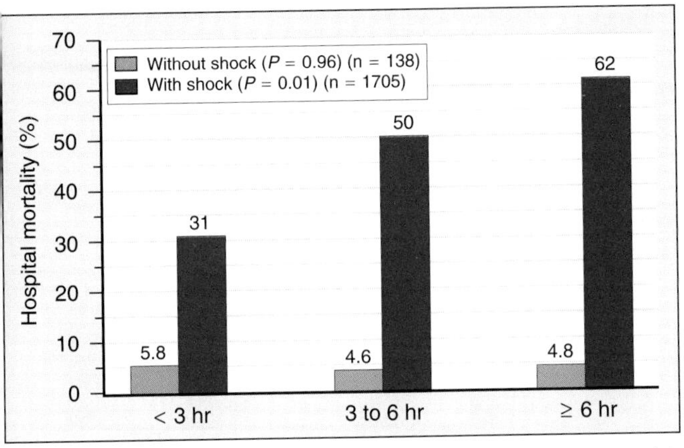

FIGURE 48–6 In-hospital mortality by time to reperfusion (symptom onset) in patients with and without shock. In this study after adjustment for baseline variables, reperfusion time was a significant predictor of mortality in patients with shock but not in patients without shock.[76]

reperfusion with thrombolytic therapy decreases with increasing delay in treatment.[77] A similar time-dependent relationship has been assumed for primary angioplasty.

There is an inherent delay in application of primary angioplasty compared with thrombolysis. The results of early randomized trials demonstrating an advantage for primary angioplasty over thrombolysis were not reproduced when some community-based registries were examined. These differences were attributed to the prolonged treatment interval to effect catheter-based reperfusion compared with thrombolysis seen in some of these registries. In the PCAT randomized trials, the mean primary angioplasty treatment delay was 26 minutes longer than the thrombolysis delay, compared with about 45 minutes relative delay in MITI and NRMI-2 registries.[2,3,10] This relative delay is an impediment to widespread application of a mechanical reperfusion strategy.

A relationship between increased mortality and prolonged treatment intervals (especially "door-to-balloon" times > 2 hours) was demonstrated in the GUSTO-IIB trial and the NRMI-2 registry.[35,78] Yet, in the same populations no survival relationship was found between time from symptom onset and reperfusion. In a series ($n = 1352$) reported by Brodie and colleagues,[79] mortality was lower when patients were reperfused early (<2 hours) but thereafter remained constant (2 to 12 hours after symptom onset). The investigators in PCAT ($n = 2635$) demonstrated increasing major adverse cardiac event rates with increasing presentation delay for thrombolysis but relatively stable event rates for primary angioplasty.[80]

An expanded concept of the mechanism of reperfusion benefit should be considered. Clearly, the earliest possible restoration of blood flow into the infarct artery is desirable. The occurrence of the most favorable outcomes with early (<2 hour) reperfusion is evident in most catheter-based reperfusion studies. This timely gain correlates with enhanced salvage of myocardium as measured by sestamibi perfusion and preservation of left ventricular function.[1,81] Myocardial salvage beyond the 2- to 3-hour window is probably modest. However, less than 20 percent of patients present early enough to achieve reperfusion in less than 2 hours.[78] Attainment of reperfusion in this early time period is more critical for patients with cardiogenic shock.[33] Moreover, in an analysis of primary PCI in 1843 patients again reported by Brodie and colleagues,[76] reperfusion time (from symptom onset) was important for the survival of patients with shock but independent of mortality in patients without shock (see Fig. 48–6).

The benefit of primary angioplasty may be less dependent on the treatment interval because of several possibilities. A consistent and high reperfusion efficacy is attained with primary angioplasty, but achievement of TIMI-3 flow decreases as treatment is delayed with thrombolysis.[82] In patients receiving thrombolysis, the complications of intracranial hemorrhage and myocardial rupture occur more frequently with longer treatment delays.[56,77] Myocardial rupture is reduced and intracranial hemorrhage is nearly eliminated with a primary angioplasty strategy.[56,57,77] Despite limited gains in myocardial salvage from primary angioplasty with later treatment, the improved patency may enhance survival by stabilizing myocardium at risk for rupture, having positive effects on ventricular remodeling, augmenting electrical stability, and providing a conduit for collateral flow.[79] The intrinsic value of infarct artery patency may be more than previously realized.

Expanding the Population for Catheter-Based Reperfusion

Only a minority of hospitals have catheterization laboratories, and even fewer offer coronary bypass surgery. The improving results of primary angioplasty (PCI) provide momentum to extend this advantage to more patients.

The prolonged temporal margin of benefit seen with a primary angioplasty strategy has created a foundation for expanding catheter-based reperfusion by transfer to capable centers. Summary evidence favoring this concept from several randomized trials (see Table 48–2) indicates a reduction in 30-day mortality (6.8 percent versus 9.6 percent, $p = 0.01$; 33 lives saved per 1000 patients treated) and adverse events (death, stroke, or reinfarction) (8.5 percent versus 15.5 percent, $p < 0.001$; 70 fewer events per 1000 treated).[19] Individually, there was a statistically insignificant reduction in mortality for each trial. In the PRAGUE-2 trial the survival benefit appeared to be limited to patients presenting more than 3 hours after symptom onset, consistent with the delayed temporal advantage of primary angioplasty.[16] In these trials, interhospital transport appeared to be safe without increasing the patient's risk. Because of rapid transport and concurrent preparation for primary angioplasty in the DANAMI-2 trial, the treatment delay for transferred patients was minimal (<15 minutes) compared with that for a group presenting at the interventional centers.[18]

An alternative approach involves increasing the number of hospitals offering primary angioplasty. Experienced operators have performed primary angioplasty at hospitals without cardiac surgery with high procedural success even in patients with cardiogenic shock. A randomized trial (C-PORT) ($n = 451$) compared primary angioplasty (70 percent stents) with thrombolysis at 11 hospitals without on-site cardiac surgery.[20] A formal development program was completed prior to the trial at all hospitals and included American College of Cardiology/American Heart Association (ACC/AHA) guidelines.[83] The composite primary endpoint (death, reinfarction, stroke) was significantly reduced at 6 weeks and 6 months (12.4 percent versus 19.9 percent, $p = 0.03$) in the angioplasty group. No patient experienced a complication from attempted angioplasty that required emergency surgery.

The risk of an interventional complication requiring surgery (dissection or closure, side branch occlusion, perforation) in the setting of infarct artery angioplasty is low in the current era of stents and GP IIb/IIIa inhibitors.[54] However, a small percentage of patients require emergency surgery because of left main or complex multivessel disease and mechanical complications of infarction. In addition, institutional and operator expertise has been shown to affect the results of primary angioplasty procedures. Analysis of data from the NRMI data base indicates that mortality is lower among patients treated with primary angioplasty compared with thrombolysis at hospitals performing at intermediate (17 to 48 per year; 4.5 percent versus 5.9 percent, $p < 0.001$) and high volumes (>49 per year; 3.4 percent versus 5.4 percent, $p < 00.1$). At low-volume (<17 per year) hospitals, there was no mortality reduction for patients undergoing angioplasty (6.2 percent versus 5.9 percent, $p = 0.58$).[84] In-hospital mortality was reduced 57 percent when angioplasty was performed by high-volume operators (defined as >10 primary angioplasty procedures per year) in an analysis of the New York State registry.[85] These and other factors must be considered if primary angioplasty is considered at an institution without on-site cardiac surgery.[83]

The optimal reperfusion strategy for patients with acute myocardial infarction continues to evolve. Many regional factors may influence decisions regarding local protocols. Increasing utilization of prehospital diagnostic and risk assessment strategies should allow appropriate triage and initiation of timely reperfusion therapy for all eligible patients.

Modern Catheter-Based Reperfusion Techniques

Glycoprotein IIb/IIIa Inhibition

There is a strong theoretical basis for utilization of GP IIb/IIIa inhibition during catheter-based reperfusion therapy. Antagonism of platelet aggregation may "passivate" the unstable mechanically injured atherosclerotic arterial wall, avert thrombus formation on acutely deployed stents, and prevent microembolization with subsequent no reflow. Abciximab was shown to improve recovery of microvascular perfusion and to enhance contractile function after stenting in a randomized study of 200 patients with acute myocardial infarction.[86]

The ReoPro in AMI Primary PTCA Organization Randomized Trial (RAPPORT) randomly assigned 483 patients to placebo or abciximab while undergoing primary balloon angioplasty.[87] The incidence of death, reinfarction, or urgent target vessel revascularization (TVR) was significantly reduced at 30 days (5.8 percent versus 11.2 percent, $p = 0.03$) and 6 months (11.6 percent versus 17.8, $p = 0.05$) with abciximab. However the primary 6-month endpoint of death, reinfarction, and any TVR was equivalent (28.1 percent versus 28.2 percent).

Despite the apparent benefits of stenting in myocardial infarction, there was concern regarding the reduced rate of TIMI-3 flow achieved by stenting compared with balloon angioplasty (89.5 percent versus 92.7 percent, $p = 0.046$) in the Stent-PAMI trial.[36] This concern was amplified by the strong trend for higher mortality in the stent group at 1 year (5.4 percent versus 3 percent, $p = 0.054$).[53] It was postulated that this phenomenon may be due to thrombus embolization by stent devices during deployment. Thus, IIb/IIIa inhibition could be an important adjunct to stenting in acute myocardial infarction.

Two trials have examined the combination of primary infarct stenting and GP IIb/IIIa inhibition. The Abciximab before Direct angioplasty and stenting in Myocardial Infarction Regarding Acute and Long-term results (ADMIRAL) trial randomly assigned 300 patients undergoing primary stenting to abciximab given before angiography or placebo.[88] Patients receiving abciximab attained a greater frequency of TIMI-3 flow before stenting (16.8 percent versus 5.4 percent, $p = 0.01$), immediately after stenting (95.1 percent versus 86.7 percent, $p = 0.04$), and at 6 months (94.3 percent versus 82.8 percent, $p = 0.04$). The primary endpoint of death, reinfarction, or urgent TVR was also significantly reduced with abciximab treatment at 30 days (6 percent versus 14.6 percent, $p = 0.01$) and 6 months (7.4 percent versus 15.9 percent, $p = 0.02$). At 6 months, abciximab therapy was associated with less reocclusion (2.9 percent versus 12.1 percent, $p = 0.04$) and enhanced left ventricular function.

The risk of subacute thrombosis (stent and PTCA) at 30 days was reduced (0.4 percent versus 1.4 percent, $p < 0.001$) by abciximab in the Controlled Abciximab and Device Investigation to Lower Late Angioplasty Complications (CADILLAC) trial.[37] However, no significant advantage for abciximab treatment was evident at 6 months although a nonsignificant reduction in ischemic TVR was seen in patients with PTCA. In addition, abciximab did not significantly affect TIMI-3 flow rates or left ventricular function.

The discrepant results of these trials may be explained by differences in inclusion criteria (8 percent with shock in ADMIRAL), different stent designs, or, perhaps more important, the timing of abciximab administration. In CADILLAC, abciximab was given after angiography, whereas patients in ADMIRAL received drug before sheath insertion. In fact, in the ADMIRAL trial 26 percent of patients had abciximab administered in the emergency room or ambulance. A large benefit was identified for an early administration strategy (Fig. 48-7).[88] It must be remembered that abciximab has been associated with a small increase in minor bleeding (nonintracranial) and thrombocytopenia.

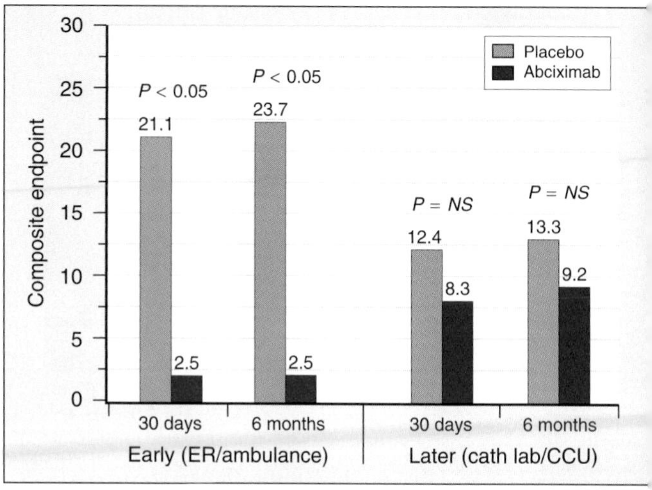

FIGURE 48–7 The incidence of the primary composite endpoint (death, reinfarction, or urgent target vessel revascularization) in the Abciximab before Direct angioplasty and stenting in Myocardial Infarction Regarding Acute and Long-term results (ADMIRAL) trial stratified by randomization and study drug administration time.[88] CCU = cardiac care unit; ER = emergency room.

Although the incremental benefits of adjunctive GP IIb/IIIa inhibition remain controversial, there is evidence supporting administration, especially early in the reperfusion process.

Primary Stent Implantation

Stents have ascended to an essential role in interventional practice. Early concerns regarding the safety of stent implantation in the presence of intracoronary thrombus have abated. High-pressure stent deployment techniques and additive antiplatelet therapy mitigated the risk of stent thrombosis and allowed utilization in acute coronary syndromes.

Suboptimal results after primary angioplasty are predictive of recurrent ischemia or reocclusion.[89] Initial use of stents was restricted to "bailout" indications, but several studies demonstrated the feasibility and safety of stents in acute myocardial infarction.[90]

Several randomized trials (Table 48–5)[36,37,91-97] have been conducted comparing primary stenting with primary balloon angioplasty. The Stent-PAMI trial reported a reduction in the 6-month combined endpoint of death, recurrent infarction and TVR related entirely to diminished TVR in the stent group (7.7 percent versus 17 percent, $p < 0.001$).[36] Stenting also reduced recurrent ischemia (9 percent versus 28 percent $p = 0.003$) and restenosis or reocclusion (17 percent versus 43 percent, $p = 0.001$). Despite a favorable influence on the combined endpoint, concern was raised regarding a trend toward increased late mortality in the stent group, possibly related to decreased TIMI-3 flow after stenting.[53] In the CADILLAC trial primary balloon angioplasty or primary stenting (newer generation device) without abciximab was compared in 1030 patients.[37] There was no significant difference in TIMI-3 flow rates (94.7 percent versus 94.5 percent) and 30-day mortality (2.5 percent versus 2.2 percent), but the 30-day TVR was significantly lower with stenting (6.0 percent versus 3.4 percent $p < 0.05$). At 6 months the combined endpoint of death, reinfarction, stroke, and ischemic TVR was significantly lower in the stent group (11.5 percent versus 20 percent, $p < 0.001$) driven by lower rates of ischemic TVR with stenting (8.3 percent versus 15.7 percent, $p < .001$). The 6-month mortality was insignificantly lower with stenting (3 percent versus 4.5 percent).

TABLE 48–5 Randomized Trials of Primary Stenting Versus Primary Angioplasty in Acute Myocardial Infarction

Reference	*n*	PTCA → Stent Crossover (%)	F/U time (mo)	MACE			Death		
				Stent	*PTCA*	*P* value	*Stent*	*PTCA*	*P* value
Zwolle[92]	227	13	6	5	20	0.0012	2	3	1
FRESCO[91]	150	0	6	9	28	0.003	0	0	—
PASTA[93]	136	10	12	22	49	0.0011	5	9	0.32
GRAMI[94]	104	25	0.2	17.3	34.6	0.002	3.8	7.7	NS
STENTIM-2[95]	211	36	6	19.8	28.2	0.14	3	1.9	NS
Stent PAMI[36]	900	15	12	17	25	<0.01	5.8	3.1	0.07
PSAAMI[97]	88	27	12	23	43	0.03	9	18	0.18
PRISAM[96]	222	1	6	—	—	—	0	0.9	—
CADILLACa*[37]	1030	18	6	11.5	20	<0.001	3	4.5	0.23
CADILLACb†[37]	1054	14	6	10.2	16.5	0.004	4.2	2.5	0.23

CADILLAC = Controlled Abciximab and Device Investigation to Lower Late Angioplasty Complications; FRESCO = Florence Randomized Elective Stenting in Acute Coronary Occlusions; F/U = follow-up; GRAMI = Gianturco-Roubin in Acute Myocardial Infarction; MACE = major adverse cardiac events—death, reinfarction, target vessel revascularization (stroke included in CADILLAC and Stent-PAMI); PAMI = Primary Angioplasty in Myocardial Infarction; PASTA = Primary Angioplasty versus STent implantation in Acute myocardial infarction; PRISAM = PRImary Stenting for Acute Myocardial infarction; PSAAMI = Primary Stenting vs. Angioplasty in Acute Myocardial Infarction; PTCA = percutaneous transluminal coronary angioplasty; STENTIM = STENT In acute Myocardial infarction.

*CADILLACa, stent alone and balloon angioplasty alone arms.

†CADILLACb, stent plus abciximab and balloon angioplasty plus abciximab arms.

A meta-analysis of the reported trials confirms the advantage of stent deployment.[98] The composite incidence of major adverse events at 6 to 12 months is significantly reduced (OR 0.52, 95 percent CI 0.44 to 0.62) without a significant difference in mortality again principally secondary to a reduction in TVR (OR 0.43, 95 percent CI 0.36 to 0.52) (Fig. 48–8). As with other PCI indications, stents should be routinely applied in acute myocardial infarction.

ADVANCES IN THE PROCESS OF REPERFUSION

There is considerable interest in developing the science of reperfusion beyond ensuring prompt and stable coronary patency. Methods for protection of microvascular integrity and preservation of the injured myocyte are evolving.

The importance of optimal myocardial perfusion and hazards of the no-reflow phenomenon have already been highlighted. Distal embolization identified by angiography during primary angioplasty was noted in 15.2 percent of patients in the Zwolle trial.[99] Procedural success (TIMI-3 flow) and perfusion (blush score) were reduced with embolization and associated with larger infarct size, lower ejection fraction, and higher 5-year mortality (44 percent versus 9 percent, $p < 0.001$).

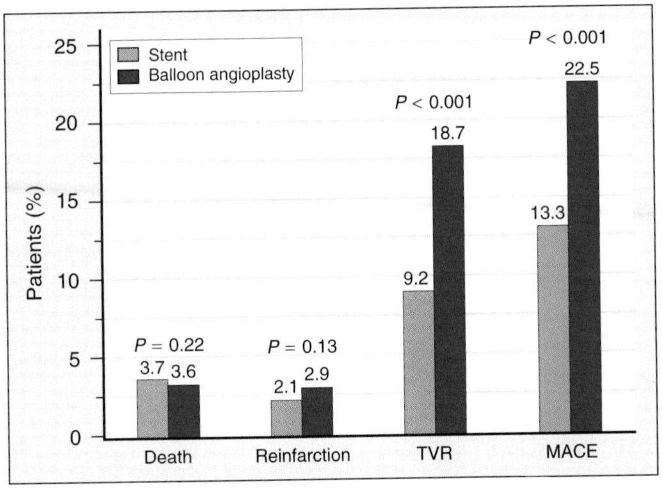

FIGURE 48–8 Results of meta-analysis comparing primary stenting with primary balloon angioplasty.[98] MACE = major adverse cardiac events including death, reinfarction, and target vessel revascularization (TVR) (stroke in Controlled Abciximab and Device Investigation to Lower Late Angioplasty Complications [CADILLAC] and Stent Primary Angioplasty in Myocardial Infarction [Stent-PAMI] trials).

In addition to pharmacological protection of the microvasculature with GP IIb/IIIa inhibition, several mechanical techniques employing thrombus removal have been reported. Kaplan and coworkers[100] reported utilization of the transluminal extraction catheter device in acute infarction with a 94 percent procedural success rate in 100 patients. However, restenosis occurred in 68 percent and this technique is limited by the large profile and complexity. Ultrasound thrombolysis has also been utilized successfully to induce patency (94 percent) in a small series.[101]

Several small series reported successful application of the AngioJet rheolytic thrombectomy catheter. This device utilizes high-velocity saline jets to create a low-pressure zone at the catheter tip through a Bernoulli effect, allowing fragmentation and aspiration of thrombus. For example, Silva and associates[102] reported a series of 79 patients with acute infarction and angiographic evidence for thrombus. Procedural success occurred in 94 percent with greater success in native arteries than venous bypass grafts. Angioplasty or stenting, or both, followed in most patients. Complications included distal embolization (10 percent) or perforation (3 percent). Beside the obvious application to patients with a large thrombus burden, utilization of this device has been reported to achieve superior outcomes in cardiogenic shock[103] and stent thrombosis,[104] in which usual catheter-based revascularization has been less successful. A randomized trial examining routine application of AngioJet thrombectomy during catheter-based reperfusion is in progress.

The X-sizer device employs helical thrombectomy and vacuum aspiration. It has been reported in a randomized trial ($n = 92$) to attain normal myocardial blush scores in a greater proportion of patients than primary stenting alone (72 percent versus 37 percent, $p = 0.006$).[105] Other thrombus removal devices using vacuum-assisted aspiration through specialized catheters have also been successfully utilized in myocardial infarction.[49,106]

Protection can also be accomplished with systems designed to prevent embolization through distal balloon occlusion and aspiration or filters designed to trap debris. The former mechanism in the form of the PercuSurge device has been reported with successful removal of thrombus and effective reperfusion in a few cases.[107] A current randomized trial is testing routine use of this device during acute infarct angioplasty. Other distal protection devices are under development and will be investigated in this setting.

Many pharmacological interventions have been proposed and investigated as methods of myocardial preservation. Considerable effort has been focused on reperfusion injury, which has been described to consist of several processes including oxygen free radical production, contraction band necrosis related to calcium overload, activation of inflammatory mediators, endothelial dysfunction, and microvascular injury contributing to no reflow.[46] Despite promising experimental data, clinical trials including those targeting neutrophil migration, free radical formation, and metabolic stabilization have failed to affect infarct size or outcomes significantly.[46,108,109]

In contrast, more favorable effects have been observed with the vasodilator adenosine, which may also work through cardioprotective mechanisms including replenishment of high-energy phosphate stores, ischemic preconditioning, free radical suppression, and platelet and neutrophil inhibition. Intracoronary adenosine reduced no reflow and improved ventricular function during primary angioplasty.[110] In the Acute Myocardial Infarction Study of Adenosine (AMISTAD) I and II trials, infarct size was significantly reduced (27 to 33 percent) by adenosine with a trend toward reduced death and heart failure in AMISTAD II.[111,112] Nicorandil, another agent with multiple effects (adenosine triphosphate-sensitive K^+ channel opener with nitrate properties) reduced no reflow and was associated with better clinical outcomes in a randomized trial involving 81 patients undergoing primary angioplasty.[113] In the COMplement inhibition in Myocardial infarction treated with Angioplasty (COMMA) trial a monoclonal antibody to the C5 terminal component of the complement cascade (pexelizumab) was tested in 814 patients undergoing primary angioplasty. Although there was no effect on the primary endpoint of infarct size, 6-month mortality was significantly lower in the antibody-treated group (3.2 percent vs, 7.4 percent, $p = 0.018$).[114]

Preliminary evidence suggests that infusion of aqueous hyperoxemic blood (oxygen partial pressure 600 to 800 mm Hg) for 60 to 90 minutes after primary angioplasty may attenuate microvascular injury and enhance myocardial salvage.[115] Induction of moderate systemic hypothermia through a heat exchange catheter in the vena cava may also reduce infarct size.[116] These and other interventions for myocardial protection during reperfusion are being tested in randomized trials.

Combining Thrombolysis and Angioplasty as Reperfusion Therapy

RESCUE ANGIOPLASTY. Despite growth in the proportion of patients undergoing primary angioplasty, in most countries the majority of patients with infarction receive thrombolytic reperfusion therapy. There remains a paucity of investigational data regarding the value of rescue angioplasty in patients who do not achieve reperfusion after thrombolysis. Observational data and early trials suggested little benefit and high mortality (>30 percent) among patients in whom attempted rescue angioplasty fails.[117] This finding is reflective of the higher risk profile in patients with failed thrombolysis and the complex management related to the uncertainty of lytic success and possible need for transfer to enable rescue procedures.

An analysis of four small randomized trials of rescue angioplasty ($n = 368$) identified a significant reduction in early severe heart failure (3.8 percent versus 11.7 percent, $p = 0.04$) and a trend toward reduced early mortality (8.5 percent versus 12.2 percent, $p = 0.26$).[118] Aggregate 1-year follow-up data from two of these trials revealed a significant survival benefit.[118] More contemporary data indicate that patients undergoing rescue intervention benefit from GP IIb/IIIa inhibition and stenting with improved procedural success and enhanced clinical outcomes.[119,120]

The difficulty of noninvasive determination of the status of infarct artery perfusion remains an important limitation of this approach. Utilization of clinical features, baseline/60-minute biomarkers, and ST segment resolution in combination as a predictive instrument may improve accuracy.[121] The role of rescue angioplasty will continue to be investigated as the concept of facilitated intervention evolves.

THE CONCEPT OF FACILITATED ANGIOPLASTY. The parallel nascent development of thrombolytic reperfusion therapy and transluminal revascularization within the catheterization laboratory invited combined application in acute myocardial infarction in an effort to optimize the arterial lumen and reduce the risk of recurrent ischemia and reocclusion. However, several trials conducted more than a decade ago demonstrated an adverse outcome for early compared with delayed angioplasty after thrombolysis with more complications (bypass surgery and bleeding), a trend for higher mortality, and no difference in left ventricular function.[83] This hazard was presumed to originate from enhanced platelet activation or extensive intramural hemorrhage, or both. Yet, advanced angioplasty techniques have improved the safety of the procedure in this setting. In a multivariate analysis of the patients in the TIMI-10B (tenecteplase [TNK] versus t-PA) and TIMI-14 (reduced dose t-PA and/or abciximab) trials, those undergoing adjunctive or delayed intervention (>60 percent stents) had a lower risk of 30-day mortality or reinfarction than patients with successful (TIMI-3 flow at 90 minutes) thrombolysis without intervention.[122]

A further impetus for revisiting a combined pharmacological and mechanical approach to reperfusion comes from an analysis of the four PAMI trials ($n = 2507$).[123] Patients (16 percent) with spontaneous reperfusion (TIMI-3 flow) on initial angiography prior to intervention had improved left ventricular function with less heart failure, hypotension, and hospital mortality. Procedural success was improved and, by multivariate analysis, TIMI-3 flow before angioplasty was an independent determinant of survival.

This information has stimulated further development of the synergistic concept of facilitated angioplasty achieving the speed advantage of pharmacological reperfusion while allowing the security of mechanical bailout and "definitive" treatment of the arterial lumen. In the Plasminogen-activator Angioplasty Compatibility Trial (PACT), patients receiving half-dose t-PA had a higher TIMI-3 flow rate (33 percent versus 15 percent with placebo) prior to angioplasty.[124] The benefits of early initiation of abciximab before primary stenting were noted in the ADMIRAL trial (see Fig. 48–7). Administration of abciximab alone before angiography resulted in 90-minute TIMI-3 flow rates of about 30 percent.[38,125] When abciximab was combined with reduced-dose (usually half) thrombolysis, the 90-minute TIMI-3 flow rates were 62 to 77 percent[38] with no increased risk of major bleeding or intracranial hemorrhage over full-dose thrombolysis. In the SPEED (Strategies for Patency Enhancement in the Emergency Department) (GUSTO IV pilot) trial, 323 patients who underwent PCI in the setting of prior combined reteplase and abciximab therapy were compared with 162 patients without intervention.[125] The patients with early PCI experienced a reduction in the composite endpoint of death, reinfarction, or urgent revascularization (5.6 percent versus 16 percent, $p = 0.001$). The risk of ischemic events or bleeding complications was also reduced with early PCI (15 percent versus 30 percent, $p = 0.001$).

Facilitated angioplasty (PCI) may augment the results of catheter-based reperfusion by enhancing myocardial salvage, the stability of the procedure, and the safety of transfer of patients. However, these benefits need to be counterbalanced by the hemorrhagic risk of combined pharmacological reperfusion therapy, especially in the elderly population.[39,40] Several trials are now in progress that will elucidate further the role of a facilitated angioplasty strategy.

The Conduct of the Primary Angioplasty (Percutaneous Coronary Intervention) Procedure

A primary interventional strategy for reperfusion in myocardial infarction is a multidisciplinary institutional commitment. Precise protocols and standards should be imposed, including mechanisms for urgent transfer to the interventional center preferably after prehospital triage utilizing

12-lead electrocardiograms. This will allow mobilization of the reperfusion team. Upon hospital arrival, evaluation should proceed in a swift and thorough manner while infarct care is begun (including aspirin, heparin, and beta blockade or nitrates as appropriate). In the PAMI trials, patients treated with precatheterization beta blockade had fewer procedural complications and lower hospital mortality (1.8 percent versus 3.7 percent, $p = 0.0035$).[126] Assessment must include acknowledgment of factors that may influence the procedure (e.g., peripheral vascular disease, renal function) with early involvement of the interventional operator in this process.

ACC/AHA guidelines for performance of primary angioplasty at hospitals without cardiac surgery have been published.[83] The importance of a formalized transfer arrangement for urgent cardiac surgery and ongoing outcomes analysis should not be underestimated.[20] Operator experience in ongoing interventional practice at a surgery center is critical to program success. Efforts to minimize the treatment interval should be diligently pursued.

In the catheterization laboratory, ongoing intensive medical care must be provided. Comprehensive protocols provide a dedicated environment where events and complications are anticipated. In most circumstances, primary angioplasty is more complicated than an elective procedure. The operator must tailor the approach to the environment of acute infarction

Preparation of both femoral access sites is a facile precautionary step. Primary angioplasty can usually be performed utilizing 6 French (6F) guide catheters and familiar guidewires, but larger guide catheters may be needed to utilize thrombectomy or distal protection devices. Attention should be paid to collateral flow during initial angiography to guide intervention in the infarct artery. Angiography of the infarct vessel can be performed with the guide catheter. Care should be taken to maintain the guidewire in the main vessel with advancement through the occlusion. An appropriately sized balloon catheter should be positioned efficiently and inflated to allow early reperfusion. In most cases, stenting should follow balloon angioplasty of the culprit lesion. Although direct stenting without predilation has been proposed as a method to minimize embolization, this practice did not reduce no reflow in one study compared with conventional stenting techniques.[127]

Heparin anticoagulation should be monitored during the procedure and adjustments made reflecting the use of GP IIb/IIIa inhibition. Thienopyridines are necessary adjuncts to stent implantation, and in the PAMI trials administration of ticlopidine prior to angiography (in addition to standard heparin and aspirin) was associated with higher preintervention TIMI-3 flow rates (20.7 percent versus 11.4 percent, $p < 0.001$).[123] The role of direct thrombin inhibitors and primary angioplasty awaits further study

Thrombectomy and distal protection devices are being tested as routine adjuncts to catheter-based reperfusion in randomized trials. The current utilization of these devices is largely based upon the operator's judgment and experience. Angiographic morphology predictive of slow or no reflow includes "cutoff" occlusion, reference diameter greater than 4 mm, floating thrombus, persistent dye stasis distal to the obstruction, thrombus more than 5 mm proximal to the occlusion, or accumulated linear thrombus more than three times the reference diameter.[128] These findings might be utilized to define circumstances for effective use of thromboembolic protective devices.

Discovery of these predictors of impaired flow should promote the use of GP IIb/IIIa inhibition and consideration of other prophylactic pharmacological measures. Giri and colleagues[129] reported less no reflow with abciximab in a consecutive case series ($n = 650$). In patients who develop angiographic evidence of no reflow (TIMI flow grade ≤2) (see Table 48–4) after primary angioplasty, epicardial vessel complications such as dissection, a suboptimal result, or spasm must be excluded. Both intracoronary adenosine[110] and intravenous nicorandil[113] reduce no reflow when given before and after intervention. Intracoronary calcium channel blockers have been reported to be effective in attenuating microvascular dysfunction during myocardial infarction.[45] Intracoronary nitroprusside resulted in improved flow compared with verapamil in a review of 68 patients with no reflow.[130] In some cases, the onset of no reflow can result in profound hemodynamic deterioration. Intracoronary epinephrine has been utilized to improve flow significantly in patients with refractory no reflow and may be appropriate treatment in patients who are hypotensive.[131] These agents are preferably administered distally in the epicardial vessels. Despite favorable effects, no agent has clearly improved clinical outcomes.[130]

Multivessel disease is encountered in 40 to 75 percent of patients undergoing reperfusion therapy.[36,37,132] The conventional approach to the patient with multivessel disease has incorporated either urgent surgery, staged angioplasty, late surgery, or noninvasive evaluation after reperfusion. The advent of modern angioplasty technology has allowed consideration of multivessel revascularization at the time of the primary angioplasty procedure. This strategy seems a logical approach in the patient with cardiogenic shock, but it should be tested against emergency bypass surgery. In the hemodynamically stable patient, multivessel disease impairs recovery of left ventricular function.[133] Multiple complex coronary lesions have been identified in approximately 40 percent of patients with acute infarction and may reflect a systemic process (inflammation, deranged lipid metabolism) affecting widespread vulnerable plaques.[132] The presence of multiple complex plaques is associated with more recurrent ischemic events. Investigation examining multivessel angioplasty during the primary procedure is lacking. Small reports suggest mixed results, and randomized trials are needed to determine the optimal revascularization strategy for patients with multivessel disease.[134,135]

The benefits of rapid reperfusion are amplified in cardiogenic shock.[33,76] If prompt reperfusion is accomplished and the patient does not improve, mechanical complications should be considered utilizing hemodynamic, ventriculographic, or echocardiographic assessment.

Intraaortic balloon counterpulsation is a necessary adjunct during reperfusion therapy of the patient with cardiogenic shock.[33] Brodie and colleagues[136] reported a reduction of adverse catheterization laboratory events in high-risk infarct patients with cardiogenic shock, heart failure, or a low (<0.30) ejection fraction. Early studies of routine counterpulsation after primary angioplasty reported reduced reocclusion and improved ventricular function. However the PAMI-2 trial identified no reduction in the risk of reocclusion, reinfarction, or death or improved ventricular function with balloon pump support of hemodynamically stable high-risk patients.[137]

The interventional team is obligated to review outcomes and modify processes continually, incorporating advances derived from investigation in the dynamic field of reperfusion therapy.

Synopsis of the Primary Angioplasty Strategy

- In comparison with thrombolysis, a primary angioplasty strategy provides a greater chance for restoring blood flow and stabilization of the infarct artery. This method increases the population that can gain effective and safe reperfusion.
- The expanded latitude of temporal benefit for primary angioplasty may mitigate the logistical constraints of this approach.

- Stents enhance the durability of the procedure. Early administration of GP IIb/IIIa inhibitors may augment the results of primary stenting.
- There is considerable promise for evolution of the science of microcirculatory and myocardial protection during infarction.

The challenge ahead is to focus on early entry of the infarct patient into a triage process that can accelerate reperfusion. Local factors are likely to influence whether a primary, facilitated, or transfer procedure is the optimal strategy.

REFERENCES

1. O'Keefe JH Jr, Bailey WL, Rutherford BD, Hartzler GO: Primary angioplasty for acute myocardial infarction in 1,000 consecutive patients. Results in an unselected population and high-risk subgroups. Am J Cardiol 72:107G, 1993.
2. Every NR, Parsons LS, Hlatky M, et al: A comparison of thrombolytic therapy with primary coronary angioplasty for acute myocardial infarction. Myocardial Infarction Triage and Intervention Investigators. N Engl J Med 335:1253, 1996.
3. Tiefenbrunn AJ, Chandra NC, French WJ, et al: Clinical experience with primary percutaneous transluminal coronary angioplasty compared with alteplase (recombinant tissue-type plasminogen activator) in patients with acute myocardial infarction: A report from the Second National Registry of Myocardial Infarction (NRMI-2). J Am Coll Cardiol 31:1240, 1998.
4. Zahn R, Schiele R, Schneider S, et al: Primary angioplasty versus intravenous thrombolysis in acute myocardial infarction: Can we define subgroups of patients benefiting most from primary angioplasty? Results from the pooled data of the Maximal Individual Therapy in Acute Myocardial Infarction Registry and the Myocardial Infarction Registry. J Am Coll Cardiol 37:1827, 2001.
5. Zahn R, Schiele R, Schneider S, et al: Decreasing hospital mortality between 1994 and 1998 in patients with acute myocardial infarction treated with primary angioplasty but not in patients treated with intravenous thrombolysis. Results from the pooled data of the Maximal Individual Therapy in Acute Myocardial Infarction (MITRA) Registry and the Myocardial Infarction Registry (MIR). J Am Coll Cardiol 36:2064, 2000.

Randomized Trials Comparing Primary Angioplasty with Thrombolysis

6. Grines CL, Browne KF, Marco J, et al: A comparison of immediate angioplasty with thrombolytic therapy for acute myocardial infarction. The Primary Angioplasty in Myocardial Infarction Study Group. N Engl J Med 328:673, 1993.
7. Gibbons RJ, Holmes DR, Reeder GS, et al: Immediate angioplasty compared with the administration of a thrombolytic agent followed by conservative treatment for myocardial infarction. The Mayo Coronary Care Unit and Catheterization Laboratory Groups. N Engl J Med 328:685, 1993.
8. Zijlstra F, de Boer MJ, Hoorntje JC, et al: A comparison of immediate coronary angioplasty with intravenous streptokinase in acute myocardial infarction. N Engl J Med 328:680, 1993.
9. GUSTO IIb Angioplasty Substudy Investigators: A clinical trial comparing primary coronary angioplasty with tissue plasminogen activator for acute myocardial infarction. The Global Use of Strategies to Open Occluded Coronary Arteries in Acute Coronary Syndromes (GUSTO IIb) Angioplasty Substudy Investigators. N Engl J Med 336:1621, 1997.
10. Weaver WD, Simes RJ, Betriu A, et al: Comparison of primary coronary angioplasty and intravenous thrombolytic therapy for acute myocardial infarction: A quantitative review. JAMA 278:2093, 1997.
11. Grines C, Patel A, Zijlstra F, et al: Primary coronary angioplasty compared with intravenous thrombolytic therapy for acute myocardial infarction: Six-month follow up and analysis of individual patient data from randomized trials. Am Heart J 145:47, 2003.
12. Zijlstra F, Hoorntje JC, de Boer MJ, et al:. Long-term benefit of primary angioplasty as compared with thrombolytic therapy for acute myocardial infarction. N Engl J Med 341:1413, 1999.
13. Schomig A, Kastrati A, Dirschinger J, et al: Coronary stenting plus platelet glycoprotein IIb/IIIa blockade compared with tissue plasminogen activator in acute myocardial infarction. Stent versus Thrombolysis for Occluded Coronary Arteries in Patients with Acute Myocardial Infarction Study Investigators. N Engl J Med 343:385, 2000.
14. Bonnefoy E, Lapostolle F, Leizorovicz A, et al: Primary angioplasty versus prehospital fibrinolysis in acute myocardial infarction: A randomised study. Lancet 360:825, 2002.
15. Widimsky P, Groch L, Zelizko M, et al: Multicentre randomized trial comparing transport to primary angioplasty vs immediate thrombolysis vs combined strategy for patients with acute myocardial infarction presenting to a community hospital without a catheterization laboratory. The PRAGUE study. Eur Heart J 21:823, 2000.
16. Widimsky P, Budesinsky T, Vorac D, et al: Long distance transport for primary angioplasty vs immediate thrombolysis in acute myocardial infarction. Final results of the randomized national multicentre trial—PRAGUE-2. Eur Heart J 24:94, 2003.
17. Grines CL, Westerhausen DR Jr, Grines LL, et al: A randomized trial of transfer for primary angioplasty versus on-site thrombolysis in patients with high-risk myocardial infarction: The Air Primary Angioplasty in Myocardial Infarction study. J Am Coll Cardiol 39:1713, 2002.
18. Moon JC, Kalra PR, Coats AJ: DANAMI-2: Is primary angioplasty superior to thrombolysis in acute MI when the patient has to be transferred to an invasive centre? Int J Cardiol 85:199, 2002.
19. Zijlstra F: Angioplasty vs thrombolysis for acute myocardial infarction: A quantitative overview of the effects of interhospital transportation. Eur Heart J 24:21, 2003.
20. Aversano T, Aversano LT, Passamani E, et al: Thrombolytic therapy vs primary percutaneous coronary intervention for myocardial infarction in patients presenting to hospitals without on-site cardiac surgery: A randomized controlled trial. JAMA 287:1943, 2002.
21. Keeley EC, Boura JA, Grines CL: Primary angioplasty versus intravenous thrombolytic therapy for acute myocardial infarction: A quantitative review of 23 randomised trials. Lancet 361:13, 2003.
22. Zijlstra F, Beukema WP, van't Hof AW, et al: Randomized comparison of primary coronary angioplasty with thrombolytic therapy in low risk patients with acute myocardial infarction. J Am Coll Cardiol 29:908, 1997.
23. Ribeiro EE, Silva LA, Carneiro R, et al: Randomized trial of direct coronary angioplasty versus intravenous streptokinase in acute myocardial infarction. J Am Coll Cardiol 22:376, 1993.
24. Grinfeld L, Berrocal D, Belardi J, et al: Fibrinolytics vs. primary angioplasty in acute myocardial infarction (FAP). J Am Coll Cardiol 27:222A, 1996.
25. Dewood MA: Direct PTCA vs. intravenous t-Pa in acute myocardial infarction: Results from a prospective randomized trial. *In* The Thrombolysis and Interventional Therapy in Acute Myocardial Infarction Symposium VI. Washington, DC, George Washington University, 1990, pp 28-29.
26. Ribichini F, Steffenino G, Dellavalle A, et al: Comparison of thrombolytic therapy and primary coronary angioplasty with liberal stenting for inferior myocardial infarction with precordial ST-segment depression: Immediate and long-term results of a randomized study. J Am Coll Cardiol 32:1687, 1998.
27. Garcia E, Elizaga J, Perez-Castellano N, et al: Primary angioplasty versus systemic thrombolysis in anterior myocardial infarction. J Am Coll Cardiol 33:605, 1999.
28. Akhras F, Abu Ousa A, Swann G: Primary coronary angioplasty or intravenous thrombolysis for patients with acute myocardial infarction? Acute and late follow-up results in a new cardiac unit. J Am Coll Cardiol 29:A235, 1997.
29. de Boer MJ, Ottervanger JP, van't Hof AW, et al: Reperfusion therapy in elderly patients with acute myocardial infarction: A randomized comparison of primary angioplasty and thrombolytic therapy. J Am Coll Cardiol 39:1723, 2002.
30. Le May MR, Labinaz M, Davies RF, et al: Stenting versus thrombolysis in acute myocardial infarction trial (STAT). J Am Coll Cardiol 37:985, 2001.
31. Kastrati A, Mehilli J, Dirschinger J, et al: Myocardial salvage after coronary stenting plus abciximab versus fibrinolysis plus abciximab in patients with acute myocardial infarction: A randomised trial. Lancet 359:920, 2002.
32. Vermeer F, Oude Ophuis AJ, vd Berg EJ, et al: Prospective randomised comparison between thrombolysis, rescue PTCA, and primary PTCA in patients with extensive myocardial infarction admitted to a hospital without PTCA facilities: A safety and feasibility study. Heart 82:426, 1999.
33. Hochman JS, Sleeper LA, Webb JG, et al: Early revascularization in acute myocardial infarction complicated by cardiogenic shock. SHOCK Investigators. Should We Emergently Revascularize Occluded Coronaries for Cardiogenic Shock. N Engl J Med 341:625, 1999.
34. GUSTO Angiographic Investigators: The effects of tissue plasminogen activator streptokinase, or both on coronary artery patency, ventricular function, and survival after acute myocardial infarction. N Engl J Med 329:1615, 1993.
35. Berger PB, Ellis SG, Holmes DR Jr, et al: Relationship between delay in performing direct coronary angioplasty and early clinical outcome in patients with acute myocardial infarction: Results from the global use of strategies to open occluded arteries in Acute Coronary Syndromes (GUSTO-IIb) trial. Circulation 100:14, 1999.
36. Grines CL, Cox DA, Stone GW, et al: Coronary angioplasty with or without stent implantation for acute myocardial infarction. Stent Primary Angioplasty in Myocardial Infarction Study Group. N Engl J Med 341:1949, 1999.
37. Stone GW, Grines CL, Cox DA, et al: Comparison of angioplasty with stenting, with or without abciximab, in acute myocardial infarction. N Engl J Med 346:957, 2002.
38. Antman EM, Giugliano RP, Gibson CM, et al: Abciximab facilitates the rate and extent of thrombolysis: Results of the thrombolysis in myocardial infarction (TIMI) 14 trial. The TIMI 14 Investigators. Circulation 99:2720, 1999.
39. ASSENT-3 Investigators: Efficacy and safety of tenecteplase in combination with enoxaparin, abciximab, or unfractionated heparin: The ASSENT-3 randomised trial in acute myocardial infarction. Lancet 358:605, 2001.
40. Lincoff AM, Califf RM, Van de Werf F, et al: Mortality at 1 year with combination platelet glycoprotein IIb/IIIa inhibition and reduced-dose fibrinolytic therapy vs conventional fibrinolytic therapy for acute myocardial infarction: GUSTO V randomized trial. JAMA 288:2130, 2002.
41. Roe MT, Ohman EM, Maas AC, et al: Shifting the open-artery hypothesis downstream: The quest for optimal reperfusion. J Am Coll Cardiol 37:9, 2001.
42. Gibson CM, Cannon CP, Daley WL, et al: TIMI frame count: A quantitative method of assessing coronary artery flow. Circulation 93:879, 1996.
43. Gibson CM, Cannon CP, Murphy SA, et al: Relationship of TIMI myocardial perfusion grade to mortality after administration of thrombolytic drugs. Circulation 101:125, 2000.
44. van 't Hof AW, Liem A, Suryapranata H, et al: Angiographic assessment of myocardial reperfusion in patients treated with primary angioplasty for acute myocardial infarction: Myocardial blush grade. Zwolle Myocardial Infarction Study Group. Circulation 97:2302, 1998.
45. Rezkalla SH, Kloner RA: No-reflow phenomenon. Circulation 105:656, 2002.
46. Verma S, Fedak PW, Weisel RD, et al: Fundamentals of reperfusion injury for the clinical cardiologist. Circulation 105:2332, 2002.
47. Agati L, Voci P, Hickle P, et al: Tissue-type plasminogen activator therapy versus primary coronary angioplasty: Impact on myocardial tissue perfusion and regional function 1 month after uncomplicated myocardial infarction. J Am Coll Cardiol 31:338, 1998.
48. Zeymer U, Schroder R, Neuhaus K: Primary PTCA accelerates myocardial reperfusion compared to thrombolysis in patients with acute myocardial infarction. Circulation 104:II-466, 2001.

49. Murakami T, Mizuno S, Takahashi Y, et al: Intracoronary aspiration thrombectomy for acute myocardial infarction. Am J Cardiol 82:839, 1998.
50. Llevadot J, Giugliano RP, McCabe CH, et al: Degree of residual stenosis in the culprit coronary artery after thrombolytic administration (Thrombolysis In Myocardial Infarction [TIMI] trials). Am J Cardiol 85:1409, 2000.
51. Veen G, de Boer MJ, Zijlstra F, Verheugt FW: Improvement in three-month angiographic outcome suggested after primary angioplasty for acute myocardial infarction (Zwolle trial) compared with successful thrombolysis (APRICOT trial). Antithrombotics in the Prevention of Reocclusion In COronary Thrombolysis. Am J Cardiol 84:763, 1999.
52. Brodie BR, Grines CL, Ivanhoe R, et al: Six-month clinical and angiographic follow-up after direct angioplasty for acute myocardial infarction. Final results from the Primary Angioplasty Registry. Circulation 90:156, 1994.
53. Grines CL, Cox DA, Stone GW, et al: Stent PAMI: 12 month results and predictors of mortality. J Am Coll Cardiol 35:402A, 2000.
54. Stone GW, Brodie BR, Griffin JJ, et al: Role of cardiac surgery in the hospital phase management of patients treated with primary angioplasty for acute myocardial infarction. Am J Cardiol 85:1292, 2000.
55. Grines CL, Marsalese DL, Brodie B, et al: Safety and cost-effectiveness of early discharge after primary angioplasty in low risk patients with acute myocardial infarction. PAMI-II Investigators. Primary Angioplasty in Myocardial Infarction. J Am Coll Cardiol 31:967, 1998.
56. Kinn JW, O'Neill WW, Benzuly KH, et al: Primary angioplasty reduces risk of myocardial rupture compared to thrombolysis for acute myocardial infarction. Cathet Cardiovasc Diagn 42:151, 1997.
57. Moreno R, Lopez-Sendon J, Garcia E, et al: Primary angioplasty reduces the risk of left ventricular free wall rupture compared with thrombolysis in patients with acute myocardial infarction. J Am Coll Cardiol 39:598, 2002.
58. Biostatistical Fact Sheet: Older Americans and Cardiovascular Diseases. Chicago, American Heart Association, 1998.
59. White HD: Thrombolytic therapy in the elderly. Lancet 356:2028, 2000.
60. Berger AK, Schulman KA, Gersh BJ, et al: Primary coronary angioplasty vs thrombolysis for the management of acute myocardial infarction in elderly patients. JAMA 282:341, 1999.
61. Thiemann DR, Coresh J, Schulman SP, et al: Lack of benefit for intravenous thrombolysis in patients with myocardial infarction who are older than 75 years. Circulation 101:2239, 2000.
62. O'Neill WW, De Boer MJ, Gibbons RJ, et al: Lessons from the pooled outcome of the PAMI, ZWOLLE, and Mayo Clinic randomized trials of primary angioplasty versus thrombolytic therapy of acute myocardial infarction. J Invasive Cardiol 10(Suppl A):4A, 1998.
63. Minai K, Horie H, Takahashi M, et al: Long-term outcome of primary percutaneous transluminal coronary angioplasty for low-risk acute myocardial infarction in patients older than 80 years: A single-center, open, randomized trial. Am Heart J 143:497, 2002.
64. Labinaz M, Sketch MH Jr, Ellis SG, et al: Outcome of acute ST-segment elevation myocardial infarction in patients with prior coronary artery bypass surgery receiving thrombolytic therapy. Am Heart J 141:469, 2001.
65. Peterson LR, Chandra NC, French WJ, et al: Reperfusion therapy in patients with acute myocardial infarction and prior coronary artery bypass graft surgery (National Registry of Myocardial Infarction-2). Am J Cardiol 84:1287, 1999.
66. Al Suwaidi J, Velianou JL, Berger PB, et al: Primary percutaneous coronary interventions in patients with acute myocardial infarction and prior coronary artery bypass grafting. Am Heart J 142:452, 2001.
67. Nguyen TT, O'Neill WW, Dixon SR, et al: Poor one year prognosis in acute myocardial infarction patients with saphenous vein grafts as the infarct related vessel treated by primary balloon angioplasty. J Am Coll Cardiol 39:309A, 2002.
68. Mattos L, Sousa A, Neto CC, et al: Primary stenting versus balloon PTCA for the treatment of acute vein graft occlusion in myocardial infarction: In-hospital results from the Brazilian Coronary Interventional Registry (CENIC). J Am Coll Cardiol 35:39A, 2000.
69. Eagle KA, Goodman SG, Avezum A, et al: Practice variation and missed opportunities for reperfusion in ST-segment-elevation myocardial infarction: Findings from the Global Registry of Acute Coronary Events (GRACE). Lancet 359:373, 2002.
70. Zahn R, Schuster S, Schiele R, et al: Comparison of primary angioplasty with conservative therapy in patients with acute myocardial infarction and contraindications for thrombolytic therapy. Maximal Individual Therapy in Acute Myocardial Infarction (MITRA) Study Group. Catheter Cardiovasc Interv 46:127, 1999.
71. Juliard JM, Himbert D, Golmard JL, et al: Can we provide reperfusion therapy to all unselected patients admitted with acute myocardial infarction? J Am Coll Cardiol 30:157, 1997.
72. Lane GE, Holmes DR: The modern strategy for cardiogenic shock. *In* Cannon CP (ed): Management of Acute Coronary Syndromes. Totowa, NJ, Humana Press, 2003, pp 603-52.
73. Barron HV, Every NR, Parsons LS, et al: The use of intra-aortic balloon counterpulsation in patients with cardiogenic shock complicating acute myocardial infarction: Data from the National Registry of Myocardial Infarction 2. Am Heart J 141:933, 2001.
74. Hochman JS, Sleeper LA, White HD, et al: One-year survival following early revascularization for cardiogenic shock. JAMA 285:190, 2001.
75. Dzavik V, Sleeper LA, Hosat S, et al: Effect of age on treatment and outcome of patients in cardiogenic shock. Eur Heart J 19:28, 1998.
76. Brodie BR, Stuckey TD, Muncy DB, et al: Importance of time-to-reperfusion in patients with acute myocardial infarction with and without cardiogenic shock treated with primary percutaneous coronary intervention. Am Heart J 145:708, 2003.
77. Newby LK, Rutsch WR, Califf RM, et al: Time from symptom onset to treatment and outcomes after thrombolytic therapy. GUSTO-1 Investigators. J Am Coll Cardiol 27:1646, 1996.
78. Cannon CP, Gibson CM, Lambrew CT, et al: Relationship of symptom-onset-to-balloon time and door-to-balloon time with mortality in patients undergoing angioplasty for acute myocardial infarction. JAMA 283:2941, 2000.
79. Brodie BR, Stuckey TD, Wall TC, et al: Importance of time to reperfusion for 30-day and late survival and recovery of left ventricular function after primary angioplasty for acute myocardial infarction. J Am Coll Cardiol 32:1312, 1998.
80. Zijlstra F, Patel A, Jones M, et al: Clinical characteristics and outcome of patients with early (<2 h), intermediate (2-4 h) and late (>4 h) presentation treated by primary coronary angioplasty or thrombolytic therapy for acute myocardial infarction. Eur Heart J 23:550, 2002.
81. Milavetz JJ, Giebel DW, Christian TF, et al: Time to therapy and salvage in myocardial infarction. J Am Coll Cardiol 31:1246, 1998.
82. Bode C, Smalling RW, Berg G, et al: Randomized comparison of coronary thrombolysis achieved with double-bolus reteplase (recombinant plasminogen activator) and front-loaded, accelerated alteplase (recombinant tissue plasminogen activator) in patients with acute myocardial infarction. The RAPID II Investigators. Circulation 94:891, 1996.
83. Smith SC Jr, Dove JT, Jacobs AK, et al: ACC/AHA guidelines of percutaneous coronary interventions (revision of the 1993 PTCA guidelines)—Executive summary. A report of the American College of Cardiology/American Heart Association Task Force on Practice Guidelines (committee to revise the 1993 guidelines for percutaneous transluminal coronary angioplasty). J Am Coll Cardiol 37:2215, 2001.
84. Magid DJ, Calonge BN, Rumsfeld JS, et al: Relation between hospital primary angioplasty volume and mortality for patients with acute MI treated with primary angioplasty vs thrombolytic therapy. JAMA 284:3131, 2000.
85. Vakili BA, Kaplan R, Brown DL: Volume-outcome relation for physicians and hospitals performing angioplasty for acute myocardial infarction in New York state. Circulation 104:2171, 2001.

Modern Catheter-Based Reperfusion Techniques

86. Neumann FJ, Blasini R, Schmitt C, et al: Effect of glycoprotein IIb/IIIa receptor blockade on recovery of coronary flow and left ventricular function after the placement of coronary-artery stents in acute myocardial infarction. Circulation 98:2695, 1998.
87. Brener SJ, Barr LA, Burchenal JE, et al: Randomized, placebo-controlled trial of platelet glycoprotein IIb/IIIa blockade with primary angioplasty for acute myocardial infarction. ReoPro and Primary PTCA Organization and Randomized Trial (RAPPORT) Investigators. Circulation 98:734, 1998.
88. Montalescot G, Barragan P, Wittenberg O, et al: Platelet glycoprotein IIb/IIIa inhibition with coronary stenting for acute myocardial infarction. N Engl J Med 344:1895, 2001.
89. Grines CL, Brodie BR, Griffin J, et al: Which primary PTCA patients may benefit form new technologies? Circulation 92:I-146, 1995.
90. Stone GW, Brodie BR, Griffin JJ, et al: Prospective, multicenter study of the safety and feasibility of primary stenting in acute myocardial infarction: In-hospital and 30-day results of the PAMI stent pilot trial. Primary Angioplasty in Myocardial Infarction Stent Pilot Trial Investigators. J Am Coll Cardiol 31:23, 1998.
91. Antoniucci D, Santoro GM, Bolognese L, et al: A clinical trial comparing primary stenting of the infarct-related artery with optimal primary angioplasty for acute myocardial infarction: Results from the Florence Randomized Elective Stenting in Acute Coronary Occlusions (FRESCO) trial. J Am Coll Cardiol 31:1234, 1998.
92. Suryapranata H, van't Hof AW, Hoorntje JC, et al: Randomized comparison of coronary stenting with balloon angioplasty in selected patients with acute myocardial infarction. Circulation 97:2502, 1998.
93. Saito S, Hosokawa G, Tanaka S, Nakamura S: Primary stent implantation is superior to balloon angioplasty in acute myocardial infarction: Final results of the primary angioplasty versus stent implantation in acute myocardial infarction (PASTA) trial. PASTA Trial Investigators. Catheter Cardiovasc Interv 48:262, 1999.
94. Rodriguez A, Bernardi V, Fernandez M, et al: In-hospital and late results of coronary stents versus conventional balloon angioplasty in acute myocardial infarction (GRAMI trial). Gianturco-Roubin in Acute Myocardial Infarction. Am J Cardiol 81:1286, 1998.
95. Maillard L, Hamon M, Khalife K, et al: A comparison of systematic stenting and conventional balloon angioplasty during primary percutaneous transluminal coronary angioplasty for acute myocardial infarction. STENTIM-2 Investigators. J Am Coll Cardiol 35:1729, 2000.
96. Kawashima A, Ueda K, Nishida Y, et al: Quantitative angiographic analysis of restenosis of primary stenting using the Wiktor stent for acute myocardial infarction: Results of the multicenter randomized PRISAM study. Circulation 100:I-856, 1999.
97. Scheller B, Hennen B, Severin-Kneib S, et al: Long-term follow-up of a randomized study of primary stenting versus angioplasty in acute myocardial infarction. Am J Med 110:1, 2001.
98. Zhu MM, Feit A, Chadow H, et al: Primary stent implantation compared with primary balloon angioplasty for acute myocardial infarction: A meta-analysis of randomized clinical trials. Am J Cardiol 88:297, 2001.
99. Henriques JP, Zijlstra F, Ottervanger JP, et al: Incidence and clinical significance of distal embolization during primary angioplasty for acute myocardial infarction. Eur Heart J 23:1112, 2002.
100. Kaplan BM, Larkin T, Safian RD, et al: Prospective study of extraction atherectomy in patients with acute myocardial infarction. Am J Cardiol 78:383, 1996.
101. Rosenschein H, Hertz I, Tenebaum-Koren E, et al: Coronary ultrasound thrombolysis in acute myocardial infarction: Results from the acute study. J Am Coll Cardiol 31:192A, 1998.
102. Silva JA, Ramee SR, Cohen DJ, et al: Rheolytic thrombectomy during percutaneous revascularization for acute myocardial infarction: Experience with the AngioJet catheter. Am Heart J 141:353, 2001.
103. Taghizadeh B, Chiu JA, Papaleo R, et al: AngioJet thrombectomy and stenting for reperfusion in acute MI complicated with cardiogenic shock. Catheter Cardiovasc Interv 57:79, 2002.
104. Silva JA, White CJ, Ramee SR, et al: Treatment of coronary stent thrombosis with rheolytic thrombectomy: Results from a multicenter experience. Catheter Cardiovasc Interv 58:11, 2003.

105. Napodano M, Reimers B, Pasquetto G, et al: Intracoronary thrombectomy improves myocardial perfusion in patients undergoing direct angioplasty: A single center randomized study. J Am Coll Cardiol 41:357A, 2003.
106. van Ommen V, Michels R, Heymen E, et al: Usefulness of the rescue PT catheter to remove fresh thrombus from coronary arteries and bypass grafts in acute myocardial infarction. Am J Cardiol 88:306, 2001.
107. Belli G, Pezzano A, De Biase AM, et al: Adjunctive thrombus aspiration and mechanical protection from distal embolization in primary percutaneous intervention for acute myocardial infarction. Catheter Cardiovasc Interv 50:362, 2000.
108. Zeymer U, Suryapranata H, Monassier JP, et al: The Na(+)/H(+) exchange inhibitor eniporide as an adjunct to early reperfusion therapy for acute myocardial infarction. Results of the evaluation of the safety and cardioprotective effects of eniporide in acute myocardial infarction (ESCAMI) trial. J Am Coll Cardiol 38:1644, 2001.
109. Faxon DP, Gibbons RJ, Chronos NA, et al: The effect of blockade of the CD11/CD18 integrin receptor on infarct size in patients with acute myocardial infarction treated with direct angioplasty: The results of the HALT-MI study. J Am Coll Cardiol 40:1199, 2002.
110. Marzilli M, Orsini E, Marraccini P, Testa R: Beneficial effects of intracoronary adenosine as an adjunct to primary angioplasty in acute myocardial infarction. Circulation 101:2154, 2000.
111. Ross AM, Gibbons RJ, Kloner RA, et al: Acute myocardial infarction study of adenosine (AMISTAD II). J Am Coll Cardiol 39:338A, 2002.
112. Mahaffey KW, Puma JA, Barbagelata NA, et al: Adenosine as an adjunct to thrombolytic therapy for acute myocardial infarction: Results of a multicenter, randomized, placebo-controlled trial: The Acute Myocardial Infarction STudy of ADenosine (AMISTAD) trial. J Am Coll Cardiol 34:1711, 1999.
113. Ito H, Taniyama Y, Iwakura K, et al: Intravenous nicorandil can preserve microvascular integrity and myocardial viability in patients with reperfused anterior wall myocardial infarction. J Am Coll Cardiol 33:654, 1999.
114. Granger C: Complement and Reduction of Infarct Size after Angioplasty or Lytics (CARDINAL) Trials. Chicago, American Heart Association, 2002.
115. Dixon SR, Bartorelli AL, Marcovitz PA, et al: Initial experience with hyperoxemic reperfusion after primary angioplasty for acute myocardial infarction: Results of a pilot study utilizing intracoronary aqueous oxygen therapy. J Am Coll Cardiol 39:387, 2002.
116. Dixon SR, Whitbourn RJ, Dae MW, et al: Induction of mild systemic hypothermia with endovascular cooling during primary percutaneous coronary intervention for acute myocardial infarction. J Am Coll Cardiol 40:1928, 2002.
117. Gibson CM, Cannon CP, Greene RM, et al: Rescue angioplasty in the thrombolysis in myocardial infarction (TIMI) 4 trial. Am J Cardiol 80:21, 1997.
118. Ellis SG, Da Silva ER, Spaulding CM, et al: Review of immediate angioplasty after fibrinolytic therapy for acute myocardial infarction: Insights from the RESCUE I, RESCUE II, and other contemporary clinical experiences. Am Heart J 139:1046, 2000.
119. Dauerman HL, Prpic R, Andreou C, et al: Angiographic and clinical outcomes after rescue coronary stenting. Catheter Cardiovasc Interv 50:269, 2000.
120. Petronio AS, Musumeci G, Limbruno U, et al: Abciximab improves 6-month clinical outcome after rescue coronary angioplasty. Am Heart J 143:334, 2002.
121. French JK, Ramanathan K, Stewart JT, et al: A score predicts failure of reperfusion after fibrinolytic therapy for acute myocardial infarction. Am Heart J 145:508, 2003.
122. Schweiger MJ, Cannon CP, Murphy SA, et al: Early coronary intervention followin pharmacologic therapy for acute myocardial infarction (the combined TIMI 10B-TIM 14 experience). Am J Cardiol 88:831, 2001.
123. Stone GW, Cox D, Garcia E, et al: Normal flow (TIMI-3) before mechanical reperfusio therapy is an independent determinant of survival in acute myocardial infarctio Analysis from the primary angioplasty in myocardial infarction trials. Circulatio 104:636, 2001.
124. Ross AM, Coyne KS, Reiner JS, et al: A randomized trial comparing primary angio plasty with a strategy of short-acting thrombolysis and immediate planned rescu angioplasty in acute myocardial infarction: The PACT trial. PACT investigators. Plas minogen-activator Angioplasty Compatibility Trial. J Am Coll Cardiol 34:1954, 1999.
125. Herrmann HC, Moliterno DJ, Ohman EM, et al: Facilitation of early percutaneous coro nary intervention after reteplase with or without abciximab in acute myocardial infarc tion: Results from the SPEED (GUSTO-4 Pilot) Trial. J Am Coll Cardiol 36:1489, 2000
126. Harjai KJ, Stone GW, Boura J, et al: Effects of prior beta-blocker therapy on clinical out comes after primary coronary angioplasty for acute myocardial infarction. Am J Cardio 91:655, 2002.
127. Sabatier R, Hamon M, Zhao QM, et al: Could direct stenting reduce no-reflow in acute coronary syndromes? A randomized pilot study. Am Heart J 143:1027, 2002.
128. Yip HK, Chen MC, Chang HW, et al: Angiographic morphologic features of infarct related arteries and timely reperfusion in acute myocardial infarction: Predictors o slow-flow and no-reflow phenomenon. Chest 122:1322, 2002.
129. Giri S, Mitchel JF, Hirst JA, et al: Synergy between intracoronary stenting and abcix imab in improving angiographic and clinical outcomes of primary angioplasty in acute myocardial infarction. Am J Cardiol 86:269, 2000.
130. Resnic FS, Wainstein M, Lee MK, et al: No-reflow is an independent predictor of deat and myocardial infarction after percutaneous coronary intervention. Am Heart J 145:4 2003.
131. Skelding KA, Goldstein JA, Mehta L, et al: Resolution of refractory no-reflow with intra coronary epinephrine. Catheter Cardiovasc Interv 57:305, 2002.
132. Goldstein JA, Demetriou D, Grines CL, et al: Multiple complex coronary plaques ir patients with acute myocardial infarction. N Engl J Med 343:915, 2000.
133. Dambrink JE, van der Schaaf RJ, Hoorntje JC, et al: Impact of multivessel disease or recovery of left ventricular function after primary angioplasty for acute myocardia infarction. J Am Coll Cardiol 41:389A, 2003.
134. Denklas AE, Orford JL, Fasseas P, et al: Multivessel percutaneous intervention for ST segment elevation myocardial infarction: The Mayo Clinic experience. J Am Col Cardiol 41:324A, 2003.
135. Roe MT, Cura FA, Joski PS, et al: Initial experience with multivessel percutaneous coronary intervention during mechanical reperfusion for acute myocardial infarction Am J Cardiol 88:170, 2001.
136. Brodie BR, Stuckey TD, Hansen C, Muncy D: Intra-aortic balloon counterpulsatior before primary percutaneous transluminal coronary angioplasty reduces catheteriza tion laboratory events in high-risk patients with acute myocardial infarction. Am Cardiol 84:18, 1999.
137. Stone GW, Marsalese D, Brodie BR, et al: A prospective, randomized evaluation of pro phylactic intraaortic balloon counterpulsation in high risk patients with acute myocar dial infarction treated with primary angioplasty. Second Primary Angioplasty ir Myocardial Infarction (PAMI-II) Trial Investigators. J Am Coll Cardiol 29:1459, 1997.

GUIDELINES *Thomas H. Lee*

Primary Percutaneous Coronary Intervention in Acute Myocardial Infarction

The American College of Cardiology and American Heart Association (ACC/AHA) updated comprehensive guidelines on percutaneous coronary interventions (PCIs) in 2001.[1] These guidelines included recommendations regarding several specific issues relevant to primary PCI. These issues were also addressed in prior ACC/AHA guidelines on acute myocardial infarction[2] and unstable angina.[3,4] The PCI guidelines use the ACC/AHA classification system for the indications (class I for generally accepted indications, class IIa when indications are controversial but the weight of evidence is supportive, class IIb when usefulness or efficacy is less well established, and class III when there is a consensus against the usefulness of the intervention). The updated guidelines use a convention for rating levels of evidence upon which recommendations have been based. *Level A* recommendations were derived from data from multiple randomized clinical trials, *level B* recommendations were derived from a single randomized trial or nonrandomized studies, and *level C* recommendations were based upon the consensus opinion of experts.

Percutaneous Coronary Intervention Without On-Site Cardiac Surgery

The guidelines note that the use of cardiac surgical backup for PCI has become less formal because of low rates of use and that some institutions use "off-site surgical backup." However, the guidelines note the greater risk associated with emergent PCI and describe specific volume thresholds for hospitals providing this service without cardiac surgical backup. The guidelines stipulate that the operators must be experienced interventionalists who regularly perform at least 75 elective PCI cases per year at a surgical center and that the institution must perform a minimum of 36 primary PCI procedures per year. The guidelines also stipulate that the procedure should be limited to patients with ST segment elevation myocardial infarction (MI) or new left bundle branch block on electrocardiography and done in a timely fashion (balloon inflation within 90 ± 30 minutes of admission). The laboratory must have written protocols in place for immediate (within 1 hour) transfer of patients to the nearest cardiac surgical facility.

Primary Percutaneous Coronary Intervention Versus Thrombolysis for Acute Transmural Myocardial Infarction

The ACC/AHA guidelines support use of PCI as an alternative to thrombolysis for acute MI (AMI) with ST segment elevation or new or presumed left bundle branch block within the first 12 hours after the onset of symptoms and afterward if such symptoms continue. As already noted, the guidelines define a performance standard for the average time from admission to balloon inflation of 90 ± 30 minutes and stipulate that the PCI should be performed by experienced operators and high-volume facilities (Table 48G–1). PCI is endorsed for a longer period (up to 36 hours after the onset of infarction) for patients who present in cardiogenic shock if the patients are younger than 75 years and the procedure can be performed within 18 hours of the onset of shock.

The guidelines do not support use of PCI for non-infarct-related arteries at the time of AMI and for patients who are asymptomatic after receiving fibrinolytic therapy within 12 hours.

Percutaneous Coronary Intervention After Thrombolysis

Coronary angiography and PCI are commonly performed after thrombolysis even though this strategy has not been studied extensively in clinical trials. Therefore, the ACC/AHA guidelines support relatively conservative use of angiography and PCI for patients after thrombolysis (Table 48G–2). PCI is considered appropriate for patients with objective evidence of recurrent infarction or ischemia and is also given support for patients with cardiogenic shock or hemodynamic instability. However, PCI is not considered routinely appropriate for patients who have successful or unsuccessful thrombolysis.

TABLE 48G–1 ACC/AHA Guidelines for Primary Percutaneous Coronary Intervention for Patients with Acute Transmural Myocardial Infarction as an Alternative to Thrombolysis

Class	Indication	Level of Evidence
Class I (indicated)	As an alternative to thrombolytic therapy in patients with AMI and ST segment elevation or new or presumed new left bundle branch block who can undergo angioplasty of the infarct artery <12 hr from the onset of ischemic symptoms or >12 hr if symptoms persist, if performed in a timely fashion (performance standard: balloon inflation within 90 ± 30 min of hospital admission) by individuals skilled in the procedure* and supported by experienced personnel in an appropriate laboratory environment.†	A
	In patients who are within 36 hr of an acute ST elevation/Q wave or new left bundle branch block MI who develop cardiogenic shock, are younger than 75 yr, and revascularization can be performed within 18 hr of the onset of shock by individuals skilled in the procedure* and supported by experienced personnel in an appropriate laboratory environment.†	A
Class IIa (good supportive evidence)	As a reperfusion strategy in candidates who have a contraindication to thrombolytic therapy.	C
Class IIb (weak supportive evidence)		
Class III (not indicated)	Elective PCI of a non–infarct-related artery at the time of acute MI (*level of evidence: C*).	C
	In patients with acute MI who	
	Have received fibrinolytic therapy within 12 hr and have no symptoms of myocardial ischemia.	
	Are eligible for thrombolytic therapy and are undergoing primary angioplasty by an inexperienced operator (individual who performs <75 PCI procedures per year).	
	Are beyond 12 hr after onset of symptoms and have no evidence of myocardial ischemia.	C

ACC/AHA = American College of Cardiology/American Heart Association; AMI = acute myocardial infarction; MI = myocardial infarction; PCI = percutaneous coronary intervention.
*Individuals who perform at least 75 PCI procedures per year.
†Centers that perform at least 200 PCI procedures per year and have cardiac surgical capability.

TABLE 48G–2 ACC/AHA Guidelines for Percutaneous Coronary Intervention After Thrombolysis

Class	Indication	Level of Evidence
Class I (indicated)	Objective evidence for recurrent infarction or ischemia (rescue PCI)	B
Class IIa (good supportive evidence)	Cardiogenic shock or hemodynamic instability	B
Class IIb (weak supportive evidence)	Recurrent angina without objective evidence of ischemia or infarction (*level of evidence: C*)	C
	Angioplasty of the infarct-related artery stenosis within hours to days (48 hr) following successful thrombolytic therapy in asymptomatic patients without clinical and/or inducible evidence of ischemia	B
Class III (not indicated)	Routine PCI within 48 hr following failed thrombolysis	B
	Routine PCI of the infarct artery stenosis immediately after thrombolytic therapy	A

ACC/AHA = American College of Cardiology /American Heart Association; PCI = percutaneous coronary intervention.

TABLE 48G–3 ACC/AHA Guidelines for Percutaneous Coronary Intervention (PCI) During Subsequent Hospital Management After Acute Therapy for Acute Myocardial Infarction Including Primary PCI

Class	Indication	Level of Evidence
Class I (indicated)	Spontaneous or provocable myocardial ischemia during recovery from infarction	C
	Persistent hemodynamic instability	C
Class IIa (good supportive evidence)	Patients with LV ejection fraction <0.4, CHF, or serious ventricular arrhythmias	C
Class IIb (weak supportive evidence)	Coronary angiography and angioplasty for an occluded infarct-related artery in an otherwise stable patient to revascularize that artery (open artery hypothesis)	C
	All patients after a non-Q-wave MI	C
	Clinical HF during the acute episode but subsequent demonstration of preserved LV function (LV ejection fraction >0.4)	C
Class III (not indicated)	PCI of the infarct-related artery within 48 to 72 hr after thrombolytic therapy without evidence of spontaneous or provocable ischemia	C

ACC/AHA = American College of Cardiology/American Heart Association; CHF = congestive heart failure; HF = heart failure; LV = left ventricular; MI = myocardial infarction.

Percutaneous Coronary Intervention Later During Hospitalization

The guidelines support use of PCI after the immediate treatment of AMI in reaction to clinical evidence of ischemia and for persistent hemodynamic instability (Table 48G–3). The ACC/AHA task force did not provide much support for use of PCI for routine care of patients who were clinically stable. However, the Treat Angina with Aggrastat and determine Cost of Therapy with an Invasive or Conservative Strategy–Thrombolysis in Myocardial Infarction 18 (TACTICS-TIMI 18) trial, which demonstrated clinical benefit from an early invasive strategy for patients with unstable angina or AMI without ST segment elevation,[5] had been presented only as an abstract at the time the guidelines were written. Thus, future revisions of these guidelines may support a lower threshold for use of PCI after AMI.

References

1. Smith SC Jr, Dove JT, Jacobs AK, et al: ACC/AHA guidelines for percutaneous coronary intervention: A report of the American College of Cardiology/American Heart Association Task Force on Practice Guidelines (Committee to Revise the 1993 Guidelines for Percutaneous Transluminal Coronary Angioplasty). J Am Coll Cardiol 37:2239i, 2001.
2. Ryan TJ, Antman EM, Brooks NH, et al: 1999 update: ACC/AHA guidelines for the management of patients with acute myocardial infarction: Executive summary and recommendations: A report of the American College of Cardiology/American Heart Association Task Force on Practice Guidelines (Committee on Management of Acute Myocardial Infarction). J Am Coll Cardiol 34:890, 1999.
3. Braunwald E, Antman EM, Beasley JW, et al: ACC/AHA guidelines for the management of patients with unstable angina and non-ST-segment elevation myocardial infarction: A report of the American College of Cardiology/American Heart Association Task Force on Practice Guidelines (Committee on the Management of Patients With Unstable Angina). J Am Coll Cardiol 36:970, 2000.
4. Braunwald E, Antman EM, Beasley JW, et al: ACC/AHA 2002 guideline update for the management of patients with unstable angina and non-ST-segment elevation myocardial infarction: Summary article: A report of the American College of Cardiology/American Heart Association Task Force on Practice Guidelines (Committee on the Management of Patients With Unstable Angina). Circulation 106:1893, 2002.
5. Cannon CP, Weinstraub WS, Demopoulos LA, et al: Comparison of early invasive and conservative strategies in patients with unstable coronary syndromes treated with the glycoprotein IIb/IIIa inhibitor tirofiban. N Engl J Med 344:1879, 2001.

CHAPTER 49

Unstable Angina and Non-ST Elevation Myocardial Infarction

Christopher P. Cannon • Eugene Braunwald

Current estimates are that 1.7 million patients with acute coronary syndromes (ACSs) are admitted each year to hospitals in the United States (see Fig. 46–1).[1] Of these, only one-quarter present with acute myocardial infarction (MI) associated with electrocardiographic ST segment elevation (Chaps. 46 and 47); three-quarters, or approximately 1.4 million patients, have unstable angina or non-ST elevation myocardial infarction (UA/NSTEMI).[1] The former is most commonly caused by acute total thrombotic occlusion of a coronary artery and urgent reperfusion is the mainstay of therapy, whereas UA/NSTEMI is usually associated with severe coronary obstruction but not total occlusion of the culprit coronary artery.[2] Among patients with UA/NSTEMI, between 40 and 60 percent have evidence of myocardial necrosis with elevated troponin.[3]

Definition and Classification

DEFINITION. The definition of unstable angina is largely based on the clinical presentation (see Chap. 45). *Stable* angina pectoris is characterized by a deep, poorly localized chest or arm discomfort (rarely described as pain) that is reproducibly associated with physical exertion or emotional stress and relieved within 5 to 15 minutes by rest or sublingual nitroglycerin, or both. In contrast, *unstable* angina is defined as angina pectoris (or equivalent type of ischemic discomfort) with at least one of three features: (1) occurring at rest (or with minimal exertion) and usually lasting more than 20 minutes (if not interrupted by nitroglycerin), (2) being severe and described as frank pain and of new onset (i.e., within 1 month), and (3) occurring with a crescendo pattern (i.e., more severe, prolonged, or frequent than previously).[4] Some patients with this pattern of ischemic discomfort, especially those with prolonged rest pain, develop evidence of myocardial necrosis on the basis of cardiac serum markers (such as creatine kinase muscle-brain fraction [CK-MB] or troponin T or I, or both) and thus have a diagnosis of NSTEMI.

CLASSIFICATION. Because UA/NSTEMI comprises such a heterogeneous group of patients, classification schemes based on clinical features are useful. A clinical classification of UA/NSTEMI (Table 49–1)[5,6] has been found to be a useful means of stratifying risk.[7] Patients are divided into three groups according to the clinical circumstances of the acute ischemic episode: primary unstable angina, secondary angina (e.g., with angina related to obvious precipitating factors such as anemia, infection, or cardiac arrhythmias), and post-MI angina. Patients are also classified according to the severity of the ischemia (acute rest pain, subacute rest pain, or new-onset severe angina). This classification has been shown to be predictive of coronary thrombus at angiography or in atherectomy specimens and in determination of prognosis.[6,7]

Because UA/NSTEMI is a clinical syndrome rather than a specific disease (much like hypertension rather than pneumococcal pneumonia), an etiological approach has been proposed.[8] There are five pathophysiological processes that may contribute to the development of UA/NSTEMI (Fig. 49–1). These are (1) plaque rupture or erosion with superimposed nonocclusive thrombus (by far the most common cause of UA/NSTEMI), (2) dynamic obstruction (i.e., coronary spasm of an epicardial artery, as in Prinzmetal angina [see Prinzmetal (Variant) Angina] or constriction of the small muscular coronary arteries), (3) progressive mechanical obstruction, (4) inflammation or infection or both, and (5) secondary unstable angina, related to increased myocardial oxygen demand or decreased supply (e.g., anemia). Individual patients may have several of these processes coexisting as the cause of their episode of UA/NSTEMI. Use of this etiological approach may help refine the diagnostic approach and help target therapeutic strategies to treat the underlying disease that precipitated the episode of UA/NSTEMI. As noted later (see Risk Stratification), several new serum markers have been shown to be effective tools in identifying these pathophysiological processes and in predicting outcome; this approach is evolving into a "multimarker strategy" for evaluation and risk stratification (Fig. 49–2; see Fig. 49–10).[9]

Pathophysiology

The pathophysiology of UA/NSTEMI involves a broad time line with three phases rather than an isolated ischemic event. Traditionally, focus had been only on the acute phase of UA/NSTEMI, whereas the true pathophysiology actually spans two or more decades before the acute clinical event and then may span more than 20 years afterward. The acute event, which usually involves thrombus formation at the site of a ruptured or eroded atherosclerotic plaque, is the clinical manifestation of a generalized and progressive disease, currently referred to as *atherothrombosis* (see Chap. 35). This new term has emerged in place of atherosclerosis because it more fully describes the pathophysiology of the disease, in which there is both progression of the atheroma (e.g., cholesterol plaque development) and disruption of the plaque with superimposed thrombosis. Thus, the full pathophysiology of an ACS event can be divided into three phases: (1) the development of the unstable plaque that ruptures, (2) the acute ischemic event, and (3) the long-term risk of recurrent coronary events that remains after the acute event. As noted in Chapter 35, inflammation can play a major role in causing plaque instability, with inflammatory cells

TABLE 49–1 Braunwald Clinical Classification of Unstable Angina or Non-ST Elevation Myocardial Infarction

Class	Definition	Death or Myocardial Infarction 1 Year* (%)
Severity		
Class I	New onset of severe angina or accelerated angina; no rest pain	7.3
Class II	Angina at rest within past month but not within preceding 48 hr (angina at rest, subacute)	10.3
Class III	Angina at rest within 48 hr (angina at rest, subacute)	10.8†
Clinical circumstances		
A (secondary angina)	Develops in the presence of extracardiac condition that intensifies myocardial ischemia	14.1
B (primary angina)	Develops in the absence of extracardiac condition	8.5
C (postinfarction angina)	Develops within 2 wks after acute myocardial infarction	18.5‡
Intensity of treatment	Patients with unstable angina may also be divided into three groups depending on whether unstable angina occurs (1) in the absence of treatment for chronic stable angina, (2) during treatment for chronic stable angina, or (3) despite maximal antiischemic drug therapy. The three groups may be designated by subscripts 1, 2, and 3, respectively.	
Electrocardiographic changes	Patients with unstable angina may be further divided into those with or without transient ST-T wave changes during pain.	

*Data from TIMI III Registry: Scirica BM, Cannon CP, McCabe CH, et al, for the Thrombolysis In Myocardial Ischemia III Registry Investigators: Prognosis in the Thrombolysis in Myocardial Ischemia III Registry according to the Braunwald unstable angina pectoris classification. Am J Cardiol 90:821, 2002.
†$p = 0.057$.
‡$p < 0.001$.
From Braunwald E: Unstable angina: A classification. Circulation 80:410, 1989.

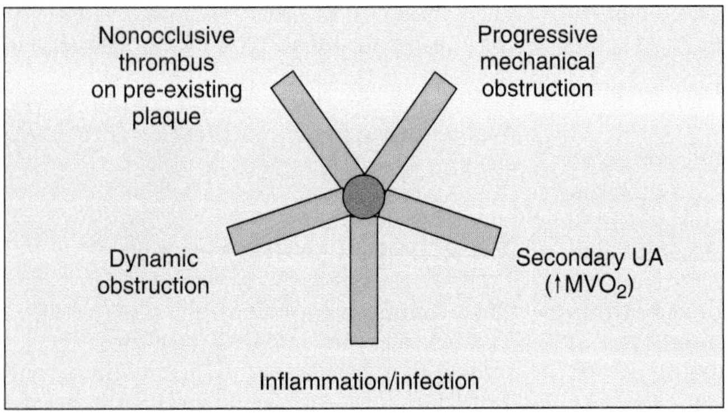

FIGURE 49–1 Schematic representation of the causes of unstable angina (UA). MVO_2 = myocardial O_2 consumption. (From Braunwald E: Unstable angina: An etiologic approach to management [editorial]. Circulation 98:2219, 1998.)

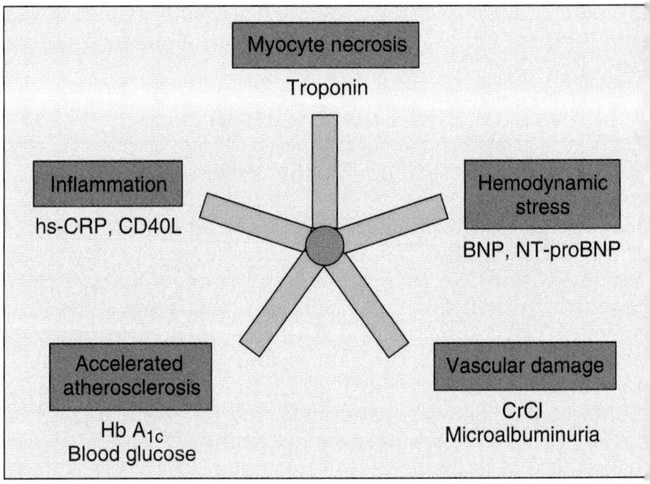

FIGURE 49–2 A multimarker strategy for evaluation of the etiology and prognosis of unstable angina or non-ST elevation myocardial infarction. Many new markers have been shown to be independent markers of an adverse prognosis. Troponin is a marker for myocyte necrosis; high-sensitivity C-reactive protein (hs-CRP) and CD40 ligand (CD40L) are markers of vascular inflammation; creatinine clearance (CrCl) and microalbuminuria are markers of vascular damage; hemoglobin (Hb) A_{1c} and blood glucose are markers of diabetes and accelerated atherosclerosis. (Adapted from Morrow DA, Braunwald E: Future of biomarkers in acute coronary syndromes: Moving toward a multimarker strategy. Circulation 108:250, 2003.)

releasing cytokines, which in turn increase the release of matrix metalloproteinases, which then make the fibrous cap thinner and more likely to rupture or erode. In parallel, inflammation can decrease the synthesis of collagen, thus further weakening the plaque and increasing the likelihood of rupture.

The acute ischemia in UA/NSTEMI can be caused by an increase in myocardial oxygen demand (e.g., precipitated by tachycardia or hypertension), more commonly by a reduction in supply (e.g., related to reduction in coronary lumen diameter by platelet-rich thrombi or vasospasm), or both. Rapid progression of the underlying coronary artery disease (CAD) has also been documented in some patients. A sequence of events can be documented in UA/NSTEMI, in which there is first a reduction in coronary sinus oxygen saturation (signifying a reduction in coronary blood flow), then ST segment depression, followed by chest discomfort.[10] Elevations in blood pressure or heart rate sometimes ensue. A patient may have a small increase in myocardial oxygen demand in conjunction with a reduction in coronary blood flow, leading to the episode of ischemia. The five major contributing causes of UA/NSTEMI are reviewed next.

THROMBOSIS (see also Chap. 80). The central role of coronary artery thrombosis in the pathogenesis of UA/NSTEMI is supported by six sets of observations:

1. At autopsy, thrombi can usually be identified at the site of a ruptured or eroded coronary plaque.[11]
2. Coronary atherectomy specimens obtained from patients with UA/NSTEMI demonstrate a high inci

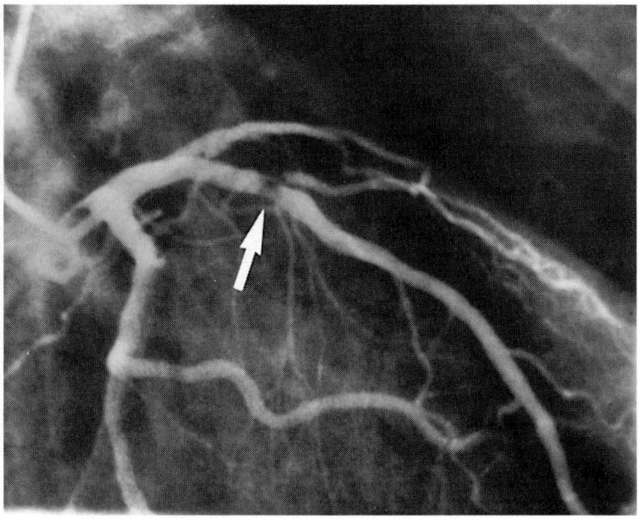

FIGURE 49–3 Coronary artery thrombus in a patient with unstable angina. A 60-year-old man presented with prolonged rest pain and transient anterior ST elevations. Coronary angiography shows an irregular hazy filling defect in the left anterior descending artery at the level of the second diagonal branch (arrow). Contrast medium surrounds the globular thrombus, which extends into the diagonal branch.

dence of thrombotic lesions compared with those obtained from patients with stable angina.[12]

3. Coronary angioscopic observations in UA/NSTEMI indicate that thrombus is frequently present.[13]
4. Coronary angiography has demonstrated ulceration or irregularities suggesting a ruptured plaque and/or thrombus in many patients (Fig. 49–3).[2] In the Thrombolysis in Myocardial Ischemia (TIMI) IIIA trial involving patients with UA/NSTEMI, 35 percent of patients had definite thrombus and an additional 40 percent had possible thrombus at angiography.[2]
5. Evidence of ongoing thrombosis has been noted with elevation of several markers of platelet activity and fibrin formation.[14,15]
6. The clinical outcome of patients with ACSs has been improved by antithrombotic therapy with aspirin,[16] unfractionated heparin (UFH) or low-molecular-weight heparin (LMWH),[17-19] platelet glycoprotein (GP) IIb/IIIa inhibitors,[20-22] or clopidogrel.[23]

PLATELET ACTIVATION AND AGGREGATION (see also Chap. 80). Platelets play a key role in the transformation of a stable atherosclerotic plaque to an unstable lesion (Fig. 49–4). With rupture or ulceration of an atherosclerotic plaque, the subendothelial matrix (e.g., collagen and tissue factor) is exposed to the circulating blood. The first step is *platelet adhesion* through the platelet GP Ib receptor by its interaction with von Willebrand factor. This is followed by *platelet activation*, which leads to (1) a shape change in the platelet (from a smooth discoid shape to a spiculated form, which increases the surface area upon which thrombin generation can occur); (2) degranulation of the alpha and dense granules, thereby releasing thromboxane A_2, serotonin, and other platelet aggregatory and chemoattractant agents; and (3) expression of GP IIb/IIIa receptors on the platelet surface with activation of the receptor, such that it can bind fibrinogen. The final step is *platelet aggregation*, i.e., the formation of the platelet plug. Fibrinogen (or von Willebrand factor) binds to the activated GP IIb/IIIa receptors of two platelets, thereby creating a growing platelet aggregate. Antiplatelet therapy is one of the cornerstones of therapy in UA/NSTEMI (see Medical Therapy) and is directed at decreasing the formation of thromboxane A_2 (aspirin), inhibiting the P2Y12 component of the adenosine diphosphate (ADP) receptor pathway of

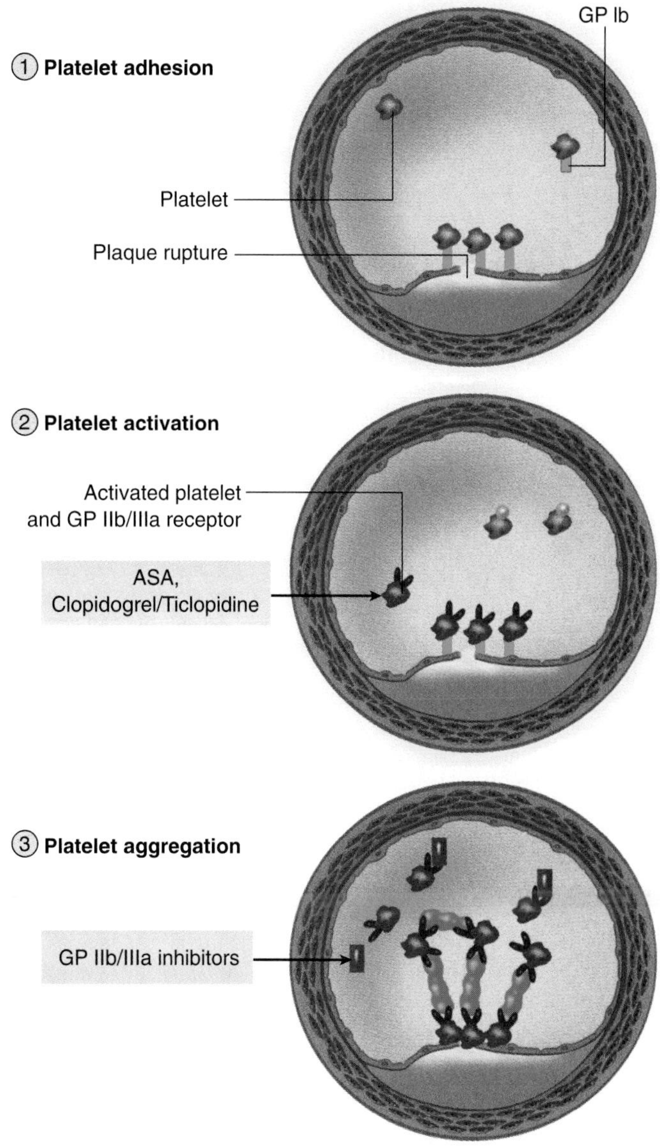

FIGURE 49–4 Primary hemostasis—process of platelet adhesion (1), activation (2), and aggregation (3) and the site of action of antiplatelet drugs. Platelets initiate thrombosis at the site of a ruptured plaque; the first step is *platelet adhesion* (1) through the glycoprotein (GP) Ib receptor in conjunction with von Willebrand factor. This is followed by *platelet activation* (2), which leads to a shape change in the platelet, degranulation of the alpha and dense granules, and expression of GP IIb/IIIa receptors on the platelet surface with activation of the receptor so that it can bind fibrinogen. The final step is *platelet aggregation* (3), in which fibrinogen (or von Willebrand factor) binds to the activated GP IIb/IIIa receptors of two platelets. Aspirin (acetylsalicylic acid [ASA]) and clopidogrel act to decrease platelet activation (see text for details), whereas the GP IIb/IIIa inhibitors inhibit the final step of platelet aggregation.

platelet activation (ticlopidine and clopidogrel),[24] and directly inhibiting platelet aggregation (GP IIb/IIIa inhibitors) (see Fig. 49–4).

SECONDARY HEMOSTASIS. Simultaneously with formation of the platelet plug, the plasma coagulation system is activated. Release of tissue factor appears to be the predominant mechanism of initiating hemostasis following plaque rupture (see Chap. 80).[25] Ultimately, factor X is activated to factor Xa, which leads to generation of thrombin (Factor IIa), which plays a central role in arterial thrombosis: (1) thrombin converts fibrinogen to fibrin in the final common pathway for clot formation, (2) it is a powerful stimulus for platelet aggregation, and (3) it activates factor XIII, which leads to cross-linking and stabilization of the fibrin clot. Thrombin molecules are incorporated into coronary thrombi and can form the nidus of rethrombosis (i.e., reocclusion or reinfarction) as the thrombus undergoes spontaneous or pharmacologically induced fibrinolysis. Accordingly, effective inhibition of thrombin and factor Xa plays an important part in the therapy of UA/NSTEMI.

CORONARY VASOCONSTRICTION. There are three settings in which the process of dynamic coronary obstruction is identified:

1. Prinzmetal variant angina, with intense focal spasm of a segment of an epicardial coronary artery, is the prototypic example.[26] It can occur in patients without coronary atherosclerosis or in patients with one or more atheromatous plaques.
2. Coronary vasoconstriction causing "microcirculatory angina," which results from constriction of the small intramural coronary resistance vessels,[27] is the second setting. Although there are no epicardial coronary artery stenoses, coronary flow is usually slowed (see Chap. 44).
3. The third and probably most common setting in which vasoconstriction occurs is that of coronary atherosclerotic plaques.[28] Vasoconstriction can occur as the result of local vasoconstrictors released from platelets, serotonin and thromboxane A_2, as well as those present within the thrombus, such as thrombin. A dysfunctional coronary endothelium, with reduced production of nitric oxide and increased release of endothelin, can also lead to vasoconstriction. Adrenergic stimuli, cold immersion, cocaine,[29] or mental stress[30] can also cause coronary vasoconstriction.

PROGRESSIVE MECHANICAL OBSTRUCTION. The fourth etiology of UA/NSTEMI is that of progressive luminal narrowing. This narrowing was most commonly seen in the setting of restenosis following percutaneous coronary intervention (PCI) in the absence of drug-eluting stents (see Chap. 52). Angiographic and atherectomy studies have demonstrated that many patients without previous intracoronary procedures have shown progressive luminal narrowing of the culprit vessel in the period preceding the onset of UA/NSTEMI that is related to rapid cellular proliferation.[31]

SECONDARY UNSTABLE ANGINA. This form of unstable angina is precipitated by an imbalance in myocardial oxygen supply and demand caused by conditions extrinsic to the coronary arteries in patients with prior coronary stenosis and chronic stable angina.[5-7] It can result from either an increase in myocardial oxygen demand, a decrease in coronary flow, or both. Conditions that increase oxygen demand include tachycardia (e.g., supraventricular tachycardia or new-onset atrial fibrillation with rapid ventricular response), fever, thyrotoxicosis, hyperadrenergic states, and elevations of left ventricular afterload such as in hypertension or aortic stenosis. Secondary unstable angina can also be due to impaired oxygen delivery, as occurs in anemia, hypoxemia (e.g., related to pneumonia or congestive heart failure), and hyperviscosity states, or hypotension. Secondary angina appears to have a worse prognosis than primary unstable angina (see Table 49–1).[7]

Clinical Presentation

The clinical profile of patients presenting with UA/NSTEMI differs from that of patients with STEMI. Women present more often with unstable angina, constituting 30 to 45 percent of patients with unstable angina in several studies,[32-34] compared with 25 to 30 percent of patients with NSTEMI and approximately 20 percent of patients with STEMI.[32,33] In comparison with the latter, patients with unstable angina also have higher rates of prior MI, angina, previous coronary revascularization, and extracardiac vascular disease.[33,3] Indeed, approximately 80 percent of patients with UA/NSTEMI have a prior history of cardiovascular disease and most have evidence of prior coronary risk factors.[36]

CLINICAL EXAMINATION. A description of "ischemic pain" is the hallmark of UA/NSTEMI (see Chap. 45). The physical examination may be unremarkable or may support the diagnosis of cardiac ischemia (see Chap. 8). Signs that suggest that the culprit artery perfuses a larger fraction of the left ventricle include diaphoresis, pale cool skin, sinus tachycardia, a third or fourth heart sound, and basilar rales on lung examination. Rarely, in UA/NSTEMI the severity of left ventricular dysfunction causes hypotension (i.e., cardiogenic shock).

ELECTROCARDIOGRAM. In UA/NSTEMI, ST depression (or transient ST elevation) and T wave changes occur in up to 50 percent of patients.[3,22,37] New (or presumably new) ST segment deviation is a specific and important measure of ischemia and prognosis. Traditionally, ST depression has been considered significant only if it was greater than 0.1 mV, which occurs in 20 to 25 percent of patients. However, an additional 20 percent of patients present with 0.05 mV ST depression,[3,37] and they have been observed to have an adverse prognosis approaching that of patients with 0.1 mV ST depression.[37,38] The worst prognosis occurs among patients with transient (i.e., <20 minutes) ST elevation, which occurs in approximately 10 percent of patients with UA/NSTEMI. T wave changes are sensitive but not as specific measures of acute ischemia unless they are marked ($\geq$0.3 mV).[22]

CONTINUOUS ELECTROCARDIOGRAPHIC MONITORING. Continuous monitoring of the electrocardiogram (ECG) can be used for two purposes in UA/NSTEMI: to monitor for arrhythmias or for recurrent ST segment deviation indicative of ischemia. For the former, telemetry of patients admitted to monitored beds can detect arrhythmias in association with the acute episode; although life-threatening arrhythmias are rare in unstable angina, they may be more common among patients with NSTEMI. For the latter goal, high-fidelity Holter monitors have been used in clinical trials to detect ST segment deviation as evidence of recurrent ischemia. In several studies, the ST segment monitoring appeared to be more sensitive than patients' symptoms and identified up to 25 percent of patients with evidence of ischemia during the first 24 hours after admission.[39,40] In addition, the presence of ST deviation is a strong marker of adverse short- and long-term outcome,[39,40] even when used in conjunction with troponins and clinical variables.[41] As with recurrent cardiac events of symptomatic ischemia or recurrent MI, silent ischemia is more frequent and prolonged in patients with NSTEMI than those with unstable angina.

CARDIAC NECROSIS MARKERS FOR DIAGNOSIS OF NSTEMI. Among patients presenting with symptoms consistent with UA/NSTEMI, elevations of markers of myocardial necrosis (i.e., CK-MB, troponin T or I) are used to identify patients with the diagnosis of NSTEMI (as opposed to UA).[4] With the use of troponins, which are both more sensitive and more specific than CK-MB, a greater percentage of patients are classified as having NSTEMI. Despite worries about the consequences of the apparent change in definition of MI, several studies have lent support to the use of these more sensitive markers, which are helpful in the assessment of prognosis.[43]

The issue of the appropriate "cut point" to define an elevated troponin level has been controversial. An important aspect is that the assay clearly discriminates truly elevated levels of troponin from false-positive results related to poor analytical performance of the assay. It has been proposed that the upper limit of normal for each specific assay be defined as the 99th percentile of a normal population of subjects[44] and meet acceptable criteria for precision of the assay at that concentration (defined as a 10 percent coefficient of variation, a measure of reproducibility from repeated testing on the same sample). Clinicians and laboratorians have debated the clinical relevance of very low-level elevation of cardiac troponin. However, studies have found that low-level elevation of cardiac troponin is associated with a higher risk of death or recurrent ischemic events[45,46] and thus support the European Society of Cardiology/American College of Cardiology proposal to ensure high accuracy at the low troponin levels.[47]

Because each assay is different, each hospital needs to review the specific cut points defined by that assay.[48] Point-of-care tests can have a positive versus negative result or provide a quantitative result, although the sensitivity and diagnostic accuracy of these tests have only recently been able to match those of current generation laboratory-based assays.

Despite increasingly accurate assays, apparent false-positive troponin elevations have been found in patients later found at coronary angiography not to have epicardial stenoses.[49] These elevations may be due to an alternative diagnosis, such as congestive heart failure, in which elevations have been observed in the absence of CAD and were associated with an adverse prognosis.[50] An analysis from the Treat Angina with Aggrastat and determine Cost of Therapy with an Invasive or Conservative Strategy (TACTICS)-TIMI 18 trial also raised a cautionary note that these troponin elevations should not be discarded as simply false positive. Patients presenting with UA/NSTEMI who had elevations of troponin but no apparent CAD on angiography were found to have a significantly worse prognosis than those who were troponin negative without coronary disease, with a 6-month rate of death or MI of 5.3 versus 0 percent, respectively.[51] This group had a prognosis similar to that of patients with documented coronary disease who were troponin negative at presentation. These data suggest that the elevations in troponin may be signs of alternative diagnoses such as heart failure that are associated with adverse outcomes.

CORONARY ARTERIOGRAPHIC FINDINGS. Patients with UA/NSTEMI enrolled in the invasive arm of TACTICS-TIMI 18 systematically underwent angiography. Thirty-four percent had critical obstruction (>50 percent luminal diameter stenosis) of three vessels, 28 percent had two-vessel disease, 26 percent had single-vessel disease, and 13 percent had no coronary stenosis greater than 50 percent.[3] Approximately 5 to 10 percent had left main stem stenosis greater than 50 percent.[3] Similar findings have been reported from registries of unselected UA/NSTEMI patients.[37,52] Women and nonwhites with UA/NSTEMI have less extensive coronary disease than their counterparts,[32,33,52,53] and patients with NSTEMI have more extensive disease than those who present with unstable angina.[33]

Approximately 15 percent of patients who present with symptoms of UA/NSTEMI have no significant coronary stenosis on coronary angiography.[32,33,37,52,53] Women and nonwhites constitute a larger proportion of such patients without epicardial coronary disease, suggesting either a difficulty in making a firm diagnosis of UA/NSTEMI in these groups or a different pathophysiological mechanism for their clinical presentation.[32-34,37,52,53] Approximately one-third of patients with UA/NSTEMI without a critical epicardial obstruction exhibit impaired coronary flow assessed angiographically, suggesting a pathophysiological role for coronary microvascular dysfunction.[54] The short-term prognosis is excellent in this group of patients.[55]

The culprit lesion in UA/NSTEMI typically exhibits an eccentric stenosis with scalloped or overhanging edges and a narrow neck.[2] These angiographic findings may represent disrupted atherosclerotic plaque, thrombus, or a combination. Features suggesting thrombus include globular intraluminal masses with a rounded or polypoid shape (see Fig. 49–3).[2] "Haziness" of a lesion has been used as an angiographic marker of possible thrombus, but this finding is less specific. Patients with angiographically visualized thrombus have impaired coronary flow and worse clinical outcomes than those without thrombus.[56]

Coronary flow as measured by the TIMI flow grade or frame count and TIMI myocardial perfusion grade have also been found to be impaired in patients with UA/NSTEMI, especially those with an elevated troponin.[56,57] Furthermore, as has been observed in patients with STEMI, abnormal tissue level perfusion is also associated with adverse outcomes in patients with UA/NSTEMI, independent of the presence of thrombus and abnormal flow in the epicardial artery.

ANGIOSCOPY AND INTRAVASCULAR ULTRASONOGRAPHY. Greater definition of the culprit lesion has been possible using angioscopy, where "white" (platelet-rich) thrombi are frequently observed, as opposed to "red" thrombi, more often seen in patients with acute ST elevation MI (Fig. 49–5).[13] Intravascular ultrasound examination identified more soft "echolucent" plaques and fewer calcified lesions among patients with unstable versus stable angina.[58]

OTHER LABORATORY TESTS. A chest roentgenogram may be useful in identifying pulmonary congestion or edema, which is more frequent in patients with NSTEMI involving a significant proportion of the left ventricle or in those with prior known left ventricular dysfunction. The presence of congestion has been shown to confer an adverse prognosis.[59]

Obtaining a serum cholesterol level and levels of its principal fractions, low-density lipoprotein (LDL) and high-density lipoprotein cholesterol, is useful in identifying an important, treatable risk factor for coronary atherothrombosis. Because serum cholesterol falls 24 hours following STEMI or UA/NSTEMI, it should be measured at the time of initial presentation. If only a later sample is obtained but the value falls into a range that warrants long-term treatment (see Chap. 39), appropriate therapy can be initiated. Other circulating markers of increased risk are discussed later. Evaluation for other secondary causes of UA/NSTEMI[5] may also be appropriate in selected patients (e.g., assessing thyroid function in patients who present with UA/NSTEMI and a persistent tachycardia).

Risk Stratification

PATHOPHYSIOLOGY OF LONG-TERM RISK FOLLOWING ACUTE CORONARY SYNDROME. An important concept that has emerged regarding the long-term risk following an ACS event is that the observed high risk of recurrent ischemic events is linked to multifocal lesions other than the culprit lesion responsible for the ACS event. Studies of coronary anatomy using angiography,[60-62] intravascular coronary ultrasonography,[63] or angioscopy[64] have shown multiple active plaques in addition to the culprit lesion (see Fig. 49–5). Thus, as aggressive interventional approaches are used successfully to treat the culprit lesion, the remaining plaques, which frequently have unstable features on angiographic or angioscopic examination, are responsible for recurrent events. The link to inflammation was also seen in one of these studies (Fig. 49–6): Multiple active plaques on angiography occurred more frequently with an increasing C-reactive protein (CRP) level.[63] This provides an important pathophysiological link between inflammation, more diffuse active coronary disease, and recurrent cardiac events in the months to years following a clinical ACS event.

NATURAL HISTORY. The short-term mortality of patients with unstable angina has been shown to be lower (1.7 percent at 30 days) than that of patients with NSTEMI or STEMI, whereas the mortality risk with the two types of MI is similar (5.1 percent for each type).[38] The early mortality risk in ACS is related to the extent of myocardial damage and resulting hemodynamic compromise.[65] In contrast, long-term outcomes—for both mortality and nonfatal events—are actually *worse* for patients with either unstable angina or NSTEMI compared with STEMI (Fig. 49–7).[38] This is probably due to

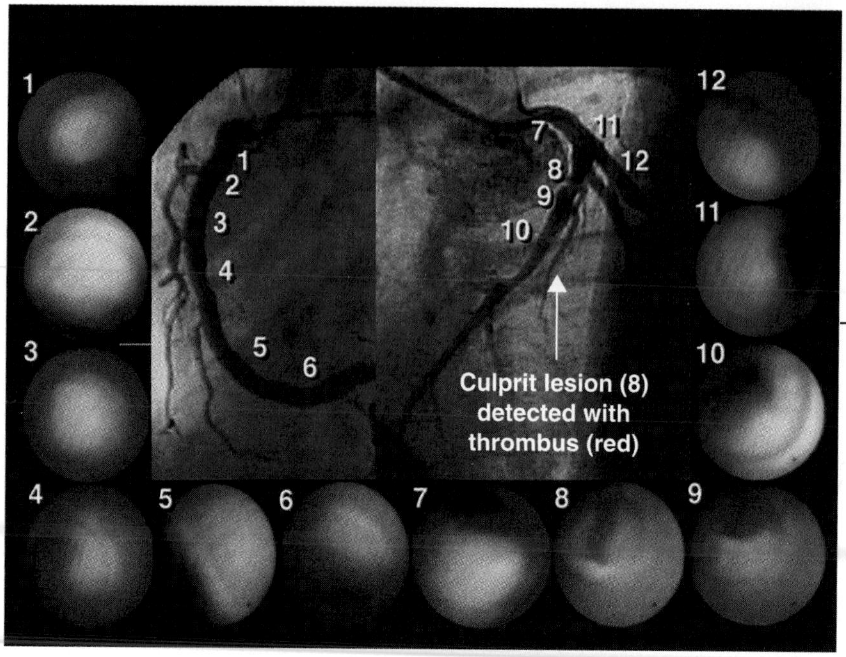

FIGURE 49–5 Evidence of multiple vulnerable plaques in a patient with acute coronary syndrome. Angiographic and angioscopic images of a 58-year-old male with anterior myocardial infarction are shown. The culprit lesion is seen in the proximal left anterior descending artery at site 8. However, other segments of the artery, which appear normal on the coronary angiogram, at angioscopy demonstrate the presence of vulnerable plaques (sites 10 to 12 and 1, 3, 4, 7). (Adapted from Asakura M, Ueda Y, Yamaguchi O, et al: Extensive development of vulnerable plaques as a pan-coronary process in patients with myocardial infarction: An angioscopic study. J Am Coll Cardiol 37:1284, 2001.)

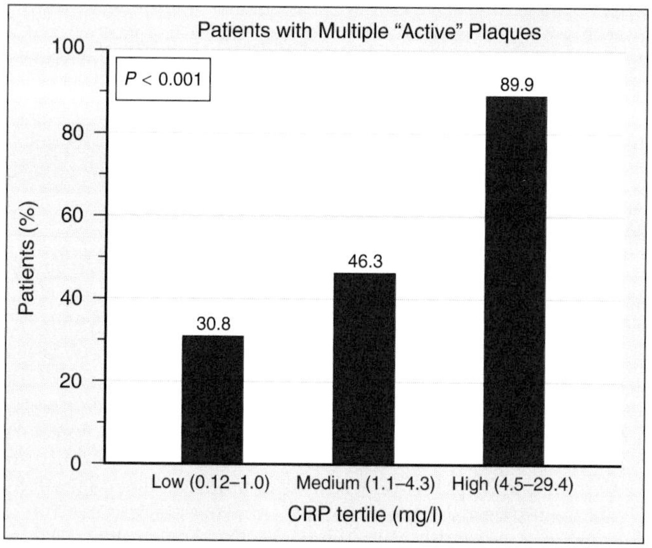

FIGURE 49–6 The level of C-reactive protein (CRP) correlated with the prevalence of multiple thrombus–containing coronary plaques in 228 patients with unstable angina or non-ST elevation myocardial infarction. (Data from Zairis MN, Papadaki OA, Manousakis SJ, et al: C-reactive protein and multiple complex coronary artery plaques in patients with primary unstable angina. Atherosclerosis 164:355, 2002.)

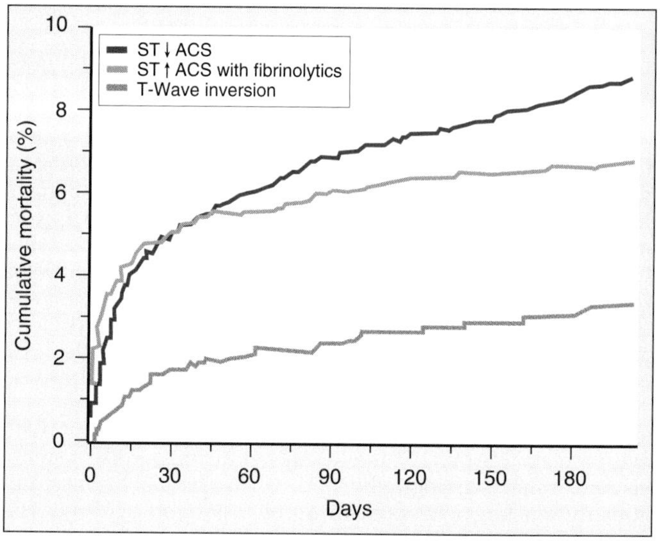

FIGURE 49–7 Kaplan-Meier curves showing mortality in patients with acute coronary syndrome (ACS) in the Global Use of Strategies to Open Occluded Coronary Arteries (GUSTO) IIb study, divided according to the electrocardiographic findings at presentation. (Adapted from Savonitto S, Ardissino D, Granger CB, et al: Prognostic value of the admission electrocardiogram in acute coronary syndromes. JAMA 281:707, 1999. Copyright 1999, American Medical Association.)

the greater extent of coronary disease and prior MI among patients with UA/NSTEMI versus STEMI.

Methods of Risk Stratification

Patients with UA/NSTEMI are a heterogeneous group, with a prognosis that ranges from an excellent outcome with modest adjustments in therapeutic regimen to one in which the risk of death or MI is high and intensive treatment is needed. Accordingly, risk stratification now plays a central role in the evaluation and management of this condition. Specific subgroups of patients, identified by clinical features, electrocardiographic findings, or cardiac (or vascular) markers are at higher risk for adverse outcomes (Table 49–2). Furthermore, these groups appear to derive greater benefit from more aggressive antithrombotic or interventional therapy, or both (see later). Clinical predictors can also be used to assist in triage of patients with unstable angina to the coronary care unit or a monitored bed. Patients determined to be at highest risk should be admitted to the coronary care unit, whereas those with intermediate or lower risk could be admitted to a monitored bed on a cardiac step-down unit. Patients sometimes referred to as at "low risk," but who are best characterized by their "low likelihood" of having an ACS, are

TABLE 49–2 Clinical Indicators of Increased Risk in Unstable Angina or Non-ST Elevation Myocardial Infarction

History
Advanced age (>70 yr)
Diabetes mellitus
Post-myocardial infarction angina
Prior peripheral vascular disease
Prior cerebrovascular disease
Clinical Presentation
Braunwald class II or III (acute or subacute rest pain)
Braunwald class B (secondary unstable angina)
Heart failure or hypotension; ventricular arrhythmias
Electrocardiogram
ST segment deviation ≥0.05 mV
T wave inversion ≥0.3 mV
Left bundle branch block
Cardiac Markers
Increased troponin T or I or creatine kinase muscle-brain (MB) fraction
Increased C-reactive protein or white blood cell count
Increased B-type natriuretic peptide
Elevated CD40 ligand
Elevated glucose or hemoglobin A_{1c}; elevated creatinine
Angiogram
Thrombus; three vessel disease; reduced ejection fraction

evaluated and managed in emergency department observation units or chest pain centers (see Chap. 45).

Clinical Variables

The aforementioned classification of unstable angina[5] (see Table 49–1) has been shown in several studies to be useful clinically in identifying high-risk patients. In the TIMI III Registry, which included 3318 consecutive patients with UA/NSTEMI, this classification was an important predictor of rate of death or MI to 1 year.[7] High-risk groups of patients with unstable angina are those with acute rest pain, those with post-MI unstable angina, and those with secondary unstable angina.

HIGH-RISK CLINICAL SUBGROUPS. Increasing age has been shown to be associated with a significant increase in adverse outcomes in patients with UA/NSTEMI.[66-68] Diabetic patients with UA/NSTEMI are at approximately 50 percent higher risk than nondiabetics.[69] Patients with extracardiac vascular disease, i.e., those with either cerebrovascular disease or peripheral arterial vascular disease, also appear to have approximately 50 percent higher rates of death or recurrent ischemic events compared with patients without previous peripheral or cerebrovascular disease, even after controlling for other differences in baseline characteristics.[70]

As with STEMI, patients with UA/NSTEMI who present with evidence of congestive heart failure (Killip Class > II) have an increased risk of death.[71] In addition, patients who develop recurrent ischemia after initial presentation have been found to be at increased risk.[72]

Risk Assessment by Electrocardiography

The admission ECG is very useful in predicting long-term adverse outcomes. In the TIMI III Registry of patients with UA/NSTEMI, independent predictors of 1-year death or MI included left bundle branch block (risk ratio 2.8), ST segment deviation greater than 0.05 mV (risk ratio 2.45), both p less than 0.001.[37] There appears to be a gradient of risk based on the degree of ST segment deviation.[73,74] In contrast, the presence of T wave changes greater than 0.1 mV was associated with a modest[73] or no increase in subsequent death or MI.[37,38]

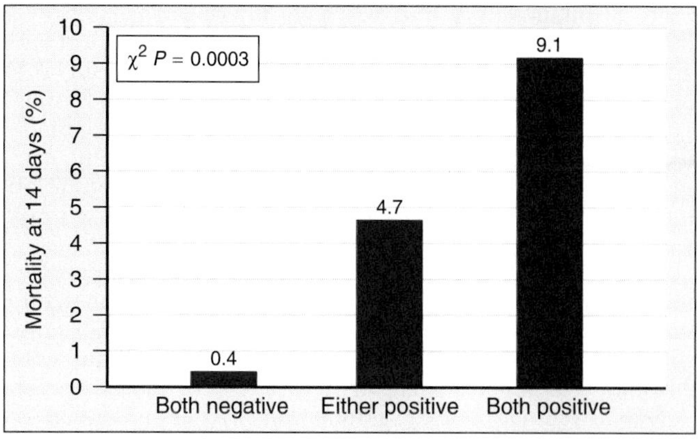

FIGURE 49–8 Use of both troponin T and C-reactive protein (CRP) to predict mortality. These data demonstrate that an elevated high-sensitivity CRP (>15.5 mg/liter in this study) and an "early positive" rapid bedside troponin T assay (defined as positive < 10 minutes) are independent predictors of increased mortality. (From Morrow DA, Rifai N, Antman EM, et al: C-reactive protein is a potent predictor of mortality independently and in combination with troponin T in acute coronary syndromes: A TIMI 11A substudy. J Am Coll Cardiol 31:1460, 1998.)

Risk Assessment by Cardiac Markers

CREATINE KINASE-MB AND THE TROPONINS. Patients with NSTEMI, defined as those with an elevated biomarker of necrosis, CK-MB, or troponin, have a worse long-term prognosis than those with unstable angina.[45,75-79] Beyond just a positive versus negative test result, there is a linear relationship between the level of troponin T or I in the blood and subsequent risk of death—the higher the troponin, the higher the mortality risk.[75] On the other hand, a higher risk of MI was observed with *lower* levels of troponin in several studies, and thus the overall rate of death or MI is equally high among patients with low or higher troponin values.[45,80] Similar results have been obtained using a bedside rapid assay for troponin T, in which time to positivity is a semiquantitative measure of serum troponin T, and related to increased mortality.[81] Thus, troponin T and troponin I are useful not only in diagnosing infarction but also in risk assessment and in targeting therapies to high-risk patients.

C-REACTIVE PROTEIN. Among the growing list of markers that appear to be useful in assessing patients with UA/NSTEMI, CRP is very promising. Elevated CRP has been related to increased risk of death, MI, or need for urgent revascularization.[80,82-84] Of note, because CRP is an acute phase reactant, it is known to be elevated by an ACS. Thus, elevated levels of CRP in patients with ACS are approximately five times higher than those of stable patients.[82,85] Among patients with negative troponin I at baseline, who overall had a 14-day mortality of only 1.5 percent, CRP was able to discriminate a high- and a low-risk group; mortality for patients with an elevated CRP was 5.8 percent versus 0.4 percent for patients without elevated CRP.[82] When using both CRP and troponin T, mortality could be stratified from 0.4 percent for patients with both markers negative to 4.7 percent if either CRP or troponin was positive to 9.1 percent if both were positive (Fig. 49–8).[82] Similar results have been seen in other studies.[80,83,84,86-89] Of note, however, in contrast to troponin, which is extremely useful in selecting patients for more aggressive treatment, CRP has not been shown in the setting of UA/NSTEMI to predict a differential benefit of a therapy.[90] CRP measured at the time of hospital discharge has been found to be a strong predictor of outcome to 3 to 12 months.[91]

Other inflammatory markers have offered consistent evidence of an association between systemic inflammation and recurrent adverse events, including serum amyloid A,[92] monocyte chemoattractant protein-1 (MCP-1),[93] and interleukin-6.[94] In addition, some of these markers of inflammation may be potential therapeutic targets, as may be the case for MCP-1.[93] Thus, these studies indicate that inflammation is related to the instability of patients and an increased risk of recurrent cardiac events.

WHITE BLOOD CELL COUNT. Another, even simpler and universally available marker of inflammation is the white blood cell (WBC) count. Several studies of patients with acute MI[95,96] and UA/NSTEMI[96-98] have observed that patients with elevated WBC counts were at higher risk of mortality and recurrent acute MI. This association was independent of CRP,[87,97] suggesting that not all the information about the influence of inflammation on outcomes is captured in one marker such as CRP.

CD40 LIGAND. Another emerging and important marker is CD40 ligand (CD40L), a member of the tumor necrosis factor-alpha family of proteins. CD40L is expressed on the platelet surface when platelets are activated and is subsequently cleaved, generating a soluble hydrolytic fragment termed sCD40L. It has been found to be both prothrombotic[99] and proinflammatory and to have a role in atherosclerotic lesion progression.[100] CD40L has been correlated with the degree of platelet activation, as measured by platelet-monocyte aggregates, and thus is a novel marker of platelet activation.[101] Studies have found that increasing levels of CD40L are associated with increased risk of death, MI, and recurrent ischemic events, independent of troponin and CRP, in patients with ACS[101,102] as well as in more stable populations of patients,[103] suggesting that this is a useful new marker of risk.

B-TYPE NATRIURETIC PEPTIDE. B-type natriuretic peptide (BNP) is a neurohormone that is synthesized in ventricular myocardium and released in response to increased wall stress.[104] It has many actions including natriuresis, vasodilation, inhibition of sympathetic nerve activity, and inhibition of the renin-angiotensin-aldosterone system. BNP has been show to be a diagnostic and prognostic marker in patients with congestive heart failure[105] and patients with acute MI.[106] BNP has now been seen to have prognostic value across the full spectrum of patients with ACS, including those with UA/NSTEMI: patients with elevated levels of BNP (>80 pg/ml) had a two- to threefold higher risk of death by 10 months.[107] This finding was confirmed in the TIMI 11 and TACTICS-TIMI 18 trials.[108,109] Together, these data suggest that measurement of BNP in patients presenting with UA/NSTEMI adds importantly to our current tools for risk stratification (see Fig. 49–2).

MYELOPEROXIDASE. Myeloperoxidase (MPO) is a hemoprotein expressed by polymorphonuclear neutrophils that possesses potent proinflammatory properties and that promotes oxidation of lipoproteins in vascular atheroma. One case-control study found an association of MPO levels with the presence of angiographically documented CAD, independent of other cardiovascular risk factors and of WBC count.[110] In patients with UA/NSTEMI, MPO serum levels were associated with increased risk for subsequent death or MI, independent of other risk factors and other cardiac markers.[111] Elevations of MPO have been seen throughout the coronary vasculature in patients with UA/NSTEMI.[112] Thus, MPO may be both a marker of inflammation, and its presence also suggests a direct role of neutrophil activation in the pathophysiology of vascular inflammation and ACS.

CREATININE. Another simple tool for risk stratification is the use of creatinine or calculation of creatinine clearance, or both. Several studies have found elevated creatinine to be associated with an adverse prognosis (see Fig. 49–2).[113-116] The risk appears to be independent of other standard risk factors, such as troponin elevation. This factor may also play a role in decreased drug clearance, in which dosages of medications such as LMWH need to be adjusted.[117]

GLUCOSE. Adverse outcomes have been seen among diabetic patients with acute MI with elevated admission glucose values compared with patients without hyperglycemia.[118] Studies have found that this association is present even among patients without a prior diagnosis of diabetes. In addition, this association was seen in patients with both STEMI and UA/NSTEMI and was independent of other baseline risk factors.[119,120] A similar association of poor glycemic control, as measured by hemoglobin A_{1c}, has been seen in other studies.[121] Thus, in patients with UA/NSTEMI, a higher baseline glucose level at the time of presentation is associated with significantly higher long-term mortality, independent of a history of diabetes, a risk factor that may be modifiable with aggressive treatment.[122]

Combined Risk Assessment Scores

Integrating all of the preceding factors, several groups have developed comprehensive risk scores that use clinical variables, findings from the ECG, and findings from serum cardiac markers.[67,68] From the Platelet Glycoprotein IIb/IIIa in Unstable Angina: Receptor Suppression Using Integrilin Therapy (PURSUIT) trial, Boersma and colleagues identified factors that were independently associated with increased mortality and with death or MI. The most important baseline determinants of higher mortality were increasing age, increasing heart rate, lower systolic blood pressure, ST segment depression, signs of heart failure, and elevated cardiac marker enzymes. The TIMI risk score identified seven independent risk factors: age older than 65 years, more than three risk factors for CAD, documented CAD at catheterization, ST deviation greater than 0.5 mm, more than two episodes of angina in the last 24 hours, aspirin within the prior week, and elevated cardiac markers. This scoring system was used to stratify the risk for patients across a 10-fold gradient of risk, from 4.7 to 40.9 percent ($p < 0.001$) (Fig. 49–9A).[67] More important, this risk score has been found to predict the response to several of the therapies used in UA/NSTEMI: patients with higher TIMI risk scores had significant reductions in events when treated with enoxaparin compared with UFH,[67] with a GP IIb/IIIa inhibitor compared with placebo,[123] and with an invasive versus conservative strategy (Fig. 49–9B).[3] With the ever-growing number of new cardiac markers (see earlier), it is expected that these comprehensive risk scores can be expanded to include these new markers as they become more widely available in clinical practice, as shown in one study using three markers in a "multimarker strategy for evaluation" (Fig. 49–10; see Fig. 49–2).

Medical Therapy

TREATMENT GOALS. The treatment objectives for patients with UA/NSTEMI are to stabilize and "passivate" the acute coronary lesion, to treat residual ischemia, and to employ long-term secondary prevention. Antithrombotic therapy (e.g., aspirin, clopidogrel, UFH or LMWH, and GP IIb/IIIa inhibitors) is used to prevent further thrombosis and allow endogenous fibrinolysis to dissolve the thrombus and reduce the degree of coronary stenosis. Antithrombotic therapy is continued in the long term to reduce the risk of developing future events or to prevent progression to complete occlusion of the coronary artery, or both. Antiischemic therapies (e.g., beta blockers, nitrates, and calcium antagonists) are used primarily to reduce myocardial oxygen demand but also appear to have effects in preventing plaque rupture, as shown in prevention of clinical events with beta

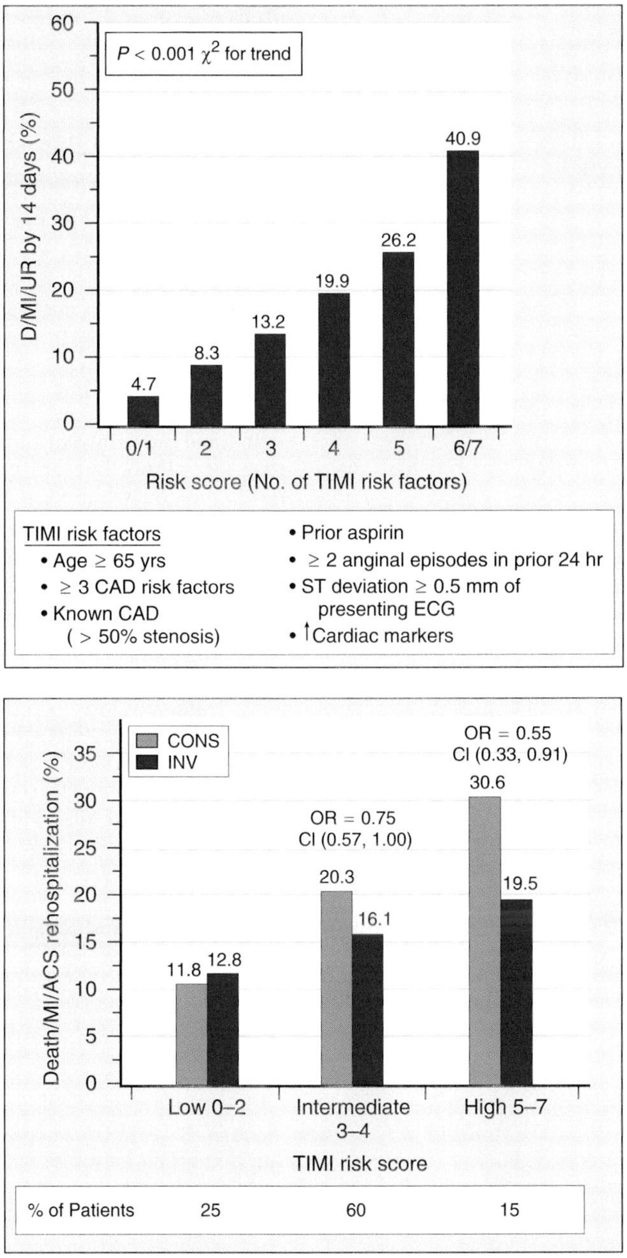

FIGURE 49–9 **A,** Thrombolysis in Myocardial Ischemia (TIMI) risk score for unstable angina or non-ST elevation myocardial infarction (UA/NSTEMI). The risk factors are shown on the right and the risk of death (D), myocardial infarction (MI), or urgent revascularization (UR) is shown along the vertical axis. **B,** Use of the TIMI risk score for UA/NSTEMI to predict the benefit of an early invasive strategy. In a prospectively defined analysis, the TIMI risk score was applied in the Treat Angina with Aggrastat and determine Cost of Therapy with an Invasive or Conservative Strategy (TACTICS)-TIMI 18 trial. As shown, 75 percent of patients had a risk score of 3 or higher, and in these patients a significant benefit of an invasive strategy was observed. ACS = acute coronary syndrome; CAD = coronary artery disease; CI = confidence interval; CONS = conservative; ECG = electrocardiogram; INV = invasive; OR = odds ratio. (**A,** Adapted from Antman EM, Cohen M, Bernink PJLM, et al: The TIMI risk score for unstable angina/non-ST elevation MI: A method for prognostication and therapeutic decision making. JAMA 284:835, 2000; **B,** data from Cannon CP, Weintraub WS, Demopoulos LA, et al: Comparison of early invasive and conservative strategies in patients with unstable coronary syndromes treated with the glycoprotein IIb/IIIa inhibitor tirofiban. N Engl J Med 344:1879, 2001.)

blockers and angiotensin-converting enzyme (ACE) inhibition. Coronary revascularization is frequently used to treat the severe stenosis of a culprit lesion, thereby preventing the thrombus from progressing and causing recurrent ischemia. After the acute event is stabilized, the many factors that led up to the event need to be reversed, i.e., treatment of atherosclerotic risk factors such as hypercholesterolemia, hypertension, and cessation of smoking, each of which contributes to stabilization of the cholesterol-laden plaque and healing of the endothelium.

General Measures

Patients with UA/NSTEMI should be admitted to a monitored bed. Continuous ECG monitoring (i.e., telemetry) is used to detect cardiac arrhythmias. Higher fidelity continuous ECG tracings can be obtained with a Holter monitor and can assess asymptomatic ST deviations as markers for ischemia. This approach has been shown to be useful in clinical trials in risk stratification with core laboratory analysis of the tracings,[41] but its usefulness "on line" in clinical practice has not been well established and deserves further study.

Bed rest is usually prescribed initially for patients with UA/NSTEMI. Ambulation as tolerated is permitted if the patient has been stable without recurrent chest discomfort for at least 12 to 24 hours or following revascularization. Means of improving the physical and emotional surroundings for the patient, such as placing the patient in a quiet atmosphere away from any emotionally taxing arguments and offering the physician's reassurance or mild sedation, may act to reduce sympathetic drive and thereby reduce ischemia. It is advisable to provide supplemental oxygen only to patients with cyanosis, extensive rales, or documented hypoxemia. Oxygen saturation determined by oxymetry is useful with supplemental oxygen administered when the arterial O_2 saturation declines below 92 percent.

Relief of chest pain is an initial goal of treatment. In patients with persistent pain despite therapy with nitrates and beta blockers (see later), morphine sulfate 1 to 5 mg intravenously is recommended. Contraindications include hypotension or prior allergy; meperidine hydrochloride can be substituted in the latter patients. With careful blood pressure monitoring, repeated doses can be administered every 5 to 30 minutes. Morphine may act as both an analgesic and anxiolytic, but its venodilatory effects may produce beneficial hemodynamic effects by reducing preload. The latter is especially useful in the setting of acute pulmonary edema. If hypotension develops after administration of morphine, supine positioning or intravenous saline should restore blood pressure, and pressors are rarely needed. If respiratory depression develops, naloxone (0.4 to 2.0 mg) may be given.

Nitrates (see also Chap. 50)

Nitrates are endothelium-independent vasodilators that both increase myocardial blood flow by coronary vasodilation and reduce myocardial oxygen demand. The latter effect is produced by venodilation, which leads to reduced myocardial preload, reduction in ventricular wall stress, and thereby reduced myocardial oxygen demand. Nitrates should initially be given sublingually or by buccal spray (0.3 to 0.6 mg) if the patient is experiencing ischemic pain. If pain persists after three sublingual tablets (or buccal sprays) given 5 minutes apart and initiation of beta blockade (see later), intravenous nitroglycerin (5 to 10 μg/min using nonabsorbing tubing) is recommended. The rate of the infusion may be increased by 10 μg/min every 3 to 5 minutes until symptoms are relieved or systolic blood pressure falls to below 100 mm Hg. Although there is no absolute maximum dose, a dose of 200 μg/min is generally used as a ceiling. Contraindications to use of nitrates are hypotension or the use of sildenafil (Viagra) or related compounds within the previous 24 to 48 hours.[124] Topical or oral nitrates can be used if the episode of pain has resolved, or they may replace intravenous nitroglycerin if the patient has been pain free for 12 to 24 hours. Dosing of nitrates depends on the formulation, but one

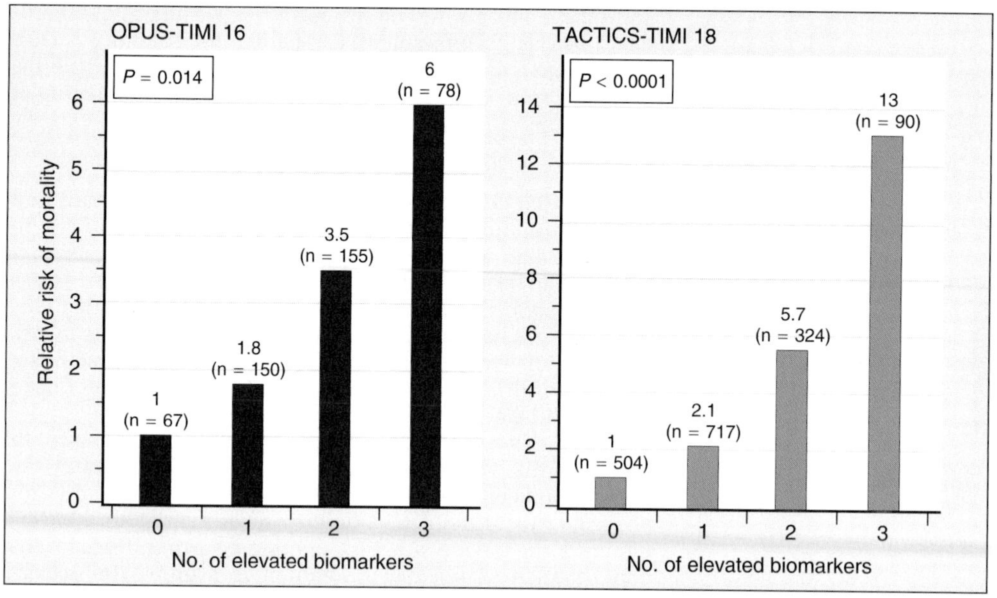

FIGURE 49–10 A multimarker strategy to predict mortality in acute coronary syndrome. Troponin I, C-reactive protein, and B-type natriuretic peptide as determinants of 30-day mortality in unstable angina or non-ST elevation myocardial infarction. Mortality is a function of the number of elevated biomarkers in two separate trials. OPUS-TIMI = Orbofiban in Patients with Unstable Coronary Syndromes–Thrombolysis in Myocardial Infarction; TACTICS-TIMI = Treat Angina with aggrastat and determine Cost of Therapy with an Invasive or Conservative Strategy–TIMI. (Adapted from Sabatine MS, Morrow DA, de Lemos JA, et al: Multimarker approach to risk stratification in non-ST elevation acute coronary syndromes: Simultaneous assessment of troponin I, C-reactive protein, and B-type natriuretic peptide. Circulation 105:1760, 2002.)

should attempt to have an 8- to 10-hour nitrate-free interval to avoid the development of tolerance.

The effect of nitrates on mortality was evaluated in the Gruppo Italiano per lo Studio della Sopravvivenza nell'Infarto Miocardico (GISSI)-3 and Fourth International Study of Infarct Survival (ISIS-4) trials for patients with suspected MI (both ST elevation and NSTEMI).[125,126] No beneficial effect on mortality was observed in the overall population or in the subgroup of patients with NSTEMI. Consequently, the goal of nitrate therapy is relief of pain; chronic nitrate therapy can frequently be tapered off in the long-term management of patients, with primary therapy being aspirin, clopidogrel, beta blockers, and so forth with sublingual or buccal nitroglycerin given as needed for new episodes of pain.

Beta Blockers (see also Chap. 50)

Several placebo-controlled trials in UA/NSTEMI have shown benefit of beta blockers in reducing subsequent MI or recurrent ischemia, or both.[127-129] Subgroup analyses of patients with non-Q-wave MI in several trials demonstrated the benefits of beta blockers (intravenous followed by oral).[130] Thus, beta blockers are recommended for patients with UA/NSTEMI who do not have contraindications to beta blockade (bradycardia, advanced atrioventricular [AV] block, persistent hypotension, known systolic dysfunction with acute pulmonary edema, history of bronchospasm). If ischemia and chest pain are ongoing, early intravenous beta blockade should be used, followed by oral beta blockade. A reduced ejection fraction, which was formerly a contraindication, has now become an *indication* for chronic beta blockade (see Chap. 23), but the dose must be escalated slowly in patients with left ventricular dysfunction, and intravenous administration should be avoided.[131]

The choice of beta blocker can be made individually on the basis of the drug's pharmacokinetics and cost and the physician's familiarity with it. However, those with intrinsic sympathomimetic activity, such as pindolol, should not be selected. Examples of doses tested in large trials include atenolol (5- to 10-mg intravenous bolus followed by 100 mg orally daily) and metoprolol (5-mg intravenous boluses, three given 2 to 5 minutes apart, followed by 50 mg orally twice daily titrated up to 100 mg twice daily).[132]

Calcium Channel Blockers (see also Chap. 50)

Calcium channel blockers have vasodilatory effects and lower blood pressure, and some (verapamil and diltiazem) also slow heart rate. They may be used in patients who have persistent or recurrent symptoms but are currently recommended only for patients who have persistent ischemia after treatment with full-dose nitrates and beta blockers or patients with contraindications to beta blockade. Such patients should be treated with heart rate–slowing calcium channel blockers (e.g., diltiazem or verapamil). Oral doses of diltiazem and verapamil range from 30 mg three times daily for the former and 80 mg three times daily for the latter to 480 mg once daily of the long-acting preparation.

In the Diltiazem Reinfarction Study, involving 576 patients with non-Q-wave MI, diltiazem reduced recurrent MI from 9.3 percent with placebo to 5.2 percent with diltiazem.[133] A pilot study using intravenous diltiazem and a larger clinical trial using long-acting diltiazem[134] in patients following thrombolytic therapy found trends toward benefit of diltiazem versus placebo. In the Danish Verapamil Infarction Trial II (DAVIT II) involving patients with suspected MI or unstable angina, of whom nearly half did not have confirmed MI, verapamil tended to reduce recurrent MI or death.[135] However, meta-analyses have found no beneficial effect of the calcium antagonist drugs as a class in reducing mortality or subsequent infarction.[136] One overview did suggest benefit of verapamil alone.[137]

In patients with acute MI with left ventricular dysfunction or congestive heart failure, a harmful effect of diltiazem was observed.[138] Nifedipine, which does not lower heart rate, has been shown to be harmful in patients with acute MI when not coadministered with a beta blocker. In contrast, no harm was observed in one study with verapamil in patients with congestive heart failure, all of whom were treated with ACE inhibitors.[139] Similarly, no harm with long-term treatment with amlodipine or felodipine[140] was observed in patients with documented left ventricular dysfunction and CAD, indicating that these vasoselective calcium antagonists may be safely used in patients with UA/NSTEMI with left ventricular dysfunction.

In summary, calcium antagonists should be used in patients with UA/NSTEMI if needed for recurrent ischemia despite beta blockade or in patients in whom beta blockade is contraindicated (e.g., bronchospasm); diltiazem should be avoided in patients with left ventricular dysfunction or congestive heart failure, or both.

Angiotensin-Converting Enzyme Inhibitors

For acute treatment, three large trials showed a 0.5 percent absolute mortality benefit of early (initiated within 24 hours)

ACE inhibition in patients with acute MI.[125,126,141] However, in the ISIS-4 study, no benefit was observed in patients without ST elevation. Thus, short-term ACE inhibition does not appear to confer any benefit for patients with UA/NSTEMI.

On the other hand, *long-term* use of ACE inhibition is beneficial in preventing recurrent ischemic events and mortality in a broad population of patients now including those with any evidence of CAD (see also Chap. 50).[142,143] It is of note that recurrent MI and the need for revascularization were reduced with captopril and enalapril in the Survival and Ventricular Enlargement (SAVE) and Studies of Left Ventricular Dysfunction (SOLVD) trials,[144,145] which has now been confirmed using ramipril and perindopril in the Heart Outcomes Prevention Evaluation (HOPE) and EURopean trial On reduction of cardiac events with Perindopril in stable coronary Artery disease (EUROPA),[142,143] suggesting an antiischemic effect of this entire class of agents.

Lipid-Lowering Therapy (see also Chap. 39)

When compared to placebo, long-term treatment with lipid-lowering therapy, especially with statins, has been shown to be beneficial in patients following acute MI and unstable angina.[146-149] In the Scandinavian Simvastatin Survival Study (4S), carried out in hypercholesterolemic patients with a history of MI *or* unstable angina, mortality was reduced by 30 percent ($p = 0.0003$) and coronary deaths were significantly reduced by 42 percent.[146] In addition, recurrent MI was significantly reduced by 37 percent ($p < 0.001$), coronary revascularization by 37 percent ($p < 0.0001$), and rehospitalization for acute cardiovascular disease by 26 percent ($p < 0.001$).[146,150] In the Long-term Intervention with Pravastatin in Ischemic Disease (LIPID) trial, involving a prespecified subgroup of more than 3200 patients with unstable angina, pravastatin therapy led to a significant 26 percent reduction in total mortality ($p = 0.004$).[151]

The National Cholesterol Education Program recommends treatment with diet and drug therapy if the LDL is greater than 100 mg/dl, with a target of reducing LDL to less than 100 mg/dl.[152] The timing of the blood sample is ideally in the first 24 hours after admission because cholesterol levels fall with acute illness. However, cholesterol should be measured at some time during admission because if it is high, therapy is warranted. Because treatment with statin drugs was associated with the benefits for mortality and cardiovascular morbidity cited earlier, these are the current first-line drugs. Additional or alternative therapy is also warranted according to the National Cholesterol Education Program (see also Chap. 39).[153]

Several pilot studies and observational studies have sought to determine whether there is an early clinical benefit of early initiation of statin therapy in ACS.[154-157] The larger, randomized Myocardial Ischaemia Reduction with Aggressive Cholesterol Lowering (MIRACL) trial found that short-term (4 months) treatment with high-dose atorvastatin (80 mg/d) reduced the primary composite endpoint of cardiac death, nonfatal MI, resuscitated sudden cardiac death, or urgent rehospitalization for recurrent ischemia by 16 percent ($p = 0.048$). The potential benefits of early aggressive statin therapy compared to placebo are also being studied in the Aggrastat to Zocor (A to Z; TIMI 21) trial.[158]

The Pravastatin or Atorvastatin Evaluation and Infection Therapy—Thrombolysis in Myocardial Infarction (PROVE IT-TIMI) 22 trial evaluated the role of intensive lipid lowering as compared with standard lipid lowering in 4162 patients within 10 days of admission for an acute coronary syndrome.[158a] Treatment with standard therapy (pravastatin, 40 mg) achieved a median LDL of 95 mg/dl (range, 79 to 113 mg/dl), while intensive therapy (atorvastatin, 80 mg) achieved a median LDL of 62 mg/dl (interquartile range, 50 to 79 mg/dl) ($p < 0.001$). The risk of death, nonfatal myocardial infarction, documented unstable angina, revascularization, or stroke was reduced by 16% ($p = 0.005$), with rates at 2 years (mean time of follow-up) falling from 26.3 percent to 22.4 percent in the standard versus intensive therapy groups. The risk of death, nonfatal myocardial infarction, or revascularization was reduced by 25 percent ($p = 0.0004$) (Fig. 49–11). In addition, all-cause mortality was reduced by 28 percent ($p = 0.07$), with 2-year mortality rates of 32 percent for standard statin therapy versus 2.2 percent for intensive therapy. Benefit emerged within 30 days postrandomization and continued throughout the 2.5 years of follow-up. Thus, this study demonstrated that (1) early use of high-dose statins following acute coronary syndrome is beneficial in reducing death or recurrent cardiac events, and (2) more intensive lipid-lowering therapy that achieved LDL cholesterol concentrations substantially below current target levels is beneficial.

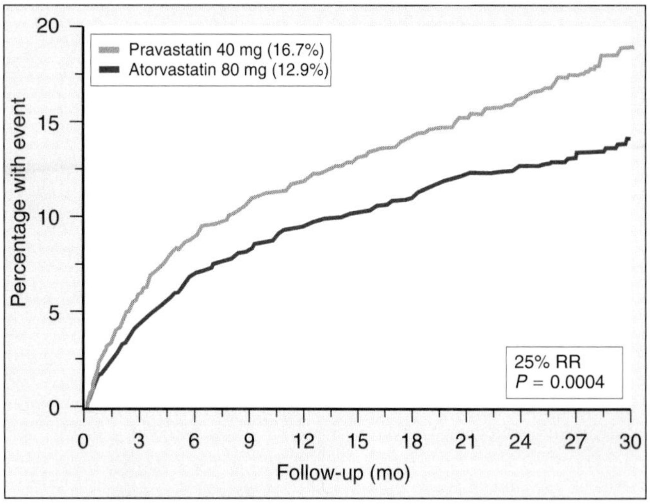

FIGURE 49–11 Results of the PROVE-IT TIMI 22 Trial showing reduction of adverse outcomes (death, nonfatal MI, or urgent revascularization) with intensive lipid lowering with atorvastatin 80 mg/day, compared to standard lipid lowering with pravastatin 40 mg/day. Rates in parentheses are at 2 years.

Beyond the issue of whether an early clinical benefit is achieved and the optimal degree of lipid lowering, studies have found that early initiation of therapy after ACS can improve long-term compliance. One study used standardized orders to ensure that all the patients are receiving appropriate guideline-recommended therapies and found an increase in the use of statins at the time of discharge and at 1-year follow-up, with 91 percent of appropriate patients receiving therapy.[159] Others have also found improved long-term treatment rates with institution of in-hospital quality improvement programs.[160]

Antithrombotic Therapy

Aspirin (see also Chap. 80)

Aspirin permanently acetylates cyclooxygenase 1, thereby blocking the synthesis of thromboxane A_2 by the platelet (Fig. 49–12). By reducing the amount of thromboxane A_2 released, which would act to stimulate other platelets, this effect decreases overall platelet aggregation at the site of the thrombus. This inhibition of cyclooxygenase is permanent, and thus the antiplatelet effects last for the lifetime of the platelets, on the order of 7 to 10 days. Several trials have demonstrated clear beneficial effects of aspirin, with a more than 50 percent reduction in the risk of death or MI in patients presenting with UA/NSTEMI (Fig. 49–13).[16,161] The benefit emerges within the first day of treatment.[161] Thus, aspirin has a dramatic effect in reducing adverse clinical

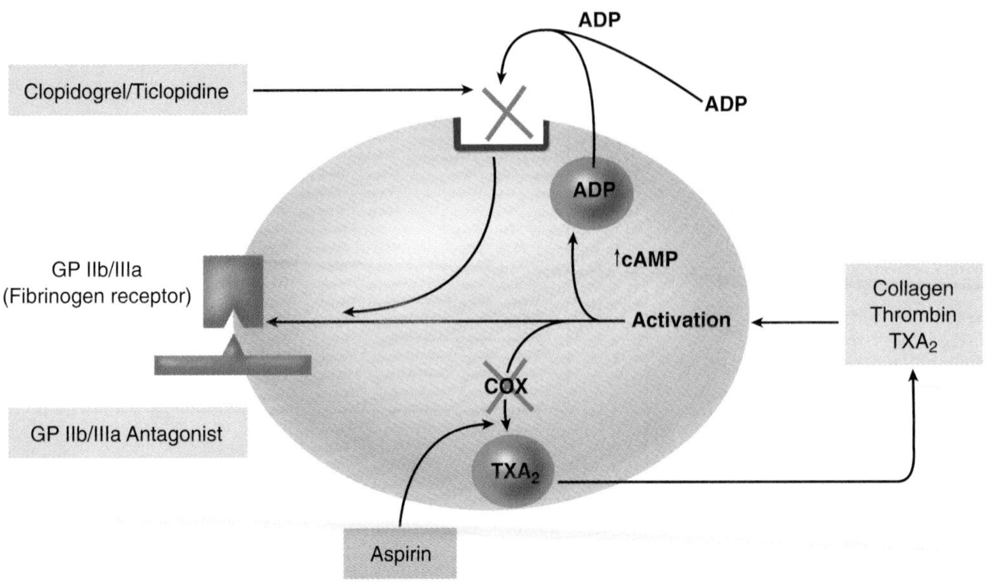

FIGURE 49–12 Mechanisms of action of antiplatelet therapies. See text and Chapter 80 for details. ADP = adenosine diphosphate; cAMP = cyclic adenosine monophosphate; COX = cyclooxygenase; GP = glycoprotein; TXA_2 = thromboxane A_2. (Adapted from Schafer AI: Antiplatelet therapy. Am J Med 101:199, 1996.)

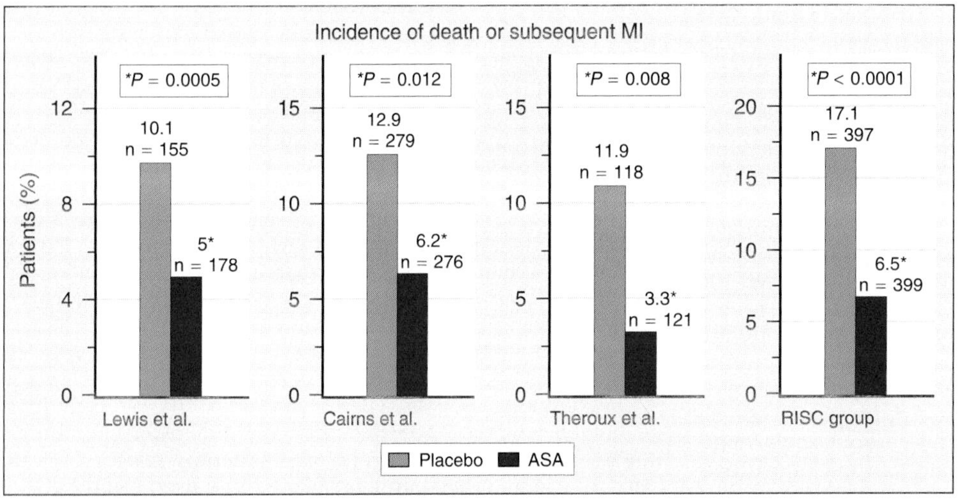

FIGURE 49–13 Four randomized trials showing the benefit of aspirin in unstable angina or non-ST elevation myocardial infarction (UA/NSTEMI). In UA/NSTEMI, the incidence of death or myocardial infarction (MI) was reduced by more than 50 percent in each of the four trials. The doses of aspirin in the four trials were 325, 1300, 650, and 75 mg/d, respectively, indicating no difference in efficacy for aspirin across these doses. ASA = acetylsalicylic acid (aspirin). (Data from Lewis HD, et al: N Engl J Med 309:396, 1983; Cairns, et al: N Engl J Med 313:1499, 1985; Theroux P, et al: N Engl J Med 319:1105, 1988; RISC Group: Lancet 349:827, 1990.)

events early in the course of treatment of UA/NSTEMI and thus is primary therapy for these patients.

The dose of aspirin in the four randomized trials ranged from 75 to 1300 mg/d, and each trial showed a roughly 50 percent reduction in death or MI.[16,161-163] In the large overview of all short- and long-term trials, there does not appear to be a dose-response effect in efficacy of aspirin.[164] In ISIS-2, a dose of 160 mg/d was shown to have a mortality benefit, and this dose is the minimum initial dose recommended.[165] In terms of safety (e.g., gastrointestinal bleeding), two observational studies have found that the rate of bleeding appears to be lower with low-dose aspirin than with medium-dose aspirin (i.e., 325 mg/d) (Table 49–3).[166,167] This was seen among patients treated with medical therapy, PCI, or coronary artery bypass graft (CABG) surgery. Thus, after an initial loading dose of 162 to 325 mg, a dose of 75 to 81 mg/d appears be appropriate for both early and long-term therapy.

During chronic therapy, aspirin resistance has been reported.[168,169] Small studies have identified 5 to 8 percent of patients who have minimal inhibition of platelet aggregation when treated with aspirin. These patients tend to have a greater risk of recurrent cardiac events.[169] No dose response has been seen with this measure of aspirin resistance. A larger study correlated outcomes at 5 years with the amount of thromboxane metabolites in the urine.[168] When patients were divided into quartiles according to the amount of thromboxane in the urine, which could be viewed as a measure of thromboxane "breakthrough" despite aspirin therapy, higher event rates were seen as the amount of thromboxane metabolites rose.[168]

Absolute contraindications for aspirin therapy are few but include documented aspirin allergy (e.g., asthma), active bleeding, or a known platelet disorder. In patients who report dyspepsia or other gastrointestinal symptoms with long-term aspirin therapy (i.e., intolerance), this would not be expected to be an acute problem for in-hospital treatment, and aspirin therapy may be considered for such patients, at least for the short term. In patients who have an allergy or who cannot tolerate aspirin, use of clopidogrel is recommended.[4]

Clopidogrel and Ticlopidine (see also Chap. 80)

Clopidogrel and ticlopidine are thienopyridine derivatives that inhibit platelet aggregation, increase bleeding time, and reduce blood viscosity by inhibiting adenosine diphosphate (ADP) action on platelet receptors.[24] They achieve their antiaggregatory action by inhibiting the binding of ADP to its platelet receptors, specifically the P_2Y_{12} component of the ADP receptor (see Fig. 49–12).[24] Blockade of this receptor not

TABLE 49–3 Major Bleeding by Aspirin Dose

Aspirin Dose (mg)	Aspirin + Placebo	Aspirin + Clopidogrel
75-100	1.9%	3.0%
100-199	2.8%	3.4%
200-325	3.7%	4.9%

Data from Peters RJ, Mehta SR, Fox KA, et al: Circulation 108:1682, 2003.

only inhibits the ADP-induced platelet activation and subsequent aggregation but also appears to decrease platelet activation by other outside stimuli (e.g., von Willebrand factor).[170] Thus, because the P_2Y_{12} receptor is part of the overall amplification of platelet activation within the platelet, inhibition of this receptor appears to have a broader effect in decreasing platelet activation than just inhibition ADP-induced aggregation.

Ticlopidine was compared with placebo (without aspirin) in a randomized trial involving 652 patients with UA/NSTEMI and was found to produce a significant 46 percent reduction in vascular death or nonfatal MI.[171] Ticlopidine has also been demonstrated to be effective in combination with aspirin for prevention of thrombosis and recurrent ischemic events in patients undergoing coronary stent implantation, a portion of whom have recently suffered UA/NSTEMI (see also Chap. 80).[172] However, ticlopidine is associated with neutropenia and thrombocytopenia in approximately 1 percent of patients and quite rarely with thrombotic thrombocytopenic purpura, which can be fatal in 25 to 40 percent of cases.[173] Thus, if ticlopidine is used, short courses (2 to 3 weeks) and biweekly monitoring of complete blood count are generally recommended.

Clopidogrel was developed to avoid these hematological complications and in clinical trials to date has not been associated with an increased incidence of neutropenia or thrombotic thrombocytopenic purpura compared with aspirin alone.[23,174,175] When added to aspirin, clopidogrel appears to be as effective as ticlopidine in preventing stent thrombosis.[176]

THE CURE TRIAL. The addition of clopidogrel to aspirin was studied in the large Clopidogrel in Unstable angina to prevent Recurrent Events (CURE) trial, in which patients were treated with aspirin (75 to 325 mg), heparin or LMWH, and other standard therapies and were randomly assigned to receive a 300-mg loading dose of clopidogrel followed by 75 mg/d.The combination of clopidogrel plus aspirin conferred a 20 percent reduction in cardiovascular death, MI, or stroke compared with aspirin alone in both low- and high-risk patients with UA/NSTEMI (Fig. 49-14).[23] Benefit was seen as early as 24 hours, with the Kaplan-Meier curves diverging after just 2 hours, indicating a very early antithrombotic and clinical effect (Fig. 49-15).[177] Moreover, the benefit continued throughout the trial's 1-year treatment period, consistent with data from the Clopidogrel for Recurrent Events During Observation (CREDO) and Clopidogrel versus Aspirin in Patients at Risk of Ischaemic Events (CAPRIE) trials showing benefit of clopidogrel through 1 and 3 years, respectively, of follow-up in patients with prior atherothrombotic disease.[174,178]

In PCI-CURE, benefit of early treatment with clopidogrel prior to PCI was also seen with a 31 percent reduction in cardiac events at 30 days and 1 year in patients.[179]

THE CREDO TRIAL. In the CREDO trial involving patients undergoing planned or likely PCI (which included approximately two-thirds of patients with ACS), patients were randomly assigned to receive a loading dose of clopidogrel (300 mg) or placebo between 3 and 24 hours before PCI. Following stenting, all patients received open-label clopidogrel for 28 days; after 28 days, patients in the pretreatment group continued on clopidogrel for 1 year, whereas the nonpretreatment group was treated with matching placebo.This study found a small but not statistically significant increase in bleeding in patients receiving clopidogrel versus placebo in addition to aspirin, heparin, and GP IIb/IIIa inhibition. Similar safety observations have been made in other studies.[179-181]

The efficacy results from CREDO also lend further support to both early and long-term use of clopidogrel in patients with UA/NSTEMI. Pretreatment with clopidogrel led to a nonsignificant 19 percent risk reduction in events; however, those given clopidogrel at least 6 hours before PCI had a 38.6 percent relative risk reduction in major events at 28 days ($p = 0.05$) compared with no reduction with treatment less than 6 hours before PCI. This emphasizes the need to initiate clopidogrel as soon as possible on admission for UA/NSTEMI, prior to any planned catheterization and possible PCI. Overall, treatment for 1 year with clopidogrel plus aspirin led to a 26.9 percent relative reduction in death, MI, or stroke compared with post-PCI clopidogrel therapy for 1 month (8.5 versus 11.5 percent [placebo], $p = 0.02$). This included an additional 37.4 percent relative reduction in major events from day 29 to 1 year with clopidogrel ($p = 0.04$). In summary, the results of PCI-CURE and CREDO support preprocedural loading and long-term therapy with clopidogrel in those scheduled or expected to undergo PCI. The significant benefits were seen with or without the concomitant use of GP IIb/IIIa inhibitors.

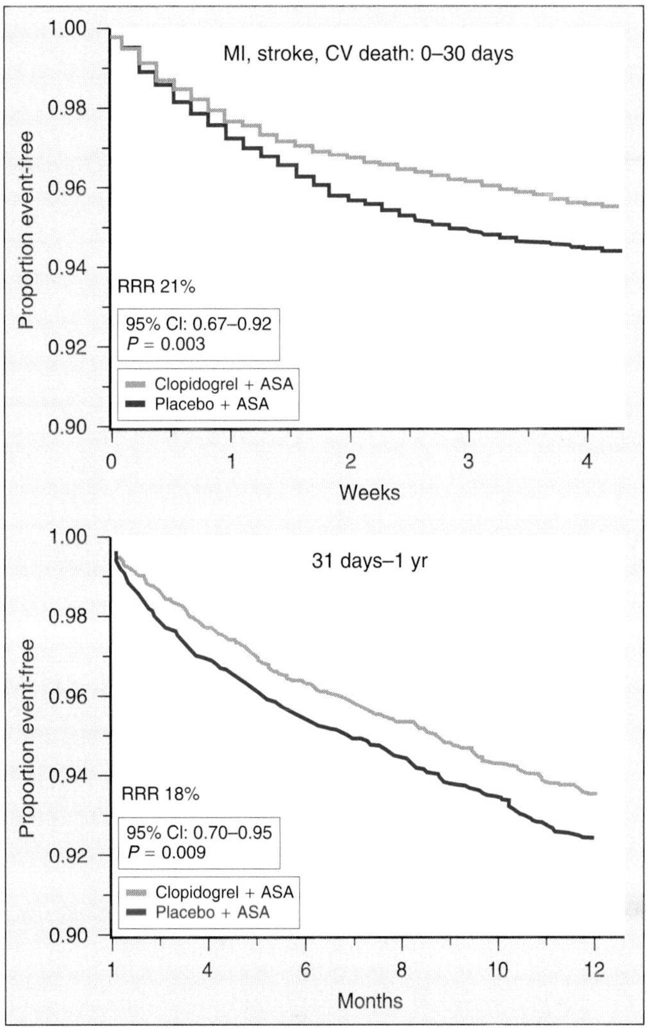

FIGURE 49–14 Benefit of the addition of clopidogrel to aspirin compared with placebo and aspirin during the first 30 days **(top)** and between 31 days and 1 year **(bottom)**. The second analysis was restricted to patients who did not experience an event during the first 31 days. ASA = acetylsalicylic acid (aspirin); CI = confidence interval; CV = cardiovascular; MI = myocardial infarction. (From Yusuf S, Mehta SR, Zhao F, et al: Early and late effects of clopidogrel in patients with acute coronary syndromes. Circulation 107:966, 2003.)

In UA/NSTEMI, the dose of clopidogrel should be an initial loading dose of 300 mg, followed by 75 mg/d. Initiation of only 75 mg/d achieves the target level of platelet inhibition after 3 to 5 days, whereas the loading dose of 300 mg achieves effective platelet inhibition within 4 to 6 hours.[182] Use of a 600-mg loading dose has been shown to achieve a steady-state level of platelet inhibition after just 2 hours.[183] This dose has been utilized in two large clinical studies and been well tolerated.[184,185] In one study, all 2159 patients received a 600-mg loading dose at least 2 hours prior to PCI and were randomly assigned to abciximab and reduced-dose heparin versus placebo and standard-dose heparin. There was no difference in outcomes between the groups at 30 days.[185] This is in contrast to 35 to 50 percent reductions seen with abciximab in other placebo-controlled trials conducted before widespread pretreatment with thienopyridines,[186-188] suggesting that the achievement of effective levels of platelet inhibition with clopidogrel before PCI is effective in reducing events. More studies are ongoing to evaluate the 600-mg loading dose.

As with aspirin, "low responders" to clopidogrel have been identified in several studies.[189,190] As with the aspirin resistance issue, defining what a low response is and determining

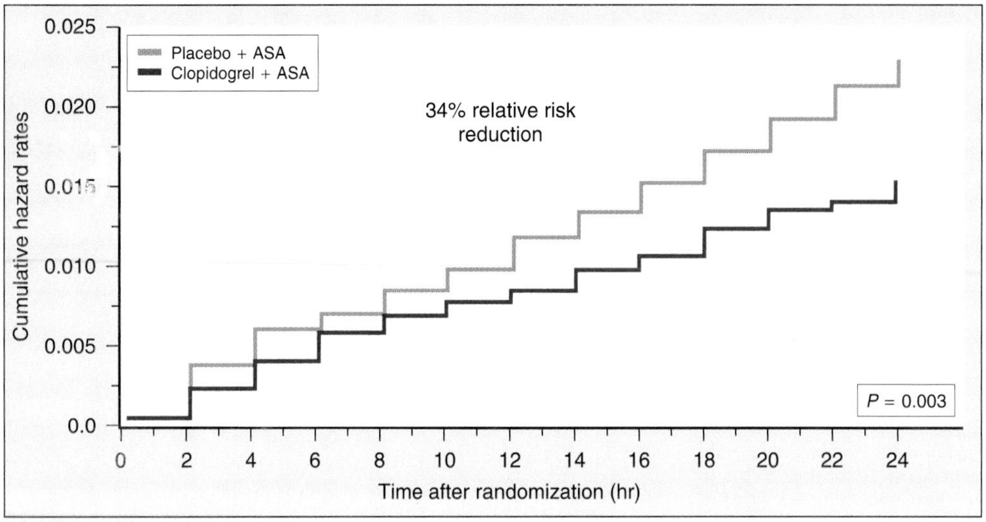

FIGURE 49–15 Effects of clopidogrel in the first 24 hours of the Clopidogrel in Unstable angina to prevent Recurrent Events (CURE) trial. ASA = acetylsalicylic acid (aspirin). (From Yusuf S, Mehta SR, Zhao F, et al: Early and late effects of clopidogrel in patients with acute coronary syndromes. Circulation 107:966, 2003.)

whether it reflects variability in the state of platelet aggregation in the patient or variability in the platelet response to the drug has been difficult using current assays. These findings have fueled interest in development of newer drugs in this class that might achieve higher levels of platelet inhibition.[24] The balance of the efficacy and safety of higher levels of inhibition with this class of drugs needs to be defined in prospective clinical trials.

Heparin (see also Chap. 80)

Anticoagulation with UFH has been a cornerstone of therapy for patients with UA/NSTEMI for over a decade on the basis of several randomized trials that found lower rates of death or MI with UFH plus aspirin compared with aspirin alone.[16,161,191,192] A meta-analysis showed a 33 percent reduction in death or MI at 2 to 12 weeks follow-up with UFH plus aspirin versus aspirin alone, although this reduction was of borderline statistical significance.[17]

Variability in the anticoagulant effects of UFH, so-called heparin resistance, is thought to be due to the heterogeneity of heparin and to the neutralization of heparin by circulating plasma factors and by proteins released by activated platelets.[193] Clinically, frequent monitoring of the anticoagulant response using the activated partial thromboplastin time (aPTT) is recommended with titrations carried out using a standardized nomogram (Table 49–4). The latter minimizes the variability in the dosing adjustments given by various physicians and has been shown to improve the achievement of a target aPTT.[194]

The level of anticoagulation that constitutes the therapeutic range is not yet firmly established. Small studies have suggested that lower aPTT values may be related to recurrent ischemic events,[195,196] suggesting that the lower limit of the target range of aPTT is at least 1.5 times the control value. On the upper boundary of the target range, higher aPTT values are associated with an increased risk of hemorrhage.[196] The lowest rate of bleeding (and mortality) in patients with STEMI treated with thrombolytic therapy was observed when the 12-hour aPTT was between 50 and 70 seconds.[196] Furthermore, in TIMI IIIB, there appeared to be no advantage in reducing ischemic events with higher levels of anticoagulation.[197]

DOSING. On the basis of available data,[198] the current optimal regimen appears to consist of weight-adjusted dosing of UFH (60 units/kg bolus and 12 units/kg/hr infusion), frequent monitoring of aPTT (every 6 hours until in the target range and every 12 to 24 hours thereafter), and titration of UFH using a standardized nomogram (see Table 49–4) with a target range of aPTT between 1.5 to 2 times the control value or approximately 50 and 70 seconds.

Low-Molecular-Weight Heparin (see also Chap. 80)

LMWHs have been widely tested as a means of improving on anticoagulation with UFH. These agents *combine* factor IIa and factor Xa inhibition and thus inhibit both the action and generation of thrombin.[199] LMWHs are obtained by depolymerization of standard UFHs and selection of those with lower molecular weight. Compared with UFH that has nearly equal anti-IIa (thrombin) and anti-Xa activity, LMWHs have increased ratios of anti-IIa to anti-Xa activity of either 2:1 (e.g., dalteparin) or 3.8:1 (e.g., enoxaparin).

LMWH has several potential advantages over UFH. First, its greater anti-factor Xa activity inhibits thrombin generation more effectively. LMWH also induces a greater release of tissue factor pathway inhibitor than UFH, and it is not neutralized by platelet factor 4.[199] LMWH has been found to induce thrombocytopenia at a lower rate than UFH.[200] Its high bioavailability allows subcutaneous administration, which provides a long duration of systemic anticoagulation so that dosing can be administered twice daily. Also, LMWH has less binding to plasma proteins (including acute phase reactant proteins) and thus has a more consistent anticoagulant effect in relation to the dose administered. Accordingly, monitoring of the level of anticoagulation (which is necessary using aPTT for UFH) is not necessary. These last two differences make LMWH a much simpler anticoagulant to administer

TABLE 49–4 Standardized Nomogram for Titration of Heparin

Initial dose: 60 U/kg bolus and 12 U/kg/hr infusion
The activated partial thromboplastin time (aPTT) should be checked and infusion adjusted at 6, 12, and 24 hr after initiation of heparin, daily thereafter, and 4 to 6 hr after any adjustment in dose.

aPTT (sec)	Change	Intravenous Infusion (U/kg/hr)
<35	60 U/kg bolus	+3
35-49	30 U/kg bolus	+2
50-70	0	0
71-90	0	−2
>100	Hold infusion for 30 min	−3

Adapted from Becker RC, Ball SP, Eisenberg P, et al: A randomized, multicenter trial of weight-adjusted intravenous heparin dose titration and point-of-care coagulation monitoring in hospitalized patients with active thromboembolic disease. Antithrombotic Therapy Consortium Investigators. Am Heart J 137:59, 1999.

han UFH. However, it should be noted that LMWHs are more affected by renal dysfunction than UFH, and a reduced dose should be considered in patients with creatinine clearance less than 30 ml/min.

CLINICAL TRIALS

There have been more than 12 randomized trials comparing LMWH with placebo[201] or UFH[18,202,203] and one comparing two different LMWHs. LMWH (plus aspirin) has been found to be effective compared with aspirin alone, leading to a 66 percent reduction in the odds of death or MI.[201,204]

In comparisons between LMWHs and UFH, heterogeneity has been seen between the LMWHs. To date, no difference was observed between dalteparin[202] or nadroparin compared with UFH.[202,203]

On the other hand, three of four trials with enoxaparin have found a significant improvement in clinical outcomes. In the Evaluation of the Safety and Efficacy of Enoxaparin in Non-ST elevation Coronary Events (ESSENCE)[18] and TIMI 11B,[19] enoxaparin conferred a significant approximately 20 percent reduction in death, MI, or recurrent ischemia compared with UFH. In both trials, patients with ST segment deviation exhibited a significant reduction in cardiac events with enoxaparin compared with UFH, whereas those without ST deviation did not.[18,19] Similarly, in the TIMI 11B troponin substudy, among patients who were CK-MB negative, those with elevations of troponin I derived a significantly greater benefit from enoxaparin versus UFH than those with negative troponins.[205] Using the TIMI risk score (see Fig. 49-9A), the benefit of enoxaparin over UFH was seen among patients with a score of 3 or higher (in both ESSENCE and TIMI 11B).[67] Thus, the clinical benefit of enoxaparin is seen among higher risk patients.

In a formal pharmacoeconomic analysis, use of enoxaparin was found to be cost effective: There was a small increase in the cost of the drug (enoxaparin versus UFH with aPTT measurements), but it was balanced by significantly lower rates of catheterization and revascularization, and thus treatment with enoxaparin led to *savings* of $1172 per patient treated.[206] Thus, both improved outcomes and lower costs were observed with in-hospital treatment with enoxaparin versus UFH. No additional benefit of continuing enoxaparin beyond hospital discharge was observed.[19] On the other hand, a more dramatic benefit of enoxaparin was seen among patients undergoing PCI.[207]

Three studies evaluated the merit of enoxaparin versus UFH among patients receiving aspirin and a GP IIb/IIIa inhibitor.[40,158,208] In one study, in which enoxaparin was administered for approximately 4 days prior to any revascularization procedure, if performed, enoxaparin led to a significant reduction in death or MI and of recurrent ischemia documented by ST segment depression on Holter monitoring.[40] In the A to Z trial, a nonsignificant trend toward improved outcomes was seen.[208] A third study (Superior Yield of the New strategy of Enoxaparin, Revascularization, GlYcoprotein IIb/IIIa inhibitors [SYNERGY]) of approximately 10,000 found no significant difference in death or myocardial infarction between enoxaparin and UFH but an increase in bleeding with enoxaparin.[208a] of the two agents in the setting of an early invasive strategy and GP IIb/IIIa inhibition. Figure 49-16 summarizes data on enoxaparin in UA/NSTEMI: a significant approximately 15 to 20 percent relative risk reduction in death or MI and of the combined endpoint of death, MI, or recurrent ischemia at 7 days.[208]

Finally, one study of 438 patients with UA/NSTEMI directly compared two LMWHs—enoxaparin and tinzaparin. The primary composite endpoint, death, MI, or recurrent angina at 7 days, was significantly lower in the enoxaparin group (12.3 percent versus 21.1 percent in the tinzaparin group, $p = 0.015$).[209] These data, combined with the multiple studies of enoxaparin versus UFH, suggest that enoxaparin has a particular benefit in UA/NSTEMI, and unless new trials with other LMWHs demonstrate a benefit over UFH, enoxaparin appears to be the LWMH (and antithrombin) of choice in UA/NSTEMI.

Because one of the purported advantages of LMWH over UFH is the greater factor Xa inhibition, research is progressing with testing of pure factor Xa inhibitors. One agent is a synthetic pentasaccharide, which has been found to be more effective than enoxaparin in prevention of deep vein thrombosis[210]; it is currently being tested in UA/NSTEMI and STEMI.

Direct Thrombin Inhibitors (see also Chap. 80)

Direct thrombin (factor IIa) inhibitors have also undergone extensive evaluation. The prototypic agent is hirudin, a naturally occurring anticoagulant from the medicinal leech. Hirudin, which is manufactured by a recombinant DNA technique, is a 65-amino-acid polypeptide that binds directly to

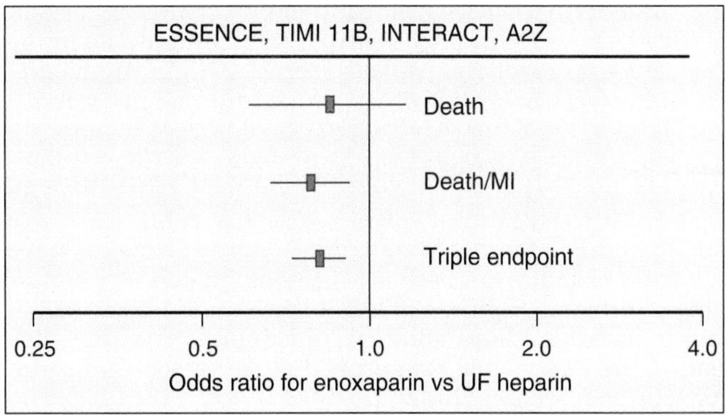

FIGURE 49–16 Meta-analysis of Thrombolysis in Myocardial Infarction (TIMI 11B), Evaluation of the Safety and Efficacy of Enoxaparin in Non-ST elevation Coronary Events (ESSENCE), Interact, and Aggrastat to Zocor (A to Z) trials comparing enoxaparin with unfractionated (UF) heparin. There is a significant reduction in the rate of death or myocardial infarction (MI) in patients treated with enoxaparin. (From Blazing MA: The A-to-Z Trial: Results of the A-Phase, investigating combined use of low-molecular-weight heparin with the glycoprotein IIb/IIIa inhibitor tirofiban. Presented at the American College of Cardiology Scientific Sessions, New Orleans, LA, March 2003.)

thrombin, independent of antithrombin. The hirudin desirudin was tested in the Global Use of Strategies to Open Occluded Coronary Arteries (GUSTO) IIb trial involving 12,142 patients with UA/NSTEMI and STEMI. In the entire cohort, the 30-day rate of death or MI tended to be lower, 8.9 versus 9.8 percent ($p = 0.06$),[35] with no difference in mortality and a modest reduction in reinfarction (5.4 versus 6.3 percent for heparin, $p = 0.04$). In the 8011 patients with UA/NSTEMI, 30-day death or MI was not significantly reduced (8.3 versus 9.1 percent, $p = 0.22$).[35]

The Organisation to Assess Strategies for Ischemic Syndromes (OASIS-2) trial[211] compared lepirudin, another form of hirudin, and UFH; cardiovascular death or MI at 7 days tended to be lower with lepirudin (3.6 versus 4.2 percent, respectively, $p = 0.08$). Major bleeding requiring transfusion was rare but more frequent with lepirudin (1.2 versus 0.7 percent for heparin, $p = 0.01$). A meta-analysis of all hirudin trials showed a modest 10 percent benefit favoring hirudin, which was not statistically significant for patients with UA/NSTEMI. Other synthetic direct thrombin inhibitors have also been tested in small trials to date (e.g., argatroban and bivalirudin), with trends toward lower rates of recurrent cardiac events and lower rates of bleeding.[212-214]

BIVALIRUDIN. This directly acting antithrombin has been tested during PCI and found to have a trend toward superior outcomes compared with UFH[215] and outcomes similar to those with the combination of UFH plus a GP IIb/IIIa inhibitor.[216] In the latter trial, only 40 percent of patients were characterized as having UA/NSTEMI, and the difference in recurrent cardiac events was numerically higher but not statistically different among this high-risk subgroup. Thus, the efficacy of bivalirudin has not been fully studied in UA/NSTEMI, but a large trial is underway. The direct thrombin inhibitors have been observed to provide a stable level of anticoagulation, as measured by aPTT,[35,217] and no episodes of thrombocytopenia have been reported for the hirudin class. Of note, lepirudin and argatroban are approved by the Food and Drug Administration for use as anticoagulants in patients with heparin-induced thrombocytopenia and associated thromboembolic disease.

Oral Anticoagulation (see also Chap. 80)

Oral anticoagulation with warfarin following ACSs has been examined in several trials, with the rationale that prolonged treatment might extend the benefit of early anticoagulation with an antithrombin agent (e.g., heparin, LMWH). Three of the initial large trials have failed to show a significant benefit of long-term warfarin plus aspirin over aspirin alone. In the OASIS-2 trial involving patients with UA/NSTEMI, the rate of cardiovascular death, MI, or stroke to 5 months was 7.6 percent for those receiving warfarin plus aspirin and 8.3 percent for those receiving aspirin alone ($p = $ NS).[218] Similarly, in the Combination Hemotherapy and Mortality Prevention (CHAMP) trial involving survivors of MI, there was no difference in the rate of all-cause mortality over an average 2.7 years of follow-up between the combination of warfarin plus aspirin and aspirin alone, but there was a higher rate of major bleeding.[219] In addition, fixed-dose warfarin plus aspirin was not better than aspirin alone in the Coumadin Aspirin Reinfarction Study (CARS).[220]

However, three subsequent trials, in addition to a post hoc analysis of OASIS-2, suggested that if a sufficient degree of anticoagulation is achieved, a benefit can be observed with the combination of aspirin plus warfarin compared with aspirin alone.[221-224] In each of these studies, the International Normalized Ratio (INR) for the warfarin (plus aspirin) treatment arm had a mean of 2.3 to 2.4, indicating a full degree of anticoagulation, compared with 1.9 in the CHAMP study, which did not find a benefit of warfarin. In the largest study,[223] 4930 patients with ACS within the prior 8 weeks were randomly assigned to warfarin alone (target INR of 2.8 to 4.2), aspirin (160 mg/d), or aspirin (75 mg/d) combined with warfarin (target INR of 2.0 to 2.5). During an average of 4 years of follow-up, death, MI, or thromboembolic cerebral stroke occurred in 20.0 percent of patients receiving aspirin, 16.7 percent of patients receiving warfarin ($p = 0.03$), and 15.0 percent of patients receiving warfarin and aspirin ($p = 0.001$). Rates of major bleeding were 0.62 percent per treatment year in both groups receiving warfarin and 0.17 percent in patients receiving aspirin ($p < 0.001$). Thus, the combination of aspirin plus warfarin is more effective than aspirin alone for long-term secondary prevention.

However, given the similar benefit seen with clopidogrel plus aspirin, the lack of need for monitoring the INR, and the frequent use of PCI and stenting in the population of patients in which clopidogrel is well established, the clinical use of aspirin plus warfarin is limited. However, among patients with another indication for warfarin, such as chronic atrial fibrillation or severe left ventricular dysfunction, who are at high risk for systemic embolization, the combination of aspirin plus warfarin would be preferable as the long-term antithrombotic strategy.[225] The combination of all three agents has not been tested to date but might portend a higher bleeding risk during long-term therapy. Use of all three agents together is sometimes needed among patients with atrial fibrillation or other strong indications for warfarin who undergo stenting. In such patients, one approach is to use aspirin (75 to 81 mg/d) and warfarin (INR 2.0 to 2.5) and to use clopidogrel for only 1 month (the period during which the risk of stent thrombosis is highest).

Research is ongoing to identify alternative oral anticoagulants. One agent, ximelagatran, an oral direct thrombin inhibitor, has been tested in patients following ACS in a dose-ranging study. Overall, the combination of ximelagatran plus aspirin reduced the rate of death, MI, or severe recurrent ischemia by 24 percent compared with aspirin, from 16.3 to 12.7 percent ($p = 0.049$).[226] Although this agent was associated with elevations of liver function tests, it is administered at a fixed dose and does not require monitoring of the level of anticoagulation, but it does require monitoring of liver function tests. Oral factor Xa inhibitors are also in early stages of development.

Glycoprotein IIb/IIIa Inhibitors (see also Chap. 80)

The GP IIb/IIIa receptor inhibitors are a potent class of antiplatelet drugs that act by preventing the final common pathway of platelet aggregation, i.e., fibrinogen-mediated cross-linkage of platelets through the GP IIb/IIIa receptor (see Fig. 49–4). These agents are potent inhibitors of platelet aggregation caused by all types of stimuli (e.g., thrombin, ADP, collagen, serotonin). Three agents are now available for use in UA/NSTEMI, abciximab, eptifibatide, and tirofiban, with the former currently approved only in patients undergoing PCI. *Abciximab* is an Fab fragment of a monoclonal antibody directed at the GP IIb/IIIa receptor. *Eptifibatide*, a synthetic heptapeptide, and *tirofiban*, a nonpeptide molecule, are antagonists of the GP IIb/IIIa receptor whose structure mimics the arginine-glycine-aspartic acid (abbreviated RGD) amino acid sequence by which fibrinogen binds to the GP IIb/IIIa receptor.

Several trials have shown benefit of IIb/IIIa inhibition in UA/NSTEMI in patients receiving predominantly medical management,[21] early interventional management,[227] or both.[20,22,228] In Platelet Receptor Inhibition for Ischemic Syndrome Management in Patients Limited by Unstable Signs and Symptoms (PRISM-PLUS), tirofiban plus heparin and aspirin significantly reduced the rate of death, MI, or refractory ischemia at 7 days compared with heparin plus aspirin.[22] Death or MI at 30 days was also significantly reduced by 30 percent, from 11.9 to 8.7 percent. In the PURSUIT trial, involving 10,948 patients, eptifibatide also significantly reduced the rate of death or MI at 30 days.[20]

There appeared to be a greater benefit of treatment when administered earlier in relation to the onset of pain, i.e., within the first 6 to 12 hours.[229] This benefit may be related in part to reduction in the amount of myocardial necrosis with early treatment.[230] In addition, GP IIb/IIIa inhibitors have been observed to lead to greater resolution of thrombus and improved coronary flow compared with aspirin and heparin alone.[56,231] Together, these data establish the pathophysiological link between the potent platelet inhibition achieved by GP IIb/IIIa inhibition, a reduction in thrombus, improvement in coronary blood flow, and consequent improvement in clinical outcome for patients.

However, the most recent trial, GUSTO-IV ACS, found no benefit and higher early mortality with the use of abciximab in high-risk UA/NSTEMI patients for whom an early conservative strategy (initial medical management) was planned.[232] The higher mortality in the 48-hour infusion group has been proposed to be due to low levels of inhibition of platelet aggregation during the infusion of abciximab at the dose tested. This proposal is in part based on data from other studies showing that during the 12-hour infusion, the level of platelet inhibition falls steadily.[233] Low levels of platelet inhibition have been found to lead to shedding of CD40L, a prothrombotic and proinflammatory protein. Thus, the failure of this agent to improve outcomes in the setting of medically managed UA/NSTEMI may have related to the pharmacodynamics of the agent at the dose tested. In meta-analyses not including GUSTO-IV ACS, largely evaluating the "small molecule" GPIIb/IIIa inhibitors, a 20 percent reduction in death or MI was observed at 30 days.[234] However, when GUSTO-IV ACS was included, the benefit of IIb/IIIa inhibition was only a 9 percent reduction in death or MI at 30 days ($p = 0.015$).

RISK STRATIFICATION TO TARGET GLYCOPROTEIN IIB/IIIA INHIBITORS. GP IIb/IIIa inhibition appears to be a treatment than can be targeted to higher risk patients. In the initial trials, it was observed that the subgroup of patients with ST segment depression or transient ST elevation had a two to three times greater absolute benefit than patients without ST changes.[22] Diabetic patients with UA/NSTEMI were found to have a 26 percent reduction in mortality with GP IIb/IIIa inhibition compared with no reduction in nondiabetics.[69]

Substudies using baseline troponin (and now other cardiac markers) have found that the benefit of GP IIb/IIIa inhibition appears to be greatest in these high-risk patients. This was first seen in the Chimeric c7E3 AntiPlatelet Therapy in Unstable angina REfractory to standard treatment (CAPTURE) trial: among patients who were troponin T positive at baseline, treatment with abciximab before PCI led to a 68 percent reduction in death or MI at 6 months compared with no significant benefit for those who were troponin T negative ($p < 0.001$).[78] These findings have been essentially duplicated with tirofiban versus heparin in the PRISM trial (Fig. 49–17)[79] and two other trials.[235,236] Similar findings were seen using the TIMI risk score to identify high-risk patients who benefit from GP IIb/IIIa inhibition.[123] These subgroups have been seen to have more thrombus at coronary angiography[57,237] and thus be at risk for microvascular embolization[238] and are subgroups in which this potent class of antithrombotic drugs would be of great benefit.

Other cardiac markers have also been able to identify patients at high risk, who derive benefit from GP IIb/IIIa inhibition. CD40L appeared to add information in addition to that provided by troponin in identifying patients who benefit; among troponin-positive patients, those with low levels of CD40L had no benefit from abciximab. Conversely, among troponin-negative patients, who overall had no benefit from abciximab in the original study,[78] those with elevated levels of CD40L had a significant reduction in events with the addition of abciximab. These data suggest that more careful identification of coronary thrombosis and platelet activation with these new cardiac markers may help identify patients in whom GP IIb/IIIa inhibitors will be of greater benefit.

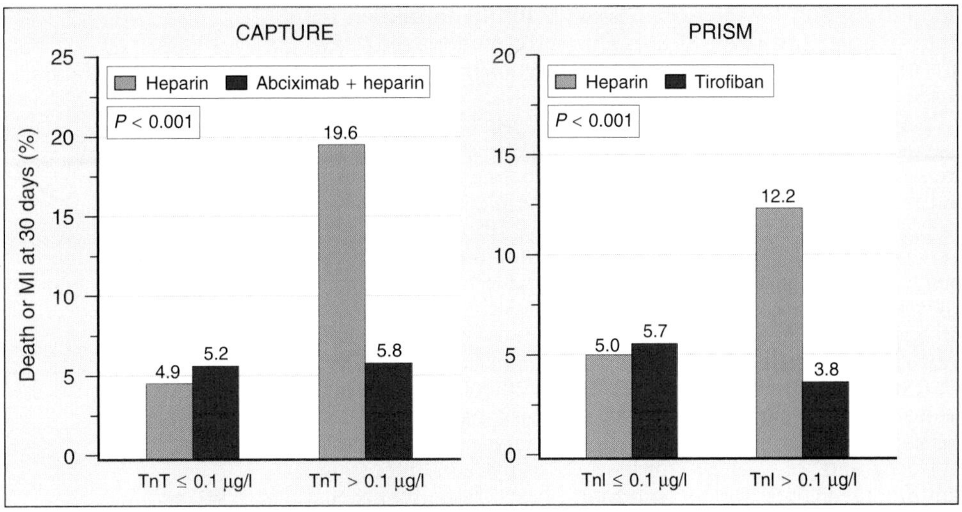

FIGURE 49–17 **Left,** Benefit of abciximab in the CAPTURE trial involving patients with refractory unstable angina treated with angioplasty in those with positive versus negative troponin T (TnT) values at study entry. **Right,** Greater benefit of tirofiban versus heparin in patients with unstable angina or non-ST elevation myocardial infarction was also seen in those with positive troponin I (TnI) values in the PRISM trial, with a nearly 70 percent reduction in death or myocardial infarction (MI) at 30 days with the IIb/IIIa inhibitor. (**Left,** Data from Hamm CW, Heeschen C, Goldmann B, et al: Benefit of abciximab in patients with refractory unstable angina in relation to serum troponin T levels. C7E3 Fab antiplatelet therapy in unstable refractory angina [CAPTURE] study investigators. N Engl J Med 340:1623, 1999; **right,** from Heeschen C, Hamm CW, Goldmann B, et al: Troponin concentrations for stratification of patients with acute coronary syndromes in relation to therapeutic efficacy of tirofiban. PRISM study investigators. Platelet Receptor Inhibition in Ischemic Syndrome Management. Lancet 354:1757, 1999.)

GLYCOPROTEIN IIB/IIIA INHIBITION AND PERCUTANEOUS CORONARY INTERVENTION. With the greater relative benefit of GP IIb/IIIa inhibitors seen in trials of patients undergoing PCI,[186,188] compared with the 9 percent overall benefit in UA/NSTEMI, many have felt that this class of drugs can be reserved for those who undergo PCI. Two meta-analyses found that the majority of the benefit in the UA/NSTEMI trials was seen in those who had early PCI (or CABG).[239] However, one aspect not accounted for in these analyses was the proportion of benefit that was achieved before the PCI procedure. In a pooled analysis of three trials, PRISM-PLUS, PURSUIT, and CAPTURE, involving 12,296 patients, there was a 34 percent relative reduction in death or MI during a period of 24 hours of medical management only (3.8 versus 2.5 percent, $p = 0.001$), with that benefit continuing up through the time of PCI.[240] Furthermore, there is evidence that initial medical treatment with a small-molecule GP IIb/IIIa inhibitor leads to clinical benefit; in the PRISM trial a significant 32 percent reduction in death, MI, or refractory ischemia at 48 hours was found, suggesting a significant clinical benefit during medical treatment alone.[21]

CORONARY ARTERY BYPASS GRAFTING. Patients who undergo CABG also appear to derive particular benefit from early treatment with GP IIb/IIIa inhibition.[241] This benefit of early GP IIb/IIIa inhibition was also seen in the meta-analysis for patients who underwent CABG within 5 days of randomization.[228] As is the case for patients undergoing PCI, the benefit of GP IIb/IIIa inhibition is observed both prior to the CABG and in the early post-CABG phase. The hypothesis is that the early antiplatelet therapy reduces the thrombus and stabilizes the patient preoperatively, thereby reducing perioperative complications.

Thus, it appears that there is benefit of GP IIb/IIIa inhibition during the phase of medical treatment as well as in patients undergoing PCI and CABG. Because patients with UA/NSTEMI are such a high-risk group, the benefit of GP IIb/IIIa inhibition has been quite dramatic, with reductions of death or MI ranging from 30 to 70 percent.[242] Thus, patients who undergo PCI should have been treated with a GP IIb/IIIa inhibitor at the time of presentation or, if not, should receive it during the procedure.

RISK-BASED VERSUS STRATEGY-BASED TARGETING OF THERAPY. The relative merits of targeting GP IIb/IIIa inhibition to the patients' risk versus the treatment strategy have been addressed in several studies. In the PRISM trial, the benefit of GP IIb/IIIa inhibition in patients with positive troponin was seen with or without revascularization,[79] suggesting that risk-based rather than intervention-based targeting of these agents may be optimal. Similar results were seen in PRISM-PLUS, using the risk score; among higher risk patients, the degree of benefit of GP IIb/IIIa inhibition was similar in those who had PCI and those who did not.[123,243] Because it is not clear at the time of presentation whether a patient will be managed with PCI, CABG, or medical therapy alone, the targeting of GP IIb/IIIa inhibition to high-risk patients appears warranted.

New data from two large observational studies provide additional support for early treatment. The National Registry of Myocardial Infarction (NRMI) included 60,770 patients with NSTEMI. Patients who received GP IIb/IIIa inhibition within 24 hours after presentation were compared with those who did not, with 10 percent of the latter group receiving GP IIb/IIIa inhibition for PCI later during the hospital course.[244] Only 25 percent of eligible patients received early GP IIb/IIIa therapy. Patients treated with early GP IIb/IIIa inhibition had 12 percent lower adjusted mortality. In addition, patients treated at hospitals with greater use of early GP IIb/IIIa inhibition also had lower adjusted mortality rates than those treated at hospitals in which GP IIb/IIIa inhibition was used less frequently.[244] A nearly identical finding has been seen in a similar analysis of the CRUSADE (Can Rapid Risk Stratification of Unstable Angina Patients Suppress Adverse Outcomes with Early Implementation of the ACC/AHA Guidelines) registry, with greater benefit in patients with positive troponin at the time of presentation.[245] These data provide support for the early use of GP IIb/IIIa inhibition in high-risk patients with NSTEMI. Currently, randomized trials are underway to study further the question of appropriate timing of GP IIb/IIIa inhibition.

SAFETY. The rate of major hemorrhage was slightly higher for patients treated with GP IIb/IIIa inhibitors than for those receiving aspirin and heparin alone. In a meta-analysis of the large placebo-controlled trials, major bleeding occurred in 2.4 percent of patients treated with GP IIb/IIIa inhibition versus 1.4 percent for placebo, *p* less than 0.0001.[228] Thrombocytopenia is an uncommon but important complication of GP IIb/IIIa inhibitors. For tirofiban in PRISM-PLUS, the rate of severe thrombocytopenia (<50,000 cells/mm^3) was 0.5 versus 0.3 percent for heparin (p = not significant)[22]; in the PURSUIT trial, thrombocytopenia (<20,000 cells/mm^3) occurred in 0.2 percent compared with less than 0.1 percent for heparin.[20] Thrombocytopenia is associated with increased bleeding and, in a smaller proportion of patients, recurrent thrombotic events.[246] This syndrome bears resemblance to heparin-induced thrombocytopenia and indicates a need to monitor platelet count daily during GP IIb/IIIa infusion.

ORAL IIB/IIIA INHIBITION. Because the benefit of intravenous GP IIb/IIIa inhibitors occurs only during the infusion, it was hypothesized that prolonged IIb/IIIa inhibition, using oral agents, might further improve outcomes. Unfortunately, five large trials failed to show any benefit of this approach.[166,247-250] In addition, a 35 percent increase in mortality was seen across all of the trials.

THROMBOLYTIC THERAPY. Because thrombolytic therapy is beneficial in the treatment of patients with acute MI presenting with ST elevation, it was thought that it might also play a role in the other ACSs in which thrombosis is involved. In TIMI IIIB, 1473 patients with UA/NSTEMI were treated with aspirin, UFH, and antiischemic therapy and were randomly assigned to receive either tissue plasminogen activator or its placebo. No differences were observed in the incidence of death, postrandomization MI, or recurrent, objectively documented ischemia through 6 weeks.[251] The proposed mechanism for an adverse effect of thrombolysis in UA/NSTEMI is a prothrombotic effect of thrombolysis.

Invasive Versus Conservative Strategies

Two general approaches to the use of cardiac catheterization and revascularization in UA/NSTEMI exist. The first is an "early invasive" strategy, involving routine early cardiac catheterization and revascularization with PCI or bypass surgery, depending on the coronary anatomy. The other is a more "conservative" approach with initial medical management with catheterization and revascularization only for recurrent ischemia either at rest or in a noninvasive stress test.

CLINICAL TRIALS

To date, nine randomized trials have studied the relative merits of an invasive strategy, involving routine cardiac catheterization with revascularization if feasible, compared with a conservative strategy in which angiography and revascularization are reserved for patients who have evidence of recurrent ischemia either at rest or on provocative testing. The first three trials failed to demonstrate a significant benefit,[251] but the subsequent six have all shown a significant benefit, including the FRagmin and Fast Revascularisation during InStability in Coronary artery disease (FRISC) II and TACTICS-TIMI 18 trials and the Randomized Intervention Trial of unstable Angina (RITA) (Fig. 49–18).[3,252,253]

In FRISC II, 2457 patients with UA/NSTEMI were randomly assigned to an invasive strategy involving coronary angiography carried out on average 4 days after randomization, thus a "delayed" invasive strategy, or a conservative strategy. The latter had strict criteria for catheterization requiring refractory angina despite maximal medical treatment or a positive ECG exercise test with greater than 0.3 mV ST depression. Accordingly, with these strict criteria in the conservative strategy, only 9 percent of patients underwent revascularization during the first 7 days. This trial found that the rate of death or MI at 6 months was significantly lower in the invasive than in the conservative group, 9.4 versus 12.1 percent, $p = 0.031$. At 1 year there was a significant reduction in mortality in the invasive compared with the conservative group (2.2 versus 3.9 percent, respectively, $p = 0.016$).[252]

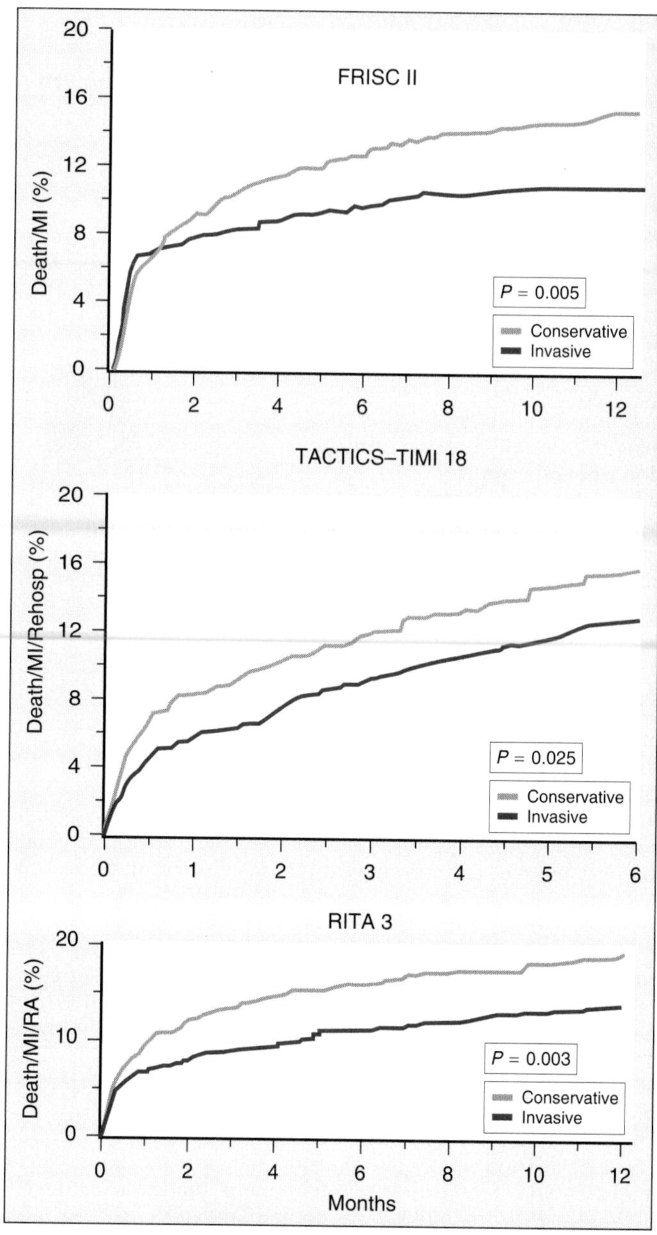

FIGURE 49–18 Kaplan-Meier event curves of three trials comparing invasive versus conservative strategies in ACA. **Top,** Probability of death or myocardial infarction (MI) according to assignment to the invasive or noninvasive strategies in the FRagmin and Fast Revascularisation during InStability in Coronary artery disease (FRISC) II trial. **Middle,** Adverse outcomes (death, MI, or rehospitalization) of both treatment groups in the Treat Angina with aggrastat and determine Cost of Therapy with an Invasive or Conservative Strategy–Thrombolysis in Myocardial Infarction (TACTICS-TIMI) 18 trial. **Bottom,** Death, MI, or refractory angina (RA) in the Randomized Intervention Trial of unstable Angina (RITA) 3 trial. (**Top,** Adapted from Wallentin L, Lagerqvist B, Husted S, et al: Outcome at 1 year after an invasive compared with a non-invasive strategy in unstable coronary artery disease: The FRISC II invasive randomized trial. Lancet 356:9, 2000; **middle,** from Cannon CP, Weintraub WS, Demopoulos LA, et al: Comparison of early invasive and conservative strategies in patients with unstable coronary syndromes treated with the glycoprotein IIb/IIIa inhibitor tirofiban. N Engl J Med 344:1879, 2001; **bottom,** adapted from Fox KAA, Poole-Wilson PA, Henderson RA, et al: Interventional versus conservative treatment for patients with unstable angina or non-ST-elevation myocardial infarction: The British Heart Foundation RITA 3 randomised trial. Lancet 360:743, 2002.)

In TACTICS-TIMI 18, all patients received aspirin, heparin, and the GP IIb/IIIa inhibitor tirofiban at the time of randomization for at least 48 hours, including more than 12 hours following PCI. The rate of death, MI, or rehospitalization for ACS at 6 months was reduced with the early invasive strategy, from 19.4 percent in the conservative group to 15.9 percent in the early invasive group, $p = 0.025$.[3] At 30 days the event rates were 10.5 percent for conservative and 7.4 percent for invasive, $p = 0.009$. Death or nonfatal MI was significantly reduced at 30 days (7.0 to 4.7 percent, respectively, $p = 0.02$) and at 6 months ($p = 0.0498$). In a prospective analysis of costs, the estimated cost per year of life gained for the invasive strategy, based on projected life expectancy, was $12,739, indicating that an early invasive strategy is very cost effective relative to other cardiac medications and interventions.[254]

RISK STRATIFICATION. The benefits of the early invasive strategy have been observed in higher risk patients, especially in those with ST segment changes who had positive troponin on admission.[3,45,252] In TACTICS-TIMI 18, a prespecified hypothesis was that there would be a significantly greater benefit in patients with positive troponin values than in those with negative values.[3] In patients with a troponin T greater than 0.01 ng/ml, there was a relative 39 percent risk reduction in the primary endpoint with the invasive versus the conservative strategy ($p < 0.001$), whereas patients with negative troponin had similar outcomes with either strategy. Death or nonfatal MI was also significantly reduced with the invasive strategy in patients with troponin T greater than 0.01 ng/ml. Similar results were obtained using a troponin T cut point of 0.1 ng/ml and with troponin I.[45]

The same findings of benefit were seen in patients with ST segment changes on admission, with a 10 percent absolute benefit in the primary endpoint in TACTICS-TIMI 18[3] compared with no benefit in those without ST segment changes on admission. Similar findings were observed in FRISC II.[252]

Using the TIMI risk score in TACTICS, there was significant benefit of the early invasive strategy in intermediate-risk (score 3 to 4) and high-risk patients (5 to 7), whereas low-risk (0 to 2) patients had similar outcomes when managed with either strategy (see Fig. 49–9B).[3] The intermediate- and high-risk groups constituted 75 percent of the total population in the trial.

TIMING OF AN INVASIVE STRATEGY. With the benefit of an early invasive strategy now well established, research has turned to the optimal timing. The Intracoronary Stenting with Antithrombotic Regimen Cooling-Off (ISAR-COOL) study found a benefit of an immediate invasive strategy with an average time to catheterization of 2 hours, compared with a delayed invasive strategy (average time to catheterization 4 days).[184] An analysis of the timing of angiography within the early invasive arm of TACTICS-TIMI failed to find any major differences in outcomes among patients who underwent protocol-mandated catheterization within the first 12 hours versus 12 to 24 hours and 24 to 48 hours.[255] Additional trials are ongoing to evaluate the optimal timing of an invasive approach, but on the basis of available data the optimal timing appears to be within the first 48 hours of presentation.

Summary: Indications for Invasive Versus Conservative Management Strategies

On the basis of multiple randomized trials, an early invasive strategy is now strongly recommended for high-risk patients with UA/NSTEMI with ST segment changes or a positive troponin (on admission or that evolves over the next 24 hours), or both. In addition, other high-risk indicators, such as recurrent ischemia and evidence of congestive heart failure, are indications for an early invasive strategy.[4] An early invasive approach appears warranted in those with cardiogenic shock on the basis of studies in acute MI.[256] In addition, an early invasive strategy in those who present with UA/NSTEMI within 6 months of a prior PCI or in patients with prior CABG is indicated.[257]

CURRENT UTILIZATION. The use of cardiac procedures varies by region around the world, although management of patients with UA/NSTEMI is shifting toward a more invasive approach worldwide. In the United States in 2003, in the CRUSADE registry of patients with high-risk UA/NSTEMI, 62 percent underwent cardiac catheterization during hospitalization, 37 percent underwent PCI, and 11 percent underwent coronary bypass surgery.[258] In the 2002 Euro Heart Survey of ACS, involving 10,484 patients admitted to 103 hospitals in 25 countries, the corresponding rates of these procedures were 52.0, 25.4, and 5.4 percent in UA/NSTEMI patients. Cardiac procedures are used more frequently in lower risk patients, not higher risk patients, as recommended in the guidelines.[259]

Noninvasive Testing

In the management of UA/NSTEMI, noninvasive testing is used (1) at presentation, usually in the emergency department to diagnose the presence or absence of CAD (in patients with a low likelihood of coronary disease) (see Chap. 45); (2) to guide further therapy as part of an early conservative strategy; (3) after medical therapy has been carried out, to evaluate the extent of residual ischemia; (4) to evaluate left ventricular function; and (5) to estimate prognosis (i.e., risk stratification).

The results from noninvasive tests that portend high risk of future cardiac events are shown in Table 49–5 (see also Chaps. 10, 16, and 50). These results are derived from studies involving patients with unstable angina, MI, and stable CAD. The marker of high risk is either evidence of ischemia on stress testing or left ventricular dysfunction (either at rest or

TABLE 49–5 Noninvasive Test Results Predicting High Risk for Adverse Outcomes

Exercise Electrocardiographic Testing
Abnormal horizontal or downsloping ST segment depression with
Onset at heart rate <120 beats/min or ≤6.5 METs
Magnitude ≥2.0 mm
Postexercise duration of ≥6 min
Depression in multiple leads
Abnormal systolic blood pressure response
With sustained decrease of >10 mm Hg or flat blood pressure response ≤130 mm Hg, associated with abnormal electrocardiogram
Other
Exercise-induced ST segment elevation
Ventricular tachycardia
Radionuclide Myocardial Perfusion Imaging
Abnormal myocardial tracer distribution in more than one coronary artery region at rest or with stress or an anterior defect that reperfuses
Abnormal myocardial distribution with increased lung uptake
Cardiac enlargement
Left Ventricular Imaging
Stress radionuclide ventriculography
Exercise EF ≤50%
Rest EF ≤35%
Fall in EF ≥10%
Stress echocardiography
Rest EF ≤35%
Wall motion score index >1

EF = ejection fraction; METs = metabolic equivalents.

Adapted from Schlant RC, Blomqvist CG, Brandenburg RO, et al: Guidelines for exercise testing. Circulation 74:653A, 1986; Guidelines for Clinical Use of Cardiac Radionuclide Imaging, December 1986. J Am Coll Cardiol 8:1471, 1986; Cheitlin MD, Alpert JS, Armstrong WF, et al: ACC/AHA Guidelines for the Clinical Application of Echocardiography. Circulation 95:1686, 1997.

stress induced). The use of angiography and revascularization for patients who had a positive stress test (i.e., evidence of ischemia) has long been assumed to be necessary and has been included in the "conservative" arms of most randomized trials.[3,251,260] A benefit of revascularization for provocable ischemia has been documented in patients with a positive ECG stress test following thrombolytic therapy for STEMI.[261]

The safety of early stress testing in patients with UA/NSTEMI has been debated, but evidence from several trials has suggested that pharmacological[262] or symptom-limited stress testing[263] is safe after a period of at least 24 to 48 hours of stabilization in patients with UA/NSTEMI.[264] A contraindication to stress testing is a recent recurrence of rest pain, especially if associated with ECG changes or other signs of instability (hemodynamic or significant arrhythmias).

The merits of various modalities of stress testing have been compared directly in relatively small series of patients (see also Chaps. 10 and 16). For most patients ECG exercise stress testing is recommended if the ECG is without significant ST segment abnormalities. If ST abnormalities exist, perfusion or echo imaging is recommended. Exercise testing is generally recommended unless the patient cannot walk sufficiently to achieve a significant workload, in which case pharmacological stress testing is recommended.

Revascularization

PERCUTANEOUS CORONARY INTERVENTION (see also Chap. 52). PCI is an effective means of reducing coronary obstruction, improving acute ischemia, and improving regional and global left ventricular function in patients with UA/NSTEMI. Current angiographic success rates are high, generally greater than 95 percent, although the presence of UA/NSTEMI or visualized thrombus is associated with an increased risk of acute complications such as abrupt closure or MI (as compared with patients with stable angina or those without visualized thrombus).[56,265] Thus, use of IIb/IIIa inhibitors, clopidogrel, bivalirudin, or other antithrombotic drugs in such patients is associated with improved acute and long-term outcomes following PCI. Use of drug-eluting stents has been shown to reduce the risk of restenosis,[266] further enhancing the overall clinical benefit of an invasive approach.

PERCUTANEOUS CORONARY INTERVENTION VERSUS CORONARY ARTERY BYPASS GRAFTING. When revascularization is required in patients with UA/NSTEMI, the choice is between PCI and CABG. More than eight trials have compared PCI and CABG in patients with ischemic heart disease, many of whom had UA/NSTEMI.[267,268] The results of these trials are reviewed in Chapter 50. On the basis of the results of these trials, CABG is recommended for patients with disease of the left main coronary artery, multivessel disease, and impaired left ventricular function. For other patients, either PCI or CABG may be suitable. PCI is associated with a slightly lower initial morbidity and mortality than CABG but a higher rate of repeated procedures; CABG is associated with more effective relief from angina.

INTRAAORTIC BALLOON COUNTERPULSATION. Intraaortic balloon counterpulsation (IABP) is an effective means of increasing diastolic coronary blood flow and reducing left ventricular afterload, which act in concert to reduce ischemia (see Chap. 25). IABP is usually reserved for patients with UA/NSTEMI who are refractory to maximal medical therapy, those with hemodynamic compromise who are awaiting cardiac catheterization, or those with very high risk coronary anatomy (e.g., left main stenosis) as a bridge to PCI or CABG. Although no randomized trials have documented the benefit of IABP, this method is effective in stabilizing patients with refractory ischemia.

Summary: Acute Management of Unstable Angina or Non-ST Elevation Myocardial Infarction

The evaluation of patients with UA/NSTEMI begins with the clinical history, ECG, and measurement of cardiac biomarkers to assess (1) the likelihood of coronary disease and (2) the patient's risk of death or recurrent cardiac events (Fig. 49–19). Patients with a low likelihood of having UA/NSTEMI should undergo a "diagnostic pathway" evaluation through serial ECGs, cardiac biomarkers, and early stress testing to evaluate for coronary disease (Fig. 49–20). This evaluation can frequently be accomplished in an emergency department observation–chest pain unit. For patients with a clinical history strongly consistent with UA/NSTEMI, those at low risk should be treated with antithrombotic therapy with aspirin, clopidogrel, either heparin or LMWH, beta blockers, and nitrates. An early conservative strategy is adequate in low-risk patients, although an invasive strategy is equally clinically beneficial. For high-risk patients (e.g., those with positive troponin, ST segment changes, TIMI risk score > 3), GP IIb/IIIa inhibition should be added to the preceding medications, and an early invasive strategy is preferred (Fig. 49–21).

Long-Term Secondary Prevention Following Unstable Angina or Non-ST Elevation Myocardial Infarction

The time of hospital discharge following UA/NSTEMI has been noted to be a "teachable moment" for the patient,[269] when the physician and staff can review and optimize the medical regimen for long-term treatment. Risk factor modification is critical and includes discussions with the patient (as appropriate to the patient's risk factors) concerning the importance of smoking cessation, achieving optimal weight, daily exercise, following an appropriate diet, good blood pressure control, tight control of hyperglycemia in diabetics, and lipid management (Table 49–6).

Five classes of drugs that have been shown in large randomized trials to improve outcomes following UA/NSTEMI are now recommended for long-term treatment. Each agent

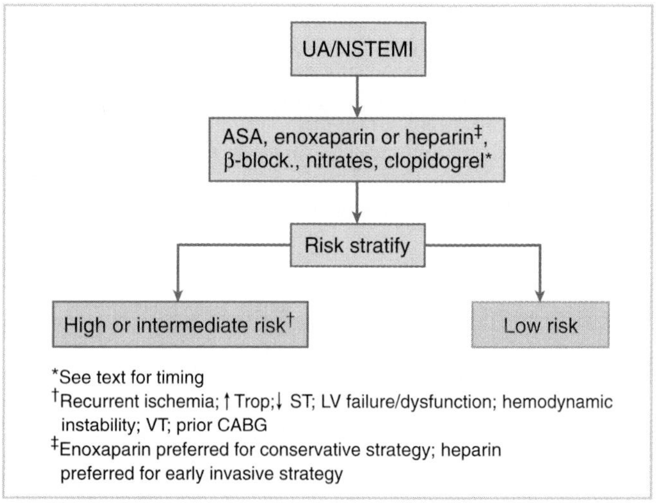

FIGURE 49–19 Algorithm for the management of patients with unstable angina or non-ST elevation myocardial infarction (UA/NSTEMI). Patients in whom the diagnosis is confirmed or suspected are treated with aspirin (ASA), heparin (enoxaparin preferred to unfractionated heparin), beta blockade, nitrates, and clopidogrel. Risk stratification is then performed, and their subsequent management is dictated by their risk category. CABG = coronary artery bypass graft; LV = left ventricular; VT = ventricular tachyarrhythmia. (From Braunwald E: Application of current guidelines to the management of unstable angina and non-ST elevation myocardial infarction. Circulation 108:III-28, 2003.)

nay contribute to long-term clinical stability in different vays. Statins[149,270] and ACE inhibitors[143,144,271] are recomnended for long-term treatment that may facilitate plaque stabilization. Beta blockers are indicated for antiischemic herapy[130,272] and may help decrease "triggers" for MI during follow-up. For antiplatelet therapy, the combination of aspirin and clopidogrel for at least a year has been shown to be beneficial[175,177] and would prevent or decrease the severity of any thrombosis if a plaque rupture does occur. Thus, a multifactorial approach to long-term medical therapy is directed toward preventing the various components of atherothrombosis.

Registry Experience

A major problem identified in clinical practice is that a large proportion of patients do not receive guideline-recommended therapies. Five large registries, in the United States and worldwide, have documented that only 80 to 85 percent of patients received aspirin.[34,66,253,273,274] In addition to guideline development and education, there is a need for specific tools to ensure that the guideline recommendations are implemented on a patient-by-patient basis. Adherence to practice guidelines has been found to be associated with improved outcomes.[269] This was first observed in UA/NSTEMI, by Giugliano and colleagues, who observed in a single-center study that patients who were treated according

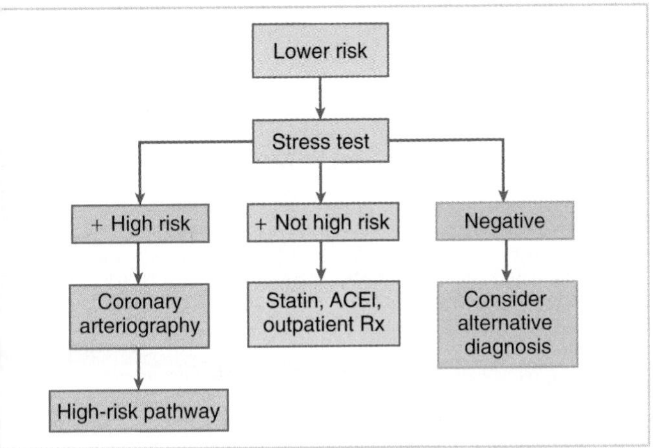

FIGURE 49–20 Management of lower risk patients with unstable angina or non-ST elevation myocardial infarction. ACEI = angiotensin-converting enzyme inhibitor. (From Braunwald E: Application of current guidelines to the management of unstable angina and non-ST elevation myocardial infarction. Circulation 108:III-28, 2003.)

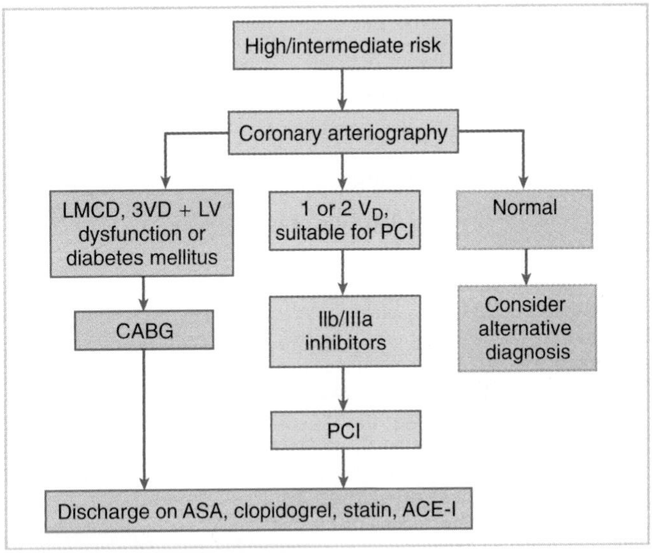

FIGURE 49–21 Management of high- and medium-risk patients with unstable angina or non-ST elevation myocardial infarction. ACE-I = angiotensin-converting enzyme inhibitor; ASA = aspirin; LMCD = left main coronary disease; LV dys = left ventricular dysfunction; VD = vessel disease. (From Braunwald E: Application of current guidelines to the management of unstable angina and non-ST elevation myocardial infarction. Circulation 108:III-28, 2003.)

TABLE 49–6 Cardiac Checklist for Unstable Angina or Non-ST Elevation Myocardial Infarction*

Cardiac Checklist—Admission		Cardiac Checklist—Discharge	
Patient Name:	**Admit Date:**	**Patient Name:**	**Admit Date:**
(First Name) (Middle Initial) (Last Name)		(First Name) (Middle Initial) (Last Name)	
Brief History:		**Brief History:**	
Medications		**Medications**	
1. Aspirin	☐	1. Aspirin	☐
2. Clopidogrel	☐	2. Clopidogrel	☐
3. Heparin (or LMWH)	☐	3. Statin	☐
4. GP IIb/IIIa inhibitor	☐	4. ACE inhibitor	☐
5. Beta blocker	☐	5. Beta blocker	☐
6. Nitrate	☐	**Interventions**	
7. ACE inhibitor	☐	6. LDL controlled to goal	☐
Interventions		7. Blood pressure controlled	☐
8. Cath/revascularization for recurrent ischemia or in intermediate and high-risk patients	☐	8. Diabetes controlled	☐
		9. Smoking cessation counseling (if applicable)	☐
Risk Factor Modification		10. Cardiac rehab/life-style change	☐
9. Cholesterol—check and treat as needed	☐		
10. Treat other risk factors (e.g., smoking)	☐		

*These simple lists serve as reminders of guideline-recommended therapies, such as aspirin, clopidogrel, heparin, or low-molecular-weight heparin. This "cardiac checklist" could be used in two ways: physicians could keep a copy on a small index card in their pocket or in their personal digital assistant (PDA) and run down the list when writing admission orders for patients, or it could be used in developing standard orders for unstable angina or non-ST elevation myocardial infarction—either printed order sheets or computerized orders. See text for details of specific indications and contraindications for medications.
ACE = angiotensin-converting enzyme; GP = glycoprotein; LDL = low-density lipoprotein; LMWH = low-molecular-weight heparin.

to the guidelines had an adjusted 1-year survival that was significantly improved compared with those who had lower compliance with guideline recommendations.[275]

Critical Pathways and Continuous Quality Improvement

Critical pathways and the process of continuous quality improvement (CQI) are means of trying to improve care.[276,277] Critical pathways are standardized protocols for the management of specific diseases (e.g., ACS) that aim to optimize and streamline care of patients.[276,278] In general, these pathways involve having standardized order sets (or computerized ones), simple pocket cards, reminders, or checklists of the appropriate therapies (see Table 49–6). The process of implementation of pathways generally involves physician and nursing education, including presentations at grand rounds, inservices, and other educational meetings throughout the institution involving the relevant caretakers. Another key part of an overall CQI effort is to monitor data on performance, i.e., utilization of guideline-recommended therapies.

Critical Pathways Improve Outcomes

There are now several well-conducted studies showing that use of critical pathways can lead to improved quality of care. The Cardiac Hospitalization Atherosclerosis Management Program (CHAMP) involved staff who assisted the physicians to ensure that all the patients were treated with appropriate guideline-recommended therapies.[269] They were able to improve the use of therapies, such as aspirin, from 78 percent before the program up to 92 percent at the time of hospital discharge. Notably, at 1-year follow-up the CHAMP program had further increased utilization, up to 94 percent of patients, whereas prior to the program compliance had actually fallen to 68 percent.[159] The same was seen for beta blocker, ACE inhibitor, and statin use.

The American College of Cardiology–sponsored Guideline Applied in Practice (GAP) Program provided important multicenter data supporting the efficacy of critical pathways.[279] They found improvement in the use of guideline-recommended therapies and procedures following implementation of their pathways: early use of aspirin and beta blockers and measurement of LDL cholesterol were all improved after implementation of the GAP quality improvement effort.[279] Most interestingly, patients for whom there was evidence in the medical records that the pathways and tools had been used had the highest rates of treatment with the recommended therapies. This finding demonstrated that having tools available for clinicians to use as reminders really can lead to improvements in the use of various therapies.

Thus, critical pathways have now been shown to lead to improvements in the quality of care and to be associated with improved outcomes. Monitoring of performance is key to ensuring that the efforts in education on guideline implementation and changes in the system actually translate into improved care.

Prinzmetal (Variant) Angina

In 1959, Prinzmetal and associates described an unusual syndrome of cardiac pain secondary to myocardial ischemia that occurs almost exclusively at rest, is not usually precipitated by physical exertion or emotional stress, and is associated with ST segment elevations on the ECG (Fig. 49–22).[280] This syndrome, now known as *Prinzmetal,* or *variant, angina* (the terms are interchangeable), may be associated with acute MI and severe cardiac arrhythmias, including ventricular tachycardia and fibrillation, as well as sudden death. A prevailing clinical impression is that Prinzmetal angina has become less frequent in North America for reasons that are unclear, but it appears to remain common in Japan.

Mechanisms

The original hypothesis of Prinzmetal and colleagues, that variant angina is the result of transient increases in coronary vasomotor tone or vasospasm, has been convincingly demonstrated by coronary angiography. Vasospasm causes a transient, abrupt, marked decrease in the diameter of an epicardial (or large septal) coronary artery resulting in severe myocardial ischemia. This event occurs in the absence of any preceding increases in myocardial O_2 demand, as reflected in an increased heart rate or blood pressure. The decrease in luminal diameter can usually be reversed by nitroglycerin, sometimes requiring large doses. Although the sites of vasospasm may correspond to areas of severe focal stenosis, in some patients with apparently normal vessels at angiography the vasospastic segments appear to occur at sites of at least minimal atherosclerotic change, as detected by intravascular ultrasonography.[281] This severe focal vasospasm should not be confused with vasoconstriction of both the large and small coronary vessels, a *normal* response to stimuli such as cold exposure. The latter response is much less intense and occurs diffusely throughout the coronary vascular bed.

Although responses to various vasoconstrictor substances, including catecholamines, thromboxane A_2, serotonin, endothelin, and arginine vasopressin, are greater in spastic segments of the coronary arteries, hypersensitivity to vasoconstrictor stimuli also occurs throughout the entire coronary tree in patients with Prinzmetal angina,[282] perhaps as a manifestation of a more generalized response to vasoactive stimuli. The precise mechanisms have not been established, but a systemic alteration in NO production or an imbalance between endothelium-derived relaxing and contracting factors has been suggested.[282,283] Impaired endothelium-dependent vasodilation in the brachial artery has been demonstrated in Prinzmetal angina,[284] and diurnal fluctuations in flow-mediated endothelium-dependent dilation in this vessel are associated with variations in the frequency of ischemic episodes.[285] Cultured skin fibroblasts obtained from patients with Prinzmetal angina have demonstrated enhanced phospholipase C (PLC) activity. Because PLC (through activating the inositol triphosphate pathway) mobilizes Ca^{2+} from intracellular stores, it may enhance contraction of smooth muscle cells.[286]

The sites of spasm in Prinzmetal angina may be adjacent to atheromatous plaque. It has been suggested that in this subgroup of patients, the basic abnormality may be hypercontractility of the arterial wall associated with the atherosclerotic process itself. Other suggested mechanisms include endothelial injury (which reverses the dilator response to a variety of stimuli, e.g., acetylcholine [see Chap. 44]) and hypercontractility of vascular smooth muscle as a result of vasoconstrictor mitogens, leukotrienes, serotonin, endothelin, angiotensin II, histamine,[287] and higher local concentrations of blood-borne vasoconstrictors in areas adjacent to neovascularized atherosclerotic plaque.

The sequelae of coronary spasm may accelerate atherosclerosis and predispose to further spasm. One mechanism may involve the release of potent vasoconstrictor substances, such as platelet-derived growth factors, in addition to activation of the coagulation system.[288] The combination of a reduction in blood flow and an increase in platelet activation and local thrombosis may accelerate atherosclerosis.[288] Histological findings in patients undergoing coronary atherectomy suggest that repetitive coronary vasospasm may provoke vascular injury and lead to the formation of neointimal hyperplasia at the initial site of spasm. In this respect, coronary spasm may have a key role in the rapid progression of coronary stenosis in some patients.[289]

Imaging with iodine-123-labeled metaiodobenzylguanidine (^{123}I-MIBG) has demonstrated regional myocardial sympathetic denervation in the area of distribution of the vessel in which vasospasm developed.[290]

Coronary spasm in patients with variant angina may induce stasis and result in the conversion of fibrinogen to fibrin in the coronary vessels, with elevated levels of both plasma fibrinogen[291] and fibrinopeptide A, an index of fibrin formation.[292] It has been reported that hypomagnesemia predisposes to variant angina,[293] and magnesium sulfate has been shown to terminate and to suppress attacks.

Clinical and Laboratory Findings

Patients with variant angina tend to be younger than patients with chronic stable angina or unstable angina secondary to coronary atherosclerosis, and many do not exhibit classical coronary risk factors except that they are often heavy cigarette smokers.[294] The anginal discomfort is often extremely severe and may be accompanied by syncope. Features associated with syncope include inferior ST segment elevation and serious arrhythmias, either AV block and asystole or ventricular tachyarrhythmias.[295-297]

Attacks of Prinzmetal angina tend to be clustered between midnight and 8 AM[292] and sometimes occur in clusters of two or three within 30 to 60 minutes. Patients studied by means of ambulatory ECG, even those without clinically apparent angina pectoris, show more frequent abnormalities in the morning. Although exercise capacity is generally well preserved in patients with Prinzmetal angina, some patients experience typical pain and ST segment elevations not only at rest but during or after exertion as well. Exertion of angina usually signifies exertion-induced vasospasm or associated fixed obstruction.

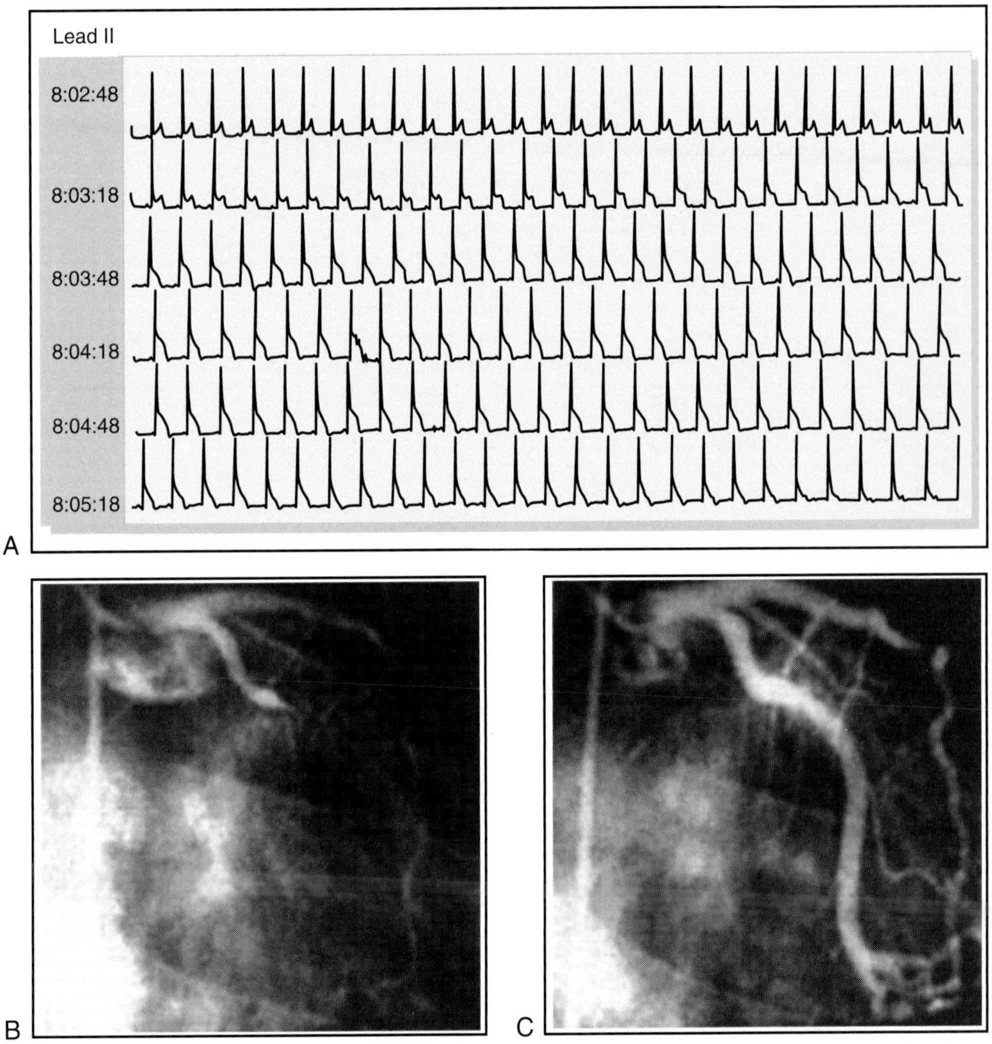

FIGURE 49–22 Findings in a 39-year-old man with Prinzmetal angina. **A,** During an episode of angina, transient ST segment elevation (in lead II) was noted on continuous telemetry. Continuous telemetric recording demonstrating dynamic ST segment elevation. **B,** Hyperventilation-induced total occlusion of the proximal left circumflex artery (visible on angiography from the right anterior oblique caudal view). **C,** Spasm that resolved with the administration of intracoronary nitroglycerine and diltiazem. The patient's symptoms were controlled with oral nitrates and calcium channel blockade during a follow-up of 2 years. (From Chen HSV, Pinto DS: Prinzmetal's angina. N Engl J Med 349:e1, 2003.)

Patients with Prinzmetal angina and severe fixed coronary obstruction may have a combination of fixed-threshold, exertion-induced angina with ST segment depression and episodes of angina at rest with ST segment elevation. Some patients appear to demonstrate a distinct relationship between emotional distress and episodes of coronary vasospasm, which is consistent with studies suggesting that a sympathovagal imbalance may precipitate spasm in patients with variant angina. In rare cases, Prinzmetal angina develops after coronary artery bypass surgery, and occasionally it appears to be a manifestation of a generalized vasospastic disorder associated with migraine and Raynaud phenomenon; it has also been reported in association with aspirin-induced asthma[298] and has been reported to be provoked by 5-fluorouracil and by cyclophosphamide (see Chaps. 62 and 83). Alcohol withdrawal may precipitate variant angina and, conversely, alcohol ingestion may prevent coronary spasm.[299]

ELECTROCARDIOGRAPHY. The key to the diagnosis of variant angina lies in the detection of episodic ST segment elevation with pain (see Fig. 49–22). In one series of patients with variant angina and normal coronary arteries monitored with a computerized 24-hour, 12-lead ECG recording and analysis system, approximately 90 percent of episodes were associated with ST segment elevation, with accompanying arrhythmias in 19 percent, but no arrhythmias were noted in the small proportion of patients with ST segment depression.[295] In some patients, episodes of ST segment depression follow episodes of ST segment elevation and are associated with T wave changes. ST segment and T wave alternans and increased QT dispersion are the result of ischemic conduction delay and may be associated with potentially lethal ventricular arrhythmias. Many patients exhibit multiple episodes of asymptomatic ST segment elevation (silent ischemia). ST segment deviations may be present in any leads.

Transient conduction disturbances may occur during episodes of ischemia.[296] Ventricular ectopic activity is more frequent during longer episodes of ischemia, is often associated with ST segment and T wave alternans, and is of ominous prognostic import. In survivors of out-of-hospital cardiac arrest without flow-limiting coronary stenoses, spontaneous or induced focal coronary spasm has been found to be associated with life-threatening ventricular arrhythmias. In some patients, reperfusion rather than ischemia itself correlates with the onset of the arrhythmias.[300] Myocardial cell damage, as reflected in the release of small quantities of CK-MB, may occur in the absence of persistent ECG changes in patients with prolonged attacks of variant angina; transient Q waves have been observed, which may be explained by a transient loss of normal cell membrane electrical activity during spasm. Q wave MI caused by coronary artery spasm in the absence of angiographically demonstrable obstructive CAD has been well documented.[301]

Exercise testing in patients with variant angina is of limited value because the response is so variable. Approximately equal numbers of patients show ST segment depression, no change in ST segments during exercise, or ST segment elevation, which reflects the presence of underlying fixed CAD in some patients, the absence of significant lesions in others, and the provocation of spasm by exercise in the remainder. Ambulatory ECG monitoring or the use of a telephone transmitter may be helpful in capturing ST segment elevation during symptomatic episodes.[302]

CORONARY ARTERIOGRAPHY. Spasm of a proximal coronary artery with resultant transmural ischemia and abnormalities in left ventricular function are the diagnostic hallmarks of Prinzmetal angina (see Fig. 49–22). Significant fixed proximal coronary obstruction of at least one major artery occurs in the majority of patients, and in them spasm usually occurs within 1 cm of this obstruction. The remainder have normal coronary arteries in the absence of ischemia. Patients with no or mild fixed coronary obstruction tend to experience a more benign course than patients with associated severe obstructive lesions.[303] The vasospastic process almost always involves large segments of the epicardial vessels at a single site, but at different times other sites may be involved. The right coronary artery is the most frequent site, followed by the left anterior descending coronary artery.[302]

PROVOCATIVE TESTS

THE ERGONOVINE TEST. Several provocative tests for coronary spasm have been developed. Of these, the ergonovine test is the most sensitive. Ergonovine maleate, an ergot alkaloid that stimulates both alpha-adrenergic and serotonergic receptors and therefore exerts a direct constrictive effect on vascular smooth muscle,[304] has been used to induce coronary artery spasm, which results in chest pain and ST segment elevation in patients with Prinzmetal angina. Occasionally, ergonovine may produce a similar response in patients with more typical effort-related anginal symptoms.[302] When administered intravenously in doses ranging from 0.05 to 0.40 mg, ergonovine provides a sensitive and specific test for provoking coronary artery spasm. The majority of patients who have a response to ergonovine do so at a dose of less than 0.20 mg.[302]

In low doses and in carefully controlled clinical situations, ergonovine is a relatively safe drug, but prolonged coronary artery spasm precipitated by ergonovine may cause MI. Occasionally, conduction disturbances develop (heart block, asystole, or severe tachyarrhythmias). Because of these hazards, it is recommended that ergonovine be administered only to patients in whom coronary arteriography has demonstrated normal or nearly normal coronary arteries and in gradually increasing doses, beginning with a very low dose. Nitrates and calcium antagonists are usually effective in providing prompt relief from drug-induced spasm, and the intracoronary route for these drugs is usually the most expeditious in patients already undergoing angiography.

The ergonovine test should be conducted only in a setting where appropriate resuscitative equipment, drugs, and personnel are readily available, usually in the cardiac catheterization laboratory, and with a catheter poised to enter the coronary arteries, so that the angiographic diagnosis of spasm can be made and intracoronary nitroglycerin administered to abolish the spasm. Absolute contraindications to ergonovine testing include pregnancy, severe hypertension, severe left ventricular dysfunction, moderate to severe aortic stenosis, and high-grade left main coronary artery stenosis. Relative contraindications include uncontrolled or unstable angina, uncontrolled ventricular arrhythmias, recent MI, and advanced CAD. Although the provocative test with ergonovine is a useful test, the drug is no longer readily available in the United States.

HYPERVENTILATION. This stimulus has also been demonstrated to provoke episodes of intense angina,[305] ST segment elevations on the ECG, angiographic evidence of coronary artery spasm, and ventricular arrhythmias. A large series documented the relative specificity of the hyperventilation test in patients with vasospastic angina.[306] Patients with positive tests had a statistically significantly greater frequency of high disease activity (five or more attacks per week), severe arrhythmias during attacks, and multivessel spasm.

ACETYLCHOLINE. Stimulation of acetylcholine receptors produces a uniform endothelium-dependent dilation of normal coronary vessels of all sizes but leads to vasoconstriction when endothelial function is impaired.[307] In patients with variant angina, intracoronary injections of acetylcholine have been shown to induce severe coronary spasm and reproduce the clinical syndrome.[308] This focal spasm should not be confused with the mild diffuse constriction that acetylcholine induces in patients with abnormal coronary endothelium. Because this method allows induction of spasm separately in the left and right coronary arteries, it is useful in patients with known multivessel disease or spasm. Acetylcholine is infused over a 1-minute period into a coronary artery in incremental doses of 10, 25, 50, and 100 μg, and doses should be separated by 5-minute intervals.

Histamine, dopamine, and serotonin can also induce coronary artery spasm. Like ergonovine and acetylcholine, these agents are capable of causing marked coronary artery spasm in patients with variant angina who have severe underlying arteriosclerotic coronary artery narrowing and in those without such fixed stenoses. Exercise, the cold pressor test, and induced alkalosis can all cause coronary spasm in patients with variant angina, but none of these tests is as sensitive as ergonovine or acetylcholine.

Management

Patients with variant angina should be urged strongly to stop smoking. The mainstay of therapy for vasospastic angina is a calcium antagonist alone or in combination with long-acting nitrates. There are several important differences between the optimal management of Prinzmetal angina and that of classical (stable and unstable) angina.

1. Patients with both variant and classical angina usually respond well to nitrates; sublingual or intravenous nitroglycerin often abolishes attacks of variant angina promptly, and long-acting nitrates are useful in preventing attacks.[309] However, the mechanisms of action of the drugs may differ in the two types of angina. As discussed in Chapter 50, in chronic (effort-induced) stable angina as well as in unstable angina, one important action of nitrates is to reduce myocardial O_2 need and another is to cause coronary vasodilation. In Prinzmetal angina, nitrates abolish or prevent myocardial ischemia *exclusively* by exerting a direct vasodilating effect on the spastic coronary arteries.
2. In patients with classical angina (stable and unstable), beta blockade is usually beneficial, but the response to these agents in patients with Prinzmetal angina is variable.[310] Some, particularly those with associated fixed lesions, exhibit a reduction in the frequency of exertion-induced angina caused primarily by augmentation of myocardial O_2 requirements. In others, however, nonselective beta adrenoreceptor blockers may actually be detrimental because blockade of $beta_2$ receptors, which subserve coronary dilation, allows unopposed alpha receptor–mediated coronary vasoconstriction to occur; in these patients, the duration of episodes of vasotonic angina may be prolonged by propranolol.
3. In contrast to the variable effectiveness of beta blockers, calcium antagonists are extremely effective in preventing the coronary artery spasm of variant angina,[311] and they should ordinarily be prescribed in maximally tolerated doses on a long-term basis. These drugs, along with long- and short-acting nitrates, are the mainstay of therapy. Because calcium antagonists act through a different mechanism than nitrates, the vasodilatory actions of these two classes of drugs may be additive. All first- and second-generation calcium antagonists have similar (approximately 90 percent) efficacy in

producing relief of symptoms,[282,312-314] and they also suppress asymptomatic ischemia. In rare instances, a patient responds to only one of these agents, and even less commonly, the simultaneous administration of two or even three calcium antagonists is required. Some patients need extremely high doses, although side effects are increased. Reports have suggested a rebound of symptoms when calcium antagonist therapy is discontinued.[314] Prolonged, in some instances life-long, treatment may be required.

4. *Prazosin*, a selective alpha adrenoreceptor blocker, has also been found to be of value in patients with Prinzmetal angina.[315] *Nicorandil*,* a vasodilator that influences coronary arterial tone by acting through potassium channel activation, appears to be effective for the treatment of vasospastic angina.[316] *Aspirin*, helpful in unstable angina, may actually *increase* the severity of ischemic episodes in patients with Prinzmetal angina because it inhibits biosynthesis of the naturally occurring coronary vasodilator prostacyclin. *ACE inhibition* has been shown to be ineffective.[317] Other novel but promising approaches to the management of vasospastic angina include troglitazone, an insulin sensitizer,[318] and in a small study of patients in whom vasospastic angina was induced by hyperventilation, the infusion of B-type (brain) natriuretic peptide was highly effective.[319] Estradiol supplementation has been reported to suppress hyperventilation-induced coronary vasospasm in women with variant angina.[320]
5. PCI and occasionally CABG may be helpful in patients with variant angina and discrete, proximal fixed obstructive lesions.[321,322] However, spasm may develop at a site different from the initial stenosis; therefore, calcium antagonists should be continued for at least 6 months following successful revascularization. PCI and coronary artery bypass surgery are *contraindicated* in patients with isolated coronary artery spasm without accompanying fixed obstructive disease.
6. Patients who have experienced ischemia-associated ventricular fibrillation who continue to manifest ischemia despite treatment should receive an implantable cardioverter-defibrillator.[323]

Prognosis

Many patients with Prinzmetal angina pass through an acute, active phase, with frequent episodes of angina and cardiac events during the first 6 months after diagnosis. In a series of 277 patients with a median follow-up of 7.5 years, recurrent angina was common (39 percent), but cardiac death and MI were relatively infrequent and occurred in 3.5 and 6.5 percent of patients, respectively.[324] The extent and severity of the underlying CAD and the activity or the tempo of the syndrome have a major effect on the incidence of late mortality and MI. Patients with variant angina in whom serious arrhythmias (ventricular tachycardia, ventricular fibrillation, high-degree AV block, or asystole) develop during spontaneous episodes of pain have a higher risk of sudden death.[325]

In most patients who survive an infarction or the initial 3- to 6-month period of frequent episodes, the condition stabilizes and symptoms and cardiac events tend to diminish with time. In patients who experience such remissions, cautious tapering of calcium antagonists may be attempted. In one series, 16 percent of patients had spontaneous remission for 3 months after withdrawal of therapy, 44 percent continued to have symptoms despite treatment with calcium antagonists and nitrates, and the other 40 percent were free of angina but receiving treatment. Remission occurred more frequently in patients without significant coronary artery stenoses and in those who stopped smoking.[326]

For reasons that are not clear, some patients, after a relatively quiescent period of months or even years, experience a recrudescence of vasospastic activity with frequent and severe episodes of ischemia. Fortunately, these patients respond to retreatment with calcium antagonists and nitrates.

*Nicorandil is not available in the United States at the time of this writing.

REFERENCES

1. American Heart Association: 2004 Heart and Stroke Statistical Update (www.americanheart.org).
2. The TIMI IIIA Investigators: Early effects of tissue-type plasminogen activator added to conventional therapy on the culprit lesion in patients presenting with ischemic cardiac pain at rest. Results of the Thrombolysis in Myocardial Ischemia (TIMI IIIA) Trial. Circulation 87:38, 1993.
3. Cannon CP, Weintraub WS, Demopoulos LA, et al: Comparison of early invasive and conservative strategies in patients with unstable coronary syndromes treated with the glycoprotein IIb/IIIa inhibitor tirofiban. N Engl J Med 344:1879, 2001.
4. Braunwald E, Antman EM, Beasley JW, et al: ACC/AHA guideline update for the management of patients with unstable angina and non-ST-segment elevation myocardial infarction-2002: Summary article: A report of the American College of Cardiology/American Heart Association Task Force on Practice Guidelines (Committee on the Management of Patients With Unstable Angina). Circulation 106:1893, 2002.
5. Braunwald E: Unstable angina: A classification. Circulation 80:410, 1989.
6. Hamm CW, Braunwald E: A classification of unstable angina—Revisited. Circulation 102:118, 2000.
7. Scirica BM, Cannon CP, McCabe CH, et al, for the Thrombolysis In Myocardial Ischemia III Registry Investigators: Prognosis in the Thrombolysis in Myocardial Ischemia III Registry according to the Braunwald unstable angina pectoris classification. Am J Cardiol 90:821, 2002.
8. Braunwald E: Unstable angina: An etiologic approach to management. Circulation 98:2219, 1998.
9. Morrow DA, Braunwald E: Future of biomarkers in acute coronary syndromes: Moving toward a multimarker strategy. Circulation 108:250, 2003.

Pathophysiology

10. Maseri A: Ischemic Heart Disease: A Rational Basis for Clinical Practice and Clinical Research. New York, Churchill Livingstone, 1995.
11. Davies MJ: The composition of coronary-artery plaques. N Engl J Med 336:1312, 1997.
12. Harrington RA, Califf RM, Holmes DR Jr, et al, for the CAVEAT Investigators: Is all unstable angina the same? Insights from the Coronary Angioplasty Versus Excisional Atherectomy Trial (CAVEAT-I). Am Heart J 137:227, 1999.
13. Nesto RW, Waxman S, Mittleman MA, et al: Angioscopy of culprit coronary lesions in unstable angina pectoris and correlation of clinical presentation with plaque morphology. Am J Cardiol 81:225, 1998.
14. Kennon S, Price CP, Mills PG, et al: The central role of platelet activation in determining the severity of acute coronary syndromes. Heart 89:1253, 2003.
15. Serebruany VL, Glassman AH, Malinin AI, et al: Enhanced platelet/endothelial activation in depressed patients with acute coronary syndromes: Evidence from recent clinical trials. Blood Coagul Fibrinolysis 14:563, 2003.
16. Theroux P, Ouimet H, McCans J, et al: Aspirin, heparin or both to treat unstable angina. N Engl J Med 319:1105, 1988.
17. Oler A, Whooley MA, Oler J, Grady D: Adding heparin to aspirin reduces the incidence of myocardial infarction and death in patients with unstable angina. A meta-analysis. JAMA 276:811, 1996.
18. Cohen M, Demers C, Gurfinkel EP, et al, for the Efficacy and Safety of Subcutaneous Enoxaparin in Non-Q-Wave Coronary Events Study Group: A comparison of low-molecular-weight heparin with unfractionated heparin for unstable coronary artery disease. N Engl J Med 337:447, 1997.
19. Antman EM, McCabe CH, Gurfinkel EP, et al: Enoxaparin prevents death and cardiac ischemic events in unstable angina/non-Q-wave myocardial infarction: Results of the Thrombolysis In Myocardial Infarction (TIMI) 11B trial. Circulation 100:1593, 1999.
20. The PURSUIT Trial Investigators: Inhibition of platelet glycoprotein IIb/IIIa with eptifibatide in patients with acute coronary syndromes. N Engl J Med 339:436, 1998.
21. The Platelet Receptor Inhibition for Ischemic Syndrome Management (PRISM) Study Investigators: A comparison of aspirin plus tirofiban with aspirin plus heparin for unstable angina. N Engl J Med 338:1498, 1998.
22. The Platelet Receptor Inhibition for Ischemic Syndrome Management in Patients Limited by Unstable Signs and Symptoms (PRISM-PLUS) Trial Investigators: Inhibition of the platelet glycoprotein IIb/IIIa receptor with tirofiban in unstable angina and non-Q-wave myocardial infarction. N Engl J Med 338:1488, 1998.
23. Clopidogrel in Unstable Angina to Prevent Recurrent Events Trial Investigators: Effects of clopidogrel in addition to aspirin in patients with acute coronary syndromes without ST-segment elevation. N Engl J Med 345:494, 2001.
24. Storey RF, Newby LJ, Heptinstall S: Effects of P2Y(1) and P2Y(12) receptor antagonists on platelet aggregation induced by different agonists in human whole blood. Platelets 12:443, 2001.
25. Badimon JJ, Lettino M, Toschi V, et al: Local inhibition of tissue factor reduces the thrombogenicity of disrupted human atherosclerotic plaques: Effects of tissue factor

pathway inhibitor on plaque thrombogenicity under flow conditions. Circulation 99:1780, 1999.
26. Prinzmetal M, Kennamer R, Merliss R, et al: A variant form of angina pectoris. Am J Med 27:375, 1959.
27. Bottcher M, Botker HE, Sonne H, et al: Endothelium-dependent and -independent perfusion reserve and the effect of L-arginine on myocardial perfusion in patients with syndrome X. Circulation 99:1795, 1999.
28. Marzilli M, Sambuceti G, Fedele S, L'Abbate A: Coronary microcirculatory vasoconstriction during ischemia in patients with unstable angina. J Am Coll Cardiol 35:327, 2000.
29. Pitts WR, Lange RA, Cigarroa JE, Hillis LD: Cocaine-induced myocardial ischemia and infarction: Pathophysiology, recognition, and management. Prog Cardiovasc Dis 40:65, 1997.
30. Strike PC, Steptoe A: Systematic review of mental stress–induced myocardial ischaemia. Eur Heart J 24:690, 2003.
31. Kaski JC: Rapid coronary artery disease progression and angiographic stenosis morphology. Ital Heart J 1:21, 2000.

Clinical Presentation

32. Hochman JS, McCabe CH, Stone PH, et al, for the TIMI Investigators: Outcome and profile of women and men presenting with acute coronary syndromes: A report from TIMI IIIB. J Am Coll Cardiol 30:141, 1997.
33. Hochman JS, Tamis JE, Thompson TD, et al: Sex, clinical presentation, and outcome in patients with acute coronary syndromes. Global Use of Strategies to Open Occluded Coronary Arteries in Acute Coronary Syndromes IIb Investigators. N Engl J Med 341:226, 1999.
34. Scirica BM, Moliterno DJ, Every NR, et al, and the GUARANTEE Investigators: Differences between men and women in the management of unstable angina pectoris (the GUARANTEE Registry). Am J Cardiol 84:1145, 1999.
35. The Global Use of Strategies to Open Occluded Coronary Arteries (GUSTO) IIb Investigators: A comparison of recombinant hirudin with heparin for the treatment of acute coronary syndromes. N Engl J Med 335:775, 1996.
36. Khot UN, Khot MB, Bajzer CT, et al: Prevalence of conventional risk factors in patients with coronary heart disease. JAMA 290:898, 2003.
37. Cannon CP, McCabe CH, Stone PH, et al, for the TIMI III Registry ECG Ancillary Study Investigators: The electrocardiogram predicts one-year outcome of patients with unstable angina and non-Q wave myocardial infarction: Results of the TIMI III Registry ECG Ancillary Study. J Am Coll Cardiol 30:133, 1997.
38. Savonitto S, Ardissino D, Granger CB, et al: Prognostic value of the admission electrocardiogram in acute coronary syndromes. JAMA 281:707, 1999.
39. Akkerhuis KM, Klootwijk PA, Lindeboom W, et al: Recurrent ischaemia during continuous multilead ST-segment monitoring identifies patients with acute coronary syndromes at high risk of adverse cardiac events; meta-analysis of three studies involving 995 patients. Eur Heart J 22:1997, 2001.
40. Goodman SG, Fitchett D, Armstrong PW, et al: Randomized evaluation of the safety and efficacy of enoxaparin versus unfractionated heparin in high-risk patients with non-ST-segment elevation acute coronary syndromes receiving the glycoprotein IIb/IIIa inhibitor eptifibatide. Circulation 107:238, 2003.
41. Jernberg T, Lindahl B, Wallentin L: ST-segment monitoring with continuous 12-lead ECG improves early risk stratification in patients with chest pain and ECG nondiagnostic of acute myocardial infarction. J Am Coll Cardiol 34:1413, 1999.
42. The Joint European Society of Cardiology/American College of Cardiology committee: Myocardial infarction redefined—A consensus document of The Joint European Society of Cardiology/American College of Cardiology committee for the redefinition of myocardial infarction. J Am Coll Cardiol 36:959, 2000.
43. Meier MA, Al-Badr WH, Cooper JV, et al: The new definition of myocardial infarction: Diagnostic and prognostic implications in patients with acute coronary syndromes. Arch Intern Med 162:1585, 2002.
44. Panteghini M, Apple FS, Christenson RH, et al: Use of biochemical markers in acute coronary syndromes. IFCC Scientific Division, Committee on Standardization of Markers of Cardiac Damage. International Federation of Clinical Chemistry. Clin Chem Lab Med 37:687, 1999.
45. Morrow DA, Cannon CP, Rifai N, et al, for the TACTICS-TIMI 18 Investigators: Ability of minor elevations of troponin I and T to predict benefit from an early invasive strategy in patients with unstable angina and non-ST elevation myocardial infarction: Results from a randomized trial. JAMA 286:2405, 2001.
46. Diderholm E, Andren B, Frostfeldt G, et al: The prognostic and therapeutic implications of increased troponin T levels and ST depression in unstable coronary artery disease: The FRISC II invasive troponin T electrocardiogram substudy. Am Heart J 143:760, 2002.
47. The Joint European Society of Cardiology/American College of Cardiology committee: Myocardial infarction redefined—A consensus document of The Joint European Society of Cardiology/American College of Cardiology committee for the redefinition of myocardial infarction. Eur Heart J 21:1502, 2000.
48. Morrow DA, Rifai N, Sabatine MS, et al: Evaluation of the AccuTnI assay for cardiac troponin I for risk assessment in acute coronary syndromes. Clin Chem 49:1396, 2003.
49. Wright SA, Sawyer DB, Sacks DB, et al: Elevation of troponin I levels in patients without evidence of myocardial injury. JAMA 278:2144, 1997.
50. Horwich TB, Patel J, MacLellan WR, Fonarow GC: Cardiac troponin I is associated with impaired hemodynamics, progressive left ventricular dysfunction, and increased mortality rates in advanced heart failure. Circulation 108:833, 2003.
51. Dokainish H, Pillai M, Murphy S, et al, for the TACTICS -TIMI 18 Investigators: Prognostic implications of elevated troponin in patients with suspected acute coronary syndromes but no epicardial coronary disease. J Am Coll Cardiol (in press).
52. Cannon CP, Johnson EB, Cermignani M, et al: Emergency department thrombolysis critical pathway reduces door-to-drug times in acute myocardial infarction. Clin Cardiol 22:17, 1999.
53. Scirica BM, Moliterno DJ, Every NR, et al, and the GUARANTEE Investigators: Racia differences in the management of unstable angina: Results from the GUARANTE Registry. Am Heart J 138:1065, 1999.
54. Diver DJ, Bier JD, Ferreira PE, et al, for the TIMI-IIIA Investigators. Clinical and arte riographic characterization of patients with unstable angina without critical coronar arterial narrowing (from the TIMI-IIIA trial). Am J Cardiol 74:531, 1994.
55. Roe MT, Harrington RA, Prosper DM, et al: Clinical and therapeutic profile of patient presenting with acute coronary syndromes who do not have significant coronary arter disease. The Platelet Glycoprotein IIb/IIIa in Unstable Angina: Receptor Suppressio Using Integrilin Therapy (PURSUIT) Trial Investigators. Circulation 102:1101, 2000.
56. Zhao X-Q, Theroux P, Snapinn SM, Sax FL, for the PRISM-PLUS Investigators: Intra coronary thrombus and platelet glycoprotein IIb/IIIa receptor blockade with tirofiba in unstable angina or non-Q-wave myocardial infarction. Angiographic results fror the PRISM-PLUS trial (Platelet Receptor Inhibition for Ischemic Syndrome Manage ment in Patients Limited by Unstable Signs and Symptoms). Circulation 100:160 1999.
57. Wong GC, Morrow DA, Murphy S, et al, for the TACTICS-TIMI 18 Study Group: Ele vations in troponin T and I are associated with abnormal tissue level perfusion: TACTICS-TIMI 18 substudy. Circulation 106:202, 2002.
58. De Servi S, Arbustini E, Marsico F, et al: Correlation between clinical and morphologi findings in unstable angina. Am J Cardiol 77:128, 1996.
59. Jaber WA, Prior DL, Marso SP, et al: CHF on presentation is associated with markedl worse outcomes among patients with acute coronary syndromes: PURSUIT trial find ings. Circulation 100(Suppl I):I-433, 1999.

Risk Stratification

60. Kerensky RA, Wade M, Deedwania P, et al: Revisiting the culprit lesion in non-Q-wav myocardial infarction. Results from the VANQWISH trial angiographic core laborator J Am Coll Cardiol 39:1456, 2002.
61. Goldstein JA, Demetriou D, Grines CL, et al: Multiple complex coronary plaques i patients with acute myocardial infarction. N Engl J Med 343:915, 2000.
62. Rioufol G, Finet G, Ginon I, et al: Multiple atherosclerotic plaque rupture in acute coro nary syndrome: A three-vessel intravascular ultrasound study. Circulation 106:80 2002.
63. Zairis MN, Papadaki OA, Manousakis SJ, et al: C-reactive protein and multipl complex coronary artery plaques in patients with primary unstable angina. Athero sclerosis 164:355, 2002.
64. Asakura M, Ueda Y, Yamaguchi O, et al: Extensive development of vulnerable plaque as a pan-coronary process in patients with myocardial infarction: An angioscopi study. J Am Coll Cardiol 37:1284, 2001.
65. Lindahl B, Diderholm E, Lagerqvist B, et al: Mechanisms behind the prognostic valu of troponin T in unstable coronary artery disease: A FRISC II substudy. J Am Co Cardiol 38:979, 2001.
66. Stone PH, Thompson B, Anderson HV, et al, for the TIMI III Registry Study Group Influence of race, sex, and age on management of unstable angina and non-Q-wav myocardial infarction: The TIMI III Registry. JAMA 275:1104, 1996.
67. Antman EM, Cohen M, Bernink PJ, et al: The TIMI risk score for unstable angina/non ST elevation MI: A method for prognostication and therapeutic decision making. JAM 284:835, 2000.
68. Boersma E, Pieper KS, Steyerberg EW, et al, for the PURSUIT Investigators: Predictor of outcome in patients with acute coronary syndromes without persistent ST-segmer elevation. Results from an international trial of 9461 patients. Circulation 101:2557 2000.
69. Roffi M, Chew DP, Mukherjee D, et al: Platelet glycoprotein IIb/IIIa inhibitors reduc mortality in diabetic patients with non-ST-segment-elevation acute coronary syn dromes. Circulation 104:2767, 2001.
70. Cotter G, Cannon CP, McCabe CH, et al: Prior peripheral arterial disease and cere brovascular disease are independent predictors of adverse outcome in patients wit acute coronary syndromes: Are we doing enough? Results from the Orbofiban i Patients with Unstable Coronary Syndromes-Thrombolysis In Myocardial Infarctio (OPUS-TIMI) 16 study. Am Heart J 145:622, 2003.
71. Khot UN, Jia G, Moliterno DJ, et al: Prognostic importance of physical examination fo heart failure in non-ST-elevation acute coronary syndromes: The enduring value c Killip classification. JAMA 290:2174, 2003.
72. Klootwijk P, Meij S, Melkert R, et al: Reduction of recurrent ischemia with abciximal during continuous ECG-ischemia monitoring in patients with unstable angina refrac tory to standard treatment (CAPTURE). Circulation 98:1358, 1998.
73. Hyde TA, French JK, Wong CK, et al: Four-year survival of patients with acute coro nary syndromes without ST-segment elevation and prognostic significance of 0.5-mn ST-segment depression. Am J Cardiol 84:379, 1999.
74. Holmvang L, Clemmensen P, Lindahl B, et al: Quantitative analysis of the admissior electrocardiogram identifies patients with unstable coronary artery disease who benefi the most from early invasive treatment. J Am Coll Cardiol 41:905, 2003.
75. Antman EM, Tanasijevic MJ, Thompson B, et al: Cardiac-specific troponin I levels t predict the risk of mortality in patients with acute coronary syndromes. N Engl J Me 335:1342, 1996.
76. Kleiman N, Lakkis N, Cannon C, et al: Prospective analysis of creatine kinase muscle brain fraction and comparison with troponin T to predict cardiac risk and benefit o an invasive strategy in patients with non-ST-elevation acute coronary syndromes. J An Coll Cardiol 40:1044, 2002.
77. Newby LK, Christenson RH, Ohman EM, et al: Value of serial troponin T measures fo early and late risk stratification in patients with acute coronary syndromes. Th GUSTO-IIa Investigators. Circulation 98:1853, 1998.
78. Hamm CW, Heeschen C, Goldmann B, et al, for the c7E3 Fab Antiplatelet Therapy ir Unstable Refractory Angina (CAPTURE) Study Investigators: Benefit of abciximab ir patients with refractory unstable angina in relation to serum troponin T levels. N Eng J Med 340:1623, 1999.

79. Heeschen C, Hamm CW, Goldmann B, et al, for the PRISM Study Investigators: Troponin concentrations for stratification of patients with acute coronary syndromes in relation to therapeutic efficacy of tirofiban. Lancet 354:1757, 1999.
80. James SK, Armstrong P, Barnathan E, et al: Troponin and C-reactive protein have different relations to subsequent mortality and myocardial infarction after acute coronary syndrome: A GUSTO-IV substudy. J Am Coll Cardiol 41:916, 2003.
81. Antman EM, Sacks DB, Rifai N, et al: Time to positivity of a rapid bedside assay for cardiac-specific troponin T predicts prognosis in acute coronary syndromes: A Thrombolysis in Myocardial Infarction (TIMI) 11A substudy. J Am Coll Cardiol 31:326, 1998.
82. Morrow DA, Rifai N, Antman EM, et al: C-reactive protein is a potent predictor of mortality independently and in combination with troponin T in acute coronary syndromes: A TIMI 11A substudy. J Am Coll Cardiol 31:1460, 1998.
83. Rebuzzi AG, Quaranta G, Liuzzo G, et al: Incremental prognostic value of serum levels of troponin T and C-reactive protein on admission in patients with unstable angina pectoris. Am J Cardiol 82:715, 1998.
84. de Winter RJ, Bholasingh R, Lijmer JG, et al: Independent prognostic value of C-reactive protein and troponin I in patients with unstable angina or non-Q-wave myocardial infarction. Cardiovasc Res 42:240, 1999.
85. Ridker PM, Rifai N, Rose L, et al: Comparison of C-reactive protein and low-density lipoprotein cholesterol levels in the prediction of first cardiovascular events. N Engl J Med 347:1557, 2002.
86. Lindahl B, Toss H, Siegbahn A, et al, for the FRISC Study Group: Fragmin during Instability in Coronary Artery Disease. Markers of myocardial damage and inflammation in relation to long-term mortality in unstable coronary artery disease. N Engl J Med 343:1139, 2000.
87. Cannon CP, McCabe CH, Wilcox RG, et al: High-sensitivity C-reactive protein is a potent predictor of long-term mortality in 3225 patients with acute coronary syndromes: Results from OPUS-TIMI 16. Circulation 102(Suppl II):II-499, 2000.
88. Lenderink T, Boersma E, Heeschen C, et al: Elevated troponin T and C-reactive protein predict impaired outcome for 4 years in patients with refractory unstable angina, and troponin T predicts benefit of treatment with abciximab in combination with PTCA. Eur Heart J 24:77, 2003.
89. Sabatine MS, Morrow DA, de Lemos JA, et al: Multimarker approach to risk stratification in non-ST elevation acute coronary syndromes: Simultaneous assessment of troponin I, C-reactive protein, and B-type natriuretic peptide. Circulation 105:1760, 2002.
90. Heeschen C, Hamm CW, Bruemmer J, Simoons ML, for the Chimeric c7E3 AntiPlatelet Therapy in Unstable angina REfractory to standard treatment trial (CAPTURE) Investigators: Predictive value of C-reactive protein and troponin T in patients with unstable angina: A comparative analysis. J Am Coll Cardiol 35:1535, 2000.
91. Biasucci LM, Liuzzo G, Grillo RL, et al: Elevated levels of C-reactive protein at discharge in patients with unstable angina predict recurrent instability. Circulation 99:855, 1999.
92. Morrow DA, Rifai N, Antman EM, et al: Serum amyloid A predicts early mortality in acute coronary syndromes: A TIMI 11A substudy. J Am Coll Cardiol 35:358, 2000.
93. de Lemos JA, Morrow DA, Sabatine MS, et al: Association between plasma levels of monocyte chemoattractant protein-1 and long-term clinical outcomes in patients with acute coronary syndromes. Circulation 107:690, 2003.
94. Lindmark E, Diderholm E, Wallentin L, Siegbahn A: Relationship between interleukin 6 and mortality in patients with unstable coronary artery disease: Effects of an early invasive or noninvasive strategy. JAMA 286:2107, 2001.
95. Barron HV, Cannon CP, Murphy SA, et al: Association between white blood cell count, epicardial blood flow, myocardial perfusion, and clinical outcomes in the setting of acute myocardial infarction: A Thrombolysis In Myocardial Infarction 10 substudy. Circulation 102:2329, 2000.
96. Cannon CP, McCabe CH, Wilcox RG, et al, for the OPUS-TIMI 16 Investigators: Association of white blood cell count with increased mortality in acute myocardial infarction and unstable angina pectoris. Am J Cardiol 87:636, 2001.
97. Sabatine MS, Morrow DA, Cannon CP, et al: Relationship between baseline white blood cell count and degree of coronary artery disease and mortality in patients with acute coronary syndromes: A TACTICS-TIMI 18 (Treat Angina with Aggrastat and determine Cost of Therapy with an Invasive or Conservative Strategy –Thrombolysis in Myocardial Infarction 18 trial) substudy. J Am Coll Cardiol 40:1761, 2002.
98. Mueller C, Neumann FJ, Roskamm H, et al: Women do have an improved long-term outcome after non-ST-elevation acute coronary syndromes treated very early and predominantly with percutaneous coronary intervention: A prospective study in 1,450 consecutive patients. J Am Coll Cardiol 40:245, 2002.
99. Andre P, Prasad KS, Denis CV, et al: CD40L stabilizes arterial thrombi by a beta3 integrin–dependent mechanism. Nat Med 8:247, 2002.
100. Schonbeck U, Sukhova GK, Shimizu K, et al: Inhibition of CD40 signaling limits evolution of established atherosclerosis in mice. Proc Natl Acad Sci USA 97:7458, 2000.
101. Heeschen C, Dimmeler S, Hamm CW, et al: Soluble CD40 ligand in acute coronary syndromes. N Engl J Med 348:1104, 2003.
102. Varo N, de Lemos JA, Libby P, et al: Soluble CD40L: Risk prediction after acute coronary syndromes. Circulation 108:1049, 2003.
103. Schonbeck U, Varo N, Libby P, et al: Soluble CD40L and cardiovascular risk in women. Circulation 104:2266, 2001.
104. Wiese S, Breyer T, Dragu A, et al: Gene expression of brain natriuretic peptide in isolated atrial and ventricular human myocardium: Influence of angiotensin II and diastolic fiber length. Circulation 102:3074, 2000.
105. Dao Q, Krishnaswamy P, Kazanegra R, et al: Utility of B-type natriuretic peptide in the diagnosis of congestive heart failure in an urgent-care setting. J Am Coll Cardiol 37:379, 2001.
106. Richards AM, Nicholls MG, Yandle TG, et al: Plasma N-terminal pro-brain natriuretic peptide and adrenomedullin: New neurohormonal predictors of left ventricular function and prognosis after myocardial infarction. Circulation 97:1921, 1998.
107. de Lemos JA, Morrow DA, Bentley JH, et al: The prognostic value of B-type natriuretic peptide in patients with acute coronary syndromes. N Engl J Med 345:1014, 2001.
108. Morrow DA, de Lemos JA, Sabatine MS, et al: Evaluation of B-type natriuretic peptide for risk assessment in unstable angina/non-ST-elevation myocardial infarction: B-type natriuretic peptide and prognosis in TACTICS-TIMI 18. J Am Coll Cardiol 41:1264, 2003.
109. Omland T, de Lemos JA, Morrow DA, et al: Prognostic value of N-terminal pro-atrial and pro-brain natriuretic peptide in patients with acute coronary syndromes. Am J Cardiol 89:463, 2002.
110. Zhang R, Brennan ML, Fu X, et al: Association between myeloperoxidase levels and risk of coronary artery disease. JAMA 286:2136, 2001.
111. Baldus S, Heeschen C, Meinertz T, et al: Myeloperoxidase serum levels predict risk in patients with acute coronary syndromes. Circulation 108:1440, 2003.
112. Buffon A, Biasucci LM, Liuzzo G, et al: Widespread coronary inflammation in unstable angina. N Engl J Med 347:5, 2002.
113. Januzzi JL, Cannon CP, DiBattiste PM, et al: Effects of renal insufficiency on early invasive management in patients with acute coronary syndromes (the TACTICS-TIMI 18 trial). Am J Cardiol 90:1246, 2002.
114. Januzzi JL Jr, Snapinn SM, DiBattiste PM, et al: Benefits and safety of tirofiban among acute coronary syndrome patients with mild to moderate renal insufficiency: Results from the Platelet Receptor Inhibition in Ischemic Syndrome Management in Patients Limited by Unstable Signs and Symptoms (PRISM-PLUS) trial. Circulation 105:2361, 2002.
115. Aviles RJ, Askari AT, Lindahl B, et al: Troponin T levels in patients with acute coronary syndromes, with or without renal dysfunction. N Engl J Med 346:2047, 2002.
116. Gibson CM, Pinto DS, Murphy SA, et al: Association of creatinine and creatinine clearance on presentation in acute myocardial infarction with subsequent mortality. J Am Coll Cardiol 42:1535, 2003.
117. Becker RC, Spencer FA, Gibson M, et al: Influence of patient characteristics and renal function on factor Xa inhibition pharmacokinetics and pharmacodynamics after enoxaparin administration in non-ST-segment elevation acute coronary syndromes. Am Heart J 143:753, 2002.
118. Malmberg K, Norhammar A, Wedel H, Ryden L: Glycometabolic state at admission: Important risk marker of mortality in conventionally treated patients with diabetes mellitus and acute myocardial infarction: Long-term results from the Diabetes and Insulin-Glucose Infusion in Acute Myocardial Infarction (DIGAMI) study. Circulation 99:2626, 1999.
119. Bhadriraju S, Cannon CP, DeFranco AC, et al: Association between blood glucose and long term mortality in patients with acute coronary syndromes in the OPUS-TIMI 16 trial. Circulation 108(Suppl 1):1475, 2003.
120. Foo K, Cooper J, Deaner A, et al: A single serum glucose measurement predicts adverse outcomes across the whole range of acute coronary syndromes. Heart 89:512, 2003.
121. Tenerz A, Nilsson G, Forberg R, et al: Basal glucometabolic status has an impact on long-term prognosis following an acute myocardial infarction in non-diabetic patients. J Intern Med 254:494, 2003.
122. Malmberg K, Ryden L, Hamsten A, et al, for the Diabetes Insulin-Glucose in Acute Myocardial Infarction (DIGAMI) Study Group. Effects of insulin treatment on cause-specific one-year mortality and morbidity in diabetic patients with acute myocardial infarction. Eur Heart J 17:1337, 1996.
123. Morrow DA, Antman EM, Snapinn SM, et al: An integrated clinical approach to predicting the benefit of tirofiban in non-ST elevation acute coronary syndromes: Application of the TIMI risk score for UA/NSTEMI in PRISM-PLUS. Eur Heart J 23:223, 2002.

Medical Therapy

124. Cheitlin MD, Hutter AM Jr, Brindis RG, et al: ACC/AHA expert consensus document. Use of sildenafil (Viagra) in patients with cardiovascular disease. American College of Cardiology/American Heart Association. J Am Coll Cardiol 33:273, 1999.
125. Gruppo Italiano per lo Studio della Sopravvivenza nell'Infarto Miocardico: GISSI-3: Effect of lisinopril and transdermal glyceryl trinitrate singly and together on 6-week mortality and ventricular function after acute myocardial infarction. Lancet 343:1115, 1994.
126. ISIS-4 Collaborative Group: ISIS-4: Randomized factorial trial assessing early oral captopril, oral mononitrate, and intravenous magnesium sulphate in 58,050 patients with suspected acute myocardial infarction. Lancet 345:669, 1995.
127. Gottlieb SO, Weisfeldt ML, Ouyang P, et al: Effect of the addition of propranolol to therapy with nifedipine for unstable angina: A randomized, double-blind, placebo-controlled trial. Circulation 73:331, 1986.
128. The Holland Interuniversity Nifedipine/Metoprolol Trial (HINT) Research Group: Early treatment of unstable angina in the coronary care unit: A randomised, double blind, placebo controlled comparison of recurrent ischaemia in patients treated with nifedipine or metoprolol or both. Br Heart J 56:400, 1986.
129. Theroux P, Taeymans Y, Morissette D, et al: A randomized study comparing propranolol and diltiazem in the treatment of unstable angina. J Am Coll Cardiol 5:717, 1985.
130. Yusuf S, Peto R, Lewis J, et al: Beta-blockade during and after myocardial infarction: An overview of the randomized trials. Prog Cardiovasc Dis 27:335, 1985.
131. Foody JM, Farrell MH, Krumholz HM: Beta-blocker therapy in heart failure: Scientific review. JAMA 287:883, 2002.
132. TIMI Study Group: Comparison of invasive and conservative strategies after treatment with intravenous tissue plasminogen activator in acute myocardial infarction. Results of the Thrombolysis in Myocardial Infarction (TIMI) Phase II Trial. N Engl J Med 320:618, 1989.
133. Gibson RS, Boden WE, Theroux P, et al, and the Diltiazem Re-Infarction Study (DRS) Group: Diltiazem and reinfarction in patients with non-Q wave myocardial infarction. Results of a double-blind, randomized, multicenter trial. N Engl J Med 315:423, 1986.
134. Boden WE, van Gilst WH, Scheldewaert RG, et al: Diltiazem in acute myocardial infarction treated with thrombolytic agents: A randomised placebo-controlled trial. Incomplete Infarction Trial of European Research Collaborators Evaluating Prognosis post-Thrombolysis (INTERCEPT). Lancet 355:1751, 2000.

135. The Danish Study Group on Verapamil in Myocardial Infarction: Effect of verapamil on mortality and major events after acute infarction (the Danish Verapamil Infarction Trial II—DAVIT II). Am J Cardiol 66:779, 1990.
136. Hennekens CH, Albert CM, Godfried SL, et al: Adjunctive drug therapy of acute myocardial infarction—Evidence from clinical trials. N Engl J Med 335:1660, 1996.
137. Pepine CJ, Faich G, Makuch R: Verapamil use in patients with cardiovascular disease: An overview of randomized trials. Clin Cardiol 21:633, 1998.
138. The Multicenter Diltiazem Postinfarction Trial Research Group: The effect of diltiazem on mortality and reinfarction after myocardial infarction. N Engl J Med 319:385, 1988.
139. Hansen JF, Hagerup L, Sigurd B, et al, for the Danish Verapamil Infarction Trial (DAVIT) Study Group. Cardiac event rates after acute myocardial infarction in patients treated with verapamil and trandolapril versus trandolapril alone. Am J Cardiol 79:738, 1997.
140. Cohn JN, Ziesche S, Smith R, et al: Effect of the calcium antagonist felodipine as supplementary vasodilator therapy in patients with chronic heart failure treated with enalapril: V-HeFT III. Vasodilator-Heart Failure Trial (V-HeFT) Study Group. Circulation 96:856, 1997.
141. Chinese Cardiac Study Collaborative Group: Oral captopril versus placebo among 13,634 patients with suspected myocardial infarction: Interim report from the Chinese Cardiac Study (CCS-1). Lancet 345:686, 1995.
142. Yusuf S, Sleight P, Pogue J, et al, for the Heart Outcomes Prevention Evaluation Study Investigators. Effects of an angiotensin-converting-enzyme inhibitor, ramipril, on cardiovascular events in high-risk patients. N Engl J Med 342:145, 2000 [published erratum appears in N Engl J Med 342:748, 2000].
143. Fox KM: Efficacy of perindopril in reduction of cardiovascular events among patients with stable coronary artery disease: Randomised, double-blind, placebo-controlled, multicentre trial (the EUROPA study). Lancet 362:782, 2003.
144. Rutherford JD, Pfeffer MA, Moye LA, et al, on behalf of the SAVE Investigators. Effects of captopril on ischemic events after myocardial infarction. Results of the Survival and Ventricular Enlargement Trial. Circulation 90:1731, 1994.
145. The SOLVD Investigators: Effect of enalapril on survival in patients with reduced left ventricular ejection fractions and congestive heart failure. N Engl J Med 325:293, 1991.
146. Scandinavian Simvastatin Survival Study Group: Randomised trial of cholesterol lowering in 4444 patients with coronary heart disease: The Scandinavian Simvastatin Survival Study (4S). Lancet 344:1383, 1994.
147. Sacks RM, Pfeffer MA, Moye LA, et al, for the Cholesterol and Recurrent Events Trial Investigators. The effect of pravastatin on coronary events after myocardial infarction in patients with average cholesterol levels. N Engl J Med 335:1001, 1996.
148. The Long-Term Intervention with Pravastatin in Ischaemic Disease (LIPID) Study Group: Prevention of cardiovascular events and death with pravastatin in patients with coronary heart disease and a broad range of initial cholesterol levels. N Engl J Med 339:1349, 1998.
149. Heart Protection Study Collaborative Group: MRC/BHF Heart Protection Study of cholesterol lowering with simvastatin in 20,536 high-risk individuals: A randomised placebo controlled trial. Lancet 360:7, 2002.
150. Pedersen TR, Kjekshus J, Berg K, et al, for the Scandinavian Simvastatin Survival Study Group: Cholesterol lowering and the use of healthcare resources. Results of the Scandinavian Simvastatin Survival Study. Circulation 93:1796, 1996.
151. Tonkin AM, Colquhoun D, Emberson J, et al: Effects of pravastatin in 3260 patients with unstable angina: Results from the LIPID study. Lancet 356:1871, 2000.
152. Executive Summary of The Third Report of The National Cholesterol Education Program (NCEP) Expert Panel on Detection, Evaluation, and Treatment of High Blood Cholesterol in Adults (Adult Treatment Panel III). JAMA 285:2486, 2001.
153. Expert Panel on Detection, Evaluation, and Treatment of High Blood Cholesterol in Adults: Summary of the second report of the National Cholesterol Education Program (NCEP) expert panel on detection, evaluation, and treatment of high blood cholesterol in adults (Adult Treatment Panel II). JAMA 269:3015, 1993.
154. Arntz HR, Agrawal R, Wunderlich W, et al: Beneficial effects of pravastatin (+/– cholestyramine/niacin) initiated immediately after a coronary event (the randomized Lipid-Coronary Artery Disease [L-CAD] Study). Am J Cardiol 86:1293, 2000.
155. Liem AH, van Boven AJ, Veeger NJ, et al: Effect of fluvastatin on ischaemia following acute myocardial infarction: A randomized trial. Eur Heart J 23:1931, 2002.
156. Aronow HD, Topol EJ, Roe MT, et al: Effect of lipid-lowering therapy on early mortality after acute coronary syndromes: An observational study. Lancet 357:1063, 2001.
157. Stenestrand U, Wallentin L: Early statin treatment following acute myocardial infarction and 1-year survival. JAMA 285:430, 2001.
158. Blazing MA, De Lemos JA, Dyke CK, et al: The A-to-Z Trial: Methods and rationale for a single trial investigating combined use of low-molecular-weight heparin with the glycoprotein IIb/IIIa inhibitor tirofiban and defining the efficacy of early aggressive simvastatin therapy. Am Heart J 142:211, 2001.
158a. Cannon CP, Braunwald E, McCabe CH, et al: Intensive versus moderate lipid lowering with statins after acute coronary syndromes. N Engl J Med 350:1495, 2004.
159. Fonarow GC, Gawlinski A, Moughrabi S, Tillisch JH: Improved treatment of coronary heart disease by implementation of a Cardiac Hospitalization Atherosclerosis Management Program (CHAMP). Am J Cardiol 87:819, 2001.
160. Jha AK, Perlin JB, Kizer KW, Dudley RA: Effect of the transformation of the Veterans Affairs Health Care System on the quality of care. N Engl J Med 348:2218, 2003.
161. The RISC Group: Risk of myocardial infarction and death during treatment with low dose aspirin and intravenous heparin in men with unstable coronary artery disease. Lancet 336:827, 1990.
162. Lewis HD, Davis JW, Archibald DG, et al: Protective effects of aspirin against acute myocardial infarction and death in men with unstable angina. N Engl J Med 309:396, 1983.
163. Cairns JA, Gent M, Singer J, et al: Aspirin, sulfinpyrazone, or both in unstable angina. N Engl J Med 313:1369, 1985.
164. Antithrombotic Trialists' Collaboration: Collaborative meta-analysis of randomise trials of antiplatelet therapy for prevention of death, myocardial infarction, and strok in high risk patients. BMJ 324:71, 2002.
165. ISIS-2 (Second International Study of Infarct Survival) Collaborative Group: Ran domised trial of intravenous streptokinase, oral aspirin, both, or neither among 17,18 cases of suspected acute myocardial infarction: ISIS-2. Lancet 2:349, 1988.
166. Topol EJ, Easton D, Harrington RA, et al: Randomized, double-blind, placebo-con trolled, international trial of the oral IIb/IIIa antagonist lotrafiban in coronary and cere brovascular disease. Circulation 108:399, 2003.
167. Peters RJ, Mehta SR, Fox KA, et al: Effects of aspirin dose when used alone or in com bination with clopidogrel in patients with acute coronary syndromes: Observation from the Clopidogrel in Unstable angina to prevent Recurrent Events (CURE) study Circulation 108:1682, 2003.
168. Eikelboom JW, Hirsh J, Weitz JI, et al: Aspirin-resistant thromboxane biosynthesis an the risk of myocardial infarction, stroke, or cardiovascular death in patients at hig risk for cardiovascular events. Circulation 105:1650, 2002.
169. Gum PA, Kottke-Marchant K, Welsh PA, et al: A prospective, blinded determination o the natural history of aspirin resistance among stable patients with cardiovascula disease. J Am Coll Cardiol 41:961, 2003.
170. Goto S, Tamura N, Eto K, et al: Functional significance of adenosine 5′-diphosphat receptor (P2Y(12)) in platelet activation initiated by binding of von Willebrand facto to platelet GP Ibalpha induced by conditions of high shear rate. Circulation 105:2531 2002.
171. Balsano F, Rizzon P, Violi F, et al, the Studio della Ticlopidina nell'Angina Instabil Group: Antiplatelet treatment with ticlopidine in unstable angina: A controlled mul ticenter clinical trial. Circulation 82:17, 1990.
172. Leon MB, Baim DS, Popma JJ, et al: A clinical trial comparing three antithrombotic drug regimens after coronary-artery stenting. Stent Anticoagulation Restenosis Study Investigators. N Engl J Med 339:1665, 1998.
173. Steinhubl SR, Tan WA, Foody JM, Topol EJ, for the EPISTENT Investigators: Incidenc and clinical course of thrombotic thrombocytopenic purpura due to ticlopidine fol lowing coronary stenting. JAMA 281:806, 1999.
174. CAPRIE Steering Committee: A randomised, blinded, trial of clopidogrel versus aspiri in patients at risk of ischaemic events (CAPRIE). Lancet 348:1329, 1996.
175. Steinhubl SR, Berger PB, Mann JT 3rd, et al: Early and sustained dual oral antiplatele therapy following percutaneous coronary intervention: A randomized controlled trial JAMA 288:2411, 2002.
176. Bhatt DL, Bertrand ME, Berger PB, et al: Meta-analysis of randomized and registry com parisons of ticlopidine with clopidogrel after stenting. J Am Coll Cardiol 39:9, 2002.
177. Yusuf S, Mehta SR, Zhao F, et al: Early and late effects of clopidogrel in patients wit acute coronary syndromes. Circulation 107:966, 2003.
178. Cannon CP, on behalf of the CAPRIE Investigators: Effectiveness of clopidogrel versus aspirin in preventing acute myocardial infarction in patients with symptomati atherothrombosis (CAPRIE trial). Am J Cardiol 90:960, 2002.
179. Mehta SR, Yusuf S, Peters RJ, et al: Effects of pretreatment with clopidogrel and aspiri followed by long-term therapy in patients undergoing percutaneous coronary inter vention: The PCI-CURE study. Lancet 358:527, 2001.
180. Topol EJ, Moliterno DJ, Herrmann HC, et al: Comparison of two platelet glycoprotei IIb/IIIa inhibitors, tirofiban and abciximab, for the prevention of ischemic events wit percutaneous coronary revascularization. N Engl J Med 344:1888, 2001.
181. Bonz AW, Lengenfelder B, Strotmann J, et al: Effect of additional temporary glycopro tein IIb/IIIa receptor inhibition on troponin release in elective percutaneous coronary interventions after pretreatment with aspirin and clopidogrel (TOPSTAR trial). J Am Coll Cardiol 40:662, 2002.
182. Helft G, Osende JI, Worthley SG, et al: Acute antithrombotic effect of a front-loadec regimen of clopidogrel in patients with atherosclerosis on aspirin. Arterioscler Thromb Vasc Biol 20:2316, 2000.
183. Muller I, Seyfarth M, Rudiger S, et al: Effect of a high loading dose of clopidogre on platelet function in patients undergoing coronary stent placement. Heart 85:92 2001.
184. Neumann FJ, Kastrati A, Pogatsa-Murray G, et al: Evaluation of prolonged antithrombotic pretreatment ("cooling-off" strategy) before intervention in patients with unstable coronary syndromes: A randomized controlled trial. JAMA 290:1593, 2003.
185. Neumann F: Intracoronary Stenting and Antithrombotic Regimen Rapid Early Action for Coronary Treatment (ISAR REACT). In: American College of Cardiology Scientific Sessions; 2003.
186. The EPISTENT Investigators: Randomised placebo-controlled and balloon-angioplasty-controlled trail to assess the safety of coronary stenting with use of platelet glycoprotein-IIb/IIIa blockade. Lancet 352:87, 1998.
187. The EPILOG Investigators: Platelet glycoprotein IIb/IIIa receptor blockade and low-dose heparin during percutaneous coronary revascularization. N Engl J Med 336:1689, 1997.
188. The ESPRIT Investigators: Novel dosing regimen of eptifibatide in planned coronary stent implantation (ESPRIT): A randomised, placebo-controlled trial. Lancet 356:2037, 2000.
189. Muller I, Besta F, Schulz C, et al: Prevalence of clopidogrel non-responders among patients with stable angina pectoris scheduled for elective coronary stent placement Thromb Haemost 89:783, 2003.
190. Gurbel PA, Bliden KP, Hiatt BL, O'Connor CM: Clopidogrel for coronary stenting: Response variability, drug resistance, and the effect of pretreatment platelet reactivity Circulation 107:2908, 2003.
191. Theroux P, Waters D, Qiu S, et al: Aspirin versus heparin to prevent myocardial infarction during the acute phase of unstable angina. Circulation 88:2045, 1993.
192. Cohen M, Adams PC, Parry G, et al, and the Antithrombotic Therapy in Acute Coronary Syndromes Research Group: Combination antithrombotic therapy in unstable rest angina and non-Q-wave infarction in nonprior aspirin users. Primary end points analysis from the ATACS trial. Circulation 89:81, 1994.

193. Hirsh J, Anand SS, Halperin JL, Fuster V: Guide to anticoagulant therapy: Heparin: A statement for healthcare professionals from the American Heart Association. Circulation 103:2994, 2001.
194. Flaker GC, Bartolozzi J, Davis V, et al: Use of a standardized nomogram to achieve therapeutic anticoagulation after thrombolytic therapy in myocardial infarction. Arch Intern Med 154:1492, 1994.
195. Anand SS, Yusuf S, Pogue J, et al: Relationship of activated partial thromboplastin time to coronary events and bleeding in patients with acute coronary syndromes who receive heparin. Circulation 107:2884, 2003.
196. Granger CB, Hirsh J, Califf RM, et al, for the GUSTO-I Investigators: Activated partial thromboplastin time and outcome after thrombolytic therapy for acute myocardial infarction: Results from the GUSTO-I Trial. Circulation 93:870, 1996.
197. Becker RC, Cannon CP, Tracy RP, et al, for the Thrombolysis in Myocardial Ischemia IIIB Investigators: Relationship between systemic anticoagulation as determined by activated partial thromboplastin time and heparin measurements and in-hospital clinical events in unstable angina and non-Q wave myocardial infarction. Am Heart J 131:421, 1996.
198. Hochman JS, Wali AU, Gavrila D, et al: A new regimen for heparin use in acute coronary syndromes. Am Heart J 138:313, 1999.
199. Hirsh J, Warkentin TE, Shaughnessy SG, et al: Heparin and low-molecular-weight heparin: Mechanisms of action, pharmacokinetics, dosing, monitoring, efficacy, and safety. Chest 119:64S, 2001.
200. Warkentin TE, Levine MN, Hirsh J, et al: Heparin-induced thrombocytopenia in patients treated with low-molecular-weight heparin or unfractionated heparin. N Engl J Med 332:1330, 1995.
201. Fragmin during Instability in Coronary Artery Disease (FRISC) Study Group: Low-molecular-weight heparin during instability in coronary artery disease. Lancet 347:561, 1996.
202. Klein W, Buchwald A, Hillis SE, et al, for the FRIC Investigators: Comparison of low-molecular-weight heparin with unfractionated heparin acutely and with placebo for 6 weeks in the management of unstable coronary artery disease. Fragmin in Unstable Coronary Artery Disease Study (FRIC). Circulation 96:61, 1997.
203. The FRAX.I.S Study Group: Comparison of two treatment durations (6 days and 14 days) of a low molecular weight heparin with a 6-day treatment of unfractionated heparin in the initial management of unstable angina or non-Q wave myocardial infarction: FRAX.I.S. (FRAXiparine in Ischaemic Syndrome). Eur Heart J 20:1553, 1999.
204. Eikelboom JW, Anand SS, Malmberg K, et al: Unfractionated heparin and low-molecular-weight heparin in acute coronary syndrome without ST elevation: A meta-analysis. Lancet 355:1936, 2000.
205. Morrow DA, Antman EM, Tanasijevic M, et al: Cardiac troponin I for stratification of early outcomes and the efficacy of enoxaparin in unstable angina: A TIMI 11B substudy. J Am Coll Cardiol 36:1812, 2000.
206. Mark DB, Cowper PA, Berkowitz SD, et al: Economic assessment of low-molecular-weight heparin (enoxaparin) versus unfractionated heparin in acute coronary syndrome patients: Results from the ESSENCE randomized trial. Circulation 97:1702, 1998.
207. Fox KA, Antman EM, Cohen M, Bigonzi F: Comparison of enoxaparin versus unfractionated heparin in patients with unstable angina pectoris/non-ST-segment elevation acute myocardial infarction having subsequent percutaneous coronary intervention. Am J Cardiol 90:477, 2002.
208. Blazing MA: The A-to-Z Trial: Results of the A-Phase, investigating combined use of low-molecular-weight heparin with the glycoprotein IIb/IIIa inhibitor tirofiban. Presented at the American College of Cardiology Scientific Sessions, New Orleans, LA, March 2003.
208a. SYNERGY Steering Committee: Superior yield of the New strategy of Enoxaparin, Revascularization and GlYcoprotein IIb/IIIa inhibitors (SYNERGY): Primary results. JAMA 2004 (in press).
209. Michalis LK, Katsouras CS, Papamichael N, et al: Enoxaparin versus tinzaparin in non-ST-segment elevation acute coronary syndromes: The EVET trial. Am Heart J 146:304, 2003.
210. Eriksson BI, Bauer KA, Lassen MR, Turpie AG: Fondaparinux compared with enoxaparin for the prevention of venous thromboembolism after hip-fracture surgery. N Engl J Med 345:1298, 2001.
211. Organisation to Assess Strategies for Ischemic Syndromes (OASIS-2) Investigators: Effects of recombinant hirudin (lepirudin) compared with heparin on death, myocardial infarction, refractory angina, and revascularisation procedures in patients with acute myocardial ischaemia without ST elevation: A randomised trial. Lancet 353:429, 1999.
212. Antman EM, McCabe CH, Braunwald E: Bivalirudin as a replacement for unfractionated heparin in unstable angina/non-ST-elevation myocardial infarction: Observations from the TIMI 8 trial. Am Heart J 143:229, 2002.
213. Kong DF, Topol EJ, Bittl JA, et al: Clinical outcomes of bivalirudin for ischemic heart disease. Circulation 100:2049, 1999.
214. Direct Thrombin Inhibitor Trialists' Collaborative Group: Direct thrombin inhibitors in acute coronary syndromes and during percutaneous coronary intervention: Design of a meta-analysis based on individual patient data. Am Heart J 141:E2, 2001.
215. Bittl JA, Strony J, Brinker JA, et al, for the Hirulog Angioplasty Study Investigators: Treatment with bivalirudin (Hirulog) as compared with heparin during coronary angioplasty for unstable or post-infarction angina. N Engl J Med 333:764, 1995.
216. Lincoff AM, Bittl JA, Harrington RA, et al: Bivalirudin and provisional glycoprotein IIb/IIIa blockade compared with heparin and planned glycoprotein IIb/IIIa blockade during percutaneous coronary intervention: REPLACE-2 randomized trial. JAMA 289:853, 2003.
217. Fuchs J, Cannon CP, and the TIMI 7 Investigators: Hirulog in the treatment of unstable angina: Results of the Thrombin Inhibition in Myocardial Ischemia (TIMI) 7 trial. Circulation 92:727, 1995.
218. The Organization to Assess Strategies for Ischemic Syndromes (OASIS) Investigators: Effects of long-term, moderate-intensity oral anticoagulation in addition to aspirin in unstable angina. J Am Coll Cardiol 37:475, 2001.
219. Fiore LD, Ezekowitz MD, Brophy MT, et al: Department of Veterans Affairs Cooperative Studies Program clinical trial comparing combined warfarin and aspirin with aspirin alone in survivors of acute myocardial infarction: Primary results of the CHAMP Study. Circulation 105:557, 2002.
220. Coumadin Aspirin Reinfarction Study (CARS) Investigators: Randomised double-blind trial of fixed low-dose warfarin with aspirin after myocardial infarction. Lancet 350:389, 1997.
221. Anand SS, Yusuf S, for the OASIS Investigators: Randomized trial of oral anticoagulation therapy in patient with acute ischemic syndromes without ST elevation: Importance of good compliance. J Am Coll Cardiol 33(Suppl A):396A, 1999.
222. van Es RF, Jonker JJ, Verheugt FW, et al: Aspirin and Coumadin after acute coronary syndromes (the ASPECT-2 study): A randomised controlled trial. Lancet 360:109, 2002.
223. Hurlen M, Abdelnoor M, Smith P, et al: Warfarin, aspirin, or both after myocardial infarction. N Engl J Med 347:969, 2002.
224. Brouwer MA, van den Bergh PJ, Aengevaeren WR, et al: Aspirin plus coumarin versus aspirin alone in the prevention of reocclusion after fibrinolysis for acute myocardial infarction: Results of the Antithrombotics in the Prevention of Reocclusion In Coronary Thrombolysis (APRICOT)-2 Trial. Circulation 106:659, 2002.
225. Loh E, Sutton MS, Wun CC, et al: Ventricular dysfunction and the risk of stroke after myocardial infarction. N Engl J Med 336:251, 1997.
226. Wallentin L, Wilcox RG, Weaver WD, et al: Oral ximelagatran for secondary prophylaxis after myocardial infarction: The ESTEEM randomised controlled trial. Lancet 362:789, 2003.

Glycoprotein IIb/IIIa Inhibitors

227. The CAPTURE Investigators: Randomised placebo-controlled trial of abciximab before and during coronary intervention in refractory unstable angina: The CAPTURE study. Lancet 349:1429, 1997 [published erratum appears in Lancet 350:744, 1997].
228. Boersma E, Harrington RA, Moliterno DJ, et al: Platelet glycoprotein IIb/IIIa inhibitors in acute coronary syndromes: A meta-analysis of all major randomised clinical trials. Lancet 359:189, 2002.
229. Bhatt DL, Topol EJ: Current role of platelet glycoprotein IIb/IIIa inhibitors in acute coronary syndromes. JAMA 284:1549, 2000.
230. Januzzi JL, Hahn SS, Chae CU, et al: Effects of tirofiban plus heparin versus heparin alone on troponin I levels in patients with acute coronary syndromes. Am J Cardiol 86:713, 2000.
231. van den Brand M, Laarman GJ, Steg PG, et al: Assessment of coronary angiograms prior to and after treatment with abciximab, and the outcome of angioplasty in refractory unstable angina patients. Angiographic results from the CAPTURE trial. Eur Heart J 20:1572, 1999.
232. The GUSTO IV-ACS Investigators: Effect of glycoprotein IIb/IIIa receptor blocker abciximab on outcome in patients with acute coronary syndromes without early coronary revascularisation: The GUSTO IV-ACS randomised trial. Lancet 357:1915, 2001.
233. Steinhubl SR, Talley JD, Braden GA, et al: Point-of-care measured platelet inhibition correlates with a reduced risk of an adverse cardiac event after percutaneous coronary intervention: Results of the GOLD (AU-Assessing Ultegra) multicenter study. Circulation 103:2572, 2001.
234. Kong DF, Califf RM, Miller DP, et al: Clinical outcomes of therapeutic agents that block the platelet glycoprotein IIb/IIIa integrin in ischemic heart disease. Circulation 98:2829, 1998.
235. Newby LK, Ohman EM, Christenson RH, et al: Benefit of glycoprotein IIb/IIIa inhibition in patients with acute coronary syndromes and troponin t-positive status: The PARAGON-B troponin T substudy. Circulation 103:2891, 2001.
236. Januzzi JL, Chai CU, Sabatine MS, Jang IK: Elevation in serum troponin I predicts the benefit of tirofiban. J Thromb Thrombolysis 11:211, 2001.
237. Heeschen C, van Den Brand MJ, Hamm CW, Simoons ML: Angiographic findings in patients with refractory unstable angina according to troponin T status. Circulation 100:1509, 1999.
238. Topol EJ, Yadav JS: Recognition of the importance of embolization in atherosclerotic vascular disease. Circulation 101:570, 2000.
239. Roffi M, Chew D, Mukherjee D, et al: Platelet glycoprotein IIb/IIIa inhibition in acute coronary syndromes. Gradient of benefit related to the revascularization strategy. Eur Heart J 23:1441, 2002.
240. Boersma E, Akkerhuis KM, Theroux P, et al: Platelet glycoprotein IIb/IIIa receptor inhibition in non-ST-elevation acute coronary syndromes: Early benefit during medical treatment only, with additional protection during percutaneous coronary intervention. Circulation 100:2045, 1999.
241. Marso SP, Bhatt DL, Roe MT, et al: Enhanced efficacy of eptifibatide administration in patients with acute coronary syndrome requiring in-hospital coronary artery bypass grafting. Circulation 102:2952, 2000.
242. Braunwald E, Antman EM, Beasley JW, et al: ACC/AHA guidelines for the management of patients with unstable angina and non-ST-segment elevation myocardial infarction: Executive summary and recommendations: A report of the American College of Cardiology/American Heart Association task force on practice guidelines (Committee on the management of patients with unstable angina). Circulation 102:1193, 2000.
243. Morrow DA, Sabatine MS, Cannon CP, Theroux P: Benefit of tirofiban among patients treated without coronary intervention: Application of the TIMI Risk Score for Unstable Angina and Non-ST Elevation MI in PRISM-PLUS. Circulation 104(Suppl II):II-782, 2001.
244. Peterson ED, Pollack CV Jr, Roe MT, et al: Early use of glycoprotein IIb/IIIa inhibitors in non-ST-elevation acute myocardial infarction: Observations from the National Registry of Myocardial Infarction 4. J Am Coll Cardiol 42:45, 2003.

245. Peterson ED: Early glycoprotein IIb/IIIa inhibition is associated with improved outcomes: A CRUSADE registry substudy. Presented at the First International Quality Improvement Summit on Acute Coronary Syndromes, Orlando, Fla, 2003.
246. Mahaffey KW, Harrington RA, Simoons ML, et al, for the PURSUIT Investigators: Stroke in patients with acute coronary syndromes: Incidence and outcomes in the Platelet glycoprotein IIb/IIIa in Unstable angina Receptor suppression using Integrilin therapy (PURSUIT) trial. Circulation 99:2371, 1999.
247. O'Neill WW, Serruys P, Knudtson M, et al, for the EXCITE Trial Investigators: Long-term treatment with a platelet glycoprotein-receptor antagonist after pecutaneous coronary revascularization. N Engl J Med 342:1316, 2000.
248. Cannon CP, McCabe CH, Wilcox RG, et al, for the OPUS-TIMI 16 Investigators: Oral glycoprotein IIb/IIIa inhibition with Orbofiban in patients with unstable coronary syndromes (OPUS-TIMI 16) trial. Circulation 102:149, 2000.
249. The SYMPHONY Investigators: Comparison of sibrafiban with aspirin for prevention of cardiovascular events after acute coronary syndromes: A randomised trial. Lancet 355:337, 2000.
250. Second Symphony Investigators: Randomized trial of aspirin, sibrafiban, or both for secondary prevention after acute coronary syndromes. Circulation 103:1727, 2001.
251. The TIMI IIIB Investigators: Effects of tissue plasminogen activator and a comparison of early invasive and conservative strategies in unstable angina and non-Q-wave myocardial infarction: Results of the TIMI IIIB Trial. Circulation 89:1545, 1994.

Invasive Versus Conservative Strategies

252. FRagmin and Fast Revascularisation during InStability in Coronary artery disease Investigators: Invasive compared with non-invasive treatment in unstable coronary-artery disease: FRISC II prospective randomised multicentre study. Lancet 354:708, 1999.
253. Fox KA, Goodman SG, Klein W, et al: Management of acute coronary syndromes. Variations in practice and outcome; findings from the Global Registry of Acute Coronary Events (GRACE). Eur Heart J 23:1177, 2002.
254. Mahoney EM, Jurkovitz CT, Chu H, et al, for the "Treat Angina with Aggrastat and Determine Cost of Therapy with an Invasive or Conservative Strategy (TACTICS)-TIMI 18" Investigators: Cost and cost-effectiveness of an early invasive versus conservative strategy for the treatment of unstable angina and non-ST elevation myocardial infarction. JAMA 288:1851, 2002.
255. McCullough PA, Gibson CM, DiBattiste PM, et al, for the TACTICS TIMI-18 Investigators: Timing of angiography and revascularization in acute coronary syndromes: An analysis from the TACTICS-TIMI 18 trial. J Interv Cardiol 17:81, 2004.
256. Hochman JS, Sleeper LA, Webb JG, et al, for the SHOCK Investigators: Early revascularization in acute myocardial infarction complicated by cardiogenic shock. N Engl J Med 341:625, 1999.
257. Kugelmass AD, Sadanandan S, Cannon CP, et al, for the TACTICS-TIMI 18 Investigators: Early invasive strategy improves outcomes in acute coronary syndrome patients with prior CABG: Results from TACTICS-TIMI 18. Circulation 104(Suppl II):II-548, 2001.
258. Bhatt DL, Greenbaum A, Roe MT, et al: An early invasive approach to acute coronary syndromes in CRUSADE: Dissociation between clinical guidelines and current practice. Circulation 106(Suppl II):II-494, 2002.
259. Sharis PJ, Cannon CP, Rogers WJ, et al: Predictors of mortality, coronary angiography, and revascularization in unstable angina pectoris and acute non-ST elevation myocardial infarction (the TIMI III Registry). Am J Cardiol 90:1154, 2002.
260. Boden WE, O'Rourke RA, Crawford MH, et al, for the Veterans Affairs Non-Q-Wave Infarction Strategies in Hospital (VANQWISH) Trial Investigators: Outcomes in patients with acute non-Q-wave myocardial infarction randomly assigned to an invasive as compared with a conservative strategy. N Engl J Med 338:1785, 1998.
261. Madsen JK, Grande P, Saunamaki K, et al, on behalf of the DANAMI Study Group: Danish multicenter randomized study of invasive versus conservative treatment in patients with inducible ischemia after thrombolysis in acute myocardial infarction (DANAMI). Circulation 96:748, 1997.
262. Heller GV, Brown KA, Landin RJ, Haber SB: Safety of early intravenous dipyridamole technetium 99m sestamibi SPECT myocardial perfusion imaging after uncomplicated first myocardial infarction. Early Post MI IV Dipyridamole Study (EPIDS). Am Heart J 134:105, 1997.
263. Larsson H, Areskog M, Areskog NH, et al: Should the exercise test (ET) be performed at discharge or one month later after an episode of unstable angina or non-Q-wave myocardial infarction? Int J Card Imaging 7:7, 1991.
264. Karha J, Cannon CP, for the TIMI Study Group: Safety of stress testing following an acute coronary syndrome. J Am Coll Cardiol (in press).
265. Kamp O, Beatt KJ, De Feyter PJ, et al: Short-, medium-, and long-term follow-up after percutaneous transluminal coronary angioplasty for stable and unstable angina pectoris. Am Heart J 117:991, 1989.
266. Moses JW, Leon MB, Popma JJ, et al: Sirolimus-eluting stents versus standard stents in patients with stenosis in a native coronary artery. N Engl J Med 349:1315, 2003.
267. The Bypass Angioplasty Revascularization Investigation (BARI) Investigators: Comparison of coronary bypass surgery with angioplasty in patients with multivessel disease. N Engl J Med 335:217, 1996.
268. Morrison DA, Sethi G, Sacks J, et al: Percutaneous coronary intervention versus coronary bypass graft surgery for patients with medically refractory myocardial ischemia and risk factors for adverse outcomes with bypass: The VA AWESOME multicenter registry: Comparison with the randomized clinical trial. J Am Coll Cardiol 39:266, 2002.
269. Fonarow GC: In-hospital initiation of statins: Taking advantage of the 'teachable moment'. Cleve Clin J Med 70:502, 504, 2003.
270. Schwartz GG, Olsson AG, Ezekowitz MD, et al: Effects of atorvastatin on early recurrent ischemic events in acute coronary syndromes: The MIRACL study: A randomized controlled trial. JAMA 285:1711, 2001.
271. Heart Outcomes Prevention Evaluation Study Investigators: Effects of ramipril on cardiovascular and microvascular outcomes in people with diabetes mellitus: Results of the HOPE study and MICRO-HOPE substudy. Lancet 355:253, 2000.
272. Shivkumar K, Schultz L, Goldstein S, Gheorghiade M: Effects of propranolol in patients entered in the Beta-Blocker Heart Attack Trial with their first myocardial infarction and persistent electrocardiographic ST-segment depression. Am Heart J 135:261, 1998.
273. Hasdai D, Behar S, Wallentin L, et al: A prospective survey of the characteristics, treatments and outcomes of patients with acute coronary syndromes in Europe and the Mediterranean basin; the Euro Heart Survey of Acute Coronary Syndromes (Euro Heart Survey ACS). Eur Heart J 23:1190, 2002.
274. Hoekstra JW, Pollack CV Jr, Roe MT, et al: Improving the care of patients with non-ST elevation acute coronary syndromes in the emergency department: The CRUSADE initiative. Acad Emerg Med 9:1146, 2002.
275. Giugliano RP, Lloyd-Jones DM, Camargo CA Jr, et al: Association of unstable angina guideline care with improved survival. Arch Intern Med 160:1775, 2000.
276. Cannon CP, O'Gara PT: Goals, design and implementation of critical pathways in cardiology. *In* Cannon CP, O'Gara PT (eds): Critical Pathways in Cardiology. Philadelphia, Lippincott Williams & Wilkins, 2001, pp 3-6.
277. Califf RM, Peterson ED, Gibbons RJ, et al: Integrating quality into the cycle of therapeutic development. J Am Coll Cardiol 40:1895, 2002.
278. Cannon CP, Hand MH, Bahr R, et al: Critical pathways for management of patients with acute coronary syndromes: An assessment by the National Heart Attack Alert Program. Am Heart J 143:777, 2002.
279. Mehta RH, Montoye CK, Gallogly M, et al, on behalf of the GAP Steering Committee of the American College of Cardiology: Improving quality of care of acute myocardial infarction: The Guideline Applied in Practice (GAP) initiative in southeast Michigan. JAMA 287:1269, 2002.

Prinzmetal (Variant) Angina

280. Prinzmetal M, Kennamer R, Merliss R, et al: Angina pectoris. I. A variant form of angina pectoris: Preliminary report. Am J Med 27:375, 1959.
281. Yamagishi M, Miyatake K, Tamai J, et al: Intravascular ultrasound detection of atherosclerosis at the site of focal vasospasm in angiographically normal or minimally narrowed coronary segments. J Am Coll Cardiol 23:352, 1994.
282. Mayer S, Hillis LD: Prinzmetal's variant angina. Clin Cardiol 21:243, 1998.
283. Cox ID, Kaski JC, Clague JR: Endothelial dysfunction in the absence of coronary atheroma causing Prinzmetal's angina. Heart 77:584, 1997.
284. Hamabe A, Takase B, Uehata A, et al: Impaired endothelium-dependent vasodilation in the brachial artery in variant angina pectoris and the effect of intravenous administration of vitamin C. Am J Cardiol 87:1154, 2001.
285. Kawano H, Motoyama T, Yasue H, et al: Endothelial function fluctuates with diurnal variation in the frequency of ischemic episodes in patients with variant angina. J Am Coll Cardiol 40:266, 2002.
286. Okumura K, Osanai T, Kosugi T, et al: Enhanced phospholipase C activity in the cultured skin fibroblast obtained from patients with coronary spastic angina: Possible role for enhanced vasoconstrictor response. J Am Coll Cardiol 36:1847, 2000.
287. Sakata Y, Komamura K, Hirayama A, et al: Elevation of the plasma histamine concentration in the coronary circulation in patients with variant angina. Am J Cardiol 77:1121, 1996.
288. Vandergoten P, Benit E, Dendale P: Prinzmetal's variant angina: Three case reports and a review of the literature. Acta Cardiol 54:71, 1999.
289. Suzuki H, Kawai S, Aizawa T, et al: Histological evaluation of coronary plaque in patients with variant angina: Relationship between vasospasm and neointimal hyperplasia in primary coronary lesions. J Am Coll Cardiol 33:198, 1999.
290. Sakata K, Miura F, Sugino H, et al: Assessment of regional sympathetic nerve activity in vasospastic angina: Analysis of iodine 123-labeled metaiodobenzylguanidine scintigraphy. Am Heart J 133:484, 1997.
291. Umemoto S, Suzuki N, Fujii K, et al: Eosinophil counts and plasma fibrinogen in patients with vasospastic angina pectoris. Am J Cardiol 85:715, 2000.
292. Ogawa H, Yasue H, Oshima S, et al: Circadian variation of plasma fibrinopeptide A level in patients with variant angina. Circulation 80:1617, 1989.
293. Igawa A, Miwa K, Miyagi Y, et al: Comparison of frequency of magnesium deficiency in patients with vasospastic angina and fixed coronary artery disease. Am J Cardiol 75:728, 1995.
294. Kim HS, Lee MM, Oh BH, et al: Variant angina is not associated with angiotensin I converting enzyme gene polymorphism but rather with smoking. Coron Artery Dis 10:227, 1999.
295. Onaka H, Hirota Y, Shimada S, et al: Clinical observation of spontaneous anginal attacks and multivessel spasm in variant angina pectoris with normal coronary arteries: Evaluation by 24-hour 12-lead electrocardiography with computer analysis. J Am Coll Cardiol 27:38, 1996.
296. Unverdorben M, Haag M, Fuerste T, et al: Vasospasm in smooth coronary arteries as a cause of asystole and syncope. Cathet Cardiovasc Diagn 41:430, 1997.
297. Tsurukawa T, Kawabata K, Miyahara K, et al: Sudden death during Holter electrocardiogram monitoring in a patient with variant angina. Intern Med 35:966, 1996.
298. Waters DD, Theroux P, Crittin J, et al: Previously undiagnosed variant angina as a cause of chest pain after coronary artery bypass surgery. Circulation 61:1159, 1980.
299. Matsuguchi T, Araki H, Nakamura N, et al: Prevention of vasospastic angina by alcohol ingestion: Report of 2 cases. Angiology 39:394, 1988.
300. Myerburg RJ, Kessler KM, Mallon SM, et al: Life-threatening ventricular arrhythmias in patients with silent myocardial ischemia due to coronary-artery spasm. N Engl J Med 326:1451, 1992.
301. Lip GY, Gupta J, Khan MM, et al: Recurrent myocardial infarction with angina and normal coronary arteries. Int J Cardiol 51:65, 1995.
302. Pepine CJ, el-Tamimi H, Lambert CR: Prinzmetal's angina (variant angina). Heart Dis Stroke 1:281, 1992.
303. Crea F: Variant angina in patients without obstructive coronary atherosclerosis: A benign form of spasm (editorial). Eur Heart J 17:980, 1996.

se of immediate-release dihy-ropyridine calcium antagonists the absence of a beta blocker appropriate (class III).

Recommendations for use of ntithrombotic therapy were vised considerably to reflect ore recent research in the 2002 pdate to the guidelines, leading an expanded role for clopido-rel and more complex tactics r use of platelet glycoprotein b/IIIa inhibitors.[2] Aspirin contin-es to be recommended for initial erapy, but the 2002 guidelines escribe class I indications for opidogrel for patients who are nable to take aspirin, for atients in whom an early nonin-rventional approach is planned, nd for patients in whom percu-neous coronary intervention CI) is planned (Table 49G–4). lopidogrel should be withheld r 5 to 7 days before elective ronary artery bypass graft ABG) surgery. The guidelines so recommend anticoagulation ith low-molecular-weight or nfractionated heparin in addi-on to antiplatelet therapy.

Glycoprotein IIb/IIIa inhibi-rs are considered in the 2002 uidelines to be clearly indicated lass I) when PCI is planned for tients receiving aspirin and eparin. If such patients are ready receiving heparin, aspirin, d *clopidogrel*, the ACC/AHA sk force considered evidence ss conclusive but still generally pportive for addition of a gly-protein IIb/IIIa inhibitor (class indication) (see Table 49G–4). ese agents also received some pport for use in high-risk bsets of patients with acute ronary syndromes even if an vasive strategy is not planned (Class IIa), but the task force thought idence was generally not favorable for their use in patients without ntinuing ischemia or other high-risk features. Abciximab was con-dered inappropriate in patients for whom PCI is not planned.

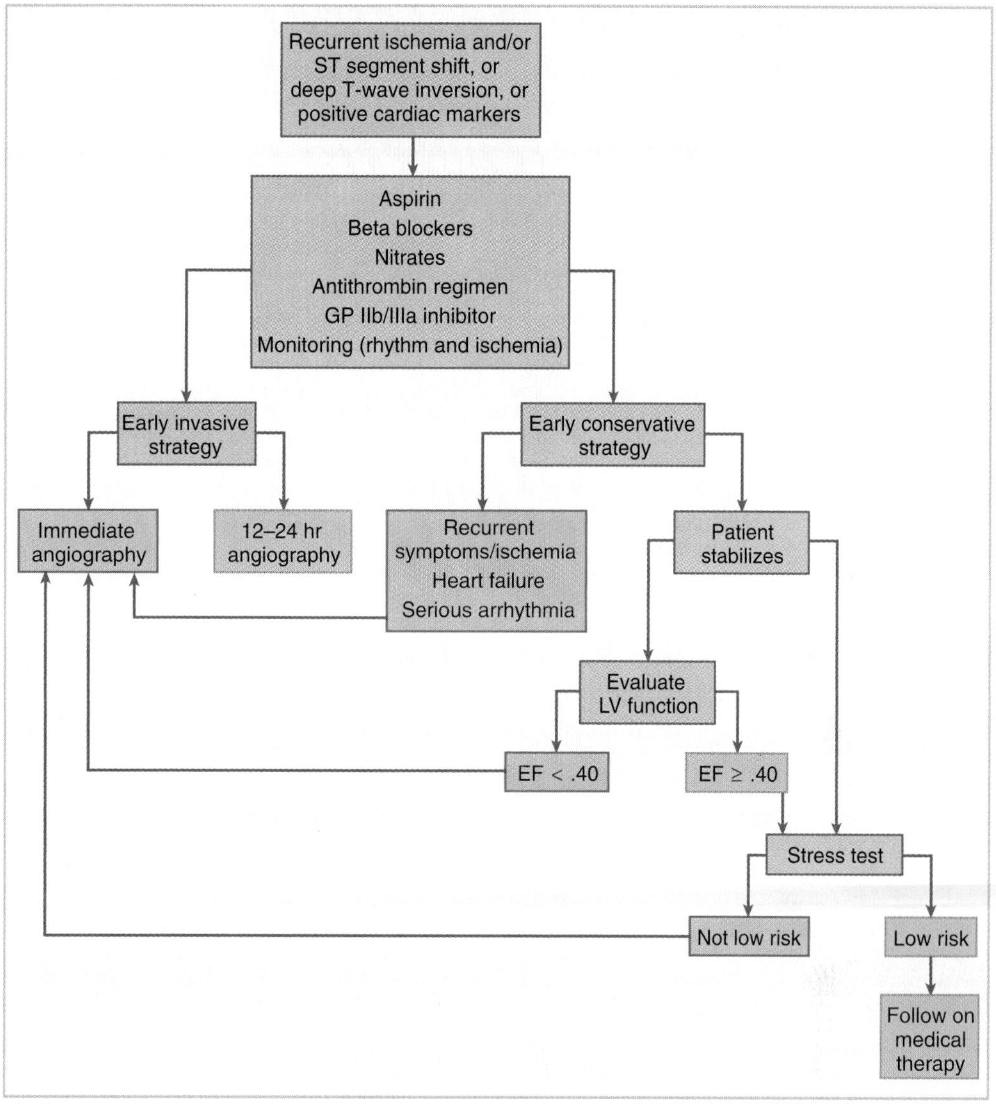

FIGURE 49G–1 Acute ischemia pathway. EF = ejection fraction; GP = glycoprotein. (From Braunwald E, Antman EM, Beasley JW, et al: ACC/AHA 2002 guideline update for the management of patients with unstable angina and non-ST-segment elevation myocardial infarction: Summary article: A report of the American College of Cardiology/American Heart Association Task Force on Practice Guidelines (Committee on the Management of Patients with Unstable Angina). J Am Coll Cardiol 36:970, 2000.

LATER RISK STRATIFICATION AND MANAGEMENT

ne ACC/AHA guidelines support early stress testing in low-risk tients (see Table 49G–1 for risk category definition); for termediate-risk patients, stress testing can be performed after they ve been free of ischemia and heart failure for a minimum of 2 to 3 ys (Table 49G–5). The first choice in noninvasive tests is exercise ectrocardiography; imaging technologies and pharmacological ress tests should be used for subsets of patients for whom exercise ectrocardiography would be expected to have a high likelihood of oviding inadequate data. Data from noninvasive tests can be used stratify patients into high-, intermediate-, and low-risk groups able 49G–6). The guidelines endorse prompt angiography without ninvasive risk stratification for patients who are not readily stabi-ed by intensive medical therapy.

The guidelines recommend an early invasive strategy for patients with acute coronary syndromes and high-risk indicators from their clinical data or noninvasive testing (Table 49G–7). In the absence of such high-risk indicators, the guidelines consider either an early conservative or early invasive strategy to be reasonable. The guidelines also provided some support for use of an early invasive strategy in patients with repeated episodes of suspected acute coronary syndrome without clear evidence for ischemia.

For patients who require coronary revascularization, the principles for choosing between CABG and PCI are similar to those used for patients with chronic stable angina. The guidelines recommend CABG over PCI for patients with significant left main coronary artery disease and for patients with multivessel disease and diminished ejection fraction or diabetes (Tables 49G–8 and 49G–9). CABG and PCI were both considered appropriate for patients with one- or two-vessel disease without proximal left anterior descending (LAD) coronary artery disease but who had large areas of myocardium in jeopardy (see Table 49G–9). The guidelines provided some support for revascularization with either CABG or PCI for patients with proximal LAD disease alone (class IIa) but did not recommend revascularization for patients without proximal LAD disease or those who had only small amounts of ischemia detected by noninvasive testing.

TABLE 49G–3 American College of Cardiology/American Heart Association Recommendations for Antiischemic Therapy

Class	Indication	Level of Evidence
Class I (indicated)	Bed rest with continuous ECG monitoring for ischemia and arrhythmia detection in patients with ongoing rest pain.	C
	NTG, sublingual tablet or spray, followed by intravenous administration, for the immediate relief of ischemia and associated symptoms.	C
	Supplemental oxygen for patients with cyanosis or respiratory distress; finger pulse oximetry or arterial blood gas determination to confirm adequate arterial oxygen saturation (SaO_2 greater than 90%) and continued need for supplemental oxygen in the presence of hypoxemia.	C
	Morphine sulfate intravenously when symptoms are not immediately relieved with NTG or when acute pulmonary congestion and/or severe agitation is present.	C
	A beta blocker, with the first dose administered intravenously if there is ongoing chest pain, followed by oral administration, in the absence of contraindications.	B
	In patients with continuing or frequently recurring ischemia when beta blockers are contraindicated, a nondihydropyridine calcium antagonist (e.g., verapamil or diltiazem) as initial therapy in the absence of severe LV dysfunction or other contraindications.	B
	An ACEI when hypertension persists despite treatment with NTG and a beta blocker in patients with LV systolic dysfunction or CHF and in ACS patients with diabetes.	B
Class IIa (good supportive evidence)	Oral long-acting calcium antagonists for recurrent ischemia in the absence of contraindications and when beta blockers and nitrates are fully used.	C
	An ACEI for all post-ACS patients.	B
	Intraaortic balloon pump (IABP) counterpulsation for severe ischemia that is continuing or recurs frequently despite intensive medical therapy or for hemodynamic instability in patients before or after coronary angiography.	C
Class IIb (weak supportive evidence)	Extended-release form of nondihydropyridine calcium antagonists instead of a beta blocker.	B
	Immediate-release dihydropyridine calcium antagonists in the presence of a beta blocker.	B
Class III (not indicated)	NTG or other nitrate within 24 hr of sildenafil (Viagra) use.	C
	Immediate-release dihydropyridine calcium antagonists in the absence of a beta blocker.	A

ACEI = angiotensin-converting enzyme inhibitor; ACS = acute coronary syndrome; CHF = congestive heart failure; ECG = electrocardiographic, LV = left ventricular; NTG nitroglycerin; SaO_2 = oxygen saturation in arterial blood.

TABLE 49G–4 American College of Cardiology/American Heart Association Guidelines for Antiplatelet and Anticoagulation Therapy

Class	Indication	Level of Evidence
Class I (indicated)	Antiplatelet therapy should be initiated promptly. ASA should be administered as soon as possible after presentation and continued indefinitely.	A
	Clopidogrel should be administered to hospitalized patients who are unable to take ASA because of hypersensitivity or major gastrointestinal intolerance.	A
	In hospitalized patients in whom an early noninterventional approach is planned, clopidogrel should be added to ASA as soon as possible on admission and administered for at least 1 mo and for up to 9 mo.	B
	In patients for whom a PCI is planned, clopidogrel should be started and continued for at least 1 mo and up to 9 mo in patients who are not at high risk for bleeding.	B
	In patients taking clopidogrel in whom elective CABG is planned, the drug should be withheld for 5 to 7 d.	B
	Anticoagulation with subcutaneous LMWH or intravenous UFH should be added to antiplatelet therapy with ASA and/or clopidogrel.	A
	A platelet GP IIb/IIIa antagonist should be administered, in addition to ASA and heparin, to patients in whom catheterization and PCI are planned. The GP IIb/IIIa antagonist may also be administered just prior to PCI.	A
Class IIa (good supportive evidence)	Eptifibatide or tirofiban should be administered, in addition to ASA and LMWH or UFH, to patients *with* continuing ischemia, elevated troponin, or other high-risk features in whom an invasive management strategy is *not* planned.	A
	Enoxaparin is preferable to UFH as an anticoagulant in patients with UA/NSTEMI, unless CABG is planned within 24 hr.	A
	A platelet GP IIb/IIIa antagonist should be administered to patients already receiving heparin, ASA, *and clopidogrel* in whom catheterization and PCI are planned. The GP IIb/IIIa antagonist may also be administered just prior to PCI.	B
Class IIb (weak supportive evidence)	Eptifibatide or tirofiban, in addition to ASA and LMWH or UFH, to patients *without* continuing ischemia who have no other high-risk features and in whom PCI is *not* planned.	A
Class III (not indicated)	Intravenous fibrinolytic therapy in patients without acute ST segment elevation, a true posterior MI, or a presumed new left bundle branch block.	A
	Abciximab administration in patients in whom PCI is not planned.	A

ASA = acetylsalicylic acid (aspirin); CABG = coronary artery bypass graft; GP = glycoprotein; LMWH = low-molecular-weight heparin; MI = myocardial infarction; PCI = pe cutaneous coronary intervention; UA/NSTEMI = unstable angina or non-ST elevation myocardial infarction; UFH = unfractionated heparin.

TABLE 49G–5 American College of Cardiology/American Heart Association Guidelines for Risk Stratification in Patients with Acute Coronary Syndromes

Class	Indication	Level of Evidence
Class I (indicated)	Noninvasive stress testing in low-risk patients (see Table 49G–1) who have been free of ischemia at rest or with low-level activity and of CHF for a minimum of 12 to 24 hr.	C
	Noninvasive stress testing in patients at intermediate risk who have been free of ischemia at rest or with low-level activity and of CHF for a minimum of 2 or 3 d.	C
	Choice of stress test is based on the resting ECG, ability to perform exercise, local expertise, and technologies available. Treadmill exercise is suitable in patients able to exercise in whom the ECG is free of baseline ST segment abnormalities, bundle branch block, LV hypertrophy, intraventricular conduction defect, paced rhythm, preexcitation, and digoxin effect.	C
	An imaging modality is added in patients with resting ST segment depression (greater than or equal to 0.10 mV), LV hypertrophy, bundle branch block, intraventricular conduction defect, preexcitation, or digoxin who are able to exercise. In patients undergoing a low-level exercise test, imaging modality may add sensitivity.	B
	Pharmacological stress testing with imaging when physical limitations (e.g., arthritis, amputation, severe peripheral vascular disease, severe COPD, general debility) preclude adequate exercise stress.	B
	Prompt angiography without noninvasive risk stratification for failure of stabilization with intensive medical treatment.	B
Class IIa (good supportive evidence)	A noninvasive test (echocardiogram or radionuclide angiogram) to evaluate LV function in patients with definite ACS who are not scheduled for coronary arteriography and left ventriculography.	C
Class IIb (weak supportive evidence)	None	
Class III (not indicated)	None	

ACS = acute coronary syndrome; CHF = congestive heart failure; COPD = chronic obstructive pulmonary disease; ECG = electrocardiogram; LV = left ventricular.

TABLE 49G–6 American College of Cardiology/American Heart Association Noninvasive Risk Stratification

High Risk (>3% Annual Mortality Rate)
1. Severe resting LV dysfunction (LVEF <0.35)
2. High-risk treadmill score (score ≤–11)
3. Severe exercise LV dysfunction (exercise LVEF <0.35)
4. Stress-induced large perfusion defect (particularly if anterior)
5. Stress-induced multiple perfusion defects of moderate size
6. Large, fixed perfusion defect with LV dilation or increased lung uptake (thallium-201)
7. Stress-induced moderate perfusion defect with LV dilation or increased lung uptake (thallium-201)
8. Echocardiographic wall motion abnormality (involving > two segments) developing at a low dose of dobutamine (≤10 mg/kg/min) or at a low heart rate (<120 beats/min)
9. Stress echocardiographic evidence of extensive ischemia

Intermediate Risk (1–3% Annual Mortality Rate)
1. Mild/moderate resting LV dysfunction (LVEF 0.35–0.49)
2. Intermediate-risk treadmill score (–11 < score <5)
3. Stress-induced moderate perfusion defect without LV dilation or increased lung intake (thallium-201)
4. Limited stress echocardiographic ischemia with a wall motion abnormality only at higher doses of dobutamine involving ≤ two segments

Low Risk (<1% Annual Mortality Rate)
1. Low-risk treadmill score (score ≥5)
2. Normal or small myocardial perfusion defect at rest or with stress
3. Normal stress echocardiographic wall motion or no change of limited resting wall motion abnormalities during stress

LV = left ventricular; LVEF = left ventricular ejection fraction.
From Table 23 in Gibbons RJ, Chatterjee K, Daley J, et al: ACC/AHA/ACP-ASIM guidelines for the management of patients with chronic stable angina. J Am Coll Cardiol 33:2092, 1999.

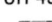

TABLE 49G–7 American College of Cardiology/American Heart Association Guidelines for Early Conservative Versus Invasive Strategies

Class	Indication	Level of Evidence
Class I (indicated)	An early invasive strategy in patients with UA/NSTEMI and any of the following high-risk indicators: Recurrent angina or ischemia at rest or with low-level activities despite intensive antiischemic therapy Elevated TnT or TnI New or presumably new ST segment depression Recurrent angina or ischemia with CHF symptoms, an S_3 gallop, pulmonary edema, worsening rales, or new or worsening MR High-risk findings on noninvasive stress testing Depressed LV systolic function (e.g., EF less than 0.40 on noninvasive study) Hemodynamic instability Sustained ventricular tachycardia PCI within 6 mo Prior CABG	A
	In the absence of these findings, either an early conservative or an early invasive strategy in hospitalized patients without contraindications for revascularization.	B
Class IIa (good supportive evidence	An early invasive strategy in patients with repeated presentations for ACS despite therapy and without evidence for ongoing ischemia or high risk.	C
Class IIb (weak supportive evidence)		
Class III (not indicated)	Coronary angiography in patients with extensive comorbidities (e.g., liver or pulmonary failure, cancer) in whom the risks of revascularization are not likely to outweigh the benefits.	C
	Coronary angiography in patients with acute chest pain and a low likelihood of ACS.	C
	Coronary angiography in patients who do not consent to revascularization regardless of the findings.	C

ACS = acute coronary syndrome; CABG = coronary artery bypass graft; CHF = congestive heart failure; EF = ejection fraction; LV = left ventricular; MR = mitral regurgitation; PCI = percutaneous coronary intervention; TnI = troponin I; TnT = troponin T; UA/NSTEMI = unstable angina or non-ST elevation myocardial infarction.

TABLE 49G–8 American College of Cardiology/American Heart Association Guidelines for Revascularization with Percutaneous Coronary Intervention and Coronary Artery Bypass Graft in Patients with Unstable Angina or Non-ST Elevation Myocardial Infarction

Class	Indication	Level of Evidence
Class I (indicated)	CABG for patients with significant left main CAD.	A
	CABG for patients with three-vessel disease; the survival benefit is greater in patients with abnormal LV function (EF less than 0.50).	A
	CABG for patients with two-vessel disease with significant proximal left anterior descending CAD and either abnormal LV function (EF less than 0.50) or demonstrable ischemia on noninvasive testing.	A
	PCI or CABG for patients with one- or two-vessel CAD without significant proximal left anterior descending CAD but with a large area of viable myocardium and high-risk criteria on noninvasive testing.	B
	PCI for patients with multivessel coronary disease with suitable coronary anatomy, with normal LV function and without diabetes.	A
	Intravenous platelet GP IIb/IIIa inhibitor in patients with UA/NSTEMI undergoing PCI.	A
Class IIa (good supportive evidence)	Repeat CABG for patients with multiple saphenous vein graft (SVG) stenoses, especially when there is significant stenosis of a graft that supplies the LAD.	C
	PCI for focal SVG lesions or multiple stenoses in poor candidates for reoperative surgery.	C
	PCI or CABG for patients with one- or two-vessel CAD without significant proximal left anterior descending CAD but with a moderate area of viable myocardium and ischemia on noninvasive testing.	B
	PCI or CABG for patients with one-vessel disease with significant proximal left anterior descending CAD.	B
	CABG with the internal mammary artery for patients with multivessel disease and treated diabetes mellitus.	B
Class IIb (weak supportive evidence)	PCI for patients with two- or three-vessel disease with significant proximal left anterior descending CAD, with treated diabetes or abnormal LV function, and with anatomy suitable for catheter-based therapy.	B
Class III (not indicated)	PCI or CABG for patients with one- or two-vessel CAD without significant proximal left anterior descending CAD or with mild symptoms or symptoms that are unlikely to be due to myocardial ischemia or who have not received an adequate trial of medical therapy and who have no demonstrable ischemia on noninvasive testing.	C
	PCI or CABG for patients with insignificant coronary stenosis (less than 50% diameter).	C
	PCI in patients with significant left main coronary artery disease who are candidates for CABG.	B

CABG = coronary artery bypass graft; CAD = coronary artery disease; EF = ejection fraction; GP = glycoprotein; LAD = left anterior descending; LV = left ventricular; PCI = percutaneous coronary intervention; UA/NSTEMI = unstable angina or non-ST elevation myocardial infarction.

TABLE 49G–9 American College of Cardiology/American Heart Association Guidelines for Mode of Coronary Revascularization for Unstable Angina or Non-ST Elevation Myocardial Infarction

Extent of Disease	Treatment	Appropriateness Class	Level of Evidence
Left main disease (≥50% stenosis), candidate for CABG	CABG PCI	I III	A C
Left main disease, not candidate for CABG	PCI	IIb	C
Three-vessel disease with EF<0.50	CABG	I	A
Multivessel disease including proximal LAD with EF<0.50 or treated diabetes	CABG PCI	I IIb	A B
Multivessel disease with EF>0.50 and without diabetes	PCI	I	A
One- or two-vessel disease without proximal LAD but with large areas of myocardial ischemia or high-risk criteria on noninvasive testing	CABG or PCI	I	B
One-vessel disease with proximal LAD	CABG or PCI	IIa	B
One- or two-vessel disease without proximal LAD with small area of ischemia or no ischemia on noninvasive testing	CABG or PCI	III*	C
Insignificant coronary stenosis	CABG	CABG or PCI	IIIC

*Class = I if severe angina persists despite medical therapy.
CABG = coronary artery bypass graft; EF = ejection fraction; LAD = left anterior descending; PCI = percutaneous coronary intervention.

Hospital Discharge and Post-Hospital Discharge Care

The ACC/AHA guidelines emphasize the importance of aggressive risk factor modification and teaching of patients about management of ischemic episodes. Class I indications for pharmacological therapy include:

- Aspirin 75 to 325 mg/d in the absence of contraindications
- Clopidogrel 75 mg/d in the absence of contraindications when aspirin is not tolerated
- The combination of aspirin and clopidogrel for 9 months after UA/NSTEMI
- Beta blockers in the absence of contraindications
- Lipid-lowering agents and diet with low-density lipoprotein (LDL) cholesterol greater than 130 mg/dl
- Lipid-lowering agents if the LDL cholesterol level after diet is greater than 100 mg/dl
- ACE inhibitors for patients with heart failure, left ventricular dysfunction, hypertension, or diabetes

Special Groups

The guidelines indicate that women with acute coronary syndromes should be managed according to the same principles as men, using the same indications for noninvasive tests and treatments. For elderly patients, the guidelines recommend that physicians weigh the patients' overall health, comorbidities, cognitive status, and life expectancy as choices are made regarding aggressiveness of management.

For patients with diabetes, the guidelines recommend CABG with internal mammary artery grafts over PCI for diabetic patients with multivessel disease who require revascularization; otherwise, management decisions should be similar to those made for nondiabetics. The task force noted that the use of stents, particularly with abciximab, may provide more favorable results in diabetics but that further data are needed before this approach can be routinely recommended.

For patients with acute coronary syndromes who have previously undergone CABG, the guidelines recommend a lower threshold for angiography because of the many potential causes of ischemia. The guidelines support use of imaging with stress testing in patients who have previously had CABG (class IIa indication).

Calcium antagonists and nitrates are recommended for patients with chest pain after cocaine use and for patients with clinical syndromes consistent with coronary spasm. In patients who have used cocaine, coronary angiography is recommended for patients whose ST segments remain elevated after such medical treatment.

References

1. Braunwald E, Antman EM, Beasley JW, et al: ACC/AHA guidelines for the management of patients with unstable angina and non-ST-segment elevation myocardial infarction: A report of the American College of Cardiology/American Heart Association Task Force on Practice Guidelines (Committee on the Management of Patients with Unstable Angina). J Am Coll Cardiol 36:970, 2000.
2. Braunwald E, Antman EM, Beasley JW, et al: ACC/AHA 2002 guideline update for the management of patients with unstable angina and non-ST-segment elevation myocardial infarction: Summary article: A report of the American College of Cardiology/American Heart Association Task Force on Practice Guidelines (Committee on the Management of Patients with Unstable Angina). Circulation 106:1893, 2002.
3. Smith SC Jr, Dove JT, Jacobs AK, et al: ACC/AHA guidelines for percutaneous coronary intervention: A report of the American College of Cardiology/American Heart Association Task Force on Practice Guidelines (Committee to Revise the 1993 Guidelines for Percutaneous Transluminal Coronary Angioplasty). J Am Coll Cardiol 37:2239i, 2001.

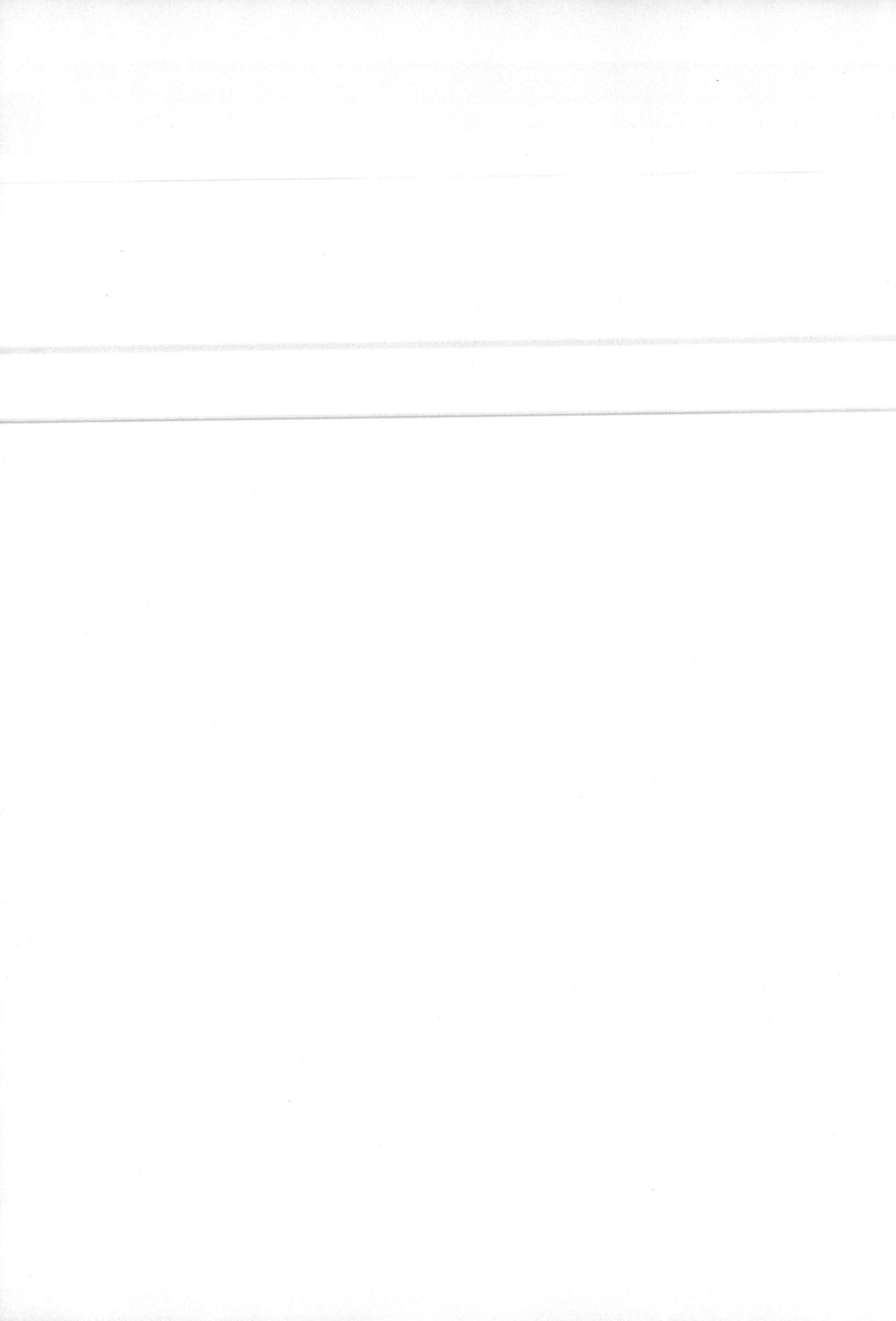

CHAPTER 50

Chronic Coronary Artery Disease

David A. Morrow • Bernard J. Gersh • Eugene Braunwald

Chronic coronary artery disease (CAD) is most commonly due to obstruction of the coronary arteries by atheromatous plaque (the pathogenesis of atherosclerosis is described in Chap. 35).[1] Factors that predispose to this condition are discussed in Chapter 36, the control of coronary blood flow in Chapter 44, acute myocardial infarction in Chapter 46, and unstable angina in Chapter 49; sudden cardiac death, another significant consequence of CAD, is presented in Chapter 33.

No uniform syndrome of signs and symptoms is initially seen in patients with CAD. Chest discomfort is usually the predominant symptom in chronic (stable) angina, unstable angina, Prinzmetal (variant) angina (see Chap. 49), microvascular angina, and acute myocardial infarction. However, syndromes of CAD also occur in which ischemic chest discomfort is absent or not prominent, such as asymptomatic (silent) myocardial ischemia, congestive heart failure, cardiac arrhythmias, and sudden death. Obstructive CAD also has many nonatherosclerotic causes, including congenital abnormalities of the coronary artery, myocardial bridging, coronary arteritis in association with the systemic vasculitides, and radiation-induced coronary disease.[2] Myocardial ischemia and angina pectoris may also occur in the *absence* of obstructive CAD, as in the case of aortic valve disease (see Chap. 57), hypertrophic cardiomyopathy, and idiopathic dilated cardiomyopathy (see Chap. 59). Moreover, CAD may coexist with these other forms of heart disease.

The Magnitude of the Problem

The importance of CAD in contemporary society is attested to by the almost epidemic number of persons afflicted (see Chap. 1). It is estimated that 13,200,000 Americans have CAD, 6,800,00 of whom have angina pectoris and 7,800,000 have had myocardial infarction.[3] Based on data from the Framingham Heart Study, the lifetime risk of developing symptomatic CAD after age 40 is 49 percent for men and 32 percent for women.[3] In 2001, CAD accounted for 54 percent of all deaths due to cardiovascular disease and was the single most frequent cause of death in American men and women, resulting in more than 1 in 5 of deaths in the United States.[3] The economic cost of CAD in the United States in 2003 is estimated at $133.2 billion.[3] Ischemic heart disease is now the leading cause of death worldwide,[4] and it is expected that the rate of CAD will only accelerate in the next decade, contributed to by aging of the population, alarming increases in the worldwide prevalence of obesity, type 2 diabetes, and the metabolic syndrome, as well as a rise in cardiovascular risk factors among younger generations.[5] The World Health Organization estimates that by 2020 the global number of deaths from CAD will have risen from 7.1 in 2002 to 11.1 million.[6]

Stable Angina Pectoris

Clinical Manifestations

CHARACTERISTICS OF ANGINA (see Chap. 7). Angina pectoris is a discomfort in the chest or adjacent areas caused by myocardial ischemia. It is usually brought on by exertion and is associated with a disturbance in myocardial function, but without myocardial necrosis. Heberden's initial description of the chest discomfort as conveying a sense of "strangling and anxiety" is still remarkably pertinent, although adjectives frequently used to describe this distress include "viselike," "constricting," "suffocating," "crushing," "heavy," and "squeezing." In other patients, the quality of the sensation is more vague and described as a mild pressure-like discomfort, an uncomfortable numb sensation, or a burning sensation. The site of the discomfort is usually retrosternal, but radiation is common and usually occurs down the ulnar surface of the left arm; the right arm and the outer surfaces of both arms may also be involved (see Fig. 7–2). Epigastric discomfort alone or in association with chest pressure is not uncommon. Anginal discomfort above the mandible or below the epigastrium is rare. Anginal "equivalents" (i.e., symptoms of myocardial ischemia other than angina), such as dyspnea, faintness, fatigue, and eructations, are common, particularly in the elderly.[7] A history of abnormal exertional dyspnea may be an early indicator of CAD even when angina is absent or no electrocardiographic (ECG) evidence of ischemic heart disease can be found. Dyspnea at rest or with exertion may be a manifestation of severe ischemia, leading to increases in left ventricular filling pressure. Nocturnal angina should raise the suspicion of sleep apnea.

The typical episode of angina pectoris usually begins gradually and reaches its maximum intensity over a period of minutes before dissipating. It is unusual for angina pectoris to reach its maximum severity within seconds, and it is characteristic that patients with angina usually prefer to rest, sit, or stop walking during episodes.

Chest discomfort while walking in the cold, uphill, or after a meal is suggestive of angina. Features suggesting the *absence* of angina pectoris include pleuritic pain, pain localized to the tip of one finger, pain reproduced by movement or palpation of the chest wall or arms, and constant pain lasting many hours or, alternatively, very brief episodes of pain lasting seconds. Pain radiating into the lower extremities is also a highly unusual manifestation of angina pectoris.

Typical angina pectoris is relieved within minutes by rest or by the use of nitroglycerin. The response to the latter is often a useful diagnostic tool, although it should be remembered that esophageal pain and other syndromes may also respond to nitroglycerin. A delay of more than 5 to 10 minutes before relief is obtained by rest and nitroglycerin suggests that the symptoms are either not due to ischemia or, alternatively, are due to severe ischemia, as with acute myocardial infarction or unstable angina. The phenomenon of "first-effort" or "warm-up" angina is used to describe the ability of some patients in whom angina develops with exertion to subsequently continue at the same or even greater level of exertion without symptoms after an intervening period of rest. This attenuation of myocardial ischemia observed with repeated exertion has been postulated to be due to ischemic preconditioning[8] and may require preceding ischemia of at least moderate intensity to induce the warm-up phenomenon.[9]

GRADING OF ANGINA PECTORIS. A system of grading the severity of angina pectoris proposed by the Canadian Cardiovascular Society has gained widespread acceptance (see Table 7–7).[10] The system is a modification of the New York Heart Association (NYHA) functional classification but allows patients to be categorized in more specific terms. Other grading systems include a specific activity scale developed by Goldman and associates[11] and an anginal "score" developed by Califf and colleagues.[12] The Goldman scale is based on the metabolic cost of specific activities and appears to be valid when used by both physicians and nonphysicians. The anginal score of Califf and coworkers integrates the clinical features and "tempo" of angina together with ECG ST and T wave changes and offers independent prognostic information above that provided by age, gender, left ventricular function, and coronary angiographic anatomy. A limitation of all of these grading systems is their dependence on accurate patient observation and patients' widely varying tolerance for symptoms. Functional estimates based on the Canadian Cardiovascular Society criteria showed a reproducibility of only 73 percent and still did not correlate well with objective measures of exercise performance.[11]

MECHANISMS. The mechanisms of cardiac pain and the neural pathways involved are poorly understood.[1] It is presumed that angina pectoris results from ischemic episodes that excite chemosensitive and mechanoreceptive receptors in the heart. Stimulation of these receptors results in the release of adenosine, bradykinin, and other substances that excite the sensory ends of the sympathetic and vagal afferent fibers. The afferent fibers traverse the nerves that connect to the upper five thoracic sympathetic ganglia and upper five distal thoracic roots of the spinal cord. Impulses are transmitted by the spinal cord to the thalamus and hence to the neocortex. Within the spinal cord, cardiac sympathetic afferent impulses may converge with impulses from somatic thoracic structures, which may be the basis for referred cardiac pain, for example, to the chest. In comparison, cardiac vagal afferent fibers synapse in the nucleus tractus solitarius of the medulla and then descend to excite the upper cervical spinothalamic tract cells, which may contribute to the anginal pain experienced in the neck and jaw.[13] Positron-emission tomographic (PET) imaging of the brain in subjects with silent ischemia suggests that failed transmission of signals from the thalamus to the frontal cortex may contribute to this phenomenon, along with impaired afferent signaling, such as that due to autonomic neuropathy.[14]

Differential Diagnosis of Chest Pain (see Table 7–3 and Fig. 7–2)

ESOPHAGEAL DISORDERS. Common disorders that may simulate or coexist with angina pectoris are gastroesophageal reflux and disorders of esophageal motility, including diffuse spasm as well as "nutcracker" esophagus, which is characterized by high-amplitude peristaltic contractions and vigorous achalasia. To compound the difficulty in distinguishing between angina and esophageal pain, both may be relieved by nitroglycerin. However, esophageal pain is often relieved by milk, antacids, foods, or, occasionally, warm liquids.

ESOPHAGEAL MOTILITY DISORDERS. Esophageal motility disorders are not uncommon in patients with retrosternal chest pain of unclear cause and should be specifically excluded or confirmed, if possible. In addition to chest pain, most such patients have dysphagia. Although barium studies may reveal motility problems, esophageal manometry may show diffuse esophageal spasm, increased pressure at the lower esophageal sphincter, and other motility disorders. Provocative pharmacological agents such as methacholine may provoke esophageal pain and manometric signs of spasm.

Both CAD and esophageal disease are common clinical entities that may coexist. Diagnostic evaluation for an esophageal disorder may be indicated in patients with CAD who have a poor symptomatic response to antianginal therapy in the absence of documentation of severe ischemia or in patients with persistent symptoms despite adequate coronary revascularization.

BILIARY COLIC. Although visceral symptoms are a common association of myocardial ischemia (particularly acute inferior myocardial infarction [see Chap. 46]), cholecystitis and related hepatobiliary disorders may also mimic ischemia and should always be considered in patients with atypical chest discomfort, particularly those with diabetes. The pain is steady, usually lasts 2 to 4 hours, and subsides spontaneously without any symptoms between attacks. It is generally most intense in the right upper abdominal area but may also be felt in the epigastrium or precordium. This discomfort is often referred to the scapula, may radiate around the costal margin to the back, or may in rare cases be felt in the shoulder and suggest diaphragmatic irritation. Ultrasonography is accurate in diagnosing gallstones and allows determination of gallbladder size and thickness and whether the bile ducts are dilated.

COSTOSTERNAL SYNDROME. In 1921, Tietze first described a syndrome of local pain and tenderness, usually limited to the anterior chest wall and associated with swelling of costal cartilage. This condition causes pain that can resemble angina pectoris. The full-blown Tietze syndrome (i.e., pain associated with tender *swelling* of the costochondral junctions) is uncommon, whereas costochondritis causing tenderness of the costochondral junctions (without swelling) is relatively common. Pain on palpation of these joints is a useful clinical sign. Local pressure should be applied routinely to the anterior chest wall during examination of a patient with suspected angina pectoris. In addition, costochondritis is usually well localized. Although palpation of the chest wall often reproduces pain in patients with various musculoskeletal conditions, it should be appreciated that chest wall tenderness may also be associated with and does not exclude symptomatic CAD.[15]

OTHER MUSCULOSKELETAL DISORDERS. Cervical radiculitis may be confused with angina. This condition may occur as a constant ache, sometimes resulting in a sensory deficit. The pain may be related to motion of the neck, just as motion of the shoulder triggers attacks of pain from bursitis. A hyperalgesic area noted by running the finger down the back and exerting pressure may lead to a suspicion of thoracic root pain. Occasionally, pain mimicking angina can be due to compression of the brachial plexus by the cervical ribs, and tendinitis or bursitis involving the left shoulder may also cause angina-like pain. Physical examination may also detect pain brought about by movement of an arthritic shoulder or a calcified shoulder tendon.

OTHER CAUSES OF ANGINA-LIKE PAIN. *Acute myocardial infarction* is usually associated with prolonged (>30 minutes), severe pain occurring at rest that, apart from duration and intensity, may be similar to angina pectoris. It is associated with characteristic ECG changes and the release of cardiac markers (see Chap. 46). Unstable angina is a severe form of angina that may also occur at rest and may not be relieved by nitroglycerin (see Chap. 49). The classic symptom

of *aortic dissection* is a severe, often sharp pain that radiates to the back (see Chap. 53).

Severe pulmonary hypertension may be associated with exertional chest pain with the characteristics of angina pectoris, and indeed, this pain is thought to be due to right ventricular ischemia that develops during exertion (see Chap. 67). Other associated symptoms include exertional dyspnea, dizziness, and syncope. Associated findings on physical examination, such as parasternal lift, a palpable and loud pulmonary component of the second sound, and right ventricular hypertrophy on the ECG, are usually readily recognized.

Pulmonary embolism is initially characterized by dyspnea as the cardinal symptom, but chest pain may also be present (see Chap. 66). Pleuritic pain suggests pulmonary infarction, and a history of exacerbation of the pain with inspiration, along with a pleural friction rub, usually helps distinguish it from angina pectoris.

The pain of *acute pericarditis* (see Chap. 64) may at times be difficult to distinguish from angina pectoris. However, pericarditis tends to occur in younger patients than angina does, and the diagnosis depends on the combination of chest pain not relieved by rest or nitroglycerin; exacerbation by movement, deep breathing, and lying flat; a pericardial friction rub; and ECG changes.

Physical Examination

Many patients with chronic CAD present with normal physical findings. Nonetheless, careful examination may reveal the presence of risk factors for coronary atherosclerosis or the consequences of myocardial ischemia.

GENERAL EXAMINATION. Inspection of the eyes may reveal a *corneal arcus*, and examination of the skin may show xanthomas. Among patients with heterozygous familial hypercholesterolemia (in whom CAD is common), the presence of a corneal arcus increases with age and, in some studies, correlates positively with levels of cholesterol and low-density lipoprotein (LDL) as well as with the prognosis. *Xanthelasma*, in which lipid deposits are intracellular, appears to be promoted by increased levels of triglycerides and a relative deficiency of high-density lipoprotein (HDL). The presence of xanthelasma is a strong marker of dyslipidemia and, often, a family history of cardiovascular disease and should provide a strong impetus for performing a comprehensive lipid profile. Retinal arteriolar changes are common in patients with CAD and diabetes mellitus or hypertension.[16] A unilateral diagonal earlobe crease is often present in younger persons with CAD and becomes bilateral with advancing age.

Blood pressure may be chronically elevated or may rise acutely (along with the heart rate) during an angina attack. Changes in blood pressure may precede (and precipitate) or follow (and be caused by) angina.

The association between peripheral vascular disease and CAD is strong and well documented.[17] This association is not confined to patients with symptomatic or clinically overt peripheral vascular disease or CAD but is also seen in asymptomatic subjects with a reduced ankle-brachial blood pressure index or evidence of early carotid disease on ultrasonography. The presence of carotid and peripheral arterial disease on palpation and auscultation increases the likelihood that chest discomfort of unclear origin is caused by CAD.

CARDIAC EXAMINATION. The physical findings of hypertrophic cardiomyopathy (see Chap. 59) or aortic valve disease (Chap. 57) suggest that angina may be due to conditions other than (or in addition to) CAD. It is often helpful to examine the heart *during* an episode of pain because ischemia may produce transient left ventricular dysfunction with a third heart sound and pulmonary rales detectable on physical examination.[18] If massage of the carotid sinus produces pain relief, the pain is probably anginal. Paradoxical splitting of the second heart sound (see Chap. 8) may occur transiently during angina and appears to be related to asynergy and prolongation of left ventricular contraction, which results in delayed closure of the aortic valve. If other obvious cardiac diseases are absent, a third or loud fourth heart sound suggests ischemia as the basis for the chest pain. A displaced ventricular impulse, particularly if dyskinetic, is a sign of significant left ventricular systolic dysfunction.

Transient apical systolic murmurs are quite common in CAD and have been attributed to reversible papillary muscle dysfunction secondary to transient myocardial ischemia. These murmurs are more prevalent in patients with extensive CAD, especially those with prior myocardial infarction and left ventricular dysfunction, and may indicate an adverse prognosis. Systolic murmurs may assume a variety of configurations (early, late, or holosystolic) and may be accentuated by exertion or during angina. A midsystolic click, often followed by a late systolic murmur produced by mitral valve prolapse (see Chap. 57), also occurs in patients with CAD. A diastolic murmur or a continuous murmur is a rare finding in CAD and has been attributed to turbulent flow across a proximal coronary artery stenosis.

Pathophysiology

Angina pectoris results from myocardial ischemia, which is caused by an imbalance between myocardial O_2 requirements and myocardial O_2 supply.[1] The former may be elevated by increases in heart rate, left ventricular wall stress, and contractility (see Chap. 19); the latter is determined by coronary blood flow and coronary arterial O_2 content (Fig. 50–1).

ANGINA CAUSED BY INCREASED MYOCARDIAL O_2 REQUIREMENTS. In this condition, sometimes termed *demand angina*, the myocardial O_2 requirement increases in the face of a constant and usually restricted O_2 supply. The increased requirement commonly stems from norepinephrine release by adrenergic nerve endings in the heart and vascular bed, a physiological response to exertion, emotion, or mental stress. Of great importance to the myocardial O_2 requirement is the *rate* at which any task is carried out. Hurrying is particularly likely to precipitate angina, as are efforts involving motion of the hands over the head. Mental stress may also precipitate angina, presumably by increased hemodynamic and catecholamine responses to stress, increased adrenergic tone, and reduced vagal activity.[19,20] The combination of physical exertion and emotion in association with sexual activity commonly precipitates angina pectoris. Anger may produce constriction of coronary arteries with preexisting narrowing without necessarily affecting O_2 demand. Other precipitants of angina include physical exertion after a heavy meal and the excessive metabolic demands imposed by chills, fever, thyrotoxicosis, tachycardia from any cause, and hypoglycemia.

ANGINA CAUSED BY TRANSIENTLY DECREASED O_2 SUPPLY. Increasing evidence suggests that not only unstable angina but also chronic stable angina may be caused by transient reductions in O_2 supply as a consequence of coronary vasoconstriction,[21] a condition that is sometimes termed *supply angina* and due to the entity of *dynamic stenosis*.[22] In the presence of organic stenoses, platelet thrombi and leukocytes may elaborate vasoconstrictor substances such as serotonin and thromboxane A_2. Also, endothelial damage in atherosclerotic coronary arteries may result in decreased production of vasodilator substances and an abnormal vasoconstrictor response to exercise and other stimuli. A variable threshold of myocardial ischemia in patients with chronic stable angina may be due to dynamic changes in peristenotic smooth muscle tone and also to constriction of arteries distal to the stenosis.[23]

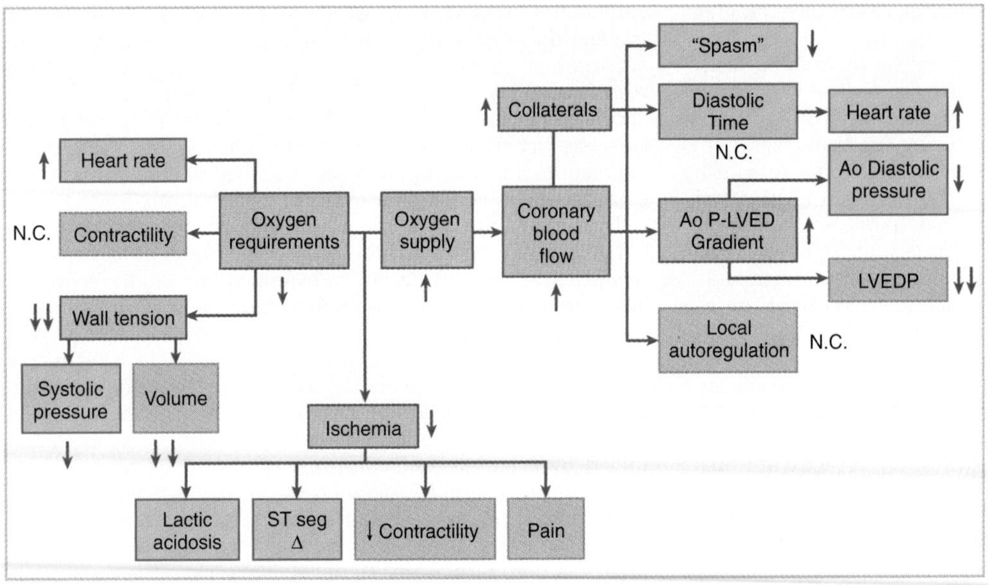

FIGURE 50–1 Factors influencing the balance between myocardial O_2 requirement **(left)** and supply **(right).** Arrows indicate effects of nitrates. In relieving angina pectoris, nitrates exert favorable effects by reducing O_2 requirements and increasing supply. Although a reflex increase in heart rate would tend to reduce the time for coronary flow, dilation of collaterals and enhancement of the pressure gradient for flow to occur as the left ventricular end-diastolic pressure (LVEDP) falls tend to increase coronary flow. Ao P-LVED = aortic pressure–left ventricular end-diastolic; LVEDP = left ventricular end-diastolic pressure; N.C. = no change. (From Frishman WH: Pharmacology of the nitrates in angina pectoris. Am J Cardiol 56:8I, 1985.)

In rare patients without organic obstructing lesions, severe dynamic obstruction occurring at rest alone can cause myocardial ischemia and result in angina (see Prinzmetal [Variant] Angina, Chap. 49). On the other hand, in patients with severe fixed obstruction to coronary blood flow, only a minor increase in dynamic obstruction is necessary for blood flow to fall below a critical level and cause myocardial ischemia.

FIXED COMPARED WITH VARIABLE-THRESHOLD ANGINA. In patients with fixed-threshold angina precipitated by increased O_2 demands with few if any dynamic (vasoconstrictor) components, the level of physical activity required to precipitate angina is relatively constant. Characteristically, these patients can predict the amount of physical activity that will precipitate angina, for example, walking up exactly two flights of stairs at a customary pace. When tested on a treadmill or bicycle, the pressure-rate product (the so-called double product, a correlate of the myocardial O_2 requirement) that elicits angina and/or ECG evidence of ischemia is relatively constant. As the activity of the left ventricle (and therefore its O_2 requirement) increases in patients with fixed-threshold, demand angina, a point is reached at which perfusion distal to a critical coronary arterial obstruction cannot supply sufficient O_2 to myocardium perfused by the obstructed artery; ischemia and angina ensue.

Most patients with variable-threshold angina have atherosclerotic coronary arterial narrowing, but dynamic obstruction caused by vasoconstriction plays an important role in causing myocardial ischemia. These patients typically have "good days," when they are capable of substantial physical activity, as well as "bad days," when even minimal activity can cause clinical and/or ECG evidence of myocardial ischemia or angina at rest. They often complain of a circadian variation in angina that is more common in the morning. Angina on exertion and sometimes even at rest may be precipitated by cold temperature,[24] emotion, and mental stress. A cold environment has been shown to increase peripheral resistance, both at rest and during exercise. The rise in arterial pressure, by augmenting myocardial O_2 requirements, lowers the threshold for the development of angina.

Postprandial angina may be a marker of severe multivessel CAD. The mechanism has not been explained, but it may be due to redistribution of coronary blood flow away from the territory supplied by severely stenosed vessels.[25] Some evidence indicates that this phenomenon is more prominent after high-carbohydrate than high-fat meals.

MIXED ANGINA. The term *mixed angina* has been proposed by Maseri and colleagues to describe the many patients who fall between the two extremes of fixed-threshold and variable-threshold angina.[26]

The pathophysiological and clinical correlations of ischemia in patients with stable CAD may have important implications for the selection of antiischemic agents, as well as for their timing. The greater the contribution from increased myocardial O_2 requirements to the imbalance between supply and demand, the greater the likelihood that beta-blocking agents will be effective, whereas nitrates and calcium-channel blocking agents, at least on theoretical grounds, are likely to be especially effective in episodes caused primarily by coronary vasoconstriction. The finding that in most patients with chronic stable angina an increase in myocardial O_2 requirement precedes episodes of ischemia, that is, that they have demand angina, argues in favor of beta blockers as essential therapeutic agents.

Noninvasive Testing

Biochemical Tests

In patients with chronic stable angina, metabolic abnormalities that are risk factors for the development of CAD are frequently detected. These abnormalities include hypercholesterolemia and other dyslipidemias (see Chap. 39), carbohydrate intolerance, and insulin resistance. All patients with established or suspected CAD warrant biochemical evaluation of total cholesterol, LDL cholesterol, HDL cholesterol, triglycerides, and fasting blood glucose.[27]

Several other biochemical markers have been shown to be associated with higher risk of future cardiovascular events (see Chap. 36). Measurement of lipoprotein Lp(a) and other lipid elements that are particularly atherogenic, such as apoprotein B and small dense LDL, appear to add to measurement of total cholesterol and LDL, but no consensus has been reached regarding routine measurement.[28] Homocysteine has also been linked to atherogenesis and to correlate with the risk of CAD; however, in aggregate, prospective studies have supported at most a modest increase in risk associated with elevated homocyst(e)ine, and have not consistently demonstrated a relationship that is independent of traditional risk factors or other biochemical markers.[29] Therefore, general screening for elevated homocyst(e)ine levels is not recommended.[30] Advances in understanding regarding the pathobiology of atherothrombosis (see Chap. 35) have generated intense interest in inflammatory biomarkers as noninvasive indicators of underlying atherosclerosis and cardiovascular risk. High-sensitivity measurement of the acute phase protein C-reactive protein (hs-CRP) has shown a strong and consistent relationship to the risk of incident cardiovascular events.[31] The prognostic value of hs-CRP is additive to traditional risk factors, including lipid screening.[32] Measurement of hs-CRP in patients judged at intermediate risk by global risk assessment (10 to 20 percent risk of CHD/10 years) may help direct further evaluation and therapy in the primary prevention of CHD (see Chap. 36) and may be useful as an independent marker of prognosis in patients with established CAD.[33]

Blood levels of cardiac markers of necrosis (e.g., cardiac troponin) are normal in patients with chronic stable angina, which serves to differentiate them from patients with acute myocardial infarction. Novel biomarkers of myocardial ischemia are currently under study and may ultimately prove valuable in the noninvasive detection of ischemia in patients with stable CAD.[34]

Resting Electrocardiogram (see Chap. 9)

The resting ECG is normal in approximately half of patients with chronic stable angina pectoris, and even patients with severe CAD may have a normal tracing at rest. A normal resting ECG suggests the presence of normal resting left ventricular function and is an unusual finding in a patient with an extensive previous infarction. The most common ECG abnormalities in patients with chronic CAD are nonspecific ST-T wave changes with or without abnormal Q waves. Numerous pitfalls must be avoided when using the *resting* ECG for the diagnosis of myocardial ischemia. In addition to myocardial ischemia, other conditions that can produce ST-T wave abnormalities include left ventricular hypertrophy and dilation, electrolyte abnormalities, neurogenic effects, and antiarrhythmic drugs. In patients with *known* CAD, however, the occurrence of ST-T wave abnormalities on the resting ECG may correlate with the severity of the underlying heart disease. This association may explain the adverse association of ST-T wave changes with prognosis in these patients. In contrast, a normal resting ECG is a more favorable long-term prognostic sign in patients with suspected or definite CAD.[35]

Interval ECGs may reveal the development of Q wave infarctions that have gone unrecognized clinically. Various conduction disturbances, most frequently left bundle branch block and left anterior fascicular block, may occur in patients with chronic stable angina, and they are often associated with impairment of left ventricular function and reflect multivessel disease and previous myocardial damage. Hence, such conduction disturbances are an indicator of a relatively poor prognosis.[18] Abnormal Q waves are relatively specific but insensitive indicators of previous myocardial infarction. Various arrhythmias, especially ventricular premature beats, may be present on the ECG, but they too have low sensitivity and specificity for CAD. Left ventricular hypertrophy on the ECG suggests a poor prognosis in patients with chronic stable angina. This finding suggests the presence of underlying hypertension, aortic stenosis, or hypertrophic cardiomyopathy and warrants further evaluation, such as echocardiography to assess left ventricular size, wall thickness, and function.

During an episode of angina pectoris, the ECG becomes abnormal in 50 percent or more of patients with normal resting ECGs. The most common finding is ST segment depression, although ST segment elevation and normalization of previous resting ST-T wave depression or inversion ("pseudonormalization") may develop. Ambulatory ECG monitoring has shown that many patients with symptomatic myocardial ischemia also have episodes of silent ischemia that would otherwise go unrecognized during normal daily activities. Although this form of ECG testing provides a quantitative estimate of the frequency and duration of ischemic episodes during routine activities, its sensitivity for detecting CAD is less than that of exercise ECG.

Noninvasive Stress Testing (see Chap. 10)

Noninvasive stress testing can provide useful and often indispensable information to establish the diagnosis and estimate the prognosis in patients with chronic stable angina.[36] However, the indiscriminate use of such tests may provide limited *incremental* information over and above that provided by the physician's detailed and thoughtful clinical assessment.[37] Appropriate application of noninvasive tests requires consideration of Bayesian principles. These principles state that the reliability and predictive accuracy of any test are defined not only by its sensitivity and specificity but also by the prevalence of disease (or pretest probability) in the population under study. A reasonable estimate of the pretest probability of CAD may be made on clinical grounds (Table 50–1).

Noninvasive testing should be performed only if the *incremental* amount of information provided by a test is likely to alter the planned management strategy. The value of noninvasive stress testing is greatest when the pretest likelihood is intermediate because the test result is likely to have the greatest effect on the posttest probability of CAD and, hence, on clinical decision making.

Exercise Electrocardiography (see Chap. 10)

DIAGNOSIS OF CORONARY ARTERY DISEASE. The exercise ECG is particularly helpful in patients with chest pain syndromes who are considered to have a moderate probability of CAD and in whom the resting ECG is normal, provided that they are capable of achieving an adequate workload.[36] Although the incremental diagnostic value of exercise testing is limited in patients in whom the estimated prevalence of CAD is either high or low, the test provides useful additional information about the degree of functional limitation in both groups of patients and about the severity of ischemia and prognosis in patients with a high pretest probability of CAD.[36] Interpretation of the exercise test should include consideration of the exercise capacity (duration and metabolic equivalents) and clinical, hemodynamic, and ECG response.[36]

The predictive value for the detection of CAD is 90 percent if typical chest discomfort occurs during exercise along with horizontal or downward-sloping ST segment depression of 1 mm or more. ST segment depression of 2 mm or more

TABLE 50–1 Pretest Likelihood of Coronary Artery Disease in Symptomatic Patients According to Age and Sex*

Age (years)	Nonanginal Chest Pain		Atypical Angina		Typical Angina	
	Men	*Women*	*Men*	*Women*	*Men*	*Women*
30-39	4	2	34	12	76	26
40-49	13	3	51	22	87	55
50-59	20	7	65	31	93	73
60-69	27	14	72	51	94	86

From Gibbons RJ, Abrams J, Chatterjee K, et al: ACC/AHA 2002 guideline update for the management of patients with chronic stable angina: A report of the American College of Cardiology/American Heart Association Task Force on Practice Guidelines (Committee to update the 1999 guidelines for the management of patients with chronic stable angina). © 2002 American College of Cardiology and American Heart Association (Available at www.acc.org/clinical/guidelines/stable/stable.pdf).

*Each value represents the percentage with significant coronary artery disease at coronary angiography.

accompanied by typical chest discomfort is virtually diagnostic of significant CAD. In the absence of typical angina pectoris, downsloping or horizontal ST segment depression of 1 mm or more has a predictive value of 70 percent for the detection of significant coronary stenosis, but the predictive value increases to 90 percent with ST segment depression of 2 mm or more. The early onset of ST segment depression during exercise, its long persistence following discontinuation of exercise, a downsloping or horizontal depression, and a low work capacity or exercise duration all are strongly associated with multivessel disease and an adverse prognosis. Exercise-induced QRS prolongation also appears to be a function of exercise-induced ischemia and is related to the extent of exercise-induced segmental contraction abnormalities.

A meta-analysis of 147 published studies involving more than 24,000 patients was performed in the process of establishing the American College of Cardiology (ACC)/American Heart Association (AHA) Guidelines on Exercise Testing (Table 50–2).[36] Wide variability in sensitivity and specificity was reported, with a mean sensitivity of 68 percent and mean specificity of 77 percent. The results of stress testing often influence the subsequent decision for angiography and create a posttest referral bias that tends to inflate sensitivity and decrease specificity. When meta-analysis is restricted to studies designed to avoid such work-up bias, the sensitivity is only 45 to 50 percent but the specificity is 85 to 90 percent.[36,38] Clinical scores (e.g., Duke Treadmill Score)[39] or more complex equations that include variables in addition to the ST segment response may improve the discrimination of angiographically significant CAD compared to the ST-segment response alone.[36,39]

A major factor contributing to the low sensitivity of exercise ECG is that many patients are incapable of reaching the level of exercise required for near-maximal effort (≥85 percent of the maximal predicted heart rate), particularly those receiving beta-adrenergic blockers; those in whom fatigue, leg cramps, or dyspnea develops; and those with musculoskeletal symptoms. ST segment changes have low specificity in patients taking digitalis and those with left ventricular hypertrophy and repolarization abnormalities. In these subsets of patients, noninvasive *imaging* with exercise or pharmacological stress testing or diagnostic coronary angiography may be indicated.

INFLUENCE OF ANTIANGINAL THERAPY. Antianginal pharmacological therapy reduces the sensitivity of exercise testing as a screening tool. Beta blockade increases the exercise duration and suppresses, diminishes, or delays the appearance of ST segment depression, and thus obscures the diagnostic interpretation of exercise testing. A negative exercise test in patients receiving antianginal drugs does not exclude significant and possibly severe CAD. Therefore if the purpose of the exercise test is to diagnose ischemia, it should be performed, if possible, in the absence of antianginal medications. Two or 3 days is required for patients receiving long-acting beta blockers. Unless the patient has severe angina, sublingual nitroglycerin for 1 or 2 days is likely to be sufficient to control symptoms if other therapy is withdrawn. For long-acting nitrates, calcium antagonists, and short-acting beta blockers, discontinuing use of the medications the day before testing usually suffices. If the purpose of the exercise test is to identify safe levels of daily activity or the extent of functional disability, or as a guide to prognosis, the test should be performed while patients are taking their usual medications.

Nuclear Cardiology Techniques (see Chap. 13)

STRESS MYOCARDIAL PERFUSION IMAGING. Exercise perfusion imaging with simultaneous ECG is superior to exercise ECG alone in detecting CAD, in identifying multivessel disease, in localizing diseased vessels, and in determining the magnitude of ischemic and infarcted myocardium. The published results of exercise single-photon emission computed tomographic (SPECT) imaging involving more than 5200 patients with angiographic documentation of the presence or absence of CAD yield an average sensitivity and specificity of 88 and 72 percent, respectively (range, 71 to 98 percent and 36 to 92 percent, respectively) (Table 50–3).[18] Referral bias may account, in part, for the low specificity of many studies, and the few studies that adjusted for referral bias report a specificity higher than 90 percent.[18] The results with thallium-201 are comparable to those obtained with ^{99m}Tc-sestamibi or ^{99m}Tc-tetrofosmin, so these agents can in general be used interchangeably for the diagnosis of CAD.[40] Perfusion imaging is also valuable for detecting myocardial viability in patients with regional or global left ventricular dysfunction, with or without Q waves.[41] Stress perfusion imaging also provides important information in regard to prognosis.[40,42]

Stress myocardial scintigraphy is particularly helpful in the diagnosis of CAD in patients with abnormal resting ECGs and those in whom ST segment responses cannot be interpreted accurately, such as patients with left ventricular hypertrophy and repolarization abnormalities, those with left bundle branch block, and those receiving digitalis. Because stress myocardial perfusion imaging is a relatively expensive test (three to four times the cost of an exercise ECG), certain issues should be considered: (1) a regular exercise ECG should always be considered first in patients with chest pain and a normal resting ECG for screening and detection of CAD[18]; (2) stress myocardial perfusion scintigraphy should *not* be used as a screening test in patients in whom the prevalence of CAD is low because the majority of abnormal tests will yield false-positive results; (3) stress perfusion imaging

TABLE 50–2 Predictive Accuracy of Exercise Electrocardiography

Grouping	Number of Studies	Total Number of Patients	Sensitivity (%)	Specificity (%)	Predictive Accuracy (%)
Meta-analysis of standard exercise test	147	24,047	68	77	73
Meta-analysis without MI	58	11,691	67	72	69
Meta-analysis without workup bias	3	>1,000	50	90	69
Meta-analysis with ST depression	22	9,153	69	70	69
Meta-analysis without ST depression	3	840	67	84	75
Meta-analysis with digoxin	15	6,338	68	74	71
Meta-analysis without digoxin	9	3,548	72	69	70
Meta-analysis with LVH	15	8,016	68	69	68
Meta-analysis without LVH	10	1,977	72	77	74

MI = myocardial infarction; LVH = left ventricular hypertrophy.

From Gibbons RJ, Balady GJ, Bricker JT, et al: ACC/AHA 2002 guideline update for exercise testing: A report of the American College of Cardiology/American Heart Association Task Force on Practice Guidelines (Committee on exercise testing). © 2002 American College of Cardiology and American Heart Association. (Available at www.acc.org/clinical/guidelines/exercise/dirIndex.htm).

TABLE 50–3 Sensitivity and Specificity of Stress Imaging*

Modality	Total Patients	Sensitivity†	Specificity†
Exercise SPECT	5272	0.88	0.72
Adenosine SPECT	2137	0.90	0.82
Exercise echocardiography	2788	0.85	0.81
Dobutamine echocardiography	2582	0.81	0.79

SPECT = single-photon emission computed tomography.
Data from Gibbons RJ, Abrams J, Chatterjee K, et al: ACC/AHA 2002 guideline update for the management of patients with chronic stable angina: A report of the American College of Cardiology/American Heart Association Task Force on Practice Guidelines (Committee to update the 1999 guidelines for the management of patients with chronic stable angina). © 2002 American College of Cardiology and American Heart Association. (Available at www.acc.org/clinical/guidelines/stable/stable.pdf).
*Without correction for referral bias.
†Weighted average pooled across individual trials.

is more sensitive in detecting CAD, especially in patients with single-vessel CAD, than is exercise ECG[43]; (4) perfusion imaging is more accurate in patients with resting ECG abnormalities and those receiving digitalis; and (5) perfusion imaging is more accurate in localizing and quantifying regions of myocardial ischemia, which is of particular importance in patients who previously had revascularization, and in determining the extent of viable myocardium in patients with left ventricular dysfunction.[18]

PHARMACOLOGICAL NUCLEAR STRESS TESTING. For patients unable to exercise adequately, especially the elderly and patients with peripheral vascular disease, pulmonary disease, arthritis, or a previous stroke, pharmacological vasodilator stress with dipyridamole or adenosine may be used.[18] In most nuclear cardiology laboratories, such patients account for approximately 40 percent of those referred for perfusion imaging. Although the diagnostic accuracy of pharmacological vasodilator stress perfusion imaging is comparable to that achieved with exercise perfusion imaging (see Table 50-3),[18] treadmill testing is preferred for patients who are capable of exercising because the exercise component of the test provides additional diagnostic and prognostic information, including ST segment changes, effort tolerance and symptomatic response, and heart rate and blood pressure response.

POSITRON EMISSION TOMOGRAPHY (see Chap. 13). PET is considered by many to be the gold standard for evaluation of myocardial viability among patients with ischemic heart disease.[40] Most commonly PET uses ^{18}F-fluorodeoxyglucose (FDG) as the metabolic marker and ^{13}N-labeled ammonia as the perfusion tracer to evaluate for mismatch between myocardial perfusion and metabolic activity. In addition to assessment of myocardial viability, PET may be used to noninvasively measure coronary flow reserve.[44]

EXERCISE RADIONUCLIDE ANGIOGRAPHY. The use of radionuclide angiography for detecting and estimating prognosis in CAD has been supplanted largely by exercise echocardiography and is now performed infrequently.[18] Echocardiography provides a more accurate assessment of exercise-induced changes in regional wall motion and systolic wall thickening, which are more specific markers of reversible ischemia than are changes in ejection fraction.

Stress Echocardiography (see Chap. 11)

EXERCISE ECHOCARDIOGRAPHY. Two-dimensional echocardiography is useful in the evaluation of patients with chronic CAD because it can assess global and regional left ventricular function in the absence and presence of ischemia, as well as detect left ventricular hypertrophy and associated valve disease. Stress echocardiography allows the detection of regional ischemia by identifying new areas of wall motion disorders. Adequate images can be obtained in more than 85 percent of patients, and the test is highly reproducible. Detection of ischemic myocardium has been enhanced with the development of systems that allow simultaneous side-by-side display of rest and postexercise images. Numerous studies have shown that exercise echocardiography can detect the presence of CAD with an accuracy that is similar to that of stress myocardial perfusion imaging and superior to exercise ECG alone (see Table 50-3).[45] Stress echocardiography is also valuable in localizing and quantifying ischemic myocardium. As with perfusion imaging, stress echocardiography also provides important prognostic information in patients with known or suspected CAD.

Indications for stress echocardiography are similar to those discussed earlier for stress myocardial perfusion imaging. Stress echocardiography is an excellent alternative to nuclear cardiology procedures. Although less expensive than nuclear perfusion imaging, stress echocardiography is more expensive and less available than exercise ECG.

PHARMACOLOGICAL STRESS ECHOCARDIOGRAPHY. In patients unable to exercise, those unable to achieve adequate heart rates with exercise, and those in whom the quality of the echocardiographic images during or immediately after exercise is poor, alternative approaches are available. The most well studied and clinically available method is dobutamine stress echocardiography. Dobutamine increases both the heart rate and contractility and produces diagnostic changes in regional wall motion and systolic wall thickening as ischemia develops. Low-dose dobutamine infusion (5 to 10 μg/kg/min) is also valuable for assessing contractile reserve in regions with hypokinetic or akinetic wall motion at rest as a means of identifying viable myocardium that may improve in function after revascularization.[46] Atropine increases the accuracy of dobutamine stress echocardiography in patients with inadequate heart rate responses, especially those taking beta blockers and those in whom second-degree heart block develops at higher atrial rates. Dobutamine stress imaging achieves diagnostic accuracy comparable to that of exercise echocardiography.

Transesophageal dobutamine stress echocardiography has been shown to be feasible, safe, and accurate for the detection of myocardial ischemia. Although not readily available for large numbers of patients, it may allow extension of dobutamine stress testing to patients with inadequate transthoracic echocardiographic imaging.[18] Poor visualization of endocardial borders in a sizable subset of patients has been a limitation of stress echocardiography. However, two developments, contrast echocardiography and harmonic imaging, have significantly improved endocardial border definition, with the potential for enhanced detection of ischemic myocardium.[47,48] Doppler tissue imaging, which allows quantification of intramural myocardial velocities, provides a more direct measure of myocardial function during stress and may provide objective, quantitative evidence of induced ischemia during stress echocardiography.[49]

STRESS ECHOCARDIOGRAPHY VERSUS STRESS NUCLEAR PERFUSION IMAGING. See Chapter 16.

Clinical Application of Noninvasive Testing

GENDER DIFFERENCES IN THE DIAGNOSIS OF CAD (see Chap. 73). On the basis of earlier studies that indicated a much higher frequency of false-positive stress test results in women than in men, it is generally accepted that ECG stress testing is not as reliable in women. However, the prevalence of CAD among women in the patient populations under study was low, and the lower positive predictive value of exercise ECG in women can be accounted for, in large part, on the basis of Bayesian principles (see Table 50-1).[36] Once men and women are stratified appropriately according to the pretest prevalence of disease, the results of stress testing are similar, although the specificity is probably slightly less in women.[36]

Exercise imaging modalities have greater diagnostic accuracy than exercise ECG in both men and women.[36] Although soft tissue attenuation artifacts, especially those caused by breast tissue, may reduce the specificity of myocardial perfusion imaging in women, these artifacts can usually be identified by experienced observers without a substantial reduction in diagnostic accuracy, and risk assessment by nuclear perfusion imaging is not diminished in women versus men.[50] In addition, the use of gated SPECT imaging has greatly improved identification of these artifacts by demonstrating that regions with apparently irreversible perfusion defects have normal wall motion, thereby enhancing diagnostic accuracy.[51]

IDENTIFICATION OF PATIENTS AT HIGH RISK. When applying noninvasive tests to the diagnosis and management of CAD, it is useful to grade the results as "negative"; "indeterminate"; "positive, not high risk"; and "positive, high risk." The criteria for high-risk findings on stress ECG, myocardial perfusion imaging, and stress echocardiography are listed in Table 50–4.

TABLE 50–4 Risk Stratification Based on Noninvasive Testing

High Risk (>3% annual mortality rate)
1. Severe resting left ventricular dysfunction (LVEF < 0.35)
2. High-risk treadmill score (score ≤ −11)
3. Severe exercise left ventricular dysfunction (exercise LVEF < 0.35)
4. Stress-induced large perfusion defect (particularly if anterior)
5. Stress-induced multiple perfusion defects of moderate size
6. Large, fixed perfusion defect with LV dilation or increased lung uptake (thallium-201)
7. Stress-induced moderate perfusion defect with LV dilation or increased lung uptake (thallium-201)
8. Echocardiographic wall motion abnormality (involving > two segments) developing at low dose of dobutamine (≤10 mg/kg/min) or at a low heart rate (<120 beats/min)
9. Stress echocardiographic evidence of extensive ischemia
Intermediate Risk (1-3% annual mortality rate)
1. Mild/moderate resting left ventricular dysfunction (LVEF = 0.35-0.49)
2. Intermediate-risk treadmill score (−11 < score < 5)
3. Stress-induced moderate perfusion defect without LV dilation or increased lung intake (thallium-201)
4. Limited stress echocardiographic ischemia with a wall motion abnormality only at higher doses of dobutamine involving ≤ two segments
Low Risk (<1% annual mortality rate)
1. Low-risk treadmill score (score ≥ 5)
2. Normal or small myocardial perfusion defect at rest or with stress*
3. Normal stress echocardiographic wall motion or no change of limited resting wall motion abnormalities during stress*

LV = left ventricular; LVEF = LV ejection fraction.

From Gibbons RJ, Abrams J, Chatterjee K, et al: ACC/AHA 2002 guideline update for the management of patients with chronic stable angina: A report of the American College of Cardiology/American Heart Association Task Force on Practice Guidelines (Committee to update the 1999 guidelines for the management of patients with chronic stable angina). © 2002 American College of Cardiology and American Heart Association. (Available at www.acc.org/clinical/guidelines/stable/stable.pdf).

*Although the published data are limited, patients with these findings will probably not be at low risk in the presence of either a high-risk treadmill score or severe resting left ventricular dysfunction (LVEF < 0.35).

Regardless of the severity of symptoms, patients with high-risk noninvasive test results have a high likelihood of CAD and, if they have no obvious contraindications to revascularization, should undergo coronary arteriography. Such patients, even if asymptomatic, are at risk for left main or triple-vessel CAD, and many have impaired left ventricular function. Hence, they are at high risk for experiencing coronary events and may be candidates for coronary revascularization. In contrast, patients with clearly negative exercise tests, regardless of symptoms, have an excellent prognosis that cannot usually be improved by revascularization. If they do not have serious symptoms, coronary arteriography is generally not indicated.

The Duke Treadmill Score (see Fig. 10–15) is an integrative tool that incorporates exercise duration, the magnitude of ST segment deviation, and exercise-induced angina, and it effectively identifies patients with a high probability of severe CAD (triple-vessel or left main CAD) at angiography and with higher mortality risk. Among groups defined by low-, moderate-, and high-risk Duke Treadmill Scores, mortality at 5 years is 3 percent, 10 percent, and 35 percent, respectively.[39]

ASYMPTOMATIC PERSONS. Exercise testing in asymptomatic individuals without known CAD is generally not recommended.[36] Exercise testing may be appropriate for asymptomatic individuals with diabetes mellitus who plan to begin vigorous exercise,[36] for those with evidence of myocardial ischemia on ambulatory ECG monitoring, or for those with severe coronary calcifications on electron-beam CT.[18]

In asymptomatic persons or in those with chest pain not likely to be angina, the pretest likelihood of CAD is low (<15 percent). In such patients, a negative exercise ECG, for practical purposes, excludes ischemic heart disease. However, if such a patient has an abnormal exercise ST segment response, several alternatives exist. If the ST segment is abnormal but not high risk (<2-mm depression) and the patient demonstrates excellent exercise capacity (i.e., to stage IV of a Bruce protocol or the equivalent), the likelihood of left main CAD or multivessel CAD is low, the prognosis is favorable, and the patient may usually be observed without further testing, although an imaging study may provide further clarification and assurance. If, however, such a patient has a high-risk positive exercise ECG, coronary angiography is usually indicated to determine whether left main CAD or severe multivessel disease with left ventricular dysfunction is present. If the patient falls into an intermediate category (a positive but not high-risk exercise test result), a stress imaging study (echocardiography or perfusion scintigraphy) may provide further information. If both studies are abnormal but not high risk, the likelihood of CAD approaches 90 percent.

PATIENTS WITH ATYPICAL ANGINA. In these patients, the pretest probability of CAD is approximately 50 percent. If two noninvasive tests are abnormal, the likelihood of CAD exceeds 95 percent; if both tests are normal, it falls below 5 percent. When test results are discordant, they should be evaluated in light of the exercise level achieved, the presence of accompanying symptoms, and whether one of the tests is positive with high risk. Thus, for example, a patient who has atypical angina and a normal exercise ECG with multiple large perfusion defects on a stress thallium-201 scintigram at a heart rate of 130 beats/min has a much greater likelihood of having CAD than one who has a normal exercise ECG and a single small perfusion defect without chest pain at a heart rate of 185 beats/min. Although the indications for performing a stress imaging test directly in such a patient without an initial exercise ECG are controversial, such an approach is reasonable if the patient with atypical angina also has multiple cardiovascular risk factors, such as smoking, hypercholesterolemia, or a positive family history of premature CAD.

PATIENTS WITH TYPICAL ANGINA. In patients with a high pretest likelihood of disease of approximately 90 percent, noninvasive testing is most valuable for estimating the extent and severity of CAD and thereby the prognosis. The development of a high-risk positive stress test points to multivessel disease and a high risk of subsequent coronary events, and unless the patient has contraindications to revascularization, coronary angiography is indicated.

Chest Roentgenogram (see Chap. 12)

The chest roentgenogram is usually within normal limits in patients with chronic stable angina, particularly if they have a normal resting ECG and have not experienced a myocardial infarction. If cardiomegaly is present, it is indicative of severe CAD with previous myocardial infarction, preexisting hypertension, or an associated nonischemic condition such as concomitant valvular heart disease or cardiomyopathy.

Computed Tomography (see Chap. 15)

Noninvasive detection of coronary artery calcification has long been possible with fluoroscopy. Such calcific deposits are diagnostic of coronary atherosclerosis.[52] Electron-beam, and now multislice cardiac, CT has emerged as a highly sensitive method for detecting coronary calcification and is being used at some centers as a screening technique for CAD. CT quantification of coronary calcium has also been proposed as a method for assessing the response to treatment of risk factors such as dyslipidemia or hypertension among individuals with suspected or established CAD.[53] The calcium score is a quantitative index of total coronary artery calcium detected by CT, and this score has been shown to be a good marker of the total coronary atherosclerotic burden.[54] However, the relationship of the coronary calcium score to subsequent cardiac events in asymptomatic persons has not been fully established.[55,56] Several other uncertainties persist as well, including (1) the value of coronary calcium screening in comparison to multiple risk factor assessment; (2) whether coronary calcium scores add incremental value beyond the standard risk factors; and (3) whether coronary calcium screening is more accurate and cost-effective in asymptomatic persons than are other established noninvasive tests or other new methods that assess atherosclerotic burden, such as inflammatory biomarkers (see Chap. 36), the ankle-brachial index, and ultrasonic carotid intimal-medial thickening.[57]

The *absence* of calcium on CT imaging is predictive of the absence of significant atherosclerotic disease in older persons, but it is possible for young people (men younger than 45 years, women younger than 55) to have obstructive CAD and, hence, a risk for future cardiac events in the absence of detectable calcification or with a low calcium score.[58] Although coronary calcification is a highly sensitive (~90 percent) finding in patients who have CAD and the presence of coronary calcification is an accurate marker of coronary atherosclerosis, the specificity of this finding for identifying patients with obstructive CAD is low (~50 percent).[57,59] In light of the poor specificity and the potential consequences of expensive and unnecessary testing as the result of false-positive results, CT is currently *not* recommended as a routine approach toward screening for obstructive CAD.[18,57] Moreover, in patients with known or suspected CAD, exercise testing is preferable to CT imaging for determining the extent of CAD and the indication for coronary angiography.[57] Selective screening of individuals at intermediate risk of CAD may be appropriate.[57] The results of ongoing investigation will guide future recommendations regarding the role of this technique in the assessment and management of CAD.

In addition to application for detection of coronary calcification, CT technology may also evolve to enable reliable noninvasive coronary angiography. In particular, the emergence of new generations of multislice spiral CT scanners has reduced the motion artifact that constitutes a critical barrier to CT becoming a viable method for coronary angiography. Preliminary data with this technology in conjunction with aggressive beta blockade to reduce heart rate during imaging show promise for detection of obstructive CAD in the major epicardial arteries.[60]

Magnetic Resonance Imaging (see Chap. 14)

Magnetic resonance imaging (MRI) is established as a valuable clinical tool for imaging the aorta and the cerebral and peripheral arterial vasculature and is emerging as a versatile noninvasive cardiac imaging modality that has multiple applications for patients with CAD.[61] At present, the clinical use of MRI for myocardial viability assessment is growing based on data demonstrating its ability to predict functional recovery after percutaneous or surgical revascularization[62] and its very good correlation with PET.[63] Specifically, delayed hyperenhancement with gadolinium identifies areas of myocardial scar, and the transmural extent of hyperenhancement is strongly inversely associated with the probability of recovery after revascularization[62] and may be useful in assessing the probability of regaining contractile function after myocardial infarction.[64] Pharmacological stress perfusion imaging with MRI also compares favorably to other methods and is being employed clinically in some centers, particularly for individuals who present limitations for other imaging modalities.[65] In these patients, MRI also offers accurate characterization of left ventricular function. New techniques are likely to lead to further improvements in MRI as a tool for stress testing.[66,67]

By virtue of its ability to visualize arteries in three dimensions and differentiate tissue constituents, MRI has received intense interest as a potential, but as yet unproven, method to characterize arterial atheroma and assess vulnerability to rupture on the basis of compositional analysis.[61,68] Characterization of arterial plaque has been achieved in the aorta and carotid arteries[69] in humans and has been shown to be predictive of subsequent vascular events.[70] Initial studies evaluating MRI coronary angiography in humans demonstrate the ability to detect stenoses in the proximal and middle of major epicardial vessels[71] or surgical bypass grafts,[72] as well as to characterize congenital coronary anomalies.[73] Analogous to CT, new MRI technology is also likely to improve myocardial definition, enhance discrimination of wall motion, and also present new methods for ischemia detection based on assessment of regional oxygen content or detection of molecular changes (e.g., phosphocreatinine and adenosine triphosphate [ATP]) during ischemia.[61] However, routine clinical use of MRI scanning of coronary plaque will require substantial additional technical developments.[61]

Catheterization, Angiography, and Coronary Arteriography

The clinical examination and noninvasive techniques described earlier are extremely valuable in establishing the diagnosis of CAD and are indispensable to an overall assessment of patients with this condition. However, currently, definitive diagnosis of CAD and precise assessment of its anatomical severity still require cardiac catheterization and coronary arteriography (see Chaps. 17 and 18). Among patients with chronic stable angina pectoris referred for coronary arteriography, approximately 25 percent each have single-, double-, or triple-vessel disease (i.e., >70 percent luminal diameter narrowing). Five to 10 percent have obstruction of the left main coronary artery, and in approximately 15 percent no critical obstruction is detectable. Newer invasive techniques such as intravascular ultrasonography (IVUS) provide a cross-sectional view of the coronary artery and have substantially enhanced the detection and quantification of coronary atherosclerosis (see Chap. 52).[74] Studies incorporating both coronary angiography and IVUS demonstrate that the severity of CAD may be underestimated by angiography alone. In addition, IVUS images provide insight regarding plaque composition, discriminating lipid-laden versus fibrous or calcified elements based on echodensity.[75] In clinical practice, IVUS is a valuable tool to assess the cross-sectional lumen dimensions and to detect coronary artery stucture and pathology. Although IVUS is used in fewer than 10 percent of percutaneous interventions, it is particularly useful when angiography provides equivocal findings, such as occult left main or ostial CAD, or when there is haziness within the vessel after coronary stent implantation.

Coronary angiographic findings differ between patients presenting with acute myocardial infarction and those with chronic stable angina. Patients with unheralded myocardial infarction have fewer diseased vessels, fewer stenoses and chronic occlusions, and less diffuse disease than do chronic stable angina patients, thus suggesting that the pathophysiological substrate and the propensity for thrombosis differ between these two groups of patients.[76] In patients with chronic angina who have a history of prior infarction, total occlusion of at least one major coronary artery is more common than in those without such a history.

CORONARY ARTERY ECTASIA AND ANEURYSMS. Patulous, aneurysmal dilation involving most of the length of a major epicardial coronary artery is present in approximately 1 to 3 percent of patients with obstructive CAD at autopsy or angiography. This angiographic lesion does not appear to affect symptoms, survival, or incidence of myocardial infarction. Most coronary artery ectasia and/or aneurysms are due to coronary atherosclerosis (50 percent), and the rest are due to congenital anomalies and inflammatory diseases such as Kawasaki disease. Despite the absence of overt obstruction, 70 percent of patients with multivessel fusiform coronary artery ectasia/aneurysms demonstrated evidence of cardiac ischemia based on cardiac lactate levels during ergometry and atrial pacing. Moreover, nitroglycerin was of no benefit.[77]

Coronary ectasia should be distinguished from discrete *coronary artery aneurysms*, which are almost never found in arteries without severe stenosis, are most common in the left anterior descending coronary artery, and are usually associated with extensive CAD.[78] These discrete atherosclerotic coronary artery aneurysms do not appear to rupture, and resection of them is not warranted.

CORONARY COLLATERAL VESSELS (see Chap. 18). Provided that they are of adequate size, collaterals may protect against myocardial infarction when total occlusion occurs. In patients with abundant collateral vessels, myocardial infarct size is smaller than in patients without collaterals, and total occlusion of a major epicardial artery may not lead to left ventricular dysfunction. In patients with chronic occlusion of a major coronary artery but without infarction, collateral-dependent myocardial segments show nearly normal baseline blood flow and O_2 consumption but severely limited flow reserve. This finding provides an explanation for the ability of collaterals to protect against resting ischemia but not exercise-induced angina.[79]

MYOCARDIAL BRIDGING. Bridging of coronary arteries (see Chap. 18) is observed at coronary angiography at a rate of less than 5 percent in otherwise angiographically normal coronary arteries and ordinarily does not constitute a hazard.[80] Occasionally, compression of a portion of a coronary artery by a myocardial bridge can be associated with clinical manifestations of myocardial ischemia during strenuous physical activity and may even result in myocardial infarction or initiate malignant ventricular arrhythmias.[80] The functional consequences of myocardial bridging may be better characterized with the use of IVUS and intracoronary Doppler measurements.[80]

LEFT VENTRICULAR FUNCTION. Left ventricular function can be assessed by means of biplane contrast ventriculography (see also Chap. 20). Global abnormalities of left ventricular systolic function are reflected by elevations in left ventricular end-diastolic and end-systolic volume and depression of the ejection fraction. These changes are, however, quite nonspecific and can occur in many forms of heart disease. Abnormalities of *regional* wall motion (hypokinesis, akinesia, or dyskinesia) are more characteristic of CAD because the latter is usually regional in distribution. Also, hyperkinetic contraction of nonischemic myocardium may compensate for hypokinetic or akinetic ischemic or necrotic myocardium, thereby maintaining normal or nearly normal global left ventricular function despite marked depression of function in one region of the ventricle.

Ventricular relaxation, as reflected in the early diastolic ventricular filling rate, may be impaired at rest in patients with chronic CAD. Diastolic filling becomes even more abnormal (slowed) during exercise, when ischemia intensifies. In patients with chronic stable angina, the frequency of elevated left ventricular end-diastolic pressure and reduced cardiac output at rest, generally attributed to abnormal left ventricular dynamics, increases with the number of vessels exhibiting critical narrowing and with the number of prior infarctions. Left ventricular end-diastolic pressure may be elevated secondary to reduced ventricular compliance, left ventricular systolic failure, or a combination of these two processes.[81] Left ventricular function (global or regional) may be normal at rest in patients with chronic CAD without previous myocardial infarction but may become abnormal during or after stress. Abnormalities of left ventricular function detected angiographically may signify irreversible damage (i.e., prior infarction) or they may indicate acute ischemia or chronic hypoperfusion sufficient to maintain viability, but not contractility of the myocardium (i.e., "myocardial hibernation") (see Chap. 19).[82] Reversibility of this form of left ventricular dysfunction in patients with CAD and chronic stable angina is reflected by improved contraction assessed angiographically after an inotropic stimulus (postextrasystolic potentiation or the infusion of a sympathomimetic amine) and is accompanied by long-term improvement after myocardial revascularization.

Left ventriculography may also show mitral valve prolapse, which occurs in up to 20 percent of patients with obstructive CAD[83] and probably results from impaired contractility of the ventricular myocardium and papillary muscles. Mitral regurgitation secondary to left ventricular dilation may be observed in patients with chronic stable angina and ischemic cardiomyopathy.

CORONARY BLOOD FLOW AND MYOCARDIAL METABOLISM. Cardiac catheterization can also document abnormal myocardial metabolism in patients with chronic stable angina. With a catheter in the coronary sinus, arterial and coronary venous lactate measurements are obtained at rest and after suitable stress, such as the infusion of isoproterenol or pacing-induced tachycardia.[84] Because lactate is a byproduct of anaerobic glycolysis, its production by the heart and subsequent appearance in coronary sinus blood is a reliable sign of myocardial ischemia.

Studies of coronary flow reserve (maximum flow divided by resting flow) and endothelial function are frequently abnormal in patients with CAD and chronic stable angina. These techniques are discussed in Chapter 44.

Natural History, Prognosis, and Risk Stratification

Data from the Framingham Study, obtained before the widespread use of aspirin, beta blockers, and aggressive modification of risk factors, showed that the average annual mortality rate of patients with chronic stable angina was 4 percent. The combination of these treatments has improved prognosis. More recent data among middle-aged men with prevalent CAD indicate an annual mortality rate of 1.7 to 3 percent and an annual rate of major ischemic events of 1.4 to 2.4 percent.[85] Clinical, noninvasive, and invasive tools

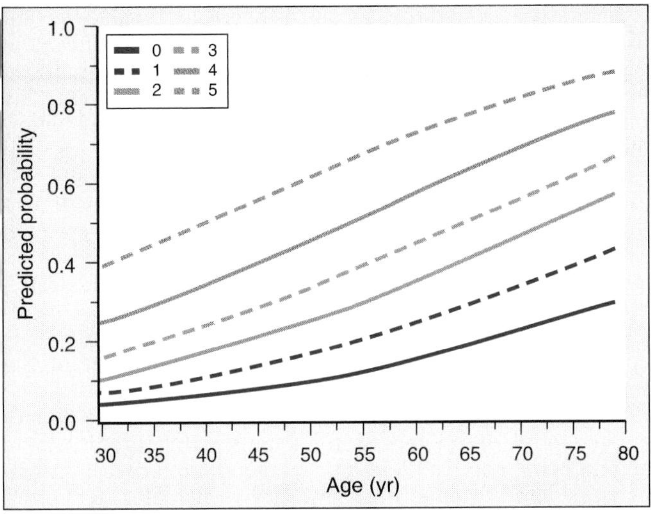

FIGURE 50–2 Nomogram showing the probability of severe (triple-vessel or left main) coronary artery disease based on a five-point clinical score assigned on the basis of the clinical variables: male gender, typical angina, history and electrocardiographic evidence of myocardial infarction, and diabetes. (Adapted from Hubbard BL, Gibbons RJ, Lapyre AC, et al: Identification of severe coronary artery disease using simple clinical parameters. Arch Intern Med 152:309-312, 1992.)

are useful in refining the estimate of risk for the individual patient with stable angina. Moreover, noninvasively acquired information is valuable in identifying patients who are candidates for invasive evaluation with cardiac catheterization.

CLINICAL AND ELECTROCARDIOGRAPHIC CRITERIA. A composite risk score based on multiple clinical variables (e.g., age, sex, diabetes, previous myocardial infarction, and the nature of the chest pain) may be quite strongly predictive of the presence of severe CAD (triple-vessel or left main CAD) and thus provide a strong indication for angiography (Fig. 50–2). Numerous studies attest to the adverse prognostic effect of congestive heart failure (based on a clinical history and/or the presence of cardiomegaly on chest radiography), previous myocardial infarction, hypertension, and advanced age in patients with stable angina pectoris.[18] A third heart sound is a useful clinical predictor of an abnormal left ventricular ejection fraction and an adverse prognosis in patients with CAD. The severity of angina, especially the tempo of intensification, is also an important predictor of outcome. On the other hand, a normal resting ECG in patients with stable angina pectoris speaks in favor of well-preserved left ventricular function and a favorable long-term prognosis.

NONINVASIVE TESTING

Exercise Electrocardiography. The prognostic importance of the treadmill exercise test was determined by several observational studies in the 1980s and early 1990s. One of the most important and consistent predictors is the maximal exercise capacity, regardless of whether it is measured by exercise duration or workload achieved or whether the test was terminated because of dyspnea, fatigue, or angina. After adjustment for age, the peak exercise capacity measured in metabolic equivalents is among the strongest predictors of mortality among men with cardiovascular disease.[86] Other factors with a poor prognosis identified in individual series of patients with chronic stable angina are described in Table 50–4 .

Stress Nuclear Myocardial Perfusion Imaging (see Chaps. 13 and 16). Although myocardial perfusion imaging was developed as a diagnostic tool for determining the presence or absence of CAD, its prognostic value is now well established.[87] In particular, the ability of myocardial perfusion SPECT to identify patients at low (<1 percent), intermediate (1 to 5 percent), or high (>5 percent) risk for future cardiac events is essential to patient management decisions. The prognostic data obtained from myocardial perfusion SPECT are incremental over the clinical and treadmill exercise data for predicting future cardiac events. Among patients with normal SPECT imaging the annual risk of death or myocardial infarction is less than 1 percent.

Echocardiography. Echocardiographic assessment of left ventricular function is one of the most valuable aspects of noninvasive imaging. Such testing is not necessary for all patients with angina pectoris, and among patients with a normal ECG and no previous history of myocardial infarction, the likelihood of preserved left ventricular systolic function is high. In contrast, among patients with a history of myocardial infarction, ST-T wave changes, or conduction defects or Q waves on the ECG, left ventricular function should be measured with echocardiography or an equivalent technique.

Evidence is increasingly demonstrating that echocardiography with exercise or pharmacological stress (dobutamine, arbutamine, or dipyridamole) is both sensitive and specific for the identification of myocardial ischemia and for risk stratification in patients with chronic stable angina.[88] The presence or absence of inducible regional wall motion abnormalities and the response of the ejection fraction to exercise appear to provide incremental prognostic information in addition to the assessment of cardiac structure and function provided by the resting echocardiogram. Moreover, a negative stress test portends a low risk for future events (<1 percent per person-year).

ANGIOGRAPHIC CRITERIA. The independent impact of multivessel disease and left ventricular dysfunction and their interaction on the prognosis of patients with CAD is well established (Fig. 50–3). The adverse effects of impaired ventricular function on prognosis are more pronounced as the number of stenotic vessels increases.[18]

Although several indices have been used to quantify the extent of severity of CAD, the simple classification of disease into single-, double-, triple-vessel, or left main CAD is the most widely used and is effective. Additional prognostic information is provided by the severity of obstruction and the location, whether proximal or distal. The concept of the gradient of risk is illustrated in Figure 50–4. Studies of treated symptomatic patients have revealed that if only one of the three major coronary arteries has more than 50 percent stenosis, the annual mortality rate is approximately 2 percent. The importance to survival of the quantity of myocardium that is jeopardized is reflected in the observation that an obstructive lesion proximal to the first septal perforating branch of the left anterior descending coronary artery was associated with a 5-year survival rate of 90 percent in comparison with 98 percent for patients with more distal lesions.[89] The survival rate of patients with isolated right CAD at 5 years appeared to be higher (96 percent) than for patients with disease of the left anterior descending coronary artery (92 percent). The overall survival of medically treated patients with left anterior descending and left circumflex CAD was not significantly different, but both were less than the survival of patients with isolated right CAD.

High-grade lesions of the left main coronary artery or its "equivalent," as defined by severe proximal left anterior descending and proximal left circumflex CAD, are particularly life threatening.[90] Mortality among medically treated patients has been reported to be 29 percent at 18 months and 43 percent at 5 years. Survival is better for patients with 50 to 70 percent stenosis (1- and 3-year survival rates of 91 and 66 percent, respectively) than for patients with a left main coronary artery stenosis greater than 70 percent (1- and 3-year survival rates of 72 and 41 percent). Furthermore, a number of characteristics found at catheterization or on noninvasive examination are predictors of an adverse prognosis in

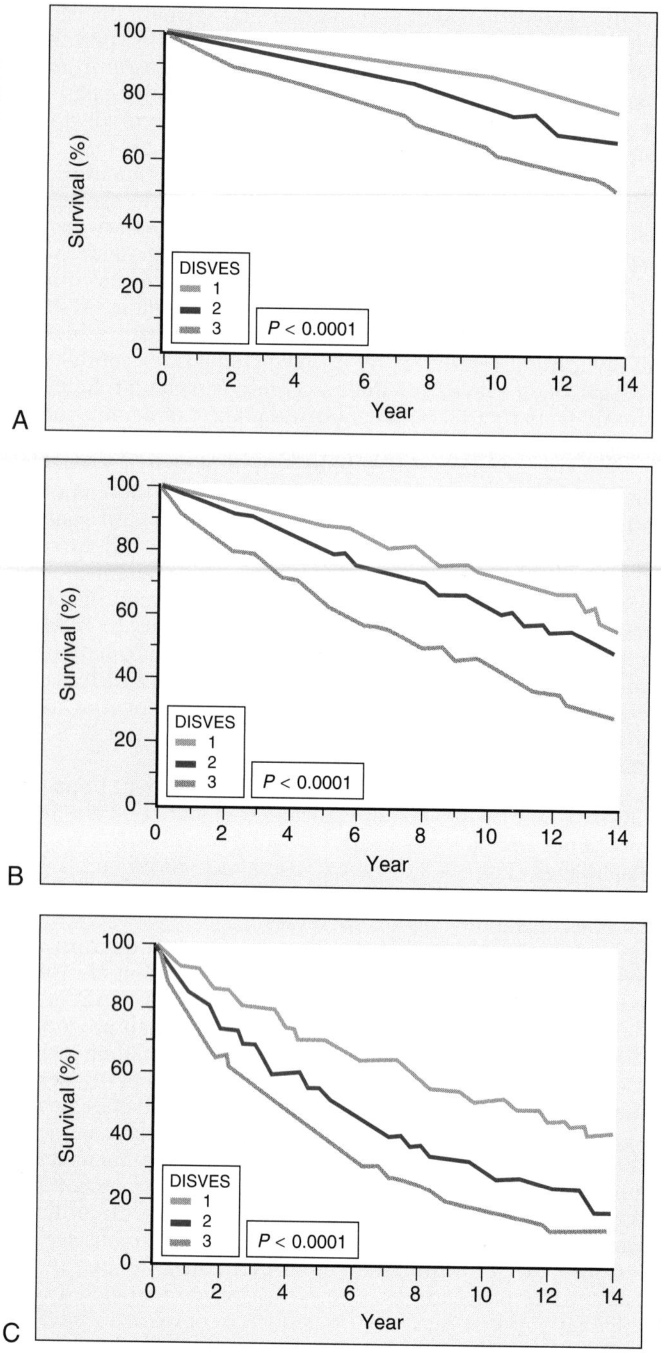

FIGURE 50–3 Graphs showing survival for medically treated CASS patients. **A,** Patients with single-, double-, or triple-vessel disease and an ejection fraction of 0.50 to 1.00 stratified by the number of diseased vessels (DISVES). **B,** Patients with single-, double-, or triple-vessel disease and an ejection fraction of 0.35 to 0.49 stratified by the number of diseased vessels. **C,** Patients with single-, double-, or triple-vessel disease and an ejection fraction of ≤0.34 stratified by the number of diseased vessels. (**A** to **C,** From Emond M, Mock MB, Davis KB, et al: Long-term survival of medically treated patients in the Coronary Artery Surgery Study [CASS] Registry. Circulation 90:2645, 1994.)

patients with 70 percent or greater left main coronary artery stenosis, including chest pain at rest, ST-T wave changes on resting ECG, cardiomegaly on chest radiography, a history of congestive heart failure, and the presence of left ventricular dysfunction at catheterization.

Limitations of Angiography. The pathophysiological significance of coronary stenoses lies in their impact on resting and exercise-induced blood flow, *and* in their potential for plaque rupture with superimposed thrombotic occlusion. It is generally accepted that a stenosis of greater than 60 percent of the luminal diameter is hemodynamically significant in that it may be responsible for a reduction in exercise-induced myocardial blood flow and cause angina and ischemia. The immediate functional significance of obstruction of "intermediate" severity (~50 percent diameter stenosis) is less well established. Coronary angiography is not a reliable indicator of the functional significance of stenosis, nor is it sensitive to the presence of thrombus. Moreover, the coronary angiographic determinants of the severity of stenosis are based on a decrease in the caliber of the lumen at the site of the lesion *relative* to adjacent reference segments, which are considered, often erroneously, to be relatively free of disease. This approach may lead to significant underestimation of the severity and extent of atherosclerosis.[74]

The most serious limitation to the routine use of coronary angiography for prognosis in patients with chronic stable angina is its inability to identify which coronary lesions can be considered to be at high risk, or "vulnerable," for future events, such as myocardial infarction or sudden death. Although it is widely accepted that myocardial infarction is the result of thrombotic occlusion at the site of plaque rupture or erosion (see Chap. 46), it is clear that it is not necessarily the plaque causing the most severe stenosis that subsequently ruptures. Lesions causing mild obstructions can rupture, thrombose, and occlude, thereby leading to myocardial infarction and sudden death. Approaches to quantifying the extent of coronary disease, inclusive of nonobstructive lesions, appear to offer additional prognostic information.[91] In contrast, arteries with severe preexisting stenoses may proceed to clinically silent complete occlusion, often without infarction, presumably because of the formation of collaterals as ischemia gradually becomes more severe.

In summary, angiographic documentation of the extent of CAD provides useful information toward assessment of the patient's risk of death and future ischemic events and is an indispensable step in the selection of patients for coronary revascularization, particularly if the interaction between the anatomical extent of disease, left ventricular function, and the severity of ischemia is taken into account. However, angiography is *not* helpful in predicting the site of subsequent plaque rupture or erosion that can precipitate myocardial infarction or sudden cardiac death. Additional tools that improve the imaging of coronary atheroma (e.g., IVUS), or the functional assessment of a stenosis (Doppler determination of coronary flow reserve) may be helpful in deciding on the flow-limiting significance of a specific lesion and the need for coronary revascularization.

Medical Management

Comprehensive management of chronic stable angina has five aspects: (1) identification and treatment of associated diseases that can precipitate or worsen angina; (2) reduction of coronary risk factors; (3) application of general and nonpharmacological methods, with particular attention toward adjustments in life style; (4) pharmacological management; and (5) revascularization by percutaneous catheter-based techniques or by coronary bypass surgery. Although discussed individually in this chapter, all five of these approaches must be considered, often simultaneously, in each patient. Among the medical therapies, three (aspirin, angiotensin-converting enzyme [ACE] inhibition, and effective lipid lowering) have been convincingly shown to reduce mortality and morbidity in patients with chronic stable angina and preserved left ventricular function. Other therapies such as nitrates, beta blockers, and calcium antagonists have been shown to improve symptomatology and exercise performance, but their effect, if any, on survival in patients with stable angina has not been demonstrated.

In stable patients with left ventricular dysfunction following myocardial infarction, data consistently indicate that ACE inhibitors and beta blockers reduce both mortality and the risk of repeat infarction, and these agents are recommended in such patients, with or without chronic angina, along with aspirin and lipid-lowering drugs.

TREATMENT OF ASSOCIATED DISEASES. Several common medical conditions that can increase myocardial O_2 demand or reduce O_2 delivery may contribute to the onset of new angina pectoris or the exacerbation of previously stable angina. These conditions include anemia, marked weight gain, occult thyrotoxicosis, fever, infections, and tachycardia. Drugs such as amphetamines and isoproterenol increase myocardial O_2 demand, as do other agents that stimulate the sympathetic nervous system. Cocaine, which can cause acute coronary spasm and myocardial infarction, is discussed in Chapter 62. In patients with CAD, heart failure, by causing cardiac dilation, mitral regurgitation, or tachyarrhythmias (including sinus tachycardia), can increase myocardial O_2 need, along with an increase in the frequency and severity of angina. Identification and treatment of these conditions are critical to the management of chronic stable angina.

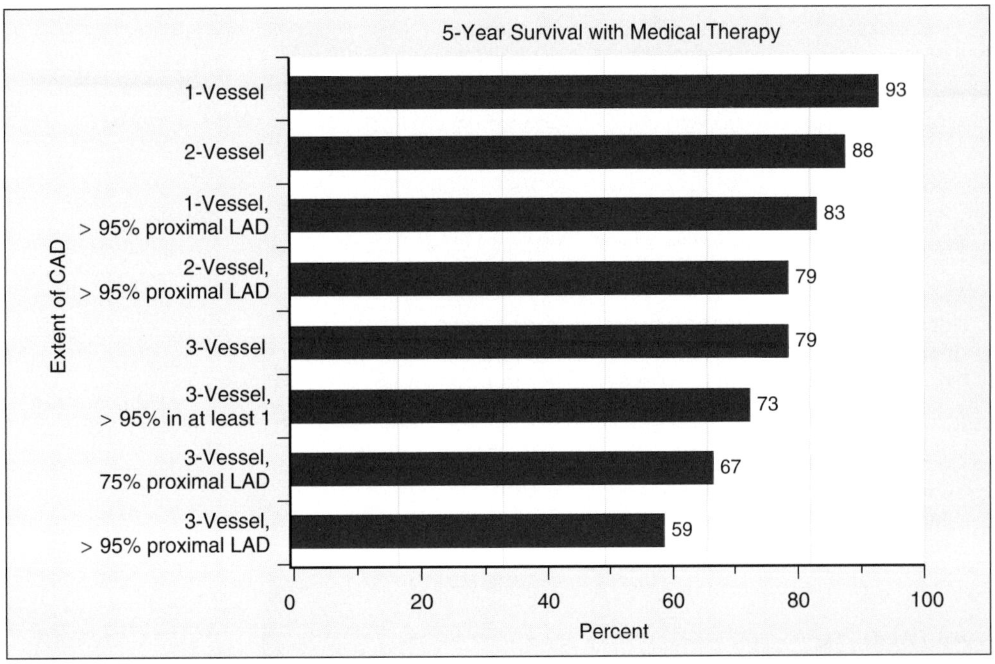

FIGURE 50–4 Angiographic extent of coronary artery disease (CAD) and subsequent survival with medical therapy. A gradient of mortality risk is established based on the number of diseased vessels and the presence and severity of disease of the proximal left anterior descending (LAD) artery. (Data from Califf RM, Armstrong PW, Carver, JR, et al: Task Force 5: Stratification of patients into high-, medium-, and low-risk subgroups for purposes of risk factor management. J Am Coll Cardiol 27:964-1047, 1996.)

Reduction of Coronary Risk Factors

HYPERTENSION (see Chaps. 37, 38, and 42). Epidemiological links between increased blood pressure and CAD severity and mortality are well established.[92] For individuals aged 40 to 70 years, the risk of ischemic heart disease doubles for each 20 mm Hg increment in systolic blood pressure across the entire range of 115 to 185 mm Hg.[93] Hypertension predisposes to vascular injury, accelerates the development of atherosclerosis, increases myocardial O_2 demand, and intensifies ischemia in patients with preexisting obstructive coronary vascular disease. Although the relationship between hypertension and CAD is linear,[93] left ventricular hypertrophy is a stronger predictor of myocardial infarction and CAD death than is the actual degree of increase in blood pressure.[94] A meta-analysis of clinical trials of treatment of mild to moderate hypertension showed a statistically significant 16 percent reduction in CAD events and mortality in patients receiving antihypertensive therapy.[95] This treatment effect is nearly twice as great in older compared with younger persons. It is logical to extend these observations on the benefits of antihypertensive therapy to patients with established CAD.[96] Moreover, the number of individuals treated to avoid one death is lower in subjects with established cardiovascular disease.[97] Therefore, blood pressure control is an essential aspect of the management of patients with chronic stable angina.

CIGARETTE SMOKING. This remains one of the most powerful risk factors for the development of CAD in all age groups (see Chap. 36). Among patients with angiographically documented CAD, cigarette smokers have a higher 5-year risk of sudden death, myocardial infarction, and all-cause mortality than do those who have stopped smoking. Moreover, smoking cessation lessens the risk of adverse coronary events in patients with established CAD.[98] Cigarette smoking may be responsible for aggravating angina pectoris other than through the progression of atherosclerosis. It may increase myocardial O_2 demand and reduce coronary blood flow by means of an alpha-adrenergically mediated increase in coronary artery tone and thereby cause acute ischemia.[99] Cigarette smoking also appears to reduce the efficacy of antianginal drugs. Smoking cessation is one of the most effective and certainly the least expensive approach to the prevention of disease progression in native vessels and bypass grafts. Strategies for smoking cessation are discussed in Chapter 43.

MANAGEMENT OF DYSLIPIDEMIA (see Chap. 39). Clinical trials in patients with established atherosclerotic vascular disease have demonstrated a significant reduction in subsequent cardiovascular events in patients with a wide range of serum cholesterol and LDL cholesterol levels who are treated with 3-hydroxy-3-methylglutaryl coenzyme A (HMG-CoA) reductase inhibitors (statins).[100-104] Angiographic trials of cholesterol lowering in patients with chronic CAD, many of whom had chronic stable angina, have shown that the effects on coronary obstruction are modest, in contrast with the substantive reduction in cardiovascular events. Several, but not all, studies have shown that statins significantly improve endothelium-mediated responses in the coronary and systemic arteries of patients with hypercholesterolemia or known atherosclerosis.[105]

Lipid-lowering with statins has been shown to reduce circulating levels of C-reactive protein[106,107] decrease thrombogenicity,[108] and favorably alter the collagen and inflammatory components of arterial atheroma;[109] these effects do not appear to correlate well with the change in serum LDL cholesterol and suggest antiatherothrombotic properties of statins.[110] These findings may explain the improvement in

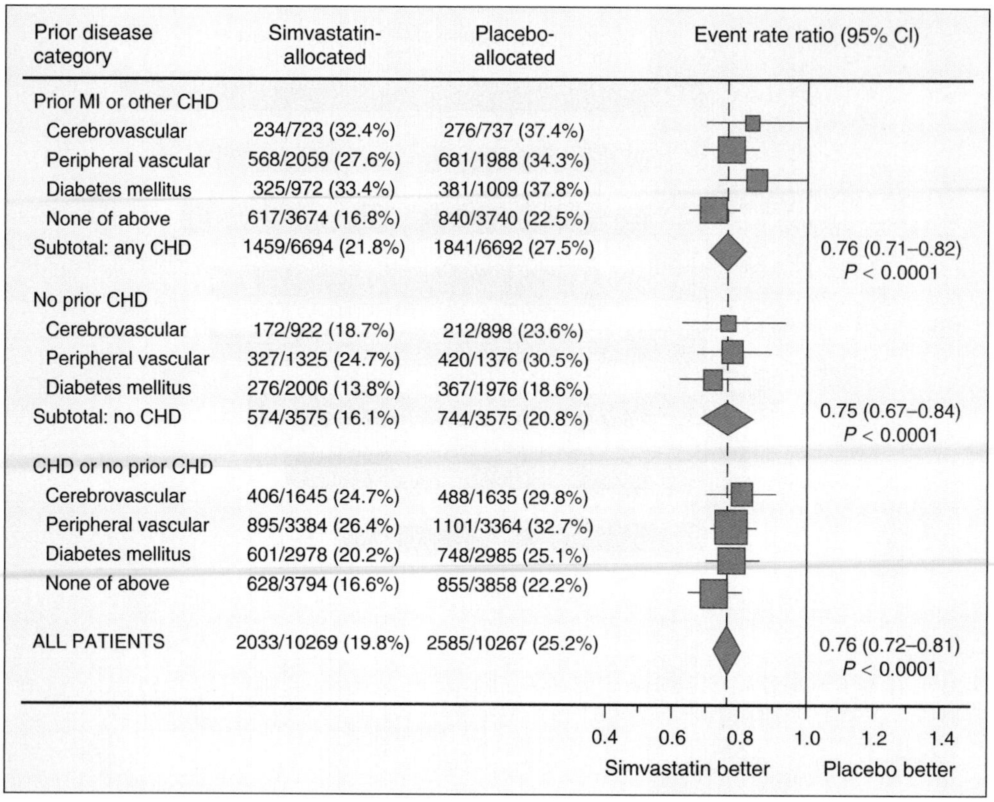
Prior disease category
Simvastatin-allocated
Placebo-allocated
Event rate ratio (95% CI)
Prior MI or other CHD
Cerebrovascular 234/723 (32.4%) 276/737 (37.4%)
Peripheral vascular 568/2059 (27.6%) 681/1988 (34.3%)
Diabetes mellitus 325/972 (33.4%) 381/1009 (37.8%)
None of above 617/3674 (16.8%) 840/3740 (22.5%)
Subtotal: any CHD 1459/6694 (21.8%) 1841/6692 (27.5%)
0.76 (0.71–0.82)
P < 0.0001
No prior CHD
Cerebrovascular 172/922 (18.7%) 212/898 (23.6%)
Peripheral vascular 327/1325 (24.7%) 420/1376 (30.5%)
Diabetes mellitus 276/2006 (13.8%) 367/1976 (18.6%)
Subtotal: no CHD 574/3575 (16.1%) 744/3575 (20.8%)
0.75 (0.67–0.84)
P < 0.0001
CHD or no prior CHD
Cerebrovascular 406/1645 (24.7%) 488/1635 (29.8%)
Peripheral vascular 895/3384 (26.4%) 1101/3364 (32.7%)
Diabetes mellitus 601/2978 (20.2%) 748/2985 (25.1%)
None of above 628/3794 (16.6%) 855/3858 (22.2%)
ALL PATIENTS 2033/10269 (19.8%) 2585/10267 (25.2%)
0.76 (0.72–0.81)
P < 0.0001
0.4 0.6 0.8 1.0 1.2 1.4
Simvastatin better
Placebo better

FIGURE 50–5 Effect of simvastatin on cardiovascular events among patients with and without coronary heart disease (CHD) in the Heart Protection Study. Among 13,386 patients with CHD enrolled in the Heart Protection Study, simvastatin (40 mg daily) reduced the risk of major vascular events (cardiovascular death, myocardial infarction [MI], stroke, or arterial revascularization) by 24 percent. CI = confidence interval. (From the Heart Protection Study Collaborative Group: MRC/BHF Heart Protection Study of cholesterol lowering with simvastatin in 20536 high risk individuals: A randomized placebo-controlled trial. Lancet 360:7-22, 2002.)

blood flow, the reduction in inducible myocardial ischemia, and the disproportionate reduction in coronary events in patients treated with statins despite small degrees of anatomical regression of atherosclerotic stenoses.

Results from secondary prevention trials of patients with a history of chronic stable angina, unstable angina, or previous myocardial infarction provide convincing evidence that effective lipid-lowering therapy significantly improves overall survival and reduces cardiovascular mortality in patients with coronary heart disease (see Chap. 39).[100-102] These effects have been demonstrated in both men and women and in the elderly[111,112] and provide a cost-effective approach to the management of large numbers of patients with chronic CAD.[113]

The National Cholesterol Education Program Guidelines (see Chap. 39)[27] advocate cholesterol-lowering therapy for all patients with coronary heart disease or extracardiac atherosclerosis to LDL levels below 100 mg/dl, and these guidelines have been adopted in recommendations from the ACC/AHA.[18] Moreover, the Heart Protection Study demonstrated an improvement in survival and reduction in future coronary events with statin therapy among individuals with diabetes, or cerebrovascular or peripheral vascular disease, as well as those with established CAD regardless of their baseline levels of cholesterol (Fig. 50–5).[104] In addition, results from the Pravastatin or Atorvastatin Evaluation and Infection Therapy (PROVE-IT)-TIMI 22 Trial demonstrated that among patients with a recent acute coronary syndrome, more aggressive lipid-lowering therapy, achieving LDL concentrations well below 100 mg/dl, provided greater protection against death or major cardiovascular events (see Fig. 49–11).[113a] These data provide additional support for aggressive cholesterol-lowering therapy among patients with established CAD.

Low HDL Cholesterol. Patients with established CAD and low levels of HDL cholesterol represent a subgroup with considerable risk for future coronary events.[114] Low HDL levels are often associated with obesity, hypertriglyceridemia, and insulin resistance and often signify the presence of small lipoprotein remnants and small dense LDL particles that are thought to be particularly atherogenic.[115] Therapy has focused on diet and exercise, as well as LDL cholesterol reduction in patients with a concomitant increase in LDL cholesterol.[27] The Veterans Affairs High-Density Lipoprotein Cholesterol Intervention Trial (VA-HIT) Study Group has demonstrated the efficacy of gemfibrozil treatment in patients with low HDL cholesterol (≤40 mg/dl) without elevations in LDL cholesterol (≤140 mg/dl) or triglycerides (mean, 160 mg/dl).[116] Gemfibrozil resulted in a 6 percent increase in HDL cholesterol and a 31 percent decrease in triglycerides, and these changes were associated with a 24 percent reduction in death, nonfatal myocardial infarction, and stroke ($p = 0.006$). The 22 percent reduction in cardiac death achieved only borderline statistical significance ($p = 0.07$).

Dyslipidemia after Myocardial Revascularization. In patients who have undergone coronary artery bypass grafting (CABG), elevation of LDL cholesterol is a risk factor for the development of saphenous vein graft occlusive disease, as well as progression of atherosclerosis in the native coronary arteries. Lipid-lowering therapy reduces mortality and acute coronary events in patients who have undergone either surgical or percutaneous revascularization,[117,118] and therapy for dyslipidemia should be given to these patients, as to all patients with chronic CAD.

ESTROGEN REPLACEMENT. A large data base derived from observational studies suggested a protective effect of hormone replacement therapy for postmenopausal women, with a 30 to 50 percent reduction in overall mortality from cardiovascular disease observed in these studies.[119] However, the major randomized, controlled secondary prevention trials have shown no cardiovascular benefit from hormone replacement therapy. Specifically, in the Heart and Estrogen/Progestin Replacement Study (HERS),[120] which randomly assigned postmenopausal women (mean age, 68 years) with established CAD to receive conjugated estrogen plus medroxyprogesterone or placebo, with a follow-up period of 4 years, no difference was seen in cumulative cardiac mortality or total cardiovascular events between the two groups despite a greater decrease in LDL cholesterol and increase in HDL cholesterol in the treatment group. The HERS-II study, which continued follow-up on unblinded therapy for an additional 2.7 years, also showed no difference between the treatment groups after 6.8 years.[121] Subsequent secondary prevention trials have added to the data indicating either no cardiovascular benefit or suggesting an increase in risk of coronary events with hormone replacement.[122-125] The increased risk of coronary heart disease among subjects treated with combined estrogen and progestin for primary prevention in the Women's Health Initiative bolsters these findings.[126] Thus, in light of the collective data from randomized clinical trials, it is *not* advised that hormone replacement therapy be initiated or continued for the purpose of secondary cardiovascular prevention in women with CAD.[18,127]

EXERCISE (see Chap. 43). The conditioning effect of exercise on skeletal muscles allows a greater workload at any level of total-body O_2 consumption. By decreasing the heart rate at any level of exertion, a higher cardiac output can be achieved at any level of myocardial O_2 consumption. The combination of these two effects of exercise conditioning permits patients with chronic stable angina to increase physical performance substantially following institution of a continuing exercise program.[128]

Most of the information about the physiological effects of exercise and their effect on prognosis in patients with CAD comes from studies on patients entered into cardiac rehabilitation programs, many of whom previously sustained a myocardial infarction.[129] Less information is available on the benefits of exercise in patients with chronic stable CAD, but nine small, randomized studies with a total of 980 patients have consistently demonstrated improved effort tolerance, O_2 consumption, and quality of life in patients undergoing exercise training.[18] Randomized trials evaluating symptom reduction and objective measures of ischemia in patients with stable CAD are few, with most supporting a reduction in symptoms or evidence of ischemia, such as with myocardial perfusion imaging.[18,128] Others have demonstrated a striking and direct relationship between the intensity of exercise and favorable changes in the morphology of obstructive lesions on angiography,[130] as well as favorable effects on vascular endothelial function thought to be mediated through expression and phosphorylation of endothelial nitric oxide synthase.[131] The question of whether exercise accelerates the development of collateral vessels in patients with chronic CAD remains unsettled.[132]

Exercise is safe if begun under supervision and increased gradually,[128,133] and if survivors of myocardial infarction can be used as a yardstick, it is probably cost-effective.[134] The psychological benefits of exercise are difficult to evaluate. However, a single nonrandomized study demonstrated significant improvement in well-being scores and positive-affect scores, as well as a reduction in disability scores, in patients in a structured exercise program.[18] In addition, exercise conditioning programs may be quite helpful in increasing the self-confidence of patients with chronic CAD. Patients who are involved in exercise programs are also more likely to be health conscious, to pay attention to diet and weight, and to discontinue cigarette smoking. For all the aforementioned reasons, patients should be urged to participate in regular exercise programs—usually walking—in conjunction with their drug therapy.[18,128]

INFLAMMATION (see Chaps. 35 and 42). Atherothrombosis has been identified as an inflammatory disease. Moreover, markers of systemic inflammation, including high-sensitivity C-reactive protein in particular, identify patients with established vascular disease who are at higher risk for death and future ischemic events.[135] Inflammation has now been identified as a potential target for therapeutic intervention in patients with CAD. Laboratory and clinical studies have provided evidence for antiinflammatory effects of established treatments aimed at other risk factors for atherogenesis (e.g., aspirin, statins, and ACE inhibitors); effects that may contribute, at least in part, to the proven clinical efficacy of these therapies.[136] For example, additional analyses from the Cholesterol and Recurrent Events (CARE) trial and the Air Force/Texas Coronary Atherosclerosis Prevention Study (AFCAPS/TexCAPS) are among the numerous studies that have demonstrated lowering of circulating levels of hs-CRP after treatment with statins.[136a] These findings lend support to the hypothesis that statins are effective in modifying the risk associated with evidence of systemic inflammation.[135,136] Other established preventive interventions, as well as novel therapeutic strategies, may also have antiinflammatory effects that could target inflammation as a risk factor in patients with CAD. ACE inhibitors, thiazolidinediones, thienopyridines, and fibric acid derivatives are among those agents that have been shown to exert antiinflammatory or immunoregulatory actions in animal models and/or in human studies.[136] Additional research is needed to clarify whether inflammation is a viable target for risk reduction in patients with stable CAD.

Additional Pharmacotherapy for Secondary Prevention

ASPIRIN (see Chaps. 42 and 80). A meta-analysis of 140,000 patients in 300 studies confirmed the prophylactic benefit of aspirin in both men and women with angina pectoris, previous myocardial infarction, or previous stroke and after bypass surgery.[137] In a Swedish trial of men and women with chronic stable angina, 75 mg of aspirin in conjunction with the beta blocker sotalol conferred a 34 percent reduction in acute myocardial infarction and sudden death.[138] In a smaller study confined to men with chronic stable angina but without a history of myocardial infarction, 325 mg of aspirin on alternate days reduced the risk of myocardial infarction during 5 years of follow-up by 87 percent.[139] Therefore, 75 to 325 mg of aspirin daily is advisable in patients with chronic stable angina but without contraindications to this drug.[18,140] Dosing at 75 to 150 mg daily appears to have comparable effects for secondary prevention to dosing at 160 to 325 mg daily[141] and may be associated with lower bleeding risk.[142]

Aspirin reduces the risk of subsequent myocardial infarction in healthy men with increased levels of C-reactive protein.[143] However, direct evidence that aspirin, administered in doses routinely used for secondary prevention, exerts antiinflammatory effects is mixed. In patients with established CAD and inducible myocardial ischemia, aspirin (300 mg/day) reduces circulating levels of C-reactive protein, macrophage colony–stimulating factor, and interleukin 6.[144] In contrast, aspirin (81 mg/day or 325 mg every third day) administered to healthy volunteers reduced measures of platelet activation but not C-reactive protein.[145] Aspirin also improves endothelial function in patients with atherosclerosis through a mechanism that may involve blockade of cyclooxygenase-dependent release of endothelium-derived constricting factors.[146]

Although warfarin has proved beneficial in patients after MI, no data support the use of chronic anticoagulation in patients with stable angina. However, a single large, randomized trial in patients with risk factors for atherosclerosis but without symptoms of angina has shown that low doses of warfarin (achieving a mean international normalized ratio [INR] of 1.47) combined with aspirin decrease the risk of coronary death and myocardial infarction when used for primary prevention in high-risk groups.[147] Any benefit of this combination must be balanced against the potential for increased bleeding, which was also noted in this study.

ASPIRIN INTERACTION WITH ACE INHIBITORS. With the increasing use of ACE inhibitors in patients with cardiovascular disease, concern has arisen about a possible adverse interaction between aspirin and these drugs. Aspirin has the potential to inhibit prostaglandin-mediated pathways of ACE inhibition, and evidence of such antagonism has been demonstrated in patients with hypertension and heart failure.[148] However, no evidence for an adverse interaction between aspirin and ACE inhibition (with ramipril) was observed in the substantially larger Heart Outcomes Prevention Evaluation (HOPE) trial.[149] Thus, current evidence supports aspirin therapy for all patients with CAD, including those taking ACE inhibitors. Ongoing clinical trials in this area will provide additional information.

CLOPIDOGREL. Another orally acting class of agents that block platelet aggregation are the thienopyridine derivatives, including clopidogrel.[150] Clopidogrel may be substituted for aspirin in patients with aspirin hypersensitivity or those who cannot tolerate aspirin (see Chap. 49). In a randomized comparison between clopidogrel and aspirin among patients with established atherosclerotic vascular disease (the Clopidogrel versus Aspirin in Patients at Risk of Ischaemic Events [CAPRIE] trial) treatment with clopidogrel resulted in a modest 8.7 percent relative reduction in the risk of vascular death, ischemic stroke, or myocardial infarction ($p = 0.043$) over 2 years.[151] Subsequent studies evaluating the addition of clopidogrel to aspirin among patients with non-ST elevation acute coronary syndromes[152] or after percutaneous coronary intervention[153] have indicated more robust risk reductions in these patient populations with CAD. Ongoing investigation will clarify the role of chronic treatment with clopidogrel for secondary prevention in patients with chronic stable angina.

BETA BLOCKERS. The value of beta blockers in reducing death and recurrent myocardial infarction in patients who have experienced a myocardial infarction is well established (see Chap. 46),[154] as is their usefulness in the treatment of angina. Whether these drugs are also of value in preventing infarction and sudden death in patients with chronic stable angina without previous infarction is uncertain, and there have been no controlled trials against placebo. However, there is no reason to assume that the favorable effects of beta blockers on ischemia and perhaps on arrhythmias should not apply to patients with chronic stable angina pectoris. Therefore, it is sensible to use these drugs when angina, hypertension, or both are present in patients with chronic CAD and when these drugs are well tolerated.

ACE INHIBITORS. Although ACE inhibitors are not indicated for the treatment of angina, these drugs appear to have important benefits in reducing the risk of future ischemic events. An unexpected and far-reaching finding from randomized trials of ACE inhibitors in postinfarct and other patients with ischemic and nonischemic causes of left ventricular dysfunction is the striking reduction in incidence of subsequent ischemic events such as myocardial infarction, unstable angina, and the need for coronary revascularization procedures.[155,156] Data from four trials including approximately 11,000 patients demonstrated a statistically significant risk reduction in myocardial infarction of 21 percent and in subsequent unstable angina of 15 percent.[156] The potentially beneficial effects of ACE inhibitors include a reduction in left ventricular hypertrophy, vascular hypertrophy, progression of atherosclerosis, plaque rupture, and thrombosis, in addition to a potentially favorable influence on myocardial O_2 supply/demand relationships and cardiac hemodynamics and a reduction in sympathetic activity.[156] Recent evidence also indicates that ACE inhibitors enhance coronary endothelial vasomotor function in patients with CAD,[157] which may contribute to enhanced myocardial blood flow during increases in myocardial demand.[158] In addition, in vitro experiments show that angiotensin II induces inflammatory changes in human vascular smooth muscle cells,[159] and treatment with ACE inhibitors can reduce signs of inflammation in animal models of atherosclerosis.[160]

These beneficial effects of ACE inhibitors on vascular structure and function should in theory extend beyond patients with left ventricular dysfunction to a much wider range of patients with CAD, including those with normal left ventricular function. This is the subject of several randomized, multicenter trials. The first of these trials to be completed provided strong evidence supporting the therapeutic benefit of ACE inhibitors. The HOPE study enrolled 9297 patients with atherosclerotic vascular disease or diabetes and at least one other CAD risk factor and randomly assigned them to receive ramipril (10 mg daily) or placebo; the mean follow-up was 5 years.[149] Eighty percent of patients had CAD, only 12 percent of whom had a myocardial infarction within 1 year after enrollment. No patient had heart failure symptoms on study entry, and echocardiograms (available for 5183 patients) demonstrated preserved left ventricular function (ejection fraction ≥0.40) in 92 percent of patients. Ramipril significantly decreased the risk of the primary composite endpoint of cardiovascular death, myocardial infarction, and stroke from 17.7 to 14.1 percent (relative risk reduction of 22 percent, $p < 0.001$). The relative decreases in cardiovascular death, myocardial infarction, and stroke were 25, 20, and 31 percent, respectively. The European Trial on Reduction of Cardiac Events with Perindopril in stable CAD (EUROPA) provided additional convincing support for the benefit of ACE inhibitors with respect to future cardiovascular events in patients with stable CAD in the absence of heart failure (Fig. 50–6).[160a] In both HOPE and EUROPA, the results were similar when examined in patient subsets defined by age, sex, known CAD, hypertension, diabetes, left ventricular function, or previous myocardial infarction. Beneficial effects were also similar in patients who were or were not taking aspirin in the HOPE trial.

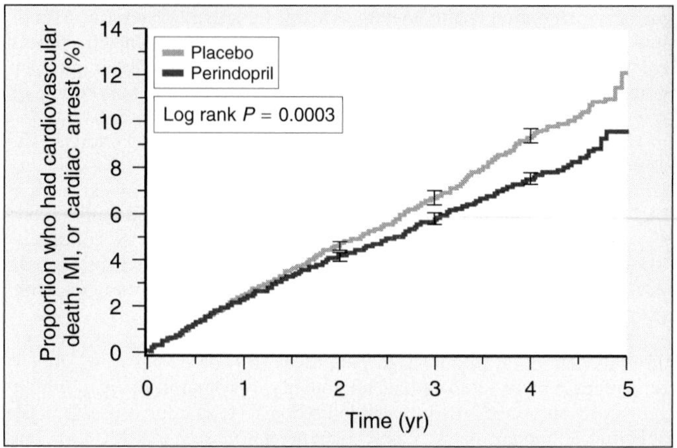

FIGURE 50–6 Kaplan-Meier time-to-event curves for the primary endpoint (cardiovascular death, myocardial infarction [MI], or cardiac arrest) with perindopril versus placebo among patients with stable coronary artery disease without apparent heart failure enrolled in the European Trial on the Reduction of Cardiac Events with Perindopril in Stable Coronary Artery Disease (EUROPA Trial). The angiotensin-converting enzyme inhibitor perindopril conferred a 20 percent relative reduction in the risk of the primary endpoint ($p = 0.0003$). (From EUROPA Investigators: Efficacy of perindopril in reduction of cardiovascular events among patients with stable coronary artery disease: Randomized double-blind, placebo-controlled, multicenter trial [the EUROPA study]. Lancet 363:782-788, 2003.)

In the 2002 AHA/ACC Guideline Update for management of patients with chronic stable angina, ACE inhibitors are recommended for all patients with CAD in conjunction with diabetes and/or left ventricular dysfunction.[18] The EUROPA study was reported after development of these guidelines. Considered together, the results of the HOPE and EUROPA studies have wide-reaching implications and suggest that patients with stable CAD, such as those enrolled in HOPE and EUROPA, should receive ACE inhibitor therapy. The role of ACE inhibition in lower risk patients with CAD is being studied in the PEACE trial.[160b]

ANTIOXIDANTS (see Chap. 42). Oxidized LDL particles are strongly linked to the pathophysiology of atherogenesis, and descriptive, prospective cohort, and case-control studies suggest that a high dietary intake of antioxidant vitamins (A, C, and beta-carotene) and flavonoids (polyphenolic antioxidants), naturally present in vegetables, fruits, tea, and wine, is associated with a decrease in coronary heart disease events.[161]

Despite this evidence for a beneficial effect of high dietary intake of antioxidant vitamins, randomized trials have not detected an advantage to treatment with supplemental beta-carotene, vitamin C, or vitamin E with respect to cardiovascular risk. Although the Cambridge Heart Antioxidant Study (CHAOS) reported a 77 percent reduction in myocardial infarction and a 47 percent reduction in all cardiovascular events among 2002 patients with angiographic CAD randomized to alpha-tocopherol compared with placebo,[162] two subsequent large, randomized, placebo-controlled trials have detected no benefit among individuals at high risk for or with established CAD.[163,164] The Heart Protection Study Collaborative Group enrolled more than 20,000 individuals with established atherosclerotic vascular disease or diabetes mellitus and found no reduction in all-cause mortality, myocardial infarction, or other vascular events with supplementation of vitamin E, vitamin C, and beta-carotene versus matched placebo during 5 years of follow-up.[164] Thus, based on present evidence, there is no basis for recommending that individuals take supplemental vitamin E, vitamin C, or beta-carotene for the purpose of treating CAD.[18]

Counseling and Changes in Life Style

The psychosocial issues faced by a patient who develops chronic stable angina for the first time are similar to, although usually less intense than, those experienced by a patient with an acute myocardial infarction. Recent data have reinforced that depressive symptoms are strongly associated with health status as reported by the patient, including the burden of symptoms and overall quality of life, independently of left ventricular function and the presence of provokable ischemia.[165] In conjunction with counseling, treatment with a selective serotonin reuptake inhibitor appears to be safe and effective in managing depression among patients with acute coronary syndromes and may be expected to be safe among patients with stable CAD.[166] Thus, efforts to evaluate and treat depression among patients with CAD is an important element of their overall management.

An important aspect of the physician's role is to counsel patients in the kinds of work they can do and in their leisure activities, eating habits, vacation plans, and the like.[167] Certain changes in life style may be helpful, such as modifying strenuous activities if they constantly and repeatedly produce angina. These changes may be minor in many instances. For example, golfing could be modified to include the use of a golf cart instead of walking. A history of CAD and stable angina is not inconsistent with the ability to continue to perform exertion, which is important not only in regard to recreational activities and life style but also for patients in whom some physical exertion is required in their employment. However, isometric activities such as weight lifting and other activities such as snow shoveling, which involves an energy expenditure between 60 and 65 percent of peak oxygen consumption, and cross-country or downhill skiing are undesirable. In addition, some activities expose the individual to the detrimental effects of cold on the O_2 demand/supply relationship, and these activities should also be avoided whenever possible.

Eliminating or reducing the factors that precipitate anginal episodes is of obvious importance. Patients learn their usual threshold by trial and error. Patients should avoid *sudden* bursts of activity, particularly after long periods of rest or after meals and in cold weather. Both chronic angina and unstable angina exhibit a circadian rhythm characterized by a lower angina threshold shortly after arising.[168] Therefore, morning activities such as showering, shaving, and dressing should be done at a slower pace and, if necessary, with the use of prophylactic nitroglycerin. The stress of sexual intercourse is approximately equal to that of climbing one flight of stairs at a normal pace or any activity that induces a heart rate of approximately 120 beats/min. With proper precautions (i.e., commencing more than 2 hours postprandially and taking an additional dose of a short-acting beta blocker 1 hour before and nitroglycerin 15 minutes before), most patients with chronic stable angina are able to continue satisfactory sexual activity. Although it is desirable to minimize the number of bouts of angina, an occasional episode is not to be feared. Indeed, unless patients occasionally reach their angina threshold, they may not appreciate the extent of their exercise capacity. Patients with stable CAD may use sildenafil but not in conjunction with nitrates.

Marked restriction in activity or even complete bed rest, in addition to drug therapy, may occasionally be necessary to control symptoms. In less critical situations, merely reducing the amount of time spent working or increasing the rest periods has a beneficial effect. For example, a long lunch break that includes a short nap may be beneficial. It may be helpful for the patient to use a face mask or scarf to cover the mouth or nose in cold weather. A hot, humid environment may also precipitate angina, and air conditioning may be a necessity rather than a luxury for patients with chronic angina. Large meals can have a similar effect if they are followed by exertion. An effort should be made to minimize emotional outbursts because they too increase myocardial O_2 requirements and sometimes induce coronary vasoconstriction. Occasionally, antianxiety drugs and sedatives or relaxation techniques using biofeedback mechanisms may be helpful.

Pharmacological Management of Angina Pectoris

Nitrates

MECHANISM OF ACTION. Even though the clinical effectiveness of amyl nitrite in angina pectoris was first described in 1867 by Brunton, organic nitrates are still the drugs most commonly used in the treatment of patients with this condition. The action of these agents is to relax vascular smooth muscle.[169] The vasodilator effects of nitrates are evident in both systemic (including coronary) arteries and veins in normal subjects and in patients with ischemic heart disease, but they appear to be predominant in the venous circulation. The venodilator effect reduces ventricular preload, which in turn reduces myocardial wall tension and O_2 requirements. The action of nitrates in reducing both preload and afterload makes them useful in the treatment of heart failure (see Fig. 50-1), as well as angina pectoris. By reducing the heart's mechanical activity, volume, and O_2 consumption, nitrates increase exercise capacity in patients with ischemic heart disease, thereby allowing a greater total-body workload to be achieved before the angina threshold is reached. In patients with stable angina, nitrates improve exercise tolerance and time to ST segment depression during treadmill exercise tests. When used in combination with calcium-channel blockers and/or beta blockers, the antianginal effects appear greater.[18]

EFFECTS ON THE CORONARY CIRCULATION (Table 50–5). Quantitative, computer-assisted measurements of coronary arterial diameter have been used to show that nitroglycerin causes dilation of epicardial stenoses. These stenoses are often eccentric lesions, and nitroglycerin causes relaxation of the smooth muscle in the wall of the coronary artery that is not encompassed by plaque. Even a small increase in a narrowed arterial lumen can produce a significant reduction in resistance to blood flow across obstructed regions.[170] Nitrates may also exert a beneficial effect in patients with impaired coronary flow reserve by alleviating the vasoconstriction caused by endothelial dysfunction.[171]

REDISTRIBUTION OF BLOOD FLOW. Studies in experimental animals with coronary obstruction have shown that nitroglycerin causes redistribution of blood flow from normally perfused to ischemic areas, particularly in the subendocardium.[172] This redistribution may be mediated in part by an increase in collateral blood flow and in part by lowering of ventricular diastolic pressure, thereby reducing subendocardial compression. Nitroglycerin appears to preferentially reduce coronary vascular resistance in viable myocardium with ischemia as detected by SPECT imaging.[173] In patients with chronic stable angina responsive to nitroglycerin, topical nitroglycerin under resting conditions alters myocardial perfusion by preferentially increasing flow to areas of reduced perfusion with little or no change in global myocardial perfusion.[174]

ANTITHROMBOTIC EFFECTS. Stimulation of guanylate cyclase by nitric oxide (NO) results in inhibitory action on platelets in addition to vasodilation. Although the antithrombotic effects of intravenous nitroglycerin have been demonstrated both in patients with unstable angina and in those with chronic stable angina, the clinical significance of these actions is not clear.[175]

CELLULAR MECHANISM OF ACTION. Nitrates have the ability to cause vasodilation regardless of whether the endothelium is intact. After entering the vascular smooth muscle cell, nitrates are converted to

TABLE 50–5 Effects of Antianginal Agents on Indices of Myocardial Oxygen Supply and Demand*

		Beta-Adrenoceptor Blockers						
		ISA		*Cardioselective*		Calcium Antagonists		
Index	**Nitrates**	***No***	***Yes***	***No***	***Yes***	***Nifedipine***	***Verapamil***	***Diltiazem***
Supply								
Coronary resistance								
Vascular tone	↓↓	↑	0	↑	0↑	↓↓↓	↓↓↓	↓↓↓
Intramyocardial diastolic tension	↓↓↓	↑	0	↑	↑	↓↓	0↑	0
Coronary collateral circulation	↑	0	0	0	0	↑	0	↑
Duration of diastole	0(↓)	↑↑↑	0↓	↑↑↑	↑↑↑	0↑(↓↓)	↑↑↑(↓)	↑↑(↓)
Demand								
Intramyocardial systolic tension								
Preload	↓↓↓	↑	0	↑	↑	↓0	↑0↓	0↓
Afterload (peripheral vascular resistance)	↓	↑	↑	↑↑	↑	↓↓	↓	↓
Contractility	0(↑)	↓↓↓	↓	↓↓↓	↓↓↓	↓(↑↑)†	↓↓(↑)†	↓(↑)†
Heart rate	0(↑)	↓↓↓	0↓	↓↓↓	↓↓↓	0(↑↑)	↓↓(↑)	↓↓(↑)

ISA = intrinsic sympathomimetic activity.

From Shub C, Vlietstra RE, McGoon MD: Selection of optimal drug therapy for the patient with angina pectoris. Mayo Clin Proc 60:539, 1985.

*↑ = Increase; ↓ = decrease; 0 = little or no definite effect. The number of arrows represents the relative intensity of effect. Symbols in parentheses indicate reflex-mediated effects.

†Effect of calcium entry on left ventricular *contractility*, as assessed in the intact animal model. The net effect on *left ventricular performance* is variable since it is influenced by alterations in afterload, reflex cardiac stimulation, and the underlying state of the myocardium.

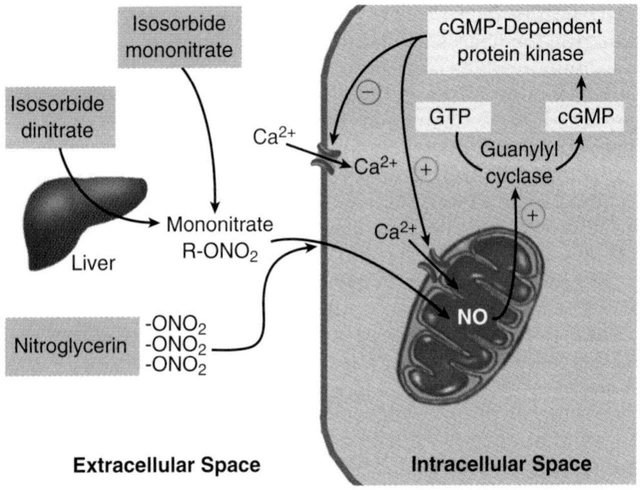

FIGURE 50–7 Mechanism of action of nitrates. Evidence exists that biotransformation of mononitrates occurs through action of mitochondrial aldehyde reductase producing nitric oxide (NO). NO activates soluble guanylyl cyclase, resulting in increased production of cyclic guanosine monophosphate (cGMP). The second messenger cGMP reduces cytoplasmic calcium (Ca^{2+}) by inhibiting inflow and stimulating mitochondrial uptake of calcium, thus mediating relaxation of smooth muscle cells and causing vasodilation. Isosorbide dinitrate is metabolized by the liver, whereas the liver is bypassed by mononitrates. GTP = guanosine triphosphate. R-ONO_2 = mononitrate. (Adapted from Gori T, Parker JD: Nitrate tolerance: A unifying hypothesis. Circulation 106:2510-2513, 2002; and Opie LH: Drugs for the Heart. 4th ed. Philadelphia, WB Saunders, 1995, p 33.)

reactive (NO) or *S*-nitrosothiols, which activate intracellular guanylate cyclase to produce cyclic guanosine monophosphate,[176] which in turn triggers smooth muscle relaxation and antiplatelet aggregatory effects (Fig. 50–7). Evidence now exists that the biotransformation of nitroglycerin occurs via mitochondrial aldehyde dehydrogenase and that inhibition of this enzyme may contribute to the development of tolerance.[177] Sulfhydryl (SH) groups appear to be required, at least as a cofactor, for both formation of NO and stimulation of guanylate cyclase, and nitroglycerin-induced vasodilation can be enhanced by prior administration of *N*-acetylcysteine, an agent that increases the availability of SH groups.[169] This action of *N*-acetylcysteine potentiates peripheral hemodynamic responses and the coronary vasodilator effect of nitroglycerin[178] and reverses the partial tolerance to the coronary vasodilator effect of nitroglycerin.

TABLE 50–6 Recommended Dosing Regimens for Long-Term Nitrate Therapy

Preparation of Agent	Dose	Schedule
Nitroglycerin*		
Ointment	0.5-2 inches	2 or 3 times daily
Buccal or transmucosal	1-3 mg	3 times daily
Transdermal patch	0.2-0.8 mg/hr	q 24 hr; remove at bedtime for 12-14 hr
Sublingual tablet	0.3-0.6 mg	As needed up to 3 doses 5 min apart
Spray	1-2 sprays	As needed up to 3 doses 5 min apart
Oral sustained release	2.5-6.5 mg	2 or 3 times daily†
Isosorbide Dinitrate*		
Oral	10-40 mg	2 or 3 times daily
Oral sustained release	80-120 mg	1 or 2 times daily (eccentric schedule)
Isosorbide 5-Mononitrate		
Oral	20 mg	2 times daily (given 7-8 hr apart)
Oral sustained release	30-240 mg	Once daily

*A 10- to 12-hour nitrate-free interval is recommended.

†Very limited data available on efficacy.

Types of Preparations and Routes of Administration (Table 50–6)

Nitroglycerin administered sublingually remains the drug of choice for the treatment of acute angina episodes and for the prevention of angina. Because sublingual administration avoids first-pass hepatic metabolism, a transient but effective concentration of the drug rapidly appears in the circulation. The half-life of nitroglycerin itself is brief, and it is rapidly converted to two inactive metabolites, both of which are found in the urine. Within 30 to 60 minutes, hepatic breakdown has abolished the hemodynamic and clinical effects. The usual sublingual dose is 0.3 to 0.6 mg, and most patients respond within 5 minutes to one or two 0.3-mg tablets. If symptoms are not relieved by a single dose, additional doses of 0.3 mg may be taken at 5-minute intervals, but no more than 1.2 mg should be used within a 15-minute period. The development of tolerance (see later) is rarely a problem with intermittent use. Sublingual nitroglycerin is especially useful when it is taken prophylactically shortly before undertaking physical activities that are likely to cause angina. When used for this purpose, it may prevent angina for up to 40 minutes.

ADVERSE REACTIONS. Adverse reactions are common and include headache, flushing, and hypotension. The last is rarely severe, but in some patients with volume depletion and in an upright posture, nitrate-induced hypotension is accompanied by a paradoxical bradycardia, consistent with a vasovagal or vasodepressor response. This reaction is more common in the elderly, who are less able to tolerate hypovolemia. Administration of nitrates before or soon after a meal, particularly in patients with a tendency toward postprandial hypotension, may augment venous pooling, preload reduction, and the extent of the fall in blood pressure after the meal. In addition, the partial pressure of O_2 in arterial blood may fall after large doses of nitroglycerin because of a ventilation-perfusion imbalance caused by inability of the pulmonary vascular bed to constrict in areas of alveolar hypoxia, thereby leading to perfusion of less hypoxic tissues. Methemoglobinemia is a rare complication of very large doses of nitrates; commonly used doses of nitrates cause small elevations of methemoglobin that are probably not of clinical significance.

PREPARATIONS (see Table 50–6)

Nitroglycerin Tablets. Nitroglycerin tablets tend to lose their potency, especially if exposed to light, and should thus be kept in dark containers. Other nitrate preparations are available in sublingual, buccal, oral, spray, and ointment forms. An oral nitroglycerin spray that dispenses metered, aerosolized doses of 0.4 mg may be better absorbed than the sublingual form in patients with dry mucosal membranes.[179] It can also be quickly sprayed onto or under the tongue. For prophylaxis, the spray should be used 5 to 10 minutes before angina-provoking activities.

Isosorbide Dinitrate. This drug is an effective antianginal agent but has low bioavailability after oral administration. It undergoes hepatic metabolism rapidly, and marked variation in plasma concentrations may be seen after oral administration. It has two metabolites (one has potent vasodilator action) that are cleared less rapidly than the parent drug and excreted unchanged in the urine. It is available in tablets for sublingual use, in chewable form, in tablets for oral use, and in sustained-release capsules.

Partial or complete nitrate tolerance (see later) develops with regimens of isosorbide dinitrate when it is administered as 30 mg three or four times daily.[180] A dosage schedule should be adopted that allows a 10- to 12-hour nitrate-free interval. If the drug is administered on a three-times-daily schedule (e.g., at 8 AM, 1 PM, and 6 PM), the antianginal benefit lasts for approximately 6 hours, and the magnitude of the antianginal benefit decreases with each successive dose.[180]

Isosorbide 5-Mononitrate. This active metabolite of the dinitrate is completely bioavailable with oral administration because it does not undergo first-pass hepatic metabolism, and it is efficacious in the treatment of chronic stable angina.[181] Plasma levels of isosorbide 5-mononitrate reach their peak between 30 minutes and 2 hours after ingestion, and the drug has a plasma half-life of 4 to 6 hours. A single 20-mg tablet still exhibits activity 8 hours after administration. Tolerance has not been demonstrated with once-a-day or eccentric dosing intervals but does occur with a twice-daily dosing regimen at 12-hour intervals. The only sustained-release preparation of isosorbide 5-mononitrate is Imdur, which is given once daily in a dose of 30 to 240 mg. Presumably, this preparation avoids tolerance by either providing a sufficiently low nitrate level or a duration of activity of 12 hours or less.

TOPICAL NITROGLYCERIN

Ointment. Nitroglycerin ointment (15 mg/inch) is efficacious when applied (most commonly to the chest) in strips of 0.5 to 2.0 inches. The delay in onset of action is approximately 30 minutes. Because this form of the drug is effective for 4 to 6 hours, it is particularly useful in patients with severe angina or unstable angina who are confined to bed and chair. Nitroglycerin ointment may also be used prophylactically after retiring by patients with nocturnal angina. Skin permeability increases with increased hydration, and absorption is also enhanced if the paste is covered with plastic whose edges are taped to the skin.

Transdermal Patches. Application of silicone gel or polymer matrix impregnated with nitroglycerin results in absorption for 24 to 48 hours at a rate determined by various methods of preparation of the patch, including a semipermeable membrane placed between the drug reservoir and the skin. The release rate of the patches varies from 0.1 to 0.8 mg per hour. Relatively low doses (0.1 to 0.2 mg/hr) may not produce sufficient plasma and tissue concentrations to sustain consistent, effective antianginal effects. Transdermal nitroglycerin therapy has been shown to increase exercise duration and maintain antiischemic effects for 12 hours after patch application throughout 30 days of therapy without significant evidence of nitrate tolerance or rebound phenomena,[182] provided that the patch is not applied for more than 12 out of 24 hours.

NITRATE TOLERANCE

A major problem with the use of nitrates is the development of nitrate tolerance, which has been demonstrated with all forms of nitrate administration delivering continuous, relatively stable blood levels of the drug.[169,180,182] Although nitrate tolerance is rapid in onset, renewed responsiveness is easily established after a short nitrate-free interval. The problem of tolerance applies to all nitrate preparations and is particularly important in patients with chronic stable angina pectoris, as opposed to those receiving short-acting courses of nitrates (e.g., unstable angina and myocardial infarction). Nitrate tolerance appears to be limited to the capacitance and resistance vessels and has not been noted in the large conductance vessels, including the epicardial coronary arteries and radial arteries, despite continuous administration of nitroglycerin for 48 hours.[183]

MECHANISMS. Several mechanisms of nitrate tolerance have been proposed.[169] Accumulating data support the hypothesis that increased generation of vascular superoxide anion ($\cdot O_2^-$) is central to the process.[184] There are multiple possible contributors to generation of oxygen free radicals, including effects of nitroglycerin on endothelial oxide synthase ("NOS uncoupling") and counterregulatory neurohormonal activation. The consequences of increased superoxide anion formation are also multiple and include plausible links to many of the proposed mechanisms of nitrate tolerance: (1) plasma volume expansion and neurohormonal activation; (2) impaired biotransformation of nitrates to NO; and (3) decreased end-organ responsiveness to NO.[184] A secondary implication of these emerging findings is that extended treatment with organic nitrates may have unfavorable consequences (free radical generation, endothelial dysfunction, and sympathetic activation) that could adversely affect long-term clinical outcomes.[184] Such data raise a cautionary note that warrants additional investigation.

MANAGEMENT. The only practical strategy to manage nitrate tolerance is to prevent it by providing a "nitrate-free" interval. The optimal interval is unknown, but with patches or ointment of nitroglycerin or preparations of isosorbide dinitrate or isosorbide 5-mononitrate, a 12-hour off period is recommended. The timing of administration should be adapted to the pattern of nitroglycerin administered by the sublingual route, which does not ordinarily result in tolerance, and even after 2 weeks of therapy, efficacy is not reduced when sublingual nitroglycerin is administered two or three times daily.[185]

NITRATE WITHDRAWAL. A common form of nitrate withdrawal (rebound) is observed in patients whose angina is intensified after discontinuation of large doses of long-acting nitrates.[186] In this situation, patients may also have heightened sensitivity to constrictor stimuli.[187] The potential for rebound can be modified by adjusting the dose and timing of administration in addition to the use of other antianginal drugs.

INTERACTION WITH SILDENAFIL. The combination of nitrates and sildenafil may cause serious, prolonged, and potentially life-threatening hypotension.[188] Nitrate therapy is an absolute contraindication to the use of sildenafil and vice versa. Patients who wish to take sildenafil should be aware of the serious nature of this adverse drug interaction and be warned about taking sildenafil within 24 hours of any nitrate preparation, including short-acting sublingual nitroglycerin tablets.

Beta-Adrenoceptor Blocking Agents

Beta-adrenoceptor blocking drugs (beta blockers) constitute a cornerstone of therapy for angina pectoris. In addition to their antiischemic properties, beta blockers are effective antihypertensives (see Chap. 38) and antiarrhythmics (see Chap. 30). They have also been shown to reduce mortality and reinfarction in patients after myocardial infarction (see Chap. 47) and to reduce mortality in patients with heart failure (see Chap. 23). This combination of actions makes them extremely useful in the management of chronic stable angina. A number of studies have shown that beta blockers, in doses that are generally well tolerated, reduce the frequency of anginal episodes and raise the anginal threshold, both when given alone and when added to other antianginal agents.

The salutary action of these drugs (which have a chemical structure resembling that of beta-adrenoceptor agonists) depends on their ability to cause competitive inhibition of the effects of neuronally released and circulating catecholamines on beta adrenoceptors (Table 50–7).[189] Beta blockade reduces myocardial O_2 requirements, primarily by slowing the heart rate; the slower heart rate in turn increases the fraction of the cardiac cycle occupied by diastole, with a corresponding increase in the time available for coronary perfusion (Fig. 50–8; see also Table 50–5). These drugs also reduce exercise-induced increases in blood pressure and limit exercise-induced increases in contractility. Thus, beta blockers reduce myocardial O_2 demand primarily during activity or excitement, when surges of increased sympathetic activity occur. In the face of impaired myocardial perfusion, the effects of beta blockers on myocardial O_2 demand may critically and favorably alter the imbalance between supply and demand, thereby resulting in the elimination of ischemia.

Beta blockers may reduce blood flow to most organs by means of the combination of unopposed alpha-adrenergic vasoconstriction and $beta_2$ receptor blockade. Complications are relatively minor, but in patients with peripheral vascular disease, the reduction in blood flow to skeletal muscles with the use of nonselective beta blockers may reduce maximal exercise capacity. In patients with preexisting left ventricular dysfunction, beta blockade may increase ventricular volume and thereby enhance O_2 demand.

Characteristics of Different Beta Blockers (Table 50–8)

SELECTIVITY. Two major subtypes of beta receptors, designated *$beta_1$* and *$beta_2$*, are present in different proportions in different tissues. $Beta_1$ receptors predominate in the heart, and stimulation of these receptors leads to an increase in heart rate, atrioventricular (AV) conduction, and contractility; release of renin from juxtaglomerular cells in the kidneys; and lipolysis in adipocytes. $Beta_2$ stimulation causes bronchodilation, vasodilation, and glycogenolysis. Nonselective beta-blocking drugs (propranolol, nadolol, penbutolol, pindolol, sotalol, timolol, carteolol) block both $beta_1$ and $beta_2$ receptors, whereas cardioselective beta blockers (acebutolol, atenolol, betaxolol, bisoprolol, esmolol, and metoprolol) block $beta_1$ receptors while having less effect on $beta_2$ receptors. Thus, cardioselective beta blockers reduce myocardial O_2 requirements while tending to not block bronchodilation, vasodilation, or glycogenolysis. However, as the doses of these drugs are increased, this cardioselectivity diminishes. Because cardioselectivity is only relative, the use of cardioselective beta blockers in doses sufficient to control angina may still cause bronchoconstriction in some susceptible patients.

Some beta blockers also cause vasodilation. Such drugs include labetalol (an alpha-adrenergic blocking agent and $beta_2$ agonist; see Chap. 38), carvedilol (with alpha- and $beta_1$-blocking activity), and bucindolol (a nonselective beta blocker that causes direct [non-alpha-adrenergic-mediated] vasodilation).[190]

ANTIARRHYTHMIC ACTIONS (see Chap. 30). Beta blockers have antiarrhythmic properties as a direct effect of their ability to block sym-

TABLE 50–7 Physiological Actions of Beta-Adrenergic Receptors

Organ	Receptor Type	Response to Stimulus
Heart		
SA node	$Beta_1$	Increased heart rate
Atria	$Beta_1$	Increased contractility and conduction velocity
AV node	$Beta_1$	Increased automaticity and conduction velocity
His-Purkinje system	$Beta_1$	Increased automaticity and conduction velocity
Ventricles	$Beta_1$	Increased automaticity, contractility, and conduction velocity
Arteries		
Peripheral	$Beta_2$	Dilation
Coronary	$Beta_2$	Dilation
Carotid	$Beta_2$	Dilation
Other	$Beta_1$	Increased insulin release Increased liver and muscle glycogenolysis
Lungs	$Beta_2$	Dilation of bronchi
Uterus	$Beta_2$	Smooth muscle relaxation

AV = atrioventricular; SA = sinoatrial.

From Abrams J: Medical therapy of stable angina pectoris. *In* Beller G, Braunwald E (eds): Chronic Ischemic Heart Disease. Atlas of Heart Disease. Vol 5. Philadelphia, WB Saunders 1995, p 7.19.

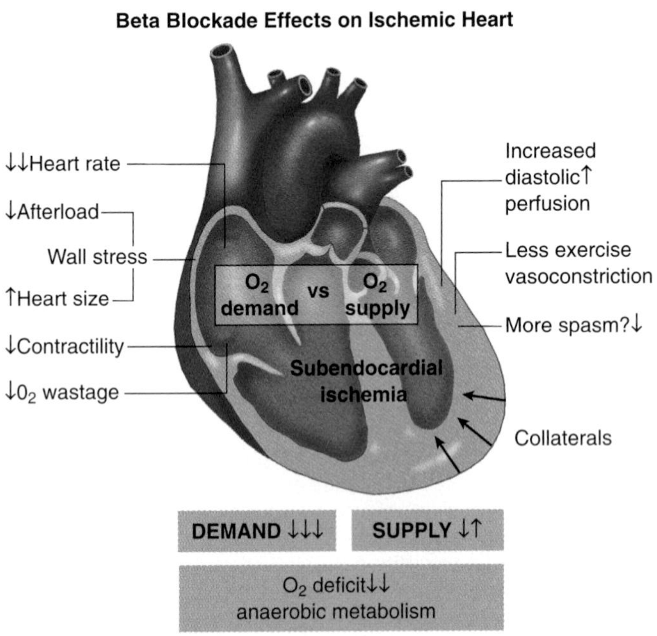

FIGURE 50–8 Effects of beta blockade on the ischemic heart. Beta blockade has a beneficial effect on ischemic myocardium unless (1) the preload rises substantially as in left-sided heart failure or (2) vasospastic angina is present, in which case spasm may be promoted in some patients. Note the proposal that beta blockade diminishes exercise-induced vasoconstriction. (Redrawn from Opie LH: Drugs for the Heart. 4th ed. Philadelphia, WB Saunders, 1995.)

pathoadrenal myocardial stimulation, which in certain situations may be arrhythmogenic.[191] Sotalol has combined class II (beta-blocking) and class III antiarrhythmic activities; it is a potentially attractive drug when it is desired to treat angina and suppress ventricular tachyarrhythmias[192] but should be used with caution in patients with left ventricular dysfunction and left ventricular hypertrophy, and it does have proarrhythmic effects.

INTRINSIC SYMPATHOMIMETIC ACTIVITY. Beta blockers with intrinsic sympathomimetic activity (ISA), such as acebutolol, bucindolol, carteolol, celiprolol, penbutolol, and pindolol, are partial beta agonists that also produce blockade by shielding beta receptors from more potent beta agonists. Pindolol and acebutolol produce low-grade beta stimulation when sympathetic activity is low (at rest), whereas these partial agonists behave more like conventional beta blockers when sympathetic activity is high. Agents with ISA may not be as effective as those without this property in reducing the heart rate or the frequency, duration, and magnitude of ambulatory ST segment changes or in increasing the duration of exercise in patients with severe angina.

POTENCY. Potency can be measured by the ability of beta blockers to inhibit the tachycardia produced by isoproterenol. All drugs are considered in reference to propranolol, which is given a value of 1.0 (see Table 50-8). Timolol and pindolol are the most potent agents, and acebutolol and labetalol are the least potent.

LIPID SOLUBILITY. The hydrophilicity or lipid solubility of beta blockers is a major determination of their absorption and metabolism. The lipid-soluble (lipophilic) beta blockers propranolol, metoprolol, and pindolol are readily absorbed from the gastrointestinal tract, are metabolized predominantly by the liver, have a relatively short half-life, and usually require administration twice or more daily to achieve continuing pharmacological effects. If either metoprolol or propranolol is administered intravenously, a much higher concentration reaches the bloodstream, and therefore intravenous dosing has much greater potency than oral dosing does. The water-soluble (hydrophilic) beta blockers (atenolol, sotalol, and nadolol) are not as readily absorbed from the gastrointestinal tract, are not as extensively metabolized, have relatively long plasma half-lives, and can be administered once daily. Water-soluble beta blockers are generally eliminated unchanged by the kidneys. Lipid-soluble agents are often preferable in patients with significant renal dysfunction for whom clearance of water-soluble agents is reduced. Greater lipid solubility is associated with greater penetration to the central nervous system and may contribute to side effects (e.g., lethargy, depression, and hallucinations) that are not clearly related to beta-blocking activity.

ALPHA-ADRENOCEPTOR BLOCKING ACTIVITY. The alpha-blocking potency of labetalol (approximately one-tenth that of phentolamine) is approximately 20 percent of its beta-blocking potency (see Table 50-8). Labetalol's combined alpha- and beta-blocking effects make it a particularly useful antihypertensive agent (see Chap. 38), and it is especially so in patients with hypertension and angina. The major side effects of labetalol are postural hypotension and retrograde ejaculation. Carvedilol is a newer beta blocker that also possesses alpha-adrenergic blocking activity with an $alpha_1$ to beta-blocking ratio of approximately 1 : 10.[190]

OXIDATION PHENOTYPE. The metabolism of metoprolol, carvedilol, and propranolol may be influenced by genetic polymorphisms or other medications.[193] The oxidative metabolism of metoprolol occurs primarily through the cytochrome P450 enzyme CYP2D6 and exhibits the debrisoquin type of genetic polymorphism; poor hydroxylators or metabolizers ($\leq$10 percent of whites) have significant prolongation of the elimination half-life of the drug in comparison to extensive hydroxylators or metabolizers. Thus, angina might be controlled by a single daily dose of metoprolol in poor metabolizers, whereas extensive metabolizers require the same dose two or three times a day.[194] If a patient exhibits an exaggerated clinical response (e.g., extreme bradycardia) following the administration of metoprolol, propranolol, or other lipid-soluble beta blockers, it may be the result of prolongation of the elimination half-life because of slow oxidative metabolism. Metabolism of metoprolol may also be altered by drugs that interact with CYP2D6.[193,195]

EFFECTS ON SERUM LIPIDS. Beta-blocker therapy (with agents lacking ISA) usually causes no significant changes in total or LDL cholesterol but increases triglycerides and reduces HDL cholesterol.[196] The most commonly studied drug has been propranolol, which can increase plasma triglyceride concentrations by 20 to 50 percent and reduce HDL cholesterol by 10 to 20 percent. Increasing $beta_1$ selectivity is associated with lesser effects on lipids. Adverse effects on the lipid profile may be more frequent with nonselective than with $beta_1$-selective blockers. The effects of these changes in serum lipids by long-term administration of beta blockers must be considered when this therapy is begun or maintained for either hypertension or angina.

DOSAGE. For optimal results, the dosage of a beta blocker should be carefully adjusted. In the case of atenolol, it is useful to start with a dose of 50 mg once daily. The usual effective dose is 50 to 100 mg daily; however, some patients benefit from up to 200 mg daily. In the case of metoprolol, it is often preferable from a perspective of the patient's compliance to use an extended-release formulation, which may be started at a dose of 100 mg once daily. Other beta blockers should be started at comparable doses. Efficacy is determined by the effect on the heart rate and symptoms, and when these are unclear, the effect on exercise performance can be evaluated by treadmill exercise testing. The resting heart rate should be reduced to between 50 and 60 beats/min, and an increase of less than 20 beats/min should occur with modest exercise (e.g., climbing one flight of stairs). Therapy with beta blockers needs to be individualized and requires repeated clinical evaluation during the initial period of drug administration.

ADVERSE EFFECTS AND CONTRAINDICATIONS. Most of the adverse effects of beta blockers occur as a consequence of the known properties of these drugs and include cardiac effects (severe sinus bradycardia, sinus arrest, AV block, reduced left ventricular contractility), bronchoconstriction, fatigue, mental depression, nightmares, gastrointestinal upset, sexual dysfunction, intensification of insulin-induced hypoglycemia, and cutaneous reactions (Table 50–9; see also Table 50–7). Lethargy, weakness, and fatigue may be caused by reduced cardiac output or may arise from a direct effect on the central nervous system.[197] Bronchoconstriction results from blockade of $beta_2$ receptors in the tracheobronchial tree. As a consequence, asthma and chronic obstructive lung disease are relative contraindications to beta blockers, even to $beta_1$-selective agents.

In patients who already have impaired left ventricular function, congestive heart failure may be intensified, an effect that can be counteracted in part by the use of digitalis or diuretics. Beginning therapy with a very low dose (e.g., metoprolol XL, 25 mg daily, for 2 weeks in patients with NYHA functional Class II) and then gradually increasing the dose over the course of several weeks has been shown to be well tolerated and beneficial in patients with idiopathic dilated cardiomyopathy and those with heart failure caused by ischemic heart disease (see Chap. 23).[198] This approach is recommended when using beta blockers in patients with angina and heart failure.

Beta blockers should be prescribed with caution in patients with cardiac conduction disease involving either the sinus node or the AV conduction system. In patients with symptomatic conduction disease, beta blockers are contraindicated unless a pacemaker is in place. In patients with asymptomatic sinus node dysfunction or first-degree AV block, beta blockers may be tolerated, but their administration requires careful observation. Pindolol, because of its ISA activity, may be preferable in this situation. Blockade of noncardiac $beta_2$ receptors inhibits catecholamine-induced glycogenolysis, so noncardioselective beta blockers can impair the defense to insulin-induced hypoglycemia. Blockade of $beta_2$ receptors also inhibits the vasodilating effects of catecholamines in peripheral blood vessels and leaves the constrictor (alpha-adrenergic) receptors unopposed, thereby enhancing vasoconstriction. Noncardioselective beta blockers may precipitate episodes of Raynaud phenomenon in patients with this condition and may cause uncomfortable coldness in the distal extremities. Reduced flow to the limbs may occur in patients with peripheral vascular disease.

Abrupt withdrawal of beta-adrenoceptor blocking agents after prolonged administration can result in increased total ischemic activity in patients with chronic stable angina. This increased ischemia may be caused by a return to the previously high levels of myocardial O_2 demand while the under-

TABLE 50–8 Pharmacokinetics and Pharmacology of Some Beta-Adrenoceptor Blockers

Characteristic	Atenolol	Metoprolol/XL	Nadolol	Pindolol	Propranolol/LA	Timolol
Extent of absorption (%)	~50	>95	~30	>90	>90	>90
Extent of bioavailability (% of dose)	~40	~50/77	~30	~90	~30/20	75
Beta-blocking plasma concentration	0.2-0.5 μg/ml	50-100 ng/ml	50-100 ng/ml	50-100 ng/ml	50-100 ng/ml	50-100 ng/ml
Protein binding (%)	<5	12	~30	57	93	~10
Lipophilicity*	Low	Moderate	Low	Moderate	High	Low
Elimination half-life (hr)	6-9	3-7	14-25	3-4	3.5 to 6/8-11	3-4
Drug accumulation in renal disease	Yes	No	Yes	No	No	No
Route of elimination	RE (mostly unchanged)	HM	RE	RE (40% unchanged and HM)	HM	RE (20% unchanged and HM)
Beta-blocker potency ratio (propranolol = 1)	1.0	1	1.0	6.0	1	6.0
Adrenergic-receptor blocking activity	β_1¶	β_1¶	β_1/β_2	β_1/β_2	β_1/β_2	β_1/β_2
Intrinsic sympathetic activity	0	0	0	+	0	0
Membrane-stabilizing activity	0	0	0	+	++	0
Usual maintenance dose	50-100 mg/d	50-100 mg b.i.d.–q.i.d./50-400 mg/d	40-80 mg/d	10-40 mg/d (b.i.d.–t.i.d.)	80-320 mg/d (b.i.d.–t.i.d.)/ 80-160 mg/d	10-30 mg b.i.d.
FDA-approved indications						
Hypertension	Yes	Yes/Yes	Yes	Yes	Yes/Yes	Yes
Angina	Yes	Yes/Yes	Yes	No	Yes/Yes	No
Post MI	Yes	Yes/No	No	No	Yes/No	Yes
Heart failure	No	Yes/Yes	No	No	No/No	No

FDA = Food and Drug Administration; HM = hepatic metabolism; ND = no data; RE = renal excretion; MI = myocardial infarction.
*Determined by the distribution ratio between octanol and water.
†Half-life of the active metabolite, diacetolol, is 12 to 15 hours.
‡Acebutolol is mainly eliminated by the liver, but its major metabolite, diacetolol, is excreted by the kidney.
§Rapid metabolism by esterases in the cytosol of red blood cells.
¶Beta$_1$ selectivity is maintained at lower doses, but beta$_2$ receptors are inhibited at higher doses.

lying atherosclerotic process has progressed,[199] but a rebound phenomenon resulting in increased beta-adrenergic sensitivity probably occurs in some patients. Occasionally, such withdrawal can precipitate unstable angina and may in rare cases even provoke myocardial infarction. Chronic beta-blocker therapy can be safely discontinued by slowly withdrawing the drug in a stepwise manner over the course of 2 to 3 weeks. If abrupt withdrawal of beta blockers is required, patients should be instructed to reduce exertion and manage angina episodes with sublingual nitroglycerin and/or substitute a calcium antagonist.

Calcium Antagonists (see Chap. 38)

The critical role of calcium ions in the normal contraction of cardiac and vascular smooth muscle is discussed in Chapter 19. Calcium antagonists are a heterogeneous group of compounds that inhibit calcium ion movement through slow channels in cardiac and smooth muscle membranes by noncompetitive blockade of voltage-sensitive L-type calcium channels (see Fig. 19–8).[200,201] The three major classes of calcium antagonists are the dihydropyridines (nifedipine is the prototype), the phenylalkylamines (verapamil is the prototype), and the modified benzothiazepines (diltiazem is the prototype). Amlodipine and felodipine are additional dihydropyridines that are among the most commonly used calcium antagonists in the United States. The two predominant effects of calcium antagonists result from blocking the entry of calcium ions and slowing recovery of the channel. Phenylalkylamines have a marked effect on recovery of the channel and thereby exert depressant effects on cardiac pacemakers and conduction, whereas dihydropyridines, which do not impair channel recovery, have little effect on the conduction system.

MECHANISM OF ACTION. The efficacy of calcium antagonists in patients with angina pectoris is related to the reduction in myocardial O_2 demand and the increase in O_2 supply that they induce (see Table 50–5).[200] The latter effect is particularly important in patients with conditions in which a prominent vasospastic or vasoconstrictor component may be present, such as Prinzmetal (variant) angina (see Chap. 49), variable-threshold angina, and angina related to impaired

Acebutolol	Labetalol	Bisoprolol	Betaxolol	Carteolol	Penbutolol	Carvedilol	Esmolol (IV)	Sotalol
~70	>90	>90	>90	>90	100	ND	ND	ND
~50	~25	80	90	85	100	~30	100	>90
0.2-2.0 μg/ml	0.7-3.0 μg/ml	0.01-0.1 μg/ml	20-50 ng/ml	40-160 ng/ml	ND	ND	0.15-2.0 μg/ml	ND
30-40	~50	30	50-60	23-30	80-98	95-98	55	0
Low	Low	Moderate	Moderate	Low	High	High	Low	Low
3-4[†]	~6	7-15	12-22	5-7	17-26	6-10	4.5 min	12
Yes[‡]	No	Yes	Yes	Yes	Yes	No	No	Yes
HM[‡]	HM	HM 50% RE 50%	HM	RE	HM	HM	§	RE
0.3	0.3	10	4	10	1	10	0.02	0.3
β_1[¶]	$\beta_1/\beta_2/\alpha_1$	β_1[¶]	β_1[¶]	β_1/β_2	β_1/β_2	$\beta_1/\beta_2/\alpha_1$	β_1[¶]	β_1/β_2
+	0	0	0	+	+	0	0	0
+	0	0	0	0	0	+	0	0
200-600 mg b.i.d.	100-400 mg b.i.d.	5-20 mg/d	5-20 mg/d	2.5-10 mg/d	10-40 mg/d	3.125-50 mg/ b.i.d.	Bolus of 500 μg/kg; infusion at 50-200 μg/kg/min	80-160 mg b.i.d.
Yes	Yes	Yes	Yes	Yes	Yes	Yes	Yes	No
No	No	No	No	No	No	No	No	No
No	No	No	No	No	No	No	Yes	No
No	No	No	No	No	No	Yes	No	No

vasodilator reserve of small coronary arteries.[202] Calcium antagonists may be effective on their own or in combination with beta-adrenoceptor blockers and nitrates in patients with chronic stable angina.[200] Several calcium antagonists are effective for the treatment of angina pectoris (Table 50–10). Each relaxes vascular smooth muscle in both the systemic arterial and coronary arterial beds. In addition, blockade of the entry of calcium into myocytes results in a negative inotropic effect, which is counteracted to some extent by peripheral vascular dilation and by activation of the sympathetic nervous system in response to drug-induced hypotension.[203] However, the negative inotropic effect must be taken into consideration in patients with significant left ventricular dysfunction.

With a rapid onset of action and metabolism by the liver, calcium antagonists have a limited bioavailability of between 13 and 52 percent and a half-life of between 3 and 12 hours. Amlodipine and felodipine are exceptions in that both drugs have long half-lives and may be administered once daily. In the case of some of the other calcium antagonists (e.g., nifedipine and diltiazem), sustained-release preparations have been shown to be effective.

ANTIATHEROGENIC ACTION. Hyperlipidemia-induced changes in the permeability of smooth muscle cells to calcium may play a role in atherogenesis; thus, the hypothesis that calcium antagonists might inhibit atherogenesis has been explored since the 1970s but not yet achieved consensus.[204] Studies of first-generation calcium antagonists showed mixed results with respect to lesion progression. Subsequent experimental work with more lipophilic second-generation calcium-channel blockers such as amlodipine have demonstrated inhibition of smooth muscle cell proliferation, migration, and ameliorated unfavorable membrane alterations.[205] In a randomized trial among patients with established CAD, treatment with amlodipine, compared with placebo, was associated with less progression of carotid atherosclerosis measured by intimal-medial thickness; however, no difference was detected in the progression of coronary atherosclerosis.[206] The role of calcium antagonists in atheroprotection is the subject of ongoing study.

First-Generation Calcium Antagonists

NIFEDIPINE. This dihydropyridine is a particularly effective dilator of vascular smooth muscle and is a more potent vasodilator than either diltiazem or verapamil. Although its in vitro actions on myocardium and specialized cardiac tissue are similar to those of other agents, the concentration required to reproduce effects on these tissues is not reached in vivo because of the early appearance of its powerful vasodilating effects. Thus, in clinical practice, the potential negative chronotropic, inotropic, and dromotropic (on AV conduction) effects of nifedipine are seldom a problem, with the exception that nifedipine has been reported to worsen heart failure in patients with preexisting chronic congestive heart failure.[207]

TABLE 50–9 Candidates for Use of Beta-Blocking Agents for Angina

Ideal Candidates
Prominent relationship of physical activity to attacks of angina
Coexistent hypertension
History of supraventricular or ventricular arrhythmias
Previous myocardial infarction
Left ventricular systolic dysfunction
Mild to moderate heart failure symptoms (NYHA functional Classes II, III)
Prominent anxiety state
Poor Candidates
Asthma or reversible airway component in chronic lung disease patients
Severe left ventricular dysfunction with severe heart failure symptoms (NYHA functional Class IV)
History of severe depression
Raynaud phenomenon
Symptomatic peripheral vascular disease
Severe bradycardia or heart block
Brittle diabetes

NYHA = New York Heart Association.
Modified from Abrams JA: Medical therapy of stable angina pectoris. *In* Beller G: Chronic Ischemic Heart Disease. *In* Braunwald E (ed): Atlas of Heart Disease. Vol 5. Philadelphia, WB Saunders, 1995, p 7.22.

The beneficial effects of nifedipine in the treatment of angina result from its capacity to reduce myocardial O_2 requirements because of its afterload-reducing effect and to increase myocardial O_2 delivery as a result of its dilating action on the coronary vascular bed (see Table 50–5). Oral nifedipine in capsule form exerts hypotensive effects within 20 minutes of administration. This immediate-release formulation is no longer recommended because of concerns regarding adverse events.[208] An extended-release formulation using the gastrointestinal therapeutic system of drug delivery (see Table 50–10) is designed to deliver 30, 60, or 90 mg of nifedipine in a single daily dose at a relatively constant rate over a 24-hour period and is useful for the treatment of chronic stable angina, Prinzmetal angina, and hypertension. Steady-state plasma levels are typically achieved within 48 hours of initiation. The efficacy of the extended-release preparation, either alone or in conjunction with beta blockers, in reducing episodes of angina and ischemia on ambulatory monitoring has been documented.[209]

Adverse Effects. These occur in 15 to 20 percent of patients and require discontinuation of medication in about 5 percent. Most adverse effects are related to systemic vasodilation and include headache, dizziness, palpitations, flushing, hypotension, and leg edema (unrelated to heart failure). Gastrointestinal side effects, including nausea, epigastric pressure, and vomiting, are noted in approximately 5 percent of patients. In rare instances, in patients with extremely severe, fixed coronary obstructions, nifedipine aggravates angina, presumably by lowering arterial pressure excessively, with subsequent reflex tachycardia. For this reason, combined treatment of angina with nifedipine and a beta blocker is particularly effective and superior to nifedipine alone.[209] Most of the adverse effects are reduced by the use of extended-release preparations.

TABLE 50–10 Pharmacokinetics of Calcium Antagonists Used Commonly for Angina Pectoris

Characteristic	Diltiazem/SR		Nicardipine	Nifedipine/SR	
Usual adult dose	IV: 0.25 mg/kg bolus, then 5-15 mg/hr Oral: 30-90 mg t.i.d.–q.i.d. SR: 60-180 mg b.i.d. CD: 120-480 mg/d		IV: 3-15 mg/hr Oral: 20-40 mg t.i.d. SR: 30-60 mg b.i.d.	Oral: 10-30 mg t.i.d. SR: 90 mg/d	
Extent of absorption (%)	80-90		100	90	
Extent of bioavailability (%)	40-70		30	65-75/86	
Onset of action	IV: 3 min Oral: 30-60 min		IV: 1 min Oral: 20 min	20 min	
Time to peak serum concentration (hr)	2-3/6-11		0.5-2.0	0.5/6	
Therapeutic serum levels (ng/ml)	50-200		30-50	25-100	
Elimination half-life (hr)	3.5/5-7		2.0-4.0	2.0-5.0	
Elimination	60% metabolized by liver; remainder excreted by kidneys		High first-pass hepatic metabolism	High first-pass hepatic metabolism	
Heart rate	↓		↑	↑↑	
Peripheral vascular resistance	↓		↓↓↓	↓↓↓	
FDA-approved indications	IR	SR		IR	SR
Hypertension	No	Yes	Yes[†]	No	Yes
Angina	Yes	Yes	Yes	Yes	Yes
Coronary spasm	Yes	No	No	Yes	Yes

CD = combination drug; CR = controlled release; FDA = Food and Drug Administration; IR = immediate release; ND = no data; SR = sustained release.
*Half-life of 4.5 to 12 hours with multiple dosing; may be prolonged in the elderly.
[†]The sustained-release formulation may preferred for hypertension.

Several clinical case-control studies of hypertension and associated reviews have suggested that *short-acting nifedipine* may cause an increase in mortality.[208] No firm data indicate that this risk applies to extended-release nifedipine or to other calcium antagonists. Although insufficient data are available to assess the long-term risks (if any) of calcium antagonists in chronic CAD, *long-acting nifedipine* should be considered an effective and safe antianginal drug for the treatment of symptomatic patients with chronic CAD who are already receiving beta blockers, with or without nitrates. Short-acting nifedipine should ordinarily be avoided.

Because of its potent vasodilator effects, nifedipine is contraindicated in patients who are hypotensive or have severe aortic valve stenosis and in patients with unstable angina who are not simultaneously receiving a beta blocker and in whom reflex-mediated increases in the heart rate may be harmful. Nifedipine (or one of the second-generation dihydropyridines) is the calcium antagonist of choice in patients with sinus bradycardia, sick sinus syndrome, or AV block (particularly if a beta-adrenoceptor blocking agent is administered concurrently and additional drug therapy for angina is indicated). This recommendation is based on the observation that in doses used clinically, nifedipine has fewer negative effects on myocardial contractility, heart rate, and AV conduction than verapamil or diltiazem.[207]

Nifedipine interacts significantly with prazosin (resulting in excessive hypotension), cimetidine, and phenytoin (resulting in increased bioavailability of nifedipine). In patients with Prinzmetal angina, abrupt cessation of nifedipine therapy may result in a rebound increase in the frequency and duration of attacks (see Chap. 49).

VERAPAMIL. Verapamil dilates systemic and coronary resistance vessels and large coronary conductance vessels. It slows the heart rate and reduces myocardial contractility. This combination of actions results in a reduction in myocardial O_2 requirement, which is the basis for the drug's efficacy in the management of chronic stable angina.

Verapamil reduces the frequency of angina and prolongs exercise tolerance in patients with symptomatic chronic CAD, and the combination of verapamil and a beta blocker provides clinical benefit that is additive.[210] When evaluated in the International Verapamil-Trandolapril Study (INVEST), a strategy combining sustained-release verapamil and trandolapril compared to atenolol and a diuretic for the treatment of patients with hypertension and CAD showed equivalent outcomes with respect to death, MI, or stroke.[210a] Despite the marked negative inotropic effects of verapamil in isolated cardiac muscle preparations, changes in contractility are modest in patients with normal cardiac function. However, in patients with cardiac dysfunction, verapamil may reduce cardiac output, increase left ventricular filling pressure, and cause clinical heart failure. In clinically useful doses, verapamil inhibits calcium influx into specialized cardiac cells, sometimes causing slowing of the heart rate and AV conduction. Therefore, it is contraindicated in patients with preexisting AV nodal disease or sick sinus syndrome, congestive heart failure, and suspected digitalis or quinidine toxicity.

The usual starting dose of verapamil for oral administration is 40 to 80 mg three times daily to a maximal dose of 480 mg daily (see Table 50-10). Sustained-release preparations of verapamil are available, and starting doses are 120 to 240 mg twice daily with a usual optimal dose range of 240 to 360 mg daily.

Verapamil interacts significantly with several other drugs. *Intravenous* verapamil should generally not be used together with a beta blocker (given intravenously or orally), nor should a beta blocker be administered *intravenously* in patients receiving oral verapamil. Both drugs can be administered orally but with caution in view of the potential for bradyarrhythmias and negative inotropic effects. The

Verapamil/SR		**Amlodipine**	**Felodipine**	**Isradipine**	**Nisoldipine**
IV: 0.075-0.15 mg/kg Oral: 80-120 mg t.i.d.–q.i.d. SR: 180-480 mg/d		Oral 2.5-10 mg/d	Oral SR: 2.5-10 mg/d	Oral CR: 2.5-10 mg b.i.d.	Oral SR: 10-40 mg/d
90		>90	>90	>90	ND
20-35		60-90	20	25	5
IV: 2-5 min Oral: 30 min		0.5-1.0 hr	2 hr	20 min	1-3 hr
IV: 3-5 min Oral: 1-2 SR: 7-9		6-12	2-5	1.5	6-12
80-300		5-20	1-5	2-10	ND
3.0-7.0*		30-50	11-16	8	7-12
85% eliminated by first-pass hepatic metabolism		Hepatic	High first-pass hepatic metabolism	High first-pass hepatic metabolism	Hepatic
↓		0	↑	0	0
↓↓		↓↓↓	↓↓↓	↓↓↓	↓↓↓
IR	SR				
Yes	Yes	Yes	Yes	Yes	Yes
Yes	No	Yes	No	No	Yes
Yes	No	Yes	No	No	No

bioavailability of verapamil is increased by cimetidine and carbamazepine, whereas verapamil may increase plasma levels of cyclosporine and digoxin and may be associated with excessive hypotension in patients receiving quinidine or prazosin. Hepatic enzyme inducers such as phenobarbital may reduce the effects of verapamil. Verapamil should not be administered in conjunction with the antiarrhythmic drug dofetilide.

Adverse effects of verapamil are noted in approximately 10 percent of patients and relate to systemic vasodilation (hypotension and facial flushing), gastrointestinal symptoms (constipation and nausea), and central nervous system reactions such as headache and dizziness. A rare side effect is gingival hyperplasia, which appears after 1 to 9 months of therapy.

DILTIAZEM. Diltiazem's actions are intermediate between those of nifedipine and verapamil. In clinically useful doses, its vasodilator effects are less profound than those of nifedipine, and its cardiac depressant action (on the sinoatrial and AV nodes and myocardium) is less than that of verapamil. This profile may explain the remarkably low incidence of adverse effects of diltiazem. Diltiazem is a systemic vasodilator that lowers arterial pressure at rest and during exertion and increases the workload required to produce myocardial ischemia, but it may also increase myocardial O_2 delivery. Although this drug causes little vasodilation of epicardial coronary arteries under basal conditions, it may enhance perfusion of the subendocardium distal to a flow-limiting coronary stenosis; it also blocks exercise-induced coronary vasoconstriction. In patients with chronic stable angina receiving maximally tolerated doses of diltiazem, the heart rate is significantly reduced at rest, but no effect on peak blood pressure is achieved during exercise, and the duration of symptom-limited treadmill exercise is prolonged.

Several sustained-release formulations of diltiazem are available for once-daily treatment of systemic hypertension and angina pectoris.[211] The usual starting dose of sustained-release formulations is 120 mg once daily up to a typical maintenance dose of 180 to 360 mg once daily. The maximum effect on blood pressure may not be observed until 14 days after starting therapy.

Diltiazem is a highly effective antianginal agent. Atenolol and diltiazem have similar efficacy in increasing nonischemic exercise duration in patients with variable-threshold angina and act primarily by slowing the resting heart rate.[212] High doses (mean dose, 340 mg) have been shown to be a relatively safe addition to maximally tolerated doses of isosorbide dinitrate and a beta blocker and cause increases in exercise tolerance and resting and exercise left ventricular ejection fraction.[211] Major side effects are similar to those of the other calcium channel blockers and are related to vasodilation, but they are relatively infrequent, particularly if the dose does not exceed 240 mg daily. As is the case with verapamil, diltiazem should be prescribed with caution for patients with sick sinus syndrome or AV block. In patients with preexisting left ventricular dysfunction, diltiazem may exacerbate or precipitate heart failure.

Diltiazem interacts with other drugs, including beta-adrenergic blocking agents (causing enhanced negative inotropic, chronotropic, and dromotropic effects), flecainide, and cimetidine (which increases the bioavailability of diltiazem), and diltiazem has been associated with increased plasma levels of cyclosporine, carbamazepine, and lithium carbonate. Diltiazem may cause excessive sinus node depression if administered with disopyramide and may reduce digoxin clearance, especially in patients with renal failure.

Second-Generation Calcium Antagonists

The second-generation calcium antagonists (nicardipine, isradipine, amlodipine, and felodipine) are mainly dihydropyridine derivatives, with nifedipine being the prototypical agent. Considerable experience has also accumulated with nimodipine, nisoldipine, and nitrendipine. These agents differ in potency, tissue specificity, and pharmacokinetics and, in general, are potent vasodilators because of greater vascular selectivity than seen with the first-generation antagonists (i.e., verapamil, nifedipine, and diltiazem).

AMLODIPINE. This agent, which is less lipid soluble than nifedipine, has a slow, smooth onset and ultra-long duration of action (plasma half-life of 36 hours). It causes marked coronary and peripheral dilation and may be useful in the treatment of patients with angina accompanied by hypertension. It may be used as a once-daily hypotensive or antianginal agent.[213] In a series of randomized, placebo-controlled studies in patients with stable exercise-induced angina pectoris, amlodipine was shown to be effective and well tolerated.[214] In two trials among patients with established CAD, amlodipine reduced the risk of major cardiovascular events.[206,214a] Amlodipine has little, if any, negative inotropic action and may be especially useful in patients with chronic angina and left ventricular dysfunction.[215]

The usual dose of amlodipine is 5 to 10 mg once daily. Downward adjustment of the starting dose is appropriate among patients with liver disease and the elderly. Significant changes in blood pressure are typically not evident until 24 to 48 hours after initiation. Steady-state serum levels are achieved at 7 to 8 days.

NICARDIPINE. This drug has a half-life similar to that of nifedipine (2 to 4 hours), but it appears to have greater vascular selectivity. Nicardipine may be used as an antianginal and antihypertensive agent and requires three-times-daily administration, although a sustained-release formulation is available for twice-daily dosing in hypertension. For chronic stable angina pectoris, it appears to be as effective as verapamil or diltiazem, and its efficacy is enhanced when combined with a beta blocker.

FELODIPINE AND ISRADIPINE. In the United States, both drugs are approved by the U.S. Food and Drug Administration (FDA) for the treatment of hypertension but not for angina pectoris. A recent study documented similar efficacy between felodipine and nifedipine in patients with chronic stable angina.[216] Felodipine has also been reported to be more vascular selective than nifedipine and to have a mild positive inotropic effect as a result of calcium-channel agonist properties. Isradipine has a longer half-life than nifedipine and demonstrates greater vascular sensitivity.

OTHER PHARMACOLOGICAL AGENTS

NICORANDIL.* Nicorandil is a nicotinamide ester that dilates peripheral and coronary resistance vessels via action on ATP-sensitive potassium channels and possesses a nitrate moiety that promotes systemic venous and coronary vasodilation. As a result of these dual actions, nicorandil reduces preload and afterload and results in an increase in coronary blood flow. In addition to these effects, nicorandil may have cardioprotective actions mediated through activation of potassium channels.[217]

Nicorandil has antianginal efficacy similar to beta blockers, nitrates, and calcium-channel blockers. In a recent randomized clinical trial ($N = 5126$), nicorandil reduced the risk of cardiac death, myocardial infarction, or hospital admission for angina (hazard ratio 0.83; $p = 0.014$) compared with placebo when added to standard antianginal therapy.[218]

METABOLIC AGENTS.† Agents aimed at increasing the metabolic efficiency of cardiac myocytes have also been studied in patients with chronic stable angina. Partial inhibitors of fatty acid oxidation appear to shift myocardial metabolism to more oxygen-efficient pathways.[219] Trimetazidine and ranolazine are agents that have been shown to inhibit fatty acid oxidation and to reduce the frequency of angina without hemodynamic effects among patients with chronic stable angina. When eval-

*This drug has not been approved by the FDA at the time of this writing.

†These agents have not been approved by the FDA at the time of this writing.

uated in patients with chronic stable angina (N = 823) taking standard doses of atenolol, amlodipine, or diltiazem, the addition of ranolazine administered twice daily increased exericise duration on treadmill testing and reduced the frequency of angina and use of nitroglycerin.[219a]

Selection of Pharmacologic Therapy for Angina Pectoris

RELATIVE ADVANTAGES OF BETA BLOCKERS AND CALCIUM ANTAGONISTS (Table 50–11). The choice between a beta blocker and a calcium-channel antagonist as initial therapy in patients with chronic stable angina is controversial because both classes of agents are effective in relieving symptoms and reducing ischemia.[18] Trials comparing beta blockers and calcium antagonists have not shown any difference in the rate of death or myocardial infarction,[18] although in some studies beta blockers appeared to have greater clinical efficacy,[220-222] and less frequent discontinuation due to side effects.[223] Because long-term administration of beta blockers has been demonstrated to prolong life in patients after acute myocardial infarction and in the treatment of hypertension, it is reasonable to consider beta blockers over calcium antagonists as the agents of choice in treating patients with chronic stable angina.[18] However, it must be recognized that beta blockers (without ISA) increase serum triglycerides and decrease HDL cholesterol with uncertain long-term consequences. In addition, these drugs may produce fatigue, depression, and sexual dysfunction. In contrast, although calcium antagonists do not show these adverse effects, their long-term administration has *not* been shown to improve long-term survival after acute myocardial infarction.[224] However, diltiazem is apparently effective in preventing severe angina and early reinfarction after non-Q-wave infarction.[225] Verapamil reduces reinfarction rates in patients post-MI[266] and, when combined with trandolapril, achieves similar outcomes to atenolol together with a diuretic for the treatment of patients with hypertension and CAD.[210a]

TABLE 50–11 Recommended Drug Therapy* (Calcium Antagonist vs. Beta Blocker) in Patients Who Have Angina in Conjunction with Other Medical Conditions

Clinical Condition	Recommended Drug
Cardiac Arrhythmia or Conduction Disturbance	
Sinus bradycardia	Nifedipine or amlodipine
Sinus tachycardia (not caused by cardiac failure)	Beta blocker
Supraventricular tachycardia	Beta blocker (verapamil)
Atrioventricular block	Nifedipine or amlodipine
Rapid atrial fibrillation	Verapamil or beta blocker
Ventricular arrhythmia	Beta blocker
Left Ventricular Dysfunction	
Heart failure	Beta blocker
Miscellaneous Medical Conditions	
Systemic hypertension	Beta blocker (calcium antagonist)
Severe preexisting headaches	Beta blocker (verapamil or diltiazem)
COPD with bronchospasm or asthma	Nifedipine, amlodipine, verapamil, or diltiazem
Hyperthyroidism	Beta blocker
Raynaud syndrome	Nifedipine or amlodipine
Claudication	Calcium antagonist
Severe depression	Calcium antagonist

COPD = chronic obstructive pulmonary disease.
*Alternatives in parentheses.

The choice of drug with which to initiate therapy is influenced by a number of clinical factors (see Table 50-11),[18] as discussed in the following:

1. Calcium antagonists are the preferred agents in patients with a history of asthma, chronic obstructive lung disease, and/or wheezing on clinical examination, in whom beta blockers, even relatively selective agents, are contraindicated.
2. Nifedipine (long acting), amlodipine, and nicardipine are the calcium antagonists of choice in patients with chronic stable angina and sick sinus syndrome, sinus bradycardia, or significant AV conduction disturbances, whereas beta blockers and verapamil should be used only with great caution in such patients. In patients with symptomatic conduction disease, neither a beta blocker nor a calcium-channel blocker should be used unless a pacemaker is in place. If a beta blocker is required in patients with asymptomatic evidence of conduction disease, pindolol, which has the greatest ISA, is useful. In the case of calcium-channel blockers in patients with conduction system disease, nifedipine or nicardipine is preferable to verapamil and diltiazem, but careful observation for deterioration of conduction is mandatory.
3. Calcium antagonists are clearly preferred in patients with suspected Prinzmetal (variant) angina (see Chap. 49); beta blockers may even aggravate angina under these circumstances.
4. Calcium antagonists may be preferred over beta blockers in patients with significant, symptomatic peripheral arterial disease because the latter may cause peripheral vasoconstriction.
5. Beta blockers should usually be avoided in patients with a history of significant depressive illness and should be prescribed cautiously for patients with sexual dysfunction, sleep disturbance, nightmares, fatigue, or lethargy.
6. The presence of moderate to severe left ventricular dysfunction in patients with angina limits the therapeutic options. The beneficial effects of beta blockers on survival in patients with left ventricular dysfunction after myocardial infarction,[154] coupled with their beneficial effects on survival and left ventricular performance in patients with heart failure,[227] has established beta blockers as the drug class of choice for the treatment of angina in patients with left ventricular dysfunction, with or without symptoms of heart failure, together with ACE inhibitors, diuretics, and digitalis. If angina persists despite beta blockade and nitrates, amlodipine can be administered.[215] Verapamil, nifedipine, and diltiazem should be avoided.
7. Short-acting nifedipine should not be used because the reflex-mediated tachycardia may aggravate ischemia.
8. Hypertensive patients with angina pectoris do well with either beta blockers or calcium antagonists because both agents have antihypertensive effects. However, beta blockers are the preferred initial agent for treating angina in such patients, as noted earlier, and an ACE inhibitor should be strongly considered for all patients with CAD with hypertension.[149]

COMBINATION THERAPY. The combination of a beta blocker, calcium antagonist, and long-acting nitrate is widely used in the management of chronic stable angina.[222] When adrenergic blockers and calcium antagonists are used together in the treatment of angina pectoris, several issues should be considered, as follows:

1. The addition of a beta blocker enhances the clinical effect of nifedipine and other dihydropyridines.
2. In patients with moderate or severe left ventricular dysfunction, sinus bradycardia, or AV conduction

disturbances, combination therapy with calcium antagonists and beta blockers either should be avoided or should be initiated with caution. In patients with AV conduction system disease, the preferred combination is a long-acting dihydropyridine and a beta blocker. The negative inotropic effects of calcium antagonists are not usually a problem in combined therapy with low doses of beta blockers but can become significant with higher doses. With such doses, amlodipine is the calcium antagonist of choice, but it should be used cautiously.
3. The combination of a dihydropyridine and a long-acting nitrate (without a beta blocker) is not an optimal combination because both are vasodilators.

Approach to Patients with Chronic Stable Angina

1. Identify and treat precipitating factors, such as anemia, uncontrolled hypertension, thyrotoxicosis, tachyarrhythmias, uncontrolled congestive heart failure, and concomitant valvular heart disease.
2. Initiate risk factor modification, physical exercise, diet, and life-style counseling. Initiate therapy with an HMG-CoA reductase inhibitor, as needed, to reduce LDL cholesterol to at least below 100 mg/dl.
3. Initiate pharmacotherapy with aspirin and a beta blocker. Strongly consider an ACE inhibitor as first-line therapy in all patients with chronic CAD.
4. Use sublingual nitroglycerin for alleviation of symptoms and for prophylaxis.
5. If angina occurs more than two or three times per week, the next step is addition of a calcium antagonist or a long-acting nitrate via dosing schedules to prevent nitrate tolerance. The decision to add a calcium antagonist or a long-acting nitrate is not based entirely on the frequency and severity of symptoms. The need to treat concomitant hypertension or the presence of left ventricular dysfunction and symptoms of heart failure may be an indication for the use of one of these agents, even in patients in whom episodes of symptomatic angina are infrequent.
6. If angina persists despite two antianginal agents (a beta blocker with either a long-acting nitrate preparation or a calcium antagonist), add the third antianginal agent.
7. Coronary angiography, with a view to considering coronary revascularization, is indicated in patients with refractory symptoms or ischemia despite optimal medical therapy; it should also be carried out in patients with "high-risk" noninvasive test results (see Table 50–4) and in those with occupations or life styles that require a more aggressive approach.

OTHER THERAPIES

SPINAL CORD STIMULATION. An option for patients with refractory angina who are not candidates for coronary revascularization is spinal cord stimulation using a specially designed electrode inserted into the epidural space. The beneficial effects of neuromodulation via this technique on pain are based on the gate theory, in which stimulation of axons in the spinal cord that do not transmit pain to the brain will reduce input to the brain from axons that do so. Irrespective of the mechanism, several observational studies have reported success rates of up to 80 percent in terms of reducing the frequency and severity of angina.[228] What is less easily explained is an apparent antiischemic effect of this technique. In a small randomized trial among patients with angina and with CAD not amenable to percutaneous coronary intervention (PCI), spinal cord stimulation was associated with similar symptom relief and long-term quality of life compared to CABG.[228,229] Mortality was lower after 6 months among those treated with spinal stimulation and comparable at 5 years between the two groups. Exercise capacity was better in the CABG group.[228] Randomized, placebo-controlled trials are impossible to perform, and this approach should be reserved for patients in whom all other treatment options have been exhausted.[230]

ENHANCED EXTERNAL COUNTERPULSATION. The use of enhanced external counterpulsation (EECP) is another promising alternative treatment of refractory angina.[231,232] EECP is generally administered as 35 1-hour treatments over 7 weeks. Observational data suggest that EECP reduces the frequency of angina and the use of nitroglycerin and improves exercise tolerance and quality of life.[232] In a randomized, double-blind, sham-controlled study of EECP for patients with chronic stable angina, active counterpulsation was associated with an increase in time to ST segment depression during exercise testing and a reduction in angina, as well as an improvement in health-related quality of life that extends to at least 1 year.[233] EECP also reduces the extent of ischemia detected with myocardial perfusion imaging.[234]

The mechanisms underlying the effects of EECP are poorly understood. Possible mechanisms include (1) durable hemodynamic changes that reduce myocardial O_2 demand; (2) improvement in myocardial perfusion due to the capacity of increased transmyocardial pressure to open collaterals; and (3) the elaboration of various substances that improve endothelial function and vascular remodeling due to augmented flow through the arterial vascular bed.[232] Lastly, the possibility of placebo effects should be recognized; most of the evidence demonstrating favorable effects of EECP are from uncontrolled studies, and data from sham-controlled studies are few.

CHELATION. Randomized trials have shown no benefit and these agents may be harmful. They have no place in the management of acute or chronic CAD.[235]

Percutaneous Coronary Intervention (see Chap. 52)

PCI, which includes percutaneous transluminal coronary angioplasty (PTCA), stenting, and related techniques, represents an important therapeutic option in the management of chronic stable angina. The practice of interventional cardiology has changed radically with increased operator experience; improved adjunctive pharmacotherapy; and advances in technology, including drug-eluting stents, distal protection devices, and devices directed at specific technical issues (e.g., thrombectomy and atherectomy catheters).[236] In line with more frequent use of percutaneous intervention for complex and/or multivessel CAD, the number of coronary interventions increased by 266 percent from 1987 to 2001.[3] Despite these advances, it must be appreciated that a dilatable lesion represents an isolated target, whereas atherosclerosis is a frequently a diffuse or multifocal process. Thus, PCI is but one aspect of a comprehensive therapeutic strategy that should vigorously address the risk factors for CAD.

PATIENT SELECTION. Improved technology and increasing operator experience have continued to expand the pool of patients with both single-vessel and multivessel disease who are candidates for PCI (and other catheter-based techniques for revascularization).[236] Factors that need to be considered in patient selection include the following:

1. The need for mechanical revascularization (surgical or catheter based) as opposed to intensification of medical therapy, including stringent risk factor modification.
2. The likelihood of successful catheter-based revascularization based on the angiographic characteristics of the lesion. Equally important are factors such as vessel size, extent of calcification, tortuosity, and relationships to side branches
3. The risk and potential consequences of acute failure of PCI, which are a function, in part, of the coronary artery anatomy (multivessel and/or diffuse disease), the percentage of viable myocardium at risk, and underlying left ventricular function.
4. The likelihood of restenosis, which has been associated with clinical (e.g., diabetes, prior restenosis) and

angiographic factors (small-vessel diameter, long-lesion length, total occlusion, and saphenous vein graft disease).

5. The need for complete revascularization based on the extent of CAD, the volume of myocardium in the distribution of the narrowed artery(ies), the severity of ischemia, and the presence or absence of left ventricular dysfunction.
6. The presence of comorbid conditions and the suitability of the patient for surgery.
7. Patient preference.

Patients with chronic stable angina who are ideal for PCI are those with significant symptoms despite intensive medical therapy, who are at low risk for complications, and in whom the likelihood of technical success is high (e.g., the patient who is younger than 70 years and has single-vessel and single-lesion CAD), the anatomical characteristics of a low risk lesion with less than 90 percent stenosis, no history of congestive heart failure, and an ejection fraction greater than 0.40. Although these characteristics define the ideal candidate, excellent technical and clinical results can still be obtained in many patients who do not fulfill these ideal criteria; newer technologies have substantially expanded the pool of suitable candidates and during the last 5 years, the majority of revascularization procedures in the United States and the United Kingdom were PCI as opposed to CABG.[3]

Features associated with an increased risk for PCI failure include advanced age, female gender, unstable angina, congestive heart failure, left main coronary artery–equivalent disease, and multivessel CAD. Diabetes mellitus in patients with multivessel disease has been associated with increased periprocedural ischemic complications and late mortality in comparison with patients without diabetes. Patients with impaired renal function, particularly those with diabetes, are also at increased risk for periprocedural morbidity and, in particular, contrast agent nephropathy.[237,238]

The ACC/AHA lesion classification criteria have been revised to reflect low, moderate, and high risk in the stent era (Table 50–12).[239,240] Factors associated with increased risk of procedural failure include the presence of total occlusion for more than 3 months old, excessive vessel tortuosity, bifurcation lesions, the presence of thrombus, the inability to protect a side branch, and degenerative vein graft lesions. The presence of the aforementioned features should be considered in weighing the risks and potential benefits of PCI.

TABLE 50–12 American College of Cardiology/American Heart Association Coronary Lesion Classification*

Low Risk
Discrete (length <10 mm)
Concentric
Readily accessible
Nonangulated segment (<45 degrees)
Smooth contour
Little or no calcification
Less than totally occlusive
Not ostial in location
No major side branch involvement
Absence of thrombus
Moderate Risk
Tubular (length 10-20 mm)
Eccentric
Moderate tortuosity of proximal segment
Moderately angulated segment (>45, <90 degrees)
Irregular contour
Moderate or heavy calcification
Total occlusions <3 mo old
Ostial in location
Bifurcation lesions requiring double guidewires
Some thrombus present
High Risk
Diffuse (length >20 mm)
Excessive tortuosity of proximal segment
Extremely angulated segments >90 degrees
Total occlusions >3 mo old and/or bridging collaterals
Inability to protect major side branches
Degenerated vein grafts with friable lesions

From Smith SC Jr, Dove JT, Jacobs AK, et al: ACC/AHA guidelines of percutaneous coronary interventions (revision of the 1993 PTCA guidelines)–executive summary. A report of the American College of Cardiology/American Heart Association Task Force on Practice Guidelines (Committee to Revise the 1993 Guidelines for Percutaneous Transluminal Coronary Angioplasty). J Am Coll Cardiol 37:2215-2239, 2001.

*Anatomic risk groups.

EARLY OUTCOME. Continued improvement in the technical aspects of PCI (predominantly coronary stenting), as well as increasing operator experience, has had a favorable impact on the rate of primary success (defined angiographically as a final stenosis diameter <20 percent in the presence of Thrombosis in Myocardial Infarction [TIMI] grade 3 flow) and the rate of reductions in complications (i.e., death, myocardial infarction, and emergency coronary bypass surgery).[241] These improvements have occurred despite broadening of the selection criteria for PCI to include higher risk patients with more complex anatomy. Current expectations for PCI, particularly with the widespread use of coronary stents, are an overall procedural success rate of at least 90 percent with a mortality of less than 1 percent, rate of Q wave myocardial infarction of less than 1.5 percent, and rate of emergency bypass surgery of 1 to 2 percent.

LONG-TERM OUTCOME. Long-term outcome after PCI is well characterized, with left ventricular function, extent of coronary disease, diabetes, and the patient's age being the major determinants of mortality risk, and restenosis at the site of intervention being a major contributor to recurrent ischemia and the need for subsequent procedures. The incidence of restenosis following balloon angioplasty is 30 to 40 percent and appears higher in certain clinical and angiographic subsets, accounting in large part for the high frequency of repeat revascularization procedures (up to 40 percent at 1 to 2 years) after angioplasty. However, contemporary datasets reflecting the widespread use of intracoronary stenting document significantly lower rates of repeat revascularization procedures at 1 year (CABG 8.6 percent and PCI 12.4 percent) than observed in the era of balloon angioplasty.[241]

STENTS (see Chap. 52). Since their entry into clinical practice in the early 1990s, stents have improved both the early and late results of PCI. In regard to the former, stents have produced a marked reduction in the need for emergency bypass surgery, and in comparison with PTCA, stents have been associated with a significant reduction in the incidence of major cardiac events after discharge.[242] These favorable results have occurred primarily through reduction in clinical restenosis and the need for repeat revascularization without translating into a reduction in death or myocardial infarction.[243] Despite the significant reduction in restenosis achieved with bare-metal stents compared with balloon angioplasty, restenosis within the stent (in-stent restenosis), occurring in 15 to 30 percent of stented lesions, has remained a limitation to long-term outcomes with PCI.[242] Drug-eluting stents (coated stents that release single or multiple bioactive agents into the surrounding tissue) have shown dramatic reductions in restenosis in patients selected for clinical trials (binary restenosis 0 to 10 percent) compared to bare-metal stents.[244] This advantage may translate into an additional decline in the need for repeat revascularization procedures after PCI, including multivessel interventions, and in patients, such as those with diabetes mellitus, who are at high risk for restenosis with bare-metal stents.[236]

CHRONIC TOTAL OCCLUSION. Chronic total occlusions are present in 20 to 40 percent of patients with angiographic documentation of CAD and are particularly frequent in patients with multivessel disease and left ventricular dysfunction, in whom a total occlusion is often a barrier to complete revascularization. The availability of newer devices, particularly guidewires dedicated to treatment of chronic total occlusions, has increased the probability of initial technical success. Nevertheless, the rate of primary success is lower (51 to 74 percent) and the rate of restenosis higher during PCI for chronic total occlusions compared with nonoccluded vessels.[245] Long-term survival appears greater and anginal symptoms are less frequent among patients with chronic total occlusions who undergo successful PCI compared with those who have failed procedures even after adjusting for differences in their baseline risk profile.[245]

RESTENOSIS. See Chapter 52.

Comparisons Between PCI and Medical Therapy

Randomized clinical trials comparing PCI to medical therapy are few in number, have involved fewer than 2000 patients (in total) with predominantly single-vessel disease, and were completed prior to routine use of coronary stenting and enhanced adjunctive pharmacotherapy.[246] In aggregate, the results of these trials have supported superior control of angina and improved exercise capacity in patients treated with angioplasty compared with medical therapy (Fig. 50–9). In addition, results from long-term follow-up in the second Randomized Intervention Treatment of Angina (RITA-2) trial indicated improved quality of life among those treated with angioplasty through 1 year of follow-up, although this benefit was attenuated by 3 years.[247] No randomized trial to date has demonstrated a reduction in death or myocardial infarction with PCI compared with medical therapy for patients with chronic stable angina. To the contrary, the RITA-2 investigators observed an excess of death and periprocedural myocardial infarction with angioplasty compared to medical therapy (6.3 percent vs. 3.3 percent; $p = 0.02$); it is worthy of note that 62 percent of the patients enrolled in RITA-2 had multivessel CAD. Among patients with stable single- or double-vessel CAD and mild symptoms (asymptomatic or Canadian Cardiovascular Society class I or II angina) and preserved left ventricular function, medical therapy, including aggressive lipid lowering, provided similar results to angioplasty with respect to a composite of cardiovascular death, need for (repeat) revascularization, myocardial infarction, or worsening angina resulting in hospitalization.[103]

Based on these best available data from randomized trials, it appears reasonable to pursue a strategy of initial medical therapy for most patients with chronic stable angina and Canadian Cardiovascular Society class I or II symptoms and reserve revascularization for those with persistent and/or more severe symptoms despite optimal medical therapy, or those with high-risk criteria on noninvasive testing, such as inducible ischemia involving a moderate or large territory of myocardium.[18] The ongoing Clinical Outcomes Utilization Revascularization and Aggressive drug Evaluation (COURAGE) trial will provide additional insight regarding the comparison of intensive medical therapy versus revascularization using contemporary technology.

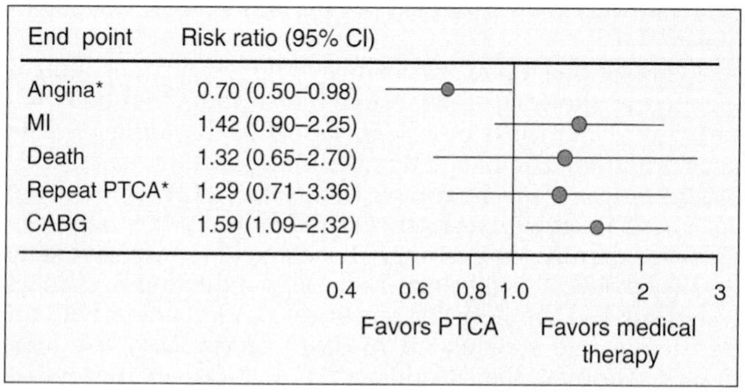
End point
Risk ratio (95% CI)
Angina*
0.70 (0.50–0.98)
MI
1.42 (0.90–2.25)
Death
1.32 (0.65–2.70)
Repeat PTCA*
1.29 (0.71–3.36)
CABG
1.59 (1.09–2.32)
0.4
0.6
0.8
1.0
2
3
Favors PTCA
Favors medical therapy

FIGURE 50–9 Relative risk of recurrent cardiac events with percutaneous transluminal coronary angioplasty (PTCA) versus medical therapy from meta-analysis of six randomized trials ($N = 1904$). Compared with medical therapy, angioplasty reduced the relative risk of recurrent angina by 30 percent. Randomized trials have not included sufficient numbers of patients for informative estimates of the effect of angioplasty on myocardial infarction (MI), death, or subsequent revascularization; however, trends in the available data do not favor angioplasty. These trials do not reflect the widespread use of coronary stenting. *Test for heterogeneity, $p < 0.0001$. CABG = coronary artery bypass grafting; CI = confidence interval. (From Bucher HC, Hengstler P, Schindler C, et al: Percutaneous transluminal coronary angioplasty versus medical therapy for treatment of non-acute coronary heart disease: A meta-analysis of randomised controlled trials. BMJ 321:73-77, 2000.)

PCI in Specific Subgroups of Patients with Chronic Stable Angina

LEFT VENTRICULAR DYSFUNCTION. Studies of balloon angioplasty in patients with chronic stable angina and left ventricular dysfunction have documented high rates of initial procedural success[248] but less complete revascularization and less favorable long-term outcomes (including survival) than in patients with normal left ventricular function. Despite advances in interventional cardiology, left ventricular dysfunction remains associated with higher in-hospital and long-term mortality after PCI.[248] Specifically, among patients with stable CAD and estimated ejection fractions of 0.40 percent or less, 0.41 to 0.49, and 0.50 or higher in the National Heart, Lung, and Blood Institute (NHLBI) Dynamic Registry, mortality at 1 year after PCI was 11.0 percent, 4.5 percent, and 1.9 percent, respectively.[248] Patients with left ventricular dysfunction are more likely to have other important factors associated with increased risk, including advanced age, diabetes mellitus, and more extensive epicardial disease. However, systolic dysfunction remains an independent predictor of mortality after PCI in the stent era.

WOMEN. Compared with men, women undergoing PCI tend to be older and to have more comorbid disease, a higher prevalence of diabetes mellitus, and more severe angina.[249] However, the extent of epicardial coronary disease is typically similar or less among women. The apparent discordance between the number of risk factors and severity of symptoms with the angiographic extent of disease has been attributed to greater abnormalities of vasomotor function and micovascular and endothelial dysfunction among women.[249] Although reports in the early 1990s demonstrated worrisome higher mortality among women undergoing PCI, subsequent studies have documented consistent reduction in the risk of early complications, despite persistent high-risk characteristics, and similar long-term outcomes compared to men.[250]

THE ELDERLY. Catheter-based revascularization is particularly attractive in the elderly because of age-related changes in cognitive function and cerebrovascular events after CABG and because of the adverse effect of coexisting disease (which is frequent in the elderly) on perioperative outcome. Nonetheless, the increased prevalence of multivessel and diffuse disease and left ventricular dysfunction in the elderly diminishes the proportion of patients likely to have significant long-term benefits in comparison to CABG. The more unfavorable coronary artery anatomy in the elderly population together with left ventricular dysfunction is reflected by he twofold to fourfold higher mortality and periprocedural :omplication rates in the elderly undergoing PCI,[251] in addi- ion to greater recurrence of angina in hospital survivors.[252] n elderly patients without ventricular dysfunction or renal nsufficiency, outcomes are comparable to those in younger ›atients. Moreover, despite a persistently high burden of :omorbidities, the rate of periprocedural complications for he elderly have decreased.[251]

The Trial of Invasive versus Medical therapy in the Eldery TIME), a randomized trial of invasive versus medical man- gement of chronic stable angina in patients 75 years of age nd older, demonstrated a trend toward an early hazard with espect to the risk of death or myocardial infarction but mproved functional outcomes among survivors of invasive nanagement.[252a] In long-term follow-up, both of these out- :omes converged between the arms so that no difference in quality of life, functional outcomes, or death/myocardial nfarction was detected (Fig 50–10). Elderly patients who vere managed medically had a significantly higher risk of najor adverse cardiac events, when rehospitalization and the need for subsequent revascularization were included (49.3 percent vs. 19.0 percent; $p < 0.001$), but no difference in death/myocardial infarction.[252a] Nonrandomized data from at least one observational study that included a propensity analysis indicate that absolute benefit of treatment with PCI compared with medical therapy may increase with age.[253]

A

B

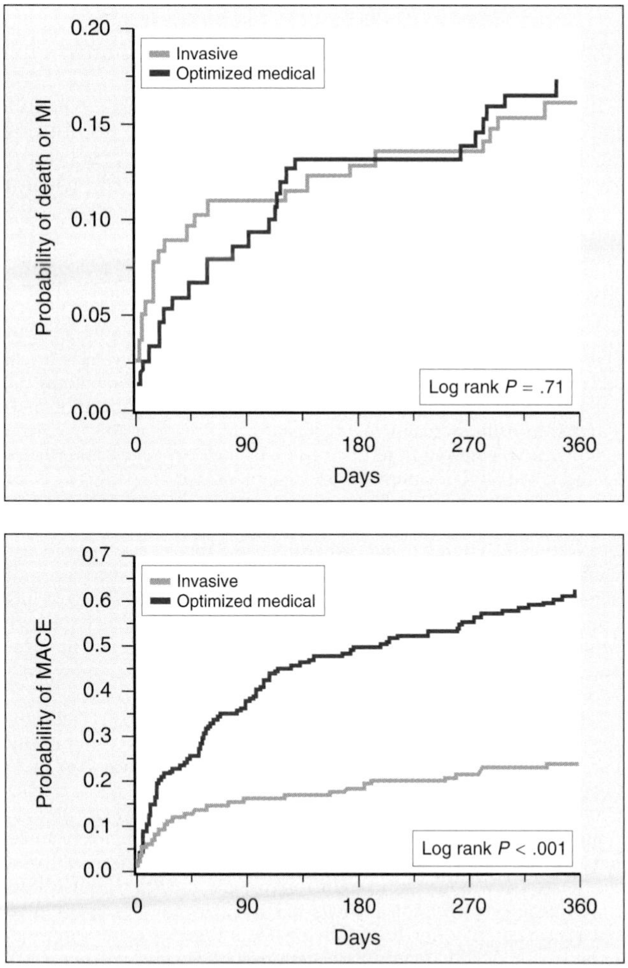

FIGURE 50–10 Results of a randomized trial of invasive versus medical manage- nent for patients (N = 282) aged 75 years or older with chronic coronary artery disease Trial of Invasive vs. Medical therapy in the Eldery [TIME] Trial). **A,** After 1 year, rates of death or nonfatal myocardial infarction were not significantly different between the wo treatment strategies. **B,** However, the rate of major adverse cardiac events (MACE; death, nonfatal myocardial infarction [MI], or hospitalization for uncontrolled symptoms or acute coronary syndrome) was significantly higher in patients randomized to a strat- egy of medical therapy. (**A** and **B,** From Pfisterer M, Buser P, Osswald S, et al: Outcome of elderly patients with chronic symptomatic coronary artery disease with an invasive vs. optimized medical treatment strategy: One-year results of the randomized TIME trial. JAMA 289:1117-1123, 2003.)

DIABETES MELLITUS. Patients with diabetes are at sub- stantially higher risk for complications after PCI. Possible explanations for the higher rate of adverse outcomes include an altered vascular biological response in diabetic patients to balloon injury and rapid progression of disease in nondilated segments. The diabetic atherosclerotic milieu is characterized by a procoagulant state, decreased fibrinolytic activity, in- creased proliferation, and inflammation.[254]

Restenosis is more frequent in diabetic patients, as is disease progression. In a study of patients referred for diag- nostic angiography 1 month or more after successful PTCA, the number of new narrowings in the arteries of diabetic patients was 22 percent higher, particularly at other sites in the artery that initially underwent PTCA. For this reason, CABG, which bypasses the majority of the vessel instead of a specific lesion, may offer a better intermediate- to long-term outcome.[255] The optimal revascularization strategy (CABG vs. PCI) for patients with diabetes and multivessel disease bears further study in the era of drug-eluting stents that have been shown to substantially reduce restenosis, including among patients with diabetes.[256,257]

PREVIOUS CORONARY BYPASS GRAFTING. CABG and PCI are often considered competitive procedures, but it is more appropriate to view them as complementary. An increasing number of patients who have had CABG and later have recurrent ischemia undergo revascularization with PCI. At the Mayo Clinic, approximately 20 percent of all PCIs are in patients who have had previous CABG.[258]

With advances in technology, the rates of initial success with PCI in venous bypass grafts have approximated those encountered for intervention in native coronaries.[259] Specifi- cally, studies indicate procedural success in more than 90 percent of lesions and mortality rates less than 2 percent. However, the incidence of periprocedural myocardial infarc- tion due to distal embolization remains higher with PCI in venous grafts compared with native coronary arteries. Restenosis in saphenous vein grafts has been reduced with the introduction of elective stenting but remains more fre- quent than in native arteries. The age of the bypass graft should be taken into consideration, because patients with older and severely diseased venous grafts may benefit from repeat CABG as an alternative to PCI.[258]

Innovative approaches to the PCI in vein graft atheroscle- rosis include catheter-based aspiration systems, in which the techniques of aspiration and filters are combined to prevent distal emboli.[260] These have provided important reductions in the risk of periprocedural myocardial infarction. Platelet glycoprotein IIb/IIIa antagonists and other newer devices, such as coronary ultrasound thrombolysis, have not yet been shown to improve outcomes.

OTHER CATHETER-BASED TECHNIQUES. Directional coronary atherectomy, rotational atherectomy, transluminal extraction catheters, thrombectomy, Excimer laser atherec- tomy, distal protection devices, and other newer catheter- based techniques are discussed in Chapter 52.

Coronary Artery Bypass Surgery

In 1964, Garrett, Dennis, and DeBakey first used CABG as a "bailout" procedure. Widespread use of the technique by Favoloro and Johnson and their respective collaborators fol- lowed in the late 1960s. Use of the internal mammary artery

(IMA) graft was pioneered by Kolessov in 1967 and by Green and colleagues in 1970.[261]

The annual number of coronary bypass operations in the United States rose steadily between 1979 and 1997, increasing by 227 percent over that period. In 2001, approximately 305,000 patients underwent coronary bypass surgery; a decline of 16 percent since 1997 that may be attributed in part to the growth of PCI.[3] Nevertheless, CABG remains one of the most frequently performed operations in the United States, resulting in the expenditure of almost $50 billion annually. CABG provides excellent short- and intermediate-term results in the management of stable CAD; its long-term results are affected by failure of venous grafts. Long-term data with totally arterial surgical revascularization are few.

Technical Considerations

When a decision has been reached to proceed with CABG, administration of beta blockers, nitrates, and calcium antagonists is continued until surgery. It is crucial to minimize perioperative damage and protect the myocardium. The most commonly used method involves a single period of aortic cross-clamping with intermittent infusion of cold cardioplegia solution. Technical modifications of traditional CABG, either using more limited incisions or eliminating cardiopulmonary bypass (CPB), or both, have been aimed at reducing the morbidity associated with this major surgery.[261] It is estimated that in 2002 approximately 20 percent of CABG was performed off-pump[262] and that this proportion is increasing. Other technical factors include the selection and method of preparation of bypass conduits, use of sutureless anastomotic devices, and the method of cardioplegia, if utilized.

MINIMALLY INVASIVE CABG. "Less invasive" or "minimally invasive" approaches may be divided into four major categories based on the approach and use of CPB. Port-access CABG is performed using limited incisions with femoral-femoral CPB and cardioplegic arrest. Port-access technology has also now enabled totally endoscopic robotically assisted CABG (TECAB) to be performed on the arrested heart.[263] Off-pump CABG is performed using a standard median sternotomy, with generally small skin incisions, and stabilization devices to reduce motion of the target vessels while anastomoses are performed without CPB. Finally, minimally invasive direct coronary artery bypass (MIDCAB) is performed through a left anterior thoracotomy without CPB.[261] Thus, off-pump approaches to CABG include both off-pump CAB (OPCAB) and MIDCAB techniques (Fig 50–11).

The potential advantages of the minimally invasive approaches include reduced postoperative patient discomfort, minimized risk of wound infection, and shorter recovery times. The avoidance of CPB may mitigate the risk of bleeding, systemic thromboembolism, renal insufficiency, myocardial stunning, stroke, and damaging neurological effects of bypass, particularly in the elderly and in patients with heavily calcified aortas.[262] Amelioration of the systemic inflammatory response that occurs after CABG using CPB is viewed as an additional advantage that may affect these clinical outcomes.[262] The "learning curve" of minimally invasive CABG has led to reports of early graft failure. In many centers, intraoperative or early postoperative angiography has been performed to assess the quality of the anastomosis. It should be emphasized that with conventional surgical techniques, the *early* patency rates of an IMA graft are excellent (98.7 percent in one large series), and less than 50 percent stenosis was noted in 91 percent of grafts.[264] Short-term clinical and angiographic outcomes suggest that the less invasive techniques can be used to achieve results comparable to traditional CABG.[265] The ultimate success of these "nontraditional" approaches to CABG will depend on long-term graft patency and the continued development of new techniques that will increase exposure to allow for more complete revascularization.

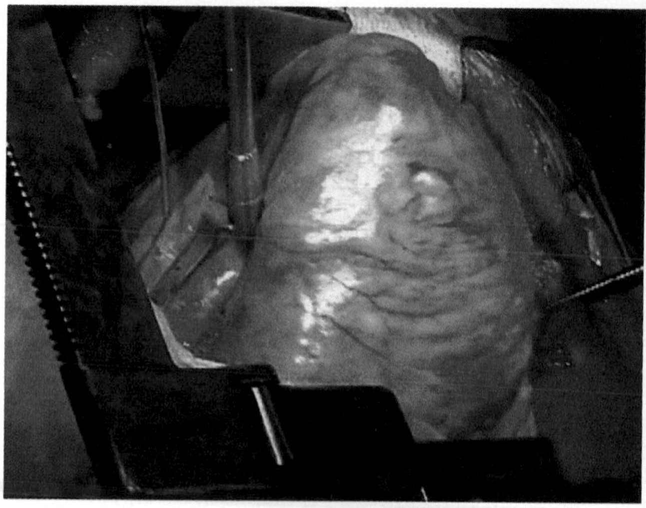

FIGURE 50–11 Off-pump coronary artery bypass grafting performed using a standard median sternotomy and a stabilization device to reduce motion of the target vessel while the anastomosis is performed without cardiopulmonary bypass. (Courtesy of Dr. Tomislav Mihaljevic.)

In addition, novel approaches to coronary revascularization may also include CABG with PCI by combining a minimally invasive coronary bypass surgical procedure on the left anterior descending coronary artery with PCI on the remaining vessels. Further experience is needed to clarify appropriate selection criteria and whether this strategy offers important advantages over multivessel bypass surgery alone.[266]

PORT-ACCESS CABG. An innovative approach to coronary revascularization is the *port-access method*, which uses small thoracotomy ports for cardiac manipulation; CPB is established by groin cannulation and an intraaortic balloon clamp for occlusion of the aorta. The two largest single-center series and the first report of the Port-Access International Registry, which documented the results of 555 bypass procedures, were encouraging.[267] Data comparing port-access to traditional CABG are few but indicate similar short-term outcomes.[268] Limitations to the use of this technique include atherosclerotic involvement of the aortic arch, high cost, long operating times due to technically very demanding surgery, and the risk of aortic dissection.[268] As a result, the port-access approach is now not widely used. However, port-access technology has enabled robotically enhanced totally endoscopic CABG to be performed and may increase in use if this new approach becomes more widely adopted.[263]

MINIMALLY INVASIVE DIRECT CABG. MIDCAB is performed through a limited left thoracotomy on the beating heart (off-pump), most commonly with grafting of the left internal thoracic artery to the left anterior descending artery. Studies of early angiographic patency have shown rates (98 percent) comparable to traditional CABG.[269] In a randomized trial comparing MIDCAB to stenting for treatment of isolated left anterior descending (LAD) artery disease, the rate of death or myocardial infarction was similar between the two groups (3 percent with stenting vs. 6 percent with MIDCAB; $p = 0.5$, $n = 220$). The need for repeated revascularization during the following 6 months was significantly higher in patients treated with coronary stenting (29 percent vs. 8 percent; $p = 0.003$).[270] In this trial, early reoperation for graft failure was necessary in 3 percent of patients and conversion to a full sternotomy was necessary in 5 percent. All grafts were patent at 6 months.[270] Outcomes were favorable (major cardiac events 7.8 percent, mortality 2.5 percent) at 1 year among 274 patients who underwent MIDCAB in an experienced center. Accumulation of operator experience appears to reduce perioperative adverse events.[271]

Limitations include the requirement that the patient can tolerate single-lung ventilation and that the operation is generally limited to revascularization of the LAD territory due to lesser accessibility of the left circumflex and right coronary arteries. The latter limitation may be successfully addressed by combined MIDCAB of the LAD with revascularization of other diseased arteries by PCI.[266] This approach has been evaluated predominantly in small observational studies; the benefit of so-called integrated coronary revascularization compared to established strategies remains to be adequately studied.

OFF-PUMP CABG. An alternative approach to revascularization on the beating heart is OPCAB, entailing a conventional median sternotomy and mechanical suction stabilizing systems. This combination enhances surgical exposure compared with MIDCAB and is particularly useful if multivessel bypass grafting is contemplated. Most surgeons consider only hemodynamic instability or severe cardiomegaly as contraindications.[262] In studies of small numbers of patients, angiographic patency rates have been documented as 99 percent at hospital discharge and 1 month and as 95 percent at 6 months.[262]

Observational data among 2223 patients who underwent OPCAB in the United Kingdom suggest better survival in analysis adjusted for baseline risk (odds ratio for CPB vs. OPCAB 1.85; 95 percent confidence interval (CI), 1.19 to 2.92).[272] The number of patients studied in randomized, controlled trials are few. A meta-analysis of nine randomized trials (<600 randomized to off-pump procedures, including MIDCAB), performed primarily in younger patients at lower risk, showed a trend toward lower risk of a composite of death, stroke, or myocardial infarction (odds ratio, 0.48; 95 percent CI, 0.21 to 1.09).[273] Generally consistent findings across randomized and observational data sets include comparable completeness of revascularization, reductions in blood loss and/or transfusion requirements, fewer wound infections, lower indices of myocardial injury, shorter duration of mechanical ventilation, and earlier hospital discharge with OPCAB.[262,274] Although trends toward neurocognitive benefits are evident, important reductions in stroke or long-term cognitive impairment with OPCAB versus traditional CABG have not yet been demonstrated.[275] Moreover, a randomized trial of OPCAB versus traditional CABG suggests that the former provides similar long-term outcomes (death, myocardial infarction, stroke, or need for reintervention) and is more cost-effective in low-risk patients,[276] but additional data regarding optimal patient selection for OPCAB are needed.

CARDIOPLEGIA

Favorable outcomes with respect to postoperative ventricular function are in large part dependent on optimal intraoperative myocardial protection.[277] Early cardioplegic techniques relied on cold crystalloid to initiate and maintain intraoperative cardiac arrest. However, blood cardioplegia facilitates myocardial aerobic metabolism, preserves myocardial high-energy phosphate stores, and reduces lactate production compared with crystalloid cardioplegia.[277] Enhancement of cardioplegia using metabolic substrates such as glutamate has also been shown to improve metabolic recovery. Other alternatives include retrograde and/or antegrade delivery, continuous versus intermittent cardioplegia, and the use of "warm" (37° C) or "tepid" (29° C) induction of cardioplegic arrest[278] and/or a terminal infusion of warm blood cardioplegia to facilitate a return to aerobic metabolism. Retrograde cardioplegia through the coronary sinus provides more uniform distribution of cardioplegic solution; many surgeons now use a combination of antegrade and retrograde perfusion. Intermittent delivery facilitates visualization of the distal anastomosis. Novel approaches with separate administration or additional additives such as sodium/hydrogen exchange inhibitors, L-arginine, insulin, or adenosine as additional myocardial protectants are under study.[277] Future advances may stem from ongoing investigation of the mediators of myocardial injury during cardioplegia and the impact of cardioplegic alternatives.[279]

Among patients with satisfactory preoperative cardiac function, a wide range of techniques have produced excellent results. For example, both cold crystalloid and warm blood cardioplegia in elective bypass surgery in patients with well-preserved preoperative ventricular function have been associated with low mortality and morbidity. This success is probably a reflection of the extent of myocardial functional reserve in those with well-preserved systolic function. In contrast, among patients with depressed left ventricular function (both acutely and chronically), it is easier to demonstrate a benefit with more specialized protocols, including the use of sanguineous cardioplegic techniques, with or without substrate enhancement, and blood cardioplegia.[277]

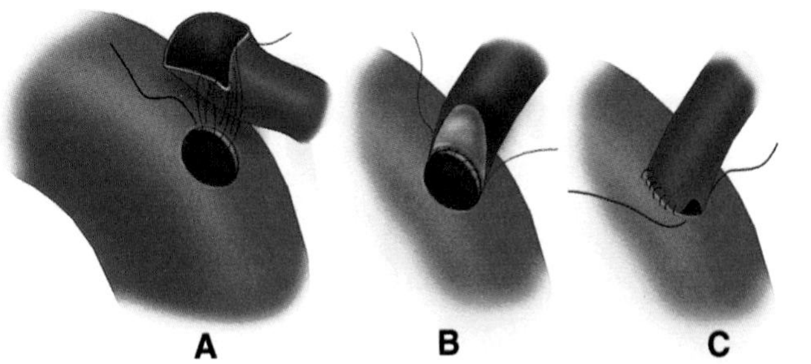

FIGURE 50–12 Aorticovenous anastomosis in a coronary artery–saphenous vein bypass graft. **A,** The technique of single cross-clamp is demonstrated. An aortotomy is created with a knife and punch Appropriate conduit length and orientation are established and a fine polypropylene suture is used in a running fashion toward and around the anastomotic heel. **B,** The conduit is carefully parachuted down onto the aorta. **C,** The suture is continued toward and around the anastomotic toe. (**A** to **C,** From Woo YJ, Gardner TJ: Myocardial revascularization with cardiopulmonary bypass. *In* Cohn LC, Edmunds LH [eds]: Cardiac Surgery in the Adult. New York, McGraw-Hill, 2003, p 597.)

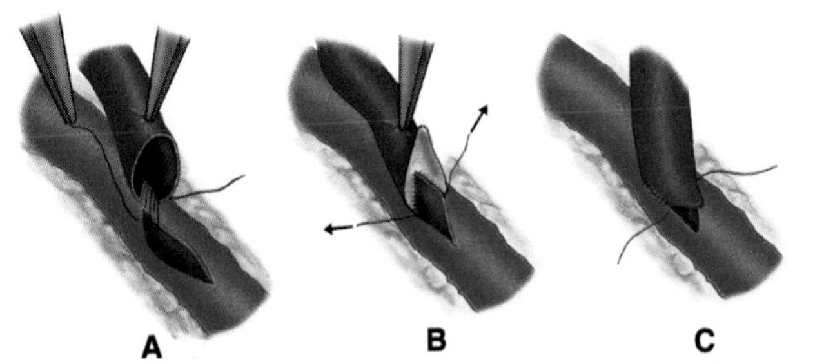

FIGURE 50–13 Venocoronary anastomosis. **A,** An initial arteriotomy is created with a knife and then extended with angled fine scissors. A fine polypropylene suture is used in a running fashion toward and around the anastomotic heel. **B,** After several throws of the suture, the conduit is carefully parachuted down onto the coronary artery. **C,** The suture is continued toward and around the anastomotic toe until the other end of the suture is reached. (From Woo YJ, Gardner TJ: Myocardia revascularization with cardiopulmonary bypass. *In* Cohn LC, Edmunds LH (eds): Cardiac Surgery in the Adult. New York: McGraw Hill, 2003, p 593.)

VENOUS CONDUITS. The saphenous vein is used mainly for distal branches of the right and circumflex coronary arteries and for sequential grafts to these vessels and diagonal branches (Figs. 50–12 and 50–13). In emergency situations, many surgeons prefer the saphenous vein to the IMA, because the saphenous vein can be harvested and grafted more rapidly. When the greater saphenous vein is not available, the lesser saphenous vein and the upper extremity veins (typically the cephalic or basilic) may be used. However, arm vein grafts are not as effective as either IMA or saphenous vein grafts. Endoscopic harvesting of saphenous vein provides improved cosmetic results and may reduce morbidity compared with open harvesting.[280] Cryopreserved homologous saphenous vein grafts and glutaraldehyde-treated umbilical veins have been used, but the patency rates are not optimal and thus these veins should be used only when there are no other alternatives.[261]

Trauma to the vein during surgical preparation can denude the endothelium, impair the intrinsic fibrinolytic activity of the saphenous vein, and damage the vessel wall, thereby predisposing to early thrombosis. Careful harvesting of the graft, with particular attention to avoidance of overdistention and the use of modified storage solutions, and inclusion of surrounding tissue to minimize manipulation of the graft have been shown to improve patency and preserve the integrity of the graft in both animal models and the clinical setting.[281-283]

Recently developed aortic-saphenous vein graft connectors enable surgeons to create the proximal anastomosis without the use of side-biting aortic clamps that may contribute to aortic injury and perioperative stroke. Early experience with sutureless connectors suggests high rates of stenosis during the first 6 months after placement; thus, although these devices have potential for substantial expansion of use in

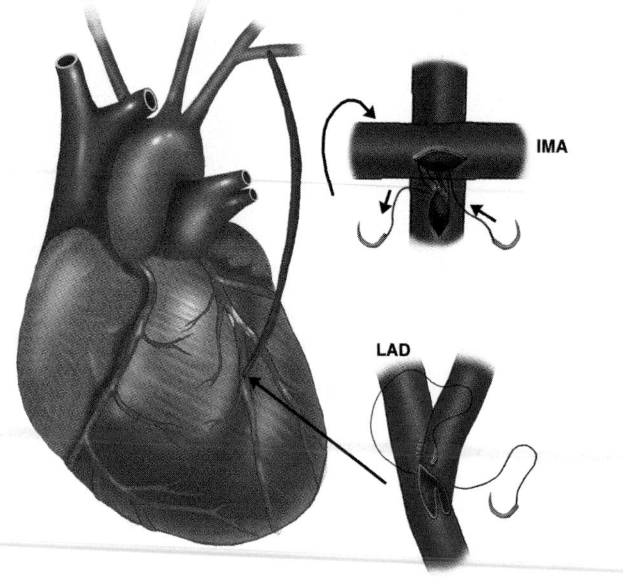

FIGURE 50–14 Internal mammary grafting consisting of an in situ left internal mammary artery (IMA) graft to the left anterior descending (LAD) artery (end to side) and diagonal branch (side to side), with the diamond anastomotic technique used for the latter. The details show the IMA pedicle rolled up over the diagonal coronary artery to facilitate exposure and the use of continuous suture. (From Jones EL: Extended use of the internal mammary–coronary artery bypass. J Card Surg 1:13, 1986.)

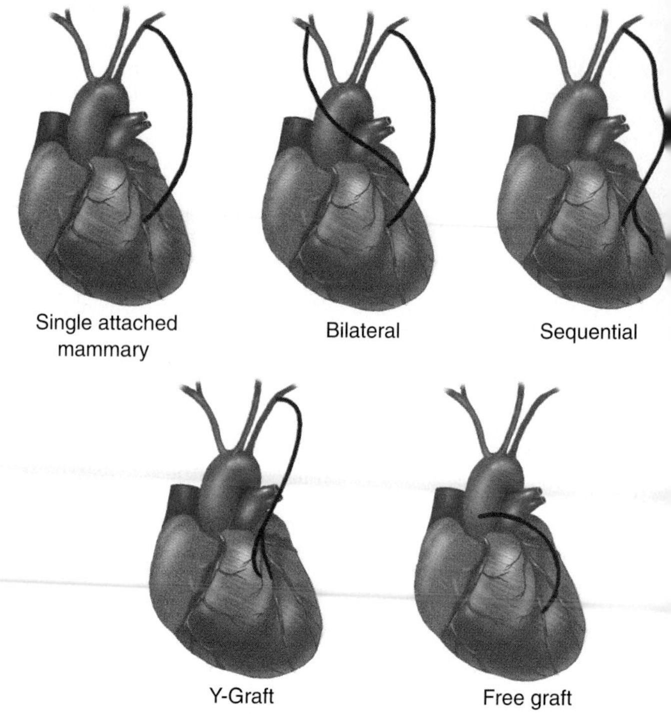

FIGURE 50–15 Different types of internal mammary artery grafts. A single attached internal mammary artery graft (either the right or left) remains attached proximally to the subclavian artery and is connected to the coronary arteries. Bilateral internal mammary artery grafts (right and left) are joined end to side to coronary arteries. Sequential internal mammary artery grafts consist of an attached or free internal mammary artery with one or more side-to-side anastomoses and one end-to-side anastomosis. The internal mammary artery Y graft has two terminal branches of either the attached or free internal mammary artery sutured to two coronary arteries. A free internal mammary graft is placed by transecting the right or left internal mammary artery near its origin in the subclavian artery and anastomosing the proximal portion of the artery to the aorta and the distal end to the coronary artery. (From Tector AJ, Schmahl TM, Canino VR: Expanding the use of the internal mammary artery to improve patency in coronary artery bypass grafting. J Thorac Cardiovasc Surg 91:9, 1986.)

conjunction with minimally invasive CABG, additional experience and long-term data are needed to clarify their role.[284]

Flow Rates. When measured at the time of surgery, flow rates through saphenous vein grafts average nearly 70 ml/min. Flow rates less than 45 ml/min—and especially less than 25 ml/min—are more frequently associated with graft closure than are higher flow rates.[285] The usefulness of measuring flow rates is enhanced by taking into account the type of conduit used and the size of the distal vasculature. If flow rates are lower than expected, reassessment of the anastomosis with a probe may be helpful. Possible causes of reduced flow include (1) subcritical obstruction of the coronary artery; (2) a technically poor anastomosis with narrowing of the lumen from kinking of the vessel or pinching at the site of anastomosis; (3) a small myocardial mass perfused by the graft; and (4) a diseased distal vascular bed.

INTERNAL MAMMARY ARTERY BYPASS GRAFTS. The IMA, also known as the internal thoracic artery, is usually remarkably free of atheroma, especially in patients younger than 65 years. When it is grafted to a coronary artery (Figs. 50–14 and 50–15), it appears to be virtually immune to the development of intimal hyperplasia, which is almost universally seen in aortocoronary vein grafts,[286] and the functional (endothelium-dependent vasodilatory) capacity of the artery remains intact.[287] The diameter of the IMA graft is usually a closer match to that of the recipient coronary artery than is the diameter of a saphenous vein.

The current standard for bypass grafting advocates routine use of the left IMA for grafting the left anterior descending coronary artery, with supplemental saphenous vein grafts to other vessels.[261] Limitations to this approach are few; the primary consideration is that the procedure is time consuming; thus, the IMA is not often used for emergency surgery.

Although the benefits of a single IMA graft over a saphenous vein graft alone are not in dispute,[288] the superiority of bilateral IMA grafts over a single IMA graft and one saphenous vein graft is less well accepted.[289] Initial enthusiasm for the use of bilateral IMA grafts was tempered by a higher rate of postoperative complications, including bleeding, wound infection, and prolonged ventilatory support. Wound infection, which has been of particular concern, remains modest in frequency (<3 percent), except among patients who are obese or diabetic or those who require prolonged ventilatory support. Subsequent series have shown that bilateral versus single IMA grafting is associated with lower rates of recurrent angina pectoris, reoperation, and myocardial infarction and improved survival in nonrandomized studies.[289] The increased technical demands and longer operative times of bilateral IMA grafting have also been a barrier to more widespread adoption but may be overcome if data supporting a survival advantage continue to accumulate.

Complications. Inadequate flow rates with evidence of myocardial ischemia in the perioperative period are rare after IMA grafts to the LAD coronary artery or its diagonal branches. Perioperative spasm is the presumed cause and can be managed by the administration of sodium nitroprusside or a combination of glyceryl trinitrate and verapamil. Other complications include an increased incidence of sternal wound infections, which is more frequent in obese patients and diabetics and after bilateral IMA implants.

OTHER CONDUITS. The success of IMA grafts has stimulated interest in the use of other arterial conduits, particularly in patients who are younger, diabetic, or hyperlipidemic or in whom the saphenous veins are unsuitable or unavailable.[261] Options for arterial grafts include the radial, right gastroepiploic, inferior epigastric, and very rarely the subscapular, intercostal, splenic, left gastric, and gastroduodenal arteries. Initial enthusiasm for use of the radial artery was blunted by reports of high reocclusion rates. More recent experience, in which attention has been paid to avoiding spasm by minimizing manipulation and the use of calcium-channel blockers, has been favorable. Early rates of patency are as high as 95 percent with mid-term patency comparable to that for IMA grafts (~85 percent at 5 years). Radial arterial grafts may be associated with fewer perioperative complications and thus preferable to the right IMA as a second arterial graft.[290] Total arterial revascularization using both IMAs and free radial or alternative arterial grafts has also gained interest. A randomized trial comparing grafting using the left IMA plus additional venous grafts versus total arterial revascularization detected no differences in the number of vessels grafted, time on CPB, or postoperative complications. At a mean follow-up of 12 months, patients managed with total arterial revascularization were less likely to have recurrent angina or to require additional revascularization.[291]

The right gastroepiploic artery can be harvested by extending the median sternotomy incision toward the umbilicus.[292] It is frequently placed as a graft to the right coronary artery, but both the circumflex and the left anterior descending coronary arteries can be grafted with this conduit. Early results demonstrated excellent patency rates, but there is a paucity of data on long-term results. Similarly, the inferior epigastric artery has been used as a free graft for coronary revascularization, with good short-term patency rates but without long-term data. Bovine IMA, Dacron, and polytetrafluoroethylene (PTFE) grafts have also been used with lower patency (~50 to 60 percent) over the mid-term. These grafts should only be used as a last resort.[261]

THE DISTAL VASCULATURE. The state of the distal coronary vasculature is important for the fate of bypass grafts. Late patency of grafts is related to coronary arterial runoff as determined by the diameter of the coronary artery into which the graft is inserted, the size of the distal vascular bed, and the severity of coronary atherosclerosis distal to the site of insertion of the graft. The highest graft patency rates are found when the lumina of the vessels distal to the graft insertion are greater than 1.5 mm in diameter, perfuse a large vascular bed, and are free of atheroma obstructing more than 25 percent of the vessel lumen. For saphenous veins, optimal patency rates are achieved with a lumen of 2.0 mm or greater.

Surgical Outcomes

The patient population undergoing CABG has been changing over time, particularly with the wider use of PCI. In comparison with the 1970s, patients undergoing CABG today are older, include a higher percentage of women, and are "sicker" in that a greater proportion have unstable angina, triple-vessel disease, previous coronary revascularization with either CABG or PCI, left ventricular dysfunction, and comorbid conditions, including hypertension, diabetes, and peripheral vascular disease. Despite the increasing risk profile of this population, outcomes with CABG have generally remained stable or improved.

OPERATIVE MORTALITY. Risk factors for death following coronary artery surgery may be separated into five categories: (1) preoperative factors related to CAD, including recent acute myocardial infarction, hemodynamic instability, left ventricular dysfunction, extensive CAD, the presence of left main CAD, and severe or unstable angina; (2) preoperative factors related to the aggressiveness of the arteriosclerotic process, as reflected in associated carotid or peripheral vascular disease; (3) preoperative biological factors (older age at surgery, diabetes mellitus, comorbidities, including pulmonary and renal disease, and perhaps female gender); (4) intraoperative factors (intraoperative ischemic damage and failure to use IMA grafts); and (5) environmental or institutional factors, including the specific surgeon and treatment protocols used. Of these factors, several variables have consistently emerged as the most potent predictors of mortality after CABG: (1) age; (2) urgency of operation; (3) prior cardiac surgery; (4) left ventricular function; (5) percent stenosis of the left main coronary artery; and (6) number of epicardial vessels with significant disease.[261]

In-hospital mortality after isolated CABG was characterized by a steady decline from 1967 to the 1980s. Despite a shift toward higher risk demographics with an older population of patients with more comorbidities being referred for CABG, early mortality continued to decline in the 1990s.[293] Specifically, during the period from 1990 to 1999, crude mortality through 30 days after CABG in the United States fell by 0.9 percent, (23.1 percent relative decrease; $p < 0.0001$). Mortality among the 503,478 CABG-only operations recorded in the Society of Thoracic Surgeons data base between 1997 and 1999 was 3.05 percent.[294] Moreover, with increasingly wide scrutiny of procedural results, it has become recognized that *absolute* rates of morbidity and mortality might not provide a fair basis for comparing institutions and individuals, unless the characteristics of the patients are considered. Several models have been developed and refined with the objective of predicting perioperative mortality.[294] Application of such models demonstrate even greater declines in CABG mortality over the past decade when adjusted for changes in risk profile.[293]

A useful perspective of long-term survival after CABG during an earlier phase in the evaluation of this therapy is provided by the most recent follow-up data (mean, 15 years) from the Coronary Artery Surgery Study (CASS) Registry. Ninety percent of patients were alive at 5 years, 74 percent at 10 years, and 56 percent at 15 years. The hazard function for death decreases rapidly after surgery to its nadir at 9 to 12 months,[295] followed by a steady increase with a doubling of the hazard ratio at 15 years in comparison to that at 5 years.

PERIOPERATIVE COMPLICATIONS

Perioperative morbidity (see Chap. 76) has increased because of a larger fraction of higher risk patients. Major morbidity (death, stroke, renal failure, reoperation, prolonged ventilation, and sternal infection) occurred in 13.4 percent through 30 days among the 503,478 CABG-only operations recorded in the Society of Thoracic Surgeons data base between 1997 and 1999.[294]

MYOCARDIAL INFARCTION. Perioperative myocardial infarction, particularly if it is associated with hemodynamic or arrhythmic complications or preexisting left ventricular dysfunction, has a major adverse effect on early and late prognosis. The reported incidence varies widely (0 to >10 percent), in large part due to heterogeneous diagnostic criteria, with an average of 3.9 percent (median 2.9 percent).[296] The cardiac troponins and myocardial creatine phosphokinase-MB (CK-MB) may be useful as markers of perioperative infarction.[297] Elevation of CK-MB more than five times the upper limit of normal is commonly considered diagnostic of myocardial infarction in this setting. Predictors of perioperative myocardial infarction in CASS were female gender, severe perioperative angina pectoris, severe stenosis of the left main coronary artery, and triple-vessel disease. Preconditioning the myocardium with short periods of ischemic stress interspersed with reperfusion increases the resistance to infarction and appears to reduce myocardial damage during cardiac surgery, but the appropriateness of this technique as a routine clinical tool has not been determined.

RESPIRATORY COMPLICATIONS. Most patients are extubated within 6 to 8 hours after undergoing CABG. Prolonged mechanical ventilation (>24 hours) is necessary in 5 to 6 percent of first-time CABGs and 10 to 11 percent of reoperations.[298] The etiology is multifactorial and includes the presence of preexisting pulmonary disease and numerous perioperative factors related directly to anesthesia, level of consciousness, CPB, incisional pain, chest tube placement, and occasionally phrenic nerve damage.[299] Severe chronic obstructive pulmonary disease, as defined by a forced expiratory volume in 1 second (FEV_1) of less than 50 percent or an FEV_1/forced vital capacity (FVC) ratio less than 0.70, is associated with a high incidence of postoperative pulmonary complications (29 percent). The left ventricular ejection fraction is also an important determinant of prolonged ventilation.[300]

Postoperative changes in pulmonary function after CABG are frequent and troublesome, but rarely serious, except in patients with preexisting chronic lung disease or the elderly.[299] A potentially serious complication is phrenic nerve injury, which may be related to cold-induced damage during myocardial protection strategies or possibly to mechanical injury while harvesting the IMA. The pulmonary consequences vary and range from an asymptomatic radiographic abnormality to severe pulmonary dysfunction requiring prolonged ventilation.[261]

BLEEDING. Impaired hemostasis and bleeding complications are an inherent risk of CABG. Reoperation for bleeding is required in 2 to 6 percent of patients and is associated with nearly threefold higher in-hospital mortality.[301] CPB causes derangement of the intrinsic coagulation and fibrinolytic systems in addition to impairing platelet function. The risk of bleeding is increased with age, a smaller body surface area, duration of CPB, reoperation, bilateral internal thoracic artery grafts, and the preoperative use of heparin, aspirin, and fibrinolytic agents. Bleeding may be reduced with aprotinin and lysine analogs such as aminocaproic acid and tranexamic acid.[302]

WOUND INFECTIONS. Major perioperative wound complications, especially mediastinitis and/or wound dehiscence, occur in 1 to 4 percent of patients and are associated with significant morbidity as well as higher mortality. This risk is substantially increased in those undergoing reoperation and by the use of double IMA grafts, particularly in diabetic patients, and it is markedly increased in obese patients. Preventive measures include careful skin preparation, increased attention to sterility in the perioperative environment, and preoperative use of antimicrobial agents. Other factors that may decrease perioperative infection include strict control of glucose in patients with diabetes and the avoidance of unnecessary blood transfusion in view of the immunosuppressive effect of the latter.[261] Successful management of deep sternal wound infection involves prompt recognition and aggressive débridement with muscle flap closure.

POSTOPERATIVE HYPERTENSION. Hypertension can occur in up to one-third of patients postoperatively. The mechanisms are unclear but may be related to increased levels of circulating catecholamines and other humoral factors in addition to vasoconstriction secondary to activation of the renin-angiotensin system. Control of postoperative hypertension is important to prevent myocardial ischemia, cardiac failure, and perioperative bleeding. Regardless of the cause, sodium nitroprusside is an effective approach to afterload reduction, and other drugs such as calcium antagonists, nitrates, and beta blockers, including short-acting esmolol, are helpful.[261]

CEREBROVASCULAR COMPLICATIONS. Neurological abnormalities following cardiac surgery are dreaded complications. Postulated mechanisms include emboli from atherosclerosis of the aorta or other large arteries, emboli possibly from the CPB machine circuit and its tubing, and intraoperative hypotension, particularly in patients with preexisting hypertension.[303] Type I injury is associated with major neurological deficits, stupor, and coma, and type II is characterized by a deterioration in intellectual function and memory.[261] The incidence of neurological abnormalities is variably estimated depending on how the deficits are defined. The incidence of stroke reported in the Society of Thoracic Surgeons data base between 1997 to 1999 was 1.63 percent and has been documented as higher in prospective studies (1.5 to 5 percent). Studies aimed at careful evaluation of neurological deficits report more frequent neurological sequelae; type I deficits have been documented in 6 percent of patients early after CABG, with short-term cognitive decline in 33 to 83 percent.[304] A prospective long-term study employing sophisticated neurocognitive testing revealed cognitive decline in 53 percent of patients at the time of hospital discharge, 36 percent at 6 weeks, and 24 percent at 6 months.[305] In regard to the neurological sequelae of CPB (including stroke, delirium, and neurocognitive dysfunction), older age in addition to other comorbid conditions (particularly diabetes) associated with atherosclerosis and intraoperative manipulation of the aorta are the more powerful predictors. In most studies, atherosclerosis of the proximal aorta has also been a strong predictor of stroke, as has the use of an intraaortic balloon pump.

ATRIAL FIBRILLATION. This arrhythmia is one of the most frequent complications of CABG. It occurs in up to 40 percent of patients, primarily within 2 to 3 days.[306] In the early postoperative period, rapid ventricular rates and loss of atrial transport may compromise systemic hemodynamics, increase the risk of embolization, and lead to a significant increase in the duration and cost of the hospital stay, and it is associated with a twofold to threefold increase in postoperative stroke. Older age, hypertension, prior atrial fibrillation, and congestive heart failure are associated with higher risk of developing atrial fibrillation after cardiac surgery.

Prophylactic use of beta blockers reduces the frequency of postoperative atrial fibrillation and should be administered routinely before and after CABG to patients without contraindications. Amiodarone is also effective in prophylaxis against postoperative atrial fibrillation and may be considered in patients at high risk for developing this dysrhythmia (see Chap. 76). Up to 80 percent of patients spontaneously revert to sinus rhythm within 24 hours without treatment other than digoxin or other agents used for controlling the ventricular rate. Most patients return to sinus rhythm by 6 weeks after surgery.

BRADYARRHYTHMIAS AND CONDUCTION DISTURBANCES. The incidence of postoperative bradyarrhythmias requiring permanent pacemaker implantation was 0.8 percent in a series of 1614 consecutive patients discharged from the hospital after coronary bypass surgery. Predictive factors were preoperative left bundle branch block, concomitant left ventricular aneurysmectomy, and older age. Most patients continued to require permanent pacemaker support during follow-up.

RENAL DYSFUNCTION. The incidence of renal failure requiring dialysis after CABG remains low (0.5 to 1.0 percent) but is associated with significantly greater morbidity and mortality.[296] A decline in renal function defined by a postoperative serum creatinine higher than 2.0 mg/dl or an increase of more than 0.7 mg/dl is more frequent (7 to 8 percent). Predictors of postoperative renal dysfunction include advanced age, diabetes, preexisting renal dysfunction, and heart failure.[307] Patients with preoperative renal dysfunction and serum creatinine higher than 2.5 mg/dl appear to be at increased risk of the need for hemodialysis and may be candidates for alternative approaches to revascularization or prophylactic dialysis.[308]

SYMPTOMATIC RESULTS. CABG is highly effective in the relief of angina and results in improved quality of life. Approximately 80 percent of patients are free of angina at 5 years and 63 percent at 10 years, but by 15 years only about 15 percent are alive and free of an ischemic event.[261] Recurrent angina is associated with a higher risk of myocardial infarction and more frequent coronary reintervention but does not appear to affect survival. The acceleration in adverse events after 5 to 15 years is due to gradual occlusion of vein grafts in addition to progressive disease in the native coronary vessels. Independent predictors of recurrence of angina are female gender, obesity, preoperative hypertension, and lack of use of the IMA as a conduit.[261] In patients with triple-vessel disease undergoing coronary bypass surgery, the completeness of revascularization was a significant determinant of the relief of symptoms at 1 year and over a 5-year period.[309] In the bypass surgery arms of recent randomized trials of PCI and CABG, recurrent angina pectoris was reported in 21.5 to 34 percent of patients at a follow-up ranging from 2 to 3 years, but (Canadian classification) grade III or IV angina was present in only 6 percent at 2.5 years.[261]

RETURN TO EMPLOYMENT. Return to full employment has been variable (35 to 80 percent) but is as high as 80 percent among those who were employed prior to undergoing CABG.[310] Patients who undergo CABG take approximately 6 weeks longer to return to work than those who are treated with PCI; however, long-term employment is similar (>80 percent) among patients treated with CABG or PCI.[310] Factors that adversely affect the prospects of patients for returning to work include advanced age, postoperative angina, job satisfaction prior to surgery, and a period of either unemployment or disability before surgery.[311]

PATENCY OF VENOUS GRAFTS. Experimental studies and observations in patients suggest that the development of disease in *venous* aortocoronary artery bypass grafts occurs in several phases. The occlusion rate, which is high in the first year, decreases substantially between the first and sixth years. Between 6 and 10 years after surgery, the attrition rate for grafts increases again. Early occlusion (before hospital discharge) occurs in 8 to 12 percent of venous grafts, and by 1 year, 15 to 30 percent of vein grafts have become occluded.[261] After the first year, the annual occlusion rate is 2 percent and rises to approximately 4 percent annually between years 6 and 10. At 10 years, approximately 50 percent of vein grafts have become occluded, and significant atherosclerosis is present in the substantial proportion of grafts remaining patent, with significant stenoses in 20 to 40 percent.[261] Patency rates with IMA grafts are superior. Predictors of graft occlusion include small target-vessel diameter and patient risk factors such as high LDL cholesterol, low HDL cholesterol, prior myocardial infarction, male gender, and active smoking.[312]

EARLY PHASE (FIRST MONTH). Technical factors that may cause thrombotic closure at the proximal or distal anastomoses include kinking because of excessive length, tension from insufficient length, poor graft flow, and inadequate distal runoff. Surgical manipulation of the saphenous vein during harvesting and preparation prior to grafting play key roles in initiating the sequence of endothelial damage with subsequent platelet and fibrin deposition leading to thrombosis.

INTERMEDIATE PHASE (1 MONTH TO 1 YEAR). Vein grafts that have been implanted in the arterial circulation for 1 month to 1 year are subject to substantial endothelial denudation and proliferation and to migration of medial cells to the intima. Migration of vascular smooth muscle cells through the internal elastic lamina into the intima may also occur.[313] This initial phase of rapid proliferation is followed after several months by a marked increase in the connective tissue matrix, which further increases intimal and medial thickness. This accelerated process of intimal hyperplasia and thickening is an early stage of atherosclerotic plaque formation and is believed to occur because of interaction between platelets and macrophages and endothelial damage. If the proliferation is severe and localized, as may occur at the site of anastomosis between the grafts and the recipient artery, total occlusion can occur within 1 year.

LATE PHASE (BEYOND 1 YEAR). Some investigators believe that the development of atherosclerosis in vein grafts, as in native arteries, is a continuum starting from platelet deposition and advancing to smooth muscle cell proliferation and finally to lipid incorporation into the plaque. By 10 years, nearly half of venous grafts patent at 5 years have become occluded.[314] Beyond the first year, particularly after 3 to 5 years, the histological appearance of occluded or obstructed coronary bypass grafts is consistent with atherosclerosis. There is clear evidence of mature lipid-laden plaque, foam cells, cholesterol clefts, ulceration, and areas of calcification with disruption of the medial layer. Late graft atherosclerosis is often characterized by an extensive thrombotic burden and marked friability of the lesions; the resultant intermittent distal embolization in turn complicates repeat revascularization procedures either by percutaneous coronary reintervention or reoperation.[315]

DETERMINATION OF GRAFT PATENCY. Although angiography is the most frequently used method for the determination of vein graft patency, the diffuseness of the atherosclerotic process, which in many patients decreases the luminal diameter of the entire vessel, may lead to an underestimation of the severity of a more focal lesion. Alternative approaches to the evaluation of vein graft patency that are being investigated include contrast-enhanced CT (see Chap. 15),[316] phase-contrast magnetic resonance angiography (see Chap. 14),[317] and transcutaneous ultrasonographic[318] and magnetic resonance measurements of angiographic flow.[72]

ARTERIAL GRAFT PATENCY. Comparative morphological and angiographic studies of IMA and saphenous vein bypass grafts that have been implanted long-term show that accelerated atherosclerosis occurs commonly in saphenous vein grafts but is extremely rare in IMA grafts. Several potential explanations may be offered for the superiority of the IMA graft. The media of the artery may derive nourishment from the lumen as well as from the vasa vasorum, and the internal elastic lamina of the IMA is uniform. Moreover, the finding that the endothelium of the IMA produces significantly more prostacyclin than that of the saphenous vein may explain the more pronounced endothelium-dependent relaxation and may allow flow-dependent autoregulation to occur. Fibrointimal proliferation occasionally develops in IMA grafts, and the resultant narrowing may be a factor in late graft closure.[261]

Clinical and angiographic outcomes are superior when IMA grafts are used compared with venous grafts. In one series, IMA grafts had patency rates of 95, 88, and 83 percent at 1, 5, and 10 years, respectively. Although comparable at 1 year, these rates are significantly higher than those observed for venous grafts at 5 and 10 years. Excellent long-term results have also been achieved with use of the right IMA as a free or sequential graft. Consistent with these angiographic findings, patients receiving an IMA graft have a decreased risk of short-term and long-term major cardiac events, including death, myocardial infarction, and reoperations, and this clinical advantage persists for up to 20 years.[261,288]

PROGRESSION OF DISEASE IN NONGRAFTED ARTERIES. Disease progression, defined as worsening of a preexisting lesion or the appearance of a new diameter narrowing of 50 percent or greater, can occur at a rate of 20 to 40 percent over 5 to 10 years in nongrafted native vessels.[319] The rate of disease progression appears highest in arterial segments already showing evidence of disease, and it is between three and six times higher in grafted native coronary arteries than in ungrafted native vessels. Disease progression is also greater in arteries with patent grafts than in arteries with occluded grafts[320] and usually occurs proximal to the site of graft insertion. These data suggest that bypassing an artery with minimal disease, even if initially successful, may ultimately be harmful to patients, who incur both the risk of graft closure and the increased risk of accelerated obstruction of native vessels. Lesions in the native vessel that are long (>10 mm) and more than 70 percent in diameter are at increased risk of progressing to total occlusion.[321]

EFFECTS OF THERAPY ON VEIN GRAFT OCCLUSION AND NATIVE VESSEL PROGRESSION

Measures aimed at enhancing long-term patency are generally directed at delaying the overall process of atherosclerosis, and thus they may have several additional benefits.[315] Secondary preventive therapy, in particular lipid-lowering treatment, is important to reducing the risk of failure of venous grafts.[282] Chronic anticoagulant therapy has *not* been shown convincingly to alter outcomes.[282] Other novel approaches, such as pretreatment of venous grafts to increase resistance to atherothrombosis, are in early stages of evaluation.[283]

ANTIPLATELET THERAPY. Several trials have demonstrated the efficacy of aspirin therapy when started 1, 7, or 24 hours preoperatively, but the benefit is lost when aspirin is started more than 48 hours postoperatively.[322] Aspirin, 80 to 325 mg daily, should be continued indefinitely. The addition of dipyridamole or warfarin in conventional doses has not been shown definitively to provide added benefit.[282] Although the effects of clopidogrel on graft patency have not been studied specifically, it is likely to be at least as effective as aspirin.

LIPID-LOWERING THERAPY. The rationale for lowering lipid levels in patients with CAD was extended to postoperative patients with at least one patent vein graft and LDL cholesterol concentrations between 130 and 175 mg/dl in the Post-Coronary Artery Bypass Graft Trial.[282] Patients who received aggressive treatment with lovastatin and, if needed, cholestyramine to decrease LDL cholesterol to less than 100 mg/dl, in comparison with "moderate" therapy resulting in an LDL cholesterol level of 134 mg/dl, had a lower rate of progressive atherosclerosis in grafts (27 vs. 39 percent; $p < 0.001$) and a lower rate of repeat revascularization procedures over a 4-year period. Similar benefits are achieved with other lipid-lowering therapies, including colestipol and niacin, and gemfibrozil. Moreover, the favorable effects of lipid-lowering on the progression of graft disease appear similar in women and men, the elderly and young, and those with and without diabetes.

SMOKING CESSATION. Strong evidence from the CASS randomized trial and other series indicates that continued smoking after bypass surgery increases mortality, the recurrence rate of angina, the need for repeat hospitalization, and repeat revascularization procedures. Not unexpectedly, continued smoking has been associated with angiographic progression of graft disease.[312]

Patient Selection

Indications for CABG consist of the need for improvement in the quality or duration of life. Patients whose angina is not adequately controlled by medical management or who have unacceptable side effects with such management should be considered for coronary revascularization. The decision to perform PCI or CABG is based partly on coronary anatomy, left ventricular function, other medical comorbidities that may affect the patient's risk for either procedure, and patient preference. Recent technological developments have enlarged the pool of patients with single-vessel or multivessel disease amenable to PCI. For patients who are suitable for

PCI and who do not fulfill the criteria of anatomy requiring surgery (e.g., left main CAD or severe triple-vessel disease and left ventricular dysfunction), PCI is generally the procedure of choice. However, if medical therapy has failed (i.e., the symptoms are severe or sufficient to impair quality of life), and the patient is not a good candidate for initial or repeat PCI, CABG should be strongly considered. This procedure is also indicated for patients with CAD, regardless of symptoms, in whom survival is likely to be prolonged, and for patients in whom noninvasive testing suggests "high risk."[261]

In making the decision about revascularization, it is important to assess the patient's prognosis (Tables 50–13 and 50–14) and how it may be affected by surgery. The key initial step is to stratify patients into categories of risk with continued medical therapy based on an analysis of clinical, noninvasive, and, in some patients, angiographic variables. This process defines the *indications* for revascularization over medical therapy and, by implication, the indications for coronary angiography in patients with chronic stable angina, as well as which *modality* of revascularization (PCI or surgery) is preferable.[18]

The four major determinants of risk in CAD are the extent of ischemia, the number of vessels diseased, left ventricular function, and the electrical substrate. The major effect of coronary revascularization is on ischemia, and the magnitude of the benefit compared with that of medical therapy is enhanced with left ventricular dysfunction, particularly in the presence of reversibly ischemic jeopardized myocardium. In this context, patients can be risk stratified according to the expected benefit of revascularization versus medical therapy. Patients with more extensive and severe CAD have an increasing magnitude of benefit from CABG over medical therapy (Figs. 50–16 and 50–17 and Table 50–15). Selection of patients for surgery is based on clinical, angiographic, and noninvasive testing characteristics that may be considered markers or, in some cases, surrogates of the three major predictors—ischemia, left ventricular function, and, to a lesser extent, arrhythmia. Other factors that must always be considered in the decision are general health and noncoronary comorbid conditions.

The appropriate use of invasive cardiovascular procedures is undergoing increasing scrutiny. It is therefore reassuring to note that in studies of coronary angiography and bypass surgery less than 4 percent of bypass procedures are

TABLE 50–13 Determinants of Adverse Prognosis in Patients with Coronary Artery Disease

Cardiac Determinants
Left ventricular dysfunction
Extent of myocardium in jeopardy
Abnormal arrhythmic substrate

Clinical and Electrocardiographic Modifying Factors
Advanced age
History of congestive heart failure
Diabetes
Rapidly accelerating angina
Resting electrocardiographic abnormalities
Left ventricular hypertrophy and hypertension
Peripheral vascular disease
Hyperlipidemia
Increased C-reactive protein (inflammation)

TABLE 50–14 Impact of Coronary Bypass Surgery on Survival in Subsets of Patients Studied in the Coronary Artery Surgery Study (CASS) Randomized Trial and Registry Studies

Category of Risk	Number of Vessels Diseased	Severity of Ischemia	Ejection Fraction	Results of Surgery on Survival
Mild	2	Mild	>0.50	Unchanged*
	3			Unchanged*
Moderate	2	Moderate to severe	>0.50	Unchanged*
	3			Improved†
	2	Mild	<0.50	Unchanged*
	3			Improved†
Severe	2	Moderate to severe	<0.50	Improved†
	3			Improved†

*Randomized trial.

†Survival improved with surgery versus medicine. In the European Coronary Surgery Trial, patients with double-vessel disease and involvement of the proximal left anterior descending coronary artery had improved survival with surgery irrespective of left ventricular function.

TABLE 50–15 Effects of Coronary Artery Bypass Grafting on Survival*

Subgroup	Medical Treatment Mortality Rate (%)	*p* Value for CABG Surgery vs. Medical Treatment
Vessel Disease		
One vessel	9.9	0.18
Two vessels	11.7	0.45
Three vessels	17.6	<0.001
Left main artery	36.5	0.004
No LAD Disease		
One or two vessels	8.3	0.88
Three vessels	14.5	0.02
Left main artery	45.8	0.03
Overall	12.3	0.05
LAD Disease Present		
One or two vessels	14.6	0.05
Three vessels	19.1	0.009
Left main artery	32.7	0.02
Overall	18.3	0.001
LV Function		
Normal	13.3	<0.001
Abnormal	25.2	0.02
Exercise Test Status		
Missing	17.4	0.10
Normal	11.6	0.38
Abnormal	16.8	<0.001
Severity of Angina		
Class 0, I, II	12.5	0.005
Class III, IV	22.4	0.001

LAD = left anterior descending artery; LV = left ventricular.

From Yusuf S, Zucker D, Peduzzi P, et al: Effect of coronary artery bypass surgery on survival: Overview of 10-year results from randomized trials by the Coronary Artery Bypass Surgery Trialists Collaboration. Lancet 344:563, 1994.

*Systematic overview of the effect of coronary artery bypass grafting (CABG) vs. medical therapy on survival based on data from the seven randomized trials comparing a strategy of initial CABG surgery with one of initial medical therapy. Subgroup results at 5 years are shown.

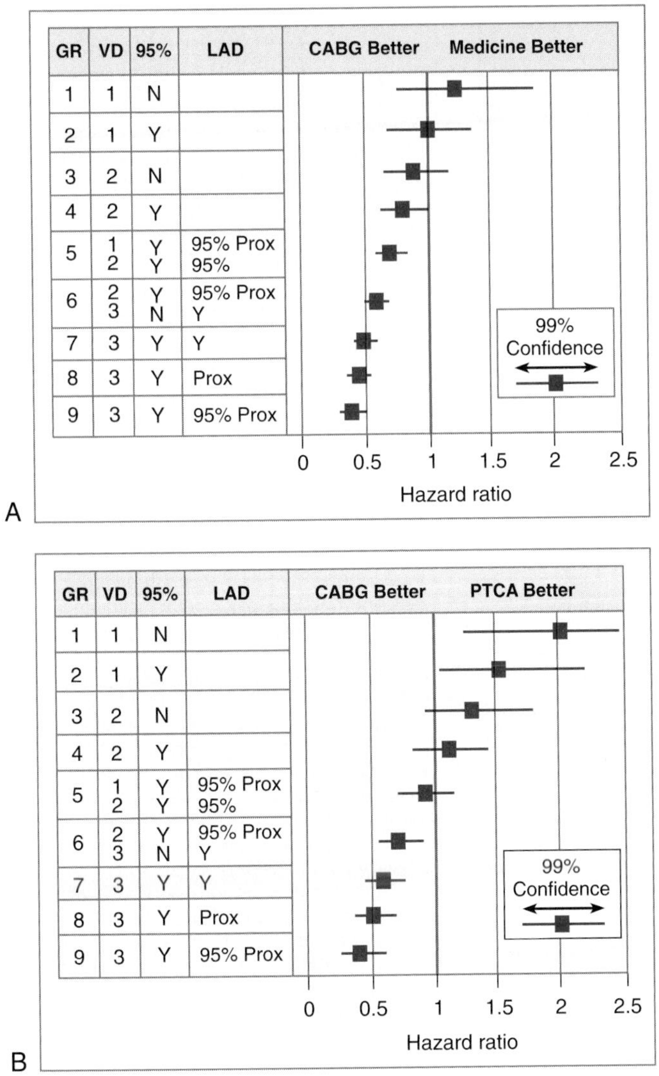

FIGURE 50–16 **A,** Adjusted hazard (mortality) ratios comparing coronary artery bypass grafting (CABG) and medical therapy for nine coronary anatomy severity groups (GR) according to the number of vessels diseased (VD), the presence or absence of a 95 percent proximal stenosis (95 percent), and involvement of the left anterior descending coronary artery (LAD). **B,** Adjusted hazard (mortality) ratios comparing CABG and percutaneous transluminal angioplasty (PTCA) for nine coronary anatomy groups according to the number of vessels diseased, the presence or absence of a 95 percent proximal stenosis, and LAD involvement. Among patients with the least severe categories of disease, 5-year survival appears to be better with PTCA (single-vessel disease without proximal stenosis and without LAD involvement), whereas for patients with triple-vessel disease and higher grade, more complex double-vessel disease, a survival benefit is noted with surgery. For other subsets of patients with double-vessel disease, no difference in survival was seen in those treated with CABG or PTCA, and many of these patients are probably similar to those included in the randomized trials. (Data from the Duke University data base. **A** and **B,** From Jones RH, Kesler K, Phillips HR III, et al: Long-term survival benefits of coronary artery bypass grafting and percutaneous transluminal angioplasty in patients with coronary artery disease. J Thorac Cardiovasc Surg 111:1013, 1996.)

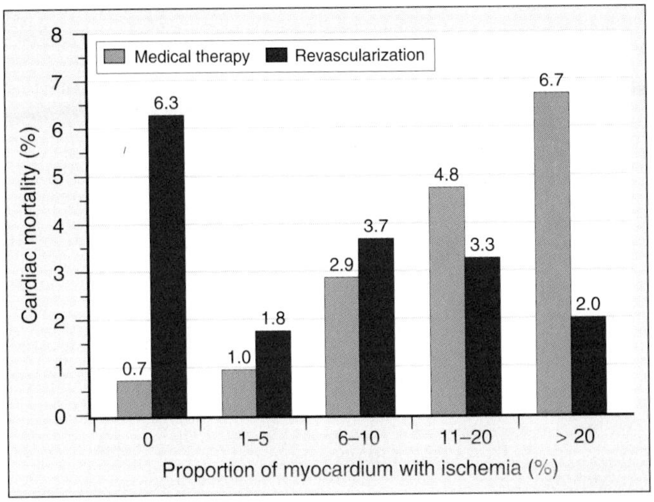

FIGURE 50–17 Rate of cardiac death among patients treated with medical therapy versus revascularization, stratified by the proportion of ischemic myocardium on stress nuclear imaging. A total of 10,627 consecutive patients without prior myocardial infarction or revascularization were followed for a mean of 1.6 years after exercise or adenosine myocardial perfusion imaging. Patients with moderate to severe ischemia who underwent percutaneous or surgical coronary revascularization within 60 days of stress imaging had lower mortality than those treated with medical therapy ($p < 0.0001$). However, those patients with no or mild ischemia had no survival advantage with revascularization. (From Hachamovitch R, Hayes SW, Friedman JD, et al: Comparison of the short-term survival benefit associated with revascularization compared with medical therapy in patients with no prior coronary artery disease undergoing stress myocardial perfusion single photon emission computed tomography. Circulation 107:2900-2906, 2003.)

considered inappropriate using criteria from an international panel.[323]

Results

In 1972, a committee of the AHA indicated that the most widely accepted indication for surgical revascularization was "significant disability from moderate to severe angina pectoris, unresponsive to optimal medical care." More than three decades later, with the development of PCI and improvements both in medical therapy of CAD and in CABG, the realization that CABG prolongs survival in subgroups of patients with either minimal or mild to moderate symptoms has shifted the emphasis toward *ischemia* instead of *symptoms alone* as the target for coronary revascularization. Consequently and appropriately, CABG is currently performed in an increasing number of patients with multivessel disease and/or left ventricular dysfunction (particularly in the face of viable jeopardized dysfunctioning myocardium). Severe ischemia and/or reversible left ventricular dysfunction provides a window of opportunity for improving survival (in comparison to medical therapy) that has resulted in an increase in the frequency of CABG in patients with unstable angina and in survivors of acute myocardial infarction. Left ventricular dysfunction, initially a relative contraindication for surgery, has become a major indication. Nonetheless, severe symptoms or even moderate symptoms that interfere with the quality of life despite adequate medical therapy remain as firm an indication for coronary revascularization (PCI or CABG) as they were for CABG three decades ago.

RELIEF OF ANGINA. CABG is highly effective in providing complete relief from angina in some patients and improvement in the severity of symptoms in most of the remainder. For example, in a series of patients who received saphenous vein grafts alone, approximately 90 percent were free of angina at 1 year. In the following 4 years, the recurrence rate was approximately 3 percent per year and 5 percent per year thereafter. Approximate rates of freedom from angina were 78 percent at 5 years, which decreased to 52 and 23 percent at 10 and 15 years, respectively.[324] Trials in which the contemporary practice of using one or more arterial grafts was prevalent demonstrate similar to superior rates of freedom from angina during short-term and mid-term follow-up.[325] The major randomized trials all have demonstrated greater relief of angina, better exercise performance, and a lower requirement for antianginal medications for surgically versus medically treated patients 5 years postoperatively.[261] Beyond 5 years, differences in symptoms between

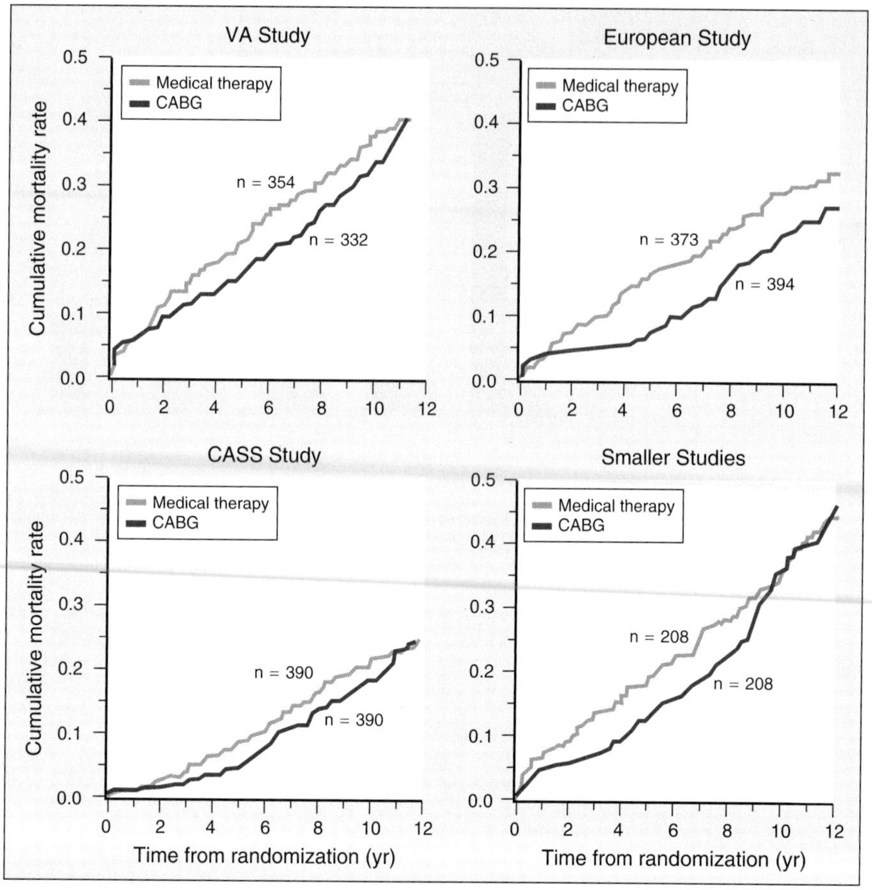

FIGURE 50–18 Survival curves of the three large randomized trials and four smaller studies combined. (From Eagle KA, Guyton RA, Davidoff R, et al: ACC/AHA guidelines for coronary artery bypass graft surgery: A report of the American College of Cardiology/American Heart Association Task Force on Practice Guidelines [Committee to Revise the 1991 Guidelines for Coronary Artery Bypass Graft Surgery]. American College of Cardiology/American Heart Association. J Am Coll Cardiol 34:1262-1347, 1999.)

patients initially treated medically and surgically are diminished, in part because of the high crossover rate from medical to surgical therapy in patients with continued symptoms and progression of disease in vein grafts and in nonbypassed vessels in the surgical group.[326] The reoperation rate for recurrence of symptoms has been reported to be in the range of 6 to 8 percent per year.

For patients with persistent angina despite adequate medical therapy or for patients who do not tolerate medications and who are not suitable candidates for PCI, CABG provides excellent symptomatic relief.[261] With increasing use of IMA grafts, long-term relief from angina and freedom from subsequent cardiac events are improved in comparison to previous patient populations who received vein grafts alone.

In summary, after 5 years, approximately three-fourths of surgically treated patients can be predicted to be free of an ischemic event, sudden death, occurrence of myocardial infarction, or the recurrence of angina; about half remain free for approximately 10 years and about 15 percent for 15 or more years. Symptomatic improvement is best maintained in patients with the most complete revascularization.

EFFECTS ON SURVIVAL. Current clinical practice has been shaped by three major randomized trials of CABG compared to meclical therapy that enrolled patients between 1972 and 1984: the Veterans Affairs (VA) Trial, the European Cardiac Society Study (ECSS), and the National Institutes of Health–supported CASS (Fig. 50–18).[261] The evidence base comprised data from 2649 patients participating in these and several smaller trials.[327] It has provided a wealth of important information but has several important limitations with respect to application to current practice as the risk profile of patients referred for surgery, as well as the available surgical and medical interventions have evolved substantially. In particular, these trials antedated the widespread use of one or two IMAs. As a result, the extent of the completeness of coronary revascularization, graft patency rates, and perioperative mortality in the VA trial fall far short of current expectations and reflect, in part, the initial learning experience of coronary bypass surgery. Moreover, although the patients allocated to initial CABG had a significantly lower mortality at 5, 7, and 10 years, 41 percent of the patients assigned to medical treatment had undergone CABG by 10 years (so-called crossovers).

The results of the trials of surgical versus medical therapy were generally highly consistent, and thus the major points guiding clinical practice may still be drawn from a meta-analysis of the results.[327] In each of the trials, a survival benefit of CABG emerged during mid-term follow-up (2 to 6 years), but this advantage eroded during long-term follow-up and remained statistically significant only in the ECSS. Considered together, the results of these trials support a 4.1 percent absolute reduction in long-term mortality (10 years) with CABG (p = 0.03). Subgroup analyses reveal several high-risk criteria that identify patients who are likely to sustain a more substantial survival benefit: (1) left main CAD; (2) single- or double-vessel disease with proximal LAD disease; (3) left ventricular systolic dysfunction; (4) a composite evaluation that indicates high risk, including severity of symptoms, high-risk exercise tolerance test, history of prior myocardial infarction, and the presence of ST depression on the resting ECG.

The only randomized data comparing CABG with medical therapy in the current era are from the Asymptomatic Cardiac Ischemia Pilot (ACIP) Study of 558 patients (Fig. 50-19).[328] This trial of angina-guided versus angina plus ischemia-guided medical therapy (using ambulatory monitoring) in comparison to revascularization by either PTCA (92 patients) or CABG (79 patients) enrolled relatively low-risk patients. After 2 years of follow-up, mortality was significantly lower among the patients assigned to routine revascularization (1.1 vs. 6.6 and 4.4 percent for the two medical groups [$p < 0.02$]), and rates of death or myocardial infarction were 12.1 percent (angina-guided medical therapy), 8.9 percent (ischemia-guided medical therapy), and 4.7 percent (coronary revascularization) ($p < 0.04$). Although this trial was designed as a pilot study and the number of patients was relatively small, the observed risk reductions were statistically significant and suggest that the benefits of revascularization in the context of current revascularization technique may be greater than previously appreciated. The trial was not designed to assess differences between PTCA and bypass surgery but does point to the need for larger, more definitive randomized trials testing current strategies of revascularization with optimal medical therapy and risk factor reduction.

Taken together, the results of all the trials and registries indicate that the "sicker" the patient (based on the severity of symptoms or ischemia, age, the number of vessels diseased, and the presence of left ventricular dysfunction), the greater the benefit of surgical over medical therapy on survival (see Figs. 50-16 and 50-17 and Table 50-15). CABG prolongs survival in patients with significant left main CAD irrespective of symptoms, in patients with multivessel disease and impaired left ventricular function, and in patients with triple-vessel disease that includes the proximal LAD coronary artery (irrespective of left ventricular function).[261] Surgical therapy has also been demonstrated to prolong life in patients with *double-vessel disease* and left ventricular dysfunction, particularly those with proximal narrowing of one or more coronary arteries and in the presence of severe angina. Although no study has documented a survival

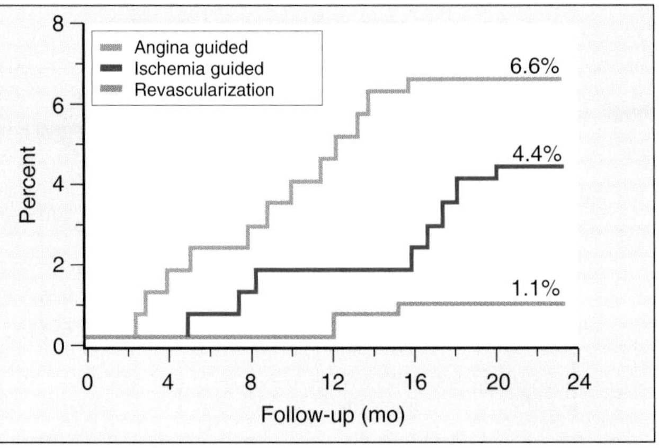

FIGURE 50–19 Two-year cumulative mortality rates for the three treatment strategies in the Asymptomatic Cardiac Ischemia Pilot (ACIP) study. Significant differences were seen between revascularization and angina-guided strategies ($p \leq 0.005$) and between revascularization and ischemia-guided strategies ($p \leq 0.05$). Angina-guided and ischemia-guided strategies were not significantly different from each other ($p = 0.34$). Similar results were noted for the endpoints of cumulative rates of death, myocardial infarction, or cardiac hospitalization. (From Davies RF, Goldberg AD, Forman S, et al: Asymptomatic Cardiac Ischemia Pilot [ACIP] study two-year follow-up: Outcomes of patients randomized to initial strategies of medical therapy versus revascularization. Circulation 95:2037, 1997.)

benefit with surgical treatment in patients with *single-vessel disease*, some evidence indicates that such patients who have impaired left ventricular function have a poor long-term survival with medical therapy. Such patients with angina or evidence of ischemia at a low or moderate level of exercise, especially those with obstruction of the proximal left anterior descending coronary artery, may benefit from coronary revascularization by either PCI or bypass surgery.

LEFT MAIN CORONARY ARTERY STENOSIS. It is widely agreed that surgical treatment improves survival in patients with left main coronary artery obstruction or its "equivalent."[261] The CASS Registry demonstrated that the superiority of revascularization was equivalent in both symptomatic and asymptomatic patients with disease affecting the left main coronary artery.

Whether a "left main–equivalent" anatomy exists that has a natural history similar to that of left main CAD is uncertain. The condition in question may consist of disease in the proximal portions of both the LAD and left circumflex coronary arteries. It is likely that significant left main coronary disease has an ominous nature because a single event (rupture of a single plaque) can cause infarction of a very large quantity of myocardium. Consequently, although combined disease of the proximal left anterior descending and circumflex coronary arteries does identify a subgroup of high-risk patients, the prognosis is not as poor as it is for patients with left main CAD.[329] Nevertheless, patients with combined stenoses of 70 percent or greater in the LAD coronary artery, before the first septal perforating branch, and in the proximal circumflex coronary artery, before the first obtuse marginal branch, who have impaired ventricular function also have improved survival and less angina following surgical revascularization than if they are treated medically, particularly in the face of left ventricular dysfunction. The median survival of surgically treated patients with left main–equivalent disease is 13.1 years versus 6.2 years for those medically treated.[261]

EFFECT ON SUBSEQUENT MYOCARDIAL INFARCTION. The major randomized trials of patients with mild to moderate angina suggested that the likelihood of occurrence of myocardial infarction after 5 to 10 years of follow-up was similar in medically and surgically treated patients. In both the VA study and the CASS, the major benefit of surgery on myocardial infarction does not appear to be mediated by a decrease in the frequency of myocardial infarction but by a decrease in the case fatality rate of patients who subsequently have infarction.[330] Potential explanations are that previous bypass surgery results in smaller infarcts caused by distal occlusions and that the bypass may enhance myocardial perfusion distal to the obstructing lesion.

Patients with Depressed Left Ventricular Function

Depressed left ventricular function is one of the most powerful predictors of perioperative and late mortality.[294] In the Society of Thoracic Surgeons data base, the mean ejection fraction among approximately 136,330 patients undergoing initial coronary bypass in 1999 was approximately 0.51, and approximately 25 percent had an ejection fraction of less than 0.45.[293] Moreover, as the population ages and the proportion undergoing reoperation increases, the number of patients with preoperative left ventricular dysfunction and clinical heart failure will increase. In the CABG Patch trial confined to patients with an ejection fraction of 0.35 or less, perioperative mortality was 3.5 percent for patients without clinical signs of heart failure versus 7.7 percent for those with NYHA Class I to IV heart failure.[331] The latter was a powerful independent predictor of increased operative mortality in patients with ventricular dysfunction and a positive signal-averaged ECG (odds ratio, 2.4; $p = 0.01$).

Although the effect of a reduced ejection fraction on operative mortality cannot be eliminated, careful attention to intraoperative metabolic, inotropic, and mechanical support, including preoperative intraaortic balloon counterpulsation in some patients, may decrease perioperative mortality in comparison with the mortality rates expected from prediction models. In addition to advances in myocardial protection for those undergoing CABG with CPB, off-pump approaches to CABG may also lead to improved surgical outcomes in this high-risk population.[332] Thus, in experienced centers, the in-hospital mortality for patients with severe left ventricular dysfunction is less than 4 percent.[333]

The powerful effect of the preoperative ejection fraction on late survival emphasizes that in the current era, the presence of left ventricular dysfunction, in association with viable myocardium, has changed from a relative contraindication to coronary bypass to a strong indication.[18] This shift in focus has been due to the realization that viable dysfunctioning myocardium may improve after coronary revascularization.[334] Indeed, the most striking survival benefits of CABG, as well as symptomatic and functional improvement, are shown by patients with seriously impaired left ventricular function in whom the prognosis of medical therapy is poor.[333] In patients with a history of congestive heart failure and multivessel (particularly triple-vessel) disease, coronary bypass surgery may also reduce the incidence of sudden cardiac death.[335] Although preoperative left ventricular dysfunction creates the potential for significant benefit, the perioperative risk should not be underestimated, particularly in the setting of clinical congestive heart failure. Selection of patients with viable myocardium supplied by a reasonable target vessel(s) for grafting appears critical in considering CABG for patients with severe left ventricular dysfunction.[336]

MYOCARDIAL HIBERNATION (see Chap. 19). Improvement in survival and left ventricular function following CABG depends on successful reperfusion of viable but noncontractile or poorly contracting myocardium.[337] Two related pathophysiological conditions have been described to explain reversible ischemic contractile dysfunction[338]: (1) myocardial stunning (prolonged but temporary postischemic ventricular dysfunction without myocardial necrosis) and (2) myocardial hibernation (persistent left ventricular dysfunction when myocardial perfusion is chronically reduced (or repetitively stunned) but sufficient to maintain the viability

TABLE 50–16 Markers of Viable Myocardium

Clinical Indicator	Diagnostic Test	Alternative Test
Diastolic wall thickness	Echo	CT, MRI
Systolic wall thickening	Echo	CT, MRI, gated SPECT
Regional wall motion	Echo	CT, MRI, gated SPECT
Regional blood flow	SPECT	PET, MRI
Myocardial metabolism	PET	SPECT
Cell membrane integrity	SPECT	PET
Contractile reserve	Dobutamine, Echo	Angiography, CT, MRI

CT = computed tomography; Echo = echocardiography; MRI = magnetic resonance imaging; PET = positron-emission tomography; SPECT = single-photon emission computed tomography.

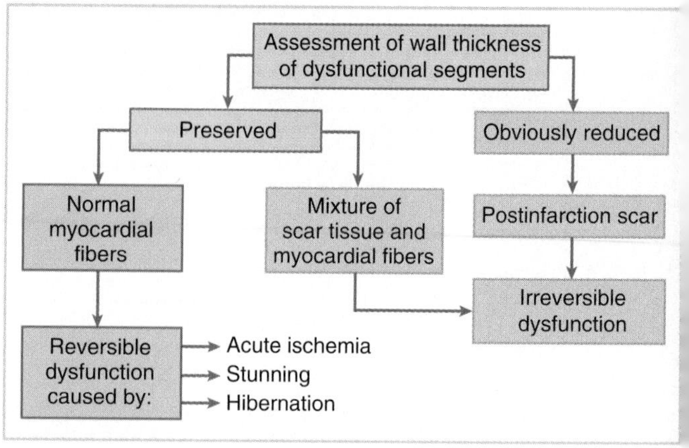

FIGURE 50–20 Flow diagram for the practical assessment of noncontractile segments of myocardial wall potentially recoverable by revascularization procedures. An obviously reduced wall thickness is indicative of a postinfarction scar. Absence of contractile function in segments of the ventricular wall with preserved wall thickness may be caused by different mechanisms. An acute ischemic cause can be excluded by the administration of sublingual nitrates. Stunning can be excluded by repeating the ventricular wall motion study several days after the last ischemic episode. Hibernating myocardium should be distinguished from a mixture of scar tissue and viable myocardial cells. (From Maseri A: Ischemic Heart Disease: A Rational Basis for Clinical Practice and Clinical Research. New York, Churchill Livingstone, 1995.)

of tissue. The reduction in myocardial contractility in hibernating myocardium conserves metabolic demands and may be protective, but more prolonged and severe hibernation may lead to severe ultrastructural abnormalities, irreversible loss of contractile units, and apoptosis.

Hibernating myocardium can cause abnormal systolic or diastolic ventricular function or both. The predominant clinical feature of myocardial ischemia in these patients may not be angina but dyspnea secondary to increased left ventricular diastolic pressure. Symptoms of heart failure resulting from chronic left ventricular dysfunction may be inappropriately ascribed to myocardial necrosis and scarring when the symptoms may, in fact, be reversed after the chronic ischemia is relieved by coronary revascularization.[334]

Detection of Hibernating Myocardium. Several clinical markers may be used to determine the likelihood that a dysfunctional myocardial segment is viable or nonviable (Table 50–16). The presence of angina and the absence of Q waves on the ECG or a history of prior myocardial infarction are useful clues. A severe reduction in the diastolic wall thickness of dysfunctional left ventricular segments is indicative of scarring. On the other hand, akinetic or dyskinetic segments with preserved diastolic wall thickness may represent a mixture of scarred and viable myocardium. A useful strategy for the assessment of dysfunctional segments has been developed by Maseri (Fig. 50–20). Although a number of imaging tools may be used for this assessment (see Chap. 16), the most readily available in most settings is low-dose dobutamine echocardiography.[339]

The term *contractile reserve* describes the ability of hibernating myocardium to exhibit augmented contractility to a suitable temporary stimulus, often causing transient improvement in the global ejection fraction. Contractile reserve underscores the fact that many hypokinetic (and even akinetic) areas of the ventricular wall are composed entirely or in part of viable, hibernating myocardium or a mixture of the latter and fibrous scar. Viable muscle is capable of responding to a sympathomimetic agent. In contrast, necrotic tissue obviously cannot be stimulated to contract by any pharmacological or hemodynamic intervention or by improved perfusion. The most common method of identifying contractile reserve is echocardiographic imaging during infusion of a low dose of dobutamine.[339] Numerous studies have demonstrated that the finding of contractile reserve by low-dose dobutamine echocardiography identifies dysfunctional but viable myocardium with the potential to improve in function after myocardial revascularization.[337]

PET (see Chap. 13) has emerged as an excellent method for demonstrating viable myocardium in patients with impaired left ventricular function. In comparative studies, PET has yielded the highest predictive accuracy of all imaging modalities in detecting dysfunctional myocardium that will improve after revascularization.[340] However, the high cost, technical difficulty, and need for a cyclotron continue to limit this technique's widespread applicability. MRI is emerging as a valuable alternative technique for assessment of myocardial viability.[63] MRI has been shown to have very good correlation with PET [63] and to predict functional recovery after percutaneous or surgical revascularization.[62] Specifically, delayed hyperenhancement with gadolinium identifies areas of myocardial scar, and the transmural extent of hyperenhancement is strongly inversely associated with the probability of recovery after revascularization[62] and may be useful in assessing the probability of regaining contractile function after myocardial infarction.[64]

Thallium-201 rest-redistribution imaging may also be used to determine whether regions with hypoperfusion at rest manifest uptake in the resting defect with time, and stress-redistribution-reinjection imaging, in which a second injection of thallium is administered, may be used to determine whether defects that do not redistribute after exercise represent fibrotic myocardium or myocardium that is severely ischemic (see Chap. 13).[40]

Prognostic Implications of Identifying Viable Myocardium. A growing body of evidence indicates that the detection of viable myocardium in patients with CAD and left ventricular dysfunction not only identifies those in whom improvement in cardiac function is likely after revascularization but also identifies a group of high-risk patients in whom revascularization improves survival (Fig 50–21).[337] Studies with PET, thallium-201, and dobutamine echocardiography have uniformly demonstrated that patients with left ventricular dysfunction and evidence of hibernating myocardium have a high mortality rate during medical therapy and appear to have a better outcome with revascularization. All these studies have limitations, including a small number of patients, the retrospective nature of the analysis, and lack of a randomized control group.[341] However, the consistency of the findings has been striking. Recent data point out that viability assessment is also helpful in the selection of patients for revascularization because patients

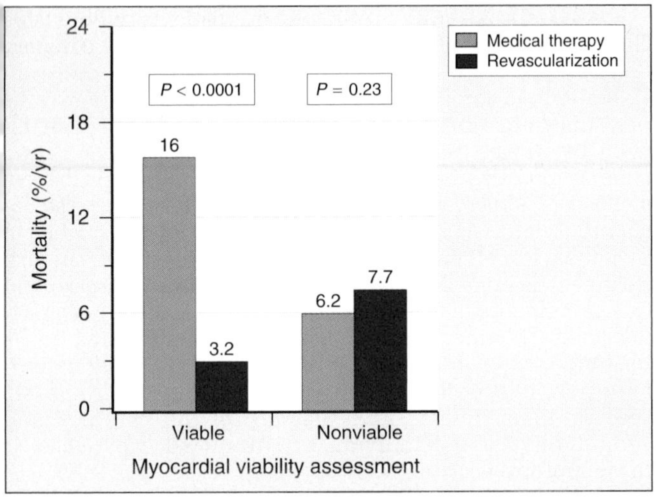

FIGURE 50–21 Meta-analysis of observational studies examining late survival with revascularization versus medical therapy for patients with coronary artery disease and left ventricular dysfunction. Analysis of results from 24 studies ($n = 3088$) demonstrated that revascularization was associated with a significant reduction in annual mortality compared with medical therapy among patients with myocardial viability. No advantage of revascularization was detected in patients without myocardial viability. (Adapted from Allman KC, Shaw LJ, Hachamovitch R, et al: Mycoardial viability testing and impact of revascularization on prognosis in patients with coronary artery disease and left-ventricular dysfunction: A meta-analysis. J Am Coll Cardiol 39:1151-1158, 2002.)

selected for revascularization on the basis of an imaging study demonstrating myocardial viability have lower operative mortality and a higher long-term survival rate than do those who have no evidence of important myocardial viability or those in whom a viability assessment is not performed.[342] Perioperative mortality in the latter patients approaches 10 percent.

The mechanisms for improved survival after revascularization in patients with hibernating myocardium may be related to improvement in left ventricular function, but it is likely that other factors are also operative, including the reduction of left ventricular remodeling, the propensity for serious arrhythmias, and the likelihood of a future fatal acute ischemic event. What remains to be established is the relationship among the extent of viability and the severity of left ventricular dysfunction and the prognostic impact of revascularization.

Surgical Treatment in Special Groups

WOMEN (see Chap. 73). Women are less likely than men to be referred for coronary angiography and subsequent revascularization.[343] In some studies, sex-based differences in referral for revascularization are explained fully by clinical factors.[344] Moreover, it has not been established whether sex-based differences represent underutilization in women, overutilization in men, or both.[343] In comparison with men, women who undergo CABG are "sicker," as defined by age, comorbid conditions, the severity of angina, and history of congestive heart failure.[249] In-hospital mortality and perioperative morbidity after CABG has remained, on average, two times higher in women compared with men. However, when adjusted for the greater risk profile of women referred for CABG, short-term mortality rates as well as long-term outcomes are similar to those for men in most, but not all studies.[345] The independent predictors of long-term prognosis in women are similar to those in men and include older age, previous coronary bypass surgery, previous myocardial infarction, and diabetes.

An excess risk of short-term mortality recently reported in younger women undergoing CABG in one study has not been well explained.[346] Smaller vessel size (as a function of smaller body surface area), a higher incidence of left ventricular hypertrophy, and hypertensive heart disease have been raised as potential contributors to higher surgical risk in women. However, these differences are reasonably expected to be more important in elderly women; the pathophysiological bases for the observed difference in younger women compared with men require further exploration.[249]

With generally similar long-term outcomes after surgical revascularization, sex should not be a significant factor in decisions regarding whether to offer CABG.[249] Newer technical approaches such as OPCAB may be particularly advantageous to women.[347]

YOUNGER PATIENTS. Patients 35 years of age or younger who undergo CABG usually have hyperlipidemia and other major risk factors for CAD. Despite the severity of the underlying disease and the rapidity of the atherosclerotic process, CABG is associated with excellent actuarial survival rates of 94 percent at 5 years and 85 percent at 10 years.[348] Nonetheless, in the CASS Registry, patients younger than 35 years had markedly impaired survival over a 15-year period in comparison with an age- and sex-matched U.S. population. This impaired survival is probably the result of progression of premature atherosclerotic disease, the presence of multiple risk factors, and the development of progressive vein graft disease. The latter underlies the current trend for the use of bilateral IMA grafts and other arterial conduits in younger patients.

THE ELDERLY. A demographic tide in combination with marked improvement in perioperative care and in the outcomes of CABG has resulted in a burgeoning population of elderly patients with extensive disease undergoing such surgery. The number of individuals older than 75 years of age in the United States is expected to quadruple in the next 50 years, with cardiovascular disease being the leading cause of morbidity and mortality in this population.[349] Many such individuals are likely to become candidates for CABG.

Older patients are sicker than their younger counterparts in that they have a greater frequency of comorbid conditions, including peripheral vascular and cerebrovascular disease, more extensive triple-vessel and left main CAD, and a higher frequency of left ventricular dysfunction and history of congestive heart failure. Not unexpectedly, these differences are translated into higher perioperative mortality and complication rates, with a sharp increase in the slope of the curve relating mortality to age seen in patients older than 70 years.[261] Despite these differences, in-hospital mortality for the elderly has declined over time to 7 to 9 percent among those undergoing CABG only and has been reported to be as low as 3 to 4 percent among the subgroup of octogenarians without significant medical comorbidities. Perioperative morbidity is greater in the elderly, with high rates of low-output syndrome, stroke, gastrointestinal complications, wound infection, and postoperative atrial fibrillation.

RENAL DISEASE. Cardiovascular disease is the major cause of mortality in patients with end-stage renal disease (ESRD) and accounts for 54 percent of deaths (see Chap. 86). Patients with ESRD, as well as those with less severe renal insufficiency, have numerous risk factors that not only accelerate the development of CAD but also complicate its medical management. These risk factors include diabetes, hypertension with left ventricular hypertrophy, both systolic and diastolic dysfunction, abnormal lipid metabolism, anemia, and increased homocysteine levels.[350] Coronary revascularization with PCI or CABG is feasible and well documented in patients with ESRD, but the mortality and complication rates are increased.[350,351] Patients with renal insufficiency (serum creatinine >2.0 mg/dl) who are not dependent on dialysis are also at higher risk of major perioperative complications, longer recovery times, and lower rates of short and mid-term survival. Observational data suggest that in patients on chronic dialysis, CABG is the preferred strategy for revascularization over PCI. However, randomized data are very few, and 30-day mortality in patients with ESRD undergoing CABG ranges from 9 to as high as 20 percent.[238]

In summary, coronary bypass surgery can be performed with an acceptable risk and a reasonable expectation of long-term benefit in carefully selected patients with ESRD. As for all high-risk situations, careful attention to patient selection is essential.

PATIENTS WITH DIABETES. In comparison with age-matched nondiabetic patients, diabetic patients with angiographically proven CAD are more likely to be women with evidence of peripheral vascular disease and a higher number of coronary occlusions. Diabetes is an important independent predictor of mortality among patients undergoing surgical revascularization. However, the benefit of CABG versus medical therapy is maintained in patients with diabetes, with a significant 44 percent relative reduction in mortality provided by surgery.[261] Patients with diabetes have smaller distal vessels judged to be poorer targets for bypass grafting. Nevertheless, the patency of arterial and venous grafts appears similar in diabetics and nondiabetic patients.[352] In the absence of new data to the contrary, patients with diabetes and multivessel disease, who are at acceptable surgical risk, should be considered as candidates for surgical revascularization.[353]

CORONARY BYPASS SURGERY IN PATIENTS WITH ASSOCIATED VASCULAR DISEASE

Management of patients with combined CAD and peripheral vascular disease involving the carotid arteries, the abdominal aorta, or the vessels of the lower extremities presents many challenges. Combined disease is becoming increasingly frequent as the population of patients under consideration for CABG ages and as technical improvements allow the application of coronary revascularization to ever more complex cases.

IMPACT OF COMBINED CAD AND PERIPHERAL VASCULAR DISEASE. Clinically apparent CAD occurs frequently in patients with peripheral vascular disease. Among patients undergoing peripheral vascular surgery, late outcomes are dominated by cardiac causes of morbidity and mortality. Conversely, in patients with CAD, the presence of peripheral vascular disease, even if asymptomatic, is associated with an adverse prognosis, presumably because of the greater total atherosclerotic burden borne by these patients.

Because patients with CAD and peripheral atherosclerosis tend to be older and have more widespread vascular disease and end-organ damage than do patients without peripheral atherosclerosis, the perioperative mortality and morbidity consequent to CABG are high and the late outcome is not as favorable.[354] In the Northern New England Cardiovascular data base, in-hospital mortality after CABG was 2.4-fold greater in patients with peripheral vascular disease than in those without it, particularly for patients with lower extremity disease.[355] In the BARI trial, approximately one-third of patients had peripheral vascular disease, among whom the risk of major complications after both bypass surgery and PTCA was markedly increased in comparison to those without peripheral vascular disease, even after controlling for baseline differences.[354] Diffuse *atheroembolism* is a particularly serious complication of CABG in patients with peripheral vascular disease and aortic atherosclerosis. It is a major cause of perioperative death, stroke, neurocognitive dysfunction, and multiorgan dysfunction after CABG.

Peripheral vascular disease is also a strong marker of an adverse long-term outcome. At any point during a 10-year period, patients in either the medical or surgical group in the CASS Registry who had peripheral vascular disease had a 25 percent greater likelihood of mortality than did those without this condition. Similarly, in the Northern New England Cardiovascular data base, the 5-year mortality remained approximately twofold greater in patients with peripheral vascular disease than in those without it, even after adjusting for other comorbid conditions, which are more frequent in patients with peripheral vascular disease.[355] In the BARI trial, patients with asymptomatic lower extremity disease, as defined by the ankle-arm index, had an almost fivefold greater mortality than did those without lower extremity arterial disease. Indeed, mortality was similar for patients with symptomatic and patients with asymptomatic lower extremity disease.

CAROTID ARTERY DISEASE. In patients with stable CAD and *carotid artery disease* in whom coronary endarterectomy is planned, exercise stress testing and consideration of coronary revascularization can ordinarily be performed after the carotid surgery. The prevalence of significant carotid disease in an increasingly elderly population coming to CABG is high—approximately 20 percent have a stenosis of 50 percent or greater, 6 to 12 percent have a stenosis of 80 percent or greater, and the percentage is higher in patients with left main CAD.[356] In patients for whom surgical treatment is considered for both carotid artery disease and CAD, the merits of a combined versus a staged approach are debated.[357] Neither strategy has been demonstrated to be unequivocally superior to the other, and an individualized approach, depending on the patient's initial condition, the severity of symptoms, the anatomy of the coronary and carotid vessels, and individual institutional experience, is most appropriate.[358]

MANAGEMENT OF PATIENTS WITH ASSOCIATED VASCULAR DISEASE. Patients with severe or unstable CAD requiring revascularization can be categorized into two groups according to the severity and instability of the accompanying vascular disease.[358] When the noncoronary vascular procedures are elective, they can generally be postponed until the cardiac symptoms have stabilized, either by intensive medical therapy or by revascularization. A combined procedure is necessary in patients with both unstable CAD and an unstable vascular condition such as frequent recurrent transient ischemic attacks or a rapidly expanding abdominal aortic aneurysm.[359] In some patients in this category, PCI offers the potential for stabilizing the patient's cardiac condition before proceeding with a definitive vascular repair. A problem is posed by the use of clopidogrel after stenting that will increase bleeding, unless surgery is performed at least 5 days after discontinuation of clopidogrel.

PATIENTS REQUIRING REOPERATION. Currently, approximately 12 percent of coronary artery procedures are reoperations, and in some centers, particularly tertiary care centers, the proportion is increasing rapidly and accounts for 20 percent of all CABG operations.[261] The major indication for reoperation is late disease of saphenous vein grafts. An added factor underlying recurrent symptoms is progression of disease in native vessels between the first and second operations.[360] Several series have emphasized the sicker preoperative status of patients undergoing reoperation, including older age, more serious comorbidity, associated valvular heart disease, and a greater prevalence of left ventricular dysfunction and greater extent of ischemic jeopardized myocardium.[361]

Not unexpectedly, the mortality associated with reoperation is significantly higher than that of initial bypass procedures. In the 1997 data base of the Society of Thoracic Surgeons, the mortality among 99,810 patients undergoing an elective first CABG procedure was 1.7 percent versus 5.2 percent for elective reoperations. For patients undergoing first operations, mortality was 2.6 percent for urgent and 6 percent for emergency procedures in comparison with 7.4 and 13.5 percent, respectively, among patients undergoing repeat bypass surgery. Indications for reoperation have not been defined by randomized trials, but in general, the same principles that apply to patients with initial disease should be followed.

Summary of Indications for Coronary Revascularization

1. Certain anatomical subsets of patients are candidates for CABG, regardless of the severity of symptoms or left ventricular dysfunction. Such patients include those with significant left main CAD and most patients with triple-vessel disease that includes the proximal LAD coronary artery, especially those with left ventricular dysfunction (ejection fraction < 0.50). Patients with chronic stable angina and double-vessel CAD with

significant proximal disease of the LAD, and either left ventricular dysfunction or high-risk findings on noninvasive testing should also be considered for CABG.[18]

2. The benefits of CABG are well documented in patients with left ventricular dysfunction and multivessel disease, regardless of symptoms. In patients whose dominant symptom is heart failure without severe angina, the benefits of coronary revascularization are less well defined, but this approach should be considered in patients who also have evidence of severe ischemia (regardless of angina symptoms), particularly in the presence of a significant extent of potentially viable dysfunctioning (hibernating) myocardium.
3. The primary objective of coronary revascularization in patients with single-vessel disease is relief of significant symptoms or objective evidence of severe ischemia. For most of these patients, PCI is the revascularization modality of choice.
4. In patients with angina who are *not* considered to be at high risk, survival is similar for surgery, PCI, and medical management.
5. All the indications discussed earlier relate to the potential benefits of surgery over medical therapy on *survival*. Coronary revascularization with PCI *or* CABG is highly efficacious in relieving symptoms and may be considered for patients with moderate to severe ischemic symptoms who are not controlled by and/or are dissatisfied with medical therapy, even if they are not in a high-risk subset. For such patients, the optimal method of revascularization is selected on the basis of left ventricular function and arteriographic findings and the likelihood of technical success.

Comparisons Between PCI and CABG

OBSERVATIONAL STUDIES. Since the catheter-based revascularizations in these comparative studies were limited largely to PTCA, this term instead of PCI is used in this section. The findings from observational studies have been largely consistent. Over a period of 1 to 5 years, the rates of mortality and nonfatal infarction were not significantly different between patients revascularized with CABG versus PTCA, but recurrent events, including angina pectoris and the need for repeat revascularization procedures, were significantly more frequent in the PTCA than the CABG group, largely as a consequence of incomplete revascularization and restenosis. Specifically, 1 year after PTCA, the recurrence of symptoms and/or the need for repeat revascularization procedures is frequent (~40 percent), and approximately 20 percent of patients are referred for CABG.

When the overall population is considered, observational data show no differences in survival. However, several subgroups of patients who may derive a survival benefit from CABG compared to PTCA are identified. These include patients with left ventricular dysfunction, probably because of the ability to achieve more complete revascularization with the CABG. In addition, CABG provided a survival benefit compared with PTCA when proximal LAD stenosis (>70 percent) was present. This finding was most evident in an analysis of 3-year survival in approximately 30,000 patients enrolled in the New York State PTCA registry.[362] In this data set, patients with single-, double-, or triple-vessel disease involving the proximal LAD had lower mortality when treated with CABG.

RANDOMIZED TRIALS

PCI VERSUS CABG IN PATIENTS WITH SINGLE-VESSEL DISEASE. Both the Lausanne trial and the Medicine, Angioplasty, or Surgery Study (MASS) trial from Brazil, which included a medical arm, were limited to patients with isolated disease of the proximal LAD coronary artery. The RITA investigators also published results for the subset of patients (45 percent) who had single-vessel disease. The results of these small trials were consistent in that over 2 to 3 years the rates of mortality and myocardial infarction were similar in the two treatment arms, as was improvement in symptoms, but at the cost of more frequent reintervention in patients treated with PTCA. At 5 years in the Lausanne trial, mortality rates and functional status were similar for the two groups; however, an excess incidence of non-Q-wave myocardial infarction was noted in patients treated with PTCA, but this complication did not affect vital status or symptomatic outcome.[363] At least one trial has now compared minimally invasive direct CABG to stenting for patients with isolated stenosis in the proximal LAD.[270] Results from this small study (N = 220) were similar to prior trials. Although patients treated with CABG were less likely to have recurrent symptoms or undergo repeat revascularization, there was no detectable difference in the risk of death or myocardial infarction with PCI versus CABG (3 percent vs. 6 percent; p = 0.5).

These results suggest that PCI and CABG are both highly effective in preventing symptoms in patients with single-vessel disease, with similar long-term survival. Moreover, technological advances in PCI since PTCA (the use of stents, first bare metal and more recently drug eluting) have achieved reductions in the frequency of reintervention among patients undergoing these procedures.

MULTIVESSEL DISEASE. At least nine published studies have compared PCI with CABG in patients with multivessel disease. Despite the heterogeneity of the trials in regard to design, methods, and the patient population enrolled, the results are generally comparable and provide a consistent perspective of CABG and PCI in selected patients with multivessel disease. A major limitation is that these trials, except for the Arterial Revascularization Therapy Study (ARTS) and the Argentine randomized trial of PTCA versus CAB surgery in multivessel disease (ERACI II) trial, were conducted before the widespread use of stents and other advances in PCI technology, as well as newer adjunctive therapy, such as clopidogrel and glycoprotein IIb/IIIa platelet inhibition. Also, these trials lacked an aggressive approach to lipid lowering in both groups of patients. In RITA, the Argentine randomized stent study (ERACI), ARTS, and the French Monocentric trials, the ability to achieve "equivalent" degrees of revascularization in the two groups was an inclusion criterion. Moreover, the majority of patients entered into the trials had well-preserved left ventricular function with a mean ejection fraction exceeding 0.50. Therefore, patients enrolled in these trials were at relatively low risk, with predominantly double-vessel disease and well-preserved left ventricular function, that is, a high proportion of patients in whom CABG surgery had *not* been previously shown to be superior to medical therapy in regard to survival. Thus, one would not expect a significant mortality difference between PCI and CABG, particularly with the relatively small sample size of the trials.[18]

The Bypass Angioplasty Revascularization Investigation (BARI) trial, conducted by the NHLBI, enrolled 1829 patients with multivessel disease in the United States and Canada. This trial is the largest of the completed randomized trials of PTCA and bypass surgery and the only trial with sufficient statistical power to detect a substantial mortality difference. At 5 years, overall survival rates were not different between the two groups (89.3 percent with CABG and 86.3 percent with PTCA; p = 0.19), nor was any difference noted in the incidence of Q wave myocardial infarction. An initially unexpected finding—but one that has subsequently been reinforced by ARTS[364] and observational data[365]—was that patients with previously treated diabetes who underwent PTCA had a 5-year mortality of 34.5 percent versus 19.4 percent for those who underwent CABG (p = 0.003) (Fig. 50-22). This advantage of CABG over PTCA among patients with diabetes became more robust by 7 years of follow-up, at which time no survival advantage was evident for patients without diabetes.[353] More rapid progression of atherosclerosis and high rates of restenosis in patients undergoing percutaneous revascularization are largely responsible for this difference. It is possible that the introduction of drug-eluting stents and more aggressive medical therapy of diabetes will reduce or eliminate this advantage of CABG over PCI in patients with diabetes.

NONFATAL OUTCOMES. Review of the nonfatal outcomes in the randomized trials reveals some differences between CABG and PCI. In each of the studies, CABG was initially associated with greater improvement in angina, which appears to be proportional to the more complete revascularization in patients with multivessel disease. Moreover, as anticipated from the observational data, repeat revascularization procedures were more frequent after PCI. This difference was less in the ARTS trial in which repeat revascularization through 1 year was performed in only 16.9 percent of patients in the stented group (Fig 50-23), contrasting

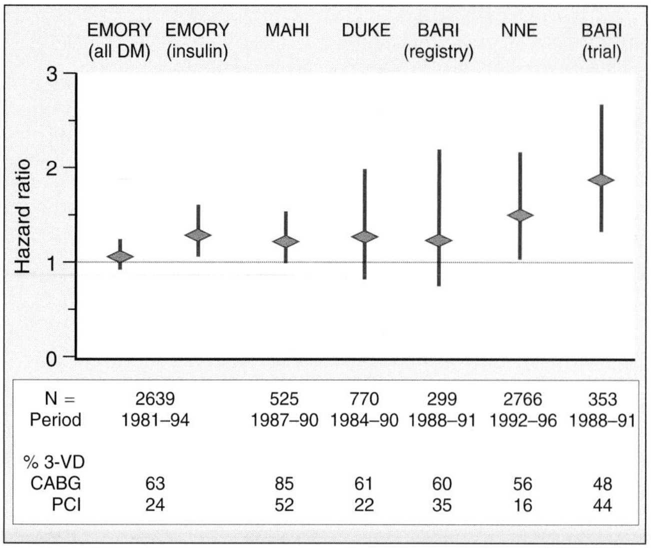

FIGURE 50–22 Five- to six-year survival after coronary artery bypass grafting (CABG) versus percutaneous coronary intervention (PCI) among patients with diabetes mellitus (DM) and multivessel coronary artery disease. Data from both observational and randomized studies show either trends toward or superior survival with CABG. All hazard ratios are adjusted with the exception of the data from the Mid America Heart Institute (MAHI). BARI = Bypass-Angioplasty Revascularization Investigation; NNE = Northern New England data base study; 3-VD = triple-vessel coronary artery disease. (Adapted from Niles NW, McGrath PD, Malenka D, et al: Survival of patients with diabetes and multivessel coronary artery disease after surgical or percutaneous revascularization: Results of a large regional prospective study. J Am Coll Cardiol 37:1008-1015, 2001.)

with 38 percent within 2 years after angioplasty in RITA-1. In the ERACI II study, results were similar to those in the ARTS trial, with only 16.8 percent of patients who had PCI with stenting requiring repeat revascularization in follow-up versus 4.8 percent of bypass surgical patients.[366] However, in the BARI trial, other measures of procedural success, including indices of the quality of life, cognitive function, and return to employment, were similar between PTCA and CABG.

Another consistent but not unexpected finding was the lower in-hospital cost for patients undergoing PCI. This initial cost advantage was sustained at 1 year in ARTS. However, the need for recurrent hospitalization and repeat revascularization procedures over the long term contributed to an increase in postdischarge cost in the PCI arms, resulting in similar overall cost over 3 to 5 years in BARI and a diminished cost advantage at 3 years in ARTS.[367,367a] A major determinant of lower cost is the presence of double-vessel disease; in comparison, patients with congestive heart failure, comorbid conditions, or diabetes are likely to accrue higher cost regardless of the procedure.[367]

The Choice Between PCI and CABG

(Figs. 50–22, 50–23, and 50–24 and Table 50–17)

Medical management of chronic CAD involves a reduction in reversible risk factors, counseling in life-style alteration, treatment of conditions that intensify angina, and pharmacological management of ischemia. When an unacceptable level of angina persists despite medical management, the patient has troubling side effects from the antiischemic drugs, and/or exhibits a "high-risk" result on noninvasive testing, the coronary anatomy should be defined to allow selection of the appropriate technique for revascularization. After elucidation of the coronary anatomy, selection of the technique of revascularization is made as follows:

SINGLE-VESSEL DISEASE. Among patients with single-vessel disease in whom revascularization is deemed necessary and the lesion is anatomically suitable, PCI is generally preferred over bypass surgery.

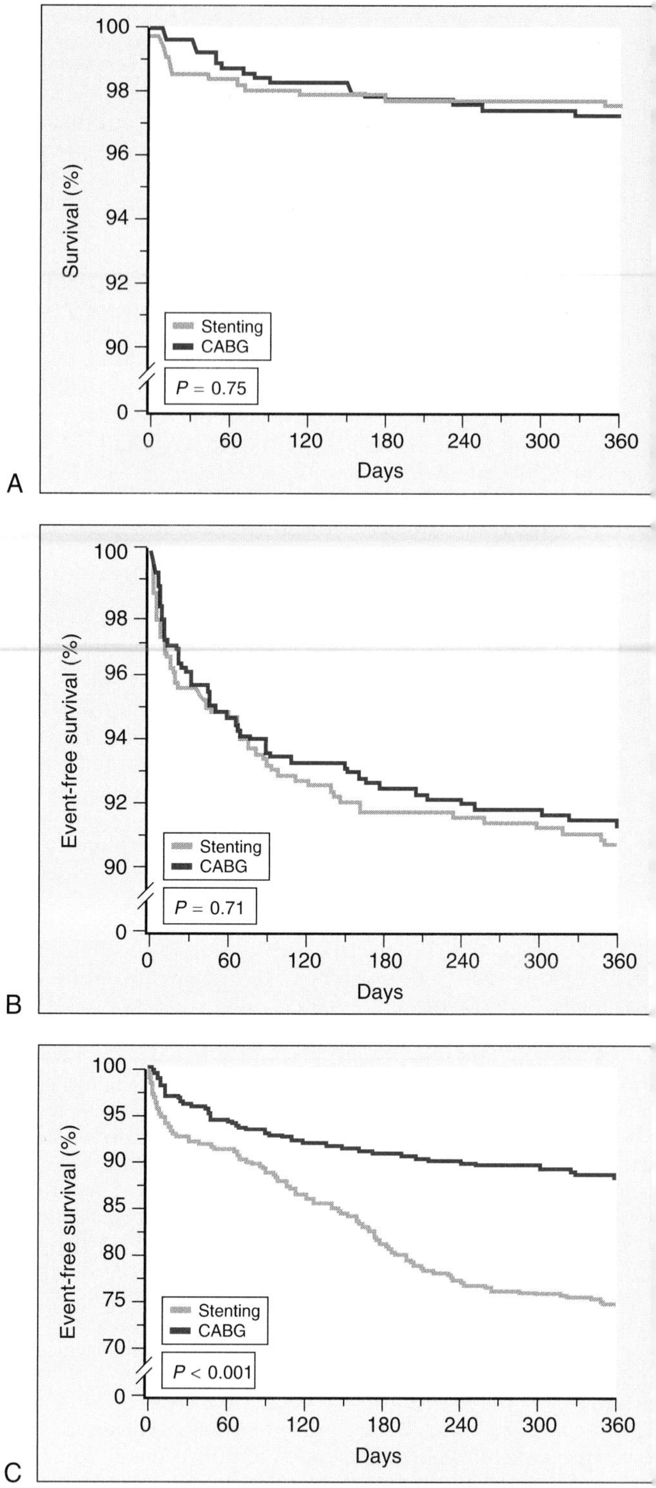

FIGURE 50–23 Outcomes among 1205 patients with multivessel coronary artery disease randomly assigned to undergo percutaneous revascularization with coronary stenting or coronary artery bypass grafting (CABG) in the Arterial Revascularization Therapies Study (ARTS). One year after the revascularization procedure, rates of death, myocardial infarction, and cerebrovascular events were not statistically different between the two revascularization strategies. However, patients undergoing initial stenting were more likely to require repeat revascularization. **A,** Actuarial survival in the stenting versus CABG groups. **B,** Kaplan-Meier estimates of survival free of myocardial infarction or cerebrovascular events. **C,** Kaplan-Meier estimates of survival free of myocardial infarction, cerebrovascular events, or repeated revascularization. (**A** to **C,** From Serruys PW, Unger F, Sousa JE, et al: Comparison of coronary artery bypass surgery and stenting for the treatment of multivessel disease. N Engl J Med 344:1117-1124, 2001.)

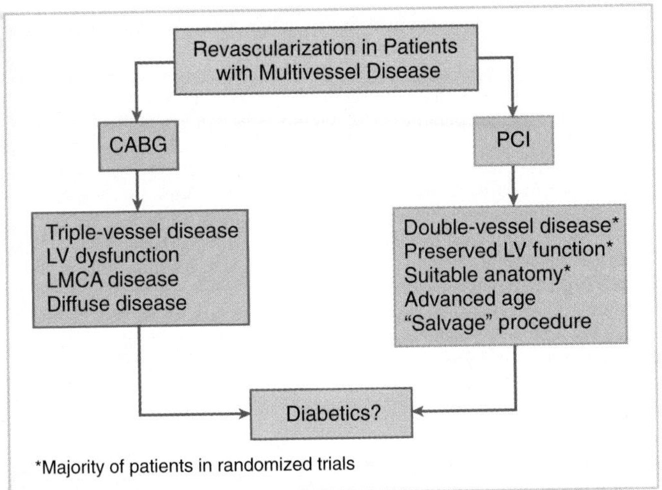

FIGURE 50–24 Indications for coronary revascularization with bypass surgery (CABG) or percutaneous coronary intervention (PCI) in patients with multivessel disease. The combination of triple-vessel disease and left ventricular (LV) dysfunction and/or left main coronary artery (LMCA) disease is primarily surgical, whereas the majority of the patients entered into the randomized trials were suitable for angioplasty on the basis of double-vessel disease, preserved LV dysfunction, and suitable anatomy. Diabetics should be treated individually.

TABLE 50–17 Comparison of Revascularization Strategies in Multivessel Disease

Advantages	Disadvantages
Percutaneous Coronary Intervention	
Less invasive	Restenosis
Shorter hospital stay	High incidence of incomplete revascularization
Lower initial cost	Relative inefficacy in patients with severe left ventricular dysfunction
Easily repeated	Less favorable outcome in diabetics
Effective in relieving symptoms	Limited to specific anatomical subsets
Coronary Artery Bypass Graft Surgery	
Effective in relieving symptoms	Cost
Improved survival in certain subsets	Morbidity
Ability to achieve complete revascularization	
Wider applicability (anatomical subsets)	

Modified from Faxon DP: Coronary angioplasty for stable angina pectoris. *In* Beller G (ed): Chronic Ischemic Heart Disease. *In* Braunwald E (ed): Atlas of Heart Disease. Vol 5. Philadelphia, WB Saunders, 1995.

MULTIVESSEL DISEASE. The first step is to decide whether a patient falls into the category of those who were included in randomized trials comparing PCI and CABG. Most of the patients included in these trials were at lower risk, as defined by double-vessel disease and well-preserved ventricular function. Moreover, several trials required that equivalent degrees of revascularization be achievable by both techniques. Most patients with chronically occluded coronary arteries were excluded, and of those who were clinically eligible, approximately two-thirds were excluded for angiographic reasons. The lack of any difference in late mortality and myocardial infarction between the two treatment arms in such patients indicates that PCI is a reasonable *initial* strategy, provided that the patient accepts the distinct possibility of symptom recurrence and need for repeat revascularization. Patients with a single localized lesion in each affected vessel and preserved left ventricular function fare best with PCI. Additional anatomical factors, such as the presence of severe proximal LAD disease, should also be considered and weigh in favor of surgery (see Fig. 50–16).

NEED FOR COMPLETE REVASCULARIZATION. Complete revascularization is an important goal in patients with left ventricular dysfunction and/or multivessel disease. The major advantage of CABG surgery over PCI is its greater ability to achieve complete revascularization, particularly in patients with triple-vessel disease. In the majority of such patients, particularly those with chronic total coronary occlusion, left ventricular dysfunction, or left main CAD, CABG is the procedure of choice. Among patients with borderline left ventricular function (ejection fraction between 0.40 and 0.50) and milder degrees of ischemia, PCI may provide adequate revascularization, even if it is not complete anatomically.

In many patients, either method of revascularization is suitable. Other factors that come into consideration include the following:

1. Access to a high-quality team and operator (surgeon or interventional cardiologist) with an excellent record of success
2. Patient preference—some patients are made anxious by the idea that after PCI they remain at risk for symptom recurrence and may require reintervention; such patients are better candidates for surgical treatment. Other patients are attracted by the less invasive nature and much more rapid recovery from PCI; these patients prefer to have PCI as their initial revascularization with the idea of "falling back" on CABG if symptoms persist and/or an excellent revascularization has not been achieved
3. Advanced patient age and comorbidity—frail, very elderly patients and those with comorbid conditions, such as cancer or serious liver disease with a limited life expectancy, but who have disabling angina, are often better candidates for PCI
4. Younger patient age—PCI is also often preferable in younger patients (<50 years of age) with the expectation that they may require CABG at some time in the future and that PCI will postpone the need for surgery; this sequence may be preferable to two operations. Patient preference is a pivotal aspect of the decision to perform PCI or CABG in these patient groups

PCI AND CABG IN DIABETIC PATIENTS (see Chap. 51). The poorer outcomes after PCI than after CABG in treated diabetic patients in the BARI trial, together with similar findings in the ARTS trial, have raised concern about whether all diabetic patients with multivessel disease should be treated surgically. This important issue has significant economic implications. Further analysis suggests that treatment of diabetic patients can be individualized, as in nondiabetic patients.

One point of debate is related to the patient selection criteria for enrollment into the trials. In the BARI Registry, in which patients were treated according to the preference of the individual physician, and in two large data base studies, poorer outcomes were noted for both CABG and PTCA in diabetics versus nondiabetics, but *among diabetics*, no survival difference was noted between PTCA and CABG.[368] Similar trends were noted in two large community studies.[369] Diabetic patients as a group in the BARI trial had a greater prevalence of triple-vessel disease, left ventricular dysfunction, and a history of congestive heart failure. It is noteworthy that in the Emory University study of diabetic patients, approximately 85 percent of those with triple-vessel disease underwent bypass surgery, whereas the use of PTCA and CABG was similar among those with double-vessel disease. A plausible explanation for the differences in results in the registry and data base studies compared to the randomized trials is that in the latter, sicker diabetic patients with triple-vessel disease and left ventricular dysfunction, by design, were treated equally with bypass surgery and PTCA, whereas in clinical practice, such patients are referred appropriately for surgery. Consistent with this notion, earlier data base studies suggest that 3- to 5-year survival after CABG in the higher-risk subgroups is superior to that obtained with PCI.

The therapeutic implications of these observations are evident. The revascularization strategy in diabetic patients should be based on the number of vessels diseased, lesion-related technical factors, the caliber of the distal vessels, and the presence or absence of left ventricular dysfunction. Most of the earlier-described comparisons between PCI and CABG involved balloon angioplasty or bare-metal stents. No comparisons between PCI using drug-eluting stents and CABG are available at this time. Since the major disadvantage of PCI prior to the development of drug-eluting stents has been the high rate of restenosis, which has now been substantially reduced, the fraction of patients referred for PCI is increasing, with a corresponding reduction in those referred for CABG. The choice between PCI with drug-eluting stents and CABG will likely revolve around the ability of each procedure to achieve complete revascularization in any given patient.

Other Surgical Procedures for Ischemic Heart Disease

CABG may be combined with surgical procedures aimed at correction of atherosclerotic disease elsewhere in the cardiovascular system, correction of mechanical complications of myocardial infarction (mitral regurgitation or ventricular septal defect), left ventricular aneurysms, and concomitant valvular heart disease. Not unexpectedly, morbidity and mortality are correspondingly increased because of the added complexity of the procedure and, in many patients who require these other procedures, the presence of underlying left ventricular dysfunction (see later).

TRANSMYOCARDIAL LASER REVASCULARIZATION. Transmyocardial laser revascularization is performed by placing a laser on the epicardial surface of the left ventricle, exposed through a lateral thoracotomy, and creating small channels from the epicardial to the endocardial surfaces. This innovative approach to the treatment of ischemic heart disease appears to improve symptoms in patients with refractory angina; however, the mechanism and magnitude of benefit remain uncertain.[370] The initial assumption was that laser-mediated channels would provide a network of functional connections between the left ventricular cavity and the ischemic myocardium. Subsequent observations demonstrating closure of the channels within hours or days despite apparent relief of symptoms have led to alternative explanations for the apparent clinical success of the procedure. These explanations include improved perfusion by stimulation of angiogenesis, a placebo effect, and an anesthetic effect mediated by the destruction of sympathetic nerves carrying pain-sensitive afferent fibers or periprocedural infarction.[371] One study evaluated sympathetic innervation with [^{11}C]hydroxyephedrine and demonstrated decreased myocardial uptake of this substance in most patients, without significant change in resting or stress myocardial perfusion, which suggests that the improvement in angina after the procedure may be partly due to sympathetic denervation.

Initial clinical studies in patients with severe CAD not amenable to a bypass procedure were promising in that most demonstrated a reduction in anginal severity and improved exercise tolerance. Several small randomized trials of transmyocardial laser revascularization resulted in improvement in comparison with maximal medical therapy. The results of one trial suggested improvement in perfusion as assessed by PET, but such improvement was not shown with thallium scintigraphy in another trial. In contrast to the positive studies, Schofield and associates reported no significant improvement in exercise time and 12-minute walking distance up to 1 year after translaser myocardial revascularization with a carbon dioxide laser, although the laser-treated patients had a modest reduction in the frequency of angina.[372] The subjective improvement in the severity of angina found in this study, in the absence of any measurable effect on myocardial perfusion or exercise tolerance, argues for a placebo effect or denervation.[371] Subsequent trials have provided mixed results with respect to the durability of symptom improvement after surgical transmyocardial laser revascularization.[373] Moreover, the failure of two sham-controlled trials of percutaneous laser myocardial revascularization to show any benefit has highlighted the impact of placebo effect in response to laser myocardial revascularization.[370] On the basis of data from the randomized trials, it would appear that the widespread use of translaser myocardial revascularization as a stand-alone method cannot be justified, but it may still have a role as an adjunctive procedure during CABG in patients who have some vessels suitable for bypass but others that are unsuitable. Because of the perioperative morbidity associated with surgical transmyocardial laser revascularization, careful selection of patients is necessary.[374] Larger sham-controlled studies of percutaneous laser myocardial revascularization are ongoing. Whether this technique will fulfill its potential as a vehicle for the delivery of angiogenic factors and other forms of gene therapy remains to be determined.

Other Manifestations of Coronary Artery Disease

Prinzmetal (Variant) Angina

See Chapter 49.

Chest Pain with Normal Coronary Arteriogram

The syndrome of angina or angina-like chest pain with a normal coronary arteriogram, often referred to as *syndrome X* (to be distinguished from the metabolic syndrome X characterized by abdominal obesity, hypertriglyceridemia, low HDL cholesterol, insulin resistance, hyperinsulinemia, and hypertension), is an important clinical entity that should be differentiated from classic ischemic heart disease caused by CAD. In this condition, the prognosis is usually excellent,[375] in contrast to the variable outcome in patients with angina caused by coronary atherosclerosis. Patients with chest pain and normal coronary arteriograms may represent as many as 10 to 20 percent of those undergoing coronary arteriography because of clinical suspicion of angina. The cause(s) of the syndrome is not conclusively defined. However, microvascular dysfunction and myocardial metabolic abnormalities have been implicated.[376] True myocardial ischemia, reflected in the production of lactate by the myocardium during exercise or pacing, is present in some of these patients; however, others have no metabolic evidence for ischemia as the cause of their discomfort. The incidence of coronary calcification on multislice CT scanning is significantly higher than that of normal controls (53 vs. 20 percent) but lower than that in patients with angina secondary to obstructive CAD (96 percent).[377]

It is postulated that the syndrome of angina pectoris with normal coronary arteries reflects a number of conditions. Included in syndrome X are patients with endothelial dysfunction or microvascular dysfunction or spasm in whom angina may be the result of ischemia.[376] This condition is frequently referred to as *microvascular angina*. In others, chest discomfort without ischemia may be due to abnormal pain perception or sensitivity.[378] Also, IVUS studies have demonstrated anatomical and physiological heterogeneity of syndrome X, with a spectrum ranging from normal coronary arteries to vessels with intimal thickening and atheromatous plaque but without critical obstructions. It is likely that some patients with syndrome X have a combination of pathobiological contributors. In addition, it is difficult to distinguish patients with syndrome X in whom chest pain is caused by ischemia from patients with noncardiac pain. Behavioral or psychiatric disorders may be evident.[379]

MICROVASCULAR DYSFUNCTION (INADEQUATE VASODILATOR RESERVE). Patients with chest pain, angiographically normal coronary arteries, and no evidence of large-vessel spasm even after an acetylcholine challenge may demonstrate an abnormally decreased capacity to reduce coronary resistance and increase coronary flow in response to stimuli such as exercise, adenosine, dipyridamole, and atrial pacing. These patients also have an exaggerated response of small coronary vessels to vasoconstrictor stimuli and an impaired response to intracoronary papaverine. In some patients, this abnormality appears to affect the smaller resistance vessels that are not visible angiographically, while the large proximal conductance vessels are normal.[380] Abnormal endothelium-dependent vasoreactivity has been associated with regional myocardial perfusion defects on SPECT and PET imaging.[381] It has been reported that patients with syndrome X also have impaired vasodilator reserve in forearm vessels and airway hyperresponsiveness, which suggests that the smooth muscle of systemic arteries and other organs may be affected in addition to that of the coronary circulation.

Endothelial dysfunction and endothelial cell activation, reported in patients with syndrome X, may participate in the release of cellular adhesion molecules, proinflammatory cytokines, and constricting mediators that induce changes in the arterial wall, resulting in microvascular dysfunction. Patients with syndrome X have been observed to have higher levels of circulating intercellular adhesion molecule-1, the vasoconstrictor endothelin-1, and the inflammatory marker hs-CRP; moreover, the level of hs-CRP appears to correlate with the severity of symptoms and burden of ischemic ECG changes.[382]

EVIDENCE FOR ISCHEMIA. Despite general acceptance that microvascular and/or endothelial dysfunction is present in many patients with syndrome X, whether ischemia is in fact the putative cause of the symptoms in these patients is not clear.[383] Studies of transmyocardial production of lactate have generated mixed results.[376,382] The development of left ventricular dysfunction and ECG or scintigraphic abnormalities during exercise in some of these patients supports an ischemic cause. However, stress echocardiography with dobutamine has failed to detect regional contraction abnormalities consistent with ischemia.[384] More sensitive techniques, such as perfusion analysis with MRI, have demonstrated that subendocardial perfusion abnormalities, in particular, may be associated with syndrome X.[385]

ABNORMAL PAIN PERCEPTION. The lack of definitive evidence of ischemia in some patients with syndrome X has focused attention on alternative nonischemic causes of cardiac-related pain, including a decreased threshold for pain perception—the so-called sensitive heart syndrome.[385] This hypersensitivity may result in an awareness of chest pain in response to stimuli such as arterial stretch or changes in heart rate, rhythm, or contractility. A sympathovagal imbalance with sympathetic predominance in some of these patients has also been postulated. At the time of cardiac catheterization, some patients with syndrome X are unusually sensitive to intracardiac instrumentation, with typical chest pain being consistently produced by direct right atrial stimulation and saline infusion.[386] Measurements of regional cerebral blood flow at rest and during chest pain suggest differential handling of afferent stimuli between patients with syndrome X and those with obstructive CAD.[378]

Clinical Features

The syndrome of angina or angina-like chest pain with normal epicardial arteries occurs more frequently in women,[385] many of whom are premenopausal, whereas obstructive CAD is found more commonly in men and postmenopausal women. Fewer than half of patients with syndrome X have typical angina pectoris; most have a variety of forms of atypical chest pain. Although the features are frequently atypical, the chest pain may nonetheless be severe and disabling. The condition may be benign in regard to survival, but it may have markedly adverse effects on the quality of life, employment, and use of health care resources.

In some patients with minimal or no CAD, an exaggerated preoccupation with personal health is associated with the chest pain, and panic disorder may be responsible in a proportion of such patients. Potts and Bass found that two-thirds of patients with chest pain and normal coronary arteries have psychiatric disorders.[379] Others have reported that the incidence of obstructive CAD is extremely low in patients with atypical chest pain who are anxious and/or depressed. The association between syndrome X and insulin resistance warrants further study.

PHYSICAL AND LABORATORY EXAMINATION. Abnormal physical findings reflecting ischemia, such as a precordial bulge, gallop sound, and the murmur of mitral regurgitation, are uncommon in syndrome X. The resting ECG may be normal, but nonspecific ST-T wave abnormalities are often observed, sometimes occurring in association with the chest pain. Approximately 20 percent of patients with chest pain and normal coronary arteriograms have positive exercise tests. However, many patients with this syndrome do not complete the exercise test because of fatigue or mild chest discomfort. Left ventricular function is usually normal at rest and during stress, unlike the situation in obstructive CAD, in which function often becomes impaired during stress.[384]

PROGNOSIS. Important prognostic information on patients with angina and either normal or nearly normal coronary arteriograms has been obtained from the CASS Registry.[387] In patients with an ejection fraction of 0.50 or more, the 7-year survival rate was 96 percent for patients with a normal arteriogram and 92 percent for those whose arteriographic study revealed mild disease (50 percent luminal stenosis). In such patients, an ischemic response to exercise was not associated with increased mortality, although a history of smoking or hypertension was. Thus, long-term survival of patients with anginal chest pain and normal coronary angiograms is excellent, markedly better than in patients with obstructive CAD and no different from that in an age-matched general population. Nonetheless, the symptoms are persistent, and most patients continue to experience chest pain that leads to repeated cardiac catheterization and hospital admission.[388]

MANAGEMENT. In patients with angina-like chest pain syndrome and normal epicardial coronary arteries, noncardiac etiologies, such as esophageal abnormalities, should be considered. In patients with syndrome X in whom ischemia can be demonstrated by noninvasive stress testing, a trial of antiischemic therapy with nitrates, calcium-channel blockers and beta blockers is logical, but the response to this therapy is variable.[388] Perhaps because of the heterogeneity of this population, studies testing these antianginal therapies have provided conflicting results. For example, beta blockers may be most effective in patients with syndrome X who also have evidence of increased sympathetic nervous activity (e.g., tachycardia and reduced heart rate variability). Calcium antagonists are effective in reducing the frequency and severity of angina and improving exercise tolerance in some patients. Sublingual nitroglycerin has shown paradoxical effects on blood flow and exercise tolerance in some studies and beneficial effects in others.[388] Alpha blockers have been demonstrated to be ineffective.

ACE inhibitors have favorable effects on endothelial function, vascular remodeling, and sympathetic tone that may be relevant to the pathophysiology of syndrome X. Preliminary data studying ACE inhibitors in this population are promising.[388] Similarly, estrogen has been shown to attenuate normal coronary vasomotor responses to acetylcholine, increase coronary blood flow, and potentiate endothelium-dependent vasodilation in postmenopausal women. Studies of estrogen replacement in postmenopausal women with syndrome X have shown improvement in symptoms and/or exercise performance; however, the role of exogenous estrogen in treatment of this group remains in question. Aimed at the altered somatic and visceral pain perception in many patients with syndrome X, imipramine (50 mg) and structured psychological intervention have been reported to be helpful in some.[389]

Oral aminophylline (an adenosine receptor blocker) may have a favorable effect on the exercise-induced chest pain threshold without any effect on exercise-induced ST segment changes.

Silent Myocardial Ischemia

The prognostic importance and the mechanisms of silent ischemia have been the subject of considerable interest for almost 30 years.[390] Patients with silent ischemia have been stratified into three categories by Cohn. The first and least common form, type I silent ischemia, occurs in totally asymptomatic patients with obstructive CAD (which may be severe). These patients *do not experience angina at any time*; indeed, some type I patients do not even experience pain in the course of myocardial infarction. Epidemiological studies of sudden death (see Chap. 33), as well as clinical and postmortem studies of patients with silent myocardial infarction and studies of patients with chronic angina pectoris, suggest that many patients with extensive coronary artery obstruction never experience angina pectoris in any of its recognized forms (stable, unstable, or variant). These patients with type I silent ischemia may be considered to have a *defective anginal warning system.* Type II silent ischemia is the form that occurs in patients with documented previous myocardial infarction.

The third and much more frequent form, designated *type III silent ischemia,* occurs in patients with the usual forms of chronic stable angina, unstable angina, and Prinzmetal angina. When monitored, patients with this form of silent ischemia exhibit some episodes of ischemia that are associated with chest discomfort and other episodes that are not—that is, episodes of silent (asymptomatic) ischemia. The *total ischemic burden* in these patients refers to the total period of ischemia, both symptomatic and asymptomatic.

AMBULATORY ELECTROCARDIOGRAPHY. The extensive use of ambulatory ECG monitoring has led to a greater appreciation of the high frequency of type III silent ischemia, occurring in up to one-third of patients with stable angina treated with appropriate therapy (Fig. 50–25).[390] It has become apparent that anginal pain is a poor indicator and underestimates the frequency of significant cardiac ischemia. Exercise-induced hemodynamic changes indicative of myocardial ischemia (increasing left ventricular end-diastolic pressure and decreasing left ventricular ejection fraction) occur in patients with CAD, regardless of the development of ischemic discomfort.

The role of myocardial O_2 demand in the genesis of myocardial ischemia has been evaluated by measuring the heart rate and blood pressure changes preceding silent ischemic events during ambulatory studies. In one series, 92 percent of all episodes were silent, and 60 to 70 percent were preceded by significant increases in heart rate or blood pressure. The circadian variations in heart rate and blood pressure also paralleled the increase in silent ischemic events. This and other studies have suggested that increases in myocardial O_2 demand have a significant role in the genesis of silent ischemia, but in other patients reductions in myocardial O_2 supply may make an important contribution to the initiation of both symptomatic and asymptomatic episodes. The mechanisms underlying the development of ischemia, as detected by ambulatory ECG and exercise testing, may be different, and in patients in the ACIP study, concordance between the ambulatory ECG and SPECT was only 50 percent. For identification of silent ischemia, the two techniques probably complement each other.

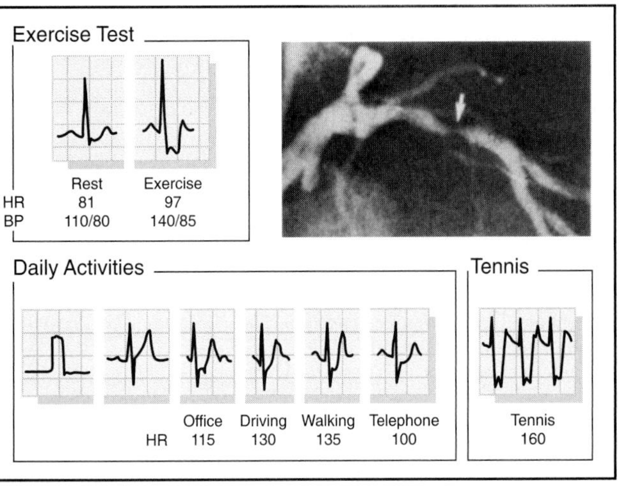

FIGURE 50–25 Ambulatory electrocardiograms and coronary angiogram of a severe left anterior descending stenosis in a patient with fatigue (but not angina) during a tennis match. In stage II of a treadmill exercise test (Bruce protocol), 4 mm of ST segment depression was seen in lead V_5. Ambulatory Holter monitoring of lead V_5 demonstrates ischemic ST segment depressions during a number of ordinary activities, such as walking and telephoning. During a game of tennis, marked ST segment depression was recorded when the patient was asymptomatic. HR = heart rate; BP = blood pressure. (From Nabel EG, Rocco MB, Selwyn AB: Characteristics and significance of ischemia detected by ambulatory electrocardiographic monitoring. Circulation 75[Suppl 5]:74, 1987.)

Transient ST segment depression of 0.1 mV or more that lasts longer than 30 seconds is a rare finding in normal subjects. Patients with known CAD show a strong correlation between such transient ST segment depression and independent measurements of impaired regional myocardial perfusion and ischemia determined by rubidium-82 uptake as measured by PET. In patients with type III silent ischemia, perfusion defects occur in the same myocardial regions during symptomatic and asymptomatic episodes of ST segment depression. Other methods of detecting silent ischemia include measurement of the left ventricular ejection fraction with a "nuclear vest," the presence of regional wall motion abnormalities, and perfusion defects on echocardiography or radionuclide scintigraphy.

Type III silent ischemia is extremely common. Analysis of ambulatory ECG recordings among patients with CAD who had both symptomatic and silent myocardial ischemia found that 85 percent of ambulant ischemic episodes occur without chest pain and 66 percent of angina reports were unaccompanied by ST segment depression.[391] Their frequency is such that it has been suggested that overt angina pectoris is merely the "tip of the ischemic iceberg." Among patients with stable CAD enrolled 1 to 6 months after hospitalization for an acute ischemic event, only 15 percent had angina with exercise, yet 28 percent had ST segment depression and 41 percent had reversible myocardial perfusion defects on thallium scintigraphy.[392] Episodes of silent ischemia have been estimated to be present in approximately one-third of all treated patients with angina, although a higher prevalence has been reported in diabetics. Episodes of ST segment depression, both symptomatic and asymptomatic, exhibit a circadian rhythm and are more common in the morning. Asymptomatic nocturnal ST segment changes are almost invariably an indicator of double- or triple-vessel CAD or left main coronary artery stenosis.

Pharmacological agents that reduce or abolish episodes of symptomatic ischemia (i.e., nitrates, beta blockers, and calcium antagonists) also reduce or abolish episodes of silent ischemia.[390]

MECHANISMS OF SILENT ISCHEMIA. It is not clear why some patients with unequivocal evidence of ischemia do not experience chest pain whereas others are symptomatic. Differences in both peripheral and central neural processing of pain have been proposed as important factors underlying silent ischemia. PET imaging of cerebral blood flow during painful versus silent ischemia has pointed toward differences in handling of afferent signals by the central nervous system.[378] Specifically, "overactive" gating of afferent signals in the thalamus may reduce the cortical activation necessary for perception of pain from the heart. Autonomic neuropathy has also been implicated as a reason for reduced sensation of pain during ischemia. Although increased release of endorphins may play a role in some patients with silent ischemia, the results of clinical studies are mixed.[390] Some researchers have suggested that antiinflammatory cytokines are at play in reducing inflammatory processes that may participate in the genesis of cardiac pain.[393]

PROGNOSIS. Although some controversy remains, ample evidence supports the view that episodes of myocardial ischemia, regardless of whether they are symptomatic or asymptomatic, are of prognostic importance in patients with CAD.[390] In asymptomatic patients (type I), the presence of exercise-induced ST segment depression has been shown to predict a fourfold to fivefold increase in cardiac mortality in comparison with patients without this finding.[394] Similarly, in patients with stable angina or prior myocardial infarction, the presence of inducible ischemia evident by ST depression or perfusion abnormalities during exercise testing is associated with unfavorable outcomes, regardless of whether symptoms are present.[395] The strength of this association is greatest when the ischemia is found to occur at a low workload. Several studies evaluating the prognostic implications of silent ischemia on ambulatory monitoring in patients with stable angina (type III) have demonstrated that the presence of myocardial ischemia on ambulatory ECG, whether silent or symptomatic, is also associated with an adverse cardiac outcome.[220,221,396] Moreover, in the ACIP study, among patients treated medically, myocardial ischemia detected by ambulatory ECG and by an abnormal exercise treadmill test were each *independently* associated with adverse cardiac outcomes.[397] However, revascularization and/or intensification of medical therapy were included as subjective elements of the composite endpoints for these studies along with death and myocardial infarction. In addition, other studies have not detected a relationship between silent ischemia on ambulatory monitoring and subsequent hard outcomes.[398]

Nevertheless, when the subgroup of patients with ischemia on stress testing is considered, silent ischemia on Holter monitoring is also a significant predictor of subsequent death or myocardial infarction. In addition, patients with ischemia on ambulatory ECG are more likely to have multivessel CAD, severe proximal stenoses, and a greater frequency of complex lesion morphology, including intracoronary thrombus, ulceration, and eccentric lesions, than are patients without evidence of ischemia on ambulatory monitoring. The presence of severe and complex CAD may partly explain the apparent independent effect of silent ischemia during ambulatory monitoring on prognosis.[399]

Whether the incremental prognostic information provided by adding an ambulatory ECG to a standard stress test justifies the cost of using this modality as a tool for widespread screening remains to be determined, but it is unlikely. Exercise ECG can identify most of the patients likely to have significant ischemia during their daily activities and remains the most important screening test for significant CAD. Many patients with type I silent ischemia have been identified because of an asymptomatic positive exercise ECG obtained following myocardial infarction. In such patients with a defective anginal warning system, it is reasonable to assume that asymptomatic ischemia has a significance similar to that of symptomatic ischemia and that their management with respect to coronary angiography and revascularization should be similar.

MANAGEMENT. Drugs that are effective in preventing episodes of symptomatic ischemia (nitrates, calcium antagonists, and beta blockers) are also effective in reducing or eliminating episodes of silent ischemia (Fig. 50–26).[390] Multiple studies have shown beta blockers to reduce the frequency, duration, and severity of silent ischemia in a dose-dependent fashion.[400] For example, in the Atenolol Silent Ischemia Study Trial (ASIST), 4 weeks of atenolol therapy decreased the number of ischemic episodes detected on ambulatory ECG (from 3.6 to 1.7; $p < 0.001$) and also the average duration (from 30 to 16.4 minutes per 48 hours; $p < 0.001$).[220] In a randomized study comparing beta blockade versus calcium-channel antagonism, metoprolol was shown to be superior to diltiazem in decreasing the mean number of ischemic episodes and the mean duration of ischemia.[401] Beta blockers may also blunt the circadian increase in ischemic events in the early morning. A combination of a beta blocker and a calcium antagonist is superior to either class of drug alone in suppressing ischemia detected by ambulatory ECG. Coronary revascularization is also effective in reducing the rate of both angina and ambulatory ischemia. In the ACIP pilot study, 57 percent of patients treated with revascularization were free of ischemia at 1 year, compared with 31 and 36 percent in the "ischemia-" and "angina-guided" strategies, respectively ($p < 0.0001$).[402] Aggressive secondary prevention with lipid-lowering therapy has also been shown to reduce ischemia on ambulatory monitoring.[403]

Although suppression of ischemia in patients with asymptomatic ischemia appears a worthwhile objective, whether treatment should be guided by symptoms or by ischemia as reflected by the ambulatory ECG has not been established. In a study of bisoprolol, nifedipine, and the combination, patients achieving complete eradication of ischemia, symptomatic and asymptomatic, were less likely to suffer death,

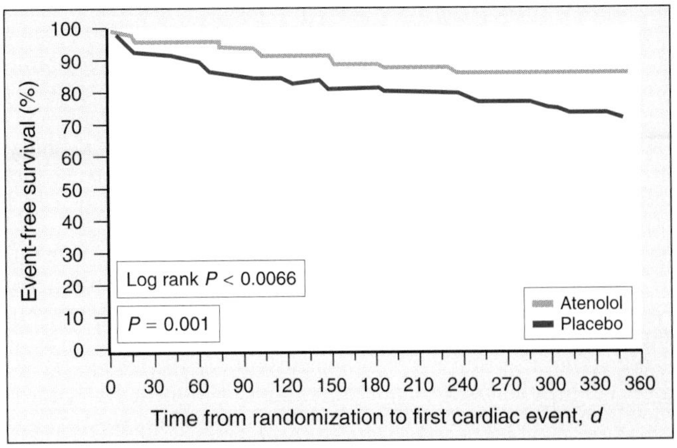

FIGURE 50–26 The Atenolol in Silent Ischemia Trial (ASIST) is the first controlled trial to demonstrate modification of cardiac risk through treatment of silent myocardial ischemia (SMI). A total of 306 asymptomatic or minimally symptomatic patients with coronary artery disease, positive exercise tests, and ambulatory electrocardiographic (ECG) episodes of SMI were randomized to receive atenolol or placebo. Ambulatory ECG monitoring was repeated at 4 weeks, and outcome was assessed after 1 year. At 4 weeks, atenolol was associated with a significant reduction in SMI. After 1 year, a significant (56 percent) relative reduction in adverse events (death, resuscitated ventricular tachycardia and fibrillation, nonfatal myocardial infarction, and unstable or worsening angina) was found when patients given atenolol were compared with those given placebo. The presence of ischemia at 4 weeks was the most important independent factor associated with adverse outcomes after 1 year. (From Bertolet BD, Pepine CJ: Silent myocardial ischemia. *In* Beller GA [ed]: Chronic Ischemic Heart Disease. *In* Braunwald E [ed]: Atlas of Heart Diseases. Vol 5. Philadelphia, WB Saunders, 1995, p 8.9.)

myocardial infarction, or angina requiring revascularization. Similarly, amelioration of all symptomatic and asymptomatic ischemia in the ASIST trial conferred an advantage with respect to the primary endpoint of death, resuscitated ventricular tachycardia or ventricular fibrillation, myocardial infarction, unstable angina, revascularization, or worsening angina.[220] However, in the ACIP trial, no differences in outcome were detected between the groups allocated to ischemia-guided versus angina-guided therapy. In contrast, the early benefits of revascularization on ischemia were associated with improved clinical outcomes. Specifically, the rate of death or myocardial infarction was 12.1 percent in the angina-guided strategy, 8.8 percent in the ischemia-guided strategy, and 4.7 percent in the revascularization strategy, and a strong reduction was also seen in recurrent hospitalizations and the revascularization strategies.[328] Patients who continue to suffer silent ischemia after revascularization may be at increased risk for recurrent cardiac events compared to those who are free of any ischemia.[404]

Heart Failure in Ischemic Heart Disease

In the current era, the leading cause of heart failure in developed countries is CAD.[405] In the United States, CAD and its complications account for two-thirds to three-fourths of all cases of heart failure. In many patients, the progressive nature of heart failure reflects the progressive nature of the underlying CAD. The term *ischemic cardiomyopathy* is used for the clinical syndrome in which one or more of the pathophysiological features just discussed result in left ventricular dysfunction and heart failure symptoms.[406] This condition is the predominant form of heart failure related to CAD. Additional complications of CAD that may become superimposed on ischemic cardiomyopathy and precipitate heart failure are the development of left ventricular aneurysm and mitral regurgitation caused by papillary muscle dysfunction.

Ischemic Cardiomyopathy

In 1970, Burch and colleagues first used the term *ischemic cardiomyopathy* to describe the condition in which CAD results in severe myocardial dysfunction, with clinical manifestations often indistinguishable from those of primary dilated cardiomyopathy (see Chap. 59). Symptoms of heart failure caused by ischemic myocardial dysfunction and hibernation, diffuse fibrosis, or multiple infarctions, alone or in combination, may dominate the clinical picture of CAD. In some patients with chronic CAD, angina may be the principal clinical manifestation at one time, but later this symptom diminishes or even disappears as heart failure becomes more prominent. Other patients with ischemic cardiomyopathy have no history of angina or myocardial infarction (type I silent ischemia), and it is in this subgroup that ischemic cardiomyopathy is most often confused with dilated cardiomyopathy.

It is important to recognize hibernating myocardium in patients with ischemic cardiomyopathy because symptoms resulting from chronic left ventricular dysfunction may be incorrectly thought to result from necrotic and scarred myocardium rather than from a reversible ischemic process. Hibernating myocardium may be present in patients with known or suspected CAD with a degree of cardiac dysfunction or heart failure not readily accounted for by previous myocardial infarctions.[407]

The outlook for patients with ischemic cardiomyopathy treated medically is quite poor, and revascularization or cardiac transplantation may be considered.[333,408] The prognosis is particularly poor for patients in whom ischemic cardiomyopathy is due to multiple myocardial infarctions, in those with associated ventricular arrhythmias, and in those with extensive amounts of hibernating myocardium. However, this last group of patients, whose heart failure, even if severe, is due to large segments of reversibly dysfunctional but viable myocardium, has a significantly better prognosis after revascularization.[333] Revascularization in this group also significantly improves heart failure symptoms. Thus, the key to management of patients with ischemic cardiomyopathy is to assess the extent of residual viable myocardium with a view to coronary revascularization of viable myocardium (see Chap. 16). Patients with little or no viable myocardium in whom heart failure is secondary to extensive myocardial infarction and/or fibrosis should be managed in a manner similar to those with dilated cardiomyopathy (see Chaps. 24 and 59). Their prognosis is poor.

Left Ventricular Aneurysm

Left ventricular aneurysm is usually defined as a segment of the ventricular wall that exhibits paradoxical (dyskinetic) systolic expansion. Chronic fibrous aneurysms interfere with ventricular performance principally through loss of contractile tissue. Aneurysms made up largely of a mixture of scar tissue and viable myocardium or of thin scar tissue also impair left ventricular function by a combination of paradoxical expansion and loss of effective contraction.[409] *False aneurysms* (pseudoaneurysms) represent localized myocardial rupture in which the hemorrhage is limited by pericardial adhesions, and they have a mouth that is considerably smaller than the maximal diameter (Fig. 50–27). True and false aneurysms may coexist, although the combination is extremely rare.

The frequency of ventricular aneurysms depends on the incidence of transmural myocardial infarction and congestive heart failure in the population studied. Left ventricular aneurysms and the need for aneurysmectomy have declined dramatically during the last 5 to 10 years in concert with the expanded use of acute reperfusion therapy in evolving myocardial infarction. More than 80 percent of left ventricular aneurysms are located anterolaterally near the apex. They

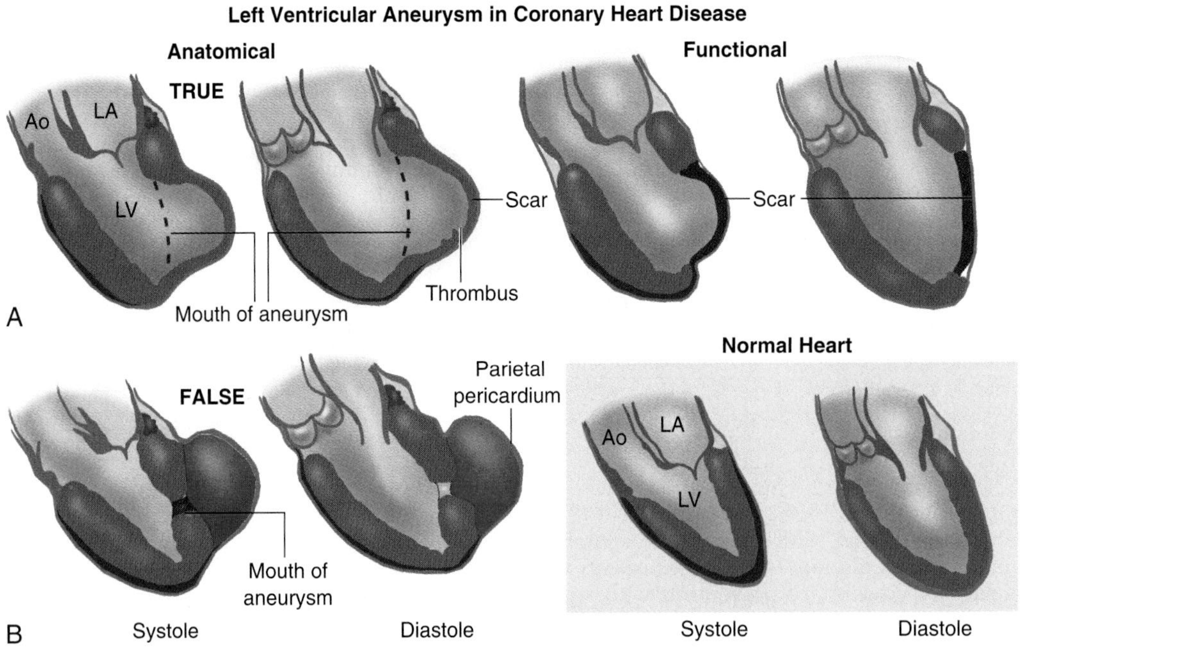

FIGURE 50–27 Hearts in systole and diastole with true and false anatomical and functional left ventricular (LV) aneurysms and healed myocardial infarction. A normal heart in systole and diastole is shown for comparison **(inset)**. A true anatomical left ventricular aneurysm **(A)** protrudes during both systole and diastole, has a mouth that is as wide as or wider than the maximal diameter, has a wall that was formerly the wall of the left ventricle, and is composed of fibrous tissue with or without residual myocardial fibers. A true aneurysm may or may not contain thrombus and almost never ruptures once the wall is healed. A false anatomical left ventricular aneurysm **(B)** protrudes during both systole and diastole, has a mouth that is considerably smaller than the maximal diameter of the aneurysm and represents a myocardial rupture site, has a wall made up of parietal pericardium, virtually always contains thrombus, and often ruptures. A functional left ventricular aneurysm protrudes during ventricular systole but not during diastole and consists of fibrous tissue with or without myocardial fibers. Ao = aorta; LA = left atrium. (From Cabin HS, Roberts WC: Left ventricular aneurysm, intraaneurysmal thrombus, and systemic embolus in coronary heart disease. Chest 77:586, 1980.)

are often associated with total occlusion of the LAD coronary artery and a poor collateral blood supply. Approximately 5 to 10 percent of aneurysms are located posteriorly. Three-fourths of patients with aneurysms have multivessel CAD.

Almost 50 percent of patients with moderate or large aneurysms have symptoms of heart failure (with or without associated angina), approximately 33 percent have severe angina alone, and approximately 15 percent have symptomatic ventricular arrhythmias that may be intractable and life threatening. Mural thrombi are found in almost half of patients with chronic left ventricular aneurysms and can be detected by angiography and two-dimensional echocardiography (see Chap. 11). Systemic embolic events in patients with thrombi and left ventricular aneurysm tend to occur early after myocardial infarction. In the Mayo Clinic series of patients with chronic left ventricular aneurysm (documented at least 1 month after infarction), subsequent systemic emboli were extremely uncommon (0.35 per 100 patient-years in patients not receiving anticoagulants).

DETECTION. Clues to the presence of aneurysm include persistent ST segment elevations on the resting ECG (in the absence of chest pain)[410] and a characteristic bulge of the silhouette of the left ventricle on a chest roentgenogram. Marked calcification of the left ventricular silhouette may be present. These findings, when clear-cut, are relatively specific, but they have limited sensitivity. Radionuclide ventriculography and two-dimensional echocardiography can demonstrate ventricular aneurysm more readily; the latter is also helpful in distinguishing between true and false aneurysms based on the demonstration of a narrow neck in relation to cavity size in the latter.[411] Color-flow echocardiographic imaging is useful in establishing the diagnosis because flow "in and out" of the aneurysm as well as abnormal flow within the aneurysm can be detected, and subsequent pulsed Doppler imaging can reveal a "to-and-fro" pattern with characteristic respiratory variation in the peak systolic velocity. MRI may be emerging as the preferred noninvasive technique for the preoperative assessment of ventricular shape, thinning, and resectability.[409]

LEFT VENTRICULAR ANEURYSMECTOMY. True ventricular aneurysms do not rupture, and operative excision is carried out to improve the clinical manifestations, most often heart failure but sometimes also angina, embolization, and life-threatening tachyarrhythmias.[409] Coronary revascularization is frequently performed along with aneurysmectomy, especially in patients in whom angina accompanies heart failure.

A large left ventricular aneurysm in a patient with symptoms of heart failure, particularly if angina pectoris is also present, is an indication for surgery. The operative mortality rate for left ventricular aneurysmectomy is approximately 8 percent (ranging from 2 to 19 percent),[412] with rates as low as 3 percent reported in more recent series.[413] Risk factors for early death include poor left ventricular function, triple-vessel disease, recent myocardial infarction, the presence of mitral regurgitation, and intractable ventricular arrhythmias.[413] The presence of angina pectoris instead of dyspnea as the dominant preoperative symptom is associated with lower operative mortality.[414] Surgery carries a particularly high risk in patients with severe heart failure, a low-output state, and akinesis of the interventricular septum, as assessed echocardiographically. Akinesis or dyskinesia of the posterior basal segment of the left ventricle and significant right coronary artery stenoses are additional risk factors.

Risk factors for late mortality following survival from surgery include incomplete revascularization, impaired systolic function of the basal segments of the ventricle and septum not involved by the aneurysm, the presence of a large aneurysm with a small quantity of residual viable myocardium, and the presence of severe cardiac failure as the initial feature.[415]

Improvement in left ventricular function has been reported in survivors of resection of left ventricular aneurysms.[416] Anterior ventricular restoration has the potential to reverse adverse remodeling, realign contractile fibers, and decrease ventricular wall stress.[417-419] By removing the abnormal mechanical burden, left ventricular aneurysmectomy has been associated with late improvement in overall systolic function and improvement in the performance of regional nonischemic myocardium in zones remote from the left ventricular aneurysm, in addition to improvement in measures of ventricular relaxation and cardiovascular neuroregulatory mechanisms.[416] A concomitant improvement in exercise performance and clinical symptoms may also occur, particularly in patients who have undergone complete revascularization. In one series, 78 percent of patients undergoing ventricular reconstruction had an improvement in symptoms, with survival of 84 percent at 5 years.[409]

New surgical approaches to the repair of left ventricular aneurysms are designed to restore normal left ventricular geometry by using an alternative method of epicardial closure and/or an endocardial patch to divide the area of the aneurysm from the remainder of the ventricular cavity (Fig. 50–28). Favorable clinical and hemodynamic results following the use of these newer techniques have been reported, with 5-year survival rates ranging from 73 to 87.5 percent and a corresponding improvement in hemodynamics and clinical symptoms.[413] In one series, 88 percent of patients treated with the endoaneurysmorrhaphy technique were in NYHA Class I or II after a mean follow-up of approximately 3.5 years.[420]

Mitral Regurgitation Secondary To Coronary Artery Disease (see Chap. 57)

Mitral regurgitation is an important cause of heart failure in some patients with CAD. Rupture of a papillary muscle or the head of a papillary muscle usually causes severe acute mitral

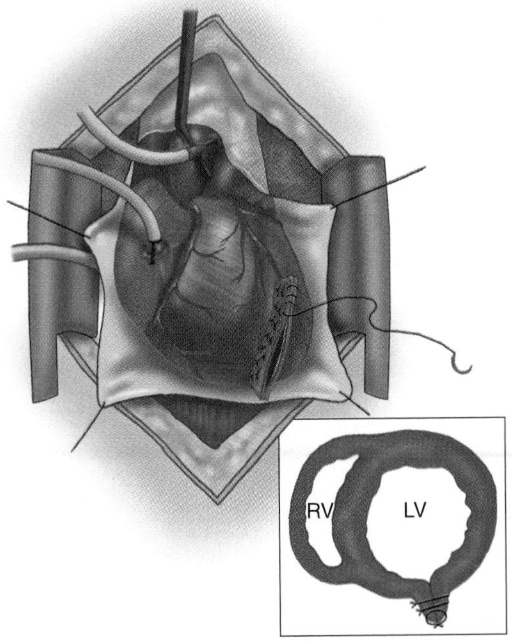

FIGURE 50–28 Linear repair technique used in left ventricular (LV) aneurysm repair. The aneurysm walls are closed in a vertical line between two layers of Teflon felt. Two layers of interrupted horizontal mattress sutures are reinforced with two layers of running sutures. RV = right ventricle. (From Glower DD, Lowe JE: Left ventricular aneurysm. *In* Cohn LC, Edmunds LH [eds]: Cardiac Surgery in the Adult. New York, McGraw-Hill, 2003, p 597.)

regurgitation in the course of acute myocardial infarction (see Chap. 57). The cause of chronic mitral regurgitation in patients with CAD is multifactorial, and the geometrical determinants are complex and include papillary muscle dysfunction from ischemia and fibrosis in conjunction with a wall motion abnormality and changes in ventricular shape in the region of the papillary muscle and/or dilation of the mitral annulus.[421,422] Enlargement of the mitral annulus at end-systole is asymmetrical, with lengthening primarily involving the posterior annular segments and leading to prolapse of leaflet tissue tethered by the posterior papillary muscle and restriction of leaflet tissue attached to the anterior leaflet. Most patients with chronic CAD and mitral regurgitation have suffered a previous myocardial infarction. Clinical features that help identify mitral regurgitation secondary to papillary muscle dysfunction as the cause of acute pulmonary edema or the cause of milder symptoms of left-sided failure include a loud systolic murmur and demonstration of a flail mitral valve leaflet on echocardiography.

In some patients with severe mitral regurgitation into a small "unprepared" left atrium, the murmur may be unimpressive or inaudible. Doppler echocardiography is helpful in assessing the severity of the regurgitation (see Chap. 11). As in mitral regurgitation of other causes, the left atrium is not usually greatly enlarged unless mitral regurgitation has been present for more than 6 months. The ECG is nonspecific, and most patients have angiographic evidence of multivessel CAD.

MANAGEMENT. In patients with severe mitral regurgitation, the indications for surgical correction, usually in association with CABG, are fairly clear-cut. Mitral valve repair, as opposed to mitral replacement, is the procedure of choice, but the decision is based on the anatomical characteristics of the structures forming the mitral valve apparatus, the urgency of the need for surgery, and the severity of left ventricular dysfunction.[423] A more complex and frequently encountered problem involves the indications for mitral valve surgery in patients undergoing coronary bypass surgery in whom the severity of mitral regurgitation is moderate.[424] The decision is based partly on the presence or absence of structural abnormalities of the mitral apparatus and the amenability of the valve to repair. Intraoperative transesophageal echocardiography is invaluable in assessing the severity of regurgitation, the reparability of the valve, and the success of the integrity of the repair after discontinuation of CPB.

The mortality associated with combined coronary bypass surgery and mitral valve placement in the 2002 Society of Thoracic Surgeons data base was 12 percent. For bypass surgery and mitral valve repair, mortality was 7 percent overall including emergency and reoperative procedures.[425] Predictors of early mortality include the need for replacement versus repair (in some but not all series) but, in addition, may include other variables such as age, comorbid conditions, the urgency of surgery, and left ventricular function.[426] Late results are strongly influenced by the pathophysiological mechanisms underlying mitral regurgitation and are poorer in patients with regurgitation resulting from annular dilation or restrictive leaflet motion than in patients with chordal or papillary muscle rupture. It is encouraging that despite the relatively high operative mortality, late survival of hospital survivors is excellent. In patients with very poor left ventricular function and dilation of the mitral annulus, mitral regurgitation can intensify the severity of left ventricular failure. In such patients, the risk of surgery is high and the benefits are less obvious, and a trial of intensive medical therapy, including afterload reduction to decrease left ventricular volume and the diameter of the annulus, may be worthwhile.

CARDIAC ARRHYTHMIAS

In some patients with CAD, cardiac arrhythmias are the dominant clinical manifestation of the disease. Various degrees and forms of ventricular ectopic activity are the most common arrhythmias in patients with CAD, but serious ventricular arrhythmias may be a major component of the clinical findings in other subgroups. The clinical presentation of arrhythmias and their management in patients with CAD are discussed in Chapter 29.

NONATHEROMATOUS CORONARY ARTERY DISEASE

Although atherosclerosis is by far the most important cause of CAD, other conditions may also be responsible. The most common causes of nonatheromatous CAD resulting in myocardial ischemia are the syndrome of angina-like pain with normal coronary arteriograms (i.e., so-called syndrome X) and Prinzmetal angina (see Chap. 49).

Nonatheromatous CAD may result from other diverse abnormalities, including congenital abnormalities in the origin or distribution of the coronary arteries (see Chap. 56). The most important of these abnormalities are anomalous origin of a coronary artery (usually the left) from the pulmonary artery, origin of both coronary arteries from either the right or the left sinus of Valsalva, and coronary arteriovenous fistula. An anomalous origin of either the left main coronary artery or right coronary artery from the aorta with subsequent coursing between the aorta and pulmonary trunk is a rare and sometimes fatal coronary arterial anomaly.[427] Coronary anomalies are reported to cause between 12 and 19 percent of sports-related deaths in U.S. high school and college athletes.[427]

MYOCARDIAL BRIDGING. This cause of systolic compression of the LAD coronary artery is a well-recognized angiographic phenomenon of questionable clinical significance.

CONNECTIVE TISSUE DISORDERS. Several inherited connective tissue disorders are associated with myocardial ischemia (see Chap. 70), including Marfan syndrome (causing aortic and coronary artery dissection), Hurler syndrome (causing coronary obstruction), homocystinuria (causing coronary artery thrombosis), Ehlers-Danlos syndrome (causing coronary artery dissection), and pseudoxanthoma elasticum (causing accelerated CAD). Kawasaki disease (the mucocutaneous lymph node syndrome) may cause coronary artery aneurysms and ischemic heart disease in children.

SPONTANEOUS CORONARY DISSECTION. This is a rare cause of myocardial infarction and sudden cardiac death.[428] Chronic dissection manifested as congestive heart failure has been described. In one series, approximately 75 percent of cases were diagnosed at autopsy, and 75 percent occurred in women, half of which were associated with a postpartum state. Some cases are associated with atherosclerosis. Hypertension has been postulated as a cause of multivessel spontaneous coronary dissection in some patients, and in others, no obvious cause has been identified. In the acute phase, thrombolytic therapy may be dangerous, but early angiography may identify patients who could benefit from stenting or bypass surgery.[429] In survivors of spontaneous coronary artery dissection, the subsequent 3-year mortality was 20 percent, but complete healing as defined angiographically may lead to a favorable outcome without intervention.[430]

CORONARY VASCULITIS. This condition resulting from connective tissue diseases or autoimmune forms of vasculitis, including polyarteritis nodosa, giant cell (temporal) arteritis, and scleroderma, is well described (see Chap. 82). Coronary arteritis is seen at autopsy in about 20 percent of patients with rheumatoid arthritis but is rarely associated with clinical manifestations. The incidence of CAD is increased in women with systemic lupus erythematosus. In patients with systemic lupus erythematosus, CAD has been attributed to a vasculitis, immune complex–mediated endothelial damage, and coronary thrombosis from antiphospholipid antibodies, as well as accelerated atherosclerosis. Giant coronary artery aneurysm associated with systemic lupus erythematosus is an unusual manifestation that has been associated with the development of acute myocardial infarction despite therapy. The antiphospholipid syndrome, which is characterized by arterial and venous thrombosis and is associated with the presence of antiphospholipid antibodies, may be associated with myocardial infarction, angina, and diffuse left ventricular dysfunction.

TAKAYASU ARTERITIS. In rare cases, (see Chap. 82) this condition is associated with angina, myocardial infarction, and cardiac failure in patients younger than 40 years of age. Coronary blood flow may be decreased by involvement of the ostia or proximal segments of the coronary arteries, but disease in distal coronary segments is rare.[431] The average age at the onset of symptoms is 24 years, and the event-free survival rate 10 years after diagnosis is approximately 60 percent. Luetic aortitis may also produce myocardial ischemia by causing coronary ostial obstruction.

POSTMEDIASTINAL IRRADIATION. The occurrence of CAD and morbid cardiac events in young persons after mediastinal irradiation is highly suggestive of a cause-and-effect relationship.[432] Pathological changes include adventitial scarring and medial hypertrophy with severe intimal atherosclerotic disease. Radiation injury may be latent and may not be manifested clinically for many years after therapy. Contributory factors include higher doses than currently administered and the presence of cardiac risk factors. Among patients without risk factors who receive an intermediate total dose of 30 and 40 Gy, the risk of cardiac death and myocardial infarction is low.

Myocardial ischemia not caused by coronary atherosclerosis can also result from embolism from infective endocarditis (see Chap. 58), implanted prosthetic cardiac valves (see Chap. 57), calcified aortic valves, mural thrombi, and primary cardiac tumors (see Chap. 63).

COCAINE (see Chap. 62). Because of its widespread use, cocaine has become a well-documented cause of chest pain, myocardial infarction, and sudden cardiac death.[433] In a population-based study of sudden death among persons 20 to 40 years old in Olmsted County over a 30-year period, a high prevalence of cocaine abuse was observed in the more recent cohort of young adults who died suddenly. The principal effects of cocaine are mediated by alpha-adrenergic stimulation, which causes an increase in myocardial O_2 demand and a reduction in O_2 supply because of coronary vasoconstriction.

Cardiac Transplant–Associated Coronary Arteriopathy

See Chapters 26 and 35.

REFERENCES

1. Maseri A: Ischemic heart disease. *In* A Rational Basis for Clinical Practice and Clinical Research. New York, Churchill Livingstone, 1995.
2. Virmani R, Forman MB: Nonatherosclerotic Ischemic Heart Disease. New York, Raven, 1989.
3. American Heart Association: Heart Disease and Stroke Statistics—2004 Update. Dallas, American Heart Association, 2004.
4. Murray CJ, Lopez AD: Mortality by cause for eight regions of the world: Global Burden of Disease Study. Lancet 349:1269-1276, 1997.
5. Bonow RO, Smaha LA, Smith SC Jr, et al: World Heart Day 2002: The international burden of cardiovascular disease—responding to the emerging global epidemic. Circulation 106:1602-1605, 2002.
6. American Heart Association: International Cardiovascular Disease Statistics. Dallas, American Heart Association, 2004.
7. Duprez DA: Angina in the elderly. Eur Heart J 17(Suppl G):8-13, 1996.
8. Bogaty P, Kingma JG Jr, Robitaille NM, et al: Attenuation of myocardial ischemia with repeated exercise in subjects with chronic stable angina: Relation to myocardial contractility, intensity of exercise, and the adenosine triphosphate–sensitive potassium channel. J Am Coll Cardiol 32:1665-1671, 1998.
9. Bogaty P, Poirier P, Boyer L, et al: What induces the warm-up ischemia/angina phenomenon: Exercise or myocardial ischemia? Circulation 107:1858-1863, 2003.
10. Campeau L: Grading of angina pectoris [letter]. Circulation 54:522-523, 1976.
11. Goldman L, Hashimoto B, Cook EF, et al: Comparative reproducibility and validity of systems for assessing cardiovascular functional class: Advantages of a new specific activity scale. Circulation 64:1227-1234, 1981.
12. Califf RM, Mark DB, Harrell FE Jr, et al: Importance of clinical measures of ischemia in the prognosis of patients with documented coronary artery disease. J Am Coll Cardiol 11:20-26, 1988.
13. Foreman RD: Mechanisms of cardiac pain. Annu Rev Physiol 61:143-167, 1999.
14. Rosen SD, Camici PG: The brain-heart axis in the perception of cardiac pain: The elusive link between ischaemia and pain. Ann Med 32:350-364, 2000.
15. Wise CM, Semble EL, Dalton CB: Musculoskeletal chest wall syndromes in patients with noncardiac chest pain: A study of 100 patients. Arch Phys Med Rehabil 73:147-149, 1992.
16. Klein R, Klein BE, Moss SE, et al: Association of ocular disease and mortality in a diabetic population. Arch Ophthalmol 117:1487-1495, 1999.
17. Eagle KA, Rihal CS, Foster ED, et al: Long-term survival in patients with coronary artery disease: Importance of peripheral vascular disease. The Coronary Artery Surgery Study (CASS) Investigators. J Am Coll Cardiol 23:1091-1095, 1994.
18. Gibbons RJ, Abrams J, Chatterjee K, et al: ACC/AHA 2002 guideline update for the management of patients with chronic stable angina—summary article: A report of the American College of Cardiology/American Heart Association Task Force on Practice Guidelines (Committee on the Management of Patients with Chronic Stable Angina). J Am Coll Cardiol 41:159-168, 2003.
19. Freedman SB, Wong CK: Triggers of daily life ischaemia. Heart 80:489-492, 1998.
20. Gullette EC, Blumenthal JA, Babyak M, et al: Effects of mental stress on myocardial ischemia during daily life. JAMA 277:1521-1526, 1997.
21. Hillis LD, Braunwald E: Coronary artery spasm. N Engl J Med 299:695-702, 1978.
22. Opie LH: The Heart: Physiology, From Cell to Circulation. 3rd ed. Philadelphia, Lippincott-Raven, 1998.
23. Maseri A, Crea F, Lanza GA: Coronary vasoconstriction: Where do we stand in 1999? An important, multifaceted but elusive role. Cardiologia 44:115-118, 1999.
24. Benhorin J, Banai S, Moriel M, et al: Circadian variations in ischemic threshold and their relation to the occurrence of ischemic episodes. Circulation 87:808-814, 1993.
25. Baliga RR, Rosen SD, Camici PG, et al: Regional myocardial blood flow redistribution as a cause of postprandial angina pectoris. Circulation 97:1144-1149, 1998.
26. Maseri A, Chierchia S, Kaski JC: Mixed angina pectoris. Am J Cardiol 56:30E-33E, 1985.
27. Expert Panel on Detection, Evaluation, and Treatment of High Blood Cholesterol in Adults: Executive Summary of the Third Report of the National Cholesterol Education Program (NCEP) Expert Panel on Detection, Evaluation, and Treatment of High Blood Cholesterol in Adults (Adult Treatment Panel III). JAMA 285:2486-2497, 2001.
28. Lamarche B, Tchernof A, Mauriege P, et al: Fasting insulin and apolipoprotein B levels and low-density lipoprotein particle size as risk factors for ischemic heart disease. JAMA 279:1955-1961, 1998.
29. The Homocysteine Studies Collaboration: Homocysteine and risk of ischemic heart disease and stroke: A meta-analysis. JAMA 288:2015-2022, 2002.
30. Malinow MR, Bostom AG, Krauss RM: Homocyst(e)ine, diet, and cardiovascular diseases: A statement for healthcare professionals from the Nutrition Committee, American Heart Association. Circulation 99:178-182, 1999.
31. Ridker PM: Clinical application of C-reactive protein for cardiovascular disease detection and prevention. Circulation 107:363-369, 2003.
32. Ridker PM, Rifai N, Rose L, et al: Comparison of C-reactive protein and low-density lipoprotein cholesterol levels in the prediction of first cardiovascular events. N Engl J Med 347:1557-1565, 2002.
33. Pearson TA, Mensah GA, Alexander RW, et al: Markers of inflammation and cardiovascular disease—application to clinical and public health practice: A statement for healthcare professionals from the Centers for Disease Control and Prevention and the American Heart Association. Circulation 107:499-511, 2003.
34. Morrow DA, de Lemos JA, Sabatine MS, et al: The search for a biomarker of cardiac ischemia. Clin Chem 49:537-539, 2003.
35. Crenshaw JH, Mirvis DM, el-Zeky F, et al: Interactive effects of ST-T wave abnormalities on survival of patients with coronary artery disease. J Am Coll Cardiol 18:413-420, 1991.
36. Gibbons RJ, Balady GJ, Bricker JT, et al: ACC/AHA 2002 guideline update for exercise testing—summary article: A report of the American College of Cardiology/American Heart Association Task Force on Practice Guidelines (Committee to Update the 1997 Exercise Testing Guidelines). Circulation 106:1883-1892, 2002.
37. Shaw LJ, Hachamovitch R, Berman DS, et al: The economic consequences of available diagnostic and prognostic strategies for the evaluation of stable angina patients: An observational assessment of the value of precatheterization ischemia. Economics of Noninvasive Diagnosis (END) Multicenter Study Group. J Am Coll Cardiol 33:661-669, 1999.
38. Froelicher VF, Lehmann KG, Thomas R, et al: The electrocardiographic exercise test in a population with reduced workup bias: Diagnostic performance, computerized interpretation, and multivariable prediction. Veterans Affairs Cooperative Study in Health Services 016 (QUEXTA) Study Group. Quantitative Exercise Testing and Angiography. Ann Intern Med 128:965-974, 1998.
39. Shaw LJ, Peterson ED, Shaw LK, et al: Use of a prognostic treadmill score in identifying diagnostic coronary disease subgroups. Circulation 98:1622-1630, 1998.
40. Beller GA, Zaret BL: Contributions of nuclear cardiology to diagnosis and prognosis of patients with coronary artery disease. Circulation 101:1465-1478, 2000.
41. Pagley PR, Beller GA, Watson DD, et al: Improved outcome after coronary bypass surgery in patients with ischemic cardiomyopathy and residual myocardial viability. Circulation 96:793-800, 1997.
42. Gibbons RJ, Hodge DO, Berman DS, et al: Long-term outcome of patients with intermediate-risk exercise electrocardiograms who do not have myocardial perfusion defects on radionuclide imaging. Circulation 100:2140-2145, 1999.
43. Ritchie J, Bateman TM, Bonow RO, et al: Guidelines for clinical use of cardiac radionuclide imaging: A report of the American Heart Association/American College of Cardiology Task Force on Assessment of Diagnostic and Therapeutic Cardiovascular Procedures, Committee on Radionuclide Imaging, developed in collaboration with the American Society of Nuclear Cardiology. Circulation 91:1278-1303, 1995.
44. Ibrahim T, Nekolla SG, Schreiber K, et al: Assessment of coronary flow reserve: Comparison between contrast-enhanced magnetic resonance imaging and positron emission tomography. J Am Coll Cardiol 39:864-870, 2002.
45. Fleischmann KE, Hunink MG, Kuntz KM, et al: Exercise echocardiography or exercise SPECT imaging? A meta-analysis of diagnostic test performance. JAMA 280:913-920, 1998.
46. Bax JJ, Poldermans D, Elhendy A, et al: Improvement of left ventricular ejection fraction, heart failure symptoms, and prognosis after revascularization in patients with chronic coronary artery disease and viable myocardium detected by dobutamine stress echocardiography. J Am Coll Cardiol 34:163-169, 1999.
47. Finkelhor RS, Pajouh M, Kett A, et al: Clinical impact of second harmonic imaging and left heart contrast in echocardiographic stress testing. Am J Cardiol 85:740-743, 2000.
48. Vlassak I, Rubin DN, Odabashian JA, et al: Contrast and harmonic imaging improves accuracy and efficiency of novice readers for dobutamine stress echocardiography. Echocardiography 19:483-488, 2002.
49. Voigt JU, Exner B, Schmiedehausen K, et al: Strain-rate imaging during dobutamine stress echocardiography provides objective evidence of inducible ischemia. Circulation 107:2120-2126, 2003.
50. Hachamovitch R, Berman DS, Kiat H, et al: Effective risk stratification using exercise myocardial perfusion SPECT in women: Gender-related differences in prognostic nuclear testing. J Am Coll Cardiol 28:34-44, 1996.
51. Taillefer R, DePuey EG, Udelson JE, et al: Comparative diagnostic accuracy of Tl-201 and Tc-99m sestamibi SPECT imaging (perfusion and ECG-gated SPECT) in detecting coronary artery disease in women. J Am Coll Cardiol 29:69-77, 1997.
52. Loecker TH, Schwartz RS, Cotta CW, et al: Fluoroscopic coronary artery calcification and associated coronary disease in asymptomatic young men. J Am Coll Cardiol 19:1167-1172, 1992.
53. Callister TQ, Raggi P, Cooil B, et al: Effect of HMG-CoA reductase inhibitors on coronary artery disease as assessed by electron-beam computed tomography. N Engl J Med 339:1972-1978, 1998.

54. Budoff MJ, Diamond GA, Raggi P, et al: Continuous probabilistic prediction of angiographically significant coronary artery disease using electron beam tomography. Circulation 105:1791-1796, 2002.
55. Detrano RC, Wong ND, Doherty TM, et al: Coronary calcium does not accurately predict near-term future coronary events in high-risk adults. Circulation 99:2633-2638, 1999.
56. Kondos GT, Hoff JA, Sevrukov A, et al: Electron-beam tomography coronary artery calcium and cardiac events: A 37-month follow-up of 5635 initially asymptomatic low-to intermediate-risk adults. Circulation 107:2571-2576, 2003.
57. O'Rourke RA, Brundage BH, Froelicher VF, et al: American College of Cardiology/American Heart Association Expert Consensus document on electron-beam computed tomography for the diagnosis and prognosis of coronary artery disease. Circulation 102:126-140, 2000.
58. Budoff MJ, Georgiou D, Brody A, et al: Ultrafast computed tomography as a diagnostic modality in the detection of coronary artery disease: A multicenter study. Circulation 93:898-904, 1996.
59. Nallamothu BK, Saint S, Bielak LF, et al. Electron-beam computed tomography in the diagnosis of coronary artery disease: A meta-analysis. Arch Intern Med 161:833-838, 2001.
60. Ropers D, Baum U, Pohle K, et al: Detection of coronary artery stenoses with thin-slice multi-detector row spiral computed tomography and multiplanar reconstruction. Circulation 107:664-666, 2003.
61. Forder JR, Pohost GM: Cardiovascular nuclear magnetic resonance: Basic and clinical applications. J Clin Invest 111:1630-1639, 2003.
62. Kim RJ, Wu E, Rafael A, et al: The use of contrast-enhanced magnetic resonance imaging to identify reversible myocardial dysfunction. N Engl J Med 343:1445-1453, 2000.
63. Klein C, Nekolla SG, Bengel FM, et al: Assessment of myocardial viability with contrast-enhanced magnetic resonance imaging: Comparison with positron emission tomography. Circulation 105:162-167, 2002.
64. Gerber BL, Garot J, Bluemke DA, et al: Accuracy of contrast-enhanced magnetic resonance imaging in predicting improvement of regional myocardial function in patients after acute myocardial infarction. Circulation 106:1083-1089, 2002.
65. Schwitter J, Nanz D, Kneifel S, et al: Assessment of myocardial perfusion in coronary artery disease by magnetic resonance: A comparison with positron emission tomography and coronary angiography. Circulation 103:2230-2235, 2001.
66. Kuijpers D, Ho KY, van Dijkman PR, et al: Dobutamine cardiovascular magnetic resonance for the detection of myocardial ischemia with the use of myocardial tagging. Circulation 107:1592-1597, 2003.
67. Kraitchman DL, Sampath S, Castillo E, et al: Quantitative ischemia detection during cardiac magnetic resonance stress testing by use of FastHARP. Circulation 107:2025-2030, 2003.
68. Fuster V, Corti R, Fayad ZA, et al: Integration of vascular biology and magnetic resonance imaging in the understanding of atherothrombosis and acute coronary syndromes. J Thromb Haemost 1:1410-1421, 2003.
69. Hatsukami TS, Ross R, Polissar NL, et al: Visualization of fibrous cap thickness and rupture in human atherosclerotic carotid plaque in vivo with high-resolution magnetic resonance imaging. Circulation 102:959-964, 2000.
70. Moody AR, Murphy RE, Morgan PS, et al: Characterization of complicated carotid plaque with magnetic resonance direct thrombus imaging in patients with cerebral ischemia. Circulation 107:3047-3052, 2003.
71. Kim WY, Danias PG, Stuber M, et al: Coronary magnetic resonance angiography for the detection of coronary stenoses. N Engl J Med 345:1863-1869, 2001.
72. Langerak SE, Vliegen HW, Jukema JW, et al: Value of magnetic resonance imaging for the noninvasive detection of stenosis in coronary artery bypass grafts and recipient coronary arteries. Circulation 107:1502-1508, 2003.
73. Taylor AM, Thorne SA, Rubens MB, et al: Coronary artery imaging in grown up congenital heart disease: Complementary role of magnetic resonance and x-ray coronary angiography. Circulation 101:1670-1678, 2000.

Catheterization, Angiography, and Coronary Arteriography

74. Schoenhagen P, Nissen S: Understanding coronary artery disease: Tomographic imaging with intravascular ultrasound. Heart 88:91-96, 2002.
75. Nair A, Kuban BD, Tuzcu EM, et al: Coronary plaque classification with intravascular ultrasound radiofrequency data analysis. Circulation 106:2200-2206, 2002.
76. Bogaty P, Brecker SJ, White SE, et al: Comparison of coronary angiographic findings in acute and chronic first presentation of ischemic heart disease. Circulation 87:1938-1946, 1993.
77. Kruger D, Stierle U, Herrmann G, et al: Exercise-induced myocardial ischemia in isolated coronary artery ectasias and aneurysms ("dilated coronopathy"). J Am Coll Cardiol 34:1461-1470, 1999.
78. Tunick PA, Slater J, Kronzon I, et al: Discrete atherosclerotic coronary artery aneurysms: A study of 20 patients. J Am Coll Cardiol 15:279-282, 1990.
79. Vanoverschelde JL, Wijns W, Depre C, et al: Mechanisms of chronic regional postischemic dysfunction in humans: New insights from the study of noninfarcted collateral-dependent myocardium. Circulation 87:1513-1523, 1993.
80. Mohlenkamp S, Hort W, Ge J, et al: Update on myocardial bridging. Circulation 106:2616-2622, 2002.
81. Mann T, Brodie BR, Grossman W, et al: Effect of angina on the left ventricular diastolic pressure-volume relationship. Circulation 55:761-766, 1977.
82. Braunwald E, Rutherford JD: Reversible ischemic left ventricular dysfunction: Evidence for the "hibernating myocardium." J Am Coll Cardiol 8:1467-1470, 1986.
83. Verani MS, Carroll RJ, Falsetti HL: Mitral valve prolapse in coronary artery disease. Am J Cardiol 37:1-6, 1976.
84. Gertz EW, Wisneski JA, Neese R, et al: Myocardial lactate metabolism: Evidence of lactate release during net chemical extraction in man. Circulation 63:1273-1279, 1981.
85. Lampe FC, Whincup PH, Wannamethee SG, et al: The natural history of prevalent ischaemic heart disease in middle-aged men. Eur Heart J 21:1052-1062, 2000.
86. Myers J, Prakash M, Froelicher V, et al: Exercise capacity and mortality among me referred for exercise testing. N Engl J Med 346:793-801, 2002.
87. Yao SS, Rozanski A: Principal uses of myocardial perfusion scintigraphy in the mar agement of patients with known or suspected coronary artery disease. Prog Cardiovas Dis 43:281-302, 2001.
88. Lee TH, Boucher CA: Clinical practice: Noninvasive tests in patients with stable coro nary artery disease. N Engl J Med 344:1840-1845, 2001.
89. Califf RM, Tomabechi Y, Lee KL, et al: Outcome in one-vessel coronary artery disease Circulation 67:283-290, 1983.
90. Caracciolo EA, Davis KB, Sopko G, et al: Comparison of surgical and medical grou survival in patients with left main coronary artery disease: Long-term CASS exper ence. Circulation 91:2325-2334, 1995.
91. Bigi R, Cortigiani L, Colombo P, et al: Prognostic and clinical correlates of angio graphically diffuse non-obstructive coronary lesions. Heart 89:1009-1013, 2003.

Medical Management

92. Jousilahti P, Vartiainen E, Tuomilehto J, et al: Sex, age, cardiovascular risk factors, an coronary heart disease: A prospective follow-up study of 14 786 middle-aged men an women in Finland. Circulation 99:1165-1172, 1999.
93. Lewington S, Clarke R, Qizilbash N, et al: Age-specific relevance of usual blood pres sure to vascular mortality: A meta-analysis of individual data for one million adult in 61 prospective studies. Lancet 360:1903-1913, 2002.
94. Devereux RB, Roman MJ: Inter-relationships between hypertension, left ventricula hypertrophy, and coronary heart disease. J Hypertens 11(Suppl):S3-S9, 1993.
95. Hebert PR, Moser M, Mayer J, et al: Recent evidence on drug therapy of mild to mod erate hypertension and decreased risk of coronary heart disease. Arch Intern Me 153:578-581, 1993.
96. Psaty BM, Lumley T, Furberg CD, et al: Health outcomes associated with various ant hypertensive therapies used as first-line agents: A network meta-analysis. JAM 289:2534-2544, 2003.
97. Ogden LG, He J, Lydick E, et al: Long-term absolute benefit of lowering blood pressur in hypertensive patients according to the JNC VI risk stratification. Hypertensio 35:539-543, 2000.
98. Critchley JA, Capewell S: Mortality risk reduction associated with smoking cessa tion in patients with coronary heart disease: A systematic review. JAMA 290:86-97 2003.
99. Czernin J, Sun K, Brunken R, et al: Effect of acute and long-term smoking on myocar dial blood flow and flow reserve. Circulation 91:2891-2897, 1995.
100. Scandinavian Simvastatin Survival Study Group: Randomised trial of cholesterc lowering in 4444 patients with coronary heart disease: The Scandinavian Simvastati Survival Study (4S). Lancet 344:1383-1389, 1994.
101. Sacks FM, Pfeffer MA, Moye LA, et al: The effect of pravastatin on coronary event after myocardial infarction in patients with average cholesterol levels. Cholesterol an Recurrent Events Trial investigators. N Engl J Med 335:1001-1009, 1996.
102. Long-Term Intervention with Pravastatin in Ischaemic Disease (LIPID) Study Grou Prevention of cardiovascular events and death with pravastatin in patients with corc nary heart disease and a broad range of initial cholesterol levels. N Engl J Me 339:1349-1357, 1998.
103. Pitt B, Waters D, Brown WV, et al: Aggressive lipid-lowering therapy compared wit angioplasty in stable coronary artery disease. Atorvastatin versus Revascularizatio Treatment Investigators. N Engl J Med 341:70-76, 1999.
104. Heart Protection Study Collaborative Group: MRC/BHF Heart Protection Study of chc lesterol lowering with simvastatin in 20,536 high-risk individuals: A randomise placebo-controlled trial. Lancet 360:7-22, 2002.
105. Dupuis J, Tardif JC, Cernacek P, et al: Cholesterol reduction rapidly improves end othelial function after acute coronary syndromes. The RECIFE (Reduction of Choles terol in Ischemia and Function of the Endothelium) trial. Circulation 99:3227-323 1999.
106. Ridker PM, Rifai N, Pfeffer MA, et al: Long-term effects of pravastatin on plasma cor centration of C-reactive protein. Circulation 100:230-235, 1999.
107. Albert MA, Danielson E, Rifai N, et al: Effect of statin therapy on C-reactive protei levels: The pravastatin inflammation/CRP evaluation (PRINCE)—a randomized tri and cohort study. JAMA 286:64-70, 2001.
108. Dangas G, Badimon JJ, Smith DA, et al: Pravastatin therapy in hyperlipidemia: Effec on thrombus formation and the systemic hemostatic profile. J Am Coll Cardiol 33:129 1304, 1999.
109. Crisby M, Nordin-Fredriksson G, Shah PK, et al: Pravastatin treatment increases co lagen content and decreases lipid content, inflammation, metalloproteinases, and ce death in human carotid plaques: Implications for plaque stabilization. Circulatio 103:926-933, 2001.
110. Rosenson RS, Tangney CC: Antiatherothrombotic properties of statins: Implications fc cardiovascular event reduction. JAMA 279:1643-1650, 1998.
111. Lewis SJ, Sacks FM, Mitchell JS, et al: Effect of pravastatin on cardiovascular even in women after myocardial infarction: The Cholesterol and Recurrent Events (CARE trial. J Am Coll Cardiol 32:140-146, 1998.
112. Shepherd J, Blauw GJ, Murphy MB, et al: Pravastatin in elderly individuals at risk c vascular disease (PROSPER): A randomised controlled trial. Lancet 360:1623-163 2002.
113. Tsevat J, Kuntz KM, Orav EJ, et al: Cost-effectiveness of pravastatin therapy for su vivors of myocardial infarction with average cholesterol levels. Am Heart J 141:72 734, 2001.
113a. Cannon CP, Braunwald E, McCabe CH, et al: Pravastatin or Atorvastatin Evaluatio and Infection Therapy (PROVE-IT)-TIMI 22 Investigators. Intensive versus modera lipid lowering with statins after acute coronary syndromes. N Engl J Med 350:149 1504, 2004.
114. Gotto AM Jr: Low high-density lipoprotein cholesterol as a risk factor in coronary hea disease: A working group report. Circulation 103:2213-2218, 2001.

15. Lamarche B, Tchernof A, Moorjani S, et al: Small, dense low-density lipoprotein particles as a predictor of the risk of ischemic heart disease in men: Prospective results from the Quebec Cardiovascular Study. Circulation 95:69-75, 1997.
16. Rubins HB, Robins SJ, Collins D, et al: Gemfibrozil for the secondary prevention of coronary heart disease in men with low levels of high-density lipoprotein cholesterol. Veterans Affairs High-Density Lipoprotein Cholesterol Intervention Trial Study Group. N Engl J Med 341:410-418, 1999.
17. Flaker GC, Warnica JW, Sacks FM, et al: Pravastatin prevents clinical events in revascularized patients with average cholesterol concentrations. Cholesterol and Recurrent Events CARE Investigators. J Am Coll Cardiol 34:106-112, 1999.
18. Serruys PW, de Feyter P, Macaya C, et al: Fluvastatin for prevention of cardiac events following successful first percutaneous coronary intervention: A randomized controlled trial. JAMA 287:3215-3222, 2002.
19. Grodstein F, Stampfer MJ, Colditz GA, et al: Postmenopausal hormone therapy and mortality. N Engl J Med 336:1769-1775, 1997.
20. Hulley S, Grady D, Bush T, et al: Randomized trial of estrogen plus progestin for secondary prevention of coronary heart disease in postmenopausal women. Heart and Estrogen/progestin Replacement Study (HERS) Research Group. JAMA 280:605-613, 1998.
21. Grady D, Herrington D, Bittner V, et al: Cardiovascular disease outcomes during 6.8 years of hormone therapy: Heart and Estrogen/progestin Replacement Study follow-up (HERS II). JAMA 288:49-57, 2002.
22. Clarke SC, Kelleher J, Lloyd-Jones H, et al: A study of hormone replacement therapy in postmenopausal women with ischaemic heart disease: The Papworth HRT atherosclerosis study. Br J Obstet Gynaecol 109:1056-1062, 2002.
23. Herrington DM, Reboussin DM, Brosnihan KB, et al: Effects of estrogen replacement on the progression of coronary-artery atherosclerosis. N Engl J Med 343:522-529, 2000.
24. Waters DD, Alderman EL, Hsia J, et al: Effects of hormone replacement therapy and antioxidant vitamin supplements on coronary atherosclerosis in postmenopausal women: A randomized controlled trial. JAMA 288:2432-2440, 2002.
25. Cherry N, Gilmour K, Hannaford P, et al: Oestrogen therapy for prevention of reinfarction in postmenopausal women: A randomised placebo-controlled trial. Lancet 360:2001-2008, 2002.
26. Rossouw JE, Anderson GL, Prentice RL, et al: Risks and benefits of estrogen plus progestin in healthy postmenopausal women: Principal results from the Women's Health Initiative randomized controlled trial. JAMA 288:321-333, 2002.
27. Mosca L, Collins P, Herrington DM, et al: Hormone replacement therapy and cardiovascular disease: A statement for healthcare professionals from the American Heart Association. Circulation 104:499-503, 2001.
28. Thompson PD, Buchner D, Pina IL, et al: Exercise and physical activity in the prevention and treatment of atherosclerotic cardiovascular disease. Circulation 107:3109-3116, 2003.
29. Jolliffe JA, Rees K, Taylor RS, et al: Exercise-based rehabilitation for coronary heart disease. Cochrane Database Syst Rev CD001800, 2004.
30. Hambrecht R, Niebauer J, Marburger C, et al: Various intensities of leisure time physical activity in patients with coronary artery disease: Effects on cardiorespiratory fitness and progression of coronary atherosclerotic lesions. J Am Coll Cardiol 22:468-477, 1993.
31. Hambrecht R, Adams V, Erbs S, et al: Regular physical activity improves endothelial function in patients with coronary artery disease by increasing phosphorylation of endothelial nitric oxide synthase. Circulation 107:3152-3158, 2003.
32. Hambrecht R, Wolf A, Gielen S, et al: Effect of exercise on coronary endothelial function in patients with coronary artery disease. N Engl J Med 342:454-460, 2000.
33. Fletcher GF, Balady GJ, Amsterdam EA, et al: Exercise standards for testing and training: A statement for healthcare professionals from the American Heart Association. Circulation 104:1694-1740, 2001.
34. Oldridge N, Furlong W, Feeny D, et al: Economic evaluation of cardiac rehabilitation soon after acute myocardial infarction. Am J Cardiol 72:154-161, 1993.
35. Ridker PM, Rifai N, Pfeffer MA, et al: Inflammation, pravastatin, and the risk of coronary events after myocardial infarction in patients with average cholesterol levels. Cholesterol and Recurrent Events (CARE) Investigators. Circulation 98:839-844, 1998.
36. Libby P, Aikawa M: Stabilization of atherosclerotic plaques: New mechanisms and clinical targets. Nat Med 8:1257-1262, 2002.
36a. Ridker PM, Rifai N, Clearfield M, et al: Air Force/Texas Coronary Atherosclerosis Prevention Study Investigators. Measurement of C-reactive protein for the targeting of statin therapy in the primary prevention of acute coronary events. N Engl J Med 344:1959-1965, 2001.
37. Antiplatelet Trialists' Collaboration: Collaborative overview of randomised trials of antiplatelet therapy: I. Prevention of death, myocardial infarction, and stroke by prolonged antiplatelet therapy in various categories of patients. BMJ 308:81-106, 1994.
38. Juul-Moller S, Edvardsson N, Jahnmatz B, et al: Double-blind trial of aspirin in primary prevention of myocardial infarction in patients with stable chronic angina pectoris. The Swedish Angina Pectoris Aspirin Trial (SAPAT) Group. Lancet 340:1421-1425, 1992.
39. Ridker PM, Manson JE, Gaziano JM, et al: Low-dose aspirin therapy for chronic stable angina: A randomized, placebo-controlled clinical trial. Ann Intern Med 114:835-839, 1991.
40. Hennekens CH, Dyken ML, Fuster V: Aspirin as a therapeutic agent in cardiovascular disease: A statement for healthcare professionals from the American Heart Association. Circulation 96:2751-2753, 1997.
41. Antithrombotic Trialists' Collaboration: Collaborative meta-analysis of randomised trials of antiplatelet therapy for prevention of death, myocardial infarction, and stroke in high-risk patients. BMJ 324:71-86, 2002.
42. Peters RJ, Mehta SR, Fox KA, et al: Effects of aspirin dose when used alone or in combination with clopidogrel in patients with acute coronary syndromes: Observations from the Clopidogrel in Unstable angina to prevent Recurrent Events (CURE) study. Circulation 108:1682-1687, 2003.
143. Ridker PM, Cushman M, Stampfer MJ, et al: Inflammation, aspirin, and the risk of cardiovascular disease in apparently healthy men. N Engl J Med 336:973-979, 1997.
144. Ikonomidis I, Andreotti F, Economou E, et al: Increased proinflammatory cytokines in patients with chronic stable angina and their reduction by aspirin. Circulation 100:793-798, 1999.
145. Feldman M, Jialal I, Devaraj S, et al: Effects of low-dose aspirin on serum C-reactive protein and thromboxane B_2 concentrations: A placebo-controlled study using a highly sensitive C-reactive protein assay. J Am Coll Cardiol 37:2036-2041, 2001.
146. Husain S, Andrews NP, Mulcahy D, et al: Aspirin improves endothelial dysfunction in atherosclerosis. Circulation 97:716-720, 1998.
147. The Medical Research Council's General Practice Research Framework. Thrombosis Prevention Trial: Randomised trial of low-intensity oral anticoagulation with warfarin and low-dose aspirin in the primary prevention of ischaemic heart disease in men at increased risk. Lancet 351:233-241, 1998.
148. Nguyen KN, Aursnes I, Kjekshus J: Interaction between enalapril and aspirin on mortality after acute myocardial infarction: Subgroup analysis of the Cooperative New Scandinavian Enalapril Survival Study II (CONSENSUS II). Am J Cardiol 79:115-119, 1997.
149. Yusuf S, Sleight P, Pogue J, et al: Effects of an angiotensin-converting-enzyme inhibitor, ramipril, on cardiovascular events in high-risk patients. The Heart Outcomes Prevention Evaluation Study Investigators. N Engl J Med 342:145-153, 2000.
150. Quinn MJ, Fitzgerald DJ: Ticlopidine and clopidogrel. Circulation 100:1667-1672, 1999.
151. CAPRIE Steering Committee: A randomised, blinded, trial of clopidogrel versus aspirin in patients at risk of ischaemic events (CAPRIE). Lancet 348:1329-1339, 1996.
152. Yusuf S, Zhao F, Mehta SR, et al: Effects of clopidogrel in addition to aspirin in patients with acute coronary syndromes without ST-segment elevation. N Engl J Med 345:494-502, 2001.
153. Steinhubl SR, Berger PB, Mann JT III, et al: Early and sustained dual oral antiplatelet therapy following percutaneous coronary intervention: A randomized controlled trial. JAMA 288:2411-2420, 2002.
154. Gottlieb SS, McCarter RJ, Vogel RA: Effect of beta-blockade on mortality among high-risk and low-risk patients after myocardial infarction. N Engl J Med 339:489-497, 1998.
155. Pfeffer MA, Braunwald E, Moye LA, et al: Effect of captopril on mortality and morbidity in patients with left ventricular dysfunction after myocardial infarction: Results of the survival and ventricular enlargement trial. The SAVE Investigators. N Engl J Med 327:669-677, 1992.
156. Lonn EM, Yusuf S, Jha P, et al: Emerging role of angiotensin-converting enzyme inhibitors in cardiac and vascular protection. Circulation 90:2056-2069, 1994.
157. Prasad A, Husain S, Quyyumi AA: Abnormal flow-mediated epicardial vasomotion in human coronary arteries is improved by angiotensin-converting enzyme inhibition: A potential role of bradykinin. J Am Coll Cardiol 33:796-804, 1999.
158. Schneider CA, Voth E, Moka D, et al: Improvement of myocardial blood flow to ischemic regions by angiotensin-converting enzyme inhibition with quinaprilat IV: A study using [15O] water dobutamine stress positron emission tomography. J Am Coll Cardiol 34:1005-1011, 1999.
159. Kranzhofer R, Schmidt J, Pfeiffer CA, et al: Angiotensin induces inflammatory activation of human vascular smooth muscle cells. Arterioscler Thromb Vasc Biol 19:1623-1629, 1999.
160. Tummala PE, Chen XL, Sundell CL, et al: Angiotensin II induces vascular cell adhesion molecule-1 expression in rat vasculature: A potential link between the renin-angiotensin system and atherosclerosis. Circulation 100:1223-1229, 1999.
160a. Fox KM: EURopean trial On reduction of cardiac events with Perindopril in stable coronary Artery disease Investigators. Efficacy of perindopril in reduction of cardiovascular events among patients with stable coronary artery disease: Randomised, double-blind, placebo-controlled, multicentre trial (the EUROPA study). Lancet 362:782-788, 2003.
160b. Pfeffer MA, Domanski M, Verter J, et al: The continuation of the Prevention of Events with Angiotensin-Converting Enzyme Inhibition (PEACE) trial. Am Heart J 142:375-377, 2001.
161. Kushi LH, Folsom AR, Prineas RJ, et al: Dietary antioxidant vitamins and death from coronary heart disease in postmenopausal women. N Engl J Med 334:1156-1162, 1996.
162. Stephens NG, Parsons A, Schofield PM, et al: Randomised controlled trial of vitamin E in patients with coronary disease: Cambridge Heart Antioxidant Study (CHAOS). Lancet 347:781-786, 1996.
163. Yusuf S, Dagenais G, Pogue J, et al: Vitamin E supplementation and cardiovascular events in high-risk patients. The Heart Outcomes Prevention Evaluation Study Investigators. N Engl J Med 342:154-160, 2000.
164. Heart Protection Study Collaborative Group. MRC/BHF Heart Protection Study of antioxidant vitamin supplementation in 20,536 high-risk individuals: A randomised placebo-controlled trial. Lancet 360:23-33, 2002.
165. Ruo B, Rumsfeld JS, Hlatky MA, et al: Depressive symptoms and health-related quality of life: The Heart and Soul Study. JAMA 290:215-221, 2003.
166. Glassman AH, O'Connor CM, Califf RM, et al: Sertraline treatment of major depression in patients with acute MI or unstable angina. JAMA 288:701-709, 2002.
167. Larson CO, Nelson EC, Gustafson D, et al: The relationship between meeting patients' information needs and their satisfaction with hospital care and general health status outcomes. Int J Qual Health Care 8:447-456, 1996.
168. Figueras J, Lidon RM: Early morning reduction in ischemic threshold in patients with unstable angina and significant coronary disease. Circulation 92:1737-1742, 1995.

Pharmacological Management of Angina Pectoris

169. Parker JD, Parker JO: Nitrate therapy for stable angina pectoris. N Engl J Med 38:520-531, 1998.
170. Brown BG, Bolson E, Petersen RB, et al: The mechanisms of nitroglycerin action: Stenosis vasodilatation as a major component of the drug response. Circulation 64:1089-1097, 1981.

171. Parker JO: Nitrates and angina pectoris. Am J Cardiol 72:3C-6C, 1993.
172. Bottcher M, Madsen MM, Randsbaek F, et al: Effect of oral nitroglycerin and cold stress on myocardial perfusion in areas subtended by stenosed and nonstenosed coronary arteries. Am J Cardiol 89:1019-1024, 2002.
173. Tadamura E, Mamede M, Kubo S, et al: The effect of nitroglycerin on myocardial blood flow in various segments characterized by rest-redistribution thallium SPECT. J Nucl Med 44:745-751, 2003.
174. Fallen EL, Nahmias C, Scheffel A, et al: Redistribution of myocardial blood flow with topical nitroglycerin in patients with coronary artery disease. Circulation 91:1381-1388, 1995.
175. Munzel T, Mulsch A, Kleschyov A: Mechanisms underlying nitroglycerin-induced superoxide production in platelets: Some insight, more questions. Circulation 106:170-172, 2002.
176. Anderson TJ, Meredith IT, Ganz P, et al: Nitric oxide and nitrovasodilators: Similarities, differences, and potential interactions. J Am Coll Cardiol 24:555-566, 1994.
177. Chen Z, Zhang J, Stamler JS: Identification of the enzymatic mechanism of nitroglycerin bioactivation. Proc Natl Acad Sci U S A 99:8306-8311, 2002.
178. Winniford MD, Kennedy PL, Wells PJ, et al: Potentiation of nitroglycerin-induced coronary dilatation by *N*-acetylcysteine. Circulation 73:138-142, 1986.
179. Parker JO, Vankoughnett KA, Farrell B: Nitroglycerin lingual spray: Clinical efficacy and dose-response relation. Am J Cardiol 57:1-5, 1986.
180. Bassan MM: The day-long pattern of the antianginal effect of long-term three times daily administered isosorbide dinitrate. J Am Coll Cardiol 16:936-940, 1990.
181. Nordlander R, Walter M: Once- versus twice-daily administration of controlled-release isosorbide-5-mononitrate 60 mg in the treatment of stable angina pectoris: A randomized, double-blind, cross-over study. The Swedish Multicentre Group. Eur Heart J 15:108-113, 1994.
182. Parker JO, Amies MH, Hawkinson RW, et al: Intermittent transdermal nitroglycerin therapy in angina pectoris. Clinically effective without tolerance or rebound. Minitran Efficacy Study Group. Circulation 91:1368-1374, 1995.
183. Jeserich M, Munzel T, Pape L, et al: Absence of vascular tolerance in conductance vessels after 48 hours of intravenous nitroglycerin in patients with coronary artery disease. J Am Coll Cardiol 26:50-56, 1995.
184. Gori T, Parker JD: Nitrate tolerance: A unifying hypothesis. Circulation 106:2510-2513, 2002.
185. May DC, Popma JJ, Black WH, et al: In vivo induction and reversal of nitroglycerin tolerance in human coronary arteries. N Engl J Med 317:805-809, 1987.
186. Przybojewski JZ, Heyns MH: Acute coronary vasospasm secondary to industrial nitroglycerin withdrawal: A case presentation and review. S Afr Med J 63:158-165, 1983.
187. Caramori PR, Adelman AG, Azevedo ER, et al: Therapy with nitroglycerin increases coronary vasoconstriction in response to acetylcholine. J Am Coll Cardiol 32:1969-1974, 1998.
188. Cheitlin MD, Hutter AM Jr, Brindis RG, et al: ACC/AHA expert consensus document: Use of sildenafil (Viagra) in patients with cardiovascular disease. American College of Cardiology/American Heart Association. J Am Coll Cardiol 33:273-282, 1999.
189. Hoffman BB: Catecholamines, sympathomimetic drugs, and adrenergic receptor antagonists. *In* Hardman JG, Limbird LE, Goodman A (eds): Goodman & Gilman's The Pharmacological Basis of Therapeutics. 10th ed. New York, McGraw-Hill, 2001, pp 215-268.
190. Frishman WH: Carvedilol. N Engl J Med 339:1759-1765, 1998.
191. Steinbeck G, Andresen D, Bach P, et al: A comparison of electrophysiologically guided antiarrhythmic drug therapy with beta-blocker therapy in patients with symptomatic, sustained ventricular tachyarrhythmias. N Engl J Med 327:987-992, 1992.
192. Hohnloser SH, Meinertz T, Stubbs P, et al: Efficacy and safety of *d*-sotalol, a pure class III antiarrhythmic compound, in patients with symptomatic complex ventricular ectopy: Results of a multicenter, randomized, double-blind, placebo-controlled dose-finding study. The *d*-Sotalol PVC Study Group. Circulation 92:1517-1525, 1995.
193. Flockhart DA, Tanus-Santos JE: Implications of cytochrome P450 interactions when prescribing medication for hypertension. Arch Intern Med 162:405-412, 2002.
194. Lennard MS: The polymorphic oxidation of beta-adrenoceptor antagonists. Pharmacol Ther 41:461-477, 1989.
195. Werner U, Werner D, Rau T, et al: Celecoxib inhibits metabolism of cytochrome P450 2D6 substrate metoprolol in humans. Clin Pharmacol Ther 74:130-137, 2003.
196. Weir MR, Moser M: Diuretics and beta-blockers: Is there a risk for dyslipidemia? Am Heart J 139:174-183, 2000.
197. Ko DT, Hebert PR, Coffey CS, et al: Beta-blocker therapy and symptoms of depression, fatigue, and sexual dysfunction. JAMA 288:351-357, 2002.
198. Gottlieb SS, Fisher ML, Kjekshus J, et al: Tolerability of beta-blocker initiation and titration in the Metoprolol CR/XL Randomized Intervention Trial in Congestive Heart Failure (MERIT-HF). Circulation 105:1182-1188, 2002.
199. Miller RR, Olson HG, Amsterdam EA, et al: Propranolol-withdrawal rebound phenomenon: Exacerbation of coronary events after abrupt cessation of antianginal therapy. N Engl J Med 293:416-418, 1975.
200. Braunwald E: Mechanism of action of calcium-channel-blocking agents. N Engl J Med 307:1618-1627, 1982.
201. Abernethy DR, Schwartz JB: Calcium-antagonist drugs. N Engl J Med 341:1447-1457, 1999.
202. Cannon RO III, Watson RM, Rosing DR, et al: Efficacy of calcium channel blocker therapy for angina pectoris resulting from small-vessel coronary artery disease and abnormal vasodilator reserve. Am J Cardiol 56:242-246, 1985.
203. Freher M, Challapalli S, Pinto JV, et al: Current status of calcium channel blockers in patients with cardiovascular disease. Curr Probl Cardiol 24:236-340, 1999.
204. Mason RP: Mechanisms of atherosclerotic plaque stabilization for a lipophilic calcium antagonist amlodipine. Am J Cardiol 88:2M-6M, 2001.
205. Tulenko TN, Sumner AE, Chen M, et al: The smooth muscle cell membrane during atherogenesis: A potential target for amlodipine in atheroprotection. Am Heart J 141:S1-S11, 2001.
206. Pitt B, Byington RP, Furberg CD, et al: Effect of amlodipine on the progression of ath erosclerosis and the occurrence of clinical events. PREVENT Investigators. Circulatio 102:1503-1510, 2000.
207. Elkayam U, Amin J, Mehra A, et al: A prospective, randomized, double-blind, crossove study to compare the efficacy and safety of chronic nifedipine therapy with that c isosorbide dinitrate and their combination in the treatment of chronic congestive hear failure. Circulation 82:1954-1961, 1990.
208. Alderman MH, Cohen H, Roque R, et al: Effect of long-acting and short-acting calciur antagonists on cardiovascular outcomes in hypertensive patients. Lancet 349:594-598 1997.
209. Parmley WW, Nesto RW, Singh BN, et al: Attenuation of the circadian patterns o myocardial ischemia with nifedipine GITS in patients with chronic stable angina. N CAP Study Group. J Am Coll Cardiol 19:1380-1389, 1992.
210. Leon MB, Rosing DR, Bonow RO, et al: Clinical efficacy of verapamil alone and com bined with propranolol in treating patients with chronic stable angina pectoris. Am Cardiol 48:131-139, 1981.
210a. Pepine CJ, Handberg EM, Cooper-DeHoff RM, et al: A calcium antagonist vs a non calcium antagonist hypertension treatment strategy for patients with coronary arter disease. The International Verapamil-Trandolapril Study (INVEST): A randomized con trolled trial. JAMA 290:2805-2816, 2003.
211. Klinke WP, Baird M, Juneau M, et al: Antianginal efficacy and safety of controlled delivery diltiazem QD versus an equivalent dose of immediate-release diltiazem TID Cardiovasc Drugs Ther 9:319-330, 1995.
212. Nadazdin A, Davies GJ: Investigation of therapeutic mechanisms of atenolol and dil tiazem in patients with variable-threshold angina. Am Heart J 127:312-317, 1994.
213. Deanfield JE, Detry JM, Lichtlen PR, et al: Amlodipine reduces transient myocardia ischemia in patients with coronary artery disease: Double-blind Circadian Anti Ischemia Program in Europe (CAPE Trial). J Am Coll Cardiol 24:1460-1467, 1994.
214. Ezekowitz MD, Hossack K, Mehta JL, et al: Amlodipine in chronic stable angina Results of a multicenter double-blind crossover trial. Am Heart J 129:527-535, 1995.
214a. Jorgensen B, Simonsen S, Endresen K, et al: Restenosis and clinical outcome i patients treated with amlodipine after angioplasty: Results from the Coronary Angio Plasty Amlodipine REStenosis Study (CAPARES). J Am Coll Cardiol 35:592-599, 2000
215. Packer M, O'Connor CM, Ghali JK, et al: Effect of amlodipine on morbidity and mor tality in severe chronic heart failure. Prospective Randomized Amlodipine Surviva Evaluation Study Group. N Engl J Med 335:1107-1114, 1996.
216. Ekelund LG, Ulvenstam G, Walldius G, et al: Effects of felodipine versus nifedipine o exercise tolerance in stable angina pectoris. Am J Cardiol 73:658-660, 1994.
217. Sato T, Sasaki N, O'Rourke B, et al: Nicorandil, a potent cardioprotective agent, act by opening mitochondrial ATP-dependent potassium channels. J Am Coll Cardio 35:514-518, 2000.
218. The IONA Study Group: Effect of nicorandil on coronary events in patients with stabl angina: The Impact of Nicorandil in Angina (IONA) randomised trial. Lancet 359:1269 1275, 2002.
219. Rupp H, Zarain-Herzberg A, Maisch B: The use of partial fatty acid oxidation inhibitor for metabolic therapy of angina pectoris and heart failure. Herz 27:621-636, 2002.
219a. Chaitman BR, Pepine CJ, Parker JO, et al: Combination Assessment of Ranolazine I Stable Angina (CARISA) Investigators. Effects of ranolazine with atenolol, amlodipine or diltiazem on exercise tolerance and angina frequency in patients with severe chroni angina: A randomized controlled trial. JAMA 291:309-316, 2004.
220. Pepine CJ, Cohn PF, Deedwania PC, et al: Effects of treatment on outcome in mildl symptomatic patients with ischemia during daily life. The Atenolol Silent Ischemi Study (ASIST). Circulation 90:762-768, 1994.
221. von Arnim T: Medical treatment to reduce total ischemic burden: Total ischemi burden bisoprolol study (TIBBS), a multicenter trial comparing bisoprolol and nifedip ine. The TIBBS Investigators. J Am Coll Cardiol 25:231-238, 1995.
222. Savonitto S, Ardissiono D, Egstrup K, et al: Combination therapy with metoprolol an nifedipine versus monotherapy in patients with stable angina pectoris: Results of th International Multicenter Angina Exercise (IMAGE) Study. J Am Coll Cardiol 27:311 316, 1996.
223. Heidenreich PA, McDonald KM, Hastie T, et al: Meta-analysis of trials comparing beta blockers, calcium antagonists, and nitrates for stable angina. JAMA 281:1927-1936 1999.
224. Ishikawa K, Nakai S, Takenaka T, et al: Short-acting nifedipine and diltiazem do no reduce the incidence of cardiac events in patients with healed myocardial infarction Secondary Prevention Group. Circulation 95:2368-2373, 1997.
225. The Multicenter Diltiazem Postinfarction Trial Research Group: The effect of diltiazer on mortality and reinfarction after myocardial infarction. N Engl J Med 319:385-392 1988.
226. The DAVIT II Investigators: Effect of verapamil on mortality and major events afte acute myocardial infarction (the Danish Verapamil Infarction Trial II—DAVIT II). Ar J Cardiol 66:779-785, 1990.
227. Gheorghiade M, Colucci WS, Swedberg K: Beta-blockers in chronic heart failure. Cir culation 107:1570-1575, 2003.
228. Mannheimer C, Eliasson T, Augustinsson LE, et al: Electrical stimulation versus coro nary artery bypass surgery in severe angina pectoris: The ESBY study. Circulatior 97:1157-1163, 1998.
229. Ekre O, Eliasson T, Norrsell H, et al: Long-term effects of spinal cord stimulation an coronary artery bypass grafting on quality of life and survival in the ESBY study. Eu Heart J 23:1938-1945, 2002.
230. Brodison A, Chauhan A: Spinal-cord stimulation in management of angina. Lance 354:1748-1749, 1999.
231. Sinvhal RM, Gowda RM, Khan IA: Enhanced external counterpulsation for refractor angina pectoris. Heart 89:830-833, 2003.
232. Bonetti PO, Holmes DR Jr, Lerman A, et al: Enhanced external counterpulsation fo ischemic heart disease: What's behind the curtain? J Am Coll Cardiol 41:1918-1925 2003.

233. Arora RR, Chou TM, Jain D, et al: The multicenter study of enhanced external counterpulsation (MUST-EECP): Effect of EECP on exercise-induced myocardial ischemia and anginal episodes. J Am Coll Cardiol 33:1833-1840, 1999.
234. Stys TP, Lawson WE, Hui JC, et al: Effects of enhanced external counterpulsation on stress radionuclide coronary perfusion and exercise capacity in chronic stable angina pectoris. Am J Cardiol 89:822-824, 2002.
235. Ernst E: Chelation therapy for coronary heart disease: An overview of all clinical investigations. Am Heart J 140:139-141, 2000.

Percutaneous Coronary Interventions

236. Popma JJ, Kuntz RE, Baim DS: A decade of improvement in the clinical outcomes of percutaneous coronary intervention for multivessel coronary artery disease. Circulation 106:1592-1594, 2002.
237. Herzog CA, Ma JZ, Collins AJ: Comparative survival of dialysis patients in the United States after coronary angioplasty, coronary artery stenting, and coronary artery bypass surgery and impact of diabetes. Circulation 106:2207-2211, 2002.
238. Szczech LA, Best PJ, Crowley E, et al: Outcomes of patients with chronic renal insufficiency in the bypass angioplasty revascularization investigation. Circulation 105:2253-2258, 2002.
239. Kastrati A, Schomig A, Elezi S, et al: Prognostic value of the modified American College of Cardiology/American Heart Association stenosis morphology classification for long-term angiographic and clinical outcome after coronary stent placement. Circulation 100:1285-1290, 1999.
240. Krone RJ, Shaw RE, Klein LW, et al: Evaluation of the American College of Cardiology/American Heart Association and the Society for Coronary Angiography and Interventions lesion classification system in the current "stent era" of coronary interventions (from the ACC-National Cardiovascular Data Registry). Am J Cardiol 92:389-394, 2003.
241. Srinivas VS, Brooks MM, Detre KM, et al: Contemporary percutaneous coronary intervention versus balloon angioplasty for multivessel coronary artery disease: A comparison of the National Heart, Lung and Blood Institute Dynamic Registry and the Bypass Angioplasty Revascularization Investigation (BARI) study. Circulation 106:1627-1633, 2002.
242. Al Suwaidi J, Berger PB, Holmes DR Jr: Coronary artery stents. JAMA 284:1828-1836, 2000.
243. Brophy JM, Belisle P, Joseph L: Evidence for use of coronary stents: A hierarchical bayesian meta-analysis. Ann Intern Med 138:777-786, 2003.
244. Sousa JE, Serruys PW, Costa MA: New frontiers in cardiology: Drug-eluting stents: I. Circulation 107:2274-2279, 2003.
245. Olivari Z, Rubartelli P, Piscione F, et al: Immediate results and one-year clinical outcome after percutaneous coronary interventions in chronic total occlusions: Data from a multicenter, prospective, observational study (TOAST-GISE). J Am Coll Cardiol 41:1672-1678, 2003.
246. Bucher HC, Hengstler P, Schindler C, et al: Percutaneous transluminal coronary angioplasty versus medical treatment for non-acute coronary heart disease: Meta-analysis of randomised controlled trials. BMJ 321:73-77, 2000.
247. Pocock SJ, Henderson RA, Clayton T, et al: Quality of life after coronary angioplasty or continued medical treatment for angina: Three-year follow-up in the RITA-2 trial. Randomized Intervention Treatment of Angina. J Am Coll Cardiol 35:907-914, 2000.
248. Keelan PC, Johnston JM, Koru-Sengul T, et al: Comparison of in-hospital and one-year outcomes in patients with left ventricular ejection fractions ≤40%, 41% to 49%, and ≥50% having percutaneous coronary revascularization. Am J Cardiol 91:1168-1172, 2003.
249. Jacobs AK: Coronary revascularization in women in 2003: Sex revisited. Circulation 107:375-377, 2003.
250. Malenka DJ, Wennberg DE, Quinton HA, et al: Gender-related changes in the practice and outcomes of percutaneous coronary interventions in Northern New England from 1994 to 1999. J Am Coll Cardiol 40:2092-2101, 2002.
251. Batchelor WB, Anstrom KJ, Muhlbaier LH, et al: Contemporary outcome trends in the elderly undergoing percutaneous coronary interventions: Results in 7,472 octogenarians. National Cardiovascular Network Collaboration. J Am Coll Cardiol 36:723-730, 2000.
252. Taddei CF, Weintraub WS, Douglas JS Jr, et al: Influence of age on outcome after percutaneous transluminal angioplasty. Am J Cardiol 84:245-251, 1999.
252a. Pfisterer M, Buser P, Osswald S, et al: Outcome of elderly patients with chronic symptomatic coronary artery disease with an invasive vs. optimized medical treatment strategy: One-year results of the randomized TIME trial. JAMA 289:1117-1123, 2003.
253. Graham MM, Ghali WA, Faris PD, et al: Survival after coronary revascularization in the elderly. Circulation 105:2378-2384, 2002.
254. Beckman JA, Creager MA, Libby P: Diabetes and atherosclerosis: Epidemiology, pathophysiology, and management. JAMA 287:2570-2581, 2002.
255. Kuntz RE: Importance of considering atherosclerosis progression when choosing a coronary revascularization strategy: The diabetes–percutaneous transluminal coronary angioplasty dilemma. Circulation 99:847-851, 1999.
256. Park SJ, Shim WH, Ho DS, et al: A paclitaxel-eluting stent for the prevention of coronary restenosis. N Engl J Med 348:1537-1545, 2003.
257. Moses JW, Leon MB, Popma JJ, et al: Sirolimus-eluting stents versus standard stents in patients with stenosis in a native coronary artery. N Engl J Med 349:1315-1323, 2003.
258. Mathew V, Clavell AL, Lennon RJ, et al: Percutaneous coronary interventions in patients with prior coronary artery bypass surgery: Changes in patient characteristics and outcome during two decades. Am J Med 108:127-135, 2000.
259. Hong MK, Mehran R, Dangas G, et al: Are we making progress with percutaneous saphenous vein graft treatment? A comparison of 1990 to 1994 and 1995 to 1998 results. J Am Coll Cardiol 38:150-154, 2001.
260. Stone GW, Rogers C, Hermiller J, et al: Randomized comparison of distal protection with a filter-based catheter and a balloon occlusion and aspiration system during percutaneous intervention of diseased saphenous vein aorto-coronary bypass grafts. Circulation 108:548-553, 2003.

Coronary Artery Bypass Surgery

261. Eagle KA, Guyton RA, Davidoff R, et al: ACC/AHA Guidelines for Coronary Artery Bypass Graft Surgery: A Report of the American College of Cardiology/American Heart Association Task Force on Practice Guidelines (Committee to Revise the 1991 Guidelines for Coronary Artery Bypass Graft Surgery). American College of Cardiology/American Heart Association. J Am Coll Cardiol 34:1262-1347, 1999.
262. Abu-Omar Y, Taggart DP: Off-pump coronary artery bypass grafting. Lancet 360:327-330, 2002.
263. Dogan S, Aybek T, Andressen E, et al: Totally endoscopic coronary artery bypass grafting on cardiopulmonary bypass with robotically enhanced telemanipulation: Report of forty-five cases. J Thorac Cardiovasc Surg 123:1125-1131, 2002.
264. Berger PB, Alderman EL, Nadel A, et al: Frequency of early occlusion and stenosis in a left internal mammary artery to left anterior descending artery bypass graft after surgery through a median sternotomy on conventional bypass: Benchmark for minimally invasive direct coronary artery bypass. Circulation 100:2353-2358, 1999.
265. de Jaegere PP, Suyker WJ: Off-pump coronary artery bypass surgery. Heart 88:313-318, 2002.
266. Cisowski M, Morawski W, Drzewiecki J, et al: Integrated minimally invasive direct coronary artery bypass grafting and angioplasty for coronary artery revascularization. Eur J Cardiothorac Surg 22:261-265, 2002.
267. Galloway AC, Shemin RJ, Glower DD, et al: First report of the Port-Access International Registry. Ann Thorac Surg 67:51-56, 1999.
268. Dogan S, Graubitz K, Aybek T, et al: How safe is the port-access technique in minimally invasive coronary artery bypass grafting? Ann Thorac Surg 74:1537-1543, 2002.
269. Oliveira SA, Lisboa LA, Dallan LA, et al: Minimally invasive single-vessel coronary artery bypass with the internal thoracic artery and early postoperative angiography: Midterm results of a prospective study in 120 consecutive patients. Ann Thorac Surg 73:505-510, 2002.
270. Diegeler A, Thiele H, Falk V, et al: Comparison of stenting with minimally invasive bypass surgery for stenosis of the left anterior descending coronary artery. N Engl J Med 347:561-566, 2002.
271. Mehran R, Dangas G, Stamou SC, et al: One-year clinical outcome after minimally invasive direct coronary artery bypass. Circulation 102:2799-2802, 2000.
272. Al-Ruzzeh S, Ambler G, Asimakopoulos G, et al: Off-pump coronary artery bypass (OPCAB) surgery reduces risk-stratified morbidity and mortality: A United Kingdom multicenter comparative analysis of early clinical outcome. Circulation 108:II1-II8, 2003.
273. Parolari A, Alamanni F, Cannata A, et al: Off-pump versus on-pump coronary artery bypass: Meta-analysis of currently available randomized trials. Ann Thorac Surg 76:37-40, 2003.
274. Puskas JD, Williams WH, Duke PG, et al: Off-pump coronary artery bypass grafting provides complete revascularization with reduced myocardial injury, transfusion requirements, and length of stay: A prospective randomized comparison of two hundred unselected patients undergoing off-pump versus conventional coronary artery bypass grafting. J Thorac Cardiovasc Surg 125:797-808, 2003.
275. Van Dijk D, Jansen EW, Hijman R, et al: Cognitive outcome after off-pump and on-pump coronary artery bypass graft surgery: A randomized trial. JAMA 287:1405-1412, 2002.
276. Nathoe HM, van Dijk D, Jansen EW, et al: A comparison of on-pump and off-pump coronary bypass surgery in low-risk patients. N Engl J Med 348:394-402, 2003.
277. Cohen G, Borger MA, Weisel RD, et al: Intraoperative myocardial protection: Current trends and future perspectives. Ann Thorac Surg 68:1995-2001, 1999.
278. Mallidi HR, Sever J, Tamariz M, et al: The short-term and long-term effects of warm or tepid cardioplegia. J Thorac Cardiovasc Surg 125:711-720, 2003.
279. Kalawski R, Majewski M, Kaszkowiak E, et al: Transcardiac release of soluble adhesion molecules during coronary artery bypass grafting: Effects of crystalloid and blood cardioplegia. Chest 123:1355-1360, 2003.
280. Kiaii B, Moon BC, Massel D, et al: A prospective randomized trial of endoscopic versus conventional harvesting of the saphenous vein in coronary artery bypass surgery. J Thorac Cardiovasc Surg 123:204-212, 2002.
281. Souza DS, Dashwood MR, Tsui JC, et al: Improved patency in vein grafts harvested with surrounding tissue: Results of a randomized study using three harvesting techniques. Ann Thorac Surg 73:1189-1195, 2002.
282. Knatterud GL, Rosenberg Y, Campeau L, et al: Long-term effects on clinical outcomes of aggressive lowering of low-density lipoprotein cholesterol levels and low-dose anti-coagulation in the post coronary artery bypass graft trial. Post CABG Investigators. Circulation 102:157-165, 2000.
283. West NE, Qian H, Guzik TJ, et al: Nitric oxide synthase (nNOS) gene transfer modifies venous bypass graft remodeling: Effects on vascular smooth muscle cell differentiation and superoxide production. Circulation 104:1526-1532, 2001.
284. Traverse JH, Mooney MR, Pedersen WR, et al: Clinical, angiographic, and interventional follow-up of patients with aortic-saphenous vein graft connectors. Circulation 108:452-456, 2003.
285. Grondin CM, Lepage G, Castonguay YR, et al: Aortocoronary bypass graft: Initial blood flow through the graft, and early postoperative patency. Circulation 44:815-819, 1971.
286. Loop FD: Internal thoracic artery grafts: Biologically better coronary arteries. N Engl J Med 334:263-265, 1996.
287. Amoroso G, Tio RA, Mariani MA, et al: Functional integrity and aging of the left internal thoracic artery after coronary artery bypass surgery. J Thorac Cardiovasc Surg 120:313-318, 2000.
288. Dabal RJ, Goss JR, Maynard C, et al: The effect of left internal mammary artery utilization on short-term outcomes after coronary revascularization. Ann Thorac Surg 76:464-470, 2003.

289. Taggart DP, D'Amico R, Altman DG: Effect of arterial revascularisation on survival: A systematic review of studies comparing bilateral and single internal mammary arteries. Lancet 358:870-875, 2001.
290. Caputo M, Reeves B, Marchetto G, et al: Radial versus right internal thoracic artery as a second arterial conduit for coronary surgery: early and midterm outcomes. J Thorac Cardiovasc Surg 126:39-47, 2003.
291. Muneretto C, Negri A, Manfredi J, et al: Safety and usefulness of composite grafts for total arterial myocardial revascularization: A prospective randomized evaluation. J Thorac Cardiovasc Surg 125:826-835, 2003.
292. Chavanon O, Durand M, Hacini R, et al: Coronary artery bypass grafting with left internal mammary artery and right gastroepiploic artery, with and without bypass. Ann Thorac Surg 73:499-504, 2002.
293. Ferguson TB Jr, Hammill BG, Peterson ED, et al: A decade of change—risk profiles and outcomes for isolated coronary artery bypass grafting procedures, 1990-1999: A Report from the STS National Database Committee and the Duke Clinical Research Institute. Society of Thoracic Surgeons. Ann Thorac Surg 73:480-489, 2002.
294. Shroyer AL, Coombs LP, Peterson ED, et al: The Society of Thoracic Surgeons: 30-day operative mortality and morbidity risk models. Ann Thorac Surg 75:1856-1864, 2003.
295. Gao D, Grunwald GK, Rumsfeld JS, et al: Variation in mortality risk factors with time after coronary artery bypass graft operation. Ann Thorac Surg 75:74-81, 2003.
296. Nalysnyk L, Fahrbach K, Reynolds MW, et al: Adverse events in coronary artery bypass graft (CABG) trials: A systematic review and analysis. Heart 89:767-772, 2003.
297. Holmvang L, Jurlander B, Rasmussen C, et al: Use of biochemical markers of infarction for diagnosing perioperative myocardial infarction and early graft occlusion after coronary artery bypass surgery. Chest 121:103-111, 2002.
298. Yende S, Wunderink R: Causes of prolonged mechanical ventilation after coronary artery bypass surgery. Chest 122:245-252, 2002.
299. Canver CC, Chanda J: Intraoperative and postoperative risk factors for respiratory failure after coronary bypass. Ann Thorac Surg 75:853-857, 2003.
300. Branca P, McGaw P, Light R: Factors associated with prolonged mechanical ventilation following coronary artery bypass surgery. Chest 119:537-546, 2001.
301. Dacey LJ, Munoz JJ, Baribeau YR, et al: Reexploration for hemorrhage following coronary artery bypass grafting: Incidence and risk factors. Northern New England Cardiovascular Disease Study Group. Arch Surg 133:442-447, 1998.
302. Pleym H, Stenseth R, Wahba A, et al: Single-dose tranexamic acid reduces postoperative bleeding after coronary surgery in patients treated with aspirin until surgery. Anesth Analg 96:923-928, 2003.
303. Taggart DP, Westaby S: Neurological and cognitive disorders after coronary artery bypass grafting. Curr Opin Cardiol 16:271-276, 2001.
304. Selnes OA, McKhann GM: Coronary artery bypass surgery and the brain. N Engl J Med 344:451-452, 2001.
305. Newman MF, Kirchner JL, Phillips-Bute B, et al: Longitudinal assessment of neurocognitive function after coronary artery bypass surgery. N Engl J Med 344:395-402, 2001.
306. Maisel WH, Rawn JD, Stevenson WG: Atrial fibrillation after cardiac surgery. Ann Intern Med 135:1061-1073, 2001.
307. Eriksen BO, Hoff KR, Solberg S: Prediction of acute renal failure after cardiac surgery: Retrospective cross-validation of a clinical algorithm. Nephrol Dial Transplant 18:77-81, 2003.
308. Durmaz I, Yagdi T, Calkavur T, et al: Prophylactic dialysis in patients with renal dysfunction undergoing on-pump coronary artery bypass surgery. Ann Thorac Surg 75:859-864, 2003.
309. Bell MR, Gersh BJ, Schaff HV, et al: Effect of completeness of revascularization on long-term outcome of patients with three-vessel disease undergoing coronary artery bypass surgery: A report from the Coronary Artery Surgery Study (CASS) Registry. Circulation 86:446-457, 1992.
310. Hlatky MA, Boothroyd D, Horine S, et al: Employment after coronary angioplasty or coronary bypass surgery in patients employed at the time of revascularization. Ann Intern Med 129:543-547, 1998.
311. Mittag O, Kolenda KD, Nordman KJ, et al: Return to work after myocardial infarction/coronary artery bypass grafting: Patients' and physicians' initial viewpoints and outcome 12 months later. Soc Sci Med 52:1441-1450, 2001.
312. Domanski MJ, Borkowf CB, Campeau L, et al: Prognostic factors for atherosclerosis progression in saphenous vein grafts: The Postcoronary Artery Bypass Graft (Post-CABG) trial. Post-CABG Trial Investigators. J Am Coll Cardiol 36:1877-1883, 2000.
313. Tsui JC, Dashwood MR: Recent strategies to reduce vein graft occlusion: A need to limit the effect of vascular damage. Eur J Vasc Endovasc Surg 23:202-208, 2002.
314. FitzGibbon GM, Leach AJ, Kafka HP, et al: Coronary bypass graft fate: Long-term angiographic study. J Am Coll Cardiol 17:1075-1080, 1991.
315. Motwani JG, Topol EJ: Aortocoronary saphenous vein graft disease: Pathogenesis, predisposition, and prevention. Circulation 97:916-931, 1998.
316. Lu B, Dai RP, Zhuang N, et al: Noninvasive assessment of coronary artery bypass graft patency and flow characteristics by electron-beam tomography. J Invasive Cardiol 14:19-24, 2002.
317. Bunce NH, Lorenz CH, John AS, et al: Coronary artery bypass graft patency: Assessment with true AST imaging with steady-state precession versus gadolinium-enhanced MR angiography. Radiology 227:440-446, 2003.
318. Chirillo F, Bruni A, Balestra G, et al: Assessment of internal mammary artery and saphenous vein graft patency and flow reserve using transthoracic Doppler echocardiography. Heart 86:424-431, 2001.
319. Hwang MH, Meadows WR, Palac RT, et al: Progression of native coronary artery disease at 10 years: Insights from a randomized study of medical versus surgical therapy for angina. J Am Coll Cardiol 16:1066-1070, 1990.
320. Kroncke GM, Kosolcharoen P, Clayman JA, et al: Five-year changes in coronary arteries of medical and surgical patients of the Veterans Administration Randomized Study of Bypass Surgery. Circulation 78:I144-I1450, 1988.
321. Pond KK, Martin GV, Every N, et al: Predictors of progression of native coronary narrowing to total occlusion after coronary artery bypass grafting. Am J Cardiol 91:971-974, A4, 2003.
322. Mangano DT: Aspirin and mortality from coronary bypass surgery. N Engl J Med 347:1309-1317, 2002.
323. Bernstein SJ, Lazaro P, Fitch K, et al: Appropriateness of coronary revascularization for patients with chronic stable angina or following an acute myocardial infarction: Multinational versus Dutch criteria. Int J Qual Health Care 14:103-109, 2002.
324. van Brussel BL, Plokker HW, Ernst SM, et al: Venous coronary artery bypass surgery: A 15-year follow-up study. Circulation 88:II87-I192, 1993.
325. Unger F, Serruys PW, Yacoub MH, et al: Revascularization in multivessel disease: Comparison between two-year outcomes of coronary bypass surgery and stenting. J Thorac Cardiovasc Surg 125:809-820, 2003.
326. Peduzzi P, Kamina A, Detre K: Twenty-two-year follow-up in the VA Cooperative Study of Coronary Artery Bypass Surgery for Stable Angina. Am J Cardiol 81:1393-1399, 1998.
327. Yusuf S, Zucker D, Peduzzi P, et al: Effect of coronary artery bypass graft surgery on survival: Overview of 10-year results from randomised trials by the Coronary Artery Bypass Graft Surgery Trialists Collaboration. Lancet 344:563-570, 1994.
328. Davies RF, Goldberg AD, Forman S, et al: Asymptomatic Cardiac Ischemia Pilot (ACIP) study two-year follow-up: Outcomes of patients randomized to initial strategies of medical therapy versus revascularization. Circulation 95:2037-2043, 1997.
329. Califf RM, Conley MJ, Behar VS, et al: "Left main equivalent" coronary artery disease: Its clinical presentation and prognostic significance with nonsurgical therapy. Am J Cardiol 53:1489, 1984.
330. Davis KB, Alderman EL, Kosinski AS, et al: Early mortality of acute myocardial infarction in patients with and without prior coronary revascularization surgery. A Coronary Artery Surgery Study Registry Study. Circulation 85:2100-2109, 1992.
331. Argenziano M, Spotnitz HM, Whang W, et al: Risk stratification for coronary bypass surgery in patients with left ventricular dysfunction: Analysis of the coronary artery bypass grafting patch trial database. Circulation. 100:II119-II124, 1999.
332. Antunes PE, de Oliveira JM, Antunes MJ: Coronary surgery with non-cardioplegic methods in patients with advanced left ventricular dysfunction: Immediate and long term results. Heart 89:427-431, 2003.
333. Lytle BW: The role of coronary revascularization in the treatment of ischemic cardiomyopathy. Ann Thorac Surg 75:S2-S5, 2003.
334. Carr JA, Haithcock BE, Paone G, et al: Long-term outcome after coronary artery bypass grafting in patients with severe left ventricular dysfunction. Ann Thorac Surg 74:1531-1536, 2002.
335. Veenhuyzen GD, Singh SN, McAreavey D, et al: Prior coronary artery bypass surgery and risk of death among patients with ischemic left ventricular dysfunction. Circulation 104:1489-1493, 2001.
336. Kleikamp G, Maleszka A, Reiss N, et al: Determinants of mid- and long-term results in patients after surgical revascularization for ischemic cardiomyopathy. Ann Thorac Surg 75:1406-1412, 2003.
337. Allman KC, Shaw LJ, Hachamovitch R, et al: Myocardial viability testing and impact of revascularization on prognosis in patients with coronary artery disease and left ventricular dysfunction: A meta-analysis. J Am Coll Cardiol 39:1151-1158, 2002.
338. Wijns W, Vatner SF, Camici PG: Hibernating myocardium. N Engl J Med 339:173-181, 1998.
339. Pasquet A, Lauer MS, Williams MJ, et al: Prediction of global left ventricular function after bypass surgery in patients with severe left ventricular dysfunction: Impact of preoperative myocardial function, perfusion, and metabolism. Eur Heart J 21:125-136, 2000.
340. Bax JJ, Wijns W, Cornel JH, et al: Accuracy of currently available techniques for prediction of functional recovery after revascularization in patients with left ventricular dysfunction due to chronic coronary artery disease: Comparison of pooled data. J Am Coll Cardiol 30:1451-1460, 1997.
341. Bonow RO: Myocardial viability and prognosis in patients with ischemic left ventricular dysfunction. J Am Coll Cardiol 39:1159-1162, 2002.
342. Kleikamp G, Maleszka A, Reiss N, et al: Determinants of mid- and long-term results in patients after surgical revascularization for ischemic cardiomyopathy. Ann Thorac Surg 75:1406-1412, 2003.
343. Schulman KA, Berlin JA, Harless W, et al: The effect of race and sex on physicians' recommendations for cardiac catheterization. N Engl J Med 340:618-626, 1999.
344. Ghali WA, Faris PD, Galbraith PD, et al: Sex differences in access to coronary revascularization after cardiac catheterization: Importance of detailed clinical data. Ann Intern Med 136:723-732, 2002.
345. Jacobs AK, Kelsey SF, Brooks MM, et al: Better outcome for women compared with men undergoing coronary revascularization: A report from the Bypass Angioplasty Revascularization Investigation (BARI). Circulation 98:1279-1285, 1998.
346. Vaccarino V, Abramson JL, Veledar E, et al: Sex differences in hospital mortality after coronary artery bypass surgery: Evidence for a higher mortality in younger women. Circulation 105:1176-1181, 2002.
347. Brown PP, Mack MJ, Simon AW, et al: Outcomes experience with off-pump coronary artery bypass surgery in women. Ann Thorac Surg 74:2113-2119, 2002.
348. Myers WO, Blackstone EH, Davis K, et al: CASS Registry long-term surgical survival. Coronary Artery Surgery Study. J Am Coll Cardiol 33:488-498, 1999.
349. Kurlansky PA, Williams DB, Traad EA, et al: Arterial grafting results in reduced operative mortality and enhanced long-term quality of life in octogenarians. Ann Thorac Surg 76:418-426, 2003.
350. Khaitan L, Sutter FP, Goldman SM: Coronary artery bypass grafting in patients who require long-term dialysis. Ann Thorac Surg 69:1135-1139, 2000.
351. Nakayama Y, Sakata R, Ura M, et al: Long-term results of coronary artery bypass grafting in patients with renal insufficiency. Ann Thorac Surg 75:496-500, 2003.
352. Schwartz L, Kip KE, Frye RL, et al: Coronary bypass graft patency in patients with diabetes in the Bypass Angioplasty Revascularization Investigation (BARI). Circulation 106:2652-2658, 2002.

353. The BARI Investigators: Seven-year outcome in the Bypass Angioplasty Revascularization Investigation (BARI) by treatment and diabetic status. J Am Coll Cardiol 35:1122-1129, 2000.
354. Rihal CS, Sutton-Tyrrell K, Guo P, et al: Increased incidence of periprocedural complications among patients with peripheral vascular disease undergoing myocardial revascularization in the bypass angioplasty revascularization investigation. Circulation 100:171-177, 1999.
355. Birkmeyer JD, Quinton HB, O'Connor NJ, et al: The effect of peripheral vascular disease on long-term mortality after coronary artery bypass surgery. Northern New England Cardiovascular Disease Study Group. Arch Surg 131:316-321, 1996.
356. Naylor AR, Mehta Z, Rothwell PM, et al: Carotid artery disease and stroke during coronary artery bypass: A critical review of the literature. Eur J Vasc Endovasc Surg 23:283-294, 2002.
357. Gansera B, Angelis I, Weingartner J, et al: Simultaneous carotid endarterectomy and cardiac surgery—additional risk factor or safety procedure? Thorac Cardiovasc Surg 51:22-27, 2003.
358. Borger MA, Fremes SE: Management of patients with concomitant coronary and carotid vascular disease. Semin Thorac Cardiovasc Surg 13:192-198, 2001.
359. Zacharias A, Schwann TA, Riordan CJ, et al: Operative and 5-year outcomes of combined carotid and coronary revascularization: Review of a large contemporary experience. Ann Thorac Surg 73:491-497, 2002.
360. Yamamuro M, Lytle BW, Sapp SK, et al: Risk factors and outcomes after coronary reoperation in 739 elderly patients. Ann Thorac Surg 69:464-474, 2000.
361. van Eck FM, Noyez L, Verheugt FW, et al: Changing profile of patients undergoing redo-coronary artery surgery. Eur J Cardiothorac Surg 21:205-211, 2002.
362. Hannan EL, Racz MJ, McCallister BD, et al: A comparison of three-year survival after coronary artery bypass graft surgery and percutaneous transluminal coronary angioplasty. J Am Coll Cardiol 33:63-72, 1999.
363. Goy JJ, Eeckhout E, Moret C, et al: Five-year outcome in patients with isolated proximal left anterior descending coronary artery stenosis treated by angioplasty or left internal mammary artery grafting: A prospective trial. Circulation 99:3255-3259, 1999.
364. Abizaid A, Costa MA, Centemero M, et al: Clinical and economic impact of diabetes mellitus on percutaneous and surgical treatment of multivessel coronary disease patients: Insights from the Arterial Revascularization Therapy Study (ARTS) trial. Circulation 104:533-538, 2001.
365. Niles NW, McGrath PD, Malenka D, et al: Survival of patients with diabetes and multivessel coronary artery disease after surgical or percutaneous coronary revascularization: Results of a large regional prospective study. Northern New England Cardiovascular Disease Study Group. J Am Coll Cardiol 37:1008-1015, 2001.
366. Rodriguez A, Bernardi V, Navia J, et al: Argentine Randomized Study: Coronary Angioplasty with Stenting versus Coronary Bypass Surgery in patients with Multiple-Vessel Disease (ERACI II): 30-day and one-year follow-up results. ERACI II Investigators. J Am Coll Cardiol 37:51-58, 2001.
367. Hlatky MA, Rogers WJ, Johnstone I, et al: Medical care costs and quality of life after randomization to coronary angioplasty or coronary bypass surgery. Bypass Angioplasty Revascularization Investigation (BARI) Investigators. N Engl J Med 336:92-99, 1997.
367a. Legrand VM, Serruys PW, Unger F, et al: Arterial Revascularization Therapy Study (ARTS) Investigators. Three-year outcome after coronary stenting versus bypass surgery for the treatment of multivessel disease. Circulation 109:1114-1120, 2004.
368. Detre KM, Guo P, Holubkov R, et al: Coronary revascularization in diabetic patients: A comparison of the randomized and observational components of the Bypass Angioplasty Revascularization Investigation (BARI). Circulation 99:633-640, 1999.
369. Weintraub WS, Stein B, Kosinski A, et al: Outcome of coronary bypass surgery versus coronary angioplasty in diabetic patients with multivessel coronary artery disease. J Am Coll Cardiol 31:10-19, 1998.
370. Saririan M, Eisenberg MJ: Myocardial laser revascularization for the treatment of end-stage coronary artery disease. J Am Coll Cardiol 41:173-183, 2003.
371. Lange RA, Hillis LD: Transmyocardial laser revascularization. N Engl J Med 341:1075-1076, 1999.
372. Schofield PM, Sharples LD, Caine N, et al: Transmyocardial laser revascularisation in patients with refractory angina: A randomised controlled trial. Lancet 353:519-524, 1999.
373. Horvath KA, Aranki SF, Cohn LH, et al: Sustained angina relief 5 years after transmyocardial laser revascularization with a CO_2 laser. Circulation 104:I81-I84, 2001.
374. Hughes GC, Landolfo KP, Lowe JE, et al: Perioperative morbidity and mortality after transmyocardial laser revascularization: Incidence and risk factors for adverse events. J Am Coll Cardiol 33:1021-1026, 1999.

Chest Pain with Normal Coronary Arteriogram

375. Lichtlen PR, Bargheer K, Wenzlaff P: Long-term prognosis of patients with angina-like chest pain and normal coronary angiographic findings. J Am Coll Cardiol 25:1013-1018, 1995.
376. Panting JR, Gatehouse PD, Yang GZ, et al: Abnormal subendocardial perfusion in cardiac syndrome X detected by cardiovascular magnetic resonance imaging. N Engl J Med 346:1948-1953, 2002.
377. Chen LC, Chen JW, Wu MH, et al: Differential coronary calcification on electron-beam CT between syndrome X and coronary artery disease in patients with chronic stable angina pectoris. Chest 120:1525-1533, 2001.
378. Rosen SD, Paulesu E, Wise RJ, et al: Central neural contribution to the perception of chest pain in cardiac syndrome X. Heart 87:513-519, 2002.
379. Potts SG, Bass CM: Psychological morbidity in patients with chest pain and normal or near-normal coronary arteries: A long-term follow-up study. Psychol Med 25:339-347, 1995.
380. Sun H, Mohri M, Shimokawa H, et al: Coronary microvascular spasm causes myocardial ischemia in patients with vasospastic angina. J Am Coll Cardiol 39:847-851, 2002.
381. Schindler TH, Nitzsche E, Magosaki N, et al: Regional myocardial perfusion defects during exercise, as assessed by three dimensional integration of morphology and function, in relation to abnormal endothelium-dependent vasoreactivity of the coronary microcirculation. Heart 89:517-526, 2003.
382. Cosin-Sales J, Pizzi C, Brown S, et al: C-reactive protein, clinical presentation, and ischemic activity in patients with chest pain and normal coronary angiograms. J Am Coll Cardiol 41:1468-1474, 2003.
383. Panza JA: Myocardial ischemia and the pains of the heart. N Engl J Med 346:1934-1935, 2002.
384. Zouridakis EG, Cox ID, Garcia-Moll X, et al: Negative stress echocardiographic responses in normotensive and hypertensive patients with angina pectoris, positive exercise stress testing, and normal coronary arteriograms. Heart 83:141-146, 2000.
385. Cannon RO III: Chest pain and the sensitive heart. Eur J Gastroenterol Hepatol 7:1161-1171, 1995.
386. Rosen SD: The pathophysiology of cardiac syndrome X—a tale of paradigm shifts. Cardiovasc Res 52:174-177, 2001.
387. Kemp HG, Kronmal RA, Vlietstra RE, et al: Seven-year survival of patients with normal or near-normal coronary arteriograms: A CASS registry study. J Am Coll Cardiol 7:479-483, 1986.
388. Kaski JC, Valenzuela Garcia LF: Therapeutic options for the management of patients with cardiac syndrome X. Eur Heart J 22:283-293, 2001.
389. Cannon RO III, Quyyumi AA, Mincemoyer R, et al: Imipramine in patients with chest pain despite normal coronary angiograms. N Engl J Med 330:1411-1417, 1994.

Silent Myocardial Ischemia

390. Cohn PF, Fox KM, Daly C: Silent myocardial ischemia. Circulation 108:1263-1277, 2003.
391. Krantz DS, Hedges SM, Gabbay FH, et al: Triggers of angina and ST-segment depression in ambulatory patients with coronary artery disease: Evidence for an uncoupling of angina and ischemia. Am Heart J 128:703-712, 1994.
392. Krone RJ, Gregory JJ, Freedland KE, et al: Limited usefulness of exercise testing and thallium scintigraphy in evaluation of ambulatory patients several months after recovery from an acute coronary event: Implications for management of stable coronary heart disease. Multicenter Myocardial Ischemia Research Group. J Am Coll Cardiol 24:1274-1281, 1994.
393. Mazzone A, Cusa C, Mazzucchelli I, et al: Increased production of inflammatory cytokines in patients with silent myocardial ischemia. J Am Coll Cardiol 38:1895-1901, 2001.
394. Laukkanen JA, Kurl S, Lakka TA, et al: Exercise-induced silent myocardial ischemia and coronary morbidity and mortality in middle-aged men. J Am Coll Cardiol 38:72-79, 2001.
395. Elhendy A, Schinkel AF, van Domburg RT, et al: Comparison of late outcome in patients with versus without angina pectoris having reversible perfusion abnormalities during dobutamine stress technetium-99m sestamibi single-photon emission computed tomography. Am J Cardiol 91:264-268, 2003.
396. Pepine CJ, Sharaf B, Andrews TC, et al: Relation between clinical, angiographic and ischemic findings at baseline and ischemia-related adverse outcomes at 1 year in the Asymptomatic Cardiac Ischemia Pilot study. ACIP Study Group. J Am Coll Cardiol 29:1483-1489, 1997.
397. Stone PH, Chaitman BR, Forman S, et al: Prognostic significance of myocardial ischemia detected by ambulatory electrocardiography, exercise treadmill testing, and electrocardiogram at rest to predict cardiac events by one year (the Asymptomatic Cardiac Ischemia Pilot [ACIP] study). Am J Cardiol 80:1395-1401, 1997.
398. Dargie HJ, Ford I, Fox KM: Total Ischaemic Burden European Trial (TIBET): Effects of ischaemia and treatment with atenolol, nifedipine SR, and their combination on outcome in patients with chronic stable angina. The TIBET Study Group. Eur Heart J 17:104-112, 1996.
399. Sharaf BL, Williams DO, Miele NJ, et al: A detailed angiographic analysis of patients with ambulatory electrocardiographic ischemia: Results from the Asymptomatic Cardiac Ischemia Pilot (ACIP) study angiographic core laboratory. J Am Coll Cardiol 29:78-84, 1997.
400. Tzivoni D, Medina A, David D, et al: Comparison between metoprolol orally osmotic once daily and metoprolol two or three times daily in suppressing exercise-induced and daily myocardial ischemia. Am J Cardiol 78:1362-1368, 1996.
401. Portegies MC, Sijbring P, Gobel EJ, et al: Efficacy of metoprolol and diltiazem in treating silent myocardial ischemia. Am J Cardiol 74:1095-1098, 1994.
402. Rogers WJ, Bourassa MG, Andrews TC, et al: Asymptomatic Cardiac Ischemia Pilot (ACIP) study: Outcome at 1 year for patients with asymptomatic cardiac ischemia randomized to medical therapy or revascularization. The ACIP Investigators. J Am Coll Cardiol 26:594-605, 1995.
403. Andrews TC, Raby K, Barry J, et al: Effect of cholesterol reduction on myocardial ischemia in patients with coronary disease. Circulation 95:324-328, 1997.
404. Zellweger MJ, Weinbacher M, Zutter AW, et al: Long-term outcome of patients with silent versus symptomatic ischemia six months after percutaneous coronary intervention and stenting. J Am Coll Cardiol 42:33-40, 2003.

Heart Failure in Ischemic Heart Disease

405. Gheorghiade M, Bonow RO: Chronic heart failure in the United States: A manifestation of coronary artery disease. Circulation 97:282-289, 1998.
406. Felker GM, Shaw LK, O'Connor CM: A standardized definition of ischemic cardiomyopathy for use in clinical research. J Am Coll Cardiol 39:210-218, 2002.
407. Schinkel AF, Bax JJ, Sozzi FB, et al: Prevalence of myocardial viability assessed by single photon emission computed tomography in patients with chronic ischaemic left ventricular dysfunction. Heart 88:125-130, 2002.
408. Baker DW, Jones R, Hodges J, et al: Management of heart failure: III. The role of revascularization in the treatment of patients with moderate or severe left ventricular systolic dysfunction. JAMA 272:1528-1534, 1994.
409. Mickleborough LL, Merchant N, Provost Y, et al: Ventricular reconstruction for ischemic cardiomyopathy. Ann Thorac Surg 75:S6-S12, 2003.

410. Candell-Riera J, Santana-Boado C, Armadans-Gil L, et al: Comparison of patients with anterior wall healed myocardial infarction with and without exercise-induced ST-segment elevation. Am J Cardiol 81:12-16, 1998.
411. Buck T, Hunold P, Wentz KU, et al: Tomographic three-dimensional echocardiographic determination of chamber size and systolic function in patients with left ventricular aneurysm: Comparison to magnetic resonance imaging, cineventriculography, and two-dimensional echocardiography. Circulation 96:4286-4297, 1997.
412. Jones RH: Is it time for a randomized trial of surgical treatment of ischemic heart failure? J Am Coll Cardiol 37:1210-1213, 2001.
413. Lundblad R, Abdelnoor M, Svennevig JL: Repair of left ventricular aneurysm: Surgical risk and long-term survival. Ann Thorac Surg 76:719-725, 2003.
414. Vural KM, Sener E, Ozatik MA, et al: Left ventricular aneurysm repair: An assessment of surgical treatment modalities. Eur J Cardiothorac Surg 13:49-56, 1998.
415. Di Mattia DG, Di Biasi P, Salati M, et al: Surgical treatment of left ventricular post-infarction aneurysm with endoventriculoplasty: Late clinical and functional results. Eur J Cardiothorac Surg 15:413-418, 1999.
416. Athanasuleas CL, Stanley AW, Buckberg GD, et al: Surgical anterior ventricular endocardial restoration (SAVER) for dilated ischemic cardiomyopathy. Semin Thorac Cardiovasc Surg 13:448-458, 2001.
417. Stanley AW Jr, Athanasuleas CL, Buckberg GD: Left ventricular remodeling and functional mitral regurgitation: Mechanisms and therapy. Semin Thorac Cardiovasc Surg 13:486-495, 2001.
418. Athanasuleas CL, Stanley AW Jr, Buckberg GD, et al: Surgical anterior ventricular endocardial restoration (SAVER) in the dilated remodeled ventricle after anterior myocardial infarction. RESTORE group. Reconstructive Endoventricular Surgery, returning Torsion Original Radius Elliptical Shape to the LV. J Am Coll Cardiol 37:1199-1209, 2001.
419. Di Donato M, Sabatier M, Dor V, et al: Effects of the Dor procedure on left ventricular dimension and shape and geometric correlates of mitral regurgitation one year after surgery. J Thorac Cardiovasc Surg 121:91-96, 2001.
420. Shapira OM, Davidoff R, Hilkert RJ, et al: Repair of left ventricular aneurysm: Long-term results of linear repair versus endoaneurysmorrhaphy. Ann Thorac Surg 63:701-705, 1997.
421. Tibayan FA, Rodriguez F, Zasio MK, et al: Geometric distortions of the mitral valvular-ventricular complex in chronic ischemic mitral regurgitation. Circulation 108(Suppl 1):II116-II121, 2003.
422. Kwan J, Shiota T, Agler DA, et al: Geometric differences of the mitral apparatus between ischemic and dilated cardiomyopathy with significant mitral regurgitation. Real-time three-dimensional echocardiography study. Circulation 107:1135-1140, 2003.
423. Gillinov AM, Wierup PN, Blackstone EH, et al: Is repair preferable to replacement for ischemic mitral regurgitation? J Thorac Cardiovasc Surg 122:1125-1141, 2001.
424. Paparella D, Mickleborough LL, Carson S, et al: Mild to moderate mitral regurgitation in patients undergoing coronary bypass grafting: Effects on operative mortality and long-term significance. Ann Thorac Surg 76:1094-1100, 2003.
425. Society of Thoracic Surgeons Database, 2002 (www.ctsnet.org).
426. Cohn LH, Rizzo RJ, Adams DH, et al: The effect of pathophysiology on the surgical treatment of ischemic mitral regurgitation: Operative and late risks of repair versus replacement. Eur J Cardiothorac Surg 9:568-574, 1995.
427. Angelini P, Velasco JA, Flamm S: Coronary anomalies: Incidence, pathophysiology, and clinical relevance. Circulation 105:2449-2454, 2002.
428. Maehara A, Mintz GS, Castagna MT, et al: Intravascular ultrasound assessment of spontaneous coronary artery dissection. Am J Cardiol 89:466-468, 2002.
429. Lane JE, Cartledge RG, Johnson JH: Successful surgical treatment of spontaneous coronary artery dissection. Curr Surg 58:316-318, 2001.
430. Longheval G, Badot V, Cosyns B, et al: Spontaneous coronary artery dissection: Favorable outcome illustrated by angiographic data. Clin Cardiol 22:374-375, 1999.
431. Endo M, Tomizawa Y, Nishida H, et al: Angiographic findings and surgical treatments of coronary artery involvement in Takayasu arteritis. J Thorac Cardiovasc Surg 125:570-577, 2003.
432. Byrd BF III, Mendes LA: Cardiac complications of mediastinal radiotherapy: The other side of the coin. J Am Coll Cardiol 42:750-751, 2003.
433. Lange RA, Hillis LD: Cardiovascular complications of cocaine use. N Engl J Med 345:351-358, 2001.

GUIDELINES *Thomas H. Lee*

Chronic Stable Angina

The American College of Cardiology and the American Heart Association (ACC/AHA) updated guidelines for management of patients with stable chest pain syndromes and known or suspected ischemic heart disease in 2002.[1] Populations addressed by these guidelines include patients with "ischemic equivalents" such as dyspnea or arm pain with exertion, and patients with ischemic heart disease who have become asymptomatic, including those who have undergone revascularization procedures. Patients with unstable ischemic syndromes are not included in these guidelines but are instead addressed in guidelines summarized in appendices to Chapter 49. As with other ACC/AHA guidelines, indications for interventions are classified into the following four groups:

- Class I—for generally accepted indications
- Class IIa—when indications are controversial, but the weight of evidence is supportive
- Class IIb—when usefulness or efficacy is less well established
- Class III—when there is consensus against the usefulness of the intervention

The guidelines use a convention for rating levels of evidence on which recommendations have been based, as follows:

- Level A—derived from data from multiple randomized clinical trials
- Level B—derived from a single randomized trial or nonrandomized studies
- Level C—based on the consensus opinion of experts

Overview

The ACC/AHA guidelines emphasize the importance of detailed symptom history, focused physical examination, and directed risk-factor assessment for patients presenting with chest pain. These data are to be used by the clinician to estimate the probability of significant coronary artery disease as low, intermediate, or high. For patients with a low probability of coronary disease (e.g., ≤5 percent), cardiovascular interventions should be limited, while noncardiac causes of chest pain should be evaluated (Fig. 50G–1). Recommended initial tests are summarized in Table 50G–1. Routine use of chest radiographs or electron-beam computed tomography (CT) is not recommended.[2]

For patients with an intermediate or high probability of coronary disease, the clinician should exclude unstable ischemic syndromes and conditions that might exacerbate or cause angina. If these are not present, then noninvasive testing should be considered to refine the diagnostic assessment of patients with an intermediate probability of coronary disease and to perform risk stratification for patients with a high probability of coronary disease (Fig. 50G–2).

The ACC/AHA guidelines do not mandate exercise testing in all such patients. Pharmacological imaging studies are recommended for patients who are unable to exercise. Exercise imaging studies are recommended for patients who have had previous coronary revascularization or whose resting electrocardiograms (ECGs) are uninterpretable. Imaging studies are also supported when the clinical evaluation and exercise ECGs have not provided sufficient information to guide management. If the results of noninvasive studies suggest a high risk for complications of coronary heart disease, then coronary angiography and revascularization should be considered.

The treatment algorithm recommended by the ACC/AHA guidelines emphasizes the importance of patient education about coronary disease; prevention of ischemia through use of nitrates, beta blockers, and calcium blockers; and prevention of progression of atherosclerosis through risk factor management (Fig. 50G–3).

The ACC/AHA guidelines require clarity from the clinician in defining the critical issues for the individual patient. For patients with a chest pain complaint of uncertain etiology, the dominant question may be whether coronary artery disease is present or absent (diagnosis). For patients with known or strongly suspected coronary disease, the focus is likely to be on the patient's risk. In these guidelines, a specific test

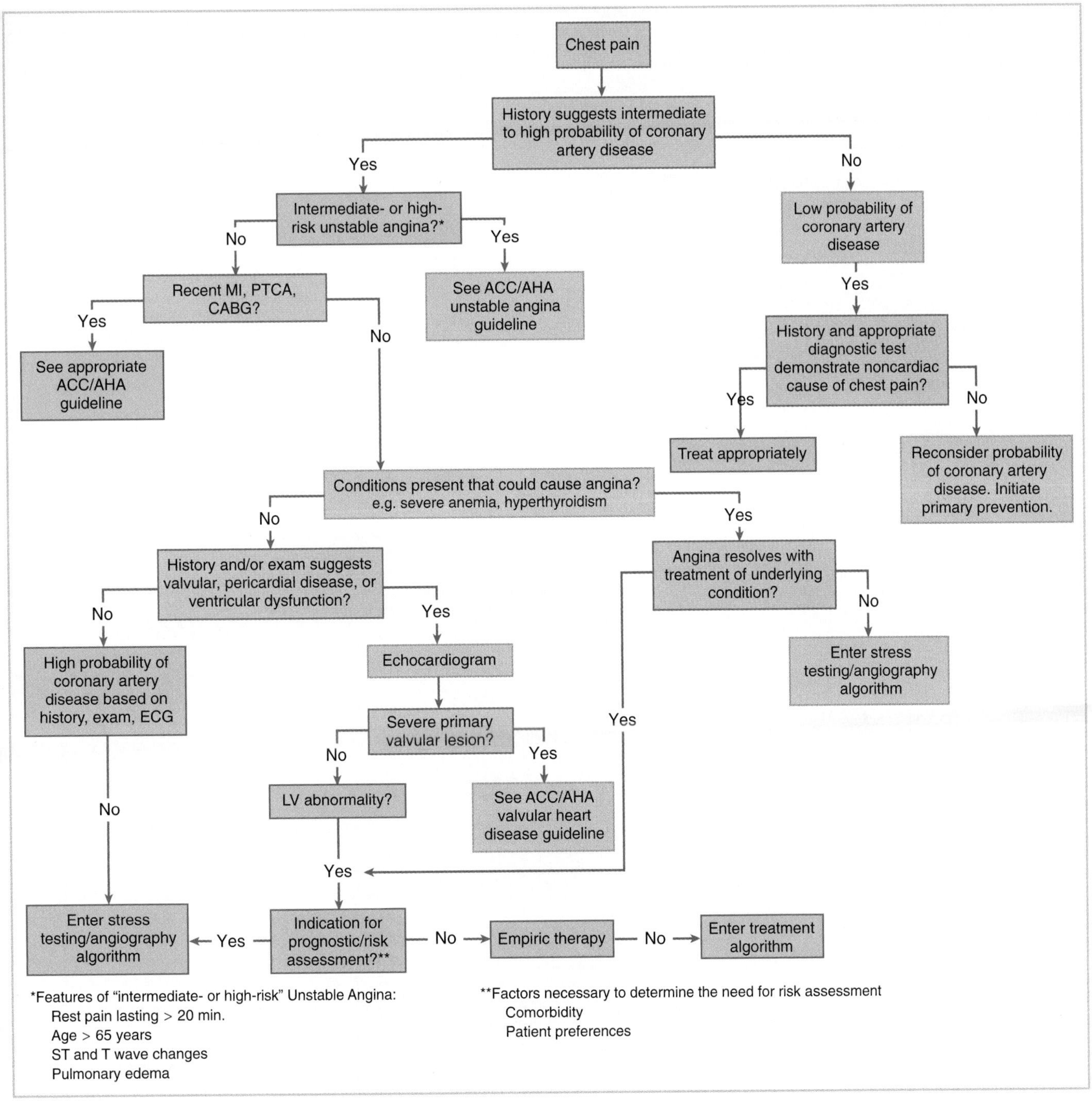

FIGURE 50G–1 Approach to the clinical assessment of chest pain. ACC = American College of Cardiology; AHA = American Heart Association; CABG = coronary artery bypass grafting; ECG = electrocardiogram; LV = left ventricular; MI = myocardial infarction; PTCA = percutaneous transluminal coronary angioplasty. (From ACC/AHA 2002 guideline update for the management of patients with chronic stable angina: A report of the American College of Cardiology/American Heart Association Task Force on Practice Guidelines [Committee to Update the 1999 Guidelines for the Management of Patients with Chronic Stable Angina]. ©2002, American College of Cardiology Foundation and the American Heart Association, p 8 [www.acc.org/clinical/guidelines/stable/stable.pdf]).

may be considered an appropriate option for addressing one or the other of these issues.

The guidelines clearly differentiate between indications for the same tests for the purpose of diagnosis and risk stratification. For example, exercise ECGs are discouraged for establishing diagnosis in patients with a high clinical probability of coronary artery disease based on age, gender, and symptoms (class IIb indication). However, exercise ECGs are strongly supported as a class I indication when used to assess prognosis in this same patient population. Thus, interpretation of these guidelines demands rigorous definition of the clinical question at hand.

DIAGNOSIS

Noninvasive Studies

Exercise Electrocardiography. Exercise testing is considered most valuable for diagnosis when the patient's other clinical data suggest an intermediate probability of coronary disease. The ACC/AHA guidelines support the use of exercise ECGs for such patients unless their baseline ECGs show abnormalities likely to render the exercise tracing uninterpretable (Table 50G–2). However, exercise ECGs were considered appropriate for patients with complete right

TABLE 50G–1 ACC/AHA Guidelines for Routine Clinical Testing in Patients with Chronic Stable Angina

Class	Indication	Evidence*
I (indicated)	1. Rest ECG in patients without an obvious noncardiac cause of chest pain 2. Rest ECG during an episode of chest pain 3. Chest radiograph in patients with signs or symptoms of congestive heart failure, valvular heart disease, pericardial disease, or aortic dissection/aneurysm 4. Hemoglobin 5. Fasting glucose 6. Fasting lipid panel	B B B C C C
IIa (good supportive evidence)	Chest radiograph in patients with signs or symptoms of pulmonary disease	B
IIb (weak supportive evidence)	1. Chest radiograph in other patients 2. Electron-beam CT	C B
III (not indicated)	none	

ACC = American College of Cardiology; AHA = American Heart Association; ECG = electrocardiogram.
*See guidelines text for definitions of level of evidence.

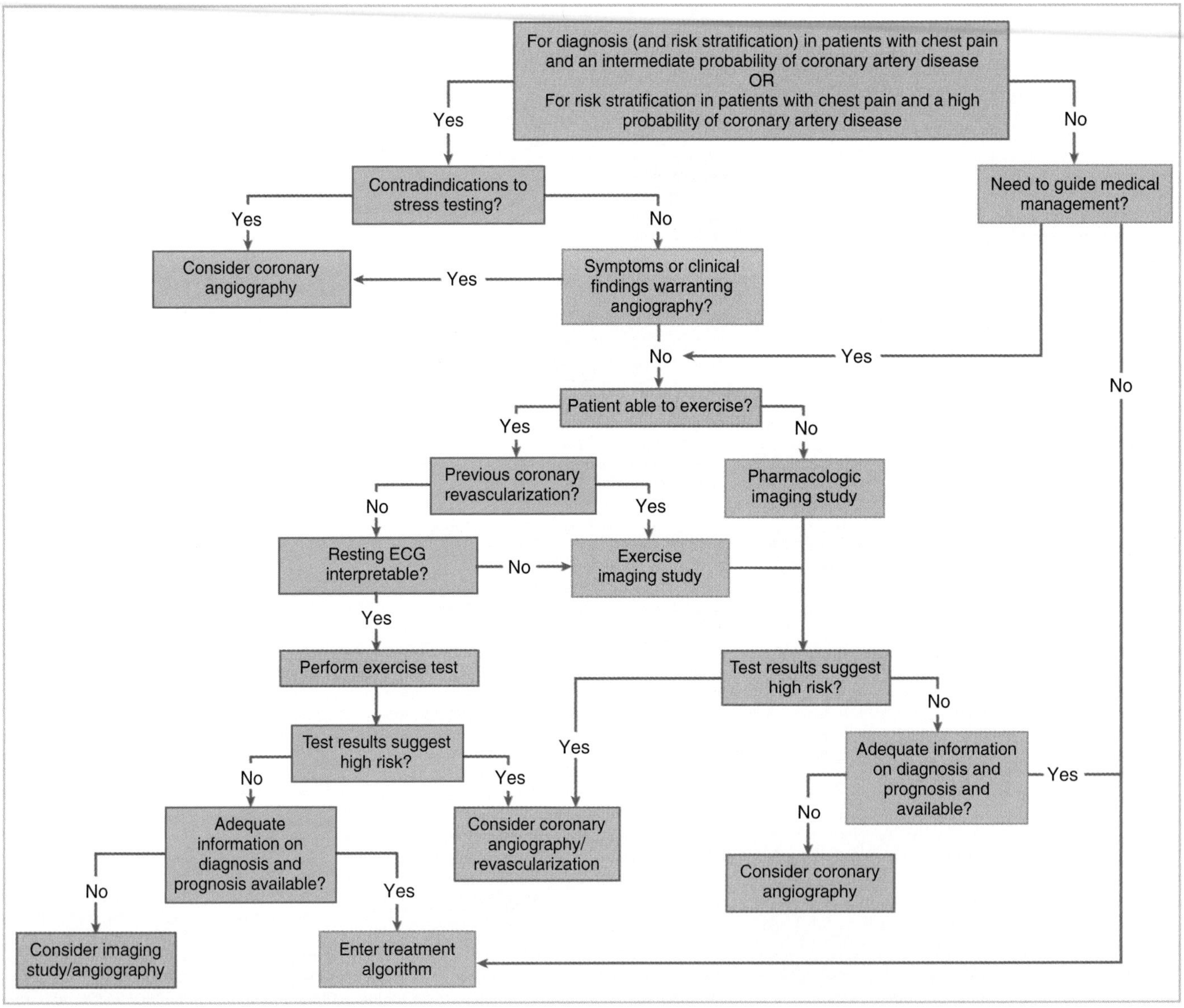

FIGURE 50G–2 Stress testing and angiography in patients with chest pain. ECG = electrocardiogram. (From ACC/AHA 2002 guideline update for the management of patients with chronic stable angina: A report of the American College of Cardiology/American Heart Association Task Force on Practice Guidleines [Committee to Update the 1999 Guidelines for the Management of Patients with Chronic Stable Angina]. ©2002, American College of Cardiology Foundation and the American Heart Association, p 9 [www.acc.org/clinical/guidelines/stable/stable.pdf]).

TABLE 50G–8 ACC/AHA Guidelines for Cardiac Stress Imaging as the Initial Test for Risk Stratification of Patients with Chronic Stable Angina Who Are Able to Exercise

Class	Indication	Evidence*
I (indicated)	1. Exercise myocardial perfusion imaging or exercise echocardiography to identify the extent, severity, and location of ischemia in patients who do not have left bundle-branch block or an electronically paced ventricular rhythm and who either have an abnormal rest ECG or are using digoxin. 2. Dipyridamole or adenosine myocardial perfusion imaging in patients with left bundle-branch block or electronically paced ventricular rhythm. 3. Exericse myocardial perfusion imaging or exercise echocardiography to assess the functional significance of coronary lesions (if not already known) in planning PCI.	B B B
IIa (good supportive evidence)		
IIb (weak supportive evidence)	1. Exercise or dobutamine echocardiography in patients with left bundle-branch block. 2. Exercise, dipyridamole, or adenosine myocardial perfusion imaging, or exercise or dobutamine echocardiography as the initial test in patients who have a normal rest ECG and who are not taking digoxin.	C B
III (not indicated)	1. Exercise myocardial perfusion imaging in patients with left bundle-branch block. 2. Exercise, dipyridamole, or adenosine myocardial perfusion imaging, or exercise or dobutamine echocardiography in patients with severe comorbidity likely to limit life expectation or prevent revascularization.	C C

ACC = American College of Cardiology; AHA = American Heart Association; ECG = electrocardiograph; PCI = percutaneous coronary intervention.
*See guidelines text for definitions of level of evidence.

TABLE 50G–9 ACC/AHA Guidelines for Cardiac Stress Imaging as the Initial Test for Risk Stratification of Patients with Chronic Stable Angina Who Are Unable to Exercise

Class	Indication	Evidence*
I (indicated)	1. Dipyridamole or adenosine myocardial perfusion imaging or dobutamine echocardiography to identify the extent, severity, and location of ischemia in patients who do not have left bundle branch block or electronically paced ventricular rhythm 2. Dipyridamole or adenosine myocardial perfusion imaging in patients with left bundle branch block or electronically paced ventricular rhythm 3. Dipyridamole or adenosine myocardial perfusion imaging or dobutamine echocardiography to assess the functional significance of coronary lesions (if not already known) in planning PCI	B B B
IIa (good supportive evidence)		
IIb (weak supportive evidence)	Dobutamine echocardiography in patients with left bundle branch block	C
III (not indicated)	Dipyridamole or adenosine myocardial perfusion imaging or dobutamine echocardiography in patients with severe comorbidity likely to limit life expectation or prevent revascularization	C

ACC = American College of Cardiology; AHA = American Heart Association; PCI = percutaneous coronary intervention.
*See guidelines text for definitions of level of evidence.

patients who are not taking digoxin, have a normal rest ECG, and are able to exercise.

The ACC/AHA guidelines support use of stress testing with either echocardiographic or radionuclide imaging to identify the severity of ischemia in patients who have ECG abnormalities precluding interpretation of the exercise tracing and for patients in whom the functional significance of coronary lesions will guide management (Tables 50G–8 and 50G–9). Dipyridamole or adenosine myocardial perfusion imaging is recommended for patients with left bundle branch block or electronically paced ventricular rhythms because of higher rates of false-positive septal perfusion defects with exercise than with either dipryridamole or adenosine. There are relatively few data on the performance of dobutamine echocardiography in this setting, so this approach is not endorsed by the guidelines for patients with left bundle branch block or electronically paced ventricular rhythms. Stress imaging studies are also supported for assessment of the functional significance of coronary lesions in planning PCI.

The guidelines discourage use of noninvasive testing for risk stratification of patients who have no symptoms of coronary disease. There were no class I or class IIa indications for use of cardiac stress imaging as an initial test for risk stratification. Supporting evidence is considered weak for use of cardiac stress imaging for asymptomatic patients with severe coronary calcification on electron-beam CT or who had undergone an exercise ECG and had inadequate tests or intermediate- or high-risk Duke treadmill scores.

Coronary Angiography

In the ACC/AHA guidelines, the decision to proceed to coronary angiography should be based on symptomatic status and risk stratification derived from clinical data and noninvasive test results. The guidelines define noninvasive findings that predict a high (>3 percent), intermediate (1 to 3 percent) and low (<1 percent) expected annual mortality rate (Table 50G–10). Coronary angiography for risk stratification and as a prelude to intervention is endorsed for patients with high-risk criteria, as well as those with disabling chronic stable angina despite medical therapy or other clinical characteristics suggesting high risk (Table 50G–11). The committee considered evidence to be generally supportive (class IIa) for coronary angiography for patients with milder angina in the setting of left ventricular dysfunction even if they do not have high-risk criteria on noninvasive testing; for

TABLE 50G–10 ACC/AHA Guideline Criteria for Noninvasive Risk Stratification

High Risk (>3% annual mortality rate)
1. Severe resting left ventricular dysfunction (LVEF <0.35)
2. High-risk treadmill score (score ≤–11)
3. Severe exercise LV dysfunction (exercise LVEF <0.35)
4. Stress-induced large perfusion defect (particularly if anterior)
5. Stress-induced multiple perfusion defects of moderate size
6. Large, fixed perfusion defect with LV dilation or increased lung uptake (thallium-201)
7. Stress-induced moderate perfusion defect with LV dilation or increased lung uptake (thallium-201)
8. Echocardiographic wall motion abnormality (involving > two segments) developing at low dose of dobutamine (≤10 mg/kg/min) or at a low heart rate (<120 beats/min)
9. Stress echocardiographic evidence of extensive ischemia
Intermediate Risk (1-3% annual mortality rate)
1. Mild/moderate resting LV dysfunction (LVEF =0.35-0.49)
2. Intermediate-risk treadmill score (–11 < score < 5)
3. Stress-induced moderate perfusion defect without LV dilation or increased lung intake (thallium-201)
4. Limited stress echocardiographic ischemia with a wall motion abnormality only at higher doses of dobutamine involving ≥ two segments
Low Risk (<1% annual mortality rate)
1. Low-risk treadmill score (score ≥5)
2. Normal or small myocardial perfusion defect at rest or with stress*
3. Normal stress echocardiographic wall motion or no change of limited resting wall motion abnormalities during stress*

ACC = American College of Cardiology; AHA = American Heart Association; LV = left ventricular; LVEF = LV ejection fraction.

From ACC/AHA 2002 guideline update for the management of patients with chronic stable angina: A report of the American College of Cardiology/American Heart Association Task Force on Practice Guidelines (Committee to Update the 1999 Guidelines for the Management of Patients with Chronic Stable Angina). ©2002, American College of Cardiology Foundation and the American Heart Association (www.acc.org/clinical/guidelines/stable/stable.pdf).

*Although the published data are limited, patients with these findings will probably not be at low risk in the presence of either a high-risk treadmill score or severe resting left ventricular dysfunction (LVEF <0.35).

TABLE 50G–11 ACC/AHA Guidelines for Coronary Angiography for Risk Stratification in Patients with Chronic Stable Angina

Class	Indication	Evidence*
I (indicated)	1. Patients with disabling (Canadian Cardiovascular Society [CCS] classes III and IV) chronic stable angina despite medical therapy	B
	2. Patients with high-risk criteria on noninvasive testing regardless of anginal severity	B
	3. Patients with angina who have survived sudden cardiac death or serious ventricular arrhythmia	B
	4. Patients with angina and symptoms and signs of CHF	C
	5. Patients with clinical characteristics that indicate a high likelihood of severe CAD	C
IIa (good supportive evidence)	1. Patients with significant LV dysfunction (ejection fraction <0.45), CCS class I or II angina, and demonstrable ischemia but < high-risk criteria on noninvasive testing	C
	2. Patients with inadequate prognostic information after noninvasive testing	C
	3. Patients with high-risk criteria suggesting ischemia on noninvasive testing	C
IIb (weak supportive evidence)	1. Patients with CCS class I or II angina, preserved LV function (ejection fraction >0.45), and < high-risk criteria on noninvasive testing	C
	2. Patients with CCS class III (not indicated) or IV angina, which with medical therapy improves to class I or II	C
	3. Patients with CCS class I or II angina but intolerance (unacceptable side effects) to adequate medical therapy	C
III (not indicated)	1. Patients with CCS class I or II angina who respond to medical therapy and who have no evidence of ischemia on noninvasive testing	C
	2. Patients who prefer to avoid revascularization	C

ACC = American College of Cardiology; AHA = American Heart Association; CHF = congestive heart failure; CAD = coronary artery disease; LV = left ventricular.

*See guidelines text for definitions of level of evidence.

asymptomatic patients with high-risk criteria; and for patients whose risk status is uncertain despite noninvasive testing.

Conversely, coronary angiography is discouraged (class III) for patients who have mild angina and no evidence of ischemia on noninvasive testing or would not undergo revascularization. There is only weak support (class IIb) for coronary angiography for patients with mild angina and good left ventricular function in the absence of high-risk criteria on noninvasive testing, for patients with severe angina whose symptoms were controlled with medical therapy, or for patients with mild angina but unacceptable side effects to adequate medical therapy.

TREATMENT

ACC/AHA guidelines for medical therapy of patients with chronic stable angina are oriented toward preventing myocardial infarction and death and reducing symptoms. When coronary revascularization has been shown to extend life, it is the recommended approach, but in many settings there are a variety of reasonable options, including medical therapy, PCI, and CABG. Cost-effectiveness and patient preference are considered important components of the decision-making process.

The guidelines assert that the goal of treatment of patients with chronic stable angina should be the complete or nearly complete

TABLE 50G–12 ACC/AHA Guidelines for Pharmacotherapy for Chronic Stable Angina

Class	Indication	Evidence*
I (indicated)	1. Aspirin in the absence of contraindications	A
	2. Beta-blockers as initial therapy in the absence of contraindications in patients with prior myocardial infarction or without prior myocardial infarction	A,B
	3. ACE inhibitor in all patients with CAD who also have diabetes and/or LV systolic dysfunction	A
	4. LDL-lowering therapy in patients with documented or suspected CAD and LDL cholesterol >130 mg/dl, with a target LDL of <100 mg/dl	A
	5. Sublingual nitroglycerin or nitroglycerin spray for the immediate relief of angina	B
	6. Calcium antagonists† or long-acting nitrates as initial therapy for reduction of symptoms when beta blockers are contraindicated	B
	7. Calcium antagonists† or long-acting nitrates in combination with beta blockers when initial treatment with beta blockers is not successful	B
	8. Calcium antagonists† and long-acting nitrates as a substitute for beta blockers if initial treatment with beta blockers leads to unacceptable side effects	C
IIa (good supportive evidence)	1. Clopidogrel when aspirin is absolutely contraindicated	B
	2. Long-acting nondihydropyridine calcium antagonists† instead of beta blockers as initial therapy	B
	3. In patients with documented or suspected CAD and LDL cholesterol 100-129 mg/dl, several therapeutic options are available: a. Lifestyle and/or drug therapies to lower LDL to <100 mg/dl b. Weight reduction and increased physical activity in persons with the metabolic syndrome c. Institution of treatment of other lipid or nonlipid risk factors; consider use of nicotinic acid or fibric acid for elevated triglycerides or low HDL cholesterol	B
	4. ACE inhibitor in patients with CAD or other vascular disease	B
IIb (weak supportive evidence)	Low-intensity anticoagulation with warfarin in addition to aspirin	B
III (not indicated)	1. Dipyridamole	B
	2. Chelation therapy	B

ACC = American College of Cardiology; AHA = American Heart Association; ACE = angiotensin-converting enzyme; CAD = coronary artery disease; LDL = low-density lipoprotein; LV = left ventricular.
*See guidelines text for definitions of level of evidence.
†Short-acting dihydropyridine calcium antagonists should be avoided.

elimination of anginal chest pain and return to normal activities, with minimal side effects. They recommend that the initial treatment of the patient should include all the elements in the following menomic:

A = Aspirin and Antianginal therapy
B = Beta blocker and Blood pressure
C = Cigarette smoking and Cholesterol
D = Diet and Diabetes
E = Education and Exercise

Pharmacological Therapy

The guidelines emphasize the importance of aspirin and beta blockers for patients with coronary disease in the absence of contraindications (Table 50G–12). Absolute contraindications to beta blockers include severe bradycardia, preexisting high degree of atrioventricular block, sick sinus syndrome, and severe, unstable left ventricular failure. Relative contraindications to beta blockers include asthma and bronchospastic disease, severe depression, and peripheral vascular disease. The guidelines note that most patients with diabetes tolerate beta blockers, although these drugs should be used with caution in patients who require insulin.

Angiotensin-converting enzyme (ACE) inhibitors are recommended (class I indication) for patients with diabetes and/or left ventricular systolic dysfunction, and evidence is considered good for their use in other patients with coronary disease (class IIa). The guidelines recommende that nitrates and calcium antagonists and nitrates should be used for symptom control but indicate that short-acting dihydropyridine calcium antagonists should be avoided. Low-density lipoprotein (LDL) cholesterol should be controlled with a target of less than 100 mg/dl (see Risk Reduction).

Several of the recommendations about pharmacological therapy may be altered in future revisions of these guidelines owing to subsequent research providing insight into the effects of these agents. For example, the guidelines give some support to use of clopidogrel only when aspirin is contraindicated (class IIa), but research on this and other antiplatelet agents is advancing rapidly so that insights into their optimal use can be expected to change in the next several years. Evidence is considered weak for anticoagulation with warfarin in addition to aspirin; since these guidelines were published, a randomized trial has shown that the combination of warfarin and aspirin were superior to aspirin alone in preventing future events but at the price of a higher rate of bleeding complications.[3] Use of dipyridamole or chelation therapy is discouraged.

For asymptomatic patients with known coronary disease (e.g., patients with prior myocardial infarction), the guidelines recommend aspirin and beta blockers in the absence of contraindications and the use of lipid-lowering therapies and ACE inhibitors as described earlier.

Risk Reduction

For patients with chronic stable angina, the ACC/AHA guidelines support intensive management of risk factors including hypertension, cigarette smoking, diabetes, LDL cholesterol, and obesity (Table 50G–13). The guidelines support use of pharmacological therapy for patients with LDL levels greater than 130 mg/dl, with a target of 100 mg/dL. For patients with coronary disease who have an LDL of 100 to 129 mg/dl, the guidelines consider several options reasonable (class IIa), including life-style modifications or drug therapies.

In changes from prior guidelines, initiation of hormone therapy for the purpose of reducing cardiovascular risk is considered inappropriate (class III), as is use of vitamins C and E supplementation, chelation therapy, garlic, acupuncture, and coenzyme Q for this purpose. Evidence to support interventions based on lipoprotein(a) and homocysteine levels are considered inconclusive.

Specific goals for key risk reduction interventions are summarized in Table 50G–14.

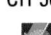

TABLE 50G–13 ACC/AHA Guidelines for Treatment of Risk Factors

Class	Indication	Evidence*
I (indicated)	1. Treatment of hypertension according to Joint National Conference VI guidelines	A
	2. Smoking cessation therapy	B
	3. Management of diabetes	C
	4. Comprehensive cardiac rehabilitation program (including exercise)	B
	5. LDL-lowering therapy in patients with documented or suspected CAD and LDL cholesterol ≥130 mg/dl, with a target LDL of <100 mg/dl	A
	6. Weight reduction in obese patients in the presence of hypertension, hyperlipidemia, or diabetes mellitus	C
IIa (good supportive evidence)	1. In patients with documented or suspected CAD and LDL cholesterol 100-129 mg/dl, several therapeutic options are available:	B
	a. Lifestyle and/or drug therapies to lower LDL to <100 mg/dl	B
	b. Weight reduction and increased physical activity in persons with the metabolic syndrome	B
	c. Institution of treatment of other lipid or nonlipid risk factors; consider use of nicotinic acid or fibric acid for elevated triglycerides or low HDL cholesterol	B
	2. Therapy to lower non-HDL cholesterol in patients with documented or suspected CAD and triglycerides >200 mg/dl, with a target non-HDL cholesterol <130 mg/dl	B
	3. Weight reduction in obese patients in the absence of hypertension, hyperlipidemia, or diabetes mellitus	C
IIb (weak supportive evidence)	1. Folate therapy in patients with elevated homocysteine levels	C
	2. Identification and appropriate treatment of clinical depression to improve CAD outcomes	C
	3. Intervention directed at psychosocial stress reduction	C
III (not indicated)	1. Initiation of hormone replacement therapy in postmenopausal women for the purpose of reducing cardiovascular risk	A
	2. Vitamins C and E supplementation	A
	3. Chelation therapy	C
	4. GarlicC	
	5. Acupuncture	C
	6. Coenzyme Q	C

ACC = American College of Cardiology; AHA = American Heart Association; CAD = coronary artery disease; HDL = high-density lipoprotein; LDL = low-density lipoprotein.
*See guidelines text for definitions of level of evidence.

TABLE 50G–14 Specific Goals for Risk Reduction Strategies in Patients with Chronic Stable Angina

Risk Factor/Strategy	Goal
Smoking	Complete cessation
Blood pressure	<140/90 or 130/85 mm Hg if heart failure or renal insufficiency; <130/85 mm Hg if diabetes
Lipid management	Primary goal: LDL <100 mg/dl Secondary goal: If triglycerides ≥200 mg/dl, then non-HDL should be <130 mg/dl
Physical activity	Minimum goal: 30 min 3 or 4 d/w Optimal goal: daily
Weight management	BMI 18.5-24.9 kg/m^2
Diabetes management	HbA1c <7%
Antiplatelet agents/anticoagulants	All patients: indefinite use of aspirin 75-325 mg per day if not contraindicated. Consider clopidogrel as an alternative if aspirin is contraindicated. Manage warfarin to international normalized ratio = 2.0 to 3.0 in patients after myocardial infarction when clinically indicated or for those not able to take aspirin or clopidogrel
ACE inhibitors	Treat all patients indefinitely after myocardial infarction; start early in stable high-risk patients (anterior myocardial infarction, previous myocardial infarction, Killip class II [S_3 gallop, rales, radiographic CHF]). Consider chronic therapy for all other patients with coronary or other vascular disease unless contraindicated. Use as needed to manage blood pressure or symptoms in all other patients
Beta blockers	Start in all post-myocardial infarction and acute patients (arrhythmia, LV dysfunction, inducible ischemia) at 5-28 days. Continue 6 mo minimum. Observe usual contraindications. Use as needed to manage angina, rhythm, or blood pressure in all patients

ACE = angiotensin-converting enzyme; LDL = low-density lipoprotein; BMI = body mass index; HbA1c = hemoglobin A1c; CHF = congestive heart failure; LV = left ventricular.

Revascularization

ACC/AHA guidelines for revascularization with PCI or CABG for patients with chronic stable angina focus on improvement of survival for patients with high clinical risk of mortality on medical therapy and on controlling symptoms in patients who have an inadequate quality of life on medical therapy. Recommendations include the use of CABG for patients with significant left main coronary artery disease and in patients with triple-vessel disease, particularly in those with abnormal left ventricular function (Table 50G–15). PCI and CABG are supported for patients with double- and triple-vessel coronary disease and who do not have treated diabetes. Revascularization is also supported for

TABLE 50G–15 ACC/AHA Guidelines for Revascularization with PCI and CABG in Patients with Stable Angina

Class	Indication	Evidence*
I (indicated)	1. CABG for patients with significant left main coronary disease	A
	2. CABG for patients with triple-vessel disease. The survival benefit is greater in patients with abnormal LV function (ejection fraction <0.50)	A
	3. CABG for patients with double-vessel disease with significant proximal LAD CAD and either abnormal LV function (ejection fraction less than 50%) or demonstrable ischemia on noninvasive testing	A
	4. Percutaneous coronary intervention for patients with double-or triple-vessel disease with significant proximal LAD CAD, who have anatomy suitable for catheter-based therapy and normal LV function and who do not have treated diabetes	B
	5. PCI or CABG for patients with single- or double-vessel CAD without significant proximal LAD CAD but with a large area of viable myocardium and high-risk criteria on noninvasive testing	B
	6. CABG for patients with single- or double-vessel CAD without significant proximal LAD CAD who have survived sudden cardiac death or sustained ventricular tachycardia	C
	7. In patients with prior PCI, CABG or PCI for recurrent stenosis associated with a large area of viable myocardium or high-risk criteria on noninvasive testing	C
	8. PCI or CABG for patients who have not been successfully treated by medical therapy and can undergo revascularization with acceptable risk	B
IIa (good supportive evidence)	1. Repeat CABG for patients with multiple saphenous vein graft stenoses, especially when there is significant stenosis of a graft supplying the LAD; it may be appropriate to use PCI for focal saphenous vein graft lesions or multiple stenoses in poor candidates for reoperative surgery	C
	2. Use of PCI or CABG for patients with single- or double-vessel CAD without significant proximal LAD disease but with a moderate area of viable myocardium and demonstrable ischemia on noninvasive testing	B
	3. Use of PCI or CABG for patients with single-vessel disease with significant proximal LAD disease	B
IIb (weak supportive evidence)	1. Compared with CABG, PCI for patients with double- or triple-vessel disease with significant proximal LAD CAD, who have anatomy suitable for catheter-based therapy, and who have treated diabetes or abnormal LV function	B
	2. Use of PCI for patients with significant left main coronary disease who are not candidates for CABG	C
	3. PCI for patients with single- or double-vessel CAD without significant proximal LAD CAD who have survived sudden cardiac death or sustained ventricular tachycardia	C
III (not indicated)	1. Use of PCI or CABG for patients with single- or double-vessel CAD without significant proximal LAD CAD, who have mild symptoms that are unlikely due to myocardial ischemia, or who have not received an adequate trial of medical therapy and a. have only a small area of viable myocardium *or* b. have no demonstrable ischemia on noninvasive testing	C
	2. Use of PCI or CABG for patients with borderline coronary stenoses (50–60% diameter in locations other than the left main coronary artery) and no demonstrable ischemia on noninvasive testing	C
	3. Use of PCI or CABG for patients with insignificant coronary stenosis (<50% diameter)	C
	4. Use of PCI in patients with significant left main coronary artery disease who are candidates for CABG	B

ACC = American College of Cardiology; AHA = American Heart Association; CAD = coronary artery disease; CABG = coronary artery bypass grafting; LAD = left anterior descending [coronary artery]; LV = left ventricular; PCI = percutaneous coronary intervention.
*See guidelines text for definitions of level of evidence.

patients with single- or double-vessel coronary disease who have a large area of viable myocardium and high-risk criteria on noninvasive testing.

The guidelines discourage use of PCI or CABG for single- or double-vessel coronary disease without significant proximal left anterior descending (LAD) coronary artery disease if they have mild symptoms or have not received an adequate trial of medical therapy, particularly if noninvasive testing data indicate either that they have only a small area of viable myocardium or have no demonstrable ischemia on noninvasive testing. PCI for patients with diabetes is considered a second-choice strategy compared with CABG.

For asymptomatic patients, the guidelines for revascularization with PCI or CABG are identical to those for other patients with chronic stable angina (see Table 50G–15), except that the following indications that were considered class IIa are regarded as weaker (class IIb) in asymptomatic patients:

Use of PCI or CABG for patients with single- or double-vessel CAD without significant proximal LAD disease but with a moderate area of viable myocardium and demonstrable ischemia on noninvasive testing

Use of PCI or CABG for patients with single-vessel disease with significant proximal LAD disease

Alternative Therapies

The guidelines do not consider alternative therapies to be sufficiently supported by evidence to warrant a class I indication for patients with chronic stable angina. Surgical laser transmyocardial revascularization is given a class IIa indication, and enhanced external counterpulsation and spinal cord stimulation are given class IIb indications.

Patient Follow-Up

The ACC/AHA guidelines recommend that patients with chronic stable angina should have follow-up evaluations every 4 to 12 months during the first year of therapy; subsequently, annual evaluations are recommended if the patient is stable and reliable enough to call when angina symptoms become worse or other symptoms occur. The guidelines urge restraint in the use of routine testing in follow-up of patients with chronic stable angina if they have not had a change in clinical status (Table 50G–16). All of the class I indications for testing are for patients who have had a significant change in clinical status, except for the use of coronary angiography for patients with marked limitations of ordinary activity despite maximal medical therapy.

TABLE 50G–16 ACC/AHA Guidelines for Echocardiography, Treadmill Exercise Testing, Stress Radionuclide Imaging, Stress Echocardiography Studies, and Coronary Angiography During Patient Follow-Up

Class	Indication	Evidence*
I (indicated)	1. Chest radiograph for patients with evidence of new or worsening CHF	C
	2. Assessment of LV ejection fraction and segmental wall motion by echocardiography or radionuclide imaging in patients with new or worsening CHF or evidence of intervening myocardial infarction by history or ECG	C
	3. Echocardiography for evidence of new or worsening valvular heart disease	C
	4. Treadmill exercise test for patients without prior revascularization who have a significant change in clinical status, are able to exercise, and do not have any of the ECG abnormalities listed in No. 5	C
	5. Stress radionuclide imaging or stress echocardiography procedures for patients without prior revascularization who have a significant change in clinical status and are unable to exercise or have one of the following ECG abnormalities: a. Preexcitation (Wolff-Parkinson-White) syndrome b. Electronically paced ventricular rhythm c. More than 1 mm of rest ST depression d. Complete left bundle branch block	C
	6. Stress radionuclide imaging or stress echocardiography procedures for patients who have a significant change in clinical status and required a stress imaging procedure on their initial evaluation because of equivocal or intermediate-risk treadmill results	C
	7. Stress radionuclide imaging or stress echocardiography procedures for patients with prior revascularization who have a significant change in clinical status	C
	8. Coronary angiography in patients with marked limitation of ordinary activity (CCS class III) despite maximal medical therapy	C
IIa (good supportive evidence)		
IIb (weak supportive evidence)	Annual treadmill exercise testing in patients who have no change in clinical status, can exercise, have none of the ECG abnormalities listed in No. 5, and have an estimated annual mortality rate >1%	C
III (not indicated)	1. Echocardiography or radionuclide imaging for assessment of LV ejection fraction and segmental wall motion in patients with a normal ECG, no history of myocardial infarction, and no evidence of CHF	C
	2. Repeat treadmill exercise testing in <3 yr in patients who have no change in clinical status and an estimated annual mortality rate <1% on their initial evaluation, as demonstrated by one of the following: a. Low-risk Duke treadmill score (without imaging) b. Low-risk Duke treadmill score with negative imaging c. Normal LV function and a normal coronary angiogram d. Normal LV function and insignificant CAD	C
	3. Stress imaging or echocardiograph procedures for patients who have no change in clinical status and a normal rest ECG, are not taking digoxin, are able to exercise, and did not require a stress imaging or echocardiographic procedure on their initial evaluation because of equivocal or intermediate-risk treadmill results	C
	4. Repeat coronary angiography in patients with no change in clinical status, no change on repeat exercise testing or stress imaging, and insignificant CAD on initial evaluation	C

ACC = American College of Cardiology; AHA = American Heart Association; CAD = coronary artery disease; CCS = Canadian Cardiovascular Society; CHF = congestive heart failure; ECG = electrocardiograph; LV = left ventricular.

*See guidelines text for definitions of level of evidence.

References

1. Gibbons RJ, Abrams J, Chatterjee K, et al: ACC/AHA 2002 guideline update for the management of patients with chronic stable angina: A report of the American College of Cardiology/American Heart Association Task Force on Practice Guidelines (Committee to Update the 1999 Guidelines for the Management of Patients with Chronic Stable Angina). 2002 (Available at www.acc.org/clinical/guidelines/stable/stable.pdf).
2. O'Rourke RA, Brundage BH, Froelicher VF, et al: American College of Cardiology/American Heart Association Expert Consensus Document on electron-beam computed tomography for the diagnosis and prognosis of coronary artery disease. Circulation 102:126-140, 2000.
3. Hurlen M, Abdelnoor M, Smith P, et al: Warfarin, aspirin, or both after myocardial infarction. N Engl J Med 347:969-974, 2002.

CHAPTER 51

Diabetes and Heart Disease

Richard W. Nesto

Scope of the Problem

People with diabetes have an increased prevalence of atherosclerosis and coronary heart disease (CHD) (see Chap. 40) and experience higher morbidity and mortality after acute coronary syndrome and myocardial infarction (MI) than people without diabetes. Diabetes has dramatic impact on outcomes following unstable angina or MI. Analyzing data collected for the Organization to Assess Strategies for Ischemic Syndromes (OASIS) Registry, Malmberg and colleagues showed that diabetes significantly increased all-cause death and the incidence of new MI, stroke, and heart failure during a 2-year mean follow-up in patients who were hospitalized for unstable angina or non-Q-wave MI.[1] In a similar study of patients hospitalized with a confirmed MI, Mukamal and colleagues found that diabetes was associated with an adjusted hazard ratio for mortality of 1.7 (95 percent confidence interval [CI] 1.2 to 2.3) compared with patients without diabetes and no previous MI.[2] In general, diabetes confers as much additional risk as having had a previous MI.

Diabetes also increases the risk of heart failure. Patients with diabetes are two to five times more likely to develop heart failure than those without diabetes,[3] and following development of heart failure, diabetic patients have higher mortality and heart failure–related morbidity.[4] The fundamental causes of heart failure are similar in diabetic and nondiabetic subjects: previous MI and the resultant loss of contracting myocardium cause most chronic congestive heart failure (CHF). Other contributors to CHF in diabetic patients include hypertension, left ventricular hypertrophy, and valvular heart disease. Although diabetes is an important risk factor for CHF, it rarely occurs independently and in fact appears to act synergistically with other risk factors.

Traditional CHD risk factors such as hypertension, dyslipidemia, and overweight and obesity cluster in patients with impaired glucose tolerance or diabetes (see discussion of metabolic syndrome in Chap. 40), but this clustering cannot account for all of the increased risk in these patients. In addition to the traditional risk factors associated with CHD and heart failure, a number of diabetes-specific risk factors contribute to the increased morbidity and mortality of coronary artery disease (CAD) in diabetes. For example, patients with diabetes have lipid-rich atherosclerotic plaque that is more vulnerable to rupture than plaque found in patients without diabetes.[5] Diabetes is associated with the presence of multiple vulnerable coronary plaques in patients undergoing catheterization for acute coronary syndromes, which may account for the increased risk of reinfarction in these patients. Platelets harvested from patients with diabetes exhibit enhanced aggregation and increased expression of activation-dependent adhesion molecules, such as glycoprotein (GP) IIb/IIIa, which contributes to thrombus formation.[6]

Changes in vascular function may also contribute to the poorer outcomes in diabetes. No reflow following successful percutaneous recanalization of an infarct-related coronary artery occurs more commonly in the presence of diabetes and/or hyperglycemia and may contribute to left ventricular dysfunction. No reflow in this circumstance probably results from platelet–endothelial cell interactions that impair microvascular function and decrease myocardial blood flow. Patients with diabetes have increased levels of plasminogen activator inhibitor type 1 (PAI-1) in plasma and in atheromas.[7,8] Elevated tissue PAI-1 could decrease fibrinolysis, increase thrombus formation, and accelerate plaque formation. Other vascular changes, including increased endothelin activity and reduced prostacyclin and nitric oxide activity, lead to abnormal control of blood flow.[9,10] The emerging recognition that CHD is part of a proinflammatory state suggests that the increased plasma C-reactive protein levels seen in people with diabetes may contribute to the increased risk.[11] Other diabetes-specific changes that occur include diabetic cardiomyopathy, which impairs myocardial performance and renders the myocardium more susceptible to and less able to recover from ischemia, and diabetic autonomic neuropathy, which results in sympathovagal imbalance and contributes to cardiovascular mortality.[12] Advanced glycation end products (AGEs) are thought to contribute to many of these diabetes-specific changes (see Chap. 40).

Medical Therapy of Acute Coronary Syndromes

A history of diabetes is important in determining the treatment of patients during and following an acute MI. However, patients with acute coronary syndromes commonly have undiagnosed diabetes and impaired glucose metabolism. In a study of 3266 patients scheduled for coronary angiography, Taubert and colleagues reported that the prevalence of previously undiagnosed diabetes was nearly 18 percent.[13] Patients with acute MI have an even higher percentage (25 to 31 percent) of previously undiagnosed diabetes.[14]

The negative interaction between diabetes and the prognosis after MI extends to patients with elevated blood glucose at the time of admission. Several studies have shown this relationship. For example, 1664 consecutively hospitalized patients with an acute MI were categorized by history of diabetes and by whether they had a blood glucose concentration greater than 198 mg/dl.[15] The patients who had a history of diabetes or who were hyperglycemic had a significantly elevated risk of in-hospital mortality compared with those without either condition. In a similar study, admission blood glucose level in nondiabetic patients independently predicted nonfatal reinfarction ($p = 0.006$), hospitalization for heart failure ($p = 0.0034$), and a major cardiovascular event ($p = 0.0042$) during the 1.5- to 2.5-year follow-up period.[16]

Antiplatelet Drugs

Studies have consistently shown that patients with either type 1 or type 2 diabetes have enhanced platelet aggregation in response to a variety of agonists.[6] This enhanced aggregability results in part from increased production of thromboxane, altered calcium and magnesium homeostasis, and increased expression of activation-dependent adhesion molecules. Endothelial dysfunction, characterized by decreased production of nitric oxide and prostacyclin, is common in diabetic individuals and enhances platelet aggregation and adhesiveness in vivo.[6] Thus, agents directed at inhibiting platelet aggregation in vivo consistently reduce the incidence of thrombotic events in nondiabetic and diabetic individuals.

Aspirin

In the Early Treatment of Diabetic Retinopathy Study (ETDRS), patients with type 1 or type 2 diabetes randomly assigned to aspirin 650 mg/day had a significantly lowered risk of MI without incurring an increase in the risk of vitreous or retinal bleeding, even in patients with retinopathy.[17] The Hypertension Optimal Treatment (HOT) trial confirmed this benefit in 1501 diabetic subjects who experienced a significant 15 percent reduction in cardiovascular events and a 36 percent reduction in MI while being treated with aspirin 75 mg/day.[17] This cardiovascular benefit resembled that seen in the nondiabetic cohort. The American Diabetes Association currently recommends enteric-coated aspirin (81 to 325 mg/day) for (1) secondary prevention in men and women with diabetes and evidence of macrovascular disease and (2) primary prevention in persons with type 1 or type 2 diabetes and additional coronary risk factors.[17]

Adenosine Diphosphate Receptor Antagonists

Ticlopidine and clopidogrel irreversibly block platelet adenosine diphosphate (ADP) receptors, preventing activation of the GP IIb/IIIa receptor and thereby inhibiting binding of fibrinogen. In the Clopidogrel versus Aspirin in Patients at Risk of Ischemic Events (CAPRIE) trial, patients who had suffered a recent MI, stroke, or had established peripheral arterial disease were randomly assigned to receive aspirin 325 mg/day or clopidogrel 75 mg/day.[18,19] During the 1.9-year follow-up, the incidence of the combined primary endpoint, stroke, MI, or vascular death, was 8.7 percent lower in the clopidogrel group than in the aspirin group. Although the incidence of the primary endpoint was higher in the nearly 4000 diabetic participants, the benefit of clopidogrel over aspirin extended to this subgroup.[19] The Clopidogrel in Unstable Angina to Prevent Recurrent Events (CURE) study tested clopidogrel plus aspirin against aspirin alone in patients with unstable angina or non-Q-wave MI. After 9 months the incidence of the primary composite endpoint (cardiovascular death, nonfatal MI, or stroke) was reduced in the clopidogrel plus aspirin group by 20 percent.[20] Subgroup analysis showed that this effect extended to the patients with diabetes.

Glycoprotein IIb/IIIa Blockers

These potent antiplatelet agents have improved outcomes in patients with unstable angina and non-Q-wave infarction and have reduced the incidence of acute ischemic events by 35 to 50 percent in patients undergoing percutaneous coronary intervention (PCI).[21] At least one of the GP IIb/IIIa inhibitors, abciximab, positively influenced long-term mortality.[21] In general, these agents appear to have equal or better efficacy in diabetic than nondiabetic patients, although most studies have not been sufficiently powered to evaluate this interaction fully. However, meta-analyses clearly show a major benefit in the diabetic population.

Four placebo-controlled trials of the use of GP IIb/IIIa blockade during PCI included detailed outcome data for the diabetic subgroups.[21] Three studies (the Evaluation of c7E3 for Prevention of Ischemic Complications [EPIC], Evaluation in PTCA to Improve Long-term Outcome with abciximab GP IIb/IIIa blockade [EPILOG], and Evaluation of Platelet Inhibition in STENTing [EPISTENT]) evaluated abciximab, and the fourth (Enhanced Suppression of the Platelet IIb/IIIa Receptor with Integrilin Therapy [ESPRIT]) tested eptifibatide. The magnitude of the reduction in acute ischemic events (death, MI, or urgent revascularization occurring within 30 days) in the active treatment group compared with the placebo group was similar in both diabetic (21 to 67 percent reduction) and nondiabetic patients (30 to 51 percent reduction). This treatment effect was durable, as indicated by the similar reductions in death or MI at 6 months in both the diabetic and nondiabetic groups. The incidence of target vessel revascularization at 6 months, a surrogate for restenosis, varied considerably between treatment groups and among trials. Thus, whether GP IIb/IIIa treatment reduces the incidence of restenosis in diabetic or nondiabetic patients remains an open issue. Long-term mortality is also reduced by abciximab in the general population, and multivariate analysis has shown that diabetes is an important factor in predicting this survival benefit.[22]

The survival benefit of GP IIb/IIIa blockade may be greater in diabetic patients treated with stents. In EPISTENT, 1-year mortality was reduced from 4.1 to 1.2 percent in stented, diabetic patients, a larger benefit than seen in the nondiabetic group (1.9 to 1.0 percent).[23] A similar reduction in 1-year mortality was found in stented, diabetic patients treated with eptifibatide in the ESPRIT trial.[24] Although these differences did not achieve statistical significance because of the studies' limited power, the results suggest that GP IIb/IIIa blockade neutralizes the mortality risk usually seen in diabetic patients following PCI. GP IIb/IIIa blockers also confer a survival benefit on diabetic patients treated for non-ST-segment elevation acute coronary syndromes. A meta-analysis of six major studies involving 6458 diabetic patients showed a reduction in 30-day mortality from 6.2 percent in the placebo group to 4.8 percent in the treated group ($p = 0.007$).[25] No benefit was seen in the 23,072 nondiabetic patients.

Part of the increased risk of thrombotic events in diabetic patients stems from their altered platelet function, including altered arachidonic acid metabolism and increased expression of activation-dependent adhesion molecules such as GP IIb/IIIa, resulting in enhanced platelet aggregation.[6] This diabetic thrombocytopathy may explain in part the greater effect of GP IIb/IIIa blockers in diabetic patients compared with nondiabetic patients. GP IIb/IIIa blockade may also improve microvascular dysfunction in acute coronary syndrome patients,[26] although the mechanism of this platelet-endothelial interaction has not yet been elucidated.

Beta-Adrenergic Blocking Agents

Overwhelming evidence exists that beta-adrenergic blocking agents (beta blockers) reduce mortality and reinfarction in patients with MI. However, the use of beta blockers in the diabetic population has been controversial because of their potential to reduce hypoglycemic symptoms, precipitate glucose intolerance, inhibit the release of insulin, and affect adversely the plasma lipid profile. Despite these concerns, treatment of diabetic patients with beta blockers following MI has reduced mortality, and the benefit in several studies exceeded that seen in the nondiabetic counterparts. Although these data derive from retrospective subgroup analyses of trials in the prethrombolytic era, they concur with more recent results. The National Cooperative Cardiovascular Project reviewed records of more than 45,000 patients who had experienced an acute MI, 26 percent of whom had diabetes. After adjusting for confounding variables, beta blocker use was associated with a lower 1-year mortality in diabetic patients without an increase in diabetes-related complications.[27]

The greater relative benefit of beta blockers in diabetic patients may derive from several factors. Beta blockers can help restore sympathovagal balance in diabetic patients with autonomic neuropathy and may decrease fatty acid utilization within the myocardium, thus reducing oxygen demand. However, despite the continuing growth of evidence regarding their efficacy and safety in the diabetic patient, beta blockers continue to be underprescribed in this group. Physicians have concerns that beta blockers can mask the warning signs of hypoglycemia, suppress glycogenolysis, interfere with insulin release, and further impair glucose tolerance in patients with diabetes. Some are also concerned that beta blockers may elevate serum triglycerides, reduce high-density lipoprotein, and increase low-density lipoprotein and thereby potentially counteract some of the widely accepted cardioprotective benefits of these drugs. However, much of the concern surrounding the use of these drugs in diabetes stems from earlier experience with noncardioselective agents in higher doses. The risk of hypoglycemia in diabetic hypertensive patients taking cardioselective beta blockers was no different from that of patients taking placebo.[28] Cardioselective agents have less tendency to worsen glycemic control than nonselective agents do, although diabetes may develop in over 20 percent of nondiabetic hypertensive patients given beta blockers.[29]

Angiotensin-Converting Enzyme Inhibitors

Angiotensin-converting enzyme (ACE) inhibitors reduce infarct size, limit ventricular remodeling, improve survival after myocardial infarction, and may be of particular benefit in patients with diabetes.[30] A post hoc analysis of one thrombolytic trial (Grupo Italiano per lo Studio della Sopravivenza nell'Infarto Miocardico-3 [GISSI-3]) revealed that early administration of lisinopril in the setting of acute MI reduced 6-week and 6-month mortality comparatively more in diabetic versus nondiabetic patients (30 versus 5 percent reduction at 6 weeks and 20 versus 0 percent at 6 months, respectively).[31] Lisinopril administration resulted in some 37 lives saved per 1000 treated diabetic patients. Another retrospective analysis, the Trandolapril Cardiac Evaluation (TRACE) study, compared the effect of oral trandolapril versus placebo in anterior MI in patients with and without diabetes.[32] Patients with diabetes experienced a greater relative improvement in survival over 5 years of follow-up than the nondiabetic cohort. Furthermore, ACE inhibition reduced by nearly 50 percent the risk of sudden death, reinfarction, and progression of CHF in patients with diabetes, whereas subjects without diabetes experienced only trends in protection against these secondary outcomes.

Many factors may explain the particular benefits of ACE inhibitors in diabetic patients with acute MI. These agents can prevent or limit remodeling of the ventricle, particularly when administered early in the course of acute MI; reduce recurrent ischemic events; and restore sympathovagal imbalance. ACE inhibitors may also improve endothelial function in diabetes, counteract reduced fibrinolysis by suppression of PAI-1 expression, and decrease insulin resistance.[33] In the Heart Outcomes Prevention Evaluation (HOPE) study, ramipril significantly reduced the rates of MI, stroke, and cardiovascular death in diabetic subjects with or without a prior history of CAD or CHF over a 5-year period when compared with placebo.[34]

Insulin

Studies have evaluated the role of strict glycemic control in diabetic patients during the acute phase of MI. The blood glucose level may increase in proportion to infarct size and hemodynamic stress in nondiabetic patients with MI as catecholamines, cortisol, and growth hormone are released. These hormones may create "transient" insulin resistance, with serum glucose returning to normal at discharge. In some cases, a very high admission glucose level out of proportion to infarct size indicates previously undiagnosed diabetes. Nevertheless, substantial evidence points to the admission glucose level as an independent predictor of early and late mortality after MI in patients with and without diabetes mellitus.[35]

Aggressive control of plasma glucose levels during the treatment of myocardial ischemia in diabetic patients can improve outcomes. In the Diabetes and Insulin-Glucose Infusion in Acute Myocardial Infarction (DIGAMI) study, 620 diabetic patients with acute MI were randomly assigned to either intensive insulin therapy (insulin-glucose infusion for 24 hours, followed by subcutaneous insulin injection for at least 3 months) or a standard glycemic control strategy.[36] Those receiving the intensive insulin regimen had a lower blood glucose level during the first hour (9.6 versus 11.7 mmol/liter, $p < 0.01$) and at discharge (8.2 versus 9.0 mmol/liter, $p < 0.01$) than the control group. During the first year of follow-up, a significant reduction in mortality was seen in the intensive insulin group compared with the conventionally treated group (19 versus 26 percent, $p = 0.027$). Mortality remained lower in the intensive control group through 3.4 years than in the conventional care group (33 versus 44 percent, $p = 0.011$).[37] Predictors of mortality were age, history of CHF, diabetes duration, admission glucose, and admission hemoglobin (Hb) A_{1c} level. The subgroup whose diabetes had been managed with diet or oral hypoglycemic drugs before infarction enjoyed the greatest survival benefit. A study of diabetic patients undergoing coronary artery bypass graft (CABG) surgery showed that continuous insulin infusion compared with subcutaneous insulin treatment reduced mortality (2.5 versus 5.3 percent, $p < 0.0001$.[38] Although no placebo group was reported, mortality in the insulin infusion group was significantly less than predicted by Society of Thoracic Surgeons risk model.

Several mechanisms may explain the findings of the DIGAMI trial. Insulin-glucose infusion may (1) increase the availability of glucose as a substrate for adenosine triphosphate (ATP) generation in cardiac muscle; (2) reduce lipolysis and decrease the generation of free fatty acids, which can impair myocardial contractility and trigger ventricular arrhythmia; and (3) shift cardiac metabolism from free fatty acid oxidation to glycolysis. In addition, tight glycemic control can reverse hyperglycemia-induced platelet reactivity and reduce the typically elevated PAI-1 activity in patients with diabetes. Part of the benefit derived from the use of insulin in the tight control arm may have resulted from the removal of any potential cardiac risk associated with the use of sulfonylureas (see later).

Infusion of glucose-insulin-potassium (GIK) solution, originally used in the 1960s and 1970s as a polarizing agent to maintain electrical stability, is regaining favor as a method to influence myocardial metabolism positively during treatment of MI, coronary revascularization procedures, and CABG surgery. A meta-analysis of nine studies including 1932 patients conducted between 1965 and 1987 concluded that GIK infusion reduced in-hospital mortality from 21 to 16.1 percent.[39] However, only two of the studies were double blind, and no information about diabetic patients was provided. In a prospective, randomized, open-label study of GIK infusion in 940 patients undergoing percutaneous transluminal coronary angioplasty (PTCA) for an acute MI, no mortality benefit was seen in the GIK group compared with the placebo group.[40] Although there seemed to be a benefit in the diabetic subgroup, in which GIK infusion reduced mortality from 12.2 to 4 percent, the small size of the subgroup and the small number of deaths prevented this effect from reaching statistical significance. In diabetic patients undergoing elective CABG surgery, GIK infusion beneficially influenced metabolism, as indicated by an elimination of myocardial extraction of nonesterified fatty acids and an increase in myocardial uptake of lactate and glucose.[41] Patients treated with GIK infusion during CABG may have a reduced prevalence of atrial fibrillation, enhanced cardiac function, and faster recovery than those who do not receive this treatment.[42] Further prospective studies are necessary to determine the long-term effect of GIK infusion in diabetic patients treated for MI or acute coronary syndromes.

Heart Failure

Heart failure, the pathophysiological state in which the heart is unable to maintain cardiac output sufficient to meet the metabolic needs of the body, and its attendant morbidity and mortality continue to be a growing problem in the United States. Although MI and hypertension are the most common risk factors associated with CHF, diabetes mellitus is also a strong and independent risk factor. In the Framingham Heart Study (Fig. 51–1), men with diabetes had an age- and risk factor–adjusted hazard ratio for CHF of 1.82 (95 percent CI = 1.28 to 2.58) compared with men without diabetes.[43] The hazard ratio in diabetic women was even larger, 3.73 (CI = 1.49 to 3.21). Patients with diabetes account for more than 33 percent of hospital admissions for heart failure, clearly a disproportionately high fraction.[44]

Not only are diabetic patients at higher risk for CHF, but the diabetic patients who develop CHF have a worse prognosis than those without diabetes. In the Studies of Left Ventricular Dysfunction (SOLVD) trials and registry, diabetic patients with symptomatic heart failure or asymptomatic left ventricular dysfunction had an increased risk of all-cause mortality (risk ratio = 1.29, CI = 1.10 to 1.50) and hospitalization for CHF (risk ratio = 1.55, CI = 1.32 to 1.82) during the average 37 months of follow-up.[4] The increased mortality was seen primarily in the diabetic patients with ischemic cardiomyopathy.[45]

Factors Responsible for the Increased Incidence of Heart Failure in Diabetic Patients

Coronary Heart Disease

As already noted, diabetes is a major risk factor for acute MI. Following an acute MI, the presence of diabetes increases the risk of developing new CHF.[1] Using the OASIS registry, which provided long-term data on 8013 patients with unstable coronary syndromes, Malmberg and colleagues showed that diabetes increases the risk of developing new CHF after hospitalization for unstable angina or non-Q-wave MI by 82 percent ($p < 0.001$; Fig. 51–2).[1] In diabetic patients with a history of previous CHD, the risk was considerably higher. The reasons for the increased incidence of CHF following an acute MI are not fully understood, but several factors may contribute. Diabetic patients may have a decreased awareness of pain or an atypical presentation of symptoms during an acute MI (Fig. 51–3).[30] These patients often delay seeking and receiving treatment, leading to more extensive and severe ischemic myocardial damage. In some cases, these patients suffer unrecognized or silent MI, creating a myocardial substrate predisposed to develop heart failure. However, the increased incidence of heart failure in diabetes cannot be accounted for solely by more extensive or severe myocardial infarctions. When the data are adjusted to account for differences in infarct size and baseline risk factors, CHF still occurs much more often in patients with diabetes than in those without the disease.

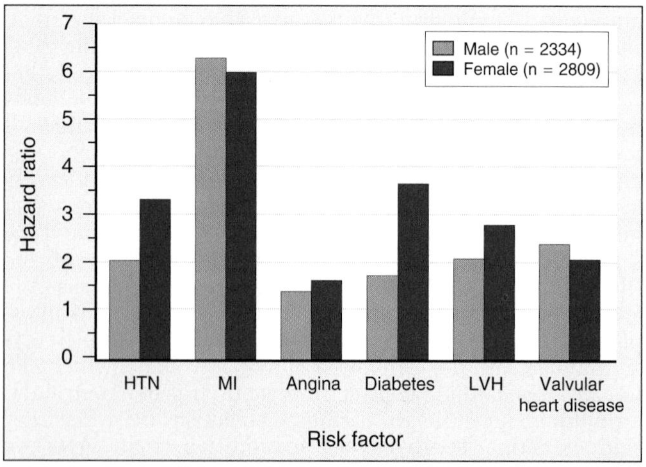

FIGURE 51–1 Risk factors for the development of heart failure in the Framingham Heart Study. In this study diabetes was defined as fasting blood glucose greater than 200 mg/dl or the use of insulin or an oral hypoglycemic agent. HTN = hypertension; LVH = left ventricular hypertrophy; MI = myocardial infarction. (From Levy D, Larson MG, Vasan RS, et al: The progression from hypertension to congestive heart failure. JAMA 275:1557, 1996.)

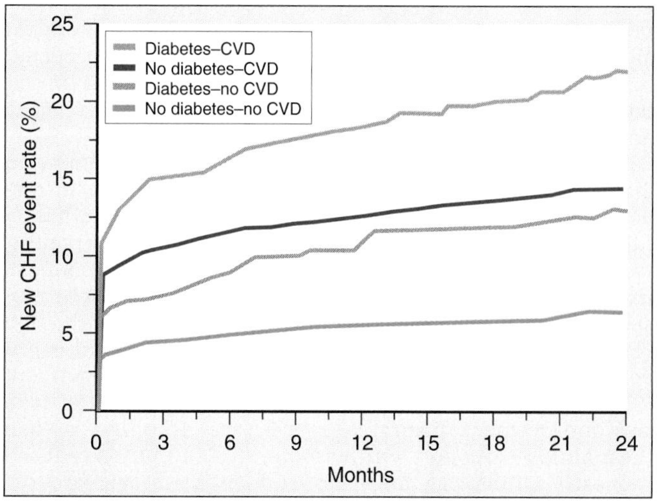

FIGURE 51–2 Heart failure is more prevalent in patients with type 2 diabetes than in those without diabetes after acute coronary syndrome. CHF = congestive heart failure; CVD = cardiovascular disease. (From Malmberg K, Yusuf S, Gerstein HC, et al: Impact of diabetes on long-term prognosis in patients with unstable angina and non-Q-wave myocardial infarction: Results of the OASIS [Organization to Assess Strategies for Ischemic Syndromes] Registry. Circulation 102:1014, 2000.)

Remodeling Following Myocardial Infarction

(see also Chap. 46)

Following a MI, the heart undergoes short- and long-term adaptation in response to the loss of contractile function, a process accentuated in diabetes. In the hours immediately after an acute MI, diabetic patients show less compensatory increase in contractility of noninfarcted myocardium than nondiabetic patients. This deficit persists over time, and thus the diabetic heart may be less capable of adapting to compensate for the loss of stroke volume than the nondiabetic heart. For example, Solomon and colleagues showed that left ventricular size increased less in diabetic patients than in nondiabetic patients in the 2 years following a MI, a difference associated with a twofold higher incidence of heart failure in the diabetic cohort.[46] The failure of the diabetic myocardium to remodel appropriately is probably due to a combination of factors associated with diabetic cardiomyopathy, including heart muscle metabolism, insufficient glucose transport, endothelial dysfunction and impaired control of myocardial blood flow, left ventricular fibrosis leading to impaired filling, and diabetic autonomic dysfunction.[30,47]

Diabetic Cardiomyopathy

The increased incidence of CHF and its poorer prognosis in diabetic patients compared with those without diabetes suggest alterations in the underlying myocardium in the diabetic patient, rendering it more susceptible to ischemia and less able to recover after an ischemic insult. Over the years, substantial evidence has accumulated that a specific, "true" diabetic cardiomyopathy distinct from ischemic injury does indeed exist. The exact prevalence, nature, and cause of cardiac dysfunction directly attributable to diabetes have given rise to considerable debate because other factors common in diabetes, such as hypertension, coronary atherosclerosis, and microvascular dysfunction, can independently impair myocardial performance (Fig. 51–4).

Epidemiological Evidence

Epidemiological studies using case-control analyses have confirmed the association between diabetes and idiopathic cardiomyopathy in men and in women, and have emphasized a possible interaction between diabetes and a history of hypertension. In men screened for the Multiple Risk Factor Intervention Trial (MRFIT) who had cardiomyopathy, diabetes was a risk factor for mortality. By combining the original Framingham Study cohort and the Framingham Offspring Study, gender-specific linear regression analysis probed the contribution of diabetes and glucose intolerance to age-adjusted echocardiographic parameters in more than 4500 men and women.[48] Diabetic individuals, particularly women, had higher heart rates, greater left ventricular wall thicknesses, and greater cardiac mass than unaffected subjects. In a reexamination of 2623 participants in the Framingham Offspring Study who had no history of myocardial infarction or heart failure, worsening glucose intolerance was associated with increasing left ventricular mass, a finding that was more significant ($p < 0.001$) in women than in men ($p = 0.054$).[48]

PATHOLOGICAL FINDINGS

Autopsy and biopsy specimens from diabetic patients with heart failure have revealed a number of morphological changes, including myocardial hypertrophy, myocyte hypertrophy, myofibril depletion, interstitial fibrosis, increased microvascular basement membrane thickness, increased matrix and basement membrane within arteriolar walls, and intramyocardial microangiopathy.[49] None of these lesions is specific to diabetes, and all can be found to some degree in cardiomyopathy of other etiologies. However, the coexistence of diabetes and other risk factors for cardiomyopathy can amplify the pathology. For example,

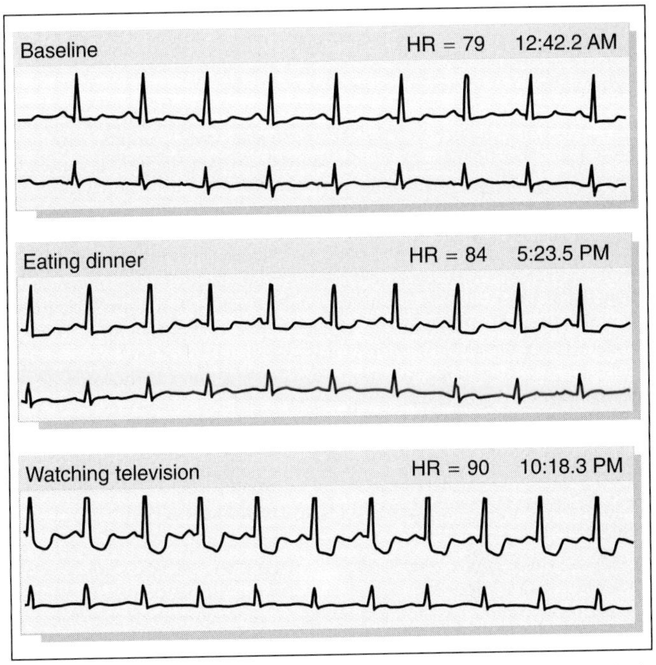

FIGURE 51–3 Holter ST segment monitoring shows no ST changes at baseline in the tracing **(top)**. Two episodes of ST depression **(middle, bottom)** are identified, demonstrating asymptomatic ischemia at rest. The lack of angina is due to cardiac autonomic neuropathy in diabetes. HR = heart rate.

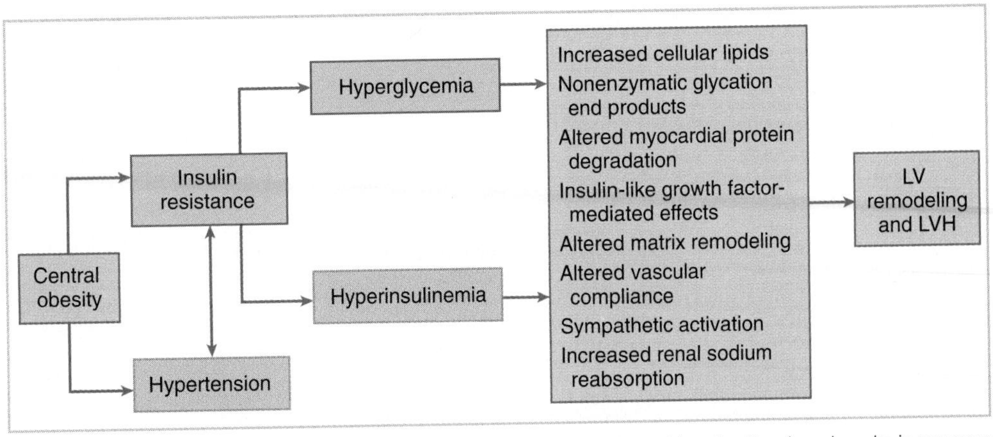

FIGURE 51–4 Central obesity is related to insulin resistance, hyperglycemia, and hyperinsulinemia and results in numerous mechanisms that may lead to remodeling of the left ventricle (LV) and left ventricular hypertrophy (LVH). Such mechanisms may also render the heart more vulnerable to maladaptive remodeling after myocardial injury. (From Rutter MK, Parise H, Benjamin EJ, et al: Impact of glucose intolerance and insulin resistance on cardiac structure and function: Sex-related differences in the Framingham Heart Study. Circulation 107:448, 2003.)

TABLE 51–1 Possible Contributors to Diabetic Cardiomyopathy

Collagen accumulation leading to decreased myocardial compliance
Accumulation of advanced glycosylation end product–modified extracellular matrix proteins causing diastolic dysfunction
Direct effects of altered energy substrate supply and utilization
Abnormal myocardial calcium handling leading to abnormal cardiac mechanics
Endothelial dysfunction characterized by decreased bioavailability of nitric oxide
Deposition of intramyocardial fat secondary to increased circulating free fatty acids
Cardiac autonomic neuropathy
Genetic abnormalities

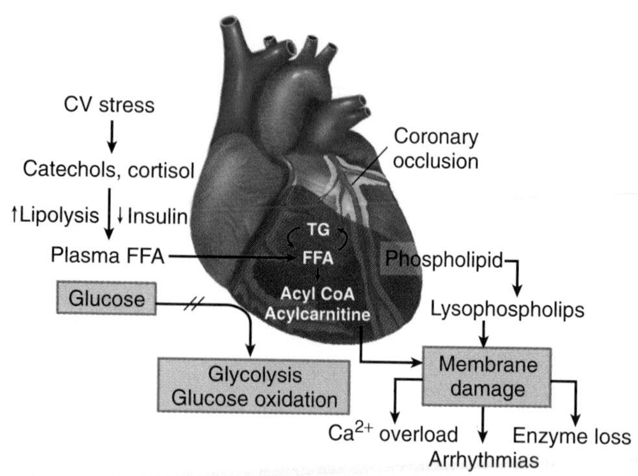

FIGURE 51–5 In the setting of insulin resistance, there is a release of free fatty acids (FFAs) from adipose tissue into the plasma. FFA becomes the dominant fuel for myocardial energy in the form of free fatty acid oxidation within cardiac myocytes. In addition, the rise in plasma free fatty acids leads to a decrease in glycolysis and glucose oxidation in these cells. Free fatty acid oxidation is a less efficient means of generating adenosine triphosphate than glucose oxidation (see text for details). CoA = coenzyme A; CV = cardiovascular; TG = triglyceride. (Adapted from Oliver MF, Opie LH: Effects of glucose and fatty acids on myocardial ischaemia and arrhythmias. Lancet 343:155, 1994.)

endomyocardial biopsy or autopsy specimens from patients with diabetes have shown that the ultrastructural changes, including capillary basement membrane thickening and interstitial and myocardial fibrosis, are accentuated by coexisting hypertension.[50]

Noninvasive methods have confirmed fibrosis as a key feature of the heart in diabetic patients without evident cardiac disease. Increased levels of collagen have been detected in patients with type 1 or type 2 diabetes, as have changes in left ventricular diastolic function.[51] Changes in left ventricular function can occur even in patients with well-controlled type 2 diabetes. One study used magnetic resonance imaging to measure left ventricular function in 12 asymptomatic normotensive newly diagnosed type 2 diabetic patients compared with 12 control subjects. The diabetic patients had normal left ventricular mass and systolic function, but all measures of left ventricular diastolic function were reduced compared with those in the control group.[52]

MECHANISMS OF DIABETIC CARDIOMYOPATHY (Table 51–1)

ADVANCED GLYCATION END PRODUCTS. Because the lesions described earlier occur together in diabetes, the metabolic derangements of diabetes account for the morphological changes seen in the diabetic heart. AGEs accumulate in tissue exposed to hyperglycemia and are implicated in the morphological changes that occur in the diabetic heart. Accumulation of AGE-modified extracellular matrix results in inelasticity of the vessel wall and could interfere with myocardial function as well. Serum levels of AGEs correlate with microvascular and renal complications in type 1 diabetes. In 52 patients with type 1 diabetes, prolongation of the isovolumic relaxation time as assessed by Doppler echocardiography correlated with serum levels of AGEs after adjustment for age, diabetes duration, renal function, blood pressure, and autonomic function parameters.[53] Experimental studies in diabetic dogs have also shown decreased left ventricular compliance associated with intramyocardial deposition of collagen in the absence of hypertrophy.[54] These data help explain the clinical observation that diabetic patients can have CHF as a result of diastolic dysfunction in the absence of hypertension or increased wall thickness, or both.

MYOCARDIAL CALCIUM HANDLING. Abnormalities in myocardial calcium handling may also contribute to abnormal cardiac mechanics in the diabetic heart. Insulin-dependent diabetes impairs sarcoplasmic reticular Ca^{2+} pump activities, which reduces the rate of calcium removal from the cytoplasm in diastole.[55] Such alterations may contribute to the increased diastolic stiffness characteristic of diabetic cardiomyopathy. Diabetes-related changes in troponin T, the contractile regulatory protein of the thin myofilament, may also contribute to both diastolic and systolic dysfunction.

MYOCARDIAL METABOLISM (Fig. 51–5). The direct effects of hyperglycemia and insulin resistance on myocardial cellular metabolism may contribute to chronic left ventricular dysfunction (cardiomyopathy) in diabetes. Altered energy substrate supply and utilization may explain some of the morphological changes seen in the diabetic heart.[56,57] Type 2 diabetes has complex effects on the energy metabolism of the heart. Normally, the heart uses nonesterified (or "free") fatty acids as its primary energy source during aerobic perfusion at normal workloads and increasingly relies on glycolysis and pyruvate oxidation during periods of ischemia or increased work. Because of reduced glucose transport into cardiac myocytes, the diabetic heart can have an exaggerated impairment in ATP generation by glycolysis during ischemia. Accumulated free fatty acids and their oxidation products may also be directly toxic to the myocardial cells and thus contribute to the development of diabetic cardiomyopathy.[57]

CORONARY MICROCIRCULATION. Not only do diabetic patients suffer more severe and diffuse CAD,[58] but also, as noted previously, the structure and function of the coronary microcirculation may be abnormal in diabetes and contribute to the development of CHF. Endothelial dysfunction, characterized by reduced synthesis or bioavailability of the potent vasodilator nitric oxide, commonly occurs in the diabetic coronary vasculature and may lead to abnormal control of blood flow (see also Chap. 40). Despite endothelial dysfunction, resting coronary blood flow in diabetic subjects is normal or even slightly elevated.[59] However, diabetic patients have reduced capacity of the myocardial circulation to vasodilate. When maximal coronary blood flow is measured during intracoronary infusion of a non-endothelium-dependent vasodilator (e.g., papaverine, dipyridamole, adenosine), diabetic subjects exhibit a smaller increase, or coronary reserve, than nondiabetic subjects.[59,60]

The angiogenic response to ischemia also appears to be impaired in diabetes. In a study of 205 diabetic and 205 nondiabetic patients undergoing coronary angiography, Abaci and coworkers[61] determined functional collateral blood vessel formation. Collateral formation was significantly less in the diabetic cohort than in the normal subjects, and the authors speculated that this observation might explain why diabetic patients have such a poor prognosis following myocardial infarction. Others have reported substantially lower capillary density in diabetic patients who had experienced a MI than in patients without diabetes (with or without a previous MI) or in diabetic patients who had not had a prior MI.[62] This failure of the diabetic heart to mount an appropriate angiogenic response following a MI may contribute to diabetic cardiomyopathy.

FAILURE OF ISCHEMIC PRECONDITIONING. Ischemic preconditioning describes the observation that short periods of transient ischemia protect the myocardium against subsequent, longer ischemic insults. Evidence of this protective effect has been shown in animal experiments[63] and in human myocardial biopsy samples.[64] Diabetes appears to eliminate ischemic preconditioning in human myocardium.[64,65] The opening of myocardial adenosine triphosphate (ATP)-sensitive potassium (K_{ATP}) channels is an essential factor in ischemic preconditioning, and the clinical use of sulfonylureas, which block K_{ATP} channels, by type 2 diabetic patients has engendered controversy, as discussed in more detail in a later section.

Reducing the Risk of Heart Failure in Diabetes

Glycemic Control

Poor glycemic control increases the risk of developing heart failure in diabetes.[66] Two studies clearly illustrate the relationship between glycemic control and the incidence of heart failure in diabetes. Iribarren and colleagues observed a group of 48,858 diabetic subjects with no history of heart failure for a median period of 2.2 years after measurement of Hb A_{1c} levels.[66] The incidence of hospitalizations for heart failure or death related to heart failure depended on baseline Hb A_{1c} in the diabetic cohort. The association was stronger in men than in women. In men, each absolute 1 percent increase in Hb A_{1c} was associated with a 12 percent increase (CI = 7 to 18 percent) in heart failure after adjustment for other factors, including use of ACE inhibitors, beta blockers, and incidence of MI during the follow-up period. In women, each absolute 1 percent increase in Hb A_{1c} was associated with a 4 percent increase (CI = −2 to 9 percent) in heart failure. A similar, although steeper, relationship was found in the United Kingdom Prospective Diabetes Study (UKPDS)[67] among 4585 participants with type 2 diabetes. During the 7.5- to 12.5-year follow-up period, each absolute 1 percent increase in average Hb A_{1c} was associated with a 16 percent increase in the incidence of heart failure ($p = 0.021$). These studies suggest that tight glycemic control might reduce the incidence of heart failure, and because no threshold was identified, the target Hb A_{1c} levels should be as close to normal as possible.

Control of Blood Pressure

Diabetes and hypertension often occur together, and this combination amplifies the morphological changes seen in diabetic cardiomyopathy. In UKPDS, systolic blood pressure was associated strongly with the incidence of nonfatal heart failure.[68] For each 10 mm Hg increase in systolic blood pressure, a 12 percent increase in the risk of heart failure ($p = 0.0028$) was observed. In the treatment phase of the study, 1148 hypertensive type 2 diabetic patients received either tight control (target blood pressure <150/85 mm Hg using either captopril or atenolol as the primary drug) or less tight control of blood pressure (target blood pressure <180/105 mm Hg avoiding the use of ACE inhibitors or beta blockers), and follow-up was for a median of 8.4 years.[69] The average blood pressure achieved in the two treatment groups was 144/82 mm Hg in the tight control group and 154/87 mm Hg in the less tight group. This small difference in average blood pressure was associated with a large difference in the incidence of heart failure—the incidence of heart failure fell by 56 percent in the tight control group compared with the less tight control group (2.77 versus 6.15 percent, $p = 0.0043$). In the tight control group, those treated with captopril or those treated with atenolol showed no difference in the incidence of heart failure (3.00 versus 2.51 percent, $p = 0.66$).[70]

The Antihypertensive and Lipid-Lowering Treatment to Prevent Heart Attack Trial (ALLHAT) addressed the issue of whether a certain class of antihypertensive drugs might more effectively reduce the incidence of heart failure in hypertensive diabetic patients.[71] In ALLHAT, a calcium channel blocker (amlodipine) or an ACE inhibitor (lisinopril) was compared with a thiazide diuretic (chlorthalidone) as first-line therapy for their ability to prevent cardiovascular events in 33,357 hypertensive subjects, 36 percent of whom were diabetic at baseline. During the average 4.9-year follow-up, the incidence of new-onset heart failure in the diabetic patients was significantly lower in the thiazide diuretic group than in either of the other treatment groups. The Second Australian National Blood Pressure Study had few diabetic patients and showed no treatment-dependent difference in the incidence of heart failure.[72]

Medical Therapy to Treat or Prevent Heart Failure in Diabetic Patients

The goals of treatment of left ventricular dysfunction and heart failure in diabetic patients are the same as those in nondiabetic patients: relief of pulmonary congestion, slowing the progression of the disease, and prolonging survival. In general, drug therapies for heart failure have similar if not better efficacy in diabetic patients than in those without the disease.

Beta-Adrenergic Blocking Agents

As noted earlier, beta blockers reduce mortality and reinfarction in diabetic patients after a MI. These benefits also extend to diabetic patients with heart failure of various severities.[73-79] The mortality benefit in patients with heart failure has been seen with nonselective beta blockers (e.g., bucindolol[73,79]), with cardioselective beta blockers (e.g., metoprolol[75]), and with a nonselective beta blocker that also blocks $alpha_1$-adrenergic receptors (carvedilol[77,80]). Beta blockers with intrinsic sympathomimetic activity, such as pindolol, may be contraindicated in patients with heart failure, particularly in diabetic patients with heart failure. Carvedilol may offer advantages in the diabetic patients because of its favorable effects on insulin sensitivity and plasma lipid profile as well as its peripheral vasodilating activity. In the Carvedilol Or Metoprolol European Trial (COMET), patients with New York Heart Association (NYHA) Class II to IV heart failure were randomly assigned to either carvedilol or metoprolol and observed for a mean of 5 years.[80] All-cause mortality was reduced by 17 percent in the carvedilol group compared with the metoprolol group. A similar benefit of carvedilol was seen in the 24 percent of the study population who were diabetic at baseline.

Angiotensin-Converting Enzyme Inhibitors

ACE inhibitors clearly and convincingly reduce the morbidity and mortality associated with left ventricular dysfunction, but the early studies lacked sufficient power to address rigorously the question of whether ACE inhibitors could influence the morbidity and mortality associated with diabetes and heart failure. Several more recent studies have addressed these questions and have shown that, indeed, ACE inhibitors are effective in diabetic patients.

In GISSI-3, lisinopril reduced 6-week and 6-month mortality in the diabetic subgroup when started within 24 hours of an acute MI but did not affect the incidence of heart failure or other signs of left ventricular dysfunction.[31] In the TRACE study,[32] patients with an enzyme-confirmed acute MI and left ventricular dysfunction (left ventricular ejection fraction ≤35 percent) present 2 to 6 days after the MI were randomly assigned to receive either the ACE inhibitor trandolapril or matching placebo. In the diabetic group, trandolapril reduced the rate of progression to severe heart failure by 62 percent ($p < 0.001$), a beneficial effect not seen in those without diabetes (Fig. 51–6).

Angiotensin II Receptor Blockers

In three major studies involving patients with chronic heart failure, angiotensin II receptor blockers (ARBs) have demonstrated rough equivalence to ACE inhibitors in preventing morbidity and mortality associated with heart failure.[81-83] However, this benefit may be smaller in the diabetic cohort.[82,83] Two studies of the ARB losartan suggest that this

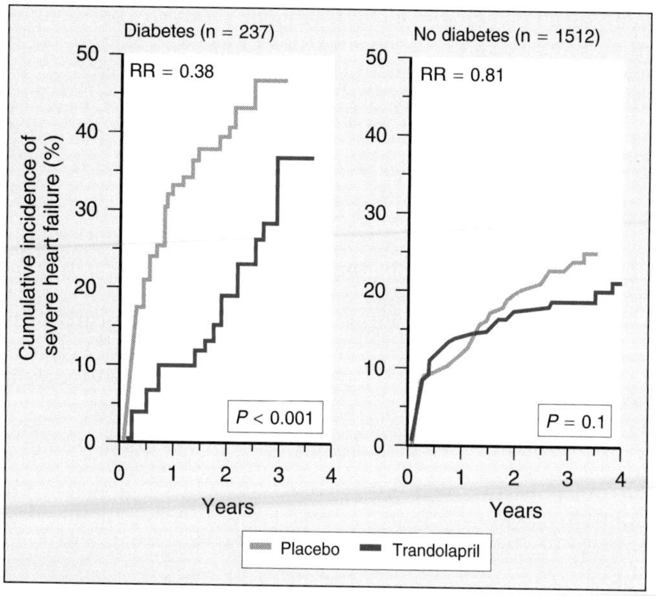

FIGURE 51–6 The Trandolapril Cardiac Evaluation (TRACE) study was carried out in patients with myocardial infarction with congestive heart failure (CHF), depressed ejection fraction, and anterior infarction. The diabetic cohort demonstrated the benefit of trandolapril in a reduction of the high incidence of early and late CHF in patients with diabetes. RR = relative risk. (From Gustafsson I, Torp-Pedersen C, Kober L, et al: Effect of the angiotensin-converting enzyme inhibitor trandolapril on mortality and morbidity in diabetic patients with left ventricular dysfunction after acute myocardial infarction. TRACE Study Group. J Am Coll Cardiol 34:83, 1999%.)

pharmacological class may prevent heart failure in type 2 diabetes. In the Reduction in Endpoints in NIDDM with the Angiotensin II Antagonist Losartan (RENAAL) study,[84] type 2 diabetic patients with nephropathy and no history of heart failure received either losartan or placebo in addition to conventional antihypertensive therapy. In addition to slowing of the progression of kidney failure over the 4-year study, the incidence of heart failure was reduced by 32 percent in the losartan group ($p = 0.005$). In the Losartan Intervention For Endpoint Reduction (LIFE) study, 1195 diabetic patients with hypertension and signs of left ventricular hypertrophy were randomly assigned either losartan or atenolol as the primary antihypertensive agent and were observed for an average of 4.7 years.[85] Not only was the incidence of the primary composite endpoint (cardiovascular death, MI, or stroke) reduced but hospitalizations for heart failure also fell by 41 percent ($p = 0.013$).

ARBs are well tolerated and have an excellent safety record. With ARBs, unlike ACE inhibitors, the incidence of cough is no higher than in patients treated with placebo and angioedema occurs rarely. However, despite these advantages, until results of clinical studies clearly demonstrate superiority or equivalence to ACE inhibitors in the treatment of heart failure, ARBs should probably be reserved for patients who are unable to tolerate ACE inhibition. Currently, only valsartan is approved for this indication

Aldosterone Antagonists

Aldosterone was traditionally thought to contribute to the pathophysiology of heart failure only through its action to increase sodium retention and potassium excretion. However, aldosterone may stimulate directly the production of inflammatory mediators, cause myocardial fibrosis, and promote endothelial dysfunction and vascular stiffening.[86,87] Evidence of the benefit of blocking aldosterone receptors was presented in the results of the Eplerenone Post-Acute Myocardial Infarction Heart Failure Efficacy and Survival Study (EPHESUS).[88] In EPHESUS, the mineralocorticoid-selective aldosterone antagonist eplerenone was added to optimal therapy (usually ACE inhibition 87 percent, beta blockade 75 percent, diuretics 60 percent, and aspirin 88 percent) in patients who had suffered a recent myocardial infarction with documented reduction in left ventricular ejection fraction and symptoms of heart failure. With this treatment, compared with placebo, the risk of death from cardiovascular causes or hospitalizations for cardiovascular causes was reduced by 13 percent ($p = 0.002$). This benefit was similar in diabetic patients, who were 32 percent of the total population of patients, but the study was not powered to evaluate the effect fully in this subgroup.

Treating Diabetes in Patients with Coronary Heart Disease, Acute Coronary Syndromes, or Heart Failure

Sulfonylureas

In the 1970s, evidence emerged that suggested that the sulfonylurea tolbutamide increased cardiovascular mortality and CAD compared with results for patients with type 2 diabetes treated with insulin. The sulfonylureas induce insulin release through a mechanism involving the blocking of K_{ATP} channels in pancreatic beta cells. The discovery that K_{ATP} channels also exist in the myocardium and that blocking them with sulfonylureas prevented ischemic preconditioning, a cardioprotective mechanism, and attenuated coronary vasodilation in animal models[63] suggested a mechanism by which these drugs might promote ischemic injury in diabetic patients. However, the results reported in the UKPDS argue strongly against a proischemic class effect of sulfonylureas. That prospective, randomized study reported the impact of tight glycemic control using a variety of treatment strategies on the incidence and severity of microvascular and macrovascular complications in newly diagnosed diabetes.[89] Patients treated with chlorpropamide or glibenclamide had a rate of myocardial infarction and sudden death over the 10-year follow-up similar to that of patients treated with insulin.

Ischemic preconditioning can be demonstrated with human myocardial biopsy samples[64] and in patients undergoing angioplasty.[90] The presence of diabetes itself appears to attenuate or eliminate ischemic preconditioning in the human heart,[64,65] and certain sulfonylureas may further inhibit this phenomenon. The discovery that cardiac and vascular K_{ATP} channels are structurally distinct from those in the pancreatic beta cells[91] stimulated studies that describe differences in specificity that sulfonylureas may exhibit toward these receptor subtypes. Although clinical extrapolation of these observations is complex, functional differences among the sulfonylureas exist that may have important implications in the treatment of diabetes in patients with CHD. For example, in a double-blind, placebo-controlled study, glibenclamide, but not glimepiride, prevented electrocardiographic evidence of ischemic preconditioning in nondiabetic patients undergoing elective balloon angioplasty of high-grade coronary artery stenoses.[90] A similar difference in response to ischemia has been reported in diabetic patients chronically treated with either glimepiride or glibenclamide.[92] Sulfonylureas may be either proarrhythmic or antiarrhythmic, depending on the presence or absence of ischemia, as a result of the role of the K_{ATP} channel in regulating the duration of the cardiac action potential.[63]

Despite these controversies, this class of hypoglycemic drugs is widely used, given the well-established benefits of improved glycemic control in preventing diabetes-related microvascular complications. However, the choice of specific sulfonylureas for patients with diabetes on the basis of the presence or absence of coronary disease remains unclear at this time.

Thiazolidinediones

Thiazolidinediones (TZDs) decrease glucose levels in type 2 diabetes by increasing the sensitivity to insulin in target tissues.[93] TZDs can increase the incidence of edema, raising concern about the use of these drugs in heart failure.[94] In addition to their glucose lowering ability, these agents induce a wide variety of effects mediated through activation of the PPAR gamma nuclear receptor on liquids, thrombosis, inflammation, and endothelial function that may benefit the cardiovascular system.[94a] An increase in the incidence of heart failure or exacerbation of symptoms has been reported for both rosiglitazone and pioglitazone, particularly when administered concomitantly with insulin.[95] Neither drug is recommended for use in patients with NYHA Class III or IV heart failure.

Metformin

Metformin (dimethylbiguanide) lowers blood glucose both by increasing insulin sensitivity and by decreasing hepatic glucose output.[96] Although epidemiological studies had suggested that the addition of metformin to sulfonylurea therapy was associated with increased mortality, a population-based cohort study involving 12,272 subjects with newly diagnosed type 2 diabetes reported significantly reduced mortality in those treated with metformin monotherapy or metformin combined with a sulfonylurea compared with the patients treated with sulfonylurea monotherapy during the average 5.1-year follow-up.[97]

Lactic acidosis is a rare but potentially life-threatening complication of metformin use, with a reported incidence of about 0.03 cases per 1000 patient-years of use and with a fatality rate of about 50 percent.[98] It occurs more commonly in patients with renal insufficiency or with tissue hypoperfusion and hypoxemia. Because patients with heart failure are at higher risk for hypoperfusion or hypoxemia, the use of metformin is contraindicated in those with CHF who require pharmacological treatment.[98]

Coronary Revascularization

Percutaneous Transluminal Coronary Angioplasty

(see also Chap. 52)

Large-scale trials generally have not shown a benefit of aggressive revascularization after thrombolytic therapy for acute myocardial infarction. Similar considerations apply to diabetic patients. Although diabetic and nondiabetic patients have similar rates of initial angioplasty success, diabetic patients have higher restenosis rates after PTCA[99] and worse long-term outcomes.[100,101]

Diabetic patients also have a higher risk of in-hospital mortality, restenosis, and long-term mortality after coronary artery stenting and atherectomy.[102] Although stenting has reduced restenosis rates in both diabetic and nondiabetic patients, diabetic patients have smaller lumina in the stented vessels and a significantly higher restenosis rate (55 versus 20 percent, $p = 0.001$) within 4 months of the procedure despite similar baseline and procedural characteristics. The mechanism underlying the increased restenosis rate in diabetes after coronary intervention is unclear. Serial intravascular ultrasonography has suggested that exaggerated intimal hyperplasia develops in diabetic patients after intervention.[103] A histological study found increased collagen-rich fibrous tissue in atherectomy specimens from diabetic patients.[104] Clinical trials of paclitaxel- and sirolimus-eluting stents have shown dramatic reductions in the restenosis rates in the general population of patients.[105,106] Although similar benefit has been observed in diabetic patients, the total number of diabetic patients studied has been small, and the studies excluded patients with multivessel disease.[107]

Coronary Artery Bypass Graft Surgery

Most studies comparing outcomes in diabetic and nondiabetic patients undergoing CABG surgery show an increased risk of postoperative death, 30-day and long-term mortality, and an increased need for subsequent reoperation in the diabetic population.[108] Although diabetic patients have a worse risk profile, tend to be older, and have more extensive CAD and poorer left ventricular function than nondiabetic patients,[109] their higher long-term mortality does not depend entirely on these factors and continues to diverge from that in nondiabetic patients during long-term follow-up. The difference probably reflects accelerated disease progression in both the nonbypassed and the bypassed native coronary vessels.

The Bypass Angioplasty Revascularization Investigation (BARI) trial, which included 641 patients with and 2962 patients without diabetes, evaluated the role of CABG in diabetic patients.[110] Five-year mortality was higher in diabetic patients. Q wave myocardial infarction occurred more frequently in diabetic patients (8 versus 4 percent). CABG significantly reduced the mortality after a myocardial infarction when compared with angioplasty, whereas no such protective effect of surgery was noted in nondiabetic patients experiencing a myocardial infarction. After 7 years, CABG showed an even more pronounced benefit over PTCA in patients with treated diabetes.[111]

Coronary Artery Bypass Graft Versus Percutaneous Transluminal Coronary Angioplasty

In general, randomized trials comparing PTCA with CABG have reported similar outcomes. However, in patients with diabetes CABG may provide better outcomes than classical PTCA, especially in patients with three-vessel disease.[112,113] The BARI trial, which randomly assigned patients with multivessel disease to CABG or PTCA, reported that bypass surgery in treated diabetic patients yielded a higher survival rate at 5 years than PTCA (81 versus 66 percent, $p = 0.003$).[113] The benefit of CABG accrued primarily in patients receiving internal mammary artery conduits. Cardiac mortality was 2.9 percent when an internal mammary artery graft was used compared with 18.2 percent when only saphenous vein grafts were used, a mortality similar to that observed with PTCA.[113] Diabetic patients undergoing stenting for multivessel disease may also have a worse outcome than those undergoing CABG. In the Arterial Revascularization Therapy Study (ARTS), the 208 patients with diabetes who underwent percutaneous revascularization had a lower 1-year survival (63 percent) than those undergoing CABG (84 percent).[114] In contrast, no difference was detected in the Veterans Affairs Angina With Extremely Serious Operative Mortality Evaluation (AWESOME) study between diabetic patients who underwent PTCA (54 percent with stents) and those who underwent CABG.[115] Survival was similar in the two groups at 30 days, 6 months, and 36 months.

Cardiovascular Autonomic Neuropathy

(see also Chap. 87)

Cardiovascular autonomic neuropathy (CAN) probably contributes to the poor prognosis of CHD and CHF in both type 1 and type 2 diabetes mellitus. The majority of patients with CAN come to clinical attention with complaints of postural hypotension, resting tachycardia, exercise intolerance, or painless myocardial ischemia or infarction. The risk for CAN depends on the duration of diabetes and the degree of glycemic control and tends to parallel the development of other end-organ disease related to diabetes such as retinopathy, nephropathy, and vasculopathy.[116] Symptoms and signs of CAN often occur relatively late in the natural history of this complication. Because reliable and quantitative noninvasive methods to assess autonomic function have become available, the diagnosis of CAN may now precede the development of symptoms. Most clinicians regard CAN as a major complication of type 1 diabetes because the challenge of managing this complication often dominates the care of these patients. CAN tends to be less fully expressed in patients with type 2 diabetes, who are typically older and have a wider variety of comorbid conditions.

DIAGNOSIS. A variety of tests can assess parasympathetic and sympathetic function in diabetes. A series of bedside maneuvers can aid in the diagnosis of CAN and differentiate the relative contribution of parasympathetic and sympathetic dysfunction in CAN. These tests use the electrocardiogram to measure beat-to-beat heart rate variation during deep breathing, at assumption of an upright posture, and during the Valsalva maneuver.[12] Tests that can detect the presence of CAN before symptoms develop include methods that assess heart rate variability during 24-hour recordings and thereby permit detection of subtle disorders in autonomic balance. Cardiac radionuclide imaging with the norepinephrine analog metaiodobenzylguanidine (MIBG) can directly image the sympathetic nerve activity of the myocardium. Diabetic individuals generally have less myocardial MIBG uptake with more pronounced regional differences from base to apex than patients without diabetes. In addition, positron-emission tomographic scanning with the sympathetic neurotransmitter analog ^{11}C-labeled hydroxyephedrine can evaluate myocardial sympathetic innervation. These noninvasive methods, alone or in combination with the standard bedside examination, can establish the presence and severity of CAN and can be used to evaluate the effects of interventions.

PREVALENCE. The reported prevalence of CAN varies with the populations studied and methods used. Regardless of this variation, CAN appears to be common in diabetes. A summary of 15 reports on CAN suggests that the prevalence is between 2.6 and 90 percent in the diabetic population, with an average prevalence of about 30 percent.[12]

PROGNOSIS. Numerous studies have documented increased mortality in diabetic patients with CAN. Maser and colleagues[117] have reviewed 15 studies involving a total of 2900 diabetic patients with and without evidence of CAN. During the follow-up period, which ranged from 0.5 to 16 years, mortality was consistently higher in the patients with CAN (30 percent) than in those without CAN at baseline (13 percent). A pooled estimate of the hazard ratio for CAN in these studies was 3.45 (CI 2.66 to 4.47, $p < 0.001$) for studies using two or more indicators of CAN and 1.20 (CI 1.02 to 1.41, $p = 0.03$) for studies using only one measure to define CAN.

The mechanisms by which CAN increases mortality remain uncertain (Table 51–2). Part of this association may derive from the high prevalence of other complications and risk factors in diabetic patients with CAN. For example, the progression of microvascular complications, such as diabetic nephropathy, appears to parallel that of CAN and can result in an increase in cardiovascular risk related to hypertension and dyslipidemia.[12] CAN may also decrease the perception of myocardial ischemia. Clinicians have long recognized that diabetic patients often experience fewer ischemic symptoms such as angina than do nondiabetic patients. Thus, compared with nondiabetic individuals with exercise-limited ischemia, diabetic individuals with CAN are less likely to be limited by angina at the time of ST segment depression.[118] Resting tachycardia, an early manifestation of parasympathetic denervation of CAN, increases myocardial oxygen demand and can place the diabetic patient with CAN closer to the ischemic threshold. In addition, CAN can cause abnormal coronary blood flow regulation. Thus, CAN may provoke ischemic episodes by upsetting the balance between myocardial supply and demand.[118]

Sudden cardiovascular death may be related to CAN in diabetic individuals. Prolongation of the QT interval in diabetic patients correlates with the degree of autonomic neuropathy and may predispose these individuals to serious arrhythmias and sudden death.[12,118] The presence of QT dispersion on the 12-lead electrocardiogram reflects dispersion of ventricular refractoriness and an increased risk for arrhythmia. In a study of 471 patients with type 2 diabetes, both QT dispersion and prolongation of the QT interval independently predicted cardiovascular and coronary mortality during the median 5.7-year follow-up.[119]

TABLE 51–2 Cardiovascular Autonomic Neuropathy and Increased Cardiovascular Morbidity and Mortality in Diabetes Mellitus—Possible Mechanisms

Impaired angina recognition
Silent ischemia and infarction
Decreased threshold for ischemia
Increased resting heart rate and blunted chronotropic response to exercise
Impaired coronary vasomotor regulation
Prolonged QT interval
Increased lethal arrhythmias and sudden death (with or without myocardial ischemia)
Abnormal diastolic and systolic function
Contributes to diabetic cardiomyopathy
Increased cardiac mass
Adversely affects the natural history of congestive heart failure
Increased perioperative risk
Increased need for hemodynamic support
Reduced hypoxia-induced respiratory drive
Alteration of normal circadian variation of sympathovagal activity
Lack of normal nighttime decrease in blood pressure
Loss of nighttime protection against myocardial infarction
Increased prevalence of other cardiovascular risk factors and other complications
Increased microvascular complications
Increased rate of progression of glomerulopathy
Increased prevalence of hypertension and dyslipidemias

REFERENCES

Scope of the Problem

1. Malmberg K, Yusuf S, Gerstein HC, et al: Impact of diabetes on long-term prognosis in patients with unstable angina and non-Q-wave myocardial infarction: Results of the OASIS (Organization to Assess Strategies for Ischemic Syndromes) Registry. Circulation 102:1014, 2000.
2. Mukamal KJ, Nesto RW, Cohen MC, et al: Impact of diabetes on long-term survival after acute myocardial infarction: Comparability of risk with prior myocardial infarction. Diabetes Care 24:1422, 2001.
3. Nichols GA, Hillier TA, Erbey JR, et al: Congestive heart failure in type 2 diabetes: Prevalence, incidence, and risk factors. Diabetes Care 24:1614, 2001.
4. Shindler DM, Kostis JB, Yusuf S, et al: Diabetes mellitus, a predictor of morbidity and mortality in the Studies of Left Ventricular Dysfunction (SOLVD) Trials and Registry. Am J Cardiol 77:1017, 1996.
5. Moreno PR, Murcia AM, Palacios IF, et al: Coronary composition and macrophage infiltration in atherectomy specimens from patients with diabetes mellitus. Circulation 102:2180, 2000.
6. Colwell JA, Nesto RW: The platelet in diabetes: Focus on prevention of ischemic events. Diabetes Care 26:2181, 2003.
7. Sobel BE, Woodcock-Mitchell J, Schneider DJ, et al: Increased plasminogen activator inhibitor type 1 in coronary artery atherectomy specimens from type 2 diabetic compared with nondiabetic patients: A potential factor predisposing to thrombosis and its persistence. Circulation 97:2213, 1998.
8. Pandolfi A, Cetrullo D, Polishuck R, et al: Plasminogen activator inhibitor type 1 is increased in the arterial wall of type II diabetic subjects. Arterioscler Thromb Vasc Biol 21:1378, 2001.
9. Cosentino F, Eto M, De Paolis P, et al: High glucose causes upregulation of cyclooxygenase-2 and alters prostanoid profile in human endothelial cells: Role of protein kinase C and reactive oxygen species. Circulation 107:1017, 2003.
10. Cardillo C, Campia U, Bryant MB, et al: Increased activity of endogenous endothelin in patients with type II diabetes mellitus. Circulation 106:1783, 2002.
11. Ford ES: Body mass index, diabetes, and C-reactive protein among U.S. adults. Diabetes Care 22:1971, 1999.
12. Vinik AI, Maser RE, Mitchell BD, et al: Diabetic autonomic neuropathy. Diabetes Care 26:1553, 2003.

Medical Therapy of Acute Coronary Syndromes

13. Taubert G, Winkelmann BR, Schleiffer T, et al: Prevalence, predictors, and consequences of unrecognized diabetes mellitus in 3266 patients scheduled for coronary angiography. Am Heart J 145:285, 2003.
14. Norhammar A, Tenerz A, Nilsson G, et al: Glucose metabolism in patients with acute myocardial infarction and no previous diagnosis of diabetes mellitus: A prospective study. Lancet 359:2140, 2002.

15. Wahab NN, Cowden EA, Pearce NJ, et al: Is blood glucose an independent predictor of mortality in acute myocardial infarction in the thrombolytic era? J Am Coll Cardiol 40:1748, 2002.
16. Norhammar AM, Ryden L, Malmberg K: Admission plasma glucose. Independent risk factor for long-term prognosis after myocardial infarction even in nondiabetic patients. Diabetes Care 22:1827, 1999.
17. Colwell JA: Aspirin therapy in diabetes. Diabetes Care 26:S87, 2003.
18. A randomised, blinded, trial of clopidogrel versus aspirin in patients at risk of ischaemic events (CAPRIE). CAPRIE Steering Committee. Lancet 348:1329, 1996.
19. Bhatt DL, Marso SP, Hirsch AT, et al: Amplified benefit of clopidogrel versus aspirin in patients with diabetes mellitus. Am J Cardiol 90:625, 2002.
20. Yusuf S, Zhao F, Mehta SR, et al: Effects of clopidogrel in addition to aspirin in patients with acute coronary syndromes without ST-segment elevation. N Engl J Med 345:494, 2001.
21. Lincoff AM: Important triad in cardiovascular medicine: Diabetes, coronary intervention, and platelet glycoprotein IIb/IIIa receptor blockade. Circulation 107:1556, 2003.
22. Kereiakes DJ, Lincoff AM, Anderson KM, et al: Abciximab survival advantage following percutaneous coronary intervention is predicted by clinical risk profile. Am J Cardiol 90:628, 2002.
23. Topol EJ, Mark DB, Lincoff AM, et al: Outcomes at 1 year and economic implications of platelet glycoprotein IIb/IIIa blockade in patients undergoing coronary stenting: Results from a multicentre randomised trial. EPISTENT Investigators. Evaluation of Platelet IIb/IIIa Inhibitor for Stenting. Lancet 354:2019, 1999.
24. Labinaz M, Madan M, O'Shea JO, et al: Comparison of one-year outcomes following coronary artery stenting in diabetic versus nondiabetic patients (from the Enhanced Suppression of the Platelet IIb/IIIa Receptor With Integrilin Therapy [ESPRIT] trial). Am J Cardiol 90:585, 2002.
25. Roffi M, Chew DP, Mukherjee D, et al: Platelet glycoprotein IIb/IIIa inhibitors reduce mortality in diabetic patients with non-ST-segment-elevation acute coronary syndromes. Circulation 104:2767, 2001.
26. Heitzer T, Ollmann I, Koke K, et al: Platelet glycoprotein IIb/IIIa receptor blockade improves vascular nitric oxide bioavailability in patients with coronary artery disease. Circulation 108:536, 2003.
27. Chen J, Marciniak TA, Radford MJ, et al: Beta-blocker therapy for secondary prevention of myocardial infarction in elderly diabetic patients. Results from the National Cooperative Cardiovascular Project. J Am Coll Cardiol 34:1388, 1999.
28. Shorr RI, Ray WA, Daugherty JR, et al: Antihypertensives and the risk of serious hypoglycemia in older persons using insulin or sulfonylureas. JAMA 278:40, 1997.
29. Gress TW, Nieto FJ, Shahar E, et al: Hypertension and antihypertensive therapy as risk factors for type 2 diabetes mellitus. N Engl J Med 342:905, 2000.
30. Nesto RW, Zarich S: Acute myocardial infarction in diabetes mellitus: Lessons learned from ACE inhibition. Circulation 97:12, 1998.
31. Zuanetti G, Latini R, Maggioni AP, et al: Effect of the ACE inhibitor lisinopril on mortality in diabetic patients with acute myocardial infarction: Data from the GISSI-3 study. Circulation 96:4239, 1997.
32. Gustafsson I, Torp-Pedersen C, Køber L, et al: Effect of the angiotensin-converting enzyme inhibitor trandolapril on mortality and morbidity in diabetic patients with left ventricular dysfunction after acute myocardial infarction. Trace Study Group. J Am Coll Cardiol 34:83, 1999.
33. McFarlane SI, Kumar A, Sowers JR: Mechanisms by which angiotensin-converting enzyme inhibitors prevent diabetes and cardiovascular disease. Am J Cardiol 91:30H, 2003.
34. Effects of ramipril on cardiovascular and microvascular outcomes in people with diabetes mellitus: Results of the HOPE study and MICRO-HOPE substudy. Lancet 355:253, 2000.
35. Capes SE, Hunt D, Malmberg K, et al: Stress hyperglycaemia and increased risk of death after myocardial infarction in patients with and without diabetes: A systematic overview. Lancet 355:773, 2000.
36. Malmberg K, Ryden L, Efendic S, et al: Randomized trial of insulin-glucose infusion followed by subcutaneous insulin treatment in diabetic patients with acute myocardial infarction (DIGAMI study): Effects on mortality at 1 year. J Am Coll Cardiol 26:57, 1995.
37. Malmberg K, Norhammar A, Wedel H, et al: Glycometabolic state at admission: Important risk marker of mortality in conventionally treated patients with diabetes mellitus and acute myocardial infarction: Long-term results from the Diabetes and Insulin-Glucose Infusion in Acute Myocardial Infarction (DIGAMI) study. Circulation 99:2626, 1999.
38. Furnary AP, Gao G, Grunkemeier GL, et al: Continuous insulin infusion reduces mortality in patients with diabetes undergoing coronary artery bypass grafting. J Thorac Cardiovasc Surg 125:1007, 2003.
39. Fath-Ordoubadi F, Beatt KJ: Glucose-insulin-potassium therapy for treatment of acute myocardial infarction: An overview of randomized placebo-controlled trials. Circulation 96:1152, 1997.
40. van der Horst IC, Zijlstra F, van't Hof AW, et al: Glucose-insulin-potassium infusion inpatients treated with primary angioplasty for acute myocardial infarction: The glucose-insulin-potassium study: A randomized trial. J Am Coll Cardiol 42:784, 2003.
41. Szabo Z, Arnqvist H, Hakanson E, et al: Effects of high-dose glucose-insulin-potassium on myocardial metabolism after coronary surgery in patients with type II diabetes. Clin Sci (Lond) 101:37, 2001.
42. Lazar HL, Chipkin S, Philippides G, et al: Glucose-insulin-potassium solutions improve outcomes in diabetics who have coronary artery operations. Ann Thorac Surg 70:145, 2000.

Heart Failure

43. Levy D, Larson MG, Vasan RS, et al: The progression from hypertension to congestive heart failure. JAMA 275:1557, 1996.
44. Reis SE, Holubkov R, Edmundowicz D, et al: Treatment of patients admitted to the hospital with congestive heart failure: Specialty-related disparities in practice patterns and outcomes. J Am Coll Cardiol 30:733, 1997.
45. Dries DL, Sweitzer NK, Drazner MH, et al: Prognostic impact of diabetes mellitus in patients with heart failure according to the etiology of left ventricular systolic dysfunction. J Am Coll Cardiol 38:421, 2001.
46. Solomon SD, St John Sutton M, Lamas GA, et al: Ventricular remodeling does not accompany the development of heart failure in diabetic patients after myocardial infarction. Circulation 106:1251, 2002.
47. Standl E, Schnell O: A new look at the heart in diabetes mellitus: From ailing to failing. Diabetologia 43:1455, 2000.

Diabetic Cardiomyopathy

48. Rutter MK, Parise H, Benjamin EJ, et al: Impact of glucose intolerance and insulin resistance on cardiac structure and function: Sex-related differences in the Framingham Heart Study. Circulation 107:448, 2003.
49. Zarich SW, Nesto RW: Diabetic cardiomyopathy. Am Heart J 118:1000, 1989.
50. Kawaguchi M, Techigawara M, Ishihata T, et al: A comparison of ultrastructural changes on endomyocardial biopsy specimens obtained from patients with diabetes mellitus with and without hypertension. Heart Vessels 12:267, 1997.
51. Picano E: Diabetic cardiomyopathy. The importance of being earliest. J Am Coll Cardiol 42:454, 2003.
52. Diamant M, Lamb HJ, Groeneveld Y, et al: Diastolic dysfunction is associated with altered myocardial metabolism in asymptomatic normotensive patients with well-controlled type 2 diabetes mellitus. J Am Coll Cardiol 42:328, 2003.
53. Berg TJ, Snorgaard O, Faber J, et al: Serum levels of advanced glycation end products are associated with left ventricular diastolic function in patients with type 1 diabetes. Diabetes Care 22:1186, 1999.
54. Avendano GF, Agarwal RK, Bashey RI, et al: Effects of glucose intolerance on myocardial function and collagen-linked glycation. Diabetes 48:1443, 1999.
55. Pierce GN, Russell JC: Regulation of intracellular Ca^{2+} in the heart during diabetes. Cardiovasc Res 34:41, 1997.
56. Taegtmeyer H, McNulty P, Young ME: Adaptation and maladaptation of the heart in diabetes: Part I. Circulation 105:1727, 2002.
57. Young ME, McNulty P, Taegtmeyer H: Adaptation and maladaptation of the heart in diabetes: Part II. Circulation 105:1861, 2002.
58. Ledru F, Ducimetiere P, Battaglia S, et al: New diagnostic criteria for diabetes and coronary artery disease: Insights from an angiographic study. J Am Coll Cardiol 37:1543, 2001.
59. McDonagh PF, Hokama JY: Microvascular perfusion and transport in the diabetic heart. Microcirculation 7:163, 2000.
60. Pitkanen OP, Nuutila P, Raitakari OT, et al: Coronary flow reserve is reduced in young men with IDDM. Diabetes 47:248, 1998.
61. Abaci A, Oguzhan A, Kahraman S, et al: Effect of diabetes mellitus on formation of coronary collateral vessels. Circulation 99:2239, 1999.
62. Yarom R, Zirkin H, Stammler G, et al: Human coronary microvessels in diabetes and ischaemia. Morphometric study of autopsy material. J Pathol 166:265, 1992.
63. Grover GJ, Garlid KD: ATP-sensitive potassium channels: A review of their cardioprotective pharmacology. J Mol Cell Cardiol 32:677, 2000.
64. Ghosh S, Standen NB, Galinianes M: Failure to precondition pathological human myocardium. J Am Coll Cardiol 37:711, 2001.
65. Ishihara M, Inoue I, Kawagoe T, et al: Diabetes mellitus prevents ischemic preconditioning in patients with a first acute anterior wall myocardial infarction. J Am Coll Cardiol 38:1007, 2001.

Reducing the Risk of Heart Failure in Diabetes

66. Iribarren C, Karter AJ, Go AS, et al: Glycemic control and heart failure among adult patients with diabetes. Circulation 103:2668, 2001.
67. Stratton IM, Adler AI, Neil HA, et al: Association of glycaemia with macrovascular and microvascular complications of type 2 diabetes (UKPDS 35): Prospective observational study. BMJ 321:405, 2000.
68. Adler AI, Stratton IM, Neil HA, et al: Association of systolic blood pressure with macrovascular and microvascular complications of type 2 diabetes (UKPDS 36): Prospective observational study. BMJ 321:412, 2000.
69. Tight blood pressure control and risk of macrovascular and microvascular complications in type 2 diabetes: UKPDS 38. BMJ 317:703, 1998.
70. Efficacy of atenolol and captopril in reducing risk of macrovascular and microvascular complications in type 2 diabetes: UKPDS 39. UK Prospective Diabetes Study Group. BMJ 317:713, 1998.
71. Major outcomes in high-risk hypertensive patients randomized to angiotensin-converting enzyme inhibitor or calcium channel blocker vs diuretic: The Antihypertensive and Lipid-Lowering Treatment to Prevent Heart Attack Trial (ALLHAT). JAMA 288:2981, 2002.
72. Wing LM, Reid CM, Ryan P, et al: A comparison of outcomes with angiotensin-converting-enzyme inhibitors and diuretics for hypertension in the elderly. N Engl J Med 348:583, 2003.
73. A trial of the beta-blocker bucindolol in patients with advanced chronic heart failure. N Engl J Med 344:1659, 2001.
74. The cardiac insufficiency bisoprolol study II (CIBIS-II): A randomised trial. Lancet 353:9, 1999.
75. Hjalmarson A, Goldstein S, Fagerberg B, et al: Effects of controlled-release metoprolol on total mortality, hospitalizations, and well-being in patients with heart failure: The Metoprolol CR/XL Randomized Intervention Trial in congestive heart failure (MERIT-HF). JAMA 283:1295, 2000.
76. Packer M, Bristow MR, Cohn JN, et al: The effect of carvedilol on morbidity and mortality in patients with chronic heart failure. N Engl J Med 334:1349, 1996.

77. Packer M, Coats AJ, Fowler MB, et al: Effect of carvedilol on survival in severe chronic heart failure. N Engl J Med 344:1651, 2001.
78. Packer M, Fowler MB, Roecker EB, et al: Effect of carvedilol on the morbidity of patients with severe chronic heart failure: Results of the carvedilol prospective randomized cumulative survival (COPERNICUS) study. Circulation 106:2194, 2002.
79. Domanski M, Krause-Steinrauf H, Deedwania P, et al: The effect of diabetes on outcomes of patients with advanced heart failure in the BEST trial. J Am Coll Cardiol 42:914, 2003.
80. Poole-Wilson PA, Swedberg K, Cleland JG, et al: Comparison of carvedilol and metoprolol on clinical outcomes in patients with chronic heart failure in the Carvedilol Or Metoprolol European Trial (COMET): Randomised controlled trial. Lancet 362:7, 2003.
81. Pitt B, Poole-Wilson PA, Segal R, et al: Effect of losartan compared with captopril on mortality in patients with symptomatic heart failure: Randomised trial—The Losartan Heart Failure Survival Study ELITE II. Lancet 355:1582, 2000.
82. Cohn JN, Tognoni G: A randomized trial of the angiotensin-receptor blocker valsartan in chronic heart failure. N Engl J Med 345:1667, 2001.
83. Pfeffer MA, Swedberg K, Granger CB, et al: Effects of candesartan on mortality and morbidity in patients with chronic heart failure: The CHARM-Overall programme. Lancet 362:759, 2003.
84. Brenner BM, Cooper ME, de Zeeuw D, et al: Effects of losartan on renal and cardiovascular outcomes in patients with type 2 diabetes and nephropathy. N Engl J Med 345:861, 2001.
85. Lindholm LH, Ibsen H, Dahlof B, et al: Cardiovascular morbidity and mortality in patients with diabetes in the Losartan Intervention For Endpoint reduction in hypertension study (LIFE): A randomised trial against atenolol. Lancet 359:1004, 2002.
86. Stier CT Jr, Chander PN, Rocha R: Aldosterone as a mediator in cardiovascular injury. Cardiol Rev 10:97, 2002.
87. Weber KT: Aldosterone in congestive heart failure. N Engl J Med 345:1689, 2001.
88. Pitt B, Remme W, Zannad F, et al: Eplerenone, a selective aldosterone blocker, in patients with left ventricular dysfunction after myocardial infarction. N Engl J Med 348:1309, 2003.

Treating Diabetes in Patients with Coronary Heart Disease, Acute Coronary Syndromes, or Heart Failure

89. Intensive blood-glucose control with sulphonylureas or insulin compared with conventional treatment and risk of complications in patients with type 2 diabetes (UKPDS 33). Lancet 352:837, 1998.
90. Klepzig H, Kober G, Matter C, et al: Sulfonylureas and ischaemic preconditioning; a double-blind, placebo-controlled evaluation of glimepiride and glibenclamide. Eur Heart J 20:439, 1999.
91. Brady PA, Terzic A: The sulfonylurea controversy: More questions from the heart. J Am Coll Cardiol 31:950, 1998.
92. Lee TM, Chou TF: Impairment of myocardial protection in type 2 diabetic patients. J Clin Endocrinol Metab 88:531, 2003.
93. Goldstein BJ: Differentiating members of the thiazolidinedione class: A focus on efficacy. Diabetes Metab Res Rev 18(Suppl 2):S16, 2002.
94. Lebovitz HE: Differentiating members of the thiazolidinedione class: A focus on safety. Diabetes Metab Res Rev 18(Suppl 2):S23, 2002.\
94a. Nesto RW, Bell D, Bonow RO, et al: Thiazolidinedione use, fluid retention, and congestive heart failure: A consensus statement from the American Heart Association and American Diabetes Associaiton. Circulation 108:2941, 2003.
95. Wooltorton E: Rosiglitazone (Avandia) and pioglitazone (Actos) and heart failure. Can Med Assoc J 166:219, 2002.
96. Libby P: Metformin and vascular protection: A cardiologist's view. Diabetes Metab 29:6S117, 2003.
97. Johnson JA, Majumdar SR, Simpson SH, et al: Decreased mortality associated with the use of metformin compared with sulfonylurea monotherapy in type 2 diabetes. Diabetes Care 25:2244, 2002.
98. Bailey CJ, Turner RC: Metformin. N Engl J Med 334:574, 1996.
99. Van Belle E, Bauters C, Hubert E, et al: Restenosis rates in diabetic patients: A comparison of coronary stenting and balloon angioplasty in native coronary vessels. Circulation 96:1454, 1997.
100. Kip KE, Alderman EL, Bourassa MG, et al: Differential influence of diabetes mellitus on increased jeopardized myocardium after initial angioplasty or bypass surgery Bypass angioplasty revascularization investigation. Circulation 105:1914, 2002.
101. Kip KE, Faxon DP, Detre KM, et al: Coronary angioplasty in diabetic patients. The National Heart, Lung, and Blood Institute Percutaneous Transluminal Coronary Angioplasty Registry. Circulation 94:1818, 1996.
102. Reginelli JP, Bhatt DL: Why diabetics are at risk in percutaneous coronary intervention and the appropriate management of diabetics in interventional cardiology. J Invasive Cardiol 14(Suppl E):2E, 2002.
103. Kornowski R, Mintz GS, Kent KM, et al: Increased restenosis in diabetes mellitus after coronary interventions is due to exaggerated intimal hyperplasia. A serial intravascular ultrasound study. Circulation 95:1366, 1997.
104. Moreno PR, Fallon JT, Murcia AM, et al: Tissue characteristics of restenosis after percutaneous transluminal coronary angioplasty in diabetic patients. J Am Coll Cardiol 34:1045, 1999.
105. Chevalier B, DeScheerder I, Gershlick A: Effect on restenosis with a paclitaxel eluting stent: Factors associated with inhibition in the ELUTES clinical study [abstract]. J Am Coll Cardiol 39:59A, 2002.
106. Serruys PW, Degertekin M, Tanabe K, et al: Intravascular ultrasound findings in the multicenter, randomized, double-blind RAVEL (RAndomized study with the sirolimus-eluting VElocity balloon-expandable stent in the treatment of patients with de novo native coronary artery Lesions) trial. Circulation 106:798, 2002.
107. Lepor NE, Madyoon H, Kereiakes D: Effective and efficient strategies for coronary revascularization in the drug-eluting stent era. Rev Cardiovasc Med 3:S38, 2002.
108. Carson JL, Scholz PM, Chen AY, et al: Diabetes mellitus increases short-term mortality and morbidity in patients undergoing coronary artery bypass graft surgery. J Am Coll Cardiol 40:418, 2002.
109. Cohen Y, Raz I, Merin G, et al: Comparison of factors associated with 30-day mortality after coronary artery bypass grafting in patients with versus without diabetes mellitus. Israeli Coronary Artery Bypass (ISCAB) Study Consortium. Am J Cardiol 81:7, 1998.
110. Detre KM, Lombardero MS, Brooks MM, et al: The effect of previous coronary-artery bypass surgery on the prognosis of patients with diabetes who have acute myocardial infarction. Bypass Angioplasty Revascularization Investigation Investigators. N Engl J Med 342:989, 2000.
111. Seven-year outcome in the Bypass Angioplasty Revascularization Investigation (BARI) by treatment and diabetic status. J Am Coll Cardiol 35:1122, 2000.
112. Niles NW, McGrath PD, Malenka D, et al: Survival of patients with diabetes and multivessel coronary artery disease after surgical or percutaneous coronary revascularization: Results of a large regional prospective study. Northern New England Cardiovascular Disease Study Group. J Am Coll Cardiol 37:1008, 2001.
113. Influence of diabetes on 5-year mortality and morbidity in a randomized trial comparing CABG and PTCA in patients with multivessel disease: The Bypass Angioplasty Revascularization Investigation (BARI). Circulation 96:1761, 1997.
114. Abizaid A, Costa MA, Centemero M, et al: Clinical and economic impact of diabetes mellitus on percutaneous and surgical treatment of multivessel coronary disease patients: Insights from the Arterial Revascularization Therapy Study (ARTS) trial. Circulation 104:533, 2001.
115. Sedlis SP, Morrison DA, Lorin JD, et al: Percutaneous coronary intervention versus coronary bypass graft surgery for diabetic patients with unstable angina and risk factors for adverse outcomes with bypass: Outcome of diabetic patients in the AWESOME randomized trial and registry. J Am Coll Cardiol 40:1555, 2002.
116. Valensi P, Huard JP, Giroux C, et al: Factors involved in cardiac autonomic neuropathy in diabetic patients. J Diabetes Complications 11:180, 1997.
117. Maser RE, Mitchell BD, Vinik AI, et al: The association between cardiovascular autonomic neuropathy and mortality in individuals with diabetes: A meta-analysis. Diabetes Care 26:1895, 2003.
118. Nesto RW, Libby P: Diabetes mellitus and the cardiovascular system. *In* Braunwald E, Zipes DP, Libby P (eds): Heart Disease. A Textbook of Cardiovascular Medicine. 6th ed. Philadelphia, WB Saunders, 2001, p 2133.
119. Cardoso CR, Salles GF, Deccache W: Prognostic value of QT interval parameters in type 2 diabetes mellitus: Results of a long-term follow-up prospective study. J Diabetes Complications 17:169, 2003.

CHAPTER 52

Percutaneous Coronary and Valvular Intervention

Jeffrey J. Popma • Richard E. Kuntz • Donald S. Baim

The use of percutaneous coronary intervention (PCI) to treat ischemic coronary artery disease (CAD) has expanded dramatically over the past two decades. From its beginning as a therapeutic novelty, PCI was performed in more than 900,000 patients in 2003 in the United States, far exceeding the number of patients undergoing coronary artery bypass graft (CABG) surgery, which peaked at 500,000 yearly and has been falling by 10 percent per year. At the same time, the procedural success, safety, and durability of PCI have improved dramatically because of continual technological improvements (e.g., drug stents, distal protection devices), refinements in periprocedural adjunctive pharmacology (e.g., glycoprotein IIb/IIIa [GP IIb/IIIa] inhibitors, alternative thrombin inhibitors), and a better understanding of early and late outcomes. These improvements support the expanded use of PCI as definitive therapy for many patients with ischemia-producing CAD.

This chapter reviews (1) the historical and current methods used for PCI, including conventional balloon angioplasty and new coronary devices; (2) the procedural outcomes and complication rates obtained with contemporary PCI methods; (3) the periprocedural pharmacological strategies to reduce acute complications and restenosis after PCI; (4) the use of drug-eluting stents and radiation brachytherapy for the prevention of restenosis; and (5) recommendations for coronary revascularization in patients with ischemic CAD, with consideration of the alternatives of medical therapy, PCI, and CABG. A discussion of the current issues in selection of patients, technical performance, and outcomes associated with percutaneous mitral and aortic valvuloplasty is also included. Primary PCI for acute coronary syndromes is the subject of Chapter 48.

HISTORICAL PERSPECTIVE

Balloon angioplasty, or percutaneous transluminal coronary angioplasty (PTCA), was first performed by Andreas Gruentzig in 1977 using a prototype, fixed-wire balloon catheter. The procedure was initially limited to the less than 10 percent of patients with symptomatic CAD who had focal noncalcified lesions of a single, proximal coronary vessel, where it was used as an alternative to CABG. As equipment design and operator experience evolved rapidly over the next decade, PCI was expanded to a broader spectrum of patients, such as those with multivessel disease, more challenging anatomy, reduced left ventricular function, and other serious comorbid medical conditions. Despite these improvements, two major complications limited the widespread use of balloon PTCA. The first was abrupt closure of the treated vessel, which occurred in 5 to 8 percent of cases and required emergency CABG for correction in 3 to 5 percent of cases. The second was the development of symptom recurrence because of restenosis of the treated segment in 15 to 30 percent of patients within 6 to 9 months after the initial procedure.

A series of new coronary devices were developed in the early 1990s that sought to improve upon the procedural outcomes achieved with balloon PTCA. Although these novel methods removed (e.g., directional, rotational, or extraction atherectomy) (Fig. 52-1), ablated (e.g., excimer laser angioplasty), or scaffolded (e.g., stents) atherosclerotic plaque, only coronary stenting consistently improved the procedural safety and late clinical outcomes compared with balloon angioplasty in the routine patients undergoing what is now referred to more broadly as PCI. Stents are currently used in more than 80 percent of PCI procedures, whereas atherectomy is used in less than 10 percent of PCI, relegated to "niche use" in patients with certain complex coronary lesions. As a result of these advances, the procedural outcome of PCI has improved substantially in the past two decades (Table 52-1).[1-7]

Balloon Percutaneous Transluminal Coronary Angioplasty

Balloon angioplasty expands the coronary lumen by stretching and tearing the atherosclerotic plaque and vessel wall and, to a lesser extent, by redistributing atherosclerotic plaque along its longitudinal axis ("footprints in the sand"). Although ischemia was generally (>90 percent) improved after balloon angioplasty alone in early series, elastic recoil of the stretched vessel wall left an average residual stenosis of 30 to 35 percent, with higher residual stenoses correlated with higher subsequent recurrence rates. Before the availability of

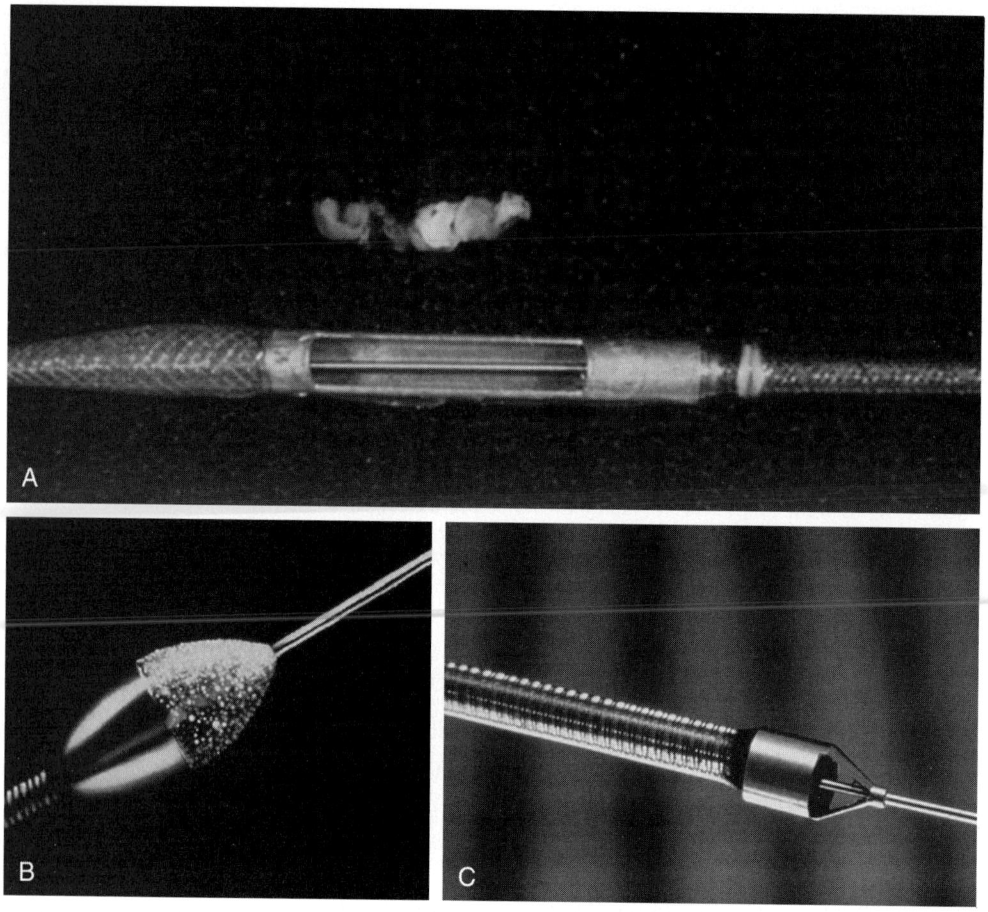

FIGURE 52–1 Atherectomy devices. **A,** Directional coronary atherectomy device alongside tissue resected. **B,** Rotational atherectomy device. **C,** Transluminal extraction catheter.

TABLE 52–1 In-Hospital Outcomes Associated with Perctaneous Intervention over Time

Variable	NHLBI-I[1]	NHLBI-II[1]	MAPS[2]	MAPS[2]	BOAT PTCA Arm[3]	STRESS PTCA Arm[4]	Benestent II PTCA Arm[5]	Cutting Balloon PTCA Arm[6]	Dynamic Registry All PCI[7]
Years of entry	1977-1981	1985-1986	1986-1987	1991	1994-1995	1991-1993	1995-1996	1994-1996	1997-1998
Number of patients	1155	1802	400	200	492	203	413	621	1559
New device use	No	No	No	Yes	"Bailout"	"Bailout"	"Bailout"	"Bailout"	64% stent
Baseline factors									
Mean age, yr	54	58	58	62	58	60	50	58	62
Women, %	25	26	29	30	24	27	23	23	32
Diabetes mellitus	9	14	19	25	14	16	13	12	26
Unstable angina, %	37	49	48	51	NA	48	45	64	43
Multivessel disease, %	25	53	100	100	NA	32	NA	NR	54
Angiographic success, %	68	91	NR	92	NA	92.6	99	NR	94
Procedure success, %	61	78	83.5	90	87	89.6	96	94.7	92
Early complications					3.3[1]	7.9[1]	7.0	2.7	4.9
Death, %	1.2	1.0	1.0	1.0	0.4	1.5	0	0	1.9
Q wave infarction, %	4.9	4.3	2.0	1.5	1.2	3.0	1.2	1.0	NR
Emergency CABG, %	5.8	3.4	5.5	1.0	2.0	4.0	0.7	1.0	1.5
Late clinical outcome	5 yr	5 yr	1 yr	1 yr	1 yr	240 d	12 mo	6 mo	NA
Any Event					31.1	23.8	23.2	15.1	NA
Death, %	4.9	8.3	NA	NA	1.6	0	1.0	0.3	NA
Q wave MI	9.7	9.1	NA	NA	1.6	0.5	1.9	1.1	NA
Revascularization, %	32.1	38.8			19.7	15.4	18.9	14.8	NA
Repeat PTCA	22.5	30.9	16.2	13.2	NA	11.4	9.4	NA	NA
CABG	15.5	13.4	13.4	8.1	NA	4.5	1.9	NA	NA

BOAT = Balloon vs Optimal Atherectomy Trial; CABG = coronary artery bypass graft; MAPS = Multivessel Angioplasty Prognosis Study; MI = myocardial infarction; NA = not applicable; NHLBI = National Heart, Lung, and Blood Institute; NR = not reported; PCI = percutaneous coronary intervention; PTCA = percutaneous transluminal coronary angioplasty; STRESS = Stent Restenosis Study.

Modified from Hirshfeld J, Ellis S, Faxon D: Recommendations for the assessment and maintenance of proficiency in coronary interventional procedures: Statement of the American College of Cardiology. J Am Coll Cardiol 31:722, 1998.

stents, the stretching process left propagating coronary dissections that resulted in abrupt vessel closure in 5 to 8 percent of patients.

Balloon angioplasty has remained an integral component of PCI, whether to dilate the vessel prior to stent placement, deploy a coronary stent, or further expand the stent after deployment. But "stand-alone" balloon angioplasty is now reserved for cases such as smaller (<2.5-mm) vessels, long (>25-mm) lesions, anastomotic stenosis in saphenous vein grafts (SVGs) in which the long-term benefits of coronary stenting are limited, or the treatment of in-stent restenosis before brachytherapy. A "provisional" stent strategy may still be used for these complex lesions, with coronary stent placement reserved for lesions with abrupt or threatened closure or suboptimal (>40 percent) residual stenosis after attempts at adequate vessel expansion with balloon angioplasty have failed. The availability of "bailout" coronary stents to treat angioplasty-induced dissection reduced the emergency CABG rate to less than 1 percent in most institutions.

Two modifications of balloon PTCA have been developed as niche devices for patients undergoing PCI. The cutting balloon (Boston Scientific, Natick, MA) is a conventional balloon that contains either three or four longitudinal microtome blades that incise the atherosclerotic plaque during balloon dilation. The cutting balloon does not reduce restenosis compared with conventional balloon angioplasty but has been approved in the United States by the Food and Drug Administration (FDA) for use in undilatable lesions.[6] The cutting balloon is also useful in patients with in-stent restenosis because the longitudinal blades prevent slippage of the balloon along the axial length of the vessel (Fig. 52-2), particularly when radiation brachytherapy is used as an adjunct. The Fx Minirail (Guidant, Santa Clara, CA) employs a similar concept by adding an additional guidewire that runs outside the balloon dilation catheter in order to score the plaque and prevent balloon slippage. These devices are used in about 10 percent of interventional procedures.

Coronary Atherectomy

Atherectomy assists with PCI by removing the obstructing atherosclerotic plaque and improving lesion wall compliance by fracturing and scoring the remaining plaque. The primary advantage of atherectomy-assisted angioplasty over balloon alone is that a larger final minimal lumen diameter can be achieved. Atherectomy use reached its peak (30 percent of interventional procedures) between 1992 and 1994 but fell dramatically after the clinical availability of coronary stents. It is estimated that 5 to 10 percent of cases currently involve the use of atherectomy devices, alone or in combination with coronary stenting.

DIRECTIONAL CORONARY ATHERECTOMY

Directional coronary atherectomy (DCA) (Guidant, Santa Clara, CA) uses a directional cutting device to remove 18 to 20 mg of tissue, with the remaining lumen gain provided by mechanical dilation by the DCA catheter and balloon angioplasty and changes in radial compliance produced by the vessel by excision of deep wall elastic components. Intravascular ultrasound studies show that a substantial amount (43 to 55 percent cross-sectional narrowing) of atherosclerotic plaque remains even after aggressive DCA.

An "optimal" DCA result is defined as a final diameter stenosis less than 10 percent, tissue removal, and the avoidance of major clinical complications (death, Q wave myocardial infarction [MI], or emergency CABG). The lowest angiographic restenosis rates are obtained in patients with discrete, native vessel lesions who undergo optimal DCA (31.4 percent) as compared with balloon PTCA (39.8 percent; $p < 0.05$) (Table 52-2).[3,8-12] More "conservative" atherectomy using smaller DCA devices and no adjunct balloon PTCA results in higher (>25 percent) residual stenosis and more complications and has no benefit over balloon PTCA. Arterial constrictive remodeling is the major cause of restenosis after DCA and can be avoided when DCA is used before stent placement. Although the strategy of debulking before stenting may lessen the chance of late restenosis, the Atherectomy before Multilink Stent Improves Lumen Gain and Clinical Outcomes Study (AMIGO) trial compared DCA followed by stent implantation with stent implantation alone in more than 800 patients and showed benefit for DCA only when very aggressive atherectomy was performed or there was a significant bifurcation stenosis involving both the parent vessel and the side branch. Accordingly, routine use of DCA before stent placement to remove atherosclerotic plaque is not recommended.

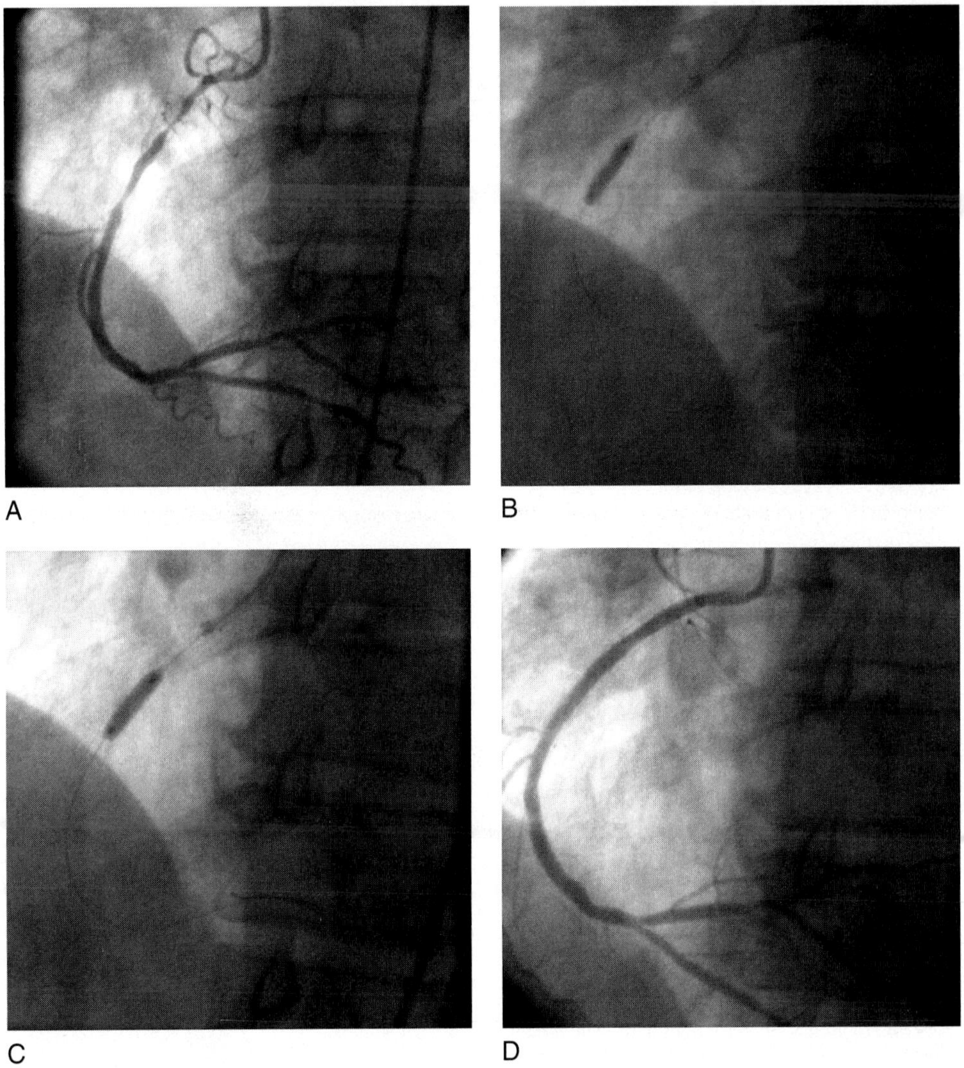

FIGURE 52-2 **A,** Sequential restenoses within a long stent within the right coronary artery. **B,** A 3.5-mm × 15-mm cutting balloon is advanced across the in-stent restenosis and inflated. **C,** The cutting balloon is positioned more proximally and a repeated inflation is performed. **D,** At the end of the cutting balloon inflation, there is a 10 percent residual stenosis. The cutting balloon limits slippage of the balloon within the stent because of the longitudinal cutting blades that score the plaque while inflating the balloon.

TABLE 52–2 Early and Late Outcome After Directional Coronary Atherectomy in Native Coronary Arteries

	CAVEAT[8]		C-CAT[9]		ABACUS[10]		BOAT[3]		START[11]		SOLD[12]
Method	***PTCA***	***DCA***	***PTCA***	***DCA***	***DCA***	***DCA + PTCA***	***PTCA***	***DCA***	***Stent***	***DCA***	***DCA + Stent***
Years of entry	1991-1992		1991-1992		1994-1995		1994-1995		1995-1997		1996-1997
Number of patients	500	512	136	138	106	108	492	497	62	60	71
Baseline factors											
Mean age, yr	59	59	55	58	62	60	58	58	62	64	57
Diabetes mellitus, %	19	19	15	17	19	21	14	14	29	22	14
Unstable angina, %	70	66	52	39	30	22	NA	NA	NR	NR	33
Procedure success, %	76	82+	88	94		99.5	87	93‡	NR	NR	96
RVD, mm	2.9	2.9	3.13	3.23	3.24	3.21	3.20	3.25	3.23	3.29	3.27
Final MLD, mm											
Baseline MLD	NR	NR	0.89	0.94	1.04	1.03	1.04	1.07	1.00	1.01	0.87
Final MLD, mm	1.80	2.02§	2.10	2.34§	2.60	2.88†	2.33	2.82§	2.80	2.89	3.47
Follow-up MLD, mm	NR	NR	1.55	1.61	1.80	1.85	1.68	1.86‡	1.89	2.18	2.57
% Diameter stenosis											
Baseline	73	71	71.5	70.6	68.7	68.0	NR	NR			74
Final	36	29	33	26§	15.0	10.8†	28.1	14.7§	14.7	12.7	0.4
Follow-up	NR	NR	48.4	48.7	32.3	33.4	45.6	40.1‡	40.1	32.1	21
Restenosis rate, %	57	50	43	46	19.6	23.6	39.8	31.4*	32.8	15.8	11
Early complications	5	11§	6	5							
Death, %	0.4	0	0	0	0	0	0.4	0	NR	NR	1.4
Q wave MI, %	2	2	0	0.7	0.9	0	1.2	2.0	NR	NR	2.8
Emergency CABG, %	2	3	4.4	1.4	0	0	2.0	1.0	NR	NR	1.4
Follow-up time	1 yr		6 mo		1 yr		1 yr		1 yr		NR
Late clinical events	42.4	38.7	29	29	18.1	21.9	24.8	21.1¶	33.9	18.3¶	NR
Death, %	0.6	2.2+	0	0.7	0	0	0.6	0.6	1.6	0	NR
Q-wave MI	1.2	2.9	1.6	0	0.9	0	1.6	2.0	NR	NR	NR
TLR, %			27.9	28.7	15.2	21.9			29	15	NR
Repeat PCI	25.9	24.4	23.3	23.5	NR	NR	NR	NR	NR	NR	NR
CABG	9.1	9.3	4.6	5.2	NR	NR	NR	NR	3.2	0	NR

ABACUS = Adjunctive Balloon Angioplasty After Coronary Atherectomy Study; BOAT = Balloon vs Optimal Atherectomy Trial; CABG = coronary artery bypass graft; CAVEAT = Coronary Angioplasty Versus Excisional Atherectomy Trial; C-CAT = Canadian Coronary Atherectomy Trial; DCA = directional coronary atherectomy; MLD = minimum lumen diameter; MI = myocardial infarction; NR = not reported; PCI = percutaneous coronary intervention; PTCA = percutaneous transluminal coronary angioplasty; RVD = reference vessel diameter; SOLD = stenting after optimal lesion debulking; START = Stent versus directional coronary Atherectomy Randomized Trial; TLR = target lesion revascularization.

*$p < 0.05$.

†$p < 0.01$.

‡$p < 0.005$.

§$p < 0.001$.

¶Target vessel failure (death, Q wave myocardial infarction, or target vessel revascularization).

In current practice, DCA is reserved for patients with noncalcified bifurcation lesions involving a large branch or in the ostium of the left anterior descending artery, particularly when there is an acute angle with the origin of the left circumflex. DCA may also be useful for the treatment of in-stent restenosis in larger vessels.

ROTATIONAL ATHERECTOMY

The rotational atherectomy (RA) device or Rotablator (Boston Scientific, Natick, MA) removes the atheromatous plaque by the differential abrasion of inelastic tissue (i.e., calcified plaque) while elastic tissue (i.e., arterial wall) is deflected away from the microscopic diamond chips on the rotating atherectomy burr. The device consists of an olive-shaped, stainless steel burr coated with diamond chips measuring 20 to 50 microns with burr diameters ranging from 1.25 to 2.50-mm. A burr about 0.7 the diameter of the reference vessel adjacent to the target lesion is spun at roughly 160,000 rpm and advanced slowly across that lesion to abrade plaque elements that intrude into the coronary lumen. This abrasion process generates 2- to 5-μm microparticles that pass through the coronary microcirculation for removal by the reticuloendothelial system. Correct technique is important to avoid slowing of rotational speed by excessive contact force between burr and lesion. Deceleration by more than 5000 rpm can lead to inadvertent stalling, burr entrapment, dissection, or vessel occlusion.[13] Two to four passes are made with each burr, with 30 to 60 seconds between passes to allow coronary perfusion. Aggressive RA (using burr-to-artery ratios of >0.7) techniques do not provide a restenosis advantage over more conservative (burr-to-artery ratio of approximately 0.7) methods and tend to increase acute procedural complications.[13] Adjunctive balloon PTCA is used in most (82 to 88 percent) cases to reduce residual percent diameter stenosis or to treat coronary dissections. RA does not appear to reduce restenosis compared with balloon angioplasty in noncalcified vessels.[14] Current RA procedures generally conclude by placement of a coronary stent within the treated segment.

RA registries have reported high (88 to 98.6 percent) procedural success rates in complex lesions. Major complications are uncommon after RA, but transient bradycardia and atrioventricular block are occasionally seen during RA, particularly during RA of the right coronary artery. In the Excimer, Rotablator, or Balloon Angioplasty for Complex Lesions (ERBAC) Study, angiographic restenosis at 6 months was similar in patients treated with RA (57 percent), excimer laser angioplasty (59 percent), or balloon PTCA (47 percent).[15] No advantage of RA over balloon angioplasty was found in noncalcified lesions.[14]

RA is currently reserved for lesions not suitable for balloon PTCA because of excess procedural risk, such as ostial and heavily calcified lesions, selected bifurcation lesions, and lesions that are undilatable with balloon PTCA (Fig. 52-3). RA may also be useful for the treatment of in-stent restenosis but should be avoided in the presence of focal or extensive dissection after balloon PTCA, visible thrombus, or extremely eccentric lesions located on the outer surface of a severe bend.

ABLATIVE LASER-ASSISTED ANGIOPLASTY

Delivery of laser energy through optical fibers can also be used to ablate atherosclerotic obstructions. Two laser systems have been used in coronary arteries: the XeCl excimer laser coronary angioplasty (ELCA) system and the holmium:yttrium aluminum garnet (Ho:YAG) laser system. The ELCA system uses laser light at 308 nm, and the Ho:YAG system uses light at a wavelength of 2100 nm. This light is delivered during a single slow (0.5 to 1.0-mm/sec) pass of the laser catheter through the lesion under fluoroscopic guidance. A concurrent saline flush through the guiding catheter removes blood and contrast medium from the coronary artery to minimize the degree of photoacoustic injury to the surrounding vessel. After successful laser passage, adjunctive balloon PTCA is needed in most (90 percent) cases to reduce the residual stenosis to below 30 percent.

Randomized trials have failed to show a reduction in restenosis associated with the use of the Ho:YAG or excimer laser system compared with balloon angioplasty in either simple or complex lesions. As a result, laser angioplasty has a limited role in PCI and is reserved for patients with in-stent restenosis, particularly those in SVGs, aortoostial SVG lesions, undilatable total occlusions, and, potentially, lesions located in friable SVGs. Laser angioplasty should be used with caution in patients with thrombus or in the presence of severe calcification.

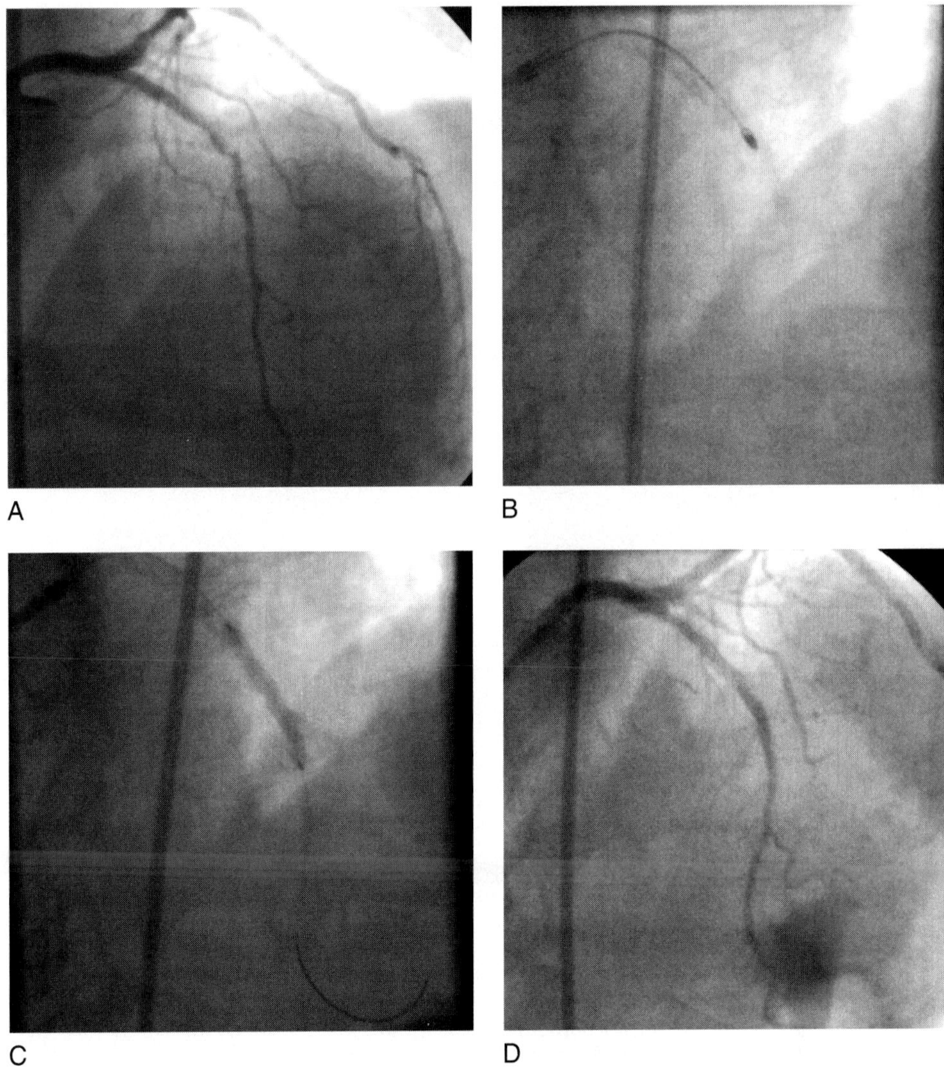

FIGURE 52–3 **A,** A heavily calcified diffuse lesion in the left anterior descending artery is generally considered undilatable with conventional balloon techniques. **B,** A 1.5-mm rotational atherectomy burr revolving at 160,000 rpm is advanced to ablate the calcified lesion. **C,** A 3.0-mm × 28-mm stent can then be advanced across the blockage and inflated to 16 atm of pressure. It is unlikely that full stent expansion could have occurred without pretreatment with rotational atherectomy. **D,** The final angiographic result shows no residual stenosis and normal flow into the distal vessel.

Catheter-Based Thrombolysis and Mechanical Thrombectomy

The presence of thrombus within the native vessel or SVG imparts a substantial risk for distal embolization, "no reflow," or other embolic complications during PCI (Fig. 52–4). Early experience with the Transluminal Extraction Catheter (TEC) (Boston Scientific, Natick, MA) showed moderate success in removing intraluminal clot, but its commercial use was limited by the need for large diameter (9 French [9F]) guiding catheters and stiffness of the device. In the mid-1990s, the Angiojet (Possis Medical, Minneapolis, MN) was introduced as a dedicated device for thrombus removal. A 4F catheter contains a high-pressure hypotube through which saline is injected through a distal tip. These high-speed saline jets are directed toward the proximal end of the catheter lumen and create intense local suction by the Venturi effect, pulling surrounding blood, thrombus, and saline into the lumen of the catheter opening and propelling the debris proximally through the catheter lumen. Repeated passes of the Angiojet may be performed until angiography shows no further evidence of thrombus (Fig. 52–5).

The Vein Graft AngioJet Study 2 (VEGAS-2) trial randomly assigned 349 patients with angiographic thrombus to treatment with the Angiojet or prolonged intraluminal urokinase consisting of a 250,000-unit bolus over a 30-minute period followed by intravenous urokinase for 6 to 30 hours.[16] The procedure success rate was higher and the complication rate was lower in patients treated with the Angiojet device.[16] The Angiojet is currently indicated in patients with moderate to large thrombus-containing native vessels or SVGs prior to definitive therapy with balloon PTCA and stents. The Angiojet should not be used in small (<2.0-mm) vessels because of the risk of perforation.

Distal Embolic Protection Devices

Although distal embolization of atherosclerotic debris was thought not to be a problem during the early years of catheter-based intervention, it is now recognized as a potential cause of distal myocardial necrosis after PCI. The first demonstration of atheroembolization was in diseased SVGs, where such embolization is now seen as the primary etiology for post-procedural cardiac enzyme elevation (17 percent of cases)

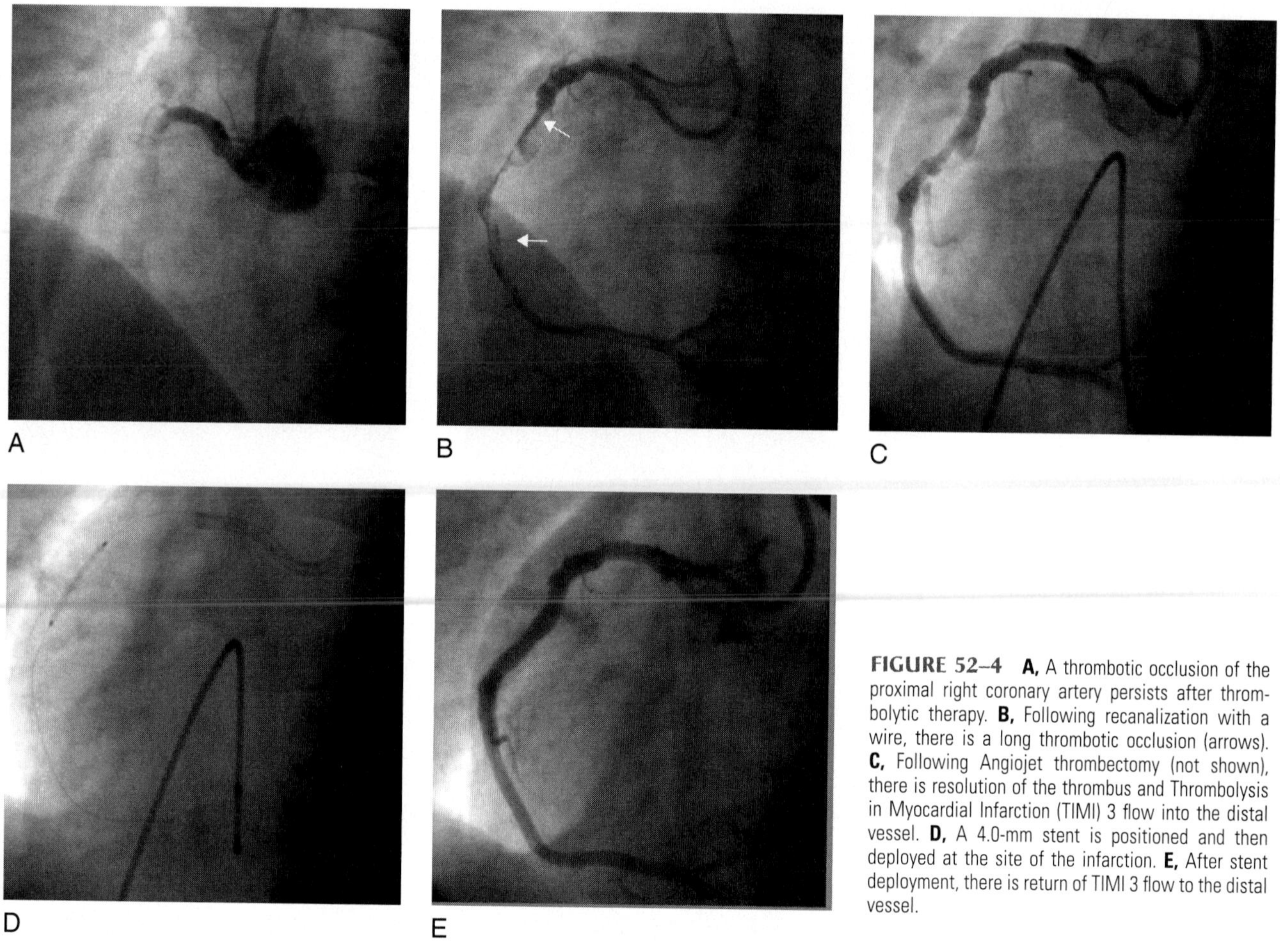

FIGURE 52–4 **A,** A thrombotic occlusion of the proximal right coronary artery persists after thrombolytic therapy. **B,** Following recanalization with a wire, there is a long thrombotic occlusion (arrows). **C,** Following Angiojet thrombectomy (not shown), there is resolution of the thrombus and Thrombolysis in Myocardial Infarction (TIMI) 3 flow into the distal vessel. **D,** A 4.0-mm stent is positioned and then deployed at the site of the infarction. **E,** After stent deployment, there is return of TIMI 3 flow to the distal vessel.

and the no-reflow phenomenon (8 percent of cases) manifest as reduced myocardial perfusion despite a patent epicardial vessel. Microvascular (arteriolar) spasm and platelet aggregation are contributory mechanisms, but only protection against distal atherosclerotic embolization has been shown to reduce the incidence of these complications.

Three classes of embolic protection devices are being evaluated. The first involves distal occlusion using a low-pressure balloon mounted on a hollow guidewire shaft. The Percusurge Guardwire (Medtronic Vascular, Santa Rosa, CA) device is passed across the target lesion and inflated to occlude flow so that any debris liberated by intervention remains trapped in the stagnant column of blood and can be aspirated before the occlusion balloon is deflated to restore antegrade flow[17] (Fig. 52–6). Preliminary data showed that embolic debris (size range between 25 μm and 2 mm) was recovered in more than 95 percent of such procedures, that the histology of the debris (cholesterol clefts, foam cells) resembled that of the treated lesion, and that the incidence of cardiac enzyme elevation was much lower (4 percent) than expected.[18] This benefit was confirmed in the 801-patient Saphenous vein graft Angioplasty Free of Emboli Randomized (SAFER) trial, in which patients undergoing SVG intervention were randomly assigned to stenting over the occlusion wire or a conventional guidewire, showing substantial reductions in 30-day major adverse clinical events (from 16.9 to 9.6 percent) and no reflow (from 8.3 to 3.3 percent) (Fig. 52–7).[17]

The second class of embolic protection devices consists of distal filters that are passed across the target lesion in their smaller collapsed state, opened to approximate the edges of the filter material against the vessel wall, and remain in place to catch any liberated embolic material larger than the filter pore size (usually 100 to 150 μm), until they are collapsed after stent deployment, thereby removing the captured embolic material from the body (Fig. 52–8).[19] This type of device has the advantages of maintaining antegrade flow during the procedure and allowing intermittent injection of contrast material to visualize underlying anatomy but the inherent disadvantage of allowing the component of debris with a diameter less than the filter pore size to pass. The first such filter to complete a pivotal clinical trial is the Embolic Protection Incorporated FilterWire (Boston Scientific, Natick, MA), which was evaluated against the Guardwire distal occlusion device in a 656-patient randomized trial (Fig. 52–9).[19] That trial showed that the distal filter was noninferior (equivalent or better) compared with the distal occlusion device in 30-day major adverse cardiac events.

The third type of embolic protection device involves proximal occlusion of the treated vessel with balloon on the tip of or just beyond the tip of the guiding catheter. With such inflow occlusion, retrograde flow generated by distal collaterals or infusion through a "rinsing" catheter can propel any liberated debris back into the lumen of the guiding catheter. Although devices of this type have thus far undergone only limited clinical testing, they have the advantage of providing protection even before the first wire is advanced across the target lesion.

Devices of all three types are also being evaluated for other anatomical and clinical situations. In native coronaries of patients experiencing acute MI, liberation of thrombus and underlying atherosclerotic debris may contribute to limited myocardial reperfusion and impaired resolution of ST

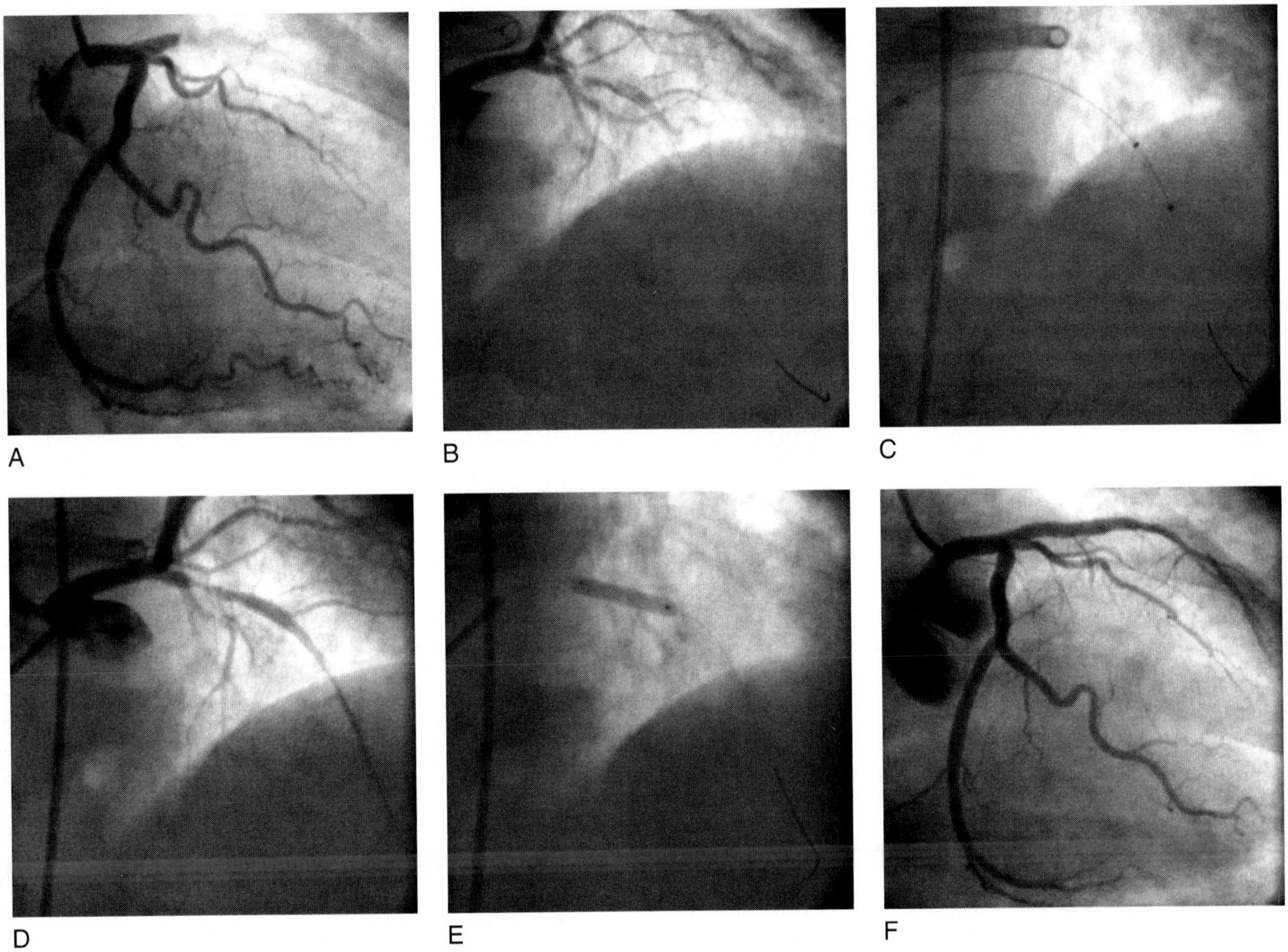

FIGURE 52–5 **A,** A thrombotic occlusion of the proximal segment of the left anterior descending artery is shown. **B,** The vessel is recanalized with a coronary guidewire. **C,** A 4F Angiojet is advanced across the lesion and multiple passes are made to relieve the stenosis. **D,** The thrombus is removed (residual stenosis shown, panels **E, A**), and a 3.5-mm stent is placed at the site of plaque rupture. **F,** There is no residual stenosis and flow is re-established into the distal left anterior descending artery.

segment elevation.[18] The Enhanced Myocardial Efficacy and Recovery by Aspiration of Liberalized Debris (EMERALD) study is a large randomized trial involving patients with acute MI in native vessels, with patients assigned to the distal occlusion device or no distal protection and nuclear imaging assessment of myocardial infarct size as the primary endpoint (Fig. 52–10). Although carotid artery stenting is still investigational, there is ample evidence from transcranial Doppler studies that stent placement is associated with cerebral embolization that probably contributes to the 3 to 5 percent incidence of postprocedural stroke. Embolic protection devices of all three types have been effective in recovering emboli and reducing the neurological complication rate, making them part of all ongoing carotid stenting protocols (see also Chap. 55).

Thus, mounting evidence indicates that distal atherosclerotic debris commonly embolizes from lesions in many vascular territories during percutaneous intervention, that it can be recovered using any of the three types of embolic protection device, and that use of those devices reduces the incidence of end-organ injury.

Total Occlusion–Crossing Devices

Many patients presenting with chronic angina have one or more coronary arteries that are completely occluded rather than just severely stenotic. The distal myocardium may still be viable as the result of inter- or intracoronary collaterals, but such collaterals are generally unable to meet increased oxygen demands during exercise or stress. Restoration of blood flow to such territories is thus an important part of any revascularization strategy. Conventional angioplasty guidewires are only 60 to 70 percent effective in crossing such occlusions, giving this anatomical subgroup the lowest success with PCI and making the presence of one or more chronic total occlusions the leading reason why patients are referred to bypass surgery instead of PCI. Slightly better results in crossing chronic total occlusions are possible with the use of stiffer and hydrophilic-coated guidewires, albeit with a concomitant increase in vessel dissection or perforation.

Considerable effort is thus being made to develop new devices for crossing total occlusions that are steerable and potent enough to make headway through the fibrous caps at either end of the occlusion (and fibrocalcific islands in between) but selective enough to minimize injury to the vessel wall. Two devices are currently approved by the FDA for this indication.

The Lumend Front Runner (Lumend, Santa Clara, CA) has a pair of mechanically openable jaws at its tip that can perform blunt microdissection to cross the total occlusion. This device can cross more than half of the total occlusions in which conventional guidewires have failed, although

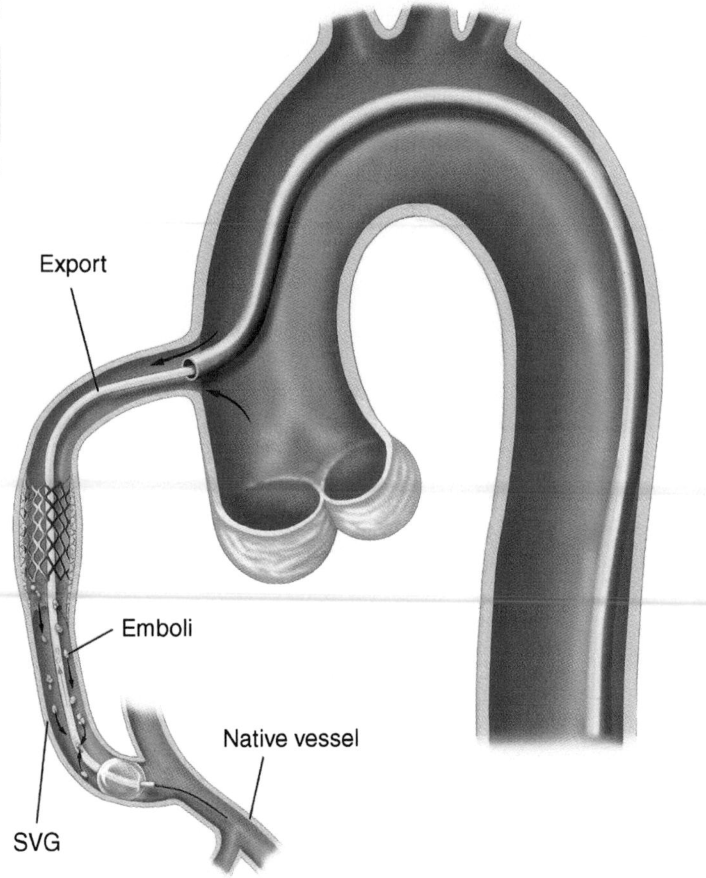

FIGURE 52–6 Key components of the Guardwire Distal Protection Balloon. The Guardwire device is advanced through the saphenous vein graft (SVG) to a distal portion of the SVG that is free of significant stenosis. The occlusion balloon is inflated and, after demonstration of occlusion, stent placement is performed within the SVG. At the end of stent deployment, an Export catheter is advanced and approximately 40 ml of blood and particulate material are removed. (From Baim D, Wahr D, George B, et al: Randomized trial of a distal embolic protection device during percutaneous intervention of saphenous vein aorto-coronary bypass grafts. Circulation 105:1285, 2002. Reproduced with permission.)

it often passes the occlusion in a subintimal dissection plane that requires guidewire use to reenter the distal true lumen.

The IntraLuminal Therapeutics SafeCross (Intraluminal Therapeutics, Kansas City, MO) guidewire is a standard size (0.014-inch) guidewire that contains a single optical fiber. This fiber carries a beam of low-coherence light to the plaque at the tip of the wire and collects the reflected light. When only amorphous plaque is ahead of the wire, that reflection falls off rapidly with increasing distance, but if the tip of the wire is near the vessel wall there is a secondary increase in reflection by the organized collagen fibers therein (i.e., a specular reflector). The system monitors the reflected signal for the presence of the vessel wall signature and alerts the operator to change directions if it is seen. If the fiber detects only plaque and mechanical advancement force is insufficient, it can be supplemented by a brief radiofrequency electrical discharge to help penetrate more fibrocalcific elements of the occlusion. This approach results in successful passage of roughly half of the total occlusions where a conventional guidewire has failed. Once the first wire has crossed the total occluded segment and entered the true lumen beyond, treatment with conventional angioplasty balloons and stents can generally be performed.

Coronary Stents

More than any other of the new devices, coronary stents have revolutionized the practice of interventional cardiology by both reducing early complications and improving late clinical outcomes in a broad array of patients. The concept of a temporary endoluminal splint to scaffold an occluded peripheral vessel was introduced by Charles Dotter nearly 40 years ago but was not practical until the first human coronary implantation was performed in 1986. Self-expanding wire mesh stents were initially used but never attained broad clinical use because of high thrombosis rates. In contrast, a series of balloon-expandable stents has been available in the United States since 1994, and because of improving designs and a large number of randomized trials demonstrating clear benefits in specific lesion subsets (Table 52–3),[4,5,20-23] these devices are now used in more than 80 percent of PCIs.

Indications

DE NOVO OR RESTENOTIC LESIONS. Randomized trials have shown that coronary stenting in relatively large (>3.0-mm), de novo native coronary vessels improves short- and long-term outcomes compared with conventional balloon PTCA. The Stent Restenosis Study (STRESS) and the Belgium Netherlands Stent (BENESTENT) trials showed that Palmaz-Schatz stent placement resulted in a 26 to 31 percent reduction in angiographic restenosis and a 27 to 31 percent lowering of 1-year clinical events compared with balloon PTCA.[4,20] The Restenosis Stent (REST) Study, a randomized trial of 383 patients with prior restenosis after balloon PTCA who were assigned to Palmaz-Schatz stenting or repeated balloon PTCA, showed that angiographic restenosis was lower in stent-treated patients than in balloon PTCA-treated patients (18 versus 32 percent, $p = 0.03$); target lesion revascularization (TLR) also occurred less often in patients treated with coronary stents (10 percent) than in patients treated with balloon PTCA alone (27 percent, $p = 0.001$).[21]

ABRUPT OR THREATENED CLOSURE AFTER BALLOON PTCA. Self-expanding and balloon-expandable coiled and slotted tube stents have been used to scaffold coronary dissections in patients with balloon PTCA–induced complications. The clinical use of coronary stents to treat procedural complications has reduced the emergency CABG rates to less than 1 percent, although clinical trials that attempted to compare prolonged balloon inflations with stent placement for abrupt closure were inconclusive because of difficulties in recruitment of patients (Fig. 52–11). Because stents are used primarily in a broad array of patients, use of stents for bailout purposes alone is uncommon and useful for suboptimal results in smaller vessels or with the development of guiding catheter or guidewire dissections.

SAPHENOUS VEIN GRAFTS. Although balloon PTCA of SVG lesions is associated with reasonably high (88 percent) procedural success rates, clinical recurrence related to restenosis or progression of disease at other SVG sites is common. The Saphenous Vein Graft De Novo (SAVED) Trial randomly assigned 220 patients with de novo SVG lesions to treatment with Palmaz-Schatz stent placement or balloon PTCA alone.[22] Stenting was associated with higher procedural success rates (92 versus 69 percent in balloon-treated patients; $p < 0.001$) at the expense of more bleeding events (17 versus 5 percent in balloon PTCA-treated patients; $p < 0.01$) because of the aggressive anticoagulation regimen used in this study. Although restenosis was not significantly lower in stent-treated patients (37 percent) than in balloon PTCA-treated patients (46 percent), freedom from significant cardiac events was better in the stent group (73 versus 58 percent in balloon PTCA-treated patients; $p = 0.03$). Stents are the pre-

TABLE 52–3 Early and Late Outcome in Randomized Trials of Coronary Stent Placement Versus Balloon Percutaneous Transluminal Coronary Angioplasty

	STRESS[4]		Benestent[20]		Benestent II[5]		REST[21]		SAVED[22]		TOSCA[23]	
Variable	*PTCA*	*Stent*	*PTCA*	*Stent*	*PTCA*	*Stent*	*PTCA*	*Stent*	*PTCA*	*Stent*	*PTCA*	*Stent*
Lesion type	De novo, native		De novo, native		De novo, native		Restenotic, native		SVGs		Chronic occlusion	
Years of entry	1991-1993		1991-1993		1995-1996		1991-1996		1993-1995		1996-1997	
Number of patients	202	205	257	259	410	413	176	178	107	108	208	202
Baseline factors												
Mean age, yr	60	60	58	57	59	50	60	59	66	66	58	58
Women, %	27	17	18	20	20	23	18	20	21	18	20	16
Diabetes mellitus	16	15	6	7	11	13	15	20	36	23	18	15
Unstable angina, %	48	47	NA	NA	40	45	22	17	77	82	25	24
Multivessel disease, %	32	36	NA	NA	NA	NA	32	33	NA	NA	NA	NA
Angiographic success, %	92.6	99.5	98.1	96.9	99	99	93.2	98.9	86	97	NA	NA
Clinical success, %s	89.6	96.1	91.1	92.7	95	96	100	100	69	92	87.9	94.6
Reference diameter, mm	2.99	3.03	3.01	2.99	2.93	2.96	3.04	3.01	3.19	3.18	3.53	3.61
Final % stenosis	35	19	33	22	8	7	30	6	32	12	38	27
Stent use, %	6.9	96.1	5.1	94.6	13.4	96.6	6.8	98.9	7.0	97	9.6	96
Early complications	0-14 d		In hospital		1 mo		In hospital		In hospital		In hospital	
Death, %	1.5	0	0	0	0.2	0	0.6	1.1	2	2	0	0
Q wave Infarction, %	3.0	2.9	0.8	1.9	1.0	1.2	0.6	2.8	1	2	NR	NR
Emergency CABG, %	4.0	2.4	1.6	1.9	0.5	0.7	0.6	1.1	4	2	0	0.5
CK-MB elevation > 3x												
Late clinical outcome	15-240 d		7 mo		12 mo		6 mo		240 d		180 d	
Death, %	0	1.5	0.4	0.8	1.0	1.0	1.1	1.1	9	7	0	0
Q wave MI	0.5	1.0	1.6	2.7	1.5	1.9	0.6	2.8	4	5	NR	NR
Revascularization, %	15.4	10.2	NA	NA	NA	NA	NA	NA	NA	NA	15.4	8.4*
Repeat PTCA	11.4	9.8	20.6	10.0	15.6	9.4	26.6	10.3	16	13	14.4	6.9
CABG	4.5	2.4	2.3	3.1	1.5	1.9	0.6	2.2	12	7	1.4	1.5
Follow-up angiography												
Restenosis, %	42.1	31.6	32	22	31	16	32	18	47	36	70	55†
Follow-up MLD	1.56	1.74	1.73	1.82	1.66	1.89	1.85	2.04	1.49	1.73	1.23	1.49
Follow-up % stenosis	49	42	43	38	17	17	47	30	51	46	61	53
Any bleeding complication	4.0	7.3	3.1	13.5	1.0	1.2	1.1	11.2	5	17	NR	NR

*$p < 0.05$.
†$p < 0.005$.
CABG = coronary artery bypass graft; CK-MB = creatine kinase with muscle and brain subunits; MLD = minimum lumen diameter; MI = myocardial infarction; NA = not applicable; NR = not reported; SAVED = Saphenous for Vein Graft Lesions de novo trial; PTCA = percutaneous transluminal coronary angioplasty; REST = Restenosis Stent Study; STRESS = Stent Restenosis Study; TOSCA = Total Occlusion Study of Canada.

ferred therapy in patients with ostial or body SVG lesions. The risk of no reflow or distal embolization is higher in patients with severe SVG friability and in those with SVG thrombus, although it is improved by the use of thrombectomy and distal embolic protection devices.

TOTAL CORONARY OCCLUSIONS. Balloon PTCA of chronic coronary occlusions is associated with reduced (47 to 69 percent) procedural success, primarily because of failure to cross with a guidewire (see Total Occlusion–Crossing Devices). Even when crossed successfully, total occlusions have a high (45 to 55 percent) incidence of restenotic recurrence, often (19 percent) as recurrent total coronary occlusion. There appears to be no significant benefit of plaque debulking for the treatment of chronic total occlusions. A number of randomized trials have shown the benefit of stent placement over balloon PTCA alone in patients with chronic occlusions. The Total Occlusion Study of Canada (TOSCA) trial randomly assigned 410 patients with native coronary occlusions to balloon PTCA or primary stenting with the heparin-coated Palmaz-Schatz stent. A reduced binary restenosis rate was found in patients treated with the heparin-coated stent (55 percent) compared with the bare metal stent (70 percent; $p < 0.0.01$).[23] In the Stenting in Chronic Coronary Occlusion (SICCO) Study, 119 patients with successful balloon PTCA of a chronic coronary occlusion were assigned to no further intervention or to Palmaz-Schatz stent placement.[24] Angiographic restenosis occurred less often in stent-treated patients (32 percent) than in patients receiving no further therapy (74 percent) ($p < 0.001$). TLR was also needed less often in stent-treated patients (22 percent) than in balloon PTCA–treated patients (42 percent) ($p = 0.025$). This benefit was sustained at late follow-up.[24]

ST SEGMENT ELEVATION MYOCARDIAL INFARCTION. When compared with thrombolytic therapy, primary balloon PTCA improves thrombolysis in myocardial infarction (TIMI) 3 flow rates and reduces the frequency of mortality, reinfarction, and stroke in patients with ST segment elevation myocardial infarction (STEMI) (see also Chap. 48). Primary balloon PTCA may be limited in this setting by recurrent in-hospital ischemia or reinfarction (10 to 15 percent), restenosis (37 to 49 percent), or late reocclusion (9 to 14 percent). Primary stenting confers advantages over balloon

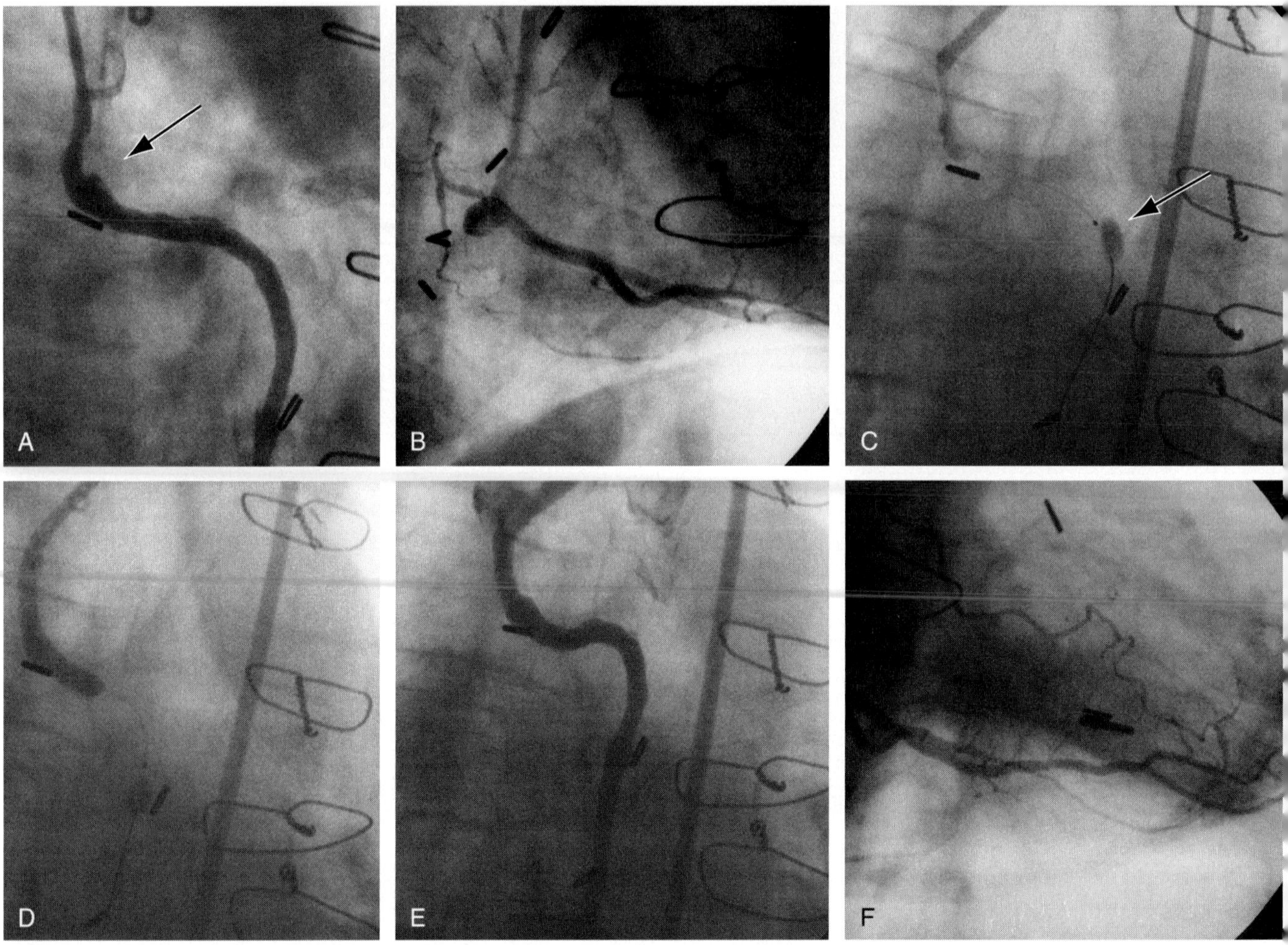

FIGURE 52–7 **A,** Degenerated saphenous vein graft (SVG) to the posterior descending artery with a diffuse stenosis in the proximal segment of the SVG (arrow). **B,** Normal distal perfusion of the SVG with demonstration of secondary and tertiary branches. Positioning of the PercuSurge balloon in the distal portion of the SVG (**C,** arrow) and a 4.0-mm stent in the proximal SVG (**D**) resulted in minimal residual stenosis (**E**) and no evidence of distal embolization (**F**).

PTCA in patients with STEMI by scaffolding the ruptured plaque and preventing the arterial remodeling that occurs with balloon angioplasty. The Primary Angioplasty in Myocardial Infarction (PAMI) stent trial randomly assigned 900 patients with acute MI to treatment with primary balloon PTCA or placement of the Palmaz-Schatz heparin-coated stent.[25] After 6 months, fewer patients in the stent group had angina (11.3 versus 16.9 percent in the balloon group; $p = 0.02$) or needed TLR (7.7 versus 17.0 percent in the balloon group; $p < 0.001$). Angiographic restenosis also occurred less often in stent-treated patients (20.3 versus 33.5 percent in balloon-treated patients; $p < 0.001$).[25]

Another study, the Controlled Abciximab and Device Investigation to Lower Late Angioplasty Complications (CADILLAC) trial, evaluated the use of abciximab and stents in a 2 × 2 factorial design in 2082 patients with STEMI.[26] At 6 months, the primary endpoint—a composite of death, reinfarction, disabling stroke, and ischemia-driven revascularization of the target vessel—had occurred in 20.0 percent of patients after PTCA, 16.5 percent after PTCA plus abciximab, 11.5 percent after stenting, and 10.2 percent after stenting plus abciximab ($p < 0.001$).[26] There was little incremental benefit associated with routine abciximab use in patients with STEMI, although another study suggested that abciximab may be useful in reducing events in high-risk patients undergoing stent placement.[27] The CADILLAC trial also found that angiographic restenosis occurred in 40.8 percent after PTCA and 22.2 percent after stenting ($p < 0.001$), and the respective rates of reocclusion of the infarct-related artery were 11.3 percent and 5.7 percent ($p = 0.01$), both independent of abciximab use.[26]

STENT DESIGNS

A number of balloon-expandable and self-expanding stents have become available for clinical use. Each stent varies with respect to its metallic composition, strut design, stent length, delivery and deployment system, and arterial surface coverage, among other factors. Although there may be differences in flexibility, ease of delivery, and side branch access among the different stent designs, randomized stent-versus-stent trials comparing various second-generation stent designs with the benchmark Palmaz-Schatz stent have generally failed to show significant differences in subacute stent thrombosis or subsequent restenosis behavior (Table 52–4).[28-32]

Because of the inherent limitations of 316L stainless steel as the major filament component of most commercially available stents, including limited radiopacity and lack of flexibility with thicker filaments, alternative alloys have been considered. Cobalt chromium appears to have better radiopacity and deliverability than stainless steel for comparable strut thicknesses. The Guidant Vision stent (Guidant, Santa Clara, CA), the Medtronic Driver stent (Medtronic Vascular, Santa Rosa, CA), and the Cordis Steeplechaser stent (Cordis, Warren, NJ) all use cobalt chromium alloys and the new generation of balloon-expandable stent and will be the platform for drug elution.

Thromboresistant stents have also been developed to reduce the occurrence of subacute thrombosis, and potentially restenosis, after PCI. The most frequently used is a heparin-coated Bx Velocity stent (Hepa-

TABLE 52–4 Early and Late Outcome in Randomized Trials of Stent Versus Stent Equivalence Trials in Native Vessels

	ASCENT[30]		Paragon[28]		NIRVANA[29]		SCORES[31]		GR-II[32]	
Variable	***PS 153***	***ML***	***Paragon***	***PS 153***	***PS 153***	***NIR***	***PS 153***	***Radius***	***PS 153***	***GR-II***
Number of patients	522	518	349	339	430	418	551	545	375	380
Lesion type	Focal, <25-mm De novo lesion 3.00-3.75-mm		Focal, <25-mm De novo or RS 3.00-4.00-mm		Focal, <25-mm De novo or RS 3.00-3.75-mm		Focal, <25-mm De novo or RS 2.75-4.35-mm		Focal, <25-mm De novo or RS 3.00-4.00-mm	
Baseline factors										
Mean age, yr	61	61	62	62	62	62	62	62	61	61
Women, %	31	33	32	32	32	30	32	30	28.5	31.3
Diabetes mellitus	20	19	21	21	22	23	19	22	22.4	23.2
Unstable angina	70	69	81	82	73	75	65	65	NR	NR
LAD location, %	44	42	41	45	40	42	38	40	43.4	39.7
Lesion length, mm	11.0	10.9	12.4	12.2	13.3	13.3	13.0	12.8	14.0	14.3
ACC/AHA B_2 or C	59	63	63	69	65	69	NR	NR	NR	NR
Maximum inflation pressure	17.1	16.7	16.7	17.1	16.6	15.5	16.8	13.3	NR	NR
Reference diameter, mm	2.94	2.95	2.97*	3.05	2.97	3.03	3.05	3.06	3.08	3.08
MLD, mm										
Baseline	1.05	1.05	1.05	1.07	1.09	1.04	0.99	1.01	1.06	1.08
Final	2.72	2.77	2.83	2.83	2.73	2.74	2.80	2.86	2.83	2.64
Follow-up	1.92	1.96	1.78	1.93	1.90	2.00	1.88	1.88	1.90	1.48
% Diameter stenosis										
Baseline	64	64	64	65	63	65	66.5	67.3	65.2	64.7
Final	10	8	6.3	8.8*	8	8	11.8	12.2	9.8	15.6
Follow-up	32	35	39.8	37.9			36.1	36.3	36.4	50.6§
Restenosis rate	22.1	16.0	29.1	23.7	22.4	19.3	18.7	24.2	20.6	47.3§
Device success, %	96.9	98.8	NR	NR	97.9	99.5	95.3	98.3‡	NR	NR
Procedural success, %s	93.9	95.7	91.9	95.5	94.3	95.4	93.5	97.0	NR	NR
30-d event rates	6.5	5.0	8.3‖	4.4	4.4	4.3	3.1	2.9	1.3	4.2
Death, %	1.1	0*	0.3	0	0.2	0	0.4	0.4	0.5	0.3
Q wave infarction, %	1.0	0.6	0.9	0.3	0.9	0.5	0.4	0.2	0.5	1.3
Emergency CABG, %	0.8	0.6	0.3	0.3	0	0.2	0.7	0.9	0.3	1.9
Subacute thrombosis, %	1.8	0.6	0.6	0.3	0.5	0.5	0.4	0.2	0.3	3.9‡
Follow-up period, mo	9 mo		6 mo		6 mo		9 mo			
TLR, %	9.8	7.7	12.0	5.9*	13.4	12.2	10.7	9.5	15.3	27.4§
Late clinical events, %	19.5	17.8	19.8	11.2†	15.3	14.1	NR	NR	17.8	29.8§
Death	2.5	1.4	2.0	1.2	0.9	1.0	1.1	1.5	2.7	2.7
Q wave MI	1.0	0.6	2.0	0.3	0.9	0.7	0.5	0.7	0.8	1.4
CABG, %	2.9	2.3	2.9	2.4	3.0	2.4	5.3	5.1	4.4	5.1
Repeat PCI, %	6.9	5.4	9.7	4.1†	8.6	7.2	11.1	10.3	10.9	22.8§

ACC/AHA = American College of Cardiology/American Heart Association; ASCENT = ACS Stent Clinical Equivalence in De Novo Lesions trial; CABG = coronary artery bypass graft; GR-II = Gianturco-Roubin stent; MI = myocardial infarction; MLD = minimal lumen diameter; NIRVANA = The NIR Vascular Advanced North American trial; NR = not reported; PS = Palmaz-Schatz stent; RS = restenotic lesion; SCORES = the Stent Comparative Restenosis Trial; TLR = target lesion revascularization.

*$p < 0.05$.

†$p < 0.01$.

‡$p < 0.005$.

§$p < 0.001$.

‖In-hospital events.

¶Balloon PTCA with "bailout" stenting.

coat, Cordis, Warren, NJ) that has been shown to have a low thrombosis rate in a number of complex subsets.[5,23,25] Silicon carbide-coated stents have also been developed with low subacute thrombosis rates.

Clinical Outcomes and Complications of Percutaneous Coronary Intervention

Anatomical (or angiographic) success after PCI is defined as the attainment of residual diameter stenosis less than 50 percent and normal TIMI 3 flow (see Chap. 18). Procedural success is defined as angiographic success without the occurrence of major complications (death, MI, or CABG) within 30 days of the procedure. Clinical success is defined as procedural success without the need for urgent repeated PCI or surgical revascularization within the first 30 days of the procedure.[33]

With stenting to control dissection and abrupt closure (and thereby to avert emergency CABG), the most common complication of current PCI is periprocedural MI. The incidence of Q wave MI remains 1 to 2 percent, and the most common events are non-Q-wave MIs as diagnosed by postprocedure

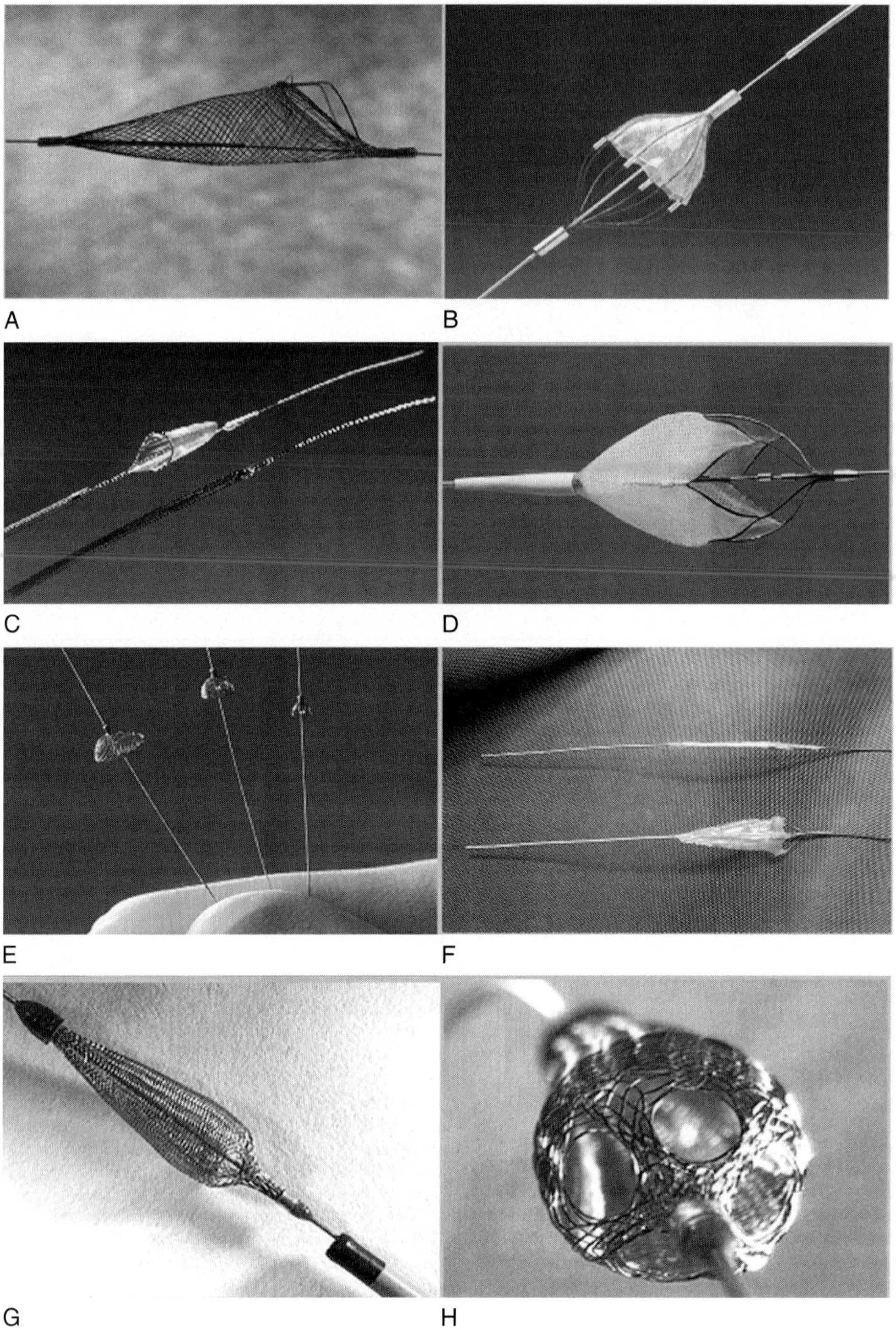

FIGURE 52–8 Filters for distal protection. **A,** The Spider filter (ev3, Minneapolis, MN). **B,** Angioguard device (Cordis, Warren, NJ). **C,** EPI Filterwire (Boston Scientific, Natick, MA). **D,** Accunet device (Guidant, Santa Clara, CA). **E,** MedNova (Abbott, Chicago, IL). **F,** Rubicon filter (Rubicon). **G** and **H,** The Interceptor filter (Medtronic Vascular, Santa Rosa, CA), in longitudinal view **(G)** and axial view **(H)**.

elevation of cardiac enzymes. Two classification systems are in use: (1) the World Health Organization (WHO) classification system, which includes a total creatine phosphokinase (CPK) isoenzyme elevation more than two times normal in association with elevation of the CPK-MB isoform and occurs after 1 to 2 percent of PCI procedures, and (2) the FDA classification system, which includes an elevation in CPK-MB of three times normal or higher after the procedure and occurs after 5 to 10 percent of procedures.[34] The incidence of such events may be significantly higher when atherectomy devices are used or in high-risk lesion subgroups, such as SVGs. Although several studies have shown that CK or CK-MB elevations over five to eight times the upper limit of normal adversely affect subsequent survival, the causal relationship of small (one to eight times normal CPK-MB) elevations to late mortality is unclear. Some studies have suggested worse long-term outcomes with even one to three times elevations of cardiac enzymes, but it is not clear whether this is a cause-and-effect relationship or just a reflection of the ability of more diffuse atherosclerotic involvement to cause both

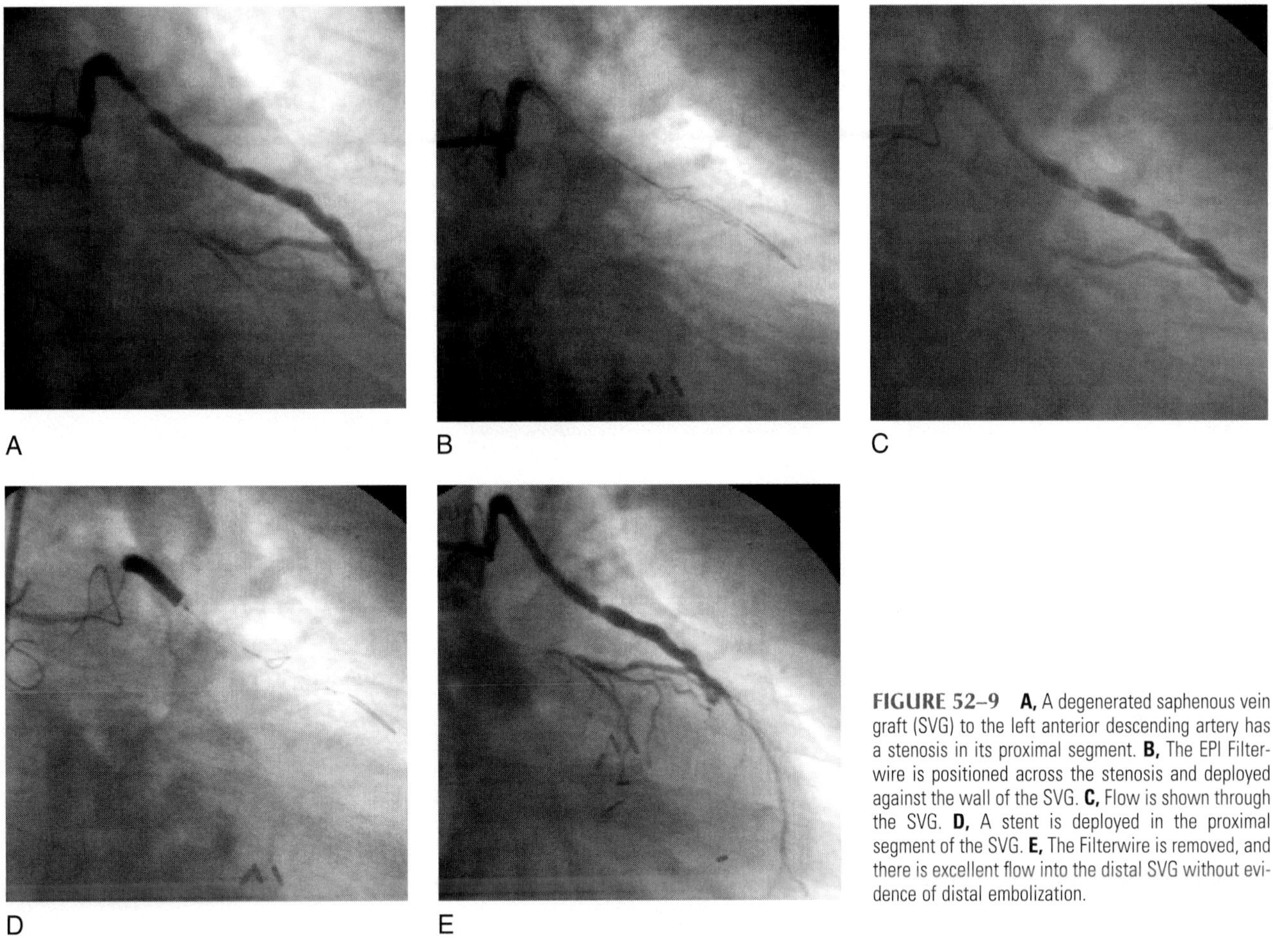

FIGURE 52–9 **A,** A degenerated saphenous vein graft (SVG) to the left anterior descending artery has a stenosis in its proximal segment. **B,** The EPI Filterwire is positioned across the stenosis and deployed against the wall of the SVG. **C,** Flow is shown through the SVG. **D,** A stent is deployed in the proximal segment of the SVG. **E,** The Filterwire is removed, and there is excellent flow into the distal SVG without evidence of distal embolization.

greater periprocedural CK elevation and worse long-term outcome.

Early procedural outcome after PCI is correlated with clinical factors, including age, unstable and Canadian Cardiovascular Society (CCS) class IV angina, congestive heart failure, cardiogenic shock, renal insufficiency, and preprocedural instability requiring intraaortic balloon pump support, among other factors. Anatomical risk variables include multivessel CAD, presence of thrombus, SVG intervention, and American College of Cardiology/American Heart Association (ACC/AHA) type C lesion morphology, including chronic total coronary occlusion. Procedural factors also affect procedure outcomes, including a higher final percent diameter stenosis, smaller minimal lumen diameter, and the presence of a residual dissection or transstenotic pressure gradient (see Chap. 18 for definitions of ACC/AHA lesion types). Procedural mortality is associated with balloon PTCA of arteries subtending 50 percent or more of the myocardium, a left ventricular ejection fraction less than 25 percent, a more severe preprocedural percent diameter stenosis, multivessel CAD, and female gender, among other factors.[35,36] The latter factors indicate a greater risk for cardiovascular collapse should abrupt vessel closure occur.

The early use of coronary stents was limited by high (3.5 to 8.6 percent) subacute thrombosis rates despite aggressive antithrombotic therapy with aspirin (>325 mg daily), dipyridamole (225 mg daily), periprocedural low-molecular-weight dextran, and an uninterrupted transition from intravenous heparin to oral warfarin. Clinical events associated with subacute thrombosis were profound, resulting in an untoward outcome (e.g., death, MI, or emergency revascularization) in virtually every such patient. Patients at high risk for subacute thrombosis included those with unstable angina, residual proximal or distal dissection, angiographic thrombus or a filling defect, in-laboratory transient or sustained abrupt closure, multiple (more than three) stent implants, smaller (<3.0-mm) vessels, total occlusions, or stent placement for failed balloon PTCA. Anatomical factors were also important contributors to subacute thrombosis after stent deployment (e.g., underdilation of the stent, proximal and distal dissections, poor inflow or outflow obstruction, <3-mm vessel diameter). Lower frequencies of subacute stent thrombosis (roughly 0.5 percent) are now achieved with optimal stent deployment and with a modern drug regimen including aspirin and a thienopyridine (ticlopidine or clopidogrel) started just after stent placement.[37]

Side branch occlusion may also occur in some patients after stent placement (6 to 14 percent), particularly in bifurcation lesions involving the origin of the side branch. The clinical importance of the side branch occlusion is related to the size of the side branch and extent of myocardium that the side branch supplies. Open-cell and coiled stent designs may provide better access to side branches than afforded by the closed-cell, tubular slotted stent designs. Stent dislodgment from the delivery catheter is an uncommon occurrence with second- and third-generation stents, but it occurred more often in the era when stents were "hand crimped" onto a balloon catheter, although generally without serious complication. Stent margin dissections can occur during stent deployment or during postdeployment stent dilation, particularly when stent dilation strategies are directed at maximizing the internal stent diameter. The availability of shorter (15-mm), noncompliant balloons allows more precise stent dilation when using high (>16 atm) pressure, thereby

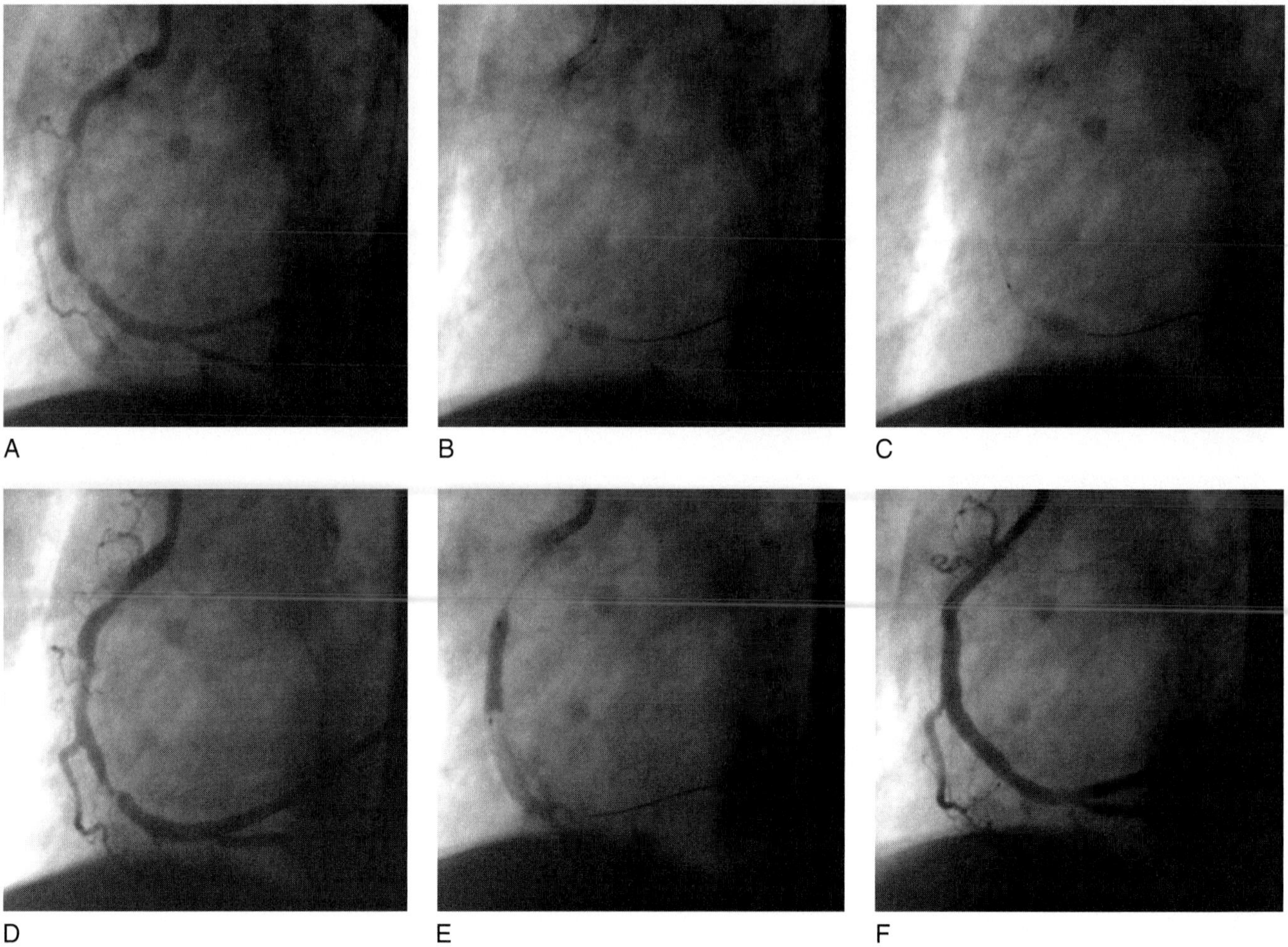

FIGURE 52–10 **A,** A thrombotic lesion causing occlusion of the middle right coronary artery (RCA) is demonstrated in a patient who experienced reperfusion after thrombolytic therapy. The vessel was at high risk for distal embolization because of the underlying thrombus burden. **B,** The Percusurge Guardwire was positioned in the distal RCA (arrow). **C,** The Export catheter (arrow) was advanced and 20 ml of blood and clot was removed before stent placement. **D,** The export catheter removed a substantial amount of thrombus. **E,** A 4.0-mm stent was placed with distal protection, and the Export catheter was again used to remove the residual thrombus. **F,** The final angiographic result demonstrated no evidence of distal embolization.

reducing the frequency of edge dissections. Coronary perforation is also an uncommon occurrence after stent deployment, but it may occur during poststent deployment dilation with an oversized balloon inflated to high pressure. No evidence indicates that higher balloon inflation pressures predispose to higher rates of stent restenosis.

Late Clinical Outcome

Clinical events after PCI are attributable to arterial renarrowing at the PTCA site, intimal hyperplasia in the region of coronary stenting, progression or instability of atherosclerotic disease at remote sites, or a combination of these events. These processes can be partially distinguished by the time of occurrence of the event, with angiographic and clinical restenosis generally developing within 6 to 9 months after balloon PTCA and death, MI, and progression of atherosclerosis occurring as a low but constant hazard (1 to 2 percent risk per year) indefinitely after the procedure. Predictors of higher risk of all-cause late mortality include advanced age, reduced left ventricular function or congestive heart failure, presence of diabetes mellitus, number of diseased vessels, inoperable disease, and severe comorbid conditions. A 95 percent 10-year survival rate can be expected in patients with single-vessel CAD and an 80 percent survival rate after PCI can be achieved in those with multivessel CAD.

The risk of restenosis after balloon PTCA depends on clinical factors, such as diabetes mellitus, unstable angina, acute MI, and prior restenosis; anatomical factors, such as total occlusions, proximal left anterior descending artery lesions, smaller vessel size, long lesions, and lesions involving an SVG; and procedural factors, such as the final minimal lumen diameter or percent diameter stenosis. Exposure to infectious agents may also predispose to the development of restenosis. Risk factors for restenosis after coronary stent placement include age, a history of diabetes, a longer lesion or total stent length, small postprocedural minimal lumen diameters, and the left anterior descending lesion location.

In-Stent Restenosis

Accumulation of neointimal tissue within the axial stent length accounts for virtually all cases of in-stent restenosis. Recurrence of symptoms may occur in 10 to 20 percent of patients within 12 months after stent implantation; after 6 to 12 months, improvements of the lumen dimensions related to scar retraction have been noted. Although some patients with multivessel CAD or multiple stent restenoses are best served by referral for CABG, the majority of patients with in-stent restenosis can be safety and effectively treated with repeated PCI, with the mechanism of benefit related to both expansion of the stent and extrusion of the tissue through the

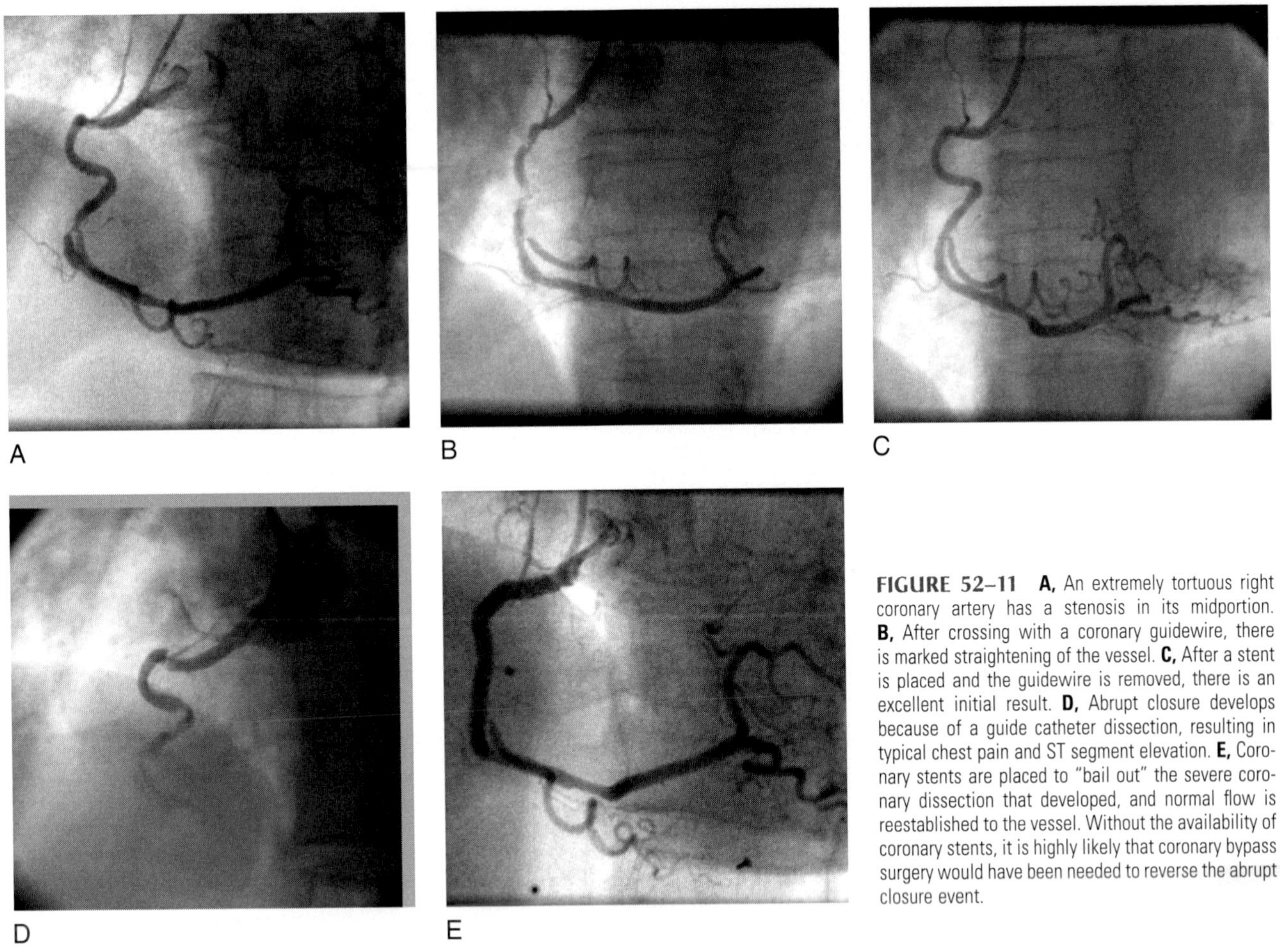

FIGURE 52–11 **A,** An extremely tortuous right coronary artery has a stenosis in its midportion. **B,** After crossing with a coronary guidewire, there is marked straightening of the vessel. **C,** After a stent is placed and the guidewire is removed, there is an excellent initial result. **D,** Abrupt closure develops because of a guide catheter dissection, resulting in typical chest pain and ST segment elevation. **E,** Coronary stents are placed to "bail out" the severe coronary dissection that developed, and normal flow is reestablished to the vessel. Without the availability of coronary stents, it is highly likely that coronary bypass surgery would have been needed to reverse the abrupt closure event.

stent struts and along its length. Early tissue recoil may also occur immediately after PCI in those with in-stent restenosis. Recurrence rates after balloon PTCA for stent restenosis ranged from 10 to 20 percent, although higher (up to 80 percent) recurrence rates have been reported depending on vessel size, pattern of restenosis (e.g., intrastent, stent margin, or remote disease), and the time to presentation.

Atheroablation by DCA, RA, or ELCA has been used in patients at "high risk" for recurrence after PCI for in-stent restenosis, but an advantage over conventional balloon PTCA alone has not been demonstrated in a prospective, randomized study. The Angioplasty versus Rotational Atherectomy for Treatment of Diffuse In-Stent Restenosis Trial (ARTIST) study was a multicenter, randomized, prospective trial with 298 patients with in-stent restenosis who were assigned to treatment with balloon angioplasty or rotablation performed using a stepped-burr approach followed by adjunctive balloon angioplasty.[38] Although restenosis rates were lower (51 percent) in the balloon angioplasty arm than in the RA arm (65 percent; $p = 0.039$),[38] these differences were related to the use of low-pressure inflations after RA that resulted in incomplete stent expansion.

"Very late" (>1 year) restenosis occurs rarely after coronary stenting in native coronary arteries. Three-year angiographic and clinical follow-up was obtained for 143 patients (147 lesions) who underwent Palmaz-Schatz stent placement in native coronaries.[39] After 14 months, TLR was necessary in only 2.1 percent of patients, whereas balloon PTCA of a new lesion was required in 7.7 percent of patients. Follow-up coronary angiography showed no further decrease in minimal lumen diameter between 6 months and 1 year (1.95-mm in both groups), as well as a significant ($p < 0.001$) improvement in minimal lumen diameter between 6 months (1.94-mm) and 3 years (2.09-mm).[39]

Radiation Brachytherapy for In-Stent Restenosis

Because in-stent restenosis is solely due to excessive neointimal proliferation within the stent, it is reasonable that local radiation therapy could retard such proliferation and reduce the chance of recurrence when an in-stent restenotic lesion is treated (Table 52–5).[40-44] Three studies have shown the value of gamma irradiation with iridium-192 (^{192}Ir) in reducing the frequency of angiographic and clinical recurrence in patients undergoing treatment for in-stent restenosis.[40-42] In the largest of these studies, the multicenter Gamma-1 trial randomly assigned 252 patients with in-stent restenosis to either ^{192}Ir intracoronary radiation or placebo after treatment of in-stent restenosis.[42] Six-month angiographic follow-up demonstrated a significant reduction of in-stent restenosis in the radiation group compared with placebo (21 percent in the gamma radiation group versus 49.5 percent in the placebo group, $p < 0.001$).[42] The beneficial effects of gamma radiation have been sustained for up to 5 years after the procedure. Gamma brachytherapy has also been shown to be particularly useful in long lesions, total occlusions, and in patients with SVG stenoses and diabetes mellitus. Its limitations are prolonged treatment times and the need for extensive shielding within the procedure room.

TABLE 52–5 Late Outcome in Randomized Trials of Radiation Brachytherapy for the Prevention of In-Stent Restenosis

	Scripps[40]		WRIST[41]		Gamma-1[42]		START[44]		INHIBIT[43]	
Variable	*Ir-192*	*PL*	*Ir-192*	*PL*	*Ir-192*	*PL*	*Sr-90*	*PL*	*P-32*	*PL*
Number of patients	26	29	65	65	131	121	244	232	166	166
Baseline factors										
Mean age, yr	70	69	63	62	58	61	61	61	62	61
Women, %	27	24	34	28	25.2	26.6	32	37	30	27
Diabetes mellitus	27	41	39	45	31.3	31.4	31	32	33	27
Lesion length, mm	12.9	11.9	28.8	26.7	19	20.3	16.3	16.0	16.9	17.9
Reference diameter, mm	2.88	2.78	2.71	2.72	2.69	2.73	2.76	2.77	2.68	2.71
MLD, mm										
Baseline	1.10	1.03	0.94	0.81	0.98	0.96	0.98	0.98	1.01	0.95
Final	2.82	2.88	2.23	2.25	2.09	2.12	1.94	1.94	1.92	1.96
Follow-up	2.43*	1.85	2.03§	1.24	1.47	1.31	1.65§	1.41	1.54*	1.38
% Diameter stenosis										
Baseline	62	62	65	70	63.3	64.6	64.2	64.2	61.9	65.2
Final	7	5	19	20	23.9	24.5	31.4	30.7	29.6	28.5
Follow-up	17*	54	30§	57	45.6	53.2	41.7§	50.1	43.3‡	51.3
Restenosis rate, %	17*	54	22§	60	32.4*	55.3	28.8§	45.2	26§	52
Stent thrombosis, %	1	0	9.2	3.5	6.3	1.6	0	0.4	3	1
Follow-up period, mo	6 mo		12 mo		9 mo		8 mo		290 d	
TLR, %	12*	45	23.0§	63.1	24.4†	42.1	13.9§	24.9	8§	26
Late clinical events, %	19*	62	35.3§	67.6	28.2*	43.8	19.1*	28.7	12§	28
Death	0	3	6.2	6.2	3.1	0.8	1.3	0.5	3	2
Q wave MI	4	0	0	0	4.6	2.5	0	0	2	0

INHIBIT = Intimal Hyperplasia Inhibition with Beta In-Stent trial; MLD = minimal lumen diameter; MI = myocardial infarction; PL = placebo; START = Stents and Radiation Therapy trial; TLR = target lesion revascularization; WRIST = Washington Radiation for In-Stent Restenosis Trial.

*$p < 0.05$.
†$p < 0.01$.
‡$p < 0.005$.
§$p < 0.001$.

Beta radiation therapy also reduces the recurrence rates in patients undergoing treatment for in-stent restenosis (Fig. 52-12).[43,44] In a multicenter, "blinded," and randomized trial 476 patients with in-stent restenosis treated with either intracoronary radiation using a $^{90}Sr/^{90}Y$ beta source or placebo for in-stent restenosis, the primary endpoint, 8-month clinically driven target vessel revascularization, was reduced from 26.8 percent in the patients assigned to placebo to 17.0 percent in patients assigned to radiation ($p = 0.015$).[44] The binary 8-month angiographic restenosis (more than 50 percent diameter stenosis) within the entire segment treated with radiation was reduced from 45.2 percent in the placebo-treated patients to 28.8 percent in the $^{90}Sr/^{90}Y$-treated patients ($p = 0.001$).[44] In another study of 332 patients with in-stent restenosis who underwent successful coronary intervention, random assignment was made to intracoronary beta radiation with a phosphorus-32 source or placebo delivered into a centering balloon catheter through an automatic afterloader.[43] The binary angiographic restenosis rate was significantly lower in the radiated group than the placebo group for the entire analyzed segment.[43] Similar results have been demonstrated with a ^{32}P beta balloon source.[45] Beta radiation is more convenient than gamma radiation, requiring shorter treatment times and less shielding in the laboratory. Its limitation is that it may have limited use in larger (>4.0-mm) vessels. Beta radiation has not proved beneficial in patients undergoing primary balloon angioplasty or provisional stenting.

Two limitations of brachytherapy were identified from these studies. Some patients developed restenosis at the margin of the treatment zone, attributable to vessel injury with incomplete radiation coverage. This limitation has been lessened by the use of longer radiation sources with a 5- to 10-mm margin proximal and distal to the regions of balloon dilation. The second limitation was the occurrence of late (>30 day) subacute stent thrombosis in patients receiving a new stent.[42] The occurrence of late vessel occlusion has been substantially reduced with the use of long-term (up to 12 months) clopidogrel administration. Indications for brachytherapy for the treatment of in-stent restenosis include early (<3 month) restenosis, recurrent restenosis, diabetes, SVG restenosis, and longer lesions.

Vascular Closure Devices

Most (90 percent) coronary interventional procedures are performed from the femoral artery using the Seldinger technique, although there is increasing use of the radial approach in obese patients, patients with a bleeding diathesis, or patients with peripheral vascular disease. At the end of the procedure, the standard approach has been to discontinue further unfractionated heparin use and allow the activated clotting time (ACT) to fall below 150 to 180 seconds. The vascular sheath was then removed and manual or mechanical external compression was applied for 10 to 30 minutes until a hemostatic plug formed over the arterial entry site. Patients were then kept at bed rest for 4 to 6 hours before ambulation and discharge. Complications at the catheter entry site occurred in 5 to 7 percent of patients and included free rebleeding, local hematoma, femoral arterial pseudoaneurysm, retroperitoneal bleeding, and femoral arteriovenous fistulas. Discomfort, prolonged hospitalization, transfusion, or even surgical repair of the femoral artery was occasionally (3 to 10 percent) required. This motivated the search for devices that could achieve immediate hemostasis at the puncture site regardless of ongoing anticoagulation, reduce subsequent complications, and allow immediate ambulation.

Several classes of approach to puncture site management have been attempted. The suture-based approach (e.g., Perclose, Sutura) is to deliver surgical suture remotely through the margins of the puncture site, knot the ends of the suture together, and slide the resulting knot down to the arterial surface to duplicate surgical closure. Initial trials showed rapid hemostasis and ambulation but with some residual complications related to incorrect placement of sutures,

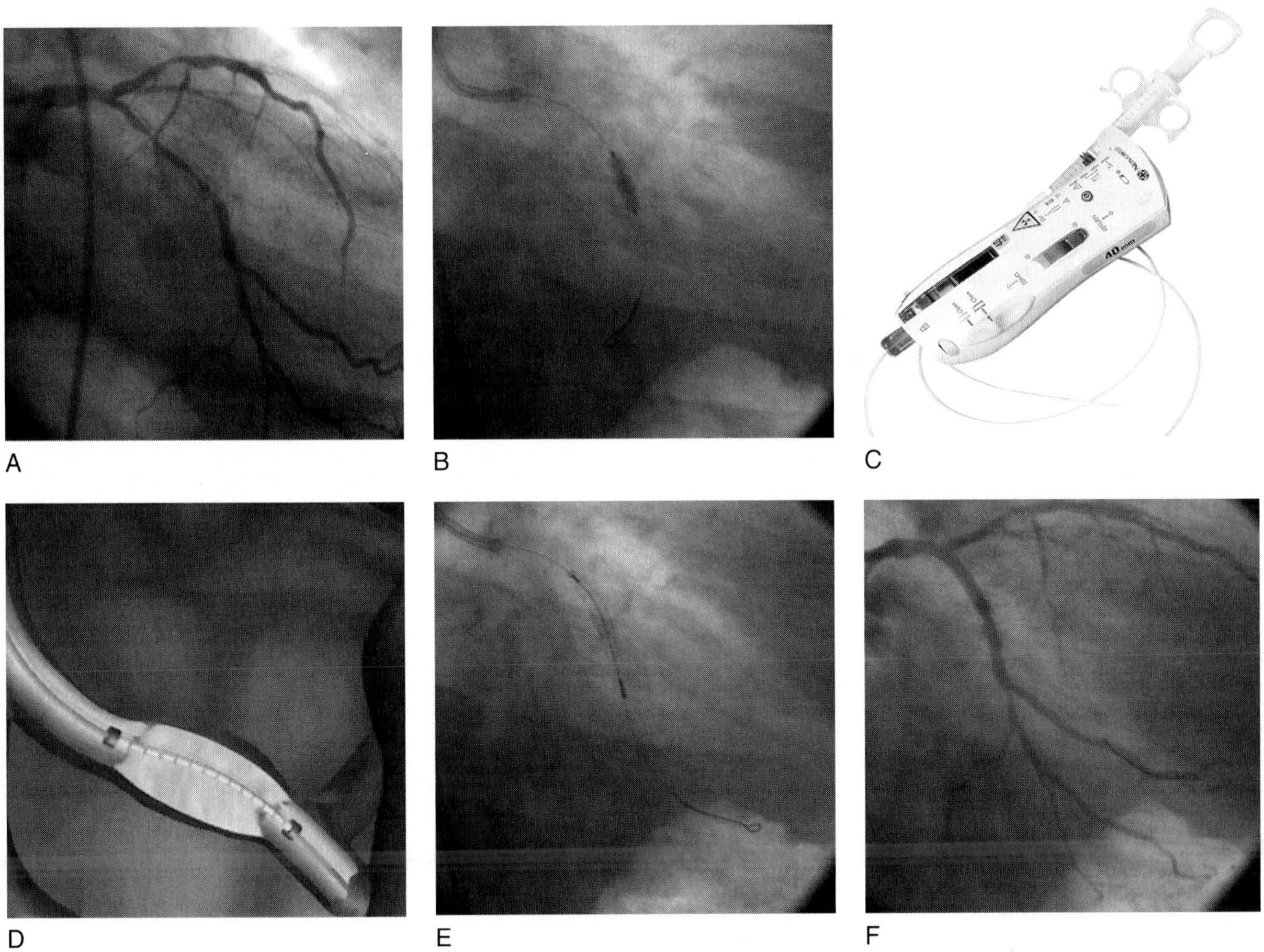

FIGURE 52–12 **A,** Restenosis after coronary stent placement in the midportion of the left circumflex coronary artery. **B,** A 3.5-mm cutting balloon was used to dilate the lesion proximally and distally. **C,** The Novoste Transfer Device uses a saline-filled syringe to advance the radiation seeds to the treatment site. The same device is used to remove the seeds at the end of the brachytherapy treatment. **D,** The Novoste delivery catheter advances $^{90}Sr/^{90}Y$ seeds to the site of angioplasty. **E,** The fluoroscopic position of the catheter is positioned to provide a 5- to 10-mm proximal and distal margin at the region of injury. **F,** The final angiographic result after radiation brachytherapy is shown.

mechanical breakage, or infection caused by the foreign body. Subsequent generations of devices have reduced the size and complexity of placement, and meticulous attention to aseptic technique or even use of prophylactic antibiotics has controlled the infection risk.

Collagen-based approaches seek to apply a small pack of purified bovine collagen to the external surface of the artery. This can be done just externally (VasoSeal, Datascope) or in conjunction with an intraarterial absorbable anchor and suture (AngioSeal, Kensey-Nash). These devices are generally easier to employ than the suture approach,[46] although correct technical placement is essential to efficacy and minimizing complications.

Procoagulant-based approaches (Vascular Solutions Duett) seek to achieve internal mechanical hemostasis temporarily with a miniature balloon-tip catheter while a liquid procoagulant (thrombin and collagen) is deposited in the soft tissue just outside the artery. Once this material is in place, the balloon can be deflated and removed, with rapid formation of the hemostatic plug following contact of the blood with the procoagulant. Incorrect deposition can lead to poor hemostasis or procoagulant deposition within the arterial lumen with production of distal limb ischemic complications.

The balance of the patient's comfort related to elimination of manual or mechanical compression and prolonged bed rest, greater staff efficiencies in not having to supervise delayed sheath removal, and the ability to facilitate outpatient procedures have made the use of one or more of the groin closure devices described previously fairly routine in catheter-based interventional procedures. Still, failure to eliminate the standard groin complications compared with manual compression and the potential for introducing unique complications such as infection and intraarterial administration of procoagulants have led other laboratories to continue to favor manual or mechanical groin compression following catheter-based intervention.

Anticoagulation During Percutaneous Coronary Intervention

(see also Chaps. 48 and 80)

PCI requires the use of one or more antiplatelet agents (e.g., aspirin, clopidogrel, and GP IIb/IIIa inhibitors) combined with some level of thrombin inhibition (e.g., intravenous heparin, low-molecular-weight heparin [LMWH], or bivalirudin) in order to prevent thrombus formation on the denuded endothelium, balloons, stents, and wires that are used to perform the PCI.

Aspirin

Aspirin is an irreversible inhibitor of the enzyme cyclooxygenase that blocks the synthesis of thromboxane A_2, a vasoconstricting agent that promotes platelet aggregation. Compared with placebo, aspirin substantially reduced periprocedural MI related to thrombotic occlusions and has been established as a standard for all patients undergoing PCI. Although the minimum effective aspirin dosage in the setting of PCI has not been established, oral or intravenous doses greater than 75 mg given at least 2 hours before the procedure appear to be effective. The inhibitory effect of aspirin occurs within 60 minutes, and its effect on platelet inhibition lasts for up to 7 days after aspirin discontinuation. It is now recognized that a substantial number of patients have aspirin resistance with standard doses of aspirin therapy.

Thienopyridine Derivatives

Thienopyridine derivatives cause irreversible platelet inhibition related to their effects on the P2Y12 adenosine diphosphate (ADP) receptor that is responsible for activation of the GP IIb/IIIa complex. Because aspirin and thienopyridine derivatives have synergistic mechanisms of action, their combination may inhibit platelet aggregation to a greater extent than either agent alone. Clopidogrel, 300 mg loading followed by 75 mg daily, or, less preferred, ticlopidine, 500 mg loading followed by 250 mg twice daily, may also be used as an alternative in aspirin-sensitive patients undergoing balloon angioplasty or coronary atherectomy.

Subacute vessel closure is a recognized complication of stent placement and occurred in 3 to 5 percent of cases in the initial stent series,[4,20] and this risk was substantially reduced with the addition of a thienopyridine derivate in addition to aspirin.[37,47] In a study of 517 high-risk patients treated with Palmaz-Schatz stents for acute MI, suboptimal angioplasty, or other high-risk clinical and anatomical features, random assignment to aspirin plus ticlopidine or anticoagulant therapy was performed after successful stent placement.[47] The primary composite endpoint of cardiac death, MI, CABG, or repeated angioplasty occurred in 6.2 percent of patients assigned to anticoagulant therapy and 1.5 percent of patients assigned to antiplatelet therapy ($p = 0.01$).[47] Subacute stent thrombosis developed in 5.4 percent of patients assigned to anticoagulant therapy and in 0.8 percent of the antiplatelet therapy group. A second study was performed in 1653 lower risk patients undergoing successful Palmaz-Schatz stent placement.[37] The Stent Anticoagulation Restenosis Study (STARS) compared the effect of aspirin, 325 mg daily; the combination of aspirin, 325 mg daily, plus ticlopidine, 500 mg daily, for 1 month; and aspirin, 325 mg daily, plus warfarin on 30-day ischemic endpoints.[37] The composite of death, TLR, angiographic thrombosis, or MI was reduced from 3.6 percent of patients assigned to aspirin only and 2.7 percent assigned to aspirin plus warfarin to 0.5 percent of those assigned to aspirin plus ticlopidine ($p < 0.001$).[37]

Ticlopidine use has been virtually abandoned because of frequent side effects and hematological toxicities with the availability of the safer thienopyridine derivative clopidogrel. Rare hematological complications have been reported with clopidogrel, including hemolytic-uremic syndrome and thrombotic thrombocytopenic purpura, but it is still considered much safer than ticlopidine. Randomized trials have shown no difference in clinical efficacy between clopidogrel and ticlopidine, with fewer side effects in patients treated with clopidogrel. Although higher (450 to 600 mg) doses of clopidogrel prior to PCI may provide additional benefit compared with conventional loading doses, additional study is needed before this is routinely recommended.

Prolonged (up to 10 days) pretreatment with clopidogrel before PCI in patients with acute coronary syndromes was associated with improved 30-day outcomes compared with patients who were not pretreated with clopidogrel,[48] although the incremental benefit of clopidogrel given just before elective PCI has not been clearly established. The combination of aspirin and clopidogrel may also be useful in preventing ischemic complications for up to 9 months after PCI in patients with acute coronary syndromes[48] and after elective angioplasty.[49] The Clopidogrel for the Reduction of Events During Observation (CREDO) trial was a randomized, double-blind, placebo-controlled trial involving 2116 patients who were to undergo elective PCI who were randomly assigned to receive a 300-mg clopidogrel loading dose or placebo 3 to 24 hours before PCI. Thereafter, all patients received clopidogrel, 75 mg/d, through day 28. From day 29 through 12 months, patients in the loading-dose group received clopidogrel, 75 mg/d, and those in the control group received placebo. Both groups received aspirin throughout the study. The 12-month incidence of the composite of death, MI, or stroke in the intent-to-treat population was reduced by 26.9 percent in patients treated with clopidogrel ($p = 0.02$).[49] Risk of major bleeding at 1 year tended to be higher in patients treated with combined clopidogrel therapy (8.8 percent with clopidogrel versus 6.7 percent with placebo; $p = 0.07$).[49]

Glycoprotein IIb/IIIa Inhibitors

Thrombin and collagen are potent platelet agonists that can cause ADP and serotonin release and activate GP IIb/IIIa fibrinogen receptors on the platelet surface. Functionally active GP IIb/IIIa activation serves as the final common pathway of platelet aggregation by binding fibrinogen and other adhesive proteins that bridge adjacent platelets.

ABCIXIMAB. The safety and efficacy of abciximab were first evaluated in the Evaluation of 7E3 for the Prevention of Ischemic Complications (EPIC) trial, a clinical study of 2099 patients at high risk for complications after PCI.[50] Patients also received aspirin 325 mg and a non-weight-adjusted, 10,000- to 12,000-IU heparin bolus prior to PCI and were then randomly assigned to treatment with placebo, a bolus of abciximab 0.25 mg/kg, or the same bolus of abciximab followed by a 12-hour abciximab infusion at 10 μg/min. Bolus and infusion abciximab was associated with a 35 percent reduction in frequency of the composite clinical endpoint, defined as death, nonfatal MI, repeated revascularization, or procedural failure (8.3 versus 12.8 percent in placebo-treated patients; $p = 0.008$).[50] Bleeding complications occurred twice as often in patients receiving abciximab, attributable to the high dose of heparin used with the procedure.

The Evaluation of PTCA to Improve Long-Term Outcome by Abciximab GP IIb/IIIa Blockade (EPILOG) trial randomly assigned 2792 "low-risk" patients who were treated with aspirin to standard-dose, weight-adjusted (100 units/kg) heparin and placebo; standard-dose, weight-adjusted heparin and abciximab; or low-dose, weight-adjusted (70 units/kg) heparin.[51] The 30-day composite event rate was significantly ($p < 0.001$) lower in patients treated with abciximab and low-dose (5.2 percent) or standard-dose (5.4 percent) heparin than in patients treated with standard-dose heparin and placebo (11.7 percent).[51] Abciximab does not reduce complication rates associated with SVG intervention. Bailout abciximab is often given during or just after PCI for the presence of residual dissection, thrombus, or suboptimal results, although its value has not been demonstrated in prospective studies.

The Evaluation of Platelet IIb/IIIa Inhibitor for Stenting Trial (EPISTENT) randomly assigned 2399 patients with ischemic CAD to stenting plus placebo, stenting plus abciximab, or balloon PTCA plus abciximab.[52] The primary 30-day endpoint, a combination of death, MI, or need for urgent revascularization, occurred in 10.8 percent of patients in the stent-plus-placebo group, 5.3 percent of patients in the stent-plus-abciximab group (hazard ratio 0.48; $p < 0.001$), and 6.9 percent of patients in the balloon-plus-abciximab group (hazard ratio 0.63; $p = 0.007$).[52] No significant differences in bleeding complications were noted among the groups. A pooled analysis also suggests that abciximab may reduce mortality in diabetic patients.

EPTIFIBATIDE. The Integrilin to Minimise Platelet Aggregation and Coronary Thrombosis-II (IMPACT-II) trial enrolled 4010 patients undergoing PCI who were randomly assigned to treatment with a single, low-dose bolus of eptifibatide (135 μg/kg) followed by a low-dose infusion (0.5 μg/kg/min for 20 to 24 hours) or the same eptifibatide bolus and a modestly higher dose infusion of 0.75 μg/kg/min for 20 to 24 hours.[53] The primary endpoint was the 30-day composite occurrence of death, MI, unplanned CABG or repeated PCI, or coronary stenting for abrupt closure. Such events occurred in 11.4 percent of patients in the placebo group versus 9.2 percent in the eptifibatide135/0.5 group ($p = 0.063$) and 9.9 percent in the eptifibatide 135/0.75 group ($p = 0.22$).[53] It is now recognized that the eptifibatide infusion dosage in the IMPACT-II trial was insufficient to provide adequate platelet inhibition during PCI.

The Enhanced Suppression of the Platelet IIb/IIIa Receptor with Integrilin Therapy (ESPRIT) study evaluated a larger double eptifibatide bolus (180 μg/kg boluses 10 minutes apart) and infusion dose (2.0 μg/kg/min for 18 to 24 hours) or placebo in a randomized study of 2064 patients undergoing stent implantation in a native coronary artery.[54] The primary endpoint was the composite of death, MI, urgent target vessel revascularization, and thrombotic bailout GP IIb/IIIa inhibitor therapy within 48 hours after randomization, and it occurred in 10.5 percent of 1024 patients receiving placebo and in 6.6 percent of patients treated with eptifibatide ($p = 0.0015$). The key 30-day secondary endpoint was also reduced, from 10.5 percent to 6.8 percent ($p = 0.0034$). Major bleeding was infrequent but arose more often with eptifibatide than placebo (1.3 percent versus 0.4 percent in placebo-treated patients; $p = 0.027$). These effects were sustained 1 year after the procedure and were effective in high-risk diabetic patients.

TIROFIBAN. Tirofiban, a nonpeptidyl tyrosine derivative, has also been evaluated for its adjunctive benefit during PCI. In the Randomized Efficacy Study of Tirofiban for Outcomes and Restenosis (RESTORE) trial that included 2139 patients undergoing PCI within 72 hours of an acute coronary syndrome, the primary 30-day composite endpoint was 16 percent lower with tirofiban treatment ($p = 0.160$), although a 38 percent relative reduction in the composite endpoint was noted at 48 hours ($p = 0.005$) and a 27 percent relative reduction at 7 days ($p = 0.022$).[55] In a larger study using the same bolus and infusion dose of tirofiban, 4809 patients were randomly assigned to receive either tirofiban or abciximab before PCI with the intent to perform stenting.[56] The primary endpoint, a composite of death, nonfatal MI, and urgent target vessel revascularization at 30 days, occurred more frequently among the patients in the tirofiban group than among patients in the abciximab group (7.6 percent versus 6.0 percent; $p = 0.038$). Subsequent studies have suggested that the tirofiban bolus dose given in this study may have been insufficient to obtain optimal anticoagulation during PCI, and larger bolus doses have been shown to improve the inhibition of platelet aggregation but have not been tested in clinical studies.

Unfractionated Heparin (see also Chap. 80)

Unfractionated heparin is the thrombin inhibitor most commonly used during PCI. "Near-patient" ACT monitoring has facilitated heparin dose titration during PCI, as the required level of anticoagulation activity is beyond the range of the activated partial thromboplastin time. Retrospective studies have related the ACT value to clinical outcome after PCI, and an analysis of 5216 patients undergoing PCI in which unfractionated heparin was used showed that an ACT in the range of 350 to 375 seconds provided the lowest composite ischemic event rate of 6.6 percent, or a 34 percent relative risk reduction in 7-day ischemic events compared with rates observed between 171 and 295 seconds by quartile analysis ($p = 0.001$).[57] Any level of ACT greater than 200 seconds was associated with no further reductions in ischemic complications with concomitant use of GP IIb/IIIa inhibitors, but bleeding complications increased incrementally at all ACTs greater than 200 seconds.[57]

Although randomized trials that have evaluated empirical and weight-adjusted heparin dosing have shown comparable results, weight-adjusted heparin dosing regimens of 50 to 70 IU/kg are now used in an attempt to avoid "overshooting" the ACT. It is generally recommended that sufficient unfractionated heparin be administered during PCI to achieve an ACT around 300 seconds if no GP IIb/IIIa inhibitor is given and more than 200 seconds if GP IIb/IIIa inhibitors are given. Routine use of intravenous heparin after PCI is no longer indicated because several randomized studies showed no benefit in reducing ischemic complications and higher access site bleeding complication rates. Early sheath removal is encouraged when the ACT falls to less than 150 to 180 seconds.

Low-Molecular-Weight Heparin

(see also Chap. 80)

An increasing number of patients with unstable angina are treated with LMWH prior to PCI, but because of difficulties monitoring anticoagulation levels with LMWH during PCI, empirical dose algorithms have been designed to guide additional anticoagulation therapy during PCI. If the last dose of enoxaparin was given less than 8 hours before PCI, no additional antithrombin is needed. If the last dose of enoxaparin was given between 8 and 12 hours, a 0.3-mg/kg bolus of intravenous enoxaparin should be given.[58] If the dose was administrated more than 12 hours before PCI, conventional anticoagulation therapy is indicated. A near-patient assay for estimating the anticoagulant activity (by estimating anti-Xa activity) with enoxaparin has been developed and is available for clinical use. The use of enoxaparin appears safe and effective when it is given in combination with tirofiban or eptifibatide during PCI.

Direct Thrombin Inhibitors

Three direct thrombin inhibitors, hirudin, bivalirudin, and argatroban, have been evaluated as alternatives to heparin during PCI. In the Hirudin in a European Trial Versus Heparin in the Prevention of Restenosis after PTCA (HELVETICA) study,[59] 1141 patients with unstable angina undergoing PCI were treated with aspirin and randomly assigned to receive a heparin bolus of 10,000 units plus infusion at 15 units/kg/hr for 24 hours; a hirudin bolus of 40 mg plus intravenous infusion at 0.2 mg/kg/hr for 24 hours; or a hirudin bolus of 40 mg, intravenous infusion at 0.2 mg/kg/hr for 24 hours, and subcutaneous infusion of 40 mg twice daily for an additional 3 days. Hirudin use was associated with a 39 percent reduction in early cardiac events ($p = 0.023$), although clinical outcomes were similar 7 months later in the three groups. A recombinant hirudin (lepirudin) bolus of 0.4 mg/kg and infusion at 0.15 mg/kg/hr are approved for use in the United States in patients with heparin-induced thrombocytopenia.

Bivalirudin (Angiomax) was compared with unfractionated heparin in a randomized trial involving 4098 patients with postinfarction or unstable angina undergoing PCI. Patients were assigned to treatment with a high-dose (175 units/kg) heparin bolus and an infusion of 15 units/kg/hr for 18 to 24 hours or to a bivalirudin bolus (1.0 mg/kg) and an infusion of 2.5 mg/kg/hr for 4 hours, followed by 0.2 mg/kg/hr for 14 to 20 hours.[60] Bivalirudin did not reduce the likelihood of in-hospital death, Q wave or non-Q-wave MI, or emergency CABG but did reduce the likelihood of bleeding complications (odds ratio of 0.4; $p < 0.001$).[60] In patients with post-MI angina, bivalirudin resulted in lower rates of major ischemic complications (9.1 versus 14.2 percent in heparin-treated patients; $p = 0.04$) and lower rates of bleeding (3.0 versus 11.1 percent in heparin-treated patients; $p < 0.001$).[60]

The Randomized Evaluation in PCI Linking Angiomax to Reduced Clinical Events (REPLACE)-2 trial randomly assigned 6010 patients undergoing PCI to receive intravenous bivalirudin (0.75 mg/kg bolus plus 1.75 mg/kg per hour for the duration of PCI), with provisional GP IIb/IIIa inhibition, or heparin (65 U/kg bolus) with planned GP IIb/IIIa inhibition (abciximab or eptifibatide).[61] The primary composite endpoint was the 30-day incidence of death, MI, urgent repeated revascularization, or in-hospital major bleeding and occurred among 9.2 percent of patients in the bivalirudin group and 10.0 percent of patients in the heparin-plus-GP IIb/IIIa group ($p = 0.32$). Bivalirudin with provisional GP IIb/IIIa blockade was statistically not inferior to heparin plus planned GP IIb/IIIa blockade during contemporary PCI with regard to suppression of acute ischemic endpoints and was associated with less bleeding. Bivalirudin may be particularly useful in patients with heparin-induced thrombocytopenia, those with excessive bleeding risk, elderly patients, and patients with renal insufficiency.

Pharmacological Approaches to Restenosis

A number of systemic agents have been used to prevent restenosis after balloon angioplasty and directional atherectomy, but none has had a consistent effect on restenosis prevention. Detailed review of the multiple trials is beyond the scope of this chapter, but a summary of ongoing evaluation of newer potential therapies may be found in Table 52–6.[62-76]

Studies that have evaluated aspirin in preventing restenosis after PCI have provided conflicting results, potentially owing to the varied dosage, timing, and duration of aspirin therapy; limited sample sizes; and incomplete angiographic follow-up. Aspirin therapy (75 to 325 mg/d) should be continued indefinitely after PCI for the secondary prevention of cardiovascular events (death, MI, or stroke) rather than for the prevention of late restenosis.

Cilostazol selectively inhibits 3′,5′-cyclic nucleotide phosphodiesterase III and has antiplatelet and vasodilating effects. Smaller studies suggest a benefit of cilostazol in preventing restenosis after coronary stenting, but one larger study failed to demonstrate a restenosis benefit of cilostazol after elective stent placement.[63] The Cilostazol for Restenosis (CREST) trial is an ongoing evaluation of 600 patients undergoing elective treatment with stent implantation treated with either aspirin and clopidogrel or aspirin, clopidogrel, and cilostazol (William Weintraub, personal communication).

Although a subgroup analysis of diabetic patients undergoing stent implantation in EPISTENT demonstrated a reduction in revascularization in diabetic patients assigned to stenting plus abciximab (8.1 percent) compared with patients receiving stenting plus placebo (16.6 percent),[77] a larger subgroup analysis in another prospective trial failed to demonstrate a difference in late outcomes in diabetic patients treated with periprocedural abciximab and tirofiban.[78] GP IIb/IIIa inhibitors are no longer recommended for the prevention of restenosis in diabetic patients undergoing stent implantation.

C-reactive protein (CRP) rises and remains elevated for up to 36 hours after stent implantation, and preprocedural elevation of CRP is an important predictor of restenosis. Although a single bolus of systemic corticosteroids does not reduce restenosis, sustained oral prednisone therapy reduced restenosis in a series of 83 patients with persistent elevation of CRP after successful stent placement,[67] reducing 6-month restenosis rates from 33 percent in placebo-treated patients to 7 percent in prednisone-treated patients.

Probucol is an antioxidant that has been shown to reduce intimal hyperplasia. Although one smaller study failed to demonstrate a reduction in angiographic restenosis after stent placement, a larger study randomly assigned 317 patients 1 month before angioplasty to treatment with placebo, probucol (500 mg), multivitamins (30,000 IU of beta carotene, 500 mg of vitamin C, and 700 IU of vitamin E), or both probucol and multivitamins—all given twice daily.[79] Restenosis rates per segment were 20.7 percent in the probucol group, 28.9 percent in the combined treatment group, 40.3 percent in the multivitamin group, and 38.9 percent in the placebo group ($p = 0.003$ for probucol versus no probucol).[79] In a subgroup of 189 patients with small (<3.0-mm) vessels in the MultiVitamins and Probucol (MVP) trial, restenosis was lower in patients treated with probucol. Although probucol has potential benefit in restenosis prevention, the prolonged pretreatment time, prolongation of the QTc interval, and unfavorable effect on high-density lipoprotein limit its clinical use. AGI-1067, a metabolically stable modification of probucol with an equipotent antioxidant effect, also has a potential beneficial effect on restenosis after stent placement.[68]

Oral rapamycin, 6 mg loading dose and 2 mg per day for 4 weeks, was given to 22 patients at high risk for restenosis after stent placement.[80] Nearly 50 percent of patients discontinued therapy because of side effects, and no reduction in the occurrence of clinical or angiographic restenosis was found.[80]

A number of studies have evaluated lipid-lowering therapy for the prevention of restenosis after coronary intervention, but none has shown a consistent reduction in restenosis. The Fluvastatin Angioplasty Restenosis (FLARE) trial found no difference in angiographic restenosis with high-dose fluvastatin use, although there was a significantly lower incidence of total death and MI was observed in 6 patients (1.4 percent) in the fluvastatin group and 17 (4.0 percent) in the placebo group (log rank $p = 0.025$).[81] A larger clinical study, the Lescol Intervention Prevention Study (LIPS), assigned patients to receive fluvastatin, 80 mg/d, or matching placebo at hospital discharge for 3 to 4 years.[82] At least one major adverse cardiac event (MACE) event occurred in 21.4 percent of patients in the fluvastatin group and 26.7 percent of patients in the placebo group ($p = 0.01$).[82] In aggregate, these findings suggest that lipid-lowering agents play a limited role in the reduction of restenosis after coronary stent placement, but their use is highly beneficial for the progression of coronary atherosclerosis and clinical events attributable to sites remote from stent placement.

Drug-Eluting Stents

In sharp contradistinction to the failed attempts to prevent restenosis with systemic drug therapy, sustained local delivery of several agents from a stent coating system (termed *drug-eluting stent system*) has been very effective at suppressing the local neointimal proliferation that causes angiographic and clinical restenosis (Table 52–7). Some drug-eluting stent systems have prevented restenosis (e.g., sirolimus, everolimus, polymer-delivered paclitaxel), whereas others have had no or a limited effect (e.g., batimastat, dexamethasone, stent-based paclitaxel) or were clinically detrimental (e.g., actinomycin D, 7-hexanoyltaxol [QP2], a taxane derivative). These studies have demonstrated the important interaction between the stent design, the presence (or absence) of a polymeric coating that is used to deliver the drug, and the types of agents that are delivered to the vessel wall.

Sirolimus

The CYPHER (Cordis, Warren, NJ) stent contains sirolimus, which is a naturally occurring antimicrobial and immunosuppressive agent that causes cytostatic inhibition of growth factor– and cytokine-stimulated cell proliferation in the G1 phase. The polymeric (Topcoat) coating on the Bx Velocity stent provides sustained release of sirolimus over a 30- to 45-day period. The CYPHER stent received CE Mark approval in Europe in April 2002 and approval by the FDA in the United States in May 2003.

TABLE 52–6 Trials of the Use of Oral Agents for the Prevention of Restenosis After Percutaneous Coronary Intervention

Author	Year	Total patients	Angio FU	Stent Use	Treatment	Pretreatment Duration	Duration of Therapy	Restenosis Rates# (%)
Cilostazol								
Tsuchikane et al[62]	1999	211	193	No	Cilostazol 200 mg qd	None	3 mo	18*
					Aspirin 250 mg qd			40
Park et al[63]	2000	409	380	Yes	Cilostazol 100 mg b.i.d.	48 hr	6 mo	23
					Ticlopidine	48 hr	1 mo	27
Kamishirado et al[64]	2002	130	111	Yes	Cilostazol 200 mg qd	48 hr	6 mo	13†
					Ticlopidine			31
Coumadin								
Garachemani et al[65]	2002	191	172	35%	Warfarin (INR = 2.5-4.0)	None	6 mo	30
					Aspirin			33
ten Berg et al[66]	2003	531	480	34%	Coumarin (INR = 2.1-4.8)	7 d	6 mo	38.9§
					Placebo			39.1
Steroids								
Versaci et al[67]	2002	83	83	Yes	Prednisolone orally with taper	None	45 d	7†
					Placebo			33
Antiinflammatory agents								
Tardif et al[68]	2003	305	NR	Yes	AGI-1067, 70 mg	14 d	4 wk	23.6
					AGI-1067, 140 mg			23.6
					AGI-1067, 280 mg			23.6
					Probucol			25.9
					Placebo			37.7
Tranilast								
Holmes et al[69]	2002	11,484		Yes	Tranilast 300 mg b.i.d.	None	1 mo	35
					Tranilast 450 mg b.i.d.		1 mo	33
					Tranilast 300 mg b.i.d.		3 mo	35
					Tranilast 450 mg b.i.d.		3 mo	32
					Placebo			33
Trapidil								
Serruys et al[70]	2001	303	269	Wallstent	Trapidil 200 mg qd	>1 hr	6 mo	31
					Placebo			24
ACE inhibitors								
Meurice et al[71]	2001	91	79	No	Quinapril 40 mg qd	None	6 mo	37
					Placebo			24
Kondo et al[72]	2001	100	99	Yes	Quinapril 10-20 mg qd	None	6 mo	12†
					Placebo			24
Angiotensin receptor blockers								
Peters et al[73]	2001	250	200	Yes	Valsartin 80 mg qd	NR	6 mo	19.2‡
					Placebo			38.6
Calcium channel antagonists								
Dens et al[74]	2001	826	646	No	Nisoldipine 40 mg qd	None	6 mo	49‖
					Placebo			55
Jorgensen et al[75]	2000	585	451	16%	Amlodipine 10 mg qd	2 wk	4 mo	28
					Placebo			28
Carvedilol								
Serruys et al[76]	2000	324	292	No	Carvedilol 12.5 mg b.i.d.	>24 hr	5 mo	23.4
					Placebo			23.9

ACE = angiotensin-converting enzyme; Angio = angiographic; FU = follow-up; INR = international normalized ratio; NR = not reported.
*$p < 0.001$.
†$p < 0.05$.
‡$p < 0.005$.
§Mean follow-up percent stenosis.
‖Restenosis defined as a loss of 50% of initial gain.
#Restenosis defined as more than 50% follow-up diameter strenosis unless indicated otherwise.

FIRST IN-HUMAN STUDIES. Sirolimus-eluting Bx Velocity stents were first implanted in 45 patients with focal native vessel disease.[83-85] In-stent minimal lumen diameter and percent diameter stenosis were essentially unchanged from the postprocedural study to the 18- to 24-month follow-up study.[86] Intravascular ultrasound–detected neointimal hyperplasia was virtually absent at 12 months in both groups (Fig. 52–13).

RAVEL. The Randomized Study with the Sirolimus-Eluting Bx Velocity Balloon-Expandable Stent (RAVEL) trial randomly assigned 238 patients with single, primary lesions located in native coronary arteries to treatment with the sirolimus stent or the bare metal stent (Table 52–8).[87] The degree of late lumen loss at 6 months was significantly lower in the sirolimus stent group (−0.01 ± 0.33-mm) than in the standard stent group (0.80 ± 0.53-mm) ($p < 0.001$). None of

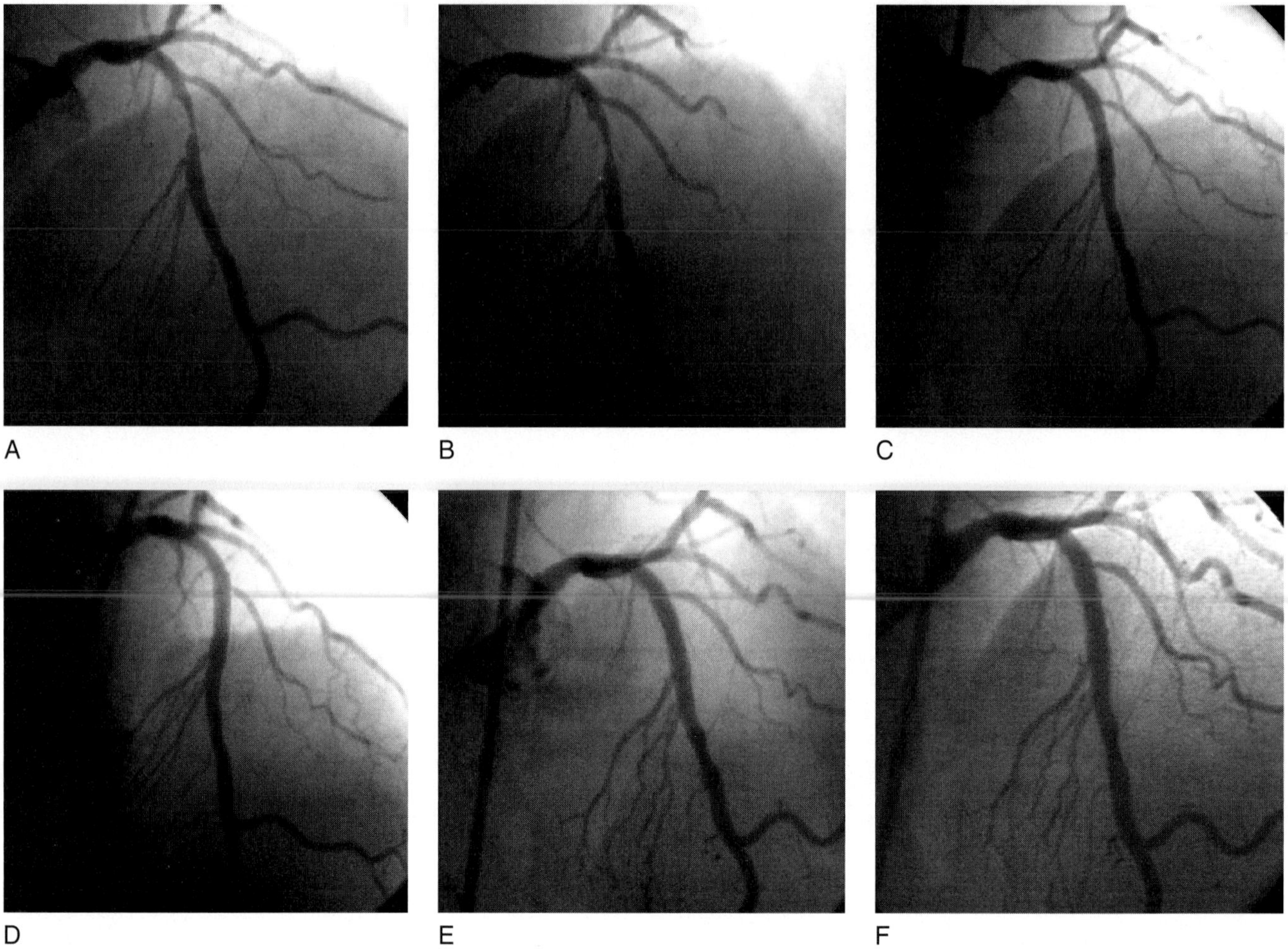

FIGURE 52–13 First in-human CYPHER stent implantation. **A,** A focal stenosis is shown in the middle left anterior descending artery. **B,** A CYPHER sirolimus-eluting stent is positioned across the stenosis. **C,** There is an excellent initial angiographic result and no residual stenosis. Follow-up angiography was performed at 4 months **(D)**, 1 year **(E)**, and 2 years after the procedure **(F)** without evidence of lumen renarrowing. This pattern of markedly reduced intimal hyperplasia was found in virtually all patients in the first in-human study. (Courtesy of Dr. Eduardo Sousa, São Paulo, Brazil.)

TABLE 52–7 Angiographic and Clinical Endpoints for Restenosis Percutaneous Coronary Intervention

Angiographic	Clinical
Binary	**Binary**
>50% follow-up diameter stenosis	Death
	Nonfatal myocardial infarction
>0.72-mm loss in lumen diameter	Revascularization
	Target vessel failure
>20% loss in gain achieved	Target vessel revascularization
Continuous	Target lesion revascularization
Follow-up minimal lumen diameter	Recurrence of angina
	Continuous
Follow-up % diameter stenosis	Exercise test duration
Late lumen loss	
Loss index	

the patients in the sirolimus stent group had restenosis, compared with 26.6 percent of those in the standard stent group ($p < 0.001$).[87] There were no episodes of stent thrombosis. During a follow-up period of up to 1 year, the overall rate of major cardiac events was 5.8 percent in the sirolimus stent group and 28.8 percent in the standard stent group ($p < 0.001$).[87] Volumetric intravascular ultrasound analysis also demonstrated a 90 percent reduction in intimal hyperplasia associated with the use of the CYPHER stent.[88]

SIRIUS. The Sirolimus-Eluting Stent in de novo Coronary Artery Lesions (SIRIUS) trial included 1058 patients with a lesion length between 15 and 30-mm and a reference diameter between 2.5 and 3.5-mm and randomly assigned them to treatment with a sirolimus-eluting stent or a bare metal stent.[89] The primary clinical endpoint in the SIRIUS trial was 8-month target vessel failure, defined as target vessel revascularization, death, or MI, and it was reduced from 21.0 percent in patients treated with bare metal stents to 8.6 percent in patients with sirolimus-eluting stents ($p < 0.001$). Target vessel revascularization was reduced from 16.6 percent with bare metal stents to 4.1 percent in patients treated with sirolimus-eluting stents ($p < 0.001$).[89] Compared with patients treated with bare metal stents, patients treated with sirolimus-eluting stents had lower rates of binary angiographic restenosis within the treated segment (36.3 percent with bare metal stents versus 8.9 percent with sirolimus-eluting stents; $p < 0.001$) and within the stent (35.4 percent with bare metal stents versus 3.2 percent with sirolimus-eluting stents; $p < 0.001$).[89]

OTHER INDICATIONS. The CYPHER stent may also be useful in patients with in-stent restenosis. Twenty-five patients with in-stent restenosis were successfully treated with the implantation of one or two sirolimus-eluting Bx Velocity stents.[90] Angiographic late loss averaged 0.07 ±

TABLE 52–8 Late Outcome in Randomized Trials of Sirolimus Eluting Stents for the Prevention of Restenosis

	RAVEL[87]		SIRIUS[89]	
Variable	***Sirolimus***	***Bare***		
Number of patients	120	118	533	525
Baseline factors				
Mean age, yr	61.8	59.7	62.1	62.4
Women, %	30	29	27	30
Diabetes mellitus	16	21	24.6	28.2
Lesion length, mm	9.6	9.6	14.4	14.4
Reference diameter, mm	2.56	2.64	2.79	2.82
MLD, mm				
Baseline	0.94	0.95	0.97	0.98
Final	2.43	2.41	2.39	2.40
Follow-up	2.42*	1.64	2.15	1.60
Late lumen loss, mm	−0.01	0.80	0.24	0.81
% Diameter stenosis				
Baseline	63.6	64.0	65.6	65.3
Final	11.9	14.0	15.8	16.1
Follow-up	14.7	36.7	23.6	43.2
Restenosis rate, %	0	26.6	8.9	36.3
Stent thrombosis, %	0	0		
Follow-up period	12 mo		9 mo	
TLR, %	0	27	4.1	16.6
Late clinical events, %	5.8	28.8	8.6	21.0
Death	2	2	0.9	0.6
Q wave MI	0	0	0.8	0.4

*$p < 0.001$.

MI = myocardial infarction; MLD = minimum lumen diameter; RAVEL = Randomized Study with the Sirolimus-Eluting Bx Velocity Balloon-Expandable Stent; SIRIUS = Sirolimus-Eluting Stent in de novo Coronary Artery Lesions; TLR = target lesion revascularization.

0.2-mm within the stent and −0.05 ± 0.3-mm within the lesion at 4 months and 0.36 ± 0.46-mm within the stent and 0.16 ± 0.42-mm within the lesion 12 months later. Only one patient had in-stent restenosis at 1-year follow-up. A second series of 16 patients with more complex recurrent in-stent restenosis in native coronary arteries (average lesion length 18.4-mm) were treated with one or more 18-mm Bx Velocity sirolimus-eluting stents.[91] Four patients had recurrent restenosis following brachytherapy, and three patients had totally occluded vessels before the procedure.[91] At 4-month follow-up, one patient had died and three patients had angiographic evidence of restenosis (one in stent and two in lesion).[91] Although there was a minimal amount of in-stent late lumen loss (averaging 0.21-mm), three patients had experienced four major adverse cardiac events by 9 months (two deaths and one acute MI necessitating repeated target vessel angioplasty).[91] One randomized trial comparing brachytherapy and the CYPHER stent in patients with in-stent restenosis is ongoing.

Paclitaxel

Paclitaxel stabilizes microtubules and prevents cell division at the M phase. In lower doses this agent may also have cytostatic effects on cell proliferation, and in higher doses it may have cytotoxic effects. Paclitaxel has been delivered to the vessel wall in two formulations—one with a polymeric coating that elutes the drug to the vessel wall over a period of 30 to 45 days (TAXUS programs, Boston Scientific, Natick, MA) and one with a spray coating of the drug on the stent that provides more rapid release (Cook, Bloomington, IN, and Guidant, Santa Clara, CA).

POLYMERIC-COATED, PACLITAXEL-ELUTING STENT: THE TAXUS STUDIES. The TAXUS I trial was a prospective, double-blind, three-center study randomly assigning 61 patients with de novo or restenotic lesions to receive an NIR stent with a polymeric coating that eluted paclitaxel or a bare metal stent (Table 52–9).[92-95] There were no cases of angiographic restenosis 6 months after the procedure, compared with 10 percent in patients treated with control stents, and these beneficial effects persisted up to 1 year after the procedure.[92] The TAXUS II study was a larger randomized trial involving 536 patients with native vessel CAD who were randomly assigned to treatment with a bare NIR Express stent, an NIR Express stent containing a slow-release vascularly compatible Translute polymeric coating that released paclitaxel, or a bare NIR Express or an NIR Express containing a moderate-release Translute polymer that released paclitaxel over a more sustained period. There was a significant reduction in the clinical and angiographic restenosis rate in patients treated with both the slow- and moderate-release formulations.[93]

Twenty-eight patients with in-stent restenosis were treated with a paclitaxel-eluting NIR stent in the TAXUS III study.[96] No subacute stent thrombosis occurred up to 12 months, but there was one late chronic total occlusion and three additional patients showed angiographic restenosis.[96] The major adverse cardiac event rate was 29 percent (eight patients; one non-Q-wave MI, one coronary artery bypass grafting, and six TLR).[96] Of the patients with TLR, one had restenosis in a bare stent implanted for edge dissection and two had restenosis in a gap between two paclitaxel-eluting stents.[96]

The TAXUS IV trial randomized 1314 patients to treatment with a bare metal or paclitaxel-coated stent. Target lesion

TABLE 52–9 Late Outcome in Randomized Trials, Patients Treated with Paclitaxel-Eluting Stents for the Prevention of Restenosis

	TAXUS-I[92]		TAXUS-II[93]				TAXUS-IV[94]		ASPECT[95]	
Variable	*SL*	*Bare*	*SL*	*Bare*	*MR*	*Bare*	*SL*	*Bare*	*High Dose*	*Placebo*
Number of patients	31	30	131	136	135	134	662	652	60	59
Baseline factors										
Mean Age, yr	66	64	62	60	59	59	63	62	58	58
Women, %	6	17	30	21	24	23	28	28	20	24
Diabetes mellitus	23	13	11	16	17	14	31	33	18	17
Lesion length, mm	10.7	11.9	10.6	10.5	10.2	10.7	14.4	14.4		
Reference diameter, mm	2.99	2.94	2.78	2.77	2.72	2.73	2.75	2.75	2.94	2.88
MLD, mm										
Baseline	1.30	1.23	1.02	1.03	0.95	0.91	0.92	0.95	0.64	0.54
Final	2.95	2.87	2.53	2.58	2.53	2.52	2.26	2.29	2.85	2.82
Follow-up	2.60	1.19	2.23	1.79	2.24	1.76	2.03	1.68	2.53*	1.79
Late lumen loss	0.36	0.71	0.31	0.79	0.30	0.77	0.23	0.61	0.29*	1.04
% Diameter stenosis										
Baseline	57	58	63.3	62.8	64.9	66.6	66.5	65.6	79.4	80.9
Final	6	10	10.9	10.2	11.0	12.0	19.1	19.1	1.8	3.8
Follow-up	14	27	19.5	31.8	18.2	33.9	26.3	39.8	14*	39
Restenosis rate, %	0	10	5.5	20.1	8.6	23.8	7.9	26.6	4*	27
Stent thrombosis, number	0	0	1	0	1	0	0.6%	0.8%	3	0
Follow-up period	12 mo		12 mo				9 mo		6 mo	
TLR, %	0	10	4.7†	12.9	3.8‡	16.0	11.3	3.0	2	2
Late clinical events, %	3	10	10.9†	22.0	9.9†	21.4	8.5	15.0	10%	5%
Death	0	0	0	1.5	0	0	1.4	1.1	0	0
Q wave MI	0	0	0.8	1.5	1.5	0.8	0.8	0.3	0	0

*$p < 0.001$.
†$p < 0.05$.
‡$p < 0.005$.
ASPECT = Asian Paclitaxel-Eluting Stent Clinical Trial; MI = myocardial infarction; MLD = minimum lumen diameter; MR = moderate release; SL = slow release; TLR = target lesion revascularization.

revascularization and angiographic restenosis were significantly reduced in patients treated with the TAXUS stent.[94]

PACLITAXEL-COATED STENTS. Another method of delivering paclitaxel by means of a spray coating was evaluated in a randomized study of 177 patients with discrete coronary lesions using low-dose paclitaxel (1.3 μg/mm²), high dose paclitaxel (3.1 μg/mm²), or control stents.[95] At follow-up, the high-dose paclitaxel group had significantly lower binary restenosis rates than control-treated patients (4 percent versus 27 percent; $p < 0.001$).[95] Intravascular ultrasonography showed a stepwise reduction in intimal hyperplasia accumulation within the stented segment in patients treated with high-dose paclitaxel .[97] The DELIVER trial was a large randomized trial that evaluated the Penta stent with paclitaxel coating and failed to demonstrate a significant benefit with a drug-eluting stent.

PACLITAXEL DERIVATIVE–ELUTING POLYMERIC SLEEVE. The Study to COmpare REstenosis rate between QueST and QuaDS-QP2 (SCORE) trial was a randomized, multicenter trial that compared QP2-eluting stents with bare metal stents in the treatment of de novo coronary lesions. This system was associated with a high (10 percent) subacute thrombosis rate, although restenosis was reduced.[98] At 6 months, three patients had TLR (20 percent). Two patients had restenosis (13.3 percent) with a minimal amount of intimal hyperplasia observed in all the segments covered by drug-eluting stents.[98] At 12 months, one patient suffered from non-Q-wave MI and 61.5 percent had angiographic restenosis.[98] Five patients with restenosis underwent DCA for recurrent in-stent restenosis.[99] Restenotic lesions from QuaDS-QP2-eluting stents at 12 months showed persistent fibrin deposition with varying degrees of inflammation.[99] These pathological changes, representing delayed healing, are usually observed up to only 3 months in human coronary arteries with stainless steel balloon-expandable stents.[99] The nonreabsorbable polymer alone may have induced chronic inflammation.[99]

Other Drug Elution Programs

Everolimus (Novartis) is another rapamycin analog that has both immunosuppressive and antiproliferative effects, and it has been submitted for FDA regulatory approval for patients with renal transplantation. Like sirolimus, everolimus inhibits the cytoplasmic phase (G1) of cell replication by inhibiting mammalian target of rapamycin (mTOR). Two programs have been proposed for the evaluation of everolimus-eluting stents. The first involves the use of a bioresorbable polymeric coating for everolimus delivery (Biosensors). The FUTURE-1 trial involving 27 patients treated with the Biosensors stent eluting everolimus and 15 patients treated with bare metal stents demonstrated no cases of restenosis in everolimus-treated patients and 9.1 percent restenosis in those treated with control metal stents with an in-stent late lumen loss of 0.10-mm. The second proposed program involves use of the Vision cobalt chromium stent (Guidant, Santa Clara, CA) with a TrueCoat polymeric coating for the elution of everolimus to the vessel wall. A randomized efficacy trial called SPIRIT FIRST is planned in Europe.

ABT-578, another rapamycin analog, has been tested in pilot studies in Australia on both the phosphylcholine (PC)-coated biodivYsio stent (Abbott Vascular, Chicago, IL) and the PC-coated cobalt chromium Driver stent (Medtronic Vascular, Santa Rosa, CA). The ENDEAVOR-II trial is the pivotal trial evaluating the Medtronic Program in Europe, commencing in the summer of 2003.

Tacrolimus elution from a ceramic coating on the Jomed was evaluated in the Endovascular Investigation Determining the Safety of a New Tacrolimus-Eluting Stent Graft (EVIDENT) and Preliminary Safety Evaluation of Nanoporous Tacrolimus-Eluting Stents (PRESENT) studies with limited results because of underdosing of the tacrolimus. The STRIDE Registry evaluated the use of dexamethasone elution from a phosphorylcholine coating in a 70-patient pilot series and reported a 13.3 percent binary restenosis rate. Although the angiographic restenosis rate was higher than expected given the noncomplex patients included in the study, the Dexamet stent received CE Mark approval in late 2002.

The value of actinomycin D elution from a polymeric coated balloon expandable stent was evaluated in the Actinomycin Eluting Stent Improves Outcomes by Reducing Neointimal Hyperplasia (ACTION) trial, but actinomycin in two doses failed to show benefit in preventing restenosis. Other agents that have been tried include Resten-NG, estrogen, and batimastat, but their effect on reducing restenosis after stent placement has not been convincing.

Indications for Percutaneous Coronary Interventions

The major value of percutaneous or surgical coronary revascularization is the relief of symptoms and signs of ischemic CAD.[33] PCI may reduce mortality and subsequent MI risk compared with medical therapy in unstable patients,[100,101] but these events are better treated with systemic therapies aimed at reducing the extent of atherosclerosis, such as lipid-lowering therapy, hypertension control, and smoking cessation.[102] In contrast, CABG prolongs life in patients in certain anatomical subsets, such as patients with left main disease, three-vessel CAD, or left anterior descending artery disease with involvement of one or two additional vessels, irrespective of left ventricular function.[103] The risks and benefits of coronary revascularization must be carefully reviewed with the patient and family members, and relative to the options of surgical bypass or continued medical therapy, before these procedures are performed. Guidelines for the performance of PCI and CABG have been published by a joint task force of the American College of Cardiology and American Heart Association.[33,103]

Asymptomatic Patients or Those with Mild Angina

Patients who are asymptomatic or have only mild symptoms are generally best treated with medical therapy unless one or more significant lesions subtend a moderate to large area of viable myocardium, the patient prefers to maintain an aggressive life style or has a high-risk occupation, and the procedure can be performed with a high chance of success and low likelihood of complications.[33] Coronary revascularization should not be performed in patients with absent or mild symptoms if only a small area of myocardium is at risk, if no objective evidence of ischemia can be found, or if the likelihood of success is low or the chance of complications is high.[33] There is no evidence that preemptive PCI of a hemodynamically insignificant "vulnerable" plaque prevents a subsequent MI.

Patients with Moderate to Severe Angina

(see Chap. 50)

Patients with CCS class II to IV angina, particularly those who are refractory to medical therapy, are suitable candidates for coronary revascularization provided that the lesion subtends a moderate to large area of viable myocardium as determined by noninvasive testing.[33] Patients who have recurrent symptoms while receiving medical therapy are candidates for revascularization even if they have a higher risk for an adverse outcome with revascularization.[33] Patients with class II to IV symptoms should not undergo revascularization without noninvasive evidence of myocardial ischemia or a trial of medical therapy, particularly if only a small region of myocardium is at risk, the likelihood of success is low, or the chance of complications is high.

Patients with Unstable Angina or Non-ST-Segment Myocardial Infarction (see Chap. 49)

Cardiac catheterization and coronary revascularization in moderate- to high-risk patients who present with unstable angina or non-ST-segment elevation MI (NSTEMI) may improve the prognosis and reduce the rate of reinfarction,[104] although two earlier studies failed to demonstrate a benefit for death or MI with the routine revascularization.[105,106] These studies were performed before the availability of GP IIb/IIIa inhibitors and coronary stents.[107]

Three subsequent trials have demonstrated benefit of routine revascularization in patients with acute coronary syndromes. The Fragmin and Fast Revascularization During Instability in Coronary Artery Disease (FRISC II) study demonstrated a 22 percent reduction ($p = 0.031$) in death or MI at 6 months in patients assigned to routine catheterization and revascularization (9.4 percent) versus those assigned to a conservative approach (12.1 percent).[108] The Treat Angina with Aggrastat and determine Cost of Therapy with an Invasive or Conservative Strategy– Thrombolysis in Myocardial Infarction 18 (TACTICS-TIMI 18) trial treated 2200 patients with NSTEMI or unstable angina with aspirin, unfractionated heparin, and intravenous tirofiban and randomly assigned patients to an early aggressive strategy with coronary arteriography and coronary revascularization within 4 to 48 hours after presentation or to a conservative strategy whereby coronary arteriography was performed only for recurrent ischemia or exercise stress testing demonstrating reversible ischemia.[100] The rate of the 6-month primary composite endpoint of death, recurrent MI, or urgent revascularization was reduced by 22 percent in patients assigned to the invasive strategy compared with the conservative strategy (15.9 percent versus 19.4 percent, respectively; $p = 0.025$).[100] The rate of death or MI at 6 months was reduced by 26 percent (7.3 percent versus 9.5 percent, respectively; $p < 0.05$).[100] These benefits were highest in patients presenting with unfavorable prognostic factors, such as rest pain, cardiac enzyme elevation, or electrocardiographic changes.[100]

The British Heart Foundation Randomized Intervention Trial of unstable Angina (RITA-3) randomly assigned 1810 patients with NSTEMI to an early intervention or conservative revascularization strategy.[101] At 4 months, 9.6 percent of patients in the intervention group had died or had MI or refractory angina, compared with 14.5 percent of patients in the conservative group (risk ratio 0.66; $p = 0.001$).[101] This difference was mainly due to a halving of refractory angina in the intervention group, as the frequency of death or MI was similar in both treatment groups.[101] Symptoms of angina were improved and use of antianginal medications significantly reduced with the interventional strategy ($p < 0.0001$).[101]

Patients with acute coronary syndromes are also excellent candidates for drug-eluting stents. The Rapamycin-Eluting Stent Evaluated At Rotterdam Cardiology Hospital (RESEARCH) registry compared 198 patients with acute coronary syndromes treated exclusively with drug-eluting stents with 301 patients with acute coronary syndromes treated with bare stents in the same time period immediately before the study.[109] The 30-day major adverse cardiac event rate was similar in both groups, with stent thrombosis occurring in 0.5 percent of patients treated with drug-eluting stents and 1.7 percent of patients treated with bare metal stents ($p = 0.4$).[109]

Options for Medical Therapy or Coronary Revascularization (see also Chap. 50)

For patients with symptomatic CAD, the clinician must decide whether medical therapy or referral for coronary revascularization by PCI or CABG would provide the better prognosis for the individual patient. A number of factors ultimately affect the decision to undertake one strategy over another, including (1) the patient's general vigor, comorbid conditions, initial symptoms, and personal preferences; (2) the coronary anatomy, number of lesions, and their location and morphology, including the presence of total occlusions; (3) left ventricular function; and (4) whether CABG has already been performed.

Percutaneous Coronary Intervention Versus Medical Therapy (see Chap. 50)

Two trials have compared medical therapy with PCI in patients with single-vessel CAD. The Veterans Administration Angioplasty Compared to Medicine (ACME) trial randomly assigned 212 patients with single-vessel coronary disease and stable angina to treatment with medical therapy or balloon PTCA. Death and MI rates were similar in both groups, but superior symptom control and a better exercise duration were shown in patients treated with balloon PTCA. The Atorvastatin Versus Revascularization Therapy (AVERT) trial compared the effect of aggressive lipid lowering with atorvastatin at 80 mg/d and coronary angioplasty in 341 patients with asymptomatic or mildly symptomatic (class I or II) CAD.[110] At an 18-month follow-up, 13 percent of medically treated patients had experienced an ischemic event compared with 21 percent of patients treated with PCI ($p = 0.048$), although more improvement in angina was shown in patients treated with PCI.

Two other trials have evaluated medical therapy with PCI in patients with more extensive CAD. The RITA-2 trial randomly assigned 1018 patients with single-vessel or multivessel disease to medical therapy or PCI. Death or definite MI occurred significantly ($p = 0.02$) more often in PCI-treated patients (6.3 percent) than in medically treated patients (3.3 percent), attributable to the occurrence of periprocedural MI. Angina improvement and exercise durations were better in the PCI group. The Asymptomatic Cardiac Ischemia Pilot (ACIP) study randomly assigned 558 patients with asymptomatic ischemia determined by stress testing and ambulatory ischemia monitoring and randomly assigned them to angina-guided therapy, angina plus ischemia–guided therapy, or revascularization using PCI or CABG. The incidence of death or MI at 2 years was significantly lower ($p < 0.01$) in patients treated with revascularization (4.7 percent) than in patients assigned to angina-guided (12.1 percent) or ischemia-guided (8.8 percent) therapy.

In aggregate, these studies suggest that patients with mild class I or II angina have a favorable prognosis whether treated with medical therapy or PCI. Angina relief is generally greater in patients treated with PCI than those receiving medical therapy. Patients with moderate to severe angina, particularly those who have not responded to medical therapy, should be considered candidates for PCI. The availability of durable treatment with drug-eluting stents may alter these paradigms in patients with documented ischemia, given that symptom recurrence is markedly reduced with these new therapies.

Percutaneous Coronary Intervention Versus Coronary Artery Bypass Graft (see Chap. 50)

At least nine randomized trials have evaluated the relative value of balloon angioplasty and CABG in patients with multivessel CAD.[103,111,112] These trials were performed before the availability of improved anticoagulation during PCI (e.g., GP IIb/IIIa inhibitors, direct thrombin inhibitors) and before the widespread use of coronary stents (i.e., bare metal or drug-eluting stents). These randomized trials had certain unavoidable design limitations, including relatively small sample sizes (127 to 1792 patients), low screened-to-recruitment ratios (limiting the generalizability of the study), and limited (1 to 5 years) follow-up. Despite these limitations, one of these studies led to a significant debate about the role of CABG in diabetic patients. The Bypass And Revascularization Investigation (BARI) found that diabetic patients assigned to PCI had a significantly ($p = 0.003$) worse survival rate (65.5 percent) than diabetic patients assigned to CABG (80.6 percent), primarily because of a reduced cardiac mortality rate (20.6 percent in PCI patients versus 5.8 percent in CABG patients; $p = 0.003$) from subsequent Q wave MI.[113] Placement of a left internal mammary artery to the left anterior descending artery appears responsible for the majority of this benefit.

With the improved outcomes associated with PCI over the past decade, a number of studies subsequently compared CABG with single-vessel or multivessel stent placement and showed that death and MI are similar in patients treated with CABG or multivessel stenting,[114-116] although one study suggested the persistence of a surgical 2-year mortality benefit in diabetic patients.[117,118] Restenosis has remained the major limitation after bare metal stenting, but with the availability of drug-eluting stents and aggressive risk factor modification after PCI, further studies are needed to evaluate the long-term outcomes of patients treated with these two therapies, particularly diabetic patients.

The ultimate choice of the method of revascularization should be made after a frank discussion with the patient about the options of revascularization. In patients with diffuse involvement of three coronary vessels, particularly in the setting of complex anatomy, including total occlusions, CABG may provide a more definitive long-term benefit, especially if one or more arterial conduits are used. In contrast, in a patient with focal lesions involving two or three large epicardial vessels, multivessel coronary stent placement may be the preferred approach as it is associated with a lower risk of Q wave MI and a shorter hospital stay than CABG. Diabetic patients with diffuse two- or three-vessel CAD may be best served with CABG.

Patients Without Options for Revascularization

Patients who suffer from substantial angina but are poor candidates for conventional revascularization have limited therapeutic options. These patients generally have a single, proximal vessel occlusion that subtends a large amount of myocardium or have undergone one or more prior CABG surgeries with stenoses of the SVGs poorly suited for conventional repeated revascularization. Patients with limited options make up approximately 4 to 12 percent of those undergoing coronary angiography; a larger percentage of patients (20 to 30 percent) have incomplete revascularization because of unsuitable coronary anatomy with surgery or percutaneous techniques.

Creation of new blood vessels in the ischemic tissue, also known as therapeutic angiogenesis, may provide symptom relief in these patients. Both surgical and percutaneous approaches have been used to improve regional blood flow to the ischemic myocardium in these patients, although these strategies vary with respect to the depth of myocardial injury, the laser-tissue interactions, the presence or absence of guidance, and the number of channels created. No such therapy has yet been proved effective in blinded clinical trials.

Percutaneous approaches to myocardial revascularization vary in the laser source, delivery catheter types, and use of guidance to direct placement of the laser channels. These techniques provide partial-thickness myocardial channels, ranging from 3 to 5-mm in depth, in contrast to the full-thickness myocardial channel produced with surgical methods. Although studies with several of the laser systems reported dramatic clinical improvement in angina severity and exercise time in open-label studies, the few placebo-controlled randomized studies performed with this group of devices have shown much of the improvement to be due to a placebo effect.[119] No such percutaneous laser myocardial revascularization systems are currently approved for use in the United States.

LOCALIZED MYOCARDIAL GENE TRANSFER. Using electromechanical localization with the Biosense system, direct intramyocardial administration of the naked plasmid VEGF-165 has been used in an attempt to stimulate angiogenesis.[120] In small series of 13 consecutive patients treated with a direct intramyocardial injection of VEGF-165, partial or complete resolution of perfusion defects seen on the sestamibi scan was observed 60 days after the procedure.[120] A multicenter placebo-controlled study evaluating this approach is ongoing.

Percutaneous Valvuloplasty

In parallel with the development of percutaneous treatments for coronary and peripheral vascular lesions, there has been an ongoing effort to provide percutaneous treatments for valvular heart disease. Percutaneous valve dilation has been used as an alternative to definitive surgical repair or replacement in selected patients with symptomatic valvular stenosis, particularly of the mitral valve. Mitral valvuloplasty is a safe and effective alternative to surgical repair in selected patients with mitral stenosis, whereas aortic valvuloplasty provides only short-term palliation and should be reserved for inoperable cases with degenerative calcific aortic stenosis. The indications and contraindications for mitral and aortic valvuloplasty are reviewed in detail elsewhere (see Chap. 57). This chapter focuses on the technical issues, selection of patients, and outcomes associated with mitral and aortic valvuloplasty.

Mitral Valvuloplasty (see also Chap. 57)

Percutaneous mitral valvuloplasty (PMV) was first performed in 1984 as an alternative to surgical mitral valve commissurotomy; subsequent reports confirmed the immediate and long-term benefits of this procedure. Although the majority of PMV procedures are performed in developing countries where rheumatic fever and valvular heart disease continue to be endemic, a few specialized centers in Western countries have developed technical expertise in PMV (Fig. 52–14).

TECHNICAL ISSUES. Several approaches for PMV have been described. The most common is transvenous or antero-grade, using a transseptal puncture to gain access to the left atrium. A balloon catheter is then floated across the mitral valve into the left ventricle. A retrograde, transarterial approach can be used to avoid the creation of a large atrial septal defect but is uncommon in clinical practice, and experience with this method is limited except for a few specialized centers.

There are several variants of the anterograde approach. With the double-balloon method, a transseptal puncture is performed and a balloon catheter is advanced across the mitral valve into the left ventricle. Two long exchange wires are then positioned in the left ventricle, and the interatrial septum is dilated with a 6- to 8-mm peripheral dilation balloon. Two mitral valvuloplasty balloons of appropriate size are advanced across the mitral valve and inflated simultaneously to split the sclerosed mitral commissures. The second technique uses the special Inoue balloon, which is a self-positioning, pressure-distensible, dumbbell-shaped balloon that locks itself into the stenotic mitral orifice and progressively dilates the orifice as the inflation pressure is increased. A stepwise dilation technique is performed to minimize the risk of mitral valve rupture and mitral regurgitation. Selection of balloon size is generally based on the patient's height, body surface area, and diameter of the mitral annulus. A mechanical valve dilator has also been used percutaneously and has the advantage of resterilization and reuse in developing countries.

Comparative studies of these two techniques have shown similar clinical success rates but shorter procedure times and higher disposable costs with the Inoue technique. The Inoue balloon has also been used in patients with severe mitral valve calcification and subvalvular fibrosis.

HEMODYNAMIC ASSESSMENT. Serial hemodynamic measurements, alone or in combination with echocardiography, may be used to evaluate the result achieved with PMV.[121] An immediate improvement in left atrial mean pressure (and reduction of the transmittal gradient) should be seen, with a gradual decrease in pulmonary artery pressure and an increase in cardiac output. Criteria for termination of the procedure include (1) a mitral valve area larger than 1 cm^2 per square meter of body surface area, (2) complete opening of at least one commissure, or (3) the appearance of an increment in mitral regurgitation. Transesophageal echocardiography may also be performed during the procedure and, in particular, may guide the transseptal puncture in patients with obscure cardiac landmarks or skeletal deformity.

PROCEDURAL OUTCOME. A favorable procedural outcome has been related to institutional volume (>25 cases per year), baseline mitral valve area (>0.5 cm^2), and the age of the patient (younger than 70 years). Procedural mortality associated with mitral valvuloplasty ranges from 0 to 3 percent in most series and is primarily related to left ventricular perforation resulting from the transseptal technique or advancement of the guidewire or balloon catheter into the left ventricle or to general comorbidity in the patient. Cerebral or coronary emboli occur in 0.5 to 5.0 percent of patients and are related to dislodgment of thromboembolic material from the left atrium or air within the dilatation apparatus, underscoring the importance of transesophageal echocardiography for detection of atrial thrombi. Severe mitral regurgitation resulting from rupture of the chordae tendineae or papillary muscle rupture may also occur. Atrial septal defects are commonly (80 percent) seen after PMV, but the magnitude of the left-to-right shunt is generally insignificant. The atrial septal defect also closes in the majority (90 to 100 percent) of cases within 3 months after PMV. Emergency surgery may be required in a minority of cases after PMV. When surgery is required for mitral regurgitation, left ven-

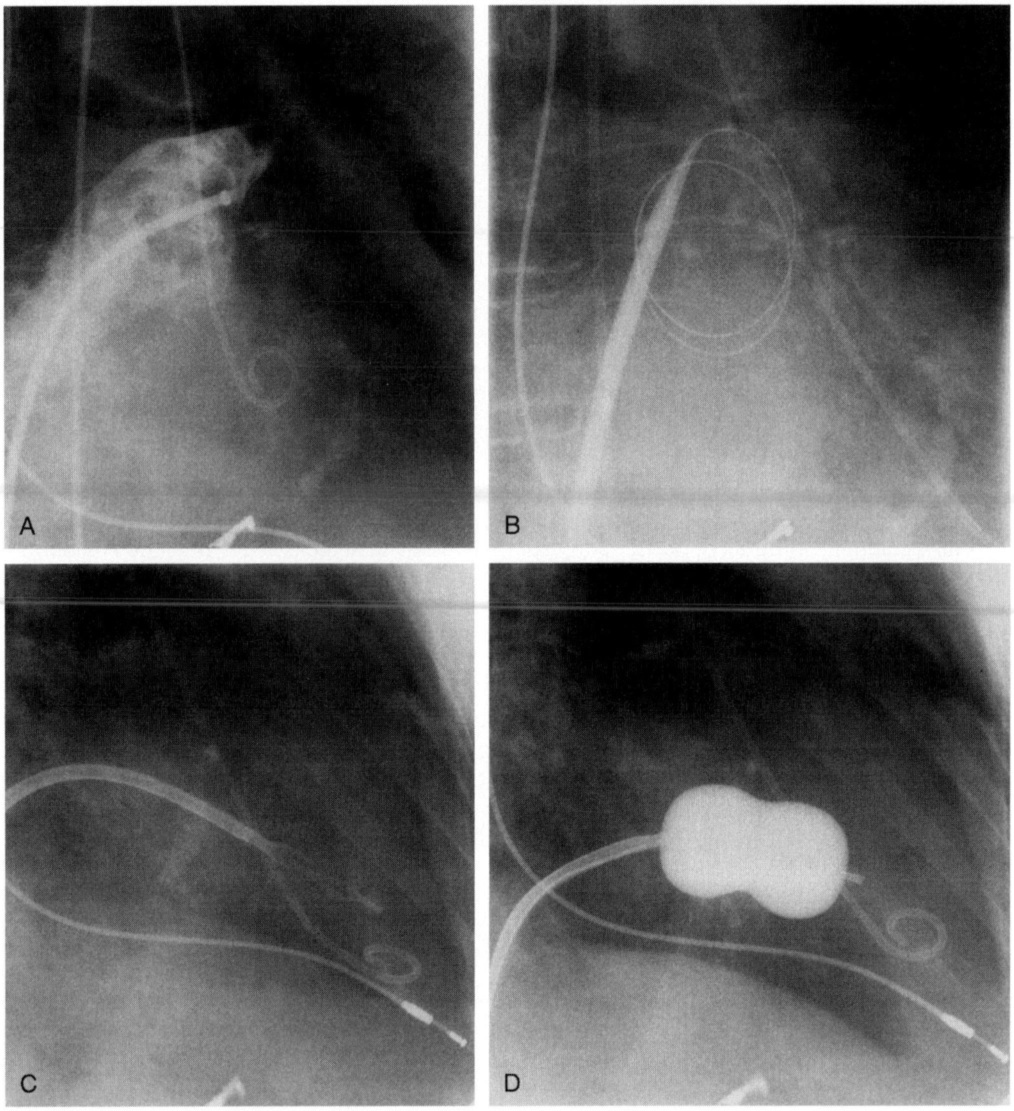

FIGURE 52–14 Mitral valvuloplasty. After transseptal puncture, a Mullins sheath is advanced into the left atrium, as demonstrated by injection of contrast medium **(A)**. An Inoue guidewire is coiled in the left atrium and an Inoue dilator is advanced across the intraatrial septum **(B)**. Advancement of the Inoue balloon dilation catheter into the left ventricle **(C)** and inflation **(D)** resulted in a successful procedure. (Courtesy of Dr. Andrew Eisenhauer.)

tricular rupture, or the development of a left-to-right shunt or as a result of a failed procedure, the mortality rate rises substantially.

LATE OUTCOME. Transthoracic echocardiography may be useful to assess the prognosis after PMV by semiquantitatively scoring leaflet mobility, valvular and subvalvular thickening, and valvular calcification. In one series of 136 patients undergoing successful PMV, the estimated 5-year mortality rate was 24 percent and the 5-year event rate (i.e., mitral valve replacement, repeated valvuloplasty, or death from cardiac causes) was 49 percent.[122] Multivariable predictors of late events after PMV were a high mitral valve echocardiographic score, an elevated left ventricular end-diastolic pressure, and a worse New York Heart Association (NYHA) functional class ($p = 0.04$).[122] Patients with fewer than two risk factors for early restenosis (echocardiographic score >8, left ventricular end-diastolic pressure >10-mm Hg, or NYHA functional Class IV) had a predicted 5-year event-free survival rate of 60 to 84 percent, whereas patients with two or three risk factors had a predicted 5-year event-free survival rate of only 13 to 41 percent.[122]

Aortic Valvuloplasty (see also Chap. 57)

The most frequent cause of acquired valvular heart disease in Western countries is degenerative calcific aortic stenosis.[121] Whereas in mitral stenosis the problem is commissural fusion, in acquired calcific stenosis the problem is rigid valve leaflets. Percutaneous aortic valvuloplasty (PAV) fractures the calcified aortic leaflets, thereby increasing their flexibility, and somewhat dilates the surrounding aortic annulus. When the annulus recoils and the leaflets recalcify, even the modest hemodynamic improvements abate (days to weeks). The long-term clinical benefit associated with PAV for calcific aortic stenosis is thus limited.

PAV is generally reserved for adult patients with severe calcific aortic stenosis who have severe comorbidities that preclude aortic valve replacement, such as patients with cardiogenic shock or other significant comorbid conditions; for patients as a "bridge" to definitive surgical correction; or for patients with severe left ventricular dysfunction (i.e., low flow, low gradient) in whom the hemodynamic response to aortic valve replacement cannot be determined (Fig. 52–15).

In the absence of these indications, definitive aortic valve replacement rather than PAV should be performed, even in elderly patients. PAV in patients with congenital aortic stenosis is discussed in Chapter 56. New percutaneous procedures are being developed to stent the calcified valve open and allow a new pericardial valve sewn with the stent to open and close with the cardiac cycle, which may allow more durable percutaneous correction of calcific aortic stenosis.[123]

TECHNICAL ISSUES. The femoral approach is most frequently used for PAV. After crossing the aortic valve with a guidewire, an extra-stiff 0.038-inch wire is inserted into the apex of the left ventricle to stabilize the balloon during inflation. In patients with severe peripheral vascular disease, a brachial approach or anterograde approach with a transseptal puncture can be used to pass a long wire through the left ventricle, across the aortic valve, and into the descending aorta. The interatrium septum is dilated with a peripheral balloon, and the PAV balloon is then advanced across the aortic valve. PAV balloons ranging in diameter between 15 and 25-mm and in length between 3 and 5 cm have variable shapes, including conventional, bifoil, trifoil, and double-sized configurations, with the proximal portion measuring 20 to 23-mm and the distal portion 15 to 18-mm.[121] The size of the balloon should not exceed 1.2 to 1.3 times the diameter of the aortic ring.

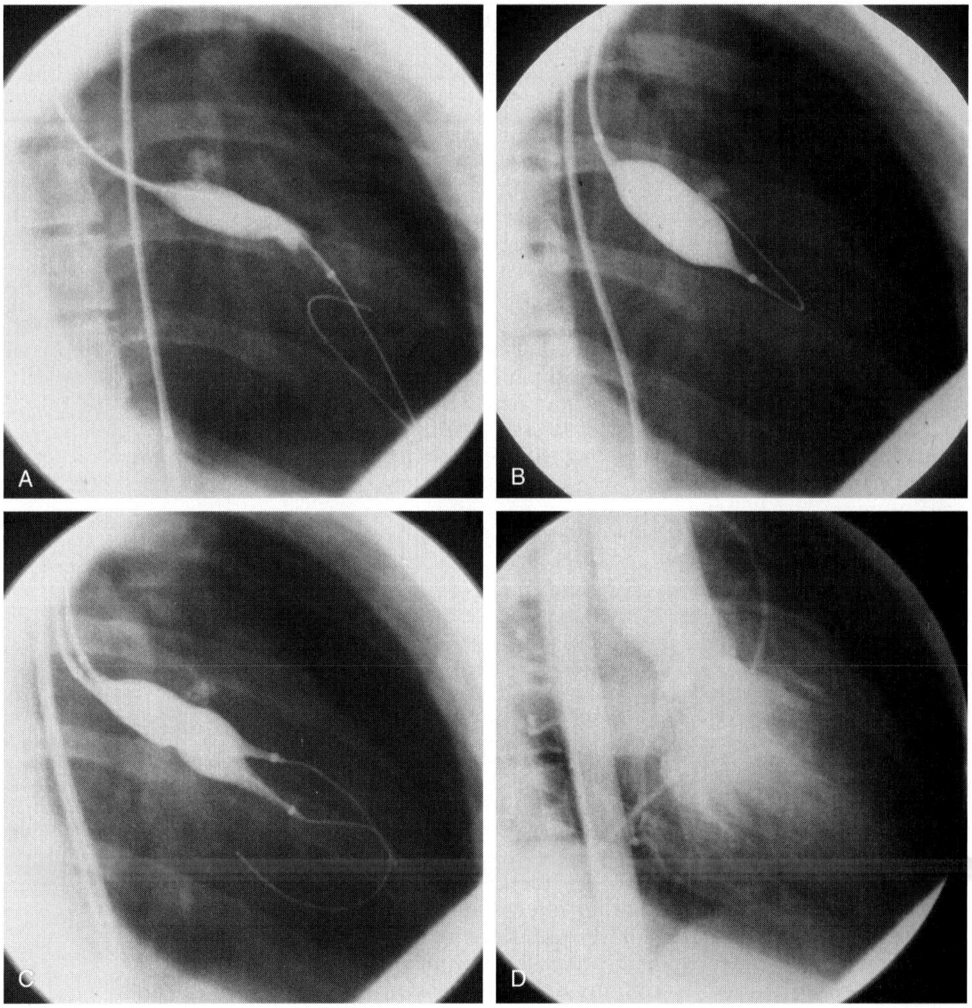

FIGURE 52–15 Aortic valvuloplasty. A 16-mm aortic valvuloplasty balloon is inflated across the aortic valve **(A)** and exchanged for a 24-mm balloon **(B)** because of a persistent gradient. To improve the aortic gradient further, two 16-mm valvuloplasty balloons are advanced across the aortic valve **(C)**. Because of the relative oversizing of the balloons to the aortic ring, aortic regurgitation results **(D)**. (Courtesy of Dr. Andrew Eisenhauer.)

HEMODYNAMIC ASSESSMENT. The transaortic valve gradient should be reduced immediately after the procedure, although little change may be noted in cardiac output. After successful dilation, 25 to 47 percent of patients obtain a final valve area larger than 1 cm^2 and 22 to 39 percent of patients achieve a valve area less than 0.7 cm^2.

PROCEDURAL SUCCESS AND COMPLICATION RATES. The clinical success rate for patients undergoing PAV ranges from 68 to 75 percent. Hospital mortality after PAV varies from 3.5 to 13.5 percent, and 20 to 25 percent of patients experience at least one complication during their hospitalization. Complications include a need for vascular access repair, embolic cerebrovascular events, aortic regurgitation, and, with the use of oversized balloons, rupture of the aortic ring. Predictors of procedural mortality include the patient's age, NYHA class, concomitant CAD, congestive heart failure, lower initial left ventricular systolic pressure, smaller final aortic valve area, lower baseline cardiac output, and the development of procedural complications. Predictors of morbidity are depressed left ventricular function, low cardiac output, diffuse coronary disease, and final valve area smaller than 0.7 cm^2.

The major limitation of PAV is the early recurrence of symptoms in most patients. The estimated incidence of late restenosis is 36 to 80 percent in the first year. Determinants of late outcomes after PAV were studied in 205 patients undergoing this procedure. The event-free survival rate, defined as survival without recurrent symptoms, repeated valvuloplasty, or aortic valve replacement, was 18 percent over the 24-month follow-up (range, 1 to 47 months). Significant predictors of event-free survival included the left ventricular ejection fraction, left ventricular and aortic systolic pressure before PAV, and percent reduction in the aortic valve pressure gradient; the pulmonary capillary wedge pressure was inversely associated with event-free survival. Although the predicted event-free survival rate for the entire group of patients was 50 percent at 1 year and 25 percent at 2 years, the probability of event-free survival at 1 year varied between 23 and 65 percent when patients were stratified according to three independent predictors: aortic systolic pressure, pulmonary capillary wedge pressure, and percent reduction in the peak aortic valve gradient. The best long-term results after valvuloplasty were observed in patients who would also have been expected to have excellent long-term results after aortic valve replacement. Repeated PAV for symptom recurrence may also be useful.

Training Standards and Proficiency in Interventional Cardiology

As the number of devices, procedures, and associated pharmacology has grown, interventional cardiology has evolved into a separate discipline in medicine. Standards for core curriculum development and procedural proficiency for interventional cardiology training programs have been established by the American College of Cardiology and by the Society for Cardiac Angiography and Intervention.[124-126] These criteria form the basis for an additional 12-month dedicated training program established under the guidelines of the American Board of Internal Medicine Accreditation Council for Graduate Medical Education. Successful completion of this training program is a prerequisite for new graduates prior to sitting for the Certification Examination for Added Qualification in Interventional Cardiology. Proficiency requirements for interventional training have become more rigorous over time, with the minimum case volume for interventional training increasing from 125 to 250 cases as the primary operator; maintenance of proficiency now requires more than 75 cases per year as the primary operator unless special circumstances are identified.[126]

Operator- and hospital-specific procedural outcomes after PCI are also collected by hospital, governmental, and managed care organizations and should be monitored to ensure quality in care of patients provided by the interventional operators. The focus on minimum volume criteria is based on studies that relate procedural outcome after PCI to both hospital and individual operator volumes. PCI complication rates are higher when the hospital procedural volume is less than 200 to 400 cases per year or individual operator volume is less than 75 to 100 coronary interventions per year. The American College of Cardiology has recommended that hospitals perform more than 200 to 400 cases per year and individual operators perform more than 75 cases per year.[33,125] Accordingly, individual institutions need to establish valid methods for peer review, including documentation of procedural success and failure rates of individual operators, minimum volume performance for the hospital and individual operators, quality of the laboratory facility, and training of the support staff. Establishment of an outcomes data base is strongly encouraged for all institutions as part of an ongoing quality assurance program.[127,128]

REFERENCES

Outcomes After Percutaneous Coronary Intervention

1. Detre K, Holubkov R, Kelsey S, et al: Percutaneous transluminal coronary angioplasty in 1985-1986 and 1977-1981. The National Heart, Lung, and Blood Institute Registry. N Engl J Med 318:265, 1988.
2. Ellis SG, Cowley MJ, Whitlow PL, et al: Prospective case-control comparison of percutaneous transluminal coronary revascularization in patients with multivessel disease treated in 1986-1987 versus 1991: Improved in-hospital and 12-month results. Multivessel Angioplasty Prognosis Study (MAPS) Group. J Am Coll Cardiol 25:1137, 1995.
3. Baim DS, Cutlip DE, Sharma SK, et al: Final results of the Balloon vs Optimal Atherectomy Trial (BOAT). Circulation 97:322, 1998.
4. Fischman DL, Leon MB, Baim DS, et al: A randomized comparison of coronary-stent placement and balloon angioplasty in the treatment of coronary artery disease. Stent Restenosis Study Investigators. N Engl J Med 331:496, 1994.
5. Serruys PW, van Hout B, Bonnier H, et al: Randomised comparison of implantation of heparin-coated stents with balloon angioplasty in selected patients with coronary artery disease (Benestent II). Lancet 352:673, 1998.
6. Mauri L, Bonan R, Weiner B, et al: Cutting balloon angioplasty for the prevention of restenosis: Results of the Cutting Balloon Global Randomized Trial. Am J Cardiol 90:1079, 2002.
7. Williams D, Holubkov R, Yeh W, et al: Percutaneous coronary intervention in the current era compared with 1985-1986: The National Heart, Lung, and Blood Institute Registries. Circulation 102:2945, 2000.

Coronary Atherectomy and Thrombectomy

8. Topol EJ, Leya F, Pinkerton CA, et al: A comparison of directional atherectomy with coronary angioplasty in patients with coronary artery disease. The CAVEAT Study Group. N Engl J Med 329:221, 1993.
9. Adelman AG, Cohen EA, Kimball BP, et al: A comparison of directional atherectomy with balloon angioplasty for lesions of the left anterior descending coronary artery. N Engl J Med 329:228, 1993.
10. Suzuki T, Hosokawa H, Katoh O, et al: Effects of adjunctive balloon angioplasty after intravascular ultrasound-guided optimal directional coronary atherectomy: The result of Adjunctive Balloon Angioplasty After Coronary Atherectomy Study (ABACAS). J Am Coll Cardiol 34:1028, 1999.
11. Tsuchikane E, Sumitsuji S, Awata N, et al: Final results of the STent versus directional coronary Atherectomy Randomized Trial (START). J Am Coll Cardiol 34:1050, 1999.
12. Moussa I, Moses J, Di Mario C, et al: Stenting after optimal lesion debulking (sold) registry. Angiographic and clinical outcome. Circulation 98:1604, 1998.
13. Whitlow PL, Bass TA, Kipperman RM, et al: Results of the study to determine rotablator and transluminal angioplasty strategy (STRATAS). Am J Cardiol 87:699, 2001.
14. Mauri L, Reisman M, Buchbinder M, et al: Comparison of rotational atherectomy with conventional balloon angioplasty in the prevention of restenosis of small coronary arteries: Results of the Dilatation vs Ablation Revascularization Trial Targeting Restenosis (DART). Am Heart J 145:847, 2003.
15. Reifart N, Vandormael M, Krajcar M, et al: Randomized comparison of angioplasty of complex coronary lesions at a single center. Excimer Laser, Rotational Atherectomy, and Balloon Angioplasty Comparison (ERBAC) Study. Circulation 96:91, 1997.
16. Kuntz R, Baim D, Cohen D, et al: A trial comparing rheolytic thrombectomy with intracoronary urokinase for coronary and vein graft thrombus (the Vein Graft AngioJet Study [VeGAS 2]). Am J Cardiol 89:326, 2002.
17. Baim D, Wahr D, George B, et al: Randomized trial of a distal embolic protection device during percutaneous intervention of saphenous vein aorto-coronary bypass grafts. Circulation 105:1285, 2002.
18. Webb J, Carere R, Virmani R, et al: Retrieval and analysis of particulate debris after saphenous vein graft intervention. J Am Coll Cardiol 34:468, 1999.
19. Stone GW, Rogers C, Hermiller J, et al: Randomized comparison of distal protection with a filter-based catheter and a balloon occlusion and aspiration system during percutaneous intervention of a diseased saphenous vein aorto-coronary bypass graft. Circulation 108:548, 2003.

Coronary Stenting

20. Serruys P, de Jaegere P, Kiemeneij F, et al: A comparison of balloon expandable stent implantation with balloon angioplasty in patients with coronary artery disease. N Engl J Med 8:489, 1994.
21. Erbel R, Haude M, Hopp H, et al: Coronary-artery stenting compared with balloon angioplasty for restenosis after initial balloon angioplasty. N Engl J Med 339:1672, 1998.
22. Savage MP, Douglas JS Jr, Fischman DL, et al: Stent placement compared with balloon angioplasty for obstructed coronary bypass grafts. Saphenous Vein De Novo Trial Investigators. N Engl J Med 337:740, 1997.
23. Buller C, Dzavik V, Carere R, et al: Primary stenting versus balloon angioplasty in occluded coronary arteries: The Total Occlusion Study of Canada (TOSCA). Circulation 100:236, 1999.
24. Sirnes PA, Golf S, Myreng Y, et al: Stenting in Chronic Coronary Occlusion (SICCO): A randomized, controlled trial of adding stent implantation after successful angioplasty. J Am Coll Cardiol 28:1444, 1996.
25. Grines C, Cox D, Stone G, et al: Coronary angioplasty with or without stent implantation for acute myocardial infarction. Stent Primary Angioplasty in Myocardial Infarction Study Group. N Engl J Med 341:1949, 1999.
26. Stone G, Grines C, Cox D, et al: Comparison of angioplasty with stenting, with or without abciximab, in acute myocardial infarction. N Engl J Med 346:957, 2002.
27. Neumann F-J, Kastrati A, Schmitt C, et al: Effect of glycoprotein IIb-IIa receptor blockade with abciximab on clinical and angiographic restenosis rates after the placement of coronary stents following acute myocardial infarction. J Am Coll Cardiol 35:915, 2000.
28. Holmes D, Lansky A, Kuntz R, et al: The PARAGON stent study: A randomized trial of a new martensitic nitinol stent versus the Palmaz-Schatz stent for treatment of complex native coronary arterial lesions. Am J Cardiol 86:1073, 2000.
29. Baim D, Cutlip D, O'Shaughnessy C, et al: Final results of a randomized trial comparing the NIR stent to the Palmaz-Schatz stent for narrowings in native coronary arteries. Am J Cardiol 87:152, 2001.
30. Baim D, Cutlip D, Midei M, et al: Final results of a randomized trial comparing the MULTI-LINK stent with the Palmaz-Schatz stent for narrowings in native coronary arteries. Am J Cardiol 87:157, 2001.
31. Han R, Schwartz R, Kobayashi Y, et al: Comparison of self-expanding and balloon-expandable stents for the reduction of restenosis. Am J Cardiol 88:253, 2001.
32. Lansky A, Roubin G, O'Shaughnessy C, et al: Randomized comparison of GR-II stent and Palmaz-Schatz stent for elective treatment of coronary stenoses. Circulation 102:1364, 2000.

Clinical Results After Percutaneous Coronary Intervention

33. Smith S, Dove J, Jacobs A, et al: ACC/AHA guidelines of percutaneous coronary interventions (revision of the 1993 PTCA guidelines)—Executive summary. A report of the American College of Cardiology/American Heart Association Task Force on Practice Guidelines (committee to revise the 1993 guidelines for percutaneous transluminal coronary angioplasty). J Am Coll Cardiol 37:2215, 2001.
34. Califf RM, Abdelmeguid AE, Kuntz RE, et al: Myonecrosis after revascularization procedures. J Am Coll Cardiol 31:241, 1998.
35. O'Conner G, Malenka D, Quiton H, et al: Multivariate prediction of in-hospital mortality after percutaneous coronary interventions in 1994-1996. J Am Coll Cardiol 34:681, 1999.
36. Moscucci M, O'Connor G, Ellis S, et al: Validation of risk adjustment models for in-hospital percutaneous transluminal coronary angioplasty on an independent data set. J Am Coll Cardiol 34:692, 1999.

37. Leon M, Baim D, Popma J, et al: A clinical trial comparing three antithrombotic-drug regimens after coronary-artery stenting. N Engl J Med 339:1665, 1998.

Treatment of In-Stent Restenosis

38. vom Dahl J, Dietz U, Haager P, et al: Rotational atherectomy does not reduce recurrent in-stent restenosis: Results of the angioplasty versus rotational atherectomy for treatment of diffuse in-stent restenosis trial (ARTIST). Circulation 105:583, 2002.
39. Kimura T, Yokoi H, Nakagawa T, et al: Three-year follow-up after implantation of metallic coronary artery stents. N Engl J Med 334:561, 1996.
40. Teirstein PS, Massullo V, Jani S, et al: Catheter-based radiotherapy to inhibit restenosis after coronary stenting. N Engl J Med 336:1697, 1997.
41. Waksman R, White R, Chan R, et al: Intracoronary gamma-radiation therapy after angioplasty inhibits recurrence in patients with in-stent restenosis. Circulation 101:2130, 2000.
42. Leon M, Teirstein P, Moses J, et al: Localized intracoronary gamma radiation therapy to inhibit the recurrence of restenosis after stenting. N Engl J Med 344:250, 2001.
43. Waksman R, Raizner A, Yeung A, et al: Use of localised intracoronary beta radiation in treatment of in-stent restenosis: The INHIBIT randomised controlled trial. Lancet 359:551, 2002.
44. Popma J, Suntharalingam M, Lansky A, et al: Randomized trial of ^{90}Sr/^{90}Y beta-radiation versus placebo control for treatment of in-stent restenosis. Circulation 106:1090, 2002.
45. Waksman R, Buchbinder M, Reisman M, et al: Balloon-based radiation therapy for treatment of in-stent restenosis in human coronary arteries: Results from the BRITE I study. Catheter Cardiovasc Interv 57:286, 2002.
46. Duffin D, Muhlestein J, Allisson S, et al: Femoral arterial puncture management after percutaneous coronary procedures: A comparison of clinical outcomes and patient satisfaction between manual compression and two different vascular closure devices. J Invasive Cardiol 13:354, 2001.

Anticoagulation During Percutaneous Coronary Intervention

47. Schomig A, Neumann FJ, Kastrati A, et al: A randomized comparison of antiplatelet and anticoagulant therapy after the placement of coronary-artery stents. N Engl J Med 334:1084, 1996.
48. Mehta S, Yusuf S, Peters R, et al: Effects of pretreatment with clopidogrel and aspirin followed by long-term therapy in patients undergoing percutaneous coronary intervention: The PCI-CURE study. Lancet 358:527, 2001.
49. Steinhubl S, Berger P, Mann J, et al: Early and sustained dual oral antiplatelet therapy following percutaneous coronary intervention: A randomized controlled trial. JAMA 288:2411, 2002.
50. The EPIC Investigators: Use of a monoclonal antibody directed against the platelet glycoprotein IIb/IIIa receptor in high-risk coronary angioplasty. The EPIC Investigation. N Engl J Med 330:956, 1994.
51. The EPILOG Investigators: Platelet glycoprotein IIb/IIIa receptor blockade and low-dose heparin during percutaneous coronary revascularization. The EPILOG Investigators. N Engl J Med 336:1689, 1997.
52. The EPISTENT Investigators: Randomised placebo-controlled and balloon-angioplasty-controlled trial to assess safety of coronary stenting with use of platelet glycoprotein-IIb/IIIa blockade. Evaluation of Platelet IIb/IIIa Inhibitor for Stenting. Lancet 352:87, 1998.
53. The IMPACT-II Investigators: Randomised placebo-controlled trial of effect of eptifibatide on complications of percutaneous coronary intervention: IMPACT-II. Integrilin to Minimise Platelet Aggregation and Coronary Thrombosis-II. Lancet 349:1422, 1997.
54. The ESPRIT Investigators: Novel dosing regimen of eptifibatide in planned coronary stent implantation (ESPRIT): A randomised, placebo-controlled trial. Lancet 356:2037, 2000.
55. The RESTORE Investigators: Effects of platelet glycoprotein IIb/IIIa blockade with tirofiban on adverse cardiac events in patients with unstable angina or acute myocardial infarction undergoing coronary angioplasty. The RESTORE Investigators. Randomized Efficacy Study of Tirofiban for Outcomes and REstenosis. Circulation 96:1445, 1997.
56. Topol E, Moliterno D, Herrmann H, et al: Comparison of two platelet glycoprotein IIb/IIIa inhibitors, tirofiban and abciximab, for the prevention of ischemic events with percutaneous coronary revascularization. N Engl J Med 344:1888, 2001.
57. Chew D, Bhatt D, Lincoff A, et al: Defining the optimal activated clotting time during percutaneous coronary intervention: Aggregate results from 6 randomized, controlled trials. Circulation 103:961, 2001.
58. Levine GN, Ferguson JJ: Low-molecular-weight heparin during percutaneous coronary interventions: Rationale, results, and recommendations. Cathet Cardiovasc Interv 60:185, 2003.
59. Serruys PW, Herrman JP, Simon R, et al: A comparison of hirudin with heparin in the prevention of restenosis after coronary angioplasty. Helvetica Investigators. N Engl J Med 333:757, 1995;.
60. Bittl JA, Strony J, Brinker JA, et al: Treatment with bivalirudin (Hirulog) as compared with heparin during coronary angioplasty for unstable or postinfarction angina. Hirulog Angioplasty Study Investigators. N Engl J Med 333:764, 1995.
61. Lincoff A, Bittl J, Harrington R, et al: Bivalirudin and provisional glycoprotein IIb/IIIa blockade compared with heparin and planned glycoprotein IIb/IIIa blockade during percutaneous coronary intervention: REPLACE-2 randomized trial. JAMA 289:853, 2003.

Systemic Approaches to Restenosis

62. Tsuchikane E, Fukuhara A, Kobayashi T, et al: Impact of cilostazol on restenosis after percutaneous coronary balloon angioplasty. Circulation 100:21, 1999.
63. Park S, Lee C, Kim H, et al: Effects of cilostazol on angiographic restenosis after coronary stent placement. Am J Cardiol 86:499, 2000.
64. Kamishirado H, Inoue T, Mizoguchi K, et al: Randomized comparison of cilostazol versus ticlopidine hydrochloride for antiplatelet therapy after coronary stent implantation for prevention of late restenosis. Am Heart J 144:303, 2002.
65. Garachemani A, Fleisch M, Windecker S, et al: Heparin and Coumadin versus acetylsalicylic acid for prevention of restenosis after coronary angioplasty. Catheter Cardiovasc Interv 55:315, 2002.
66. ten Berg J, Kelder J, Suttorp M, et al: A randomized trial assessing the effect of coumarins started before coronary angioplasty on restenosis: Results of the 6-month angiographic substudy of the Balloon Angioplasty and Anticoagulation Study (BAAS). Am Heart J 145:58, 2003.
67. Versaci F, Gaspardone A, Tomai F, et al: Immunosuppressive Therapy for the Prevention of Restenosis after Coronary Artery Stent Implantation (IMPRESS Study). J Am Coll Cardiol 40:1935, 2002.
68. Tardif J, Gregoire J, Schwartz L, et al: Effects of AGI-1067 and probucol after percutaneous coronary interventions. Circulation 107:552, 2003.
69. Holmes D, Savage M, La Blanche J, et al: Results of Prevention of REStenosis with Tranilast and its Outcomes (PRESTO) trial. Circulation 106:1243, 2002.
70. Serruys P, Foley D, Pieper M, et al: The TRAPIST Study. A multicentre randomized placebo controlled clinical trial of trapidil for prevention of restenosis after coronary stenting, measured by 3-D intravascular ultrasound. Eur Heart J 22:1938, 2001.
71. Meurice T, Bauters C, Hermant X, et al: Effect of ACE inhibitors on angiographic restenosis after coronary stenting (PARIS): A randomised, double-blind, placebo-controlled trial. Lancet 357:1321, 2001.
72. Kondo J, Sone T, Tsuboi H, et al: Effect of quinapril on intimal hyperplasia after coronary stenting as assessed by intravascular ultrasound. Am J Cardiol 87:443, 2001.
73. Peters S, Gotting B, Trummel M, et al: Valsartan for prevention of restenosis after stenting of type B2/C lesions: The VAL-PREST trial. J Invasive Cardiol 13:93, 2001.
74. Dens J, Desmet W, Coussement P, et al: Usefulness of Nisoldipine for prevention of restenosis after percutaneous transluminal coronary angioplasty (results of the NICOLE study). NIsoldipine in COronary artery disease in LEuven. Am J Cardiol 87:28, 2001.
75. Jorgensen B, Simonsen S, Endresen K, et al: Restenosis and clinical outcome in patients treated with amlodipine after angioplasty: Results from the Coronary AngioPlasty Amlodipine REStenosis Study (CAPARES). J Am Coll Cardiol 35:592, 2000.
76. Serruys P, Foley D, Hofling B, et al: Carvedilol for prevention of restenosis after directional coronary atherectomy: Final results of the European carvedilol atherectomy restenosis (EUROCARE) trial. Circulation 101:1512, 2000.
77. Lincoff A, Califf RM, Moliterno D, et al: Complementary clinical benefits of coronary artery stenting and blockade of platelet glycoprotein IIb-IIIa receptors. N Engl J Med 341:319, 1999.
78. Roffi M, Moliterno D, Meier B, et al: Impact of different platelet glycoprotein IIb/IIIa receptor inhibitors among diabetic patients undergoing percutaneous coronary intervention: Do Tirofiban and ReoPro Give Similar Efficacy Outcomes Trial (TARGET) 1-year follow-up. Circulation 105:2730, 2002.
79. Tardif JC, Cote G, Lesperance J, et al: Probucol and multivitamins in the prevention of restenosis after coronary angioplasty. Multivitamins and Probucol Study Group. N Engl J Med 337:365, 1997.
80. Brara P, Moussavian M, Grise M, et al: Pilot trial of oral rapamycin for recalcitrant restenosis. Circulation 107:1722, 2003.
81. Serruys P, Foley D, Jackson G, et al: A randomized placebo-controlled trial of fluvastatin for prevention of restenosis after successful coronary balloon angioplasty; final results of the fluvastatin angiographic restenosis (FLARE) trial. Eur Heart J 20:58, 1999.
82. Serruys P, de Feyter P, Macaya C, et al: Fluvastatin for prevention of cardiac events following successful first percutaneous coronary intervention: A randomized controlled trial. JAMA 287:3215, 2002.

Drug-Eluting Stents

83. Sousa JE, Costa MA, Abizaid AC, et al: Sustained suppression of neointimal proliferation by sirolimus-eluting stents: One-year angiographic and intravascular ultrasound follow-up. Circulation 104:2007, 2001.
84. Degertekin M, Serruys P, Foley D, et al: Persistent inhibition of neointimal hyperplasia after sirolimus-eluting stent implantation: Long-term (up to 2 years) clinical, angiographic, and intravascular ultrasound follow-up. Circulation 106:1610, 2002.
85. Rensing B, Vos J, Smits P, et al: Coronary restenosis elimination with a sirolimus eluting stent: First European human experience with 6-month angiographic and intravascular ultrasonic follow-up. Eur Heart J 22:2125, 2001.
86. Sousa J, Costa M, Sousa A, et al: Two-year angiographic and intravascular ultrasound follow-up after implantation of sirolimus-eluting stents in human coronary arteries Circulation 107:381, 2003.
87. Morice M, Serruys P, Sousa J, et al: A randomized comparison of a sirolimus-eluting stent with a standard stent for coronary revascularization. N Engl J Med 346:1773, 2002.
88. Serruys P, Degertekin M, Tanabe K, et al: Intravascular ultrasound findings in the multicenter, randomized, double-blind RAVEL (RAndomized study with the sirolimus-eluting VElocity balloon-expandable stent in the treatment of patients with de novo native coronary artery Lesions) trial. Circulation 106:798, 2002.
89. Moses J, Leon M, Popma J, et al: Angiographic and clinical outcomes after a sirolimus-eluting stent compared to a standard stent in patients with complex coronary stenoses. N Engl J Med 349:1315, 2003.
90. Sousa J, Costa M, Abizaid A, et al: Sirolimus-eluting stent for the treatment of in-stent restenosis: A quantitative coronary angiography and three-dimensional intravascular ultrasound study. Circulation 107:24, 2003.
91. Degertekin M, Regar E, Tanabe K, et al: Sirolimus-eluting stent for treatment of complex in-stent restenosis. The first clinical experience. J Am Coll Cardiol 41:184, 2003.

92. Grube E, Silber S, Hauptmann K, et al: TAXUS I: Six- and twelve-month results from a randomized, double-blind trial on a slow-release paclitaxel-eluting stent for de novo coronary lesions. Circulation 107:38, 2003.
93. Colombo A, Drzewiecki J, Banning A, et al: Randomized study to assess the effectiveness of slow- and moderate-release polymer-based paclitaxel-eluting stents for coronary artery lesions Circulation 108:788, 2003.
94. Stone C, Ellis SG, Cox DA, et al: A polymer-based, paclitaxel-eluting stent in patients with coronary artery disease. N Engl J Med 350:221, 2004.
95. Park S, Shim W, Ho D, et al: A paclitaxel-eluting stent for the prevention of coronary restenosis. N Engl J Med 348:1537, 2003.
96. Tanabe K, Serruys P, Grube E, et al: TAXUS III trial: In-stent restenosis treated with stent-based delivery of paclitaxel incorporated in a slow-release polymer formulation. Circulation 107:559, 2003.
97. Hong M, Mintz G, Lee C, et al: Paclitaxel coating reduces in-stent intimal hyperplasia in human coronary arteries: A serial volumetric intravascular ultrasound analysis from the Asian Paclitaxel-Eluting Stent Clinical Trial (ASPECT). Circulation 107:517, 2003.
98. Liistro F, Stankovic G, Di Mario C, et al: First clinical experience with a paclitaxel derivate-eluting polymer stent system implantation for in-stent restenosis: Immediate and long-term clinical and angiographic outcome. Circulation 105:1883, 2002.
99. Virmani R, Liistro F, Stankovic G, et al: Mechanism of late in-stent restenosis after implantation of a paclitaxel derivate-eluting polymer stent system in humans. Circulation 106:2649, 2002.

Indications for Coronary Revascularization

100. Cannon C, Weintraub W, Demopoulos L, et al: Comparison of early invasive and conservative strategies in patients with unstable coronary syndromes treated with the glycoprotein IIb/IIIa inhibitor tirofiban. N Engl J Med 344:1879, 2001.
101. Fox K, Poole-Wilson P, Henderson R, et al: Interventional versus conservative treatment for patients with unstable angina or non-ST-elevation myocardial infarction: The British Heart Foundation RITA 3 randomised trial. Randomized Intervention Trial of unstable Angina. Lancet 360:743, 2002.
102. Popma J, Sawyer M, Selwyn A, et al: Lipid-lowering therapy after coronary revascularization. Am J Cardiol 86(4 Suppl 2):18H, 2000.
103. Eagle K, Guyton R, Davidoff R, et al: ACC/AHA Guidelines for Coronary Artery Bypass Surgery. J Am Coll Cardiol 34:1262, 1999.
104. Braunwald E, Antman E, Beasley J, et al: ACC/AHA 2002 guideline update for the management of patients with unstable angina and non-ST-segment elevation myocardial infarction—Summary article: A report of the American College of Cardiology/American Heart Association task force on practice guidelines (Committee on the Management of Patients With Unstable Angina). J Am Coll Cardiol 40:1366, 2002.
105. Anderson H, Cannon C, Stone P, et al: One year results of the Thrombolysis In Myocardial Infarction (TIMI) IIIB clinical trial: A randomized comparison of tissue-type plasminogen activator versus placebo and early invasive versus early conservative strategies in unstable angina and non-Q-wave myocardial infarction. J Am Coll Cardiol 26:1643, 1995.
106. Boden WE, O'Rourke RA, Crawford MH, et al: Outcomes in patients with acute non-Q-wave myocardial infarction randomly assigned to an invasive as compared with a conservative management strategy. Veterans Affairs Non-Q-Wave Infarction Strategies in Hospital (VANQWISH) Trial Investigators. N Engl J Med 338:1785, 1998.
107. Boden W: "Routine invasive" versus "selective invasive" approaches to non-ST-segment elevation acute coronary syndromes management in the post-stent/platelet inhibition era. J Am Coll Cardiol 41(4 Suppl S):113S, 2003.
108. The FRISC-II Investigators: Invasive compared with non-invasive treatment in unstable coronary artery disease: FRISC II prospective randomised multcentre study. Lancet 354:708, 1999.
109. Lemos P, Lee C, Degertekin M, et al: Early outcome after sirolimus-eluting stent implantation in patients with acute coronary syndromes. Insights from the Rapamycin-Eluting Stent Evaluated At Rotterdam Cardiology Hospital (RESEARCH) registry. J Am Coll Cardiol 41:2093, 2003
110. Pitt B, Waters D, Brown W: Aggressive lipid lowering compared with angioplasty in stable coronary artery disease. N Engl J Med 341:70, 1999.

Coronary Artery Bypass Surgery Versus Percutaneous Coronary Intervention

111. Solomon AJ, Gersh BJ: Management of chronic stable angina: medical therapy, percutaneous transluminal coronary angioplasty, and coronary artery bypass graft surgery. Lessons from the randomized trials. Ann Intern Med 128:216, 1998.
112. Pocock S, Henderson R, Rickards A, et al: Meta-analysis of randomized trials comparing coronary angioplasty with bypass surgery. Lancet 346:1184, 1995.
113. Detre KM, Lombardero MS, Brooks MM, et al: The effect of previous coronary-artery bypass surgery on the prognosis of patients with diabetes who have acute myocardial infarction. Bypass Angioplasty Revascularization Investigation Investigators. N Engl J Med 342:989, 2000.
114. Diegeler A, Thiele H, Falk V, et al: Comparison of stenting with minimally invasive bypass surgery for stenosis of the left anterior descending coronary artery. N Engl J Med 347:561, 2002.
115. de Feyter P, Serruys P, Unger F, et al: Bypass surgery versus stenting for the treatment of multivessel disease in patients with unstable angina compared with stable angina. Circulation 105:2367, 2002.
116. Serruys PW, Unger F, Sousa JE, et al: Comparison of coronary-artery bypass surgery and stenting for the treatment of multivessel disease. N Engl J Med 344:1117, 2001.
117. The SOS Investigators: Coronary artery bypass surgery versus percutaneous coronary intervention with stent implantation in patients with multivessel coronary artery disease (the Stent or Surgery trial): A randomised controlled trial. Lancet 360:965, 2002;.
118. Unger F, Serruys P, Yacoub M, et al: Revascularization in multivessel disease: Comparison between two-year outcomes of coronary bypass surgery and stenting. J Thorac Cardiovasc Surg 125:809, 2003.
119. Stone G, St Goar F, Taussig A, et al: First experience with hybrid percutaneous transmyocardial laser revascularization and angioplasty in patients with lesions at high risk for restenosis: Results of a phase I feasibility study. Am Heart J 142:679, 2001.
120. Vale PR, Losordo D, Milliken CE, et al: Left ventricular electromechanical mapping to assess efficacy of phVEGF165 gene transfer for therapeutic angiogenesis in chronic myocardial ischemia. Circulation 102:965, 2000.

Aortic and Mitral Valvuloplasty

121. Vahanian A: Valvuloplasty. *In* Topol E (ed): Textbook of Cardiovascular Medicine. Philadelphia, Lippincott-Raven, 1998, pp 2155-2175.
122. Cohen DJ, Kuntz RE, Gordon SP, et al: Predictors of long-term outcome after percutaneous balloon mitral valvuloplasty. N Engl J Med 327:1329, 1992.
123. Cribier A, Eltchaninoff H, Bash A, et al: Percutaneous transcatheter implantation of an aortic valve prosthesis for calcific aortic stenosis: First human case description. Circulation 106:3006, 2002.

Institutional and Operator Proficiency

124. Pepine C, Babb J, Brinker J, et al: Guidelines for training in adult cardiovascular medicine. Core Cardiology Training Symposium (COCATS). Task Force 3: Training in cardiac catheterization and interventional cardiology. J Am Coll Cardiol 25:14, 1995.
125. Hirshfeld J, Banas J, Brundage B, et al: American College of Cardiology training statement on recommendations for the structure of an optimal adult interventional cardiology training program: A report of the American College of Cardiology task force on clinical expert consensus documents. J Am Coll Cardiol 34:2141, 1999.
126. Hirshfeld J, Ellis S, Faxon D: Recommendations for the assessment and maintenance of proficiency in coronary interventional procedures: Statement of the American College of Cardiology. J Am Coll Cardiol 31:722, 1998.
127. Shaw R, Anderson H, Brindis R, et al: Development of a risk adjustment mortality model using the American College of Cardiology-National Cardiovascular Data Registry (ACC-NCDR) experience: 1998-2000. J Am Coll Cardiol 39:1104, 2002.
128. Bashore T, Bates E, Berger P, et al: American College of Cardiology/Society for Cardiac Angiography and Interventions Clinical Expert Consensus Document on cardiac catheterization laboratory standards. A report of the American College of Cardiology Task Force on Clinical Expert Consensus Documents. J Am Coll Cardiol 37:2170, 2001.

GUIDELINES *Thomas H. Lee*

Percutaneous Coronary and Valvular Intervention

The American College of Cardiology/American Heart Association (ACC/AHA) updated guidelines for percutaneous coronary interventions (PCIs) in 2001.[1] Recommendations from these guidelines for use of PCI in the setting of acute myocardial infarction are summarized in the appendix to Chapter 48. Guidelines for use of percutaneous valvular interventions were published by the ACC/AHA in 1998[2] and are summarized in the appendix to Chapter 57. Therefore, this appendix focuses on recommendations relevant to use of PCI for stable ischemic heart disease and for unstable angina without acute myocardial infarction.

These guidelines use the ACC/AHA classification system for the indications (class I for generally accepted indications, class IIa when indications are controversial but the weight of evidence is supportive, class IIb when usefulness or efficacy is less well established, and class III when there is consensus against the usefulness of the intervention). The guidelines also use a convention for rating levels of evidence upon which recommendations have been based. *Level A* recommendations were derived from data from multiple randomized clinical trials, *level B* recommendations were derived from a single randomized trial or nonrandomized studies, and *level C* recommendations were based upon the consensus opinion of experts.

The guidelines acknowledged variability in outcomes of PCI in different populations, with particular attention to poorer outcomes in patients with diabetes mellitus. The committee concluded that much of the increase in adverse outcomes in women and elderly people was due to comorbidities; thus, with rare exception, separate recommendations for subgroups defined by gender and age were not developed.

Institutional and Operator Competence

These guidelines gave considerable attention to institutional and physician-specific factors associated with better outcomes and lower complication rates, such as higher procedure volume. Citing an ACC Training Statement,[3] the guidelines recommend that physicians undergo a 3-year comprehensive cardiac training program with 12 months of training in diagnostic catheterization during which the trainee performs 300 diagnostic catheterizations, including 200 as the primary operator. Interventional training requires a fourth year of training including more than 250 interventional procedures, a volume level that is also required for physicians to be eligible for the American Board of Internal Medicine certifying examination in interventional cardiology.

Institutions must have a system for quality measurement and improvement that includes valid peer review. The guidelines recommend that credentials committees should evaluate physician outcomes and cite benchmarks for unadjusted mortality (0.9 percent) and need for emergency coronary artery bypass surgery (<3.0 percent). The guidelines favor performance of PCI by higher volume operators (>75 cases per year) with advanced technical skills (e.g., subspecialty certification) at high-volume centers (>400 cases per year) associated with an on-site cardiovascular surgical program, except in underserved areas that are geographically far removed from major centers (Table 52G–1).

Despite technical improvements that have decreased the intensity of surgical "backup" coverage for PCI at many institutions, the guidelines continue to recommend that elective PCI should not be performed in facilities without on-site cardiac surgery.

Indications

The most recent guidelines for PCI differ from previous versions in that they no longer make recommendations based upon the number of diseased vessels. The guidelines assume that the operator can perform either single-vessel or multivessel PCI with a high likelihood of initial success and low risk. Therefore, recommendations are based upon the patient's clinical condition, specific coronary lesion morphology and anatomy, left ventricular function, and associated medical conditions.

The guidelines assert that the majority of patients with coronary disease who are asymptomatic or have mild angina should be treated medically. However, for patients with moderate or severe ischemia and few symptoms, revascularization with PCI or coronary artery bypass graft (CABG) surgery is considered reasonable and considered class I

TABLE 52G–1 Recommendations for Percutaneous Coronary Intervention Institutional and Operator Volumes at Centers with On-Site Cardiac Surgery

Operator Volume	Minimal Institutional Volume (200-400 Procedures Annually)	Optimal Institutional Volume (>400 Procedures Annually)
Low (<75 procedures annually)	Class IIb (an institution with a volume of <200 procedures per year, unless in a region that is underserved because of geography, should carefully consider whether it should continue to offer the service)	Class IIa (ideally, operators with annual procedure volume <75 should work only at institutions with an activity level of >600 procedures per year)
Acceptable (≥75 procedures annually)	Class IIa	Class I

TABLE 52G–2 ACC/AHA Recommendations for Percutaneous Coronary Intervention in Asymptomatic Patients or Patients with Class I Angina

Class	Indication	Level of Evidence
Class I (indicated)	Patients who do not have treated diabetes with asymptomatic ischemia or mild angina with one or more significant lesions in one or two coronary arteries suitable for PCI with a high likelihood of success and a low risk of morbidity and mortality. The vessels to be dilated must subtend a large area of viable myocardium.	B
Class IIa (good supportive evidence)	The same clinical and anatomical requirements as for class I, except the myocardial area at risk is of moderate size or the patient has treated diabetes.	B
Class IIb (weak supportive evidence)	Patients with asymptomatic ischemia or mild angina with > three coronary arteries suitable for PCI with a high likelihood of success and a low risk of morbidity and mortality. The vessels to be dilated must subtend at least a moderate area of viable myocardium. In the physician's judgment, there should be evidence of myocardial ischemia by ECG exercise testing, stress nuclear imaging, stress echocardiography or ambulatory ECG monitoring, or intracoronary physiological measurements.	B
Class III (not indicated)	Patients with asymptomatic ischemia or mild angina who do not meet the criteria as listed under class I or class II and who have: Only a small area of viable myocardium at risk. No objective evidence of ischemia. Lesions that have a low likelihood of successful dilation. Mild symptoms that are unlikely to be due to myocardial ischemia. Factors associated with increased risk of morbidity or mortality. Left main disease. Insignificant disease <50%.	C

ACC/AHA = American College of Cardiology/American Heart Association; ECG = electrocardiographic; PCI = percutaneous coronary intervention.

or II in appropriateness (Table 52G–2). PCI is considered inappropriate when the amount of viable myocardium at risk is small, when symptoms are unlikely to be due to ischemia, or when there is a high risk of complications.

For patients with more severe angina, the threshold for performing PCI is lower (Table 52G–3). PCI is considered appropriate in patients with single-vessel or multivessel disease if a moderate or large area of viable myocardium is at risk, the procedure has a high likelihood of success, and the risk of complications is low. PCI is considered inappropriate if patients have minimal myocardium at risk or a high risk of complications or if they have significant left main disease and are candidates for CABG.

For patients who have had CABG, the guidelines are supportive of an aggressive approach to detecting and addressing ischemia detected soon after surgery (Table 52G–4). Usually, such ischemia represents graft failure, often related to thrombosis, which can be corrected with PCI. When ischemia occurs 1 to 12 months after surgery, the etiology is usually perianastomotic graft stenosis, which also responds well to PCI. In contrast, PCI for chronic vein occlusions is characterized by lower success and higher complication rates, and thresholds for PCI are therefore higher when patients have ischemia more than 1 year after CABG.

Adjunctive Technologies

Intravascular ultrasonography can be used to facilitate deployment of coronary stents, but the guidelines do not consider it necessary for all stent procedures (Table 52G–5). The guidelines recommend that it be considered for use (class IIa) in high-risk procedures, such as those with multiple stents, impaired Thrombolysis in Myocardial Infarction (TIMI) grade flow or coronary flow reserve, and marginal angiographic appearance.

The guidelines similarly recommend a narrow role for assessment of coronary flow velocity and coronary vasodilator reserve. This tool might have a role in assessment of the physiological effects of intermediate coronary stenosis (30 to 70 percent luminal narrowing in patients with angina symptoms, class IIa), but the guidelines were dubious about its value in patients who had undergone successful PCI (Table 52G–6).

Management Issues

Recommendations for use of medications in patients undergoing PCI electively and with acute myocardial infarction are summarized in Table 52G–7. Antiplatelet therapy with aspirin and clopidogrel are considered class I indications for all patients, whereas warfarin is inappropriate except in patients with other indications for this medication. Glycoprotein IIb/IIIa inhibitors were considered clearly appropriate for patients undergoing PCI for severe or unstable angina but less clearly so (class II) for patients with class I angina. Unfractionated heparin was considered appropriate during PCI; the role of low-molecular-weight heparin was considered unresolved.

During long-term follow-up of patients after PCI, the guidelines do not endorse routine exercise testing of asymptomatic patients. If patients are symptomatic, the guidelines recommend that they undergo stress imaging studies in order to localize disease.

TABLE 52G–3 ACC/AHA Recommendations for Patients with Moderate or Severe Symptoms (Angina Class II to IV, Unstable Angina or Non-ST-Elevation Myocardial Infarction) with Single- or Multivessel Coronary Disease Receiving Medical Therapy

Class	Indication	Level of Evidence
Class I (indicated)	Patients with one or more significant lesions in one or more coronary arteries suitable for PCI with a high likelihood of success and low risk of morbidity or mortality. The vessel(s) to be dilated must subtend a moderate or large area of viable myocardium and have high risk.	B
Class IIa (good supportive evidence)	Patients with focal saphenous vein graft lesions or multiple stenoses who are poor candidates for reoperative surgery.	C
Class IIb (weak supportive evidence)	Patient has one or more lesions to be dilated with reduced likelihood of success or the vessel(s) subtends a less than moderate area of viable myocardium. Patients with two- or three-vessel disease, with significant proximal LAD CAD and treated diabetes or abnormal LV function.	C
Class III (not indicated)	Patient has no evidence of myocardial injury or ischemia on objective testing and has not had a trial of medical therapy or has Only a small area of myocardium at risk. All lesions or the culprit lesion to be dilated with morphology with a low likelihood of success. A high risk of procedure-related morbidity or mortality.	C
	Patients with insignificant coronary stenosis (e.g., <50% diameter).	C
	Patients with significant left main CAD who are candidates for CABG.	B

ACC/AHA = American College of Cardiology/American Heart Association; CABG = coronary artery bypass graft; CAD = coronary artery disease; LAD = left anterior descending; LV = left ventricular; PCA = percutaneous coronary intervention.

TABLE 52G–4 ACC/AHA Recommendations for Percutaneous Coronary Intervention with Prior Coronary Artery Bypass Graft

Class	Indication	Level of Evidence
Class I (indicated)	Patients with early ischemia (usually within 30 d) after CABG.	B
Class IIa (good supportive evidence)	Patients with ischemia occurring 1 to 3 yr postoperatively and preserved LV function with discrete lesions in graft conduits.	B
	Disabling angina secondary to new disease in a native coronary circulation. (If angina is not typical, the objective evidence of ischemia should be obtained.)	B
	Patients with diseased vein grafts >3 yr following CABG.	B
Class IIb (weak supportive evidence)		
Class III (not indicated)	PCI to chronic total vein graft occlusions.	B
	Patients with multivessel disease, failure or multiple SVGs, and impaired LV function.	B

ACC/AHA = American College of Cardiology/American Heart Association; CABG = coronary artery bypass graft; LV = left ventricular; SVG = saphenous vein graft.

TABLE 52G–5 ACC/AHA Recommendations for Coronary Intravascular Ultrasonography

Class	Indication	Level of Evidence
Class I (indicated)		
Class IIa (good supportive evidence)	Assessment of the adequacy of deployment of coronary stents, including the extent of stent apposition and determination of the minimum luminal diameter within the stent.	B
	Determination of the mechanism of stent restenosis (inadequate expansion versus neointimal proliferation) and to enable selection of appropriate therapy (plaque ablation versus repeated balloon expansion).	B
	Evaluation of coronary obstruction at a location difficult to image by angiography in a patient with a suspected flow-limiting stenosis.	C
	Assessment of a suboptimal angiographic result following PCI.	C
	Diagnosis and management of coronary disease following cardiac transplantation.	C
	Establishing presence and distribution of coronary calcium in patients for whom adjunctive rotational atherectomy is contemplated.	C
	Determination of plaque location and circumferential distribution for guidance of directional coronary atherectomy.	B
Class IIb (weak supportive evidence)	Determining extent of atherosclerosis in patients with characteristic anginal symptoms and a positive functional study with no focal stenoses or mild CAD on angiography.	C
	Preinterventional assessment of lesional characteristics and vessel dimensions as a means to select an optimal revascularization device.	C
Class III (not indicated)	When angiographic diagnosis is clear and no interventional treatment is planned.	C

ACC/AHA = American College of Cardiology/American Heart Association; CAD = coronary artery disease; PCI = percutaneous coronary intervention.

TABLE 52G–6 Recommendations for Intracoronary Physiological Measurements

Class	Indication	Level of Evidence
Class I (indicated)		
Class IIa (good supportive evidence)	Assessment of the physiological effects of intermediate coronary stenoses (30% to 70% luminal narrowing) in patients with anginal symptoms. Coronary pressure or Doppler velocimetry may also be useful as an alternative to performing noninvasive functional testing (e.g., when the functional study is absent or ambiguous) to determine whether an intervention is warranted.	B
Class IIb (weak supportive evidence)	Evaluation of the success of percutaneous coronary revascularization in restoring flow reserve and to predict the risk of restenosis.	C
	Evaluation of patients with anginal symptoms without an apparent angiographic culprit lesion.	C
Class III (not indicated)	Routine assessment of the severity of angiographic disease in patients with a positive, unequivocal noninvasive functional study.	C

TABLE 52G–7 ACC/AHA Recommendations for Pharmacological Management of Patients Undergoing Percutaneous Coronary Intervention*

Drugs	Clinical Status: *Class I Angina*	*Class II-IV Angina, Unstable Angina, NSTEMI*	*Transmural MI*: *Acute Phase MI*	*After Thrombolysis*	*Hospital Management Phase*
Aspirin	I	I	I	I	I
Ticlopidine, clopidogrel (in conjunction with stenting)	I (to be given 24-48 hours before planned stenting, if possible)	I	I	I	I (2-4 weeks after stent placement)
Warfarin	III (in patients without atrial fibrillation or other pre-existing clinical indications)	III	III	II	I (patients with anterior myocardial wall motion abnormalities or left ventricular thrombus)
Glycoprotein IIb/IIIa inhibitors	II	I	II	I	III
Unfractionated heparin	I	I	I	II	III

ACC/AHA = American College of Cardiology/American Heart Association; MI = myocardial infarction; NSTEMI = non–ST-segment elevation myocardial infarction.

*Roman numerals indicate ACC/AHA class indication.

References

1. Smith SC Jr, Dove JT, Jacobs AK, et al: ACC/AHA guidelines for percutaneous coronary intervention: A report of the American College of Cardiology/American Heart Association Task Force on Practice Guidelines (Committee to Revise the 1993 Guidelines for Percutaneous Transluminal Coronary Angioplasty). J Am Coll Cardiol 37:2239i, 2001.
2. Bonow RO, Carabello B, de Leon AC Jr, et al: ACC/AHA guidelines for the management of patients with valvular heart disease: Executive summary: A report of the American College of Cardiology/American Heart Association Task Force on Practice Guidelines (Committee on Management of Patients with Valvular Heart Disease). Circulation 98:1949, 1998.
3. Hirshfeld JW Jr, Banas JS Jr, Brudage BH, et al: American College of Cardiology training statement on recommendations for the structure of an optimal adult interventional cardiology training program: A report of the American College of Cardiology Task Force on Clinical Expert Consensus Documents. J Am Coll Cardiol 34:2141, 1999.

CHAPTER 53

Diseases of the Aorta

Eric M. Isselbacher

The Normal Aorta

Function

The aorta is the largest and strongest artery in the body, carrying roughly 200 million liters of blood through the body in an average lifetime. Three layers comprise the aorta: the thin inner layer, or *intima;* a thick middle layer, or *media;* and a rather thin outer layer, the *adventitia* (see Chap. 35). The strength of the aorta lies in the media, which is composed of laminated but intertwining sheets of elastic tissue arranged in a spiral manner that affords maximum tensile strength. Indeed, as thin as it is, experimentally the aortic wall can withstand the pressure of thousands of millimeters of mercury without bursting. In contrast to smaller muscular arteries, the aortic media contains multiple layers of elastic laminae (see Chap. 35). It is this tremendous accretion of elastic tissue that gives the aorta not only tensile strength but also distensibility and elasticity, which serve a vital circulatory role. The endothelium-lined aortic intima is a thin, delicate layer and is easily traumatized. The adventitia contains mainly collagen and carries the important vasa vasorum, which nourish the outer half of the aortic wall, including much of the media.

Ventricular systole distends the aorta by the force of the blood ejected from the left ventricle. In this manner, part of the kinetic energy generated by the contracting left ventricle is converted into potential energy stored in the aortic wall. Then, during diastole, this potential energy is transformed back into kinetic energy as the aortic walls recoil and propel the blood in the aortic lumen distally into the arterial bed. Thus, the aorta plays an essential role in maintaining forward circulation of the blood in diastole after it is delivered into the aorta by the left ventricle during systole. The pulse wave itself, with its milking effect, is transmitted along the aorta to the periphery at a speed of about 5 m/sec. This speed is much faster than the velocity of the intraluminal blood itself, which travels at only 40 to 50 cm/sec.

The systolic pressure developing within the aorta is a function of the volume of blood ejected into the aorta, the compliance or distensibility of the aorta, and resistance to blood flow. This resistance depends primarily on the tone of the peripheral muscular arteries and arterioles and, to a slight extent, on the inertia of the column of blood in the aorta when systole commences.

In addition to its conductance and pumping functions, the aorta also plays a role in indirectly controlling systemic vascular resistance and heart rate. Pressure-responsive receptors, analogous to those in the carotid sinus, lie in the ascending aorta and aortic arch and send afferent signals to the vasomotor center in the brain stem by way of the vagus nerves. An increase in intraaortic pressure causes reflex bradycardia and a reduction in systemic vascular resistance, whereas a decrease in intraaortic pressure increases the heart rate and vascular resistance.

Anatomical Considerations

The aorta is divided anatomically into thoracic and abdominal components. The thoracic aorta is further divided into the *ascending, arch,* and *descending* segments, and the abdominal aorta consists of *suprarenal* and *infrarenal* segments.

The ascending aorta is some 5 cm long and has two distinct segments. The lower segment is the *aortic root,* which begins at the level of the aortic valve and extends to the sinotubular junction. This portion of the ascending aorta is the widest and measures about 3.5 cm. The bases of the aortic leaflets are supported by the aortic root, from which the three sinuses of Valsalva bulge outward to allow for full excursion of the aortic valve leaflets during systole. In addition, the two coronary artery trunks arise from these sinuses of Valsalva. The upper tubular segment of the ascending aorta begins at the sinotubular junction and rises to join the aortic arch. Normally, the ascending aorta sits just to the right of midline, with its proximal portion lying within the pericardial cavity.

The arch of the aorta gives rise to all the brachiocephalic arteries. From the ascending aorta, the arch courses slightly leftward in front of the trachea and then proceeds posteriorly to the left of the trachea and esophagus. The pulmonary artery bifurcation and right pulmonary artery lie inferior to the arch, as does the left lung.

The descending thoracic aorta begins in the posterior mediastinum to the left of the vertebral column and gradually courses in front of the vertebral column as it descends, where it occupies a position immediately behind the esophagus. Distally, it passes through the diaphragm, usually at the level of the 12th thoracic vertebra.

The point at which the aortic arch joins the descending aorta is called the *aortic isthmus.* The aorta is especially vulnerable to trauma at this site because it is here that the relatively mobile portion of the aorta—the ascending aorta and arch—becomes relatively fixed to the thoracic cage by the pleural reflections, the paired intercostal arteries, and the left subclavian artery. Coarctations of the aorta also localize to this region.

The abdominal aorta continues from the thoracic aorta, gives rise to the mesenteric and renal arteries, and ends at its bifurcation into common iliac arteries at the level of the fourth lumbar vertebra.

Aging of the Aorta

As discussed, the elastic properties of the aorta contribute crucially to its normal function. However, the elasticity and distensibility of the aorta decline with age. Such changes occur even in normal healthy adults. The loss of elasticity and aortic compliance probably accounts for the increase in pulse pressure commonly seen in elderly persons and is accompanied by slow but progressive dilatation of the aorta.[1] This loss of aortic elasticity with aging is accelerated among persons with hypertension, hypercholesterolemia, or coronary artery disease, as compared with control subjects. Conversely, among healthy athletes, aortic elasticity is higher than in their age-matched controls.

Histologically, the aging aortic wall exhibits fragmentation of elastin with a concomitant increase in collagen that results in an increased collagen-to-elastin ratio, which contributes to the loss of aortic distensibility observed physiologically. Experimental animal data suggest that impairment of vasa vasorum flow to the aortic wall results in stiffening of the aorta with similar histological changes and may therefore be one cause of the degenerative changes seen with age.[2]

In animals, loss of aortic distensibility directly affects the mechanical performance of the left ventricle, with increases noted in left ventricular systolic pressure and wall tension and in end-diastolic pressure and volume. Furthermore, reduced aortic compliance causes a 20 to 40 percent increase in myocardial oxygen consumption to maintain a given stroke volume.[3] Over time, the changes in aortic compliance seen with age may cause clinically important alternations in cardiac function.

Examination of the Aorta

Unless the aorta is abnormally enlarged, the only location in which it can be palpated is the abdomen. The ease with which it can be felt depends largely on body habitus and pulse pressure: It is readily felt in thin individuals. It may be quite sensitive to palpation. Auscultation is usually unrevealing in patients with aortic diseases, except for occasional bruits at sites of narrowing of the aorta or its arterial branches. Diseases of the aortic root and proximal ascending aorta sometimes involve the aortic valve, with resultant aortic regurgitation that may be detectable on auscultation. Regurgitant murmurs secondary to root dilatation rather than primary valvular disease are often loudest along the right rather than the left sternal border.

Chest radiography and fluoroscopy are valuable and simple procedures for assessing the aorta. Normally, the ascending aorta is not visible on the direct anteroposterior chest radiograph. The aorta appears as a "knob" in the superior mediastinum just to the left of the vertebral column. The lateral border of the descending thoracic aorta can often be found to the left of the spine. On the lateral chest radiograph, the aortic root and proximal ascending aorta are visible as an indistinct shadow in the middle of the mediastinum arising from the base of the heart. The left anterior oblique projection best demonstrates the ascending aorta and arch.

A number of imaging modalities are available for diagnostic examination of the aorta, including aortography, computed tomography (CT), magnetic resonance imaging (MRI), and both transthoracic echocardiography (TTE) and transesophageal echocardiography (TEE). The respective utility of these imaging modalities is discussed here in the context of specific aortic diseases.

Aortic Aneurysms

The term *aortic aneurysm* refers to a pathological dilatation of the normal aortic lumen involving one or several segments. One useful criterion defines aortic aneurysm as a permanent localized dilation of the aorta having a diameter at least 1.5 times that of the expected normal diameter of that given aortic segment, although no definition is universally accepted. Aneurysms are usually described in terms of their location, size, morphologic appearance, and origin. The morphology of an aortic aneurysm is typically either *fusiform,* which is the more common shape, or *saccular.* A fusiform aneurysm has a fairly uniform shape, with symmetrical dilation that involves the full circumference of the aortic wall. Saccular aneurysms, on the other hand, have more localized dilation that appears as an outpouching of only a portion of the aortic wall. In addition, the aorta may have a *pseudoaneurysm* or *false aneurysm,* which is not actually an aneurysm at all, but rather a well-defined collection of blood and connective tissue outside the vessel wall. This defect may result from a contained rupture of the aortic wall.

The presence of an aortic aneurysm may be a marker of more diffuse aortic disease. Overall, up to 13 percent of all patients in whom an aortic aneurysm is diagnosed have multiple aneurysms, with 25 to 28 percent of those with thoracic aortic aneurysms having concomitant abdominal aortic aneurysms. For this reason, a patient in whom an aortic aneurysm is discovered should undergo examination of the entire aorta for the possible presence of other aneurysms.

Abdominal Aortic Aneurysms

Abdominal aortic aneurysms are much more common than thoracic aortic aneurysms. Age is an important risk factor. The incidence of abdominal aortic aneurysm rises rapidly after 55 years of age in men and 70 years of age in women, and abdominal aortic aneurysms occur 5 to 10 times more frequently in men than women. Men 65 years of age and older screened by ultrasonography have a prevalence of abdominal aortic aneurysms of 4 to 9 percent. The true prevalence of abdominal aortic aneurysms is difficult to determine, as there may be as much as a 10-fold variation depending on the diagnostic criteria, the imaging modality used, and the age, gender distribution, and baseline risk of the population examined.[4] Nevertheless, the incidence of abdominal aneurysms appears to have increased two- to threefold in recent decades. Some of the increase may reflect more widespread screening than in the past and more frequent use of abdominal CT scanning, which may reveal aortic aneurysms as incidental findings, for other diagnostic purposes. However, these data likely reflect, at least in part, a true increase in disease incidence.

The large majority of abdominal aortic aneurysms arise below the renal arteries and are known as *infrarenal* aneurysms. Only a small minority, known as *suprarenal aneurysms*, arise between the level of the diaphragm and the renal arteries. As a result of flow disturbance through the aneurysmal aortic segment, blood may stagnate along the walls and thus allow the formation of mural thrombus. Such thrombus, as well as atherosclerotic debris, may embolize and compromise the circulation of distal arteries. However, rupture poses the major risk of abdominal aortic aneurysms. When rupture does occur, 80 percent rupture into the left retroperitoneum, which may contain the rupture, whereas most of the remainder rupture into the peritoneal cavity and cause uncontrolled hemorrhage and rapid circulatory collapse.

ETIOLOGY AND PATHOGENESIS (see also Chap. 35). A number of risk factors favor the development of aneurysms. Smoking is most strongly associated with abdominal aortic aneurysms, followed by age, hypertension, hyperlipidemia, and atherosclerosis.[5] Gender and genes also influence aneurysm formation. Men are 10 times more likely than women to have an abdominal aortic aneurysm of 4.0 cm or greater.[6] However, women with aneurysms have a risk of rupture significantly higher than men. Those with a family history (first-degree relative) of abdominal aortic aneurysm have an increased risk of 13 to 32 percent compared with the 2 to 5 percent risk in the general population. In addition, those with familial aneurysms tend to be younger and have higher rates of rupture than those with sporadic aneurysms. Given the results of pedigree analysis and the fact that single gene defects have not yet been identified, the increased risk is probably polygenic.[7]

The aortic wall resists expansion because of the strength of its extracellular matrix, notably elastin and collagen. Degradation of these structural proteins, due to any of a number of factors, in turn weakens the aortic wall and allows aneurysms to develop. As the aorta then widens, tension in the vessel wall rises in accordance with Laplace law, which states that tension is proportional to the product of pressure and radius. Further widening results in even greater wall tension, which in turn leads to acceleration of aneurysm enlargement. A vicious cycle ensues in which the dilatation often progresses rapidly.

Classically, atherosclerosis has been considered the underlying cause of abdominal aortic aneurysms. The infrarenal abdominal aorta is most affected by the atherosclerotic process and is similarly the most common site of abdominal aneurysm formation; only a fraction of abdominal aortic aneurysms are suprarenal, and these tend to arise as an extension of a thoracic (thoracoabdominal) aneurysm. The atherosclerotic process less often involves the thoracic aorta. Atherosclerotic disease of the aorta may produce either stenotic obstruction, a process that tends to be confined to the infrarenal abdominal aorta, or aneurysmal dilatation; why one process should predominate over the other in any given individual, however, is unknown.

Although aortic atherosclerosis clearly contributes to the process, ongoing research supports a multifactorial pathogenesis of abdominal aortic aneurysms. Genetic, environmental, hemodynamic, and immunological factors all appear to play a role in the development and progressive growth of aneurysms. Moreover, although it was once thought that atherosclerotic and inflammatory abdominal aortic aneurysms were distinct conditions, it now appears that their underlying pathophysiology is actually similar, with inflammatory aneurysms simply representing an extreme of atherosclerotic aneurysms.

Inflammation within the aortic wall has been implicated in the degradation of the extracellular matrix. There is histological evidence of inflammatory infiltrates—in particular macrophages and T lymphocytes—within the media and adventitia of aneurysms. This may represent a primary inflammatory response whose target antigens within the aortic wall are unknown. Infection is one possible causal factor, with a number of studies identifying viral or bacterial antigens within aneurysm wall tissue. For example, a large proportion of men with abdominal aortic aneurysms have evidence of infection with *Chlamydia pneumoniae*. Moreover, the titer of IgA and the titer of IgG both have been found to correlate with more rapid expansion of aneurysms.[8] The infiltration with macrophages and T lymphocytes in turn results in local production of proteolytic enzymes that degrade aortic elastin, collagen, and other matrix proteins. It should be noted, however, that there is also some competing protein synthesis, so ultimately the process is one of a dynamic balance between protein degradation and synthesis that leads to remodeling of the aortic wall. T lymphocytes may induce smooth muscle cell apoptosis within the aneurysm wall. Since smooth muscle cells produce elastin and collagen, the loss of cellularity may lead to impaired maintenance and repair of the extracellular matrix in the face of ongoing degradation.[9]

Matrix metalloproteinases are zinc- and calcium-dependent enzymes that are produced by smooth muscle and inflammatory cells, and several of these proteinases may participate in abdominal aortic aneurysm formation. Indeed, certain matrix metalloproteinases can degrade elastin and collagen, primary components of the aortic extracellular matrix. The levels of some matrix metalloproteinases (e.g., MMP-9, MMP-2, MMP-14) are significantly elevated in the walls of aneurysms compared with control aortas. Moreover, in one study, the levels of MMP-9 messenger RNA expression was fourfold higher in large (5.0 to 6.9 cm) than in small (3.0-4.9 cm) aneurysms.[10] Circulating levels of MMP-9 are elevated in at least 50 percent of patients with abdominal aortic aneurysms, and levels decrease after open or endovascular aneurysm repair. The evidence linking the matrix metalloproteinases to aneurysm formation is, however, more than just circumstantial. In fact, in an experimental mouse model of aneurysm formation in which MMP-2 and MMP-9 levels are increased, both MMP-2 and MMP-9 knockout mice resisted aneurysm formation.[11] Reduced levels of metalloproteinases inhibitors, known as TIMPs (tissue inhibitors of metalloproteinases), in the walls of aneurysms may promote matrix breakdown by MMPs as well.

Pharmacological inhibition of proteolysis may slow the growth of aneurysms. The tetracyclines inhibit matrix metalloproteinases through a mechanism unrelated to their antibiotic activity. In animal models of abdominal aortic aneurysms, treatment with either doxycycline or tetracycline derivatives without antibiotic activity has reduced aortic wall production of MMP-9, led to preservation of medial elastin, and reduced aneurysmal expansion. In one murine model, doxycycline administration reduced aneurysm growth by 33 to 66 percent at circulating doxycycline levels similar to those achieved in humans at standard doses.[12] The early data in human trials is encouraging. Curci and colleagues found that preoperative treatment with oral doxycycline resulted in a fivefold reduction in the amount of MMP-9 expressed within aneurysm wall tissue resected at surgery.[13] A multicenter group led by Robert Thompson has reported a phase II trial demonstrating the safety of prolonged 6-month administration of doxycycline (100 mg bid) to subjects with abdominal aortic aneurysms. Their findings also showed that therapy is associated with a gradual reduction in plasma MMP-9 levels.[14] In a relatively small trial of 92 subjects, roxithromycin therapy for 28 days reduced the rate of aneurysm expansion by 44 percent in the first year, although by only 5 percent in the second year of follow-up.[15] As discussed earlier, *C. pneumoniae* may contribute to the inflammatory process underlying aneurysm formation. Because doxycycline is effective in the treatment of *C. pneumoniae* infection as well, this may provide another mechanism by which the drug might slow aneurysm expansion.

In addition to the matrix metalloproteinases, several other proteinases, including plasminogen activators, serine elastases, and cathepsins, may contribute to the formation of aneurysms. Cathepsins S and K are potent elastases overexpressed in human atheromas. Increased levels of cathepsin S have been demonstrated in both atherosclerotic plaques and aneurysms. On the other hand, patients with wider aortas have lower levels of cystatin C, an endogenous cathepsin S inhibitor, compared with control subjects.[16]

CLINICAL MANIFESTATIONS. The majority of abdominal aortic aneurysms are asymptomatic and discovered incidentally on routine physical examination or on imaging studies ordered for other indications. Younger patients (50 years old or younger), however, are several times more likely to be symptomatic at the time of diagnosis.[17] Among these patients, pain is the most frequent complaint and is usually located in the hypogastrium or lower part of the back. The pain is usually steady, has a gnawing quality, and may last for hours to days at a time. In contrast to musculoskeletal back pain, movement does not affect aneurysm pain, although patients may be more comfortable in certain positions, such as with the legs drawn up.

RUPTURED ANEURYSM. The development of new or worsening pain, often of sudden onset, may herald expansion or impending rupture of an aneurysm. This pain is characteristically constant, severe, and located in the back or lower part of the abdomen, sometimes with radiation into the groin, buttocks, or legs. Actual rupture is associated with abrupt

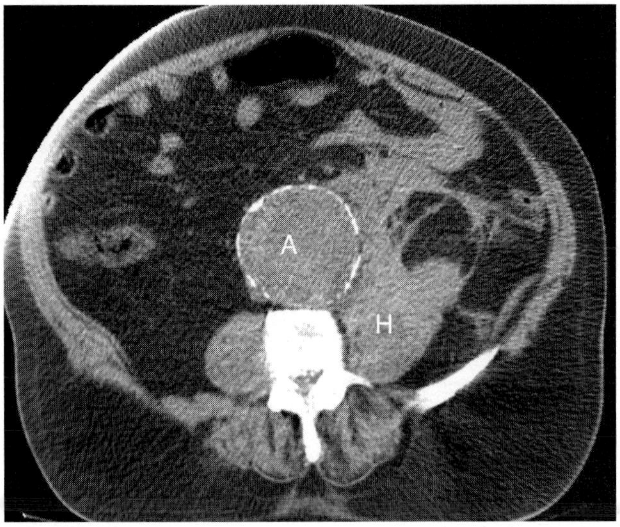

FIGURE 53–1 A non-contrast-enhanced computed tomography scan of the abdomen revealing a ruptured infrarenal abdominal aortic aneurysm. The aneurysm (A) is large, measuring 8.7 cm in greatest diameter, and its wall is well defined by the intimal calcification. The high-attenuation material (approximately 50 Hounsfield units) extending from the aneurysm into the left perirenal space is consistent with hemorrhage (H).

onset of back pain along with abdominal pain and tenderness. Most patients have a palpable, pulsatile abdominal mass, and many are hypotensive when initially seen. However, this familiar triad of abdominal/back pain, a pulsatile abdominal mass, and hypotension—recognized as pathognomonic of a ruptured abdominal aortic aneurysm—is seen in as few as one-third of cases.[18] Moreover, a ruptured aneurysm may mimic other acute abdominal conditions, such as renal colic, diverticulitis, or a gastrointestinal hemorrhage, and may therefore be initially misdiagnosed in as many as 30 percent of cases.

Patients who suffer rupture of an abdominal aortic aneurysm (Fig. 53–1) are critically ill. Hemorrhagic shock and its complications may ensue rapidly. Retroperitoneal hemorrhage may be signaled by hematomas in the flanks and groin. Rupture into the abdominal cavity may result in abdominal distention, whereas rupture into the duodenum is manifested as massive gastrointestinal hemorrhage.

PHYSICAL EXAMINATION. Many aneurysms can be detected on physical examination, although even large aneurysms may be difficult or impossible to detect in obese individuals.[19] When palpable, a pulsatile mass extending variably from the xiphoid process to the umbilicus may be appreciated. Because of difficulty distinguishing the abdominal aorta from surrounding structures by palpation, the size of an aneurysm tends to be overestimated on physical examination. Moreover, it may be difficult to differentiate a tortuous, ectatic aorta from true aneurysmal dilatation. Aneurysms are often sensitive to palpation and may be quite tender if rapidly expanding or about to rupture. Although tender aneurysms should be examined cautiously, no risk is known to be associated with palpation of the abdominal aorta.[20]

Associated occlusive arterial disease is sometimes present in the femoral pulses and distal pulses in the legs and feet. Bruits arising from associated narrowed arteries can be heard over the aneurysm. Occasionally, an arteriovenous fistula is formed by spontaneous rupture into the inferior vena cava, iliac vein, or renal vein and can cause a syndrome of hemodynamic collapse and acute high-output cardiac failure.

DIAGNOSIS AND SIZING. Several diagnostic imaging modalities are currently used for detecting, sizing, and serially monitoring abdominal aortic aneurysms, as well as for precise definition of the aortic anatomy preoperatively. Abdominal ultrasonography is perhaps the most practical way to screen for abdominal aortic aneurysms. It can visualize an aneurysm in the transverse and longitudinal planes, has a sensitivity of 87 to 99 percent (depending on the segment involved),[21] and can accurately define aneurysm size to within ±0.3 cm, but it is limited by less reliable measurements of the suprarenal aorta and significant interobserver variability. Its major advantages are that it is relatively inexpensive, is noninvasive, and does not require the use of a contrast agent. However, because ultrasonography is limited in its ability to visualize the cephalic or pelvic extent of disease or define the associated mesenteric and renal arterial anatomy, it is insufficient for planning operative repair.

Computed tomography is an extremely accurate method for both diagnosing aortic aneurysms (Fig. 53–2A) and sizing them to within ±0.2 cm. CT has an advantage over ultrasonography in that it can better define the shape and extent of the aneurysm as well as the local anatomical relationships of the visceral and renal vessels. Its disadvantages are that the procedure is more expensive and less widely available than ultrasonography, and it also requires the use of ionizing radiation and intravenous contrast. Although CT may therefore be less practical than ultrasonography as a screening tool, its high accuracy in sizing aneurysms makes it an excellent modality for serially monitoring changes in aneurysm size. It is important to note that CT measurements of aneurysm size tend to be larger than ultrasonographic measurements by an average of 0.27 cm.[22] Spiral (helical) CT, which permits three-dimensional display of the aorta and its branches, provides more comprehensive evaluation of the anatomy of an abdominal aortic aneurysm and information regarding renal, mesenteric, or iliac arterial occlusive disease and thus may be sufficient for preoperative evaluation of abdominal aneurysms (see Fig. 53–2B).

Magnetic resonance angiography (MRA) is also an alternative for the preoperative evaluation of aortic aneurysms. On conventional spin-echo MRI, flowing blood appears as a signal void, but with the use of MRA, blood has a bright appearance and vessels can be visualized in a projective fashion, similar to traditional angiography. Moreover, because tomographic images are reconstructed to create a three-dimensional image, the aorta can be visualized from a series of projections to facilitate appreciation of anatomical relationships. MRA is extremely accurate in determining aneurysm size, and it correctly defines the proximal extent of disease and iliofemoral involvement in more than 80 percent of cases.[23]

Aortography may underestimate aneurysm size in the presence of nonopacified mural thrombus lining the aneurysm walls, but it nevertheless remains an excellent technique for defining the suprarenal extent of the aneurysm and any associated renal, mesenteric, or iliofemoral arterial disease. Its disadvantages are that it is expensive, it is an invasive procedure with inherent risks, and it requires the use of intraarterial contrast and ionizing radiation. Preoperative aortography is now used only in selected cases, as CT and MRA provide sufficient information in most cases.

Many practitioners currently recommend the use of screening ultrasonography only for patients at high risk, in particular those with a family history of abdominal aortic aneurysm or those older than 60 years who have a history of smoking or hypertension. However, an important, but not fully resolved, issue is the potential utility of routine screening of asymptomatic patients for the presence of abdominal aneurysms. The largest and most definitive trial to date is the recent report of the Multicentre Aneurysm Screening Study Group, which provides a 4-year cost-effective analysis based on the results of a controlled trial in which a population-based sample of 67,800 men (aged 65-74 years) were randomized to an invitation to ultrasonography screening or to a control group not offered screening.[24] Eighty percent accepted the invitation for screening. Men found to have an abdominal aortic aneurysm of 3 cm or greater were followed with serial ultrasonographic scans for a mean of 4 years. Surgery was considered when the diameter reached 5.5 cm or greater, grew more than 1 cm per year, or became tender. There were 65 deaths related to the aneurysm in the invited

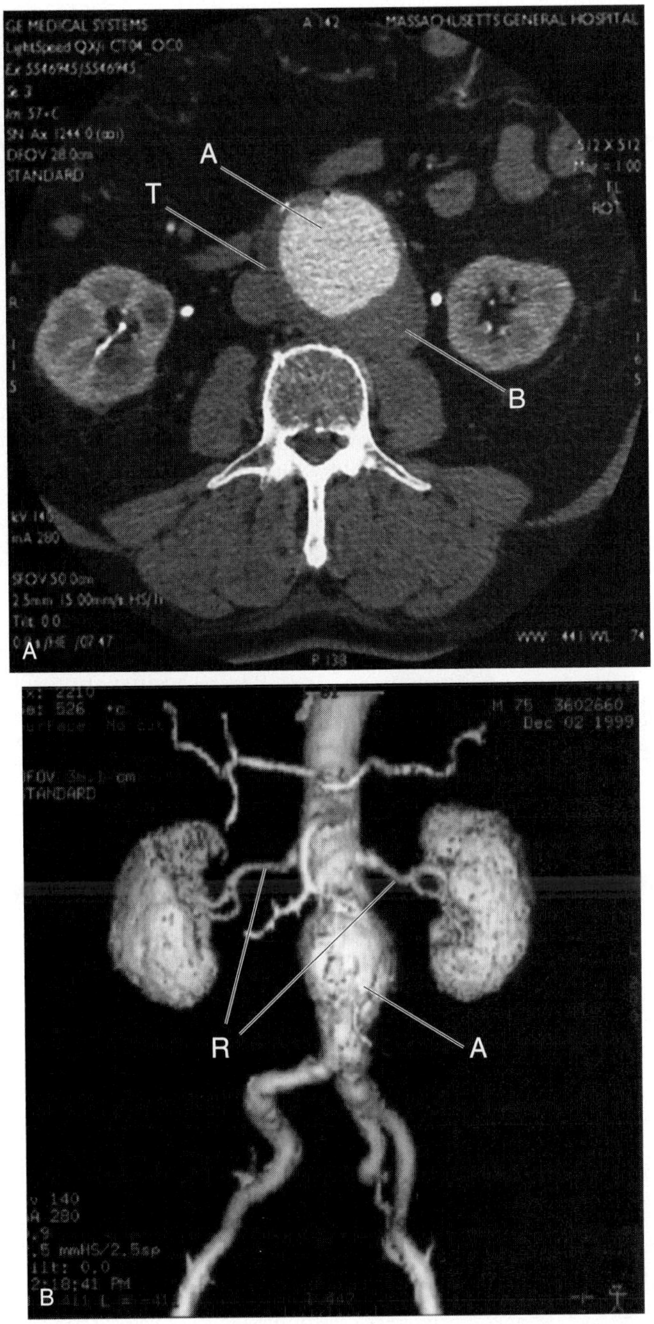

FIGURE 53–2 **A,** Axial contrast-enhanced computed tomography (CT) scan showing a 6.6-cm abdominal aortic aneurysm (A) lined with mural thrombus (T). Blistering of the aneurysm (B) is indicative of a weakened aortic wall and suggests impending rupture. **B,** Three-dimensional shaded-surface display of the same CT scan. This anteroposterior projection demonstrates that the aneurysm (A) is infrarenal and displays its anatomical relationship to surrounding structures, including the renal arteries (R) proximally and the aortic bifurcation distally. (Courtesy of John A. Kaufman, M.D., Division of Vascular Radiology, Massachusetts General Hospital, Boston.)

group, compared with 113 in the control group, yielding an estimated risk reduction of 42 percent. After 4 years, the cost was estimated to be $57,000 per quality-adjusted life year gained; it was expected to fall to $14,200 at 10 years. Screening of 710 subjects was required to prevent one death. The authors conclude that at 4 years, the cost-effectiveness of screening for abdominal aortic aneurysm is acceptable and is likely to become increasingly favorable over time. However, one important question left unanswered by this study is the cost-effectiveness of screening women for abdominal aneurysms. Another British study addressed the potential utility of repeated screening for abdominal aneurysms.[25] The investigators followed 223 65-year-old men who had abdominal aortic diameters of less than 2.6 cm at baseline with repeated ultrasonographic evaluations at 5 and 12 years. None of those who survived the 12-year interval had any clinically significant increase in the mean aortic diameter, and none of those who died did so from a ruptured abdominal aneurysm. The authors conclude that a normal ultrasonogram at age 65 effectively excludes the risk of a clinically significant aneurysm for life.

NATURAL HISTORY. The paramount concern in managing abdominal aortic aneurysms is their tendency to rupture. Mortality from rupture is quite high: Among the participants in the United Kingdom Small Aneurysm Trial who suffered a ruptured abdominal aneurysm, 25 percent died before reaching a hospital and 51 percent died in the hospital without undergoing surgery. The operative mortality rate for the 13 percent undergoing surgery was 46 percent (compared with 4 to 6 percent for elective surgery), yielding an overall 30-day survival of just 11 percent.[26] To prevent the associated mortality, surgical repair is the therapy of choice for aneurysms considered to be at significant risk of rupture.

It is well established that the risk of rupture increases with aneurysm size. The United Kingdom Small Aneurysm Trial found that aneurysms smaller than 4.0 cm have a 0.3 percent annual risk of rupture, those 4.0 to 4.9 cm have a 1.5 percent annual risk of rupture, and those 5.0 to 5.9 cm have a 6.5 percent annual risk of rupture.[26] For aneurysms 6.0 cm or larger, the risk of rupture rises sharply, although an exact risk cannot be estimated. Although abdominal aneurysms are less prevalent among women than men, when present they rupture three times more frequently among women and at a smaller aortic diameter (mean diameter of 5.0 cm among women versus 6.0 cm among men). Rupture is also more common among current smokers and those with hypertension.[26]

Because 80 percent of abdominal aortic aneurysms expand over time, with as many as 15 to 20 percent expanding rapidly (>0.5 cm/yr), the risk of rupture may concomitantly increase with time. Accordingly, the ability to predict rates of aortic aneurysm expansion would be useful in estimating the risk of future rupture. Although the mean rate of abdominal aortic aneurysm expansion is thought to approximate 0.4 cm per year, the rates of expansion within a population are extremely variable. Expansion rates even vary within one individual over time, as would be expected given the "vicious cycle" of aneurysm growth explained earlier. Baseline aneurysm size is perhaps the best predictor of aneurysm expansion rate, with larger aneurysms expanding more rapidly than small ones, probably as a consequence of the Laplace law. A rapid rate of expansion apparently also predicts aneurysm rupture, especially abdominal aneurysms 5.0 cm or greater in diameter. Many surgeons therefore consider both large size and rapid expansion to be indications for repair.

Management

SURGICAL TREATMENT. The goal of treating abdominal aortic aneurysms is to prolong life by preventing rupture. The decision to operate must weigh the natural history of the aneurysm and life expectancy of the patient against the anticipated morbidity and mortality of the proposed surgical procedure. Operative mortality is 4 to 6 percent overall for elective aneurysm repair and as low as 2 percent in low-risk patients. However, operative mortality rises to 19 percent for urgent aortic repair and reaches 50 percent for repair of a ruptured aneurysm. Aneurysm size remains the primary indicator for repair of asymptomatic aneurysms, and for many years there has been debate on the minimum aneurysm diameter that necessitates surgery. Recently, two large-scale clinical trials investigating this very question have been completed.

The United Kingdom Small Aneurysm Trial[27] randomized 1090 patients aged 60 to 76 years with small aortic aneurysms (diameter 4.0 to 5.5 cm) to either early elective surgery or regular ultrasonographic surveillance. They found no long-term difference in survival between the early-surgery group and the surveillance group, although after 8 years, total mortality was slightly lower in the early-surgery group. However, since the operative mortality rate in this trial was 5.8 percent, some practitioners have questioned whether there may have been a survival benefit from early surgery had the operative mortality rate been lower. However, a similar trial known as the Aneurysm Detection and Management (ADAM) Veterans Affairs Cooperative Study[28] has suggested otherwise. In ADAM 1136, patients with small asymptomatic aneurysms (diameter 4.0 to 5.4 cm) were randomized to undergo immediate surgical repair or surveillance at 6-month intervals by ultrasonography or CT scanning. Despite a remarkably low operative mortality rate of 2.1 percent, after a mean follow-up of 5 years there was no difference in survival between the two groups. Collectively, these trials suggest that surgery is not indicated in most instances for patients with asymptomatic aneurysms less than 5.5 cm in size. However, it should be recognized that the subjects randomized to the surveillance arms of these trials have careful clinical follow-up with both medical management and regular surveillance imaging to monitor the aneurysm. Such careful follow-up does not always take place in general practice settings outside a trial. Another important limitation is that these two study populations consisted almost entirely of men (United Kingdom Aneurysm Trial, 78 percent; ADAM, 99 percent), and since the risk of aneurysm rupture is greater and occurs at smaller diameters in women than in men, these results may well not be equally applicable to women.[29]

Surgical repair of abdominal aortic aneurysms consists of opening of the aneurysm and insertion of a synthetic prosthesis, usually fabricated of Dacron or expanded polytetrafluoroethylene (Gore-Tex). Sometimes, a simple tube graft is all that is necessary, although frequently the operation must be carried distally into one or both of the iliac arteries to excise the aneurysm completely. In the case of large aneurysms, much of the aneurysm wall may be left in situ ("intrasaccular approach of Creech"), thereby reducing the need for extensive dissection and thus decreasing aortic cross-clamping time.

A less invasive alternative to open surgery for repair of abdominal aortic aneurysms is the use of percutaneously implanted, expanding endovascular stent-grafts (see Chap. 55 and Figs. 53–3 and 53–4). The device consists of a collapsible prosthetic tube graft that is inserted remotely (e.g., via the femoral artery), advanced transluminally across the aneurysm under fluoroscopic guidance, and then secured at both its proximal and distal ends with an expandable stent attachment system. For aortic aneurysm repair, the stent-graft serves to bridge the region of the aneurysm, thereby excluding it from the circulation while allowing aortic blood flow to continue distally through the prosthetic stent-graft lumen. In some cases, stent-grafts are bifurcated, with two arms on the distal end designed to extend into the common iliac arteries when these vessels are aneurysmal as well. The rate of successful stent-graft implantation in several recent series ranged from 78 to 94 percent,[30-32] with some outcome variability resulting from differing definitions of procedural success. Despite these promising results, only 30 to 60 percent of patients

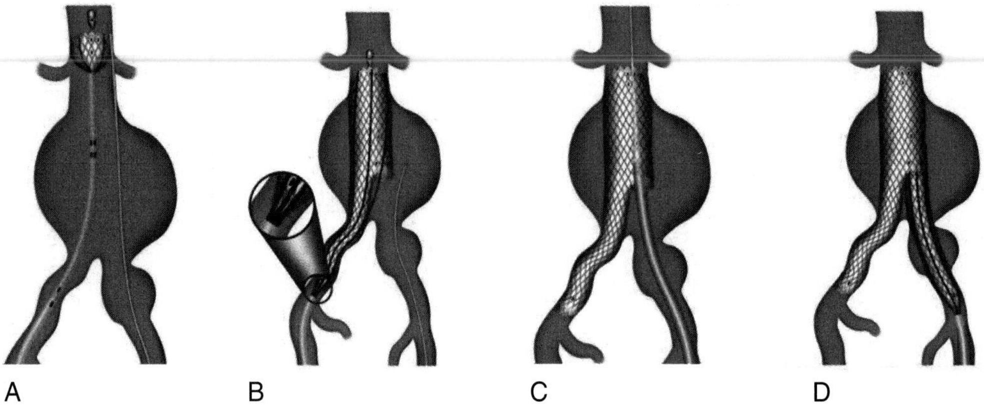

FIGURE 53–3 Diagram of deployment of an aortic stent graft. **A,** The catheter placement and proximal stabilization are achieved via right femoral access. **B,** The body and right limb of the stent graft are positioned and deployed. **C,** The cannula for deployment of the left limb of the graft is placed via left femoral access. **D,** The left limb of the graft is deployed, completing the endovascular repair of the aortic aneurysm with left iliac involvement. (Courtesy of Medtronics Corporation.)

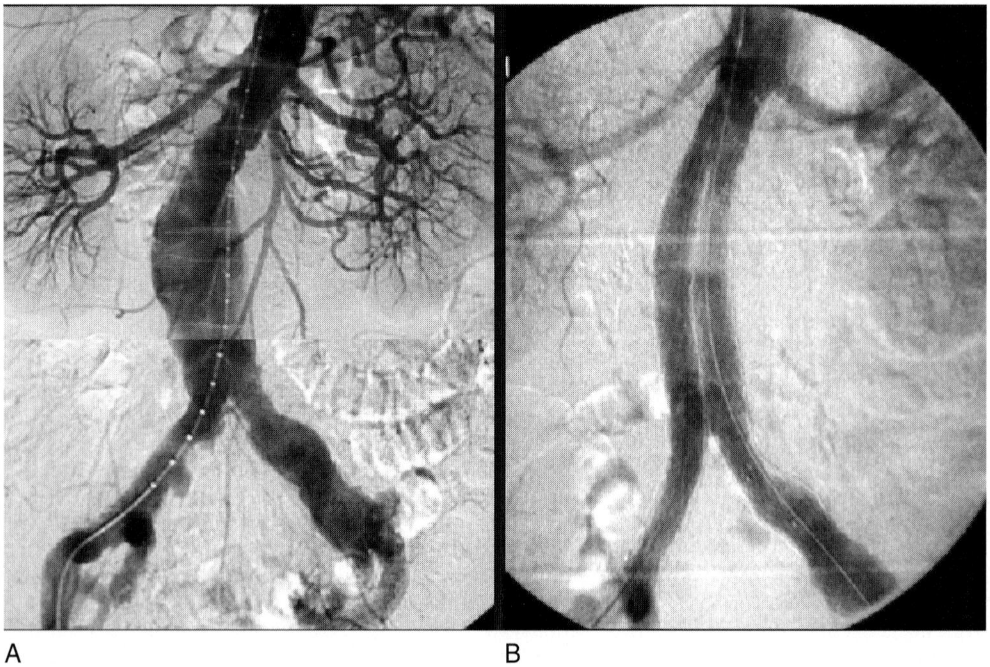

FIGURE 53–4 Angiographic views of an infrarenal abdominal aortic aneurysm with bi-iliac involvement treated by stent grafting before **(A)** and following **(B)** deployment of the aortic stent graft. (Courtesy of Dr. Edwin Graveraux, Brigham and Women's Hospital, Boston.)

with abdominal aortic aneurysms have aneurysm anatomy suitable for endovascular repair. Moreover, the long-term outcomes of endovascular repair versus conventional surgical repair are not yet known. One of the major technical difficulties associated with the stent-graft technique that has yet to be overcome is the frequent occurrence of *endoleaks,* which are seen angiographically as persistent contrast flow into the aneurysm sac because of failure to completely exclude the aneurysm from the aortic circulation. Such endoleaks, if left untreated, may leave the patient at continued risk for aneurysm expansion or rupture.[33] Therefore, at present, the use of stent-grafts for endovascular repair of abdominal aortic aneurysms has generally been limited to a subset of patients, typically older patients or those at high operative risk.

ASSESSING OPERATIVE RISK (see Chap. 77). Because patients with abdominal aortic aneurysms in almost all cases have atherosclerosis, their high likelihood of concomitant coronary, renal, and cerebrovascular arterial disease significantly increases the risk of major vascular surgery. Indeed, half of all perioperative deaths from aneurysm repair result from myocardial infarction. In addition, in one study, routine coronary arteriography in patients undergoing aneurysm repair revealed severe revascularizable coronary artery disease in 18 percent of all patients, including an 8 percent incidence in patients without prior symptoms of coronary ischemia.[34] Moreover, among those with angiographically significant coronary artery disease, about half have multivessel disease.

Several studies have demonstrated that cardiac scintigraphy is an effective means of identifying patients at highest risk for perioperative ischemic events (see Chaps. 9, 13, and 77). Patients with reversible perfusion defects in multiple segments of myocardium are at highest risk, and it is in this subgroup that coronary angiography is likely to be most helpful. The safety of nuclear imaging with pharmacological stress in such patients has been well established. Although exercise scintigraphy is also a useful screening method, many patients with vascular disease fail to achieve an adequate heart rate because of limited exercise capacity. Other useful techniques for preoperative evaluation of myocardial ischemia include dobutamine stress echocardiography and electrocardiographic exercise testing in patients with a normal baseline electrocardiogram and adequate exercise tolerance.

Selective preoperative evaluation to identify the presence and severity of coronary artery disease in patients with clinical markers of coronary artery disease has been widely advocated, and some investigators further suggest screening those with strong cardiac risk factors despite the absence of clinical evidence of coronary artery disease. Although patients found to have significant revascularizable coronary artery disease are presumed to benefit from preoperative coronary revascularization with selective coronary artery bypass surgery or angioplasty, at present this conclusion remains unproven. Data available from nonrandomized studies of patients with significant coronary artery disease undergoing vascular surgery do demonstrate lower mortality for those who have undergone coronary bypass surgery. Furthermore, a randomized study has demonstrated that the long-term outcome of patients with combined peripheral vascular disease and high-risk coronary artery disease is improved by coronary artery revascularization in patients with three-vessel coronary disease.[35] As is the case for coronary artery bypass surgery, no data are yet available to confirm that preoperative percutaneous coronary revascularization for significant coronary stenoses decreases the risk from major vascular surgery.

In addition to such preoperative screening and potential coronary revascularization, the use of perioperative invasive hemodynamic monitoring and careful perioperative surveillance for evidence of ischemia may further reduce operative risk secondary to cardiac ischemic events. Furthermore, myocardial ischemia and perhaps myocardial infarction may be prevented by using beta-adrenergic blockers perioperatively (see Chap. 77).

Late Survival. A review of late survival following abdominal aortic aneurysm repair among almost 2500 patients revealed 1-, 5-, and 10-year survival rates of 93, 63, and 40 percent, respectively.[18]

MEDICAL MANAGEMENT. Risk factor modification is fundamental in the medical management of abdominal aortic aneurysms. Hypercholesterolemia and hypertension should be carefully controlled. Most patients with abdominal aortic aneurysms are cigarette smokers, and given the increased risk of aneurysm rupture among active smokers, the habit must be discontinued. Beta blockers have long been considered an important therapy for reducing the risk of aneurysm expansion and rupture, and both animal and human studies support such a role. Brophy and coworkers demonstrated that propranolol delays the development of aneurysms in a mouse model prone to spontaneous aortic aneurysms.[36] Interestingly, it appears that the drug's efficacy in this model may have been independent of reductions in blood pressure or diminution of the rate of left ventricular ejection (dP/dt) and, instead, may have resulted from changes in connective tissue metabolism and the structure of the aortic wall. In humans, the data are mixed. Several trials have shown that treatment with propranolol has no significant impact on the rate of growth of smaller aneurysms (less than 4 cm in diameter), but decreases the rate of growth of larger aneurysms (4.0 to 5.0 cm in diameter, or larger) by 50 percent or more.[37] Therefore beta blockers should be recommended for patients with larger aneurysms managed medically.

When following an abdominal aortic aneurysm 4.0 cm in size or larger, careful routine follow-up is indicated to detect either rapid expansion (≥0.5 cm/yr) or an increase in size to 5.5 cm or larger, either of which is an indication for surgery. CT scanning every 6 months, perhaps as frequently as every 3 months for those at higher risk, has been advocated as an effective method of follow-up in such patients. CT scanning is preferable to ultrasonography for monitoring aneurysm growth because CT measurements of aneurysm size are more accurate.

Thoracic Aortic Aneurysms

Thoracic aortic aneurysms are much less common than aneurysms of the abdominal aorta. Thoracic aneurysms are classified by the portion of aorta involved, i.e., the ascending, arch, or descending thoracic aorta. This anatomical distinction is important because the etiology, natural history, and treatment of thoracic aneurysms differ for each of these segments. In modern series aneurysms of the ascending aorta occur most commonly (60 percent), followed by aneurysms of the descending aorta (40 percent), whereas arch aneurysms (10 percent) and thoracoabdominal aneurysms (10 percent) occur less often. *Thoracoabdominal aortic aneurysm* refers to descending thoracic aneurysms that extend distally to involve the abdominal aorta. Sometimes, the entire aorta may be ectatic, with localized aneurysms seen at sites in both the thoracic and abdominal aorta.

ETIOLOGY AND PATHOGENESIS. Aneurysms of the ascending thoracic aorta most often result from cystic medial degeneration (or cystic medial necrosis). Histologically, cystic medial degeneration has the appearance of smooth muscle cell drop-out and elastic fiber degeneration, with the presence in the media of cystic spaces filled with mucoid material. Although these changes occur most frequently in the ascending aorta, some cases may involve the entire aorta.

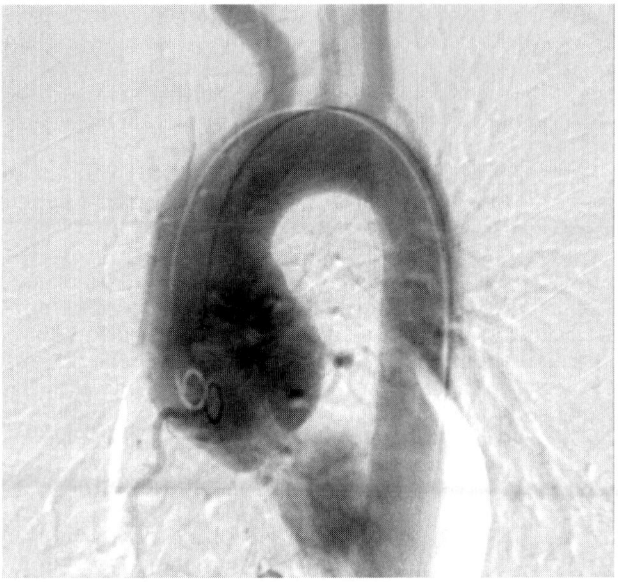

FIGURE 53–5 Left anterior oblique digital-subtraction aortogram in a man with annuloaortic ectasia and aneurysmal dilatation of the ascending thoracic aorta. The bulbous, pear-shaped aortic root can easily be seen. The aorta tapers to a normal diameter before the aortic arch, which is normal in size. Also of note, some contrast material is seen within the left ventricle, signifying the presence of aortic regurgitation.

The histological changes lead to weakening of the aortic wall, which in turn results in the formation of a fusiform aneurysm. Such aneurysms often involve the aortic root and may consequently result in aortic regurgitation: The term *annuloaortic ectasia* (Fig. 53–5) is often used to describe this condition (see later).

Cystic medial necrosis occurs to some extent with aging and is accelerated by hypertension.[38] At younger ages, cystic medial degeneration is classically associated with Marfan syndrome and can be associated with other connective tissue disorders as well, such as the Ehlers-Danlos syndrome. The Marfan syndrome (see Chap. 70) is an autosomal dominant heritable disorder of connective tissue that has been discovered to be due to mutations in one of the genes for fibrillin-1, a structural protein that is the major component of microfibrils of elastin. These mutations result in a decrease in the amount of elastin in the aortic wall, together with a loss of elastin's normally highly organized structure. As a consequence, from an early age a marfanoid aorta exhibits markedly abnormal elastic properties and increased systemic pulse wave velocities, and over time the aorta exhibits progressively increasing degrees of stiffness and dilatation.

But cystic medial degeneration is also seen in patients with ascending thoracic aortic aneurysms who do not have overt connective tissue disorders. It has long been suspected that some patients who have annuloaortic ectasia and proven cystic medial degeneration without the classic phenotypic manifestations of the Marfan syndrome may, in fact, have a variation, or *forme fruste,* of the Marfan syndrome. Indeed, increasing evidence suggests that many of these patients also have a genetic mutation that may account for cystic medial degeneration. Moreover, it is now recognized that although cases of thoracic aortic aneurysms in the absence of overt connective tissue disorders may be sporadic, they are often familial in nature and are now referred to as the *familial thoracic aortic aneurysm syndrome.*

In an analysis using the large database of patients treated at Yale, Coady and colleagues identified those with a familial pattern of thoracic aortic aneurysms and compared them with both sporadic cases and those with the Marfan syndrome. At least 19 percent of patients had a family history of a thoracic aortic aneurysm. The mean age of presentation for patients with familial syndromes was 57 years, which was significantly younger than sporadic cases (64 years) but older than the Marfan syndrome cases (25 years). Most pedigrees suggested an autosomal dominant mode of inheritance, but some suggested a recessive mode and possibly X-linked inheritance as well.[39] Biddinger and colleagues investigated the families of 158 patients referred for surgical repair or thoracic aortic aneurysms or dissections and found that first-degree relatives of probands had a higher risk (risk ratio [RR] 1.8 for fathers and sisters, RR 10.9 for brothers) of thoracic aortic aneurysms or sudden death compared with control subjects.[40]

Milewicz and colleagues have identified a mutation on 3p24.2-25 that can cause both isolated and familial thoracic aortic aneurysms. Although there appears to be dominant inheritance, there is marked variability in the expression and penetrance of the disorder, such that some inherit and pass on the gene but show no manifestation. Pathological evaluation of the aorta and these families reveals cystic medial degeneration.[41] Recently, two studies of familial thoracic aortic aneurysm syndromes have successfully mapped the mutations to at least two different chromosomal loci, but some families mapped to neither of these, suggesting at least a third locus.[38,42] As more families are studied, the extent of genetic heterogeneity is likely to become more evident. Indeed, the fact that there is such variable expression and penetrance suggests that this may be a polygenic condition.

Some cases of ascending thoracic aortic aneurysms are associated with an underlying bicuspid aortic valve (see Chap. 57). In fact, the risks of aortic dilatation, aneurysm, and dissection are significantly increased among those with a bicuspid aortic valve. Historical teaching attributed such aneurysms to "poststenotic dilatation" of the ascending aorta, but the data suggest otherwise. Nistri and colleagues found that 52 percent of young people with normally functioning bicuspid aortic valves have echocardiographic evidence of aortic dilatation. Dilatation occurred most frequently at the level of the tubular portion of the ascending aorta (44 percent), but the 20 percent had dilatation at the level of sinuses.[43] In a community sample, Nkomo and colleagues demonstrated that bicuspid aortic valve is associated with a dilated aorta regardless of the presence or absence of hemodynamically significant valve dysfunction.[44]

Cystic medial degeneration appears to be the underlying cause of the aortic aneurysms associated with bicuspid aortic valve. Indeed, 75 percent of patients with bicuspid aortic valve undergoing aortic valve replacement surgery have biopsy-proven significant cystic medial necrosis of the ascending aorta, compared with only 14 percent of patients with tricuspid aortic valves undergoing similar surgery.[45] Inadequate production of fibrillin-1 during embryogenesis may result in both the bicuspid aortic valve and a weakened aortic wall.[46] In addition, among those with bicuspid aortic valve, deficient microfibrillar elements within the aortic wall may cause smooth muscle cell detachment, matrix metalloproteinase release, matrix disruption, and cell death.[47] No single gene responsible for bicuspid aortic valve has yet been identified, and it is likely genetically heterogeneous. Moreover, in the study by Nistri and colleagues, 48 percent of patients with bicuspid valves had aortic dimensions equal to those of control subjects, so it appears that not all are at increased risk.[43]

ATHEROSCLEROSIS. Atherosclerotic aneurysms infrequently occur in the ascending aorta and, when they do, tend to be associated with diffuse aortic atherosclerosis. Aneurysms in the aortic arch are often contiguous with aneurysms of the ascending or descending aorta. They may be due to atherosclerotic disease, cystic medial degeneration, and syphilis or other infections. The predominant cause of aneurysms of the descending thoracic aorta is atherosclerosis. These aneurysms tend to originate just distal to the origin of the left subclavian artery and may be either fusiform or saccular. The pathogenesis of such atherosclerotic aneurysms in the thoracic aorta may resemble that of abdominal aneurysms but has not been extensively examined.

SYPHILIS. Syphilis was once a common cause of ascending thoracic aortic aneurysm, but today it has become a rarity in most major medical centers as a result of aggressive antibiotic treatment of the disease in its early stages. The latent period from initial spirochetal infection to aortic complications may range from 5 to 40 years but is most commonly 10 to 25 years. During the secondary phase of the disease, spirochetes directly infect the aortic media, most commonly involving the ascending aorta. The infection and attendant inflammatory response destroys the muscular and elastic medial elements, which undergo replacement by fibrous tissue that frequently calcifies. Weakening of the aortic wall from medial destruction results in progressive aneurysmal dilatation. In addition, the infection may spread into the aortic root, and the subsequent root dilation may result in aortic regurgitation.

INFECTIOUS AORTITIS. Infectious aortitis is a rare cause of aortic aneurysm that can result from a primary infection of the aortic wall causing aortic dilation with the formation of fusiform or saccular aneurysms. More commonly, infected, or mycotic, aneurysms arise secondarily from an infection occurring in a preexisting aneurysm of another cause. When an infected aneurysm involves the ascending aorta, it is often the consequence of direct spread from aortic valve bacterial endocarditis.

Several other causes of thoracic aortic aneurysms are discussed in detail elsewhere in this or other chapters, including giant cell arteritis (see Chap. 82), aortic trauma (see Chap. 65), and aortic dissection (see below). Note that the clinical features, natural history, and treatment of thoracic aneurysms discussed here apply specifically to nondissecting thoracic aortic aneurysms.

CLINICAL MANIFESTATIONS. At least half the patients with thoracic aortic aneurysms are asymptomatic at the time of diagnosis, with such aneurysms typically discovered as incidental findings on a routine physical examination, chest radiograph, or CT scan. When patients do experience symptoms, the symptoms tend to reflect either a vascular consequence of the aneurysm or a local mass effect. Vascular consequences include aortic regurgitation from dilatation of the aortic root, often associated with secondary congestive heart failure, or thromboembolism causing stroke, lower extremity ischemia, renal infarction, or mesenteric ischemia. A local mass effect from an ascending or arch aneurysm may cause superior vena cava syndrome as a result of obstruction of venous return via compression of the superior vena cava or innominate vein. Aneurysms of the arch or descending aorta may compress the trachea (Fig. 53–6) or main stem bronchus and produce tracheal deviation, wheezing, cough, dyspnea (with symptoms that may be positional), hemoptysis, or recurrent pneumonitis. Compression of the esophagus can produce dysphagia, and compression of the recurrent laryngeal nerve can cause hoarseness. Chest pain or back pain occur in one-quarter of cases of nondissecting aneurysms and result from direct compression of other intrathoracic structures or the chest wall, or from erosion into adjacent bone. Typically, such pain is steady, deep, boring, and at times severe.

As with abdominal aortic aneurysms, the most worrisome consequence of thoracic aneurysms is leakage or rupture. Rupture is accompanied by the dramatic onset of excruciating pain, often in the region where less severe pain had previously existed. Rupture occurs most commonly into the left intrapleural space or the mediastinum and is manifested as hypotension. Less often, an aneurysm of the descending thoracic aorta ruptures into the adjacent esophagus (an aortoesophageal fistula), which causes life-threatening hematemesis. Acute aneurysm expansion, which may herald rupture, can cause similar pain. Thoracic aneurysms can also be accompanied by aortic dissection, as discussed in detail later in this chapter.

DIAGNOSIS AND SIZING. Many thoracic aneurysms are readily visible on chest radiographs (Fig. 53–7) and are characterized by widening of the mediastinal silhouette, enlargement of the aortic knob, or displacement of the trachea from the midline. Unfortunately, smaller aneurysms, especially saccular ones, may not be evident on the chest radiograph; therefore, this technique cannot exclude the diagnosis of aortic aneurysm.

Aortography had long been the preferred modality for the preoperative evaluation of thoracic aortic aneurysms and for precise definition of the anatomy of the aneurysm and great vessels (see Fig. 53–5). However, as is the case for abdominal aortic aneurysms, CT and MRA are now often sufficient in most cases to define both aortic and branch vessel anatomy. Both contrast-enhanced CT scanning (Fig. 53–8) and MRI very accurately detect and size thoracic aortic aneurysms. When aneurysms involve the aortic root, MRA is preferable to CT scanning, as CT images the root less well and is less accurate in sizing its diameter. When patients have a tortuous thoracic aorta, which is often the case among the elderly, one should use caution in using axial images to measure the aortic diameter. The axial images often cut through the descending aorta off-axis, resulting in a falsely large aortic diameter. When the axial data are reconstructed into three-dimensional images (i.e., CT angiography), one can measure the tortuous aorta in true cross section and obtain an accurate diameter. Such three-dimensional imaging should then always be used to follow such patients over time.

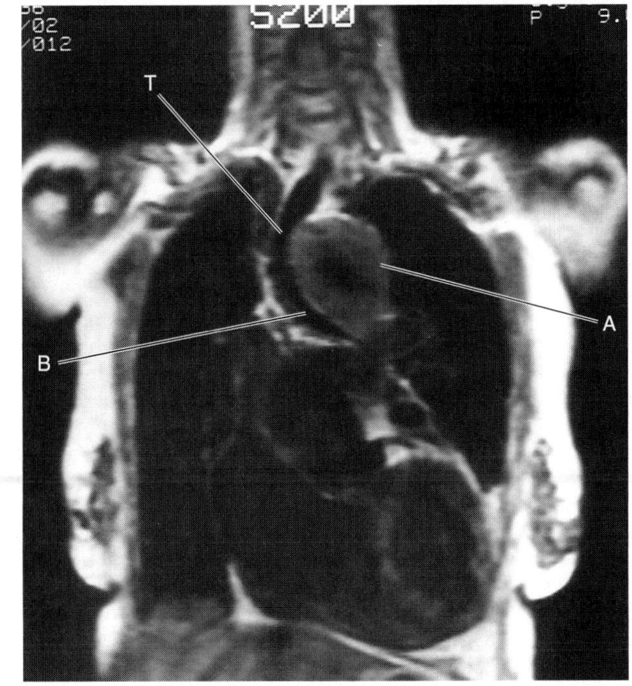

FIGURE 53–6 Magnetic resonance imaging scan in the coronal projection of a large thoracic aortic aneurysm in an elderly woman with dyspnea and cough. In this view, the markedly dilated aortic arch (A) is compressing the trachea (T) and causing rightward tracheal deviation. The aneurysm is also compressing the left main stem bronchus (B). In addition, all four cardiac chambers are dilated, consistent with the patient's known idiopathic dilated cardiomyopathy

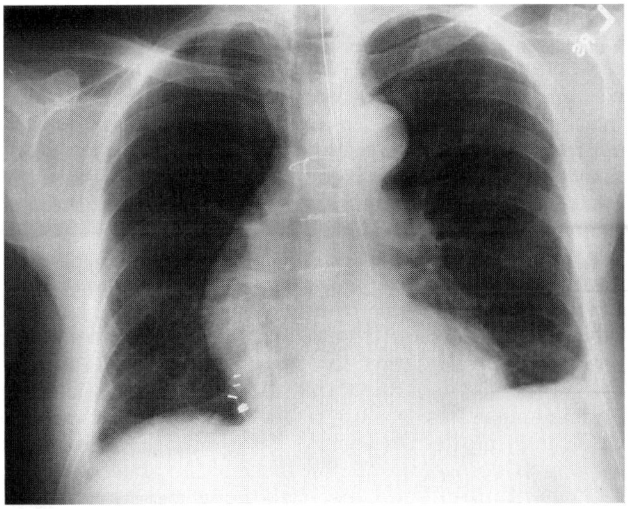

FIGURE 53–7 Chest radiograph of a patient with a very large aneurysm of the ascending thoracic aorta. Evident are both marked widening of the mediastinum and an abnormal aortic contour.

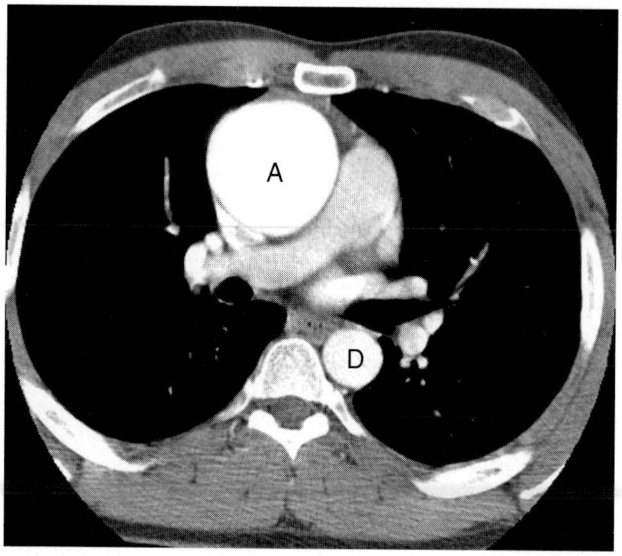

FIGURE 53–8 Contrast-enhanced computed tomography scan of the chest at the level of the right pulmonary artery demonstrating a 6.5-cm ascending thoracic aortic aneurysm (A).The descending aorta (D) is normal in caliber.

TTE is an excellent modality for imaging the aortic root, which is important for patients with the Marfan syndrome, but it is not able to visualize the middle or distal ascending aorta well in many cases and is particularly limited in its ability to examine the descending thoracic aorta. Therefore, among patients other than those with the Marfan syndrome, TTE should not be used for diagnosing thoracic aneurysms. TEE, on the other hand, can visualize the entire thoracic aorta quite well and therefore has become widely used for detection of aortic dissection. However, given that TEE is a semi-invasive procedure, CT and MR are usually preferred imaging techniques in the evaluation of nondissecting thoracic aneurysms. (The advantages and disadvantage of each imaging modality are discussed later in greater detail.)

NATURAL HISTORY. Defining the natural history of thoracic aortic aneurysms has been challenging for a number of reasons. Both the origin and the location of a thoracic aneurysm can affect its rate of growth and propensity for dissection or rupture. The presence or absence of aneurysm symptoms is another important predictor inasmuch as symptomatic patients have a much poorer prognosis than do those without symptoms, in large part because the onset of new symptoms is frequently a harbinger of rupture or death. Finally, during the recent decades in which it has been routine to image aneurysms serially to document growth and size, surgery has typically been performed when aneurysms have been large enough to be considered at high risk for rupture. Those patients whose large aneurysms have been managed without surgery are often elderly or have important comorbidities, thus increasing their mortality irrespective of the aneurysm.

Perhaps the best data currently available on the natural history of thoracic aortic aneurysms come from a longitudinal study recent reported by Davies and colleagues from the Yale group in which 304 patients with thoracic aortic aneurysms at least 3.5 cm in size were followed for a mean of more than 31 months.[48] The mean rate of growth for all thoracic aneurysms was 0.1 cm/yr. The rate of growth was significantly greater for aneurysms of the descending aorta (0.19 cm/yr), however, than for those of the ascending aorta (0.07 cm/yr). In addition, dissected thoracic aneurysms grew significantly more rapidly (0.14 cm/yr) than did nondissected ones (0.09 cm/yr), and patients with Marfan syndrome also had higher growth rates. The mean rate of rupture or dissection was only 2 percent per year for aneurysms less than 5 cm in diameter, rose slightly to 3 percent per year for aneurysms 5.0 to 5.9 cm, but increased sharply to 7 percent per year for aneurysms 6.0 cm or larger. In a multivariate logistic regression analysis of the predictors of dissection or rupture, the relative risk associated with an aneurysm diameter of 5.0 to 5.9 cm was 2.5; with an aneurysm diameter of 6.0 cm or larger, 5.2; with Marfan syndrome, 3.7; and with female gender, 2.9. In addition, concomitant vascular disease or abdominal aortic aneurysm were univariate predictors of both dissection/rupture and mortality. Other natural history studies focused on thoracic and thoracoabdominal aneurysms have found that the odds of rupture are increased by chronic obstructive pulmonary disease (COPD) (RR, 3.6), advanced age (RR, 2.6/decade), and aneurysm-related pain (RR, 2.3).[49]

As with abdominal aneurysms, initial size is an important predictor of the rate of thoracic aneurysm growth. Dapunt and colleagues[50] monitored 67 patients with thoracic aortic aneurysms by serial CT scanning and found that the only independent predictor of rapid expansion (>0.5 cm/yr) was an initial aortic diameter larger than 5.0 cm. Aneurysms that were 5.0 cm or smaller grew more slowly than did those larger than 5.0 cm. Unfortunately, even when controlling for initial aneurysm size, substantial variation was still seen in individual aneurysm growth rates, thus rendering such mean growth rates of little value in predicting aneurysm growth for a given patient. More helpful, however, was the finding that growth rates among small aneurysms were more consistent, with only 1 of 25 aneurysms 4.0 cm or smaller at baseline showing rapid growth.

Rupture or acute dissection are the major complications of thoracic aortic aneurysms and can be fatal. Fewer than half of patients with rupture may arrive at the hospital alive; mortality at 6 hours is 54 percent and at 24 hours reaches 76 percent.[51]

Management

SURGICAL TREATMENT. The optimal timing of surgical repair of thoracic aortic aneurysms remains uncertain for several reasons. First, as noted earlier, the data available on the natural history of thoracic aneurysms are limited, especially with respect to the outcomes of surgical intervention. Second, with the high incidence of coexisting cardiovascular disease in this population, many patients die of other cardiovascular diseases before their aneurysms ever rupture. Finally, significant risks are associated with thoracic aortic surgery, particularly in the arch and descending aorta, which in many cases may outweigh the potential benefits of aortic repair.

We currently recommend surgery when aneurysms of the ascending thoracic aorta reach 5.5 cm or larger and those of the descending thoracic aorta reach 6.0 cm or larger, or perhaps 6.0 and 7.0 cm or larger, respectively, in patients at high operative risk. Indications for surgery in patients with smaller aneurysms include a rapid rate of expansion, associated significant aortic regurgitation, or the presence of aneurysm-related symptoms. In patients with the Marfan syndrome, bicuspid aortic valve, or a familial thoracic aortic aneurysm syndrome, given their higher risk of dissection and rupture, we often recommend repair of ascending thoracic aneurysms when they reach only 5.0 cm in size. Surgery can be considered even sooner (e.g., 4.5 cm) in Marfan syndrome patients at especially high risk, such as those with rapid and progressive aortic dilatation, those with a family history of the Marfan syndrome plus aortic dissection, or women planning pregnancy.[52] Finally, if patients require aortic valve replacement for a dysfunctional bicuspid valve, we recommend replacement of the ascending aorta if its diameter is 4 cm or larger, given that they are now recognized to be at high risk for postoperative aortic dissection.[53,54] Of course, the aggressiveness with which surgical repair is undertaken in any case should be appropriately influenced by the general condition of the individual patient.

Thoracic aortic aneurysms are generally resected and replaced with a prosthetic sleeve of appropriate size. Cardiopulmonary bypass is necessary for the removal of ascending aortic aneurysms, and partial bypass to support the circulation distal to the aneurysm while the aortic site being repaired is cross-clamped is often advisable when resecting descending thoracic aortic aneurysms. The use of such adjuncts is less important, however, than the nature and extent of the aneurysm in determining the incidence of postoperative complications.

The use of a composite graft consisting of a Dacron tube with a prosthetic aortic valve sewn into one end (known as a *composite aortic repair* or the *Bentall procedure*) is generally the method of choice in treating ascending thoracic aneurysms involving the root and associated with significant aortic regurgitation. The valve and graft are sewn directly into the aortic annulus, and the coronary arteries are then reimplanted into the Dacron aortic graft (Fig. 53–9). The operative risk for mortality is about 5 percent.[55] For patients with structurally normal aortic valve leaflets whose aortic regurgitation is secondary to dilatation of the root, David and colleagues have successfully repaired the native valve either by reimplanting it within a Dacron graft or by remodeling of the aortic root. By avoiding valve replacement, it is expected that this procedure, when successful, will eliminate the long-term risks associated with a prosthetic valve and reduce the risk for repeat valve surgery. In a series of 151 patients with aortic root aneurysms who underwent valve-sparing surgery, 67 percent had mild or no aortic regurgitation during the first 8 years of follow-up, with only 2 percent developing severe aortic regurgitation.[56]

Aneurysms of the aortic arch can be successfully excised surgically, but the procedure remains particularly challenging. Neurological damage is a major cause of morbidity and mortality from aortic arch repair and typically results from embolization of atherosclerotic debris or as a consequence of global ischemic injury during antegrade circulatory arrest. The brachiocephalic vessels must be removed from the aortic arch before its resection and then reimplanted into the prosthetic tube graft arch after its interposition. Traditionally, the surgical procedure involves removing and then reimplanting the brachiocephalic vessels en bloc (i.e., as an island of native aortic tissue containing the three branch-vessels), after which normal cerebral perfusion is restored. Recently, however, several novel surgical techniques have been introduced to reduce the hypothermic circulatory arrest times and embolic events by placing a multilimbed prosthetic arch graft, to which each arch vessel is in turn anastomosed individually (Fig. 53–10).

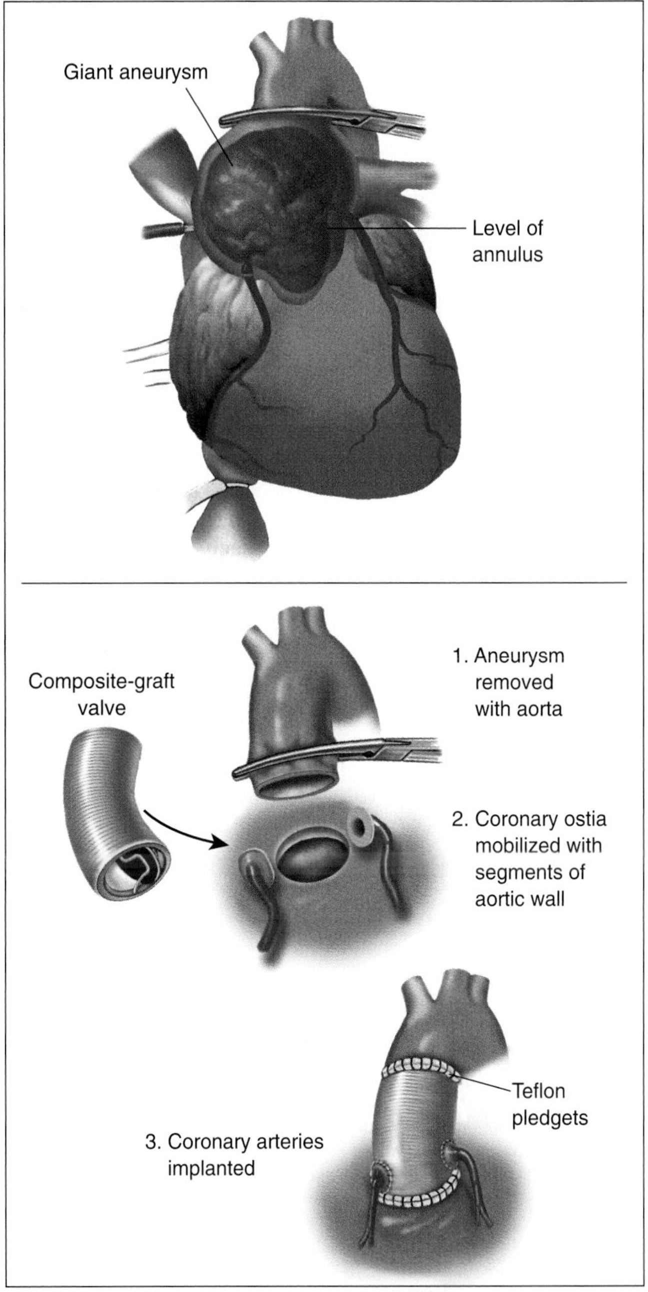

FIGURE 53–9 Technique for the composite graft replacement of an aneurysm of the ascending aorta. **Top,** The aneurysm is shown involving the sinuses of Valsalva. The patient is maintained on total cardiopulmonary bypass. **Bottom,** The composite graft is shown, with a low-profile, tilting disc aortic prosthesis attached to its inferior end. (1) The aneurysm is resected with the native aortic valve. (2) The coronary ostia have been excised and mobilized with a button of aortic wall. (3) The composite graft has been secured in place with Teflon felt reinforcement for the suture line. The coronary artery ostia are then reimplanted directly into the graft.

Three methods of cerebral protection have been used for aortic arch surgery. The traditional method has been the use of profound hypothermic circulatory arrest with arrest of cerebral perfusion. The hypothermia is intended to reduce the cerebral metabolic rate by cooling to 10°C to 13°C. The simplicity of the technique, however, is offset by the high incidence of stroke and temporary neurological dysfunction. In 1990, the use of retrograde cerebral perfusion via a superior vena cava cannula was introduced as an adjunct for cerebral protection during hypothermic arrest. It was originally suggested that this technique would improve outcomes by providing nutrients and oxygen to the brain and to flush out both air and particulate matter from the cerebral and carotid arteries that would otherwise embolize. More extensive studies have shown that there is, in fact, no metabolic benefit to the brain from retrograde cerebral perfusion and several studies have shown no improvement in outcomes.[57,58] More recently, the technique of selective antegrade cerebral perfusion has been introduced, in which perfusion cannulae inserted directly into the cerebral vessels allows perfusion of the brain through all but brief periods during the procedure. Indeed, the use of the multilimbed prosthetic aortic graft makes selective antegrade cerebral perfusion easier and more effective. This technique allows for a longer time of safe circulatory arrest, which is of greater importance in more complex arch procedures. The available data suggest that selective antegrade cerebral perfusion does not reduce the risk of stroke but does significantly reduce the incidence of temporary neurological dysfunction.[58] Historically, for aortic arch repair, the rates of mortality and stroke were as high as 6 to 20 percent and 4 to 11 percent, respectively, but with the use of these modern techniques in experienced hands, the rates are as low as 4 percent and 2 percent, respectively.[59]

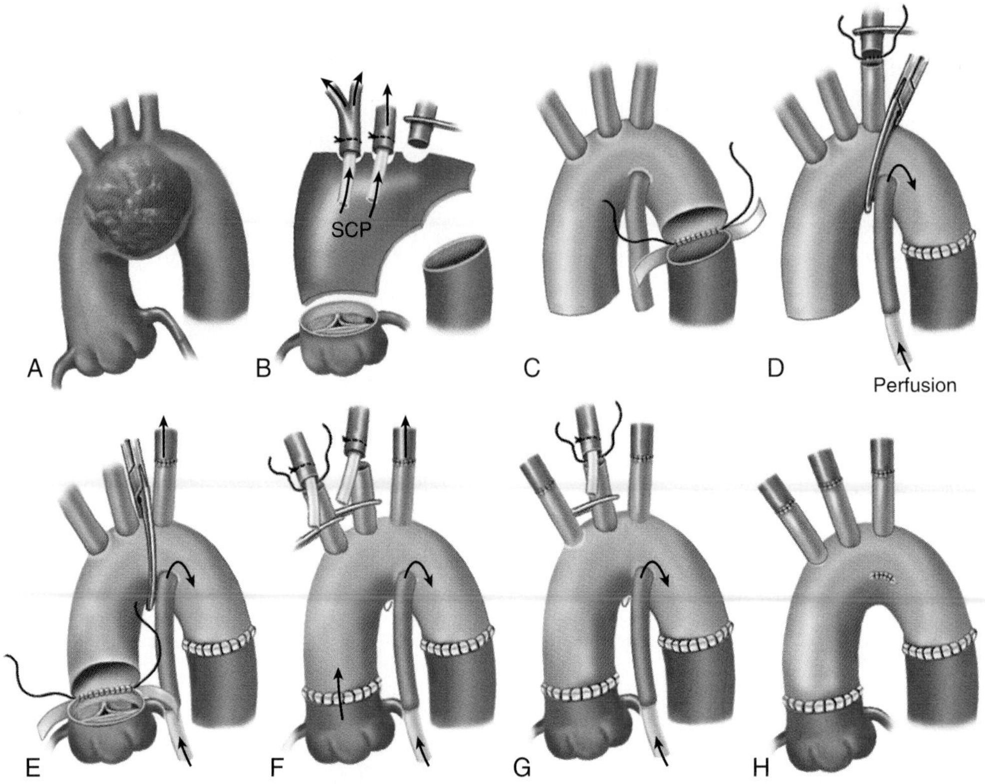

FIGURE 53–10 **A-H,** Surgical technique for total arch replacement with a branched aortic graft. Following initiation of circulatory arrest, the aneurysm is transected in the ascending aorta and where it meets the proximal descending aorta. The branched graft is anastomosed at its distal end. The graft proximal to the fourth limb is clamped and perfusion is restored through this limb to the distal circulation. The third limb is anastomosed to the left subclavian artery and flow to this vessel is restored. Then, the proximal end of the graft is anastomosed to the stump of the ascending aorta, flow is restored to the remaining arch vessels, and the fourth branch is then resected. (Adapted from Kazui T, Washiyama N, Muhammad BAH, et al: Improved results of atherosclerotic arch aneurysm operations with a refined technique. J Thorac Cardiovasc Surg 121:491, 2001.)

Many of the patients undergoing surgical repair of a thoracic aortic aneurysm have multiple aortic segments involved. Such widespread aneurysmal dilatation of the aorta presents a particular challenge to the surgeon and often precludes surgery. Although it is possible to successfully replace virtually the entire diseased thoracic aorta, attempts to replace the ascending, arch, and descending thoracic aorta in one surgery carry increased risks. An alternative strategy is the use of a staged procedure, known as the "elephant trunk" technique, in which the ascending aorta and arch are replaced initially, whereas the descending aorta is replaced at a later date. Use of the elephant trunk technique has been shown to facilitate such extensive surgical procedures and reduce the associated risks.[60]

Elective surgical repair of ascending and descending thoracic aortic aneurysms in large centers is associated with mortality rates of 3 to 10 percent and 5 to 14 percent, respectively. Major complications include stroke and hemorrhage. A catastrophic complication of resection of descending thoracic aortic aneurysms is postoperative paraplegia secondary to interruption of the blood supply to the spinal cord. The incidence of paraplegia has been as high as 13 to 17 percent, but in most modern series is 5 to 6 percent. A number of methods have been proposed to reduce the likelihood of paraplegia, although none has proved to be consistently safe and effective. One of the more promising techniques involves regional hypothermic protection of the spinal cord with epidural cooling during surgical repair of the aorta, which has reduced the frequency of spinal cord complications to 3 percent (compared with a historical control of 20 percent) in one large series by Cambria and colleagues.[61] The use of cerebrospinal fluid drainage was similarly shown to reduce the rate of paraplegia to 3 percent in a recent randomized trial by Coselli and colleagues.[62] Other important techniques that may also reduce the risk of spinal cord injury include the reimplantation of patent critical intercostal arteries, the use of intraoperative somatosensory-evoked potential monitoring, and maintenance of distal aortic perfusion during surgery with the use of atriofemoral (left heart) bypass to the distal aorta during the proximal anastomosis.[63] Controlled trials might better clarify the efficacy of such techniques.

An alternative approach to the surgical management of descending thoracic aneurysms is the use of a transluminally placed endovascular stent-graft (see Chap. 55). This technique has the advantage of being far less invasive than surgery with potentially fewer postoperative complications and a lower morbidity rate. Dake and coworkers reported the results of a large series in which "first-generation" endovascular stentgrafts were implanted in 103 patients with thoracic aortic aneurysms, only 62 (60 percent) of whom were judged to be reasonable candidates for traditional surgical aortic repair.[64] Complete thrombosis of the aortic aneurysm was achieved in 83 percent of patients, but rates of early stroke and paraplegia were 3 and 7 percent, respectively. The authors suggest that with newer and more refined devices together with more precise stent-graft deployment, the overall success rates should rise and complication rates fall. Although still experimental at present, such a device may in the future have an important role in the management of patients who are at risk for aortic rupture but are otherwise poor surgical candidates. Unfortunately, the curvilinear nature of the ascending aorta and arch makes application of similar techniques to aneurysms of these proximal aortic segments far more challenging.

Complications of associated atherosclerosis, such as myocardial infarction, cerebrovascular accidents, and renal failure, often arise under the massive physiological stress of aortic surgery. The most frequent causes of early postoperative death are myocardial infarction, congestive heart failure, stroke, renal failure, hemorrhage, respiratory failure, and sepsis. Advanced age, emergency surgery, prolonged aortic cross-clamp time, extent of the aneurysm, diabetes, prior aortic surgery, aneurysm symptoms, and intraoperative hypotension are the most important factors determining perioperative morbidity and mortality. Many patients with atherosclerotic aneurysms are heavy smokers, and pulmonary complications following surgery are common. The left lung may be severely traumatized by compression during resection of large aneurysms of the descending thoracic aorta, a complication that can seriously jeopardize the patient's survival, particularly in the setting of underlying pulmonary disease.

MEDICAL MANAGEMENT. The long-term impact of medical therapy on aneurysm growth and survival in patients with typical atherosclerotic thoracic aneurysms has not been examined. However, Shores and colleagues examined the efficacy of beta blockers in adult patients with the Marfan syndrome[65] (see Chap. 70). They randomized 70 patients to treatment with propranolol versus no beta blocker therapy and monitored them over a 10-year period. The treated group showed a significantly slower rate of aortic dilatation, fewer adverse clinical endpoints (death, aortic dissection, aortic regurgitation, aortic root larger than 6 cm), and significantly lower mortality from the 4-year point onward. Although this study examined only the effect of beta blockade in patients with the Marfan syndrome, it follows logically that medical therapy to reduce dP/dt and control blood pressure is essential to the treatment of thoracic aortic aneurysms, both for patients with smaller aneurysms being monitored serially and for patients who have undergone aortic aneurysm repair.

Aortic Dissection

Acute aortic dissection is an uncommon but potentially catastrophic illness that occurs with an incidence of approximately 2.9/100,000/yr with at least 7000 cases per year in the United States.[66] Early mortality is as high as 1 percent per hour if untreated,[66] but survival may be significantly improved by the timely institution of appropriate medical and/or surgical therapy. Prompt clinical recognition and definitive diagnostic testing are therefore essential in the management of patients with aortic dissection.

Aortic dissection is believed to begin with the formation of a tear in the aortic intima that directly exposes an underlying diseased medial layer to the driving force (or pulse pressure) of intraluminal blood (Fig. 53–11A). This blood penetrates the diseased medial layer and cleaves the media longitudinally, thereby dissecting the aortic wall. Driven by persistent intraluminal pressure, the dissection process extends a variable length along the aortic wall, typically antegrade (driven by the forward force of aortic blood flow) but sometimes retrograde from the site of the intimal tear. The blood-filled space between the dissected layers of the aortic wall becomes the false lumen. Shear forces may lead to further tears in the intimal flap (the inner portion of the dissected aortic wall) and produce exit sites or additional entry sites for blood flow into the false lumen. Distention of the false lumen with blood may cause the intimal flap to bow into the true lumen and thereby narrow its caliber and distort its shape.

Alternatively, aortic dissection may begin with rupture of the vasa vasorum within the aortic media; that is, with the development of an intramural hematoma (see Fig. 53–11B). Local hemorrhage then secondarily ruptures through the intimal layer and creates the intimal tear and aortic dissection. Since in autopsy series as many as 13 percent of aortic dissections do not have an identifiable intimal tear, at least in a minority of cases independent medial hemorrhage does appear to be the primary cause of dissection. On the other hand, one might argue that the lack of an intimal tear in these patients indicates they do not, in fact, have classic aortic dissection but rather have intramural hematoma of the aorta, a closely related condition (see later).

CLASSIFICATION. Most classification schemes for aortic dissection are based on the fact that the vast majority of aortic dissections originate in one of two locations: (1) the ascending aorta, within several centimeters of the aortic valve, and (2) the descending aorta, just distal to the origin of the left subclavian artery at the site of the ligamentum arteriosum. Sixty-five percent of intimal tears occur in the ascending aorta, 20 percent in the descending aorta, 10 percent in the aortic arch, and 5 percent in the abdominal aorta.

Three major classification systems are used to define the location and extent of aortic involvement, as defined in Table 53–1 and depicted in Figure 53–12: (1) DeBakey types I, II, and III; (2) Stanford types A and B; and (3) the anatomical categories "proximal" and "distal." All three schemes share the same basic principle of distinguishing aortic dissections with and without ascending aortic involvement for prognostic and therapeutic reasons; in general, surgery is indicated for dissections involving the ascending aorta, whereas medical management is reserved for dissections without ascending aortic involvement. Accordingly, because both DeBakey types I and II involve the ascending aorta, they are grouped together for simplicity in the Stanford (type A) and anatomical (proximal) classification systems, irrespective of the site of intimal tear. Less experienced clinicians will sometimes misclassify as type A dissections that begin in the aortic arch and progress distally, but since the ascending aorta is not involved, such cases should, in fact, be classified as type B. Aortic dissections confined to the abdominal aorta, although quite uncommon, are best categorized as type B or distal dissections. Proximal or type A dissections occur in about two-thirds of cases, with distal dissections comprising the remaining one-third.

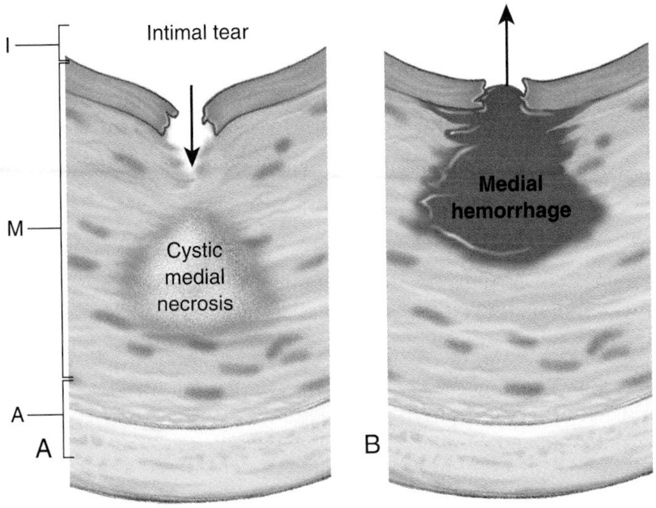

FIGURE 53–11 Proposed mechanisms of initiation of aortic dissection. A = adventitia; I = intima; M = media.

TABLE 53–1 Commonly Used Classification Systems to Describe Aortic Dissection

Type	Site of Origin and Extent of Aortic Involvement
DeBakey	
Type I	Originates in the ascending aorta, propagates at least to the aortic arch and often beyond it distally
Type II	Originates in and is confined to the ascending aorta
Type III	Originates in the descending aorta and extends distally down the aorta or, rarely, retrograde into the aortic arch and ascending aorta
Stanford	
Type A	All dissections involving the ascending aorta, regardless of the site of origin
Type B	All dissections not involving the ascending aorta
Descriptive	
Proximal	Includes DeBakey types I and II or Stanford type A
Distal	Includes DeBakey type III or Stanford type B

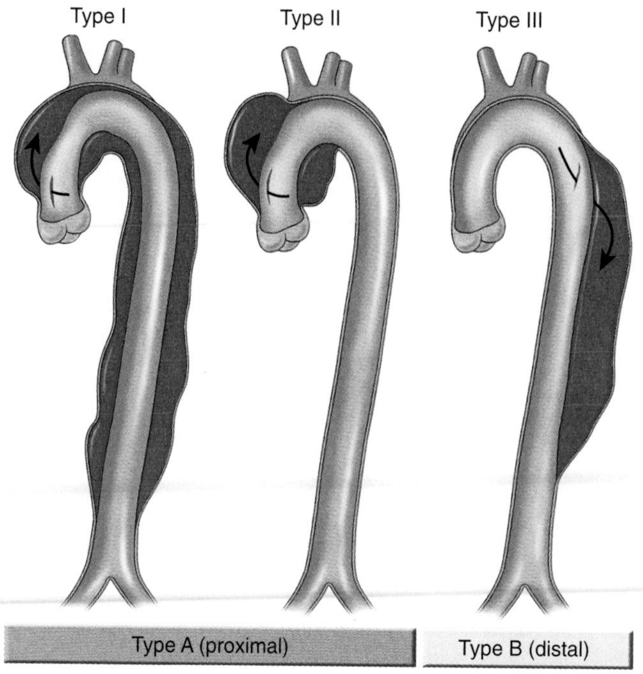

FIGURE 53–12 Commonly used classification systems for aortic dissection. (Refer to Table 53–1 for definitions.)

In addition to its location, aortic dissection is also classified according to its duration, defined as the length of time from symptom onset to medical evaluation. The mortality from dissection and its risk of progression decrease progressively over time, which makes therapeutic strategies for longstanding aortic dissections quite different from those seen acutely. A dissection present less than 2 weeks is defined as "acute," whereas those present 2 weeks or more are defined as "chronic" because the mortality curve for untreated aortic dissections begins to level off at 75 to 80 percent at this time. At diagnosis, the large majority of aortic dissections are acute.

ETIOLOGY AND PATHOGENESIS. Cystic medial degeneration, as described earlier, is the chief predisposing factor in aortic dissection. Therefore, any disease process or other condition that undermines the integrity of the elastic or muscular components of the media predisposes the aorta to dissection. Cystic medial degeneration is an intrinsic feature of several hereditary defects of connective tissue, most notably the Marfan and Ehlers-Danlos (see Chap. 70) syndromes, and is also common among patients with bicuspid aortic valve. In addition to their propensity for thoracic aortic aneurysms, patients with the Marfan syndrome are indeed at high risk for aortic dissection, especially proximal dissection, at a relatively young age. In fact, the Marfan syndrome accounts for 5 percent of all aortic dissections.[67]

In the absence of the Marfan syndrome, only a minority of cases of aortic dissection have histologically classic cystic medial degeneration. Nevertheless, the degree of medial degeneration found in most other cases of aortic dissection still tends to be qualitatively and quantitatively much greater than expected as part of the aging process. Although the cause of such medial degeneration remains unclear, advanced age and hypertension appear to be two of the most important factors.

The peak incidence of aortic dissection is in the sixth and seventh decades of life, with men affected twice as often as women. About three-quarters of patients with aortic dissection have a history of hypertension. [67] A bicuspid aortic valve is a well-established risk factor for proximal aortic dissection and occurs in 5 to 7 percent of aortic dissections. As is the case with ascending thoracic aortic aneurysms, the risk of aortic dissection appears to be independent of the severity of the bicuspid valve stenosis. Certain other congenital cardiovascular abnormalities predispose the aorta to dissection, including coarctation of the aorta. Rarely, aortic dissection complicates arteritis involving the aorta (see Chap. 82), particularly giant cell arteritis. A number of reports describe aortic dissection in association with cocaine abuse, typically among young, black, and hypertensive men. However, cocaine likely accounts for less than 1 percent of cases of aortic dissection and the mechanisms by which it causes dissection remain speculative.[68]

An unexplained relationship exists between pregnancy and aortic dissection (see Chap. 74). About half of all aortic dissections in women younger than 40 years occur during pregnancy, typically in the third trimester and also occasionally in the early postpartum period. The increases in blood volume, cardiac output, and blood pressure seen in late pregnancy may contribute to the risk, although this explanation cannot account for postpartum occurrence. Women with the Marfan syndrome and a dilated aortic root are at particular risk for acute aortic dissection during pregnancy,[69] and in some cases, diagnosis of the Marfan syndrome is first made when such women are evaluated for peripartum aortic dissection.

Direct trauma to the aorta may also cause aortic dissection. Blunt trauma tends to cause localized tears, hematomas, or frank aortic transection (see Chap. 65) and only rarely causes classic aortic dissection. Iatrogenic trauma, on the other hand, is associated with true aortic dissection and accounts for 5 percent of cases.[70] Both intraarterial catheterization and the insertion of intraaortic balloon pumps may induce aortic dissection, probably from direct trauma to the aortic intima. Cardiac surgery also entails a very small risk (0.12 to 0.16 percent) of acute aortic dissection. The majority of these dissections are discovered intraoperatively and repaired at that time, although 20 percent are detected only after a delay. In addition, aortic dissection sometimes occurs late (months to years) after cardiac surgery; in fact, as many as 18 percent of those with acute aortic dissection have a history of prior cardiac surgery. Of cardiac surgical patients, those undergoing aortic valve replacement have the highest risk for aortic dissection as a late complication. The association with aortic valve surgery may occur because many such patients had surgery to replace dysfunctional bicuspid aortic valves. As discussed earlier, cystic medial degeneration often accompanies this condition and can predispose them to subsequent dissection. Von Kodolitsch and colleagues have found that patients with a dilated ascending aorta together with aortic regurgitation or a thinned aortic wall at the time of aortic valve replacement are most likely to have such a late aortic dissection.[71] This association argues for an aggressive approach in replacing even a mildly dilated ascending aorta at the time of bicuspid aortic valve replacement, as discussed earlier.

Clinical Manifestations

SYMPTOMS. Much of the data presented regarding the clinical manifestations of aortic dissection are from the older clinical series of Slater and DeSanctis[72] and Spittel and colleagues,[73] as well as from a more recent series from the International Registry of Acute Aortic Dissection (IRAD), which studied 464 consecutive patients with acute aortic dissection from 12 international referral centers.[67] By far the most common initial symptom of acute aortic dissection is pain, which is found in up to 96 percent of cases, whereas the large majority of those without pain are found to have chronic dissections. The pain is typically severe and of sudden onset and is as severe at its inception as it ever becomes, in contrast to the pain of myocardial infarction, which usually has a crescendo-like onset and is not as intense. In fact, the pain of aortic dissection may be all but unbearable in some instances and force the patient to writhe in agony, fall to the ground, or pace restlessly in an attempt to gain relief. Several features of the pain should arouse suspicion of aortic dissection. The quality of the pain as described by the patient is often morbidly appropriate to the actual event, with adjectives such as "tearing," "ripping," "sharp," and "stabbing" frequently used in more than half the cases. In fact, it is not uncommon to hear descriptors that are collectively almost diagnostic of aortic dissection, but quite unlike the symptoms of myocardial ischemia or infarction, such as someone "stabbed me in the chest with a knife" or "hit me in the back with an ax."

Another important characteristic of the pain of aortic dissection is its tendency to migrate from its point of origin to other sites, generally following the path of the dissection as it extends through the aorta. However, such migratory pain is described in as few as 17 percent of cases. The location of pain may be quite helpful in suggesting the location of the aortic dissection because localized symptoms tend to reflect involvement of the underlying aorta. Spittell and colleagues found that when the location of chest pain was anterior only (or if the most severe pain was anterior), more than 90 percent of patients had involvement of the ascending aorta. Conversely, when the chest pain was interscapular only (or when the most severe pain was interscapular), more than 90 percent of patients had involvement of the descending thoracic aorta (i.e., DeBakey type I or III). The presence of any pain in the neck, throat, jaw, or face strongly predicted involvement of the ascending aorta, whereas pain anywhere in the back, abdomen, or lower extremities strongly predicted involvement of the descending aorta.[73] In rare cases, the presenting pain is only pleuritic in nature, owing to acute pericarditis that results from hemorrhage into the pericardial space from the dissected ascending aorta. In such cases, the underlying diagnosis may be overlooked if one does not search for other symptoms or signs that might suggest the presence of aortic dissection.

Less common symptoms at initial evaluation, occurring with or without associated chest pain, include congestive heart failure (7 percent), syncope (13 percent), cerebrovascular accident (6 percent), ischemic peripheral neuropathy, paraplegia, and cardiac arrest or sudden death. The presence of acute congestive heart failure in this setting is almost invariably due to severe aortic regurgitation induced by a proximal aortic dissection (discussed later). Patients with syncope have been found to have a higher rate of mortality than those without syncope and are more likely to have cardiac tamponade or stroke. However, when the complications of cardiac tamponade and stroke are excluded, syncope alone does not increase mortality.[74] On occasion, a patient presents with acute chest pain, and the initial imaging study reveals hemopericardium yet fails to demonstrate an aortic dissection. In such a scenario, unless another diagnosis, such as tumor metastatic to the pericardium, is evident, one must still suspect the presence of acute aortic dissection (or contained aortic rupture). Ideally, such a patient would be taken presumptively to the operating room or, at the very least, immediately undergo additional imaging with other modalities to confirm the diagnosis.[75]

PHYSICAL FINDINGS. Although extremely variable, findings on physical examination generally reflect the location of aortic dissection and the extent of associated cardiovascular involvement. In some cases, physical findings alone may be sufficient to suggest the diagnosis, whereas in other cases, such pertinent physical findings may be subtle or absent, even in the presence of extensive aortic dissection. Hypertension is seen in 70 percent of patients with distal aortic dissection but in only 36 percent with proximal dissection. Hypotension, on the other hand, occurs much more commonly among those with proximal than with distal aortic dissection (25 and 4 percent, respectively). True hypotension is usually the result of cardiac tamponade, acute severe aortic regurgitation, intrapleural rupture, or intraperitoneal rupture. Dissection involving the brachiocephalic vessels may result in "pseudohypotension," an inaccurate measurement of blood pressure caused by compromise or occlusion of the brachial arteries.

The physical findings most typically associated with aortic dissection—pulse deficits, the murmur of aortic regurgitation, and neurological manifestations—are more characteristic of proximal than distal dissection. Reduced or absent pulses in patients with acute chest pain strongly suggest the presence of aortic dissection. Such pulse abnormalities are present in about 30 percent of proximal aortic dissections and occur throughout the arterial tree, but they are seen in only 15 percent of distal dissections, where they usually involve the femoral or left subclavian artery. The presence of pulse deficits predicts an increased risk for adverse outcomes.[76] Impaired pulses, and similarly, visceral ischemia, result from extension of the dissection flap into a branch artery with compression of the true lumen by the false channel (Fig. 53–13), which diminishes blood flow in the aortic true lumen because of narrowing or obliteration by the distended false lumen (occurring most commonly in the descending or abdominal aorta); impaired pulses may also result from proximal obstruction of flow caused by a mobile portion of the intimal flap overlying the branch vessel's orifice. Whichever the cause, the pulse deficits in aortic dissection may be transient, secondary to decompression of the false lumen by distal reentry into the true lumen or secondary to movement of the intimal flap away from the occluded orifice.

Aortic regurgitation is an important feature of proximal aortic dissection, with the murmur of aortic regurgitation detected in one-third of cases. When present in patients with distal dissection, aortic regurgitation generally antedates the dissection and may be the result of preexisting dilation of the aortic root from the underlying aortic pathologic condition, such as cystic medial degeneration. The murmur of aortic regurgitation may wax and wane, the intensity varying directly with the height of the arterial blood pressure. Depending on the severity of the regurgitation, other peripheral signs of aortic incompetence may be present, such as collapsing pulses and a wide pulse pressure. In some cases, however, congestive heart failure secondary to severe acute aortic regurgitation may occur with little or no murmur and no peripheral signs of aortic runoff.

The acute aortic regurgitation associated with proximal aortic dissection, which occurs in one-half to two-thirds of such cases, may result from any of several mechanisms (Fig. 53–14). First, the dissection may dilate the aortic root, thereby widening the sinotubular junction from which the aortic leaflets hang so that the leaflets are unable to coapt properly in diastole (incomplete closure). Second, the dissection may extend into the aortic root and detach one or more aortic leaflets from their commissural attachments at the sinotubular junction, thereby resulting in diastolic leaflet prolapse. Not infrequently, both incomplete closure and leaflet prolapse are present at the same time. Finally, in the setting of an extensive or circumferential intimal tear the unsupported intimal flap may prolapse into the left ventricular outflow tract, occasionally appearing as frank intimal intussusception, and produce severe aortic regurgitation.

Neurological manifestations occur in as many as 6 to 19 percent of all aortic dissections and accompany proximal dissection more frequently. Cerebrovascular accidents may occur in 3 to 6 percent when the innominate or left common

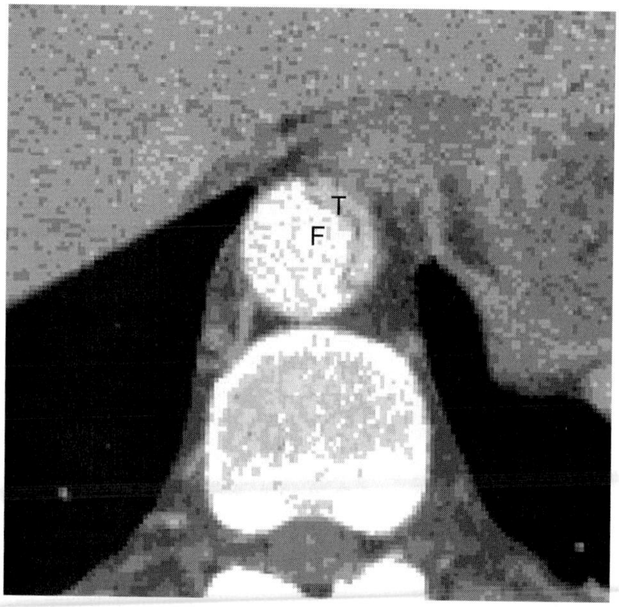

A

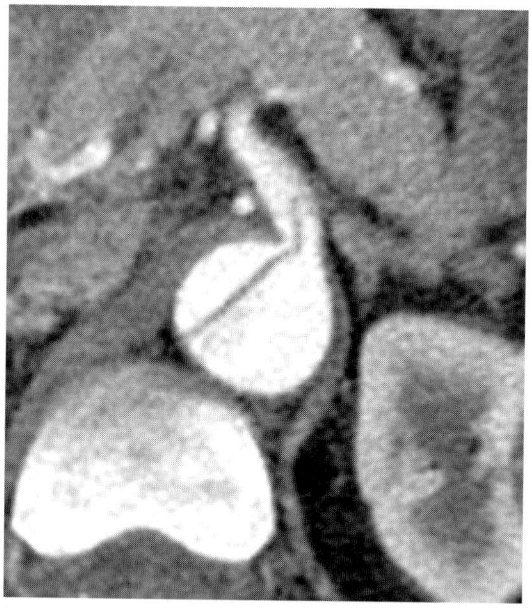

B

FIGURE 53–13 Mechanisms of compromised perfusion of branch arteries due to aortic dissection. **A,** The branch artery still originates from the true lumen, but the true lumen (T) is markedly compressed by the false lumen (F) throughout the cardiac cycle, resulting in low pressure and reduced flow within the true lumen and its branches. **B,** The intimal flap of the aortic dissection extends into the ostium of a branch artery, potentially narrowing or obstructing it.

carotid arteries are directly involved. Less often, patients may have altered consciousness or even coma. When spinal artery perfusion is compromised, ischemic spinal cord damage may produce paraparesis or paraplegia.

In a small minority, about 1 to 2 percent, of cases, a proximal dissection flap may involve the ostium of a coronary artery and cause acute myocardial infarction. Because most proximal dissections arise above the right sinus of Valsalva, retrograde extension into the aortic root more often affects the right coronary artery than the left, which explains why these myocardial infarctions tend to be inferior in location. Unfortunately, when secondary myocardial infarction does occur, its symptoms may complicate the clinical picture by obscuring symptoms of the primary aortic dissection. Most worrisome is the possibility that in the setting of electrocardiographic evidence of myocardial infarction, the underlying aortic dissection may go unrecognized. Moreover, the consequences of such a misdiagnosis in the era of thrombolytic therapy can be catastrophic. In a review of the literature, Kamp and colleagues described an early mortality rate of 71 percent (many from cardiac tamponade) among 21 patients with aortic dissection treated with thrombolysis.[77] It thus remains essential that when evaluating patients with acute myocardial infarction, particularly inferior infarctions, one carefully consider the possibility of an underlying aortic dissection before thrombolytic or anticoagulant therapy is instituted. Although some physicians feel reassured that performing a chest radiograph before the institution of thrombolysis is adequate to exclude the diagnosis of dissection, studies have shown it is not sufficient.

Extension of aortic dissection into the abdominal aorta can cause other vascular complications. Compromise of one or both renal arteries occurs in about 5 to 8 percent and can lead to renal ischemia or frank infarction and, eventually, severe hypertension and acute renal failure. Mesenteric ischemia and infarction are also occasional and potentially lethal complications of abdominal dissection seen in 3 to 5 percent of cases. In addition, aortic dissection may extend into the iliac arteries and cause diminished femoral pulses (12 percent) and acute lower extremity ischemia. If in such cases, the associated chest pain is minimal or absent, the pulse deficit and ischemic peripheral neuropathy may be mistaken for a peripheral embolic event.

Additional clinical manifestations of aortic dissection include the presence of small pleural effusions, seen more commonly on the left side. The effusion typically arises secondary to an inflammatory reaction around the involved aorta, but in some cases larger effusions may result from hemothorax caused by a transient rupture or leak from a descending dissection. Several rarely encountered clinical manifestations of aortic dissection include hoarseness, upper airway obstruction, rupture into the tracheobronchial tree with hemoptysis, dysphagia, hematemesis from rupture into the esophagus, superior vena cava syndrome, pulsating neck masses, Horner syndrome, and unexplained fever. Other rare findings associated with the presence of a continuous murmur include rupture of the aortic dissection into the right atrium, into the right ventricle, or into the left atrium with secondary congestive heart failure.

A variety of conditions can mimic aortic dissection, including myocardial infarction or ischemia, pericarditis, pulmonary embolism, acute aortic regurgitation without dissection, nondissecting thoracic or abdominal aortic aneurysms, or mediastinal tumors.

LABORATORY FINDINGS. Chest radiography is included in the discussion of clinical manifestations of aortic dissection rather than the discussion of diagnostic techniques because an abnormal incidental finding on a routine chest radiograph may first raise clinical suspicion of aortic dissection (Fig. 53–15). Moreover, although chest radiography may help support a diagnosis of suspected aortic dissection, the findings are nonspecific and rarely diagnostic. The results of chest radiography therefore add to the other available clinical data used in deciding whether suspicion of aortic dissection warrants proceeding to a more definitive diagnostic study.

The most common abnormality seen on a chest radiograph in cases of aortic dissection is widening of the aortic silhouette, which appears in 81 to 90 percent of cases. Less often, nonspecific widening of the superior mediastinum is seen. If calcification of the aortic knob is present, separation of the intimal calcification from the outer aortic soft tissue border by more than 1.0 cm—the "calcium sign"—is suggestive, although not diagnostic, of aortic dissection. Comparison of the current chest radiograph with a previous study may reveal acute changes in the aortic or mediastinal silhouettes that would otherwise have gone unrecognized. Pleural effusions are common, typically occur on the left side, and are more often associated with dissection involving the descending aorta. Although the majority of patients with aortic dissection have one or more of these radiographic abnormalities, the remainder, up to 12 percent, have chest radiographs that appear unremarkable. Therefore, a normal chest radiograph can never exclude the presence of aortic dissection.

Electrocardiographic findings in patients with aortic dissection are nonspecific. One-third of electrocardiograms show changes consistent with left ventricular hypertrophy, whereas another third are normal. Nevertheless, obtaining an electrocardiogram is diagnostically important for two reasons: (1) in cases of aortic dissection, nonspecific chest pain and the absence of ischemic ST segment and T wave changes on electrocardiogram may argue against the diagnosis of myocardial ischemia and thereby prompt consideration of other chest pain syndromes, including aortic dissection, and (2) in patients with proximal dissection, the electrocardiogram may reveal acute myocardial infarction when the dissection flap has involved a coronary artery.

Because of the variable extent of aortic, branch vessel, and cardiac involvement occurring with aortic dissection, the signs and symptoms associated with the condition occur sporadically. Consequently, the presence or absence of aortic dissection cannot be diagnosed accurately in most cases on the basis of symptoms and clinical findings alone. In the series of Spittell and associates,[73] of all aortic dissections (without a known diagnosis), the initial clinical diagnosis was aortic dissection in only 62 percent, and the other 38 percent of patients were initially thought to have myocardial ischemia, congestive heart failure, nondissecting aneurysms of the thoracic or abdominal aorta, symptomatic aortic stenosis, pulmonary embolism, and so forth. Among this 38 percent in whom aortic dissection went undiagnosed at initial evaluation, nearly two-thirds of patients had their aortic dissection detected incidentally while undergoing a diagnostic procedure for other clinical questions, and in

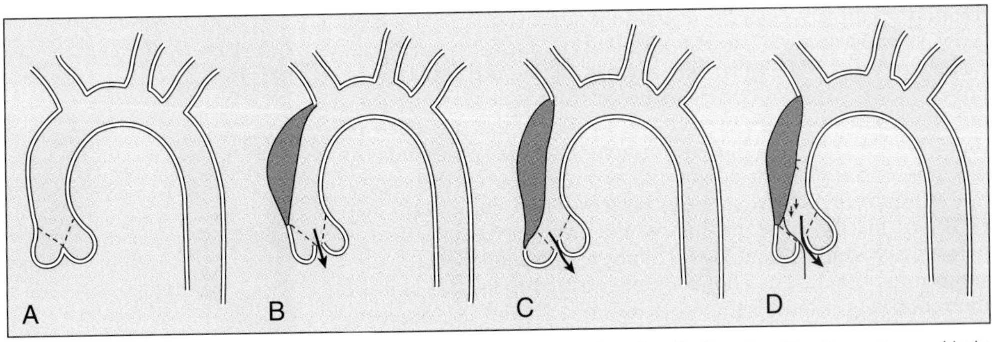

FIGURE 53–14 Mechanisms of aortic regurgitation in proximal aortic dissection. **A,** Normal aortic valve anatomy, with the leaflets suspended (dotted lines) from the sinotubular junction. **B,** A type A dissection dilates the ascending aorta, which in turn widens the sinotubular junction from which the aortic leaflets hang so that the leaflets are unable to coapt properly in diastole (incomplete closure). Aortic regurgitation (arrow) results. **C,** A type A dissection extends into the aortic root and detaches an aortic leaflet from its commissural attachment to the sinotubular junction. Diastolic leaflet prolapse results. **D,** In the setting of an extensive or circumferential intimal tear, the unsupported intimal flap may prolapse across the aortic valve and into the left ventricular outflow tract and prevent normal leaflet coaptation.

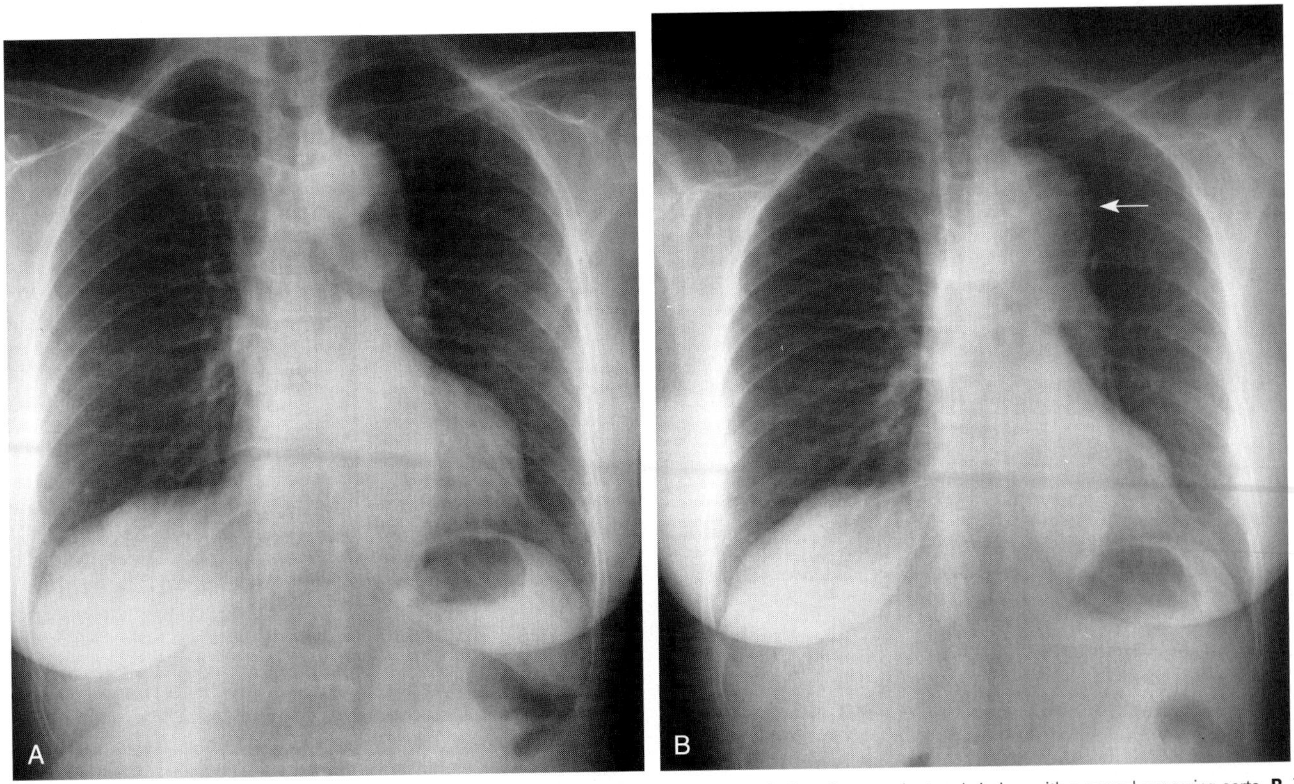

FIGURE 53–15 Chest radiograph of a patient with aortic dissection. **A,** The patient's baseline study from 3 years prior to admission, with a normal-appearing aorta. **B,** The chest radiograph upon admission, which is remarkable for the interval enlargement of the aortic knob (arrow). The patient was found to have a proximal aortic dissection. (From Isselbacher EM: Aortic dissection. *In* Creager, MA [ed]: Atlas of Vascular Disease. 2nd ed. Philadelphia, Current Medicine, 2003.)

nearly one-third, the aortic dissection remained undiagnosed until necropsy. Given the clinical challenge that detection of aortic dissection presents, physicians should remain vigilant for any risk factors, symptoms, and signs consistent with aortic dissection if a timely diagnosis is to be made.

DIAGNOSTIC TECHNIQUES. Once the diagnosis of aortic dissection is suspected on clinical grounds, it is essential to confirm the diagnosis both promptly and accurately. The diagnostic modalities currently available for this purpose include aortography, contrast-enhanced CT, MRI, and TTE or TEE. Each modality has certain advantages and disadvantages with respect to diagnostic accuracy, speed, convenience, risk, and cost, but none is appropriate in all situations.

When comparing the four imaging modalities, one must begin by considering what diagnostic information is needed. First and foremost, the study must confirm or refute the diagnosis of aortic dissection. Second, it must determine whether the dissection involves the ascending aorta (i.e., proximal or type A) or is confined to the descending aorta or arch (i.e., distal or type B). Third, if possible, it should identify a number of the anatomical features of the dissection, including its extent, the sites of entry and reentry, the presence of thrombus in the false lumen, branch vessel involvement by the dissection, the presence and severity of aortic regurgitation, the presence or absence of pericardial effusion, and any coronary artery involvement by the intimal flap. Unfortunately, no single imaging modality provides all of this anatomical detail. The choice of diagnostic modalities should therefore be guided by the clinical scenario and by targeting information that will best assist patient management.

Aortography. Retrograde aortography was the first accurate diagnostic technique for evaluating suspected aortic dissection. The diagnosis of aortic dissection is based on direct angiographic signs, including visualization of two lumina or an intimal flap (considered diagnostic), as in Figure 53–16, or on indirect signs (considered suggestive), such as deformity of the aortic lumen, thickening of the aortic walls, branch vessel abnormalities, and aortic regurgitation.

Aortography had long been considered the diagnostic standard for the evaluation of aortic dissection because for several decades it was the only accurate method of diagnosing aortic dissection antemortem, although its true sensitivity could not be defined. However, the more recent introduction of alternative diagnostic modalities has shown that aortography is not as sensitive as previously thought. Prospective studies have found that for the diagnosis of aortic dissection, the sensitivity of aortography is 88 percent and falls to only 77 percent when the definition of aortic dissection included intramural hematoma with noncommunicating dissection.[78] The specificity of aortography is 94 percent. False-negative aortograms occur because of thrombosis of the false lumen, equal and simultaneous opacification of both the true and false lumina, or the presence of an intramural hematoma.

Important advantages of aortography include its ability to delineate the extent of the aortic dissection, including branch vessel involvement (Fig. 53-17). It is also useful in detecting some of the major complications of aortic dissection, such as the presence of aortic regurgitation, and is often useful in revealing patency of the coronary arteries. In addition to the limited sensitivity of aortography, other disadvantages are the inherent risks of the invasive procedure, the risks associated with the use of contrast material, and the time needed to complete the study, both in assembling an angiography team and the long duration of the procedure. Finally, aortography requires that potentially unstable patients travel to the angiography suite.

Computed Tomography. In contrast-enhanced CT scanning, aortic dissection is diagnosed by the presence of two distinct aortic lumina, either visibly separated by an intimal flap (Fig. 53–18) or distinguished by a differential rate of contrast opacification. Spiral (helical) CT scanning, which is now used routinely, permits three-dimensional display of the aorta and its branches (Fig. 53–19), has improved the accuracy of CT in diagnosing aortic dissection, as well as in defining anatomical features. Several series have found that spiral CT scanning has both a sensitivity and specificity for acute aortic dissection of 96 to 100 percent (see Chap. 14).

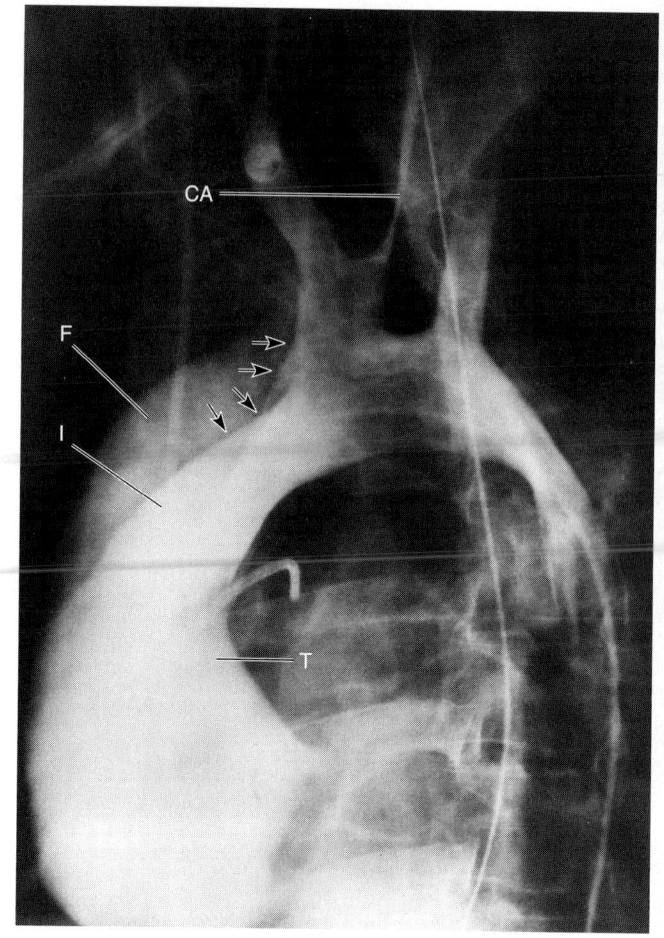

FIGURE 53–16 Aortogram in the left oblique view demonstrating proximal aortic dissection and its associated cardiovascular complications. The true lumen (T) and false lumen (F) are separated by the intimal flap (I), which is faintly visible as a radiolucent line following the contour of the pigtail catheter. The true lumen is better opacified than the false lumen, and two planes of the intimal flap can be distinguished (arrows). The branch vessels are opacified, along with marked narrowing of the right carotid artery (CA), which suggests that its lumen is compromised by the dissection. (From Isselbacher EM: Aortic dissection. *In* Creager MA [ed.]: Atlas of Vascular Disease. 2nd ed. Philadelphia, Current Medicine, 2003.)

Computed tomography scanning has the advantage that, unlike aortography, it is noninvasive. However, it does require the use of an intravenous contrast agent. Most hospitals are equipped with a readily accessible CT scanner available on an emergency basis. CT is also helpful in identifying the presence of thrombus in the false lumen and in detecting pericardial effusion. The use of CT angiography (three-dimensional reconstruction of axial CT data) permits assessment of branch vessel compromise in both the thoracic and abdominal segments. A disadvantage of CT scanning is that the site of intimal tear is rarely identified. CT scanning also cannot reliably detect the presence of aortic regurgitation.

Magnetic Resonance Imaging. The use of MRI has particular appeal for diagnosing aortic dissection in that it is entirely noninvasive and does not require the use of intravenous contrast material or ionizing radiation. Furthermore, MRI produces high-quality images in the transverse, sagittal, and coronal planes, as well as in a left anterior oblique view that displays the entire thoracic aorta in one plane (see Chap. 14). The availability of these multiple views facilitates the diagnosis of aortic dissection and determination of its extent

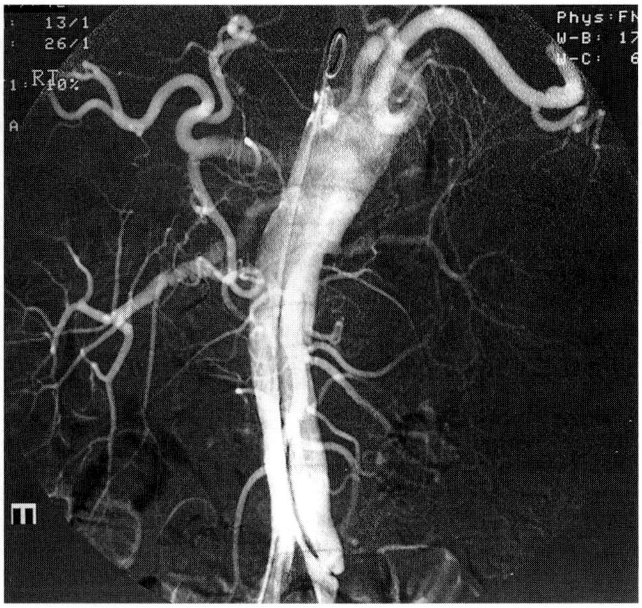

FIGURE 53–17 Digital subtraction angiogram of the abdominal aorta, in a patient with a distal thoracic aortic dissection, to assess the status of renal perfusion. This study confirmed the presence of an intimal flap extending down into the left common iliac artery. The celiac axis, superior mesenteric artery, and right renal artery are widely patent and fill from the true lumen. The left renal artery fills from the false lumen, with the intimal flap involving the ostium of the artery and impairing distal flow. As a consequence, there is minimal contrast excretion by the left kidney compared to the right.

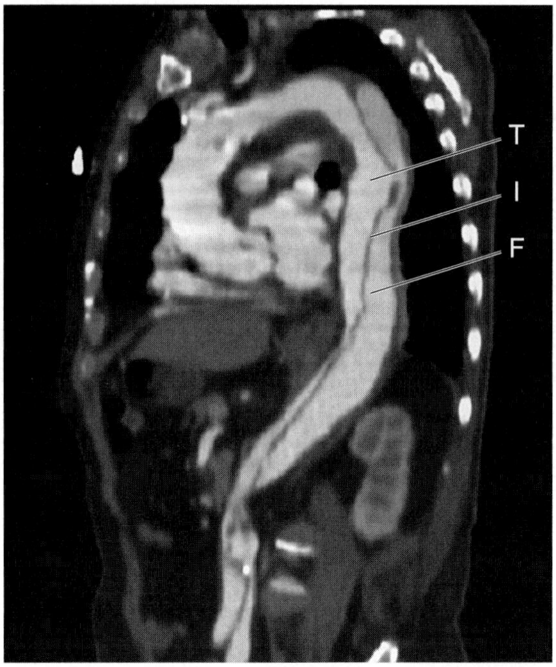

FIGURE 53–19 Computed tomography (CT) for diagnosing aortic dissection. Shown is a contrast-enhanced spiral CT scan of the chest at the level of the pulmonary artery showing an intimal flap (I) in the descending thoracic aorta separating the two lumina in a type B aortic dissection. F = false lumen; T = true lumen.

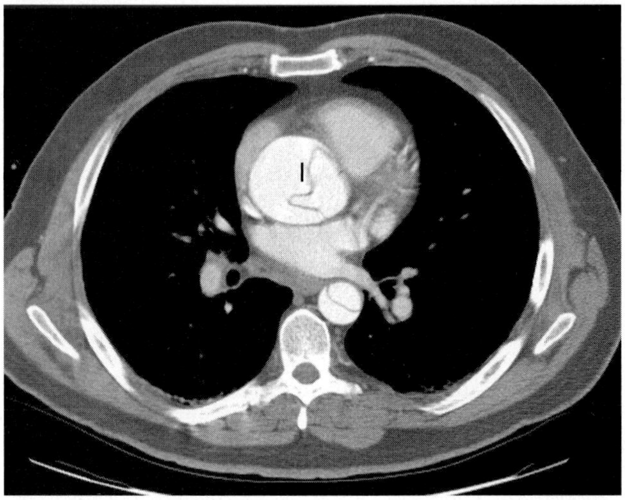

FIGURE 53–18 Computed tomography (CT) for diagnosing aortic dissection. Shown is a contrast-enhanced spiral CT scan of the chest at the level of the right pulmonary artery showing an intimal flap (I) in both the ascending and descending thoracic aorta separating the two lumina in a type B aortic dissection. (Reprinted with permission from Isselbacher EM: Aortic dissection. *In* Creager MA [ed]: Atlas of Vascular Disease. 2nd ed. Philadelphia, Current Medicine, 2003.)

and in many cases reveals the presence of branch vessel involvement.

Magnetic resonance imaging has been found to have both a sensitivity and a specificity of approximately 98 percent. Furthermore, use of the cine-MRI technique in a subset of these patients showed 85 percent sensitivity for detecting aortic regurgitation. Intravenous administration of gadolinium yields a magnetic resonance angiogram, which can be used to define the patency of aortic branch vessels. Still, MRI does have a number of disadvantages. It is contraindicated in patients with pacemakers or implantable defibrillators and certain types of vascular clips. MRI provides only limited images of branch vessels (unless gadolinium is used) and does not consistently identify the presence of aortic regurgitation. In most hospitals, magnetic resonance scanners are not readily available on an emergency basis. Many patients with aortic dissection are hemodynamically unstable, often intubated or receiving intravenous antihypertensive medications with arterial pressure monitoring, but magnetic resonance scanners limit the presence of many monitoring and support devices in the imaging suite and also limit patient accessibility during the lengthy study. Understandably, concern for the safety of unstable patients has led many physicians to conclude that the use of MRI is relatively contraindicated for unstable patients.

Echocardiography. Echocardiography is well suited for the evaluation of patients with suspected aortic dissection because it is readily available in most hospitals, it is noninvasive and quick to perform, and the full examination can be completed at the bedside. The echocardiographic finding considered diagnostic of an aortic dissection is the presence of an undulating intimal flap within the aortic lumen that separates the true and false channels. Reverberations and other artifacts can cause linear echodensities within the aortic lumen that mimic aortic dissection; to distinguish an intimal flap definitively from such artifacts, the flap should be identified in more than one view, it should have motion independent of that of the aortic walls or other cardiac structures, and a differential in color Doppler flow patterns should be noted between the two lumina. In cases in which the false lumen is thrombosed, displacement of intimal calcification or thickening of the aortic wall may suggest aortic dissection.

TRANSTHORACIC ECHOCARDIOGRAPHY. TTE has a sensitivity of 59 to 85 percent and a specificity of 63 to 96 percent for the diagnosis of aortic dissection. Such poor sensitivity significantly limits the general utility of this technique. Furthermore, image quality is often adversely affected by obesity,

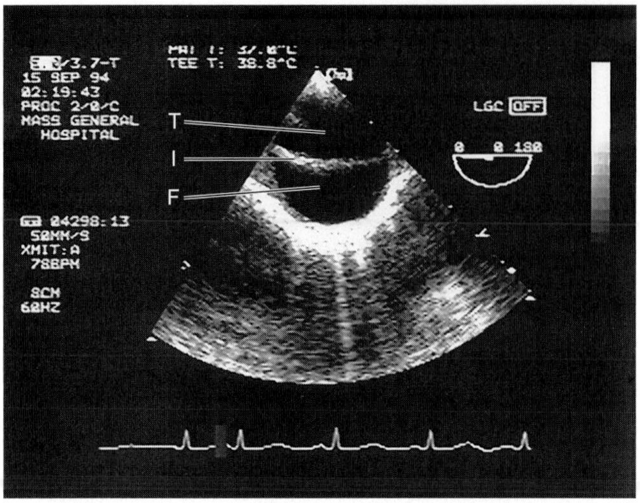

FIGURE 53–20 Cross-sectional transesophageal echocardiogram of the descending thoracic aorta demonstrating aortic dissection. The aorta is dilated. Evident is an intimal flap (I) dividing the true lumen (T) anteriorly and the false lumen (F) posteriorly. The true lumen fills during systole and is therefore seen bowing slightly into the false lumen in this systolic image.

emphysema, mechanical ventilation, or small intercostal spaces.

TRANSESOPHAGEAL ECHOCARDIOGRAPHY. The proximity of the esophagus to the aorta enables TEE to overcome many of the limitations of transthoracic imaging and permits the use of higher frequency ultrasonography, which provides better anatomical detail (Figs. 53–20 and 53–21). The examination is generally performed at the bedside with the patient under sedation or light general anesthesia and typically requires 10 to 15 minutes to complete. The procedure does not require arterial access nor intravenous contrast or ionizing radiation. Relative contraindications include known esophageal disease such as strictures or tumors. The incidence of important side effects (such as hypertension, bradycardia, bronchospasm, or rarely, esophageal perforation) is much less than 1 percent. One important disadvantage of TEE is its limited ability to visualize the distal ascending aorta and proximal arch because of interposition of the air-filled trachea and main stem bronchus.

The results of large prospective studies have demonstrated that the sensitivity of TEE for aortic dissection is 98 to 99 percent, whereas the sensitivity for detecting an intimal tear (Fig. 53–22) is 73 percent. Furthermore, TEE detects both aortic regurgitation and pericardial effusion in 100 percent of cases. The specificity of TEE for the diagnosis of aortic dissection is less well defined but is likely in the range of 94 to 97 percent.

In addition to its high sensitivity for detecting aortic dissection, TEE can provide other important information useful to the surgeon. Some surgeons want to know preoperatively whether the intimal flap involves the ostia of the coronary arteries, but this determination has traditionally required the performance of coronary angiography. Ballal and colleagues performed TEE on 34 patients with aortic dissection, 7 of whom had coronary artery involvement confirmed at surgery.[79] In six of these seven patients, TEE identified the intimal flap extending into the coronary ostia. However, TEE delineates only the very proximal portions of the coronary arteries, so when assessment of coronary atherosclerosis is necessary, coronary angiography is still required (see later).

Among patients with suspected aortic dissection, the diagnosis is excluded in as many as two-thirds of cases, which yields a group of patients with a chest pain syndrome of unknown origin. Among patients determined not to have aortic dissection, TEE identifies alternative cardiovascular diagnoses (e.g., other aortic abnormalities or evidence of acute myocardial infarction or ischemia) in 66 to 73 percent.[80]

Selecting an Imaging Modality. Each of the four imaging modalities has particular advantages and disadvantages. In selecting among them, one must consider the accuracy as well as the safety and availability of each test. Given their extremely high sensitivity and specificity and ability to provide three-dimensional images, CT angiography and MRA are considered the current standards for evaluating aortic dissection. The four imaging modalities described earlier differ in their ability to detect complications associated with dissection, so the specific diagnostic information sought by the treating physician and/or surgeon should have a bearing on the procedure chosen.

Both the accessibility of imaging studies and the time required to complete them are key considerations given the high rate of early mortality associated with unoperated proximal aortic dissection. Aortography can only rarely be performed on an emergency basis, because it often requires assembly of an angiography team and is subject to the risks associated with an invasive procedure and use of a contrast agent. MRI is also generally unavailable on an emergency basis and poses the risk of limited patient monitoring and accessibility during the lengthy procedure. CT scanning is more readily available in most emergency departments and is quickly completed. TEE is also readily available in most larger centers and can be completed quickly at the bedside, which makes it ideal for evaluating unstable patients. Among the centers in the IRAD, CT was used most often (63 percent) as the imaging study of first choice, with TEE performed first about half as often (32 percent).[81] Aortography and MRI were rarely used as the initial imaging modality (4 percent and 1 percent, respectively).

In a setting in which all these imaging modalities are available, CT should be considered first in the evaluation of suspected aortic dissection in light of its accuracy, safety, speed, and convenience. When CT identifies a type A aortic dissection, the patient may be taken directly to the operating room, where TEE can then be performed to assess the anatomy and competence of the aortic valve without unduly delaying surgery. However, in cases of suspected aortic dissection in which aortic valve disease is suspected or the patient is unstable, TEE may be the initial procedure of choice.

Despite its relative disadvantages, aortography still plays an important role when clear definition of the anatomy of the branch vessels is essential for management. Performance of aortography should also be considered when a definitive diagnosis is not made by one or more of the other imaging modalities.

In the final analysis, each institution must determine its own best diagnostic approach to the evaluation of suspected aortic dissection and base it on available human and material resources and the speed with which such resources can be mobilized. The level of skill and experience of those who carry out each diagnostic procedure should also enter into the choice of diagnostic modality.

The Role of Coronary Angiography. The importance of assessing the status of coronary artery patency before surgical repair of acute aortic dissection continues to be controversial. Some surgeons believe that obtaining this information before surgery is essential, whereas others are content to assess the coronary arteries intraoperatively. Two types of coronary artery involvement must be considered in the setting of aortic dissection. The first is acute proximal coronary narrowing or occlusion as a result of the dissection itself, often caused by occlusion of the coronary ostia by the intimal flap. The second is the possible presence of chronic atherosclerotic coronary artery disease, which, although generally independent of the dissection process, may complicate its surgical management.

In some cases, coronary involvement by the intimal flap is self-evident if the electrocardiogram shows evidence of acute myocardial ischemia or infarction. Should this acute process not be clinically evident, however, TEE can effectively define the patency of the proximal coronary arteries in a majority of cases. Aortography may also reveal such coronary artery involvement. More comprehensive evaluation requires the performance of coronary angiography; however, this study may be risky in patients with aortic dissection and often prolongs the time to aortic repair by several hours. Moreover, catheterization of the coronary arteries is sometimes unsuccessful in patients with proximal dissection and a dilated root, in which case the added procedural delay offers no potential benefit. In addition, such proximal coronary obstructions can usually be readily identified at the time of surgery.

Chronic coronary artery disease is seen in about one-quarter of patients with aortic dissection. Identifying the presence of this underlying coronary disease is beyond the capability of any of the four imaging modalities discussed earlier. Furthermore, accurately defining such atherosclerotic disease intraoperatively is challenging, although Rizzo and coworkers have suggested probing of the proximal coronary arteries, epicardial palpation, and angioscopy as possible means to identify coronary stenoses.[82]

The impact of unrecognized coronary artery disease on outcome is not certain. In a 10-year review examining 54 patients undergoing urgent aortic repair, Kern and colleagues found that only 1 of 27 patients with a proximal dissection had a perioperative myocardial infarction; this patient had a prior history of coronary artery disease.[83] In addition, Rizzo and associates observed that among patients in whom unrecognized coronary artery disease was discovered at autopsy, none died of coronary ischemia but several died of aortic rupture.[82] Lastly, Penn and colleagues studied 122 consecutive patients undergoing emergency aortic repair and found no difference in in-hospital mortality between patients who had preoperative angiography and those who did not.[84] Accordingly, we and others recommend avoiding preoperative coronary angiography unless a specific indication exists, such as a known history of coronary artery disease, prior coronary artery bypass grafting, or the presence of ischemic electrocardiographic changes. Conversely, Creswell and coauthors reported good outcomes when performing combined aortic repair and coronary artery bypass grafting in patients with underlying coronary artery disease and therefore argue that all stable patients with acute proximal dissec-

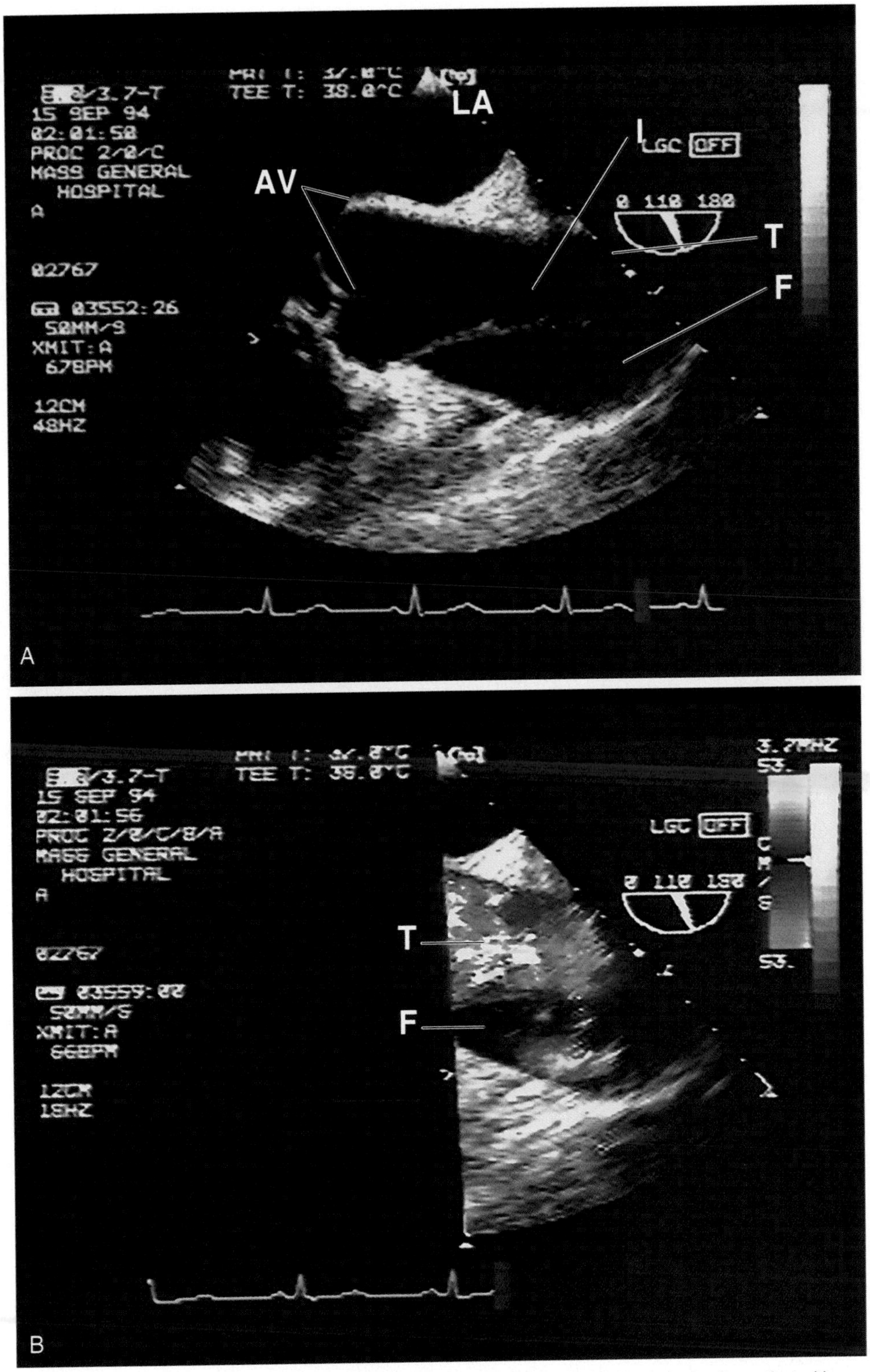

FIGURE 53–21 Transesophageal echocardiogram of the proximal ascending aorta in long-axis view in a patient with proximal aortic dissection. **A,** The left atrium (LA) is closest to the transducer. The aortic valve (AV) is seen on the left in this view, with the ascending aorta extending to the right. Within the proximal aorta is an intimal flap (I) that originates just at the level of the sinotubular junction above the right sinus of Valsalva. The true lumen (T) and the false lumen (F) are separated by the intimal flap. **B,** The addition of color flow Doppler in the same view confirms the presence of two distinct lumina. The true lumen (T) fills completely with brisk blood flow (bright blue color), while at the same time minimal retrograde flow (dark orange) is seen in the false lumen (F).

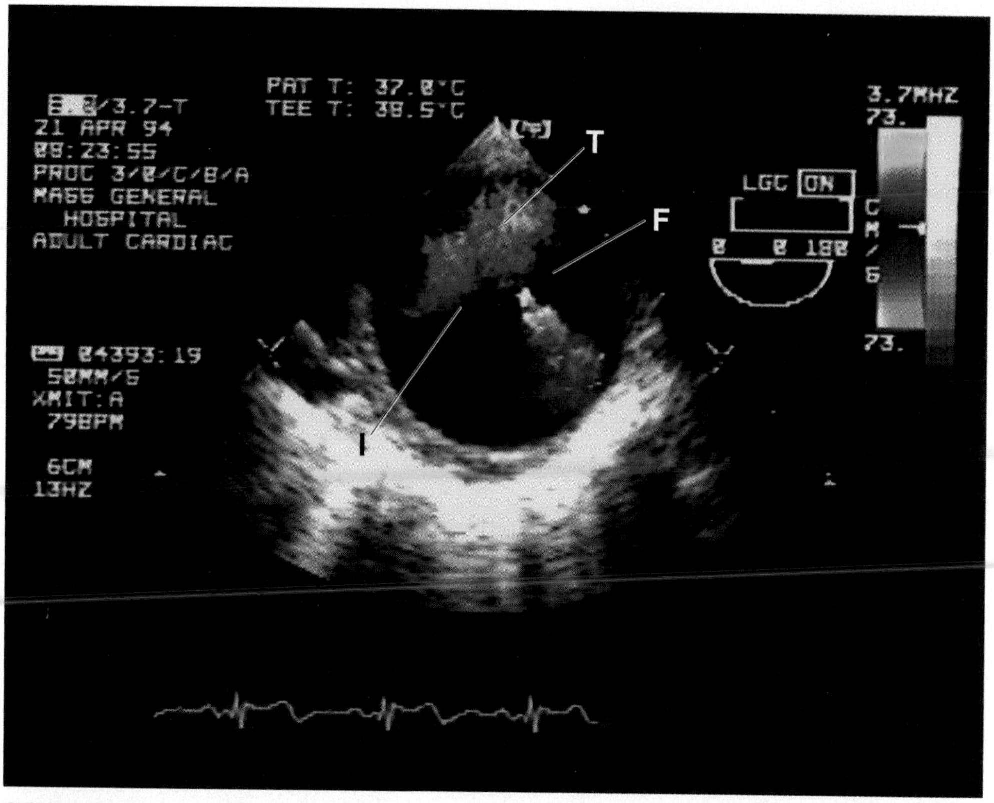

FIGURE 53–22 Cross-sectional transesophageal echocardiogram of a descending aortic dissection demonstrating a site of intimal tear. Blood flow (in orange) is evident in the true lumen (T) during systole, while a narrow jet of high-velocity blood (in blue) crosses into the false lumen (F) through a tear in the intimal flap (I).

tion should undergo preoperative coronary angiography.[85] While the debate continues unresolved, the trend in the literature has been a retreat from the routine performance of coronary angiography in cases of acute aortic dissection.

Management

Therapy for aortic dissection aims to halt progression of the dissecting hematoma because lethal complications arise not from the intimal tear itself but rather from the subsequent course taken by the dissecting aorta, such as vascular compromise or aortic rupture. Without treatment, aortic dissection has a high mortality rate. In a collective review of long-term survival in patients with untreated aortic dissection, more than 25 percent of all patients died within the first 24 hours after the onset of dissection, more than 50 percent died within the first week, more than 75 percent died within 1 month, and more than 90 percent died within 1 year.

The first surgical approach to aortic dissection was a fenestration procedure in which the dissected aorta was incised and a distal communication created between the true and false channels, thereby decompressing the false lumen. This procedure is, in fact, still used by some surgeons in selected cases of dissection involving the descending aorta to relieve limb, renal, or mesenteric ischemia. Definitive surgical therapy was pioneered by DeBakey and colleagues in the early 1950s. Its purpose is to excise the intimal tear, obliterate the false channel by oversewing the aortic edges, reconstitute the aorta directly or with the interposition of a synthetic graft, and in the case of proximal dissection, restore aortic valve competence either by resuspension of the displaced aortic leaflets or by prosthetic aortic valve replacement.

Aggressive medical treatment of aortic dissection was first advocated by Wheat and colleagues in the 1960s. The authors established reduction of systolic blood pressure and diminution of the rate of left ventricular ejection (dP/dt) as the two primary goals of pharmacological therapy. Originally introduced for patients too ill to withstand surgery, medical therapy is now the initial treatment for virtually all patients with aortic dissection before definitive diagnosis and furthermore serves as the primary long-term therapy in a subset of patients, particularly those with distal dissections.

IMMEDIATE MEDICAL MANAGEMENT. All patients in whom acute aortic dissection is strongly suspected should immediately be placed in an acute care setting for hemodynamic stabilization and monitoring of blood pressure, cardiac rhythm, and urine output. Two large-bore intravenous catheters should be inserted for intravenous medications and fluid resuscitation if necessary. An arterial line should be placed, preferably in the right arm so that it remains functional during surgery when the aorta is cross-clamped. However, in cases in which the blood pressure is significantly greater on the left than on the right, the arterial line should be placed on the left. In patients with a lower likelihood of dissection who are hemodynamically stable, an automatic blood pressure cuff should suffice.

A central venous or pulmonary arterial line to monitor central venous or pulmonary artery wedge pressure and cardiac output should be considered in patients with hypotension or congestive heart failure. Femoral lines and blood gas studies should be avoided if possible to conserve these sites for bypass cannulation during potential aortic repair. If a femoral line must be placed urgently, the opposite groin site should be protected from needle puncture.

BLOOD PRESSURE REDUCTION. Initial therapeutic goals include the elimination of pain and reduction of systolic blood pressure to 100 to 120 mm Hg (mean of 60 to 75 mm Hg) or the lowest level commensurate with adequate vital organ (cardiac, cerebral, renal) perfusion. Simultaneously, beta-blocking agents should be administered as well, regardless of whether pain or systolic hypertension is present. The use of long-acting medications should be avoided in patients who are surgical candidates because they may complicate intraoperative arterial pressure management. Pain, which may itself exacerbate hypertension and tachycardia, should be promptly treated with intravenous morphine sulfate.

For the acute reduction of arterial pressure, the potent vasodilator sodium nitroprusside is very effective. It is initially infused at 20 μg/min with the dosage titrated upward, as high as 800 μg/min, according to the blood pressure response. When used alone, however, sodium nitroprusside can actually cause an increase in dP/dt, which in turn may potentially contribute to propagation of the dissection. Therefore, concomitant beta-blocking treatment is essential. For those patients with acute or chronic renal insufficiency, intravenous fenoldopam may be preferable to sodium nitroprusside.[86]

To reduce dP/dt acutely, an intravenous beta blocker should be administered in incremental doses until evidence of satisfactory beta blockade is noted, usually indicated by a heart rate of 60 to 80 beats/min in the acute setting. Because propranolol was the first generally available beta blocker, it has been used most widely in treating aortic dissection. However, it is believed that other noncardioselective beta blockers are equally effective. Propranolol should be administered in intravenous doses of 1 mg every 3 to 5 minutes until the desired effect is achieved, although the maximum initial dose should not exceed 0.15 mg/kg (or approximately 10 mg). To maintain adequate beta blockade, as evidenced by the heart rate, additional propranolol should be given intravenously every 4 to 6 hours, or administered as a continuous infusion.

Labetalol, which acts as both an alpha- and a beta-adrenergic receptor blocker, can be especially useful in the setting of aortic dissection because it effectively lowers both dP/dt and arterial pressure. The initial dose of labetalol is 20 mg, administered intravenously over a 2-minute period, followed by additional doses of 40 to 80 mg every 10 to 15 minutes (up to a maximum total dose of 300 mg) until the heart rate and blood pressure have been controlled. Maintenance dosing can then be achieved with a continuous intravenous infusion starting at 2 mg/min and titrating up to 5 to 10 mg/min.

The ultra-short-acting beta blocker esmolol may be particularly useful in patients with labile arterial pressure, especially if surgery is planned, because use of this drug can be abruptly discontinued if necessary. It is administered as a 500 μg/kg intravenous bolus followed by continuous infusion at 50 μg/kg/min and titrated up to 200 μg/kg/min. Esmolol can also be useful as a means to test beta blocker safety and tolerance in patients with a history of obstructive pulmonary disease who may be at uncertain risk for bronchospasm from beta blockade. In such patients, a cardioselective beta blocker, such as atenolol or metoprolol, can be considered.

When contraindications exist to the use of beta blockers—including sinus bradycardia, second- or third-degree atrioventricular block, congestive heart failure, or bronchospasm—other agents to reduce arterial pressure and dP/dt should be considered. Calcium channel antagonists, which are effective in managing hypertensive crisis, are used on occasion in the treatment of aortic dissection. The combined vasodilator and negative inotropic effects of both diltiazem and verapamil make these agents well suited for the treatment of aortic dissection. Moreover, these agents may be administered intravenously. Nifedipine has the advantage that it can be given immediately by the sublingual route while other medications are being prepared. A key limitation of nifedipine, however, is that it has little negative chronotropic or inotropic effect.

Refractory hypertension may result when a dissection flap compromises one or both of the renal arteries, thereby causing the release of large amounts of renin. In this situation, the most efficacious antihypertensive may be the intravenous angiotensin-converting enzyme (ACE) inhibitor enalaprilat, which is administered initially in doses of 0.625 to 1.25 mg every 6 hours and then titrated upward if necessary to a maximum of 5 mg every 6 hours.

In the event that a patient with suspected aortic dissection has significant hypotension, rapid volume expansion should be considered given the possible presence of cardiac tamponade or aortic rupture. Before initiating aggressive treatment of such hypotension, however, the possibility of *pseudohypotension*, which occurs when arterial pressure is being measured in an extremity where the circulation is selectively compromised by the dissection, should be carefully excluded. If vasopressors are absolutely required for refractory hypotension, norepinephrine (Levophed) or phenylephrine (Neo-Synephrine) is preferred. Dopamine should be reserved for improving renal perfusion and used only at very low doses, given that it may raise dP/dt.

Once appropriate medical therapy has been initiated and the patient sufficiently stabilized, a definitive diagnostic study should be promptly undertaken. If a patient remains unstable, TEE is preferred because it can be performed at the bedside in the emergency department or intensive care unit, thereby allowing both monitoring and therapeutic intervention to continue uninterrupted. When a patient with a strongly suspected dissection becomes extremely unstable, aortic rupture or cardiac tamponade is likely and the patient should go directly to the operating room rather than delaying surgery for diagnostic imaging. In such situations, intraoperative TEE can be used both to confirm the diagnosis and to guide surgical repair.

MANAGEMENT OF CARDIAC TAMPONADE. Cardiac tamponade frequently complicates acute proximal aortic dissection and is one of the most common mechanisms of death in these patients. It is often the cause of hypotension when patients have aortic dissection, and pericardiocentesis is commonly performed in this setting in an effort to stabilize patients while they await definitive surgical repair. In a retrospective series, however, we found that pericardiocentesis may be harmful rather than beneficial in this setting because it can precipitate hemodynamic collapse and death rather than stabilize the patient as intended.[87] Seven patients in this series were relatively stable initially (six hypotensive, one normotensive). Three of four who underwent successful pericardiocentesis died suddenly between 5 and 40 minutes after the procedure due to acute pulseless electrical activity. In contrast, none of the three patients without pericardiocentesis died before surgery. It may be that in such patients, the increase in intraaortic pressure that follows pericardiocentesis causes a closed communication between the false lumen and pericardial space to reopen, thereby leading to recurrent hemorrhage and lethal cardiac tamponade.

Therefore, when a patient with acute aortic dissection complicated by cardiac tamponade is relatively stable, the risks of pericardiocentesis probably outweigh the benefits and *every effort should be made to proceed as urgently as possible to the operating room for direct surgical repair of the aorta with intraoperative drainage of the hemopericardium.* However, when patients have pulseless electrical activity or marked hypotension, an attempt to resuscitate the patient with pericardiocentesis is warranted and may indeed be successful. A prudent strategy in such cases is to aspirate only enough pericardial fluid to raise blood pressure to the lowest acceptable level.

Definitive Therapy

Despite minor variations from center to center, a reasonable consensus regarding definitive therapy for aortic dissection has evolved over the past several decades. All practitioners agree that surgical therapy is superior to medical therapy for acute proximal dissection. With even limited progression of a proximal dissection, patients may suffer the potentially devastating consequences of aortic rupture or cardiac tamponade, acute aortic regurgitation, or neurological compromise. Thus, by controlling this risk, immediate surgical repair promises a better outcome. Occasional patients with proximal dissection who refuse surgery or for whom surgery is contraindicated (e.g., by age or prior debilitating illness) may

TABLE 53–2 Indications for Definitive Surgical and Medical Therapy in Aortic Dissection

Surgical

Treatment of choice for acute proximal dissection
Treatment for acute distal dissection complicated by the following:
- Progression with vital organ compromise
- Rupture or impending rupture (e.g., saccular aneurysm formation)
- Retrograde extension into the ascending aorta
- Dissection in the Marfan syndrome

Medical

Treatment of choice for uncomplicated distal dissection
Treatment for stable, isolated arch dissection
Treatment of choice for stable chronic dissection (uncomplicated dissection presenting 2 weeks or later after onset)

be treated successfully with medical therapy with a 30-day survival rate of up to 42 percent.[67]

Patients suffering acute distal aortic dissection, on the other hand, are at significantly lower risk of early death from complications of the dissection than are those with proximal dissection. Furthermore, because patients with distal dissection tend to be older and have a relatively increased prevalence of advanced atherosclerosis or cardiopulmonary disease, their surgical risk is often considerably higher. A large retrospective series involving patients from both Duke and Stanford universities has, by multivariate analysis, shown that medical therapy provides an outcome equivalent to that of surgical therapy in patients with uncomplicated distal dissection. As a consequence, medical therapy for such patients is favored. An important exception is that when distal dissection is complicated by vital organ or limb ischemia, uncontrolled pain, rapid expansion, medical therapy yields poor results and surgery is therefore recommended.

Patients with chronic aortic dissection have, through self-selection, survived the early period of highest mortality, and whether treated medically or surgically, their subsequent hospital survival rate is approximately 90 percent. Accordingly, medical therapy is recommended for the management of all stable patients with chronic proximal and distal dissection, again unless complicated by rupture, aneurysm formation, aortic regurgitation, arterial occlusion, or extension or recurrence of dissection.

SURGICAL MANAGEMENT. Generally advocated indications for definitive surgical therapy are summarized in Table 53–2. Surgical candidacy should be determined whenever possible at the start of the patient's evaluation because this option guides the selection of diagnostic studies. Surgical risk for all patients is increased by age, comorbid disease (especially pulmonary emphysema), aneurysm leakage, cardiac tamponade, shock, or vital organ compromise as a result of such conditions as myocardial infarction, cerebrovascular accident, and in particular, preexisting renal failure.

Preoperative mortality in patients with acute dissection ranges from 3 percent when surgery is expedited to as high as 20 percent when the preoperative evaluation is more prolonged. These data reinforce the need for prompt diagnosis and repair to prevent even minimal progression of the dissection, which might lead to further complications.

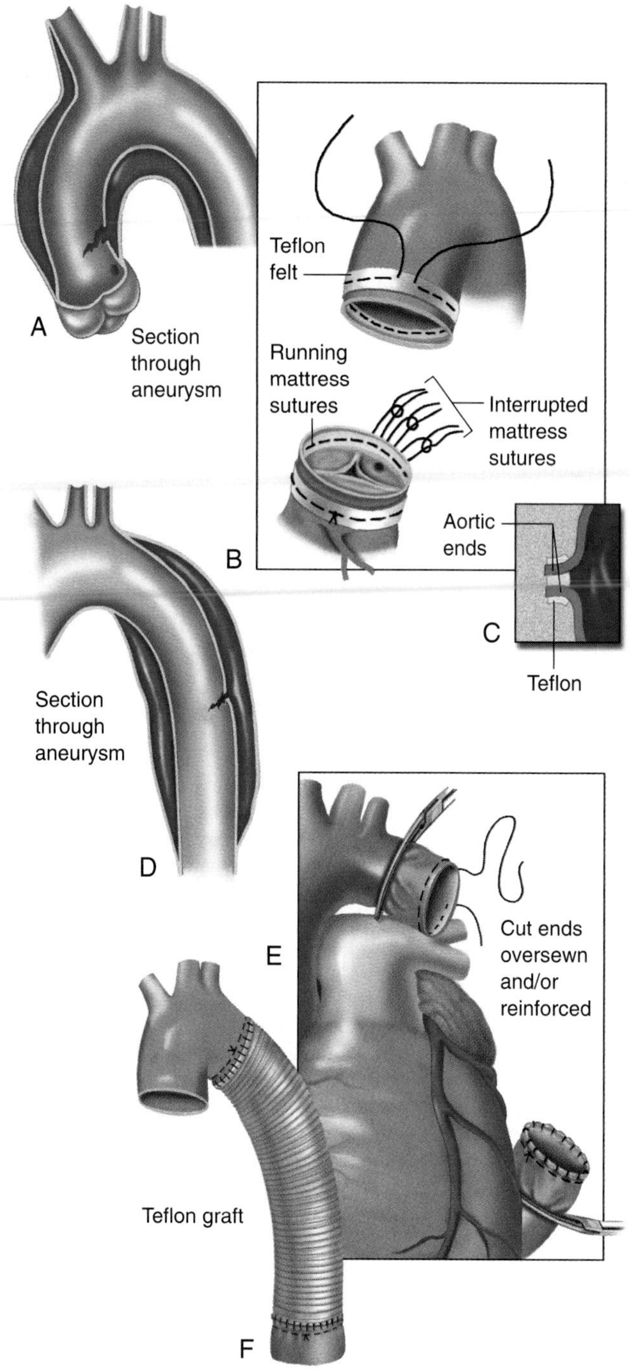

FIGURE 53–23 Several steps in the surgical repair of proximal **(A, B,** and **C)** and distal **(D, E,** and **F)** aortic dissections. **A** and **D,** Dissections and intimal tears. **B,** The aorta has been transected, and the ends of the aorta have been oversewn to obliterate the false lumen and buttressed with Teflon felt to prevent the sutures from tearing through the fragile tissue. **C,** The aortic ends are brought together in such a way that the Teflon is again used to reinforce the suture line between the two ends of the aorta and between the aorta and a sleeve graft, if such a graft is necessary for reconstitution of the aorta. **E,** Resection of a distal dissection, with a Teflon graft interposed in **F.** (**D, E,** and **F** from Austen WG, DeSanctis RW: Surgical treatment of dissecting aneurysm of the thoracic aorta. N Engl J Med 272:1314, 1965.)

The usual objectives of definitive surgical therapy include resection of the most severely damaged segment of aorta, excision of the intimal tear when possible, and obliteration of entry into the false lumen by suturing of the edges of the dissected aorta both proximally and distally. After the diseased segment containing the intimal tear is resected, typically a segment of the ascending aorta in proximal dissections or the proximal descending aorta in distal dissections, aortic continuity is then reestablished by interposing a prosthetic sleeve graft between the two ends of the aorta (Fig. 53–23).

Importantly, several studies have demonstrated that the immediate and long-term survival of patients treated surgically was not significantly affected by failure to excise the intimal tear. Some patients with proximal dissection have an intimal tear located in the aortic arch. Because surgical repair of the arch may increase the morbidity and mortality associated with the procedure and because resection of the tear may not necessarily improve mortality,[88] many surgeons elect not to repair the arch if the sole purpose of surgery is resection of the intimal tear. However, with improvements in surgical technique during the last decade, several groups suggest that even these challenging lesions can be resected with favorable results.[89]

When aortic regurgitation complicates aortic dissection, simple decompression of the false lumen is sometimes all that is required to allow resuspension of the aortic leaflets and restoration of valvular competence. More often, however, preservation of the aortic valve requires approximation of the two layers of dissected aortic wall and resuspension of the commissures with pledgeted sutures. In this setting, the use of intraoperative TEE may be particularly helpful to the surgeon in guiding aortic valve repair.[90] This resuspension technique has had favorable results with a fairly low incidence of recurrent aortic regurgitation in long-term follow-up. Preserving the aortic valve in this fashion may avoid the complications associated with prosthetic valve replacement, especially the requirement for oral anticoagulation, which may pose an added risk in patients prone to future aortic rupture.

Prosthetic aortic valve replacement is sometimes necessary, however, either because attempts at valve repair are unsuccessful or in the setting of preexisting valvular disease or Marfan syndrome. Many surgeons are aggressive about replacing the aortic valve if it appears that even moderate aortic regurgitation will remain after the leaflets are resuspended and choose to avoid the risk of having to replace the aortic valve at some later date in a second operation through a diseased aorta. When the proximal aorta is fragile or badly torn, most surgeons use a composite prosthetic graft (described earlier) for replacement of both the ascending aorta and the aortic valve together. The operative procedure for aortic dissection is technically demanding. The wall of the diseased aorta is often friable, and the repair must be performed with meticulous care. Use of Teflon felt to buttress the wall and prevent sutures from tearing through the fragile aorta is essential (see Fig. 53-23). Determining the sources of vital organ perfusion distal to the surgical site by diagnostic imaging studies may be of critical importance. For example, if one or both renal arteries are supplied by the false lumen and are not going to be directly corrected surgically, the surgeon may leave communication between the true and false channels distal to the site of aortic repair so that renal perfusion is not jeopardized.

Complications. Bleeding, infection, pulmonary failure, and renal insufficiency constitute the most common early complications of surgical therapy. Spinal cord ischemia with paraplegia caused by inadvertent interruption of the blood supply from the anterior spinal or intercostal arteries is an uncommon but dreaded consequence of descending thoracic aortic repair. Late complications include progressive aortic regurgitation if the aortic valve has not been replaced, localized aneurysm formation, and recurrent dissection at the original site or at a secondary site. With modern operative techniques, 30-day surgical survival rates for proximal and distal dissections are 74 and 69 percent, respectively.[67]

Newer Surgical Techniques. As a modification of more standard operative techniques, many surgeons now use tissue glues to appose permanently the dissected aortic layers to both eliminate the false lumen and to strengthen friable aortic tissue in order to improve the anastomoses. After resection of the diseased aortic segment, this glue is used in place of pledgeted sutures to seal the false lumen of the aortic stumps, before implantation of the Dacron prosthesis. The glue not only hardens and reinforces the fragile dissected aortic tissue but may also simplify the operation, facilitate resuspension of the aortic valve, and potentially reduce the incidence of late aortic root aneurysm formation.[91] Although some reports have shown favorable morbidity and mortality with the use of these new techniques, others suggest that glue use may result in late complications of tissue necrosis,[92] particularly if the glue is used improperly. Before the use of tissue glue can be widely adopted, a direct comparison with standard operative techniques is needed.

Endovascular Techniques. One of the more promising avenues of investigation is the use of endovascular techniques for treating high-risk patients with aortic dissection. For example, because patients with renal or visceral artery compromise from dissection have had operative mortality rates exceeding 50 percent, alternative management strategies are desirable. Two endovascular techniques have been used in many centers to manage patients with acute vascular complications secondary to aortic dissection. The first is balloon fenestration of the intimal flap, which involves crossing an intact intimal flap with a wire, passing a balloon-tipped catheter over the wire, and then expanding the balloon to tear a hole in the intimal flap. The hole acts as a site of reentry to allow blood to flow from the false into the true lumen, thereby decompressing the distended false lumen. The second technique involves percutaneous stenting of an affected arterial branch whose flow has been compromised by the dissection process. Slonim and coauthors reported the use of percutaneous management of ischemic complications of aortic dissection in a series of 22 patients.[93] Sixteen patients were treated with endovascular stents, three with balloon fenestration of the intimal flap, and three with fenestration in combination with stenting of the aorta or its branches; revascularization with clinical success was achieved in all 22 patients, with excellent long-term outcomes. In comparing our recent 10-year experience with a previously reported 30-year experience, we found that current methods of peripheral vascular intervention have reduced the overall mortality of dissection-associated branch vessel occlusion from 51 percent to 23 percent.[94] In the large IRAD series of acute aortic dissection, 3.2 percent of patients were treated with percutaneous fenestration procedures.[67]

More recently, intraluminal stent-grafts placed percutaneously by the transfemoral catheter technique have been introduced as a potential alternative to aortic repair. This procedure aims to close the site of entry into the false lumen (intimal tear), decompress and promote thrombosis of the false lumen, and relieve any obstruction of branch vessels that may accompany the dissection. It is hoped that this approach will reduce the morbidity and mortality of aortic dissection and reduce the risk of subsequent aneurysm formation. Nienaber and colleagues compared the use of stent-graft placement with standard surgical repair in a group of 24 patients with subacute or chronic type B aortic dissection and a patent false lumen.[95] No procedural complications occurred among the 12 patients undergoing stent-graft treatment, and when compared with the surgical group, the stent-graft group had a significantly shorter hospital stay, lower rate of morbidity, and lower 1-year postprocedural mortality rate. Dake and colleagues inserted stent-grafts in the descending thoracic aortas of 19 patients with acute aortic dissection and a patent false lumen who suffered from obstruction of branch vessels, acute aortic rupture, or persistent back pain.[96] Endovascular stent-graft deployment was successful in all cases, with complete thrombosis of the false lumen in 79 percent and partial thrombosis in the remaining 21 percent. Restoration of flow to ischemic arterial branches with relief of corresponding symptoms occurred in 76 percent of obstructed branches. The results of these two series are extremely promising, but larger studies with more patients and longer follow-up will be required before stent-graft therapy becomes an accepted therapy for aortic dissection.

DEFINITIVE MEDICAL MANAGEMENT. As discussed earlier, we prefer medical therapy for stable patients with uncomplicated acute distal dissection (see Table 53-2) given that the 30-day survival rate for those with distal dissection treated medically is 92 percent.[67] However, surgery (or percutaneous intervention) clearly must be performed in cases of medical management failure, such as in the presence of rupture or impending rupture, progression of the dissection with vital organ compromise, an inability to control pain with medicines, or retrograde progression of a type B dissection into the ascending aorta. Because of the extreme difficulty of surgery to repair the aortic arch when it is involved by the dissection, medical therapy is also usually advocated for type B dissections that either originate in the arch or extend retrograde into the arch. Operative therapy is again reserved for patients with serious complications. Medical therapy is also generally recommended for patients with chronic aortic dissection, whether proximal or distal, unless late complications of the dissection, such as aortic regurgitation or localized aneurysm formation, necessitate surgery.

Severe hypertension is relatively common during the period of hospitalization after acute aortic dissection and may occur even in patients without a history of significant hypertension. In the past, some practitioners have argued that such refractory hypertension should be considered an indication for aortic repair, as it might increase the risk of early complications. In a retrospective analysis, however, we found that although almost two-thirds of our patients with distal dissections required the administration of four or more antihypertensive medications to control refractory hypertension early in their hospitalization, there was no increase in adverse events as compared with patients without such hypertension, and surgery is generally not necessary in this setting.[97] The etiology for this hypertensive response is unclear but it may reflect a marked increase in sympathetic tone triggered by the severe inflammation of the aortic wall that accompanies dissection. In our experience, renal ischemia rarely caused hypertension, so in the absence of a fall in urine output or a rise in serum creatinine, renal artery imaging is typically not necessary. Furthermore, the severe hypertension usually improves 5 to 7 days after onset of the aortic dissection, allowing a reduction in antihypertensive therapy.

When patients with type B aortic dissection are managed medically, in addition to the reduction in dP/dt and heart rate, a second goal is to monitor the patient vigilantly for any evidence of branch arterial compromise, with the most lethal consequence being mesenteric ischemia. Unfortunately, the clinical features of mesenteric ischemia may be subtle initially and therefore go unrecognized, and by the time they have become clinically obvious, organ damage may be irreversible. Adding to the challenge of this condition is the fact that in as many as half such cases,[98] imaging studies such as urgent CT scanning may show patent mesenteric vessels arising from the true lumen with no evidence of the dissection flap extending into the branches. However, often a large false lumen is distended with blood and compresses a small true lumen throughout most of the cardiac cycle, markedly reducing antegrade flow through the true lumen to the mesenteric vessels and resulting in nonobstructive ischemia (see Fig. 53–13). In this setting, a strong clinical suspicion and a low threshold for surgical or percutaneous intervention are the keys to preventing a catastrophic outcome.

Long-Term Therapy and Late Follow-Up

Late follow-up of patients leaving the hospital with treated aortic dissection shows an actuarial survival rate not much worse than that of individuals of comparable age without dissection. No significant differences are seen among discharged patients when comparing proximal versus distal dissection, acute versus chronic dissection, or medical versus surgical treatment.[99] Five-year survival rates for all these groups (among discharged patients) are typically 75 to 82 percent. Thus, the initial success of surgical or medical therapy is usually sustained on long-term follow-up. Late complications include aortic regurgitation, recurrent dissection, and aneurysm formation or rupture. The presence of a persistently patent false lumen is one of the strongest predictors of adverse late outcomes, including more rapid aortic dilatation, a greater likelihood of requiring subsequent aortic surgery, and late mortality.[100,101]

Long-term medical therapy to control hypertension and reduce dP/dt is indicated for all patients who have sustained an aortic dissection, regardless of whether their in-hospital definitive treatment was surgical or medical. Indeed, one study found that late aneurysm rupture after aortic dissection was 10 times more common in patients with poorly controlled hypertension than in those with controlled blood pressure,[102] which dramatically demonstrates the importance of aggressive lifelong antihypertensive therapy. Systolic blood pressure should be maintained at or below 130 mm Hg. The preferred agents are beta blockers or, if contraindicated, other agents with a negative inotropic as well as a hypotensive effect, such as verapamil or diltiazem. Pure vasodilators, such as dihydropyridine calcium channel antagonists or hydralazine, may cause an increase in dP/dt and should therefore be used only in conjunction with adequate beta blockade. ACE inhibitors are attractive antihypertensive agents for treating aortic dissection and may be of particular benefit in patients with some degree of renal ischemia as a consequence of the dissection.

Up to 29 percent of late deaths following surgery result from rupture of either the dissecting aneurysm or another aneurysm at a remote site. Moreover, the incidence of subsequent aneurysm formation at a site remote from the surgical repair is 17 to 25 percent, with these remote aneurysms accounting for many of the rupture-related deaths. The mean time interval from primary aortic dissection to the appearance of subsequent aneurysms is 18 months, with the majority appearing within 2 years. Many such aneurysms occur from dilatation of the residual false lumen in the more distal aortic segments not resected at the time of surgery. Because the dissected aneurysm wall is relatively thin and consists of only the outer half of the original aortic wall, these aneurysms rupture more frequently than do typical atherosclerotic thoracic aneurysms. Thus, an aggressive approach to treating such late-appearing aneurysms may be indicated.

The high incidence of late aneurysm formation and rupture emphasizes both the diffuse nature of the aortic disease process in this population and the tremendous importance of careful follow-up. The primary goal of long-term surveillance is the early detection of aortic lesions that might require subsequent surgical intervention, such as the appearance of new aneurysms or rapid aneurysm expansion, progression or recurrence of dissection, aortic regurgitation, or peripheral vascular compromise.

Follow-up evaluation of patients after aortic dissection should include careful and repeated physical examinations, periodic chest radiographs, and serial aortic imaging with CT, MRI, or TEE. We generally prefer CT for serially monitoring of these patients because it is completely noninvasive and provides excellent anatomical detail that may be exceedingly helpful in evaluating interval changes. Patients are at highest risk immediately after hospitalization and during the first 2 years, with the risk progressively declining thereafter. It is therefore important to have more frequent early follow-up; for example, patients can be seen and imaged at 3 and 6 months initially and then return every 6 months for 2 years, after which time they can be reevaluated at 6- to 12-month intervals, depending on the given patient's risk.

Atypical Aortic Dissection

In aortic dissection as classically described, two other diseases of the aorta are closely related, *intramural hematoma* of the aorta and *penetrating atherosclerotic ulcer* of the aorta. These two conditions share with aortic dissection many of the predisposing risk factors and initial symptoms, and indeed, both may lead to either classic aortic dissection or aortic rupture. In light of their clinical similarities, it is appropriate to consider classic aortic dissection and its variants collectively among the "acute thoracic aortic syndromes," a category that also includes traumatic aortic transection and rupture, contained rupture (pseudoaneurysm), or acute expansion of thoracic aortic aneurysms.

INTRAMURAL HEMATOMA. Intramural hematoma is an acute aortic syndrome that is essentially a hemorrhage contained within the medial layer of the aortic wall but—unlike classic aortic dissection—without an evident tear in the intima or active communication between the hematoma and the aortic lumen. Hence, some practitioners have termed it *aortic dissection without intimal rupture.* The actual causes of intramural hematoma remain debatable. Historically, it has been presumed that intramural hematoma results from rupture of the vasa vasorum within the aortic wall. Others have argued, however, that the hematoma results from a tear in the intima (too small to visualize) that permits transient blood flow from the lumen into the aortic wall, which then thromboses to form a hematoma rather than a false lumen. The hematoma can be localized or discrete, but more often the hemorrhage extends for a variable distance by dissecting along the outer media beneath the adventitia.

Clinically, intramural hematoma can be indistinguishable from true aortic dissection. The risk factors, signs, and symptoms associated with intramural hematoma resemble those seen in classic aortic dissection, and it is therefore impossible to predict on clinical grounds (without an imaging study) whether a patient with suspected aortic dissection has a classic aortic dissection or intramural hematoma. Indeed, a significant minority—historically 10 percent to 17 percent—of apparent aortic dissection cases are diagnosed as intramural hematoma. Furthermore, many of the acute complications of aortic dissection such as aortic insufficiency, rupture into the pericardium, pleural and pericardial effusions, and branch vessel occlusion also occur with intramural hematoma, raising the question of whether intramural hematoma is just a morphological variant of aortic dissection or a distinct clinical entity with a different course and prognosis.

On axial imaging studies (i.e., CT, MRI, and TEE) intramural hematoma appears as a crescentic or sometimes circumferential thickening of the aortic wall, with no evidence of flow within the hematoma. The appearance of the thickened wall, especially in the ascending aorta, is often subtle on TEE, so the reader must be vigilant when clinical suspicion is high. CT scanning is the modality that best demonstrates the intramural hematoma. On a non-contrast-enhanced CT scan (see Fig. 53–24A) it appears as a continuous, crescentic, high-attenuation area along the aortic wall without evidence of an intimal tear, false lumen, or associated intimal atherosclerotic ulcer. This first examination is followed by a contrast-enhanced CT scan (see Fig. 53–24B), which demonstrates failure of the intramural hematoma to enhance (appearing as a darker crescentic thickening of the aortic wall), thereby excluding communication with the aortic lumen. In some cases, it may be challenging to distinguish intramural hematoma from aortic dissection with thrombosis of the false lumen or from mural thrombus within an aortic aneurysm. With an intramural hematoma, however, the aortic lumen retains its overall size and round shape, unlike the case with aortic dissection or a thrombus-lined aneurysm.

Conversely, intramural hematoma is often not detected by catheter-based contrast aortography, because this technique images the aortic lumen itself—which, in this case, appears normal—and not the aortic wall where the abnormality lies. During the years that contrast aortography was the standard imaging technique for suspected aortic dissection, intramural hematomas often went clinically unrecognized. In fact, the sensitivity of aortography for detecting intramural hematoma is as low as 19 percent[103]; therefore, although a negative aortogram can exclude the presence of classic aortic dissection, it does not reliably exclude the important variant of intramural hematoma.

Although intramural hematoma is now recognized as pathoanatomically distinct from classic aortic dissection, its natural history is still debated. When followed with serial imaging studies, it can have four possible courses: the hematoma may persist (although its thickness may change); it may be reabsorbed, so that the appearance of the aortic wall

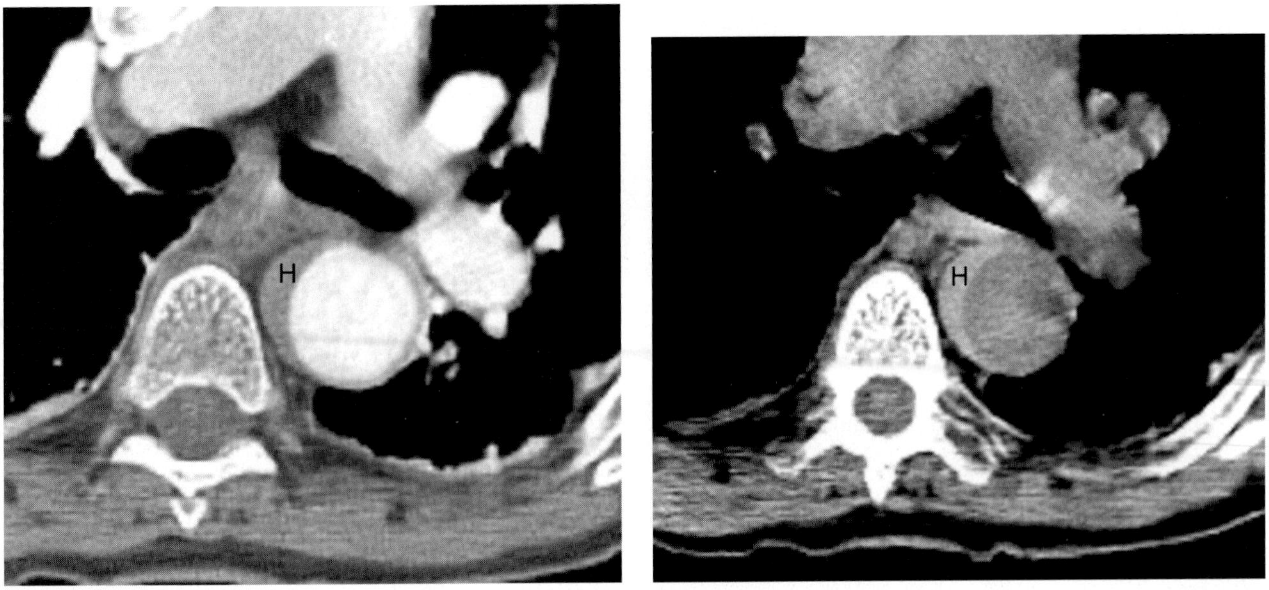

A B

FIGURE 53–24 Intramural hematoma of the descending thoracic aorta. **A,** An axial contrast-enhanced computed tomography (CT) scan at the level of the pulmonary artery demonstrating crescentic dark thickening of the aortic wall (H) that does not enhance, confirming the presence of an intramural hematoma. Note that neither the size nor the shape of the aortic lumen is distorted the way it would typically be in the presence of a classic aortic dissection. **B,** On a non-contrast-enhanced CT scan there is crescentic thickening of the aortic wall that is of increased density (H) compared with blood in the lumen, consistent with an intramural hematoma of the aorta.

returns to normal; it may lead to an aortic aneurysm; or it may convert to a classic aortic dissection, with the development of a typical intimal flap and flow in a false lumen.

In the 1990s, several retrospective reports described the outcomes of intramural hematoma, but the study samples were small. More recently, Sawhney and colleagues[104] performed a review of 160 patients from 11 studies reporting outcomes of aortic intramural hematoma and found that proximal intramural hematoma was associated with a mortality rate of 47 percent when managed medically compared with 24 percent when managed surgically. On the other hand, distal intramural hematoma was associated with a mortality rate of 13 percent with medical management compared with 15 percent with surgical repair. These rates are similar to those for classic aortic dissection as reported by the IRAD[67]: 58 percent for proximal aortic dissection when managed medically compared with 26 percent when managed surgically, and 11 percent for distal aortic dissection with medical management compared with 31 percent with surgical repair. Consequently, most treatment centers currently accept a general management strategy for aortic intramural hematoma similar to that used for classic aortic dissection: proximal aortic involvement is treated surgically[105] and distal aortic involvement is managed medically. Physicians should have a low threshold for proceeding to surgery in patients with distal disease if symptoms persist or evidence of progression is seen, however. Medical management should therefore include serial imaging studies to monitor progression or regression of the intramural hematoma.

It should be noted that several recent reports have suggested that the outcomes associated with proximal intramural hematoma may be more benign than with classic aortic dissection, with a large proportion of patients surviving with medical therapy alone. For example, Song and coworkers[106] reported in-hospital mortality rates for medically managed proximal and distal intramural hematoma of only 7 percent and 1 percent, respectively, both of which are substantially lower than the rates of 47 percent and 13 percent, respectively, reported by Sawhney and coworkers.

How can such dramatic differences be reconciled? It may be that the samples studied were not comparable. In fact, in Song's series, 29 percent of apparent aortic dissection cases were diagnosed as intramural hematoma, a proportion about double what other investigators have reported. It is therefore possible that in this series, more "subtle" cases of intramural hematoma, which would go undetected in other hospitals and which are likely to be associated with a lower risk of progression or rupture, were identified and included. There may in fact be a continuum of risk for intramural hematoma rather than an absolute risk. The morphological features that distinguish intramural hematoma from classic aortic dissection, such as the absence of a patent false lumen, suggest that intramural hematomas are somewhat less likely to rupture. However, factors that increase aortic wall stress, such as large aortic diameters and thick hematomas, could increase the risk of rupture or dissection. Indeed, one recent study of acute intramural hematoma[107] found that a maximum aortic diameter 50 mm or larger was an independent predictor of progression, whereas in another study of patients with distal intramural hematoma managed medically,[108] both a maximum aortic diameter of 40 mm or larger and a maximum aortic wall thickness of 10 mm or larger were independent predictors of progression. These findings confirm that some patients with intramural hematoma may be at considerably lower risk than others, suggesting that baseline differences in patient characteristics could substantially influence outcomes. However, until further studies help to better define those patients at very low risk, we still recommend the strategy of routine aortic surgery for proximal intramural hematoma.[109]

PENETRATING ATHEROSCLEROTIC ULCER. Penetrating atherosclerotic ulcer, first defined in the modern literature in 1986, is an ulceration of an atherosclerotic lesion of the aorta that penetrates the internal elastic lamina and allows hematoma formation within the media of the aortic wall (Fig. 53–25). Although such ulcerations usually occur in the descending thoracic aorta, they may also localize in the arch or rarely in the ascending aorta. The hematoma that results from a penetrating atherosclerotic ulcer usually remains localized or extends several centimeters in length, but a classic false lumen typically does not develop. However, some cases of intramural hematoma of the aorta may in fact result from small penetrating atherosclerotic ulcers that have escaped detection on imaging studies but are later identified at the time of surgery.[110]

Atherosclerotic aortic ulcers penetrate through the media in one-quarter of cases to cause aortic pseudoaneurysms or less often through the adventitia to cause transmural aortic rupture. Rarely, a penetrating atherosclerotic ulcer may progress to an extensive classic aortic dissection. Over time, penetrating atherosclerotic ulcers frequently lead to the late formation of saccular or fusiform aortic aneurysms.

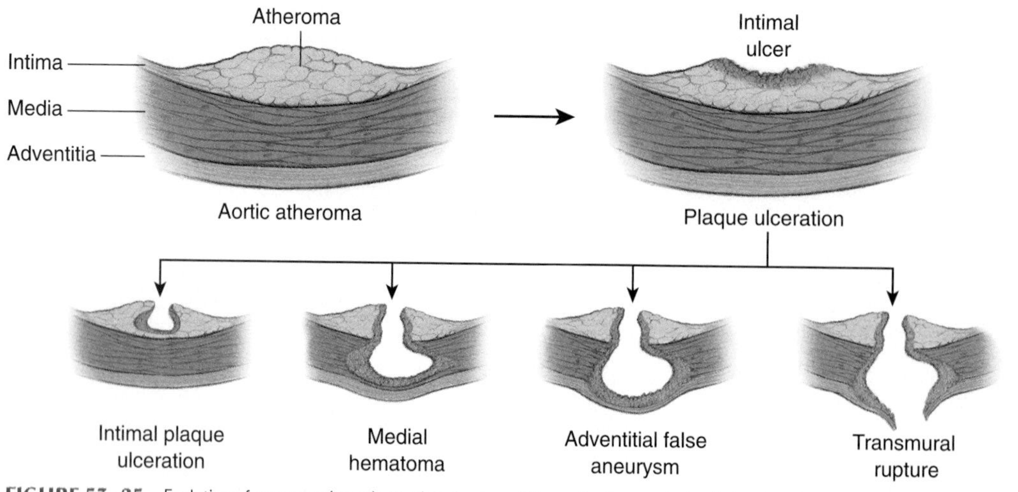

FIGURE 53–25 Evolution of a penetrating atherosclerotic ulcer of the aorta. Once an intimal ulcer has formed, it may then progress to a variable depth. Penetration through the intima causes a medial hematoma, while penetration through the media leads to the formation of a pseudoaneurysm, and perforation through the adventitial layer results in aortic rupture. (From Stanson AW, Kazmier FJ, Hollier LH, et al: Penetrating atherosclerotic ulcers of the thoracic aorta: Natural history and clinicopathological correlations. Ann Vasc Surg 1:15, 1986.)

Patients in whom penetrating atherosclerotic ulcers develop tend to be elderly with a history of hypertension and smoking. The majority have evidence of other atherosclerotic cardiovascular disease and as many as half also have a history of a preexisting abdominal or thoracic aortic aneurysm. Initial symptoms include chest and back pain similar to that of aortic dissection, and the majority are hypertensive at initial evaluation. However, since penetrating atherosclerotic ulcers tend to be localized, the vascular compromise or aortic regurgitation that often complicates aortic dissection does not develop.

Chest radiographs often demonstrate a dilated descending thoracic aorta as well as left-sided or bilateral pleural effusions. Aortography had been the diagnostic standard for detecting a penetrating atherosclerotic ulcer, with the lesion appearing as a contrast-filled outpouching in the descending aorta in the absence of an intimal flap or false lumen. However, penetrating atherosclerotic ulcers are now particularly well visualized with the use of CT or MRA (Fig. 53–26), in which the lesion appears as a focal ulceration with thickening of the aortic wall and consistent with an associated intramural hematoma. TEE may identify the presence of a culprit atherosclerotic ulcer in the setting of a visible intramural hematoma, but making the diagnosis is more difficult than with the above mentioned imaging modalities.

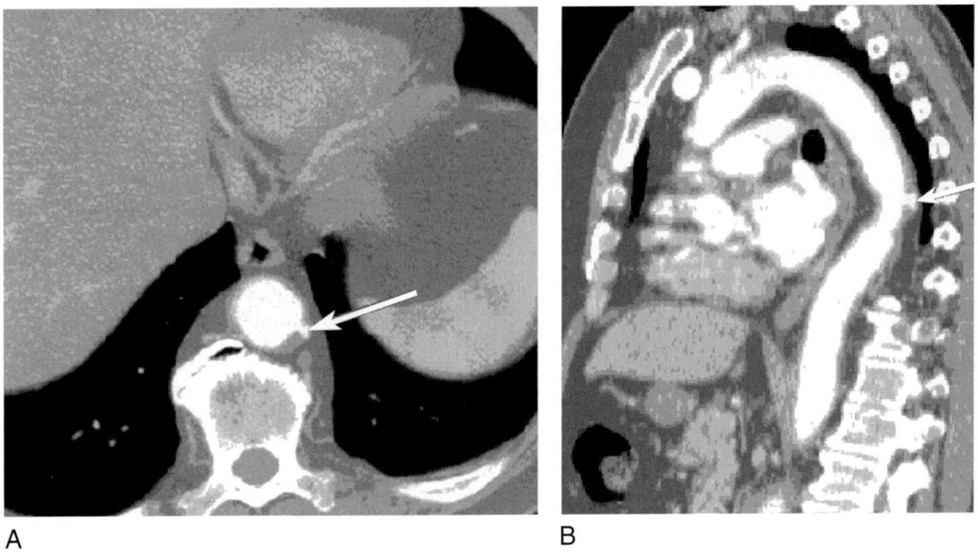

FIGURE 53–26 Contrast-enhanced CT scan through the distal descending aorta demonstrating the presence of a penetrating atherosclerotic ulcer. **A,** An axial image showing a small discrete ulcer (arrow) penetrating the aortic intima and producing a very localized hematoma within the aortic wall. **B,** Computed tomography angiogram in the same patient showing how the ulcer (arrow) projects out from the lumen of the distal descending aorta.

The natural history of a penetrating atherosclerotic ulcer remains largely unclear, and likely differs significantly between patients presenting with symptoms (i.e., acute aortic syndrome) versus without symptoms (i.e., an incidental finding). Coady and colleagues found that the risk of rupture and 1-year mortality are greater among patients with penetrating atherosclerotic ulcer than among those with aortic dissection.[111] At present, no definitive treatment strategy has been agreed upon. Certainly, patients who are hemodynamically unstable or who have evidence of pseudoaneurysm formation or transmural rupture should undergo urgent surgical repair. Continued or recurrent pain, distal embolization, and progressive aneurysmal dilation are also indications for surgery. However, it remains unclear if otherwise stable patients with distal penetrating atherosclerotic ulcers should undergo surgery or can be safely managed medically, as in the case of classic aortic dissection. In a study by Tittle and colleagues[112] of 26 patients with penetrating atherosclerotic ulcer, there was no difference in the 1- or 5-year survival between surgical and medical management strategies, suggesting that surgery may not improve the otherwise poor prognosis. On the other hand, there is growing optimism that transluminal placement of an endovascular stent-graft may become a lower risk alternative to surgery in such patients.

Ganaha and coworkers[113] recently examined the outcomes of 31 patients with penetrating atherosclerotic ulcers, of whom 17 were managed medically, whereas 8 underwent surgical repair and the other 6 underwent stent-grafting for evidence of aortic rupture or impending rupture. Importantly, there was no significant difference in early survival among the three strategies. The authors compared patients with a progressive in-hospital course—defined as aortic rupture, hematoma expansion, or appearance of a distinct false lumen—to those with a stable course. Uncontrolled pain and an enlarging pleural effusion were both highly predictive of a progressive course. CT findings associated with a progressive rather than a stable course included maximum diameter of the ulcer (21 mm versus 12 mm, respectively), maximum depth of the ulcer (14 mm versus 7 mm, respectively), and an ulcer located in the proximal third of the descending aorta rather than more distal. Using these various markers, about half of the patients in their study would have been considered low-risk for a progressive course. We recommend treating patients with such uncomplicated conditions with antihypertensive medications and close monitoring with serial imaging studies, similar to the management of a patient with a distal aortic dissection.

Aortic Trauma

See Chapter 65.

Aortic Atheroembolic Disease

See Chapter 54.

Acute Aortic Occlusion

Acute aortic occlusion is an infrequent, but potentially catastrophic, condition with an early mortality rate of 31 to 52 percent. It is caused by either embolic occlusion of the infrarenal aorta at the bifurcation, known as a "saddle embolus," or acute thrombosis of the abdominal aorta. At least 95 percent of aortic emboli originate from the left side of the heart, typically as a thrombus from the left atrium secondary to atrial fibrillation, particularly in the setting of rheumatic mitral stenosis, or from the left ventricle secondary to myocardial infarction, aneurysm, or dilated cardiomyopathy. Less common cardiac sources of emboli include atrial myxoma, prosthetic valve thrombus, and acute bacterial or fungal endocarditis. Primary thrombosis accounts for the remaining 35 to 92 percent of acute aortic occlusions. Seventy-five to 80 percent of thrombotic aortic occlusions occur in the setting of underlying severe aortoiliac occlusive disease and are frequently precipitated by a low-flow state secondary to heart failure or dehydration. In patients without aortoiliac occlusive disease, a hypercoagulable state may precipitate thrombosis of an abdominal aortic aneurysm and lead to aortic occlusion.[114]

Acute aortic occlusion is in most cases heralded by the sudden onset of excruciating bilateral lower extremity pain, usually radiating from the midportion of the thigh distally and associated with weakness, numbness, and paresthesias. Nonclassic manifestations include sudden onset of bilateral lower extremity weakness, severe hypertension from renal artery involvement, and abdominal pain from mesenteric ischemia. Persistent ischemia may lead to myonecrosis with secondary hypotension, hyperkalemia, myoglobinuria, and acute tubular necrosis. If perfusion is not reestablished within hours, death is almost inevitable.

DIAGNOSIS. Physical examination reveals cold pale extremities that are cyanotic and often exhibit a mottled, reticulated, and reddish blue appearance that may progress to the blue-black color of gangrene. Pulses are notably absent below the abdominal aorta, and capillary refill is absent. Signs of ischemic neuropathy are present and include symmetrical weakness, loss of all modalities of sensation (usually with demarcation at the level of the midthigh), and diminished or absent deep tendon reflexes. When neurological symptoms predominate, patients are often mistakenly thought to have spinal cord infarction or compression and their ischemic symptoms may initially be overlooked. In fact, as many as 11 to 17 percent of such patients first undergo neurological or neurosurgical evaluation before the vascular cause is recognized.

The diagnosis of acute aortic occlusion is confirmed by aortography. While some practitioners suggest that all stable patients should undergo the procedure, others advise prompt surgical intervention without angiography if the diagnosis is strongly suspected, since added delays increase the likelihood of irreversible ischemic damage to the limbs. Aortography is desirable in the presence of concomitant abdominal pain, hypertension, or anuria to evaluate the possibility of renal and mesenteric arterial involvement.

MANAGEMENT. Once a clinical diagnosis of acute aortic occlusion is made, intravenous heparin therapy should be initiated while the patient awaits immediate surgery. A saddle embolus can be removed by using Fogarty balloon-tipped catheters inserted through a transfemoral arterial approach under local anesthesia. If the embolus cannot be retrieved with Fogarty catheters, removal by direct transabdominal aortotomy is undertaken. Patients with thrombotic occlusion generally undergo either direct aortic reconstruction or revascularization with aortofemoral or axillofemoral bypass. The operative mortality rate for acute aortic occlusion is 31 to 40 percent and as high as 85 percent among patients with severe left ventricular dysfunction or a hypercoagulable state. Limb salvage rates are as high as 98 percent. Lifelong anticoagulant therapy is necessary after surgery in almost all cases to prevent recurrent emboli.

Aortoarteritis Syndromes

See Chapters 54 and 82.

Bacterial Infections of the Aorta

Infected aortic aneurysms are rare, with as few as one case per year reported from large medical centers. In an effort to avoid confusion with infections truly of fungal origin, the term *infected aneurysm* has gradually replaced the original designation, *mycotic aneurysm*, used by Osler to define localized dilation in the wall of the aorta caused by sepsis. Although saccular aneurysms are seen most commonly, infections can also cause fusiform and false aneurysms. In a minority of cases, infection may arise in a preexistent aortic aneurysm, typically atherosclerotic ones. Rarely, one may encounter nonaneurysmal bacterial aortitis.

PATHOGENESIS. Aortic infection can arise by several mechanisms. A septic embolus from bacterial endocarditis was once the most common cause but has become rare in the era of efficacious antibiotic treatment of septicemia. Contiguous spread of infection from adjacent sites is also infrequently seen. The most common cause of an infected aneurysm is direct deposition of circulating bacteria in a diseased, atherosclerotic, or traumatized aortic intima, after which organisms penetrate the aortic wall through breeches in intimal integrity to cause microbial arteritis. In some cases, aortic infections occur in patients with impaired immunity as a consequence of chronic disease, immunosuppressive therapy, or immune deficiency, whereas in other cases, the infection is introduced from distant surgical sites or via intraaortic catheterization procedures.[115]

MICROBIOLOGY. Although virtually any organism can infect the aorta, certain bacteria seem to have a proclivity for this site. *Staphylococcus aureus* and *Salmonella* species are consistently the most frequently identified organisms.[115,116] *Salmonella* commonly infects atherosclerotic arteries but can also adhere to a normal aortic wall and directly penetrate an intact intima. Other gram-positive organisms, particularly *Pneumococcus*, and gram-negative organisms can also cause infected aortic aneurysms. *Pseudomonas, Bacteroides fragilis, Campylobacter fetus, Neisseria gonorrhoeae*, and fungal infections are seen less often. Aortic infections with unusual organisms now occur with increasing frequency in the overtly immunocompromised population.

CLINICAL MANIFESTATIONS. Most patients with infected aortic aneurysm are febrile, with extremely high fevers and rigors being common. Symptoms can arise from localized expansion of an infected aneurysm, which is palpable in as many as 50 percent of patients and almost always tender. A tender and pulsatile abdominal mass in a febrile patient should therefore be considered an infected aneurysm until proved otherwise.

Leukocytosis and an elevated erythrocyte sedimentation rate are present in most cases. When positive, blood cultures are helpful in suggesting the diagnosis and identifying the pathogen. In any patient with fever of unknown origin and documented *Salmonella* bacteremia, an arterial source of infection should be considered. The absence of positive blood cultures, however, does not exclude the diagnosis of infected aortic aneurysm, because cultures have been found to be negative in 25 percent of cases.

Although abdominal ultrasonography may identify the presence of an aortic aneurysm, CT scanning is superior in demonstrating associated pathological findings suggestive of an infectious cause. Sometimes the aorta is normal in size when bacterial aortitis is first evaluated, however, so lack of aneurysmal dilation does not exclude the diagnosis. In such cases, if a patient's fever, leukocytosis, and pain persist, follow-up imaging should be performed because the aorta can rapidly dilate during the course of the infection. Aortography can also be used to make the diagnosis and is sometimes performed preoperatively to assist in surgical planning.

The natural history of infected aortic aneurysms is that of expansion and eventual rupture, with extremely rapid progression. *Salmonella* and other gram-negative infections have a greater tendency to early rupture and death. Overall mortality from infected aortic aneurysms is more than 50 percent, despite advances in therapy.

MANAGEMENT. Infected aortic aneurysms require treatment with intravenous antibiotics and most often surgical excision. The standard surgical approach involves resection of the infected aneurysm and infected retroperitoneal tissue, oversewing of the native aorta as stumps, and restoration of distal perfusion by placement of an extraanatomical bypass graft tunneled through unaffected tissue planes to avoid placing a graft in a contaminated region. Antibiotic therapy must be continued postoperatively for at least 6 weeks. Several reports suggest that in selected patients with localized infection and no gross pus, an effective and simpler surgical approach is in situ reconstruction of the aorta with a prosthetic graft[117] or cryopreserved arterial allograft.[118]

Primary Tumors of the Aorta

Primary tumors of the aorta are quite rare, although as a result of improvements in noninvasive imaging techniques, the frequency of reports of such tumors has increased significantly over the past two decades. Most are diagnosed in the seventh to eighth decades of life. The thoracic aorta and abdominal aorta are involved with equal frequency. In several cases, aortic tumors have appeared in association with previously inserted Dacron aortic grafts. Histologically, the majority of primary aortic tumors are classified as sarcomas, with the malignant fibrous histiocytoma subtype especially common.

The majority of primary aortic tumors arise in the intima and grow along the intimal surface and into the aortic lumen to form polypoid masses (often with superimposed thrombus), but they tend to not invade the aortic wall.[119] Intimal tumors may be characterized by symptoms of vascular obstruction from narrowing of the aortic lumen or, more typically, by signs and symptoms of peripheral embolization identical to those of atherothrombotic emboli. Emboli are commonly a mixture of tumor and thrombus, and the correct diagnosis may remain obscure until histological analysis of an embolectomy specimen is completed. Less commonly, aortic tumors arise in the medial or adventitial layers of the aortic wall. Such tumors tend to not invade the aortic lumen but, instead, behave as aggressive mass lesions and cause constitutional symptoms or back pain.

Since primary aortic tumors are so uncommon and their features nonspecific, the diagnosis is rarely considered before surgical exploration or necropsy. However, several imaging modalities can be helpful in suggesting the diagnosis. Aortography demonstrates narrowing of the lumen or an intraluminal filling defect in the presence of an intimal tumor, but it may be negative if the tumor is adventitial. Intraaortic biopsy of an intraluminal aortic mass with intravascular biopsy forceps guided by aortography has been reported.[120] CT scanning can detect intimal tumors but may not easily differentiate these masses from protruding atheromas. MRI may better define both the tumor anatomy and the extent of invasion. Finally, the ability of TEE to image the aortic intima may make it especially useful in the detection of intimal tumors of the thoracic aorta (Fig. 53–27).

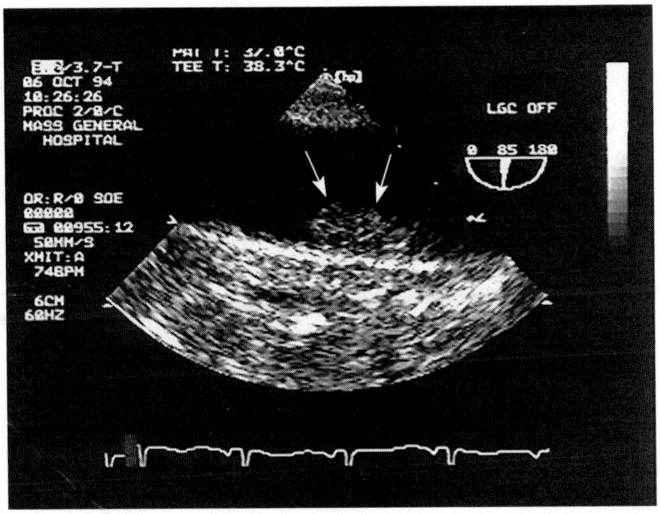

FIGURE 53–27 Transesophageal echocardiogram in a long-axis view of the descending thoracic aorta demonstrating a primary tumor of the aorta (arrows) protruding into the lumen. The tumor, 3.5 cm in length, involves the intimal layer but does not appear to be invading any farther into the aortic wall.

Treatment of primary aortic tumors has met with little success. Because the majority of patients initially have metastatic disease, surgical approaches are often only palliative, to prevent further embolization. Many patients die secondary to the consequences of multiple emboli to vital organs. Of those undergoing surgical therapy, the large majority die within days to months postoperatively.

Acknowledgment

The author wishes to gratefully acknowledge the contributions of Drs. Kim A. Eagle, Roman W. DeSanctis, and Eve E. Slater to previous versions of this chapter in earlier editions of this text.

REFERENCES

1. Fleishmann D, Hastie TJ, Dannegger FC, et al: Quantitative determination of age-related geometric changes in the normal abdominal aorta. J Vasc Surg 33:97, 2001.
2. Stefanadis C, Vlachopoulos C, Karayannacos P, et al: Effect of vasa vasorum flow on structure and function of the aorta in experimental animals. Circulation 91:2669, 1995.
3. Kelly RP, Tunin R, Kass DA: Effect of reduced aortic compliance on cardiac efficiency and contractile function of in situ canine left ventricle. Circ Res 71:490, 1992.
4. Wanhainen A, Bjork M, Boman K, et al: Influence of diagnostic criteria on the prevalence of abdominal aortic aneurysm. J Vasc Surg 34:229, 2001.
5. Lederle FA, Johnson GR, Wilson SE, et al: Prevalence and associations of abdominal aortic aneurysm detected through screening. Aneurysm Detection and Management (ADAM) Veterans Affairs Cooperative Study Group. Ann Intern Med 126:441, 1997.
6. Lederle FA, Johnson GR, Wilson SE, et al: Abdominal aortic aneurysm in women. J Vasc Surg 34:122, 2001.
7. Davies MJ: Aortic aneurysm formation: Lessons from human studies and experimental models. Circulation 98:193, 1998.
8. Lindholt JS, Juul S, Ashton HA, Scott RAP: Indicators of infection *Chlamydia pneumoniae* are associated with expansion of abdominal aortic aneurysm. J Vasc Surg 34:212, 2001.
9. Henderson EL, Geng Y-J, Sukhova GK, et al: Death of smooth muscle cells and expression of mediators of apoptosis by T lymphocytes in human abdominal aortic aneurysms. Circulation 99:96, 1999.
10. McMillan WD, Tamarina NA, Cipollone M, et al: Size matters: The relationship between MMP-9 expression and aortic diameter. Circulation 96:2228, 1997.
11. Longo GM, Xiong W, Greiner TC, et al: Matrix metalloproteinases 2 and 9 work in concert to produce aortic aneurysms. J Clin Invest 110:625, 2002.
12. Prall AK, Longo M, Mayhan WG, et al: Doxycycline in patients with abdominal aortic aneurysms and in mice: Comparison of serum levels and effect on aneurysm growth in mice. J Vasc Surg 35:923, 2002.
13. Curci JA, Mao D, Bohner DG, et al: Preoperative treatment with doxycycline reduces aortic wall expression and activation of matrix metalloproteinases in patients with abdominal aortic aneurysms. J Vasc Surg 31:325, 2000.
14. Baxter BT, Pearce WH, Waltke EA, et al: Prolonged administration of doxycycline in patients with small asymptomatic abdominal aortic aneurysms: Report of a prospective (phase II) multicenter study. J Vasc Surg 36:1, 2002.
15. Vammen S, Lindholt JS, Ostergaard L, et al: Randomized double-blind trial of roxithromycin for prevention of abdominal aortic aneurysm expansion. Br J Surg 88:1066, 2001.
16. Shi G-P, Sukhova GK, Grubb A: Cystatin C deficiency in human atherosclerosis and aortic aneurysms. J Clin Invest 104:1191, 1999.
17. Muluk SC, Gertler JP, Brewster DC, et al: Presentation and patterns of aortic aneurysms in young patients. J Vasc Surg 20:880, 1994.
18. Kiell CS, Ernst CB: Advances in the management of abdominal aortic aneurysm. Adv Surg 26:73, 1993.
19. Lederle FA, Simel DL: Does this patient have abdominal aortic aneurysm? JAMA 281:77, 1999.
20. Fink HA, Lederle FA, Roth CS, et al: The accuracy of physical examination to detect aortic aneurysms. Arch Intern Med 160:833, 2000.
21. Lindholt JS, Vammen S, Juul S, et al: The validity of ultrasonographic scanning as screening method for abdominal aortic aneurysm. Eur J Vasc Endovasc Surg 17:472, 1999.
22. Lederle FA, Wilson SE, Johnson GR, et al: Variability in measurement of abdominal aortic aneurysms. J Vasc Surg 21:945, 1995.
23. Petersen MJ, Cambria RP, Kaufman JA, et al: Magnetic resonance angiography in the preoperative evaluation of abdominal aortic aneurysms. J Vasc Surg 21:891, 1995.
24. Multicentre Aneurysm Screening Study Group: Multicentre aneurysm screening study (MASS): Cost-effectiveness analysis of screening for abdominal aortic aneurysms based on four year results from a randomised controlled trial. BMJ 325:1135, 2002.
25. Crow P, Shaw E, Earnshaw JJ, et al: A single normal ultrasonographic scanning at age 65 years rules out significant aneurysm disease for life in men. Br J Surg 88:941, 2001.
26. Brown LC, Powell JT: Risk factors for aneurysm rupture in patients kept under ultrasound surveillance. UK Small Aneurysm Trial Participants. Ann Surg 230:289, 1999.

27. The United Kingdom Small Aneurysm Trial Participants: Long-term outcomes of immediate repair compared with surveillance of small abdominal aortic aneurysms. N Engl J Med 346:1445, 2002.
28. Lederle FA, Wilson ES, Johnson GR, et al: Immediate repair compared with surveillance of small abdominal aortic aneurysms. N Engl J Med 346:1437, 2002.
29. Thompson RW: Detection and management of small aortic aneurysms. N Engl J Med 346:1484, 2002.
30. Brewster DC, Geller SC, Kaufman JA, et al: Initial experience with endovascular aneurysm repair: Comparison of early results with outcome of conventional open repair. J Vasc Surg 27:992, 1998.
31. Blum U, Voshage G, Lammer J, et al: Endoluminal stent-grafts for infrarenal abdominal aortic aneurysms. N Engl J Med 336:13, 1997.
32. Zarins CK, White RA, Schwarten D, et al: AneuRx stent graft versus open surgical repair of abdominal aortic aneurysms: Multicenter prospective clinical trial. J Vasc Surg 29:292, 1999.
33. Finlayson SR, Birkmeyer JD, Fillinger MF, et al: Should endovascular surgery lower the threshold for repair of abdominal aortic aneurysms? J Vasc Surg 29:973, 1999.
34. Kioka Y, Tanabe A, Kotani Y, et al: Review of coronary artery disease in patients with infrarenal abdominal aortic aneurysm. Circulation 66:1110, 2002.
35. Rihal CS, Eagle KA, Mickel MC, et al: Surgical therapy for coronary artery disease among patients with combined coronary artery and peripheral vascular disease. Circulation 91:46, 1995.
36. Brophy C, Tilson JE, Tilson MD: Propranolol delays the formation of aneurysms in the male blotchy mouse. J Surg Res 44:687, 1988.
37. The Propranolol Aneurysm Trial Investigators: The propranolol for small abdominal aortic aneurysms: Results of a randomized trial. J Vasc Surg 35:72, 2002.
38. Guo D, Hasham S, Kuang S-Q, et al: Familial thoracic aortic aneurysms and dissections. Circulation 103:2461, 2001.
39. Coady MA, Davis RR, Roberts M, et al: Familial patterns of thoracic aortic aneurysms. Arch Surg 134:361, 1999.
40. Biddinger A, Rocklin M, Coselli J, Milewicz DM: Familial thoracic aortic dilatations and dissections: A case control study. J Vasc Surg 25:506, 1997.
41. Milewicz DM, Chen H, Park E-S, et al: Reduced penetrance and variable expressivity of familial thoracic aneurysms/dissections. Am J Cardiol 82:474, 1998.
42. Vaughan CJ, Casey M, He J, et al: Identification of a chromosome 11q23.2-q24 locus for familial aortic aneurysm disease, a genetically heterogeneous disorder. Circulation 103:2469, 2001.
43. Nistri S, Sorbo MD, Marin M, et al: Aortic root dilatation in young men with normally functioning bicuspid aortic valves. Heart 82:19, 1999.
44. Nkomo VT, Enriquez-Sarano M, Ammash NM, et al: Bicuspid aortic valve associated with aortic dilatation: A community-based study. Arterioscler Thromb Vasc Biol 23:351, 2003.
45. DeSa M, Moshkovitz Y, Butany J, David TE: Histologic abnormalities of the ascending aorta and pulmonary trunk in patients with bicuspid aortic valve disease: Clinical relevance to the Ross procedure. J Thorac Cardiovasc Surg 118:588, 1999.
46. Huntington K, Hunter AGW, Chan K-L: A prospective study to assess the frequency of familial clustering of congential bicuspid aortic valve. J Am Coll Cardiol 30:1809, 1997.
47. Fedak PWM, Verma S, David T, et al: Clinical and pathophysiological implications of a bicuspid aortic valve. Circulation 106:900, 2002.
48. Davies RR, Goldstein LJ, Coady MA, et al: Yearly rupture or dissection rates for thoracic aortic aneurysms: Simple prediction based on size. Ann Thorac Surg 73:17, 2002.
49. Griepp RB, Ergin A, Gall JD, et al: Natural history of descending thoracic and thoracoabdominal aneurysms. Ann Thorac Surg 67:1927, 1999.
50. Dapunt OE, Galla JD, Sadeghi AM, et al: The natural history of thoracic aortic aneurysms. J Thorac Cardiovasc Surg 107:1323, 1994.
51. Johansson G, Markström U, Swedenborg J: Ruptured thoracic aortic aneurysms: A study of incidence and mortality rates. J Vasc Surg 21:985, 1995.
52. Devereux RB, Roman MJ: Aortic disease in Marfan's syndrome. N Engl J Med 340:1358, 1999.
53. Sundt TM, Mora BN, Moon MR, et al: Options for repair of a bicuspid aortic valve and ascending aortic aneurysm. Ann Thorac Surg 69;1333, 2000.
54. Russo CF, Massett S, Garatti A, et al: Aortic complications after bicuspid aortic valve replacement: Long-term results. Ann Thorac Surg 74:S1773, 2002.
55. Gott VL, Gillinov AM, Pyeritz RE, et al: Aortic root replacement: Risk factor analysis of a seventeen-year experience with 270 patients. J Thorac Cardiovasc Surg 109:536, 1995.
56. David TE, Ivanov J, Armstrong S, et al: Aortic valve-sparing operations in patients with aneurysms of the aortic root or ascending aorta. Ann Thorac Surg 74:S1758, 2002.
57. Moon MR, Sundt TM: Influence of retrograde cerebral perfu-sion during aortic arch procedures. Ann Thorac Surg 74:426, 2002.
58. Hagl C, Ergin MA, Galla JD, et al: Neurologic outcome after ascending aorta-aortic arch operations: Effect of brain protection technique in high-risk patients. J Thorac Cardiovasc Surg 121:1107, 2001.
59. Kazui T, Washiyama N, Muhammad BAH, et al: Improved results of atherosclerotic arch aneurysm operations with a refined technique. J Thorac Cardiovasc Surg 121:491, 2001.
60. Estera AL, Miller CC, Porat EE, et al: Staged repair of extensive aortic aneurysms. Ann Thorac Surg 74:S1803, 2002.
61. Cambria RP, Davison JK, Zannetti S, et al: Clinical experience with epidural cooling for spinal cord protection during thoracic and thoracoabdominal aneurysm repair. J Vasc Surg 25:234, 1997.
62. Coselli JS, LeMaire SA, Koksoy C, et al: Cerebrospinal fluid drainage reduces paraplegia following thoracoabdominal aortic aneurysm repair: Results of a randomized clinical trial. J Vasc Surg 35:635, 2002.
63. Coselli JS, Conkin LD, LeMaire SA: Thoracoabdominal aortic aneurysm repair: Review and update of current strategies. Ann Thorac Surg 74:S1881, 2002.
64. Dake MD, Miller DC, Mitchell RS, et al: The "first generation" of endovascular stent-grafts for patients with aneurysms of the descending thoracic aorta. J Thorac Cardiovasc Surg 116:689, 1998.
65. Shores J, Berger KR, Murphy EA, Pyeritz RE: Progression of aortic dilatation and the benefit of long-term β-adrenergic blockade in Marfan's syndrome. N Engl J Med 330:1335, 1994.
66. Meszaros I, Morocz J, Szlavi J, et al: Epidemiology and clinicopathology of aortic dissection: A population-based longitudinal study over 27 years. Chest 117:1271, 2000.
67. Hagan PG, Nienaber CA, Isselbacher EM, et al: International Registry of Acute Aortic Dissection (IRAD): New insights into an old disease. JAMA 283:897, 2000.
68. Eagle KA, Isselbacher EM, DeSanctis W: Cocaine-related aortic dissection in perspective. Circulation 105:1529, 2002.
69. Elkayam U, Ostzega E, Shotan A, Mehra A: Cardiovascular problems in pregnant women with the Marfan syndrome. Ann Intern Med 123:117, 1995.
70. Januzzi JL, Sabatine MS, Eagle KA, et al: Iatrogenic aortic dissection. Am J Cardiol 89:623, 2002.
71. von Kodolitsch Y, Simic O, Schwartz A, et al: Predictors of proximal aortic dissection at the time of aortic valve replacement. Circulation 100(Suppl 2):287, 1999.
72. Slater EE, DeSanctis RW: The clinical recognition of dissecting aortic aneurysm. Am J Med 60:625, 1976.
73. Spittell PC, Spittell JA Jr, Joyce JW, et al: Clinical features and differential diagnosis of aortic dissection: Experience with 236 cases (1980 through 1990). Mayo Clin Proc 68:642, 1993.
74. Nallamothu BK, Mahta RH, Saint S, et al: Syncope in acute aortic dissection: Diagnostic, prognostic, and clinical implications. Am J Med 133:468, 2002.
75. Kim MH, Eagle KA, Isselbacher EM: Bayesian persuasion. Circulation 100:e68, 1999.
76. Bossone E, Rampoldi V, Nienaber CA, et al: Usefulness of pulse deficits to predict in-hospital complications and mortality in patients with acute type A aortic dissection. Am J Cardiol 89:851, 2002.
77. Kamp TJ, Goldschmidt-Clermont PJ, Brinker JA, Resar JR: Myocardial infarction, aortic dissection, and thrombolytic therapy. Am Heart J 128:1234, 1994.
78. Bansal RC, Chandrasekaran K, Ayala K, Smith D: Frequency and explanation of false negative diagnosis of aortic dissection by aortography and transesophageal echocardiography. J Am Coll Cardiol 25:1393, 1995.
79. Ballal RS, Nanda NC, Gatewood R, et al: Usefulness of transesophageal echocardiography in assessment of aortic dissection. Circulation 84:1903, 1991.
80. Armstrong WF, Bach DS, Carey LM, et al: Clinical and echocardiographic findings in patients with suspected acute aortic dissection. Am Heart J 136:1051, 1998.
81. Moore AG, Eagle KA, Bruckman D, et al: Choice of computed tomography, transesophageal echocardiography, magnetic resonance imaging, and aortography in acute aortic dissection: International Registry of Acute Aortic Dissection (IRAD). Am J Cardiol 89:1235, 2002.
82. Rizzo RJ, Aranki SF, Aklog L, et al: Rapid noninvasive diagnosis and surgical repair of acute ascending aortic dissection. J Thorac Cardiovasc Surg 108:567, 1994.
83. Kern MJ, Serota H, Callicoat P, et al: Use of coronary arteriography in the preoperative management of patients undergoing urgent repair of the thoracic aorta. Am Heart J 119:143, 1990.
84. Penn MS, Smedira N, Lytle B, Brener SJ: Does coronary angiography before emergency aortic surgery affect in-hospital mortality? J Am Coll Cardiol 35:889, 2000.
85. Creswell LL, Kouchoukos NT, Cox JL, Rosenbloom M: Coronary artery disease in patients with type A aortic dissection. Ann Thorac Surg 59:585, 1995.
86. Murphy MB, Murray C, Shorten GD: Fenoldopam: A selective peripheral dopamine-receptor agonist for the treatment of hypertension. N Engl J Med 345:1548, 2001.
87. Isselbacher EM, Cigarroa JE, Eagle KA: Cardiac tamponade complicating proximal aortic dissection: Is pericardiocentesis harmful? Circulation 90:2375, 1994.
88. Sabik JF, Lytle BW, Blackstone EH, et al: Long-term effectiveness of operations for ascending aortic dissections. J Thorac Cardiovasc Surg 119:946, 2000.
89. Hirotani T, Kameda T, Kumamoto T, Shirota S: Results of a total aortic arch replacement of an acute aortic arch dissection. J Thorac Cardiovasc Surg 120:686, 2000.
90. Movsowitz HD, Levine RA, Hilgenberg AD, Isselbacher EM: Transesophageal echocardiographic description of the mechanisms of aortic regurgitation in acute type A aortic dissection: Implications for aortic valve repair. J Am Coll Cardiol 36:884, 2000.
91. Bavaria JE, Brinster DR, Gorman RC, et al: Advances in the treatment of acute type a dissection: An integrated approach, Ann Thorac Surg 74:S1848, 2002.
92. Kazui T, Washiyama N, Bashar AHM, et al: Role of biologic glue repair of proximal aortic dissection in the development of early and midterm redissection of the aortic root. Ann Thorac Surg 72:509, 2001.
93. Slonim SM, Nyman U, Semba CP, et al: Aortic dissection: Percutaneous management of ischemic complications with endovascular stents and balloon fenestration. J Vasc Surg 23:241, 1996.
94. Lauterbach SE, Cambria RP, Brewster DC, et al: Contemporary management of aortic branch compromise resulting from acute aortic dissection. J Vasc Surg 33:1185, 2001.
95. Nienaber CA, Fattori R, Lund G, et al: Nonsurgical reconstruction of thoracic aortic dissection by stent-graft placement. N Engl J Med 340:1539, 1999.
96. Dake MD, Kato N, Mitchell RS, et al: Endovascular stent-graft placement for the treatment of acute aortic dissection. N Engl J Med 340:1546, 1999.
97. Januzzi JL, Sabatine MS, Choi JC, et al: Refractory systemic hypertension following type B aortic dissection. Am J Cardiol 88:686, 2001.
98. Neri E, Sassi S, Massetti M, et al: Nonocclusive intestinal ischemia in patients with acute aortic dissection. J Vasc Surg 36:738, 2002.
99. Doroghazi RM, Slater EE, DeSanctis RW, et al: Long-term survival of patients with treated aortic dissection. J Am Coll Cardiol 3:1026, 1984.

100. Fattori R, Bacchi-Reggiani L, Bertaccini P, et al: Evolution of aortic dissection after surgical repair. Am J Cardiol 86:868, 2000.
101. Bernard Y, Zimmermann H, Chocron S, et al: False lumen patency as a predictor of late outcome in aortic dissection. Am J Cardiol 87:1378, 2001.
102. Neya K, Omoto R, Kyo S, et al: Outcome of Stanford type B acute aortic dissection. Circulation 86(Suppl 2):1, 1992.
103. Vilacosta I, San Roman JA, Ferreiros J, et al: Natural history and serial morphology of aortic intramural hematoma: A novel variant of aortic dissection. Am Heart J 134:495, 1997.
104. Sawhney NS, DeMaria AN, Blanchard DG: Aortic intramural hematoma: An increasingly recognized and potentially fatal entity. Chest 120:1340, 2001.
105. von Kodolitsch Y, Csosz SK, Koschyk DH, et al: Intramural hematoma of the aorta: Predictors of progression to dissection and rupture. Circulation 107:1158, 2003.
106. Song J-K, Kim H-S, Song JM, et al: Outcomes of medically treated patients with aortic intramural hematoma. Am J Med 113:244, 2002.
107. Kaji S, Nishigami K, Akasaka T, et al: Prediction of progression or regression of type A aortic intramural hematoma by computed tomography. Circulation 100(suppl II):II281, 1999.
108. Sueyoshi E, Imada T, Sakamoto I, et al: Analysis of predictive factors for progression of type B aortic intramural hematoma with computed tomography. J Vasc Surg 35:1179, 2002.
109. Isselbacher EM: Intramural hematoma of the aorta: Should we let down our guard? Am J Med 113:181, 2002.
110. Muluk SC, Kaufman JA, Torchiana DF, et al: Diagnosis and treatment of thoracic aortic intramural hematoma. J Vasc Surg 24:1022, 1996.
111. Coady MA, Rizzo JA, Hammond GL, et al: Penetrating ulcer of the thoracic aorta: How do we recognize it? How do we manage it? J Vasc Surg 27:1006, 1998.
112. Tittle SL, Lynch RJ, Cole PE, et al: Midterm follow-up of penetrating ulcer and intramural hematoma of the aorta. J Thorac Cardiovasc Surg 123:1051, 2002.
113. Ganaha F, Miller DC, Sugimoto K, et al: Prognosis of aortic intramural hematoma with and without penetrating atherosclerotic ulcer: A clinical and radiological analysis. Circulation 106:342, 2002.
114. Babu SC, Shah PM, Nitahara J: Acute aortic occlusion: Factors that influence outcome. J Vasc Surg 21:567, 1995.
115. Muller BT, Wegener OR, Grabitz K, et al: Mycotic aneurysms of the thoracic and abdominal aorta and iliac arteries: Experience with anatomic and extra-anatomic repair in 33 cases. J Vasc Surg 33:106, 2001.
116. Williamson WK, Keller FS: SCVIR annual meeting film panel session: Diagnosis and discussion of Case 4. J Vasc Interv Radiol 12:544, 2001.
117. Oderich GS, Panneton JM, Bower TC, et al: Infected aortic aneurysms: Aggressive presentation, complicated early outcome, and durable results. J Vasc Surg 34:900, 2001.
118. Leseche G, Castier Y, Petit M-D, et al: Long-term results of cryopreserved arterial allograft reconstruction in infected prosthetic grafts and mycotic aneurysms of the abdominal aorta. J Vasc Surg 34:616, 2001.
119. Khan A, Jilani F, Kaye S, Greenberg BR: Aortic wall sarcoma with tumor emboli and peripheral ischemia: Case report with review of literature. Am J Clin Oncol 20:73, 1997.
120. Ronaghi AH, Roberts AC, Rosenkrantz H: Intraaortic biopsy of a primary aortic tumor. J Vasc Interv Radiol 5:777, 1994.

CHAPTER 54

Peripheral Arterial Diseases

Mark A. Creager • Peter Libby

The term *peripheral arterial disease* (PAD) generally refers to atherosclerosis that obstructs the blood supply to the lower or upper extremities. The term *peripheral vascular disease* has less specificity because it encompasses a group of diseases affecting blood vessels, including not only PAD but also vasculitis, vasospasm, venous thrombosis, venous insufficiency, and lymphatic disorders.

Traditionally, cardiologists have devoted most of their efforts to the diagnosis and treatment of arterial disease of the coronary tree. Although cardiology training and practice often accord a place to diseases of the aorta, focus on the disease of the peripheral arteries has lagged. PAD strongly correlates with risk of major cardiovascular events, since it frequently associates with coronary and cerebral atherosclerosis. Moreover, symptoms of PAD, including intermittent claudication, jeopardize quality of life and independence for many patients. In contrast to coronary artery afflictions, PAD is commonly underdiagnosed and undertreated. Thus, practitioners of cardiology have increasing interest in the diagnosis and management of PAD. This chapter provides a framework for the approach to the diagnosis and management of the patient with PAD.

Epidemiology

The prevalence of PAD varies depending on the population studied, the diagnostic method used, and whether symptoms are included to derive estimates. Most epidemiological studies have used a noninvasive measurement, the ankle/brachial index (ABI), to diagnose PAD. The ABI is the ratio of the ankle to brachial systolic blood pressure and is described in greater detail later in this chapter. In relatively large population-based studies conducted in the United States, Europe, and the Middle East, the prevalence of PAD based on abnormal ABI ranged from 4.6 to 29 percent (Table 54–1).[1-5] In a free-living population, PAD was detected in less than 3 percent of persons younger than 60 years of age, but in more than 20 percent of those 75 years and older and 27 percent greater in men than in women.[6] In other studies, however, women had similar or greater prevalence of PAD. These aggregate data indicate that some 8 to 10 million individuals in the United States have PAD.

Questionnaires specifically designed to elicit symptoms of intermittent claudication can assess the prevalence of symptomatic disease in these populations. Estimates have varied depending on the age and gender of the population but generally indicate that only one-third to one-half of patients with PAD have symptoms of claudication. Overall, the estimated prevalence of claudication ranges from 1.0 to 4.5 percent of a population typically older than 40 years of age.[1,2] The prevalence and incidence of claudication increase with age and are greater in men than in women in most but not all studies (Fig. 54–1).[1,2,6]

There is less information regarding the incidence of critical limb ischemia, but it is estimated at 400 to 450 per million population per year.[1] The incidence of amputation ranges from 112 to 250 per million population per year.

Contribution of Risk Factors (see Chap. 36)

The well-known modifiable risk factors associated with coronary atherosclerosis also contribute to atherosclerosis of the peripheral circulation. Cigarette smoking, diabetes mellitus, dyslipidemia, hypertension, and hyperhomocysteinemia increase the risk of PAD (Table 54–2). Data derived from several observational studies (including the Edinburgh Artery Study, the Framingham Heart Study, and the Cardiovascular Health Study, among others) indicates a two- to fivefold increase in the risk of developing PAD in smokers.[1,2,7] Approximately 84 to 90 percent of patients with claudication are current or ex-smokers.[8] Progression of disease to critical limb ischemia and limb loss is more likely to occur in patients who continue to smoke than in those who stop.[9] Smoking can even increase the risk of developing PAD more than it does coronary artery disease. Patients with diabetes mellitus often have extensive and severe PAD and a greater propensity for vascular calcification.[10] Involvement of the femoral and popliteal arteries resembles that of nondiabetic persons, but distal disease affecting the tibial and peroneal arteries occurs more fre-

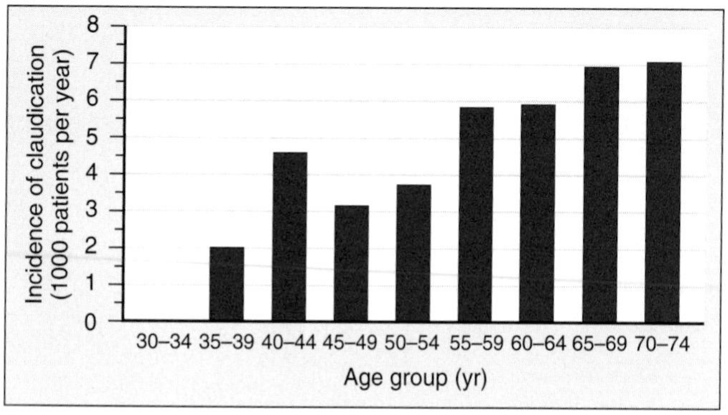

FIGURE 54–1 Age-related incidence of intermittent claudication derived from large population-based studies. (From Dormandy JA, Rutherford RB: Management of peripheral arterial disease (PAD), TASC Working Group. J Vasc Surg 31:51, 2000.)

TABLE 54–2 Risk of Peripheral Arterial Disease in Persons with Modifiable Risk Factors

Risk Factor	Estimated Relative Risk
Cigarette smoking	2.0-5.0
Diabetes mellitus	3.0-4.0
Hypertension	1.1-2.2
Hypercholesterolemia (per 40-50 mg/dl increase in total cholesterol)	1.2-1.4
Fibrinogen (per 0.7 g/liter increase in fibrinogen)	1.35
C-reactive protein	2.1
Hyperhomocysteinemia	2.0-3.2

TABLE 54–1 The Prevalence of Peripheral Arterial Disease

Study/Location	Population (No.)	Age (years)	Prevalence (%)
San Diego	613	38-82	11.7
The Jerusalem Lipid Research Clinic Prevalence Study	1592	≥35	4.6
The Edinburgh Artery Study	1592	55-74	9.0
The Cardiovascular Health Study	5084	≥65	12.4
The Rotterdam Study	7715	≥55	19.1
The Limburg PAOD Study	3650	40-78	12.4
The Strong Heart Study	4549	45-74	5.3
The PARTNERS Program	6979	50-69*; ≥70	29
The Framingham Offspring Study	3313	≥40	3.6

*Age 50-69 plus diabetes or cigarette smoking.

quently.[11] The risk of developing PAD increases two- to fourfold in patients with diabetes mellitus.[7] Among patients with PAD, diabetic patients are more likely to have an amputation than nondiabetic patients.

Abnormalities in lipid metabolism also are associated with an increased prevalence of PAD. Elevations in total or low-density lipoprotein (LDL) cholesterol increase the risk of developing PAD and claudication in some studies but not in others.[7,12,13] The odds ratio for developing claudication in the Framingham Heart Study was 1.2 for each 40 mg/dl increase in total cholesterol.[14] In a cohort of patients participating in a Lipid Research Clinic protocol, however, no association was found between LDL cholesterol and PAD based on a multiple logistic regression analysis that included cigarette smoking, blood pressure, glucose, and obesity.[6] Hypertriglyceridemia independently predicts risk for PAD.[7] Increased levels of lipoprotein(a) impart a twofold increased risk of developing PAD, with higher levels associated with a greater risk for critical limb ischemia.[15]

Hypertension increased the risk of claudication in the Framingham and the Framingham Offspring Studies, and the risk increased proportionally with the severity of hypertension.[5,16] Similarly, in the Edinburgh Artery Study, elevations in systolic blood pressure correlated with PAD. In the Limburg study, diastolic hypertension was associated with PAD.[17] However, not all epidemiological studies have found a link between hypertension and PAD.

Hyperhomocysteinemia increases the risk of developing atherosclerosis (see Chap. 36). In a meta-analysis of studies relating homocysteine level to atherosclerotic disease, the odds ratio for PAD in patients with increased homocysteine levels was 6.8.[18] Some 30 to 40 percent of patients with PAD have high levels of homocysteine. The plasma levels of B complex vitamins, including folate, cobalamin, and pyridoxal 5′ phosphate, all inversely relate to plasma homocysteine concentration, and patients taking B vitamin supplements have a lower risk of vascular disease.[19]

Fibrinogen levels also correlate with risk of developing PAD.[5,20] In the Edinburgh Artery Study, the risk for developing PAD increased 35 percent over 5 years for each 0.70 g/liter increase in fibrinogen.[21] Patients with PAD have elevated levels of C-reactive protein, a serological marker of systemic inflammation. In the Physicians' Health Study, the relative risk of developing PAD among men in the highest quartile for C-reactive protein concentrations was 2.5 (see Chap. 36).[13,22]

The risk of developing PAD and intermittent claudication increases progressively with the burden of contributing factors. In the Framingham study, the probability of claudication in a 70-year-old man whose only risk factor was smoking versus nonsmoking was 2.5 percent versus 0.8 percent per 4 years. In a 70-year-old male smoker who was also hypertensive, hypercholesterolemic, and diabetic, the risk increased to 24 percent per 4 years (Fig. 54–2).[14] Similar observations apply to women.

Pathobiology

Heterogeneity of Blood Vessels in Different Circulatory Beds

Atherosclerosis preferentially affects certain locations in the circulation. As discussed in Chapter 35, atheromatous lesions tend to form at flow dividers and branch points in arteries and usually spare veins. Recent progress has increased the understanding of the link between hydrodynamics of the circulation and the cellular and molecular mechanisms of atherosclerosis, and the atheroprotective functions of vascular wall cells. Chapter 35 discusses the focality of atherosclerosis in terms of local hemodynamic differences. Other questions remain, however: Are blood vessels intrinsically different in particular regions of the circulation? Do regional variations in the propensity for atherosclerosis merely depend on the external hemodynamic forces that impinge upon them? Indeed, vessels in different beds have distinct

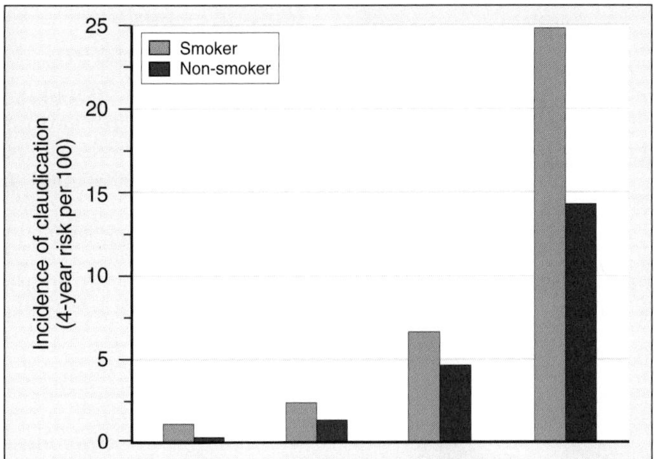

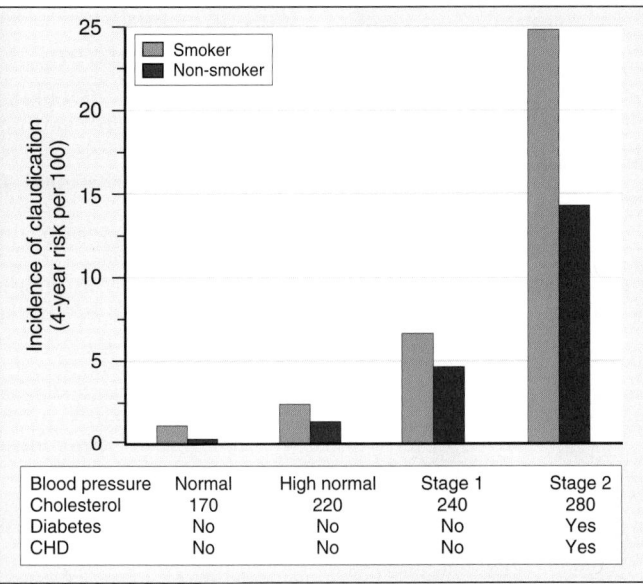

Blood pressure	Normal	High normal	Stage 1	Stage 2
Cholesterol	170	220	240	280
Diabetes	No	No	No	Yes
CHD	No	No	No	Yes

FIGURE 54–2 The incidence of intermittent claudication in the Framingham Heart Study in smokers and nonsmokers is compounded by an increased burden of risk factors. (From Murabito JM, D'Agostino RB, Silbershatz H, Wilson WF: Intermittent claudication: A risk profile from the Framingham Heart Study. Circulation 96:44, 1997.)

morphological, physiological, and pharmacological features, indicating intrinsic heterogeneity. Recent advances help us to understand the biological basis of differences among blood vessels. This section considers, in turn, new information regarding the development of blood vessels related to arterial heterogeneity, differences in functions of blood vessels depending on the circulatory bed, and finally, whether the mechanisms leading to clinical manifestations of arterial disease vary from one circulatory bed (e.g., the coronary circulation) and other arteries (e.g., the carotid, the aorta, or the femoral).

Developmental Biology of the Heterogeneity Among Blood Vessels

Endothelial cells have a common origin but acquire bed-specific characteristics during development.[23] The endothelial cells that form the inner lining of all blood vessels arise during embryogenesis from regions known as the blood islands, located on the embryo's periphery. Angioblasts, the predecessors of the endothelial cells, share this site with the precursors of blood cells. Despite arising from the same site, cells display considerable heterogeneity even during embryological and early postnatal development. Although endothelial cells presumably derive from a common precursor, the signals they encounter during vessel development differ. As rudimentary blood vessels begin to form, endothelial precursors interact with surrounding cells. The interchange permits spatial and temporal gradients of various stimuli and their receptors on the endothelial cells, leading to this cell type's heterogeneity in the adult.

Recent evidence has indicated that the cells that make up various compartments of the arterial wall can originate from bone marrow during postnatal life as well as from their traditional embryological sources. In particular, peripheral blood appears to contain endothelial precursor cells that may help the repair of areas of endothelial desquamation. Moreover, in injured or transplanted arteries, smooth muscle cells of apparent bone marrow origin can take up residence in the intima or media.[24,25] The endothelial progenitor cells bear characteristic markers such as CD133, CD34, and vascular endothelial growth factor receptor-2.[26]

Differential expression of endothelial genes in various types of blood vessels depends on transcriptional regulation by the local environment. For example, the promoter region of the gene that encodes von Willebrand factor directs expression in the endothelium of brain and heart microvessels but not in larger arteries. Indeed, co-culture of endothelial cells with cardiac myocytes, but not other cell types, could selectively activate a von Willebrand factor gene promoter construct.[27] Likewise, endothelial nitric oxide synthase gene activity in the heart shows bed-specific regulation.[28] Members of the EPH family of tyrosine kinase receptors and their ligands, known as ephrins, display heterogeneous expressions in arterial versus venous endothelial cells during development.[29] In the adult, arterial endothelial and smooth muscle cells, but not venous vascular cells, express EphrinB2.[30] This finding supports a stable lineage difference between cells that make up arteries and veins. These examples illustrate the molecular diversity of cells' location in the circulation. Phage display techniques have begun to substantiate the in vivo significance of vascular cell heterogeneity in atherogenesis.[31,32]

Smooth Muscle Cells Derive from Several Local Sources During Development

In contrast to endothelial cells thought to derive from a common precursor, smooth muscle cells can arise from many sources.[33] After endothelial cells form tubes, the rudimentary precursor of blood vessels, they recruit the cells that will become smooth muscle, or pericytes (smooth muscle-like cells associated with microvessels). In the descending aorta and arteries of the lower body, the regional mesoderm serves as the source of smooth muscle precursors. The mesodermal cells in somites give rise to the smooth muscle cells that invest much of the distal aorta and its branches. In arteries of the upper body, however, smooth muscle cells can actually derive from a completely different germ layer, neurectoderm rather than mesoderm. Before the neural tube closes, neurectodermal cells migrate and become the precursors of smooth muscle cells in the ascending aorta and some of its branches, including the carotid arteries (Fig. 54–3).[34] Smooth muscle cells in the coronary arteries derive from mesoderm, but in a special way. The precursors of coronary artery smooth muscle cells arise from yet another embryological source, a structure known as the *proepicardial organ*.[35]

As in the case of endothelial cells, smooth muscle cells show molecular heterogeneity early during development.[36] For example, the promoter of a characteristic smooth muscle gene, known as SM22, drives gene expression in venous but not arterial smooth muscle cells during embryogenesis.[37] A specific transcription factor known as dHAND signals the recruitment of mesenchyme by endothelial cells in an anatomically heterogeneous manner during development. In particular, dHAND regulation participates selectively in recruitment of mesenchyme in upper body blood vessels versus those of the more caudal portions of the embryo.[38] A CArG box-dependent enhancer within the regulatory regions of the cysteine-rich protein 1 gene directs this protein's expression in arterial but not venous or visceral smooth muscle cells.[39] These findings also point to molecular distinctions between the cells that compose different types of vessels.

Clinical Implications of Vascular Developmental Biology

Far from being of mere theoretical concern, the developmental biology of the arterial tree has important clinical implications in terms of issues that arise in daily practice. The distinct embryonic origins of smooth muscle cells in various arteries can help explain why some regions of the arterial tree have particular predilection to atherogenesis. Although local hydrodynamics doubtless control the expression of genes that protect against or promote atherogenesis (see Chap. 35), the cellular substrate acted on by biomechanical forces varies, as described earlier.

Curiously, certain regions of the arterial tree develop intimal "cushions" early in life. These cushions consist of regions of intimal expansion populated by smooth muscle cells and extracellular matrix (Fig. 54–4). Two regions of intimal cushion formation of particular consequence for cardiologists include the proximal left anterior descending coronary artery and the carotid siphon.[40,41] The intimal cushion in the proximal left anterior descending coronary artery begins to form even during intrauterine life. It progresses rapidly in early postnatal life, leading to intimal cushions in the proximal left anterior coronary artery in all humans by 2 years of age. It remains unclear to what extent lineage

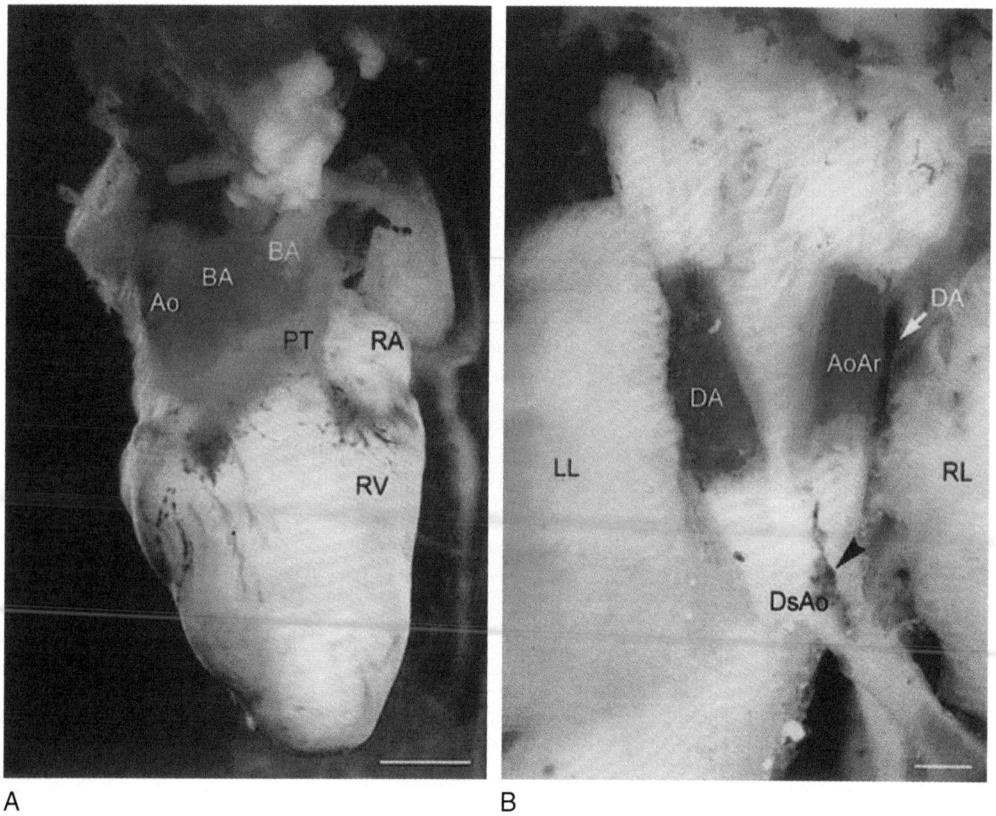

FIGURE 54–3 **Left,** Anterior view of an embryonic chick heart in which cells of neural crest origin stain blue. Note the focal localization of cells derived from neural crest in the great arteries as well as the cardiac innervation plexus spread over the ventricles. Ao = aorta; BA = brachiocephalic artery; PT = pulmonary trunk; RA = right atrium; RV = right ventricle. Bar = 750 μm. **Right,** Posterior view of a chicken embryo heart-lung whole-mount similarly tagged. Note the sharp demarcation in the localization of the blue neural crest-derived cells in the aortic arch (AoAr) and dorsal aorta (DA) before they unite to form the descending aorta (DsAo). The arrowhead indicates neural crest–derived neural tissue. LL and RL indicate left and right lung, respectively. Bar = 250 μm. (From Bergwerff M, Verberne ME, DeRuiter MC, et al: Neural crest cell contribution to the developing circulatory system. Circ Res 82:221, 1998.)

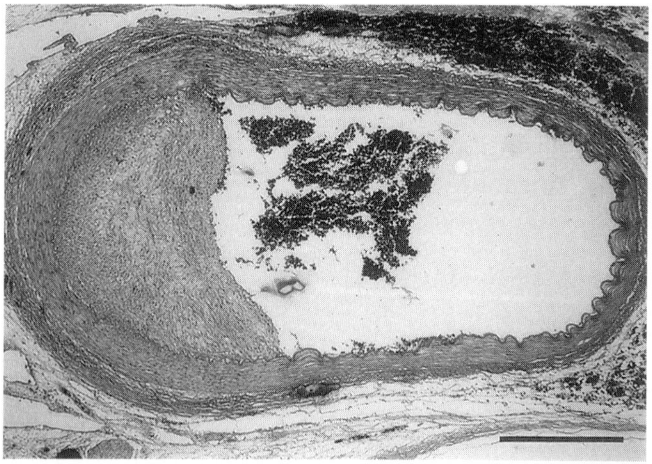

FIGURE 54–4 An intimal cushion shown in a cross-section through the internal carotid artery of a 10-week-old male infant. Areas where intimal cushions form in early life tend to develop atheroma more commonly in later years. The bar shows 0.5 mm. (From Weniger WJ, Muller GB, Reiter C, et al: Intimal hyperplasia of the infant parasellar carotid artery: A potential developmental factor in atherosclerosis and SIDS. Circ Res 85:970, 1999.)

differences versus local hemodynamic forces contribute to the formation of these intimal cushions in arteries prone to develop atherosclerosis. These cushions of smooth muscle and connective tissue form the "soil" in which atheromatous lesions can grow in later life.[42]

Heterogeneity in Vascular Functions

The functions of blood vessels differ in various regions of the circulation, as evidenced by preferential effects on select vascular beds of many vasoactive drugs commonly used in the practice of cardiology. Nitrates dilate both arteries and veins, whereas other vasodilators, such as hydralazine, act primarily as arterial vasodilators. The well-recognized differences in the clinical outcomes of saphenous vein and internal mammary artery bypass grafts furnish another example of clinically relevant heterogeneity among vessels. Internal mammary arteries release more nitric oxide than do saphenous veins. In addition, saphenous veins produce more vasoconstrictor endothelial-derived cyclooxygenase products than do internal mammary arteries. Such differences can help to explain the superior clinical outcomes with internal mammary grafts versus autologous venous bypass grafts.

Indeed, the reactions of blood vessels or vascular cells from various regions of the circulation sometimes differ directionally. The pulmonary vasoconstrictive versus systemic vasodilator response to hypoxia, or the disparate response of the cerebral versus systemic arterial circulation to carbon dioxide furnish commonly encountered examples. Neurectoderm-derived smooth muscle cells in upper body blood vessels grow in response to transforming growth factor-beta, but mesenchymal-derived smooth muscle cells from lower body arteries may actually show growth inhibition when exposed to this mediator. Perhaps the different embryonic origins of smooth muscle cells in the ascending versus descending aorta explain why certain gene defects express themselves primarily in the ascending aorta. In cases of Marfan syndrome, for example, the fibrillin mutation characteristically involves the ascending aorta first (see Chap. 70). Likewise, in cases of Williams syndrome, the genetic defect affects elastin throughout the body, yet the vascular phenotype of these patients manifests primarily in the supravalvular portion of the ascending aorta just where smooth muscle cells of neurectodermal origin reside (see Fig. 54–3).

Heterogeneity of the Clinical Manifestations of Arterial Disease

The Pathobiological Determinants of Atherosclerosis in Youth (PDAY) study collected arterial specimens from Americans younger than 35 years of age who died of noncardiac causes. This study found that fatty streaks and raised arterial lesions localize initially in the dorsal portion of the abdominal aorta. Involvement of the thoracic aorta with fatty streaks or early atheroma follows lesion formation in the abdominal aorta (see Chap. 35). The PDAY data suggest that the formation of coronary atheroma actually lags behind the development of fatty lesions in the aorta.[43,44] Interventions that lower lipids, however, benefit the coronary, carotid, and femoral arteries, although intimal changes in one bed do not necessarily track well with changes in another in a given individual.[45,46]

The most dreaded clinical consequences of atherosclerosis include thrombosis, the cause of most myocardial infarctions and many strokes. A physical disruption of the atherosclerotic plaque causes most fatal coronary events. The role of plaque disruption as a cause of thrombosis in other arterial beds has received less attention. The above discussion has highlighted the developmental and anatomical reasons that coronary arteries differ from peripheral arteries. In addition, the hemodynamic stresses impinging on lesions in the coronary versus the peripheral arterial tree differ. Notably, most coronary artery flow occurs during diastole, whereas the peak pressure and flow in peripheral arteries occurs during systole. Thus, the underlying mechanism of the thrombotic complications of atheroma might well differ in the coronary versus peripheral arteries. Yet, commonalties also exist that link the fundamental mechanisms of stenosis formation, plaque instability, and thrombosis in the coronary and peripheral arteries. Constrictive remodeling, or a failure of compensatory enlargement, appears to cause stenosis in the femoral as well as coronary arteries.[47] Intravascular ultrasound elastography shows that both femoral and coronary arteries harbor atheromata of the fibro-fatty or fibrous variety.[48] Importantly, inflammation appears to occur in disrupted plaques in the carotid as it does in the coronary circulations.[49] These pathoanatomical findings agree well with studies of serum markers of inflammation that show greater incidence of PAD in individuals with higher levels of biomarkers of inflammation, such as C-reactive protein or soluble intercellular adhesion molecule-1.[22,50]

In the aorta, mural thrombi seldom develop into occlusive clots because of the high flow. Nonetheless, aortic plaques frequently rupture, and aortic thrombi are recognized as a clinically important source of embolic disease (Fig. 54–5). Plaques in the aorta encounter high "hoop" (circumferential) stress, due to the large radius, according to the Laplace relationship. This difference may account for the common finding of multiple disrupted plaques in the atherosclerotic aorta (see Fig. 54–5). Recent evidence suggests that plaque rupture also underlies symptoms of carotid artery disease. Features associated with vulnerability of coronary plaques, such as ulcerated plaque with superimposed thrombus, occur frequently in carotid plaques as detected by magnetic resonance imaging.[51] Features such as abundance of foam cells and thinned fibrous caps can help distinguish symptomatic from asymptomatic carotid plaques. As in the unstable coronary plaque, there is infiltration with inflammatory cells and activation of these cells (determined by expression of the histocompatibility antigen HLA-DR). The proportion of active inflammatory cells is consistently higher in the ruptured plaque than in the asymptomatic plaques of similar degree of stenosis.[49]

An independent line of clinical evidence supports a commonality in the mechanisms of complication shared by carotid and coronary arteries. One large study dichotomized patients with symptomatic carotid artery lesions into those with or without irregularity of the carotid lesion by angiography. Over 10 years of follow-up, patients with irregular carotid lesions had a greater than twofold higher cumulative incidence of non-stroke vascular death (mostly due to coronary events) than did those presenting with smooth lesions.[52] Nonvascular deaths and the risk factors assessed in this study did not differ between groups. Similar mechanisms are likely

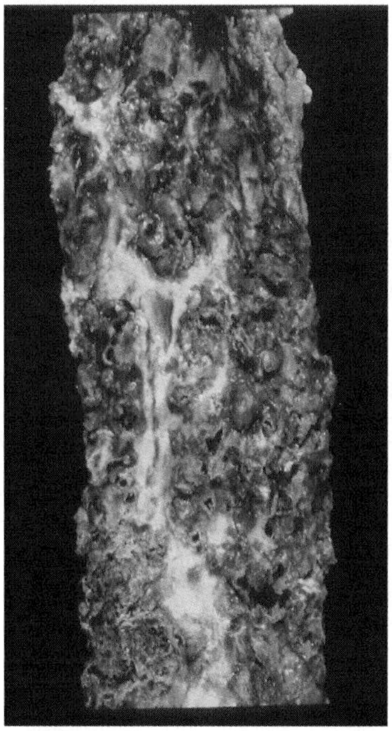

FIGURE 54–5 Atherosclerotic aorta of a patient with atheroemboli. There are multiple, protruding, shaggy atheromas with superimposed mural thrombi. (Courtesy of R.N. Mitchell, MD, PhD, Department of Pathology, Brigham and Women's Hospital, Boston, MA.)

to account for acute thromboses in peripheral arteries, although detailed investigations are not available. Despite the considerable biological and functional heterogeneity among arterial beds, the mechanisms causing the most important clinical manifestations appear similar.

Pathophysiology of Limb Ischemia

Pathophysiological considerations in patients with PAD must take into account the balance of circulatory supply of nutrients to the skeletal muscle and the oxygen and nutrient demand of the skeletal muscle (Table 54–3).

Factors Regulating Blood Supply (see Chap. 44)

The primary determinant of inadequate blood supply to the extremity is a flow-limiting lesion of a conduit artery. Flow through an artery is directly proportional to perfusion pressure and inversely proportional to

TABLE 54–3 Pathophysiological Considerations in Peripheral Arterial Disease

Factors regulating blood supply to limb
Flow-limiting lesion (stenosis severity, inadequate collateral vessels)
Impaired vasodilation (decreased nitric oxide and reduced responsiveness to vasodilators)
Accentuated vasoconstriction (thromboxane, serotonin, angiotensin II, endothelin, norepinephrine)
Abnormal rheology (reduced red blood cell deformability, increased leukocyte adhesivity, platelet aggregation, microthombosis, increased fibrinogen)
Altered skeletal muscle structure and function
Axonal denervation of skeletal muscle
Loss of type II, glycolytic fast twist fibers
Impaired mitochondrial enzymatic activity

the vascular resistance. If atherosclerosis causes a stenosis, flow through the artery is reduced, as described in the Poiseuille equation, in which

$$Q = \frac{\Delta P \pi r^4}{8 \eta l},$$

where ΔP is the pressure gradient across the stenosis, r is the radius of the residual lumen, η is blood viscosity, and l is the length of the vessel affected by the stenosis. As the severity of a stenotic lesion increases, flow becomes progressively reduced. The pressure gradient across the stenosis increases in a nonlinear manner, emphasizing the importance of a stenosis at high blood flow rates. Usually, a blood pressure gradient exists at rest if the stenosis reduces the lumen diameter by more than 50 percent, because as distorted flow develops there is loss of kinetic energy. A stenosis that does not cause a pressure gradient at rest may cause a gradient during exercise, when blood flow rises consequent to higher cardiac output and decreased vascular resistance. Thus, as flow through a stenosis increases, distal perfusion pressure is not maintained. Also, as the metabolic demand of exercising muscle outstrips its blood supply, local metabolites, including adenosine, nitric oxide, potassium, and hydrogen ion, accumulate and peripheral resistance vessels dilate. This results in a further drop of perfusion pressure, since the stenosis limits flow. In addition, intramuscular pressure rises during exercise and may exceed the arterial pressure distal to an occlusion, causing blood flow to cease. Flow through collateral blood vessels is usually adequate to meet the resting metabolic needs of the skeletal muscle tissue but is not enough during exercise.

Functional abnormalities in vasomotor reactivity also may interfere with blood flow. Vasodilator capability of both conduit and resistance vessels is reduced in patients with peripheral atherosclerosis. Normally, arteries dilate in response to pharmacological and biochemical stimuli, such as acetylcholine, serotonin, thrombin, or bradykinin, as well as to shear stress induced by increases in blood flow. This vasodilator response results from the release of biologically active substances from the endothelium, particularly nitric oxide. The vascular relaxation of a conduit vessel that occurs after a flow stimulus, such as that induced by exercise, may facilitate the delivery of blood to exercising muscles in healthy persons. Endothelium-dependent vasodilation subsequent to flow or pharmacological stimuli is impaired in the atherosclerotic femoral arteries and calf resistance vessels of patients with PAD. This failure of vasodilation might prevent an increase in nutritive blood supply to exercising muscle, since endothelium-derived nitric oxide can contribute to hyperemic blood volume after an ischemic stimulus.[53] Several studies have suggested that L-arginine, the precursor for endothelium-derived nitric oxide, increases muscle blood flow and improves claudication distance in patients with PAD, further supporting the contention that endothelium-dependent vasodilation is abnormal in these individuals.[54-56] No large trials have as yet established the clinical benefits of L-arginine, however. It is not known whether vasodilator function with respect to prostacyclin, adenosine, or ion-channels is abnormal in atherosclerotic peripheral arteries. Endogenous vasoconstrictor substances such as prostanoids and other lipid mediators, thrombin, serotonin, angiotensin II, endothelin, and norepinephrine may interfere with vasodilation.

Skeletal Muscle Structure and Metabolic Function

Electrophysiological and histopathological examination has found evidence of partial axonal denervation of the skeletal muscle in legs affected by PAD. There is preservation of type I, oxidative slow twitch fibers, but a loss of type II, or glycolytic, fast twitch fibers in the skeletal muscle of patients with PAD.[57] The loss of type II fibers correlates with decreased muscle strength and reduced exercise capacity. In skeletal muscle distal to PAD, there is a shift to anaerobic metabolism earlier during exercise and it persists longer after cessation of exercise. Patients with claudication have increased lactate release and accumulation of acylcarnitines during exercise, indicative of ineffective oxidative metabolism.[57] Moreover, mitochondrial respiratory activity and phosphocreatine and adenosine triphosphate recovery time decrease in the calf muscles of PAD patients as assessed after submaximal exercise by ^{31}P magnetic resonance spectroscopy.[58]

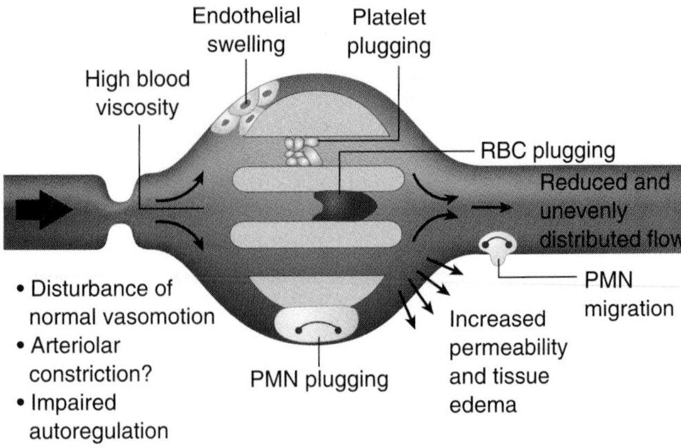

FIGURE 54–6 Schematic representation of potential pathophysiological mechanisms that lead to microvascular obstruction in patients with critical limb ischemia. (From Brevetti G, Corrado S, Marone VD, et al: Microcirculation and tissue metabolism in peripheral arterial disease. Clin Hemorheol Microcirc 21:245, 1999.)

Pathophysiology of Critical Limb Ischemia

Abnormalities in the microcirculation contribute to the pathophysiology of critical limb ischemia. Patients with severe limb ischemia have a reduced number of perfused skin capillaries.[59] Other potential causes of decreased capillary perfusion in this condition include reduced red blood cell deformability, increased leukocyte adhesivity, platelet aggregates, fibrinogen, microthrombosis, excessive vasoconstriction, and interstitial edema (Fig. 54–6). Intravascular pressure may also decrease because of precapillary arteriolar dilation due to locally released vasoactive metabolites.[60]

Clinical Presentation

Symptoms

The cardinal symptoms of PAD include intermittent claudication and rest pain. The term *claudication* is derived from the Latin word *claudicare*, "to limp." Intermittent claudication is characterized by a pain, ache, sense of fatigue, or other discomfort that occurs in the affected muscle group with exercise, particularly walking, and resolves with rest. Claudication occurs when skeletal muscle oxygen demand during effort exceeds blood oxygen supply and results from activation of local sensory receptors by accumulation of lactate or other metabolites. The location of the symptom often relates to the site of the most proximal stenosis. Buttock, hip or thigh claudication typically occurs in patients with obstruction of the aorta and iliac arteries. Calf claudication characterizes femoral and popliteal artery stenoses. The gastrocnemius muscle consumes more oxygen during walking than other muscle groups in the leg and hence causes the most frequent symptom reported by patients. Ankle or pedal claudication occurs in patients with tibial and peroneal artery disease. Similarly, stenoses of the subclavian, axillary, or brachial arteries may cause shoulder, biceps, or forearm claudication, respectively. Symptoms should resolve several minutes after cessation of effort. Calf and thigh pain that occurs at rest, such as nocturnal cramps, should not be confused with claudication and is not a symptom of PAD. The history obtained from persons reporting claudication should note the walking distance, speed, and incline that precipitate claudication. This baseline assessment evaluates disability and provides an initial qualitative measure with which to determine stability, improvement, or deterioration during subsequent encounters with the patient. Symptoms other than claudication can limit functional capacity.[61] Patients with PAD walk more slowly and have less walking endurance than patients who do not have PAD.[62,63]

Several questionnaires have been developed to assess the presence and severity of claudication. The Rose Questionnaire was developed initially to diagnose both angina and intermittent claudication in epidemiological surveys. It questions whether the patient develops pain in either calf with walking and whether the pain occurs at rest, while walking at an ordinary or hurried pace, or when walking uphill. There have been several modifications in this questionnaire, including the Edinburgh Claudication Questionnaire and the San Diego Claudication Questionnaire,[64,65] both of which are more sensitive and specific in comparison to a physician's diagnosis of intermittent claudication based on walking distance, walking speed, and nature of symptoms. A more recently validated instrument, the Walking Impairment Questionnaire, asks a series of questions and develops a point score based on walking distance, walking speed, and nature of symptoms.[66]

Limb claudication occasionally results from nonatherosclerotic causes of arterial occlusive disease (Table 54–4). Several of these are discussed later in the chapter and include arterial embolism, vasculitides such as thromboangiitis obliterans, Takayasu arteritis, giant cell arteritis, aortic coarctation, fibromuscular dysplasia, irradiation, or extravascular compression due to arterial entrapment or adventitial cyst (see Chap. 82).

Several nonvascular causes of exertional leg pain should be considered in patients who present with symptoms suggestive of intermittent claudication (see Table 54–4). Lumbosacral radiculopathy resulting from degenerative joint disease, spinal stenosis, and herniated disks can cause pain in the buttock, hip, thigh, calf, and/or foot with walking, often after very short distances, or even with standing. The term *neurogenic pseudoclaudication* has been used to describe this symptom. Lumbosacral spine disease and PAD both preferentially affect the elderly, and hence may coexist in the same individual. Arthritis of the hips and knees also provokes leg pain with walking. Typically, the pain localizes to the affected joint and can be elicited on physical examination through palpation and range of motion maneuvers. Rarely, skeletal muscle disorders such as myositis can cause exertional leg pain. Muscle tenderness, an abnormal neuromuscular examination finding, elevated skeletal muscle enzyme levels, and a normal pulse examination finding should distinguish myositis from PAD. McArdle syndrome, in which there is a deficiency of skeletal muscle phosphorylase, can cause symptoms mimicking the claudication of PAD. Patients with chronic venous insufficiency sometimes report leg discomfort with exertion, which is designated *venous claudication*. Venous hypertension during exercise increases arterial resistance in the affected limb and limits blood flow. In the case of venous insufficiency, elevated extravascular pressure caused by interstitial edema further diminishes capillary perfusion. A physical examination demonstrating peripheral edema, venous stasis pigmentation, and occasionally venous varicosities will identify this unusual cause of exertional leg pain.

TABLE 54–4 Differential Diagnosis of Exertional Leg Pain

Vascular causes
Atherosclerosis
Thrombosis
Embolism
Vasculitis
Thromboangiitis obliterans
Takayasu arteritis
Giant cell arteritis
Aortic coarctation
Fibromuscular dysplasia
Irradiation
Extravascular compression
Arterial entrapment (e.g., popliteal artery entrapment, thoracic outlet syndrome)
Adventitial cysts
Nonvascular causes
Lumbosacral radiculopathy
Degenerative arthritis
Spinal stenosis
Herniated disc
Arthritis
Hips, knees
Venous insufficiency
Myositis
McArdle syndrome

Rest pain occurs in patients with critical limb ischemia in whom the available blood supply does not adequately meet the resting metabolic needs of the tissue. Typically, patients complain of pain or paresthesias in the foot or toes of the affected extremity. This discomfort worsens upon leg elevation and improves with leg dependency, as might be anticipated by the respective effects of gravity on perfusion pressure. The pain can be particularly severe at sites of skin fissuring, ulceration, or necrosis. Often the skin is very sensitive and even the weight of bedclothes or sheets elicits pain. Patients may sit on the edge of the bed and dangle their legs to alleviate the discomfort. Patients with ischemic or diabetic neuropathy can experience little or no pain despite the presence of severe ischemia.

Critical limb and digital ischemia can result from arterial occlusions other than those caused by atherosclerosis. These include vasculitides, such as thromboangiitis obliterans, connective tissue disorders such as systemic lupus erythematosus and scleroderma, vasospasm, atheromatous embolism, and acute arterial occlusion caused by thrombosis or embolism (see later). Acute gouty arthritis, trauma, and sensory neuropathies such as that caused by diabetes mellitus, lumbosacral radiculopathies, and reflex sympathetic dystrophy can cause foot pain. Leg ulcers also occur in patients with venous insufficiency and sensory neuropathies, particularly that related to diabetes. These ulcers are easily distinguished from arterial ulcers. The venous ulcer usually localizes near the medial malleolus and has an irregular border and a pink base with granulation tissue. Venous ulcers produce milder pain than arterial ulcers. Neurotrophic ulcers occur where there is pressure or trauma, usually on the sole of the foot. These ulcers are deep, frequently infected, and usually not painful because of the loss of sensation (Fig. 54–7, right panel).

Physical Findings

A careful vascular examination includes palpation of pulses and auscultation of accessible arteries for bruits. Pulses that are readily palpable in healthy individuals include the brachial, radial, and ulnar arteries of the upper extremity and the femoral, popliteal, dorsalis pedis, and posterior tibial arteries of the lower extremities. The aorta also can be palpated in asthenic persons. A decreased or absent pulse provides insight into the location of arterial stenoses. For example, a normal right femoral pulse but absent left femoral

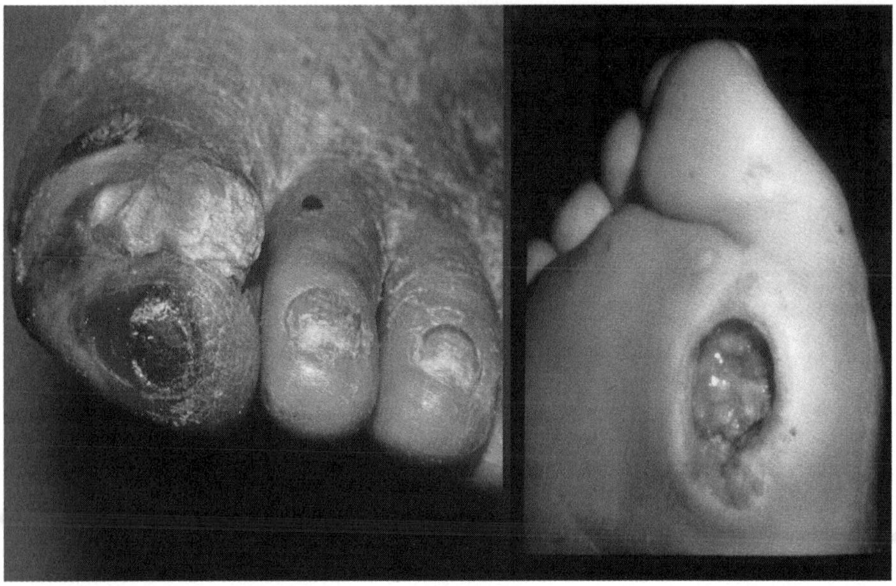

FIGURE 54–7 **Left,** A typical arterial ulcer. It is a discrete, circumscribed, necrotic ulcer located on the great toe. **Right,** A trophic ulcer in a patient with diabetes mellitus. It is located on the volar surface of the foot beneath the head of the first metatarsal bone, a typical area of pressure; its base has granulation tissue.

pulse suggests the presence of left iliofemoral arterial stenosis. A normal femoral artery pulse but absent popliteal artery pulse would indicate a stenosis in the superficial femoral artery or proximal popliteal artery. Similarly, disease of the anterior and posterior tibial arteries can be inferred when the popliteal artery pulse is present but the dorsalis pedis and posterior tibial pulses, respectively, are not palpable. Bruits are often indicative of accelerated blood flow velocity and flow disturbance at sites of stenosis. A stethoscope should be used to auscultate the supraclavicular and infraclavicular fossae for evidence of subclavian artery stenosis, the abdomen, flank, and pelvis for evidence of stenoses in the aorta and its branch vessels, and each groin for evidence of femoral artery stenoses. Pallor can be elicited on the soles of the feet of some patients with PAD by performing a maneuver in which the feet are elevated above the level of the heart and the calf muscles are exercised by repeated dorsiflexion and plantar flexion of the ankle. The legs are then placed in the dependent position and the time to the onset of hyperemia and venous distention is measured. Each of these variables depends on the rate of blood flow, which in turn reflects the severity of stenosis and adequacy of collateral vessels.

The legs of patients with chronic aortoiliac disease may show muscle atrophy. Additional signs of chronic low-grade ischemia include hair loss, thickened and brittle toenails, smooth and shiny skin, and subcutaneous fat atrophy of the digital pads. Patients with severe limb ischemia have cool skin and may also have petechiae, persistent cyanosis or pallor, dependent rubor, pedal edema resulting from prolonged dependency, skin fissures, ulceration, or gangrene. Arterial ulcers typically have a pale base with irregular borders and usually involve the tips of the toes or the heel of the foot, or develop at sites of pressure (see Fig. 54–7, left panel). These ulcers vary in size and may be as small as 3 to 5 mm.

Categorization

Classification of patients with PAD depends on the severity of the symptoms and abnormalities detected on physical examination. Categorization of the clinical manifestations of PAD improves communication among professionals caring for these patients and provides a structure for defining guidelines for therapeutic interventions. Fontaine described one widely used scheme that classified patients in one of four stages progressing from asymptomatic to critical limb ischemia (Table 54–5). Several professional vascular societies have adopted a contemporary, more descriptive classification that includes asymptomatic patients, three grades of claudication, and three grades of critical limb ischemia ranging from rest pain alone to minor and major tissue loss (Table 54–6).[67]

Testing

Segmental Pressure Measurement and Ankle/Brachial Indices

The measurement of systolic blood pressure along selected segments of each extremity furnishes one of the most useful and simplest noninvasive tests to evaluate the presence and severity of stenoses in the peripheral arteries. In the lower extremities, pneumatic cuffs are placed on the upper and lower portions of the thigh, the calf, above the ankle, and often over the metatarsal area of the foot. Likewise, in the upper extremity, pneumatic cuffs

TABLE 54–5 Fontaine Classification of Peripheral Arterial Disease

Stage	Symptoms
I	Asymptomatic
II	Intermittent claudication
IIa	Pain-free, claudication walking >200 m
IIb	Pain-free, claudication walking <200 m
III	Rest and nocturnal pain
IV	Necrosis, gangrene

TABLE 54–6 Clinical Categories of Chronic Limb Ischemia

Grade	Category	Clinical Description
	0	Asymptomatic, not hemodynamically correct
I	1	Mild claudication
	2	Moderate claudication
	3	Severe claudication
II	4	Ischemic rest pain
	5	Minor tissue loss: nonhealing ulcer, focal gangrene with diffuse pedal ulcer
III	6	Major tissue loss extending above transmetatarsal level, functional foot no longer salvageable

Adapted from Rutherford RB, Baker JD, Ernst C, et al. Recommended standards for reports dealing with lower extremity ischemia: Revised version. J Vasc Surg 26:517, 1997.

TABLE 54–7 Leg Segmental Pressure Measurements in a Patient with Bilateral Calf Claudication

Brachial Artery	152/84	
	Right leg	*Left leg*
Upper thigh	160	162
Lower thigh	110	140
Calf	108	100
Ankle	64	78
Ankle/brachial index	0.42	0.51

are placed on the upper arm over the biceps, on the forearm below the elbow, and at the wrist. Systolic blood pressure at each respective limb segment can be measured by first inflating the pneumatic cuff to suprasystolic pressure and then determining the pressure at which blood flow occurs during cuff deflation. The onset of flow can be assessed by placing a Doppler ultrasound flow probe over an artery distal to the cuff. In the lower extremities, it is most convenient to place the Doppler probe on the foot over the posterior tibial artery as it courses inferior and posterior to the medial malleolus or over the dorsalis pedis artery on the dorsum of the metatarsal arch. In the upper extremities, the Doppler probe can be placed over the brachial artery in the antecubital fossa or over the radial and ulnar arteries at the wrist.

Left ventricular contraction imparts kinetic energy to blood, which is maintained throughout the large and medium-sized vessels. Systolic blood pressure in the more distal vessels may be higher than in the aorta and proximal vessels because of reflection of blood pressure waves.[68] A stenosis can cause loss of pressure energy as a result of increased frictional forces and flow disturbance at the site of the stenosis. Approximately 90 percent of the cross-sectional area of the aorta must be narrowed before a pressure gradient develops. In smaller vessels, such as the iliac and femoral arteries, a 70 to 90 percent decrease in cross-sectional area will cause a resting pressure gradient sufficient to decrease systolic blood pressure distal to the stenosis. Taking into consideration the precision of this noninvasive method and the variability in blood pressure over even short periods of time, a blood pressure gradient in excess of 20 mm Hg between successive cuffs is generally used as evidence of arterial stenosis in the lower extremity, whereas a 10 mm Hg gradient is indicative of a stenosis between sequential cuffs in the upper extremity. Systolic blood pressure in the toes and fingers approximates 60 percent of the systolic blood pressure at the ankle and wrist, respectively, as pressure diminishes further in the smaller distal vessels.

Table 54–7 gives examples of leg segmental pressure measurements in a patient with bilateral calf claudication. In the right leg, there are pressure gradients between upper and lower thigh and between the calf and ankle. These are indicative of stenoses in the superficial femoral artery and in the tibioperoneal arteries. In the left leg, there are pressure gradients between the upper and lower thigh, between the lower thigh and calf, and between the calf and ankle. These are indicative of stenoses in the superficial femoral and popliteal arteries and in the tibioperoneal arteries.

Ankle/Brachial Index

Determination of the ABI furnishes a simplified application of leg segmental blood pressure measurements readily used at the bedside. This index is the ratio of the systolic blood pressure measured at the ankle to the systolic blood pressure measured at the brachial artery. A pneumatic cuff placed around the ankle is inflated to suprasystolic pressure and subsequently deflated, while the onset of flow is detected with a Doppler ultrasound probe placed over the dorsalis pedis and posterior tibial arteries, thus denoting ankle systolic blood pressure. Brachial artery systolic pressure can be assessed in a routine manner, using either a stethoscope to listen for the first Korotkoff sound or a Doppler probe to listen for the onset of flow during cuff deflation. The normal ABI should be 1.0 or greater. However, recognizing the variability intrinsic to sequential blood pressure measurements, an ABI of less than 0.90 is considered abnormal and is 95 percent sensitive for angiographically verified peripheral arterial stenosis.[1] The ABI is often used to gauge the severity of PAD. Patients with symptoms of leg claudication often have ABIs ranging from 0.5 to 0.8, and patients with critical limb ischemia usually have an ABI of less than 0.5. The ABI correlates inversely with walking distance and speed. Fewer than 40 percent of patients whose ABI is less than 0.40 can complete a 6-minute walk.[69] In patients with skin ulcerations, an ankle pressure of less than 55 mm Hg would predict poor ulcer healing.

One limitation of leg blood pressure recordings is that they cannot be used reliably in patients with calcified vessels, as might occur in persons with diabetes mellitus or renal insufficiency. The calcified vessel cannot be compressed during inflation of the pneumatic cuff and therefore the Doppler probe indicates continuous blood flow, even when the mercury manometer records pressure in excess of 250 mm Hg.

Treadmill Exercise Testing

Treadmill exercise testing serves to evaluate the clinical significance of peripheral arterial stenoses and to provide objective evidence of the patient's walking capacity. The initial claudication distance is defined as the point at which symptoms of claudication first develop and the absolute claudication distance is when the patient is no longer able to continue walking because of severe leg discomfort. This standardized and more objective measurement of walking capacity supplements the patient's history and thus provides a quantitative assessment of the patient's disability as well as a metric that can be monitored after therapeutic interventions.

Treadmill exercise protocols use a motorized treadmill that incorporates fixed or progressive speeds and angles of incline. A fixed workload test usually maintains a constant grade of 12 percent and speed of 1.5 to 2.0 miles per hour. A progressive, or graded, treadmill protocol typically maintains a constant speed of 2 miles per hour while the grade is gradually increased by 2 percent every 2 to 3 minutes. Reproducibility of repeated treadmill test results is reportedly better with progressive than with constant grade protocols.[70]

Treadmill testing provides a means to determine whether arterial stenoses contribute to the patient's symptoms of exertional leg pain. During exercise, blood flow through a stenosis increases as vascular resistance falls in the exercising muscle. According to Poiseuille's Law, described previously, the pressure gradient across the stenosis increases in direct proportion to flow. Thus, ankle and brachial systolic blood pressures are measured under resting conditions before treadmill exercise, within 1 minute after exercise, and repeatedly until baseline values are reestablished. Normally, the blood pressure increase that occurs during exercise should be the same in both upper and lower extremities, maintaining a constant ABI of 1.0 or greater. In the presence of peripheral arterial stenoses, the ABI decreases, because the increase in blood pressure that is observed in the arm is not matched by a comparable increase in ankle blood pressure. A 25 percent or greater decrease in ABI after exercise in a patient whose walking capacity is limited by claudication is considered diagnostic, implicating PAD as a cause of the patient's symptoms.

Many patients with PAD also have coronary atherosclerosis. The addition of cardiac monitoring to the exercise protocol may provide adjunctive information regarding the presence of myocardial ischemia. A workload sufficient to increase myocardial oxygen demand and provoke myocardial ischemia may not be achieved in patients whose exercise capacity is limited by claudication. Nonetheless, electrocardiographic changes, particularly during low levels of treadmill exercise, may provide evidence of severe coronary artery disease.

Pulse Volume Recording

The pulse volume recording graphically illustrates the volumetric change in a segment of the limb that occurs with each pulse. Plethysmographic instruments, typically utilizing strain gauges or pneumatic cuffs, are used to transduce volumetric changes in the limb, which can be displayed on a graphic recorder. These transducers are strategically placed along the limb to record the pulse volume in its different segments, such as the thigh, calf, ankle, metatarsal region, and toes or the upper arm, forearm, and fingers. The normal pulse volume contour is influenced by both local arterial pressure and vascular wall distensibility and resembles a blood pressure waveform. It consists of a sharp systolic upstroke, rising rapidly to a peak, a dicrotic notch, and a concave downslope that drops off gradually toward the baseline.[71] The contour of the pulse wave changes distal to a stenosis. There is loss of the dicrotic notch, a slower rate of rise, a more rounded peak, and a slower descent. The amplitude becomes lower with increasing severity of disease, and the pulse wave may not be recordable at all in the critically ischemic limb. Segmental analysis of the pulse wave may indicate the location of an arterial stenosis, which is likely to be sited in the artery between a normal and an abnormal pulse volume recording. The pulse volume wave also provides information regarding the integrity of blood flow when blood pressure measurements cannot be accurately obtained because of noncompressible vessels.

Doppler Ultrasonography

Continuous wave and pulsed wave Doppler systems transmit and receive high-frequency ultrasound signals. The Doppler frequency shift caused by moving red blood cells varies directly with the velocity of blood flow. Typically, the perceived frequency shift is between 1 and 20 kHz and is within the audible range of the human ear. Therefore, placement of a Doppler probe along an artery enables the examiner to hear whether blood flow is present and the vessel is patent. Processing and graphically recording the Doppler signal permits a more detailed analysis of the frequency components.

Doppler instruments can be used without or with gray scale imaging to evaluate an artery for the presence of stenoses. The Doppler probe is positioned at approximately a 60-degree angle over the common femoral, superficial femoral, popliteal, dorsalis pedis, and posterior tibial arteries. The normal Doppler waveform has three components: a rapid forward flow component during systole, a transient flow reversal during early diastole, and a slow antegrade component during late diastole. The Doppler waveform becomes altered if the probe is placed distal to an arterial stenosis and is characterized by deceleration of systolic flow, loss of the early diastolic reversal, and diminished peak frequencies. Arteries in a limb with critical ischemia may not show any Doppler frequency shift. As with pulse volume recordings, a change from a normal to an abnormal Doppler waveform as the artery is interrogated more distally provides inferential evidence of the location of a stenosis.[71,72]

Duplex Ultrasound Imaging

Duplex ultrasound imaging provides a direct, noninvasive means of assessing both the anatomic characteristics of peripheral arteries and the functional significance of arterial stenoses. The methodology incorporates gray scale B-mode ultrasound imaging, pulsed Doppler velocity measurements, and color coding of the Doppler-shift information (Fig. 54–8). Real-time ultrasonography scanners emit and receive high-frequency sound waves, typically ranging from 2 to 10 mHz, to construct an image. The acoustic properties of the vascular wall differ from those of the surrounding tissue, enabling them to be imaged easily. Atherosclerotic plaque may be present and visible on gray scale images. Pulsed wave Doppler systems emit ultrasound beams at precise times and can therefore sample the reflected ultrasound waves at specific depths, enabling the examiner to determine the blood cell velocity within the lumen of the artery. By positioning the pulsed Doppler beam at a known angle, the examiner can calculate blood flow velocity according to the following equation:

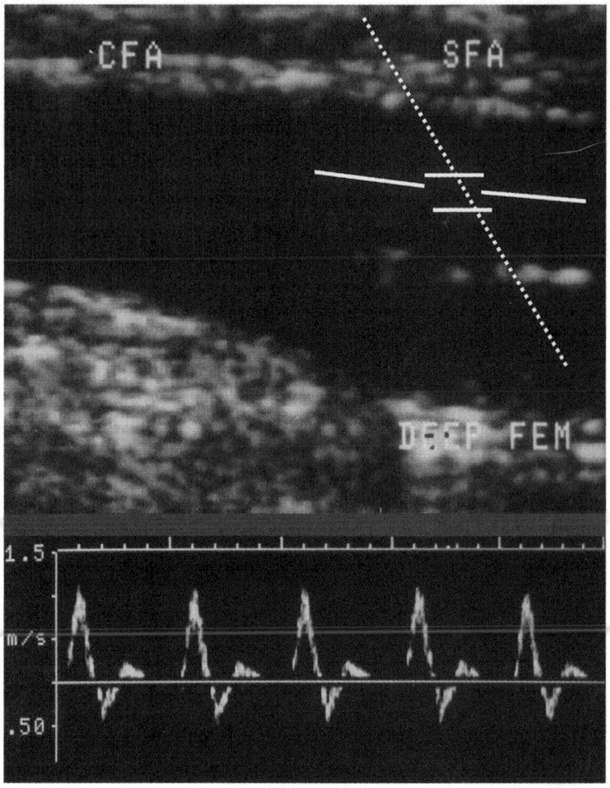

FIGURE 54–8 Duplex ultrasonogram of the common femoral artery bifurcation into the superficial and deep femoral arteries. The **upper image** shows a normal gray scale image of the artery in which the intima is not thickened and the lumen is widely patent. The **lower image** is a recording of the pulse Doppler velocity sampled from the superficial femoral artery. The triphasic profile is apparent, the envelope is thin, and the peak systolic velocity is within normal limits.

$$Df = 2VF\cos\theta/C,$$

where Df is the frequency shift, V is the velocity, F is the frequency of the transmitted sound, θ is the angle between the transmitted sound and the velocity vector, and C is the velocity of sound and tissue. For optimal measurements, the angle of the pulsed Doppler beam should be less than 60 degrees. With color Doppler, the frequency shift information within the entire field sampled by the ultrasound beam can be superimposed on the gray scale image. This provides a composite real-time display of flow velocity within the vessel.

Color-assisted duplex ultrasound imaging is an effective means of localizing peripheral arterial stenoses (Fig. 54–9). Normal arteries have laminar flow, with the highest velocity at the center of the artery. The corresponding color image is usually homogeneous, with relatively constant hue and intensity. In the presence of an arterial stenosis, blood flow velocity increases through the narrowed lumen. As the velocity increases, there is progressive desaturation of the color display, and flow disturbance distal to the stenosis causes changes in hue and color. Pulsed Doppler velocity measurements can be made along the length of the artery and particularly at areas of flow abnormalities suggested by the color images. A twofold or greater increase in peak systolic velocity at the site of an atherosclerotic plaque indicates a 50 percent or greater diameter stenosis (see Fig. 54–9). A threefold increase in velocity suggests 75 percent or greater stenosis. An occluded artery generates no Doppler signal. Using contrast angiography as a reference standard, duplex ultrasound imaging for identifying sites of arterial stenoses has approximately a 95 percent specificity and an 80 to 90 percent sensitivity.[73,74]

Magnetic Resonance Angiography

Magnetic resonance angiography (MRA) can noninvasively visualize the aorta and the peripheral arteries (see Chaps. 14 and 53). A detailed description of the instrumentation and technique is beyond the scope of this chapter. The resolution of the vascular anatomy with gadolinium-enhanced MRA approaches that of conventional contrast digital subtraction angiography (Fig. 54–10). Comparative studies have reported sensitivities of 93 to 100 percent and specificity of 96 to 100 percent for the aorta, iliac, femoropopliteal, and tibioperoneal arteries.[74-79] MRA currently has greatest utility for the evaluation of symptomatic patients to assist decision-making before endovascular and surgical intervention or in patients at risk for renal, allergic, or other complications during conventional angiography.

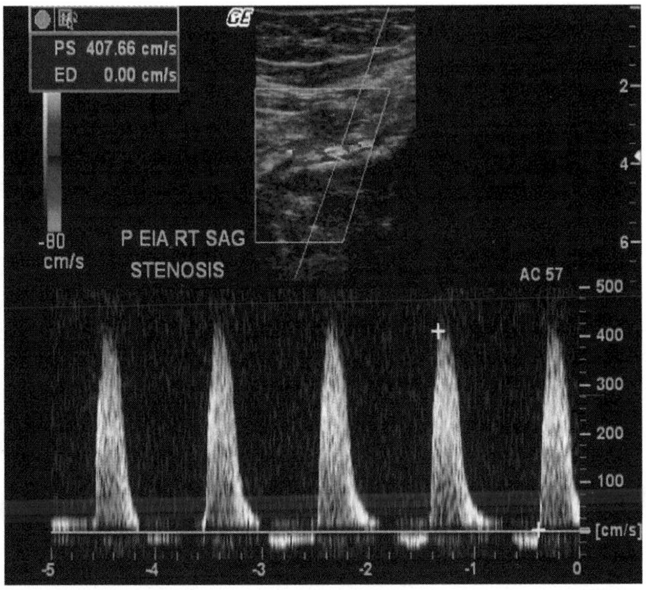

FIGURE 54–9 Duplex ultrasonogram of the external iliac artery. The **upper image** shows a color image of the artery in which there is heterogeneity and desaturation of color indicative of high-velocity flow through a stenosis. The **lower image** is a recording of the pulse Doppler velocity sampled from the right external iliac artery. The peak velocity of 350 cm/sec is elevated. These features are consistent with a significant stenosis.

Computed Tomographic Angiography

Computed tomographic angiography (CTA) utilizes intravenous administration of radiocontrast material to opacify and visualize the aorta and peripheral arteries (see Chap. 15). New computed tomography scanners using multidetector technology can acquire up to 16 simultaneous cross-sectional images displayed with maximal intensity projection. This advance permits imaging of peripheral arteries with excellent spatial resolution over a relatively short period of time and using reduced amount of radiocontrast (Fig. 54–11).[80] Images can be displayed in three dimensions and rotated to optimize visualization of arterial stenoses. Compared to conventional contrast angiography, the sensitivity and specificity for occlusions reported for CTA using single detector technology are 94 to 100 percent and 98 to 100 percent, respectively. For stenoses greater than 75 percent, the sensitivity is 73 to 88 percent and the specificity is 94 to 100 percent.[81] The use of newer generation multidetector scanners improves this accuracy.[80,82]

Experience with CTA is still relatively limited compared to that of MRA and conventional intraarterial angiography. CTA offers an advantage over MRA in that it can be used in patients with stents, metal clips, and pacemakers, although it also has the disadvantage of requiring radiocontrast and ionizing radiation.

Contrast Angiography (see Chap. 18)

Conventional angiography, using a radioiodinated or other contrast agent, is indicated for evaluation of the arterial anatomy prior to a revascularization procedure. It still has occasional utility when the diagnosis is in doubt. Most contemporary angiography laboratories use digital subtraction techniques following intraarterial administration of contrast

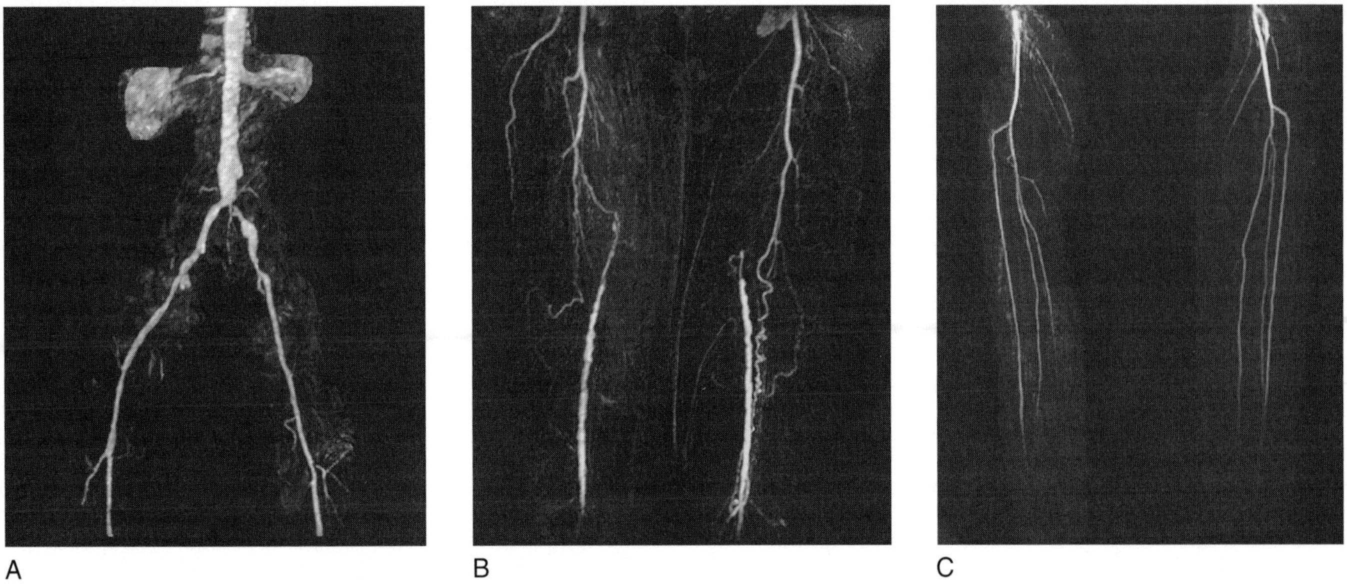

FIGURE 54–10 Gadolinium-enhanced two-dimensional magnetic resonance angiogram of the aorta and both legs, extending from the thighs to above the ankle. **A,** Aortoiliac atherosclerosis with stenosed left common iliac artery. **B,** Bilateral superficial femoral artery occlusion with reconstitution of the distal portion of the right and left superficial femoral arteries. **C,** The anterior tibial, posterior tibial, and peroneal arteries, which are patent in each leg.

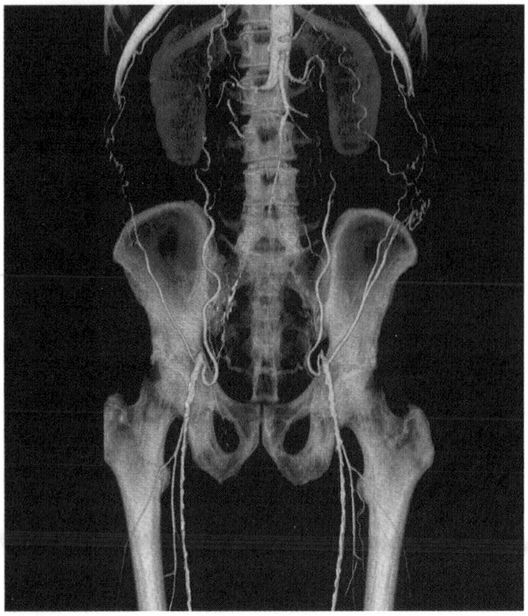

FIGURE 54–11 Computed tomographic angiogram of a patient with complete occlusion of the aorta and both iliac arteries. There is reconstitution of the common femoral arteries. (Courtesy of the 3D and Image Processing Center of Brigham and Women's Hospital, Boston, MA.)

material to enhance resolution. Evaluation of the aorta and the peripheral arteries generally uses retrograde transfemoral catheterization. Injection of the radiocontrast material into the aorta permits visualization of the aorta and iliac arteries, and injection of contrast material into the iliofemoral segment of the involved leg permits optimal visualization of the femoral, popliteal, tibial, and peroneal arteries (Fig. 54–12). In patients with aortic occlusion, catheterization of the femoral arteries is not feasible. The aorta can be approached by brachial or axillary artery cannulation or, if necessary, directly by a translumbar approach.

Prognosis

Patients with PAD have an increased risk for adverse cardiovascular events as well as the risk of limb loss and impaired quality of life.[2,12,83,84] Patients with PAD frequently have concomitant coronary artery disease and cerebrovascular disease.[1,85,86] The relative prevalence of each of these manifestations of atherosclerosis depends, in part, on the diagnostic criteria used to establish their diagnosis. In the Clopidogrel vs. Aspirin in Patients at Risk of Ischemic Events (CAPRIE) trial, 21 percent of the patients with PAD had a history of myocardial infarction and 26 percent had angina.[85] Patients with abnormal ABIs are twice as likely as those with normal ABIs to have a history of myocardial infarction, angina, congestive heart failure, or cerebrovascular ischemia.[1] Approximately 15 to 25 percent of patients with peripheral artery disease have significant carotid artery stenoses as detected by duplex ultrasonography. The risk of death from cardiovascular causes increases 2.5- to sixfold in patients with PAD, and their annual mortality rate is 4.3 to 4.9 percent.[1,87] The risk of death is greatest in those with the most severe PAD, and mortality correlates with decreasing ABI (Fig. 54–13). Approximately 25 percent of patients with critical limb ischemia die within 1 year, and the 1-year mortality rate among patients who have undergone amputation for PAD may be as high as 45 percent.[1,88]

Approximately 25 percent of patients with claudication develop worsening symptoms. Clinical progression to critical limb ischemia occurs in 7.5 to 8.0 percent of patients with claudication in the first year after diagnosis and in approximately 2.2 percent each year thereafter.[89] Both smoking and diabetes mellitus independently predict progression of disease.[1] Of patients with PAD, the risk of amputation in those with diabetes mellitus is at least 12-fold higher than in nondiabetic persons.[90]

Treatment

The goals of treatment for PAD include reduction in cardiovascular morbidity and mortality as well as improvement in quality of life by decreasing symptoms of claudication, eliminating rest pain, and preserving limb viability.[5] Therapeutic considerations, therefore, include risk factor modification by lifestyle measures and pharmacological therapy to reduce the risk of adverse cardiovascular events, such as myocardial infarction, stroke, and death. Symptoms of claudication can improve with pharmacotherapy or exercise rehabilitation, whereas optimal management of critical limb ischemia often includes endovascular interventions or surgical reconstruction to improve blood supply and maintain limb viability.[1,2,91]

Risk Factor Modification (see Chaps. 39 and 42)

Lipid-lowering therapy reduces the risk of adverse cardiovascular events in patients with coronary artery disease. Secondary prevention trials with statins documented reduced risk of nonfatal myocardial infarction or death from coronary artery disease by 24 to 34 percent (see Chap. 39). The recent Heart Protection Study found that lipid-lowering therapy with simvastatin reduced the risk of adverse cardiovascular outcomes by 25 percent in patients with atherosclerosis, including more than 6700 patients with PAD (Fig. 54–14).[92] The National Cholesterol Education Program Adult Treatment Panel III designated PAD a "coronary risk equivalent," hence the current recommendations for lipid-lowering therapy in patients with PAD. Such patients should receive diet and drug therapy to achieve a target LDL cholesterol level of 100 mg/dl or less.[93]

Several clinical trials have found that lipid-lowering therapy with diet, niacin, binding resins, or clofibrate reduces the progression of femoral artery atherosclerosis. In one study, the addition of probucol to cholestyramine did not affect femoral atherosclerosis.[94] Lipid-lowering therapy may also reduce the incidence or severity of claudication. The Program on the Surgical Control of the Hyperlipidemia (POSCH) found that partial ileal bypass surgery, a surgical procedure that lowers cholesterol levels, reduced the incidence of intermittent claudication or critical limb ischemia by 34 percent and reduced the risk for developing an abnormal ABI by 44 percent.[95] A post hoc analysis of the Scandinavian Simvastatin Survival Study (4S) found that simvastatin, as compared with placebo, reduced the risk of developing new or worsening claudication by 38 percent.[96]

Prospective trials have found that statins improve walking distance in patients with PAD.[97-99] In the Treatment of Peripheral Atherosclerotic Disease with Moderate or Intensive Lipid Lowering (TREADMILL) trial, atorvastatin (80 mg) increased pain-free walking distance by more than 60 percent as compared with 38 percent increase with placebo (Fig. 54-15).[98] Also, patients treated with statins have superior leg functioning as assessed by walking speed and distance compared to those not so treated.[100]

Smoking Cessation

Prospective trials examining the benefits of smoking cessation are lacking. However, observational evidence unequivocally supports the notion that cigarette smoking increases the risk of atherosclerosis and its clinical sequelae. Nonsmokers with PAD have lower rates of myocardial infarction and mortality than those who have smoked or continue to smoke, and

PAD patients who discontinue smoking have approximately twice the 5-year survival rate of those who continue to smoke.[8] Smoking cessation also lowers the risk of developing critical limb ischemia.

Treatment of Diabetes

(see Chaps. 40 and 51)

Aggressive treatment of diabetes decreases the risk for microangiopathic events such as nephropathy and retinopathy; however, only limited data support the benefit of aggressive treatment of diabetes on the clinical manifestations of atherosclerosis (see Chap. 40). In the Diabetes Control and Complications Trial (DCCT), which involved patients with type 1 diabetes mellitus, a post-hoc analysis found that intensive insulin therapy, as compared with usual care, caused a nonsignificant 42 percent reduction in cardiovascular events, including a 22 percent reduction in events related to PAD.[101] Also, after 6 years, the rate of growth of carotid intima–media thickness was less in the intensive treatment group, indicating a favorable effect on atherosclerosis progression.[102] The United Kingdom Prospective Diabetes Study (UKPDS) of patients with type 2 diabetes mellitus found that intensive treatment with sulfonylureas or insulin was associated with a 16 percent reduction in myocardial infarction, a finding of borderline statistical significance, and a trend for a decrease in the incidence of death or amputation from PAD.[103]

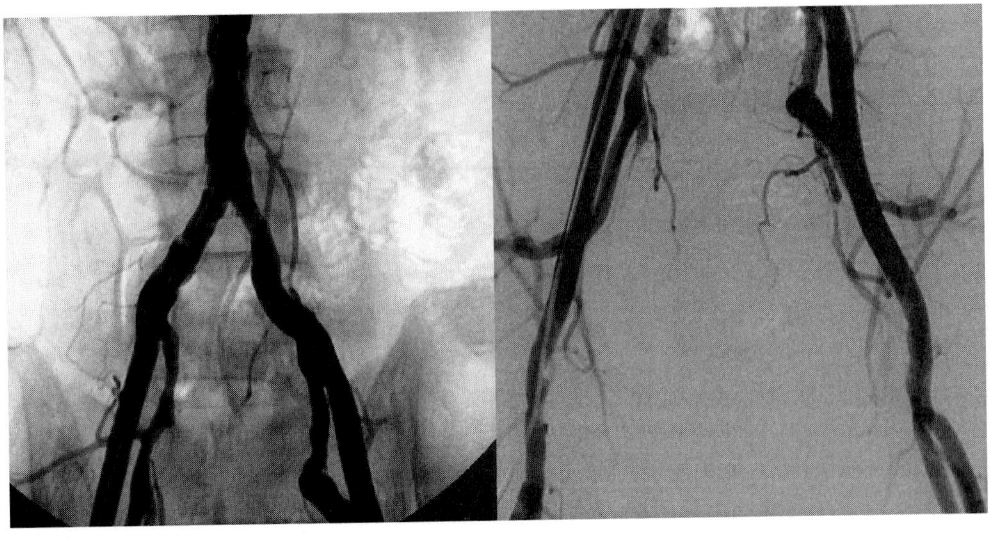

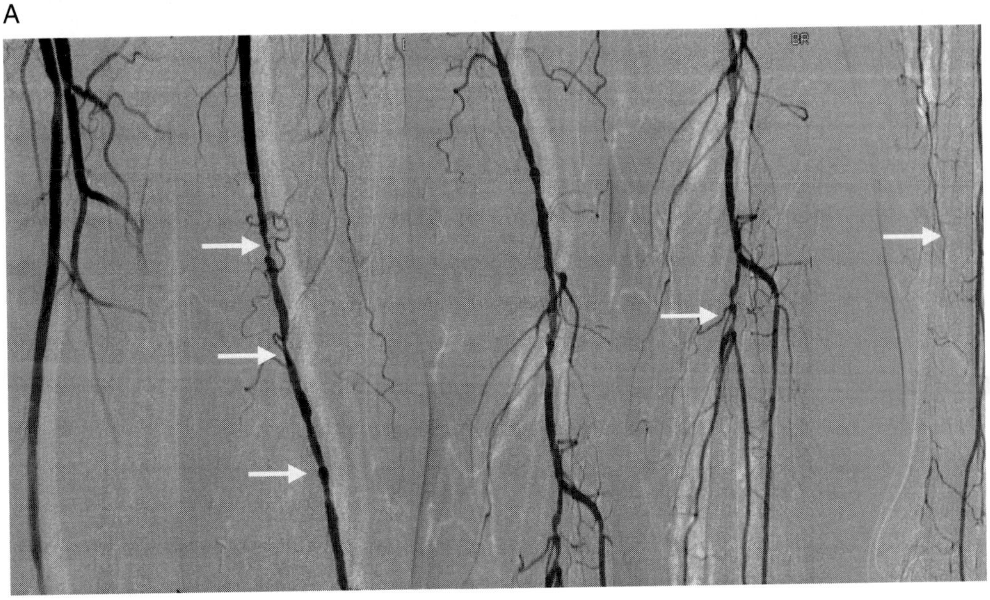

FIGURE 54–12 Angiogram of a patient with disabling left calf claudication. **A,** The aorta and bilateral common iliac arteries are patent. **B,** The left superficial femoral artery has multiple stenotic lesions (arrows). There is a significant stenosis of the left tibioperoneal trunk and left posterior tibial artery (arrows).

Blood Pressure Control

Antihypertensive therapy reduces the risk of stroke, coronary artery disease, and vascular death. In the Appropriate Blood Pressure Control in Diabetes (ABCD) trial, intensive blood pressure control to levels approximating 128/75 mm Hg substantially reduced cardiovascular events as compared with moderate blood pressure control in patients with PAD.[104] It is not known whether antihypertensive therapy prevents the progression of PAD. Treatment of hypertension might decrease perfusion pressure to extremities already compromised by peripheral arterial stenoses. In addition, concern has been raised regarding the potential adverse affects of beta-adrenergic receptor blockers on peripheral blood flow and symptoms of claudication or critical limb ischemia. Beta-adrenergic blocking agents worsen claudication in some trials but not in others. A meta-analysis that included 11 studies of beta-blocker therapy, as compared with placebo, in patients with intermittent claudication found no significant impairment on walking capacity.[105] Beta-blocking drugs reduce the risk of myocardial infarction and death in patients with coronary artery disease, a problem affecting many patients with PAD.[106] Thus, if clinically indicated for other conditions, these drugs should not be withheld in patients with PAD. The balance of evidence supports treatment of hypertension in patients with PAD according to established clinical guidelines (see Chap. 38).[107]

Angiotensin-converting enzyme inhibitors reduce cardiovascular events in patients with atherosclerosis. In the Heart Outcomes Prevention Evaluation study (HOPE), the angiotensin-converting enzyme inhibitor ramipril decreased the risk for vascular death, myocardial infarction, or stroke by 22 percent. Forty-four percent of the patients enrolled in the HOPE trial had evidence of PAD as manifested by an ABI less than 0.9. Ramipril reduced cardiovascular events in the patients with PAD to a comparable degree as in those without PAD (Fig. 54–16).[108]

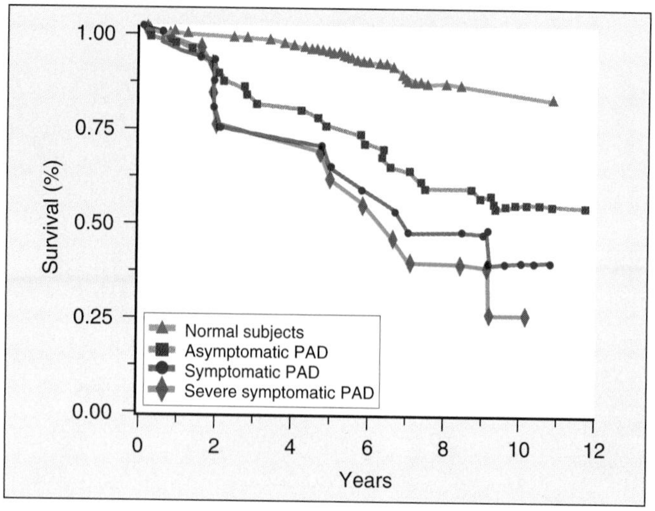

FIGURE 54–13 Survival rates of patients with peripheral arterial disease (PAD) derived from a population-based study. PAD was diagnosed by measuring the ankle/brachial index. Just the presence of PAD, even in the absence of symptoms, was associated with decreased survival. Survival was poorest in patients with symptoms. (From Criqui M, Langer RD, Fronek A, et al: Mortality over a period of 10 years in patients with peripheral arterial disease. N Engl J Med 326:381, 1992.)

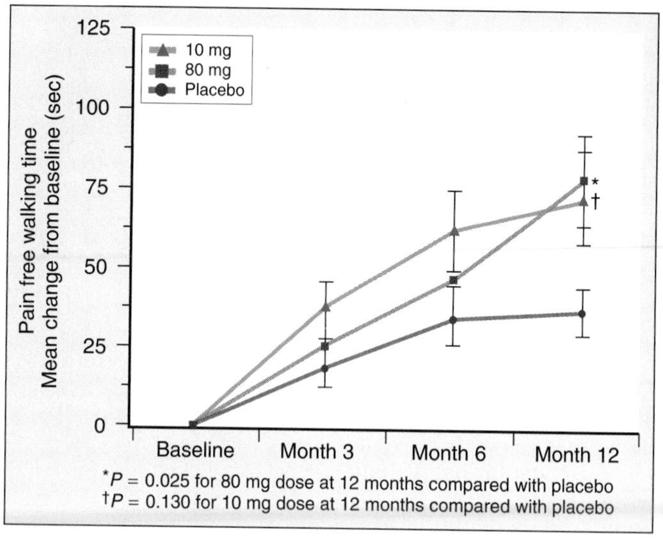

FIGURE 54–15 In the TREADMILL Study, lipid-lowering therapy with atorvastatin improved pain-free walking time in patients with intermittent claudication. (From Mohler ER 3rd, Hiatt Wr, Creager MA: Cholesterol reduction with atorvastatin improves walking distance in patients with arterial artery disease. Circulation 108:1481, 2003.)

Antiplatelet Therapy

Substantial evidence supports the use of antiplatelet agents to reduce adverse cardiovascular outcome in patients with atherosclerosis. A meta-analysis that included approximately 135,000 high-risk patients with atherosclerosis, including those with acute and prior myocardial infarction, stroke, and transient cerebrovascular ischemia, and other high-risk groups, including those with PAD, found that antiplatelet therapy yielded a 22 percent odds reduction for subsequent vascular death, myocardial infarction, or stroke (see Chap. 80).[109] Among the 9214 patients with PAD included in this analysis, antiplatelet therapy reduced the risk of myocardial infarction, stroke, or death by 22 percent (Fig. 54–17).[109] The CAPRIE trial compared clopidogrel with aspirin in terms of efficacy in preventing ischemic events in patients with recent myocardial infarction, recent ischemic stroke, or PAD. Overall, there was 8.7 percent relative risk reduction for

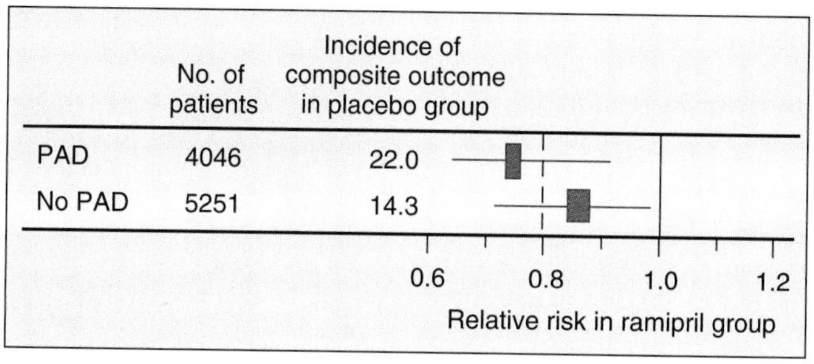

FIGURE 54–16 The relative risk of adverse cardiovascular events in the patients with and without peripheral arterial disease (PAD) according to treatment with the angiotensin-converting enzyme inhibitor ramipril in the Heart Outcomes Prevention Evaluation (HOPE) study. (Modified from Yusuf S, Sleight P, Pogue J, et al: Effects of an angiotensin-converting enzyme inhibitor, ramipril, on cardiovascular events in high-risk patients. The Heart Outcomes Prevention Evaluation Study Investigators [published erratum appears in N Engl J Med 342:748, 2000]. N Engl J Med 342:145, 2000.)

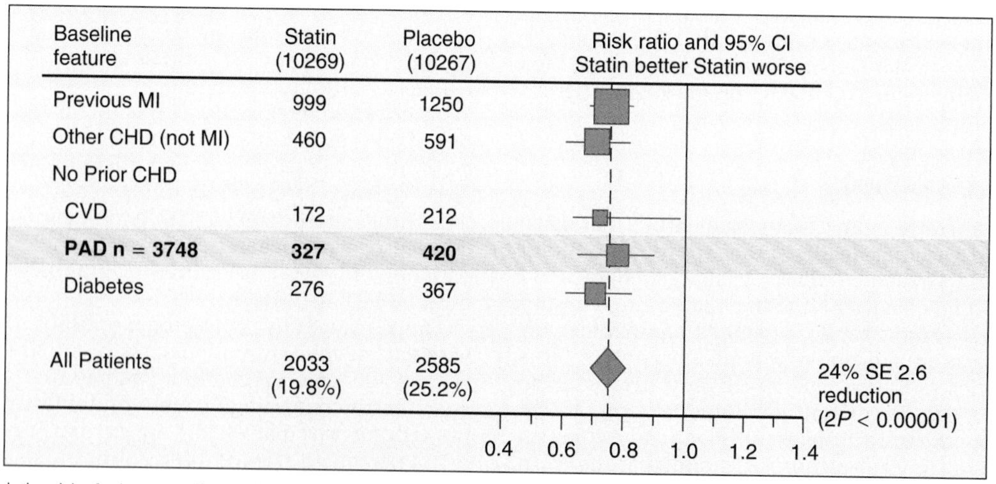

FIGURE 54–14 Relative risk of adverse cardiovascular events in participants in the Heart Protection Study based on treatment with statin or placebo. Included in this study were 6700 patients with peripheral arterial disease (PAD), including 3748 patients who had no prior coronary heart disease, in whom there was an approximate 24 percent risk reduction of vascular events. CHD = congestive heart disease; MI = myocardial infarction. (From MRC/BHF: Heart Protection Study of cholesterol lowering with simvastatin in 20,536 high-risk individuals: A randomized placebo-controlled trial. Lancet 360:7, 2002.)

myocardial infarction, ischemic stroke, or vascular death in the group treated with clopidogrel.[85] Notably, among the 6452 patients in the PAD subgroup, clopidogrel treatment reduced adverse cardiovascular events by 23.8 percent (Fig. 54–18).

Antiplatelet therapy also prevents occlusion in the peripheral circulation after revascularization procdures. Of approximately 3000 patients with peripheral arterial procedures previously analyzed by the Antiplatelet Trialists Collaboration, the odds reduction for arterial or graft occlusion by antiplatelet therapy, primarily aspirin or aspirin plus dipyridamole, was 43 percent. Ticlopidine improved long-term patency of peripheral saphenous vein bypass grafts.[110] Several studies suggested that ticlopidine improves claudication or reduces the need for reconstructive vascular surgery, but these observations will require confirmation in additional clinical trials.

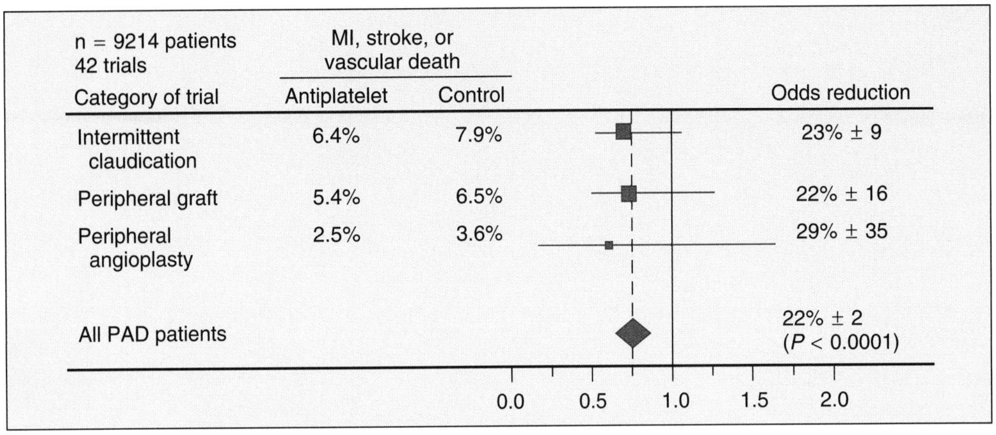

n = 9214 patients
42 trials
MI, stroke, or vascular death
Category of trial
Antiplatelet
Control
Odds reduction
Intermittent claudication
6.4%
7.9%
23% ± 9
Peripheral graft
5.4%
6.5%
22% ± 16
Peripheral angioplasty
2.5%
3.6%
29% ± 35
All PAD patients
22% ± 2
(P < 0.0001)
0.0
0.5
1.0
1.5
2.0

FIGURE 54–17 The effect of antiplatelet therapy on cardiovascular events in patients with peripheral arterial disease (PAD) based on the Antiplatelet Trialists' Collaboration. The odds ratios are shown for patients with claudication, infrainguinal bypass grafts, and percutaneous transluminal angioplasty. MI = myocardial infarction. (From Antithrombotic Trialists' Collaboration: Collaborative meta-analysis of randomised trials of antiplatelet therapy for prevention of death, myocardial infarction, and stroke in high risk patients. BMJ 324:71, 2002.)

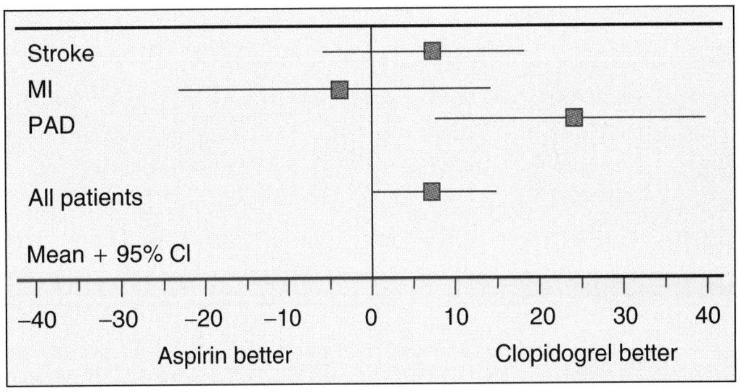

FIGURE 54–18 The relative risk reduction in adverse cardiovascular events in the Clopidogrel vs. Aspirin in Patients at Risk for Ischemic Events (CAPRIE) study. Patients with peripheral arterial disease (PAD) who received placebo had a 24 percent risk reduction compared with those receiving aspirin. (From CAPRIE Steering Committee: A randomised, blinded trial of clopidogrel versus aspirin in patients at risk of ischaemic events (CAPRIE). Lancet 348:1329, 1996.)

Pharmacotherapy

The development of effective pharmacotherapy for treating symptoms of PAD has lagged substantially behind pharmacotherapy for treating coronary artery disease. Published consensus guidelines for conducting clinical trials of pharmacological agents for treatment of patients with PAD should provide common ground for the objective evaluation of new drugs.[111] Most studies of vasodilator therapy have failed to demonstrate any efficacy in patients with intermittent claudication. Several pathophysiological explanations may account for the failure of vasodilator therapy in patients with PAD. During exercise, resistance vessels distal to a stenosis dilate in response to ischemia. Vasodilators would have minimal, if any, effect on these endogenously dilated vessels but would decrease resistance in other vessels and create a relative steal phenomenon, reducing blood flow and perfusion pressure to the affected leg. Moreover, in contrast to their effects on myocardial oxygen consumption in patients with coronary artery disease (due to afterload reduction), vasodilators do not reduce skeletal muscle oxygen demand.

In the United States, the Food and Drug Administration has approved two drugs, pentoxifylline (Trental) and cilostazol (Pletal), for treating claudication in patients with PAD. Additional drugs have been approved by licensing bodies in Europe, Asia, and South America. Pentoxifylline is a xanthine derivative used to treat patients with intermittent claudication. Its action is thought to be mediated via its hemorheological properties, including its ability to decrease blood viscosity and improve erythrocyte flexibility. It may have antiinflammatory and antiproliferative effects.[112,113] Two meta-analyses of randomized placebo-controlled trials of pentoxifylline found that it increased initial claudication distance by approximately 20 to 30 meters and absolute claudication distance by approximately 45 to 50 meters.[114,115]

Cilostazol is a quinolinone derivative that inhibits phosphodiesterase III, thereby decreasing cyclic adenosine monophosphate degradation and increasing its concentration in platelets and blood vessels. Although cilostazol inhibits platelet aggregation and causes vasodilation in experimental animals, its mechanism of action in patients with PAD is not known.[116] Several trials have reported that cilostazol improves absolute claudication distance by 40 to 50 percent as compared with placebo (Fig. 54-19).[117-119] Quality of life measures, assessed by the Medical Outcomes Scale (SF-36) and Walking Impairment Questionnaire, also demonstrated improvement. One study also found that absolute walking distance improves more with cilostazol than with either pentoxifylline or placebo, with the latter two having equivalent efficacy.[120] An advisory from the Food and Drug Administration stated that cilostazol should not be used in patients with congestive heart failure, since other phosphodiesterase III inhibitors have been shown to decrease survival in these patients.[121] The effect of cilostazol on cardiac morbidity and mortality is not known.

Other classes of drugs have been studied or are currently under investigation for treatment of either claudication or critical limb ischemia. These include serotonin (5HT-2) antagonists, calcium channel blockers, L-arginine, carnitine derivatives, vasodilator prostaglandins, and angiogenic growth factors. Naftidrofuryl, a serotonin-antagonist, has been reported to have improved symptoms of claudication in some trials and is currently available for use in Europe.[122] L-Arginine, the precursor for endothelium-derived nitric oxide, was found to have improved claudication distance after 3 weeks of intravenous therapy.[54] A nutritional bar enriched with L-arginine improved claudication time in a small study, but a large clinical trial did not confirm this observation.[56] Propionyl L-carnitine, a cofactor for fatty acid metabolism, has been reported to improve claudication, particularly in patients whose baseline maximum walking distance is less than 250 meters.[123,124]

Therapy with vasodilator prostaglandins has been investigated in patients with intermittent claudication and in those with critical limb ischemia. Intravenous administration of prostaglandin E_1 (PGE_1) or its precursor and oral administration of prostacyclin analogs improved claudication distance in preliminary trials.[125-127] A phase III study with the oral

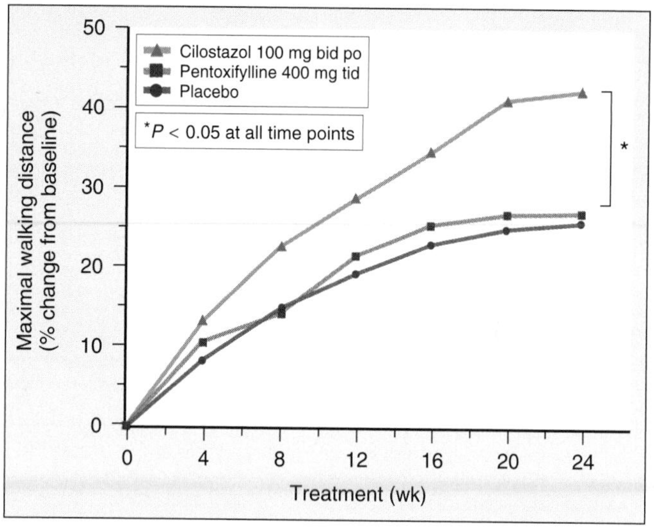

FIGURE 54–19 The effect of cilostazol, compared with pentoxifylline and placebo, on maximal walking distance. (From Dawson DL, Cutler BS, Hiatt WR, et al: A comparison of cilostazol and pentoxifylline for treating intermittent claudication. Am J Med 109:523, 2000.)

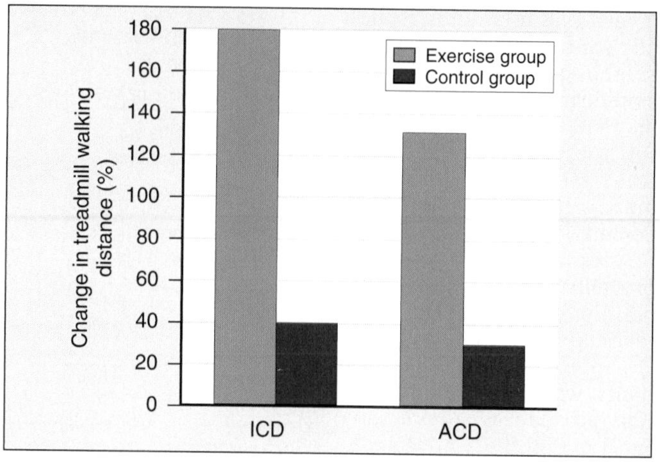

FIGURE 54–20 The effect of supervised exercise training on peak treadmill exercise time in patients with intermittent claudication. ACD = absolute claudication difference; ICD = initial claudication distance. (Adapted from Gardner AW, Poehlman ET: Exercise rehabilitation programs for the treatment of claudication pain. A meta-analysis. JAMA 274:975, 1995.)

prostacyclin derivative beraprost found no improvement in walking distance in patients with intermittent claudication.[128] In a large trial of 1560 patients with critical limb ischemia, PGE_1 administered intravenously for up to 28 days reduced the composite endpoint of death, major amputation, persistence of critical limb ischemia, acute myocardial infarction, and stroke at the time of hospital discharge from 73 to 64 percent, but its effect on this outcome did not differ significantly from the effect of placebo at the 6-month timepoint.[129] Most of the benefit of PGE_1 in this trial was related to recovery from leg ischemia.

The therapeutic use of angiogenic growth factors has engendered considerable enthusiasm. Administration of basic fibroblast growth factor and vascular endothelial growth factor as protein or gene therapy increases collateral blood vessel development, capillary number, and blood flow in experimental models of hindlimb ischemia. Gene transfer of human plasmid phVEGF165 by intraarterial catheter-based technique or by intramuscular injection into the ischemic extremity improved collateral blood vessel development in small case series.[130] Also, one recent study found that intramuscular administration of bone marrow–derived mononuclear cells to induce angiogenesis improved ABI, rest pain, and pain-free walking time in patients with chronic limb ischemia.[131] To date, few placebo-controlled clinical trials have evaluated angiogenic growth factors in patients with either claudication or critical limb ischemia. Intramuscular delivery of $AdVEGF_{121}$, an adenovirus encoding the 121 isoform of vascular endothelial growth factor, did not improve walking time or ABI in patients with claudication.[132] Intrafemoral artery administration of recombinant fibroblast growth factor-2 modestly improved maximal walking time but not ABI in patients with claudication.[133] Other studies are in progress.

Exercise Rehabilitation

Supervised exercise rehabilitation programs improve symptoms of claudication in patients with PAD. Meta-analyses of controlled studies of exercise rehabilitation found that supervised exercise programs increase the average distance walked to the onset of claudication by 180 percent and the maximal distance walked by 120 to 150 percent (Fig. 54–20).[134,135] The greatest benefit occurred when sessions were at least 30 minutes in duration, sessions occurred at least three times per week for 6 months, and walking was used as the mode of exercise. Postulated mechanisms through which exercise training improves claudication include formation of collateral vessels and improvement in endothelium-dependent vasodilation, hemorheology, muscle metabolism, and walking efficiency.[136] Studies in experimental models of hindlimb ischemia have suggested that regular exercise increases the development of collateral blood vessels.[136] Expression of angiogenic factors is increased by exercise, particularly in hypoxic tissue.[137,138] Exercise training may improve endothelium-dependent vasodilation in patients with PAD, as it does in patients with coronary atherosclerosis and in the peripheral circulation of patients with congestive heart failure.[139-141] Improvement in calf blood flow has not been demonstrated consistently in patients with claudication after exercise training, although one study found that maximal calf blood flow increased commensurate with improvement in walking distance.[136,142] To date, no imaging studies have demonstrated increased collateral blood vessels after exercise training in patients with PAD.

The benefits of exercise training in patients with PAD may result from changes in skeletal muscle function, such as increased muscle mitochondrial enzyme activity, ATP production rate, and lactate production. In patients with PAD, improvement in exercise performance is associated with a decrease in plasma and skeletal muscle short chain acylcarnitine concentrations, which indicate improvement in oxidative metabolism, and increased peak oxygen consumption.[57] Training may also enhance biomechanical performance, enabling patients to walk more efficiently with less energy expenditure.

Percutaneous Transluminal Angioplasty and Stents (see Chap. 55)

Peripheral Arterial Surgery

Surgical revascularization is generally indicated to improve quality of life in patients with disabling claudication on maximal medical therapy and to relieve rest pain and preserve limb viability in patients with critical limb ischemia not amenable to percutaneous interventions. The specific operation must take into account the anatomic location of the arterial lesions and the presence of comorbid conditions. The surgical procedure is planned after identification of the arterial obstruction by imaging, ensuring that there is sufficient arterial inflow to and outflow from the graft to maintain patency. A preoperative evaluation to assess the risk of vascular surgery should be performed, since many of these patients have coexisting coronary artery disease. Guidelines for this evaluation have been established and are beyond the scope of this chapter (see Chap. 77).[143]

Aorta–bifemoral bypass is the most frequent operation for patients with aortoiliac disease. Typically, a knitted or woven prosthesis made of Dacron or polytetrafluoroethylene (PTFE) is anastomosed proximally to the aorta and distally to each common femoral artery. Occasionally, the iliac artery is used for the distal anastomosis, to maintain antegrade flow into at least one hypogastric artery. A meta-analysis of aortic bifurcation grafts based on 23 studies reported from 1970 to 1996 noted that 5 and 10-year limb patency rates were 91 percent and 87 percent for patients with claudication, respectively, and were 88 percent and 82 percent for patients with critical limb ischemia, respectively.[144] Patency rates appear to be lower in younger than in older patients, and this may result from more aggressive atherosclerosis in the aorta and outflow vessels in these younger patients.[145] Among the more recent series in the meta-analysis, operative morbidity and mortality rates were 8.3 percent and 3.3 percent, respectively.[144]

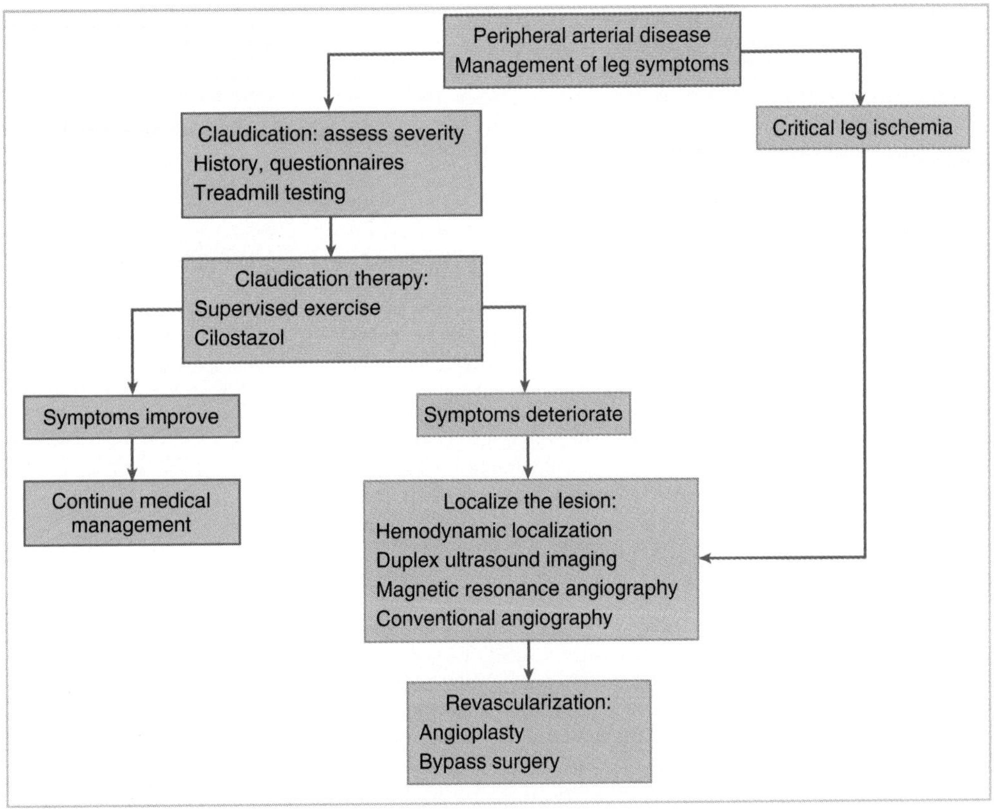

FIGURE 54–21 Management algorithm for the treatment of symptomatic peripheral arterial disease (PAD). (From Hiatt WR: Medical treatment of peripheral arterial disease and claudication. N Engl J Med 344:1608, 2001.) See also Fig. 55–1 for an aggressive scheme for life-style limiting claudication.

Extra-anatomic surgical reconstructive procedures for aortoiliac disease include axillo-bifemoral bypass, ilio-bifemoral bypass, and femoral-femoral bypass. These bypass grafts, made of Dacron or PTFE, circumvent the aorta and iliac arteries and are generally utilized in high-risk patients with critical limb ischemia.[146] Long-term patency rates are inferior to those of aorto-bifemoral bypass procedures. Five-year patency rates for axillo-bifemoral bypass operations range from 50 to 70 percent, and for femoral-femoral bypass grafts from 70 to 80 percent. The operative mortality rate for extra-anatomic bypass procedures is 3 to 5 percent, reflecting, in part, the serious comorbid conditions and advanced atherosclerosis of many of the patients who undergo these procedures.

Reconstructive surgery for infrainguinal arterial disease includes femoral-popliteal and femoral-tibial or femoral-peroneal artery bypass. In situ or reversed autologous saphenous veins or synthetic grafts made of PTFE are used for the infrainguinal bypass. Patency rates for autologous saphenous vein bypass grafts exceed those with PTFE grafts.[1,2,147,148] Also, patency rates are better for grafts in which the distal anastomosis is placed in the popliteal artery above the knee as compared with below the knee.[1] Five-year primary patency rates for femoral-popliteal reconstruction in patients with claudication are approximately 80 percent and 75 percent for autogenous vein grafts or PTFE grafts, respectively, and in patients with critical limb ischemia are approximately 65 percent and 45 percent, respectively. For femoral-below knee bypass, including tibioperoneal artery reconstruction, the 5-year patency rates for saphenous vein grafts in patients with claudication or critical limb ischemia are comparable to those for femoral-popliteal above knee grafts and range from 60 to 80 percent. The 5-year patency rate for PTFE grafts in the infrapopliteal position is considerably inferior, approximating 65 percent in patients with claudication and 33 percent in patients with critical limb ischemia. The operative mortality rate for infrainguinal bypass operations is 1 to 2 percent.

Graft stenoses can result from technical errors at the time of surgery, such as retained valve cuffs or intimal flap or valvotome injury; from fibrous intimal hyperplasia, usually within 6 months of surgery; or from atherosclerosis, usually occurring within the vein graft at least 1 to 2 years after surgery. Institution of graft surveillance protocols using color-assisted duplex ultrasonography has enabled the identification of graft stenoses, prompting graft revision and avoiding complete graft failure.[2] Graft outcome is improved as a result of routine ultrasonographic surveillance. Also, antithrombotic agents, including antiplatelet drugs and coumarin derivatives, improve graft patency. Several studies have suggested that antiplatelet drugs may be more effective in preserving synthetic grafts, whereas coumarin derivates may be more effective for vein bypass grafts.[149,150]

A management algorithm for treating symptomatic PAD is illustrated in Figure 54-21.

Vasculitis

See Chapter 82.

Thromboangiitis Obliterans

Thromboangiitis obliterans (TAO) is a segmental vasculitis that affects the distal arteries, veins, and nerves of the upper and lower extremities. It typically occurs in young persons who smoke. A patient with characteristics of TAO was described initially by von Winiwater in 1879.[151] Leo Buerger coined the term *thromboangiitis obliterans* and described its pathology in 11 amputated limbs.[152]

Pathology and Pathogenesis

Thromboangiitis obliterans primarily affects the medium and small vessels of the arms, including the radial, ulnar, palmar, and digital arteries, and their counterparts in the legs, including the tibial, peroneal, plantar, and digital arteries. Involvement can extend to the cerebral, coronary, renal, mesenteric, aortoiliac, and pulmonary arteries.[153-155] The pathological findings include an occlusive, highly cellular thrombus incorporating polymorphonuclear leukocytes, microabscesses, and occasionally multinucleated giant cells.[156] The inflammatory infiltrate can also affect the vascular wall, but the internal elastic membrane remains intact. In the chronic phase of the disease, the thrombus becomes organized and the vascular wall becomes fibrotic.

The precise cause of TAO is not known. Tobacco use or exposure is present in virtually every patient. Potential immunological mechanisms include increased cellular sensitivity to type I and type III collagen or the presence of antiendothelial cell antibodies. CD4 T cells have been identified in cellular infiltrates of vessels of patients with TAO.[157,158] The prevalence of anticardiolipin antibodies may be increased, particularly among the more severely affected patients.[159] Decreased endothelium-dependent vasodilation to acetylcholine can occur in both affected and unaffected limbs of patients with TAO, raising the possibility that reduced bioavailability of nitric oxide contributes to the disorder.[160]

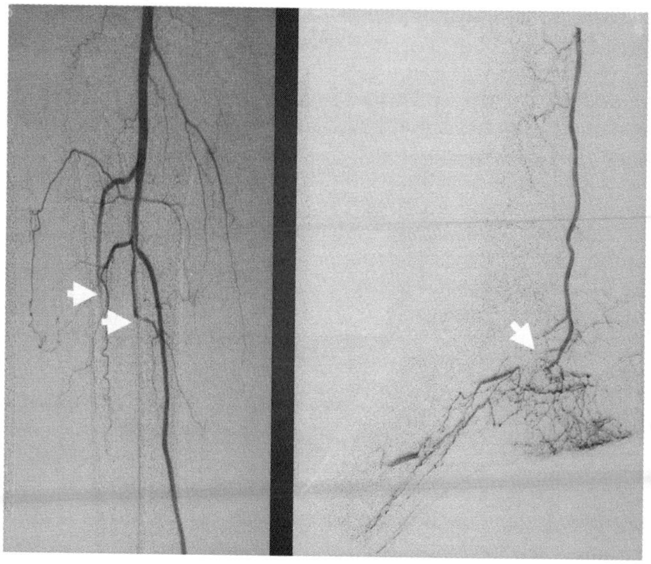

FIGURE 54–22 Angiogram of a young woman with thromboangiitis obliterans. The **left panel** demonstrates occlusion of the anterior tibial and peroneal arteries (arrows). The **right panel** demonstrates an occlusion of the distal portion of the posterior tibial artery (arrow) with bridging collateral vessels.

Clinical Presentation

The prevalence of TAO is greater in Asia than in North America or Western Europe. In the United States, TAO occurs in approximately 13 per 100,000 population.[156] Most patients with TAO develop symptoms before 45 years of age, and 75 to 90 percent are men. Patients can have claudication of the hands, forearms, feet, or calves. The majority of patients with TAO present with rest pain and digital ulcerations. Often more than one extremity is affected. Raynaud phenomenon occurs in approximately 45 percent of patients, and superficial thrombophlebitis, which may be migratory, occurs in approximately 40 percent of patients.

The radial, ulnar, dorsalis pedis, and posterior tibial pulses may be absent if the corresponding vessel is involved. The clinical characteristics of critical limb ischemia and ischemic digital ulcerations are described earlier in this chapter. The Allen test result is abnormal in two-thirds of patients.[156] To perform the Allen test, both radial and ulnar arteries are compressed while the hand is clenched and then opened. This maneuver causes palmar blanching. Release of compression from either pulse should normally produce palmar erythema if the palmar arches are patent. If these are occluded, pallor persists on the side where compression is maintained. The distal aspects of the extremities may have discrete, tender, erythematous subcutaneous cords, indicating a superficial thrombophlebitis .

Diagnosis

No specific laboratory tests other than biopsy can diagnose TAO. Most tests, therefore, require exclusion of other diseases that might have similar clinical presentations, including autoimmune diseases, such as scleroderma or systemic lupus erythematosus, hypercoagulable states, diabetes, or acute arterial occlusion due to embolism. Acute phase indicators, such as the erythrocyte sedimentation rate or C-reactive protein, are usually normal. Serum immunological markers, including antinuclear antibodies and rheumatoid factor, should not be present, and serum complement levels should be normal. If clinically indicated, a proximal source of embolism should be excluded by cardiac and vascular ultrasonography or by arteriography. Arteriography of an affected limb supports the diagnosis of TAO if there is segmental occlusion of small and medium-size arteries, absence of atherosclerosis, and corkscrew collateral vessels circumventing the occlusion (Fig. 54–22). These same findings, however, can occur in patients with scleroderma, systemic lupus erythematosus, mixed connective tissue disease, and antiphospholipid antibody syndrome. The pathognomonic test is a biopsy showing the classic pathological findings. This procedure is rarely indicated, and biopsy sites may fail to heal because of severe ischemia. The diagnosis, therefore, usually depends on an age of onset younger than 45 years, a history of tobacco use, physical examination demonstrating distal limb ischemia, exclusion of other diseases, and, if necessary, angiographic demonstration of typical lesions.[161]

Treatment

The cornerstone of treatment is cessation of tobacco use.[162] Patients without gangrene who stop smoking rarely require amputation.[163,164] In contrast, one or more amputations may ultimately be required in 40 to 45 percent of those patients with TAO who continue to smoke.

Several drugs can benefit patients with TAO. The prostacyclin analogue iloprost, administered 6 hours per day for 28 days, was more effective than aspirin in relieving rest pain and healing ulcers.[165] In a multicenter trial, however, oral iloprost administered for 8 weeks had no greater effect than placebo in healing ulcers, although there was somewhat more effective relief of pain at low doses.[166] Cyclophosphamide improved symptoms but not the angiographic appearance of TAO in one study.[167] A naked plasmid DNA-encoding vascular endothelial growth factor (phVEGF 165) was administered intramuscularly into seven limbs of six patients with TAO, with subsequent healing of ulcers in three to five limbs and relief of rest pain in two others.[168]

Vascular reconstructive surgery is usually not a viable option because of the segmental nature of this disease and involvement of distal vessels. An autogenous saphenous vein bypass graft can be considered if a target vessel for the distal anastomosis is available. Long-term patency rates are better in ex-smokers than in smokers.[169]

Takayasu Arteritis and Giant Cell Arteritis

See Chapter 82.

Acute Limb Ischemia

Acute limb ischemia occurs when an arterial occlusion suddenly reduces blood flow to the arm or leg. The metabolic needs of the tissue outstrip perfusion, placing limb viability in jeopardy. The clinical presentation of patients with acute limb ischemia relates to the location of the arterial occlusion and the resulting decrease in blood flow. Depending on the severity of ischemia, patients may note disabling claudication or pain at rest. Pain may develop over a short period and is manifest in the affected extremity distal to the site of obstruction. It is not necessarily confined to the foot or toes, or hand or fingers, as is usually the case in chronic limb ischemia. Concurrent ischemia of peripheral nerves causes sensory loss and motor dysfunction.

The physical findings can include absence of pulses distal to the occlusion, cool skin, pallor, delayed capillary return and venous filling, diminished or absent sensory perception, and muscular weakness or paralysis. This constellation of symptoms and signs is often recalled as the five Ps, *p*ain, *p*ulselessness, *p*allor, *p*aresthesias, and *p*aralysis.

Prognosis

Comorbid cardiovascular disorders are usually found in patients who present with acute limb ischemia and may even be responsible for the event. Therefore, long-term prognosis is limited in this population.[170] The 5-year survival rate after acute limb ischemia caused by thrombosis approximates 45 percent and after embolism is less than 20 percent.[171] The 1-month survival rate in persons older than 75 years of age with acute limb ischemia approximates 40 percent.[172] The risk of limb loss depends on the severity of the ischemia and the elapsed time before a revascularization procedure is undertaken.

A classification scheme that takes into consideration the severity of ischemia and the viability of the limb, along with related neurological findings and Doppler signals, has been developed by the Society for Vascular Surgery and the International Society for Cardiovascular Surgery (Table 54–8).[67] A viable limb, category 1, is not immediately threatened, has neither sensory nor motor abnormalities, and has blood flow detectable by Doppler. Threatened viability, category 2, indicates that the severity of ischemia will cause limb loss unless the blood supply is restored promptly. The category is subdivided into marginally and immediately threatened limbs, the latter characterized by pain, sensory deficits, and muscular weakness. Arterial blood flow cannot be detected by Doppler. Irreversible limb ischemia leading to tissue loss and requiring amputation, category 3, is characterized by loss of sensation, paralysis, and the absence of Doppler-detected blood flow in both arteries and veins distal to the occlusion.

Pathogenesis

The causes of acute limb ischemia include arterial embolism, thrombosis in situ, dissection, and trauma. Most arterial emboli arise from thrombotic sources in the heart. Atrial fibrillation complicating valvular heart disease, congestive heart failure, coronary artery disease, and hypertension accounts for approximately 50 percent of cardiac emboli to the limbs. Other sources include rheumatic or prosthetic cardiac valves, ventricular thrombus resulting from myocardial infarction or left ventricular aneurysm, paradoxical embolism of venous thrombi through the intraatrial or intraventricular communications, and cardiac tumors such as left atrial myxomas. Aneurysms of the aorta or peripheral arteries may harbor thrombi, which subsequently embolize to more distal arterial sites, usually lodging at branch points where the artery decreases in size.

Thrombosis in situ occurs in atherosclerotic peripheral arteries, infrainguinal bypass grafts, peripheral artery aneurysms, and normal arteries of patients with hypercoagulable states. In patients with peripheral atherosclerosis, thrombosis in situ may complicate plaque rupture, causing acute arterial occlusion and limb ischemia, in a manner analogous to that which occurs in coronary arteries in patients with acute myocardial infarction. Thrombosis complicating popliteal artery aneurysms is a much more common complication than rupture and may account for 10 percent of cases of acute limb ischemia in elderly men.[1,173] Acute thrombotic occlusion of a normal artery is unusual but may occur in patients with procoagulant disorders such as antiphospholipid antibody syndrome, activated protein C resistance (Factor V Leiden), deficiency of protein C or S, heparin-induced thrombocytopenia, essential thrombocythemia, and hyperhomocysteinemia. One of the most common causes of acute limb ischemia is thrombotic occlusion of an infrainguinal bypass graft, as discussed previously.

Diagnostic Tests

The history and physical examination usually establish the diagnosis of acute limb ischemia. Time available for diagnostic tests is often limited, and diagnostic tests should not delay urgent revascularization procedures if limb viability is immediately threatened. The pressure in the affected limb and corresponding ABI can be measured if flow is detectable by Doppler ultrasonography. A Doppler probe can be used to

TABLE 54–8 Clinical Categories of Acute Limb Ischemia (Modified from the SVS/ISCVS Classification)

		Findings		Doppler Signals	
Category	**Description/Prognosis**	***Sensory loss***	***Muscle weakness***	***Arterial***	***Venous***
I. Viable	Not immediately threatened	None	None	audible	Audible
II. Threatened					
a. Marginally	Salvageable if promptly treated	Minimal (toes) or none	None	(Often) inaudible	Audible
b. Immediately	Salvageable with immediate revascularization	More than toes, rest pain	Mild, moderate	(Usually) inaudible	Audible
III. Irreversible	Major tissue loss or permanent nerve damage inevitable	Profound, anesthetic	Profound, paralysis (rigor)	Inaudible	Inaudible

Adapted from Rutherford RB, Baker JD, Ernst C, et al. Recommended standards for reports dealing with lower extremity ischemia: revised version. J Vasc Surg 26:517, 1997.

detect the presence of blood flow in peripheral arteries, particularly when pulses are not palpable. Color-assisted duplex ultrasonography can be used to determine the site of occlusion. It is particularly applicable to evaluate the patency of infrainguinal bypass grafts. Contrast arteriography demonstrates the site of occlusion and provides an anatomic guide for revascularization.

Treatment

Analgesic medications should be administered to reduce pain. For patients with acute leg ischemia, the bed should be positioned such that the feet are lower than chest level, thereby increasing limb perfusion pressure via gravitational effects. This can be accomplished by putting blocks under the posts at the head of the bed. Efforts should be made to reduce pressure on the heels, on bony prominences, and between the toes by appropriate placement of soft material on the bed, such as sheep skin, and between the toes, such as lamb's wool. The room should be kept warm to prevent cold-induced cutaneous vasoconstriction.

Heparin is administered intravenously as soon as the diagnosis of acute limb ischemia is made. The dose should be sufficient to increase the partial thromboplastin time by 1.5 to 2.5 times control values to prevent thrombus propagation or recurrent embolism. It is not known whether low-molecular-weight heparin would be as effective as unfractionated heparin in patients with acute limb ischemia.

Catheter-directed intraarterial thrombolysis is an initial treatment option for patients presenting with category I and IIA acute limb ischemia, if there is no contraindication to thrombolysis.[174-176] Catheter-based thrombolysis can also be considered for patients with more severe limb ischemia who are considered a high risk for surgical intervention. Long-term patency after thrombolysis is greater in patients with category I and II critical limb ischemia than in those with category III, in native arteries than in grafts, and in vein grafts than in prosthetic grafts.[176] Identification and repair of a graft stenosis after successful thrombolysis improves long-term graft patency.[176,177] Thrombolytic regimens have employed streptokinase, urokinase, recombinant tissue plasminogen activator, and reteplase. The duration of catheter-based thrombolytic therapy should generally not exceed 48 hours to achieve optimal benefit and limit the risk of bleeding. Percutaneous, catheter-based, mechanical thrombectomy can be used alone or in addition to pharmacological thrombolysis to treat patients with acute limb ischemia.[175,178]

Urgent revascularization is indicated for patients presenting with category IIB and early category III acute limb ischemia. The procedure depends on the nature and location of the arterial occlusion. Thromboembolectomy can be attempted in patients whose acute limb ischemia is caused by systemic embolism.[179] If thromboembolectomy is neither feasible nor successful, then surgical reconstruction, bypassing the occluded area, should be performed. These techniques were discussed previously in this chapter.

Five prospective randomized trials, comprising 1283 patients, have compared the benefits and risks of thrombolysis and surgical reconstruction in patients presenting with acute limb ischemia (Table 54–9).[180] The Surgery versus Thrombolysis for Ischemia of the Lower Extremity (STILE) trial compared thrombolysis with either recombinant tissue plasminogen activator or urokinase to surgery after native artery or graft occlusion in patients with limb ischemia of less than 6 months' duration. The trial was stopped prematurely after enrollment of 393 patients. The composite outcome of death, ongoing or recurrent ischemia, major amputation, and major morbidity occurred in 62 percent of the group randomized to thrombolysis compared with 36 percent of those randomized to surgery. Of those patients who had symptoms for less than 14 days, however, amputation-free survival at 6 months was greater in the patients treated with thrombolysis than in those treated with surgery.[181] In the Thrombolysis or Peripheral Arterial Study (TOPAS), intraarterial thrombolysis with urokinase was compared to surgery in 554 patients with acute limb ischemia of less than 14 days. Amputation-free survival at 6 and 12 months was 72 and 65 percent, respectively, in the thrombolysis group and 75 and 70 percent, respectively, in the surgery group.[182] Taken together, the findings from these trials would suggest that catheter-based thrombolysis is an appropriate initial option in patients with category I and IIA acute limb ischemia of less than 7 days' duration, whereas surgical revascularization would be more appropriate for those with category IIB and early III acute limb ischemia and in those whose symptoms have been present for more than 7 days (Fig. 54–23).

Atheroembolism

Atheroembolism refers to the occlusion of arteries resulting from detachment and embolization of atheromatous debris, including fibrin, platelets, cholesterol crystals, and calcium fragments. Other terms include *atherogenic embolism* and *cholesterol embolism*. Atheroemboli originate most frequently from shaggy protruding atheromas of the aorta and less frequently from atherosclerotic branch arteries. The atheroemboli typically occlude small downstream arteries and arterioles of the extremities, brain, eye, kidneys, or mesentery.[183,184]

The prevalence of atheroembolism in the general population is not known. Most affected individuals are males who are older than 60 years of age with clinical evidence of atherosclerosis. The Dutch National Pathology Information System reported an incidence of atheroemboli in 6.2 patients per million per year, and atheroemboli were present in 0.3 percent of autopsy cases.[185] In autopsy series of persons over the age of 60, the incidence of atheroembolism has ranged from 0.8 to 2.4 percent.

Pathogenesis

The risk of atheroembolism is greatest in patients with aortic atherosclerosis characterized by large protruding atheromas (see Fig. 54–5). There is a strong association between large

TABLE 54–9 Comparison of Catheter-Directed Thrombolysis and Surgical Revascularization in Treatment of Limb Ischemia

		Catheter Directed Thrombolysis			Surgical Revascularization		
Study	Results at	*Patients*	*Limb Salvage (%)*	*Mortality (%)*	*Patients*	*Limb Salvage (%)*	*Mortality (%)*
Rochester	12 mo	57	82	16	57	82	42
STILE[181]	6 mo	248	88	6	144	89	8
TOPAS[182]	12 mo	272	85	20	272	86	17

Adapted from Dormandy JA, Rutherford RB: Management of peripheral arterial disease (PAD), TASC Working Group. J Vasc Surg 31:S1, 2000.

aortic plaques identified by ultrasonography and previous embolic disease.[186-188] Similarly, identification of large protruding atheromas by transesophageal echocardiography predicts future embolic events.[186,189,190] Approximately 50 percent of atheroemboli involve vessels in the lower extremities.

Catheter manipulation causes a large proportion of atheroemboli.[191] Similarly, surgical manipulation of the aorta during cardiac or vascular operations precipitates atheroembolism in 2 to 3 percent of patients.[192] Controversy remains as to whether anticoagulants or thrombolytic drugs contribute to atheroembolism.[183,184,190,193,194] In the Stroke Prevention and Atrial Fibrillation (SPAF) study, atheroembolism occurred in 0.7 percent per patient-year in those patients assigned to adjusted-dose warfarin.[195] In the French Study of Aortic Plaques in Stroke Group, no patient receiving warfarin developed clinical evidence of atheroembolism.[189] Muscle biopsies at the time of coronary artery bypass surgery in patients with recent myocardial infarction detected atheroemboli in 14 percent of patients who received thrombolysis and 10 percent of those who did not.[196]

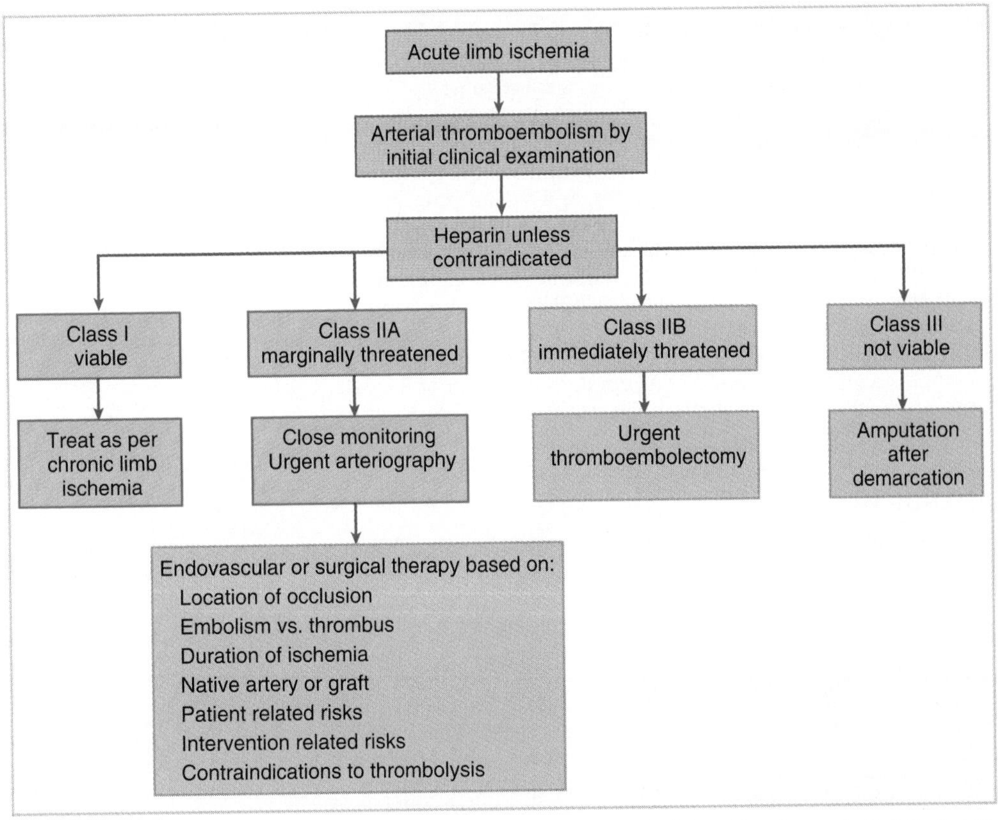

FIGURE 54–23 Management algorithm for the treatment of acute limb ischemia. (Adapted from Dormandy JA, Rutherford RB: Management of peripheral arterial disease (PAD). TASC Working Group. J Vasc Surg 31:S1, 2000.)

Clinical Presentation

The most notable clinical features of atheroembolism to the extremities includes painful cyanotic toes, resulting in the appellation *blue-toe syndrome* (Fig. 54–24). Livedo reticularis occurs in approximately 50 percent of patients. Local areas of erythematous or violaceous discoloration may be present on the lateral aspects of the feet and the soles and also on the calves. Other findings include digital and foot ulcerations, nodules, purpura, and petechiae. Pedal pulses are typically present, since the emboli tend to lodge in the more distal digital arteries and arterioles. Symptoms and signs indicating additional organ involvement with atheroemboli should be sought. Fundoscopy can visualize Hollenhorst plaques in patients with visual loss secondary to retinal ischemia or infarction. Renal involvement manifested by increased blood pressure and azotemia commonly occurs in patients with peripheral atheroemboli. Patients also sometimes have evidence of mesenteric or bladder ischemia and splenic infarction.

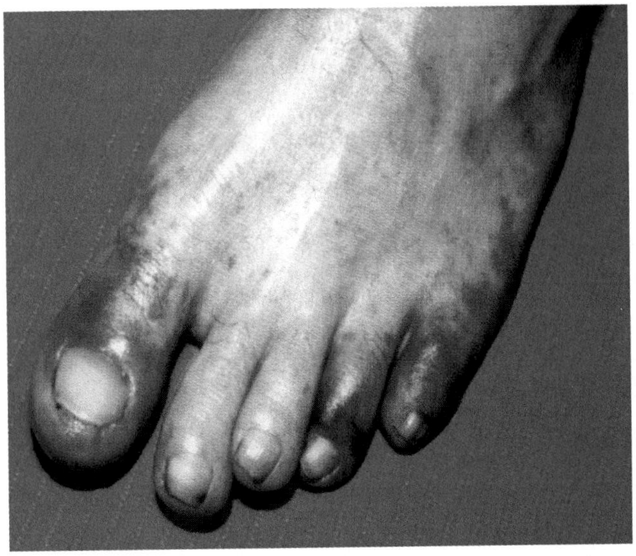

FIGURE 54–24 Atheroemboli to the foot, or "blue toe syndrome." There is cyanotic discoloration of the first, fourth, and fifth toes, as well as localized areas of violaceous discoloration along the lateral aspect of the foot.

The clinical setting and findings are usually sufficient to diagnose atheroembolism. However, some of the manifestations of atheroemboli may be present with other diseases. As discussed previously, critical limb ischemia occurs in patients with severe peripheral atherosclerosis, and acute limb ischemia is a consequence of thromboembolism, each of which would be characterized by an abnormal pulse examination. Hypersensitivity vasculitides secondary to connective tissue diseases, infections, drugs, polyarteritis nodosa, or cryoglobulinemia, for example, may manifest with multisystem organ damage and cutaneous findings of purpura, ulcers, and digital ischemia similar to those findings that result from atheroemboli (see Chap. 82). Procoagulant disorders such as antiphospholipid antibody syndrome, heparin-induced thrombocytopenia, and myeloproliferative disorders such as essential thrombocythemia can cause digital artery thrombosis with resultant digital ischemia, cyanosis, and ulceration.

Laboratory studies that are consistent with atheroembolism include an elevated erythrocyte sedimentation rate, eosinophilia, and eosinophiluria. Other findings may include anemia, thrombocytopenia, hypocomplementemia, and azotemia. Imaging of the aorta with transesophageal echocardiography, magnetic resonance angiography, and computed tomography may identify sites of severe atherosclerosis and shaggy atheroma indicative of a source for atheroemboli.[197] The only definitive test for atheroembolism is pathological confirmation by skin or muscle biopsy. Pathognomonic findings include elongated needle-shaped clefts in small arteries, which are caused by cholesterol crystals, often accompanied by inflammatory infiltrates composed of lymphocytes and possibly giant cells and eosinophils, intimal thickening, and perivascular fibrosis.

Treatment

There is no definitive treatment for atheroembolism. Analgesics should be administered for pain. Local foot care should be provided as described previously for patients with acute limb ischemia. It may be necessary to excise or amputate necrotic areas.

Patients with this condition are subject to recurrent atheroembolic events. Risk factor modification, such as lipid-lowering therapy and smoking cessation, can have favorable effects on overall outcome from atherosclerosis, but it is not known whether such intervention will prevent recurrent atheroembolism. The use of antiplatelet drugs to prevent recurrent atheroembolism remains controversial.[184,188] It is reasonable, however, to administer antiplatelet agents even in the absence of strong clinical evidence of efficacy, since the agents will prevent other adverse cardiovascular events in patients with atherosclerosis. The use of warfarin also engenders controversy, and some investigators have even suggested that anticoagulants precipitate atheroemboli.[183,184,186,193] Others have found that warfarin reduces atheroembolic events, particularly in patients with mobile aortic atheroma.[190,194] The use of corticosteroids to treat atheroembolism also remains controversial.[184]

Surgical removal of the source should be considered in patients with atheroembolism, particularly in those in whom it recurs. Surgical procedures include excision and replacement of affected portions of the aorta, endarterectomy, and bypass operations. Operative intervention is targeted to the site of the aorta, iliac, or femoral arteries where there is aneurysm formation or obvious shaggy friable atherosclerotic plaque. Often, the aorta is diffusely affected by severe atherosclerosis and it is not possible to identify the precise segment that is responsible for atheroembolism. In addition, many of these patients are elderly and have coexisting coronary artery disease, which increases the risk of major vascular operations.

REFERENCES

General Considerations and Epidemiology

1. Dormandy JA, Rutherford RB: Management of peripheral arterial disease (PAD). TASC Working Group. J Vasc Surg 31:S1, 2000.
2. ACC/AHA Guidelines for the Management of Peripheral Arterial Disease. J Am Coll Cardiol. In press. Available at http://www.acc.org/xxx.
3. Meijer WT, Hoes AW, Rutgers D, et al: Peripheral arterial disease in the elderly: The Rotterdam Study. Arterioscler Thromb Vasc Biol 18:185, 1998.
4. Hirsch AT, Criqui MH, Treat-Jacobson D, et al: Peripheral arterial disease detection, awareness, and treatment in primary care. JAMA 286:1317, 2001.
5. Murabito JM, Evans JC, Nieto K, et al: Prevalence and clinical correlates of peripheral arterial disease in the Framingham Offspring Study. Am Heart J 143:961, 2002.
6. Criqui MH: Peripheral arterial disease—epidemiological aspects. Vasc Med 6(Suppl 1):3, 2001.
7. Beckman J, Creager M: Risk factors. *In* Creager M (ed): Management of Peripheral Arterial Disease. London, ReMEDICA Publishing, 2000, pp 19-42.
8. Lu J, Creager MA: The relationship of cigarette smoking to peripheral arterial disease. Rev Cardiovasc Med. In press.
9. Doyle J, Creager MA: Pharmacotherapy and behavioral intervention for peripheral arterial disease. Rev Cardiovasc Med 4:18, 2003.
10. Beckman JA, Creager MA, Libby P: Diabetes and atherosclerosis: Epidemiology, pathophysiology, and management. JAMA 287:2570, 2002.
11. Jude EB, Oyibo SO, Chalmers N, Boulton AJ: Peripheral arterial disease in diabetic and nondiabetic patients: A comparison of severity and outcome. Diabetes Care 24:1433, 2001.
12. Criqui MH, Denenberg JO, Langer RD, Fronek A: The epidemiology of peripheral arterial disease: Importance of identifying the population at risk. Vasc Med 2:221, 1997.
13. Ridker PM, Stampfer MJ, Rifai N: Novel risk factors for systemic atherosclerosis: A comparison of C-reactive protein, fibrinogen, homocysteine, lipoprotein(a), and standard cholesterol screening as predictors of peripheral arterial disease. JAMA 285:2481, 2001.
14. Murabito JM, D'Agostino RB, Silbershatz H, Wilson WF: Intermittent claudication: A risk profile from The Framingham Heart Study. Circulation 96:44, 1997.
15. Cheng SW, Ting AC, Wong J: Lipoprotein (a) and its relationship to risk factors and severity of atherosclerotic peripheral vascular disease. Eur J Vasc Endovasc Surg 14:17, 1997.
16. Kannel WB: The demographics of claudication and the aging of the American population. Vasc Med 1:60, 1996.
17. Hooi JD, Kester AD, Stoffers HE, et al: Incidence of and risk factors for asymptomatic peripheral arterial occlusive disease: A longitudinal study. Am J Epidemiol 153:666, 2001.
18. Boushey CJ, Beresford SA, Omenn GS, Motulsky AG: A quantitative assessment of plasma homocysteine as a risk factor for vascular disease. Probable benefits of increasing folic acid intakes. JAMA 274:1049, 1995.
19. Graham IM, Daly LE, Refsum HM, et al: Plasma homocysteine as a risk factor for vascular disease. The European Concerted Action Project. JAMA 277:1775, 1997.
20. Smith FB, Lowe GD, Lee AJ, et al: Smoking, hemorheologic factors, and progression of peripheral arterial disease in patients with claudication. J Vasc Surg 28:129, 1998.
21. Smith FB, Lee AJ, Hau CM, et al: Plasma fibrinogen, haemostatic factors and prediction of peripheral arterial disease in the Edinburgh Artery Study. Blood Coagul Fibrinolysis 11:43, 2000.
22. Ridker PM, Cushman M, Stampfer MJ, et al: Plasma concentration of C-reactive protein and risk of developing peripheral vascular disease. Circulation 97:425, 1998.

Pathophysiology of PAD

23. Aird WC: Endothelial cell heterogeneity. Crit Care Med 31:S221, 2003.
24. Shimizu K, Sugiyama S, Aikawa M, et al: Host bone-marrow cells are a source of donor intimal smooth-muscle-like cells in murine aortic transplant arteriopathy. Nat Med 7:738, 2001.
25. Saiura A, Sata M, Hirata Y, et al: Circulating smooth muscle progenitor cells contribute to atherosclerosis. Nat Med 7:382, 2001.
26. Hristov M, Erl W, Weber PC: Endothelial progenitor cells: Mobilization, differentiation, and homing. Arterioscler Thromb Vasc Biol 23:1185, 2003.
27. Aird WC, Edelberg JM, Weiler-Guettler H, et al: Vascular bed-specific expression of an endothelial cell gene is programmed by the tissue microenvironment. J Cell Biol 138:1117, 1997.
28. Guillot PV, Guan J, Liu L, et al: A vascular bed-specific pathway. J Clin Invest 103:799, 1999.
29. Adams RH, Wilkinson GA, Weiss C, et al: Roles of ephrinB ligands and EphB receptors in cardiovascular development: Demarcation of arterial/venous domains, vascular morphogenesis, and sprouting angiogenesis. Genes Develop 13:295, 1999.
30. Shin D, Garcia-Cardena G, Hayashi S, et al: Expression of ephrinB2 identifies a stable genetic difference between arterial and venous vascular smooth muscle as well as endothelial cells, and marks subsets of microvessels at sites of adult neovascularization. Dev Biol 230:139, 2001.
31. Tomlinson JE, Topper JN: New insights into endothelial diversity. Curr Atheroscler Rep 5:223, 2003.
32. Liu C, Bhattacharjee G, Boisvert W, et al: In vivo interrogation of the molecular display of atherosclerotic lesion surfaces. Am J Pathol 163:1859, 2003.
33. Majesky MW: Vascular smooth muscle diversity: Insights from developmental biology. Curr Atheroscler Rep 5:208, 2003.
34. Bergwerff M, Gittenberger-de Groot AC, Wisse LJ, et al: Loss of function of the Prx1 and Prx2 homeobox genes alters architecture of the great elastic arteries and ductus arteriosus. Virchows Arch 436:12, 2000.
35. Lu J, Landerholm TE, Wei JS, et al: Coronary smooth muscle differentiation from proepicardial cells requires rhoA-mediated actin reorganization and p160 rho-kinase activity. Dev Biol 240:404, 2001.
36. Miano JM: Mammalian smooth muscle differentiation: Origins, markers and transcriptional control. Results Probl Cell Differ 38:39, 2002.
37. Li L, Liu Z, Mercer B, et al: Evidence for serum response factor-mediated regulatory networks governing SM22alpha transcription in smooth, skeletal, and cardiac muscle cells. Dev Biol 187:311, 1997.
38. Yamagishi H, Olson EN, Srivastava D: The basic helix-loop-helix transcription factor, dHAND, is required for vascular development [review]. J Clin Invest 105:261, 2000.
39. Lilly B, Olson EN, Beckerle MC: Identification of a CArG box–dependent enhancer within the cysteine-rich protein 1 gene that directs expression in arterial but not venous or visceral smooth muscle cells. Dev Biol 240:531, 2001.
40. Ikari Y, McManus BM, Kenyon J, Schwartz SM: Neonatal intima formation in the human coronary artery. Arterioscler Thromb Vasc Biol 19:2036, 1999.
41. Weninger WJ, Muller GB, Reiter C, et al: Intimal hyperplasia of the infant parasellar carotid artery: A potential developmental factor in atherosclerosis and SIDS. Circ Res 85:970, 1999.
42. Schwartz SM: The intima: A new soil. Circ Res 85:877, 1999.

43. Rainwater DL, McMahan CA, Malcom GT, et al: Lipid and apolipoprotein predictors of atherosclerosis in youth: Apolipoprotein concentrations do not materially improve prediction of arterial lesions in PDAY subjects. The PDAY Research Group. Arterioscler Thromb Vasc Biol 19:753, 1999.
44. Strong JP, Malcom GT, Oalmann MC, Wissler RW: The PDAY Study: Natural history, risk factors, and pathobiology. Pathobiological Determinants of Atherosclerosis in Youth. Ann N Y Acad Sci 811:226, 1997.
45. de Groot E, Jukema JW, Montauban van Swijndregt AD, et al: B-mode ultrasound assessment of pravastatin treatment effect on carotid and femoral artery walls and its correlations with coronary arteriographic findings: A report of the Regression Growth Evaluation Statin Study (REGRESS). J Am Coll Cardiol 31:1561, 1998.
46. Zhao XQ, Yuan C, Hatsukami TS, et al: Effects of prolonged intensive lipid-lowering therapy on the characteristics of carotid atherosclerotic plaques in vivo by MRI: A case-control study. Arterioscler Thromb Vasc Biol 21:1623, 2001.
47. Vink A, Schoneveld AH, Borst C, Pasterkamp G: The contribution of plaque and arterial remodeling to de novo atherosclerotic luminal narrowing in the femoral artery. J Vasc Surg 36:1194, 2002.
48. de Korte CL, Pasterkamp G, van der Steen AF, et al: Characterization of plaque components with intravascular ultrasound elastography in human femoral and coronary arteries in vitro. Circulation 102:617, 2000.
49. Carr SC, Farb A, Pearce WH, et al: Activated inflammatory cells are associated with plaque rupture in carotid artery stenosis. Surgery 122:757, discussion 763, 1997.
50. Pradhan AD, Rifai N, Ridker PM: Soluble intercellular adhesion molecule–1, soluble vascular adhesion molecule-1, and the development of symptomatic peripheral arterial disease in men. Circulation 106:820, 2002.
51. Yuan C, Zhang SX, Polissar NL, et al: Identification of fibrous cap rupture with magnetic resonance imaging is highly associated with recent transient ischemic attack or stroke. Circulation 105:181, 2002.
52. Rothwell PM, Villagra R, Gibson R, et al: Evidence of a chronic systemic cause of instability of atherosclerotic plaques. Lancet 355:19, 2000.

Pathophysiology of Limb Ischemia

53. Meredith IT, Currie KE, Anderson TJ, et al: Postischemic vasodilation in human forearm is dependent on endothelium-derived nitric oxide. Am J Physiol 270:H1435, 1996.
54. Böger RH, Bode-Böger SM, Thiele W, et al: Restoring vascular nitric oxide formation by L-arginine improves the symptoms of intermittent claudication in patients with peripheral arterial occlusive disease. J Am Coll Cardiol 32:1336, 1998.
55. Schellong SM, Boger RH, Burchert W, et al: Dose-related effect of intravenous L-arginine on muscular blood flow of the calf in patients with peripheral vascular disease: A H215O positron emission tomography study. Clin Sci (Colch) 93:159, 1997.
56. Maxwell AJ, Anderson BE, Cooke JP: Nutritional therapy for peripheral arterial disease: A double-blind, placebo-controlled, randomized trial of HeartBar. Vasc Med 5:11, 2000.
57. Hiatt WR: Pathophysiology. *In* Creager M (ed): Management of Peripheral Arterial Disease. London, ReMEDICA Publishing Limited, 2000, pp 43-56.
58. Pipinos II, Shepard AD, Anagnostopoulos PV, et al: Phosphorus 31 nuclear magnetic resonance spectroscopy suggests a mitochondrial defect in claudicating skeletal muscle. J Vasc Surg 31:944, 2000.
59. Bollinger A, Hoffmann U, Franzeck UK: Microvascular changes in arterial occlusive disease: Target for pharmacotherapy. Vasc Med 1:50, 1996.
60. Brevetti G, Corrado S, Martone VD, et al: Microcirculation and tissue metabolism in peripheral arterial disease. Clin Hemorheol Microcirc 21:245, 1999.
61. McDermott MM, Mehta S, Greenland P: Exertional leg symptoms other than intermittent claudication are common in peripheral arterial disease. Arch Intern Med 159:387, 1999.
62. McDermott MM, Fried L, Simonsick E, et al: Asymptomatic peripheral arterial disease is independently associated with impaired lower extremity functioning: The women's health and aging study. Circulation 101:1007, 2000.

Testing for PAD

63. McDermott MM, Liu K, Guralnik JM, et al: The ankle brachial index independently predicts walking velocity and walking endurance in peripheral arterial disease. J Am Geriatr Soc 46:1355, 1998.
64. Leng GC, Fowkes FG: The Edinburgh Claudication Questionnaire: An improved version of the WHO/Rose Questionnaire for use in epidemiological surveys. J Clin Epidemiol 45:1101, 1992.
65. Criqui MH, Denenberg JO, Bird CE, et al: The correlation between symptoms and non-invasive test results in patients referred for peripheral arterial disease testing. Vasc Med 1:65, 1996.
66. Coyne KS, Margolis MK, Gilchrist KA, et al: Evaluating effects of method of administration on Walking Impairment Questionnaire. J Vasc Surg 38:296, 2003.
67. Rutherford RB, Baker JD, Ernst C, et al: Recommended standards for reports dealing with lower extremity ischemia: Revised version. J Vasc Surg 26:517, 1997.
68. Nichols WW, O'Rourke MF: Wave reflections. *In* Nichols WW, O'Rourke MF (eds): McDonald's Blood Flow in Arteries. 4th ed. London, Arnold, 1998, pp 201-222.
69. McDermott MM, Greenland P, Liu K, et al: The ankle brachial index is associated with leg function and physical activity: The Walking and Leg Circulation Study. Ann Intern Med 136:873, 2002.
70. Chaudhry H, Holland A, Dormandy J: Comparison of graded versus constant treadmill test protocols for quantifying intermittent claudication. Vasc Med 2:93, 1997.
71. Creager MA: Clinical assessment of the patient with claudication: The role of the vascular laboratory. Vasc Med 2:231, 1997.
72. Gale SS, Scissons RP, Salles-Cunha SX, et al: Lower extremity arterial evaluation: Are segmental arterial blood pressures worthwhile? J Vasc Surg 27:831, discussion 838, 1998.
73. Pemberton M, London NJ: Colour flow duplex imaging of occlusive arterial disease of the lower limb. Br J Surg 84:912, 1997.
74. Visser K, Hunink MG: Peripheral arterial disease: Gadolinium-enhanced MR angiography versus color-guided duplex US—a meta-analysis. Radiology 216:67, 2000.
75. Poon E, Yucel EK, Pagan-Marin H, Kayne H: Iliac artery stenosis measurements: Comparison of two-dimensional time-of-flight and three-dimensional dynamic gadolinium-enhanced MR angiography. AJR Am J Roentgenol 169:1139, 1997.
76. Ho KY, de Haan MW, Kessels AG, et al: Peripheral vascular tree stenoses: Detection with subtracted and nonsubtracted MR angiography. Radiology 206:673, 1998.
77. Quinn SF, Sheley RC, Semonsen KG, et al: Aortic and lower-extremity arterial disease: Evaluation with MR angiography versus conventional angiography. Radiology 206:693, 1998.
78. Rofsky NM, Johnson G, Adelman MA, et al: Peripheral vascular disease evaluated with reduced-dose gadolinium-enhanced MR angiography. Radiology 205:163, 1997.
79. Nelemans PJ, Leiner T, de Vet HC, van Engelshoven JM: Peripheral arterial disease: Meta-analysis of the diagnostic performance of MR angiography. Radiology 217:105, 2000.
80. Rubin GD, Schmidt AJ, Logan LJ, Sofilos MC: Multi-detector row CT angiography of lower extremity arterial inflow and runoff: Initial experience. Radiology 221:146, 2001.
81. Rieker O, Duber C, Schmiedt W, et al: Prospective comparison of CT angiography of the legs with intraarterial digital subtraction angiography. AJR Am J Roentgenol 166:269, 1996.
82. Rubin GD: MDCT imaging of the aorta and peripheral vessels. Eur J Radiol 45(Suppl 1):S42, 2003.

Prognosis of PAD

83. Belch JJ, Topol EJ, Agnelli G, et al: Critical issues in peripheral arterial disease detection and management: A call to action. Arch Intern Med 163:884, 2003.
84. Ouriel K: Peripheral arterial disease. Lancet 358:1257, 2001.
85. A randomised, blinded, trial of clopidogrel versus aspirin in patients at risk of ischaemic events (CAPRIE). CAPRIE Steering Committee. Lancet 348:1329, 1996.
86. Ness J, Aronow WS: Prevalence of coexistence of coronary artery disease, ischemic stroke, and peripheral arterial disease in older persons, mean age 80 years, in an academic hospital-based geriatrics practice. J Am Geriatr Soc 47:1255, 1999.
87. Criqui MH, Denenberg JO: The generalized nature of atherosclerosis: How peripheral arterial disease may predict adverse events from coronary artery disease. Vasc Med 3:241, 1998.
88. Criqui M, Langer RD, Fronek A, et al: Mortality over a period of 10 years in patients with peripheral arterial disease. N Engl J Med 326:381, 1992.
89. Leng GC, Lee AJ, Fowkes FG, et al: Incidence, natural history and cardiovascular events in symptomatic and asymptomatic peripheral arterial disease in the general population. Int J Epidemiol 25:1172, 1996.
90. Diabetes-related amputations of lower extremities in the Medicare population—Minnesota, 1993-1995. MMWR Morb Mortal Wkly Rep 47:649, 1998.

Management of PAD

91. Hiatt WR: Medical treatment of peripheral arterial disease and claudication. N Engl J Med 344:1608, 2001.
92. MRC/BHF Heart Protection Study of cholesterol lowering with simvastatin in 20,536 high-risk individuals: A randomised placebo-controlled trial. Lancet 360:7, 2002.
93. Executive Summary of the Third Report of the National Cholesterol Education Program (NCEP) Expert Panel on Detection, Evaluation, and Treatment of High Blood Cholesterol in Adults (Adult Treatment Panel III). JAMA 285:2486, 2001.
94. Walldius G, Erikson U, Olsson AG, et al: The effect of probucol on femoral atherosclerosis: The Probucol Quantitative Regression Swedish Trial (PQRST). Am J Cardiol 74:875, 1994.
95. Buchwald H, Bourdages HR, Campos CT, et al: Impact of cholesterol reduction on peripheral arterial disease in the Program on the Surgical Control of the Hyperlipidemias (POSCH). Surgery 120:672, 1996.
96. Pedersen TR, Kjekshus J, Pyorala K, et al: Effect of simvastatin on ischemic signs and symptoms in the Scandinavian simvastatin survival study (4S). Am J Cardiol 81:333, 1998.
97. Aronow WS, Nayak D, Woodworth S, Ahn C: Effect of simvastatin versus placebo on treadmill exercise time until the onset of intermittent claudication in older patients with peripheral arterial disease at six months and at one year after treatment. Am J Cardiol 92:711, 2003.
98. Mohler ER 3rd, Hiatt WR, Creager MA: Cholesterol reduction with atorvastatin improves walking distance in patients with peripheral arterial disease. Circulation 108:1481, 2003.
99. Mondillo S, Ballo P, Barbati R, et al: Effects of simvastatin on walking performance and symptoms of intermittent claudication in hypercholesterolemic patients with peripheral vascular disease. Am J Med 114:359, 2003.
100. McDermott MM, Guralnik JM, Greenland P, et al: Statin use and leg functioning in patients with and without lower-extremity peripheral arterial disease. Circulation 107:757, 2003.
101. Effect of intensive diabetes management on macrovascular events and risk factors in the Diabetes Control and Complications Trial. Am J Cardiol 75:894, 1995.
102. Nathan DM, Lachin J, Cleary P, et al: Intensive diabetes therapy and carotid intima-media thickness in type 1 diabetes mellitus. N Engl J Med 348:2294, 2003.
103. Intensive blood-glucose control with sulphonylureas or insulin compared with conventional treatment and risk of complications in patients with type 2 diabetes (UKPDS 33). UK Prospective Diabetes Study (UKPDS) Group [published erratum appears in Lancet 354:602, 1999]. Lancet 352:837, 1998.
104. Mehler PS, Coll JR, Estacio R, et al: Intensive blood pressure control reduces the risk of cardiovascular events in patients with peripheral arterial disease and type 2 diabetes. Circulation 107:753, 2003.

105. Radack K, Deck C: Beta-adrenergic blocker therapy does not worsen intermittent claudication in subjects with peripheral arterial disease: A meta-analysis of randomized controlled trials. Arch Intern Med 151:1769, 1991.
106. Freemantle N, Cleland J, Young P, et al: Beta blockade after myocardial infarction: Systematic review and meta regression analysis. BMJ 318:1730, 1999.
107. Chobanian AV, Bakris GL, Black HR, et al: The Seventh Report of the Joint National Committee on Prevention, Detection, Evaluation, and Treatment of High Blood Pressure: The JNC 7 Report. JAMA 289:2560, 2003.
108. Yusuf S, Sleight P, Pogue J, et al: Effects of an angiotensin-converting-enzyme inhibitor, ramipril, on cardiovascular events in high-risk patients. The Heart Outcomes Prevention Evaluation Study Investigators [published erratum appears in N Engl J Med 342:748, 2000]. N Engl J Med 342:145, 2000.
109. Antithrombotic Trialists' Collaboration: Collaborative meta-analysis of randomised trials of antiplatelet therapy for prevention of death, myocardial infarction, and stroke in high risk patients. BMJ 324:71, 2002.
110. Becquemin JP: Effect of ticlopidine on the long-term patency of saphenous-vein bypass grafts in the legs. Etude de la Ticlopidine apres Pontage Femoro-Poplite and the Association Universitaire de Recherche en Chirurgie. N Engl J Med 337:1726, 1997.
111. Labs KH, Dormandy JA, Jaeger KA, et al: Transatlantic Conference on Clinical Trial Guidelines in Peripheral Arterial Disease: Clinical trial methodology. Basel PAD Clinical Trial Methodology Group. Circulation 100:e75, 1999.
112. Hansen PR, Holm AM, Qi JH, et al: Pentoxifylline inhibits neointimal formation and stimulates constrictive vascular remodeling after arterial injury. J Cardiovasc Pharmacol 34:683, 1999.
113. Chen YM, Wu KD, Tsai TJ, Hsieh BS: Pentoxifylline inhibits PDGF-induced proliferation of and TGF-beta-stimulated collagen synthesis by vascular smooth muscle cells. J Mol Cell Cardiol 31:773, 1999.
114. Hood SC, Moher D, Barber GG: Management of intermittent claudication with pentoxifylline: Meta-analysis of randomized controlled trials. CMAJ 155:1053, 1996.
115. Girolami B, Bernardi E, Prins MH, et al: Treatment of intermittent claudication with physical training, smoking cessation, pentoxifylline, or nafronyl: A meta-analysis. Arch Intern Med 159:337, 1999.
116. Ikeda Y: Antiplatelet therapy using cilostazol, a specific PDE3 inhibitor. Thromb Haemost 82:435, 1999.
117. Money SR, Herd JA, Isaacsohn JL, et al: Effect of cilostazol on walking distances in patients with intermittent claudication caused by peripheral vascular disease. J Vasc Surg 27:267, discussion 274, 1998.
118. Beebe HG, Dawson DL, Cutler BS, et al: A new pharmacological treatment for intermittent claudication: Results of a randomized, multicenter trial. Arch Intern Med 159:2041, 1999.
119. Regensteiner JG, Ware JE Jr, McCarthy WJ, et al: Effect of cilostazol on treadmill walking, community-based walking ability, and health-related quality of life in patients with intermittent claudication due to peripheral arterial disease: Meta-analysis of six randomized controlled trials. J Am Geriatr Soc 50:1939, 2002.
120. Dawson DL, Cutler BS, Hiatt WR, et al: A comparison of cilostazol and pentoxifylline for treating intermittent claudication. Am J Med 109:523, 2000.
121. Cohn JN, Goldstein SO, Greenberg BH, et al: A dose-dependent increase in mortality with vesnarinone among patients with severe heart failure. Vesnarinone Trial Investigators. N Engl J Med 339:1810, 1998.
122. Barradell LB, Brogden RN: Oral naftidrofuryl: A review of its pharmacology and therapeutic use in the management of peripheral occlusive arterial disease. Drugs Aging 8:299, 1996.
123. Brevetti G, Diehm C, Lambert D: European multicenter study on propionyl-L-carnitine in intermittent claudication. J Am Coll Cardiol 34:1618, 1999.
124. Hiatt WR, Regensteiner JG, Creager MA, et al: Propionyl-L-carnitine improves exercise performance and functional status in patients with claudication. Am J Med 110:616, 2001.
125. Belch JJ, Bell PR, Creissen D, et al: Randomized, double-blind, placebo-controlled study evaluating the efficacy and safety of AS-013, a prostaglandin E1 prodrug, in patients with intermittent claudication. Circulation 95:2298, 1997.
126. Boger RH, Bode-Boger SM, Thiele W, et al: Restoring vascular nitric oxide formation by L-arginine improves the symptoms of intermittent claudication in patients with peripheral arterial occlusive disease. J Am Coll Cardiol 32:1336, 1998.
127. Lievre M, Morand S, Besse B, et al: Oral Beraprost sodium, a prostaglandin I(2) analogue, for intermittent claudication: A double-blind, randomized, multicenter controlled trial. Beraprost et Claudication Intermittente (BERCI) Research Group. Circulation 102:426, 2000.
128. Mohler ER 3rd, Hiatt WR, Olin JW, et al: Treatment of intermittent claudication with beraprost sodium, an orally active prostaglandin I2 analogue: A double-blinded, randomized, controlled trial. J Am Coll Cardiol 41:1679, 2003.
129. ICAI Study Group: Prostanoids for chronic critical leg ischemia: A randomized, controlled, open-label trial with prostaglandin E1. Ischemia Cronica degli Arti Inferiori. Ann Intern Med 130:412, 1999.
130. Baumgartner I, Pieczek A, Manor O, et al: Constitutive expression of phVEGF165 after intramuscular gene transfer promotes collateral vessel development in patients with critical limb ischemia. Circulation 97:1114, 1998.
131. Tateishi-Yuyama E, Matsubara H, Murohara T, et al: Therapeutic angiogenesis for patients with limb ischaemia by autologous transplantation of bone-marrow cells: A pilot study and a randomised controlled trial. Lancet 360:427, 2002.
132. Rajagopalan S, Mohler ER 3rd, Lederman RJ, et al: Regional angiogenesis with vascular endothelial growth factor in peripheral arterial disease: A phase II randomized, double-blind, controlled study of adenoviral delivery of vascular endothelial growth factor 121 in patients with disabling intermittent claudication. Circulation 108:1933, 2003.
133. Lederman RJ, Mendelsohn FO, Anderson RD, et al: Therapeutic angiogenesis with recombinant fibroblast growth factor-2 for intermittent claudication (the TRAFFIC study): A randomised trial. Lancet 359:2053, 2002.
134. Gardner AW, Poehlman ET: Exercise rehabilitation programs for the treatment of claudication pain: A meta-analysis. JAMA 274:975, 1995.
135. Leng GC, Fowler B, Ernst E: Exercise for intermittent claudication. Cochrane Database Syst Rev CD000990, 2000.
136. Stewart KJ, Hiatt WR, Regensteiner JG, Hirsch AT: Exercise training for claudication. N Engl J Med 347:1941, 2002.
137. Hoppeler H: Vascular growth in hypoxic skeletal muscle. Adv Exp Med Biol 474:277, 1999.
138. Gustafsson T, Puntschart A, Kaijser L, et al: Exercise-induced expression of angiogenesis-related transcription and growth factors in human skeletal muscle. Am J Physiol 276:H679, 1999.
139. Hambrecht R, Wolf A, Gielen S, et al: Effect of exercise on coronary endothelial function in patients with coronary artery disease. N Engl J Med 342:454, 2000.
140. Hambrecht R, Fiehn E, Weigl C, et al: Regular physical exercise corrects endothelial dysfunction and improves exercise capacity in patients with chronic heart failure. Circulation 98:2709, 1998.
141. Brendle DC, Joseph LJ, Corretti MC, et al: Effects of exercise rehabilitation on endothelial reactivity in older patients with peripheral arterial disease. Am J Cardiol 87:324, 2001.
142. Gardner AW, Katzel LI, Sorkin JD, et al: Exercise rehabilitation improves functional outcomes and peripheral circulation in patients with intermittent claudication: A randomized controlled trial. J Am Geriatr Soc 49:755, 2001.
143. Eagle KA, Berger PB, Calkins H, et al: ACC/AHA guideline update for perioperative cardiovascular evaluation for noncardiac surgery—executive summary a report of the American College of Cardiology/American Heart Association Task Force on Practice Guidelines (Committee to Update the 1996 Guidelines on Perioperative Cardiovascular Evaluation for Noncardiac Surgery). Circulation 105:1257, 2002.
144. de Vries SO, Hunink MG: Results of aortic bifurcation grafts for aortoiliac occlusive disease: A meta-analysis. J Vasc Surg 26:558, 1997.
145. Reed AB, Conte MS, Donaldson MC, et al: The impact of patient age and aortic size on the results of aortobifemoral bypass grafting. J Vasc Surg 37:1219, 2003.
146. Biancari F, Lepantalo M: Extra-anatomic bypass surgery for critical leg ischemia: A review. J Cardiovasc Surg (Torino) 39:295, 1998.
147. Abbott WM, Green RM, Matsumoto T, et al: Prosthetic above-knee femoropopliteal bypass grafting: Results of a multicenter randomized prospective trial. Above-Knee Femoropopliteal Study Group. J Vasc Surg 25:19, 1997.
148. Illig KA, Green RM: Prosthetic above-knee femoropopliteal bypass. Semin Vasc Surg 12:38, 1999.
149. Dorffler-Melly J, Koopman MM, Adam DJ, et al: Antiplatelet agents for preventing thrombosis after peripheral arterial bypass surgery. Cochrane Database Syst Rev CD000535, 2003.
150. Dorffler-Melly J, Buller H, Koopman M, Prins M: Antithrombotic agents for preventing thrombosis after infrainguinal arterial bypass surgery. Cochrane Database Syst Rev 4:CD000536, 2003.

Thromboangiitis Obliterans

151. von Winiwater F: Ueber eine eighenthumliche Form von Endarteritis und Endophlebitis mit Gangran des Fusses. Arch Klin Chir 23:202, 1879.
152. Buerger L: Thromboangiitis obliterans: A study of the vascular lesions leading to presenile spontaneous gangrene. Am J Med Sci 136:567, 1908.
153. Donatelli F, Triggiani M, Nascimbene S, et al: Thromboangiitis obliterans of coronary and internal thoracic arteries in a young woman. J Thorac Cardiovasc Surg 113:800, 1997.
154. Lie JT: Visceral intestinal Buerger's disease. Int J Cardiol 66(Suppl 1):S249, 1998.
155. Michail PO, Filis KA, Delladetsima JK, et al: Thromboangiitis obliterans (Buerger's disease) in visceral vessels confirmed by angiographic and histological findings. Eur J Vasc Endovasc Surg 16:445, 1998.
156. Olin JW: Thromboangiitis obliterans (Buerger's disease). N Engl J Med 343:864, 2000.
157. Lee T, Seo JW, Sumpio BE, Kim SJ: Immunobiologic analysis of arterial tissue in Buerger's disease. Eur J Vasc Endovasc Surg 25:451, 2003.
158. Eichhorn J, Sima D, Lindschau C, et al: Antiendothelial cell antibodies in thromboangiitis obliterans. Am J Med Sci 315:17, 1998.
159. Maslowski L, McBane R, Alexewicz P, Wysokinski WE: Antiphospholipid antibodies in thromboangiitis obliterans. Vasc Med 7:259, 2002.
160. Makita S, Nakamura M, Murakami H, et al: Impaired endothelium-dependent vasorelaxation in peripheral vasculature of patients with thromboangiitis obliterans (Buerger's disease). Circulation 94:II211, 1996.
161. Shionoya S: Diagnostic criteria of Buerger's disease. Int J Cardiol 66(Suppl 1):S243, 1998.
162. Jaff MR: Thromboangiitis Obliterans (Buerger's Disease). Curr Treat Options Cardiovasc Med 2:205, 2000.
163. Olin JW: Thromboangiitis obliterans (Buerger's disease). *In* Rutherford RB (ed): Vascular Surgery. 4th ed. Philadelphia, WB Saunders, 2000, pp 350-364.
164. Shigematsu H, Shigematsu K: Factors affecting the long-term outcome of Buerger's disease (thromboangiitis obliterans). Int Angiol 18:58, 1999.
165. Fiessinger JN, Schafer M: Trial of iloprost versus aspirin treatment for critical limb ischaemia of thromboangiitis obliterans. The TAO Study. Lancet 335:555, 1990.
166. Oral iloprost in the treatment of thromboangiitis obliterans (Buerger's disease): A double-blind, randomised, placebo-controlled trial. The European TAO Study Group [published erratum appears in Eur J Vasc Endovasc Surg 16):456, 1998]. Eur J Vasc Endovasc Surg 15:300, 1998.
167. Saha K, Chabra N, Gulati SM: Treatment of patients with thromboangiitis obliterans with cyclophosphamide. Angiology 52:399, 2001.
168. Isner JM, Baumgartner I, Rauh G, et al: Treatment of thromboangiitis obliterans (Buerger's disease) by intramuscular gene transfer of vascular endothelial growth factor: Preliminary clinical results. J Vasc Surg 28:964, 1998.

169. Sasajima T, Kubo Y, Inaba M, et al: Role of infrainguinal bypass in Buerger's disease: An eighteen-year experience. Eur J Vasc Endovasc Surg 13:186, 1997.

Acute Limb Ischemia

170. Dormandy J, Heeck L, Vig S: The fate of patients with critical leg ischemia. Semin Vasc Surg 12:142, 1999.
171. Aune S, Trippestad A: Operative mortality and long-term survival of patients operated on for acute lower limb ischaemia. Eur J Vasc Endovasc Surg 15:143, 1998.
172. Braithwaite BD, Davies B, Birch PA, et al: Management of acute leg ischaemia in the elderly. Br J Surg 85:217, 1998.
173. Ascher E, Markevich N, Schutzer RW, et al: Small popliteal artery aneurysms: Are they clinically significant? J Vasc Surg 37:755, 2003.
174. Working Party on Thrombolysis in the Management of Limb Ischemia: Thrombolysis in the management of lower limb peripheral arterial occlusion—a consensus document. Am J Cardiol 81:207, 1998.
175. Ouriel K: Acute arterial occlusion. Curr Treat Options Cardiovasc Med 2:255, 2000.
176. Thrombolysis in the management of lower limb peripheral arterial occlusion—a consensus document. J Vasc Interv Radiol 14:S337, 2003.
177. Semba CP, Murphy TP, Bakal CW, et al: Thrombolytic therapy with use of alteplase (rt-PA) in peripheral arterial occlusive disease: Review of the clinical literature. The Advisory Panel. J Vasc Interv Radiol 11:149, 2000.
178. Kasirajan K, Gray B, Beavers FP, et al: Rheolytic thrombectomy in the management of acute and subacute limb-threatening ischemia. J Vasc Interv Radiol 12:413, 2001.
179. Dormandy J, Heeck L, Vig S: Acute limb ischemia. Semin Vasc Surg 12:148, 1999.
180. Berridge DC, Kessel D, Robertson I: Surgery versus thrombolysis for acute limb ischaemia: Initial management. Cochrane Database Syst Rev CD002784, 2002.
181. Results of a prospective randomized trial evaluating surgery versus thrombolysis for ischemia of the lower extremity. The STILE trial. Ann Surg 220:251, 1994.
182. Ouriel K, Veith FJ, Sasahara AA: A comparison of recombinant urokinase with vascular surgery as initial treatment for acute arterial occlusion of the legs. Thrombolysis or Peripheral Arterial Surgery (TOPAS) Investigators. N Engl J Med 338:1105, 1998.

Atheroembolism

183. Tunick PA, Kronzon I: Embolism from the aorta: Atheroemboli and thromboemboli. Curr Treat Options Cardiovasc Med 3:181, 2001.
184. Smyth JS, Scoble JE: Atheroembolism. Curr Treat Options Cardiovasc Med 4:255, 2002.
185. Moolenaar W, Lamers CB: Cholesterol crystal embolization in the Netherlands. Arch Intern Med 156:653, 1996.
186. Kronzon I, Tunick PA: Atheromatous disease of the thoracic aorta: Pathologic and clinical implications. Ann Intern Med 126:629, 1997.
187. Spittell PC, Seward JB, Hallett JW Jr: Mobile thrombi in the abdominal aorta in cases of lower extremity embolic arterial occlusion: Value of extended transthoracic echocardiography. Am Heart J 139:241, 2000.
188. Tunick PA, Kronzon I: Atheromas of the thoracic aorta: Clinical and therapeutic update. J Am Coll Cardiol 35:545, 2000.
189. The French Study of Aortic Plaques in Stroke Group: Atherosclerotic disease of the aortic arch as a risk factor for recurrent ischemic stroke. N Engl J Med 334:1216, 1996.
190. Ferrari E, Vidal R, Chevallier T, Baudouy M: Atherosclerosis of the thoracic aorta and aortic debris as a marker of poor prognosis: benefit of oral anticoagulants. J Am Coll Cardiol 33:1317, 1999.
191. Fukumoto Y, Tsutsui H, Tsuchihashi M, et al: The incidence and risk factors of cholesterol embolization syndrome, a complication of cardiac catheterization: A prospective study. J Am Coll Cardiol 42:211, 2003.
192. Kolh PH, Torchiana DF, Buckley MJ: Atheroembolization in cardiac surgery: The need for preoperative diagnosis. J Cardiovasc Surg (Torino) 40:77, 1999.
193. Bols A, Nevelsteen A, Verhaeghe R: Atheromatous embolization precipitated by oral anticoagulants. Int Angiol 13:271, 1994.
194. Dressler FA, Craig WR, Castello R, Labovitz AJ: Mobile aortic atheroma and systemic emboli: Efficacy of anticoagulation and influence of plaque morphology on recurrent stroke. J Am Coll Cardiol 31:134, 1998.
195. Blackshear JL, Zabalgoitia M, Pennock G, et al: Warfarin safety and efficacy in patients with thoracic aortic plaque and atrial fibrillation. SPAF TEE Investigators. Stroke Prevention and Atrial Fibrillation. Transesophageal echocardiography. Am J Cardiol 83:453, A9, 1999.
196. Blankenship JC, Butler M, Garbes A: Prospective assessment of cholesterol embolization in patients with acute myocardial infarction treated with thrombolytic vs conservative therapy. Chest 107:662, 1995.
197. Vaduganathan P, Ewton A, Nagueh SF, et al: Pathologic correlates of aortic plaques, thrombi and mobile "aortic debris" imaged in vivo with transesophageal echocardiography. J Am Coll Cardiol 30:357, 1997.

CHAPTER 55

Endovascular Treatment of Noncoronary Obstructive Vascular Disease

Andrew C. Eisenhauer • Kenneth Rosenfield

Noncoronary arterial disease, otherwise known as peripheral artery disease (PAD), is increasingly recognized for its high prevalence and clinical importance (see Chap. 54). As the population ages and the number of people with both symptomatic and asymptomatic PAD grows, physicians and patients alike are developing more awareness of the ramifications of PAD, including its associated morbidity and power to predict mortality. Percutaneous transluminal angioplasty (PTA) was initially developed as treatment for PAD, although it is the explosion of its use for treatment of coronary artery disease (CAD) that has fueled the commercial development and academic interest in catheter-based techniques in general. The resulting major improvements in technology and results, combined with patient demand for less invasive therapies, has provided impetus for their extended use in PAD. The widespread availability of high-resolution noninvasive diagnostic imaging, capable of accurately identifying disease and distinguishing lesions amenable to less invasive treatment, has further lowered the threshold for considering treatment for symptomatic PAD.

Although surgery has been the historical mainstay of revascularization therapy for PAD, percutaneous vascular intervention now provides patients with a less invasive, effective modality for the treatment of atheromatous disease over a wide spectrum of anatomical and clinical situations. Catheter-based intervention can provide symptomatic relief of claudication and amelioration of limb ischemia. It can be used for definitive therapy of stenosis in the renal, brachiocephalic, and carotid arteries. In addition, effective methods have been developed to treat aneurysmal disease and venous conditions percutaneously. Nonetheless, establishing recommendations for therapy in PAD can be more complex than in CAD, owing to the wide range of available options (surgical, endovascular, medical, or combination therapy), the involvement of multiple different end-organs, and the relative paucity of definitive data in this rapidly evolving field. Given these complexities, the clinician, whose focus is on providing the optimal treatment strategy, must be knowledgeable about the disease state and aware of the full range of options. In complicated cases, the patient may benefit from the input of physicians from multiple specialties.

Interventions for Atherosclerotic Disease

For Lower Extremity Claudication or Limb Salvage

Intermittent claudication involving the lower extremities is commonly caused by stenosis or occlusion of the iliac, femoral, or infrapopliteal vessels (see Chap. 54). Although first-line therapy has included aggressive risk factor modification and exercise training, life-style–limiting claudication, rest pain, or tissue loss can dictate more aggressive investigation and therapy. The goals of therapy for lower extremity obstructive disease are symptomatic relief of claudication and, in more advanced cases, limb salvage. Although surgical therapy has been reserved historically for patients with limb-threatening ischemia and rest pain, the availability of endovascular therapies has lowered the threshold for intervention. Because most percutaneous interventions have low procedural risk, patients with life-style–limiting claudication are now often considered for angiographic investigation and intervention. In addition, percutaneous treatment usually preserves the surgical option, should it be needed subsequently. An increasingly informed patient population will, given the choice, often opt for less invasive therapies, accepting results that may be less durable or even less effective than those associated with a more invasive approach. For the clinician treating patients with lower extremity vascular disease, improvement in functional capacity and quality of life, as well as long-term results, are important in weighing the value of potential treatments. Evaluation of a patient with lower extremity symptoms requires awareness of the variable manifestations of PAD. In some instances, patients and even physicians misconstrue hip discomfort and other symptoms of claudication as those of "arthritis," or as a normal component of aging. Some patients unintentionally self-restrict their activities to avoid ischemic pain: their symptoms abate because they no longer exercise. These patients are akin to the patient with exertional angina who limits his or her activity to below the angina threshold.

Though progression from claudication to limb-threatening ischemia is relatively uncommon—occurring in only 10 to 20 percent of claudicants—even asymptomatic PAD is associated with significant morbidity (see Chap. 54). The U.S. National Institutes of Health suggest that peripheral arterial disease results in more than 60,000 hospitalizations annually, with an average length of stay greater than 11 days.[1] Approximately 1 to 2 percent of people aged 45 to 69 years have clinical evidence of intermittent claudication, and risk factors for lower extremity disease include tobacco use, diabetes mellitus, hyperlipidemia, and systolic hypertension (see Chap. 54). Smoking appears to be the greatest modifiable risk factor and one of the most potent—perhaps even more so than in association with coronary atherosclerosis.

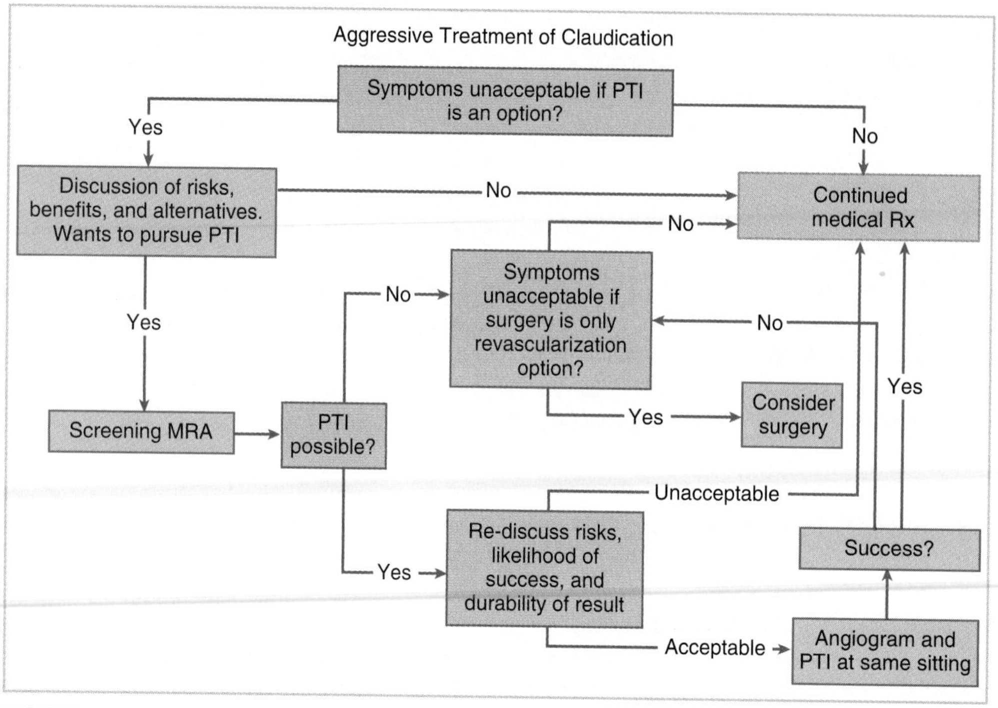

FIGURE 55–1 A strategy for aggressive treatment of claudication. The strategy is based on assessment of symptoms and frank discussion with patients about the risks and benefits of available therapies. In the current era, noninvasive diagnostic imaging is used not to make a diagnosis but to ascertain the anatomical suitability for intervention and to assess the patient's procedural risk profile. MRA = magnetic resonance angiography; PTI = percutaneous transluminal intervention; Rx = treatment. See also Figure 54–21 for a management scheme for less life-style limiting claudication.

Noninvasive functional testing, such as pulse volume recordings and segmental Doppler pressures (ankle-brachial index) with or without exercise, is helpful in confirming the presence of obstructive disease and estimating its level and severity. The broad indications for lower extremity angiography of any kind, noninvasive or invasive, include symptoms of PAD where, if the angiogram demonstrates a suitable anatomic situation, surgery or PTA would be undertaken. Recent advances in axial imaging techniques (both magnetic resonance [MR] angiography and computed tomography [CT] angiography) now enable remarkable definition of the vascular anatomy. These studies are now frequently obtained to confirm the diagnosis and to help formulate a strategy and approach to revascularization. Invasive angiography is necessary when the results from axial imaging are ambiguous. For critical limb ischemia, anatomical definition is required to plan therapy in nearly all cases. In the case of claudication, imaging should be performed as outlined in Figure 55–1.

The goals of revascularization include not only limb salvage and wound healing but also relief of exertional symptoms. The likelihood of clinical success, the durability, and the technical approach vary according to anatomical site. These aspects are best considered separately for aortoiliac, femoropopliteal, and infrapopliteal segments.

Aortoiliac Obstruction

Obstructive disease in the aorta and iliac vessels is usually atherosclerotic in origin, and treatment for both sites, typically labeled *inflow vessels* to the leg, is similar. Many patients with aortoiliac disease have concomitant femoral and tibial obstructive disease. In these patients with multilevel disease, correction of hemodynamically significant inflow lesions is usually undertaken as the first stage in revascularization. In some cases, aortoiliac treatment alone may result in symptomatic improvement by increasing the proximal pressure head and thus collateral blood flow to the distal extremity.

Perhaps more so than for any other vascular territory in the body, the preferred mode of revascularization of the aortoiliac vessels has shifted over the past 15 years from predominantly surgical to nearly all percutaneous. This change in strategy is based on both the less invasive nature of PTA and its short- and long-term success, which are comparable to that of more high-risk surgical bypass.[2,3] Furthermore, the primary use of stents, as opposed to balloon angioplasty alone, has gained enormous popularity in the aortoiliac (and other) vessels, due to generally superior angiographic and hemodynamic results and the paucity of complications associated with stents. Insufficient data exist to support or reject the strategy of primary stenting. One trial did suggest that patency rates (~70 percent) and clinical success rates (~78 percent) at 2 years are similar to stenting when excellent angiographic and hemodynamic results are obtained from balloon angioplasty alone.[4] This has led some to favor a strategy of "provisional stenting," wherein stents are reserved for cases of failed balloon angioplasty. However, in the single trial comparing the two strategies, nearly half of the patients (43 percent) randomized to receive balloon alone crossed over to receive stents. Moreover, a meta-analysis of all trials published after 1990 suggests that both immediate success rate (96 vs. 91 percent) and 4-year patency (77 vs. 65 percent for stenoses) are superior for stenting versus balloon alone.[2] These data support the strategy of primary stenting when treating aortoiliac lesions. Long lesions, diffuse disease, and occlusions, in particular, benefit from primary stenting. Since stented segments that restenose can be treated successfully with repeat angioplasty, long-term patency may be even greater when one includes secondary procedures. Finally, with regard to type of stent selected (balloon-expandable vs. self-expanding; stainless steel vs. nitinol), there are insufficient data to recommend one over another; however, recent experience suggests that nitinol may offer advantages in placement accuracy and long-term patency for self-expanding stents over that achieved with stainless steel in the past.[5]

Although endovascular therapy is the preferred initial therapy for focal aortoiliac stenosis, the approach to diffusely diseased vessels and total occlusions is more controversial. Early studies demonstrated poor technical results and high complication rates. However, the advent of hydrophilic guidewires and other technical advances have enabled recanalization of occluded iliac segments with a greater than 80 percent rate of primary success, independent of location (external, internal, or common iliac artery); secondary patency rates at 6 years are as high as 80 percent. There is general agreement that stents should be used primarily (not provisionally) when treating occlusions. The same is true of a subset of patients with stenotic or occlusive disease that involves the terminal aorta, extends into its bifurcation, and compromises the origins of the common iliac arteries. These patients do well with reconstruction of the bifurcation using stents.

The most serious complications of endovascular aortoiliac repair remain distal embolization, with rates ranging from 4 to 7 percent,[6] and arterial perforation or rupture, which is rare. Routine treatment with covered stents is now possible for the latter. Based on these improved outcomes, percutaneous treatment is generally attempted for short occlusions and for longer iliac stenosis or occlusions that are technically suitable (Fig. 55–2). Total occlusions of the abdominal aorta are more often treated surgically, though thrombolysis followed by PTA remains an option.

Pretreatment before PTA with therapies that dissolve or remove thrombus, such as thrombolytic therapy, rheolytic thrombectomy, and suction thrombectomy, can reduce embolic complications in thrombus-containing lesions. Distal embolic protection devices have also been used for the same purpose. Although individual reports and small series show favorable outcomes in selected cases, further delineation of the specific indications is required for these adjunct therapies. Finally, covered stents are now used for iliac artery lesions with associated aneurysm or anatomical complexities, further extending the applicability of percutaneous therapy.

In summary, PTA and stenting represent appropriate first-line therapy for aortoiliac obstructive disease. They offer durability similar to that of surgical reconstruction, with less risk and at reduced cost. In the small percentage of patients in whom patency cannot be maintained, surgery remains an option. The availability of these effective and less invasive techniques has lowered the threshold at which intervention can be offered to patients with aortoiliac disease who are disabled by claudication or limb ischemia (Table 55–1).

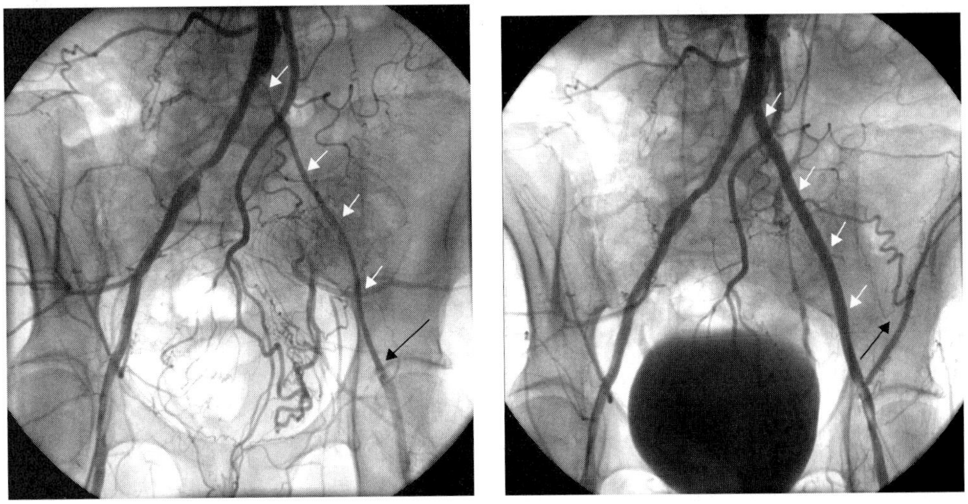
A B

FIGURE 55–2 Iliac stenting. **A** shows a severe long segment disease of the left common and external iliac arteries (white arrows). The black arrow shows the level of collateral inflow and the resulting mixing opacified and unopacified blood. This patient was treated with predilation and a single balloon-expandable stent placed at the origin of the left common iliac artery (white arrows). This was followed by implantation of a self-expanding stent in the remainder of the vessel. **B** shows wide patency of that vessel and reversal of flow to antegrade in the collateral vessel (black arrow). This patient's claudication was abolished.

TABLE 55–1 Recent Results of Iliac Artery Stent Placement*

Lead Author	Reference	Year	No. of Patients	Lesions Treated	Percent with Occlusions	Technical Success (%)	Ankle-Brachial Index		Mean Lesion Length (cm)	Stent Used	Primary Patency at 2 Years (%)	Cumulative Patency at 2 Years (%)
							Before	*After*				
Reyes	16	1997	59	61	100	92	0.51	0.9	10	SES	73	88
Dyet	17	1997	72	72	100	93	NA	NA	6.7	BES, SES	85	85
Murphy	15	1998	65	90	31	97	0.62	0.9	5.6	BES, SES	69	80
Tetleroo	4	1998	143	187	9	NA	0.78	NA	NA	BES	NA	71.3
Powell	14	2000	87	210	NA	97	0.56	0.75	NA	Various	43	72
Saha	12	2001	50	61	4	97	NA	NA	NA	BES, SES	97	100
Timaran	13	2001	189	247	NA	97	NA	NA	NA	BES, SES	NA	
Haulon	7	2002	106	212	NA	100	NA	NA	NA	BES/SES	79.4	97.7
Siskin	8	2002	42	59	8.5	95	0.68	0.99	NA	BES/SES	72	88
Mohamed	9	2002	24	48	42	100	NA	NA	5.2	BES/SES	58	84
Reekers	10	2002	126	143	10	100	0.67	0.92	3.3	BES	84†	89†
Funovics	11	2002	78	94	100	96	NA	NA	6.2	Various	74.5	88.8

BES = balloon-expandable stainless steel; SES = self-expanding stainless steel; SEN = self-expanding nitinol; SESG = self-expanding stent graft; NA = not assessed or reported.

*Historical and contemporary results of iliac artery stent placement. The difficulty in determining the literature is that these reports of experience include patients with widely varying degrees of disease and incorporate a variety of stent types and techniques. Nevertheless, cumulative 2-year patency is approximately 90% in most series.

†At 12 months.

Prior experience has shown little difference between the results of endovascular therapy for the superficial femoral (SFA) and popliteal arteries. Accordingly, these two vessels traditionally are considered together with respect to indications and results. The SFA, particularly within the adductor canal of the thigh, has a tremendous propensity to accumulate atherosclerotic plaque. Whether this is due to the inherent physical stresses and flow patterns specific to this vessel (low flow vessel, high resistance bed), the presence of a natural collateral (the profunda femoris artery), or other undefined factors is not known. In the current era, procedural success for femoropopliteal recanalization exceeds 90 percent. The advent of hydrophilic guidewires and catheters has greatly enhanced the ability to traverse femoropopliteal occlusions, which now can be treated successfully in 80 to 90 percent of cases. Even though hydrophilic wires and other technological advances have improved acute success, the rate of restenosis remains more than twofold that of iliac disease and far exceeds what would be expected considering the size (mean lumen diameter, 5 to 6 mm) of the SFA.

A variety of adjunct technologies has been used in an attempt to improve long-term patency. Debulking devices, such as directional atherectomy, excimer laser, and rotational atherectomy, although sometimes enhancing acute success and providing a better angiographic result, have failed to demonstrate a reduction in restenosis. Newer debulking devices, which are more aggressive and "thorough" in their tissue removal, have not been evaluated yet for long-term efficacy.

Though it had been hoped that stent placement would offer advantages over balloon angioplasty, as it does in the coronary circulation, initial reports of long-term results were disappointing. Restenosis rates after 6 months were in the 30 to 70 percent range, with poorer results associated with longer lesions, total occlusions, and more distal disease. However, following recanalization, there was little evidence to support the superiority of endovascular stents over balloon angioplasty alone in this anatomical locale.

However, the advent of flexible thin-strutted nitinol self-expanding stents improved the clinically perceived rates of restenosis following long-segment SFA recanalization and stenting have improved. Given the past moderate rates of procedural success with femoropopliteal intervention, percutaneous treatment has been relatively neglected in the treatment of claudication, and many believed it was unsatisfactory for the treatment of limb-threatening ischemia. Traditionally, it has been reserved for claudicants with isolated short-segment disease and those with limb-threatening ischemia believed to be at high risk for surgical therapy.

Recognition is increasing that a great potential advantage of endovascular therapy is that restenosis or occlusion of previously successfully treated limbs seldom results in greater clinical deterioration than simply a return to the preprocedure state. In contrast, occlusion of surgical bypasses can worsen ischemia. Thus, the use of endovascular approaches to recanalize and stent diffuse SFA disease is reemerging.

In addition, the development of stent coatings containing drugs such as rapamycin may further reduce the incidence of renarrowing to that approaching the patency of surgical bypass. In a randomized series of long-segment SFA disease patients, those receiving rapamycin-coated nitinol self-expanding stents developed much less intimal thickening and no restenosis at 6 months.[18] Of additional interest, the control group that received identical but noncoated stents had only 23 percent restenosis—suggesting that stent design may also influence the success of the treatment of long-segment SFA disease. Although it is likely that longer follow-up and additional studies will demonstrate that drug-eluting stents do not abolish restenosis completely, these initial findings have engendered tremendous interest in the development of recanalization technologies to treat the long-segment chronic total occlusion.

Because it is the rule rather than the exception for lower extremity arterial disease of the SFA to present with chronic total occlusion, there is renewed interest in both the treatment of long-segment disease and the recanalization of chronic total occlusions, especially with the excimer laser. Scheinert and colleagues have reported 411 lesions in 318 patients successfully recanalized with the excimer laser. The success achieved in this group was remarkable when one considers the mean lesion length was 19.4 cm.[19,20] Table 55–2 summarizes recently reported femoropoliteal interventional studies.

How is one to decide on the best treatment for his or her patient today? Unfortunately, there is scant evidence on which to base this decision. Surgical revascularization and its initial technologies were developed long before balloon angioplasty and other catheter-based technologies emerged, and surgery thus became the traditional or gold standard. However, "traditional" does not necessarily mean "superior," and "new" does not necessarily mean "better." We lack prospective, randomized series or surgery versus catheter-based intervention to permit valid comparisons.

Adherents of surgical technique particularly point to the superior durability and primary patency of autologous saphenous vein bypass as well as poorer technical success and long-term patency of endovascular recanalization and/or stenting. They note that salvage of critically ischemic limbs probably requires reconstitution of unobstructed "straight-line" flow to the foot (i.e., through revascularized native arteries or bypass grafts and not via collaterals).

Interventionalists remark that their ability to recanalize the long-segment chronic total occlusion has improved rival surgical technical success rates and that if straight-line perfusion can be achieved with endovascular technique, the results can be hemodynamically equivalent. They further note that interventional procedure-related cardiac mortality is rare and interventional therapy, because of its minimally invasive nature, should be considered a *course* of treatment and not judged by the surgical primary patency standard. In addition, angiographic restenosis may play a less critical role in the follow-up of *endovascular* treatment of critical limb ischemia—when applied properly, there is little or no surgical dissection and disruption of native anatomy. Thus, slowly developing restenosis may afford time for the continued development of collaterals and, after giving the distal tissues time to heal, closure of the revascularized segment may be less consequential than the original occlusion.

Those who advocate the medical treatment of claudication point to the success of exercise programs, ongoing research into new palliative drugs, the increasingly documented benefits of aggressive risk factor modification, and the complete lack of "procedure-related mortality" with medical treatment alone as a demonstration of the need for conservatism in the treatment of claudicants (see Chap. 54). In many instances, either surgery or interventional techniques can ameliorate the patient's symptoms. The decision regarding the most appropriate therapy can be made by the patient and the physician, taking into account the risks and discomforts of the proposed procedure, its probable durability and reproducibility, the degree to which a procedure closes the door to other therapies, the magnitude of life-style limitation, and the individual patient's tolerance for risk.

The treatment of femoropopliteal disease now stands at a new threshold. The advent of new stent design, better recanalization techniques, and the promise of drug-eluting

TABLE 55–2 Recent Results of Femoropopliteal Interventions*

Lead Author	Reference	Year	No. of Patients	Lesions Treated	Percent with Occlusions	Technical Success (%)	Ankle-Brachial Index		Mean Lesion Length (cm)	Devices Used Primarily	Primary Success† (%)	Duration (mo)	Cumulative Success† (%)	Duration (mo)
							Before	After						
Gray	21	1997	55	58	NA	NA	0.48	0.71	16.5	SES, BES	22	24	46	24
Martin	22	1999	68	NA	6	100	NA	NA	NA	PTA	NA	—	57	24
Kessel	23	2000	20	NA	—	95	0.6	1	17	SG	29	12	64	12
Conroy	24	2000	48	61	100	100	NA	NA¶	13.5	SES, Some BES	47	12	79	12
Cheng	25	2001	55	69	NA	92	NA	NA	13.8	SEN, SES	53.8	24	72.1	24
Gordon	26	2001	57	71	100	NA	0.59	0.86	14.4	SES	38.2	24	76.2	24
Scheinert	19	2001	318	411	100	83	0.62	NA	19.4	LPTA, some SEN	33.6†	12	75.9	12
Lofberg	27	2001	92	121	47	88	NA	NA	NA	PTA	27	60	34	60
Bauermeister	28	2001	35	NA	100	100	0.25	0.87	22	SG§	73.2	12	82.6	12
Duda	18	2002	36	36	57	100	NA	NA	8.5	DEN vs. SEN	100/77	6	NA	—
Steinkamp	29	2002	312	312	100	91.7	0.56	0.88	7.5	LPTA, some SEN	61.5	24	90.2	24
Gray	30	2002	23	NA	84	88	0.54	0.84	6.2	LPTA	33	24	75	24
Jamsen	31	2002	173	218	NA	83.5	NA	NA	NA	PTA	25	60	4.1	60
Cho	5	2003	40	40	100	100	0.61	0.93	NA	SEN	NA	—	NA	—
Becquemin	32	2003	251	277	NA	90	0.52	NA	2.5	BES vs. PTA	65/67‡	12	NA	—
Jahnke	33	2003	52	63	83	100	0.54	0.89	10.9	SG	74.1	24	83.2	24

BES = balloon-expandable stainless steel; SES = self-expanding stainless steel; SEN = self-expanding nitinol; DEN = drug-eluting nitinol; PTA = percutaneous transluminal (balloon) angioplasty; LPTA = excimer laser-assisted PTA; SG = stent graft; NA = not assessed or reported.

*Summary of reports of femoropopliteal interventions from the literature. A wide variety of anatomical situations are represented here, including many with chronic long-segment total occlusions. Of note is that primary patency of 2 years, when reported, is considerably lower than that for iliac interventions yet cumulative patency ranges from approximately 75% to 90%. This emphasizes the need for both postprocedure surveillance and consideration of the performance of a femoral intervention when embarking on a course of therapy.

†Clinical or objective patency.

‡Angiographic patency (<50% stenosis) in mandatory stent group vs. PTA with selective stenting group.

§Devices placed surgically.

¶Average increase of 0.26.

stents will provide many more effective treatment options for patients (Figs. 55–3 through 55–6).

Infrapopliteal Obstruction

PAD is typically a diffuse process involving multiple arterial levels and segments. Thus, when disease is seen in the proximal vessels, significant occlusive disease is often seen in the three infrapopliteal arteries (anterior tibial, peroneal, and posterior tibial). Similarly, when infrapopliteal narrowing is present, one is likely to find coexisting proximal disease. Rarely, stenosis may be isolated to one or more vessels below the knee. Revascularization considerations below the knee must take into account the extent, severity, and distribution of disease in more proximal vessels. Indeed, for patients with claudication and compromised outflow, correction of coexisting disease in a proximal vessel is often sufficient in and of itself to achieve symptomatic relief. This differs from patients with critical limb ischemia, in whom lesion healing generally requires restoration of uninterrupted patency of at least one vessel to the foot. In the absence of severe and flow-limiting proximal disease, significant disease of all three crural vessels is usually required to provoke symptomatic calf claudication or higher grades of ischemia (rest pain or tissue loss).

Traditionally, revascularization for vessels below the knee has been reserved for patients with rest pain; limbs threatened by ulcers, infection, or gangrene; or symptoms at very low levels of exertion. Until recently, the preferred mode of treatment has been surgical bypass. However, paradigms that challenge the traditional approach are emerging with respect to both indications and mode of revascularization. Dramatic technological advances and incremental experience now allow for routine and uncomplicated access to vessels in the infrapopliteal distribution. Although the relative advantages of catheter-based arterial revascularization have been more clearly established for lesions in more proximal vessels, numerous studies have now confirmed the feasibility, safety, and efficacy of tibial PTA. Infrapopliteal PTA was initially limited to patients with critical limb ischemia who were at high risk for bypass graft surgery; those who had no saphenous vein available for bypass conduit; or those with more proximal interventions in whom improving distal runoff might help maintain overall vessel patency. In these patients, the less invasive approach is now preferred routinely over higher risk surgical intervention. Primary success rates are generally 80 to 95 percent, and cumulative 2-year patency rates can approximate 75 percent (Table 55–3). More important, limb salvage rates of percutaneous intervention have now been demonstrated to rival those of surgical reconstruction.[36,38,39] Even in diabetic patients, in whom skepticism regarding small-vessel intervention previously prevailed, balloon angioplasty can effectively salvage ischemic limbs.[41,42]

The safe and effective reconstruction achieved with the percutaneous approach in this higher-risk cohort has caused a shift in the management of patients who have critical limb ischemia due to infrapopliteal disease. When anatomically feasible, an initial attempt at PTA is now considered a reasonable and appropriate strategy for revascularization in *all* patients, even those who are suitable candidates for infrapopliteal bypass (Figs. 55–7 and 55–8). The exception to this may be in patients with more extensive disease, in whom long-term outcomes may be hampered by restenosis rates as high as 40 to 60 percent. Rotational atherectomy or excimer laser angioplasty can be useful as adjunctive therapy in lesions that have unfavorable morphology, such as total occlusion, heavy calcification, and/or ostial location. Previous studies with rotational atherectomy have shown it to be useful acutely, though data on long-term follow-up are no more favorable than balloon angioplasty alone. Though wide-ranging use may not be appropriate, selected patients (particularly those with limited surgical options) clearly benefit from these "niche" devices.[30]

Strategies for revascularization must reflect the limitations of technology but also must be considered in the context of the patient's overall clinical condition. Selection of a higher-risk open surgical procedure based on anticipation of better long-term patency should be tempered by the knowledge that shorter-term patency established by less risky percutaneous means is often adequate to salvage the extremity. In many instances, critical limb ischemia does not recur once the extremity has healed, even in the face of restenosis or reocclusion. The optimal strategy is one that is safest and most likely to provide both acute improvement and—to the greatest extent possible—long-term benefit.

The changing paradigm for revascularization also relates to the indications for intervention in patients with symptomatic but less critical infrapopliteal disease. The traditionally high threshold for intervention was maintained largely due to the associated risk and invasive nature of the surgical approach. Currently, however, a lower threshold for intervention may be considered. Specifically, in the subset of patients who claudicate solely due to infrapopliteal disease, favorable acute and intermediate term patency and clinical results have been achieved using PTA.[39] Such a strategy should be limited to patients with severe symptoms (Rutherford category 3) and straightforward anatomy. Infrapopliteal PTA may also be useful in claudicants undergoing proximal revascularization (either with surgery or PTA), in whom the runoff is severely impaired. When tibial outflow is a major

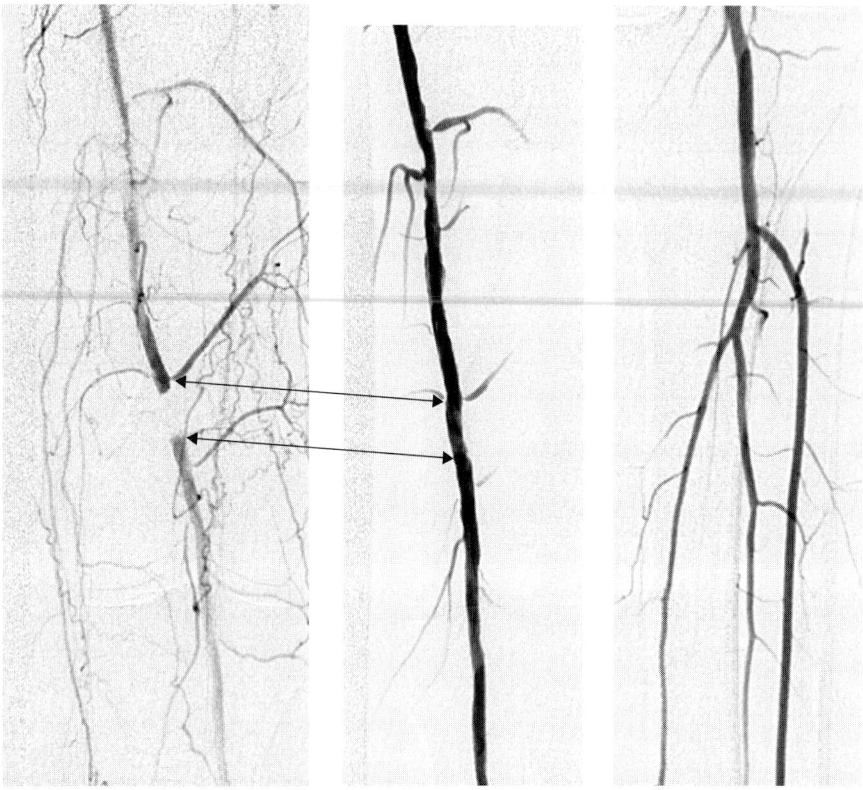

FIGURE 55–3 The result of recanalization and balloon dilation of a short-segment femoropopliteal occlusion. In **A,** a digital subtraction angiogram illustrates the area of total occlusion and compares it to that in **B,** showing the results of balloon dilation only. Both areas are indicated by the double-ended black arrows. **C** shows an intact three-vessel runoff without evidence of distal embolization.

TABLE 55–3 Results of Tibial Artery Interventions*

Lead Author	Reference	Year	No. of Patients	Lesions Treated	Percent with Occlusions	Technical Success (%)	Ankle-Brachial Index *Before*	Ankle-Brachial Index *After*
Sivananthan	34	1994	38	73	24	96	NA	NA
Varty	35	1995	38	40	17	98	0.55	0.84
Dorros	36	1998	312	657	27	98	NA	NA
Desgranges	37	2000	33	NA	NA	82	NA	NA
Soder	38	2000	60	72	35	84/61†	NA	NA
Dorros	39	2001	235	529	28.9	92	NA	NA
Tsetis	40	2002	12	13	100	92.3	0.35	0.68

PTA = percultaneous transluminal (balloon) angioplasty; VPTA = vibrational PTA; NA = not assessed or reported.

*Summary of recent literature on tibial artery interventions. Most reports are those of review of single-center experience and procedural results. The 2001 report of Dorros and associates deserves special mention: It is of long-term follow-up of event-free survival and limb salvage.

†Stenosis/occlusion.

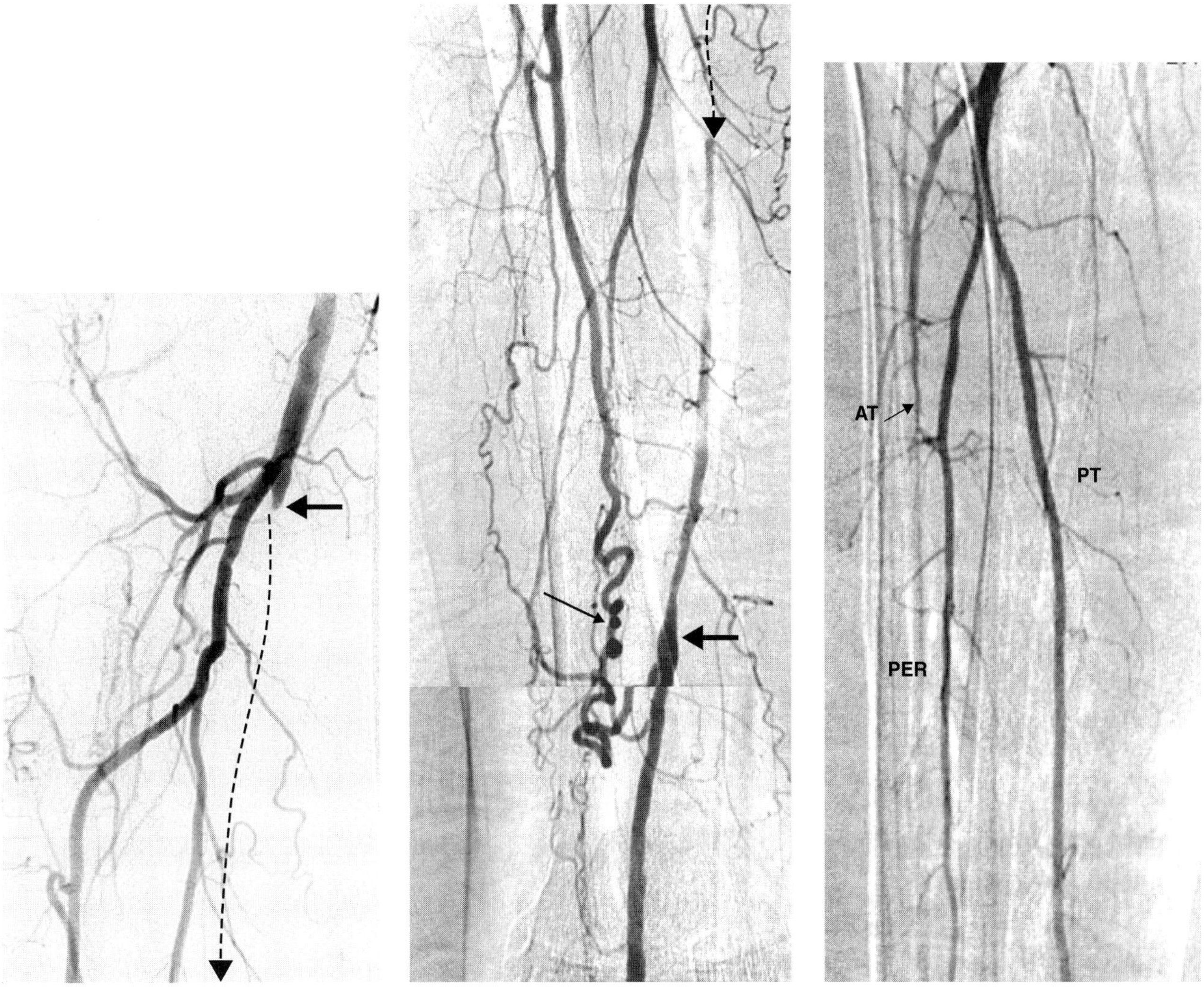

A B C

FIGURE 55–4 A long-segment chronic total occlusion. In contrast to the short-segment disease in Figure 55-3, this requires recanalization from the origin of the superficial femoral artery (SFA) (**A,** thick arrow) along the path of the SFA (dashed arrow) continuing to the level of the most significant collateral inflow and reconstitution of the vessel **(B)**. **C** shows the crural vessels and demonstrates occlusion of the anterior tibial (AT) with patent peroneal (PER) and posterior tibial (PT) runoff.

Mean Lesion Length (cm)	Primary Device	Primary Patency		Cumulative Patency		Event-Free Survival		Limb Salvage	
		Percent	*Duration (mo)*	*Percent*	*Duration (mo)*	*Percent*	*Duration (mo)*	*Percent*	*Duration (mo)*
NA	PTA	NA	—	NA	—	NA	—	NA	—
1	PTA	59	24	68	24	NA	—	77	12
NA	PTA	NA	—	NA	—	NA	—	NA	—
NA	PTA	66	12	77	12	94	12	91	12
NA	PTA	68/48†	10	56	18	NA	—	80	18
NA	PTA	NA	—	NA	—	31	60	91	60
7	VPTA	NA	—	NA	—	NA	—	NA	—

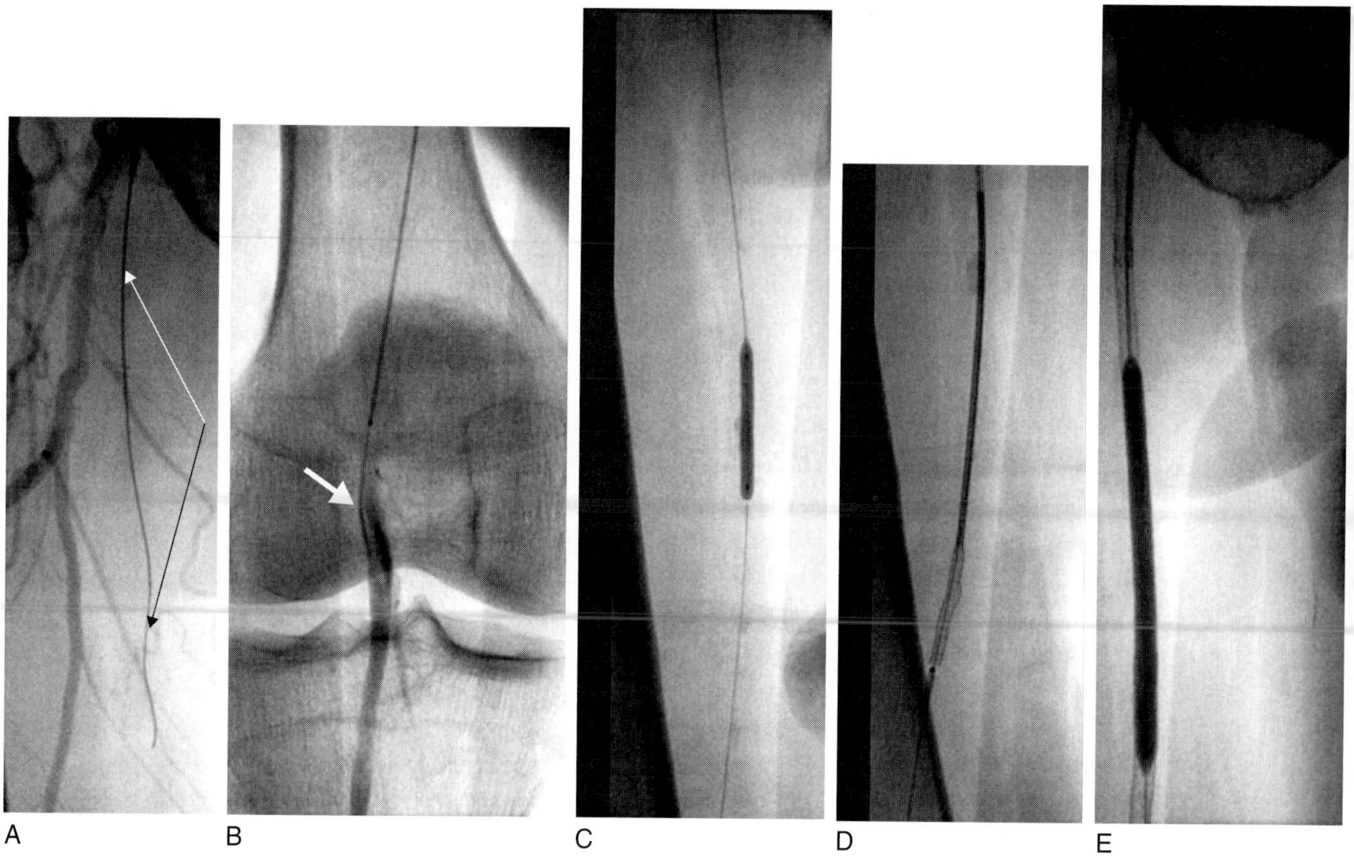

FIGURE 55–5 Recanalization of this lesion was accomplished from the contralateral approach using a hydrophilic guidewire advanced into the occluded segment **(A)**. Once the guidewire is free in the distal vessel, a small catheter is passed over the wire and a contrast agent injection is made to confirm the intravascular position **(B)**. This is followed by "pre"-dilation **(C)**, self-expanding stent placement from distal to proximal **(D)**, and, finally, "post"-dilation to the appropriate size **(E)**

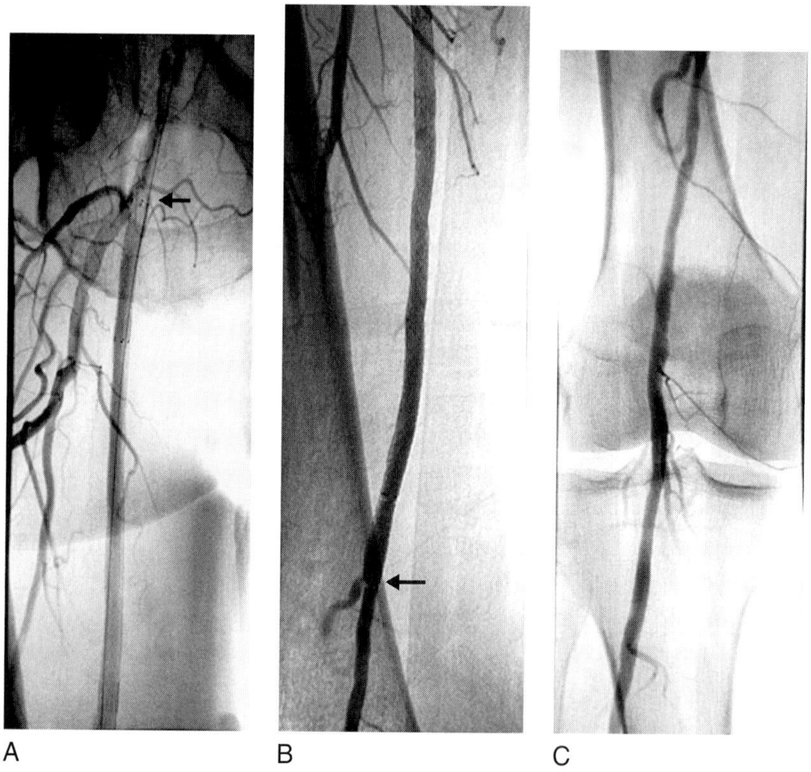

FIGURE 55–6 Recanalization of this long-segment occlusion and stenting from the origin of the superficial femoral artery (SFA) in **A** (arrow) to the level of collateral reconstitution in **B** (arrow) resulted in reconstitution of the normal anatomy, return of pedal pulses, and healing of digital ulcers. Care was taken to preserve the collateral vessel ostia so that, in the event of restenosis, collateral pathways are reestablished. This anatomy should be contrasted with total occlusion of the SFA but short-segment disease shown in Figure 55-3. These cases illustrate the anatomical variations that commonly occur and emphasize the difficulty in characterizing the true extent of disease in patients with total occlusions of this vessel.

determinant of long-term patency, recanalizing the runoff vessels may provide a benefit. In any case, when performing PTA for critical limb ischemia or claudication, particular care must be taken not to compromise subsequent surgical options. For example, disruption of a distal, previously uncompromised vessel may prohibit subsequent bypass to that site. Although this is a rare occurrence, a thoughtful strategy is required to avoid "burning a bridge" to a subsequent surgical intervention.

In summary, optimal management of patients with lower extremity arterial occlusive disease and associated symptoms

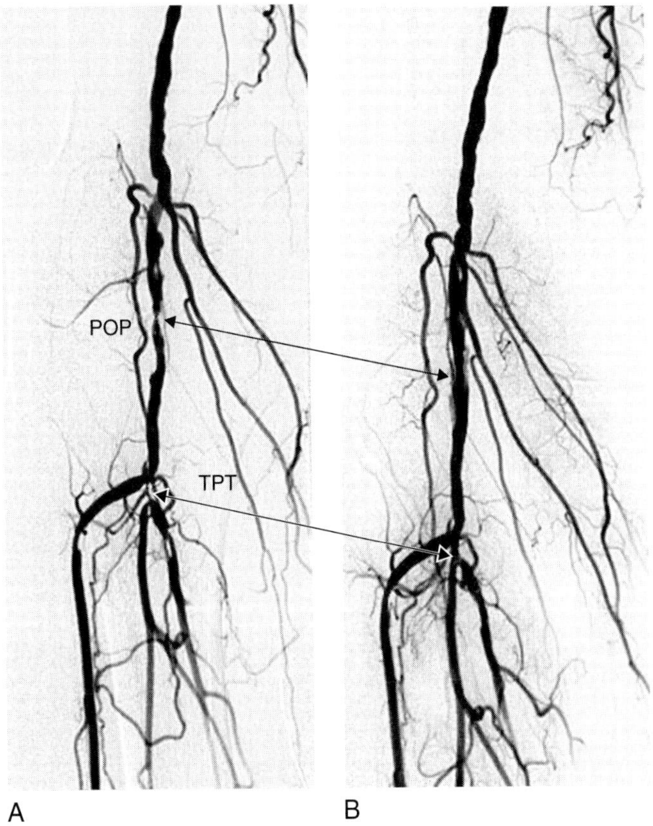

FIGURE 55–7 Intervention in tibial disease. Lesions in the below-knee popliteal artery **(A)** and in the very short tibioperoneal trunk **(B)** were identified and successfully treated with percutaneous transluminal angioplasty.

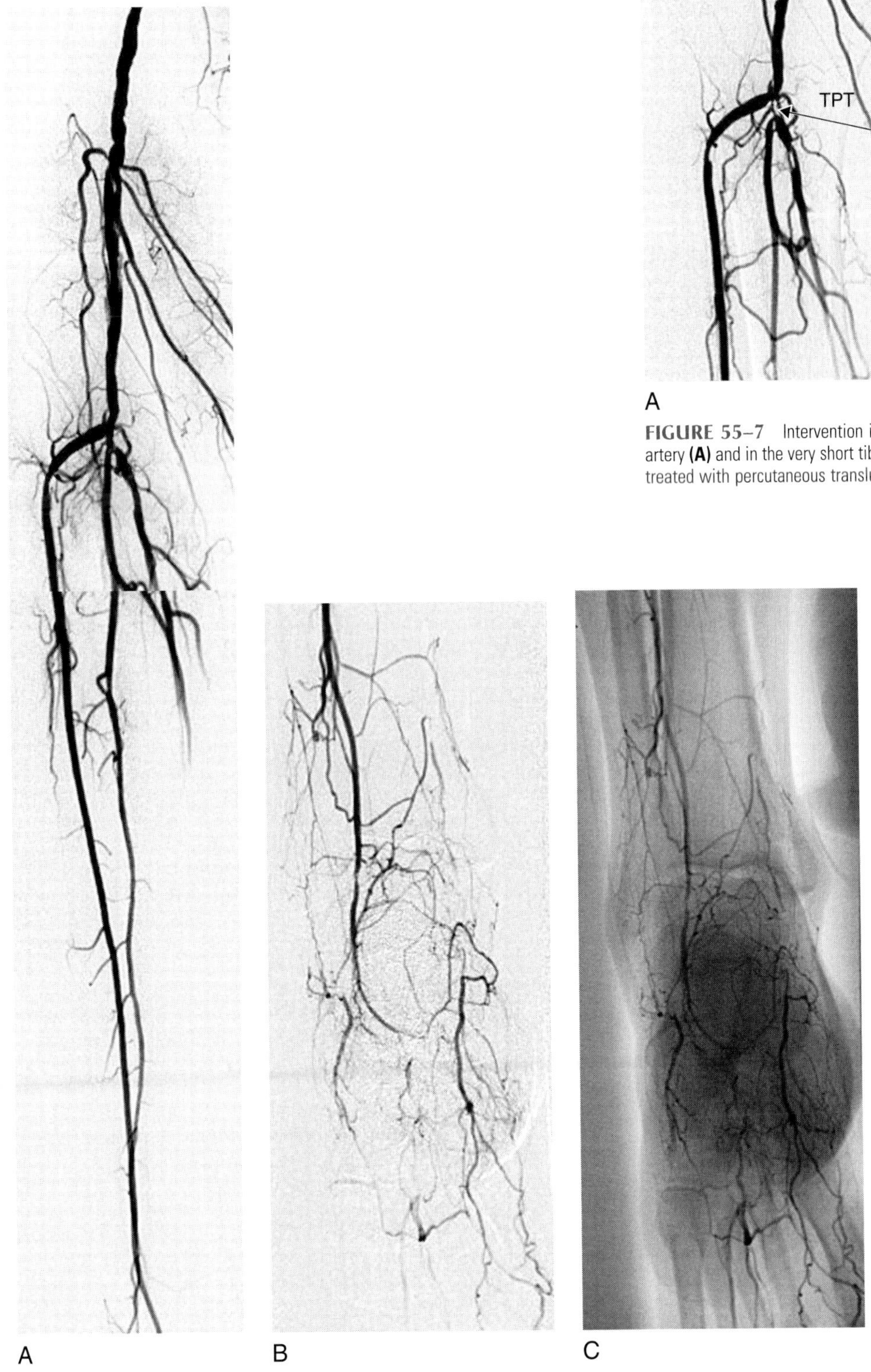

FIGURE 55–8 **A** shows a composite angiogram from the patient in Figure 55-7 demonstrating the intact anterior tibial runoff in the calf. The peroneal normally attenuates by the level of the malleoli and, in this case, the posterior tibial is also occluded. **B** and **C** show the pedal circulation in both digital subtraction angiography and native views. Though "straight-line" flow to the foot was reconstituted and the patient's ulcers healed, the evident diffuse small-vessel disease in the pedal vessels still places the foot in long-term jeopardy. Careful surveillance and compulsive continuing medical management are critical in this group of patients, even in the context of technical procedural success.

requires the input of practitioners knowledgeable of the capabilities of both percutaneous and surgical revascularization. If their disease is anatomically suitable, patients should be considered for percutaneous endovascular treatment. The physician must provide a frank discussion of the risks, potential symptomatic benefit, and durability of the proposed intervention. For patients with claudication, there is little evidence to suggest that an early and aggressive revascularization alters the natural history of lower extremity occlusive disease. Thus, treatment should be guided by the patient's degree of impairment and personal wishes. Limb-threatening ischemia, in contrast, should be treated promptly, utilizing the modality that will provide the most complete revascularization with the lowest procedural risk. For example, endovascular treatment of isolated iliac occlusive disease is often equivalent hemodynamically and may be preferable to surgery. Infrainguinal disease that is diffuse or associated with long-segment femoral obstruction has traditionally been addressed with saphenous vein bypass. However, given the coexistence of coronary disease with peripheral vascular disease, a less invasive endovascular approach may be a preferable first step in a given patient. Generally, the greater the patient's comorbidity, the more likely one is to turn to a percutaneous approach.

Determination of optimal strategy in the future will likely be based on accumulating evidence and data, wherein patient and lesion characteristics, functional outcome measures, and cost analyses will be standardized to enable comparison among pure endovascular, pure surgical, and combined percutaneous and surgical approaches.[43] As the short- and long-term outcomes of catheter-based interventions continue to improve, it is likely that these techniques will be used in an increasing number of patients presenting with either claudication or critical limb ischemia.

Regardless of initial treatment strategy, a key determinant of the long-term outcome is the requirement for intensive follow-up surveillance. Although surveillance strategies for surgical bypass grafts have been developed, no formal guidelines exist for monitoring patients following percutaneous therapy. However, there is general agreement that these individuals should be subjected to regular evaluation, examination of the affected limb, and noninvasive testing. Early and prompt reintervention is indicated for restenosis to maximize the chances of long-term symptom relief, wound healing, and integrity of the limb.

For Visceral Ischemia

Renal Artery Obstructive Disease

Renovascular disease is an important and often unrecognized contributor to renal insufficiency, refractory hypertension, and overall cardiovascular mortality. However, because not all patients with angiographic evidence of renovascular disease are hypertensive or have renal dysfunction, patient selection for more invasive therapy requires careful consideration. Additionally, since the clinical syndrome associated with this anatomical diagnosis can resemble that of more common clinical diagnoses, such as isolated essential hypertension, a renovascular cause may not be considered. The onset of diastolic hypertension after the age of 55 years, refractory or malignant hypertension, resistant hypertension in a previously well-controlled patient, and/or an increasing serum creatinine level should alert the clinician and prompt further diagnostic testing. Unfortunately, modalities such as angiotensin-converting enzyme (ACE) inhibitor–induced venous plasma renin sampling and intravenous urography have insufficient sensitivity and specificity to provide a reliable screening and diagnostic tool.[44] Although post-ACE renal scintigraphy has high levels of sensitivity and specificity in some patient subsets, its utility is limited by lower sensitivity and specificity in patients with bilateral disease or abnormal renal function.[45] Duplex renal artery ultrasound,[46] spiral CT,[47] and more recently, MR angiography[46] all have been used in the noninvasive assessment of the renal vasculature with high degrees of accuracy. Although these modalities vary in their sensitivity and specificity, ultimately one's clinical conviction regarding the diagnosis must weigh heavily in the decision to pursue angiographic evaluation, because none of the techniques allows assessment of the functional significance of a renovascular lesion. Furthermore, even the traditional reference standard, contrast angiography, has considerable intraobserver and interobserver variability.[48,49] Determining the functional significance of an anatomical finding remains one of the greatest challenges of renal intervention. Nevertheless, significant renal artery obstruction is associated with an adverse prognosis in patients with atherosclerosis.[50]

After establishing the anatomical diagnosis of renal artery stenosis, one must consider the most appropriate management. The goals of treatment, both surgical and percutaneous, for renal artery stenosis include preservation of renal function, improved control of hypertension, and prevention of hemodialysis. Improvement in blood pressure control and reduction in the number of antihypertensive medications is common, but complete resolution of hypertension is unusual because concomitant essential hypertension often coexists. To the extent that severe renal artery disease can cause renal dysfunction, the identification and treatment of functionally significant renal artery stenosis could have major health benefits.[51] A major question remaining is whether percutaneous renal revascularization can slow, delay, or prevent deterioration in renal function and subsequent hemodialysis.

Historical data from the surgical literature support treatment of patients with both unilateral and bilateral renal artery stenosis. Although anatomical revascularization may allow improved antihypertensive management and preserve renal parenchymal function, how does percutaneous therapy compare to surgery? This question has particular importance, given the advanced age of many patients with atherosclerotic disease and the significant perioperative morbidity and operative mortality rates of up to 6 percent associated with surgical therapy. Only one randomized, controlled study has compared surgical therapy versus balloon angioplasty for unilateral atherosclerotic renal artery stenosis.[52] The authors reported slightly lower primary patency rates in the balloon angioplasty group, as one may expect in the prestent era. However, secondary patency was 90 percent in the PTA group and 97 percent in the surgical group, with comparable improvement in blood pressure and similar likelihood of improvement or stabilization in renal function after intervention. Even in the prestent era, the results of percutaneous intervention compared favorably to those of surgery.[53,54]

The availability of stents and the associated technological improvements that facilitate secure delivery of devices to the target site have led to more predictable and hemodynamically favorable results in renal revascularization. In spite of technical success rates in excess of 95 percent using stents, not all patients undergoing this procedure enjoy a clinical benefit. Thus, the presence of arterial stenosis does not guarantee a causal relationship to the patient's coexisting hypertension or renal insufficiency. In addition, patients with renovascular disease are commonly afflicted by other nephrotoxic conditions, including diabetes, essential hypertension, atheroemboli, and medication-related insults. Thus, the outcome of intervention in patients with isolated renovascular disease differs from that in candidates with renal artery stenosis and concomitant renal parenchymal disease. For this reason, it is likely that the desired clinical outcome of

TABLE 55–4 Clinical and/or Historical Factors Influencing the Degree of Suspicion of Renal Artery Stenosis*

Type of Influence	Effects	
Indication	Hypertension of recent onset or newly refractory Mildly elevated creatinine level (≤2.5) without diabetes Increasing creatinine on ACE inhibitor Disparate renal size (1 normal, 1 small) Pulmonary edema not explained by cardiac dysfunction	*The presence of any two is indication for determining renovascular anatomy*
Increases	Coronary atherosclerosis Claudication Known aortic branch vessel (brachiocephalic/mesenteric) atherosclerosis Abdominal bruit Known atherosclerotic abdominal aortic aneurysm Mild proteinuria without diabetes	
Decreases	Normal creatinine Severely elevated creatinine level (>3.5 mg/dl) Diabetes *with* evidence of nephropathy/retinopathy Severe (nephrotic range) proteinuria Longstanding stable hypertension Bilateral atrophic kidneys	

ACE = angiotensin-converting enzyme.
*Current potential indications for investigating the anatomical presence of renal artery stenosis and intervening if it is found. In our laboratories, the presence of any two with the indications in concert is cause for anatomical definition of the renal arteries. The intensity of this set of indications is augmented by the presence of the factors causing increases and is reduced in the presence of mitigating factors causing decreases.

improved blood pressure, with concomitant reduction in requirement for antihypertensive medications, is seen in only two-thirds of patients treated with stenting for renovascular disease.

This discrepancy between anatomical result and clinical outcome remains a challenge for the clinician who must assess the potential efficacy of a proposed renal artery intervention. How can one determine if revascularizing one of two kidneys will achieve the intended goals? The Dutch Renal Artery Stenosis Intervention Cooperative Study Group performed a study to determine whether an aggressive approach with invasive therapy is superior to that of "provisional" angioplasty. The group, consisting of some 26 centers, prospectively studied 106 patients with difficult-to-control hypertension, unilateral atherosclerotic renal artery stenosis (>50 percent decrease in luminal diameter), and a serum creatinine of less than 2.3 mg/dl, randomizing between angioplasty and best medical therapy.[55] The results suggested little advantage of angioplasty over medical therapy in the control of hypertension based on an intention-to-treat analysis. However, several issues severely limited the utility of this investigation, including the small sample size; inclusion of patients with only moderate renal artery stenoses; failure to use vascular stents; high percentage (44 percent) of cross-over to balloon angioplasty among patients in the control arm; and the authors' focus on the effect of therapy on blood pressure control to the exclusion of effect on renal function.

Many investigators and clinicians believe the routine use of vascular stents improves the results. Harden and associates studied patients with both bilateral and unilateral renal artery stenosis. Although the number of patients investigated was small, evidence suggested a slowing of renal impairment after stenting.[56] Additionally, when the entire renal mass is involved ("global renal ischemia"), the response is more dramatic: Renal intervention in patients with severe (>75 percent) bilateral disease or unilateral disease in a solitary kidney uniformly improves or stabilizes renal function and preserves kidney size.[57]

In summary, percutaneous treatment of renovascular disease offers a safe, flexible, and effective therapy that is preferable to open surgical revascularization. Renal artery stenting can ameliorate hypertension, can improve or stabilize renal function, and may delay the need for hemodialysis in appropriately selected patients. Controversy remains regarding the appropriate threshold for intervention in patients with severe unilateral renal artery stenosis, associated with normal renal function and only modest hypertension that is reasonably controlled. Future randomized trials and the adoption of uniform reporting standards will hopefully shed light on this issue.[58,59] Lastly, the advent of distal protection devices to limit atheroembolic complications may further improve safety and renal parenchymal preservation. The current recommended systematic approach to the investigation and treatment of this condition is outlined in Table 55–4 and Figures 55–9 and 55–10, and examples of complex renal intervention are shown in Figures 55–11 through 55–13.

Mesenteric Ischemia

The clinical syndrome of mesenteric ischemia is surprisingly uncommon, given the high frequency of atherosclerotic disease of the aorta and the common finding of aorto-ostial stenosis of the visceral vessels. It is likely that the rarity of the clinical syndrome reflects the good collateralization and redundancy of the visceral circulation with multiple pathways from the superior mesenteric artery and the inferior mesenteric artery. In addition, there are clearly lesser degrees of ischemia, often misdiagnosed, that manifest with moderate postprandial discomfort, bloating, or gas rather than the full-blown syndrome of delayed postprandial pain, vomiting, food avoidance, and weight loss. Even in advanced cases, multiple other etiologies for the manifest of weight loss and abdominal pain are often entertained before "intestinal angina" comes into focus as the diagnosis of exclusion. Evidence of significant obstruction of two or more of these vessels is often found when classic symptoms and endoscopy suggest bowel ischemia.[60] With the advent of MR angiography imaging, it is now possible to make the "anatomical" diagnosis without resorting to invasive angiography.[61] When the symptoms are classic, the anatomical findings severe, and the alternative pathological explanations few, the diagnosis is confirmed and revascularization is in order. As might be expected, however, this patient group has a high incidence of CAD, and surgical mortality and morbidity ranges from 5 to 8 percent,[62-65] with the highest incidence of complications

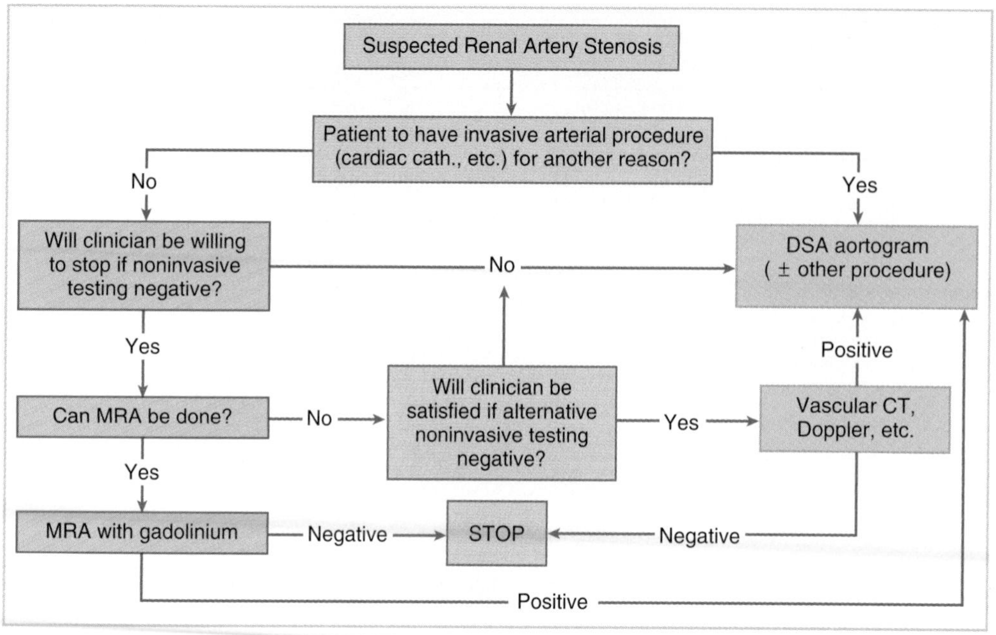

FIGURE 55–9 The approach to the anatomical evaluation of renal artery stenosis. Once stenosis is suspected, if the patient is to have another invasive arterial procedure, noninvasive imaging is deferred and a low-volume digital subtraction aortogram (DSA) is done at the time of that procedure. In other cases, the clinician should assess whether a negative noninvasive test would be sufficient evidence to acquit the renal arteries. If so, noninvasive testing should be performed. If not, consideration should be given to DSA and selective angiography. cath = catheterization; MRA = magnetic resonance angiography.

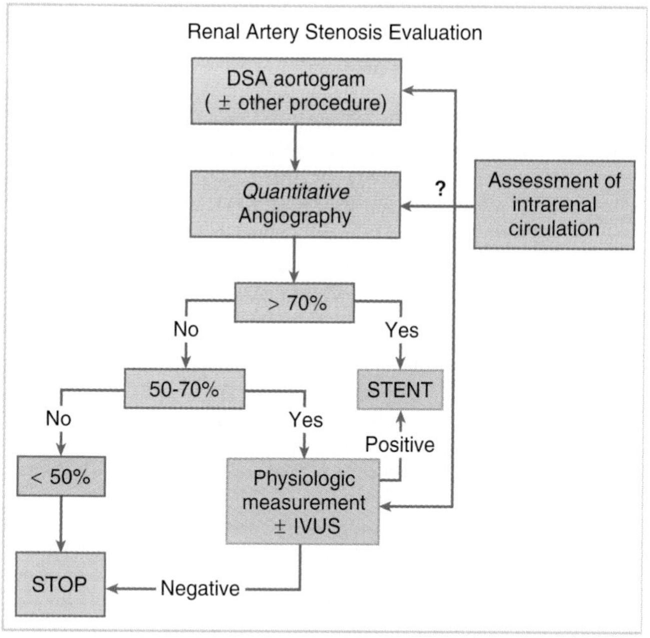

FIGURE 55–10 The approach to the angiographic evaluation and treatment of renal artery stenosis. Once a digital subtraction aortogram (DSA) is performed confirming the presence of renovascular disease, quantitative angiography and objective evaluation of the severity of stenosis should be performed. Very severe (>70 percent diameter stenosis) lesions are subjected to revascularization and mild lesions (<50 percent diameter stenosis) are not. We believe that the intermediate lesion should be assessed with physiological evaluation and/or an additional anatomical documentation of severity such as intravascular ultrasound (IVUS). The absence of translesional flow acceleration or a pressure gradient should mitigate the desire to intervene.

occurring in patients older than 70 years of age.[64] Mortality for operation on *acute* mesenteric ischemia is an order of magnitude higher.[66] In view of these risks, the clinician must have a high degree of diagnostic certainty before commending the patient to surgery for chronic mesenteric ischemia.

Obstructions of the visceral vessels are similar to those of the renal arteries, and the technical considerations for PTA and stent placement are similar to those for renal artery intervention. The endovascular approach circumvents the need for general anesthesia, and the operative trauma associated with open surgery and, it is believed, will result in a lower acute mortality and morbidity.[67-69]

As is true for the evaluation of alternative therapies in most other peripheral vascular beds, there is no side-by-side comparison of surgery versus endovascular treatment for chronic mesenteric ischemia. Interpretation of the literature, which reports successful case series of both surgical and interventional treatment, is confounded by the obvious case selection and other inherent biases. Interventional treatment offers a clear alternative for the management of chronic visceral ischemia that may have advantages over surgery, especially in those patients with advanced age or additional increased risk of morbidity and mortality (Figs. 55–14 and 55–15).

For Cerebral Ischemia

Brachiocephalic and Subclavian Obstructive Disease

Once considered rare, brachiocephalic and subclavian artery obstructions have received increased attention due to the use of internal mammary conduits for coronary bypass surgery. Subclavian steal syndrome arises due to reversal of flow in the vertebral artery as blood is shunted into the brachial circulation. Symptoms of dizziness, syncope, and vertigo are most common along with extremity claudication in the ipsilateral limb. In coronary-subclavian steal, there is reversal of flow within the left internal mammary artery because of proximal subclavian stenosis. These patients often come to clinical attention with myocardial ischemia. Although some clinical improvement may be seen with conservative therapy, relief of the anatomical obstruction is usually necessary.[70]

Balloon angioplasty for subclavian artery stenosis was described in the early 1980s, with subsequent reports showing that acute success and patency rates at follow-up were comparable to surgery. Furthermore, there was a low rate of complications and infrequent mortality.[71,72] There was initial concern about the potential for distal embolization and stroke, uncertain long-term patency, and difficulty in treating total occlusions. This concern, in conjunction with continued improvements in anesthetic and operative technique, short hospital stays, and early discharge, has led many practitioners to continue to regard surgery as the standard therapy against which endovascular methods must be compared.

Vascular stents have become the endovascular treatment of choice for atherosclerotic obstructive disease of branches of

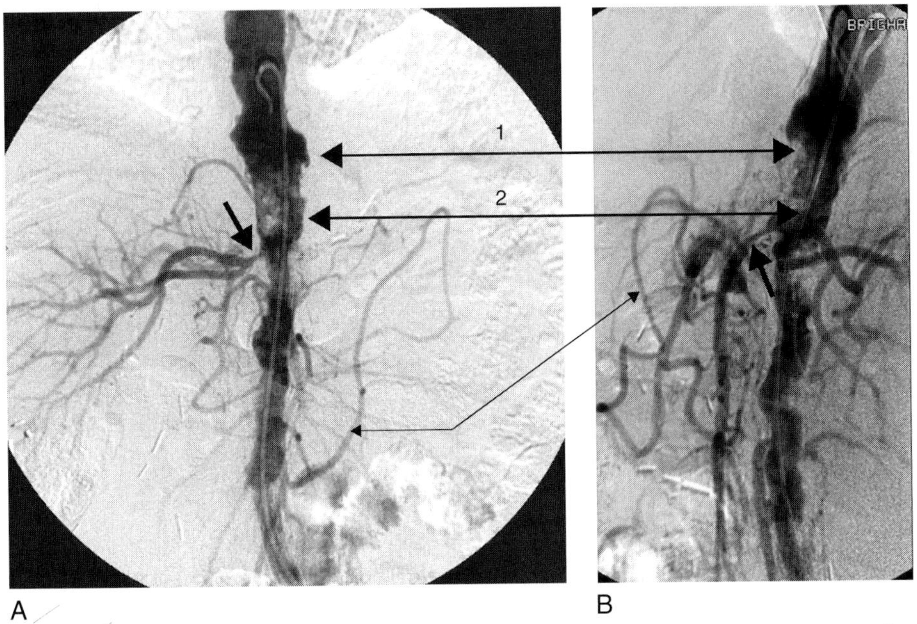

FIGURE 55–11 The anatomical complexity in treatment of advanced renovascular disease. **A** shows an anteroposterior aortogram in a patient with refractory hypertension and monthly hospitalizations for hypertensive crises and pulmonary edema. Initially, this patient was to have aortic and renovascular surgery, but on exploration, the aorta was so calcified that no operative approach was deemed feasible. Medical therapy was elected, but after continued refractory hypertension, aortography and intervention were performed. Between levels 1 and 2, shown by the double-headed arrows, an eccentric atherosclerotic excrescence produced a pressure gradient of between 30 and 50 mm Hg. In addition, there was an intrinsic ostial renal artery stenosis indicated by the single thick arrow in **A.** In **B** the thick arrow shows an origin stenosis of the superior mesenteric artery, and the thin arrow projecting into both panels identifies the marginal artery collaterals filling the mesenteric circulation.

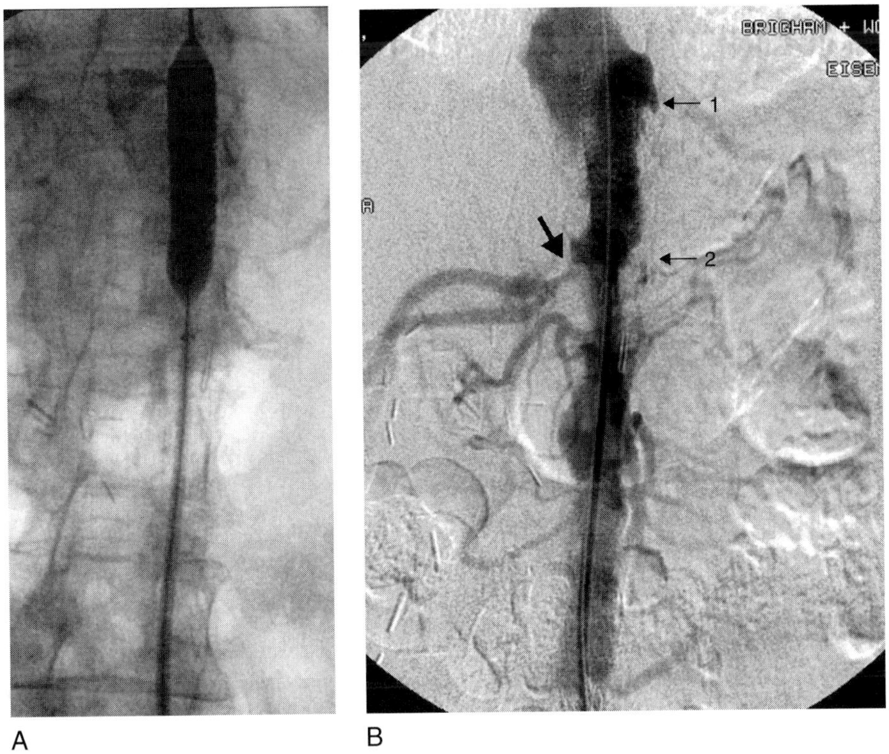

FIGURE 55–12 **A,** Balloon postdilation of a 14-mm self-expanding stent. **B,** This stent obliterated the translesional gradient from position 1 to position 2, yet the intrinsic renal artery stenosis remained (thick arrow).

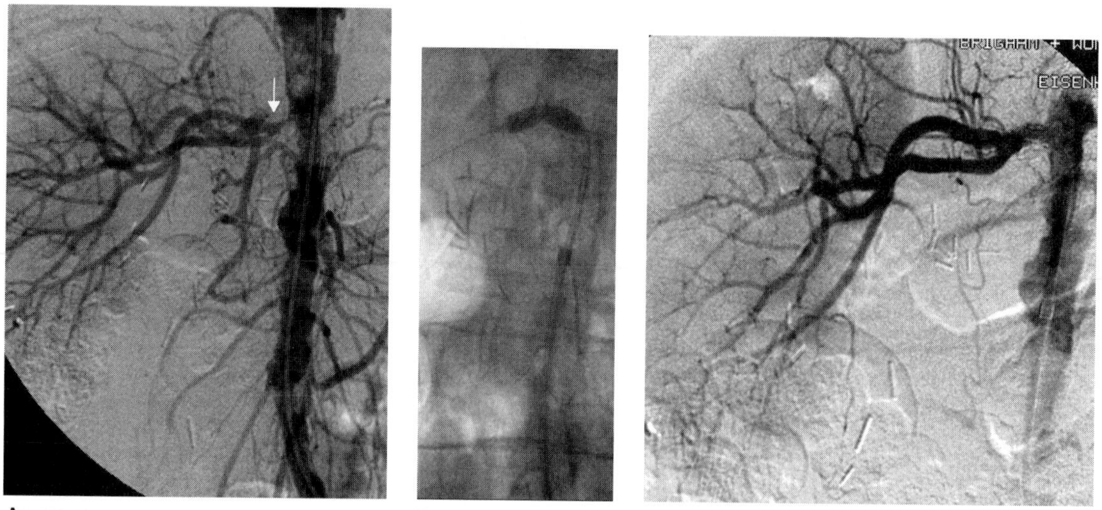

A B C

FIGURE 55–13 Selective balloon and stent placement in this vessel. **A,** The initial stenosis. **B,** Balloon-expandable stent placement. **C,** Selective angiography demonstrating resolution of the stenosis. Final hemodynamic measurements showed no pressure gradient from the thoracic aorta and downstream of the renal stent. This patient tolerated the procedure well, had mild improvement in the serum creatinine level, but most significantly was no longer refractory to antihypertensive medications, and her blood pressure control prevented further hospitalizations for hypertensive crises and pulmonary edema.

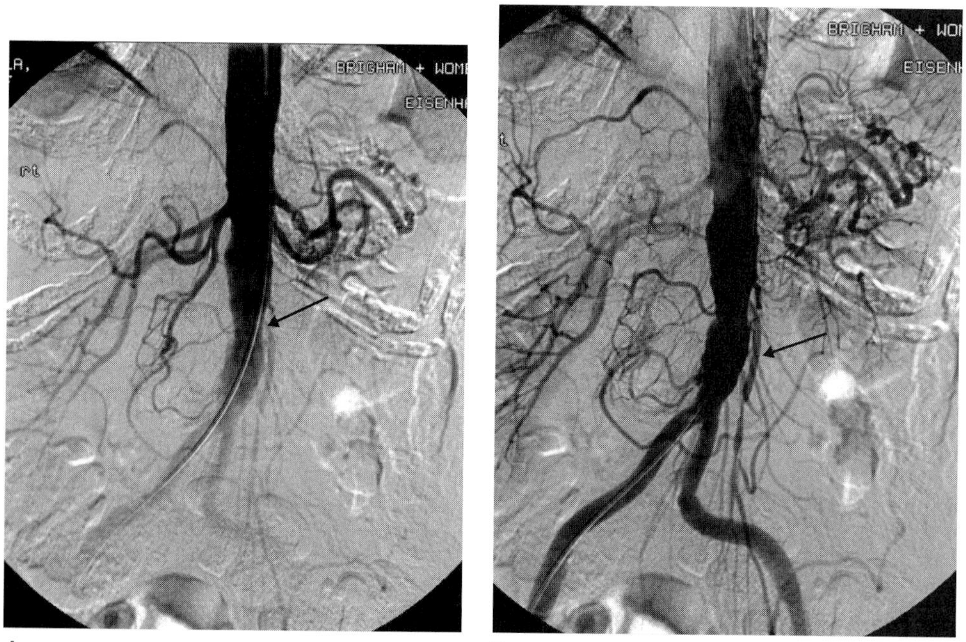

A B

FIGURE 55–14 Visceral angiogram from a patient with postprandial abdominal pain, weight loss, and abdominal bruits. Of note is that this projection does not demonstrate the origins of the celiac or superior mesenteric arteries, though in **A,** early in the run, the thin arrow indicates a stenosis at the origin of the inferior mesenteric artery. Then, from a later frame, **B** shows the origins of the renal arteries; though potentially not seen in absolute profile, they appear unobstructed.

the aorta, including the subclavian and carotid arteries. However, long-term patency and clinical data for percutaneous treatment of the subclavian/brachiocephalic vessels are limited. An evaluation of the reports of surgery versus angioplasty/stenting of this condition has been published, compiling technical success (the ability to perform the planned procedure yielding target lesion revascularization and survival to discharge), patient death, stroke, and patency of the treated segment.[73] There was no uniformity or standardization for evaluation or reporting of complications in the studies in which stenting was performed; however, adverse events were reported in approximately 6 percent of patients.[73] Similarly, the overall incidence of postprocedure complications such as vascular access difficulty, hemorrhage, pseudoaneurysm, transfusion, or contrast-mediated transient renal insufficiency is not known. Of the patients represented in the reports, technical success was achieved in 97 percent. No strokes or deaths occurred. Follow-up data were available in about two-thirds of technically successful cases at a mean duration of 16.8 months. Occlusion or restenosis was reported in 6 percent. Following publication of this review, there were editorials from interventionalists suggesting broadening the horizons of interventional therapy[74] and from surgeons advising to proceed with caution.[75]

The reports of vascular stenting continue to suggest that perioperative strokes are quite uncommon. Al-Mubarak and colleagues reported no strokes in their series of 38 patients,[71] and strokes occurred in only 0.9 percent of subclavian procedures described by Henry and coworkers.[72] In addition, treatment failures, when they occurred, were limited to totally occluded arteries. Primary patency ranged from 94 percent at 20 months to 75 percent at 8 years; with overall patency of 100 percent at 20 months to 90 percent at 8 years.[71]

There have been some conflicting reports regarding the efficacy of stent implantation. There are concerns about not only long-term patency but also durability of the stent owing to wire fracture at the site of flexion and compression.[76] Motarjeme reported disappointing patency rates for

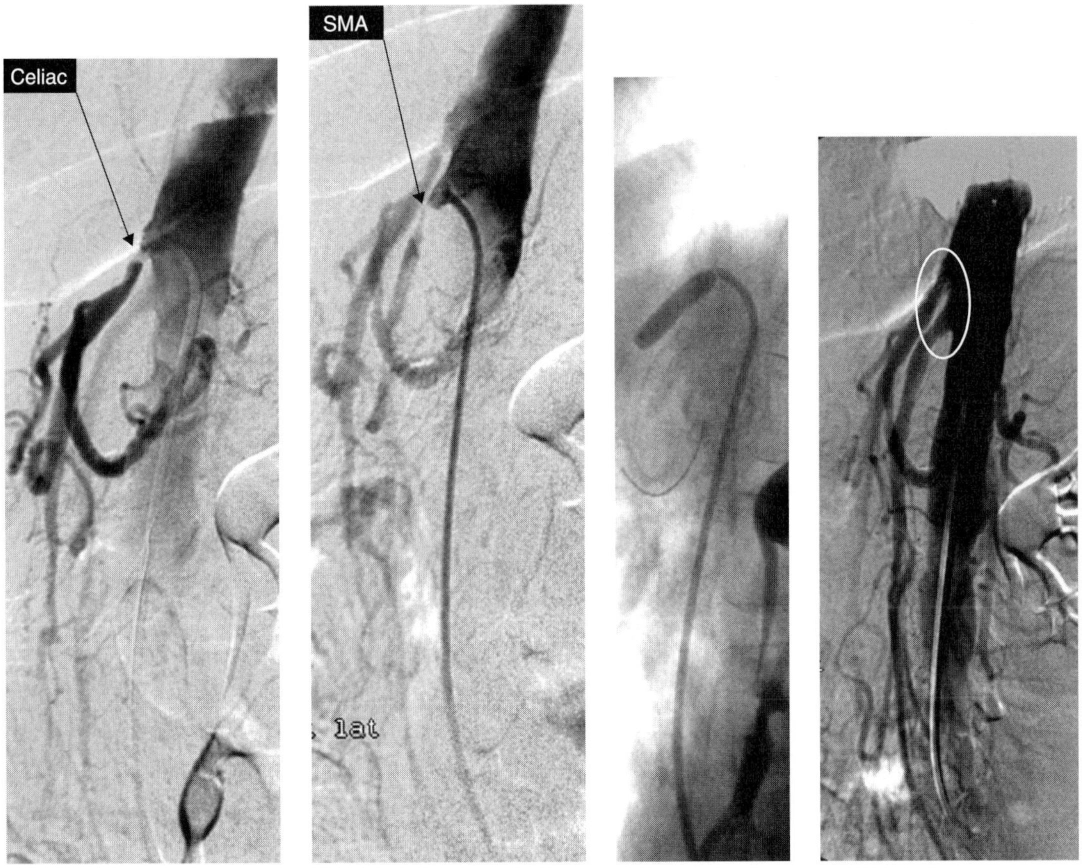

A B C D

FIGURE 55–15 The selective evaluation of the celiac and superior mesenteric arteries (SMA) in the lateral projection of the patient in Figure 55–21. Both these vessels proved to be critically stenosed (**A** and **B**) and were treated interventionally (**C**), restoring wide patency to both as outlined in **D**. The patient's symptoms abated, and she began to gain weight.

balloon angioplasty alone in a group of patients with total occlusions of the subclavian,[77] whereas Henry and associates reported good short and intermediate results in both those who underwent angioplasty alone and those who had angioplasty and stenting.[72] A European series reviewed 115 patients with subclavian disease who were treated percutaneously.[78] The procedures were performed between 1984 and 1998, and all patients after January 1, 1996, routinely received balloon-expandable stents. Successful revascularization was achieved in 98 patients. There were no periprocedural deaths, 1 patient had a transient ischemic attack (TIA) from the left vertebral artery, and 2 patients had emboli (one to the renal artery and 1 to the mesenteric artery). All 3 patients recovered completely from these events. Although patency rates were significantly higher at 1 year in the stented group compared with those treated only with angioplasty (95 vs. 76 percent), by 4 years of follow-up there was more restenosis in the stented patients.[78] Furthermore, in a multivariate model, predictors of restenosis in this study included lesion length, residual stenosis after angioplasty, and stent implantation.[78] However, this analysis was limited by the large difference in patient numbers in the two groups (26 in the stented group vs. 72 in the angioplasty group) and because stents were placed only in patients treated after 1996. By that time technological advances had made it easier to open totally occluded vessels that were previously rarely successfully treated percutaneously. Thus, many of these lesions in the stent group had other factors increasing their risk of restenosis and would not have been successfully treated percutaneously before the introduction of stents.

It remains unlikely that the near future will produce a large well-designed trial comparing surgical and interventional treatment of patients with brachiocephalic and subclavian disease. At present, experience and examination of the literature support the consideration of a primary percutaneous approach in most patients with symptomatic obstructive disease (Fig. 55–16; also see Fig. 55–22).

Carotid Disease

Stroke and its associated debilitation is one of the most dreaded threats to health. As a result, prophylactic surgical therapy for significant carotid stenosis was embraced by both patients and physicians, and carotid endarterectomy became one of the most commonly performed procedures by vascular surgeons. Now, developing endovascular technology has allowed the expansion of available treatment modalities for cerebrovascular disease. Although catheter-based therapy may offer a less invasive alternative to carotid endarterectomy, controversy still exists regarding where and when the endovascular treatment of cerebrovascular disease should be applied.

The goals of treating carotid artery disease are to prevent disabling stroke and to prolong life. All therapies should be judged ultimately on their ability to achieve these endpoints rather than surrogate ones. Planning mechanical treatment for cerebrovascular disease requires knowledge of the natural history of the problem. In the Dutch TIA trial, 3000 patients with a history of recent TIA were randomized to treatment with low or moderate dose aspirin.[79] After 36 months, the risk of nonfatal stroke was 5.7 percent in the low-dose group and 6.9 percent in the high-dose group. Thus the risk of stroke in unselected aspirin-treated patients is 3 percent per year after an index event. Given the concerning natural history of cerebrovascular disease and the unknown effects of carotid endarterectomy, several randomized trials were organized to determine whether endarterectomy had benefits over medical therapy for both symptomatic and asymptomatic disease. In the early 1990s, European Carotid Endarterectomy Surgery

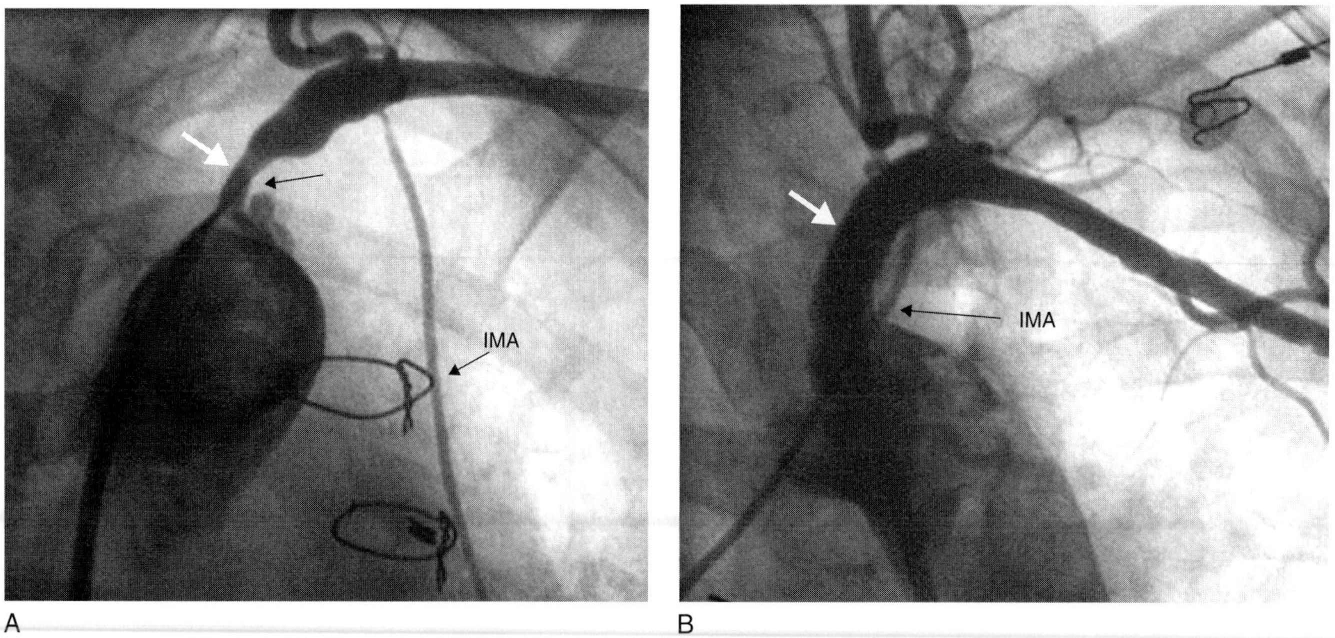

FIGURE 55–16 The treatment of proximal subclavian disease. In **A,** a severe stenosis at the origin of the left subclavian artery is identified (thick white arrow). This is in association with an atherosclerotic ulcer (thin black arrow). The internal mammary artery (IMA) is indicated. Following balloon dilation and stent placement **(B),** the subclavian artery is widely patent and the IMA is preserved.

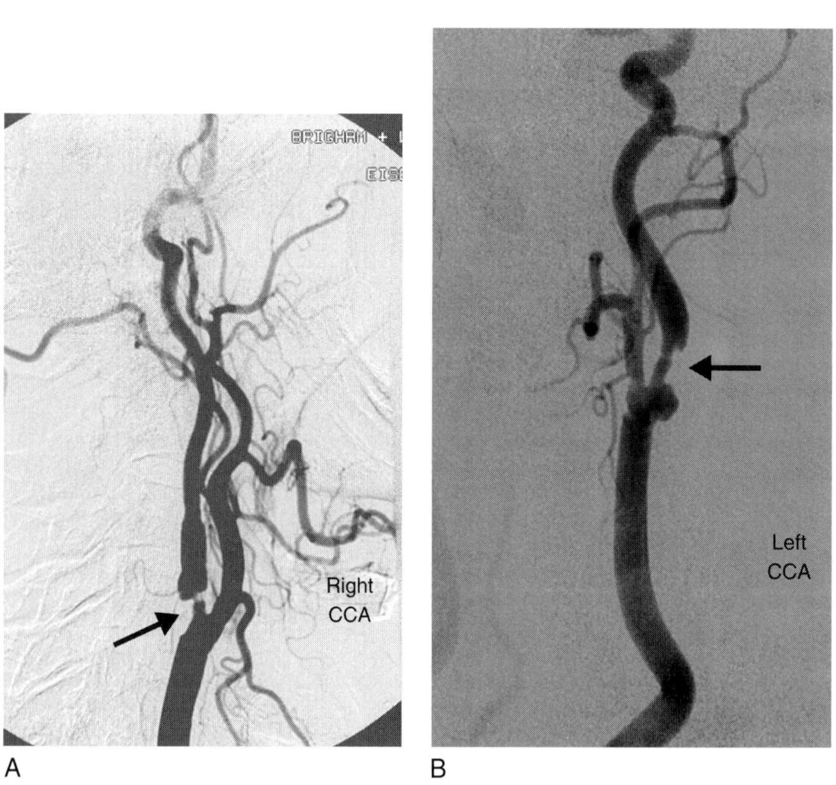

FIGURE 55–17 Selective digital subtraction angiograms of the cervical carotid artery (CCA) in a patient with disseminated atherosclerosis and severe bilateral internal carotid obstruction. This patient had a recent right hemisphere transient ischemic attack, and the stenosis at the origin of the right internal carotid artery (**A,** arrow) is extremely severe. In **B,** the left carotid angiogram demonstrates a severe stenosis (arrow), but one with a lesser degree of obstruction than the contralateral artery.

Trialists (ECST)[80] enrolled patients with 70 to 99 percent carotid stenosis within 180 days of an ipsilateral TIA. Patients were randomized to medical versus surgical therapy, yielding a 21.9 percent risk of stroke at 36 months for the medically treated group and a 12.3 percent risk in the surgically treated group. The North American Symptomatic Carotid Endarterectomy Trial (NASCET) randomized patients with 70 to 99 percent stenosis and ipsilateral TIA symptoms within 120 days of randomization to medical or surgical therapy.[81] The 30-day follow-up favored medical therapy with a 5.8 percent rate of all stroke and death in the surgical group and a 3.6 percent risk in the medical group. Similarly, the major stroke rate was increased more than twofold to 2.1 percent in the surgical group. As in the ECST data, the 36-month death rate did not differ significantly between groups in the NASCET study (12.7 vs. 9.9 percent, surgical vs. medical), with most of these deaths related to cardiovascular causes. However, the 36-month total stroke rate (9 vs. 26 percent) and major stroke rate (2.5 vs. 13.1 percent, surgical vs. medical) were significantly less in the surgical group. The results of this study have served as the gold standard for treatment of symptomatic carotid disease and clearly suggest that surgical endarterectomy stabilizes the index lesion. Similar data have been developed for severe asymptomatic stenoses,[82] albeit with results that are less compelling compared to those in patients with symptomatic disease.

Although these randomized trials suggest that high-quality carotid endarterectomy, despite procedural risk, decreases long-term incidence of ipsilateral stroke in patients with severe carotid stenoses, endarterectomy has not been shown to prolong life. The patients in these studies were carefully selected to avoid confounding conditions, and many with significant comorbidities were excluded—such as those with atrial fibrillation, severe symptomatic coronary disease, recent myocardial

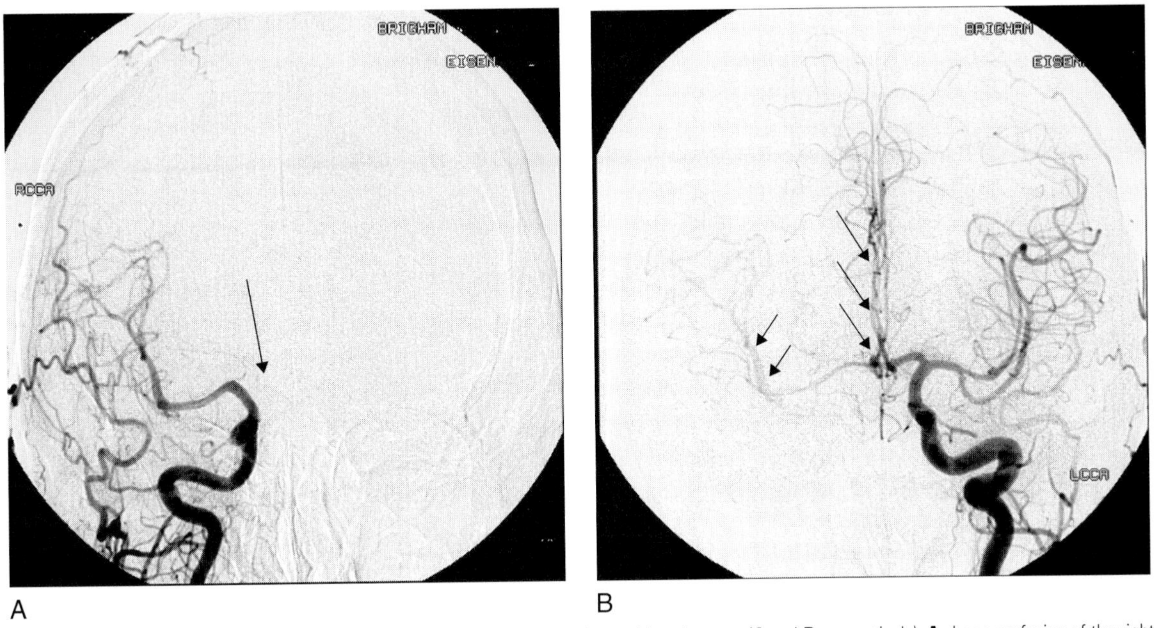

FIGURE 55–18 The corresponding anteroposterior (Townes) view of the right and left carotid angiograms (**A** and **B,** respectively). **A** shows perfusion of the right middle cerebral territory only, and no flow is seen into the anterior cerebral vessel, the expected location of which is delineated by the arrow. In contrast, **B** shows the injection of the left carotid artery and demonstrates filling of both hemispheres, including the right anterior cerebral (three long arrows) and middle cerebral (two short arrows) territories.

infarction, past ipsilateral carotid endarterectomy, ipsilateral disabling stroke, age older than 79 years, or life expectancy less than 5 years. To participate, institutions and surgeons had to demonstrate acceptably low rates of complications and stroke in their surgical patients.

Clearly, for endarterectomy to have achieved those benefits in the populations studied, the strokes *prevented* by the operation must significantly exceed the strokes *caused* by the operation. Similarly, operative mortality could obliterate any benefit of surgery. In NASCET, carotid endarterectomy was associated with a 6.5 percent complication rate of combined stroke and death, with about 0.9 percent of death not related to stroke. Most strokes in NASCET resulted from thromboembolism within 6 hours of the procedure. These perioperative strokes were mostly ipsilateral to the carotid endarterectomy and were attributed to thrombus formation at a denuded arterial site. The longer term results of NASCET showed that although there was no mortality benefit, the reduction in stroke ipsilateral to the endarterectomy during the operative and 3-year follow-up period favored endarterectomy. After the perioperative period, the risk of ipsilateral major stroke was almost zero,

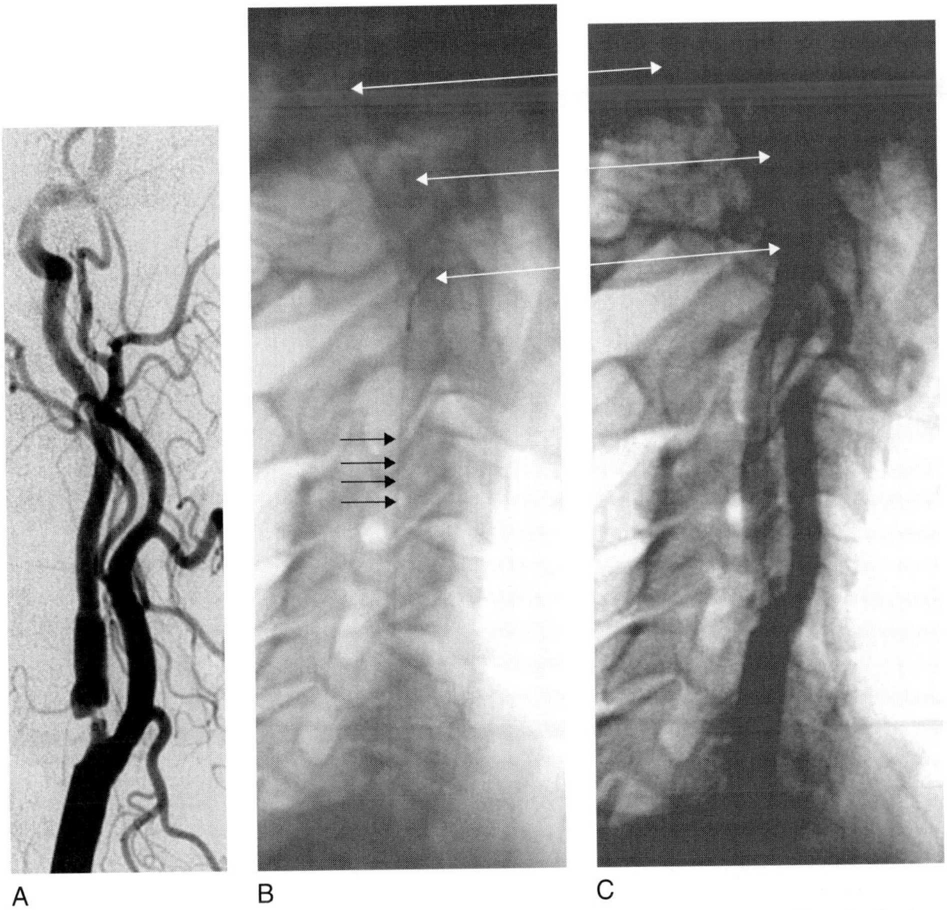

FIGURE 55–19 **A,** The prestenting angiogram; the right carotid is repeated. **B** and **C** illustrate the Filterwire distal protection device in place. In **B,** the four short arrows indicate the body of the guidewire, with the uppermost horizontal arrow indicating the distal portion of the guidewire; the middle horizontal arrow showing the end of the cone of the distal protection device; and the lowermost horizontal arrow showing the hoop supporting the entry into the conically shaped microporous membrane of the distal protection device. **C** is an unsubtracted angiogram with the device in place, demonstrating distal perfusion through the membrane of this device.

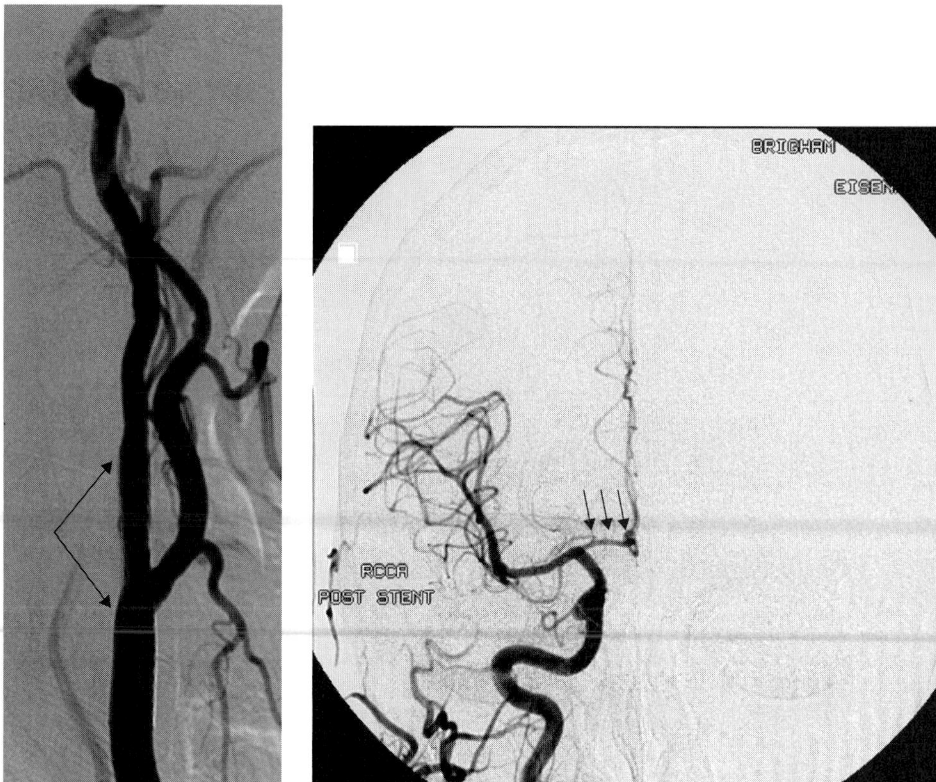

A B

FIGURE 55–20 **A** illustrates the results of stent placement; the extent of the stent is indicated by the arrows, and wide patency of the carotid has been restored. **B** shows a poststenting right carotid angiogram illustrating renewed vigorous flow into the anterior cerebral artery in this hemisphere (three arrows).

implying that strokes occurring outside the perioperative period are *not* under the influence of the operation or surgical technique.[83,84] The large size of the trial and the relatively low adverse event rates indicated that small absolute differences in these rates could have obliterated the statistical benefit of endarterectomy. Indeed, subsequent analysis of operative stroke rates in the general population at the NASCET-participating hospitals suggested the reported rates were unusually low.[85] On balance, however, the randomized surgical data demonstrate that once a perioperative stroke is avoided, endarterectomy is a durable prophylaxis against ipsilateral stroke.

Endovascular Carotid Treatment

It was a logical evolution of endovascular technique to consider its potential in extracranial cerebrovascular disease. Given the results of the randomized surgical trials, this extension encountered a number of conceptual and ethical hurdles. First, was it ethical to extend a new and untested therapy to a clinical situation in which there was already another therapy shown to be superior to medical treatment alone? Because of this consideration, early endovascular efforts were not extended to every patient whose clinical characteristics matched those in the NASCET, the European Carotid Endarterectomy Surgery Trial (ECST), or the Asymptomatic Carotid Atherosclerosis Study (ACAS). Instead, stenting was first offered to patients who were at high risk. They would have been ineligible for the surgical trials but had carotid *lesions* similar to those benefiting from surgical revascularization. Results were encouraging, but the rate of periprocedure central nervous system events did not appear to be *identical* to those in the NASCET population. Alternative possibilities advanced to explain these results were that the endovascular technique was responsible or that the incongruent outcomes were the result of the inclusion of high-risk patients not studied in the surgical trials.

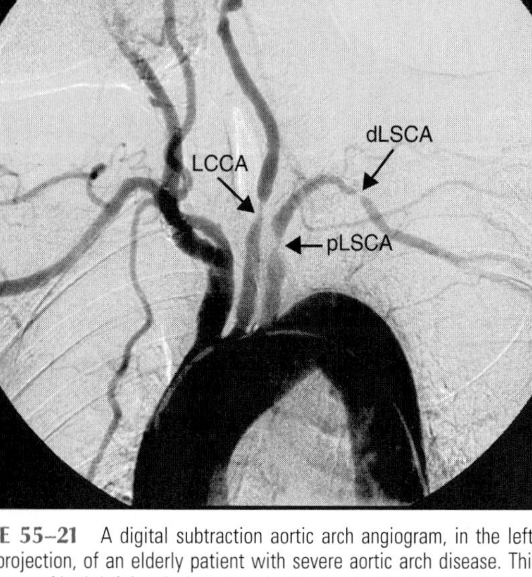

FIGURE 55–21 A digital subtraction aortic arch angiogram, in the left anterior oblique projection, of an elderly patient with severe aortic arch disease. This patient had evidence of both left hemisphere transient ischemic attacks and left arm claudication. This case illustrates the ability to treat complex aortic arch vessel disease with interventional technique. dLSCA = distal left subcavian artery; LCCA = left common carotid artery; pLSCA = proximal left subclavian artery.

Currently, experience with carotid stenting is accumulating. Some early publications suggested a high rate of procedural complications. However, Roubin and associates reported the complications of TIA, stroke, myocardial infarction, and death in their first series of patients treated with carotid stenting.[86] The 5.7 percent procedural stroke incidence corresponds to an overall stroke and death rate at 30 days of 5.8 percent in the surgically treated group in NASCET—certainly suggesting clinical equipoise. Five-year follow-up results of 528 patients[87] undergoing carotid stenting showed a 1.6 percent fatal stroke and nonstroke death rate at 30 days. The major stroke rate was 1 percent and the minor stroke rate was 4.8 percent. The overall 30-day stroke and death rate was 7.4 percent ($n = 43$). Over the course of follow-up there was a 3-year freedom from stroke rate of 92 ± 1 percent. Of particular note is the learning curve that is appar-

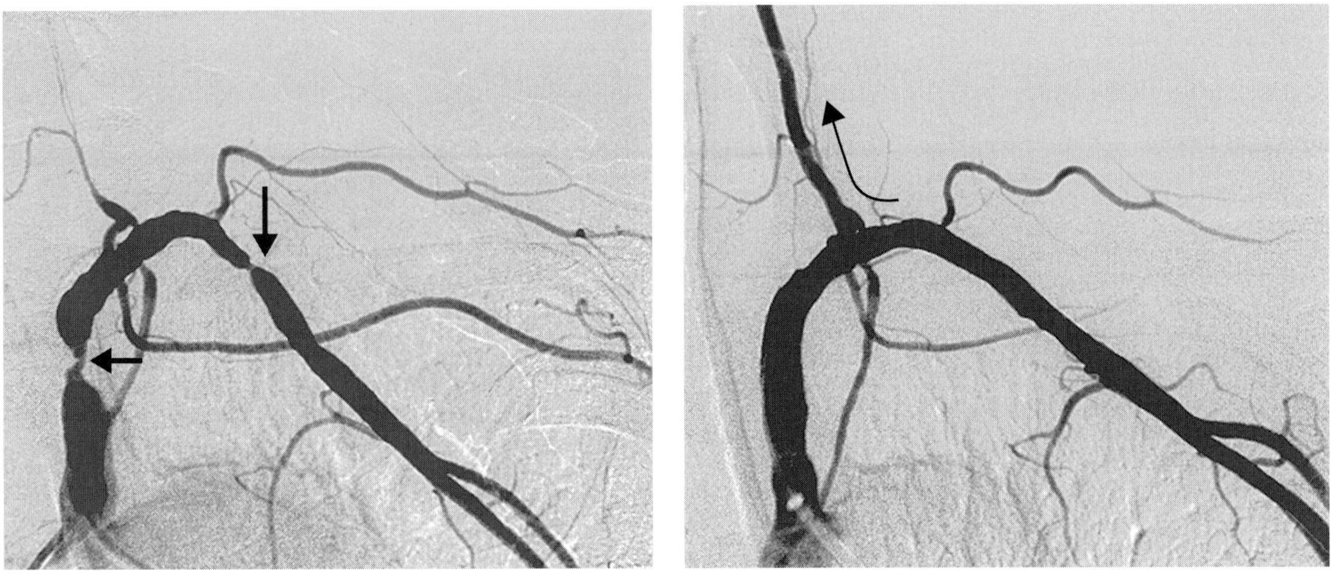

A B

FIGURE 55–22 **A,** A selective digital subtraction angiogram of the left subclavian. This study shows a stenosis proximal to the origin of the left vertebral and left internal mammary artery (horizontal black arrow) and a severe stenosis distal to the left vertebral, internal mammary, and thyrocervical trunk. Treatment of the distal lesion without relief of the proximal obstruction would potentially exacerbate the subclavian steal, and thus both lesions require treatment. **B,** A repeat subclavian angiogram after placement of proximal and distal stents. In **A** and **B,** the injection technique was similar, yet **B** shows antegrade flow in the left vertebral, indicated by the curved black arrow in **B**. Because of the potential for external compression, a self-expanding stent with appropriate postdilation was used to treat the more distal subclavian lesion.

ent in the application of this technology—over the 5-year study period, the 30-day minor stroke rate significantly improved from 7.1 percent for the first year to 3.1 percent for the fifth year.

The International Society for Carotid Artery Treatment has compiled an ongoing voluntary, self-reported registry of procedures performed outside of formal trials.[88,89] This registry also discloses a learning, or experience, curve, with the highest rates of major stroke and death (~3 percent each) occurring in centers that have performed procedures on fewer than 50 patients. Overall, however, in this patient group, the reported rates of TIA and minor stroke in 1999 were less than 3 percent, major stroke 1.35 percent, and death less than 1 percent. An additional report[90] of 8612 procedures describes 2.3 percent TIA, 2.5 percent minor stroke, and 1.32 percent major stroke, for a summed ischemic complication rate of 6.12 percent. The overall procedural mortality was 0.72 percent. Of course, these are self-reported registry data and not independently collected or adjudicated, as would be the case in prospective, randomized studies. However, these data suggest the rate of complications that is likely to be encountered in practice.

The Carotid and Vertebral Artery Transluminal Angioplasty Study (CAVATAS) provided the first prospective, randomized comparative data on patients with cerebrovascular disease randomized to endovascular or surgical treatment.[91] In this study, the mortality was equivalent in both arms and the neurovascular event rates were statistically similar. The major stroke and death rate was 5.9 percent among the surgical patients and 6.4 percent among the angioplasty patients (10 percent and 9.9 percent for any stroke lasting >7days within 30 days of treatment). All deaths in the endovascular group were due to fatal strokes, but there was only one fatal stroke in the surgical arm. The high event rate in both arms of CAVATAS led to criticism of both carotid endarterectomy and endovascular intervention in this trial.[92] In a small randomized series comparing carotid stenting and endarterectomy, there were no strokes in either the surgical or the endovascular stent groups, and only one death in the surgical group.[93] Though the rate of adverse events did not differ between the groups, the small size of this study raises the question of whether it had sufficient power to prove equivalence of the techniques. As of this writing, these are the only peer-reviewed reports of direct comparisons of carotid endarterectomy with endovascular technique. However, the results of the high-risk randomized trial of Stenting and Angioplasty with (embolic) Protection in Patients at High Risk for Endarterectomy (SAPPHIRE) trial, comparing stenting to endarterectomy in high-risk patients, have been presented in abstract form. This trial, although designed as an equivalency study, surprisingly indicated an advantage of endovascular therapy over carotid endarterectomy with regards to the primary endpoint of stroke, death, or myocardial infarctin at 30 days. One-year data, recently reported but not peer reviewed, indicate a persistent advantage to stenting at 1 year, with favorable rates of combined ipsilateral stroke and death compared to the surgical approach.

Carotid Intervention and Embolic Debris

The key to the overall benefit of any carotid procedure is the *avoidance of the periprocedural stroke.* Both stenting and endarterectomy appear to stabilize the area of the lesion effectively. The trade-off versus medical therapy alone is the exchange of procedure-related strokes in the short term with spontaneous lesion–related strokes in the follow-up period.

The recognition that the avoidance of periprocedure stroke is critical and that distal emboli are potentially disastrous, combined with the desire to improve percutaneous methods of treating obstructive carotid atherosclerosis, has underscored the need to identify risk factors to optimize patient selection. Neurological deficits can be predicted by the presence of symptomatic lesion, a lesion length greater than 11.2 mm, and the absence of hypercholesterolemia.[94] The lesion length was thought to predict stroke because the treatment of long stenoses required more manipulations, longer stents, and multiple postdilations after stent placement. It was postulated that the postdilation surface provided a prothrombotic area immediately following intervention; thromboembolic stroke was an implicated outcome. In addition, neurological complications of endovascular treatment were found in one study to be predicted by advanced age (>80 years) and long (>10 mm) or multiple (>1 lesion separated by normal vessel wall) stenoses.[95] The incidence of stroke in patients younger than 80 years was 5.6 percent, whereas in those 80 years or older, the incidence was 19.2 percent.

However, thrombotic debris is not the only cause of embolic stroke. Evidence of carotid plaque embolization as a result of stenting and PTA was reported by Manninen and colleagues.[96,97] The results of stenting, including postdilation when necessary ($n = 9$) and PTA ($n = 10$), were compared in situ in human cadavers, and embolic debris was detected in equal amounts for both types of interventions. Histological analysis of the debris determined that it was composed primarily of atherosclerotic plaque constituents. Observations of the postintervention surfaces with intravascular ultrasound and MR imaging led the investigators to postulate that the smoother stent surface could be preferable to the post-PTA surface. Additional ex vivo studies have confirmed that embolic debris is commonly released during endovascular plaque manipulation at many stages.[98] Ohki,[99] Rapp,[100] and their associates found that embolic debris was released from all specimens.

Clinically, Doppler evidence of emboli is found in 30 to 40 percent of symptomatic patients and 4 to 20 percent of asymptomatic patients, and it has been said that microembolization is universal. The clinical consequences of embolic showers likely depend on the size and number of emboli and the nature of the distal vascular bed.[101] Thus, the major concern associated with balloon angioplasty and stenting of carotid lesions has been the periprocedural complications that arise due to embolic debris and not the long-term outcome.[102]

Distal Embolization Protection (see also Chap. 52)

The determination that distal embolization is both dire and common during endovascular carotid procedures has prompted a search for devices and techniques to limit its occurrence. Devices that employ distal balloon occlusion, the distal positioning of a porous filter, and proximal occlusion with aspiration all have been developed.[103] Henry and coworkers[104] were first to report use of balloon occlusion and aspiration for carotid applications in high-risk patients. Carotid occlusion was well tolerated in all but 1 of the 48 patients; intolerance was due to the presence of multiple severe carotid lesions and poor collateralization. Analysis of debris retrieved in a similar patient population[105] revealed particle sizes ranging from 50 to 2500 μm in diameter composed of atherothrombotic material—fresh thrombus, old thrombus, lipoid masses, fibrous particles, and calcified particles.

Technical reports of experience with distal embolic protection devices report aggregate rates of periprocedural stroke and death from 2 to 5 percent.[106-110] The use of the devices can be associated with difficult placement distal to the lesion, distal carotid spasm, or difficulty in protection device retrieval through stents. Debris is often grossly visible, and histological analysis of the particulate routinely demonstrates typical components of atherosclerotic plaque. Although occlusion balloons currently have a more favorable, lower crossing profile, they do not allow flow and are not tolerated by all patients. Filters provide distal perfusion and, in doing so, not only benefit the target organ but also allow better visualization for stent placement. Although there are no randomized studies and the technology continues to evolve rapidly, carotid stenting distal cerebral protection appears safe, and further investigation with such devices is warranted. Recent peer-reviewed procedural results of carotid intervention are outlined in Table 55–5.

Though it is an evolving technology, carotid stenting offers an appealing, less invasive modality with benefits comparable to surgical endarterectomy. With increasing operator experience and use of increasingly effective distal embolization protection devices and antiplatelet therapy, endovascular techniques will undoubtedly advance rapidly. Large-scale randomized, controlled trials and registries, some currently ongoing, will ultimately determine relative advantages of surgical and endovascular approaches to carotid disease. For the present, endarterectomy remains the reference standard. Refinements of endovascular technique will be led by devices that mitigate distal embolization; reports suggest that these devices are clearly effective in reducing the incidence of

TABLE 55–5 Recent Carotid Intervention Series*

Lead Author	Reference	Year	Protected (P), Unprotected (U), or Mixed (M)	*N*	TIA (%)	Minor Stroke (%)	Major Stroke %	All Stroke (%)	Death (%)	MACE (%)
Wholey	90	2000	M	8612	2.3	2.5	1.32	—	—	6.12
Shawl	112	2000	U	170	—	—	—	2.9	0	2.9‡
Roubin	86	2001	U	528	—	4.8	1	—	1.6	7.4
Spence	92	2001	U	—	—	—	—	—	—	9.9
Brooks	93	2001	U	53	1.9	—	—	—	0	1.9
Dietz	107	2001	P	43	—	—	—	—	—	5
Reimers	110	2001	P	86	—	1.2	—	—	—	2.3
Henry	104	2002	M	315	1.3	1.3	1.6	4.2	0.3	4.5
Schluter	108	2002	P	93	2.1	—	—	3.1	—	5.2
Al-Mubarak	109	2002	P	162	—	1	—	—	1	2
Mean†										**4.72**
Range										**1.9–9.9%**

MACE = major adverse cardiac event; TIA = transient ischemic attack.

*A recent published series of carotid artery interventions. Of note is that the mean MACE rate is <5%, ranging from 1.9% to 9.9%. Major stroke appears rare in the series in which embolic protection is used.

†Mean of all studies, not weighted by patient numbers.

‡Excludes death.

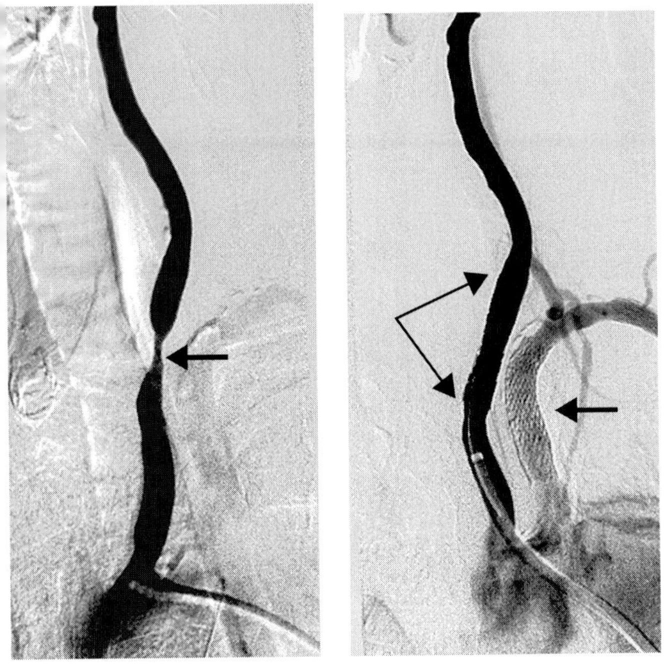

FIGURE 55–23 A, A selective digital subtraction angiogram of the left common carotid. This reveals a severe stenosis of the intrathoracic portion of the left common carotid, which was treated with a single-balloon expandable stent. The stented segment is between the two long arrows. Wide patency was restored. The large horizontal arrow in **B** shows the previously stented left subclavian. The patient's arm claudication and transient ischemic attacks were successfully treated by this procedure.

symptomatic embolization. However, the reduction in risk is likely influenced by the overall risk of the patients being studied. Elderly patients, for example, have an excess risk of distal embolization, whereas those who are younger are at lesser risk. Thus the immediate effectiveness of carotid stenting with embolic protection depends on the risk profile of the patients for whom it is employed. The risk of adverse outcomes of carotid stenting in the current literature is from 2 to 10 percent, and future stent systems and embolic protection devices should be expected to perform within that range as we work to improve the results of carotid revascularization. At present, the global experience with carotid stenting, both with and without distal protection, suggests clinical equivalence to carotid endarterectomy as neurovascular interventions to prevent stroke in the several years after the procedure.[111] The very long-term effects on prevention of stroke and death and the more subtle influences on cognitive function will require further investigation. However, the clinical practice of carotid intervention will likely advance in light of the accumulating experience in support of its safety and efficacy (Figs. 55–17 through 55–23).

Interventions for Venous Disease

For Extremity Venous Thrombosis

Unlike atherosclerotic arterial obstructive disease, the major presenting obstructive element in venous obstruction is thrombus. Thus, dissolution or removal of the offending thrombus is the most evident goal of interventions for extremity venous thrombosis. Yet underlying the thrombus is almost always a predisposing factor such as a hypercoagulable state, external obstruction, venous stricture, scarring, or an indwelling foreign body. As a result, the treatment of venous thrombosis comprises not only the removal of thrombus but also attempt to correct the underlying predisposition(s). For most patients, anticoagulation and/or thrombolytic therapy are the mainstays of therapy (see Chap. 66). Both systemic and catheter-directed thrombolysis have achieved some success. Mechanical thrombectomy, balloon venoplasty, and stenting all have been reported, yet compelling data supporting the use of catheter-directed therapy are limited.

Despite the reports of experience, the data do not support the *routine* use of catheter-directed thrombolysis in the treatment of lower extremity deep venous thrombosis. Because of the suggestion of a reduction in the incidence of postthrombotic syndrome with lysis compared to anticoagulation alone and because of the suggestion of reduced major bleeding, catheter-directed therapy seems reasonable to apply in patients at higher risk for the complications of systemic lysis and in those who have a large thrombus burden and/or a high risk of developing a postthrombotic syndrome. In addition, more interventional concepts are emerging. There are reports of experience with rheolytic thrombectomy[113] or mechanical clot disruption. Additional experience with stents suggests that in cases where there is residual venous obstruction from scarring or external compression, relief of that obstruction with self-expanding stents may be important to maintain venous patency and prevent recurrent thrombosis. This is particularly true when the initial insult, such as an indwelling port infusion catheter, has been removed. Balloon venoplasty is also increasingly used to provide temporary relief of venous obstruction to facilitate the placement of transvenous pacing and/or defibrillator leads. Thus, the selective application of catheter-based thrombolysis, thrombectomy, and venous stenting is appropriate based on individual circumstances.

For Central Venous Obstruction

Superior vena cava (SVC) syndrome results from the obstruction of the blood flow in the SVC (see Chap. 83). Pathological processes from contiguous structures can compress or directly invade the SVC. Superimposed venous thrombosis may contribute to the development of SVC syndrome in up to 50 percent of patients. Historically, SVC syndrome was most frequently caused by direct tumor compression. Currently, the use of indwelling venous access catheters, coupled with the improved survival of chemotherapy patients, is increasing the occurrence of "nonmalignant" SVC syndrome in patients whose cancers have been cured. The explosion in the use of the automatic implantable cardioverter-defibrillator and sophisticated multilead pacing systems has increased the incidence and recognition of this condition.

Percutaneous Treatment

Medical and surgical options for the treatment of SVC obstruction are well established (see Chap. 83). Since the initial description of successful percutaneous treatment of SVC syndrome in the adult, the use of angioplasty alone was limited by a high rate of initial failure and early restenosis due to recoil of highly elastic SVC wall. Stenting therefore quickly gained acceptance in this area of vascular intervention after it was first reported in the 1980s.

Stenting in malignant SVC syndrome rapidly improves symptoms. Patients report almost immediate resolution of headache, visual disturbances, and other central nervous system symptoms. Dyspnea, cough, and edema usually resolve within 1 to 3 days but occasionally may take up to 1 week. Stenting results in complete resolution of symptoms in 68 to 100 percent of patients with malignant SVC syndrome.[114] In the largest series, 76 consecutive patients with

SVC syndrome were treated with stents and compared with historical control of patients treated with radiation. Procedural success was 100 percent, and all patients had improvement of symptoms within 48 hours. Ninety percent of patients treated with a stent had no symptoms of SVC obstruction at the time of death compared with 12 percent of patients treated with radiation.[114] The recurrence rate of SVC syndrome after percutaneous intervention has been reported between 0 and 45 percent.[115,116] Many pathophysiological mechanisms of recurrence have been documented. Acute stent thrombosis can develop shortly after stent placement in patients on insufficient anticoagulation or antiplatelet therapy; tumor ingrowth through stent struts had been reported; and intimal hyperplasia or fibrous scarring can occur. Stent length oversizing may prevent recurrence of SVC syndrome due to stent edge overgrowth; however, it may increase risk of SVC stent thrombosis or restenosis. The highest recurrence rate of SVC syndrome has been reported in patients with total SVC occlusion, but repeated procedures in these patients are uniformly successful, with additional stent placement, angioplasty, and/or thrombolysis used alone or in combination

Superior Vena Cava Syndrome of Nonmalignant Etiology

In the developed world, SVC syndrome of nonmalignant etiology ("benign" SVC syndrome) is usually iatrogenic in origin and it is most frequently due to indwelling intravenous catheters and pacing leads. Complications of pacemaker lead placement such as venous thrombosis or stenosis occurs in up to 30 percent of patients. Only a few patients, however, become symptomatic, but the presence of multiple leads, retention of severed lead(s), and previous lead infection may increase the risk of SVC syndrome. The largest series of percutaneous therapy in benign SVC syndrome included 16 patients. Ten patients had SVC syndrome due to the indwelling catheter, 2 due to the pacemaker wire, and 1 each due to goiter, fibrous mediastinitis, heart-lung transplant, and spontaneous thrombosis. The patency rate in 13 patients who were followed for a mean of 17 months was 85 percent.[117] Similar results can be expected in patients with SVC syndrome associated with central venous infusion catheters. Ideally, interventional treatment should also include removal of the inciting lead or catheter.

SVC stenting is a low-risk procedure that provides fast and durable symptomatic relief in malignant caval obstruction, often in combination with chemotherapy or radiation to provide patients with benefit of life prolongation together with effective symptom control. In patients with SVC syndrome of nonmalignant etiology, based on mid-term follow-up results, stenting is the treatment of choice. Surgical therapy should be reserved for patients with benign SVC syndrome refractory to percutaneous therapy. Only a few patients are likely to become truly refractory because most patients with recurrent SVC syndrome can be treated successfully with repeated percutaneous intervention (Figs. 55–24 through 55–26).

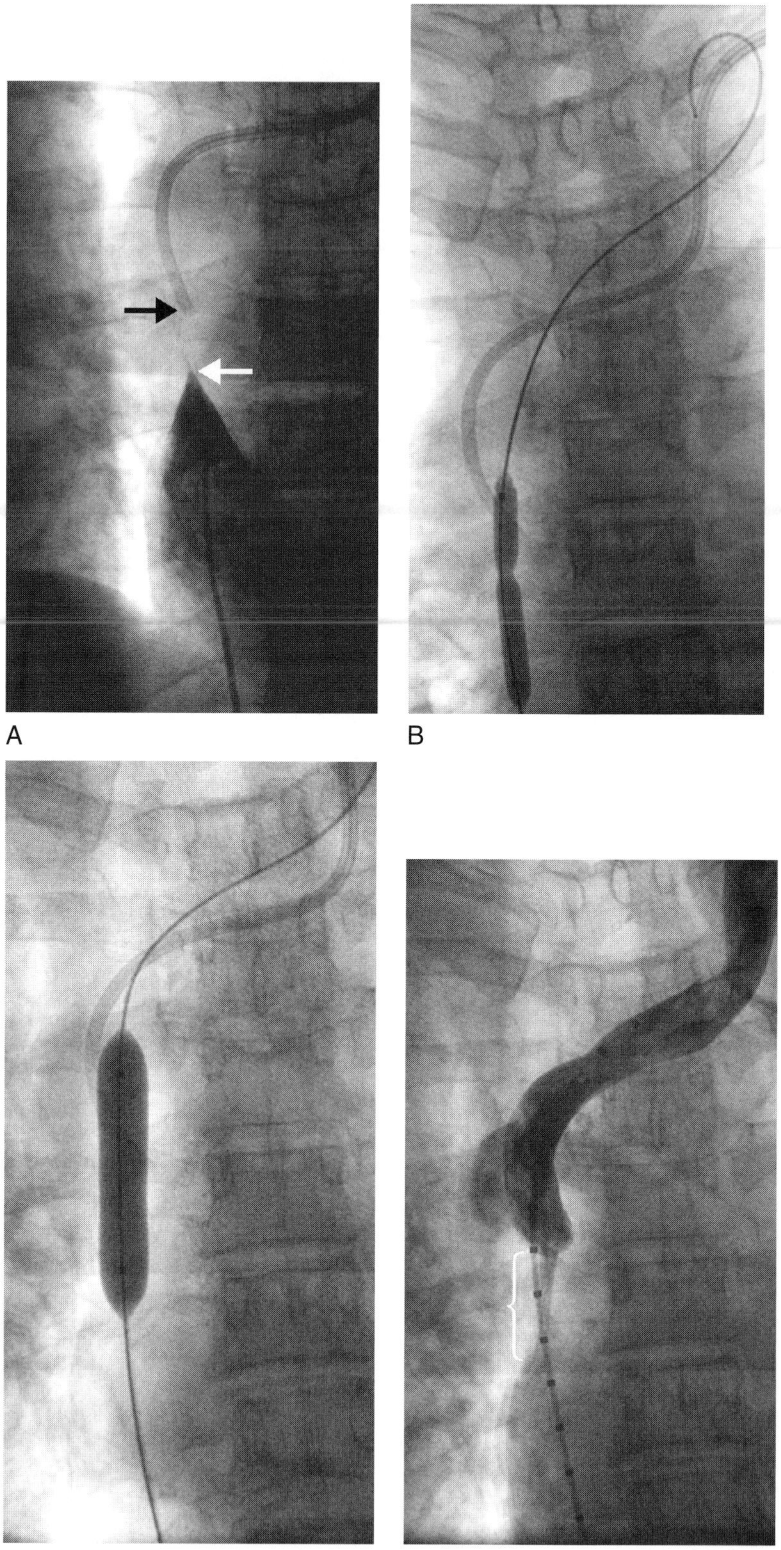

FIGURE 55–24 Superior vena cava (SVC) syndrome and its treatment in a middle-aged woman with an indwelling port access catheter who had received chemotherapy for breast cancer. Though these catheters allow potentially sclerosing agents to be given into the central circulation, the position of the catheter tip along the wall of the SVC likely induces an inflammatory reaction and fibrous scarring. In this case the catheter tip, identified by the black arrow in **A,** ends at an area of complete occlusion of the superior vena cava. Injection of contrast agent into the right atrial–SVC junction shows the SVC to be completely occluded at that point (horizontal white arrow, **A**). This total occlusion was pierced with a hydrophilic guidewire, and a series of balloon dilations were performed. **B** shows the first dilation with a small balloon indicating an indentation in that balloon. This was likely the nidus of the complete occlusion. Successive dilations with up to a 10-mm balloon **(C)** were successful, but given the fibrous and elastic nature of these venous obstructions, there is severe elastic recoil. **D** demonstrates a venogram performed with a catheter across the total occlusion and shows the reestablishment of a small channel (bracket) between the SVC and the right atrium. Stenting is required to ensure wide and durable patency; however, the indwelling port access catheter may be entrapped by the placement of a stent.

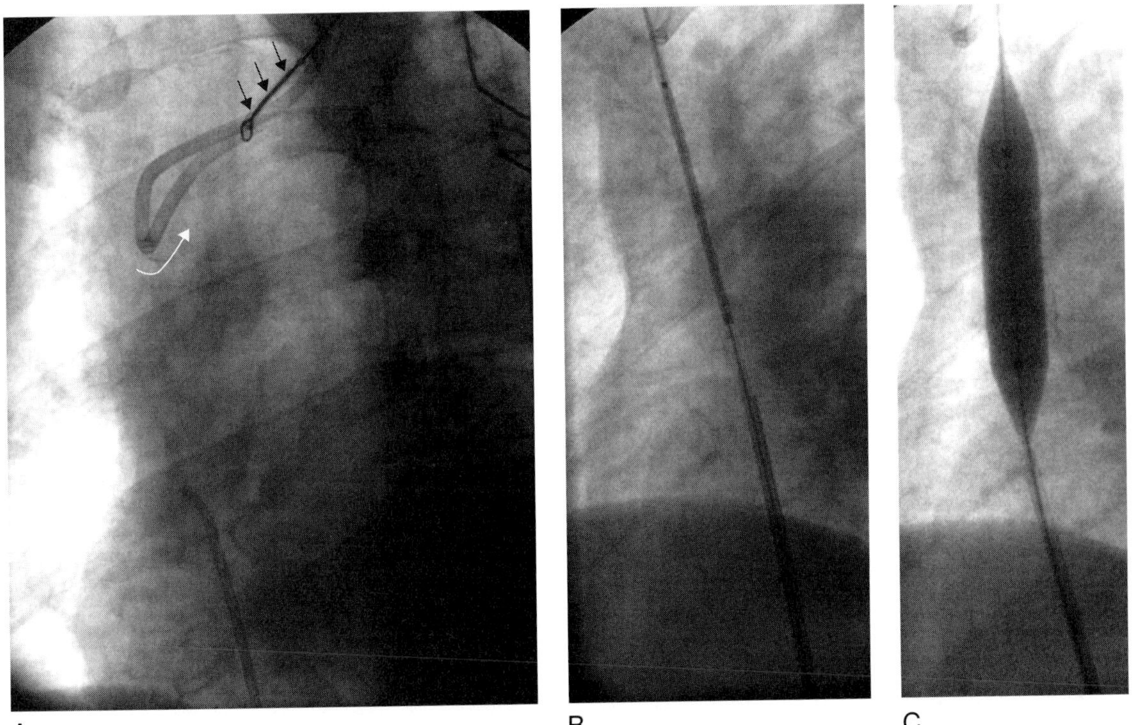

FIGURE 55–25 An option for stenting in the presence of an indwelling port access catheter. When indwelling pacing or implantable cardioverter-defibrillator leads traverse the cavoatrial junction, these leads must be removed before being trapped between stents and the vascular wall. In this case, the end of the port access catheter was snared from the left brachial approach (**A,** three short arrows) and the tip withdrawn by doubling it over in the superior vena cava (white arrow). From below, a large self-expanding nitinol stent **(B)** was positioned in the area of residual stenosis, deployed, and postdilated with a 14-mm balloon **(C)**.

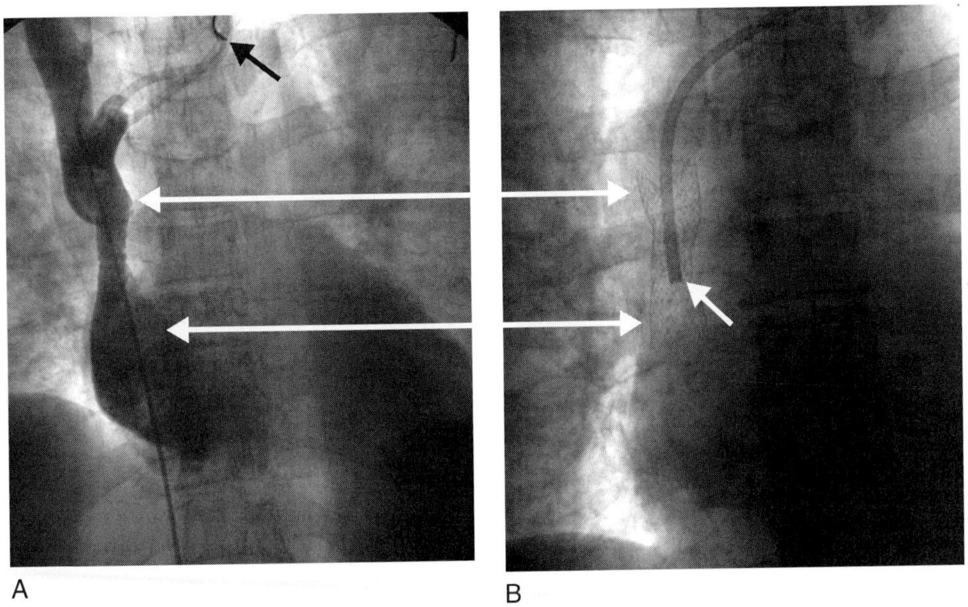

FIGURE 55–26 Final result from stent placement. In **A,** an injection into the superior vena cava shows free flow of contrast agent into the right atrium via the stented segment (delineated by the uppermost and lowermost horizontal arrows). The end of the indwelling port access catheter can still be seen trapped by the snare in **A** (black arrow). The tip of this catheter was repositioned within the stented segment (**B,** white arrow). The patient's symptoms were completely resolved, and the use of the port access catheter was preserved.

Conclusion

Though the specific tools and techniques vary, the theme of endovascular intervention is similar across many vascular territories. In general, vascular stenting has become the mainstay of percutaneous revascularization for relief of symptoms. The challenge for the future will be to continue to improve the long-term durability of endovascular therapy and to explore its potential for preventing the complications of progressive vascular disease.

1. U.S. Department of Health and Human Services: Chartbook on Cardiovascular, Lung and Blood Diseases: Morbidity and Mortality. Bethesda, National Heart, Blood, and Lung Institute, National Institutes of Health, 1994.

Aortoiliac Obstruction

2. Bosch JL, Hunink MG: Meta-analysis of the results of percutaneous transluminal angioplasty and stent placement for aortoiliac occlusive disease. Radiology 204:87-96, 1997.
3. Wilson SE, Wolf GL, Cross AP: Percutaneous transluminal angioplasty versus operation for peripheral arteriosclerosis: Report of a prospective randomized trial in a selected group of patients. J Vasc Surg 9:1-9, 1989.
4. Tetteroo E, van der Graaf Y, Bosch JL, et al: Randomised /comparison of primary stent placement versus primary angioplasty followed by selective stent placement in patients with iliac artery occlusive disease. Dutch Iliac Stent Trial study group. Lancet 351:1153-1159, 1998.
5. Cho L, Roffi M, Mukherjee D, et al: Superficial femoral artery occlusion: Nitinol stents achieve better flow and reduce the need for medications than balloon angioplasty alone. J Invasive Cardiol 15:198-200, 2003.
6. Henry M, Amor M, Ethevenot G, et al: Percutaneous endoluminal treatment of iliac occlusions: Long-term follow-up of 105 patients. J Endovasc Surg 5:228-235, 1998.
7. Haulon S, Mounier-Vehier C, Gaxotte V, et al: Percutaneous reconstruction of the aortoiliac bifurcation with the "kissing stents" technique: Long-term follow-up in 106 patients. J Endovasc Ther 9:363-368, 2002.
8. Siskin GP, Englander M, Roddy S, et al: Results of iliac artery stent placement in patients younger than 50 years of age. J Vasc Interv Radiol 13:785-790, 2002.
9. Mohamed F, Sarkar B, Timmons G, et al: Outcome of "kissing stents" for aortoiliac atherosclerotic disease, including the effect on the non-diseased contralateral iliac limb. Cardiovasc Intervent Radiol 25:472-475, 2002.
10. Reekers JA, Vorwerk D, Rousseau H, et al: Results of a European multicentre iliac stent trial with a flexible balloon expandable stent. Eur J Vasc Endovasc Surg 24:511-515, 2002.
11. Funovics MA, Lackner B, Cejna M, et al: Predictors of long-term results after treatment of iliac artery obliteration by transluminal angioplasty and stent deployment. Cardiovasc Intervent Radiol 25:397-402, 2002.
12. Saha S, Gibson M, Torrie EP, et al: Stenting for localised arterial stenoses in the aorto-iliac segment. Eur J Vasc Endovasc Surg 22:37-40, 2001.
13. Timaran CH, Stevens SL, Freeman MB, Goldman MH: External iliac and common iliac artery angioplasty and stenting in men and women. J Vasc Surg 34:440-446, 2001.
14. Powell RJ, Fillinger M, Bettmann M, et al: The durability of endovascular treatment of multisegment iliac occlusive disease. J Vasc Surg 31:1178-1184, 2000.
15. Murphy TP, Khwaja AA, Webb MS: Aortoiliac stent placement in patients treated for intermittent claudication. J Vasc Interv Radiol 9:421-428, 1998.
16. Reyes R, Maynar M, Lopera J, et al: Treatment of chronic iliac artery occlusions with guide wire recanalization and primary stent placement. J Vasc Interv Radiol 8:1049-1055, 1997.
17. Dyet JF, Gaines PA, Nicholson AA, et al: Treatment of chronic iliac artery occlusions by means of percutaneous endovascular stent placement. J Vasc Interv Radiol 8:349-353, 1997.

Femoropopliteal Obstruction

18. Duda SH, Pusich B, Richter G, et al: Sirolimus-eluting stents for the treatment of obstructive superficial femoral artery disease: Six-month results. Circulation 106:1505-1509, 2002.
19. Scheinert D, Biamino G: Femoropopliteal occlusions: Experience with peripheral excimer laser angioplasty. Curr Interv Cardiol Rep 3:130-138, 2001.
20. Scheinert D, Laird JR Jr., Schroder M, et al: Excimer laser-assisted recanalization of long, chronic superficial femoral artery occlusions. J Endovasc Ther 8:156-166, 2001.
21. Gray BH, Sullivan TM, Childs MB, et al: High incidence of restenosis/reocclusion of stents in the percutaneous treatment of long-segment superficial femoral artery disease after suboptimal angioplasty. J Vasc Surg 25:74-83, 1997.
22. Martin DR, Katz SG, Kohl RD, Qian D: Percutaneous transluminal angioplasty of infrainguinal vessels. Ann Vasc Surg 13:184-187, 1999.
23. Kessel DO, Wijesinghe LD, Robertson I, et al: Endovascular stent-grafts for superficial femoral artery disease: Results of 1-year follow-up. J Vasc Interv Radiol 10:289-296, 1999.
24. Conroy RM, Gordon IL, Tobis JM, et al: Angioplasty and stent placement in chronic occlusion of the superficial femoral artery: Technique and results. J Vasc Interv Radiol 11:1009-1020, 2000.
25. Cheng SW, Ting AC, Wong J: Endovascular stenting of superficial femoral artery stenosis and occlusions: Results and risk factor analysis. Cardiovasc Surg 9:133-140, 2001.
26. Gordon IL, Conroy RM, Arefi M, et al: Three-year outcome of endovascular treatment of superficial femoral artery occlusion. Arch Surg 136:221-228, 2001.
27. Lofberg AM, Karacagil S, Ljungman C, et al: Percutaneous transluminal angioplasty of the femoropopliteal arteries in limbs with chronic critical lower limb ischemia. J Vasc Surg 34:114-121, 2001.
28. Bauermeister G: Endovascular stent-grafting in the treatment of superficial femoral artery occlusive disease. J Endovasc Ther 8:315-320, 2001.
29. Steinkamp HJ, Wissgott C, Rademaker J, et al: Short (1–10 cm) superficial femoral artery occlusions: Results of treatment with excimer laser angioplasty. Cardiovasc Intervent Radiol 25:388-396, 2002.
30. Gray BH, Laird JR, Ansel GM, Shuck JW: Complex endovascular treatment for critical limb ischemia in poor surgical candidates: A pilot study. J Endovasc Ther 9:599-604, 2002.
31. Jamsen TS, Manninen HI, Jaakkola PA, Matsi PJ: Long-term outcome of patients with claudication after balloon angioplasty of the femoropopliteal arteries. Radiology 225:345-352, 2002.
32. Becquemin JP, Favre JP, Marzelle J, et al: Systematic versus selective stent placement after superficial femoral artery balloon angioplasty: A multicenter prospective randomized study. J Vasc Surg 37: 487-494, 2003.
33. Jahnke T, Andresen R, Muller-Hulsbeck S, et al: Hemobahn stent-grafts for treatment of femoropopliteal arterial obstructions: Midterm results of a prospective trial. J Vasc Interv Radiol 14:41-51, 2003.

Infrapopliteal Obstruction

34. Sivananthan UM, Browne TF, Thorley PJ, Rees MR: Percutaneous transluminal angioplasty of the tibial arteries. Br J Surg 81:1282-1285, 1994.
35. Varty K, Bolia A, Naylor AR, et al: Infrapopliteal percutaneous transluminal angioplasty: A safe and successful procedure. Eur J Vasc Endovasc Surg 9:341-345, 1995.
36. Dorros G, Jaff MR, Murphy KJ, Mathiak L: The acute outcome of tibioperoneal vessel angioplasty in 417 cases with claudication and critical limb ischemia. Cathet Cardiovasc Diagn 45:251-256, 1998.
37. Desgranges P, Kobeiter K, d'Audiffret A, et al: Acute occlusion of popliteal and/or tibial arteries: The value of percutaneous treatment. Eur J Vasc Endovasc Surg 20:138-145, 2000.
38. Soder HK, Manninen HI, Jaakkola P, et al: Prospective trial of infrapopliteal artery balloon angioplasty for critical limb ischemia: Angiographic and clinical results. J Vasc Interv Radiol 11:1021-1031, 2000.
39. Dorros G, Jaff MR, Dorros AM, et al: Tibioperoneal (outflow lesion) angioplasty can be used as primary treatment in 235 patients with critical limb ischemia: Five-year follow-up. Circulation 104:2057-2062, 2001.
40. Tsetis DK, Michalis LK, Rees MR, et al: Vibrational angioplasty in the treatment of chronic infrapopliteal arterial occlusions: Preliminary experience. J Endovasc Ther 9:889-895, 2002.
41. Hanna GP, Fujise K, Kjellgren O, et al: Infrapopliteal transcatheter interventions for limb salvage in diabetic patients: Importance of aggressive interventional approach and role of transcutaneous oximetry. J Am Coll Cardiol 30:664-669, 1997.
42. Faglia E, Mantero M, Caminiti M, et al: Extensive use of peripheral angioplasty, particularly infrapopliteal, in the treatment of ischaemic diabetic foot ulcers: Clinical results of a multicentric study of 221 consecutive diabetic subjects. J Intern Med 252:225-232, 2002.
43. Bakal CW, Cynamon J, Sprayregen S: Infrapopliteal percutaneous transluminal angioplasty: What we know. Radiology 200:36-43, 1996.

Renal Artery Obstructive Disease

44. Lenz T, Kia T, Rupprecht G, et al: Captopril test: Time over? J Hum Hypertens 13:431-435, 1999.
45. Olin JW, Novick AC: Renovascular disease. *In* Young JR, et al (eds): Peripheral Vascular Diseases. St. Louis, CV Mosby, 1996, pp 321-342.
46. Leung DA, Hoffman U, Pfammatter T, et al: Magnetic resonance angiography versus duplex sonography for diagnosis renovascular disease. Hypertension 33:726-731, 1999.
47. Johnson PT, Halpern EJ, Kuszyk BS, et al: Renal artery stenosis: CT angiography—comparison of real-time volume-rendering and maximal intensity projection algorithms. Radiology 211:337-343, 1999.
48. van Jaarsveld BC, Pieterman H, vanDijk LC, et al: Inter-observer variability in the angiographic assessment of renal artery stenosis. J Hypertens 17:1731-1736, 1999.
49. Schreij G, deHaan MW, Oei TK, et al: Interpretation of renal angiography by radiologists. J Hypertens 17:1737-1741, 1999.
50. Conlon PJ, Little MA, Pieper K, Mark DB: Severity of renal vascular disease predicts mortality in patients undergoing coronary angiography. Kidney Int 60:1490-1497, 2001.
51. Caps MT, Erissinotto C, Zierler RE, et al: Prospective study of atherosclerotic disease progression in the renal artery. Circulation 98:2866-2872, 1998.
52. Weibull H, Bergquist P, Bergentz SE, et al: Percutaneous transluminal renal angioplasty versus surgical reconstruction of atherosclerotic renal artery stenosis: A prospective randomized study. J Vasc Surg 18:841-852, 1993.
53. Eisenhauer AC: Atherosclerotic renovascular disease: Diagnosis and treatment. Curr Opin Nephrol Hypertens 9:659-668, 2000.
54. Safian RD, Textor SC: Renal artery stenosis. N Engl J Med 344:431-442, 2001.
55. van Jaarsveld BC, Krijnen P, Pieterman H, et al: The effect of balloon angioplasty on hypertension in atherosclerotic renal artery stenosis. N Engl J Med 342:1007-1014, 2000.
56. Harden PN, Macleod MJ, Rodger RSC, et al: Effect of renal artery stenting on progression of renovascular renal failure. Lancet 349:1133-1136, 1997.
57. Watson PS, Hadjipetrou P, Cox SV, et al: Effect of renal artery stenting on renal function and size in patients with atherosclerotic renovascular disease. Circulation 102:1671-1677, 2000.
58. Rundback JH, Murphy TP, Cooper C, Weintraub JL: Chronic renal ischemia: Pathophysiologic mechanisms of cardiovascular and renal disease. J Vasc Interv Radiol 13:1085-1092, 2002.
59. Rundback, JH, Sacks D, Kent KC, et al: Guidelines for the reporting of renal artery revascularization in clinical trials. J Vasc Interv Radiol 13:959-974, 2002.

Mesenteric Ischemia

60. Matsumoto AH, Tegtmeyer CJ, Fitzcharles EK, et al: Percutaneous transluminal angioplasty of visceral arterial stenoses: Results and long-term clinical follow-up. J Vasc Interv Radiol 6:165-174, 1995.
61. Chow LC, Chan FP, Li KC: A comprehensive approach to MR imaging of mesenteric ischemia. Abdom Imaging 27:507-516, 2002.
62. Mateo RB, O'Hara PJ, Hertzer NR, et al: Elective surgical treatment of symptomatic chronic mesenteric occlusive disease: Early results and late outcomes. J Vasc Surg 29:821-831, 1999; discussion 832.
63. Kihara TK, Blebea J, Anderson KM, et al: Risk factors and outcomes following revascularization for chronic mesenteric ischemia. Ann Vasc Surg 13:37-44, 1999.

64. Park WM, Cherry KJ Jr., Chua HK, et al: Current results of open revascularization for chronic mesenteric ischemia: A standard for comparison. J Vasc Surg 35:853-859, 2002.
65. Leke MA, Hood DB, Rowe VL, et al: Technical consideration in the management of chronic mesenteric ischemia. Am Surg 68:1088-1092, 2002.
66. Park WM, Gloviczki P, Cherry KJ Jr., et al: Contemporary management of acute mesenteric ischemia: Factors associated with survival. J Vasc Surg 35:445-452, 2002.
67. Maspes F, Mazzetti di Pietralata G, Gandini R, et al: Percutaneous transluminal angioplasty in the treatment of chronic mesenteric ischemia: Results and 3 years of follow-up in 23 patients. Abdom Imaging 23:358-363, 1998.
68. Cognet F, Bensalem D, Dranssart M, et al: Chronic mesenteric ischemia: Imaging and percutaneous treatment. Radiographics 22:863-879, 2002; discussion 879-880.
69. Matsumoto AH, Angle JF, Spinosa DJ, et al: Percutaneous transluminal angioplasty and stenting in the treatment of chronic mesenteric ischemia: Results and long-term followup. J Am Coll Surg 194(1 Suppl): S22-S31, 2002.

Brachiocephalic and Subclavian Obstructive Disease

70. Eisenhauer AC: Subclavian and innominate revascularization: Surgical therapy versus catheter-based intervention. Curr Interv Cardiol Rep 2:101-110, 2000.
71. Al-Mubarak N, Liu MW, Dean LS, et al: Immediate and late outcomes of subclavian artery stenting. Cathet Cardiovasc Intervent 46:169-172, 1999.
72. Henry M, Amor M, Henry I, et al: Percutaneous transluminal angioplasty of the subclavian arteries. J Endovasc Surg 6:33-41, 1999.
73. Hadjipetrou P, Cox S, Piemonte T, Eisenhauer A: Percutaneous revascularization of atherosclerotic obstruction of aortic arch vessels. J Am Coll Cardiol 33:1238-1245, 1999.
74. White CJ: The times they are a-changin'. J Am Coll Cardiol 33:1246-1247, 1999.
75. Hollier LH: Combining endovascular and surgical techniques: The best of both worlds. J Endovasc Surg 5:333-334, 1998.
76. Phipp LH, Scott DJ, Kessel D, Robertson I: Subclavian stents and stent-grafts: Cause for concern? J Endovasc Surg 6: 223-226, 1999.
77. Motarjeme A: Percutaneous transluminal angioplasty of supra-aortic vessels. J Endovasc Surg 3:171-181, 1996.
78. Schillinger M, Haumer M, Schillinger S, et al: Risk stratification for subclavian artery angioplasty: Is there an increased rate of restenosis after stent implantation? J Endovasc Ther 8:550-557, 2001.

Carotid and Distal Embolic Protection

79. The Dutch TIA Trial Study Group: A comparison of two doses of aspirin (30 mg vs. 283 mg a day) in patients after a transient ischemic attack or minor stroke. N Engl J Med 325:1261-1266, 1991.
80. Randomised trial of endarterectomy for recently symptomatic carotid stenosis: Final results of the MRC European Carotid Surgery Trial (ECST). Lancet 351:1379-1387, 1998.
81. NASCET Collaborators: Beneficial effect of carotid endarterectomy in symptomatic patients with high-grade carotid stenosis. N Engl J Med 325:445-453, 1991.
82. Endarterectomy for asymptomatic carotid artery stenosis. Executive Committee for the Asymptomatic Carotid Atherosclerosis Study. JAMA 273:1421-1428, 1995.
83. Barnett HJ, Taylor DW, Eliasziw M, et al: Benefit of carotid endarterectomy in patients with symptomatic moderate or severe stenosis. North American Symptomatic Carotid Endarterectomy Trial Collaborators. N Engl J Med 339:1415-1425, 1998.
84. Ferguson GG, Eliasziw M, Barr HW, et al: The North American Symptomatic Carotid Endarterectomy Trial : Surgical results in 1415 patients. Stroke 30:1751-1758, 1999.
85. Wennberg DE, Lucas FL, Birkmeyer JD, et al: Variation in carotid endarterectomy mortality in the Medicare Population: Trial hospitals, volume and patient characteristics. JAMA 279:1278-1281, 1998.
86. Roubin GS, Iyer SS, Vitek J: Carotid artery stenting: rationale, indications, technique. *In* Heuser R (ed): Peripheral Vascular Stenting for Cardiologists. New York, Martin Dunitz, 1999, pp 67-117.
87. Roubin GS, New G, Iyer SS, et al: Immediate and late clinical outcomes of carotid artery stenting in patients with symptomatic and asymptomatic carotid artery stenosis: A 5-year prospective analysis. Circulation 103:532-537, 2001.
88. Wholey MH, Wholey M, Bergeron P, et al: Current global status of carotid artery stent placement. Cathet Cardiovasc Diagn 44:1-6, 1998.
89. Wholey MH, Wholey MH, Eles G: Clinical experience in cervical carotid artery stent placement: Carotid and neurovascular intervention. 1:2-9, 1998.
90. Wholey MH, Wholey M, Mathias K, et al: Global experience in cervical carotid artery stent placement. Cathet Cardiovasc Interv 50:160-167, 2000.
91. Veith FJ, Amor M, Ohki T, et al: Current status of carotid bifurcation angioplasty and stenting based on a consensus of opinion leaders. J Vasc Surg 33:S111, 2001.
92. Spence D, Eliasziw M: Endarterectomy or angioplasty for treatment of carotid stenosis? Lancet 357:1722-1723, 2001.
93. Brooks WH, McClure RR, Jones MR, et al: Carotid angioplasty and stenting versus carotid endarterectomy: Randomized trial in a community hospital. J Am Coll Cardiol 38:1589-1595, 2001.
94. Qureshi AI, Luft AR, Janardhan V, et al: Identification of patients at risk for periprocedural neurological deficits associated with carotid angioplasty and stenting. Stroke 31:376-382, 2000.
95. Mathur A, Roubin GS, Iyer SS, et al: Predictors of stroke complicating carotid artery stenting. Circulation 97: 1239-1245, 1998.
96. Manninen HI, Rasanen H, Vanninen RL, et al: Human carotid arteries: Correlation of intravascular US with angiographic and histopathologic findings. Radiology 206:65-74, 1998.
97. Manninen HI, Rasanen HT, Vanninen RL, et al: Stent placement versus percutaneous transluminal angioplasty of human carotid arteries in cadavers in situ: Distal embolization and findings at intravascular US, MR imaging, and histopathologic analysis. Radiology 212:483-492, 1999.
98. Coggia M, Goeau-Brissonniere O, Duval JL, et al: Embolic risk of the different stages of carotid bifurcation balloon angioplasty: An experimental study. J Vasc Surg 31:550-557, 2000.
99. Ohki T, Marin ML, Lyon RT, et al: Ex vivo human carotid artery bifurcation stenting: Correlation of lesion characteristics with embolic potential. J Vasc Surg 27:463-471, 1998.
100. Rapp JH, Pan XM, Sharp FR, et al: Atheroemboli to the brain: size threshold for causing acute neuronal cell death. J Vasc Surg 32:68-76, 2000.
101. Markus H: Monitoring embolism in real time. Circulation 102:826-828, 2000.
102. Ohki T, Veith FJ: Carotid stenting with and without protection devices: Should protection be used in all patients? Semin Vasc Surg 13:144-152, 2000.
103. Macdonald S, Gaines PA: Current concepts of mechanical cerebral protection during precutaneous carotid intervention. Vasc Med 8:25-32, 2003.
104. Henry M, Amor M, Henry I, et al: Carotid stenting with cerebral protection: First clinical experience using the PercuSurge GuardWire system. J Endovasc Surg 6:321-331, 1999.
105. Kownator S, et al: Relationship between the structure of the plaque and the importance of embolization during carotid angioplasty. J Am Coll Cardiol 35(Suppl A):67, 2000.
106. Henry M, Henry I, Klonaris C, et al: Benefits of cerebral protection during carotid stenting with the PercuSurge GuardWire system: Midterm results. J Endovasc Ther 9:1-13, 2002.
107. Dietz A, Berkefeld J, Theron JG, et al: Endovascular treatment of symptomatic carotid stenosis using stent placement: Long-term follow-up of patients with a balanced surgical risk/benefit ratio. Stroke 32:1855-1859, 2001.
108. Schluter M, Tubler T, Mathey DG, Schofer J: Feasibility and efficacy of balloon-based neuroprotection during carotid artery stenting in a single-center setting. J Am Coll Cardiol 40:890-895, 2002.
109. Al-Mubarak N, Colombo A, Gaines PA, et al: Multicenter evaluation of carotid artery stenting with a filter protection system. J Am Coll Cardiol 39:841-846, 2002.
110. Reimers B, Corvaja N, Moshiri S, et al: Cerebral protection with filter devices during carotid artery stenting. Circulation 104:12-15, 2001.
111. Wholey MH, Al-Mubarak N, Wholey M: Fifth-year update of carotid artery stenting global registry: What have we learned? J Am Coll Cardiol 30H, 2002.
112. Shawl F, Kadro W, Domanski MJ, et al: Safety and efficacy of elective carotid artery stenting in high-risk patients. J Am Coll Cardiol 35:1721-1728, 2000.

Peripheral Venous Disease and Superior Vena Cava Syndrome

113. Kasirajan K, Gray B, Ouriel K: Percutaneous AngioJet thrombectomy in the management of extensive deep venous thrombosis. J Vasc Interv Radiol 12:179-185, 2001.
114. Nicholson AA, Ettles DF, Arnold A, et al: Treatment of malignant superior vena cava obstruction: Metal stents or radiation therapy. J Vasc Interv Radiol 8:781-788, 1997.
115. Crowe MT, Davies CH, Gaines PA: Percutaneous management of superior vena cava occlusions. Cardiovasc Intervent Radiol 18:367-372, 1995.
116. Gross CM, Kramer J, Waigand J, et al: Stent implantation in patients with superior vena cava syndrome. AJR Am J Roentgenol 169:429-432, 1997.
117. Kee ST, Kinoshita L, Razavi MK, et al: Superior vena cava syndrome: Treatment with catheter-directed thrombolysis and endovascular stent placement. Radiology 206:187-193, 1998.

PART VII

Diseases of the Heart, Pericardium, and Pulmonary Vasculature Bed

CHAPTER 56

Congenital Heart Disease

Gary D. Webb • Jeffrey F. Smallhorn • Judith Therrien • Andrew N. Redington

This chapter has been written for the practicing cardiologist and is compatible with the existing expert management recommendations[1-3] for the care of adult patients with congenital cardiac defects. These guidelines are available on the Internet at www.cachnet.org, at www.achd-library.com, and at www.isaccd.org. For the occasions when more detailed information is needed, the reader is referred to other sources.[4-9]

Congenital cardiovascular disease is defined as an abnormality in cardiocirculatory structure or function that is present at birth, even if it is discovered much later. Congenital cardiovascular malformations usually result from altered embryonic development of a normal structure or failure of such a structure to progress beyond an early stage of embryonic or fetal development. The aberrant patterns of flow created by an anatomical defect may, in turn, significantly influence the structural and functional development of the remainder of the circulation. For instance, the presence in utero of mitral atresia may prohibit normal development of the left ventricle, aortic valve, and ascending aorta. Similarly, constriction of the fetal ductus arteriosus may result in right ventricular dilation and tricuspid regurgitation in the fetus and newborn, or it may contribute importantly to the development of pulmonary arterial aneurysms in the presence of a ventricular septal defect (VSD) and absent pulmonary valve, or it may result in an alteration in the number and caliber of fetal and newborn pulmonary vascular resistance vessels.

Postnatal events can markedly influence the clinical presentation of a specific "isolated" malformation. Infants with Ebstein malformation of the tricuspid valve may improve dramatically as the magnitude of tricuspid regurgitation diminishes with the normal fall in pulmonary vascular resistance after birth; and infants with pulmonary atresia or severe stenosis may not become cyanotic until normal spontaneous closure of a patent ductus arteriosus (PDA) occurs. Ductal constriction many days after birth also may be a central factor in some infants in the development of coarctation of the aorta. Still later in life, patients with a VSD may experience spontaneous closure of the abnormal communication or may develop right ventricular outflow tract obstruction and/or aortic regurgitation or pulmonary vascular obstructive disease. These selected examples serve to emphasize that anatomical and physiological changes in the heart and circulation can continue indefinitely from prenatal life in association with any specific congenital cardiocirculatory lesion.

INCIDENCE. The true incidence of congenital cardiovascular malformations is difficult to determine accurately, partly because of difficulties in definition. About 0.8 percent of live births are complicated by a cardiovascular malformation. This figure does not take into account what may be the two most common cardiac anomalies: the congenital, functionally normal bicuspid aortic valve and prolapse of the mitral valve.

Specific defects can show a definite gender preponderance: PDA, Ebstein anomaly of the tricuspid valve, and atrial septal defect (ASD) are more common in females, whereas aortic valve stenosis, coarctation of the aorta, hypoplastic left heart, pulmonary and tricuspid atresia, and transposition of the great arteries (TGA) are more common in males.

Extracardiac anomalies occur in about 25 percent of infants with significant cardiac disease, and their presence may significantly increase mortality. The extracardiac anomalies are often multiple. One-third of infants with both cardiac and extracardiac anomalies have some established syndrome.

ADULT PATIENT. Thanks to the great successes of pediatric cardiac care, the overall number of adult patients with congenital heart disease (CHD) is now greater than the number of pediatric cases. In 2000, there were about 485,000 American adults with moderately complex to very complex CHD. There were another 300,000 patients with simple forms of CHD, for a total population of 785,000 adult CHD patients in the United States. The 485,000 moderately to very complex patients are at significant risk of premature mortality, reoperation, or future complications of their conditions and their treatments. Many patients, especially those with moderately to very complex conditions, should see a specialist. At present, there are not enough such practitioners or facilities to always make this possible. Adult patients should have been taught in adolescence about their condition, their future outlook, and the possibility of further surgery and complications if appropriate, and they also should have been advised about their responsibilities in ensuring self-care and professional surveillance. Copies of operative reports should accompany patients being transferred for adult care and other key documents from the pediatric file.

Table 56–1 shows a listing of the types of patients who should be considered "simple" and suitable for community care. Tables 56–2 and 56–3 show the diagnoses for "moderately complex" and "very complex" patients. The moderately and very complex patients should be monitored throughout their life.

CHD in the adult is not simply a continuation of the childhood experience. The patterns of many lesions change in adult life. Arrhythmias are more frequent and of a different character. Cardiac chambers often enlarge, and ventricles tend to develop systolic dysfunction. Bioprosthetic valves, prone to early failure in childhood, last longer when implanted at an older age. The comorbidities that tend to develop in adult life often become important factors needing attention. As a result, the needs of these adult CHD patients are often best met by a physician or a team familiar with both pediatric and adult cardiology issues. Congenital heart surgery and interventional catheterization procedures should be performed at centers with adequate surgical and institu-

TABLE 56–1 Types of Adult Patients with Simple Congenital Heart Disease*

Native disease Isolated congenital aortic valve disease Isolated congenital mitral valve disease (except parachute valve, cleft leaflet) Isolated patent foramen ovale or small atrial septal defect Isolated small ventricular septal defect (no associated lesions) Mild pulmonic stenosis
Repaired conditions Previously ligated or occluded ductus arteriosus Repaired secundum or sinus venosus atrial septal defect without residua Repaired ventricular septal defect without residua

From Webb G, Williams R, Alpert J, et al: 32nd Bethesda Conference: Care of the Adult with Congenital Heart Disease, October 2-3, 2000. J Am Coll Cardiol 37:1161-1198, 2001.

*These patients can usually be cared for in the general medical community.

TABLE 56–2 Types of Adult Patients with Congenital Heart Disease of Moderate Severity*

Aorto–left ventricular fistulas
Anomalous pulmonary venous drainage, partial or total
Atrioventricular septal defects (partial or complete)
Coarctation of the aorta
Ebstein anomaly
Infundibular right ventricular outflow obstruction of significance
Ostium primum atrial septal defect
Patent ductus arteriosus (not closed)
Pulmonary valve regurgitation (moderate to severe)
Pulmonic valve stenosis (moderate to severe)
Sinus of Valsalva fistula/aneurysm
Sinus venosus atrial septal defect
Subvalvular or supravalvular aortic stenosis (except HOCM)
Tetralogy of Fallot
Ventricular septal defect with Absent valve or valves Aortic regurgitation Coarctation of the aorta Mitral disease Right ventricular outflow tract obstruction Straddling tricuspid/mitral valve Subaortic stenosis

HOCM = hypertrophic obstructive cardiomyopathy.

From Webb G, Williams R, Alpert J, et al: 32nd Bethesda Conference: Care of the Adult with Congenital Heart Disease, October 2-3, 2000. J Am Coll Cardiol 37:1161-1198, 2001.

*These patients should be seen periodically at regional adult congenital heart disease centers.

TABLE 56–3 Types of Adult Patients with Congenital Heart Disease of Great Complexity*

Conduits, valved or nonvalved
Cyanotic congenital heart (all forms)
Double-outlet ventricle
Eisenmenger syndrome
Fontan procedure
Mitral atresia
Single ventricle (also called *double inlet* or *outlet*, *common* or *primitive*)
Pulmonary atresia (all forms)
Pulmonary vascular obstructive diseases
Transposition of the great arteries
Tricuspid atresia
Truncus arteriosus/hemitruncus
Other abnormalities of atrioventricular or ventriculoarterial connection not included above (i.e., crisscross heart, isomerism, heterotaxy syndromes, ventricular inversion)

From Webb G, Williams R, Alpert J, et al: 32nd Bethesda Conference: Care of the Adult with Congenital Heart Disease, October 2-3, 2000. J Am Coll Cardiol 37:1161-1198, 2001.

*These patients should be seen regularly at adult congenital heart disease centers.

tional volumes of congenital heart cases at any age. Echocardiographic studies, diagnostic heart catheterizations, electrophysiological studies, and magnetic resonance imaging (MRI) and other imaging of complex cases are best done where qualified staff have relevant training, experience, and equipment. Patient care ideally should be multidisciplinary. Special cardiology and echocardiography skills are essential, but individuals with other special training, experience, and interest should also be accessible. These include congenital heart surgeons and their teams, nurses, reproductive health staff, mental health professionals, medical imaging technicians, respiratory consultants, and others.

Etiology

Congenital cardiac malformations can occur with mendelian inheritance directly as a result of a genetic abnormality, be strongly associated with an underlying genetic disorder (e.g., trisomy), be related directly to the effect of an environmental toxin (e.g., alcohol), or result from an interaction between multifactorial genetic and environmental systems too complex to allow a single specification of cause (e.g., CHARGE syndrome [see Syndromes in Congenital Heart Disease]). The latter group is shrinking as new genetic research identifies new genetic abnormalities underlying many conditions.

GENETIC. A single gene mutation can be causative in the familial forms of ASD with prolonged atrioventricular (AV) conduction, mitral valve prolapse, VSD, congenital heart block, situs inversus, pulmonary hypertension, and the syndromes of Noonan, LEOPARD, Ellis-van Creveld, and Kartagener (see Syndromes in Congenital Heart Disease). The genes responsible for several defects have either been mapped (e.g., long-QT syndrome, Holt-Oram syndrome) or identified (e.g., Marfan syndrome, hypertrophic cardiomyopathy, supravalvular aortic stenosis). Contiguous gene defects on the long arm of chromosome 22 likely underlie the conotruncal malformations of DiGeorge and velocardiofacial syndromes. At present, fewer than 15 percent of all cardiac malformations can be accounted for by chromosomal aberrations or genetic mutations or transmission (see Chap. 69).

The finding that, with some exceptions, only one of a pair of monozygotic twins is affected by CHD indicates that most cardiovascular malformations are not inherited in a simple manner. However, this observation may have led, in the past, to an underestimation of genetic contribution, because most recent twin studies reveal more than double the incidence of heart defects in monozygotic twins but usually in only one of the pair. Family studies indicate a 2-fold to 10-fold increase in the incidence of CHD in siblings of affected patients or in the offspring of an affected parent. Malformations often are concordant or partially concordant within families. Routine fetal cardiac screening seems a worthwhile investigation in such circumstances.

ENVIRONMENTAL. Maternal rubella, ingestion of thalidomide and isotretinoin early during gestation, and chronic maternal alcohol abuse are environmental insults known to interfere with normal cardiogenesis in humans. Rubella syndrome consists of cataracts, deafness, microcephaly, and, either singly or in combination, PDA, pulmonary valve and/or arterial stenosis, and ASD. Thalidomide exposure is associated with major limb deformities and, occasionally, with cardiac malformations without a predilection for a specific lesion. Tricuspid valve anomalies are associated with ingestion of lithium during pregnancy. The fetal alcohol syndrome consists of microcephaly, micrognathia, microphthalmia, prenatal growth retardation, developmental delay, and cardiac defects (often defects of the ventricular septum) occur in about 45 percent of affected infants.

Prevention

Physicians who deal with pregnant women should be aware of known teratogens as well as drugs that may have a functional rather than a structural damaging influence on the fetal and newborn heart and circulation, and they should recognize that for many drugs, information about their teratogenic potential is inadequate. Similarly, appropriate radiological equipment and techniques for reducing gonadal and fetal radiation exposure should always be used to reduce the potential hazards of this likely cause of birth defects.

Detection of genetic abnormalities is becoming an increasing reality for many problems. Fetal cells are obtained from amniotic fluid or chorionic villus biopsy. Many fetuses in whom CHD is detected will undergo genetic testing, and fetal echo is frequently indicated when a chromosomal abnormality is diagnosed for other reasons. Many social, religious, and legal considerations influence whether termination of pregnancy is performed under these circumstances, but the improved outcomes for even the most complex CHDs frequently mandate against the cardiac condition being used as the sole reason. Immunization of children with rubella vaccine has been one of the most effective preventive strategies against fetal rubella syndrome and its associated congenital cardiac abnormalities.

Anatomy and Embryology

Embryology

NORMAL CARDIAC DEVELOPMENT. During the first month of gestation, the primitive, straight cardiac tube is formed, comprising the sinuatrium (most cephalad), the primitive ventricle, the bulbus cordis, and the truncus arteriosus (most caudad) in series. In the second month of gestation, this tube doubles over on itself to form two parallel pumping systems, each with two chambers and a great artery. The two atria develop from the sinuatrium, the AV canal is divided by the endocardial cushions into tricuspid and mitral orifices, and the right and left ventricles develop from the primitive ventricle and bulbus cordis. Differential growth of myocardial cells causes the straight cardiac tube to bear to the right, and the bulboventricular portion of the tube doubles over on itself, bringing the ventricles side by side. Migration of the AV canal to the right and of the ventricular septum to the left serves to align each ventricle with its appropriate AV valve. At the distal end of the cardiac tube, the bulbus cordis divides into a subaortic muscular conus and a subpulmonary muscular conus; the subpulmonary conus elongates and the subaortic conus resorbs, allowing the aorta to move posteriorly and connect with the left ventricle.

ABNORMAL DEVELOPMENT. A host of anomalies can result from defects in this basic developmental pattern. Double-inlet left ventricle is observed if the tricuspid orifice does not align over the right ventricle. The various types of persistent truncus arteriosus result from failure of the truncus to divide into main pulmonary artery and aorta. Double-outlet anomalies of the right ventricle are produced by failure of either the subpulmonary or subaortic conus to resorb, whereas resorption of the subpulmonary instead of the subaortic conus may lead to TGA.

ATRIA. The primitive sinuatrium is separated into right and left atria by the downgrowth from its roof of the septum primum toward the AV canal, thereby creating an inferior interatrial ostium primum opening. Numerous perforations form in the anterosuperior portion of the septum primum as the septum secundum begins to develop to the right of the former. The coalescence of these perforations forms the ostium secundum. The septum secundum completely separates the atrial chambers except for a central opening—the fossa ovalis—that is covered by tissue of the septum primum, forming the valve of the foramen ovale.

Fusion of the endocardial cushions anteriorly and posteriorly divides the AV canal into tricuspid and mitral inlets. The inferior portion of the atrial septum, the superior portion of the ventricular septum, and portions of the septal leaflets of both the tricuspid and mitral valves are formed from the endocardial cushions. The integrity of the atrial septum depends on growth of the septum primum and septum secundum and proper fusion of the endocardial cushions. ASDs and various degrees of AV defect are the result of developmental deficiencies of this process.

VENTRICLES. Partitioning of the ventricles occurs as cephalic growth of the main ventricular septum results in its fusion with the endocardial cushions and the infundibular or conus septum. Defects in the ventricular septum may occur owing to a deficiency of septal substance; malalignment of septal components in different planes preventing their fusion; or an overly long conus, keeping the septal components apart. Isolated defects probably result from the first mechanism, whereas the latter two appear to generate the VSDs in tetralogy of Fallot and transposition complexes.

PULMONARY VEINS. These structures arise from the primitive foregut and are drained early in embryogenesis by channels from the splanchnic plexus to the cardinal and umbilicovitelline veins. An outpouching from the posterior left atrium forms the common pulmonary vein, which communicates with the splanchnic plexus establishing pulmonary venous drainage to the left atrium. The umbilicovitelline and anterior cardinal vein communications atrophy as the common pulmonary vein is incorporated into the left atrium. Anomalous pulmonary venous connections to the umbilicovitelline (portal) venous system or to the cardinal system (superior vena cava) result from failure of the common pulmonary vein to develop or establish communications to the splanchnic plexus. Cor triatriatum results from a narrowing of the common pulmonary vein to left atrial junction.

GREAT ARTERIES. The truncus arteriosus is connected to the dorsal aorta in the embryo by six pairs of aortic arches. Partition of the truncus arteriosus into two great arteries is a result of the fusion of tissue arising from the back wall of the vessel and the truncus septum. Rotation of the truncus coils the aortopulmonary septum and creates the normal spiral relation between aorta and pulmonary artery. Semilunar valves and their related sinuses are created by absorption and hollowing out of tissue at the distal side of the truncus ridges. Aortopulmonary septal defect and persistent truncus arteriosus represent various degrees of partitioning failure.

Although the six aortic arches appear sequentially, portions of the arch system and dorsal aorta disappear at different times during embryogenesis. The first, second, and fifth sets of paired arches regress completely. The proximal portions of the sixth arches become the right and left pulmonary arteries, and the distal left sixth arch becomes the ductus arteriosus. The third aortic arch forms the connection between internal and external carotid arteries, and the left fourth arch becomes the arterial segment between left carotid and subclavian arteries. The proximal portion of the right subclavian artery forms from the right fourth arch. An abnormality in regression of the arch system in a number of sites can produce a wide variety of arch anomalies, whereas a failure of regression usually results in a double aortic arch malformation.

Normal Cardiac Anatomy

The key to understanding CHD is an appreciation of the segmental approach to the diagnosis of both simple and complex lesions.

CARDIAC SITUS. This refers to the status of the atrial appendages. The normal left atrial appendage is a finger-like structure with a narrow base and no guarding crista. On the other hand, the right atrial appendage is broad based and has a guarding crista and pectinate muscles. *Situs solitus* or *inversus* refers to hearts with both a morphological left and right atrium. *Situs ambiguous* refers to hearts with two morphological left or right atrial appendages. These are dealt with in the section on isomerism and have implications with regard to associated intracardiac and extracardiac abnormalities.

ATRIOVENTRICULAR CONNECTIONS. This refers to the connections between the atria and ventricles. The AV connections are said to be concordant if the morphological left atrium is connected to a morphological left ventricle via the mitral valve, with the morphological right atrium connecting to the morphological right ventricle via a tricuspid valve. They are said to be discordant in other circumstances, such as in congenitally corrected TGA (cc-TGA).

VENTRICULOARTERIAL CONNECTIONS. This refers to the connections between the semilunar valve and the ventricles. Ventriculoarterial concordance occurs when the morphological left ventricle is connected to the aorta, while the morphological right ventricle is connected to the pulmonary artery. Ventriculoarterial discordance is when the morphological left ventricle is connected to the pulmonary artery, with the aorta being connected to the morphological right ventricle. Double-outlet right ventricle is where more than 50 percent of both great arteries are connected to the morphological right ventricle. A single-outlet heart is where there is only one great artery that is connected to the heart.

ATRIA. The assignment of either a morphological left or right atrium is determined by the morphology of the atrial appendages and not by the status of the systemic or pulmonary venous drainage. Although the pulmonary veins usually drain to a morphological left atrium, and the systemic veins drain into a morphological right atrium, this is not always the case.

ATRIOVENTRICULAR VALVES. The morphological mitral valve is a bileaflet valve with the anterior leaflet in fibrous continuity with the noncoronary cusp of the aortic valve. The mitral valve leaflets are supported by two papillary muscle groups located in the anterolateral and posteromedial positions. Each papillary muscle supports the adjacent part of both valve leaflets, with considerable variation in the morphology of the papillary muscles.

The tricuspid valve is a trileaflet valve, although it can frequently be difficult to identify all three leaflets. With close inspection, the commissural chordae that arise from the papillary muscles may permit the identification of the three leaflets. The three leaflets occupy a septal anterior, superior, and inferior position. The commissures between the leaflets are the anterior septal, anterior inferior, and inferior. The papillary muscles supporting the valve leaflets arise mostly from the trabeculoseptomarginalis and its apical ramifications.

MORPHOLOGICAL RIGHT VENTRICLE. The morphological right ventricle is a triangular-shaped structure with an inlet, trabecular, and outlet component. The inlet component of the right ventricle has attachments from the septal leaflet of the tricuspid valve. Inferior to this is the moderator band, which arises at the base of the trabeculoseptomarginalis, with extensive trabeculations toward the apex of the right ventricle. The outlet component of the right ventricle consists of a fusion of three structures, that is, the infundibular septum separating the aortic from the pulmonary valve, the ventriculoinfundibular fold separating the tricuspid valve from the pulmonary valve, and finally the anterior and posterior limbs of the trabeculoseptomarginalis.

MORPHOLOGICAL LEFT VENTRICLE. The morphological left ventricle is an elliptical-shaped structure with a fine trabecular pattern, with absent septal attachments of the mitral valve in the normal heart. It consists of an inlet portion containing the mitral valve and a tension apparatus, with an apical trabecular zone that is characterized by fine trabeculations and an outlet zone that supports the aortic valve.

SEMILUNAR VALVES. The aortic valve is a trileaflet valve with the left and right cusps giving rise to the left and right coronary arteries, respectively, with the noncoronary cusp lacking a coronary artery connection. Of note, the noncoronary cusp is in fibrous continuity with the anterior leaflet of the mitral valve. The aortic valve has a semilunar attachment to the junction of the ventricular outlet and its great arteries. The aortic cusps have a main core of fibrous tissue with endocardial linings on each surface. The cusps are thickened at the midpoint to form a nodule. The characteristics of the pulmonary valve are similar to its aortic counterpart, noting the absence of the coronary ostia arising at the superior portion of the sinuses.

AORTIC ARCH AND PULMONARY ARTERIES. In the normal heart the aortic arch usually points to the left with the first branch, the innominate artery, giving rise to the right carotid and subclavian artery. In general, the left carotid and left subclavian arteries arise separately from the aortic arch. By definition the ascending aorta is proximal to the origin of the innominate artery, with the transverse aortic arch being from the innominate artery to the origin of the left subclavian artery. The aortic isthmus is the area between the left subclavian artery and a PDA or ligamentum arteriosum.

SYSTEMIC VENOUS CONNECTIONS. In the normal heart the left and right innominate veins form the superior vena cava, which connects to the roof of the right atrium. The inferior vena cava connects to the inferior portion of the morphological right atrium, with hepatic veins joining the inferior vena cava prior to its insertion into the atrium. The coronary veins drain into the flow of the coronary sinus, with the latter running in the posterior AV groove and terminating in the right atrium. The inferior vena cava is guarded by the eustachian valve, which may vary in size between different hearts.

PULMONARY VENOUS DRAINAGE IN THE NORMAL HEART. The pulmonary veins drain to the left-sided atrium. There are usually three pulmonary veins arising from the trilobed right lung and two pulmonary veins from the bilobed left lung. The pulmonary veins drain into the left atrium in superior and inferior locations. There is a short segment of extraparenchymal pulmonary vein prior to it disappearing into the adjacent hila of the lungs.

Fetal and Transitional Circulations

(Fig. 56–1)

CHD is being diagnosed with increasing frequency during fetal life. Our ability to modify the evolution of structural (by fetal intervention) and physiological (by drug therapy) heart disease is increasing. Knowledge of the changes in cardiocirculatory structure, function, and metabolism that occur during fetal development is more important today than at any time in the past.

FETAL CIRCULATORY PATHWAYS. Dynamic alterations occur in the circulation during the transition from fetal to neonatal life when the lungs take over the function of gas exchange from the placenta. The fetal circulation consists of parallel pulmonary and systemic pathways in contrast to the "in series" circuit of the normal postnatal circulation. Oxygenated blood returns from the placenta through the

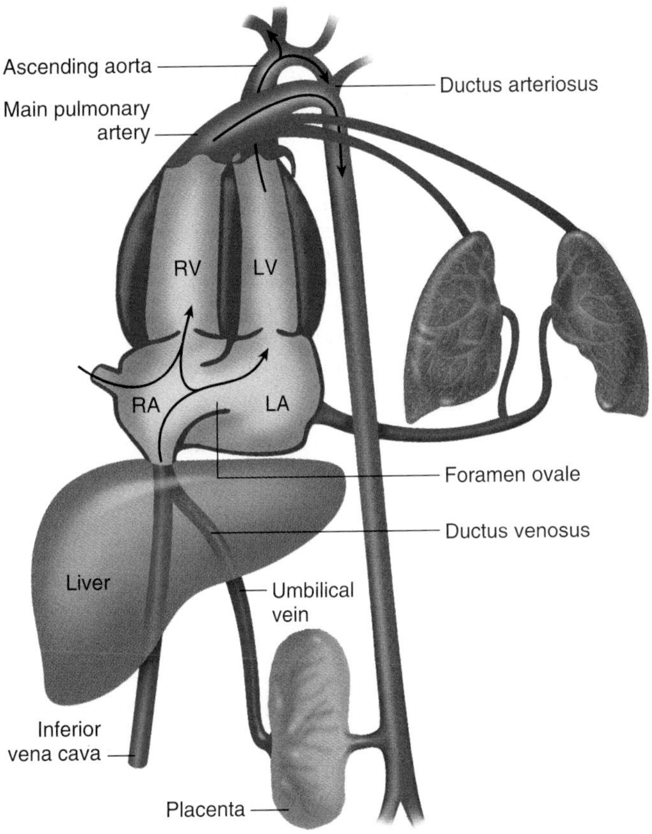

FIGURE 56–1 The fetal circulation, with arrows indicating the directions of flow. A fraction of umbilical venous blood enters the ductus venosus and bypasses the liver. This relatively highly oxygenated blood flows across the foramen ovale to the left side of the heart, preferentially perfusing the coronary arteries, head, and upper trunk. The output of the right ventricle flows preferentially across the ductus arteriosus and circulates to the placenta, as well as to the abdominal viscera and lower trunk. (Courtesy of Dr. David Teitel.)

umbilical vein and enters the portal venous system. A variable amount of this stream bypasses the hepatic microcirculation and enters the inferior vena cava by way of the ductus venosus. Inferior vena caval blood is from the ductus venosus, hepatic veins, and lower body venous drainage and is partly deflected across the foramen ovale into the left atrium. Almost all superior vena caval blood passes directly through the tricuspid valve, entering the right ventricle. Most of the blood that reaches the right ventricle bypasses the high-resistance, unexpanded lungs and passes through the ductus arteriosus into the descending aorta. The right ventricle contributes about 55 percent and the left 45 percent to the total fetal cardiac output. The major portion of blood ejected from the left ventricle supplies the brain and upper body, with lesser flow to the coronary arteries; the balance passes across the aortic isthmus to the descending aorta, where it joins with the large stream from the ductus arteriosus before flowing to the lower body and back to the placenta.

FETAL PULMONARY CIRCULATION. In fetal life, the alveoli are fluid filled, and the pulmonary arteries and arterioles have relatively thick walls and a small lumen, similar to arteries in the systemic circulation. The low pulmonary blood flow in the fetus (7 to 10 percent of the total cardiac output) is the result of high pulmonary vascular resistance. Fetal pulmonary vessels are highly reactive to changes in oxygen tension or in the pH of blood perfusing them as well as to a number of other physiological and pharmacological influences.

EFFECTS OF CARDIAC MALFORMATIONS ON THE FETUS. Although fetal somatic growth may be unimpaired, the hemodynamic effects of many cardiac malformations can alter the development and structure of the fetal heart and circulation. For example, while lesions associated with left-to-right shunts in postnatal life rarely influence fetal cardiac development directly, regurgitant AV valves can lead to chamber dilation, hydrops, and fetal death. Ventricular obstructive lesions (e.g., aortic valve stenosis) may variably lead to hypertrophy, dilation, and failure. The secondary effects of congenital lesions are also important. Reduced flow through the left heart can result in aortic hypoplasia and coarctation. Reduced antegrade pulmonary blood flow is associated with pulmonary artery hypoplasia. These effects rarely affect the fetal circulation overtly, however, and often only become exposed as problems after birth as the ductus arteriosus closes.

FUNCTION OF THE FETAL HEART. Compared with the adult heart, the fetal and newborn heart is unique with respect to its ultrastructural appearance, its mechanical and biochemical properties, and its autonomic innervation. During late fetal and early neonatal development there is maturation of the excitation-contraction coupling process and changes in the biochemical composition of the heart's energy-utilizing myofibrillar proteins and of adenosine triphosphate and creatine phosphate energy-producing proteins. Moreover, fetal and neonatal myocardial cells are small in diameter and reduced in density, so that the young heart contains relatively more noncontractile mass (primarily mitochondria, nuclei, and surface membranes) than later in postnatal life. As a result, force generation and the extent and velocity of shortening are decreased, and stiffness and water content of ventricular myocardium are increased in the fetal and early newborn periods. The fetal heart is surrounded by fluid-filled rather than air-filled lungs. As a result, the fetal and neonatal heart has limited ability to increase cardiac output in the presence of either a volume load or a lesion that increases resistance to emptying. Ultimately cardiac output is much more dependent on changes in heart rate, explaining why bradycardia is so poorly tolerated by the fetal circulation. Tachycardia can also rapidly lead to heart failure in the fetus, whether due to the hemodynamic issues discussed earlier or a manifestation of energy-substrate utilization.

CHANGES AT BIRTH. Inflation of the lungs at the first inspiration produces a marked reduction in pulmonary vascular resistance. The reduced extravascular pressure and increased alveolar oxygen content, as fluid is removed from the lungs and replaced by air, leads to pulmonary vasodilation and recruitment. As a result, pulmonary artery pressure falls, and pulmonary blood flow increases greatly, raising left atrial pressure and closing the flap valve of the foramen ovale. Conversely, systemic vascular resistance rises. This is related to loss of the low-resistance placental circulation and gradual closure of the ductus arteriosus. It is also related to a sudden increase in arterial blood oxygen tension, consequent to the lack of mixing of oxygenated and deoxygenated blood that characterizes the fetal milieu. In healthy, mature infants, the ductus arteriosus is profoundly constricted at 10 to 15 hours and is closed functionally by 72 hours, with total anatomical closure following within a few weeks by a process of thrombosis, intimal proliferation, and fibrosis. Preterm infants have a high incidence of persistent patency of the ductus arteriosus because of an immaturity of those mechanisms responsible for constriction.

The ductus venosus, ductus arteriosus, and foramen ovale remain potential channels for blood flow after birth. Thus, persistent patency of the ductus venosus is capitalized on during balloon atrial septostomy performed via the umbilical vein. Lesions producing right or left atrial volume or pressure overload can stretch the foramen ovale and render incompetent the flap valve mechanism for its closure. Anomalies that depend on patency of the ductus arteriosus for preserving pulmonary or systemic blood flow remain latent until the ductus arteriosus constricts. A common example is the rapid intensification of cyanosis observed in infants with tetralogy of Fallot when the magnitude of pulmonary hypoperfusion is unmasked by spontaneous closure of the ductus arteriosus. Moreover, increasing evidence shows that ductal constriction is a key factor in the postnatal development of coarctation of the aorta and is clearly the most important factor governing the presentation in babies with a duct-dependent systemic circulation. The management of these conditions is discussed in the appropriate sections.

NEONATE AND INFANT. Most management decisions in patients with significant CHD occur during the first few months of life. An increase in the prenatal diagnosis of major congenital heart defects has resulted in earlier admission and intervention in the neonate with CHD. These neonates are, in general, healthier than in the past owing to the administration of prostaglandins at the time of delivery, thus maintaining hemodynamic stability. With improved surgery and interventional catheterization techniques, many of these neonates undergo early intervention. There has been a trend toward complete repair in the neonate and young infant due to an improvement in myocardial preservation and surgical techniques. In most major cardiac centers, the surgical mortality for this age group is in the range of 2 to 4 percent, which is an improvement on the results of the past, where a palliative procedure often preceded a complete repair.

With increasing experience in this age group, the focus has now shifted from mortality to morbidity. Because the expectation is that most of these neonates and young infants will survive into their adult years, their neurodevelopmental outcome has become as important as the results of the cardiac intervention. Ongoing research in this age group will provide increasing data as to the benefit of early intervention in neonates and infants with CHD.

CHILD AND ADOLESCENT. The rapid somatic growth rates of infancy and adolescence are periods of rapid hemodynamic change. Stenotic lesions that may be relatively slowly progressive throughout early childhood need more frequent surveillance during adolescence. Childhood and adolescence is a time to begin educating the patient, not just the parents, about their heart disease, and the responsibilities that go with it. Issues such as the need for compliance with medications, avoidance of smoking and illicit drug use, and pregnancy and contraception counseling are by no means exclusively issues of the adult with CHD, and increasingly require discussion in the pediatric cardiac clinic.

Indeed, the early teenage years should be regarded as part of the transition process prior to transfer to adult follow-up. The whole area of the follow-up of adults with newly discovered or previously treated CHD is a burgeoning new subspecialty that will require careful planning to ensure adequate resources for the increasing number of adult "graduates" of pediatric programs. A coordinated approach with specialists in an affiliated adult congenital clinic is clearly desirable.

ADULT. Patients and often family members should understand their cardiac condition[10] both in terms of what has been done so far and what could happen in the future. This is important for a young patient graduating into the adult world. Patients need information and should become partners in their own care.

Potential long-term complications in adults with CHD (such as arrhythmias, ventricular failure, conduit obstruction and endocarditis) should be explained to patients who are at relatively high risk. The possible need for future therapy—medical (antiarrhythmics, anticoagulation, heart failure therapy), catheter based (valve dilation, stents, arrhythmia ablation), or surgical (redo surgery, transplantation)—should be discussed if the patient may require them in the short or intermediate future. Day-to-day issues of concern for these young adults need to be addressed, such as exercise prescriptions,[11,12] driving restrictions, and traveling limitations. Many young people with CHD need advice regarding career choices, entering the work force, insurability, and life expectancy.

Many will want to start a family, and reproductive issues will need to be addressed. Discussion of appropriate contraception methods for any given patient should be offered. Counseling prior to conception as to the risk to the mother and the fetus for any given pregnancy should be done by specialized physicians. They will take into account the maternal cardiac anatomy, maternal functional status, maternal life expectancy, risk of CHD transmission to the offspring, and risk of premature birth. High-risk patients (e.g., Marfan with aortic root dilation, severe pulmonary hypertension, New York Heart Association [NYHA] Class III or IV, and severe aortic stenosis) must be advised against pregnancy. Intermediate-risk patients (e.g., cyanotic, mechanical valve and other warfarin [Coumadin]-requiring patients, left ventricular outflow tract obstruction, moderate-to-severe left ventricular dysfunction) need to know that pregnancy, although possible, may be complicated and that they will require careful follow-up.[13,14]

Last but not least, comorbidities such as obesity, smoking, high blood pressure, diabetes, and high cholesterol level add new levels of complexity to these adults as they age and must be part of the mandate of the patient's cardiologist.

Pathological Consequences of Congenital Cardiac Lesions

Congestive Heart Failure

Although the basic mechanisms of cardiac failure are similar for all ages, the common causes, time of onset, and often the approach to treatment vary with age (see Chaps. 20 to 25). The development of fetal echocardiography has allowed the diagnosis of intrauterine cardiac failure. The cardinal findings of *fetal heart failure* are scalp edema, ascites, pericardial effusion, and decreased fetal movements. In *preterm infants*, especially of less than 1500 gm birth weight, persistent patency of the ductus arteriosus is the most common cause of cardiac decompensation, and other forms of structural heart disease are rare. In *full-term newborns*, the earliest important causes of heart failure are the hypoplastic left heart and aortic coarctation syndromes, sustained tachyarrhythmia, cerebral or hepatic arteriovenous fistula, and myocarditis. Among the lesions commonly producing heart failure *beyond age 1 to 2 weeks*, when diminished pulmonary vascular resistance allows substantial left-to-right shunting, are VSDs and AV septal defects, TGA, truncus arteriosus, and total anomalous pulmonary venous connection. *Infants younger than 1 year* who have cardiac malformations account for 80 to 90 percent of pediatric patients who develop congestive failure. In *older children*, heart failure often is due to acquired disease or is a complication of open-heart surgical procedures. In the acquired category are rheumatic and endomyocardial diseases, infective endocarditis, hematological and nutritional disorders, and severe cardiac arrhythmias.

The distinction between left and right heart failure is less obvious in infants than in the older children or adults. Conversely, augmented filling or elevated pressure of the right ventricle in infants reduces left ventricular compliance disproportionately when compared with older children or adults and gives rise to signs of both systemic and pulmonary venous congestion.

Care of infants with heart failure must include careful consideration of the underlying structural or functional disturbance. The general aims of treatment are to achieve an increase in cardiac performance, augment peripheral perfusion, and decrease pulmonary and systemic venous congestion. In many conditions, medical management cannot control the effects of the abnormal loads imposed by a host of congenital cardiac lesions. Under these circumstances, cardiac diagnosis and interventional catheter or operative intervention may be urgently required.

Congestive heart failure is not common in adult congenital heart practice, although prevention of myocardial dysfunction is a common concern. The adult patient with CHD develops heart failure in the presence of a substrate (e.g., myocardial dysfunction, valvular regurgitation) and a precipitant (e.g., sustained arrhythmia, pregnancy, hyperthyroidism). Patients prone to congestive failure include those with long-standing volume loads (e.g., valvular regurgitation and left-to-right shunts), those with a primary depression of myocardial function (e.g., systemic right ventricles, ventricles damaged during surgery or because of late treatment of ventricular overload). Treatment depends on a clear understanding of the elements contributing to decompensation and addressing each of the treatable components. The greatest success is achieved when the main elements can be eliminated. When this is not possible, standard palliative adult heart failure regimens are applied and may include angiotensin-converting enzyme (ACE) inhibitors,[15,16] angiotensin receptor blockers, beta blockers,[17] diuretics, resynchronization pacing,[18] transplantation,[19,20] and other novel therapies.

Cyanosis

DEFINITION. *Central cyanosis* refers to arterial oxygen desaturation resulting from the shunting or mixing of systemic venous blood into the arterial circulation. The magnitude of shunting/mixing and the amount of pulmonary blood flow determine the severity of desaturation.

MORPHOLOGY. Cardiac defects that result in central cyanosis can be divided into two categories: (1) those with increased pulmonary blood flow or (2) those with decreased pulmonary blood flow (Table 56–4).[21]

PATHOPHYSIOLOGY. Hypoxemia increases renal production of erythropoietin, which in turn stimulates bone marrow production of circulating red blood cells, enhancing oxygen-carrying capacity. Secondary erythrocytosis should be present in all cyanotic patients since it is a physiological response to tissue hypoxia. The improved tissue oxygenation that results from this adaptation may be sufficient to reach a new equilibrium at a higher hematocrit. However, adaptive failure can occur if the increased whole blood viscosity rises so much that it impairs oxygen delivery.

TABLE 56–4 Cardiac Defects Causing Central Cyanosis

Transposition of the great arteries	Ebstein's anomaly
Tetralogy of Fallot	Eisenmenger physiology
Tricuspid atresia	Critical pulmonary stenosis or atresia
Truncus arteriosus	Functionally single ventricle
Total anomalous pulmonary venous return	

Note 5 Ts and 2 Es.

Hyperviscosity Syndrome. Erythrocytosis, by virtue of increasing whole blood viscosity, may cause hyperviscosity symptoms, including headaches, faintness, dizziness, fatigue, altered mentation, visual disturbances, paresthesias, tinnitus and myalgias. Iron deficiency, a common finding in cyanotic adult patients if repeated phlebotomies or excessive bleeding occurs, may cause hyperviscosity symptoms at hematocrit levels well below 65 percent. The patient usually experiences the same hyperviscosity symptoms each time (e.g., headache, visual disturbances, fatigue), and they must be relieved by phlebotomy to qualify as hyperviscosity symptoms.

Hematological. Hemostatic abnormalities have been documented in cyanotic patients with erythrocytosis and can occur in up to 20 percent of patients. A bleeding tendency can be mild and superficial, leading to easy bruising, skin petechiae, and mucosal bleeding, or it can be moderate or life-threatening with hemoptysis or intracranial, gastrointestinal, or postoperative bleeding. An elevated prothrombin and partial thromboplastin time; decreased levels of factors V, VII, VIII, and IX; qualitative and quantitative platelet disorders; and increased fibrinolysis all have been implicated.[22]

Central Nervous System. Neurological complications including cerebral hemorrhage can occur secondary to hemostatic defects and can be seen in patients taking anticoagulants. Patients with right-to-left shunts may be at risk for paradoxical cerebral emboli, especially if they are iron deficient. A brain abscess should be suspected in a cyanotic patient with a new or different headache or new neurological symptoms. Air filters should be used in peripheral/central venous lines in cyanotic patients to avoid paradoxical emboli through a right-to-left shunt.

Renal. Renal dysfunction can manifest itself as proteinuria, hyperuricemia, or renal failure. Pathological studies at the level of the glomeruli show evidence of vascular abnormalities as well as increased cellularity and fibrosis.[23] Hyperuricemia is common and is thought to be due mainly to the decreased reabsorption of uric acid rather than to overproduction with erythrocytosis. Urate nephropathy, uric acid nephrolithiasis, and gouty arthritis may occur.

Arthritic. Rheumatological complications include gout and especially hypertrophic osteoarthropathy, which is thought to be responsible for the arthralgias and bone pain affecting up to one-third of patients. In patients with right-to-left shunting, megakaryocytes released from the bone marrow can bypass the lung. The entrapment of megakaryocytes in the systemic arterioles and capillaries induces the release of platelet-derived growth factor, promoting local cell proliferation. New osseous formation with periostitis ensues and gives rise to arthralgia and bony pain.

INTERVENTIONAL OPTIONS AND OUTCOMES

Physiological Repair. Physiological repair results in total or near-total anatomical and physiological separation of the pulmonary and systemic circulations in complex cyanotic lesions that leads to relief of cyanosis. Such procedures should be performed whenever feasible.

Palliative Surgical Intervention. Palliative surgical interventions can be performed in patients with cyanotic lesions to increase pulmonary blood flow while allowing cyanosis to persist. Palliative surgical shunts are summarized in Table 56–5. Blalock-Taussig, central, and Glenn (also called *cavopulmonary*) shunts are still in use today. Blalock-Taussig shunts seldom caused pulmonary hypertension and were less prone to causing pulmonary artery distortion. Glenn shunts have the advantage of increasing pulmonary flow without imposing a volume load on the systemic ventricle. Glenn shunts require low pulmonary artery pressures to work, and they are associated with the development over time of pulmonary arteriovenous fistulas, which can worsen cyanosis.

TABLE 56–5 Palliative Systemic-to-Pulmonary Shunts

Arterial
Blalock-Taussig shunt (subclavian artery to PA)
Classic—end-to-side, no or reduced ipsilateral arm pulses
Current—side-to-side tubular grafts, preserved arm pulses
Central shunt (side-to-side tubular graft, aorta to PA)
Potts shunt (descending aorta to LPA)
Waterston shunt (ascending aorta to RPA)
Venous
Glenn shunt (SVC to ipsilateral PA without cardiac or other PA connection)
Bidirectional cavopulmonary (Glenn) shunt (end-to-side SVC to LPA and RPA shunt)

PA = pulmonary artery; LPA = left PA; RPA = right PA; SVC = superior vena cava.

Transplantation (see Chap. 26). Transplantation of heart, one or both lungs with surgical cardiac repair, and heart-lung transplantation have been performed in cyanotic patients with or without palliation who were no longer candidates for other forms of intervention. Pulmonary vascular obstructive disease precludes isolated heart transplantation. An increasing number of CHD patients with previous palliation and ventricular failure are successfully undergoing cardiac transplantation.[24] Timing of transplantation in these patients remains difficult.

OTHER MANAGEMENT

Phlebotomy. The goal of phlebotomy is symptom control. When patients have troubling symptoms of hyperviscosity, are iron replete, and are not dehydrated, removal of 250 to 500 ml of blood over 30 to 45 minutes should be performed with concomitant quantitative volume replacement. The procedure may be repeated every 24 hours until symptomatic improvement occurs or the hemoglobin level has fallen too far.[25] Phlebotomy is not indicated for asymptomatic patients. The only indication for prophylactic phlebotomy is in the preoperative patient when the hematocrit is higher than 65 percent to reduce the chances of perioperative bleeding.

Iron Replacement. If iron deficiency anemia is found or anticipated, iron supplements should be prescribed. Cyanotic patients should be helped to avoid iron deficiency, which can cause functional deterioration and is associated with an increased risk of stroke.

Bleeding Diathesis. Platelet transfusions, fresh frozen plasma, vitamin K, cryoprecipitate, and desmopressin can be used to treat severe bleeding. Given the inherent tendency to bleed, aspirin, heparin, and warfarin should be avoided unless the risks of treatment are outweighed by the risks of nontreatment. Likewise, nonsteroidal antiinflammatory drugs should be avoided to prevent bleeding.

Gouty Arthritis. Symptomatic hyperuricemia and gouty arthritis can be treated as necessary with colchicine, probenecid, antiinflammatory drugs, or allopurinol.

REPRODUCTIVE ISSUES. Pregnancy in cyanotic CHD (excluding Eisenmenger syndrome) results in a 32 percent incidence of maternal cardiovascular complications and a 37 percent incidence of fetal prematurity. Pregnant women with a resting oxygen saturation greater than 85 percent fare better than women with an oxygen saturation less than 85 percent.[13]

FOLLOW-UP ISSUES. All cyanotic patients should be followed by a CHD cardiologist, and particular attention should be paid to the underlying heart condition; symptoms of hyperviscosity; systemic complications of cyanosis; change in exercise tolerance; change in saturation levels; and prophylaxis against endocarditis, influenza, and pneumococcal infections. In stable cyanotic patients, yearly follow-up is recommended and should include annual flu shots, periodic pneumococcal vaccination, yearly blood work (complete blood count, ferritin, clotting profile, renal function, uric acid), and regular echo Doppler studies.

Pulmonary Hypertension

Pulmonary hypertension is a common accompaniment of many congenital cardiac lesions, and the status of the pulmonary vascular bed is often the principal determinant of the clinical manifestations, the course, and whether corrective treatment is feasible (see Chap. 67). Increases in pulmonary arterial pressure result from elevations of pulmonary blood flow and/or resistance, the latter sometimes caused by an increase in vascular tone but usually the result of underdevelopment and/or obstructive/obliterative structural changes within the pulmonary vascular bed. Although pulmonary hypertension usually affects the entire pulmonary vascular bed, it may occur focally. For example, unilateral pulmonary hypertension may occur in an overshunted lung (the other lung perhaps protected and fed by a cavopulmonary Glenn shunt), or in lung segments supplied by aortopulmonary collateral flow.

Pulmonary vascular resistance normally falls rapidly immediately after birth, owing to the onset of ventilation and subsequent release of hypoxic pulmonary vasoconstriction. Subsequently, the medial smooth muscle of pulmonary arterial resistance vessels thins gradually. This latter process often is delayed by several months in infants with large aortopulmonary or ventricular communications, at which time levels of pulmonary vascular resistance are still somewhat elevated. In patients with high pulmonary arterial pressures from birth, failure of normal growth of the pulmonary circulation may occur, and anatomical changes in the pulmonary vessels in the form of proliferation of intimal cells and intimal and medial thickening often progress, so that in an older child or adult vascular resistance ultimately may become relatively fixed by obliterative changes in the pulmonary vascular bed. The causes of pulmonary vascular obstructive disease remain unknown, although increased pulmonary arterial blood pressure, elevated pulmonary venous pressure, erythrocytosis, systemic hypoxia, acidemia, and the nature of the bronchial circulation all have been implicated. Quite likely, injury to pulmonary vascular endothelial cells initiates a cascade of events that involve the release or activation of factors that alter the extracellular matrix, induce hypertrophy, cause proliferation of vascular smooth muscle cells, and promote connective tissue protein synthesis. Considered together, these may permanently alter vessel structure and function.

MECHANISMS OF DEVELOPMENT. Intimal damage appears to be related to shear stresses because endothelial cell damage occurs at high shear rates. A reduction in pulmonary arteriolar lumen size due to either thickened medial muscle or vasoconstriction increases the velocity of flow. Shear stress also increases as blood viscosity rises; therefore, infants with hypoxemia and high hematocrit levels as well as increased pulmonary blood flow are at increased risk of developing pulmonary vascular disease. In patients with left-to-right shunts, pulmonary arterial hypertension, if not present in infancy or childhood, may never occur or may not develop until the third or fourth decade or later. Once developed, intimal proliferative changes with hyalinization and fibrosis are not reversible by repair of the underlying cardiac defect. In severe pulmonary vascular obstructive disease, arteriovenous malformations may develop and predispose to massive hemoptysis.

Most vexing is the variability among patients with the same or similar cardiac lesions in both the time of appearance and the rate of progression of their pulmonary vascular obstructive process. Although genetic influences may be operative (an example is the apparent acceleration of pulmonary vascular disease in patients with CHD and trisomy 21), evidence is now accumulating for important prenatal and postnatal modifiers of the pulmonary vascular bed that appear, at least in part, to be lesion dependent. Thus, a quantitative variability exists in the pulmonary vascular bed related to the number, not just the size and wall structure, of arterial vessels within the pulmonary circulation.

Modeling of the blood vessels occurs proximal to and within terminal bronchioles (preacinar and intraacinar vessels, respectively) continuously from before birth. The intraacinar vessels, in particular, increase in size and number from late fetal life throughout childhood, with minimal muscularization of their walls. The ensuing increase in the cross-sectional area of the pulmonary arterial circulation allows the cardiac output to rise substantially without an increase in pulmonary arterial pressure. If, however, the presence of a cardiac lesion interferes with the normal growth and multiplication of these peripheral arteries, the resulting elevation of pulmonary vascular resistance may first be related to failure of the intraacinar pulmonary circulation to develop fully, and then secondarily to the morphological changes of obliterative vascular disease—medial thickening, intimal proliferation, hyalinization and fibrosis, angiomatoid and plexiform lesions, and ultimately, arterial necrosis.

Eisenmenger Syndrome

DEFINITION. *Eisenmenger syndrome,* a term coined by Paul Wood, is defined as pulmonary vascular obstructive disease that develops as a consequence of a large preexisting left-to-right shunt such that pulmonary artery pressures approach systemic levels and the direction of the flow becomes bidirectional or right-to-left. Congenital heart defects that can result in Eisenmenger syndrome include "simple" defects such as ASD, VSD, and PDA as well as more "complex" defects such as AV septal defect, truncus arteriosus, aortopulmonary window, and univentricular heart. The high pulmonary vascular resistance is usually established in infancy (by age 2 years, except in ASD) and is present sometimes from birth.

NATURAL HISTORY OF THE UNOPERATED PATIENT. Patients with defects that allow free communication between the pulmonary and systemic circuits at the aortic or ventricular levels usually have a fairly healthy childhood and gradually become overtly cyanotic during their second or third decade. Exercise intolerance (dyspnea and fatigue) is proportional to the degree of hypoxemia or cyanosis. In the absence of complications, these patients generally have an excellent to good functional capacity up to their third decade[26,27] and thereafter usually experience a slowly progressive decline in their physical abilities. Most patients survive to adulthood,[27-29] with a reported 77 percent and 42 percent survival rate at 15 and 25 years of age, respectively.[27]

Congestive heart failure in patients with Eisenmenger syndrome usually occurs after 40 years of age.[26] The most common modes of death are sudden death (~30 percent), congestive heart failure (~25 percent), and hemoptysis (~15 percent). Pregnancy, perioperative mortality after noncardiac surgery, and infectious causes (brain abscesses and endocarditis) account for most of the remainder.[26,27,29]

CLINICAL MANIFESTATIONS. Patients can present with the following complications: those related to their cyanotic state; palpitations in nearly half the patients (atrial fibrillation/flutter in 35 percent, ventricular tachycardia in up to 10 percent); hemoptysis in about 20 percent; pulmonary thromboembolism, angina, syncope, and endocarditis in about 10 percent each; and congestive heart failure.[26] Hemoptysis is usually due to bleeding bronchial vessels or pulmonary infarction. Physical examination reveals central cyanosis and clubbing of the nail beds. Patients with Eisenmenger PDA can have pink nail beds on the right (> left) hand and cyanosis and clubbing of both feet, so-called differential cyanosis. This occurs because venous blood shunts through the ductus and enters the aorta distal to the subclavian arteries. The jugular venous pressure in patients with Eisenmenger syndrome can be normal or elevated, especially with prominent v waves when tricuspid regurgitation is present. Signs of pulmonary hypertension—a right ventricular heave, palpable and loud P_2, and a right-sided S_4—are typically present. In many patients, a pulmonary ejection click and a soft and scratchy systolic ejection murmur, attributable to dilation of the pulmonary trunk, and a high-pitched decrescendo diastolic murmur of pulmonary regurgitation (Graham Steell) are audible. Peripheral edema is absent until right-sided heart failure ensues.

LABORATORY INVESTIGATIONS

Electrocardiography (ECG). Peaked P waves consistent with right atrial overload and evidence of right ventricular hypertrophy with right axis deviation are the rule. Atrial arrhythmias can be present.

Chest Radiography. Dilated central pulmonary arteries with rapid tapering of the peripheral pulmonary vasculature are the radiographic hallmarks of Eisenmenger syndrome. Pulmonary artery calcification may be seen and is diagnostic of long-standing pulmonary hypertension. Eisenmenger syndrome due to VSD or PDA usually has a normal or slightly increased cardiothoracic ratio. Eisenmenger syndrome due to an ASD typically has a large cardiothoracic ratio due to right atrial and ventricular dilation, along with an inconspicuous aorta. Calcification of the duct may be seen in Eisenmenger PDA.

Echocardiography. The intracardiac defect should be seen readily along with bidirectional shunting. A pulmonary hypertensive PDA is not easily seen. Evidence of pulmonary hypertension is found. Assessment of pulmonary right ventricular function adds prognostic value.

Cardiac Catheterization. Cardiac catheterization not only provides direct measurement of the pulmonary artery pressure, documenting the existence of severe pulmonary hypertension, but also can allow assessment of reactivity of the pulmonary vasculature. Administration of pulmonary arterial vasodilators (O_2, nitric oxide, prostaglandin I_2 [epoprostenol]) can discriminate between patients in whom surgical repair is contraindicated and those with reversible pulmonary hypertension who may benefit from surgical repair. Radiographic contrast material may cause hypotension and worsening cyanosis and should be used cautiously.

Open-Lung Biopsy. Open-lung biopsy should be considered only when the reversibility of the pulmonary hypertension is uncertain from the hemodynamic data. An expert opinion will determine the severity of the changes, often using the Heath-Edwards classification.

INDICATIONS FOR INTERVENTION. The underlying principle of clinical management in patients with Eisenmenger syndrome is to avoid any factors that may destabilize the delicately balanced physiology. In general, an approach of nonintervention has been traditionally recommended, although research in the treatment of pulmonary hypertension may alter this approach in the future. The main interventions, therefore, are directed toward preventing complications (e.g., flu shots to reduce the morbidity of respiratory infections) or to restore the physiological balance (e.g., iron replacement for iron deficiency, antiarrhythmic management of atrial arrhythmias, diuretics for right-sided heart failure). As a general rule, the first episode of hemoptysis should be considered an indication for investigation. Bed rest is usually recommended; and, although usually self-limiting, each such episode should be regarded as potentially life threatening, and a treatable cause should be sought. When patients are severely incapacitated from severe hypoxemia or congestive heart failure, the main intervention available is lung (plus repair of the cardiac defect) or, with somewhat better results, heart-lung transplantation. This is generally reserved for individuals without contraindications who are thought to have a 1-year survival of less than 50 percent. Such assessment is fraught with difficulty because of the unpredictability of the time course of the disease and the risk of sudden death.

Noncardiac surgery should be performed only when absolutely necessary because of its high associated mortality.[30] Eisenmenger syndrome patients are particularly vulnerable to alterations in hemodynamics induced by anesthesia or surgery, such as a minor decrease in systemic vascular resistance that can increase right-to-left shunting and possibly potentiate cardiovascular collapse. Local anesthesia should be used whenever possible. Avoidance of prolonged fasting and especially dehydration, the use of antibiotic prophylaxis when appropriate, and careful intraoperative monitoring are recommended. The choice of general versus epidural-spinal anesthesia is controversial.[31] An experienced cardiac anesthetist with an understanding of Eisenmenger syndrome physiology should administer anesthesia. Additional risks of surgery include excessive bleeding, postoperative arrhythmias, and deep venous thrombosis with paradoxical emboli. An “air filter” or “bubble trap” should be used for most intravenous lines in cyanotic patients. Early ambulation is recommended. Postoperative care in an intensive care unit setting is optimal.

INTERVENTIONAL OPTIONS AND OUTCOMES

Oxygen. Supplemental nocturnal oxygen has recently been shown to have no impact on exercise capacity or on survival in adult patients with Eisenmenger syndrome.[32] Supplemental oxygen during commercial air travel is often recommended, but the scientific basis for this recommendation is lacking.[33]

Transplantation. Lung transplant may be undertaken in association with repair of existing cardiovascular defect(s). Alternatively, heart-lung transplantation may be required if the intracardiac anatomy is not correctable. The 1-year survival rate for adults undergoing lung transplantation with primary intracardiac repair is 55 percent. The 1-year survival rate after heart-lung transplantation is 70 percent.[34] These procedures offer the best hope to individuals with end-stage CHD who are confronting death and have an intolerable quality of life.

INVESTIGATIONAL OPTIONS[35,36]

Calcium-Channel Blockers. The chronic use of nifedipine in a small group of patients with Eisenmenger syndrome demonstrated a small but significant increase in exercise tolerance and a decrease in pulmonary vascular resistance, especially in children. This therapy is still considered investigational and should be prescribed only in a clinical research setting. Indeed with the advent of newer therapies that may have a more direct role on the pulmonary vasculature, there are fewer proponents for their use.

ACE Inhibitors. Data available[37] on a highly selected group of 10 patients with cyanotic CHD showed no change in oxygen saturation despite a subjective improvement in functional capacity. Proponents of the use of ACE inhibitors in these patients argue that, by decreasing systemic vascular resistance, one improves the cardiac output and thus oxygen delivery.[37] The counterargument is that these agents are potentially dangerous because they lower systemic vascular resistance without changing pulmonary vascular resistance and lead to an increase in right-to-left shunting. The use of this medication remains highly experimental and again should be administered only within the boundaries of a study trial guided by rigorous monitoring.

Prostacyclin. There are two reports of the use of long-term prostacyclin therapy for patients with Eisenmenger syndrome. In 20 patients (9 ASDs, 7 VSDs, 4 TGAs, 3 PDAs, 3 partial anomalous pulmonary venous drainage, and 1 aortopulmonary window), the chronic infusion of prostacyclin led to an improvement in hemodynamics after a 1-year period of therapy.[38] Pulmonary arterial pressure was reduced from 77 ± 20 to 61 ± 5 mm Hg ($p < 0\ .01$), and pulmonary vascular resistance decreased from 25 ± 13 to 12 ± 7 units ($p < 0.01$). Exercise capacity also improved from 408 ± 149 meters to 460 ± 99 meters during a 6-minute walk. Eight of the 12 patients listed for transplantation were removed from the active transplant list because of persistent clinical and hemodynamic improvement. One patient with an ASD initially believed to be inoperable improved enough that her ASD was closed with a device. A subsequent study of McLaughlin and associates evaluated 33 patients with secondary forms of pulmonary hypertension, 7 of whom had CHD. In these patients mean pulmonary arterial pressure decreased by 18 percent over a mean 1-year follow-up.[39]

Endothelin Receptor Antagonists. A large randomized North American trial of a nonselective endothelin receptor antagonist (Bosentan) has been recently completed in patients with pulmonary hypertension. There was a statistically significant increase in exercise tolerance in the entire cohort.[40] Fourteen patients in that study had congenital cardiac disease (11 in the Bosentan group and 3 in the placebo group). In this subgroup there was an increase of 46 meters traveled in a 6-minute walk test compared with 7.7 meters in the placebo group (personal communication, 2003). The results of two small studies of Bosentan in patients with Eisenmenger syndrome are pending. Given the high levels of endothelin in patients with congenital cardiac disease, it would seem logical to evaluate this therapy more rigorously in a larger prospective trial.

Sildenafil (Viagra) is another promising agent. Despite biological plausibility and early reports of benefit of sildenafil in pulmonary hypertension, at present there are little data to warrant its use outside a clinical trial. The results of a large multicenter trial of sildenafil in primary and secondary forms of pulmonary artery hypertension is anticipated.

FOLLOW-UP. Patient education is critical. Avoidance of over-the-counter medications, dehydration, smoking, high-altitude exposure, and excessive physical activity should be stressed. Avoidance of pregnancy is of paramount importance. Annual flu shots and use of endocarditis prophylaxis together with proper skin hygiene (avoidance of nail biting) are recommended. A yearly assessment of complete blood cell count and uric acid, creatinine, and ferritin levels should be done to monitor treatable causes of deterioration.

Cardiac Arrhythmias

In teenagers and young adults, most arrhythmias (see Chap. 32) encountered are in association with previously operated CHD. Arrhythmias can be a major clinical challenge in adolescent and adult congenital heart patients. They are the most frequent reason for emergency department visits and hospital admissions, and they are usually recurrent and may worsen or become less responsive to treatment with time. Treatment may be challenging.

ATRIAL ARRHYTHMIAS. Atrial flutter and, to a lesser degree, atrial fibrillation are most common. Atrial flutter tends to reflect right atrial, and atrial fibrillation left atrial abnormalities. Atrial flutter in such patients is often atypical in appearance and behavior and is better called intraatrial reentrant tachycardia. Recognition of atrial flutter can be difficult, and the observer will need to be vigilant in recognizing 2:1 conduction masquerading as sinus rhythm. Recurrence is likely and should not necessarily be assumed to represent failure of the management strategy. The conditions in which atrial flutter is most likely are Mustard/Senning repairs of TGA,[41-43] repaired or unrepaired ASDs,[44-46] repaired tetralogy of Fallot,[47] Ebstein anomaly of the tricuspid valve,[48-50] and after a Fontan operation.[51-53] Atrial flutter may reflect hemodynamic deterioration in patients who have had Mustard, Senning, tetralogy of Fallot, or Fontan repairs. Its arrival is usually associated with more symptoms and functional limitation.

The pharmaceutical agents most commonly used in therapy are warfarin, beta blockers, amiodarone, sotalol, propafenone, and digoxin. As a rule, patients with good ventricular function can receive sotalol or propafenone, whereas those with depressed ventricular function should receive amiodarone. Other therapies, including pacemakers, ablative procedures,[47,54,55] and innovative surgery,[56-59] are being both applied and refined. Sustained ventricular tachycardia[47,60-62] or ventricular fibrillation occurs less often, usually in the setting of ventricular dilation, dysfunction, and scarring. Although sudden death is common in several conditions,[63,64] the mechanism is poorly understood.

VENTRICULAR TACHYCARDIA. This arrhythmia can be seen as a manifestation of proarrhythmic effects of various agents; in patients with acute myocardial injury or infarction; and in CHD patients with severe ventricular dysfunction. In particular, sustained VT has been seen in patients with repaired tetralogy of Fallot, where it is seen as a manifestation of hemodynamic problems requiring repair; as a reflection of right ventricular dilation and dysfunction[61,62]; and in relation to ventricular scarring.

SUDDEN DEATH. In contrast to adults, children seldom die suddenly and unexpectedly of cardiovascular disease. Nonetheless, sudden death has been reported with arrhythmias, aortic stenosis, hypertrophic obstructive cardiomyopathy, primary pulmonary hypertension, Eisenmenger syndrome, myocarditis, congenital complete heart block, primary endocardial fibroelastosis, and when there are undiagnosed anomalies of the coronary arteries. Sudden death is more frequent in older patients with postoperative heart disease,[63-65] particularly after atrial switch procedures,[65] and repair of tetralogy of Fallot.[63,64]

ATRIOVENTRICULAR BLOCK. First-degree AV block is commonly seen in patients with AV septal defects, the older ASD patient, Ebstein, and complete TGA (D-TGA).[41-43] Complete heart block may develop in patients with cc-TGA[66] and may develop postoperatively in other patients. When pacing is required, epicardial leads are usually placed in cyanotic patients. Many adult patients with CHD are prone to problems of vascular access because of prior surgeries and pacing leads.

INFECTIVE ENDOCARDITIS

Infective endocarditis complicating CHD is uncommon before 2 years of age, except in the immediate postoperative period. The list of those conditions not requiring antibiotic prophylaxis is shorter than for those requiring it and is limited to patients before and after closure of a secundum ASD, after closure of a PDA, after spontaneous closure of a muscular and sometimes a perimembranous VSD, and in those with unoperated or operated anomalous pulmonary venous drainage in whom there is no residual hemodynamic abnormality.

CHEST PAIN

Angina pectoris is an uncommon symptom of cardiac disease in young infants and children, although it probably explains the irritability and crying during or after feeding in babies with coronary ischemia resulting from anomalous origin of the coronary artery from the pulmonary artery. In older children and young adults with severe left or right ventricular outflow tract obstruction and pulmonary hypertension, chest pain commonly follows effort and may be identical to effort angina of coronary artery disease in older adults. A sensation of chest discomfort or cardiac awareness is frequently interpreted as pain by the parents of children with cardiac arrhythmias. Careful questioning serves to identify palpitations rather than pain as the symptom and often elicits an additional history of anxiety, pallor, and sweating. Pain caused by pericarditis is commonly of acute onset and associated with fever, and can be identified by specific physical, radiographic, and echocardiographic findings. Most commonly, late postoperative chest pain is musculoskeletal in origin and may be reproduced on upper extremity movement or by palpation. Finally, children and adults may suffer chest pain of nonspecific form owing to anxiety, with or without hyperventilation.

SYNDROMES IN CONGENITAL HEART DISEASE[67]

ALCAPA SYNDROME. The acronym stands for *a*nomalous *l*eft *co*ronary *a*rtery arising from the *p*ulmonary *a*rtery. It is also called *Bland-White-Garland syndrome*.

ALAGILLE SYNDROME. This is a hereditary syndrome consisting of intrahepatic cholestasis, characteristic facies, butterfly-like vertebral anomalies, and varying degrees of peripheral pulmonary artery stenoses or diffuse hypoplasia of the pulmonary artery and its branches. It is associated with deletion in chromosome 20p.

CATCH-22. This is a syndrome that is due to microdeletion at chromosome 22q11 resulting in a wide clinical spectrum. CATCH stands for *c*ardiac defect, *a*bnormal facies, *t*hymic hypoplasia, *c*left palate, and *h*ypocalcemia. Cardiac defects include conotruncal defects such as interrupted aortic arch, tetralogy of Fallot, truncus arteriosus, and double-outlet right ventricle. It is also known as *DiGeorge syndrome* and *velocardiofacial syndrome*.

CHARGE ASSOCIATION. This anomaly is characterized by the presence of coloboma or choanal atresia and three of the following defects: CHD, nervous system anomaly or mental retardation, genital abnormalities, ear abnormality, or deafness. Congenital heart defects seen in the CHARGE association are tetralogy of Fallot with or without other cardiac defects, AV septal defect, double-outlet right ventricle, double-inlet left ventricle, TGA, interrupted aortic arch, and others.

DOWN SYNDROME. This is the most common malformation caused by trisomy 21. Most of the patients (95 percent) have complete trisomy of chromosome 21; some have translocation or mosaic forms. The phenotype is diagnostic (short stature, characteristic facial appearance, mental retardation, brachydactyly, atlantoaxial instability, and thyroid and white blood cell disorders). Congenital heart defects are frequent, AV septal defect and VSD being the most common. Mitral valve prolapse and aortic regurgitation may be present. Patients with Down syndrome are prone to earlier and more severe pulmonary vascular disease than otherwise expected as a result of the lesions identified.

ELLIS–VAN CREVELD SYNDROME. This is an autosomal recessive syndrome in which common atrium, primum ASD, and partial AV septal defect are the most common cardiac lesions.

HOLT-ORAM SYNDROME. This is an autosomal dominant syndrome consisting of radial abnormalities of the forearm and hand associated with secundum ASD (most common), VSD, or, rarely, other cardiac malformations.

LEOPARD SYNDROME. This autosomal dominant condition includes *l*entigines, *E*CG abnormalities, *o*cular hypertelorism, *p*ulmonary stenosis, *a*bnormal genitalia, *r*etardation of growth, and *d*eafness. Rarely, cardiomyopathy or complex CHD may be present.

NOONAN SYNDROME. This is an autosomal dominant syndrome, phenotypically somewhat similar to Turner syndrome but with a normal chromosomal complement. It is associated with congenital cardiac anomalies, especially dysplastic pulmonary valve stenosis, pulmonary artery stenosis, and ASD. Hypertrophic cardiomyopathy is less common. Congenital lymphedema is a commonly associated anomaly that may be unrecognized.

RUBELLA SYNDROME. This is a wide spectrum of malformations caused by rubella infection early in pregnancy, including cataracts, retinopathy, deafness, CHD, bone lesions, and mental retardation. The spectrum of congenital heart lesions is wide and includes pulmonary artery stenosis, PDA, tetralogy of Fallot, and VSD.

SCIMITAR SYNDROME. This is a constellation of anomalies including total or partial anomalous pulmonary venous connection (PAPVC) of the right lung to the inferior vena cava, often associated with hypoplasia of the right lung and right pulmonary artery. The lower portion of the right lung (sequestered lobe) tends to receive its arterial supply from the abdominal aorta. The name of the syndrome derives from the appearance on posteroanterior chest radiograph of the shadow formed by the anomalous pulmonary venous connection that resembles a Turkish sword, or scimitar.

SHONE COMPLEX (SYNDROME). This is an association of multiple levels of left ventricular inflow and outflow obstruction (subvalvular and valvular left ventricular outflow tract obstruction, coarctation of the aorta, and mitral stenosis [parachute mitral valve and supramitral ring]).

TURNER SYNDROME. This is a clinical syndrome due to the 45 XO karyotype in about 50 percent of cases, with various other X chromosome abnormalities comprising the remainder. There is a characteristic but variable phenotype, an association with congenital cardiac anomalies, especially postductal coarctation of the aorta and other left-sided obstructive lesions, as well as PAPVC without ASD. The female phenotype varies with the age of presentation and is somewhat similar to that of Noonan syndrome.

WILLIAMS SYNDROME. This is a congenital syndrome of heterogeneous cause, often sporadic, occasionally autosomal dominant, associated with infantile hypercalcemia, characteristic phenotype, and CHD, especially supravalvular aortic stenosis and multiple peripheral pulmonary stenoses.

Evaluation of the Patient with Congenital Heart Disease

Physical Examination

Although the advances in technology have profoundly improved our diagnostic abilities, there is still a role for detailed clinical examination in the assessment and follow-up of unoperated, palliated, and repaired CHD. The relevant findings pertaining to specific abnormalities are outlined in the appropriate sections that follow, but some general principles bear consideration (see Chap. 8).

PHYSICAL ASSESSMENT. One should assess both cardiac and visceral situs and not assume the heart will be left sided. The presence of characteristic facial or somatic features of an underlying syndrome may be a strong clue to the type of heart disease (e.g., Williams, Noonan, Down) at any age. Central cyanosis can be difficult to diagnose clinically when mild but should be actively excluded by oximetry in any patient with suspected CHD. It is also important to perform careful surveillance of the chest wall for scars in older patients and adults, who do not always know or report the type and sequence of their surgical interventions. The thin chest wall of children and many young adults with CHD facilitates the detection of chamber enlargement by palpation, as well as the detection of systolic or diastolic thrills.

The infant or child with hemodynamically significant heart disease may show signs of failure to thrive. Simply put, the infant or child is underweight, small, or both. The weight and height should therefore be plotted sequentially against normal growth curves appropriate to race, sex, and underlying syndrome (e.g., Down syndrome growth chart). The manifestations of "heart failure" vary with age and underlying problem. In children, peripheral edema is rare, but intercostal recession, nasal flaring, and grunting with respiration are signs of congestive heart failure. In small children, liver size and pulsatility are an excellent barometer of cardiac function, reflecting right atrial pressure, right ventricular filling time, and diastolic dysfunction or tricuspid regurgitation. The jugular venous pressure is difficult to assess in young children but is a fundamental part of the examination of the older child, teenager, and adult.

Examination of the upper and lower limb peripheral pulses is important at any age. Delay, absence, or reduction of a pulse is an important clue to the presence of arterial obstruction and its site. The left brachial pulse is often compromised by surgery for coarctation, and blood pressure measurements should not be taken in only the left arm. Similarly, other palliative procedures (Blalock-Taussig shunt, interposition grafts) may affect either or both upper limb pulses. It is always important to assess the femoral and carotid pulses in addition to the upper limb pulses in such patients. The pulse volume and character also provide important information regarding severity of obstructive or regurgitant left heart disease. A low-volume pulse (usually with a narrow pulse pressure) reflects a low cardiac output. Pulsus alternans signifies severe systemic ventricular dysfunction. Pulsus paradoxus points to cardiac tamponade.

In adolescents and adults, the jugular venous pressure examination is often very important. It may give indication of cardiac decompensation, cardiac chamber hypertrophy or noncompliance, valvular regurgitation or stenosis, arrhythmia or conduction disturbance, cardiac tamponade, pericardial constriction, and other phenomena.

AUSCULTATION. The rules of auscultation follow those developed for acquired heart disease. However, cardiac and vascular malposition may significantly affect the appreciation of heart sounds and murmurs. For example, in TGA treated by an atrial switch procedure, the aorta remains anterior to the pulmonary artery. Consequently the aortic component of the second sound can be exceptionally loud, and the pulmonary component may be virtually inaudible, making it difficult to assess the pulmonary artery pressure under such circumstances. Conversely, when there is a valved conduit between the right ventricle and pulmonary artery, the pulmonary closure sound may be extremely loud, even though the pulmonary artery diastolic pressure is low. This is because the conduit is frequently "stuck" to the chest wall, facilitating sound transmission to the stethoscope placed just above it. Calcification of semilunar valves is relatively unusual in childhood and early adult life, making the differentiation of valve stenosis from subvalve or supravalve narrowing, by the presence of an ejection click, more precise in these patients. The differentiation of multiple murmurs is sometimes a challenge. There may be several causes of systolic and/or diastolic murmurs in an individual, and supplementary clinical information may be required to establish their significance in some cases. It is important to auscultate over the entire anterior and posterior chest wall. The continuous murmurs of aorto-aortic collateral arteries in coarctation may be audible only between the shoulder blades posteriorly, for example, and similarly the presence of a localized distal pulmonary artery stenosis or the presence of an aortopulmonary collateral artery may be detected only in a very localized area of the chest wall, particularly in adults.

Electrocardiogram

The ECG remains an important tool in the assessment of CHD (see Chap. 9). Heart rhythm and rate as well as AV conduction can be evaluated. The dominant theme that runs through ECGs in CHD is the prevalence of right heart disease. This often takes the form of right axis deviation along with right atrial and right ventricular hypertrophy. Right ventricular hypertrophy may reflect pulmonary hypertension, right ventricular outflow tract obstruction, or a subaortic right ventricle. Incomplete right bundle branch block often indicates right ventricular hypertrophy due to pressure (e.g., pulmonary hypertension or pulmonary stenosis) or volume (e.g., ASD) overload. Right ventricular volume overload is likely when the r′ in V_1 is less than 7 mm. Very wide QRS complexes should be seen as possible manifestations of very dilated and dysfunctional ventricles, most specifically in patients with repaired tetralogy, complete right bundle branch block, and severe pulmonary regurgitation. The ECG may be uninterpretable in patients with abnormal cardiac or visceral situs unless it is clear where the leads were placed.

Atrial flutter (often in an atypical form—so-called intra-atrial reentrant tachycardia) is much more common in young patients than is atrial fibrillation. First-degree block is often seen in AV septal defects, cc-TGA, and Ebstein anomaly. Complete heart block is most often seen in patients with cc-TGA, as well those with older VSD repairs.

Left atrial overload may reflect increased pulmonary blood flow as well as AV valve dysfunction and myocardial failure. Left axis deviation should make one think of AV septal defect, a univentricular heart, and a hypoplastic right ventricle. Deep q waves in the left chest leads can be caused by left ventricular volume overload in a young person with aortic or mitral regurgitation. Pathological Q waves can be evidence of the anomalous origin of the left coronary from the pulmonary artery.

Chest Radiograph

The chest radiograph is another valuable tool for the discerning physician caring for patients with congenital heart defects (see Chap. 12). Although more recent technologies have rightly attracted much attention, there is value in learning how to interpret the chest radiograph. Some teaching points can be made that may anchor the interpretation of chest radiographs of some CHD patients. In the following sections are provided a number of clinical and radiographic differential diagnoses.

CRITERIA FOR SHUNT VASCULARITY. These include (1) uniformly distributed vascular markings with absence of the normal lower lobe vascular predominance; (2) right descending pulmonary artery diameter that exceeds 17 mm; and (3) a pulmonary artery branch that is larger than its accompanying bronchus (best noted in the right parahilar area). Prominent vascularity is apparent only if the pulmonary-to-systemic flow ratio is greater than 1.5 to 1.0. As a rule, cardiac enlargement usually implies a shunt greater than 2.5 to 1.0. Anemia, pregnancy, thyrotoxicosis, and a pulmonary AV fistula may mimic shunt vascularity.

CYANOTIC PATIENTS WITH SHUNT VASCULARITY. This group includes single ventricle with transposition, persistent truncus arteriosus, tricuspid atresia without significant pulmonary outflow obstruction, total anomalous pulmonary venous connection, double-outlet right ventricle, and a common atrium.

CYANOTIC PATIENTS WITH A VSD AND NORMAL OR DECREASED PULMONARY VASCULARITY. This group includes tetralogy of Fallot; tricuspid atresia with pulmonary stenosis; single ventricle and pulmonary stenosis; D-TGA with pulmonary stenosis; cc-TGA with pulmonary stenosis; double-outlet right ventricle with pulmonary stenosis; pulmonary atresia; and asplenia syndrome.

CAUSES OF RETROSTERNAL FILLING ON LATERAL CHEST RADIOGRAPH. These include right ventricular dilation, TGA, ascending aortic aneurysm, and noncardiovascular masses (e.g., lymphoma, thymoma, teratoma, and thyroid).

CAUSES OF A STRAIGHT LEFT HEART BORDER. These include right ventricular dilation, left atrial dilation, cc-TGA, pericardial effusion, Ebstein anomaly, and congenital absence of the left pericardium.

CARDIOVASCULAR DISEASES ASSOCIATED WITH SCOLIOSIS. These include cyanotic CHD, Eisenmenger syndrome, Marfan syndrome, and occasionally mitral prolapse.

CAUSES OF LARGE CENTRAL PULMONARY ARTERIES. These include increased pulmonary flow (main pulmonary artery and branches), increased pulmonary pressure (main pulmonary artery and branches), pulmonary stenosis (main and left pulmonary artery), and idiopathic dilation of the pulmonary artery (main pulmonary artery).

SITUS SOLITUS WITH CARDIAC DEXTROVERSION. Situs solitus with cardiac dextroversion is associated with CHD in more than 90 percent of cases. Up to 80 percent have a congenitally corrected transposition with a high incidence of associated VSD, pulmonary stenosis, and tricuspid atresia. *Situs inversus with dextrocardia* carries a low incidence of CHD, whereas *situs inversus with levocardia* is virtually always associated with severe CHD.

Cardiovascular MRI

Cardiac MRI in adolescents and adults with CHD has become of ever-increasing importance in the past decade (see Chap. 14). MRI is able to circumvent the echocardiographic problem of suboptimal visualization of the heart in adult patients, especially those who have had surgery. This technique can now generate information never previously available and also more easily or more accurately than by other means. New MRI image acquisition methods are faster and provide improved temporal and spatial resolution. Major advances in hardware design, new pulse sequences, and faster image reconstruction techniques now permit rapid high-resolution imaging of complex cardiovascular anatomy. MRI can produce quantitative measures of ventricular volumes, mass, and ejection fraction. MRI can quantify blood flow in any vessel.

Cardiac MRI is of particular value when transthoracic echocardiography cannot provide the needed diagnostic information; as an alternative to diagnostic cardiac catheterization; and for MRI's unique capabilities such as tissue imaging, myocardial tagging, and vessel-specific flow quantification. The value of MRI over echocardiography in the evaluation of the right ventricle is becoming increasingly appreciated. The capability of MRI to assess the right ventricle is of great importance since the right ventricle is a key component of many of the more complex CHD lesions. In addition, MRI can evaluate valve regurgitation, postoperative systemic and pulmonary venous pathways, Fontan pathways, and the great vessels. MRI should be considered the main imaging modality in adolescents and adults with repaired tetralogy of Fallot, TGA, Fontan procedure, and diseases of the aorta. In the near future, we will see real-time MRI to allow MR-guided interventional procedures, and molecular imaging that will further expand MRI's capabilities.

Transthoracic Echocardiography (see Chap. 11)

FETAL ECHOCARDIOGRAPHY

General Considerations. Fetal echocardiography has graduated from being a special area of interest to some pediatric cardiologists to one of standard care. As early as 16 weeks' gestation excellent images of the fetal cardiac structures can be obtained by the transabdominal route, along with an appreciation of cardiac and placental physiology through the use of Doppler technology. Transvaginal ultrasound is a newer approach that permits the echocardiographer to obtain images at around 13 to 14 weeks' gestation. Although it has some application for cases with a higher risk of recurrent CHD (e.g., obstructive left-sided lesions), its accuracy has yet to be determined. This is in part due to the limited number of views that are possible due to a relatively fixed position of the transducer. Although there are specific indications for fetal echocardiographic scanning, the highest number of cases arise from anatomical or functional abnormalities detected at routine obstetrical screening. A routine anatomical screen has become a standard of care in many obstetrical practices throughout the world. As a result there has been a tremendous push by pediatric fetal echocardiographers to improve the standard of routine screening of the prenatal heart. There has been a rapid rise in the number of abnormalities that are detected by general obstetrical ultrasonographers that are subsequently referred in a timely manner to the pediatric cardiologist and echocardiographer.

Impact of Fetal Echocardiography. Most major structural congenital heart defects are now accurately categorized through fetal echocardiography. Once the abnormalities are identified families and obstetrical caregivers can be counseled as to the impact of the abnormality to the fetus and the family. Decisions appropriate to the individual family and fetus can then be made. Although termination of pregnancy is one of the consequences of prenatal diagnosis, it is not the main objective.[68] In fact data are starting to appear in the literature indicating that prenatal diagnosis of some major cardiac malformations has a direct impact on outcome, from a survival, morbidity, and cost outcome.[69] This is in part due to the fact that when a prenatal diagnosis is made, subsequent caregivers are prepared for the immediate postnatal effects of the defect. For example, in hypoplastic left heart syndrome and other duct-dependent lesions prostaglandin E_1 can be started immediately after birth, hopefully in a hospital within or attached to a pediatric cardiology facility.

Fetal echocardiography has also permitted us to understand more about the evolution of certain congenital cardiac malformations. For example, although the fetal heart is fully formed by the time a prenatal scan is performed, there is a tremendous growth of the cardiac structures that still has to occur. Therefore, in some circumstances a cardiac chamber that may appear only mildly hypoplastic at 16 weeks' gestation may be profoundly affected at the time of birth. This has a major impact on the management of the newborn as well as the counseling process at 16 weeks' gestation.

Direct Fetal Intervention. The next step is direct intervention for specific cardiac lesions. This has initially involved obstructive lesions, thus far mainly being limited to the left ventricle. The rationale behind this therapy is based on the notion that the relief of obstructive outflow tract lesions will permit growth of the affected ventricle, potentially changing a neonatal pathway from univentricular to biventricular. Cardiac surgery to the fetus is also a future option, and indeed there is already a considerable amount of research on the impact of this in fetal animal models.

SEGMENTAL APPROACH[70,71] TO ECHOCARDIOGRAPHY IN CONGENITAL HEART DISEASE. The following four echocardiographic steps of segmental analysis are crucial in any patient with CHD. Starting from a standard subcostal view, one should determine the position of the apex, the situs of the atria, as well as the AV and ventriculoarterial relationships.

1. *Apex Position.* From a standard subcostal view, determine if the apex of the heart is pointing to the right (dextrocardia), to the left (levocardia), or to the middle (mesocardia).

2. *Situs of the Atria* (Fig. 56–2). The right and left atria differ morphologically with regard to their appendages. A morphological right atrium has a broad right atrial appendage, whereas a morphological left atrium has a narrow left atrial appendage. Right and left atrial appendages, however, are difficult to visualize by transthoracic echocardiography, and one often has to rely on abdominal situs to determine the atrial situs. Atrial situs follows abdominal situs in about 70 to 80 percent of the cases. From a standard subcostal view with the probe pointing at a right angle to the spine, one can visualize the abdominal aorta as well as the inferior vena cava and the spine at the back. When the aorta is to the left of the spine and the inferior vena cava to the right of the spine, there is abdominal situs solitus and, in all probability, corresponding atrial situs solitus (meaning the morphological right atrium is on the right side and the morphological left atrium is on the left side). When the aorta is to the right of the spine and the inferior vena cava is to the left of the spine, there is abdominal situs inversus and, in all probability, corresponding atrial situs inversus (morphological right atrium on the left side and morphological left atrium on the right side). When both the aorta and inferior vena cava are to the left of the spine, there is abdominal as well as atrial left isomerism (two morphological left atria). When both the aorta and inferior vena cava are to the right of the spine, there is abdominal as well as atrial right isomerism (two morphological right atria).

3. Atrioventricular Relationship. Once the situs of the atria is determined, one has to assess the position of the ventricles in relation to the atria. The morphological right ventricle has four characteristic features that distinguish it from the morphological left ventricle: (1) a trabeculated apex, (2) a moderator band, (3) septal attachment of the tricuspid valve, and (4) lower (apical) insertion of the tricuspid valve. The tricuspid valve is always "attached" to the morphological right ventricle. The morphological left ventricle has the following characteristics: (1) a smooth apex, (2) no moderator band, (3) no septal attachment of the mitral valve, and (4) higher (basal) insertion of the mitral valve. The mitral valve is always "attached" to the morphological left ventricle. Once the position of the ventricles is determined, one can then establish the AV relationship. When the morphological right atrium empties into to the morphological right ventricle, and the morphological left atrium empties into to the morphological left ventricle, there is AV concordance. When the morphological right atrium empties into to the morphological left ventricle, and the morphological left atrium empties into to the morphological right ventricle, there is AV discordance. When both atria empty into one ventricle (right or left), it is called a *double-inlet* (right or left) *ventricle*.

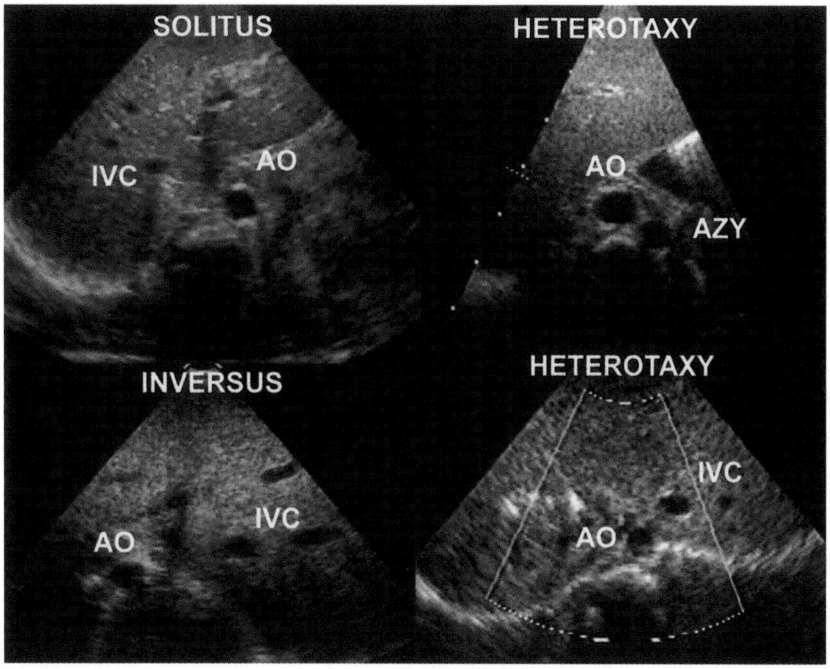

FIGURE 56–2 Montage of the different types of situs as seen by a subcostal echocardiographic scan. Note that situs solitus and inversus are just the mirror image of each other. The upper right picture is in the setting of heterotaxy with an interrupted intrahepatic inferior vena cava, with azygos continuation on the left. This is seen more frequently in left atrial isomerism. The lower right picture is also in the setting of heterotaxy with an intrahepatic inferior vena cava that is positioned closer to the aorta that in solitus or inversus. Note also the midline liver. This pattern is seen more commonly in right atrial isomerism. AO = aorta; AZY = azygos; IVC = inferior vena cava.

4. Ventriculoarterial Relationship. Once the AV relationship has been determined, one should assess the position of the great arteries in relation to the ventricles. The pulmonary artery can be distinguished by: its early branching pattern into the left and right pulmonary arteries; the pulmonary valve is always "attached" to the pulmonary artery. Similarly, the aorta can be distinguished by its "candy cane" shape and the take-off of its three head and neck vessels (innominate, carotid, and subclavian arteries). The aortic valve is always "attached" to the aorta. Once the position of the great arteries is determined, one can then establish the ventriculoarterial relationship. When the morphological right ventricle ejects into to the pulmonary artery, and the morphological left ventricle ejects into to the aorta, there is ventriculoarterial concordance. When the morphological right ventricle ejects into to the aorta, and the morphological left ventricle ejects into to the pulmonary artery, there is ventriculoarterial discordance. When both great arteries are exiting from one ventricle (right or left), it is called *double-outlet* (right or left) *ventricle*.

Once segmental analysis has been completed, one can then proceed to the usual echocardiographic windows to determine the nature of the specific lesions as well as their hemodynamic relevance.

ECHOCARDIOGRAPHY IN THE NEONATE AND INFANT. Echocardiography is of immense value in differentiating between heart disease and lung disease in newborns. Indeed, it has become the standard for the diagnosis of virtually all cardiovascular malformations. Most neonates and infants are now referred directly after ultrasound study for operative repair, without intervening cardiac catheterization. It is simpler to list those lesions where it cannot be used as the sole mode of investigation prior to making a management decision.[72] For example, in pulmonary atresia and VSD with multiple aortopulmonary collaterals, echocardiography is used as an adjunct to angiocardiography. Echocardiography provides details about the intracardiac pathology, whereas angiocardiography is necessary to delineate the sources of pulmonary blood supply. In pulmonary atresia with intact ventricular septum, the presence or absence of a right ventricular dependent coronary circulation is best assessed by angiocardiography. Apart from these two lesions, there are few other preoperative decisions that cannot be made by echocardiography alone in the newborn and infant. Postoperative management is different, particularly for those defects that are on Fontan track where precise hemodynamic measurements are of key importance in the decision process.

Transesophageal echocardiography (TEE) is usually unnecessary for the preoperative evaluation of the neonate or infant with heart disease. This technique has now become a standard in the immediate postoperative period for the evaluation of residual anatomical or functional abnormalities. Newer techniques such as tissue Doppler and three-dimensional (3D) echocardiography are starting to be applied to this age group and will add important additional information in the future.

ECHOCARDIOGRAPHY IN THE OLDER CHILD AND ADOLESCENT. This technique still plays a key role in the diagnosis and follow-up of the older child and adolescent with congenital or acquired heart disease. As many of the patients underwent surgery in the neonatal or infant periods they often have suboptimal ultrasound windows that necessitate other modes of investigation, especially magnetic resonance angiography (MRA). The application of newer technologies such as tissue Doppler and 3D echocardiography are already possible in this population and provide additional information that has thus far not been obtainable from standard techniques. For example, force-frequency relationships have been obtained in postoperative patients to try and predict the optimal heart rates to maintain maximum cardiac efficiency. On the other hand 3D echocardiography can provide new insights into AV valve function[73] that have not been possible from standard 2D techniques. In the future, 3D echocardiography may replace some TEE procedures.

ECHOCARDIOGRAPHY IN THE ADULT. Advances in cardiac ultrasonography now allow comprehensive noninvasive assessment of cardiovascular structure and function in adults with CHD. Because of its widespread availability, easy use, and quick interpretation, transthoracic echocardiography remains the technique of choice for the initial diagnosis and for follow-up in adults with CHD. The general initial approach to the diagnosis of CHD by transthoracic echocardiography starts with a segmental approach to ascertain the relative position of the various cardiac chambers. Once the segmental approach has been completed, a more lesion-specific approach can then be carried out, as discussed in the individual lesion sections.

Transesophageal Echocardiography

DIAGNOSTIC ASSESSMENT. TEE offers a better 2D resolution than transthoracic echocardiography. This is especially important in adult patients with multiple previous cardiac operations, when adequate transthoracic windows are often difficult to obtain.

TEE should be used whenever transthoracic echo does not provide adequate 2D, color, or Doppler information. TEE should be considered in the setting of the conditions discussed in the following sections.

Secundum Atrial Septal Defect. Use TEE for assessment of device closure feasibility, measuring ASD size, assessing adequacy of margins for device anchoring, and ruling out anomalous pulmonary venous connection.

Mitral Regurgitation. Use TEE for preoperative evaluation of mitral valve leaflet morphology and suitability for mitral valve repair versus replacement.

Ebstein Anomaly. Use TEE for preoperative assessment of tricuspid valve morphology and the potential for tricuspid valve repair.[74]

Fontan. Use TEE when right atrial clot is suspected on clinical grounds or by transthoracic echocardiography, or when circuit obstruction is suspected.

Precardioversion. For any patient who is not anticoagulated, presenting with atrial flutter or fibrillation longer than 24 hours, TEE should be performed prior to chemical or electrical cardioversion. Patients with a Fontan circuit should undergo TEE irrespective of the duration of atrial tachyarrhythmia to rule out a right or left atrial thrombus.

GUIDANCE OF THERAPEUTIC INTERVENTION. TEE can be instrumental in helping guide therapy at the time of transcatheter or surgical procedures. TEE is particularly helpful in the following situations.

Percutaneous Device Closure. TEE is performed at the time of transcatheter ASD closure to assist ASD-stretched balloon sizing and device deployment, unless intracardiac echocardiography (ICE) (see later) is available.

Intraoperative and Postoperative Assessment. TEE is often required for the intraoperative and postoperative assessment of the adult patient undergoing congenital cardiac surgery. It has a particular role in the intraoperative assessment of adequacy of valve repair. A TEE service by an experienced echocardiographer is an essential requirement for centers performing adult congenital cardiac surgery.

Three-Dimensional Echocardiography

DIAGNOSTIC ASSESSMENT. Presently, 3D echocardiography is not being widely used for the adult with CHD. However, with the expected improvement in technology that will permit real-time 3D echocardiography, its clinical applications will widen. By providing unique imaging planes and projections of the septa and AV and semilunar valves, 3D echocardiography offers the potential to enhance the understanding of complex cardiac anatomy.[75] It will also permit volumetric analyses independent of geometric assumptions, which will make it a particularly useful method for the assessment of the irregularly shaped, and thus problematic, right ventricle.[76]

Intracardiac Echocardiography

Intracardiac echocardiography (ICE) uses lower frequency transducers that have been miniaturized and mounted into catheters capable of percutaneous insertion into the heart. ICE not only provides high-resolution 2D and hemodynamic data with full Doppler capabilities but also eliminates the need for general anesthesia, which is often required for TEE.

CURRENT APPLICATIONS

Percutaneous ASD Device Closure. ICE supports percutaneous ASD device closure by adequately sizing the defect and by assisting device positioning[77] while avoiding the need for general anesthesia.

Electrophysiological Studies. ICE facilitates electrophysiological procedures by guiding transseptal puncture, enabling endocardial visualization, and ensuring electrode/tissue contact at the time of ablative procedures.[78]

Cardiac Catheterization

With the development of cross-sectional echocardiography, and the subsequent introduction of MRI and fast computed tomographic (CT) methods, truly diagnostic cardiac catheterization is a thing of the past for both children and adults. "Diagnostic" catheterization is reserved for resolving unanswered questions from the less-invasive techniques and measuring hemodynamics. A good example of this is the assessment of major aortopulmonary collateral arteries in tetralogy with pulmonary atresia, where their presence and distribution may be shown beautifully by MRA, but cardiac catheterization is required to demonstrate the presence of communications with the central pulmonary arteries and measure the pressure within them. There is no adequate substitute for cardiac catheterization to measure ventricular end-diastolic pressures or pulmonary artery pressures and resistance with the precision required to plan for, or to assess, the Fontan circulation. Such diagnostic testing may also be needed to evaluate possible coronary artery disease, especially prior to heart surgery.

THERAPEUTIC CATHETERIZATION. Balloon atrial septostomy was the first catheter intervention that proved useful in treating CHD, and it remains the standard initial palliation in many infants with D-TGA unless the arterial switch operation is performed immediately. Many transcatheter techniques are now used successfully to treat CHD: blade atrial septostomy; device or coil closure of PDA; closure of ASD and patent foramen ovale; transluminal balloon dilation of pulmonary and aortic valve stenosis; radiofrequency perforation of pulmonary valve atresia; balloon-expandable intravascular stents for right ventricular outflow tract, pulmonary artery, aortic coarctation, and other vascular stenoses; and device occlusion of unwanted collateral vessels and AV fistulas. These have all become treatments of choice in some centers with these capabilities. Some are universally accepted as standard of care (e.g., balloon pulmonary valvuloplasty), whereas debate continues for other interventions (e.g., unoperated coarctation).[79,80] Going along with the extraordinary expansion of interventional techniques for the treatment of structural abnormalities, ablative techniques for the treatment of tachycardias are now performed routinely in centers with congenital heart electrophysiology programs and are crucial to the management of the adult with operated and unoperated CHD, where arrhythmias are such a burden in terms of their morbidity, as well as a significant cause of late mortality. The indications, outcomes, and current status of each of these techniques are discussed in detail in the sections concerning specific lesions that follow.

Specific Cardiac Defects

Left-to-Right Shunts

Atrial Septal Defect

MORPHOLOGY. There are four types of ASDs or interatrial communications: ostium primum, ostium secundum, sinus venosus, and coronary sinus defects (Fig. 56–3A and D). (Ostium primum is discussed in the section on AV septal defect.) Ostium secundum defects occur from either excessive resorption of the septum primum or from deficient growth of the septum secundum and are occasionally associated with anomalous pulmonary venous connection (<10 percent). Sinus venosus defect of the superior vena cava type occurs at the cardiac junction of the superior vena cava, giving rise to a superior vena cava connected to both atria, and almost always associated with anomalous pulmonary venous connection (right >> left). Sinus venosus–inferior vena cava-type defects are very uncommon, and abut the junction of the inferior vena cava, inferior to the fossa ovalis. Coronary sinus septal defects are rare and arise from an opening of its wall with the left atrium, allowing left-to-right atrial shunting.

PATHOPHYSIOLOGY. In any type of ASD, the degree of left-to-right atrial shunting depends on the size of the defect and the relative diastolic filling properties of the two ventricles. Any condition causing reduced left ventricular compliance (e.g., systemic hypertension, cardiomyopathy, or myocardial infarction) or increased left atrial pressure (mitral stenosis and/or regurgitation) tends to increase the left-to-right shunt. If similar forces are present in the right heart, this will diminish the left-to-right shunt and promote right-to-left shunting.

NATURAL HISTORY. A large ASD (pulmonary artery blood flow relative to systemic blood flow [Qp/Qs] > 2.0/1.0) may cause congestive heart failure and failure to thrive in an infant or child. An undetected ASD with a significant shunt (Qp/Qs > 1.5/1.0) probably causes symptoms over time in adolescence or adulthood, and symptomatic patients usually become progressively more limited as they age. Effort dyspnea is seen in about 30 percent of patients by the third decade and more than 75 percent of patients by the fifth decade.[81] Supraventricular arrhythmias (atrial fibrillation or flutter) and right-sided heart failure develop by 40 years of age in about 10 percent of patients and become more prevalent with aging.[82] Paradoxical embolism resulting in a transient ischemic attack or stroke can call the diagnosis to attention. The development of pulmonary hypertension, although probably not as common as originally thought,[82] can occur at an early age. If pulmonary hypertension is severe, a second causative diagnosis should be sought. Life expectancy is clearly reduced, although not as severely as was quoted in earlier papers, since only patients with large ASDs were reported.

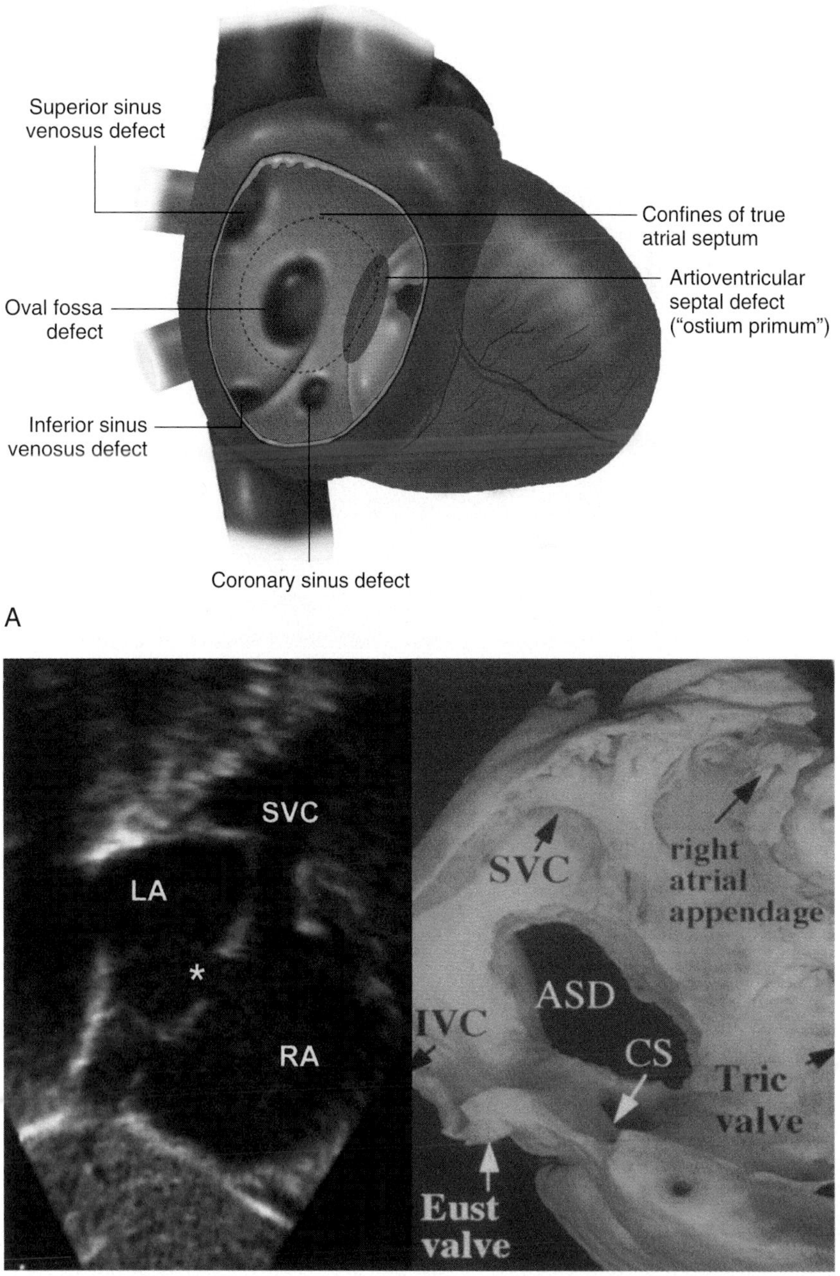

FIGURE 56–3 **A,** Schematic diagram outlining the different types of interatrial shunting that can be encountered. Note that only the central defect is suitable for device closure. **B,** Subcostal right anterior oblique view of a secundum atrial septal defect (asterisk) that is suitable for device closure. The right panel is a specimen as seen in a similar view, outlining the landmarks of the defect. *Continued*

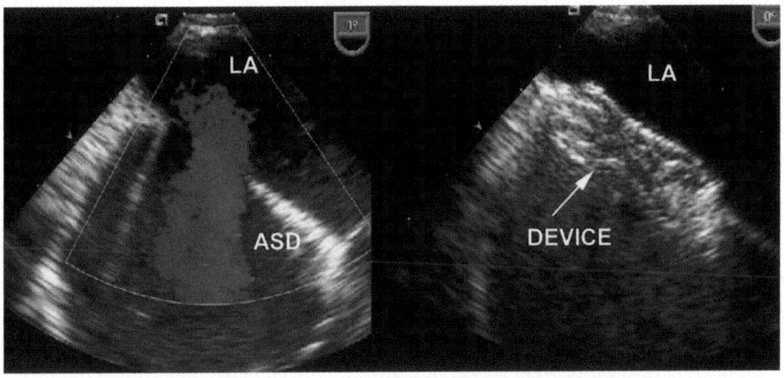

C

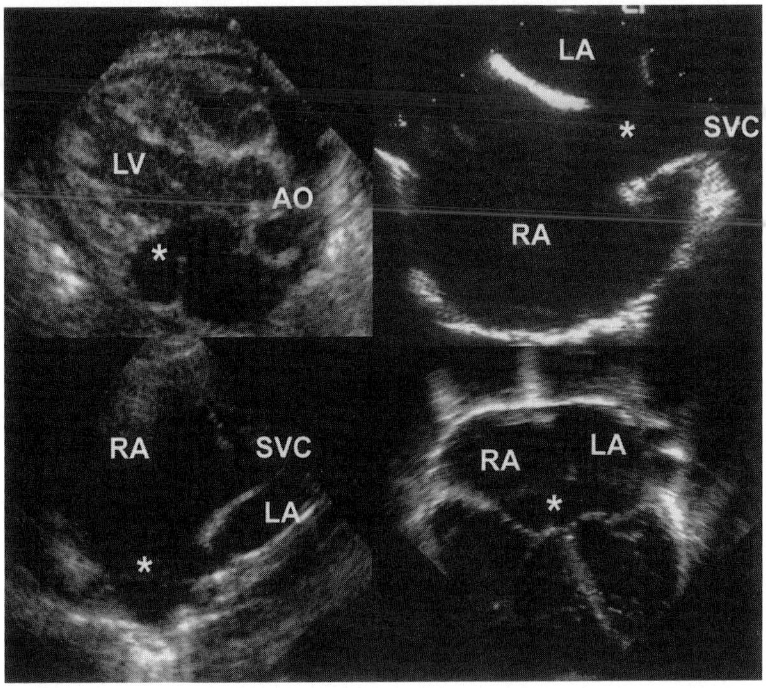

D

FIGURE 56–3, cont'd **C,** The left image is a transesophageal echocardiogram with color flow before device closure, whereas the right side shows postrelease of an Amplatzer device. **D,** Montage of interatrial communications that are not atrial septal defects (asterisks) and therefore not suitable for device closure. The upper left is a coronary sinus defect, due to unroofing; the top right is a superior sinus venosus defect; the bottom left is an inferior sinus venosus defect; and the bottom right is an atrial septal defect in the setting of an atrioventricular septal defect. AO = aorta; ASD = atrial septal defect; CS = coronary sinus; Eust = eustachian; IVC = inferior vena cava; LA = left atrium; LV = left ventricle; RA = right atrium; SVC = superior vena cava; Tric = tricuspid.

CLINICAL FEATURES

Pediatrics. Most children are asymptomatic, and the diagnosis is made following the discovery of a murmur. Occasionally, increased pulmonary blood flow may be so great that congestive heart failure, recurrent chest infections, chronic wheeze, or even pulmonary hypertension may necessitate closure in infancy. Spontaneous closure of an ASD may occur within the first year of life. Even quite substantial defects diagnosed in the neonatal period (<7 mm) may reduce in size and not require later intervention. Thus, in asymptomatic children with isolated secundum ASD, intervention is usually deferred so that elective device closure becomes an option if indicated.

Adults. The most common presenting symptoms in adults are exercise intolerance (exertional dyspnea and fatigue) and palpitations (typically from atrial flutter, atrial fibrillation, or sick sinus syndrome). Right ventricular failure can be the presenting symptom in older patients. The presence of cyanosis should alert one to the possibility of shunt reversal and Eisenmenger syndrome or, alternatively, to a prominent eustachian valve directing inferior vena cava flow to the left atrium via a secundum ASD or sinus venosus ASD of the inferior vena cava type.

On examination, there is "left atrialization" of the jugular venous pressure (A wave = V wave). A hyperdynamic right ventricular impulse may be felt at the left sternal border at the end of expiration or in the subxyphoid area on deep inspiration. A dilated pulmonary artery trunk may be palpated in the second left intercostal space. A wide and fixed split of S_2 is the auscultatory hallmark of ASD, although not always present. A systolic ejection murmur, usually grade 2 and often scratchy, is best heard at the second left intercostal space and a mid-diastolic rumble, from increased flow through the tricuspid valve, may be present at the left lower sternal border. When right ventricular failure occurs, a pansystolic murmur of tricuspid regurgitation is usual.

LABORATORY INVESTIGATIONS

ECG. Sinus rhythm or atrial fibrillation or flutter may be present. The QRS axis is typically rightward in secundum ASD. Negative P waves in the inferior leads indicate a low atrial pacemaker often seen in sinus venosus–superior vena cava-type defects, which are located in the area of the sinoatrial node and render it deficient. Complete right bundle branch block appears as a function of age. Tall R or R′ waves in V_1 often indicate pulmonary hypertension.

Chest Radiography. The classic radiographic features are of cardiomegaly (from right atrial and ventricular enlargement), dilated central pulmonary arteries with pulmonary plethora indicating increased pulmonary flow, and a small aortic knuckle (reflecting a chronic low cardiac output state).

Echocardiography. Transthoracic echocardiography documents the type(s) and size (defect diameter) of the ASD(s), the direction(s) of the shunt (see Fig. 56–3B) and sometimes the presence of anomalous pulmonary venous return. The functional importance of the defect can be estimated by the size of the right ventricle, the presence or absence of right ventricular volume overload (paradoxical septal motion), and the calculation of Qp/Qs. Indirect measurement of the pulmonary artery pressure can be obtained from the Doppler velocity of the tricuspid regurgitation jet. TEE permits better visualization of the interatrial septum and is usually required when device closure is contemplated, partly to ensure that pulmonary venous drainage is normal.

INDICATIONS FOR INTERVENTION. In asymptomatic children, the decision to intervene is based on the presence of right-sided heart dilation and a significant ASD (>5 mm) that shows no sign of spontaneous closure. Shunt fractions are now rarely measured and are reserved for "borderline" cases. Hemodynamically insignificant ASDs (Qp/Qs < 1.5) do not require closure, with the possible exception of trying to prevent paradoxical emboli in older patients after a stroke. "Significant" ASDs (Qp/Qs > 1.5, or ASDs associated with right ventricular volume overload) should be closed, especially if device closure is available and appropriate.[83,84] For patients with pulmonary hypertension (pulmonary artery pressure > ⅔ systemic arterial blood pressure, or pulmonary arteriolar resistance > ⅔ systemic arteriolar resistance), closure can be recommended if there is a net left-to-right shunt of at least 1.5:1, evidence of pulmonary artery reactivity when challenged with a pulmonary vasodilator (e.g., oxygen or nitric oxide), or evidence on lung biopsy (rarely required) that pulmonary arterial changes are potentially reversible.

INTERVENTIONAL OPTIONS AND OUTCOMES

Device Closure. Device closure of secundum ASDs percutaneously under fluoroscopy and TEE or with intracardiac echo guidance[83] is the therapy of choice when appropriate (see Fig. 56–3C).[85] Indications for device closure are the same as for surgical closure, but the selection criteria are stricter. Depending on the device, this technique is available only for patients with a secundum ASD with a stretched diameter of less than 36 mm and with adequate rims to enable secure deployment of the device. Anomalous pulmonary venous connection or proximity of the defect to the AV valves or coronary sinus or systemic venous drainage usually precludes the use of this technique. It is a safe and effective procedure in experienced hands, with major complications (e.g., device embolization, atrial perforation) occurring in less than 1 percent of patients, and clinical closure achieved in more than 80 percent of patients. Device closure of an ASD improves functional status in symptomatic patients and exercise capacity in asymptomatic and symptomatic patients,[86] but long-term follow-up data are not available.

Surgery. Device closure is not an option for those with sinus venosus or ostium primum defects or with secundum defects with unsuitable anatomy. Surgical closure of ASDs can be performed by primary suture closure or using a pericardial or synthetic patch. The procedure is usually performed via a midline sternotomy, but the availability of an inframammary or minithoracotomy approach to a typical secundum ASD should be made known to cosmetically sensitive patients. Surgical mortality in the adult without pulmonary hypertension should be less than 1 percent. Surgical closure of an ASD improves functional status and exercise capacity in symptomatic patients[87] and improves (but usually does not normalize) survival and improves or eliminates congestive heart failure, especially when patients are operated on at an earlier age. However, surgical closure of ASD in adult life does not prevent atrial fibrillation/flutter or stroke, especially when patients are operated on after the age of 40 years.[88] The role of a concomitant Cox/maze procedure in patients with a prior history of atrial flutter/fibrillation is unclear (see Chap. 30).[89]

REPRODUCTIVE ISSUES. Pregnancy is well tolerated in patients after ASD closure. Pregnancy is also well tolerated in women with unrepaired ASDs, but the risk of paradoxical embolism is increased (still only to a very low risk) during pregnancy as well as in the postpartum period. Pregnancy is contraindicated in Eisenmenger syndrome because of the high maternal (≤50 percent) and fetal (≤60 percent) mortality.

FOLLOW-UP ISSUES. Most children with isolated secundum defect can be discharged to the care of their family physician 6 months after complete closure is confirmed, no matter whether surgical or by device. They do not require any special precautions or endocarditis prophylaxis. Patients with sinus venosus defect are at risk of developing caval and/or pulmonary vein stenosis and should be kept under intermittent review. Patients who have had surgical or device repair as adults, patients with atrial arrhythmias preoperatively or postoperatively, and patients with ventricular dysfunction should remain under long-term cardiology surveillance.

Atrioventricular Septal Defect

TERMINOLOGY. The terms *atrioventricular septal defect, atrioventricular canal defect,* and *endocardial cushion defect* can be used interchangeably to describe this group of defects. The variable components of these lesions are explained in the following sections.

MORPHOLOGY. The basic morphology of AV septal defect is common to all types and is independent of the presence or absence of an ASD or VSD.[72,90-92] These common features (Figs. 56–4 and 56–5) are absence of the muscular AV septum (resulting in the AV valves being at the same level on echo); inlet/outlet disproportion (resulting in an elongated left ventricular outflow tract, the so-called goose-neck deformity); abnormal lateral rotation of the posteromedial papillary muscle; and abnormal configuration of the AV valves. The left AV valve is a trileaflet valve made of superior and inferior bridging leaflets separated by a mural leaflet. The space between the superior and inferior leaflets as they bridge the interventricular septum is called the *cleft* in the left AV valve. The bridging leaflets may be completely adherent to the crest of the interventricular septum, free floating, or attached by chordal apparatus.

PARTITIONED VERSUS COMPLETE ATRIOVENTRICULAR SEPTAL DEFECTS. A *partitioned* orifice is one where the superior and inferior leaflets are joined together by a connecting tongue of tissue as they bridge the interventricular septum. This partitions the valve into a separate left and right orifice. A *common* AV valve orifice is one where there is no such connecting tongue, resulting in one large orifice that encompasses the left- and right-sided components. Interatrial (ostium primum) and interventricular defects are common in AV septal defect.

The left ventricular outflow tract is elongated and predisposes to subaortic stenosis. The papillary muscles are closer together than normal. The term *unbalanced AV septal defect* refers to cases where one ventricle is hypoplastic. This is seen

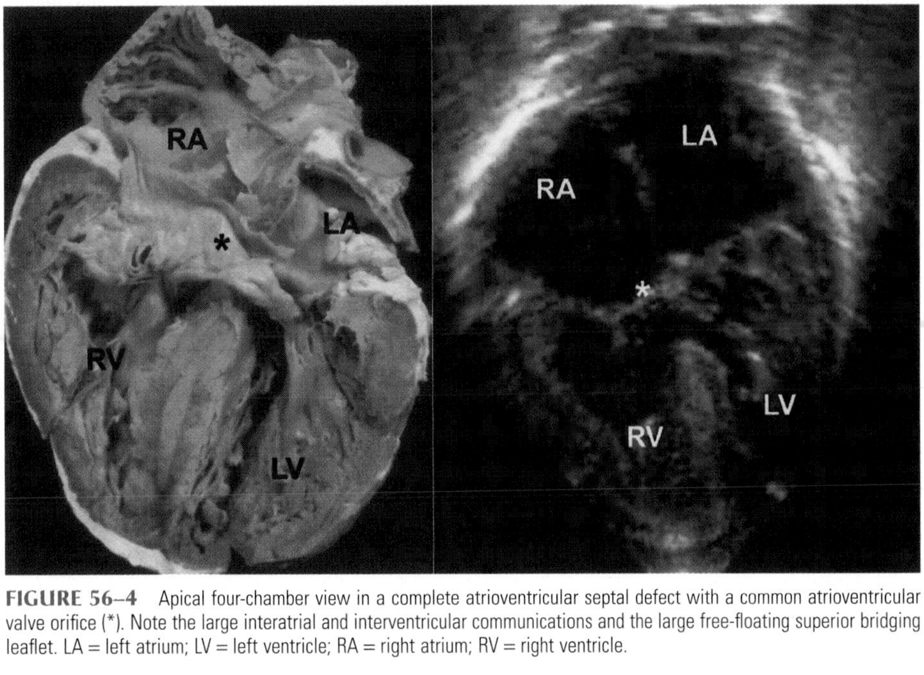

FIGURE 56–4 Apical four-chamber view in a complete atrioventricular septal defect with a common atrioventricular valve orifice (*). Note the large interatrial and interventricular communications and the large free-floating superior bridging leaflet. LA = left atrium; LV = left ventricle; RA = right atrium; RV = right ventricle.

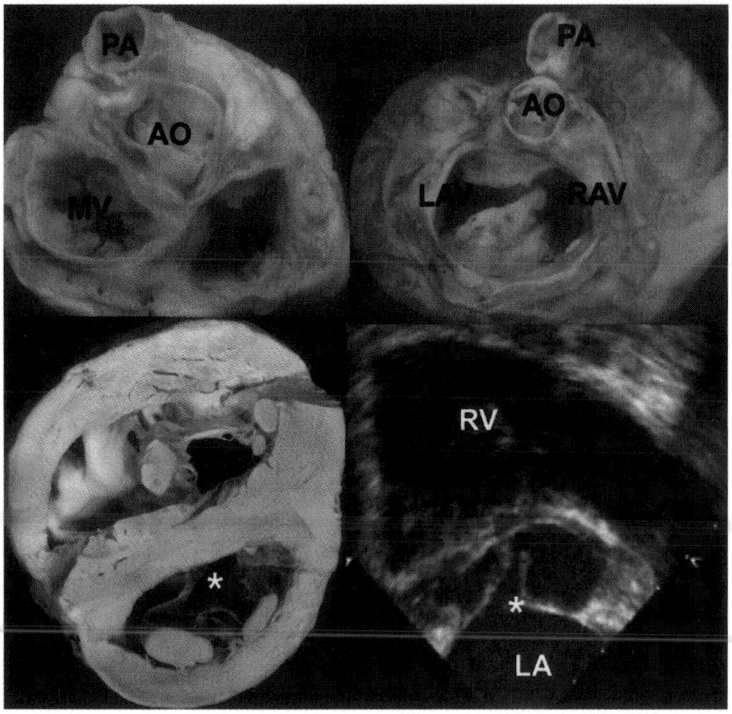

FIGURE 56–5 Montage comparing the normal atrioventricular junction to that seen in an atrioventricular septal defect. The upper left picture is the normal atrioventricular junction as seen from above. Note the normal morphology of the mitral and tricuspid valve, with the aorta wedged between them. The upper right picture is a similar view in an atrioventricular septal defect. Note the unwedged aorta, the trileaflet left atrioventricular valve, and the cleft between the superior and inferior bridging leaflets. The lower left picture is a specimen of an atrioventricular septal defect demonstrating the cleft. The lower right picture is an echo showing the cleft. AO = aorta; LA = left atrium; LAV = left atrioventricular valve; MV = mitral valve; PA = pulmonary artery; RAV = right atrioventricular valve; RV = right ventricle; TV = tricuspid valve.

more commonly in patients with heterotaxy and those with left-sided obstructive defects.

PATHOPHYSIOLOGY

Native. The pathophysiology of those with an isolated shunt at atrial level (commonly referred to as a *primum ASD*) is similar to that of a large secundum ASD, with unrestricted left-to-right shunting through the primum ASD, leading to right-sided atrial and ventricular volume overload. Chronic left AV valve regurgitation may produce left-sided ventricular and atrial volume overload. Complete AV septal defect has a greater degree of left-to-right shunting from the primum ASD as well as the nonrestrictive VSD, which triggers earlier left ventricular dilation as well as a greater degree of pulmonary hypertension.

After Correction. Residual significant left AV valve regurgitation may occur and cause significant left atrial as well as left ventricular dilation. Left AV valve stenosis from overzealous repair of the valve may also occur. The long, narrow left ventricular outflow tract of AV septal defect promotes left ventricular outflow tract obstruction and leads to subaortic stenosis in about 5 percent of patients.

NATURAL HISTORY. Patients with an isolated primum ASD have a course similar to that of those with large secundum ASDs, although symptoms may appear sooner when significant left AV valve regurgitation is present. Patients are usually asymptomatic until their third or fourth decade, but progressive symptoms related to congestive heart failure, atrial arrhythmias, complete heart block, and variable degrees of pulmonary hypertension develop in virtually all of them by the fifth decade.[93,94]

Most patients with complete AV septal defect have had surgical repair in infancy. Infants present with dyspnea, congestive heart failure, and failure to thrive. When presenting unrepaired, most adults have established pulmonary vascular disease. Patients with Down syndrome have a propensity to develop pulmonary hypertension at an even earlier age than do other patients with AV septal defect.

CLINICAL ISSUES

Down Syndrome. Down syndrome occurs in 35 percent of patients with AV septal defect. These patients more commonly have a complete AV septal defect with a common AV valve orifice and a large associated VSD. They often present in infancy with pulmonary hypertension. Clinical features are cardiomegaly, a right ventricular heave, and a pulmonary outflow tract murmur. If there is associated AV valve regurgitation, there is a pansystolic murmur.

Non-Down Syndrome. Clinical presentation depends on the presence and size of the ASD and the VSD and on the competence of the left AV valve. A large left-to-right shunt gives rise to symptoms of heart failure (exertional dyspnea or fatigue) or pulmonary vascular disease (exertional syncope, cyanosis). In adulthood, palpitations from atrial arrhythmias are common. Cardiac findings on physical examination for patients with an isolated shunt at atrial level are similar to those of patients with secundum ASD, with the important addition of a prominent left ventricular apex and pansystolic murmur when significant left AV valve regurgitation is present. Cases with a primum ASD and a restrictive VSD have similar findings, but with the addition of a pansystolic VSD murmur heard best at the left sternal border. Complete AV septal defects have a single S_1 (common AV valve), a mid-diastolic murmur from augmented AV valve inflow, and findings of pulmonary hypertension and/or a right-to-left shunt.

LABORATORY INVESTIGATIONS

ECG. Most patients have first-degree AV block and left axis deviation. Complete AV block and/or atrial fibrillation/flutter can be present in older patients. Partial or complete right bundle branch block is usually associated with right ventricular dilation or prior surgery.

Chest Radiography. If unrepaired, this demonstrates cardiomegaly with right atrial and right ventricular prominence with increased pulmonary vascular markings. In those cases with a small interatrial communication and left AV valve regurgitation, there is cardiomegaly due to left ventricular enlargement and normal pulmonary vascular markings. Findings of Eisenmenger syndrome are also possible. When repaired, the study may be normal with sternal wires.

Echocardiography. This has replaced angiography in assessing virtually all cases with AV septal defect.[72,90,91] The cardinal and common features discussed in the morphology section are readily recognized by echocardiography. In the four-chamber view the AV valve(s) appear at the same level, irrespective of the presence or absence of a VSD. The typical inferior ASD and the posteriorly positioned VSD will be sought. The degree of associated AV valve regurgitation, the left-to-right shunt from left ventricle to right atrium, and the estimated right ventricular systolic pressure should be assessed. When using the right AV valve to assess right ventricular pressure, care must be taken to ensure that the jet is not contaminated by an obligatory left ventricle-right atrial shunt.

Cardiac Catheterization. In general this technique has been replaced by echocardiography for the evaluation of patients with an AV septal defect. The one role it still has is in the evaluation of the patient who presents late and may have associated pulmonary vascular disease.

Open-Lung Biopsy. This should be considered only when the reversibility of pulmonary hypertension is uncertain from the hemodynamic data.

INDICATIONS FOR INTERVENTION. The patient with an unoperated or newly diagnosed AV septal defect and significant hemodynamic defects requires surgical repair. Equally, patients with persistent left AV valve regurgitation (or stenosis from previous repair) causing symptoms, atrial arrhythmia or deterioration in ventricular function, or patients with significant subaortic obstruction (a gradient ≥50 mm Hg at rest) require surgical intervention.[83]

In the presence of severe pulmonary hypertension (pulmonary artery pressure > ⅔ systemic blood pressure or pulmonary arteriolar resistance > ⅔ systemic arteriolar resistance), there must be a net left-to-right shunt of at least 1.5:1.0, evidence of pulmonary artery reactivity when challenged with a pulmonary vasodilator (e.g., oxygen, nitric oxide, and/or prostaglandins), or lung biopsy evidence that pulmonary arterial changes are potentially reversible (Heath-Edwards grade ≤ II-III) before surgical intervention can be carried out.

INTERVENTIONAL OPTIONS AND OUTCOMES

Isolated Shunt at Atrial Level (Primum Atrial Septal Defect). Pericardial patch closure of the primum ASD with concomitant suture (with or without annuloplasty) of the "cleft" left AV valve is usually performed. When left AV valve repair is not possible, replacement may be necessary. In the short term, the results of repair of partial AV septal defect are similar to those following closure of secundum ASD,[95-97] but sequelae of left AV ("mitral") valve regurgitation,[96-101] subaortic stenosis[102,103] and AV block may develop or progress.

Complete Atrial Septal Defect. The "staged approach" (pulmonary artery banding followed by intracardiac repair) has been supplanted by primary intracardiac repair in infancy. The goals of intracardiac repair are ventricular and atrial septation with adequate mitral and tricuspid reconstruction. Both single- and double-patch techniques[104] to close ASDs and VSDs have been described with comparable results. Occasionally, left AV valve replacement is necessary when valve repair is not possible. The long-term results of repair of complete AV septal defect are not well known, but similar problems as with partial AV septal defect are likely.

REPRODUCTIVE ISSUES. Pregnancy is well tolerated in patients with complete repair and no significant residual lesions. Women in NYHA Classes I and II with unoperated isolated primum ASD usually tolerate pregnancy very well. Pregnancy is contraindicated in Eisenmenger syndrome because of the high maternal (≤50 percent) and fetal (≤60 percent) mortality.

FOLLOW-UP ISSUES. All patients require periodic follow-up by an expert cardiologist because of the possibility of the postoperative complications, which include patch dehiscence or residual septal defects (1 percent), the development of complete heart block (3 percent), late atrial fibrillation/flutter, left AV valve dysfunction,[96-101] and subaortic stenosis.[102,103] Left AV valve regurgitation requires reoperation in at least 10 percent of patients.[105] Subaortic stenosis develops or progresses in 5 to 10 percent of patients after repair, particularly in patients with primum ASD, especially if the left AV ("mitral") valve has been replaced. Particular attention should be paid to those patients with pulmonary hypertension preoperatively.[106] Antibiotic prophylaxis is needed in most patients after repair, given the common occurrence of residual "mitral" regurgitation.

Isolated Ventricular Septal Defect

MORPHOLOGY. The ventricular septum can be divided into three major components—inlet, trabecular, and outlet—all abutting on a small membranous septum lying just underneath the aortic valve. VSDs (Fig. 56–6) are classified into three main categories according to their location and margins (Fig. 56–7). *Muscular* VSDs are bordered entirely by myocardium and can be trabecular, inlet, or outlet in location. *Membranous* VSDs often have inlet, outlet, or trabecular extension and are bordered in part by fibrous continuity between the leaflets of an AV valve and an arterial valve. *Doubly committed* subarterial VSDs are more common in Asian patients, are situated in the outlet septum, and are bordered by fibrous continuity of the aortic and pulmonary valves.[107] This section deals with VSDs occurring in isolation from major associated cardiac anomalies.

PATHOPHYSIOLOGY. A *restrictive* VSD is a defect that produces a significant pressure gradient between the left ventricle and the right ventricle (pulmonary/aortic systolic pressure ratio < 0.3) and is accompanied by a small (<1.4/1.0) shunt. A *moderately restrictive* VSD is accompanied by a moderate shunt (Qp/Qs = 1.4 to 2.2/1.0) with a pulmonary/aortic systolic pressure ratio less than 0.66. A large or *nonrestrictive* VSD is accompanied by a large shunt (Qp/Qs > 2.2) and a pulmonary/aortic systolic pressure ratio greater than

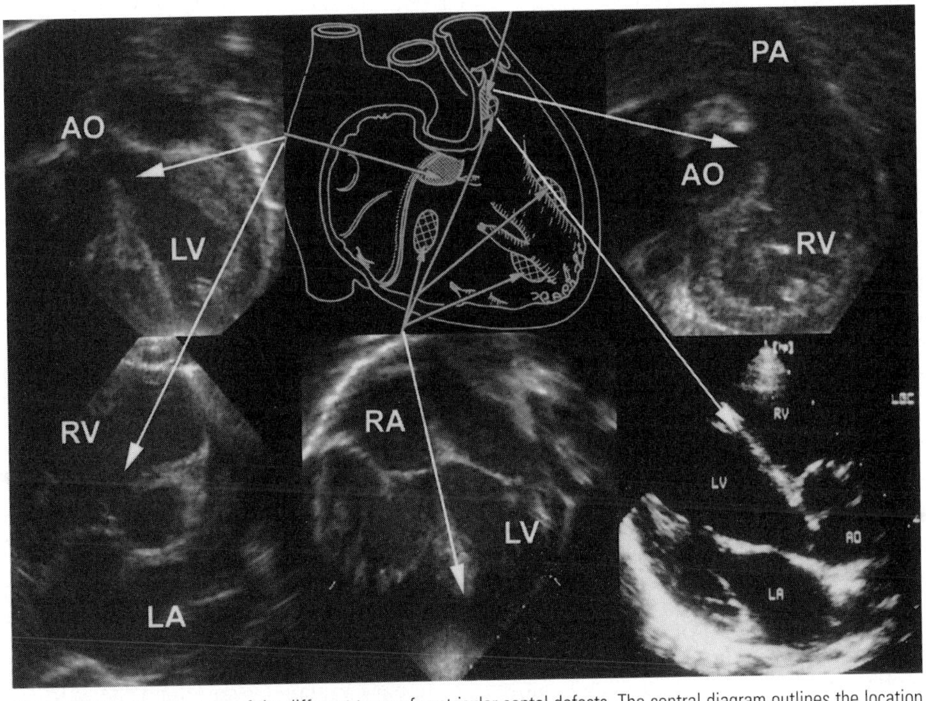

FIGURE 56–6 Montage of the different types of ventricular septal defects. The central diagram outlines the location of the various types of defects as seen from the right ventricle. The two left images show a perimembranous ventricular septal defect as seen in the five-chamber and short-axis views. Note the defect is roofed by the aorta and is next to the tricuspid valve. The bottom middle echocardiogram is a muscular apical defect. The upper right image is a right anterior oblique view in a doubly committed ventricular septal defect. The lower right is a short-axis view showing an outlet ventricular septal defect with prolapse of the right coronary cusp. AO = aorta; LV = left ventricle; PA = pulmonary artery; RA = right atrium; RV = right ventricle.

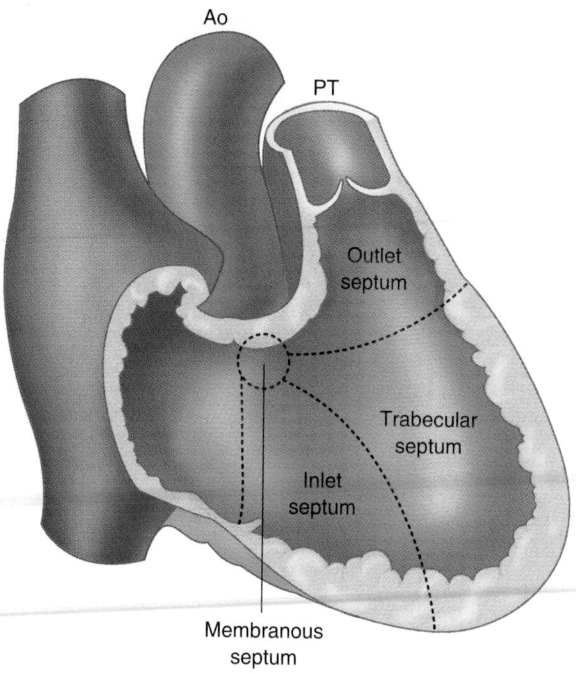

FIGURE 56–7 Four components of the ventricular septum shown here from the right ventricular aspect are now described by Anderson and associates as inlet and outlet components of the right ventricle because these areas do not correspond to septal structures as initially suggested. Ao = aorta; PT = pulmonary trunk. (Modified from Anderson RH, Becker AE, Lucchese E, et al: Morphology of Congenital Heart Disease. Baltimore, University Park Press, 1983.)

0.66. An *Eisenmenger VSD* has a systolic pressure ratio of 1.0 and Qp/Qs less than 1:1, a net right-to-left shunt.[83]

NATURAL HISTORY. A *restrictive* VSD does not cause significant hemodynamic derangement[108] and may close spontaneously during childhood and sometimes in adult life. Small VSDs pose an ongoing and relatively high risk of endocarditis. A perimembranous defect in an immediately subaortic position, or any doubly committed VSD, may be associated with progressive aortic regurgitation.[109] Late development of subaortic and subpulmonary stenosis (see double-chambered right ventricle) as well as the formation of a left ventricular to right atrial shunt all are well described and should be excluded at follow-up.[110] A *moderately restrictive* VSD imposes a hemodynamic burden on the left ventricle, which leads to left atrial and ventricular dilation and dysfunction as well as a variable increase in pulmonary vascular resistance. A large or nonrestrictive VSD features left ventricular volume overload early in life with a progressive rise in pulmonary artery pressure and a fall in left-to-right shunting. In turn, this leads to higher pulmonary vascular resistance and to Eisenmenger syndrome.

CLINICAL FEATURES

Pediatrics. Neonatal presentation with a murmur is increasingly frequent. Most of these patients have a restrictive defect, the murmur becoming apparent only as the pulmonary vascular resistance falls. Paradoxically, those infants with large nonrestrictive defects tend to present later. This is because equalization of pressures across the defect obviates the generation of a pansystolic murmur. Instead, pulmonary blood flow increases progressively as the pulmonary vascular resistance falls. Presentation with breathlessness, congestive heart failure, and failure to thrive in the 2nd and 3rd months of life is usual. At that time a pulmonary ejection murmur and a mitral rumble may be heard, reflecting increased pulmonary flow and pulmonary venous return. Cyanosis is rare in early childhood, and if present, other causes of a raised pulmonary vascular resistance should be excluded (e.g., mitral stenosis or coexisting lung pathology).

Medical management of the symptomatic infant is directed at improving symptoms prior to surgery, or "buying time" while spontaneous closure, or diminution in size, occurs. Treatment with diuretics is universally accepted, and increasingly, the successful use of ACE inhibition is being reported.

Adults. Most adult patients with a small *restrictive* VSD are asymptomatic. Physical examination reveals a harsh or high frequency pansystolic murmur, usually grade 3 to 4/6, heard with maximal intensity at the left sternal border in the 3rd or 4th intercostal space. Patients with a *moderately restrictive* VSD often present with dyspnea in adult life perhaps triggered by atrial fibrillation. Physical examination typically reveals a displaced cardiac apex with a similar pansystolic murmur as well as an apical diastolic rumble and third heart sound at the apex from the increased flow through the mitral valve. Patients with large *nonrestrictive* Eisenmenger VSDs present with central cyanosis and clubbing of the nail beds. Signs of pulmonary hypertension—a right ventricular heave, palpable and loud P_2, and a right-sided S_4—are typically present. A pulmonary ejection click, a soft and scratchy systolic ejection murmur, and a high-pitched decrescendo diastolic murmur of pulmonary regurgitation (Graham Steell) may be audible. Peripheral edema usually reflects right-sided heart failure.

LABORATORY INVESTIGATIONS

ECG. The ECG mirrors the size of the shunt and the degree of pulmonary hypertension. Small, *restrictive* VSDs usually produce a normal tracing. *Moderate*-sized VSDs produce a broad notched P wave characteristic of left atrial overload as well as evidence of left ventricular volume overload, namely deep Q and tall R waves with tall T waves in leads V_5 and V_6, and perhaps eventually atrial fibrillation. Following repair, the ECG is usually normal with right bundle branch block.

Chest Radiography. The chest radiograph reflects the magnitude of the shunt as well as the degree of pulmonary hypertension. A *moderate*-sized shunt causes signs of left ventricular dilation with some pulmonary plethora.

Echocardiography. Transthoracic echocardiography can identify the location, size, and hemodynamic consequences of the VSD as well as any associated lesions (aortic regurgitation, right ventricular outflow tract obstruction, or left ventricular outflow tract obstruction).

Cardiac Catheterization. Cardiac catheterization may be required when the hemodynamic significance of a VSD is questioned or when assessment of pulmonary artery pressures and resistances is needed. In some centers therapeutic catheterization is performed for percutaneous closure (see later).

INDICATIONS FOR INTERVENTION. The presence of a significant VSD (the symptomatic patient shows a Qp/Qs > 1.5/1.0; pulmonary artery systolic pressure > 50 mm Hg; increased LV and LA size, or deteriorating left ventricular function) in the absence of irreversible pulmonary hypertension warrants surgical closure. If severe pulmonary hypertension (see ASD section) is present, closure is seldom feasible. Other relative indications for VSD closure include the presence of a perimembranous or outlet VSD with more than mild aortic regurgitation[111] and a history of recurrent endocarditis.

In children, the presence of a nonrestrictive VSD, or a smaller VSD with significant symptoms failing to respond to medication, are indications for surgical or device closure. Elective surgery is usually performed between 3 and 9 months of age. Some patients have pulmonary hypertension. If pulmonary arteriolar resistance is less than 7 Wood units, closure can be safely undertaken if there is a net left-to-right shunt of at least 1.5/1.0, strong evidence of pulmonary reactivity when challenged with a pulmonary vasodilator (oxygen, nitric oxide), or lung biopsy evidence that pulmonary artery changes are reversible (rarely required).

INTERVENTIONAL OPTIONS AND OUTCOMES

Surgery. Surgical closure by direct suture or with a patch has been used for more than 50 years with a low perioperative mortality—even in adults—and a very high closure rate. VSDs should be closed by congenital heart surgeons. Patch leaks are not uncommon but seldom need reoperation.

Device Closure. Successful transcatheter device closure of trabecular (muscular) and perimembranous VSDs has recently been reported. Trabecular VSDs have proven more amenable to this technique because of their relatively straightforward anatomy and muscular rim to which the device attaches well. The closure of perimembranous VSDs is technically more challenging due to its proximity to valve structures and requires careful patient selection.[112] It should be performed only in centers with appropriate expertise. No long-term follow-up is available.

REPRODUCTIVE ISSUES. Pregnancy is well tolerated in women with small or moderate VSD and in women with repaired VSDs. Pregnancy is contraindicated in Eisenmenger syndrome because of high maternal (≤50 percent) and fetal (≤60 percent) mortality.

FOLLOW-UP ISSUES. For patients with good to excellent functional class and good left ventricular function prior to surgical closure, life expectancy after surgical correction is close to normal. The risk of progressive aortic regurgitation is reduced after surgery, as is the risk of endocarditis, unless a residual VSD persists. Yearly cardiac evaluation is suggested for patients with right ventricular outflow tract obstruction, left ventricular outflow tract obstruction, and aortic regurgitation not undergoing surgical repair; patients with Eisenmenger syndrome; and adults with significant atrial or ventricular arrhythmias. Cardiac surveillance is also recommended for patients who had late repair of moderate or large defects, which are often associated with left ventricular impairment and elevated pulmonary artery pressure at the time of surgery.

Patent Ductus Arteriosus

MORPHOLOGY. The ductus arteriosus derives from the left sixth primitive aortic arch and connects the proximal left pulmonary artery to the descending aorta, just distal to the left subclavian artery.[113]

PATHOPHYSIOLOGY. The ductus is widely patent in the normal fetus, carrying unoxygenated blood from the right ventricle through the descending aorta to the placenta, where the blood is oxygenated. Functional closure of the ductus from vasoconstriction occurs shortly after a term birth, whereas anatomical closure from intimal proliferation and fibrosis takes several weeks to complete. Some patients have "ductus-dependent" physiology as neonates. This means their circulation is dependent on the ductus for pulmonary blood flow such as in severe aortic coarctation, hypoplastic left heart syndrome, and sometimes D-TGA. If spontaneous closure of the ductus occurs in such neonates, clinical deterioration and death usually follow.

Isolated PDAs, the subject of this section, are often categorized according to the degree of left-to-right shunting, which is determined by both the size and length of the duct and the difference between systemic and pulmonary vascular resistances, as follows:

- Silent: tiny PDA detected only by nonclinical means (usually echo)
- Small: continuous murmur common; Qp/Qs < 1.5:1.0
- Moderate: continuous murmur common; Qp/Qs = 1.5 to 2.2:1.0
- Large: Qp/Qs > 2.2:1.0
- Eisenmenger: continuous murmur absent; substantial pulmonary hypertension, differential hypoxemia, and differential cyanosis

NATURAL HISTORY

Premature Infants. Patency of a ductus arteriosus is common in a preterm infant who lacks the normal mechanisms for postnatal ductal closure because of immaturity. A PDA is thus an expected finding in a premature infant, and delayed spontaneous closure of the ductus may be anticipated if the infant does not succumb to other problems.

Full-Term Infant. In a full-term newborn, patency of a ductus is a true congenital malformation. Occasionally, some full-term newborns have persistent patency of the ductus arteriosus because their relative hypoxemia contributes to vasodilation of the channel. This includes infants born at high altitude; those with congenital malformations causing hypoxemia; or malformations in which ductal flow supplies the systemic circulation, such as hypoplastic left heart syndrome, interrupted aortic arch, or aortic coarctation.

Children and Adults. Children and adults with *silent* PDAs are detected by nonclinical means, usually echocardiography, and face virtually no long-term complications. An exception occurs if the patient's murmur is inaudible because of obesity or other somatic factors. A *small* ductus accompanied by a small shunt does not cause a significant hemodynamic derangement but may predispose to endarteritis, especially when a murmur is present. A *moderate-sized* duct and shunt pose a volume load on the left atrium and ventricle with resultant left ventricular dilation and dysfunction and perhaps eventual atrial fibrillation. A *large* duct results initially in left ventricular volume overload but develops a progressive rise in pulmonary artery pressures and eventually irreversible pulmonary vascular changes by 2 years of age (Eisenmenger syndrome).

CLINICAL FEATURES

Premature Infants. Most preterm infants with a birth weight less than 1500 gm have a PDA, and about one-third have a large enough shunt to cause significant cardiopulmonary deterioration. Clinical findings in these patients include bounding peripheral pulses, an infraclavicular and interscapular systolic murmur (occasionally a continuous murmur), precordial hyperactivity, hepatomegaly, and either multiple episodes of apnea and bradycardia or ventilator dependence.

Full-Term Infants, Children, and Adults. A *small* audible duct usually causes no symptoms but may rarely present as an endovascular infection. Physical examination may reveal a grade 1 or 2 continuous murmur peaking in late systole and best heard in the 1st or 2nd left intercostal space. Patients with a *moderate-sized* duct may present with dyspnea or palpitations from atrial arrhythmias. A louder continuous or "machinery" murmur in the 1st or 2nd left intercostal space is typically accompanied by a wide systemic pulse pressure from aortic diastolic runoff into the pulmonary trunk and signs of left ventricular volume overload, such as a displaced left ventricular apex and sometimes a left-sided S_3 (meaningful in adults only). With a moderate degree of pulmonary hypertension, the diastolic component of the murmur disappears, leaving a systolic murmur. Adults with a *large* uncorrected PDA eventually present with a short systolic ejection murmur, hypoxemia in the feet more than the hands (differential cyanosis), and Eisenmenger physiology.

LABORATORY INVESTIGATIONS IN PREMATURE INFANTS

ECG. This may be normal or demonstrate right or left ventricular hypertrophy or both, depending on the amount of left-to-right shunting and the degree of associated pulmonary hypertension.

Chest Radiography. This may demonstrate cardiomegaly and increased pulmonary vascular markings that may be difficult to interpret in the setting of hyaline membrane disease.

Echocardiography. This is the key to diagnosis. The ductus arteriosus can be imaged in its entirety and its size estimated. Doppler demonstrates the shunt and permits an accurate assessment of mean pulmonary artery pressure. This is achieved from calculating the mean left-to-right spectral trace and subtracting it from the mean blood pressure. Measurements of the left atrial and left ventricular size provide indirect evidence of the magnitude of left-to-right shunting.

LABORATORY INVESTIGATIONS IN FULL-TERM INFANTS, CHILDREN, AND ADULTS

ECG. The ECG reflects the size and degree of shunting occurring through the duct. A *small* duct produces a normal ECG. A *moderate* duct may show left ventricular volume overload with broad, notched P waves together with deep Q waves, tall R waves, and peaked T waves in V_5 and V_6. A *large* duct produces findings of right ventricular hypertrophy.

Chest Radiography. A *small* duct produces a normal chest radiograph. A *moderate*-sized duct causes moderate cardiomegaly with left-sided heart enlargement, a prominent aortic knuckle, and increased pulmonary perfusion. Ring calcification of the ductus may be seen through the soft tissue density of the aortic arch or pulmonary trunk in older adults. The large PDA produces an Eisenmenger appearance with a prominent aortic knuckle.

Echocardiography. This determines the presence, size, and degree of shunting and the physiological consequences of the shunt. The PDA is seen with difficulty in an Eisenmenger context. A bubble study shows the communication.

INDICATIONS FOR INTERVENTION

Premature Infants. Treatment of preterm infants with a PDA varies with the magnitude of shunting and the severity of hyaline membrane disease because the ductus may contribute importantly to mortality in infants with respiratory distress syndrome. Intervention in an asymptomatic infant with a small left-to-right shunt is unnecessary because the PDA almost invariably undergoes spontaneous closure. Those infants who demonstrate unmistakable signs of a significant ductal left-to-right shunt during the course of the respiratory distress syndrome are often unresponsive to medical measures to control congestive heart failure and require closure of the PDA to survive. These infants are best treated by pharmacological inhibition of prostaglandin synthesis with indomethacin or ibuprofen to constrict and close the ductus.[114] Surgical ligation is required in the estimated 10 percent of infants who are unresponsive to indomethacin.

Full-Term Infants. In the clinical settings in which the ductus preserves pulmonary blood flow, the inevitable spontaneous closure of the vessel is associated with profound clinical deterioration and often death. Undesirable ductal closure may be reversed medically within the first 4 or 5 days of life by an infusion of prostaglandin E_1. By dilating the constricted ductus arteriosus, a temporary increase should occur in arterial blood oxygen tension and saturation and correction of acidemia.

Children and Adults. Closure of an isolated, clinically detectable PDA, in the absence of irreversible pulmonary hypertension, is often recommended. There is no debate about the desirability of closing a hemodynamically important PDA. There is debate about closing a PDA strictly to reduce the risk of endarteritis. The risk of endarteritis in a patient with a silent PDA is considered negligible, and closure of such ducts is seldom recommended for that reason. In the presence of severe pulmonary hypertension (see ASD section), closure is seldom indicated. Contraindications to ductal closure include irreversible pulmonary hypertension or active endarteritis.[83]

INTERVENTIONAL OPTIONS AND OUTCOMES

Transcatheter Treatment (Fig. 56–8). Over the past 20 years, the efficacy and safety of transcatheter device closure for ducts smaller than 8 mm have been established with complete ductal closure achieved in more than 85 percent of patients by 1 year following device placement at a mortality rate of less than 1 percent.[115] In centers with appropriate resources and experience, transcatheter device occlusion should be the method of choice for ductal closure.[115,116]

Surgical Treatment. Surgical closure, by ductal ligation and/or division, has been performed for more than 50 years with a marginally greater closure rate than device closure but somewhat greater morbidity and mortality. Immediate clinical closure (no shunt audible on physical examination) is achieved in more than 95 percent of patients. Surgical closure is a low-risk procedure in children. Surgical mortality in adults is 1.0 to 3.5 percent and relates to the presence of pulmonary arterial hypertension and difficult ductal morphology (calcified or aneurysmal) often seen in adults. Surgical closure should be reserved for those in whom the PDA is too large for device closure or at centers without access to device closure.

REPRODUCTIVE ISSUES. Pregnancy is well tolerated in women with silent and small PDA or in patients who were asymptomatic prior to pregnancy. In the woman with a hemodynamically important PDA, pregnancy may precipitate or worsen heart failure. Pregnancy is contraindicated in Eisenmenger syndrome because of the high maternal (≤50 percent) and fetal (≤60 percent) mortality.

FOLLOW-UP ISSUES. Patients with device occlusion or after surgical closure should be examined periodically for possible recanalization. Silent residual shunts may be found by transthoracic echocardiography.[117] The risk of late endarteritis from a clinically silent residual shunt after device implantation or surgical closure is low, and the need for endocarditis prophylaxis in such patients is uncertain. Endocarditis prophylaxis is recommended for 6 months following PDA device closure or for life if any residual defect persists.

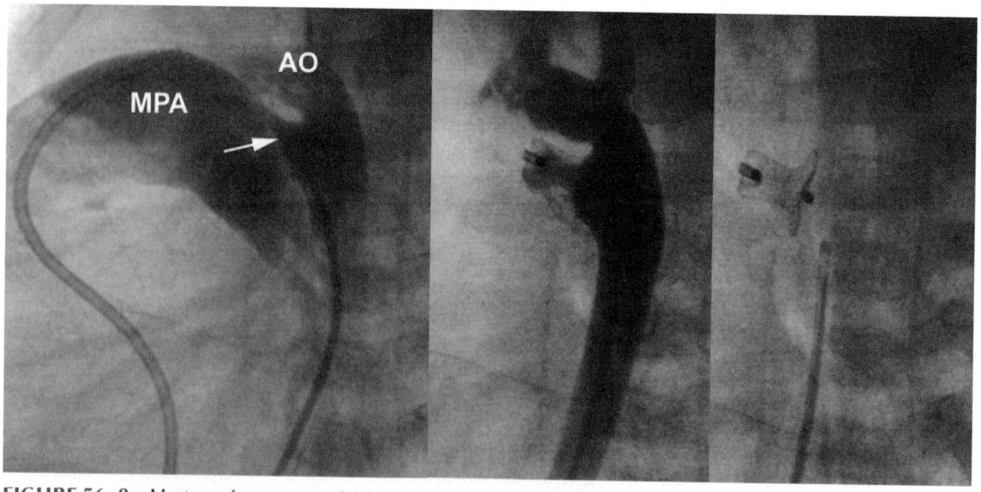

FIGURE 56–8 Montage of a patent arterial duct, before and after device occlusion. AO = aorta; MPA = main pulmonary artery.

Patients with a silent PDA probably do not require endocarditis prophylaxis or follow-up.

Persistent Truncus Arteriosus

MORPHOLOGY. Persistent truncus arteriosus is an anomaly in which a single vessel forms the outlet of both ventricles and gives rise to the systemic, pulmonary, and coronary arteries. It is always accompanied by a VSD, and frequently with a right-sided aortic arch. The truncal valve is usually tricuspid but is quadricuspid in about one-third of patients. Truncal valve regurgitation and truncal valve stenosis are each seen in 10 to 15 percent of patients. There can be a single coronary artery.

Truncus malformations can be classified either anatomically according to the mode of origin of pulmonary vessels from the common trunk or from a functional point of view, based on the magnitude of blood flow to the lungs. In the common type (type I) of truncus arteriosus, a partially separate pulmonary trunk of variable length exists and gives rise to left and right pulmonary arteries. In type II, each pulmonary artery arises separately but close to the other from the posterior aspect of the truncus. In type III, each pulmonary artery arises from the lateral aspect of the truncus. Less commonly, one pulmonary artery branch may be absent, with aortopulmonary collateral arteries supplying the lung that does not receive a pulmonary artery branch from the truncus.

PATHOPHYSIOLOGY. Pulmonary blood flow is governed by the size of the pulmonary arteries and the pulmonary vascular resistance. In infancy, pulmonary blood flow is usually excessive because pulmonary vascular resistance is not greatly increased. Thus, in the neonate, only minimal cyanosis is present. With time, pulmonary vascular resistance increases, relieving the left ventricular volume load but at the price of increasing cyanosis. When pulmonary vascular resistance reaches systemic levels, Eisenmenger physiology and bidirectional shunting occur. Significant truncal valve regurgitation produces a volume load on both right and left ventricles because of the biventricular origin of the truncal artery.

NATURAL HISTORY. Most deaths from congestive heart failure occur before 1 year of age. Unoperated patients who survive past 1 year most likely present with established pulmonary hypertension. The prevalence of truncal valve regurgitation increases with age, causing biventricular heart failure and increasing susceptibility to endocarditis.

CLINICAL FEATURES

Pediatrics. Infants with truncus arteriosus usually present with mild cyanosis coexisting with the cardiac findings of a large left-to-right shunt. This is the result of excessive pulmonary blood flow due to a low pulmonary vascular resistance. Symptoms of heart failure and poor physical development usually appear in the first weeks or months of life. The most frequent physical findings include cardiomegaly, collapsing peripheral pulses, a loud single second heart sound, a harsh systolic murmur preceded by an ejection click, and a low-pitched mid-diastolic rumbling murmur and bounding pulses. A decrescendo diastolic murmur suggests associated truncal valve regurgitation.

DiGeorge syndrome may be seen with truncus arteriosus. Facial dysmorphism, a high incidence of extracardiac malformations (particularly of the limbs, kidneys, and intestine), atrophy or absence of the thymus gland, T-lymphocyte deficiency, and a predilection to infection also may be features of the clinical presentation.

The physical findings are different if pulmonary blood flow is restricted by a high pulmonary vascular resistance: Cyanosis is prominent, and only a short systolic murmur may be heard in association with an ejection click. Pulmonary vascular obstruction usually does not restrict pulmonary blood flow before 1 year of age.

Adults. Adults presenting with an unrepaired truncus arteriosus have Eisenmenger syndrome and its typical findings.

LABORATORY INVESTIGATIONS (UNREPAIRED)

ECG. This demonstrates biventricular hypertrophy with strain as the pulmonary resistance rises.

Chest Radiography. This demonstrates cardiomegaly with prominent pulmonary arterial markings and by unusually high hilar areas. A right aortic arch occurs in 50 percent of cases.

Echocardiography (Fig. 56–9). In most cases, 2D echocardiography provides a complete diagnosis. The study should demonstrate the overriding truncal root, the origin of the pulmonary arteries, the number of truncal cusps, the origin of the coronary arteries, the functional status of the truncal valve, and VSD size.

Cardiac Catheterization and Angiography. This is rarely necessary and in fact carries a risk of both morbidity and mortality. In general, significant arterial desaturation in the absence of branch pulmonary artery stenosis indicates that the lesion cannot be repaired.

INDICATIONS FOR INTERVENTION. Early surgical intervention is indicated in all cases within the first 2 months of life. In the presence of severe pulmonary hypertension (see ASD section), surgical intervention is usually not performed.

INTERVENTIONAL OPTIONS AND OUTCOMES. Operation consists of closure of the VSD, leaving the aorta arising from the left ventricle; excision of the pulmonary arteries from their truncus origin; and a valve-containing prosthetic conduit or aortic homograft valve conduit between the right ventricle and the pulmonary arteries to establish circulatory continuity.[118] Truncal valve insufficiency is a challenging problem and may require valve replacement or repair.[119]

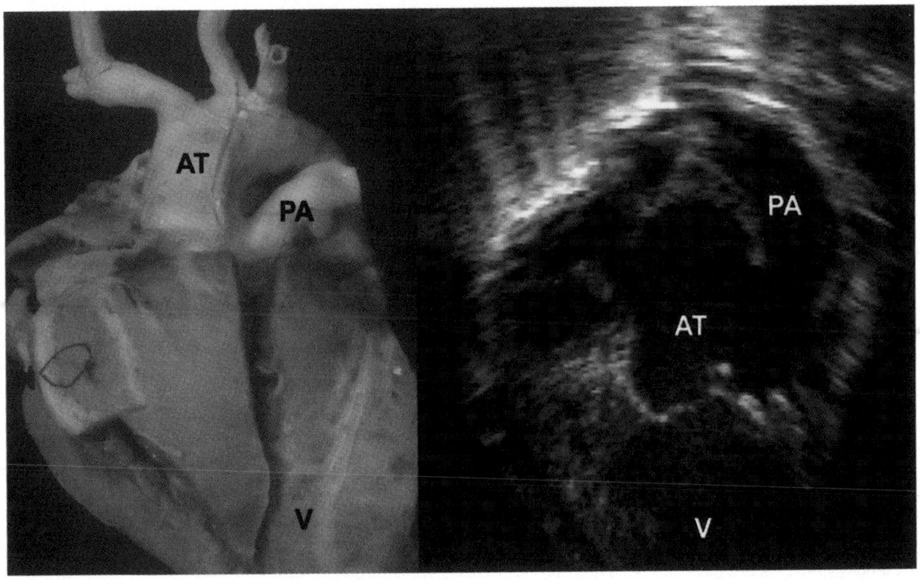

FIGURE 56–9 View of the origin of the pulmonary artery in truncus arteriosus. Note the lateral origin of the pulmonary artery. AT = ascending trunk; PA = pulmonary artery; V = ventricle.

Important risk factors for perioperative death are severe truncal valve regurgitation, interrupted aortic arch, coronary artery anomalies, and age at operation older than 100 days. Patients with only one pulmonary artery are especially prone to early development of severe pulmonary vascular disease.

REPRODUCTIVE ISSUES. Patients with a repaired truncus arteriosus and no hemodynamically important residual lesions should tolerate pregnancy well. Patients with significant conduit obstruction and/or important truncal valve regurgitation need prepregnancy counseling, with correction of the lesions prior to pregnancy and/or careful follow-up throughout pregnancy. Pregnancy is contraindicated in patients with Eisenmenger syndrome, given its 50 percent maternal mortality.

FOLLOW-UP ISSUES. Patients operated on early (<1 year of age) generally do well. However, conduit change is often indicated within the first few years after repair as the patient outgrows its size.[118] Those cases with significant truncal valve stenosis and/or regurgitation may eventually require truncal valve replacement. Patients operated on late (>1 year of age) require careful follow-up for any signs of pulmonary hypertension progression. Endocarditis prophylaxis is required in all patients.

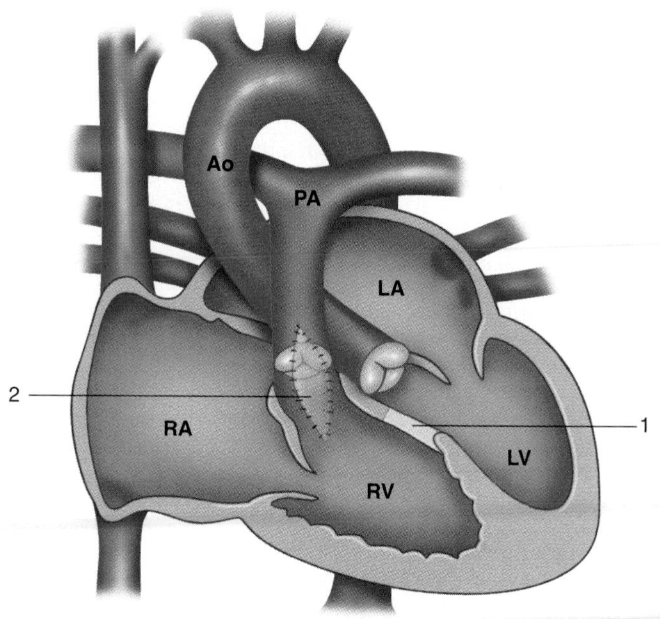

FIGURE 56–11 Diagrammatic representation of the surgical repair of tetralogy of Fallot. 1, Patch closure of ventricular septal defect; 2, right ventricular outflow/main pulmonary artery outflow patch (transannular patch). RA = right atrium; RV = right ventricle; LA = left atrium; LV = left ventricle; Ao = aorta; PA = pulmonary artery. (From Mullins CE, Mayer DC: Congenital Heart Disease: A Diagrammatic Atlas. New York, Wiley-Liss, 1988.)

Cyanotic Heart Disease

Tetralogy of Fallot (Including Tetralogy with Pulmonary Atresia)

MORPHOLOGY (Figs. 56–10 and 56–11). The four components of tetralogy of Fallot are an outlet VSD, obstruction to right ventricular outflow, overriding of the aorta (< 50 percent), and right ventricular hypertrophy. The fundamental abnormality contributing to each of these features is anterior and cephalad deviation of the outlet septum, which is malaligned with respect to the trabecular septum. Tetralogy may also coexist with an AV septal defect. Right ventricular outflow tract obstruction is variable. There is often a stenotic, bicuspid pulmonary valve with supravalvular hypoplasia. The dominant site of obstruction is usually at the subvalve level. In some cases the outflow tract is atretic, and the heart can be diagnosed as having tetralogy of Fallot with pulmonary atresia (also known as *complex pulmonary atresia* when major aortopulmonary collateral arteries are present). The management and outcome for patients with major aortopulmonary collateral arteries are significantly different from those with less extreme forms of tetralogy and are discussed separately at the end of this section.

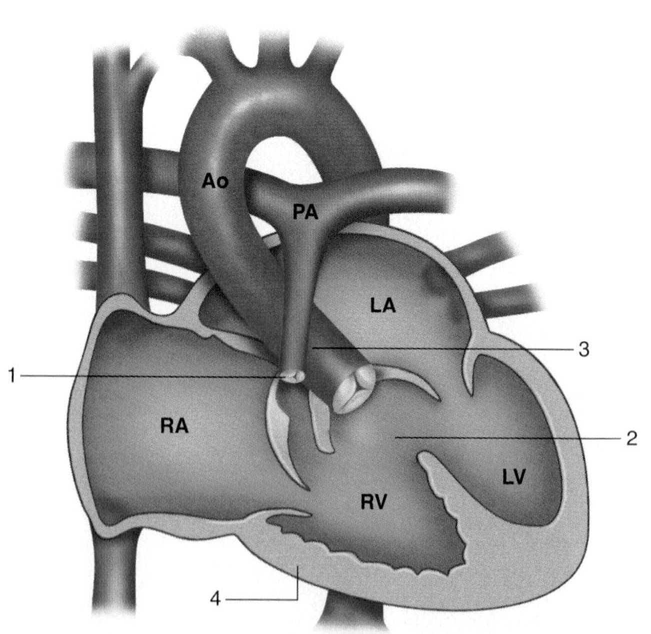

FIGURE 56–10 Diagrammatic representation of tetralogy of Fallot. 1, Pulmonary stenosis; 2, ventricular septal defect; 3, overriding aorta; 4, right ventricle hypertrophy. RA = right atrium; RV = right ventricle; LA = left atrium; LV = left ventricle; Ao = aorta; PA = pulmonary artery. (From Mullins CE, Mayer DC: Congenital Heart Disease: A Diagrammatic Atlas. New York, Wiley-Liss, 1988.)

Associated Anomalies. A right aortic arch occurs in about 25 percent of patients, and abnormalities of the course of the coronary arteries occur in approximately 5 percent. The most common anomaly is when the anterior descending artery originates from the right coronary artery and may course anteriorly to cross the infundibulum of the right ventricle. Absent pulmonary valve syndrome is a rare form of tetralogy in which stenosis and regurgitation of the right ventricular outflow tract is due to a markedly stenotic pulmonary valve ring with poorly formed or absent valve leaflets. The pulmonary arteries are markedly dilated or aneurysmal. This may produce airway compression at birth, a poor prognostic feature.

PATHOPHYSIOLOGY. In the absence of alternative sources of pulmonary blood flow, the degree of cyanosis reflects the severity of right ventricular outflow tract obstruction and the level of systemic vascular resistance. There is right-to-left shunting across the VSD. A tetralogy "spell" is an acute fall in arterial saturation and it may be life threatening. Its treatment is aimed at relieving obstruction and increasing (e.g., with norepinephrine) systemic resistance. Relief of hypoxic pain with morphine, intravenous propranolol, and systemic vasoconstriction (e.g., squatting) usually reverses the cyanosis.

NATURAL HISTORY. Progressive hypoxemia in the first years of life is expected. Survival to adult life is rare without palliation or correction. The presence of additional sources of blood supply (see later) modifies the rate of progression of cyanosis and its complications.

CLINICAL FEATURES

Unoperated Patients. There is variable cyanosis. A right ventricular impulse and systolic thrill are often palpable along the left sternal border. An early systolic ejection sound that is aortic in origin may be heard at the lower left sternal border and apex; the second heart sound is usually single. The intensity and duration of the systolic ejection murmur vary inversely with the severity of obstruction—the opposite of the relation that exists in patients with pulmonary stenosis and an intact ventricular septum. With extreme outflow tract stenosis or pulmonary atresia and during an attack of paroxysmal hypoxemia, no murmur or only a very short, faint murmur may be detected. A continuous murmur faintly audible over the anterior or posterior chest reflects flow through enlarged bronchial collateral vessels.

After Surgery, Palliated. Progressive cyanosis with its complications can result from worsening right ventricular outflow tract obstruction, gradual stenosis and occlusion of palliative aortopulmonary shunts, or the development of pulmonary hypertension (sometimes seen after Waterston or Potts shunts). Progressive aortic dilation and aortic regurgitation are becoming increasingly recognized. Central cyanosis and clubbing are invariably present.

After Surgery, Repaired. After intracardiac repair more than 85 percent of patients are asymptomatic on follow-up,[120] although objective testing may demonstrate a marked reduction in maximal performance.[121] Palpitations from atrial and ventricular arrhythmias and exertional dyspnea from progressive right ventricular dilation secondary to chronic pulmonary regurgitation or severe residual right ventricular outflow tract obstruction occur in 10 to 15 percent of patients at 20 years after initial repair. An ascending aortic aneurysm and progressive aortic regurgitation from a dilated aortic root can also be present.[122] There may be a parasternal right ventricular lift and a soft and delayed P_2 with a low-pitched diastolic murmur from pulmonary regurgitation. A systolic ejection murmur from right ventricular outflow tract obstruction, a high-pitched diastolic murmur from aortic regurgitation, and a pansystolic murmur from a VSD patch leak can also be heard.

Tetralogy of Fallot with Pulmonary Atresia and Major Aortopulmonary Collateral Arteries. This subgroup represents one of the greatest challenges in CHD. The aim of unifocalization surgery is to amalgamate all the sources of pulmonary blood flow and to establish unobstructed right ventricular-to-pulmonary artery continuity while achieving a normal pulmonary artery pressure and a closed ventricular septum.[123] If an adequate number of segments can be unifocalized in an unobstructed fashion, then coincident intracardiac repair can be contemplated. When this is not possible, a combined interventional catheterization and surgical approach is required.[124] Balloon dilation and stenting of stenosed arteries and anastomoses can "rehabilitate" segmental supply and allow subsequent VSD closure, or if already closed, reduce right ventricular pressure.

LABORATORY INVESTIGATIONS

ECG. Right axis deviation with right ventricular and right atrial hypertrophy is common. In adults with repaired tetralogy of Fallot, a complete right bundle branch block following repair has been the rule. QRS width may reflect the degree of right ventricular dilation.[61,125] A QRS duration 180 milliseconds or longer is a risk factor for sustained ventricular tachycardia and sudden death.

Chest Radiography. Characteristically, there is a normal-sized boot-shaped heart (*coeur en sabot*) with prominence of the right ventricle and a concavity in the region of the underdeveloped right ventricular outflow tract and main pulmonary artery. The pulmonary vascular markings are typically diminished, and the aortic arch may be on the right side (25 percent). The ascending aorta is often prominent.

Echocardiography (Fig. 56–12). A complete diagnosis can usually be established by echo-Doppler alone. The study should identify the malaligned and nonrestrictive VSD and overriding aorta (<50 percent override) and the presence and degree of right ventricular outflow tract obstruction (infundibular, valvular, and/or pulmonary arterial stenosis). It is rare that any other investigations are required prior to corrective surgery. The exception to this rule is when there are additional sources of pulmonary blood flow. In patients with *repaired* tetralogy of Fallot, residual pulmonary stenosis and regurgitation, residual VSD, right and left ventricular sizes and function, aortic root size, and the degree of aortic regurgitation should be assessed.

Cardiac Catheterization and Angiocardiography. Although echocardiography, MRA, and fast CT may delineate the presence and proximal course of the pulmonary blood vessels, the preoperative assessment of tetralogy with pulmonary atresia with major aortopulmonary collateral arteries must include delineation of the arterial supply to both lungs by selective catheterization and angiography to show the course and segmental supply from the collateral arteries and central pulmonary arteries. Major aortopulmonary collateral arteries usually arise from the descending aorta at the level of the tracheal bifurcation.

MRI. The goals of MRI examination after tetralogy of Fallot repair include the quantitative assessment of left and particularly right ventricular volumes, stroke volumes and ejection fraction; imaging of the anatomy of the right ventricular outflow tract, the pulmonary arteries, the aorta and

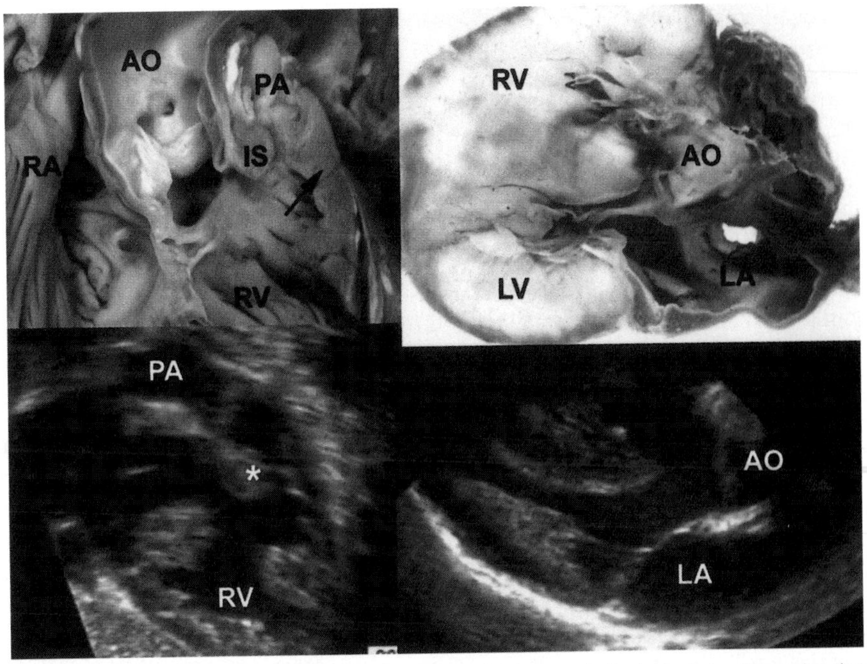

FIGURE 56–12 Montage of tetralogy of Fallot. The two left images are in the right anterior oblique view that demonstrates the anteriorly deviated infundibular septum and the ventricular septal defect. The arrow on the specimen points to the hypertrophied septoparietal trabeculations. The right images demonstrate the overriding aorta and the ventricular septal defect. AO = aorta; IS = infundibular septum; LA = left atrium; PA = pulmonary artery; RA = right atrium; RV = right ventricle.

aortopulmonary collaterals; and quantifying pulmonary, aortic, and tricuspid regurgitation.

INDICATIONS FOR INTERVENTION

Children. Symptomatic infants are now repaired at any age, and elective repair in asymptomatic infants during the first 6 months is advocated by many.[126,127] This is often at the expense of a transannular patch enlargement of the right ventricular outflow tract, which may be a risk factor for later failure. Marked hypoplasia of the pulmonary arteries, small body size, and prematurity are relative contraindications for early corrective operation, and these patients may be successfully palliated by balloon dilation of the right ventricular outflow tract and pulmonary arteries.

Adults, Unoperated. For unoperated adults, surgical repair is still recommended because the results are gratifying and the operative risk is comparable to pediatric series provided there is no serious coexisting morbidity.[128]

Palliated. Palliation was seldom intended as a permanent treatment strategy, and most of these patients should undergo surgical repair. In particular, palliated patients with increasing cyanosis and erythrocytosis (from gradual shunt stenosis or development of pulmonary hypertension), left ventricular dilation, or aneurysm formation in the shunt should undergo intracardiac repair with takedown of the shunt unless irreversible pulmonary hypertension has developed.

Repaired. The following situations *may* warrant intervention after repair: a residual VSD with a shunt greater than 1.5/1.0; residual pulmonary stenosis (either the native right ventricular outflow or valved conduit if one is present) with right ventricular pressure ⅔ or more of systemic pressure; or severe pulmonary regurgitation associated with substantial right ventricular dilation/dysfunction, exercise intolerance, or sustained arrhythmias.[83] The development of major cardiac arrhythmias, most commonly atrial flutter/fibrillation or sustained ventricular tachycardia, usually reflects hemodynamic deterioration and should be treated accordingly. Surgery is occasionally necessary for significant aortic regurgitation associated with symptoms and/or progressive left ventricular dilation and for aortic root enlargement of 55 mm or more. Rapid enlargement of a right ventricular outflow tract aneurysm needs surgical attention.

INTERVENTIONAL OPTIONS

Surgery. Reparative surgery involves closing the VSD with a Dacron patch and relieving the right ventricular outflow tract obstruction. The latter may involve resection of infundibular muscle, and insertion of a right ventricular outflow tract or transannular patch—a patch across the pulmonary valve annulus that disrupts the integrity of the pulmonary valve and causes important pulmonary regurgitation. When an anomalous coronary artery crosses the right ventricular outflow tract and precludes transection of the latter, an extracardiac conduit is placed between the right ventricle and pulmonary artery, bypassing the right ventricular outflow tract obstruction. A patent foramen ovale or secundum ASD is closed. Additional treatable lesions such as muscular VSDs, PDA, and aortopulmonary collaterals should also be addressed at the time of surgery.

Reoperation is necessary in 10 to 15 percent of patients after reparative surgery over a 20-year follow-up.[47] For persistent right ventricular outflow tract obstruction, resection of residual infundibular stenosis or placement of a right ventricular outflow or transannular patch, with or without pulmonary arterioplasty, can be performed. Occasionally, an extracardiac valved conduit may be necessary. Pulmonary valve replacement (either homograft or xenograft) is used to treat severe pulmonary regurgitation. Concomitant tricuspid valve annuloplasty may be performed for moderate or severe tricuspid regurgitation. Concomitant cryoablation should often be performed at the time of surgery for patients with either preexisting atrial or ventricular arrhythmias.[129]

Interventional. Significant branch pulmonary artery stenosis can be managed with balloon dilation and usually stent insertion. A catheter-delivered pulmonary bioprosthesis is being developed.

INTERVENTIONAL OUTCOMES. The overall survival of patients who have had initial operative repair is excellent, provided the VSD has been closed and the right ventricular outflow tract obstruction has been relieved. A 25-year survival of 94 percent has been reported.[130] Pulmonary valve replacement for chronic pulmonary regurgitation or right ventricular outflow tract obstruction after initial intracardiac repair can be done safely with a mortality rate of 1 percent.[131] Pulmonary valve replacement, when performed for significant pulmonary regurgitation, leads to an improvement in exercise tolerance as well as right ventricular dimension and function.[132] Sudden death can occur. Ventricular tachycardia can arise at the site of the right ventriculotomy, from VSD patch sutures, or from the right ventricular outflow tract. Patients at high risk for sudden death include those with right ventricular dilation and a QRS duration of 180 milliseconds or more on their ECG.[61] Moderate to severe left ventricular dysfunction is another risk factor for sudden death.[133] The reported incidence of sudden death is approximately 5 percent, which accounts for approximately one-third of late deaths over the first 20 years of follow-up.

FOLLOW-UP. All patients should have expert cardiology follow-up every 1 to 2 years.

Fontan Procedure–Requiring Lesions

The next four sections describe lesions usually or often treated with a Fontan procedure. These include tricuspid atresia, hypoplastic left heart syndrome, double-inlet ventricle, and isomerism. *Fontan procedure* has become a generic term to describe a palliative surgical procedure that redirects the systemic venous return directly to the pulmonary arteries without passing through a subpulmonary ventricle. It is performed in patients having a "functionally single" ventricle or when an intracardiac repair is not possible even though there are two good-sized ventricles. Although undoubtedly imperfect, the Fontan circuit restores an in-series pulmonary-to-systemic circulation, removing the chronic volume load of the systemic ventricle previously supporting a parallel circuit of pulmonary and systemic circulations. The earliest iteration of the Fontan procedure was a simple "atriopulmonary" connection, whereby the right atrium or its appendage was anastomosed to the pulmonary arteries. Because of the long-term problems of atrial dilation, arrhythmia, and thrombosis, this procedure has been abandoned in favor of hemodynamically superior versions. In the early 1990s the total cavopulmonary anastomosis was introduced. This consisted of a direct, end-to-side superior cavopulmonary anastomosis (bidirectional Glenn operation) in combination with an intraatrial baffle or tube connection of the inferior vena cava to the underside of the confluent pulmonary arteries. More recently the inferior vena cava has been directed to the pulmonary arteries via an extracardiac conduit, completely excluding the atrium from the circuit. It remains to be seen whether these modifications will have the desired effect of reducing late morbidity, and all patients will require regular and careful review in special centers.

Tricuspid Atresia (Absent Right Atrioventricular Connection)

MORPHOLOGY. *Classic tricuspid atresia* is best described as absence of the right AV connection (Figs. 56–13 and 56–14). Consequently, there must be an ASD. There is usually hypoplasia of the morphological right ventricle, which communicates to the dominant ventricle via a VSD. Patients may be subdivided into those with concordant ventriculoarterial connections and normally related great arteries (70 to 80 percent of cases) and those with discordant connections, where the aorta arises from the small right ventricle and is fed via the VSD. Associated lesions in the latter group include subaortic stenosis and aortic arch anomalies.

PATHOPHYSIOLOGY. The clinical picture and management are dominated by issues related to the ventriculoarterial connections. All patients have "mixing" of atrial blood, and their degree of cyanosis is governed by the amount of pulmonary blood flow. Patients with concordant ventriculoarterial connections tend to be more cyanosed (depending on the size of the VSD), whereas those with discordant connections are pinker and tend to develop heart failure (because the unobstructed pulmonary circulation arises directly from the left ventricle). Some present with a critical reduction of systemic blood flow, because of obstruction at the VSD and/or associated aortic arch anomalies, and behave much like hypoplastic left heart syndrome.

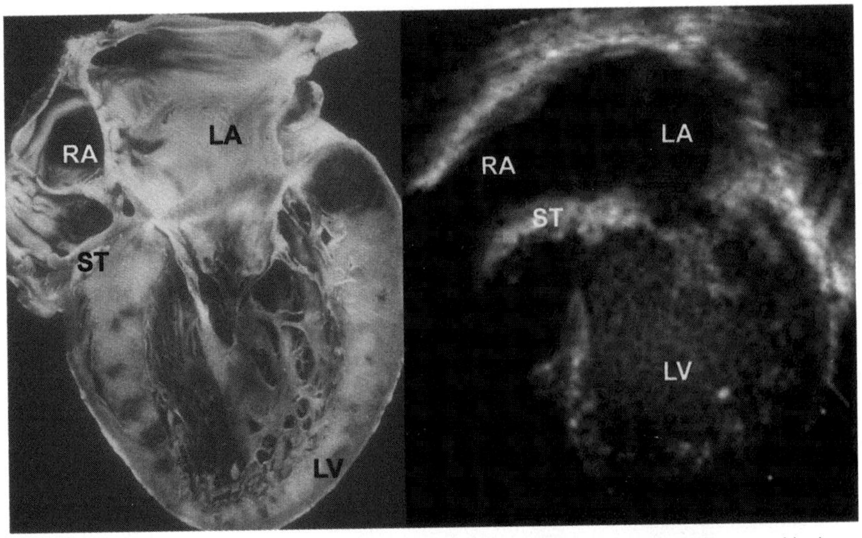

FIGURE 56–13 Apical four-chamber view in univentricular connection of left ventricular type with absent right connection (tricuspid atresia). Note the wedge of sulcus tissue in the floor of the right atrium. LA = left atrium; LV = left ventricle; RA = right atrium; ST = sulcus tissue.

LABORATORY INVESTIGATIONS

ECG. There is often left axis deviation, right atrial enlargement, and left ventricular hypertrophy. Left atrial enlargement may be present if pulmonary flow is high.

Chest Radiography. There is usually situs solitus, levocardia, and a left-sided aortic arch. The heart size and pulmonary vascular markings vary with the amount of pulmonary blood flow. The main pulmonary trunk is inapparent. There is a right aortic arch in 25 percent.

Echocardiogram. This establishes the full segmental diagnosis. The size of the ASD, VSD, and aortic arch all must be carefully assessed.

Cardiac Catheterization. This is rarely required for initial diagnosis or management. It can be useful to assess the degree of subaortic stenosis (by assessing the change in left ventricle-to-aortic pressure gradient while performing a dobutamine challenge) and is mandatory to measure the pulmonary artery pressure and resistance prior to venopulmonary connections.

MANAGEMENT OPTIONS. In those with concordant ventriculoarterial connections and severe cyanosis, a systemic-to-pulmonary shunt is performed in the first 6 to 8 weeks of life, and in older children, a primary bidirectional Glenn procedure can be considered. In infants with discordant arterial connections, early palliation ranges from pulmonary artery banding to reduce pulmonary blood flow when there is no subaortic narrowing, to a full Norwood stage 1 procedure in those presenting with severe stenosis and a hypoplastic ascending aorta and arch.

The aim of early palliation is to prepare for a Fontan procedure. This should be performed only when there is good ventricular function, unobstructed systemic blood flow, and minimal AV valve regurgitation. Candidates for these corrective procedures must also have normal pulmonary vascular resistance and a low pulmonary resistance, a mean pulmonary artery pressure less than 15 mm Hg, and pulmonary arteries of adequate size.

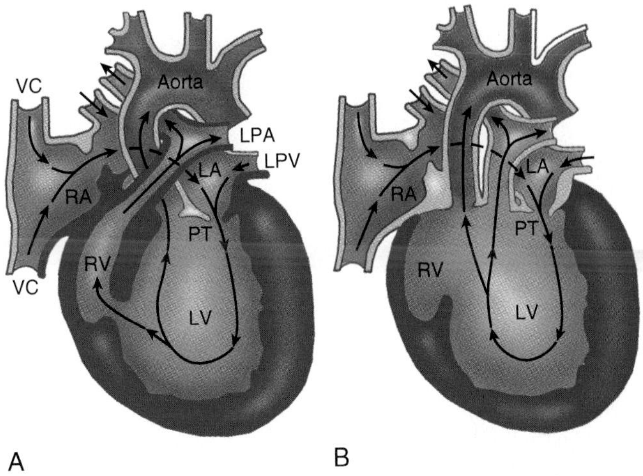

FIGURE 56–14 **A,** Tricuspid atresia with normally related great arteries, a small ventricular septal defect, diminutive right ventricular chamber, and narrowed outflow tract. **B,** An example of tricuspid atresia and complete transposition of the great arteries in which the left ventricular chamber is essentially a common ventricle, with the aorta arising from an infundibular component (RV) of the common ventricle. VC = vena cava; RA = right atrium; LA = left atrium; RV = right ventricle; LV = left ventricle; LPV = left pulmonary vein; LPA = left pulmonary artery; PT = pulmonary trunk. (**A** and **B,** Modified from Edwards JE, Burchell HB: Congenital tricuspid atresia: Classification. Med Clin North Am 33:1177, 1949.)

Hypoplastic Left Heart Syndrome

DEFINITION. *Hypoplastic left heart syndrome* is a generic term used to describe a group of closely related cardiac anomalies characterized by underdevelopment of the left cardiac chambers, in association with atresia or stenosis of the aortic and/or the mitral orifices, and hypoplasia of the aorta. The term should be restricted to those with normally connected hearts with concordant AV and ventriculoarterial connections. Hypoplastic left heart syndrome (Fig. 56–15) is characterized by duct-dependent systemic blood flow and so tends to present with severe symptoms within the first week of life, as ductal constriction occurs. Untreated, the disease is almost uniformly fatal in infancy. In the past, many infants would present with severe acidemic circulatory collapse, but this is becoming less frequent as fetal ultrasound screening for cardiac anomalies becomes more generally available and successful. Fetal diagnosis allows for a planned delivery and institution of prostaglandin therapy from birth and has now been proven to reduce subsequent preoperative morbidity

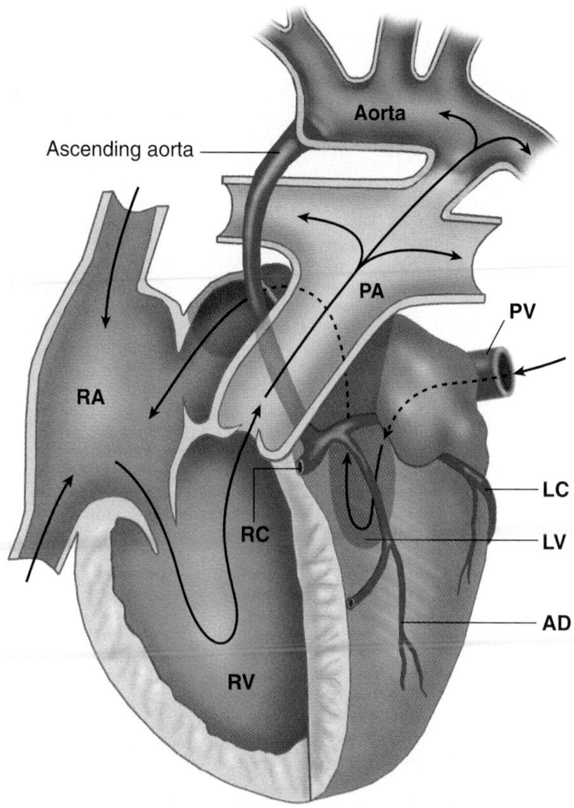

FIGURE 56–15 Hypoplastic left heart with aortic hypoplasia, aortic valve atresia, and a hypoplastic mitral valve and left ventricle. AD = anterior descending; RA = right atrium; RV = right ventricle; RC = right coronary artery; PA = pulmonary artery; PV = pulmonary vein; LC = left circumflex. (From Neufeld HN, Adams P Jr, Edwards JE, et al: Diagnosis of aortic atresia by retrograde aortography. Circulation 25:278, 1962.)

and perioperative mortality during the first stage of surgical repair.

PATHOPHYSIOLOGY. It remains uncertain whether hypoplastic left heart syndrome reflects a primary myocardial disease or is a consequence of a structural or hemodynamic abnormality. There is no doubt that in some patients, an apparently isolated dilated cardiomyopathy in early fetal life may evolve (as a result of a subsequent lack of left ventricular growth) into hypoplastic left heart syndrome later in gestation. Congenital structural abnormalities clearly play a significant role as well. This is exemplified by the effect of isolated valvular stenosis to produce a continuum of hypoplastic left heart syndrome to critical aortic stenosis with a normal-sized left ventricle. It is likely therefore that hypoplastic left heart syndrome is multifactorial in origin.

CLINICAL FEATURES. The diagnosis should be considered in any infant with the sudden onset of circulatory collapse and severe lactic acidosis. As such, it must be distinguished from neonatal sepsis and metabolic disorders. Until excluded, any child presenting in this way should be treated with prostaglandin, which may have a dramatic positive effect if there is an underlying cardiac abnormality and little effect if there is not.

LABORATORY INVESTIGATIONS

ECG. This frequently shows right axis deviation, right atrial and ventricular enlargement, and ST and T wave abnormalities in the left precordial leads.

Chest Radiography. This usually shows some cardiac enlargement shortly after birth, but with clinical deterioration there may be marked cardiomegaly and increased pulmonary venous and arterial vascular markings.

Echocardiography (Fig. 56–16). Cross-sectional echocardiography provides a full segmental diagnosis. In its classic form, the left ventricular cavity is small, with a diminutive mitral valve. The myocardium may be thinned or be of normal thickness, but the endocardium is usually thickened, consistent with endocardial fibroelastosis. There may be fistulous communications between the left ventricular cavity and the coronary arteries, a feature much more likely when the mitral valve is patent rather than atretic. The aortic root is usually diminutive, less than 4 to 5 mm in diameter at the level of the sinuses of Valsalva and narrowed in its ascending portion. The aortic arch is usually larger, but there is often a juxtaductal coarctation. The duct varies in size according to treatment, and assessment of this and the size of the interatrial communication are crucial to management. There may be profound desaturation and rapid demise (because of a combination of reduced pulmonary blood flow and pulmonary edema) in children with an intact atrial septum or restrictive patent foramen ovale.

MANAGEMENT OPTIONS. Early treatment with prostaglandin is mandatory. Those presenting in shock require paralysis, mechanical ventilation, and inotropic support. Crucial to managing these patients is maintenance of a balanced pulmonary and systemic blood flow. The cardiac output is fixed and is distributed according to the relative magnitude of the systemic and pulmonary vascular resistance. Thus, measures to elevate the pulmonary resistance (by imposing hypercapnia or by alveolar hypoxia) and reduce the systemic resistance (using vasodilators) are frequently required.

Surgical Treatment. Staged surgical management now provides long-term palliation to most patients with hypoplastic left heart syndrome. The first stage, often referred to as the *Norwood procedure*, now has many versions, but its essence is the creation of an unobstructed communication between the right ventricle and an unobstructed aorta. The right ventricular to aortic connection is accomplished by direct connection between the transected proximal pulmonary trunk and ascending aorta, usually with a patch extending around the augmented aortic arch. Pulmonary blood flow is established via a systemic-to-pulmonary shunt, or the more recently introduced right ventricle-to-pulmonary artery conduit. The

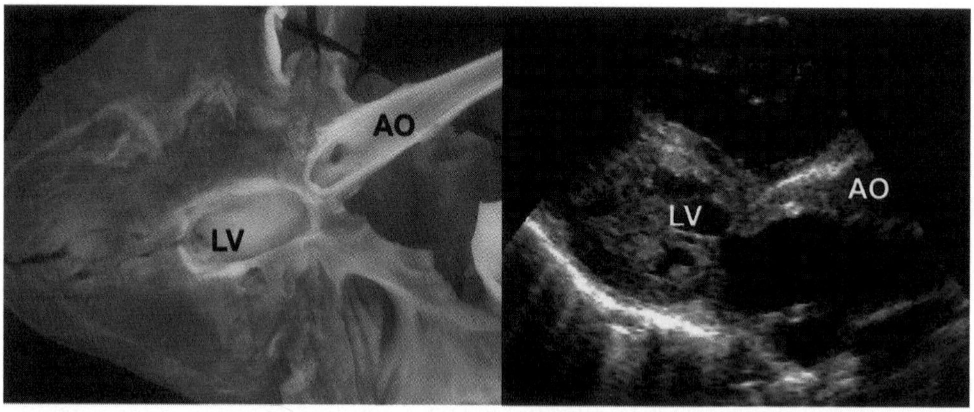

FIGURE 56–16 Long-axis view of the left ventricle and aorta in hypoplastic left heart syndrome. Note the associated endocardial fibroelastosis in the specimen. AO = aorta, LV = left ventricle.

PDA is ligated and a large interatrial communication is created. Early results of this procedure were poor, but survival rates higher than 85 percent have recently been published. Institutional variations, the interval mortality, and those unsuitable to progress to stage 2 must also be taken into account, however, and in some centers, the preferred operation is cardiac transplantation.

Stage 2 consists of an end-to-side superior vena cava-to-pulmonary artery connection (bidirectional Glenn procedure) or a hemi-Fontan (incorporating the roof of the atrium into the pulmonary artery anastomosis. This is performed at approximately 6 months of age as an intermediate step before stage 3, a Fontan operation.

ADULT ISSUES. The survivors of the earliest attempts at staged Norwood palliation are just now entering adult life. Their issues are likely to be common to all late survivors of Fontan palliation.[134]

Double-Inlet Ventricle

DEFINITION. Double-inlet connection falls under the umbrella of univentricular AV connections. These hearts are defined by having more than 50 percent of both AV connections connected to a dominant ventricle. In practice this usually means the whole of one and greater than 50 percent of the alternative junction is connected to either a left or right ventricle. When there is a common junction, then more than 75 percent of the junction must be connected to the dominant ventricle.

MORPHOLOGY. In about 75 percent of patients, the dominant ventricle is a left ventricle that is separated from the right ventricle by a VSD. In 20 percent the dominant ventricle is a right ventricle and the small, incomplete ventricle is of left ventricular apical morphology. In only 5 percent of cases is there truly only one ventricle in the ventricular mass. In double-inlet left ventricle the most common ventriculoarterial connection is discordant. Thus the aorta arises from the small right ventricle and is fed via the VSD, and the generally unobstructed pulmonary artery arises from the left ventricle. Aortic and aortic arch anomalies are frequent in these patients.

PATHOPHYSIOLOGY. The basic circulatory physiology of *double-inlet left ventricle* is identical to that of tricuspid atresia. There is common mixing of systemic and pulmonary venous blood, which is then ejected from the left ventricle into the pulmonary artery (with discordant connections) or aorta (with concordant connections). In the former, the blood must pass through the VSD to gain egress to the aorta. Subaortic stenosis, aortic hypoplasia, and arch anomalies are therefore common. In *double-inlet right ventricle*, it is those patients with concordant ventriculoarterial connections who are at particular risk of systemic outflow obstruction. One or the other or both of the two AV valves (when present) may be stenotic, atretic, or regurgitant. Under these circumstances the integrity of the atrial septum becomes important. If there is left or right atrial outflow obstruction, then a septectomy or septostomy will be required.

CLINICAL FEATURES. When there is critical reduction of systemic outflow, infants may be duct dependent and present with acidemic shock. Conversely, when pulmonary blood flow is reduced, presentation may be with severe cyanosis or with duct-dependent pulmonary blood flow. Other patients may not present in the neonatal period and will develop heart failure because of increased pulmonary blood flow. Patients undergo the same surgical algorithms as those with tricuspid atresia and so ultimately will undergo a Fontan operation. Their clinical issues are typical of any patient after this procedure.

LABORATORY INVESTIGATIONS

ECG. This is highly variable. Ventricular hypertrophy appropriate to the dominant ventricle is expected.

Chest Radiography. This is similarly variable and rarely diagnostic.

Echocardiography (Fig. 56–17). A full segmental diagnosis should be possible in all patients. Particular attention should be paid to defining AV valve anomalies and the presence and anatomy of any subaortic obstruction. This may develop, even if not present at birth, and should be part of the routine surveillance of these patients.

INDICATIONS AND OPTIONS FOR INTERVENTION. Survival without intervention may be prolonged, but at the expense of increasing cyanosis (when there is restriction to pulmonary blood flow) or pulmonary vascular disease (when there is unrestricted pulmonary blood flow). Those born with restricted systemic blood flow require urgent surgical intervention, usually undergoing a Norwood-type repair to establish the pulmonary valve as the unobstructed systemic outflow tract. Pulmonary artery banding is only offered to those infants with pulmonary overcirculation, heart failure, and unobstructed systemic outflow. Subsequently, and sometimes as the primary procedure, a bidirectional Glenn anastomosis is performed as a prelude to a Fontan procedure.

FOLLOW-UP. These patients should be reviewed frequently and in a center conversant with the issues of the Fontan operation.

Isomerism

DEFINITION. For the purposes of describing the cardiac manifestations, isomerism describes the situation where both atrial appendages have either left or right anatomical features (i.e., bilateral right or bilateral left atrial appendages).

MORPHOLOGY. There have been many attempts to describe hearts with complex abnormalities of visceral and atrial situs, whereby normal lateralization is lost. Terms such as *heterotaxy, asplenia,* and *polysplenia* fail to adequately describe either the visceral or cardiac manifestations with enough precision. The left atrial appendage is characterized by its tubular shape and pectinate muscles confined to the

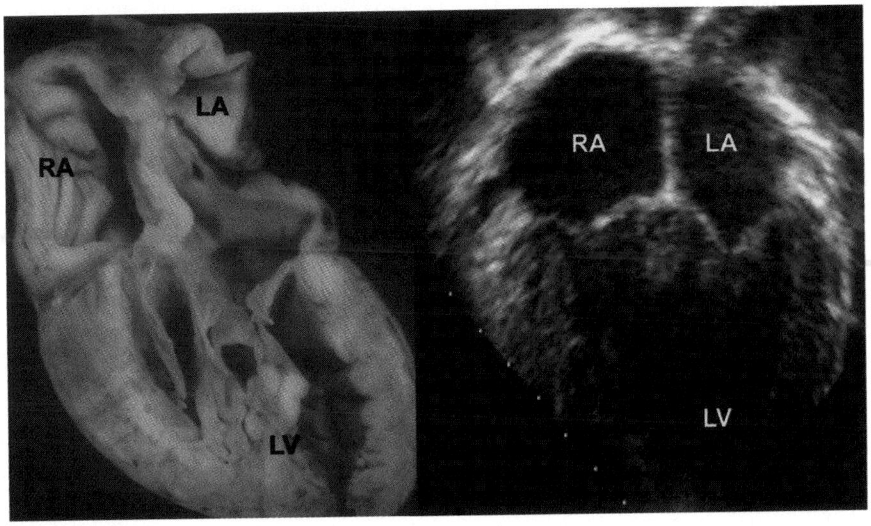

FIGURE 56–17 Apical four-chamber view in a double-inlet univentricular connection of left ventricular type with two atrioventricular valves. LA = left atrium; LV = left ventricle; RA = right atrium.

appendage. The pectinate muscles of the triangular right atrial appendage extend from its broad junction with the atrium, to extend around the vestibule or AV junction. Thus the arrangement of the atria (be it usual, mirror image, right or left isomerism) can be defined independent of the venous anatomy.

In left isomerism it is not unusual to have a biventricular AV connection, with separate AV junctions. A common junction (with an AV septal defect) is seen in approximately 30 percent of cases of left isomerism and more than 90 percent of hearts with isomerism of the right atrial appendages. Concordant ventriculoarterial connections predominate in left isomerism, and a double-outlet right ventricle with an anterior aorta is most frequently seen when there is right isomerism. The venous connections are very variable. These variations significantly affect the clinical and interventional management of these patients.

Isomerism of the Right Atrial Appendages

CLINICAL FEATURES. Bilateral "right-sidedness" results in a pattern of visceral abnormalities sometimes described as asplenia syndrome. The liver is midline, both lungs are trilobed with symmetrically short bronchi on the chest radiograph, and the spleen is hypoplastic or absent. The latter mandates immunization against pneumococcal infection and continuous penicillin prophylaxis against gram-positive sepsis. The diagnosis can be inferred from the bronchial pattern on the chest radiograph but most often is established by cross-sectional echocardiography because of early presentation with severe CHD. Abdominal scanning shows ipsilateral arrangement of the aorta and an anterior inferior vena cava. The intracardiac anatomy is most often that of an AV septal defect with varying degrees of right ventricular dominance, and frequently there is associated double-outlet right ventricle with an anterior aorta and subpulmonary stenosis or atresia. Thus cyanosis is the most common presentation. The inferior vena cava may connect to either right atrium, and superior vena cavae are often lateralized and separate. It is the pulmonary venous drainage that is crucial to the presentation and outcome of these children. By definition, the pulmonary veins are draining anomalously to one or other right atrium, but frequently this is indirect and/or obstructed. Adequate repair of the latter is fundamental to the outcome of these children, who almost uniformly ultimately require a Fontan procedure.

MANAGEMENT OPTIONS AND OUTCOMES. Initial palliation is usually directed toward regulating pulmonary blood flow and dealing with anomalies of pulmonary venous connection. Subsequently these patients (even when there are equal-sized ventricles) are treated along a Fontan algorithm. This is because repair of complete AV septal defect in the setting of abnormal ventriculoarterial connections is technically difficult or impossible. Thus a unilateral, or bilateral superior cavopulmonary anastomosis is performed at approximately 6 months of age, followed when possible by a Fontan procedure when aged 2 to 4 years.

The long-term outcome of surgery for right isomerism, however, has been poor. Improved early palliation and a staged approach toward the Fontan procedure have led to improved results. The prognosis for these infants, particularly when there is obstruction to pulmonary venous return, must remain guarded.

Isomerism of the Left Atrial Appendages

CLINICAL FEATURES. These patients have bilateral "left-sidedness." Hence they have two left lungs and bronchi, tend to have polysplenia, and frequently have malrotation of the gut. The cardiac abnormalities tend to be less severe than those of right isomerism. These patients are particularly prone to develop atrial arrhythmias, since the normal sinoatrial node is a right atrial structure and is usually absent in these patients. The ECG often shows an abnormal P wave axis, or wandering pacemaker. The anatomical diagnosis is usually established by echocardiography. The abdominal great vessels are both to the right or left of the spine, as with right isomerism, but in left isomerism the vein is a posterior azygos vein that continues to connect to a left- or right-sided superior vena cava. The intrahepatic inferior vena cava is absent in 90 percent, and under these circumstances the hepatic veins drain directly to the atria. The pulmonary venous connection needs to be defined precisely prior to any surgical intervention. Pulmonary arteriovenous malformations are not infrequently seen in patients with left isomerism. These can lead to cyanosis in unoperated or operated patients. The intracardiac anatomy varies from essentially normal to very complex. Again, AV septal defect (partial and complete) is overrepresented but with less frequent ventricular imbalance and abnormalities of ventriculoarterial connection.

MANAGEMENT OPTIONS. A biventricular repair is achieved in many more of these patients, albeit with the need for complex atrial baffle surgery to separate the systemic and pulmonary venous returns. The long-term outcome for patients with left isomerism is therefore much better than for those with right isomerism. The issues are very much those related to the type of surgery, but monitoring for arrhythmia needs to be even more intense than usual.

The Fontan Patient (Fig. 56–18)

BACKGROUND. As stated in the introduction to this section, such is the uncertain nature of the Fontan circulation, and the frequency of its failure,[135,136] that all patients should be followed regularly in a specialized center for CHD, and new symptoms should prompt early re-evaluation in such a center.

Since its description for the surgical management of tricuspid atresia in 1971, the Fontan procedure has become the definitive palliative surgical treatment when a biventricular repair is not possible. The principle is diversion of the systemic venous return directly to the pulmonary arteries without passing through a subpulmonary ventricle. Over the years, many modifications of the original procedure have been described and performed, namely, direct atriopulmonary connection, total cavopulmonary connection, and extracardiac conduit. Fenestration (5-mm diameter) of the Fontan circuit into the left atrium is sometimes performed at the time of surgery in high-risk patients, permitting right-to-left shunting and decompression of the Fontan circuit.

PATHOPHYSIOLOGY. Elevation of the central venous pressure and a reduced cardiac output (sometimes at rest[137] but always on exercise[138]) are inevitable consequences of the Fontan procedure. Small adverse changes in ventricular function (particularly diastolic), circuit efficiency (elevated pulmonary resistance, obstruction, thrombosis), or the onset of arrhythmia, all potentially lead to major symptomatic deterioration.

Although it is reasonable to describe patients after the Fontan procedure as existing in a form of chronic heart failure (since their right atrial pressure must be high), this is seldom due to marked systolic dysfunction.[139] Indeed, a small elevation in ventricular diastolic pressure may be much more harmful. Thus it may be incorrect to treat these patients with traditional heart failure medications. In a randomized, blinded placebo-controlled study, ACE inhibition failed to improve functional performance, and some indices worsened.[140]

The more "steamlined" Fontan circulations (total cavopulmonary anastomosis, extracardiac conduit) that exclude the right atrium from the circulation have demonstrably better fluid dynamic properties and improved functional performance.[138] Physical obstruction at surgical anastomoses, the distal pulmonary arteries, or pulmonary veins (often due to compression by a dilated right atrium) all reduce circulatory efficiency, however. Similarly, elevated pulmonary arteriolar resistances have adverse effects. This is because the pulmonary vascular resistance is the single biggest contributor to impairment of venous return and elevation of venous pressure. Relatively little is known about pulmonary vascular resistance late after the procedure, but it has recently been shown to be elevated in a significant number of patients and to be reactive to inhaled nitric oxide, suggesting pulmonary endothelial dysfunction.[141]

CLINICAL FEATURES. The majority of patients (~90 percent) present with functional Class I to II at 5 years' follow-up after a Fontan procedure.[136,142,143] Progressive deterioration of functional status with time is the rule.[136,142-144] Supraventricular arrhythmias such as atrial tachycardia, flutter, and fibrillation are common. Physical examination in an otherwise uncomplicated patient reveals an elevated, usually nonpulsatile jugular venous pulse (10 cm above the sternal angle and needed to provide the hydrostatic pressure to drive cardiac output through the pulmonary circulation), a quiet apex, a normal S_1, and a single S_2 (the pulmonary artery having been tied off). A heart murmur should not be present, and its identification suggests the presence of systemic AV valve regurgitation or subaortic obstruction. Generalized edema may be a sign of protein-losing enteropathy.

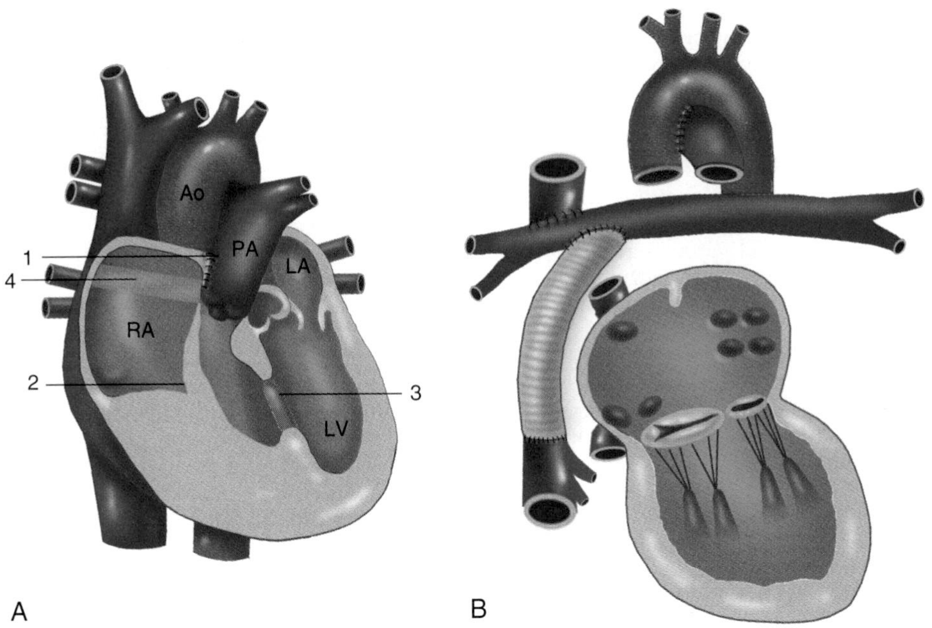

FIGURE 56–18 Modification of the Fontan operation. **A,** Direct atriopulmonary connection (1) for tricuspid valve atresia (2); ventricular septal defect, oversewn (3); patch closure of atrial septal defect (4). **B,** Extracardiac conduit made of a Dacron graft bypassing the right atrium, connecting the inferior vena cava to the inferior aspect of the right pulmonary artery. Superior vena cava is anastomosed to the superior aspect of the right pulmonary artery. RA = right atrium; LA = left atrium; LV = left ventricle; Ao = aorta; PA = pulmonary artery. (**A,** From Mullins CE, Mayer DC: Congenital Heart Disease: A Diagrammatic Atlas. New York, Wiley-Liss, 1988; and **B,** From Marcelletti C: Inferior vena cava–pulmonary artery extracardiac conduit: A new form of right heart bypass. J Thorac Cardiovasc Surg 100:228-232, 1990.)

COMPLICATIONS AND SEQUELAE

Arrhythmia. Although often associated with marked symptomatic decline, atrial arrhythmias tend to reflect the consequences of the abnormalities of ventricular function and circulatory efficiency described earlier. The massively dilated right atrium after an atriopulmonary connection is commonly associated with atrial flutter and fibrillation. With new-onset arrhythmia, hemodynamic abnormalities and atrial/venous thrombosis—which may develop within 2 hours of arrhythmia onset—should be actively excluded prior to therapy. Atrial flutter/fibrillation is common (15 to 20 percent at 5 years' follow-up)[51,52,145,146] and increases with duration of follow-up.[51-53] Atrial flutter/fibrillation carries significant morbidity, can be associated with profound hemodynamic deterioration, and needs prompt medical attention. The combination of atrial incisions and multiple suture lines at the time of Fontan surgery combined with increased right atrial pressure and size probably explains the high incidence of atrial arrhythmias in such patients. Patients at greater risk for atrial tachyarrhythmias are those who were operated on at an older age, with poor ventricular function, systemic AV valve regurgitation, or increased pulmonary artery pressure. It has been suggested that the exclusion of the right atrium from elevated systemic venous pressure (as in total cavopulmonary connection or extracardiac conduit) leads to a decrease in the incidence of atrial arrhythmias. This apparent benefit may, however, be due exclusively to the shorter length of follow-up in this group of patients. Sinus node dysfunction and complete heart block can occur and require pacemaker insertion.

Thrombosis and Stroke. The reported incidence of thromboembolic complications in the Fontan circuit varies from 6 to 25 percent, depending on the diagnostic method used and the length of follow-up.[147-149] Thrombus formation may relate to the presence of supraventricular arrhythmias, right atrial dilation, right atrial "smoke," and the presence of artificial material used to construct the Fontan circuit.[147-149] Accordingly, a similar incidence of thrombus formation had been reported for all types of Fontan circuits. Systemic arterial embolism in patients with and without a fenestrated Fontan has also been reported. Protein C deficiency has been reported in these patients and may explain in part their propensity to thromboembolism.

Protein-Losing Enteropathy. Protein-losing enteropathy, defined as severe loss of serum protein into the intestine, occurs in 4 to 13 percent of patients after a Fontan procedure.[145,150,151] Patients present with generalized edema, ascites, pleural effusion, and/or chronic diarrhea. Protein-losing enteropathy is thought to result principally from chronically elevated systemic venous pressure causing intestinal lymphangiectasia with consequent loss of albumin, protein, lymphocytes, and immunoglobulin into the gastrointestinal tract. The diagnosis is confirmed by finding low serum albumin and protein, low plasma alpha$_1$-antitrypsin level and lymphocyte counts, and, most important, a high alpha$_1$-antitrypsin stool clearance. It carries a dismal prognosis, with a 5-year survival of 46 to 59 percent.[150,151]

Right Pulmonary Vein Compression/Obstruction. Right pulmonary vein obstruction/compression can occur from the enlarged right atrium or atrial baffle bulging into the left atrium and can lead to increased pulmonary artery pressure with further dilation of the right atrium. It should be sought.

Pulmonary thromboembolism is increasingly recognized[147-149,152] and will elevate central venous pressure. There is continuing debate as to the role of anticoagulation, antiplatelet therapy, or both in the long-term management of these patients, but most receive some form of therapy.[153-155]

Fontan Obstruction. Stenosis or partial obstruction of the Fontan connection leads to exercise intolerance, atrial tachyarrhythmias, and right-sided heart failure. Sudden total obstruction can present as sudden death.

Ventricular Dysfunction and Valvular Regurgitation. Progressive deterioration of systemic ventricular function, with or without progressive AV valve regurgitation, is common. Patients with morphological systemic right ventricles may fare less well than those with morphological left ventricles.

Hepatic Dysfunction. Mildly raised hepatic transaminase levels from hepatic congestion are frequent but seldom clinically important. Cirrhosis apparently due to chronic venous hypertension has been described.

Cyanosis. Worsening cyanosis may relate to worsening of ventricular function, the development of venous collateral channels draining to the left atrium, or the development of pulmonary arteriovenous malformations (especially if a classic Glenn procedure remains as part of the Fontan circulation).

LABORATORY INVESTIGATIONS

ECG. Sinus rhythm, atrial flutter, junctional rhythm, or complete heart block may be present. The QRS complex reflects the basic underlying cardiac anomaly. In patients with tricuspid atresia, left axis deviation is the norm. In patients with univentricular hearts, the conduction pattern varies widely and depends on the morphology and relative position of the rudimentary chamber.

Chest Radiography. Mild bulging of the right lower heart border from a dilated right atrium is often seen in patients with an atriopulmonary connection.

Echocardiography. The presence or absence of right atrial stasis, thrombus, patency of a fenestration, and Fontan circuit obstruction should be sought. Superior and inferior vena cavae biphasic and pulmonary artery triphasic flow patterns suggest unobstructed flow in the Fontan circuit, whereas a mean gradient between the Fontan circuit and the pulmonary artery of 2 mm Hg or more may represent significant obstruction. Assessment of the pulmonary venous flow pattern is important in detecting pulmonary vein obstruction (right pulmonary vein > left pulmonary vein) sometimes caused by an enlarged right atrium (often ~ 80 × 60 mm in adults with atriopulmonary connections). Concomitant assessment of systemic ventricular function and AV valve regurgitation can be readily accomplished. TEE may be required if there is inadequate visualization of the Fontan anastomosis or to exclude thrombus in the right atrium.

Diagnostic Catheterization. Complete heart catheterization is advised if surgical reintervention is planned or if adequate assessment of the hemodynamics is not obtained by noninvasive means.

MRI. The objectives of MRI in Fontan patients include assessment of the pathways from the systemic veins to the pulmonary arteries for obstruction and thrombus; detection of Fontan baffle fenestration or leaks; evaluation of the pulmonary veins for compression; assessing systemic ventricular volume, mass, and ejection fraction; imaging of the systemic ventricular outflow tract for obstruction; and quantitative assessment of the AV and semilunar valve(s) for regurgitation, the aorta for obstruction or an aneurysm, and for aortopulmonary, systemic venous, or systemic-to-pulmonary venous collateral vessels.

MANAGEMENT OPTIONS AND OUTCOMES. Patient selection is of utmost importance and has a major impact on clinical outcome. Long-term survival in "ideal" candidates is 81 percent at 10 years,[142] compared with 60 to 71 percent in "all comers."[144] Death occurs mostly from congestive heart failure and atrial arrhythmias. The Fontan procedure remains a palliative, not curative, procedure. A more radical approach to the failing Fontan circulation including surgical revision of the circuit to an extracardiac conduit, in combination with a Cox/maze procedure and, frequently, simultaneous epicardial pacemaker insertion, has recently been shown to provide good early palliation.[59,59,156-159] Ultimately cardiac transplantation is likely to be required by many of these patients.[150]

Arrhythmias. Atrial tachyarrhythmias are quite difficult to manage and should quickly raise the thought of long-term warfarin therapy. When atrial flutter/fibrillation are present, an underlying hemodynamic cause should always be sought, and, in particular, evidence for obstruction of the Fontan circuit needs to be sought. Prompt attempts should be made to restore sinus rhythm. Antiarrhythmic medications, alone or combined with an epicardial antitachycardia pacing device, and radiofrequency catheter ablation techniques have had limited success. Surgical conversion from an atriopulmonary Fontan to a total cavopulmonary connection with concomitant atrial cryoablation therapy at the time of surgery has been reported with good short-term success.[59,158,159] Epicardial pacemaker insertion for sinus node dysfunction and/or complete heart block may be necessary. Epicardial AV sequential pacing should be employed whenever possible.

Anticoagulant Therapy. The use of prophylactic long-term anticoagulation is contentious. It is recommended that patients with a history of documented arrhythmias, fenestration in the Fontan connection, or spontaneous contrast (smoke) in the right atrium on echocardiography be anticoagulated.[153,154] For established thrombus, thrombolytic therapy versus surgical removal of the clot and conversion of the Fontan circuit have been described, both with high mortality rates.

Protein-Losing Enteropathy. Treatment modalities include a low-fat, high-protein, medium-chain triglyceride diet to reduce intestinal lymphatic production; albumin infusions to increase intravascular osmotic pressure; and/or the introduction of diuretics, afterload-reducing agents, and positive inotropic agents to lower central venous pressure. Most often these therapies are ineffective and should not be continued if indeed tried at all. Catheter-based interventions such as balloon dilation of pathway obstruction or creation of an atrial fenestration as well as surgical interventions from conversion or takedown of the Fontan circuit to cardiac transplantation have also been advocated. Other reportedly effective treatment modalities include subcutaneous heparin, octreotide treatment, and prednisone therapy. All therapies have a similar approximately 50 percent failure rate.[151,160]

Right Pulmonary Vein Compression/Obstruction. When hemodynamically significant, Fontan conversion to a total cavopulmonary connection or extracardiac conduit may be recommended.

Fontan Obstruction. Surgical revision of obstructed right atrium to pulmonary artery or superior and inferior vena cavae to pulmonary artery connections is recommended, usually to an extracardiac Fontan. Alternatively, balloon angioplasty with or without stenting may be used when appropriate and feasible.

Ventricular Failure and Valvular Regurgitation. ACE inhibitors are of unproven benefit, do not appear to enhance exercise capacity, and may cause clinical deterioration. Patients with systemic AV valve regurgitation may require AV valve repair or replacement. Cardiac transplantation should also be considered.

Cyanosis. In the setting of a fenestrated Fontan, surgical or preferably transcatheter closure of the fenestration can be attempted. Pulmonary arteriovenous fistulas from a classic Glenn may be improved by surgical conversion to a bidirectional Glenn connection.

FOLLOW-UP ISSUES. Close and expert follow-up is recommended with particular attention to ventricular function and systemic AV valve regurgitation. The development of atrial tachyarrhythmia should instigate a search for possible obstruction at the Fontan anastomosis, right pulmonary vein obstruction, or thrombus within the right atrium.

Total Anomalous Pulmonary Venous Connection

DEFINITION. This describes the situation where all pulmonary veins fail to drain directly to the left atrium. As a result, all of the systemic and pulmonary venous return drains to the right atrium, albeit using varied routes.

MORPHOLOGY (Fig. 56–19). The anatomical varieties of total anomalous pulmonary venous connection may be subdivided, depending on the level of the abnormal drainage. The anomalous connection is most often supradiaphragmatic, connecting via a vertical vein to the left brachiocephalic vein, direct to the right atrium, to the coronary sinus, or directly to the superior vena cava. In about 10 to 15 percent the site of connection is below the diaphragm. The anomalous trunk then connects into the portal vein or one of its tributaries, the ductus venosus, or, rarely, to the hepatic or other abdominal veins.

PATHOPHYSIOLOGY. The physiological consequences and, accordingly, the clinical picture depend on the size of the interatrial communication and on the magnitude of the pulmonary vascular resistance. When the interatrial communication is small, systemic blood flow is severely limited with right-sided heart failure. Obstruction to pulmonary venous return and pulmonary venous hypertension are invariably present in patients with infradiaphragmatic anomalous pulmonary venous connection.

NATURAL HISTORY. Most patients with total anomalous pulmonary venous connection have symptoms during the first year of life, and 80 percent die before 1 year of age if not treated. The presence of obstruction in the pulmonary venous pathway or at the atrial septum leads to earlier presentation. When the obstruction is severe, neonatal presentation with severe cyanosis and cardiovascular collapse may occur. This is incompatible with survival without urgent surgical intervention.

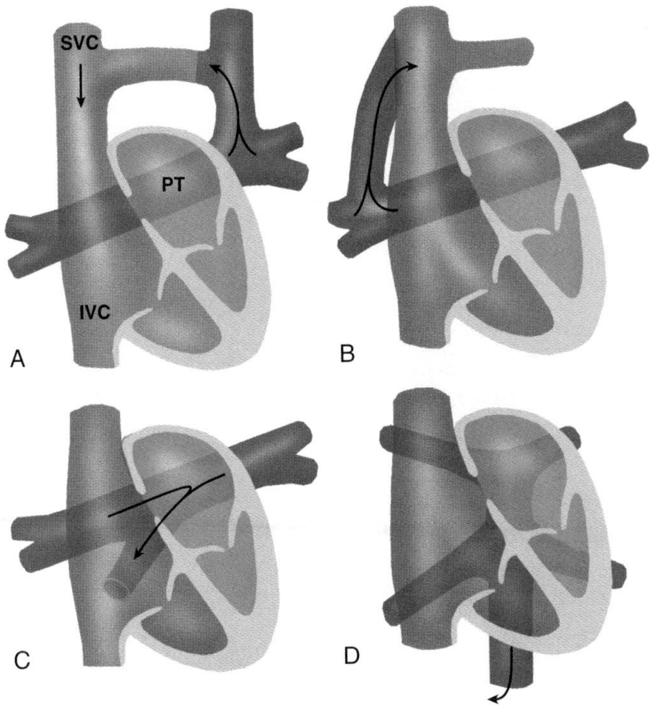

FIGURE 56–19 Anatomical types of total anomalous pulmonary venous return: supracardiac, in which the pulmonary veins drain either via the vertical vein to the anomalous vein **(A)** or directly to the superior vena cava (SVC) with the orifice close to the orifice of the azygos vein **(B)**. **C,** Drainage into the right atrium via the coronary sinus. **D,** Infracardiac drainage via a vertical vein into the portal vein or the inferior vena cava (IVC). PT = pulmonary trunk. (**A** to **D,** From Stark J, deLeval M: Surgery for Congenital Heart Defects. 2nd ed. Philadelphia, WB Saunders, 1994, p 330.)

CLINICAL FEATURES. Symptomatic infants with total anomalous pulmonary venous connection present with signs of heart failure and/or cyanosis. Infants with pulmonary venous obstruction present with the early onset of severe dyspnea, pulmonary edema, cyanosis, and right-sided heart failure. When unobstructed, cyanosis may be minimal and go undetected. On auscultation there is usually a fixed, widely split second heart sound with an accentuated pulmonic component.

LABORATORY INVESTIGATIONS

ECG. This usually shows right axis deviation and right atrial and right ventricular hypertrophy.

Chest Radiography. In the unrepaired patient, this usually shows cardiomegaly with increased pulmonary blood flow. The right atrium and ventricle are dilated and hypertrophied, and the pulmonary artery segment is enlarged. The so-called "figure-of-8" or "snowman" heart is due to enlargement of the heart and the presence of a dilated right superior vena cava, innominate vein, and left vertical vein.

Echocardiography (Fig. 56–20). This will usually show marked enlargement of the right ventricle and a small left atrium. It is usually possible to demonstrate the entire pathway of pulmonary venous drainage, and cardiac catheterization (which may be hazardous) is almost never performed now. An echo-free space representing the pulmonary venous confluence can usually be seen behind the left atrium. The drainage of all four pulmonary veins and their connections must be identified.

MRI. Although not often used, especially in infants, MRI may be helpful to delineate the site of connections of total anomalous pulmonary venous return, when there are multiple mixed sites, in older children, and to detect stenosis in postoperative patients.

INDICATIONS FOR INTERVENTION. Medical therapy, other than mechanical ventilation, has a limited role in the symptomatic infant, and corrective surgery should be performed as soon as possible. In asymptomatic children without pulmonary hypertension, surgery can be deferred to 3 to 6 months of age.

INTERVENTIONAL OPTIONS AND OUTCOMES. Occasionally an urgent balloon atrial septostomy is required to increase systemic blood flow prior to surgery. Otherwise, interventional catheterization is restricted to attempts at relieving postoperative pulmonary venous stenosis, although this is often unrewarding. Historically, surgical repair of restenosis was also disappointing. However, the sutureless technique, whereby the pulmonary veins are opened widely into the retroatrial space, has markedly improved the results of such surgery. Adult patients have almost always had surgical repair in childhood. As a rule, they function normally and are not too prone to arrhythmias or other problems. They are seen as low- to moderate-risk adults.

FOLLOW-UP. Early follow-up should be frequent and aimed at early detection of stenosis of the pulmonary veins or the surgical anastomosis. If not present within the first year, stenosis is rare, but annual follow-up during childhood is required.

Transposition Complexes

The key anatomical feature that characterizes this group of diagnoses is ventriculoarterial discordance. This is most commonly seen in the context of AV concordance, also known as

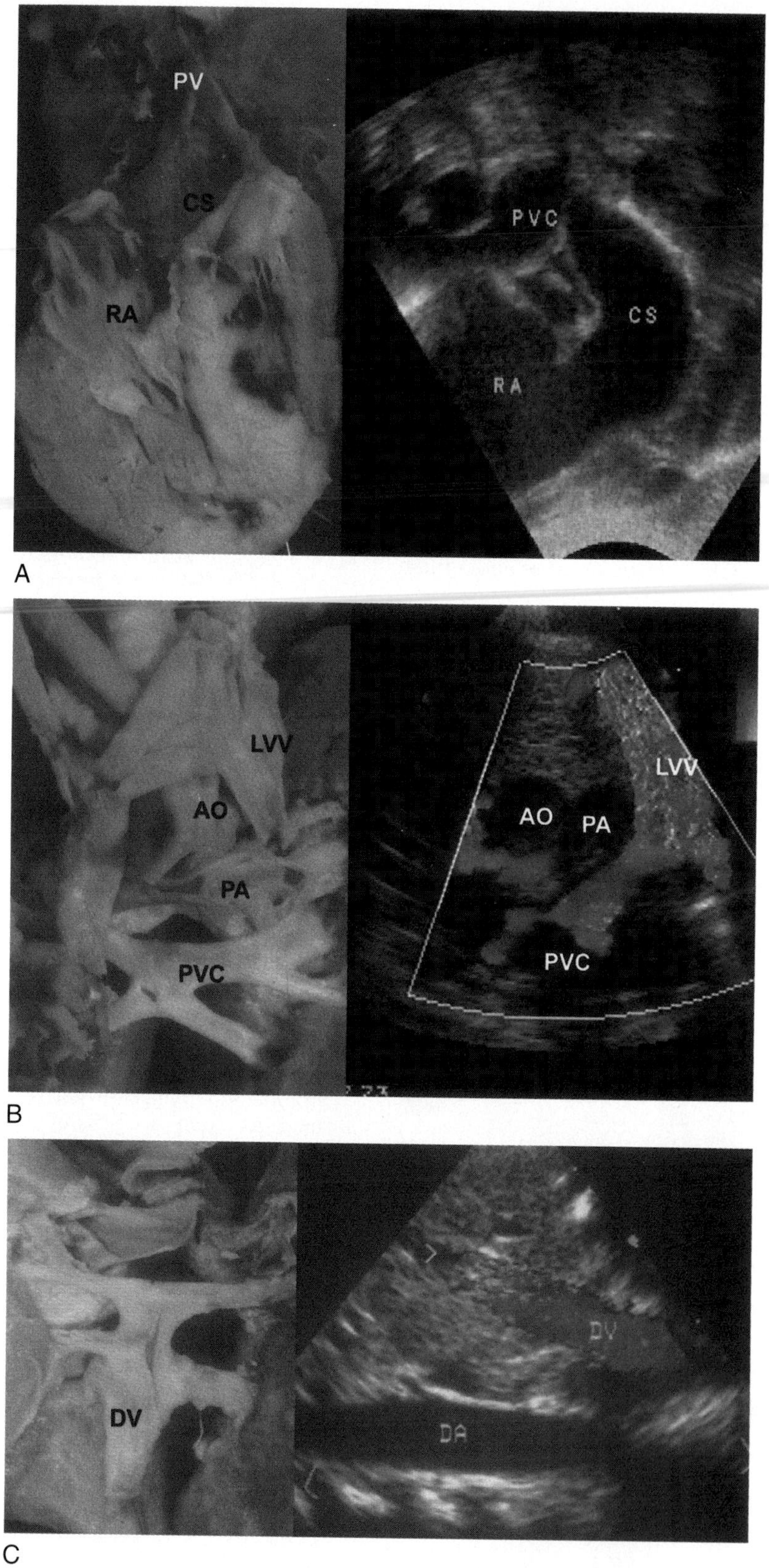

FIGURE 56–20 **A,** Subcostal view demonstrating total anomalous pulmonary drainage to the coronary sinus. Note the dilated coronary sinus in both images. The echocardiogram also demonstrates an associated confluence that connects to the coronary sinus. **B,** Suprasternal view demonstrating total anomalous pulmonary venous drainage to a left vertical vein. Note the direction of flow in the vertical vein that differentiates it from a left superior vena cava. **C,** Total anomalous pulmonary venous drainage below the diaphragm. The specimen shows the pulmonary veins as they enter the confluence, whereas the echocardiogram demonstrates the descending veins as it enters the liver. Note the direction of flow is away from the heart. CS = coronary sinus; PVC = pulmonary venous confluence; RA = right atrium; DA = descending aorta; DV = descending vein; AO = aorta; LVV = left vertical vein; PA = pulmonary artery.

complete transposition or *D-TGA*. The second condition that is discussed in this section is the combination of ventriculoarterial discordance with AV discordance, commonly referred to as *congenitally corrected TGA* or *L-TGA*. More complex arrangements are not considered here.

Complete Transposition of the Great Arteries

DEFINITION AND NATURAL HISTORY. This is a common and potentially lethal form of heart disease in newborns and infants. The malformation consists of the origin of the aorta from the morphological right ventricle and that of the pulmonary artery from the morphological left ventricle. Consequently, the pulmonary and systemic circulations are connected in parallel rather than the normal in-series connection. In one circuit, systemic venous blood passes to the right atrium, the right ventricle, and then to the aorta. In the other, pulmonary venous blood passes through the left atrium and ventricle to the pulmonary artery. This situation is incompatible with life unless mixing of the two circuits occurs.

Approximately two-thirds of patients have no major associated abnormalities (*"simple" transposition*) and one-third have associated abnormalities (*"complex" transposition*). The most common associated abnormalities are VSD and pulmonary/subpulmonary stenosis. It is increasingly being diagnosed in utero.[161] Without treatment, about 30 percent of these infants die within the first week of life, and 90 percent die within the first year.

MORPHOLOGY. Some communication between the two circulations must exist after birth to sustain life; otherwise, unoxygenated systemic venous blood is directed inappropriately to the systemic circulation and oxygenated pulmonary venous blood is directed to the pulmonary circulation. Almost all patients have an interatrial communication, blood flow across which governs the amount of desaturation. Two-thirds have a PDA, and about one-third have an associated VSD.

PATHOPHYSIOLOGY. The degree of tissue hypoxia, the nature of the associated cardiovascular anomalies, and the anatomical and functional status of the pulmonary vascular bed determine the clinical course.

The anatomical arrangement results in two separate and parallel circulations. The systemic arterial oxygen saturation is governed by the amount of blood exchanged between the two circulations. Infants with D-TGA are particularly susceptible to the early development of pulmonary vascular obstructive disease even in the absence of a PDA and with an intact ventricular septum.

CLINICAL FEATURES

Pediatric. Average birth weight and size of infants born with complete transposition of the great arteries are greater than normal. The usual clinical manifestations are dyspnea and cyanosis from birth, progressive hypoxemia, and congestive heart failure. The most severe cyanosis and hypoxemia are observed in infants who have only a small patent foramen ovale or ductus arteriosus and an intact ventricular septum, or in those infants with relatively reduced pulmonary blood flow because of left ventricular outflow tract obstruction. With a large PDA or a large VSD, cyanosis can be minimal, and heart failure is usually the dominant problem after the first few weeks of life. Cardiac murmurs are of little diagnostic significance.

The 2D echocardiogram should establish the complete diagnosis, including the coronary artery pattern. Prenatal detection is possible and favorably modifies neonatal morbidity and mortality. Ultrasound imaging has become a standard procedure to guide catheter placement and manipulation during balloon atrial septostomy and to assess the anatomical adequacy of the septostomy.

MANAGEMENT OPTIONS. Dilation of the duct by prostaglandin E_1 in the early neonatal period improves the arterial saturation by enhancing mixing. There is a frequent misconception that significant mixing occurs at ductal level. This is incorrect; the effect of prostaglandin is to increase pulmonary blood flow, and by so doing to increase left atrial pressure, and increase mixing at atrial level. This is usually as a prelude to the creation or enlargement of an interatrial communication by a balloon or blade atrial septostomy. Surgical atrial septectomy is seldom required now.

Surgery. Although balloon atrial septostomy is often life saving, it is palliative prior to "corrective" surgery. Atrial redirection procedures were developed in the 1950s and 1960s but were replaced by the arterial switch operation, which became widely adopted in the 1980s.[162]

Atrial Switch (Fig. 56–21). The most common surgical procedure in patients who are currently adults is the atrial switch operation. Patients will have had either a Mustard or a Senning procedure. Blood is redirected at the atrial level using a baffle made of Dacron or pericardium (Mustard operation) or atrial flaps (Senning operation), achieving physiological correction. Systemic venous return is diverted through the mitral valve into the subpulmonary left ventricle, and the pulmonary venous return is rerouted through the tricuspid valve into the subaortic right ventricle. By virtue of this repair, the morphological right ventricle is left to support the systemic circulation.

Palliative Atrial Switch. Uncommonly, in patients with a large VSD and established pulmonary vascular disease, a palliative atrial switch operation is done to improve oxygenation. The VSD is left open or enlarged at the time of atrial baffle surgery. These patients resemble patients with Eisenmenger VSDs and should be managed as such.

Arterial Switch Operation (Fig. 56–22). In this operation, the arterial trunks are transected and reanastomosed to the contralateral root. If present, a VSD is closed. The coronary arteries must be transposed to the neoaorta. This is the most

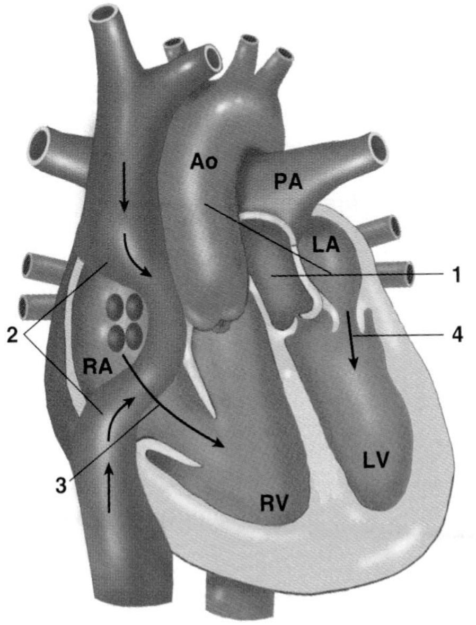

FIGURE 56–21 Diagrammatic representation of atrial switch surgery (Mustard/Senning procedure). Superior vena cava (SVC) and inferior vena cava (IVC) blood is redirected into the morphological left ventricle (LV), which pumps blood into the pulmonary artery (PA), whereas the pulmonary venous blood flow is rerouted to the morphological right ventricle (RV), which empties into the aorta (Ao). RA = right atrium; LA = left atrium; 1 = transposition of the great arteries; 2 = atrial baffles; 3 = pulmonary vein blood flow through tricuspid valve to RV; 4 = IVC and SVC blood flow through mitral valve to LV. (From Mullins CE, Mayer DC: Congenital Heart Disease: A Diagrammatic Atlas. New York, Wiley-Liss, 1988.)

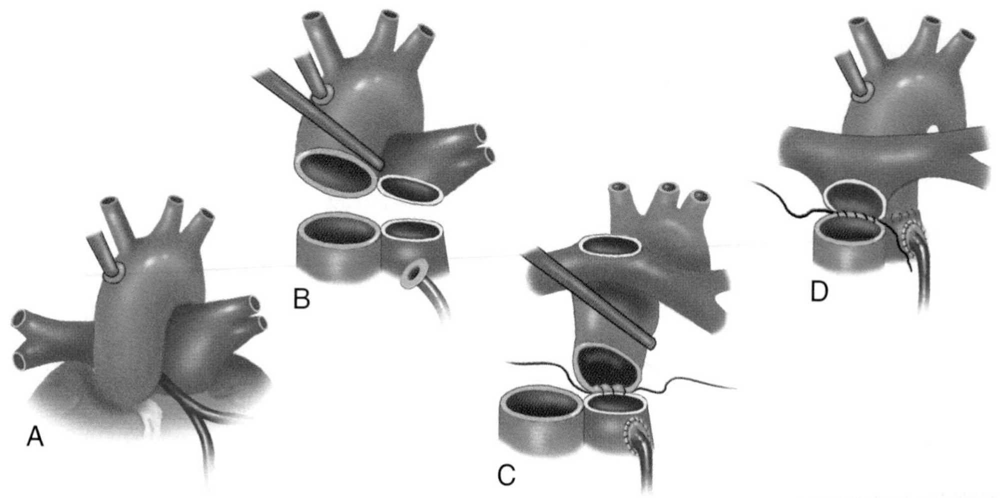

FIGURE 56–22 Complete transposition of the great arteries, corrected by a modified arterial switch operation **(A)**. The aorta and pulmonary artery are transected, and the orifices of the coronary arteries are excised with a rim of adjacent aortic wall **(B)**. The aorta is brought under the bifurcation of the pulmonary artery, and the pulmonary artery and the aorta are anastomosed without necessitating graft interposition. The coronary arteries are transferred to the pulmonary artery **(C)**. The mobilized pulmonary artery is directly anastomosed to the proximal aortic stump **(D)**. (**A** to **D,** From Stark J, deLaval M: Surgery for Congenital Heart Defects. New York, Grune & Stratton, 1983, p 379.)

challenging part of the procedure and accounts for most of the mortality. Nonetheless, this rate has fallen to less than 2 percent in most large centers.[162,163] The major advantages of the arterial switch procedure, when compared with the atrial switch procedure, are restoration of the left ventricle as the systemic pump and the potential for long-term maintenance of sinus rhythm.

Follow-up studies after the arterial switch operation have demonstrated good left ventricular function and normal exercise capacity.[163,164] Potential sequelae of the operation include coronary occlusion, supravalvular pulmonary stenosis (which may be treated by either reoperation or balloon angioplasty), supravalvular aortic stenosis, and neoaortic regurgitation, usually mild.[165-167] Long-term patency and growth of the coronary arteries appear satisfactory.

Rastelli Procedure. Infants with TGA plus a VSD and left ventricular outflow tract obstruction may require an early systemic-to-pulmonary artery anastomosis when a pronounced diminution in pulmonary blood flow exists. A later corrective procedure for these patients bypasses the left ventricular outflow obstruction with an extracardiac prosthetic conduit between the right ventricle and the distal end of a divided pulmonary artery and uses an intracardiac ventricular baffle to tunnel the left ventricle to the aorta.

MANAGEMENT OUTCOMES

Atrial Switch. After atrial baffle surgery, most patients who reach adulthood are in NYHA Classes I and II,[41,168,169] but abnormalities of ventricular filling, due to the abnormal atrial pathways, may be of more direct importance to functional capacity than right ventricular performance issues in many.[170] Some present with symptoms of congestive heart failure (2 to 15 percent). Echocardiographic evidence of moderate or severe systemic right ventricular dysfunction is present in up to 40 percent of patients. Relative right ventricular ischemia (supply-demand mismatch) is thought to perhaps play a role in systemic right ventricular dysfunction.[171-173] More than mild systemic tricuspid regurgitation is present in 10 to 40 percent, both reflecting and exacerbating right ventricular dysfunction. Palpitations and near-syncope/syncope from rhythm disturbances is fairly common. Atrial flutter occurs in 20 percent of patients by 20 years of age, and sinus node dysfunction is seen in half of the patients by that time.[42,174-176] These rhythm disturbances are a consequence of direct and indirect atrial and sinus node damage at the time of atrial baffle surgery.[177]

A shortened life expectancy is the rule, with 70 to 80 percent survival at 20 to 30 years' follow-up.[41] Patients with "complex" TGA in general fare much worse than those with "simple" TGA. Sudden cardiac death occurs in about 5 percent of these patients and may relate to systemic right ventricular dysfunction, the presence of atrial flutter, and pulmonary hypertension. Significant pulmonary vascular disease can develop over time and relates to older age at the time of atrial switch operation, particularly in patients with a substantial VSD, as well as in those with long-standing left-to-right shunts through a baffle leak. Superior vena cava or inferior vena cava baffle obstruction often goes undetected because collateral drainage through the azygos vein prevents systemic venous congestion. Pulmonary venous baffle obstruction causes elevated pulmonary artery pressure, and patients can present with dyspnea and pulmonary venous congestive features.

Physical examination of a patient whose condition is otherwise uncomplicated reveals a right ventricular parasternal lift, a normal S_1, a single S_2 (P_2 is not heard because of its posterior location), a pansystolic murmur from tricuspid regurgitation if present (best heard at the left lower sternal border, but not increasing with inspiration), and a right-sided S_3 when severe systemic ventricular dysfunction is present.

Arterial Switch. Data on clinical presentation in adults who have undergone the arterial switch procedure are lacking, because most patients have not yet reached adulthood. Clinical arrhythmia promises to be less of a problem in this group of patients.[165,178] Concerns about the development of supra-neopulmonary artery stenosis, ostial coronary artery disease, and progressive neoaortic valve regurgitation remain to be addressed over the long-term. Cardiac examination in uncomplicated patients is normal.

Rastelli. Progressive right ventricular-to-pulmonary artery conduit obstruction can cause exercise intolerance or right ventricular angina. Left ventricular tunnel obstruction can present as dyspnea or syncope. Conduit replacement is inevitably required in surviving patients. Physical examination in uncomplicated patients reveals, in contrast to atrial switches, no right ventricular lift, an ejection systolic murmur from the conduit, and two components to the S_2.

LABORATORY INVESTIGATIONS

ECG. Sinus bradycardia or junctional rhythm (without a right atrial overload pattern) with evidence of marked right ventricular hypertrophy is characteristically present in patients after the atrial switch procedure. The ECG is typically normal in patients after the arterial switch procedure. The ECG typically shows right bundle branch block after a Rastelli procedure.

Chest Radiography. On the posteroanterior film, a narrow vascular pedicle with an oblong cardiac silhouette ("egg on side") is typically seen in patients after the atrial switch procedure. On the lateral view, the anterior aorta is seen to fill the retrosternal space. For the arterial switch, normal mediastinal borders are present despite the Lecompte maneuver. After the Rastelli procedure, the chest radiograph is normal unless the conduit becomes calcified or a nonhomograft prosthesis is employed.

Echocardiography. After the atrial switch procedure, parallel great arteries are the hallmark of TGA (Fig. 56–23). They are best visualized from a parasternal long-axis view (running side by side) or from a parasternal short-axis view (seen *en face*, with the aorta anterior and rightward).[179] Qualitative assessment of systemic right ventricular function, the degree of tricuspid regurgitation, and the presence or absence of subpulmonary left ventricular obstruction (dynamic or fixed) is possible. Assessment of baffle leak or obstruction (Fig. 56–24) is best done using color and Doppler flow imaging. Normal baffle flow should be phasic in nature and vary with respiration, with a peak velocity less than 1 meter per second. After arterial switch, neoaortic valve regurgitation, supra-neopulmonary valve stenosis, and segmental wall motion abnormality from ischemia due to coronary ostial stenosis should be sought. In patients who have undergone the Rastelli operation, left ventricular-to-aorta tunnel obstruction as well as right ventricular-to-pulmonary artery conduit degeneration (stenosis/regurgitation) must be sought.

MRI. The major role of MRI in patients with atrial switch is to evaluate the baffles and systemic right ventricular volume and ejection fraction. As a rule, MRI reports better right ventricular size and function than does echo. For patients who are claustrophobic or have a pacemaker, a high-quality radionuclide angiogram with volume estimates will serve as a substitute. MRI can evaluate issues in arterial switch and Rastelli patients as well.

Cardiac Catheterization. Diagnostic cardiac catheterization may be required for assessing the presence or severity of systemic/pulmonary baffle obstruction, baffle leak, and pulmonary hypertension; coronary ostial stenosis; or tunnel or conduit obstruction when not diagnosed by noninvasive means.

INDICATIONS FOR REINTERVENTION. After the *atrial switch procedure*, severe symptomatic right ventricular dysfunction may warrant surgical treatment in the form of a *two-stage arterial switch* procedure[180-184] or cardiac transplantation. Tricuspid valve replacement is rarely performed for severe systemic (tricuspid) AV valve regurgitation if due to a flail leaflet or cusp perforation providing right ventricular function is adequate. A baffle leak resulting in a significant left-to-right shunt (>1.5/1.0), any right-to-left shunt, or attributable symptoms requires surgical or transcatheter closure. Superior vena cava or inferior vena cava pathway obstruction may require intervention. Superior vena cava stenosis is usually benign, whereas inferior vena cava stenosis may be life threatening. Balloon dilation of superior vena cava or inferior vena cava stenosis is an option in expert hands. Stenting usually relieves the stenosis completely.

Pathway obstruction after the Senning operation is usually more amenable to balloon dilation and stenting. Pulmonary venous obstruction, although usually seen early and reoperated on in childhood, may present in adulthood. Symptomatic bradycardia warrants permanent pacemaker implantation, whereas tachyarrhythmias may require catheter ablation, an antitachycardia pacemaker device, or medical therapy. After an atrial switch, transvenous pacing leads must traverse the upper limb of the baffle to enter the morphological left ventricle. Active fixation is required because coarse trabeculation is absent in the morphological left ventricle. Transvenous pacing should be avoided in patients with residual intracardiac communications because paradoxical emboli can occur.

After an *arterial switch procedure*, significant right ventricular outflow tract obstruction at any level (gradient > 50 mm Hg or right-to-left ventricular pressure ratio > 0.6) may require surgical or catheter augmentation of the right ventricular outflow tract.[21] Myocardial ischemia from coronary artery obstruction may require coronary artery bypass grafting, preferably with arterial conduits. Significant neoaortic valve regurgitation may warrant aortic valve replacement.

In patients who have had the *Rastelli procedure*, significant right ventricle-to-pulmonary artery conduit stenosis (>50 mm Hg withdrawal gradient or mean echo gradient) or significant regurgitation necessitates conduit replacement.

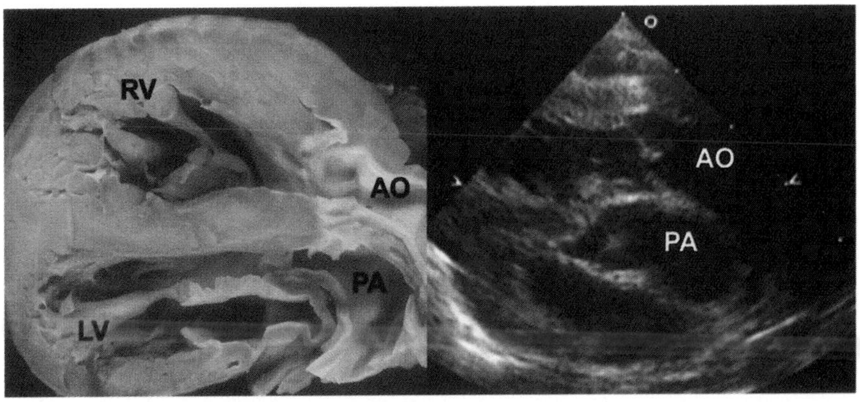

FIGURE 56–23 Parasternal long-axis view in transposition of the great arteries. Note the parallel nature of the aorta and pulmonary artery. AO = aorta; LV = left ventricle; PA = pulmonary artery; RV = right ventricle.

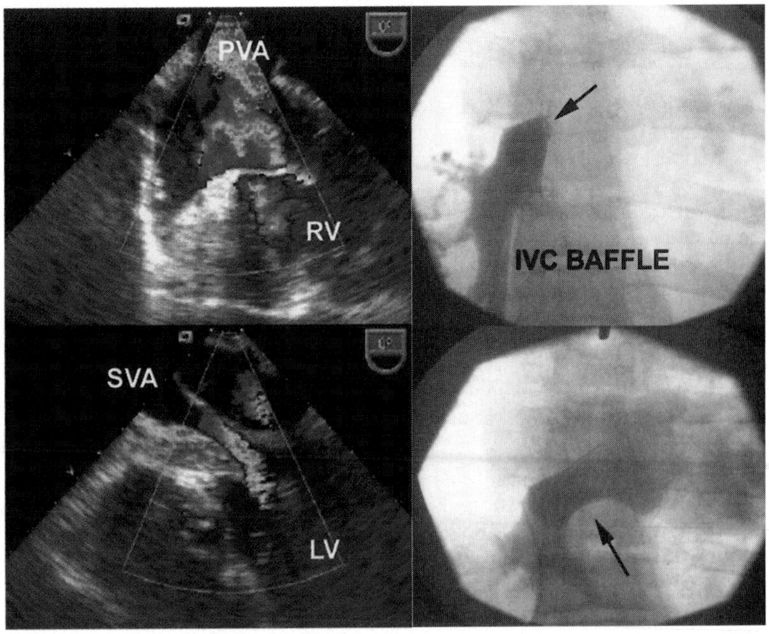

FIGURE 56–24 Montage of post-Mustard cases. The angiogram on the right upper panel shows complete obstruction of the inferior limb of the systemic venous baffle, whereas the lower right panel is the same case after stenting. The upper left image is a transesophageal echocardiogram showing the pulmonary venous baffle with some mild flow acceleration in its midpoint. The lower left panel shows the systemic venous baffle at its left ventricular end. LV = left ventricle; PVA = pulmonary venous atrium; RV = right ventricle; SVA = systemic venous atrium; IVC = inferior vena cava.

Subaortic obstruction across the left ventricle-to-aorta tunnel necessitates left ventricle-to-aorta baffle reconstruction. A significant residual VSD (shunt > 1.5/1.0) may require surgical closure.

Patients with clinical deterioration and a palliative atrial switch should be considered for lung or heart-lung transplantation.

REINTERVENTION OPTIONS

Medical Therapy. The role of afterload reduction with ACE inhibitors to preserve systemic right ventricular function is unknown. In light of the effects of these drugs on dysfunctional systemic left ventricles, it seems logical to assume that similar beneficial effects on systemic right ventricles may occur.[15,16]

Two-Stage Arterial Switch. Patients with symptomatic, severe systemic (right) ventricular dysfunction with or without severe systemic (tricuspid) AV valve regurgitation, following an atrial switch procedure, may require consideration of a conversion procedure to an arterial switch (two-stage arterial switch)[181-183] or heart transplantation. The two-stage arterial switch, or switch-conversion procedure, consists of banding the pulmonary artery in the first stage to induce subpulmonary left ventricular hypertrophy and "train" the left ventricle to support systemic pressure. Once left ventricular systolic pressure is more than 75 percent of systemic pressure and the left ventricular mass is considered adequate, in the second stage the atrial baffles and the pulmonary band are taken down, the atrial septum is reconstructed, and the great arteries are switched, leaving the morphological left ventricle as the systemic ventricle. This procedure is still experimental in adults, with little data available to assess its short- and long-term efficacy.

Cardiac Transplantation. Heart transplantation should be considered as an alternative, given its relatively good 5- to 10-year survival.

REPRODUCTIVE ISSUES. Severe systemic ventricular dysfunction or intractable arrhythmias may be a contraindication to pregnancy, and baffle obstruction should, ideally, be relieved before childbearing.

FOLLOW-UP. Regular follow-up by physicians with special expertise in CHD is recommended.

Atrial Switch. Serial follow-up of systemic right ventricular function is warranted. MRI is best, followed by radionuclide angiography and perhaps by echocardiography. Asymptomatic baffle obstruction should be sought with echocardiography or MRI. Regular Holter monitoring is recommended to diagnose unacceptable bradyarrhythmias or tachyarrhythmias.

Arterial Switch. Regular follow-up with echocardiography is recommended.

Rastelli. Regular follow-up with echocardiography is warranted given the inevitability of conduit degeneration over time.

Congenitally Corrected Transposition of the Great Arteries

DEFINITION. This term describes hearts in which there are discordant AV connections in combination with discordant ventriculoarterial connections.[185]

MORPHOLOGY (Fig. 56–25). cc-TGA is a rare condition, accounting for less than 1 percent of all CHD. When there is the usual atrial arrangement, systemic venous blood passes from the right atrium through a mitral valve to a left ventricle and then to the posteriorly located pulmonary artery. Pulmonary venous blood passes from the left atrium through a tricuspid valve to a left-sided right ventricle and then to an anterior, left-sided aorta. The circulation is thus "physiologically" corrected, but the morphological right ventricle supports the systemic circulation. Associated anomalies occur in up to 95 percent of patients and consist of VSD (75 percent), pulmonary or subpulmonary stenosis (75 percent), and left-sided (tricuspid and often "Ebstein-like") valve anomalies (>75 percent).

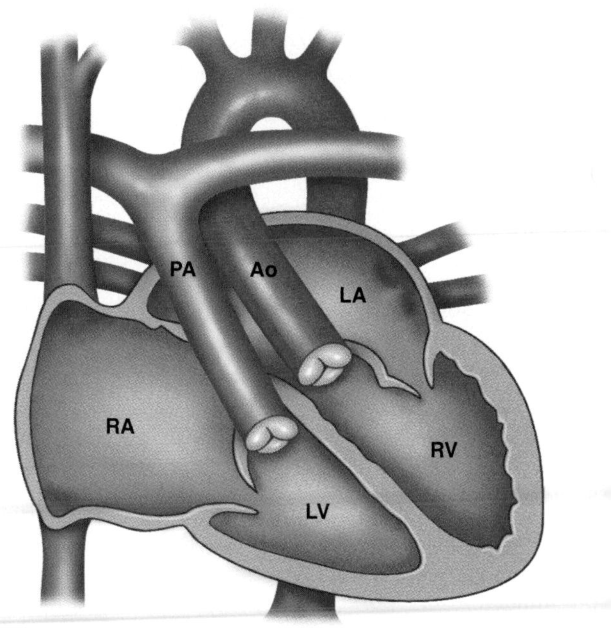

FIGURE 56–25 Diagrammatic representation of congenitally corrected transposition of the great arteries. RA = right atrium; RV = right ventricle; LA = left atrium; LV = left ventricle; Ao = aorta; PA = pulmonary artery. (From Mullins CE, Mayer DC: Congenital Heart Disease: A Diagrammatic Atlas. New York, Wiley-Liss, 1988.)

Because of the inherently abnormal conduction system, 5 percent of patients with cc-TGA are born with congenital complete heart block.

PATHOPHYSIOLOGY. Patients with no associated abnormalities ("isolated" cc-TGA) can exceptionally survive until the seventh or eighth decade.[186] Progressive systemic (tricuspid) AV valve regurgitation and systemic (right) ventricular dysfunction tend to occur from the fourth decade onward, whereas atrial tachyarrhythmias are more common from the fifth decade onward.[187] In addition to those born with congenital complete heart block, acquired complete AV block continues to develop at a rate of 2 percent per year, concentrated mainly at the time of cardiac surgery. Patients with associated anomalies (VSD, pulmonary stenosis, left-sided [tricuspid] valve anomaly) often have undergone surgical palliation (systemic-to-pulmonary artery shunt for cyanosis) or repair of the associated anomalies (see surgical procedures), but a significant number of patients are naturally balanced by a combination of their VSD and subpulmonary left ventricular outflow tract obstruction. While cyanosed they often remain well, with no intervention for many years.[188]

CLINICAL FEATURES

Unoperated. Patients with no associated defects (≤5 percent) can be asymptomatic until late adulthood. Dyspnea, exercise intolerance from developing congestive heart failure, and palpitations from supraventricular arrhythmias most often arise in the fifth or sixth decade.[189] Patients with well-balanced VSD and pulmonary stenosis can present with paradoxical emboli or cyanosis, especially if pulmonary stenosis is severe. Physical examination of a patient whose condition is otherwise uncomplicated reveals a somewhat more medial apex due to the side-by-side orientation of the two ventricles. The A_2 is often palpable in the 2nd left intercostal space due to the anterior location of the aorta. A single S_2 (A_2) is heard, with P_2 often being silent due to its variably posterior location. The murmur of an associated VSD or of left AV valve regurgitation may be heard. The murmur of pulmonary stenosis radiates upward and to the right, given the rightward direction of the main pulmonary artery. If there is complete heart block, cannon "*a* waves" with an S_1 of variable intensity are present.

VSD Patch and Left Ventricular-to-Pulmonary Artery Conduit Repair. Most patients are in functional Class I at 5 to 10 years after surgery despite the common development of tricuspid regurgitation and systemic right ventricular dysfunction after surgical repair. Dyspnea, exercise intolerance, and palpitations from supraventricular arrhythmia often occur in the fourth decade. Complete heart block may complicate surgery in an additional 25 percent. Physical examination reflects the basic cardiac malformation with or without residual coexisting anomalies.

LABORATORY INVESTIGATIONS

ECG. An abnormal direction of initial (septal) depolarization from right to left causes reversal of the precordial Q wave pattern (Q waves are often present in the right precordial leads and absent in the left). First-degree AV block occurs in about 50 percent, and complete AV block occurs in up to 25 percent of patients. Atrial arrhythmias may be seen.

Chest Radiography. Characteristically reveals absence of the normal pulmonary artery segment in favor of a smooth convexity of the left supracardiac border produced by the left-sided ascending aorta. The main pulmonary trunk is medially displaced and absent from the cardiac silhouette; the right pulmonary hilum is often prominent and elevated compared with the left, producing a right-sided "waterfall" appearance.

Echocardiography (Fig. 56–26). Echocardiography permits the identification of the basic malformation as well as any associated anomalies. The morphological left ventricle is characterized by its smooth endocardial surface and is guarded by a bileaflet AV (mitral) valve with no direct septal attachment. The morphological right ventricle is recognized by its apical trabeculation and moderator band and is guarded by a trileaflet apically displaced AV valve (tricuspid valve) with direct attachment to the septum. The AV valves therefore show reversed offsetting, a strong clue to the diagnosis. Ebstein-like malformation of the left (tricuspid) AV valve is defined by excessive (>8 mm/m^2 BSA) apical displacement of the left (tricuspid) AV valve, with or without dysplastic features.

MRI. The major role of MRI in cc-TGA patients is to evaluate the systemic right ventricular volume and ejection fraction. It does so better than echocardiography can at present. For claustrophobic or pacemaker patients, a high-quality radionuclide angiogram with volume estimates serves as a substitute. MRI can evaluate other issues as well, including conduit function and AV valve regurgitation.

Cardiac Catheterization. This is rarely required for diagnosis but may be indicated prior to surgical repair, to demonstrate the coronary artery anatomy as well as ventricular end-diastolic and pulmonary artery pressures.

INDICATIONS FOR INTERVENTION AND REINTERVENTION. If moderate or severe systemic (tricuspid, left) AV valve regurgitation develops, valve replacement should be considered. Left AV valve replacement should be performed before systemic right ventricular function deteriorates, namely at an ejection fraction of 45 percent or more.[190,191] When tricuspid regurgitation is associated with poor systemic (right) ventricular function, the double-switch procedure should perhaps be considered.[192-195] Patients with end-stage symptomatic heart failure should be referred for cardiac transplantation. The presence of a hemodynamically significant VSD (Qp/Qs > 1.5:1.0) or residual VSD with significant native or postsurgical (conduit) pulmonary outflow tract stenosis (echo mean or catheter gradient > 50 mm Hg) may require surgical correction. Left AV valve replacement at the time of VSD and pulmonary stenosis surgery should be considered if concomitant left AV valve regurgitation is present. Pacemaker implantation is usual when complete AV block is present. The optimal pacing modality is DDD. Active fixation electrodes are required, owing to the lack of apical trabeculation in the morphological left ventricle. Transvenous pacing should be avoided if there are intracardiac shunts because paradoxical emboli may occur. Epicardial leads are preferred under these circumstances.

INTERVENTIONAL OPTIONS

Medical Therapy. ACE inhibitor or beta-blocker therapy for patients with systemic ventricular dysfunction may be intuitive, but the role of such agents has not yet been demonstrated.

Conduit Replacement. This is inevitably required in survivors of this type of initial surgery.

Tricuspid Valve Replacement. For significant regurgitation, this is preferable to tricuspid valve repair.[190] Valve repair is usually unsuccessful because of the abnormal, often Ebstein-like anatomy of the valve.

Double-Switch Procedure. This procedure has been successfully performed in children. It should be considered for patients with severe tricuspid regurgitation and systemic ventricular dysfunction.[192] Its purpose is to relocate the left ventricle into the systemic circulation and the right ventricle into the pulmonary circulation, achieving physiological correction. An atrial switch procedure (Mustard or Senning), together with either an arterial switch procedure (when pulmonary stenosis is not present) or a Rastelli-type repair, the so-called Ilbawi procedure[196] (left ventricle tunneled to aorta and right ventricle-to-pulmonary artery valved conduit when VSD and pulmonary stenosis are present), can be performed after adequate left ventricular retraining, leaving the regurgitant tricuspid valve and failing right ventricle on the pulmonary side.

Cardiac Transplantation. Patients with deteriorating systemic (right) ventricular function should be treated aggressively with medical therapy but may need to be considered for transplantation.

INTERVENTIONAL OUTCOMES. After conduit repair and VSD patching, the median survival of patients reaching adulthood is 40 years.[197] The usual causes of death are sudden (presumed arrhythmic) or, more commonly, progressive systemic right ventricular dysfunction with systemic (tricuspid) AV valve regurgitation. The major predictor of poor outcome

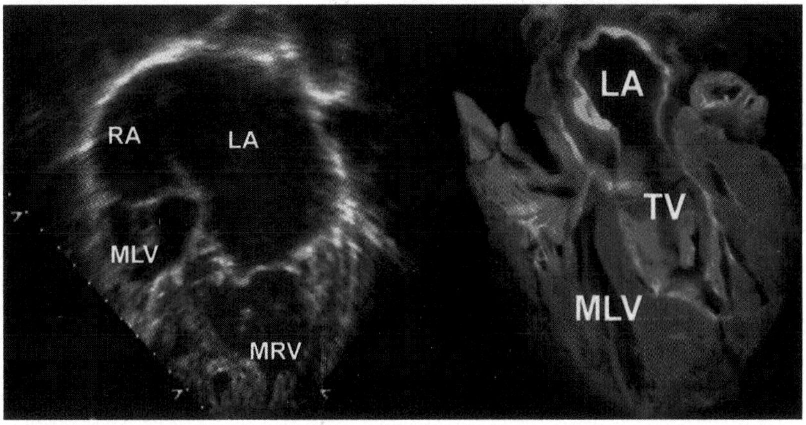

FIGURE 56–26 Four-chamber view in congenitally corrected transposition with dysplasia and displacement of the morphological left-sided tricuspid valve. LA = left atrium; MLV = morphological left ventricle; MRV = morphological right ventricle; RA = right atrium; TV = tricuspid valve.

is the presence of left AV (tricuspid) valve regurgitation.[197] Reoperation is common (15 to 25 percent), with left AV valve replacement usually being the primary reason. Data in adults using the double-switch procedure are lacking, and this procedure should be considered experimental in this patient population.

FOLLOW-UP. All patients should have at least annual cardiology follow-up with an expert in the care of patients with congenital cardiac defects. Regular assessment of systemic (tricuspid) AV valve regurgitation by serial echocardiographic studies and systemic ventricular function by MRI or radionuclide angiography should be done. Holter recording can be useful if paroxysmal atrial arrhythmias or transient complete AV block is suspected.

Double-Outlet Right Ventricle

DEFINITION. The term *double-outlet right ventricle* describes hearts in which more than 50 percent of both semilunar valves arise from the morphological right ventricle. It may coexist with any form of atrial arrangement or AV connection and is independent of infundibular (conal) anatomy.

MORPHOLOGY (Fig. 56–27). There are few morphological descriptors that have invoked more discussion and controversy than double-outlet right ventricle. The definition given earlier is flawed but pragmatic.[198] To some extent this anatomical definition is less important than the understanding of the relationship between the great vessels and the VSD, and the anatomy of the outlets to the great vessels, both of which are crucial determinants of clinical presentation and management.

CLINICAL FEATURES. There are three main categories of double-outlet right ventricle: (1) double-outlet right ventricle with a subaortic VSD, (2) double-outlet right ventricle with a subpulmonary VSD, and (3) double-outlet right ventricle with a noncommitted VSD.

When present, the anatomy of the infundibular septum further modifies the hemodynamics. Taking double-outlet right ventricle with a *subaortic VSD* as an example, where the aorta and its semilunar valve is closest to, or overriding, the trabecular septum, anterior deviation of the outlet septum causes subpulmonary stenosis, and the clinical scenario and management algorithm are similar or identical to that of tetralogy of Fallot. Conversely, if the outlet septum is deviated posteriorly, there will be subaortic stenosis, often with a coexisting abnormality of the aortic arch. The presentation and management of this variation are therefore entirely different. If there is no deviation of the outlet septum, and no outlet obstruction, the clinical scenario will be that of a simple VSD. Double-outlet right ventricle with a *subpulmonary VSD* (Taussig-Bing anomaly) can be considered along with TGA. This is because the usual position of the pulmonary artery (posterior and leftward to the aorta) means that the streaming of deoxygenated and oxygenated blood is similar to that of transposition, even though most of the pulmonary valve is connected to the right ventricle. Anterior deviation of the outlet septum causes subaortic stenosis and aortic anomalies, and posterior deviation causes subpulmonary stenosis and limits pulmonary blood flow. It is also important to recognize double-outlet right ventricle with a *noncommitted VSD*. This defines hearts in which the VSD is remote from the outlets. Surgical management may be particularly difficult.

ASSOCIATED LESIONS. More than half of patients with double-outlet right ventricle have associated anomalies of the AV valves. Mitral valve atresia associated with a hypoplastic left ventricle is common. Ebstein anomaly of the tricuspid valve, complete AV septal defect, and overriding or straddling of either AV valve may occur.[199]

LABORATORY INVESTIGATIONS. Because of the diversity of underlying anatomies, discussion of the ECG and radiographic features is not included here.

Echocardiography. This is the mainstay of diagnosis. The commitment of the semilunar valves to the ventricles is ascertained. When present, deviation of the outlet septum beneath a semilunar valve likely has implications for downstream development. For example, when there is subaortic stenosis, the echocardiographic examination is incomplete until abnormalities of the aorta and arch have been excluded. Preoperative evaluation must also take account of potential AV valve anomalies and straddling in particular.

INDICATIONS FOR INTERVENTION. The goals of operative treatment are to establish left ventricle-to-aorta continuity, create adequate right ventricle-to-pulmonary continuity, and repair associated lesions. Palliative surgery is reserved for those in whom biventricular repair is not possible and in those with markedly reduced pulmonary blood flow. In the latter, an aortopulmonary shunt may be placed to temporize prior to complete correction. For the remainder, complete repair is now performed as a primary procedure in the majority.[200] In double-outlet right ventricle with a subaortic VSD, repair is accomplished by creating an intraventricular baffle that conducts left ventricular blood to the aorta. If there is coexisting subpulmonary stenosis, the repair is similar to that of tetralogy of Fallot. When the VSD is subpulmonary, but without subpulmonary stenosis, repair is accomplished by closure of the VSD and arterial switch. Subpulmonary stenosis frequently is present in double-outlet right ventricle with a subpulmonary VSD. In these cases the aorta is connected to the left ventricle using an intraventricular baffle, and a

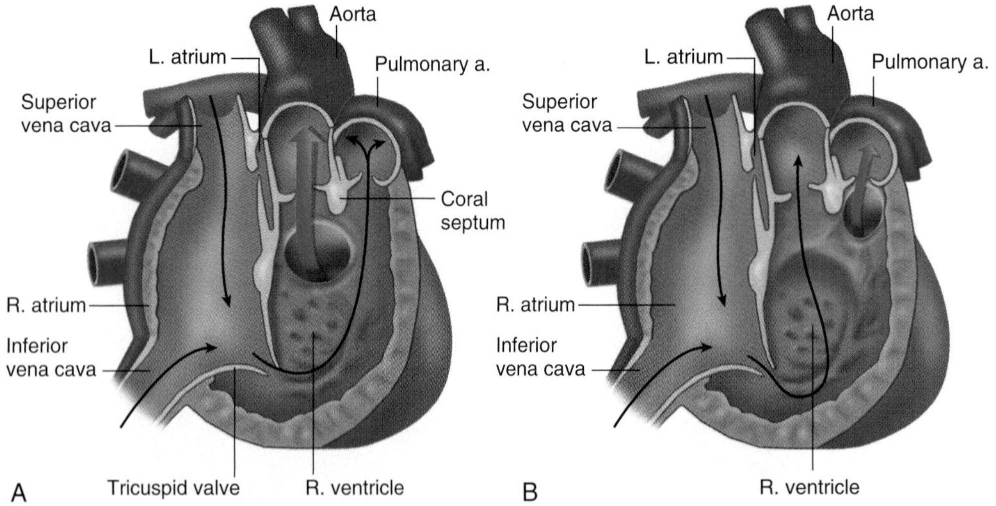

FIGURE 56–27 Double-outlet right ventricle with side-by-side relation of great arteries is illustrated in both panels. **A,** A subaortic ventricular septal defect below the crista supraventricularis favors delivery of left ventricular blood to the aorta. **B,** Subpulmonary location of the ventricular septal defect above the crista favors streaming to the pulmonary trunk. (**A** and **B,** From Castañeda A, Jonas RA, Mayer JE, et al: Cardiac Surgery of the Neonate and Infant. Philadelphia, WB Saunders, 1994, p 446.)

right ventricle-to-pulmonary artery conduit is placed to complete the repair (Rastelli procedure). Classic surgical approaches cannot be used when the VSD is remote and uncommitted to either semilunar orifice.[201] Occasionally the VSD can be baffled toward the aorta, but when this is not possible, the right ventricle may be used as the systemic ventricle. This requires a Mustard or Senning atrial redirection procedure, closure of the VSD, and placement of a conduit between the left ventricle and the pulmonary trunk.

INTERVENTIONAL OPTIONS AND OUTCOMES. The late follow-up of the surgical procedures described earlier (e.g., tetralogy of Fallot repair, arterial switch, Rastelli) tend to be less satisfactory when there is double-outlet right ventricle than when performed for more classic indications.[200,202,203] The development of subaortic stenosis is more likely because of the abnormal geometry of the left ventricular outflow tract that often results after correction.[204] Similarly, right ventricle-to-pulmonary conduit obstruction is more likely because of the spatial difficulties imposed on placement of the conduit, with respect to the position on the right ventricle and the sternum. Because of these considerations, the options for catheter interventions are often fairly limited. However, recurrent arch obstruction and distal pulmonary artery obstruction are amenable to balloon dilation with or without stenting.

FOLLOW-UP. All of these patients require at least annual review by a congenital heart cardiologist.

Ebstein Anomaly

MORPHOLOGY (Fig. 56–28). The common feature in all cases of Ebstein anomaly is apical displacement of the septal tricuspid leaflet in conjunction with leaflet dysplasia. Many, but not all, have associated displacement of the posterior mural leaflet, with the anterior leaflet never being displaced. Although the anterior leaflet is never displaced apically, it may be adherent to the free wall of the right ventricle, causing right ventricular outflow tract obstruction. The displacement of the tricuspid valve results in "atrialization" (functioning as an atrial chamber) of the inflow tract of the right ventricle and consequently produces a variably small, functional right ventricle. Associated anomalies include patent foramen ovale or ASD in approximately 50 percent of patients, accessory conduction pathways in 25 percent (usually right sided), and, occasionally, varying degrees of right ventricular outflow tract obstruction, VSD, aortic coarctation, PDA, or mitral valve disease.

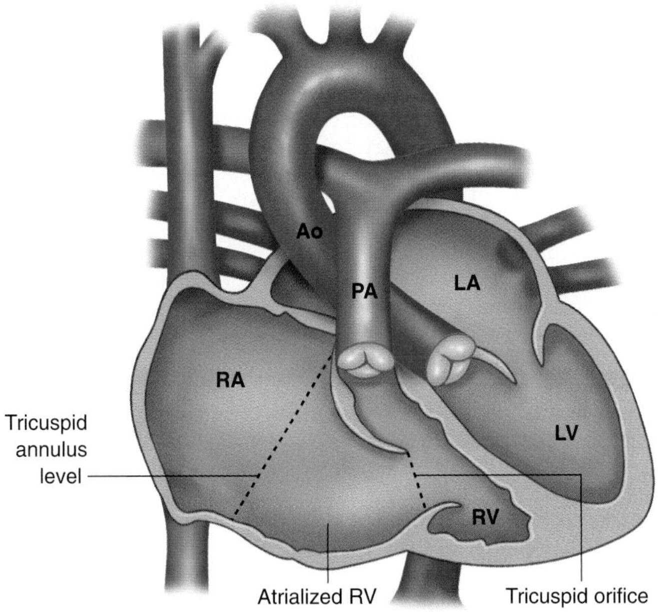

FIGURE 56–28 Diagrammatic representation of Ebstein anomaly. RA = right atrium; RV = right ventricle; LA = left atrium; LV = left ventricle; Ao = aorta; PA = pulmonary artery. (From Mullins CE, Mayer DC: Congenital Heart Disease: A Diagrammatic Atlas. New York, Wiley-Liss, 1988.)

PATHOPHYSIOLOGY. Varying degrees of tricuspid regurgitation (or exceptionally tricuspid stenosis) result from the abnormal tricuspid leaflet morphology with consequent further right atrial enlargement. Right ventricular volume overload from significant tricuspid regurgitation and infundibular dilation can also be present. Right-to-left shunting through a patent foramen ovale or ASD occurs if the right atrial pressure exceeds the left atrial pressure (which is often the case when severe tricuspid regurgitation is present).

NATURAL HISTORY. The natural history of patients with Ebstein anomaly depends on its severity.[205] When the tricuspid valve deformity and dysfunction are extreme, death in utero from hydrops fetalis is the norm. When the tricuspid valve deformity is severe, symptoms usually develop in newborn infants. Patients with moderate tricuspid valve deformity and dysfunction usually develop symptoms during late adolescence or young adult life. Adults with Ebstein anomaly can occasionally remain asymptomatic throughout their life if the anomaly is mild—exceptional survival to the ninth decade has been reported.

CLINICAL ISSUES

Pediatrics. With severe tricuspid valve deformity, newborns and infants present with failure to thrive and right-sided congestive heart failure. Most other pediatric patients who present after the neonatal period remain asymptomatic until late adolescence or early adult life.

Adults. Most adult patients present with exercise intolerance (exertional dyspnea and fatigue), palpitations of supraventricular origin, or cyanosis from a right-to-left shunt at atrial level. Occasionally, a paradoxical embolus resulting in a transient ischemic attack or stroke can call attention to the diagnosis. Right-sided cardiac failure from severe tricuspid regurgitation and right ventricular dysfunction is possible. Sudden death (presumed to be arrhythmic in nature) is described. Physical examination typically reveals an unimpressive jugular venous pressure because of the large and compliant right atrium and atrialized right ventricle; a widely split S_1 with a loud tricuspid component (the "sail sound"); a widely split S_2 from the right bundle branch block; and a right-sided third heart sound. A pansystolic murmur increasing on inspiration from tricuspid regurgitation is best heard at the lower left sternal border. Cyanosis from a right-to-left shunt at the atrial level may or may not be present.

LABORATORY INVESTIGATIONS

ECG. The ECG presentation of Ebstein anomaly varies widely. Low voltage is typical. Peaked P waves in leads II and V_1 reflect right atrial enlargement. The PR interval is usually prolonged, but a short PR interval and a delta wave from early activation through an accessory pathway can be present. An rsr′ pattern consistent with right ventricular conduction delay is typically seen in lead V_1, and right bundle branch block is common in adults. Atrial flutter and fibrillation are common. The ECG may be normal.

Chest Radiography. A rightward convexity from an enlarged right atrium and atrialized right ventricle coupled with a leftward convexity from a dilated infundibulum give the heart a "water bottle" appearance on chest radiograph. Cardiomegaly, highly variable in degree, is the rule. The aorta and the pulmonary trunk are inconspicuous. The pulmonary vasculature is usually normal to reduced.

Echocardiography (Fig. 56–29). The diagnosis of Ebstein anomaly is usually made by echocardiography. Apical displacement of the septal leaflet of the tricuspid valve by

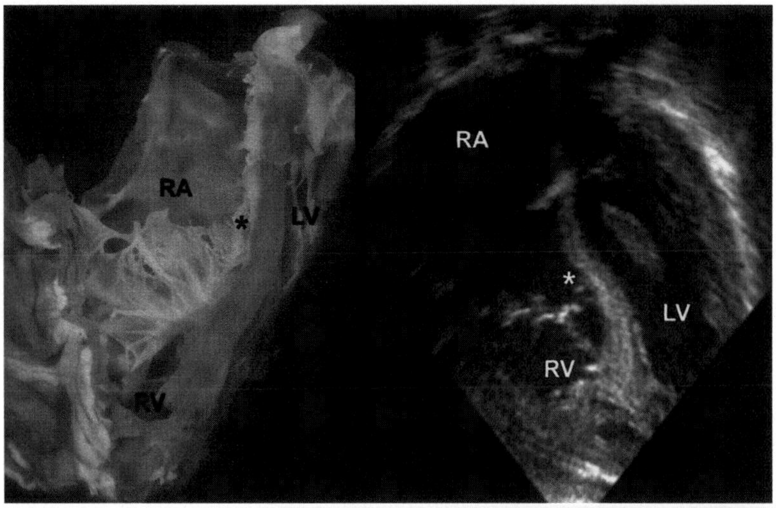

FIGURE 56–29 Apical four-chamber view in Ebstein malformation of the tricuspid valve. Note the significant displacement of the septal tricuspid valve leaflet (asterisk), with associated valve dysplasia. LV = left ventricle; RA = right atrium; RV = right ventricle.

8 mm/m^2 or more, combined with an elongated sail-like appearance of the anterior leaflet, confirms the diagnosis. The size of the atrialized portion of the right ventricle (identified between the tricuspid annulus and the ventricular attachment of the tricuspid valve leaflets) and the systolic performance of the functional right ventricle can be estimated. The degree of tricuspid regurgitation (and more rarely stenosis) can be assessed. Associated defects such as ASDs as well as the presence and direction of shunting can also be identified.

Angiography. Cardiac catheterization is required mainly when concomitant coronary artery disease is suspected and to determine if pulmonary artery pressures are elevated. When performed, selective right ventricular angiography shows the extent of tricuspid valve displacement, the size of the functional right ventricle, and configuration of its outflow tract.

MRI. This investigation can offer insights into functional right ventricular volume and function.

INDICATIONS FOR INTERVENTION. Indications for intervention include substantial cyanosis, right-sided heart failure, deteriorating functional capacity (NYHA ≥ class III), and perhaps the occurrence of paradoxical emboli. Recurrent supraventricular arrhythmias not controlled by medical or ablation therapy, and asymptomatic substantial cardiomegaly (cardiothoracic ratio >65 percent) are relative indications.[206]

INTERVENTIONAL OPTIONS. Tricuspid valve repair when feasible is preferable to tricuspid valve replacement. The feasibility of tricuspid valve repair depends primarily on the experience and skill of the surgeon, as well as on the adequacy of the anterior leaflet of the tricuspid valve to form a monocusp valve. Tricuspid valve repair is possible when the edges of the anterior leaflet of the tricuspid valve are not severely tethered down to the myocardium and when the functional right ventricle is of adequate size (>35 percent of the total right ventricle).[74] If the tricuspid valve is not repairable, valve replacement will be necessary, usually with a bioprosthetic tricuspid valve. For "high-risk" patients (those with severe tricuspid regurgitation, an inadequate functional right ventricle [because of size or function], and/or chronic supraventricular arrhythmias), a bidirectional cavopulmonary connection can be added to reduce right ventricular preload if pulmonary artery pressures are low.[207] Occasionally a Fontan operation may be the best option in patients with tricuspid stenosis and/or a hypoplastic right ventricle. A concomitant right atrial or biatrial maze procedure at the time of surgery should be considered in patients with chronic atrial flutter/fibrillation.[58] If an accessory pathway is present, this should be mapped and obliterated either at the time of surgical repair or preoperatively in the catheter laboratory. An atrial communication, if present, should be closed.

With satisfactory valve repair, with or without plication of the atrialized right ventricle or bidirectional cavopulmonary connection, the medium-term prognosis is excellent.[50,208] Late arrhythmias can occur.[209] With valve replacement, results are less satisfactory. Valve re-replacement may be necessary because of a failing bioprosthesis or a thrombosed mechanical valve.

REPRODUCTIVE ISSUES. In the absence of maternal cyanosis, right-sided heart failure, or arrhythmias, pregnancy is usually well tolerated.[210]

FOLLOW-UP ISSUES. All patients with Ebstein anomaly should have regular follow-up, the frequency being dictated by the severity of their disease. Particular attention should be paid to patients with cyanosis, substantial cardiomegaly, poor right ventricular function, and recurrent atrial arrhythmias. Patients with substantial tricuspid regurgitation following tricuspid valve repair need close follow-up, as do patients with recurrent atrial arrhythmias, degenerating bioprostheses, or dysfunctional mechanical valves.

Valvular and Vascular Conditions

Left Ventricular Outflow Tract Lesions (Fig. 56–30)

COARCTATION OF THE AORTA

Aortic arch obstruction may be divided into (1) localized coarctation in close proximity to a PDA or ligamentum, (2) tubular hypoplasia of some part of the aortic arch system, and (3) aortic arch interruption.

Localized Aortic Coarctation

MORPHOLOGY. This lesion consists of a localized shelf in the posterolateral aortic wall opposite the ductus arteriosus. A neonatal presentation is more often associated with a shelf plus transverse aortic arch and isthmic hypoplasia, whereas with a later presentation these areas are larger.[211,212]

CLINICAL FEATURES. Coarctation occurs two to five times more commonly in males, and there is a high degree of association with gonadal dysgenesis (Turner syndrome) and bicuspid aortic valve. Other common associated anomalies include VSD and mitral stenosis or regurgitation. Additional lesions have an impact on outcome.[213]

NEONATES. Rapid, severe obstruction in infancy is a prominent cause of left ventricular failure and systemic hypoperfusion. Heart failure in this setting is due to a sudden increase in left ventricular wall stress after closure of the arterial duct. Substantial left-to-right shunting across a patent foramen ovale and pulmonary venous hypertension secondary to heart failure cause pulmonary arterial hypertension. Because little or no aortic obstruction existed during fetal life, the collateral circulation in the newborn period is often poorly developed. In these infants, peripheral pulses characteristically are weak throughout the body until left ventricular function is improved with medical management; a significant pressure difference then develops between the arms and the legs, allowing detection of a pulse discrepancy. Cardiac murmurs are nonspecific in infancy and commonly are derived from associated lesions.

ECG. This shows right axis deviation and right ventricular hypertrophy.

Chest Radiography. This shows generalized cardiomegaly and pulmonary arterial and venous engorgement.

Echocardiography (Fig. 56–31A). This demonstrates the posterior shelf and the degree of associated isthmic and/or transverse arch hypoplasia. Doppler echocardiography is helpful if the ductus is closed or partially restrictive and demonstrates a high-velocity jet during systole and diastole. On the other hand, if the ductus is widely patent, then the usual right-to-left shunting makes the Doppler assessment invalid, because the distal pressure then reflects the high pulmonary artery pressure. With associated tubular hypoplasia, Doppler-derived gradients provide higher and less reliable values compared with those obtained by blood pressure or catheterization measurements.[214,215]

MRA. Although this is the gold standard for evaluation of the aortic arch in the older child and adult, it is usually unnecessary in the neonate and infant.[216]

Management usually involves prostaglandin therapy in an attempt to reopen or maintain patency of a ductus arteriosus. After prostaglandin E_1 infusion to dilate the ductus arteriosus, the pressure difference may be obliterated across the site of coarctation because the fetal flow pattern is reestablished. This has the additional benefit of improving renal perfusion, which in turn helps reverse the frequently associated metabolic acidosis.

Intervention in this age group usually involves surgical relief of the obstruction with excision of the area of coarctation and extended end-to-end repair or end-to-side anastomosis with absorbable sutures to allow remodeling of the aorta with time.[217] Subclavian flap aortoplasty, which was employed extensively in the past, is now less popular than the earlier-mentioned procedures. It is generally believed that balloon dilation does not play a role in management in this age group. Early surgery is associated with a lower incidence of long-term hypertension.[217]

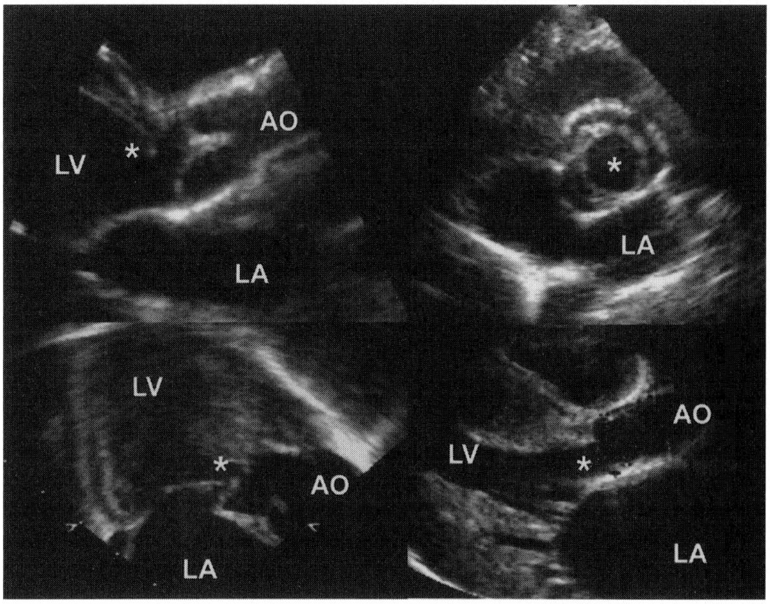

FIGURE 56–30 Montage demonstrating the different types of left ventricular outflow tract obstruction (asterisks). The upper left image shows isolated fibromuscular obstruction, the upper right stenosis due to a bicuspid aortic valve, the lower left due to chordal apparatus from the anterior mitral leaflet, and the lower right due to tunnel narrowing at the valve, annular, and subvalve level. AO = aorta; LA = left atrium; LV = left ventricle.

INFANTS AND CHILDREN

Presentation. Most infants and children with isolated coarctation are asymptomatic, with the findings of reduced femoral pulses and/or hypertension being detected during routine medical care of the pediatric patient. Heart failure is uncommon because the left ventricle has a chance to become hypertrophied, thus maintaining a normal wall stress. Complaints of headache, cold extremities, and claudication with exercise may be noted in the older child and adolescent.

A midsystolic murmur over the anterior chest, back, and spinous processes is most frequent, becoming continuous if the lumen is sufficiently narrowed to result in a high-velocity jet across the lesion throughout the cardiac cycle. Additional systolic and continuous murmurs over the lateral thoracic wall may reflect increased flow through dilated and tortuous collateral vessels, which are commonly not heard until later childhood.

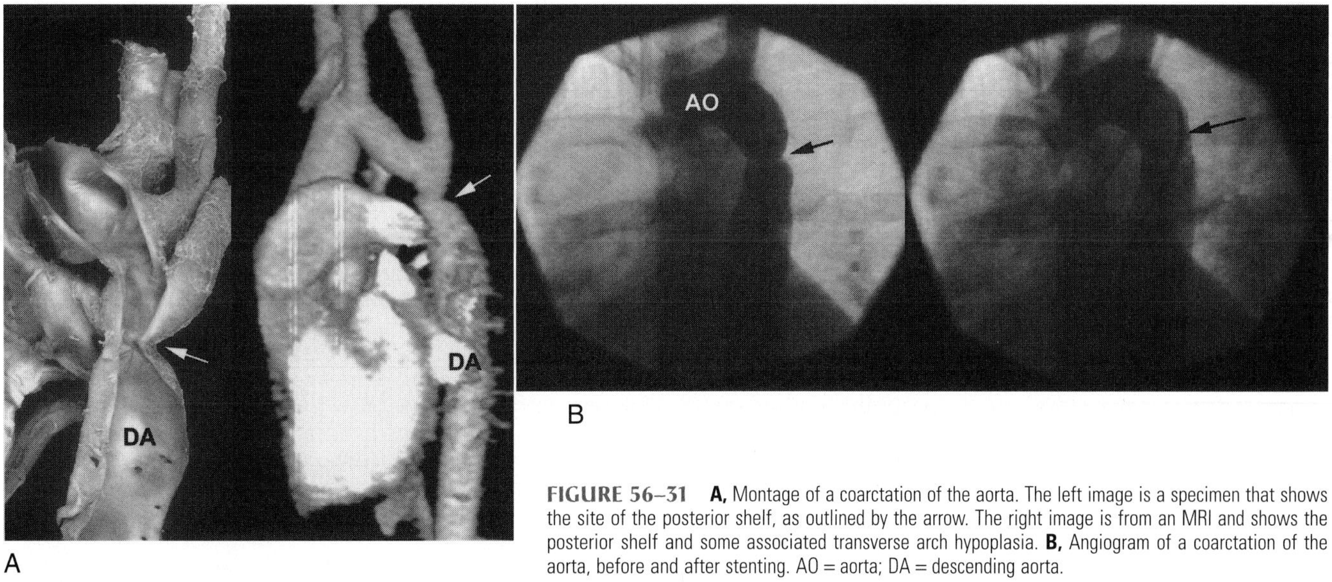

FIGURE 56–31 **A,** Montage of a coarctation of the aorta. The left image is a specimen that shows the site of the posterior shelf, as outlined by the arrow. The right image is from an MRI and shows the posterior shelf and some associated transverse arch hypoplasia. **B,** Angiogram of a coarctation of the aorta, before and after stenting. AO = aorta; DA = descending aorta.

ECG. This reveals left ventricular hypertrophy of various degrees, depending on the height of arterial pressure above the obstruction and the patient's age. Coexisting right ventricular hypertrophy usually implies a complicated lesion.

Chest Radiography. The characteristic posteroanterior film feature is the so-called figure-3 configuration of the proximal descending thoracic aorta due to both prestenotic and poststenotic dilation. Rib notching (unilateral or bilateral, second to ninth ribs) is present in 50 percent of cases. Rib notching is unilateral if the right or left subclavian arteries arise from the aorta distal to the coarctation. Rib notching is noted as an erosion of the undersurface of a posterior rib, usually at its outer third, with a sclerotic margin.

Echocardiography. This demonstrates a posterior shelf, a well-expanded isthmus and transverse aortic arch (in most cases), and a high-velocity continuous jet through the coarctation site. Of interest there is a slow upstroke on the abdominal aortic velocity profile when compared to that seen in the ascending aorta.

MRI. This provides detailed information in this age group and may be performed prior to intervention, particularly if balloon dilation is the treatment of choice. This is the best tool for post-intervention imaging and has become routine in many centers.[216]

Angiocardiography. This is reserved for delineating the coarctation at the time of balloon dilation.

Primary management in those cases with a well-expanded isthmus and transverse aortic arch invariably involves balloon dilation.[218] Surgery is usually reserved for cases where there is associated arch hypoplasia that requires a patch, as well as coarctation resection.

Paradoxical hypertension of short duration is often noted in the immediate postoperative period, a phenomenon much less common after balloon angioplasty. A resetting of carotid baroreceptors and increased catecholamine secretion appears to be responsible for the initial phase of postoperative systemic hypertension, with a later, second phase of prolonged elevation of systolic and particularly diastolic blood pressure related to activation of the renin-angiotensin system. A necrotizing panarteritis of the small vessels of the gastrointestinal tract of uncertain cause occasionally complicates the course of recovery.

Recoarctation. The risk of recurrent narrowing after repair of coarctation in infancy is 5 to 10 percent. Such narrowing is best screened for with Doppler ultrasonography, with MRI being the gold standard for imaging. Clinical decisions to intervene are usually based on a cuff blood pressure difference between the right arm and leg (for a left aortic arch and normal innominate artery). Although there are no hard and fast rules for absolute blood pressure difference, it has been common practice to reintervene when the blood pressure difference is more than 25 to 30 mm Hg, in the presence of systemic hypertension. Although Doppler measurements can detect the presence of a recurrent obstruction, this technique provides an overestimation of the blood pressure–measured gradients due to the phenomenon of pressure recovery.[214] Recoarctation is usually addressed with balloon dilation if the obstruction is relatively localized. In the presence of long-segment narrowings, surgical intervention may be necessary, with the use of patch augmentation of the hypoplastic segment. More recently in the adolescent or adult, balloon-expandable stents have been employed with good success.[219] This has the advantage of avoiding the risk of potential neurological damage in post-intervention cases that invariably have poorly developed collaterals.

Long-Term Complications. In those patients who survive the first 2 years of life, complications of juxtaductal coarctation are uncommon before the second or third decade.[220-222] The chief hazards to patients with coarctation result from severe hypertension and include the development of cerebral aneurysms and hemorrhage, hypertensive encephalopathy, rupture of the aorta, left ventricular failure, and infective endocarditis. Systemic hypertension in the absence of residual coarctation has been observed in resting or exercise-stressed patients postoperatively and appears to be related to the duration of preoperative hypertension.[11,223] Life-long observation is desirable because of the late onset of hypertension in some postoperative patients.

ADULTS. Although much of the previous material is also relevant in the adult, there are some differences in the issues faced by adult patients. *Complex coarctation* is used to describe coarctation in the presence of other important intracardiac anomalies (e.g., VSD, left ventricular outflow tract obstruction, and mitral stenosis) and is usually detected in infancy. *Simple coarctation* refers to coarctation in the absence of such lesions. It is the most common form detected de novo in adults. Associated abnormalities include bicuspid aortic valve in most cases; intracranial aneurysms (most commonly of the circle of Willis) in up to 10 percent; and acquired intercostal artery aneurysms. One definition of *significant coarctation* requires a gradient greater than 20 mm Hg across the coarctation site at angiography with or without proximal systemic hypertension. A second definition of significant coarctation requires the presence of proximal hypertension in the company of echocardiographic or angiographic evidence of aortic coarctation. If there is an extensive collateral circulation, there may be minimal or no pressure gradient and acquired aortic atresia.

Death in patients who do not undergo repair is usually due to heart failure (usually > 30 years of age), coronary artery disease, aortic rupture/dissection, concomitant aortic valve disease, infective endarteritis/endocarditis, or cerebral hemorrhage.[224,225] Of Turner syndrome patients, 35 percent have aortic coarctation.

Clinical Features. Patients can be asymptomatic, or they can present with minimal symptoms of epistaxis, headache, and leg weakness on exertion or more serious symptoms of congestive heart failure, angina, aortic stenosis, aortic dissection, or unexplained intracerebral hemorrhage. Leg claudication (pain) is rare unless there is concomitant abdominal aortic coarctation (Somerville J, personal communication, 1998). A thorough clinical examination reveals upper limb systemic hypertension as well as a differential systolic blood pressure of at least 10 mm Hg (brachial > popliteal artery pressure). Radial-femoral pulse delay is evident unless significant aortic regurgitation coexists. Auscultation may reveal an interscapular systolic murmur emanating from the coarctation site and a widespread crescendo-decrescendo systolic murmur throughout the chest wall from intercostal collateral arteries. Fundoscopic examination can reveal "corkscrew" tortuosity of retinal arterioles.

INTERVENTIONAL OUTCOMES

Surgical. After surgical repair of simple coarctation, the obstruction is usually relieved with minimal mortality (1 percent). Paraplegia due to spinal cord ischemia is uncommon (0.4 percent) and may occur in patients who do not have well-developed collateral circulation. The prevalence of recoarctation reported in the literature varies widely, from 7 to 60 percent depending on the definition used, the length of follow-up, and the age at surgery. The appropriateness of the surgical repair for a given anatomy is probably the main factor dictating the chance of recoarctation rather than the type of surgical repair itself.[226] True aneurysm formation at the site of coarctation repair is also a well-recognized entity, with a reported incidence between 2 and 27 percent.[227-229] Aneurysms are particularly common after Dacron patch aortoplasty and usually occur in the native aorta opposite the patch. Late dissection at the repair site is rare, but false aneurysms, usually at the suture line, can occur. Long-term follow-up after surgical correction of coarctation of the aorta still reveals an increased incidence of premature cardiovascular disease and death.[230,231]

Transcatheter. After balloon dilation (Fig. 56–31B), aortic dissection, restenosis, and aneurysm formation at the site of coarctation all have been documented.[232-236] These complications may well be reduced if stents are used.[219] The significance of aneurysm formation is often unknown, and longer-term data are needed.[237]

Prior hypertension resolves in up to 50 percent of patients but may recur later in life, especially if the intervention is performed at an older age.[230,231] In some of these patients this may be essential hypertension, but a hemodynamic basis should be sought and blood pressure control should be attained. Systolic hypertension is also common with exercise and is not a surrogate marker for recoarctation of the aorta.[11] It may be related to residual arch hypoplasia or to increased renin and catecholamine activity from residual functional abnormalities of the precoarctation vessels. The criteria for and significance of exertional systolic hypertension are controversial.[11] Late cerebrovascular events occur, notably in those patients undergoing repair as adults and in those with residual hypertension. Endocarditis or endarteritis can occur at the coarctation site or on intracardiac lesions; and if this occurs at the coarctation site, embolic manifestations are restricted to the legs.

FOLLOW-UP. All patients should have follow-up examination every 1 to 3 years. Particular attention should be directed toward residual hypertension; heart failure; intracardiac disease, such as an associated bicuspid aortic valve, which can become stenotic or regurgitant later in life; or an ascending aortopathy sometimes seen in the presence of bicuspid aortic valve. Complications at the site of repair such as restenosis and aneurysm formation should also be sought using clinical examination, chest radiography, echocardiography, and periodic MRI or CT scanning. Patients with Dacron patch repair should probably undergo an MRI[238] or spiral CT examination every 3 to 5 years or so to detect subclinical aneurysm formation. Hemoptysis from a leaking or ruptured aneurysm is a serious complication requiring immediate investigation and surgery. New or unusual headaches raise the possibility of berry aneurysms. Endocarditis prophylaxis is recommended for any residual turbulent flow.

AORTIC ARCH HYPOPLASIA

MORPHOLOGY. The aortic isthmus, the portion of the aorta between the left subclavian artery and the ductus arteriosus, should be narrowed in the fetus and newborn. The lumen of the aortic isthmus is about two-thirds that of the ascending and descending portions of the aorta until age 6 to 9 months, when the physiological narrowing disappears. Pathological tubular hypoplasia of the aortic arch usually is noted in the aortic isthmus and is most commonly associated with presentation of aortic coarctation in the newborn period. Despite this, there is a small group of cases where the arch obstruction is due primarily to tubular hypoplasia, usually involving both the aortic isthmus and transverse aortic arch (between the innominate and subclavian artery). These cases usually present early on in life with similar findings to those with a severe coarctation of the aorta. As with the latter, they are duct dependent and may also be associated with other left-sided obstructive lesions.

MANAGEMENT OPTIONS. Provided the other left-sided structures are formed well enough to sustain life, the management involves arch reconstruction with a patch, in a similar fashion to those cases undergoing a Norwood procedure for hypoplastic left heart syndrome. If the left-sided structures are hypoplastic, then palliative surgery with a Norwood procedure or cardiac transplantation are the two treatments of choice.

Complex Coarctation. In some instances the coarctation of the aorta is part of a more complex spectrum of lesions. This can be seen in cases with double-outlet right ventricle, cc-TGA, D-TGA, functionally single ventricle, truncus arteriosus, and AV septal defect. In these cases the decision process involves not only the coarctation repair but the management of the associated lesion(s). In the current era, the general trend is to complete repair of the intracardiac lesion at the same time as the arch repair.

SINUS OF VALSALVA ANEURYSM AND FISTULA

MORPHOLOGY. The malformation consists of a separation, or lack of fusion, between the media of the aorta and the annulus fibrosus of the aortic valve. The receiving chamber of a right aortic sinus aortocardiac fistula is usually the right ventricle, but occasionally, when the noncoronary cusp is involved, the fistula drains into the right atrium. Five to 15 percent of aneurysms originate in the posterior or noncoronary sinus. The left aortic sinus is seldom involved. Associated anomalies are common and include a VSD, bicuspid aortic valve, and aortic coarctation.

CLINICAL FEATURES. The deficiency in the aortic media appears to be congenital. Reports in infants are exceedingly rare and are infrequent in children, because progressive aneurysmal dilation of the weakened area develops but may not be recognized until the third or fourth decade of life, when rupture into a cardiac chamber occurs.[239-241] A congenital aneurysm of an aortic sinus of Valsalva, particularly the right coronary sinus, is an uncommon anomaly that occurs three times more often in males. An unruptured aneurysm usually does not produce a hemodynamic abnormality. Rarely, myocardial ischemia may be caused by coronary arterial compression. Rupture is often of abrupt onset, causes chest pain, and creates continuous arteriovenous shunting and acute volume loading of both right and left heart chambers, which promptly results in heart failure. An additional complication is infective endocarditis, which may originate either on the edges of the aneurysm or on those areas in the right side of the heart that are traumatized by the jetlike stream of blood flowing through the fistula.

The presence of this anomaly should be suspected in a patient with a combination of chest pain of sudden onset, resting or exertional dyspnea, bounding pulses, and a loud, superficial, continuous murmur accentuated in diastole when the fistula opens into the right ventricle, as well as a thrill along the right or left lower sternal border. The physical findings can be difficult to distinguish from those produced by a coronary arteriovenous fistula.

LABORATORY INVESTIGATIONS

ECG. This may show biventricular hypertrophy, or it may be normal.

Chest Radiography. This may demonstrate generalized cardiomegaly and usually heart failure.

Echocardiography. Studies based on 2D and pulsed Doppler echocardiography may detect the walls of the aneurysm and disturbed flow within the aneurysm or at the site of perforation, respectively. TEE may provide more precise information than the transthoracic approach.[242,243]

Cardiac Catheterization. This reveals a left-to-right shunt at the ventricular or, less commonly, the atrial level; the diagnosis may be established definitively by retrograde thoracic aortography.

MANAGEMENT OPTIONS AND OUTCOMES. Preoperative medical management consists of measures to relieve cardiac failure and to treat coexistent arrhythmias or endocarditis, if present. At operation, the aneurysm is closed and amputated, and the aortic wall is reunited with the heart, either by direct suture or with a prosthesis. Every effort should be made to preserve the aortic valve in children because patch closure of the defect combined with prosthetic valve replacement greatly enhances the risk of operation in small patients. Rarely, device closure of the ruptured aneurysm has been attempted.[244]

VASCULAR RINGS

MORPHOLOGY. The term *vascular ring* is used for those aortic arch or pulmonary artery malformations that exhibit an abnormal relation with the esophagus and trachea, often causing dysphagia and/or respiratory symptoms.[245]

DOUBLE AORTIC ARCH (Fig. 56–32). The most common vascular ring is produced by a double aortic arch in which both the right and left fourth embryonic aortic arches persist. In the most common type of double aortic arch, there is a left ligamentum arteriosum or occasionally a ductus arteriosus. Although both arches may be patent at the time of diagnosis, invariably the left arch distal to the left subclavian artery is atretic and is connected to the descending aorta by a fibrous remnant that completes the ring. In the setting where both arches are patent, the right arch is usually larger than the left. This usually occurs as an isolated lesion, with the respiratory symptoms being caused by tracheal compression and frequently associated laryngomalacia, usually in the neonate and young infant.

RIGHT AORTIC ARCH. A right aortic arch with a left ductus or ligamentum arteriosum connecting the left pulmonary artery and the upper part of the descending aorta is the next most important vascular ring seen. Although all with this lesion have a vascular ring, not all cases are symptomatic. Indeed those patients who are symptomatic usually have an associated diverticulum of Kommerrell.[246] This is a large outpouching at the distal takeoff of the left subclavian artery from the descending aorta. It is the combination of the diverticulum and the ring that causes the airway compression.

ANOMALOUS ORIGIN OF A RIGHT SUBCLAVIAN ARTERY. This is one of the most common abnormalities of the aortic arch that is encountered. Although the aberrant right subclavian artery runs posterior to the esophagus it does not form a vascular ring unless there is an associated right-sided ductus or ligamentum to complete the ring. During adulthood about 5 percent of patients with an aberrant right subclavian artery (and a left ductus) develop symptoms due to rigidity of the aberrant vessel.

RETROESOPHAGEAL DESCENDING AORTA. This is a rarer but more problematic type of vascular ring. In this setting there may be either an ascending left and descending right, or an ascending right and descending left, aorta. The retroesophageal component of the descending aorta causes the tracheal compression, in conjunction with the left- or right-sided ligamentum.[247,248]

PULMONARY ARTERY SLING. This is usually made up of the left pulmonary artery arising from the right pulmonary artery and runs posterior to the trachea but anterior to the esophagus. This is usually seen in isolation and is associated with significant hypoplasia of the bronchial tree, which is the predominant cause of the airway symptoms.

CLINICAL FEATURES. The symptoms produced by vascular rings depend on the tightness of anatomical constriction of the trachea and esophagus and consist principally of respiratory difficulties including stridor, cyanosis (especially with feeding), and dysphagia. Not all patients with a vascular ring are symptomatic, and cases with an aberrant left subclavian artery are frequently detected at the time of evaluation for associated CHD. Although most patients with a true ring and some airway compression present early on in life, others present later on with dysphagia, with others escaping diagnosis forever.

LABORATORY INVESTIGATIONS

ECG. This appears normal unless associated cardiovascular anomalies are present.

Chest Radiography. If there is evidence of a right aortic arch in a symptomatic patient, then a vascular ring should be suspected. In some instances there is evidence of some airway narrowing. The barium esophagogram is a useful screening procedure. Prominent posterior indentation of the esophagus is observed in many of the common vascular ring arrangements, although the pulmonary artery vascular sling produces an anterior indentation.

Echocardiography. This is a very sensitive tool for evaluating the laterality of the aortic arch, including a detailed assessment of the associated brachiocephalic vessels.[249] In general if there is normal branching of the innominate artery, to the right for a left aortic arch and to the left for a right, along with the correct "sidedness" of the descending aorta, then a vascular ring can be excluded. *Most cases with a double aortic arch* have a dominant right arch, with the descending aorta appearing to dip posteriorly as it runs behind the esophagus. A patent ductus or ligamentum can usually be identified by echocardiography. When both arches are patent, a frontal plane sweep from inferior to superior demonstrates both patent arches, as well as their brachiocephalic vessels. *A right aortic arch with an aberrant left subclavian artery* is suspected when it is not possible to identify normal branching of the left-sided innominate artery. *A retroesophageal descending aorta* should be suspected when the ascending aorta and its brachiocephalic arteries are readily identified but there is difficulty in identifying the descending aorta as it traverses behind the esophagus. *A left pulmonary artery sling* is suspected when the normal branching pattern of pulmonary arteries cannot be identified. In this setting color Doppler permits the identification of the left pulmonary artery as it arises from the right pulmonary artery and runs in a posterior and leftward direction.

MRI and CT. MRI and CT play a major role in the evaluation of patients with a vascular ring. In fact MRA has become the gold standard for the evaluation of the aorta and its branches. The only disadvantage for infants is that it often requires general anesthesia to achieve a successful examination. On the other hand, spiral CT is a technique that is fast and provides better definition of the affected airways. This latter technique is particularly valuable for patients with a pulmonary artery sling, where the vascular ring plays a secondary role to the airway abnormalities. The advantages of these techniques are that, unlike echocardiog-

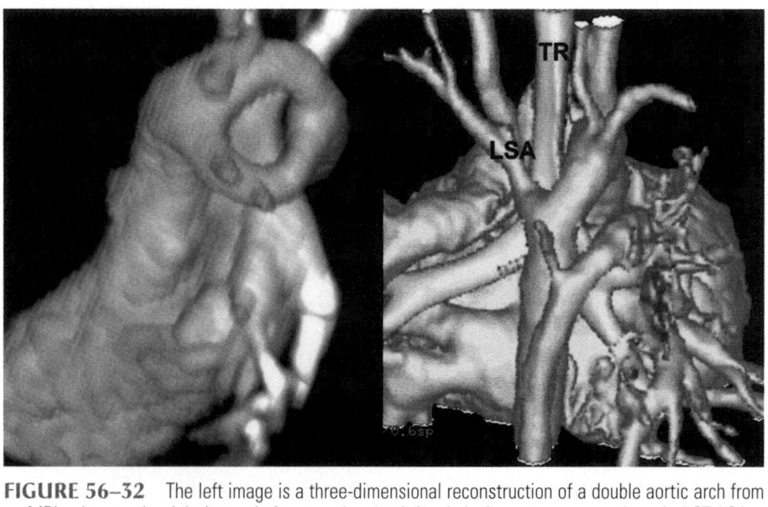

FIGURE 56–32 The left image is a three-dimensional reconstruction of a double aortic arch from an MRI, whereas the right image is from an aberrant left subclavian artery as seen by spiral CT. LSA = left subclavian artery; TR = trachea.

raphy, they permit a precise assessment of the more posterior vascular structures and their relationships to the esophagus and airways. These techniques are particularly valuable in the more complex forms, such as a retroesophageal descending aorta.

Management Options and Outcomes. The severity of symptoms and the anatomy of the malformation are the most important factors in determining treatment. Patients, particularly infants, with respiratory obstruction require prompt surgical intervention.[250] A left thoracotomy is the surgical approach in most patients with a vascular ring. For the most common vascular rings such as a double aortic arch or aberrant left subclavian artery, the combination of a chest radiograph, barium swallow, and echocardiogram is all that is necessary prior to surgical intervention.

Operative repair of the double aortic arch requires division of the minor arch (usually the left) and the ligamentum. Patients with a right aortic arch and a left ductus or ligamentum arteriosum require division of the ductus or ligamentum and/or ligation and division of the left subclavian artery, which is the posterior component of the ring. Video-assisted thoracoscopy holds promise as an alternative to open thoracotomy for management.[251,252] In patients with a pulmonary artery vascular sling, operation consists of detachment of the left pulmonary artery at its origin and anastomosis to the main pulmonary artery directly or by way of a conduit with its proximal end brought anterior to the trachea.

CONGENITAL AORTIC VALVE STENOSIS

GENERAL CONSIDERATIONS. We deal here only with this condition in newborns and children, since the adult presentation is dealt with in Chapter 52. Congenital aortic valve stenosis is a relatively common anomaly. Congenital aortic valve stenosis occurs much more frequently in males, with a gender ratio of 4:1. Associated cardiovascular anomalies have been noted in as many as 20 percent of patients. PDA and coarctation of the aorta occur most frequently with aortic valve stenosis; all three of these lesions may coexist.

MORPHOLOGY. The basic malformation consists of thickening of valve tissue with various degrees of commissural fusion. The valve most commonly is bicuspid. In some patients, the stenotic aortic valve is unicuspid and dome shaped, with no or one lateral attachment to the aorta at the level of the orifice. In infants and young children with severe aortic stenosis, the aortic valve annulus may be relatively underdeveloped. This lesion forms a continuum with the hypoplastic left heart syndrome and the aortic atresia and hypoplasia complexes. Secondary calcification of the valve is rare in childhood. When the obstruction is hemodynamically significant, concentric hypertrophy of the left ventricular wall and dilation of the ascending aorta occur.

NEONATAL PRESENTATION. The newborn presentation is often similar to that seen with other obstructive left-sided lesions, such as coarctation of the aorta or interrupted aortic arch. They present with heart failure and are dependent on ductal patency for survival. There is a frequent association with varying degrees of left ventricular hypoplasia, mitral valve abnormalities, and endocardial fibroelastosis. With the advent of good prenatal screening, many are detected before birth, with deliveries being performed in a high-risk obstetrical unit attached to a congenital heart facility. The decision process around single versus biventricular repair is a complex one and beyond the scope of this chapter. Suffice it to say there are formulas that have been derived to assist the pediatric cardiologist in the decision process.[253]

Clinical Findings. The newborns generally have weak pulses throughout, signs of heart failure, and often little in the way of murmurs, despite the severe left ventricular outflow tract obstruction.

ECG. This usually shows right ventricular dominance with evidence of diffuse ST wave changes due to left ventricular strain.

Chest Radiography. This usually shows cardiomegaly due to a large right ventricle and varying degrees of pulmonary edema.

Echocardiography. This is currently the diagnostic test of choice. It usually shows a poorly contracting left ventricle with varying degrees of endocardial fibroelastosis and frequently hypoplasia of the left ventricle and aortic root. Doppler assessment of gradients are often unreliable due to poor left ventricular function. The presence of right ventricular hypertension and tricuspid valve regurgitation are common associated findings.

Management. Prostaglandin therapy is instituted in this patient population to maintain the fetal circulation with retrograde ductal flow that permits coronary and cerebral perfusion. The nature of further treatment depends on whether the left ventricle and aortic root are believed to be of a sufficient size to support a biventricular repair. If so, balloon dilation is rapidly becoming the treatment of choice,[254] though surgical intervention is still preferred by some.[255] If the left heart structures are believed to be too small to sustain life, then either cardiac transplantation or a Norwood procedure can be undertaken.[253]

PRESENTATION BEYOND THE NEWBORN PERIOD. The diagnosis is invariably made following the detection of a murmur. Occasionally heart failure ensues, usually in the first 1 to 2 months of life when there is a rapid progression of the obstruction and lack of left ventricular mass to maintain a normal wall stress. The natural history studies performed several years ago demonstrated that more rapid progression of aortic valve stenosis is more likely to happen within the first 2 years of life, following which the rate of progressive obstruction is more uniform.[256,257]

Clinical Findings. In general the children are asymptomatic, having normal peripheral pulses if the stenosis is less severe and low-volume, slow-rising pulses when it progresses. Exercise fatigue and chest pain are rare complaints and occur only when the stenosis is severe. With severe stenosis there is systolic thrill in the same area that can also be felt in the suprasternal notch and carotid arteries. Beyond the newborn period there is usually an ejection click at the apex that precedes the murmur. The second heart sound is usually normal in children. There is an ejection systolic murmur heard along the left sternal border, with radiation into the right infraclavicular area. Associated aortic regurgitation may be heard.

ECG. Left ventricular hypertrophy with or without strain are the hallmark features.

Chest Radiography. Overall heart size is normal, or the degree of enlargement is slight in most children with congenital aortic valve stenosis.

Echocardiography. 2D echocardiography provides detailed information about the morphology of the valve, the left ventricular function, and the presence of associated left-sided lesions. Doppler echocardiography can be used to determine the severity of stenosis and the presence or absence of associated aortic regurgitation. Doppler provides peak instantaneous gradients that are higher than the peak-to-peak gradients determined from cardiac catheterization.[258,259] The importance of this lies in the fact that the natural history studies and clinical decision-making have thus far been based on peak-to-peak catheterization gradients in the infant, child, and adolescent. Valve areas are usually not calculated in this age group because there are no good data to support their use in pediatric patients. Mean gradients as derived from Doppler and catheterization correlate closely, but again there is lack of data to support their use in clinical decision-making. Some data exist that convert the Doppler-derived mean gradients to peak to peak, with the addition of the pulse pressure as obtained from blood pressure measurements. Whatever absolute number is chosen to work with, the additional finding of left ventricular hypertrophy on ECG and echocardiography provide supportive data regarding timing for intervention. There is general agreement in the pediatric population that a peak-to-peak gradient of 60 mm Hg or more probably warrants intervention.

Diagnostic Cardiac Catheterization. Cardiac catheterization is now rarely used to establish the site and severity of obstruction to left ventricular outflow. Instead, catheterization is undertaken when therapeutic interventional balloon aortic valvuloplasty is indicated.

Management Options. In this current era balloon dilation has almost completely replaced primary surgical valvotomy in children.

FOLLOW-UP. Follow-up studies indicate that aortic valvotomy is a safe and effective means of palliative treatment with excellent relief of symptoms. Aortic insufficiency can occasionally be progressive and require valve replacement.[260-262] Moreover, after commissurotomy, the valve leaflets remain somewhat deformed, and it is likely that further degenerative changes, including calcification, will lead to significant stenosis in later years. Thus, prosthetic aortic valve replacement is required in approximately 35 percent of patients within 15 to 20 years of the original operation. For those children and adolescents requiring aortic valve replacement, the surgical options include replacement with a mechanical aortic valve, an aortic homograft, or a pulmonary autograft in the aortic position. Accumulating evidence shows that the pulmonary autograft may ultimately be preferable to the aortic homograft. In the pulmonary autograft, called the *Ross procedure*, the patient's pulmonary valve is removed and used to replace the diseased aortic valve, and the right ventricular outflow tract is reconstructed with a pulmonary valve homograft.[262,263] We consider it likely that the Ross procedure will emerge as the approach of choice in the future,[263] although caution is needed when applied to patients with bicuspid aortic valve and aortic regurgitation.[264] This surgical approach can be applied from neonatal through to adult life. Neither homografts nor autografts require anticoagulation.

SUBAORTIC STENOSIS

MORPHOLOGY

Discrete Fibromuscular. This lesion consists of a ridge or fibrous ring encircling the left ventricular outflow tract at varying distances from the aortic valve.[265] The subvalvular fibrous process usually extends onto the aortic valve cusps and almost always makes contact with the ventricular aspect of the anterior mitral leaflet at its base. In other cases with fibrous discontinuity between the mitral and aortic valves, it forms more of a tunnel obstruction.

Focal Muscular. Rarely there is no fibrous element, but rather a focal muscular obstruction on the crest of the interventricular septum, which differs from cases with hypertrophic cardiomyopathy.

Hypoplasia of the Left Ventricular Outflow Tract. In some cases, valvular and subvalvular aortic stenoses coexist with hypoplasia of the aortic valve annulus and thickened valve leaflets, producing a tunnel-like narrowing of the left ventricular outflow tract. Additional findings often include a small ascending aorta.

Discrete Subaortic Stenosis and VSD. This combination is frequently encountered in the pediatric age group, with the fibromuscular component often being absent at the initial echocardiographic evaluation. The association should be suspected in those VSDs with some associated anterior malalignment of the aorta and a more acute aortoseptal angle.[266] These hearts frequently develop subpulmonary stenosis. In a different subset of patients with aortic arch interruption and a VSD, there is muscular subaortic stenosis due to posterior deviation of the infundibular septum.

Complex Subaortic Stenosis. Various anatomical lesions other than a discrete ridge may produce subaortic stenosis. Among these are abnormal adherence of the anterior leaflet of the mitral valve to the septum and the presence in the left ventricular outflow tract of accessory endocardial cushion tissue.[267,268] These are frequently associated with a "cleft in the anterior mitral valve leaflet," which is to be differentiated from that seen in an AV septal defect. These types of obstruction are seen more commonly in those cases with abnormalities of the ventriculoarterial connection in association with a VSD (e.g., double-outlet right ventricle, transposition, and VSD).

CLINICAL FEATURES. These types of obstruction are usually identified as secondary lesions in those cases with associated VSDs, with or without abnormalities of the ventriculoarterial connections or aortic arch obstruction. In general the substrate for left ventricular outflow tract obstruction is present, though in some cases actual physiological obstruction is absent. In other cases the patients are referred with a systolic murmur for evaluation. In the those cases with a gradient across their left ventricular outflow tract, there is an ejection systolic murmur heard along the lower left sternal border with the absence of an ejection click.

LABORATORY INVESTIGATIONS

ECG. In those with associated defects the ECG reflects the major abnormality rather than the associated left ventricular outflow tract obstruction. With isolated forms of left ventricular outflow tract obstruction, there may be left ventricular hypertrophy when the obstruction is significant.

Chest Radiography. This is usually unhelpful in these cases.

Echocardiography. Echocardiography is the current standard diagnostic tool in this lesion.[269] Not only can it permit an accurate delineation of the mechanisms of obstruction but it provides detailed data regarding associated lesions. In all forms the parasternal long-axis view is key to providing an accurate diagnosis. The presence of mitral aortic discontinuity, the relationship of a fibromuscular ridge to the aortic valve, the presence of accessory obstructive tissue, and the dimensions of the aortic annulus and root all are well imaged in this view. As well, color-flow mapping permits the identification of associated aortic valve regurgitation and provides hemodynamic evidence of the site of onset of obstruction. The extension of a fibromuscular ridge onto the anterior mitral leaflet is best appreciated in the apical five-chamber view. As well, this provides the best site for pulsed or continuous-wave Doppler assessment of the maximum gradient across the left ventricular outflow tract. In the older patient TEE plays an important role in delineating the pathology.[270]

Cardiac Catheterization. This technique is no longer of importance in evaluating this lesion. Although balloon dilation has been attempted, it is generally believed that this is a surgical lesion.

MRI. In general, MRI is unnecessary unless there are problems obtaining the needed information by echocardiography.

INTERVENTIONAL OPTIONS. Surgical intervention is indicated either at the time of the repair of the underlying primary lesion or in those cases with discrete obstruction when the obstruction is severe enough to raise concerns.

Discrete Subaortic Stenosis (Fibrous and Muscular). The rate of progression is varied and may be slow.[271] In general the approach to the latter group has been to intervene when there is a mean gradient across the left ventricular outflow tract of greater than 30 mm Hg to avoid future aortic leaflet damage.[272] Surgery involves a fibromectomy, with care to avoid damage to the aortic valve or to create a traumatic VSD.[273] There is a recurrence rate of subaortic stenosis requiring reoperation in up to 20 percent of cases. In some the recurrence is in the form of a fibrous ridge, whereas in others there is acquired pathology of the aortic valve in the form of stenosis as well as regurgitation. Reoperation may involve just repeat resection of a recurrent fibrous ridge, or it may involve surgery for the aortic valve in those cases with significant aortic regurgitation.

Complex Forms of Left Ventricular Outflow Tract Obstruction and an Intact Ventricular Septum. In cases with an intact ventricular septum the indications for intervention are similar to those cases with discrete obstruction. The difference lies in the fact that the surgical approach has to be modified according to the underlying pathology. Resection of any fibromuscular component or accessory tissue (provided it is not a primary support mechanism for the mitral valve), a valve-sparing Konno operation, and, in those cases with a hypoplastic aortic annulus, a classic Konno procedure with aortic valve replacement, are the potential surgical options.[274,275]

Left Ventricular Outflow Tract Obstruction and Complex Forms of CHD. In general, surgery to the left ventricular outflow tract is part of the general repair of the lesion and is not dependent on the precise degree of obstruction across this site.

OUTCOMES. Immediate complications related to surgery include complete AV block, creation of a VSD, or mitral regurgitation from intraoperative damage to the mitral valve apparatus. Long-term complications include recurrence of fibromuscular subvalvular left ventricular outflow tract obstruction (up to 20 percent). Clinically important aortic regurgitation is not uncommon (up to 25 percent of patients). In some cases with predominant acquired aortic valve stenosis, balloon dilation has been the treatment of choice.

FOLLOW-UP. Particular attention should be paid to patients with residual or recurrent subaortic stenosis or those with an associated bicuspid aortic valve or important aortic regurgitation because they are most likely to require surgery eventually. Patients with bioprosthetic aortic valves in the aortic position (following the Konno procedure) or the pulmonary position (following the Ross-Konno procedure) need close follow-up. Endocarditis prophylaxis should be used for prosthetic valves or in the presence of any residual lesions.

SUPRAVALVULAR AORTIC STENOSIS

MORPHOLOGY. Three anatomical types of supravalvular aortic stenosis are recognized, although some patients may have findings of more than one type. Most common is the hourglass type, in which marked thickening and disorganization of the aortic media produce a constricting annular ridge at the superior margin of the sinuses of Valsalva. The membranous type is the result of a fibrous or fibromuscular semicircular diaphragm with a small central opening stretched across the lumen of the aorta. Diffuse hypoplasia of the ascending aorta characterizes the third type.

Because the coronary arteries arise proximal to the site of outflow obstruction in supravalvular aortic stenosis, they are subjected to the elevated pressure that exists within the left ventricle. These vessels often are dilated and tortuous, and premature coronary arteriosclerosis has been described. Moreover, if the free edges of some or all of the aortic cusps adhere to the site of supravalvular stenosis, coronary artery inflow may be compromised. The left ventricle may have a "ballerina foot" configuration, which can result in muscular left ventricular outflow tract obstruction, particularly when associated with significant supravalvular obstruction.

CLINICAL FEATURES. The clinical picture of supravalvular obstruction differs in major respects from that observed in the other forms of aortic stenosis. Chief among these differences is the association of supravalvular aortic stenosis with idiopathic infantile hypercalcemia, a disease that occurs in the first years of life and can be associated with deranged vitamin D metabolism.

WILLIAMS SYNDROME. The designation *supravalvular aortic stenosis syndrome, Williams syndrome*, or *Williams-Beuren syndrome* has been applied to the distinctive picture produced by coexistence of the cardiac and a multisystem disorder.[276] Beyond infancy in these patients, a challenge with vitamin D- or calcium-loading tests unmasks abnormalities in the regulation of circulating 25-hydroxyvitamin D. Infants with Williams syndrome often exhibit feeding difficulties, failure to thrive, and gastrointestinal problems in the form of vomiting, constipation, and colic. The entire spectrum of clinical manifestations includes auditory hyperacusis, inguinal hernia, a hoarse voice, and a typical personality that is outgoing and engaging. Other manifestations of this syndrome include intellectual impairment, "elfin facies", narrowing of peripheral systemic and pulmonary arteries, strabismus, and abnormalities of dental development consisting of microdontia, enamel hypoplasia, and malocclusion.

Many medical conditions can complicate the course of Williams syndrome, including systemic hypertension, gastrointestinal problems, and urinary tract abnormalities. In an older child or adult, progressive joint limitation and hypertonia may become a problem. Adult patients are usually handicapped by their developmental disabilities.

Williams syndrome was previously considered to be nonfamilial; however, a number of families in which parent-to-child transmission of Williams syndrome has occurred have now been identified. All of these families show a parent and child to be affected with Williams syndrome, including one instance of male-to-male transmission. This supports autosomal dominant inheritance as the likely pattern, with most cases of Williams syndrome probably occurring as the result of a new mutation. New information indicates that a genetic defect for supravalvular aortic stenosis is located in the same chromosomal subunit as elastin on chromosome 7q11.23.[277] Elastin is an important component of the arterial wall, but precisely how mutations in elastin genes cause the phenotypes of supravalvular aortic stenosis is not known.

FAMILIAL AUTOSOMAL DOMINANT PRESENTATION. Occasionally the aortic anomaly and peripheral pulmonary arterial stenosis are also found in familial and sporadic forms not associated with the other features of the syndrome.[278] Affected patients have normal intelligence and are normal in facial appearance. Genetic studies suggest that when the anomaly is familial, it is transmitted as autosomal dominant with variable expression. Some family members may have peripheral pulmonary stenosis either as an isolated lesion or in combination with the supravalvular aortic anomaly.

CLINICAL FEATURES. Patients with Williams syndrome are intellectually challenged (Fig. 56–33). The typical appearance is similar to that of the elfin facies observed in the severe form of idiopathic infantile hypercalcemia and is characterized by a high prominent forehead, stellate or lacy iris patterns, epicanthal folds, underdeveloped bridge of the nose and mandible, overhanging upper lip, strabismus, and anomalies of dentition. Recognition of this distinctive appearance, even in infancy, should alert the physician to the possibility of underlying multisystem disease. In addition, a positive family history in a patient with a normal appearance and clinical signs suggesting left ventricular outflow obstruction should lead to the suspicion of either supravalvular aortic stenosis or hypertrophic obstructive cardiomyopathy.

Studies of the natural history of the principal vascular lesions in these patients—supravalvular aortic stenosis and peripheral pulmonary artery stenosis[279]—indicate that the aortic lesion is usually progressive, with an increase in the

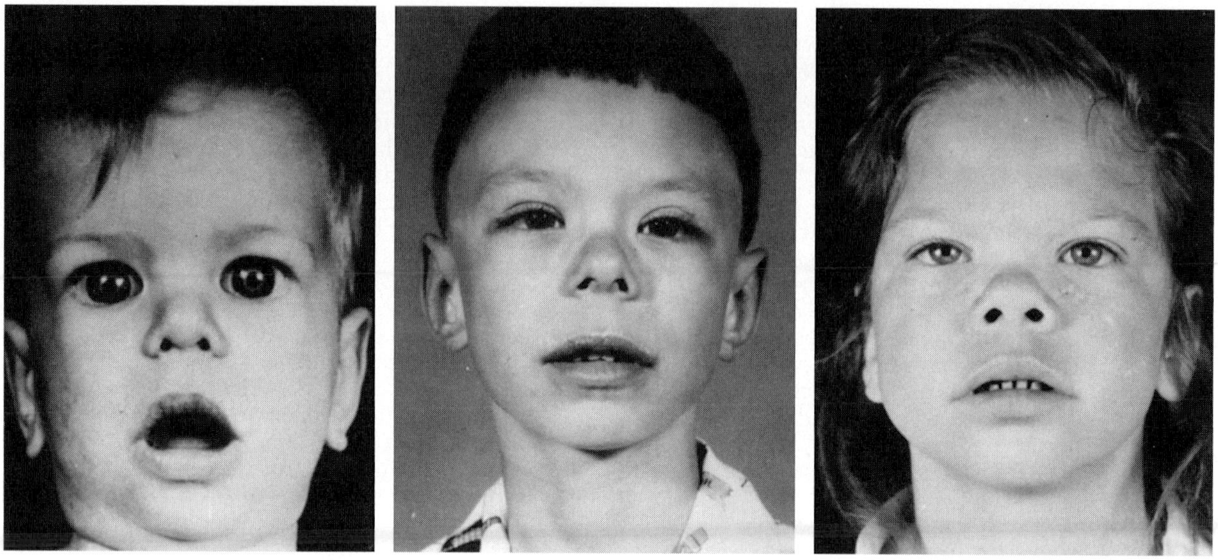

FIGURE 56–33 Typical elfin facies in three patients with supravalvular aortic stenosis. (From Friedman WF, Kirkpatrick SE: Congenital aortic stenosis. *In* Adams FH, Emmanouilides GC, Riemenschneider TA, et al [eds]: Moss' Heart Disease in Infants, Children, and Adolescents. 4th ed. Baltimore, Williams & Wilkins, 1989.)

intensity of obstruction related often to poor growth of the ascending aorta. In contrast, the patients with pulmonary branch stenosis, whether associated with the aortic lesion or not, tend to show no change or a reduction in right ventricular pressure with time.[280,281]

With few exceptions, the major *physical findings* resemble those observed in patients with aortic valve stenosis. Among these exceptions are accentuation of aortic valve closure due to elevated pressure in the aorta proximal to the stenosis, an absent ejection click, and the especially prominent transmission of a thrill and murmur into the jugular notch and along the carotid vessels. The narrowing of the peripheral pulmonary arteries may produce a late systolic or continuous murmur heard best in the lung fields and usually are accentuated by inspiration. Another hallmark of supravalvular aortic stenosis is that the systolic pressure in the right arm is usually higher than in the left arm. This pulse disparity may relate to the tendency of a jet stream to adhere to a vessel wall (Coanda effect) and selective streaming of blood into the innominate artery.

LABORATORY INVESTIGATIONS

ECG. This usually reveals left ventricular hypertrophy when obstruction is severe. Biventricular or even right ventricular hypertrophy may be found if there is significant narrowing of peripheral pulmonary arteries.

Chest Radiography. In contrast to valvular and discrete subvalvular aortic stenosis, poststenotic dilation of the ascending aorta is absent.

Echocardiography. This is a valuable technique for localizing the site of obstruction to the supravalvular area.[282] Most often the sinuses of Valsalva are dilated, and the ascending aorta and arch appear small or of normal size. The diameter of the aortic annulus is always greater than that of the sinotubular junction. Doppler examination determines the location of obstruction but usually overestimates the gradient compared with that obtained at cardiac catheterization. This results from the obstruction being lengthy, and the Doppler gradient is overestimated due to the phenomena of pressure recovery.

Angiocardiography. In most cases, this is necessary to define an accurate hemodynamic gradient across the left ventricular outflow tract, as well as to determine the status of the coronary arteries. Usually it also involves an assessment of the branch pulmonary arteries as well as the brachiocephalic, renal, and mesenteric arteries, all of which can be stenotic. Because of the nature of the anatomical defect, transcatheter balloon angioplasty, with or without stenting, is not an effective treatment option.

INTERVENTIONAL OPTIONS AND OUTCOMES. Surgical intervention for the supravalvular aortic stenosis has been successful in most cases with good medium and long-term results.[283,284] A variety of surgical procedures may be performed, all of which are tailored to the type of pathology. The use of a Y patch, resection with end-to-end anastomosis, or a Ross procedure are the main techniques employed. Additional lesions, including coronary ostial stenosis, aortic valvuloplasty, and subaortic resection, may be necessary in some cases.

The cardiac prognosis is very good, with some patients requiring further surgery for recurrent supravalvular stenosis.[279,285] As peripheral pulmonary artery stenosis tends to improve with time, there is a reluctance to attempt intervention, either surgical or via balloon angioplasty. Long-term behavioral and intellectual problems persist.[285]

Congenital Mitral Valve Anomalies

CONGENITAL MITRAL STENOSIS

MORPHOLOGY. Anatomical types of mitral stenosis include the parachute deformity of the valve, in which shortened chordae tendineae converge and insert into a single large papillary muscle; thickened leaflets with shortening and fusion of the chordae tendineae; an anomalous arcade of obstructing papillary muscles; accessory mitral valve tissue; and a supravalvar circumferential ridge or "ring" of connective tissue arising at the base of the atrial aspect of the mitral leaflets.[286] Associated cardiac defects are common, including endocardial fibroelastosis, coarctation of the aorta, PDA, and left ventricular outflow tract obstruction. There is also an association between persistence of the left superior vena cava and obstructive left-sided lesions.[287]

CLINICAL FEATURES. In most cases the findings are incidental at the time of evaluation of another left-sided obstructive lesion, such as coarctation of the aorta or aortic valve stenosis. The classic auscultatory findings seen with rheumatic mitral valve stenosis are often absent in the congenital form. Typical findings include a normal S_1, a mid-diastolic murmur with or without some presystolic accentuation, and no opening snap.

LABORATORY INVESTIGATIONS

ECG. In milder forms this is usually normal, or there may be left atrial overload, with or without right ventricular hypertrophy due to associated pulmonary hypertension.

Chest Radiography. This is normal in milder forms, with evidence of pulmonary edema in those cases with more severe obstruction.

Echocardiography. The 2D echocardiography, combined with Doppler studies, usually provides a complete analysis of the anatomy and function of congenital mitral stenosis.[288] The status of the papillary muscles is best appreciated in the precordial short-axis view. In patients with two papillary muscles, they are usually closer together than is seen in the normal heart. The precordial long-axis view permits identification of a supravalvular mitral ring as well as the degree of mobility of the valve leaflets. Color flow Doppler allows identification of the level of the obstruction, as well as the presence of mitral valve regurgitation. Pulsed or continuous-wave Doppler provides an accurate assessment of the mean gradient across the mitral valve. The advantage of the pressure half-time lies in the fact that it is independent of cardiac output, unlike the mean gradient across the mitral valve. Due to more rapid heart rates in children, the pressure half-time is of less value.

INTERVENTIONAL OPTIONS AND OUTCOMES. In asymptomatic cases clinical and echocardiographic follow-up is all that is necessary. If the patient starts to develop pulmonary hypertension or symptoms, surgical intervention is usually indicated. Mitral valve balloon dilation[289] is not as successful as it is in rheumatic mitral valve stenosis. Surgery usually involves removing a supramitral ring if present, splitting papillary muscles and fused chordal apparatus in those cases with more common forms of congenital mitral stenosis. In general, surgical intervention provides temporary relief, with many operated cases requiring valve replacement later in life.[290,291]

CONGENITAL MITRAL REGURGITATION

MORPHOLOGY

Isolated Congenital Mitral Valve Regurgitation. This is usually due to either an isolated cleft of the anterior mitral valve leaflet[292] or as the result of leaflet dysplasia. In these cases there is evidence of shortened chordae in conjunction with dysplastic valve leaflets. In those with an isolated mitral valve *cleft*, the deficiency in the anterior mitral leaflet points toward the left ventricular outflow tract, unlike those cases with an AV septal defect. In general, the larger the cleft in the anterior mitral leaflet, the greater the degree of regurgitation.

In cases with a *dysplastic* mitral valve the chordal apparatus is shortened with varying degrees of dysplasia of the leaflets. Other anatomical lesions such as mitral valve arcade resulting in regurgitation are usually part of a more generalized abnormality of the left side of the heart.

Complex Congenital Mitral Valve Regurgitation. This is seen more frequently in association with abnormalities of the ventriculoarterial connection, such as double-outlet right ventricle, transposition and VSD, and corrected transposition. In the first two it is frequent to have a cleft in the anterior mitral valve leaflet with some chordal support apparatus that renders the valve less regurgitant than in those cases with an isolated cleft. In cc-TGA the morphological mitral valve may have an associated cleft, be dysplastic, or have multiple papillary muscles, all of which increase the tendency for it to be regurgitant.

CLINICAL FEATURES. The presence of symptoms relates to the severity of the regurgitation in those cases where the pathology is isolated to the valve. Exercise intolerance, combined with a pansystolic murmur at the apex, with or without a mid-diastolic murmur, are the cardinal clinical features.

LABORATORY INVESTIGATIONS

ECG. This is either normal or demonstrates left atrial and left ventricular hypertrophy.

Chest Radiography. This demonstrates cardiomegaly predominantly involving the left ventricle and atrium.

Echocardiography. Doppler and 2D echocardiography provide an accurate evaluation of the mechanisms and degree of valvular regurgitation.[288,292] The cleft in the anterior mitral valve leaflet is best seen in the precordial short-axis view, pointing toward the left ventricular outflow tract. Patients with a dysplastic mitral valve lack mobility of the valve leaflets and have shortened chordae. Color Doppler interrogation helps in locating the site of regurgitation. The severity of regurgitation is assessed in the standard fashion. The 3D echocardiography permits a comprehensive evaluation of the mechanisms of regurgitation, with additional information being obtained regarding commissural length, leaflet area, and sites of regurgitation from color flow Doppler.

Angiocardiography and MRI. These procedures are seldom helpful in management planning.

INTERVENTIONAL OPTIONS AND OUTCOMES. This depends on the severity of regurgitation and its impact on left ventricular function. Surgery should not be delayed until the patients become symptomatic. Surgery involves suture of an isolated cleft, with or without associated commissuroplasties. In those cases with a dysplastic mitral valve, leaflet extension in conjunction with an annuloplasty and commissuroplasty usually results in effective control of the regurgitation in the short and medium term.[293] Despite this, many of these patients most likely end up with a mitral valve replacement at some stage in the future. Attempted surgical repair, rather than replacement, is important in the pediatric age group, because it permits temporary relief that allows the child to grow such that future surgery can be done into a larger mitral annulus. When required, mitral valve replacement has had a good short- and medium-term outcome in those cases where repair is not possible.[294]

Right Ventricular Outflow Tract Lesions

PERIPHERAL PULMONARY ARTERY STENOSIS (Fig. 56–34)

Right ventricular outflow tract is a term that applies to those patients with both peripheral pulmonary artery stenosis and an intact ventricular septum. It excludes those with an associated VSD, which is dealt with in the sections on tetralogy

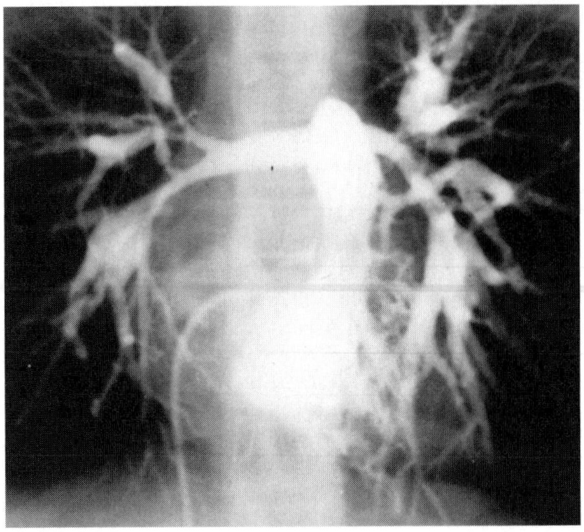

FIGURE 56–34 Right ventricular angiocardiogram showing numerous sites of peripheral pulmonic stenosis and poststenotic dilation of the peripheral pulmonic arteries.

of Fallot and pulmonary atresia with a ventricular septal defect. Also excluded is Noonan syndrome, which is dealt with in the subsequent section on pulmonary valve stenosis.

ETIOLOGY

Rubella Syndrome. The most important cause of significant pulmonary artery stenoses producing symptoms in newborns used to be intrauterine rubella infection. Other cardiovascular malformations commonly found in association with congenital rubella include PDA, pulmonary valve stenosis, and ASD. Generalized systemic arterial stenotic lesions also may be a feature of the rubella embryopathy, which may involve large and medium-sized vessels such as the aorta and coronary, cerebral, mesenteric, and renal arteries. Cardiovascular lesions are but one manifestation of intrauterine rubella infection because cataracts, microphthalmia, deafness, thrombocytopenia, hepatitis, and blood dyscrasias are also common. The clinical picture in infants with rubella syndrome depends on the severity of the cardiovascular lesions and the associated abnormalities.

Williams Syndrome. Peripheral pulmonary artery stenosis is also associated with supravalvular aortic stenosis in patients with Williams syndrome, which is discussed in the section on supravalvular aortic stenosis.[295]

Alagille Syndrome. Peripheral pulmonary artery stenosis is a component of this syndrome, with some cases having a *JAG1* mutation.[296]

Isolated Branch Pulmonary Artery Stenosis. This is encountered mainly in the proximal left pulmonary artery and is invariably related to a sling of ductal tissue that causes stenosis when the ductus arteriosus closes after birth. In most cases this is fairly mild, but a significant obstruction resulting in failure of distal growth of the left pulmonary artery may also be seen.

MORPHOLOGY. Apart from the isolated form mentioned earlier, the stenoses are usually diffuse and bilateral and extend into the mediastinal, hilar, and intraparenchymal pulmonary arteries.

CLINICAL FEATURES. The degree of obstruction is the principal determinant of clinical severity. The type of obstruction determines the feasibility of intervention. Most patients are asymptomatic. An ejection systolic murmur heard at the upper left sternal border and well transmitted to the axillae and back is most common. There is no pulmonary ejection click. The pulmonic component of the second heart sound may be accentuated and is loud only if there is proximal pulmonary hypertension. A continuous murmur is often audible in patients with significant branch stenosis. The murmurs in the lung fields are typically increased by inspiration.

LABORATORY INVESTIGATIONS

ECG. Right ventricular hypertrophy is seen when obstruction is severe. Left axis deviation with counterclockwise orientation of the frontal QRS vector is common in rubella syndrome and when there is also supravalvular aortic stenosis.

Chest Radiography. Mild or moderate stenosis usually produces normal findings. Detectable differences in vascularity between regions of the lungs or dilated pulmonary artery segments are uncommon. When obstruction is bilateral and severe, right atrial and ventricular enlargement may be seen.

Echocardiography. Echocardiography is helpful in making the diagnosis and excluding associated lesions; however, it is limited in its ability to image the distal pulmonary arteries beyond the hilum of the lung. Right ventricular pressure assessment may be predicted if there is associated tricuspid valve regurgitation.

MRI and Spiral CT. These are valuable diagnostic tests because they permit a more distal evaluation of the branch pulmonary arteries. The advantage of spiral CT in young children is that it can be performed without the need for heavy sedation or even general anesthesia. Although most patients require cardiac catheterization and angiography, these other techniques are excellent for the initial evaluation and for following the progress of the lesions.

Radionuclide Quantitative Lung Perfusion Scan. This is valuable in those cases with unilateral stenosis to determine whether intervention is necessary. Similar flow estimates can now be obtained by MRI.

Cardiac Catheterization and Angiocardiography. This permits the assessment of right ventricular pressure and the pressures in the pulmonary arterial tree. Angiocardiography is the key to precisely assessing the extent and severity of the stenoses.

INTERVENTIONAL OPTIONS AND OUTCOMES. For those cases with isolated left pulmonary artery stenosis where there is less than 30 percent of flow to the lung, balloon dilation with or without stent insertion is effective in relieving the obstruction. In those cases with more diffuse bilateral stenoses, the indications for intervention depend on the right ventricular pressure. As the natural history of diffuse peripheral pulmonary artery stenosis in Williams syndrome is one of potential regression over time, intervention is in general reserved for those cases with systemic or suprasystemic right ventricular pressure. Intervention is also dependent in part on the extent of the stenosis and the dilation capability of the lesions, with or without stenting.[297-299] In some cases, several attempts at dilation are required to achieve any improvement in vessel caliber. High-pressure balloons are usually needed, but some lesions cannot be dilated even with such balloons. Recently, improved results have been reported using "cutting" balloons, which may facilitate dilation in an otherwise undilatable stenosis. As a rule, surgery has little to offer those patients with diffuse peripheral pulmonary artery stenoses and can indeed make the situation worse.

SUPRAVALVULAR RIGHT VENTRICULAR OUTFLOW TRACT OBSTRUCTION

Supravalvular right ventricular outflow tract obstruction seldom occurs in isolation. It can occur in tetralogy of Fallot, Williams syndrome, Noonan syndrome, VSD, or arteriohepatic dysplasia (Alagille syndrome). Supravalvular right ventricular outflow tract obstruction can progress in severity and should be monitored. Dilation of the pulmonary trunk is not a feature of subvalvular and supravalvular right ventricular outflow tract obstruction. Intervention is recommended when the peak gradient across the right ventricular outflow tract is more than 50 mm Hg at rest or when the patient is symptomatic.

PULMONARY STENOSIS WITH INTACT VENTRICULAR SEPTUM (Figs. 56–35 and 56–36)

This lesion exists as a continuum, ranging from those patients with isolated valvular stenosis to others where there is complete atresia of the pulmonary outflow tract. There are two modes of presentation. The first presents in the neonatal period, usually with associated pathology of the tricuspid valve, right ventricle, and/or coronary arteries. The second mode of presentation is beyond the neonatal period, when the valvular stenosis is usually isolated. Some cases with severe stenosis diagnosed in utero can present with valvular atresia at the time of birth.

MORPHOLOGY. The pulmonary valve may vary from a well-formed trileaflet valve with varying degrees of commissural fusion to an imperforate membrane. If stenosis is present, the right ventricle is usually of normal size or only mildly hypoplastic. Those patients with an imperforate valve and a patent infundibulum invariably have a larger right ventricular volume than cases with both infundibular and valve atresia.

CLINICAL FEATURES

Neonate with Critical Pulmonary Valve Stenosis. The neonate presents with central cyanosis due to right-to-left shunting at the atrial level and depends on a prostaglandin infusion to maintain the patency of the ductus arteriosus. Auscultatory findings include a single second heart sound, no ejection click, and a murmur that, when present, is due to tricuspid valve regurgitation.

Infant and Child. In cases beyond the newborn period the referral is usually for the assessment of a cardiac murmur. This may be detected within the first few weeks of life, more commonly at the routine 6-week postnatal visit or later. These patients usually have an ejection click and a second heart sound that moves with respiration but with a soft pulmonary component. There is an ejection murmur of varying intensity and duration heard best in the pulmonary area.

Adult. Adults with isolated mild to moderate right ventricular outflow tract obstruction of any type are usually asymptomatic. Patients with severe right ventricular outflow tract obstruction may present with exertional fatigue, dyspnea, lightheadedness, and chest discomfort (right ventricular angina). Physical examination may reveal a prominent jugular A wave, a right ventricular lift, and possibly a thrill in the 2nd left interspace. Auscultation reveals a normal S_1, a single or split S_2 with a diminished P_2 (unless the obstruction is supravalvular in which case the intensity of the P_2 is normal or increased), and a systolic ejection murmur best heard in the 2nd left intercostal space. When the pulmonary valve is thin and pliable, a systolic ejection click will be heard which decreases on inspiration. As the severity of the pulmonary stenosis progresses, the interval between S_1 and the systolic ejection click becomes shorter, S_2 becomes widely split, P_2 diminishes or disappears, and the systolic ejection murmur lengthens and peaks later in systole, often extending beyond A_2. An ejection click seldoms occur with dysplastic pulmonary stenosis. Cyanosis may be present when a patent foramen ovale or ASD permits right-to-left shunting.

Adult patients with trivial and mild valvular right ventricular outflow tract obstruction do not become worse with time. Moderate valvular right ventricular outflow tract obstruction can progress in 20 percent of unoperated patients,[300] especially in adults because of calcification of the valve, and may require intervention. Some of these patients can also become symptomatic, particularly in later life, because of atrial arrhythmias resulting from right ventricular pressure overload and tricuspid regurgitation. Patients with severe valvular right ventricular outflow tract obstruction will have had balloon or surgical valvotomy to survive to adult life. Long-term survival in patients with repaired pulmonary valve stenosis is similar to that of the general population, with excellent to good functional class at long-term follow-up in most patients. A few patients have severe pulmonary regurgitation.

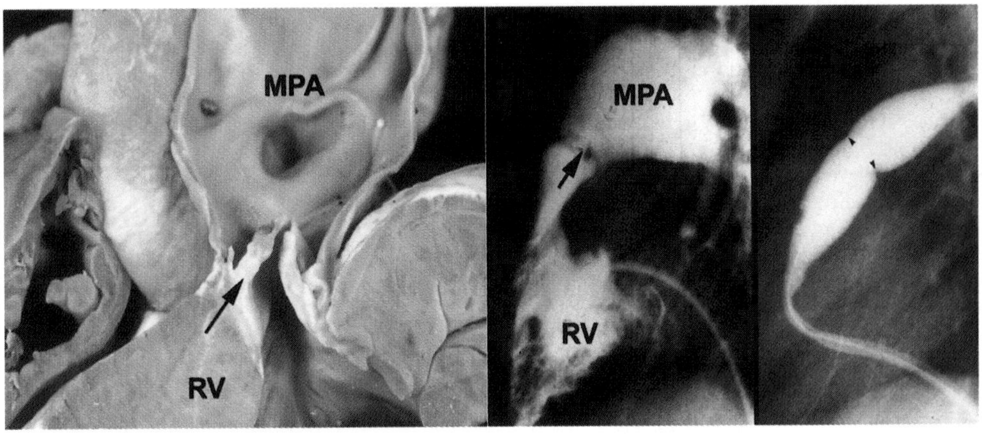

FIGURE 56–35 Montage of pulmonary valve stenosis demonstrating typical pathology (**left**, arrow) with a thickened pulmonary valve and obstruction due to commissural fusion. Note the post-stenotic dilation. The angiogram demonstrates a case before (**middle**, arrow) and during (**right**) balloon dilation. MPA = main pulmonary artery; RV = right ventricle.

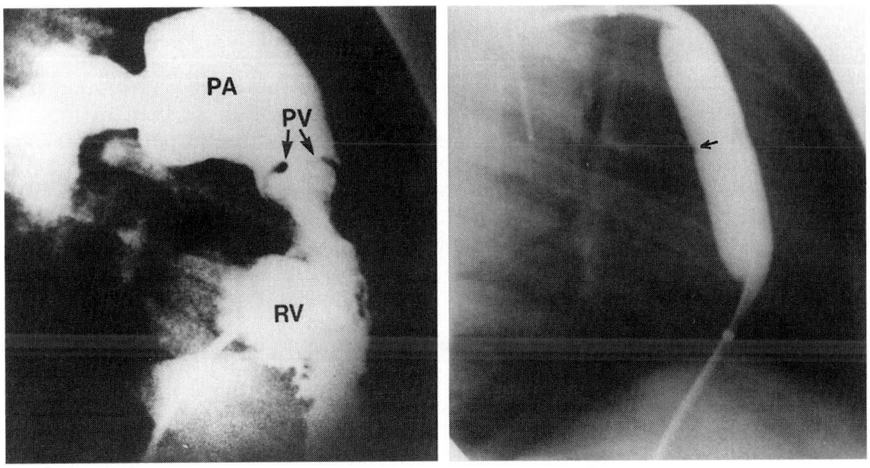

FIGURE 56–36 Right ventriculogram (RV) in the lateral projection (left) from a patient with valvular pulmonic stenosis. The pulmonary valve (PV) is thickened and domes in systole (arrows). Poststenotic dilation of the pulmonary artery (PA) is seen. At the right, successful balloon valvuloplasty shows almost complete disappearance of the stenotic waist (arrow). (Courtesy of Dr. Thomas G. DiSessa.)

LABORATORY INVESTIGATIONS

ECG. *In the newborn* period this may show left axis deviation and left ventricular dominance in those cases with significant right ventricular hypoplasia. Other patients may have a normal QRS axis. Right atrial overload is present in those with increased right atrial pressure. *In the infant, child, and adult* the findings are dependent on the severity of the stenosis. In milder cases the ECG should be normal. As the stenosis progresses, evidence of right ventricular hypertrophy appears. Severe stenosis is seen in the form of a tall R wave in lead V_4R or V_1 with a deep S wave in V_6. A tall QR wave in the right precordial leads with T wave inversion and ST segment depression (right ventricular "strain") reflects very severe stenosis. When an rSR′ pattern is observed in lead V_1 (20 percent of patients), lower right ventricular pressures are found than in patients with a pure R wave of equal amplitude. Right atrial overload is associated with moderate to severe pulmonary stenosis.

Chest Radiography. *In the neonate* this demonstrates pulmonary oligemia with a prominent right heart border in those with associated tricuspid valve regurgitation. *In the infant, child, and adult* with mild or moderate pulmonary stenosis, chest radiography often shows a heart of normal size and normal pulmonary vascularity. Poststenotic dilation of the main and left pulmonary arteries is often seen. Right atrial and right ventricular enlargement are observed in patients with severe obstruction and right ventricular failure. The pulmonary vascularity is usually normal in the absence of a right-to-left atrial shunt but may be reduced in patients with severe stenosis and right ventricular failure.

Echocardiography. Combined 2D echocardiographic and continuous-wave Doppler examination characterizes the anatomical valve abnormality and its severity and has essentially eliminated the requirement for diagnostic cardiac catheterization. Invasive studies are currently used for balloon valvuloplasty.

Right ventricular size is currently best assessed indirectly from the tricuspid annular dimension. In the absence of a VSD there is an excellent correlation between the two. Right ventricular pressure can be assessed indirectly from the tricuspid regurgitation gradient. Tricuspid valve morphology and function and the status of the interatrial septum all need to be addressed.

INTERVENTIONAL OPTIONS AND OUTCOMES

Neonate. In the neonate, prostaglandin E_1 is instituted in those cases with ductal dependency. Following this, balloon dilation is performed in those with stenosis, whereas radiofrequency perforation in conjunction with dilation may be undertaken in those with pulmonary valve atresia. If relief of the obstruction is successful, then the prostaglandins are slowly weaned to determine if the right ventricle is large enough to support the circulation. If not, a systemic-to-pulmonary artery shunt is necessary early in the management. In those cases with a normal-sized right ventricle, no further therapy is usually necessary in the future, since there is a very low recurrence rate of stenosis. Newborns with isolated pulmonary stenosis do well after relief of the stenosis.

Infant and Older Child. Balloon dilation of the pulmonary valve is the therapeutic procedure of choice with excellent short- and medium-term results.

Adults. Balloon valvuloplasty is recommended when the gradient across the right ventricular outflow tract is greater than 50 mm Hg at rest[206] or when the patient is symptomatic. Intermediate- and long-term outcomes are excellent.[301]

DYSPLASTIC PULMONARY VALVE STENOSIS

MORPHOLOGY. In pulmonary valve stenosis due to valvular dysplasia the obstruction is caused not by commissural fusion but by a combination of thickened and dysplastic pulmonary valve leaflets in combination with varying degrees of supravalvular pulmonary stenosis. The supravalvular stenosis is classically at the distal part of pulmonary valve sinuses, and there is usually no poststenotic pulmonary artery dilation. This entity is associated with Noonan syndrome, which in turn may be associated with hypertrophic cardiomyopathy.

CLINICAL FEATURES. In most cases, the diagnosis is made either during an evaluation of a systolic murmur or in a child with dysmorphic features who is undergoing clinical evaluation. Children with Noonan syndrome have short stature, webbed necks, and broad-shaped chests in a fashion similar to Turner syndrome. Although this syndrome does not have an associated chromosomal abnormality, it may be familial and affects both sexes equally. A unique association in the newborn is pulmonary lymphangiectasia. The auscultatory finding that differentiates the dysplastic valves from simple pulmonary valve stenosis is the lack of an ejection click. The other features of the murmur are similar to that described in pulmonary valve stenosis.

ECG. The ECG is helpful in that patients with dysplastic pulmonary stenosis frequently have a leftward QRS axis, particularly when associated with hypertrophic cardiomyopathy. The remainder of the ECG is similar to that seen in pulmonary valve stenosis.

Chest Radiography. The findings are similar to typical pulmonary valve stenosis, apart from the lack of post-stenotic pulmonary trunk dilation, even in the presence of severe obstruction. In those with pulmonary lymphangiectasia the chest radiograph has a ground-glass appearance, which can be difficult to differentiate from pulmonary venous obstruction.

Echocardiography. This demonstrates a thickened fleshy pulmonary valve, lack of post-stenotic dilation, and varying degrees of supravalvular pulmonary stenosis. The associated diagnosis of hypertrophic cardiomyopathy can be confirmed or excluded. If the initial echocardiogram does not demonstrate hypertrophic cardiomyopathy, then further studies should be performed throughout childhood and adolescence, particularly in those cases with left axis deviation.

INTERVENTIONAL OPTIONS AND OUTCOMES

Cardiac Catheterization and Angiography. Although the results of balloon valvuloplasty are less rewarding than those with stenosis due to commissural fusion, it is worth attempting this before considering surgical intervention. There has been varied success, with many cases having some reduction in gradient that can delay surgery.

Surgical Intervention. If balloon valvuloplasty fails, then surgical intervention is indicated. This usually involves a partial valvectomy in conjunction with patch repair of the supravalvular stenosis.

Outcomes. Adequate relief of the right ventricular outflow tract obstruction results in an excellent outlook, with the greatest long-term risk factor being the presence of hypertrophic cardiomyopathy.

SUBPULMONARY RIGHT VENTRICULAR OUTFLOW TRACT OBSTRUCTION (ANOMALOUS MUSCLE BUNDLES OR A DOUBLE-CHAMBERED RIGHT VENTRICLE)

MORPHOLOGY. A double-chambered right ventricle is formed by right ventricular obstruction due to anomalous muscle bundles.[302,303] Although this can occur in isolation, it is more frequently part of a combination of lesions that includes right ventricular muscle bundles, a perimembranous-outlet VSD, and subaortic stenosis with or without aortic valve prolapse.

CLINICAL FEATURES. Most cases are discovered as an incidental finding during the evaluation of a VSD.[304] In some cases there may be only an ejection systolic murmur. If the obstruction is isolated, then there is an ejection systolic murmur heard best in the upper left sternal border. If the VSD is the predominant lesion, the right ventricular outflow tract murmur may not be appreciated. Before the routine use of echocardiography, the diagnosis was often made during follow-up for a VSD when the pansystolic murmur decreased in intensity and a systolic ejection murmur emerged. The patients are usually pink unless there is progression of the subpulmonary stenosis in the setting of a VSD. The diagnosis may be more problematic in adults.[305,306]

LABORATORY INVESTIGATIONS

ECG. The ECG is similar to those with isolated pulmonary valve stenosis beyond the newborn period. In cases with a nonrestrictive VSD and mild subpulmonary stenosis, the ECG typically shows biventricular hypertrophy due to a left-to-right shunt and associated pulmonary hypertension. If the stenosis is more severe, right ventricular hypertrophy will be seen. Those with a restrictive VSD may have a normal ECG or left ventricular hypertrophy, the latter of which is replaced with right ventricular hypertrophy if the subpulmonary stenosis increases in severity.

Chest Radiography. This is usually normal in those with isolated subpulmonary stenosis, whereas those with a VSD may have increased or reduced pulmonary blood flow, depending on the severity of the obstruction.

Echocardiography. Doppler and 2D echocardiography usually provide a complete diagnosis.[304] The level of subpulmonary obstruction is appreciated best in a combination of subcostal right anterior oblique and precordial short-axis views. These views permit the identification of the relationship of the VSD to the muscle bundles, as well as the degree of anterior malalignment of the infundibular septum in those with a VSD. The precordial short-axis view is the best position to evaluate the presence of possible subaortic stenosis and aortic cusp prolapse. Color and pulsed or continuous-wave Doppler evaluation usually allows differentiation of the VSD flow jet from that originating from the muscle bundles. This permits an accurate assessment of the hemodynamic effect of the subpulmonary obstruction.

Cardiac Catheterization and Angiocardiography. This technique is rarely necessary.[304] In older patients where the echocardiographic images of the subpulmonary region may be suboptimal, a combination of MRA[307] and echocardiography is all that is generally needed.

MANAGEMENT OPTIONS AND OUTCOMES. Management is dictated by the severity of the subpulmonary stenosis and the presence of associated defects. In those patients with isolated subpulmonary stenosis, surgery is indicated when the right ventricular pressure is more than 60 percent of systemic. This involves resection of the muscle bundles through the right atrium. For those cases with an associated VSD, the decision is based on the size of the VSD, the degree of associated subaortic stenosis, the presence of aortic valve prolapse, and the severity of the subpulmonary stenosis. These patients tend to have a progressive disease, so many cases that are followed conservatively for several years will eventually require surgery.[306] In general, the outcome is excellent with a low rate of recurrence after surgical resection of obstructive muscle bundles.[308] Infrequently, recurrence of the subaortic obstruction may occur.

Miscellaneous Lesions

Cor Triatriatum

MORPHOLOGY. In this malformation, failure of resorption of the common pulmonary vein results in a left atrium divided by an abnormal fibromuscular diaphragm into a posterosuperior chamber receiving the pulmonary veins and an anteroinferior chamber giving rise to the left atrial appendage and leading to the mitral orifice.[309] The communication between the divided atrial chambers may be large, small, or absent, depending on the size of the opening(s) in the diaphragm, which determines the degree of obstruction to pulmonary venous return. Elevations of both pulmonary venous pressure and pulmonary vascular resistance may result in severe pulmonary artery hypertension.

CLINICAL FEATURES. Cor triatriatum may be detected as an incidental finding in a patient who has an echocardiogram for another reason. In general these represent the unobstructed form that requires no early intervention. Cases with more severe obstruction present in a fashion similar to patients with congenital pulmonary vein stenosis.

LABORATORY INVESTIGATIONS

ECG. In unobstructed cases this is normal, whereas in those with significant obstruction there is right ventricular hypertrophy due to the associated pulmonary hypertension.

Chest Radiography. This may be normal in those with mild obstruction or demonstrate pulmonary edema with significant obstruction.

Echocardiography. The diagnosis is established by 2D or TEE, with further insight from 3D reconstruction.[310] The obstructive diaphragm is visualized in the parasternal long- and short-axis and four-chamber views and can be distinguished from a supravalvular mitral ring by its position superior to the left atrial appendage, which forms part of the distal chamber. Also present is diastolic fluttering of the mitral leaflets and high-velocity flow detected by Doppler examination in the distal atrial chamber and at the mitral orifice.

Cardiac Catheterization and Angiocardiography. This technique is usually unnecessary with the advent of echocardiography and MRI.

MANAGEMENT OPTIONS AND OUTCOMES. Surgical resection of the membrane is the treatment of choice for patients with significant obstruction.[311] This results in symptom relief and a reduction of pulmonary artery pressure. In general the outcome following surgery is very good. With the advent of more routine echocardiography a subset of cases with typical but nonobstructive forms has been recognized.[312] Thus far these cases appear to remain asymptomatic, with an infrequent need for surgical intervention.

Pulmonary Vein Stenosis

Congenital pulmonary vein stenosis may occur as a focal stenosis at the atrial junction or generalized hypoplasia of one or more pulmonary veins. The incidence of associated cardiac malformations is extremely high, including VSD, ASD, tetralogy of Fallot, tricuspid and mitral atresia, and AV septal defect.[313] In other cases the pulmonary vein stenosis is acquired after surgical intervention for total anomalous pulmonary venous connection. Children frequently present with recurrent respiratory infections, whereas adults exhibit exercise intolerance. Pulmonary hypertension is one of the consequences of pulmonary vein stenosis, whether it is congenital or acquired. In those cases with unilateral pulmonary vein stenosis, clinical symptoms are frequently absent because there is pulmonary blood flow redistribution away from the affected lung.

LABORATORY INVESTIGATIONS

ECG. The ECG is usually normal unless there is evidence of pulmonary hypertension, in which case right ventricular hypertrophy may be seen.

Chest Radiography. With unilateral pulmonary vein stenosis there is oligemia of the affected lung and increased flow to the contralateral side. If the obstruction is bilateral, then pulmonary edema is seen.

Echocardiography. This can usually exclude or confirm the diagnosis of pulmonary vein stenosis. Assessment of pulmonary artery pressure from tricuspid or pulmonary valve regurgitation is possible. Doppler color flow assessment of the right- and left-sided pulmonary veins is the best screening tool.[314] If there is evidence of turbulence or aliasing in the color flow pattern, then spectral analysis with pulsed Doppler will help confirm the diagnosis. Usually pulmonary venous flow is low velocity and phasic. If the pattern is high velocity and turbulent, there is disturbed pulmonary venous flow. Absolute Doppler gradients may or may not be helpful for two reasons. First, the absolute velocity is dependent on the amount of pulmonary blood flow to that segment of lung. Second, it is often difficult to obtain a parallel line of interrogation of the pulmonary veins that will impact on gradient assessment. The absolute velocity is less important than the diagnosis of pulmonary vein stenosis and its effect on pulmonary artery pressure.

MRI (Fig. 56–37). This technique has now become the gold standard for the diagnosis of pulmonary vein stenosis. This permits a detailed assessment of the pulmonary veins. Velocity assessment is now possible, though this is in the actual veins themselves rather than at the venoatrial junction, which is the site assessed by Doppler echocardiography.

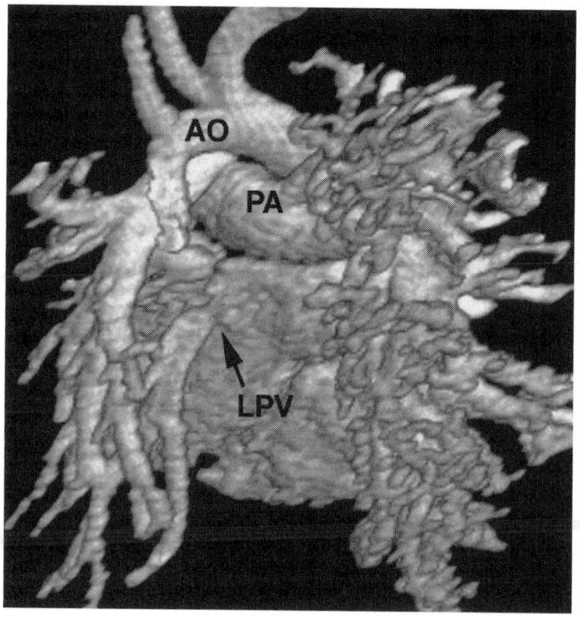

FIGURE 56–37 Three-dimensional MRI demonstrating stenosis of the left lower lobe pulmonary vein. AO = aorta; LPV = left pulmonary vein; PA = pulmonary artery.

Cardiac Catheterization and Angiography. In general a combination of echocardiography and MRI makes invasive procedures unnecessary.

MANAGEMENT OPTIONS AND OUTCOMES. If the patient has unilateral pulmonary vein stenosis and normal pulmonary artery pressure, no treatment may be necessary. Continued follow-up is important because this is often a progressive disease that can subsequently affect both sides. In cases with bilateral stenoses the outlook in the past was believed to be hopeless, with a virtually 100 percent mortality. Stents usually provided only temporary relief. More recently a pericardial reflection procedure using native tissue has resulted in some early success in this lesion. This involves using native atrial tissue to form a pocket around the surgically resected stenotic region.[201,315]

Partial Anomalous Pulmonary Venous Connection

MORPHOLOGY. This refers to those conditions where part or all of one lung drains to a site other than the left atrium. Sinus venosus defects have PAPVC typically from the right upper and middle lobe pulmonary veins to the superior vena cava.[316] PAPVC may be directed to a left vertical vein, to the superior vena cava at the level of or above the right pulmonary artery, to the azygos vein, or to the coronary sinus. PAPVC to the inferior vena cava (scimitar syndrome) may have associated hypoplasia of the right lung, pulmonary sequestration, and abnormal collateral supply to the sequestered segment. It can be seen in some patients (<10 percent) with a secundum ASD, as well as in association with many other forms of CHD. PAPVC to the right atrium has the pulmonary veins lying in the normal position; however, there is deviation of the septum primum to the left with absence of the septum secundum. This type of lesion is seen more frequently in hearts with visceral heterotaxy.

CLINICAL FEATURES. In the absence of associated anomalies, the physiological disturbance is determined by the number of anomalous veins and their site of connection, the presence and size of an ASD, and the state of the pulmonary vascular bed. In the usual patient with isolated partial pulmonary venous connection, the hemodynamic state and physical findings are similar to those in ASD.

LABORATORY INVESTIGATIONS

ECG. In isolated cases findings similar to a secundum ASD may be seen.

Chest Radiography. Isolated cases shows cardiomegaly involving the right ventricle with increased pulmonary vascular markings. In scimitar syndrome there is invariably right lung hypoplasia, with a secondary shift of the heart into the right thorax and a right-sided scimitar sign that represents the anomalous pulmonary vein.

Echocardiography. If there is a significant left-to-right shunt, then there is right ventricular volume overload with paradoxical interventricular septal motion.[317] A dilated coronary sinus is seen in PAPVC to the coronary sinus. In scimitar syndrome the abnormal pulmonary vein can be seen from the subcostal position during evaluation of the inferior vena cava.[318,319] There may be associated stenosis of the pulmonary vein. The suprasternal position permits identification of a left vertical vein, and in general it is possible in children to identify the number of connecting veins on that side. Abnormal venous drainage to the right superior vena cava may be more difficult to identify, unless a systematic approach is undertaken. The suprasternal frontal plane view allows the identification of those veins that connect just above the right pulmonary artery. Those that connect just behind the right pulmonary artery, either into the superior vena cava or the azygos, can be identified with a right anterior oblique view of the superior vena cava, whether from the subcostal position or a high right parasternal location. In adults, TEE may also be useful in detecting PAPVC.[320]

MRI. Although TEE can be used in older patients with a poorer ultrasound window with a considerable degree of accuracy,[320] it is less invasive to obtain the data using MRI.[321] This provides superb images of the connecting veins that can be seen more distally to their connections with the hilum of the lung. The pulmonary-to-systemic flow ratio can be calculated, obviating the need for hemodynamic evaluation. The pulmonary-to-systemic flow ratio can also be calculated by radionuclide techniques.

MANAGEMENT OPTIONS. In cases with a volume-loaded right ventricle, surgical intervention should be considered. Surgery is not needed when a single anomalously draining vein has not produced right ventricular volume loading. Surgery is typically performed at a similar time to an ASD at around 3 to 5 years of age. The type of surgery depends on the location of the drainage[322,323] but in general consists of reconnecting the abnormal vein(s) to the left atrium, either directly in the case of a left vertical vein or via a baffle in most other instances. In scimitar syndrome occlusion of the collateral arteries may be necessary as well as redirection of the pulmonary veins.

OUTCOMES. In general patients with repaired PAPVC have a good outcome similar to patients with an isolated ASD. What is unclear is the exact patency rate of the veins that are reconnected or baffled back to the left atrium. Patients with scimitar syndrome fare well if the lesion is relatively isolated but do poorly if there is significant associated intracardiac pathology.

Pulmonary Arteriovenous Fistula

Abnormal development of the pulmonary arteries and veins in a common vascular complex is responsible for this uncommon congenital anomaly. A variable number of pulmonary arteries communicate directly with branches of the pulmonary veins. Most patients have an associated Weber-Osler-Rendu syndrome; associated problems include bronchiectasis and other malformations of the bronchial tree, as well as absence of the right lower lobe. Pulmonary AV fistulas may also complicate classic Glenn shunts used in the palliation of cyanotic CHD and are believed to be due to the absence of "hepatic factor" in the venous blood feeding the superior vena cava–pulmonary artery connection. The amount of right-to-left shunting depends on the extent of the fistulous communications and may result in cyanosis. Paradoxical emboli or a brain abscess may cause major neurological deficits.[324,325] Patients with hereditary hemorrhagic telangiectasia often are anemic owing to repeated blood loss and may have less obvious cyanosis because of anemia. Systolic and continuous murmurs may be audible over areas of the fistula. Rounded opacities of various sizes in one or both lungs on chest radiography may suggest the presence of the lesion.

LABORATORY INVESTIGATIONS. Echocardiography is helpful in the initial diagnostic process with the use of a saline contrast injection into a systemic vein.[326] With pulmonary arteriovenous malformations there is early pulmonary venous return to the left atrium, but not as quickly as for patients with a patent foramen ovale or ASD and right-to-left atrial shunting. More recently CT and MRI techniques have provided valuable diagnostic information.[327,328] Pulmonary angiography reveals the site and extent of the abnormal communication.

MANAGEMENT OPTIONS. Unless the lesions are widespread throughout both lungs, surgical treatment aimed at removing the lesions with preservation of healthy lung tissue commonly is indicated to avoid the complications of massive hemorrhage,[324] bacterial endocarditis, and rupture of arteriovenous aneurysms. Transcatheter balloon or plug or coil occlusion embolotherapy may prove to be the therapeutic procedure of choice in some patients.[329]

Coronary Arteriovenous Fistula

MORPHOLOGY. A coronary arteriovenous fistula is a communication between one of the coronary arteries and a cardiac chamber or vein. The right coronary artery (or its branches) is the site of the fistula in about 55 percent of patients; the left coronary artery is involved in about 35 percent; and both coronary arteries are involved in a few. Connections between the coronary system and a cardiac chamber appear to represent persistence of embryonic intertrabecular spaces and sinusoids. Most of these fistulas drain into the right ventricle, right atrium, or the coronary sinus. Coronary to pulmonary artery fistulas are an occasional and usually incidental finding in the adult coronary angiography suite.

CLINICAL FEATURES. The shunt through the fistula is usually small and myocardial blood flow is not compromised. Potential complications include pulmonary hypertension and congestive heart failure if a large left-to-right shunt exists, bacterial endocarditis, rupture or thrombosis of the fistula or of an associated arterial aneurysm, and myocardial ischemia distal to the fistula due to a "myocardial steal."

Most pediatric patients are asymptomatic and are referred because of a cardiac murmur that is loud, superficial, and continuous at the lower or midsternal border. The site of maximal intensity of the murmur is related to the site of drainage and is usually away from the 2nd left intercostal space—the classic site of the continuous murmur of persistent ductus arteriosus.

LABORATORY INVESTIGATIONS

ECG. This is usually normal unless there is a large left-to-right shunt.

Chest Radiography. Radiographic findings often are normal and seldom show selective chamber enlargement.

Echocardiography. Coronary artery fistulas are now recognized with a high degree of accuracy with the advent of routine coronary artery evaluation during most pediatric echocardiography examinations. A significantly enlarged feeding coronary artery can be detected, and the entire course and site of entry of the arteriovenous fistula can be traced by Doppler color flow mapping. The shunt entry site is characterized by a continuous turbulent systolic and diastolic flow pattern. Multiplane TEE also accurately defines the origin, course, and drainage site of the fistula.

Cardiac Catheterization and Angiocardiography. If echocardiography demonstrates a significant coronary artery fistula, then hemodynamic evaluation is warranted. Standard retrograde thoracic aortography, balloon occlusion angiography of the aortic root with a 45-degree caudal tilt of the frontal camera ("laid back" aortogram), or coronary arteriography can be used reliably to identify the size and anatomical features of the fistulous tract.[330]

MANAGEMENT OPTIONS AND OUTCOMES. Small fistulas have an excellent long-term prognosis.[331] Untreated larger fistulas may predispose the individual to premature coronary artery disease in the affected vessel. Coil embolization at the time of cardiac catheterization is rapidly becoming the treatment of choice.[332] Surgical treatment is still required in some instances.[333]

REFERENCES

1. Therrien J, Somerville J, Webb G, et al: Canadian Cardiovascular Society Consensus Conference 2001 update: Recommendations for the Management of Adults with Congenital Heart Disease, Parts I, II, III. Can J Cardiol 17:940-959; 1029-1050; 1135-1158, 2001.
2. Deanfield J, Thaulow E, Warnes C, et al: Task Force on the Management of Grown-Up Congenital Heart Disease ESoC, ESC Committee for Practice Guidelines: Management of grown-up congenital heart disease. Eur Heart J 24:1035-1084, 2003.
3. Webb G, Williams R, Alpert J, et al: 32nd Bethesda Conference: Care of the Adult with Congenital Heart Disease, October 2-3, 2000. J Am Coll Cardiol 37:1161-1198, 2001.
4. Gatzoulis MA, Webb GD, Daubeney PE: Diagnosis and Management of Adult Congenital Heart Disease. Philadelphia, Churchill Livingstone, 2003.
5. Emmanouilides GC, Allen HD, Gutgesell HP, et al: Clinical Synopsis of Moss and Adams Heart Disease in Infants, Children, and Adolescents: Including the Fetus and Young Adult. Baltimore, Williams & Wilkins, 1998.
6. Anderson RH, Baker E, Macartney F, et al: Paediatric Cardiology. 2nd ed. London, Churchill Livingstone, 2002.
7. Nadas AS, Fyler DC: Pediatric Cardiology. 3rd ed. Philadelphia, WB Saunders, 1972.
8. Park MK: Pediatric Cardiology for Practitioners. 3rd ed. St. Louis, Mosby, 1996.
9. Garson A Jr, Bricker JT, Fisher DJ, et al: The Science and Practice of Pediatric Cardiology. 2nd ed. Baltimore, Williams & Wilkins, 1998.
10. Dore A, De Guise P, Mercier LA: Transition of care to adult congenital heart centres: What do patients know about their heart condition? Can J Cardiol 18:141-146, 2002.
11. Swan L, Goyal S, Hsia C, et al: Exercise systolic blood pressures are of questionable value in the assessment of the adult with a previous coarctation repair. Heart 89:189-192, 2003.
12. Graham TP Jr, Bricker JT, James FW, Strong WB: 26th Bethesda Conference: Recommendations for Determining Eligibility for Competition in Athletes with Cardiovascular Abnormalities. Task Force 1: Congenital Heart Disease. J Am Coll Cardiol 24:867-873, 1994.
13. Siu SC, Sermer M, Colman JM, et al: Cardiac Disease in Pregnancy (CARPREG) Investigators: Prospective multicenter study of pregnancy outcomes in women with heart disease. Circulation 104:515-521, 2001.
14. Siu SC, Colman JM: Heart disease and pregnancy. Heart 85:710-715, 2001.
15. Hechter SJ, Fredriksen PM, Liu P, et al: Angiotensin-converting enzyme inhibitors in adults after the Mustard procedure. Am J Cardiol 87:660-663, 2001.
16. Lester SJ, McElhinney DB, Viloria E, et al: Effects of losartan in patients with a systemically functioning morphologic right ventricle after atrial repair of transposition of the great arteries. Am J Cardiol 88:1314-1316, 2001.
17. Laer S, Mir TS, Behn F, et al: Carvedilol therapy in pediatric patients with congestive heart failure: A study investigating clinical and pharmacokinetic parameters. Am Heart J 143:916-922, 2002.
18. Rodriguez-Cruz E, Karpawich PP, Lieberman RA, Tantengco MV: Biventricular pacing as alternative therapy for dilated cardiomyopathy associated with congenital heart disease. Pacing Clin Electrophysiol 24:235-237, 2001.
19. Odim J, Laks H, Burch C, et al: Transplantation for congenital heart disease. Adv Cardiac Surg 12:59-76, 2000.
20. Pigula FA, Gandhi SK, Ristich J, et al: Cardiopulmonary transplantation for congenital heart disease in the adult. J Heart Lung Transplant 20:297-303, 2001.
21. Therrien J, Warnes C, Daliento L, et al: Canadian Cardiovascular Society Consensus Conference 2001 update: Recommendations for the Management of Adults with Congenital Heart Disease: Part III. Can J Cardiol 17:1135-1158, 2001.
22. Tempe DK, Virmani S: Coagulation abnormalities in patients with cyanotic congenital heart disease. J Cardiothorac Vasc Anesth 16:752-765, 2002.
23. Perloff JK, Latta H, Barsotti P: Pathogenesis of the glomerular abnormality in cyanotic congenital heart disease. Am J Cardiol 86:1198-1204, 2000.

24. Lamour JM, Addonizio LJ, Galantowicz ME, et al: Outcome after orthotopic cardiac transplantation in adults with congenital heart disease. Circulation 100(Suppl):5, 1999.
25. Thorne S: Management of polycythaemia in adults with cyanotic congenital heart disease. Heart 79:315-316, 1998.

Eisenmenger Syndrome

26. Daliento L, Somerville J, Presbitero P, et al: Eisenmenger syndrome: Factors relating to deterioration and death. Eur Heart J 19:1845-1855, 1998.
27. Saha A, Balakrishnan KG, Jaiswal PK, et al: Prognosis for patients with Eisenmenger syndrome of various aetiology. Int J Cardiol 45:199-207, 1994.
28. Vongpatanasin W, Brickner ME, Hillis LD, Lange RA: The Eisenmenger syndrome in adults. Ann Intern Med 128:745-755, 1998.
29. Corone S, Davido A, Lang T, Corone P: [Outcome of patients with Eisenmenger syndrome. Apropos of 62 cases followed-up for an average of 16 years]. [French]. Arch Mal Coeur Vaiss 85:521-526, 1992.
30. Ammash NM, Connolly HM, Abel MD, Warnes CA: Noncardiac surgery in Eisenmenger syndrome. J Am Coll Cardiol 33:222-227, 1999.
31. Martin JT, Tautz TJ, Antognini JF: Safety of regional anesthesia in Eisenmenger's syndrome. Reg Anesth Pain Med 27:509-513, 2002.
32. Sandoval J, Aguirre JS, Pulido T, et al: Nocturnal oxygen therapy in patients with the Eisenmenger syndrome. Am J Respir Crit Care Med 164:1682-1687, 2001.
33. Harinck E, Hutter PA, Hoorntje TM, et al: Air travel and adults with cyanotic congenital heart disease. Circulation 93:272-276, 1996.
34. Waddell TK, Bennett L, Kennedy R, et al: Heart-lung or lung transplantation for Eisenmenger syndrome. J Heart Lung Transplant 21:731-737, 2002.
35. Berman EB, Barst RJ: Eisenmenger's syndrome: Current management. Prog Cardiovasc Dis 45:129-138, 2002.
36. Granton JT, Rabinovitch M: Pulmonary arterial hypertension in congenital heart disease. Cardiol Clin 20:441-457, 2002.
37. Hopkins WE, Kelly DP: Angiotensin-converting enzyme inhibitors in adults with cyanotic congenital heart disease. Am J Cardiol 77:439-440, 1996.
38. Rosenzweig EB, Kerstein D, Barst RJ: Long-term prostacyclin for pulmonary hypertension with associated congenital heart defects. Circulation 99:1858-1865, 1999.
39. McLaughlin VV, Genthner DE, Panella MM, et al: Compassionate use of continuous prostacyclin in the management of secondary pulmonary hypertension: A case series. Ann Intern Med 130:740-743, 1999.
40. Rubin LJ, Badesch DB, Barst RJ, et al: Bosentan therapy for pulmonary arterial hypertension. N Engl J Med 346:896-903, 2002.

Cardiac Arrhythmias

41. Wilson NJ, Clarkson PM, Barratt-Boyes BG, et al: Long-term outcome after the Mustard repair for simple transposition of the great arteries: 28-year follow-up. J Am Coll Cardiol 32:758-765, 1998.
42. Puley G, Siu S, Connelly M, et al: Arrhythmia and survival in patients > 18 years of age after the Mustard procedure for complete transposition of the great arteries. Am J Cardiol 83:1080-1084, 1999.
43. Myridakis DJ, Ehlers KH, Engle MA: Late follow-up after venous switch operation (Mustard procedure) for simple and complex transposition of the great arteries. Am J Cardiol 74:1030-1036, 1994.
44. Gatzoulis MA, Freeman MA, Siu SC, et al: Atrial arrhythmia after surgical closure of atrial septal defects in adults. N Engl J Med 340:839-846, 1999.
45. Murphy JG, Gersh BJ, McGoon MD, et al: Long-term outcome after surgical repair of isolated atrial septal defect: Follow-up at 27 to 32 years. N Engl J Med 323:1645-1650, 1990.
46. Konstantinides S, Geibel A, Olschewski M, et al: A comparison of surgical and medical therapy for atrial septal defect in adults. N Engl J Med 333:469-473, 1995.
47. Oechslin EN, Harrison DA, Harris L, et al: Reoperation in adults with repair of tetralogy of Fallot: Indications and outcomes. J Thorac Cardiovasc Surg 118:245-251, 1999.
48. Gentles TL, Calder AL, Clarkson PM, Neutze JM: Predictors of long-term survival with Ebstein's anomaly of the tricuspid valve. Am J Cardiol 69:377-381, 1992.
49. Giuliani ER, Fuster V, Brandenburg RO, Mair DD: Ebstein's anomaly: The clinical features and natural history of Ebstein's anomaly of the tricuspid valve. Mayo Clin Proc 54:163-173, 1979.
50. Augustin N, Schmidt-Habelmann P, Wottke M, et al: Results after surgical repair of Ebstein's anomaly. Ann Thorac Surg 63:1650-1656, 1997.
51. Fishberger SB, Wernovsky G, Gentles TL, et al: Factors that influence the development of atrial flutter after the Fontan operation. J Thorac Cardiovasc Surg 113:80-86, 1997.
52. Gelatt M, Hamilton RM, McCrindle BW, et al: Risk factors for atrial tachyarrhythmias after the Fontan operation. J Am Coll Cardiol 24:1735-1741, 1994.
53. Peters NS, Somerville J: Arrhythmias after the Fontan procedure. Br Heart J 68:199-204, 1992.
54. Downar E, Harris L, Kimber S, et al: Ventricular tachycardia after surgical repair of tetralogy of Fallot: Results of intraoperative mapping studies. J Am Coll Cardiol 20:648-655, 1992.
55. Balaji S, Johnson TB, Sade RM, et al: Management of atrial flutter after the Fontan procedure. J Am Coll Cardiol 23:1209-1215, 1994.
56. Bonchek LI, Burlingame MW, Worley SJ, et al: Cox/maze procedure for atrial septal defect with atrial fibrillation: Management strategies. Ann Thorac Surg 55:607-610, 1993.
57. Sandoval N, Velasco VM, Orjuela H, et al: Concomitant mitral valve or atrial septal defect surgery and the modified Cox-maze procedure. Am J Cardiol 77:591-596, 1996.
58. Theodoro DA, Danielson GK, Porter CJ, Warnes CA: Right-sided maze procedure for right atrial arrhythmias in congenital heart disease. Ann Thorac Surg 65:149-153, 1998.
59. Mavroudis C, Backer CL, Deal BJ, Johnsrude CL: Fontan conversion to cavopulmonary connection and arrhythmia circuit cryoblation. J Thorac Cardiovasc Surg 115:547-556, 1998.
60. Harrison DA, Harris L, Siu SC, et al: Sustained ventricular tachycardia in adult patients late after repair of tetralogy of Fallot. J Am Coll Cardiol 30:1368–1373, 1997.
61. Gatzoulis MA, Till JA, Somerville J, Redington AN: Mechanoelectrical interaction in tetralogy of Fallot: QRS prolongation relates to right ventricular size and predicts malignant ventricular arrhythmias and sudden death. Circulation 92:231-237, 1995.
62. Berul CI, Hill SL, Geggel RL, et al: Electrocardiographic markers of late sudden death risk in postoperative tetralogy of Fallot children. J Cardiovasc Electrophysiol 8:1349-1356, 1997.
63. Murphy JG, Gersh BJ, Mair DD, et al: Long-term outcome in patients undergoing surgical repair of tetralogy of Fallot. N Engl J Med 329:593-599, 1993.
64. Nollert G, Fischlein T, Bouterwek S, et al: Long-term survival in patients with repair of tetralogy of Fallot: 36-year follow-up of 490 survivors of the first year after surgical repair. J Am Coll Cardiol 30:1374-1383, 1997.
65. Oechslin EN, Harrison DA, Connelly MS, et al: Mode of death in adults with congenital heart disease. Am J Cardiol 86:1111-1116, 2000.
66. Huhta JC, Maloney JD, Ritter DG, et al: Complete atrioventricular block in patients with atrioventricular discordance. Circulation 67:1374-1377, 1983.
67. Colman JM, Oechslin E: Adapted from Abbreviations and Glossary, Canadian Consensus Conference on Adult Congenital Heart Disease, 1996. Can J Cardiol 14:395-452, 1996.
68. Bull C: Current and potential impact of fetal diagnosis on prevalence and spectrum of serious congenital heart disease at term in the UK. British Paediatric Cardiac Association. Lancet 354:1242-1247, 1999.
69. Bonnet D, Coltri A, Butera G, et al: Detection of transposition of the great arteries in fetuses reduces neonatal morbidity and mortality. Circulation 99:916-918, 1999.
70. Van Praagh R: The segmental approach to diagnosis in congenital heart disease. *In* Bergsma D (ed): Birth Defects: Original Article Series. Baltimore, Williams & Wilkins, 1972.
71. Shinebourne EA, Macartney FJ, Anderson RH: Sequential chamber localization: Logical approach to diagnosis in congenital heart disease. Br Heart J 38:327-340, 1976.
72. Sittiwangkul R, Ma RY, McCrindle BW, et al: Echocardiographic assessment of obstructive lesions in atrioventricular septal defects. J Am Coll Cardiol 38:253-261, 2001.
73. Sugeng L, Spenser KT, Mor-Avi V, et al: Dynamic three-dimensional color-flow Doppler: An improved technique for the assessment of mitral regurgitation. Echocardiography 20:265, 2003.
74. Shiina A, Seward JB, Tajik AJ, et al: Two-dimensional echocardiographic-surgical correlation in Ebstein's anomaly: Preoperative determination of patients requiring tricuspid valve plication vs. replacement. Circulation 68:534-544, 1983.
75. Marx GR, Sherwood MC: Three-dimensional echocardiography in congenital heart disease: A continuum of unfulfilled promises? No. A presently clinically applicable technology with an important future? Yes. Pediatr Cardiol 23:266-285, 2002.
76. Heusch A, Rubo J, Krogmann ON, Bourgeois M: Volumetric analysis of the right ventricle in children with congenital heart defects: Comparison of biplane angiography and transthoracic 3-dimensional echocardiography. Cardiol Young 9:577-584, 1999.
77. Jan SL, Hwang B, Lee PC, et al: Intracardiac ultrasound assessment of atrial septal defect: Comparison with transthoracic echocardiographic, angiocardiographic, and balloon-sizing measurements. Cardiovasc Intervent Radiol 24:84-89, 2001.
78. Bruce CJ, Friedman PA: Intracardiac echocardiography. Eur J Echocardiogr 2:234-244, 2001.
79. Cowley CG, Lloyd TR: Interventional cardiac catheterization advances in nonsurgical approaches to congenital heart disease. Curr Opin Pediatr 11:425-432, 1999.
80. Hornung TS, Benson LN, McLaughlin PR: Catheter interventions in adult patients with congenital heart disease. Curr Cardiol Rep 4:54-62, 2002.

Atrial Septal Defect

81. Campbell M: Natural history of atrial septal defect. Br Heart J 32:820-826, 1970.
82. Craig RJ, Selzer A: Natural history and prognosis of atrial septal defect. Circulation 37:805-815, 1968.
83. Therrien J, Dore A, Gersony W, et al: Canadian Cardiovascular Society: CCS Consensus Conference 2001 update: Recommendations for the management of adults with congenital heart disease: Part I. Can J Cardiol 17:940-959, 2001.
84. Attie F, Rosas M Granados N, et al: Surgical treatment for secundum atrial septal defects in patients older than 40 years old: A randomized clinical trial. J Am Coll Cardiol 38:2035-2042, 2001.
85. Mullen MJ, Dias BF, Walker F, et al: Intracardiac echocardiography guided device closure of atrial septal defects. J Am Coll Cardiol 41:285-292, 2003.
86. Du ZD, Hijazi ZM, Kleinman CS, et al: Comparison between transcatheter and surgical closure of secundum atrial septal defect in children and adults: Results of a multicenter nonrandomized trial. J Am Coll Cardiol 39:1836-1844, 2002.
87. Brochu MC, Baril JF, Dore A, et al: Improvement in exercise capacity in asymptomatic and mildly symptomatic adults after atrial septal defect percutaneous closure. Circulation 106:1821-1826, 2002.
88. Helber U, Baumann R, Seboldt H, et al: Atrial septal defect in adults: Cardiopulmonary exercise capacity before and 4 months and 10 years after defect closure. J Am Coll Cardiol 29:1345-1350, 1997.
89. McCarthy PM, Gillinov AM, Castle L, et al: The Cox-maze procedure: The Cleveland Clinic experience. Semin Thorac Cardiovasc Surg 12:25-29, 2000.

Atrioventricular Septal Defect

90. Lange A, Mankad P, Walayat M, et al: Transthoracic three-dimensional echocardiography in the preoperative assessment of atrioventricular septal defect morphology. Am J Cardiol 85:630-635, 2000.
91. Smallhorn JF: Cross-sectional echocardiographic assessment of atrioventricular septal defect: Basic morphology and preoperative risk factors. Echocardiography 18:415-432, 2001.
92. Suzuki K, Ho SY, Anderson RH, Becker AE, et al: Morphometric analysis of atrioventricular septal defect with common valve orifice. J Am Coll Cardiol 31:217-223, 1998.

93. Ostium primum defect: Factors causing deterioration in the natural history. Br Heart J 27:413-419, 1965.
94. Hynes JK, Tajik AJ, Seward JB, et al: Partial atrioventricular canal defect in adults. Circulation 66:284-287, 1982.
95. Barnett MG, Chopra PS, Young WP: Long-term follow-up of partial atrioventricular septal defect repair in adults. Chest 94:321-324, 1988.
96. Burke RP, Horvath K, Landzberg M, et al: Long-term follow-up after surgical repair of ostium primum atrial septal defects in adults. J Am Coll Cardiol 27:696-699, 1996.
97. Bergin ML, Warnes CA, Tajik AJ, Danielson GK: Partial atrioventricular canal defect: Long-term follow-up after initial repair in patients ≥ 40 years old. J Am Coll Cardiol 25:1189-1194, 1995.
98. Pearl JM, Laks H: Intermediate and complete forms of atrioventricular canal. Semin Thorac Cardiovasc Surg 9:8-20, 1997.
99. Hanley FL, Fenton KN, Jonas RA, et al: Surgical repair of complete atrioventricular canal defects in infancy: Twenty-year trends. J Thorac Cardiovasc Surg 106:387-394, 1993.
100. Michielon G, Stellin G, Rizzoli G, et al: Left atrioventricular valve incompetence after repair of common atrioventricular canal defects. Ann Thorac Surg 60(Suppl):9, 1995.
101. Bando K, Turrentine MW, Sun K, et al: Surgical management of complete atrioventricular septal defects: A twenty-year experience. J Thorac Cardiovasc Surg 110:1543-1552, 1995.
102. Van Arsdell GS, Williams WG, Boutin C, et al: Subaortic stenosis in the spectrum of atrioventricular septal defects: Solutions may be complex and palliative. J Thorac Cardiovasc Surg 110:1534-1541, 1995.
103. DeLeon SY, Ilbawi MN, Wilson WR Jr, et al: Surgical options in subaortic stenosis associated with endocardial cushion defects. Ann Thorac Surg 52:1076-1082, 1991.
104. Mavroudis C, Backer CL: The two-patch technique for complete atrioventricular canal. Semin Thorac Cardiovasc Surg 9:35-43, 1997.
105. El Najdawi EK, Driscoll DJ, Puga FJ, et al: Operation for partial atrioventricular septal defect: A forty-year review. J Thorac Cardiovasc Surg 119:880-889, 2000.
106. Kameyama T, Ando F, Okamoto F, et al: Long term follow-up of atrioventricular valve function after repair of atrioventricular septal defect. Ann Thorac Cardiovasc Surg 5:101-106, 1999.

Ventricular Septal Defect

107. Perloff J: Ventricular septal defect. *In* The Clinical Recognition of Congenital Heart Disease. 4th ed. Philadelphia, WB Saunders, 1999, pp 467-489.
108. Gabriel HM, Heger M, Innerhofer P, et al: Long-term outcome of patients with ventricular septal defect considered not to require surgical closure during childhood. J Am Coll Cardiol 39:1066-1071, 2002.
109. Neumayer U, Stone S, Somerville J: Small ventricular septal defects in adults. Eur Heart J 19:1573-1582, 1998.
110. Eroglu AG, Oztunc F, Saltik L, et al: Evolution of ventricular septal defect with special reference to spontaneous closure rate, subaortic ridge and aortic valve prolapse. Pediatr Cardiol 24:31-35, 2003.
111. Eroglu AG, Oztunc F, Saltik L, et al: Aortic valve prolapse and aortic regurgitation in patients with ventricular septal defect. Pediatr Cardiol 24:36-39, 2003.
112. Arora R, Trahan V, Kumar A, et al: Transcatheter closure of congenital ventricular septal defects: Experience with various devices. J Intervent Cardiol 16:83-91, 2003.

Patent Ductus Arteriosus

113. Perloff J: Patent ductus arteriosus. *In* The Clinical Recognition of Congenital Heart Disease. 4th ed. Philadelphia, WB Saunders, 1999, pp 467-489.
114. Van Overmeire B, Smets K, Lecoutere D, et al: A comparison of ibuprofen and indomethacin for closure of patent ductus arteriosus. N Engl J Med 343:674-681, 2000.
115. Galal MO: Advantages and disadvantages of coils for transcatheter closure of patent ductus arteriosus. J Intervent Cardiol 16:157-163, 2003.
116. Landzberg MJ: Transcatheter occlusion: The treatment of choice for the adult with patent ductus arteriosus. Circulation 84(Suppl II):67, 1999.
117. Bennhagen RG, Benson LN: Silent and audible persistent ductus arteriosus: An angiographic study. Pediatr Cardiol 24:27-30, 2003.
118. Dearani JA, Danielson GK, Puga FJ, et al: Late follow-up of 1095 patients undergoing operation for complex congenital heart disease utilizing pulmonary ventricle to pulmonary artery conduits. Ann Thorac Surg 75:399-410, 2003.
119. Mavroudis C, Backer CL: Surgical management of severe truncal insufficiency: Experience with truncal valve remodeling techniques. Ann Thorac Surg 72:396-400, 2001.

Tetralogy of Fallot

120. Hokanson JS, Moller JH: Adults with tetralogy of Fallot: Long-term follow-up. Cardiol Rev 7:149-155, 1999.
121. Graham TP Jr: Management of pulmonary regurgitation after tetralogy of Fallot repair. Curr Cardiol Rep 4:63-67, 2002.
122. Niwa K, Perloff JK, Bhuta SM, et al: Structural abnormalities of great arterial walls in congenital heart disease: Light and electron microscopic analyses. Circulation 103:393-400, 2001.
123. Reddy VM, McElhinney DB, Amin Z, et al: Early and intermediate outcomes after repair of pulmonary atresia with ventricular septal defect and major aortopulmonary collateral arteries: Experience with 85 patients. Circulation 101:1826-1832, 2000.
124. Mair DD, Puga FJ: Management of pulmonary atresia with ventricular septal defect. Curr Treat Options Cardiovasc Med 5:409-415, 2003.
125. Abd El Rahman MY, Abdul-Khaliq H, Vogel M, et al: Relation between right ventricular enlargement, QRS duration, and right ventricular function in patients with tetralogy of Fallot and pulmonary regurgitation after surgical repair. Heart 84:416-420, 2000.
126. Alexiou C, Mahmoud H, Al Khaddour A, et al: Outcome after repair of tetralogy of Fallot in the first year of life. Ann Thorac Surg 71:494-500, 2001.
127. Parry AJ, McElhinney DB, Kung GC, et al: Elective primary repair of acyanotic tetralogy of Fallot in early infancy: Overall outcome and impact on the pulmonary valve. J Am Coll Cardiol 36:2279-2283, 2000.
128. Hu DC, Seward JB, Puga FJ, et al: Total correction of tetralogy of Fallot at age 40 years and older: Long-term follow-up. J Am Coll Cardiol 5:40-44, 1985.
129. Therrien J, Siu SC, Harris L, et al: Impact of pulmonary valve replacement on arrhythmia propensity late after repair of tetralogy of Fallot. Circulation 103:2489-2494, 2001.
130. Nollert G, Fischlein T, Bouterwek S, et al: Long-term results of total repair of tetralogy of Fallot in adulthood: 35 years follow-up in 104 patients corrected at the age of 18 or older. Thorac Cardiovasc Surgeon 45:178-181, 1997.
131. Yemets IM, Williams WG, Webb GD, et al: Pulmonary valve replacement late after repair of tetralogy of Fallot. Ann Thorac Surg 64:526-530, 1997.
132. Vliegen HW, van Straten A, de Roos A, et al: Magnetic resonance imaging to assess the hemodynamic effects of pulmonary valve replacement in adults late after repair of tetralogy of fallot. Circulation 106:1703-1707, 2002.
133. Ghai A, Silversides C, Harris L, et al: Left ventricular dysfunction is a risk factor for sudden cardiac death in adults late after repair of tetralogy of Fallot. J Am Coll Cardiol 40:1675-1680, 2003.
134. Mahle WT, Spray TL, Wernovsky G, et al: Survival after reconstructive surgery for hypoplastic left heart syndrome: A 15-year experience from a single institution. Circulation 102(Suppl):41, 2000.

Fontan Patient

135. Gentles TL, Mayer JE Jr, Gauvreau K, et al: Fontan operation in five hundred consecutive patients: Factors influencing early and late outcome. J Thorac Cardiovasc Surg 114:376-391, 1997.
136. Gentles TL, Gauvreau K, Mayer JE Jr, et al: Functional outcome after the Fontan operation: Factors influencing late morbidity. J Thorac Cardiovasc Surg 114:392-403, 1997.
137. Senzaki H, Masutani S, Kobayashi J, et al: Ventricular afterload and ventricular work in fontan circulation: Comparison with normal two-ventricle circulation and single-ventricle circulation with Blalock-Taussig shunts. Circulation 105:2885-2892, 2002.
138. Rosenthal M, Bush A, Deanfield J, Redington A: Comparison of cardiopulmonary adaptation during exercise in children after the atriopulmonary and total cavopulmonary connection Fontan procedures. Circulation 91:372-378, 1995.
139. Milanesi O, Stellin G, Colan SD, et al: Systolic and diastolic performance late after the Fontan procedure for a single ventricle and comparison of those undergoing operation at <12 months of age and at >12 months of age. Am J Cardiol 89:276-280, 2002.
140. Kouatli AA, Garcia JA, Zellers TM, et al: Enalapril does not enhance exercise capacity in patients after Fontan procedure. Circulation 96:1507-1512, 1997.
141. Khambadkone S, Li J, de Leval MR, et al: Basal pulmonary vascular resistance and nitric oxide responsiveness late after Fontan-type operation. Circulation 107:3204-3208, 2003.
142. Fontan F, Kirklin JW, Fernandez G, et al: Outcome after a "perfect" Fontan operation. Circulation 81:1520-1536, 1990.
143. Gates RN, Laks H, Drinkwater DC, et al: The Fontan procedure in adults. Ann Thorac Surg 63:1085-1090, 1997.
144. Driscoll DJ, Offord KP, Feldt RH, et al: Five- to fifteen-year follow up after Fontan operation. Circulation 85:469-496, 1992.
145. Durongpisitkul K, Porter CJ, Cetta F, et al: Predictors of early- and late-onset supraventricular tachyarrhythmias after Fontan operation. Circulation 98:1099-1107, 1998.
146. Gewillig M, Wyse RK, de Leval MR, Deanfield JE: Early and late arrhythmias after the Fontan operation: Predisposing factors and clinical consequences. Br Heart J 67:72-79, 1992.
147. Shirai LK, Rosenthal DN, Reitz BA, et al: Arrhythmias and thromboembolic complications after the extracardiac Fontan operation. J Thorac Cardiovasc Surg 115:499-505, 1998.
148. Balling G, Vogt M, Kaemmerer H, et al: Intracardiac thrombus formation after the Fontan operation. J Thorac Cardiovasc Surg 119:52, 2000.
149. Coon PD, Rychik J, Novello RT, et al: Thrombus formation after the Fontan operation. Ann Thorac Surg 71:1990-1994, 2001.
150. Brancaccio G, Carotti A, D'Argenio P, et al: Protein-losing enteropathy after Fontan surgery: Resolution after cardiac transplantation. J Heart Lung Transplant 22:484-486, 2003.
151. Mertens L, Hagler DJ, Sauer U, et al: Protein-losing enteropathy after the Fontan operation: An international multicenter study. PLE Study Group. J Thorac Cardiovasc Surg 115:1063-1073, 1998.
152. Varma C, Warr MR, Hendler AL, et al: Prevalence of "silent" pulmonary emboli in adults after the Fontan operation. J Am Coll Cardiol 41:2252-2258, 2003.
153. Monagle P, Cochrane A, McCrindle B, et al: Thromboembolic complications after Fontan procedures: The role of prophylactic anticoagulation. J Thorac Cardiovasc Surg 115:493-498, 1998.
154. Jacobs ML, Pourmoghadam KK, Geary EM, et al: Fontan's operation: is aspirin enough? Is Coumadin too much? Ann Thorac Surg 73:64-68, 2002.
155. Seipelt RG, Franke A, Vazquez-Jimenez JF, et al: Thromboembolic complications after Fontan procedures: Comparison of different therapeutic approaches. Ann Thorac Surg 74:556-562, 2002.
156. Deal BJ, Mavroudis C, Backer CL: Beyond Fontan conversion: Surgical therapy of arrhythmias including patients with associated complex congenital heart disease. Ann Thorac Cardiovasc Surg 76:542-553; Discussion 553-554, 2003.
157. Mavroudis C, Deal BJ, Backer CL: Arrhythmia surgery in association with complex congenital heart repairs excluding patients with Fontan conversion. Semin Thorac Cardiovasc Surg Pediatr Card Surg Annu 6:33-50, 2003.
158. Deal BJ, Mavroudis C, Backer CL, et al: Impact of arrhythmia circuit cryoablation during Fontan conversion for refractory atrial tachycardia. Am J Cardiol 83:563-568, 1999.

159. Mavroudis C, Backer CL, Deal BJ, et al: Total cavopulmonary and Maze procedure for patients with failure of the Fontan operation. Thorac Cardiovasc Surgeon 122:863-871, 2001.
160. Feldt RH, Driscoll DJ, Offord KP, et al: Protein-losing enteropathy after the Fontan operation. J Thorac Cardiovasc Surg 112:672-680, 1996.

Transposition Complexes

161. Bonnet D, Coltri A, Butera G, et al: [Prenatal diagnosis of transposition of great vessels reduces neonatal morbidity and mortality]. [French]. Arch Mal Coeur Vaiss 92:637-640, 1999.
162. Williams W, McCrindle B, Ashburn DA, et al: Congenital Heart Surgeon's Society: Outcome of 829 neonates with complete transposition of the great arteries 12-17 years after repair. Eur J Cardiothorac Surg 24:1-9, 2003.
163. Rehnstrom P, Gilljam T, Sudow G, Berggren H: Excellent survival and low complication rate in medium-term follow-up after arterial switch operation for complete transposition. Scand Cardiovasc J 37:104-106, 2003.
164. Hovels-Gurich HH, Kunz D, Seghaye M, et al: Results of exercise testing at a mean age of 10 years after neonatal arterial switch operation. Acta Paediatr 92:190-196, 2003.
165. Losay J, Touchot A, Serraf A, et al: Late outcome after arterial switch operation for transposition of the great arteries. Circulation 104(Suppl):6, 2001.
166. Yoshizumi K, Yagihara T, Uemura H: Approach to the neoaortic valve for replacement after the arterial switch procedure in patients with complete transposition. Cardiol Young 11:666-669, 2001.
167. Legendre A, Losay J, Touchot-Kone A, et al: [Prevalence and diagnosis of coronary lesions after arterial switch]. [French]. Arch Mal Coeur Vaiss 96:485-488, 2003.
168. Wells WJ, Blackstone E: Intermediate outcome after Mustard and Senning procedures: A study by the Congenital Heart Surgeons Society. Semin Thorac Cardiovasc Surg Pediatr Card Surg Annu 3:186-197, 2000.
169. Connelly M, Walters JE, McLaughlin PR, et al: Functional capacity in adult patients with Mustard operation. J Am Coll Cardiol 25:378A, 1995.
170. Derrick GP, Narang I, White PA, et al: Failure of stroke volume augmentation during exercise and dobutamine stress is unrelated to load-independent indexes of right ventricular performance after the Mustard operation. Circulation 102(Suppl):9, 2000.
171. Hauser M, Bengel FM, Kuhn A, et al: Myocardial blood flow and flow reserve after coronary reimplantation in patients after arterial switch and Ross operation. Circulation 103:1875-1880, 2001.
172. Lubiszewska B, Gosiewska E, Hoffman P, et al: Myocardial perfusion and function of the systemic right ventricle in patients after atrial switch procedure for complete transposition: Long-term follow-up. J Am Coll Cardiol 36:1365-1370, 2000.
173. Millane T, Bernard EJ, Jaeggi E, et al: Role of ischemia and infarction in late right ventricular dysfunction after atrial repair of transposition of the great arteries. J Am Coll Cardiol 35:1661-1668, 2000.
174. Gelatt M, Hamilton RM, McCrindle BW, et al: Arrhythmia and mortality after the Mustard procedure: A 30-year single-center experience. J Am Coll Cardiol 29:194-201, 1997.
175. Gewillig M, Cullen S, Mertens B, et al: Risk factors for arrhythmia and death after Mustard operation for simple transposition of the great arteries. Circulation 84(Suppl):92, 1991.
176. Rhodes LA, Wernovsky G, Keane JF, et al: Arrhythmias and intracardiac conduction after the arterial switch operation. J Thorac Cardiovasc Surg109:303-310, 1995.
177. Gatzoulis MA, Walters J, McLaughlin PR, et al: Late arrhythmia in adults with the Mustard procedure for transposition of great arteries: A surrogate marker for right ventricular dysfunction? Heart 84:409-415, 2000.
178. Haas F, Wottke M, Poppert H, Meisner H: Long-term survival and functional follow-up in patients after the arterial switch operation. Ann Thorac Surg 68:1692-1697, 1999.
179. Mahoney LT, Knoedel DL, Skorton DJ: Echocardiographic postoperative assessment of patients with transposition of the great arteries. J Cardiovasc Ultrasound Allied Tech 12:545-557, 1999.
180. Daebritz SH, Tiete AR, Sachweh JS, et al: Systemic right ventricular failure after atrial switch operation: Midterm results of conversion into an arterial switch. Ann Thorac Surg 71:1255-1259, 2001.
181. Chang AC, Wernovsky G, Wessel DL, et al: Surgical management of late right ventricular failure after Mustard or Senning repair. Circulation 86(Suppl):9, 1992.
182. Cochrane AD, Karl TR, Mee RB: Staged conversion to arterial switch for late failure of the systemic right ventricle. Ann Thorac Surg 56:854-861, 1993.
183. van Son JA, Reddy VM, Silverman NH, Hanley FL: Regression of tricuspid regurgitation after two-stage arterial switch operation for failing systemic ventricle after atrial inversion operation. J Thorac Cardiovasc Surg 111:342-347, 1996.
184. Carrel T, Pfammatter JP: Complete transposition of the great arteries: Surgical concepts for patients with systemic right ventricular failure following intraatrial repair. Thorac Cardiovasc Surgeon 48:224-227, 2000.

Congenitally Corrected Transposition of the Great Arteries

185. Webb GD, McLaughlin PR, Gow RM, et al: Transposition complexes. Cardiol Clin 11:651-664, 1993.
186. Roffi M, de Marchi SF, Seiler C: Congenitally corrected transposition of the great arteries in an 80-year-old woman. Heart 79:622-623, 1998.
187. Kafali G, Elsharshari H, Ozer S, et al: Incidence of dysrhythmias in congenitally corrected transposition of the great arteries. Turk J Pediatr 44:219-223, 2002.
188. Rutledge JM, Nihill MR, Fraser CD, et al: Outcome of 121 patients with congenitally corrected transposition of the great arteries. Pediatr Cardiol 23:137-145, 2002.
189. Presbitero P, Somerville J, Rabajoli F, et al: Corrected transposition of the great arteries without associated defects in adult patients: Clinical profile and follow up. Br Heart J 74:57-59, 1995.
190. Beauchesne LM, Warnes CA, Connolly HM, et al: Outcome of the unoperated adult who presents with congenitally corrected transposition of the great arteries. J Am Coll Cardiol 40:285-290, 2002.
191. van Son JA, Danielson GK, Huhta JC, et al: Late results of systemic atrioventricular valve replacement in corrected transposition. J Thorac Cardiovasc Surg 109:642-652, 1995.
192. Duncan BW, Mee RB, Mesia CI, et al: Results of the double-switch operation for congenitally corrected transposition of the great arteries. Eur J Cardiothorac Surg 24:11-19, 2003.
193. Imai Y: Double-switch operation for congenitally corrected transposition. Adv Cardiac Surg 9:65-86, 1997.
194. Karl TR, Weintraub RG, Brizard CP, et al: Senning plus arterial switch operation for discordant (congenitally corrected) transposition. Ann Thorac Surg 64:495-502, 1997.
195. Prieto LR, Hordof AJ, Secic M, et al: Progressive tricuspid valve disease in patients with congenitally corrected transposition of the great arteries. Circulation 98:997-1005, 1998.
196. Ilbawi MN, Ocampo CB, Allen BS, et al: Intermediate results of the anatomic repair for congenitally corrected transposition. Ann Thorac Surg 73:594-599, 2002.
197. Graham TP Jr, Bernard YD, Mellen BG, et al: Long-term outcome in congenitally corrected transposition of the great arteries: A multi-institutional study. J Am Coll Cardiol 36:255-261, 2000.

Double-Outlet Right Ventricle

198. Anderson RH: Double-outlet right ventricle. Eur J Cardiothorac Surg 22:853, 2002.
199. Anderson RH, McCarthy K, Cook AC: Continuing medical education: Double-outlet right ventricle. Cardiol Young 11:329-344, 2001.
200. Brown JW, Ruzmetov M, Okada Y, et al: Surgical results in patients with double-outlet right ventricle: A 20-year experience. Ann Thorac Surg 72:1630-1635, 2001.
201. Lacour-Gayet F, Zoghbi J, Serraf AE, et al: Surgical management of progressive pulmonary venous obstruction after repair of total anomalous pulmonary venous connection. J Thorac Cardiovasc Surg 117:679-687, 1999.
202. Belli E, Serraf A, Lacour-Gayet F, et al: Biventricular repair for double-outlet right ventricle: Results and long-term follow-up. Circulation 98(Suppl):5, 1998.
203. Aoki M, Forbess JM, Jonas RA, et al: Result of biventricular repair for double-outlet right ventricle. J Thorac Cardiovasc Surg 107:338-349, 1994.
204. Rychik J, Jacobs ML, Norwood WI: Early changes in ventricular geometry and ventricular septal defect size following Rastelli operation or intraventricular baffle repair for conotruncal anomaly: A cause for development of subaortic stenosis. Circulation 90:II13-19, 1994.
205. Celermajer DS, Bull C, Till JA, et al: Ebstein's anomaly: Presentation and outcome from fetus to adult. J Am Coll Cardiol 23:170-176, 1994.
206. Therrien J, Gatzoulis M, Graham T, et al: Canadian Cardiovascular Society Consensus Conference 2001 update: Recommendations for the Management of Adults with Congenital Heart Disease: Part II. Can J Cardiol 17:1029-1050, 2001.
207. Chauvaud S, Fuzellier JF, Berrebi A, et al: Bi-directional cavopulmonary shunt associated with ventriculo and valvuloplasty in Ebstein's anomaly: Benefits in high-risk patients. Eur J Cardiothorac Surg 13:514-519, 1998.
208. Chauvaud S: Ebstein's malformation: Surgical treatment and results. Thorac Cardiovasc Surgeon 48:220-223, 2000.
209. Chauvaud SM, Brancaccio G, Carpentier A: Cardiac arrhythmia in patients undergoing surgical repair of Ebstein's anomaly. Ann Thorac Surg 71:1547-1552, 2001.
210. Almange C: [Ebstein anomaly and pregnancy]. [French]. Arch Mal Coeur Vaiss 95:525, 2002.

Coarctation of the Aorta

211. Aluquin VP, Shutte D, Nihill MR, et al: Normal aortic arch growth and comparison with isolated coarctation of the aorta. Am J Cardiol 91:502-505, 2003.
212. Bharati S, Lev M: The surgical anatomy of the heart in tubular hypoplasia of the transverse aorta (preductal coarctation). J Thorac Cardiovasc Surg 91:79-85, 1986.
213. Levine JC, Sanders SP, Colan SD, et al: The risk of having additional obstructive lesions in neonatal coarctation of the aorta. Cardiol Young 11:44-53, 2001.
214. De Mey S, Segers P, Coomans I, et al: Limitations of Doppler echocardiography for the post-operative evaluation of aortic coarctation. J Biomechan 34:951-960, 2001.
215. Lim DS, Ralston MA: Echocardiographic indices of Doppler flow patterns compared with MRI or angiographic measurements to detect significant coarctation of the aorta. Echocardiography 19:55-60, 2002.
216. Godart F, Labrot G, Devos P, et al: Coarctation of the aorta: Comparison of aortic dimensions between conventional MR imaging, 3D MR angiography, and conventional angiography. Eur Radiol 12:2034-2039, 2002.
217. Seirafi PA, Warner KG, Geggel RL, et al: Repair of coarctation of the aorta during infancy minimizes the risk of late hypertension. Ann Thorac Surg 66:1378-1382, 1998.
218. Ovaert C, Benson LN, Nykanen D, Freedom RM: Transcatheter treatment of coarctation of the aorta: A review. Pediatr Cardiol 19:27-44, 1998.
219. Zabal C, Attie F, Rosas M, et al: The adult patient with native coarctation of the aorta: Balloon angioplasty or primary stenting? Heart 89:77-83, 2003.
220. Bouchart F, Dubar A, Tabley A, et al: Coarctation of the aorta in adults: Surgical results and long-term follow-up. Ann Thorac Surg 70:1483-1488, 2000.
221. Toro-Salazar OH, Steinberger J, Thomas W, et al: Long-term follow-up of patients after coarctation of the aorta repair. Am J Cardiol 89:541-547, 2002.
222. von Kodolitsch Y, Aydin MA, Koschyk DH, et al: Predictors of aneurysmal formation after surgical correction of aortic coarctation. J Am Coll Cardiol 39:617-624, 2002.
223. O'Sullivan JJ, Derrick G, Darnell R: Prevalence of hypertension in children after early repair of coarctation of the aorta: A cohort study using casual and 24-hour blood pressure measurement. Heart (British Cardiac Society) 88:163-166, 2002.
224. Jenkins NP, Ward C: Coarctation of the aorta: Natural history and outcome after surgical treatment. QJM 92:365-371, 1999.
225. Campbell M: Natural history of coarctation of the aorta. Br Heart J 32:633-640, 1970
226. Messmer BJ, Minale C, Muhler E, von Bernuth G: Surgical correction of coarctation in early infancy: Does surgical technique influence the result? Ann Thorac Surg 52:594-600, 1991.

227. Ala-Kulju K, Jarvinen A, Maamies T, et al: Late aneurysms after patch aortoplasty for coarctation of the aorta in adults. Thorac Cardiovasc Surg 31:301-306, 1983.
228. Hehrlein FW, Mulch J, Rautenburg HW, et al: Incidence and pathogenesis of late aneurysms after patch graft aortoplasty for coarctation. J Thorac Cardiovasc Surg 92:226-230, 1986.
229. Maron BJ, Humphries JO, Rowe RD, Mellits ED: Prognosis of surgically corrected coarctation of the aorta: A 20-year postoperative appraisal. Circulation 47:119-126, 1973.
230. Bergdahl L, Bjork VO, Jonasson R: Surgical correction of coarctation of the aorta: Influence of age on late results. J Thorac Cardiovasc Surg 85:532-536, 1983.
231. Clarkson PM, Nicholson MR, Barratt-Boyes BG, et al: Results after repair of coarctation of the aorta beyond infancy: A 10- to 28-year follow-up with particular reference to late systemic hypertension. Am J Cardiol 51:1481-1488, 1983.
232. Siblini G, Rao PS, Nouri S, et al: Long-term follow-up results of balloon angioplasty of postoperative aortic recoarctation. Am J Cardiol 81:61-67, 1998.
233. Ebeid MR, Prieto LR, Latson LA: Use of balloon-expandable stents for coarctation of the aorta: Initial results and intermediate-term follow-up. J Am Coll Cardiol 30:1847-1852, 1997.
234. Yetman AT, Nykanen D, McCrindle BW, et al: Balloon angioplasty of recurrent coarctation: A 12-year review. J Am Coll Cardiol 30:811-816, 1997.
235. McCrindle BW, Jones TK, Morrow WR, et al: Acute results of balloon angioplasty of native coarctation versus recurrent aortic obstruction are equivalent. Valvuloplasty and Angioplasty of Congenital Anomalies (VACA) Registry Investigators. J Am Coll Cardiol 28:1810-1817, 1996.
236. Rothman A: Interventional therapy for coarctation of the aorta. Curr Opin Cardiol 13:66-72, 1998.
237. Harrison DA, McLaughlin PR, Lazzam C, et al: Endovascular stents in the management of coarctation of the aorta in the adolescent and adult: One-year follow-up. Heart 85:561-566, 2001.
238. Therrien J, Thorne SA, Wright A, et al: Repaired coarctation: A "cost-effective" approach to identify complications in adults. J Am Coll Cardiol 35:997-1002, 2000.

Sinus of Valsalva Aneurysm and Fistula

239. Barragry TP, Ring WS, Moller JH, Lillehei CW: 15- to 30-year follow-up of patients undergoing repair of ruptured congenital aneurysms of the sinus of Valsalva. Ann Thorac Surg 46:515-519, 1988.
240. Dong C, Wu QY, Tang Y: Ruptured sinus of Valsalva aneurysm: A Beijing experience. Ann Thorac Surg 74:1621-1624, 2002.
241. Perry LW, Martin GR, Galioto FM Jr, Midgley FM: Rupture of congenital sinus of Valsalva aneurysm in a newborn. Am J Cardiol 68:1255-1256, 1991.
242. Pasteuning WH, Roukema JA, van Straten AH, et al: Rapid hemodynamic deterioration because of acute rupture of an aneurysm of the sinus of Valsalva: The importance of echocardiography in early diagnosis. J Am Soc Echocardiogr 15:1108-1110, 2002.
243 Shah RP, Ding ZP, Ng AS, Quek SS: A ten-year review of ruptured sinus of Valsalva: Clinicopathological and echo-Doppler features. Singapore Med J 42:473-476, 2001.
244. Fedson S, Jolly N, Lang RM, Hijazi ZM: Percutaneous closure of a ruptured sinus of Valsalva aneurysm using the Amplatzer Duct Occluder. Cathet Cardiovasc Intervent 58:406-411, 2003.
245. Edwards JE: Anomalies of the derivatives of the aortic arch system. Med Clin North Am 32:925, 1948.
246. van Son JA, Konstantinov IE: Burckhard F: Kommerell and Kommerell's diverticulum. Tex Heart Instit J 29:109-112, 2002.
247. Edwards JE: Retro-esophageal segment of the left aortic arch, right ligamentum arteriosum and right descending aorta causing a congenital vascular ring about the trachea and esophagus. Proc Mayo Clin 23:108, 1948.
248. Philip S, Chen SY, Wu MH, et al: Retroesophageal aortic arch: Diagnostic and therapeutic implications of a rare vascular ring. Int J Cardiol 79:133-141, 2001.
249. Parikh SR, Ensing GJ, Darragh RK, Caldwell RL: Rings, slings and such things: Diagnosis and management with special emphasis on the role of echocardiography. J Am Soc Echocardiogr 6:1-11, 1993.
250. Sebening C, Jakob H, Tochtermann U, et al: Vascular tracheobronchial compression syndromes: Experience in surgical treatment and literature review. Thorac Cardiovasc Surgeon 48:164-174, 2000.
251. Mihaljevic T, Cannon JW, del Nido PJ: Robotically assisted division of a vascular ring in children. J Thorac Cardiovasc Surg 125:1163, 2003.
252. Decampli WM: Video-assisted thoracic surgical procedures in children. Semin Thorac Cardiovasc Surg Pediatr Card Surg Annu 1:61, 1998.

Congenital Aortic Valve Stenosis

253. Lofland GK, McCrindle BW, Williams WG, et al: Critical aortic stenosis in the neonate: A multi-institutional study of management, outcomes, and risk factors. Congenital Heart Surgeons Society. J Thorac Cardiovasc Surg 121:10-27, 2001.
254. McCrindle BW, Blackstone EH, Williams WG, et al: Are outcomes of surgical versus transcatheter balloon valvotomy equivalent in neonatal critical aortic stenosis? Circulation 104(Suppl):8, 2001.
255. Weber HS, Mart CR, Myers JL: Transcarotid balloon valvuloplasty for critical aortic valve stenosis at the bedside via continuous transesophageal echocardiographic guidance. Cathet Cardiovasc Intervent 50:326-329, 2000.
256. Lakier JB, Lewis AB, Heymann MA, et al: Isolated aortic stenosis in the neonate: Natural history and hemodynamic considerations. Circulation 50:801-808, 1974.
257. Nishimura RA, Pieroni DR, Bierman FZ, et al: Second natural history study of congenital heart defects: Pulmonary stenosis—echocardiography. Circulation 87(Suppl):9, 1993.
258. Barker PC, Ensing G, Ludomirsky A, et al: Comparison of simultaneous invasive and noninvasive measurements of pressure gradients in congenital aortic valve stenosis. J Am Soc Echocardiogr 15:1496-1502, 2002.
259. Lemler MS, Valdes-Cruz LM, Shandas RS, Cape EG: Insights into catheter/Doppler discrepancies in congenital aortic stenosis. Am J Cardiol 83:1447-1450, 1999.
260. Alexiou C, McDonald A, Langley SM, et al: Aortic valve replacement in children: Are mechanical prostheses a good option? Eur J Cardiothorac Surg 17:125-133, 2000.
261. Bacha EA, Satou GM, Moran AM, et al: Valve-sparing operation for balloon-induced aortic regurgitation in congenital aortic stenosis. J Thorac Cardiovasc Surg 122:162-168, 2001.
262. Ohye RG, Gomez CA, Ohye BJ, et al: The Ross/Konno procedure in neonates and infants: Intermediate-term survival and autograft function. Ann Thorac Surg 72:823-830, 2001.
263. Al Halees Z, Pieters F, Qadoura F, et al: The Ross procedure is the procedure of choice for congenital aortic valve disease. J Thorac Cardiovasc Surg 123:437-441, 2002.
264. Favaloro R, Stutzbach P, Gomez C, et al: Feasibility of the Ross procedure: Its relationship with the bicuspid aortic valve. J Heart Valve Dis 11:375-382, 2002.
265. Tentolouris K, Kontozoglou T, Trikas A, et al: Fixed subaortic stenosis revisited: Congenital abnormalities in 72 new cases and review of the literature. Cardiology 92:4-10, 1999.
266. Bezold LI, Smith EO, Kelly K, et al: Development and validation of an echocardiographic model for predicting progression of discrete subaortic stenosis in children. Am J Cardiol 81:314-320, 1998.
267. Cohen L, Bennani R, Hulin S, et al: Mitral valvar anomalies and discrete subaortic stenosis. Cardiol Young 12:138-146, 2002.
268. McElhinney DB, Reddy VM, Silverman NH, Hanley FL: Accessory and anomalous atrioventricular valvar tissue causing outflow tract obstruction: Surgical implications of a heterogeneous and complex problem. J Am Coll Cardiol 32:1741-1748, 1998.
269. Sigfusson G, Tacy TA, Vanauker MD, Cape EG: Abnormalities of the left ventricular outflow tract associated with discrete subaortic stenosis in children: An echocardiographic study. J Am Coll Cardiol 30:255-259, 1997.
270. Sharma S, Stamper T, Dhar P: The usefulness of transesophageal echocardiography in the surgical management of older children with subaortic stenosis. Echocardiography 13:653, 1996.
271. Oliver JM, Gonzalez A, Gallego P, et al: Discrete subaortic stenosis in adults: Increased prevalence and slow rate of progression of the obstruction and aortic regurgitation. J Am Coll Cardiol 38:835-842, 2001.
272. Coleman DM, Smallhorn JF, McCrindle BW, et al: Postoperative follow-up of fibromuscular subaortic stenosis. J Am Coll Cardiol 24:1558-1564, 1994.
273. Serraf A, Zoghby J, Lacour-Gayet F, et al: Surgical treatment of subaortic stenosis: A seventeen-year experience. J Thorac Cardiovasc Surg 117:669-678, 1999.
274. Jahangiri M, Nicholson IA, del Nido PJ, et al: Surgical management of complex and tunnel-like subaortic stenosis. Eur J Cardiothorac Surg 17:637-642, 2000.
275. Caldarone CA: Left ventricular outflow tract obstruction: The role of the modified Konno procedure. Semin Thorac Cardiovasc Surg Pediatr Card Surg Annu 6:98, 2003.
276. Garcia RC, Friedman WF, Kaback MM, Rowe RD: Idiopathic hypercalcemia and supravalvular aortic stenosis: Documentation of a new syndrome. N Engl J Med 271:117, 1964.
277. Metcalfe K, Rucka AK, Smoot L, et al: Elastin: mutational spectrum in supravalvular aortic stenosis. Eur J Hum Genet 8:955-963, 2000.
278. Vaideeswar P, Shankar V, Deshpande JR, et al: Pathology of the diffuse variant of supravalvar aortic stenosis. Cardiovasc Pathol 10:33-37, 2001.
279. Eronen M, Peippo M, Hiippala A, et al: Cardiovascular manifestations in 75 patients with Williams syndrome. J Med Genet 39:554-558, 2002.
280. Giddins NG, Finley JP, Nanton MA, Roy DL: The natural course of supravalvar aortic stenosis and peripheral pulmonary artery stenosis in Williams's syndrome. Br Heart J 62:315-319, 1989.
281. Wren C, Oslizlok P, Bull C: Natural history of supravalvular aortic stenosis and pulmonary artery stenosis. J Am Coll Cardiol 15:1625-1630, 1990.
282. Brand A, Keren A, Reifen RM, et al: Echocardiographic and Doppler findings in the Williams syndrome. Am J Cardiol 63:633-635, 1989.
283. McElhinney DB, Petrossian E, Tworetzky W, et al: Issues and outcomes in the management of supravalvar aortic stenosis. Ann Thorac Surg 69:562-567, 2000.
284. Stamm C, Kreutzer C, Zurakowski D, et al: Forty-one years of surgical experience with congenital supravalvular aortic stenosis. J Thorac Cardiovasc Surg 118:874-885, 1999.
285. Einfeld SL, Tonge BJ, Rees VW: Longitudinal course of behavioral and emotional problems in Williams syndrome. Am J Ment Retard 106:73-81, 2001.

Congenital Mitral Valve Anomalies

286. Ruckman RN, Van Praagh R: Anatomic types of congenital mitral stenosis: Report of 49 autopsy cases with consideration of diagnosis and surgical implications. Am J Cardiol 42:592-601, 1978.
287. Agnoletti G, Annecchino F, Preda L, Borghi A: Persistence of the left superior caval vein: Can it potentiate obstructive lesions of the left ventricle? Cardiol Young 9:285-290, 1999.
288. Banerjee A, Kohl T, Silverman NH: Echocardiographic evaluation of congenital mitral valve anomalies in children. Am J Cardiol 76:1284-1291, 1995.
289. Patel JJ, Munclinger MJ, Mitha AS, Patel N: Percutaneous balloon dilatation of the mitral valve in critically ill young patients with intractable heart failure. Br Heart J 73:555-558, 1995.
290. Serraf A, Zoghbi J, Belli E, et al: Congenital mitral stenosis with or without associated defects: An evolving surgical strategy. Circulation 102(Suppl):71, 2000.
291. Agarwal S, Airan B, Chowdhury UK, et al: Ventricular septal defect with congenital mitral valve disease: Long-term results of corrective surgery. Indian Heart J 54:67-73, 2002.
292. Tamura M, Menahem S, Brizard C: Clinical features and management of isolated cleft mitral valve in childhood. J Am Coll Cardiol 35:764-770, 2000.
293. Zias EA, Mavroudis C, Backer CL, et al: Surgical repair of the congenitally malformed mitral valve in infants and children. Ann Thorac Surg 66:1551-1559, 1998.
294. Erez E, Kanter KR, Isom E, et al: Mitral valve replacement in children. J Heart Valve Dis 12:25-29, 2003.

295. Kim YM, Yoo SJ, Choi JY, et al: Natural course of supravalvar aortic stenosis and peripheral pulmonary arterial stenosis in Williams' syndrome. Cardiol Young 9:37-41, 1999.
296. McElhinney DB, Krantz ID, Bason L, et al: Analysis of cardiovascular phenotype and genotype-phenotype correlation in individuals with a *JAG1* mutation and/or Alagille syndrome. Circulation 106:2567-2574, 2002.
297. Trivedi KR, Benson LN: Interventional strategies in the management of peripheral pulmonary artery stenosis. J Intervent Cardiol 16:171-188, 2003.
298. Rothman A, Levy DJ, Sklansky MS, et al: Balloon angioplasty and stenting of multiple intralobar pulmonary arterial stenoses in adult patients. Cathet Cardiovasc Intervent 58:252-260, 2003.
299. Rosales AM, Lock JE, Perry SB, Geggel RL: Interventional catheterization management of perioperative peripheral pulmonary stenosis: Balloon angioplasty or endovascular stenting. Cathet Cardiovasc Intervent 56:272-277, 2002.
300. Hayes CJ, Gersony WM, Driscoll DJ, et al: Second natural history study of congenital heart defects. Results of treatment of patients with pulmonary valvar stenosis. Circulation 87(Suppl):37, 1993.
301. Chen CR, Cheng TO, Huang T, et al: Percutaneous balloon valvuloplasty for pulmonic stenosis in adolescents and adults. N Engl J Med 335:21-25, 1996.
302. Alva C, Ortegon J, Herrera F, et al: Types of obstructions in double-chambered right ventricle: Mid-term results. Arch Med Res 33:261-264, 2002.
303. Alva C, Ho SY, Lincoln CR, et al: The nature of the obstructive muscular bundles in double-chambered right ventricle. J Thorac Cardiovasc Surg 117:1180-1189, 1999.
304. Singh M, Agarwala MK, Grover A, et al: Clinical, echocardiographic, and angiographic profile of patients with double-chambered right ventricle: Experience with 48 cases. Angiology 50:223-231, 1999.
305. Lascano ME, Schaad MS, Moodie DS, Murphy D Jr: Difficulty in diagnosing double-chambered right ventricle in adults. Am J Cardiol 88:816-819, 2001.
306. McElhinney DB, Chatterjee KM, Reddy VM: Double-chambered right ventricle presenting in adulthood. Ann Thorac Surg 70:124-127, 2000.
307. Kilner PJ, Sievers B, Meyer GP, Ho SY: Double-chambered right ventricle or sub-infundibular stenosis assessed by cardiovascular magnetic resonance. J Cardiovasc MR 4:373-379, 2002.
308. Hachiro Y, Takagi N, Koyanagi T, et al: Repair of double-chambered right ventricle: Surgical results and long-term follow-up. Ann Thorac Surg 72:1520-1522, 2001.

Cor Triatriatum

309. Marin-Garcia J, Tandon R, Lucas RV Jr, Edwards JE: Cor triatriatum: Study of 20 cases. Am J Cardiol 35:59-66, 1975.
310. Roldan FJ, Vargas-Barron J, Espinola-Zavaleta N, et al: Cor triatriatum dexter: Transesophageal echocardiographic diagnosis and 3-dimensional reconstruction. J Am Soc Echocardiogr 14:634-636, 2001.
311. Oglietti J, Cooley DA, Izquierdo JP, et al: Cor triatriatum: Operative results in 25 patients. Ann Thorac Surg 35:415-420, 1983.
312. Dauphin C, Lusson JR, Motreff P, et al: Left intra-atrial membrane without pulmonary vein obstruction: Benign condition of progressive evolution? Apropos of 7 cases. [French]. Arch Mal Coeur Vaiss 91:615-621, 1998.
313. Breinholt JP, Hawkins JA, Minich LA, et al: Pulmonary vein stenosis with normal connection: Associated cardiac abnormalities and variable outcome. Ann Thorac Surg 68:164-168, 1999.
314. Ha JW, Chung N, Yoon J, et al: Pulsed wave and color Doppler echocardiography and cardiac catheterization findings in bilateral pulmonary vein stenosis. J Am Soc Echocardiogr 11:393-396, 1998.
315. Caldarone CA, Najm HK, Kadletz M, et al: Relentless pulmonary vein stenosis after repair of total anomalous pulmonary venous drainage. Ann Thorac Surg 66:1514-1520, 1998.
316. Oliver JM, Gallego P, Gonzalez A, et al: Sinus venosus syndrome: Atrial septal defect or anomalous venous connection? A multiplane transoesophageal approach. Heart 88:634-638, 2002.
317. Wong ML, McCrindle BW, Mota C, Smallhorn JF: Echocardiographic evaluation of partial anomalous pulmonary venous drainage. J Am Coll Cardiol 26:503-507, 1995.
318. Gao YA, Burrows PE, Benson LN, et al: Scimitar syndrome in infancy. J Am Coll Cardiol 22:873-882, 1993.
319. Shibuya K, Smallhorn JE, McCrindle BW: Echocardiographic clues and accuracy in the diagnosis of scimitar syndrome. J Am Soc Echocardiogr 9:174-181, 1996.
320. Ammash NM, Seward JB, Warnes CA, et al: Partial anomalous pulmonary venous connection: Diagnosis by transesophageal echocardiography. J Am Coll Cardiol 29:1351-1358, 1997.
321. Ferrari VA, Scott CH, Holland GA, et al: Ultrafast three-dimensional contrast-enhanced magnetic resonance angiography and imaging in the diagnosis of partial anomalous pulmonary venous drainage. J Am Coll Cardiol 37:1120-1128, 2001.
322. Hijii T, Fukushige J, Hara T: Diagnosis and management of partial anomalous pulmonary venous connection: A review of 28 pediatric cases. Cardiology 89:148-151, 1998.
323. Brown JW, Ruzmetov M, Minnich DJ, et al: Surgical management of scimitar syndrome: An alternative approach. J Thorac Cardiovasc Surg 125:238-245, 2003.
324. Swanson KL, Prakash UB, Stanson AW: Pulmonary arteriovenous fistulas: Mayo Clinic experience, 1982-1997. Mayo Clin Proc 74:671-680, 1999.
325. Gonzalez VR: Pulmonary arteriovenous fistula in childhood. Z Kinderchir 40:101, 1985.
326. Gudavalli A, Kalaria VG, et al: Intrapulmonary arteriovenous shunt: Diagnosis by saline contrast bubbles in the pulmonary veins. J Am Soc Echocardiogr 15:1012-1014, 2002.
327. Tsunezuka Y, Sato H, Tsukioka T: Strategy for 3-D computed tomography diagnosis and treatment of small pulmonary arteriovenous fistula. Scand Cardiovasc J 34:90-91, 2000.
328. Berthezene Y, Howarth NR, Revel D: Pulmonary arteriovenous fistula: Detection with magnetic resonance angiography. Eur Radiol 8:1403-1404, 1998.
329. Grady RM, Sharkey AM, Bridges ND: Transcatheter coil embolisation of a pulmonary arteriovenous malformation in a neonate. Br Heart J 71:370-371, 1994.

Coronary Arteriovenous Fistula

330. Hofbeck M, Wild F, Singer H: Improved visualisation of a coronary artery fistula by the "laid-back" aortogram. Br Heart J 70:272-273, 1993.
331. Sherwood MC, Rockenmacher S, Colan SD, Geva T: Prognostic significance of clinically silent coronary artery fistulas. Am J Cardiol 83:407-411, 1999.
332. Okubo M: Outcomes of transcatheter embolization in the treatment of coronary artery fistulas. Cathet Cardiovasc Intervent 52:510, 2001.
333. Kamiya H, Yasuda T, Nagamine H, et al: Surgical treatment of congenital coronary artery fistulas: 27 years' experience and a review of the literature. J Cardiac Surg 17:173-177, 2002.

CHAPTER 57

Valvular Heart Disease

Robert O. Bonow • Eugene Braunwald

During the last quarter century, remarkable changes in the evaluation and management of patients with valvular heart disease have resulted in improvement in patient outcomes that would have been unfathomable to earlier generations of physicians. Advances in surgical approaches and interventional cardiology procedures, coupled with innovation in noninvasive imaging and understanding of the natural history of these conditions, have resulted in enhanced diagnosis and more scientific selection of patients for therapeutic interventions, which are now performed at relatively low risk. Despite the continually expanding information base and the development of clinical practice guidelines,[1,2] many aspects of the diagnostic evaluation and indications for intervention remain uncertain or controversial. Hence, clinical knowledge, experience, and judgment on the part of the practitioner remain the key components of the management of patients with cardiac valvular disease.

Mitral Stenosis

Etiology and Pathology

The predominant cause of mitral stenosis (MS) is rheumatic fever (see Chap. 81),[1,3] and rheumatic involvement is present in 99 percent of stenotic mitral valves excised at the time of mitral valve replacement (MVR). Approximately 25 percent of all patients with rheumatic heart disease have pure MS, and an additional 40 percent have combined MS and mitral regurgitation (MR).[4] Two-thirds of all patients with rheumatic MS are women.[1]

Rheumatic fever results in four forms of fusion of the mitral valve apparatus leading to stenosis: (1) commissural, (2) cuspal, (3) chordal, and (4) combined.[5] Thickening of the commissures alone occurs in 30 percent of patients, of the cusps alone in 15 percent, and of the chordae tendineae alone in 10 percent; in the remaining patients, thickening of more than one of these structures is involved. Characteristically, mitral valve cusps fuse at their edges, and fusion of the chordae tendineae results in thickening and shortening of these structures. The leaflets exhibit fibrous obliteration and revascularization. The stenotic mitral valve is typically funnel shaped (Fig. 57–1), and the orifice is frequently shaped like a "fish mouth" or buttonhole, with calcium deposits in the valve leaflets sometimes extending to involve the valve ring, which may become severely thickened. The thickened leaflets may be so adherent and rigid that they cannot open or shut, reducing or rarely even abolishing the first heart sound (S_1) and leading to combined MS and MR. When rheumatic fever results exclusively or predominantly in contraction and fusion of the chordae tendineae, with little fusion of the valvular commissures, dominant MR results.[5]

A debate continues about whether the anatomical changes in severe MS result from a smoldering rheumatic process or whether, once the valve has been deformed by the initial episode, the constant trauma produced by the turbulent blood flow leads to progressive fibrosis, thickening, and calcification of the valve apparatus.[6] Probably both processes are involved. Enlargement of the left atrium and resultant elevation of the left main stem bronchus, calcification of the left atrial wall, development of mural thrombi, and obliterative changes in the pulmonary vascular bed (see Chap. 67) all may result from chronic rheumatic MS.

Far less frequently, MS is congenital in etiology, and this form is observed almost exclusively in infants and young children (see Chap. 56). Rarely, MS is a complication of malignant carcinoid, systemic lupus erythematosus, rheumatoid arthritis, the mucopolysaccharidoses of the Hunter-Hurler phenotype, Fabry disease, and Whipple disease. Amyloid deposits may occur on rheumatic valves and contribute to the obstruction to left atrial emptying. Methysergide therapy is an unusual but documented cause of MS. Atrial septal defect is associated with MS, generally of rheumatic origin, in Lutembacher syndrome (see Chap. 56). A number of conditions may simulate MS: obstruction to left atrial outflow may be caused by a left atrial tumor, particularly myxoma (see Chap. 63); ball-valve thrombus in the left atrium (usually associated with MS); infective endocarditis with large vegetations; and a congenital membrane in the left atrium, i.e., cor triatriatum (see Chap. 56). These conditions may simulate MS. Although calcification of the mitral annulus usually causes MR, MS may result when subvalvular or intravalvular extension is extensive.

Pathophysiology

In normal adults, the cross-sectional area of the mitral valve orifice is 4 to 6 cm^2.

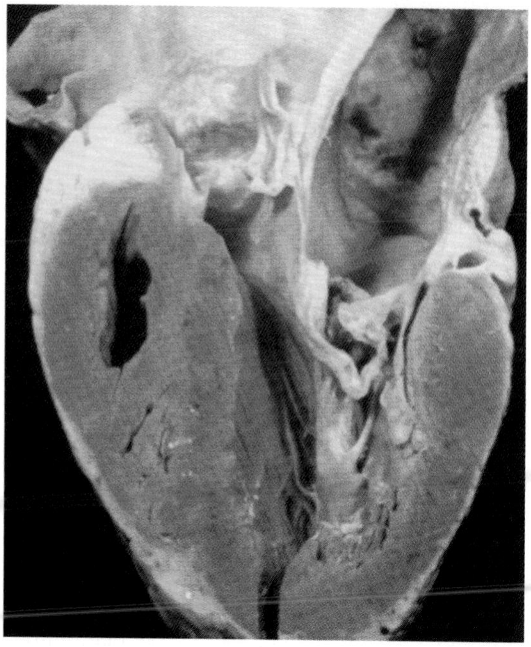

FIGURE 57–1 Rheumatic mitral stenosis. There are severe valvular changes, including marked fibrosis and calcification of the mitral valve leaflets and severe chordal thickening and fusion into pillars of fibrous tissue. (From Becker AE, Anderson RH [eds]: Cardiac Pathology: An Integrated Text and Colour Atlas. New York, Raven Press, 1983, p 4.3.)

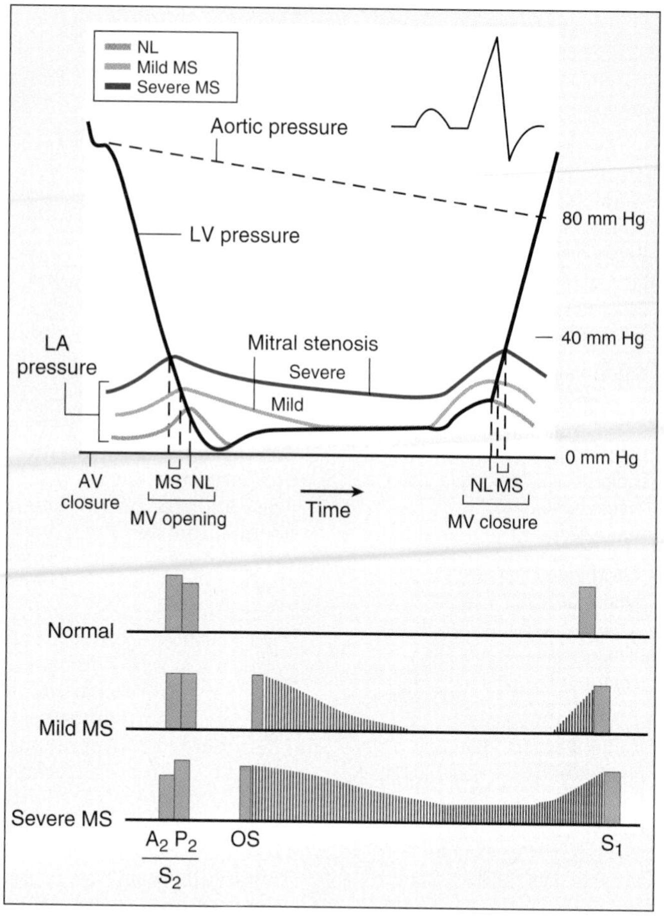

FIGURE 57–2 Schematic representation of left ventricular (LV), aortic, and left atrial (LA) pressures, showing normal relationships and alterations with mild and severe mitral stenosis (MS). Corresponding classic auscultatory signs of MS are shown at the bottom. Compared with mild MS, with severe MS the higher left atrial *v* wave causes earlier pressure crossover and earlier mitral valve (MV) opening, leading to a shorter time interval between aortic valve (AV) closure and the opening snap (OS). The higher left atrial end-diastolic pressure with severe MS also results in later closure of the mitral valve. With severe MS, the diastolic rumble becomes longer and there is accentuation of the pulmonic component (P_2) of the second heart sound (S_2) in relation to the aortic component (A_2).

When the orifice is reduced to approximately 2 cm^2, which is considered to represent *mild* MS, blood can flow from the left atrium to the left ventricle only if propelled by a small, although abnormal, pressure gradient. When the mitral valve opening is reduced to 1 cm^2, which is considered to represent *critical* MS,[3] a left atrioventricular pressure gradient of approximately 20 mm Hg (and, therefore, in the presence of a normal left ventricular diastolic pressure, a mean left atrial pressure of ≈25 mm Hg) is required to maintain normal cardiac output at rest (Fig. 57–2; see also Fig. 17–14). The elevated left atrial pressure, in turn, raises pulmonary venous and capillary pressures, resulting in exertional dyspnea. The first bouts of dyspnea in patients with MS are usually precipitated by tachycardia resulting from exercise, emotional stress, sexual intercourse, infection, or atrial fibrillation, all of which increase the rate of blood flow across the mitral orifice and result in further elevation of the left atrial pressure.[1,3,7]

To assess the severity of obstruction of the mitral valve (and, for that matter, of any valve), both the transvalvular pressure gradient and the transvalvular flow rate must be measured (see Chap. 17).[8] The latter is a function not only of the cardiac output but also of the heart rate. An increase in heart rate shortens diastole proportionately more than systole and diminishes the time available for flow across the mitral valve. Therefore, at any given level of cardiac output, tachycardia augments the transmitral valvular pressure gradient and elevates left atrial pressures further.[1] This explains the sudden occurrence of dyspnea and pulmonary edema in previously asymptomatic patients with MS who develop atrial fibrillation with a rapid ventricular rate. It also accounts for the equally rapid improvement in these patients when the ventricular rate is slowed by cardiac glycosides, beta-blocking agents, and/or heart rate–slowing calcium antagonists, even when the transvalvular flow rate per minute remains constant. Hydraulic considerations dictate that at any given orifice size the transvalvular pressure gradient is a function of the square of the transvalvular flow rate.[9] Thus, a doubling of flow rate quadruples the pressure gradient, so that a stress such as exercise in patients with moderate or severe MS causes a marked elevation of left atrial pressure.[10] Pregnancy, hypervolemia, and hyperthyroidism all increase mitral valve flow and thereby the transvalvular pressure gradient. Hence, it is common for the first clinical manifestation of MS in young women to occur during pregnancy.

Atrial contraction augments the presystolic transmitral valvular gradient by approximately 30 percent in patients with MS. Withdrawal of atrial transport when atrial fibrillation develops reduces cardiac output by about 20 percent.

Although the Gorlin formula has been the benchmark for evaluating stenotic valvular orifices since 1951,[9] there is increasing evidence that valvular orifices are not rigid and that, in fact, as transvalvular flow increases, the orifice becomes distended (see Chap. 17). Accordingly, it has been proposed that stenosis can also be expressed as valvular resistance, the quotient of the mean transvalvular pressure gradient, and the mean transvalvular flow.

INTRACARDIAC AND INTRAVASCULAR PRESSURES

Left Atrial and Right Heart Pressures. In patients with MS and sinus rhythm, mean left atrial pressure is elevated, and the left atrial pressure pulse generally exhibits a prominent atrial contraction (*a*) wave and a gradual pressure decline after mitral valve opening (*y* descent). In patients with mild to moderate MS without elevated pulmonary vascular resistance, pulmonary arterial pressure may be normal or only minimally elevated at rest but rises during exercise. However, in patients with severe MS and those in whom the pulmonary vascular resistance is significantly increased, pulmonary arterial pressure is elevated when the patient is at rest. In rare patients with extremely elevated pulmonary vascular resistance, pulmonary arterial pressure may exceed systemic arterial pressure. Further elevations of left atrial and pulmonary vascular pressures occur during exercise and/or tachycardia. With moderately elevated pulmonary arterial pressure (systolic pressure 30 to 60 mm Hg), right ventricular performance is usually maintained. However, a greater elevation of pulmonary arterial pressure represents a serious impedance to emptying of the right ventricle. Hence, patients with MS and severe pulmonary hypertension commonly fail to exhibit normal elevation of the right ventricular ejection fraction during exercise and ultimately may develop right ventricular dysfunction and dilation at rest, with accompanying tricuspid regurgitation (TR).

Left Ventricular Diastolic Pressure. This pressure is normal in patients with isolated MS; however, coexisting MR, aortic valve lesions, systemic hypertension, ischemic heart disease, and cardiomyopathy all may be responsible for elevations of left ventricular diastolic pressure. In approximately 85 percent of patients with isolated MS, the left ventricular end-diastolic volume is within the normal range, whereas it is reduced in the remaining patients. In approximately 25 percent of patients with isolated MS, the ejection fraction and other ejection indices of systolic performance (see Chap. 20) are below normal,[11] most likely resulting in part from chronic reduction in preload and elevated afterload. Regional hypokinesis is common, perhaps caused by extension of the scarring process from the mitral valve into the adjacent posterior basal myocardium or by associated ischemic heart disease. Leftward displacement of the interventricular septum secondary to more rapid early filling of the right ventricle may be responsible for a reduction of left ventricular compliance (left ventricular stiffening).[7] The left ventricular mass is usually normal but may be slightly reduced.[12]

The bulk of available evidence suggests that other than the posterior basal myocardium, left ventricular contractility is normal or only slightly impaired in the majority of patients with isolated MS. Most patients with MS have a normal elevation of ejection fraction and a reduction of end-systolic volume during exercise,[11] although ejection fraction does not increase normally with exercise in a subset of patients. In these latter patients, the normal increase in left ventricular diastolic volume during exercise fails to occur, resulting in reduced stroke volume and ejection fraction responses to exercise.[11] Associated ischemic heart disease is not common but may occur[1,13] and contribute to myocardial dysfunction in some patients.

Pulmonary Hypertension. Pulmonary hypertension in patients with MS results from (1) passive backward transmission of the elevated left atrial pressure; (2) pulmonary arteriolar constriction, which presumably is triggered by left atrial and pulmonary venous hypertension (reactive pulmonary hypertension); and (3) organic obliterative changes in the pulmonary vascular bed, which may be considered to be a complication of longstanding and severe MS (see Chap. 67).[6,7] In time, severe pulmonary hypertension results in right-sided heart failure, with dilation of the right ventricle and its annulus and secondary tricuspid and sometimes pulmonic regurgitation (PR). These changes in the pulmonary vascular bed may also exert a protective effect; the elevated precapillary resistance makes the development of symptoms of pulmonary congestion less likely by tending to prevent blood from surging into the pulmonary capillary bed and damming up behind the stenotic mitral valve, although this protection occurs at the expense of a reduced cardiac output. In patients with severe MS, pulmonary vein–bronchial vein shunts occur. Their rupture may cause hemoptysis. Patients with severe MS manifest a reduction in pulmonary compliance, an increase in the work of breathing, and a redistribution of pulmonary blood flow from the base to the apex.

Clinical and Hemodynamic Features. At any given severity of stenosis, the clinical picture is dictated largely by the levels of cardiac output and pulmonary vascular resistance. The response to a given degree of mitral obstruction may be characterized at one end of the hemodynamic spectrum by a normal cardiac output and a high left atrioventricular pressure gradient or, at the opposite end of the spectrum, by a markedly reduced cardiac output and low transvalvular pressure gradient. Thus, in some patients with moderately severe MS (mitral valve area = 1.0 to 1.5 cm^2), cardiac output at rest may be normal and rises normally during exertion. In these patients, the high transvalvular pressure gradient with exertion causes marked elevation of left atrial and pulmonary capillary pressures. This leads to severe pulmonary congestion during exertion. In contrast, in most patients with severe MS, cardiac output rises subnormally during exertion, thus reducing the pulmonary venous pressure and the severity of symptoms of pulmonary congestion more than would be the case if the cardiac output rose normally. In patients with severe MS (mitral valve area $\leq$ 1.0 cm^2), particularly when pulmonary vascular resistance is elevated, cardiac output is usually depressed at rest and may fail to rise at all during exertion. These patients frequently have severe weakness and fatigue secondary to a low cardiac output.

Left Atrial Changes. The combination of mitral valve disease and atrial inflammation secondary to rheumatic carditis causes (1) left atrial dilation, (2) fibrosis of the atrial wall, and (3) disorganization of the atrial muscle bundles. The last leads to disparate conduction velocities and inhomogeneous refractory periods. Premature atrial activation, due either to an automatic focus or to reentry, may stimulate the left atrium during the vulnerable period and thereby precipitate atrial fibrillation. The development of this arrhythmia correlates independently with the severity of the MS, the degree of left atrial dilation, and the height of the left atrial pressure.[14] Atrial fibrillation is often episodic at first but then becomes more persistent. Atrial fibrillation per se causes diffuse atrophy of atrial muscle, further atrial enlargement, and further inhomogeneity of refractoriness and conduction. These changes, in turn, lead to irreversible atrial fibrillation.

Clinical Manifestations

History

The principal symptom of MS is exertional dyspnea, largely the result of reduced pulmonary compliance. Dyspnea may be accompanied by cough and wheezing. Vital capacity is reduced, presumably owing to the presence of engorged pulmonary vessels and interstitial edema. Patients who have critical obstruction to left atrial emptying and dyspnea with ordinary activity (New York Heart Association [NYHA] Class III) generally have orthopnea as well and are at risk of experiencing attacks of frank pulmonary edema. The latter may be precipitated by effort, emotional stress, respiratory infection, fever, sexual intercourse, pregnancy, or atrial fibrillation with a rapid ventricular rate or other tachyarrhythmia. Indeed, pulmonary edema may be caused by any condition that increases flow across the stenotic mitral valve, either by increasing total cardiac output or by reducing the time available for blood flow across the mitral orifice to occur. In patients with a markedly elevated pulmonary vascular resistance, right ventricular function is often impaired.[7,15]

MS is a slowly progressive disease, and many patients remain seemingly asymptomatic merely by readjusting their life styles to a more sedentary level. Exercise testing may be useful in selected asymptomatic patients to determine functional status in an objective manner and may be combined with Doppler echocardiography (see later) to assess exercise hemodynamics.

HEMOPTYSIS. In his seminal paper 50 years ago, Wood differentiated between several kinds of *hemoptysis* complicating MS, as follows[16]:

1. Sudden hemorrhage. Although the hemorrhage is often profuse, it is only rarely life threatening. It results from the rupture of thin-walled, dilated bronchial veins, usually as a consequence of a sudden rise in left atrial pressure. With persistence of pulmonary venous hypertension, the walls of these veins thicken appreciably. This form of hemoptysis tends to disappear as MS progresses.
2. Blood-stained sputum associated with attacks of paroxysmal nocturnal dyspnea.
3. Pink, frothy sputum characteristic of acute pulmonary edema with rupture of alveolar capillaries.
4. Pulmonary infarction, a late complication of MS associated with heart failure.
5. Blood-stained sputum complicating chronic bronchitis. The edematous bronchial mucosa in patients with chronic MS increases the likelihood of chronic

bronchitis, which is a common complication of MS, particularly in Great Britain.

CHEST PAIN. A small percentage, perhaps 15 percent, of patients with MS experience chest discomfort that is indistinguishable from angina pectoris. This symptom may be caused by severe right ventricular hypertension secondary to the pulmonary vascular disease or by concomitant coronary atherosclerosis.[1,13] Rarely, chest pain may be secondary to coronary obstruction caused by coronary embolization. In many patients, however, a satisfactory explanation for the chest pain cannot be uncovered even after complete hemodynamic and angiographic studies.

SYSTEMIC EMBOLISM. Before the advent of surgical treatment, this serious complication of MS developed in at least 20 percent of patients at some time during the course of their disease.[17] Before the era of anticoagulant therapy and surgical treatment, approximately 25 percent of all fatalities in patients with mitral valve disease were secondary to systemic embolism. The tendency for development of systemic embolization correlates directly with the patient's age and the size of the left atrial appendage and inversely with the cardiac output[17,18]; 80 percent of patients with MS in whom systemic emboli develop are in atrial fibrillation. When embolization occurs in patients in sinus rhythm, the possibility of transient atrial fibrillation or underlying infective endocarditis should be considered. There is no simple correlation between the incidence of embolism on the one hand and the size of the mitral orifice on the other. Indeed, embolism may be the first symptom of MS and may occur in patients with mild MS even before the development of dyspnea.

Because thrombi are found in the left atrium at operation in only a few patients with a history of recent embolism, it is likely that only fresh clots are discharged. Approximately half of all clinically apparent emboli are found in the cerebral vessels. Coronary embolism may lead to myocardial infarction and/or angina pectoris, and renal emboli may be responsible for the development of systemic hypertension. Emboli are recurrent and multiple in approximately 25 percent of patients who develop this complication. Rarely, massive thrombosis develops in the left atrium, resulting in a pedunculated ball-valve thrombus, which may suddenly aggravate obstruction to left atrial outflow when a specific body position is assumed or may cause sudden death. Similar consequences occur in patients with free-floating thrombi in the left atrium. These two conditions are usually characterized by variability in the physical findings, often on a positional basis. They are extremely hazardous and require surgical treatment, often as an emergency.

INFECTIVE ENDOCARDITIS (see Chap. 58). This complication tends to occur *less frequently* on rigid, thickened, calcified valves and is therefore more common in patients with mild MS than those with severe MS.

OTHER SYMPTOMS. Compression of the left recurrent laryngeal nerve by a greatly dilated left atrium, enlarged tracheobronchial lymph nodes, and a dilated pulmonary artery may cause hoarseness (Ortner syndrome). A history of repeated hemoptysis is common in patients with pulmonary hemosiderosis. Systemic venous hypertension, hepatomegaly, edema, ascites, and hydrothorax all are signs of severe MS with elevated pulmonary vascular resistance and right-sided heart failure.

Physical Examination

Patients with severe MS, a low cardiac output, and systemic vasoconstriction may exhibit the so-called mitral facies, characterized by pinkish-purple patches on the cheeks. The *arterial pulse* is usually normal, but in patients with a reduced stroke volume, the pulse may be small in volume. The *jugular venous pulse* usually exhibits a prominent *a* wave in patients with sinus rhythm and elevated pulmonary vascular resistance. In patients with atrial fibrillation, the *x* descent of the jugular venous pulse disappears, and there is only one crest, a prominent *v* or *c-v* wave, per cardiac cycle. *Palpation* of the cardiac apex usually reveals an inconspicuous left ventricle; the presence of either a palpable presystolic expansion wave or an early diastolic rapid filling wave speaks strongly against serious MS. A readily palpable, tapping S_1 suggests that the anterior mitral valve leaflet is pliable. When the patient is in the left lateral recumbent position, a diastolic thrill of MS may be palpable at the apex. Often a right ventricular lift is felt in the left parasternal region in patients with pulmonary hypertension. A markedly enlarged right ventricle may displace the left ventricle posteriorly and produce a prominent apex beat that can be confused with a left ventricular lift. A loud pulmonic closure sound (P_2) may be palpable in the second left intercostal space in patients with MS and pulmonary hypertension.

AUSCULTATION

The auscultatory features of MS (see Fig. 57–2) include an accentuated first heart sound (S_1) with prolongation of the Q-S_1 interval, correlating with the level of the left atrial pressure. Accentuation of S_1 occurs when the mitral valve leaflets are flexible. It is caused, in part, by the rapidity with which left ventricular pressure rises at the time of mitral valve closure as well as by the wide closing excursion of the leaflets. Marked calcification and/or thickening of the mitral valve leaflets reduces the amplitude of S_1, probably because of diminished motion of the leaflets. As pulmonary arterial pressure rises, closure of the pulmonic valve (P_2) at first becomes accentuated and widely transmitted and can often be readily heard at both the mitral and the aortic areas. With further elevation of pulmonary arterial pressure, splitting of the second heart sound (S_2) narrows because of reduced compliance of the pulmonary vascular bed, and this shortens the "hangout interval." Finally, S_2 becomes single and accentuated. Other signs of severe pulmonary hypertension include a nonvalvular pulmonic ejection sound that diminishes during inspiration, owing to dilation of the pulmonary artery; a systolic murmur of TR; a Graham Steell murmur of PR; and a fourth heart sound (S_4) originating from the right ventricle. A third heart sound (S_3) originating from the left ventricle is absent in patients with MS unless significant MR or aortic regurgitation (AR) coexists.

The *opening snap* (OS) of the mitral valve is caused by a sudden tensing of the valve leaflets after the valve cusps have completed their opening excursion. The OS occurs when the movement of the mitral dome into the left ventricle suddenly stops. It is most readily audible at the apex, using the diaphragm of the stethoscope. The OS can usually be differentiated from P_2 because the OS occurs later, unless right bundle branch block is present. The mitral valve cannot be totally rigid if it produces an OS, which is usually accompanied by an accentuated S_1. Calcification confined to the tip of the mitral valve leaflets does not preclude an OS, although calcification of both the body and the tip does. The mitral OS follows A_2 by 0.04 to 0.12 second; this interval varies inversely with the left atrial pressure. A short A_2-OS interval is a reliable indicator of severe MS.

THE DIASTOLIC MURMUR OF MS. This murmur is a low-pitched, rumbling murmur, best heard at the apex, with the bell of the stethoscope and with the patient in the left lateral recumbent position. When this murmur is soft, it is limited to the apex, but when louder, it may radiate to the left axilla or the lower left sternal area. Although the intensity of the diastolic murmur is not closely related to the severity of stenosis, the *duration* of the murmur is a guide to the severity of mitral valve narrowing. The murmur persists for as long as the left atrioventricular pressure gradient exceeds approximately 3 mm Hg. The murmur usually commences immediately after the OS. In mild MS, the early diastolic murmur is brief, but in the presence of sinus rhythm it resumes in presystole (see Fig. 57–2). In severe MS, the murmur is holodiastolic, with presystolic accentuation while sinus rhythm is maintained.

The *diastolic rumbling murmur* of MS is heard best with the patient lying in the left lateral decubitus position. It may be masked by the presence of a thick chest wall, pulmonary emphysema, and a low cardiac output with a low flow rate across the mitral valve. This murmur may be sharply localized and thus missed unless palpation is used to detect the apex of the left ventricle and to pinpoint the area at which auscultation should be carried out. In so-called silent MS, there is usually marked right ventricular enlargement. Consequently, the right ventricle occupies the cardiac apex, the left ventricle is rotated posteriorly, and cardiac output is reduced, so that the murmur either is not audible at all or can be heard only in the mid or posterior axillary line. In addition to placing the patient in the left lateral position, auscultation of the murmur is facilitated during expiration after having the patient do a few sit-ups, walk up a flight of stairs, or other maneuvers described later.

Dynamic Auscultation (see Chap. 8). The diastolic murmur and OS of MS are often reduced during inspiration and augmented during expiration, which is the opposite of what occurs when these findings are secondary to tricuspid stenosis. During inspiration, the A_2-OS interval widens, and three sequential sounds (A_2, P_2, and OS) may be audible. Sudden standing and the resultant reduction of venous return lower the left atrial pressure and widen the A_2-OS interval; this maneuver is useful in distinguishing an A_2-OS combination from a split S_2, which narrows on standing. In contrast, the A_2-OS interval is significantly narrowed during exercise as left atrial pressure rises. The diastolic rumbling murmur of MS is reduced during the strain of a Valsalva maneuver and in any condition in which transmitral valve flow rate declines. Amyl nitrite inhalation, coughing, isometric or isotonic exercise, and sudden squatting all are useful in accentuating a faint or equivocal murmur of MS.

Differential Diagnosis. The *Carey Coombs murmur* of acute rheumatic fever is a sign of active mitral valvulitis and can be confused with the murmur of MS. The Carey Coombs murmur is a soft early diastolic murmur, usually varies from day to day, and is higher pitched than the diastolic rumbling murmur of established MS. In pure, severe MR—indeed, in any condition in which flow across a nonstenotic mitral valve is increased (e.g., a ventricular septal defect)—there may also be a short diastolic murmur following an S_3. *Left atrial myxoma* may produce auscultatory findings similar to those in rheumatic valvular MS (see Chap. 63). A diastolic rumble may also be present in some patients with hypertrophic cardiomyopathy, caused by early diastolic flow into the hypertrophied, nondistensible left ventricle.

A high-frequency early systolic murmur is audible along the lower left sternal border in one-third of patients with MS. This should be distinguished from the apical (often holosystolic or late systolic) murmur of MR. In addition, a *pansystolic murmur of TR* and an S_3 originating from the right ventricle may be audible in the 4th intercostal space in the left parasternal region in patients with severe MS. These signs, which are secondary to pulmonary hypertension, may be confused with the findings of MR. However, the inspiratory augmentation of the murmur and of the S_3 and the prominent *v* wave in the jugular venous pulse aid in establishing that the murmur originates from the tricuspid valve. A high-pitched decrescendo diastolic murmur along the left sternal border in patients with MS and pulmonary hypertension is usually due to concomitant AR but occasionally represents a Graham Steell murmur of pulmonary regurgitation. The latter, when present, characteristically increases during inspiration.

Laboratory Examination

ELECTROCARDIOGRAPHY (see Chap. 9). The electrocardiogram (ECG) is relatively insensitive for detecting mild MS, but it does show characteristic changes in moderate or severe obstruction. Left atrial enlargement (P wave duration in lead II ≥ 0.12 second and/or a P wave axis between +45 and −30 degrees) is a principal ECG feature of MS and is found in 90 percent of patients with significant MS and sinus rhythm. The ECG signs of left atrial enlargement correlate more closely with left atrial volume than with left atrial pressure and often regress following successful valvotomy. Atrial fibrillation usually develops in the presence of preexisting ECG evidence of left atrial enlargement and is related to the size of the chamber, the extent of fibrosis of the left atrial myocardium, the duration of atriomegaly, and the age of the patient.

Whether or not there is ECG evidence of right ventricular hypertrophy depends largely on the height of right ventricular systolic pressure. Approximately half of all patients with right ventricular systolic pressures between 70 and 100 mm Hg manifest the ECG criteria for right ventricular hypertrophy, including both a mean QRS axis greater than 80 degrees in the frontal plane and an R:S ratio greater than 1.0 in lead V_1. Other patients with this degree of pulmonary hypertension have no frank evidence of right ventricular hypertrophy, but the R:S ratio fails to increase from the right to the midprecordial leads. When right ventricular systolic pressure is higher than 100 mm Hg in patients with isolated or predominant MS, ECG evidence of right ventricular hypertrophy is found quite consistently.

The *QRS axis in the frontal plane* correlates roughly with the severity of valve obstruction and with the level of pulmonary vascular resistance in patients with pure MS. Thus, a mean frontal axis between 0 and +60 degrees suggests that the mitral valve area is greater than 1.3 cm^2, whereas an axis of more than 60 degrees suggests that the valve area is less than 1.3 cm^2. In patients in whom pulmonary vascular resistance exceeds 650 $dyne \cdot sec^{-1} \cdot cm^{-5}$, the mean axis is usually greater than +110 degrees. In patients whose pulmonary artery systolic pressure approaches systemic levels, the mean axis averages +150 degrees.

RADIOLOGICAL FINDINGS (see Figs. 12–17 and 12–19). Although their cardiac silhouette may be normal in the frontal projection, patients with hemodynamically significant MS almost invariably have evidence of left atrial enlargement on the lateral and left anterior oblique views. Extreme left atrial enlargement rarely occurs in pure MS; when it is present, MR is usually severe. Enlargement of the pulmonary artery, right ventricle, and right atrium (as well as the left atrium) is commonly seen in patients with severe MS. Occasionally, calcification of the mitral valve is evident on the chest roentgenogram, but, more commonly, fluoroscopy is required to detect valvular calcification.

Radiological changes in the lung fields indirectly reflect the severity of MS. Interstitial edema, an indication of severe obstruction, is manifested as Kerley B lines (dense, short, horizontal lines most commonly seen in the costophrenic angles). This finding is present in 30 percent of patients with resting pulmonary arterial wedge pressures lower than 20 mm Hg and in 70 percent of patients with pressures higher than 20 mm Hg. Severe, longstanding mitral obstruction often results in Kerley A lines (straight, dense lines ≤ 4 cm in length running toward the hilum) as well as the findings of pulmonary hemosiderosis and rarely of parenchymal ossification. Pulmonary edema is seldom evident.

ANGIOGRAPHY. Angiograms exposed in the right and left anterior oblique projections afford the best views of the mitral valve. Although contrast material should ideally be injected into the left atrium, it is often possible to achieve good visualization of the left side of the heart by injecting a large volume of contrast material into the main pulmonary artery. Such angiograms provide an assessment of left atrial size, may demonstrate thickening and reduced motion of the valve leaflets, and outline large intraluminal thrombi. Left ventriculography makes possible simultaneous assessment of left ventricular contractile function and of the subvalvular mitral apparatus. However, echocardiography has largely superseded angiography in the evaluation of patients with MS or suspected MS.

ECHOCARDIOGRAPHY (see Chap. 11). Echocardiography is now the cornerstone of the diagnostic assessment of patients with MS. Two-dimensional transthoracic or transesophageal echocardiograms of a thickened, calcified, stenotic rheumatic valve demonstrate increased acoustic impedance and fusion of the mitral valve leaflets and poor leaflet separation in diastole (Fig. 57–3; see also Figs. 11–50 to 11–52). In mild MS, in which some leaflet mobility is preserved, the anterior leaflet may demonstrate diastolic doming. The leaflets fail to close normally in mid-diastole and may not reopen widely during atrial contraction when sinus rhythm is present. The left atrium is usually enlarged, and in isolated MS the left ventricular cavity is normal or reduced in size. Two-dimensional echocardiography may be helpful in recognizing left atrial thrombus preoperatively and in assessing mitral valve calcification and left ventricular contractility.[19] With progressive thickening and fibrosis of the

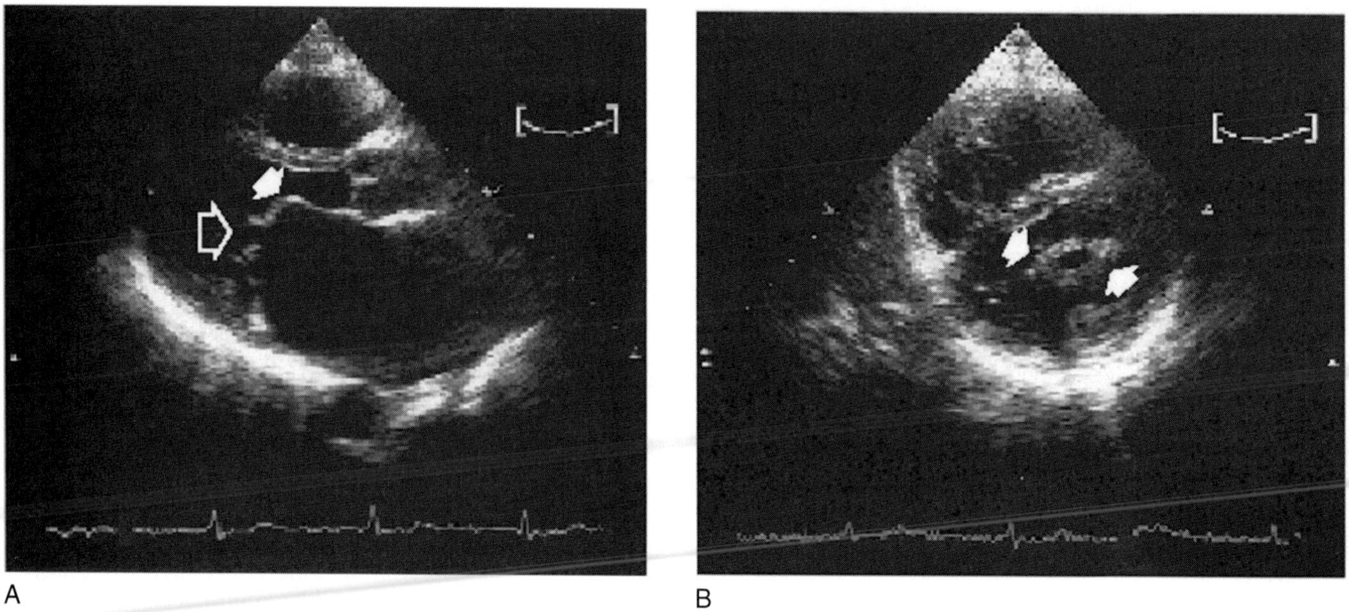

FIGURE 57–3 Two-dimensional transthoracic parasternal long-axis **(A)** and short-axis **(B)** views of the mitral valve and its orifice during diastole, demonstrating leaflet thickening, the "fish mouth" appearance of the valve in the short axis (white arrows), and doming of the anterior leaflet in the long axis (white arrow). The subvalvular apparatus is not severely thickened. The open arrow indicates narrowed mitral valve orifice. (From Bach DS: Rheumatic mitral stenosis. N Engl J Med 337:31, 1997.)

leaflets, the orifice becomes fixed and can then often be imaged directly and measured. Two-dimensional echocardiography also provides information on the pliability of the leaflets, the extent of valvular calcification, thickening of the subvalvular apparatus, and fusion and retraction of the chordae tendineae, as well as calcification of the mitral annulus. This technique allows determination of left ventricular size and function and can also evaluate the aortic valve. The two-dimensional echocardiogram is helpful in determining whether the patient with MS is a suitable candidate for balloon mitral valvuloplasty (see Figs. 11–50 and 11–51). Transesophageal two-dimensional echocardiography provides images of the mitral valve that are superior to those obtained by transthoracic imaging and is more sensitive in detecting left atrial thrombus. Pedunculated and free-floating thrombi are also usually readily detected by this technique, as are atrial myxomas. Transesophageal echocardiography is necessary when the transthoracic signal is inadequate.

Doppler echocardiography is the most accurate noninvasive technique available for quantifying the severity of MS (see Fig. 11–54).[19] The pulmonary arterial pressure also can be estimated from the TR velocity signal.[20,21] Color-flow Doppler imaging can enhance the accuracy of the Doppler data by determining whether MR, AR, and other valvular abnormalities coexist.

In most patients with MS, a detailed echocardiographic examination, including two-dimensional echocardiography (transthoracic or transesophageal), a Doppler study, and color-flow Doppler imaging, can usually provide sufficient information to develop a therapeutic plan without the need for cardiac catheterization (see later).[22]

Exercise Testing with Doppler Echocardiography. Exercise testing is useful in many patients with MS to ascertain the level of physical conditioning and to elicit covert cardiac symptoms. The exercise test can be combined with Doppler echocardiography to assess exercise hemodynamics,[1] usually with the Doppler examination performed at rest after termination of exercise (see Fig. 11–54). Exercise Doppler testing is helpful in the following situations: (1) to confirm that the asymptomatic patient has satisfactory effort tolerance and has no symptoms during workloads equivalent to activities of normal living; (2) to assess pulmonary artery systolic pressure during exercise; and (3) to evaluate exercise hemodynamics in symptomatic patients who appear to have only mild MS on resting measurements.

Management

Medical Treatment

Patients with MS due to rheumatic heart disease should receive penicillin prophylaxis for beta-hemolytic streptococcal infections and prophylaxis for infective endocarditis (see Chaps. 58 and 81). Anemia and infections should be treated promptly and aggressively in patients with valvular heart disease. Adolescents and young adults with severe MS should be advised to avoid entering occupations requiring strenuous exertion. Asymptomatic patients with moderate MS should be reevaluated yearly.[1] Heavy exertion is contraindicated in symptomatic patients.

In symptomatic patients with mitral valve disease, considerable improvement occurs with the administration of oral diuretics and the restriction of sodium intake. Digitalis glycosides do not alter the hemodynamics and usually do not benefit patients with MS and sinus rhythm, but these drugs are of value in slowing the ventricular rate in patients with atrial fibrillation and in treating patients with right-sided heart failure. Hemoptysis is managed by measures designed to reduce pulmonary venous pressure, including sedation, assumption of the upright position, and aggressive diuresis. Beta-blocking agents and rate-slowing calcium antagonists may increase exercise capacity by reducing heart rate in patients with sinus rhythm and especially in patients with atrial fibrillation.[1]

Anticoagulant therapy is helpful in preventing venous thrombosis and pulmonary embolism in patients who have experienced one or more previous pulmonary embolic episodes; in patients who are at high risk of systemic embolization, i.e., with persistent or transient atrial fibrillation (especially elderly patients > 70 years of age); and in those with previous systemic emboli. Treatment with warfarin, to maintain the international normalized ratio

(INR) between 2.0 and 3.0, is indicated in such patients.[23,24] However, no firm evidence exists that anticoagulant therapy reduces the incidence of pulmonary or systemic embolism in patients in sinus rhythm in whom such episodes have not previously occurred. Although current guidelines do not recommend anticoagulation in patients in sinus rhythm, this may be considered in patients with extreme left atrial enlargement (>50 to 55 mm).[1,25]

TREATMENT OF ARRHYTHMIAS. Frequent premature atrial contractions often presage atrial fibrillation. The administration of antiarrhythmic agents (see Chap. 30) may be effective in preventing this complication. However, once atrial fibrillation has developed, these agents may be ineffective in restoring sinus rhythm because of the pathological changes that predispose to atrial fibrillation and that develop in the atrium secondary to the arrhythmia itself. After electrical cardioversion, sinus rhythm can often be maintained with antiarrhythmic agents, especially in young patients with mild MS but without marked left atrial enlargement who have been in atrial fibrillation less than 6 months.

Immediate treatment of atrial fibrillation should include intravenous heparin followed by oral warfarin. The ventricular rate should be slowed with intravenous digoxin and a beta-blocking agent or rate-slowing calcium antagonist. An effort should be made to reestablish sinus rhythm by a combination of pharmacological treatment and cardioversion. If cardioversion is planned in a patient who has had atrial fibrillation for more than 24 hours before the procedure, anticoagulation with warfarin for more than 3 weeks is indicated. Alternatively, if a transesophageal echocardiogram shows no atrial thrombus, immediate cardioversion can be carried out using intravenous heparin.[26] Paroxysmal atrial fibrillation and repeated conversions, spontaneous or induced, carry the risk of embolization. In patients who cannot be converted or maintained in sinus rhythm, digitalis should be used to maintain the ventricular rate at rest at approximately 60 beats/min. If this is not possible, small doses of a beta-blocking agent, such as atenolol (25 mg daily) or metoprolol (50 to 100 mg daily), may be added. Beta blockers are particularly helpful in preventing rapid ventricular responses that develop during exertion. Multiple repeat cardioversions are *not* indicated if the patient fails to sustain sinus rhythm while on adequate doses of an antiarrhythmic.

Patients with chronic atrial fibrillation who undergo open mitral valve repair or replacement may undergo the maze procedure (atrial compartment operation). More than 80 percent of patients undergoing this procedure can be maintained in sinus rhythm postoperatively and can regain normal atrial function,[27-29] including a satisfactory success rate in those with massive left atrial enlargement (>65 mm).[28]

NEED FOR CATHETERIZATION. There has been considerable debate concerning the need for routine cardiac catheterization in determining whether valvotomy is indicated.[1] A careful clinical evaluation and noninvasive assessment, particularly using two-dimensional and Doppler echocardiography, can provide sufficient information to permit an informed decision in the majority of patients. Preoperative catheterization is recommended for the following patients with MS: (1) patients who have a discrepancy between clinical and echocardiographic findings; hemodynamic measurements during exercise are often useful in these patients; (2) patients who have associated chronic obstructive pulmonary disease in whom it is important to determine the contribution of MS to the symptoms; (3) patients in whom left atrial myxoma should be excluded; (4) patients who have angina pectoris or angina-like chest pain in whom associated coronary artery disease must be excluded; and (5) men older than 40 years of age and women older than 50 years of age who have risk factors for coronary artery disease or a positive stress test and in whom surgery is planned; it is important to ascertain whether or not bypass grafting is indicated for those patients at risk of having coexisting coronary artery disease. Critical narrowing of one or more coronary vessels occurs in approximately 25 percent of all adults with severe MS.[1] This finding is more common in men older than 45 years of age who have angina and risk factors for coronary artery disease.

Natural History

The development of effective surgical treatment has obscured our understanding of the natural history of MS and, for that matter, of all valvular lesions. Although few meaningful data are available, it appears that in temperate zones, such as the United States and Western Europe, patients who develop acute rheumatic fever have an asymptomatic period of approximately 15 to 20 years before symptoms of MS develop. It then takes approximately 5 to 10 years for most patients to progress from mild disability (i.e., early NYHA Class II) to severe disability (i.e., NYHA Class III or IV). The progression is much more rapid in patients in tropical and subtropical areas, in Polynesians, and in Alaskan Inuit. Both economic and genetic conditions may play a role. In India, critical MS may be present in children as young as 6 to 12 years of age. In North America and Western Europe, however, symptoms develop more slowly and occur most commonly between 45 and 65 years of age.[1] Serial echocardiographic data regarding hemodynamic progression in patients with MS who have not undergone surgery demonstrate considerable interpatient variability, but on average the mitral valve area decreases by 0.09 cm^2 per year.[30]

Natural history data obtained In the *presurgical era* indicate that symptomatic patients with MS have a poor outlook. Olesen reported 5-year survival rates of 62 percent among patients with MS in NYHA Class III but only 15 percent among those in Class IV.[31] Recent data confirm these results in the current era; Horstkotte and associates[32] reported a 5-year survival rate of 44 percent in patients with symptomatic MS who refused valvotomy (Fig. 57–4).

Valvotomy

Indications

Patients with MS who are asymptomatic or minimally symptomatic frequently remain so for years. However, once moderate symptoms develop (NYHA Class II), if the stenosis is not relieved mechanically, the disease may progress relatively rapidly, as already discussed (see Fig. 57–4). Valvotomy (percutaneous balloon mitral valvuloplasty [BMV] or

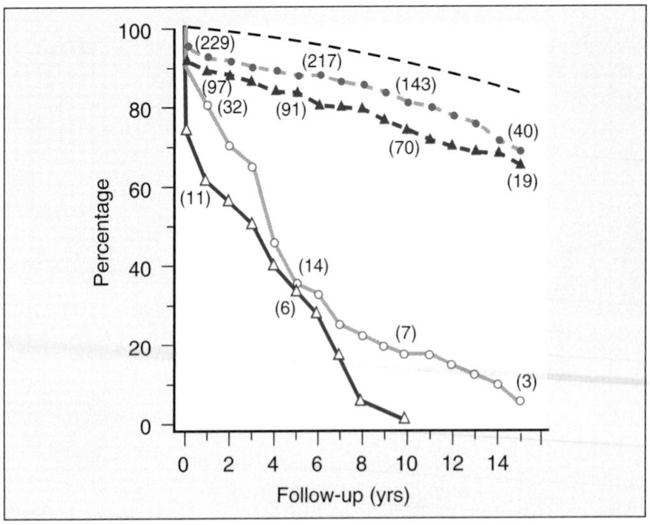

FIGURE 57–4 Natural history of 159 patients with isolated mitral stenosis (solid blue line) or mitral regurgitation (solid purple line) who were not operated on (even though the operation was indicated) compared with patients treated with valve replacement for mitral stenosis (dashed blue line) or mitral regurgitation (dashed purple line). The expected survival rate in the absence of mitral valve disease is indicated by the upper curve (dashed black line). (From Horstkotte D, Niehues R, Strauer BE: Pathomorphological aspects, aetiology, and natural history of acquired mitral valve stenosis. Eur Heart J 12[Suppl]:55-60, 1991.)

surgical valvotomy) should therefore be carried out in symptomatic patients with moderate to severe MS (i.e., a mitral valve orifice area < ≈1.0 cm^2/m^2 body surface area [BSA] or < 1.5 to 1.7 cm^2 in normal-sized adults). It is also indicated in patients with mild stenosis (orifice area 1.0 to 1.5 cm^2/m^2 BSA) who are symptomatic during ordinary activity and who develop pulmonary arterial systolic pressures exceeding 60 mm Hg or mean pulmonary capillary wedge pressures exceeding 25 mm Hg during exercise.[1,2]

Treatment must be individualized. For instance, mechanical relief of obstruction might well be deferred in a retired, mildly symptomatic, sedentary septuagenarian with a mitral valve orifice area of 0.8 cm^2/m^2 BSA. On the other hand, a 30-year-old laborer whose family's economic well-being depends on his continued physical exertion might be an excellent candidate for mechanical relief of obstruction, although his mitral valve orifice size is 1.2 cm^2/m^2 BSA. However, there is no evidence that valvotomy improves the prognosis of patients with no or only slight functional impairment. Therefore, valvotomy is *not* ordinarily indicated in patients who are entirely asymptomatic. Because of the high rate of recurrence, mechanical relief of obstruction is also indicated in patients with MS who have had a previous systemic embolism,[2] even if they are otherwise asymptomatic and even though there is no *definitive* evidence that the incidence of recurrent emboli will be significantly reduced. Anticoagulants should be administered to such patients up to the time of the procedure.

BALLOON MITRAL VALVOTOMY (see Chap. 52)
This percutaneous technique consists of advancing a small balloon flotation catheter across the interatrial septum (after transseptal puncture), enlarging the opening, advancing a large (23- to 25-mm) hourglass-shaped balloon (the Inoue balloon), and inflating it within the orifice (Fig. 57–5).[33-36] Alternatively, two smaller (15- to 20-mm) balloons may be employed.[33,35,36] A third technique involves retrograde, nontransseptal dilation of the mitral valve in which the balloon is positioned across the mitral valve using a steerable guide wire.[37] Commissural separation and fracture of nodular calcium appear to be the mechanisms responsible for improvement in valvular function. In several series, the hemodynamic results of BMV have been quite favorable (Fig. 57–6), with reduction of the transmitral pressure gradient from an average of approximately 18 to 6 mm Hg, a small (average 20 percent) increase in cardiac output, and an average doubling of the calculated mitral valve area from 1.0 to 2.0 cm^2. Although the double-balloon technique may result in a slightly greater valve opening, the clinical outcomes of the two approaches are similar.[33,35,36] Improvement in exercise tolerance has paralleled the favorable hemodynamic changes.

Results are especially impressive in younger patients without severe valvular thickening or calcification (see Fig. 57–3).[38] Elevated pulmonary vascular resistance declines rapidly, although usually not completely.[39] The reported mortality rate has ranged from 1 to 2 percent. Complications include cerebral emboli and cardiac perforation, each in approximately 1 percent of patients, and the development of MR severe enough to require operation in another 2 percent (≈15 percent develop lesser, but still undesirable, degrees of MR).

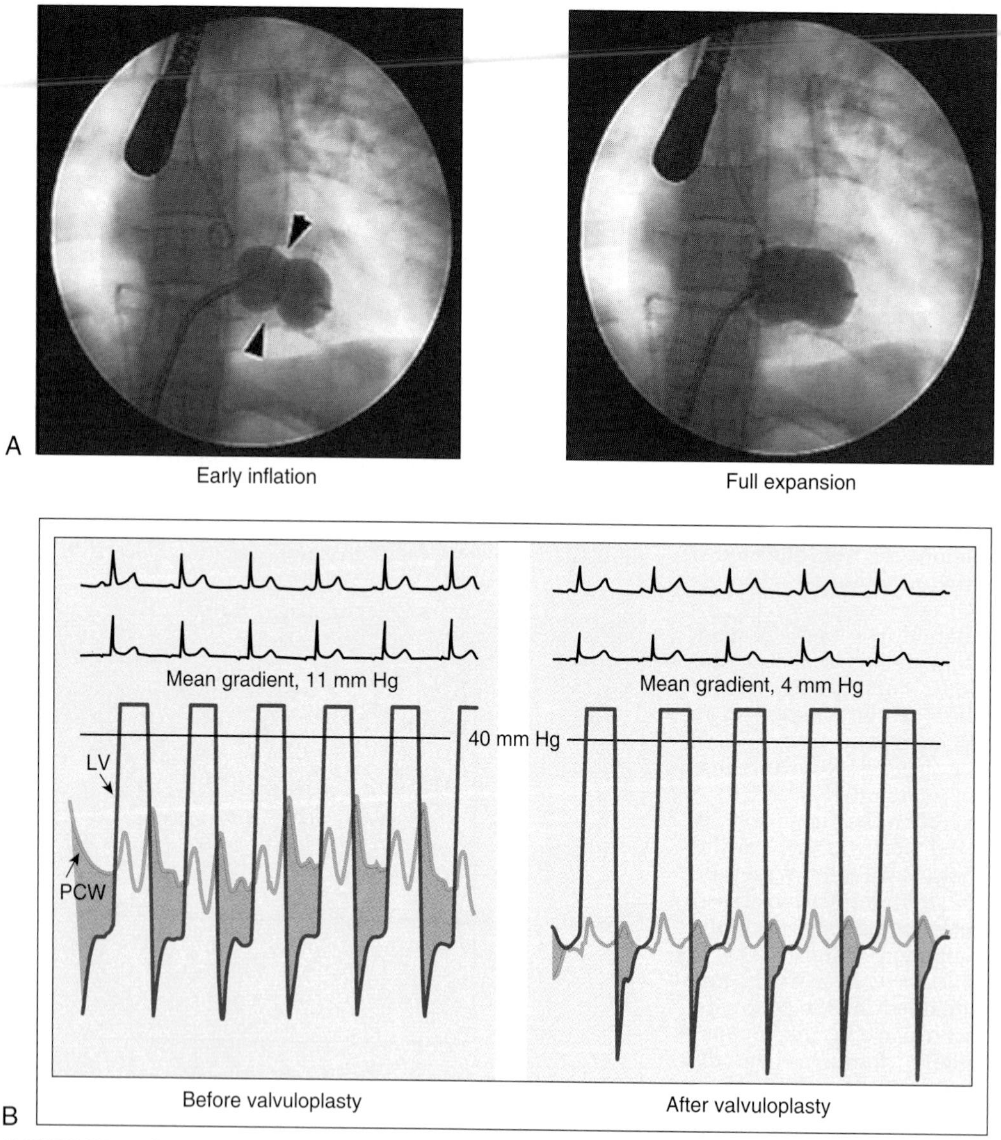

FIGURE 57–5 Percutaneous balloon mitral valvotomy (BMV) for mitral stenosis using the Inoue technique. **A,** The catheter is advanced into the left atrium via the transseptal technique and guided antegrade across the mitral orifice. As the balloon is inflated, its distal portion expands first and is pulled back so that it fits snugly against the orifice. With further inflation, the proximal portion of the balloon expands to center the balloon within the stenotic orifice (left panel). Further inflation expands the central "waist" portion of the balloon (right panel), resulting in commissural splitting and enlargement of the orifice. **B,** Successful BMV results in significant increase in mitral valve area, as reflected by reduction in the diastolic pressure gradient between left ventricle (magenta) and pulmonary capillary wedge (blue) pressure, as indicated by the shaded area. (From Delabays A, Goy JJ: Images in clinical medicine: Percutaneous mitral valvuloplasty. N Engl J Med 345:e4, 2001.)

Approximately 5 percent of patients are left with a small residual atrial septal defect, but this closes or decreases in size in the majority. Rarely, the defect is large enough to cause right-sided heart failure. Results are surgeon dependent and patients should be referred to experienced teams.

The indications for BMV are the same as those for surgical valvotomy (discussed later). A combination of significant symptoms and documented MS generally serves as the indication. Detailed two-dimensional and Doppler echocardiographic studies are indicated before a decision is made. Left atrial thrombus must be excluded by echocardiography.

An echocardiographic scoring system has been found to be particularly valuable in patient selection and has been widely adopted.[34,38,40,41] Leaflet rigidity, leaflet thickening, valvular calcification, and subvalvular disease are each scored from 0 to 4 (Table 57–1). Rigid, thickened valves with extensive subvalvular fibrosis and calcification lead to suboptimal results. A score of 8 or less is usually associated with an excellent immediate and long-term result, whereas scores exceeding 8 are associated with less impressive results (Fig. 57–7), including the risk of development of MR.[40] Significant valvular calcification[38] and coexisting MR[41,42] are additional important predictors of an adverse outcome. Transesophageal echocardiography provides a precise assessment of mitral valve structure and function and evaluation of accompanying MR and left atrial thrombus (a contraindication to BMV).[43] It also

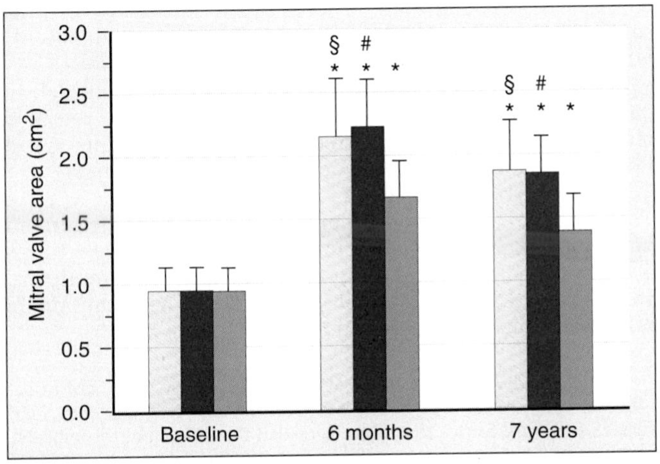

FIGURE 57–6 Mitral valve area before and 6 months and 7 years after valvotomy in a prospective, randomized trial of balloon mitral valvotomy (BMV, yellow bars), open surgical mitral commissurotomy (OMC, purple bars) and closed mitral commissurotomy (CMC, blue bars). At 6 months and 7 years, the results of BMV were equivalent to those of OMC, and superior to those of CMC. (From Farhat MB, Ayari M, Maatouk F, et al: Percutaneous balloon versus surgical closed and open mitral commissurotomy: Seven-year follow-up results of a randomized trial. Circulation 97:245, 1998.)

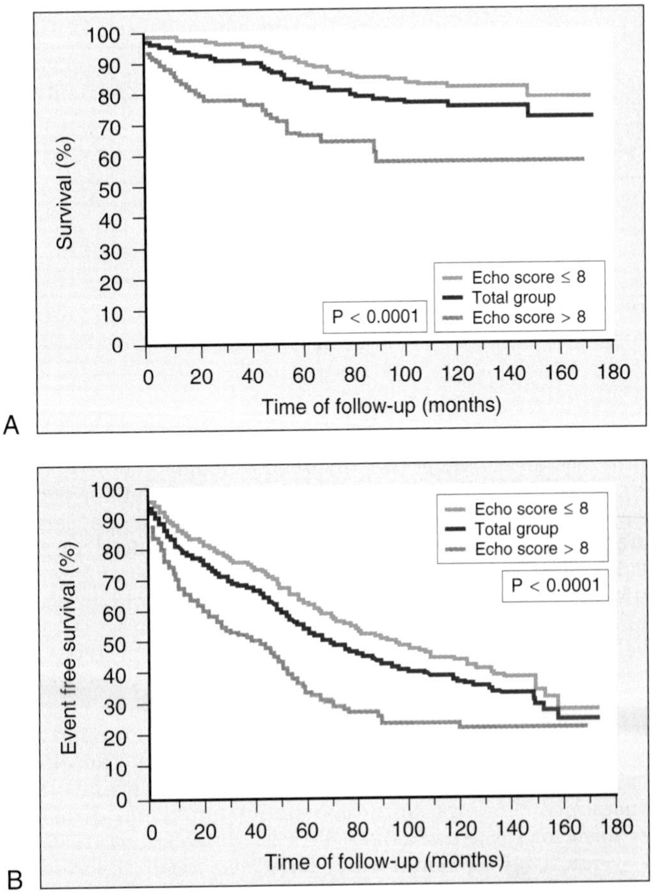

FIGURE 57–7 Long-term survival **(A)** and event-free survival **(B)** after balloon mitral valvotomy for 879 patients who were stratified by baseline echocardiographic morphology score: ≤ 8 (blue line) or > 8 (gold line). Patients with the lower echo score had a significantly better outcome initially and over the next 12 to 13 years. (From Palacios IF, Sanchez PL, Harrell LC, et al: Which patients benefit from percutaneous mitral balloon valvuloplasty? Prevalvuloplasy and postvalvuloplasty variables that predict long-term outcome. Circulation 105:1465, 2002.)

TABLE 57–1 Determinants of the Echocardiographic Mitral Valve Score

Grade	Mobility	Subvalvular Thickening	Thickening	Calcification
1	Highly mobile valve with only leaflet tips restricted	Minimal thickening just below the mitral leaflets	Leaflets near normal in thickness (4-5 mm)	A single area of increased echo brightness
2	Leaflet mid and base portions have normal mobility	Thickening of chordal structures extending up to one third of the chordal length	Midleaflets normal, considerable thickening of margins (5-8 mm)	Scattered areas of brightness confined to leaflet margins
3	Valve continues to move forward in diastole, mainly from the base	Thickening extending to the distal third of the chords	Thickening extending through the entire leaflet (5-8 mm)	Brightness extending into the midportion of the leaflets
4	No or minimal forward movement of the leaflets in diastole	Extensive thickening and shortening of all chordal structures extending down to the papillary muscles	Considerable thickening of all leaflet tissue (>8-10 mm)	Extensive brightness throughout much of the leaflet tissue

From Wilkens GT, Wyeman AL, Abscal VM, et al: Percutaneous balloon dilatation of the mitral valve: An analysis of echocardiographic variables related to outcome and the mechanism of dilatation. Br Heart J 60:299, 1988.

TABLE 57–2 Approaches to Mechanical Relief of Mitral Stenosis

Approach	Advantages	Disadvantages
Closed surgical valvotomy	Inexpensive Relatively simple Good hemodynamic results in selected patients Good long-term outcome	No direct visualization of valve Only feasible with flexible, noncalcified valves Contraindicated if MR > 2+ Surgical procedure with general anesthesia
Open surgical valvotomy	Visualization of valve allows directed valvotomy Concurrent annuloplasty for MR is feasible	Best results with flexible, noncalcified valves Surgical procedure with general anesthesia
Valve replacement	Feasible in all patients regardless of extent of valve calcification or severity of MR	Surgical procedure with general anesthesia Effect of loss of annular-papillary muscle continuity on LV function Prosthetic valve Chronic anticoagulation
Balloon mitral valvotomy	Percutaneous approach Local anesthesia Good hemodynamic results in selected patients Good long-term outcome	No direct visualization of valve Only feasible with flexible, noncalcified valves Contraindicated if MR > 2+

LV = left ventricular; MR = mitral regurgitation.
From Otto CM: Valvular Heart Disease. 2nd ed. Philadelphia, WB Saunders, 2004, p 296.

provides an accurate assessment of outcome. Three-dimensional echocardiography has also been found to be useful in assessing indications for BMV.[44] The findings on echocardiography affect the outcome of both open and closed surgical valvotomy in a similar manner. A prospective randomized trial in which patients with severe MS were randomized to undergo BMV, closed surgical valvotomy, or open surgical valvotomy resulted in similar clinical results from BMV and the open surgical technique that were superior to the results of the closed surgical valvotomy.[37] Indeed, after 7 years, mitral valve area was equivalent in the BMV and open surgical groups, both significantly greater than in the closed valvotomy group (see Fig. 57–6).[37] In patients with favorable anatomical findings, survival without functional disability or need for surgery or repeat BMV is 75 percent or greater at 7 years.[33-37] Excellent results have also been reported in children[45,46] and adolescents[47] in developing nations, where patients tend to be younger. These young patients usually have quite pliable valves, which are ideal for BMV.

Percutaneous BMV is the procedure of choice in patients who have symptomatic, hemodynamically severe stenosis with an echocardiographic score of 8 or less and without left atrial thrombus.[34,38,40,41] The lower cost and morbidity are obvious advantages. BMV can also be the initial procedure in patients with symptomatic, severe MS and less favorable valves (echocardiographic score > 8 and/or dense calcification on fluoroscopic or ultrasound examination).[34,38,41] However, the failure rate is considerable in these patients, and they may require surgical treatment, most often MVR. BMV also has acceptable results in patients with accompanying mild or moderate AR[43] and in those with mitral restenosis after surgical valvotomy.[48] It may also be used in patients with less favorable valves, including patients with restenosis after a previous BMV,[13] who are unsuitable for surgery because of very high risk. These include very elderly, frail patients; patients with associated severe ischemic heart disease; patients in whom MS is complicated by pulmonary, renal, or neoplastic disease; women of childbearing age in whom valve replacement is undesirable; and pregnant women with MS.[49,50] Patients with atrial fibrillation have a worse clinical and hemodynamic outcome with BMV than those in sinus rhythm[51]; the arrhythmia by itself does not unfavorably influence outcome, but is a marker for other clinical and morphological features associated with inferior results of BMV. BMV is contraindicated in patients with severe MR or AR and should probably not be used in patients with stenotic bioprosthetic valves.

Because the cost of the balloon catheter is deemed high in countries with restricted financial resources, a reusable metallic valvulotome has been devised. Early results are at least as good as those achieved with balloon catheters.[52]

SURGICAL VALVOTOMY

Three operative approaches are available for the treatment of rheumatic MS: (1) closed mitral valvotomy using a transatrial or transventricular approach[53]; (2) open valvotomy, i.e., valvotomy carried out under direct vision with the aid of cardiopulmonary bypass; and (3) MVR (Table 57–2).

CLOSED MITRAL VALVOTOMY. This procedure is performed without cardiopulmonary bypass but with the aid of a transventricular dilator. It is an effective operation, provided that MR, atrial thrombosis, or valvular calcification is not serious and that chordal fusion and shortening are not severe. Echocardiography is useful in selecting suitable candidates for this procedure by identifying patients without valvular calcification or dense fibrosis. If possible, closed mitral valvotomy should be carried out with "pump standby"; if the surgeon is unable to achieve a satisfactory result, the patient can be placed on cardiopulmonary bypass and the valvotomy carried out under direct vision or the valve replaced.

On average, the mitral valve area is increased by 1.0 cm^2, with only 20 to 30 percent of patients requiring MVR within 15 years.[54] In one large series,[53] the hospital mortality rate was 1.5 percent, and 0.3 percent of patients developed severe MR. Marked symptomatic improvement occurred in 86 percent of survivors. The actuarial survival rate was 89.5 percent after 18 years. Patients undergoing closed valvotomy for restenosis had a 6.7 percent mortality rate. Long-term follow-up has shown that the results are best if the operation is carried out before chronic atrial fibrillation and/or heart failure has occurred, but complication rates are higher when valves are calcified and/or severely thickened.

Closed mitral valvotomy is rarely used in the United States today, having been replaced by BMV, which is of greater effectiveness in patients who are candidates for closed mitral valvotomy.[37] Closed mitral valvotomy is more popular in developing nations, where the expense of open-heart surgery and even of balloon catheters for BMV is an important factor and where patients with mitral valve disease are younger and therefore have more pliable valves. But even in these nations, closed mitral valvotomy is being displaced by BMV.

OPEN VALVOTOMY. Most surgeons in North America and Western Europe now prefer to carry out *direct-vision* or *open valvotomy.* This operation is most frequently performed in patients with MS whose mitral valves are too distorted or calcified for BMV. Cardiopulmonary bypass is established, and to obtain a dry, quiet heart, body temperature is usually lowered, the heart is arrested, and the aorta is occluded intermittently.

Thrombi are removed from the left atrium and its appendage, and the latter is often amputated to remove a potential source of postoperative emboli. The commissures are incised, and, when necessary, fused chordae tendineae are separated, the underlying papillary muscle is split, and the valve leaflets are débrided of calcium. Mild or even moderate MR may be corrected. Left atrial and ventricular pressures are measured after bypass has been discontinued to confirm that the valvotomy has, in fact, been effective. When it has not been effective, another attempt can be made. When repair is not possible—most commonly owing to severe distortion and calcification of the valve and subvalvular apparatus with accompanying regurgitation that cannot be corrected—MVR should be carried out. In patients with atrial fibrillation, conversion to sinus rhythm is done at the completion of the operation. Open valvotomy is feasible and successful in more than 80 percent of patients referred for this procedure, with an operative mortality of 1 percent, a rate of reoperation for valve replacement of 0 to 16 percent at 36 to 53 months, and 10-year actuarial survival rates of 81 to 100 percent.[54]

In general, open valvotomy provides better hemodynamic relief of mitral valve obstruction than does the closed procedure, and the risk of dislodging thrombi from the atrium or calcium from the mitral valve is also less. Left atrial size, the need for mitral or tricuspid annuloplasty, and the presence of left atrial thrombus are all "risk factors" for a less than optimal outcome after open mitral valvotomy. Although a contemporary control series of medically and surgically treated patients is not available (nor is it likely ever to be), valvotomy appears to prolong survival substantially in patients with MS (see Fig. 57–4).

MITRAL RESTENOSIS. Mitral valvotomy, whether percutaneous or operative and whether open or closed, is *palliative* rather than curative, and even when successful, this procedure merely "turns the clock back." (The generally more effective open valvotomy and BMV turn the clock back further than does the closed valvotomy.) Thus, successful valvotomy does not result in a normal mitral valve but rather in one resembling the valve as it existed perhaps a decade earlier. Because the valve is not normal postoperatively, turbulent flow usually persists in the paravalvular region, and the resultant trauma may well play a role in restenosis. These changes are analogous to the gradual development of obstruction in a congenitally bicuspid aortic valve and are *not* usually the result of recurrent rheumatic fever.

On clinical grounds alone, i.e., based on the reappearance of symptoms, the incidence of "restenosis" has been estimated to range widely (from 2 to 60 percent). Recurrence of symptoms is usually *not* due to restenosis but may be due to one or more of the following conditions: (1) an inadequate first operation with residual stenosis; (2) the presence or development of MR, either at operation or as a consequence of infective endocarditis; (3) the progression of aortic valve disease; and (4) the development of coronary artery disease. True restenosis occurs in less than 20 percent of patients who are followed for 10 years.[1]

Thus, in properly selected patients, mitral valvotomy, however performed—balloon angioplasty, closed or open valvotomy—is a low-risk procedure that results in a significant increase in the size of the mitral orifice and favorably alters the clinical course of an otherwise progressive disease. Pulmonary arterial pressure falls promptly and decisively when mitral obstruction is effectively relieved. Most patients maintain clinical improvement for 10 to 15 years of follow-up. When a second procedure is required because of symptomatic deterioration, the valve is usually calcified and more seriously deformed than at the time of the first operation, and adequate reconstruction may not be possible. Accordingly, MVR is often necessary at that time.

Indications for Mitral Valve Replacement

This procedure is often required in patients with combined MS and moderate or severe MR; in those with extensive commissural calcification, severe fibrosis, and subvalvular fusion; and in those who have undergone previous valvotomy. The operative mortality rate following isolated MVR ranges from 3 to 8 percent in most centers and averaged 6.04 percent in the large data base of 16,105 such operations for patients with MS and/or MR reported in the Society of Thoracic Surgeons National Database (Table 57–3).[55] As described later, structural deterioration of bioprosthetic valves may occur. Also, the hazards of lifelong anticoagulant treatment in patients with mechanical prostheses must be considered. Therefore, the threshold for operation should be higher in patients in whom preoperative evaluation suggests that MVR may be required than in patients in whom valvotomy alone appears to be indicated.

MVR is indicated in two groups of patients with MS whose valves are not suitable for valvotomy: (1) those with a mitral valve area less than 1.5 cm^2 in NYHA Class III or IV; and (2) those with severe MS (mitral valve area < 1.0 cm^2), NYHA Class II, and severe pulmonary hypertension (pulmonary artery systolic pressure > 70 mm Hg).[1] Since the operative

TABLE 57–3 Operative Mortality Rates Following Valve Replacement and Repair

Operative Category	Number*	Operative Mortality* (%)	Number†	Operative Mortality† (%)
AVR (isolated)	26,317	4.3	32,968	4.0
MVR (isolated)	13,936	6.4	16,105	6.04
Multiple valve replacement	3,840	9.6	—	—
AVR + CAB	22,713	8.0	32,538	6.8
MVR + CAB	8,788	15.3	10,925	13.3
Multiple valve replacement + CAB	1,424	18.8		
AVR + any valve repair	938	7.4		
MVR + any valve repair	1,266	12.5		
Aortic valve repair	597	5.9		
Mitral valve repair	4,167	3.0		
Tricuspid valve repair	144	13.9		
AVR + aortic aneurysm repair	1,723	9.7		

AVR = aortic valve replacement; CAB = coronary artery bypass; MVR = mitral valve replacement.
*Modified from Jamieson WRE, Edwards FH, Schwartz M, et al: Risk stratification for cardiac valve replacement. National Cardiac Surgery Database, Ann Thorac Surg 67:943, 1999.
†Modified from Edwards FH, Peterson ED, Coombs LP, et al: Prediction of operative mortality after valve replacement surgery. J Am Coll Cardiol 37:885, 2001.

TABLE 57–4 Causes of Acute and Chronic Mitral Regurgitation

Acute	*Chronic*
Mitral Annulus Disorders Infective endocarditis (abscess formation) Trauma (valvular heart surgery) Paravalvular leak due to suture interruption (surgical technical problems or infective endocorditis)	**Inflammatory** Rheumatic heart disease Systemic lupus erythematosus Scleroderma
Mitral Leaflet Disorders Infective endocarditis (perforation or interfering with valve closure by vegetation) Trauma (tear during percutaneous balloon mitral valvotomy or penetrating chest injury) Tumors (atrial myxoma) Myxomatous degeneration Systemic lupus erythematosus (Libman-Sacks lesion)	**Degenerative** Myxomatous degeneration of mitral valve leaflets (Barlow click-murmur syndrome, prolapsing leaflet, mitral valve prolapse) Marfan syndrome Ehlers-Danlos syndrome Pseudoxanthoma elasticum Calcification of mitral valve annulus
Rupture of Chordae Tendineae Idiopathic, e.g., spontaneous Myxomatous degeneration (mitral valve prolapse, Marfan syndrome, Ehlers-Danlos syndrome) Infective endocarditis Acute rheumatic fever Trauma (percutaneous balloon valvotomy, blunt chest trauma)	**Infective** Infective endocarditis affecting normal, abnormal, or prosthetic mitral valves
Papillary Muscle Disorders Coronary artery disease (causing dysfunction and rarely rupture) Acute global left ventricular dysfunction Infiltrative diseases (amyloidosis, sarcoidosis) Trauma	**Structural** Ruptured chordae tendineae (spontaneous or secondary to myocardial infarction, trauma, mitral valve prolapse, endocarditis) Rupture or dysfunction of papillary muscle (ischemia or myocardial infarction) Dilation of mitral valve annulus and left ventricular cavity (congestive cardiomyopathies, aneurysmal dilation of the left ventricle) Hypertrophic cardiomyopathy Paravalvular prosthetic leak
Primary Mitral Valve Prosthetic Disorders Porcine cusp perforation (endocarditis) Porcine cusp degeneration Mechanical failure (strut fracture) Immobilized disc or ball of the mechanical prosthesis	**Congenital** Mitral valve clefts or fenestrations Parachute mitral valve abnormality in association with Endocardial cushion defects Endocardial fibroelastosis Transposition of the great arteries Anomalous origin of the left coronary artery

Data from Jutzy KR, Al-Zaibag M: Acute mitral and aortic valve regurgitation. *In* Al-Zaibag M, Duran CMG (eds): Valvular Heart Disease. New York, Marcel Dekker, 1994, pp 345-362 (left column); and Haffajee CI: Chronic mitral regurgitation. *In* Dalen JE. Alpert JS (eds): Valvular Heart Disease. 2nd ed. Boston, Little, Brown, 1987, p 112 (right column).

mortality risk may be quite high (10 to 20 percent) in patients in NYHA Class IV, operation should be carried out before patients reach this stage if possible. On the other hand, even such high-risk patients should not be denied operation unless they have comorbid conditions that preclude surgery or a satisfactory outcome.

Mitral Regurgitation

Etiology and Pathology

The mitral valve apparatus involves the mitral leaflets per se, chordae tendineae, papillary muscles, and mitral annulus. Abnormalities of any of these structures may cause MR.[56,57] The major causes of MR include mitral valve prolapse (MVP), rheumatic heart disease, infective endocarditis, annular calcification, cardiomyopathy, and ischemic heart disease (Table 57–4). Specific aspects of the MVP syndrome, the most important cause of significant MR in the United States, are discussed in a separate section. Less common causes of MR include collagen vascular diseases, trauma, the hypereosinophilic syndrome, carcinoid, and exposure to certain appetite suppressant drugs.

Abnormalities of Valve Leaflets

MR due to predominant involvement of the valve leaflets occurs in patients with chronic rheumatic heart disease. However, in contrast to MS, this lesion is more frequent in men than in women. It is a consequence of shortening, rigidity, deformity, and retraction of one or both mitral valve cusps and is associated with shortening and fusion of the chordae tendineae and papillary muscles. MVP involves both leaflets and chordae and may also affect the annulus. Infective endocarditis can cause MR by perforating valve leaflets (see Chap. 58); vegetations can prevent leaflet coaptation, and valvular retraction during the healing phase of endocarditis can cause MR. Destruction of the mitral valve leaflets can also occur in patients with penetrating and nonpenetrating trauma (see Chap. 65).

Abnormalities of the Mitral Annulus

DILATION. In a normal adult, the mitral annulus measures approximately 10 cm in circumference. It is soft and flexible, and contraction of the surrounding left ventricular muscle during systole causes the annular constriction that contributes importantly to valve closure. MR secondary to dilation of the mitral annulus can occur in any form of heart disease characterized by dilation of the left ventricle, especially dilated cardiomyopathy (Fig. 57–8; see also Fig. 11–57). Left ventricular submitral aneurysm has been reported as a cause of annular MR in sub-Saharan Africa and appears to be due to a congenital defect in the posterior portion of the annulus. Diagnosis by transesophageal echocardiography and surgical repair have been reported.

CALCIFICATION. Idiopathic (degenerative) calcification of the mitral annulus is one of the most common cardiac abnormalities found at autopsy; in most hearts it is of little functional consequence. However, when severe (see Fig. 12-21), it may be an important cause of MR,[57,58] and, in contrast to MR secondary to rheumatic fever, it is more common in women than in men. The development of degenerative calcification of the mitral annulus shares common risk factors with atherosclerosis, including systemic hypertension, hypercholesterolemia, and diabetes.[59] Hence, mitral annular calcification is associated with coronary[60] and carotid[61] atherosclerosis and identifies patients at higher risk for cardiovascular morbidity and mortality.[59] Annular calcification may also be accelerated by an intrinsic defect in the fibrous skeleton of the heart, as occurs in Marfan and Hurler syndromes. In these two latter syndromes, the mitral annulus is not only calcified but also dilated, further contributing to MR. The incidence of mitral annular calcification is also increased in patients who have chronic renal failure with secondary hyperparathyroidism. The annulus may also become thick, rigid, and calcified secondary to rheumatic involvement; when this process is severe, it also can interfere with valve closure.

With severe annular calcification, a rigid, curved bar or ring of calcium encircles the mitral orifice (see Fig. 12–21), and calcific spurs may project into the adjacent left ventricular myocardium. The calcification may immobilize the basal portion of the mitral leaflets, preventing their normal excursion in diastole and coaptation in systole, and aggravating the MR that results from loss of the normal sphincteric action of the mitral ring. Rarely, obstruction to left ventricular filling may occur when severe calcification encroaches on or protrudes into the mitral orifice. In patients with severe calcification, the conduction system may be invaded by calcium, leading to atrioventricular and/or intraventricular conduction defects. Calcification of the aortic valve cusps is an associated finding in approximately 50 percent of patients with severe mitral annular calcification, but this rarely causes aortic stenosis (AS). Occasionally, calcific deposits extend into the coronary arteries.

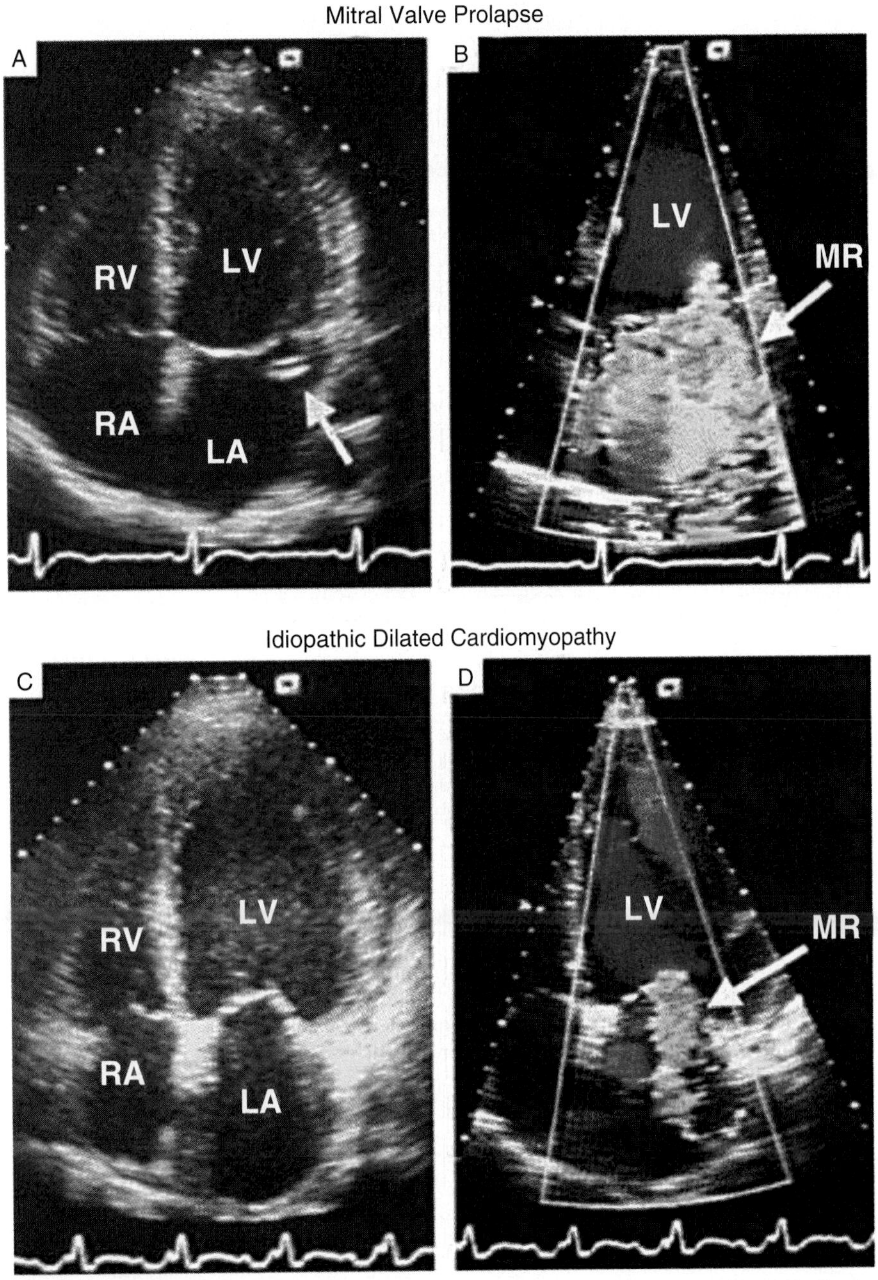

FIGURE 57–8 Echocardiographic long-axis images in two patients with mitral regurgitation (**A** and **C**) with color Doppler images of the same patients (**B** and **D**). The top panels were obtained in a 46-year-old man with mitral valve prolapse and a partial flail posterior leaflet (arrow in **A**). The left ventricle (LV) is not dilated but the left atrium (LA) is enlarged, and there is severe mitral regurgitation (MR). The bottom images were obtained in a patient with dilated cardiomyopathy, demonstrating left ventricular dilation, normal mitral valve leaflets, and moderate MR. RA = right atrium; RV = right ventricle. (From Otto CM: Evaluation and management of chronic mitral regurgitation. N Engl J Med 345:740, 2001.)

Abnormalities of the Chordae Tendineae. Such abnormalities are important causes of MR. Lengthening and rupture of the chordae tendineae are cardinal features of the MVP syndrome (Fig. 57–8).[62] The chordae may be congenitally abnormal; rupture may be spontaneous ("primary") or may occur as a consequence of infective endocarditis, trauma, rheumatic fever, or, rarely, osteogenesis imperfecta or relapsing polychondritis. In most patients, no cause for chordal rupture is apparent other than increased mechanical strain. Chordae to the posterior leaflet rupture more frequently than those to the anterior leaflet. Patients with idiopathic rupture of mitral chordae tendineae frequently exhibit pathological fibrosis of the papillary muscles. It is possible that the dysfunction of the papillary muscles may cause stretching and ultimately rupture of the chordae tendineae. Chordal rupture may also result from acute left ventricular dilation, regardless of the cause. Depending on the number of chordae involved in rupture and the rate at which rupture occurs, the resultant MR may be mild, moderate, or severe and acute, subacute, or chronic.

Involvement of the Papillary Muscles. Diseases of the left ventricular papillary muscles are a frequent cause of MR. Because these muscles are perfused by the terminal portion of the coronary vascular bed, they are particularly vulnerable to ischemia, and any disturbance in coronary perfusion may result in papillary muscle dysfunction. When ischemia is transient, it results in temporary papillary muscle dysfunction and may cause transient episodes of MR that are sometimes associated with attacks of angina pectoris. When ischemia of papillary muscles is severe and prolonged, it causes papillary muscle dysfunction and scarring, as well as chronic MR. The posterior papillary muscle, which is supplied by the posterior descending branch of the right coronary artery, becomes ischemic and infarcted more frequently than does the anterolateral papillary muscle; the latter is supplied by diagonal branches of the left anterior descending coronary artery and often by marginal branches from the left circumflex artery as well. Ischemia of the papillary muscles is caused most commonly by coronary atherosclerosis, but it may also occur in patients with severe anemia, shock, coronary arteritis of any cause, or an anomalous left coronary artery. MR occurs frequently in patients with healed myocardial infarcts[63] and is caused by dyskinesis of the left ventricular myocardium at the base of a papillary muscle.

Left ventricular dilation of any cause, including ischemia, can alter the spatial relationships between the papillary muscles and the chordae tendineae and thereby result in MR.[64] Although *necrosis of a papillary muscle* is a frequent complication of myocardial infarction, frank rupture is far less common; the latter is usually fatal because of the extremely severe MR that it produces (see Chap. 46). However, rupture of one or two of the apical heads of a papillary muscle results in a lesser degree of MR and thus makes survival possible, usually following surgical therapy.

Some degree of MR is found in approximately 30 percent of patients with coronary artery disease who are being considered for coronary artery bypass surgery. In these patients, MR is secondary to ischemic damage to the papillary muscles and/or dilation of the mitral valve ring. In most of these patients, MR is mild; however, in the small percentage with severe MR (3 percent in one large series of patients with coronary artery disease proved by coronary arteriography), it is associated with a poor prognosis.[65,66] The incidence and severity of regurgitation vary inversely with the left ventricular ejection fraction and directly with the left ventricular end-diastolic pressure. MR occurs in approximately 20 percent of patients following acute myocardial infarction and, even when mild, is associated with a higher risk of adverse outcomes.

Various other disorders of the papillary muscles may also be responsible for the development of MR (see Table 57–4). These include congenital malposition of the muscles; absence of one papillary muscle, resulting in the so-called parachute mitral valve syndrome; and involvement or infiltration of the papillary muscles by a variety of processes, including abscesses, granulomas, neoplasms, amyloidosis, and sarcoidosis.

Other causes of MR, discussed in greater detail elsewhere, include obstructive hypertrophic cardiomyopathy (see Chap. 59), hypereosinophilic syndrome, endomyocardial fibrosis, trauma affecting the leaflets and/or papillary muscles (see Chap. 65), Kawasaki disease (see Chap. 56), left atrial myxoma (see Chap. 63), and various congenital anomalies, including cleft anterior leaflet and ostium secundum atrial septal defect (see Chap. 56).

Pathophysiology

Because the regurgitant mitral orifice is functionally in parallel with the aortic valve, the impedance to ventricular emptying is reduced in patients with MR. Consequently, MR enhances left ventricular emptying. Almost 50 percent of the regurgitant volume is ejected into the left atrium before the aortic valve opens. The volume of MR flow depends on a combination of the instantaneous size of the regurgitant orifice and the (reverse) pressure gradient between the left ventricle and the left atrium.[1,57] Both the orifice size and the pressure gradient are labile. Left ventricular systolic pressure, and therefore the left ventricular–left atrial gradient, depends on systemic vascular resistance, and in patients in whom the mitral annulus has normal flexibility, the cross-sectional area of the mitral annulus may be altered by many interventions. Thus, increase of both preload and afterload and depression of contractility increase left ventricular size and enlarge the mitral annulus and thereby the regurgitant orifice. When ventricular size is reduced by treatment with positive inotropic agents, diuretics, and particularly vasodilators, the regurgitant orifice size decreases, and the volume of regurgitant flow declines,[67,68] as reflected in the height of the *v* wave in the left atrial pressure pulse and in the intensity and duration of the systolic murmur. Conversely, left ventricular dilation, regardless of cause, may increase MR.

LEFT VENTRICULAR COMPENSATION. The left ventricle initially compensates for the development of *acute* MR in part by emptying more completely and in part by increasing preload, i.e., by use of the Frank-Starling principle. Because *acute* MR reduces both late systolic ventricular pressure and radius, left ventricular wall tension declines markedly (and proportionately to a greater extent than left ventricular pressure), permitting a reciprocal increase in both the extent and the velocity of myocardial fiber shortening, leading to a reduced end-systolic volume (Fig. 57–9). As regurgitation, particularly severe regurgitation, becomes chronic, the left ventricular end-diastolic volume increases and the end-systolic volume returns to normal. By means of the Laplace principle (which states that myocardial wall tension is related to the product of intraventricular pressure and radius), the increased ventricular end-diastolic volume increases wall tension to normal or supranormal levels in the so-called chronic compensated stage of severe MR.[57] The resultant increase in left ventricular end-diastolic volume and mitral annular diameter may create a vicious circle in which "MR begets more MR." In patients with chronic MR, both left ventricular end-diastolic volume and mass are increased; i.e., typical volume overload (eccentric) hypertrophy develops. However, the degree of hypertrophy is often not proportionate to the degree of left ventricular dilation, so that the ratio of left ventricular mass to end-diastolic volume may be less than normal.[57,69] Nonetheless, the reduced afterload permits maintenance of ejection fraction in the normal to supranormal range. The reduced left ventricular afterload allows a

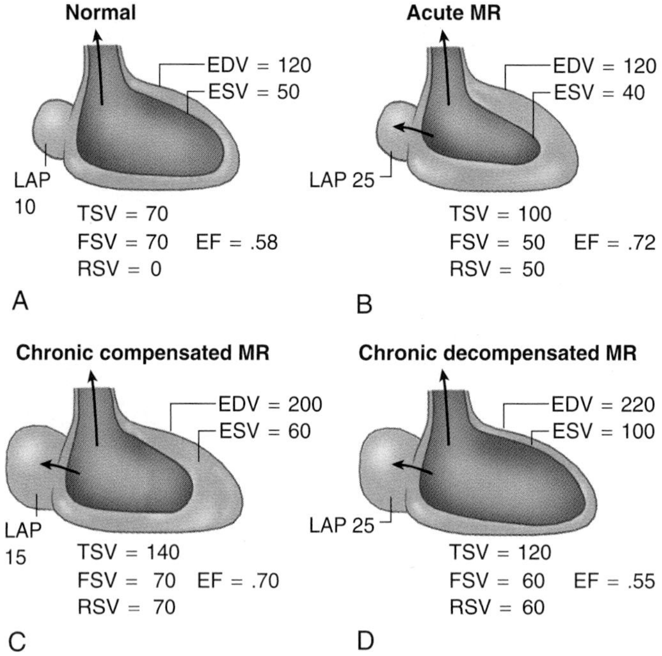

FIGURE 57–9 Three phases of mitral regurgitation (MR) are depicted and compared with normal physiology **(A)**. In acute MR **(B)**, an increase in preload and a decrease in afterload cause an increase in end-diastolic volume (EDV) and a decrease in end-systolic volume (ESV), producing an increase in total stroke volume (TSV). However, forward stroke volume (FSV) is diminished because 50 percent of the TSV regurgitates as the regurgitant stroke volume (RSV), resulting in an increase in left atrial pressure (LAP). In the chronic compensated phase **(C)**, eccentric hypertrophy has developed, and EDV is now increased substantially. Afterload has returned toward normal as the radius term of the LaPlace relationship increases with the increase in EDV. Normal muscle function and a large increase in EDV permit a substantial increase in TSV from the acute phase. This, in turn, permits a normal FSV. Left atrial enlargement now accommodates the regurgitant volume at lower LAP. Ejection fraction (EF) remains greater than normal. In the chronic decompensated phase **(D)**, muscle dysfunction has developed, impairing ejection fraction, diminishing both TSV and FSV. EF, although still "normal," has decreased to 0.55, and LAP is reelevated because less volume is ejected during systole, causing a higher ESV. (From Carabello BA: Progress in mitral and aortic regurgitation. Curr Probl Cardiol 28:553, 2003.)

greater proportion of the contractile energy of the myocardium to be expended in shortening than in tension development and explains how the left ventricle can adapt to the load imposed by MR.

The eccentric ventricular hypertrophy that accompanies the elevated end-diastolic volume of chronic MR is secondary to new sarcomeres laid down in parallel. A shift to the right (greater volume at any pressure) occurs in the left ventricular diastolic pressure-volume curve in patients with chronic MR. With decompensation, chamber stiffness increases, raising the diastolic pressure at any volume.

In most patients with severe primary MR, compensation is maintained for years, but in some patients the prolonged hemodynamic overload ultimately leads to myocardial decompensation. End-systolic volume, preload, and afterload all rise, whereas ejection fraction and stroke volume decline. In such patients, there is evidence of neurohormonal activation[70-71a] and elevation of circulating proinflammatory cytokines.[72] Plasma natriuretic peptide levels also increase in response to the volume load, more so in patients with symptomatic decompensation,[70] and a depressed ratio of phosphocreatine/adenosine triphosphate has been reported in patients with MR and severe decompensation.[73] It is not clear whether this is the cause or a marker of heart failure in these patients.

Coronary flow rates may be increased in patients with severe MR,[74] but the increases in myocardial oxygen consumption (MVO_2) are relatively modest compared to patients with AS and AR, because myocardial fiber shortening, which is elevated in patients with MR, is not one of the principal determinants of MVO_2. One of these determinants, mean left ventricular wall tension, may actually be reduced in patients with MR, whereas the other two, contractility and heart rate, may be little affected. Thus patients with MR have a low incidence of clinical manifestations of myocardial ischemia compared with the much higher incidence occurring in those with AS and AR, conditions in which MVO_2 is greatly augmented.

ASSESSMENT OF MYOCARDIAL CONTRACTILITY IN MITRAL REGURGITATION. Because the ejection phase indices of myocardial contractility are inversely correlated with afterload, patients with early MR (with reduced left ventricular afterload) often exhibit elevations in ejection phase indices of myocardial contractility, such as ejection fraction, fractional fiber shortening, and velocity of circumferential fiber shortening.[1,57] Many patients ultimately develop symptoms because of elevated left atrial and pulmonary venous pressures related to the regurgitant volume, and they may do so with no change in these ejection phase indices, which remain elevated. However, in other patients, major symptoms reflect serious contractile dysfunction, at which time ejection fraction, fiber shortening, and mean velocity of circumferential fiber shortening have declined to *low-normal* or *below-normal* levels (see Fig. 57–9). As MR persists, the reduction in afterload, which increases myocardial fiber shortening and the earlier mentioned ejection phase indices, is opposed by the impairment of myocardial function characteristic of severe chronic diastolic overload. However, even in patients with overt heart failure secondary to MR, the ejection fraction and fiber shortening may be only modestly reduced.[75] Therefore, values in the *low-normal* range for the ejection phase indices of myocardial performance in patients with chronic MR may actually reflect impaired myocardial function, whereas moderately reduced values (e.g., ejection fraction of 0.40 to 0.50) generally signify severe, often irreversible, impairment of contractility,[76,77] identifying patients who may do poorly after surgical correction of the MR (Fig. 57–10). An ejection fraction of less than 0.35 in patients with severe MR usually represents advanced myocardial dysfunction; such patients are high operative risks and may not experience satisfactory improvement following MVR.

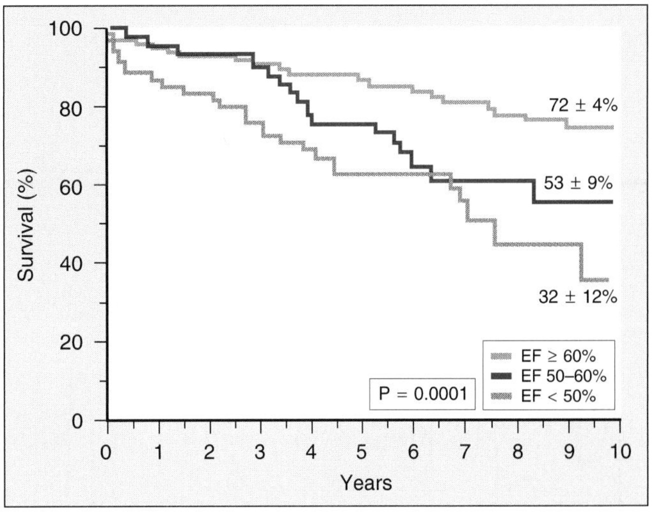

FIGURE 57–10 Graph of the late survival of patients who underwent surgical correction of mitral regurgitation as a function of the preoperative echocardiographic ejection fraction (EF). (From Enriquez-Sarano M, Tajik AJ, Schaff HV, et al: Echocardiographic prediction of survival after surgical correction of organic mitral regurgitation. Circulation 90:833, 1994.)

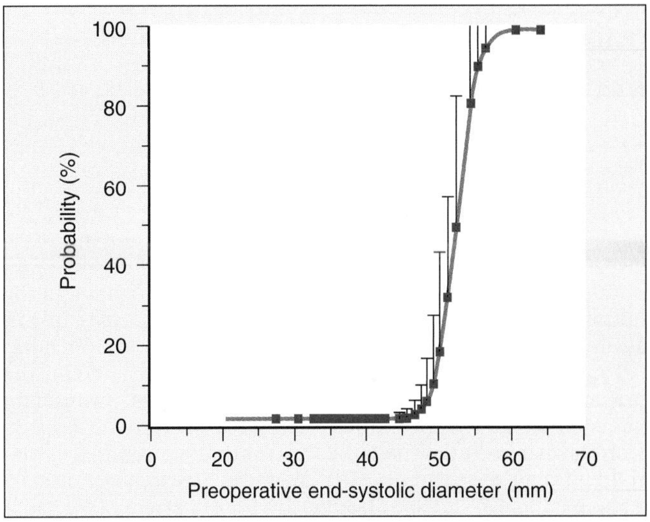

FIGURE 57–11 The probability of postoperative death or persistence of severe heart failure in patients with mitral regurgitation plotted against preoperative echocardiographic end-systolic diameter. As end-systolic diameter exceeded 45 mm, the incidence of a poor postoperative outcome increased abruptly. (From Wisenbaugh T, Skudicky D, Sareli P: Prediction of outcome after valve replacement for rheumatic mitral regurgitation in the era of chordal preservation. Circulation 89:191, 1994.)

End-Systolic Volume.. Preoperative myocardial contractility is an important determinant of the risk of operative death, of cardiac failure perioperatively, and of the level of left ventricular function postoperatively. Therefore, it is not surprising that the end-systolic pressure/volume (or stress/dimension) relation has emerged as a useful index for evaluating left ventricular function in patients with MR.[78] Indeed, the simple measurement of end-systolic volume or diameter has been found to be a useful predictor of function and survival following mitral valve surgery.[1,56,76-79] The outcome is excellent until the end-systolic diameter exceeds approximately 45 mm or 26 mm/m^2 (Fig. 57–11),[79] although even lower values of end-systolic climension have been associated with impaired postoperative ejection fraction.[76]

HEMODYNAMICS. Effective (forward) *cardiac output* is usually depressed in severely symptomatic patients with MR,

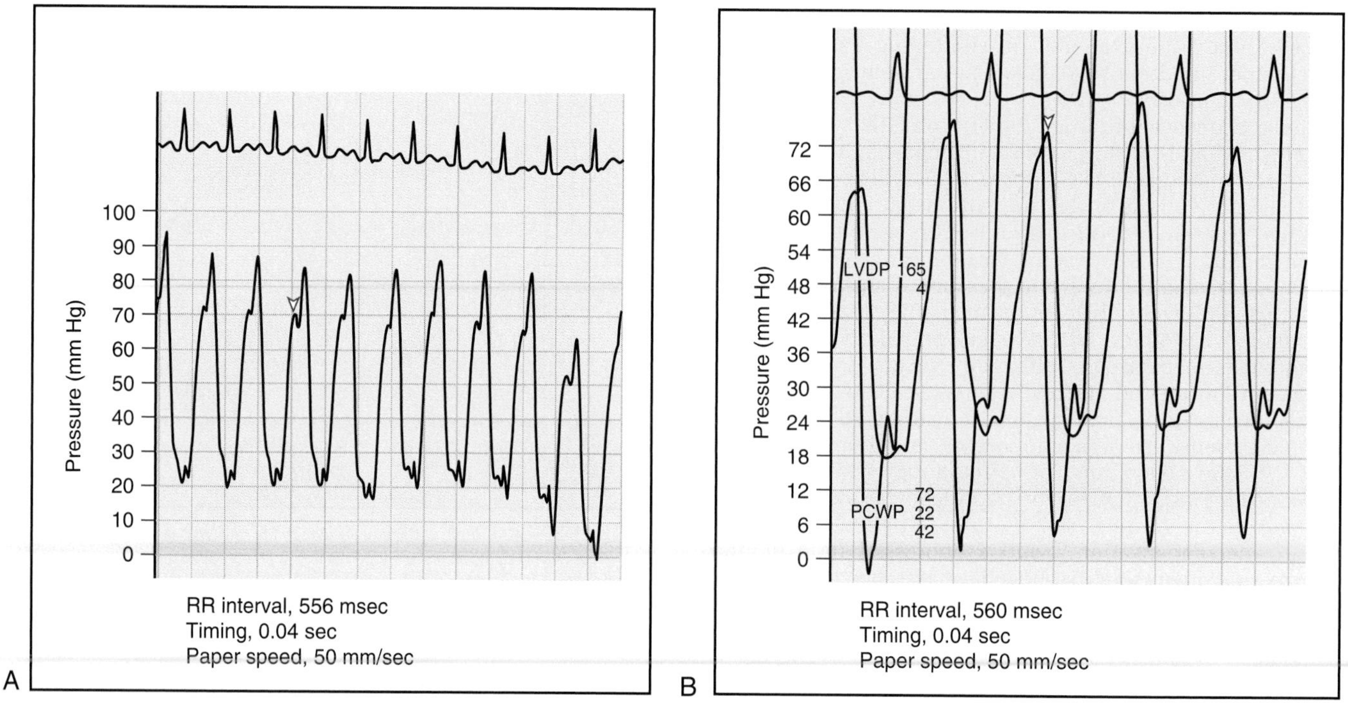

FIGURE 57–12 Hemodynamic tracings in a 45-year-old woman with acute mitral regurgitation from bacterial endocarditis. **A,** Pulmonary artery pressure. **B,** Simultaneous left ventricular diastolic pressure (LVDP) and pulmonary capillary wedge pressure (PCWP). The PCWP demonstrates a markedly elevated "v" wave (arrowhead, **B**) that transmits to the pulmonary artery pressure (arrowhead, **A**). (Adapted from Wisse B, Sniderman AD: Severe mitral regurgitation. N Engl J Med 343:1386, 2000.)

whereas *total* left ventricular output (the sum of forward and regurgitant flow) is usually elevated until quite late in the patient's course. The cardiac output achieved during exercise, not the regurgitant volume, is the principal determinant of functional capacity.[80] The atrial contraction (*a*) wave in the left atrial pressure pulse is usually not as prominent in MR as in MS, but the *v* wave is characteristically much taller because it is inscribed during ventricular systole, when the left atrium is being filled with blood from the pulmonary veins as well as from the left ventricle. Occasionally, backward transmission of the tall *v* wave into the pulmonary arterial bed may result in an early diastolic "pulmonary arterial *v* wave" (Fig. 57–12; see also Fig. 17–5). In patients with pure MR, the *y* descent in the pulmonary capillary pressure pulse is particularly rapid as the distended left atrium empties rapidly during early diastole. However, in patients with combined MS and MR, the *y* descent is gradual. Although a left atrioventricular pressure gradient persisting throughout diastole signifies the presence of significant associated MS, a brief early diastolic gradient may occur in patients with isolated, severe MR as a result of the rapid flow of blood across a normal-sized mitral orifice early in diastole, often accompanied by an early diástolic murmur at the apex.

LEFT ATRIAL COMPLIANCE

The compliance of the left atrium (and pulmonary venous bed) is an important determinant of the hemodynamic and clinical picture in patients with severe MR. Three major subgroups of patients with severe MR based on left atrial compliance have been identified and are characterized as follows:

Normal or Reduced Compliance. In this subgroup, there is little enlargement of the left atrium but marked elevation of the mean left atrial pressure (Fig. 57–13), particularly of the *v* wave, and pulmonary congestion is a prominent symptom. Severe MR usually develops acutely, as occurs with rupture of the chordae tendineae, infarction of one of the heads of a papillary muscle, or perforation of a mitral leaflet as a consequence of trauma or endocarditis. In patients with acute MR, the left atrium initially operates on the steep portion of its pressure-volume curve with a marked rise in pressure for a small increase in volume. Sinus rhythm is usually present; after the passage of weeks or a few months, the left atrial wall becomes hypertrophied, is capable of contracting vigorously, and facilitates left ventricular filling. The thicker atrium is less compliant than normal, which further increases the height of the *v* wave. Thickening of the walls of the pulmonary veins and proliferative changes in the pulmonary arteries, as well as marked elevations of pulmonary vascular resistance and pulmonary artery pressure, usually develop over the course of 6 to 12 months after the onset of acute, severe MR.

Markedly Increased Compliance. At the opposite end of the spectrum from patients in the first group are those with severe, longstanding MR with massive enlargement of the left atrium and normal or only slightly elevated left atrial pressure (see Fig. 57–13). The atrial wall contains only a small remnant of muscle surrounded by fibrous tissue. Longstanding MR in these patients has altered the physical properties of the left atrial wall and thereby displaced the atrial pressure-volume curve to the right, allowing a normal or almost-normal pressure to exist in a greatly enlarged left atrium. Pulmonary arterial pressure and pulmonary vascular resistance may be normal or only slightly elevated at rest. Atrial fibrillation and a low cardiac output are almost invariably present.

Moderately Increased Compliance. This, the most common subgroup, consists of patients between the ends of the spectrum represented by the first and second groups. These patients have severe, chronic MR and exhibit variable degrees of enlargement of the left atrium, associated with significant elevation of the left atrial pressure, and these two factors (in association with age) determine the likelihood that atrial fibrillation will ensue.

Clinical Manifestations

History

The nature and severity of symptoms in patients with chronic MR are functions of a combination of interrelated factors including the severity of MR; the rate of its progression; the level of left atrial, pulmonary venous, and pulmonary arterial pressures; the presence of episodic or chronic atrial tachyarrhythmias; and the presence of associated valvular, myocardial, or coronary artery disease. Symptoms may occur with preserved left ventricular contractile function in patients with chronic MR who have severely elevated pulmonary venous pressures or atrial fibrillation. In other

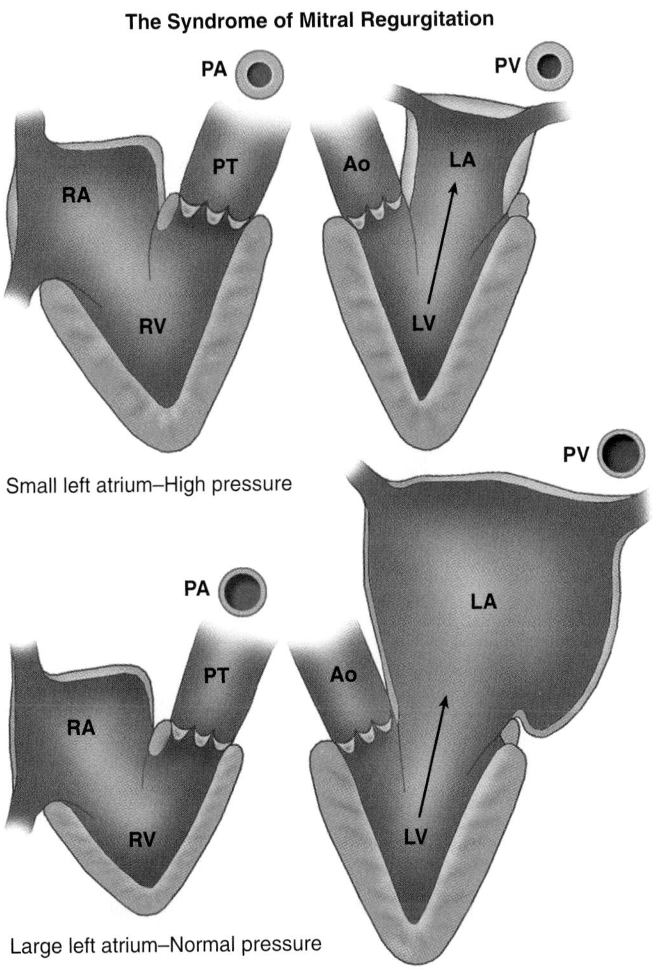

FIGURE 57–13 Diagram depicting the two extremes of the spectrum in pure mitral regurgitation. When severe mitral regurgitation appears suddenly in individuals with previously normal or near-normal hearts (top), the left atrium (LA) is relatively small and the high pressure within it is reflected back into the pulmonary vessels and right ventricle (RV). The anatomical indicator of this latter physiological event is severe hypertrophy of the LA and RV walls and marked intimal proliferation and medial hypertrophy of the pulmonary arteries (PA), arterioles, and veins (PV). At the other extreme, in patients with severe chronic mitral regurgitation (bottom), the LA cavity is of giant size and its wall is thin. It is thus able to "absorb" the left ventricular (LV) pressure without reflecting it back into the pulmonary vessels or RV. As a consequence, pulmonary vessels remain normal, and the RV wall does not thicken. PT = pulmonary trunk; RA = right atrium. (From Roberts WC, Dangel JC, Bulkley BH: Nonrheumatic valvular cardiac disease: A clinicopathologic survey of 27 different conditions causing valvular dysfunction. Cardiovasc Clin 5:403, 1973.)

patients, symptoms herald left ventricular decompensation. In patients with rheumatic MR, the time interval between the initial attack of rheumatic fever and the development of symptoms tends to be longer in patients than in those with MS and often exceeds two decades. Hemoptysis and systemic embolization are less common in patients with isolated or predominant MR than in those with MS. The development of atrial fibrillation affects the course adversely but perhaps not as dramatically as in MS. On the other hand, chronic weakness and fatigue secondary to a low cardiac output are more prominent features in MR.

Most patients with MR of rheumatic origin have only mild disability, unless regurgitation progresses as a result of chronic rheumatic activity, infective endocarditis, or rupture of the chordae tendineae. However, the indolent course of MR may be deceptive. By the time that symptoms secondary to a reduced cardiac output and/or pulmonary congestion become apparent, serious and sometimes even irreversible left ventricular dysfunction may have developed.

In patients with severe, chronic MR who have a greatly enlarged left atrium and relatively mild left atrial hypertension (patients with increased left atrial compliance [second subgroup], described earlier), pulmonary vascular resistance does not usually rise markedly. Instead, the major symptoms, fatigue and exhaustion, are related to the depressed cardiac output. Right-sided heart failure, characterized by congestive hepatomegaly, edema, and ascites, is prominent in patients with acute MR, elevated pulmonary vascular resistance, and pulmonary hypertension. Angina pectoris is rare unless coronary artery disease coexists.

NATURAL HISTORY. This is variable and depends on a combination of the volume of regurgitation, the state of the myocardium, and the cause of the underlying disorder. Asymptomatic patients with mild primary MR usually remain in a stable state for many years. Severe regurgitation develops in only a small percentage of these patients, most commonly because of intervening infective endocarditis or rupture of the chordae tendineae. In patients with mild MR related to MVP, the rate of progression in severity of MR is highly variable; in most patients progression is gradual unless a ruptured chordae or flail leaflet supervenes.[81] Regurgitation tends to progress more rapidly in patients with connective tissue diseases, such as Marfan syndrome, than in those with chronic MR of rheumatic origin. Acute rheumatic fever is a frequent cause of isolated, severe MR in adolescents in developing nations, and these patients often have a rapidly progressive course.

Because the natural history of severe MR has been altered greatly by surgical intervention, it is difficult now to predict the course of patients who receive medical therapy alone. However, Horstkotte and associates[32] reported a 5-year survival of only 30 percent in patients who were candidates for operation (presumably because of symptoms) but who declined (see Fig. 57–4). Among patients with severe MR resulting from flail leaflets, Ling and Enriquez-Sarano[82] reported an annual mortality rate of 6.3 percent; at 10 years 90 percent died or underwent surgical correction. This latter series included many patients who were initially symptomatic or had left ventricular dysfunction or atrial fibrillation and thus might be considered to be a higher risk. However, even among asymptomatic patients with initially normal left and right ventricular ejection fractions,[83] severe MR is associated with a high rate of symptoms or left ventricular dysfunction requiring surgery, and surgery is nearly unavoidable over the course of 10 years (Fig. 57–14).

Physical Examination

Palpation of the arterial pulse is helpful in differentiating AS from MR, both of which may produce a prominent systolic murmur both at the base of the heart and at the apex. The carotid arterial upstroke is sharp in severe MR and delayed in AS; the volume of the pulse may be normal or reduced in the presence of heart failure. The cardiac impulse, like the arterial pulse, is brisk and hyperdynamic. It is displaced to the left, and a prominent left ventricular filling wave is frequently palpable. Systolic expansion of the enlarged left atrium may result in a late systolic thrust in the parasternal region, which may be confused with right ventricular enlargement.

AUSCULTATION

With severe, chronic MR due to defective valve cusps, S_1, produced by mitral valve closure, is usually diminished. Wide splitting of S_2 is common and results from the shortening of left ventricular ejection and an earlier A_2 as a consequence of reduced resistance to left ventricular outflow. In patients with MR who have severe pulmonary hypertension, P_2 is louder than A_2. The abnormal increase in the flow rate across the mitral orifice during the rapid filling phase is often associated with an S_3, which should not be interpreted as a feature of heart failure in these patients, and this may be accompanied by a brief diastolic rumble.

The *systolic murmur* is the most prominent physical finding; it must be differentiated from the systolic murmur of AS, TR, and ventricular septal defect. In most patients with severe MR, the systolic murmur commences immediately after the soft S_1 and continues beyond and may obscure the A_2 because of the persisting pressure difference between the left ventricle and left atrium after aortic valve closure. The holosystolic murmur of chronic MR is usually constant in intensity, blowing, high-pitched, and loudest at the apex with radiation to the left axilla and left infrascapular area. However, radiation toward the sternum or the aortic area may occur with abnormalities of the posterior leaflet and is particularly common in patients with MVP involving this leaflet. The murmur shows little change even in the presence of large beat-to-beat variations of left ventricular stroke volume, as occur in atrial fibrillation. This contrasts with most midsystolic (ejection) murmurs, such as in AS, which vary greatly in intensity with stroke volume and therefore with the duration of diastole. There is little correlation between the intensity of the systolic murmur and the severity of MR. Indeed, in patients with severe

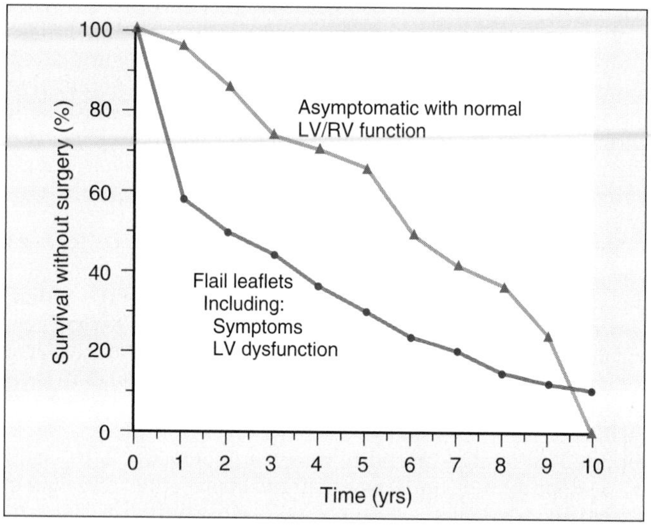

FIGURE 57–14 Two series examining the natural history of patients with severe mitral regurgitation (MR), including a series of patients with flail mitral leaflets reported by Ling and associates (magenta), many of whom were symptomatic, had atrial fibrillation, or had evidence of left ventricular (LV) dysfunction, and a second series reported by Rosen and associates (blue) who initially were asymptomatic with normal LV and right ventricular (RV) function. Although the patients with flail leaflets had a steeper initial attrition rate, both series demonstrated that patients with severe MR have a very low likelihood of remaining stable and asymptomatic over the course of 10 years. (Adapted from Ling LH, Enriquez-Sarano M, Seward JB, et al: Clinical outcome of mitral regurgitation due to flail leaflet. N Engl J Med 335:1417, 1996; and Rosen SF, Borer JS, Hochreiter C, et al: Natural history of the asymptomatic patient with severe mitral regurgitation secondary to mitral valve prolapse and normal right and left ventricular performance. Am J Cardiol 74:374, 1994.)

MR due to left ventricular dilation, acute myocardial infarction, or paraprosthetic valvular regurgitation, or in those who have marked emphysema, obesity, chest deformity, or a prosthetic heart valve, the systolic murmur may be barely audible or even absent, a condition referred to as *silent MR*.

The murmur of MR may be holosystolic, late systolic, or early systolic. When the murmur is confined to late systole, the regurgitation is usually not severe and may be secondary to prolapse of the mitral valve or to papillary muscle dysfunction. These causes of MR are frequently associated with a normal S_1 because initial closure of the mitral valve cusps may be unimpaired. The late systolic murmur of papillary muscle dysfunction is particularly variable; it may become accentuated or holosystolic during acute myocardial ischemia and often disappears when ischemia is relieved. A midsystolic click preceding a mid to late systolic murmur and the response of that murmur to a number of maneuvers, helps establish the diagnosis of MVP. Early systolic murmurs are typical of *acute* MR. When the left atrial v wave is markedly elevated in acute MR, the murmur may diminish or disappear in late systole as the reverse pressure gradient declines. As noted previously, a short, low-pitched diastolic murmur following S_3 may be audible in patients with severe MR, even without accompanying MS.

Dynamic Auscultation. The holosystolic murmur of MR varies little during respiration. However, sudden standing and amyl nitrite inhalation usually diminish the murmur (Table 57–5), whereas squatting augments it. The late systolic murmur of MVP behaves in the opposite direction, decreasing in duration with squatting and increasing in duration with standing. The holosystolic MR murmur is reduced during the strain of the Valsalva maneuver and shows a left-sided response (i.e., a transient overshoot that occurs six to eight beats following release of the strain). The murmur of MR is usually intensified by isometric exercise, differentiating it from the systolic murmurs of valvular AS and hypertrophic obstructive cardiomyopathy, both of which are reduced by this intervention. The murmur of MR caused by left ventricular dilation *decreases* in intensity and duration following effective therapy with cardiac glycosides, diuretics, rest, and particularly vasodilators.

Differential Diagnosis. The holosystolic murmur of MR resembles that produced by a ventricular septal defect. However, the latter is usually loudest at the sternal border rather than the apex and is often accompanied by a parasternal, rather than an apical, thrill. The murmur of MR may also be confused with that of TR, but the latter is usually heard best along the left sternal border, is augmented during inspiration, and is accompanied by a prominent v wave and y descent in the jugular venous pulse.

When the chordae tendineae to the posterior leaflet of the mitral valve rupture, the regurgitant jet is often directed anteriorly, so that it impinges on the atrial septum adjacent to the aortic root and causes a systolic murmur that is most prominent at the base of the heart. This murmur can be confused with that of AS. On the other hand, when the chordae tendineae to the anterior leaflet rupture, the jet is usually directed to the posterior wall of the left atrium, and the murmur may be transmitted to the spine or even to the top of the head.

Patients with rheumatic disease of the mitral valve exhibit a spectrum of abnormalities, ranging from pure MS to pure MR. The presence of an S_3, a rapid left ventricular filling wave and left ventricular impulse on palpation, and a soft S_1 all favor predominant MR. In contrast, an accentuated S_1, a prominent OS with a short A_2-OS interval, and a soft, short

TABLE 57–5 Effect of Various Interventions on Systolic Murmurs

Intervention	Hypertrophic Obstructive Cardiomyopathy	Aortic Stenosis	Mitral Regurgitation	Mitral Valve Prolapse
Valsalva	↑	↓	↓	↑ or ↓
Standing	↑	↑ or unchanged	↓	↑
Handgrip or squatting	↓	↓ or unchanged	↑	↓
Supine position with legs elevated	↓	↑ or unchanged	Unchanged	↓
Exercise	↑	↑ or unchanged	↓	↑
Amyl nitrite	↑↑	↑	↓	↑
Isoproterenol	↑↑	↑	↓	↑

Modified from Paraskos JA: Combined valvular disease. *In* Dalen JE, Alpert JS, Rahimtoola SH (eds): Valvular Heart Disease. 3rd ed. Philadelphia, Lippincott Williams & Wilkins, 2000, p 332.

↑↑ = markedly increased.

systolic murmur all point to predominant MS. Elucidation of the predominant valvular lesion may be complicated by the presence of a holosystolic murmur of TR in patients with pure MS and pulmonary hypertension; this murmur may sometimes be heard at the apex when the right ventricle is greatly enlarged and may therefore be mistaken for the murmur of MR.

Laboratory Examination

ELECTROCARDIOGRAPHY. The principal ECG findings are left atrial enlargement and atrial fibrillation. ECG evidence of left ventricular enlargement occurs in about one-third of patients with severe MR. Approximately 15 percent of patients exhibit ECG evidence of right ventricular hypertrophy, a change that reflects the presence of pulmonary hypertension of sufficient severity to counterbalance the hypertrophied left ventricle of MR.

RADIOLOGICAL FINDINGS. Cardiomegaly with left ventricular enlargement, and particularly with left atrial enlargement, is a common finding in patients with chronic, severe MR (see Fig. 12–20). Although the left atrium may be severely enlarged, there is little correlation between left atrial size and pressure. Interstitial edema with Kerley B lines is frequently seen in patients with acute MR or with progressive left ventricular failure.

In patients with combined MS and MR, overall cardiac enlargement and particularly left atrial dilation are prominent findings. However, it is often difficult to determine which lesion is predominant from the plain chest roentgenogram because distinguishing between right and left ventricular enlargement may not be possible. Predominant MS is suggested by relatively mild cardiomegaly (principally straightening of the left cardiac border) and significant changes in the lung fields, whereas predominant MR is more likely when the heart is greatly enlarged and the changes in the lungs are relatively inconspicuous. Chronic MR is almost always the dominant lesion when the left atrium is aneurysmally dilated. *Calcification of the mitral annulus,* an important cause of MR in the elderly, is most prominent in the posterior third of the cardiac silhouette. The lesion is best visualized on chest films exposed in the lateral or right anterior oblique projections, in which it appears as a dense, coarse, C-shaped opacity (see Fig. 12–21).

ECHOCARDIOGRAPHY (see Chap. 11). In patients with severe MR, *two-dimensional echocardiography* shows enlargement of the left atrium and left ventricle, with increased systolic motion of both chambers. The underlying cause of the regurgitation, e.g., rupture of chordae tendineae, MVP (see Fig. 11–61), rheumatic mitral disease, a flail leaflet (see Fig. 57–8A), vegetations (see Chap. 58), and left ventricular dilation (see Fig. 57–8B; see also Fig. 11–57) can often be determined on the transthoracic echocardiogram. It may also show calcification of the mitral annulus as a band of dense echoes between the mitral apparatus and the posterior wall of the heart. This technique is also useful for estimating the hemodynamic consequences of MR; in patients with left ventricular dysfunction, end-diastolic and end-systolic volumes are increased and the ejection fraction and shortening rate may decline.

Doppler echocardiography in MR characteristically reveals a high-velocity jet in the left atrium during systole.[84] Quantitative assessment of the severity of MR has been challenging. The severity of the regurgitation is a function of the distance from the valve that the jet can be detected (see Fig. 11–56) and the size of the left atrium. Qualitative assessment using either color-flow Doppler imaging and pulsed techniques correlates reasonably well with angiographic methods in estimating the severity of MR. However, color-flow jet areas are significantly influenced by the cause of the regurgitation and jet eccentricity, thus limiting the accuracy of this approach.

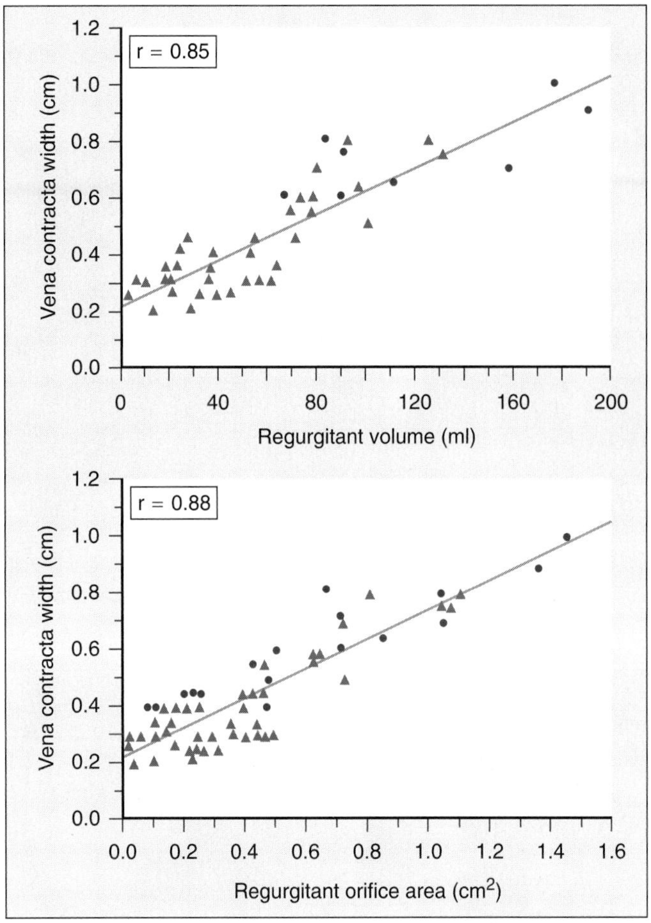

FIGURE 57–15 Linear regression plot showing good correlation between biplane vena contracta width and regurgitant volume (top) and regurgitant orifice area (bottom). Blue triangles indicate central jets and magenta circles indicate eccentric jets. (From Hall SA, Brickner E, Willen DL, et al: Assessment of mitral regurgitation severity by Doppler color-flow mapping of the vena contracta. Circulation 95:636, 1997.)

Quantitative methods to measure regurgitant fraction, regurgitant volume and regurgitant orifice area have greater accuracy in comparison with angiography (see Figs. 11–35 and 11–60),[84,85] and echocardiographic criteria to grade severity of MR have been developed (see Table 11–3).[85a] The vena contracta, defined as the narrowest cross-sectional areas of the regurgitant jet as mapped by color-flow Doppler echocardiography, also predicts the severity of MR (Fig. 57–15).[86,87] The proximal isovelocity surface area method[84] estimates MR severity with isovelocity hemispheric shells as regurgitant flow accelerates toward the mitral orifice. This latter method has not gained widespread acceptance because it is time consuming and has a number of technical limitations. Reversal of flow in the pulmonary veins during systole[88] and a high peak mitral inflow velocity[89] are also useful signs of severe MR. A mitral valve regurgitant index[90] has also been proposed to measure the severity of MR, which incorporates six variables, each graded on a scale from 0 to 3.

Doppler echocardiography is also an important tool to estimate the pulmonary artery systolic pressure and to determine the presence and severity of associated AR or TR.

Transesophageal echocardiography (see Fig. 11–58) is superior to transthoracic echocardiography in assessing the detailed anatomy of the regurgitant mitral valve and in assessing severity of MR.[91,92] Therefore, this technique is useful when the transthoracic image is suboptimal and also when determining whether mitral valve repair is feasible or whether MVR is necessary.[92a] Three-dimensional transthoracic echocardiography and three-dimensional color

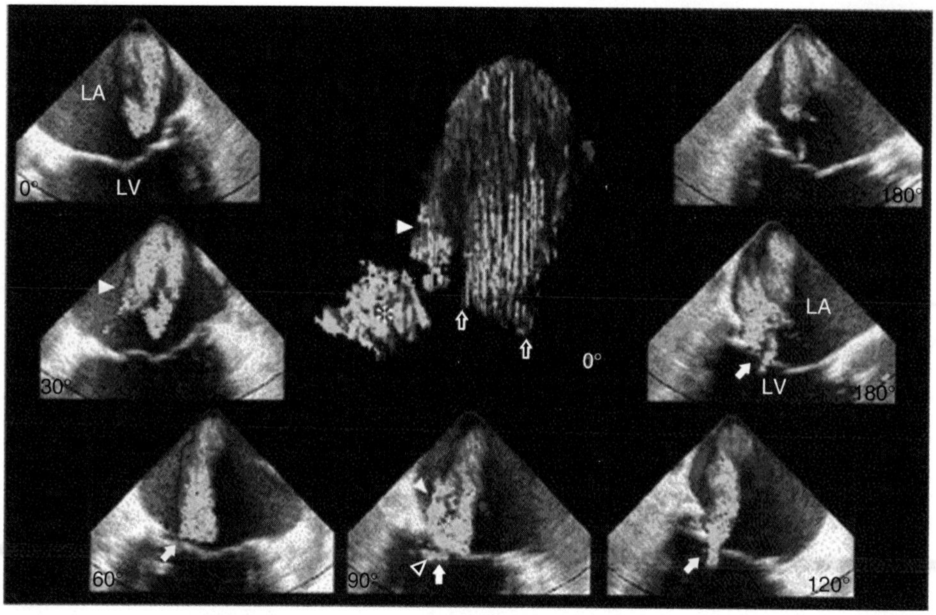

A

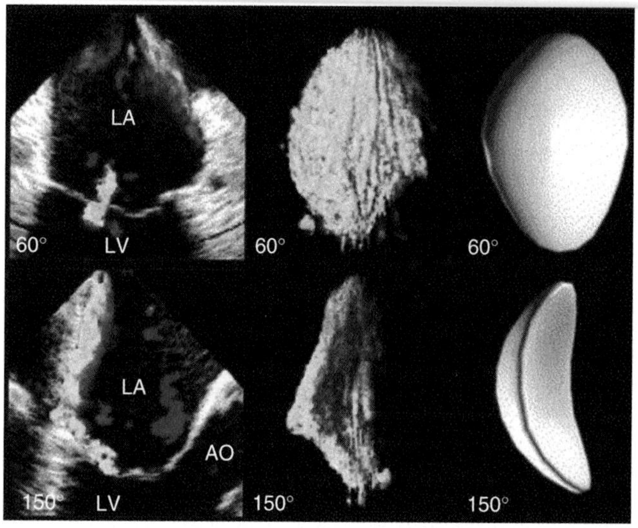

B

FIGURE 57–16 Three-dimensional color Doppler examination of the mitral valve. **A,** Central jet in a patient with moderate-to-severe mitral regurgitation (MR). The origin of the jet can be visualized (arrows) from multiple views from 60 to 150 degrees. The open arrows in the three-dimensional reconstruction show the extension of the regurgitant orifice, which consists of a large linear coaptation defect of the commissures. **B,** Eccentric MR jet with a "spoon" pattern in a patient with anterior leaflet prolapse. The two-dimensional view at 60 degrees can visualize only a portion of the jet at its origin. The two objects at the right represent surface reconstructions of jet geometry. LA = left atrium; LV = left ventricle. (From De Simone R, Glombitza G, Vahl CF, et al: Three-dimensional color Doppler: A clinical study in patients with mitral regurgitation. J Am Coll Cardiol 33:1646, 1999.)

Doppler[93] have also been reported to help elucidate the mechanism of MR (Fig. 57–16; see also Fig. 11–59).

Exercise echocardiography is helpful in determining severity of MR and hemodynamic abnormalities (such as pulmonary hypertension) during exercise.[94] This is a useful, objective means to evaluate symptoms in patients who appear to have only mild MR at rest and, alternatively, to determine functional status and dynamic changes in hemodynamics in patients who otherwise appear stable and asymptomatic.

Radionuclide Angiography (see Chap. 13). Although echocardiography is the imaging method most suited for routine evaluation of structure, function, and MR severity, gated blood pool nuclear imaging or first-pass angiography may be helpful in instances in which the echo images are suboptimal, there is a discrepancy between the clinical and the echocardiographic information, or there is a need for more precise measurement of left ventricular ejection fraction.[1] In addition, right ventricular function can be assessed, and the regurgitant fraction can be estimated from the ratio of left ventricular to right ventricular stroke volume. In patients with MR and impaired left ventricular function, the ejection fraction fails to rise normally during exercise. Radionuclide angiograms are useful for interval follow-up, and progressive decreases in resting ejection fraction into the low-normal range, or progressive increases in left ventricular end-diastolic and/or end-systolic volume, often suggest that surgical treatment is necessary (discussed later).

Left Ventricular Angiocardiography. The prompt appearance of contrast material in the left atrium following its injection into the left ventricle indicates the presence of MR. The injection should be rapid enough to permit left ventricular opacification but slow enough to avoid the development of premature ventricular contractions, which can induce spurious regurgitation.

The regurgitant volume can be determined from the difference between the total left ventricular stroke volume, estimated by angiocardiography, and the simultaneous measurement of the effective forward stroke volume by the Fick method. In patients with severe MR, the regurgitant volume may approach, and even exceed, the effective forward stroke volume. Qualitative but clinically useful estimates of the severity of MR may be made by cineangiographic observation of the degree of opacification of the left atrium and pulmonary veins following the injection of contrast material into the left ventricle.

The cause of the regurgitation (e.g., prolapse of the mitral valve) and a flail leaflet can often be distinguished by angiography, but this assessment has largely been superceded by echocardiography in most institutions. MR secondary to rheumatic heart disease is characterized angiographically by a central regurgitant jet and by thickened leaflets that exhibit reduced motion. In regurgitation due to other causes, particularly dilation or calcification of the mitral annulus or ruptured chordae tendineae and papillary muscles, the systolic jet may be eccentric, and the valves consist of thin filaments that display excessive motion.

Magnetic Resonance Imaging (see Chap. 14). Cardiac magnetic resonance imaging (MRI) provides accurate measurements of regurgitant flow that correlate well with quantitative Doppler imaging.[95] It is also the most accurate noninvasive technique for measuring ventricular end-diastolic volume, end-systolic volume, and mass. Detailed visualization of mitral valve structure and function is obtained more reliably with echocardiography.

Management

Medical Treatment

The role of pharmacological therapy for MR remains a subject of uncertainty and some debate. Although there is no doubt that afterload reduction therapy is indicated and, indeed, may be lifesaving, in patients with *acute* MR, the indications for such therapy in patients with *chronic* MR are much less clear. Because afterload is not excessive in most patients with chronic MR, in whom systolic shortening is facilitated by the reduced systolic wall stress, systemic vasodilator therapy to reduce afterload further may not provide additional benefit. Acute administration of nitroprusside, nifedipine, and

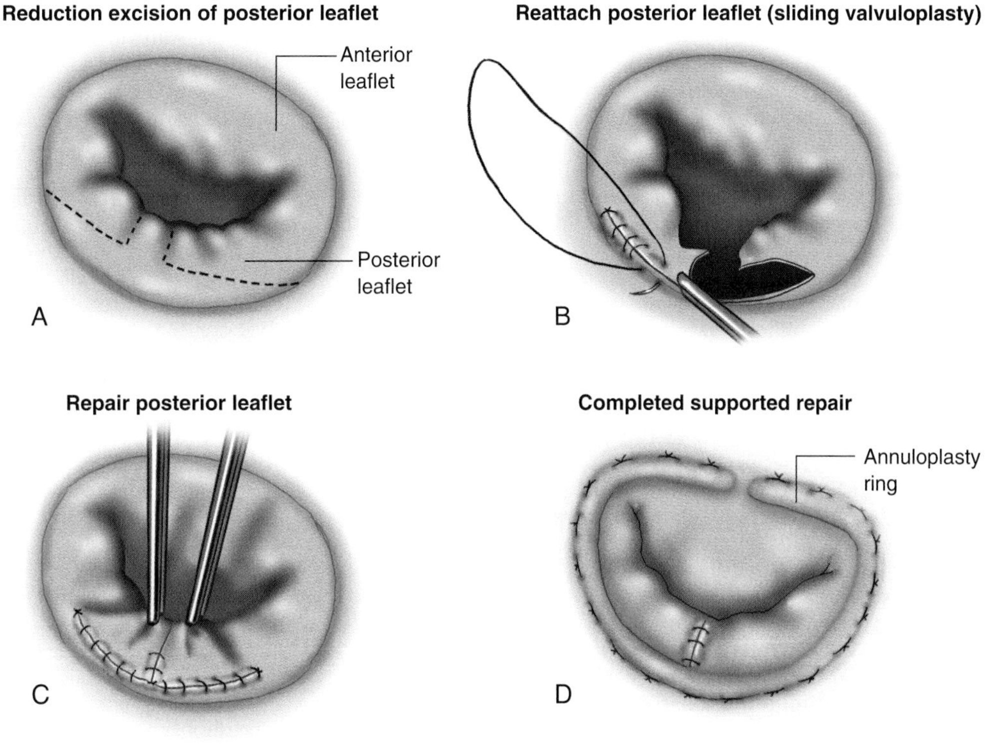

FIGURE 57–17 Mitral valve repair (**A** to **D**) employing reduction excision and reattachment of the posterior leaflet with implantation of an annuloplasty ring. (From Doty DB [ed]: Cardiac Surgery: Operative Technique. St. Louis, Mosby–Year Book, 1997, p 259.)

angiotensin-converting enzyme (ACE) inhibitors to severely symptomatic patients has been demonstrated to alter hemodynamics favorably in some studies, but these effects may not pertain to asymptomatic patients with preserved systolic function. Several small studies of chronic therapy with ACE inhibitors, ranging from 4 weeks to 6 months have failed to provide evidence of hemodynamic benefit,[96] and there are no long-term studies, and no randomized trials, with which to make definitive recommendations. One study investigating oral enalapril treatment in 12 patients with MVP and chronic MR did demonstrate over the course of 6 months that ACE inhibition resulted in significant reductions in end-diastolic and end-systolic volumes and in ventricular mass, along with a significant increase in ejection fraction.[97] It is noteworthy, however, that the mean systolic blood pressure at baseline was 136 ± 15 mm Hg (which was reduced significantly by enalapril), indicating that a high proportion of these patients were hypertensive and that the improvement in left ventricular volume and function was related to blood pressure control. Currently, there is a lack of convincing data that ACE inhibitors affect left ventricular volumes or systolic function favorably in the absence of symptoms or hypertension, and current guidelines do not recommend the use of these agents for chronic therapy.[1,2] An exception would be those patients with severe chronic MR, with symptoms or left ventricular dysfunction (or both) who are not candidates for surgery because of age or other comorbidities. These patients should receive standard, aggressive management for heart failure with ACE inhibitors and beta-adrenergic blocking agents (see Chap. 23).

The accumulating experimental data suggest that beta-blocking drugs may be more beneficial than ACE inhibitors in preserving or improving left ventricular function.[57,71,98,99] Although conceptually attractive, at present there are no clinical data with which to justify chronic beta-blocker therapy.

As do all patients with valvular lesions, patients with MR require appropriate prophylaxis to prevent infective endocarditis (see Chap. 58). All patients with atrial fibrillation, paroxysmal or chronic, should receive chronic anticoagulation.

Surgical treatment should be considered for patients with functional disability and/or for patients with no symptoms or only mild symptoms but with progressively deteriorating left ventricular function or progressively increasing left ventricular dimensions as documented by noninvasive studies.[1,2] The indications for surgery are discussed subsequently.

In patients considered for surgery, two-dimensional transthoracic or transesophageal echocardiography with Doppler echocardiography and color-flow Doppler imaging provide detailed assessment of mitral valve structure and function. However, left-heart catheterization, left ventricular angiocardiography, and coronary arteriography are indicated for the following: (1) in evaluating a discrepancy between echocardiographic findings and the clinical picture; (2) in detecting and assessing the severity of any associated valvular lesions; and (3) in determining the presence and assessing the extent of coronary artery disease.

Surgical Treatment

Without surgical treatment, the prognosis for patients with MR and heart failure is poor (see Fig. 57–4). When operative treatment is being considered, the chronic and often slowly but relentlessly progressive nature of MR must be weighed against the immediate risks and long-term uncertainties attendant on surgery, especially if MVR is required. Surgical mortality depends on the patient's clinical and hemodynamic status (particularly the function of the left ventricle); on the presence of comorbid conditions such as renal, hepatic, or pulmonary disease; and on the skill and experience of the surgical team.[55] The decision to replace or to reconstruct the valve (Fig. 57–17) is of critical importance. Replacement involves the operative risk, as well as the risks of thromboembolism and anticoagulation in patients receiving mechanical prostheses; of late structural valve deterioration in patients receiving bioprostheses; and of late mortality, especially in patients with associated coronary artery disease who require coronary artery bypass grafting (see Table 57–3). Surgical mortality does not depend significantly on *which* of the currently used tissue or mechanical valve prostheses is selected.

Mitral valve repair consists of reconstruction of the valve, which usually is accompanied by an mitral annuloplasty employing a rigid or a flexible prosthetic ring (see Fig. 57–17).[100-103a] Prolapsed valves causing severe MR are usually treated with resection of the prolapsing segment with plication and reinforcement of the annulus. Replacing, reimplanting, elongating, or shortening of chordae tendineae; splitting the papillary muscles; and repairing the subvalvular apparatus have been successful in selected patients with pure or predominant MR in whom subvalvular pathology contributes to the MR.[100-104] Reconstruction of the mitral valve is most often successful in (1) children and adolescents with pliable valves; (2) adults with MR secondary to MVP; (3) annular dilation; (4) papillary muscle secondary to ischemia, dysfunction, or rupture; or (5) chordal rupture and perforation of a mitral leaflet due to infective endocarditis. These procedures are less likely to be successful in older patients with the rigid, calcified, deformed valves of rheumatic heart disease or those with severe subvalvular chordal thickening, mitral annular calcification, and major loss of leaflet substance. Many of the latter patients require MVR, which is also usually the procedure of choice for patients with badly scarred mitral valves who have previously undergone mitral valve repair. Young patients in developing countries who have severe rheumatic MR in the absence of active carditis may undergo successful repair.

Ischemic MR following rupture of a papillary muscle head during acute myocardial infarction may be managed by reattaching the papillary muscle to adjacent myocardium or by MVR. Episodic MR due to transient ischemia is often eliminated by coronary revascularization, whereas moderate to severe, chronic MR secondary ischemic heart disease usually requires MVR or repair.[105,106] Ischemic MR secondary to severe annular dilation may be treated by direct or ring annuloplasty. Annuloplasty is also successful in many patients with significant functional MR resulting from dilated cardiomyopathy.[107-109]

Although MVR with a mechanical or bioprosthesis has been used successfully in treating MR for almost four decades,[110] there has been some dissatisfaction with the results of this operation. First, left ventricular function often deteriorates following this procedure, contributing to early and late mortality and late disability. The increase in afterload consequent to abolishing the low impedance leak was first believed to be responsible, but now it is clear that the loss of annular-chordal-papillary muscle continuity (Fig. 57–18) interferes with left ventricular geometry, volume, and function in patients who have undergone MVR. This does not occur after mitral valve reconstruction. Indeed, animal experiments have shown convincingly that the normal function of the mitral valve apparatus "primes" the left ventricle for normal contraction and that contraction is prevented when operation causes discontinuity of this apparatus.[57] There is evidence from animal experiments and from human patients that preservation of the papillary muscle and its chordal attachments to the mitral annulus is beneficial to postoperative left ventricular function, after both mitral valve reconstruction[76] and in MVR. Thus, preservation of these tissues, whenever possible, is now considered a critical feature of MVR.[111,112]

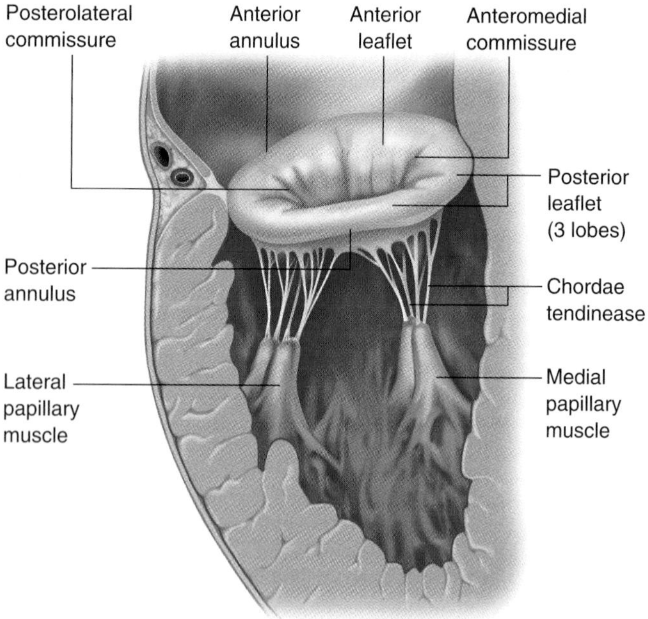

FIGURE 57–18 Continuity of the mitral apparatus and the left ventricular myocardium. Mitral regurgitation (MR) may be caused by any condition that affects the leaflets or the structure and function of the left ventricle. Similarly, a surgical procedure that disrupts the mitral apparatus in an attempt to correct MR has adverse effects on left ventricular geometry, volume, and function. (From Otto CM: Evaluation and management of chronic mitral regurgitation. N Engl J Med 345:740, 2001.)

A second disadvantage of MVR results from the prosthesis itself. This includes thromboembolism or hemorrhage associated with mechanical prostheses, late mechanical dysfunction of bioprostheses, and the risk of infective endocarditis with all prostheses. For these reasons, increasing efforts are being made to reconstruct the mitral valve whenever possible, especially in patients with isolated or predominant MR.[100-103] The Society of Thoracic Surgeons National Database Committee reported an operative mortality rate of less than 2 percent in 3309 patients undergoing isolated mitral valve repair in 2002.[113] This compares favorably to the 6 percent operative mortality for the 4064 patients undergoing isolated MVR.

Intraoperative transesophageal color-flow Doppler mapping is extremely useful in assessing the adequacy of mitral valve repair.[114] In a few patients with persistent severe MR in whom the operative results are unsatisfactory, the problem can usually be corrected immediately, or, if necessary, the valve can be replaced. Left ventricular outflow tract obstruction due to systolic anterior motion of the mitral valve occurs in 5 to 10 percent of patients following mitral valve repair. The causes are not clear, but they may include excess valvular tissue with severe leaflet redundancy and/or an interventricular septum bulging into a small left ventricle. These complications may also be recognized intraoperatively by transesophageal echocardiography. Treatment with volume-loading and beta-blocking agents is often helpful. The obstruction usually disappears with time; if it does not, reoperation and re-repair or MVR may be necessary.

Progressive decrease in the prevalence of rheumatic heart disease (involving severely damaged valves that often are not suitable for reconstructive surgery) and a simultaneous increase in degenerative causes of MR (including MVP and rupture of chordae tendineae) as well as in ischemic MR are increasing the number of patients in whom reconstruction is carried out.[76,114a] In many centers in the United States, approximately two-thirds of all patients requiring operation for pure or predominant MR now receive reconstructive procedures, and the remainder undergo MVR. However, at the current time, the Society of Thoracic Surgeons National Cardiac Surgery Database indicates that most patients in the United States undergoing mitral valve surgery receive MVR rather than repair.[113,114a] Mitral valve repair is technically a more demanding procedure than is MVR, with a distinct learning curve for the surgeon. Furthermore, some regurgitant valves, particularly those that are thickened, severely deformed, calcified, and partly stenotic, are not suitable for reconstruction, and patients with these valves require MVR.[65,66,110,115] In addition, MR recurs after valve repair in a subset of patient with degenerative valve disease.[116]

Minimally invasive surgical techniques utilizing a small, low, asymmetrical sternotomy or anterior thoracotomy[117,118] and percutaneous cardiopulmonary bypass,[119] although quite demanding technically, have been found to be less traumatic and can be employed for both valve repair and replacement. This approach has been reported to reduce cost, improve cosmetic results, and shorten the recovery time.[120] However, it also is technically difficult and is successfully performed by only a few cardiac surgeons.

SURGICAL RESULTS. Mortality rates of 3 to 9 percent are now common in many centers for patients with pure or predominant MR (NYHA Class II or III) who undergo elective isolated MVR. The Society of Thoracic Surgeons National Database Committee reported an overall operative mortality rate of 6.04 percent in 16,105 patients undergoing isolated MVR between 1994 and 1997 (see Table 57–3); this compares with 4 percent for isolated aortic valve replacement (AVR) and 2 to 3 percent for isolated mitral valve repair.[55,113] The combination of MVR with coronary artery bypass grafting was associated with a mortality rate of 13.3 percent during this same period. The mortality rate is higher (≤25 percent) in older patients with severe left ventricular dysfunction, especially when MR is secondary to myocardial ischemia, when pulmonary or renal function is impaired, or when the operation must be carried out as an emergency. Age per se is no barrier to successful surgery; MVR can be performed in patients older than 75 years of age if their general health status is adequate; however, surgery in these patients has a higher risk than in younger patients.[76]

Surgical treatment substantially improves survival in patients with symptomatic MR. Preoperative factors such as age less than 60 years, NYHA Class II, a cardiac index exceeding 2.0 liter/min/m^2, a left ventricular end-diastolic pressure less than 12 mm Hg, and a normal ejection fraction and end-systolic volume all correlate with excellent immediate and long-term survival rates. Both preoperative ejection fraction (see Fig. 57–10) and end-systolic diameter (see Fig. 57–11) are important predictors of short-term and long-term outcomes.[76,77] Excellent survival is observed in patients with end-systolic diameters less than 45 mm and ejection fractions of 0.60 or more. Intermediate outcomes are seen in patients with end-systolic diameters between 45 and 52 mm and ejection fractions between 0.50 and 0.60. Poor outcomes are associated with values beyond these limits.

A large proportion of operative survivors have improved clinical status, quality of life, and exercise tolerance following valve replacement or repair. Severe pulmonary hypertension is reduced, left ventricular end-diastolic volume and mass decrease, and coronary flow reserve increases.[74] Depressed contractile function improves, especially if the papillary muscles and chordal attachment to the annulus remain intact.[121] However, patients with MR who have marked left ventricular dysfunction preoperatively sometimes remain symptomatic with a depressed ejection fraction despite a technically satisfactory surgical procedure.[76] Indeed, progressive left ventricular dysfunction and death from heart failure may occur in adults. Recovery of left ventricular function is much better in children.[122] Long-term survival in patients with predominant MR who undergo MVR may be poorer than in those with pure MS or with mixed stenotic and regurgitant lesions, presumably because left ventricular dysfunction may be quite advanced and largely irreversible by the time patients with pure MR develop serious symptoms. Ten-year survival was 76 percent in patients in NYHA Class I or II versus 48 percent in patients in Class III or IV.[123] Thus, every effort should be made to operate on patients before they develop serious symptoms. However, even though operating on patients with MR is clearly desirable before they develop marked left ventricular dysfunction[1,57,76] and despite the limitations of the results of surgical treatment, operation is still indicated in most patients with left ventricular dysfunction because conservative therapy has little to offer. Postoperative survival rates are lower in patients in atrial fibrillation than those in sinus rhythm.[124] As with patients with MS, the arrhythmia by itself does not unfavorably influence outcome but is a marker for older age and other clinical and hemodynamic features associated with less optimal results.

The cause of MR also plays an important role in the outcome following surgical treatment.[65,66,101-105,107,108] In patients in whom mitral dysfunction is secondary to ischemic heart disease, the 5-year survival rate is about 40 percent, whereas in patients with rheumatic MR it is approximately 75 percent. Occlusive coronary artery disease coexisting with, but not the primary cause of, mitral dysfunction requires simultaneous coronary artery bypass grafting and mitral valve repair or replacement[125] and is associated with decreased perioperative and long-term postoperative survival (Fig. 57–19). However, some improvement resulting from mitral valve repair or replacement can be expected even in patients with MR secondary to ischemic heart disease who

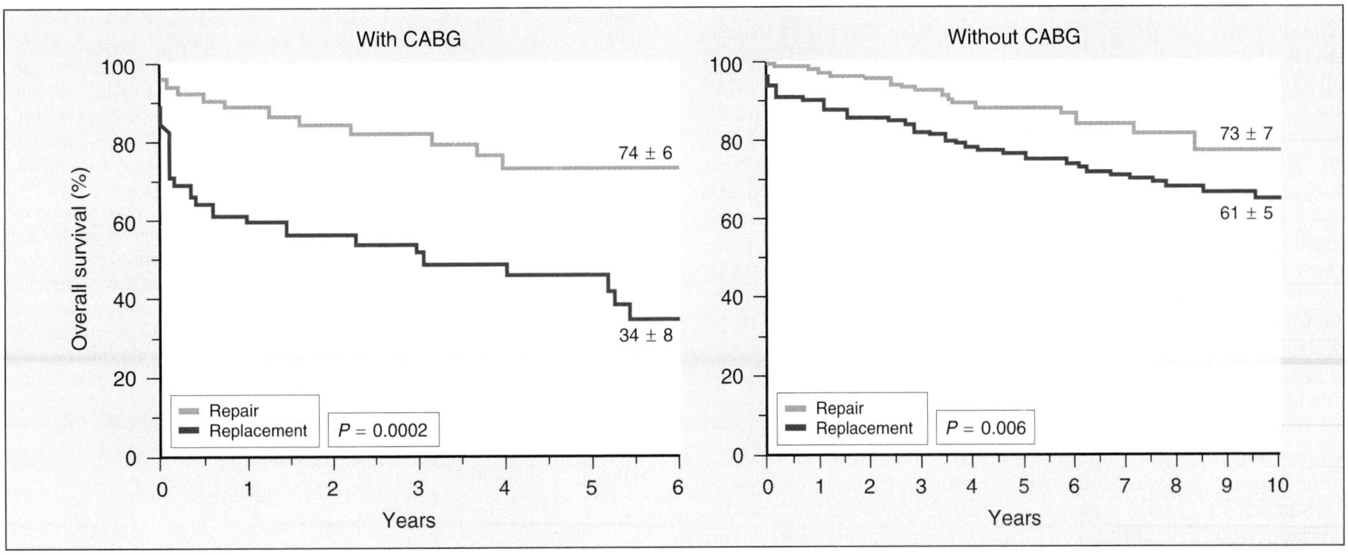

FIGURE 57–19 Plots of overall survival compared for mitral repair and replacement groups in patients who had **(left)** or did not have **(right)** associated coronary artery bypass grafting (CABG). Note that the outcome is better with repair than with replacement in both groups and that the outcome is worse in patients who underwent CABG and mitral valve replacement. (From Enriquez-Sarano M, Schaff HV, Orszulak TA, et al: Valve repair improves the outcome of surgery for mitral regurgitation: A multivariate analysis. Circulation 91:1022, 1995.)

have not responded to medical treatment and now have congestive heart failure, as long as the cardiac index exceeds 1.8 liter/min/m^2 and the ejection fraction is greater than 0.30. When left ventricular dysfunction is more severe, however, the risk of perioperative death becomes very high.[66]

INDICATIONS FOR OPERATION

The threshold for surgical treatment of MR is declining for several reasons. These include the reductions in operative mortality, the improvements in both mitral valve reconstructive procedures and procedures involving prosthetic valves, and the recognition of the poor long-term results in many patients whose MR is corrected only after a long history of symptoms, impaired left ventricular function, atrial fibrillation, or pulmonary hypertension.

A detailed echocardiographic examination should be carried out to assess the likelihood that mitral valve repair, rather than replacement, is possible. In addition, the difference in outcome between these procedures should be weighed when deciding whether or not to proceed. Asymptomatic patients (NYHA Class I) should be considered for mitral valve reconstruction only if they have left ventricular dysfunction (ejection fraction ≤ 0.60 and/or left ventricular end-systolic diameter ≤ 45 mm).[1] Class I patients with normal left ventricular function should be followed clinically and by echocardiography every 6 to 12 months. Rarely, they *may* be considered for operation if atrial fibrillation or pulmonary hypertension is present. At times, a careful history and performance of an exercise test often reveal that these patients are not truly asymptomatic.[1,94] Patients with severe MR who are asymptomatic, who perform well on an exercise test, and who have excellent ventricular function (ejection fraction > 0.70, end-systolic diameter < 40 mm, end-systolic volume < 40 ml/m^2) can be followed by echocardiography every 6 to 12 months. However, operation may be considered even in asymptomatic patients if they are younger than 70 years of age, if they are likely to be candidates for mitral valve repair, and if ventricular function (as reflected by end-systolic diameter and ejection fraction) shows *progressive* deterioration. If MVR is likely to be necessary, a higher threshold for clinical and hemodynamic impairment should be employed than if valve reconstruction is contemplated. Because of the higher operative mortality, older patients (>75 years of age) should, in general, undergo surgery only if they are symptomatic.

In asymptomatic patients with severe MR, a lower threshold for surgery may be entertained in patients with progressive enlargement of the left atrium (>45 to 50 mm) in whom successful mitral valve repair appears highly likely. A number of centers are moving toward a more aggressive surgical approach in which surgery is recommended to *all* patients with severe MR, independent of symptoms of left ventricular function. Such a recommendation should be considered *only* in centers in which the surgical experience indicates that the patient will undergo successful mitral valve repair with a high degree of certainty. Unfortunately, successful mitral valve repair cannot be guaranteed, and even in the best of circumstances, with this approach some young asymptomatic patients will be subjected to the risks of prosthetic valves prematurely and unnecessarily.

Patients with severe MR and moderate or severe symptoms (NYHA Classes II, III, and IV) should generally be considered for surgery. One exception is a patient in whom echocardiography suggests that MVR will be required and whose ejection fraction is less than 0.30. Because of the high risk of operation in these patients, medical therapy is usually advised, but the outcome is poor in any event. However, when mitral valve repair appears possible, even patients with serious left ventricular dysfunction may be considered for operation.[107-109]

ACUTE MITRAL REGURGITATION

The causes of acute MR are shown at the top of Table 57–4. They are diverse and represent acute manifestations of disease processes that may, under other circumstances, cause chronic MR. Especially important causes of acute MR are spontaneous rupture of chordae tendineae, infective endocarditis with disruption of valve leaflets or chordal rupture, ischemic dysfunction or rupture of a papillary muscle, and malfunction of a prosthetic valve.

One major hemodynamic difference between acute and chronic MR derives from the differences in left atrial compliance, as illustrated in Figure 57–13. Acute, severe MR causes a marked reduction of forward stroke volume, a slight reduction of end-systolic volume, and an increase in end-diastolic volume. Patients who develop acute, severe MR usually have a normal-sized left atrium (normal or reduced left atrial compliance [first subgroup]). The left atrial pressure rises abruptly, which often leads to pulmonary edema, marked elevation of pulmonary vascular resistance, and right-sided heart failure.

Because the *v* wave is markedly elevated in patients with acute, severe MR, the reverse pressure gradient between the left ventricle and left atrium declines at the end of systole, and the murmur may be decrescendo rather than holosystolic, ending well before A_2. It is usually lower pitched and softer than the murmur of chronic MR. A left-sided S_4 is frequently found.[130] Pulmonary hypertension, which is common in patients with acute MR, may increase the intensity of P_2 and the murmurs of pulmonary and TR may also develop along with a right-sided S_4. In patients with severe, acute MR, a *v* wave (late systolic pressure rise) in the pulmonary artery pressure pulse (see Fig. 57–12; see also Fig. 17–5) may rarely cause premature closure of the pulmonary valve, an early P_2, and paradoxical splitting of S_2. Acute MR, even if severe, often does not increase overall cardiac size, as seen on the chest roentgenogram, and may produce only mild left atrial enlargement despite marked elevation of left atrial pressure. In addition, the echocardiogram may show little increase in the internal diameter of either the left atrium or the left ventricle, but increased systolic motion of the left ventricle is prominent. Characteristic features on Doppler echocardiography are the severe jet of MR and elevation of the pulmonary artery systolic pressure.

Medical Management of Acute Mitral Regurgitation. Afterload reduction with afterload reducing agents is of particular importance in treating patients with acute MR. Intravenous nitroprusside may be lifesaving in patients with acute MR due to rupture of the head of a papillary muscle that occurs during an acute myocardial infarction. It may permit stabilization of the patient's condition and thereby allow coronary arteriography and surgery to be performed with the patient in optimal condition. In patients with acute MR who are hypotensive, an inotropic agent such as dobutamine should be administered with the nitroprusside. Intraaortic balloon counterpulsation may be necessary to stabilize the patient as preparations for surgery are made.

Surgical Treatment of Acute Mitral Regurgitation. Emergency surgical treatment may be required for patients with acute left ventricular failure caused by acute MR. Emergency surgery is associated with higher mortality rates than is elective surgery for chronic MR. However, unless patients with acute, severe MR and heart failure are treated aggressively, a fatal outcome is almost certain. If patients with MR secondary to acute myocardial infarction can be stabilized by medical treatment, it is preferable to defer operation until 4 to 6 weeks after the infarction. Vasodilator treatment may be useful during this period. However, medical management should not be prolonged if multisystem (renal and/or pulmonary) failure develops. Intraaortic balloon counterpulsation may be required to stabilize the patient preoperatively. Surgical mortality rates are also higher in patients with acute MR and refractory heart failure (NYHA Class IV), in those in whom a previously implanted prosthetic valve must be replaced because of thromboembolism or valve dysfunction, and in those with active infective endocarditis (of either a natural or a prosthetic valve). Despite the higher surgical risks, the efficacy of early operation has been established in patients with infective endocarditis complicated by medically uncontrollable congestive heart failure and/or recurrent emboli (see Chap. 58). Because fungal endocarditis responds poorly to medical management, the practice now is to recommend valve replacement in these patients *before* the onset of heart failure or embolization.

Mitral Valve Prolapse Syndrome

Etiology and Pathology

DEFINITION. The MVP syndrome has been given many names, including the *systolic click-murmur syndrome, Barlow syndrome, billowing mitral cusp syndrome, myxomatous mitral valve syndrome, floppy valve syndrome,* and *redundant cusp syndrome.*[126-129] It is a variable clinical syndrome that results from diverse pathogenic mechanisms of one or more portions of the mitral valve apparatus, valve leaflets, chordae tendineae, papillary muscle, and valve annulus. The MVP syndrome is one of the most prevalent cardiac valvular abnormalities and was previously thought to affect as much as 5 to 15 percent of the population.[130,131] It now appears likely that overdiagnosis occurred in many individuals, perhaps because of the absence of rigorous echocardiographic criteria. Using such criteria (to be discussed), a community-based study showed that MVP syndrome occurred in only 2.4 percent of the population.[131] The syndrome is twice as frequent in women as in men. However, serious MR occurs more frequently in older men (>50 years) with MVP than in young women with this disorder.

Normally, the mitral valve billows slightly into the left atrium, and an exaggerated finding should be termed *billowing mitral valve.* A "floppy valve" is regarded as an extreme form of billowing. MR occurs when the leaflet edges of the valve do not coapt. With chordal rupture, the prolapsed mitral valve is "flail," which is almost always associated with severe MR. Obviously, these conditions blend into one another, and it is often difficult to distinguish among them.

The criteria for the diagnosis of MVP have been divided into three groups (Table 57–6): (1) major criteria, the presence of one or more of which establishes the diagnosis of MVP; (2) minor criteria, the presence of which cannot be discounted and should raise the suspicion of MVP but which by themselves are not sufficient to establish the diagnosis; and (3) other findings not shown in Table 57–6, which, although often present in patients with MVP, are nonspecific. Superior displacement of the mitral valve leaflets by more than 2 mm above the plane of the annulus is an important two-dimensional echocardiographic criterion,[131,132] and systolic displacement of one or both mitral leaflets into the left atrium in the *parasternal view* improves the specificity of this finding (see Fig. 11–61). The latter criterion avoids overdiagnosis, which may occur with posterior bowing of the mitral valve on M-mode echocardiography and even in the four-chamber view on two-dimensional echocardiography.

TABLE 57–6 Diagnostic Criteria in Mitral Valve Prolapse

Major Criteria
Auscultation
Mid to late systolic clicks and late systolic murmur or "whoop" alone or in combination at the cardiac apex
Two-dimensional echocardiogram
Marked superior systolic displacement of mitral leaflets (≥2 mm above annulus) with coaptation point at or superior to annular plane
Mild to moderate superior systolic displacement of mitral leaflets with
Chordal rupture
Doppler mitral regurgitation
Annular dilation
Echocardiogram plus auscultation
Mild to moderate superior systolic displacement of mitral leaflets with
Prominent mid to late systolic clicks at the cardiac apex
Apical late systolic or holosystolic murmur in the young patient
Late systolic "whoop"
Minor Criteria
Auscultation
Loud S_1 with an apical holosystolic murmur
Two-dimensional echocardiogram
Isolated mild to moderate superior systolic displacement of the posterior mitral leaflet
Moderate superior systolic displacement of both mitral leaflets
Echocardiogram plus history of
Mild to moderate superior systolic displacement of mitral leaflets with
Focal neurologic attacks or amaurosis fugax in the young patient
First-degree relatives with major criteria

Modified from Perloff JK, Child JS, Edwards JE: New guidelines for the clinical diagnosis of mitral valve prolapse. Am J Cardiol 57:1124, 1986.

ETIOLOGY. Most frequently, MVP occurs as a primary condition that is not associated with other diseases. However, it has also been associated with many conditions. MVP occurs quite commonly in heritable disorders of connective tissue that increase the size of the mitral leaflets and apparatus, including Marfan syndrome (see Chap. 70), Ehlers-Danlos syndrome (see Chap. 70), osteogenesis imperfecta, pseudoxanthoma elasticum, periarteritis nodosa, myotonic dystrophy, von Willebrand disease, hyperthyroidism, and congenital malformations such as Ebstein anomaly of the tricuspid valve, atrial septal defect of the ostium secundum variety, Holt-Oram syndrome, and hypertrophic cardiomyopathy. There may be a higher incidence of MVP in patients with an asthenic habitus and various congenital thoracic deformities, including "straight back" syndrome, pectus excavatum, and a shallow chest. These associations have not been proved using rigorous echocardiographic criteria, and, with the exception of connective tissue disorders, it is not clear how many of these are chance associations.

PATHOLOGY (Fig. 57–20). Findings include myxomatous proliferation of the mitral valve, in which the spongiosa component of the valve (i.e., the middle layer of the leaflet composed of loose, myxomatous material) is unusually prominent,[129,132,133] and the quantity of acid mucopolysaccharide is increased (see Fig. 57–20).[134] Electron microscopy shows a haphazard arrangement of cells with disruption and with fragmentation of collagen fibrils.

In mild cases, the valvular myxoid stroma is enlarged on histological examination, but the leaflets are grossly normal. However, with increasing quantities of myxoid stroma, the leaflets become grossly abnormal, redundant, and prolapsed. Regions of endothelial disruption are common and are possible sites of endocarditis or thrombus formation. The severity of MR depends on the extent of the prolapse. The cusps of the mitral valve, the chordae tendineae, and the annulus all may be affected by myxomatous proliferation. Degeneration of collagen and myxomatous changes within the central core of the chordae tendineae, with associated decreases in tensile strength,[62,133] are primarily responsible for chordal rupture, which often occurs and may intensify the severity of MR. Increased chordal tension resulting from the enlarged area of the valve cusps may play a contributory role. Myxomatous changes in the annulus may result in annular dilation and calcification, further contributing to the severity of MR.

Myxomatous proliferation, although most commonly affecting the mitral valve, has also been described in the tricuspid, aortic, and pulmonic valves, particularly in patients

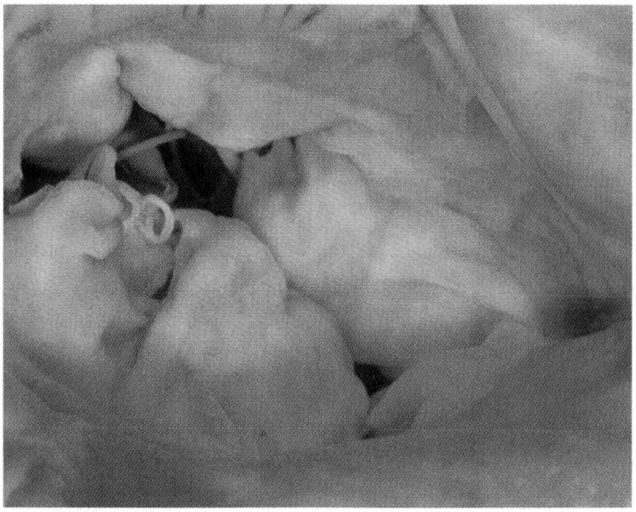

A

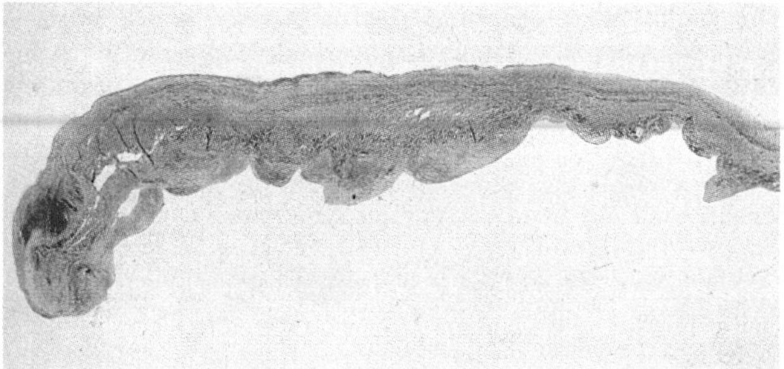

B

FIGURE 57–20 **A,** Myxomatous mitral valve in a patient with severe mitral regurgitation, viewed from the left atrium. The surface area of the valve is increased, with increased folding of the valve surface. Individual scallops of the posterior leaflet are enlarged and redundant. **B,** Histological section of posterior valve leaflet from a patient with mitral valve prolapse. The valve is thickened with marked myxomatous proliferation and interruption of the fibrosa and atrialis by the spongiosa tissue. There are extensive deposits of acid mucopolysaccharides (blue-green staining) expanding the spongiosa and extending into the fibrosa. (From Becker AE, Anderson RH [eds]: Cardiac Pathology: An Integrated Text and Colour Atlas. New York, Raven Press, 1983, pp 4.8 and 4.11.)

with Marfan syndrome, and may lead to regurgitation of these valves as well as the mitral valve.

The MVP syndrome can coexist with rheumatic MS, and it may develop following mitral valvotomy. *Ischemic heart disease* and MVP are both common disorders and sometimes coexist. MVP may also occur secondary to papillary muscle dysfunction. In some patients, MVP has been documented to develop for the first time *following* myocardial infarction. It has been proposed that MVP may *cause* myocardial ischemia by increasing tension on the base of the involved muscle, which may contribute to symptoms in some patients. During systole, the tips of the papillary muscles move basally instead of apically.

Clinical Manifestations

MVP syndrome appears to exhibit a strong hereditary component[126] and in some patients is transmitted as an autosomal dominant trait with varying penetrance. The clinical presentations of the MVP syndrome are diverse. The condition has been observed in patients of all ages and in both sexes. Despite the overestimation of the prevalence in the population referred to earlier, MVP is the most common cause of isolated MR requiring surgical treatment in the United States[128,132] and the most common cardiac condition predisposing patients to infective endocarditis (see Chap 58).[135] Echocardiographic evidence of MVP has been found in most patients with Marfan syndrome and in many of their first-degree relatives.

History

Most patients with MVP are asymptomatic and remain so throughout their lives. In many instances, otherwise asymptomatic patients with MVP suffer from undue anxiety, perhaps precipitated by their having been informed of the presence of heart disease. Although early studies called attention to an "MVP syndrome" with a characteristic systolic nonejection click and various nonspecific symptoms, such as fatigability, palpitations, postural orthostasis, and neuropsychiatric symptoms, as well as symptoms of autonomic dysfunction, these associations have not been confirmed in carefully controlled studies.[132] How, and even whether, these symptoms relate to the presence of MVP is not clear.

Patients may complain of syncope, presyncope, palpitations, chest discomfort, and, when MR is severe, symptoms of diminished cardiac reserve. Chest discomfort may be typical of angina pectoris but is more often atypical in that it is prolonged, not clearly related to exertion, and punctuated by brief attacks or severe stabbing pain at the apex. The discomfort may be secondary to abnormal tension on papillary muscles. In patients with MVP and severe MR, the symptoms of the latter (fatigue, dyspnea, and exercise limitation) are present. Patients with MVP may also develop symptomatic arrhythmias (to be discussed).

Physical Examination

The body weight is often low, and the habitus may be asthenic. Blood pressure is usually normal or low; orthostatic hypotension may be present. As already mentioned, patients with MVP have a higher than expected prevalence of straight back syndrome, scoliosis, and pectus excavatum.[129] MR ranges from nonexistent to severe.

AUSCULTATION

The auscultatory findings unique to the MVP syndrome are best elicited with the diaphragm of the stethoscope. The patient should be examined in the supine, left decubitus, and sitting positions. The most important finding is a nonejection systolic click at least 0.14 second after S_1.[136] This can be differentiated from a systolic ejection click because it occurs *after* the beginning of the carotid pulse upstroke. Occasionally, multiple mid and late systolic clicks are audible, most readily along the lower left sternal border. The clicks are believed to be produced by sudden tensing of the elongated chordae tendineae and of the prolapsing leaflets. They are often, although not invariably, followed by a mid to late crescendo systolic murmur that continues to A_2. This murmur is similar to that produced by papillary muscle dysfunction, which is readily understandable because both result from mid to late systolic MR. In general, the duration of the murmur is a function of the severity of the MR. When the murmur is confined to the latter portion of systole, MR usually is not severe. However, as MR becomes more severe, the murmur commences earlier and ultimately becomes holosystolic.

It is important to emphasize the variability of the physical findings in the MVP syndrome. Some patients exhibit both a midsystolic click and a mid to late systolic murmur; others present with only one of these two findings; still others have only a click on one occasion and only a murmur on another, both on a third examination, and no abnormality at all on a fourth. Conditions other than MVP cause midsystolic clicks; these include tricuspid valve prolapse, atrial septal aneurysms, and extracardiac causes.

Dynamic Auscultation. The auscultatory findings are exquisitely sensitive to physiological and pharmacological interventions, and recognition of the changes induced by these interventions is of great value in the diagnosis of the MVP syndrome (Fig. 57–21 and Table 57–5). The mitral valve begins to prolapse when the reduction of left ventricular volume during systole reaches a critical point at which the valve leaflets no longer coapt; at that instant, the click occurs and the murmur commences. Any maneuver that decreases left ventricular volume, such as a reduction of impedance to left ventricular outflow, a reduction in venous

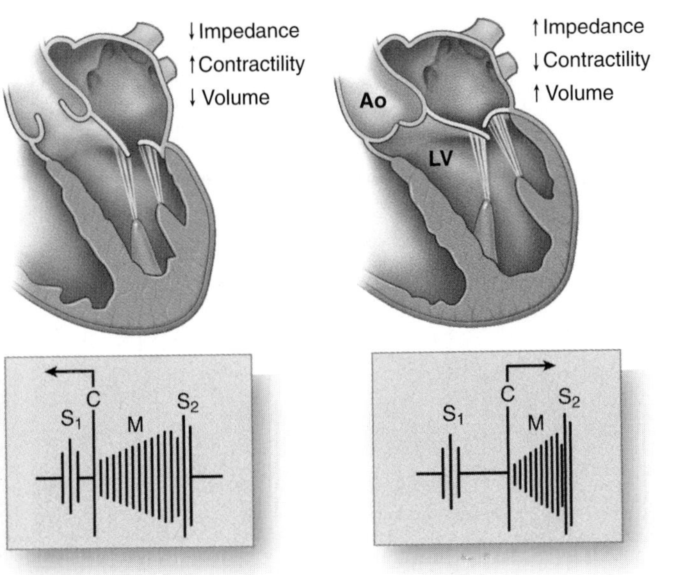

FIGURE 57–21 Dynamic auscultation in mitral valve prolapse. Any maneuver that decreases left ventricular (LV) volume (e.g., decreased venous return, tachycardia, decreased outflow impedance, increased contractility) worsens the mismatch in size between the enlarged mitral valve and LV chamber, resulting in prolapse earlier in systole and movement of the click (C) and murmur (M) toward the first heart sound (S_1). Conversely, maneuvers that increase LV volume (e.g., increased venous return, bradycardia, increased outflow impedance, decreased contractility) delay the occurrence of prolapse, resulting in movement of the click and murmur toward the second heart sound (S_2). Ao = aorta. (Adapted from O'Rourke RA, Crawford MH: The systolic click-murmur syndrome: Clinical recognition and management. Curr Probl Cardiol 1:9, 1976.)

return, tachycardia, or an augmentation of myocardial contractility, results in an earlier occurrence of prolapse during systole. As a consequence, the click and onset of the murmur move closer to S_1. When prolapse is severe and/or left ventricular size is markedly reduced, prolapse may begin with the onset of systole. As a consequence, the click may not be audible, and the murmur may be holosystolic. On the other hand, when left ventricular volume is augmented by an increase in the impedance to left ventricular emptying, an increase in venous return, a reduction of myocardial contractility, or bradycardia, both the click and the onset of the murmur will be delayed.

During the straining phase of the Valsalva maneuver, on sudden standing, and early during the inhalation of amyl nitrite, cardiac size decreases, and both the click and the onset of the murmur occur earlier in systole. In contrast, a sudden change from the standing to the supine position, leg-raising, squatting, maximal isometric exercise, and, to a lesser extent, expiration delay the click and the onset of the murmur. During the overshoot phase of the Valsalva maneuver (i.e., six to eight cycles following release) and with prolongation of the R-R interval, either following a premature contraction or in atrial fibrillation, the click and onset of the murmur are usually delayed, and the intensity of the murmur is reduced. Maneuvers that elevate arterial pressure, such as isometric exercise, increase the intensity of the click and murmur. In general, when the onset of the murmur is delayed, both its duration and intensity are diminished, reflecting a reduction in the severity of MR.

The response to several interventions may be helpful in differentiating obstructive hypertrophic cardiomyopathy from MVP (see Chap. 59). During the strain of the Valsalva maneuver, the murmur of hypertrophic cardiomyopathy increases in intensity, whereas the murmur of MVP becomes longer but usually not louder. The murmur of hypertrophic cardiomyopathy becomes louder after amyl nitrite inhalation, whereas that of MVP does not. Following a premature beat, the murmur of hypertrophic cardiomyopathy increases in intensity and duration, whereas that due to MVP usually remains unchanged or decreases.

Laboratory Examination

ELECTROCARDIOGRAPHY. The ECG is usually normal in asymptomatic patients with MVP. In a minority of asymptomatic patients and in many symptomatic patients, the ECG shows inverted or biphasic T waves and nonspecific ST segment changes in leads II, III, and aVf and occasionally in the anterolateral leads as well.

ARRHYTHMIAS. A spectrum of arrhythmias have been observed in patients with MVP. These include atrial and ventricular premature contractions and supraventricular and ventricular tachyarrhythmias,[132,137] as well as bradyarrhythmias due to sinus node dysfunction or varying degrees of atrioventricular block. The mechanism of the arrhythmias is not clear. Diastolic depolarization of muscle fibers in the anterior mitral leaflet in response to stretch has been demonstrated experimentally, and the abnormal stretch of the prolapsed leaflet may be of pathogenetic significance.

Paroxysmal supraventricular tachycardia is the most common sustained tachyarrhythmia in patients with MVP and may be related to what may be an increased incidence of left atrioventricular bypass tracts. The incidence of MVP among patients with Wolff-Parkinson-White syndrome is increased. There is also an increased association between MVP and prolongation of the QT interval, and this association may play a role in the pathogenesis of serious ventricular arrhythmias. Patients with MVP have an increased incidence of abnormal late potentials on signal-averaged ECGs, as well as reduced heart rate variability.

ECHOCARDIOGRAPHY (see Chap. 11). Echocardiography plays a key role in the diagnosis of MVP and has been most useful in the delineation of this syndrome (Fig. 57–22; see also Figs. 11–61 and 11–62).[138] The most common finding on M-mode echocardiography is abrupt posterior movement of the posterior leaflet or of both mitral leaflets in midsystole with the leaflet interface greater than 2 mm posterior to the C-D line. This movement occurs simultaneously with the systolic click. An alternate finding is pansystolic posterior prolapse of one or both leaflets, giving rise to a U- or hammock-shaped configuration 3 mm or more posterior to the C-D segment.

To establish the diagnosis, the two-dimensional echocardiogram must show that one or both mitral valve leaflets billow by at least 2 mm into the left atrium during systole in the long-axis view.[131,132,139] Thickening of the involved leaflet to greater than 5 mm supports the diagnosis. Findings of more severe myxomatous disease include increased leaflet area, leaflet redundancy, chordal elongation and annular dilation (see Fig. 57–22; see also Fig. 11–61). These findings are also helpful in identifying patients at significant risk for developing severe MR or infective endocarditis (Table 57–7). The mitral annular diameter is often abnormally increased. Transesophageal echocardiography provides additional details regarding integrity of the mitral valve apparatus, such as rupture of chordae tendineae. In MR secondary to MVP, the echocardiogram also provides valuable information regarding left ventricular size and function.

The variability in physical findings in this syndrome, already commented on, extends to the echocardiogram. Thus, some patients have a systolic click with or without a murmur and show no evidence of MVP on the echocardiogram. Conversely, the echocardiographic findings of MVP may be observed in patients without a click or murmur. Others have both the typical echocardiographic and auscultatory features. The echocardiographic findings of MVP have been reported to occur in a large number of first-degree relatives of patients with established MVP. Two-dimensional echocardiography has also revealed prolapse of the tricuspid and aortic valves in approximately 20 percent of patients with MVP.[132] Conversely, however, prolapse of the tricuspid and aortic valves occurs *uncommonly* in patients without prolapse of the mitral valve.

Doppler echocardiography frequently reveals mild MR that is not always associated with an audible murmur. Color-flow Doppler echocardiography is useful in identifying the

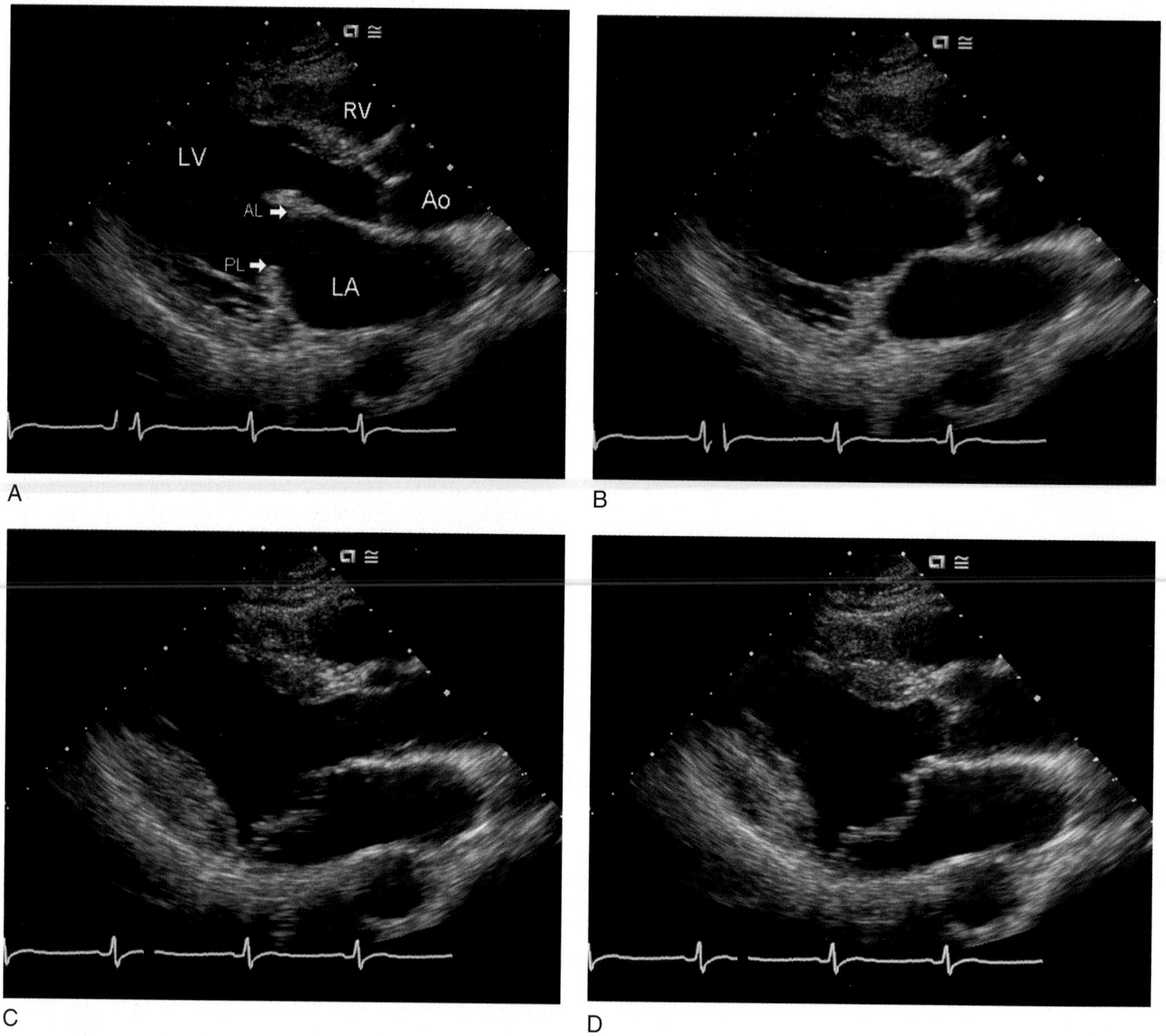

FIGURE 57–22 Parasternal long-axis two-dimensional echocardiographic images in a 41-year-old man with mitral valve prolapse and auscultatory findings of a midsystolic click and mitral regurgitation (MR). **A,** End-diastolic image. The mitral valve leaflets are severely thickened, and the anterior leaflet (AL) is elongated. **B** to **D,** Serial images from early systole to midsystole, demonstrating bileaflet prolapse, Color-flow imaging in this patient demonstrated severe MR. Patients with these findings are at increased risk of complications, such as infective endocarditis, systemic emboli, and heart failure. Ao = aorta; LA = left atrium; LV = left ventricle; PL = posterior leaflet; RV = right ventricle.

TABLE 57–7 Predictors of Clinical Outcome in Mitral Valve Prolapse

	Survival	Valve Surgery	Arrbythmias/Sudden Death	Endocarditis
Age	+++*	+++	–	–
Gender	++	++	–	–
Leaflet thickness or redundancy	+++	+++	++++	++++
Severity of mitral regurgitation	++++	++++	++++	++++
Systolic click	+	–	–	–
Left ventricular dilation	+	++++	++	–
Left atrial dilation	–	++	+	–

From Otto CM: Valvular Heart Disease. 2nd ed. Philadelphia, WB Saunders, 2004, p 376.

*The symbols indicate the relative predictive value of each variable for the listed clinical outcomes on a scale of no predictive value (–) to strongly predictive (++++).

location and severity of the regurgitant jets. MR is moderate or severe in about 10 percent of patients with MVP, most commonly in men older than 50 years of age.[140]

STRESS SCINTIGRAPHY. The differential diagnosis between two common conditions—MVP associated with atypical chest pain and ECG abnormalities and primary coronary artery disease associated with MVP—may be aided by exercise ECG. However, myocardial perfusion scintigraphy using thallium-201 or sestamibi during pharmacological exercise stress (see Chap. 13) is more specific. When findings are normal, i.e., when there is no evidence of stress-induced regional myocardial ischemia, the diagnosis of MVP unrelated to ischemic heart disease is favored.

ANGIOGRAPHY. The configuration of the left ventriculogram during systole is helpful in confirming the diagnosis of MVP. The right anterior oblique projection is most useful for defining the posterior leaflet of the mitral valve, and the left anterior oblique projection is most useful for studying the anterior leaflet. The most helpful sign is extension of the mitral leaflet tissue inferiorly and posteriorly to the point of attachment of the mitral leaflets to the mitral annulus. Angiography may also reveal scalloped edges of the leaflets, reflecting redundancy of tissue. Other abnormalities noted on angiography of some patients with MVP include dilation, decreased systolic contraction, and calcification of the mitral annulus and poor contraction of the basal portion of the left ventricle.

MAGNETIC RESONANCE IMAGING AND CARDIAC COMPUTED TOMOGRAPHY. These advanced imaging techniques can help in determining the extent of MVP and left ventricular function in patients with suboptimal echocardiographic examinations (see Fig. 15–11). MRI is also useful for evaluating the presence and severity of MR.

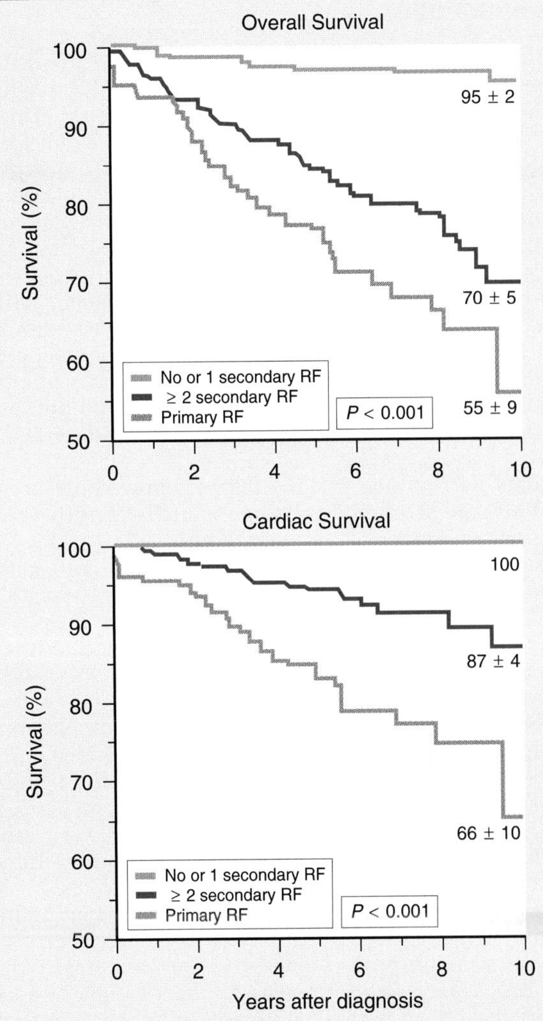

FIGURE 57–23 Survival in patients with mitral valve prolapse according to categories of baseline risk factors (RFs). Primary RFs were moderate-to-severe mitral regurgitation (MR) and ejection fraction less than 0.50. Secondary RFs were mild MR, left atrium larger than 40 mm, flail leaflet, atrial fibrillation, and age older than 50 years. (Adapted from Avierinos JF, Gersh BJ, Melton LJ, et al: Natural history of asymptomatic mitral valve prolapse in the community. Circulation 106:1355, 2002.)

NATURAL HISTORY

The outlook for patients with MVP in general is excellent; most remain asymptomatic for many years without any change in clinical or laboratory findings.[1,126,131,141,142] Zuppiroli and associates monitored 316 patients with MVP for an average of more than 8 years; 70 percent were women and 29 percent had familial MVP.[141] Serious complications (cardiac death, need for cardiac surgery, acute infective endocarditis, or cerebral embolic events) occurred at a rate of only 1 per 100 patient years, and 4 percent of patients died during the 8 years. In contrast, Avierinos and colleagues[143] observed a much more aggressive natural history in 833 patients with MVP, with a 19 percent mortality rate at 10 years and a 20 percent rate of MVP-related events, including heart failure, atrial fibrillation, cerebrovascular events, arterial thromboembolism, and endocarditis. The apparent differences between these two series can be reconciled by the finding in the latter series that patients with MVP could be risk stratified on the basis of several factors (Fig. 57-23).[143] The primary risk factors were moderate to severe MR and/or left ventricular ejection fraction less than 0.50, and secondary risk factors included mild MR, left atrial dimension greater than 40 mm, flail leaflet, and age older than 50 years. Patients with a primary risk factor had excessive mortality and morbidity, as did those with two or more secondary risk factors.[143] The data of Zuppiroli and coworkers[141] are concordant with these observations, since their patients had a high likelihood of dying or having MVP-related complications if they were men (17 percent with events), were older than 45 years of age (15 percent), or had a holosystolic murmur (67 percent) or left atrial dimension greater than 40 mm (50 percent). In keeping with these findings, other series that have reported a lower prevalence of adverse sequelae of MVP[131,144] have included relatively fewer patients with these risk factors. Variables associated with an adverse outcome are summarized in Table 57-7.

Progressive MR with gradual increase in left atrial and left ventricular size, atrial fibrillation, pulmonary hypertension, and the development of congestive heart failure is the most frequent serious complication,[1,141] occurring in about 15 percent of patients over a 10- to 15-year period. Patients with the MVP syndrome are also at risk of developing infective endocarditis.[135] Both severe MR and endocarditis develop more frequently in patients with both murmurs and clicks than in those with an isolated click, in patients with thickened (>5-mm diameter) and redundant mitral valve leaflets, and in men older than 50 years of age (see Table 57-7). In many patients, rupture of chordae tendineae is responsible for the precipitation and/or intensification of the MR.[81] Infective endocarditis often aggravates the severity of MR and therefore the need for surgical treatment.

Acute hemiplegia, transient ischemic attacks, cerebellar infarcts, amaurosis fugax, and retinal arteriolar occlusions have been reported to occur more frequently in patients with MVP syndrome, suggesting that cerebral emboli are unusually common in this condition.[132,143] It has been proposed that these neurological complications are associated with loss of endothelial continuity and tearing of the endocardium overlying the myxomatous valve, which initiates platelet aggregation and the formation of mural platelet-fibrin complexes. Although it has been proposed that embolization secondary to MVP may be a significant cause for unexplained strokes in young people without cerebrovascular disease, a large case-control study showed no association between MVP and ischemic neurological events in persons younger than 45 years of age.[144]

Mitral Valve Prolapse and Sudden Death. The relation between the MVP syndrome and sudden death is not clear. However, the best evidence suggests that MVP increases the risk of sudden death slightly,[126,129,132,145,146] especially in patients with severe MR or severe valvular deformity, and those with complex ventricular arrhythmias, QT interval prolongation, and a history of syncope and palpitations.

Management

Patients with the physical findings of MVP (and those without such findings who have been given the diagnosis) should have two-dimensional and color-flow Doppler echocardiography. This procedure should also be performed in first-degree relatives of patients with MVP.[1] The diagnosis of MVP requires definitive echocardiographic findings, and overdiagnosis and incorrect "labeling" have been a major problem with this condition. *Asymptomatic patients* (or those whose principal complaint is anxiety), with no arrhythmias evident on a routine extended ECG tracing and without evidence of MR, have an excellent prognosis. They should be reassured about the favorable prognosis and be encouraged to engage in normal life styles but should have follow-up examinations every 3 to 5 years. This should include a two-dimensional echocardiogram and a color-flow Doppler study.

Patients with a long systolic murmur may show progression of MR and should be evaluated more frequently, at intervals of approximately 12 months. *Endocarditis prophylaxis* is advisable for patients with a typical click and systolic murmur and in those with only a click who have the characteristic echocardiographic features of MVP. Prophylaxis does *not* appear to be necessary for patients with a midsystolic click without a systolic murmur or without typical echocardiographic findings (see Chap. 58).[1]

Patients with a history of palpitations, lightheadedness, dizziness, or syncope or those who have ventricular arrhythmias or QT prolongation on a routine ECG should undergo ambulatory (24-hour) ECG monitoring and/or exercise ECG to detect arrhythmias. Because of the risk, albeit very low, of sudden death, further electrophysiological studies may be carried out to characterize arrhythmias if they exist. Beta-adrenergic blockers are useful in the treatment of palpitations secondary to frequent premature ventricular contractions and for self-terminating episodes of supraventricular tachycardia. These drugs may also be useful in the treatment of chest discomfort, both in patients with associated coronary artery disease and in those with normal coronary vessels in whom the symptoms may be due to regional ischemia secondary to MVP. Radiofrequency ablation of atrioventricular bypass tracts is useful for frequent or prolonged episodes of supraventricular tachycardia.

Aspirin should be given to patients with MVP who have had a documented focal neurological event and in whom no other cause, such as a left atrial thrombus or atrial fibrillation, is apparent.

Patients with MVP and severe MR should be treated similarly to other patients with severe MR and may require mitral valve surgery. Reconstructive surgery without valve replacement is usually possible (see Fig. 57–17).[100-102,103a,104] Therefore, the threshold for surgical treatment in these patients is lower than in patients with MR in whom MVR may be necessary, providing that patients are referred to a surgical team with established success in mitral valve repair. Most mitral valve reconstructions for MR are now carried out in patients with MVP. Resection of the most deformed leaflet segment, usually the middle scallop of the posterior leaflet, and insertion of an annuloplasty ring to reduce the dilated annulus is the most commonly employed procedure. Repair or anterior leaflet prolapse is more challenging. Rupture of the chordae tendineae to the anterior leaflet can sometimes be treated by chordal transfer from the posterior leaflet. In other patients, shortening of the chordae tendineae and/or papillary muscle is necessary. The average operative mortality is 2 to 3 percent,[113] and long-term studies demonstrate excellent durability of mitral valve repair in most patients.[100-102] However, MR recurs in a subset of patients,[116,147] at which point it is usually necessary to perform MVR.

Coronary arteriography should be performed in patients with angina pectoris on effort and/or ischemic ECG changes or those with abnormalities on a stress myocardial perfusion scan. Treatment should take into account both the responsiveness of symptoms to medical management and the coronary anatomy.

Although this discussion has focused attention on complications of the MVP syndrome, it should not be forgotten that, on the whole, this is a benign condition and that the vast majority of patients with this syndrome remain asymptomatic for their entire lives and require, at most, observation every few years and reassurance.

Aortic Stenosis

Etiology and Pathology

Obstruction to left ventricular outflow is localized most commonly at the aortic valve and is discussed in this section. However, obstruction may also occur above the valve (supravalvular stenosis) or below the valve (discrete subvalvular stenosis) (see Chap. 56), or it may be caused by hypertrophic obstructive cardiomyopathy (see Chap. 59). Valvular AS has three principal causes: congenital, rheumatic, and degenerative (Fig. 57–24). Valvular AS *without accompanying mitral valve disease* is more common in men than in women, rarely occurs on a rheumatic basis, and is usually either congenital or degenerative in origin.[1,148,149]

CONGENITAL AORTIC STENOSIS (see Chap. 56). Congenital malformations of the aortic valve may be unicuspid, bicuspid, or tricuspid, or there may be a dome-shaped diaphragm. *Unicuspid valves* produce severe obstruction in infancy and are the most frequent malformations found in fatal valvular AS in children younger than 1 year of age. Congenitally *bicuspid valves* may be stenotic with commissural fusion at birth, but more often they are not responsible for serious narrowing of the aortic orifice during childhood. Their abnormal architecture induces turbulent flow, which traumatizes the leaflets and leads to fibrosis, increased rigidity, calcification of the leaflets, and narrowing of the aortic orifice in adulthood (see Fig. 57–24B).[148] With fibrosis and immobilization of the valve, in some patients a congenitally bicuspid valve may become purely or predominantly regurgitant. Infective endocarditis developing on a congenitally bicuspid valve may also lead to severe regurgitation.

Bicuspid aortic valves often have familial clustering consistent with an autosomal dominant inheritance with incomplete penetrance,[150,151] such that echocardiographic screening of first-degree relatives is justified. Bicuspid valves are also often associated with dilation of the ascending aorta[151,152] related to accelerated degeneration of the aortic media.[153] In some cases, this may progress to frank aneurysm formation. Dilation of the aortic root is another cause for development of AR in patients with bicuspid valves.

A third form of a congenitally malformed valve is *tricuspid,* with the cusps of unequal size and some commissural fusion. Although many of these valves retain normal function throughout life, it has been postulated that the turbulent flow produced by the mild congenital architectural abnormality may lead to fibrosis and ultimately to calcification and stenosis. Tricuspid stenotic aortic valves in adults may be congenital, rheumatic, or degenerative in origin.

ACQUIRED AORTIC STENOSIS. Rheumatic AS results from adhesions and fusions of the commissures and cusps and vascularization of the leaflets of the valve ring, leading

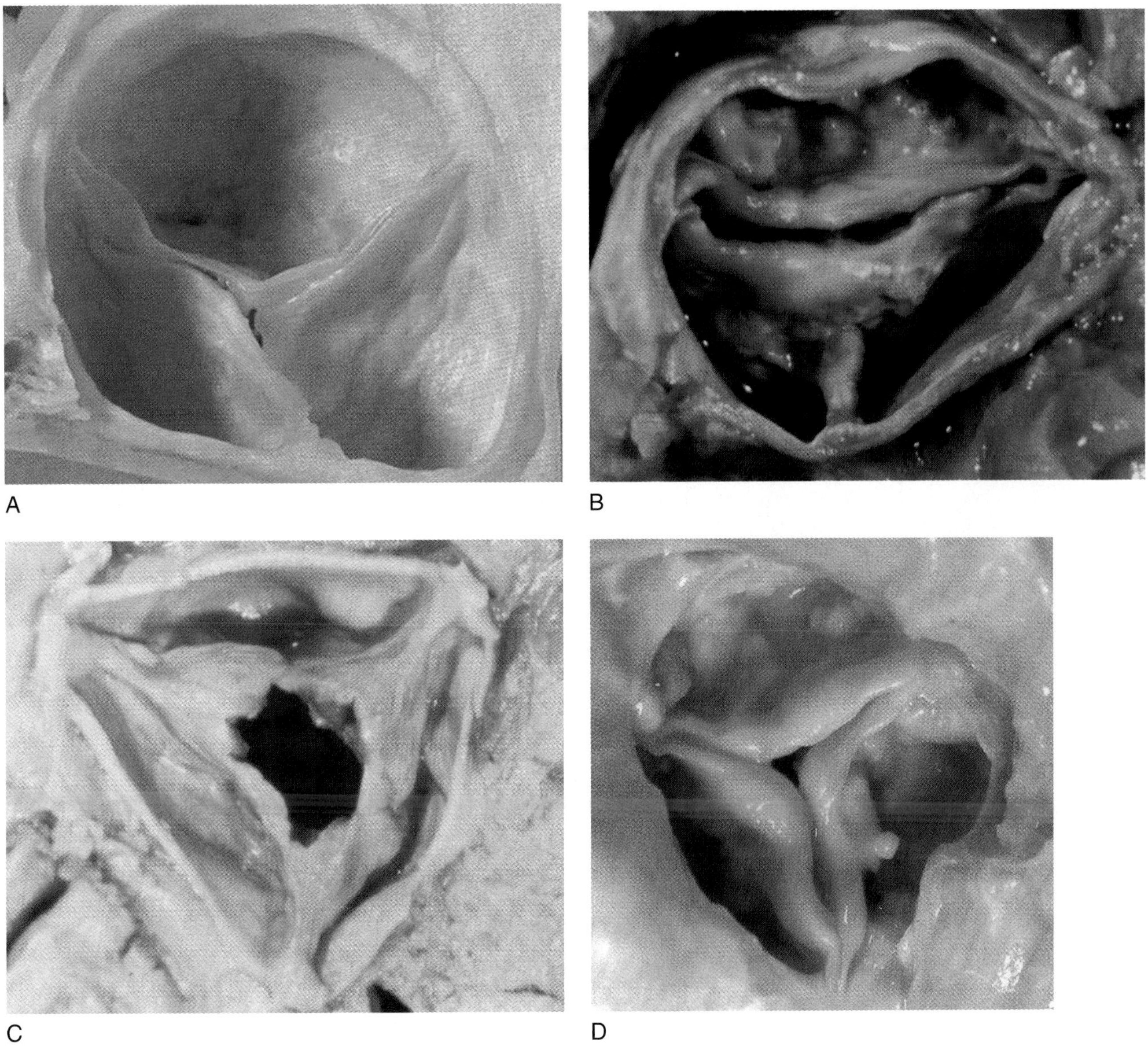

FIGURE 57–24 Major types of aortic valve stenosis. **A,** Normal aortic valve. **B,** Congenital bicuspid aortic stenosis. A false raphe is present at 6 o'clock. **C,** Rheumatic aortic stenosis. The commissures are fused with a fixed central orifice. **D,** Calcific degenerative aortic stenosis. (**A** and **D,** From Manabe H, Yutani C [eds]: Atlas of Valvular Heart Disease. Singapore, Churchill Livingstone, 1998, pp 6 and 131; **B** and **C,** Courtesy of William C. Roberts, MD.)

to retraction and stiffening of the free borders of the cusps. Calcific nodules develop on both surfaces, and the orifice is reduced to a small round or triangular opening (see Fig. 57–24C). As a consequence, the rheumatic valve is often regurgitant as well as stenotic. The heart frequently exhibits other stigmata of rheumatic disease, especially mitral valve involvement. With the decline in rheumatic fever in industrialized nations, rheumatic AS is decreasing in frequency.

Age-related degenerative calcific (formerly termed *senile*) AS is now the most common cause of AS in adults and the most frequent reason for AVR in patients with AS.[154] In a population-based echocardiographic study, 2 percent of persons 65 years of age or older had frank calcific AS, whereas 29 percent exhibited age-related aortic valve sclerosis without stenosis, defined by Otto and colleagues as irregular thickening of the aortic valve leaflets detected by echocardiography without significant obstruction and believed to represent a milder and/or earlier disease process.[155] Although once considered to represent the result of years of normal mechanical stress on an otherwise normal valve, the evolving concept is that the degenerative process represents proliferative and inflammatory changes, with lipid accumulation, upregulation of ACE activity, and infiltration of macrophages and T lymphocytes,[154,156-159] ultimately leading to bone formation[160,161] in a manner analogous to vascular calcification. Progressive calcification, initially along the flexion lines at their bases, leads to immobilization of the cusps (see Fig. 57–24D). This process rarely leads to significant AR.

Age-related AS or degenerative calcific AS shares common risk factors with mitral annular calcification,[59-61] and the two conditions often coexist. The risk factors for the development of calcific AS are similar to those for vascular atherosclerosis and include elevated serum levels of LDL cholesterol and Lp(a), diabetes, smoking, and hypertension.[162-164] Not surprisingly, age-related aortic valve sclerosis is associated with an increased risk of cardiovascular death and myocardial

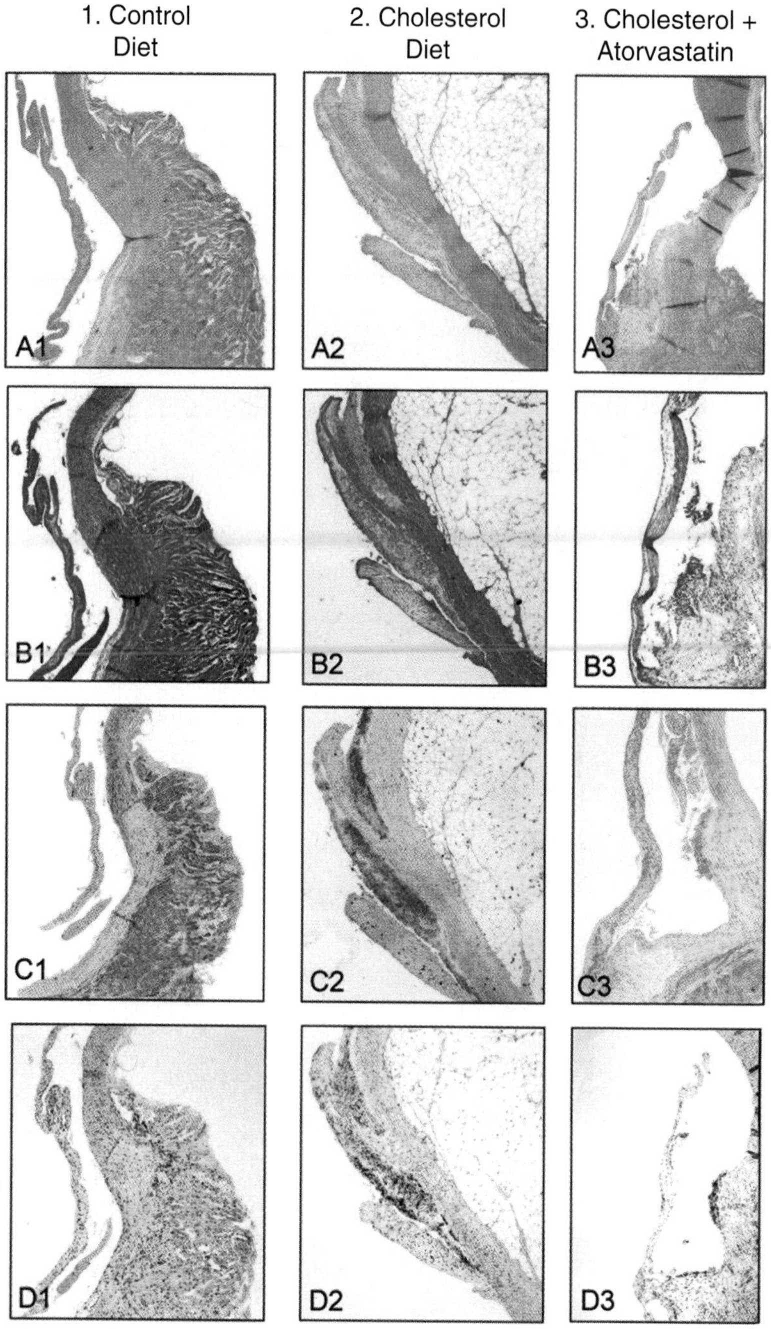

FIGURE 57–25 Light microscopy of rabbit aortic valves from a rabbit fed a conventional diet **(left column)**, one fed a high-cholesterol diet **(middle column)**, and one fed a high-cholesterol diet and treated with atorvastatin **(right column)**. In each panel, the aortic valve leaflet is positioned to the left with the aorta on the right. **A1-A3,** Hematoxylin and eosin stain. **B1-B3,** Masson trichrome stain for collagen (blue stain). **C1-C3,** Macrophage RAM-11 stain for macrophages and foam cells. **D1-D3,** Stain for proliferating cell nuclear antigen. The high-cholesterol diet results in cellular proliferation and macrophage and foam cell infiltration. These changes are prevented with atorvastatin. (From Rajamannan NM, Subramanian M, Sebo T, et al: Atorvastatin inhibits hypercholesterolemia-induced cellular proliferation and bone matrix production in the rabbit aortic valve. Circulation 105:2660, 2002.)

infarction.[155] Moreover, retrospective studies have linked treatment with HMG-CoA reductase (statin) medications with a lower rate of progression of calcific AS,[165-167] and this effect has been confirmed prospectively in an animal model of hypercholesterolemia (Fig. 57–25).[168] Hence, there is growing consensus that "degenerative" calcific AS shares many pathophysiological features with atherosclerosis and that aggressive prevention measures may retard (and perhaps even prevent) this process.[154,169,170] Whether similar preventive strategies might be used at an early age in patients with bicuspid valves to slow progressive to severe AS awaits further study.

In *atherosclerotic* aortic valve stenosis, severe atherosclerosis involves the aorta and other major arteries; this form of AS occurs most frequently in patients with severe hypercholesterolemia and is observed in children with homozygous type II hyperlipoproteinemia.[171]

Calcific AS is observed in a number of other conditions, including Paget disease of bone[172] and end-stage renal disease. *Rheumatoid involvement* of the valve is a rare cause of AS and results in nodular thickening of the valve leaflets and involvement of the proximal portion of the aorta. *Ochronosis* with alkaptonuria is another rare cause of AS.[173]

Hemodynamically significant AS leads to severe concentric left ventricular hypertrophy, with heart weights as great as 1000 gm. The interventricular septum often bulges into and encroaches on the right ventricular cavity. When left ventricular failure supervenes, the ventricle dilates, the left atrium enlarges, and changes secondary to left atrial hypertension occur in the pulmonary vascular bed, the right side of the heart, and the systemic venous bed. Isolated AS may produce significant pulmonary hypertension,[174] but this is less common than in patients with associated mitral valve disease.

Pathophysiology (Fig. 57–26)

The left ventricle responds to *sudden* severe obstruction to outflow by dilation and reduction of stroke volume. However, in adults with AS, the obstruction usually develops and increases gradually over a prolonged period. In infants and children with congenital AS, the valve orifice shows little change as the child grows, thereby intensifying the relative obstruction quite gradually. Left ventricular function can be well maintained in experimentally produced, gradually developing subcoronary AS in animals. In the experimental model, as well as in children and adults with chronic, severe AS, left ventricular output is maintained by the presence of left ventricular hypertrophy, which may sustain a large pressure gradient across the aortic valve for many years without a reduction in cardiac output, left ventricular dilation, or the development of symptoms. Critical obstruction to left ventricular outflow is usually characterized by (1) a peak systolic pressure gradient exceeding 50 mm Hg in the presence of a normal cardiac output or (2) an effective aortic orifice area (calculated by the Gorlin formula [see Chap. 17]) less than about 0.8 cm^2 in an average-sized adult, i.e., 0.5 cm^2/m^2 of BSA (less than about one-fourth of the normal aortic orifice of 3.0 to 4.0 cm^2). An aortic valve orifice of 1.0 to 1.5 cm^2 is considered moderate stenosis, and an orifice of 1.5 to 2.0 cm^2 is referred to as *mild stenosis.*

As contraction of the left ventricle becomes progressively more isometric, the left ventricular pressure pulse exhibits a rounded, rather than flattened, summit. The elevated left ventricular end-diastolic pressure, which is characteristic of severe AS, often reflects diminished compliance of the hypertrophied left ventricular wall.

In patients with severe AS, large *a* waves usually appear in the left atrial pressure pulse because of the combination of enhanced contraction of a hypertrophied left atrium and diminished left ventricular compliance. Atrial contraction plays a particularly important role in filling of the left ventricle in AS. It raises left ventricular end-diastolic pressure without causing a concomitant elevation of mean left atrial pressure. This "booster pump" function of the left atrium prevents the pulmonary venous and capillary pressures from rising to levels that would produce pulmonary congestion, while at the same time maintaining left ventricular end-diastolic pressure at the elevated level necessary for effective contraction of the hypertrophied left ventricle. Loss of appropriately timed, vigorous atrial contraction, as occurs in atrial fibrillation or atrioventricular dissociation, may result in rapid clinical deterioration in patients with severe AS.

Although the *cardiac output* at rest is within normal limits in most patients with severe AS, it often fails to rise normally during exertion. Late in the course of the disease, the cardiac output, stroke volume, and therefore the left ventricular–aortic pressure gradient all decline, whereas the mean left atrial, pulmonary capillary, pulmonary arterial, right ventricular systolic and diastolic, and right atrial pressures rise, often sequentially. As a consequence of pulmonary hypertension and/or bulging of the hypertrophied septum into the right ventricular cavity, the *a* wave in the right atrial pressure pulse becomes prominent.

Left ventricular end-diastolic volume usually remains normal until late in the course of severe AS, but left ventricular mass increases in response to the chronic pressure overload, resulting in an increase in the mass/volume ratio. However, the increase in mass may not be as great as that seen with aortic AR or combined AS and AR.

Gender differences in the response of the left ventricle to AS have been reported.[175] Women more frequently exhibit normal or even supernormal ventricular performance and a smaller, thicker walled, concentrically hypertrophied left ventricle with diastolic dysfunction (to be discussed) and normal or even subnormal systolic wall stress. Men more frequently have eccentric left ventricular hypertrophy, excessive systolic wall stress, systolic dysfunction (Fig. 57–27), and ventricular dilation.

MYOCARDIAL FUNCTION IN AORTIC STENOSIS

When the aorta is suddenly constricted in experimental animals, left ventricular pressure rises, wall stress increases significantly, and both the extent and the velocity of shortening decline. As pointed out in Chapter 21, the development of ventricular hypertrophy is one of the principal mechanisms by which the heart adapts to such an increased hemodynamic burden.[149] The increased systolic wall stress induced by AS leads to parallel replication of sarcomeres and concentric hypertrophy. The increase in left ventricular wall thickness is often sufficient to counterbalance the increased pressure, so that peak systolic wall tension returns to normal or remains normal if the obstruction develops slowly. An inverse correlation between wall stress and ejection fraction has been described in patients with AS. This suggests that the depressed ejection fraction and velocity of fiber shortening that occur in *some* patients are a consequence of inadequate wall thickening, resulting in "afterload mismatch." In others, the lower ejection fraction is secondary to a true depression of contractility; in this group, surgical treatment is less effective. Thus, both increased afterload and altered contractility are operative to varying extents in depressing left ventricular performance. To evaluate myocardial function in patients with AS, the ejection phase indices, such as ejection fraction and myocardial fiber shortening, should be related to the existing wall tension.

Diastolic Properties (see Chap. 20). Although ventricular hypertrophy is a key adaptive mechanism to the pressure load imposed by AS, it has an adverse pathophysiological consequence; i.e., it increases diastolic stiffness.[149] As a result, greater intracavitary pressure is required for ventricular filling. Some patients with AS manifest an increase in stiffness of the left ventricle (increased *chamber* stiffness) owing simply to increased muscle mass with no alteration in the diastolic properties of each unit of

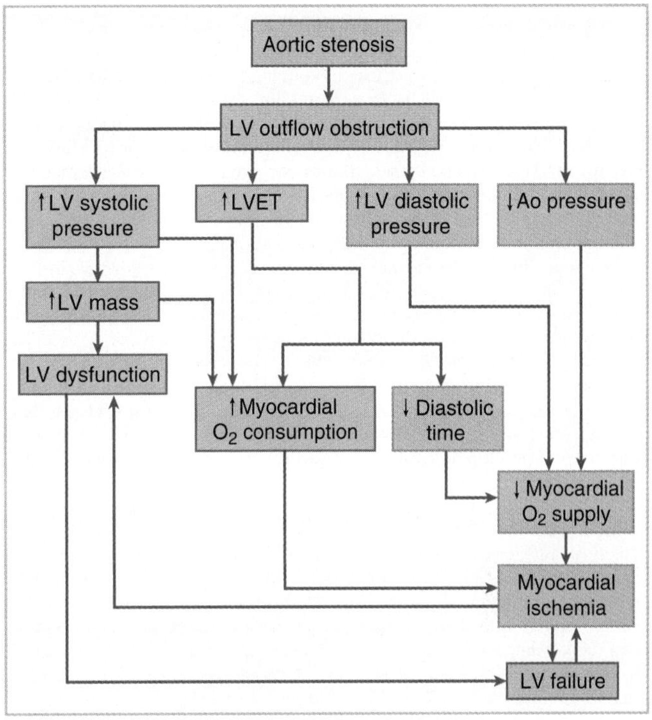

FIGURE 57–26 Pathophysiology of aortic stenosis. Left ventricular (LV) outflow obstruction results in an increased LV systolic pressure, increased LV ejection time (LVET), increased LV diastolic pressure, and decreased aortic (Ao) pressure. Increased LV systolic pressure with LV volume overload increases LV mass, which may lead to LV dysfunction and failure. Increased LV systolic pressure, LV mass, and LVET increase myocardial oxygen (O_2) consumption. Increased LVET results in a decrease of diastolic time (myocardial perfusion time). Increased LV diastolic pressure and decreased Ao diastolic pressure decrease coronary perfusion pressure. Decreased diastolic time and coronary perfusion pressure decrease myocardial O_2 supply. Increased myocardial O_2 consumption and decreased myocardial O_2 supply produce myocardial ischemia, which further deteriorates LV function. (From Boudoulas H, Gravanis MB: Valvular heart disease. *In* Gravanis MB [ed]: Cardiovascular Disorders: Pathogenesis and Pathophysiology. St. Louis, CV Mosby, 1993, p 64.)

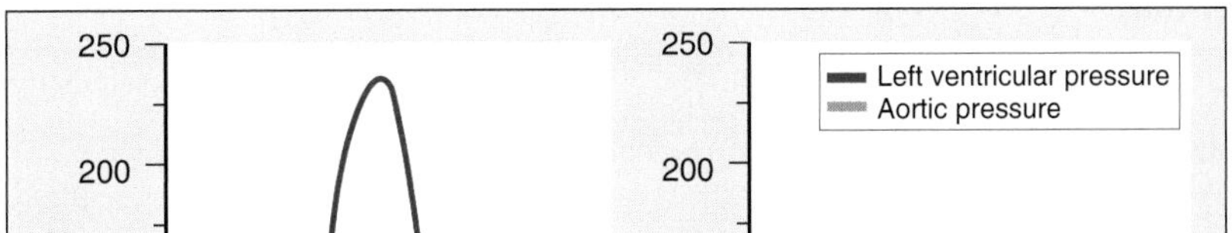

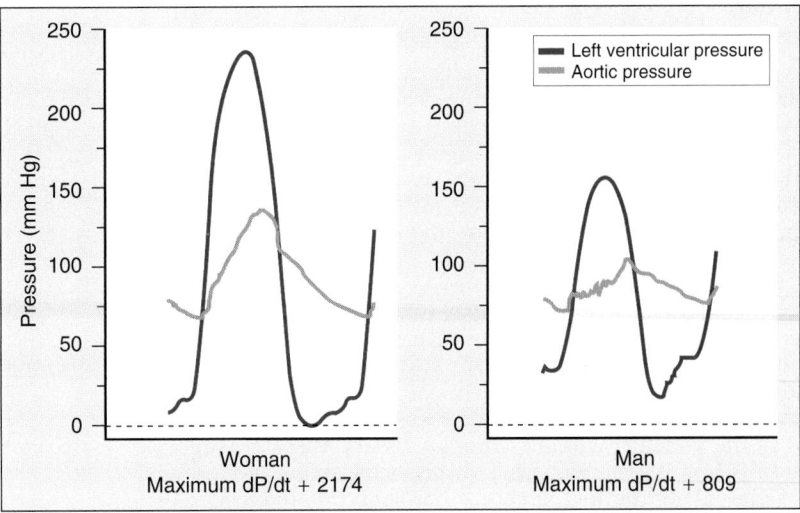

FIGURE 57–27 The difference in pressure-generating capabilities of the left ventricle in an 83-year-old woman and a 60-year-old man with a similar degree of aortic stenosis is shown. dP/dt = rate of pressure increase. (From Carroll JD, Carroll EP, Feldman T, et al: Sex-associated differences in left ventricular function in aortic stenosis of the elderly. Circulation 86:1099, 1992.)

myocardium (normal *muscle* stiffness); others exhibit increases in both chamber and muscle stiffness. This increased stiffness, however produced, contributes to the elevation of ventricular diastolic filling pressure at any level of ventricular diastolic volume and may be responsible for flash pulmonary edema in patients with AS. Diastolic dysfunction may revert toward normal with regression of hypertrophy following surgical relief of AS.

Cardiac Structure. In adults with AS, both myocardial cellular hypertrophy and relative and absolute increases in connective tissue occur. An increase in the total collagen volume of the myocardium along with increased myocardial gene expression for collagens I and III and fibronectin is related to activation of the cardiac renin-angiotensin system.[176] This likely contributes to the altered diastolic properties just discussed. The collagen and fibronectin gene expression correlate directly with the left ventricular end-diastolic pressure and inversely with the ejection fraction.[176] Reduction in renin-angiotensin activation parallels regression of hypertrophy after relief of AS.[177]

Changes in the myocardial ultrastructure in patients with severe AS include unusually large nuclei, loss of myofibrils, accumulation of mitochondria, large cytoplasmic areas devoid of contractile material, and proliferation of fibroblasts and collagen fibers in the interstitial space. The depression of myocardial function that occurs late in the course of the disease may well be related to these morphological alterations.

Ischemia. In patients with AS, coronary blood flow at rest is elevated in absolute terms but is normal when corrections are made for myocardial mass.[178] Reduced coronary blood flow reserve may produce inadequate myocardial oxygenation in patients with severe AS, even in the absence of coronary artery disease. The hypertrophied left ventricular muscle mass, the increased systolic pressure, and the prolongation of ejection all elevate myocardial oxygen consumption. The abnormally heightened pressure compressing the coronary arteries may exceed the coronary perfusion pressure, and the shortening of diastole interferes with coronary blood flow, thus leading to an imbalance between myocardial oxygen supply and demand.[179] Myocardial perfusion is also impaired by the relative decrease in myocardial capillary density as myocardial mass increases and by the elevation of left ventricular end-diastolic pressure, which lowers the aortic–left ventricular pressure gradient in diastole (i.e., the coronary perfusion pressure gradient). This underperfusion may be responsible for the development of subendocardial ischemia,[178] especially during tachycardia.

Myocardial ischemia in patients with severe AS and normal coronary arteries may also develop secondary to high systolic and diastolic stresses caused by inadequate ventricular hypertrophy and the reduced coronary flow reserve just described.[180] Metabolic evidence of myocardial ischemia, i.e., lactate production, can be demonstrated when myocardial oxygen needs are stimulated by exercise or by isoproterenol in patients with AS, even in the absence of coronary artery narrowing.[148]

Clinical Manifestations

History

In the natural history of adults with AS, a long latent period exists during which there is gradually increasing obstruction and an increase in the pressure load on the myocardium while the patient remains asymptomatic. The cardinal manifestations of acquired AS are angina pectoris, syncope, exertional dyspnea, and ultimately heart failure.[148,181] These commence most commonly in the fifth or sixth decades of life in patients with congenital or rheumatic AS and in the seventh through ninth decades in those with degenerative calcific AS.

Angina occurs in approximately two-thirds of patients with critical AS (about half of whom have associated significant coronary artery obstruction).[148] It usually resembles the angina observed in patients with coronary artery disease, in that it is commonly precipitated by exertion and relieved by rest. In patients without coronary artery disease, angina results from the combination of the increased oxygen needs of the hypertrophied myocardium and the reduction of oxygen delivery secondary to the excessive compression of coronary vessels (as discussed previously).[179] In patients with coronary artery disease, angina is caused by a combination of the epicardial coronary artery obstruction in combination with the oxygen imbalance characteristic of AS. Rarely, angina results from calcium emboli to the coronary vascular bed.

Syncope is most commonly due to the reduced cerebral perfusion that occurs during exertion when arterial pressure declines consequent to systemic vasodilation in the presence of a fixed cardiac output. Syncope has also been attributed to malfunction of the baroreceptor mechanism in severe AS, as well as to a vasodepressor response to a greatly elevated left ventricular systolic pressure during exercise. Premonitory symptoms of syncope are common. Exertional hypotension may also be manifested as "graying out" spells or dizziness on effort. Syncope at rest may be due to transient ventricular fibrillation, from which the patient recovers spontaneously; to transient atrial fibrillation with loss of the atrial contribution to left ventricular filling, which causes a precipitous decline in cardiac output; or to transient atrioventricular block due to extension of the calcification of the valve into the conduction system. Exertional dyspnea with orthopnea, paroxysmal nocturnal dyspnea, and pulmonary edema reflect varying degrees of pulmonary venous hypertension. These are relatively late symptoms in patients with AS, and their presence for more than 5 years should suggest the possibility of associated mitral valvular disease.

Because cardiac output is usually well maintained for many years in patients with severe AS, marked fatigability, debilitation, peripheral cyanosis, and other clinical manifestations of a low cardiac output are usually not prominent until quite late in the course of the disease. Other late findings in patients with isolated AS include atrial fibrillation, pulmonary hypertension, and systemic venous hypertension. Although AS may be responsible for sudden death, this usually occurs in patients who had previously been symptomatic (see Chap. 33).

In patients in whom the obstruction remains unrelieved, the prognosis is poor once these symptoms are manifested. Survival curves show that the interval from the onset of symptoms to the time of death is approximately 2 years in patients with heart failure, 3 years in those with syncope, and 5 years in those with angina (Fig. 57–28).

Gastrointestinal bleeding may develop in patients with severe AS, often associated with angiodysplasia (most commonly of the right colon) or other vascular malformations. This complication arises from shear stress–induced platelet aggregation with reduction in high-molecular-weight

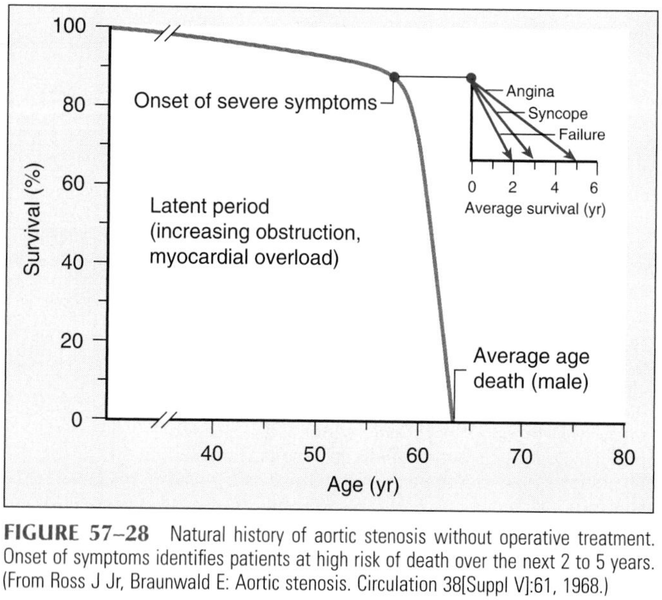

FIGURE 57–28 Natural history of aortic stenosis without operative treatment. Onset of symptoms identifies patients at high risk of death over the next 2 to 5 years. (From Ross J Jr, Braunwald E: Aortic stenosis. Circulation 38[Suppl V]:61, 1968.)

multimers of von Willebrand factor and increases in proteolytic subunit fragments. These abnormalities correlate with the severity of AS and are correctable by AVR.[182,183]

Infective endocarditis is a greater risk in younger patients with milder valvular deformity than in older patients with rock-like calcific aortic deformities. Cerebral emboli resulting in stroke or transient ischemic attacks may be due to microthrombi on thickened bicuspid valves. Calcific AS may cause embolization of calcium to various organs, including the heart, kidneys, and brain. Abrupt loss of vision has been reported when calcific emboli occlude the central retinal artery.[148]

Physical Examination (Table 57–8)

The arterial pulse characteristically rises slowly and is small and sustained (pulsus parvus et tardus). In the late stage of AS, systolic and pulse pressures are both reduced. However, in patients with mild AS with associated AR and in older patients with an inelastic arterial bed, both systolic and pulse pressures may be normal or even increased. A systolic pressure exceeding 200 mm Hg is rare in patients with critical AS. The anacrotic notch and coarse systolic vibrations are felt most readily in the carotid arterial pulse, producing the so-called carotid shudder. Simultaneous palpation of the apex and carotid arteries reveals a lag in the latter in patients with severe AS. Although left ventricular alternans occurs commonly in patients who have AS with left ventricular dysfunction, obstruction of the aortic valve may prevent its recognition in the peripheral arterial pulse. The jugular venous pulse usually shows prominent *a* waves, reflecting reduced right ventricular compliance consequent to pulmonary hypertension or hypertrophy of the ventricular septum. With pulmonary hypertension and secondary right ventricular failure and TR, *v* or *c-v* waves may become prominent.

The cardiac impulse is sustained and becomes displaced inferiorly and laterally with left ventricular failure. Presystolic distention of the left ventricle (i.e., a prominent precordial *a* wave) is often both visible and palpable. A hyperdynamic left ventricle suggests concomitant AR and/or MR. A systolic thrill is usually best appreciated when the patient leans forward during full expiration. It is palpated most readily in the second left intercostal space on either side of the sternum or in the suprasternal notch and is frequently transmitted along the carotid arteries. A systolic thrill is quite specific for severe AS.

Rarely, right ventricular failure with systemic venous congestion, hepatomegaly, and edema precedes left ventricular failure. This is probably caused by the so-called Bernheim effect, which results when the hypertrophied ventricular septum bulges into and encroaches on the right ventricular cavity and leads to impairment of right ventricular filling. In such cases, the jugular venous pressure is elevated, and the *a* wave is prominent.

AUSCULTATION (see Table 57–8)

S_1 is normal or soft and S_4 is prominent, presumably because atrial contraction is vigorous and the mitral valve is partially closed during presystole. S_2 may be single because calcification and immobility of the aortic valve make A_2 inaudible, because P_2 is buried in the prolonged aortic ejection murmur, or because prolongation of left ventricular systole makes A_2 coincide with P_2. Paradoxical splitting of S_2, which suggests associated left bundle branch block or left ventricular dysfunction, may also occur. In patients with left ventricular failure and secondary pulmonary hypertension, P_2 may become accentuated. When the aortic valve is rigid, which is the usual finding in adults with severe AS, A_2 may be inaudible, but when the valve is flexible, as may occur in patients with congenital AS, A_2 may be snapping and accentuated.

An aortic ejection sound occurs simultaneously with the halting upward movement of the aortic valve. Like an audible A_2, this sound is dependent on mobility of the valve cusps and disappears when they become severely calcified. Thus, it is common in children and young

TABLE 57–8 Differential Diagnosis of Aortic Stenosis: Physical Findings

Type of Stenosis	Maximum Murmur and Thrill	Aortic Election Sound	Aortic Component of Second Sound	Regurgitant Diastolic Murmur	Arterial Pulse
Acquired, nonrheumatic or rheumatic	Second right sternal border to neck; may be at apex in the aged	Uncommon	Decreased or absent	Common	Delayed upstroke: anacrotic notch; ± small amplitude
Hypertrophic, subaortic	Fourth left sternal border to apex (± regurgitant systolic murmur at apex)	Rare	Normal or decreased	Very rare	Brisk upstroke, sometimes bisferiens
Congenital, valvular	Second right sternal border to neck (along left sternal border in some infants)	Very common in children, disappearing with decrease in valve mobility with age	Normal or increased in children; decreased with decrease in valve mobility with age	Uncommon in children: not uncommon in adults	Delayed upstroke: anacrotic notch; ± small amplitude
Congenital, subvalvular	Discrete: like valvular; tunnel: left sternal border	Rare	Not helpful (normal, increased, decreased, or absent)	Almost all	
Congenital, supravalvular	First right sternal border to neck and sometimes to medial aspect of right arm; occasionally greater in neck than in chest	Rare	Normal or decreased	Uncommon	Rapid upstroke in right carotid, delayed in left carotid, right arm pulse pressure greater than left

From Levinson GF: Aortic stenosis. *In* Dalen JE, Alpert JS (eds): Valvular Heart Disease. 2nd ed. Boston, Little, Brown, 1987, p 202.

adults with congenital AS but is rare in adults with acquired calcific AS and rigid valves. The ejection sound occurs approximately 0.06 second after the onset of S_1.

The *systolic murmur* of AS is usually late peaking and heard best at the base of the heart but is often well transmitted both along the carotid vessels and to the apex. Cessation of the murmur before A_2 is usually helpful in differentiating it from a pansystolic mitral murmur. However, the systolic murmur may be mistaken for a pansystolic murmur because it may end with S_2, which represents pulmonic valve closure, whereas the pansystolic murmur is soft or even inaudible. In patients with calcified aortic valves, the systolic murmur is loudest at the base of the heart, but high-frequency components selectively radiate to the apex (the so-called Gallavardin phenomenon), where it may actually be more prominent and where it may be mistaken for the murmur of MR. Frequently, there is a "quiet area" between the base and apex where the murmur is diminished in intensity, supporting the erroneous impression that the apical and basal murmurs have different origins. In general, the more severe the stenosis, the longer the duration of the murmur and the more likely that it peaks later in systole. Findings on physical examination (including a delay in the carotid upstroke, a loud, long systolic murmur, and a single S_2) all correlate with severe stenosis.[184]

Patients with degenerative aortic sclerosis may have severe valvular calcification; however, obstruction may be mild or absent because the commissural fusion characteristic of congenital and rheumatic AS is not present. The nonfused, calcified cusps vibrate freely, resulting in a softer and more musical murmur that is more prominent at the apex than the murmur of congenital or rheumatic AS. High-pitched decrescendo diastolic murmurs secondary to AR are common in many patients with dominant AS.

When the left ventricle fails and the stroke volume falls, the systolic murmur of AS becomes softer; rarely, it disappears altogether. The slow rise in the arterial pulse is more difficult to recognize. Stated simply, with left ventricular failure, the clinical picture changes from typical AS to that of severe left ventricular failure with a low cardiac output. Thus, occult AS may be a cause of intractable heart failure, and critical AS should be ruled out by echocardiography in patients with severe heart failure of unknown cause because operative treatment may be life saving and may result in substantial clinical improvement.

Dynamic Auscultation (see Table 57-5). The intensity of the systolic murmur varies from beat to beat when the duration of diastolic filling varies, as in atrial fibrillation or following a premature contraction. This characteristic is helpful in differentiating AS from MR, in which the murmur is usually unaffected. The murmur of valvular AS is augmented by squatting, which increases stroke volume. It is reduced in intensity during the strain of the Valsalva maneuver and when standing, which reduce transvalvular flow.

Laboratory Examination

ELECTROCARDIOGRAPHY. The principal ECG change is left ventricular hypertrophy, which is found in approximately 85 percent of patients with severe AS. The absence of left ventricular hypertrophy does not exclude the presence of critical AS, and the correlation between the absolute ECG voltages in precordial leads and the severity of obstruction is poor in adults but is quite good in children with congenital AS. T wave inversion and ST segment depression in leads with upright QRS complexes are common. ST segment depressions greater than 0.2 mV in patients with AS (left ventricular "strain") suggest that severe ventricular hypertrophy is present. Occasionally, a "pseudoinfarction" pattern is present, characterized by a loss of R waves in the right precordial leads. There is evidence of left atrial enlargement in more than 80 percent of patients with severe, isolated AS. The principal manifestation is prominent late negativity of the P wave in lead V_1 rather than an increased duration in lead II, suggesting hypertrophy rather than dilation. Atrial fibrillation is an uncommon and late sign of pure AS, and its presence in a patient who does not appear to have end-stage aortic disease should suggest coexisting mitral valvular disease.

The extension of calcific infiltrates from the aortic valve into the conduction system may cause various forms and degrees of atrioventricular and intraventricular block in 5 percent of patients with calcific AS. Such conduction defects are more common in patients who have associated mitral annular calcification.

RADIOLOGICAL FINDINGS (see Figs. 12–8 and 12–23). Routine radiological examination may be normal in patients with critical AS. The heart is usually of normal size or slightly enlarged, with a rounding of the left ventricular border and apex, unless regurgitation or left ventricular failure is present and causes substantial cardiomegaly. Poststenotic dilation of the ascending aorta is a common finding. Marked aortic dilation suggests either a bicuspid valve or associated AR. Calcification of the aortic valve is found in almost all adults with hemodynamically significant AS, but it is more readily detected on fluoroscopy, cardiac computed tomography (see Fig. 15–11), or echocardiography than on roentgenography. The absence of calcium in the aortic valve region on careful fluoroscopic examination in a patient older than 35 years of age essentially rules out severe valvular AS. The converse is not true, however, and in patients older than 65 years of age with degenerative AS, severe calcification of the aortic valve may occur with no or only mild obstruction. The left atrium may be slightly enlarged in patients with severe AS, and there may be radiological signs of pulmonary venous hypertension. However, when left atrial enlargement is marked, the presence of associated mitral valvular disease should be suspected.

CARDIAC CATHETERIZATION AND ANGIOGRAPHY. As two-dimensional echocardiography usually defines left ventricular function, aortic valve morphology and mobility, and hemodynamic severity of AS, the principal role of the cardiac catheterization laboratory in patients with AS is to determine whether there is coexistent coronary artery disease in patients being considered for surgery. There is some hazard associated with the rapid injection of a large volume of contrast material into a high-pressure left ventricle, and therefore left ventriculography is usually not advisable in patients with AS and critical obstruction. Angiographic studies of the left ventricle and aortic valve in these patients are best performed by injecting contrast material into the pulmonary artery and filming in the 30-degree right anterior oblique and 60-degree left anterior oblique projections. These examinations often make it possible to ascertain the number of cusps of the stenotic valve and to demonstrate doming of a thickened valve and a systolic jet.

Hemodynamic assessment of AS by cardiac catheterization is not routinely necessary. However, careful hemodynamic study to determine severity of AS (see Chap. 17) is indicated when echocardiographic data are equivocal or of suboptimal quality, when there is a discrepancy between clinical information and echocardiographic findings, and when AS is associated with low cardiac output and impaired left ventricular function.[1,22] In the latter situation, hemodynamic assessment of AS severity at rest and during maneuvers to increase flow across the aortic valve (such as a dobutamine infusion) can provide information that is critical in making difficult management decisions regarding the indications for surgery (discussed subsequently).

ECHOCARDIOGRAPHY (see Chap. 11 and Figs. 11–63 to 11-68). Echocardiography has become the most important laboratory technique for evaluating and following patients with AS and selecting them for operation.

The normal range of opening of the aortic valve is 1.6 to 2.6 cm. Two-dimensional transthoracic echocardiography is helpful in detecting valvular calcification, in outlining the valve leaflets, and sometimes in determining the severity of the stenosis by imaging the orifice.[185] The orifice may be more clearly defined by transesophageal echocardiography (see Fig. 11–67), which offers a more precise short-axis view of the aortic valve.[186] Two-dimensional echocardiography is invaluable in detecting associated mitral valve disease, in assessing aortic root diameter in patients with bicuspid valves, and in assessing left ventricular systolic performance, diastolic function, dilation, and hypertrophy. Evolving three-dimensional echocardiographic methods hold promise for assessing aortic valve structure and mobility and quantifying the severity of AS.[187]

Doppler echocardiography allows calculation of the left ventricular–aortic pressure gradient from the systolic aortic valve velocity signal[188,189] using a modified Bernoulli (continuity) equation (see Figs. 11–30 and 11–65) and the continuity equation (see Figs. 11–34 and 11–68). The gradients noninvasively determined by this method correlate well with those determined by left-heart catheterization. The effective aortic valve orifice areas can also be derived from the Doppler examination.[190,191] Doppler methods can overestimate the severity of AS because of the phenomenon of pressure recovery distal to a stenosis (which has less effect on catheter-based measurements). The magnitude of this effect can be calculated and used to correct the measurements to yield accurate assessment of AS severity.[189,191,192]

Color-flow Doppler imaging is helpful in detecting and determining the severity of AR (which coexists in ≈75 percent of patients with predominant AS) and in estimating pulmonary artery pressure. Indeed, in most patients the echocardiographic examination provides the important hemodynamic information required for patient management, and under most circumstances cardiac catheterization is not essential (except to determine the status of the coronary arteries).[188-191] In patients with left ventricular dysfunction and low cardiac output, assessing the severity of AS can be enhanced by assessing hemodynamic changes during dobutamine infusion (discussed subsequently).

MAGNETIC RESONANCE IMAGING (see Chap. 14). Cardiac MRI is useful in assessing left ventricular volume, function, and mass, especially in settings in which this information cannot be obtained readily from echocardiography. MRI may also be useful in quantifying the severity of AS (see Fig. 14–13).[193,194]

NATURAL HISTORY

In contrast to MS, which leads to symptoms almost immediately after its development, patients with severe AS may be asymptomatic for many years despite the presence of severe obstruction.[1,148,181] The systolic pressure gradient may exceed 150 mm Hg, and the peak left ventricular systolic pressure may reach approximately 300 mm Hg with relatively little increase in overall heart size on radiological examination and with normal left ventricular end-diastolic and end-systolic volumes.

Patients with severe, chronic AS tend to be free of cardiovascular symptoms until relatively late in the course of the disease. Thus, there is a long latent period during which mortality and morbidity are quite low.[1,148,181] However, obstruction is progressive and often insidious, with the aortic valve area decreasing by an average of 0.12 cm^2 per year in one study,[195] associated with an average increase in aortic jet velocity of 0.32 m/sec per year and a mean gradient of 7 mm Hg per year. The rate of progression is highly variable and difficult to predict in individual patients. When symptoms develop, the valve area is, on average, 0.6 cm^2, but the severity of stenosis alone does not determine the presence or severity of symptoms. A patient may develop symptoms with a valve area of 1.0 cm^2, whereas another may remain symptom free with a valve area of 0.6 cm^2 and high systolic pressure gradients. However, the severity of AS does have predictive power regarding the likelihood that symptoms will develop with time. Most patients with peak aortic valve velocities greater than 4 m/sec experience symptom onset over the course of 3 to 4 years (Fig. 57–29),[195,197] particularly if there is evidence of severe valvular calcification or increasing severity of AS on serial examinations. Thus, the combination of high aortic jet velocity, severe valvular calcification, and increasing severity of stenosis identifies individual patients with a high likelihood of requiring surgery within a few years.

Once patients with AS develop angina pectoris or syncope, the average survival is 1 to 3 years (see Fig. 57–28).[1,148,149,196,197] Among symptomatic patients with severe AS, the outlook is poorest when the left ventricle has failed and the cardiac output and transvalvular gradient are both low.

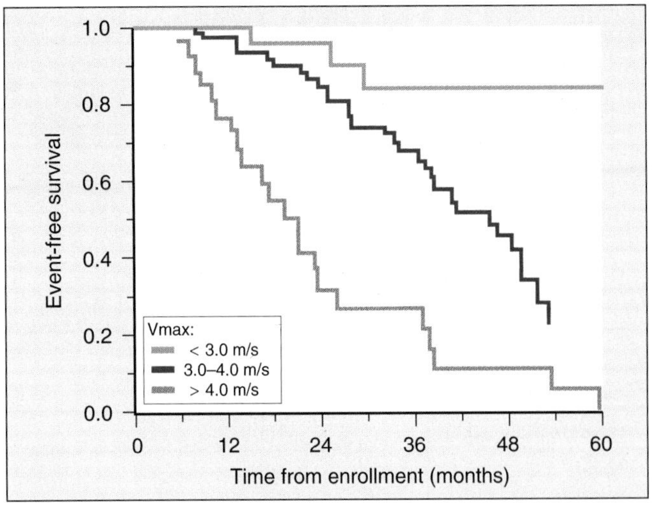

FIGURE 57–29 Natural history of asymptomatic patients with aortic stenosis. Initial aortic jet velocity (Vmax) stratifies patients according to the likelihood that symptoms requiring valve replacement will develop over time. The majority of "events" in this series were onset of symptoms warranting aortic valve replacement. (From Otto CM, Burwarsh IG, Legget ME, et al: A prospective study of asymptomatic valvular aortic stenosis: Clinical, echocardiographic, and exercise predictors of outcome. Circulation 95:2262, 1997.)

Asymptomatic patients have an excellent prognosis.[1,148,149] Sudden death, like syncope, in patients with severe AS may be due to cerebral hypoperfusion followed by arrhythmia. Although severe AS is a potentially lethal disease, death (even when sudden) usually occurs in *symptomatic* patients. A number of authors who have followed asymptomatic patients with critical AS have found that sudden death is extremely rare in this group (Table 57–9). Of 449 asymptomatic patients with critical AS, only 4 (<1 percent) died suddenly while still asymptomatic (certainly not higher than the mortality from operation).[1]

Management

Medical Treatment

Patients with known severe AS who are asymptomatic should be advised to report *promptly* the development of any symptoms possibly related to AS. Patients with critical obstruction should be cautioned to avoid vigorous athletic and physical activity. However, such restrictions do not apply to patients with mild obstruction. The need for infective endocarditis prophylaxis should be explained (see Chap 58). Because of the gradual increase in the severity of obstruction, noninvasive assessment of this finding by Doppler echocardiography should be carried out at intervals. Doppler-derived gradients have been shown to increase by 4 to 8 mm Hg per year[195] and valve areas to decrease by 0.2 to 0.3 cm^2 per year. In patients with mild obstruction, these measurements should be repeated every 2 years. In asymptomatic patients with severe obstruction, repeat echocardiography should be carried out every 6 to 12 months, with particular attention to detecting changes in left ventricular function. As patients may tailor their life styles to minimize symptoms or may ascribe fatigue and dyspnea to deconditioning or aging, they may not recognize early symptoms as important warning signals. Exercise testing may be helpful in apparently asymptomatic patients to detect covert symptoms, limited exercise capacity, and abnormal blood pressure responses.[1,195,198] Exercise stress testing should be absolutely avoided in symptomatic patients.

Symptomatic patients with severe AS are usually operative candidates, because medical therapy has little to offer. However, medical therapy may be necessary in patients who are considered to be inoperable (usually because of comorbid

TABLE 57–9 Studies of the Natural History of Asymptomatic Patients with Aortic Stenosis

Study, Year	Number of Patients	Mean Follow-up (Year)	Severity of Aortic Stenosis	Sudden Death Without Symptoms (no. of Patients)	Comments
Chizner et al, 1980	8	5.7	AVA < 1.1 cm^2	0	Retrospective study
Turina et al, 1987	17	2.0	AVA < 0.9 cm^2	0	Retrospective study
Horstkotte and Loogen, 1988	35	"years"	AVA = 0.4-0.8 cm^2	3	Retrospective study
Kelley et al, 1988	51	1.5	PV = 3.5-5.8 m/s	0	Prospective study
Pellikka et al, 1990	113	1.7	PV > 4.0 m/s	0	Prospective study
Faggiano et al, 1992	37	2.0	AVA = 0.85 ± 0.15 cm^2	0	Prospective study
Otto et al, 1997	114	2.5	PV = 3.6 ± 0.6 m/s	0	Prospective study
Rosenhek et al, 2000	106	2.3	PV > 4 m/s	1	Prospective study
Total	499	2.1		4	Average risk of sudden death ~0.4%/yr

AVA = aortic valve area; PV = peak instantaneous velocity.

Updated from Bonow RO, Carabello BA, de Leon AC, et al: ACC/AHA guidelines for the management of patients with valvular heart disease. J Am Coll Cardiol 32:1486, 1998.

conditions that preclude surgery). Digitalis glycosides are indicated if the ventricular volume is increased or the ejection fraction is reduced. Although diuretics are beneficial when there is abnormal accumulation of fluid, they must be used with caution because hypovolemia may reduce the elevated left ventricular end-diastolic pressure, lower cardiac output, and produce orthostatic hypotension. ACE inhibitors should be used with caution but are beneficial in treating patients with symptomatic left ventricular systolic dysfunction who are not candidates for surgery. They should be initiated at low doses and increased slowly to target doses, avoiding hypotension. Beta-adrenergic blockers can depress myocardial function and induce left ventricular failure and should be avoided in patients with AS.

Atrial flutter or fibrillation occurs in fewer than 10 percent of patients with severe AS, perhaps because of the late occurrence of left atrial enlargement in this condition. When such an arrhythmia is observed in a patient with AS, the possibility of associated mitral valvular disease should be considered. When atrial fibrillation occurs, the rapid ventricular rate may cause angina pectoris. The loss of the atrial contribution to ventricular filling and a sudden fall in cardiac output may cause serious hypotension. Therefore, atrial fibrillation should be treated promptly, usually with cardioversion, and a search for previously unrecognized mitral valvular disease should be undertaken. Adults with severe AS who are being considered for surgical therapy should undergo coronary arteriography. Left-heart catheterization is also indicated if there is a discrepancy between the clinical picture and the echocardiographic findings.[22]

Surgical Treatment

INDICATIONS FOR OPERATION

Children. The indications for surgery, as well as the techniques and results of operation, depend on the patient's age, the type of valvular deformity, and the function of the left ventricle. In children and adolescents with noncalcific congenital AS, who most commonly have bicuspid aortic valves, simple commissural incision under direct vision usually leads to substantial hemodynamic improvement with low risk (i.e., a mortality rate of <1 percent) (see Chap. 56). Therefore, this procedure (or now, more commonly, balloon aortic valvuloplasty [BAV]) is indicated not only in symptomatic patients but also in asymptomatic children and adolescents with severe AS,[1] which is often defined as a calculated effective orifice less than 0.8 cm^2 or 0.5 cm^2/m^2 BSA. Despite the salutary hemodynamic results following this procedure, the valve is not rendered entirely normal anatomically. The turbulent blood flow through the valve may subsequently lead to further deformation, calcification, the development of regurgitation, and restenosis after 10 to 20 years, probably requiring reoperation and valve replacement later.

Adults. In most adults with calcific AS, AVR is the surgical treatment of choice. Satisfactory long-term valvular function cannot usually be restored even by careful sculpturing procedures under direct vision, although this may be possible in a small number of selected individuals.[199] AVR should, in general, be performed in adults who have hemodynamic evidence of severe obstruction (aortic valve orifice < 1.0 cm^2 or < 0.6 cm^2/m^2 BSA) and whose symptoms are believed to result from AS. AVR should also be carried out in asymptomatic patients with *progressive* left ventricular dysfunction or a hypotensive response to exercise.[1,2,198] Although a prospective, randomized, controlled study has not been done, the long-term mortality in asymptomatic patients with critical AS and left ventricular dysfunction who undergo operation appears to be lower than that in medically treated patients who do not undergo operation.[1,2] AVR is also indicated in patients with severe stenosis who are undergoing another cardiovascular operation (e.g., coronary artery bypass grafting or surgery on the aorta or another heart valve).[1] As prosthetic valves and surgical skills continue to improve, it is likely that patients with severe AS will become candidates for operation at progressively earlier stages in the natural history of their disease,[200] and many cardiologists have already begun to lower the threshold for AVR based on severity of AS alone. Currently, however, we do *not* recommend prophylactic replacement of a critically narrow calcific aortic valve in *asymptomatic* adults unless they have progressive left ventricular dysfunction or abnormal hemodynamic responses to exercise.

Aortic Stenosis with Left Ventricular Dysfunction. Surgical risk is higher in patients with impaired left ventricular function (ejection fraction < 0.35).[201-206] However, their prognosis is poor without operation, overall survival is improved with AVR, and many patients in this group have significant clinical and functional recovery following AVR.[201-207] Hence, AVR should generally be offered to these patients. Even octogenarians with left ventricular dysfunction can have improved survival after AVR, although their operative risks are higher.[202,204,208] Exceptions are patients with advanced congestive heart failure or left ventricular dysfunction that can be related to previous myocardial infarction rather than to AS. In acutely ill patients with decompensated heart failure, nitroprusside has been reported to be safe and effective in rapidly improving hemodynamics[209] and may be used in bridging critically ill patients to AVR.

Aortic Stenosis with Low Gradient and Low Cardiac Output. Patients with critical AS, severe left ventricular dysfunction, and low cardiac output (and hence, a low transvalvular pressure gradient) often create diagnostic dilemmas for the clinician because their clinical presentation and hemodynamic data may be indistinguishable from those of patients with a dilated cardiomyopathy and a calcified valve that is not stenotic.[149,210] As aortic valve velocities and estimates of aortic valve area are dependent on flow, an important method for distinguishing between these two conditions is to reassess hemodynamics during transient increases in flow, usually by increasing cardiac output with dobutamine during Doppler echocardiography or cardiac catheterization (Fig. 56–30).[205,206,211] Patients with severe AS manifest an increase in valve gradient and no change in valve area during dobutamine, whereas those without AS manifest an increase in calculated valve area. Dobutamine echocardiography also provides evidence of myocardial contractile reserve, which is an important predictor of operative risk and improvement in left ventricular function and survival after AVR in these patients.[205,206]

RESULTS. Successful replacement of the aortic valve results in substantial clinical and hemodynamic improvement in patients with AS, AR, or combined lesions. In patients without frank left ventricular failure, the operative risk ranges from 2 to 5 percent in most centers, and in patients younger than 70 years of age, the operative risk has been reported to be as low as 1 percent. The Society of Thoracic Surgeons National Database Committee reported an overall operative mortality rate of 4 percent in 32,968 patients undergoing isolated AVR and 6.8 percent in 32,538 patients undergoing AVR and coronary artery bypass grafting (see Table 57–3).[55]

Risk factors causing a higher mortality rate include a high NYHA class, impairment of left ventricular function, advanced age, and the presence of associated coronary artery disease. The 10-year actuarial survival rate of hospital survivors in surgically treated patients is approximately 85 percent.[1,212] Risk factors for late death include higher preoperative NYHA class, advanced age, concomitant untreated coronary artery disease, preoperative impaired left ventricular function, preoperative ventricular arrhythmias, and associated significant AR.

Although age is an important determinant of risk, there is increasing experience in most surgical centers in performing AVR in symptomatic patients older than 70 or even 80 years of age with calcific AS.[208,213,214] The results of AVR are often quite satisfactory in this age group, with improved quality of life and survival, Therefore, advanced age per se, though adding to the risk, should not be considered a contraindication to operation. Particular attention must be directed to the adequacy of hepatic, renal, and pulmonary functions in these patients.

Symptoms of pulmonary congestion (exertional dyspnea) and of myocardial ischemia (angina pectoris) are relieved in almost every patient. Hemodynamic results of AVR are also impressive; elevated end-diastolic and end-systolic volumes show significant reduction. Impaired ventricular performance returns to normal more frequently in patients with AS than in those with AR or MR. However, the finding that the strongest predictor of postoperative left ventricular dysfunction is preoperative dysfunction[1,148,149] suggests that patients should, if possible, be operated on *before* left ventricular

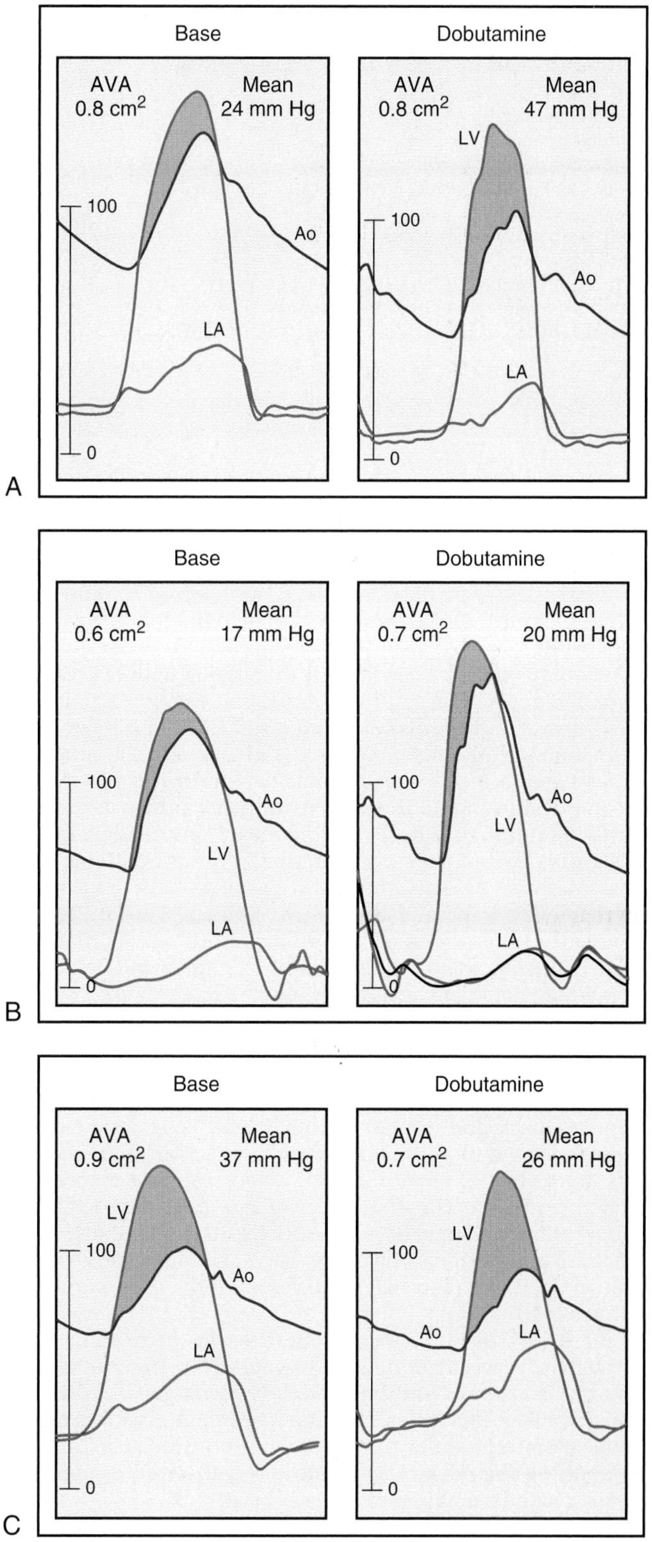

FIGURE 57–30 Hemodynamic tracings from three patients with left ventricular dysfunction, low cardiac output, and low aortic valve gradient, demonstrating three different responses to dobutamine. **A,** Increase in cardiac output and in mean aortic valve gradient from 24 to 47 mm Hg. Aortic valve area (AVA) remained 0.8 cm^2. This patient underwent successful valve replacement. **B,** Increase in cardiac output and minimal increase in mean pressure gradient from 17 to 20 mm Hg. The final calculated aortic valve area was 0.7 cm^2. The patient was found to have only minimal aortic stenosis (AS) at the time of surgery. **C,** No change in cardiac output, with decrease in mean pressure gradient from 37 to 26 mm Hg in response to dobutamine, and the test was terminated because of hypotension. The patient was found to have severe AS at the time of surgery. Ao = aortic; LA = left atrial; LV = left ventricular. (From Nishimura RA, Grantham A, Connolly HM, et al: Low-output, low-gradient aortic stenosis in patients with depressed left ventricular systolic function: The clinical utility of the dobutamine challenge in the catheterization laboratory. Circulation 106:809, 2002.)

TABLE 57–10 Predictors of Poor Outcome after Aortic Valve Replacement for Aortic Stenosis

Advanced age (>70 yr)
Female gender
Emergent surgery
Coronary artery disease
Previous coronary artery bypass grafting surgery
Hypertension
Left ventricular dysfunction (ejection fraction < 0.45 or 0.50)
Heart failure
Atrial fibrillation
Concurrent mitral valve replacement or repair
Renal failure

Adapted from Otto CM: Valvular Heart Disease. 2nd ed. Philadelphia, WB Saunders, 2004, p 227.

function becomes seriously impaired. The increased left ventricular mass is reduced toward (but not to) normal within 18 months after AVR in patients with AS,[215,216] with further reduction over the next several years.[217] Myocyte hypertrophy regresses as well. Coronary flow reserve[218,219] and diastolic function[216] also demonstrate considerable improvement after AVR.

When operation is carried out in patients with critical AS, frank left ventricular failure, a depressed ejection fraction, or a low cardiac output (and hence a reduced transaortic pressure gradient), the operative risk is higher, and the mortality rate ranges from 8 to 20 percent, depending on the skill of the surgical team and the severity of heart failure.[202-206] Obviously, performing surgery before heart failure develops is desirable, but emergency operation, even in patients with heart failure, is sometimes life saving. In view of the extremely poor prognosis of such patients who are treated medically, unless serious comorbid conditions exist that preclude surgery, there is usually little choice but to advise immediate mechanical relief of obstruction.

In patients with AS and obstructive coronary artery disease (a relatively common combination), AVR and myocardial revascularization should be performed together.[220] Although the risk of AVR is increased when accompanied by coronary artery bypass grafting (see Table 57–3),[55] the surgical risk increases even more when severe coronary artery disease is left untreated. The ability to avoid serious myocardial ischemia in the perioperative period is a major factor that has served to reduce operative mortality in these patients. Characteristics of patients that have been shown to increase the risk of AVR, as reported in different series, are shown in Table 57–10.

There has been increasing interest in performing AVR through a very small incision, generally a transverse sternotomy, so-called "minimally invasive surgery." Although the advantages (shorter hospital stay, less tissue damage, better cosmetic results) are clear, the procedure is technically demanding and the mortality rate may actually be higher than when a standard approach is employed.[221,222]

Percutaneous Treatment of Aortic Stenosis (see Chap. 52)

BAV represents an increasingly attractive alternative to aortic valvotomy in children, adolescents, and young adults with congenital noncalcific AS (see Chap. 56),[1,223] but its value is quite limited in adults with calcific AS.[1] A series of balloon dilation catheters are advanced along a guidewire positioned at the left ventricular apex. Fracture of calcified nodules, separation of fused commissures, and stretching of the aortic valve ring are responsible for the relief of obstruction. Although the response of adult patients with calcific AS varies considerably, BAV initially results in relief of obstruction in most patients, with valve areas initially increasing from approximately 0.5 to 0.8 cm^2 and the mean transvalvular gradient declining from approximately 55 to 29 mm Hg. Left ventricular ejection fraction tends to rise in patients with depressed left ventricular function who undergo BAV. In addition to the procedural mortality (3 percent), another 6 percent of patients develop serious complications such as myocardial perforation, myocardial infarction, and severe AR.

The major disadvantage of BAV in adults with critical calcified AS is restenosis due to scarring, which occurs in about 50 percent of patients within 6 months. Symptoms lessen in severity in most patients but recur in approximately 30 percent by 6 months. The 1-month and 1-year mortality rates are unacceptably high, related to the restenosis rate and the fact that the average increase in aortic valve area is slight.

Although the overall intermediate-term results (6 to 12 months) of BAV have been disappointing, the procedure does have a limited role in the management of severe calcific AS in selected patients who are not surgical candidates,[1] such as patients with cardiogenic shock due to critical AS, patients with severe heart failure who are at extremely high operative risk as a "bridge" to AVR, patients with severe comorbid conditions that preclude surgery, and patients with critical AS who refuse surgical treatment. Under most circumstances, patients with critical AS who require an urgent noncardiac operation should undergo the noncardiac operation; preoperative BAV has a very limited role in such patients. In adults with calcific AS, BAV is *not* a substitute for surgery (as BMV may be in patients with MS). In addition, nitroprusside may be a more available and effective therapy for short-term management of patients with severe heart failure,[209] but greater clinical experience with nitroprusside is needed before recommendations can be made regarding its use in this setting.[209a]

Newer percutaneous methods for implantation of prosthetic valves in seriously ill patients who are not candidates for surgery are under development.[224] Limited clinical experience has been reported to date.[225]

Aortic Regurgitation

Etiology And Pathology

AR may be caused by primary disease of the aortic valve leaflets and/or the wall of the aortic root (Fig. 57–31). Among patients with *pure* AR who undergo valve replacement, the percentage with aortic root disease has been increasing steadily during the past few decades. This now represents the most common etiology and accounts for more than 50 percent of all such patients in some series.[57,226]

Valvular Disease

Rheumatic fever is a common cause of primary disease of the aortic valve that leads to regurgitation.[57,226] The cusps become infiltrated with fibrous tissues and retract, a process that prevents cusp apposition during diastole and usually leads to regurgitation into the left ventricle through a defect in the center of the valve (see Fig. 57–24C). The associated fusion of the commissures may restrict the opening of the valve, resulting in combined AS and AR; some associated mitral valve involvement is also common. Other primary valvular causes of AR include calcific AS in the elderly, in which some degree (usually mild) of AR is present in 75 percent of patients; *infective endocarditis* (see Chap. 58), in which the infection may destroy or cause perforation of a leaflet, or the vegetations may interfere with proper coaptation of the cusps; and *trauma* that results in a tear of the ascending aorta, in which loss of commissural support can cause prolapse of an aortic cusp. Although the most common complication of a congenitally *bicuspid valve* in adults is stenosis, incomplete closure and/or prolapse of a bicuspid valve may also cause isolated regurgitation or a combination of stenosis and regurgitation.[151,227] Progressive AR may occur in patients with a large ventricular septal defect as well as in patients with membranous subaortic stenosis (see Chap. 56) and as a complication of percutaneous aortic balloon valvotomy and radiofrequency catheter ablation.[228] Progressive regurgitation may also occur in patients with myxomatous proliferation of the aortic valve. An increasingly common cause of valvular AR is structural deterioration of a bioprosthetic valve.

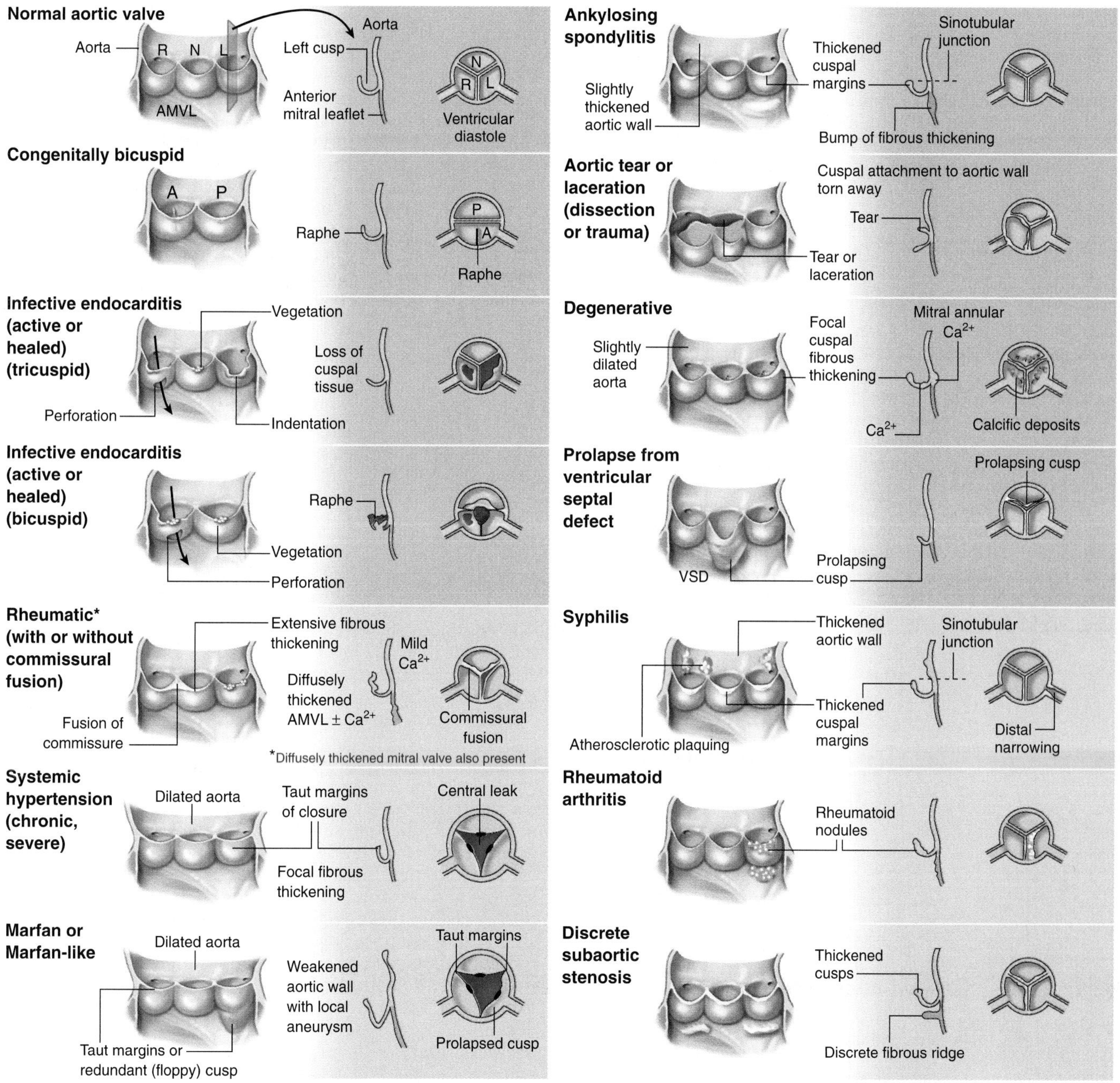

FIGURE 57–31 Diagram of various causes of pure aortic regurgitation. AMVL = anterior mitral valve leaflet; A = anterior; P = posterior; VSD = ventricular septal defect. (From Waller BF: Rheumatic and nonrheumatic conditions producing valvular heart disease. Cardiovasc Clin 16:30-31, 1986.)

Less common causes of AR include various forms of congenital AR, such as unicommissural and quadricuspid valves, or rupture of a congenitally fenestrated valve, particularly in the presence of hypertension. Other less common causes of AR occur in association with systemic lupus erythematosus, rheumatoid arthritis, ankylosing spondylitis, Jaccoud arthropathy, Takayasu disease, Whipple disease, Crohn disease, and, in the past, use of certain anorectic drugs. Isolated congenital AR is an uncommon lesion on necropsy studies, but, when present, is usually associated with a bicuspid valve.

Aortic Root Disease (see Chap. 53)

AR secondary to marked dilation of the ascending aorta is now more common than primary valve disease in patients undergoing AVR for pure AR.[57,226] The conditions responsible for aortic root disease include age-related (degenerative) aortic dilation, cystic medial necrosis of the aorta (either isolated or associated with classic Marfan syndrome), aortic dilation related to bicuspid valves, aortic dissection, osteogenesis imperfecta, syphilitic aortitis, ankylosing spondylitis, Behçet syndrome, psoriatic arthritis, arthritis associated with ulcerative colitis, relapsing polychondritis, Reiter syndrome, giant cell arteritis, and systemic hypertension, as well as exposure to some appetite-suppressant drugs.

When the aortic annulus becomes greatly dilated, the aortic leaflets separate, and AR may ensue. Dissection of the diseased aortic wall may occur and aggravate the AR. Dilation of the aortic root may also have secondary effects on the aortic valve because dilation causes tension and bowing of the individual cusps, which may thicken, retract, and become too short to close the aortic orifice. This leads to intensification of the AR, further dilating the ascending aorta and thus leading to a vicious circle in which, as is the case for MR, "regurgitation begets regurgitation."

AR, regardless of its cause, produces dilation and hypertrophy of the left ventricle, dilation of the mitral valve ring, and sometimes hypertrophy and dilation of the left atrium. Endocardial pockets frequently develop in the left ventricular cavity at sites of impact of the regurgitant jet.

Chronic Aortic Regurgitation

Pathophysiology (Fig. 57–32)

In contrast to MR, in which a fraction of the left ventricular stroke volume is ejected into the low-pressure left atrium, in AR the entire left ventricular stroke volume is ejected into a high-pressure chamber, i.e., the aorta (although the low aortic diastolic pressure does facilitate ventricular emptying during early systole). In MR, especially acute MR, the reduction of wall tension (i.e., reduced afterload) allows more complete systolic emptying; in AR, the increase in left ventricular end-diastolic volume (i.e., increased preload) provides hemodynamic compensation.[1,57,229]

Severe AR may occur with a normal effective forward stroke volume and a normal ejection fraction (forward plus regurgitant stroke volume/end-diastolic volume), together with an elevated left ventricular end-diastolic volume, pressure, and stress (Fig. 57–33).[57,230] In accord with Laplace's law (which indicates that wall tension is related to the product of the intraventricular pressure and radius divided by wall thickness), left ventricular dilation also increases the left ventricular systolic tension required to develop any level of systolic pressure. This leads to eccentric hypertrophy, with replication of sarcomeres in series and elongation of myocytes and myocardial fibers. In compensated AR, there is sufficient wall thickening so that the ratio of ventricular wall thickness to cavity radius remains normal. This maintains or returns end-diastolic wall stress to normal levels. Thus, in AR there is an increase in both preload and afterload. Left ventricular systolic function is maintained through the combination of chamber dilation and hypertrophy.[57,230] AR contrasts with AS, in which there is pressure overload (concentric) hypertrophy with replication of sarcomeres largely in parallel and an increased ratio of wall thickness to radius, but like AS there is an increase in interstitial connective tissue.[176,216,231] In AR, left ventricular mass is usually greatly increased, often to levels even higher than in isolated AS and sometimes exceeding 1000 gm (Fig. 57–34). As AR persists and increases in severity over time, wall thickening fails to keep pace with the hemodynamic load and end-systolic wall stress rises. At this point, the afterload mismatch results in a decline in systolic function, and ejection fraction falls.[57,229]

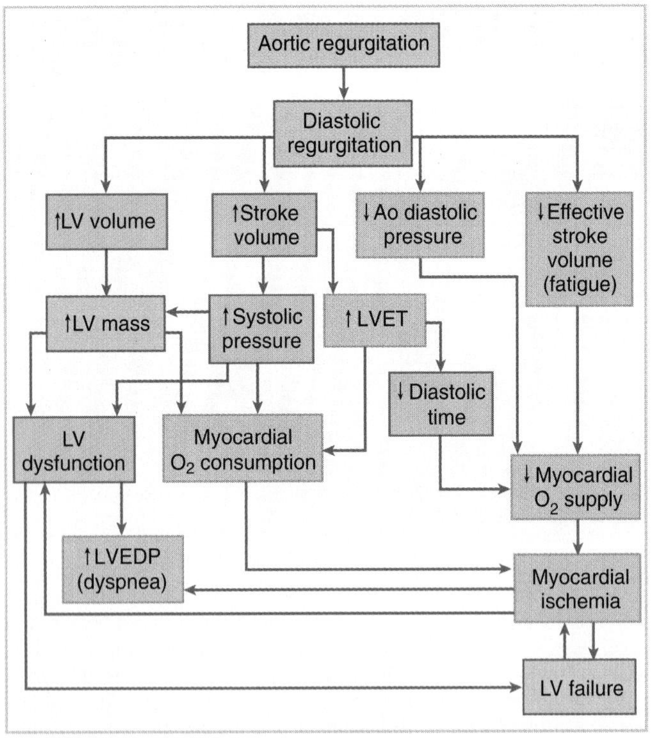

FIGURE 57–32 Pathophysiology of aortic regurgitation. Aortic regurgitation results in an increased left ventricular (LV) volume, increased stroke volume, increased aortic (Ao) systolic pressure, and decreased effective stroke volume. Increased LV volume results in an increased LV mass, which may lead to LV dysfunction and failure. Increased LV stroke volume increases systolic pressure and prolongation of LV ejection time (LVET). Increased LV systolic pressure results in a decrease in diastolic time. Decreased diastolic time (myocardial perfusion time), diastolic aortic pressure, and effective stroke volume reduce myocardial O_2 supply. Increased myocardial O_2 consumption and decreased myocardial O_2 supply produce myocardial ischemia, which further deteriorates LV function. LVEDP = LV end-diastolic pressure. (From Boudoulas H, Gravanis MB: Valvular heart disease. *In* Gravanis MB [ed]: Cardiovascular Disorders: Pathogenesis and Pathophysiology. St. Louis, CV Mosby, 1993, p 64.)

Patients with severe chronic AR have the largest end-diastolic volumes of those with any form of heart disease (resulting in so-called cor bovinum). However, end-diastolic pressure is not uniformly elevated (i.e., left ventricular compliance is often increased [see Fig. 57–33]).

In the more severe cases of AR, the regurgitant flow may exceed 20 liter/min, so that the total left ventricular output at rest approaches 25 liter/min, a level that can be achieved acutely only by a trained endurance runner during maximal exercise. Thus, the adaptive response to gradually increasing, chronic AR permits the ventricle to function as an effective high-compliance pump, handling a large stroke volume, often with little increase in filling pressure. During exercise, peripheral vascular resistance declines, and with an increase in heart rate, diastole shortens and the regurgitation per beat decreases,[1,232] facilitating an increment in effective (forward) cardiac output without substantial increases in end-diastolic volume and pressure. The ejection fraction and related ejection phase indices are often within normal limits, both at rest and during exercise, even though myocardial function, as reflected in the slope of the end-systolic pressure-volume relationship, is depressed.[233]

LEFT VENTRICULAR FUNCTION. As the left ventricle decompensates, interstitial fibrosis increases, compliance declines, and left ventricular end-diastolic pressure and volume rise (see Fig. 57–33). In advanced stages of decompensation, left atrial, pulmonary artery wedge, pulmonary arterial, right ventricular, and right atrial pressures rise and the effective (forward) cardiac output falls, at first during exercise and then at rest. The normal decline in end-systolic volume or the rise in ejection fraction fails to occur during exercise. Symptoms of heart failure, particularly those secondary to pulmonary congestion, develop.

MYOCARDIAL ISCHEMIA. When *acute* AR is induced experimentally, myocardial oxygen requirements rise substantially, secondary to an increase in wall tension. In patients with chronic, severe AR, total myocardial oxygen requirements are also augmented by the increase in left ventricular mass. Because the major portion of coronary blood flow occurs during diastole, when arterial pressure is lower than normal in AR, coronary perfusion pressure is reduced.[232] Studies in experimentally induced AR have shown a reduction in coronary flow reserve with a change in forward coronary flow from diastole to systole. The result—a combination of increased oxygen demand and reduced supply—sets the stage for the development of myocardial ischemia, especially during exercise. Thus, patients with severe AR exhibit a reduction of coronary reserve, which may be responsible for myocardial ischemia, which in turn may play a role in the deterioration of left ventricular function.

Clinical Manifestations

HISTORY
In patients with chronic, severe AR, the left ventricle gradually enlarges while the patient remains asymptomatic.[57,230] Symptoms of reduced cardiac reserve or myocardial ischemia develop, most often in the fourth or fifth decade and usually only *after* considerable cardiomegaly and myocardial dysfunction have occurred. The principal complaints of exertional dyspnea, orthopnea, and paroxysmal nocturnal dyspnea usually develop gradually. Angina pectoris is prominent late in the course; nocturnal angina may be troublesome and is often accompanied by diaphoresis that occurs when the heart rate slows and arterial diastolic pressure falls to extremely low levels. Patients with severe AR often complain of an uncomfortable awareness of the heartbeat, especially on lying down, and disagreeable thoracic pain due to pounding of the heart against the chest wall. Tachycardia, occurring with emotional stress or exertion, may cause troubling palpitations and head pounding. Premature ventricular contractions are particularly distressing because of the great heave of the volume-loaded left ventricle during the postextrasystolic beat. These complaints may be present for many years before symptoms of overt left ventricular dysfunction develop.

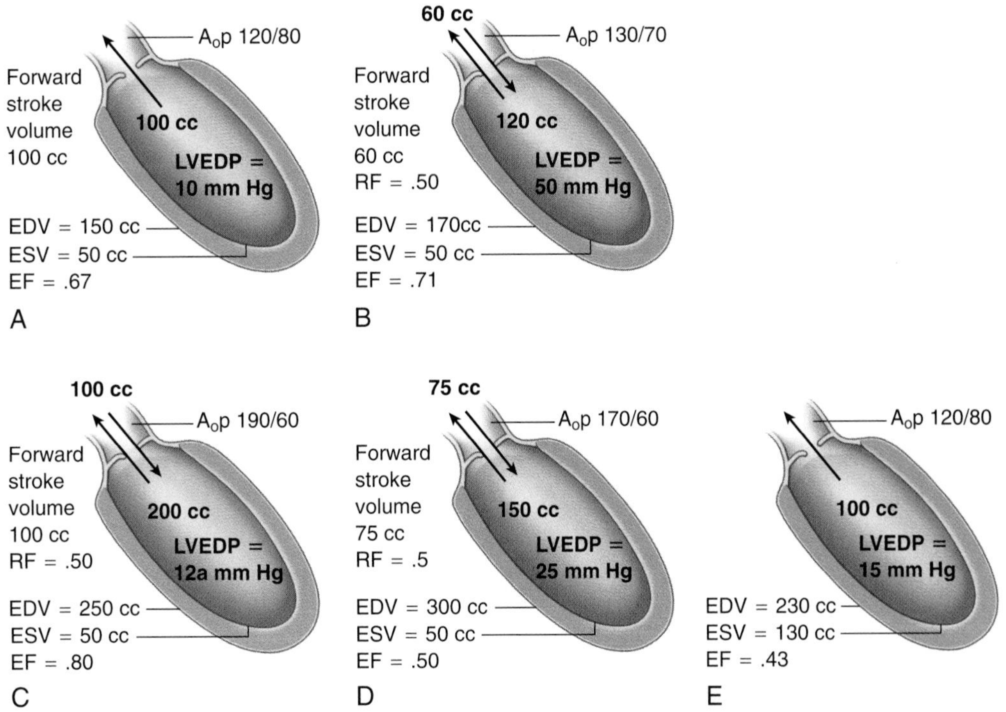

FIGURE 57–33 Hemodynamics of aortic regurgitation. **A,** Normal conditions. **B,** The hemodynamic changes that occur in severe acute aortic regurgitation. Although total stroke volume is increased, forward stroke volume is reduced. Left ventricular end-diastolic pressure (LVEDP) rises dramatically. **C,** Hemodynamic changes occurring in chronic compensated aortic regurgitation are shown. Eccentric hypertrophy produces increased end-diastolic volume (EDV), which permits an increase in total as well as forward stroke volume. The volume overload is accommodated and left ventricular filling pressure is normalized. Ventricular emptying and end-systolic volume (ESV) remain normal. **D,** In chronic decompensated aortic regurgitation, impaired left ventricular emptying produces an increase in end-systolic volume and a fall in ejection fraction (EF), total stroke volume, and forward stroke volume. There is further cardiac dilation and reelevation of left ventricular filling pressure. **E,** Immediately following valve replacement, preload estimated by EDV decreases, as does filling pressure. ESV also is decreased, but to a lesser extent. The result is an initial fall in EF. Despite these changes, elimination of regurgitation leads to an increase in forward stroke volume. A_0p = aortic pressure; RF = regurgitant fraction. (From Carabello BA: Aortic regurgitation: Hemodynamic determinants of prognosis. *In* Cohn LH, DiSesa VJ [eds]: Aortic Regurgitation: Medical and Surgical Management. New York, Marcel Dekker, 1986.)

PHYSICAL EXAMINATION (see Chap. 8)
In patients with chronic, severe AR, the head frequently bobs with each heartbeat (*de Musset sign*), and the pulses are of the "water-hammer" or collapsing type with abrupt distention and quick collapse (*Corrigan pulse*). The arterial pulse is often prominent and can be best appreciated by palpation of the radial artery with the patient's arm elevated. A *bisferiens pulse* may be present and is more readily recognized in the brachial and femoral arteries than in the carotid arteries. A variety of auscultatory findings provide confirmation of a wide pulse pressure. *Traube sign* (also known as "pistol shot sounds") refers to booming systolic and diastolic sounds heard over the femoral artery, *Müller sign* consists of systolic pulsations of the uvula, and *Duroziez sign* consists of a systolic murmur heard over the femoral artery when it is compressed proximally and a diastolic murmur when it is compressed distally. Capillary pulsations (*Quincke sign*) can be detected by pressing a glass slide on the patient's lip, by transmitting a light through the patient's fingertips, or by exerting gently pressure on the tip of a fingernail.

Systolic arterial pressure is elevated, and diastolic pressure is abnormally low. *Hill sign* refers to popliteal cuff systolic pressure exceeding brachial cuff pressure by more than 60 mm Hg. Korotkoff sounds often persist to zero even though intraarterial pressure rarely falls below 30 mm Hg.[230] The point of change in Korotkoff sounds, i.e., the muffling of these sounds in phase IV, correlates with the diastolic pressure. As heart failure develops, peripheral vasoconstriction may occur and arterial diastolic pressure may rise. This finding should not be interpreted as the presence of mild AR.

The apical impulse is diffuse and hyperdynamic and is displaced laterally and inferiorly; there may be systolic retraction over the parasternal region. A rapid ventricular filling wave is often palpable at the apex. The augmented stroke volume may create a *systolic* thrill at the base of the heart or suprasternal notch and over the carotid arteries.[230] In many patients, a carotid shudder is palpable.

AUSCULTATION
The PR interval may be prolonged, causing a soft S_1. A_2 may be normal or accentuated when AR is due to disease of the aortic root but is soft or absent when the valve is causing AR. P_2 may be obscured by the early diastolic murmur. Thus, S_2 may be absent or single or exhibit narrow or paradoxical splitting. A systolic ejection sound, presumably related to abrupt distention of the aorta by the augmented stroke volume, is frequently audible. An S_3 gallop correlates with an increased left ventricular end-diastolic volume.[230] Its development may be a sign of impaired left ventricular function, which is useful in identifying patients with severe regurgitation who are candidates for surgical treatment.

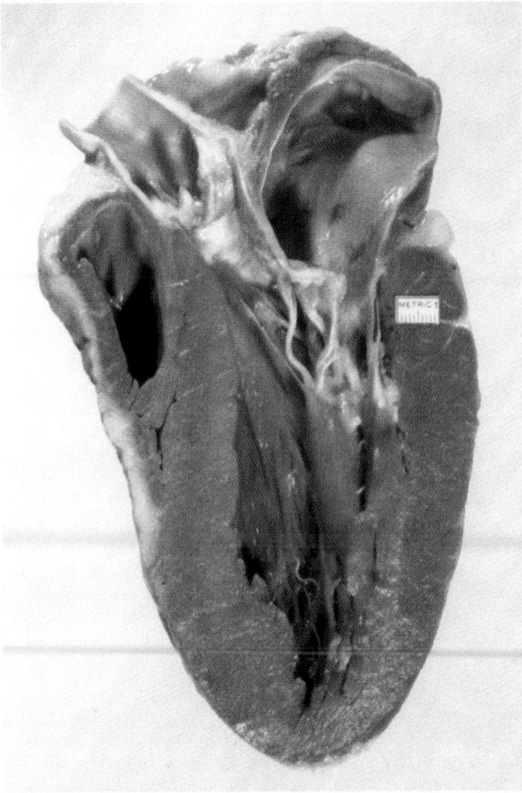

FIGURE 57–34 Heart of a young man with chronic aortic regurgitation who died suddenly, demonstrating both left ventricular dilation and marked left ventricular hypertrophy. (Courtesy of William C. Roberts, MD.)

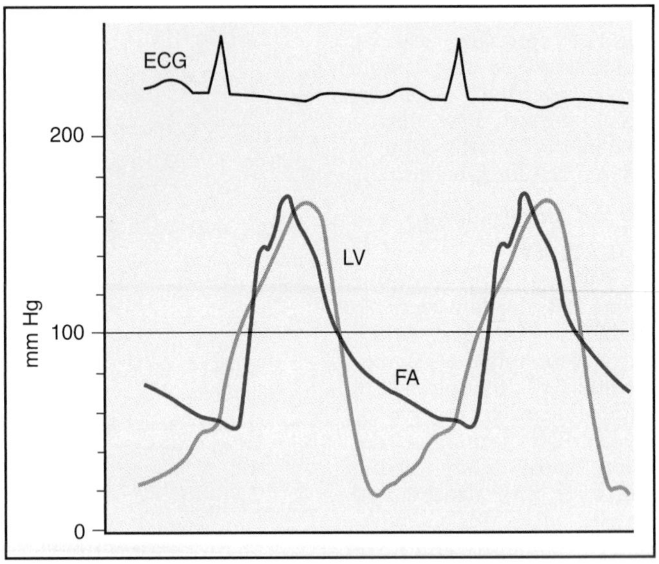

FIGURE 57–35 Pressure curves obtained from a 63-year-old man with symptoms of left ventricular (LV) failure and a loud decrescendo diastolic murmur. The femoral arterial (FA) pressure tracing demonstrates a widened pulse pressure of 115 mm Hg and equalization with LV pressure late in diastole. The LV pressure curve exhibits a steady pressure increase throughout diastole, culminating in a markedly elevated end-diastolic pressure of 45 mm Hg. These findings are indicative of severe aortic regurgitation. ECG = electrocardiogram.

The aortic regurgitant murmur, the principal physical finding of AR,[230,234] is one of high frequency that begins immediately after A_2. It may be distinguished from the murmur of PR by its earlier onset, i.e., immediately after A_2 rather than after P_2, and usually by the presence of a widened pulse pressure. The murmur is heard best with the diaphragm of the stethoscope while the patient is sitting up and leaning forward, with the breath held in deep exhalation. In severe AR, the murmur reaches an early peak and then has a dominant decrescendo pattern throughout diastole.

The severity of the regurgitation correlates better with the *duration* than with the *intensity* of the murmur. In mild AR, the murmur may be limited to early diastole and is typically high pitched and blowing. In severe AR, the murmur is holodiastolic and may have a rough quality. When the murmur is musical ("cooing dove" murmur), it usually signifies eversion or perforation of an aortic cusp. In patients with severe AR and left ventricular decompensation, equilibration of aortic and left ventricular pressures in late diastole (Fig. 57–35) abolishes the late diastolic component of the regurgitant murmur. When regurgitation is caused by primary valvular disease, the diastolic murmur is heard best along the left sternal border in the 3rd and 4th intercostal spaces. However, when it is due mainly to dilation of the ascending aorta, the murmur is often more readily audible along the right sternal border.[230]

Many patients with chronic AR have a harsh systolic outflow murmur caused by the increased total left ventricular stroke volume and ejection rate, and this often radiates to the carotid vessels.[230] The systolic murmur is often more readily audible than the diastolic murmur. It may be higher pitched and less rasping than the murmur of AS but is often accompanied by a systolic thrill. Palpation of the carotid pulses will elucidate the cause of the systolic murmur and differentiate it from the murmur of AS.

A mid and late diastolic apical rumble, the *Austin Flint murmur*, is common in severe AR and may occur in the presence of a normal mitral valve. This murmur appears to be created by rapid antegrade flow across a mitral orifice that is narrowed by the rapidly rising left ventricular diastolic pressure caused by severe aortic reflux impinging on the anterior leaflet of the mitral valve. The Austin Flint murmur may be difficult to differentiate from that due to MS, but the presence of an OS and a loud S_1 in MS and the absence of these findings in AR are helpful clues. As the left ventricular end-diastolic pressure rises, the Austin Flint murmur commences and terminates earlier.

Dynamic Auscultation. The diastolic murmur of AR may be accentuated when the patient sits up and leans forward or by interventions that raise the arterial pressure, such as squatting or isometric exercise. The intensity of the murmur is reduced by interventions that lower the systolic pressure, such as inhalation of amyl nitrite or the strain of the Valsalva maneuver. The Austin Flint murmur, like the murmur of AR, is augmented by isometric exercise and administration of vasopressors and is reduced by amyl nitrite inhalation.

Laboratory Examination

ELECTROCARDIOGRAM. *Chronic,* severe AR results in left-axis deviation and a pattern of left ventricular diastolic volume overload, characterized by an increase in initial forces (prominent Q waves in leads I, aVL, and V_3 through V_6) and a relatively small wave in lead V_1. With the passage of time, these initial forces diminish, but the total QRS amplitude increases. The T waves may be tall and upright in the left precordial leads early in the course, but, more commonly they are inverted, with ST segment depressions. A left ventricular "strain" pattern correlates with the presence of dilation and hypertrophy.[235] Left intraventricular conduction defects occur late in the course and are usually associated with left ventricular dysfunction. The ECG is not an accurate predictor of the severity of AR or cardiac weight. When AR is caused by an inflammatory process, prolongation of the PR interval may be present.[230]

RADIOLOGICAL FINDINGS (see Fig. 12–22). Cardiac size is a function of the duration and severity of regurgitation and the state of left ventricular function. In acute AR, there may be minimal cardiac enlargement, but marked enlargement is a common finding in chronic AR. Typically, the left ventricle enlarges in an inferior and leftward direction, causing a significant increase in the long axis but sometimes causing little or no increase in the transverse diameter of the heart. Calcification of the aortic valve is uncommon in patients with pure AR but is often present in patients with combined AS and AR. Distinct left atrial enlargement in the absence of heart failure suggests associated mitral valve disease. Dilation of the ascending aorta is usually more marked than in AS and may involve the entire aortic arch, including the aortic knob. Severe aneurysmal dilation of the aorta suggests that aortic root disease (e.g., Marfan syndrome, cystic medial necrosis, or annuloaortic ectasia) is responsible for the AR. Linear calcifications in the wall of the ascending aorta are seen in syphilitic aortitis but are nonspecific and are observed in degenerative disease as well.

ANGIOGRAPHY. For angiographic assessment of AR, contrast material should be injected rapidly (i.e., 25 to 35 ml/sec) into the aortic root, and filming should be carried out in the right and left anterior oblique projections. Opacification may be improved by filming during a Valsalva maneuver. In acute AR, there is only a slight increase in ventricular end-diastolic volume, but with the passage of time both the end-diastolic volume and the thickness of the ventricular wall increase, usually in parallel.

ECHOCARDIOGRAPHY (see Figs. 11–69 to 11–72 and Table 11–4). This technique is helpful in identifying the cause of AR. The echocardiogram may show thickening of the valve cusps, congenital abnormalities, prolapse of the valve, a flail leaflet, vegetations, or dilation of the aortic root. Two-dimensional studies are useful for the measurement of left ventricular end-diastolic and end-systolic dimensions, volumes, shortening fraction, ejection fraction, and mass.[232] These measurements, when made serially, are of great value in selecting the optimal time for surgical intervention. Although transthoracic imaging is usually satisfactory, transesophageal echocardiography often provides more detail.

High-frequency fluttering of the anterior leaflet of the mitral valve during diastole is an important echocardiographic finding in both acute and chronic AR (see Fig. 11–72); however, it does not develop when the mitral valve is rigid, as occurs with rheumatic involvement. This sign, which, unlike the Austin Flint murmur, occurs even in mild AR, results from the movement imparted to the anterior leaflet of the mitral valve by the jet of blood regurgitating from the aorta.

Doppler echocardiography and color-flow Doppler imaging are the most sensitive and accurate noninvasive techniques in the diagnosis and evaluation of AR. They readily detect mild degrees of AR that may be inaudible on physical examination. Both the aortic regurgitant orifice size and the aortic regurgitant flow can be estimated quantitatively (Fig. 57–36; see also Figs. 11–66 and 11–67 and Table 11–4).[236-240] Serial studies permit determination of the progression of regurgitation and its effect on the left ventricle.

RADIONUCLIDE IMAGING (see Chap. 13). In most patients, echocardiography provides the needed information regarding severity of AR and the status of the left ventricle. Radionuclide angiography is useful when the echo images are suboptimal, there is a discrepancy between the clinical and the echocardiographic information, or there is a need for more precise measurement of left ventricular ejection fraction.[1] This technique provides an accurate noninvasive assessment of the severity of AR by allowing determination of the regurgitant fraction and of the left ventricular/right ventricular stroke volume ratio. This measurement is nonspecific because the ratio is increased by the presence of associated MR and reduced by tricuspid or pulmonary regurgitation. However, in the absence of these complicating lesions, a left ventricular/right ventricular stroke volume ratio of 2.0 or more denotes severe AR. Radionuclide angiography is also of value in the assessment of left ventricular function during exercise in patients with AR.[233] Serial measurements are useful in the early detection of deterioration of left ventricular function.

MAGNETIC RESONANCE IMAGING (see Fig. 14–12B). Cardiac MRI provides accurate measurements of regurgitant volumes and the regurgitant orifice in AR. It is the most accurate noninvasive technique for assessing left ventricular end-systolic volume, diastolic volume, and mass (see Chap. 14).

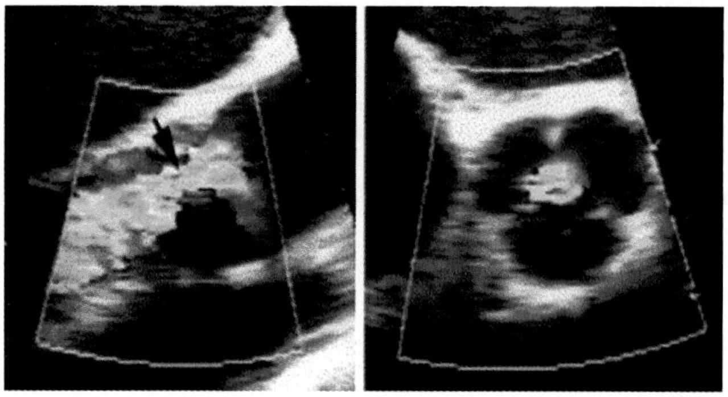

A B

FIGURE 57–36 Transesophageal color Doppler imaging of the aortic regurgitant jet. **A,** Long-axis view. The black arrow indicates the vena contracta, the narrowest portion of the jet located at or just distal to its orifice. The width (in millimeters) of the vena contracta correlates well with volumetric measurement of regurgitant fraction and regurgitant volume. **B,** Short-axis view in the same patient. (From Willett DL, Hall SA, Jessen ME, et al: Assessment of aortic regurgitation by transesophageal color Doppler imaging of the vena contracta: Validation against an intraoperative aortic flow probe. J Am Coll Cardiol 37:1450, 2001.)

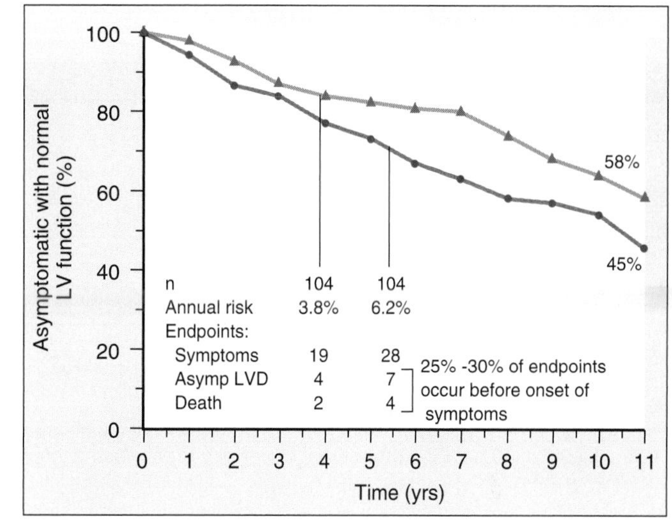

FIGURE 57–37 Natural history of chronic asymptomatic aortic regurgitation in patients with normal left ventricular (LV) ejection fraction at rest, in the series reported by Bonow and associates (blue line) and Borer and colleagues (magenta line), each enrolling 104 patients. At 11 years, 45 to 58 percent of patients remained asymptomatic with normal LV function, such that the risk of developing symptoms, LV dysfunction, or death is roughly 4 to 6 percent per year. The endpoints encountered in these series are indicated. The majority of patients who deteriorated developed symptoms leading to aortic valve replacement. However, 25 to 30 percent of the endpoints, either asymptomatic LV dysfunction (Asymp LVD) or death, occurred without warning symptoms. (Adapted from Bonow RO, Lakatos E, Maron BJ, et al: Serial long-term assessment of the natural history of asymptomatic patients with chronic aortic regurgitation and normal left ventricular systolic function. Circulation 84:1625, 1991; and Borer JS, Hochreiter C, Herrold EM, et al: Prediction of indications for valve replacement among asymptomatic and minimally symptomatic patients with chronic aortic regurgitation and normal left ventricular performance. Circulation 97:525, 1998.)

Management

NATURAL HISTORY OF CHRONIC AORTIC REGURGITATION

Moderately severe or even severe chronic AR may be associated with a generally favorable prognosis for many years. Among asymptomatic patients with severe AR and normal left ventricular ejection fractions, more than 45 percent remain asymptomatic with normal left ventricular function at 10 years (Fig. 57–37),[229,241,242] with an average rate of developing symptoms or left ventricular systolic dysfunction less than 6 percent per year (Table 57–11).[1] The likelihood of sudden death in these asymptomatic patients is less than 0.5 percent per year. However, as is the case for AS, once the patient becomes symptomatic, the downhill course becomes rapidly progressive. Congestive heart failure, punctuated by episodes of acute pulmonary edema, and sudden death may occur, usually in previously symptomatic patients who have considerable left ventricular dilation. Data compiled in the presurgical era indicate that without surgical treatment, death usually occurs within 4 years after the development of angina pectoris and within 2 years after the onset of heart failure. Dujardin and colleagues have confirmed these findings in the current era, demonstrating that 4-year survival without surgery in patients with NYHA Class III or IV symptoms is approximately 30 percent (Fig. 57–38).[244]

Gradual deterioration of left ventricular function may occur even during the asymptomatic period, and some patients may develop significant impairment of systolic function before the onset of symptoms. Numerous surgical series over the past two decades indicate that depressed left ventricular ejection fraction is among the most important determinants of mortality after AVR, particularly when ventricular dysfunction is irreversible and does not improve after operation.[1] Left ventricular dysfunction is more likely to be reversible if detected early before ejection fraction becomes severely depressed, before the left ventricle becomes markedly dilated, and before significant symptoms develop; it is therefore important to intervene surgically before these changes have become irreversible.[1,57,229,245]

TABLE 57–11 Natural History of Aortic Regurgitation

Asymptomatic Patients with Normal LV Systolic Function	
Progression to symptoms and or LV dysfunction	<6%/yr
Progression to asymptomatic LV dysfunction	<3.5%/yr
Sudden death	<0.2%/yr
Asymptomatic Patients with LV Systolic Dysfunction	
Progression to cardiac symptoms	>25%/yr
Symptomatic Patients	
Mortality rate	>10%/yr

LV = left ventricular.

From Bonow RO, Carabello B, de Leon AC Jr, et al: ACC/AHA guidelines for the management of patients with valvular heart disease. J Am Coll Cardiol 32:1486, 1988.

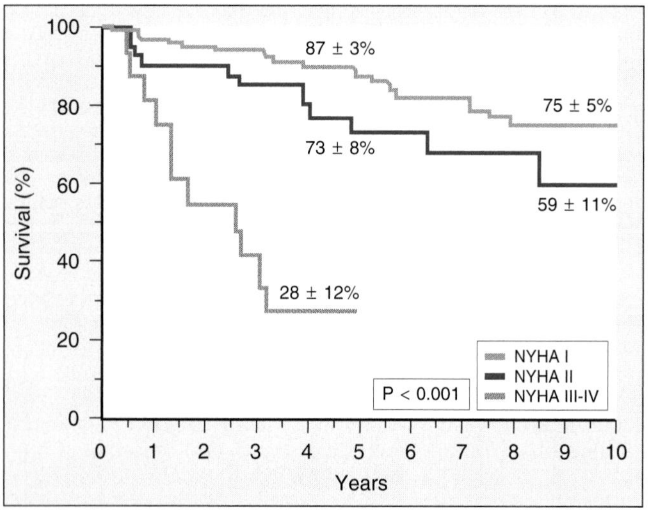

FIGURE 57–38 Survival without surgery in 242 patients with chronic aortic regurgitation, demonstrating the importance of symptoms in determining outcome. Patients with New York Heart Association (NYHA) Class III or IV symptoms had a survival of only 28 percent at 4 years. In contrast, the 10-year survival in patients in Class I was 75 percent, which was identical to that of an age-matched normal population (75 percent). (From Dujardin KS, Enriquez-Sarano M, Schaff HV, et al: Mortality and morbidity of aortic regurgitation in clinical practice: A long-term follow-up study. Circulation 99:1851, 1999.)

MEDICAL TREATMENT

All patients with AR of any severity should receive antibiotic prophylaxis for infective endocarditis (see Chap. 58). Patients with mild or moderate AR who are asymptomatic with normal or only minimally increased cardiac size require no therapy but should be followed clinically and by echocardiography every 12 or 24 months. Asymptomatic patients with chronic, severe AR and normal left ventricular function should be examined at intervals of approximately 6 months. In addition to clinical examination, serial echocardiographic assessments of left ventricular size and ejection fraction should be made. Left-heart catheterization and aortography are usually not necessary but may be useful in patients whose noninvasive test results are inconclusive or discordant with clinical findings.[1] Similarly, other noninvasive tests such as radionuclide angiography or cardiac MRI have an important role primarily when echocardiographic information is not adequate. Patients with mild to moderate AR and those with severe AR with normal ejection fractions and only mild ventricular dilation may engage in aerobic forms of exercise. However, patients with AR who have limitations of cardiac reserve and/or evidence of declining left ventricular function should not engage in vigorous sports or heavy exertion. Systemic arterial diastolic hypertension, if present, should be treated because it increases the regurgitant flow; vasodilating agents such as nifedipine or ACE inhibitors are preferred, and beta-blocking agents should be used with great caution. Atrial fibrillation and bradyarrhythmias are poorly tolerated and should be prevented if possible. If these arrhythmias occur, they must be treated promptly and vigorously.

Vasodilator Therapy. Patients with chronic AR and evidence of significant volume overload (increased end-diastolic dimension or volume) should be considered for vasodilator therapy. Short-term studies spanning 6 months to 2 years have demonstrated beneficial hemodynamic effects of oral hydralazine, nifedipine, felodipine, and ACE inhibitors.[229,246,247] One study followed asymptomatic patients with severe AR for 6 years, comparing the effects of nifedipine (69 patients) and digoxin (74 patients) on left ventricular function and symptoms.[248] Nifedipine delayed the need for operation: at 6 years, 85 percent of patients receiving nifedipine remained asymptomatic with normal left ventricular ejection fraction, compared with only 65 percent of patients receiving digoxin (Fig. 57–39).

Thus, vasodilator therapy is indicated for patients with chronic, severe AR and normal left ventricular systolic function.[1] This therapy should not be used in place of AVR in patients who fulfill the indications for surgery (discussed subsequently), except in circumstances in which AVR cannot be performed because of comorbidities or patient preference.

Symptomatic Patients. AVR is the treatment of choice in symptomatic patients. Chronic medical therapy may be necessary in some patients who refuse surgery or are considered to be inoperable because of comorbid conditions. These patients should receive an aggressive heart failure regimen (see Chap. 23) with ACE inhibitors (and perhaps other vasodilators), digoxin, diuretics, and salt restriction, but beta blockers should be avoided. Even though nitroglycerin and other nitrates are not as helpful in relieving anginal pain in patients with AR as they are in patients with coronary artery disease or AS, they are worth a trial.

In patients who are candidates for surgery but who have severely decompensated left ventricular dysfunction, vasodilator therapy may be particularly helpful in stabilizing patients while preparing for operation. Such patients also respond, at least temporarily, to treatment with digitalis glycosides, salt restriction, and diuretics.

SURGICAL TREATMENT

Indications for Operation. Because of their excellent prognosis in the short and medium term, operative correction

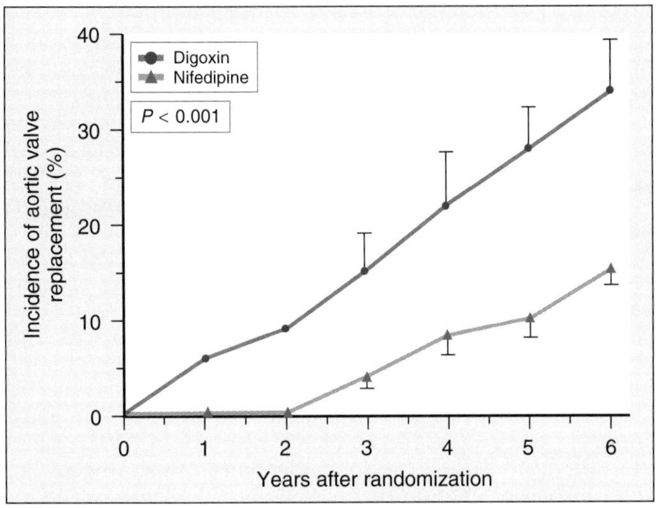

FIGURE 57–39 Randomized clinical trial of nifedipine versus digoxin in asymptomatic patients with chronic aortic regurgitation and normal left ventricular (LV) function. Data indicate the cumulative actuarial incidence of progression to aortic valve replacement because of development of symptoms or decrease in LV ejection fraction to below 50 percent. (From Scognamiglio R, Rahimtoola SH, Fasoli G, et al: Nifedipine in asymptomatic patients with severe aortic regurgitation and normal left ventricular function. N Engl J Med 331:689, 1994.)

should be deferred in patients with chronic, severe AR who are asymptomatic, have good exercise tolerance, *and* have an ejection fraction greater than 50 percent *without* severe left ventricular dilation (i.e., an end-diastolic diameter < 70 mm and an end-systolic diameter < 50 mm). Similarly, in the absence of obvious contraindications or serious comorbidity, surgical treatment is advisable for symptomatic patients with severe AR and for asymptomatic patients with an ejection fraction less than 0.50 and severe left ventricular dilation (end-diastolic diameter > 75 mm or end-systolic diameter > 55 mm).[1] Between these two ends of the clinical-hemodynamic spectrum are many patients in whom it may be quite difficult to balance the immediate risks of operation and the continuing risks of an implanted prosthetic valve on the one hand against the hazards of allowing a severe volume overload to damage the left ventricle on the other.[57,229,233,249]

Since severe symptoms (NYHA Class III or IV) and left ventricular dysfunction with an ejection fraction less than 0.50 are independent risk factors for poor postoperative survival (Fig. 57–40), surgery should be carried out in NYHA Class II patients before severe left ventricular dysfunction has developed.[1,249-252] Even after successful correction of AR, patients with severe left ventricular dysfunction may have persistent cardiomegaly and depressed left ventricular function.[229,249,251-253] Such patients often exhibit histological changes in the left ventricle, including massive fiber hypertrophy and increased interstitial fibrous tissue. Therefore, it is highly desirable to operate on patients *before* irreversible left ventricular changes have occurred.

Because AR has complex effects on both preload and afterload, the selection of appropriate indices of ventricular contractility to identify patients for operation is challenging. The relationship between end-systolic wall stress and ejection fraction or percent fractional shortening is a useful measurement,[241] as are more load-independent measures of left ventricular contractility.[254] However, in the absence of such complex measurements, *serial* changes in ventricular end-diastolic and end-systolic volumes or dimensions can be used to detect *relative* deterioration of ventricular function.[229] Although left ventricular end-diastolic volume and the ejection phase indices such as ejection fraction and ventricular

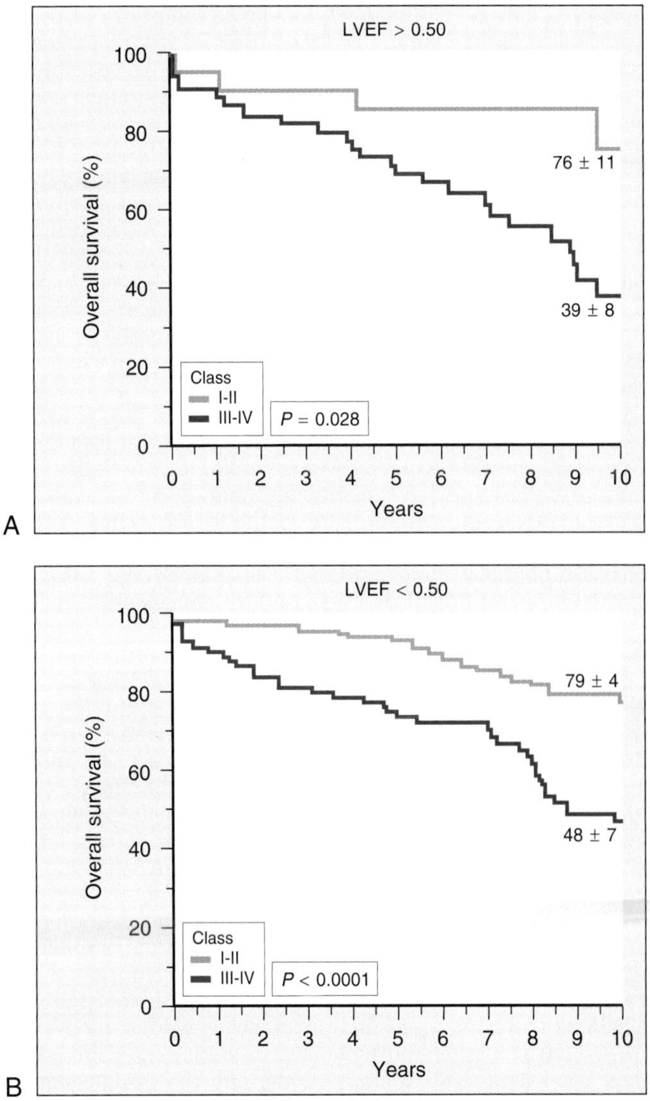

FIGURE 57–40 Long-term postoperative survival in patients with aortic regurgitation, stratified according to the severity of preoperative symptoms and preoperative left ventricular ejection fraction (LVEF). Patients with New York Heart Association (NYHA) Class III or IV symptoms experienced significantly worse survival than those with Class I or II symptoms whether the echocardiographic LVEF was higher than 0.50 **(A)** or less than 0.50 **(B)** without associated coronary artery disease. (From Klodas E, Enriquez-Sarano M, Tajik AJ, et al: Optimizing timing of surgical correction in patients with severe aortic regurgitation: Role of symptoms. J Am Coll Cardiol 30:746, 1997.)

fraction shortening are strongly influenced by loading conditions, they are nonetheless useful empirical predictors of postoperative function.

Serial echocardiograms or radionuclide ventriculograms should be obtained to detect changes in left ventricular size and function in asymptomatic patients with severe AR. Both techniques allow repeated evaluation of ejection fraction and end-systolic volume (or dimensions) both at rest and during exercise.[241] Impaired left ventricular function at *rest* is the basis for selecting patients for operation; normal left ventricular function at rest with failure of the ejection fraction to rise normally with *exercise* is not considered an indication for surgery per se but is an early warning sign that portends impaired function at rest.[1,233]

Asymptomatic patients with severe AR but normal left ventricular function have an excellent prognosis and do not warrant prophylactic operation (see Table 57–11).[1] On average, less than 6 percent of patients per year require operation because of the development of symptoms or of left ventricular dysfunction. The end-systolic diameter determined by two-dimensional echocardiography is valuable in predicting outcome in asymptomatic patients. Patients with severe AR and an end-systolic diameter less than 40 mm almost invariably remain stable and can be followed without immediate surgery. However, patients with an end-systolic diameter greater than 50 mm Hg have a 19 percent likelihood per year of developing symptoms of left ventricular dysfunction,[229] and those with an end-systolic diameter greater than 55 mm have an increased risk of irreversible left ventricular dysfunction if they are not operated on. Postoperative function and survival in this latter group are determined by severity of symptoms, severity of left ventricular dysfunction, and the *duration* of left ventricular dysfunction.[229]

In summary, the following considerations apply to the selection of patients with chronic AR for surgical treatment. Operation should be *deferred* in asymptomatic patients with normal and stable left ventricular function and should be *recommended* in symptomatic patients. In asymptomatic patients with left ventricular dysfunction, a decision should be based not on a single abnormal measurement but rather on several observations of depressed performance and impaired exercise tolerance, carried out at intervals of 2 to 4 months. If evidence of left ventricular dysfunction is borderline or is not consistent, continued close follow-up is indicated. If abnormalities are progressive or consistent (i.e., the left ventricular ejection fraction declines to the range of 0.50 to 0.55, the left ventricular end-systolic diameter rises to 55 mm or greater, or the left ventricular end-diastolic dimension rises to 75 mm or greater), operation should be strongly considered even in asymptomatic patients. The threshold for operation may be lower when the surgeon believes that AVR will not be necessary, but this prediction may be difficult. Symptomatic patients with severe AR who have normal, mildly depressed, or moderately depressed left ventricular function should be operated on. Patients with severely impaired left ventricular function (ejection fraction < 0.25) are at high surgical risk and have a guarded prognosis even after successful AVR. However, their outlook is also extremely poor when they receive medical therapy alone, and their management should be considered on an individual basis.

The indications for surgery in patients with severe AR secondary to aortic root disease are similar to those in patients with primary valvular disease. However, progressive expansion of the aortic root and/or a diameter greater than 50 mm by echocardiography with any degree of regurgitation is also an indication for surgery in patients with aortic root disease.[1]

As is the case for patients with other valvular lesions, adult surgical candidates who may have underlying coronary artery disease, based on symptoms, age, gender, and risk factors, should undergo preoperative coronary arteriography. Those with coronary artery stenoses should undergo revascularization at the time of AVR.

Operative Procedures. Because an increasing proportion of patients with severe, isolated AR coming to operation now have primary aortic root rather than primary valvular disease, an increasing number can be treated surgically by correcting the dilated aortic root.[103a,255,256] One of two annuloplasty procedures may be employed—an encircling suture of the aorta or a subcommissural annuloplasty. Aneurysmal dilation of the ascending aorta requires excision, replacement with a graft that includes a prosthetic valve, and reimplantation of the coronary arteries.[257]

In some patients with aortic root disease, the native valve can be spared when the aortic root is replaced or repaired (Fig. 57–41). Occasionally, when a leaflet has been torn from its attachments to the aortic annulus by trauma, surgical repair without replacement may be possible. In patients with AR secondary to prolapse of an aortic leaflet, aortic cusp resuspension or cusp resection may be employed. When AR is caused by leaflet perforation resulting from healed infective endocarditis, a pericardial patch can be used for repair.[227,258]

AVR is required for most patients with severe AR due to primary valve disease (as opposed to aortic root disease) and for many patients with combined AS and AR. Because the aortic annulus in patients with severe AR is usually not as narrow as it is in patients with AS, a larger prosthetic valve can be inserted, and mild postoperative obstruction to left ventricular outflow is less of a problem than it is in some patients with AS. In general, the risks and results of AVR in patients with AR are similar to those in patients with AS, with a large percentage of patients exhibiting striking improvement in symptoms. Reductions in heart size and in left ventricular diastolic volume and mass occur in most patients.[229] Exceptions are patients who are in NYHA Class III or IV heart failure and/or patients who have severe left ventricular dysfunction preoperatively.[215,250,252] As is true for patients with AS, the operative risk of AVR for patients with AR depends on the general condition of the patient, the state of left ventricular function, and the skill and experience of the surgical team. The mortality rate ranges from 3 to 8 percent in most medical centers (see Table 57–3). A late mortality of approximately 5 to 10 percent per year is observed in survivors who had marked cardiac enlargement and/or prolonged left ventricular dysfunction preoperatively. Follow-up studies have shown both early rapid and then slower long-term reductions of ventricular mass, ejection fraction, myocyte hypertrophy, and ventricular fibrous content following relief of AR.[216] By extending the indications for operation to symptomatic patients with normal left ventricular function as well as to asymptomatic patients with left ventricular dysfunction, both early and late results are improving.[252] With the continued improvement of surgical techniques and results, it will likely become possible to extend the recommendation for operative treatment to asymptomatic patients with severe regurgitation and normal cardiac function. However, given the risks of operation and the long-term complications of presently available prosthetic valves, we do not believe that the time for such a policy has yet arrived.

ACUTE AORTIC REGURGITATION

Acute AR is caused most commonly by infective endocarditis, aortic dissection, or trauma. The characteristic features of acute AR are tachycardia and an increase in left ventricular diastolic pressures. In contrast to the pathophysiological events in chronic AR just described, in which the left ventricle is able to adapt to the increased hemodynamic load, in acute AR the regurgitant volume fills a ventricle of normal size that cannot accommodate the combined large regurgitant volume and inflow from the left atrium. Because the ability of total stroke volume to rise acutely is limited, forward stroke volume declines. The sudden increase in left ventricular filling causes the left ventricular diastolic pressure to rise rapidly above left atrial pressure during early diastole (see Fig. 57-33),[259] causing the mitral valve to close prematurely in diastole. Premature closure of the mitral valve protects the pulmonary venous bed from backward transmission of the greatly elevated end-diastolic pressure unless it is accompanied by diastolic MR.[260] Premature closure of the mitral valve, together with tachycardia that also shortens diastole, reduces the time interval during which the mitral valve is open. The tachycardia may compensate for the reduced forward stroke volume and left ventricular and aortic *systolic* pressures may exhibit little change. However, severe acute AR may cause profound hypotension and cardiogenic shock. In light of the limited ability of the left ventricle to tolerate acute, severe AR, patients with this valvular lesion often develop clinical manifestations of sudden cardiovascular collapse, including weakness, severe dyspnea, and profound hypotension secondary to the reduced stroke volume and elevated left atrial pressure. In some patients, the aortic diastolic pressure equilibrates with the elevated left ventricular diastolic pressure.

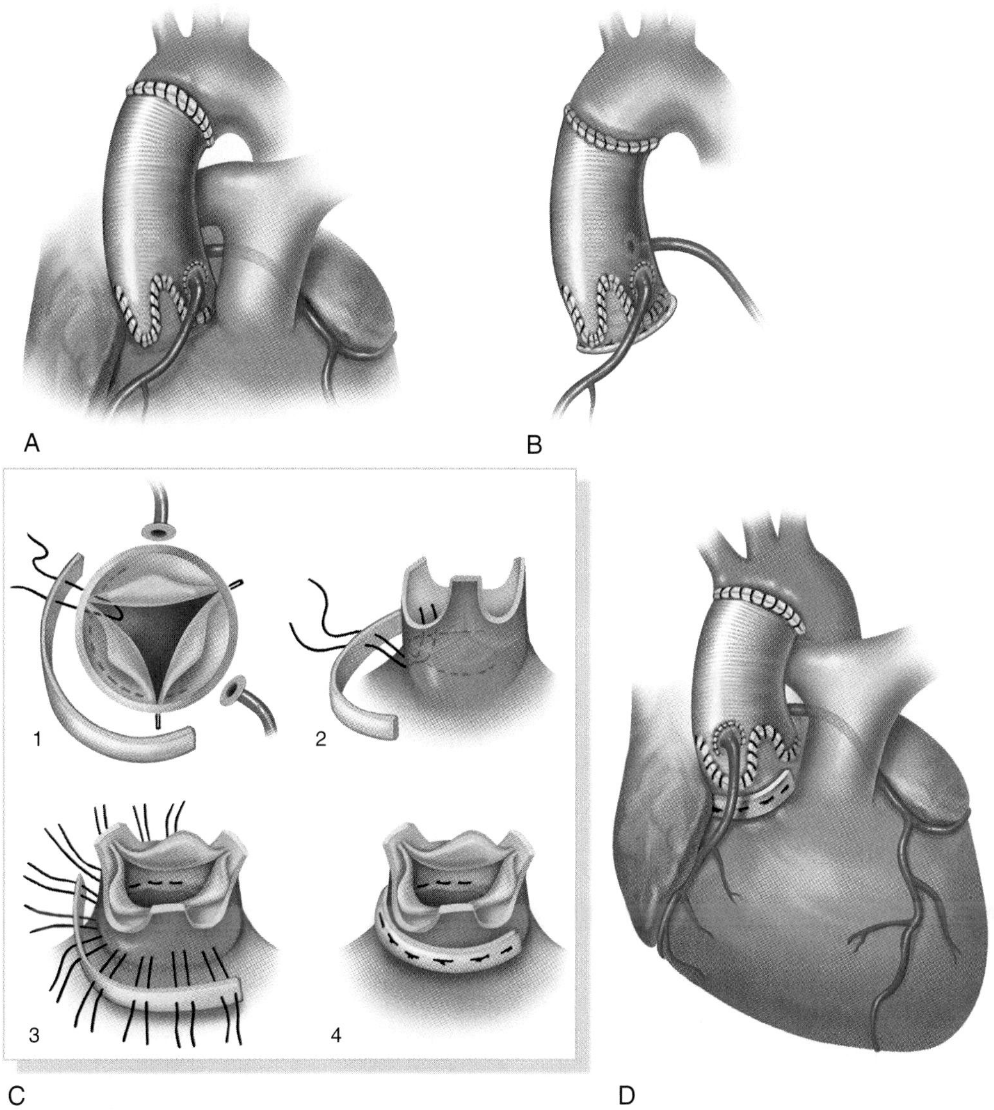

FIGURE 57–41 Repair of aortic regurgitation caused by aortic root dilation. **A,** Remodeling of the aortic root with replacement of all three aortic sinuses. **B,** Reimplantation of the aortic valve in patients with annuloaortic ectasia and aortic root aneurysm. **C** and **D,** Aortic annuloplasty in patients with annuloaortic ectasia. (From David TE: Aortic root aneurysms: Remodeling or composite replacement? Ann Thorac Surg 64:1564, 1997.)

PHYSICAL EXAMINATION. Patients with acute, severe AR appear gravely ill, with tachycardia, severe peripheral vasoconstriction and cyanosis, and sometimes pulmonary congestion and edema. The peripheral signs of AR are often not impressive and certainly not as dramatic as in patients with chronic AR. Duroziez murmur, Traube sign over the peripheral arteries, and bisferiens pulses are usually *absent* in acute AR. The normal or only slightly widened pulse pressure may lead to serious underestimation of the severity of the valvular lesion. The left ventricular impulse is normal or nearly so, and the rocking motion of the chest characteristic of chronic AR is not apparent. S_1 may be soft or absent because of premature closure of the mitral valve,[259] and the sound of mitral valve closure in mid or late diastole is occasionally audible. However, closure of the mitral valve may be incomplete, and diastolic MR may occur. Evidence of pulmonary hypertension, with an accentuated P_2, S_3, and S_4, is frequently present.

The early diastolic murmur of acute AR is lower pitched and shorter than that of chronic AR, because as left ventricular diastolic pressure rises, the (reverse) pressure gradient between the aorta and the left ventricle is rapidly reduced. A systolic murmur is common, resulting in "to and fro" sounds. The Austin Flint murmur is often present but is brief and ceases when left ventricular pressure exceeds left atrial pressure in diastole. With premature diastolic closure of the mitral valve, the presystolic portion of the Austin Flint murmur is eliminated.

LABORATORY EXAMINATION

Electrocardiography. In *acute* AR, the ECG may or may not show left ventricular hypertrophy, depending on the severity and duration of the regurgitation. However, nonspecific ST segment and T wave changes are common.

Radiological Findings. In acute AR, there is often evidence of marked pulmonary venous hypertension and pulmonary edema. The cardiac silhouette is usually remarkably normal, although left atrial enlargement may be present and, depending on the cause of the AR, there may be enlargement of the ascending aorta.

Echocardiography. In *acute* AR, the echocardiogram reveals a reduction in amplitude of the opening movement, premature closure, and delayed opening of the mitral valve.[259] Left ventricular end-diastolic dimensions are not markedly increased, and fractional shortening is normal. This contrasts with the findings in chronic AR, in which end-diastolic dimensions and wall motion are increased. Occasionally, with equilibration of aortic and left ventricular pressures in diastole, premature opening of the aortic valve may be detected.

MANAGEMENT OF ACUTE AORTIC REGURGITATION. Since early death due to left ventricular failure is frequent in patients with *acute, severe* AR despite intensive medical management, prompt surgical intervention is indicated. Even a normal ventricle cannot sustain the burden of acute, severe volume overload; therefore, the risk of *acute* AR is much greater than that of chronic AR.[259] While the patient is being prepared for surgery, treatment with an intravenous positive inotropic agent (dopamine or dobutamine) and/or a vasodilator (nitroprusside) is often necessary. The agent and dosage should be selected on the basis of arterial pressure (see Chap. 23). Beta-blocking agents and intraaortic balloon counterpulsation are contraindicated, because either lowering the heart rate or augmenting peripheral resistance during diastole can lead to rapid hemodynamic decompensation. In hemodynamically stable patients with acute AR secondary to active infective endocarditis, operation may be deferred to allow 5 to 7 days of intensive antibiotic therapy. However, AVR should be undertaken at the earliest sign of hemodynamic instability or if echocardiographic evidence of diastolic closure of the mitral valve develops.

Tricuspid, Pulmonic, and Multivalvular Disease

Tricuspid Stenosis

Etiology and Pathology

Tricuspid stenosis (TS) is almost always rheumatic in origin.[261] Other causes of obstruction to right atrial emptying are unusual and include congenital tricuspid atresia (see

Chap. 56); right atrial tumors, which may produce a clinical picture suggesting rapidly progressive TS (see Chap. 63)[262]; and the carcinoid syndrome (see Chap. 59),[263] which more frequently produces TR. Rarely, obstruction to right ventricular inflow can be due to endomyocardial fibrosis, tricuspid valve vegetations,[264] a pacemaker lead,[265] or extracardiac tumors.

Most patients with rheumatic tricuspid valve disease present with TR or a combination of stenosis and regurgitation. Isolated rheumatic TS is uncommon and *almost* never occurs as an isolated lesion but generally accompanies mitral valve disease.[1,261,266] In many patients with TS, the aortic valve is also involved (i.e., trivalvular stenosis is present). TS is found at autopsy in about 15 percent of patients with rheumatic heart disease but is of clinical significance in only about 5 percent.[261] Organic tricuspid valve disease is more common in India, Pakistan, and other developing nations near the equator than in North America or Western Europe. The anatomical changes of rheumatic TS resemble those of MS, with fusion and shortening of the chordae tendineae and fusion of the leaflets at their edges, producing a diaphragm with a fixed central aperture.[261] However, valvular calcification is rare. As is the case with MS, TS is more common in women. The right atrium is often greatly dilated in TS, and its walls are thickened. There may be evidence of severe passive congestion, with enlargement of the liver and spleen.

TABLE 57–12 Clinical and Laboratory Features of Rheumatic Tricuspid Stenosis

History
Progressive fatigue, edema, anorexia
Minimal orthopnea, paroxysmal nocturnal dyspnea
Rheumatic fever in two-thirds of patients
Female preponderance
Pulmonary edema and hemoptysis are rare
Physical Findings
Signs of multivalvular involvement
Diastolic rumble at lower left sternal border, increasing in intensity with inspiration
Often confused with mitral stenosis
Peripheral cyanosis
Neck vein distention, with prominent *v* waves and slow *y* descent
Absent right ventricular lift
Associated murmurs of mitral and aortic valve disease
Hepatic pulsation
Ascites, peripheral edema
Laboratory Findings
Electrocardiogram: tall right atrial P waves and no right ventricular hypertrophy
Chest roentgenogram: a dilated right atrium without an enlarged pulmonary artery segment
Echocardiography: diastolic doming of tricuspid valve leaflet.

Modified from Ockene IS: Tricuspid valve disease. *In* Dalon JE. Alpert JS (eds): Valvular Heart Disease. 2nd ed. Boston, Little, Brown, 1987, pp 356, 390.

Pathophysiology

A diastolic pressure gradient between the right atrium and ventricle—the hemodynamic expression of TS—is augmented when the transvalvular blood flow increases during inspiration or exercise and is reduced when the blood flow declines during expiration. A relatively modest diastolic pressure gradient (i.e., a mean gradient of only 5 mm Hg) is usually sufficient to elevate mean right atrial pressure to a level that results in systemic venous congestion and, unless sodium intake has been restricted or diuretics have been given, is associated with jugular venous distention, ascites, and edema.

In patients with sinus rhythm, the right atrial *a* wave may be very tall and may even approach the level of the right ventricular systolic pressure. Resting cardiac output is usually markedly reduced and fails to rise during exercise. This accounts for the normal or only slightly elevated left atrial, pulmonary arterial, and right ventricular systolic pressures, despite the presence of accompanying mitral valvular disease.

A *mean* diastolic pressure gradient across the tricuspid valve as low as 2 mm Hg is sufficient to establish the diagnosis of TS. However, exercise, deep inspiration, and the rapid infusion of fluids or the administration of atropine may greatly enhance a borderline pressure gradient in a patient with TS. Therefore, when this diagnosis is suspected, right atrial and ventricular pressures should be recorded simultaneously, using two catheters or a single catheter with a double lumen, with one lumen opening on either side of the tricuspid valve. The effects of respiration on any pressure difference should be examined.

Clinical Manifestations (Table 57–12)

HISTORY. The low cardiac output characteristic of TS causes fatigue, and patients often complain of discomfort due to hepatomegaly, swelling of the abdomen, and anasarca. The severity of these symptoms, which are secondary to an elevated systemic venous pressure, is out of proportion to the degree of dyspnea. Some patients complain of a fluttering discomfort in the neck, caused by giant *a* waves in the jugular venous pulse. Despite the coexistence of MS, the symptoms characteristic of this valvular lesion (i.e., severe dyspnea, orthopnea, and paroxysmal nocturnal dyspnea) are usually mild or absent in the presence of severe TS because the latter prevents surges of blood into the pulmonary circulation behind the stenotic mitral valve. Indeed, the *absence* of symptoms of pulmonary congestion in a patient with obvious MS should suggest the possibility of TS.

PHYSICAL EXAMINATION. Because of the high frequency with which MS occurs in patients with TS and the similarity in the physical findings between the two valvular lesions, the diagnosis of TS is commonly missed. The physical findings are mistakenly attributed to MS, which is more common and may be more obvious. Therefore, a high index of suspicion is required to detect the tricuspid valvular lesion. In the presence of sinus rhythm, the *a* wave in the jugular venous pulse is tall, and a presystolic hepatic pulsation is often palpable. The *y* descent is slow and barely appreciable. The lung fields are clear, and despite engorged neck veins and the presence of ascites and anasarca, the patient may be comfortable while lying flat. Thus, the diagnosis of TS may be suspected from inspection of the jugular venous pulse in a patient with MS but without clinical evidence of pulmonary hypertension. This suspicion is strengthened when a diastolic thrill is palpable at the lower left sternal border, particularly if the thrill appears or becomes more prominent during inspiration.

The auscultatory findings of the accompanying MS are usually prominent and often overshadow the more subtle signs of TS. A tricuspid OS may be audible but is often difficult to distinguish from a mitral OS. However, the tricuspid OS usually follows the mitral OS and is localized to the lower left sternal border, whereas the mitral OS is usually most prominent at the apex and radiates more widely. The diastolic murmur of TS is also commonly heard best along the lower left parasternal border in the 4th intercostal space and is usually softer, higher pitched, and shorter in duration than the murmur of MS. The presystolic component of the TS murmur has a scratchy quality and a crescendo-decrescendo configuration that diminishes before S_1. The diastolic murmur and OS of

TS are both augmented by maneuvers that increase transtricuspid valve flow, including inspiration, the Müller maneuver, assumption of the right lateral decubitus position, leg raising, inhalation of amyl nitrite, squatting, and isotonic exercise. They are reduced during expiration or the strain of the Valsalva maneuver and return to control levels immediately (i.e., within two or three beats) after Valsalva release.

Laboratory Examination

ELECTROCARDIOGRAM. In the absence of atrial fibrillation in a patient with valvular heart disease, TS is suggested by the presence of ECG evidence of right atrial enlargement (see Chap. 9). The P wave amplitude in leads II and V_1 exceeds 0.25 mV. Because most patients with TS have mitral valvular disease, the EGG signs of biatrial enlargement are commonly found. The amplitude of the QRS complex in lead V_1 may be reduced by the dilated right atrium.

RADIOLOGICAL FINDINGS. The key radiological finding is marked cardiomegaly with conspicuous enlargement of the right atrium (i.e., prominence of the right heart border), which extends into a dilated superior vena cava and azygos vein, but without conspicuous dilation of the pulmonary artery. The vascular changes in the lungs characteristic of mitral valvular disease may be masked, with little or no interstitial edema or vascular redistribution, but left atrial enlargement may be present.

Angiography carried out following injection of contrast material into the right atrium and filming in the 30-degree right anterior oblique projection characteristically shows thickening and decreased mobility of the leaflets, a diastolic jet through the constricted orifice, and thickening of the normal atrial wall.

ECHOCARDIOGRAM (see Chap. 11). The echocardiographic changes of the tricuspid valve in TS resemble those observed in the mitral valve in MS. Two-dimensional echocardiography characteristically shows diastolic doming of the leaflets (especially the anterior tricuspid valve leaflet), thickening and restricted motion of the other leaflets, reduced separation of the tips of the leaflets, and reduction in diameter of the tricuspid orifice. Transesophageal echocardiography allows added delineation of the details of valve structure. Doppler echocardiography shows a prolonged slope of antegrade flow and compares well with cardiac catheterization in the quantification of TS and in the assessment of associated TR.[267] Doppler evaluation of TS has largely replaced the need for catheterization to assess severity.[266]

MANAGEMENT

Although the fundamental approach to the management of severe TS is surgical treatment, intensive sodium restriction and diuretic therapy may diminish the symptoms secondary to the accumulation of excess salt and water. A preparatory period of diuresis may diminish hepatic congestion and thereby improve hepatic function sufficiently to diminish the risks of subsequent operation.

Most patients with TS have coexisting valvular disease that requires surgery. In patients with combined TS and MS, the former must *not* be corrected alone because pulmonary congestion or edema may ensue. Surgical treatment of TS should be carried out at the time of mitral valve repair or replacement in patients with TS in whom the mean diastolic pressure gradient exceeds 5 mm Hg and the tricuspid orifice is less than approximately 2.0 cm^2. The final decision concerning surgical treatment is often made at the operating table.

Because TS is almost always accompanied by some TR, simple finger fracture valvotomy may not result in significant hemodynamic improvement but may merely substitute severe regurgitation for stenosis. However, open valvotomy in which the stenotic tricuspid valve is converted into a functionally bicuspid valve may result in substantial improvement. The commissures between the anterior and septal leaflets and between the posterior and septal leaflets are opened. It is not advisable to open the commissure between the anterior and posterior leaflets for fear of producing severe regurgitation. If open valvotomy does not restore reasonably normal valve function, the tricuspid valve may have to be replaced.[268] A large porcine bioprosthesis is preferred to a mechanical prosthesis in the tricuspid position because of the high risk of thrombosis of the latter and the longer durability of bioprostheses in the tricuspid than in the mitral or aortic positions. The feasibility of tricuspid balloon valvuloplasty has been demonstrated, and this procedure may be combined with mitral balloon valvuloplasty.[269]

Tricuspid Regurgitation

Etiology and Pathology (Table 57–13)

The most common cause of TR is not intrinsic involvement of the valve itself (i.e., primary TR) but rather *dilation of the right ventricle* and of the tricuspid annulus causing secondary (functional) TR. This may be a complication of right ventricular failure of any cause. It is observed in patients with right ventricular hypertension secondary to any form of cardiac or pulmonary vascular disease, most commonly mitral valve disease.[261] In general, a systolic right ventricular systolic pressure greater than 55 mm Hg causes functional TR.[1] TR can also occur secondary to right ventricular infarction,[261] congenital heart disease (see Chap. 56) (e.g., pulmonic stenosis (PS) and pulmonary hypertension secondary to Eisenmenger syndrome), primary pulmonary hypertension, and, rarely, cor pulmonale. In infants, TR may complicate right ventricular failure secondary to neonatal pulmonary diseases and pulmonary hypertension with persistence of the

TABLE 57–13 Causes and Mechanisms of Pure Tricuspid Regurgitation

Causes

- Anatomically ABNORMAL valve
  - Rheumatic
  - Nonrheumatic
    - Infective endocarditis
    - Ebstein anomaly
    - Floppy (prolapse)
    - Congenital (non-Ebstein)
    - Carcinoid
    - Papillary muscle dysfunction
    - Trauma
    - Connective tissue disorders (Marfan)
    - Rheumatoid arthritis
    - Radiation injury
- Anatomically NORMAL valve (functional)
  - Elevated right ventricular systolic pressure (dilated annulus)

Mechanisms

Condition	*Leaflet Area*	*Annular Circumference*	*Leaflet Insertion*
Floppy	↑	↑	Normal
Ebstein anomaly	↑	↑	Abnormal
Pulmonary/right ventricular systolic hypertension	Normal	↑	Normal
Papillary muscle dysfunction	Normal	Normal	Normal
Carcinoid	↓ /Normal	Normal	Normal
Rheumatic	↓ /Normal	Normal	Normal
Infective endocarditis	↓ /Normal	Normal	Normal

Modified from Waller BF: Rheumatic and nonrheumatic conditions producing valvular heart disease. *In* Frankl WS, Brest AN (eds): Cardiovascular Clinics: Valvular Heart Disease: Comprehensive Evaluation and Management. Philadelphia, FA Davis, 1989, pp 35, 95.

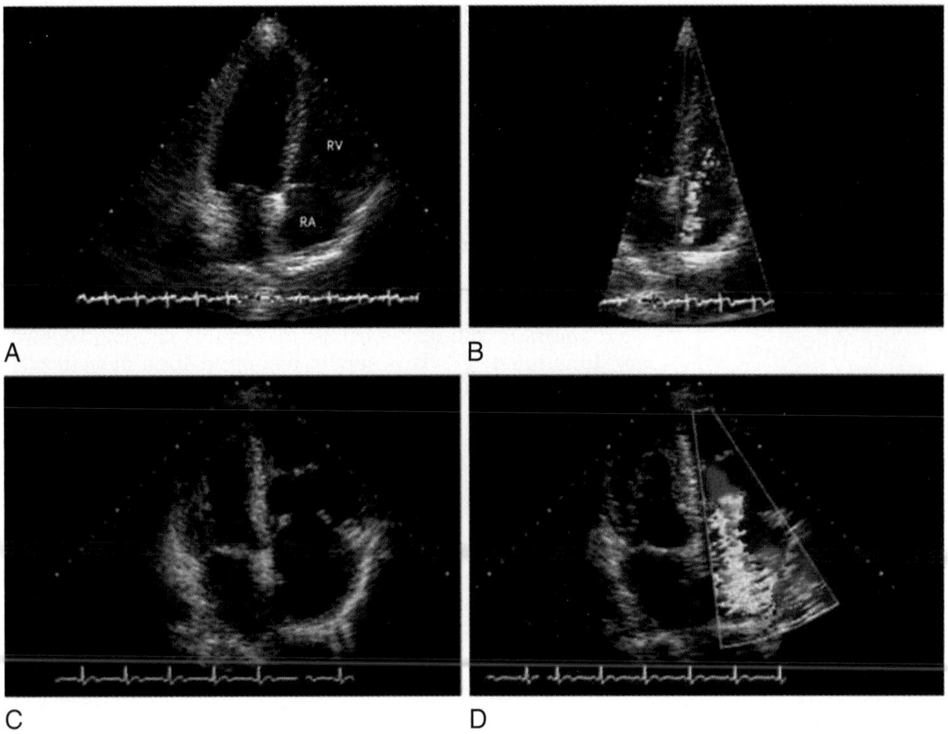

FIGURE 57–42 Tricuspid regurgitation (TR) caused by carcinoid involvement of the tricuspid valve. Serial two-dimensional echocardiograms **(A** and **C)** and color Doppler studies **(B** and **D)**, separated by 3 years are shown. After 3 years, there is severe thickening and fixation of the tricuspid leaflets **(C)**, leading to severe TR and associated right ventricular (RV) and right atrial (RA) enlargement. (From Møller JE, Connolly HM, Rubin J, et al: Factors associated with progression of carcinoid heart disease. N Engl J Med 348:1005, 2003.)

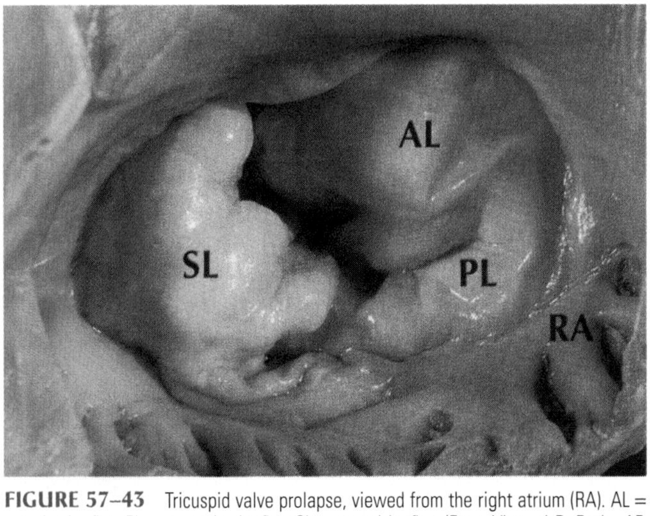

FIGURE 57–43 Tricuspid valve prolapse, viewed from the right atrium (RA). AL = anterior leaflet; PL = posterior leaflet; SL = septal leaflet. (From Virmani R, Burke AP, Farb A: Pathology of valvular heart disease. *In* Rahimtoola SH [ed]: Valvular Heart Disease. *In* Braunwald E [series ed]: Atlas of Heart Diseases. Vol 11. Philadelphia, Current Medicine, 1997, p 1.17.)

fetal pulmonary circulation. In all of these cases, TR reflects the presence of, and in turn aggravates, severe right ventricular failure. Functional TR may diminish or disappear as the right ventricle decreases in size with the treatment of heart failure. TR can also occur as a consequence of dilation of the annulus in Marfan syndrome, in which right ventricular dilation secondary to pulmonary hypertension is not present.

A variety of disease processes can affect the tricuspid valve apparatus *directly* and lead to regurgitation (primary TR). Thus, organic TR may occur on a congenital basis, as part of *Ebstein anomaly,* in atrioventricular canal, and when the tricuspid valve is involved in the formation of an aneurysm of the ventricular septum, or in corrected transposition of the great arteries,[270] or it may occur as an isolated congenital lesion. Rheumatic fever may involve the tricuspid valve directly.[266] When this occurs, it usually causes scarring of the valve leaflets and/or chordae tendineae, leading to limited leaflet mobility and either isolated TR or a combination of TR and TS. Rheumatic involvement of the mitral, and often aortic, valves coexist.

TR or the combination of TR and TS is an important feature of the *carcinoid syndrome* (Fig. 57–42), which leads to focal or diffuse deposits of fibrous tissue on the endocardium of the valvular cusps and cardiac chambers and on the intima of the great veins and coronary sinus (see Chap. 59).[263,271,272] The white, fibrous carcinoid plaques are most extensive on the right side of the heart, where they are usually deposited on the ventricular surfaces of the tricuspid valve and cause the cusps to adhere to the underlying right ventricular wall, thereby producing TR (see Fig. 57–42). Endomyocardial fibrosis with shortening of the tricuspid leaflets and chordae tendineae is an important cause of TR in tropical Africa (see Chap. 59). TR may result from prolapse of the tricuspid valve caused by myxomatous changes in the valve and chordae tendineae (Fig. 57–43); prolapse of the mitral valve is usually present in these patients as well.[261] Prolapse of the tricuspid valve occurs in about 20 percent of all patients with MVP. Tricuspid valve prolapse may also be associated with atrial septal defect. Other causes of TR include penetrating and nonpenetrating trauma, dilated cardiomyopathy, infective endocarditis (particularly staphylococcal endocarditis in narcotic addicts), and following surgical excision of the tricuspid valve in patients with infective endocarditis that is unresponsive to medical management. Less common causes of TR include cardiac tumors (particularly right atrial myxoma), transvenous pacemaker leads,[273] repeated endomyocardial biopsy in a transplanted heart,[274] endomyocardial fibrosis, methysergide-induced valvular disease, exposure to fenfluramine-phentermine,[275] and systemic lupus erythematosus involving the tricuspid valve.

Clinical Manifestations

HISTORY. In the absence of pulmonary hypertension, TR is generally well tolerated. However, when pulmonary hypertension and TR coexist, cardiac output declines and the manifestations of right-sided heart failure become intensified. Thus, the symptoms of TR result from a reduced cardiac output and from ascites, painful congestive hepatomegaly, and massive edema. Occasionally, patients have throbbing pulsations in the neck, which intensify on effort and are due to jugular venous distention, and systolic pulsations of the eyeballs have also been described. In the many patients with TR who have mitral valve disease, the symptoms of the latter usually predominate. Symptoms of pulmonary congestion may abate as TR develops, but they are replaced by weakness, fatigue, and other manifestations of a depressed cardiac output.

PHYSICAL EXAMINATION. Evidence of weight loss and cachexia, cyanosis, and jaundice are often present on inspection in patients with severe TR. Atrial fibrillation is common. There is jugular venous distention,[261] the normal *x* and *x′* descents disappear, and a prominent systolic wave, i.e., a *c-v* wave (or *s* wave), is apparent. The descent of this wave, the *y* descent, is sharp and becomes the most prominent feature of the venous pulse (unless there is coexisting TS, in which case it is slowed). A venous systolic thrill and murmur in the neck may be present in patients with severe TR. The right ventricular impulse is hyperdynamic and thrusting in quality. Systolic pulsations of an enlarged, tender liver are commonly present initially. However, in patients with chronic TR and congestive cirrhosis, the liver may become firm and nontender.[276] Ascites and edema are frequent.

Auscultation. This usually reveals an S_3 originating from the right ventricle, which is accentuated by inspiration. When TR is associated with and secondary to pulmonary hypertension, P_2 is accentuated as well. When TR occurs in the presence of pulmonary hypertension, the systolic murmur is usually high-pitched, pansystolic, and loudest in the 4th intercostal space in the parasternal region but occasionally is loudest in the subxiphoid area. When TR is mild, the murmur may be short. When TR occurs in the absence of pulmonary hypertension (e.g., in infective endocarditis or following trauma), the murmur is usually of low intensity and limited to the first half of systole. When the right ventricle is greatly dilated and occupies the anterior surface of the heart, the murmur may be prominent at the apex and difficult to distinguish from that produced by MR.

The response of the systolic murmur to respiration and other maneuvers is of considerable aid in establishing the diagnosis of TR. The murmur is characteristically augmented during inspiration (Carvallo sign). However, when the failing ventricle can no longer increase its stroke volume in the recumbent or sitting positions, the inspiratory augmentation may be elicited by standing. The murmur also increases during the Müller maneuver (forced inspiration against a closed glottis), exercise, leg-raising, and hepatic compression. It demonstrates an immediate overshoot after release of the Valsalva strain but is reduced in intensity and duration in the standing position and during the strain of the Valsalva maneuver. Increased atrioventricular flow across the tricuspid orifice in diastole may cause a short, early diastolic flow rumble in the left parasternal region following S_3. Tricuspid valve prolapse, like MVP, causes nonejection systolic clicks and late systolic murmurs. However, in tricuspid valve prolapse, these findings are more prominent at the lower left sternal border. With inspiration, the clicks occur later, and the murmurs intensify and become shorter in duration.

Laboratory Examination

ELECTROCARDIOGRAM. This is usually nonspecific and characteristic of the lesion causing TR. Incomplete right bundle branch block, Q waves in lead V_1, and atrial fibrillation are commonly found.

RADIOLOGICAL FINDINGS. In patients with functional TR, marked cardiomegaly is usually evident, and the right atrium is prominent. Evidence of elevated right atrial pressure may include distention of the azygos vein and the presence of a pleural effusion. Ascites with upward displacement of the diaphragm may be present. Systolic pulsations of the right atrium may be present on fluoroscopy.

ECHOCARDIOGRAM (see Fig. 11–73). The goal of echocardiography is to detect TR, estimate its severity, and assess pulmonary arterial pressure and right ventricular function.[267] In patients with TR secondary to dilation of the tricuspid annulus, the right atrium, right ventricle, and tricuspid annulus all are usually greatly dilated on echocardiography. There is evidence of right ventricular diastolic overload with paradoxical motion of the ventricular septum similar to that observed in atrial septal defect. Exaggerated motion and delayed closure of the tricuspid valve are evident in patients with Ebstein anomaly. Prolapse of the tricuspid valve due to myxomatous degeneration may be evident on echocardiography.[261] Echocardiographic indications of tricuspid valve abnormalities, especially TR by Doppler examination, can be detected in most patients with carcinoid heart disease.[271] In patients with TR due to endocarditis, echocardiography may reveal vegetations on the valve or a flail valve. Transesophageal echocardiography enhances detection of TR.

Doppler echocardiography is a sensitive technique for visualizing the TR jet. The magnitude of TR can be quantified using techniques similar to those used to evaluate MR (Fig. 57–44).[266,277-279] Contrast echocardiography also improves detection of TR and can trace regurgitant microbubbles into the inferior vena cava and hepatic veins.[266,278,279]

HEMODYNAMIC FINDINGS. The right atrial and right ventricular end-diastolic pressures are often elevated in TR, whether the condition is due to organic disease of the tricuspid valve or is secondary to right ventricular systolic overload. The right atrial pressure tracing usually reveals absence of the *x* descent and a prominent *v* or *c-v* wave ("ventricularization" of the atrial pressure). Absence of these findings essentially excludes moderate or severe TR.[280] As the severity of TR increases, the contour of the right atrial pressure pulse increasingly resembles that of the right ventricular pressure pulse. A rise or no change in right atrial pressure on deep inspiration, rather than the usual fall, is a characteristic finding. Determination of the pulmonary arterial (or right ventricular) systolic pressure may be helpful in deciding whether the TR is primary (i.e., due to disease of the valve or its supporting structures) or functional (i.e., secondary to right ventricular dilation). A pulmonary arterial or right ventricular systolic pressure less than 40 mm Hg favors a primary cause, whereas a pressure greater than 55 mm Hg suggests that TR is secondary.

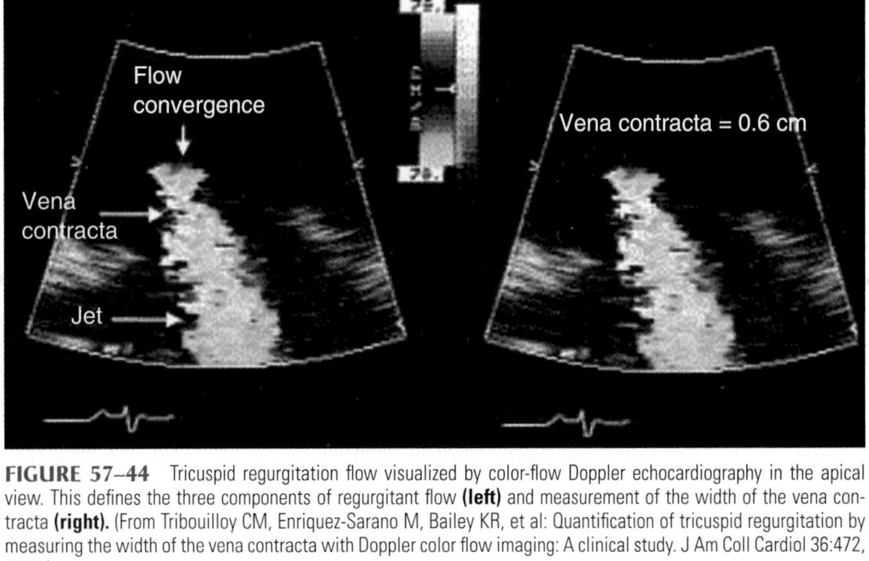

FIGURE 57–44 Tricuspid regurgitation flow visualized by color-flow Doppler echocardiography in the apical view. This defines the three components of regurgitant flow **(left)** and measurement of the width of the vena contracta **(right).** (From Tribouilloy CM, Enriquez-Sarano M, Bailey KR, et al: Quantification of tricuspid regurgitation by measuring the width of the vena contracta with Doppler color flow imaging: A clinical study. J Am Coll Cardiol 36:472, 2000.)

TR in the absence of pulmonary hypertension usually is well tolerated and may not require surgical treatment. Indeed, both human patients and experimental animals with normal pulmonary arterial pressure may tolerate total excision of the tricuspid valve as long as right ventricular systolic pressure is normal. Dilation of the right side of the heart usually occurs months or years after tricuspid valvectomy (usually carried out for acute infective endocarditis). *Surgical treatment* of acquired regurgitation secondary to annular dilation was greatly improved with development of annuloplasty techniques, with or without an annuloplasty ring. Annuloplasty without insertion of a prosthetic ring (the so-called DeVega annuloplasty) has also been found to be effective in patients with annular dilation. This technique is now widely employed.[281,282] This reduces but does not always eliminate TR.[266]

At the time of mitral valve surgery in patients with TR secondary to pulmonary hypertension, the severity of the regurgitation should be assessed by palpation of the tricuspid valve. In addition, it should be determined whether the TR is secondary to pulmonary hypertension, in which case the valve is normal, or whether it is secondary to rheumatic fever. Patients with mild TR usually do not require surgical treatment[261]; pulmonary vascular pressures decline following successful mitral valve surgery, and the mild TR tends to disappear. Excellent results have been reported in patients with moderate TR with the use of suture annuloplasty of the posterior (unsupported) portion of the annulus. Patients with severe TR and primary rheumatic tricuspid valve disease with commissural fusion require valvotomy and ring annuloplasty. The latter is also employed for TR secondary to annular dilation. A surgical mortality rate of 13.9 percent has been reported (see Table 57-3).[283] If these procedures do not provide a good functional result at the operating table (as assessed by transesophageal echocardiography), valve replacement using a large porcine mitral heterograft may be required.

When organic disease of the tricuspid valve (Ebstein anomaly or carcinoid heart disease) causes TR severe enough to require surgery, valve replacement is usually needed. The risk of thrombosis of mechanical prostheses is greater in the tricuspid than in the mitral or aortic positions, presumably because pressure and flow rates are lower in the right side of the heart. For this reason, the artificial valve of choice for the tricuspid position in adults is a large porcine heterograft. Anticoagulants are not required, and a graft durability of more than 10 years has been established.

In treating the difficult problem of tricuspid endocarditis in heroin addicts, total excision of the tricuspid valve *without immediate replacement* can generally be tolerated by these patients, who usually do not have associated pulmonary hypertension. When antibiotic therapy is unsuccessful, valvular replacement frequently results in reinfection or continued infection. Therefore, diseased valvular tissue should be excised to eradicate the endocarditis, and antibiotic treatment can then be continued. Initially, most patients tolerate loss of the tricuspid valve without great difficulty. Later, right ventricular dysfunction usually occurs. A bioprosthetic valve may therefore be inserted 6 to 9 months after valve excision and control of the infection.

Pulmonic Valve Disease

Etiology and Pathology

PULMONIC STENOSIS. The *congenital* form is the most common cause of PS.[266] Manifestations in children and adults are discussed in Chapter 56. *Rheumatic* inflammation of the pulmonic valve is uncommon, is usually associated with involvement of other valves, and rarely leads to serious deformity. *Carcinoid* plaques, similar to those involving the tricuspid valve, are often present in the outflow tract of the right ventricle of patients with malignant carcinoid. The plaques result in constriction of the pulmonic valve ring, retraction and fusion of the valve cusps, and either PS or the combination of PS and PR (Fig. 57–45).[263,271,272] Obstruction in the region of the pulmonic valve may be extrinsic to the valve apparatus and may be produced by cardiac tumors or by aneurysm of the sinus of Valsalva.

Management of congenital PS focuses on balloon dilation (see Chaps. 52 and 56).

PULMONIC REGURGITATION. By far the most common cause of PR is dilation of the valve ring secondary to pulmonary hypertension (of any etiology) or to dilation of the pulmonary artery, either idiopathic or consequent to a connective tissue disorder such as Marfan syndrome. The second most common cause of PR is infective endocarditis. Less frequently, PR is iatrogenic and is induced at the time of surgical treatment of congenital PS or tetralogy of Fallot.[284,285] PR may also result from various lesions that directly affect the pulmonic valve. These include congenital malformations such as absent, malformed, fenestrated, or supernumerary leaflets. These anomalies may occur as isolated lesions but more often are associated with other congenital anomalies, particularly tetralogy of Fallot, ventricular septal defect, and pulmonic valvular stenosis. Less common causes include trauma, carcinoid syndrome,[263] rheumatic involvement, injury produced by a pulmonary artery flow-directed catheter, syphilis, and chest trauma.

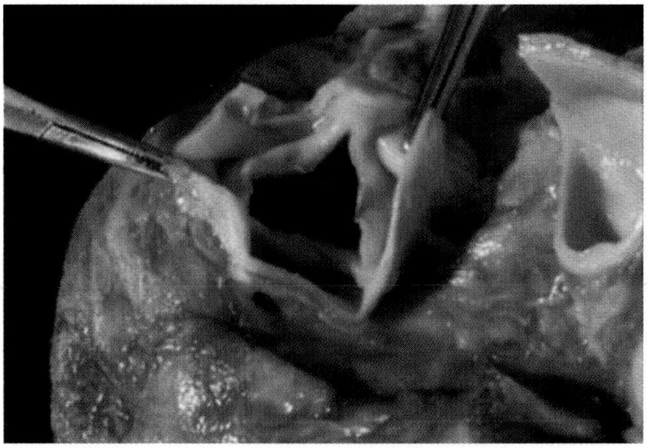

FIGURE 57–45 Carcinoid heart disease. The pulmonary valve is viewed from above. (From Kulke MH, Mayer RJ: Carcinoid tumors. N Engl J Med 340:858, 1999.)

Clinical Manifestations

Like TR, isolated PR causes right ventricular volume overload and may be tolerated for many years without difficulty unless it complicates, or is complicated by, pulmonary hypertension. In this case, PR is usually accompanied by and aggravates right ventricular failure. Patients with PR caused by infective endocarditis who develop septic pulmonary emboli and pulmonary hypertension often exhibit severe right ventricular failure. In most patients, the clinical manifestations of the primary disease are severe and usually overshadow the PR, which often results only in incidental auscultatory findings. *Physical examination* reveals a hyperdynamic right ventricle that produces palpable systolic pulsations in the left parasternal area and an enlarged pulmonary artery that often results in systolic pulsations in the 2nd left intercostal space. Sometimes systolic and diastolic thrills are felt in the same area. A tap reflecting pulmonic valve closure is usually easily palpable in the 2nd intercostal space in patients with pulmonary hypertension and secondary PR.

Auscultation. P_2 is not audible in patients with congenital absence of the pulmonic valve; however, this sound is accentuated in patients with PR secondary to pulmonary hypertension. There may be wide splitting of S_2 caused by prolongation of right ventricular ejection accompanying the augmented right ventricular stroke volume. A nonvalvular systolic ejection click due to the sudden expansion of the pulmonary artery by the augmented right ventricular stroke volume frequently initiates a midsystolic ejection murmur, most prominent in the 2nd left intercostal space. An S_3 and S_4 originating from the right ventricle are often audible, most readily in the 4th intercostal space at the left parasternal area, and are augmented by inspiration.

In the absence of pulmonary hypertension, the diastolic murmur of PR is low pitched and usually heard best at the 3rd and 4th left intercostal spaces adjacent to the sternum. The murmur commences when pressures in the pulmonary artery and right ventricle diverge, approximately 0.04 second after P_2. It is diamond shaped and brief, reaching a peak intensity when the gradient between these pressures is maximal and ending with equilibration of the pressures. The murmur becomes louder during inspiration.

When systolic pulmonary arterial pressure exceeds approximately 55 mm Hg, dilation of the pulmonic annulus results in a high-velocity regurgitant jet that is responsible for the *Graham Steell murmur* of PR. (Doppler ultrasonography reveals pulmonary regurgitation at much lower pulmonary arterial pressures.) The Graham Steell murmur is a high-pitched, blowing, decrescendo murmur beginning immediately after P_2 and is most prominent in the left parasternal region in the 2nd to 4th intercostal spaces. Thus, although it resembles the murmur of AR, it is usually accompanied by severe pulmonary hypertension, i.e., an accentuated P_2 or fused S_2, an ejection sound, and a systolic murmur of TR, and not by a widened arterial pulse pressure. Sometimes a low-frequency presystolic murmur is present, i.e., a right-sided Austin Flint murmur originating from the tricuspid valve.

The Graham Steell murmur of PR secondary to pulmonary hypertension usually increases in intensity with inspiration, exhibits little change after amyl nitrite inhalation or vasopressor administration, is diminished during the Valsalva strain, and returns to baseline intensity almost immediately after release of the Valsalva strain. This murmur resembles and may be confused with the diastolic blowing murmur of AR. However, indicator dilution studies and aortography have established that a diastolic blowing murmur along the left sternal border in patients with rheumatic heart disease and pulmonary hypertension (even in the *absence* of peripheral signs of AR) is usually due to AR rather than PR.

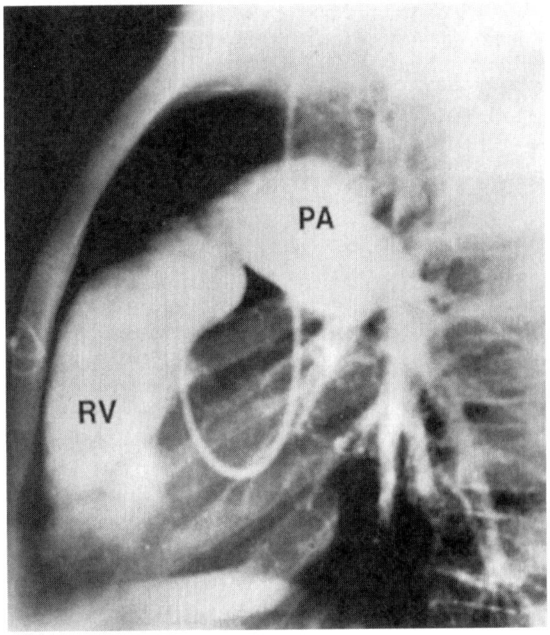

FIGURE 57–46 Pulmonic valvular regurgitation. Contrast material has been injected into the main pulmonary artery (PA) and has regurgitated back into an enlarged right ventricle (RV). (From Carlsson E, Gross R, Holt RG: The radiological diagnosis of cardiac valvular insufficiency. Circulation 55:921, 1977.)

Laboratory Examination

ELECTROCARDIOGRAM. In the absence of pulmonary hypertension, PR often results in an ECG that reflects right ventricular diastolic overload, i.e., an rSr (or rsR) configuration in the right precordial leads. PR secondary to pulmonary hypertension is usually associated with ECG evidence of right ventricular hypertrophy.

RADIOLOGICAL AND ANGIOGRAPHIC FINDINGS. Both the pulmonary artery and the right ventricle are usually enlarged, but these signs are nonspecific. Fluoroscopy may demonstrate pronounced pulsation of the main pulmonary artery. PR can be diagnosed by observing opacification of the right ventricle following injection of contrast material into the main pulmonary artery (Fig. 57–46). The diagnosis is supported by noting superimposition of the pulmonary arterial and right ventricular pressure curves during mid and late diastole. Indicator dilution studies with injections into the pulmonary artery and sampling from the right ventricle, as well as intracardiac phonocardiography, can also be helpful in establishing the diagnosis in mild cases.

ECHOCARDIOGRAM. Two-dimensional echocardiography shows right ventricular dilation and, in patients with pulmonary hypertension, right ventricular hypertrophy as well. Right ventricular function can be evaluated. Abnormal motion of the septum characteristic of volume overload of the right ventricle in diastole and/or septal flutter may be evident. The motion of the pulmonic valve may point to the cause of the PR. Absence of *a* waves and systolic notching of the posterior leaflet suggest pulmonary hypertension; large *a* waves indicate PS. PR can be detected by contrast echocardiography. The pulsed Doppler technique is also extremely accurate in detecting PR and in helping to estimate its severity. Abnormal Doppler signals in the right ventricular outflow tract with velocity sustained throughout diastole are generally observed in patients in whom PR is caused by dilation of the valve ring secondary to pulmonary hypertension. When the velocity falls during diastole, the pulmonary artery pressure is usually normal, and the regurgitation is caused by an abnormality of the valve itself.

MAGNETIC RESONANCE IMAGING. Cardiac MRI is helpful is assessing pulmonary artery dilation, imaging the regurgitant jet, and evaluating right ventricular function (see Fig. 14–12A).

MANAGEMENT

PR alone is seldom severe enough to require specific treatment. Cardiac glycosides are useful in the management of right ventricular dilation or failure. Treatment of the primary condition, such as infective endocarditis, or the lesion responsible for the pulmonary hypertension, such as surgery for mitral valvular disease, often ameliorates the PR. Surgical treatment directed specifically at the pulmonic valve (e.g., in patients in whom surgical correction of tetralogy of Fallot has caused severe PR[284,285]) is required only occasionally because of intractable right heart failure. Under such circumstances, valve replacement may be carried out, preferably with a porcine bioprosthesis or a pulmonary allograft.[286-288]

Multivalvular Disease

Multivalvular involvement is caused most frequently by rheumatic fever, and various clinical and hemodynamic syndromes can be produced by different combinations of valvular abnormalities. Marfan syndrome and other connective tissue disorders may cause multivalve prolapse and dilation, resulting in multivalvular regurgitation. Degenerative calcification of the aortic valve may be associated with degenerative mitral annular calcification and cause AS and MR. Different pathological conditions may affect two valves in the same patient, such as infective endocarditis on the aortic valve causing AR and ischemia causing MR. Development of PR and TR secondary to dilation of the pulmonic valve ring and tricuspid annulus, as a consequence of pulmonary hypertension secondary to mitral and/or aortic valvular disease, was discussed previously, as was the combination of organic rheumatic tricuspid and mitral valvular disease.

In patients with multivalvular disease, the clinical manifestations depend on the relative severities of each of the lesions. When the valvular abnormalities are of approximately equal severity, clinical manifestations produced by the more proximal (upstream) of the two valvular lesions (i.e., the mitral valve in patients with combined mitral and aortic valvular disease and the tricuspid valve in patients with combined tricuspid and mitral valvular disease) are generally more prominent than those produced by the distal lesion. Thus, the proximal lesion tends to mask the distal lesion.

It is important to recognize multivalvular involvement preoperatively because failure to correct all significant valvular disease at the time of operation increases mortality considerably. In patients with multivalvular disease, the relative severity of each lesion may be difficult to estimate by clinical examination and noninvasive techniques because one lesion may mask the manifestations of the other. For this reason, patients suspected of having multivalvular involvement and who are being considered for surgical treatment should undergo right- and left-sided cardiac catheterization and angiography. These studies are in addition to careful clinical examination and a noninvasive work-up, with emphasis on two-dimensional and Doppler echocardiography. If there is any question concerning the presence of significant AS in patients undergoing mitral valve surgery, the aortic valve should be inspected because overlooking this condition can lead to a high perioperative mortality. Similarly, it is useful to palpate the tricuspid valve at the time of mitral valve surgery.

Mitral Stenosis and Aortic Regurgitation

Approximately two-thirds of patients with severe MS have an early blowing diastolic murmur along the left sternal border with a normal pulse pressure. In about 90 percent of these patients, the murmur is due to mild or moderate AR and is usually of little clinical importance. However, approximately 10 percent of patients with MS have severe rheumatic AR,[289] which can generally be recognized by the usual signs of AR (i.e., a widened pulse pressure, left ventricular dilation and increased wall motion on echocardiography, and signs of left ventricular enlargement on radiological and ECG examinations).

In keeping with the general observation that a proximal lesion may mask a distal lesion, significant AR may be missed in patients with severe MS. The widened pulse pressure, in particular, may be absent. On the other hand, MS may be missed or, conversely, may be falsely diagnosed on clinical examination of patients with obvious AR. An accentuated S_1 and an OS in a patient with AR should suggest the possibility of mitral valvular disease. However, an Austin Flint murmur is often inappropriately considered to be the diastolic rumbling murmur of MS. These two murmurs may be distinguished at the bedside by means of amyl nitrite inhalation, which diminishes the Austin Flint murmur but augments the murmur of MS; isometric handgrip and squatting augment both the diastolic murmur of AR and the Austin Flint murmur. Echocardiography, particularly pulsed Doppler echocardiography, is of decisive value in detecting MS and MR.

Since double-valve replacement is associated with increased short-term and long-term risks,[290] balloon mitral valvotomy can be the first procedure. If this causes left ventricular dilation, AVR can follow. Alternatively, open mitral valvotomy and AVR can be performed at the same time.[1]

Mitral Stenosis and Aortic Stenosis

The left ventricle of a patient with these two lesions is usually small, stiff, and hypertrophied. When severe MS and AS coexist, the former masks many of the manifestations of the latter.[289] The cardiac output tends to be reduced more than in patients with isolated AS. The reduced cardiac output lowers both the transaortic valvular pressure gradient and the left ventricular systolic pressure, diminishes the incidence of angina pectoris, and retards the development of aortic valvular calcification and left ventricular hypertrophy. On the other hand, clinical manifestations associated with MS, such as pulmonary congestion and hemoptysis, atrial fibrillation, and systemic embolization, occur more frequently in patients with coexisting MS and AS than in those with isolated AS.

On physical examination, an S_4, (which is common in patients with pure AS) is usually not present. The midsystolic murmur characteristic of AS may be reduced in intensity and duration because the stroke volume is reduced by the MS. The ECG may fail to demonstrate left ventricular hypertrophy, but left atrial enlargement is common. The chest roentgenogram is usually typical of MS except that calcium may be present in the region of the aortic valve, and left ventricular enlargement may occur (see Fig. 12–5). The two-dimensional and Doppler echocardiograms are of the greatest value because stenosis of both valves may be evident. However, the low cardiac output characteristic of the combined lesions may reduce the transvalvular pressure gradients estimated by Doppler echocardiography.

It is vital to recognize the presence of hemodynamically significant aortic valvular disease (i.e., stenosis and/or regurgitation) preoperatively in patients who are to undergo mitral valvotomy. This procedure may be hazardous because it can impose a sudden hemodynamic load on the left ventricle that had previously been protected by the MS and may lead to acute pulmonary edema. Balloon mitral valvotomy and AVR may be the treatment of choice.

Aortic Stenosis and Mitral Regurgitation

This combination of lesions is usually caused by rheumatic heart disease, although AS may be congenital and MR may be due to MVP. The combination of severe AS and MR is a hazardous one, but fortunately it is relatively uncommon. Obstruction to left ventricular outflow augments the volume of MR flow, whereas the presence of MR diminishes the ventricular preload necessary for maintenance of the left ventricular stroke volume in patients with AS.[289] The result is a reduced forward cardiac output and marked left atrial and pulmonary venous hypertension. The development of atrial fibrillation (due to left atrial enlargement) has an adverse hemodynamic effect in the presence of AS. The physical findings may be confusing because it may be difficult to recognize two distinct systolic murmurs. On echocardiography and roentgenography, the left atrium and ventricle are usually larger than in isolated AS. In patients with severe AS and MR, both valves must usually be treated surgically by AVR and, if possible, by mitral valve repair.[290]

Aortic Regurgitation and Mitral Regurgitation

This relatively frequent combination of lesions[289] may be caused by rheumatic heart disease, by prolapse of both the aortic and the mitral valves due to myxomatous degeneration, or by dilation of both annuli in patients with connective tissue disorders. The left ventricle is usually greatly dilated. The clinical features of AR usually predominate, and it is sometimes difficult to determine whether the MR is due to organic involvement of this valve or to dilation of the mitral valve ring secondary to left ventricular enlargement. When both valvular leaks are severe, this combination of lesions is poorly tolerated. The normal mitral valve ordinarily serves as a "back-up" to the aortic valve, and premature (diastolic) closure of the mitral valve limits the volume of reflux that occurs in patients with acute AR. With severe combined regurgitant lesions, regardless of the cause of the mitral lesion, blood may reflux from the aorta through both chambers of the left side of the heart into the pulmonary veins. Physical and laboratory examinations usually show evidence of both lesions. An S_3 and a brisk arterial pulse are frequently present. The relative severity of each lesion can be assessed best by Doppler echocardiography and contrast angiography. This combination of lesions leads to severe left ventricular dilation.

MR that occurs in patients with AR secondary to left ventricular dilation often regresses following AVR alone. If severe, the MR may be corrected by annuloplasty at the time of AVR. An intrinsically normal mitral valve that is regurgitant because of a dilated annulus should not be replaced.

Surgical Treatment of Multivalvular Disease

Combined AVR and MVR is usually associated with a higher risk and poorer survival than is replacement of either of the valves alone.[291,292] The operative risk of double-valve replacement is about 70 percent higher than it is for single-valve replacement. The Society of Thoracic Surgeons National Database Committee reported an overall operative mortality rate of 9.6 percent for multiple (usually double) valve replacement in 3840 patients, compared with 4.3 percent and 6.4 percent for isolated AVR and MVR, respectively (see Table 57–3).[283] The long-term survival depends strongly on the preoperative functional status.[292] Patients operated on for combined AR and MR have poorer outcomes than patients receiving double-valve replacement for any of the other combinations of lesions, presumably because both AR and MR may produce irreversible left ventricular damage. Mitral repair or balloon valvotomy in combination with AVR is preferable to double-valve replacement and should be carried out whenever possible.[290] Risk factors that reduce long-term survival after double-valve replacement include advanced age, higher NYHA class, lower left ventricular ejection fraction, greater left ventricular enlargement, and accompanying ischemic heart disease requiring coronary artery bypass grafting.[292]

Given the higher risks, a higher threshold is required for multivalvular versus single-valve surgery. Thus, patients are generally advised not to undergo multivalvular surgery until they reach late NYHA Class II or III, unless there is evidence of declining left ventricular function. Despite a detailed noninvasive and invasive work-up, the decision to treat more than one valve is often made by palpation or by direct inspection at the operating table.

Three-Valve Disease

Hemodynamically significant disease involving the mitral, aortic, and tricuspid valves is uncommon. Patients with trivalvular disease may present in advanced heart failure with marked cardiomegaly, and surgical correction of all three valvular lesions is imperative. However, triple-valve replacement is a long and complex operation. Early in the experience with this procedure, the mortality rate was 20 percent for patients in NYHA Class III and 40 percent for patients in Class IV. More recently, the mortality rate has declined, but, nevertheless, triple-valve replacement should be avoided if possible. In many patients with trivalvular disease, it is possible to replace the aortic valve, repair the mitral valve, and perform a tricuspid annuloplasty or valvuloplasty.

Patients who survive triple-valve replacement surgery usually show substantial clinical improvement during the early postoperative period, and postoperative catheterization studies show marked reductions in pulmonary arterial and capillary pressures. However, some patients die of arrhythmias or congestive heart failure in the late postoperative period despite three normally functioning prostheses. The cause of cardiac failure in this situation is not known, but it may be related to intraoperative myocardial ischemia, microemboli from the multiple prostheses, or continued subclinical episodes of rheumatic myocarditis.

When multiple prosthetic valves must be inserted, it is logical to select either two bioprostheses or two mechanical prostheses for the left side of the heart. If the patient is to be exposed to the hazards of anticoagulants for one mechanical prosthesis, it seems unreasonable to add the potential risks of early failure of a bioprosthesis. However, if two mechanical prostheses are selected for the left side of the heart, the use of a bioprosthesis in the tricuspid position is suggested.

Prosthetic Cardiac Valves

The first successful replacements of cardiac valves in the human were accomplished by Nina Braunwald and colleagues,[293] Harken and coworkers,[294] and Starr and Edwards[295] in 1960. Two major groups of artificial (prosthetic) valves are currently available in models designed for both the atrioventricular (mitral and tricuspid) and the aortic positions: mechanical prostheses and bioprostheses (tissue valves). The major differences are related to the risk of thromboembolism (higher with mechanical valves) and the risk of structural deterioration of the prosthesis (higher with bioprostheses).

Mechanical Prostheses

Mechanical prosthetic valves are classified into three major groups: caged-ball, tilting-disc and bileaflet valves. The *Starr-Edwards* caged-ball valve, the oldest prosthetic valve in continuous use (Fig. 57–47A), has the longest record of predictable performance of any artificial valve.[296-299] The poppet is made of silicone rubber, the cage of Stellite alloy, and the sewing ring of Teflon/polypropylene cloth. A disadvantage is its bulky cage design. Therefore, the Starr-Edwards valve is not suitable for the mitral position in patients with a small left ventricular cavity or for the aortic position in those with a small aortic annulus or those requiring a valve–aortic arch composite graft. In a small number of patients, this valve induces hemolysis, which may be greatly exaggerated and become clinically important if a perivalvular leak develops. When they are small, Starr-Edwards valves may cause mild obstruction, and the incidence of thromboembolism is slightly higher than with the tilting-disc valve or bileaflet valve.[1,297,298]

The bileaflet valves are widely employed; these are less bulky, have a lower profile than the caged-ball valve, and are therefore superior hemodynamically. The *St. Jude* bileaflet valve (Fig. 57–47D), currently the most widely used prosthesis worldwide, is coated with pyrolytic carbon and has two semicircular discs that pivot between open and closed positions without the need for supporting struts.[299,300] It has favorable flow characteristics and causes a lower transvalvular pressure gradient at any outer diameter and cardiac output than the caged-ball or tilting-disc valves.[297] The St. Jude valve appears to have particularly favorable hemodynamic characteristics in the smaller sizes; therefore, it is especially useful in children. Thrombogenicity in the mitral position *may* be less than that associated with other prosthetic valves.[296,297] However, as with other mechanical prostheses, lifelong anticoagulation is needed.[1] A variation of the St. Jude valve, the *CarboMedics* prosthesis (Fig. 57–47E), is also a bileaflet valve composed of pyrolytic carbon with a titanium housing that can be rotated so as to avoid interference with disc excursion by subvalvular tissue.[301]

There are two principal tilting disc valves in current use. The *Omniscience* valve (Fig. 57–47B), the successor to the *Lillehei-Kaster* pivoting-disc valve, consists of a titanium valve housing with a polyester knit sewing ring in which a pyrolytic disc is suspended. In the open position, the disc swings to an angle of 80 degrees, providing a large central flow orifice. A closely related valve is the *Medtronic-Hall* valve (Fig. 57–47C), which has a Teflon sewing ring and titanium housing; its thin, carbon-coated pivoting disc has a central perforation that allows improved hemodynamics. Thrombogenicity appears to be quite low[296,297] (less than one episode per 100 patient-years in the mitral position), and mechanical performance is excellent over the long term. Both the bileaflet and the tilting-disc valves are associated with small (5 to 10 ml/beat) obligatory (normal) regurgitation. All have distinctive auscultatory features (Fig. 57–48).

DURABILITY AND THROMBOGENICITY. All mechanical prosthetic valves have an excellent record of durability, up to 40 years for the Starr-Edwards valve. In the mitral position, perivalvular regurgitation appears to occur more frequently with mechanical than with tissue valves.[302] Thrombosis and thromboembolism risks are greater with any mechanical valve in the mitral than in the aortic position, and higher doses of warfarin are generally recommended for mitral prostheses.[1,303] However, patients with any *mechanical* prosthesis, regardless of design or site of placement, require long-term anticoagulation and aspirin administration because of the hazard of thromboembolism, which is greatest in the first postoperative year. Without anticoagulants and aspirin, the incidence of thromboembolism is threefold to sixfold higher than when proper doses of these medications are

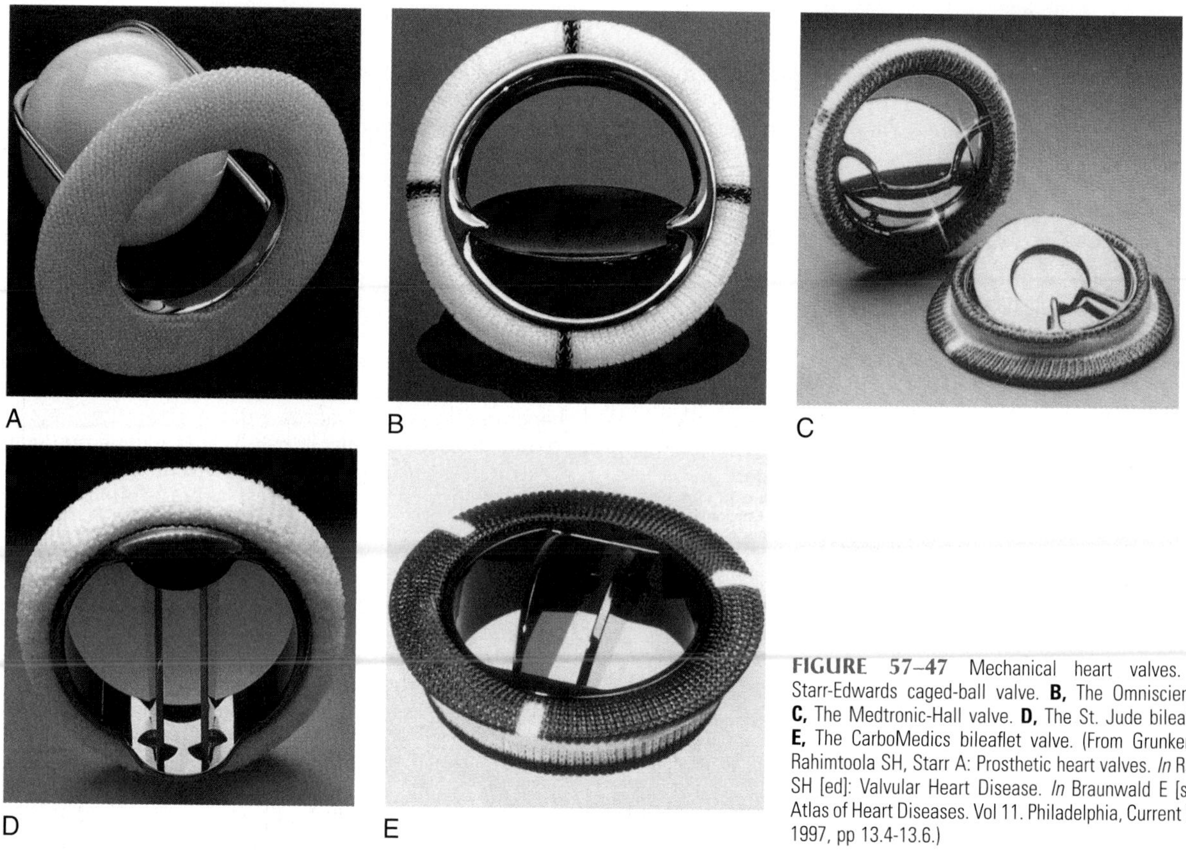

FIGURE 57–47 Mechanical heart valves. **A,** The Starr-Edwards caged-ball valve. **B,** The Omniscience valve. **C,** The Medtronic-Hall valve. **D,** The St. Jude bileaflet valve. **E,** The CarboMedics bileaflet valve. (From Grunkemeier GL, Rahimtoola SH, Starr A: Prosthetic heart valves. *In* Rahimtoola SH [ed]: Valvular Heart Disease. *In* Braunwald E [series ed]: Atlas of Heart Diseases. Vol 11. Philadelphia, Current Medicine, 1997, pp 13.4-13.6.)

Type of Valve	Aortic Prosthesis		Mitral Prosthesis	
	Normal findings	Abnormal findings	Normal findings	Abnormal findings
Caged-Ball (Starr–Edwards)	OC, S_1, CC, P_2, SEM	Aortic diastolic murmur; Decreased intensity of opening or closing click	CC, OC, S_2, SEM	Low-frequency apical diastolic murmur; High-frequency holosystolic murmur
Single-Tilting-Disc (Björk–Shiley or Medtronic–Hall)	OC, S_1, CC, P_2, SEM, DM	Decreased intensity of closing click	CC, OC, S_2, DM	High-frequency holosystolic murmur; Decreased intensity of closing click
Bileaflet-Tilting-Disc (St. Jude Medical)	OC, S_1, CC, P_2, SEM	Aortic diastolic murmur; Decreased intensity of closing click	CC, OC, S_2, DM	High-frequency holosystolic murmur; Decreased intensity of closing click
Heterograft Bioprosthesis (Hancock or Carpentier–Edwards)	S_1, AC, P_2, SEM	Aortic diastolic murmur	MC, S_2 MO, SEM, DM	High-frequency holosystolic murmur

FIGURE 57–48 Auscultatory characteristics of various prosthetic valves in the aortic and mitral positions, with schematic diagrams of normal findings and descriptions of abnormal findings. OC = opening click; CC = closing click; SEM = systolic ejection murmur; DM = diastolic murmur; AC = aortic closure; MC = mitral valve closure; MO = mitral opening. (From Vongpatanasin W, Hillis LD, Lange RA: Prosthetic heart valves. N Engl J Med 335:407, 1996.)

administered. Rarely, thrombosis of the mechanical valve occurs. This may be a fatal event, but when nonfatal, it interferes with prosthetic valve function.

Warfarin should begin about 2 days after operation, and the INR should be in the range of 2.0 to 3.0 for patients with the bileaflet disc and the Medtronic-Hall valve in the aortic position. The INR should be between 2.5 and 3.5 for patients at higher risk for thrombosis (e.g., atrial fibrillation, previous thromboembolism) as well as for patients with other mechanical valves in the aortic position and for *all* valves in the mitral position (see Chap. 80).[1] This relatively conservative approach reduces the risk of anticoagulant hemorrhage but does not appear to be associated with a greater frequency of thromboembolism than an INR of 3.0 to 4.0, which was used in the past.[303-305] Antiplatelet agents without anticoagulants do not provide adequate protection. However, the addition of aspirin, 80 to 150 mg daily, together with warfarin may reduce the risk of thromboembolism and should be given to all patients with prosthetic valves.[1] Although this approach does increase the risk of bleeding slightly,[306,307] there is a favorable risk-to-benefit profile.[307]

Prosthetic valve thrombosis should be suspected by the sudden appearance of dyspnea and muffled sounds or new murmurs on auscultation (see Fig. 57–48). This serious complication is diagnosed by transesophageal two-dimensional and Doppler echocardiography. Treatment consists of infusion of a thrombolytic agent for 24 to 72 hours, heparin, and aspirin. Surgery is required for nonresponders and for patients with mobile thrombi.[1,308]

It must be recognized that (1) the administration of warfarin carries its own mortality and morbidity, i.e., serious hemorrhage, estimated at 0.2 and 2.2 episodes per 100 patient-years, respectively; and (2) despite treatment with anticoagulants, the incidence of thromboembolic complications with the best mechanical prosthesis is still about 0.2 fatal complications and 1.0 to 2.0 nonfatal complications per 100 patient-years for aortic valves and 2.0 to 3.0 nonfatal complications for mitral valves. Valve thrombosis, a particularly hazardous complication, occurs at an incidence of about 0.1 percent per year in the aortic position and 0.35 percent per year in the mitral position. Thrombosis of mechanical prostheses in the tricuspid position is quite high, and for this reason bioprostheses are preferred at this site. The incidence of embolization in patients who have experienced repeated emboli from a prosthetic valve despite anticoagulants may be reduced by replacement with a tissue valve.

Mechanical prostheses regularly cause mild hemolysis, but this is not severe enough to be of clinical importance unless the patient develops periprosthetic regurgitation.

Tissue Valves

Tissue valves (bioprostheses) have been developed primarily to overcome the risk of thromboembolism that is inherent in all mechanical prosthetic valves and the attendant hazards and inconvenience of permanent anticoagulant therapy.[309] The first tissue valves to be widely used were chemically sterilized aortic homografts (allografts) obtained from cadavers. However, these had a high incidence of breakdown within 3 years, and antibiotic-treated, cryopreserved, frozen, irradiated homografts were then developed. These homografts are more durable, but, although they have many desirable properties, their use has been restricted by the problems inherent in their procurement (discussed later).

PORCINE HETEROGRAFTS. Stented porcine aortic heterografts were developed for both the mitral and the aortic positions and have been in wide clinical use since 1965.[296,297] The semirigid stents facilitate implantation and maintain the three-dimensional relationship between the leaflets. Three porcine heterografts are widely used today.[310-313] The *Hancock* valve (Fig. 57–49A) is fixed and preserved in glutaraldehyde and is mounted on a Dacron cloth–covered flexible polypropylene strut. In the smaller aortic models, the right coronary cusp is replaced by a posterior cusp from another valve to reduce obstruction resulting from the septal shelf of the valve.[310,313] The *Carpentier-Edwards* valve (Fig. 57–49B) is pressure fixed, preserved in glutaraldehyde, and mounted on a Teflon-covered strut so as to minimize the septal shelf.[311,313] The Medtronic *Intact* valve (Fig. 57–49C) is also glutaraldehyde treated but at a fixation pressure of zero and with toluidine in an attempt to inhibit calcium deposition.[312] The hemodynamic profiles of the porcine heterografts are similar to those of comparably sized low-profile mechanical prostheses.

During the first 3 postoperative months, while the sewing ring becomes endothelialized, the thromboembolic rate is high enough that anticoagulation is extremely desirable. Thereafter, anticoagulants are not required for porcine valves in the aortic position, and the thromboembolic rate is approximately one or two episodes per 100 patient-years without these drugs.[1,296,297] When these valves have been placed in the mitral position in patients who are in sinus rhythm, who do not have heart failure or thrombus in the left atrium or the left atrial appendage, and who do not have a history of embolism preoperatively, anticoagulants are not needed after the first 3 postoperative months, and the thromboembolic rate is also approximately one or two episodes per 100 patient-years. This rate is comparable to that observed in patients with the St. Jude or other mechanical valves who are receiving anticoagulants and are therefore subject to the risks of hemorrhage. It is unlikely that any MVR can be associated with a thromboembolic rate much below 0.5 episode per 100 patient-years because some of the emboli in patients with longstanding mitral disease are derived from the left atrium rather than from the valve itself. In patients undergoing MVR with a bioprosthesis who have experienced a previous embolism, in whom thrombus is found in the left atrium at operation, or who remain in atrial fibrillation postoperatively (about one-third of all patients receiving MVR), the hazard of thromboembolism and the need for anticoagulants persist. This negates the principal advantage of the tissue valves, and mechanical prostheses would appear to be preferable to bioprostheses in these patients.

Durability. The major problem with porcine bioprostheses is their limited durability (Fig. 57–50). Cuspal tears, degeneration, fibrin deposition, disruption of the fibrocollagenous structure, perforation, fibrosis, and calcification sufficiently severe to require reoperation begin to appear in some patients in the fourth or fifth postoperative year, and by 10 years the rate of primary tissue failure averages 30 percent. It then accelerates, and by 15 years postoperatively the actuarial *freedom* from bioprosthetic primary tissue failure has ranged from 30 to 60 percent in several series. Hypercholesterolemia has been shown to contribute to prosthesis calcification and degeneration,[314,315] suggesting that secondary prevention strategies may slow down this process.

Structural valve deterioration is more frequent in patients with bioprostheses in the mitral than in the aortic position,[302] presumably because of the higher closing pressure. With the passage of time, it is anticipated that many of the currently implanted valves will likely fail, especially in younger patients, and essentially all valves implanted into patients younger than 60 years of age may have to be replaced ultimately. Fortunately, however, these valves usually do not fail suddenly (as is often the case for structural failure or thrombosis of mechanical prostheses). Re-replacement of a bioprosthetic valve should be carried out when significant and/or progressive structural deterioration is evident but before operation becomes an emergency. The second operation, when carried out on an elective basis, may be associated with a surgical mortality rate of 10 to 15 percent.

Color Doppler echocardiography with two-dimensional imaging is extremely helpful in the early detection of bioprosthetic valve malfunction. Transesophageal echocardiography is more sensitive than transthoracic imaging in detecting bioprosthetic valve deterioration. Even patients without new murmurs or other physical findings of valve dysfunction should have routine echocardiographic studies to look for early bioprosthetic valve dysfunction every year for 5 to 6 years after valve replacement and every 6 months after that.

The rate of structural valve failure is age dependent and is significantly lower in patients older than 65 years than in younger patients, especially in the aortic position (Fig. 57–51A). In patients older than 65 years undergoing AVR with a porcine bioprosthesis, the rate of structural deterioration is less than 10 percent at 10 years.[1,302,310,312] Valve failure is prohibitively rapid in children and in adults younger than 35 to 40 years of age. Therefore, bioprostheses are *not* advisable in these age groups. On the other hand, degeneration is rare when these valves are implanted into patients older than 70 years of age.[1,310,312] Bioprostheses also have been reported to have extremely limited durability in patients with chronic renal failure, but recent studies have called this into question (discussed subsequently).

Prosthetic valve endocarditis is a serious, often grave illness (see Chap. 58).

STENTLESS PORCINE XENOGRAFTS. Since the stent adds to the obstruction and thereby increases stress on the leaflets, stentless valves have been developed for the aortic position (see Fig. 57–49)[316] and are now being used increasingly, especially in patients with small aortic roots.[317] These include the Toronto SPV stentless valve (St. Jude Medical valve),[318,319] the Edwards stentless valve,[320] and the Medtronic

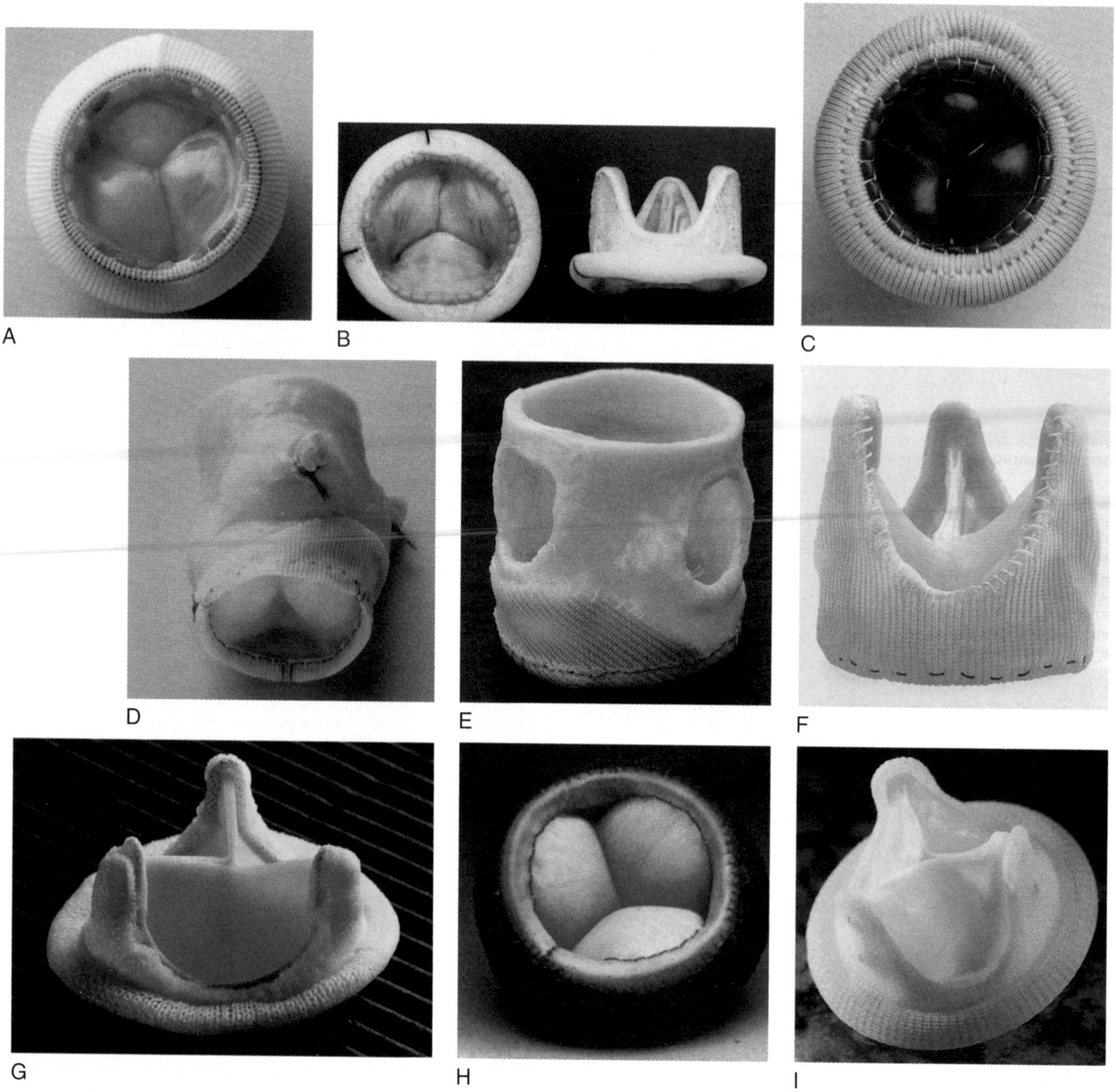

FIGURE 57–49 Bioprosthetic valves. The **top row** shows stented porcine valves: **A,** Hancock porcine valve; **B,** Carpentier-Edwards porcine valve; and **C,** Medtronic Intact porcine valve. The **middle row** shows stentless valves: **D,** Medtronic Freestyle stentless valve; **E,** Edwards Prima stentless valve; and **F,** St. Jude Medical Toronto SPV stentless valve. The **bottom row** shows pericardial valves: **G,** Carpentier-Edwards pericardial valve; **H,** Sorin Pericarbon pericardial valve; and **I,** Autologous pericardial valve. (From Grunkemeier GL, Rahimtoola SH, Starr A: Prosthetic heart valves. *In* Rahimtoola SH [ed]: Valvular Heart Disease. *In* Braunwald E [series ed]: Atlas of Heart Diseases. Vol 11. Philadelphia, Current Medicine, 1997, pp 13.9-13.13.)

Freestyle valve.[316] These valves have been reported to have more physiological flow and lower transvalvular gradients than stented porcine valves, with the potential for enhanced regression of left ventricular hypertrophy and improved left ventricular function. Although the early experience tends to confirm this,[321-323] it is yet uncertain whether this translates into improved outcomes in terms of survival and long-term prosthesis durability. It is hoped that the slightly improved hemodynamics provided by the stentless valves will translate into better valve longevity than that of valves mounted on stents.

PERICARDIAL (XENOGRAFT) AORTIC VALVES. Bovine pericardial valves, unlike porcine valves, are fabricated rather than harvested directly (see Fig. 57–49). Although the first generation of these valves had a high rate of premature structural deterioration, the current generation of stented bovine pericardial prostheses has been demonstrated to have good long-term durability that appears to be equivalent or better than that of the porcine bioprosthesis.[324,325] As with the stented porcine valves, the rate of structural deterioration is extremely low in individuals aged 70 years or older (Fig. 57–51B).[326] There is a greater risk for the development of stenosis in the mitral position.[327]

HOMOGRAFT (ALLOGRAFT) AORTIC VALVES. These are harvested from cadavers, often along with kidneys, usually within 24 hours of donor death. They are sterilized

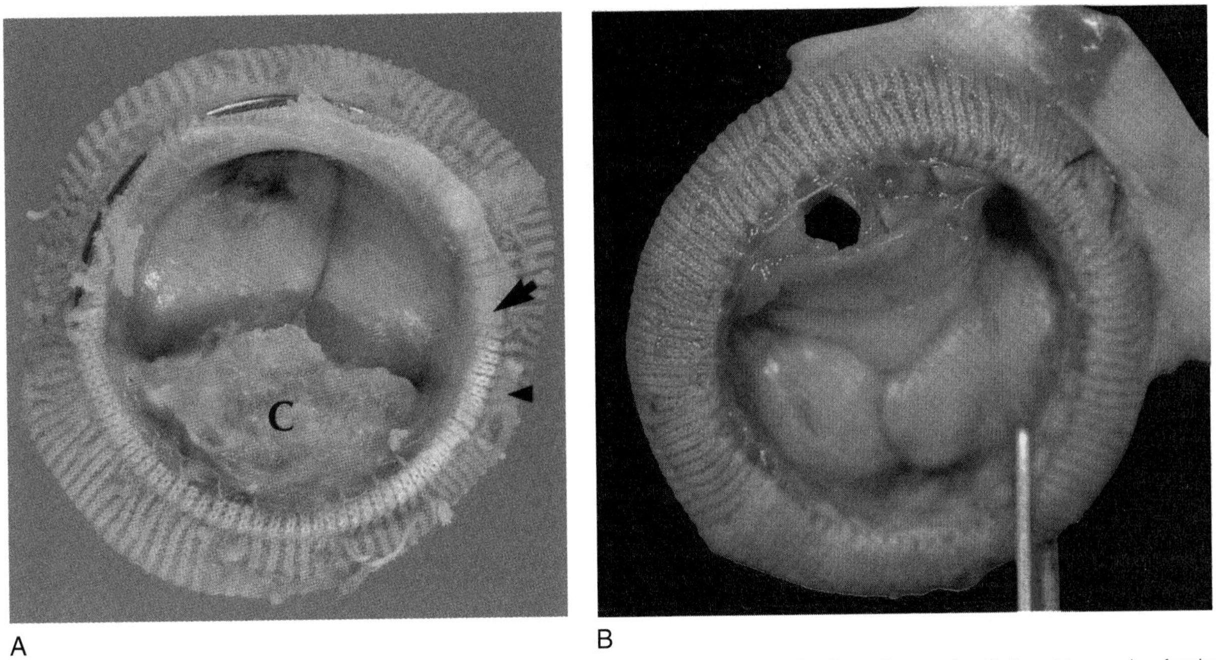

A B

FIGURE 57–50 Structural deterioration of bioprosthetic valves. **A,** Valve failure related to mineralization and collagen degeneration. **B,** Cuspal tears and perforations. These processes may occur independently, or they may be synergistic. (**A,** From Virmani R, Burke AP, Farb A: Pathology of valvular heart disease. *In* Rahimtoola SH [ed]: Valvular Heart Disease. *In* Braunwald E [series ed]: Atlas of Heart Diseases. Vol 11. Philadelphia, Current Medicine, 1997, p 1.26; **B,** From Manabe H, Yutani C [eds]: Atlas of Valvular Heart Disease. Singapore, Churchill Livingstone, 1998, p 158.)

with antibiotics and cryopreserved for long periods at −196°C. They are inserted directly, usually in the aortic position, *without* being placed into a prosthetic stent. In the aortic position, the isolated valve is implanted in the subcoronary position, or the valve and a portion of attached aorta are implanted as a root replacement, with reimplantation of the coronary arteries into the graft. Homograft hemodynamics are superior to those of stented porcine valves and similar to those of stentless porcine valves.[328] Like porcine xenografts, their thrombogenicity is low, but cryopreserved valves appear to have similar issues with structural deterioration,[329] with evidence that this rate is reduced with the use of freshly harvested valves, approximate matching of donor's and patient's ages, and use of the root replacement technique. The subcoronary technique is associated with a higher incidence of prosthetic AR and reoperation.[329-331] Homograft aortic valves have an extremely low rate of infection and are indicated for patients with native or prosthetic valve endocarditis. They are difficult to use when the aortic root and ascending aorta are greatly enlarged, and availability is often limited.

PERICARDIAL AUTOGRAFT VALVES. The patient's own pericardium is inserted into a frame on the operating table and is inserted into either the aortic or the mitral position (see Fig. 57–49I). Long-term durability appears to be excellent; in 267 patients undergoing isolated AVR, the 14-year actuarial freedom of need for re-replacement because of structural valve dysfunction was 85 percent (94 percent in patients > 65 years of age).

PULMONARY AUTOGRAFTS. In this operation, the Ross procedure, the patient's own pulmonary valve and adjacent main pulmonary artery are removed and used to replace the diseased aortic valve and often the neighboring aorta, with reimplantation of the coronary arteries into the graft.[333] A human pulmonary or aortic homograft is then inserted into the pulmonary position. The autograft is nonthrombogenic.[334] In children and adolescents, there is evidence that the autograft grows along with the patient.[335] The risk of endocarditis is low, anticoagulants are not required, and, perhaps most important, the long-term durability appears to be excellent. A high incidence of pulmonary homograft stenosis has been reported in some series,[336,337] which may represent a postoperative inflammatory reaction. The pulmonary artery tissue adapts to the aortic pressure and usually does not dilate.[338] However, this procedure should not be performed in patients with bicuspid valves and dilated aortic roots, because the implanted pulmonary artery tissue exposed to the higher aortic pressures may also undergo degenerative changes leading to significant dilation of the autograft.[339] A subcoronary technique, in which the pulmonary autograft is inserted without a root replacement, may circumvent this problem.[340]

The pulmonary autograft is the replacement valve of choice in children, adolescents, and younger adults who have a long (>20-year) life expectancy, particularly young women who wish to become pregnant. However, its use has been limited because the operation is technically much more demanding than a simple AVR. The procedure should be carried out only by experienced surgeons.

Hemodynamics of Valve Replacements

The most commonly used prosthetic valves, i.e., mechanical prostheses and stented porcine or pericardial xenografts, have an effective in vitro orifice size that is *smaller* than the normal valve at the same site. Unstented porcine xenografts, homografts, and pulmonary autografts do not have this problem. After implantation, tissue ingrowth and endothelialization reduce the size of the effective orifice even more. Therefore, the prosthetic valves that are currently available must be considered to be mildly stenotic. However, postoperative hemodynamic measurements of the mechanical prostheses show reasonably good function, with effective mitral valve orifice areas averaging 1.7 to 2.0 cm^2 and mitral valve gradients of 4 to 8 mm Hg at rest. The cloth-covered Starr-Edwards valve appears to be intrinsically slightly more stenotic than the Medtronic-Hall or Omniscience tilting-disc valves. The bileaflet St. Jude and CarboMedics valves, in turn, may be slightly superior to the Medtronic-Hall or Omniscience valve. In hemodynamic studies, the stented porcine mitral valves

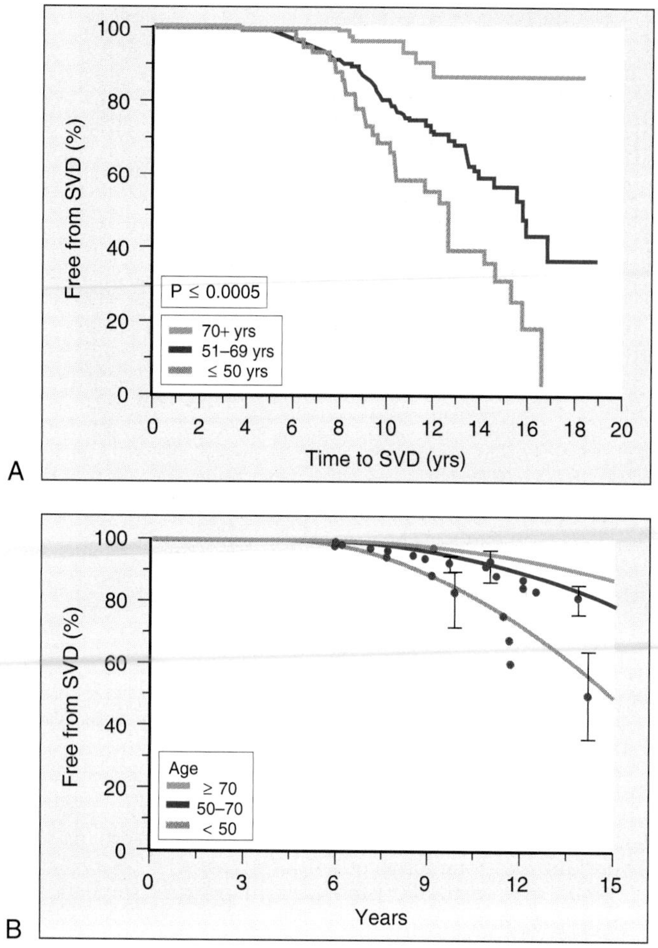

FIGURE 57–51 Estimates of freedom from structural valve deterioration (SVD) for patients undergoing porcine **(A)** and bovine pericardial **(B)** aortic valve replacement who are stratified according to age. (**A,** From Cohn LH, Collins JJ Jr, Rizzo RJ, et al: Twenty-year follow-up of the Hancock modified orifice porcine aortic valve. Ann Thorac Surg 66:S30, 1998; **B,** From Banbury MK, Cosgrove DM, White JA, et al: Age and valve size effect on the long-term durability of the Carpentier-Edwards aortic pericardial bioprosthesis. Ann Thorac Surg 72:753, 2001.)

behave in a manner similar to mechanical prosthetic valves of the same diameter. *Serious* hemodynamic obstruction of an artificial valve in the mitral position is quite uncommon, unless the valve (most commonly the Starr-Edwards valve) is placed into a small left ventricular cavity or into an unusually small mitral annulus or the prosthesis chosen is of inappropriate size.

The problem of prosthetic valve stenosis may be more serious in patients who undergo AVR for AS. The annulus into which the prosthesis is inserted in these patients is usually smaller than it is in patients with AR, and the surgeon may be forced to select an artificial valve that is relatively small. As a consequence, AVR may not abolish obstruction in patients with AS, but the "prosthesis-patient mismatch"[341] may merely convert severe to mild or moderate obstruction. When the smaller models of the stented porcine xenograft or mechanical prosthesis are placed into the aortic position, effective orifice areas of about 1.1 to 1.3 cm^2 are common. In such patients, peak transvalvular gradients as high as 40 mm Hg during exercise have been recorded. In patients with a small annulus, a stentless bioprosthesis valve has better hemodynamic performance that a stented valve.[342] The poor late results observed in a few patients undergoing replacement of stenotic aortic valves may possibly be related to the moderate stenosis of the prosthesis,[343] although the impact of prosthesis-patient mismatch on survival remains controversial.[344-344b] In patients with AS who do not exhibit clinical improvement postoperatively, it is important to evaluate the function of both the prosthetic valve and the left ventricle. Rarely, reoperation to correct a malfunctioning prosthesis may be necessary.

Selection of an Artificial Valve

Most comparisons of mechanical and bioprosthetic valves indicate similar overall results in terms of early and late mortality, prosthetic valve endocarditis and other complications, and the need for reoperation, at least for the first 5 years postoperatively. As indicated, there appear to be no significant differences insofar as hemodynamics are concerned, except that patients with an unusually small left ventricular cavity or mitral or aortic annulus may have better results with the low-profile (tilting-disc) St. Jude or Carbomedics prosthesis or a tissue valve. Patients with a small aortic annulus may be better candidates for unstented homografts, heterografts, or pulmonary autografts. In general, patient outcome after valve surgery is related more to preoperative factors, such as age, left ventricular function, associated coronary artery disease, and comorbid conditions, than to the prosthesis itself.

The major task in selecting an artificial valve is to weigh the advantage of durability and the disadvantages of the risks of thromboembolism and anticoagulant treatment inherent in mechanical prostheses on the one hand with the advantage of low thrombogenicity and the disadvantage of abbreviated durability of bioprostheses on the other. Hammermeister and associates[302] have compared the 15-year outcome in 575 men who were randomized to undergo MVR or AVR with either a mechanical or bioprosthetic valve. Patients undergoing AVR with a mechanical valve had better survival than those receiving the bioprosthesis (Fig. 57–52), principally because of the higher rate of structural deterioration of the bioprosthesis (especially in patients < 65 years of age). Much of the increased mortality in patients receiving the tissue valve was related to reoperation (which is associated with about twice the mortality of the initial procedure). The prosthetic valve did not influence survival after MVR, nor the probability of developing other valve-related complications, including endocarditis, valve thrombosis, and systemic embolism. As anticipated, anticoagulant-related bleeding was higher in patients receiving mechanical valves. Patients with mechanical valves also had a higher incidence of perivalvular regurgitation in the mitral position (see Fig. 11–79) and a trend for this complication in the aortic position. In the Edinburgh randomized trial, which also compared a mechanical with a porcine xenograft valve,[345] 20-year outcome data demonstrated no difference in overall mortality, but survival with the original prosthesis and survival without major valve-related adverse events (except bleeding) were significantly better with mechanical valves. Retrospective cohort analyses are in agreement with the results of these trials.[346,347] Therefore, mechanical prostheses, usually of the bileaflet variety, are the valves of choice in most patients younger than 65 years of age.

However, the following groups of patients should receive bioprostheses: (1) patients with coexisting disease who are prone to hemorrhage and who therefore tolerate anticoagulants poorly, such as those with bleeding disorders, intestinal polyposis, and angiodysplasia; (2) patients who are likely to be noncompliant with permanent anticoagulant treatment, who are unwilling to take anticoagulants on a regular basis, or who live in developing nations and cannot be monitored; (3) patients older than 65 years of age in whom bioprosthetic valves deteriorate slowly (see Fig. 57–51), who are unlikely to outlive their bioprostheses, and who because of their age may also be at greater risk of hemorrhage while taking anticoagulants; (4) patients with a small aortic annulus in whom an unstented (free) bioprosthetic graft may provide superior hemodynamics; and (5) younger patients (<40 years of age), especially women wishing to bear children, who require AVR and in whom a pulmonary autograft may be preferable. However, the technical difficulties associated with the last procedure must be taken into account.

Special Situations

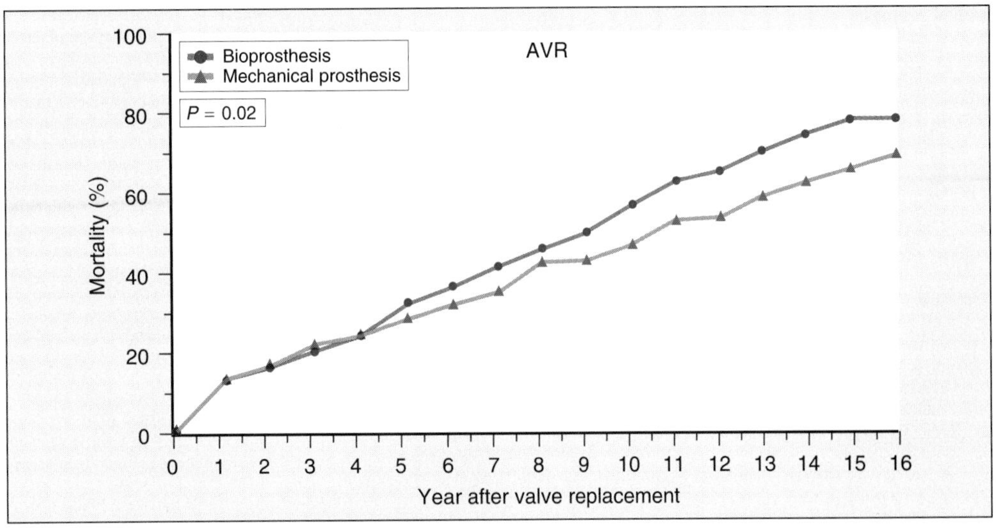

FIGURE 57–52 Mortality after aortic valve replacement (AVR) with the Björk-Shiley and porcine valves from the Department of Veterans Affairs trial. (From Hammermeister KE, Sethi GK, Henderson WG, et al: Outcomes 15 years after valve replacement with a mechanical versus a bioprosthetic valve: Final report of the Veterans Affairs randomized trial. J Am Coll Cardiol 36:1152, 2000.)

PREGNANCY (see Chap. 74). Women with artificial valves can tolerate the hemodynamic burden of pregnancy well, but the hypercoagulable state of pregnancy increases the risk of thromboembolism in pregnant patients with mechanical prostheses. Anticoagulation must not be interrupted, although an increased risk of fatal fetal hemorrhage occurs in women in whom anticoagulants are continued. There is also a risk of fetal malformation caused by the probable teratogenic effect of warfarin, but this risk is low (1.6%).[348] Although these problems represent rationales for the use of tissue valves in all women of childbearing age,[349] their limited durability in young adults makes their use unacceptable. Therefore, unless a pulmonary autograft can be employed (for patients who require AVR), every effort should be made to defer valve replacement until after childbirth. In pregnant women with critical MS or AS, balloon valvuloplasty should be considered, and, if at all possible, mitral valve repair instead of replacement should be undertaken for patients with MR. Women of childbearing potential who have a mechanical prosthesis should be counseled against pregnancy. When a woman who already has a mechanical prosthetic valve becomes pregnant, the risk to the fetus if the mother receives oral anticoagulants appears to be lower than the risk to the mother if anticoagulants are discontinued. Therefore, coumarin derivatives should be continued and the INR maintained between 2.0 and 3.0 until 2 weeks before expected delivery, at which time the patient should be switched to intravenous heparin.[1,25,350] Heparin should be discontinued at the onset of labor but may be restarted, along with coumarin, several hours after delivery. Alternatively, warfarin may be briefly interrupted at the 38th week of gestation and planned cesarean section carried out.[349] There are no data on the safety and effectiveness of low-molecular-weight heparin in pregnant patients with mechanical prosthetic valves, and this agent cannot be recommended in these patients.[348,351] Low-molecular-weight heparin is not approved for this use, and additional precautions have been added to the warning labels.

NONCARDIAC SURGERY. When noncardiac surgery is required in patients with prosthetic valves who are receiving anticoagulants, the risk is minimal when the anticoagulant is stopped 1 to 3 days preoperatively and for a similar period postoperatively. It may be desirable, however, to protect the patient with low-molecular-weight dextran during the perioperative period and to resume anticoagulation rapidly with intravenous heparin.

PATIENTS DESTINED TO RECEIVE ANTICOAGULANTS. Patients with earlier implantation of a mechanical prosthesis, chronic atrial fibrillation with an enlarged left atrium, a history of thromboembolism, or a thrombus in the left atrium at operation, and who therefore are destined to receive anticoagulants, should receive a mechanical valve prosthesis because the potential advantage of a tissue valve is negated.[1]

CHILDREN AND PATIENTS RECEIVING CHRONIC HEMODIALYSIS. The high incidence of bioprosthetic valve failure in children and adolescents virtually prohibits their use in these groups. In young adults between the ages of 25 and 35 years, the failure of bioprosthetic valves is somewhat higher than it is in older adults; this serves as a relative, but not an absolute, contraindication to their use in this age group.

In children, a mechanical prosthesis (generally the St. Jude valve) with its favorable hemodynamics and established durability is preferred despite the disadvantages inherent in the need for anticoagulants in this age group. Similarly, mechanical valve prostheses should be used in patients with chronic renal failure and/or hypercalcemia. Alternatively, if an experienced surgical team is available and the patient requires an AVR, a pulmonary autograft is an excellent alternative.

Previous studies indicated a high rate of bioprosthetic structural deterioration in patients receiving chronic renal dialysis. However, subsequent studies have reported no difference in survival of patients with a bioprosthesis or a mechanical valve, coupled with an unacceptably high rate of stroke and major bleeding in patients with the mechanical valves.[352,353] Although current guidelines recommend mechanical valves in these patients, this clearly is an area in which physician judgment is important for individual patients.

TRICUSPID POSITION. The risk of thrombosis for all valves is highest in the tricuspid position because of the lower pressures and velocity of blood flow. This complication appears to be highest for tilting-disc valves, intermediate for caged-ball valves, and lowest for bioprostheses, which are the valves of choice as tricuspid replacements. Fortunately, bioprostheses exhibit a much slower rate of mechanical deterioration in the tricuspid position than in the mitral or aortic positions.

REFERENCES

1. Bonow RO, Carabello B, de Leon AC, et al: ACC/AHA guidelines for the management of patients with valvular heart disease: A report of the American College of Cardiology/American Heart Association Task Force on Practice Guidelines (Committee on Management of Patients with Valvular Heart Disease). J Am Coll Cardiol 32:1486, 1998.
2. Iung B, Gohlke-Barwolf C, Tornos P, et al: Recommendations on the management of the asymptomatic patient with valvular heart disease. Eur Heart J 23:1253, 2002.

3. Rahimtoola SH, Durairaj A, Mehra A, et al: Current evaluation and management of patients with mitral stenosis. Circulation 106:1183, 2002.
4. Waller B, Howard J, Fess S: Pathology of mitral valve stenosis and pure mitral regurgitation: I. Clin Cardiol 17:330, 1994.
5. Filgner CL, Reichenbach DD, Otto CM: Pathology and etiology of valvular heart disease. *In* Otto CM (ed): Valvular Heart Disease. 2nd ed. Philadelphia, WB Saunders, 2004, pp 30-33.
6. Dalen JE, Fenster PE: Mitral stenosis. *In* Alpert JS, Dalen JE, Rahimtoola SH (eds): Valvular Heart Disease. 3rd ed. Philadelphia, Lippincott Williams & Wilkins, 2000, pp 75-83.
7. Otto CM: Mitral stenosis. *In* Otto CM (ed): Valvular Heart Disease. 2nd ed. Philadelphia, WB Saunders, 2004, pp 252-255.
8. Grossman W: Profiles in valvular heart disease. *In* Baim DS, Grossman W (eds): Cardiac Catheterization, Angiography and Interventions. 6th ed. Baltimore, Lippincott, Williams & Wilkins, 2000, pp 735-756.
9. Gorlin R, Gorlin SG: Hydraulic formula for calculation of the area of stenotic mitral valve, other cardiac valves, and central circulatory shunts. Am Heart J 41:1, 1951.
10. Braunwald E, Turi ZG: Pathophysiology of mitral valve disease. *In* Wells FC, Shapiro LM (eds): Mitral Valve Disease. 2nd ed. London, Butterworths, 1996, pp 28-36.
11. Choi BW, Bacharach SL, Barbour DJ, et al: Left ventricular systolic dysfunction, diastolic filling characteristics, and exercise cardiac reserve in mitral stenosis. Am J Cardiol 75:526, 1995.
12. Stefanadis C, Dernellis J, Stratos C, et al : Effects of balloon mitral valvuloplasty on left atrial function in mitral stenosis as assessed by pressure-area relation. J Am Coll Cardiol 32:159, 1998.
13. Pathan AZ, Mahdi NA, Leon MN, et al: Is redo percutaneous mitral balloon valvuloplasty (PMV) indicated in patients with post-PMV mitral restenosis? J Am Coll Cardiol 34:49, 1999.
14. Moreyra AE, Wilzon AC, Deac R, et al: Factors associated with atrial fibrillation in patients with mitral stenosis: A cardiac catheterization study. Am Heart J 135:138-145, 1998.
15. Leatham A: Assessment of mitral valve function: Clinical presentation, assessment, and prognosis. *In* Wells FC, Shapiro LM (eds): Mitral Valve Disease. 2nd ed. London, Butterworths, 1996, pp 37-46.
16. Wood P: An appreciation of mitral stenosis. BMJ 1:1051,1113, 1954.
17. Chiang CW, Lo SK, Kuo CT, et al: Noninvasive predictors of systemic embolism in mitral stenosis: An echocardiographic and clinical study of 500 patients. Chest 106:396, 1994.
18. Chiang CW, Lo SK, Ko YS, et al: Predictors of systemic embolism in patients with mitral stenosis: A prospective study. Ann Intern Med 128:885, 1998.
19. Shapiro LM: Echocardiography of the mitral valve. *In* Wells FC, Shapiro LM (eds): Mitral Valve Disease. 2nd ed. London, Butterworths, 1996, pp 47-50.
20. Sagie A, Freitas N, Chen MH, et al: Echocardiographic assessment of mitral stenosis and its associated valvular lesions in 205 patients and lack of association with mitral valve prolapse. J Am Soc Echocardiogr 10:141, 1997.
21. Faletr F, Pezzano JA, Fusc R, et al: Measurement of mitral valve area in mitral stenosis: Four echocardiographic methods compared with direct measurement of anatomic orifices. J Am Coll Cardiol 28:1190, 1996.
22. Popovic AD, Thomas JD, Neskovic AN, et al: Time-related trends in the preoperative evaluation of patients with valvular stenosis. Am J Cardiol 80:1464, 1997.
23. Prystowsky EN, Benson DW Jr, Fuster V, et al: Management of patients with atrial fibrillation: A Statement for Healthcare Professionals. From the Subcommittee on Electrocardiography and Electrophysiology. Circulation 93:1262, 1996.
24. Fuster V, Ryden L, Asinger RW, et al: ACC/AHA/ESC guidelines for the management of patients with atrial fibrillation: Executive summary. J Am Coll Cardiol 38:1231, 2001.
25. Gohlke-Barwolf C, Acar J, Oakley C, et al: Guidelines for the prevention of thromboembolic events in valvular heart disease. Eur Heart J 16:1230, 1995.
26. Manning WJ, Silverman DI, Keighley CS, et al: Transesophageal echocardiographically facilitated early cardioversion from atrial fibrillation using short-term anticoagulation: Final results of a prospective 4.5 year study. J Am Coll Cardiol 25:1354, 1995.
27. Kawaguchi AT, Kosakai Y, Sasako Y, et al : Risks and benefits of combined maze procedure for atrial fibrillation with organic heart disease. J Am Coll Cardiol 28:985, 1996.
28. Yuda S, Nakatini S, Isobe F, et al: Comparative efficacy of the maze procedure for restoration of atrial contraction in patients with and without giant left atrium associated with mitral valve disease. J Am Coll Cardiol 31,1097, 1998.
29. Nakajima H, Kobayashi J, Bando K, et al: The effect of cryo-maze procedure on early and intermediate-term outcome in mitral valve disease: Case-matched study. Circulation 106:I-46, 2002.
30. Sagie A, Freitas N, Padial LR, et al: Doppler echocardiographic assessment of long-term progression of mitral stenosis in 103 patients: Valve area and right heart disease. J Am Coll Cardiol 28:472, 1996.
31. Olesen KH: The natural history of 271 patients with mitral stenosis under medical treatment. Br Heart J 24:349, 1962.
32. Horstkotte D, Niehues R, Strauer BE: Pathomorphological aspects, aetiology, and natural history of acquired mitral valve stenosis. Eur Heart J 12(Suppl):55, 1991.
33. Orrange E, Kawanishi DT, Lopez BM, et al: Actuarial outcome after catheter balloon commissurotomy in patients with mitral stenosis. Circulation 95:382, 1997.
34. Hernandez R, Banuelos C, Alfonso F, et al: Long-term clinical and echocardiographic follow-up after percutaneous mitral valvuloplasty with the Inoue balloon. Circulation 99:1580, 1999.
35. Iung B, Garbarz E, Michaud P, et al: Late results of percutaneous mitral commissurotomy in a series of 1024 patients—Analysis of late clinical deterioration: Frequency, anatomic findings, and predictive factors. Circulation 99:3273, 1999.
36. Kang DH, Park SW, Song JK, et al: Long-term clinical and echocardiographic outcome of percutaneous mitral valvuloplasy: Randomized comparison of Inoue and double-balloon techniques. J Am Coll Cardiol 35:169, 2000.
37. Farhat MB, Ayari M, Maatzouk F, et al: Percutaneous balloon versus surgical closed and open mitral commissurotomy: Seven-year follow-up results of a randomized trial. Circulation 97:245, 1998.
38. Cannan CR, Nishimura RA, Reeder GS, et al: Echocardiographic assessment of commissural calcium: A simple predictor of outcome after percutaneous mitral balloon valvotomy. J Am Coll Cardiol 29:175, 1997.
39. Gomez-Hospital JA, Cequier A, Romero PV, et al: Partial improvement in pulmonary function after successful percutaneous balloon mitral valvotomy. Chest 117:643, 2000.
40. Padial LR, Abascal VM, Moreno PR, et al: Echocardiography can predict the development of severe mitral regurgitation after percutaneous mitral valvuloplasty by the Inoue technique. Am J Cardiol 83:1210, 1999.
41. Palacios IF, Sanchez PL, Harrell, et al: Which patients benefit from percutaneous mitral balloon valvuloplasty? Prevalvuloplasy and postvalvuloplasty variables that predict long-term outcome. Circulation 105:1465, 2002.
42. Zhang HP, Yen GS, Allen JW, et al: Comparison of late results of balloon valvotomy in mitral stenosis with versus without mitral regurgitation. Am J Cardiol 81:51, 1998.
43. Mazur W, Parilak LD, Kaluza G, et al: Balloon valvuloplasty for mitral stenosis. Curr Opin Cardiol 14:95, 1999.
44. Applebaum R, Kasliwal R, Kanojia A, et al: Utility of three-dimensional echocardiography during balloon mitral valvuloplasty. J Am Coll Cardiol 32:1405, 1998.
45. Joseph PK, Bhat A, Francis B, et al: Percutaneous transvenous mitral commissurotomy using an Inoue balloon in children with rheumatic mitral stenosis. Int J Cardiol 62:19, 1997.
46. Kothari SS, Kamath P, Juneja R, et al: Percutaneous transvenous mitral commissurtomy using Inoue balloon in children less than 12 years. Cathet Cardiovasc Diagn 43:408, 1998.
47. Zaki A, Salama M, El Masry M, Elhendy A: Five-year follow-up after percutaneous balloon mitral valvuloplasty. Am J Cardiol 83:735, 1999.
48. Iung B, Garbarz E, Michaud P, et al: Percutaneous mitral commissurotomy for restenosis after surgical commissurotomy: Late efficacy and implications for patient selection. J Am Coll Cardiol 35:1295, 2000.
49. Ben Farat M, Gamra H, Betbout F, et al: Percutaneous balloon mitral commissurotomy during pregnancy. Heart 77:564, 1997.
50. de Souza JAM, Martinez EE, Ambrose JA, et al: Percutaneous balloon mitral valvuloplasty in comparison with open mitral valve commissurotomy for mitral stenosis during pregnancy. J Am Coll Cardiol 37:900, 2001.
51. Leon MN, Harrell LC, Simosa HF, et al: Mitral balloon valvotomy for patients with mitral stenosis and atrial fibrillation: Immediate and long-term results. J Am Coll Cardiol 34:1145, 1999.
52. Cribier A, Elchaninoff H, Koning R, et al: Percutaneous mechanical mitral commissurotomy with a newly designed metallic valvulotome: Immediate results of the initial experience in 153 patients. Circulation 99:793, 1999.
53. English T: Closed mitral valvotomy. *In* Wells FC, Shapiro LM (eds): Mitral Valve Disease. 2nd ed. London, Butterworths, 1996, pp 107-113.
54. Otto CM: Surgical and percutaneous intervention for mitral stenosis. *In* Otto CM (ed): Valvular Heart Disease. 2nd ed. Philadelphia, WB Saunders, 2004, pp 272-276.
55. Edwards FH, Peterson ED, Coombs LP, et al: Prediction of operative mortality after valve replacement surgery. J Am Coll Cardiol 37:885, 2001.

Mitral Regurgitation

56. Otto CM: Evaluation and management of chronic mitral regurgitation. N Engl J Med 345:740, 2001.
57. Carabello BA: Progress in mitral and aortic regurgitation. Curr Probl Cardiol 28:553, 2003.
58. Mann JM, Davies MJ: The pathology of the mitral valve. *In* Wells FC, Shapiro LM (eds): Mitral Valve Disease. 2nd ed. London, Butterworths, 1996, pp 16-27.
59. Fox CS, Vasan RS, Parise H, et al: Mitral annular calcification predicts cardiovascular morbidity and mortality: The Framingham Heart Study. Circulation 107:1492, 2003.
60. Jeon DS, Atar S, Brasch AV, et al: Association of mitral annulus calcification, aortic valve sclerosis, and aortic root calcification with abnormal myocardial perfusion single-photon emission tomography in subjects <65 years old. J Am Coll Cardiol 38:1988, 2001.
61. Adler Y, Fink N, Tame D, et al: Association between mitral annulus calcification and carotid atherosclerotic disease. Stroke 29:1833, 1998.
62. Barber JE, Ratliff NB, Cosgrove DM, et al: Myxomatous mitral valve chordae: I. Mechanical properties. J Heart Valve Dis 10:320, 2001.
63. Lamas GA, Mitchell GF, Flaker GC, et al: Clinical significance of mitral regurgitation after acute myocardial infarction. Survival and Ventricular Enlargement Investigators. Circulation 96:827, 1997.
64. Otsuji Y, Handschumacher MD, Schwammenthal E, et al: Insights from three-dimensional echocardiography into the mechanism of functional mitral regurgitation: Direct in vivo demonstration of altered leaflet tethering geometry. Circulation 96:1999, 1997.
65. Thourani VH, Weintraub WS, Guyton RA, et al: Outcomes and long-term survival for patients undergoing mitral valve repair versus replacement: Effect of age and concomitant coronary artery bypass grafting. Circulation 108:298, 2003.
66. Dahlberg PS, Orszulak TA, Mullany CJ, et al: Late outcome of mitral valve surgery for patients with coronary artery disease. Ann Thorac Surg 76:1539, 2003.
67. 126. Rosario LB, Stevenson LW, Solomon SD, et al: The mechanism of decrease in dynamic mitral regurgitation during heart failure treatment: Importance of reduction in the regurgitant orifice size. J Am Coll Cardiol 32:1819, 1998.
68. Kizilbash AM, Willett DL, Brickner ME, et al: Effects of afterload reduction on vena contracta width in mitral regurgitation. J Am Coll Cardiol 32:427, 1998.
69. Carabello BA: Concentric versus eccentric remodeling. J Card Fail 8(Suppl):S258, 2002.
70. Sutton TM, Stewart RAH, Gerber IL, et al: Plasma natriuretic peptide levels increase with symptoms and severity of mitral regurgitation. J Am Coll Cardiol 41:2280, 2003.

71. Tallaj J, Hankes GH, Holland M, et al: Beta$_1$-adrenergic receptor blockade attenuates angiotensin II-mediated catecholamine release into the cardiac interstitium in mitral regurgitation. Circulation 108:225, 2003.
71a. Mehta RH, Supiamo MA, Oral H, et al: Compared with control subjects, the systemic sympathetic nervous system is activated in patients with mitral regurgitation. Am Heart J 145:1078, 2003.
72. Oral H, Sivasubramanian N, Dyke DB, et al: Myocardial proinflammatory cytokine expression and left ventricular remodeling in patients with chronic mitral regurgitation. Circulation 107:831, 2003.
73. Conway MA, Bottomley PA, Ouwerkerk R, et al: Mitral regurgitation: Impaired systolic function, eccentric hypertrophy, and increased severity are linked to lower phosphocreatine/ATP ratios in humans. Circulation 97:1716, 1998.
74. Akasaka T, Yoshida K, Hozumi T, et al: Restricted coronary flow reserve in patients with mitral regurgitation improves after mitral reconstructive surgery. J Am Coll Cardiol 32:1923, 1998.
75. Timmis SB, Kirsh MM, Montgomery DG, Starling MR: Evaluation of left ventricular ejection fraction as a measure of pump performance in patients with chronic mitral regurgitation. Cathet Cardiovasc Intervent 49:290, 2000.
76. Enriquez-Sarano M, Schaff HV, Tajik AJ, et al: Chronic mitral regurgitation. *In* Alpert JS, Dalen JE, Rahimtoola SH (eds): Valvular Heart Disease. 3rd ed. Philadelphia, Lippincott Williams & Wilkins, 2000, pp 113-142.
77. Matsumura T, Ohtaki E, Tanaka K, et al: Echocardiographic prediction of left ventricular dysfunction after mitral valve repair for mitral regurgitation as an indicator to decide the optimal timing of repair. J Am Coll Cardiol 42:458, 2003.
78. Flemming MA, Oral H, Rothman ED, et al: Echocardiographic markers for mitral valve surgery to preserve left ventricular performance in mitral regurgitation. Am Heart J 140:476, 2000.
79. Wisenbaugh T, Skudicky D, Sareli P: Prediction of outcome after valve replacement for rheumatic mitral regurgitation in the era of chordal preservation. Circulation 89:191, 1994.
80. Leung DY, Griffin BP, Snader CE, et al: Determinant of functional capacity in chronic mitral regurgitation unassociated with coronary artery disease or left ventricular dysfunction. Am J Cardiol 79:914, 1997.
81. Enriquez-Sarano M, Basmadjian AJ, Rossi A, et al: Progression of mitral regurgitation: A prospective Doppler echocardiographic study. J Am Coll Cardiol 34:1137, 1999.
82. Ling LH, Enriquez-Sarano M. Long-term outcomes of patients with flail mitral valve leaflets. Coron Artery Dis 11:3, 2000.
83. Rosen SF, Borer JS, Hochreiter C, et al: Natural history of the asymptomatic patient with severe mitral regurgitation secondary to mitral valve prolapse and normal right and left ventricular performance. Am J Cardiol 74:374, 1994.
84. Heinle SK, Grayburn PA: Doppler echocardiographic assessment of mitral regurgitation. Coron Artery Dis 11:11, 2000.
85. Dujardin KS, Enriquez-Sarano M, Bailey KR, et al: Grading of mitral regurgitation by quantitative Doppler echocardiography: Calibration by left ventricular angiography in routine clinical practice. Circulation 96:3409, 1996.
85a. Zoghbi WA, Enriquez-Sarano M, Foster E, et al: Recommendations for evaluation of the severity of native valvular regurgitation with two-dimensional and Doppler echocardiography. J Am Soc Echocardiogr 16:777, 2003.
86. Zhou X, Jones M, Shiota T, et al: Vena contracta imaged by Doppler color-flow mapping predicts the severity of eccentric mitral regurgitation better than color jet area: A chronic animal study. J Am Coll Cardiol 30:1393, 1997.
87. Hall SA, Brickner ME, Willett DL, et al: Assessment of mitral regurgitation severity by Doppler color-flow mapping of the vena contracta. Circulation 95:636, 1997.
88. Enriquez-Sarano M, Dujardin KS, Tribouilloy CM, et al: Determinants of pulmonary venous flow reversal in mitral regurgitation and its usefulness in determining the severity of regurgitation. Am J Cardiol 83:535, 1999.
89. Thomas L, Foster E, Schiller NB: Peak mitral inflow velocity predicts mitral regurgitation severity. J Am Coll Cardiol 31:174, 1998.
90. Thomas L, Foster E, Hoffman JIE, et al: The mitral regurgitation index: An echocardiographic guide to severity. J Am Coll Cardiol 33:2016, 1999.
91. Enriquez-Sarano M, Freeman WK, Tribouilloy CM, et al : Functional anatomy of mitral regurgitation: Accuracy and outcome implications of transesophageal echocardiography. J Am Coll Cardiol 34:1129, 1999.
92. Pu M, Thomas JD, Vandervoort PM, et al : Comparison of quantitative and semiquantitative methods for assessing regurgitation by transesophageal echocardiography. Am J Cardiol 87:66, 2001.
92a. Omram AS, Woo A, David TE, et al: Intraoperative transesophageal echocardiography accurately predicts mitral valve anatomy and suitability for repair. J Am Soc Echocardiogr 15:950, 2002.
93. De Simone R, Glombitza G, Vahl CF, et al: Three-dimensional color Doppler: A clinical study in patients with mitral regurgitation. J Am Coll Cardiol 33:1646, 1999.
94. Armstrong GP, Griffin BP: Exercise echocardiographic assessment in severe mitral regurgitation. Coron Artery Dis 11:23, 2000.
95. Kizilbash AM, Hundley WG, Willett DL, et al: Comparison of quantitative Doppler with magnetic resonance imaging for assessment of the severity of mitral regurgitation. Am J Cardiol 81:792, 1998.
96. Høst U, Kelbaek H, Hildebrant P, et al: Effect of ramipril on mitral regurgitation secondary to mitral valve prolapse. Am J Cardiol 80:655, 1997.
97. Tischler MD, Rowan M, LeWinter MM: Effect of enalapril therapy on left ventricular mass and volumes in asymptomatic chronic, severe, mitral regurgitation secondary to mitral valve prolapse. Am J Cardiol 82:242, 1998.
98. Nemoto S, Hamawaki M, De Freitas G, et al : Differential effects of the angiotensin-converting enzyme inhibitor lisinopril versus the beta-adrenergic receptor blocker atenolol on hemodynamics and left ventricular contractile function in experimental mitral regurgitation. J Am Coll Cardiol 40:149, 2002.
99. Perry GJ, Wei CC, Hankes GH, et al: Angiotensin II receptor blockade does not improve left ventricular function and remodeling in subacute mitral regurgitation in the dog. J Am Coll Cardiol 39:1374, 2002.
100. Gillinov AM, Cosgrove DM, Blackstone EH, et al: Durability of mitral valve repair for degenerative disease. J Thorac Cardiovasc Surg 116:734, 1998.
101. Braunberger E, Deloche A, Berregi A, et al: Very long-term results (>20 years) of valve repair with Carpentier's techniques in nonrheumatic mitral valve insufficiency. Circulation 104:I-8, 2001.
102. Mohty D, Orszulak TA, Schaff HV, et al: Very long-term survival and durability of mitral valve repair for mitral valve prolapse. Circulation 104:I-1, 2001.
103. Chauvand S, Fuzellier JF, Berrebi A, et al : Long-term (29 years) results of reconstructive surgery in rheumatic mitral valve insufficiency. Circulation 104:I-12, 2001.
103a. Yacoub MH, Cohn LH: Novel approaches to cardiac valve repair: From structare to function (two parts). Circulation 109:942 and 1064, 2004.
104. Phillips MR, Daly RC, Schaff HV, et al: Repair of anterior leaflet mitral valve prolapse: Chordal replacement versus chordal shortening. Ann Thorac Surg 69:25, 2000.
105. von Oppell UO, Stemmet F, Braink J, et al: Ischemic mitral valve repair surgery. J Heart Valve Dis 9:64, 2000.
106. Gillinov AM, Wierup PN, Blackstone EH, et al: Is repair preferable to replacement for ischemic mitral regurgitation? J Thorac Cardiovasc Surg 122:1125, 2001.
107. Bolling SF, Pagani FD, Deeb GM, Bach DS: Intermediate-term outcome of mitral reconstruction in cardiomyopathy. J Thorac Cardiovasc Surg 115:381, 1998.
108. Chen FY, Adams DH, Aranki SF, et al: Mitral valve repair in cardiomyopathy. Circulation 98:III-124, 1998.
109. Bishay ES, McCarthy PM, Cosgrove DM, et al: Mitral valve surgery in patients with severe left ventricular dysfunction. Eur J Cardiothorac Surg 17:213, 2000.
110. Remadi JP, Baron O, Roussel C, et al: Isolated mitral valve replacement with St. Jude medical prosthesis—Long-term results: A follow-up of 19 years. Circulation 103:1542, 2001.
111. Reardon MJ, David TE: Mitral valve replacement with preservation of the subvalvular apparatus. Curr Opin Cardiol 14:104, 1998.
112. Yun KL, Sintek CF, Miller DC, et al: Randomized trial of partial versus complete chordal preservation methods of mitral valve replacement: A preliminary report. Circulation 100:II-90, 1999.
113. Society of Thoracic Surgeons National Cardiac Surgery Database. Accessed December 10, 2003. (http://www.ctsnet.org/file/STSNationalDatabaseSpring2003ExecutiveSummary.pdf)
114. Click RL, Schaff HV: Intraoperative transesophageal echocardiography: 5-year prospective review of impact on surgical management. Mayo Clin Proc 75:241, 2000.
114a. Savage EB, Ferguson TB Jr, DiSesa VJ: Use of mitral valve repair: Analysis of contemporary United States experience reported to the Society of Thoracic Surgeons National Cardiac Database. Ann Thorac Surg 75:820, 2003.
115. Grossi EA, Galloway AC, Miller JS, et al: Valve repair versus replacement for mitral insufficiency: When is a mechanical valve still indicated? J Thorac Cardiovasc Surg 115:389, 1998.
116. Flameng W, Herijgers P, Bogaerts K: Recurrence of mitral valve regurgitation after mitral valve repair in degenerative valve disease. Circulation 107:1609, 2003.
117. Loulmet DF, Carpentier A, Cho PW, et al: Less invasive techniques for mitral valve surgery. J Thorac Cardiovasc Surg 115:772, 1998.
118. Gillinov AM, Cosgrove DM: Minimally invasive mitral valve surgery: Mini-sternotomy with extended transseptal approach. Semin Thorac Cardiovasc Surg 11:206, 1999.
119. Greelish JP, Cohn LH, Leacche M, et al: Minimally invasive mitral valve repair suggests earlier operations for mitral valve disease. J Thorac Cardiovasc Surg 126:365, 2003.
120. Letsou GV, Reardon MJ: Minimally invasive valve surgery. Curr Opin Cardiol 13:105, 1998.
121. Goldfine H, Aurigemma GP, Zile MR, et al: Left ventricular length–force-shortening relations before and after surgical correction of chronic mitral regurgitation. J Am Coll Cardiol 31:180, 1998.
122. Krishman US, Gersony WW, Berman-Rosenzweig E, Apfel HD: Late left ventricular function after surgery for children with chronic symptomatic mitral regurgitation. Circulation 96:4280, 1997.
123. Tribouilloy CM, Enriquez-Sarano M, Schaff HV, et al: Impact of preoperative symptoms on survival after surgical correction of organic mitral regurgitation: Rationale for optimizing surgical indications. Circulation 99:400, 1999.
124. Lim E, Barlow CW, Hosseinpour AR, et al: Influence of atrial fibrillation on outcome following mitral valve repair. Circulation 104:I-59, 2001.
125. Gillinov AM, Faber C, Houghtaling PL, et al: Repair versus replacement for degenerative mitral valve disease with coexisting ischemic heart disease. J Thorac Cardioavasc Surg 125:1197, 2003.

Mitral Valve Prolapse Syndrome

126. Devereux RB: Recent developments in the diagnosis and management of mitral valve prolapse. Curr Opin Cardiol 10:107, 1995.
127. David TE, Omran A, Armstrong S, et al: Long-term results of mitral valve repair for myxomatous disease with and without chordal replacement with expanded polytetrafluoroethylene sutures. J Thorac Cardiovasc Surg 115:1279, 1998.
128. Cohn LH, Couper GS, Aranki SF, et al: Long-term results of mitral valve reconstruction for the regurgitating myxomatous mitral valve. J Thorac Cardiovasc Surg 107:143, 1994.
129. O'Rourke RA: Syndrome of mitral valve prolapse. *In* Alpert JS, Dalen JE, Rahimtoola SH (eds): Valvular Heart Disease. 3rd ed. Philadelphia, Lippincott Williams & Wilkins, 2000, pp 157-182.
130. Nishimura RA, McGoon MD: Perspectives on mitral valve prolapse. N Engl J Med 341:48, 1999.
131. Freed LA, Benjamin EJ, Levy D, et al: Mitral valve prolapse in the general population: The benign nature of the echocardiographic features in the Framingham Heart Study. J Am Coll Cardiol 40:1298, 2002.

132. Otto CM: Mitral valve prolapse. *In* Otto CM (ed): Valvular Heart Disease. 2nd ed. Philadelphia, WB Saunders, 2004, pp 368-387.
133. Becker AE, Davies MJ: Pathomorphology of mitral valve prolapse. *In* Boudoulas H, Wooley CF (eds): Mitral Valve: Floppy Mitral Valve, Mitral Valve Prolapse, Mitral Valvular Regurgitation. 2nd ed. Armonk, NY, Futura, 2000, pp 91-114.
134. Grande-Allen KJ, Griffin BP, Calabro A, et al: Myxomatous mitral valve chordae: II. Selective elevation of glycosaminoglycan content. J Heart Valve Dis 10:325, 2001.
135. Mylonakis E, Calderwood SB: Infective endocarditis in adults. N Engl J Med 345:1318, 2001.
136. Fontana MF: Mitral valve prolapse and floppy mitral valve: Physical examination. *In* Boudoulas H, Wooley CF (eds): Mitral Valve: Floppy Mitral Valve, Mitral Valve Prolapse, Mitral Valvular Regurgitation. 2nd ed. Armonk, NY, Futura, 2000, pp 283-304.
137. Schaal SF: Mitral valve prolapse: Cardiac arrhythmias and electrophysiological correlates. *In* Boudoulas H, Wooley CF (eds): Mitral Valve: Floppy Mitral Valve, Mitral Valve Prolapse, Mitral Valvular Regurgitation. 2nd ed. Armonk, NY, Futura, 2000, pp 409-430.
138. Malkowski MJ, Pearson AC: The echocardiographic assessment of the floppy mitral valve: An integrated approach. *In* Boudoulas H, Wooley CF (eds): Mitral Valve: Floppy Mitral Valve, Mitral Valve Prolapse, Mitral Valvular Regurgitation. 2nd ed. Armonk, NY, Futura, 2000, pp 231-252.
139. Langholz D, Mackin WJ, Wallis DE, et al: Transesophageal echocardiographic assessment of systolic mitral leaflet displacement among patients with mitral valve prolapse. Am Heart J 135:197, 1998.
140. Fukuda N, Oki T, Iuchi A, et al: Predisposing factors for severe mitral regurgitation in idiopathic mitral valve prolapse. Am J Cardiol 76:503, 1995.
141. Zuppiroli A, Rinaldi M, Kramer-Fox R, et al: Natural history of mitral valve prolapse. Am J Cardiol 75:1028, 1995.
142. Boudoulas H, Kolibash AJ, Wooley CF: Floppy mitral valve, mitral valve prolapse, mitral valvular regurgitation: Natural history. *In* Boudoulas H, Wooley CF (eds): Mitral Valve: Floppy Mitral Valve, Mitral Valve Prolapse, Mitral Valvular Regurgitation. 2nd ed. Armonk, NY, Futura, 2000, pp 503-540.
143. Avierinos JF, Gersh BJ, Melton LJ, et al: Natural history of asymptomatic mitral valve prolapse in the community. Circulation 106:1355, 2002.
144. Gilon D, Buonanno FS, Joffe MM, et al: Lack of evidence of an association between mitral valve prolapse and stroke in young patients. N Engl J Med 341:8, 1999.
145. Boudoulas H, Wooley CF: Floppy mitral valve/Mitral valve prolapse: Sudden death. *In* Boudoulas H, Wooley CF (eds): Mitral Valve: Floppy Mitral Valve, Mitral Valve Prolapse, Mitral Valvular Regurgitation. 2nd ed. Armonk, NY, Futura, 2000, pp 431–448.
146. Corrado D, Basso C, Rizzoli G, et al: Does sports activity enhance the risk of sudden death in adolescents and young adults? J Am Coll Cardiol 42:1959, 2003.
147. Gillinov AM, Cosgrove DM, Lytle BW, et al: Reoperation for failure of mitral valve repair. J Thorac Cardiovasc Surg 113:467, 1997.

Aortic Stenosis

148. Levinson GE, Alpert JS. Aortic stenosis. *In* Alpert JS, Dalen JE, Rahimtoola SH (eds): Valvular Heart Disease. 3rd ed. Philadelphia, Lippincott Williams & Wilkins, 2000, pp 183-211.
149. Carabello BA: Aortic stenosis. N Engl J Med 346:677, 2002.
150. Huntington K, Hunter AGW, Chan KL: A prospective study to assess the frequency of familial clustering of congenital bicuspid aortic valve. J Am Coll Cardiol 30:1809, 1997.
151. Fedak PWM, Verma S, David TE: Clinical and pathophysiological implications of a bicuspid aortic valve. Circulation 106:900, 2002.
152. Keane MG, Wiegers SE, Plappert T, et al. Bicuspid aortic valves are associated with aortic dilatation out of proportion to coexistent valvular lesions. Circulation 102:III-35, 2000.
153. Nataatmadja M, West M, West J, et al: Abnormal extracellular matrix protein transport associated with increased apoptosis of vascular smooth muscle cells in Marfan syndrome and bicuspid aortic valve thoracic aortic aneurysm. Circulation 108:II-329, 2003.
154. Rajamannan NM, Gersh B, Bonow RO: Calcific aortic stenosis: From bench to bedside—Emerging clinical and cellular concepts. Heart 89:1, 2003.
155. Otto CM, Lind BK, Kitzman DW, et al: Association of aortic valve sclerosis with cardiovascular mortality and morbidity in the elderly. N Engl J Med 341:142, 1999.
156. Olsson M, Thyberg J, Nilsson J: Presence of oxidized low-density lipoproteins in nonrheumatic stenotic aortic valves. Arterioscler Thromb Vasc Biol 19:1218, 1999.
157. Ghaisas NK, Foley JB, O'Briain DS, et al: Adhesion molecules in nonrheumatic aortic valve disease: Endothelial expression, serum levels, and effects of valve replacement. J Am Coll Cardiol 36:2257, 2000.
158. Galante A, Pietroiusti A, Vellini M, et al: C-reactive protein is increased in patients with degenerative aortic valvular stenosis. J Am Coll Cardiol 38:1078, 2001.
159. O'Brien KD, Shavelle DM, Caulfield MT, et al: Association of angiotensin-converting enzyme with low-density lipoprotein in aortic valvular lesions and in human plasma. Circulation 106:2224, 2002.
160. Mohler ER, Gannon F, Reynolds C, et al: Bone formation and inflammation in cardiac valves. Circulation 103:1522, 2001.
161. Rajamannan NM, Subramaniam M, Rickard D, et al : Human aortic valve calcification is associated with an osteoblast phenotype. Circulation 107:2181, 2003.
162. Stewart BF, Siscovick D, Lind BK, et al: Clinical factors associated with calcific aortic valve disease. J Am Coll Cardiol 29:630, 1997.
163. Palta S, Pai AM, Gill K, et al: New insights into the progression of aortic stenosis: Implications for secondary prevention. Circulation 101:2497, 2000.
164. Peltier M, Trojette F, Enriquez-Sarano M, et al: Relation between cardiovascular risk factors and nonrheumatic severe calcific aortic stenosis among patients with a three-cuspid aortic valve. Am J Cardiol 91:97, 2003.
165. Novaro GM, Iong IY, Pearce GL, et al: Effect of hydoxymethylglutaryl coenzyme A reductase inhibitors on the progression of calcific aortic stenosis. Circulation 104:2205, 2001.
166. Shavelle DM, Takasu J, Budoff MJ, et al: HMG CoA reductase inhibitor (statin) and aortic valve calcium. Lancet 359:1125, 2002.
167. Bellamy MF, Pellikka PA, Klarich KW, et al: Association of cholesterol levels, hydoxymethylglutaryl coenzyme-A reductase inhibitor treatment, and progression of aortic stenosis in the community. J Am Coll Cardiol 40:1723, 2002.
168. Rajamannan NM, Subramanian M, Sebo T, et al: Atorvastatin inhibits hypercholesterolemia-induced cellular proliferation and bone matrix production in the rabbit aortic valve. Circulation 105:2660, 2002.
169. Alpert JS: Aortic stenosis: A new face for an old disease. Arch Intern Med 163:1769, 2003.
170. Chan C: Is aortic stenosis a preventable disease? J Am Coll Cardiol 42:593, 2003.
171. Kawaguchi A, Miyatake K, Yutani C, et al: Characteristic cardiovascular manifestations in homozygous and heterozygous familial hypercholesterolemia. Am Heart J 137:410, 1999.
172. Hultgren HN: Osteitis deformans (Paget's disease) and calcific disease of the heart valves. Am J Cardiol 81:1461, 1998.
173. Hangaishi M, Taguchi J, Ikari Y, et al: Aortic valve stenosis in alkaptonuria. Circulation 98:1148, 1998.
174. Malouf JF, Enriquez-Sarano M, Pellikka PA, et al: Severe pulmonary hypertension in patients with severe aortic stenosis: Clinical profile and prognostic implications. J Am Coll Cardiol 40:789, 2002.
175. Legget ME, Kuusisto J, Healy NL, et al: Gender differences in left ventricular function at rest and with exercise in asymptomatic aortic stenosis. Am Heart J 131:94, 1996.
176. Fielitz J, Hein S, Mitrovic V, et al: Activation of the cardiac renin-angiotensin system and increased myocardial collagen expression in human aortic valve disease. J Am Coll Cardiol 37:1443, 2001.
177. Walther T, Schubert A, Falk V, et al: Left ventricular reverse remodeling after surgical therapy for aortic stenosis: Correlation to renin-angiotensin system gene expression. Circulation 106:I-23, 2002.
178. Rajappan K, Rimoldi OE, Dutka DP, et al: Mechanisms of coronary microcirculatory dysfunction in patients with aortic stenosis and angiographically normal coronary arteries. Circulation 105:470, 2002.
179. Gould KL, Carabello BA: Why angina in aortic stenosis with normal coronary arteriograms? Circulation 107:3121, 2003.
180. Julius BK, Spillmann M, Vassalli G, et al: Angina pectoris in patients with aortic stenosis and normal coronary arteries. Circulation 95:892, 1997.
181. Carabello BA: Evaluation and management of patients with aortic stenosis. Circulation 105:1746, 2002.
182. Pareti FI, Lattuada A, Bressi C, et al: Proteolysis of von Willebrand factor and shear stress-induced platelet aggregation in patients with aortic stenosis. Circulation 102:1290, 2000.
183. Vincentelli A, Susen S, Le Tourneau T, et al: Acquired von Willebrand syndrome in aortic stenosis. N Engl J Med 343:349, 2003.
184. Munt B, Legget ME, Kraft CD, et al: Physical examination in valvular aortic stenosis: Correlation with stenosis severity and prediction of clinical outcome. Am Heart J 137:298, 1999.
185. Okura H, Yoshida K, Hozumi T, et al: Planimetry and transthoracic two-dimensional echocardiography in noninvasive assessment of aortic valve area in patients with valvular aortic stenosis. J Am Coll Cardiol 30:753, 1997.
186. Kim KS, Maxted W, Nanda NC, et al: Comparison of multiplane and biplane transesophageal echocardiography in the assessment of aortic stenosis. Am J Cardiol 79:436, 1997.
187. Gilon D, Capre EG, Handschumacher MD, et al: Effect of three-dimensional valve shape on the hemodynamics of aortic stenosis: Three-dimensional echocardiographic stereolthography and patient studies. J Am Coll Cardiol 40:1479, 2002.
188. Leborgne L, Tribouilloy C, Otmani A, et al: Comparative value of Doppler echocardiography and cardiac catheterization in the decision to operate on patients with aortic stenosis. Int J Cardiol 65:163, 1998.
189. Baumgartner H, Stefenelli T, Niederberger J, et al: "Overestimation" of catheter gradients by Doppler ultrasound in patients with aortic stenosis: A predictable manifestation of pressure recovery. J Am Coll Cardiol 33:1655, 1999.
190. Garcia D, Pibarot P, Dumesnil JG, et al: Assessment of aortic valve stenosis severity: A new index based on the energy loss concept. Circulation 101:765, 2000.
191. Garcia D, Dumesnil JG, Durand LG, et al: Discrepancies between catheter and Doppler estimates of valve effective orifice area can be predicted from the pressure recovery phenomenon: Practical implications with regard to quantification of aortic stenosis severity. J Am Coll Cardiol 41:435, 2003.
192. Levine RA, Schwammenthal E: Stenosis is in the eye of the observer: Impact of pressure recovery on assessing aortic valve area. J Am Coll Cardiol 41:443, 2003.
193. John AS, Dill T, Brandt RR, et al: Magnetic resonance to assess the aortic valve area in aortic stenosis. J Am Coll Cardiol 42:519, 2003.
194. Caruthers SD, Lin SJ, Brown P, et al: Practical value of cardiac magnetic resonance imaging for clinical quantification of aortic valve stenosis: Comparison with echocardiography. Circulation 208:2236, 2003.
195. Otto CM, Burwarsh IG, Legget ME, et al: A prospective study of asymptomatic valvular aortic stenosis: Clinical, echocardiographic, and exercise predictors of outcome. Circulation 95:2262, 1997.
196. Iivanainian AM, Lindroos M, Tilvis R, et al: Natural history of aortic valve stenosis of varying severity in the elderly. Am J Cardiol 78:97, 1996.
197. Rosenhek R, Porenta G, Lang I, et al: Predictors of outcome in severe, asymptomatic aortic stenosis. N Engl J Med 343:611, 2000.
198. Amato MCM, Moffa PJ, Ramires JAF: Treatment decision in asymptomatic aortic valve stenosis: Role of exercise testing. Heart 86:381, 2001.
199. Weinschelbaum E, Stutzbach P, Oliva M, et al: Manual débridement of the aortic valve in elderly patients with degenerative aortic stenosis. J Thorac Cardiovasc Surg 87:1157, 1999.

200. Braunwald E: Aortic valve replacement: An update at the turn of the millennium. Eur Heart J 21:1032-1033, 2000.
201. Connolly HM, Oh JK, Orszulak TA, et al: Aortic valve replacement for aortic stenosis with severe left ventricular dysfunction: Prognostic indicators. Circulation 95:2395, 1997.
202. Connolly HM, Oh JK, Schaff HV, et al: Severe aortic stenosis with low transvalvular gradient and severe left ventricular dysfunction: Result of aortic valve replacement in 52 patients. Circulation 101:1940, 2000.
203. Rahimtoola SH: Severe aortic stenosis with low systolic gradient: The good and bad news. Circulation 101:1892, 2000.
204. Pereira JJ, Lauer MS, Bashir M, et al: Survival after aortic valve replacement for severe aortic stenosis with low transvalvular gradients and severe left ventricular dysfunction. J Am Coll Cardiol 39:1356, 2002.
205. Monin JL, Monchi M, Gest V, et al: Aortic stenosis with severe left ventricular dysfunction and low transvalvular pressure gradients: Risk stratification by low-dose dobutamine echocardiography. J Am Coll Cardiol 37:2102, 2001.
206. Monin JL, Quere JP, Monchi M, et al: Low-gradient aortic stenosis: Operative risk stratification and predictors for long-term outcome—A multicenter study using dobutamine stress hemodynamics. Circulation 108:319, 2003.
207. Powell DE, Tunick PA, Rosenzweig BP, et al: Aortic valve replacement in patients with aortic stenosis and severe left ventricular dysfunction. Arch Intern Med 160:1337, 2000.
208. Jolobe O: Surgery for aortic stenosis in severely symptomatic patients older than 80 years: Experience in a single UK centre. Heart 83:583, 2000.
209. Khot UN, Novaro GM, Popovic ZB, et al: Nitroprusside in critically ill patients with left ventricular dysfunction and aortic stenosis. N Engl J Med 348:1756, 2003.
209a. Rahimtoola SH: The year in valvular heart disease. J Am Coll Cardiol 43:491, 2004.
210. Zile MR, Gaasch WH: Heart failure in aortic stenosis: Improving diagnosis and treatment. N Engl J Med 348:1735, 2003.
211. Nishimura RA, Grantham A, Connolly HM, et al: Low-output, low-gradient aortic stenosis in patients with depressed left ventricular systolic function: The clinical utility of the dobutamine challenge in the catheterization laboratory. Circulation 106:809, 2002.
212. Kivdal P, Bergström R, Hörte LG, et al: Observed and relative survival after aortic valve replacement. J Am Coll Cardiol 35:747, 2000.
213. Asimakopoulous G, Edwards MB, Taylor KM: Aortic valve replacement in patients 80 years of age and older: Survival and cause of death on 1100 cases. Collective results from the UK Heart Valve Registry. Circulation 96:3403, 1997.
214. Sundt TM, Bailey MS, Moon MR, et al: Quality of life after aortic valve replacement at the age of > 80 years. Circulation 102:III-70, 2000.
215. De Paulis R, Sommariva L, Colagrande L, et al: Regression of left ventricular hypertrophy after aortic valve replacement for aortic stenosis with different valve substitutes. J Thorac Cardiovasc Surg 116:590, 1998.
216. Lamb HJ, Beyerbacht HP, de Roos A, et al : Left ventricular remodeling early after aortic valve replacement: Differential effects on diastolic function in aortic valve stenosis and aortic regurgitation. J Am Coll Cardiol 40:2182, 2002.
217. Khan SS, Siegel RJ, DeRobertis MA, et al: Regression of hypertrophy after Carpentier-Edwards pericardial aortic valve replacement. Ann Thorac Surg 69:531, 2000.
218. Hildek-Smtih DJR, Shapiro LM: Coronary flow reserve improves after aortic valve replacement for aortic stenosis: An adenosine transthoracic echocardiography study. J Am Coll Cardiol 36:1889, 2000.
219. Rajappan K, Rimoldi OE, Camici PG, et al: Functional changes in coronary microcirculation after valve replacement in patients with aortic stenosis. Circulation 107:3170, 2003.
220. Gall S Jr, Lowe JE, Wolfe WG, et al: Efficacy of the internal mammary artery in combined aortic valve replacement coronary artery bypass grafting. J Thorac Surg 69:524, 2000.
221. Cohn LH: Minimally invasive aortic valve surgery: Technical considerations and results with the parasternal approach. J Card Surg 13:302, 1998.
222. Bouchard D, Perrault LP, Carrier M, et al: Ministernotomy for aortic valve replacement: A study of the preliminary experience. Can J Surg 43:39-42, 2000.
223. Galal O, Rao PS, Al-Fadley F, Wilson AD: Follow-up result of balloon aortic valvuloplasty in children with special reference to causes of late aortic insufficiency. Am Heart J 133:418, 1997.
224. Boudjemline Y, Bonhoeffer P: Steps toward percutaneous aortic valve replacement. Circulation 105:775, 2002.
225. Cribier A, Eltchanioff H, Bash A, et al: Percutaneous transcatheter implantation of an aortic valve prosthesis for calcific aortic stenosis: First human case description. Circulation 106:3006, 2002.

Aortic Regurgitation

226. Rahimtoola SH: Aortic regurgitation. *In* Rahimtoola SH (ed): Valvular Heart Disease. Atlas of Heart Diseases. Vol. 11. Braunwald E (series ed). Philadelphia, Current Medicine, 1997, p 7.9.
227. Casselman FP, Gillinov AR, Kasirajan V, et al: Intermediate-term durability of bicuspid aortic valve repair for prolapsing leaflet. Eur J Cardiothorac Surg 15:302, 1999.
228. Olsson A, Darpo B, Bergfeldt L, Rosenqvist M: Frequency and long-term follow-up of valvar insufficiency caused by retrograde aortic radiofrequency catheter ablation procedures. Heart 81:292, 1999.
229. Bonow RO: Chronic aortic regurgitation: Role of medical therapy and optimal timing for surgery. Cardiol Clin 16:449, 1998.
230. Bonow RO: Chronic aortic regurgitation. *In* Alpert JS, Dalen JE, Rahimtoola SH (eds): Valvular Heart Disease. 3rd ed. Philadelphia, Lippincott Williams & Wilkins, 2000, pp 245-268.
231. Borer JS, Truter S, Herrold EM, et al: Myocardial fibrosis in chronic aortic regurgitation: Molecular and cellular responses to volume overload. Circulation 105:1837, 2002.
232. Otto CM: Aortic regurgitation. *In* Otto CM (ed): Valvular Heart Disease. 2nd ed. Philadelphia, WB Saunders, 2004, pp 302-335.
233. Borer JS, Bonow RO: Contemporary approach to aortic and mitral regurgitation. Circulation 108:2432, 2003.
234. Choudhry NK, Etchells EE: Does this patient have aortic regurgitation? JAMA 281:2231, 1999.
235. Chen J, Okin PM, Roman MJ, et al: Combined rest and exercise electrocardiographic repolarization findings in relation to structural and functional abnormalities in asymptomatic aortic regurgitation. Am Heart J 132:343, 1996.
236. Tribouilloy CM, Enriquez-Sarano M, Fett SL, et al: Application of the proximal flow convergence method to calculate the effective regurgitant orifice area in aortic regurgitation. J Am Coll Cardiol 32:1032, 1998.
237. Shiota T, Jones M, Agler DA, McDonald RW: New echo cardiographic windows for quantitative determination of aortic regurgitation volume using color Doppler flow convergence and vena contracta. Am J Cardiol 83:1064, 1999.
238. Tribouilloy CM, Enriquez-Sarano M, Bailey KR, et al: Assessment of severity of aortic regurgitation using the width of the vena contracta: A clinical color Doppler imaging study. Circulation 102:558, 2000.
239. Willett DL, Hall SA, Jessen ME, et al: Assessment of aortic regurgitation by transesophageal color Doppler imaging of the vena contracta: Validation against an intraoperative aortic flow probe. J Am Coll Cardiol 37:1450, 2001.
240. Zoghbi WA, Enriquez-Sarano M, Foster E, et al: Recommendations for evaluation of the severity of native valvular regurgitation with two-dimensional and Doppler echocardiography. J Am Soc Echocardiogr 16:777, 2003.
241. Borer JS, Hochreiter C, Herrold EM, et al: Prediction of indications for valve replacement among asymptomatic or minimally symptomatic patients with chronic aortic regurgitation and normal left ventricular performance. Circulation 97:525, 1998.
242. Tarasoutchi F, Grinberg M, Spina GS, et al: Ten-year clinical laboratory follow-up after application of a symptom-based therapeutic strategy to patients with severe chronic aortic regurgitation of predominant rheumatic etiology. J Am Coll Cardiol 41:1316, 2003.
243. Pohost GM, Hung L, Doyle M: Clinical use of cardiovascular magnetic resonance. Circulation 12:647, 2003.
244. Dujardin KS, Enriquez-Sarano M, Schaff HV et al: Mortality and morbidity of aortic regurgitation in clinical practice: A long-term follow-up study. Circulation 99:1851, 1999.
245. Klodas E, Enriquez-Sarano M, Tajik AJ, et al: Aortic regurgitation complicated by extreme left ventricular dilatation: Long-term outcome after surgical correction. J Am Coll Cardiol 27:670, 1996.
246. Sondergaard L, Aldershvile J, Hildebrandt P, et al: Vasodilatation with felodipine in chronic asymptomatic aortic regurgitation. Am Heart J 139:667, 2000.
247. Alehan D, Ozkutlu S: Beneficial effects of 1-year captopril therapy in children with chronic aortic regurgitation who have no symptoms. Am Heart J 135:598, 1998.
248. Scognamiglio R, Rahimtoola SH, Fasoli G, et al: Nifedipine in asymptomatic patients with severe aortic regurgitation and normal left ventricular function. N Engl J Med 331:689, 1994.
249. Klodas E, Enriquez-Sarano M, Tajik AJ, et al: Optimizing timing of surgical correction in patients with severe aortic regurgitation: Role of symptoms. J Am Coll Cardiol 30:746, 1997.
250. Borer JS: Aortic valve replacement for the asymptomatic patient with aortic regurgitation: A new piece of the strategic puzzle. Circulation 106:2637, 2002.
251. Tornos MO, Olona M, Permanyer-Miralda G, et al: Heart failure after aortic valve replacement for aortic regurgitation: Prospective 20-year study. Am Heart J 136:681, 1998.
252. Turina J, Stark T, Seifert B, et al: Predictors of the long-term outcome after combined aortic and mitral valve surgery. Circulation 100:II-48, 1999.
253. Chaliki HP, Mohty D, Avierinos JF, et al: Outcomes after aortic valve replacement in patients with severe aortic regurgitation and markedly reduced left ventricular function. Circulation 106:2687, 2002.
254. Devlin WH, Petrusha J, Briesmiester K, et al: Impact of vascular adaptation to chronic aortic regurgitation on left ventricular performance. Circulation 99:1027, 1999.
255. Odell JA, Orszulak TA: Surgical repair and reconstruction of valvular lesions. Curr Opin Cardiol 10:135, 1995.
256. Burkhart HM, Zehr KJ, Schaff HV, et al: Valve-preserving aortic root reconstruction: A comparison of techniques. J Heart Valve Dis 12:62, 2003.
257. David TE: Aortic valve repair in patients with Marfan syndrome and ascending aorta aneurysms due to degenerative disease. J Cardiovasc Surg 9(Suppl):182, 1994.
258. Leyh RG, Schmidtke C, Sievers HH, et al: Opening and closing characteristics of the aortic valve after different types of valve-preserving surgery. Circulation 100:2153, 1999.
259. Alpert JS: Acute aortic insufficiency. *In* Alpert JS, Dalen JE, Rahimtoola SH (eds): Valvular Heart Disease. 3rd ed. Philadelphia, Lippincott Williams & Wilkins, 2000, pp 269-289.
260. Eusebio J, Louie EK, Edwards DC, et al: Alterations in transmitral flow dynamics in patients with early mitral valve closure and aortic regurgitation. Am. Heart J 128:941, 1994.

Tricuspid, Pulmonic, and Multivalvular Disease

261. Ewy GA: Tricuspid valve disease. *In* Alpert JS, Dalen JE, Rahimtoola SH (eds): Valvular Heart Disease. 3rd ed. Philadelphia, Lippincott Williams & Wilkins, 2000, pp 377-392.
262. Ananthasubramaniam K, Farha A: Primary right atrial angiosarcoma mimicking acute pericarditis, pulmonary embolism, and tricuspid stenosis. Heart 81:556, 1999.
263. Møller JE, Connolly HM, Rubin J, et al: Factors associated with progression of carcinoid heart disease. N Engl J Med 348:1005, 2003.
264. Hagers Y, Koole M, Schoors D, Van Camp G: Tricuspid stenosis: A rare complication of pacemaker-related endocarditis. J Am Soc Echocardiogr 13:66, 2000.
265. Heaven DJ, Henein MY, Sutton R: Pacemaker lead related to tricuspid stenosis: A report of two cases. Heart 83:351, 2000.
266. Otto CM: Right-sided valve disease. *In* Otto CM (ed): Valvular Heart Disease. 2nd ed. Philadelphia, WB Saunders, 2004, pp 415-436.

267. Ha JW, Chung N, Jang Y, Rim SJ: Tricuspid stenosis and regurgitation: Doppler and color-flow echocardiography and cardiac catheterization findings. Clin Cardiol 23:51, 2000.
268. Del Campo C, Sherman JR: Tricuspid valve replacement: Results comparing mechanical and biological prostheses. Ann Thorac Surg 69:1295, 2000.
269. Bahl VK, Chandra S, Mishra S: Concurrent balloon dilatation of mitral and tricuspid stenosis during pregnancy using an Inoue balloon. Int J Cardiol 59:199, 1997.
270. Prieto LR, Hordof AJ, Secic M, et al: Progressive tricuspid valve disease in patients with congenitally corrected transposition of the great arteries. Circulation 98:997, 1998.
271. Kulke MH, Mayer RJ: Carcinoid tumors. N Engl J Med 858, 1999.
272. Simula DV, Edwards WD, Tazelaar HD, et al: Surgical pathology of carcinoid heart disease: A study of 139 valves from 75 patients spanning 20 years. Mayo Clin Proc 77:139, 2002.
273. Paniagua D, Aldrich HR, Lieberman EH, et al: Increased prevalence of significant tricuspid regurgitation in patients with transvenous pacemaker leads. Am J Cardiol 82:1130, 1998.
274. Reynertson MD, Kundur R, Mullen GM, et al: Asymmetry of right ventricular enlargement in response to tricuspid regurgitation. Circulation 100:465, 1999.
275. Jick H, Vasilakis C, Weinrauch LA, et al: A population-based study of appetite suppressant drugs and the risk of cardiac valve regurgitation. N Engl J Med 339:719, 1998.
276. Naschitz JE, Goldstein L, Zuckerman E, et al: Benign course of congestive cirrhosis associated with tricuspid regurgitation: Does pulsatility protect against complications of venous hypertension? J Clin Gastroenterol 30:213, 2000.
277. Kemp WE Jr, Kerins DM, Shyr Y, Byrd BF III: Optimal Albunex dosing for enhancement of Doppler tricuspid regurgitation spectra. Am J Cardiol 79:232, 1997.
278. Grossmann G, Giesler M, Stein M, et al: Quantification of mitral and tricuspid regurgitation by the proximal flow convergence method using two-dimensional colour Doppler and colour Doppler M-mode: Influence of the mechanism of regurgitation. Int J Cardiol 66:299, 1998.
279. Tribouilloy CM, Enriquez-Sarano M, Bailey KR, et al: Quantification of tricuspid regurgitation by measuring the width of the vena contracta with Doppler color-flow imaging: A clinical study. J Am Coll Cardiol 36:472, 2000.
280. Pitts WR, Lange RA, Cigarroa JE, Hillis LD: Predictive value of prominent right atrial v waves in assessing the presence and severity of tricuspid regurgitation. Am J Cardiol 83:617, 1999.
281. Sugimoto T, Okada M, Ozaki N, et al: Long-term evaluation of treatment for functional tricuspid regurgitation with regurgitant volume: Characteristic differences based on primary cardiac lesion. J Thorac Cardiovasc Surg 117:463, 1999.
282. Bajzer CT, Stewart WJ, Cosgrove DM, et al: Tricuspid valve surgery and intraoperative echocardiography: Factors affecting survival, clinical outcome, and echocardiographic success. J Am Coll Cardiol 32:1023, 1998.
283. Jamieson WRE, Edwards FH, Schwartz M, et al: Risk stratification for cardiac valve replacement. National Cardiac Surgery Database. Ann Thorac Surg 67:943, 1999.
284. Discigil B, Dearani JA, Puga FJ, et al: Late pulmonary valve replacement after repair of tetralogy of Fallot. J Thorac Cardiovasc Surg 121:344, 2001.
285. Helbing WA, de Roos A: Optimal imaging in assessment of right ventricular function in tetralogy of Fallot with pulmonary regurgitation. Am J Cardiol 82:1561, 1998.
286. Balaguer JM, Byrne JG, Cohn LH: Orthotopic pulmonic valve replacement with a pulmonary homograft as an interposition graft. J Card Surg 11:417, 1996.
287. Conte S, Jashari R, Eyskens B, et al: Homograft valve insertion for pulmonary regurgitation late after valveless repair of right ventricular outflow tract obstruction. Eur J Cardiothorac Surg 15:143, 1999.
288. Connolly HM, Schaff HV, Mullany CJ, et al: Carcinoid heart disease: Impact of pulmonary valve replacement in right ventricular function and remodeling. Circulation 106:I-51, 2002.
289. Paraskos JA: Combined valve disease. *In* Alpert JS, Dalen JE, Rahimtoola SH (eds): Valvular Heart Disease. 3rd ed. Philadelphia, Lippincott Williams & Wilkins, 2000, pp 291-337.
290. Gillinov AM, Blackstone EH, Cosgrove DM, et al: Mitral valve repair with aortic valve replacement in superior to double valve replacement. J Thorac Cardiovasc Surg 125:1372, 2003.
291. John S, Ravikumar E, John CN, Bashi VV: 25-year experience with 456 combined mitral and aortic valve replacement for rheumatic heart disease. Ann Thorac Surg 69:1167, 2000.
292. Turina J, Stark T, Seifert B, et al: Predictors of the long-term outcome after combined aortic and mitral valve surgery. Circulation 100:II-48, 1999.

Prosthetic Cardiac Valves

293. Braunwald NS, Cooper TS, Morrow AG: Complete replacement of the mitral valve. J Thorac Cardiovasc Surg 40:1, 1960.
294. Harken DE, Soroff MS, Taylor MC: Partial and complete prostheses in aortic insufficiency. J Thorac Cardiovasc Surg 40:744, 1960.
295. Starr A, Edwards ML: Mitral replacement: Clinical experience with a ball-valve prosthesis. Ann Surg 154:726, 1961.
296. Grunkemeier GL, Rahimtoola SH, Starr A: Prosthetic heart valves. *In* Rahimtoola SH (ed): Valvular Heart Disease. Atlas of Heart Diseases. Vol. 11. Braunwald E (series ed). Philadelphia, Mosby, 1997, pp 13.1-13.27.
297. Grunkemeier GL, Li HH, Naftel DC, et al: Long-term performance of heart valve prostheses. Curr Probl Cardiol 25:73, 2000.
298. Rahimtoola SH: Choice of prosthetic heart valve for adult patients. J Am Coll Cardiol 41:893, 2003.
299. Murday AJ, Hochstitzky A, Mansfield J, et al: A prospective controlled trial of St. Jude versus Starr Edwards aortic and mitral valve prostheses. Ann Thorac Surg 76:66, 2003.
300. Emery RW, Erickson CA, Arom KV, et al: Replacement of the aortic valve in patients under 50 years of age: Long-term follow up of the St. Jude medical prosthesis. Ann Thorac Surg 75:1815, 2003.
301. Jamieson WR, Fradet GJ, Miyagishima RT, et al: CarboMedics mechanical prosthesis: Performance at eight years. J Heart Valve Dis 9:678, 2000.
302. Hammermeister KE, Sethi GK, Henderson WG, et al: Outcomes 15 years after valve replacement with a mechanical versus a bioprosthetic valve: Final report of the Veterans Affairs randomized trial. J Am Coll Cardiol 36:1152, 2000.
303. Cannegieter SC, Rosendaal FR, Wintzen AR, et al: Optimal oral anticoagulant therapy in patients with mechanical heart valves. N Engl J Med 333:11, 1995.
304. Acar J, Iung B, Boissel JP, et al: AREVA, multicenter randomized comparison of low-dose versus standard-dose anticoagulation in patients with mechanical prosthetic heart valves. Circulation 94:2107, 1996.
305. Meschengieser SS, Fondevila CG, Frontroth J, et al: Low-intensity oral anticoagulation plus low-dose aspirin versus high-intensity oral anticoagulation alone: A randomized trial in patients with mechanical prosthetic heart valves. J Thorac Cardiovasc Surg 113:910, 1997.
306. Laffort P, Roudaut R, Roques X, et al: Early and long-term (one-year) effects of the association of aspirin and oral anticoagulant on thrombi and morbidity after replacement of the mitral valve with the St. Jude medical prosthesis: A clinical and transesophageal echocardiographic study. J Am Coll Cardiol 35:739, 2000.
307. Massel D, Little SH: Risks and benefits of adding anti-platelet therapy to warfarin among patients with prosthetic heart valves: A meta-analysis. J Am Coll Cardiol 37:569, 2001.
308. Lengyel M, Fuster V, Keltai M, et al: Guidelines for management of left-sided prosthetic valve thrombosis: A role for thrombolytic therapy. Consensus Conference on Prosthetic Valve Thrombosis. J Am Coll Cardiol 30:1521, 1997.
309. Schoen FJ, Levy RJ: Tissue heart valves: Current challenges and future research perspectives. J Biomed Mater Res 47:439, 1999.
310. Cohn LH, Collins JJ Jr, Rizzo RJ, et al: Twenty-year follow-up of the Hancock modified orifice porcine aortic valve. Ann Thorac Surg 66:S30, 1998.
311. Jamieson WR, Burr LH, Miyagishima RT, et al: Actuarial versus actual freedom from structural valve deterioration with the Carpentier-Edwards porcine bioprosthesis. Can J Cardiol 15:973, 1999.
312. Jamieson WRE, Lemieux MD, Sullivan JA, et al: Medtronic intact porcine bioprosthesis experience to twelve years. Ann Thorac Surg 71:S278, 2001.
313. Jamieson WR, David TE, Feindel CM, et al: Performance of the Carpentier-Edwards SAV and Hancock-II porcine bioprostheses in aortic valve replacement. J Heart Valve Dis 11:424, 2002.
314. Nollert G, Miksch J, Kreuzer E, et al: Risk factors for atherosclerosis and the degeneration of pericardial valves after aortic valve replacement. J Thorac Cardiovasc Surg 126:965, 2003.
315. Farivar RS, Cohn LS: Hypercholesterolemia is a risk factor for bioprosthetic valve calcification and explantation. J Thorac Cardiovasc Surg 126:969, 2003.
316. Westaby S, Jin XY, Katsumata T, Arifi A: Valve replacement with a stentless bioprosthesis: Versatility of the porcine aortic root. J Thorac Cardiovasc Surg 116:477, 1998.
317. Hvass U, Palatianos GM, Frassani R, et al: Multicenter study of stentless valve replacement in the small aortic root. J Thorac Cardiovasc Surg 117:267, 1999.
318. Yun KL, Sintek CF, Fletcher AD, et al: Aortic valve replacement with the Freestyle stentless prosthesis: Five year experience. Circulation 100:II-17,1999.
319. Dellgren G, Feindel CM, Bos J, et al: Aortic valve replacement with the Toronto SPV: Long-term clinical and hemodynamic results. Eur J Cardiothorac Surg 21:698, 2002.
320. Dossche K, Vanerman H, Daernen W, et al: Edwards stentless aortic valve xenograft: Early results of a multicenter clinical trial. Thorac Cardiovasc Surgeon 44:11, 1996.
321. Walther T, Falk V, Langebartels G, et al: Prospective randomized evaluation of stentless versus conventional biological aortic valves: Impact on early regression of left ventricular hypertrophy. Circulation 100:II-6, 1999.
322: Collinson J, Henein M, Flather M, et al: Valve replacement for aortic stenosis in patients with poor left ventricular function: Comparison of early changes with stented and stentless valves. Circulation 100:II-1, 1999.
323. Pibarot P, Dumesnil JG, Jobin J et al: Hemodynamic and physical performance during maximal exercise in patients with an aortic bioprosthetic valve: Comparison of stentless versus unstented bioprostheses. J Am Coll Cardiol 34:1609, 1999.
324. Le Tourneau T, Savoye C, McFadden EP, et al : Mid-term comparative follow-up after aortic valve replacement with Carpentier-Edwards and Pericarbon pericardial prostheses. Circulation 100:II-11, 1999.
325. Banbury MK, Cosgrove DM, Thomas JD, et al: Hemodynamic stability during 17 years of the Carpentier-Edwards aortic pericardial bioprosthesis. Ann Thorac Surg 73:1460, 2002.
326. Banbury MK, Cosgrove DM, White JA, et al: Age and valve size effect on the long-term durability of the Carpentier-Edwards aortic pericardial bioprosthesis. Ann Thorac Surg 72:753, 2001.
327. Aupart MR, Neville PH, Hammami S, et al: Carpentier-Edwards pericardial valves in the mitral position: Ten-year follow-up. J Thorac Cardiovasc Surg 113:492, 1997.
328. Eriksson MA, Kallner G, Rosfors S, et al: Hemodynamic performance of cryopreserved aortic homograft valves during midterm follow-up. J Am Coll Cardiol 32:1002, 1998.
329. Lund O, Chandrasekaran V, Grocott-Mason R, et al: Primary aortic valve replacement with allografts over twenty-five years: Valve-related and procedure-related determinants of outcome. J Thorac Cardiovasc Surg 117:77, 1999.
330. Willems TP, Takkenberg JJM, Sterberg WE, et al: Human tissue valves in the aortic position: Determinants of reoperation and valve regurgitation. Circulation 103:1515, 2001.
331. Palka P, Harrocks S, Lange A, et al: Primary aortic valve replacement with cryopreserved aortic allograft: An echocardiographic follow-up study of 570 patients. Circulation 105:61, 2002.
332. Frater RWM, Furlong P, Cosgrove CM, et al: Long-term durability and patient functional status of the Carpentier-Edwards Perimount Pericardial Bioprosthesis in the aortic position. J Heart Valve Dis 7:48, 1998.
333. Chambers JC, Somerville J, Stone S, Ross DN: Pulmonary autograft procedure for aortic valve disease: Long-term results of the pioneer series. Circulation 96:2206, 1997.
334. Santini F, Dyke C, Edwards S, et al: Pulmonary autograft versus homograft replacement of the aortic valve: A prospective randomized trial. J Thorac Cardiovasc Surg 113:894, 1997.

335. Elkins RC, Knott-Craig CJ, Ward KE, Lane MM: The Ross operation in children: 10-year experience. Ann Thorac Surg 65:496, 1998.
336. Carr-White GS, Kilner PJ, Hon JK, et al: Incidence, location, pathology, and significance of pulmonary homograft stenosis after the Ross operation. Circulation 104:I-16, 2001.
337. Laforest I, Dumesnil JG, Briand M, et al: Hemodynamic performance at rest and during exercise after aortic replacement: Comparison of pulmonary autografts versus aortic homografts. Circulation 106:I-57, 2002.
338. Carr-White GS, Afoke A, Birks EJ, et al: Aortic root characteristics of human pulmonary autografts. Circulation 102:III-15, 2000.
339. Luciani GB, Casali G, Favaro A, et al: Fate of the aortic root late after Ross operation. Circulation 108:II-61, 2003.
340. Schmidtke C, Bechtel JF, Noetzold A, et al: Up to seven years of experience with the Ross procedure in patients >60 years of age. J Am Coll Cardiol 36:117, 2000.
341. Rahimtoola SH: Valve prosthesis-patient mismatch: An update. J Heart Valve Dis 7:207, 1998.
342. Yun KL, Jamieson WR, Vurr LH, et al. Prosthesis-patient mismatch: Hemodynamic comparison of stented and stentless valves. Semin Thorac Cardiovasc Surg 11:98, 1999.
343. Rao V, Jamieson WR, Ivanov J, et al: Prosthesis-patient mismatch affects survival after aortic valve replacement. Circulation 102(Suppl III):III-5, 2000.
344. Blackstone EH, Cosgrove DM, Jamieson WR, et al: Prosthesis size and long-term survival after aortic valve replacement. J Thorac Cardiovasc Surg 126:783, 2003.
344a. Blais C, Dumensil JG, Baillot R, et al: Impact of valve prosthesis-patient mismatch on short-term mortality after aortic value replacement. Circulation 108:983, 2003.
344b. Pibarot P, Dumensil JG: Hemodynamic and clinical impact of prosthesis-patient mismatch in the aortic position and its prevention. J Am Coll Cardiol 36:1131, 2000.
345. Oxenham H, Bloomfield P, Wheatley DJ, et al: Twenty-year comparison of a Björk-Shiley mechanical heart valve with porcine bioprostheses. Heart 89:715, 2003.
346. Peterseim DS, Cen YY, Cheruvu S, et al: Long-term outcome after biologic versus mechanical aortic valve replacement in 841 patients. J Thorac Cardiovasc Surg 117:890, 1999.
347. Cohen G, David TE, Ivanov J, et al: The impact of age, coronary artery disease, and cardiac comorbidity on late survival after bioprosthetic aortic valve replacement. J Thorac Cardiovasc Surg 117:273, 1999.
348. Hung L, Rahimtoola SH: Prosthetic heart valves and pregnancy. Circulation 107:1240, 2003.
349. Vitale N, De Feo M, De Santo LS, et al: Dose-dependent fetal complications of warfarin in pregnant women with mechanical heart valves. J Am Coll Cardiol 33:1637, 1999.
350. Elkayam U: Pregnancy through a prosthetic heart valve. J Am Coll Cardiol 33:1642, 1999.
351. Hirsh J, Fuster V, Ansell J, et al: American Heart Association/American College of Cardiology Foundation guide to warfarin therapy. Circulation 107:1692, 2003.
352. Lucke JC, Samy RN, Atkins BZ, et al: Results of valve replacement with mechanical valves and biological prostheses in chronic renal dialysis patients. Ann Thorac Surg 64:129, 1997.
353. Herzog CA, Ma JZ, Collins AJ: Long-term survival of dialysis patients in the United States with prosthetic heart valves: Should ACC/AHA practice guidelines on valve selection be modified? Circulation105:1336, 2002.

GUIDELINES *Thomas H. Lee*

Management of Valvular Heart Disease

The American College of Cardiology and the American Heart Association (ACC/AHA) published guidelines for management of patients with valvular heart disease in 1998.[1] Other recommendations for these conditions were included in ACC/AHA guidelines for use of echocardiography,[2] ACC guidelines for assessment of athletes with cardiovascular abnormalities,[3] and AHA guidelines on cardiovascular assessment of master athletes.[4] As is the case for other ACC/AHA guidelines, the indications for various tests and procedures are divided into the following classes.

Class I: conditions for which there is evidence and/or general agreement that a given procedure or treatment is useful and effective

Class II: conditions for which there is conflicting evidence and/or a divergence of opinion about the usefulness/efficacy of a procedure or treatment

- Class IIa: weight of evidence/opinion is in favor of usefulness/efficacy
- Class IIb: usefulness/efficacy is less well established by evidence/opinion

Class III: conditions for which there is evidence and/or general agreement that the procedure/treatment is not useful/effective, and in some cases may be harmful

Some material from these guidelines is presented elsewhere in this book. Guidelines for prevention and treatment of infective endocarditis are summarized in the appendix to Chapter 58. Guidelines for management of anticoagulation in pregnancy are included in the appendix to Chapter 74.

The guidelines emphasize that the clinical assessment should be based on the patient's symptomatic status and findings from the physical examination. The chest radiograph and electrocardiogram (ECG), if normal, can often provide reassurance that a murmur is clinically insignificant. Echocardiography should be considered after assessment of these more routine data, and the guidelines consider echocardiography to be inappropriate (Class III) for evaluation of murmurs that experienced observers consider innocent or functional. In contrast, echocardiography was considered appropriate even in asymptomatic patients with murmurs suggesting significant valvular disease or with other signs or symptoms of cardiovascular disease (Table 57G–1).

TABLE 57G–1 ACC/AHA Guidelines for Echocardiography of Valvular Heart Disease in Adults

Indication	Class I	Class IIa	Class IIb	Class III
Echocardiography in asymptomatic patients with cardiac murmurs	1. Diastolic or continuous murmurs 2. Holosystolic or late systolic murmurs 3. Grade 3 or greater midsystolic murmurs	1. Murmurs associated with abnormal physical findings on cardiac palpation or auscultation 2. Murmurs associated with an abnormal ECG or chest radiograph		1. Grade 2 or softer midsystolic murmur identified as innocent or functional by an experienced observer 2. To detect "silent" aortic regurgitation or mitral regurgitation in patients without cardiac murmurs, then recommend endocarditis prophylaxis
Echocardiography in symptomatic patients with cardiac murmurs	1. Symptoms or signs of congestive heart failure, myocardial ischemia, or syncope 2. Symptoms or signs consistent with infective endocarditis or thromboembolism	Symptoms or signs likely due to noncardiac disease with cardiac disease not excluded by standard cardiovascular evaluation		Symptoms or signs of noncardiac disease with an isolated midsystolic "innocent" murmur

ACC = American College of Cardiology; AHA = American Heart Association; ECG = electrocardiogram.

Transthoracic echocardiography is endorsed in the ACC/AHA guidelines as the first-line test for diagnosis and follow-up of patients with mitral stenosis; transesophageal echocardiography was considered to have a potential role (Class IIa) for detection of left atrial thrombus in patients being considered for percutaneous mitral balloon valvotomy or cardioversion (Table 57G–2).

Anticoagulation was recommended for patients with mitral stenosis if they had a history of atrial fibrillation or a prior embolic event, but the guidelines were not strongly supportive of anticoagulation on the basis of left atrial dimension greater than 55 mm alone. Surgical therapy with valvotomy, valve repair, or valve replacement is indicated for patients with moderate or severe mitral stenosis (valve area < 1.5 cm²) and New York Heart Association (NYHA) functional Class III or IV, with the choice of the procedure dictated by the anatomy. Balloon valvotomy was also endorsed for patients who were NYHA Class II. For patients with mild or no symptoms of mitral stenosis, balloon valvotomy was considered reasonably appropriate (Class IIa) in the presence of pulmonary hypertension in the absence of left atrial thrombus or moderate to severe mitral regurgitation.

TABLE 57G–2 ACC/AHA Guidelines for Management of Patients with Mitral Stenosis

Indication	Class I	Class IIa	Class IIb	Class III
Echocardiography in mitral stenosis	1. Diagnosis of MS, assessment of hemodynamic severity (mean gradient, mitral valve area, pulmonary artery pressure), and assessment of right ventricular size and function 2. Assessment of valve morphology to determine suitability for percutaneous mitral balloon valvotomy 3. Diagnosis and assessment of concomitant valvular lesions 4. Reevaluation of patients with known MS with changing symptoms or signs	1. Assessment of hemodynamic response of mean gradient and pulmonary artery pressures by exercise Doppler echocardiography in patients when there is a discrepancy between resting hemodynamics and clinical findings	1. Reevaluation of asymptomatic patients with moderate to severe MS to assess pulmonary artery pressure	1. Routine reevaluation of the asymptomatic patient with mild MS and stable clinical findings
Transesophageal echocardiography in mitral stenosis		1. Assess for presence or absence of left atrial thrombus in patients being considered for percutaneous mitral balloon valvotomy or cardioversion 2. Evaluate mitral valve morphology and hemodynamics when transthoracic echocardiography provides suboptimal data		1. Routine evaluation of mitral valve morphology and hemodynamics when complete transthoracic echocardiographic data are satisfactory
Anticoagulation in mitral stenosis	1. Patients with atrial fibrillation, paroxysmal or chronic 2. Patients with a prior embolic event		1. Patients with severe MS and left atrial dimension ≥ 55 mm by echocardiography	All other patients with MS
Cardiac catheterization in mitral stenosis	Perform percutaneous mitral balloon valvotomy in properly selected patients	1. Assess severity of MR in patients being considered for percutaneous mitral balloon valvotomy when clinical and echocardiographic data are discordant 2. Assess pulmonary artery, left atrial, and left ventricular diastolic pressure when symptoms and/or estimated pulmonary artery pressure are discordant with the severity of MS by 2D and Doppler echocardiography 3. Assess hemodynamic response of pulmonary artery and left atrial pressures to stress when		1. Assess mitral valve hemodynamics when 2D and Doppler echocardiographic data are concordant with clinical findings

TABLE 57G–2 ACC/AHA Guidelines for Management of Patients with Mitral Stenosis—cont'd

Indication	Class I	Class IIa	Class IIb	Class III
		clinical symptoms and resting hemodynamics are discordant		
Percutaneous mitral balloon valvotomy	1. Symptomatic patients (NYHA Classes II–IV), moderate or severe MS (mitral valve area ≤ 1.5 cm²) and valve morphology favorable for percutaneous balloon valvotomy in the absence of left atrial thrombus or moderate to severe MR	1. Asymptomatic patients with moderate or severe MS (mitral valve area < 21.5 cm²) and valve morphology favorable for percutaneous balloon valvotomy who have pulmonary hypertension (pulmonary artery systolic pressure > 50 mm Hg at rest or 60 mm Hg with exercise) in the absence of left atrial thrombus or moderate to severe MR 2. Patients with NYHA Class III or IV symptoms, moderate or severe MS (mitral valve area < 1.5 cm²), and a nonpliable calcified valve who are at high risk for surgery in the absence of left atrial thrombus or moderate to severe MR	1. Asymptomatic patients, moderate or severe MS (mitral valve area < 21.5 cm²) and valve morphology favorable for percutaneous balloon valvotomy who have new onset of atrial fibrillation in the absence of left atrial thrombus or moderate to severe MR 2. Patients in NYHA Class III or IV, moderate or severe MS (mitral valve area ≤ 1.5 cm²), and a nonpliable calcified valve who are low-risk candidates for surgery	Patients with mild MS
Mitral valve repair for MS	1. Patients with NYHA Class III or IV symptoms, moderate or severe MS (mitral valve area ≤ 1.5 cm²), and valve morphology favorable for repair if percutaneous mitral balloon valvotomy is not available 2. Patients with NYHA Class III or IV symptoms, moderate or severe MS (mitral valve area ≤ 1.5 cm²), and valve morphology favorable for repair if a left atrial thrombus is present despite anticoagulation 3. Patients with NYHA Class III or IV symptoms, moderate or severe MS (mitral valve area ≤ 1.5 cm²), and a nonpliable or calcified valve with the decision to proceed with either repair or replacement made at the time of the operation		1. Patients in NYHA Class I, moderate or severe MS (mitral valve area ≤ 1.5 cm²), and valve morphology favorable for repair who have had recurrent episodes of embolic events on adequate anticoagulation	1. Patients with NYHA Classes I–IV symptoms and mild MS
Mitral valve replacement for mitral stenosis	1. Patients with moderate or severe MS (mitral valve area ≤ 1.5 cm²) and NYHA Class III or IV symptoms who are not considered candidates for percutaneous balloon valvotomy or mitral valve repair	1. Patients with severe MS (mitral valve area ≤ 1 cm²) and severe pulmonary hypertension (pulmonary artery systolic pressure > 60–80 mm Hg) with NYHA Class I or II symptoms who are not considered candidates for percutaneous balloon valvotomy or mitral valve repair		

ACC = American College of Cardiology; AHA = American Heart Association; MS = mitral stenosis; 2D = two-dimensional; NYHA = New York Association; MR = mitral regurgitation.

The ACC/AHA guidelines consider echocardiography appropriate for diagnosis of acute or chronic mitral regurgitation, as well as annual or semiannual surveillance of left ventricular function in patients with severe mitral regurgitation even if asymptomatic (Table 57G–3). Serial use of chest radiographs and ECGs are considered to be of less value. In asymptomatic patients with mild mitral regurgitation and no evidence of left ventricular dysfunction, the guidelines recommend yearly evaluations to detect worsening symptomatic status but do not support annual echocardiography. Transesophageal echocardiography is considered most appropriate for intraoperative guidance and when transthoracic studies are inadequate.

Cardiac catheterization is usually performed as a prelude to surgery in patients with mitral regurgitation. Coronary angiography is not considered routinely necessary in the ACC/AHA guidelines in patients younger than 35 years of age if there is no clinical suspicion of coronary artery disease. Left ventriculography and hemodynamic assessment are appropriate only when noninvasive studies do not provide adequate information to guide management.

TABLE 57G–3 ACC/AHA Guidelines for Management of Patients with Mitral Regurgitation

Indication	Class I	Class IIa	Class IIb	Class III
Transthoracic echocardiography in mitral regurgitation	1. For baseline evaluation to quantify severity of MR and LV function in any patient suspected of having MR 2. For delineation of mechanism of MR 3. For annual or semiannual surveillance of LV function (estimated by ejection fraction and end-systolic dimension) in asymptomatic severe MR 4. To establish cardiac status after a change in symptoms 5. For evaluation after MVR or mitral valve repair to establish baseline status			1. Routine follow-up evaluation of mild MR with normal LV size and systolic function
Transesophageal echocardiography in mitral regurgitation	1. Intraoperative transesophageal echocardiography to establish anatomical basis for MR and to guide repair 2. For evaluation of MR patients in whom transthoracic echocardiography provides nondiagnostic images regarding severity of MR, mechanism of MR, and/or status of LV function			1. In routine follow-up or surveillance of patients with native valve MR
Coronary angiography in mitral regurgitation	1. When mitral valve surgery is contemplated in patients with angina or previous myocardial infarction 2. When mitral valve surgery is contemplated in patients with ≥1 risk factor for CAD 3. When ischemia is suspected as an etiological factor in MR		1. To confirm noninvasive tests in patients not suspected of having CAD	1. When mitral valve surgery is contemplated in patients aged <35 years and there is no clinical suspicion of CAD
Left ventriculography and hemodynamic measurements in mitral regurgitation	1. When noninvasive tests are inconclusive regarding severity of MR, LV function, or the need for surgery 2. When there is a discrepancy between clinical and noninvasive findings regarding severity of MR			1. In patients in whom valve surgery is not contemplated

TABLE 57G–3 ACC/AHA Guidelines for Management of Patients with Mitral Regurgitation—cont'd

Indication	Class I	Class IIa	Class IIb	Class III
Mitral valve surgery in nonischemic severe mitral regurgitation	1. Acute symptomatic MR in which repair is likely 2. Patients with NYHA Class II, III, or IV symptoms with normal LV function defined as ejection fraction > 0.60 and end-systolic dimension < 45 mm 3. Symptomatic or asymptomatic patients with mild LV dysfunction, ejection fraction 0.50–0.60, and end-systolic dimension 45–50 mm 4. Symptomatic or asymptomatic patients with moderate LV dysfunction, ejection fraction 0.30–0.50, and/or end-systolic dimension 50–55 mm	1. Asymptomatic patients with preserved LV function and atrial fibrillation 2. Asymptomatic patients with preserved LV function and pulmonary hypertension (pulmonary artery systolic pressure > 50 mm Hg at rest or > 60 mm Hg with exercise) 3. Asymptomatic patients with ejection fraction 0.50–0.60 and end-systolic dimension < 45 mm and asymptomatic patients with ejection fraction > 0.60 and end-systolic dimension 45–55 mm 4. Patients with severe LV dysfunction (ejection fraction < 0.30 and/or end-systolic dimension > 55 mm) in whom chordal preservation is highly likely	1. Asymptomatic patients with chronic MR with preserved LV function in whom mitral valve repair is highly likely 2. Patients with mitral valve prolapse and preserved LV function who have recurrent ventricular arrhythmias despite medical therapy	1. Asymptomatic patients with preserved LV function in whom significant doubt about the feasibility of repair exists

ACC = American College of Cardiology; AHA = American Heart Association; MR = mitral regurgitation; LV = left ventricular; MVR = mitral valve replacement; CAD = coronary artery disease; NYHA = New York Heart Association.

Surgery is considered appropriate for acute symptomatic mitral regurgitation and for patients with chronic severe mitral regurgitation and symptoms of congestive heart failure, even if they have normal left ventricular function. Even if patients are asymptomatic, surgery is appropriate when patients have mild or worse left ventricular dysfunction (ejection fraction 0.50 to 0.60 and/or end-systolic dimension 50 to 55 mm).

Mitral Valve Prolapse

Recommendations on use of echocardiography for patients with mitral valve prolapse were presented in ACC/AHA guidelines on echocardiography (Table 57G–4).[2] These guidelines emphasize that the diagnosis of mitral valve prolapse should be made by physical examination; echocardiography should be used primarily for evaluation of mitral regurgitation and ventricular compensation. Echocardiography is also considered appropriate for *excluding* the diagnosis of mitral valve prolapse in patients who have been given the diagnosis inappropriately. Serial use of echocardiography in stable patients with mild or no regurgitation is discouraged.

In general, asymptomatic athletes with mitral valve prolapse need not have any restrictions, but 2001 AHA guidelines recommended restriction of patients to low-intensity competitive sports (such as golf and bowling) if any of the following are present: (1) history of syncope, judged probably arrhythmogenic in origin; (2) family history of sudden death due to mitral valve prolapse; (3) repetitive supraventricular or complex ventricular tachyarrhythmias, particularly if exacerbated by exercise; (4) moderate to severe mitral regurgitation; and (5) prior embolic event.[4]

Antibiotic prophylaxis is considered appropriate for patients with the characteristic click-murmur complex or with echocardiographic evidence of mitral prolapse with regurgitation. Daily aspirin therapy is recommended for patients who have had cerebral transient ischemic attacks and for patients younger than 65 years of age who have atrial fibrillation without other complicating factors. Warfarin therapy is recommended for poststroke patients and older patients with atrial fibrillation accompanied by hypertension, mitral regurgitation, or a history of heart failure.

Aortic Stenosis

Doppler echocardiography is a highly appropriate test for diagnosis and assessment of aortic stenosis and for evaluation of left ventricular function in patients with this condition. The guidelines commented that yearly echocardiograms may be helpful for management of asymptomatic patients with severe aortic stenosis, but recommended intervals of 2 and 5 years for asymptomatic patients with moderate and mild aortic stenosis, respectively.

The ACC/AHA guidelines indicated that exercise testing of asymptomatic patients could be performed safely and provide useful information but emphasized the need for supervision by an experienced physician with close monitoring of blood pressure and the ECG. The Task Force on Acquired Valvular Heart Disease of the 26th Bethesda Conference recommended that competitive athletes with severe aortic stenosis be advised to limit activity to relatively low levels.[3]

The guidelines discourage catheterization solely for the purposes of confirming information available from noninvasive tests (Table 57G–5). Coronary angiography is considered appropriate in the ACC/AHA guidelines for patients with possible coronary artery disease and may be needed to assess the severity of stenosis in symptomatic patients when other data are not conclusive.

TABLE 57G–4 ACC/AHA Guidelines for Management of Patients with Mitral Valve Prolapse

Indication	Class I	Class IIa	Class IIb	Class III
Echocardiography in MVP	1. Diagnosis, assessment of hemodynamic severity of MR, leaflet morphology, and ventricular compensation in patients with physical signs of MVP 2. To exclude MVP in patients who have been given the diagnosis when there is no clinical evidence to support the diagnosis	1. To exclude MVP in patients with first-degree relatives with known myxomatous valve disease 2. Risk stratification in patients with physical signs of MVP or known MVP		1. To exclude MVP in patients in the absence of physical findings suggestive of MVP or a positive family history 2. Routine repetition of echocardiography in patients with MVP with mild or no regurgitation and no changes in clinical signs or symptoms
Antibiotic endocarditis prophylaxis for patients with MVP undergoing procedures associated with bacteremia	1. Patients with characteristic systolic click-murmur complex 2. Patients with isolated systolic click and echocardiographic evidence of MVP and MR	1. Patients with isolated systolic click, echocardiographic evidence of high-risk MVP		1. Patients with isolated systolic click and equivocal or no evidence of MVP
Aspirin and oral anticoagulants in MVP	1. Aspirin therapy for cerebral transient ischemic attacks 2. Warfarin therapy for patients aged ≥ 65 years, in atrial fibrillation with hypertension, MR murmur, or history of heart failure 3. Aspirin therapy for patients aged < 65 years in atrial fibrillation with no history of MR, hypertension, or heart failure 4. Warfarin therapy for poststroke patients	1. Warfarin therapy for transient ischemic attacks despite aspirin therapy 2. Aspirin therapy for poststroke patients with contraindications to anticoagulants	1. Aspirin therapy for patients in sinus rhythm with echocardiographic evidence of high-risk MVP	

ACC = American College of Cardiology; AHA = American Heart Association; MVP = mitral valve prolapse; MR = mitral regurgitation.

Aortic valve replacement is considered indicated in virtually all symptomatic patients with severe aortic stenosis, and the ACC/AHA guidelines were generally supportive (Class IIa) of this procedure for patients who were asymptomatic despite severe aortic stenosis but had evidence of left ventricular systolic dysfunction or exertional hypotension. However, valve replacement for asymptomatic patients was otherwise discouraged. Aortic balloon valvotomy was given qualified support only as a "bridge" to surgery in hemodynamically unstable patients who could not undergo immediate aortic valve replacement.

Aortic Regurgitation

Doppler echocardiography is a highly appropriate test for diagnosis and serial assessment of patients with aortic regurgitation (Table 57G–6). For new patients in whom the chronic nature of the lesion is uncertain, the guidelines support repeating the physical examination and echocardiogram 2 to 3 months after the initial evaluation to ensure that rapid progression is not underway. Asymptomatic patients with mild aortic regurgitation, normal left ventricular function, and little or no left ventricular dilation can be seen on an annual basis, and echocardiography can be performed every 2 to 3 years in the absence of changes in symptoms. However, the guidelines support echocardiography every 6 to 12 months for patients with severe aortic regurgitation and significant left ventricular dilation, such as end-diastolic dimension greater than 60 mm. For patients with even more advanced left ventricular dilation, echocardiography as often as every 4 to 6 months is endorsed.

Exercise testing is considered appropriate for assessment of functional capacity in patients in whom the history is not definitive, but the impact of this test on management was not otherwise strongly supported by the ACC/AHA guidelines. Radionuclide angiography was endorsed as an alternative to echocardiography for assessment of left ventricular volume and function. However, the ACC/AHA guidelines emphasized that there is no need for serial testing with both technologies. The guidelines also note that exercise ejection fraction has not been shown to have incremental value in the management of patients.

The ACC/AHA guidelines considered vasodilator therapy appropriate in patients with hypertension or left ventricular dysfunction, even if the patients were asymptomatic. However, the guidelines do not endorse vasodilator therapy in normotensive patients with normal left ventricular function and mild aortic regurgitation. The guidelines emphasize that vasodilator therapy is not an alternative to surgery for patients who are appropriate candidates for valve replacement.

TABLE 57G–5 ACC/AHA Guidelines for Management of Patients with Aortic Valve Stenosis

Indication	Class I	Class IIa	Class IIb	Class III
Echocardiography in aortic stenosis	1. Diagnosis and assessment of severity of aortic stenosis 2. Assessment of LV size, function, and/or hemodynamics 3. Reevaluation of patients with known aortic stenosis with changing symptoms or signs 4. Assessment of changes in hemodynamic severity and ventricular compensation in patients with known aortic stenosis during pregnancy 5. Reevaluation of asymptomatic patients with severe aortic stenosis	1. Reevaluation of asymptomatic patients with mild to moderate aortic stenosis and evidence of LV dysfunction or hypertrophy		1. Routine reevaluation of asymptomatic adult patients with mild aortic stenosis having stable physical signs and normal LV size and function
Cardiac catheterization in aortic stenosis	1. Coronary angiography before aortic valve replacement in patients at risk for coronary artery disease 2. Assessment of severity of aortic stenosis in symptomatic patients when aortic valve replacement is planned or when noninvasive tests are inconclusive or there is a discrepancy with clinical findings regarding severity of aortic stenosis or need for surgery		1. Assessment of severity of aortic stenosis before aortic valve replacement when noninvasive tests are adequate and concordant with clinical findings and coronary angiography is not needed	1. Assessment of LV function and severity of aortic stenosis in asymptomatic patients when noninvasive tests are adequate
Aortic valve replacement in aortic stenosis	1. Symptomatic patients with severe aortic stenosis 2. Patients with severe aortic stenosis undergoing coronary artery bypass surgery 3. Patients with severe aortic stenosis undergoing surgery on the aorta or other heart valves	1. Patients with moderate aortic stenosis undergoing coronary artery bypass surgery or surgery on the aorta or other heart valves 2. Asymptomatic patients with severe aortic stenosis and • Left ventricular systolic dysfunction, or • Abnormal response to exercise (e.g., hypotension)	1. Asymptomatic patients with severe aortic stenosis and • Ventricular tachycardia, or • Marked or excessive LV hypertrophy, or • Valve area < 0.6 cm^2	1. Prevention of sudden death in asymptomatic patients with none of the findings listed in NYHA Class II
Aortic balloon valvotomy in adults with aortic stenosis		1. A "bridge" to surgery in hemodynamically unstable patients who are at high risk for aortic valve replacement	1. Palliation in patients with serious comorbid conditions 2. Patients who require urgent noncardiac surgery	1. An alternative to aortic valve replacement

ACC = American College of Cardiology; AHA = American Heart Association; MVP = mitral valve prolapse; LV = left ventricular; NYHA = New York Heart Association.

Cardiac catheterization is not routinely needed to confirm the diagnosis or assess the severity of aortic regurgitation when echocardiographic studies are adequate. The most common appropriate indication for cardiac catheterization is the performance of coronary angiography as a prelude to surgery. Aortic valve replacement is considered clearly appropriate in patients with severe (NYHA Class III or IV) symptoms, progressive left ventricular dilation, mild-to-moderate left ventricular dysfunction, or declining exercise tolerance. The guidelines were not supportive of surgery solely because of a decline in ejection fraction during exercise.

TABLE 57G–6 ACC/AHA Guidelines for Management of Patients with Aortic Regurgitation

Indication	Class I	Class IIa	Class IIb	Class III
Echocardiography in aortic regurgitation	1. Confirm presence and severity of acute aortic regurgitation 2. Diagnosis of chronic aortic regurgitation in patients with equivocal physical findings 3. Assessment of etiology of regurgitation (including valve morphology and aortic root size and morphology) 4. Assessment of LV hypertrophy, dimension (or volume), and systolic function 5. Semiquantitative estimate of severity of aortic regurgitation 6. Reevaluation of patients with mild, moderate or severe regurgitation with new or changing symptoms 7. Reevaluation of LV size and function in asymptomatic patients with severe regurgitation 8. Reevaluation of asymptomatic patients with mild, moderate, or severe regurgitation and enlarged aortic root			1. Yearly reevaluation of asymptomatic patients with mild to moderate regurgitation with stable physical signs and normal or near-normal LV chamber size
Exercise testing in chronic aortic regurgitation	1. Assessment of functional capacity and symptomatic responses in patients with a history of equivocal symptoms	1. Evaluation of symptoms and functional capacity before participation in athletic activities 2. Prognostic assessment before aortic valve replacement in patients with LV dysfunction	1. Exercise hemodynamic measurements to determine the effect of aortic regurgitation on LV function 2. Exercise radionuclide angiography for assessing LV function in asymptomatic or symptomatic patients	1. Exercise echocardiography or dobutamine stress echocardiography for assessing LV function in asymptomatic or symptomatic patients
Radionuclide angiography in aortic regurgitation	1. Initial and serial assessment of LV volume and function at rest in patients with suboptimal echocardiograms or equivocal echocardiographic data 2. Serial assessment of LV volume and function at rest when serial echocardiograms are not used 3. Assessment of LV volume and function in asymptomatic patients with moderate to severe regurgitation when echocardiographic evidence of declining LV function is suggestive but not definitive 4. Confirmation of subnormal LV ejection fraction before recommending surgery in an asymptomatic patient with borderline echocardiographic evidence of LV dysfunction 5. Assessment of LV volume and function in patients with moderate to severe regurgitation when clinical assessment and echocardiographic data are discordant		1. Routine assessment of exercise ejection fraction 2. Quantification of AR in patients with unsatisfactory echocardiograms	1. Quantification of AR in patients with satisfactory echocardiograms 2. Initial and serial assessment of LV volume and function at rest in addition to echocardiography
Vasodilator therapy for chronic aortic regurgitation	1. Chronic therapy in patients with severe regurgitation who have symptoms and/or LV dysfunction when surgery is not recommended because of additional cardiac or noncardiac factors			1. Long-term therapy in asymptomatic patients with mild to moderate AR and normal LV systolic function 2. Long-term therapy in

TABLE 57G–6 ACC/AHA Guidelines for Management of Patients with Aortic Regurgitation—cont'd

Indication	Class I	Class IIa	Class IIb	Class III
	2. Long-term therapy in asymptomatic patients with severe regurgitation who have LV dilation but normal systolic function 3. Long-term therapy in asymptomatic patients with hypertension and any degree of regurgitation 4. Long-term ACE inhibitor therapy in patients with persistent LV systolic dysfunction after AVR 5. Short-term therapy to improve the hemodynamic profile of patients with severe heart failure symptoms and severe LV dysfunction before proceeding with AVR			asymptomatic patients with LV systolic dysfunction who are otherwise candidates for valve replacement 3. Long-term therapy in symptomatic patients with either normal LV function or mild to moderate LV systolic dysfunction who are otherwise candidates for valve replacement
Cardiac catheterization in chronic aortic regurgitation	1. Coronary angiography before AVR in patients at risk for CAD 2. Assessing severity of regurgitation when noninvasive tests are inconclusive or discordant with clinical findings regarding severity of regurgitation or need for surgery 3. Assessing LV function when noninvasive tests are inconclusive or discordant with clinical findings regarding LV dysfunction and need for surgery in patients with severe AR		1. Assessment of LV function and severity of regurgitation before AVR when noninvasive tests are adequate and concordant with clinical findings and coronary angiography is not needed	1. Assessment of LV function and severity of regurgitation in asymptomatic patients when noninvasive tests are adequate
Aortic valve replacement in chronic severe aortic regurgitation	1. Patients with NYHA Class III or IV symptoms and preserved LV systolic function, defined as normal ejection fraction at rest (ejection fraction ≥ 0.50) 2. Patients with NYHA Class II symptoms and preserved LV systolic function (ejection fraction ≥ 0.50 at rest) but with progressive LV dilation or declining ejection fraction at rest on serial studies or declining effort tolerance on exercise testing 3. Patients with Canadian Heart Association Class II or greater angina with or without CAD 4. Asymptomatic or symptomatic patients with mild to moderate LV dysfunction at rest (ejection fraction 0.25–0.49) 5. Patients undergoing coronary artery bypass surgery or surgery on the aorta or other heart valves	1. Patients with NYHA Class II symptoms and LV systolic function (ejection fraction ≥ 0.50 at rest) with stable LV size and systolic function on serial studies and stable exercise tolerance 2. Asymptomatic patients with normal LV systolic function (ejection fraction > 0.50) but with severe LV dilation (diastolic dimension > 75 mm or end-systolic dimension > 55 mm; consider lower threshold values for patients of small stature)	1. Patients with severe LV dysfunction (ejection fraction < 0.25) 2. Asymptomatic patients with normal systolic function at rest (ejection fraction > 0.50) and progressive LV dilation when the degree of dilation is moderately severe (end-diastolic dimension 70–75 mm, end-systolic dimension 50–55 mm) 3. Asymptomatic patients with normal systolic function at rest (ejection fraction > 0.50) but with decline in ejection fraction during exercise radionuclide angiography	1. Asymptomatic patients with normal systolic function at rest (ejection fraction > 0.50) but with decline in ejection fraction during stress echocardiography 2. Asymptomatic patients with normal systolic function at rest (ejection fraction > 0.50) and LV dilation when degree of dilation is not severe (end-diastolic dimension < 70 mm, end-systolic dimension < 50 mm)

ACC = American College of Cardiology; AHA = American Heart Association; LV = left ventricular; AR = aortic regurgitation; ACE = angiotensin-converting enzyme; AVR = aortic value replacement; CAD = coronary artery disease; NYHA = New York Heart Association.

Other Valvular Disease

Tricuspid valve annuloplasty is an appropriate procedure for patients with severe tricuspid regurgitation and pulmonary hypertension in patients who are undergoing surgery for mitral valve disease but not considered appropriate in patients without pulmonary artery systolic pressure of 60 mm Hg or more (Table 57G–7). The ACC/AHA guidelines otherwise offer no recommendations regarding treatment of multiple valve disease.

Anorectic Drugs

The ACC/AHA task force did not consider it possible to offer definitive diagnostic and treatment guidelines for patients who have

TABLE 57G–7 ACC/AHA Guidelines for Management of Patients with Other Valvular Heart Disease

Indication	Class I	Class IIa	Class IIb	Class III
Recommendations for surgery for tricuspid regurgitation	1. Annuloplasty for severe TR and pulmonary hypertension in patients with mitral valve disease requiring mitral valve surgery	1. Valve replacement for severe TR secondary to diseased/ abnormal tricuspid valve leaflets not amenable to annuloplasty or repair 2. Valve replacement or annuloplasty for severe TR with mean pulmonary artery pressure < 60 mm Hg when symptomatic	1. Annuloplasty for mild TR in patients with pulmonary hypertension secondary to mitral valve disease requiring mitral valve surgery	1. Valve replacement or annuloplasty for TR with pulmonary artery systolic pressure < 60 mm Hg in the presence of a normal mitral valve, in asymptomatic patients, or in symptomatic patients who have not received a trial of diuretic therapy
Patients who have used anorectic drugs (fenfluramine or dexfenfluramine or the combination of fenfluramine-phentermine or dexfenfluramine-phentermine)	1. Discontinuation of the anorectic drug(s) 2. Cardiac physical examination 3. Echocardiography in patients with symptoms, heart murmurs, or associated physical findings 4. Doppler echocardiography in patients for whom cardiac auscultation cannot be performed adequately because of body habitus	1. Repeat physical examination in 6–8 mo for those without murmurs	1. Echocardiography in all patients before dental procedures in the absence of symptoms, heart murmurs, or associated physical findings	1. Echocardiography in all patients without heart murmurs
Follow-up strategy of patients with prosthetic heart valves	1. History, physical examination ECG, chest radiograph echocardiogram, complete blood count, serum chemistries, and INR (if indicated) at first postoperative outpatient evaluation. (this evaluation should be performed 3–4 wk after hospital discharge) 2. Radionuclide angiography or magnetic resonance imaging to LV function if result of echocardiography is unsatisfactory 3. Routine follow-up visits at yearly intervals with earlier reevaluations for change in clinical status		1. Routine serial echocardiograms at time of annual follow-up visit in absence of change in clinical status	1. Routine serial fluoroscopy
Valve replacement with a mechanical prosthesis	1. Patients with expected long life spans 2. Patients with a mechanical prosthetic valve already in place in a different position than the valve to be replaced	1. Patients in renal failure, on hemodialysis, or with hypercalcemia (Class II rather than IIa) 2. Patients requiring warfarin therapy because of risk factors for thromboembolism 3. Patients ≤65 years for AVR and ≤70 years for MVR	1. Valve re-replacement for thrombosed biological valve	1. Patients who cannot or will not take warfarin therapy
Valve replacement with a bioprosthesis	1. Patients who cannot or will not take warfarin therapy 2. Patients ≥65 years needing AVR who do not have risk factors for thromboembolism	1. Patients considered to have possible compliance problems with warfarin therapy 2. Patients >70 years needing MVR who do not have risk factors for thromboembolism	1. Valve re-replacement for thrombosed mechanical valve 2. Patients <65 years	1. Patients in renal failure, on hemodialysis, or with hypercalcemia 2. Adolescent patients who are still growing

ACC = American College of Cardiology; AHA = American Heart Association; TR = tricuspid regurgitation; ECG = electrocardiogram; LV = left ventricular; AVR = aortic valve replacement; MVR = mitral valve replacement.

received anorectic drugs beyond recommending discontinuation of these agents and careful periodic examinations. The guidelines recommended echocardiography only in patients with cardiovascular symptoms, heart murmurs, or a body habitus that hindered an effective examination.

VALVULAR DISEASE IN YOUNG ADULTS

For adolescents and young adults with aortic stenosis, ACC/AHA guidelines recommend a lower threshold for exercise testing and cardiac catheterization to assess the risk of participation in athletics (Table 57G–8). In this population, balloon valvotomy is an effective and appropriate option. Since this procedure has little morbidity and mortality, the indications for intervention are more liberal in younger patients than in adults. The indications for management of chronic aortic regurgitation and mitral valve disease are similar to those for older adult patients. Pulmonic valvotomy is considered an appropriate intervention for patients who are symptomatic due to pulmonic stenosis and for asymptomatic patients with a peak valve gradient greater than 50 mm.

PATIENTS WITH PROSTHETIC HEART VALVES

The ACC/AHA guidelines recommend that the international normalized ratio (INR) be maintained between 2.0 and 3.0 for patients with bileaflet mechanical valves and Medtronic-Hall valves and between 2.5 and 3.5 for other disc valves and Starr-Edward valves (Table 57G–9). Aspirin therapy was considered appropriate for patients with aortic or mitral valve bioprostheses and no risk factors for thromboembolism.

The ACC/AHA guidelines indicate that admission to the hospital to give heparin before noncardiac surgery or dental care is usually unnecessary. They recommend that heparin be reserved for patients who have had a recent thrombosis or embolus, those with demonstrated thrombotic problems when previously off therapy, those with the Björk-Shiley valve, and those with three or more risk factors for thromboembolism.

After prosthetic valve implantation, asymptomatic patients need be seen only at 1-year intervals (see Table 57G–7). Routine serial echocardiograms were not strongly endorsed (Class IIb).

The ACC/AHA guidelines offer general recommendations to guide the selection of bioprosthetic versus mechanic valves. Bioprostheses are considered inappropriate in patients in renal failure, on hemodialysis, or with hypercalcemia or in adolescent patients who are still growing.

TABLE 57G–8 ACC/AHA Guidelines for Management of Valvular Heart Disease in Adolescents and Young Adults

Indication	Class I	Class IIa	Class IIb	Class III
Diagnostic evaluation of the adolescent or young adult with aortic stenosis*	1. ECG* 2. Echo-Doppler study	1. Graded exercise test† 2. Cardiac catheterization† for evaluation of gradient	1. Chest radiograph*	1. Coronary arteriography in the absence of history suggestive of concomitant CAD
Aortic balloon valvotomy in the adolescent or young adult (≤21 yr) with normal cardiac output	1. Symptoms of angina, syncope, and dyspnea on exertion, with catheterization peak gradient ≥ 50 mm Hg‡ 2. Catheterization peak gradient > 60 mm Hg 3. New-onset ischemic or repolarization changes on ECG at rest or with exercise (ST depression, T wave inversion over left precordium) with a gradient > 50 mm Hg)‡	1. Catheterization peak gradient > 50 mm Hg if patient wants to play competitive sports or desires to become pregnant		1. Catheterization gradient < 50 mm Hg without symptoms or ECG changes
Aortic valve surgery (replacement with mechanical valve, homograft, or pulmonary autograft) in the adolescent or young adult with chronic aortic regurgitation	1. Onset of symptoms 2. Asymptomatic patients with LV systolic dysfunction (ejection fraction < 0.50) on serial studies 1–3 months apart 3. Asymptomatic patients with progressive LV enlargement (end-diastolic dimension > 4 SD above normal)		1. Moderate AS (gradient >40 mm Hg) (peak-to-peak gradient at cardiac catheterization) 2. Onset of ischemic or repolarization abnormalities (ST depression, T wave inversion) over left precordium at rest	
Mitral valve surgery in the adolescent or young adult with congenital mitral regurgitation with severe MR	1. NYHA Class III or IV symptoms 2. Asymptomatic patients with LV systolic dysfunction (ejection fraction ≤ 0.60)	1. NYHA Class II symptoms with preserved LV systolic function if valve repair rather than replacement is likely	1. Asymptomatic patients with preserved LV systolic function in whom valve replacement is highly likely	

TABLE 57G–8 ACC/AHA Guidelines for Management of Valvular Heart Disease in Adolescents and Young Adults—cont'd

Indication	Class I	Class IIa	Class IIb	Class III
Mitral valve surgery in the adolescent or young adult with congenital mitral stenosis	1. Symptomatic patients (NYHA Class III or IV) and mean mitral valve gradient > 10 mm Hg on Doppler echocardiography	1. Mildly symptomatic patients (NYHA Class II) and mean mitral valve gradient > 10 mm Hg on Doppler echocardiographic study 2. Systolic pulmonary artery pressure 50 to 60 mm Hg with a mean mitral valve gradient ≥ 10 mm Hg	1. New-onset atrial fibrillation or multiple systemic emboli while receiving adequate anticoagulation	
Intervention in the adolescent or young adult with pulmonic stenosis (balloon valvotomy or surgery)	1. Patients with exertional dyspnea, angina, syncope, or presyncope 2. Asymptomatic patients with normal cardiac output (estimated clinically or determined by catheterization) and right ventricular to pulmonary artery peak gradient > 50 mm Hg	1. Asymptomatic patients with normal cardiac output (estimated clinically or determined by catheterization) and right ventricular to pulmonary artery peak gradient 40–49 mm Hg	1. Asymptomatic patients with normal cardiac output (estimated clinically or determined by catheterization) and right ventricular to pulmonary artery peak gradient 30–39 mm Hg	1. Asymptomatic patients with normal cardiac output (estimated clinically or determined by catheterization) and right ventricular to pulmonary artery peak gradient < 30 mm Hg

ACC = American College of Cardiology; AHA = American Heart Association; ECG = electrocardiogram; LV = left ventricular; CAD = coronary artery disease; AS = aortic stenosis; MR = mitral regurgitation; NYHA = New York Heart Association.

*Yearly if echo-Doppler gradient > 36 mm Hg (velocity ≥ 3 m/sec); every 2 years if echo-Doppler gradient < 36 mm Hg (peak velocity < 3 m/sec).

†If echo-Doppler gradient > 36 mm Hg (velocity > 3 m/sec) and patient interested in athletic participation or if clinical findings and echo-Doppler are disparate.

‡If gradient < 50 mm Hg, other causes of symptoms should be explored.

From Bonow RO, Carabello B, de Leon AC Jr, et al: ACC/AHA guidelines for the management of patients with valvular heart disease: Executive summary. A report of the American College of Cardiology/American Heart Association Task Force on Practice Guidelines (Committee on Management of Patients with Valvular Heart Disease). Circulation 98:1949-1984, 1998.

TABLE 57G–9 ACC/AHA Recommendations for Appropriate (Class I) Antithrombotic Therapy in Patients with Prosthetic Heart Valves

Indication	Medication	Target	Class
First 3 months after valve replacement	Warfarin	INR 2.5-3.5	I
≥3 months after valve replacement			
Mechanical valve			
AVR and no risk factor*			
Bileaflet valve or Medtronic Hall valve	Warfarin	INR 2-3	I
Other disk valves or Starr-Edwards valve	Warfarin	INR 2.5-3.5	I
AVR plus risk factor*	Warfarin	INR 2.5-3.5	I
MVR	Warfarin	INR 2.5-3.5	I
Bioprosthesis			
AVR and no risk factor*	Aspirin	80-100 mg/day	I
AVR and risk factor*	Warfarin	INR 2-3	I
MVR and no risk factor*	Aspirin	80-100 mg/day	I
MVR and risk factor*	Warfarin	INR 2.5-3.5	I

ACC = American College of Cardiology; AHA = American Heart Association; AVR = atrial valve replacement; MVR = mitral valve replacement; INR = international normalized ratio.

*Risk factors: atrial fibrillation, LV dysfunction, previous thromboembolism, and hypercoagulable condition.

References

1. Bonow RO, Carabello B, de Leon AC Jr, et al: ACC/AHA guidelines for the management of patients with valvular heart disease: Executive summary: A report of the American College of Cardiology/American Heart Association Task Force on Practice Guidelines (Committee on Management of Patients With Valvular Heart Disease). Circulation 98:1949-1984, 1998.
2. Cheitlin MD, Alpert JS, Armstrong WF, et al: ACC/AHA guidelines for the clinical application of echocardiography: A report of the American College of Cardiology/American Heart Association Task Force on Practice Guidelines (Committee on Clinical Application of Echocardiography). Circulation 95:1686-1744, 1997.
3. Cheitlin MD, Douglas PS, Parmley WW: 26th Bethesda Conference: Recommendations for Determining Eligibility for Competition in Athletes with Cardiovascular Abnormalities. Task Force 2: Acquired Valvular Heart Disease. J Am Coll Cardiol 24:874-880, 1994.
4. Maron BJ, Araujo GS, Thompson PD, et al: Recommendations for preparticipation screening and the assessment of cardiovascular disease in masters athletes. An advisory for healthcare professionals from the Working Groups of the World Heart Federation, the International Federation of Sports Medicine, and the American Heart Association Committee on Exercise, Cardiac Rehabilitation, and Prevention. Circulation 103:327-334, 2001.

CHAPTER 58

Infective Endocarditis

Adolf W. Karchmer

Infective endocarditis (IE) is a microbial infection of the endothelial surface of the heart. The characteristic lesion, the vegetation, is a variably sized amorphous mass of platelets and fibrin in which abundant microorganisms and moderate inflammatory cells are enmeshed. Heart valves are most commonly involved; however, infection may occur at the site of a septal defect or on chordae tendineae or mural endocardium. Infection of arteriovenous shunts, arterioarterial shunts (patent ductus arteriosus), or coarctation of the aorta, although actually an endarteritis, is clinically and pathologically similar to IE. Many species of bacteria and fungi, mycobacteria, rickettsiae, chlamydiae, and mycoplasmas cause IE; nevertheless, streptococci, staphylococci, enterococci, and fastidious gram-negative coccobacilli cause the majority of cases of IE.

The terms *acute* and *subacute* are often used to describe IE. Acute IE arises with marked toxicity and progresses over days to several weeks to valvular destruction and metastatic infection. In contrast, subacute IE evolves over weeks to months with only modest toxicity and rarely causes metastatic infection. Acute IE is caused typically, although not exclusively, by *Staphylococcus aureus*, whereas the subacute syndrome is more likely to be caused by viridans streptococci, enterococci, coagulase-negative staphylococci, or gram-negative coccobacilli.

EPIDEMIOLOGY

The incidence of IE remained relatively stable from 1950 through 1987 at about 4.2 per 100,000 patient-years. During the early 1980s, the yearly incidence of IE per 100,000 population was 2.0 in the United Kingdom and Wales and 1.9 in the Netherlands.[1] A higher incidence was noted from 1984 through 1999; 5.9 and 11.6 episodes per 100,000 population were reported from Sweden and metropolitan Philadelphia, respectively.[2,3] Injection drug abuse accounted for approximately half of the cases in Philadelphia. Endocarditis usually occurred more frequently in men; gender-derived ratios range from 1.6 to 2.5. The age-specific incidence of endocarditis increased progressively after 30 years of age and exceeded 14.5 to 30 cases per 100,000 person-years in the sixth through eighth decades of life.[3] From 36 to 75 percent of patients with native valve endocarditis (NVE) have predisposing conditions: rheumatic heart disease, congenital heart disease, mitral valve prolapse, degenerative heart disease, asymmetrical septal hypertrophy, or intravenous (IV) drug abuse.[2] From 7 to 25 percent of cases involve prosthetic valves.[2,3] Predisposing conditions cannot be identified in 25 to 47 percent of patients. The nature of predisposing conditions and, in part, the microbiology of IE correlate with the age of patients (Table 58-1).

CHANGE IN PATIENTS WITH INFECTIVE ENDOCARDITIS. The median age of patients has gradually increased from 30 to 40 years of age in the preantibiotic and early antibiotic eras to 47 to 69 years in recent decades.[2] Rheumatic fever with subsequent rheumatic heart disease in children and young adults has been markedly reduced in developed countries. Acquired valvular disease emerges as a risk for IE as patients enjoy greater longevity. In addition, during their later years, many of these patients require valve replacement, which places them at greater risk for endocarditis. The increasing life span of the general population results in the emergence of degenerative heart disease as a major substrate for IE. Finally, nosocomial endocarditis arises with increased frequency among elderly people, who experience high rates of hospitalization for underlying illnesses.[4]

Groups of Patients

CHILDREN. The incidence of IE among hospitalized children ranges from 1 in 4500 to 1 in 1280.[1] In the Netherlands, IE was noted in 1.7 and 1.2 per 100,000 male and female children younger than 10 years, respectively.[1] IE has been noted in neonates with increasing frequency. Among neonates, IE typically involves the tricuspid valve of structurally normal hearts and is associated with very high mortality rates. It is likely that many of these episodes arise as a consequence of infected IV and right-heart catheters as well as cardiac surgery.[5]

The vast majority of children with IE occurring after the neonatal period have identifiable structural cardiac abnormalities (see Table 58-1). In some series, rheumatic heart disease was an infrequent predisposition for IE (≤4 percent).[5] Congenital heart abnormalities, particularly those involving the aortic valve; ventricular septal defects; tetralogy of Fallot; and other complex structural anomalies associated with cyanosis are found in 75 to 90 percent of cases. Of children with IE on congenital defects, 50 percent develop infection after cardiac surgery; in these children, infection frequently involves prosthetic valves, valved conduits, or synthetic patches.[5] Secundum atrial septal defects are not associated with an increased risk for IE, nor is patent ductus arteriosus or pulmonic stenosis after repair.[6] Since 1990, mitral valve prolapse has been recognized to predispose to IE in children; it, generally in association with a regurgitant murmur, was the predisposing cardiac abnormality in 15 percent and 5 percent of cases in two series.

The clinical features and echocardiographic findings of IE in children are similar to those noted among adults with NVE or prosthetic valve endocarditis (PVE), respectively.

ADULTS. *Mitral valve prolapse* (MVP) has emerged as a prominent predisposing structural cardiac abnormality and in adults accounts for 7 to 30 percent of native valve endocarditis (NVE) in cases not related to drug abuse or nosocomial infection.[1] The frequency of MVP in IE is not entirely a direct reflection of risk but rather arises because of the frequency of the lesion in the general population, 2.4 percent of community-based samples.

The relative risk of endocarditis among patients with MVP ranges from 3.5 to 8.2. This increased risk of endocarditis is largely confined to patients with prolapse, thickened valve leaflets (>5 mm), and mitral

TABLE 58–1 Predisposing Conditions and Microbiology of Native Valve Endocarditis

Conditions and Microbiology	Children (%)		Adults (%)	
	Neonates	2 mo-15 yr	15-60 yr	>60 yr
Predisposing conditions				
RHD		2-10	25-30	8
CHD	28	75-90*	10-20	2
MVP		5-15	10-30	10
DHD			Rare	30
Parenteral drug abuse			15-35	10
Other			10-15	10
None	72†	2-5	25-45	25-40
Microbiology				
Streptococci	15-20	40-50	45-65	30-45
Enterococci		4	5-8	15
S. aureus	40-50	25	30-40	25-30
Coagulase-negative staphylococci	10	5	3-5	5-8
GNB	10	5	4-8	5
Fungi	10	1	1	Rare
Polymicrobial	4		1	Rare
Other			1	2
Culture negative	4	0-15	3-10	5

CHD = congenital heart disease; DHD = degenerative heart disease; GNB = gram-negative bacteria, frequently *Hemophilus* species, *Actinobacillus actinomycetemcomitans*, *Cardiobacterium hominis*; MVP = mitral valve prolapse; RHD = rheumatic heart disease.

*50% of cases follow surgery and may involve implanted devices and foreign material.

†Often tricuspid valve IE.

regurgitation murmur. Risk is also increased among men and patients older than 45 years (see Chap. 57). Among patients with MVP and a systolic murmur, the incidence of IE is 52 per 100,000 person-years, compared with a rate of 4.6 per 100,000 person-years among those with prolapse and no murmur or among the general population. The microbiology of IE engrafted on MVP is similar to that of NVE that is not associated with drug abuse. Similarly, the mortality rate of 14 percent approximates that of NVE in general.

Rheumatic heart disease was the predisposing cardiac lesion for IE in 20 to 25 percent of cases in the 1970s and 1980s. In reports from hospitals in North America and Europe in the 1980s, rheumatic heart disease predisposed to IE in only 7 and 18 percent of cases.[2] In patients with rheumatic heart disease, endocarditis occurs most frequently on the mitral valve, a site at which women are more commonly infected. The aortic valve is the next most common site for IE; infection in this setting occurs more commonly in men.

Congenital heart disease is the substrate for IE in 10 to 20 percent of younger adults and 8 percent of older adults. Among adults, the common predisposing lesions are patent ductus arteriosus, ventricular septal defect, and bicuspid aortic valve, the latter particularly found among older men (>60 years).[2]

Infection with *human immunodeficiency virus* (HIV), unless associated with endocarditis-prone behavior, i.e., IV drug abuse, is not a significant risk factor for IE. Among HIV-infected persons who are not IV drug abusers, IE is caused not only by organisms typical of NVE but also by organisms that are uniquely associated with bacteremia in this population, i.e., *Salmonella* spp. and *Streptococcus pneumoniae*. Notably, 40 percent of cases were nosocomial.[7]

In settings where NVE among adults is not skewed dramatically by infection occurring among IV drug abusers and nosocomial disease, the microbiology is notably similar to that shown in Table 58–1.[2] *Coxiella burnetii*, an uncommon cause of IE in the United States, caused 3 percent of all cases in the United Kingdom from 1976 to 1985 and is a prominent cause of IE in France.[8] *Bartonella* species have emerged as a significant cause of IE, accounting for 3 percent of cases in one report.[9]

INTRAVENOUS DRUG ABUSERS. The risk for IE among IV drug abusers, 2 to 5 percent per patient-year, is estimated to be several fold greater than that of patients with rheumatic heart disease or prosthetic valves.[10] In one study, IE was diagnosed in 74 (6.4 percent) of 1150 IV drug abusers who were hospitalized during 12 months. In metropolitan Philadelphia, 5.3 of a total of 11.6 cases of IE per 100,000 population were attributed to injection drug abuse. From 65 to 80 percent of cases of IE in this population occur in men, who typically range in age from 27 to 37 years.[11-13]

Endocarditis occurring in IV drug abusers has a unique propensity to infect right heart valves.[10-13] In clinical series, distribution of valve involvement is tricuspid in 46 to 78 percent, mitral in 24 to 32 percent, and aortic in 8 to 19 percent (as many as 16 percent of patients have infection at multiple sites).[11] In IV drug abusers, the valves were normal before infection in 75 to 93 percent of patients.[10,11] The remaining patients have preexisting aortic or mitral valve abnormalities, resulting primarily from rheumatic heart disease, congenital heart disease, or prior episodes of IE. IV drug abuse is a risk factor for recurrent NVE.

MICROBIOLOGY. The microbiology of IE occurring in IV drug abusers is unique in several respects (Table 58–2). In contrast to the etiology of NVE among adults in general, *S. aureus* causes more than 50 percent of these infections overall and 60 to 70 percent of those involving the tricuspid valve. The well-established predilection for *S. aureus* to infect normal as well as abnormal left heart valves is noted in addicts. Although the phenomenon of *S. aureus* infection of normal tricuspid valves is not unique to addicts, the high frequency is characteristic.[10] Streptococcal and enterococcal infection of previously abnormal mitral or aortic valves in addicts is comparable to that noted generally in NVE. In contrast, infection of right and left heart valves by *Pseudomonas aeruginosa* and other gram-negative bacilli and left heart valves by fungi occurs with increased frequency among drug abusers. In addition, unusual organisms, some of which are probably related to injection of contaminated materials, cause endocarditis in these patients, e.g., *Corynebacterium* species, *Lactobacillus, Bacillus cereus,* and nonpathogenic *Neisseria* species. Polymicrobial endocarditis accounts for 3 to 5 percent of cases of IE.

The clinical manifestations of IE in IV drug abusers depend on the valve or valves involved and, to a lesser degree, on the infecting organism. Tricuspid valve endocarditis, particularly when caused by *S. aureus,* arises with pleuritic chest pain, shortness of breath, cough, and hemoptysis. In 65 to 75 percent of patients, chest roentgenograms reveal abnormalities related to septic pulmonary emboli. Murmurs of tricuspid regurgitation are noted in less than half of these patients. Infection of the aortic or mitral valve in addicts clinically resembles IE seen in other patients. That caused by *S. aureus* generally arises as acute endocarditis with marked systemic toxicity. Symptoms and signs of left-sided heart failure, neurological injury, systemic emboli, metastatic infections, and the classical peripheral stigmata of IE are strongly associated with left-sided endocarditis.[10,11]

Infection with HIV has been noted in 27 to 73 percent of IV drug abusers with IE (see Chap. 61).[11-13] Among drug

TABLE 58–2 Microbiology of Endocarditis Associated with Intravenous Drug Abuse

Organisms	Number of Cases (%) of Endocarditis in Drug Addicts*			
	Right-Sided† *N* = 346	*Left-Sided*† *N* = 204	*Total*‡ *N* = 675	*Spain (1977-1993)*§ *N* = 1529
Streptococci‖	17 (5)	31 (15)	80 (12)	131 (8.5)
Enterococci	7 (2)	49 (24)	59 (9)	21 (1)
Staphylococcus aureus	267 (77)	47 (23)	396 (57)	1138 (74)
Coagulase-negative staphylococci	—	—		44 (3)
Gram-negative bacilli¶	17 (5)	26 (13)	45 (7)	23 (1.5)
Fungi (predominantly *Candida* species)	—	25 (12)	26 (4)	18 (1)
Polymicrobia/miscellaneous	28 (8)	20 (10)	49 (7)	48 (3)
Culture negative	10 (3)	6 (3)	20 (3)	106 (7)

*Ten patients with right- and left-sided IE are counted twice.
†Data from references 10 and Levine DP, Crane LR, Zervos MJ: Bacteremia in narcotic addicts at the Detroit Medical Center. Infectious endocarditis: A prospective comparative study. Rev Infect Dis 8:374, 1986. Hecht SR, Berger M: Right-sided endocarditis in intravenous drug users: Prognostic features in 102 episodes. Ann Intern Med 17:560, 1992.
‡Data from references 10, 11, and Sandre RM, Shafran SD: Infective endocarditis: Review of 135 cases over 9 years. Clin Infect Dis 22:276-286, 1996.
§Data from reference 7.
‖Includes viridans streptococci, *Streptococcus bovis*, other non-group A groupable streptococci, *Abiotrophia* species (nutritionally variant streptococci).
¶*P. aeruginosa*, *S. marcescens*, and Enterobacteriaceae.

abusers with IE, HIV serostatus does not significantly modify the clinical presentation, microbiology, complications, and overall survival. However, among HIV-infected drug abusers with IE, the risk of death is increased among those with a CD4 count less than 200/mm^3.[12,13]

PROSTHETIC VALVE ENDOCARDITIS. Epidemiological studies suggest that PVE constitutes 10 to 30 percent of all cases of IE in developed countries.[3,12] In metropolitan Philadelphia, 0.94 cases of IE per 100,000 population involved prosthetic valves. In six studies that observed patients undergoing valve surgery between 1965 and 1995, the cumulative incidence of PVE estimated actuarially ranged from 1.4 to 3.1 percent at 12 months and 3.0 to 5.7 percent at 5 years.[14-17] The risk of PVE over time, however, is not uniform. The risk is greatest during the initial 6 months after valve surgery (particularly during the initial 5 to 6 weeks) and thereafter declines to a lower but stable risk (0.2 to 0.35 percent per year).[14-17]

PVE has been called "early" when symptoms begin within 60 days of valve surgery and "late" with onset thereafter. These terms were established to distinguish PVE that arose early as a complication of valve surgery from infection that became symptomatic later and was more likely to be community acquired. In fact, many cases with onset between 60 days and 1 year after surgery are likely to be nosocomial and, despite their delayed presentation, derive from events during the surgical admission. Studies to identify risk factors for PVE have not resulted in a coherent picture. Data suggest that, during the initial months after valve implantation, mechanical prostheses are at greater risk of infection than bioprosthetic valves but that after 12 months the risk of infection of bioprostheses exceeds that of mechanical valves.[14-16] By 5 years after valve surgery, the rates of PVE for the two valve types are comparable.[17] Patients with antecedent NVE, particularly if the disease is active, are at increased risk for PVE.[14-16]

Microbiology. The microbiology of PVE is relatively predictable and reflects in part the presumed nosocomial or community acquisition of infection (Table 58–3). Coagulase-negative staphylococci, which when speciated are primarily *Staphylococcus epidermidis*, are the predominant causes of PVE diagnosed within 60 days after surgery. *S. aureus*, gram-negative bacilli, diphtheroids (particularly *Corynebacterium jeikeium*), and fungi (particularly *Candida* species) are also common causes of PVE during this period. Occasional cases of nosocomial PVE caused by *Legionella* species, atypical mycobacteria, mycoplasma, and fungi other than *Candida* have been reported.

TABLE 58–3 Microbiology of Prosthetic Valve Endocarditis 1975-1994

Organisms	Number of Cases (%)* with Time of Onset After Valve Surgery		
	<2 mo *N* = 144	*2-12 mo* *N* = 31	*>12 mo* *N* = 194
Streptococci†	2 (1)	3 (9)	61 (31)
Pneumococci	—	—	—
Enterococci	12 (8)	4 (12)	22 (11)
Staphylococcus aureus	32 (22)	4 (12)	34 (18)
Coagulase-negative staphylococci	47 (33)	11 (32)	22 (11)
Fastidious gram-negative coccobacilli (HACEK group)‡	—	—	11 (6)
Gram-negative bacilli	19 (13)	1 (3)	11 (6)
Fungi, *Candida* species	12 (8)	4 (12)	3 (1)
Polymicrobial/miscellaneous	4 (3)	2 (6)	9 (5)
Diphtheroids	9 (6)	—	5 (3)
Culture negative	7 (5)	2 (6)	16 (8)

Adapted from Karchmer AW: Infections of prosthetic valves and intravascular devices. *In* Mandell GL, Bennett JE, Dolin R (eds): Principles and Practice of Infectious Disease. 5th ed. New York, Churchill Livingstone, 2000, pp 907-917.
*Data from reference 90.
†Includes viridans streptococci, *Streptococcus bovis*, other non-group A groupable streptococci, *Abiotrophia* species (nutritionally variant streptococci).
‡Includes *Hemophilus* species, *Actinobacillus actinomycetemcomitans*, *Cardiobacterium hominis*, *Eikenella* species, and *Kingella kingae*.

Pathology. The intracardiac pathology of PVE differs notably from the largely leaflet-confined pathology of NVE. Infection on mechanical prostheses commonly extends beyond the valve ring into the annulus and periannular tissue as well as the mitral-aortic intravalvular fibrosa, resulting in ring abscesses, septal abscesses, fistulous tracts, and dehiscence of the prosthesis with hemodynamically significant paravalvular regurgitation and conduction disturbances. In autopsy experience with 74 patients, which is clearly biased toward the most severe pathology, annular invasion was noted in 85 percent, myocardial abscess in 32 percent, and valve obstruction by vegetation overgrowth, a phenomenon of PVE at the mitral site, in 19 percent.[18] Erosion through the aortic annulus to cause pericarditis occurred in 5 percent (Fig. 58–1).[18]

In clinical series encompassing 85 patients, the rate of annulus invasion was 42 percent, myocardial abscess 14 percent, valve obstruction 4 percent, and pericarditis 2 percent.[18] Bioprosthetic valve IE may result in invasive disease, comparable to that noted when PVE involves mechanical valves, as well as leaflet destruction. Among 85 patients with bioprosthetic PVE, 29 (59 percent) of 49 with infection within a year after surgery had invasive disease, in contrast to only 9 (25 percent) of 36 patients with infection occurring more than 1 year postoperatively. In surgically treated bioprosthetic IE, invasion was confirmed in 15 of 19 cases (79 percent) with onset in the initial 12 months after surgery but in only 22 of 71 bioprostheses (31 percent) when infection began more than 12 months after surgery.[19] Aortic site and clinical onset within a year of valve surgery were significantly correlated with an increased risk of invasive infection.

Signs and symptoms in patients developing PVE within 60 days of cardiac surgery may be obscured by surgery or other postoperative complications. Peripheral signs of endocarditis (5 to 14 percent) and central nervous system emboli (10 percent) occur less frequently in these patients than in those with PVE occurring later after surgery. Among patients with later onset PVE, congestive heart failure (CHF) occurs in 40 percent, cerebrovascular complications in 26 to 28 percent, and peripheral signs in 15 to 28 percent.[18,20]

HEALTH CARE–ASSOCIATED ENDOCARDITIS. Health care–associated endocarditis includes true nosocomial IE as well as IE arising in the community setting as a direct consequence of long-term indwelling devices, e.g., central venous lines, tunneled lines, and hemodialysis catheters. Hospital-acquired endocarditis unrelated to concurrent cardiac surgery makes up 5 to 29 percent of all cases of IE in various series.[4] Health care–associated IE has a predilection for abnormal native cardiac valves, normal valves including the tricuspid, transvenous pacemakers and defibrillators, and prosthetic valves.[1,17] Hemodialysis-associated *S. aureus* bacteremia is commonly associated with metastatic seeding of deep tissue sites including cardiac valves; in fact, hemodialysis is independently associated with *S. aureus* IE.[21] Infected intravascular devices and catheters give rise to 45 to 65 percent of the bacteremia that results in nosocomial IE.[4] Right-sided endocarditis was found in 5 and 7 percent of patients with central venous catheters extending into or near the right atrium and those with flow-directed pulmonary artery catheters, respectively.

The onset of health care–associated IE is usually acute, and although a changing murmur may be heard, other classical signs of endocarditis are infrequent. Mortality rates among these patients, many of whom are elderly and have serious underlying diseases, are high (40 to 56 percent).[4]

MICROBIOLOGY. Gram-positive cocci are the predominant cause of nosocomial IE. Among 82 episodes from two series, *S. aureus* caused 55 percent, coagulase-negative staphylococci 10 percent, enterococci 16 percent, streptococci 7 percent, *Candida* species 4 percent, and gram-negative bacilli 5 percent; 3 percent were culture negative.

Catheter-associated *S. aureus* bacteremia occurs with sufficient frequency to be the predominant predisposing factor for health care–associated IE.[4,21,22] In a meta-analysis of catheter-related *S. aureus* bacteremia, the mean rate of subsequent endocarditis or other deep-seated infection after short-course treatment was 6.1 percent.[21] However, when 69 patients with catheter-related *S. aureus* bacteremia were studied with transesophageal echocardiography (TEE), 16 (23 percent) were found to have IE. Only seven of the IE episodes would have been diagnosed without information from the TEE.[22] Patients with *S. aureus* catheter-related bacteremia who have abnormal heart valves, prosthetic valves, or persisting fever or bacteremia for 3 days after catheter removal and initiation of therapy are at high risk for IE.

Given the relatively high risk of IE in patients with *S. aureus* catheter-related bacteremia and its morbidity, these patients should be evaluated by echocardiography. Two decision analysis studies concluded that the most cost-effective management would proceed directly to TEE to establish the presence or absence of IE.[23,24] If, however, transthoracic echocardiography (TTE) is performed initially and is nondiagnostic, the evaluation should proceed to TEE.

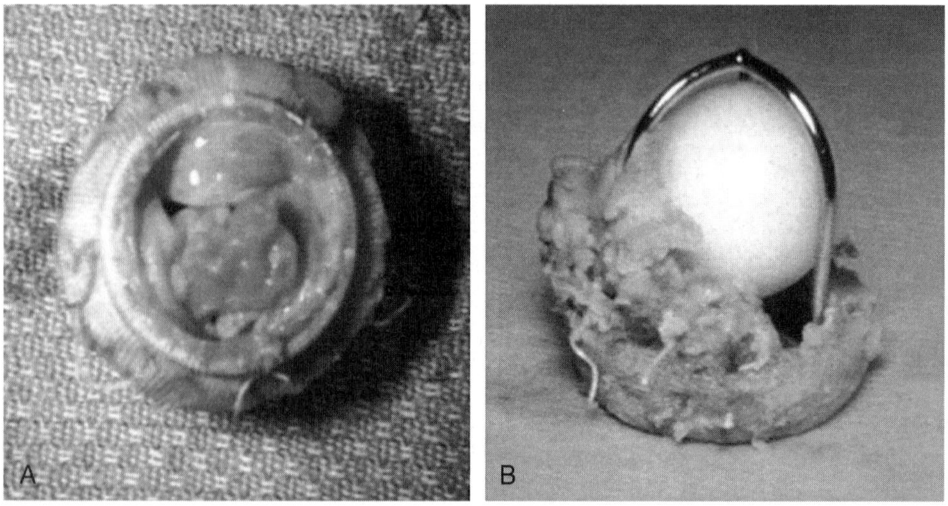

FIGURE 58–1 **A,** A large vegetation caused by *Candida albicans* partially occludes the orifice of a bioprosthetic valve removed from the mitral position. **B,** A Starr-Edwards prosthesis removed from the aortic position, where this large vegetation related to *Aspergillus* infection partially obstructed the outflow tract but also allowed regurgitation by preventing valve closure. (**A,** From Karchmer AW: Infections of prosthetic heart valves. *In* Korzeniowski OM [ed]: Cardiovascular Infection, vol x, Atlas of Infectious Diseases. Philadelphia, Churchill Livingstone, 1998, p 5.7.)

Etiological Microorganisms

VIRIDANS STREPTOCOCCI. These streptococci, which cause 30 to 65 percent of NVE cases unrelated to drug abuse, are normal inhabitants of the oropharynx, characteristically produce alpha hemolysis when grown on sheep blood agar, and are usually nontypable using the Lancefield system. Using earlier taxonomy, the species causing streptococcal NVE were distributed as follows: *Streptococcus mitior* (31 percent of cases), *Streptococcus sanguis* (24 percent), *Streptococcus bovis* (27 percent), *Streptococcus mutans* (7 percent), *Streptococcus milleri* (4 percent), *Streptococcus faecalis* (now *Enterococcus faecalis*) (7 percent), and *Streptococcus salivarius* and other species (2 percent). Another study, adjusted for the new taxonomy, has reported a similar distribution of streptococci causing IE. Nutritional variant organisms that require media supplemented with either pyridoxal hydrochloride or L-cysteine for growth and were previously speciated as *Streptococcus adjacens* or *Streptococcus defectivus* cause 5 percent of cases of streptococcal NVE. These organisms have been reclassified into a new genus, *Abiotrophia*.[25]

The viridans streptococci, other than the nutritionally variant organisms, had been in general highly susceptible to penicillin (minimum inhibitory concentration [MIC] ≤ 0.1 μg/ml for 83 percent) and are killed in an enhanced manner (synergistically) by penicillin plus gentamicin.[25]

***STREPTOCOCCUS BOVIS* AND OTHER STREPTOCOCCI.** *S. bovis* and other group D streptococci, part of the gastrointestinal tract normal flora, cause 25 to 40 percent of the episodes of streptococcal NVE.[3] Although superficially resembling the enterococci, these organisms can be easily distinguished by their biochemical characteristics. The distinction is important because group D streptococci are highly penicillin susceptible, in contrast to the relative penicillin resistance of enterococci. *S. bovis* type I NVE is frequently associated with coexistent colonic polyps or malignancy.

Group A streptococci, which can infect normal valves, cause rare episodes of endocarditis. Among IV drug abusers, group A streptococci have caused tricuspid valve IE similar to that noted with *S. aureus*. Group B organisms, *Streptococcus agalactiae*, are part of the normal flora of the mouth, genital tract, and gastrointestinal tract. Group B streptococci infect normal and abnormal valves and cause a morbid NVE syndrome with a high incidence of systemic emboli and septic musculoskeletal complications (arthritis, discitis, osteomyelitis).[26] Group G streptococci also produce a destructive, highly morbid left-sided NVE. The *S. milleri* group, now divided into three species—*Streptococcus intermedius*, *Streptococcus constellatus*, and *Streptococcus anginosus*—are highly pyogenic organisms that cause destructive infections and IE, similar to those caused by *S. aureus*. Although both beta-hemolytic streptococci (group A, B, C, and G) and the *S. milleri* group are invasive tissue-destroying organisms, they cause different IE syndromes.[27] IE caused by beta-hemolytic streptococci often occurs in the absence of valvular disease, has a rapid onset, and frequently results in extracardiac complications. That caused by *S. milleri* more likely occurs in the setting of valvular disease and arises less aggressively with fewer extracardiac complications. Both, however, are associated with frequent intracardiac complications, and 65 percent of patients require surgical intervention often early during therapy. Mortality rates are higher for IE caused by beta-hemolytic streptococci versus *S. milleri*, 27 and 14 percent, respectively.

***STREPTOCOCCUS PNEUMONIAE*.** Although pneumococcal bacteremia occurs frequently, *S. pneumoniae* accounts for only 1 to 3 percent of NVE cases.[28] When causing IE, *S. pneumoniae* frequently involves a previously normal aortic valve and progresses rapidly with valve destruction, myocardial abscess formation, and acute CHF.[29] The diagnosis of IE is often delayed until intracardiac complications or systemic emboli are evident. The clinical presentation, complications, and outcome of endocarditis caused by penicillin-susceptible and penicillin-resistant *S. pneumoniae* are similar. Almost half of the patients require cardiac surgery because of valve dysfunction, heart failure, or persisting fever. Mortality (35 percent) is related to left-sided heart failure and not to the penicillin susceptibility of the infecting strain.[27]

ENTEROCOCCI. *E. faecalis* and *Enterococcus faecium* cause 85 and 10 percent of cases of enterococcal IE, respectively. Enterococci, which are part of the normal gastrointestinal flora and cause genitourinary tract infection, account for 5 to 15 percent of cases of NVE and a similar percentage of PVE cases (see Tables 58–2 and 58–3).[18] Cases occur in young women as a consequence of genitourinary tract manipulation or infection and in older, predominantly male patients, who have the urinary tract as a likely portal of entry. Enterococci infect either normal or previously abnormal valves and arise as either acute or subacute IE.

Enterococci are overtly resistant to cephalosporins, semisynthetic penicillinase-resistant penicillins (oxacillin and nafcillin), and therapeutic concentrations of aminoglycosides. Most enterococci have been inhibited by modest concentrations of the cell wall–active antibiotics—penicillin, ampicillin, vancomycin, and teicoplanin (not licensed in the United States). Bactericidal antienterococcal activity can be achieved by combining an inhibitory cell wall–active agent and streptomycin or gentamicin. This bactericidal activity, called *synergy*, is essential for optimal treatment of enterococcal IE. Strains of enterococci that are highly resistant to penicillin and ampicillin, resistant to vancomycin, or highly resistant to all aminoglycosides have been identified as causes of IE. These resistant strains of enterococci may be unresponsive to standard antienterococcal agents and defy development of a synergistic bactericidal regimen. The antibiotic susceptibility of any enterococcus causing IE must be thoroughly evaluated if optimal therapy is to be assured.

STAPHYLOCOCCI. The coagulase-positive staphylococci are a single species, *S. aureus*. Of the 13 species of coagulase-negative staphylococci that colonize humans, 1, *S. epidermidis*, has emerged as an important pathogen in the setting of implanted devices and hospitalized patients. Coagulase-negative staphylococci on the surface of foreign devices have altered phenotypes, including increased resistance to the bactericidal effects of many antibiotics.

Antibiotic Resistance. In excess of 90 percent of *S. aureus* cases, whether acquired in the hospital or community, produce beta-lactamase and thus are resistant to penicillin, ampicillin, and the ureidopenicillins. These organisms are, however, susceptible to the penicillinase-resistant beta-lactam antibiotics (oxacillin, nafcillin, cefazolin, and other first-generation cephalosporins). Methicillin-resistant strains of *S. aureus* are prevalent in nosocomial settings and among some nonhospitalized populations (IV drug abusers, nursing home residents, persons hospitalized or incarcerated within the prior 6 to 12 months) and must be considered when selecting initial empirical therapy for IE.[21] Coagulase-negative staphylococci frequently produce beta-lactamase; furthermore, strains causing community-acquired infections are frequently methicillin susceptible, whereas those causing nosocomial infections, including IE, are commonly methicillin resistant.[30] Coagulase-negative staphylococci may not always phenotypically express methicillin resistance (a property called *heteroresistance*). Consequently, special testing may be required to detect this resistance.[30] Although most staphylococci, including most strains that are resistant to methicillin, remain susceptible to the glycopeptide antibiotics, vancomycin and teicoplanin, strains of *S. aureus* and coagulase-negative staphylococci with reduced susceptibility (and occasionally overt resistance) to glycopeptides have emerged as pathogens.[21]

Clinical Features. *S. aureus* is a major cause of IE in all population groups (see Tables 58–1 and 58–2). *S. aureus* IE is characterized by a highly toxic febrile illness, frequent focal metastatic infection, and a 30 to 50 percent rate of CHF and central nervous system complications.[21] A cerebrospinal fluid polymorphonuclear pleocytosis, with or without *S. aureus* cultured from the cerebrospinal fluid, is common. Heart murmurs are heard in 30 to 45 percent of patients on initial evaluation and are ultimately heard in 75 to 85 percent as a consequence of intracardiac damage. The mortality rate in nonaddicts with left-sided *S. aureus* endocarditis ranges from 16 to 65 percent overall and increases in those older than 50 years, in those with significant underlying diseases, and when IE is complicated by a major neurological event, valve dysfunction, or CHF.[21,31,32] Among addicts, left-sided *S. aureus* IE resembles that in nonaddicts. In contrast, in patients with IE limited to the tricuspid valve, complications are rare and mortality rates are only 2 to 4 percent.[11] Tricuspid staphylococcal IE occasionally results in overwhelming septic pulmonary emboli, pyopneumothorax, and severe respiratory insufficiency.

Coagulase-Negative Staphylococci. These are a major cause of PVE, particularly during the initial year after valve surgery, an important cause of nosocomial IE, and the cause of 3 to 8 percent of NVE cases, usually in the setting of prior valve abnormalities (see Tables 58–1 and 58–2).[30] The vast majority of coagulase-negative staphylococci causing PVE, when speciated, are *S. epidermidis*. In contrast, when infection involves native valves, only 50 percent of isolates are *S. epidermidis*.[30] *Staphylococcus lugdunensis*, a coagulase-negative species, has caused highly destructive, often fatal NVE and PVE. *S. lugdunensis* IE is usually community acquired, and the organism is often susceptible to many antistaphylococcal antibiotics, including penicillin.

GRAM-NEGATIVE BACTERIA. Organisms of the so-called HACEK group (*Hemophilus parainfluenzae*, *Hemophilus aphrophilus*, *Actinobacillus actinomycetemcomitans*, *Cardiobacterium hominis*, *Eikenella corrodens*, and *Kingella kingae*), which are part of the upper respiratory tract and oropharyngeal flora, infect abnormal cardiac valves, causing subacute NVE, and cause PVE that occurs a year or more after valve surgery.[33,34] In NVE, the HACEK organisms have been associated with large vegetations and a high incidence of systemic emboli.[33,34] Among the HACEK group, in descending order, *Actinobacillus actinomycetemcomitans*, *Cardiobacterium hominis*, *Hemophilus aphrophilus*, and *Hemophilus parainfluenzae* are the most common causes of IE. Although fastidious and slow growing, HACEK organisms are usually detected in blood cultures after 5 days of incubation; occasionally more prolonged incubation is required.[34]

P. aeruginosa is the gram-negative bacillus that most commonly causes endocarditis. The Enterobacteriaceae, despite causing frequent episodes of bacteremia, are implicated in only sporadic cases of IE.

Neisseria gonorrhoeae, a common cause of IE during the preantibiotic era, rarely causes endocarditis today.[35] Gonococci, similar to pneumococci, infect the aortic valve of young patients, resulting in valve destruction, abscess formation, and a probable need for valve replacement.[33-35] Although they are generally susceptible to ceftriaxone, antibiotic resistance is widespread among *N. gonorrhoeae*; accordingly, treatment must be based upon the susceptibility of the implicated isolate. Other *Neisseria* species (nongonococcal, nonmeningococcal) cause rare episodes of IE, usually in the setting of preexisting valvulopathy.[34]

OTHER ORGANISMS. *Corynebacterium* species, often called diphtheroids, although often contaminants in blood cultures, cannot be ignored when isolated from multiple blood cultures. Prolonged incubation of blood cultures is often required to isolate these slow-growing, fastidious organisms from patients with IE. They are an important cause of PVE occurring during the initial year after valve surgery and a surprisingly common cause of endocarditis involving abnormal valves.[18,35,36] *Listeria monocytogenes,* a small gram-positive rod, causes occasional cases of IE involving abnormal left heart valves and prosthetic devices,[35] most commonly in immune-compromised patients. *Tropheryma whippelii,* the cause of Whipple disease, has caused a cryptic afebrile form of IE with associated arthralgias but without diarrhea as well as valvular disease as part of typical Whipple disease.[37] The diagnosis has been established by identification of the organism in macrophages in resected valves using periodic acid–Schiff stain or by polymerase chain reaction (PCR).[34,38] Valve involvement may complicate Whipple disease more frequently than recognized. IE caused by *T. whippelii* often does not fulfill the Duke criteria for diagnosis (Table 58–4); thus, detection requires a high index of suspicion.[34,37]

The rickettsia *C. burnetii* infects humans after inhalation of desiccated materials from infected livestock or pets or contact with infected parturient animals. At variable intervals after acute infection by *C. burnetii* (Q fever), persons with abnormal mitral or aortic valves, particularly those with prosthetic valves, who have not been able to eradicate the organism develop very insidious subacute IE.[8,39] Endocarditis-prone patients with acute Q fever should receive prolonged antibiotic treatment with doxycycline plus hydroxychloroquine to prevent IE.[39] IE commonly arises with low-grade fever, fatigue, weight loss, and CHF. Hepatosplenomegaly, digital clubbing, and an immune complex vasculitis–induced purpuric rash are not uncommon. Vegetations are small, have smooth surfaces, and are not uniformly visible. On pathological examination, the vegetations of Q fever IE are nodular with a smooth surface (compared with other causes of IE) and the organisms are detected by immunohistological or Gimenez stains nearly exclusively within macrophages or by PCR.[34] The diagnosis is typically based on high antiphase I immunoglobulin G antibody titers to phase I *C. burnetii* antigens plus immunoglobulin A antibody or on demonstration of the organism in excised cardiac valves by immunohistological or Gimenez staining.[8]

Bartonella quintana and *Bartonella henselae*, which together may cause 3 percent of NVE, can be isolated from blood cultures by prolonged incubation and special techniques. In the absence of special culturing efforts, PCR detection of genetic material in excised vegetations, or serological testing, many cases would have been "culture negative."[9,34] *B. henselae*, which causes cat-scratch disease and in the HIV-infected population bacillary angiomatosis and hepatic peliosis, causes IE in patients with prior valve injury and cat exposure. In contrast, *B. quintana*, the agent of trench fever, causes IE largely in homeless people who are exposed to body lice and commonly occurs in the absence of prior valvular disease.[34] *Bartonella* IE arises insidiously; diagnosis is often delayed, and CHF and systemic emboli frequently complicate infection.[9,34] *Bartonella* infection destroys valve tissue and therapy commonly requires valve surgery.[34,40] On the basis of serological testing, *Chlamydia* species have been suggested as the cause of frequent episodes of IE. Because of the extensive serological cross-reaction between *Chlamydia* and *Bartonella*, many of these episodes have actually been *Bartonella* IE.[9,34]

FUNGI. *Candida albicans,* nonalbicans *Candida* species, *Histoplasma*, and *Aspergillus* species are the most common of the many fungal organisms identified as causing IE.[38] Unusual so-called emerging

TABLE 58–4 Diagnosis of Infective Endocarditis (Modified Duke Criteria)

Definitive Infective Endocarditis
Pathological criteria
- Microorganisms: demonstrated by culture or histology in a vegetation, *or* in a vegetation that has embolized, *or* in an intracardiac abscess, *or*
- Pathological lesions: vegetation or intracardiac abscess present, confirmed by histology showing active endocarditis

Clinical criteria, using specific definitions listed below
- Two major criteria, *or*
- One major and three minor criteria, *or*
- Five minor criteria

Possible Infective Endocarditis
One major criterion and one minor criterion or three minor criteria

Rejected
Firm alternative diagnosis for manifestations of endocarditis, *or*
Sustained resolution of manifestations of endocarditis, with antibiotic therapy for 4 days or less, *or*
No pathological evidence of infective endocarditis at surgery or autopsy, after antibiotic therapy for 4 days or less

Criteria for Diagnosis of Infective Endocarditis
Major criteria
Positive blood culture
- Typical microorganism for infective endocarditis from two separate blood cultures
  - Viridans streptococci, *Streptococcus bovis*, HACEK group *or* *Staphylococcus aureus* or community-acquired enterococci in the absence of a primary focus, *or*
- Persistently positive blood culture, defined as recovery of a microorganism consistent with infective endocarditis from:
  - Blood cultures (≥2) drawn more than 12 hr apart, *or*
  - All of three or a majority of four or more separate blood cultures, with first and last drawn at least 1 hr apart
- Single positive blood culture for *coxiella burnetii* or antiphase I IgG antibody titer >1:800

Evidence of endocardial involvement
- Positive echocardiogram
  - (TEE advised for PVE or complicated IE)
  - Oscillating intracardiac mass, on valve or supporting structures, *or* in the path of regurgitant jets, *or* on implanted material, in the absence of an alternative anatomical explanation, *or*
  - Abscess, *or*
  - New partial dehiscence of prosthetic valve, *or*
- New valvular regurgitation (increase or change in preexisting murmur not sufficient)

Minor criteria
Predisposition: predisposing heart condition *or* intravenous drug use
Fever ≥38.0°C (100.4°F)
Vascular phenomena: major arterial emboli, septic pulmonary infarcts, mycotic aneurysm, intracranial hemorrhage, conjunctival hemorrhages, Janeway lesions
Immunological phenomena: glomerulonephritis, Osler nodes, Roth spots, rheumatoid factor
Microbiological evidence: positive blood culture but not meeting major criterion as noted previously* *or* serologic evidence of active infection with organism consistent with infective endocarditis

IE = infective endocarditis; IgG = immunoglobulin G; PVE = prosthetic valve endocarditis; TEE = transesophageal echocardiography.

Adapted from Durack DT, Lukes AS, Bright DK: New criteria for diagnosis of infective endocarditis: Utilization of specific echocardiographic findings. Am J Med 96:200, 1994; modified per Li JS, Sexton DJ, Mick N, et al: Proposed modifications to the Duke criteria for the diagnosis of infective endocarditis. Clin Infect Dis 30:633, 2000.

*Excluding single positive cultures for coagulase-negative staphylococci and organisms that do not cause endocarditis commonly.

fungi and molds account for 25 percent of cases. Among 269 cases of fungal IE described between 1965 and 1995, 25 percent were nosocomial.[41] Risk factors include previous valve surgery, antibiotic use, injection drug abuse, intravascular catheters, surgery other than cardiac, and immunocompromised state. The last three have increased, and virtually all patients have two or more risk factors. Fever, new or changing murmurs, systemic embolization including major limb artery occlusion, neurological abnormalities, and heart failure are common symptoms. Blood cultures are positive commonly when IE is caused by *Candida* species but rarely when caused by mycelial organisms. Culture and histological examination of vegetations yield a microbiological diagnosis in 75 and 95 percent of cases, respectively, and 65 percent of embolic vegetations from peripheral arteries are diagnostic.

Pathogenesis

The interactions between the human host and selected microorganisms that culminate in IE involve the vascular endothelium, hemostatic mechanisms, the host immune system, gross anatomical abnormalities in the heart, surface properties of microorganisms, enzyme and toxin production by microorganisms, and peripheral events that initiate bacteremia. Each component of these interactions is in itself complex, influenced by many factors and not fully elucidated. These complex interactions result in a pathogenetic sequence wherein microorganisms adhere to valve surfaces, become persistent at the site of adherence, proliferate to cause local damage and vegetation growth, and ultimately disseminate hematogenously. Detailed in vitro and in vivo studies, aided by genetic manipulations, have begun to elucidate the pathogenesis of IE caused by viridans streptococci and *S. aureus*.[42] The rarity of endocarditis in spite of frequent transient asymptomatic and symptomatic bacteremia indicates that the intact endothelium is relatively resistant to infection. Endothelial damage results in platelet-fibrin deposition, which in turn is more receptive to colonization by bacteria than is the intact endothelium. It is hypothesized that platelet-fibrin deposition occurs spontaneously in persons with valvular disease and that these deposits, called nonbacterial thrombotic endocarditis (NBTE), are the sites at which microorganisms adhere during bacteremia to initiate IE.[43]

DEVELOPMENT OF NONBACTERIAL THROMBOTIC ENDOCARDITIS. Two major mechanisms appear pivotal in the formation of NBTE: endothelial injury and a hypercoagulable state. NBTE has been found in 1.3 percent of patients at autopsy and is more common with increasing age and in patients with malignancy, disseminated intravascular coagulation, uremia, burns, systemic lupus erythematosus, valvular heart disease, and intracardiac catheters.[44] NBTE deposits are found at the valve closure contact line on the atrial surfaces of the mitral and tricuspid valves and on the ventricular surfaces of the aortic and pulmonic valves, the sites of infected vegetations in patients with IE.

Three hemodynamic circumstances may injure the endothelium, initiating NBTE: (1) a high-velocity jet striking endothelium, (2) flow from a high- to a low-pressure chamber, and (3) flow across a narrow orifice at high velocity. Flow through a narrowed orifice, as a consequence of the Venturi effect, deposits bacteria maximally at the low-pressure sink immediately beyond an orifice or at the site where a jet stream strikes a surface. These are the same sites where NBTE forms as a result of hemodynamic circumstances. The superimposition of NBTE formation and preferential deposition of bacteria helps to explain the distribution of infected vegetations.[45]

CONVERSION OF NONBACTERIAL THROMBOTIC ENDOCARDITIS TO INFECTIVE ENDOCARDITIS. Bacteremia is the initiating event that ultimately converts NBTE to IE. The frequency and magnitude of bacteremia associated with daily activities and health care procedures appear related to specific mucosal surfaces and skin, the density of colonizing bacteria, the disease state of the surface, and the extent of the local trauma. Bacteremia rates are highest for events that traumatize the oral mucosa, particularly the gingiva, and progressively decrease with procedures involving the genitourinary tract and the gastrointestinal tract. A diseased mucosal surface—particularly one that is infected—is associated with an increased risk of bacteremia.

For viable circulating microorganisms to reach NBTE, they must be resistant to the complement-mediated bactericidal activity of serum.

The adherence of microorganisms to the NBTE or to apparently intact valve endothelium is a pivotal early event in the development of IE. Redundant interacting bacterial surface molecules mediate adherence to host extracellular matrix molecules on valve endothelium or NBTE. Collectively, these bacterial molecules are known as microbial surface components recognizing adhesive matrix molecules (MSCRAMMs). Streptococci that produce surface polysaccharides called glucans or dextran cause endocarditis more frequently than strains that do not produce dextran. Dextran on the surface of streptococci can be shown to mediate adherence to platelet fibrin lattices and injured valves and to facilitate development of endocarditis in experimental models.[42,44] Dextran production, however, is not universal among the major microbial causes of IE; thus, other mechanisms of adherence are likely. For example, Fim A protein of *Streptococcus parasanguis*, which belongs to a family of oral mucosal adhesins in viridans streptococci, facilitates adherence to fibrin and development of experimental endocarditis.[42]

Fibronectin, an important factor in the pathogenesis of IE, has been identified in lesions on heart valves and is produced by endothelial cells, platelets, and fibroblasts in response to vascular injury; a soluble form binds to exposed subendothelial collagen. Receptors for fibronectin, MSCRAMMs, are present on the surface of *S. aureus*; viridans streptococci; group A, C, and G streptococci; enterococci; *S. pneumoniae*; and *C. albicans*. Fibronectin has numerous binding domains and thus can bind simultaneously to fibrin, collagen, cells, and microorganisms and facilitate adherence of bacteria to the valve at the site of injury or NBTE. Fibronectin binding proteins A and B in *S. aureus* are critical in the induction of experimental endocarditis. Clumping factor (or fibrinogen-binding surface protein) of *S. aureus* also mediates the binding of these organisms to platelet fibrin thrombi and to aortic valves in models of endocarditis.[42] The glycocalyx or slime on the surface of *S. epidermidis* does not appear to function as an adhesin but may render organisms more virulent by enhancing their ability to avoid eradication by host defenses.

The mechanism by which virulent organisms colonize and infect intact valvular endothelium is less clearly understood. In elderly people, degenerative valve sclerosis may be associated with local inflammation, which in turn may promote endothelial cell binding of fibronectin and other extracellular matrix molecules. Particulate material injected during IV drug abuse might stimulate similar endothelial events. These endothelial changes could promote *S. aureus* adherence through MSCRAMMs to apparently normal valves.[42] Binding of *S. aureus* fibronectin-binding protein is required for the invasion of intact endothelial cells.[42] Multiplication of the organism intracellularly results in cell death, which in turn disrupts the endothelial surface and initiates formation of platelet-fibrin deposits and additional sites for bacterial adherence.

After adherence to NBTE or the endothelium, bacteria must persist and multiply if IE is to develop. Resistance of viridans streptococci and *S. aureus* to platelet antimicrobial proteins is associated with increased ability to cause experimental endocarditis.[42] Persistence and multiplication result in a complex dynamic process during which the infected vegetation increases in size by platelet-fibrin aggregation, microorganisms multiply and are shed into the blood, and vegetation fragments embolize. Staphylococcal and streptococcal surface proteins bind to platelets and promote aggregation and growth of the vegetation. Organisms that bind and aggregate platelets are more virulent in experimental models.[42] In addition, both streptococci and staphylococci increase local procoagulant activity by inducing fibrin-adherent monocytes to elaborate tissue factor (a tissue thromboplastin that binds to activated factor VII to initiate clotting).[42] Also, *S. aureus* can induce tissue factor production by endothelial cells, which would facilitate endocarditis development on normal valves.[42] Multiple replications of this cycle from adherence to multiplication and platelet-fibrin deposition result in clinical IE.

Pathophysiology

Aside from the constitutional symptoms of infection, which are probably mediated by cytokines, the clinical manifestations of IE result from (1) the local destructive effects of intracardiac infection; (2) the embolization of bland or septic fragments of vegetations to distant sites, resulting in infarction or infection; (3) the hematogenous seeding of remote sites during continuous bacteremia; and (4) an antibody response to the infecting organism with subsequent tissue injury caused by deposition of preformed immune complexes or antibody-complement interaction with antigens deposited in tissues.

The intracardiac consequences of IE range from trivial, characterized by an infected vegetation with no attendant tissue damage, to catastrophic, when infection is locally destructive or extends beyond the valve leaflet. Distortion or perforation of valve leaflets, rupture of chordae tendineae, and perforations or fistulas between major vessels and cardiac chambers or between chambers themselves as a consequence of burrowing infection may result in CHF that is progressive (Fig. 58–2).[46-48] Infection, particularly that involving the aortic valve or prosthetic valves, may extend into paravalvular tissue and result in abscesses and persistent fever related to antibiotic-unresponsive infection, disruption of the conduction system with electrocardiographic conduction abnormalities and clinically relevant arrhythmias, or purulent pericarditis.[48] Large vegetations, particularly at the mitral valve, can result in functional valvular stenosis and hemodynamic deterioration.[18,49] In general, intracardiac complications involving the aortic valve evolve more rapidly than those associated with the mitral valve; nevertheless, the progression is highly variable and unpredictable in individual patients.

Embolization of fragments from vegetations producing symptoms by infection or infarction is clinically evident in 11 to 43 percent of patients.[45,50-52] However, pathological evidence of emboli at autopsy is found more frequently (45 to 65 percent). Pulmonary emboli, which are often septic, occur in 66 to 75 percent of IV drug abusers with tricuspid valve IE.[10,11] The persistent bacteremia of IE, with or without septic emboli, may result in metastatic infection in any organ or tissue. These infections, which may vary in size from small miliary to large abscesses, may be manifest as local signs and symptoms or as persistent fever during therapy. IE caused by virulent organisms, particularly *S. aureus* or beta-hemolytic streptococci, is complicated more frequently by metastatic infection than that due to avirulent bacteria, e.g., viridans streptococci.[21,27] Metastatic abscesses are often small and miliary. Metastatic infection assumes particular importance when the required therapy is more than the antibiotics indicated for IE or when these infections constitute a focus that engenders relapse.

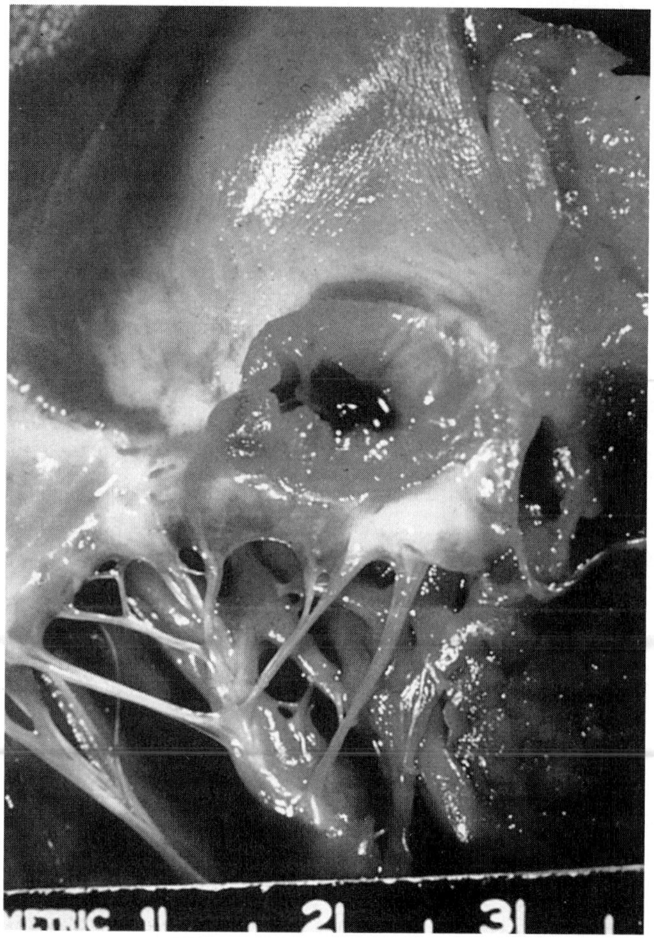

FIGURE 58–2 A normal valve with a large, bulky vegetation caused by *Staphylococcus aureus* infection. Clot is present centrally in the vegetation, obscuring a valve fenestration.

Clinical Features

The interval between the presumed initiating bacteremia and the onset of symptoms of IE is estimated to be less than 2 weeks in more than 80 percent of patients with NVE. Interestingly, in some patients with intraoperative or perioperative infection of prosthetic valves, the incubation period may be prolonged (2 to 5 or more months).[18]

Fever is the most common symptom and sign in patients with IE (Table 58–5). Fever may be absent or minimal in elderly persons or in those with CHF, severe debility, or chronic renal failure and occasionally in patients with NVE caused by coagulase-negative staphylococci.[30,53] *Heart murmurs* are noted in 80 to 85 percent of patients with NVE and are emblematic of the lesion predisposing to IE. Murmurs are commonly not audible in patients with tricuspid valve IE. Similarly, in acute NVE caused by *S. aureus,* murmurs are heard in only 30 to 45 percent of patients on initial evaluation but are ultimately noted in 75 to 85 percent. The new or changing murmurs (alterations unrelated to heart rate or cardiac output but rather regurgitant murmurs indicative of valve dysfunction) are relatively infrequent in subacute NVE and are more prevalent in acute IE and PVE.[18] They are frequently important harbingers of CHF. *Enlargement of the spleen* is noted in 15 to 50 percent of patients and is more common in subacute IE of long duration.

TABLE 58–5 Clinical Features of Infective Endocarditis

Symptoms	Percent	Signs	Percent
Fever	80-85	Fever	80-90
Chills	42-75	Murmur	80-85
Sweats	25	Changing/new murmur	10-40
Anorexia	25-55	Neurological abnormalities†	30-40
Weight loss	25-35	Embolic event	20-40
Malaise	25-40	Splenomegaly	15-50
Dyspnea	20-40	Clubbing	10-20
Cough	25	Peripheral manifestation	
Stroke	13-20	Osler nodes	7-10
Headache	15-40	Splinter hemorrhage	5-15
Nausea/vomiting	15-20	Petechiae	10-40
Myalgia/arthralgia	15-30	Janeway lesion	6-10
Chest pain*	8-35	Retinal lesion/Roth spots	4-10
Abdominal pain	5-15		
Back pain	7-10		
Confusion	10-20		

*More common in intravenous drug abusers.
†Central nervous system.

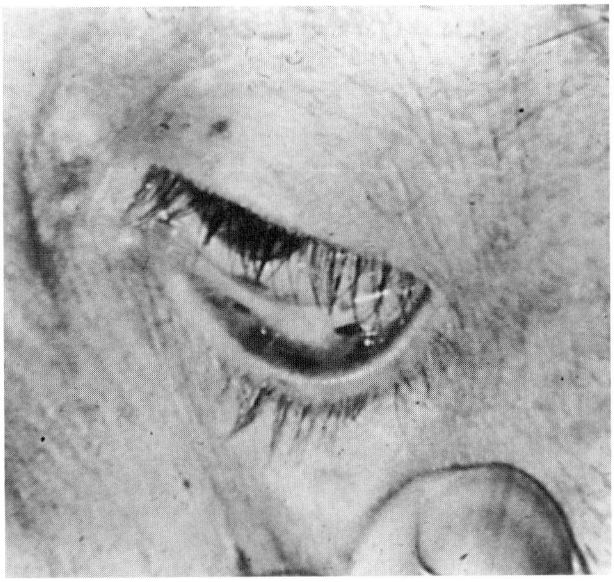

FIGURE 58–3 Conjunctival petechiae in a patient with infective endocarditis. (From Kaye D: Infective Endocarditis. Baltimore, University Park Press, 1976.)

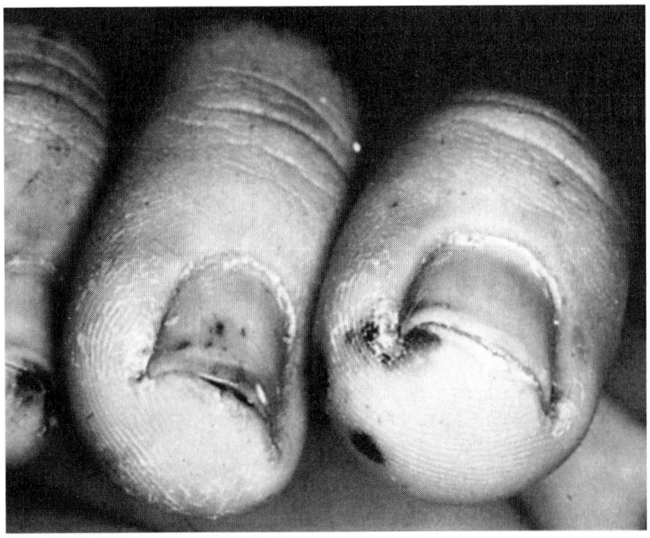

FIGURE 58–4 Subungual hemorrhages (splinter hemorrhages) and digital petechiae in a patient with infective endocarditis. (From Korzeniowski OM, Kaye D: Infective endocarditis. *In* Braunwald E [ed]: Heart Disease. 4th ed. Philadelphia, WB Saunders, 1992, p 1087.)

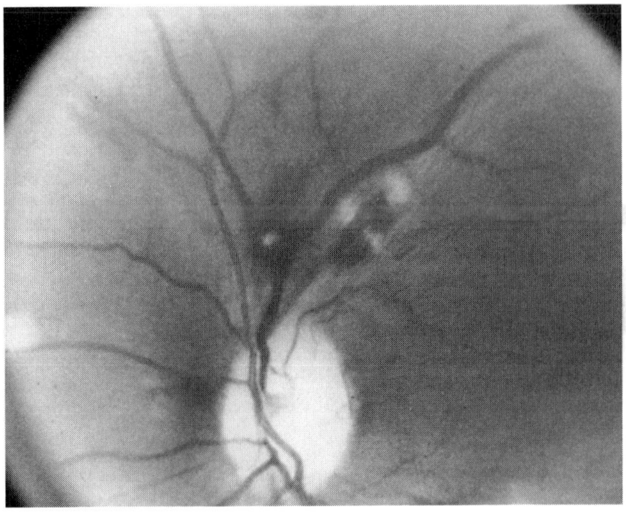

FIGURE 58–5 Roth spot (retinal hemorrhage with a clear center) in a patient with infective endocarditis. (From Korzeniowski OM, Kaye D: Infective endocarditis. *In* Braunwald E [ed]: Heart Disease. 4th ed. Philadelphia, WB Saunders, 1992, p 1087.)

The classical peripheral manifestations of IE are encountered less frequently today and are absent in IE restricted to the tricuspid valve.[10,54] *Petechiae* (Fig. 58–3), the most common of these manifestations, are found on the palpebral conjunctiva, the buccal and palatal mucosa, and the extremities. They are not specific for endocarditis even on the conjunctiva. *Splinter* or *subungual hemorrhages* (Fig. 58–4) are dark red, linear, or occasionally flame-shaped streaks in the nail bed of the fingers or toes. Distal lesions are probably due to trauma, whereas the more proximal ones are more likely to be related to IE. *Osler nodes* are small, tender subcutaneous nodules that develop in the pulp of the digits or occasionally more proximally in the fingers and persist for hours to several days. These, too, are not pathognomonic for IE. Janeway lesions are small erythematous or hemorrhagic macular nontender lesions on the palms and soles and are the consequence of septic embolic events. Roth spots (Fig. 58–5), oval retinal hemorrhages with pale centers, are infrequent findings in patients with IE. They have been noted in patients with collagen-vascular disease and hematological disorders, including severe anemia.

Musculoskeletal symptoms, unrelated to focal infection, are relatively common in patients with IE. These include arthralgias and myalgias, occasional true arthritis with nondiagnostic but inflammatory synovial fluid findings, and prominent back pain without evidence of vertebral body, disc space, or sacroiliac joint infection. In patients with arthritis or back pain, focal infection must be excluded because additional therapy may be required.

Systemic emboli are among the most common clinical sequelae of IE, occurring in up to 40 percent of patients, and are frequent subclinical events found only at autopsy.[45,50-52,54] Emboli often antedate diagnosis. Although embolic events may occur during or after antimicrobial therapy, the incidence decreases promptly during administration of effective antibiotic therapy.[53,55] Embolic splenic infarction may cause left upper quadrant abdominal pain and left shoulder pain. Renal emboli may occur asymptomatically or with flank pain and may cause gross or microscopic hematuria. Embolic stroke syndromes, predominantly involving the middle cerebral artery territory, occur in 15 to 20 percent of patients with NVE and PVE.[18] Coronary artery emboli are common findings at autopsy but rarely result in transmural infarction. Emboli to the extremities may produce pain and overt ischemia, and those to mesenteric arteries may cause abdominal pain, ileus, and guaiac-positive stools.

Neurological symptoms and signs occur in 30 to 40 percent of patients with IE, are more frequent when IE is caused by *S. aureus*, and are associated with increased mortality rates.[50,56,57] Embolic stroke is the most common and clinically important of the neurological manifestations. Intracranial hemorrhage occurs in 5 percent of patients with IE. Bleeding results from rupture of a mycotic aneurysm, rupture of an artery related to septic arteritis at the site of embolic occlusion, or hemorrhage into an infarct.[58] Mycotic aneurysms, with or without rupture, occur in 2 to 10 percent of patients with IE; approximately half of these involve intracranial arteries (Fig. 58–6). Cerebritis with microabscesses complicates IE caused by invasive pathogens such as *S. aureus*, but large brain abscesses are rare. Purulent meningitis complicates some episodes of IE caused by *S. aureus* or *S. pneumoniae*, but more typically the cerebrospinal fluid has an aseptic profile.[29,56] Other neurological manifestations include severe headache (a potential clue to a mycotic aneurysm), seizure, and encephalopathy.

Heart murmurs complicating IE are primarily the result of valve destruction or distortion or rupture of chordae tendineae. Intracardiac fistulas, myocarditis, or coronary artery embolization may occasionally contribute to the genesis of CHF, as obviously can underlying cardiac disease. In the absence of surgery to correct valvular dysfunction, CHF, particularly that related to aortic insufficiency, is associated with very high mortality rates.[46]

Renal insufficiency as a result of immune complex–mediated glomerulonephritis occurs in less than 15 percent of patients with IE. Azotemia as a result of this process may develop or progress during initial therapy; it usually improves with continued administration of effective antibiotic therapy. Focal glomerulonephritis and embolic renal infarcts cause hematuria but rarely result in azotemia. Renal dysfunction in patients with IE is most commonly a manifestation of impaired hemodynamics or toxicities associated with antimicrobial therapy (interstitial nephritis or aminoglycoside-induced injury).

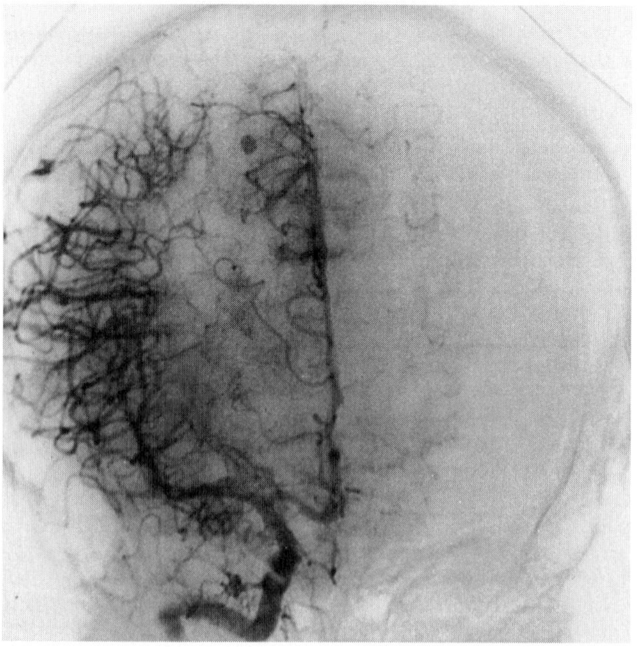

FIGURE 58–6 An irregular mycotic aneurysm of the middle cerebral artery lies laterally on the cerebral cortex. A second aneurysm is projected just lateral to the anterior cerebral artery.

Diagnosis

The symptoms and signs of endocarditis are often constitutional and, when localized, often result from a complication of IE rather than reflect the intracardiac infection itself (see Table 58–5). Consequently, if physicians are to avoid overlooking the diagnosis of IE, a high index of suspicion must be maintained. The diagnosis must be investigated when patients with fever present with one or more of the cardinal elements of IE: a predisposing cardiac lesion or behavior pattern, bacteremia, embolic phenomenon, and evidence of an active endocardial process. Because patients with prosthetic heart valves are always at risk for PVE, the presence of fever or new prosthesis dysfunction at any time warrants considering this diagnosis. In patients at risk for endocarditis, concurrent illnesses or iatrogenic events may create clusters of symptoms and signs that superficially mimic IE and require careful consideration to arrive at a correct diagnosis. Even when the illness seems typical of endocarditis, the definitive diagnosis requires positive blood cultures or positive cultures (or histology or PCR recovery of a microorganism's DNA) from the vegetation or embolus. There are many culture-negative mimics of IE: atrial myxoma, acute rheumatic fever, systemic lupus erythematosus or other collagen-vascular disease, marantic endocarditis, the antiphospholipid syndrome, carcinoid syndrome, renal cell carcinoma with increased cardiac output, and thrombotic thrombocytopenic purpura.

The modified Duke criteria provide a schema that facilitates evaluating patients for endocarditis (see Table 58–4).[59,60] Clinical and laboratory data, including echocardiography, should be collected in a manner that allows one to assess the presence or absence of the listed major and minor criteria. Finding evidence of two major or one major plus three minor or five minor criteria establishes a clinical diagnosis of "definite endocarditis," whereas finding one major plus one minor or three minor criteria indicates "possible endocarditis." When used judiciously over the entire evaluation, i.e., not limited to initial findings, these criteria are sensitive and specific for the diagnosis of IE (see Table 58–4).[59-61] Erroneous rejection of the diagnosis of endocarditis is unlikely. When these diagnostic criteria are used to guide therapy, patients who are categorized with possible endocarditis should be treated as if they have IE. Requiring at least one major criterion or three minor criteria to designate possible endocarditis reduces the potential for overdiagnosis (failure to reject the diagnosis) and the likelihood of treating uninfected patients.[60]

To use bacteremia caused by coagulase-negative staphylococci or diphtheroids (organisms that may cause IE but more often contaminate blood cultures) to support the diagnosis of endocarditis, blood cultures must be persistently positive or the organisms recovered in several sporadically positive cultures must be proved to represent a single clone.[59,60] These considerations are embodied in the diagnostic criteria (see Table 58–4).[57-59]

ECHOCARDIOGRAPHY. Inclusion of echocardiographic evidence of endocardial infection in these criteria recognizes the high sensitivity of two-dimensional echocardiography with color Doppler, especially if multiplanar TEE and TTE are combined, and the relative infrequency of false-positive studies when experienced operators use specific definitions for vegetations.[61,62] Although the sensitivity of TEE to detect vegetations in patients with suspected IE ranges from 85 to 95 percent (or higher if a follow-up study is performed), a negative study result does not preclude the diagnosis or the need for therapy if the clinical suspicion is high.[62] The likelihood of a false-negative result can be reduced to 5 to 10 percent if TEE is repeated, especially if the study is biplanar or multiplanar.[61,62] Thus, these studies help to preclude the diagnosis when the clinical suspicion is low.[61,62] Nevertheless, when the clinical suspicion is high, even these highly sensitive tests cannot preclude the diagnosis. In addition, because the echocardiogram cannot distinguish healed vegetations and valvular masses from actively infected vegetations, these guidelines are vulnerable to misidentifying as culture-negative IE the vegetations that complicate marasmus, malignancy, cryptic collagen-vascular disease, or the antiphospholipid antibody syndrome.

ESTABLISHING THE MICROBIAL CAUSE. A microbial cause of IE is established by recovering the infecting agent from the blood or by identifying it in surgically removed vegetations or embolic material. In detecting the bacteremia of IE, there is no advantage to obtaining blood cultures in relationship to fever or from arterial blood (as opposed to venous blood). In patients who have not received prior antibiotics and who will ultimately have blood culture-positive IE, it is likely that 95 to 100 percent of all cultures obtained will be positive and that one of the first two cultures will be positive in at least 95 percent of patients. Prior antibiotic therapy is a major cause of blood culture–negative IE, particularly when the causative microorganism is highly antibiotic susceptible. At least 35 percent of cases of culture-negative IE can be attributed to prior antimicrobial therapy.[63] After subtherapeutic antibiotic exposure, the time required for reversion to positive cultures is directly related to the duration of antimicrobial therapy and the susceptibility of the causative agent; days to a week or more may be required.

OBTAINING BLOOD CULTURES. Three separate sets of blood cultures, each from a separate venipuncture, obtained over 24 hours, are recommended to evaluate patients with suspected endocarditis.[61] Each set should include two flasks, one containing an aerobic medium and the other containing thioglycollate broth (anaerobic medium), into each of which at least 10 ml of blood should be placed.[64]

For optimal processing, the laboratory should be advised that endocarditis is a possible diagnosis and which, if any, unusual bacteria are suspected (*Legionella* species, *Bartonella* species, HACEK organisms). If a clinically stable patient has received an antimicrobial agent during the past several weeks, it is prudent to delay therapy so that repeated cultures can be obtained on successive days.[64] If fungal endocarditis is suspected, blood cultures should be obtained using the lysis-centrifugation method. The laboratory should be asked to save the organism causing endocarditis until successful therapy has been completed. Serological tests are occasionally used to make the presumptive etiological diagnosis of endocarditis caused by *Brucella* species, *Legionella* species, *Bartonella* species, *C. burnetii*, or *Chlamydia* species. By special techniques, including PCR, these agents and others that are difficult to recover in blood culture can be identified in blood or vegetations.[8,38,61,65]

Sustained bacteremia is typical of IE. In evaluating positive blood cultures, sustained bacteremia (persisting over 1 hour) should be distinguished from transient bacteremia. When several blood cultures obtained over 24 hours or more are positive, the diagnosis of IE must be considered. The identity of the organism is also helpful in determining the intensity with which the diagnosis is entertained. Organisms can be divided into those that commonly cause IE, those that rarely cause IE, and the intermediate-behaving organisms, e.g., enterococci and *S. aureus*, which, when in the blood, may or may not indicate IE. Finally, the presence or absence of alternative sources for the bacteremia aids in the assessment of bacteremia.

Laboratory Tests

Many other tests are inevitably performed in the evaluation of patients with suspected IE. Hematological parameters are commonly abnormal. Anemia, with normochromic normocytic red blood cell indices, a low serum iron level, and low serum iron-binding capacity, is found in 70 to 90 percent of patients. Anemia worsens with increased duration of illness and thus in acute IE may be absent. In subacute IE, the white blood cell count is usually normal; in contrast, a leukocytosis with increased segmented granulocytes is common in acute IE. Thrombocytopenia occurs only rarely.

The *erythrocyte sedimentation rate* (ESR) is elevated (average approximately 55 mm/hr) in almost all patients with IE; the exceptions are those with CHF, renal failure, or disseminated intravascular coagulation. Other tests often indicate immune stimulation or inflammation (see Pathophysiology): circulating immune complexes, rheumatoid factor, quantitative immune globulin determinations, cryoglobulins, and C-reactive protein. Although the results of these tests parallel disease activity, the tests are costly and not efficient ways to diagnose IE or monitor response to therapy. Measurement of circulating immune complexes and complement may be useful in evaluating for azotemia related to diffuse immune complex glomerulonephritis.

The *urinalysis* result is often abnormal, even when renal function remains normal. Proteinuria and microscopic hematuria are noted in 50 percent of patients.

Echocardiography (see also Chap. 11)

Evaluation of patients with clinically suspected IE by this technique frequently allows morphological confirmation of infection and increasingly aids in decisions about management.[62,66] Echocardiography should not be used as a screening test for IE in unselected patients with positive blood cultures or in patients with fevers of unknown origin when the clinical probability is low.[61,67] Nevertheless, echocardiographic evaluation should be performed in most patients with clinically suspected IE, especially those with negative blood cultures.[61] Although many patients with NVE involving the aortic or mitral valve can be imaged adequately by TTE, TEE using biplane or multiplane technology with incorporated color flow and continuous as well as pulsed Doppler is the state of the art.[67-69] TEE allows visualization of smaller vegetations and provides improved resolution compared with TTE. Not only is TEE the preferred approach in patients with clinically suspected IE in whom TTE is suboptimal, it is also the procedure of choice for imaging the pulmonic valve, patients with PVE (especially at the mitral site), and patients who are at high risk for intracardiac complications or those with signs of persistent or invasive infection despite adequate antimicrobial therapy.[61,68-70]

A decision analysis evaluation of echocardiography for diagnosis of NVE in patients with bacteremia suggests that, assuming the diagnostic enhancement of TEE over TTE is 15 percent, the most cost-effective strategy (yielding optional quality-adjusted life-years) is as follows: (1) if prior probability of IE is less than 2 percent, treat for bacteremia without echocardiography; (2) if prior probability is 2 to 4 percent, use TTE; and (3) if prior probability is 5 to 45 percent, use TEE initially in lieu of TTE. If the prior probability of IE is greater than 45 percent, therapy without echocardiography is cost effective, although studies may still be desirable to evaluate for complications and other risks.[24] The high frequency of IE patients with a high prior probability of endocarditis results in studies that demonstrate that data from TEE rarely alter clinical management plans built on data from TTE.[67,68]

TEE becomes pivotal when TTE is a technically inadequate study, when PVE is sought, and when the clinical prior probability is medium.

Another cost-effectiveness analysis suggests that in patients with clinically uncomplicated catheter-associated *S. aureus* bacteremia, evaluation with TEE to determine duration of antibiotic therapy (4 versus 2 weeks, i.e., treatment of endocarditis or not) is more cost effective than empirical selection of either duration of therapy.[23] The strategy of diagnosing IE by TTE to be followed by TEE if negative was not evaluated, but given the anticipated prior probability of IE (≥6 percent) it would probably be more costly.

The sensitivity of TTE for the detection of vegetations in NVE is approximately 65 percent. In contrast, in NVE, the sensitivity of TEE for vegetation detection ranges from 85 to 95 percent.[62] In patients with PVE, TTE is limited by the shadowing effect of the prostheses, especially in the mitral position, and its diagnostic sensitivity is reduced to 15 to 35 percent. In contrast, the sensitivity of TEE for detecting vegetations in PVE involving mechanical or bioprosthetic devices in the aortic or mitral position ranged from 82 to 96 percent.[70,71]

Despite the sensitivity of TEE in detecting vegetations in patients with proven IE, echocardiography does not itself provide a definite diagnosis. Vegetations and valve dysfunction may be demonstrated, but determination of causality requires clinical or direct anatomical and microbiological confirmation. Infectious vegetations cannot be distinguished on the echocardiogram from marantic lesions, nor can vegetations be distinguished from thrombus or pannus on prostheses. Furthermore, it is usually not possible to distinguish active from healed vegetations in NVE.[72] Thickened valves, ruptured chordae or valves, valve calcification, and nodules may be mistaken for vegetations, indicating the specificity limitations of isolated echocardiography.

Valve dysfunction caused by tissue disruption, leaflet perforation, or large obstructing vegetations can be visualized and quantitated by echocardiogram with Doppler. Some degree of regurgitation by Doppler is almost universal early in the course of NVE and PVE and does not necessarily predict progressive hemodynamic deterioration. Extension of infection beyond the valve leaflet into surrounding tissue results in abscesses in various areas of the annulus or adjacent structures, mycotic aneurysms of the sinus of Valsalva or mitral valve, intracardiac fistulas, and purulent pericarditis. Myocardial abscesses are more readily detected by TEE than TTE in patients with NVE or PVE.[70,71] The sensitivity and specificity for abscess detection were 28 percent and 98 percent for TTE, compared with 87 percent and 95 percent for TEE. TEE is also more sensitive and accurate than TTE for recognizing subaortic invasive disease and valve perforations.[73]

MAGNETIC RESONANCE AND COMPUTED TOMOGRAPHIC IMAGING. These techniques have identified paravalvular extension of infection, aortic root aneurysms, and fistulas; however, their utility relative to echocardiography has not been established.

SCINTIGRAPHY. Efforts to identify vegetations and intracardiac abscess in patients with IE and in animal models have used scintigraphy with gallium-67 citrate, indium-111-labeled granulocytes, and indium-111-labeled platelets. These efforts have not been sufficiently sensitive or anatomically localizing to be useful clinically.[74]

Treatment

Two major objectives must be achieved to treat IE effectively. The infecting microorganism in the vegetation must be eradicated. Failure to accomplish this results in relapse of infection. Also, invasive, destructive intracardiac and focal extracardiac complications of infection must be resolved if morbidity and mortality are to be minimized. The second objective often exceeds the capacity of effective antimicrobial therapy and requires cardiac or other surgical intervention.

Bacteria in vegetations multiply to population densities approaching 10^9 to 10^{10} organisms per gram of tissue, become metabolically dormant, and are difficult to eradicate. Clinical experience and animal model experiments suggest that optimal therapy should use bactericidal antibiotics or antibiotic combinations rather than bacteriostatic agents. In addition, antibiotics reach the central areas of avascular vegetations by passive diffusion. To reach effective antibiotic concentrations in vegetations, high serum concentrations must be achieved, and penetration by some agents is limited even then. Parenteral antimicrobial therapy is used whenever feasible in order to achieve suitable serum antibiotic concentrations and to avoid the potentially erratic absorption of orally administered therapy. Treatment is continued for prolonged periods to ensure eradication of dormant microorganisms.

In selecting antimicrobial therapy for patients with IE, one must consider the ability of potential agents to kill the causative organism as well as the MIC and minimum bactericidal concentration (MBC) of these antibiotics for the organism. The MIC is the lowest concentration that inhibits growth, and the MBC is the lowest concentration that decreases a standard inoculum of organisms 99.9 percent during 24 hours. For the vast majority of streptococci and staphylococci, the MIC and MBC of penicillins, cephalosporins, or vancomycin are the same or differ by only a factor of 2 to 4. Organisms for which the MBC for these antibiotics is 10-fold or greater than the MIC are occasionally encountered. This phenomenon has been termed *tolerance*.[66] Most of the tolerant strains are simply killed more slowly than nontolerant strains, and with prolonged incubation (48 hours) their MICs and MBCs are similar. Enterococci exhibit what superficially appears to be tolerance when tested against penicillins and vancomycin; however, these organisms are, in fact, not killed by these agents but are merely inhibited, even after longer incubation times. Enterococci can be killed by the combined activity of selected penicillins or vancomycin and an aminoglycoside. This enhanced antibiotic activity of the combination against enterococci, if of sufficient magnitude, is called *synergy* or a *synergistic bactericidal* effect.[66] A similar effect can be seen with these combinations against streptococci and staphylococci.

A synergistic bactericidal effect is required for optimal therapy of enterococcal endocarditis and has been used to achieve more effective therapy or effective short-course therapy of IE caused by other organisms. Tolerance in streptococci or staphylococci, although demonstrable in vivo, in animal model experiments has not been correlated with decreased cure rates or delayed responses to treatment with penicillins, cephalosporins, or vancomycin. Accordingly, the presence of tolerance in streptococci or staphylococci has not required combination therapy, and, in fact, regimens are designed using the MICs of these organisms.[75]

The regimens recommended for the treatment of IE caused by specific organisms are designed to provide high concentrations of antibiotics in serum and deep in vegetations that exceed the organism's MIC throughout most of the interval between doses. Although antibiotic concentrations in vegetations of patients with IE have been measured infrequently, the success of the recommended regimens suggests that this goal has been achieved. Accordingly, for optimal therapy, it is important that the recommended regimens be followed carefully.

Antimicrobial Therapy for Specific Organisms

The antimicrobial therapy for endocarditis should not only eradicate the causative agent but also do so while causing little or no toxicity. Therapy for a given patient requires modification to accommodate end-organ dysfunction, existing allergies, and other anticipated toxicities. With the exception of staphylococcal endocarditis, the antimicrobial regimens recommended for the treatment of NVE and PVE are similar,

TABLE 58–6 Treatment for Native Valve Endocarditis Caused by Penicillin-Susceptible Viridans Streptococci and *Streptococcus bovis* (Minimum Inhibitory Concentration ≤0.1 μg/ml)*

Antibiotic	Dosage and Route†	Duration (wk)
Aqueous penicillin G	12-18 million units/24 hr IV either continuously or every 4 hr in six equally divided doses	4
Ceftriaxone	2 gm once daily IV or IM	4
Aqueous penicillin G	12-18 million units/24 hr IV either continuously or every 4 hr in six equally divided doses	2
plus Gentamicin	1 mg/kg IM or IV every 8 hr	2
Vancomycin	30 mg/kg/24 hr IV in two equally divided doses, not to exceed 2 gm/24 hr unless serum levels are monitored	4

Modified from Wilson WR, Karchmer AW, Dajani AS, et al: Antibiotic treatment of adults with infective endocarditis due to streptococci, enterococci, staphylococci, and HACEK microorganisms. JAMA 274:1706, 1995. Copyright 1995 American Medical Association.

*For nutritionally variant streptococci (*Streptococcus adjacens, Streptococcus defectivus*), see Table 58–8.

†Dosages given are for patients with normal renal function. Vancomycin and gentamicin doses must be reduced for treatment of patients with renal dysfunction. Vancomycin and gentamicin doses are calculated using ideal body weight (men = 50 kg + 2.3 kg per inch over 5 feet; women = 45.5 kg + 2.3 kg per inch over 5 feet).

although more prolonged treatment is often advised for PVE.[18,74]

PENICILLIN-SUSCEPTIBLE VIRIDANS STREPTOCOCCI OR *STREPTOCOCCUS BOVIS*. Four regimens provide highly effective, comparable therapy for patients with endocarditis caused by penicillin-susceptible streptococci and *S. bovis* (Table 58–6). The 4-week regimens yield bacteriological cure rates of 98 percent among patients who complete therapy. Treatment with the synergistic combination of penicillin plus gentamicin for 2 weeks is as effective in selected cases as treatment with the 4-week regimens. The combination regimen is recommended for patients who have uncomplicated NVE and who are not at increased risk for aminoglycoside toxicity. Patients with endocarditis caused by nutritionally variant streptococci (*Abiotrophia* species), endocarditis involving a prosthetic valve, or endocarditis complicated by a mycotic aneurysm, myocardial abscess, perivalvular infection, or an extracardiac focus of infection should not be treated with this short-course regimen.

From 2 to 8 percent of viridans streptococci and *S. bovis* causing endocarditis are highly resistant to streptomycin (MIC >2000 μg/ml) and are not killed synergistically by penicillin plus streptomycin. These highly streptomycin-resistant strains are, however, killed synergistically by penicillin plus gentamicin. Consequently, unless a causative streptococcus can be evaluated to preclude high-level resistance to streptomycin, gentamicin is recommended for use in the short-course combination regimen.[76] Ceftriaxone 2 gm once daily plus either gentamicin (3 mg/kg) or netilmicin (4 mg/kg) given as a single daily dose for 14 days has effectively treated endocarditis caused by penicillin-susceptible streptococci.[77] Nevertheless, experience with single daily doses of aminoglycosides in the treatment of IE is limited, and these regimens are not currently recommended. The *Abiotrophia* species are generally more resistant to penicillin than other viridans streptococci.[25] Patients with endocarditis caused by these organisms are treated with regimens recommended for enterococcal endocarditis (see Table 58–8); however, outcome remains unsatisfactory.

For the treatment of streptococcal endocarditis in patients with a history of immediate allergic reactions (urticarial or anaphylactic reactions) to a penicillin or cephalosporin antibiotic, vancomycin is recommended (see Table 58–6). Patients with other forms of penicillin allergy (delayed maculopapular skin rash) may be treated cautiously with the ceftriaxone regimen (see Table 58–6) or with cefazolin, 2 gm IV every 8 hours for 4 weeks.

For patients with PVE caused by penicillin-susceptible streptococci, treatment with 6 weeks of penicillin is recommended, with gentamicin given during the initial 2 weeks.[18]

RELATIVELY PENICILLIN-RESISTANT STREPTOCOCCI. Four weeks of high-dose parenteral penicillin plus an aminoglycoside (primarily gentamicin for the reasons noted previously) during the initial 2 weeks are recommended for treatment of patients with endocarditis caused by streptococci with MICs for penicillin between 0.2 and 0.5 μg/ml (Table 58–7). Patients who cannot tolerate penicillin because of immediate hypersensitivity reactions can be treated with vancomycin alone. For those with nonimmediate penicillin hypersensitivity, effective treatment can be accomplished either with vancomycin alone or by adding gentamicin to the initial 2 weeks of the ceftriaxone regimen (see Table 58–6). Patients with endocarditis caused by streptococci that are highly resistant to penicillin (MIC > 0.5 μg/ml) should be treated with one of the regimens recommended for enterococcal endocarditis (Table 58–8).

***STREPTOCOCCUS PYOGENES*, *STREPTOCOCCUS PNEUMONIAE*, AND GROUP B, C, AND G STREPTOCOCCI.** Endocarditis caused by these streptococci has been either refractory to antibiotic therapy or associated with extensive valvular damage. Penicillin G in a dose of 3 million units IV every 4 hours for 4 weeks is recommended for the treatment of group A streptococcal endocarditis.

IE caused by group G, C, or B streptococci is more difficult to treat than that caused by penicillin-susceptible viridans streptococci. Consequently, the addition of gentamicin to the first 2 weeks of a 4-week regimen using high doses of penicillin is often advocated (see Table 58-7).[26,27] Early cardiac surgery to correct intracardiac complications is needed in almost half of these cases and may improve outcome.[26,27]

In selecting treatment for pneumococcal IE, both antibiotic resistance in the infecting strain and coexisting meningitis are important considerations.[28] The treatment of IE caused by penicillin-susceptible pneumococci (MIC = 0.6 μg/ml) with or without concomitant meningitis is penicillin G 4 million units IV every 4 hours, ceftriaxone 2 gm IV every 12 hours, or cefotaxime 4 gm IV every 6 hours. In the absence of meningitis, these regimens are effective for IE caused by pneumococci that are relatively penicillin resistant (MIC 0.1 to 1.0 μg/ml). If IE, including that

TABLE 58–7 Treatment for Native Valve Endocarditis Caused by Strains of Viridans Streptococci and *Streptococcus bovis* Relatively Resistant to Penicillin G (Minimum Inhibitory Concentration >0.1 μg/ml and <0.5 μg/ml)

Antibiotic	Dosage and Route*	Duration (wk)
Aqueous penicillin G	18 million units/24 hr IV either continuously or every 4 hr in six equally divided doses	4
plus Gentamicin	1 mg/kg IM or IV every 8 hr	2
Vancomycin	30 mg/kg/24 hr IV in two equally divided doses, not to exceed 2 gm/24 hr unless serum levels are monitored	4

*Dosages are for patients with normal renal function; see Table 58–6 footnote.

Modified from Wilson WR, Karchmer AW, Dajani AS, et al: Antibiotic treatment of adults with infective endocarditis due to streptococci, enterococci, staphylococci, and HACEK microorganisms. JAMA 274:1706, 1995. Copyright 1995 American Medical Association.

TABLE 58–8 Standard Therapy for Endocarditis Caused by Enterococci*

Antibiotic	Dosage and Route†	Duration (wk)
Aqueous penicillin G	18-30 million units/24 hr IV given continuously or every 4 hr in six equally divided doses	4-6
plus Gentamicin	1 mg/kg IM or IV every 8 hr	4-6
Ampicillin	12 gm/24 hr IV given continuously or every 4 hr in six equally divided doses	4-6
plus Gentamicin	1 mg/kg IM or IV every 8 hr	4-6
Vancomycin‡	30 mg/kg/24 hr IV in two equally divided doses not to exceed 2 gm/24 hr unless serum levels are monitored	4-6
plus Gentamicin	1 mg/kg IM or IV every 8 hr	4-6

Modified from Wilson WR, Karchmer AW, Dajani AS, et al: Antibiotic treatment of adults with infective endocarditis due to streptococci, enterococci, staphylococci, and HACEK microorganisms. JAMA 274:1706, 1995. Copyright 1995 American Medical Association.

*All enterococci causing endocarditis must be tested for antimicrobial susceptibility in order to select optimal therapy. These regimens are for treatment of endocarditis caused by enterococci that are susceptible to vancomycin or ampicillin and not highly resistant to gentamicin. These may also be used for treatment of endocarditis caused by penicillin-resistant (minimum inhibitory concentration >0.5) viridans streptococci and nutritionally variant streptococci (*S. defectivus, S. adjacens*), or enterococcal prosthetic valve endocarditis.

†Dosages are for patients with normal renal function. See Table 58–6, footnote.

‡Cephalosporins are not alternatives to penicillin/ampicillin in penicillin-allergic patients.

complicated by meningitis, is caused by a penicillin-resistant (MIC = 2.0 μg/ml) or cefotaxime-resistant (MIC = 2.0 μg/ml) pneumococcus, therapy with ceftriaxone 2 gm IV every 12 hours (or cefotaxime 4 gm IV every 4 hours) plus vancomycin 15 mg/kg IV every 12 hours is preferred. Heart failure rather than penicillin resistance is associated with mortality.

ENTEROCOCCI. Optimal therapy for enterococcal endocarditis requires synergistic bactericidal interaction of an antimicrobial targeted against the bacterial cell wall (penicillin, ampicillin, or vancomycin) and an aminoglycoside that is able to exert a lethal effect (primarily streptomycin or gentamicin). High-level resistance, defined as the inability of high concentrations of streptomycin (2000 μg/ml) or gentamicin (500 to 2000 μg/ml) to inhibit the growth of an enterococcus, is predictive of the agent's inability to exert this lethal effect and participate in the bactericidal synergistic interaction in vitro and in vivo. The standard regimens recommended for the treatment of enterococcal endocarditis (see Table 58–8) are designed to achieve bactericidal synergy. Synergistic combination therapy has resulted in cure rates of approximately 85 percent, compared with 40 percent with single-agent, nonbactericidal treatment.

Some authorities prefer gentamicin doses of 1.5 mg/kg every 8 hours; however, because this dose may be associated with an increased frequency of nephrotoxicity, others advocate doses of 1 mg/kg every 8 hours. Peak serum gentamicin concentrations of approximately 5 and 3.5 μg/ml are sought with these doses, respectively. In the absence of high-level resistance to streptomycin in a causative strain, streptomycin, 7.5 mg/kg intramuscularly (IM) or IV every 12 hours to achieve a peak serum concentration of approximately 20 μg/ml, can be substituted for gentamicin in the standard regimens. For patients allergic to penicillin, the vancomycin-aminoglycoside regimen (see Table 58-8) is recommended; alternatively, patients can be desensitized to penicillin. Desensitization may be desirable when preexisting renal dysfunction favors avoiding the potentially more nephrotoxic vancomycin-aminoglycoside combination. Cephalosporins are not effective in the treatment of enterococcal endocarditis. Therapy is administered for 4 to 6 weeks, with the longer course used to treat patients with IE that was symptomatic for more than 3 months, with complicated disease, and with enterococcal PVE. During treatment, careful clinical follow-up of patients and aminoglycoside levels is required to prevent nephrotoxicity and ototoxicity.

In the largest series to date, of 93 patients treated for enterococcal IE (66 with NVE, 27 with PVE), 75 (81 percent) were cured, 15 (16 percent) died, and 3 (3 percent) relapsed.[78] Cure was achieved with a median duration of cell wall-active antimicrobial therapy and aminoglycoside therapy of 42 and 15 days, respectively. In 39 patients who were cured, aminoglycosides were administered for 21 days or less. These favorable outcomes with regimens using foreshortened courses of aminoglycosides suggest that the aminoglycoside component of combination therapy can be reduced if toxicity becomes significant.

All enterococci causing endocarditis must be evaluated carefully in order to select effective therapy (Table 58-9). The strain causing endocarditis must be tested for high-level resistance to both streptomycin and gentamicin as well as to determine its susceptibility to penicillin, ampicillin, and vancomycin. If the strain is either resistant to achievable serum

TABLE 58–9 Strategy for Selecting Therapy for Enterococcal Endocarditis Caused by Strains Resistant to Components of the Standard Regimen 1

I. Ideal therapy includes a cell wall–active agent plus an effective aminoglycoside to achieve bactericidal synergy

II. Cell wall–active antimicrobial
   A. Determine MIC for ampicillin and vancomycin; test for beta-lactamase production (nitrocefin test)
   B. If ampicillin and vancomycin susceptible, use ampicillin
   C. If ampicillin resistant (MIC ≥ 16 μg/ml) and vancomycin susceptible, use vancomycin
   D. If beta-lactamase produced, use vancomycin or consider ampicillin-sulbactam
   E. If ampicillin resistant and vancomycin resistant (MIC ≥ 16 μg/ml), consider teicoplanin*
   F. If ampicillin resistant and highly resistant to vancomycin and teicoplanin (MIC ≥ 256 μg/ml), see IV C, D

III. Aminoglycoside to be used with cell wall–active antimicrobial
   A. If no high-level resistance to streptomycin (MIC < 2000 μg/ml) or gentamicin (MIC < 500-2000 μg/ml), use gentamicin or streptomycin
   B. If high-level resistance to gentamicin (MIC > 500-2000 μg/ml), test streptomycin. If no high-level resistance to streptomycin, use streptomycin
   C. If high-level resistance to gentamicin and streptomycin, omit aminoglycoside therapy; use prolonged therapy (8-12 wk) with cell wall–active antimicrobial if the organism is susceptible (see II A-E) or alternative therapy (see IV C, D)

IV. Alternative regimens and approaches
   A. Single-drug therapy (see III C) and surgical intervention
   B. Consider ampicillin, vancomycin (or teicoplanin), and gentamicin (or streptomycin) based on absence of high-level resistance
   C. Consider quinupristin/dalfopristin therapy for infective endocarditis caused by susceptible *Enterococcus faecium* and surgical intervention
   D. Consider linezolid therapy with or without surgical intervention
   E. Treatment with fluoroquinolones, rifampin, or trimethoprim-sulfamethoxazole of questionable efficacy
   F. Daptomycin active in vitro against vancomycin resistant enterococci but no clinical data for this entity

MIC = minimum inhibitory concentration.

*Not approved by the Food and Drug Administration for use in the United States; may be available by compassionate-use protocol.

concentrations of the cell wall-active agent or highly resistant to the aminoglycosides, synergy and optimal therapy cannot be obtained with a standard regimen that includes the inactive antimicrobial. Furthermore, high-level resistance to gentamicin predicts resistance to all other aminoglycosides except streptomycin. These susceptibility data allow selection of a bactericidal synergistic regimen, if one is possible, or alternative treatment (see Table 58-9).[46]

STAPHYLOCOCCI. More than 90 percent of coagulase-positive and coagulase-negative staphylococci are penicillin resistant. Methicillin resistance is common among coagulase-negative staphylococci and is increasingly frequent among *S. aureus*. Methicillin-resistant strains are resistant to all beta-lactam antibiotics but usually remain susceptible to vancomycin. Rare staphylococci have reduced susceptibility or resistance to vancomycin. Among staphylococci killed by cell wall–active antibiotics, the bactericidal effects of these agents can be enhanced by aminoglycosides. Combinations of semisynthetic penicillinase-resistant penicillins or vancomycin with rifampin do not result in predictable bactericidal synergism; nevertheless, rifampin has unique activity against staphylococcal infections that involve foreign material.[18] Staphylococcal infections involving prosthetic heart valves are treated differently from NVE caused by the same species (Table 58–10).[18,30,75]

STAPHYLOCOCCAL NATIVE VALVE ENDOCARDITIS. The semisynthetic penicillinase-resistant penicillins are the cornerstones of the treatment of endocarditis caused by methicillin-susceptible staphylococci. When patients have a penicillin allergy that does not induce urticaria or anaphylaxis, a first-generation cephalosporin can be used. The synergistic interaction of beta-lactam antibiotics with an aminoglycoside has not increased the cure rates for staphylococcal endocarditis; however, treatment with these combinations has modestly accelerated the eradication of staphylococci in vegetations and from the blood. To achieve this potential benefit, gentamicin may be added to beta-lactam antibiotic therapy for *S. aureus* during the initial 3 to 5 days of treatment.[75] More prolonged administration of gentamicin has been associated with nephrotoxicity and should be avoided. The role for combination therapy is less well defined in NVE caused by coagulase-negative staphylococci; pooled data suggest improved cure rates with combination therapy.[30]

In IV drug addicts, methicillin-susceptible *S. aureus* endocarditis that is uncomplicated and limited to the right heart valves has been effectively treated with 2 weeks of semisynthetic penicillinase-resistant penicillin (but not vancomycin) plus an aminoglycoside (doses as noted in Table 58-10). However, some patients with right-sided *S. aureus* during the initial week of treatment develop signs suggesting left-sided infection; these patients are not candidates for abbreviated therapy.

Endocarditis caused by methicillin-resistant staphylococci requires treatment with vancomycin (see Table 58-10). Trimethoprim-sulfamethoxazole treatment of right-sided endocarditis caused by *S. aureus* susceptible to this antimicrobial has been only moderately successful. Truly suitable alternatives to vancomycin are not available. Methicillin-resistant staphylococci are usually susceptible to linezolid and daptomycin; however, experience using either agent for treatment of endocarditis is limited. Teicoplanin, a glycopeptide antibiotic similar to vancomycin but not available in the United States, has been considered a possible alternative; however, some strains of *S. aureus* have become resistant to teicoplanin.[79]

Teicoplanin is initiated at a dose of 6 mg/kg twice daily for 3 to 4 days until a trough serum concentration of 20 to 30 μg/ml is achieved; thereafter, for optimal results this trough concentration should be maintained using a daily 10 mg/kg dose. If the methicillin-resistant strain is susceptible to gentamicin, the aminoglycoside can be used in combination with vancomycin to enhance activity against these organisms. However, the frequency of renal toxicity may also be increased by this combination. The addition of rifampin to vancomycin for treatment of methicillin-resistant *S. aureus* NVE has not been beneficial. Right-sided endocarditis caused by methicillin-resistant *S. aureus* is not treated with a 2-week regimen.

STAPHYLOCOCCAL PROSTHETIC VALVE ENDOCARDITIS. Staphylococcal infections of prosthetic heart valves should be treated with three antibiotics in combination. Rifampin provides unique antistaphylococcal activity when infection involves foreign bodies. However, rifampin-resistant staphylococci rapidly emerge when rifampin is used alone or in combination with vancomycin or beta-lactam antibiotics to treat staphylococcal PVE.[18] Consequently, staphylococcal PVE is treated with two antimicrobials plus rifampin.[18] I prefer to delay rifampin therapy briefly until treatment with two effective antistaphylococcal agents has been administered for 48 hours.

For PVE caused by methicillin-resistant staphylococci, treatment is initiated with vancomycin plus gentamicin, with rifampin added if the organism is susceptible to gentamicin. If the organism is resistant to gentamicin, an alternative aminoglycoside to which the organism is susceptible should be sought. Alternatively, if the organism is resistant to all aminoglycosides, a quinolone to which it is susceptible may be used in lieu of an aminoglycoside.[18] For treatment of PVE caused by methicillin-susceptible staphylococci, a semisyn-

TABLE 58–10 Treatment for Staphylococcal Endocarditis in the Absence of Prosthetic Material

Antibiotic	Dosage and Route*	Duration
Methicillin-susceptible staphylococci†		
Nafcillin or oxacillin	2 gm IV every 4 hr	4-6 wk
With optional addition of gentamicin	1 mg/kg IM or IV every 8 hr	3-5 d
Cefazolin (or other first-generation cephalosporins in equivalent dosages)‡	2 gm IV every 8 hr	4-6 wk
With optional addition of gentamicin	1 mg/kg IM or IV every 8 hr	3-5 d
Vancomycin‡	30 mg/kg/24 hr IV in two equally divided doses, not to exceed 2 gm/24 hr unless serum levels are monitored	4-6 wk
Methicillin-resistant staphylococci		
Vancomycin	30 mg/kg/24 hr IV in two equally divided doses, not to exceed 2 gm/24 hr unless serum levels are monitored	4-6 wk

Modified from Wilson WR, Karchmer AW, Dajani AS, et al: Antibiotic treatment of adults with infective endocarditis due to streptococci, enterococci, staphylococci, and HACEK microorganisms. JAMA 274:1706, 1995. Copyright 1995 American Medical Association.

*Dosages are for patients with normal renal function. See Table 58–6, footnote.

†For treatment of endocarditis caused by penicillin-susceptible staphylococci (minimum inhibitory concentration ≤ 0.1 μg/ml), aqueous penicillin G (18-24 million units/24 hr) can be used for 4-6 wk instead of nafcillin or oxacillin.

‡Cefazolin, other first-generation cephalosporins, or vancomycin may be used in selected penicillin-allergic patients.

TABLE 58–11 Treatment of Staphylococcal Endocarditis in the Presence of a Prosthetic Valve or Other Prosthetic Material

Antibiotic	Dosage and Route*	Duration (wk)
Regimen for Methicillin-Resistant Staphylococci		
Vancomycin	30 mg/kg/24 hr IV in two equally divided doses, not to exceed 2 gm/24 hr unless serum levels are monitored	≥6
plus		
Rifampin *and* gentamicin†	300 mg PO every 8 hr 1.0 mg/kg IM or IV every 8 hr	≥6 2
Regimen for Methicillin-Susceptible Staphylococci		
Nafcillin or oxacillin	2 gm IV every 4 hr	≥6
plus		
Rifampin *and* gentamicin†	300 mg PO every 8 hr 1.0 mg/kg IM or IV every 8 hr	≥6 2

Modified from Wilson WR, Karchmer AW, Dajani AS, et al: Antibiotic treatment of adults with infective endocarditis due to streptococci, enterococci, staphylococci, and HACEK microorganisms. JAMA 274:1706, 1995. Copyright 1995 American Medical Association.

*Dosages are for patients with normal renal function. See Table 58–6, footnote.

†Use during initial 2 wk of treatment. If strain is gentamicin resistant, see text for alternatives.

TABLE 58–12 Treatment for Endocarditis Caused by HACEK Microorganisms*

Antibiotic	Dosage and Route†	Duration (wk)
Ceftriaxone‡	2 gm once daily IV or IM	4
Ampicillin	12 gm/24 hr IV given continuously or every 4 hr in six equally divided doses	4
plus		
Gentamicin	1 mg/kg IM or IV every 8 hr	4

Modified from Wilson WR, Karchmer AW, Dajani AS, et al: Antibiotic treatment of adults with infective endocarditis due to streptococci, enterococci, staphylococci, and HACEK microorganisms. JAMA 274:1706, 1995. Copyright 1995 American Medical Association.

*HACEK microorganisms are *Hemophilus parainfluenzae, Hemophilus aphrophilus, Actinobacillus actinomycetemcomitans, Cardiobacterium hominis, Eikenella corrodens*, and *Kingella* species.

†Dosages are for those with normal renal function. See Table 58–6, footnote.

‡Cefotaxime or ceftizoxime in comparable doses may be substituted for ceftriaxone.

thetic penicillinase-resistant penicillin should be substituted for vancomycin in the combination regimen (Table 58–11).

Patients with a nonimmediate penicillin allergy can be treated with a first-generation cephalosporin in lieu of the semisynthetic penicillin. PVE caused by coagulase-negative staphylococci that occurs within the initial year after valve placement is often complicated by perivalvular extension of infection, and valve replacement surgery is often required to eradicate infection and maintain suitable valve function.[18] Patients with *S. aureus* PVE have frequent intracardiac complications and exceptionally high mortality rates. Cure of *S. aureus* PVE is significantly more likely if early surgical intervention is combined with appropriate combination antimicrobial therapy.[80,81]

***HEMOPHILUS PARAINFLUENZAE, HEMOPHILUS APHROPHILUS, ACTINOBACILLUS ACTINOMYCETEMCOMITANS, CARDIOBACTERIUM HOMINIS, EIKENELLA CORRODENS,* AND *KINGELLA KINGAE* (HACEK ORGANISMS).** Endocarditis caused by the HACEK group has in the past been treated with ampicillin administered alone or in combination with gentamicin. Occasional HACEK organisms that are ampicillin resistant by virtue of beta-lactamase production have been isolated. Given the marked susceptibility of both beta-lactamase–producing and non-beta-lactamase-producing HACEK strains to third-generation cephalosporins, ceftriaxone or a comparable third-generation cephalosporin is recommended for treatment of NVE or PVE caused by these organisms (Table 58-12).[75] For endocarditis caused by strains that do not produce beta-lactamase, ampicillin combined with gentamicin can be used in lieu of ceftriaxone (see Table 58-12).

OTHER PATHOGENS. Antimicrobial therapy for patients with IE caused by unusual organisms is based on limited clinical experience and data from animal models and in vitro studies. Amphotericin at full doses, often combined with 5-fluorocytosine, is recommended for treatment of *Candida* endocarditis. Several patients with *Candida* NVE and PVE without intracardiac complications are reported to have been cured by prolonged treatment with fluconazole.[82] Nevertheless, surgical intervention shortly after beginning amphotericin treatment remains the standard treatment for *Candida* endocarditis.[41,83] Prolonged or indefinite fluconazole administration has been advocated for patients treated either medically or surgically.[82,83] Although they have been used infrequently to treat IE, liposomal formulations of amphotericin may be useful because they are less toxic than amphotericin desoxycholate. New echinocandin and azole agents may also offer alternatives for acute and suppressive therapy.

The antimicrobial susceptibility of corynebacteria causing endocarditis must be carefully evaluated. Many remain susceptible to penicillin, vancomycin, and aminoglycosides. Strains susceptible to aminoglycosides are killed synergistically by penicillin in combination with an aminoglycoside. *C. jeikeium,* although often resistant to penicillin and aminoglycosides, is killed by vancomycin. NVE or PVE caused by *Corynebacterium* species can be treated with the combination of penicillin plus an aminoglycoside or vancomycin, contingent on the susceptibilities of the causative strain.

The Enterobacteriaceae (*Escherichia coli* and *Klebsiella, Enterobacter, Serratia,* and *Proteus* species) are highly susceptible to third-generation cephalosporins, imipenem, and aztreonam. One of these antimicrobial agents in high doses is combined with an aminoglycoside to treat IE caused by Enterobacteriaceae.

C. burnetii IE is difficult to eradicate. Prolonged therapy (at least 4 years) using doxycycline (100 mg twice daily) or another tetracycline combined with a quinolone has been advocated. Treatment with doxycycline combined with hydroxychloroquine for 18 to 48 months (mean 31 months, median 26 months) may be more effective than longer courses of doxycycline plus a quinolone.[34,84] Surgery is important in effective treatment.

CULTURE-NEGATIVE ENDOCARDITIS. Special studies to diagnose IE caused by fastidious bacteria and other organisms must be performed (see Diagnosis). Thereafter, unless clinical or epidemiological clues suggest an etiological diagnosis, the recommended treatment for culture-negative NVE is ampicillin plus gentamicin (see standard regimen for enterococcal endocarditis, Table 58–8); because in the absence of confounding antibiotic therapy enterococci and staphylococci are unlikely causes of culture-negative NVE, ceftriaxone could be used in this regimen instead of ampicillin. For patients with culture-negative PVE, vancomycin is added to this regimen.[18] Mortality rates are lower for patients who have culture-negative endocarditis and who had received antibiotics before blood cultures were obtained and those who become afebrile during the initial week of antimicrobial treatment.[85] Marantic endocarditis should be carefully considered when treating patients for culture-negative IE. Surgical intervention should be considered for those who do not fully respond to empirical antimicrobial therapy. If surgical intervention is undertaken, a detailed microbiological and pathological examination of excised material must be performed to establish an etiologic diagnosis.

TIMING THE INITIATION OF ANTIMICROBIAL THERAPY. Current cost-containment pressures frequently result in initiation of antimicrobial therapy for suspected endocarditis immediately after blood cultures have been obtained. This practice is appropriate in the treatment of patients with acute IE that is highly destructive and rapidly progressive and of patients presenting with hemodynamic decompensation requiring urgent or emergent surgical intervention. Immediate therapy may have a favorable impact on outcome in these patients. In contrast, precipitous initiation of therapy in hemodynamically stable patients with suspected subacute endocarditis does not prevent early complications and may, by compromising subsequent blood cultures, obscure the etiological diagnosis of endocarditis. In the latter patients, it is prudent to delay antibiotic therapy briefly pending the results of the initial blood cultures. If these cultures are not positive promptly, this delay provides an important opportunity to obtain additional blood cultures without the confounding effect of empirical treatment. This opportunity is particularly important when patients have received antibiotics recently.

MONITORING THERAPY FOR ENDOCARDITIS. Patients must be carefully monitored during therapy and for several months thereafter. Failure of antimicrobial therapy, myocardial or metastatic abscess, emboli, hypersensitivity to antimicrobial agents, and other complications of therapy (catheter-related infection, thrombophlebitis) or intercurrent illness may be manifested by persistent or recurrent fever. Adverse reactions occur in 33 percent of patients treated for IE with beta-lactam antimicrobials, especially penicillin and ampicillin. The reactions include fever, rash, and neutropenia; they are increasingly frequent after 15 days of therapy.[86] Clinical events may indicate a need for potentially life-saving revision of antimicrobial therapy or adjunctive surgical therapy.

The serum concentration of vancomycin or aminoglycosides should be measured periodically. Periodic measurement allows dose adjustment to ensure optimal therapy and avoid adverse events. In addition, renal function should be monitored in patients receiving these two antimicrobials, and the complete blood count should be checked at least weekly in patients receiving high-dose beta-lactam antibiotics or vancomycin.

Repeated blood cultures should be obtained during the initial days of therapy or if fever persists to determine whether the bacteremia has been controlled. In patients with recrudescent fever after treatment, prompt cultures are essential to assess possible relapse of endocarditis.

OUTPATIENT ANTIMICROBIAL THERAPY. Technical advances allowing safe administration of complex antimicrobial regimens, combined with well-developed home care systems that provide supplies and monitor outpatient treatment, make it feasible to treat patients with endocarditis on an outpatient basis. Doing so can significantly reduce the cost of therapy. However, only patients who have responded to initial therapy and are free of fever, who are not experiencing threatening complications, who will be compliant with therapy, and who have a home situation that is physically suitable should be considered for outpatient treatment. Because most threatening complications of IE occur during the initial 2 weeks of therapy, some have suggested that treatment during this period be administered in the inpatient setting or an outpatient setting that provides daily physician oversight.[87] Furthermore, patients being treated at home must be apprised of the potential complications of endocarditis, instructed to seek advice promptly when encountering unexpected or untoward clinical events, and have assiduous clinical and laboratory monitoring. Finally, outpatient therapy must not result in compromises of antimicrobial therapy leading to suboptimal treatment.

Surgical Treatment of Intracardiac Complications

Cardiac surgical intervention has an increasingly important role in the treatment of intracardiac complications of endocarditis. Retrospective data suggest that mortality is unacceptably high when these complications are treated with antibiotics alone, whereas mortality is reduced when treatment combines antibiotics and surgical intervention.[46,88,89,89a] Accordingly, these complications have become indications for cardiac surgery (Table 58–13).

TABLE 58–13 Cardiac Surgery in Patients with Infective Endocarditis

Indications
Moderate to severe congestive heart failure caused by valve dysfunction
Unstable prosthesis, prosthesis orifice obstructed
Uncontrolled infection despite optimal antimicrobial therapy
Unavailable effective antimicrobial therapy: endocarditis caused by fungi, *Brucellae, Pseudomonas aeruginosa* (aortic or mitral valves)
Staphylococcus aureus PVE with an intracardiac complication
Relapse of PVE after optimal therapy
Fistula to pericardial sac
Relative Indications*
Perivalvular extension of infection, intracardiac fistula, myocardial abscess with persistent fever
Poorly responsive *S. aureus* NVE (aortic or mitral valves)
Relapse of NVE after optimal antimicrobial therapy
Culture-negative NVE or PVE with persistent fever (≥10 d)
Large (>10 mm diameter) hypermobile vegetation (with or without prior arterial embolus)
Endocarditis caused by highly antibiotic-resistant enterococci

NVE = native valve endocarditis; PVE = prosthetic valve endocarditis.
*Surgery commonly required for optimal outcome.

VALVULAR DYSFUNCTION. Medical therapy of NVE that is complicated by moderate to severe (New York Heart Association [NYHA] Class III and IV) CHF related to new or worsening valvular dysfunction results in mortality rates of 50 to 90 percent. Survival rates for a similar group of patients treated with antibiotics and cardiac surgery are 60 to 80 percent.[46,88] Although survival rates among surgically treated patients with PVE complicated by valvular dysfunction and CHF are 45 to 85 percent, few PVE patients with these complications are alive at 6 months when treated with antibiotics alone.[17-19] Worsening aortic valve incompetence is associated with more severe and more rapidly progressive CHF than is mitral valve incompetence. Hence, patients with aortic valve endocarditis not only account for the majority of surgically treated patients but also require surgery on a more urgent basis when heart failure supervenes. Severe mitral valve insufficiency, nevertheless, results in inexorable heart failure and ultimately requires surgical intervention. Doppler echocardiography and color flow mapping indicating significant valvular regurgitation during the initial week of endocarditis treatment do not reliably predict the patients who require valve replacement during active endocarditis. Alternatively, despite the absence of significant valvular regurgitation on early echocardiography, marked CHF may still develop. Thus, decisions about surgical intervention should be made by integrating clinical data and echocardiographic findings obtained during careful serial monitoring. On occasion, very large vegetations on the mitral valve, particularly a mitral valve prosthesis, result in significant obstruction and require surgery.[18]

UNSTABLE PROSTHESES. Dehiscence of an infected prosthetic valve is a manifestation of perivalvular infection and often results in hemodynamically significant valvular dysfunction. Surgical intervention is recommended for PVE patients with these complications.[18] The risk of invasive infection is increased among patients with onset of PVE within the year after valve implantation and those with infection of an aortic valve prosthesis. Endocarditis in these patients is often caused by invasive antimicrobial-resistant organisms; consequently, the benefit of combined medical-surgical therapy is enhanced further. Patients who appear clinically stable but who have overtly unstable and hypermobile prostheses, a finding indicative of dehiscence in excess of 40 percent of the circumference, are likely to experience progressive valve instability and warrant surgical treatment. Occasional patients with PVE caused by noninvasive, highly antibiotic-susceptible organisms, e.g., streptococci, despite a favorable clinical course during antibiotic therapy, late in treatment experience minor valve dehiscence without prosthesis instability or hemodynamic deterioration. Surgical treatment of these patients can be deferred unless clear indications arise.

UNCONTROLLED INFECTION OR UNAVAILABLE EFFECTIVE ANTIMICROBIAL THERAPY. Surgical intervention has improved the outcome of several forms of endocarditis when maximal antibiotic therapy fails to eradicate infection or, in some instances, even to suppress bacteremia. Amphotericin B is inadequate therapy for fungal endocarditis, including that caused by *Candida* species, and surgical intervention is recommended shortly after initiation of full doses of antifungal therapy. Endocarditis caused by some gram-negative bacilli, e.g., *P. aeruginosa*, *Achromobacter xylosoxidans*, may not be eradicated by maximum tolerable antibiotic therapy and may require surgical excision of the infected tissue to achieve cure. Similarly, standard therapy of endocarditis caused by *Brucella* species includes surgery because medical therapy is rarely successful.[61] Surgical intervention is recommended when patients with enterococcal endocarditis caused by a strain resistant to synergistic bactericidal therapy do not respond to initial therapy or relapse. Perivalvular invasive infection is in some instances a form of ineradicable infection. Relapse of PVE after optimal antimicrobial therapy reflects invasive disease or the difficulty in eradicating infection involving foreign devices. Patients with relapse of PVE are treated surgically.[28] In contrast, patients with NVE that relapses, unless it is associated with a highly resistant microorganism or demonstrable perivalvular infection, are often treated again with an intensified, prolonged course of antimicrobial therapy.

***S. AUREUS* PROSTHETIC VALVE ENDOCARDITIS.** Among 129 patients who had *S. aureus* PVE and who were culled from large retrospective general series of PVE, the crude mortality rate for those treated with antibiotics alone and with antibiotics plus surgery was 73 and 25 percent, respectively.[31,81,90,91] Although management strategy is undoubtedly distorted by selection bias—the most ill patients often being denied surgery—the outcomes are alarming. The overall mortality rate in 33 cases of *S. aureus* PVE treated at a single institution was 42 percent.[81] In the latter cases, when a multivariate model was used for analysis to adjust for confounding variables, the presence of intracardiac complications was associated with a 13.7-fold increased risk of death, and surgical intervention during active disease was accompanied by a 20-fold reduction in mortality. These findings do not change when the data are restricted to patients surviving a week of treatment (to correct for rejection from surgery because of imminent death) and reanalyzed. These data suggest that surgical treatment can improve outcome. Although the occurrence of central nervous system emboli is often considered to limit the opportunity for surgical intervention, in fact, appropriately timed surgery remains the preferred treatment. Thus, surgical intervention is recommended for *S. aureus* PVE with intracardiac complication and may benefit even patients with uncomplicated *S. aureus* PVE.[18,81,90]

PERIVALVULAR INVASIVE INFECTION. NVE at the aortic site and PVE are most commonly associated with perivalvular invasion with abscess or intracardiac fistula formation.[18] Invasive infection occurs in 10 to 14 percent of patients with NVE and 45 to 60 percent of those with PVE.[18] Persistent, otherwise unexplained fever despite appropriate antimicrobial therapy or pericarditis in patients with aortic valve endocarditis suggests infection extending beyond the valve leaflet. New-onset and persistent electrocardiographic conduction abnormalities, although not a sensitive indicator of perivalvular infection (28 to 53 percent), are relatively specific (85 to 90 percent).[92,93] TEE is superior to TTE for detecting invasive infection in patients with NVE and PVE. Doppler and color flow Doppler or contrast two-dimensional echocardiography optimally defines fistulas. Abscesses suspected but not detected by initial and repeated TEE may be detected by magnetic resonance imaging, including magnetic resonance angiography. Cardiac catheterization adds little to these imaging studies and is not recommended unless coronary angiography is needed.

In patients with endocarditis complicated by perivalvular extension of infection, cardiac surgery should be considered to débride invasive infection, ablate abscesses, and reconstruct anatomical damage. Surgery is warranted in patients with invasive disease that significantly disrupts cardiac structures, that is associated with CHF, that results in instability of a prosthetic valve, or that renders infection uncontrolled (persistent fever). However, it is likely that increasingly sensitive imaging techniques will elucidate invasive infections that do not require immediate surgery. Sporadic case reports of medically treated invasive infection suggest that these infections will be small, structurally nonsignificant abscesses in which the cavity is open to the circulatory stream.

LEFT-SIDED *S. AUREUS* ENDOCARDITIS. Because this infection is difficult to control, highly destructive, and associated with high mortality (25 to 47 percent), some investigators have suggested that these patients should be considered for surgical treatment when the response to antimicrobial therapy is not prompt and complete.[89] Also, patients with *S. aureus* NVE (aortic or mitral valve) and vegetations that are visible by TTE are at increased risk for arterial emboli and death and should be considered for surgery.[32] In contrast, IV drug abusers with *S. aureus* endocarditis limited to the tricuspid or pulmonary valves often experience prolonged fever during antimicrobial therapy; nevertheless, the vast majority of these patients respond to antimicrobial therapy and do not require surgery.

UNRESPONSIVE CULTURE-NEGATIVE ENDOCARDITIS. Patients who have culture-negative endocarditis and who experience unexplained persistent fever during empirical antimicrobial therapy, particularly those with PVE, should be considered for surgical intervention. If endocarditis is not marantic, persistent fever in these patients is likely to represent either unrecognized perivalvular infection or ineffective antimicrobial therapy. Causative organisms can be seen or cultured from valve-vegetation specimens in 40 to 70 percent of these patients.[91] Molecular techniques can identify additional pathogens.[65]

LARGE VEGETATIONS (>10 MM) AND THE PREVENTION OF SYSTEMIC EMBOLI. Although it was not demonstrated in all studies, in pooled data and meta-analysis, systemic embolization was increased in patients with vegetations greater than 10 mm versus those with smaller or no detectable vegetations, 33 to 37 percent versus 19 percent.[94] Larger mitral valve vegetations (>10 mm), particularly those on the anterior mitral valve leaflet, and vegetation mobility are uniquely associated with systemic emboli.[52,94-96] Although a relationship may exist between vegetation characteristics—including size, mobility, and extent (number of leaflets involved)—and embolic complications, the implications for surgical intervention are not clear. Yet to be performed are analyses examining embolic complications or outcome and vegetation characteristics but adjusted for valve dysfunction, perivalvular invasion by infection, organism, and infection site. Nevertheless, some researchers have concluded that vegetation characteristics alone might warrant surgery to prevent arterial emboli. This recommendation can be questioned, as can the recommendation for valve surgery after two major arterial emboli.[61]

In deciding to intervene with cardiac surgery to prevent arterial emboli, many factors must be considered carefully. The rate of systemic or cerebral emboli in patients with NVE and PVE decreases during the course of effective antibiotic therapy.[55,97] Also, it is not clear that surgical intervention reduces the frequency of systemic emboli.[46] Finally, the risks of morbidity and mortality caused by cerebral and coronary emboli, the major events to be prevented, must be compared with the immediate and long-term risks of valve replacement surgery or, if feasible, vegetectomy and valve repair. These risks include perioperative mortality, recrudescent endocarditis on the prosthesis, thromboembolic complications, early and late valve dysfunction requiring repeated valve replacement, the hazards of warfarin anticoagulation (including its contraindication during pregnancy), and the risk and morbidity of late-onset PVE.[85] Vegetation size alone is rarely an indication for surgery. The clinical findings and echocardiographic evidence for other intracardiac complications must be weighed against the immediate and remote hazards of cardiac surgery, including the possibility of valve preservation by vegetectomy and valve repair, when recommending therapy.[61] Thus, the risk for systemic embolization as related to vegetation size or prior systemic embolus is not an independent indication for surgical intervention but is only one of many factors to be considered when planning treatment.[55,61,97]

Repair of Intracardiac Defects

TECHNIQUES. New surgical techniques to address severe tissue destruction in NVE and PVE have been developed. Although these are beyond the scope of this discussion, examples include valve composite graft replacement of the aortic root, use of sewing skirts attached to the prostheses, and homograft replacement of the aortic valve and root with coronary artery reimplantation. Furthermore, repair of the mitral valve in patients with acute or healed endocarditis avoids the need for insertion of prosthetic materials and the associated hazards. Although tricuspid valvulectomy without valve replacement has been advocated for treatment of uncontrolled tricuspid valve infection in IV drug abusers at high risk for recidivism and recurrent endocarditis, the likelihood of refractory right-sided heart failure with time after valvulectomy makes tricuspid valve repair preferable. Cardiac transplantation has been used to salvage an occasional patient with refractory endocarditis.

TIMING OF SURGICAL INTERVENTION. When endocarditis is complicated by valvular regurgitation and significant impairment of cardiac function, surgical intervention before the development of severe intractable hemodynamic dysfunction is recommended, regardless of the duration of antimicrobial therapy.[98] Postoperative mortality correlates with the severity of preoperative hemodynamic dysfunction; consequently, this approach is justified.[94] In patients who have valvular dysfunction and in whom infection is controlled and cardiac function is compensated, surgery may be delayed until antimicrobial therapy has been completed. If infection is not controlled, surgery should be performed promptly. Similarly, if a patient who requires valve replacement in the near future has a large vegetation, indicating a high risk for systemic embolization, early cardiac surgery is appropriate (see Large Vegetations and the Prevention of Systemic Emboli).

More specific recommendations for timing of surgery have been presented.[88] Strong clinical evidence suggested emergent (same day) surgery for acute aortic regurgitation with mitral valve preclosure, sinus of Valsalva rupture into the right heart, and fistula to the pericardial sac; urgent (1 to 2 days) surgery for valve obstruction, unstable prosthesis, acute aortic or mitral regurgitation with heart failure (NYHA Class III to IV), septal perforation, perivalvular extension of infection, and no effective antimicrobial therapy; and early elective surgery for progressive paravalvular regurgitation, valve dysfunction and persistent fever, and fungal (mold or complicated yeast) IE.

To avoid worsening of neurological status or death in patients who have sustained recent neurological injury, the timing of surgical intervention may require modification. Among patients who have had a nonhemorrhagic embolic stroke, exacerbation of cerebral dysfunction occurs during cardiac surgery in 44 percent of cases when the interval between the stroke and surgery is 7 days or less, in 17 percent when the interval is 8 to 14 days, and in 10 percent or less when more than 2 weeks has elapsed. After hemorrhagic intracerebral events, the risk for neurological worsening or death with cardiac surgery persists at 20 percent even after 1 month.[99] Thus, when the response of IE to antimicrobial therapy and hemodynamic status permit, delaying cardiac surgery for 2 to 3 weeks after a significant embolic infarct and at least a month after intracerebral hemorrhage (with prior repair of a mycotic aneurysm) has been recommended.[99,100]

DURATION OF ANTIMICROBIAL THERAPY AFTER SURGICAL INTERVENTION. Inflammatory changes and bacteria visible with Gram stain have been found in vegetations removed from patients who received most or all of the standard antibiotic therapy recommended for endocarditis caused by a specific microorganism. In fact, in patients who had successfully completed standard recommended antibiotic therapy for IE—29 of 53 (55 percent) still taking antibiotics, 7 of 15 (47 percent) without antibiotics for less than a month, and 4 of 18 (22 percent) without antibiotics for 1 to 6 months—the valve or vegetation removed surgically contained visible bacteria on Gram stain or histological examination. Cultures of these valves or vegetations yielded bacteria in 5, 0, and 1 instance, respectively.[91] If valve cultures are negative, visible bacteria do not indicate that antimicrobial therapy has failed or that a full course of antibiotic therapy is needed postoperatively. The duration of antimicrobial therapy after surgery depends on the length of preoperative therapy, the antibiotic susceptibility of the causative organism, the presence of paravalvular invasive infection, and the culture status of the vegetation. In general, for endocarditis caused by relatively antibiotic-responsive organisms with negative cultures of operative specimens, preoperative plus postoperative therapy should at least equal a full course of recommended therapy; for patients with prostheses sewn into a débrided abscess cavity or with positive intraoperative cultures, a full course of therapy should be given postoperatively. Patients with PVE should receive a full course of antimicrobial therapy postoperatively when organisms are seen in resected material.[18]

Treatment of Extracardiac Complications

SPLENIC ABSCESS. Three to 5 percent of patients with IE develop a splenic abscess.[50] Although splenic defects can be identified by ultrasonography and computed tomography, these tests usually cannot reliably discriminate between abscess and infarct. Persistent fever and progressive enlargement of the lesion during antimicrobial therapy suggest that it is an abscess, which can be confirmed by percutaneous needle aspiration. Successful therapy of splenic abscesses generally requires drainage, which can sometimes be accomplished by percutaneous placement of a catheter. In patients with numerous splenic abscesses or in whom percutaneous drainage is unsuccessful, splenectomy is required.[61] Splenic abscesses should be treated effectively before valve replacement surgery. If they are not treated effectively before cardiac surgery, splenectomy should be performed as soon thereafter as surgical risks permit.[61]

MYCOTIC ANEURYSMS AND SEPTIC ARTERITIS. From 2 to 10 percent of patients with endocarditis have mycotic aneurysms; in 1 to 5 percent, the aneurysms involve cerebral vessels. Cerebral mycotic aneurysms occur at the branch points in cerebral vessels, are generally located distally over the cerebral cortex, and are found most commonly in branches of the middle cerebral artery. The aneurysms arise either from occlusion of vessels by septic emboli with secondary arteritis and vessel wall destruction or from bacteremic seeding of the vessel wall through the vasa vasorum. *S. aureus* is commonly implicated in the former and viridans streptococci in the latter.[58] Many patients with mycotic aneurysms or septic arteritis present with devastating intracranial hemorrhage. Focal deficits from embolic events, persistent focal headache, unexplained neurological deterioration or focal neurological abnormalities, or sterile meningeal irritation (cerebrospinal fluid pleocytosis) may be premonitory symptoms. Cerebral angiography is required to evaluate patients with subarachnoid hemorrhage, and this or magnetic resonance or spiral computed tomographic angiography has been recommended for patients experiencing premonitory symptoms, especially if cardiac surgery or anticoagulant therapy is planned.[61] Although rupture may occur at any point before or during antibiotic therapy, aneurysms that leak or rupture do so most commonly before or during early treatment.

Mycotic aneurysms may resolve during antimicrobial therapy[61]; however, when anatomically feasible, aneurysms that have ruptured should be repaired surgically.[101] Aneurysms that have not leaked should be monitored angiographically during antimicrobial therapy. Surgery should be considered for a single lesion that enlarges during or after antimicrobial therapy. Anticoagulant therapy should be avoided in patients with a persisting mycotic aneurysm. On rare occasions, persistent stable aneurysms may rupture after completion of standard antimicrobial therapy; however, there is no accurate estimation of risk for late rupture, and recommendations for surgical intervention are arbitrary. Nevertheless, prevailing opinion favors, whenever possible without serious neurological injury, the resection of single aneurysms that persist after therapy.[101] The potential existence of occult aneurysms in patients without neurological symptoms or in those who have had a nondiagnostic angiographic evaluation is not considered a contraindication to anticoagulant therapy after completion of antimicrobial therapy.

Extracranial mycotic aneurysms should be managed as outlined for cerebral aneurysms. Those that leak, are expanding during therapy, or persist after therapy should be repaired. Particular attention should be given to aneurysms that involve intraabdominal arteries, rupture of which could result in life-threatening hemorrhage.[61]

ANTICOAGULANT THERAPY. Patients with PVE involving devices that would usually warrant maintenance anticoagulation are continued on anticoagulant therapy.[18] Anticoagulation is not initiated as prophylaxis against IE-related thromboembolism in either patients with PVE involving devices that do not usually require this therapy or patients with NVE. Neither aspirin nor anticoagulant therapy has been shown to prevent embolization, and either might contribute to intracranial hemorrhage, particularly in the presence of a recent cerebral infarct or a mycotic aneurysm. Anticoagulant therapy in patients with NVE is limited to patients for whom there is a clear indication for this therapy and for whom there is not a known increased risk for intracranial hemorrhage. If central nervous system complications occur in patients who have IE and who are receiving anticoagulant therapy, anticoagulation should be reversed immediately.[18]

Response to Therapy

Within a week after initiation of effective antimicrobial therapy, almost 75 percent of patients with IE, including those with PVE, are afebrile and 90 percent have defervesced by the end of the second week of treatment.[18,46,97,102] The duration of fever during therapy is longer in patients with IE related to *S. aureus* or *P. aeruginosa* and culture-negative IE as well as IE characterized by microvascular phenomena and major embolic complications.[46,102] Persistence or recurrence of fever more than 7 to 10 days after initiation of antibiotic therapy identified patients with increased mortality rates and with complications of infection or therapy.[18,102] Patients with prolonged or recurrent fever should be evaluated for intracardiac complications, focal extracardiac septic complications, intercurrent nosocomial infections, recurrent pulmonary emboli (patients with right-sided IE), drug-associated fever, additional underlying illnesses, and, if appropriate, in-hospital substance abuse.

Blood cultures should be repeated in search of persistent bacteremia or the presence of additional pathogens, e.g., previously unrecognized polymicrobial IE. The antimicrobial susceptibility of the causative organism should be reevaluated, as should the adequacy of antibiotic therapy. Drug reactions have accounted for fever in 17 to 28 percent of these patients. Drug fever attributed to the antimicrobial therapy itself may warrant revision of treatment if a suitable alternative is available. In the absence of effective alternative therapy, treatment can be continued despite drug fever if the antimicrobial is not causing significant end-organ toxicity. In 33 to 45 percent of patients, persistent fever was associated with significant intracardiac complications, many of which required surgical intervention.[102]

Many clinical and laboratory features of IE are slow to resolve despite effective antimicrobial therapy. Systemic emboli occur during the early weeks of treatment, although with decreasing frequency.[55] The increased ESR and anemia may not be corrected until after therapy has been completed.

Mortality rates for large series of patients with NVE treated between 1975 and 1993 ranged from 16 to 27 percent.[1,91] Death from IE has been associated with increased age (>65 to 70 years old), underlying diseases, infection involving the aortic valve, development of CHF, renal failure, and central nervous system complications.[1,102a] The treatment of heart failure related to valve dysfunction by early surgical intervention has decreased the mortality associated with CHF, but subsequent neurological events and septic complications, e.g., uncontrolled infection and myocardial abscess, have accounted for a larger proportion of deaths and have been associated with high mortality rates.[50]

Mortality rates among patients with IE caused by viridans streptococci and *S. bovis* have ranged from 4 to 16 percent.[1] Higher mortality rates are reported with left-sided NVE caused by other organisms: enterococci, 15 to 25 percent[1]; *S. aureus*, 25 to 47 percent[1,30]; nonviridans streptococci (groups B, C, and G), 13 to 50 percent[26,27]; *C. burnetii*, 5 to 37 percent[20,76,82]; *P. aeruginosa*, Enterobacteriaceae, and fungi, greater than 50 percent.[33]

In a retrospective study of patients with NVE with NYHA Class III or IV heart failure or invasive uncontrolled infection, only 9 percent of patients treated surgically died, compared with 51 percent of those treated with antibiotics alone.[46] Mortality rates among patients with active NVE who were treated surgically have ranged from 5 to 26 percent.[103-107] Severity of heart failure, abscess, *S. aureus* infection, and decreased renal function (possibly related to heart failure) have been associated with increased postoperative mortality.[105] Nevertheless, survival rates of 85 percent can be achieved when patients with paravalvular abscesses undergo meticulous débridement and reconstructive cardiac surgery.[108]

In a large retrospective study of patients with complicated left-sided NVE, the mortality rate was 25 percent, and in a multivariate analysis the following variables were independent predictors of mortality and could be assigned a weighted mortality risk score (discrete score): abnormal mental status (4), Charlson comorbidity score = 2 (3), moderate to severe CHF (3), bacterial etiology other than viridans streptococci (*S. aureus* = 6, other = 8), and medical therapy without valve surgery (5). The model was verified in an independent cohort and the 6-month mortality rate could be predicted by total point score: less than or equal to 6 points, 6 percent; 7 to 11 points, 17 percent; 12 to 15 points, 31 percent; more than 15 points, 63 percent.[102a,109]

Outcome for patients with PVE, as contrasted with NVE, has been less desirable. Before 1980, mortality rates among patients with onset less than 60 days after surgery and later onset PVE averaged 70 and 45 percent, respectively. With the recognition that PVE was frequently complicated by invasive infection and that patients would benefit from surgical intervention, mortality rates have decreased to 33 to 45 percent, with lower rates in later onset cases.[18,108] Long-term survival was adversely affected by the presence of moderate or severe heart failure at discharge. Survival rates after aggressive surgery for PVE ranged from 75 to 85 percent and were not related to time of onset after cardiac surgery.[19,106,107]

Among patients with NVE (nonaddicts) discharged after medical or medical-surgical therapy, long-term survival was 88 percent at 5 years and 81 percent at 10 years.[91] Among patients treated surgically for NVE, survival at 5 years ranged from 70 to 80 percent.[104,107] Among patients with PVE treated surgically, survival rates at 4 to 6 years ranged from 50 to 82 percent.[19,107]

RELAPSE AND RECURRENCE. Relapse of IE usually occurs within 2 months of discontinuing antibiotic treatment. Of patients who have NVE caused by penicillin-susceptible viridans streptococci and who receive a recommended course of therapy, less than 2 percent suffer relapse. From 8 to 20 percent of patients with enterococcal IE experience relapse after standard therapy. Patients with IE caused by *S. aureus*, Enterobacteriaceae, or fungi are more likely to experience overt failure of therapy rather than relapse; nevertheless, 4 percent of patients with *S. aureus* IE suffer relapse. Relapse of fungal endocarditis at long intervals after treatment has been reported. Relapse occurs in 10 percent of patients with PVE overall and in 6 to 15 percent of those treated surgically.

Among nonaddicts with an initial episode of NVE or PVE, 4.5 to 7 percent experience one or more additional episodes.[91] Among these patients, recurrent IE shares the clinical and microbiological features and response to therapy noted in primary episodes of IE. IV drug abuse is now the most common predisposing factor for recurrent IE (43 percent of patients).

Prevention

Viridans streptococci, a common cause of NVE and late-onset PVE, are the primary target for prophylaxis used in conjunction with procedures involving the oral cavity, respiratory tract, or esophagus. Procedures involving the genitourinary and gastrointestinal tracts commonly precede the development of enterococcal endocarditis. Accordingly, the prophylaxis for endocarditis used in conjunction with procedures involving these mucosal surfaces is targeted against enterococci. When incision and drainage of infected skin or soft tissue infections are undertaken, prophylaxis is focused on *S. aureus.*

Procedures for which IE prophylaxis is recommended or not recommended have been identified by the American Heart Association and others (see Table 58G–1).[109,110] Although prophylaxis is advised for all at-risk patients who undergo dental procedures that cause gingival bleeding, extractions are the most strongly associated with subsequent IE. Because endocarditis has been reported only rarely in association with other gastrointestinal endoscopic procedures with or without biopsy, prophylaxis is not routinely recommended in this situation. Prophylaxis is not recommended with routine cardiac catheterization or TEE.[109,110]

On the basis of their frequency among patients with endocarditis compared with the general population, lesions have been assigned to high, intermediate, low, and negligible risk categories (Table 58–14).[110-113] Rheumatic heart disease is currently a less common predisposition for IE in most of the developed countries; however, the attack rate of IE among persons with rheumatic valvular disease approaches that with prosthetic valves and suggests that these lesions also entail a high risk.

The risk of IE for patients with MVP and the resulting role of prophylaxis among these patients have been controversial. MVP has been identified frequently among patients with IE. However, the risk of endocarditis among patients with MVP and a murmur of mitral regurgitation is still relatively low. It is 5- to 10-fold higher than that in the general population but 100-fold less than that among patients with rheumatic valvular heart disease. As a result, MVP with a murmur of mitral regurgitation or mitral valve thickening and prolapse defines a patient with an intermediate risk for IE and one for whom prophylaxis against endocarditis is recommended.

GENERAL METHODS. The incidence of IE can be significantly reduced by total surgical correction of some congenital lesions that otherwise predispose patients to IE, e.g., patent ductus arteriosus, ventricular septal defect, and pulmonary stenosis.[6,112] The incidence of IE remains high among patients who have undergone surgical correction of other major congenital defects, especially those involving a stenotic aortic valve.[6] Patients with persisting as well as many corrected congenital lesions and those with acquired valvular heart disease who remain at risk for IE should be given written material about their predisposing lesion, their risk for endocarditis, and the recommended antibiotic prophylaxis.

Maintaining good oral hygiene, which decreases the frequency of bacteremia that accompanies daily activities (chewing, brushing teeth), may be a more important preventive than procedure-focused chemoprophylaxis.[111] Oral hygiene and dental health should be addressed before prosthetic valves are placed electively.

Among patients at risk for IE, some activities or procedures likely to induce bacteremia should be avoided. Oral irrigating devices, which may produce bacteremia even in patients with normal gingiva, are not recommended. Similarly, the use of central intravascular catheters and urinary catheters should be minimized. Infections associated with bacteremia must be treated promptly and if possible eradicated before the involved tissues are incised or manipulated.

CHEMOPROPHYLAXIS. The widely promulgated recommendations of antimicrobial prophylaxis for endocarditis are based on circumstantial evidence supplemented by studies of prophylaxis in animal models. Studies suggest that prophylactic antibiotics prevent endocarditis by inhibiting growth of the bacteria adherent to NBTE sufficiently to allow their subsequent complete elimination by host defenses.[110,114] Experimental studies that mimic single-dose amoxicillin prophylaxis in humans suggest that adequate margins of efficacy are present after a single prophylactic dose. Nevertheless, because a more sustained inhibitory effect can be achieved through a postprocedure dose of antibiotics, this is recommended for patients in the high-risk group.[109,115]

Clinical studies supporting the efficacy of antibiotic prophylaxis for endocarditis are limited. A retrospective study of patients who had prosthetic valves and who underwent dental and surgical procedures suggested that antibiotic prophylaxis prevented PVE. However, a large case-control study failed to identify dental procedures as a risk for IE among persons with valvular abnormalities and questioned the

TABLE 58–14 Relative Risk of Infective Endocarditis Associated with Preexisting Cardiac Disorders

Relatively High Risk	Intermediate Risk	Very Low or Negligible Risk*
Prosthetic heart valves†	Mitral valve prolapse with regurgitation (murmur) or thickened valve leaflets	Mitral valve prolapse without regurgitation (murmur) or thickened valve leaflets
Previous infective endocarditis†		
Cyanotic congenital heart disease†	Pure mitral stenosis	
Patent ductus arteriosus	Tricuspid valve disease	Trivial valvular regurgitation on echocardiography without structural abnormality
Aortic regurgitation	Pulmonary stenosis	
Aortic stenosis	Asymmetrical septal hypertrophy	
Mitral regurgitation	Bicuspid aortic valve or calcific aortic sclerosis with minimal hemodynamic abnormality	Isolated atrial septal defect (secundum)
Mitral stenosis and regurgitation		Arteriosclerotic plaques
Ventricular septal defect		Coronary artery disease
Coarctation of the aorta	Degenerative valvular disease in elderly patients	Cardiac pacemaker, implanted defibrillators
Surgically repaired intracardiac lesion with residual hemodynamic abnormality or prosthetic device	Surgically repaired intracardiac lesions with minimal or no hemodynamic abnormality, less than 6 mo after operation	Surgically repaired intracardiac lesions, with minimal or no hemodynamic abnormality, more than 6 mo after operation (atrial septal defect, ventricular septal defect, patent ductus arteriosus, pulmonary stenosis)
Surgically constructed systemic-pulmonary shunts†		
		Prior coronary bypass graft surgery
		Prior Kawasaki disease or rheumatic fever without valvular dysfunction

Adapted from Durack DT: Prevention of infective endocarditis. N Engl J Med 332:38, 1995; and Dajani AS, Taubert KA, Wilson W, et al: Prevention of bacterial endocarditis: Recommendations of the American Heart Association from the Committee on Rheumatic Fever, Endocarditis, and Kawasaki Disease, Council on Cardiovascular Disease in the Young. JAMA 277:1794, 1997. Copyright 1997 American Medical Association.

*Prophylaxis against endocarditis not recommended.

†Lesions considered at highest risk for endocarditis.

TABLE 58–15 Regimens for Prophylaxis Against Endocarditis: Use with Dental, Oral, and Upper Respiratory Tract Procedures

Setting	Regimen*
Standard regimen†	Amoxicillin 3.0 gm PO 1 hr before procedure, then 1.5 gm 6 hr after initial dose
Amoxicillin/penicillin-allergic patients	Erythromycin ethylsuccinate 800 mg, or erythromycin stearate 1.0 gm, PO 2 hr before procedure, then half the dose 6 hr after initial dose *OR* Clindamycin 300 mg PO 1 hr before procedure and 150 mg 6 hr after initial dose
Patients unable to take oral medications	Ampicillin 2.0 gm IM or IV 30 min before procedure, then either ampicillin 1.0 g IM or IV, or amoxicillin 1.5 gm PO, 6 hr after initial dose
Ampicillin/amoxicillin/penicillin-allergic patients unable to take oral medications	Clindamycin 300 mg IV 30 min before procedure, then 150 mg 6 hr after initial dose
Patients considered at highest risk and not candidates for standard regimen	Use standard regimen for genitourinary and gastrointestinal procedures
Ampicillin/amoxicillin/penicillin-allergic patients considered at highest risk	Use regimen for allergic patients undergoing genitourinary and gastrointestinal procedures

*Dosages for adults. Initial pediatric dosages are as follows: Ampicillin or amoxicillin, 50 mg/kg; clindamycin, 10 mg/kg; erythromycin ethylsuccinate or erythromycin stearate, 20 mg/kg; gentamicin, 2.0 mg/kg; and vancomycin, 20 mg/kg. Follow-up doses should be one-half the initial dose. **Total pediatric dose should not exceed total adult dose.**

†Generally recommended for patients at highest risk including those with prosthetic heart valves; physician may elect more vigorous regimens.

Adapted from Dajani AS, Bisno AL, Chung KJ, et al: Prevention of bacterial endocarditis: Recommendations of the American Heart Association. JAMA 264:2919, 1990. Copyright 1990 American Medical Association.

TABLE 58–16 Regimens for Prophylaxis Against Endocarditis: Use with Genitourinary and Gastrointestinal (Except Esophageal) Procedures

Setting	Antibiotic	Regimen*
High-risk patients	Ampicillin plus gentamicin	Ampicillin 2.0 gm IV/IM plus gentamicin 1.5 mg/kg within 30 min of procedure, repeat ampicillin 1.0 gm IV/IM or give amoxicillin 1.0 gm PO 6 hr later
High-risk, penicillin-allergic patients	Vancomycin plus gentamicin	Vancomycin 1.0 gm IV over 1-2 hr plus gentamicin 1.5 mg/kg IM/IV infused or injected 30 min before procedure. No second dose recommended
Moderate-risk patients	Amoxicillin or ampicillin	Amoxicillin 2.0 gm PO 1 hr before procedure or ampicillin 2.0 gm IM/IV 30 min before procedure
Moderate-risk, penicillin-allergic patients	Vancomycin	Vancomycin 1.0 gm IV infused over 1-2 hr and completed within 30 min of procedure

*Dosing for children: ampicillin 50 mg/kg IV/IM, vancomycin 20 mg/kg IV, gentamicin 1.5 mg/kg IV/IM (children's doses should not exceed adult doses).

Adapted from Dajani AS, Taubert KA, Wilson W, et al: Prevention of bacterial endocarditis: Recommendations by the American Heart Association from the Committee on Rheumatic Fever, Endocarditis, and Kawasaki Disease, Council on Cardiovascular Disease in the Young. JAMA 277:1794-1801, 1997.

benefit of antibiotic prophylaxis for these procedures.[116] Failures of antibiotic prophylaxis unrelated to resistant bacteria have also been noted.[110]

Risk-benefit and cost-benefit analyses have raised significant questions about antibiotic prophylaxis for patients with MVP. Unless both the cost and risks of prophylaxis are very low, the cost per case of IE prevented is high and mortality or morbidity may not be reduced. From a population perspective, prophylaxis in low- to intermediate-risk settings may not be cost or risk beneficial, and prophylaxis might be reserved for patients who have high-risk cardiac lesions and who are undergoing high-risk procedures.[116] Expert committees are currently reassessing guidelines for endocarditis prophylaxis.

Even if antibiotic prophylaxis is effective as well as safe and inexpensive, only a small percentage of the cases are preventable. For example, only 55 to 75 percent of patients with NVE have preexisting endocarditis-prone valvular disease, and many are not aware of the lesion before the onset of NVE.[110,111] In addition, among patients with IE, only a small fraction (5 percent) had both a known valve lesion and a procedure within 30 days of onset of IE that would have warranted prophylaxis.[111] Nevertheless, the morbidity and mortality associated with IE are used to justify prophylaxis (Table 58–15 shows for regimens used for dental and upper respiratory tract procedures; Table 58–16 shows regimens for genitourinary and gastrointestinal procedures) in patients who have high- and intermediate-risk cardiac lesions (see Table 58–14) and who are to undergo bacteremia-inducing procedures. Penicillin-resistant flora may emerge among patients who are receiving continuous penicillin for prevention of rheumatic fever or repetitive courses of antibiotics for serial dental procedures. Consequently, a nonpenicillin prophylaxis regimen is preferred for these patients. Initiation of prophylaxis several days before a procedure encourages the emergence of antibiotic-resistant organisms at the mucosal site and is not recommended.

REFERENCES

Epidemiology

1. van der Meer JTM, Thompson J, Valkenburg HA, Michel MF: Epidemiology of bacterial endocarditis in the Netherlands. I. Patient characteristics. Arch Intern Med 152:1863, 1992.

2. Hogevik H, Olaison L, Andersson R, et al: Epidemiologic aspects of infective endocarditis in an urban population: A 5-year prospective study. Medicine (Baltimore) 74:324-339, 1995.
3. Hoen B, Alla F, Selton-Suty C, et al: Changing profile of infective endocarditis: Results of a 1-year survey in France. JAMA 288:75, 2002.
4. Fernandez-Guerrero ML, Verdejo C, Azofra J, de Gorgolas M: Hospital-acquired infectious endocarditis not associated with cardiac surgery: An emerging problem. Clin Infect Dis 20:16, 1995.
5. Baltimore RS: Infective endocarditis in children. Pediatr Infect Dis J 11:907, 1992.
6. Morris CD, Reller MD, Menashe VD: Thirty-year incidence of infective endocarditis after surgery for congenital heart defect. JAMA 279:599, 1998.
7. Miro JM, del Rio A, Mestres CA: Infective endocarditis in intravenous drug abusers and HIV-1 infected patients. Infect Dis Clin North Am 16:273, 2002.
8. Stein A, Raoult D: Q fever endocarditis. Eur Heart J 16(Suppl B):19, 1995.
9. Raoult D, Fournier PE, Drancourt M, et al: Diagnosis of 22 new cases of *Bartonella* endocarditis. Ann Intern Med 125:646, 1996.
10. Sande MA, Lee BL, Mills J, et al: Endocarditis in intravenous drug users. *In* Kaye D (ed): Infective Endocarditis. 2nd ed. New York, Raven Press, 1992, p 345.
11. Mathew J, Addai T, Anand A, et al: Clinical features, site of involvement, bacteriologic findings, and outcome of infective endocarditis in intravenous drug users. Arch Intern Med 155:1641, 1995.
12. Pulvirenti JJ, Kerns E, Benson C, et al: Infective endocarditis in injection drug users: Importance of human immunodeficiency virus serostatus and degree of immunosuppression. Clin Infect Dis 22:40, 1996.
13. Ribera E, Miro JM, Cortes E, et al: Influence of human immunodeficiency virus 1 infection and degree of immunosuppression in the clinical characteristics and outcome of infective endocarditis in intravenous drug users. Arch Intern Med 158:2043, 1998.
14. Arvay A, Lengyel M: Incidence and risk factors of prosthetic valve endocarditis. Eur J Cardiothorac Surg 2:340, 1988.
15. Calderwood SB, Swinski LA, Waternaux CM, et al: Risk factors for the development of prosthetic valve endocarditis. Circulation 72:31, 1985.
16. Agnihotri AK, McGiffin DC, Galbraith AJ, O'Brien MF: Surgery for acquired heart disease. J Thorac Cardiovasc Surg 110:1708, 1995.
17. Karchmer AW, Longworth DL: Infections of intracardiac devices. Infect Dis Clin North Am 16:477, 2002.
18. Karchmer AW: Infections of prosthetic heart valves. *In* Waldvogel F, Bisno AL (eds): Infections Associated with Indwelling Medical Devices. Washington, DC, American Society for Microbiology, 2000, pp 145-172.
19. Lytle BW, Priest BP, Taylor PC, et al: Surgery for acquired heart disease: Surgical treatment of prosthetic valve endocarditis. J Thorac Cardiovasc Surg 111:198, 1996.
20. Chastre J, Trouillet JL: Early infective endocarditis on prosthetic valves. Eur Heart J 16(Suppl B):32, 1995.
21. Petti CA, Fowler VG Jr: *Staphylococcus aureus* bacteremia and endocarditis. Infect Dis Clin North Am 16:413, 2002.
22. Fowler VG Jr, Li J, Corey GR, et al: Role of echocardiography in evaluation of patients with *Staphylococcus aureus* bacteremia: Experience in 103 patients. J Am Coll Cardiol 30:1072, 1997.
23. Rosen AB, Fowler VG Jr, Corey GR, et al: Cost-effectiveness of transesophageal echocardiography to determine the duration of therapy for intravascular catheter-associated *Staphylococcus aureus* bacteremia. Ann Intern Med 130:810, 1999.
24. Heidenreich PA, Masoudi FA, Maini B, et al: Echocardiography in patients with suspected endocarditis: A cost-effectiveness analysis. Am J Med 107:198, 1999.
25. Bouvet A: Human endocarditis due to nutritionally variant streptococci: *Streptococcus adjacens* and *Streptococcus defectivus*. Eur Heart J 16(Suppl B):24, 1995.
26. Baddour LM, Infectious Diseases Society of America Emerging Infections Network: Infective endocarditis caused by β-hemolytic streptococci. Clin Infect Dis 26:66, 1998.
27. Lefort A, Lortholary O, Casassus P, et al: Comparison between adult endocarditis due to beta-hemolytic streptococci (serogroups A, B, C, and G) and *Streptococcus milleri*: A multi-center study in France. Arch Intern Med 162:2450, 2002.
28. Martinez E, Miro JM, Almirante B, et al: Effect of penicillin resistance of *Streptococcus pneumoniae* on the presentation, prognosis, and treatment of pneumococcal endocarditis in adults. Clin Infect Dis 35:130, 2002.
29. Aronin SI, Mukherjee SK, West JC, Cooney EL: Review of pneumococcal endocarditis in adults in the penicillin era. Clin Infect Dis 26:165, 1998.
30. Whitener C, Caputo GM, Weitekamp MR, Karchmer AW: Endocarditis due to coagulase-negative staphylococci: Microbiologic, epidemiologic, and clinical considerations. Infect Dis Clin North Am 7:81, 1993.
31. Roder BL, Wandall DA, Frimodt-Moller N, et al: Clinical features of *Staphylococcus aureus* endocarditis: A 10-year experience in Denmark. Arch Intern Med 159:462, 1999.
32. Fowler VG Jr, Sanders LL, Kong LK, et al: Infective endocarditis due to *Staphylococcus aureus*: 59 prospectively identified cases with follow-up. Clin Infect Dis 28:106, 1999.
33. Hessen MT, Abrutyn E: Gram-negative bacterial endocarditis. *In* Kaye D (ed): Infective Endocarditis. 2nd ed. New York, Raven Press, 1992, p 251.
34. Brouqui P, Raoult D: Endocarditis due to rare and fastidious bacteria. Clin Microbiol Rev 14:177, 2001.
35. Berbari EF, Cockerill FR III, Steckelberg J: Infective endocarditis due to unusual or fastidious microorganisms. Mayo Clin Proc 72:532, 1997.
36. Petit AIC, Bok JW, Thompson J, et al: Native-valve endocarditis due to CDC coryneform group ANF-3: Report of a case and review of corynebacterial endocarditis. Clin Infect Dis 19:897, 1994.
37. Fenollar F, Lepidi H, Raoult D: Whipple's endocarditis: Review of the literature and comparisons with Q fever, *Bartonella* infection, and blood culture–positive endocarditis. Clin Infect Dis 33:1309, 2001.
38. Gubler JGH, Kuster M, Dutly F, et al: Whipple endocarditis without overt gastrointestinal disease: Report of four cases. Ann Intern Med 131:112, 1999.
39. Fenollar F, Fournier PE, Carrieri MP, et al: Risk factors and prevention of Q fever endocarditis. Clin Infect Dis 33:312, 2001.
40. Raoult D, Fournier PE, Vandenesch F, et al: Outcome and treatment of *Bartonella* endocarditis. Arch Intern Med 163:226, 2003.
41. Ellis ME, Al-Abdely H, Sandridge A, et al: Fungal endocarditis: Evidence in the world literature, 1965-1995. Clin Infect Dis 32:50, 2001.

Pathogenesis and Pathophysiology

42. Moreillon P, Que YA, Bayer AS: Pathogenesis of streptococcal and staphylococcal endocarditis. Infect Dis Clin North Am 16:297, 2002.
43. Weinstein L, Schlesinger JJ: Pathoanatomic, pathophysiologic and clinical correlations in endocarditis (first of two parts). N Engl J Med 291:832, 1974.
44. Livornese LL Jr, Korzeniowski OM: Pathogenesis of infective endocarditis. *In* Kaye D (ed): Infective Endocarditis. 2nd ed. New York, Raven Press, 1992, p 19.
45. Weinstein L, Schlesinger JJ: Pathoanatomic, pathophysiologic and clinical correlations in endocarditis (second of two parts). N Engl J Med 291:1122, 1974.
46. Croft CH, Woodward W, Elliott A, et al: Analysis of surgical versus medical therapy in active complicated native valve infective endocarditis. Am J Cardiol 51:1650, 1983.
47. Watanabe G, Haverich A, Speier R, et al: Surgical treatment of active infective endocarditis with paravalvular involvement. J Thorac Cardiovasc Surg 107:171, 1994.
48. Baumgartner FJ, Omari BO, Robertson JM, et al: Annular abscesses in surgical endocarditis: Anatomic, clinical and operative features. Ann Thorac Surg 70:442, 2000.
49. Douglas JL, Dismukes WE: Surgical therapy of infective endocarditis on natural valves. *In* Kaye D (ed): Infective Endocarditis. 2nd ed. New York, Raven Press, 1992, p 397.
50. Mansur AJ, Grinberg M, Lamos da Luz P, Bellotti G: The complications of infective endocarditis: A reappraisal in the 1980's. Arch Intern Med 152:2428, 1992.
51. Steckelberg JM, Murphy JG, Wilson WR: Management of complications of infective endocarditis. *In* Kaye D (ed): Infective Endocarditis. 2nd ed. New York, Raven Press, 1992, p 435.
52. DiSalvo G, Habib G, Pergola V, et al: Echocardiography predicts embolic events in infective endocarditis. J Am Coll Cardiol 37:1077, 2001.

Clinical Features and Diagnosis

53. Werner GS, Schulz R, Fuchs JB, et al: Infective endocarditis in the elderly in the era of transesophageal echocardiography: Clinical features and prognosis compared with younger patients. Am J Med 100:90, 1996.
54. Crawford MH, Durack DT: Clinical presentation of infective endocarditis. Cardiol Clin 21:159, 2003.
55. Steckelberg JM, Murphy JG, Ballard D, et al: Emboli in infective endocarditis: The prognostic value of echocardiography. Ann Intern Med 114:635, 1991.
56. Roder BL, Wandall DA, Espersen F, et al: Neurologic manifestations in *Staphylococcus aureus* endocarditis: A review of 260 bacteremic cases in nondrug addicts. Am J Med 102:379, 1997.
57. Gagliardi JP, Nettles RE, McCarty DE, et al: Native valve infective endocarditis in elderly and younger adult patients: Comparison of clinical features and outcomes with use of the Duke criteria and the Duke endocarditis data base. Clin Infect Dis 26:1165, 1998.
58. Masuda J, Yutani C, Waki R, et al: Histopathological analysis of the mechanisms of intracranial hemorrhage complicating infective endocarditis. Stroke 23:843, 1992.
59. Durack DT, Lukes AS, Bright DK: New criteria for diagnosis of infective endocarditis: Utilization of specific echocardiographic findings. Am J Med 96:200, 1994.
60. Li JS, Sexton DJ, Mick N, et al: Proposed modifications to the Duke criteria for the diagnosis of infective endocarditis. Clin Infect Dis 30:633, 2000.
61. Bayer AS, Bolger AF, Taubert KA, et al: Diagnosis and management of infective endocarditis and its complications. Circulation 98:2936, 1998.
62. Sochowski RA, Chan KL: Implication of negative results on a monoplane transesophageal echocardiographic study in patients with suspected infective endocarditis. J Am Coll Cardiol 21:216, 1993.
63. Hoen B, Selton-Suty C, Lacassin F, et al: Infective endocarditis in patients with negative blood cultures: Analysis of 88 cases from a one-year nationwide survey in France. Clin Infect Dis 20:501, 1995.
64. Towns ML, Reller LB: Diagnostic methods current best practices and guidelines for isolation of bacteria and fungi in infective endocarditis. Infect Dis Clin North Am 16:363, 2002.
65. Lisby G, Gutschik E, Durack DT: Molecular methods for diagnosis of infective endocarditis. Infect Dis Clin North Am 16:393, 2002.
66. Bayer AS, Scheld WM: Endocarditis and intravascular infections. *In* Mandell GL, Bennett JE, Dolin R (eds): Principles and Practice of Infectious Diseases. Philadelphia, Churchill Livingstone, 2000, pp 857-902.
67. Lindner JR, Case RA, Dent JM, et al: Diagnostic value of echocardiography in suspected endocarditis: An evaluation based on the pretest probability of disease. Circulation 93:730, 1996.
68. Roe MT, Abramson MA, Li J, et al: Clinical information determines the impact of transesophageal echocardiography on the diagnosis of infective endocarditis by the Duke criteria. Am Heart J 139:945, 2000.
69. Daniel WG, Mugge A: Transesophageal echocardiography. N Engl J Med 332:1268, 1995.
70. Morguet AJ, Werner GS, Andreas S, Kreuzer H: Diagnostic value of transesophageal compared with transthoracic echocardiography in suspected prosthetic valve endocarditis. Herz 20:390, 1995.
71. Daniel WG, Mugge A, Grote J, et al: Comparison of transthoracic and transesophageal echocardiography for detection of abnormalities of prosthetic and bioprosthetic valves in the mitral and aortic positions. Am J Cardiol 71:210, 1993.
72. Vuille C, Nidorf M, Weyman AE, Picard MH: Natural history of vegetations during successful medical treatment of endocarditis. Am Heart J 128:1200, 1994.

73. DeCastro S, Cartoni D, d'Amati G, et al: Diagnostic accuracy of transthoracic and multiplane transesophageal echocardiography for valvular perforation in acute infective endocarditis: Correlation with anatomic findings. Clin Infect Dis 30:826, 2000.
74. Sachdev M, Peterson GE, Jollis JG: Imaging techniques for diagnosis of infective endocarditis. Infect Dis Clin North Am 16:319, 2002.

Treatment

75. Wilson WR, Karchmer AW, Dajani AS, et al: Antibiotic treatment of adults with infective endocarditis due to streptococci, enterococci, staphylococci, and HACEK microorganisms. JAMA 274:1706, 1995.
76. Roberts SA, Lang SDR, Ellis-Pegler RB: Short-course treatment of penicillin-susceptible viridans streptococcal infective endocarditis with penicillin and gentamicin. Infect Dis Clin Pract 2:191, 1993.
77. Sexton DJ, Tenenbaum MJ, Wilson WR, et al: Ceftriaxone once daily for four weeks compared with ceftriaxone plus gentamicin once daily for two weeks for treatment of endocarditis due to penicillin-susceptible streptococci. Clin Infect Dis 27:1470, 1998.
78. Olaison L, Schadewitz K, The Swedish Society for Infectious Diseases Quality Assurance Study Group for Endocarditis: Enterococcal endocarditis in Sweden, 1995-1999: Can shorter therapy with aminoglycosides be used? Clin Infect Dis 34:159, 2002.
79. Mainardi JL, Shlaes DM, Goering RV, et al: Decreased teicoplanin susceptibility of methicillin-resistant strains of *Staphylococcus aureus*. J Infect Dis 171:1646, 1995.
80. Sett SS, Hudon MPJ, Jamieson WRE, Chow AW: Prosthetic valve endocarditis: Experience with porcine bioprostheses. J Thorac Cardiovasc Surg 105:428, 1993.
81. John MVD, Hibberd PL, Karchmer AW, et al: *Staphylococcus aureus* prosthetic valve endocarditis: Optimal management and risk factors for death. Clin Infect Dis 26:1302, 1998.
82. Nguyen MH, Nguyen ML, Yu VL, et al: *Candida* prosthetic valve endocarditis: Prospective study of six cases and review of the literature. Clin Infect Dis 22:262, 1996.
83. Nasser RM, Melgar GR, Longworth DL, Gordon SM: Incidence and risk of developing fungal prosthetic valve endocarditis after nosocomial candidemia. Am J Med 103:25, 1997.
84. Raoult D, Houpikian P, Tissot Dupont H, et al: Treatment of Q fever endocarditis: Comparison of 2 regimens containing doxycycline and ofloxacin or hydroxychloroquine. Arch Intern Med 159:167, 1999.
85. Tunkel AR, Kaye D: Endocarditis with negative blood cultures. N Engl J Med 326:1215, 1992.
86. Olaison L, Berlin L, Hogevik H, Alestig K: Incidence of β-lactam-induced delayed hypersensitivity and neutropenia during treatment of infective endocarditis. Arch Intern Med 159:607, 1999.
87. Andrews MM, von Reyn CF: Patient selection criteria and management guidelines for outpatient parenteral antibiotic therapy for native valve infective endocarditis. Clin Infect Dis 33:203, 2001.
88. Olaison L, Pettersson G: Current best practices and guidelines indications for surgical intervention in infective endocarditis. Cardiol Clin 21:235, 2003.
89. Bishara J, Leibovici L, Gartman-Israel D, et al: Long-term outcome of infective endocarditis: The impact of early surgical intervention. Clin Infect Dis 33:1636, 2001.
89a. Vikram HR, Buenconsejo J, Hasbun R, Quagliarello VJ: Impact of valve surgery on 6-month mortality in adults with complicated, left-sided native valve endocarditis: A propensity analysis. JAMA 290:3207, 2003.
90. Karchmer AW: Infections of prosthetic valves and intravascular devices. *In* Mandell GL, Bennett JE, Dolin R (eds): Principles and Practice of Infectious Diseases. New York, Churchill Livingstone, 2000, pp 907-913.
91. Morris AJ, Drinkovic D, Pottumarthy S, et al: Gram stain, culture, and histopathological examination findings for heart valves removed because of infective endocarditis. Clin Infect Dis 36:697, 2003.
92. Blumberg EA, Karalis DA, Chandrasekaran K, et al: Endocarditis-associated paravalvular abscess. Do clinical parameters predict the presence of abscess? Chest 107:898, 1995.
93. Meine TJ, Nettles RE, Anderson DJ, et al: Cardiac conduction abnormalities in endocarditis defined by the Duke criteria. Am Heart J 142:280, 2001.
94. Tischler MD, Vaitkus PT: The ability of vegetation size on echocardiography to predict clinical complications: A meta-analysis. J Am Soc Echocardiogr 10:562, 1997.
95. Cabell CH, Pond KK, Peterson GE, et al: The risk of stroke and death in patients with aortic and mitral valve endocarditis. Am Heart J 142:75, 2001.
96. Mangoni ED, Adinolfi LE, Tripodi MF, et al: Risk factors for "major" embolic events in hospitalized patients with infective endocarditis. Am Heart J 146:311, 2003.
97. Davenport J, Hart RG: Prosthetic valve endocarditis 1976-1987: Antibiotics, anticoagulation, and stroke. Stroke 21:993, 1990.
98. Reinhartz O, Herrmann M, Redling F, Zerkowski HR: Timing of surgery in patients with acute infective endocarditis. J Cardiovasc Surg 37:397, 1996.
99. Eishi K, Kawazoe K, Kuriyama Y, et al: Surgical management of infective endocarditis associated with cerebral complications: Multicenter retrospective study in Japan. J Thorac Cardiovasc Surg 110:1745, 1995.
100. Gillinov AM, Shah RV, Curtis WE, et al: Valve replacement in patients with endocarditis and acute neurologic deficit. Ann Thorac Surg 61:1125, 1996.
101. Phuong LK, Link M, Wijdicks E: Management of intracranial infections aneurysms: A series of 16 cases. Neurosurgery 51:1145, 2002.
102. Lederman MM, Sprague L, Wallis RS, Ellner JJ: Duration of fever during treatment of infective endocarditis. Medicine (Baltimore) 71:52, 1992.
102a. Hasbun R, Vikram HR, Barakat LA, et al: Complicated left-side native valve endocarditis in adults: Risk classification for mortality. JAMA 289:1933, 2003.
103. Acar J, Michel PL, Varenne O, et al: Surgical treatment of infective endocarditis. Eur Heart J 16(Suppl B):94, 1995.
104. Amrani M, Schoevaerdts JC, Eucher P, et al: Extension of native aortic valve endocarditis: Surgical considerations. Eur Heart J 16(Suppl B):103, 1995.
105. Mullany CJ, Chua YL, Schaff HV, et al: Early and late survival after surgical treatment of culture-positive active endocarditis. Mayo Clin Proc 70:517, 1995.
106. d'Udekem Y, David TE, Feindel CM, et al: Long-term results of surgery for active infective endocarditis. Eur J Cardiothorac Surg 11:46, 1997.
107. Alexiou C, Langley SM, Stafford H, et al: Surgery for active culture-positive endocarditis: Determinants of early and late outcome. Ann Thorac Surg 69:1448, 2000.
108. d'Udekem Y, David TE, Feindel CM, et al: Long-term results of operation for paravalvular abscess. Ann Thorac Surg 62:48, 1996.
109. Dajani AS, Taubert KA, Wilson W, et al: Prevention of bacterial endocarditis: Recommendations by the American Heart Association, from the Committee on Rheumatic Fever, Endocarditis, and Kawasaki Disease, Council on Cardiovascular Diseases in the Young. JAMA 277:1794, 1997.

Prevention

110. Durack DT: Prevention of infective endocarditis. N Engl J Med 332:38, 1995.
111. van der Meer JTM, Thompson J, Valkenburg HA, Michel MF: Epidemiology of bacterial endocarditis in the Netherlands. II. Antecedent procedures and use of prophylaxis. Arch Intern Med 152:1869, 1992.
112. DeGevigney G, Pop C, Delahaye JP: The risk of infective endocarditis after cardiac surgical and interventional procedures. Eur Heart J 16(Suppl B):7, 1995.
113. Spirito P, Rapezzi C, Bellone P, et al: Infective endocarditis hypertrophic cardiomyopathy. Circulation 99:2132, 1999.
114. Blatter M, Francioli P: Endocarditis prophylaxis: From experimental models to human recommendation. Eur Heart J 16(Suppl B):107, 1995.
115. Fluckiger U, Moreillon P, Blaser J, et al: Simulation of amoxicillin pharmacokinetics in humans for the prevention of streptococcal endocarditis in rats. Antimicrob Agents Chemother 38:2846, 1994.
116. Strom BL, Abrutyn E, Berlin JA, et al: Dental and cardiac risk factors for infective endocarditis: A population-based, case-control study. Ann Intern Med 129:761, 1998.

GUIDELINES *Thomas H. Lee*

Infective Endocarditis

The American Heart Association issued guidelines for antibiotic prophylaxis to prevent infective endocarditis in 1997[1] and a scientific statement with recommendations for diagnosis and management of this condition in 1998.[2] Other guidelines with recommendations relevant to this condition include American College of Cardiology/American Heart Association (ACC/AHA) guidelines for management of valvular heart disease published in 1998[3] and guidelines for use of echocardiography published in 1997.[4]

Prevention

The 1997 AHA guidelines for antibiotic prophylaxis to prevent endocarditis represented a major departure from prior recommendations by emphasizing that most cases are not attributable to an invasive procedure. According to these guidelines, patients with preexisting cardiac disease should be divided into high-, moderate-, and negligible-risk categories on the basis of their potential outcomes if endocarditis develops (see Table 58–14). For dental work, for example, antibiotic prophylaxis is recommended just for patients with high- and moderate-risk cardiac conditions who are undergoing higher risk procedures (Table 58G–1). For nondental procedures, endocarditis prophylaxis is recommended just for high-risk patients undergoing high-risk procedures (see Table 58–14); this strategy is considered optional for medium-risk patients. Antibiotic regimens are described in Table 58–16.

The 1998 ACC/AHA guidelines for patients with valvular heart disease[3] are consistent with these recommendations, with a few caveats. The ACC/AHA guidelines recommend antibiotic prophylaxis for patients with hypertrophic cardiomyopathy only when there is latent or resting obstruction. In addition, the ACC/AHA committee expressed concern that an increased risk for endocarditis may exist

TABLE 58G–1 Dental Procedures and Endocarditis Prophylaxis
Endocarditis Prophylaxis Recommended for Patients with High- and Moderate-Risk Cardiac Conditions (see Tables 58–14 and 58–15)
Dental extractions
Periodontal procedures including surgery, scaling and root planning, probing, and recall maintenance
Dental implant placement and reimplantation of avulsed teeth
Endodontic (root canal) instrumentation or surgery only beyond the apex
Subgingival placement of antibiotic fibers or strips
Initial placement of orthodontic bands but not brackets
Intraligamentary local anesthetic injections
Prophylactic cleaning of teeth or implants where bleeding is anticipated
Endocarditis Prophylaxis not Recommended
Restorative dentistry* (operative and prosthodontic) with or without retraction cord†
Local anesthetic injections (nonintraligamentary)
Intracanal endodontic treatment; after placement and build-up
Placement of rubber dams
Postoperative suture removal
Placement of removable prosthodontic or orthodontic appliances
Taking of oral impressions
Fluoride treatments
Taking of oral radiographs
Orthodontic appliance adjustment
Shedding of primary teeth

From Dajani AS, Taubert KA, Wilson W, et al: Prevention of bacterial endocarditis: Recommendations by the American Heart Association. Circulation 96:358, 1997.

*This includes restoration of decayed teeth (filling cavities) and replacement of missing teeth.

†Clinical judgment may indicate antibiotic use in selected circumstances that may create significant bleeding.

for some patients with mitral valve prolapse without regurgitation; hence, this group was not willing to state that antibiotic prophylaxis was inappropriate for such patients. Finally, the ACC/AHA guidelines specified that antibiotic prophylaxis was not necessary in patients with physiological mitral regurgitation in the absence of a murmur.

Indications for Echocardiography

Echocardiography is strongly supported in virtually all patients with suspected or known infective endocarditis, but the 1997 ACC/AHA guidelines on echocardiography[4] do not recommend transesophageal echocardiography (TEE) as the initial test of choice in the diagnosis of native valve endocarditis (Table 58G–2). The guidelines urge use of TEE when specific questions are not adequately addressed by an initial transthoracic echocardiography (TTE) evaluation, such as if the TTE is of poor quality, if the TTE is negative despite a high clinical suspicion of endocarditis, if a prosthetic valve is involved, and if there is a high suspicion such as in a patient with staphylococcal bacteremia or in an elderly patient with valvular abnormalities that make diagnosis by TTE difficult.

Diagnosis of prosthetic valve endocarditis with TTE is more difficult than diagnosis of endocarditis of native valves. Thus, the ACC/AHA guidelines suggest a lower threshold for performance of TEE in patients with prosthetic valves and suspected endocarditis (see Table 58G–2).

Surgery for Active Endocarditis

The ACC/AHA guidelines for valvular heart disease support performance of surgery for patients with life-threatening congestive heart failure or cardiogenic shock related to active endocarditis. Indications for surgery for patients with stable endocarditis are considered less clear (see Table 58G–2).

TABLE 58G–2 ACC/AHA Guidelines for Prevention, Evaluation, and Treatment of Endocarditis

Indication	Class I	Class IIa	Class IIb	Class III
Antibiotic endocarditis prophylaxis for patients with mitral valve prolapse undergoing procedures associated with bacteremia	1. Patients with characteristic systolic click-murmur complex 2. Patients with isolated systolic click and echocardiographic evidence of MVP and MR	1. Patients with isolated systolic click, echocardiographic evidence of high-risk MVP		1. Patients with isolated systolic click and equivocal or no evidence of MVP
Echocardiography in infective endocarditis: native valves	1. Detection and characterization of valvular lesions, their hemodynamic severity, and/or ventricular compensation* 2. Detection of vegetations and characterization of lesions in patients with congenital heart disease in whom infective endocarditis is suspected 3. Detection of associated abnormalities (e.g., abscesses, shunts)* 4. Re-evaluation studies in complex endocarditis (e.g., virulent organism, severe hemodynamic lesion, aortic valve involvement, persistent fever or bacteremia, clinical change, or symptomatic deterioration) 5. Evaluation of patients with high clinical suspicion of culture-negative endocarditis*	1. Evaluation of bacteremia without a known source* 2. Risk stratification in established endocarditis*	1. Routine re-evaluation in uncomplicated endocarditis during antibiotic therapy	1. Evaluation of fever and nonpathological murmur without evidence of bacteremia

TABLE 58G–2 ACC/AHA Guidelines for Prevention, Evaluation, and Treatment of Endocarditis—cont'd

Indication	Class I	Class IIa	Class IIb	Class III
Echocardiography in infective endocarditis: prosthetic valves	1. Detection and characterization of valvular lesions, their hemodynamic severity, and/or ventricular compensation* 2. Detection of associated abnormalities (e.g., abscesses, shunts)* 3. Re-evaluation in complex endocarditis (e.g., virulent organism, severe hemodynamic lesion, aortic valve involvement, persistent fever or bacteremia, clinical change, or symptomatic deterioration) 4. Evaluation of suspected endocarditis and negative cultures* 5. Evaluation of bacteremia without a known source*	1. Evaluation of persistent fever without evidence of bacteremia or new murmur*	1. Routine re-evaluation in uncomplicated endocarditis during antibiotic therapy*	1. Evaluation of transient fever without evidence of bacteremia or new murmur
Surgery for native valve endocarditis (criteria also apply to repaired mitral and aortic allograft or autograft valves)	1. Acute AR or MR with heart failure 2. Acute AR with tachycardia and early closure of the mitral valve 3. Fungal endocarditis 4. Evidence of annular or aortic abscess, sinus or aortic true or false aneurysm 5. Evidence of valve dysfunction and persistent infection after a prolonged period (7 to 10 d) of appropriate antibiotic therapy, as indicated by presence of fever, leukocytosis, and bacteremia, provided there are no noncardiac causes for infection	1. Recurrent emboli after appropriate antibiotic therapy 2. Infection with gram-negative organisms or organisms with a poor response to antibiotics in patients with evidence of valve dysfunction	1. Mobile vegetations >10 mm	1. Early infections of the mitral valve that can probably be repaired 2. Persistent pyrexia and leukocytosis with negative blood cultures
Surgery for prosthetic valve endocarditis (criteria exclude repaired mitral and aortic allograft or autograft valves)	1. Early prosthetic valve endocarditis (first 2 mo or less after surgery) 2. Heart failure with prosthetic valve dysfunction 3. Fungal endocarditis 4. Staphylococcal endocarditis not responding to antibiotic therapy 5. Evidence of paravalvular leak, annular or aortic abscess, sinus or aortic true or false aneurysm, fistula formation, or new-onset conduction disturbances 6. Infection with gram-negative organisms or organisms with a poor response to antibiotics	1. Persistent bacteremia after a prolonged course (7 to 10 d) of appropriate antibiotic therapy without noncardiac causes for bacteremia 2. Recurrent peripheral embolus despite therapy	1. Vegetation of any size on or near the prosthesis	

ACC/AHA = American College of Cardiology/American Heart Association; AR = aortic regurgitation; MR = mitral regurgitation; MVP = mitral valve prolapse.

From Bonow RO, Carabello B, de Leon AC Jr, et al: ACC/AHA guidelines for the management of patients with valvular heart disease: Executive summary. A report of the American College of Cardiology/American Heart Association Task Force on Practice Guidelines (Committee on Management of Patients With Valvular Heart Disease). Circulation 98:1949, 1998; and Cheitlin MD, Alpert JS, Armstrong WF, et al: ACC/AHA guidelines for the clinical application of echocardiography: A report of the American College of Cardiology/American Heart Association Task Force on Practice Guidelines (Committee on Clinical Application of Echocardiography). Circulation 95:1686, 1997.

*Transesophageal echocardiography may provide incremental value in addition to information obtained by transthoracic imaging.

References

1. Dajani AS, Taubert KA, Wilson W, et al: Prevention of bacterial endocarditis: Recommendations by the American Heart Association. Circulation 96:358, 1997.
2. Bayer AS, Bolger AF, Taubert KA, et al: Diagnosis and management of infective endocarditis and its complications. Circulation 98:2936, 1998.
3. Bonow RO, Carabello B, de Leon AC Jr, et al: ACC/AHA guidelines for the management of patients with valvular heart disease: Executive summary: A report of the American College of Cardiology/American Heart Association Task Force on Practice Guidelines (Committee on Management of Patients With Valvular Heart Disease). Circulation 98:1949, 1998.
4. Cheitlin MD, Alpert JS, Armstrong WF, et al: ACC/AHA guidelines for the clinical application of echocardiography: A report of the American College of Cardiology/American Heart Association Task Force on Practice Guidelines (Committee on Clinical Application of Echocardiography). Circulation 95:1686, 1997.

CHAPTER 59

The Cardiomyopathies

Joshua Wynne • Eugene Braunwald

The cardiomyopathies constitute a group of disorders in which the dominant feature is direct involvement of the heart muscle itself. They are distinctive because they are *not* the result of pericardial, hypertensive, congenital, or valvular diseases. Although the diagnosis of cardiomyopathy requires the exclusion of these etiological factors, the features of cardiomyopathy are often sufficiently distinctive—both clinically and hemodynamically—to allow a definitive diagnosis to be made. With increasing awareness of this condition, along with improvements in diagnostic techniques, cardiomyopathy is being recognized as a significant cause of morbidity and mortality. Whether the result of improved recognition or of other factors, the incidence and prevalence of heart failure related to cardiomyopathy appear to be increasing.[1] Although coronary artery disease is the most common cause of congestive heart failure (accounting for more than two-thirds of all cases), we avoid using the term *ischemic cardiomyopathy* in this setting because the primary problem is in the coronary arteries and not the heart muscle itself. Nevertheless, some use this imprecise term to describe the condition in which coronary artery disease causes multiple infarctions, diffuse fibrosis, or severe ischemia that leads to left ventricular dilation with congestive heart failure; it may or may not be associated with angina pectoris (see Chap. 50).

A variety of schemes have been proposed for classifying the cardiomyopathies. The most widely recognized classification is that promulgated jointly by the World Health Organization (WHO) and the International Society and Federation of Cardiology (ISFC) (Table 59–1).[2] In the WHO/ISFC classification, the cardiomyopathies are classified on the basis of their predominant pathophysiological features; other diseases that affect the myocardium but that are associated with a particular cardiac disorder or are part of a generalized systemic disorder are termed *specific cardiomyopathies* (in the previous WHO/ISFC classification, they were termed *specific heart muscle diseases*).[2]

Three basic types of functional impairment have been described (Table 59–2 and Fig. 59–1): (1) *dilated* cardiomyopathy (DCM), the most common form, accounting for the majority of cardiomyopathies and characterized by ventricular dilation, contractile dysfunction, and often symptoms of congestive heart failure; (2) *hypertrophic* cardiomyopathy (HCM), recognized by inappropriate left ventricular hypertrophy, often with asymmetrical involvement of the interventricular septum, with preserved or enhanced contractile function until late in the course of the disease; and (3) *restrictive* cardiomyopathy (RCM), the least common form in Western countries, marked by impaired diastolic filling and in some cases with endocardial scarring of the ventricle.[3] The distinction between the three major functional categories is not absolute, and often there is overlap; in particular, patients with HCM also have increased wall stiffness (as a consequence of the myocardial hypertrophy) and thus manifest some of the features of an RCM.[2] Two less common forms of cardiomyopathy are recognized: *arrhythmogenic right ventricular cardiomyopathy* (ARVC) and *unclassified*; the latter includes fibroelastosis, systolic dysfunction with minimal dilation, and isolated ventricular noncompaction, an unusual disease marked by prominent endocardial thickening with prominent trabeculations and deep recesses.[4] Furthermore, ventricular dilation and systolic heart failure may occur late in the course of HCM and bear a resemblance to DCM.

Examples of what have been termed *specific cardiomyopathies* include valvular cardiomyopathy, hypertensive cardiomyopathy, and inflammatory cardiomyopathy (myocarditis with cardiac dysfunction) (see Table 59–1 and Chap. 60).[2]

Endomyocardial Biopsy

Evaluation of some patients suspected of suffering from a cardiomyopathy has been facilitated by the use of endomyocardial biopsy.[5] Using a flexible bioptome, the clinician may obtain tissue samples from the right ventricle (and left ventricle when required) through a transvenous (or transarterial) approach with ease and safety (see Chap. 17). The availability of disposable transfemoral bioptomes has further facilitated endomyocardial biopsy. Two-dimensional echocardiography may help guide the placement of the bioptome and reduce or eliminate radiation exposure. Endomyocardial biopsy results in a small tissue sample (average size 1 to 2 mm), and multiple samples (usually four or more) are required because pronounced topographical variations may be found within the myocardium. Which patients should be subjected to biopsy remains controversial, but there is general agreement that biopsy may be of benefit in certain specific situations.[6] There is little debate about its clinical utility in detecting infiltrative disorders of the myocardium and in monitoring for anthracycline cardiotoxicity and cardiac transplant rejection.[5,7]

Although on occasion endomyocardial biopsy may identify a specific etiological agent in an individual patient with cardiac disease of uncertain cause, the clinical utility of routine biopsy in cardiomyopathy is limited (particularly because no definitive pattern has been found in DCM) (Fig. 59-2).[8] It has been estimated that a specific etiological diagnosis is obtained by biopsy in fewer than 10 percent of patients with cardiomyopathy[8] and a treatable disease is found even less often.

DALLAS CRITERIA. Interpretation of biopsy specimens had been plagued by a high degree of interobserver variability; the adoption of a generally accepted set of histological definitions, the *Dallas criteria,* has improved agreement.[8] Nevertheless, there continues to be a lack of agreement about the diagnostic usefulness of any scheme that utilizes conventional histological findings—including the Dallas criteria—to evaluate a process as complex as

TABLE 59–1 Classification of the Cardiomyopathies

Disorder	Description
Dilated cardiomyopathy	Dilation and impaired contraction of the left or both ventricles. Caused by familial-genetic, viral, and/or immune, alcoholic-toxic, or unknown factors or is associated with recognized cardiovascular disease.
Hypertrophic cardiomyopathy	Left and/or right ventricular hypertrophy, often asymmetrical, which usually involves the interventricular septum. Mutations in sarcoplasmic proteins cause the disease in many patients.
Restrictive cardiomyopathy	Restricted filling and reduced diastolic size of either or both ventricles with normal or near-normal systolic function. Is idiopathic or associated with other disease (e.g., amyloidosis, endomyocardial disease).
Arrhythmogenic right ventricular cardiomyopathy	Progressive fibrofatty replacement of the right, and to some degree left, ventricular myocardium. Familial disease is common.
Unclassified cardiomyopathy	Diseases that do not fit readily into any category. Examples include systolic dysfunction with minimal dilation, mitochondrial disease, and fibroelastosis.
Specific Cardiomyopathies	
Ischemic cardiomyopathy	Arises as dilated cardiomyopathy with depressed ventricular function not explained by the extent of coronary artery obstructions or ischemic damage.
Valvular cardiomyopathy	Arises as ventricular dysfunction that is out of proportion to the abnormal loading conditions produced by the valvular stenosis and/or regurgitation.
Hypertensive cardiomyopathy	Arises with left ventricular hypertrophy with features of cardiac failure related to systolic or diastolic dysfunction.
Inflammatory cardiomyopathy	Cardiac dysfunction as a consequence of myocarditis.
Metabolic cardiomyopathy	Includes a wide variety of causes, including endocrine abnormalities, glycogen storage disease, deficiencies (such as hypokalemia), and nutritional disorders.
General systemic disease	Includes connective tissue disorders and infiltrative diseases such as sarcoidosis and leukemia.
Muscular dystrophies	Includes Duchenne, Becker-type, and myotonic dystrophies.
Neuromuscular disorders	Includes Friedreich ataxia, Noonan syndrome, and lentiginosis.
Sensitivity and toxic reactions	Includes reactions to alcohol, catecholamines, anthracyclines, irradiation, and others.
Peripartal cardiomyopathy	First becomes manifest in the peripartum period, but it is probably a heterogeneous group.

Derived from Richardson, P McKenna W, Bristow M, et al: Report of the 1995 World Health Organization/International Society and Federation of Cardiology Task Force on the Definition and Classification of Cardiomyopathies. Circulation 93:841, 1996. Copyright 1996, American Heart Association.

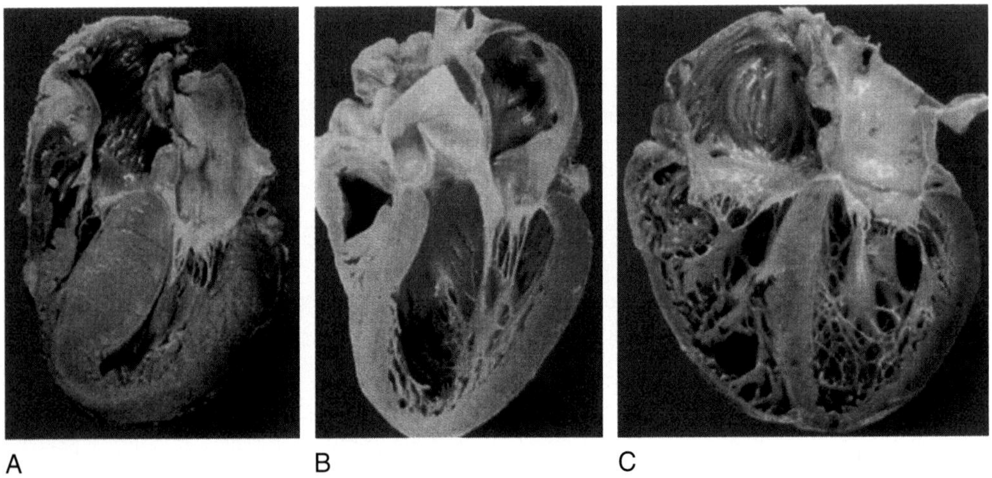

FIGURE 59–1 Gross pathological specimens of the cardiomyopathies. **A,** Hypertrophic cardiomyopathy, showing a marked increase in myocardial mass and preferential hypertrophy of the interventricular septum. **B,** Normal heart, with normal left ventricular dimensions and thickness. **C,** Dilated cardiomyopathy, showing marked increase in chamber size. Atrial enlargement is also evident in both cardiomyopathies (A and C). (From Seidman JG, Seidman C: The genetic basis for cardiomyopathy: From mutation identification to mechanistic paradigms. Cell 104:557, 2001.)

TABLE 59–2 Functional Classification of the Cardiomyopathies

Dilated	Restrictive	Hypertrophic
Symptoms		
Congestive heart failure, particularly left sided Fatigue and weakness Systemic or pulmonary emboli	Dyspnea, fatigue Right-sided congestive heart failure Signs and symptoms of systemic disease, e.g., amyloidosis, iron storage disease	Dyspnea, angina pectoris Fatigue, syncope, palpitations
Physical Examination		
Moderate to severe cardiomegaly; S_3, S_4 Atrioventricular valve regurgitation, especially mitral	Mild to moderate cardiomegaly; S_3 or S_4 Atrioventricular valve regurgitation; inspiratory increase in venous pressure (Kussmaul sign)	Mild cardiomegaly Apical systolic thrill and heave; brisk carotid upstroke S_4 common Systolic murmur that increases with Valsalva maneuver
Chest Roentgenogram		
Moderate to marked cardiac enlargement, especially left ventricular Pulmonary venous hypertension	Mild cardiac enlargement Pulmonary venous hypertension	Mild to moderate cardiac enlargement Left atrial enlargement
Electrocardiogram		
Sinus tachycardia Atrial and ventricular arrhythmias ST segment and T wave abnormalities Intraventricular conduction defects	Low voltage Intraventricular conduction defects Atrioventricular conduction defects	Left ventricular hypertrophy ST segment and T wave abnormalities Abnormal Q waves Atrial and ventricular arrhythmias
Echocardiogram		
Left ventricular dilation and dysfunction Abnormal diastolic mitral valve motion secondary to abnormal compliance and filling pressures	Increased left ventricular wall thickness and mass Small or normal-sized left ventricular cavity Normal systolic function Pericardial effusion	Asymmetrical septal hypertrophy (ASH) Narrow left ventricular outflow tract Systolic anterior motion (SAM) of the mitral valve Small or normal-sized left ventricle
Radionuclide Studies		
Left ventricular dilation and dysfunction (RVG)	Infiltration of myocardium (^{201}Tl) Small or normal-sized left ventricle (RVG) Normal systolic function (RVG)	Small or normal-sized left ventricle (RVG) Vigorous systolic function (RVG) Asymmetrical septal hypertrophy (RVG or ^{201}Tl)
Cardiac Catheterization		
Left ventricular enlargement and dysfunction Mitral and/or tricuspid regurgitation Elevated left- and often right-sided filling pressures Diminished cardiac output	Diminished left ventricular compliance "Square root sign" in ventricular pressure recordings Preserved systolic function Elevated left- and right-sided filling pressures	Diminished left ventricular compliance Mitral regurgitation Vigorous systolic function Dynamic left ventricular outflow gradient

RVG = radionuclide ventriculogram; ^{201}Tl = thallium-201.

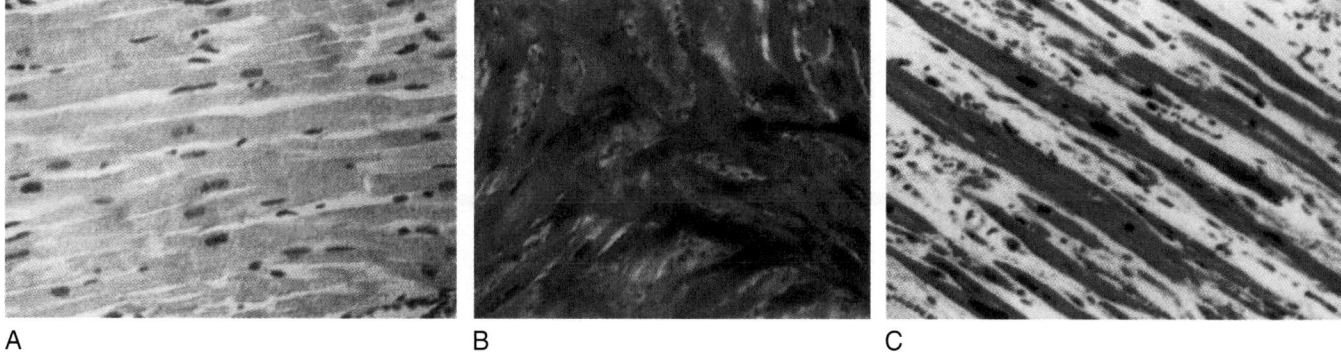

A B C

FIGURE 59–2 Histopathology of hypertrophic and dilated cardiomyopathy. **A,** The normal architecture of healthy myocardium shows orderly alignment of myocytes with minimal interstitial fibrosis. **B,** Hypertrophic cardiomyopathy, demonstrating marked enlargement and disarray of myocytes (red) with increased interstitial fibrosis (blue). **C,** Dilated cardiomyopathy, showing hypertrophy and degeneration of myocytes (dark red) without disarray. There is an increase in interstitial fibrosis (pale pink). Stains: A and C, hematoxylin and eosin; B, Masson trichrome. (From Seidman JG, Seidman C: The genetic basis for cardiomyopathy: From mutation identification to mechanistic paradigms. Cell 104:557, 2001.)

inflammatory cardiomyopathy.[9] It is hoped that newer immunohistochemical and molecular biological techniques (such as the polymerase chain reaction or in situ hybridization techniques to detect viral infection of the heart) may expand further the diagnostic utility of endomyocardial biopsy.[10]

Dilated Cardiomyopathy

Idiopathic Dilated Cardiomyopathy

DCM is a syndrome characterized by cardiac enlargement and impaired systolic function of one or both ventricles (see Figs. 59–1 and 59–2). Although it was formerly called congestive cardiomyopathy, the term *dilated cardiomyopathy* is now preferred because the earliest abnormality is usually ventricular enlargement and systolic contractile dysfunction, with the signs and symptoms of congestive heart failure often (but not invariably) developing later. In an occasional patient, the predominant finding is that of contractile dysfunction with only a minimally dilated left ventricle. In the WHO/ISFC classification scheme, this variant of DCM is placed in the *unclassified* cardiomyopathy group. Conversely, apparently normal elite athletes may demonstrate considerable ventricular enlargement with *normal* systolic performance. It is presumed that this is a physiological adaptation to intense athletic training and does not appear to represent a disease state, although the long-term consequences are not fully known.

The incidence of DCM is reported to be 5 to 8 cases per 100,000 population per year and appears to be increasing, although the true figure is probably higher as a consequence of underreporting of mild or asymptomatic cases.[11] It occurs almost three times more frequently in blacks and males as in whites and females, and this difference does not appear to be related solely to different degrees of hypertension, cigarette smoking, or alcohol use. Survival in blacks and males appears to be worse than in whites and females.[12]

Although the cause is not definable in many cases, more than 75 specific diseases of heart muscle can produce the clinical manifestations of DCM. It is likely that this condition represents a final common pathway that is the end result of myocardial damage produced by a variety of cytotoxic, metabolic, immunological, familial, and infectious mechanisms. Alcohol, for example, may lead to severe cardiac dysfunction and may produce clinical, hemodynamic, and pathological findings identical to those present in idiopathic DCM.

NATURAL HISTORY. The natural history of DCM is not well established. Many patients have minimal or no symptoms, and the progression of the disease in these patients is unclear, although there is some evidence that the long-term prognosis is not good. Nevertheless, in symptomatic patients the course is usually one of progressive deterioration, with 10 to 50 percent of patients with heart failure succumbing within a year, depending on the cohort of patients under study.[13] It has been estimated that the annual mortality rate for a typical patient with heart failure is about 11 to 13 percent.[14] A minority of patients with recent-onset DCM—perhaps about a quarter—improve spontaneously, even some sick enough initially to be considered for cardiac transplantation.

PROGNOSIS. A variety of clinical predictors of patients at enhanced risk for dying of DCM have been identified, including the presence of a protodiastolic (S_3) gallop, ventricular arrhythmias, advanced age, and the failure of the myopathic ventricle to respond to inotropic stimulation (Table 59–3).[15] However, the predictive reliability of any single feature is not high, and it may be difficult to predict with any accuracy the clinical course and outcome in an individual patient. Nevertheless, greater ventricular enlargement and worse dysfunction tend to correlate with poorer prognosis, particularly if the right ventricle is dilated and dysfunctional as well.[16]

Cardiopulmonary exercise testing can also provide useful prognostic information (see Chap. 10). Marked limitation of exercise capacity manifested by reduced maximal systemic oxygen uptake (especially when below 10 to 12 ml/kg/min) is a reliable predictor of mortality and is used widely as an indicator for consideration of cardiac transplantation (see Chap. 26).

Pathology

MACROSCOPIC EXAMINATION. This usually reveals enlargement and dilation of all four cardiac chambers; the ventricles are more dilated than the atria (see Fig. 59–1). Although the thickness of the ventricular wall is increased in some cases, the degree of hypertrophy is often less than might be expected given the severe dilation present. The development of left ventricular hypertrophy appears to have a protective or beneficial role in DCM, presumably because it reduces systolic wall stress and thus protects against further cavity dilation. The cardiac valves are intrinsically normal, and intracavitary thrombi, particularly in the ventricular apex, are not uncommon. The coronary arteries are usually normal. The right ventricle is preferentially involved in some cases of DCM, sometimes on a familial basis.

HISTOLOGICAL EXAMINATION. Microscopic study reveals extensive areas of interstitial and perivascular fibrosis, particularly involving the left ventricular subendocardium (see Fig. 59–2). Small areas of necrosis and cellular infiltrate are seen on occasion, but these are typically not prominent features. There is marked variation in myocyte size; some myocardial cells are hypertrophied, and others are atrophied. No viruses or other etiological agents have been identified with any regularity in tissue from patients with DCM. Particularly disappointing has been the failure to identify any immunological, histochemical, morphological, ultrastructural, or microbiological marker that might be used to establish the diagnosis of idiopathic DCM or to clarify its cause.

TABLE 59–3 Factors Associated with an Adverse Outcome in Dilated Cardiomyopathy

Clinical	Noninvasive	Invasive
NYHA Class III/IV	Low LV ejection fraction	High LV filling pressures
Increasing age	Marked LV dilation	
Low exercise peak oxygen consumption	Low LV mass	
Marked intraventricular conduction delay	≥Moderate mitral regurgitation	
Complex ventricular arrhythmias	Abnormal diastolic function	
Abnormal signal-averaged ECG	Abnormal contractile reserve	
Evidence of excessive sympathetic stimulation	Right ventricular dilation or dysfunction	
Protodiastolic gallop (S_3)		

ECG = electrocardiogram; LV = left ventricular; NYHA = New York Heart Association.

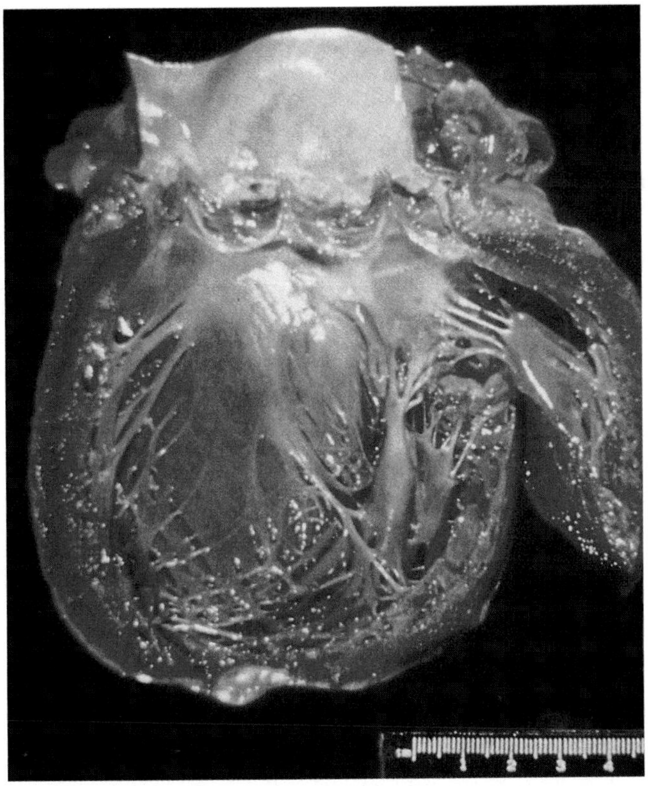

FIGURE 59–3 Gross pathology of dilated cardiomyopathy. Prominent ventricular dilatation is apparent in this heart, which has been opened so that the interior of the left ventricle can be seen. Wall thickness is normal, but the shape of the heart has become more globular. (From Kasper EK, Hruban RH, Baughman KL: Idiopathic dilated cardiomyopathy. *In* Abelmann WH, Braunwald E [eds.]. Atlas of Heart Diseases. Vol 2. Cardiomyopathies, Myocarditis, and Pericardial Disease. Philadelphia, Current Medicine, 1995, pp 3.1-3.18.)

TABLE 59–4 Molecular Defects Linked to the Various Cardiomyopathies

	Cardiomyopathy		
Genomic Defect	***Hypertrophic***	***Dilated***	***Restrictive***
Sarcomere			
Myosin heavy chain	M	M	
Myosin essential light chain	M		
Myosin regulatory light chain	M		
Cardiac actin	M	M	
Troponin T	M/D	D	
Troponin I	M		M
Alpha-tropomyosin	M	M	
Myosin-binding protein C	M/D		
Titin/titin-related Protein			
Titin	M	M/D	
Telethonin (T-cap)		M	
Z-disk-associated Proteins			
Muscle LIM domain protein		M	
Sarcolemma Cytoskeleton			
Dystrophin		D	
Beta-sarcoglycan		D/Dup	
Delta-sarcoglycan		M	
Alpha-dystrobrevin		M	
Metavinculin		D	
Intermediate Filaments			
Desmin		M	
Lamin A/C		M	

D = deletion; Dup = duplication; M = missense.

Adapted from Chien KR: Genotype, phenotype: Upstairs, downstairs in the family of cardiomyopathies. J Clin Invest 111:175, 2003.

Etiology

About a fourth of the cases of congestive heart failure in the United States are due to DCM; most of the remainder are caused by the sequelae of coronary artery disease or, less frequently, hypertensive heart disease.[11] More than half of all patients with the clinical picture of DCM have no identifiable etiology apparent despite rigorous evaluation and are therefore considered to have *idiopathic* DCM.[17] It is likely that this condition represents a common expression of myocardial damage that has been produced by a variety of as yet unestablished myocardial insults. Although the cause or causes remain unclear, interest has centered on three possible basic mechanisms of damage: (1) familial and genetic factors, (2) viral myocarditis and other cytotoxic insults, and (3) immunological abnormalities (Fig. 59–3).

GENETICS. Familial linkage of DCM occurs more commonly than is often appreciated. It is thought that about 25 to 30 percent of patients with DCM have an inherited form of the disease that is the result of a genetic mutation.[18] Some asymptomatic relatives of patients with DCM have subclinical left ventricular enlargement or dysfunction, or both, that may progress to overt symptomatic DMC.[19] Most familial cases demonstrate autosomal dominant transmission. More than a dozen chromosomal loci have been identified, and more are likely to be found (Table 59–4).[20] Familial DCM results from mutations in genes that encode cytoskeletal, nuclear membrane, or contractile proteins, including desmin, titin, and troponin T.[20–23] One unique form is due to mutations in the lamin A/C gene and is associated with conduction defects, variable skeletal muscle involvement, and reduced survival to adulthood.[24] Another variant affects phospholamban and leads to myocellular calcium dysregulation.[25]

However, familial DCM is genetically quite heterogeneous, and autosomal recessive and X-linked inheritance have been found as well.[26] One form of familial X-linked DCM is due to a deletion in the promoter region and the first exon of the gene that codes for the protein dystrophin, a component of the cytoskeleton of myocytes.[27] This has fueled speculation that a resulting deficiency of cardiac dystrophin is the cause of the associated DCM (see also Chap. 85).[28] Mutations involving mitochondrial DNA have been reported as well.[29]

Whether any of the patients without apparent familial linkage has a genetic predisposition to DCM remains unknown. There is great interest in using molecular genetic techniques to identify markers of disease susceptibility in asymptomatic carriers at risk for the eventual development of overt clinical DCM. An example of such a marker may be the angiotensin-converting enzyme DD genotype that is associated with an adverse clinical course in patients with DCM.[30] Even where there is no evidence of familial linkage, the failing heart demonstrates a variety of alterations in the gene and protein expression of various contractile proteins.[11]

SEQUELA OF VIRAL MYOCARDITIS (see also Chap. 60). Wide speculation exists that an episode of subclinical viral myocarditis initiates an autoimmune reaction that culminates in the development of full-blown DCM.[31] Although this hypothesis is inviting, it remains controversial.[32] In some patients who exhibit the clinical features of DCM, endomyocardial biopsy reveals evidence of an inflammatory myocarditis. The reported frequency of evidence of an inflammatory infiltrate in DCM varies widely and undoubtedly depends largely on selection of patients and the criteria used for diagnosis; using rigorous criteria, only about 15 percent (or less) of patients with DCM have biopsy evidence of myocarditis.[32] Other evidence favoring the concept that DCM is a postviral disorder includes the presence of high antibody viral titers, viral-specific RNA sequences, and apparent viral particles in patients with "idiopathic" DCM.[33] Similarly, the polymerase chain reaction generally has confirmed the presence of viral remnants in the myocardium of some patients with cardiomyopathy.[34]

AUTOIMMUNITY. Abnormalities of both humoral and cellular immunity have been found in patients with DCM,[9,35] although the findings have not been completely reproducible. It has been postulated that viral components may be incorporated into the cardiac sarcolemma, only to serve as an antigenic source that directs the immune response to attack the myocardium. On the other hand, there is speculation that antibodies might be the *result* of myocardial damage rather than the cause.[36] There appears to be an association with specific human leukocyte antigen (HLA) class II antigens (particularly DR4), suggesting that abnormalities of immunoregulation may play a role in DCM.[37] Circulating antimyocardial antibodies to a variety of antigens (including the myosin heavy chain, the beta adrenoceptor, the muscarinic receptor, sarcolemmal sodium-potassium adenosine triphosphatase, laminin, and mitochondrial proteins) have been identified.[38,39] Additional evidence for the significance of circulating antimyocardial antibodies comes from the demonstration of short- and intermediate-term clinical improvement in the manifestations of heart failure in some but not all patients treated with immunoadsorption and elimination of anti-beta$_1$-adrenergic receptor antibodies.[40–42] Conversely, a randomized trial of immune globulin in recent-onset DCM showed no benefit.[9] Thus, the precise role of either humoral or cellular immunomodulation in the pathogenesis of DCM remains unestablished.[43]

PROINFLAMMATORY CYTOKINES. A variety of proinflammatory cytokines such as tumor necrosis factor-alpha (TNF-alpha) (and the related TNF-alpha converting enzyme) are expressed in DCM and may play a role in producing contractile dysfunction; whether viral infection, autoimmune abnormalities, or other factors induce their expression is unknown.[44–46] Additional support for an etiological role of TNF-alpha in the contractile dysfunction of DCM is that the inhibition of its production by pentoxifylline results in symptomatic and functional improvement.[47] Similarly, the vasoconstrictor peptide endothelin is increased in decompensated DCM and has been implicated as a cause of the heightened vascular tone that accompanies congestive heart failure.[48,49]

OTHER POTENTIAL CAUSES. A variety of other possible causes have been proposed, although none is accepted as *the* cause of DCM. Thus, endocrine abnormalities as well as the effects of chemicals or toxins have been suggested as possible etiological factors. It has been suggested that microvascular hyperreactivity (spasm) and decreased coronary flow reserve may lead to myocellular necrosis and scarring, with resultant heart failure.[50] Apoptosis, or programmed cell death, has been demonstrated in the hearts of patients with DCM and ARVC, although there is some controversy regarding these findings in DCM.[49,51,52]

From a clinical standpoint, the more important causes of nonidiopathic DCM include alcohol and cocaine abuse (see Chap. 62),[53] human immunodeficiency virus (HIV) infection (see Chap. 61), metabolic abnormalities, and the cardiotoxicity of anticancer drugs (especially doxorubicin) (see Chap. 83).

Clinical Manifestations

HISTORY. Although patients of any age may be affected, DCM is most common in middle age and is more frequent in men than in women. Symptoms usually develop gradually in patients with DCM. Some patients are asymptomatic and yet have left ventricular dilation for months or even years. This dilation may be recognized clinically only later when symptoms develop or when routine chest roentgenography demonstrates cardiomegaly. A relatively small number of patients develop symptoms of heart failure for the first time after recovery from what appears to be a systemic viral infection. In still others, severe heart failure develops acutely during an episode of myocarditis; although some recovery occurs, chronic manifestations of diminished cardiac reserve persist and heart failure reappears months or years later. It is important to question the patient and family carefully about alcohol consumption because excessive alcohol consumption is a major cause of DCM, and its cessation may result in substantial clinical improvement.[54]

The most striking symptoms of DCM are those of left ventricular failure (see Chap. 22). Fatigue and weakness related to diminished cardiac output are common. Right-sided heart failure is a late and ominous sign and is associated with a particularly poor prognosis. Chest pain occurs in a minority of patients and may suggest concomitant ischemic heart disease. The demonstrated reduction in the vasodilator reserve of the coronary microvasculature in DCM suggests that subendocardial ischemia may play a role in the genesis of chest pain that occurs despite angiographically normal coronary arteries.[55] Chest pain secondary to pulmonary embolism and abdominal pain secondary to congestive hepatomegaly are frequent in the late stages of illness.

PHYSICAL EXAMINATION (see also Chaps. 8 and 22). Examination usually reveals variable degrees of cardiac enlargement and findings of congestive heart failure. The systolic blood pressure is usually normal or low, and the pulse pressure is narrow, reflecting a diminished stroke volume. *Pulsus alternans* is common when severe left ventricular failure is present. Cheyne-Stokes breathing may be present and is associated with a poor prognosis. The jugular veins are distended when right-sided heart failure appears, but on initial presentation most patients do not have evidence of this. Prominent a and v waves may be visible. Grossly pulsatile jugular veins with prominent regurgitant waves indicate the presence of tricuspid valvular regurgitation; this is usually a late and often ominous finding. The liver may be engorged and pulsatile. Peripheral edema and ascites are present when right-sided heart failure is advanced.

The precordium usually reveals left and, occasionally, right ventricular impulses, but the heaves are not sustained as they are in patients with ventricular hypertrophy. The apical impulse is usually displaced laterally, reflecting left ventricular dilation. A presystolic a wave may be palpable on occasion and is generated in a manner similar to that of a presystolic (S_4) gallop heard on auscultation. The second heart sound (S_2) is usually normally split, although paradoxical splitting may be detected in the presence of left bundle branch block, an electrocardiographic (ECG) finding that is not unusual in DCM. If pulmonary hypertension is present, the pulmonary component of S_2 may be accentuated and the splitting may be narrow. Presystolic gallop sounds (S_4) are common and often precede the development of overt congestive heart failure. Ventricular gallops (S_3) are the rule when cardiac decompensation occurs, and a summation gallop is heard when there is concomitant tachycardia.[56]

Systolic murmurs are common and are usually due to mitral or, less commonly, tricuspid valvular regurgitation. Mitral regurgitation results from enlargement and abnormal motion of the mitral annulus and distortion of the geometry of the subvalvular apparatus; ventricular dilation by itself plays a lesser role.[57] Gallop sounds and regurgitant murmurs can often be elicited or intensified by isometric handgrip exercise with its attendant enhancement of systemic vascular resistance and impedance to left ventricular outflow. Systemic emboli resulting from dislodgement of intracardiac thrombi from the left atrium and ventricle and pulmonary emboli that originate in the venous system of the legs are common late complications.

NONINVASIVE LABORATORY EXAMINATIONS. To identify potentially reversible causes of DCM, several basic screening biochemical tests are indicated, including determination of levels of serum phosphorus (hypophosphatemia), serum calcium (hypocalcemia), and serum creatinine and urea nitrogen (uremia); thyroid function studies (hypothyroidism and hyperthyroidism); and iron studies (hemochromatosis). It is prudent to test for HIV as well because this infection is an important and often unrecognized cause of congestive heart failure (see Chap. 61). Although not particularly useful for the diagnosis of DCM, elevated troponin T levels are predictive of a worse clinical course than normal levels.[58] The *chest roentgenogram* usually reveals generalized cardiomegaly and pulmonary vascular redistribution; interstitial and alveolar edema are less common on initial presentation. Pleural effusions may be present, and the azygos vein and superior vena cava may be dilated when right-sided heart failure supervenes.

Electrocardiography. The electrocardiogram often shows sinus tachycardia when heart failure is present. The entire spectrum of atrial and ventricular tachyarrhythmias may be seen. Poor R wave progression and intraventricular conduction abnormalities, especially left bundle branch block, are common.[59] Anterior Q waves may be present when there is extensive left ventricular fibrosis, even without a discrete myocardial scar or evidence of coronary artery disease. ST segment and T wave abnormalities are common, as are P wave changes, especially left atrial abnormality. Ambulatory monitoring demonstrates the ubiquity of ventricular arrhythmias, with the majority of monitored patients with DCM exhibiting nonsustained ventricular tachycardia.[60] There is no consensus that complex or frequent ventricular arrhythmias predict sudden (presumably arrhythmic) death, although they do appear to predict *total* mortality.[60] Perhaps ventricular arrhythmias as detected on ambulatory monitoring are a marker for the extent of myocardial damage in DCM and therefore are associated with sudden death without necessarily being its cause. In occasional cases, particularly in children, recurrent or incessant supraventricular or ventricular tachyarrhythmias may actually be the cause (rather than the result) of ventricular dysfunction.[61] In those cases, restoration of sinus rhythm or slowing of the heart rate may reverse the cardiomyopathy.[62]

Echocardiography. Two-dimensional and Doppler forms of echocardiography are useful in assessing the degree of impairment of left ventricular function and for excluding concomitant valvular or pericardial disease (see Chap. 11). In addition to examining all four cardiac valves for evidence of structural or functional abnormalities, echocardiography allows evaluation of the size of the ventricular cavity and thickness of the ventricular walls. A pericardial effusion is occasionally present. Doppler studies are useful in delineating the severity of mitral (and tricuspid) regurgitation. Patients with a pattern of left ventricular filling that simulates that seen with restrictive cardiomyopathies appear to have more advanced disease. Combining echocardiography with dobutamine infusion may identify patients with left ventricular dysfunction related to coronary artery disease by demonstrating provocable differences in regional wall motion and thus distinguish them from patients with idiopathic DCM. Furthermore, patients who demonstrate substantial contractile reserve with dobutamine infusion experience a better prognosis than those who do not.[63]

RADIONUCLIDE IMAGING. Current techniques using newer radionuclides and imaging protocols for *myocardial perfusion stress imaging* are quite reliable in making the differentiation of an ischemic from a nonischemic etiology of heart failure.[64] Like echocardiography, *radionuclide ventriculography* reveals increased end-diastolic and end-systolic left ventricular volumes, reduced ejection fraction in one or both ventricles, and wall motion abnormalities (see Chap. 13); it is used most commonly when echocardiography is technically suboptimal.

In most patients it is not necessary to carry out serial studies or batteries of noninvasive tests to observe patients with DCM and evaluate their response to treatment; adjustments in pharmacological therapies are usually based on routine bedside clinical features and symptomatic response.

CARDIAC CATHETERIZATION AND ANGIOCARDIOGRAPHY. Only certain patients with DCM require cardiac catheterization (particularly those with chest pain and a suspicion of ischemic disease or patients thought to have a treatable systemic disease such as sarcoidosis or hemochromatosis, in which myocardial biopsy is an important part of the catheterization procedure).[65] When cardiac catheterization is carried out, the left ventricular end-diastolic and pulmonary artery wedge pressures are usually elevated. Modest degrees of pulmonary arterial hypertension are common. Advanced cases may demonstrate right ventricular dilation and failure as well, with resultant elevation of the right ventricular end-diastolic, right atrial, and central venous pressures.

Left ventriculography demonstrates enlargement of this chamber, typically with a diffuse reduction in wall motion. Segmental wall motion abnormalities are not uncommon and may simulate the angiographic findings in ischemic heart disease. However, prominent localized wall motion disturbances are more characteristic of ischemic heart disease, whereas diffuse global dysfunction is more typical of DCM. The ejection fraction is reduced and the end-systolic volume is increased as a result of the impairment of left ventricular contractility. Sometimes left ventricular thrombi may be visualized within the left ventricle as intracavitary filling defects. Mild mitral regurgitation is often present. On occasion, it may be difficult to distinguish left ventricular dilation secondary to severe mitral regurgitation related to intrinsic mitral valve disease from DCM with secondary mitral regurgitation.

Coronary arteriography usually reveals normal vessels, although coronary vasodilator capacity may be impaired. This examination may be of particular value in excluding coronary artery disease in patients with abnormal Q waves on the electrocardiogram or regional left ventricular wall motion abnormalities on noninvasive evaluation. Coronary arteriography, when necessary, thus helps to distinguish between myocardial infarction as a result of obstructive coronary artery disease and extensive localized myocardial fibrosis secondary to severe DCM in the absence of coronary artery obstruction.

Management

Because the cause of idiopathic DCM, by definition, is unknown, specific therapy is not possible. Treatment, therefore, is for heart failure, as discussed in Chapters 23 and 24. Most patients should be treated with standard therapy, consisting of diuretics as needed for symptoms, angiotensin-converting enzyme inhibition, and beta-adrenergic blockade. Digoxin is considered a second-line agent, and the optimal dose is one that achieves a serum level of 0.5 to 0.8 ng/ml, as higher levels are associated with a small increase in mortality.[66]

Many of the therapeutic approaches are directed at modifying the results of the long-term activation of two interrelated systems, the adrenergic and renin-angiotensin systems. Physical, dietary, and pharmacological interventions may help to control symptoms; regular physical exercise (as tolerated) increases exercise capacity by improving endothelial dysfunction and augmenting blood flow in skeletal muscles.[67] Patients with left ventricular dysfunction not infrequently have sleep apnea, and treatment of those with obstructive sleep apnea with continuous positive airway pressure leads to an improvement in ventricular function, at least in part by reducing the increased afterload that results from the associated hypertension. Only cardiac transplantation (see Chap. 26) and specific pharmacological therapy (the vasodilators hydralazine plus nitrates, the angiotensin-converting enzyme inhibitor enalapril, the beta adrenoceptor blockers carvedilol and metoprolol, and the aldosterone receptor blocker spironolactone) have been shown to prolong life, but substantial progress has been made, with a nearly 50 percent reduction in heart failure mortality in the past decade![68]

CALCIUM ANTAGONISTS. Because of the possible link between DCM, microvascular circulatory abnormalities, and abnormal myocardial calcium handling, there has been interest in the use of calcium antagonists. These agents have generally been well tolerated when used in patients with DCM, although myocardial depression is an important potential side effect of the calcium antagonists as a group. Unfortunately, combining a calcium antagonist with traditional standard therapy does not appear to have substantial clinical benefit, nor does it reduce further the mortality in DCM. At present, the routine use of calcium antagonists in DCM is considered nonstandard and not first-line therapy.[69]

IMMUNOSUPPRESSIVES. In patients with chronic heart failure secondary to DCM and lymphocytic infiltrate on myocardial biopsy, treatment with corticosteroids and immunosuppressive agents had been advocated in the past. Unfortunately, such therapy does *not* appear to have a clinically important impact on mortality or progression to cardiac transplantation or on symptoms, exercise performance, or ejection fraction (except in the short term and perhaps in specific subgroups of DCM patients, such as those with HLA upregulation found on myocardial biopsy specimens).[70] In addition, it may be associated with significant complications.[71] Routine clinical use of immunosuppressive therapy thus cannot be recommended at present, at least until the subsets of DCM patients most likely to respond to such therapy can be identified.

BIVENTRICULAR PACING ("RESYNCHRONIZATION") (see Chaps. 24 and 31)

SURGICAL TREATMENT Surgical repair of a structurally normal but functionally incompetent mitral valve has been attempted in an increasing number of patients with DCM and prominent atrioventricular valvular regurgitation.[72] Although surgery was previously thought to be contraindicated because of the degree of preexisting cardiac dysfunction and damage (especially when valve replacement rather than repair was undertaken), some patients have shown symptomatic improvement, at least over the intermediate term.[73] The utility of left ventricular assist devices for end-stage DCM has been demonstrated (Chap. 25).[74] In appropriately selected patients, cardiac transplantation should be considered (see Chap. 26).

Alcoholic Cardiomyopathy

Chronic excessive consumption of alcohol may be associated with congestive heart failure, hypertension, cerebrovascular accidents, arrhythmias, and sudden death; it is the major cause of secondary, nonischemic DCM in the Western world and accounts for upward of one-third of all cases of DCM.[75] It is estimated that two-thirds of the adult population use alcohol to some extent, and more than 10 percent are heavy users.[76] Therefore, it is not surprising that alcoholic cardiomyopathy is a major problem. Ceasing alcohol consumption early in the course of alcoholic cardiomyopathy may halt the progression of or even reverse left ventricular contractile dysfunction. This is unlike the situation in nonalcoholic cardiomyopathy, which is often marked by progressive clinical deterioration.[77,78]

The consumption of alcohol may result in myocardial damage by three mechanisms: (1) a presumed direct toxic effect of alcohol or its metabolites; (2) nutritional effects, most commonly in association with thiamine deficiency that leads to beriberi heart disease (see Chap. 22); and (3) rarely, toxic effects related to additives in the alcoholic beverage (cobalt). There had been speculation that alcohol caused myocardial damage only through dietary deficiencies, but it is now clear that alcoholic cardiomyopathy occurs in the absence of nutritional deficiencies.

Typical Oriental beriberi may coexist with alcoholic cardiomyopathy, although it is no longer noted with any frequency. The distinguishing features of each include peripheral vasodilation and high-output heart failure, often right sided, in the former and reduced contractility with typically left-sided low-output failure in the latter.

The precise mechanisms of cardiac depression produced by alcohol are undetermined, but a direct toxic effect on striated muscle is likely (particularly because alcoholics often demonstrate concomitant skeletal myopathy and cardiomyopathy).[79] In acute studies, alcohol and its metabolite acetaldehyde have been shown to interfere with a number of membrane and cellular functions that involve the transport and binding of calcium, mitochondrial respiration, myocardial lipid metabolism, myocardial protein synthesis, and signal transduction.[80] The role that other associated electrolyte imbalances (hypokalemia, hypophosphatemia, hypomagnesemia) may play in alcohol-mediated damage has not been settled.

Because not all alcoholics develop cardiomyopathy, the relationship between the development of cardiac dysfunction and dose of alcohol is complex and probably multifactorial. There appears to be a genetic predisposition to the development of cardiomyopathy because alcoholics with the DD genotype of the angiotensin-converting enzyme are 16 times more likely to develop cardiac dysfunction than those without.[81] The cumulative dose of alcohol appears to be important in the eventual development of cardiomyopathy, and some data suggest that more moderate alcohol consumption may actually have a protective effect against the development of cardiac dysfunction and death.[82,83]

PATHOLOGY. The gross and microscopic pathological findings are nonspecific and similar to those observed in idiopathic DCM, with interstitial fibrosis, myocytolysis, evidence of small-vessel coronary artery disease, and myocyte hypertrophy.[75] Electron microscopy shows enlarged and disorganized mitochondria, with large glycogen-containing vacuoles.

Clinical Manifestations

Alcoholic cardiomyopathy most commonly occurs in men 30 to 55 years of age who have been heavy consumers of whisky, wine, or beer, usually for more than 10 years.[75] Female alcoholics who develop cardiomyopathy appear to have a lower cumulative lifetime dose of alcohol than men.[77] Although alcoholic cardiomyopathy may be observed in the homeless, malnourished, "skid row" alcoholic man, many patients are well-nourished individuals of middle and even upper socioeconomic status without liver disease or peripheral neuropathy. Accordingly, unless a high index of suspicion is maintained, it may be easy to miss a history of alcohol abuse. Persistent questioning of the patient and particularly the relatives of patients with unexplained cardiomegaly or cardiomyopathy is often required to elicit a history of alcoholism.

It is frequently possible to demonstrate mild depression of cardiac function in chronic alcoholics even before cardiac dysfunction becomes clinically manifest. Abnormalities of both systolic function (reduced ejection fraction) and diastolic function (increased myocardial wall stiffness) have been demonstrated in alcoholic patients without cardiac symptoms by a variety of invasive and noninvasive techniques.[84] Although overt alcoholic liver disease and cardiac involvement usually do not occur together, even cirrhotic patients without signs or symptoms of heart disease often have demonstrable evidence of asymptomatic myocardial disease.

The development of symptoms may be insidious, although some patients have acute and florid left-sided congestive heart failure. A paroxysm of atrial fibrillation is a relatively frequent initial presenting finding. More advanced cases demonstrate biventricular failure, with left ventricular dysfunction usually dominating. Dyspnea, orthopnea, and paroxysmal nocturnal dyspnea are frequently observed. Palpitations may be present and are usually due to supraventricular tachyarrhythmias. Syncope may occur as well and may be the result of supraventricular, or more likely ventricular, tachyarrhythmias. Angina pectoris does not occur unless there is concomitant coronary artery disease or aortic stenosis, although atypical chest pain may be seen.

PHYSICAL EXAMINATION. The cardiac findings resemble those seen in idiopathic DCM. Examination usually reveals a narrow pulse pressure, often with an elevated diastolic pressure secondary to excessive peripheral vasoconstriction. There is cardiomegaly, and protodiastolic (S3) and presystolic (S4) gallop sounds are common. An apical systolic murmur of mitral regurgitation is often found. The severity of right-sided heart failure varies, but jugular venous distention and peripheral edema are common. A concomitant skeletal muscle myopathy involving the shoulder and pelvic girdle is a frequent finding, and the degree of muscle weakness and histological abnormality in the skeletal muscles parallels that in the heart.[79]

LABORATORY EXAMINATION. The chest roentgenogram in advanced cases demonstrates considerable cardiac enlargement, pulmonary congestion, and pulmonary venous hypertension (see Chap. 12). Pleural effusions are often seen. ECG abnormalities are common and frequently are the only indication of alcoholic heart disease during the preclinical phase. Alcoholic patients without other evidence of heart disease are often seen after developing palpitations, chest discomfort, or syncope, typically after a binge of alcohol consumption on a weekend (particularly during the year-end holiday season). This has been dubbed the "holiday heart syndrome." The most common arrhythmia observed is atrial fibrillation, followed by atrial flutter and frequent ventricular premature contractions. Alcohol consumption may predispose to atrial flutter or fibrillation even in nonalcoholics. Hypokalemia may play a role in the genesis of some of these arrhythmias. Supraventricular arrhythmias are also frequently observed in patients with overt alcoholic cardiomyopathy. Sudden unexpected death is not uncommon in young adult alcoholics, and it is likely that ventricular fibrillation is responsible.

Atrioventricular conduction disturbances (most commonly first-degree heart block), bundle branch block, left ventricular hypertrophy, poor R wave progression across the precordium, and repolarization abnormalities are common ECG findings. Prolongation of the QT interval is noted frequently. ST segment and T wave changes are often restored to normal within several days after cessation of alcohol consumption.

The hemodynamic findings observed at cardiac catheterization and the assessment of left ventricular function by noninvasive methods (echocardiography and isotope angiography) resemble those in idiopathic DCM.

MANAGEMENT. The key to the long-term treatment of alcoholic cardiomyopathy is a reduction of alcohol consumption (and preferably abstinence) as early in the course of the disease as possible.[83] This may be quite effective in improving the signs and symptoms of congestive heart failure.[85] The prognosis in patients who continue to drink heavily is poor,[54] particularly if they have been symptomatic for a long time.

The management of acute episodes of congestive heart failure is similar to that of idiopathic DCM. For patients with severe congestive heart failure, it is prudent to administer thiamine on the chance that beriberi may be contributing to the heart failure. Whether to use chronic anticoagulation (as is often considered in idiopathic DCM) is a difficult question; we usually do not prescribe warfarin unless there are unequivocal and pressing indications because of the increased risk of bleeding related to noncompliance, trauma, and over-anticoagulation because of hepatic dysfunction.

COBALT CARDIOMYOPATHY

A previously unrecognized syndrome of severe congestive heart failure appeared in the mid-1960s, first in Canada and subsequently in the United States and Europe.[86] The disease was found in people who drank a particular brand of beer to which cobalt sulfate had been added as a foam stabilizer. Since cobalt was removed from the process, no more cases of the disease have been reported.

Arrhythmogenic Right Ventricular Cardiomyopathy (see also Chap. 32)

This unique cardiomyopathy (which is also called arrhythmogenic right ventricular dysplasia) is marked by myocardial cell loss with partial or total replacement of right ventricular muscle by adipose and fibrous tissue; apoptosis appears to be a principal cause of the cell death (Fig. 59–4).[87-89] ARVC is associated with reentrant ventricular tachyarrhythmias of right ventricular origin (producing a left bundle branch block configuration in the QRS complex)[90] that are often precipitated by an exercise-induced discharge of catecholamines and are a harbinger of sudden death.[88] In about one-third of the cases there is autosomal dominant inheritance of the disease,[91] and several distinct genetic mutations have been reported, including a mutation in the gene coding for the cardiac ryanodine receptor (hRYR2).[92] Another variant, found on the Greek island of Naxos, is inherited as a recessive trait but with a high degree of penetrance.[93]

ARVC is distinct from the *Uhl anomaly,* which is marked by extreme thinning of the ventricular wall.[94] The diagnosis of AVRC is based on a constellation of clinical, ECG, histological, and echocardiographic findings.[95,96] Typical features include the appearance of clinical manifestations in adolescence or early adulthood, male predominance, normal physical examination, inverted T waves in the right precordial ECG leads, symptoms of palpitations and syncope, and a risk of sudden death.[96,97] In some patients with ventricular arrhythmias of no evident cause, clinically subtle right ventricular dysplasia may be responsible.

Noninvasive and invasive evaluations demonstrate a dilated, poorly contractile right ventricle, usually with a normal left ventricle, although variable degrees of left ventricular involvement have been seen.[95,98] When left-sided involvement is present, the risk of sudden death is increased.[99] Magnetic resonance imaging (MRI) is of particular value in identifying patients with this condition[100] who in other regards may appear to be completely normal (Fig. 59–5).

MANAGEMENT. Antiarrhythmic therapy, especially with beta adrenoceptor blockers, sotalol, or amiodarone, is often effective in controlling the arrhythmias.[88] The arrhythmias may be related to abnormalities of regional right ventricular sympathetic innervation and a reduced density of beta-adrenergic receptors or impaired presynaptic catecholamine reuptake, as has been demonstrated by noninvasive scintigraphy.[101] Cryo- or catheter-based radiofrequency ablation of the presumed arrhythmogenic focus has been successful in resolving the ventricular arrhythmia in some patients unresponsive to or intolerant of antiarrhythmic drug therapy.[102] Insertion of an implantable cardioverter-defibrillator (ICD) or cardiac transplantation is reserved for patients with indications for these procedures (see Chaps. 26 and 31).[88,97]

Hypertrophic Cardiomyopathy

Although HCM was first described more than a century ago, the unique features of HCM were not studied systematically until the late 1950s.[103,104] The characteristic finding is inappropriate myocardial hypertrophy that occurs in the absence of an obvious cause for the hypertrophy (e.g., aortic stenosis or systemic hypertension), often predominantly involving the interventricular septum of a nondilated left ventricle that shows hyperdynamic systolic function (Fig. 59–6).[105,106] A distinctive clinical feature was soon recognized in some patients with HCM—a dynamic pressure gradient in the subaortic area that divided the left ventricle into a high-pressure apical region and a lower pressure subaortic region (Fig. 59–7A).[103] Although subsequent studies have shown that only a minority of patients (perhaps a fourth)[105–108] demonstrate this outflow gradient, its unique features attracted much attention and led to a myriad of terms (more than 75) used to describe the disease (among the more popular terms were *idiopathic hypertrophic subaortic* stenosis[103] and *muscular subaortic stenosis*).[109] The term *hypertrophic cardiomyopathy* is now preferred because most patients do not have an outflow gradient or "stenosis" of the left ventricular outflow tract.[106] Because hypertrophy typically occurs in the absence of a pressure gradient, the characteristic distinguishing feature of HCM is myocardial hypertrophy that is out of proportion to the hemodynamic load.

characterized by abnormal stiffness of the left ventricle with resultant impaired ventricular filling. This abnormality in relaxation produces increased left ventricular end-diastolic pressure with resulting pulmonary congestion and dyspnea, the most common symptoms in HCM, despite typically hyperdynamic left ventricular systolic function. The overall prevalence of HCM is low: about 0.2 percent (1 in 500) of the general population and 0.5 percent of unselected patients referred for an echocardiographic examination.[105] It may be the most common genetically transmitted cardiac disorder.[106]

Pathology

MACROSCOPIC EXAMINATION. This typically discloses a marked increase in myocardial mass, and the ventricular cavities are small (see Figs. 59–1 and 59–6).[104] The left ventricle is usually more involved in the hypertrophic process than the right, but variable degrees of right-sided involvement may be seen.[110] The atria are dilated and often hypertrophied, reflecting the high resistance to filling of the ventricles caused by diastolic dysfunction and the effects of atrioventricular valve regurgitation. The pattern and extent of left ventricular hypertrophy in HCM vary greatly from patient to patient, and a characteristic feature is heterogeneity in the amount of hypertrophy evident in different regions of the left ventricle. A feature found in most patients with HCM is disproportionate involvement of the interventricular septum and anterolateral wall compared with the posterior segment of the free wall of the left ventricle.[106] When hypertrophy is largely localized to the anterior septum, the process has been called asymmetrical septal hypertrophy (ASH). A wide variety of other patterns of hypertrophy may be seen, and about 30 percent of patients show only localized and relatively mild hypertrophy in a single region of the ventricle.[104,106]

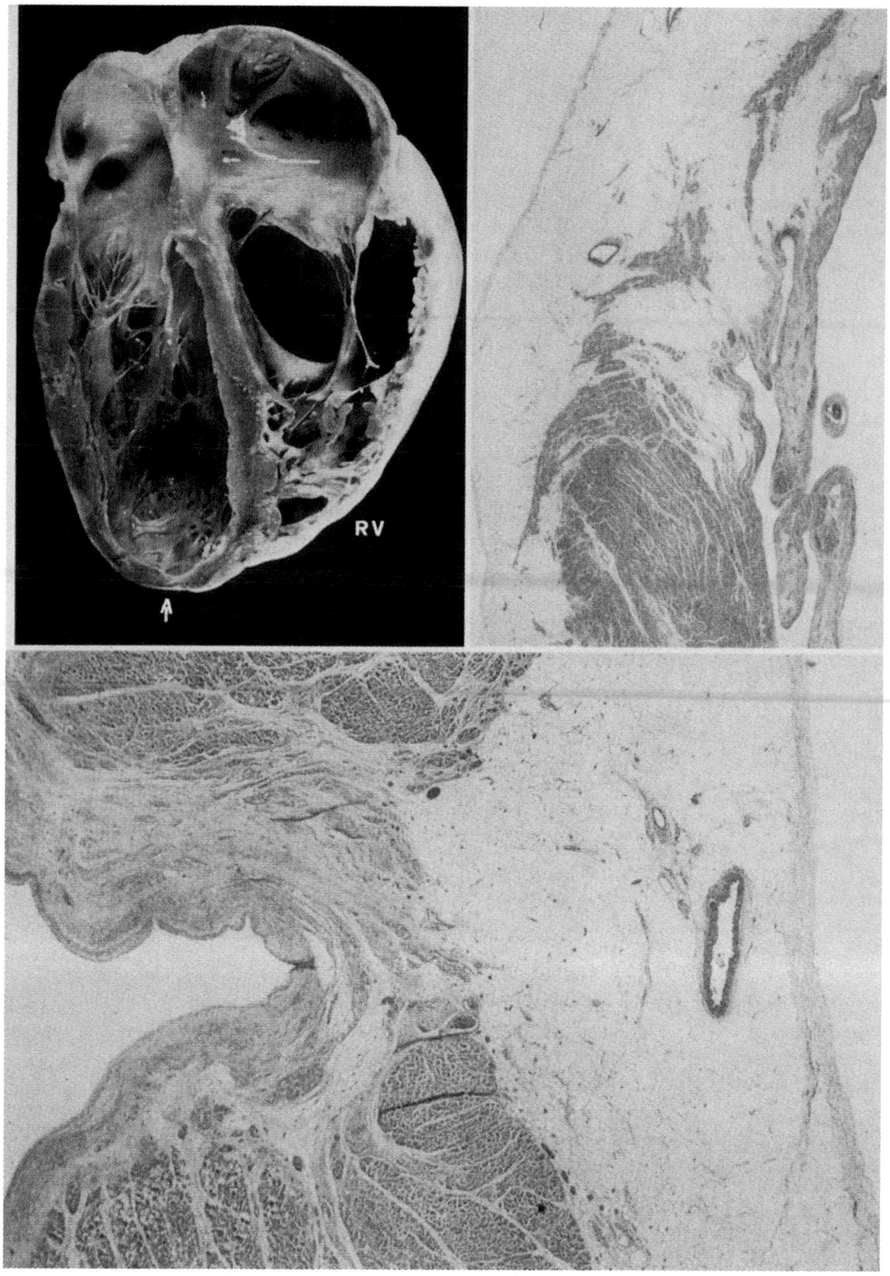

FIGURE 59–4 **Top left,** Postmortem pathological section of heart (four-chamber) in a patient with arrhythmogenic right ventricular cardiomyopathy and biventricular involvement. Severe widespread fatty infiltration of right ventricular (RV) wall is present; an apical aneurysm is present at the left ventricular level (arrow). **Top right,** Histological section at level of RV inflow (hematoxylin and eosin, ×2.5). Severe transmural fibrofatty infiltration of RV wall is present, compatible with RV dysplasia. **Bottom,** Histological section at the level of the left ventricle (outflow) (hematoxylin and eosin, ×2.5) shows focal severe fibrofatty infiltration with myocellular atrophy, compatible with left ventricular involvement. (From Pinamonti B, Pagnan L, Bussani R, et al: Right ventricular dysplasia with biventricular involvement. Circulation 98:1943-1945, 1998. Copyright 1998, American Heart Association.)

Morphological evidence of the disease is found in about one-fourth of the first-degree relatives of a patient with HCM; in many of the relatives the disease is milder than in the propositus, the degree of hypertrophy is less and is more localized, and outflow gradients are usually lacking. Symptoms are often absent or minimal, and the disease is detected only by echocardiography.

The physiological characteristics of HCM differ substantially from those of DCM. The most characteristic pathophysiological abnormality in HCM is *diastolic* rather than systolic dysfunction (see Chaps. 20 and 22).[104] Thus, HCM is

Differentiation of the "physiological" hypertrophy that occurs in some highly trained athletes from that seen in HCM may be difficult. Elite athletes may demonstrate left ventricular wall thicknesses up to 16 mm in the absence of HCM (normal <12 mm) along with marked ECG abnormalities.[104,111] Features that may permit differentiation of the two are the abnormal response of Doppler ultrasound–derived indices of diastolic function in response to isometric handgrip, the identification of HCM in a relative, or the simple demonstration of exceptional exercise capacity on cardiopulmonary exercise testing in normal elite athletes.[106,112]

Some patients with HCM have substantial hypertrophy in unusual locations, such as the posterior portion of the septum, the posterobasal free wall, and the midventricular level.[104] The degree of hypertrophy is dynamic in most patients and changes over time; prominent hypertrophy is rarely found in infants, and the typical patient develops hypertrophy during adolescence.[108] Development of the morphological features of HCM is unusual after the age of about 18 years,[106] although when it does occur later it is seen especially with a mutation of cardiac myosin-binding protein C.[113] There is usually an inverse relationship between the extent of hypertrophy in HCM and age. Whether this is due to premature death of younger patients with greater hypertrophy or progressive reduction in the extent of hypertrophy is unknown.[106] About 5 to 10 percent of patients eventually develop a "burned-out" phase of HCM that resembles DCM and is marked by myocardial wall thinning, ventricular dilation, systolic dysfunction, and progressive congestive heart failure.[104] Clinically silent remodeling of the ventricle may produce subtle regression of hypertrophy in some patients.[104]

Other morphological abnormalities include enlargement and elongation of the mitral valve leaflets and, in rare cases, anomalous papillary muscle insertion directly into the anterior mitral valve leaflet.[106,114,115]

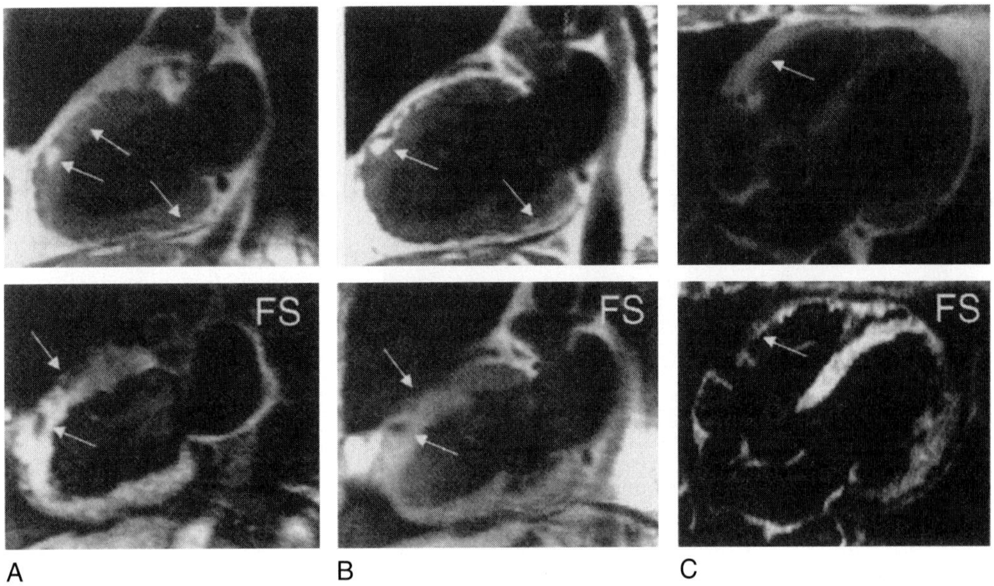

FIGURE 59–5 Magnetic resonance images before (upper panels) and after (lower panels) the application of a special imaging algorithm (fat saturation, FS) to highlight areas of fat deposition in a patient with biventricular involvement by arrhythmogenic right ventricular cardiomyopathy. The arrows (upper panels) point to areas of fatty infiltration of the anterior and inferior left (**A** and **B**) and right (**C**) ventricular myocardium. Fatty infiltration is confirmed (lower panels) by the special FS algorithm as black areas that are highlighted by arrows. (From McCrohon JA, John AS, Lorenz CH, et al: Images in cardiovascular medicine. Left ventricular involvement in arrhythmogenic right ventricular cardiomyopathy. Circulation 105:1394, 2002. Copyright 2002, American Heart Association.)

APICAL HYPERTROPHIC CARDIOMYOPATHY. A variant with predominant involvement of the apex is common in Japan and is estimated to represent a fourth of Japanese patients with HCM.[116] In other parts of the world, apical HCM is less common (<10 percent in one large Western center).[115] Typical features include a characteristic spade-like configuration of the left ventricle during angiographic study, giant negative T waves in the precordial ECG leads, absence of an intraventricular pressure gradient, mild symptoms, and a generally benign course with low mortality.[117] Nevertheless, complications may be seen, with atrial fibrillation the most common.[118]

HYPERTROPHIC CARDIOMYOPATHY IN ELDERLY PEOPLE. HCM may on occasion arise in elderly people and often demonstrates unique features, including an especially small left ventricular cavity but with relatively mild hypertrophy. Other findings include marked anterior displacement of the mitral valve, extensive submitral (annular) calcification in some patients, a left ventricular outflow gradient, and late appearance of symptoms.[119]

Gross cardiac morphological features similar to those in HCM may be seen in infants of diabetic mothers and in patients with a variety of other conditions,[104] including hyperparathyroidism, neurofibromatosis, generalized lipodystrophy, lentiginosis, pheochromocytoma, Friedreich ataxia, and Noonan syndrome. Rarely, the findings may be simulated by amyloid, glycogen storage disease, or tumor involvement of the septum.

HISTOLOGY. Microscopic findings in HCM are distinctive, with myocardial hypertrophy and gross disorganization of the muscle bundles, resulting in a characteristic whorled pattern (see Fig. 59-2); abnormalities are found in the cell-to-cell arrangement (disarray) (see Fig. 59-6) and disorganization of the myofibrillar architecture within a given cell.[120] Fibrosis is usually prominent and may be extensive enough to produce grossly visible scars. Foci of disorganized cells are often interspersed between areas of hypertrophied but otherwise normal-appearing muscle cells. Interstitial (matrix) connective tissue elements are increased. Although abnormally arranged cardiac muscle cells were initially considered specific for HCM, it is now recognized that they may be found in a variety of congenital and acquired heart conditions. What is unique about the disarray in HCM is its ubiquity and frequency. Almost all HCM patients have some degree of disarray, and most have involvement of 5 percent or more of the myocardium; in general, a third or more of the myocardium demonstrates disarray.[104,106,120] In contrast, disarray in non-HCM patients (when it occurs) usually involves less than 5 percent of the myocardium.[108] In an experimental model of HCM, myocardial regions with prominent disarray demonstrate regional contractile dysfunction related in part to the structural abnormalities themselves (as a result of the attendant abnormal geometry and length of the myocardial fibers).[121]

Abnormal intramural coronary arteries, with a reduction in the size of the lumen and thickening of the vessel wall, are common in HCM.[120] The prominence of abnormal intramural coronary arteries in areas of extensive myocardial fibrosis is consistent with the hypothesis that these abnormalities may be responsible for the development of myocardial ischemia that appears to be central to many of the clinical manifestations of HCM, including angina pectoris, arrhythmias, and sudden death.[104,106]

Etiology

Genetics of Hypertrophic Cardiomyopathy (see also Chap. 70)

Familial HCM occurs as an autosomal dominant mendelian-inherited disease at least 50 percent of the time.[122] It is thought that some if not all of the sporadic forms of the disease are due to spontaneous mutations.[123] At least 10 different genes are associated with HCM (Fig. 59–8; see Table 59–4).[124] All of the genes encode cardiac sarcomere proteins, including components of the thick or thin filaments that have contractile, regulatory, or structural functions.[11,20,113,124] More than 150 different mutations have been discovered thus far, and most are of the missense type.[104,113.,125] It is clear that more genetic defects are yet to be identified. The precise mechanism by which the various genetic mutations culminate in the morphological and clinical features of HCM is speculative at present, but all of the mutations probably cause abnormal force generation with an attendant hypertrophic response.[11,108,126,127] The ultimate manifestations of the resulting cardiomyopathy are probably the end result of a variety of interacting factors.[20,124,128] Thus, various sarcomeric mutations (such as of troponin T, tropomyosin, or the beta-myosin heavy chain [MHC] gene) can culminate in *either* HCM or DCM (see Table 59–4),[20,22] although in some cases the apparent DCM may simply reflect the burned-out phase of HCM.[129] An occasional family with familial HCM is affected by more than one mutation.[123]

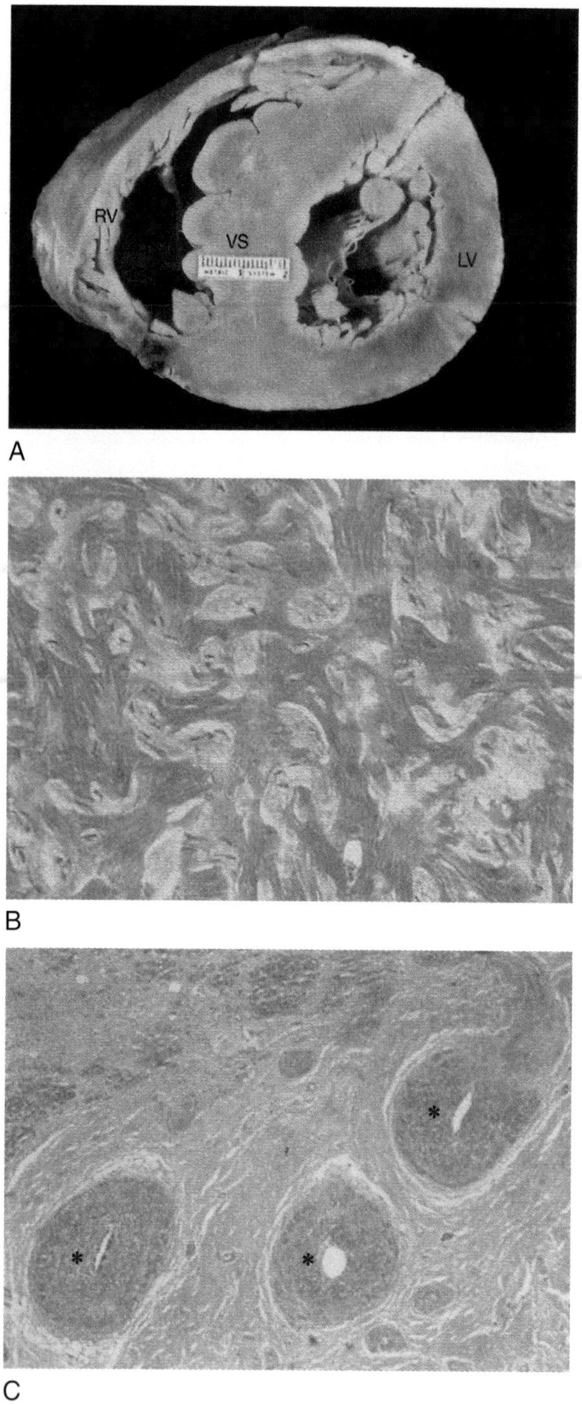

FIGURE 59–6 Morphological features of hypertrophic cardiomyopathy. **A,** Gross heart specimen of a 13-year-old male athlete with disproportionate thickening of the interventricular septum (VS) compared with the left ventricular (LV) free wall. **B,** Histological specimen showing marked cellular disarray with hypertrophied cells arranged in a chaotic pattern. **C,** Histological specimen showing several abnormal intramural coronary arteries, with markedly thickened walls and narrowed lumina. RV = right ventricle; hematoxylin and eosin stain in B and C; original magnifications ×50. (Adapted from Maron BJ: Hypertrophic cardiomyopathy. Curr Probl Cardiol 18:637, 1993, with permission of Mosby, Inc.)

The genetic basis of HCM was first reported by Seidman and Seidman, who reported the existence of a disease gene located on chromosome 14q11-12.[18] Subsequently they found this to be the gene encoding beta cardiac MHC. Sequencing of this gene in one family with HCM revealed that the abnormality was caused by a gene duplication in which the alpha and beta MHC genes were fused and present in an extra copy. In the second family, there was a point mutation in the beta MHC sequence that altered the myosin's arginine to glutamine. Both of these mutations affect the polypeptides crucial to the structure of myofibrils and might be responsible for the myocyte and myofibrillar disarray characteristic of familial HCM. Other disease loci that have been identified include chromosome 1q32 (encoding troponin T), chromosome 19p13 (encoding troponin I), chromosome 15q22 (encoding alpha-tropomyosin), chromosome 11p11 (encoding myosin-binding protein C), chromosomes 3p21 and 12q23-p21 (encoding essential and regulatory myosin light chains), and chromosome 15q14 (encoding actin).[18,122,130] A missense mutation of the gene that encodes a subunit of the adenosine monophosphate–activated protein kinase (*PRKAG2*) is associated with the Wolff-Parkinson-White syndrome, conduction abnormalities, and apparent left ventricular hypertrophy,[131] but this condition is due to glycogen accumulation within myocytes and thus should be regarded as a metabolic storage disease rather than a form of HCM.[104]

Most cases of familial HCM are caused by one of three mutant genes.[104] It is estimated that about 35 to 50 percent are due to mutations of the cardiac MHC gene, 15 to 25 percent due to mutations of myosin-binding protein C, 15 to 20 percent due to mutations of the cardiac troponin T gene, less than 5 percent due to mutations of the tropomyosin gene, and the remainder due to mutations of other genes.[132] There is wide variation in the phenotypic expression of a specific mutation of a given gene, with variability in clinical symptoms and the degree as well as time course of appearance of hypertrophy.[104] Of particular interest are mutations of the troponin T gene that typically result in only modest (or no) hypertrophy but indicate a poor prognosis and a high risk of sudden death (although at least one mutation has a favorable prognosis).[133,134] Several other "malignant" mutations have been described that involve the beta-MHC and tropomyosin.[135,136] Conversely, certain genes and mutations are felt to be associated with a more favorable prognosis, although the concept of a mutation-specific clinical outcome has been challenged.[137] In some patients with an abnormal gene and no echocardiographic evidence of HCM, the electrocardiogram is abnormal. Thus, otherwise unexplained abnormalities of the electrocardiogram in first-degree relatives of patients with HCM may be indicative of a carrier or preclinical state.[138]

Despite the substantial insights that molecular genetic studies have provided into the fundamental mechanisms responsible for HCM, DNA analysis for mutant genes is not yet routinely available for clinical use, although it is anticipated that it will become available in the future.[104,111] In addition, many clinicians do not adequately discuss the genetic implications of HCM with their patients, at least in part because the typical cardiologist manages only a small number of patients with HCM.[139]

Pathophysiology

SYSTOLE. Since the initial descriptions of HCM, the feature that has attracted the greatest attention is the dynamic pressure gradient across the left ventricular outflow tract (see Fig. 59–7).[103,107,139,140] Although this pressure gradient was initially attributed to a muscular sphincter action in the subaortic region or was believed by some to be an artifact,[109] it is now considered to be related to further narrowing of an already small outflow tract (narrowed by prominent septal hypertrophy and possibly abnormal location of the mitral valve) by systolic anterior motion of often elongated mitral valve leaflets against the hypertrophied septum.

There continues to be considerable controversy about the cause and significance of the outflow gradient.[109] Central to the disagreement is whether there is true obstruction to left ventricular ejection or whether the pressure gradient is simply the consequence of vigorous ventricular emptying.[141] It is now agreed that true mechanical impediment to left ventricular ejection occurs when outflow gradients are present and is the result of distal portions of the mitral valve apparatus moving anteriorly across the outflow tract and making contact with the ventricular septum in midsystole.[106,139,141] There continues to be controversy about the fundamental cause of the distinctive mitral valve systolic movement. Central to the controversy is whether the valve apparatus is displaced anteriorly because of Venturi effects and as a result of the increased ejection velocities produced by the abnormal left ventricular outflow tract orientation and geometry or whether it is *pushed* into the outflow tract as a consequence of ejection.

The pressure overload that results from the outflow gradient appears to play some role in the development of ventricular hypertrophy in HCM, perhaps involving TNF-alpha, because both myocyte hypertrophy and TNF-alpha levels are reduced after successful reduction of the gradient by septal ablation.[142,143]

DIASTOLE. Most patients with HCM demonstrate abnormalities of diastolic function (see Chaps. 20 and 21) at rest or with stress, whether or not a pressure gradient is present and whether or not they are symptomatic.[144] These abnormalities of global diastolic filling are largely independent of the extent and distribution of myocardial hypertrophy; patients with mild and apparently localized hypertrophy may demonstrate prominent diastolic dysfunction, suggesting that the myopathic process occurs in ventricular regions that are not macroscopically hypertrophied.[116] Diastolic dysfunction in turn leads to increased ventricular filling pressure despite a normal or small left ventricular cavity and appears to result from abnormalities of left ventricular relaxation and distensibility, at least in part as a direct result of the altered protein expression that occurs in many HCM patients as a consequence of genetic mutations.[145] Early diastolic filling is impaired when relaxation is prolonged, perhaps related to abnormal calcium kinetics, subendocardial ischemia, or the abnormal loading conditions found in HCM.[146] Late diastolic filling is altered when left ventricular distensibility is impaired; as a consequence, filling pressures rise. HCM may cause abnormal distensibility of the ventricle because of fibrosis or cellular disorganization.

MYOCARDIAL ISCHEMIA. Myocardial ischemia is common and multifactorial in HCM (Table 59–5).[147] Major causes include impaired vasodilator reserve (perhaps related to the thickened and narrowed small intramural coronary arteries found in HCM)[148]; increased oxygen demand, especially in patients with outflow gradients; and elevated filling pressures with resultant subendocardial ischemia.[147,149,150] In children, compression of intramyocardial segments of the left anterior descending coronary artery (so-called myocardial bridge) has been reported to predispose to myocardial ischemia and sudden death, but this has been contested.[151]

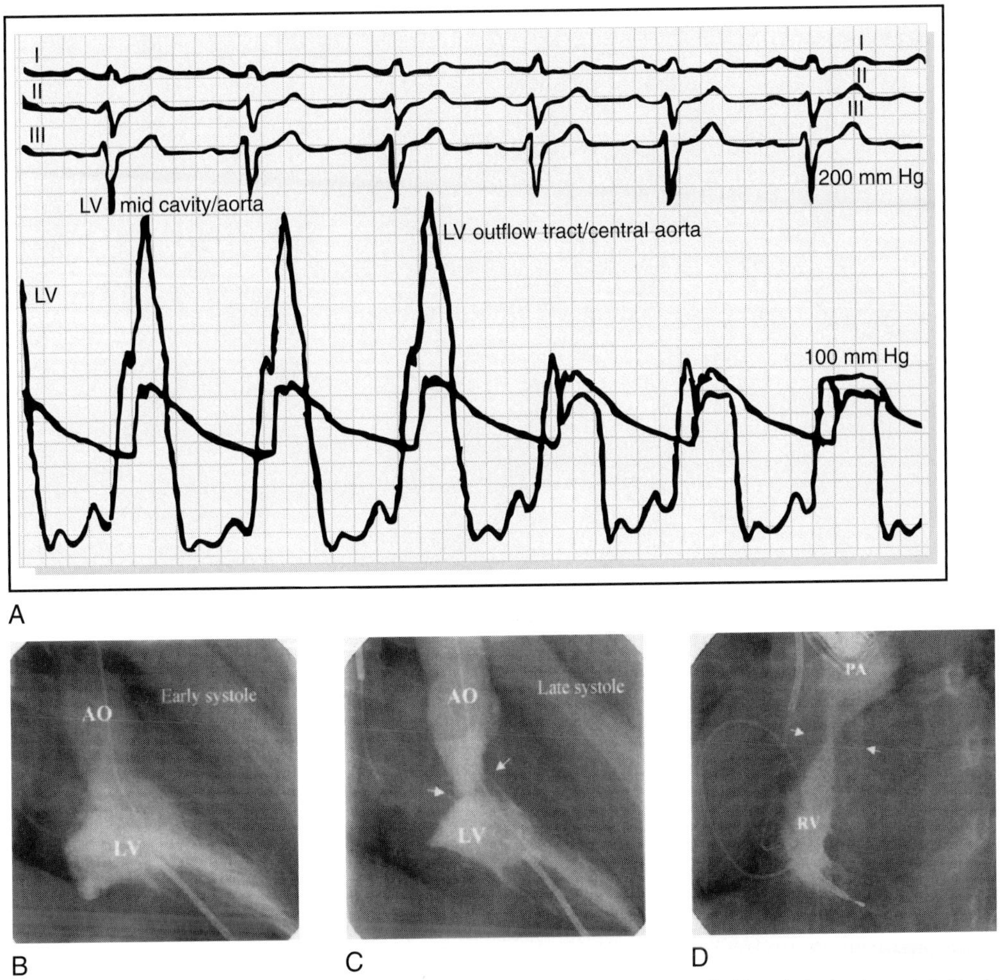

FIGURE 59–7 Hemodynamic and angiographic findings in hypertrophic cardiomyopathy with biventricular involvement. **A,** Simultaneous pressure recordings from the mid left ventricular (LV) cavity and aorta show a 100 mm Hg gradient. The aortic tracing shows a "spike-and-dome" pattern related to systolic anterior movement of the anterior leaflet of the mitral valve. The subaortic location of the gradient is confirmed as the LV catheter is pulled back from the midcavity (left) to the subaortic outflow tract (right). **B** and **C,** Left ventriculogram in the right anterior oblique projection. Arrows show systolic anterior mitral valve movement in late systole with attendant obstruction of the outflow tract. **D,** Right ventriculogram in the left lateral projection showing massive hypertrophy of the right ventricular (RV) outflow area (arrows) with an "hourglass" configuration. AO = aorta; PA = pulmonary artery. (From Doshi SN, Kim MC, Sharma SK, et al: Images in cardiovascular medicine. Right and left ventricular outflow tract obstruction in hypertrophic cardiomyopathy. Circulation 106:e3, 2002. Copyright 2002, American Heart Association.)

TABLE 59–5 Possible Mechanisms for Ischemia in Hypertrophic Cardiomyopathy

Increased Myocardial Oxygen Demand	Reduced Myocardial Perfusion
Myocardial hypertrophy	Small vessel disease
Diastolic dysfunction	Abnormal vascular responses
Myocyte disarray	Myocardial bridges
Left ventricular outflow obstruction	Increased coronary vascular resistance
Arrhythmias	

From McKenna WJ, Behr ER: Hypertrophic cardiomyopathy: Management, risk stratification, and prevention of sudden death. Heart 87:169, 2002.

Clinical Manifestations

HISTORY. The majority of patients with HCM are asymptomatic or only mildly symptomatic[105,140,152] and often are identified during screening of relatives of a patient with HCM. Unfortunately, the first clinical manifestation of the disease in such individuals may be sudden death. The disease is identified most often in adults in their fourth and fifth decades; it occurs more often than is commonly suspected in elderly patients. The condition has been observed at necropsy in stillborns and both clinically and

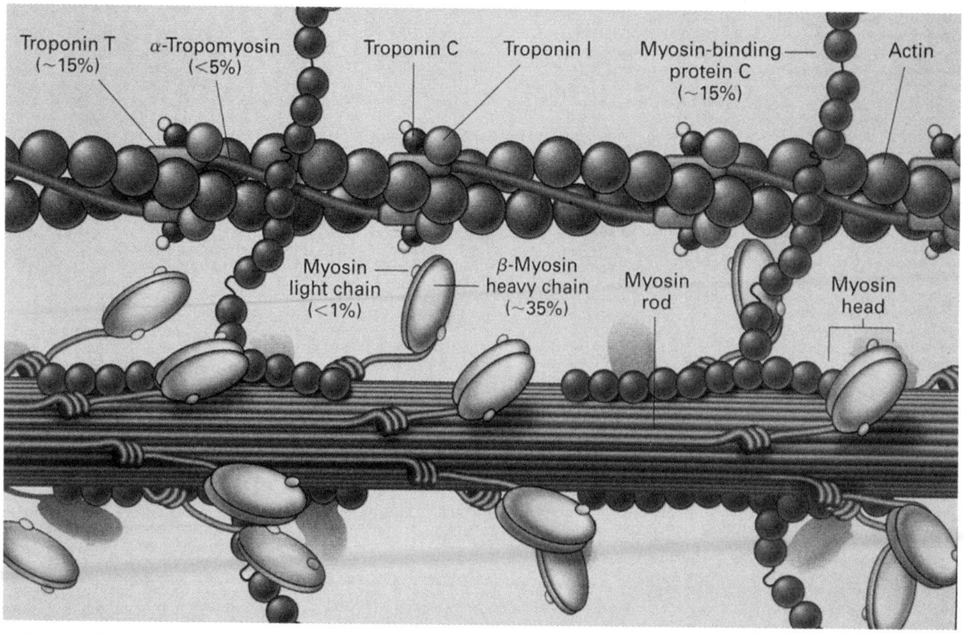

FIGURE 59–8 Drawing showing components of the sarcomere and mutations in hypertrophic cardiomyopathy. Cardiac contraction occurs when calcium binds the troponin complex (subunits C, I, and T) and alpha-tropomyosin. Actin stimulates ATPase activity in the globular myosin head and results in the production of force along actin filaments. Cardiac myosin-binding protein C binds myosin and modulates contraction. In hypertrophic cardiomyopthy, mutations may impair these and other protein interactions, result in ineffectual contraction, and produce hypertrophy. Percentages represent the estimated frequency with which a mutation causes hypertrophic cardiomyopathy. (From Spirito P, Seidman C, McKenna WJ, et al: The management of hypertophic cardiomyopathy. N Engl J Med 336:775, 1997. Copyright 1997, Massachusetts Medical Society.)

pathologically in octogenarians and is distinguished among cardiovascular diseases by its potential for clinical presentation during any phase of life.[104,140,152,153] The importance of recognizing this disorder in children at the earliest possible time is highlighted by the higher mortality rate in younger patients; death is often sudden and unexpected.[107,140] When HCM is first diagnosed in older patients, several features are distinctive and are in contrast to findings in younger patients: generally mild degrees of left ventricular hypertrophy, frequent demonstration of outflow gradients, and appearance of marked symptoms late in life (typically after age 55).[104,152] A particularly high index of suspicion of this condition must be maintained to make the clinical diagnosis in elderly people because their symptoms may easily be confused with those of coronary artery or aortic valve disease. Because syncope and sudden death have been associated with competitive sports and severe exertion in patients with HCM, it is important to diagnose this condition so that these activities may be proscribed. It appears that HCM may be more commonly unrecognized and undiagnosed in the black population than in the white population.[154]

The clinical picture varies considerably, ranging from the asymptomatic relative of a patient with recognized HCM who has a slightly abnormal echocardiogram but no other overt manifestation of the disease to the patient with incapacitating symptoms.[140] A general relationship exists between the extent of hypertrophy and the severity of symptoms, but the relationship is not absolute, and some patients have severe symptoms with only mild and apparently localized hypertrophy and vice versa. A complex interaction occurs between left ventricular hypertrophy, the left ventricular pressure gradient, diastolic dysfunction, and myocardial ischemia, which accounts for the great variability in symptoms from patient to patient.

The most common symptom is *dyspnea,* occurring in up to 90 percent of symptomatic patients. It is largely a consequence of the elevated left ventricular diastolic (and therefore left atrial and pulmonary venous) pressure, which results principally from impaired ventricular filling owing to diastolic dysfunction.[107,133,139,140] Angina pectoris (found in about three-fourths of symptomatic patients), fatigue, presyncope, and syncope are also common. Palpitations, paroxysmal nocturnal dyspnea, overt congestive heart failure, and dizziness are found less frequently, although severe congestive heart failure culminating in death may be seen. Exertion tends to exacerbate many of the symptoms. A variety of mechanisms may contribute to the production of angina pectoris (see Table 59–5). It is at least in part the result of an imbalance between oxygen supply and demand as a consequence of the greatly increased myocardial mass.[107] Abnormalities of the small coronary arteries may contribute to myocardial ischemia, particularly during exertion, and perhaps 20 percent of older patients with HCM may have concomitant atheromatous obstructive coronary artery disease. Transmural infarction may occur in the absence of narrowing of the extramural coronary arteries. Impaired diastolic relaxation may produce subendocardial ischemia as a result of prolonged maintenance of wall tension with a concomitant slower than normal decrease in the impedance to coronary blood flow. Syncope may result from inadequate cardiac output with exertion or from cardiac arrhythmias. Near-syncopal ("graying out") spells that occur in the erect posture and that can be relieved by immediately lying down are common.[140] However, in contrast to valvular aortic stenosis, syncope or near-syncope may not be an ominous finding in adult patients with HCM; some patients have a history of such episodes dating back many years without clinical deterioration.[105] In children and adolescents, however, presyncope and syncope identify patients at increased risk for sudden death (see Natural History).

PHYSICAL EXAMINATION. This may be normal (except for an S_4; see later), especially in asymptomatic patients without pressure gradients, those with mild hypertrophy, and those with the apical variant of HCM, but findings are usually prominent in patients with a left ventricular outflow tract pressure gradient.[103,104] The apical precordial impulse is often displaced laterally and is usually abnormally forceful and diffuse. Because of decreased left ventricular compliance, a prominent presystolic apical impulse that results from forceful atrial systole is often present.[140] This may result in a double apical impulse as a result of the prominent a wave. A more characteristic but less frequently recognized abnormality is a triple apical beat, the third impulse consisting of a late systolic bulge that occurs when the heart is almost empty and is performing near-isometric contraction.[140] The jugular venous pulse may demonstrate a prominent a wave, reflecting diminished right ventricular compliance secondary to massive hypertrophy of the ventricular septum. The carotid pulse typically rises briskly and then declines in midsystole as the gradient develops, followed by a secondary rise.[140] This may be appreciated on physical examination but can be demonstrated more clearly by means of indirect carotid pulse tracings. It is identical to the "spike-and-dome" configuration seen on direct arterial pressure recordings obtained during cardiac catheterization (see Fig. 59–7).

AUSCULTATION. The S_1 is normal and is often preceded by an S_4 that corresponds to the apical presystolic impulse. The S_2 is usually normally split. In some patients, however, it is narrowly split and in others, particularly those with severe outflow gradients, paradoxical splitting may be noted.[140] An S_3 may be present but does not have the same ominous significance as in patients with valvular aortic stenosis. Systolic ejection sounds related to rapid acceleration of blood flow may be found on occasion. The auscultatory hallmark of HCM associated with an outflow gradient is a systolic murmur that typically is harsh and crescendo-decrescendo in configuration; it usually commences well after S_1 and is best heard between the apex and the left sternal border.[140] It often radiates well to the lower sternal border, the axillae, and the base of the heart but not into the neck vessels. In patients with large gradients, the murmur usually reflects both left ventricular outflow tract turbulence and concomitant mitral regurgitation.[133,155] Accordingly, the murmur is often more holosystolic and blowing at the apex and in the axillae (because of mitral regurgitation) and midsystolic and harsher along the lower sternal border (because of turbulent flow across the narrowed outflow tract).[115]

The systolic murmur is labile in intensity and duration, and a variety of maneuvers may be used to augment or suppress it (Table 59–6).[133,140] A diastolic rumbling murmur, reflecting increased transmitral flow, may occur in patients with marked mitral regurgitation. The murmur of aortic regurgitation is observed in a minority of patients. It may develop after operation to correct the outflow gradient or following infective endocarditis.[156]

DIFFERENTIATION FROM VALVULAR AORTIC STENOSIS. It is important to emphasize the features of the physical examination that permit differentiation of HCM from fixed orifice obstruction, most commonly related to valvular aortic stenosis (see Chap. 57). The character of the carotid pulse and features of the murmur are most useful in this regard. Because there is obstruction to left ventricular emptying from the beginning of systole with fixed valvular stenosis, the carotid upstroke is slowed and of low amplitude (pulsus parvus et tardus). With HCM, initial ejection of blood from the left ventricle is actually enhanced, and therefore the arterial upstroke is brisk. The murmur of HCM, as opposed to that of aortic stenosis, can be reliably identified by its increase with the Valsalva maneuver and during standing from a squatting position and its decrease during squatting from a standing position, passive leg elevation, and handgrip (see Table 59–6).[115] Other features that may be helpful but are of less importance are the location of the murmur (it radiates along the carotid arteries in valvular aortic stenosis but not in HCM) and the presence and location of a systolic thrill when present (not uncommon and most prominent when present in the second right intercostal space in valvular aortic stenosis versus uncommon and in the fourth interspace along the left sternal border in HCM).

TABLE 59–6 Effects of Interventions on Outflow Gradient and Systolic Murmur in Hypertrophic Cardiomyopathy

Intervention	Contractility	Preload	Afterload
Increase in Gradient and Murmur			
Valsalva maneuver (during strain)	—	↓	↓
Standing	—	↓	—
Postextrasystole	↑	↑	—
Isoproterenol	↑	↓	↓
Digitalis	↑	↓	—
Amyl nitrite	— then ↑	↓ then ↑	↓
Nitroglycerin	—	↓	↓
Exercise	↑	↑	↑
Tachycardia	↑	↓	—
Hypovolemia	↑	↓	↓
Decrease in Gradient and Murmur			
Müller maneuver	—	↑	↑
Valsalva overshoot	—	↑	↑
Squatting	—	↑	↑
Alpha-adrenoceptor stimulation (phenylephrine)	—	—	↑
Beta-adrenoceptor blockade	↓	↑	—
General anesthesia	↓	—	—
Isometric handgrip	—	—	↑

↑ = increase; ↓ = decrease; — = no major change.

ELECTROCARDIOGRAM. This is usually abnormal in HCM and invariably so in symptomatic patients with left ventricular outflow tract gradients, showing a wide variety of patterns.[157] Entirely normal electrocardiograms are seen in only 15 to 25 percent of patients and are usually found in the presence of only localized left ventricular hypertrophy.[104] The most common abnormalities are ST segment and T wave abnormalities, followed by evidence of left ventricular hypertrophy, with QRS complexes that are tallest in the midprecordial leads.[132,158] Unfortunately, these findings are nonspecific and may be seen as well in completely healthy individuals, especially highly trained athletes in whom the abnormalities may reflect athletic conditioning itself. Only a modest relationship exists between the magnitude of left ventricular hypertrophy on electrocardiography and the degree of hypertrophy found on echocardiography.[104] Giant negative T waves in the midprecordial leads of Japanese patients are characteristic of HCM involving the apex,[115,117] but such a pattern in whites may be found with HCM involving segments other than the apex. Prominent Q waves are relatively common, occurring in 20 to 50 percent of patients.[158] The Q wave abnormalities often involve the inferior (II, III, aV_F) or precordial (V_2 to V_6) leads, or both.[132] A variety of other ECG abnormalities may occur, including abnormal electrical axis (usually left axis deviation) and P wave abnormalities (usually left atrial abnormality). Accessory atrioventricular pathways have been found in HCM, although they are uncommon. Clinically significant abnormalities of atrioventricular conduction are uncommon but may cause syncope.

ARRHYTHMIAS (see Chap. 32). Although hemodynamic or ischemic mechanisms may play a role in the death of some patients with HCM (particularly the young), many deaths, particularly those that are known to have been sudden, are probably due to ventricular tachycardia or fibrillation.[159]

Supraventricular tachyarrhythmias are common in HCM and may be found in one-fourth to one-half of patients.[160] Because of the systolic and diastolic abnormalities in this disorder, rhythm disturbances are less well tolerated. Atrial fibrillation is the most common sustained arrhythmia and eventually occurs in almost a quarter of patients; it increases in incidence with age and is associated with left atrial enlargement.[152,161] It is reasonably well tolerated by about one-third of patients but may be associated with embolic stroke, progressive congestive heart failure, and death.[162]

Ventricular arrhythmias are common in patients with HCM, occurring in more than three-fourths of patients undergoing continuous ambulatory ECG monitoring. Runs of nonsustained ventricular tachycardia are found in about one-fourth of patients with HCM, although sustained monomorphic tachycardia is uncommon.[160] In some it is a harbinger of subsequent sudden death; however, its overall predictive value in identifying patients at high risk for sudden death is limited. Treadmill testing may expose arrhythmias that are not present at rest, although continuous ambulatory monitoring is superior in detecting repetitive ventricular tachyarrhythmias. The signal-averaged electrocardiogram has not proved to be helpful in identifying patients at increased risk for sustained or lethal ventricular arrhythmia, nor has the degree of QT dispersion.[160,163] Reduced heart rate variability on ambulatory monitor recordings, a predictor of increased sudden death risk after myocardial infarction, appears to be less useful in risk stratification in patients with HCM and is not widely used.

ELECTROPHYSIOLOGICAL TESTING. The role of electrophysiological studies in identifying patients with HCM at increased risk for sudden death is controversial; despite earlier enthusiasm, it is now generally believed that it is of limited predictive value.[105,159,160] These studies may identify a variety of abnormalities in HCM patients; they induce polymorphic ventricular tachycardia in many patients with HCM, but such a response is generally believed to be nonspecific and does not identify high-risk patients.[105] Unfortunately, unlike its utility in ischemic heart disease, the predictive value of the more typical inducible sustained ventricular arrhythmias during electrophysiological testing is low in HCM. Aggressive stimulation protocols are required to induce a sustained arrhythmia in high-risk HCM patients,[159] often resulting in arrhythmias in low-risk patients as well. Tilt-table testing has shown an abnormal response consisting of an early decrease in cardiac output in some patients with HCM and a history of syncope, perhaps related to an abnormality in baroreceptor function.[164]

CHEST ROENTGENOGRAM. The findings on radiographic examination are variable; the cardiac silhouette may range from normal to markedly increased, and in most cases of apparent "cardiomegaly" the enlarged cardiac silhouette is the result of left ventricular hypertrophy or left atrial enlargement, or both.[115] Left atrial enlargement is observed frequently, especially when significant mitral regurgitation is present. Aortic root enlargement and valvular calcification are not seen unless associated diseases are present, although calcification of the mitral annulus is common in HCM.

ECHOCARDIOGRAPHY. Because echocardiography combines the attributes of high resolution and no known risk, it has been widely used in the evaluation of HCM.[115] It is useful in the study of patients with suspected HCM and also in the screening of relatives of HCM patients. The echocardiogram is of value in identifying and quantifying morphological features (i.e., distribution of septal hypertrophy), functional aspects (e.g., hypercontractile left ventricle), and (when combined with Doppler recordings) hemodynamic findings (e.g., magnitude of outflow gradient) (see Chap. 11).

Left Ventricular Hypertorphy. The cardinal echocardiographic feature of HCM is left ventricular hypertrophy (Fig. 59–9).[104] Although the characteristic feature is hypertrophy of the septum and anterolateral free wall, the echocardiogram is useful in identifying involvement of other left ventricular locations, including portions of the free wall and the apex.[106,165,166] Considerable variability exists in the degree and pattern of hypertrophy; in most patients, there is variation in the extent of hypertrophy from one left ventricular region to another.[104] Maximal hypertrophy of the septum often occurs midway between the base and apex of the left ventricle. The finding of a thickened septum that is at least 1.3 to 1.5 times the thickness of the posterior wall when measured in diastole just before atrial systole has been the time-honored criterion for the diagnosis of ASH.[133] The septum not only is relatively thicker than the posterior wall but also is typically at least 15 mm in thickness (normal < 12 mm). Although the average wall thickness detected on echocardiography is about 20 mm (i.e., almost twice normal), there is great variation, ranging from very mild hypertrophy (13 to 15 mm) to massive hypertrophy (60 mm).[104]

Outflow Tract Obstruction. A second echocardiographic feature often found in HCM is narrowing of the left ventricular outflow tract,[155] which is formed by the interventricular septum anteriorly and the anterior leaflet of the mitral valve posteriorly. The mitral valve leaflets may be abnormally large and elongated and are associated with abnormal left ventricular outflow tract geometry that culminates in the production of a pressure gradient.[115] This abnormal geometry is causally related to the mitral regurgitation that accompanies an outflow gradient; the degree of mitral regurgitation correlates with the extent of anterior and posterior leaflet malcoaptation.[167] When HCM is associated with a pressure gradient, there is abnormal systolic anterior motion of the anterior leaflet and occasionally the posterior leaflet of the mitral valve. A close relationship exists between the degree of systolic anterior motion and attendant mitral regurgitation with the magnitude of the outflow gradient.[155] Prolonged interventricular septal contact of the mitral apparatus is limited to HCM with resting pressure gradients, and a close temporal relationship exists between the onset of the pressure gradient and the onset of septal apposition of the mitral apparatus.

Three explanations have been offered for *systolic anterior motion*: (1) the mitral valve is *pulled* against the septum by contraction of abnormally oriented papillary muscles and elongated leaflets, (2) the mitral valve is *pushed* against the septum (perhaps by the left ventricular posterior wall) because of its abnormal position in the outflow tract, and (3) the mitral valve is drawn toward the septum because of the lower pressure that occurs as blood is ejected at a high velocity through a narrowed outflow tract (Venturi effect).[168] In a minority of cases (less than 15 percent), one or both papillary muscles insert anomalously directly into the anterior mitral leaflet, causing a long area of midventricular narrowing that results in an intraventricular pressure gradient.[114] Systolic anterior motion of the mitral valve and dynamic left ventricular gradients are not pathognomonic of HCM but may be found in a variety of other conditions,[104] including hypercontractile states, left ventricular hypertrophy, transposition of the great arteries, and infiltration of the septum.

OTHER ECHOCARDIOGRAPHIC FINDINGS. The following may be present: (1) a small left ventricular cavity; (2) reduced septal motion and thickening during systole, particularly of the upper septum (presumably because of the disarray of the myofibrillar architecture and abnormal contractile function); (3) normal or increased motion of the posterior wall; (4) a reduced rate of closure of the mitral valve in middiastole secondary to a decrease in left ventricular compliance or abnormal transmittal diastolic flow; (5) mitral valve prolapse; and (6) partial systolic closure or, more commonly, coarse systolic fluttering of the aortic valve related to turbulent blood flow in the outflow tract. The echocardiographic findings that accompany a left ventricular outflow tract gradient (systolic anterior motion of the mitral valve and partial closure of the aortic valve) may be quite labile, and provocative measures such as the Valsalva maneuver, pharmacologically induced vasodilation with amyl nitrite, stimulation of contractility with isoproterenol, or an induced premature ventricular contraction may be required to precipitate the findings.[115]

Abnormalities of diastolic function (see Chaps. 20 and 21) may be demonstrated by echocardiography and Doppler recordings in about 80 percent of patients with HCM, independent of the presence or absence of a systolic pressure gradient. Because the septum is typically hypokinetic, the rate of left ventricular filling is determined primarily by the rate of free wall thinning. Little relationship exists between the extent of hypertrophy and the severity of abnormalities of diastolic function.

RADIONUCLIDE SCANNING (see Chap. 13). Thallium-201 myocardial imaging, particularly when tomographic imaging (single-photon emission computed tomography [SPECT]) is performed (see Chap. 13), permits direct determination of the relative thicknesses of the septum and free wall and may be of particular value when technical constraints limit the reliability of echocardiographic evaluation in a given patient with presumed HCM. Reversible thallium defects, presumably indicative of ischemia, may be seen in HCM in the absence of obstructive coronary artery disease.[160] They may be found in adult patients with HCM and in young patients with a history of sudden death or syncope, suggesting that myocardial ischemia is playing some etiological role.[160] Fixed defects, probably indicative of myocardial scarring, occur primarily in patients with impaired systolic function (similar patchy defects can be demonstrated in hypertrophied myocardial segments by MRI in the majority of HCM patients).[169] Gated radionuclide ventriculography with blood pool labeling permits the evaluation of not only the size but also the motion of the septum and left ventricle. As with the echocardiogram, abnormal diastolic filling of the ventricle has been observed in patients with HCM (both with and without gradients) by computer analysis of the blood pool scan.[170] Because of the ease and availability of transthoracic and transesophageal echocardiography, this technique is not widely used in the evaluation of HCM.

MAGNETIC RESONANCE IMAGING (see Chap. 14). This technique may be useful for identifying HCM in cases in which the standard echocardiogram is technically inadequate and can distinguish between different causes of increased wall thickness (i.e., hypertrophy versus infiltration).[171] MRI supplemented by the contrast agent gadolinium leads to a pattern of hyperenhancement of the myocardial images in the majority of patients with HCM, presumably reflecting myocardial fibrosis or cellular disarray, or both[172] There is more hyperenhancement in patients at the highest risk for premature death, and it is hoped that the technique may aid in risk stratification of patients with HCM.[173]

Hemodynamics and Angiography

CARDIAC CATHETERIZATION. Cardiac catheterization is not required for the diagnosis of HCM because noninvasive evaluation almost always suffices; it is reserved for situations where concomitant coronary artery disease is a consideration or when invasive modalities of therapy (e.g., pacemaker, percutaneous septal ablation, surgery) are being considered.[115] It discloses diminished diastolic left ventricular compliance and in some patients a systolic pressure gradient within the body of the left ventricle, which is separated from a subaortic chamber by the thickened septum and the anterior leaflet of the mitral valve that abuts the septum (see Fig. 59–7). The pressure gradient may be quite labile and may vary between 0 and 175 mm Hg in the same patient under different conditions (see later).[140] The arterial pressure tracing may demonstrate a spike-and-dome configuration similar to the carotid pulse recording (Fig. 59–10). As a consequence of diminished left ventricular compliance, the mean and particularly the a wave in the left atrial pressure pulse and the left ventricular end-diastolic pressures are usually elevated. Artifactual outflow gradients may occur if the left ventricular catheter becomes entrapped in the trabeculae of a markedly hypertrophied left ventricle.[109] Proper technique and choice of catheters with side holes should clarify the mechanism of such gradients. Cardiac output may be depressed in patients with longstanding severe gradients, but in the majority of patients it is normal; occasionally it is elevated.

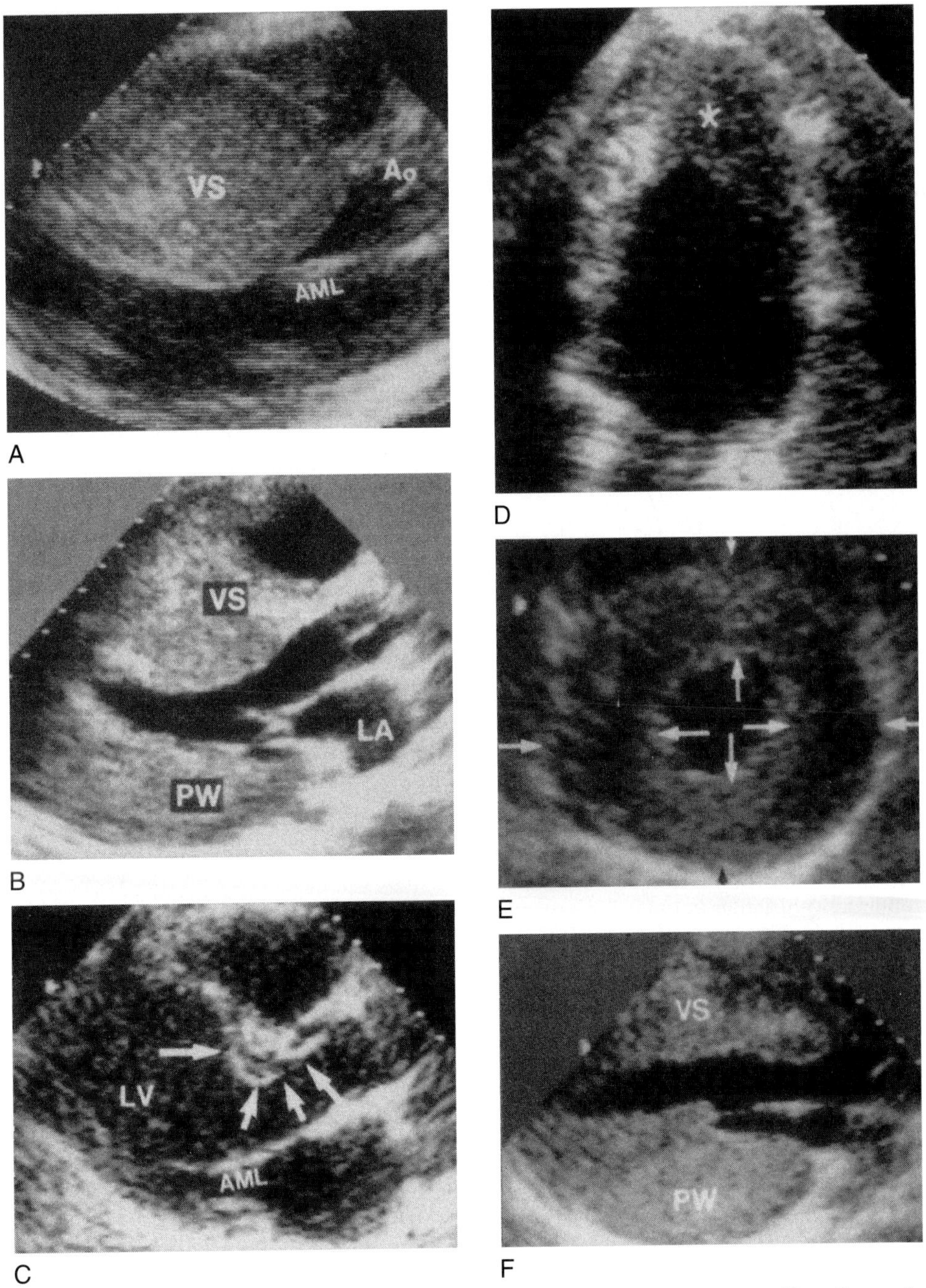

FIGURE 59–9 Heterogeneity in the pattern and extent of left ventricular wall thickening in hypertrophic cardiomyopathy (HCM) as shown by echocardiography. **A,** Massive hypertrophy of the ventricular septum (VS) with wall thickness greater than 50 mm. **B,** Distal VS thickening greater than proximal VS. **C,** Localized VS hypertrophy, confined to the immediate subaortic region. **D,** Apical HCM, with hypertrophy confined to the apex (asterisk). **E,** Concentric hypertrophy, with relatively similar thickening of VS and free wall (paired arrows). **F,** Inverted pattern of hypertrophy, with disproportionate posterior wall (PW) hypertrophy compared with the VS. A, B, C, and F = long-axis views; D = apical view; E = short-axis view. Calibration marks are 1 cm apart. Ao = aorta; AML = anterior mitral leaflet; LA = left atrium; LV = left ventricle. (From Klues HG, Schiffers A, Maron BJ: Phenotypic spectrum and patterns of left ventricular hypertrophy in hypertrophic cardiomyopathy: Morphologic observations and significance as assessed by two-dimensional echocardiography in 600 patients. J Am Coll Cardiol 26:1699, 1995.)

Hemodynamic abnormalities in HCM are not limited to the left side of the heart. Approximately one-fourth of patients demonstrate pulmonary hypertension, which is usually mild but in some cases may be moderate to severe.[140] This is due (at least in part) to elevated mean left atrial pressures as a consequence of diminished left ventricular compliance. A pressure gradient in the right ventricular outflow tract occurs in approximately 15 percent of patients who have obstruction to left ventricular outflow[174] and appears to result from markedly hypertrophied right ventricular tissue (see Fig. 59–7).[110]

LABILITY OF GRADIENT. A feature characteristic of HCM is the variability and lability of the left ventricular outflow gradient (see Table 59–6 and Fig. 59–10).[103,107,140,175] A given patient may demonstrate a large outflow tract pressure

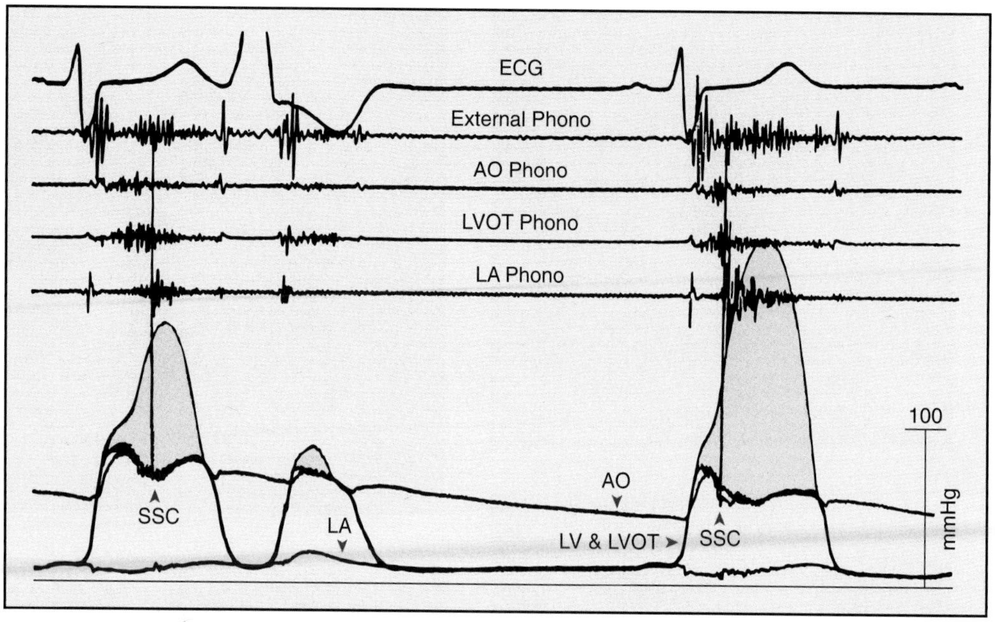

FIGURE 59–10 Hypertrophic cardiomyopathy with intracardiac pressure and phonocardiographic (phono) recordings from aorta (AO), left ventricle (LV), left ventricular outflow tract (LVOT), and left atrium (LA). Note the marked accentuation of the murmur and gradient (shaded) (in the third cycle) after a premature ventricular contraction with failure of the aortic pulse pressure to rise in the post-premature ventricular contraction beat (Brockenbrough-Braunwald sign). ECG = electrocardiogram; SSC = systolic anterior motion of the mitral valve septal contact. (From Murgo JP: Systolic ejection murmurs in the era of modern cardiology: What do we really know? J Am Coll Cardiol 32:1596, 1998.)

gradient on one occasion but have none at another time. In some patients without a resting gradient, it may be temporarily provoked. Three basic mechanisms are involved in the production of dynamic gradients, all of which act by reducing ventricular volume and presumably accentuate the apposition of the anterior mitral leaflet against the septum: (1) increased contractility, (2) decreased preload, and (3) decreased afterload.[107] In a minority of patients with HCM—perhaps about 5 percent of patients—the gradient is midventricular and may be intensified by increased contractility, which exerts a direct muscular sphincter action.[115] The stimuli that provoke or intensify left ventricular outflow tract gradients in HCM generally improve myocardial performance in normal subjects and in patients with most other forms of heart disease. Conversely, reductions in contractility or increases in preload or afterload, which increase left ventricular dimensions, reduce or abolish the left ventricular outflow gradient.

Alterations in the magnitude of the gradient are reflected by changes in the findings on physical examination, noninvasive tests, and left-sided heart catheterization. *This dynamic characteristic of HCM distinguishes it from the discrete forms of obstruction to ventricular outflow.*[140] An increase in the gradient is usually associated with a louder murmur, a longer ejection period with a more characteristic spike-and-dome configuration in the carotid pulse, and more flagrant echocardiographic evidence of systolic anterior motion of the anterior mitral leaflet. In some patients, the intensity of the murmur may *not* track with the gradient, perhaps because in many cases the murmur reflects mitral regurgitation (at least in part).[103]

A number of bedside procedures may be useful in the evaluation of suspected HCM.[140] Perhaps the most helpful is sudden standing from a squatting position.[115] Squatting results in an increase in venous return and an increase in aortic pressure, which increases ventricular volume, diminishing the gradient and decreasing the intensity of the murmur. Sudden standing has the opposite effects and results in accentuation of the gradient and the murmur.

VALSALVA MANEUVER. This is another useful bedside technique for eliciting or exacerbating the gradient.[115] After a transient increase in arterial pressure that usually lasts for four or five cardiac cycles after the onset of the strain and coincident with an increase in heart rate, the arterial systolic and pulse pressures and ventricular volume decline and the gradient (and murmur) increases. After release of the strain, a compensatory overshoot of arterial pressure and venous return with cardiac slowing occur, all of which increase ventricular volume and reduce the magnitude of the gradient and the murmur. Occasional patients may show paradoxical attenuation of the systolic murmur despite an increase in the pressure gradient, presumably related to a critical reduction in stroke volume. Inhalation of amyl nitrite also intensifies the murmur and the abnormality of the arterial pulse. Passive leg elevation, handgrip, and sudden squatting from a standing position attenuate the murmur of HCM.

POST-EXTRASYSTOLIC CHANGES. One of the most potent stimuli for enhancing the gradient is *post-extrasystolic potentiation* (see Chap. 19), which may occur after a spontaneous premature contraction or be induced by mechanical stimulation with a catheter. The resultant increase in contractility in the beat after the extrasystole is so marked that it outweighs the otherwise salutary effect of increased ventricular filling caused by the compensatory pause and produces an increase in the gradient and often of the murmur as well. A characteristic change often occurs in the directly recorded arterial pressure tracing, which, in addition to displaying a more marked spike-and-dome configuration, exhibits a pulse pressure that fails to increase as expected or actually decreases (the so-called Brockenbrough-Braunwald phenomenon) (see Fig. 59-10). This is one of the more reliable signs of dynamic obstruction of the left ventricular outflow tract. In some patients, the post-extrasystolic murmur is attenuated despite an increase in the outflow gradient, apparently because in this setting the murmur (a hybrid of outflow tract turbulence and mitral regurgitation) is mirroring to a greater degree changes in the severity of mitral regurgitation rather than changes in the outflow tract gradient.

POSITIVE INOTROPIC AGENTS. Digitalis glycosides and the beta adrenoceptor agonist isoproterenol augment the gradient because they increase myocardial contractility, whereas nitroglycerin and amyl nitrite exaggerate the gradient by decreasing arterial pressure and ventricular volume.[140] The ingestion of alcoholic beverages may exacerbate the outflow pressure gradient by producing systemic vasodilation. Hypovolemia (as a result of hemorrhage or overly aggressive diuresis) may also provoke overt obstruction to left ventricular outflow. The intensity of the murmur and the left ventricular outflow gradient may be decreased by beta adrenoceptor blockade, although the effect of the latter is often not dramatic and is of greatest hemodynamic benefit in protecting against the *increase* in the gradient that may be provoked by exercise. In most patients the severity of mitral regurgitation and the intensity of the apical blowing regurgitant murmur vary with the degree of obstruction of left ventricular outflow.[155]

ANGIOGRAPHY. Left ventriculography shows a hypertrophied ventricle; when an outflow gradient is present, the anterior leaflet of the mitral valve moves anteriorly during systole and encroaches on the outflow tract. Associated with this motion of the leaflet is mitral regurgitation, which is a constant finding in patients with gradients. The left ventricular cavity is often small, and systolic ejection is typically vigorous, resulting in virtual obliteration of the cavity at end systole (see Fig. 59-7), although the apparent hypercontractile state may relate more to reduced afterload (low end-systolic wall stress) than to enhanced inotropy. The papillary muscles are often prominent and may fill the left ventricular cavity in late systole. In patients with apical involvement, the extensive hypertrophy may convey a spade-like configuration to the left ventricular angiogram.[115]

It may be helpful to supplement angiographic evaluation of the left ventricle with simultaneous right ventriculography in a cranially angulated left anterior oblique projection to obtain optimal visualization of the size, shape, and configuration of the interventricular septum. The left septal surface either is flat or bulges into the left ventricular cavity at its middle or lower portion, in contrast to the normal findings of the septum curving toward the right ventricle.

In patients older than 45 years, obstructive coronary artery disease may be present, although the symptoms of ischemic pain are indistinguishable from those of patients with normal coronary angiograms and HCM. The left anterior descending and septal perforator coronary arteries may demonstrate phasic narrowing and associated abnormalities of coronary blood flow.[148,176]

Natural History

The clinical course in HCM is varied; in many patients symptoms are absent or mild, remain stable, and in some instances improve over a period of 5 to 10 years. The annual mortality is around 3 percent in adults seen in large referral centers but probably closer to 1 percent when all patients with HCM are included (Fig. 59–11).[104,177] The risk of sudden death is higher in children, perhaps as high as 6 percent per year.[104,152,159,160] Clinical deterioration (aside from sudden death) is usually slow. Although symptoms do not bear a predictable relationship to the severity or even the presence of a gradient, patients with gradients are more likely to develop eventual clinical deterioration than those without gradients.[177,178] The percentage of severely symptomatic patients increases with age. The onset of atrial fibrillation may lead to an increase in symptoms, although it is well tolerated in about a third of patients.[105,162] Conversion to sinus rhythm by pharmacological or electrical cardioversion should be attempted, although maintenance of sinus rhythm may be difficult.[105] Patients who develop atrial fibrillation ordinarily should be started on long-term therapy with oral anticoagulants.[104,162]

Progression of HCM to left ventricular dilation and dysfunction without a gradient (i.e., DCM) occurs in 5 to 10 percent of patients.[104,160] It appears to result, at least in part, from wall thinning and scar formation as a consequence of myocardial ischemia caused by small-vessel coronary artery disease and abnormal coronary vasodilator reserve (Fig. 59–12), although in some patients it appears to be genetically determined.[115,129] It is more likely to occur in patients with marked septal hypertrophy and generally is associated with a poor prognosis. The extent of left ventricular hypertrophy in adults usually remains stable over time, although a majority of children demonstrate increasing degrees of hypertrophy (often considerable) and adult patients (mainly women) appear to experience a very gradual degree of regression of hypertrophy over time (Fig. 59–13).[179] Whether this is the result of ventricular remodeling or an artifact related to the premature death of patients with more severe hypertrophy is unknown at present. In some children, the findings of HCM may develop despite a previous normal echocardiogram; this is not common in adults, but it may be seen in particular with

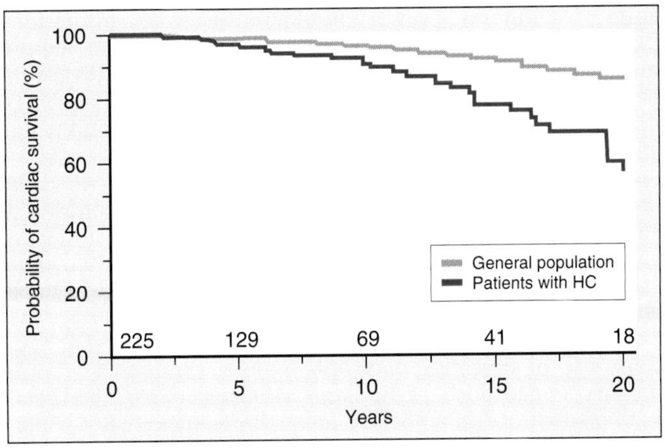

FIGURE 59–11 Kaplan-Meier survival curve of 225 community-based patients with hypertrophic cardiomyopathy (HC) and age-matched control subjects. The numbers above the horizontal axis refer to the number of patients at each follow-up period. The annual total mortality rate of the patients with HC was 1.3 percent. (From Kofflard MJ, Ten Cate FJ, van der Lee C, et al: Hypertrophic cardiomyopathy in a large community-based population: Clinical outcome and identification of risk factors for sudden cardiac death and clinical deterioration. J Am Coll Cardiol 41:987, 2003.)

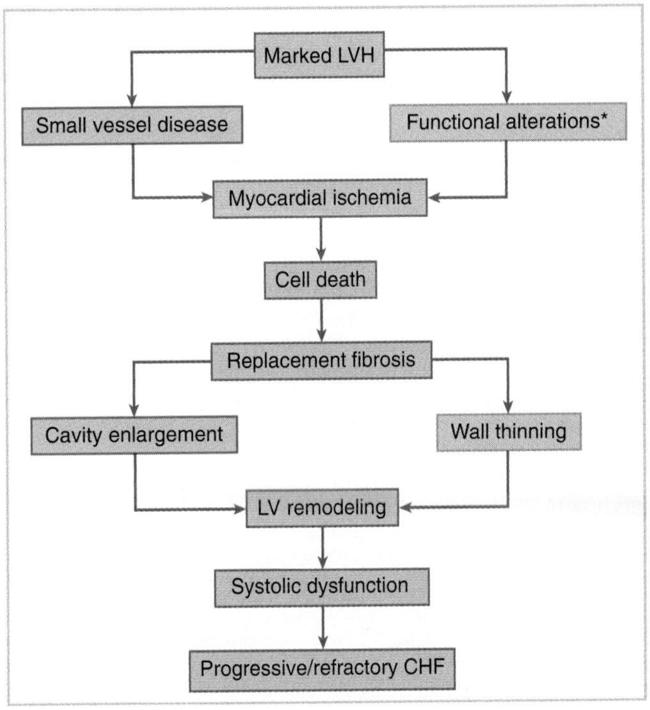

FIGURE 59–12 Hypothetical model for the pathogenesis of the end-stage phase of hypertrophic cardiomyopathy. Asterisk designates the following possibilities: (1) enhanced myocardial oxygen requirements and reduced myocardial capillary density relative to marked left ventricular (LV) hypertrophy (LVH) and (2) increased diastolic wall tension and coronary vascular resistance resulting from abnormal LV relaxation and impaired filling. CHF = congestive heart failure. (Modified from Maron BJ, Spirito P: Implications of left ventricular remodeling in hypertrophic cardiomyopathy. Am J Cardiol 81:1339-1344, 1998.)

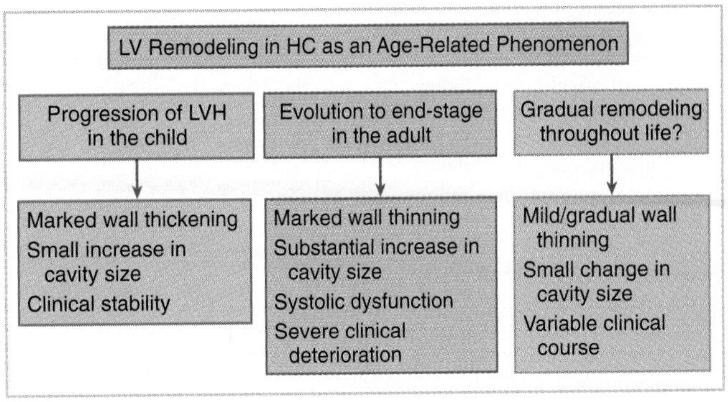

FIGURE 59–13 Patterns of left ventricular (LV) remodeling in the natural history of hypertrophic cardiomyopathy (HC). LVH = left ventricular hypertrophy. (From Maron BJ, Spirito P: Implications of left ventricular remodeling in hypertrophic cardiomyopathy. Am J Cardiol 81:1339-1344, 1998.)

the cardiac myosin-binding protein C mutation.[113] Its occurrence emphasizes that a single normal echocardiogram does *not* exclude HCM in a child or adolescent; cellular disarray and the attendant risk of sudden death may be present even in the absence of left ventricular hypertrophy. It furthermore suggests that apparently normal but at-risk postadolescent relatives of patients with HCM continue to be screened with periodic echocardiograms, perhaps at 5-year intervals.[104,160]

Many patients with HCM survive to old age, and about a quarter of all patients with diagnosed HCM are older than 75 years.[152] In such elderly HCM patients, outflow gradients are common (occurring in about 40 percent), but findings of advanced heart failure are relatively uncommon.[104]

SUDDEN DEATH. Death is most often sudden in HCM and may occur in previously asymptomatic patients, in individuals who were unaware they had the disease, and in patients with an otherwise stable course.[153,159] There is difficulty in identifying the patients at particular risk for sudden death.[180] Nevertheless, the features that most reliably identify the 10 to 20 percent of HCM patients at high risk include prior cardiac arrest or sustained ventricular tachycardia; multiple and repetitive episodes of nonsustained ventricular tachycardia[181]; young age (<30 years) at diagnosis (especially in those with extreme left ventricular hypertrophy and wall thicknesses greater than or equal to 30 mm on echocardiography); a family history of HCM with sudden death (so-called malignant family history); an abnormal blood pressure response to exercise especially in patients younger than 50 years (presumably related to subendocardial ischemia with attendant transient left ventricular systolic dysfunction)[182]; and genetic abnormalities associated with increased prevalence of sudden death (Table 59–7).[105,166,183] Prognosis correlates with the degree of hypertrophy, and patients with extreme hypertrophy (>30 mm) have almost a 40 percent risk of sudden death over a 20-year period.[165]

The presence (and severity) of an outflow tract gradient has modest predictive power for the risk of death (although not necessarily sudden), and a resting gradient on Doppler echocardiography of greater than 30 mm Hg is associated with about 1.6-fold increase in risk.[178] The degree of functional limitation and symptoms in general do not correlate with the risk of death, although syncope (especially in the young) does appear to be associated with an increased risk of sudden death.[177] It is presumed that sudden death in most patients is due to a ventricular arrhythmia, although atrial arrhythmias may play a role in sensitizing the heart so that ventricular arrhythmias appear subsequently. Bradyarrhythmias and disease of the atrioventricular conduction system may also play some role in sudden death.

TABLE 59–7 Factors Associated with an Adverse Outcome in Hypertrophic Cardiomyopathy

History of sudden cardiac death
Family history of premature death
"Malignant" causal mutations
"Malignant" modifier genes
History of syncope
Magnitude of LV hypertrophy
Extent of myocyte disarray
Extent of interstitial fibrosis
Early onset of disease
Myocardial ischemia on perfusion tomography
Abnormal blood pressure response to exercise
Nonsustained VT on Holter monitor
LV outflow tract obstruction

LV = left ventricular; VT = ventricular tachycardia.

Adapted from Marian AJ: On predictors of sudden cardiac death in hypertrophic cardiomyopathy. J Am Coll Cardiol 41:994, 2003.

Despite the difficulty in identifying patients at high risk for sudden death, the *absence* of a variety of characteristics (including the absence of severe symptoms, malignant family history, nonsustained ventricular tachycardia, marked hypertrophy, marked left atrial dilation, and abnormal blood pressure response to exercise) identifies a low-risk group that comprises more than half of all patients with HCM and requires little in the way of routine therapy.[105,166] Patients with mild hypertrophy, for example, with wall thicknesses less than 19 mm, experienced almost no sudden death mortality in one large study that spanned 20 years![165] Although avoidance of intense physical exertion is probably appropriate in this group, participation in recreational sports activities is not believed to be contraindicated.[105]

Children. The mechanism of death may be different in children with HCM because spontaneous ventricular arrhythmias and inducibility on electrophysiological testing are much less common than in adults.[154] Hemodynamic mechanisms may be involved, because younger patients are more likely to demonstrate abnormal changes in peripheral vascular resistance in response to exercise.[160,184]

Competitive Sports. Guidelines for participation in competitive sports have been developed; strenuous exertion should probably be proscribed in all patients with HCM whether or not symptoms are prominent, especially if high-risk clinical characteristics are present. Unsuspected HCM is the most common abnormality found at autopsy in young competitive athletes who die suddenly.[154] Cardiovascular screening before participation in competitive sports may identify asymptomatic patients with dormant HCM and appears to reduce the frequency of unexpected sudden death, although whether large-scale screening of athletes is administratively feasible or cost effective is not clear.[185]

Why some athletes with HCM die suddenly and others are able to continue to compete without limitation or death is not known. It has been speculated that the extent and severity of myocardial disarray may play an important role in determining prognosis, although this is not a finding that is ordinarily or easily obtainable in a living patient. Patients with marked hypertrophy are at increased risk.[159]

Pregnancy is usually well tolerated, although there is some increase in the relative risk of maternal mortality, especially in women known to be at increased risk.[186]

Management

Management of patients with HCM is directed toward alleviation of symptoms, prevention of complications, and reduction in the risk of death (Fig. 59–14). Most patients should undergo a risk assessment stratification that includes a full history and physical examination, two-dimensional echocardiography, 24- to 48-hour ambulatory (Holter) monitoring, and treadmill or bicycle exercise testing.[104]

Whether asymptomatic patients should receive drug therapy is not established because no adequate controlled studies are available.[105,109,187] Digitalis glycosides should generally be avoided unless atrial fibrillation or systolic dysfunction develops.[140] Diuretics were previously thought to be contraindicated to avoid precipitating or worsening the outflow gradient. More recent experience indicates that cautious use of diuretics may help reduce symptoms of pulmonary congestion, particularly when they are combined with beta-adrenergic blockers or calcium antagonists.[160] Beta-adrenergic agonists may improve diastolic filling but should not be used because they may produce ischemia and usually worsen the outflow gradient.[140] The majority of patients with HCM require only medical management, and at least half of all significantly symptomatic patients are improved with drug therapy.[107] Invasive interventions are needed in only 5 to 10 percent of patients and then only in patients with

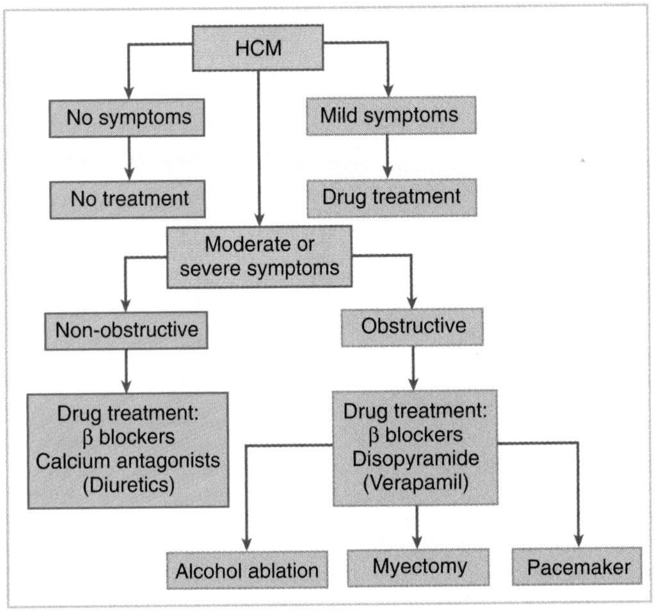

FIGURE 59–14 Clinical management algorithm for patients with hypertrophic cardiomyopathy (HCM). (From McKenna WJ, Behr ER: Hypertrophic cardiomyopathy: Management, risk stratification, and prevention of sudden death. Heart 87:169, 2002.)

outflow gradients who remain severely symptomatic despite optimal medical therapy.[105]

BETA ADRENOCEPTOR BLOCKERS. These drugs are the mainstay of medical therapy of HCM.[107,160] With their use, angina, dyspnea, and presyncope may all be improved. In patients with resting or provocable gradients, beta adrenoceptor blockade may prevent the increase in outflow obstruction that accompanies exertion, although resting gradients are largely unchanged.[105] The drugs reduce the determinants of myocardial oxygen consumption and thus angina pectoris and perhaps exert an antiarrhythmic action as well. Angina pectoris generally responds more favorably to treatment with a beta adrenoceptor blocker than does dyspnea. It has been suggested that beta adrenoceptor blockade may prevent sudden death and reduce mortality in HCM, and accordingly some use prophylactic beta adrenoceptor blockade therapy even in asymptomatic patients.[186] However, its efficacy for this purpose has not been established.[159] Beta adrenoceptor blockade also blunts the heart's chronotropic response, thus limiting the demand for increased myocardial oxygen delivery.[107] Beta adrenoceptor blockade was previously thought to have a beneficial effect on diastolic ventricular filling, but it now appears that any benefit is simply the consequence of a slower heart rate.[107] The overall clinical response to beta adrenoceptor blockade is variable, and only about one-third to two-thirds of patients experience symptomatic improvement. If beta adrenoceptor blockers are discontinued, they should probably be withdrawn slowly to avoid rebound adrenergic hypersensitivity.

CALCIUM ANTAGONISTS. These are an alternative to beta adrenoceptor blockade in the management of HCM; most of the experience has been with verapamil, with more limited use of nifedipine, diltiazem, and amlodipine.[104] No clear consensus exists as to whether therapy should be initiated first with a beta adrenoceptor blocker or a calcium antagonist, although verapamil is often effective in improving symptoms in patients who have not responded to beta adrenoceptor blockade. Exercise performance in particular may be improved when patients are changed from a beta adrenoceptor blocker to verapamil. Both the hypercontractile systolic function and the abnormalities of diastolic filling may be related to abnormal calcium kinetics,[145] and drugs that block the inward transport of calcium across the myocardial cell membrane may be able to rectify both abnormalities. Indeed, in an animal model of familial HCM, diltiazem prevented the development of the morphological features of HCM.[188]

Verapamil has been the most widely used calcium antagonist in this condition. Its use was suggested, at least in part, by the observation that it produces a protective and beneficial effect in the hereditary cardiomyopathy of the Syrian hamster, a condition marked by intracellular calcium overload in which propranolol is ineffective.[189] Although the vasodilator effects of verapamil should not be helpful in HCM, it appears that by depressing myocardial contractility, verapamil can decrease the left ventricular outflow gradient when given intravenously or orally. Perhaps more important from a symptomatic point of view, verapamil improves diastolic filling in HCM, at least in part by reducing asynchronous regional diastolic performance.[190] It also improves regional myocardial blood flow in some patients, which may contribute to the improvement in diastolic behavior.[191]

Although variable clinical responses have been reported with verapamil, about two-thirds or more of patients show increased exercise capacity and an improved symptomatic status. Sustained symptomatic improvement has been noted with the long-term administration of verapamil in ambulatory patients, although important adverse effects, including sudden death, have been observed in a small fraction of patients so treated.[105] Complications with verapamil include suppression of sinus node automaticity and inhibition of atrioventricular conduction, vasodilation, and negative inotropic effects.[160] These side effects may culminate in hypotension, pulmonary edema, and death; antiarrhythmic agents, especially quinidine, may exacerbate the deleterious hemodynamic effects of verapamil. Because of these adverse effects, it has been suggested that verapamil should not be used, or should be used only with extreme caution, in patients with high left ventricular filling pressure or symptoms of paroxysmal nocturnal dyspnea or orthopnea.[105] Unfortunately, these are usually the patients in greatest need of therapy.

The experience with other calcium channel blockers is limited. *Nifedipine* has been used in HCM, and it may have theoretical advantages over verapamil because it causes less depression of atrioventricular conduction. This may be counteracted by its more potent vasodilator action. Nifedipine may alleviate the chest pain in HCM patients. However, it should be recognized that the potent vasodilator effects of nifedipine may lead to systemic hypotension and an increase in the outflow gradient,[105] and in high doses it may depress left ventricular function. *Diltiazem* has also shown beneficial effects in HCM, producing improved diastolic function and reducing ischemia, although, like verapamil and nifedipine, it may cause an increase in the outflow gradient and a worrisome elevation of pulmonary capillary pressure.[192]

The combination of a beta adrenoceptor blocker and a calcium antagonist may be effective in patients who respond inadequately to monotherapy, although there are only anecdotal reports of the superiority of combination therapy.[105,107]

OTHER DRUGS. Disopyramide, an antiarrhythmic drug that alters calcium kinetics, has produced symptomatic improvement and a reduction or abolition of the pressure gradient in patients with HCM as a consequence of depression of left ventricular systolic performance and a reduction in ejection acceleration.[193] Particularly when combined with a beta-adrenergic blocker, it appears to be particularly efficacious in reducing outflow gradients.[140] However, long-term experience with disopyramide is limited, particularly in asymptomatic patients and those without outflow gradients, and the initial benefits appear to decrease with time.[105] Beta adrenoceptor blockers, calcium antagonists, and the conventional antiarrhythmic agents do not appear to suppress serious ventricular arrhythmias or reduce the frequency of supraventricular arrhythmias. However, amiodarone is effective in the treatment of both supraventricular[105] and ventricular tachyarrhythmias in HCM. Although there is some belief that amiodarone improves prognosis in HCM, only limited and inconclusive data are available.[105,106,159,194] Experience with sotalol is limited. We do *not* favor empirical use of amiodarone (or other antiarrhythmic agents for that matter) in unselected patients with HCM, and we worry about possible proarrhythmic effects and potential toxicity, including sudden death.

Atrial fibrillation should usually be pharmacologically or electrically converted because of the hemodynamic consequences of the loss of the atrial contribution to ventricular filling in this disorder. Amiodarone is thought to reduce the recurrence rate after successful cardioversion (based on limited data).[104] Anticoagulants should be given to patients with atrial fibrillation when no contraindication exists.[161] Infective endocarditis may occur in about 5 percent of patients but appears to be limited to those with an outflow gradient; accordingly, appropriate antibiotic prophylaxis is indicated in this group.[195] The infection usually occurs on the aortic valve or mitral apparatus, on the endocardium, or at the site of the contact lesion on the septum; thus, chronic endocardial trauma may provide a nidus for subsequent infection.

EXERCISE. Strenuous exercise should be avoided because of the risk of sudden death; almost half of deaths in HCM occur during or just after physical activity.[166] Even though many individuals with subclinical HCM exercise vigorously, the threat of sudden death is sufficiently real that competitive sports are proscribed in patients with marked hypertrophy or other factors believed to be associated with increased risk (see Table 59–7).

DDD PACING. Insertion of a dual-chamber DDD pacemaker may be useful in some patients with an outflow gradient and severe symptoms, especially elderly patients,[196,197] but it is likely that no more than 10 percent of HCM patients are candidates. Symptoms are generally improved, and the gradient appears to be reduced by an average of about 25 percent, although better symptomatic and hemodynamic results appear to follow surgery. Benefits have been described even after termination of pacing, suggesting a modification of myocardial properties. The long-term utility of pacing, however, is not known at present, and a substantial placebo effect has been demonstrated.[196,198–200] The benefit of pacing in patients without a resting outflow gradient is even more equivocal, and its use in this setting is generally not recommended at present.

ICD IMPLANTATION (see Chap. 31). In high-risk patients (especially the minority of HCM patients with sustained monomorphic ventricular tachycardia) or those with aborted sudden death, an ICD should be inserted,[201] although it may be less beneficial in HCM than in other conditions (such as coronary artery disease) with aborted sudden death.[202] Nevertheless, appropriate ICD discharges occurred in almost a quarter of the high-risk HCM patients in one large study and more than 40 percent of the subset of patients who had a device inserted for secondary prevention (i.e., after a prior cardiac arrest or spontaneous, sustained ventricular tachycardia), suggesting its efficacy in preventing sudden death.[159] However, there continues to be uncertainty about the characterization of what precisely constitutes high-risk status in consideration for ICD insertion; certainly, patients with a prior cardiac arrest or spontaneous sustained hemodynamically unstable ventricular tachycardia qualify.[201,202]

ALCOHOL SEPTAL ABLATION. A number of patients with resting or provocable outflow gradients have derived benefit (at least over the medium term) from intentional infarction of a portion of the interventricular septum by the infusion of alcohol into a selectively catheterized septal artery, with attendant reduction of the outflow gradient and mitral regurgitation, improvement in ventricular relaxation, regression of hypertrophy, and reduction in symptoms (Figs. 59–15 and 59–16).[107,203–207] Reported results of percutaneous septal reduction therapy vary from a somewhat inferior degree of gradient reduction when compared with surgical myotomy-myectomy to equivalent results, although exercise parameters may be better with surgery.[156,208,209] Both procedures improve diastolic ventricular filling.[210] It may take weeks to months for the full benefits of the procedure to become manifest.[211] Complications of the percutaneous technique include the frequent development of right bundle branch block, the precipitation of procedure-related complete heart block in half the patients, and the need for permanent pacing in about a quarter (although rates as low as 5 percent have been reported by one high-volume center).[211,212] The use of myocardial contrast echocardiography appears to improve the success rate of the procedure and reduce the need for permanent pacing after the procedure.[213] The mortality rate from the procedure in experienced centers is low (0 to 4 percent).[211,214,215]

SURGICAL TREATMENT. A number of surgical procedures aimed at reducing the outflow gradient have been developed. They are used most commonly in markedly symptomatic patients with gradients at rest greater than 50 mm Hg who have not responded well to medical management; such patients constitute less than 5 percent of all HCM patients.[104-106]

Myotomy-Myectomy. The most widely used operation for HCM consists of incising and resecting about 5 gm of the hypertrophied septum using a transaortic approach (the operation has been called the Morrow procedure, named after the cardiac surgeon who developed the technique).[106,216] Left transventricular as well as combined transaortic and left ventricular approaches have also been used successfully.

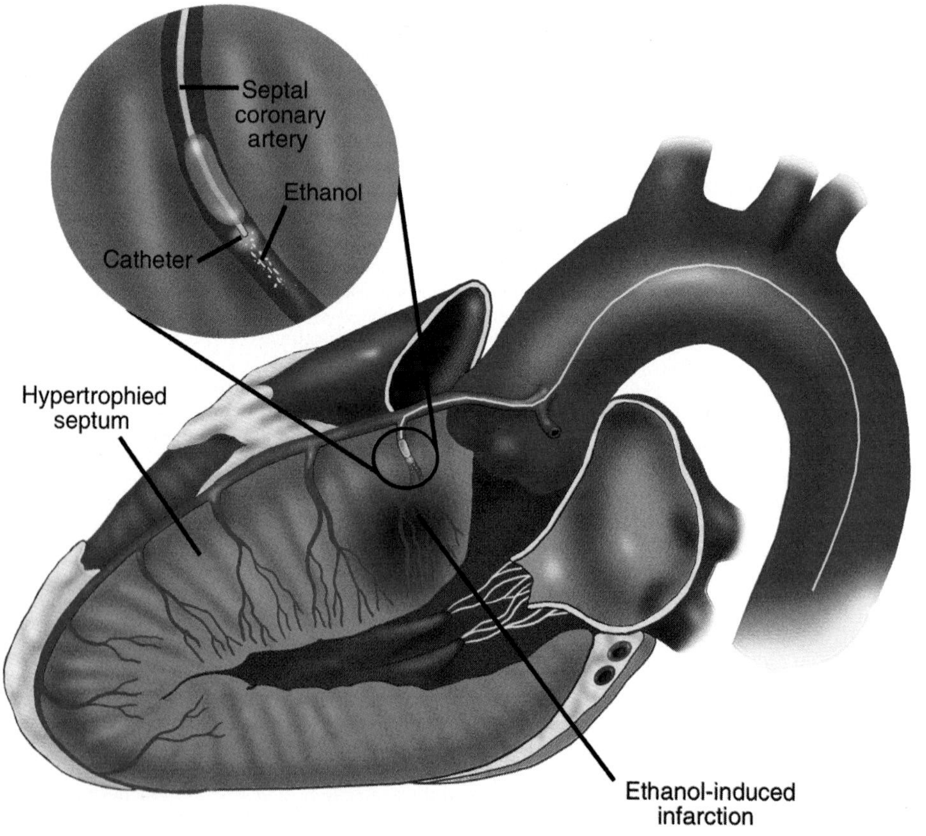

FIGURE 59–15 Drawing demonstrating technique of ethanol infusion into a septal artery in hypertrophic cardiomyopathy. The insert shows a balloon occluding the septal artery and the alcohol-induced septal infarction. (From Braunwald E: Hypertrophic cardiomyopathy—The benefits of a multidisciplinary approach. N Engl J Med 347:1306, 2002.)

Operative management is facilitated by intraoperative echocardiography, and operative mortality at large centers is in the range of 2 to 3 percent or even less.[104,141,174,216] Surgery often relieves the obstruction (Fig. 59–17) as well as the mitral regurgitation.[155,211,216] Patients older than 65 as well as younger than 10 years have undergone successful operations; the operative risk is higher in older patients.[141]

Surgery results in long-term improvement in symptoms and exercise capacity in most (70 to 90 percent) patients.[104,107,211,216] Significant aortic regurgitation is an uncommon complication of the transaortic valve approach, although mild aortic regurgitation is not uncommon.[156] Myotomy-myectomy may be combined with other necessary operative procedures (particularly coronary artery bypass grafting), although the surgical risk is increased.[141] There has been enthusiasm for combining septal myotomy-myectomy with plication of the anterior leaflet of the mitral valve and reconstruction of the submitral valvular apparatus.[114,141]

Mitral Valve Replacement. Although performed less commonly than myotomy-myectomy, mitral valve replacement or repair (sometimes performed simultaneously with septal resection) has been used by some surgeons to treat HCM.[104] The rationale for this operation is that it abolishes obstruction by preventing systolic anterior motion of the mitral valve or corrects for intrinsic anatomical abnormalities of the mitral valve. It appears to be of particular value in patients with less than severe (<18 mm) hypertrophy of the upper septum or other atypical septal morphology, in those with previous myotomy-myectomy with persistent severe symptoms and obstruction, and in patients with intrinsic mitral valve disease (particularly the rare patients with HCM in whom the papillary muscles insert directly into the mitral valve leaflets).[114,141,155] In appropriate candidates not responding to maximal standard medical and surgical therapy, cardiac transplantation may be considered; this is usually required only for patients who have entered the dilated phase of HCM and have intractable symptoms of congestive heart failure.[217]

CHOICE OF THERAPY

Pharmacological therapy is the first line of treatment for symptomatic patients with HCM.[160,186] Beta adrenoceptor blockers, verapamil, and diltiazem are often used for patients without an outflow gradient (the so-called nonobstructive form), and beta adrenoceptor blockers and disopyramide are often preferred for those with a gradient.[140] A major challenge is the choice of subsequent therapy for patients who remain severely symptomatic despite maximal and optimal medical treatment, at least in part because of the paucity of studies comparing different treatment strategies.[191,195] For patients without an outflow gradient, the only established treatment option is medical because none of the interventional approaches (DDD pacing, septal ablation, or myotomy-myectomy) has an established role at this time.[195]

For severely symptomatic patients with an outflow gradient, there is no clear consensus about which intervention to choose when medical therapy has failed. Nevertheless, there are some general considerations that may be helpful in making this determination.

DDD PACING. Although the true benefit of pacing for symptom relief in HCM[196,197] is uncertain (see discussion earlier), it may be an appropriate addition to medical therapy in specific persistently symptomatic patients, including those with (1) an independent need for permanent pacing, such as those with symptomatic sinus node dysfunction or conducting system disease; (2) symptomatic or worrisome bradycardia that would otherwise preclude more aggressive treatment with pharmacological agents such as beta adrenoceptor blockers; (3) contraindications to surgery or septal ablation, including advanced age, comorbidities, or disinclination; or (4) lack of easy accessibility to a medical center skilled in septal ablation or surgery.

SEPTAL ABLATION[206]. Concern about two complications—one observed and the other theoretical—has tempered to some degree the enthusiasm for percutaneous septal ablation. A minority of patients develop heart block after the procedure and require permanent pacing. The theoretical concern is that the "therapeutic" myocardial infarction that results from the infusion of alcohol and is the mechanism of septal ablation creates myocardial scar tissue that may lead to subsequent malignant ventricular arrhythmias and sudden death. In view of these issues, septal ablation may be a preferred option for severely symptomatic patients with "obstructive" HCM if they (1) already have a pacemaker (or,

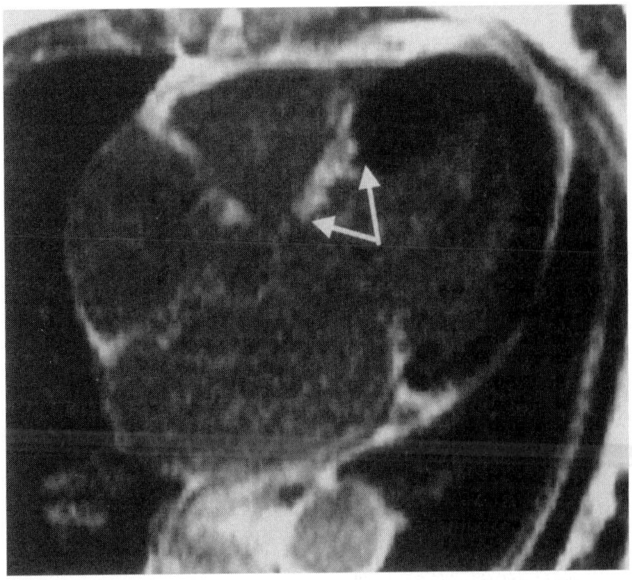

FIGURE 59–16 Magnetic resonance image after gadolinium-diethylenetriamine-pentaacetic acid contrast that demonstrates hyperenhancement (arrows) of the area of the interventricular septum that had undergone previous ablation by transcatheter alcohol infusion. (From Sievers B, Moon JC, Pennell DJ: Images in cardiovascular medicine. Magnetic resonance contrast enhancement of iatrogenic septal myocardial infarction in hypertrophic cardiomyopathy. Circulation 105:1018, 2002. Copyright 2002, American Heart Association.)

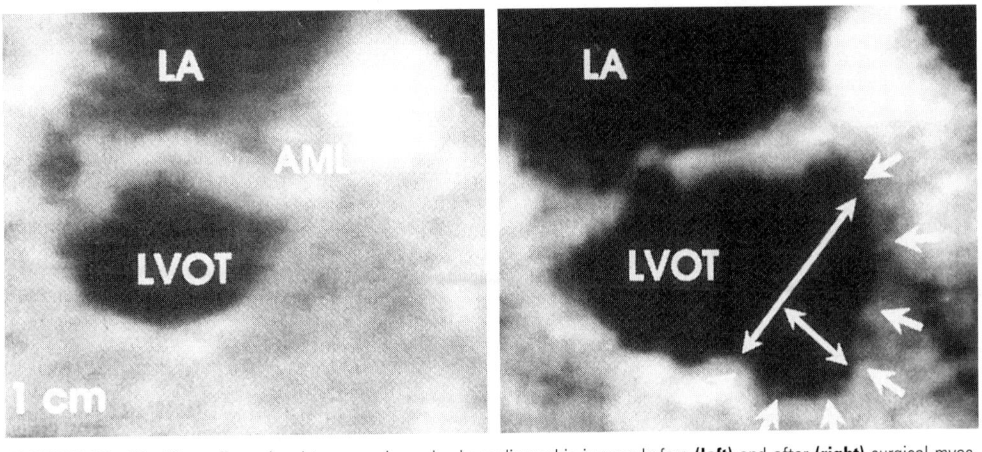

FIGURE 59–17 Three-dimensional transesophageal echocardiographic images before **(left)** and after **(right)** surgical myectomy of the left ventricular outflow tract (LVOT) in a patient with hypertrophic cardiomyopathy. The maximal width and depth of the myectomy trough are marked by large arrows. Small arrows indicate limits of myectomy trough. LA = left atrium. (From Franke A, Schondube FA, Kuhl HP, et al: Quantitative assessment of the operative results after extended myectomy and surgical reconstruction of the subvalvular mitral apparatus in hypertrophic obstructive cardiomyopathy using dynamic three-dimensional transesophageal echocardiography. J Am Coll Cardiol 31:1641, 1998.)

even better, an ICD) in place or (2) have concomitant medical conditions, advanced age, prior sternotomy, or other relative contraindications to surgery. As more favorable experience is gained with this procedure, it is being used increasingly in place of surgery in centers with skilled operators.

SURGERY. Although only a minority of patients require surgery for drug-refractory HCM,[191] it is the time-honored approach, with a 40-year experience that has demonstrated its efficacy and relative safety. It remains the "gold standard" for treating persistently symptomatic patients.[104] For these reasons, it should probably be the preferred option in younger patients, where the relatively short period of follow-up of septal ablation (3 to 5 years[331]) raises some concerns regarding long-term results. It should also be employed in failures of septal ablation.

Restrictive and Infiltrative Cardiomyopathies

Of the three major functional categories of the cardiomyopathies (dilated, hypertrophic, and restrictive), RCM is the least common form in Western countries, although nonidiopathic forms of RCM such as endomyocardial disease (Table 59–8) are common in specific geographical regions of the world.[3,218] The hallmark of the RCMs is abnormal diastolic function; the ventricular walls are excessively rigid and impede ventricular filling. Systolic function, on the other hand, is often unimpaired, even in many cases with extensive infiltration of the myocardium.[218,219] Thus, RCM bears some functional resemblance to constrictive pericarditis, which is also characterized by normal or nearly normal systolic function but abnormal ventricular filling (see Chap. 64).[218] Differentiation of the two conditions is mandatory because of the potential for successful surgical treatment of constriction.[3]

TABLE 59–8 Classification of Types of Restrictive Cardiomyopathy According to Cause

Myocardial
Noninfiltrative
Idiopathic cardiomyopathy*
Familial cardiomyopathy
Hypertrophic cardiomyopathy
Scleroderma
Pseudoxanthoma elasticum
Diabetic cardiomyopathy
Infiltrative
Amyloidosis*
Sarcoidosis*
Gaucher disease
Hurler disease
Fatty infiltration
Storage Disease
Hemochromatosis
Fabry disease
Glycogen storage disease
Endomyocardial
Endomyocardial fibrosis*
Hypereosinophilic syndrome
Carcinoid heart disease
Metastatic cancers
Radiation*
Toxic effects of anthracycline*
Drugs causing fibrous endocarditis (serotonin, methysergide, ergotamine, mercurial agents, busulfan)

From Kushwaha S, Fallon JT, Fuster V: Restrictive cardiomyopathy. N Engl J Med 336:267, 1997. Copyright 1997, Massachusetts Medical Society.

*These conditions are more likely than the others to be encountered in clinical practice.

A variety of specific pathological processes may result in RCM, although the cause often remains unknown. Myocardial fibrosis (Fig. 59–18), infiltration, or endomyocardial scarring is usually responsible for the abnormal diastolic behavior; in the idiopathic variety there is often histological evidence of myocyte hypertrophy.[218,220] Myocardial involvement with amyloid (often in the setting of multiple myeloma) is a common cause of RCM, although it can be caused by a variety of other conditions (see Table 59–8). An occasional patient with a plasma cell dyscrasia may present with RCM related not to the deposition of amyloid fibrils into the myocardium but rather that of light chains.[221] Some patients may manifest the clinical features of an RCM and yet exhibit the pathological findings of left ventricular hypertrophy and fibrosis[3]; certainly, ventricular hypertrophy, especially HCM, can cause diminished ventricular compliance, but not RCM per se. RCM on occasion is inherited and has been found in association with mutations of the gene encoding troponin I (see Table 59–4); in some cases there may be an associated skeletal muscle disease.[218,222]

HEMODYNAMICS. The clinical and hemodynamic features of restrictive heart disease simulate those of chronic constrictive pericarditis; endomyocardial biopsy, CT, and radionuclide angiography may be particularly useful in differentiating the two diseases by demonstrating myocardial scarring or infiltration (on biopsy) or thickening of the pericardium (on CT and MRI).[3] With the use of these modalities, exploratory thoracotomy should rarely be required; nevertheless, if the differentiation between constriction and RCM cannot be established with certainty, surgical exploration is in order.[218,223] The characteristic hemodynamic feature in both conditions is a deep and rapid early decline in ventricular pressure at the onset of diastole, with a rapid rise to a plateau in early diastole (although this finding is absent in some patients with RCM).[218] This dip and plateau has been termed the *square root sign* and is manifested in the atrial pressure tracing as a prominent *y* descent followed by a rapid rise and plateau. The *x* descent may also be rapid, and the combination results in the characteristic M or W waveform in the atrial pressure tracing.[218] The a wave is prominent and often of the same amplitude as the v wave. Both systemic and pulmonary venous pressures are elevated, although patients with restrictive heart disease typically have left ventricular filling pressures that exceed right ventricular filling pressure by more than 5 mm Hg; this difference is accentuated by exercise, fluid challenge, and Valsalva maneuver (although not all patients demonstrate this finding).[218]

In this respect, they differ from patients with constrictive pericarditis, in whom diastolic pressures are similar in both ventricles, usually differing by no more than 5 mm Hg. The pulmonary artery systolic pressure is often greater than 50 mm Hg in patients with RCM but is lower in constrictive pericarditis.[218] Furthermore, the plateau of the right ventricular diastolic pressure is usually at least one-third of the peak right ventricular systolic pressure in patients with constrictive pericarditis, whereas it is frequently lower in RCM.[218]

CLINICAL MANIFESTATIONS. Exercise intolerance is frequent because of the inability of patients with RCM to increase their cardiac output by tachycardia without further compromising ventricular filling. Weakness and dyspnea are often prominent. Exertional chest pain may be prominent in some patients but is usually absent. Particularly in advanced cases, the central venous pressure is elevated, with attendant peripheral edema, enlarged liver, ascites, and anasarca. *Physical examination* may reveal jugular venous distention and an S_3, S_4, or both. An inspiratory increase in venous pressure may be seen (Kussmaul sign). However, in contrast to

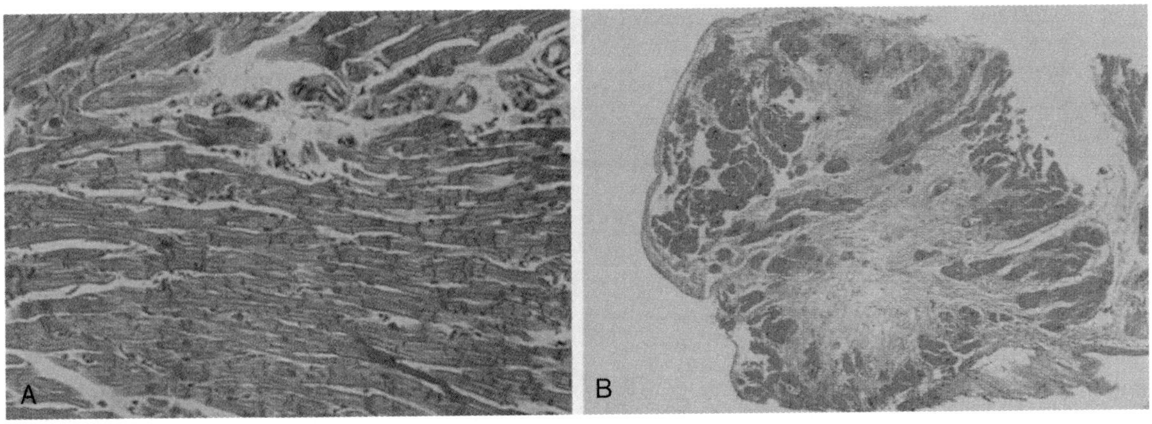

FIGURE 59–18 Endomyocardial biopsy specimens from patients with idiopathic restrictive cardiomyopathy. **A,** This histological specimen (hematoxylin and eosin, ×250) shows myocytes with slight hypertrophy but is otherwise normal. **B,** Another specimen (hematoxylin and eosin, ×40), from another patient, shows marked interstitial fibrosis, which may also occur in idiopathic restrictive cardiomyopathy. (From Kushwaha SS, Fallon JT, Fuster V: Restrictive cardiomyopathy. N Engl J Med 336:267, 1997. Copyright 1997, Massachusetts Medical Society.)

constrictive pericarditis, the apex impulse is usually palpable in RCM.[218]

LABORATORY STUDIES. The *electrocardiogram* often shows atrial fibrillation.[219] Various ancillary laboratory findings in addition to endomyocardial biopsy, CT, and MRI (see Chaps. 14 and 15) may be useful in distinguishing between constrictive and restrictive disease. Although pericardial calcification that is visible on the chest radiograph is neither absolutely sensitive nor specific for constrictive pericarditis (see Chap. 64), its presence in a patient in whom the differential diagnosis rests between RCM and constrictive pericarditis lends strong support to the latter diagnosis. The *echocardiogram* may demonstrate thickening of the left ventricular wall and an increase of left ventricular mass in patients with infiltrative disease causing RCM. The atria are almost always dilated.[219] The pattern of filling of the left ventricle differs in the two conditions, as can be demonstrated by transthoracic and transesophageal Doppler ultrasonography supplemented by tissue Doppler measurements.[218,223,224] Patients with RCM have an increased early left ventricular filling velocity, decreased atrial filling velocity, and decreased isovolumetric relaxation time.[218]

The prognosis in RCM is variable; usually it is one of relentless symptomatic progression and high mortality.[219,225] No specific therapy (other than symptomatic) is available for the idiopathic form of RCM, but several of the secondary forms may benefit from targeted treatment regimens (e.g., the cardiomyopathy related to iron overload, which is improved by removal of the iron, and Fabry disease, in which enzyme replacement therapy has demonstrated efficacy).[226,227]

Amyloidosis

ETIOLOGY AND TYPES. Amyloidosis is a disease complex that results from deposition of unique twisted beta-pleated sheet fibrils formed from various proteins by several different pathogenic mechanisms. Amyloid may be found in almost any organ, but clinically evident disease does not appear unless infiltration is extensive. Several classification systems have been used to characterize the different clinical presentations of amyloidosis. The condition with the traditional designation of *primary amyloidosis* is now known to be caused by the production of an amyloid protein composed of portions of immunoglobulin light chain (designated *AL*) by a monoclonal population of plasma cells, often as a consequence of multiple myeloma.[228] Secondary amyloidosis (also known as reactive systemic) is due to the production of a non-immunoglobulin protein termed *AA*.

Familial Amyloidosis. This condition, inherited as an autosomal dominant trait, results from the production of a variant prealbumin serum carrier protein termed *transthyretin*; more than 80 different point mutations have been described so far.[228] It generally occurs in one of three clinical presentations: progressive neuropathy, cardiomyopathy, or nephropathy.[229] The cardiomyopathic variant typically has involvement limited to the heart and is four times more common in blacks than in whites because of a genetic variant that is found in 4 percent of the black population.[230]

Senile Systemic Amyloidosis. This form of amyloid is due to the production of either an atrial natriuretic-like protein or transthyretin and is becoming increasingly common as the average age of the population increases. Scattered deposits of amyloid localized to the aorta or atria are virtually ubiquitous in individuals older than 80 and may predispose to the development of atrial fibrillation.[231] Small deposits of amyloid may often be found in the pulmonary vessels or the vessels of other organs as well.

Cardiac Amyloidosis

Involvement of the heart is a common finding and is the most frequent cause of death in amyloidosis associated with an immunocyte dyscrasia.[232] Clinically apparent heart disease is present in one-third of patients,[233] although the heart is virtually always involved when studied pathologically.[234] In secondary amyloidosis, on the other hand, clinically significant cardiac involvement is uncommon; the myocardial deposits are typically small and perivascular and usually do not result in significant myocardial dysfunction.[235] Familial amyloidosis is associated with overt cardiac involvement in about one-fourth of the afflicted patients, usually late in the course of the disease, and often dominated by conducting system disease.[236] The clinical course is usually dominated by neurological or renal dysfunction, although death is due to heart failure or arrhythmia about half the time. Cardiac involvement in senile amyloidosis varies from small atrial deposits that do not result in functional impairment to extensive ventricular involvement with resultant cardiac failure.[231]

Cardiac amyloidosis occurs more commonly in men than in women, and it is rare before the age of 40 years. Even in the familial form, the onset of clinical cardiac disease usually does not occur before the age of 35 years and generally occurs much later in life.

PATHOLOGY. The pathological findings often include mild atrial enlargement, usually without significant ventricular dilation. The walls of both ventricles are typically firm, rubbery, noncompliant, and thickened. Amyloid is present between the myocardial fibers, often with extensive deposition in the papillary muscles. Endocardial involvement of the atria and ventricles is frequent, and disease limited to the atria may be seen.[231] Amyloidosis often results in focal thickening of or deposits on the cardiac valves, but these abnormalities do not appear to interfere with valvular function other than to produce murmurs. The intramural coronary arteries and veins frequently contain amyloid deposits in the media and adventitia, occasionally compromising the lumina of the vessels and reducing coronary flow reserve.[231,237]

CLINICAL MANIFESTATIONS. Involvement of the cardiovascular system by amyloidosis occurs in four general forms that may overlap:

1. The most common presentation of cardiac amyloidosis is that of RCM.[217] The restrictive physiology results not only from the physical presence of amyloid infiltrates in the myocardium but also from direct depression of diastolic function by circulating immunoglobulin light chains.[238] Right-sided findings dominate the clinical presentation; peripheral edema is a prominent finding, whereas paroxysmal nocturnal dyspnea and orthopnea are absent. Myopathic involvement produces the characteristic diastolic dip and plateau (square root sign) in the ventricular pressure pulse that may simulate constrictive pericarditis. In contrast to the accelerated early left ventricular diastolic filling found in constrictive pericarditis, cardiac amyloidosis is marked by an impaired rate of early diastolic filling.
2. A second common presentation is congestive heart failure related to systolic dysfunction, which is usually a late finding in cardiac amyloidosis.[239] Hemodynamic evidence of restriction of ventricular filling may not be prominent in these patients. In some patients amyloid deposition in the atria may be responsible for loss of atrial transport function despite the maintenance of electrical "sinus" rhythm, with the production of congestive heart failure. The course of this form of the disease is often one of relentless progression, usually poorly responsive to treatment. Angina pectoris occurs on occasion despite angiographically normal coronary arteries.
3. Orthostatic hypotension occurs in about 10 percent of cases. Although it is most likely due to amyloid infiltration of the autonomic nervous system or blood vessels, or both, amyloid deposition in the heart and adrenals may contribute to the pathogenesis of this variant.[240] Hypovolemia as a result of the nephrotic syndrome secondary to renal amyloidosis may worsen the postural hypotension. Frank syncope is common in amyloidosis, is often multifactorial in etiology, and is associated with emotional or physical stress.[241] When exertional, it is a dire prognostic sign, and most patients die within 3 months.[239]
4. An abnormality of cardiac impulse formation and conduction is the fourth and least common mode of presentation and may result in arrhythmias and conduction disturbances.[242] Sudden death, presumably arrhythmic in origin, is relatively common and may be preceded by episodes of syncope.[241,243]

PHYSICAL EXAMINATION. This often reveals congestive heart failure, especially right sided; a systolic murmur caused by atrioventricular valvular regurgitation may be present. Jugular venous distention, a protodiastolic gallop, hepatomegaly, peripheral edema, and a narrow pulse pressure are found in patients presenting with RCM. An S_4 is uncommon, presumably because of amyloid infiltration of the atrium with attendant reduced systolic function of the atrial myocardium.[244] Patients are typically normotensive or hypotensive; even previously hypertensive individuals usually have a fall in blood pressure as the disease progresses.

NONINVASIVE TESTING. The *chest roentgenogram* usually shows cardiomegaly in patients with systolic dysfunction, although heart size may be normal in patients with the restrictive form.[239] Pulmonary congestion may be prominent in patients with congestive heart failure. The *electrocardiogram* is often abnormal; the most characteristic feature is diffusely diminished voltage. Bundle branch block and abnormal axis deviation are common, although some patients have significant conducting system disease despite a normal QRS on ECG study.[237,242] Myocardial infarction is often simulated because of small or absent R waves in right precordial leads or, less frequently, by Q waves in the inferior leads.[239] Arrhythmias, particularly atrial fibrillation, are common and may be related to amyloid infiltration of the atrium.[231] Complex ventricular arrhythmias are found frequently in patients with cardiac amyloidosis and may be a harbinger of sudden death. The *signal-averaged electrocardiogram* can help to identify patients at increased risk for sudden death.[243] Various forms of atrioventricular conduction defects are often seen and may be associated with increased mortality, although significant infrahisian block may be apparent only on *electrophysiological testing.*[242] Abnormalities of atrioventricular conduction appear to be particularly common in familial amyloidosis with polyneuropathy. Sinus node involvement is common, and the clinical and ECG features of the sick sinus syndrome may be present (see Chap. 29).

Echocardiography (see Chap. 11). In advanced cases this most commonly reveals increased thickness of the walls of the ventricles, small ventricular chambers, dilated atria, and thickening of the interatrial septum (Fig. 59–19). Left ventricular dysfunction may be seen, especially in advanced cases, but systolic function is often surprisingly normal.[237,244] Early, unsuspected cardiac involvement may be detectable only by echocardiography or Doppler ultrasonography, although in some cases echocardiography may be falsely normal. Although the cardiac valves may be thickened, they usually move normally.[234] A pericardial effusion is common but rarely results in tamponade.[244] The appearance of the thickened cardiac walls is often distinctive on two-dimensional echocardiography, demonstrating a granular sparkling texture, presumably related to the amyloid deposit.[234,244] In some cases the pattern of increased wall thickness is nonuniform and may resemble HCM. Echocardiographic demonstration of thick left ventricular walls with concomitant low voltage on the electrocardiogram appears to distinguish cardiac amyloidosis from pericardial disease or left ventricular hypertrophy, and this distinctive voltage/mass ratio is characteristic of myocardial infiltration by amyloid (especially AL amyloid).[236] Doppler ultrasonography and radionuclide ventriculography routinely demonstrate abnormalities of diastolic function and, by estimating the degree of cardiac involvement by amyloid, provide prognostic information.[234,244]

Imaging. *Scintigraphy* with technetium-99m pyrophosphate and other agents that bind to calcium is often strongly positive with prominent amyloid involvement (Fig. 59–20), although in some patients it is falsely negative.[245] Positive scans tend to correlate with extensive cardiac involvement. Scanning with indium-labeled antimyosin antibody may also detect cardiac amyloid involvement, as may MRI.[171,246] Scanning with specialized agents has shown sympathetic denervation in patients with cardiac amyloidosis.[245]

DIAGNOSIS. Whereas two or three decades ago the clinical diagnosis of systemic amyloidosis was made correctly ante mortem in only about one-fourth of cases, with more recent clinical awareness of the disease and the utilization of *biopsy techniques* the diagnosis is now made before death in the majority of patients. An abdominal fat aspirate has been the single most useful diagnostic procedure, combining the attributes of ease of performance, sensitivity, and safety.[232,247]

Biopsy of rectum, gingiva, bone marrow, liver, kidney, and various other tissues has also been used. Endomyocardial biopsy of the right or left ventricles may be helpful in establishing the diagnosis of cardiac amyloidosis (Fig. 59–21) if the abdominal fat aspirate is negative.[232] Immunohistochemical staining of tissue samples is important to distinguish systemic senile, familial, and primary forms of amyloidosis in otherwise equivocal presentations because prognosis and management differ in the various forms[232]; unsuspected hereditary amyloidosis is found in almost 10 percent of patients thought to have the primary (AL) form.[228]

MANAGEMENT. The treatment of cardiac amyloidosis is generally unsatisfactory, although there has been some improvement in survival and functional state with the use of alkylating agents in primary (AL) amyloidosis.[248] However, the median survival is less than a year, and it is the rare patient (<5 percent) who survives for more than 5 years.[249,250] Digitalis glycosides should be used with caution because patients with cardiac amyloidosis appear to be sensitive to digitalis preparations.[251] Nevertheless, the glycosides have been used with success to control the ventricular rate in atrial fibrillation.[239] The calcium antagonists are also said to be problematic in cardiac amyloidosis and may lead to exacerbation of congestive heart failure symptoms because of an enhanced negative inotropic effect. Insertion of a permanent pacemaker may be beneficial in the short term in patients with symptomatic conducting system disease.[252] Careful use of low doses of diuretics and vasodilators may afford some symptomatic benefit, but there is a risk of hypotension and hypoperfusion with use of these agents.[218,233,239] In patients with atrial standstill related to amyloid infiltration, anticoagulation may be appropriate even in the absence of atrial arrhythmias because there is some risk of thrombus formation, presumably as a consequence of stasis in the atrium. The rare patient with a plasma cell dyscrasia and RCM caused by light-chain deposition may improve with chemotherapy.[221]

Autologous bone marrow stem cell transplantation is being used with increasing frequency in primary (AL) amyloidosis, but patients with advanced cardiac amyloidosis or multiorgan involvement do not appear to reap much benefit.[253] However, selected patients (especially those with early and mild cardiac involvement) may derive some benefit from stem cell transplantation. A small number of patients have undergone cardiac transplantation, with poor long-term results (39 percent survival at 4 years in one study and 30 percent at 5 years in another) because of progressive amyloidosis in other organs or recurrence in the transplanted heart, although a few carefully selected patients have shown long-term survival and functional improvement.[218,254] No therapy is effective for the senile form, but survival is about 10 times longer than in the primary form (60 versus 6 months for patients with congestive heart failure).[244,249]

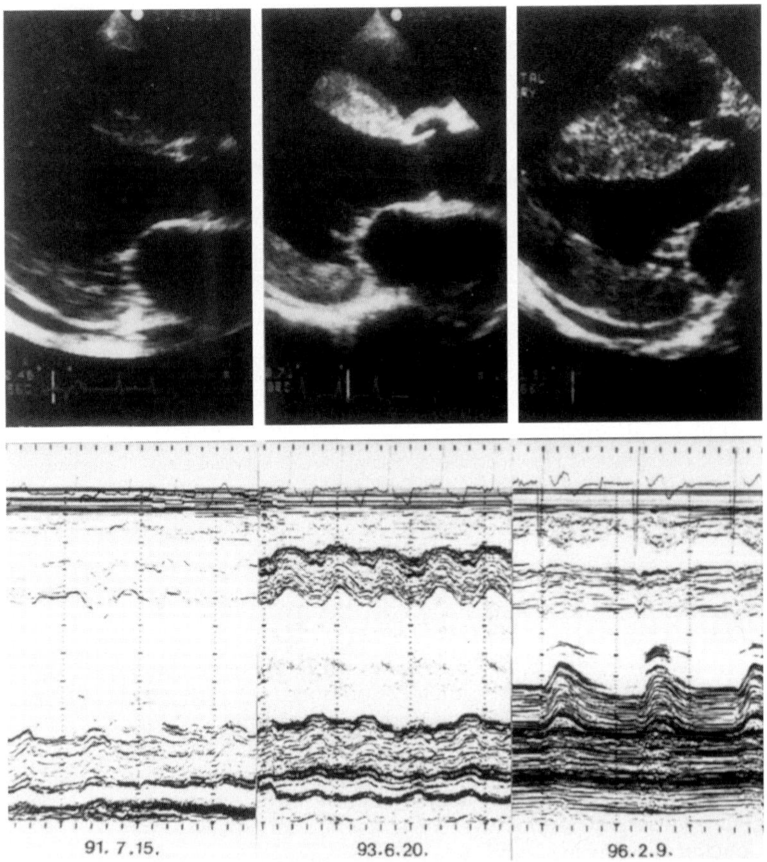

FIGURE 59–19 Serial echocardiographic findings in a patient developing cardiac amyloidosis. **Top,** Serial two-dimensional echocardiographic findings. Note the thickening of all myocardial walls and valves. **Bottom,** Serial M-mode echocardiography shows gradual increase of interventricular septal, left ventricular posterior wall, and right ventricular wall thickness. The date of the study is shown at the bottom (year.month.day). (From Youn H, Chae JS, Lee KY, et al: Images in cardiovascular medicine: Amyloidosis with cardiac involvement. Circulation 97:2093, 1998. Copyright 1998, American Heart Association.)

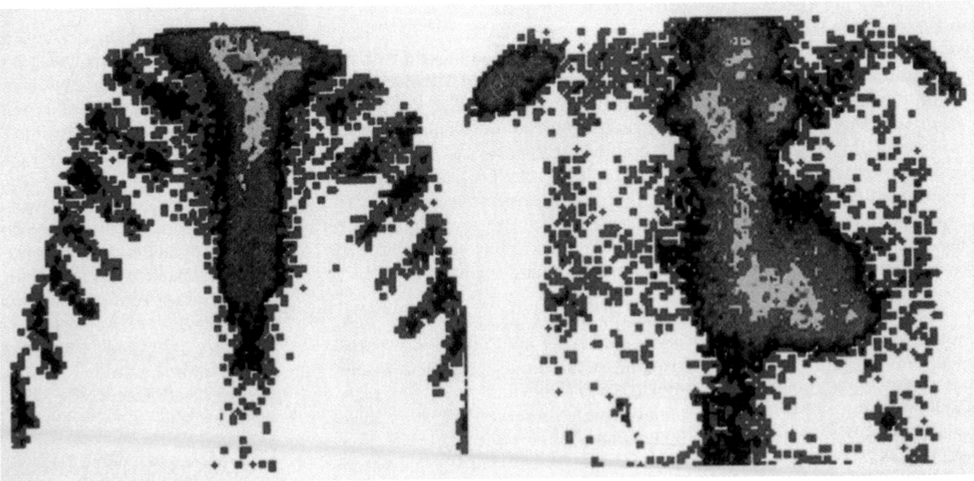

FIGURE 59–20 Nuclear scan using ^{99}Tc-methylene diphosphonate that binds to the calcium-binding site of amyloid. **Left,** Control patient, with normal uptake in bones. **Right,** Patient with familial amyloidosis, showing striking uptake by cardiac involvement. (From Singer R, Schnabel A, Strasser RH: Restrictive cardiomyopathy in familial amyloidosis TTR-Arg-50. Circulation 107:643, 2003. Copyright 2003, American Heart Association.)

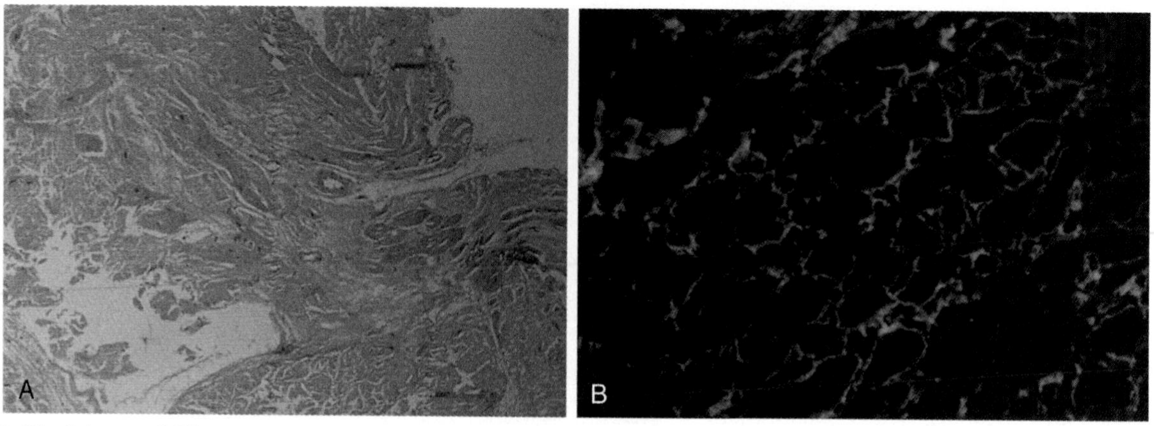

FIGURE 59–21 Endomyocardial biopsy specimens from patients with cardiac amyloidosis. **A,** This histological section (hematoxylin and eosin, ×250) shows interstitial deposition of amyloid fibrils in a specimen from the right ventricle. **B,** Immunofluorescent stain (×400) shows lambda light chains. (From Kushwaha SS, Fallon JT, Fuster V: Restrictive cardiomyopathy. N Engl J Med 336:267, 1997. Copyright 1997, Massachusetts Medical Society.)

Inherited Infiltrative Disorders Causing Restrictive Cardiomyopathy

The intramyocardial accumulation or infiltration of an abnormal metabolic product typically produces a restrictive picture with impaired diastolic ventricular filling. Systolic impairment may be seen as well but is not invariably found. A variety of infiltrative diseases, often inherited, may result in this hemodynamic picture, including the glycogenoses, the mucopolysaccharidoses, Fabry disease, and Gaucher disease.

FABRY DISEASE

This condition, also known as angiokeratoma corporis diffusum universale, is an X-linked recessive disorder of glycosphingolipid metabolism resulting from a deficiency of the lysosomal enzyme alpha-galactosidase A that is caused by one of more than 160 mutations.[227,255,256] Some mutations result in no detectable alpha-galactosidase A activity and widespread manifestations throughout the body, whereas others produce some degree of enzyme activity with attendant atypical variants of Fabry disease with involvement limited solely to the myocardium.[227,255,257] The disease is characterized by an intracellular accumulation of glycosphingolipids (especially globotriaosylceramide) with prominent involvement of the skin and kidneys as well as the myocardium in the classical form. *Histological examination* often reveals widespread involvement of the myocardium, vascular endothelium, conducting tissues, and valves, particularly the mitral valve (Fig. 59–22). The major clinical manifestations result from the accumulation of the glycolipid substrate in endothelial cells, with eventual occlusion of small arterioles.[227] The accumulation of the glycolipid occurs in the lysosomes of the cardiac tissues and is responsible for the multiple cardiovascular manifestations of Fabry disease.

CARDIAC FINDINGS. These typically include angina pectoris and myocardial infarction caused by accumulation of lipid moieties in coronary endothelial cells, but coronary arteries are usually angiographically normal. There is increased left ventricular wall thickness producing diastolic dysfunction that is usually mild, generally preserved left ventricular systolic function, and clinically unimportant mitral regurgitation.[258] Preclinical cardiac involvement (i.e., before the development of increased wall thickness) may be suggested by abnormal myocardial tissue Doppler measurements of myocardial contraction and relaxation.[259] Symptomatic cardiovascular involvement occurs eventually in most affected males, whereas female carriers are usually asymptomatic or only minimally symptomatic.[255] Systemic hypertension, mitral valve prolapse, and congestive heart failure are common clinical manifestations. ECG abnormalities may include a short PR interval, atrioventricular block, ST segment and T wave abnormalities, left ventricular hypertrophy, and QRS prolongation.[255,260] The echocardiogram usually reveals increased left ventricular wall thickness as a result of glycolipid deposition, which may simulate HCM.[256] Differentiation from other hypertrophic or restrictive processes (such as cardiac amyloidosis) may not be possible on echocardiographic grounds but may be possible with MRI (Fig. 59–23). Endomyocardial biopsy may be of considerable value in making a definitive diagnosis, as is low plasma alpha-galactosidase A activity.[260] Differentiation from HCM is important because enzyme replacement therapy for Fabry disease is safe and effective.[261] It reduces the accumulated stores of globotriaosylceramide from the heart and other tissues and produces symptomatic, clinical, and echocardiographic improvement (Fig. 59–24).[227]

GAUCHER DISEASE

Gaucher disease is an uncommon inherited disorder of glycosyl ceramide metabolism. It is secondary to a deficiency of the enzyme beta-glucosidase and results in accumulation of cerebrosides in the spleen, liver, bone marrow, lymph nodes, brain, and myocardium. Diffuse interstitial infiltration of the left ventricle by cells laden with cerebroside produces reduced left ventricular compliance and cardiac output. Clinical evidence of cardiac involvement is uncommon but when present it is characterized by left ventricular dysfunction, hemorrhagic pericardial effusion, increased left ventricular wall mass, and thickening and calcification of the left-sided valves.[262,263] Enzyme replacement therapy and liver transplantation may produce a reduction in tissue infiltration by cerebrosides with attendant clinical improvement.[262,264]

HEMOCHROMATOSIS

Hemochromatosis is characterized by excessive deposition of iron in a variety of parenchymal tissues (heart, liver, gonads, and pancreas). It may occur (1) as a familial (autosomal recessive) or idiopathic disorder, (2) in association with a defect in hemoglobin synthesis resulting in ineffective erythropoiesis, (3) in chronic liver disease, and (4) with excessive oral or parenteral intake of iron (or blood transfusions) over many years.[226] Although patients who have iron deposits in the myocardium almost always have deposits in other organs (e.g., liver, spleen, pancreas, bone marrow), the severity of myocardial involvement varies widely and only roughly parallels that in other organs. Cardiac involvement leads to a mixed DCM-RCM pattern with both systolic and diastolic dysfunction, often with associated arrhythmias.[265,266] Myocardial damage is thought to be due to direct tissue toxicity of the free iron moiety rather than simply to tissue infiltration.[267] Although cirrhosis and hepatocellular carcinoma are the most common causes of death, cardiac mortality is an important additional concern (especially in the group of patients—usually men—who present at a young age) and accounts for a third of the mortality.[267,268]

PATHOLOGICAL FINDINGS. These consist of a dilated heart with thickened ventricular walls. Myocardial iron deposits are found within the sarcoplasmic reticulum and are most common in the subepicardial region, followed by the subendocardial region, and are least common in the midmyocardial wall. They are more extensive in ventricular than in atrial myocardium. Involvement of the cardiac conducting system is common. Myocardial degeneration and fibrosis may also occur.

The severity of myocardial dysfunction is proportional to the quantity of iron present in the myocardium.[269] Extensive deposits of cardiac iron (particularly those grossly visible at postmortem examination) are invariably associated with cardiac dysfunction.

CLINICAL MANIFESTATIONS. These vary widely, depending on the extent of myocardial involvement. Some patients remain asymptomatic despite echocardiographic evidence of myocardial involvement, which is expressed initially as increased left ventricular wall thickness and later as chamber enlargement and contractile dysfunction.[269] In such cases, a variety of noninvasive techniques (CT and especially MRI) may demonstrate early subclinical myocardial involvement in which treatment is most effective.[226] Symptomatic cardiac involvement is usually associated with ECG abnormalities, including ST segment and T wave abnormalities, as well as supraventricular arrhythmias[265]; these ECG changes correlate with the degree of iron deposit in the heart.

Cardiac involvement is usually evident from the clinical and echocardiographic features; endomyocardial biopsy may be useful to confirm (but not exclude) the diagnosis. The diagnosis is aided by finding an elevated plasma iron level, a normal or low total iron-binding capacity, and markedly elevated values for serum ferritin, urinary iron, liver iron, and especially saturation of transferrin.[269] Repeated phlebotomies or the use of the chelating agent desferrioxamine may be clinically beneficial.[226,267,270]

GLYCOGEN STORAGE DISEASES

Patients may demonstrate cardiac involvement in type II, III, IV, and V glycogen storage disease, but survival to adulthood is unusual except in type III (glycogen debranching enzyme deficiency).[271] Cardiac involvement is marked most commonly by often clinically silent apparent left ventricular hypertrophy on the electrocardiogram and echocardiogram, but some patients develop overt cardiac dysfunction, arrhythmias, and a pattern of DCM.[226,267,270,272,273]

SARCOIDOSIS

Sarcoidosis is a granulomatous disorder of unknown cause, characterized by multisystem involvement. Infiltration of the lungs, reticuloendothelial system, and skin usually dominates the clinical picture, but virtually any tissue may be affected. The most important manifestation results from

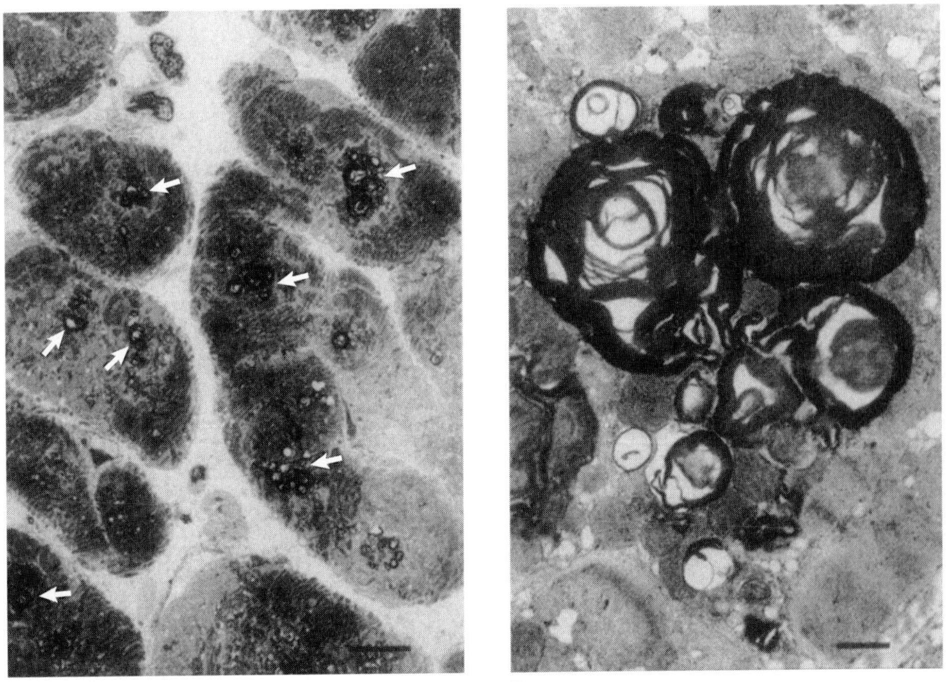

A B

FIGURE 59–22 Transmission electron micrographs of left ventricular endomyocardial biopsy specimen of a patient with Fabry disease, showing at low **(A)** and high **(B)** magnification the perinuclear vacuoles (arrows) that consist of single membrane-bound vesicles containing concentric, lamellar, electron-dense figures, typical of glycolipid storage disease. A, ×1250 (scale bar represents 10 mm); B, ×11,000 (scale bar represents 1 μm). (From Pieroni M, Chimenti C, Ricci R, et al: Early detection of Fabry cardiomyopathy by tissue Doppler imaging. Circulation 107:1978, 2003. Copyright 2003, American Heart Association.)

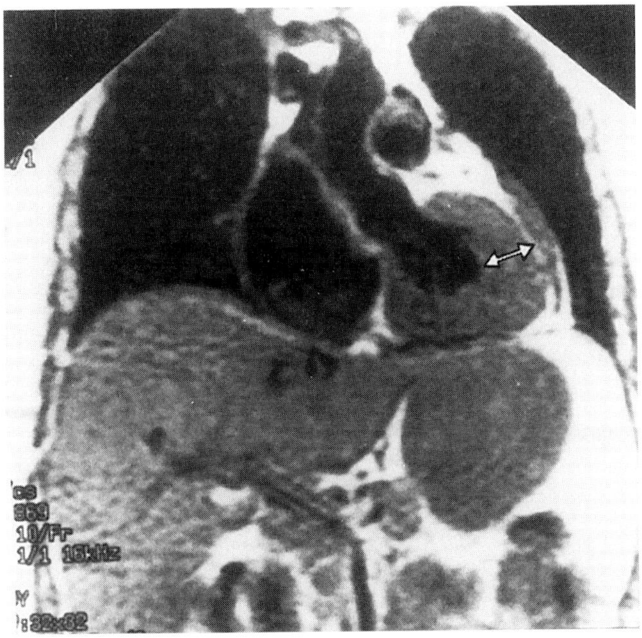

FIGURE 59–23 Cardiac magnetic resonance imaging (T1-weighted spin echo) in Fabry disease, showing marked ventricular thickening (arrow). Coronal view. (From Cantor WJ, Butany J, Iwanochko M, Liu P: Restrictive cardiomyopathy secondary to Fabry's disease. Circulation 98:1457, 1998. Copyright 1998, American Heart Association.)

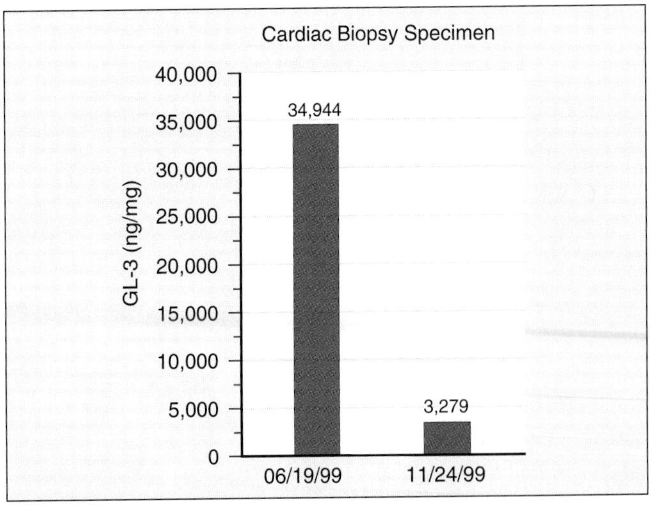

FIGURE 59–24 Marked decline in myocardial tissue levels of globotriaosylceramide (GL-3) in a patient with Fabry disease who was treated with enzyme replacement therapy. (From Waldek S: PR interval and the response to enzyme-replacement therapy for Fabry's disease. N Engl J Med 348:1186, 2003. Copyright 2003, Massachusetts Medical Society.)

pulmonary involvement. This often leads to diffuse fibrosis that may result in fatal right-sided heart failure. Primary cardiac involvement is not often recognized clinically, although it may be demonstrated at autopsy in 20 to 30 percent of cases, most of which demonstrate generalized sarcoidosis.[274,275]

Clinical manifestations of sarcoid heart disease are present in less than 5 percent of patients, although myocardial involvement may result in heart block, congestive heart failure, ventricular arrhythmias, and sudden death.[276,277] Myocardial sarcoidosis may have restrictive as well as congestive features because cardiac infiltration by sarcoid granulomas results not only in increased stiffness of the ventricular wall but also in diminished systolic contractile function.[278]

PATHOLOGY. The typical pathological feature is the presence of noncaseating granulomas, which occur in many organs (Fig. 59–25). They infiltrate the myocardium and may eventually form fibrotic scars. The granulomas may involve any region of the heart, although the left ventricular free wall and the interventricular septum are the most common sites, and extensive granulomas and scar tissue in the cephalad portion of the interventricular septum are constant findings in patients with abnormalities of the conduction system.[279] Cardiac infiltration may range from a few scattered lesions to extensive involvement. Because of the variable cardiac involvement, myocardial biopsy may be positive in as few as 20 percent of patients, and therefore a negative biopsy by no means excludes the diagnosis.[65] Transmural involvement may be seen, and large portions of the ventricular wall may be replaced by scar tissue, which may lead to aneurysm formation.[275] Although involvement of small coronary artery branches may be found in sarcoidosis, the larger conductance vessels are uninvolved.

CLINICAL MANIFESTATIONS. Sudden death is the most feared and unfortunately one of the more common manifestations of cardiac sarcoidosis. Conduction disturbances and congestive heart failure are common manifestations of symptomatic involvement in nonfatal cases, but many patients are asymptomatic despite extensive cardiac involvement.[276] Syncope is common and may reflect paroxysmal arrhythmias or conduction disturbances.[278] Atrial and ventricular arrhythmias, especially ventricular tachycardia, are observed frequently.[280] Although cor pulmonale as a consequence of pulmonary sarcoidosis accounts for some of the symptoms of heart failure, many symptoms are caused by direct myocardial involvement by granulomas and scar tissue, and patients show the clinical features of RCM or DCM, or both.[280] Cardiac dysfunction is often severe and progressive. Occasionally, patients with extensive involvement develop overt left ventricular aneurysms. Symptoms of myocardial sarcoid may be present for variable lengths of time; however, the disease may progress rapidly to death, and in some patients the interval from the onset of cardiac symptoms to death is measured in months.[276] In others, survival may be considerably longer.[278,281]

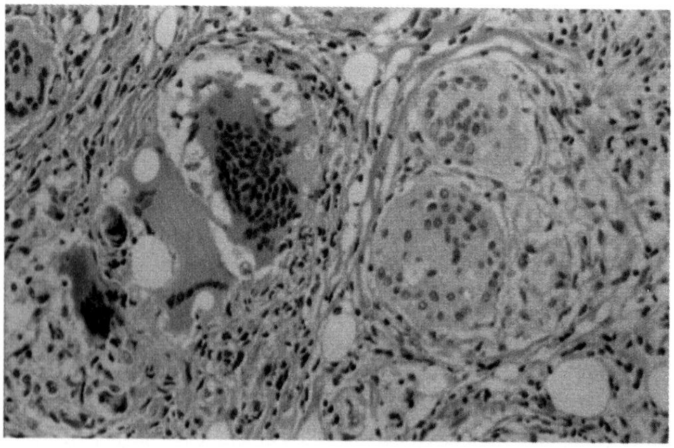

FIGURE 59–25 Typical histological findings in sarcoidosis, demonstrating many noncaseating granulomas with giant cells in skin biopsy specimen. (From Shindo T, Kurihara H, Ohishi N, et al: Images in cardiovascular medicine. Cardiac sarcoidosis. Circulation 97:1306, 1998. Copyright 1998, American Heart Association.)

The *physical examination* may reveal findings of extracardiac sarcoid or may be totally normal. A systolic murmur reflecting mitral regurgitation is common. This appears to be more the result of left ventricular dilation than of direct sarcoid involvement of the papillary muscles.

The *electrocardiogram* is frequently abnormal and most commonly demonstrates T wave abnormalities.[275] Sarcoidosis appears to have an affinity for involvement of the atrioventricular junction and bundle of His, and thus varying degrees of intraventricular or atrioventricular block are common.[274] With extensive myocardial involvement, pathological Q waves may appear and simulate myocardial infarction (Fig. 59–26). Characteristic echocardiographic features include left ventricular dilation and dysfunction, often with regional wall motion abnormalities suggestive of ischemic heart disease; wall thinning and increased echogenicity are sometimes observed.[275,276] A small to moderate-sized pericardial effusion may be found.[280]

DIAGNOSIS. In many cases the diagnosis may be suspected in patients with bilateral hilar lymphadenopathy on chest roentgenogram in whom there is clinical or ECG evidence of myocardial disease. Endomyocardial biopsy may be useful in establishing the diagnosis, although the nonuniform involvement of the heart by sarcoidosis means that a negative biopsy does not exclude the diagnosis.[65,274] The *echocardiogram* demonstrates diffuse and often regional left ventricular wall motion abnormalities in patients with clinical cardiac involvement.[276] *Myocardial imaging* with thallium-201 or technetium-99m sestamibi may be helpful in demonstrating segmental perfusion defects that result from sarcoid infiltration of the myocardium.[274,276] Imaging may also indicate the presence of right ventricular hypertrophy in patients with right ventricular overload related to pulmonary

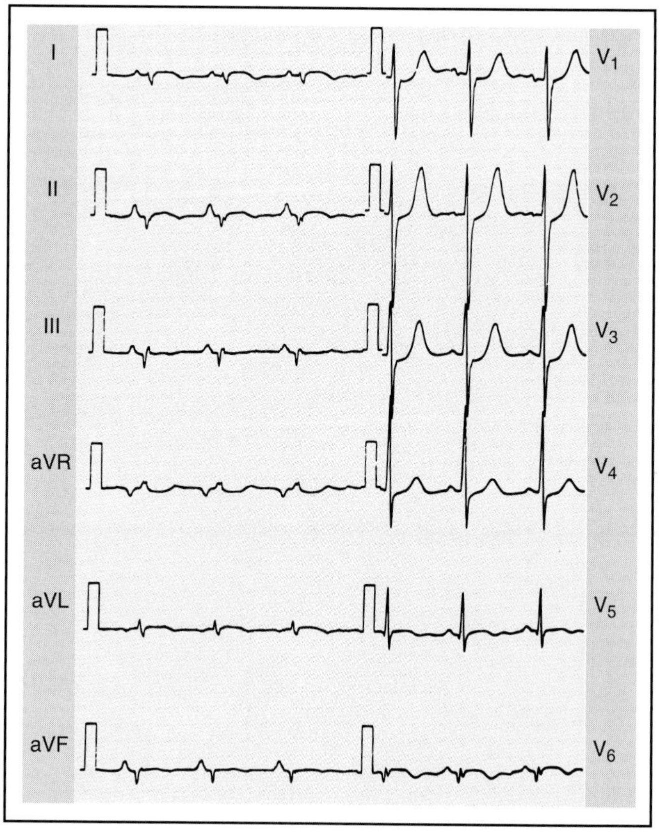

FIGURE 59–26 Electrocardiogram of a patient with cardiac sarcoidosis shows abnormal Q wave in leads II and III and aVF and ST segment elevation in V_5 and V_6. (From Shindo T, Kurihara H, Ohishi N, et al: Images in cardiovascular medicine: Cardiac sarcoidosis. Circulation 97:1306, 1998. Copyright 1998, American Heart Association.)

fibrosis and pulmonary hypertension. Uptake of technetium pyrophosphate, gallium, and labeled antimyosin antibody may aid in the diagnosis, as may MRI.[275,276,282,283]

MANAGEMENT. The treatment of myocardial sarcoidosis is difficult. Arrhythmias are often refractory to antiarrhythmic drugs. Permanent pacing may be helpful in patients with involvement of the atrioventricular conduction system. Although the matter is not settled, corticosteroids may be of some benefit in treating the conduction disturbances, arrhythmias, and myocardial dysfunction of sarcoidosis, with a suggestion of improved survival.[275,280,281] It has been suggested that further benefit may be derived from the addition of hydroxychloroquine, methotrexate, or cyclophosphamide. Because the risk of sudden death appears to be greatest in patients with extensive myocardial involvement, it may be reasonable to attempt to halt the progression of the disease with corticosteroids before irreversible fibrosis occurs.[281] Insertion of an ICD may be considered in appropriate patients at high risk for sudden death.[280] Heart or heart-lung transplantation has been used in selected patients with intractable heart failure, although recurrent sarcoid involvement of the transplanted heart can occur.[218,280]

Endomyocardial Disease

DEFINITION AND PATHOGENESIS. Endomyocardial disease (EMD) is a common form of RCM that is typically found in a geographical distribution near the equator. It is most frequent in equatorial Africa and is encountered with less frequency in South America, Asia, and nontropical countries, including the United States.[284] It is marked by intense endocardial fibrotic thickening of the apex and subvalvular regions of one or both ventricles that results in obstruction to inflow of blood into the respective ventricle, thus producing restrictive physiology.[285] For many years it had been thought that there are two variants of the disease, one occurring principally in tropical countries (termed *endomyocardial fibrosis* [EMF] or Davies disease) and the other in temperate countries (called Löffler endocarditis parietalis fibroplastica or the hypereosinophilic syndrome). However, despite the pathological similarities, there are important contrasts in clinical presentation that challenge the concept of a single disease process.[286] In addition to the geographical differences, the temperate form of the disease is a more aggressive and rapidly progressive disorder, affecting principally males, and is associated with hypereosinophilia, thromboembolic phenomena, and generalized arteritis. EMF, conversely, occurs in younger patients and has an inconstant association with an intense eosinophilia.[285,287]

DIFFERENCES BETWEEN LÖFFLER ENDOCARDITIS AND ENDOMYOCARDIAL FIBROSIS. Part of the thesis that Löffler endocarditis and EMF are different phases of a single disease is based on a theory of pathogenesis involving the toxic effect of eosinophils on the heart.[284] Under this formulation, an initial hypereosinophilia of whatever cause results in damage to the myocardium that produces the first phase of EMD: a necrotic phase, marked by an intense myocarditis, rich in eosinophils, and with an associated arteritis (i.e., Löffler endocarditis). This initial phase occurs within the first few months of illness. It may be followed by a thrombotic stage, occurring about a year after initial presentation, during which the myocarditis has receded, nonspecific thickening of the myocardium is beginning, and there is a variable degree of superimposed thrombus formation.[286] The putative last stage is one of fibrosis, presenting all of the features of EMF. The three stages—necrotic, thrombotic, and fibrotic—have been defined on the basis of postmortem material, and it is not suggested by proponents of the unified pathogenesis hypothesis that each patient with advanced disease (manifested by EMF) has necessarily passed through the earlier phases.

ROLE OF EOSINOPHILS. The possible role of eosinophils in the production of the cardiac abnormalities has intrigued investigators for years.[284] Eosinophils may damage tissues by direct invasion or by the release of toxic substances. The presence of degranulated eosinophils in the peripheral blood of patients with Löffler endocarditis suggests that the protein constituents of the eosinophil's granule may be cardiotoxic, first producing the necrotic phase of EMD, followed by the thrombotic and fibrotic phases after the disappearance of the initial eosinophilia.[284,288]

There is now, however, increasing speculation that this continuum occurs only in the temperate countries, and the endemic EMF found in tropical countries is a distinct and separate disease because a constant link with eosinophilia has been difficult to document, despite the frequency of parasitic diseases.[284,285,289] Other etiological factors have been implicated; the fibrosis of tropical EMF has been linked to the higher levels of cerium and lower concentrations of magnesium that apparently are found in endemic areas.[284,286,290,291]

Because the clinical manifestations of EMD demonstrate geographical and clinical differences, Löffler endocarditis and EMF are discussed separately, even though they are likely to be part of the same disease continuum.

Löffler Endocarditis: The Hypereosinophilic Syndrome

Marked eosinophilia of any cause may be associated with EMD. The typical patient who presents with Löffler endocarditis is a man in his fourth decade who lives in a temperate climate and has the hypereosinophilic syndrome (i.e., persistent eosinophilia with 1500 eosinophils/mm^3 for at least 6 months or until death, with evidence of organ involvement).[287,292] Cardiac involvement in the hypereosinophilic syndrome is the rule, occurring in the majority of patients.[292,293] Hypereosinophilia and cardiac involvement are also seen in the Churg-Strauss syndrome, which is differentiated by asthma or allergic rhinitis and a necrotizing vasculitis.[294] The cause of the eosinophilia in most patients with Löffler endocarditis is unknown, although in some it may be the result of leukemia, or it may be reactive (i.e., secondary to various parasitic, allergic, granulomatous, hypersensitivity, or neoplastic disorders).[292]

PATHOLOGY. In the hypereosinophilic syndrome, a variety of organs are usually involved besides the heart, including the lungs, bone marrow, and brain.[287] Cardiac involvement is often biventricular, with mural endocardial thickening of the inflow portions and apex of the ventricles.[288,293] Histological findings include variable degrees of (1) an acute inflammatory eosinophilic myocarditis involving the myocardium and endocardium; (2) thrombosis, fibrinoid change, and inflammatory reaction involving small intramural coronary vessels; (3) mural thrombosis, often containing eosinophils; and (4) fibrotic thickening of up to several millimeters.[293]

CLINICAL MANIFESTATIONS. The principal clinical features include weight loss, fever, cough, rash, and congestive heart failure. Although early cardiac involvement may be asymptomatic, overt cardiac dysfunction occurs in more than half of the patients and may be right or left sided, or both.[287] Cardiomegaly, often without overt symptoms of congestive heart failure, may be present, and the murmur of mitral regurgitation is common. Systemic embolism is frequent and may lead to neurological and renal dysfunction. Death is usually due to congestive heart failure, often with associated renal, hepatic, or respiratory dysfunction.[292]

LABORATORY EXAMINATION. The *chest roentgenogram* may reveal cardiomegaly and pulmonary congestion or, less commonly, pulmonary infiltrates. The *electrocardiogram* most commonly shows nonspecific ST segment and T wave abnormalities.[292] Arrhythmias, especially atrial fibrillation, and conduction defects, particularly right bundle branch block, may also be present.

The *echocardiogram* commonly demonstrates localized thickening of the posterobasal left ventricular wall, with absent or markedly limited motion of the posterior leaflet of the mitral valve.[287] There may be obliteration of the apex by thrombus.[293] Enlargement of the atria may be seen,[292] along with Doppler ultrasound evidence of atrioventricular regurgitation. Systolic function often is well preserved, in keeping with the restrictive picture seen in this condition.

The hemodynamic consequences of the dense endocardial scarring seen in Löffler endocarditis are those of an RCM, with abnormal diastolic filling resulting from increased stiffness of the ventricles and a reduction in the size of the ventricular cavity by organized thrombus.[287,293] Atrioventricular valvular regurgitation may occur because of involvement of the supporting apparatus of the mitral or tricuspid valves. *Cardiac catheterization* reveals markedly elevated ventricular filling pressures, and there may be evidence of tricuspid or mitral regurgitation. A characteristic feature on angiocardiography is largely preserved systolic function with obliteration of the apex of the ventricles. The diagnosis is often confirmed by percutaneous endomyocardial biopsy, but the biopsy is not invariably positive.[287]

MANAGEMENT. Medical therapy during the course of early Löffler endocarditis and surgical therapy during the later phases of fibrosis may have a positive effect on symptoms and survival.[292] Corticosteroids appear to have a beneficial effect on acute myocarditis and together with cytotoxic drugs (hydroxyurea in particular) may improve survival substantially.[218] A limited number of patients not responding to standard therapy have responded to treatment with interferon.[288,292] Routine cardiac therapy with digitalis, diuretics, afterload reduction, and anticoagulation as indicated are adjuncts in the management of these patients.[287,292] Surgical therapy appears to offer significant palliation of symptoms when the fibrotic stage has been reached.[295]

Endomyocardial Fibrosis

EMF occurs most commonly in tropical and subtropical Africa, particularly Uganda and Nigeria.[296] It is characterized by fibrous endocardial lesions of the inflow of the right or left ventricle or both and often involves the atrioventricular valves, resulting in regurgitation.[297] It is a relatively frequent cause of heart failure and death in equatorial Africa, accounting for about a quarter of all of the cases of congestive heart failure.[298]

Although most prominent in Africa, it is also found in tropical and subtropical regions in the rest of the world, typically within 15 degrees of the equator, including India, Brazil, Colombia, and Sri Lanka.[284,290] EMF is most common in specific ethnic groups, notably the Rwanda tribe in Uganda, and in people of low socioeconomic status.[296,299] The disease is equally frequent in both sexes, and, although most common in children and young adults, its reported age range is 4 to 70 years. It is most common in blacks, but cases have been reported occasionally in whites in temperate climates, rarely in the absence of prior residence in tropical areas.

PATHOLOGY. A pericardial effusion, which may be quite large, may be present. The heart is normal in size or slightly enlarged, but massive four-chamber cardiomegaly does not occur. The right atrium is often dilated, and in patients with severe right ventricular involvement there may be substantial enlargement of this chamber.[285] Indentation of the right border of the heart above the apex as a result of apical scarring may occur.

Combined right and left ventricular disease occurs in about half the cases, with pure left ventricular involvement occurring in 40 percent and pure right ventricular involvement in the remaining 10 percent. When affected, the right ventricle exhibits extensive dense fibrous thickening of the inflow tract and apex, with involvement of the papillary muscles and chordae tendineae. Involvement of the right ventricle may lead to obliteration of the apex, with a mass of thrombus and fibrous tissue filling the cavity.[297] The tricuspid valve is often distorted by the fibrous process involving the supporting structures. Right atrial thrombi occur commonly. Left ventricular involvement is similar, with fibrosis extending from the apex up the inflow portion of the left ventricle to the posterior mitral valve leaflet. The anterior leaflet of the mitral valve and the outflow portion of the left ventricle are usually spared. Thrombi often overlie the endocardial lesions, and widely distributed endocardial calcific deposits may occur.[300] The epicardial coronary arteries are free of obstructive lesions.

Histological Findings. Microscopically, the involved endocardium demonstrates a thick layer of collagen tissue on top of a layer of loosely arranged connective tissue.[301] Septa composed of fibrous and granulation tissue extend for variable distances into the myocardium. Interstitial edema is often present, but there is no prominent cellular infiltration. Small patches of fibroelastosis may occur in both ventricular outflow tracts beneath the semilunar valves but are thought to be a secondary phenomenon related to local trauma rather than a result of the basic pathological process. The intramural coronary arteries may show medial degeneration, fibrosis, and fibrin deposits.

CLINICAL MANIFESTATIONS. Because EMF may involve both ventricles or either ventricle selectively, symptoms vary. Left-sided involvement results in symptoms of pulmonary congestion, whereas predominant right-sided disease may present features of an RCM and therefore simulate constrictive pericarditis. There is often regurgitation of one or both atrioventricular valves. The onset of the disease is usually insidious, but it is sometimes ushered in by an acute febrile illness. Rarely, the disease appears to stabilize; although survival for up to 12 years has been observed, EMF is usually relentlessly progressive. Death is due to progressive myocardial failure, often associated with pulmonary congestion, infection, infarction, or sudden, unexpected cardiovascular collapse, presumably arrhythmic in origin. Survival appears to be unrelated to the site of predominant involvement (right or left ventricle), although patients presenting in advanced right-sided failure have a worse prognosis than other patients.[302]

RIGHT VENTRICULAR ENDOMYOCARDIAL FIBROSIS

Pure or predominant right ventricular involvement is characterized by fibrous obliteration of the right ventricular apex that diminishes the capacity of this chamber.[297] The fibrosis often extends to the supporting apparatus of the tricuspid valve, resulting in tricuspid regurgitation. Clinical manifestations in patients with right-sided involvement include an elevated jugular venous pressure, a prominent v wave, and a rapid *y* descent. A protodiastolic gallop sound may be heard along the lower sternal border, reflecting right ventricular dysfunction.[284] The liver is usually large and pulsatile, and ascites, splenomegaly, and peripheral edema are common. Pulmonary congestion is not present in the absence of left-sided involvement, and the pulmonary artery and pulmonary capillary wedge pressures are normal.[284] A pericardial effusion, which is sometimes quite large, may be present. The right atrium is often enlarged, sometimes massively so.

LABORATORY FINDINGS. The *electrocardiogram* is usually abnormal, with diminished QRS voltage (probably resulting from the presence of a pericardial effusion), ST segment and T wave abnormalities, and findings suggestive of right-sided enlargement, especially a qR pattern in lead V_1. Supraventricular arrhythmias are common.[284] The *chest roentgenogram* demonstrates cardiac enlargement, usually with gross prominence of the right atrium and a pericardial effusion. Calcification in the walls of the right or, less commonly, the left ventricle may be seen.[284] *Echocardiography* may demonstrate right ventricular thickening, obliteration of the apex, dilated atrium, strong echoes emanating from the endocardial surface, and abnormal septal motion in patients with tricuspid regurgitation.[284,297] At *angiography* the right ventricular apex is characteristically not visualized because of obliteration by the fibrous endocardium, but tricuspid regurgitation, right atrial enlargement, and filling defects in the right atrium caused by intraatrial thrombi are sometimes seen. Early angiographic changes that may be present before advanced disease develops include a change in the endocardial appearance, small apical filling defects, and mild tricuspid regurgitation.

LEFT VENTRICULAR ENDOMYOCARDIAL FIBROSIS

With predominant *left-sided* involvement, the EMF invades the apex of the ventricle and usually the chordae tendineae or the posterior mitral valve leaflet as well, leading to mitral regurgitation.[297] The associated murmur may be confined to late systole, as is characteristic of the papillary muscle dysfunction type of murmur, or it may be pansystolic. Findings of pulmonary hypertension may be prominent. A protodiastolic gallop is commonly heard.

LABORATORY FINDINGS The *electrocardiogram* usually shows ST segment and T wave abnormalities.[297] QRS voltage may be diminished in the presence of a pericardial effusion, although left ventricular hypertrophy may be present. There may be findings of left atrial abnormality. As with right-sided involvement, atrial fibrillation is often present and is a marker of increased mortality.[303] *Echocardiographic features* include increased echoreflectivity of the endocardium, preserved systolic wall motion in the presence of apical obliteration, dilated atrium, variable degrees of pericardial effusion, and Doppler ultrasound evidence of mitral regurgitation.[297] *Cardiac catheterization* often reveals pulmonary hypertension, with elevated left ventricular filling pressures and a reduced cardiac index. The left ventriculogram usually shows mitral regurgitation, and a filling defect related to an intracavitary thrombus within the ventricle may be present (Fig. 59–27). Coronary arteriography does not reveal obstructive disease.

BIVENTRICULAR ENDOMYOCARDIAL FIBROSIS

This form of EMF occurs more frequently than either isolated right- or left-sided disease.[295,297] If there is more than minimal right ventricular involvement, severe pulmonary hypertension does not occur and the right-sided findings dominate the clinical presentation. Typical patients with biventricular involvement may have the features of right ventricular EMF, with only a mitral regurgitant murmur to suggest left ventricular involvement. Systemic embolization may occur in up to 15 percent of patients; infective endocarditis is even less frequent and is found in less than 2 percent.

DIAGNOSIS This is based on the presence in an individual of the typical clinical and laboratory features, particularly angiography, from the appropriate geographical area. Eosinophilia may be present and may or may not reflect associated parasitic infestation.[286,296,299] Endomyocardial biopsy may occasionally be helpful in establishing the diagnosis. However, this risks dislodging a mural thrombus, with resultant embolization, and left-sided biopsy is *not* recommended. In addition, because the disease is often focal, the biopsy may miss the pathological process, particularly if a right ventricular biopsy is performed in a patient with isolated left-sided disease.

MANAGEMENT The medical treatment of EMF is often difficult and not particularly effective. In patients with advanced disease, the outlook is poor, with 35 to 50 percent 2-year mortality. Substantially better survival may be seen in less symptomatic patients who have milder forms of the disease. Digitalis glycosides may be helpful in controlling the ventricular rate in patients with atrial fibrillation,[284] but the response of congestive symptoms to treatment is disappointing, and the development of atrial fibrillation is a sign of poor prognosis.[303] Although diuretics may be useful in the early stages of the disease, they are not particularly helpful in the treatment of massive ascites in the setting of advanced right-sided heart failure and tricuspid regurgitation.[284] When EMD has reached the fibrotic stage, surgery offers the possibility of symptomatic improvement and is the treatment of choice.[295,304] Operative excision of the fibrotic endocardium and replacement of the mitral or tricuspid valves, or both, have led to substantial symptomatic improvement, especially with predominant left-sided involvement.[218,297,304] Postoperative catheterization has provided objective evidence of hemodynamic improvement with a reduction in ventricular filling pressures, an increase in cardiac output, and normalization of the angiographic appearance.[304] Operative mortality has been high, between 15 and 25 percent in the larger series,[218,295] although it appears to be lower if valve replacement can be avoided. Long-term results suggest that surgery is at best palliative, with recurrent fibrosis, continued functional limitation, and cumulative mortality limiting the overall success of an operative approach.[295]

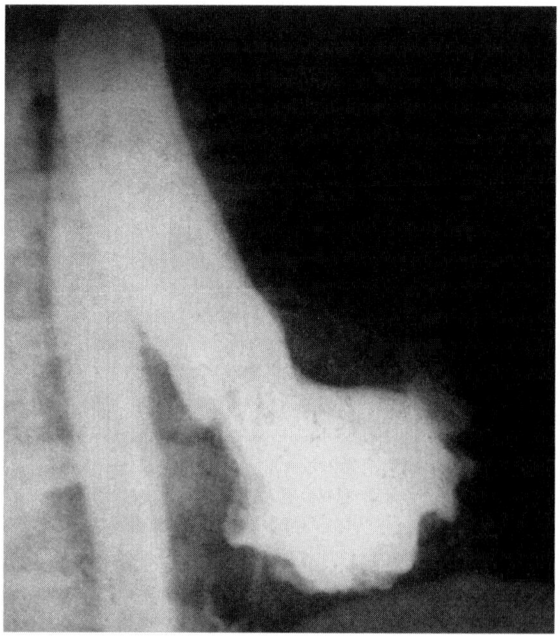

FIGURE 59–27 Left ventricular angiogram of a patient with left ventricular involvement by endomyocardial fibrosis. There is lobulated obliteration of the apex of the ventricle. (From Krishnamoorthy KM: Images in cardiology: Angiographic features of endomyocardial fibrosis. Heart 85:12, 2001.)

Carcinoid Heart Disease (see also Chap. 57)

ETIOLOGY. The carcinoid syndrome is caused by a metastasizing carcinoid tumor and is characterized by cutaneous flushing, diarrhea, bronchoconstriction, and endocardial plaques composed of a unique type of fibrous tissue. The vasomotor, bronchoconstrictor, and cardiac manifestations are related to the tumor's release of serotonin and other circulating humoral substances secreted by the tumor.[305] Virtually all patients develop diarrhea and flushing, and cardiac abnormalities are found on echocardiography in more than half; clinically apparent and severe usually right-sided disease is seen in a fourth of patients.[306,307]

Sixty to 90 percent of tumors arise in the small bowel and appendix, and the rest originate in other areas of the gastrointestinal tract and bronchus.[307] Carcinoid tumors of the ileum are the most likely to metastasize, with involvement of the regional lymph nodes and liver. Usually only carcinoid tumors that invade the liver result in carcinoid heart disease.[305] The cardiac lesions appear to be related to large circulating quantities of serotonin and its degradation product (5-hydroxyindolacetic acid), and patients with progressive cardiac disease tend to have higher levels than those without.[305] Hepatic metastases apparently allow large quantities of tumor products to reach the heart. The preferential right-sided involvement is presumably related to inactivation of the offending humoral substance or substances by the lungs.[308] In 5 to 10 percent of cases, significant left-sided valvular disease develops,[306] related in some to passage of blood directly from the right to the left side of the heart through a patent foramen ovale or less commonly to tumor involvement of the lungs.[309]

PATHOLOGY. The characteristic pathological findings are fibrous plaques that involve the "downstream" aspect of the tricuspid and pulmonic valves, the endocardium of the cardiac chambers, and the intima of the venae cavae, pulmonary artery, and coronary sinus. The fibrous tissue in the plaques results in structural and functional distortion of the valves, leading to both stenosis and regurgitation.[306,310] Histologically, the plaques consist of deposits of fibrous tissue located superficially on the endocardium, often with extension into the underlying layers. Identical morphological features have been found in some patients treated with the anorectic drugs fenfluramine and dexfenfluramine.[306] Ultrastructural and immunohistochemical studies have demonstrated that the plaques are composed of smooth muscle cells embedded in a stroma rich in acid mucopolysaccharides and collagen. Metastatic involvement of the myocardium itself is uncommon, but when it occurs, it may involve either ventricle.[311]

CLINICAL MANIFESTATIONS. Physical examination reveals a systolic murmur of tricuspid regurgitation along the left sternal border, which is a virtually ubiquitous finding; in some cases, there may be a concomitant murmur of pulmonic stenosis or regurgitation, or both.[306]

The *chest roentgenogram* is normal in half of the patients, but it may reveal enlargement of the heart and pleural effusions or nodules; the pulmonary artery trunk is typically of normal size, without evidence of poststenotic dilation as occurs in congenital pulmonic stenosis. No specific *ECG* pattern is diagnostic of carcinoid heart disease. Right atrial enlargement may be seen on occasion, but ECG evidence of right ventricular hypertrophy is usually lacking. Nonspecific ST segment and T wave abnormalities and sinus tachycardia are the most common findings, although severely symptomatic patients usually have low QRS voltage. *Echocardiography* may reveal tricuspid or pulmonary valve thickening, along with right atrial and right ventricular dilation; small pericardial effusions are present in a minority.[312]

MANAGEMENT. In patients with mild congestive heart failure, therapy includes digitalis and diuretics. Symptomatic improvement and perhaps improved survival have been noted with the use of somatostatin analogs and chemotherapy, but neither appears to slow or prevent the development of progressive cardiac disease in patients with carcinoid.[305] *Balloon valvuloplasty* of the right-sided valves has produced symptomatic improvement in some patients with stenotic tricuspid or pulmonary valves, although others have developed recurrent symptoms despite initially "successful" valvuloplasty.[307] *Surgical replacement* of the tricuspid or pulmonary valves, or both, and pulmonic valvotomy or valvectomy result in symptomatic improvement and a reduction in right ventricular dilation in severely symptomatic patients with serious valvular dysfunction, although the operative mortality is high.[306,308,309] The long-term mortality remains high regardless of treatment modality, with half the patients dead within 1 to 2 years.[308]

ENDOCARDIAL FIBROELASTOSIS

This condition is found principally in fetuses and infants and is characterized by collagen and elastin deposition, ventricular hypertrophy, and diffuse endocardial thickening.[313] The cause is unclear but endocardial fibroelastosis (EFE) is seen in association with viral infections (especially mumps), metabolic disorders, autoimmune disease, and congenital left-sided obstructive lesions.[313-315] It shares many of the clinical features of DCM and usually progresses to severe congestive heart failure and subsequent death.[316,317] EFE may be suggested on echocardiography by strong reflections from the endocardial surface of the ventricular myocardium, but such an appearance may also be seen in association with survivable left-sided lesions that do not imply the dire prognosis ordinarily associated with a diagnosis of EFE.[314]

Obesity and Heart Disease (see Chap. 79)

Diabetic Cardiomyopathy (see Chap. 51)

REFERENCES

1. Parmley WW: Surviving heart failure: Robert L. Frye lecture. Mayo Clin Proc 75:111, 2000.
2. Richardson P, McKenna W, Bristow M, et al: Report of the 1995 World Health Organization/International Society and Federation of Cardiology Task Force on the Definition and Classification of Cardiomyopathies. Circulation 93:841, 1996.
3. Artz G, Wynne J: Restrictive cardiomyopathy. Curr Treat Options Cardiovasc Med 2:431, 2000.
4. Oechslin EN, Attenhofer Jost CH, Rojas JR, et al: Long-term follow-up of 34 adults with isolated left ventricular noncompaction: A distinct cardiomyopathy with poor prognosis. J Am Coll Cardiol 36:493, 2000.
5. Veinot JP: Diagnostic endomyocardial biopsy pathology: Secondary myocardial diseases and other clinical indications—A review. Can J Cardiol 18:287, 2002.
6. Frustaci A, Pieroni M, Chimenti C: The role of endomyocardial biopsy in the diagnosis of cardiomyopathies. Ital Heart J 3:348, 2002.
7. Veinot JP: Diagnostic endomyocardial biopsy pathology—General biopsy considerations, and its use for myocarditis and cardiomyopathy: A review. Can J Cardiol 18:55, 2002.
8. Arbustini E, Gavazzi A, Dal Bello B, et al: Ten-year experience with endomyocardial biopsy in myocarditis presenting with congestive heart failure: Frequency, pathologic characteristics, treatment and follow-up. G Ital Cardiol 27:209, 1997.
9. McNamara DM, Holubkov R, Starling RC, et al: Controlled trial of intravenous immune globulin in recent-onset dilated cardiomyopathy. Circulation 103:2254, 2001.
10. Kuhl U, Lauer B, Souvatzoglu M, et al: Antimyosin scintigraphy and immunohistologic analysis of endomyocardial biopsy in patients with clinically suspected myocarditis—Evidence of myocardial cell damage and inflammation in the absence of histologic signs of myocarditis. J Am Coll Cardiol 32:1371, 1998.

Dilated Cardiomyopathy

11. Braunwald E, Bristow MR: Congestive heart failure: Fifty years of progress. Circulation 102:IV14, 2000.
12. Dries DL, Exner DV, Gersh BJ, et al: Racial differences in the outcome of left ventricular dysfunction. N Engl J Med 340:609, 1999.
13. Deedwania PC: The key to unraveling the mystery of mortality in heart failure: An integrated approach. Circulation 107:1719, 2003.
14. Konstam MA: Progress in heart failure management? Lessons from the real world. Circulation 102:1076, 2000.
15. Drozdz J, Krzeminska-Pakula M, Plewka M, et al: Prognostic value of low-dose dobutamine echocardiography in patients with idiopathic dilated cardiomyopathy. Chest 121:1216, 2002.
16. Sun JP, James KB, Yang XS, et al: Comparison of mortality rates and progression of left ventricular dysfunction in patients with idiopathic dilated cardiomyopathy and dilated versus nondilated right ventricular cavities. Am J Cardiol 80:1583, 1997.
17. Felker GM, Hu W, Hare JM, et al: The spectrum of dilated cardiomyopathy. The Johns Hopkins experience with 1,278 patients. Medicine (Baltimore) 78:270, 1999.
18. Seidman JG, Seidman C: The genetic basis for cardiomyopathy: From mutation identification to mechanistic paradigms. Cell 104:557, 2001.
19. Crispell KA, Hanson EL, Coates K, et al: Periodic rescreening is indicated for family members at risk of developing familial dilated cardiomyopathy. J Am Coll Cardiol 39:1503, 2002.
20. Chien KR: Genotype, phenotype: Upstairs, downstairs in the family of cardiomyopathies. J Clin Invest 111:175, 2003.
21. Itoh-Satoh M, Hayashi T, Nishi H, et al: Titin mutations as the molecular basis for dilated cardiomyopathy. Biochem Biophys Res Commun 291:385, 2002.
22. Li D, Czernuszewicz GZ, Gonzalez O, et al: Novel cardiac troponin T mutation as a cause of familial dilated cardiomyopathy. Circulation 104:2188, 2001.
23. Wang X, Osinska H, Dorn GW 2nd, et al: Mouse model of desmin-related cardiomyopathy. Circulation 103:2402, 2001.
24. Taylor MR, Fain PR, Sinagra G, et al: Natural history of dilated cardiomyopathy due to lamin A/C gene mutations. J Am Coll Cardiol 41:771, 2003.
25. Haghighi K, Kolokathis F, Pater L, et al: Human phospholamban null results in lethal dilated cardiomyopathy revealing a critical difference between mouse and human. J Clin Invest 111:869, 2003.
26. Sinagra G, Di Lenarda A, Brodsky GL, et al: New insights into the molecular basis of familial dilated cardiomyopathy. Ital Heart J 2:280, 2001.
27. Feng J, Yan JY, Buzin CH, et al: Comprehensive mutation scanning of the dystrophin gene in patients with nonsyndromic X-linked dilated cardiomyopathy. J Am Coll Cardiol 40:1120, 2002.
28. Vatta M, Stetson SJ, Perez-Verdia A, et al: Molecular remodelling of dystrophin in patients with end-stage cardiomyopathies and reversal in patients on assistance-device therapy. Lancet 359:936, 2002.
29. Arbustini E, Diegoli M, Fasani R, et al: Mitochondrial DNA mutations and mitochondrial abnormalities in dilated cardiomyopathy. Am J Pathol 153:1501, 1998.
30. Abraham MR, Olson LJ, Joyner MJ, et al: Angiotensin-converting enzyme genotype modulates pulmonary function and exercise capacity in treated patients with congestive stable heart failure. Circulation 106:1794, 2002.
31. Luppi P, Rudert WA, Zanone MM, et al: Idiopathic dilated cardiomyopathy: A superantigen-driven autoimmune disease. Circulation 98:777, 1998.
32. Frustaci A, Chimenti C, Calabrese F, et al: Immunosuppressive therapy for active lymphocytic myocarditis: Virological and immunologic profile of responders versus nonresponders. Circulation 107:857, 2003.
33. Fujioka S, Kitaura Y, Ukimura A, et al: Evaluation of viral infection in the myocardium of patients with idiopathic dilated cardiomyopathy. J Am Coll Cardiol 36:1920, 2000.
34. Bowles NE, Ni J, Marcus F, et al: The detection of cardiotropic viruses in the myocardium of patients with arrhythmogenic right ventricular dysplasia/cardiomyopathy. J Am Coll Cardiol 39:892, 2002.
35. Limas CJ: Cardiac autoantibodies in dilated cardiomyopathy: A pathogenetic role? Circulation 95:1979, 1997.
36. Pohlner K, Portig I, Pankuweit S, et al: Identification of mitochondrial antigens recognized by antibodies in sera of patients with idiopathic dilated cardiomyopathy by two-dimensional gel electrophoresis and protein sequencing. Am J Cardiol 80:1040, 1997.
37. McKenna CJ, Codd MB, McCann HA, et al: Idiopathic dilated cardiomyopathy: Familial prevalence and HLA distribution. Heart 77:549, 1997.
38. Liu HR, Zhao RR, Jiao XY, et al: Relationship of myocardial remodeling to the genesis of serum autoantibodies to cardiac beta(1)-adrenoceptors and muscarinic type 2 acetylcholine receptors in rats. J Am Coll Cardiol 39:1866, 2002.
39. Baba A, Yoshikawa T, Ogawa S: Autoantibodies produced against sarcolemmal Na-K-ATPase: Possible upstream targets of arrhythmias and sudden death in patients with dilated cardiomyopathy. J Am Coll Cardiol 40:1153, 2002.
40. Muller J, Wallukat G, Dandel M, et al: Immunoglobulin adsorption in patients with idiopathic dilated cardiomyopathy. Circulation 101:385, 2000.
41. Staudt A, Bohm M, Knebel F, et al: Potential role of autoantibodies belonging to the immunoglobulin G-3 subclass in cardiac dysfunction among patients with dilated cardiomyopathy. Circulation 106:2448, 2002.
42. Wallukat G, Muller J, Hetzer R: Specific removal of beta1-adrenergic autoantibodies from patients with idiopathic dilated cardiomyopathy. N Engl J Med 347:1806, 2002.
43. Pankuweit S, Portig I, Maisch B: Pathophysiology of cardiac inflammation: Molecular mechanisms. Herz 27:669, 2002.
44. Tsutamoto T, Wada A, Matsumoto T, et al: Relationship between tumor necrosis factor-alpha production and oxidative stress in the failing hearts of patients with dilated cardiomyopathy. J Am Coll Cardiol 37:2086, 2001.
45. Zwaka TP, Manolov D, Ozdemir C, et al: Complement and dilated cardiomyopathy: A role of sublytic terminal complement complex-induced tumor necrosis factor-alpha synthesis in cardiac myocytes. Am J Pathol 161:449, 2002.
46. Parthenakis FI, Patrianakos A, Prassopoulos V, et al: Relation of cardiac sympathetic innervation to proinflammatory cytokine levels in patients with heart failure secondary to idiopathic dilated cardiomyopathy. Am J Cardiol 91:1190, 2003.
47. Skudicky D, Bergemann A, Sliwa K, et al: Beneficial effects of pentoxifylline in patients with idiopathic dilated cardiomyopathy treated with angiotensin-converting enzyme inhibitors and carvedilol: Results of a randomized study. Circulation 103:1083, 2001.

48. Bristow MR: Why does the myocardium fail? Insights from basic science. Lancet 352(Suppl 1):SI8, 1998.
49. Kanoh M, Takemura G, Misao J, et al: Significance of myocytes with positive DNA in situ nick end-labeling (TUNEL) in hearts with dilated cardiomyopathy: Not apoptosis but DNA repair. Circulation 99:2757, 1999.
50. van den Heuvel AF, van Veldhuisen DJ, van der Wall EE, et al: Regional myocardial blood flow reserve impairment and metabolic changes suggesting myocardial ischemia in patients with idiopathic dilated cardiomyopathy. J Am Coll Cardiol 35:19, 2000.
51. Steenbergen C, Afshari CA, Petranka JG, et al: Alterations in apoptotic signaling in human idiopathic cardiomyopathic hearts in failure. Am J Physiol 284:H268, 2003.
52. Wencker D, Chandra M, Nguyen K, et al: A mechanistic role for cardiac myocyte apoptosis in heart failure. J Clin Invest 111:1497, 2003.
53. Lange RA, Hillis LD: Cardiovascular complications of cocaine use. N Engl J Med 345:351, 2001.
54. Nicolas JM, Fernandez-Sola J, Estruch R, et al: The effect of controlled drinking in alcoholic cardiomyopathy. Ann Intern Med 136:192, 2002.
55. Nikolaidis LA, Doverspike A, Huerbin R, et al: Angiotensin-converting enzyme inhibitors improve coronary flow reserve in dilated cardiomyopathy by a bradykinin-mediated, nitric oxide–dependent mechanism. Circulation 105:2785, 2002.
56. Wynne J: The clinical meaning of the third heart sound. Am J Med 111:157, 2001.
57. Yiu SF, Enriquez-Sarano M, Tribouilloy C, et al: Determinants of the degree of functional mitral regurgitation in patients with systolic left ventricular dysfunction: A quantitative clinical study. Circulation 102:1400, 2000.
58. Sato Y, Yamada T, Taniguchi R, et al: Persistently increased serum concentrations of cardiac troponin T in patients with idiopathic dilated cardiomyopathy are predictive of adverse outcomes. Circulation 103:369, 2001.
59. Grunig E, Benz A, Mereles D, et al: Prognostic value of serial cardiac assessment and familial screening in patients with dilated cardiomyopathy. Eur J Heart Fail 5:55, 2003.
60. Saxon LA, De Marco T: Arrhythmias associated with dilated cardiomyopathy. Card Electrophysiol Rev 6:18, 2002.
61. Umana E, Solares CA, Alpert MA: Tachycardia-induced cardiomyopathy. Am J Med 114:51, 2003.
62. Luchsinger JA, Steinberg JS: Resolution of cardiomyopathy after ablation of atrial flutter. J Am Coll Cardiol 32:205, 1998.
63. Pratali L, Picano E, Otasevic P, et al: Prognostic significance of the dobutamine echocardiography test in idiopathic dilated cardiomyopathy. Am J Cardiol 88:1374, 2001.
64. Danias PG, Ahlberg AW, Clark BA 3rd, et al: Combined assessment of myocardial perfusion and left ventricular function with exercise technetium-99m sestamibi gated single-photon emission computed tomography can differentiate between ischemic and nonischemic dilated cardiomyopathy. Am J Cardiol 82:1253, 1998.
65. Uemura A, Morimoto S, Hiramitsu S, et al: Histologic diagnostic rate of cardiac sarcoidosis: Evaluation of endomyocardial biopsies. Am Heart J 138:299, 1999.
66. Rathore SS, Curtis JP, Wang Y, et al: Association of serum digoxin concentration and outcomes in patients with heart failure. JAMA 289:871, 2003.
67. Hambrecht R, Fiehn E, Weigl C, et al: Regular physical exercise corrects endothelial dysfunction and improves exercise capacity in patients with chronic heart failure. Circulation 98:2709, 1998.
68. Bristow MR: Beta-adrenergic receptor blockade in chronic heart failure. Circulation 101:558, 2000.
69. Abraham WT, Wagoner LE: Medical management of mild-to-moderate heart failure before the advent of beta blockers. Am J Med 110(Suppl 7A):47S, 2001.
70. Wojnicz R, Nowalany-Kozielska E, Wojciechowska C, et al: Randomized, placebo-controlled study for immunosuppressive treatment of inflammatory dilated cardiomyopathy: Two-year follow-up results. Circulation 104:39, 2001.
71. Garg A, Shiau J, Guyatt G: The ineffectiveness of immunosuppressive therapy in lymphocytic myocarditis: An overview. Ann Intern Med 129:317, 1998.
72. Rothenburger M, Rukosujew A, Hammel D, et al: Mitral valve surgery in patients with poor left ventricular function. Thorac Cardiovasc Surg 50:351, 2002.
73. Bolling SF, Pagani FD, Deeb GM, et al: Intermediate-term outcome of mitral reconstruction in cardiomyopathy. J Thorac Cardiovasc Surg 115:381, 1998.
74. Rose EA, Gelijns AC, Moskowitz AJ, et al: Long term use of a left ventricular assist device for end-stage heart failure. N Engl J Med 345:1435, 2001.

Alcoholic Cardiomyopathy

75. Piano MR: Alcoholic cardiomyopathy: Incidence, clinical characteristics, and pathophysiology. Chest 121:1638, 2002.
76. Reid MC, Fiellin DA, O'Connor PG: Hazardous and harmful alcohol consumption in primary care. Arch Intern Med 159:1681, 1999.
77. Fernandez-Sola J, Estruch R, Nicolas JM, et al: Comparison of alcoholic cardiomyopathy in women versus men. Am J Cardiol 80:481, 1997.
78. Gavazzi A, De Maria R, Parolini M, et al: Alcohol abuse and dilated cardiomyopathy in men. Am J Cardiol 85:1114, 2000.
79. Preedy VR, Patel VB, Reilly ME, et al: Oxidants, antioxidants and alcohol: Implications for skeletal and cardiac muscle. Front Biosci 4:e58, 1999.
80. Duan J, McFadden GE, Borgerding AJ, et al: Overexpression of alcohol dehydrogenase exacerbates ethanol-induced contractile defect in cardiac myocytes. Am J Physiol 282:H1216, 2002.
81. Fernandez-Sola J, Nicolas JM, Oriola J, et al: Angiotensin-converting enzyme gene polymorphism is associated with vulnerability to alcoholic cardiomyopathy. Ann Intern Med 137:321, 2002.
82. Walsh CR, Larson MG, Evans JC, et al: Alcohol consumption and risk for congestive heart failure in the Framingham Heart Study. Ann Intern Med 136:181, 2002.
83. Wynne J: Stirred, not shaken. Ann Intern Med 136:247, 2002.
84. Lazarevic AM, Nakatani S, Neskovic AN, et al: Early changes in left ventricular function in chronic asymptomatic alcoholics: Relation to the duration of heavy drinking. J Am Coll Cardiol 35:1599, 2000.
85. Guillo P, Mansourati J, Maheu B, et al: Long-term prognosis in patients with alcoholic cardiomyopathy and severe heart failure after total abstinence. Am J Cardiol 79:1276, 1997.
86. Barceloux DG: Cobalt. J Toxicol Clin Toxicol 37:201, 1999.

Arrhythmogenic Right Ventricular Cardiomyopathy

87. Burke AP, Farb A, Tashko G, et al: Arrhythmogenic right ventricular cardiomyopathy and fatty replacement of the right ventricular myocardium: Are they different diseases? Circulation 97:1571, 1998.
88. Gemayel C, Pelliccia A, Thompson PD: Arrhythmogenic right ventricular cardiomyopathy. J Am Coll Cardiol 38:1773, 2001.
89. Thiene G, Basso C, Calabrese F, et al: Pathology and pathogenesis of arrhythmogenic right ventricular cardiomyopathy. Herz 25:210, 2000.
90. Pinski SL: The right ventricular tachycardias. J Electrocardiol 33(Suppl):103, 2000.
91. Hamid MS, Norman M, Quraishi A, et al: Prospective evaluation of relatives for familial arrhythmogenic right ventricular cardiomyopathy/dysplasia reveals a need to broaden diagnostic criteria. J Am Coll Cardiol 40:1445, 2002.
92. Danieli GA, Rampazzo A: Genetics of arrhythmogenic right ventricular cardiomyopathy. Curr Opin Cardiol 17:218, 2002.
93. Protonotarios N, Tsatsopoulou A, Anastasakis A, et al: Genotype-phenotype assessment in autosomal recessive arrhythmogenic right ventricular cardiomyopathy (Naxos disease) caused by a deletion in plakoglobin. J Am Coll Cardiol 38:1477, 2001.
94. Kilinc M, Akdemir I, Sivasli E: A case with Uhl's anomaly presenting with severe right heart failure. Acta Cardiol 55:367, 2000.
95. Naccarella F, Naccarelli G, Fattori R, et al: Arrhythmogenic right ventricular dysplasia: Cardiomyopathy current opinions on diagnostic and therapeutic aspects. Curr Opin Cardiol 16:8, 2001.
96. Nava A, Bauce B, Basso C, et al: Clinical profile and long-term follow-up of 37 families with arrhythmogenic right ventricular cardiomyopathy. J Am Coll Cardiol 36:2226, 2000.
97. Corrado D, Buja G, Basso C, et al: Clinical diagnosis and management strategies in arrhythmogenic right ventricular cardiomyopathy. J Electrocardiol 33(Suppl):49, 2000.
98. Patel VV, Ferrari VA, Narula N, et al: Right ventricular dysplasia in an asymptomatic young man: An uncommon case with biventricular involvement and no known family history. J Am Soc Echocardiogr 14:317, 2001.
99. Le Guludec D, Gauthier H, Porcher R, et al: Prognostic value of radionuclide angiography in patients with right ventricular arrhythmias. Circulation 103:1972, 2001.
100. Di Cesare E: MRI of the cardiomyopathies. Eur J Radiol 38:179, 2001.
101. Wichter T, Schafers M, Rhodes CG, et al: Abnormalities of cardiac sympathetic innervation in arrhythmogenic right ventricular cardiomyopathy: Quantitative assessment of presynaptic norepinephrine reuptake and postsynaptic beta-adrenergic receptor density with positron emission tomography. Circulation 101:1552, 2000.
102. Borger van der Burg AE, de Groot NM, van Erven L, et al: Long-term follow-up after radiofrequency catheter ablation of ventricular tachycardia: A successful approach? J Cardiovasc Electrophysiol 13:417, 2002.

Hypertrophic Cardiomyopathy

103. Braunwald E, Morrow AG, Cornell WP, et al: Idiopathic hypertrophic subaortic stenosis: Clinical, hemodynamic and angiographic manifestations. Am J Med 29:924, 1960.
104. Maron BJ: Hypertrophic cardiomyopathy: A systematic review. JAMA 287:1308, 2002.
105. Spirito P, Seidman CE, McKenna WJ, et al: The management of hypertrophic cardiomyopathy. N Engl J Med 336:775, 1997.
106. Maron BJ: Hypertrophic cardiomyopathy. Lancet 350:127, 1997.
107. Braunwald E, Seidman CE, Sigwart U: Contemporary evaluation and management of hypertrophic cardiomyopathy. Circulation 106:1312, 2002.
108. Marian AJ, Roberts R: The molecular genetic basis for hypertrophic cardiomyopathy. J Mol Cell Cardiol 33:655, 2001.
109. Criley JM: Unobstructed thinking (and terminology) is called for in the understanding and management of hypertrophic cardiomyopathy. J Am Coll Cardiol 29:741, 1997.
110. Mozaffarian D, Caldwell JH: Right ventricular involvement in hypertrophic cardiomyopathy: A case report and literature review. Clin Cardiol 24:2, 2001.
111. Sharma S, Maron BJ, Whyte G, et al: Physiologic limits of left ventricular hypertrophy in elite junior athletes: Relevance to differential diagnosis of athlete's heart and hypertrophic cardiomyopathy. J Am Coll Cardiol 40:1431, 2002.
112. Sharma S, Elliott PM, Whyte G, et al: Utility of metabolic exercise testing in distinguishing hypertrophic cardiomyopathy from physiologic left ventricular hypertrophy in athletes. J Am Coll Cardiol 36:864, 2000.
113. Niimura H, Bachinski LL, Sangwatanaroj S, et al: Mutations in the gene for cardiac myosin-binding protein C and late-onset familial hypertrophic cardiomyopathy. N Engl J Med 338:1248, 1998.
114. Maron BJ, Nishimura RA, Danielson GK: Pitfalls in clinical recognition and a novel operative approach for hypertrophic cardiomyopathy with severe outflow obstruction due to anomalous papillary muscle. Circulation 98:2505, 1998.
115. Wigle ED: Cardiomyopathy: The diagnosis of hypertrophic cardiomyopathy. Heart 86:709, 2001.
116. Reddy V, Korcarz C, Weinert L, et al: Apical hypertrophic cardiomyopathy. Circulation 98:2354, 1998.
117. Sakamoto T: Apical hypertrophic cardiomyopathy (apical hypertrophy): An overview. J Cardiol 37(Suppl 1):161, 2001.
118. Eriksson MJ, Sonnenberg B, Woo A, et al: Long-term outcome in patients with apical hypertrophic cardiomyopathy. J Am Coll Cardiol 39:638, 2002.
119. Niimura H, Patton KK, McKenna WJ, et al: Sarcomere protein gene mutations in hypertrophic cardiomyopathy of the elderly. Circulation 105:446, 2002.
120. Varnava AM, Elliott PM, Sharma S, et al: Hypertrophic cardiomyopathy: The interrelation of disarray, fibrosis, and small vessel disease. Heart 84:476, 2000.

121. Usyk TP, Omens JH, McCulloch AD: Regional septal dysfunction in a three-dimensional computational model of focal myofiber disarray. Am J Physiol 281:H506, 2001.
122. Mogensen J, Klausen IC, Pedersen AK, et al: Alpha-cardiac actin is a novel disease gene in familial hypertrophic cardiomyopathy. J Clin Invest 103:R39, 1999.
123. Richard P, Charron P, Carrier L, et al: Hypertrophic cardiomyopathy. Distribution of disease genes, spectrum of mutations, and implications for a molecular diagnosis strategy. Circulation 107:2227, 2003.
124. Chung MW, Tsoutsman T, Semsarian C: Hypertrophic cardiomyopathy: From gene defect to clinical disease. Cell Res 13:9, 2003.
125. Maron BJ, Moller JH, Seidman CE, et al: Impact of laboratory molecular diagnosis on contemporary diagnostic criteria for genetically transmitted cardiovascular diseases: Hypertrophic cardiomyopathy, long-QT syndrome, and Marfan syndrome: A statement for healthcare professionals from the Councils on Clinical Cardiology, Cardiovascular Disease in the Young, and Basic Science, American Heart Association. Circulation 98:1460, 1998.
126. Marian AJ: Pathogenesis of diverse clinical and pathological phenotypes in hypertrophic cardiomyopathy. Lancet 355:58, 2000.
127. McNally EM: Beta-myosin heavy chain gene mutations in familial hypertrophic cardiomyopathy: The usual suspect? Circ Res 90:246, 2002.
128. Fatkin D, McConnell BK, Mudd JO, et al: An abnormal Ca(2+) response in mutant sarcomere protein–mediated familial hypertrophic cardiomyopathy. J Clin Invest 106:1351, 2000.
129. Konno T, Shimizu M, Ino H, et al: A novel missense mutation in the myosin binding protein-C gene is responsible for hypertrophic cardiomyopathy with left ventricular dysfunction and dilation in elderly patients. J Am Coll Cardiol 41:781, 2003.
130. Moolman JA, Reith S, Uhl K, et al: A newly created splice donor site in exon 25 of the MyBP-C gene is responsible for inherited hypertrophic cardiomyopathy with incomplete disease penetrance. Circulation 101:1396, 2000.
131. Arad M, Benson DW, Perez-Atayde AR, et al: Constitutively active AMP kinase mutations cause glycogen storage disease mimicking hypertrophic cardiomyopathy. J Clin Invest 109:357, 2002.
132. Roberts R, Sigwart U: New concepts in hypertrophic cardiomyopathies, Part I. Circulation 104:2113, 2001.
133. Ho CY, Lever HM, DeSanctis R, et al: Homozygous mutation in cardiac troponin T: Implications for hypertrophic cardiomyopathy. Circulation 102:1950, 2000.
134. Anan R, Shono H, Kisanuki A, et al: Patients with familial hypertrophic cardiomyopathy caused by a Phe110Ile missense mutation in the cardiac troponin T gene have variable cardiac morphologies and a favorable prognosis. Circulation 98:391, 1998.
135. Ackerman MJ, VanDriest SL, Ommen SR, et al: Prevalence and age-dependence of malignant mutations in the beta-myosin heavy chain and troponin T genes in hypertrophic cardiomyopathy: A comprehensive outpatient perspective. J Am Coll Cardiol 39:2042, 2002.
136. Jongbloed RJ, Marcelis CL, Doevendans PA, et al: Variable clinical manifestation of a novel missense mutation in the alpha-tropomyosin (TPM1) gene in familial hypertrophic cardiomyopathy. J Am Coll Cardiol 41:981, 2003.
137. Van Driest SL, Ackerman MJ, Ommen SR, et al: Prevalence and severity of "benign" mutations in the beta-myosin heavy chain, cardiac troponin T, and alpha-tropomyosin genes in hypertrophic cardiomyopathy. Circulation 106:3085, 2002.
138. Charron P, Dubourg O, Desnos M, et al: Diagnostic value of electrocardiography and echocardiography for familial hypertrophic cardiomyopathy in a genotyped adult population. Circulation 96:214, 1997.
139. van Langen IM, Birnie E, Leschot NJ, et al: Genetic knowledge and counselling skills of Dutch cardiologists: Sufficient for the genomics era? Eur Heart J 24:560, 2003.
140. Braunwald E. Lambrew CT, Rickoff SD, et al. Idiopathic hypertrophic subaortic stenosis. I. A description of the disease based upon an analysis of 64 patients. Circulation 30(Suppl 4):3, 1964
141. Sherrid MV, Chaudhry FA, Swistel DG: Obstructive hypertrophic cardiomyopathy: Echocardiography, pathophysiology, and the continuing evolution of surgery for obstruction. Ann Thorac Surg 75:620, 2003.
142. Nagueh SF, Stetson SJ, Lakkis NM, et al: Decreased expression of tumor necrosis factor-alpha and regression of hypertrophy after nonsurgical septal reduction therapy for patients with hypertrophic obstructive cardiomyopathy. Circulation 103:1844, 2001.
143. Mazur W, Nagueh SF, Lakkis NM, et al: Regression of left ventricular hypertrophy after nonsurgical septal reduction therapy for hypertrophic obstructive cardiomyopathy. Circulation 103:1492, 2001.
144. Nagueh SF, Bachinski LL, Meyer D, et al: Tissue Doppler imaging consistently detects myocardial abnormalities in patients with hypertrophic cardiomyopathy and provides a novel means for an early diagnosis before and independently of hypertrophy. Circulation 104:128, 2001.
145. Michele DE, Gomez CA, Hong KE, et al: Cardiac dysfunction in hypertrophic cardiomyopathy mutant tropomyosin mice is transgene-dependent, hypertrophy-independent, and improved by beta-blockade. Circ Res 91:255, 2002.
146. Knollmann BC, Kirchhof P, Sirenko SG, et al: Familial hypertrophic cardiomyopathy–linked mutant troponin T causes stress-induced ventricular tachycardia and Ca^{2+}-dependent action potential remodeling. Circ Res 92:428, 2003.
147. Lazzeroni E, Picano E, Morozzi L, et al: Dipyridamole-induced ischemia as a prognostic marker of future adverse cardiac events in adult patients with hypertrophic cardiomyopathy. Echo Persantine Italian Cooperative (EPIC) Study Group, Subproject Hypertrophic Cardiomyopathy. Circulation 96:4268, 1997.
148. Krams R, Kofflard MJ, Duncker DJ, et al: Decreased coronary flow reserve in hypertrophic cardiomyopathy is related to remodeling of the coronary microcirculation. Circulation 97:230, 1998.
149. Takemura G, Takatsu Y, Fujiwara H: Luminal narrowing of coronary capillaries in human hypertrophic hearts: An ultrastructural morphometrical study using endomyocardial biopsy specimens. Heart 79:78, 1998.
150. Kyriakidis M, Triposkiadis F, Dernellis J, et al: Effects of cardiac versus circulatory angiotensin-converting enzyme inhibition on left ventricular diastolic function and coronary blood flow in hypertrophic obstructive cardiomyopathy. Circulation 97:1342, 1998.
151. Mohiddin SA, Begley D, Shih J, et al: Myocardial bridging does not predict sudden death in children with hypertrophic cardiomyopathy but is associated with more severe cardiac disease. J Am Coll Cardiol 36:2270, 2000.

Clinical Manifestations

152. Maron BJ, Casey SA, Poliac LC, et al: Clinical course of hypertrophic cardiomyopathy in a regional United States cohort. JAMA 281:650, 1999.
153. Maron BJ, Olivotto I, Spirito P, et al: Epidemiology of hypertrophic cardiomyopathy–related death: Revisited in a large non-referral-based patient population. Circulation 102:858, 2000.
154. Maron BJ, Carney KP, Lever HM, et al: Relationship of race to sudden cardiac death in competitive athletes with hypertrophic cardiomyopathy. J Am Coll Cardiol 41:974, 2003.
155. Yu EH, Omran AS, Wigle ED, et al: Mitral regurgitation in hypertrophic obstructive cardiomyopathy: Relationship to obstruction and relief with myectomy. J Am Coll Cardiol 36:2219, 2000.
156. Nagueh SF, Ommen SR, Lakkis NM, et al: Comparison of ethanol septal reduction therapy with surgical myectomy for the treatment of hypertrophic obstructive cardiomyopathy. J Am Coll Cardiol 38:1701, 2001.
157. Maron BJ: The electrocardiogram as a diagnostic tool for hypertrophic cardiomyopathy: Revisited. Ann Noninvasive Electrocardiol 6:277, 2001.
158. Runquist LH, Nielsen CD, Killip D, et al: Electrocardiographic findings after alcohol septal ablation therapy for obstructive hypertrophic cardiomyopathy. Am J Cardiol 90:1020, 2002.
159. Maron BJ, Shen WK, Link MS, et al: Efficacy of implantable cardioverter-defibrillators for the prevention of sudden death in patients with hypertrophic cardiomyopathy. N Engl J Med 342:365, 2000.
160. McKenna WJ, Behr ER: Hypertrophic cardiomyopathy: Management, risk stratification, and prevention of sudden death. Heart 87:169, 2002.
161 Maron BJ, Olivotto I, Bellone P, et al: Clinical profile of stroke in 900 patients with hypertrophic cardiomyopathy. J Am Coll Cardiol 39:301, 2002.
162. Olivotto I, Cecchi F, Casey SA, et al: Impact of atrial fibrillation on the clinical course of hypertrophic cardiomyopathy. Circulation 104:2517, 2001.
163. Maron BJ, Leyhe MJ, 3rd, Casey SA, et al: Assessment of QT dispersion as a prognostic marker for sudden death in a regional nonreferred hypertrophic cardiomyopathy cohort. Am J Cardiol 87:114, 2001.
164. Manganelli F, Betocchi S, Ciampi Q, et al: Comparison of hemodynamic adaptation to orthostatic stress in patients with hypertrophic cardiomyopathy with or without syncope and in vasovagal syncope. Am J Cardiol 89:1405, 2002.
165. Spirito P, Bellone P, Harris KM, et al: Magnitude of left ventricular hypertrophy and risk of sudden death in hypertrophic cardiomyopathy. N Engl J Med 342:1778, 2000.
166. Elliott PM, Poloniecki J, Dickie S, et al: Sudden death in hypertrophic cardiomyopathy: Identification of high risk patients. J Am Coll Cardiol 36:2212, 2000.
167. Schwammenthal E, Nakatani S, He S, et al: Mechanism of mitral regurgitation in hypertrophic cardiomyopathy: Mismatch of posterior to anterior leaflet length and mobility. Circulation 98:856, 1998.
168. Sherrid MV, Gunsburg DZ, Moldenhauer S, et al: Systolic anterior motion begins at low left ventricular outflow tract velocity in obstructive hypertrophic cardiomyopathy. J Am Coll Cardiol 36:1344, 2000.
169. Choudhury L, Mahrholdt H, Wagner A, et al: Myocardial scarring in asymptomatic or mildly symptomatic patients with hypertrophic cardiomyopathy. J Am Coll Cardiol 40:2156, 2002.
170. Losi MA, Betocchi S, Manganelli F, et al: Pattern of left ventricular filling in hypertrophic cardiomyopathy. Assessment by Doppler echocardiography and radionuclide angiography. Eur Heart J 19:1261, 1998.
171. Fattori R, Rocchi G, Celletti F, et al: Contribution of magnetic resonance imaging in the differential diagnosis of cardiac amyloidosis and symmetric hypertrophic cardiomyopathy. Am Heart J 136:824, 1998.
172. Moon JC, McKenna WJ, McCrohon JA, et al: Toward clinical risk assessment in hypertrophic cardiomyopathy with gadolinium cardiovascular magnetic resonance. J Am Coll Cardiol 41:1561, 2003.
173. Kim RJ, Judd RM: Gadolinium-enhanced magnetic resonance imaging in hypertrophic cardiomyopathy. In vivo imaging of the pathologic substrate for premature cardiac death? J Am Coll Cardiol 41:1568, 2003.
174. Fananapazir L, McAreavey D: Therapeutic options in patients with obstructive hypertrophic cardiomyopathy and severe drug-refractory symptoms. J Am Coll Cardiol 31:259, 1998.
175. Kizilbash AM, Heinle SK, Grayburn PA: Spontaneous variability of left ventricular outflow tract gradient in hypertrophic obstructive cardiomyopathy. Circulation 97:461, 1998.
176. de Gregorio C, Recupero A, Grimaldi P, et al: Noninvasive assessment of intramyocardial coronary flow in hypertrophic cardiomyopathy by high-resolution Doppler echocardiography. Ital Heart J 3:615, 2002.
177. Kofflard MJ, Ten Cate FJ, van der Lee C, et al: Hypertrophic cardiomyopathy in a large community-based population: Clinical outcome and identification of risk factors for sudden cardiac death and clinical deterioration. J Am Coll Cardiol 41:987, 2003.
178. Maron MS, Olivotto I, Betocchi S, et al: Effect of left ventricular outflow tract obstruction on clinical outcome in hypertrophic cardiomyopathy. N Engl J Med 348:295, 2003.
179. Maron BJ, Casey SA, Hurrell DG, et al: Relation of left ventricular thickness to age and gender in hypertrophic cardiomyopathy. Am J Cardiol 91:1195, 2003.
180. Doevendans PA: Hypertrophic cardiomyopathy: Do we have the algorithm for life and death? Circulation 101:1224, 2000.
181. Marian AJ: On predictors of sudden cardiac death in hypertrophic cardiomyopathy. J Am Coll Cardiol 41:994, 2003.

182. Ciampi Q, Betocchi S, Lombardi R, et al: Hemodynamic determinants of exercise-induced abnormal blood pressure response in hypertrophic cardiomyopathy. J Am Coll Cardiol 40:278, 2002.
183. Atiga WL, Fananapazir L, McAreavey D, et al: Temporal repolarization lability in hypertrophic cardiomyopathy caused by beta-myosin heavy-chain gene mutations. Circulation 101:1237, 2000.
184. Yasui K, Shibata T, Nishizawa T, et al: Response of the stroke volume and blood pressure of young patients with nonobstructive hypertrophic cardiomyopathy to exercise. Jpn Circ J 65:300, 2001.
185. Pelliccia A, Di Paolo FM, Maron BJ: The athlete's heart: Remodeling, electrocardiogram and preparticipation screening. Cardiol Rev 10:85, 2002.
186. Ostman-Smith I, Wettrell G, Riesenfeld T: A cohort study of childhood hypertrophic cardiomyopathy: Improved survival following high-dose beta-adrenoceptor antagonist treatment. J Am Coll Cardiol 34:1813, 1999.

Management

187. Autore C, Conte MR, Piccininno M, et al: Risk associated with pregnancy in hypertrophic cardiomyopathy. J Am Coll Cardiol 40:1864, 2002.
188. Semsarian C, Ahmad I, Giewat M, et al: The L-type calcium channel inhibitor diltiazem prevents cardiomyopathy in a mouse model. J Clin Invest 109:1013, 2002.
189. Paquette F, Jasmin G, Dumont L: Cardioprotective efficacy of verapamil and mibefradil in young UM-X7.1 cardiomyopathic hamsters. Cardiovasc Drugs Ther 13:525, 1999.
190. Pacileo G, De Cristofaro M, Russo MG, et al: Hypertrophic cardiomyopathy in pediatric patients: Effect of verapamil on regional and global left ventricular diastolic function. Can J Cardiol 16:146, 2000.
191. Petkow Dimitrow P, Krzanowski M, Nizankowski R, et al: Effect of verapamil on systolic and diastolic coronary blood flow velocity in asymptomatic and mildly symptomatic patients with hypertrophic cardiomyopathy. Heart 83:262, 2000.
192. Sugihara H, Taniguchi Y, Ito K, et al: Effects of diltiazem on myocardial perfusion abnormalities during exercise in patients with hypertrophic cardiomyopathy. Ann Nucl Med 12:349, 1998.
193. Sherrid MV, Pearle G, Gunsburg DZ: Mechanism of benefit of negative inotropes in obstructive hypertrophic cardiomyopathy. Circulation 97:41, 1998.
194. Cecchi F, Olivotto I, Montereggi A, et al: Prognostic value of non-sustained ventricular tachycardia and the potential role of amiodarone treatment in hypertrophic cardiomyopathy: Assessment in an unselected non-referral based patient population. Heart 79:331, 1998.
195. Spirito P, Rapezzi C, Bellone P, et al: Infective endocarditis in hypertrophic cardiomyopathy: Prevalence, incidence, and indications for antibiotic prophylaxis. Circulation 99:2132, 1999.
196. Maron BJ, Nishimura RA, McKenna WJ, et al: Assessment of permanent dual-chamber pacing as a treatment for drug-refractory symptomatic patients with obstructive hypertrophic cardiomyopathy. A randomized, double-blind, crossover study (M-PATHY). Circulation 99:2927, 1999.
197. Nagueh SF, Lakkis NM, Middleton KJ, et al: Changes in left ventricular diastolic function 6 months after nonsurgical septal reduction therapy for hypertrophic obstructive cardiomyopathy. Circulation 99:344, 1999.
198. Nishimura RA, Trusty JM, Hayes DL, et al: Dual-chamber pacing for hypertrophic cardiomyopathy: A randomized, double-blind, crossover trial. J Am Coll Cardiol 29:435, 1997.
199. Linde C, Gadler F, Kappenberger L, et al: Placebo effect of pacemaker implantation in obstructive hypertrophic cardiomyopathy. Am J Cardiol 83:903, 1999.
200. Erwin JP 3rd, Nishimura RA, Lloyd MA, et al: Dual chamber pacing for patients with hypertrophic obstructive cardiomyopathy: A clinical perspective in 2000. Mayo Clin Proc 75:173, 2000.
201. Elliott PM, Sharma S, Varnava A, et al: Survival after cardiac arrest or sustained ventricular tachycardia in patients with hypertrophic cardiomyopathy. J Am Coll Cardiol 33:1596, 1999.
202. Primo J, Geelen P, Brugada J, et al: Hypertrophic cardiomyopathy: Role of the implantable cardioverter-defibrillator. J Am Coll Cardiol 31:1081, 1998.
203. Seggewiss H, Gleichmann U, Faber L, et al: Percutaneous transluminal septal myocardial ablation in hypertrophic obstructive cardiomyopathy: Acute results and 3-month follow-up in 25 patients. J Am Coll Cardiol 31:252, 1998.
204. Kim JJ, Lee CW, Park SW, et al: Improvement in exercise capacity and exercise blood pressure response after transcoronary alcohol ablation therapy of septal hypertrophy in hypertrophic cardiomyopathy. Am J Cardiol 83:1220, 1999.
205. Park TH, Lakkis NM, Middleton KJ, et al: Acute effect of nonsurgical septal reduction therapy on regional left ventricular asynchrony in patients with hypertrophic obstructive cardiomyopathy. Circulation 106:412, 2002.
206. Gietzen FH, Leuner CJ, Obergassel L, et al: Role of transcoronary ablation of septal hypertrophy in patients with hypertrophic cardiomyopathy, New York Heart Association functional class III or IV, and outflow obstruction only under provocable conditions. Circulation 106:454, 2002.
207. Braunwald E. Hypertrophic cardiomyopathy: The benefits of a multidisciplinary approach. N Engl J Med 347:1306, 2002
208. Firoozi S, Elliott PM, Sharma S, et al: Septal myotomy-myectomy and transcoronary septal alcohol ablation in hypertrophic obstructive cardiomyopathy. A comparison of clinical, haemodynamic and exercise outcomes. Eur Heart J 23:1617, 2002.
209. Qin JX, Shiota T, Lever HM, et al: Outcome of patients with hypertrophic obstructive cardiomyopathy after percutaneous transluminal septal myocardial ablation and septal myectomy surgery. J Am Coll Cardiol 38:1994, 2001.
210. Sitges M, Shiota T, Lever HM, et al: Comparison of left ventricular diastolic function in obstructive hypertrophic cardiomyopathy in patients undergoing percutaneous septal alcohol ablation versus surgical myotomy/myectomy. Am J Cardiol 91:817, 2003.
211. Maron BJ: Role of alcohol septal ablation in treatment of obstructive hypertrophic cardiomyopathy. Lancet 355:425, 2000.
212. Seggewiss H: Percutaneous transluminal septal myocardial ablation: A new treatment for hypertrophic obstructive cardiomyopathy. Eur Heart J 21:704, 2000.
213. Faber L, Ziemssen P, Seggewiss H: Targeting percutaneous transluminal septal ablation for hypertrophic obstructive cardiomyopathy by intraprocedural echocardiographic monitoring. J Am Soc Echocardiogr 13:1074, 2000.
214. Seggewiss H: Current status of alcohol septal ablation for patients with hypertrophic cardiomyopathy. Curr Cardiol Rep 3:160, 2001.
215. Lakkis NM, Nagueh SF, Dunn JK, et al: Nonsurgical septal reduction therapy for hypertrophic obstructive cardiomyopathy: One-year follow-up. J Am Coll Cardiol 36:852, 2000.
216. Brunner-La Schonbeck MH, Rocca HP, Vogt PR, et al: Long-term follow-up in hypertrophic obstructive cardiomyopathy after septal myectomy. Ann Thorac Surg 65:1207, 1998.
217. Obeid AI, Maron BJ: Apical hypertrophic cardiomyopathy developing at a relatively advanced age. Circulation 103:1605, 2001.

Restrictive and Infiltrative Cardiomyopathies

218. Kushwaha SS, Fallon JT, Fuster V: Restrictive cardiomyopathy. N Engl J Med 336:267, 1997.
219. Ammash NM, Seward JB, Bailey KR, et al: Clinical profile and outcome of idiopathic restrictive cardiomyopathy. Circulation 101:2490, 2000.
220. Angelini A, Calzolari V, Thiene G, et al: Morphologic spectrum of primary restrictive cardiomyopathy. Am J Cardiol 80:1046, 1997.
221. Nakamura M, Satoh M, Kowada S, et al: Reversible restrictive cardiomyopathy due to light-chain deposition disease. Mayo Clin Proc 77:193, 2002.
222. Mogensen J, Kubo T, Duque M, et al: Idiopathic restrictive cardiomyopathy is part of the clinical expression of cardiac troponin I mutations. J Clin Invest 111:209, 2003.
223. Palka P, Lange A, Donnelly JE, et al: Differentiation between restrictive cardiomyopathy and constrictive pericarditis by early diastolic Doppler myocardial velocity gradient at the posterior wall. Circulation 102:655, 2000.
224. Rajagopalan N, Garcia MJ, Rodriguez L, et al: Comparison of new Doppler echocardiographic methods to differentiate constrictive pericardial heart disease and restrictive cardiomyopathy. Am J Cardiol 87:86, 2001.
225. Felker GM, Thompson RE, Hare JM, et al: Underlying causes and long-term survival in patients with initially unexplained cardiomyopathy. N Engl J Med 342:1077, 2000.
226. Hoffbrand AV: Diagnosing myocardial iron overload. Eur Heart J 22:2140, 2001.
227. Frustaci A, Chimenti C, Ricci R, et al: Improvement in cardiac function in the cardiac variant of Fabry's disease with galactose-infusion therapy. N Engl J Med 345:25, 2001.
228. Lachmann HJ, Booth DR, Booth SE, et al: Misdiagnosis of hereditary amyloidosis as AL (primary) amyloidosis. N Engl J Med 346:1786, 2002.
229. Puille M, Altland K, Linke RP, et al: ^{99m}Tc-DPD scintigraphy in transthyretin-related familial amyloidotic polyneuropathy. Eur J Nucl Med Mol Imaging 29:376, 2002.
230. Jacobson DR, Pastore RD, Yaghoubian R, et al: Variant-sequence transthyretin (isoleucine 122) in late-onset cardiac amyloidosis in black Americans. N Engl J Med 336:466, 1997.
231. Rocken C, Peters B, Juenemann G, et al: Atrial amyloidosis: An arrhythmogenic substrate for persistent atrial fibrillation. Circulation 106:2091, 2002.
232. Gertz MA, Rajkumar SV: Primary systemic amyloidosis. Curr Treat Options Oncol 3:261, 2002.
233. Wald DS, Gray HH: Restrictive cardiomyopathy in systemic amyloidosis. Q J Med 96:380, 2003.
234. Trikas A, Rallidis L, Hawkins P, et al: Comparison of usefulness between exercise capacity and echocardiographic indexes of left ventricular function in cardiac amyloidosis. Am J Cardiol 84:1049, 1999.
235. Sinha MK, Lachmann HJ, Kuriakose B, et al: An unusual cause of progressive heart failure. Lancet 357:1498, 2001.
236. Dubrey SW, Cha K, Skinner M, et al: Familial and primary (AL) cardiac amyloidosis: Echocardiographically similar diseases with distinctly different clinical outcomes. Heart 78:74, 1997.
237. Mueller PS, Edwards WD, Gertz MA: Symptomatic ischemic heart disease resulting from obstructive intramural coronary amyloidosis. Am J Med 109:181, 2000.
238. Liao R, Jain M, Teller P, et al: Infusion of light chains from patients with cardiac amyloidosis causes diastolic dysfunction in isolated mouse hearts. Circulation 104:1594, 2001.
239. Gertz MA, Lacy MQ, Dispenzieri A: Amyloidosis. Hematol Oncol Clin North Am 13:1211, 1999.
240. Pelo E, Da Prato L, Ciaccheri M, et al: Familial amyloid polyneuropathy with genetic anticipation associated to a gly47glu transthyretin variant in an Italian kindred. Amyloid 9:35, 2002.
241. Chamarthi B, Dubrey SW, Cha K, et al: Features and prognosis of exertional syncope in light-chain associated AL cardiac amyloidosis. Am J Cardiol 80:1242, 1997.
242. Reisinger J, Dubrey SW, Lavalley M, et al: Electrophysiologic abnormalities in AL (primary) amyloidosis with cardiac involvement. J Am Coll Cardiol 30:1046, 1997.
243. Dubrey SW, Bilazarian S, LaValley M, et al: Signal-averaged electrocardiography in patients with AL (primary) amyloidosis. Am Heart J 134:994, 1997.
244. Cacoub P, Axler O, De Zuttere D, et al: Amyloidosis and cardiac involvement. Ann Med Interne (Paris) 151:611, 2000.
245. Tanaka M, Hongo M, Kinoshita O, et al: Iodine-123 metaiodobenzylguanidine scintigraphic assessment of myocardial sympathetic innervation in patients with familial amyloid polyneuropathy. J Am Coll Cardiol 29:168, 1997.
246. Lekakis J, Dimopoulos M, Nanas J, et al: Antimyosin scintigraphy for detection of cardiac amyloidosis. Am J Cardiol 80:963, 1997.
247. Arbustini E, Verga L, Concardi M, et al: Electron and immuno-electron microscopy of abdominal fat identifies and characterizes amyloid fibrils in suspected cardiac amyloidosis. Amyloid 9:108, 2002.
248. Kyle RA, Gertz MA, Greipp PR, et al: A trial of three regimens for primary amyloidosis: Colchicine alone, melphalan and prednisone, and melphalan, prednisone, and colchicine. N Engl J Med 336:1202, 1997.

249. Grogan M, Gertz MA, Kyle RA, et al: Five or more years of survival in patients with primary systemic amyloidosis and biopsy-proven cardiac involvement. Am J Cardiol 85:664, 2000.
250. Sanchorawala V, Wright DG, Seldin DC, et al: Low-dose continuous oral melphalan for the treatment of primary systemic (AL) amyloidosis. Br J Haematol 117:886, 2002.
251. Jacobson DR, Ittmann M, Buxbaum JN, et al: Transthyretin Ile 122 and cardiac amyloidosis in African-Americans. 2 case reports. Tex Heart Inst J 24:45, 1997.
252. Mathew V, Olson LJ, Gertz MA, et al: Symptomatic conduction system disease in cardiac amyloidosis. Am J Cardiol 80:1491, 1997.
253. Comenzo RL, Gertz MA: Autologous stem cell transplantation for primary systemic amyloidosis. Blood 99:4276, 2002.
254. Dubrey SW, Burke MM, Khaghani A, et al: Long term results of heart transplantation in patients with amyloid heart disease. Heart 85:202, 2001.
255. Linhart A, Magage S, Palecek T, et al: Cardiac involvement in Fabry disease. Acta Paediatr Suppl 91:15, 2002.
256. Yoshitama T, Nakao S, Takenaka T, et al: Molecular genetic, biochemical, and clinical studies in three families with cardiac Fabry's disease. Am J Cardiol 87:71, 2001.
257. Perrot A, Osterziel KJ, Beck M, et al: Fabry disease: Focus on cardiac manifestations and molecular mechanisms. Herz 27:699, 2002.
258. Linhart A, Palecek T, Bultas J, et al: New insights in cardiac structural changes in patients with Fabry's disease. Am Heart J 139:1101, 2000.
259. Pieroni M, Chimenti C, Ricci R, et al: Early detection of Fabry cardiomyopathy by tissue Doppler imaging. Circulation 107:1978, 2003.
260. Sachdev B, Takenaka T, Teraguchi H, et al: Prevalence of Anderson-Fabry disease in male patients with late onset hypertrophic cardiomyopathy. Circulation 105:1407, 2002.
261. Eng CM, Guffon N, Wilcox WR, et al: Safety and efficacy of recombinant human alpha-galactosidase A—Replacement therapy in Fabry's disease. N Engl J Med 345:9, 2001.
262. Torloni MR, Franco K, Sass N: Gaucher's disease with myocardial involvement in pregnancy. Sao Paulo Med J 120:90, 2002.
263. George R, McMahon J, Lytle B, et al: Severe valvular and aortic arch calcification in a patient with Gaucher's disease homozygous for the D409H mutation. Clin Genet 59:360, 2001.
264. Schiffmann R, Brady RO: New prospects for the treatment of lysosomal storage diseases. Drugs 62:733, 2002.
265. Strobel JS, Fuisz AR, Epstein AE, et al: Syncope and inducible ventricular fibrillation in a woman with hemochromatosis. J Interv Card Electrophysiol 3:225, 1999.
266. Yalcinkaya S, Kumbasar SD, Semiz E, et al: Sustained ventricular tachycardia in cardiac hemochromatosis treated with amiodarone. J Electrocardiol 30:147, 1997.
267. Britton RS, Leicester KL, Bacon BR: Iron toxicity and chelation therapy. Int J Hematol 76:219, 2002.
268. Yang Q, McDonnell SM, Khoury MJ, et al: Hemochromatosis-associated mortality in the United States from 1979 to 1992: An analysis of multiple-cause mortality data. Ann Intern Med 129:946, 1998.
269. Anderson LJ, Holden S, Davis B, et al: Cardiovascular T2-star (T2*) magnetic resonance for the early diagnosis of myocardial iron overload. Eur Heart J 22:2171, 2001.
270. Barton JC, McDonnell SM, Adams PC, et al: Management of hemochromatosis. Hemochromatosis Management Working Group. Ann Intern Med 129:932, 1998.
271. Toda G, Yoshimuta T, Kawano H, et al: Glycogen storage disease associated with left ventricular aneurysm in an elderly patient. Jpn Circ J 65:462, 2001.
272. Lee PJ, Deanfield JE, Burch M, et al: Comparison of the functional significance of left ventricular hypertrophy in hypertrophic cardiomyopathy and glycogenosis type III. Am J Cardiol 79:834, 1997.
273. Cuspidi C, Sampieri L, Pelizzoli S, et al: Obstructive hypertrophic cardiomyopathy in type III glycogen-storage disease. Acta Cardiol 52:117, 1997.
274. Sharma OP: Diagnosis of cardiac sarcoidosis: An imperfect science, a hesitant art. Chest 123:18, 2003.
275. Shimada T, Shimada K, Sakane T, et al: Diagnosis of cardiac sarcoidosis and evaluation of the effects of steroid therapy by gadolinium-DTPA-enhanced magnetic resonance imaging. Am J Med 110:520, 2001.
276. Yazaki Y, Isobe M, Hiramitsu S, et al: Comparison of clinical features and prognosis of cardiac sarcoidosis and idiopathic dilated cardiomyopathy. Am J Cardiol 82:537, 1998.
277. Pisani B, Taylor DO, Mason JW: Inflammatory myocardial diseases and cardiomyopathies. Am J Med 102:459, 1997.
278. Okura Y, Dec GW, Hare JM, et al: A clinical and histopathologic comparison of cardiac sarcoidosis and idiopathic giant cell myocarditis. J Am Coll Cardiol 41:322, 2003.
279. Veinot JP, Johnston B: Cardiac sarcoidosis—An occult cause of sudden death: A case report and literature review. J Forensic Sci 43:715, 1998.
280. Shabetai R: Sarcoidosis and the heart. Curr Treat Options Cardiovasc Med 2:385, 2000.
281. Yazaki Y, Isobe M, Hiroe M, et al: Prognostic determinants of long-term survival in Japanese patients with cardiac sarcoidosis treated with prednisone. Am J Cardiol 88:1006, 2001.
282. Mana J: Magnetic resonance imaging and nuclear imaging in sarcoidosis. Curr Opin Pulm Med 8:457, 2002.
283. Vignaux O, Dhote R, Duboc D, et al: Detection of myocardial involvement in patients with sarcoidosis applying T2-weighted, contrast-enhanced, and cine magnetic resonance imaging: Initial results of a prospective study. J Comput Assist Tomogr 26:762, 2002.
284. Andy JJ, Ogunowo PO, Akpan NA, et al: Helminth associated hypereosinophilia and tropical endomyocardial fibrosis (EMF) in Nigeria. Acta Trop 69:127, 1998.
285. Berenguer A, Plancha E, Munoz Gil J: Right ventricular endomyocardial fibrosis and microfilarial infection. Int J Cardiol 87:287, 2003.
286. Andy JJ: Aetiology of endomyocardial fibrosis (EMF). West Afr J Med 20:199, 2001.
287. Karnak D, Kayacan O, Beder S, et al: Hypereosinophilic syndrome with pulmonary and cardiac involvement in a patient with asthma. CMAJ 168:172, 2003.
288. Baratta L, Afeltra A, Delfino M, et al: Favorable response to high-dose interferon-alpha in idiopathic hypereosinophilic syndrome with restrictive cardiomyopathy—Case report and literature review. Angiology 53:465, 2002.
289. Barbosa MM, Lamounier JA, Oliveira EC, et al: Short report: Endomyocardial fibrosis and cardiomyopathy in an area endemic for schistosomiasis. Am J Trop Med Hyg 58:26, 1998.
290. Kumari KT, Ravikumar A, Kurup PA: Accumulation of glycosaminoglycans associated with hypomagnesaemia in endomyocardial fibrosis in Kerala: Possible involvement of dietary factors. Indian Heart J 49:49, 1997.
291. Eapen JT, Kartha CC, Valiathan MS: Cerium levels are elevated in the serum of patients with endomyocardial fibrosis (EMF). Biol Trace Elem Res 59:41, 1997.
292. Corssmit EP, Trip MD, Durrer JD: Löffler's endomyocarditis in the idiopathic hypereosinophilic syndrome. Cardiology 91:272, 1999.
293. Puvaneswary M, Joshua F, Ratnarajah S: Idiopathic hypereosinophilic syndrome: Magnetic resonance imaging findings in endomyocardial fibrosis. Australas Radiol 45:524, 2001.
294. McGavin CR, Marshall AJ, Lewis CT: Churg-Strauss syndrome with critical endomyocardial fibrosis: 10 year survival after combined surgical and medical management. Heart 87:E5, 2002.
295. Moraes F, Lapa C, Hazin S, et al: Surgery for endomyocardial fibrosis revisited. Eur J Cardiothorac Surg 15:309, 1999.
296. Freers J, Masembe V, Schmauz R, et al: Endomyocardial fibrosis syndrome in Uganda. Lancet 355:1994, 2000.
297. Berensztein CS, Pineiro D, Marcotegui M, et al: Usefulness of echocardiography and Doppler echocardiography in endomyocardial fibrosis. J Am Soc Echocardiogr 13:385, 2000.
298. Amoah AG, Kallen C: Aetiology of heart failure as seen from a national cardiac referral centre in Africa. Cardiology 93:11, 2000.
299. Rutakingirwa M, Ziegler JL, Newton R, et al: Poverty and eosinophilia are risk factors for endomyocardial fibrosis (EMF) in Uganda. Trop Med Int Health 4:229, 1999.
300. Canesin MF, Gama RF, Smith DL, et al: Endomyocardial fibrosis associated with massive calcification of the left ventricle. Arq Bras Cardiol 73:499, 1999.
301. Radhakumary C, Kumari TV, Kartha CC: Endomyocardial fibrosis is associated with selective deposition of type I collagen. Indian Heart J 53:486, 2001.
302. Barretto AC, Mady C, Oliveira SA, et al: Clinical meaning of ascites in patients with endomyocardial fibrosis. Arq Bras Cardiol 78:196, 2002.
303. Barretto AC, Mady C, Nussbacher A, et al: Atrial fibrillation in endomyocardial fibrosis is a marker of worse prognosis. Int J Cardiol 67:19, 1998.
304. Schneider U, Jenni R, Turina J, et al: Long-term follow up of patients with endomyocardial fibrosis: Effects of surgery. Heart 79:362, 1998.
305. Moller JE, Connolly HM, Rubin J, et al: Factors associated with progression of carcinoid heart disease. N Engl J Med 348:1005, 2003.
306. Kulke MH, Mayer RJ: Carcinoid tumors. N Engl J Med 340:858, 1999.
307. Di Luzio S, Rigolin VH: Carcinoid heart disease. Curr Treat Options Cardiovasc Med 2:399, 2000.
308. Connolly HM, Schaff HV, Mullany CJ, et al: Carcinoid heart disease: Impact of pulmonary valve replacement in right ventricular function and remodeling. Circulation 106:I51, 2002.
309. Connolly HM, Schaff HV, Mullany CJ, et al: Surgical management of left-sided carcinoid heart disease. Circulation 104:I36, 2001.
310. Simula DV, Edwards WD, Tazelaar HD, et al: Surgical pathology of carcinoid heart disease: A study of 139 valves from 75 patients spanning 20 years. Mayo Clin Proc 77:139, 2002.
311. Pandya UH, Pellikka PA, Enriquez-Sarano M, et al: Metastatic carcinoid tumor to the heart: Echocardiographic-pathologic study of 11 patients. J Am Coll Cardiol 40:1328, 2002.
312. Denney WD, Kemp WE, Jr., Anthony LB, et al: Echocardiographic and biochemical evaluation of the development and progression of carcinoid heart disease. J Am Coll Cardiol 32:1017, 1998.
313. Nield LE, Silverman ED, Taylor GP, et al: Maternal anti-Ro and anti-La antibody-associated endocardial fibroelastosis. Circulation 105:843, 2002.
314. Mahle WT, Weinberg PM, Rychik J: Can echocardiography predict the presence or absence of endocardial fibroelastosis in infants <1 year of age with left ventricular outflow obstruction? Am J Cardiol 82:122, 1998.
315. Ni J, Bowles NE, Kim YH, et al: Viral infection of the myocardium in endocardial fibroelastosis. Molecular evidence for the role of mumps virus as an etiologic agent. Circulation 95:133, 1997.
316. Jaeggi ET, Hamilton RM, Silverman ED, et al: Outcome of children with fetal, neonatal or childhood diagnosis of isolated congenital atrioventricular block. A single institution's experience of 30 years. J Am Coll Cardiol 39:130, 2002.
317. Nield LE, Silverman ED, Smallhorn JF, et al: Endocardial fibroelastosis associated with maternal anti-Ro and anti-La antibodies in the absence of atrioventricular block. J Am Coll Cardiol 40:796, 2002.

CHAPTER 60

Myocarditis

Kenneth Lee Baughman • Joshua Wynne

Myocarditis is one of the most challenging diagnoses in cardiology. The entity is rarely recognized, the pathophysiology is poorly understood, there is no commonly accepted diagnostic gold standard, and all current treatment is controversial. Primary myocarditis is presumed to be due to either an acute viral infection or a postviral autoimmune response. Secondary myocarditis is myocardial inflammation caused by a specific pathogen. These pathogens include bacteria, spirochetes, rickettsia, fungi, protozoa, drugs, chemicals, physical agents, and other inflammatory diseases such as systemic lupus erythematosus. We will first review primary myocarditis and then consider secondary causes.

Primary Myocarditis

Many viruses can cause myocarditis (Table 60–1), including those with RNA and DNA cores. As the ability to diagnose viral myocarditis has expanded with molecular techniques, an increasingly large number of viruses have been associated with cardiac inflammation and dilated cardiomyopathy. Historically, the RNA core virus Coxsackie has been identified most frequently as responsible for myocardial or pericardial inflammation. Coxsackie virus is a member of the picornavirus family, which also includes echovirus and polioviruses. Other responsible RNA core viruses include influenza (orthomyxovirus). Responsible DNA core viruses include adenovirus, herpesvirus (varicella zoster, cytomegalovirus, and Epstein-Barr virus), and poxvirus (variola and vaccinia).[1,2]

Pathophysiology

A viral infection of the heart follows a standard progression (Fig. 60–1). Most viral pathogens enter the body through the upper respiratory or gastrointestinal tract. Susceptibility to viral infection in humans is increased by malnutrition, exercise, age (young and old), stress, and hormones.[3,4] There are undoubtedly genetic susceptibilities that alter the autoimmune response to viral infections.

The typical viral infection produces a systemic viremia and associated vascular response on days 0 to 3. During this interval, the pathogenic virus can invade the myocardium and replicate in the myocyte, causing myocytolysis. In days 5 to 10 there is a generalized macrophage and IgM antibody response associated with a histological inflammatory infiltrate.[5] An antigen-specific IgG antibody response peaks by day 14 and is associated with histological evidence of myofiber dropout and interstitial fibrosis. Each of these sequential pathophysiological stages are reviewed in further detail.

DAYS 0 THROUGH 3. The offending virus enters the upper respiratory or gastrointestinal tract and replicates, causing typical symptoms. The virus then escapes the initial portal of entry immunological response and is transported in the bloodstream to other target organs. The infection in the lungs or gut initiates a cytokine response, which may activate the cardiac immune process. The invading viral pathogen must have a mechanism by which it can enter the cardiac cell. Coxsackie virus and adenovirus share a common receptor (Coxsackie adenoviral receptor, or CAR), which serves as the docking site for the pathogenic virus.[6] Coreceptors must be present for the virus to invade the myocardium. Once the coreceptor has facilitated the binding of the virus to the CAR, the virus is transported into the myocardial cell. Once in the cell, the virus can influence cell function and present myosin-like antigens (epitopes) on the cell surface.[7]

Nuclear Factor (NF) [κ] B. NF [κ] B is an intracellular transcription factor that, when activated by cytokines, viruses, oxidants, and protein kinase, induces the production of cytokines, intracellular adhesion molecules (ICAM), and inducible nitric oxide, which are involved in the inflammatory response to viral myocarditis.[8]

DAYS 3 THROUGH 14. Dendritic cells and macrophages are present in normal myocardium and are responsible for the initial antigen-independent response to viral invasion. These immune-response cells release cytokines, interleukins, perforin, reactive oxygen species, proteases, tumor necrosis factor (TNF), and regulatory growth factors, such as transforming growth factor-beta. Dendritic cells and macrophages ingest viral agents for subsequent processing.

The viral peptide fragments, or exposed myocardial membrane antigens, are processed in the Golgi apparatus and transported to the cell surface.[3,4] These epitopes are presented to T cells in collaboration with the major histocompatibility complex (MHC) antigen, ICAM-1, as well as costimulatory signals provided by various molecules, including CD40 (a member of the TNF superfamily).

TABLE 60–1 Infectious Causes of Myocarditis

Viral	**Fungal**
Adenovirus	*Actinomyces*
Arbovirus (dengue fever, yellow fever)	*Aspergillus*
Arenavirus (Lassa fever)	*Blastomyces*
Coxsackie virus	*Candida*
Cytomegalovirus	*Coccidioides*
Echovirus	*Cryptococcus*
Encephalomyocarditis virus	*Histoplasma*
Epstein-Barr virus	*Nocardia*
Hepatitis B	*Sporothrix*
Herpesvirus	
Human immunodeficiency virus-1	**Rickettsial**
Influenza virus	Rocky Mountain spotted fever
Mumps virus	Q fever
Poliomyelitis virus	Scrub typhus
Rabies	Typhus
Respiratory syncytial virus	
Rubella virus	**Spirochetal**
Rubeola virus	*Borrelia* (Lyme disease and relapsing fever)
Vaccinia virus	*Leptospira*
Varicella virus	Syphilis
Variola virus	
	Helminthic
Bacterial	*Cysticercus*
Brucellosis	*Echinococcus*
Clostridia	*Schistosoma*
Diphtheria	*Toxocara* (visceral larva migrans)
Francisella (tularemia)	*Trichinella*
Gonococcus	
Haemophilus	**Protozoal**
Legionella	*Entamoeba*
Meningococcus	*Leishmania*
Mycobacterium (tuberculosis, avium-intracellulare, leprae)	*Trypanosoma* (Chagas disease)
Mycoplasma	Toxoplasmosis
Pneumococcus	
Psittacosis	
Salmonella	
Staphylococcus	
Streptococcus	
Tropheryma whippleii (Whipple disease)	

From Pisani B, Taylor D, Mason J: Inflammatory myocardial disease and cardiomyopathies. Am J Med 102:459, 1997.

The first wave of response to myocarditis is brief and is determined by the cardiotropic features of the virus as well as by the nonspecific immune response from natural killer cells, cytokines, interferon, Fas/Fas ligand, TNF, matrix metalloproteinase, elastase, endothelium, interleukins, and proteins such as perforin and apolipoprotein J/clusterin.[9-14]

The second wave of response is immunological in nature. There is initially a nonspecific IgM and macrophage response driven by activation of local macrophages and dendritic cells. Upon activation, the CD4 T cells proliferate and differentiate into effector lymphocytes and macrophages.[5] Associated with this activation is the release of cytokines, including interferon-gamma, TNF, interleukin (IL)-2, IL-3, IL-4, IL-5, IL-6, and IL-10.[9,10] Cytokines have several functions, including further proliferation and differentiation of B-lymphocytes to produce antibodies, and proliferation and differentiation of T lymphocytes (both CD4 and CD8 cells) to attract additional macrophages, lymphocytes, and other cells to the antigen-producing area. CD8 lymphocytes attach to myocytes with appropriate antigens and lyse the cell, destroying cytoplasm and nucleus. Antibodies against the myocyte enhance lysis on the activated T cell. Ultimately, the immunological response is determined by the development of TH 1 (CD4) and TH 2 (CD8) cells specific for the antigen presented and production of IgG antibodies.[15] Neutralizing antiviral antibodies and infiltrating macrophages begin to clear the virus from the myocardium within 5 to 10 days after infection. As the antibody-producing B-lymphocytes increase, their T lymphocytic counterparts decrease over the course of several weeks.

The epitope responsible for the long-term autoimmune attack on patients with virally induced cardiomyopathy is unknown. It is considered that the Coxsackie B3 virus may have a similar antigen construct to myosin. Alternatively, damage to the myocyte membrane may expose myosin, which may then contribute to the autoimmune process. Most patients with viral myocarditis clear the virus and the infected cells with minimal fibrosis and no functional deterioration in their myocardium. Other patients display a variety of responses, varying from a transient depression of myocardial function to slow evolution of a dilated cardiomyopathy.[16]

NITRIC OXIDE

The nitric oxide (NO) system may have beneficial or adverse effects in cases of myocarditis.

Furchgott demonstrated that the vascular endothelium produces a relaxing factor, subsequently named NO.[17] Three forms of NO exist in humans; endothelial cell NO (type III), macrophage NO (type II), and neuronal NO (type I). NO is an intercellular messenger that can influence vessel relaxation, platelet adhesion, and endothelial cell as well as smooth muscle cell proliferation. Inducible NO synthase (NOS) and endothelial NOS have been studied in normal and failing hearts. In normal hearts, both forms of NOS are low. In heart failure, endothelial NOS is increased and localized in the subendocardial myocytes.[18] In failing hearts with myocarditis, inducible NOS is increased in macrophages.

Nitric oxide may enhance or suppress myocardial function. Coxsackie virus B3 produces a protease IIA that cleaves dystrophin on the cardiac membrane. Dystrophin is an integral membrane glycoprotein that, when disrupted, can interfere with mechanical force generation and result in altered membrane permeability, both of which may contribute to decreased myocardial function. Viral infections result in stimulation of interferon-alpha and interferon-gamma. These cytokines induce the production of NOS by macrophages, and increased NO indeed both depresses viral replication and inhibits protease IIA, preventing myocardial dysfunction.[19,20] Excess inducible NOS, however, results in peroxynitrite, a free radical that can cause cell death. NO also stimulates cGMP, which inhibits sarcolemmal L type calcium channels, which decreases the filament response to calcium. Therefore, excess NO can depress myocardial function.[21]

DAY 14 AND BEYOND. For many years, the etiology of the progression of myocarditis to dilated cardiomyopathy has been investigated but poorly understood. There are now data to suggest that this progression may be due to viral persistence, apoptosis, autoimmune, and/or structural effects.

Viral Persistence. Molecular cardiology techniques, including detection of viral RNA by slot-blot probe hybridization, in situ probe hybridization, or polymerase chain reaction (PCR) has allowed the demonstration of persistent virus particles in patients with dilated cardiomyopathy and acute myocarditis.[22,23] Viral persistence, even without the ability to multiply, can induce dilated cardiomyopathy when matched with an activated immune system.[22] In addition to the myocardium, there is a suggestion that the skeletal muscle system may serve as a reservoir for viral infection. The patient with a skeletal infection may be asymptomatic or have symptoms of peripheral muscle infection overwhelmed by symptoms from the heart.

Apoptosis. Apoptosis may be induced by viral-mediated proteases or differentially expressed genes (Nip 21) involved in cell death by activation of a caspase pathway.[24] In addition, cytokines have been demonstrated to remain elevated for greater than 80 days, even though they first appear by 3 days and peak by 7 days after infection.[25] Cytokine expression can depress cardiac function or induce apoptosis.

Immune Responses. Myosin and Coxsackie virus capsid protein share approximately 40% identity in their amino acid sequences. This may account for the molecular mimicry that directs immunological cells against myocytes. In some patients, it is likely that the autoimmune antibody mechanism induced does not autoregulate after the clearance of the virus. This continued immune activation and myosin destruction may cause myocardial dysfunction and vasospasm.

A final mechanism of acute and chronic myocardial damage is coronary microvascular spasm, resulting in myocyte necrosis, fibrosis, calcification, and ultimately, cardiac dilation.[26] Viruses associated with viral myocarditis also can infect endothelial cells. Endothelial cell antibodies have been identified in viral myocarditis and can contribute to microvascular spasm due to interruption of endothelial cell function or nitric oxide production.[26]

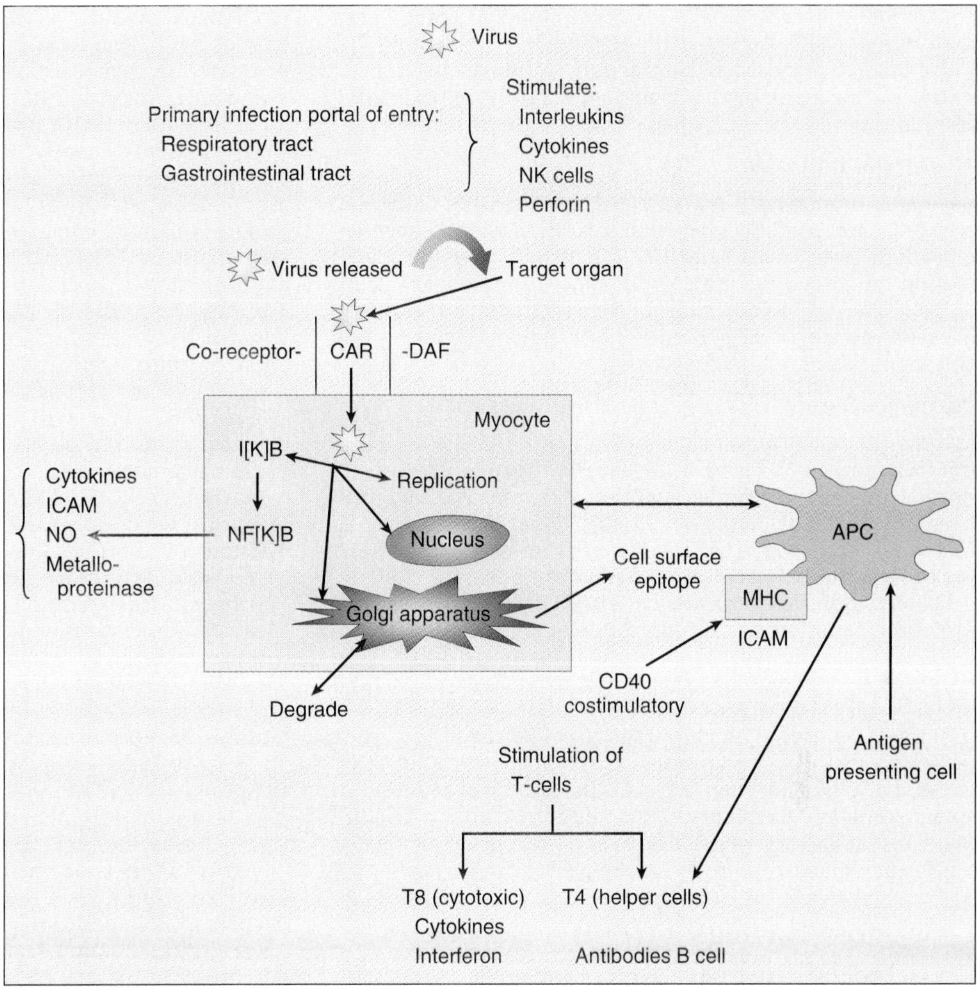

FIGURE 60–1 Pathophysiology of viral myocarditis. The virus enters the body through the respiratory or gastrointestinal tract stimulating a systemic immune response. The virus enters the myocytes through the CAR (Coxsackie adenoviral receptor) with coreceptors including DAF (decay accelerating factor). Once in the myocyte, the virus replicates and is transmitted to the nucleus, where it redirects cell activity and is released to the cell surface, where the virus can escape to infect additional cells. Dendritic cells and macrophages ingest foreign elements, including viruses, causing further enhancement of the immune response. Antigen-presenting cells expressing MHC (major histocompatibility complex) and associated with coreceptors ICAM and CD40 couple with infected myocytes displaying antigen (epitope) on their surface. The APC (antigen presenting cell) then stimulates cytotoxic cells capable of ingesting the myocyte surface or antibody-producing cells, which affect cell function or enhance membrane damage by cytotoxic cells. NK = natural killer; NO = nitric oxide.

Clinical Manifestations

Patients with myocarditis can develop a more spherical left ventricle, which is less efficient in myocardial contraction and mitral valve leaflet malcoaptation, causing additional myocardial functional deterioration.

Signs

In patients with viral myocarditis, the illness begins with the initial viral infection. The symptoms of the viral illness are due to the virus and its portal of entry (upper respiratory or gastrointestinal tract). After the viral illness, which may be unappreciated by the patient, there is a delay of days to weeks before cardiac symptoms appear, including congestive heart failure, arrhythmia (sometimes leading to sudden cardiac death), or embolic events. The latter are not infrequent in patients with acute inflammatory states because of the procoagulant effects of cytokines combined with decreased cardiac function and blood stasis.

Symptoms and signs of myocarditis and subsequent cardiac dysfunction may be protean. Symptoms include fatigue, dyspnea, chest pain (which may be pleuritic due to concomitant pericarditis), and palpitations. Signs can include sinus tachycardia, a diminished first heart sound due to decreased myocardial contraction, gallops, murmurs of mitral or tricuspid insufficiency, and, rarely, a pericardial friction rub.

Myocardial Infarction

Several authors have reported patients presenting with what appears to be an acute myocardial infarction with ST-segment elevation, positive CK and CK MB bands, and focal wall motion abnormalities (but with normal coronary arteriograms) due to myocarditis as demonstrated on endomyocardial biopsy.[27,28] Importantly, most patients' wall motion abnormalities normalized over time.[27]

Microaneurysms

Myocarditis may produce single or multiple ventricular microaneurysms.[29] These patients are characterized by (1) normal overall ventricular function, (2) nonsustained ventricular tachycardia, and (3) left heart biopsies demonstrating histological myocarditis in which standard right heart endomyocardial biopsies are infrequently positive.

Ventricular Tachycardia. Patients with myocarditis have also been reported to develop refractory ventricular tachycardia, torsade de pointes, or sudden cardiac death.[30,31] No prospective randomized trials have evaluated the natural history and spontaneous resolution of these arrhythmias. Immunosuppressive therapy has been utilized in some patients presenting with these arrhythmias when no other cause could be identified. Myocarditis has been reported in some athletes succumbing to sudden cardiac death.[32] Recently, refractory atrial fibrillation has been associated with inflammatory infiltrates in the atrium.[33]

Laboratory Findings

Electrocardiogram. The electrocardiogram is almost always abnormal in patients with myocarditis and may display changes of acute injury. More typical, however, are the presence of nonspecific ST-T wave changes. Any form of atrial or ventricular arrhythmia can be demonstrated, including atrial or ventricular premature beats, atrial or ventricular tachycardia, and atrioventricular fibrillation. In addition, patients with myocarditis may display atrial, ventricular, or intraventricular conduction delays.

Chest X-Ray. The cardiothoracic ratio is usually normal, particularly early in the illness before the development of a cardiomyopathy. Progressive compromise of left ventricular function may result in cardiomegaly. Elevation of filling pressures, regardless of the heart size, may result in findings of congestive heart failure including cephalization of blood flow or overt pulmonary edema.

Blood Studies. There are no characteristic findings on routine laboratory studies to confirm the diagnosis of myocarditis, although the white blood cell count is usually elevated.

Biomarkers of Myonecrosis. Myocardial enzymes are usually not elevated unless the patient presents acutely and displays a rapid deterioration. Cardiac specific troponin I elevation may be found in up to a third of patients, compared with less than 10% displaying CK elevations.[34] Patients with elevated enzyme levels tended to have symptoms of less than 1 month's duration.

Autoantibodies. Other immune markers have been evaluated as a means to confirm the diagnosis of myocarditis. Antibodies have been demonstrated to sarcolemma, myolemma, alpha-myosin, mitochondrial, and endothelial antigens. A number of cytokines have been demonstrated to be elevated in patients with progressive heart failure, including TNF, IL-6, and IgG3.[35,36]

NONINVASIVE STUDIES. Noninvasive imaging techniques have been used in an attempt to diagnose myocarditis, including echocardiography, nuclear scans, and magnetic resonance imaging (MRI). Echocardiography may help to identify patients with fulminant myocarditis at presentation. These patients usually have normal diastolic volumes and increased ventricular wall thickness (likely due to inflammation associated with interstitial edema).[37] Antimyosin scanning (when compared with endomyocardial biopsy) demonstrates a sensitivity of 83 percent, specificity of 53 percent, and a negative predictive value of 92 percent.[38] Gallium scanning demonstrates a sensitivity of only 36 percent but a specificity of 98 percent.[39] MRI has been used more recently; sensitivities of 100 percent and specificity between 90 and 100 percent have been claimed (Fig. 60–2).[40] These MRI data will require confirmation, particularly as most studies were accompanied by a limited number of histological analyses.

ENDOMYOCARDIAL BIOPSY. Because of the inadequacy of noninvasive means to establish the diagnosis of myocarditis, a histological diagnosis has been considered necessary to establish a secure diagnosis (which is especially important during clinical trials of therapeutic agents). The National Heart, Lung and Blood Institute Workshop reported that "idiopathic dilated cardiomyopathy is believed frequently to be a sequela of viral myocarditis, and the distinction between the two conditions is often obscured in clinical studies."[41] Studies have reported the frequency of finding myocarditis in patients presenting with cardiomyopathy or new-onset congestive heart failure who were submitted to endomyocardial biopsy to vary between 0 and 63 percent.[42,43] This variance reflects the lack of established histological criteria for myocarditis in most early studies. Later series, using standardized criteria, have displayed a prevalence between 9 and 15 percent.[44] In addition, some patients have improvement in their ejection fraction despite having negative biopsy findings for myocarditis, suggesting that they may have had myocarditis that was not histologically documented. Those with myocarditis more often have had a preceding flu-like illness,

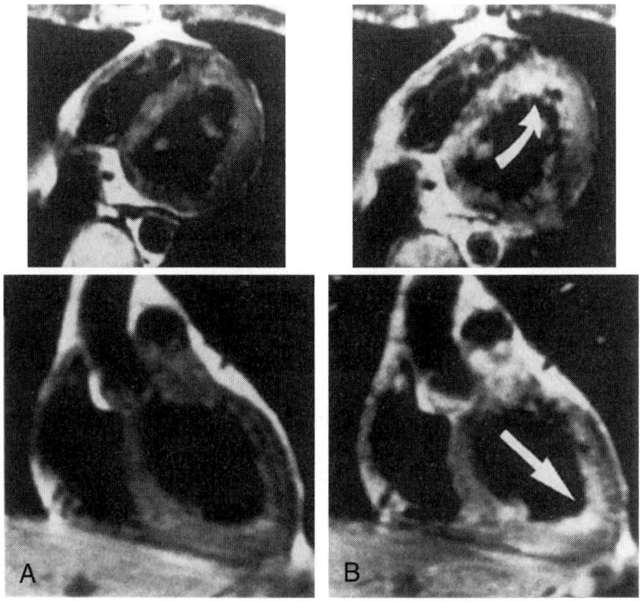

FIGURE 60–2 **A,** Precontrast T1-weighted transaxial **(upper)** and coronal **(lower)** magnetic resonance images through the left ventricle in a patient with myocarditis. **B,** Postcontrast magnetic resonance images at the same levels after contrast injection. Note enhancement of the myocardial signal in the septum and apical region (arrows). (From Matsouka H, Hamada M, Honda T, et al: Evaluation of acute myocarditis and pericarditis by Gd-DTPA enhanced magnetic resonance imaging. Eur Heart J 15:283, 1994.)

are younger, and are less frequently male, as compared with patients with idiopathic or ischemic cardiomyopathy.[44]

HISTOLOGICAL CRITERIA FOR MYOCARDITIS

In 1986, eight expert cardiac pathologists met in Dallas, Texas to establish a histopathological definition and classification for myocarditis. This classification scheme has subsequently been termed the "Dallas criteria" and has been utilized as the standard for the histological diagnosis in all subsequent studies of myocarditis (Fig. 60-3).[45] The authors defined myocarditis as "a process characterized by an inflammatory infiltrate of the myocardium with necrosis and/or degeneration of adjacent myocytes not typical of ischemic damage associated with coronary artery disease." Criteria were established to diagnose myocarditis, borderline myocarditis, or no myocarditis in the initial biopsy specimens.

Myocarditis requires an inflammatory infiltrate and damage to adjacent myocytes confirmed by light microscopy. The myocardial inflammation, both by amount and distribution, can be characterized as mild, moderate, or severe and focal, confluent, or diffuse, respectively. Similarly, the type of inflammatory infiltrate is subclassified as lymphocytic, neutrophilic, eosinophilic, giant cell, granulomatous, or mixed. Borderline myocarditis "implies the inflammatory infiltrate is too sparse, or damage to the myocyte is not demonstrable by light microscopy or both."[45] *Borderline myocarditis* does not allow an unequivocal diagnosis of myocarditis to be established, and the panel suggested re-biopsy in these cases.

Despite these seemingly straightforward criteria, subsequent publications have documented substantial interobserver and intraobserver variability. Although the endomyocardial biopsy has been considered to be the gold standard, studies have demonstrated the difficulty in making the diagnosis of myocarditis because of its focal nature.[46] Endomyocardial biopsies were performed in postmortem hearts from patients who had died from myocarditis, and the ability to establish the diagnosis was assessed. With only one biopsy of the endomyocardium in these patients with known myocarditis, histological confirmation was possible in only 17 to 28 percent of patients. With more than five biopsies, approximately two-thirds of patients had a histological diagnosis of myocarditis established. Inclusion of borderline myocarditis increased the yield by an additional 10 to 15 percent. Therefore, with approximately five biopsies, the potential to make the diagnosis of myocarditis or borderline myocarditis (when it is present) is approximately 75 to 80 percent.

Additional studies can be performed on each histological biopsy specimen to enhance the potential to establish the diagnosis of myocarditis. Common leukocyte antigen staining ensures that the mononuclear cells present in the specimen are of white cell origin. Mononuclear cells can

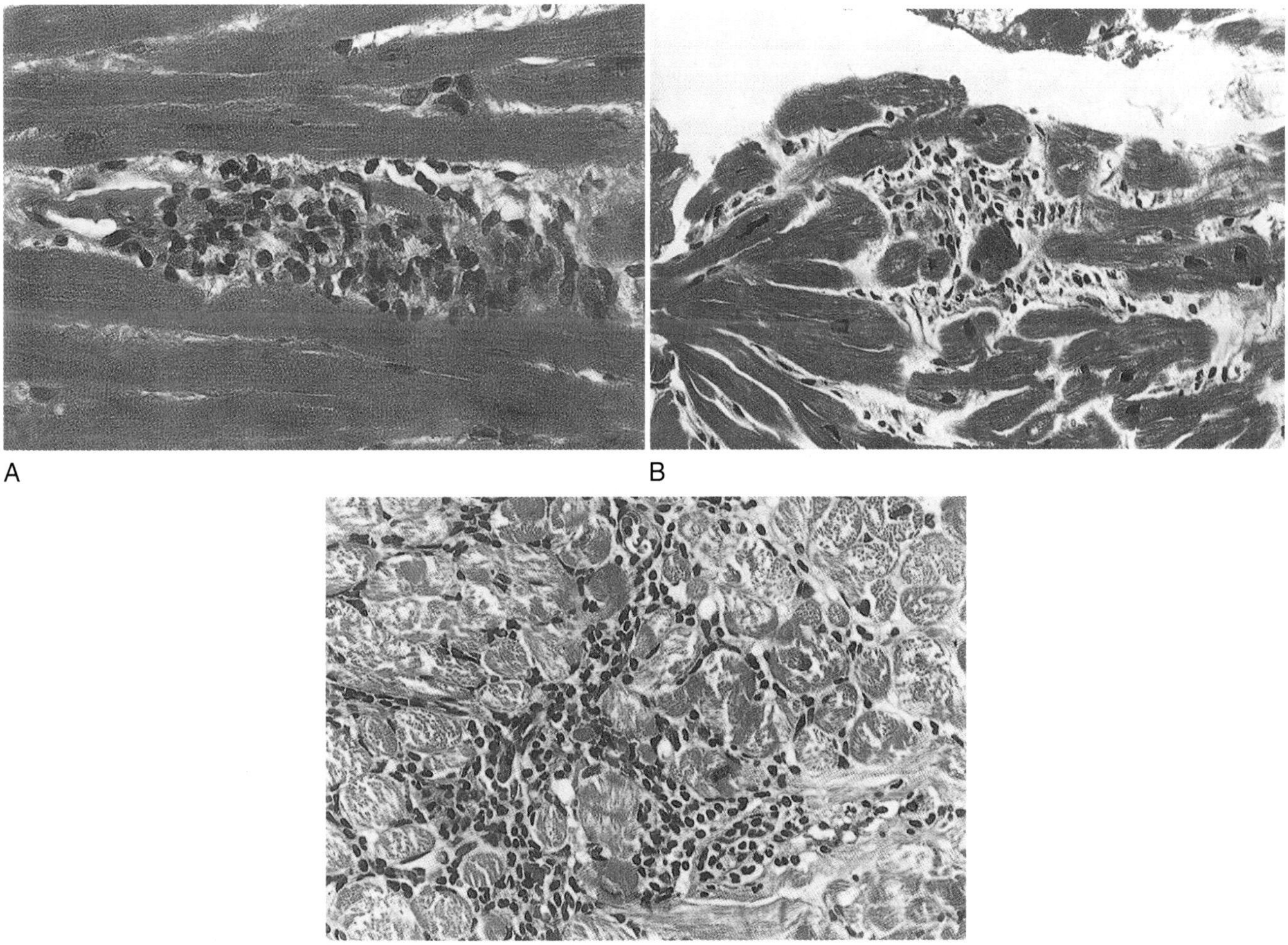

FIGURE 60–3 The diagnosis of myocarditis requires histological examination of myocardial tissue. This tissue can be obtained through endomyocardial biopsy of the interventricular septum. **A,** In this sample, longitudinally oriented myocytes are engulfed centrally by lymphocytes causing destruction of myocardial tissue. Often, sites examined immediately adjacent to the involved myofibrils appear normal. On initial biopsy, active myocarditis is defined as an inflammatory infiltrate of the myocardium with necrosis or degeneration of myocytes not typical of the ischemic changes associated with coronary artery disease. **B,** Borderline myocarditis (Dallas criteria). Borderline myocarditis is diagnosed when the inflammatory infiltrate is sparse or when myocyte damage is not demonstrated under light microscopy. This specimen demonstrates a limited mononuclear cell infiltrate not resulting in myocyte necrosis. Heart tissue from patients with idiopathic dilated cardiomyopathy reveals increased interstitial cellularity associated with myocyte hypertrophy and interstitial fibrosis (common features of myocardial response to stress). **C,** Some features of subtle myocyte degenerative changes that reflect irreversible myocyte damage. In addition to frank myocyte necrosis (see part **A**), this figure demonstrates a focus of interstitial inflammatory cells surrounding individual myocytes and small myocyte clusters. Myocytes with inflammatory cells immediately adjacent to their plasma membrane contain membrane vacuoles and irregular surface outlines. These morphological changes are similar to those noted in experimental postviral murine myocarditis during the early phases of myocyte injury. (From Herskowitz A, Ansari AA: Myocarditis. *In* Abelmann WH [ed]: Cardiomyopathies, myocarditis and pericardial disease. *In* Braunwald E [series ed]. Atlas of Heart Diseases. Vol. 2. Philadelphia, Current Medicine, 1995.)

represent myocyte nuclei, endothelial cells, or fibrous tissue. Major histocompatibility complex (MHC) antigens should be expressed in patients when there is immune upregulation. MHC class I molecules are present to some extent in virtually all nucleated cells, whereas MHC class II molecules are confined to immune system cells. In cases of myocarditis, both MHC class I and II antigens are markedly upregulated and have been used by some investigators as surrogates for the Dallas criteria for myocarditis, because MHC upregulation is more diffuse than histological inflammatory infiltrates.[47] Other histological markers of immune upregulation are being investigated, including CD40 antigen expression, NK cell and perforin upregulation, and apoptosis.[48-50]

The spontaneous improvement of some patients with Dallas criteria–negative myocarditis, the difficulties noted in establishing the histological diagnosis of myocarditis in patients with known myocarditis, and the subsequent demonstration of causative viruses by PCR in patients with histologically negative myocarditis have confirmed how rudimentary the reliance on inflammatory infiltrates or myocyte destruction has been to establish a diagnosis of myocarditis.

Antibodies are produced against important portions of the myocyte membrane (myosin, laminin, beta receptor) and mitochondria (adenine nucleotide translocator and branched chain ketoacid dehydrogenase), which may well contribute to cardiac dysfunction in this population.[51,52]

Clinical Pathological Classification of Myocarditis

In 1991, we proposed a classification system for primary (postviral) myocarditis that included fulminant, acute, (subacute) chronic active, and chronic persistent myocarditis, much as had been previously accepted for acute hepatitis (Table 60–2).[53] Patients with secondary myocarditis were excluded from this histopathological classification, including those with peripartum cardiomyopathy, human immunodeficiency virus (HIV)-related myocarditis, sarcoidosis, systemic lupus erythematosus, and ischemia with inflammation. Patients with primary myocarditis were differentiated based on their onset of illness, left ventricular function at the time of presentation, endomyocardial biopsy findings at presentation, and clinical and histological outcomes.

FULMINANT MYOCARDITIS. Patients with fulminant myocarditis have a distinct onset of the condition, usually within days of the well-identified viral illness. They present with severe left ventricular dysfunction, often cardiogenic shock requiring pressors or artificial mechanical support.[54] The left ventricles are usually not dilated, but rather thick-walled, likely a manifestation of interstitial edema. Endomyocardial biopsies in the fulminant category are unequivocally positive with severe inflammatory infiltrates and myocyte necrosis. Despite their severe decompensation at presentation, these patients typically either recover completely or die within a period of 2 weeks. Survivors show histological resolution of their myocarditis, and their hearts return to normal size and function in follow-up.

SUBACUTE MYOCARDITIS. Patients with subacute myocarditis have an indistinct onset of the disease with no clearly defined initial viral illness. They present with moderately severe ventricular dysfunction but usually mild dilation. Their biopsies reveal active or borderline myocarditis, and evidence of inflammation is often difficult to find. These patients have incomplete recovery or go on to develop progressive dilated cardiomyopathy despite complete resolution by biopsy of any inflammation. This group may have viral persistence based on the work of other investigators.

CHRONIC ACTIVE MYOCARDITIS. Patients with this form of myocarditis typically have distinctive features. Their onset is indistinct and similar to that of subacute myocarditis and they present with similar degrees of moderate left ventricular dysfunction and mild left ventricular dilation. Their biopsies at presentation and in follow-up reveal a combination of active myocarditis and active healing. Over the course of these patients' illnesses (usually 2 to 3 years), this pattern of inflammation and scarring persists and the patients ultimately develop a nondilated restrictive cardiomyopathy (see Chap. 59) with evidence of giant cell formation.

CHRONIC PERSISTENT MYOCARDITIS. Patients with chronic persistent myocarditis are usually submitted to biopsy because of non-heart failure–related symptoms of atypical chest pain or palpitations. They have no distinct onset to their illness and usually have a history of many months or years of cardiac complaints. They have no left ventricular dysfunction despite having active or borderline myocarditis on biopsy. Their clinical history is one of continued symptomatology and persistently normal left ventricular function despite ongoing inflammation.

PROGNOSIS. A follow-up study of patients with fulminant myocarditis reveals that once past the initial presentation, these patients do well and have virtually no cardiac-related morbidity or mortality (Fig. 60–4).[54] Patients with subacute myocarditis, whether meeting Dallas criteria or displaying borderline myocarditis have the same relatively poor prognosis as those with dilated cardiomyopathy. Interestingly, the rate of presentation of patients with fulminant myocarditis remained relatively constant over time, whereas the number of patients presenting with acute myocarditis declined over the period of case collection.[54] The latter finding is a mirror image of the frequency of nonpolio enteroviral infections documented by the Centers for Disease Control and Prevention over the same time interval. This suggests that there is a correlation between enteroviral infections and subacute myocarditis, which appears not to be present in patients with fulminant myocarditis. In view of their excellent long-term recovery, patients with fulminant myocarditis must be supported with whatever means necessary to provide them an opportunity to recover. This may include pressors, intraaortic balloon counterpulsation, or left ventricular assist device.[55]

TABLE 60–2 Histopathological Myocarditis Classification*

	Fulminant	Subacute	Chronic Active	Chronic Persistent
Onset	Distinct	Indistinct	Indistinct	Indistinct
Left ventricular function	Severe dysfunction	Moderate dysfunction	Moderate dysfunction	No dysfunction
Biopsy	Multiple foci	Active or borderline	Active or borderline	Active or borderline
Clinical history	Recovery or death	Incomplete dilated cardiomyopathy	Restrictive cardiomyopathy	Normal left ventricular function
Histological outcome	Complete resolution	Complete resolution	Giant cells-fibrosis	Ongoing

*Primary myocarditis is classified by clinical presentation, initial left ventricular (LV) size and function, results of endomyocardial biopsy, clinical outcome, and histological outcome into the following categories: fulminant, subacute, chronic active, and chronic persistent myocarditis. Other forms of myocarditis include giant cell myocarditis and eosinophilic myocarditis.

From Lieberman EB, Hutchins GM, Herskowitz A, et al: Clinicopathologic description of myocarditis. J Am Coll Cardiol 18:1617, 1991.

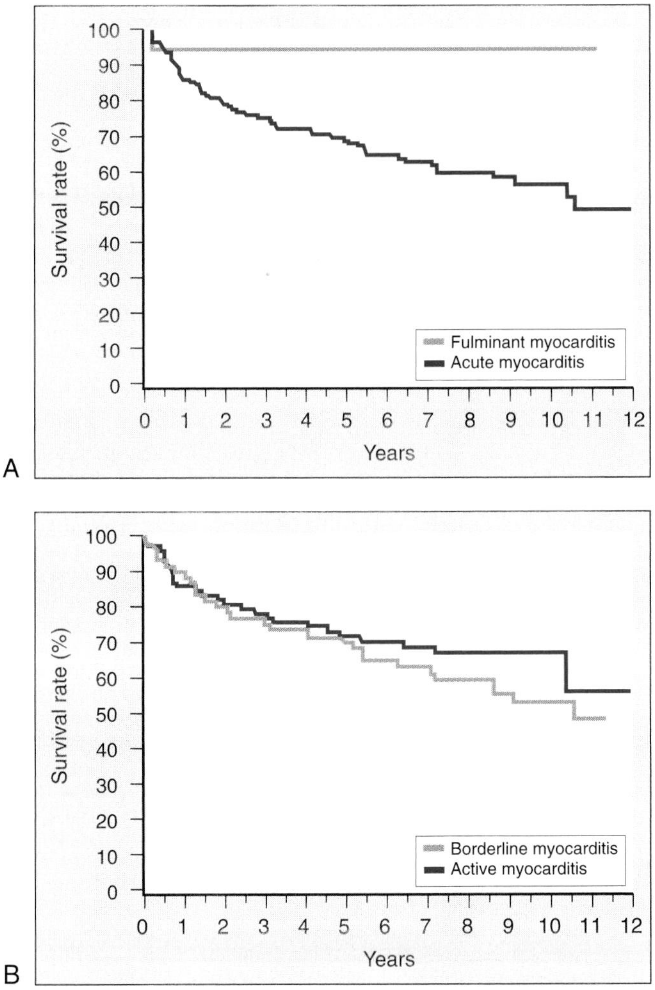

FIGURE 60–4 **A,** Unadjusted transplantation-free survival according to clinicopathological classification. Patients with fulminant myocarditis were significantly less likely to die or require heart transplantation during follow-up than were patients with acute myocarditis ($p = 0.05$ by the log-rank test). **B,** Unadjusted transplantation-free survival according to the Dallas histopathological criteria. Long-term survival did not differ significantly according to the degree of inflammation on biopsy ($p = 0.38$ by the log-rank test). (Modified from McCarthy RE 3rd, Boehmer JP, Hruban RH, et al: Long-term outcome of fulminant myocarditis as compared with acute (nonfulminant) myocarditis. N Engl J Med 342:690, 2000.)

RISKS OF ENDOMYOCARDIAL BIOPSY

In our experience, approximately 6% of those with new-onset congestive heart failure or dilated cardiomyopathy have a complication with myocardial biopsy.[56] Approximately one-half of these complications are related to venous access and the remainder to the biopsy procedure itself. Access complications include inadvertent arterial puncture, pneumothorax, vasovagal reaction, or bleeding after sheath removal.

Complications associated with the procedure include arrhythmias, cardiac conduction abnormalities, and heart perforation. Heart perforation can cause pericardial tamponade and, rarely, death. Patients with perforation report pain, which otherwise should not be experienced during the procedure. These patients may deteriorate rapidly, in part due to their degree of myocardial decompensation at the initiation of the procedure, and the rapid accumulation of blood in the pericardial space. Additionally, the rapid accumulation of blood in the pericardial space can form a clot acutely, which may interfere with pericardial evacuation attempted percutaneously. Patients who cannot be immediately resuscitated by percutaneous pericardiocentesis should have open chest evacuation of the hematoma. This requires coordination with cardiovascular surgery and preparation in the laboratory for the occurrence of these rare, but expected, complications.

The use of ultrasonographically guided techniques to identify the internal jugular vein and/or guide in vein cannulation improves the success rate and decreases the complication rate and access time.[57] The complication rate with biopsies via the femoral vein is at least equivalent to that experienced with a jugular venous procedure. Performance of left ventricular biopsies shares similar perforation complication rates, despite the greater wall thickness of the left ventricle.

Treatment

The treatment of myocarditis is controversial, and no specific therapeutic regimen has been established. All patients with myocarditis should limit their physical activity, receive standard heart failure therapy, have their arrhythmia suppressed (if indicated), and avoid vascular spasm. There have been no studies of exercise compared with rest in the management of patients with myocarditis. In animal models, acute exercise in the face of an active viral infection increases viral replication and shortens survival.[2] Patients therefore are advised to moderately limit their activities. Although activities of daily living are allowed, patients should not "work up a sweat" in sustained physical exertion. Patient should be treated for heart failure with appropriate medications, as outlined in other chapters. This includes diuretics to lower symptomatic preload excess, afterload reduction therapy (particularly with angiotensin-converting enzyme inhibitors), and beta blockers for both arrhythmia management and in hopes of improving myocardial function. Because vascular spasm is a component of myocarditis, agents that precipitate or exacerbate vascular spasm should be avoided. This may include the use of digoxin.

It has been hypothesized from animal models that calcium channel blockers are beneficial, by preventing microvascular spasm or inhibiting nitric oxide production, decreasing viral replication, decreasing T-cell activation, and diminishing interleukin production; however, there are no adequate studies upon which to base recommendations.[58] Beta blockers can stabilize myocardial membranes and prevent arrhythmia, provide antioxidants, or stimulate interleukins.[59] Angiotensin-converting enzyme inhibitors can decrease oxygen demand, protein synthesis, cardiac mass, fibrosis, inflammation, and free radical injury and, through bradykinin, dilate coronary arteries.[60]

Immunosuppressive Therapy

Immunosuppressive therapy has been proposed to treat myocarditis and new-onset cardiomyopathy in both children and adults. As hypothesized in animal models, immunoglobulin may provide an antibody to the specific virus responsible for the illness or cause a nonspecific immune response with downregulation of cytokines. Although early studies in children and adults were encouraging, the data were not from prospective, randomized trials and not all patients were submitted to endomyocardial biopsy; furthermore, the immunoglobulin treatment was not controlled.[61]

Ultimately, a multicenter prospective randomized trial in patients with new-onset cardiomyopathy (less than 6 months) and symptomatic congestive heart failure was performed.[62] All 62 patients were biopsied and only 16 percent had histological Dallas criteria myocarditis. The improvement in the ejection fraction for both treated and control groups was substantial, with a baseline ejection fraction of 25 percent rising to 41 percent in the short term and 42 percent at 1-year follow-up. The responses in both the immunoglobulin-treated and standard populations were statistically identical, and the 1-year survival rates were 92 and 88 percent, respectively. Thus, intravenous immunoglobulin therapy does *not* appear to be beneficial for adult patients with new-onset cardiomyopathy and presumed myocarditis.

Immunosuppressive therapy has been studied more extensively than any other form of treatment for myocarditis. In 1984, a compilation of 82 patients with biopsy-proven myocarditis culled from nine series was published.[63] Forty-nine of the 82 patients were reported to improve on immunosuppressive therapy (60 percent), whereas 33 percent reported no significant change and 5 percent deteriorated. Of note, however, only 1 of 21 patients (5 percent) with an acute presentation appeared to respond, whereas 20 of 22 patients with chronic disease states (91 percent) responded with an improvement in symptoms. This observation is in keeping with later reports of the inadvisability of treatment of patients with fulminant myocarditis with immunosuppressive therapy compared with the potential benefit in those with an immune complex–driven depression of heart function.

Based on these observations, two important prospective randomized trials were conducted. Parillo at the National Institutes of Health reported in 1989 the response of 102 patients with established dilated cardiomyopathy to prednisone treatment.[64] Although there was an initial improvement in the prednisone group, particularly in patients with "reactive" heart biopsies, by 9 months the increase in ejection fraction had reversed. Therefore, there seems little benefit to treating patients with an established cardiomyopathy with immunosuppressive therapy.

THE MYOCARDITIS TREATMENT TRIAL

The results of an international trial termed the Myocarditis Treatment Trial (Fig. 60–5) were reported in 1995.[65] The investigators evaluated 2233 candidates with a clinical syndrome compatible with myocarditis. Two hundred and fourteen had compatible biopsies with Dallas criteria myocarditis determined by local pathologists' interpretation. Of the 214 potential candidates for the trial, 30 were excluded with ejection fractions greater than 45 percent, 44 patients met other exclusion criteria, and 29 declined enrollment. The trial was, therefore, based on evaluation of 111 patients, with only 64 percent confirmed as having myocarditis on review by the expert panel of pathologists. Treatment was randomized to placebo versus prednisone and cyclosporin. (An initial treatment arm using prednisone and azathioprine was terminated because of low enrollment.) At 1 and 5 years of follow-up, there was no difference in survival (80 and 44 percent, respectively, for both groups combined). There was also no difference in heart function in the treated or placebo group at 28 weeks. The treated group showed an increase in ejection fraction from 24 to 34 percent, and the control group went from 26 to 32 percent.

Despite the negative results of this trial, the authors indicated that patients who responded appeared to have higher initial ejection fractions and a shorter duration of illness. The Myocarditis Treatment Trial had a sobering effect on the subsequent evaluation of myocarditis in the United States and markedly diminished the enthusiasm for endomyocardial biopsy.

OTHER TRIALS OF IMMUNOSUPPRESSIVE THERAPY

Additional data may help identify a population of patients with myocarditis who may benefit from immunosuppressive therapy. In 1984, it was suggested in a pre-Dallas criteria retrospective review that patients with more chronic forms of inflammation appear to respond more favorably to immunosuppressive therapy.[63] We evaluated 20 patients with biopsy-proven myocarditis or borderline myocarditis.[66] Both groups were treated with prednisone and azathioprine for 6 to 8 weeks and underwent repeat endomyocardial biopsy, right heart catheterization, and echocardiogram. Patients with borderline myocarditis had a greater increase in their ejection fractions in follow-up and more dramatic improvement in heart rate–corrected velocity of circumferential fiber shortening by echocardiography.

Another author recently reported the results of 84 patients with presumed myocarditis of 202 patients with cardiomyopathy evaluated by endomyocardial biopsy.[67] Patients with myocarditis were defined by demonstration of upregulation of the HLA antigen by endomyocardial biopsy rather than Dallas criteria. These patients were randomized to receive immunosuppression or a placebo. The primary endpoint of the trial (i.e., death, transplant, or hospitalization) was no different in the treated patients compared with the placebo group. The ejection fraction in the immunosuppressive group increased from 24 to 36 percent, however, while it remained virtually constant (25-27 percent) in the control group. Additionally, at the 3-month follow-up clinical improvement was noted in 72 percent of immunosuppressed patients but only 31 percent of control subjects. In another important recent trial, Italian investigators found myocarditis in 112 of 652 patients with new-onset cardiomyopathy submitted to biopsy.[68] Forty-one of these 112 patients had progressive congestive heart failure despite standard medical treatment for heart failure. These 41 patients were treated with prednisone and azathioprine. The authors noted that 20 patients responded and 21 had no response. The responders increased their ejection fraction from 26 to 47 percent and showed healed myocarditis on repeat biopsy. The 20 nonresponders showed a progressive histological evolution to dilated cardiomyopathy; 12 remained unchanged, while 3 underwent cardiac transplantation and 5 died. Cardiac autoantibodies were present in 90 percent of patients who responded and 0 percent of the nonresponders. On the other hand, viral genome was present in 85 percent of the nonresponders (enterovirus, Epstein-Barr virus, influenza A virus, and parvovirus-B19). The three responders with viral genome were all positive for hepatitis C.

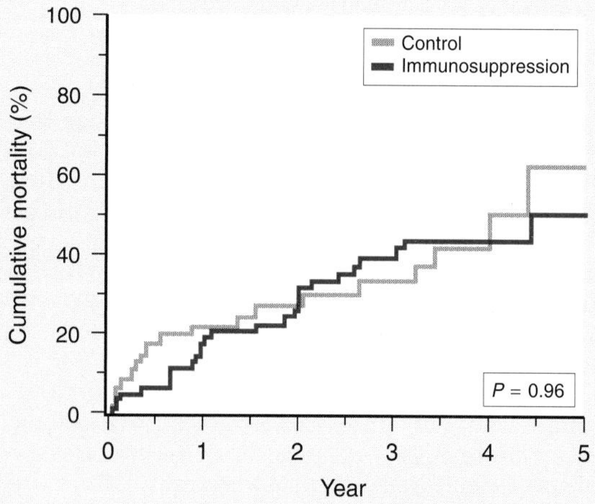

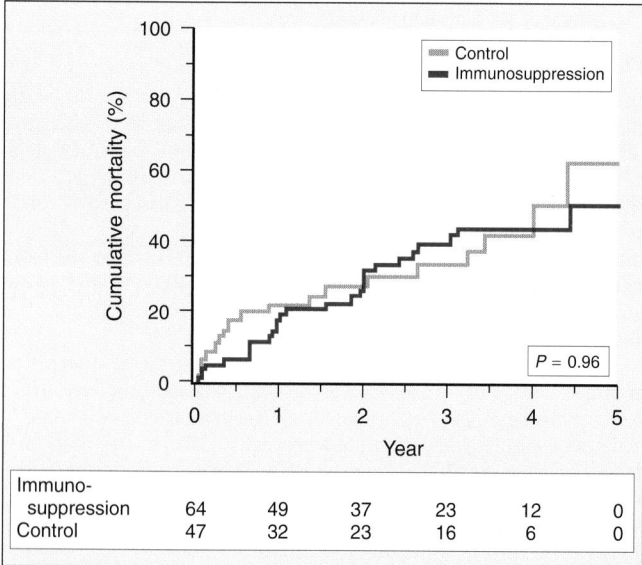

	0	1	2	3	4	5
Immuno-suppression	64	49	37	23	12	0
Control	47	32	23	16	6	0

FIGURE 60–5 Actuarial mortality (defined as deaths and cardiac transplantations) in the immunosuppression and control groups. The numbers of patients at risk are shown at the bottom. There was no significant difference in mortality between the two groups. (Modified from Mason JW, O'Connell JB, Herskowitz A, et al: A clinical trial of immunosuppressive therapy for myocarditis. The Myocarditis Treatment Trial Investigators. N Engl J Med 333:269, 1995.)

The findings summarized indicate that patients with fulminant myocarditis should not be treated with immunosuppressive therapy, as their clinical course usually is one of spontaneous recovery. Patients with fulminant myocarditis, in particular, may require short-term support with intraaortic balloon counterpulsation or left ventricular assist devices. A number of case reports have documented the efficacy of this therapeutic option.[69,70] Recently, use of percutaneous cardiopulmonary support has been reported, and current trials are ongoing that compare intraaortic balloon counterpulsation with this form of cardiopulmonary support. Patients with well-established dilated cardiomyopathies do not respond to immunosuppressive therapy. There is undoubtedly a group with chronic myocardial inflammation who do respond to immunosuppressive therapy. Current data suggest that these patients have an active immune process and do not have viral persistence. Undoubtedly, our ability to identify this group of patients will improve with future investigation of endomyocardial biopsies and autoantibodies. Currently, immunosuppression therapy cannot be recommended for patients without histological confirmation of myocarditis, and then only in those who have failed to improve on standardized heart failure treatment.

Immunoabsorption of circulating antibodies in patients with myocarditis and/or dilated cardiomyopathy has been evaluated.[71] Short-term and intermediate-term studies have demonstrated the efficacy of this form of treatment, and larger prospective randomized trials are pending.

Finally, some investigators have suggested that antiviral vaccines to combat heart disease may be technologically possible, concentrating on frequently encountered viruses, including Coxsackie, adenovirus, and enteroviruses.[72]

In summary, myocarditis remains an important entity and may be a precursor to dilated cardiomyopathy in an unknown number of patients. Endomyocardial biopsy remains the key to establishing the diagnosis. Only now is our understanding of the pathophysiology adequate to allow evaluation of appropriate methods of treatment.

Giant Cell Myocarditis

CLINICAL FEATURES. Giant cell myocarditis is a relatively rare form of myocarditis first described in 1905. By 1997, only 80 cases had been reported, usually at autopsy.[73] Affected patients have an average age of 43 years, but infants as young as 6 weeks and adults as old as 88 years have been affected with the disorder. Approximately 90 percent are white. Men and women are equally affected. Patients present with rapidly progressive congestive heart failure or arrhythmias. The arrhythmias may be difficult-to-control ventricular arrhythmias or, less frequently, complete heart block. Rarely, patients present as if they are in the throes of an acute myocardial infarction.

Nearly 20 percent of patients have some other autoimmune disease, including Hashimoto thyroiditis, rheumatoid arthritis, myasthenia gravis, Takayasu arteritis, alopecia, vitiligo, pernicious anemia, Crohn disease, ulcerative colitis, idiopathic thrombocytopenic purpura, orbital myositis, and celiac disease.[74-76] The histological entity can also be associated with drug reactions and eosinophils,[77] but it is unclear whether the survival characteristics are similar for this category.[73]

Diagnosis. Patients are diagnosed by endomyocardial biopsy. The pathological assessment reveals widespread serpiginous necrosis and multifocal inflammation consisting of lymphocytes, histiocytes, and eosinophils (Fig. 60–6). Multinucleated giant cells without granuloma (particularly at the margins in the areas of myocyte necrosis) are found and characterize the condition histologically. There are conflicting reports as to whether the T cells are primarily CD4 (helper) or CD8 (cytotoxic) cells.[73] Endomyocardial biopsy has a sensitivity of approximately 80 percent in establishing the diagnosis of giant cell myocarditis in patients who are affected.[78]

Patients with giant cell myocarditis must be evaluated for bacterial, fungal, protozoal, and cytomegaloviral infection. These patients must be differentiated from those with cardiac sarcoidosis. The clinical presentation is usually dramatically different.[79,80] Patients with giant cell myocarditis have rapidly progressive symptomatology, whereas those with sarcoidosis (absent sudden cardiac death and heart block) usually present in a less abrupt fashion. Patients with giant cell myocarditis are usually white and sarcoidosis patients are usually black. Sarcoidosis patients usually present more frequently with syncope and less profound congestive heart failure. Their prognosis is much better than that of patients with giant cell myocarditis. Histologically, patients with sarcoidosis and giant cell myocarditis both have giant cells; however, only in the former case are noncaseating granulomas seen. Patients with giant cell myocarditis have myocyte destruction and, by most studies, cytotoxic CD8 cells. Sarcoidosis patients tend to have an interstitial disease without myocyte necrosis.[80]

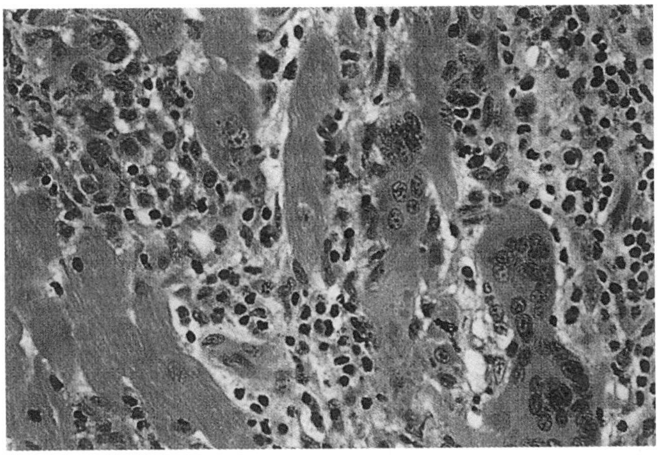

FIGURE 60–6 Giant cell myocarditis. A mixed inflammatory infiltrate, multinucleated giant cells, and extensive myocyte damage. (From Winters GL, McManus BM: Myocarditis. *In* Silver MD, et al [eds]: Cardiovascular Pathology. 3rd ed. New York, Churchill Livingstone, 2001, p 269.

PROGNOSIS. The survival of patients with giant cell myocarditis is markedly limited. In a multicenter natural history study reported by Cooper, the average survival was only 5.5 months from the onset of symptoms.[73] Cooper and others have reported an improvement in prognosis with immunosuppressive therapy. In Cooper's original study, the survival with no immunosuppressive agents was only 3 months. With use of corticosteroids alone, the survival was only 3.8 months. Additional immunosuppressive therapy (combining cyclosporin, azathioprine, or OKT_3) improved the survival to 12.3 months.[81] A subsequent report found the transplant-free survival to be 33 months in patients with combined therapy compared with patients receiving no immunosuppression. Case reports have suggested that high-dose multidrug immunosuppressive treatment may be beneficial, even to the point of including OKT_3, cyclosporin, azathioprine, and corticosteroids.[82,83] These observations are preliminary, and patients with giant cell myocarditis should be entered into the ongoing treatment trial to determine the most effective management strategy. Unfortunately, the small number of patients affected makes such a trial difficult to conduct.

Some patients are so severely affected that they will need support with a left ventricular assist device or intraaortic balloon counterpulsation as a "bridge" to transplant.[84] Thirty-eight patients with giant cell myocarditis have been reported to undergo cardiac transplantation.[85] Nine of the 38 patients had recurrence of giant cells in their endomyocardial biopsies, usually associated with rejection. This recurrence may appear up to 9 years after the transplant, but on average occurs approximately 3 years afterward. The recurrence of giant cells is usually responsive to immunosuppressive therapy in the transplanted population.

Arrhythmogenic Right Ventricular Dysplasia

Arrhythmogenic right ventricular dysplasia is discussed in Chapter 32.

Specific Agents Causing Myocarditis

Secondary Viral Myocarditis

A large number of viral pathogens cause human myocarditis. As the ability to diagnose viral causes by molecular analysis of endomyocardial biopsies has expanded, our appreciation of the frequency of myocarditis causing acute and chronic left ventricular dysfunction is increasing. The pathophysiology of secondary myocarditis is not well established but, as with primary myocarditis, is assumed to be a combination of direct viral toxicity and autoimmune damage. The pathological condition varies, depending on the cardiotrophic nature of the viral agent as well as the inflammatory and immune response, but includes lymphocytic infiltrates with myocyte damage and varying degrees of hypertrophy and fibrosis. Electrocardiographic abnormalities are common and include arrhythmias, heart block, and interventricular conduction delays. Noninvasive studies of patients with viral myocarditis document the severity of the associated left ventricular compromise and presence or absence of pericarditis. Treatment is symptomatic in most cases and is outlined in the previous section. Fortunately, most patients with secondary myocarditis resolve their illness spontaneously; however, most if not all viral agents may cause cardiomyopathy and fatalities.

HUMAN IMMUNODEFICIENCY VIRUS. See Chapter 61.

COXSACKIE VIRUS (see Primary Myocarditis)**.** Both Coxsackie viruses A and B can produce myocarditis, although infection with coxsackie virus B is more common. Coxsackie virus B is the most frequent cause of viral myocarditis, causing more than half the cases.[86,87]

Although most infections are benign, self-limited, and subclinical, Coxsackie viral myocarditis appears to be particularly virulent in the neonate, child, and young adult. In most infections in adults, the other clinical manifestations of viral involvement predominate, such as pleurodynia, myalgia, upper respiratory tract symptoms, and arthralgias. Severe cases in the adult are characterized by myopericardial involvement with pleuritic or pericarditic chest pain, palpitations, and fever. Patients with overt myocardial involvement develop congestive heart failure with cardiomegaly and pulmonary edema.

Most patients recover completely within weeks, although the electrocardiogram (ECG) and ventricular function may require months to return to normal. Rarely, Coxsackie viral myocarditis is fatal in adults. Some patients become symptomatic after resolution of the infection, and they may present years later with dilated cardiomyopathy.[88]

Treatment. Patients with myocarditis are predisposed to ventricular and atrial thrombi due to procoagulant effects of cytokines and vascular stasis. Anticoagulation is recommended unless patients have associated pericarditis, which increases the risk for hemorrhagic pericardial tamponade.

CYTOMEGALOVIRUS. Unrecognized infection with cytomegalovirus is extremely common in childhood, and the majority of the adult population have antibodies to cytomegalovirus.[89] Primary infection after the age of 35 years is uncommon, and generalized infection usually occurs only in immunosuppressed patients with neoplastic disease, after transplantation, or with HIV infection.[90] The diagnosis of cytomegaloviral myocarditis can be suggested by the presence of viral inclusions in myocardial biopsy specimens and confirmed by the detection of viral DNA in the myocardium.[90]

VIRAL HEPATITIS. Clinical cardiac involvement in patients with hepatitis is rare; an occasional patient may develop fulminant myocarditis with congestive heart failure, hypotension, and death.[91] There are contested data implicating hepatitis C viral infection as an etiological factor in at least some cases of dilated cardiomyopathy.[92-94] The ventricles may be dilated with petechial hemorrhages. Hemorrhage into the myocardium may be a conspicuous finding.[91]

Symptomatic myocarditis is generally observed in the first to third week of illness. Patients may have dyspnea, palpitations, and anginal chest pain; fatalities have been reported.[91]

INFLUENZA. Although clinically apparent myocarditis is rare in patients with influenza, the presence of preexisting cardiovascular disease greatly increases the risk of morbidity and mortality.[95] During epidemics, 5 to 10 percent of infected patients may experience cardiac symptoms.[96]

Cardiac involvement typically occurs within 4 days to 2 weeks of the onset of the illness and may be severe, sometimes contributing to mortality.[97,98] Death may be associated with massive hemorrhagic pulmonary edema due to viral or bacterial involvement of the lungs.

MUMPS. Myocardial involvement during the course of mumps is rarely recognized.[99] The hearts of only a few patients with mumps have undergone postmortem examination, and they have been found to be both dilated and hypertrophied. Histologically, there is diffuse interstitial fibrosis, with infiltration of mononuclear cells and areas of focal necrosis.[99,100] There is speculation that prior mumps myocarditis may be involved in the development of endocardial fibroelastosis.[100] Cardiac involvement is usually unrecognized clinically, and the diagnosis of myocarditis is based on nonspecific ECG changes.[99]

RUBELLA AND RUBEOLA. Congenital cardiovascular lesions may develop in the offspring when the mother contracts rubella during the first trimester of pregnancy, with persistent ductus arteriosus and pulmonary artery maldevelopment as prominent anomalies. Rare cases of postgestational myocarditis occur, with attendant conduction defects and heart failure.[101]

Overt myocarditis is rare in patients with rubeola, although transient ECG abnormalities have been reported.[102] Congestive heart failure occurs on rare occasions, and its appearance is a poor prognostic sign, often indicating a fatal outcome.

VARICELLA. Clinical myocarditis is a rare finding in patients with varicella, although unsuspected myocarditis is common in cases of fatal varicella. Occasionally, a patient may develop overt clinical evidence of myocarditis with congestive heart failure.[103] Histological findings include rare but characteristic intranuclear inclusion bodies within the myocardial cells, along with interstitial edema, cellular infiltrates, and myonecrosis.[104]

VARIOLA AND VACCINIA. Cardiac involvement after smallpox is rare, although several cases of myocarditis associated with acute cardiac failure and death have been reported. Myocarditis with pericardial effusion and congestive heart failure has also been observed as a complication of smallpox vaccination; an immunological mechanism has been suggested, and dramatic responses to corticosteroids have been reported.[105]

OTHER VIRUSES

Other viruses causing myocarditis include the following:

Dengue[106,107]
Infectious mononucleosis[108]
Lassa fever[109]
Poliomyelitis[110]
Respiratory syncytial virus[111-113]
Enterovirus-71[114]
Parvovirus B19[115]

RICKETTSIAL MYOCARDITIS. The rickettsial diseases are frequently associated with evidence of myocardial involvement but usually it is subclinical. Transient ST segment and T wave alterations are commonly observed. The circulatory collapse that may accompany these diseases is largely a manifestation of abnormalities of the peripheral vascular bed, but a myocardial component may also be present. The basic histopathological process is a vasculitis with a periarterial interstitial infiltrate.

Other rickettsial pathogens causing myocarditis include Q fever,[116,117] Rocky Mountain spotted fever,[118] and scrub typhus.[119,120]

Bacterial Myocarditis

Virtually any bacterial agent can cause myocardial dysfunction. This occurs because of direct bacterial invasion, microabscess formation, or toxins elaborated by the pathogen. Other clinical manifestations of the infection mask or delay the appreciation of myocardial involvement, which may include atrial or ventricular arrhythmias, heart block, left or biventricular heart failure, pericarditis, or circulatory collapse. The clinician must always be alert for cardiac involvement during systemic bacterial infections.

CLOSTRIDIAL INFECTION. Cardiac involvement is common in patients with clostridial infections with multiple organ involvement. The myocardial damage results from the toxin elaborated by the bacteria but the precise actions of the toxin remain to be elucidated.[121] The pathological findings are distinctive, with gas bubbles present in the myocardium. Areas of degenerated muscle fibers are apparent, but an inflammatory infiltrate is usually absent.[121] *Clostridium perfringens* may cause myocardial abscess formation with myocardial perforation and resultant purulent pericarditis.

DIPHTHERIA. Myocardial involvement is one of the more serious complications of diphtheria and occurs in up to one half of cases.[122,123] Indeed, myocardial involvement is the most common cause of death in this infection and half of the fatal cases demonstrate cardiac involvement.[124] Cardiac damage is due to the liberation by the diphtheria bacillus of a toxin that inhibits protein synthesis by interfering with the transfer of amino acids from soluble RNA to polypeptide chains under construction. The toxin appears to have a particular affinity for the cardiac conducting system.

Because of the serious effects of the toxin on the myocardium, antitoxin should be administered as rapidly as possible.[124] Antibiotic therapy is of less urgency. The development of complete atrioventricular block is an ominous complication and mortality is high despite insertion of a transvenous pacemaker.[125]

STREPTOCOCCAL INFECTION. The most commonly detected cardiac finding after beta-hemolytic streptococcal infection is acute rheumatic fever, which is discussed in detail in Chapter 81.

Involvement of the heart by the streptococcus may produce a myocarditis that is distinct from acute rheumatic carditis. It is characterized by an interstitial infiltrate composed of mononuclear cells with occasional polymorphonuclear leukocytes; the infiltrate may be focal or diffuse and may be localized to the subendocardial or perivascular region. There may be small areas of myocardial necrosis. ECG abnormalities, including prolongation of the PR and QT intervals, occur frequently. Although these abnormalities are rarely associated with other clinical manifestations of myocardial involvement, sudden death, conduction disturbances, and arrhythmias may occur.

TUBERCULOSIS. Involvement of the myocardium by *Mycobacterium tuberculosis* (not as a complication of tuberculous pericarditis) is rare, particularly since the introduction of drugs effective against tuberculosis.[126,127] Most cases of myocardial tuberculosis are clinically silent and are diagnosed only at autopsy. Tuberculous involvement of the myocardium occurs by means of hematogenous or lymphatic spread or directly from contiguous structures and may cause nodular, miliary, or diffuse infiltrative disease. It may lead to arrhythmias, including atrial fibrillation and ventricular tachycardia, complete atrioventricular block, congestive heart failure, left ventricular aneurysms, and sudden death.[126,128,129]

WHIPPLE DISEASE. Although overt involvement is rare, intestinal lipodystrophy, or Whipple disease, is not uncommonly associated with cardiac involvement and periodic acid-Schiff-positive macrophages can be found in the myocardium, pericardium, and heart valves of patients with this disorder.[130,131] Coronary artery lesions, with smooth muscle necrosis, panarteritis, and medial scarring, can be seen. Electron microscopy has demonstrated rod-shaped structures in the myocardium similar to those found in the small intestine, and these represent the causative agent of the disease, *Tropheryma whippleii,* an agent related to the actinomycetes.[130] There may be an associated inflammatory infiltrate and foci of fibrosis. The valvular fibrosis may be severe enough to result in aortic regurgitation and mitral stenosis. Although usually asymptomatic, nonspecific ECG changes are most common; systolic murmurs, pericarditis, complete heart block, and even overt congestive heart failure may occur.[10] The cardiac manifestations of Whipple disease can be overshadowed by the prominent gastrointestinal symptoms that often are present, or it can be unappreciated.[132] Antibiotic therapy appears to be effective in treating the basic disease, but relapses can occur, often more than 2 years after initial diagnosis.

Other Bacteria

Other bacterial causes of myocarditis include the following:

- Brucellosis[133]
- Chlamydia[134,135]
- Legionnaires disease[136]
- Meningococcal infection[137,138]
- *Mycoplasma pneumoniae* infection[139,140]
- Psittacosis[141]
- Salmonellosis[142,143]

Spirochetal Infections

LYME CARDITIS. Lyme disease is caused by a tickborne spirochete (*Borrelia burgdorferi*).[144] It usually begins during the summer months with a characteristic rash (erythema chronicum migrans), followed in weeks to months by neurological, joint, or cardiac involvement. Although some clinical manifestations may persist for years,[144,145] the majority of patients (90 percent) have no long-term sequelae.[145a]

About 10 percent of patients with Lyme disease develop evidence of transient cardiac involvement, the most common manifestation being variable degrees of atrioventricular block[146-149] at the level of the atrioventricular node. Syncope due to complete heart block is frequent with cardiac involvement because often there is an associated depression of ventricular escape rhythms. Ventricular tachycardia occurs uncommonly.[146] Diffuse ST segment and T wave abnormalities are transient; usually asymptomatic, left ventricular dysfunction may be found in some patients, although cardiomegaly or symptoms of congestive heart failure are rare.[147,150] A positive gallium scan can point to suspected cardiac involvement in this disease. The demonstration of spirochetes in myocardial biopsies of some patients with Lyme carditis suggests that the cardiac manifestations are due to a direct effect, although there is speculation that immune-mediated mechanisms may be involved as well.[151]

Treatment. The value of specific therapy in cases of Lyme carditis remains uncertain, and even without therapy the disease is usually self-limited, with complete recovery the rule.[152] Nevertheless, it is thought that treating the early manifestations of the disease will prevent development of late complications.[144] Patients with second-degree or complete heart block should be hospitalized and undergo continuous ECG monitoring. Temporary transvenous pacing may be required for a week or longer in patients with high-grade block. Although the efficacy of antibiotics is not established, they are used routinely in patients with Lyme carditis. Intravenous antibiotics (ceftriaxone, 2 gm, or penicillin G, 20 million units daily for 14 days) are suggested, although oral antibiotics (doxycycline, 100 mg twice daily, or amoxicillin, 500 mg three times daily for 14 to 21 days) can be used when there is only mild cardiac involvement (first-degree atrioventricular block of less than 40 msec duration).[152] Whether antiinflammatory agents (salicylates, corticosteroids) can ameliorate heart block is not clear.

OTHER SPIROCHETAL INFECTIONS CAUSING MYOCARDITIS. Other spirochetal infections include leptospirosis (Weil disease[153-155]), relapsing fever,[156] and syphilis.[157]

Fungal Infections of the Heart

Cardiac fungal infections occur most frequently in patients with malignant disease and/or those receiving chemotherapy, corticosteroids, radiation, or immunosuppressive therapy. Cardiac surgery, intravenous drug abuse, and infection with HIV are also predisposing factors for fungal cardiac involvement. Cardiac involvement may be associated with myocardial seeding by hematogenous dissemination but may also be due to direct myocardial extension from pulmonary or mediastinal infection. Rarely, coronary obstruction can occur due to fungal mycelia.

ASPERGILLOSIS. Myocardial involvement is not uncommon in patients with generalized aspergillosis, and when it occurs it is usually fatal.[158] Rarely, myocardial involvement may appear to be primary, typically after cardiac surgery. However, it is being encountered increasingly in the immunocompromised patient.[159] On pathological examination, myocardial necrosis and infarction caused by thrombosis of vessels that contain fungal mycelia are commonly seen, along with myocardial abscesses and pericardial involvement. The ECG may be normal in the face of significant myocardial damage, but T wave changes may be present. The diagnosis of *Aspergillus* infection is often difficult.[160] Identification of *Aspergillus* through open-lung biopsy, aspiration lung biopsy, transtracheal aspiration, or bronchial brush technique may be successful. Treatment is difficult and usually unsuccessful.

OTHER FUNGAL INFECTIONS. Other fungal infections causing myocarditis include the following:

Actinomycosis[160]
Blastomycosis[161]
Candidiasis[162,163]
Coccidioidomycosis[164]
Cryptococcosis[165]
Histoplasmosis[166]
Mucormycosis[167,168]

Protozoal Myocarditis

Trypanosomiasis (Chagas Disease)

Chagas disease is caused by the protozoan *Trypanosoma cruzi.* The major cardiovascular manifestation is an extensive myocarditis that typically becomes evident years after the initial infection. The disease is prevalent in Central and South America, particularly in Brazil, Argentina, and Chile, where it constitutes a major public health problem (Fig. 60–7). Upward of 20 million people are thought to be infected with the parasite and an estimated 100 million are at risk of infection.[169,170] In rare cases, the disease can be found in nonendemic areas as a consequence of transfusion with contaminated blood products; somewhat more common is emigration of patients with the disease to nonendemic areas.[171]

NATURAL HISTORY. The natural history of Chagas disease is characterized by three phases: acute, latent, and chronic. During the acute phase, the disease is transmitted to humans (usually younger than 20 years of age) through the bite of a reduviid bug (subfamily Triatominae), which harbors the parasite in its gastrointestinal tract.[169-172] This insect acquires the disease from feeding on infected animals, including the armadillo, raccoon, opossum, and skunk as well as domestic dogs and cats. The reduviid bug, popularly known in Argentina as *vinchuca,* meaning "to let oneself drop," lives in the walls and roofs of houses and, during nocturnal feedings, drops from the ceiling onto the sleeping person below. The bug then often bites the person around the eyes, and infection of the human host occurs when the trypanosomes in the animal's feces gain entry through abraded skin or through the conjunctivae.[169] Occasionally, this results in unilateral periorbital edema and swelling of the eyelid, termed the *Romaña sign,* whereas entry through the skin may result in a lesion called a *chagoma.*[169,172] Transmission can occur through blood transfusions; unfortunately, adequate screening to preclude transfusion-related disease is not possible in many areas due to financial and logistical constraints.[169]

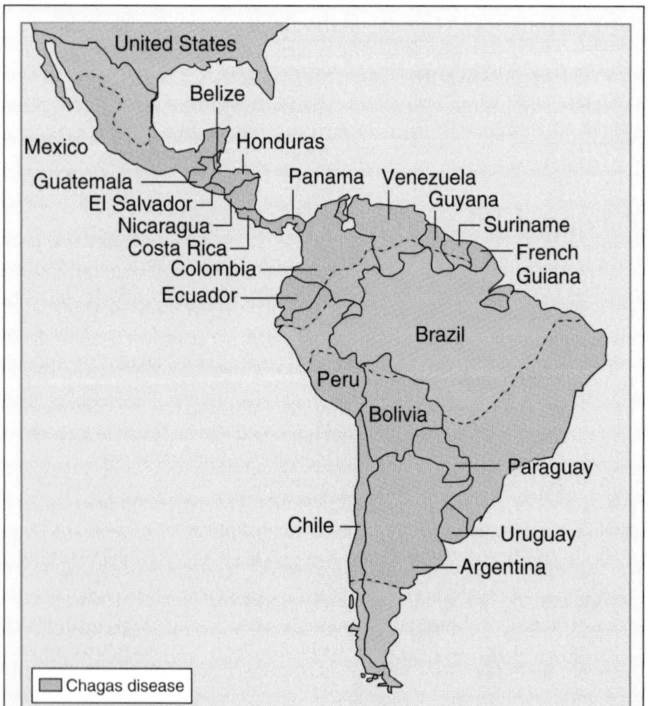

FIGURE 60–7 Distribution of Chagas disease in the Americas. (Modified from Acquatella H: Chagas' disease. *In* Abelmann WH, Braunwald E [eds]: Atlas of Heart Diseases. Vol. 2. Cardiomyopathies, Myocarditis, and Pericardial Disease. Philadelphia, Current Medicine, 1995, pp 8.1-8.18.)

ACUTE TRYPANOSOMIASIS. After inoculation, the protozoa multiply and then migrate widely throughout the body. In less than 10 percent of cases an acute illness occurs; this acute illness is fatal in about 10 percent of patients.[171,172] Pathological examination during the acute phase often reveals parasites in the cardiac fibers with a marked cellular infiltrate, particularly around cardiac cells that have ruptured and released the parasites.[172] Involvement may extend into the endocardium, resulting in thrombus formation, and into the epicardium, resulting in pericardial effusion. The pathogenesis of the myocardial lesions of acute Chagas disease appears to relate in large part to immune lysis by antibody and cell-mediated immunity directed against antigens released from *T. cruzi*–infected cells, which become adsorbed onto the surface of infected and noninfected host cells.[169] *T. cruzi* parasite growth can be regulated by inducible NOS activation and cytokine production.[173]

Clinical Manifestations. Clinical manifestations include fever, muscle pains, sweating, hepatosplenomegaly, myocarditis with congestive heart failure, pericardial effusion, and, occasionally, meningoencephalitis.[169,172] Most patients recover, and their symptoms resolve over several months. Young children most commonly develop clinical acute disease and generally are more seriously ill than adults.

LATENT AND CHRONIC TRYPANOSOMIASIS. The disease then enters a latent phase without clinical symptoms; however, there is evidence of early and progressive subclinical cardiomyopathy. ECG changes often appear at this stage and are a marker for the eventual clinical heart disease and increased mortality to become evident later. At an average of 20 years after the initial (and usually unrecognized) infestation, approximately 30 percent of infected individuals develop findings of chronic Chagas disease, the manifestations of which cover a wide spectrum from asymptomatic but seropositive patients through those with ECG abnormalities to those with advanced disease characterized by cardiomegaly, congestive heart failure, arrhythmias, thromboembolic phenomena, atypical chest pain, right bundle branch block, and sudden death.[171] In the advanced stage, cardiac dilation typically involves all the cardiac chambers, although right-sided enlargement may predominate.[171]

PATHOGENESIS. The central paradox in the pathogenesis of this disorder is the poor correlation between the level of parasitemia and the severity of disease.[174] It is not unusual to be unable to detect parasites in patients dying of Chagas disease,[175] although evidence of prior infection may be detected more frequently by the much more sensitive PCR technique.[176] *T. cruzi* antigen is frequently found in biopsy specimens of the heart from patients with chronic Chagas heart disease.[176] An autoimmune etiological mechanism has been proposed, and this may explain the lack of correlation of parasitemia with disease severity.[174,176,177] Based on animal models, it appears that self-reactive cytotoxic T lymphocytes develop after the initial infection and produce various cytokines.[174] A more vigorous Th 1 immune response and production of interferon-gamma against *T. cruzi* antigens can differentiate patients with cardiac involvement.[178,179] This response results in the lysis of normal host cells, perhaps related to cross-reacting antigens of *T. cruzi* and striated muscle.[171,180] A variety of antibodies against myocyte sarcoplasmic reticulum, laminin, and other constituents (most recently the cardiac beta receptor) have also been implicated in the pathogenesis of Chagas myocarditis.[181] It is thought that the acute phase results in the release from parasite-modified host cells of self-components that are immunogenic.[171] Another hypothesis suggests that cardiac parasympathetic denervation leads to eventual chronic Chagas disease.[171]

PATHOLOGY. Nerves and autonomic ganglia are frequently abnormal, and megaesophagus and megacolon may occur; less commonly, there is dilation of the stomach, duodenum, ureter, and bronchi. Different strains of *T. cruzi* may account for the geographical differences in the expression of Chagas disease; megaesophagus and megacolon are common in Brazil but quite uncommon in Central America and Mexico, and megaesophagus is unusual in Venezuela.[169] Lesions of the cardiac nerves are routinely found in patients with chronic Chagas disease, with evidence of cardiac parasympathetic denervation.[169] Pathological cardiac findings include cardiac enlargement with dilation and hypertrophy of all cardiac chambers. In more than half the patients, the left (and occasionally right) ventricular apex is thin and bulging, resembling an aneurysm.[182] Thrombus formation is frequent and may fill much of the apex; the right atrium also frequently contains thrombus. It has been suggested that these characteristic apical aneurysms (Fig. 60–8) may be the result of intravascular platelet aggregation leading to focal myocardial necrosis.[176]

The microscopic findings are principally those of extensive fibrosis, particularly of the left ventricle.[171,183] A chronic cellular infiltrate composed of lymphocytes, plasma cells, and macrophages often is present.[169] Increases in arteriole and capillary diameters have been reported.[183] Preferential involvement of the right bundle branch and the anterior fascicle of the left bundle branch by inflammatory and fibrotic changes explains the frequent occurrence of right bundle branch and left anterior fascicular block.[169] The basement membranes of capillaries, vascular smooth muscle cells, and myocytes are thickened.[176] It is unusual to be able to find parasites in the myofibers of autopsied patients.[182]

Clinical Manifestations. Clinical manifestations include anginal chest pain, symptomatic conducting system disease, and sudden death; chronic progressive heart failure, often predominantly right-sided, is the rule in advanced cases.[171] Thus, although pulmonary congestion is occasionally noted, the usual findings include fatigue due to diminished cardiac output, peripheral edema, ascites, and hepatic congestion. Tricuspid regurgitation is often present, particularly in patients with severe right-sided heart failure, although mitral regurgitation is frequently present as well. The S_2 is widely split, often with an accentuated pulmonic component, reflecting the combined effects of right bundle branch block and pulmonary hypertension. Autonomic dysfunction is common, with marked abnormalities in the expected reflex changes in heart rate produced by various maneuvers. Deaths result most commonly from pump failure or occur suddenly. Apical aneurysms and left ventricular dilation place patients at high risk for sudden death.[184]

Laboratory Findings. The chest radiograph often demonstrates severe cardiomegaly, with or without pulmonary venous hypertension. The serum aldolase level is usually elevated.[185] ECG abnormalities are the rule late in the course of the disease, particularly in patients who are seroreactive to *T. cruzi* antigen. Right bundle branch block, left anterior hemiblock, atrial fibrillation, and ventricular premature depolarizations are the most common findings in patients with chronic Chagas disease.[164,186] ST segment and T wave abnormalities also are common, as are Q waves; P wave abnormalities and atrioventricular block are seen less frequently.[169] Early in the disease, the ECG may be normal or nearly so. Administration of the antiarrhythmic agent ajmaline may precipitate the appearance of ECG abnormalities and thus identify patients with as yet clinically silent cardiac involvement.[169] Furthermore, electrophysiological testing of asymptomatic patients, even those with normal ECGs, may demonstrate abnormalities of the conducting system in many.

VENTRICULAR ARRHYTHMIAS. These are a prominent feature of chronic Chagas disease.[169,176,177] Frequent ventricular premature depolarizations, often with multiple morphologies, are seen frequently, and bouts of ventricular tachycardia can occur.[187] Ventricular arrhythmias are particularly common during and after exercise,[169] occurring in the majority of patients subjected to stress ECG testing (including some without any other clinical evidence of cardiac involvement). Ventricular tachycardia induced by electrophysiological testing is most common in patients with evidence of conduction abnormalities on the ECG, low ejection fraction, and apical left ventricular aneurysm, and may predict sudden death.[188] Syncope and sudden death due to ventricular fibrillation are constant threats and may develop

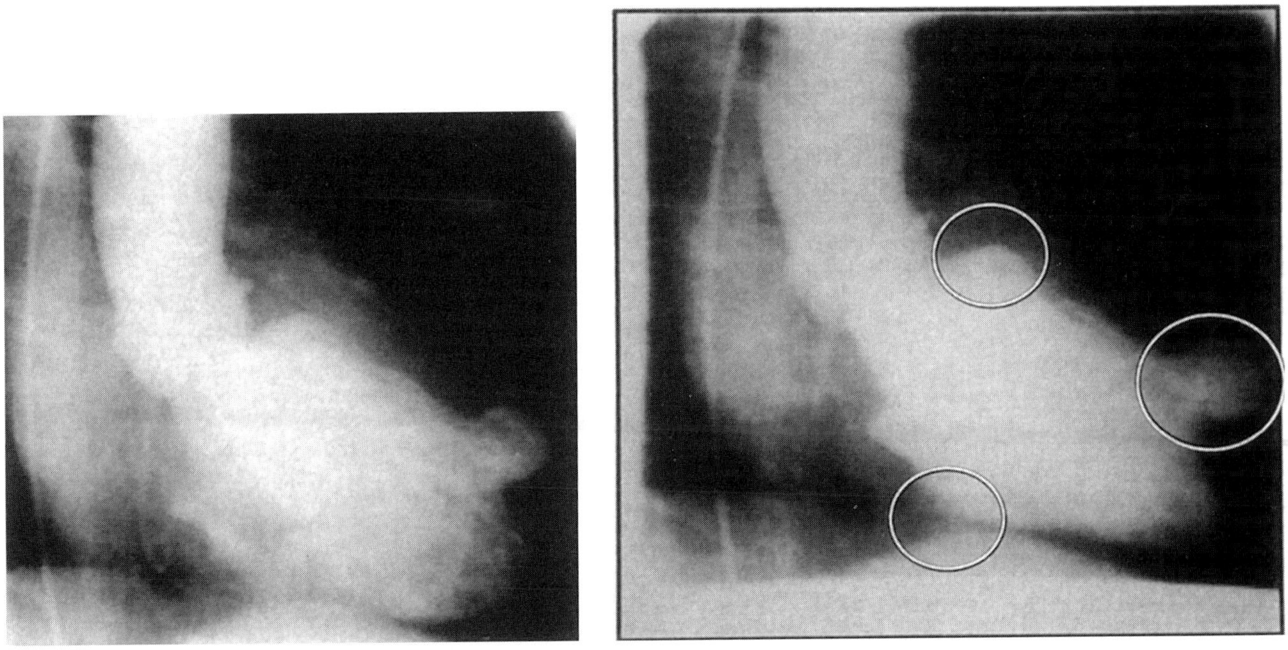

FIGURE 60–8 Left ventriculogram in the right anterior oblique view of a 55-year-old woman with chronic Chagas disease. Multiple left ventricular aneurysms are noted in anterobasal, anterior, and inferior aspects of left ventricle **(right, circled)**. (From Venegoni P, Bhatia HS: Chagas disease and ventricular arrhythmias. Circulation 96:1363, 1997. Copyright 1997, American Heart Association.)

even before cardiomegaly or heart failure.[169,189] Sinus bradycardia can also be seen, even in patients with severe heart failure when a tachycardia would be expected, presumably related to cardiac autonomic dysfunction.[169] Atrial arrhythmias, including atrial fibrillation (often with a slow ventricular response), also can occur.[169] Thromboembolic phenomena are a frequent complication, occurring in more than 50 percent of the patients.[190]

Noninvasive Imaging. The echocardiographic findings in advanced cases are those of a dilated cardiomyopathy with increased end-diastolic and end-systolic volumes and reduced ejection fraction, often with enlargement of the left atrium and right ventricle.[169] Diastolic filling of the left ventricle is frequently abnormal, even in patients without other clinical or echocardiographic evidence of cardiac involvement. In the majority of advanced cases, the echocardiographic appearance is distinctive, with left ventricular posterior wall hypokinesis and relatively preserved interventricular septal motion; an apical aneurysm is often seen on two-dimensional echocardiography. Ten to 15 percent of asymptomatic patients demonstrate apical dyskinesis. Dobutamine echocardiography may unmask chronotropic incompetence and limited myocardial contractural reserve in patients without overt heart disease.[191]

Radionuclide ventriculography may, like echocardiography, demonstrate right or left ventricular wall motion abnormalities in the absence of an overall depression of global ventricular function. Perfusion scanning with thallium-201 may show fixed defects (corresponding to areas of fibrosis) as well as evidence of reversible ischemia.[192] MRI can identify morphological and functional aspects of cardiac involvement; with the use of gadolinium as a contrast medium, it can identify patients with more active myocardial disease.[193]

Left ventricular cineangiography in advanced cases shows a dilated, hypokinetic left ventricle with one large or several apical aneurysms (Fig. 60–8) containing intracavitary thrombus, often with evidence of mitral regurgitation.[169] Coronary angiography is usually normal, although abnormalities of the coronary microcirculation have been suggested as a cause of the clinical manifestations of Chagas disease.

Serodiagnosis. The complement-fixation test (Machado-Guerreiro test) is useful in diagnosis; it has high sensitivity and specificity for the identification of chronic Chagas disease.[169] Also used in diagnosis are the indirect immunofluorescent antibody test, the enzyme-linked immunosorbent assay, and the hemagglutination test.[169] Perhaps the most widely used test in endemic areas is the detection of parasites in the blood of patients with chronic Chagas disease (which occurs in upward of 50 percent of cases) by means of xenodiagnosis.[194] The patient is bitten by reduviid bugs bred in the laboratory; the subsequent identification of parasites in the intestine of the insect is proof of infection in the human host.

MANAGEMENT. The treatment of Chagas disease remains difficult; although slowly progressive at first, once cardiac decompensation develops, there is usually a rapid and inexorable progression to death, which is usually due to arrhythmia, although congestive failure and systemic thromboembolism account for additional mortality.[195] Patients at greatest risk of mortality are those with left ventricular enlargement and especially those with impaired left ventricular function.[186,189] Patients with Chagas disease may respond to beta blockade, and there is some evidence that captopril, early in the course of disease, may alleviate disease in animal models.[196] Major efforts are aimed at interrupting transmission of the parasite to humans; such vector control methods have been generally successful.[169] They may prevent not only the initial infection but also reinfection that may play a role in determining the severity of the resulting cardiomyopathy.

Amiodarone appears to be effective in controlling the ventricular arrhythmias frequently seen in patients with Chagas disease, although whether this translates into improved survival remains to be established.[195] Implantable cardioverter defibrillators are useful, and the indications are similar to those in patients with life-threatening arrhythmias associated with other causes (see Chap. 31),[197] but this is not a practical option for the vast majority of patients (owing to financial constraints). Anticoagulation may be of some benefit in preventing recurrent thromboembolic episodes.[190] Although antiparasitic agents such as nifurtimox, benzimidazole, and itraconazole are effective in reducing parasitemia and are useful in acute disease, no evidence indicates that they are efficacious in curing the late phases of the disease.[169,198] A promising avenue of approach appears to be immunoprophylaxis, although a clinically useful vaccine is not yet available. Heart transplantations have been performed in a few patients, but the results so far appear to be inferior to those found in patients with other conditions, and neoplasms as well as episodes of parasitemia and recurrent Chagas disease may be a problem.[199-201]

Other protozoal causes of myocarditis include African trypanosomiasis,[202] toxoplasmosis,[203,204] and malaria.[205,206]

Metazoal Myocardial Diseases

ECHINOCOCCUS (HYDATID CYST). *Echinococcus* is endemic in many sheep-raising areas of the world, particularly Argentina, Uruguay, New Zealand, Greece, North Africa, and Iceland, but cardiac involvement in patients with hydatid disease is uncommon, occurring in less than 2 percent of cases.[207] The usual host of *Echinococcus granulosus* is the dog, but humans may serve as intermediate hosts (rather than the sheep, the usual intermediate host) if they accidentally ingest ova from contaminated dog feces.

When cardiac involvement is present, the cysts usually are intramyocardial in the interventricular septum or left ventricular free wall (Fig. 60–9); involvement of the right ventricle or atrium may occur.[207] Involvement of the tricuspid valve can be seen on occasion; in most cases, a single cardiac cyst is present.

A myocardial cyst can degenerate and calcify, develop daughter cysts, or rupture. Rupture of the cyst is the most dreaded complication; rupture into the pericardium can result in acute pericarditis, which may progress to chronic constrictive pericarditis.[207] Rupture into the cardiac chambers can result in systemic or pulmonary emboli.[208] Rapidly progressive pulmonary hypertension can occur with rupture of right-sided cysts, with subsequent embolization of hundreds of scolices into the pulmonary circulation. The liberation of hydatid fluid into the circulation can produce profound, fatal circulatory collapse due to an anaphylactic reaction to the protein constituents of the fluid.[207]

Symptoms depend on the location, size, and integrity of the cyst; patients may be asymptomatic or in profound circulatory collapse. It is estimated that only about 10 percent of patients with cardiac hydatid cysts have clinical manifestations.[207] The ECG may reflect the location of the cyst: T-wave changes and loss of QRS voltage can occur with left ventricular involvement, whereas atrioventricular conduction defects or right bundle branch block can be seen with involvement of the interventricular septum. Chest pain is usually due to rupture of the cyst into the pericardial space with resultant pericarditis. Large cystic masses sometimes produce right-sided obstruction.[207]

Diagnosis. Recognition of an echinococcal cyst of the heart is a relatively simple matter if there is evidence of cysts in other organs, particularly the liver and lung. However, a cardiac cyst can be an isolated, solitary finding. The chest radiograph frequently shows an abnormal cardiac silhouette or a calcified lobular mass adjacent to the left ventricle.[201] Although computed tomography (CT) and MRI may aid in the detection and localization of heart cysts, two-dimensional echocardiography is thought to be the best choice (see Fig. 60–9).[207] Eosinophilia, present in some patients, is a useful adjunctive finding. The Casoni skin test is not very helpful because both false-positive and false-negative results occur. Serological tests, including hemagglutination and complement fixation, may be more useful, but their predictive accuracy is limited.[207]

Management. Until recently, treatment for hydatid disease was limited to surgical excision.[209] Experience suggests that the benzimidazole derivatives mebendazole and albendazole are somewhat useful in the medical management of this disease.[207,210] Despite the availability of drug therapy, adjunctive surgical excision is generally recommended, even for asymptomatic patients, because of the significant risk of rupture of the cyst and its attendant serious and sometimes fatal consequences.[207] The surgical results generally have been favorable.[211]

TRICHINOSIS. Infestation with *Trichinella spiralis* is a common human finding. Mild myocarditis has been said to be a frequent finding, but recent data suggest that clinically detectable cardiac involvement occurs in only a minority of patients.[212] Symptomatic involvement is uncommon and may be responsible for the majority of fatalities.[213] Less frequently, death is due to pulmonary embolism secondary to venous thrombosis or neurological complications.

Although the parasite can invade the heart, it does not usually encyst there, and it is rare to find larvae or larval fragments in the myocardium. Nonetheless, pathological findings at autopsy can be impressive. The heart may be dilated and flabby, and a pericardial effusion may be present.[212] A prominent focal infiltrate composed of lymphocytes and eosinophils is commonly found, with occasional microthrombi in the intramural arterioles. Areas of muscle degeneration and necrosis are present.

Clinical Manifestations. Myocarditis is usually mild and goes unnoticed, but in occasional cases it is manifested by congestive heart failure and chest pain, usually appearing around the third week of the disease, when the general constitutional symptoms are abating. Physical examination findings may be normal, or there may be gross cardiomegaly with severe congestive heart failure. Sudden death can occur, usually in the fourth to eighth week of the illness.

Electrocardiographic abnormalities are detected in about 10 percent of patients with trichinosis and parallel the time course of clinical cardiac involvement, initially appearing in the second or third week and usually resolving by the seventh week of the illness. The most common ECG abnormalities are repolarization abnormalities and ventricular premature complexes.[212] The ECG changes usually resolve completely.

The diagnosis is usually based on the demonstration of a positive indirect immunofluorescent antibody test in a patient with the clinical features of trichinosis. Eosinophilia, when present, is a supportive finding. The skin test is usually but not invariably positive. Treatment is with anthelmintics and corticosteroids; dramatic improvement in cardiac function has been reported after their use.

Other metazoal causes of myocarditis include visceral larva migrans[214,215] and schistosomiasis.[216]

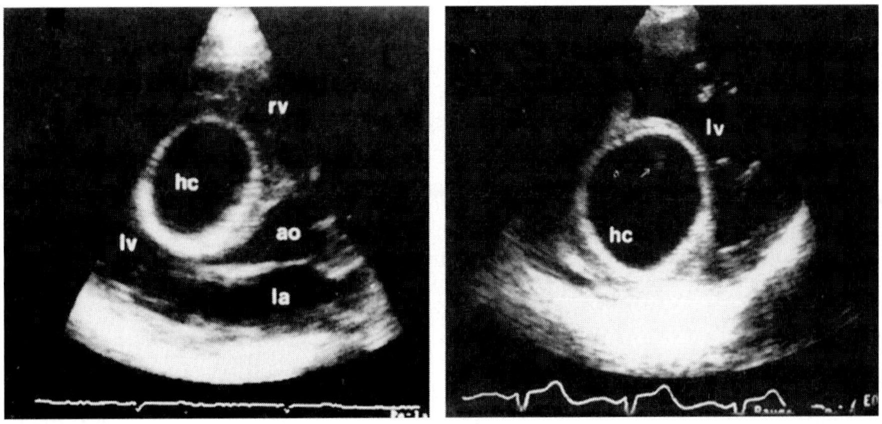

FIGURE 60–9 Involvement of interventricular septum by a hydatid cyst. **Left,** Transthoracic two-dimensional echocardiogram of parasternal long-axis view showing a 3-cm diameter hydatid cyst (hc) in the upper ventricular septum. **Right,** Transesophageal echocardiography showing a hydatid cyst (hc) having a rounded and well-contrasted capsule. ao = aorta; la = left atrium; lv = left ventricle; rv = right ventricle. (From Aupetit J, Ritz B, Ferrini M, et al: Images in cardiovascular medicine: Hydatid cyst of the interventricular septum. Circulation 95:2325, 1997. Copyright 1997, American Heart Association.)

Toxic, Chemical, Immune, and Physical Damage to the Heart

A wide variety of substances other than infectious agents can act on the heart and damage the myocardium. In some cases, the damage is acute, transient, and associated with evidence of an inflammatory myocardial infiltrate with myocyte necrosis (e.g., with the arsenicals and lithium); in other cases, a hypersensitivity reaction occurs, without prominent evidence of necrosis (e.g., with sulfonamides). Other agents that damage the myocardium can lead to chronic changes with resulting histological evidence of fibrosis and a clinical picture of a dilated cardiomyopathy. Furthermore, many offending stimuli are associated with both acute and chronic phases (e.g., alcohol, doxorubicin). The extent of myocardial damage often is related to the dose and rate of exposure to the toxin.

Numerous chemicals and drugs (both industrial and therapeutic) can lead to cardiac damage and dysfunction. Several physical agents (e.g., radiation and excessive heat) can also contribute to myocardial damage.

Toxic Agents

The cardiac effects of ethanol, cocaine, amphetamines, catecholamines, ergot, appetite suppressants, and Taxol are discussed in Chapter 62. The effects of the antineoplastic agents daunorubicin, cyclophosphamide, and 5-fluorouracil are discussed in Chapter 83. The cardiac effects of tricyclic antidepressants and phenothiazines are discussed further in Chapter 84.

TRICYCLIC ANTIDEPRESSANTS. Although sinus tachycardia, postural hypotension, disturbances in rhythm, abnormalities of atrioventricular conduction, and even sudden death can be seen in patients taking tricyclic antidepressants, particularly when they are taken as an overdose, important depression of left ventricular function usually does not occur, even in patients with preexisting heart disease.[217] There has been concern when using tricyclic antidepressants in patients with prior myocardial infarction and/or preexisting ventricular arrhythmias because these agents have a class I antiarrhythmic effect, prolong the QT interval, and might be proarrhythmic in these settings. The selective serotonin reuptake inhibitors are remarkably free of cardiovascular toxicity and do not appear to depress ventricular function.[217] They may produce side effects by interacting with the metabolism of drugs mediated through the cytochrome-P450 enzyme system.

PHENOTHIAZINES. The phenothiazines are associated with a variety of cardiac disturbances, including ECG changes, atrial and ventricular arrhythmias, and sudden death.[218,219] Postural hypotension can also be seen. The cardiac effects are largely dose dependent. ECG abnormalities can be observed with as little as 200 mg of thioridazine per day and consist of lengthening of the QT interval and T wave changes. Prolongation of the QT interval can set the stage for the emergence of ventricular arrhythmias, particularly torsades de pointes.[218,219] Higher doses may lead to frank T wave inversion and increased amplitude of the U wave. Changes in the P wave, QRS complex, and ST segment are usually absent. The ECG abnormalities and arrhythmias resolve with discontinuation of the drug, usually within 48 hours. An occasional patient requires temporary ventricular pacing.

Pathological changes in the hearts of patients who have received phenothiazines and who have died suddenly include the deposition of acid mucopolysaccharide between muscle bundles in periarteriolar regions as well as the conduction system, with myofibrillar degeneration and endothelial proliferation in the smaller blood vessels, although a direct causal relationship between drug administration and cardiomyopathic changes is only inferential. A variety of explanations have been invoked for the apparent cardiac damage, including direct toxic effects of the phenothiazines on the myocardium, stimulation of higher autonomic centers, and changes in circulating or myocardial levels of catecholamines.

CARBON MONOXIDE. Both acute and chronic carbon monoxide toxicity can occur. Although central nervous system findings usually dominate the clinical presentation, significant and occasionally fatal cardiac abnormalities have been reported, although some investigators have found no precipitation of arrhythmias following exposure.[220,221] Because carbon monoxide has a higher affinity for hemoglobin than does oxygen, reduced amounts of oxygen are delivered to the tissues. Thus, the cardiac toxicity may be partially caused by myocardial hypoxia, but a direct toxic effect of the gas on myocardial mitochondria may play an even more important role.[222] The histological features include focal areas of necrosis, most marked in the subendocardium. Focal perivascular infiltrates and punctate hemorrhages are also seen.[222]

Cardiac involvement can appear promptly after exposure or it can be delayed for up to several days. Palpitations, sinus tachycardia, and various arrhythmias, including ventricular extrasystoles and atrial fibrillation, are common.[223] Bradycardia and atrioventricular block can occur in more severe cases.[223] In patients with ischemic heart disease, angina pectoris and myocardial infarction can be precipitated. ECG ST segment and T wave abnormalities are quite common. Transient right and/or left ventricular wall motion abnormalities can be present.[222] Administration of 100 percent oxygen, bed rest, and surveillance for serious rhythm or conduction abnormalities usually permit rapid recovery.

Other Agents

Other toxic, chemical, immune, and physical agents that can be damaging to the heart include the following:

- Interferon-alpha[224]
- Interleukin-2[225]
- Clozapine[226]
- Emetine[227]
- Methysergide[228]
- Chloroquine[229]
- Antimony compounds[230,231]
- Lithium[232,233]
- Hydrocarbons[234,235]
- Lead[236]
- Hypocalcemia[237,238]
- Hypophosphatemia[239,240]
- Hypomagnesemia[241,242]
- Wasp stings[243]
- Snake bite[244,245]
- Arsenic[246]
- Carnitine[247,248]
- Selenium[249,250]
- Scorpion sting[251,252]
- Ephedra[253,254]

Hypersensitivity

Allergic reactions to a variety of agents can involve the myocardium. A number of drugs (most commonly the sulfonamides, hydrochlorothiazide, the penicillins, and methyldopa) or other sensitizers may lead to an allergic myocarditis (Table 60–3), characterized by peripheral eosinophilia and a perivascular infiltration of the myocardium by eosinophils, lymphocytes, and histiocytes; necrosis is seen on occasion.[255] Hypersensitivity myocarditis is rarely recognized clinically and is often first discovered at postmortem examination, although it is occasionally diagnosed on endomyocardial biopsy.[256] Most patients who have hypersensitivity myocarditis are not critically ill, but nevertheless may die suddenly, presumably as a consequence of an arrhythmia. Patients with hypersensitivity may develop an arteritis, and acute myocardial infarction rarely occurs.[257] An occasional patient has intense eosinophilic infiltration of the myocardium of no obvious cause, with prominent necrosis evident and findings of hemodynamic collapse; some of these patients have undiagnosed hypersensitivity myocarditis.[255] Because of the potential for significant deleterious effects, a high index of suspicion for this condition should be maintained. Therapy includes discontinuation of the offending agent and corticosteroids and/or immunosuppression therapy in severe cases.

TABLE 60–3 Principal Drugs Capable of Causing Hypersensitivity Myocarditis

Antibiotics	**Antiinflammatory**
Amphotericin B	Indomethacin
Ampicillin	Oxyphenbutazone
Chloramphenicol	Phenylbutazone
Penicillin	
Tetracycline	**Diuretics**
Streptomycin	Acetazolamide
	Chlorthalidone
Sulfonamides	Hydrochlorothiazide
Sulfadiazine	Spironolactone
Sulfisoxazole	
	Others
Anticonvulsants	Amitriptyline
Phenindione	Methyldopa
Phenytoin	Sulfonylureas
Carbamazepine	Tetanus toxoid
Antituberculous	
Isoniazid	
Paraaminosalicylic acid	

From Kounis NG, Zavras GM, Soufras GD, Kitrou MP: Hypersensitivity myocarditis. Ann Allergy 62:71, 1989.

METHYLDOPA. Although hepatitis is the most frequently encountered serious adverse reaction to methyldopa, sudden and unexpected death has been reported in a number of patients found at necropsy to have had an unsuspected myocarditis.[258] The histological findings have the characteristics of an allergic myocarditis, showing an interstitial inflammatory infiltrate with abundant eosinophils, vasculitis, and focal myocardial necrosis. ECG changes include sinus bradycardia, sinus pauses, and first- and second-degree atrioventricular block.

PENICILLIN. Allergic reactions to penicillin are fairly common, but myocardial involvement is rare.[259] Histological findings consist of a perivascular and interstitial infiltrate composed of eosinophils and mononuclear cells. Both myocardial infarction and pericarditis may occur and account for some of the ECG changes.[259] Transient ECG changes may be the only manifestation of cardiac involvement, with sinus tachycardia, ST segment elevation, and T wave inversion.

SULFONAMIDES. Use of sulfonamides can result in myocardial damage owing to a hypersensitivity vasculitis as well as a myocarditis.[255] In fatal cases, eosinophilic myocarditis, sometimes with granulomas, can be demonstrated.[258] Although usually clinically silent, myocardial involvement can produce severe and even fatal congestive heart failure. ECG changes are usually absent, but nonspecific ST segment and T wave abnormalities are sometimes seen.

TETRACYCLINE. Allergic reactions to antibiotics of the tetracycline class include fever, tachycardia, and first-degree atrioventricular block. Postmortem findings include cardiac dilation, fibrinoid muscle cell degeneration, and a diffuse interstitial and perivascular infiltrate.[255]

Physical Agents

RADIATION (see Chap. 83). The use of radiation therapy can result in a variety of cardiac complications, which are usually chronic and include pericarditis with effusion, tamponade, or constriction; coronary artery fibrosis and myocardial infarction; valvular abnormalities; myocardial fibrosis; and conduction disturbances.[260] Although the heart has been regarded as one of the organs more resistant to the effects of radiation, the clinical significance of radiation-induced heart disease is greater than often appreciated.[258] Although radiation probably results in some degree of tissue damage in all patients, clinically significant cardiac involvement occurs in the minority of patients, usually long after the radiation treatment has ended.[260] Radiation-induced cardiac damage is related to the dose of radiation, the mass of heart irradiated, and the dose schedule of the radiation.

The late cardiac damage that may follow irradiation appears to result from a long-lasting injury of the capillary endothelial cells, which leads to cell death, capillary rupture, and microthrombi.[260,261] Because of this damage to the microvasculature, ischemia results and is followed by myocardial fibrosis. In addition to microvascular damage, the major epicardial coronary arteries can become narrowed, especially at the ostia.[261,262]

Only an occasional patient manifests acute clinical cardiac abnormality with radiation therapy; typically, this consists of acute pericarditis. A mild, transient, asymptomatic depression of left ventricular function is sometimes seen early after radiation therapy. The more common clinical expressions of radiation heart disease occur months or years after the exposure. The pericardium is the most common site of clinical involvement, with findings of chronic pericardial effusion or pericardial constriction (see Chap. 64).[260] Myocardial damage occurs less frequently and is characterized by myocardial fibrosis with or without endocardial fibrosis or fibroelastosis. Left and/or right ventricular dysfunction at rest or with exercise appears to be a common, albeit usually asymptomatic, finding 5 to 20 years after radiation therapy, especially in patients in whom the now-outmoded technique of a single anteroposterior port was used.[260] Occasional patients develop usually asymptomatic left-sided (and rarely right-sided) valvular regurgitation (or on occasion stenosis) that sometimes requires valve replacement, particularly when associated with calcification of the mitral or aortic valves.[261,263,264] Often there is a latent period of a decade or more between the radiation exposure and the development of valvular deformity.[261] ECG abnormalities, heart block, accelerated atherosclerosis, and a variety of arrhythmias may be seen months or years after therapeutic radiation, although usually they are of limited clinical significance.[260,262,265]

Heat Stroke

Heat stroke results from failure of the thermoregulatory center following exposure to high ambient temperature. It is manifested principally by hyperpyrexia, renal insufficiency, disseminated intravascular coagulation, and central nervous system dysfunction.[266] However, cardiovascular abnormalities (usually ECG) appear to be common; pulmonary edema and transient right and/or left ventricular dysfunction may occur, along with hypotension and circulatory collapse. Pathological changes include dilation of the right side of the heart, particularly the right atrium. Hemorrhages of the subendocardium and the subepicardium are frequently seen at necropsy and often involve the interventricular septum and posterior wall of the left ventricle. Histological findings include degeneration and necrosis of muscle fibers as well as interstitial edema. Factors that have been implicated as possible causes of myocardial damage include direct thermal injury, myocardial hypoxia resulting from circulatory collapse, decreased coronary blood flow, and metabolic abnormalities resulting from widespread injury to other organs.

Sinus tachycardia is invariably present,[266] whereas atrial and ventricular arrhythmias usually are absent. Transient prolongation of the QT interval may be seen along with ST segment and T wave abnormalities. It can take up to several months for these repolarization abnormalities to resolve. Serum enzyme levels can be elevated and may reflect myocardial damage, at least in part, although concomitant rhabdomyolysis often is present.

Hypothermia

Low temperature can also result in myocardial damage.[267] Cardiac dilation can occur, with epicardial petechiae and subendocardial hemorrhages. Microinfarcts are found in the ventricular myocardium, presumably related to abnormalities in the microcirculation. The lesions are not caused by the low temperature per se but appear to be the result of the circulatory collapse, hemoconcentration, capillary slugging, and depressed cellular metabolism that accompany hypothermia. Clinical manifestations of hypothermia include sinus bradycardia, conduction disturbances, atrial (and occasionally ventricular) fibrillation, hypotension, a fall in cardiac output, reversible myocardial depression, and a characteristic deflection of the terminal portion of the QRS pattern (Osborn wave).[263] Treatment includes core warming (often utilizing extracorporeal blood warming), cardiopulmonary resuscitation, and management of pulmonary, hematological, and renal complications.[268,269] Notwithstanding its potential cardiac risks, mild therapeutic hypothermia appears to improve neurological outcome after cardiac arrest and is a currently accepted practice.

REFERENCES

Primary Myocarditis

1. Abelmann WH: Virus and the heart. Circulation 44:950, 1971.
2. Woodruff JF: Viral myocarditis: A review. Am J Pathol 101:425, 1980.
3. Kawai C: From myocarditis to cardiomyopathy: Mechanisms of inflammation and cell death: Learning from the past for the future. Circulation 99:1091, 1999.
4. Liu PP, Mason JW: Advances in the understanding of myocarditis. Circulation 104:1076, 2001.
5. Lange LG, Schreiner GF: Immune mechanisms of cardiac disease. N Engl J Med 330:112, 1994.
6. Liu PP, Opavsky MA: Viral myocarditis: Receptors that bridge the cardiovascular with the immune system? Circ Res 86:253, 2000.
7. Knowlton KU, Badorff C: The immune system in viral myocarditis: Maintaining the balance. Circ Res 85:559, 1999.
8. Liu PP, Le J, Nian M: Nuclear factor-kappaB decoy: Infiltrating the heart of the matter in inflammatory heart disease. Circ Res 89:850, 2001.
9. Eriksson U, Kurrer MO, Schmitz N, et al: Interleukin-6-deficient mice resist development of autoimmune myocarditis associated with impaired upregulation of complement C3. Circulation 107:320, 2003.
10. Watanabe K, Nakazawa M, Fuse K, et al: Protection against autoimmune myocarditis by gene transfer of interleukin-10 by electroporation. Circulation 104:1098, 2001.
11. Seko Y, Kayagaki N, Seino K, et al: Role of Fas/FasL pathway in the activation of infiltrating cells in murine acute myocarditis caused by Coxsackievirus B3. J Am Coll Cardiol 39:1399, 2002.
12. Bryant D, Becker L, Richardson J, et al: Cardiac failure in transgenic mice with myocardial expression of tumor necrosis factor-alpha. Circulation 97:1375, 1998.
13. Li J, Schwimmbeck PL, Tschope C, et al: Collagen degradation in a murine myocarditis model: Relevance of matrix metalloproteinase in association with inflammatory induction. Cardiovasc Res 56:235, 2002.
14. McLaughlin L, Zhu G, Mistry M, et al: Apolipoprotein J/clusterin limits the severity of murine autoimmune myocarditis. J Clin Invest 106:1105, 2000.
15. Opavsky MA, Penninger J, Aitken K, et al: Susceptibility to myocarditis is dependent on the response of alphabeta T lymphocytes to coxsackieviral infection. Circ Res 85:551, 1999.
16. Mendes LA, Picard MH, Dec GW, et al: Ventricular remodeling in active myocarditis. Myocarditis Treatment Trial. Am Heart J 138:303, 1999.
17. Finkel MS: Nitric oxide and viral cardiomyopathy. Circulation 102:2162, 2000.
18. Fukuchi M, Hussain SN, Giaid A: Heterogeneous expression and activity of endothelial and inducible nitric oxide synthases in end-stage human heart failure: Their relation to lesion site and beta-adrenergic receptor therapy. Circulation 98:132, 1998.
19. Badorff C, Fichtlscherer B, Rhoads RE, et al: Nitric oxide inhibits dystrophin proteolysis by coxsackieviral protease 2A through S-nitrosylation: A protective mechanism against enteroviral cardiomyopathy. Circulation 102:2276, 2000.
20. Lowenstein CJ, Hill SL, Lafond-Walker A, et al: Nitric oxide inhibits viral replication in murine myocarditis. J Clin Invest 97:1837, 1996.
21. Zaragoza C, Ocampo C, Saura M, et al: The role of inducible nitric oxide synthase in the host response to Coxsackievirus myocarditis. Proc Natl Acad Sci U S A 95:2469, 1998.
22. Wessely R, Henke A, Zell R, et al: Low-level expression of a mutant coxsackieviral cDNA induces a myocytopathic effect in culture: An approach to the study of enteroviral persistence in cardiac myocytes. Circulation 98:450, 1998.
23. Li Y, Bourlet T, Andreoletti L, et al: Enteroviral capsid protein VP1 is present in myocardial tissues from some patients with myocarditis or dilated cardiomyopathy. Circulation 101:231, 2000.

24. Zhang HM, Yanagawa B, Cheung P, et al: Nip21 gene expression reduces coxsackievirus B3 replication by promoting apoptotic cell death via a mitochondria-dependent pathway. Circ Res 90:1251, 2002.
25. Shioi T, Matsumori A, Sasayama S: Persistent expression of cytokine in the chronic stage of viral myocarditis in mice. Circulation 94:2930, 1996.
26. Sole MJ, Liu P: Viral myocarditis: A paradigm for understanding the pathogenesis and treatment of dilated cardiomyopathy. J Am Coll Cardiol 22:99A, 1993.

Clinical Manifestations

27. Angelini A, Calzolari V, Calabrese F, et al: Myocarditis mimicking acute myocardial infarction: Role of endomyocardial biopsy in the differential diagnosis. Heart 84:245, 2000.
28. Sarda L, Colin P, Boccara F, et al: Myocarditis in patients with clinical presentation of myocardial infarction and normal coronary angiograms. J Am Coll Cardiol 37:786, 2001.
29. Chimenti C, Calabrese F, Thiene G, et al: Inflammatory left ventricular microaneurysms as a cause of apparently idiopathic ventricular tachyarrhythmias. Circulation 104:168, 2001.
30. Badorff C, Zeiher AM, Hohnloser SH: Torsade de pointes tachycardia as a rare manifestation of acute enteroviral myocarditis. Heart 86:489, 2001.
31. Theleman KP, Kuiper JJ, Roberts WC: Acute myocarditis (predominately lymphocytic) causing sudden death without heart failure. Am J Cardiol 88:1078, 2001.
32. Maron BJ, Shirani J, Poliac LC, et al: Sudden death in young competitive athletes: Clinical, demographic, and pathological profiles. JAMA 276:199, 1996.
33. Frustaci A, Chimenti C, Bellocci F, et al: Histological substrate of atrial biopsies in patients with lone atrial fibrillation. Circulation 96:1180, 1997.
34. Smith SC, Ladenson JH, Mason JW, et al: Elevations of cardiac troponin I associated with myocarditis: Experimental and clinical correlates. Circulation 95:163, 1997.
35. Torre-Amione G, Kapadia S, Benedict C, et al: Proinflammatory cytokine levels in patients with depressed left ventricular ejection fraction: A report from the Studies of Left Ventricular Dysfunction (SOLVD). J Am Coll Cardiol 27:1201, 1996.
36. Toyozaki T, Hiroe M, Saito T, et al: Levels of soluble Fas in patients with myocarditis, heart failure of unknown origin, and in healthy volunteers. Am J Cardiol 81:798, 1998.
37. Felker GM, Boehmer JP, Hruban RH, et al: Echocardiographic findings in fulminant and acute myocarditis. J Am Coll Cardiol 36:227, 2000.
38. Dec GW, Palacios I, Yasuda T, et al: Antimyosin antibody cardiac imaging: Its role in the diagnosis of myocarditis. J Am Coll Cardiol 16:97, 1990.
39. O'Connell JB, Henkin RE, Robinson JA, et al: Gallium-67 imaging in patients with dilated cardiomyopathy and biopsy-proven myocarditis. Circulation 70:58, 1984.
40. Laissy JP, Messin B, Varenne O, et al: MRI of acute myocarditis: A comprehensive approach based on various imaging sequences. Chest 122:1638, 2002.
41. Manolio TA, Baughman KL, Rodeheffer R, et al: Prevalence and etiology of idiopathic dilated cardiomyopathy (summary of a National Heart, Lung, and Blood Institute workshop). Am J Cardiol 69:1458, 1992.
42. Dec GW Jr, Palacios IF, Fallon JT, et al: Active myocarditis in the spectrum of acute dilated cardiomyopathies: Clinical features, histologic correlates, and clinical outcome. N Engl J Med 312:885, 1985.
43. Felker GM, Hu W, Hare JM, et al: The spectrum of dilated cardiomyopathy. The Johns Hopkins experience with 1,278 patients. Medicine (Baltimore) 78:270, 1999.
44. Felker GM, Thompson RE, Hare JM, et al: Underlying causes and long-term survival in patients with initially unexplained cardiomyopathy. N Engl J Med 342:1077, 2000.
45. Aretz HT, Billingham ME, Edwards WD, et al: Myocarditis: A histopathologic definition and classification. Am J Cardiovasc Pathol 1:3, 1987.
46. Chow LH, Radio SJ, Sears TD, et al: Insensitivity of right ventricular endomyocardial biopsy in the diagnosis of myocarditis. J Am Coll Cardiol 14:915, 1989.
47. Herskowitz A, Ahmed-Ansari A, Neumann DA, et al: Induction of major histocompatibility complex antigens within the myocardium of patients with active myocarditis: A nonhistologic marker of myocarditis. J Am Coll Cardiol 15:624, 1990.
48. Seko Y, Takahashi N, Ishiyama S, et al: Expression of costimulatory molecules B7-1, B7-2, and CD40 in the heart of patients with acute myocarditis and dilated cardiomyopathy. Circulation 97:637, 1998.
49. Satoh M, Nakamura M, Satoh H, et al: Expression of tumor necrosis factor-alpha–converting enzyme and tumor necrosis factor-alpha in human myocarditis. J Am Coll Cardiol 36:1288, 2000.
50. Alter P, Jobmann M, Meyer E, et al: Apoptosis in myocarditis and dilated cardiomyopathy: Does enterovirus genome persistence protect from apoptosis? An endomyocardial biopsy study. Cardiovasc Pathol 10:229, 2001.
51. Neumann DA, Rose NR, Ansari AA, et al: Induction of multiple heart autoantibodies in mice with coxsackievirus B3- and cardiac myosin-induced autoimmune myocarditis. J Immunol 152:343, 1994.
52. Limas CJ, Goldenberg IF, Limas C: Autoantibodies against beta-adrenoceptors in human idiopathic dilated cardiomyopathy. Circ Res 64:97, 1989.
53. Lieberman EB, Hutchins GM, Herskowitz A, et al: Clinicopathologic description of myocarditis. J Am Coll Cardiol 18:1617, 1991.
54. McCarthy RE 3rd, Boehmer JP, Hruban RH, et al: Long-term outcome of fulminant myocarditis as compared with acute (nonfulminant) myocarditis. N Engl J Med 342:690, 2000.
55. Aoyama N, Izumi T, Hiramori K, et al: National survey of fulminant myocarditis in Japan: Therapeutic guidelines and long-term prognosis of using percutaneous cardiopulmonary support for fulminant myocarditis (special report from a scientific committee). Circ J 66:133, 2002.
56. Deckers JW, Hare JM, Baughman KL: Complications of transvenous right ventricular endomyocardial biopsy in adult patients with cardiomyopathy: A seven-year survey of 546 consecutive diagnostic procedures in a tertiary referral center. J Am Coll Cardiol 19:43, 1992.
57. Denys BG, Uretsky BF, Reddy PS: Ultrasound-assisted cannulation of the internal jugular vein: A prospective comparison to the external landmark-guided technique. Circulation 87:1557, 1993.

Treatment of Primary Myocarditis

58. Wang WZ, Matsumori A, Yamada T, et al: Beneficial effects of amlodipine in a murine model of congestive heart failure induced by viral myocarditis: A possible mechanism through inhibition of nitric oxide production. Circulation 95:245, 1997.
59. Nishio R, Shioi T, Sasayama S, et al: Carvedilol increases the production of interleukin-12 and interferon-gamma and improves the survival of mice infected with the encephalomyocarditis virus. J Am Coll Cardiol 41:340, 2003.
60. Rezkalla SH, Raikar S, Kloner RA: Treatment of viral myocarditis with focus on captopril. Am J Cardiol 77:634, 1996.
61. Bozkurt B, Villaneuva FS, Holubkov R, et al: Intravenous immune globulin in the therapy of peripartum cardiomyopathy. J Am Coll Cardiol 34:177, 1999.
62. McNamara DM, Holubkov R, Starling RC, et al: Controlled trial of intravenous immune globulin in recent-onset dilated cardiomyopathy. Circulation 103:2254, 2001.
63. Kereiakes DJ, Parmley WW: Myocarditis and cardiomyopathy. Am Heart J 108:1318, 1984.
64. Parrillo JE, Cunnion RE, Epstein SE, et al: A prospective, randomized, controlled trial of prednisone for dilated cardiomyopathy. N Engl J Med 321:1061, 1989.
65. Mason JW, O'Connell JB, Herskowitz A, et al: A clinical trial of immunosuppressive therapy for myocarditis. The Myocarditis Treatment Trial Investigators. N Engl J Med 333:269, 1995.
66. Jones SR, Herskowitz A, Hutchins GM, et al: Effects of immunosuppressive therapy in biopsy-proved myocarditis and borderline myocarditis on left ventricular function. Am J Cardiol 68:370, 1991.
67. Wojnicz R, Nowalany-Kozielska E, Wojciechowska C, et al: Randomized, placebo-controlled study for immunosuppressive treatment of inflammatory dilated cardiomyopathy: Two-year follow-up results. Circulation 104:39, 2001.
68. Frustaci A, Chimenti C, Calabrese F, et al: Immunosuppressive therapy for active lymphocytic myocarditis: Virological and immunologic profile of responders versus nonresponders. Circulation 107:857, 2003.
69. Kato S, Morimoto S, Hiramitsu S, et al: Use of percutaneous cardiopulmonary support of patients with fulminant myocarditis and cardiogenic shock for improving prognosis. Am J Cardiol 83:623, 1999.
70. Rockman HA, Adamson RM, Dembitsky WP, et al: Acute fulminant myocarditis: Long-term follow-up after circulatory support with left ventricular assist device. Am Heart J 121:922, 1991.
71. Felix SB, Staudt A, Landsberger M, et al: Removal of cardiodepressant antibodies in dilated cardiomyopathy by immunoadsorption. J Am Coll Cardiol 39:646, 2002.
72. Hofling K, Kim KS, Leser JS, et al: Progress toward vaccines against viruses that cause heart disease. Herz 25:286, 2000.
73. Cooper LT Jr, Berry GJ, Shabetai R: Idiopathic giant-cell myocarditis: Natural history and treatment. Multicenter Giant Cell Myocarditis Study Group Investigators. N Engl J Med 336:1860, 1997.
74. Nash CL, Panaccione R, Sutherland LR, et al: Giant cell myocarditis, in a patient with Crohn's disease, treated with etanercept—a tumour necrosis factor-alpha antagonist. Can J Gastroenterol 15:607, 2001.
75. Hyogo M, Kamitani T, Oguni A, et al: Acute necrotizing eosinophilic myocarditis with giant cell infiltration after remission of idiopathic thrombocytopenic purpura. Intern Med 36:894, 1997.
76. Frustaci A, Cuoco L, Chimenti C, et al: Celiac disease associated with autoimmune myocarditis. Circulation 105:2611, 2002.
77. Daniels PR, Berry GJ, Tazelaar HD, et al: Giant cell myocarditis as a manifestation of drug hypersensitivity. Cardiovasc Pathol 9:287, 2000.
78. Shields RC, Tazelaar HD, Berry GJ, et al: The role of right ventricular endomyocardial biopsy for idiopathic giant cell myocarditis. J Card Fail 8:74, 2002.
79. Okura Y, Dec GW, Hare JM, et al: A clinical and histopathologic comparison of cardiac sarcoidosis and idiopathic giant cell myocarditis. J Am Coll Cardiol 41:322, 2003.
80. Litovsky SH, Burke AP, Virmani R: Giant cell myocarditis: An entity distinct from sarcoidosis characterized by multiphasic myocyte destruction by cytotoxic T cells and histiocytic giant cells. Mod Pathol 9:1126, 1996.
81. Menghini VV, Savcenko V, Olson LJ, et al: Combined immunosuppression for the treatment of idiopathic giant cell myocarditis. Mayo Clin Proc 74:1221, 1999.
82. Frustaci A, Chimenti C, Pieroni M, et al: Giant cell myocarditis responding to immunosuppressive therapy. Chest 117:905, 2000.
83. Pinderski LJ, Fonarow GC, Hamilton M, et al: Giant cell myocarditis in a young man responsive to T-lymphocyte cytolytic therapy. J Heart Lung Transplant 221:818, 2002.
84. Davies RA, Veinot JP, Smith S, et al: Giant cell myocarditis: Clinical presentation, bridge to transplantation with mechanical circulatory support, and long-term outcome. J Heart Lung Transplant 21:674, 2002.
85. Scott RL, Ratliff NB, Starling RC, et al: Recurrence of giant cell myocarditis in cardiac allograft. J Heart Lung Transplant 20:375, 2001.

Secondary Myocarditis

86. Pisani B, Taylor DO, Mason JW: Inflammatory myocardial diseases and cardiomyopathies. Am J Med 102:459, 1997.
87. Hyypia T: Etiological diagnosis of viral heart disease. Scand J Infect Dis 88:25, 1993.
88. Remes J, Helin M, Vaino P, et al: Clinical outcome and left ventricular function 23 years after acute coxsackievirus myopericarditis. Eur Heart J 11:182, 1990.
89. Lowry RW, Adam E, Hu C, et al: What are the implications of cardiac infection with cytomegalovirus before heart transplantation? J Heart Lung Transplant 13:122, 1994.
90. Partanen J, Nieminen MS, Krogerus L, et al: Cytomegalovirus myocarditis in transplanted heart verified by endomyocardial biopsy. Clin Cardiol 14:847, 1991.
91. Ursell PC, Habib A, Sharma P, et al: Hepatitis B virus and myocarditis. Hum Pathol 15:481, 1984.
92. Prati D, Poli F, Farma E, et al: Multicenter study on hepatitis C virus infection in patients with dilated cardiomyopathy. J Med Virol 58:116, 1999.

93. Dalekos GN, Achenbach K, Christodoulou D, et al: Idiopathic dilated cardiomyopathy: Lack of association with hepatitis C virus infection. Heart 80:270, 1998.
94. Frustaci A, Calabrese F, Chimenti C, et al: Lone hepatitis C virus myocarditis responsive to immunosuppressive therapy. Chest 122:2611, 2002.
95. Craver RD, Sorrells K, Gohd R: Myocarditis with influenza B infection. Pediatr Infect Dis J 16:629, 1997.
96. Kaji M, Kuno H, Turu T, et al: Elevated serum myosin light chain I in influenza patients. Intern Med 40:594, 2001.
97. McGregor D, Henderson S: Myocarditis, rhabdomyolysis and myoglobinuric renal failure complicating influenza in a young adult. N Z Med J 110:237, 1997.
98. Agnino A, Schena S, Ferlan G, et al: Left ventricular pseudoaneurysm after acute influenza A myocardiopericarditis. J Cardiovasc Surg 43:203, 2002.
99. Ozkutlu S, Soylemezoglu O, Calikoglu AS, et al: Fatal mumps myocarditis. Jpn Heart J 30:109, 1989.
100. Kabakus N, Aydinoglu H, Yekeler H, Arslan IN: Fatal mumps nephritis and myocarditis. J Trop Pediatr 45:358, 1999.
101. Frustaci A, Abdulla AK, Caldarulo M, et al: Fatal measles myocarditis. Cardiologia 35: 347, 1990.
102. Degen JA: Visceral pathology in measles. Am J Med Sci 194:104, 1937.
103. Alter P, Grimm W, Maisch B: Varicella myocarditis in an adult. Heart 85:E2, 2001.
104. Tsintsof A, Delprado WJ, Keogh AM: Varicella zoster myocarditis progressing to cardiomyopathy and cardiac transplantation. Br Heart J 70:93, 1993.
105. Matthews AW, Griffiths ID: Post-vaccinial pericarditis and myocarditis. Br Heart J 36:1043, 1974.
106. Kabra SK, Juneja R, Madhulika, et al: Myocardial dysfunction in children with dengue haemorrhagic fever. Natl Med J India 11:59, 1998.
107. Wali JP, Biswas A, Chandra S, et al: Cardiac involvement in dengue haemorrhagic fever. Int J Cardiol 64:31, 1998.
108. Hebert MM, Yu C, Towbin JA, et al: Fatal Epstein-Barr virus myocarditis in a child with repetitive myocarditis. Pediatr Pathol Lab Med 15:805, 1995.
109. Cummins D, Bennett D, Fisher-Hoch SP, et al: Electrocardiographic abnormalities in patients with Lassa fever. J Trop Med Hyg 92:350, 1989.
110. Hildes JA, Schaberg A, Alcock AUW: Cardiovascular collapse in acute poliomyelitis. Circulation 12:986, 1955.
111. Thomas JA, Raroque S, Scott WA, et al: Successful treatment of severe dysrhythmias in infants with respiratory syncytial virus infections: Two cases and a literature review. Crit Care Med 25:880, 1997.
112. Olesch CA, Bullock AM: Bradyarrhythmia and supraventricular tachycardia in a neonate with RSV. J Paediatr Child Health 34:199, 1998.
113. Huang M, Bigos D, Levine M: Ventricular arrhythmia associated with respiratory syncytial viral infection. Pediatr Cardiol 19:498, 1998.
114. Ho M, Chen E, Hsu K, et al: An epidemic of enterovirus 71 infection in Taiwan. N Engl J Med 341:13, 1999.
115. Schowengerdt K, Ni J, Denfield S, et al: Association of parvovirus B19 genome in children with myocarditis and cardiac allograft rejection. Circulation 96:3549, 1997.
116. Fournier PE, Etienne J, Harle JR, et al: Myocarditis, a rare but severe manifestation of Q fever: Report of 8 cases and review of the literature. Clin Infect Dis 32:1440, 2001.
117. Raoult D, Tissot-Dupont H, Foucault C, et al: Q fever 1985-1998: Clinical and epidemiologic features of 1,383 infections. Medicine (Baltimore) 79:109, 2000.
118. Marin-Garcia J, Barrett FF: Myocardial function in Rocky Mountain spotted fever: Echocardiographic assessment. Am J Cardiol 51:341, 1983.
119. Yotsukura M, Aoki N, Fukuzumi N, et al: Review of a case of Tsutsugamushi disease showing myocarditis and confirmation of rickettsia by endomyocardial biopsy. Jpn Circ J 55:149, 1991.
120. Tsay RW, Chang FY: Serious complications in scrub typhus. J Microbiol Immunol Infect 31:240, 1998.
121. Stevens DL, Troyer BE, Merrick DT, et al: Lethal effects and cardiovascular effects of purified alpha- and theta-toxins from *Clostridium perfringens*. J Infect Dis 157:272, 1988.
122. Kadirova R, Kartoglu HU, Strebel PM: Clinical characteristics and management of 676 hospitalized diphtheria cases, Kyrgyz Republic, 1995. J Infect Dis 181(Suppl 1):S110, 2000.
123. Loukoushkina EF, Bobko PV, Kolbasova EV, et al: The clinical picture and diagnosis of diphtheritic carditis in children. Eur J Pediatr 157:528, 1998.
124. Havaldar PV, Patil VD, Siddibhavi BM, et al: Fulminant diptheretic myocarditis. Indian Heart J 41:265, 1989.
125. Dung NM, Kneen R, Kiem N: Treatment of severe diphtheritic myocarditis by temporary insertion of a cardiac pacemaker. Clin Infect Dis 35:1425, 2002.
126. O'Neill PG, Rokey R, Greenberg S, et al: Resolution of ventricular tachycardia and endocardial tuberculoma following antituberculosis therapy. Chest 100:1467,1991.
127. Afzal A, Keohane M, Keeley E, et al: Myocarditis and pericarditis with tamponade associated with disseminated tuberculosis. Can J Cardiol 16:4, 2000.
128. Chan AC, Dickens P: Tuberculous myocarditis presenting as sudden cardiac death. Forensic Sci Int 57:45, 1992.
129. Alkhuja S, Miller A: Tuberculosis and sudden death: A case report and review. Heart & Lung 30:388, 2001.
130. Silvestry FE, Kim B, Pollack BJ, et al: Cardiac Whipple disease: Identification of Whipple bacillus by electron microscopy of a patient before death. Ann Intern Med 126:214, 1997.
131. Elkins C, Shuman TA, Pirolo JS: Cardiac Whipple's disease without digestive symptoms. Ann Thorac Surg 67:250, 1999.
132. Mooney EE, Kenan DJ, Sweeney EC, et al: Myocarditis in Whipple's disease: An unsuspected cause of symptoms and sudden death. Mod Pathol 10:524, 1997.
133. Jubber AS, Gunawardana DR, Lulu AR: Acute pulmonary edema in *Brucella* myocarditis and interstitial pneumonitis. Chest 97:1008, 1990.
134. Schinkel A, Bax J, van der Wall E, et al: Echocardiographic follow-up of *Chlamydia psittaci* myocarditis. Chest 117:1203, 2000.
135. Bachmaier K, Neu N, de la Maza L, et al: Chlamydia infections and heart disease linked through antigenic mimicry. Science 283:5406, 1999.
136. Armengol S, Domingo C, Mesalles E: Myocarditis: A rare complication during Legionella infection. Int J Cardiol 37:418, 1992.
137. Garcia NS, Castelo JS, Ramos V, et al: Frequency of myocarditis in cases of fatal meningococcal infection in children: Observations on 31 cases studied at autopsy. Rev Soc Bras Med Trop 32:517, 1999.
138. Sandler MA, Pincus PS, Weltman MD, et al: Meningococcaemia complicated by myocarditis: A report of 2 cases. S Afr Med J 75:391, 1989.
139. Agarwala BN, Ruschhaupt DG: Complete heart block from *Mycoplasma pneumoniae* infection. Pediatr Cardiol 12:233, 1991.
140. Hofner G, Hofbeck M, Koch A, et al: Intrapericardial hemorrhage as a manifestation of mycoplasma pneumoniae infection. Kardiol 86:423, 1997.
141. Odeh M, Oliven A: Chlamydial infections of the heart. Eur J Clin Microbiol Infect Dis 11:885, 1992.
142. Neuwirth C, François C, Laurent N, et al: Myocarditis due to *Salmonella virchow* and sudden infant death. Lancet 354:1004, 1999.
143. Lu M, Ji B, Ouyang K: Clinical and laboratory studies with typhoid fever in 178 patients. Hunan Yi Ke Da Xue Xue Bao 22:15, 1997.

Spirochetal, Fungal, and Protozoal Myocarditis

144. Sangha O, Phillips CB, Fleischmann KE, et al: Lack of cardiac manifestations among patients with previously treated Lyme disease. Ann Intern Med 128:346, 1998.
145. Hajjar R, Kradin R: Weekly clinicopathological exercises. Case 17-2002: A 55-year-old man with second degree atrioventricular block and chest pain. N Engl J Med 346:1732, 2002.
145a. Nowakowski JN, Nadelman RB, Sell R, et al: Long-term follow-up of patients with culture-confirmed Lyme disease. Am J Med 115:91, 2003.
146. Haywood GA, O'Connell S, Gray HH: Lyme carditis: A United Kingdom perspective. Br Heart J 70:15, 1993.
147. Asch ES, Bujak DI, Weiss M, et al: Lyme disease: An infectious and postinfectious syndrome. J Rheumatol 21:454, 1994.
148. Ledford DK: Immunologic aspects of vasculitis and cardiovascular disease. JAMA 278:1962, 1997.
149. Nagi KS, Joshi R, Thakur RK: Cardiac manifestations of Lyme disease: A review. Can J Cardiol 12:503, 1996.
150. Rees DH, Keeling PJ, McKenna WJ, et al: No evidence to implicate *Borrelia burgdorferi* in the pathogenesis of dilated cardiomyopathy in the United Kingdom. Br Heart J 71:459, 1994.
151. Stanek G, Klein J, Bittner R, et al: Isolation of *Borrelia burgdorferi* from the myocardium of a patient with long-standing cardiomyopathy. N Engl J Med 322:249, 1990.
152. Rahn DW, Malawista SE: Lyme disease: Recommendations for diagnosis and treatment. Ann Intern Med 14:472, 1991.
153. Rajajee S, Shankar J, Dhattatri L: Pediatric presentations of leptospirosis. Indian J Pediatr 69:10, 2002.
154. Singh SS, Vijayachari P, Sinha A, et al: Clinico-epidemiological study of hospitalized cases of severe leptospirosis. Indian J Med Res 109:94, 1999.
155. Rajiv C, Manjuran RJ, Sudhayakumar N, et al: Cardiovascular involvement in leptospirosis. Indian Heart J 48:691, 1996.
156. Mekasha A: Louse-borne relapsing fever in children. J Trop Med Hyg 95:206, 1992.
157. Chino M, Minami T, Nishikawa K: Ruptured ventricular aneurysm in secondary syphilis. Lancet 342:935, 1993.
158. Berarducci L, Ford K, Olenick S, et al: Invasive intracardiac aspergillosis with widespread embolization. J Am Soc Echocardiogr 6:539, 1993.
159. Rueter F, Hirsch HH, Kunz F: Late *Aspergillus fumigatus* endomyocarditis with brain abscess as a lethal complication after heart transplantation. J Heart Lung Transplant 21:1242, 2002.
160. Bashour TT, Gord C, Baladi N, et al: Intracardiac actinomycosis. Am Heart J 133:467, 1997.
161. Serody JS, Mill MR, Detterbeck FC, et al: Blastomycosis in transplant recipients: Report of a case and review. Clin Infect Dis 16:54, 1993.
162. Parker JC: The potentially lethal problem of cardiac candidosis. Am J Clin Pathol 73:356, 1980.
163. Franklin WG, Simon AB, Sodeman TM: Candida myocarditis without valvulitis. Am J Cardiol 38:924, 1976.
164. Faul JL, Hoang K, Schmoker J, et al: Constrictive pericarditis due to coccidioidomycosis. Ann Thorac Surg 68:1407, 1999.
165. Lafont A, Wolff M, Marche C, et al: Overwhelming myocarditis due to *Cryptococcus neoformans* in an AIDS patient. Lancet 2:1145, 1987.
166. Kirchner SG, Hernanz-Schulman M, Stein SM, et al: Imaging of pediatric mediastinal histoplasmosis. Radiographics 11:365, 1991.
167. Jackman JD Jr, Simonsen RL: The clinical manifestations of cardiac mucormycosis. Chest 101:1733, 1992.
168. Virmani R, Connor DH, McAllister HA: Cardiac mucormycosis: A report of five patients and review of 14 previously reported cases. Am J Clin Pathol 78:42, 1982.
169. Hagar JM, Rahimtoola SH: Chagas' heart disease. Curr Probl Cardiol 20:825, 1995.
170. Rassi A Jr, Rassi A, Little WC: Chagas' heart disease. Clin Cardiol 23:883, 2000.
171. Rossi MA, Bestetti RB: The challenge of chagasic cardiomyopathy: The pathologic roles of autonomic abnormalities, autoimmune mechanisms and microvascular changes, and therapeutic implications. Cardiology 86:1, 1995.
172. Parada H, Carrasco HA, Anez N, et al: Cardiac involvement is a constant finding in acute Chagas' disease: A clinical, parasitological and histopathological study. Int J Cardiol 60:49, 1997.
173. Machado F, Martins G, Aliberti J, et al: *Trypanosoma cruzi*-infected cardiomyocytes produce chemokines and cytokines that trigger potent nitric oxide-dependent trypanocidal activity. Circulation 102:3003, 2000.

174. Reis MM, Higuchi M, de la Benvenuti LA, et al: An in situ quantitative immunohistochemical study of cytokines and IL-2R+ in chronic human chagasic myocarditis: Correlation with the presence of myocardial *Trypanosoma cruzi* antigens. Clin Immunol Immunopathol 83:165, 1997.
175. Anez N, Carrasco H, Parada H, et al: Myocardial parasite persistence in chronic chagasic patients. Am J Trop Med Hyg 60:726, 1999.
176. Bellotti G, Bocchi EA, de Moraes AV, et al: In vivo detection of *Trypanosoma cruzi* antigens in hearts of patients with chronic Chagas' heart disease. Am Heart J 131:301, 1996.
177. Bestetti RB, Muccillo G: Clinical course of Chagas' heart disease: A comparison with dilated cardiomyopathy. Int J Cardiol 60:187, 1997.
178. Cunha-Neto E, Kalil J: Heart-infiltrating and peripheral T cells in the pathogenesis of human Chagas' disease cardiomyopathy. Autoimmunity 34:187, 2001.
179. Gomes JA, Bahia-Oliveira LM, Rocha MO, et al: Evidence that development of severe cardiomyopathy in human Chagas' disease is due to a Th 1-specific immune response. Infect Immun 71:1185, 2003.
180. Higuchi MD, Ries MM, Aiello VD, et al: Association of an increase in CD8+ T cells with the presence of *Trypanosoma cruzi* antigens in chronic, human, chagasic myocarditis. Am J Trop Med Hyg 56:485, 1997.
181. Sterin-Borda L, Gorelik G, Postan M, et al: Alterations in cardiac beta-adrenergic receptors in chagasic mice and their association with circulating beta-adrenoceptor-related autoantibodies. Cardiovasc Res 41:116, 1999.
182. Rossi MA: Comparison of Chagas' heart disease to arrhythmogenic right ventricular cardiomyopathy. Am Heart J 129:626, 1995.
183. Higuchi ML, Fukasawa S, De Brito T, et al: Different microcirculatory and interstitial matrix patterns in idiopathic dilated cardiomyopathy and Chagas' disease: A three dimensional confocal microscopy study. Heart 82:279, 1999.
184. Bestetti RB, Dalbo CM, Arruda CA, et al: Predictors of sudden cardiac death for patients with Chagas' disease: A hospital-derived cohort study. Cardiology 87:481, 1996.
185. Carrasco HA, Alarçon M, Olmos L, et al: Biochemical characterization of myocardial damage in chronic Chagas' disease. Clin Cardiol 20:865, 1997.
186. Bestetti RB, Dalbo CM, Freitas QC, et al: Noninvasive predictors of mortality for patients with Chagas' heart disease: A multivariate stepwise logistic regression study. Cardiology 84:261, 1994.
187. Martinelli F, De Siqueira S, Moreira H: Probability of occurrence of life-threatening ventricular arrhythmias in Chagas' disease versus non-Chagas' disease. Pacing Clin Electrophysiol 23:1944, 2000.
188. de Paola AA, Gomes JA, Terzian AB, et al: Ventricular tachycardia during exercise testing as a predictor of sudden death in patients with chronic chagasic cardiomyopathy and ventricular arrhythmias. Br Heart J 74:293, 1995.
189. Carrasco HA, Parada H, Guerrero L, et al: Prognostic implications of clinical, electrocardiographic and hemodynamic findings in chronic Chagas' disease. Int J Cardiol 43:27, 1994.
190. Braga JC, Labrunie A, Villaca F, et al: Thromboembolism in chronic Chagas' heart disease. Rev Paul Med 113:862, 1995.
191. Acquatella H, Perez JE, Condado JA, et al: Limited myocardial contractile reserve and chronotropic incompetence in patients with chronic Chagas' disease: Assessment by dobutamine stress echocardiography. J Am Coll Cardiol 3:22, 1999.
192. Marin-Neto JA, Marzullo P, Marcassa C, et al: Myocardial perfusion abnormalities in chronic Chagas' disease as detected by thallium-201 scintigraphy. Am J Cardiol 69:780, 1992.
193. Kalil Filho R, de Albuquerque CP: Magnetic resonance imaging in Chagas' heart disease. Rev Paul Med 113:880, 1995.
194. Ferreira AW, de Avila SD: Laboratory diagnosis of Chagas' heart disease. Rev Paul Med 113:767, 1995.
195. de Paola AA, Gondin AA, Hara V, et al: Medical treatment of cardiac arrhythmias in Chagas' heart disease. Rev Paul Med 113:858, 1995.
196. Leon J, Wang K, Engman D: Captopril ameliorates myocarditis in acute experimental Chagas disease. Circulation 107:2264, 2003.
197. Muratore C, Rabinovich R, Iglesias R, et al: Implantable cardioverter defibrillators in patients with Chagas' disease: Are they different from patients with coronary disease? Pacing Clin Electrophysiol 20:194, 1997.
198. Apt W, Aguilera X, Arribada A, et al: Treatment of chronic Chagas' disease with itraconazole and allopurinol. Am J Trop Med Hyg 59:133, 1998.
199. Bocchi EA, Bellotti G, Mocelin AO, et al: Heart transplantation for chronic Chagas' heart disease. Ann Thorac Surg 61:1727, 1996.
200. Bocchi EA, Fiorelli A: The paradox of survival results after heart transplantation for cardiomyopathy caused by *Trypanosoma cruzi*. Ann Thorac Surg 71:6, 2001.
201. Bocchi EA, Higuchi ML, Vieira ML, et al: Higher incidence of malignant neoplasms after heart transplantation for treatment of chronic Chagas' heart disease. J Heart Lung Transplant 17:399, 1998.
202. Tsala Mbala P, Blackett K, Mbonifor CL, et al: Functional and immunologic involvement in human African trypanosomiasis caused by *Trypanosoma gambiense*. Bull Soc Pathol Exot Filiales 81:490, 1988.
203. Duffield JS, Jacob AJ, Miller HC: Recurrent, life-threatening atrioventricular dissociation associated with *Toxoplasma* myocarditis. Heart 76:453, 1996.
204. Montoya JG, Jordan R, Lingamneni S, et al: Toxoplasmic myocarditis and polymyositis in patients with acute acquired toxoplasmosis diagnosed during life. Clin Infect Dis 24:676, 1997.
205. Vuong PN, Richard F, Snounou G, et al: Development of irreversible lesions in the brain, heart, and kidneys following acute and chronic murine malaria infection. Parasitology 119:543, 1999.
206. Bethell DB, Phuong PT, Phuong CX, et al: Electrocardiographic monitoring in severe falciparum malaria. Trans R Soc Trop Med Hyg 90:266, 1996.
207. Salih OK, Celik SK, Topcuoglu MS, et al: Surgical treatment of hydatid cysts of the heart: A report of 3 cases and a review of the literature. Can J Surg 41:321, 1998.
208. Benomar A, Yahyaoui M, Birouk N, et al: Middle cerebral artery occlusion due to hydatid cysts of myocardial and intraventricular cavity cardiac origin: Two cases. Stroke 25:886, 1994.
209. Miralles A, Bracamonte L, Pavie A, et al: Cardiac echinococcosis: Surgical treatment and results. J Thorac Cardiovasc Surg 107:184, 1994.
210. Franchi C, Di Vico B, Teggi A: Long-term evaluation of patients with hydatidosis treated with benzimidazole carbamates. Clin Infect Dis 29:304, 1999.
211. Ozer N, Aytemir K, Kuru G, et al: Hydatid cyst of the heart as a rare cause of embolization: Report of 5 cases and review of published reports. J Am Soc Echocardiogr 14:299, 2001.
212. Lazarevic AM, Neskovic AN, Goronja M, et al: Low incidence of cardiac abnormalities in treated trichinosis: A prospective study of 62 patients from a single-source outbreak. Am J Med 107:18, 1999.
213. Compton SJ, Celum CL, Lee C, et al: Trichinosis with ventilatory failure and persistent myocarditis. Clin Infect Dis 16:500, 1993.
214. Dao AH, Virmani R: Visceral larva migrans involving the myocardium: Report of two cases and review of literature. Pediatr Pathol 6:449, 1986.
215. Abe K, Shimokawa H, Kubota T, et al: Myocarditis associated with visceral larva migrans due to *Toxocara canis*. Intern Med 41:706, 2002.
216. Morris W, Knauer CM: Cardiopulmonary manifestations of schistosomiasis. Semin Respir Infect 12:159, 1997.

Toxic, Chemical, and Physical Damage

217. Feenstra J, Grobbee DE, Remme WJ, et al: Drug-induced heart failure. J Am Coll Cardiol 33:1152, 1999.
218. Le Blaye I, Donatini B, Hall M, et al: Acute overdosage with thioridazine: A review of the available clinical exposure. Vet Hum Toxicol 35:147, 1993.
219. Schmidt W, Lang K: Life-threatening dysrhythmias in severe thioridazine poisoning treated with physostigmine and transient atrial pacing. Crit Care Med 25:1925, 1997.
220. Vanoli E, De Ferrari GM, Stramba-Badiale M, et al: Carbon monoxide and lethal arrhythmias in conscious dogs with healed myocardial infarction. Am Heart J 117:348, 1989.
221. Dahms TE, Younis LT, Wiens RD, et al: Effects of carbon monoxide exposure in patients with documented cardiac arrhythmias. J Am Coll Cardiol 21:442, 1993.
222. McMeekin JD, Finegan BA: Reversible myocardial dysfunction following carbon monoxide poisoning. Can J Cardiol 3:118, 1987.
223. Marius-Nunez AL: Myocardial infarction with normal coronary arteries after acute exposure to carbon monoxide. Chest 97:491, 1990.
224. Angulo MP, Navajas A, Galdeano JM, et al: Reversible cardiomyopathy secondary to alpha-interferon in an infant. Pediatr Cardiol 20:293, 1999.
225. Goel M, Flaherty L, Lavine S, et al: Reversible cardiomyopathy after high-dose interleukin-2 therapy. J Immunother 11:225, 1992.
226. La Grenade L, Graham D, Trontell A: Myocarditis and cardiomyopathy associated with clozapine use in the United States. N Engl J Med 345:224, 2001.
227. Ho PC, Dweik R, Cohen MC: Rapidly reversible cardiomyopathy associated with chronic ipecac ingestion. Clin Cardiol 21:780, 1998.
228. Silberstein SD: Methysergide. Cephalalgia 18:421, 1998.
229. Iglesias Cubero G, Rodriguez Reguero JJ, Rojo Ortega JM: Restrictive cardiomyopathy caused by chloroquine. Br Heart J 69:451, 1993.
230. Sundar S, Sinha PR, Agrawal NK, et al: A cluster of cases of severe cardiotoxicity among kala-azar patients treated with a high-osmolarity lot of sodium antimony gluconate. Am J Trop Med Hyg 59:139, 1998.
231. Ortega-Carnicer J, Alcazar R, De la Torre M, et al: Pentavalent antimonial-induced torsades de pointes. J Electrocardiol 30:143, 1997.
232. Groleau G: Lithium toxicity. Emerg Med Clin North Am 12:511, 1994.
233. Terao T, Abe H, Abe K: Irreversible sinus node dysfunction induced by resumption of lithium therapy. Acta Psychiatr Scand 93:407, 1996.
234. Gerhardt RT: Acute halon (bromochlorodifluoromethane) toxicity by accidental and recreational inhalation. Am J Emerg Med 14:675, 1996.
235. Brady WJ Jr, Stremski E, Eljaiek L, et al: Freon inhalational abuse presenting with ventricular fibrillation. Am J Emerg Med 12:533, 1994.
236. Kopp SJ, Barron JT, Tow JP: Cardiovascular actions of lead and relationship to hypertension: A review. Environ Health Perspect 78:91, 1988.
237. Kudoh C, Tanaka S, Marusaki S, et al: Hypocalcemic cardiomyopathy in a patient with idiopathic hypoparathyroidism. Intern Med 31:561, 1992.
238. Feldman AM, Fivush B, Zahka KG, et al: Congestive cardiomyopathy in patients on continuous ambulatory peritoneal dialysis. Am Kidney Dis 11:76, 1988.
239. Claudius I, Sachs C, Shamji T: Hypophosphatemia-induced heart failure. Am J Emerg Med 20:369, 2002.
240. Davis SV, Olichwier KK, Chakko SC: Reversible depression of myocardial performance in hypophosphatemia. Am J Med Sci 295:183, 1988.
241. Kurnik BR, Marshall J, Katz SM: Hypomagnesemia-induced cardiomyopathy. Magnesium 7:49, 1988.
242. Riggs JE, Klingberg WG, Flink EB, et al: Cardioskeletal mitochondrial myopathy associated with chronic magnesium deficiency. Neurology 42:128, 1992.
243. Wagdi P, Mehan VK, Burgi H, et al: Acute myocardial infarction after wasp stings in a patient with normal coronary arteries. Am Heart J 128:820, 1994.
244. Lalloo DG, Trevett AJ, Nwokolo N, et al: Electrocardiographic abnormalities in patients bitten by taipans (*Oxyuranus scutellatus canni*) and other elapid snakes in Papua New Guinea. Trans R Soc Trop Med Hyg 91:53, 1997.
245. Kurnik D, Haviv Y, Kochva E: A snake bite by the burrowing asp, *Atractaspis engaddensis*. Toxicon 37:223, 1999.
246. Hall JC, Harruff R: Fatal cardiac arrhythmia in a patient with interstitial myocarditis related to chronic arsenic poisoning. South Med J 82:1557, 1989.
247. Paulson DJ: Carnitine deficiency-induced cardiomyopathy. Mol Cell Biochem 180:33, 1998.
248. Ergur AT, Tanzer F, Cetinkaya O: Serum-free carnitine levels in children with heart failure. J Trop Pediatr 45:168, 1999.

249. Huttunen JK: Selenium and cardiovascular diseases: An update. Biomed Environ Sci 10:220, 1997.
250. Levy JB, Jones HW, Gordon AC: Selenium deficiency, reversible cardiomyopathy and short-term intravenous feeding. Postgrad Med J 70:235, 1994.
251. Kumar EB, Soomro RS, al Hamdani A, et al: Scorpion venom cardiomyopathy. Am Heart J 123:725, 1992.
252. Gueron M, Ilia R, Sofer S: Scorpion venom cardiomyopathy. Am Heart J 125:1816, 1993.
253. Haller CA, Jacob P 3rd, Benowitz NL: Pharmacology of ephedra alkaloids and caffeine after single-dose dietary supplement use. Clin Pharmacol Ther 71:421, 2002.
254. Samen KD, Link MS, Homoud MK, et al: Adverse cardiovascular events temporally associated with ma huang, an herbal source of ephedrine. Mayo Clin Proc 77:12, 2002.
255. Burke AP, Saenger J, Mullick F, et al: Hypersensitivity myocarditis. Arch Pathol Lab Med 115:764, 1991.
256. Getz MA, Subramanian R, Logemann T, et al: Acute necrotizing eosinophilic myocarditis as a manifestation of severe hypersensitivity myocarditis: Antemortem diagnosis and successful treatment. Ann Intern Med 115:201, 1991.
257. Galiuto L, Enriquez S, Reeder G, et al: Eosinophilic myocarditis manifesting as myocardial infarction: Early diagnosis and successful treatment. Mayo Clin Proc 72:603, 1997.
258. Webster J, Koch HF: Aspects of tolerability of centrally acting antihypertensive drugs. J Cardiovasc Pharmacol 27 (Suppl 3):S49, 1996.
259. Garty BZ, Offer I, Livni E, et al: Erythema multiforme and hypersensitivity myocarditis caused by ampicillin. Ann Pharmacother 28:730, 1994.
260. Loyer EM, Delpassand ES: Radiation-induced heart disease: Imaging features. Semin Roentgenol 28:321, 1993.
261. Gyenes G, Fornander T, Carlens P, et al: Detection of radiation-induced myocardial damage by technetium-99m sestamibi scintigraphy. Eur J Nucl Med 24:286, 1997.
262. Orzan F, Brusca A, Gaita F, et al: Associated cardiac lesions in patients with radiation-induced complete heart block. Int J Cardiol 39:151, 1993.
263. Veeragandham RS, Goldin MD: Surgical management of radiation-induced heart disease. Ann Thorac Surg 65:1014, 1998.
264. Hering D, Faber L, Horstkotte D: Echocardiographic features of radiation-associated valvular disease. Am J Cardiol 92:226, 2003.
265. Khan MH, Ettinger SM: Post mediastinal radiation coronary artery disease and its effect on arterial conduits. Catheter Cardiovasc Inter 52:242, 2001.
266. Dematte JE, O'Mara K, Buescher J, et al: Near-fatal heat stroke during the 1995 heat wave in Chicago. Ann Intern Med 129:173, 1998.
267. Danzl DF, Pozos RS: Accidental hypothermia. N Engl J Med 331:1756, 1994.
268. Walpoth BH, Walpoth-Aslan BN, Mattle HP, et al: Outcome of survivors of accidental deep hypothermia and circulatory arrest treated with extracorporeal blood warming. N Engl J Med 337:1500, 1997.
269. Lazar HL: The treatment of hypothermia. N Engl J Med 337:1545, 1997.

CHAPTER 61

Cardiovascular Abnormalities in HIV-Infected Individuals

Stacy D. Fisher • Steven E. Lipshultz

BACKGROUND

Infection with the human immunodeficiency virus (HIV) is one of the leading causes of acquired heart disease and specifically of symptomatic heart failure (Table 61-1). Cardiac complications of HIV infection tend to occur late in the disease and are therefore becoming more prevalent in our society as therapy and longevity improve.[1-5] Complicated drug therapies for HIV infection have sustained life but may lead to accelerated cardiovascular risk and atherosclerotic disease.[1,6]

Some 42 million adults and children are living with HIV or the acquired immunodeficiency syndrome (AIDS); 5 million more became infected in 2002.[7] The 2- to 5-year incidence of symptomatic heart failure ranges from 4 to 28 percent,[3,4] suggesting a prevalence of symptomatic HIV-related heart failure between 4 million and 5 million cases worldwide. Among HIV-infected children up to 10 years of age, 25 percent die with chronic cardiac disease,[8] and 28 percent experience serious cardiac events after an AIDS-defining illness.[9] The incidence of new HIV infection in the United States has decreased substantially over the last 5 years. Deaths related to HIV infection decreased 42 percent in 1996 to 1997 and 20 percent in 1997 to 1998 because of improved antiretroviral therapies and better identification and treatment of opportunistic infections. An estimated 3.1 million HIV-related deaths occurred worldwide in 2002, 15,000 in North America and 2.4 million in sub-Saharan Africa. Early in the epidemic, HIV infections were chiefly found in homosexual males; however, now most new cases occur in injection drug users and heterosexual partners of infected persons. Minority groups are overrepresented.[7]

A range of cardiac abnormalities (see Table 61–1) associated with HIV infection has been suggested by autopsy study; the conditions, in order of frequency, were pericardial effusion, lymphocytic interstitial myocarditis, dilated cardiomyopathy (frequently with myocarditis), infective endocarditis, and malignancy (myocardial Kaposi sarcoma and B-cell immunoblastic lymphoma).[10]

Left Ventricular Systolic Dysfunction (see Chap. 21)

CLINICAL PRESENTATION. In HIV-infected patients, concurrent pulmonary infections, pulmonary hypertension, anemia, portal hypertension, malnutrition, or malignancy can alter or confuse the characteristic signs that define heart failure in other populations. Thus, patients with left ventricular systolic dysfunction can be asymptomatic or can present with New York Heart Association Class III or IV heart failure.

Echocardiography is a useful test to assess left ventricular systolic function in this population and, in addition to uncovering left ventricular dysfunction, often reveals either low to normal wall thickness or left ventricular hypertrophy and a dilated left ventricular chamber.[2] Echocardiography should be performed in any patient at elevated cardiovascular risk, with any clinical manifestations of cardiovascular disease, or with unexplained or persistent pulmonary symptoms or viral coinfections at baseline and every 1 to 2 years or as clinically indicated.[6,11]

Electrocardiography (ECG) can reveal nonspecific conduction defects or repolarization changes. In one multicenter trial, 57 percent of asymptomatic HIV-infected individuals had baseline abnormalities on ECG, including supraventricular and ventricular ectopic beats.[12] The chest radiograph has low sensitivity and specificity for congestive heart failure in patients with HIV infection. Brain natriuretic peptide levels in small studies of HIV-infected patients and large populations of patients without HIV infection have been shown to correlate inversely with left ventricular ejection fraction and can be useful in the differential diagnosis of congestive cardiomyopathy in this population.[13]

Patients with encephalopathy are more likely to die of congestive heart failure than those without encephalopathy (hazard ratio 3.4).[14] HIV persists in reservoir cells in the myocardium and the cerebral cortex, even after antiretroviral therapy. These cells seem to play an important role in the development and progression of cardiomyopathy and encephalopathy. Reservoir cells may hold HIV on their surfaces for extended periods of time and cause progressive tissue damage by chronic release of cytotoxic cytokines.[15]

INCIDENCE. A 4-year observational study of 296 patients with a spectrum of HIV-related disease found 44 (15 percent) with dilated cardiomyopathy (fractional shortening <28 percent, with global left ventricular hypokinesis), 13 (4 percent) with isolated right ventricular dysfunction (right ventricle larger than left ventricle on standard two-dimensional views), and 12 (4 percent) with borderline left ventricular dysfunction (left ventricular end-systolic diameter >58 mm but fractional shortening >28 percent, or global dysfunction reported by one or two but not all three observers) (Fig. 61–1). Dilated cardiomyopathy was strongly associated with a CD4 count of less than 100 cells/ml.[4]

Left ventricular dysfunction is a common consequence of HIV infection in children. In a study of 205 children infected with HIV

TABLE 61–1 HIV-Associated Cardiovascular Disease

Type	Possible Etiologies	Incidence/Prevalence	Diagnosis	Treatment
Dilated cardiomyopathy	*Drug related:* cocaine, AZT, IL-2, doxorubicin, interferon *Infectious:* HIV, toxoplasma, coxsackievirus group B, EBV, CMV, adenovirus *Metabolic or endocrine:* selenium or carnitine deficiency, anemia, hypocalcemia, hypophosphatemia, hyponatremia, hypokalemia, hypoalbuminemia, hypothyroidism, growth hormone deficiency, adrenal insufficiency, hyperinsulinemia, hemochromatosis, pheochromocytoma, sarcoidosis, amyloidosis *Cytokines:* TNF-alpha, nitric oxide, TGF-beta, endothelin-I, interleukins *Immunodeficiency:* CD4 < 100 *Autoimmune*	Up to 8% of asymptomatic patients Up to 25% of autopsy cases Systolic > diastolic	Chest radiograph findings: nonspecific conduction abnormalities, PVCs, PACs Echocardiogram findings: low-normal LV wall thickness, increased LV mass, dilated LV, systolic LV dysfunction Possible laboratory studies: Troponin T, brain natiuretic peptide level, CD4 count, viral load, viral PCR, toxoplasma serology, thyroid-stimulating hormone, growth hormone, cortisol, carnitine, selenium, serum ACE, vanillylmandelic acid, amyloid, urine analysis, stress testing, myocardial biopsy, cardiac catheterization	Diuretics, digoxin, ACE inhibitors, beta blockers ***Adjunctive treatment in HIV+ patients*** Treatment of infection Nutritional replacement IVIg Intensify antiretroviral therapy ***Follow-up*** Serial echocardiograms
Pericardial effusion	*Bacteria: Staphylococcus, Streptococcus, Proteus, Nocardia, Klebsiella, Enterococcus, Listeria, Mycobacterium* *Viral pathogens:* HIV, HSV,CMV, adenovirus, echovirus *Other pathogens: Cryptococcus, Toxoplasma, Histoplasma* *Malignancy:* Kaposi sarcoma, lymphoma, capillary leak/wasting/malnutrition *Hypothyroidism* *Immunodeficiency* *Uremia*	11%/yr Spontaneous resolution in 42% of affected patients Approximately 30% increase in 6-mo mortality	Pericardial rub on examination Echocardiogram Fluid analysis for Gram stain and culture, malignant cells Associated pleural and peritoneal fluid analysis Pericardial biopsy	Treatment of underlying cause Pericardiocentesis Pericardial window ***Follow-up*** Serial echocardiograms Intensify antiretroviral therapy
Infective endocarditis	*Autoimmune* *Bacteria: Staphlococcus aureus* or *Staphylococcus epidermidis, Salmonella, Streptococcus, Hemophilus parainfluenzae, Pseudallescheria boydii,* HASEK *Fungal: Aspergillus fumigatus, Candida, Cryptococcus neoformans*	6% Increased incidence in IVDA regardless of HIV status	Blood cultures Echocardiogram	IV antibiotics Valve replacement
Nonbacterial thrombotic endocarditis	Valvular damage, vitamin C deficiency, malnutrition, wasting, DIC, hypercoagulable state, prolonged acquired immunodeficiency	Rare, but clinically relevant emboli in 42% of cases	Echocardiogram	Anticoagulation, treat vasculitis or underlying illness
Malignancy	Kaposi sarcoma, non-Hodgkin lymphoma, leiomyosarcoma Low CD4 count, prolonged immunodeficiency HHV-8, EBV	Approximately 1% incidence Usually metastatic in HIV+ patients	Echocardiogram, biopsy	Chemotherapy possible

TABLE 61–1 HIV-Associated Cardiovascular Disease—cont'd

Type	Possible Etiologies	Incidence/Prevalence	Diagnosis	Treatment
Right ventricle and pulmonary disease	Recurrent pulmonary infections, pulmonary arteritis, microvascular pulmonary emboli		ECG, echocardiogram Right heart catheterization	Diuretics Treat underlying lung infection or disease ± anticoagulation
Primary pulmonary HTN	Plexogenic pulmonary arteriopathy	0.5%	ECG, echocardiogram Right heart catheterization	Anticoagulation Vasodilators Prostacycline analogs
Vasculitis	Drug therapy with antibiotics and antiretrovirals	Increasing incidence	Clinical diagnosis	Systemic corticosteroids Withdrawal of causative drug
Accelerated atherosclerosis	Protease inhibitors, atherogenesis with virus-infected macrophages, chronic inflammation	Up to 8% prevalence	Stress testing Echocardiogram Lipid profile	Minimize risk factors
Autonomic dysfunction	CNS disease Drug therapy, prolonged immunodeficiency, malnutrition	Increased in patients with CNS disease	Tilt-table test Holter monitor	Procedural precautions
Arrhythmias	Drug therapy, pentamidine, autonomic dysfunction		ECG—long QT Holter monitor	Discontinue drug Procedural precautions
Lipodystrophy	Drug therapy: Protease inhibitors		Echocardiogram Lipid profile Cardiac catheterization Coronary calcium score	Lipid therapy: beware of drug interactions Aerobic exercise Altered antiretroviral therapy

ACE = angiotensin-converting enzyme; AZT = azidothymidine; CMV = cytomegalovirus; CNS = central nervous system; DIC = disseminated intravascular coagulation; EBV = Epstein-Barr virus; ECG = electrocardiogram; HHV = human herpesvirus; HIV = human immunodeficiency virus; HSV = herpes simplex virus; HTN = hypertension; IL-2 = interleukin-2; IVDA = intravenous drug abuse; IVIg = intravenous immunoglobulin; LV = left ventricular; PAC = premature atrial complex; PCR = polymerase chain reaction; PVC = premature ventricular complex; TGF = transforming growth factor; TNF = tumor necrosis factor.

by maternal-fetal transmission (enrolled at a median age of 22 months and observed with echocardiography every 4 to 6 months and ECG, Holter monitoring, and chest radiography every year), the prevalence of decreased left ventricular function (fractional shortening ≤ 28 percent) was 5.7 percent. The 2-year cumulative incidence was 15.3 percent.[3] The cumulative incidence of symptomatic congestive heart failure or the use of cardiac medications, or both, was 10 percent over 2 years.[3]

Global estimates of HIV-infected people ranged from 33.4 million to 120 million worldwide between the years 1998 and 2000. If there was a 10 percent incidence of symptomatic congestive heart failure over the 2 years, 3.34 million to 12 million cases of congestive heart failure would have presented during a 2-year interval.

PATHOGENESIS. A wide variety of possible etiologic agents have been postulated in HIV-related cardiomyopathy (see Table 61–1), including myocardial infection with HIV itself, opportunistic infections, viral infections, autoimmune response to viral infection, cardiotoxicity from therapeutic or illicit drugs, nutritional deficiencies, cytokine overexpression, and many others.

MYOCARDITIS (see Chap. 60). Myocarditis is perhaps the best studied of the possible causes. Dilated cardiomyopathy can be related to a direct action of HIV on the myocardial tissue or to proteolytic enzymes or cytokine mediators induced by HIV alone or in conjunction with coinfecting viruses.[16,17] *Toxoplasma gondii*, coxsackievirus group B, Epstein-Barr virus, cytomegalovirus, adenovirus, and HIV in myocytes have been found in biopsy specimens.

Autopsy and biopsy results have revealed only scant and patchy inflammatory cell infiltrates in the myocardium.[10,18] HIV can clearly infect myocardial interstitial cells but not the cardiac myocyte. Increased numbers of infected interstitial cells have been found in patients with confirmed myocarditis in which proteolytic enzymes or increased levels of tumor necrosis factor-alpha (TNF-α) or interleukin may injure the myocytes. Increased levels of TNF-α, inducible nitric oxide synthase, and interleukin-6 in affected patients and experimental models have been reported.[18]

Notably, HIV-related cardiomyopathy is often not associated with any specific opportunistic infection, and approximately 40 percent of patients have not experienced any opportunistic infection before the onset of cardiac symptoms.[10]

CYTOKINE ALTERATIONS. HIV infection increases the production of TNF-α, which alters intracellular calcium homeostasis and increases nitric oxide production, transforming growth factor-beta, and endothelin-1 upregulation.[14] Nitric oxide induced in high levels has been shown experimentally to have a negative inotropic effect and to be cytotoxic to myocytes.

In one study, HIV-infected individuals with dilated cardiomyopathy were much more likely to have myocarditis and had a broader spectrum of viral infections than HIV-negative patients with idiopathic dilated cardiomyopathy. Also, levels of TNF-α and induced nitric oxide synthase were higher in myocytes from the HIV-infected patients with dilated cardiomyopathy (particularly those with viral coinfections) and levels varied inversely with the CD4 count. Immunodeficiency may favor the selection of viral variants of increased pathogenicity or enhance the cardiovirulence of viral strains.[14,18]

NUTRITIONAL DEFICIENCIES. Nutritional deficiencies are common in HIV infection, particularly in late-stage disease. Poor absorption and diarrhea both lead to electrolyte imbalances and deficiencies in elemental nutrients. Deficiencies of trace elements have been associated with cardio-

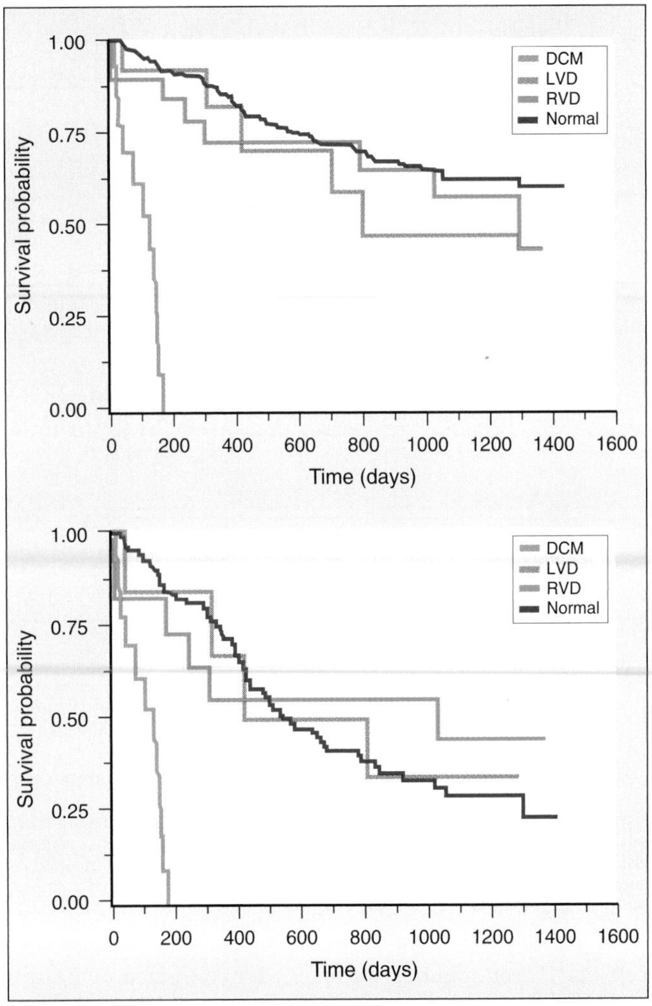

FIGURE 61–1 **Top,** Survival curves for 296 HIV-infected patients with structurally normal hearts, dilated cardiomyopathy (DCM), left ventricular dysfunction (LVD), or right ventricular dysfunction (RVD). **Bottom,** Time to death related to AIDS in 81 patients with CD4+ cell counts less than 20×10^6 cells/liter. (From Currie PF, Jacob AJ, Foreman AR, et al: Heart muscle disease related to HIV infection: Prognostic implications. Br Med J 309:1605, 1994.)

myopathy. For example, selenium deficiency increases the virulence of coxsackievirus to cardiac tissue.[10] Selenium replacement reverses cardiomyopathy and restores left ventricular function in nutritionally depleted patients. Levels of vitamin B_{12}, carnitine, and growth and thyroid hormone can also be altered in HIV disease; all have been associated with left ventricular dysfunction.

PATHOGENESIS IN CHILDREN. In children with vertically transmitted HIV infection, two mechanisms of pathogenesis have been described. One is dilation of the left ventricle with a reduction in the ratio of thickness to end-systolic dimension of the ventricle. The other is concentric hypertrophy of the muscle; with dilation, the ratio of thickness to end-systolic dimension remains normal or is increased.[2]

COURSE OF DISEASE. Patients with asymptomatic left ventricular dysfunction (fractional shortening <28 percent, with global left ventricular hypokinesis) may have transient disease by echocardiographic criteria. In one serial echocardiographic study, three of six patients with abnormal fractional shortening had normal readings after a mean of 9 months. The three with persistently depressed left ventricular function died within 1 year of baseline.[10]

PROGNOSIS. Mortality in HIV-infected patients with cardiomyopathy is increased, independent of CD4 count, age, sex, and risk group. The median survival to AIDS-related death was 101 days in patients with left ventricular dysfunction and 472 days in patients with a normal heart at a similar stage of infection (see Fig. 61–1).[4] Isolated right ventricular dysfunction or borderline left ventricular dysfunction did not place patients at risk.

In the Pediatric Pulmonary and Cardiovascular Complications of Vertically Transmitted HIV Infection (P^2C^2 HIV) study of children with vertically transmitted HIV infection (median age 2.1 years), 5-year cumulative survival was 64 percent.[9] Mortality was higher in children with baseline depressed left ventricular fractional shortening or increased left ventricular dimension, thickness, mass, wall stress, heart rate, or blood pressure. Decreased left ventricular fractional shortening and increased wall thickness were also predictive of survival after adjustment for age, height, CD4 count, HIV RNA copy number, clinical center, and encephalopathy.[2,9] Fractional shortening was abnormal for up to 3 years before death, whereas wall thickness identified a population at risk only 18 to 24 months before death. Thus, in children, fractional shortening may be a useful long-term predictor and wall thickness a useful short-term predictor of mortality.[19] Postmortem cardiomegaly was associated with echocardiographic evidence of increased left ventricular mass and documented chronically increased heart rate prior to death but not with anemia, encephalopathy, or HIV viral load.[20]

Rapid-onset congestive heart failure has a grim prognosis in HIV-infected adults and children, with over half of patients dying from primary cardiac failure within 6 to 12 months of presentation.[2,10] Chronic-onset heart failure may respond better to medical therapy in this population of patients.

THERAPY. Therapy for dilated cardiomyopathy associated with HIV infection is generally similar to therapy for nonischemic cardiomyopathy and includes diuretics, digoxin, beta blockers, aldosterone antagonists, and angiotensin-converting enzyme inhibitors as tolerated. No studies have investigated the efficacy of specific cardiac therapeutic regimens other than intravenous immunoglobulin.[19]

Opportunistic or other infections should be sought aggressively and treated with the potential to improve or resolve the cardiomyopathy. Right ventricular biopsy may be useful in identifying infectious causes of failure in order to institute targeted therapy.[6,11] However, right ventricular biopsy is probably underused.

After medical therapy is begun, serial echocardiographic studies should be performed at 4-month intervals (Fig. 61–2).[11] Monitoring recommendations for testing and timing of follow-up are based on studies relating impairment of fractional shortening to a worse prognosis. If function continues to worsen or the clinical course deteriorates, a biopsy should be considered. Patients with congestive heart failure who have not responded to 2 weeks of medical therapy may benefit from cardiac catheterization and endomyocardial biopsy, which may reveal lymphocytic infiltrates suggesting myocarditis or treatable opportunistic infections (by special stains), permitting aggressive therapy of an underlying pathogen. Tissue should be evaluated for the presence of abnormal mitochondria that could suggest benefit from an antiretroviral "drug holiday." Angiography should be selectively performed if there are risk factors for atherosclerotic disease or suggestive clinical symptoms.[11]

Intravenous immunoglobulins have had some success in acute congestive cardiomyopathy and nonspecific myocarditis in patients who are not infected with HIV.[21] Immunoglobulin therapy is beneficial in Kawasaki disease, an immunologically mediated illness with cardiac dysfunction resembling that seen with HIV disease. Monthly immunoglobulin infusions in HIV-infected pediatric patients have been associated with minimized left ventricular dysfunction, an increase in left ventricular wall thickness, and a

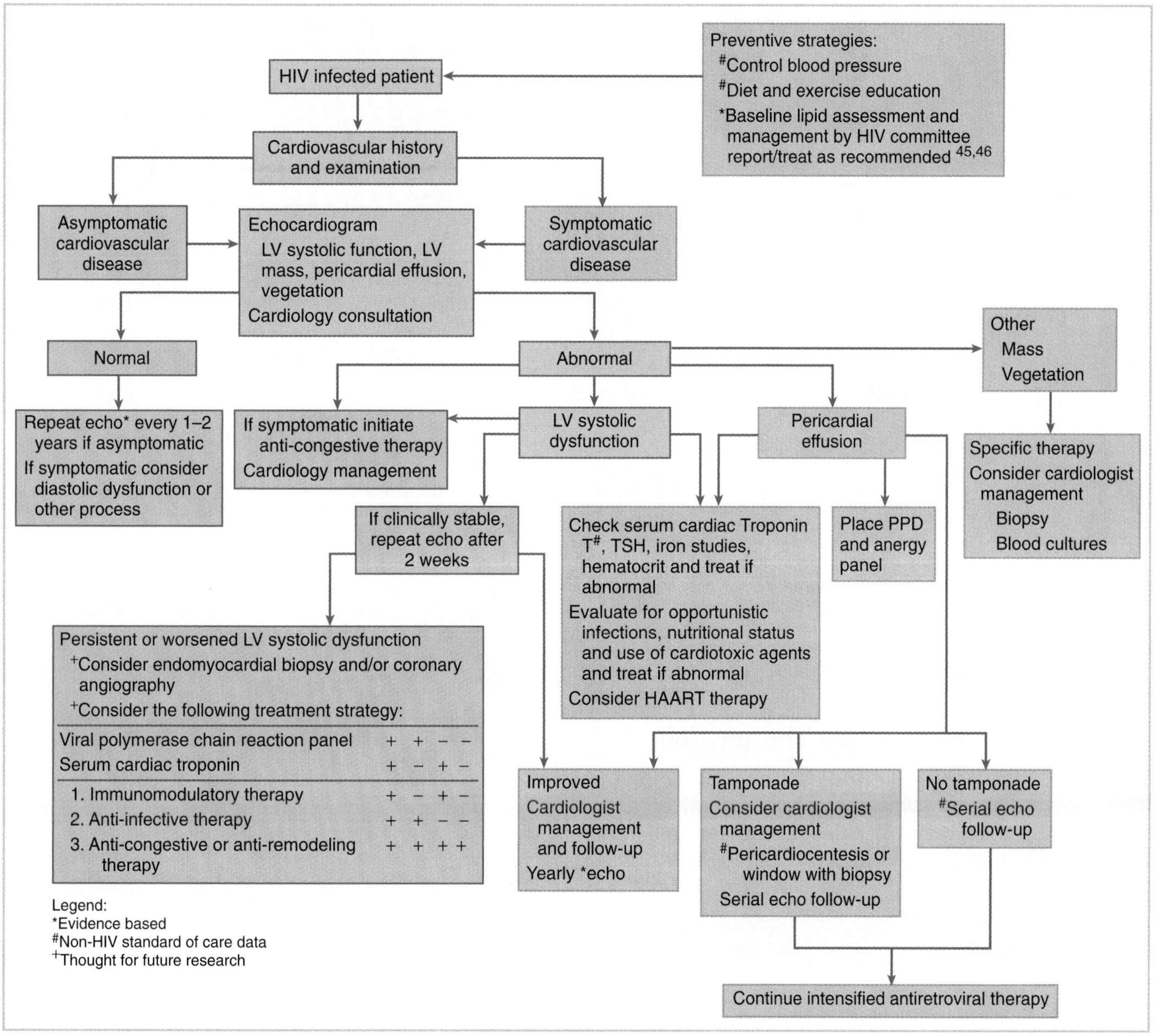

FIGURE 61–2 Cardiac dysfunction in HIV-infected patients. HAART = highly active antiretroviral therapy; LV = left ventricular; PPD = purified protein derivative; TSH = thyroid-stimulating hormone. (From Dolin R, Masur H, Saag MS [eds]: AIDS Therapy. 2nd ed. New York, Churchill Livingstone, 2003, p 817.)

reduction in peak left ventricular wall stress (Fig. 61–3), suggesting that both impaired myocardial growth and left ventricular dysfunction can be immunologically mediated.[19]

The apparent efficacy of immunoglobulin therapy may be the result of immunoglobulins removing cardiac autoantibodies or dampening the secretion or effects of cytokines and cellular growth factors. Immunomodulatory therapy may be helpful in special circumstances or in children with declining left ventricular function.

Patients should be evaluated for nutritional status and any with deficiencies should receive supplements. Supplementation with selenium, carnitine, multivitamins, or all three can be helpful, especially in anorexic patients or those with wasting or diarrhea syndromes.

Solid organ orthotopic heart transplantation has been reported in one HIV-infected man believed to have anthracycline-related cardiomyopathy, with 24 months of follow-up. His course has been complicated by more frequent and higher grade episodes of rejection than average but otherwise relatively uneventful and productive.[22] Liver and kidney transplantation in this population has also now been reported with greater frequency and generally acceptable outcomes. Transplantation therapy is not currently widely available but is an area of active consideration and discussion.

ANIMAL MODELS. Chronic pathogenic simian immunodeficiency virus (SIV) infection in rhesus macaques resulted in significant depression of left ventricular ejection fraction and extensive coronary arteriopathy suggestive of a cell-mediated immune response.[23] Notably, two-thirds of chronically infected macaques that died of SIV had myocardial pathology with lymphocytic myocarditis in 9 of 15 and coronary arteriopathy in 9 of 15 (6 alone and 3 in combination with myocarditis). Coronary arteriopathy was associated with evidence of vessel occlusion and recanalization, with associated areas of myocardial necrosis in four macaques. Two animals had marantic endocarditis and one had a left ventricular mural thrombus on pathological examination. Macaques with cardiac pathology were emaciated to a greater extent than macaques with SIV and similar periods of infection who did not experience cardiac pathology.

Transgenic mouse models with cardiac pathological changes have been created and may help to evaluate the impact of environmental factors, therapeutic or illicit drugs, or drug combinations in both the etiology and therapy of HIV-associated myocarditis.[24]

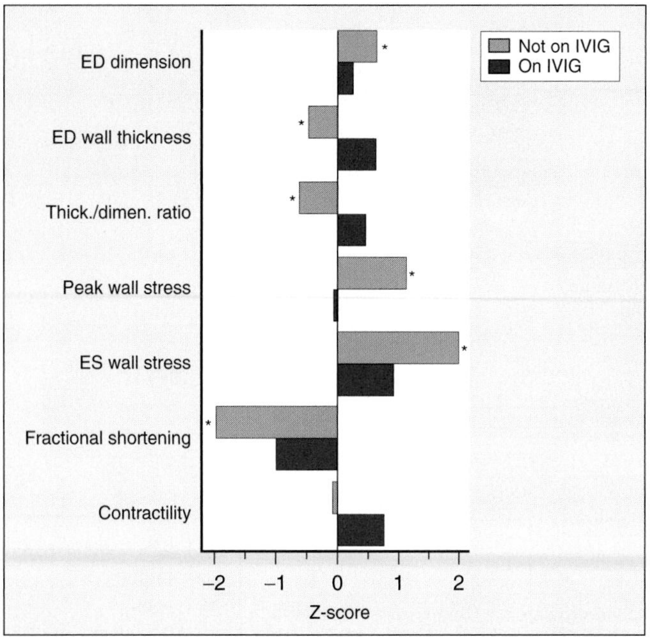

FIGURE 61–3 Mean echocardiographically measured cardiac dimensions in patients taking intravenous immunoglobulin (IVIG) and patients not taking it. All measurements are presented as age- or body surface area–adjusted Z scores. ED = end diastolic; ES = end systolic. (From Lipshultz SE, Orav EJ, Sanders SP, et al: Immunoglobulins and left ventricular structure and function in pediatric HIV infection. Circulation 92:2220, 1995. Copyright 1995, American Heart Association.)

Left Ventricular Diastolic Dysfunction

Clinical and echocardiographic findings suggest that diastolic dysfunction is relatively common in long-term survivors of HIV infection. Left ventricular diastolic dysfunction may precede systolic dysfunction.[11]

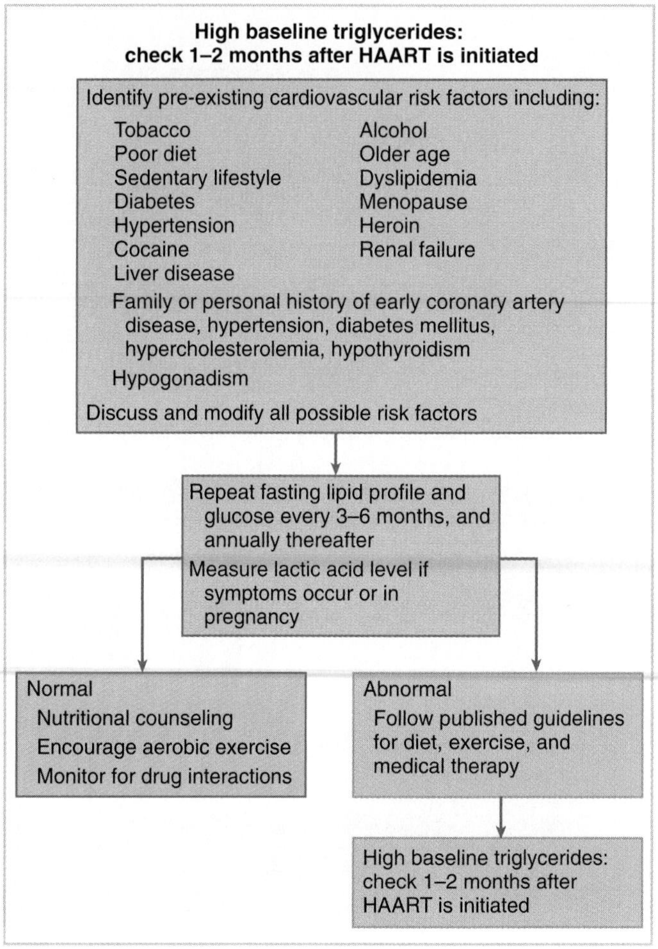

FIGURE 61–4 Cardiovascular considerations when initiating highly active antiretroviral therapy (HAART).

Pericardial Effusion (see Chap. 64)

CLINICAL PRESENTATION. HIV-infected patients with pericardial effusions generally have a lower CD4 count than those without effusions, marking more advanced disease.[10,16] Effusions are generally small and asymptomatic.

INCIDENCE. Asymptomatic pericardial effusions are common in HIV-infected patients. The 5-year Prospective Evaluation of Cardiac Involvement in AIDS (PRECIA) study found that 16 of 231 patients (59 subjects with asymptomatic HIV, 62 with AIDS-related complex, and 74 with AIDS) developed pericardial effusions.[16] Three subjects had an effusion on enrollment and 13 developed effusions during follow-up (12 of them had AIDS). Pericardial effusions were small (maximum pericardial space <10 mm at end diastole) in 80 percent and asymptomatic in 87 percent of patients with effusion. The incidence of pericardial effusion among those with AIDS was 11 percent per year.[16] The prevalence of effusion in AIDS patients rises over time, reaching a mean in asymptomatic patients of about 22 percent after 25 months of follow-up.[16]

HIV infection should be suspected whenever young patients have pericardial effusion or tamponade. In a retrospective series of cardiac tamponade cases in a city hospital, 13 of 37 patients (35 percent) had HIV infection.[10]

PATHOGENESIS. Pericardial effusion may be related to an opportunistic infection, metabolic abnormality, or malignancy (see Table 61–1), but most often a clear etiology is not found. The effusion is often part of a generalized serous effusive process also involving pleural and peritoneal surfaces. This "capillary leak" syndrome may be related to enhanced cytokine production in the later stages of HIV disease. Other causes can include uremia from HIV-associated nephropathy or drug nephrotoxicity. Fibrinous pericarditis with or without effusion is also well described, constituting 9 percent of cardiac lesions found in AIDS patients in one autopsy series.[16]

COURSE OF DISEASE AND PROGNOSIS. Effusion markedly increases mortality. For example, in the PRECIA study, it nearly tripled the risk of death among AIDS patients (Fig. 61–4).[16] Also, 2 of 16 patients with effusions developed pericardial tamponade. Pericardial effusion may, however, resolve spontaneously in up to 42 percent of patients.[10,16] Mortality was still markedly increased in patients who had an effusion.

MONITORING AND THERAPY. Screening echocardiography is recommended in HIV-infected individuals regardless of the stage of disease.[11] All HIV-infected patients with evidence of heart failure, Kaposi sarcoma, tuberculosis, or other pulmonary infections should have baseline echocardiography and ECG testing.[11] Patients should undergo pericardiocentesis if they have pericardial effusion and clinical signs of tamponade such as elevated jugular venous pressure, dyspnea, hypotension, persistent tachycardia, and pulsus paradoxus or echocardiographic signs of tamponade such as valvular inflow respiratory variation by continuous-wave Doppler study, septal bounce, right ventricular diastolic collapse, and a large effusion.

Patients with pericardial effusion without tamponade should be evaluated for treatable opportunistic infections such as tuberculosis and for malignancy. Highly active antiretroviral therapy (HAART) should be considered if therapy has not already been instituted. Repeated echocardiography is recommended after 1 month, or sooner if clinical symptoms direct (see Fig. 61–2).

Infective Endocarditis (see Chap. 58)

Injection drug users are at greater risk than the general population for infective endocarditis, chiefly of right-sided heart valves. Surprisingly, HIV-infected patients may not have a higher incidence of endocarditis than people with similar risk behaviors.

As the autoimmune response to bacterial endocarditis is often largely responsible for valvular destruction associated with endocarditis, variations in the course of the disease in HIV-infected patients may occur. For example, HIV-infected patients have a higher risk of developing salmonella endocarditis than immunocompetent patients because they are more likely to develop salmonella bacteremia during salmonella infection. However, they respond better to antibiotic therapy and may be less likely to sustain valvular damage because of their impaired immune response.[10,25]

Common organisms associated with endocarditis in HIV-infected patients include *Staphylococcus aureus* and *Salmonella* species. Fungal endocarditis with organisms such as *Aspergillus fumigatus*, *Candida* species, and *Cryptococcus neoformans* are more common in intravenous drug users with HIV than in those without it and again may be responsive to therapy (see Table 61–1).[10]

Fulminant courses of infective endocarditis with high mortality can occur in late-stage AIDS patients with poor nutritional status and severely compromised ability to fight infection, but several cases have been successfully treated with antibiotic therapy. Operative indications in HIV-infected patients with endocarditis include hemodynamic instability, failure to sterilize cultures after appropriate intravenous antibiotics, and severe valvular destruction in patients with a reasonable life expectancy after recovery from surgery.

Nonbacterial Thrombotic Endocarditis

Nonbacterial thrombotic endocarditis (or marantic endocarditis) involves large friable sterile vegetations that form on the cardiac valves. These lesions have been associated with disseminated intravascular coagulation and systemic embolization. Lesions are rarely diagnosed ante mortem; among patients who do receive the diagnosis, clinically relevant emboli occur in an estimated 42 percent of cases.[26] In the early HIV epidemic, several case series suggested a high incidence of this uncommon disorder; however, few cases have since been reported, and almost none have been found in prospective series. Marantic endocarditis should be suspected in any patient with systemic embolization, yet it should be considered rare in AIDS patients.

Treatment of nonbacterial thrombotic endocarditis should focus on reducing the underlying disease state causing coagulation abnormalities or valvular endothelial damage, or both. An anticoagulation risk-benefit assessment must be made on an individual basis.

Cardiovascular Malignancy

(see Chap. 63)

Malignancy affects many AIDS patients, generally in the later stages of disease. Cardiac malignancy is usually metastatic disease.

Kaposi sarcoma (angiosarcoma) is associated with human herpesvirus 8 and affects up to 35 percent of AIDS patients, particularly homosexuals, with an incidence inversely related to the CD4 count. Autopsy studies found that 28 percent of HIV-infected patients with widespread Kaposi sarcoma had cardiac involvement and rarely described it as a primary cardiac tumor.[27] Kaposi sarcoma has not been found invading the coronary arteries but is often an endothelial cell neoplasm with a predilection in the heart for subpericardial fat around the coronaries.[27]

Kaposi sarcoma involving the heart is generally an incidental finding at autopsy, rarely causing cardiac symptoms. Specific symptoms can be related to pericardial effusion associated with the epicardial location of the tumor. Pericardial fluid in patients with cardiac Kaposi sarcoma is typically serosanguineous without malignant cells or infection.[27] Kaposi sarcoma is difficult to treat. Most affected patients die from opportunistic infections related to the advanced stage of immunodeficiency rather than from the malignancy. Protease inhibitor use has significantly decreased the incidence of Kaposi sarcoma from the reported incidence in the pre-HAART era.[28]

Primary cardiac malignancy associated with HIV infection is generally due to cardiac lymphoma. Non-Hodgkin lymphomas are 25 to 60 times more common in HIV-infected individuals. They are the first manifestation of AIDS in up to 4 percent of new cases.[29] Patients with primary cardiac lymphoma can present with dyspnea, right-sided heart failure, biventricular failure, chest pain, or arrhythmias.[29] Cardiac lymphoma is associated with rapid progression to cardiac tamponade, symptoms of congestive heart failure, myocardial infarction, tachyarrhythmias, conduction abnormalities, or superior vena cava syndrome. Pericardial fluid typically reveals malignant cells but can be histologically normal. Systemic multiagent chemotherapy with and without concomitant radiation or surgery has been beneficial in some patients, but, overall, the prognosis is poor.[29] HAART has not substantially affected the incidence of HIV-related non-Hodgkin lymphomas.[28]

Leiomyosarcoma, associated with Epstein-Barr virus, is a rare, malignant tumor of smooth muscle origin with an increased incidence in children with AIDS. Leiomyosarcomas are largely noncardiac and often involve the arterial wall.[27] An intracardiac mass in late-stage HIV infection is associated with a uniformly poor prognosis.

Isolated Right Ventricular Disease

Isolated right ventricular hypertrophy with or without right ventricular dilation is relatively uncommon in HIV-infected individuals and is generally related to pulmonary disease that increases pulmonary vascular resistance (see Chap. 67). Possible causes include multiple bronchopulmonary infections, pulmonary arteritis from the immunological effects of HIV disease, or microvascular pulmonary emboli caused by thrombus or contaminants in injected drugs.

Pulmonary Hypertension

Primary pulmonary hypertension has been described in a disproportionate number of HIV-infected individuals, primarily in case reports. Primary pulmonary hypertension is estimated to occur in about 0.5 percent of hospitalized AIDS patients.[30,31] In one series of pulmonary hypertension associated with right ventricular hypertrophy and failure, clinical findings included dyspnea on exertion, hypoxemia, restrictive lung disease with decreased diffusing lung capacity for carbon monoxide, and right ventricular hypertrophy on ECG.[32]

Plexogenic pulmonary arteriopathy characterized by remodeling of the pulmonary vasculature with intimal fibrosis and replacement of normal endothelial structure was frequently demonstrated on lung histology. All of these patients had clear lung fields on examination and chest radiography and normal perfusion scans.

Pulmonary hypertension is often explained by lung infections, venous thromboembolism, or left ventricular dysfunction. Pulmonary hypertension found on screening echocardiography or right heart catheterization warrants further examination for treatable pulmonary infections.

Primary pulmonary hypertension has been reported in HIV-infected patients without a history of thromboembolic disease, intravenous drug use, or pulmonary infections associated with HIV.[30-33] One autopsy and one biopsy specimen revealed precapillary muscular pulmonary artery and arteriole medial hypertrophy, fibroelastosis, and eccentric intimal fibrosis without direct viral infection of pulmonary artery cells. This finding suggests mediator release from infected cells elsewhere. Primary pulmonary hypertension has also been found in hemophiliacs receiving lyophilized factor VIII, intravenous drug users, and patients with left ventricular dysfunction, obscuring any relationship with HIV.[31] It may be that HIV causes endothelial damage and mediator-related vasoconstriction of the pulmonary arteries.

In a study of 82 patients with HIV and pulmonary arterial hypertension, the CD4 count was independently associated with survival and pulmonary hypertension was the direct cause of death in 72 percent. Survival rates at 1, 2, and 3 years were 73, 60, and 47 percent, respectively. Survival rates in New York Heart Association functional Class III-IV patients at the time of diagnosis were 60, 45, and 28 percent.[32]

Therapy includes anticoagulation (on the basis of individual risk-benefit analysis) and vasodilator agents as tolerated. Safe and effective therapy has been reported using treprostinil (subcutaneous prostacyclin analog)[33] and epoprostenol in combination with antiretroviral agents.

Vasculitis

Vasculitis is being reported more often in HIV-infected patients (see Chap. 82).[34] It should be suspected in patients with fever of unknown origin, unexplained multisystem disease, unexplained arthritis or myositis, glomerulonephritis, peripheral neuropathy (especially mononeuritis multiplex), or unexplained gastrointestinal, cardiac, or central nervous system ischemia. Many types of vasculitis have been described in HIV-infected patients (see Table 61–1). Successful immunomodulatory therapy, chiefly with systemic corticosteroid therapy, has been described.

Accelerated Atherosclerosis

Accelerated atherosclerosis has been observed in young HIV-infected individuals without traditional coronary risk factors (see Chaps. 35 and 36).[35-37] Significant coronary lesions were discovered at autopsy in HIV-positive subjects 23 to 32 years of age who died unexpectedly. Cytomegalovirus was present in two of eight patients, and hepatitis B virus was found in two of eight patients. None had evidence of cocaine use.

Premature cerebrovascular disease is common in AIDS patients. An 8 percent stroke prevalence in AIDS patients was estimated in an autopsy study in the 1980s. Of the patients with stroke, 4 of 13 had evidence of cerebral emboli and 3 of those 4 had a clear cardiac source of embolus.

Protease inhibitor therapy significantly alters lipid metabolism and can be associated with premature atherosclerotic disease. Angiographically proven advanced symptomatic coronary artery disease has been reported in three men younger than 40 treated with protease inhibitors.[35] Chronic inflammatory states have also been associated with premature atherosclerotic vascular disease.

The benefits of protease inhibitor therapy and specifically HAART overall, however, have clearly been shown for morbidity and mortality endpoints with no short-term evidence of increased cardiovascular mortality.[1] Lipodystrophy including fat redistribution with increased truncal obesity, increased triglycerides and elevated small dense low-density lipoprotein, and glucose intolerance should still be recognized and treated because of an elevated 10-year cardiovascular risk.[6,11,36] Risk stratification based on traditional risk factors plus diet, alcohol intake, physical exercise, hypertriglyceridemia, cocaine use, heroin use, thyroid disease, renal disease, and hypogonadism should be considered for long-term cardiac preventive care (see Fig. 61–4).

Autonomic Dysfunction

Early clinical signs of autonomic dysfunction in HIV-infected patients include syncope and presyncope, diminished sweating, diarrhea, bladder dysfunction, and impotence (see Chap. 87). In one study, heart rate variability, Valsalva ratio, cold pressor testing, and hemodynamic responses to isometric exercise, tilt-table testing, and standing showed that autonomic dysfunction occurred in patients with AIDS-related complex and was pronounced in AIDS patients. Patients with HIV-associated nervous system disease had the greatest abnormalities in autonomic function (Fig. 61–5).[38,39]

Complications of Therapy for HIV

Potent antiretroviral medications and HAART, which generally combines three or more agents and usually includes a protease inhibitor, have clearly increased the life span and quality of life of HIV-infected patients.[1] However, protease inhibitors, particularly when used in combination therapy or in HAART, are associated with lipodystrophy, fat wasting and redistribution, metabolic abnormalities, hyperlipidemia, insulin resistance, and increased atherosclerotic risk (see Fig. 61–4). HIV-infected patients treated with protease inhibitors have reported substantial decreases in total body fat with peripheral lipodystrophy (fat wasting of the face, limbs, and buttocks) and relative conservation or enhancement of central adiposity (truncal obesity, breast enlargement, and "buffalo hump") compared with patients who have not received protease inhibitors. Lipid alterations associated with protease

CHAPTER 62

Toxins and the Heart

Richard A. Lange • L. David Hillis

A number of toxins can affect the cardiovascular system. This chapter considers the toxins most commonly encountered in the practice of adult cardiology, with the exception of chemotherapeutic agents, a topic discussed in Chapter 83. The toxins discussed here include agents where exposure is primarily volitional (e.g., alcohol and cocaine) as well as toxins encountered in the environment (e.g., heavy metals).

Ethanol

Some two-thirds of Americans occasionally consume ethanol, and approximately 10 percent are considered heavy consumers. Although the ingestion of a moderate amount of ethanol (usually defined as 3 to 9 drinks per week) appears to be associated with a reduced risk of cardiovascular disease, the consumption of excessive amounts has the opposite effect. When ingested in substantial amounts, ethanol may cause ventricular systolic and/or diastolic dysfunction, systemic arterial hypertension, angina pectoris, arrhythmias, and even sudden cardiac death.

Effects of Ethanol on Myocellular Structure and Function

Ethanol may cause myocardial damage via several mechanisms (Table 62–1).[1,2] First, ethanol and its metabolites, acetaldehyde and acetate, may exert a direct toxic effect on the myocardium. Second, deficiencies of certain vitamins (e.g., thiamine), minerals (e.g., selenium), or electrolytes (e.g., magnesium, phosphorus, or potassium) that sometimes occur in heavy ethanol consumers may adversely affect myocardial function. Third, certain substances that are sometimes added to alcoholic beverages, such as lead (often found in "moonshine" alcohol) or cobalt, may be toxic to the myocardium.

Ethanol impairs excitation-contraction, mitochondrial oxidative phosphorylation, and cardiac contractility by adversely affecting the function of the sarcolemmal membrane, sarcoplasmic reticulum, mitochondria, and contractile proteins. Electron microscopic studies of the hearts of experimental animals in close temporal proximity to heavy ethanol ingestion demonstrate dilated sarcoplasmic reticula and swollen mitochondria, with fragmented cristae and glycogen-filled vacuoles. With sustained exposure to ethanol, myofibrillar degeneration and replacement fibrosis appear. In addition to the effects of ethanol on the myocardial contractile apparatus, acute or chronic consumption may adversely influence myofibrillar protein synthesis. Microscopically, the hearts of chronic heavy consumers of ethanol manifest an increased accumulation of collagen in the extracellular matrix as well as increased intermolecular cross-links.

Effects of Ethanol on Organ Function

Chronic heavy ethanol ingestion may induce left ventricular diastolic and/or systolic dysfunction. Diastolic dysfunction, which is caused at least in part by interstitial fibrosis of the myocardium,[3] is often demonstrable in heavy consumers of ethanol even in the absence of symptoms or obvious signs. About half of asymptomatic chronic alcoholics have echocardiographic evidence of left ventricular hypertrophy with preserved systolic performance. By Doppler echocardiography, the left ventricular relaxation time often is prolonged, the peak early diastolic velocity decreases, and the acceleration of early diastolic flow slows—all manifestations of left ventricular diastolic dysfunction. Abnormal increases in left ventricular filling pressure during volume or pressure loading may be observed.

Ethanol may induce asymptomatic left ventricular systolic dysfunction even when it is ingested by healthy individuals in relatively small quantities, as occurs in subjects who are considered only "social" drinkers.[4] As many as 30 percent of asymptomatic chronic alcoholics have echocardiographic evidence of left ventricular systolic dysfunction.[5] With continued heavy ethanol ingestion, these subjects often develop symptoms and signs of congestive heart failure, which is due to a dilated cardiomyopathy. In fact, ethanol abuse is the leading cause of nonischemic dilated cardiomyopathy in industrialized countries, accounting for approximately half of those diagnosed with this entity. The likelihood of developing an ethanol-induced dilated cardiomyopathy correlates with the amount of ethanol consumed in a lifetime. Most men who develop an ethanol-induced dilated cardiomyopathy have consumed more than 80 gm of ethanol (i.e., 1 liter of wine, 8 standard-sized beers, or one-half pint of hard liquor) per day for at least 5 years.[6] Women appear even more susceptible to

TABLE 62–1 Mechanisms of Ethanol-Induced Myocardial Injury

• **Direct toxic effects** *Uncoupling of the excitation/contraction system* *Reduced calcium sequestration in sarcoplasmic reticulum* *Inhibition of sarcolemmal ATP-dependent Na^+/K^+ pump* *Reduction in mitochondrial respiratory ratio* *Altered substrate utilization* *Increased interstitial/extracellular protein synthesis*
• **Toxic effect of metabolites** *Acetaldehyde* *Ethyl esters*
• **Nutritional or trace metal deficiencies** *Thiamine* *Selenium*
• **Electrolyte disturbances** *Hypomagnesemia* *Hypokalemia* *Hypophosphatemia*
• **Toxic additives** *Cobalt* *Lead*

ATP = adenosine triphosphate.

ethanol's cardiotoxic effects, in that they may develop a dilated cardiomyopathy following the consumption of a smaller amount of ethanol per day and per lifetime when compared to their male counterparts.[7]

With abstinence from ethanol, left ventricular systolic and diastolic function often improve[8,9]; the earlier in the course of ethanol consumption that abstinence is initiated, the more pronounced the benefit. Even subjects with markedly symptomatic ethanol-induced dilated cardiomyopathy may manifest a substantial improvement in left ventricular systolic function and symptoms of heart failure with complete abstinence or a dramatic reduction in ethanol consumption. Although most of this improvement occurs in the first 6 months of abstinence, it often continues for as long as 2 years of observation.

Although many heavy ethanol consumers develop a dilated cardiomyopathy, others do not, thereby suggesting individual variability in susceptibility to ethanol's cardiotoxic effects. In this regard, some studies have suggested that genetic polymorphisms in the angiotensin-converting enzyme (ACE) gene may play a role in the development of ethanol-induced dilated cardiomyopathy. Subjects who are homozygous for the deletion polymorphism of the ACE gene (so-called DD) have increased plasma and cardiac levels of ACE. In the absence of ethanol consumption, these homozygous individuals reportedly have increased risk of developing left ventricular hypertrophy and idiopathic dilated cardiomyopathy. Similarly, alcoholics who are homozygous for this deletion polymorphism appear more likely to develop a dilated cardiomyopathy than alcoholic subjects without it.[10]

Ethanol and Systemic Arterial Hypertension

It is estimated that ethanol is of etiologic importance in as many as 11 percent of men with hypertension. Individuals who consume more than two drinks per day are 1.5 to 2 times more likely to have hypertension when compared to age- and gender-matched nondrinkers.[11,12] This effect is dose related and is most prominent when the daily ethanol intake exceeds five drinks (i.e., 30 gm of ethanol).[13,14] "Social" ethanol consumption is associated with a modest rise in systolic arterial pressure, whereas heavy consumption may lead to a substantial increase. Although the mechanism by which ethanol induces a rise in systemic arterial pressure is poorly understood, previous studies have demonstrated that ethanol consumption increases plasma levels of catecholamines, renin, and aldosterone, each of which may cause systemic arterial vasoconstriction. In individuals with ethanol-induced hypertension, a normalization of systemic arterial pressure often follows abstinence.

Ethanol and Lipid Metabolism

Ethanol consumption inhibits the oxidation of free fatty acids by the liver, which stimulates hepatic triglyceride synthesis and the secretion of very low-density lipoprotein cholesterol. Most commonly, therefore, ethanol consumption causes hypertriglyceridemia. In addition, it may cause an increase in the serum concentrations of total cholesterol and its low-density lipoprotein (LDL) component. Regular ethanol consumption increases the serum concentration of HDL cholesterol. Subjects with hyperlipidemia should be encouraged to limit their ethanol intake.[15]

Coronary Artery Disease

Heavy ethanol use is associated with an increased incidence of atherosclerotic coronary artery disease and resultant cardiovascular morbidity and mortality. This increase may result, at least in part, from classic coronary risk factors common in heavy ethanol consumers, such as systemic arterial hypertension, an increased left ventricular muscle mass (with concomitant diastolic and/or systolic dysfunction), and hypertriglyceridemia. In addition, heavy ethanol drinkers often smoke cigarettes. In contradistinction, mild to moderate ethanol intake (two to seven drinks per week) appears to be associated with a decreased risk of cardiovascular morbidity and mortality in both men and women. This reduced risk of cardiovascular morbidity and mortality among consumers of moderate amounts of ethanol—when compared with nondrinkers or heavy consumers—is supported by numerous retrospectively and prospectively conducted studies. The French were noted to have a reduced incidence of coronary artery disease when compared to inhabitants of other countries with similar dietary habits (the so-called French paradox).[16] Although this diminished incidence initially was attributed to the antioxidant and antithrombotic properties of red wine, similar findings subsequently were reported in mild to moderate consumers of other alcoholic beverages and in other study populations.[17] Several prospectively performed cohort studies have demonstrated that drinkers of moderate amounts of ethanol are 40 to 70 percent less likely to manifest coronary artery disease or ischemic stroke when compared to nondrinkers or heavy consumers.[17-22] Some studies have suggested that the consumption of all alcoholic beverages exerts such an effect,[17] whereas others have reported that this so-called cardioprotection is strongest with the consumption of wine.[23] The mechanism(s) by which the consumption of moderate amounts of ethanol reduces cardiovascular risk appear to be multifactorial, in that moderate consumption exerts several beneficial effects, including (1) an increase in the serum concentrations of HDL cholesterol and apolipoprotein AI; (2) inhibition of platelet aggregation; (3) a decreased serum fibrinogen concentration; (4) increased antioxidant activity (from the phenolic compounds and flavonoids contained in red wine); and (5) improved fibrinolysis (resulting from increased concentrations of endogenous tissue plasminogen activator and a concomitant decrease in endogenous plasminogen activator inhibitor activity) (Fig. 62–1).[15,24,25]

Some studies have suggested that the cardioprotective effects of moderate ethanol intake are manifest only in those who are at increased risk for coronary artery disease (i.e.,

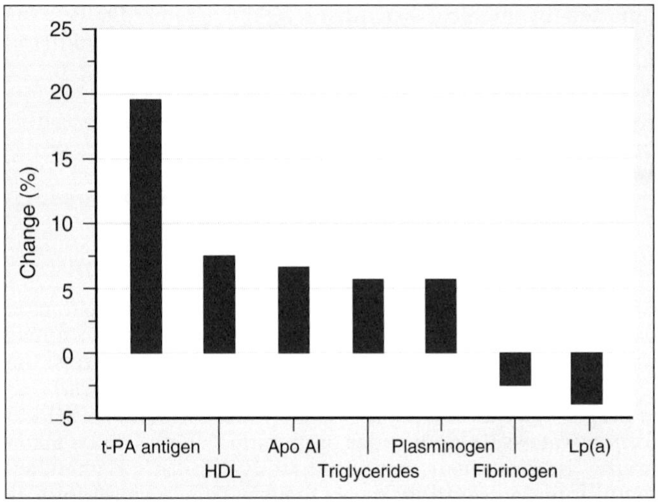

FIGURE 62–1 Percentage change in various blood variables caused by the ingestion of 30 gm of ethanol daily.[15] The ingestion of ethanol, 30 gm daily, for 1 to 9 weeks was associated with increased serum concentrations of tissue type plasminogen activator (t-PA) antigen, high-density lipoprotein (HDL) cholesterol, apolipoprotein AI (Apo AI), serum triglycerides, and serum plasminogen, as well as decreased concentrations of serum fibrinogen and lipoprotein (a) [Lp(a)]. The reduced risk of cardiovascular events seen in subjects who consume moderate amounts of ethanol may be due, at least in part, to these beneficial changes in blood variables.

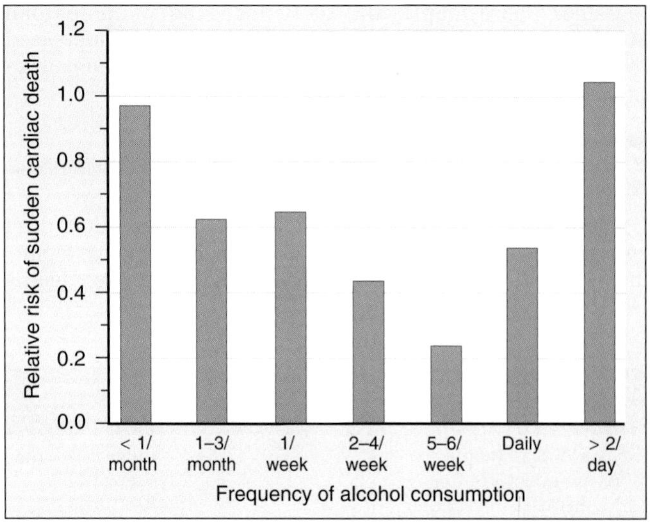

FIGURE 62–3 Ethanol consumption and the risk of sudden cardiac death among U.S. male physicians.[29] In comparison to those who had less than 1 drink per month (far left bar), those who consumed small or moderate amounts of ethanol (middle bars) had a reduced risk of sudden cardiac death. In contrast, those who consumed at least two drinks per day (far right bar) had an increased risk.

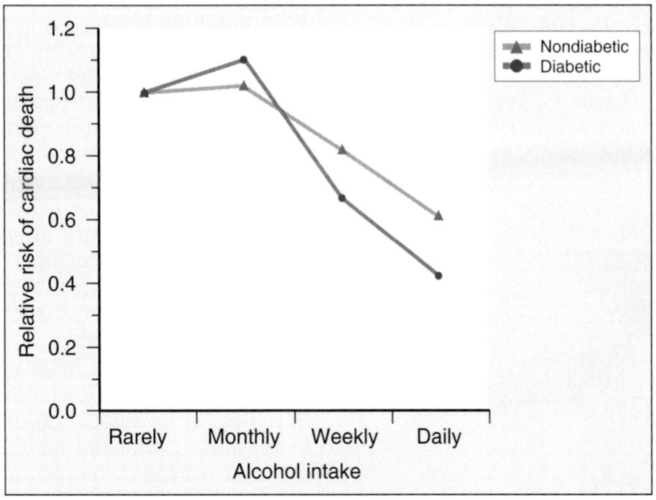

FIGURE 62–2 Ethanol consumption and relative risk of cardiac death according to diabetic status, with data from The Physicians Health Study.[28] Light to moderate alcohol consumption is associated with similar risk reductions in cardiac death among diabetic and nondiabetic men.

those > 50 to 60 years of age,[20] men with an LDL cholesterol concentration > 200 mg/dl,[26] and women with multiple risk factors for atherosclerosis).[20] Other studies have demonstrated that light to moderate ethanol consumption is associated with similar risk reductions in coronary artery disease among diabetic and nondiabetic men and women (Fig. 62–2).[27,28]

In subjects without known cardiac disease, the decrease in cardiovascular mortality associated with moderate ethanol intake results largely from a reduction in the incidence of sudden death (Fig. 62–3). Of the more than 21,000 men in the Physicians Health Study, those who consumed two to four or five or six drinks per week had a significantly reduced risk of sudden death (relative risks, 0.40 and 0.21, respectively) when compared to those who rarely or never drank.[29] In contrast, heavy ethanol consumption (i.e., six or more drinks per day) or binge drinking was associated with an increased risk of sudden death.

In survivors of myocardial infarction (MI), moderate ethanol consumption appears to reduce subsequent mortality.[19,30] In the setting of an acute MI, the recent ingestion of ethanol does not appear to reduce infarct size or the propensity for the subsequent appearance of an arrhythmia or heart failure.[31]

Arrhythmias

Ethanol consumption is associated with a variety of atrial and ventricular arrhythmias,[32,33] most commonly (1) atrial or ventricular premature beats, (2) supraventricular tachycardia, (3) atrial flutter, (4) atrial fibrillation, (5) ventricular tachycardia, or (6) ventricular fibrillation. The most common ethanol-induced arrhythmia is atrial fibrillation.[33] Ethanol is etiologically important in about one-third of subjects with new-onset atrial fibrillation; in those younger than 65 years of age, it may be responsible for as many as two-thirds of subjects. Most episodes occur after binge drinking, usually on weekends or holidays; hence, the term *holiday heart.* Electrophysiological testing in humans without cardiac disease has shown that ethanol enhances the vulnerability to the induction of atrial flutter and atrial fibrillation. The treatment of these ethanol-induced arrhythmias is abstinence.

Ethanol may be arrhythmogenic via several mechanisms. In many ethanol consumers, concomitant factors may predispose to arrhythmias, including cigarette smoking, electrolyte disturbances, metabolic abnormalities, or sleep apnea. Acute ethanol ingestion induces a diuresis, which is accompanied by the concomitant urinary loss of sodium, potassium, and magnesium. The presence of myocardial interstitial fibrosis, ventricular hypertrophy, cardiomyopathy, and autonomic dysfunction also may enhance the likelihood of dysrhythmias.

Sudden Death

Heavy ethanol consumption associates with an increased incidence of sudden death, irrespective of the presence of coronary artery disease. The incidence of ethanol-induced sudden death increases with age and the amount of ethanol ingested. For example, the daily ingestion of more than 80 gm of ethanol is associated with a threefold increased incidence of mortality when compared to a daily consumption of a lesser amount.

Cocaine

Cocaine is currently the most commonly used illicit drug among subjects seeking care in hospital emergency departments, and it is the most frequent cause of drug-related deaths reported by medical examiners in the United States.[34] Its widespread use is attributable to (1) its ease of administration, (2) the ready availability of relatively pure drug, (3) its relatively low cost, and (4) the misperception that its recreational use is safe. As cocaine abuse has increased in prevalence, the number of cocaine-related cardiovascular complications, including angina pectoris, MI, cardiomyopathy, and sudden death, has increased (Table 62–2).

TABLE 62–2 Cardiovascular Complications of Cocaine Use

Myocardial ischemia	Pulmonary edema
Angina pectoris	Myocarditis
Myocardial infarction	Endocarditis
Sudden death	Aortic dissection
Arrhythmias	

TABLE 62–3 Pharmacokinetics of Cocaine According to the Route of Administration

Route of Administration	Onset of Action	Peak Effect	Duration of Action
Inhalation (smoking)	3-5 sec	1-3 min	5-15 min
Intravenous	10-60 sec	3-5 min	20-60 min
Intranasal or other mucosal	1-5 min	15-20 min	60-90 min

Pharmacology and Mechanisms of Action

Cocaine (benzoylmethylecgonine) is an alkaloid extracted from the leaf of the *Erythroxylon coca* bush, which grows primarily in South America. It is available in two forms: the hydrochloride salt and the "freebase." Cocaine *hydrochloride* is prepared by dissolving the alkaloid in hydrochloric acid to form a water-soluble powder or granule, which can be taken orally, intravenously, or intranasally (so-called chewing, mainlining, or snorting, respectively). The *freebase* form is manufactured by processing the cocaine with ammonia or sodium bicarbonate (baking soda). Unlike the hydrochloride form, freebase cocaine is heat stable, so that it can be smoked. It is known as "crack" because of the popping sound it makes when heated.

Cocaine hydrochloride is well absorbed through all mucous membranes; therefore, users may achieve a high blood concentration with intranasal, sublingual, intravaginal, or rectal administration. The route of administration determines the rapidity of onset and duration of action (Table 62–3). The euphoria associated with smoking crack cocaine occurs within seconds and is short lived. Crack cocaine is considered the most potent and addictive form of the drug. Cocaine is metabolized by serum and liver cholinesterases to water-soluble metabolites (primarily benzoylecgonine and ecgonine methyl ester), which are excreted in the urine. Since cocaine's serum half-life is only 45 to 90 minutes, it is detectable in blood or urine only for several hours after its use. However, its metabolites are detectable in blood or urine for 24 to 36 hours after its administration.

When applied locally, cocaine acts as an anesthetic by virtue of its inhibition of membrane permeability to sodium during depolarization, thereby blocking the initiation and transmission of electrical signals. When given systemically, it blocks the presynaptic reuptake of norepinephrine and dopamine, thereby producing an excess of these neurotransmitters at the site of the postsynaptic receptor (Fig. 62–4). In short, cocaine acts as a powerful sympathomimetic agent.

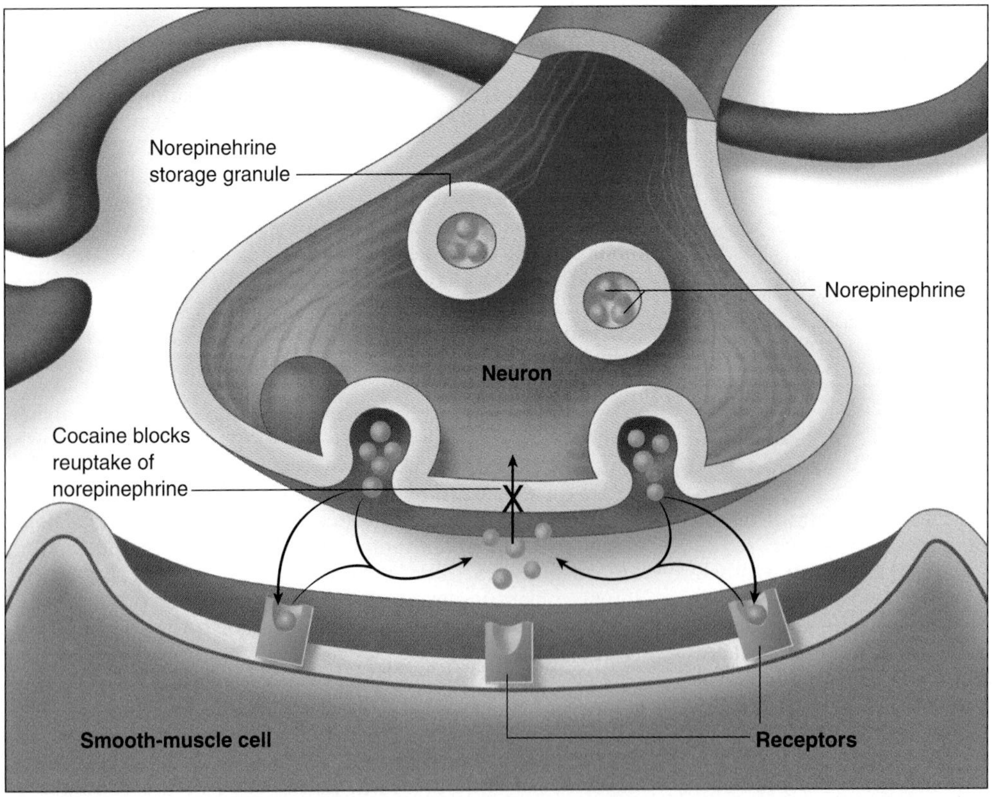

FIGURE 62–4 The mechanism by which cocaine alters sympathetic tone. Cocaine blocks the reuptake of norepinephrine by the preganglionic neuron (X), resulting in excess amounts of this neurotransmitter at receptor sites at the postganglionic site.

Cocaine-Related Myocardial Ischemia and Infarction

In 1982, Coleman and associates reported an association between cocaine use and myocardial ischemia and infarction. Subsequently, numerous reports have described cocaine-related myocardial ischemic events. In one survey of 10,085 adults, aged 18 to 45 years, 25 percent of nonfatal MI were attributed to cocaine use.[35] Cocaine-related myocardial ischemia or infarction may result from (1) increased myocardial oxygen demand in the setting of a limited or fixed oxygen supply; (2) marked coronary arterial vasoconstriction; and (3) enhanced platelet aggregation and thrombus formation (Fig. 62–5).

By virtue of its sympathomimetic effects, cocaine increases the three major determinants of myocardial oxygen demand: heart rate, left ventricular wall tension, and left ventricular contractility. At the same time, the ingestion of even small amounts of the drug causes vasoconstriction of the epicardial coronary arteries (so-called inappropriate vasoconstriction) in that the myocardial oxygen supply decreases as demand increases.[36] Cocaine induces vasoconstriction in normal and diseased coronary arterial segments, but its vasoconstrictive effect is particularly marked in the latter.[37] As a result, cocaine users with atherosclerotic coronary artery disease are probably at an especially high risk for an ischemic event after cocaine use. Cocaine-induced coronary arterial vasoconstriction primarily results from the stimulation of coronary arterial alpha-adrenergic receptors, since it is reversed by phentolamine (an alpha-adrenergic antagonist)[36] and exacerbated by propranolol (a beta-adrenergic antagonist).[38] In addition, cocaine causes increased endothelial production of endothelin (a potent vasoconstrictor) and decreased production of nitric oxide (a potent vasodilator), which also may promote vasoconstriction.

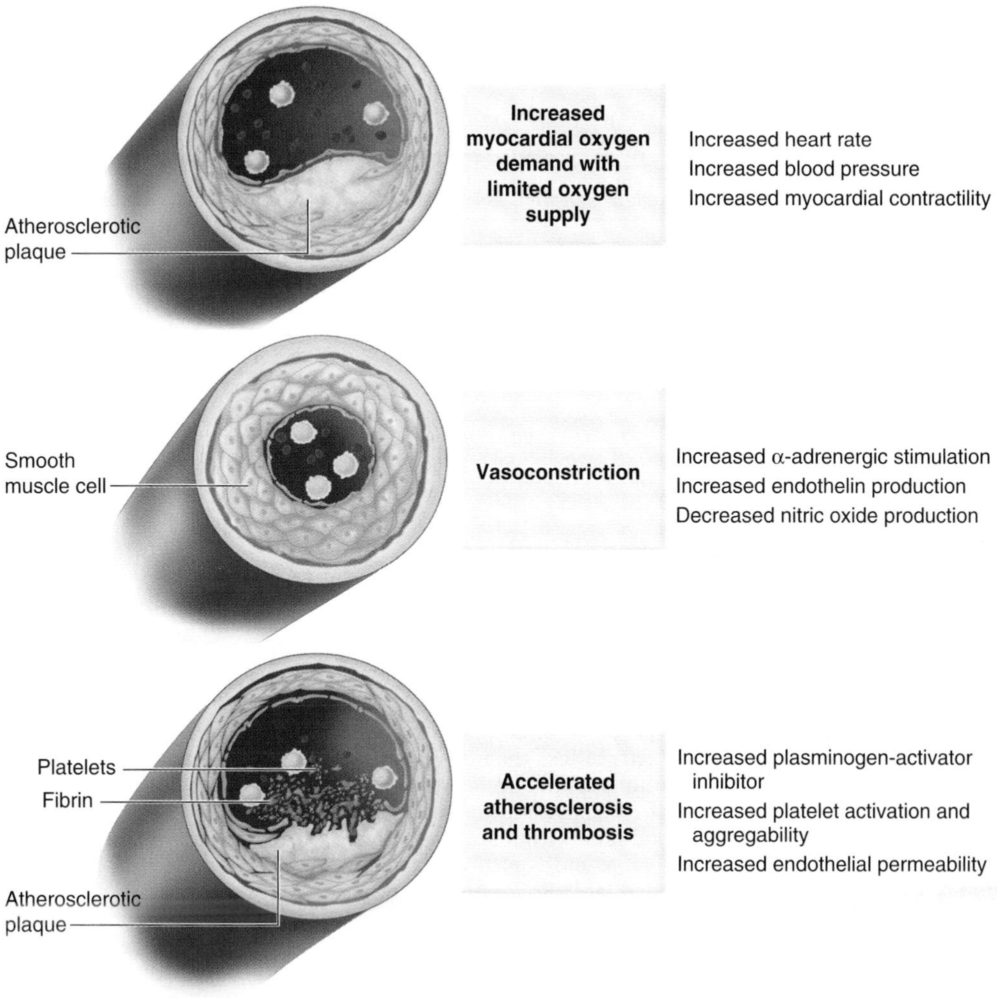

FIGURE 62–5 Mechanisms by which cocaine may induce myocardial ischemia or infarction. Cocaine may induce myocardial ischemia or infarction by increasing the determinants of myocardial oxygen demand in the setting of limited oxygen supply **(top)**, causing intense coronary arterial vasoconstriction **(middle)**, or inducing accelerated atherosclerosis and thrombosis **(bottom)**.

Cocaine use is associated with enhanced platelet activation and aggregability[39] as well as an increased concentration of plasminogen activator inhibitor,[40] which may promote thrombus formation. The presence of premature atherosclerotic coronary artery disease, which has been observed in postmortem studies of long-term cocaine users, may provide a nidus for thrombus formation. In vitro studies have shown that cocaine causes structural abnormalities in the endothelial cell barrier, increasing its permeability to LDL and enhancing the expression of endothelial adhesion molecules and leukocyte migration, all of which are associated with atherogenesis.

Chest pain is the most common cardiovascular complaint of patients seeking medical assistance following cocaine use. Approximately 6 percent of those who come to the emergency department with cocaine-associated chest pain have enzymatic evidence of myocardial necrosis.[41] Most subjects with cocaine-related MI are young, nonwhite, male cigarette smokers without other risk factors for atherosclerosis who have a history of repeated cocaine use (Table 62–4). Similar to cocaine, cigarette smoking induces coronary arterial vasoconstriction through an alpha-adrenergic mechanism. The deleterious effects of cocaine on myocardial oxygen supply and demand are exacerbated substantially by concomitant cigarette smoking: following concomitant cocaine use and smoking, heart rate and systemic arterial pressure increase markedly, and coronary arterial vasoconstriction is more intense than with either alone.[42]

The risk of MI is increased 24-fold during the 60 minutes after cocaine use by subjects considered at low risk for infarction.[43] The occurrence of MI after cocaine use appears unrelated to the amount ingested, its route of administration, and the frequency of its use: cocaine-related infarction has been reported with doses ranging from 200 to 2000 mg, after ingestion by all routes, and in habitual as well as first-time users. About half the patients with cocaine-related MI have no angiographic evidence of atherosclerotic coronary artery disease.[43] Therefore, when subjects with no or few risk factors for atherosclerosis, particularly those who are young or have a history of substance abuse, present with acute MI, urine and blood samples should be analyzed for cocaine and its metabolites.

TABLE 62–4 Characteristics of Patients with Cocaine-Induced Myocardial Infarction

- **Dose of cocaine**
  5 or 6 lines (150 mg) to as much as 2 gm
  Serum concentration, 0.01 to 1.02 mg/liter
- **Frequency of use**
  Reported in chronic, recreational, and first-time users
- **Route of administration**
  Occurs with all routes of administration
  75% of reported myocardial infarctions occurred after intranasal use
- **Age**
  Mean, 34 (range, 17-71) yr
  20% are < 25 yr
- **Gender**
  80%-90% male
- **Timing**
  Often within minutes of cocaine use
  Reported as late as 5-15 hr after use

Cardiovascular complications resulting from cocaine-related MI are relatively uncommon, with ventricular arrhythmias occurring in 4 to 17 percent, congestive heart failure in 5 to 7 percent, and death in less than 2 percent.[34] This low incidence of complications is due, at least in part, to the young age and absence of extensive multivessel coronary artery disease of most patients with cocaine-related infarction. If complications develop, most occur within 12 hours of presentation to the hospital.[44] Following hospital discharge, continued cocaine use and recurrent chest pain are common, and occasionally a patient has recurrent nonfatal or fatal MI.

Most subjects with cocaine-related myocardial ischemia or infarction have chest pain within an hour of cocaine use, at a time when the blood cocaine concentration is highest. However, an occasional individual notes the onset of symptoms several hours after the administration of the drug, when the blood cocaine concentration is low or even undetectable. With cocaine ingestion, the diameter of the coronary arteries decreases as the drug concentration increases. Then, as the drug concentration declines, the vasoconstriction resolves. Thereafter, as the concentrations of cocaine's major metabolites (benzoylecgonine and ecgonine methyl ester) rise, "delayed" (i.e., recurrent) coronary arterial vasoconstriction occurs,[45] thereby providing an explanation of why myocardial ischemia or infarction has been reported to occur several hours after drug use.

Cocaethylene

In individuals who use cocaine in temporal proximity to the ingestion of ethanol, hepatic transesterification leads to the production of a unique metabolite, cocaethylene. Cocaethylene is often detected postmortem in subjects who are presumed to have died of cocaine and ethanol toxicity. Similar to cocaine, cocaethylene blocks the reuptake of dopamine at the synaptic cleft, thereby possibly potentiating the systemic toxic effects of cocaine. In experimental animals, in fact, cocaethylene is more lethal than cocaine.[46] In humans, the combination of cocaine and ethanol has been shown to cause a substantial increase in myocardial oxygen demand. The concomitant use of cocaine and ethanol is associated with a higher incidence of disability and death than either agent alone.[47] Individuals presumably dying of a combined cocaine-ethanol overdose have been found to have much lower blood cocaine concentrations than those presumably dying of a cocaine overdose alone, thereby suggesting an additive or synergistic effect of ethanol on the catastrophic cardiovascular events induced by cocaine.

Cocaine-Induced Myocardial Dysfunction

Long-term cocaine abuse has been associated with left ventricular hypertrophy and systolic dysfunction. Several reports have described dilated cardiomyopathy in long-term cocaine abusers, and others have described profound but reversible myocardial depression after binge cocaine use. Bertolet and colleagues found that 7 percent of long-term chronic users without cardiac symptoms had radionuclide ventriculographic evidence of left ventricular systolic dysfunction.[48]

Cocaine may adversely affect left ventricular systolic function by several mechanisms.[34] First, as noted previously, cocaine may induce myocardial ischemia or infarction. Second, the profound repetitive sympathetic stimulation induced by cocaine is similar to that observed in patients with pheochromocytoma—either may induce a cardiomyopathy and characteristic microscopic changes of subendocardial contraction band necrosis. Third, the concomitant administration of adulterants or infectious agents may cause myocarditis, which has been seen on occasion in intravenous cocaine users studied at postmortem. Fourth, studies in experimental animals have shown that cocaine alters cytokine production in the endothelium and in circulating leukocytes, induces the transcription of genes responsible for changes in the composition of myocardial collagen and myosin, and induces myocyte apoptosis.

Aside from the effects of long-term cocaine use on myocardial performance, it may cause an acute deterioration of left ventricular systolic and/or diastolic function. In some subjects, this deterioration may be caused by metabolic and/or acid-base disturbances that accompany cocaine intoxication, whereas in others it may be caused by a direct toxic effect of the drug. Pitts and coworkers demonstrated that an intracoronary infusion of cocaine (in an amount sufficient to produce a concentration in coronary sinus blood similar in magnitude to the peripheral blood concentration found in abusers presumably dying of cocaine intoxication) had a deleterious effect on left ventricular systolic and diastolic function.[49] It seems feasible that cocaine or its metabolites alter the manner in which myocytes handle calcium.

Arrhythmias

Cardiac dysrhythmias may occur with cocaine use (Table 62–5), but the precise arrhythmogenic potential of the drug is poorly defined. In many instances, the dysrhythmias ascribed to cocaine occur in the setting of profound hemodynamic or metabolic derangements, such as hypotension, hypoxemia, seizures, or MI. Nonetheless, because of cocaine's sodium-channel–blocking properties and its ability to enhance sympathetic activation, it is considered a likely

TABLE 62–5 Cardiac Dysrhythmias and Conduction Disturbances Reported with Cocaine Use

Sinus tachycardia	Ventricular tachycardia
Sinus bradycardia	Ventricular fibrillation
Supraventricular tachycardia	Asystole
Bundle branch block	Torsade de pointes
Complete heart block	Brugada pattern (right bundle branch block with ST segment elevation in leads V_1 to V_3)
Accelerated idioventricular rhythm	

cause of cardiac arrhythmias.[50] The development of lethal arrhythmias with cocaine use may require an underlying substrate of abnormal myocardium: studies in experimental animals have shown that cocaine precipitates ventricular arrhythmias only in the presence of myocardial ischemia or infarction. In humans, life-threatening arrhythmias and sudden death in association with cocaine use occur most often in those with myocardial ischemia or infarction or in those with nonischemic myocellular damage. Long-term cocaine use is associated with increased left ventricular mass and wall thickness,[51] a known risk factor for ventricular dysrhythmias. In some cocaine users, such an increased mass may provide the substrate for arrhythmias.

Cocaine may affect the generation and conduction of cardiac impulses by several mechanisms. First, its sympathomimetic properties may increase ventricular irritability and lower the threshold for fibrillation. Second, it inhibits action potential generation and conduction (i.e., it prolongs the QRS and QT intervals) as a result of its sodium-channel–blocking effects. In so doing, it acts in a manner similar to that of a class I antiarrhythmic agent. Third, cocaine increases the intracellular calcium concentration, which may result in afterdepolarizations and triggered ventricular arrhythmias. Fourth, it reduces vagal activity, thereby potentiating its sympathomimetic effects.

Endocarditis

Although the intravenous administration of any illicit drug is associated with an increased risk of bacterial endocarditis, the intravenous use of cocaine appears to be accompanied by a greater risk of endocarditis than the intravenous administration of other drugs.[52] The reason for this enhanced risk of endocarditis in intravenous cocaine users is unknown, but several hypotheses have been proposed. The increase in heart rate and systemic arterial pressure that accompanies cocaine use may induce valvular injury that predisposes to bacterial invasion. Cocaine's immunosuppressive effects may increase the risk of infection. The manner in which cocaine is manufactured as well as the adulterants that are often present in it may increase the risk of endocarditis. In contradistinction to the endocarditis associated with other drugs, the endocarditis of cocaine users more often involves the left-sided cardiac valves.

Aortic Dissection

Aortic dissection or rupture has been temporally related to cocaine use; therefore, it should be considered as a possible cause of chest pain in cocaine users (see Chap. 53). In one study of 38 patients with acute aortic dissection, 14 (37 percent) were related to cocaine use, with an average interval from cocaine use to the onset of symptoms of 12 (range, 0 to 24) hours.[53] Dissection probably results from a cocaine-induced increase in systemic arterial pressure. In addition to aortic rupture, the cocaine-related rupture of mycotic and intracerebral aneurysms has been reported.

Amphetamines

Amphetamines were prescribed previously for the treatment of obesity, attention deficit disorder, and narcolepsy; at present, their use is strictly limited. The most frequently abused amphetamines are dextroamphetamine, methcathinone, methamphetamine, methylphenidate, ephedrine, propylhexedrine, phenmetrazine, and 3,4-methylenedioxymethamphetamine (MDMA, also known as *ecstasy*). *Ice* is a freebase form of methamphetamine that can be inhaled, smoked, or injected. Since amphetamines are sympathomimetic agents, their use has been associated with systemic arterial hypertension, MI, and lethal arrhythmias.[54] Similar to cocaine, amphetamines may induce intense coronary arterial vasoconstriction with or without thrombus formation.[55] Finally, subjects with dilated cardiomyopathy following repetitive amphetamine use have been described.

Catecholamines

Catecholamines, administered exogenously or secreted by a neuroendocrine tumor (e.g., pheochromocytoma or neuroblastoma), may produce acute myocarditis (with focal myocardial necrosis and inflammation), cardiomyopathy, tachycardia, and arrhythmias. Similar abnormalities have been described with the excessive use of beta-adrenoceptor agonist inhalants and methylxanthines in patients with severe pulmonary disease.[56] The secretion of large amounts of endogenous catecholamines, as may occur in subjects with subarachnoid hemorrhage, has been associated with the appearance of transient left ventricular apical dyskinesis and electrocardiographic (ECG) T wave inversions anteriorly. This entity, known as *takotsubo cardiomyopathy*, spontaneously resolves when catecholamine secretion abates.[57]

Several mechanisms may be responsible for the acute and chronic myocardial damage associated with catecholamines. They may exert a direct toxic effect on the myocardium through changes in autonomic tone, enhanced lipid mobility, calcium overload, free radical production, or increased sarcolemmal permeability. Alternatively, myocardial damage may be secondary to a sustained increase in myocardial oxygen demand and/or decrease in myocardial oxygen supply (the latter due to catecholamine-induced coronary arterial vasoconstriction or platelet aggregation).

Inhalants

The inhalants may be classified as organic solvents, organic nitrites (such as amyl nitrite or amyl butyl), and nitrous oxide. The organic solvents include toluene (airplane glue), Freon, kerosene, gasoline, carbon tetrachloride, acrylic paint sprays, shoe polish, degreasers, nail polish remover, typewriter correction fluid, adhesives, and lighter fluid. These solvents are most often inhaled by children or young adolescents. Acute or chronic inhalant use occasionally has been reported to induce cardiac abnormalities, most commonly dysrhythmias; rarely, inhalant use has been associated with myocarditis, MI,[58] and sudden death.[59] The inhalation of freon, for example, has been shown to sensitize the myocardium to catecholamines; in these individuals, fatal arrhythmias have been reported to occur when the user is startled during inhalation.[60]

Antiretroviral Agents (Protease Inhibitors)

Subjects treated with protease inhibitors have been observed to have severe hypertriglyceridemia (serum triglycerides > 1000 mg/dl) and marked elevations in lipoprotein(a) (see Chaps. 39 and 61).[61] Not surprisingly, therefore, patients who are maintained on these agents have an increased risk of atherosclerosis.[62] Dilated cardiomyopathy in association with zidovudine use has been reported.[63,64] In mice, zidovudine produces a cardiomyopathy, with pathologic changes demonstrable in the mitochondria,[65] and similar ultrastructural mitochondrial changes have been observed in myocardial biopsy specimens from HIV-infected patients treated with this agent. In one individual, zidovudine's discontinuation resulted in a reversal of cardiac dysfunction.

Ergotamine and Serotonin Agonists

Two medications used to treat subjects with migraine headaches, ergotamine and sumatriptan, have been associated with acute MI. Ergotamine causes vasoconstriction of intracerebral and extracranial arteries; rarely, its use has been associated with coronary arterial vasospasm and acute MI.[66] Its vasoconstrictor effects are exaggerated by concomitant caffeine ingestion or beta-adrenergic blocker use. Sumaptriptan, a selective 5-hydroxytryptamine agonist, also exerts its therapeutic effects by inducing cerebral arterial vasoconstriction. Several patients have been reported in whom coronary vasospasm and acute MI occurred following the administration of therapeutic doses of sumatriptan,[67] some of which were complicated by ventricular tachycardia or ventricular fibrillation and sudden cardiac death.[68]

Appetite Suppressants

Exposure to the appetite suppressants, fenfluramine or dexfenfluramine, alone or in combination with phentermine, has been implicated in the pathogenesis of certain valvular abnormalities. Fenfluramine (Pondimin), a sympathomimetic amine, promotes the release of serotonin and blocks its neuronal uptake; dexfenfluramine (Redux) is the dextroisomer of fenfluramine. Phentermine (Adipex, Fastin, Ionamin) is a noradrenergic central nervous system stimulant.

The association of appetite suppressant use and valvular abnormalities was first described in 1997, when subjects receiving the combination of fenfluramine and phentermine were noted to have unusual valvular morphology and resultant regurgitation of both left- and right-sided heart valves. All had aortic and/or mitral regurgitation, and half had tricuspid regurgitation.[69] Echocardiographic and histopathological findings resembled those described in patients with carcinoid or ergotamine-induced valvular heart disease. Grossly, the aortic and mitral valve leaflets and chordae tendineae were thickened and had a glistening white appearance. Histologically, leaflet architecture was intact; a plaque-like encasement of the leaflets and chordal structures was noted; and proliferative myofibroblasts surrounded by an abundant extracellular matrix were observed. As a result of these observations, the manufacturer withdrew fenfluramine and dexfenfluramine from the market. Since no valvular abnormalities have been associated with the use of phentermine alone, it is still available.

The risk of valvular heart disease associated with exposure to fenfluramine or dexfenfluramine, alone or in combination with phentermine, has been addressed in several studies, with the prevalence of valvular regurgitation varying from less than 1 percent to as much as 26 percent.[70-73] This apparent wide-ranging risk is attributable to differences in study type, patient populations, varying definitions of regurgitation, and differing durations of treatment with these agents. The prevalence of "significant" valvular regurgitation appears to be related directly to the duration of exposure to the anorectic agents.[72] In most subjects, the valvular abnormalities stabilize or improve after the agents are discontinued.[74]

Currently, it is recommended that all persons exposed to fenfluramine or dexfenfluramine for any period of time, alone or in combination with other agents, should undergo a thorough cardiovascular assessment to determine the presence or absence of cardiopulmonary symptoms or signs. Those with symptoms or signs suggestive of valvular disease (e.g., dyspnea or a new murmur) should undergo echocardiographic evaluation.

Pergolide (Permax)

Pergolide is a dopamine receptor agonist that is used in the treatment of subjects with Parkinson disease. During pergolide treatment, a small number of individuals have developed cardiac valvulopathy. In some of them, the symptoms or signs of valvulopathy improved with discontinuation of the drug, whereas others necessitated valve replacement surgery. Pathologically, the excised valves appeared similar morphologically and microscopically to the valvulopathy associated with the carcinoid syndrome or the use of ergot alkaloids.

Paclitaxel (Taxol) and Other Chemotherapeutic Drugs

A number of agents used in cancer chemotherapy can cause cardiac toxicity, a subject considered in detail in Chapter 83. For example, up to 29 percent of patients who receive paclitaxel as a chemotherapeutic agent develop transient asymptomatic bradycardia.[75] More substantial cardiac disturbances, including atrioventricular block, left bundle branch block, ventricular tachycardia, or myocardial ischemia, occur in up to 5 percent of subjects. When paclitaxel is given in combination with doxorubicin, the risk of cardiotoxicity may be higher: some reports have suggested that heart failure developed in as many as 20 percent of patients treated with this combination. Other chemotherapeutic agents that may cause cardiac dysfunction include doxorubicin, cyclophosphamide, trastuzumab (Herceptin),[76] and 5-fluorouracil.[77] The latter also may cause myocardial ischemia or infarction, which is thought to be caused by coronary arterial vasospasm.[78]

Environmental Exposures

Cobalt

In the mid-1960s, an acute and fulminant form of dilated cardiomyopathy was described in heavy beer drinkers. It was suggested that the cobalt chloride, which was added to the beer as a foam stabilizer, was the causative agent[79]; therefore, its addition was discontinued. Subsequently, this acute and severe form of cardiomyopathy disappeared. More recently, several reports of dilated cardiomyopathy after occupational exposure to cobalt have appeared; in these individuals, high concentrations of cobalt were demonstrated in endomyocardial biopsy specimens.[80]

Lead

Patients with lead poisoning typically have complaints that are referable to the gastrointestinal and central nervous systems. On occasion, subjects with lead poisoning have ECG abnormalities, atrioventricular conduction defects, and overt congestive heart failure; rarely, myocardial involvement may contribute to or be the principal cause of death.[81]

Mercury

Occupational exposure to metallic mercuric vapors may cause systemic arterial hypertension and myocardial failure.[82] Although some studies have suggested that a high mercury content of fish may counteract the beneficial effects of its n-3 fatty acids, thereby increasing the risk of atherosclerotic cardiovascular disease,[83,84] more recent assessments have not supported an association between total mercury exposure and the risk of coronary artery disease.[85]

Antimony

Various antimony compounds previously have been used in the treatment of patients with schistosomiasis. Their use is often associated with ECG abnormalities, including prolongation of the QT interval and T wave flattening or inversion.[86] Rarely, chest pain, bradycardia, hypotension, ventricular arrhythmias, and sudden death have been reported.

Arsenic

Arsenic exposure typically occurs from pesticide poisoning. Its cardiac manifestations include pericardial effusion, myocarditis, and various ECG abnormalities, including QT interval prolongation with T wave inversion.[87]

Carbon Monoxide

Carbon monoxide has a higher affinity for hemoglobin than does oxygen; as a result, elevated blood concentrations of carbon monoxide lead to reduced tissue oxygen delivery. Although central nervous system symptoms are the predominant manifestations of carbon monoxide poisoning, cardiac toxicity may occur because of myocardial hypoxia or a direct toxic effect of the gas on myocardial mitochondria. Such cardiac involvement may appear promptly after carbon monoxide exposure, or it may be delayed for several days. Sinus tachycardia and various arrhythmias, including ventricular extrasystoles and atrial fibrillation, are common; bradycardia and atrioventricular block may occur in more severe cases. Angina pectoris[88,89] or MI[90] may be precipitated by carbon monoxide exposure in patients with or without[91,92] underlying coronary artery disease. ECG ST segment and T wave abnormalities occur commonly, and transient ventricular dysfunction may occur. The administration of 100 percent oxygen or treatment in a hyperbaric oxygen chamber usually results in rapid recovery.

REFERENCES

Ethanol

1. Patel VB, Why HJ, Richardson PJ, et al: The effects of alcohol on the heart. Adverse Drug React Toxicol Rev 16:15, 1997.
2. Preedy VR, Patel VB, Why HJ, et al: Alcohol and the heart: Biochemical alterations. Cardiovasc Res 31:139, 1996.
3. Lazarevic AM, Nakatani S, Neskovic AN, et al: Early changes in left ventricular function in chronic asymptomatic alcoholics: Relation to the duration of heavy drinking. J Am Coll Cardiol 35:1599, 2000.
4. Kelbaek H, Gjorup T, Brynjolf I, et al: Acute effects of alcohol on left ventricular function in healthy subjects at rest and during upright exercise. Am J Cardiol 55:164, 1985.
5. Urbano-Marquez A, Estruch R, Fernandez-Sola J, et al: The greater risk of alcoholic cardiomyopathy and myopathy in women compared with men. JAMA 274:149, 1995.
6. Wilke A, Kaiser A, Ferency I, et al: [Alcohol and myocarditis]. Herz 21:248, 1996.
7. Fernandez-Sola J, Estruch R, Nicolas JM, et al: Comparison of alcoholic cardiomyopathy in women versus men. Am J Cardiol 80:481, 1997.
8. Masani F, Kato H, Sasagawa Y, et al: [An echocardiographic study of alcoholic cardiomyopathy after total abstinence]. J Cardiol 20:627, 1990.
9. Nicolas JM, Fernandez-Sola J, Estruch R, et al: The effect of controlled drinking in alcoholic cardiomyopathy. Ann Intern Med 136:192, 2002.
10. Fernandez-Sola J, Nicolas JM, Oriola J, et al: Angiotensin-converting enzyme gene polymorphism is associated with vulnerability to alcoholic cardiomyopathy. Ann Intern Med 137:321, 2002.
11. Klatsky AL: Alcohol and cardiovascular disease—more than one paradox to consider. Alcohol and hypertension: Does it matter? Yes. J Cardiovasc Risk 10:21, 2003.
12. Klatsky AL, Friedman GD, Siegelaub AB, et al: Alcohol consumption and blood pressure: Kaiser-Permanente Multiphasic Health Examination data. N Engl J Med 296:1194, 1977.
13. Thadhani R, Camargo CA Jr, Stampfer MJ, et al: Prospective study of moderate alcohol consumption and risk of hypertension in young women. Arch Intern Med 162:569, 2002.
14. Fuchs FD, Chambless LE, Whelton PK, et al: Alcohol consumption and the incidence of hypertension: The Atherosclerosis Risk in Communities Study. Hypertension 37:1242, 2001.
15. Rimm EB, Williams P, Fosher K, et al: Moderate alcohol intake and lower risk of coronary heart disease: Meta-analysis of effects on lipids and haemostatic factors. BMJ 319:1523, 1999.
16. Renaud S, de Lorgeril M: Wine, alcohol, platelets, and the French paradox for coronary heart disease. Lancet 339:1523, 1992.
17. Mukamal KJ, Conigrave KM, Mittleman MA, et al: Roles of drinking pattern and type of alcohol consumed in coronary heart disease in men. N Engl J Med 348:109, 2003.
18. Thun MJ, Peto R, Lopez AD, et al: Alcohol consumption and mortality among middle-aged and elderly U.S. adults. N Engl J Med 337:1705, 1997.
19. Muntwyler J, Hennekens CH, Buring JE, et al: Mortality and light to moderate alcohol consumption after myocardial infarction. Lancet 352:1882, 1998.
20. Fuchs CS, Stampfer MJ, Colditz GA, et al: Alcohol consumption and mortality among women. N Engl J Med 332:1245, 1995.
21. Gaziano JM, Gaziano TA, Glynn RJ, et al: Light-to-moderate alcohol consumption and mortality in the Physicians' Health Study enrollment cohort. J Am Coll Cardiol 35:96, 2000.
22. Camargo CA Jr, Stampfer MJ, Glynn RJ, et al: Moderate alcohol consumption and risk for angina pectoris or myocardial infarction in U.S. male physicians. Ann Intern Med 126:372, 1997.
23. Gronbaek M, Becker U, Johansen D, et al: Type of alcohol consumed and mortality from all causes, coronary heart disease, and cancer. Ann Intern Med 133:411, 2000.
24. Booyse FM, Parks DA: Moderate wine and alcohol consumption: Beneficial effects on cardiovascular disease. Thromb Haemost 86:517, 2001.
25. Mukamal KJ, Jadhav PP, D'Agostino RB, et al: Alcohol consumption and hemostatic factors: Analysis of the Framingham offspring cohort. Circulation 104:1367, 2001.
26. Hein HO, Suadicani P, Gyntelberg F: Alcohol consumption, serum low-density lipoprotein cholesterol concentration, and risk of ischaemic heart disease: Six-year follow-up in the Copenhagen male study. BMJ 312:736, 1996.
27. Solomon CG, Hu FB, Stampfer MJ, et al: Moderate alcohol consumption and risk of coronary heart disease among women with type 2 diabetes mellitus. Circulation 102:494, 2000.
28. Ajani UA, Gaziano JM, Lotufo PA, et al: Alcohol consumption and risk of coronary heart disease by diabetes status. Circulation 102:500, 2000.
29. Albert CM, Manson JE, Cook NR, et al: Moderate alcohol consumption and the risk of sudden cardiac death among U.S. male physicians. Circulation 100:944, 1999.
30. Mukamal KJ, Maclure M, Muller JE, et al: Prior alcohol consumption and mortality following acute myocardial infarction. JAMA 285:1965, 2001.
31. Mukamal KJ, Muller JE, Maclure M, et al: Lack of effect of recent alcohol consumption on the course of acute myocardial infarction. Am Heart J 138:926, 1999.
32. Greenspon AJ, Schaal SF: The "holiday heart": Electrophysiologic studies of alcohol effects in alcoholics. Ann Intern Med 98:135, 1983.
33. Menz V, Grimm W, Hoffmann J, et al: Alcohol and rhythm disturbance: The holiday heart syndrome. Herz 21:227, 1996.

Cocaine

34. Lange RA, Hillis LD: Cardiovascular complications of cocaine use. N Engl J Med 345:351, 2001.
35. Qureshi AI, Suri MF, Guterman LR, et al: Cocaine use and the likelihood of nonfatal myocardial infarction and stroke: Data from the Third National Health and Nutrition Examination Survey. Circulation 103:502, 2001.
36. Lange RA, Cigarroa RG, Yancy CW Jr, et al: Cocaine-induced coronary artery vasoconstriction. N Engl J Med 321:1557, 1989.
37. Flores ED, Lange RA, Cigarroa RG, et al: Effect of cocaine on coronary artery dimensions in atherosclerotic coronary artery disease: Enhanced vasoconstriction at sites of significant stenoses. J Am Coll Cardiol 16:74, 1990.
38. Lange RA, Cigarroa RG, Flores ED, et al: Potentiation of cocaine-induced coronary vasoconstriction by beta-adrenergic blockade. Ann Intern Med 112:897, 1990.
39. Kugelmass AD, Oda A, Monahan K, et al: Activation of human platelets by cocaine. Circulation 88:876, 1993.
40. Moliterno DJ, Lange RA, Gerard RD, et al: Influence of intranasal cocaine on plasma constituents associated with endogenous thrombosis and thrombolysis. Am J Med 96:492, 1994.
41. Hollander JE, Hoffman RS, Burstein JL, et al: Cocaine-associated myocardial infarction: Mortality and complications. Cocaine-Associated Myocardial Infarction Study Group. Arch Intern Med 155:1081, 1995.
42. Moliterno DJ, Willard JE, Lange RA, et al: Coronary artery vasoconstriction induced by cocaine, cigarette smoking, or both. N Engl J Med 330:454, 1994.
43. Mittleman MA, Mintzer D, Maclure M, et al: Triggering of myocardial infarction by cocaine. Circulation 99:2737, 1999.
44. Weber JE, Shofer FS, Larkin GL, et al: Validation of a brief observation period for patients with cocaine-associated chest pain. N Engl J Med 348:510, 2003.
45. Brogan WC III, Lange RA, Glamann DB, et al: Recurrent coronary vasoconstriction caused by intranasal cocaine: Possible role for metabolites. Ann Intern Med 116:556, 1992.
46. Hearn WL, Rose S, Wagner J, et al: Cocaethylene is more potent than cocaine in mediating lethality. Pharmacol Biochem Behav 39:531, 1991.
47. Randall T: Cocaine, alcohol mix in body to form even longer lasting, more lethal drug. JAMA 267:1043, 1992.
48. Bertolet BD, Freund G, Martin CA, et al: Unrecognized left ventricular dysfunction in an apparently healthy cocaine abuse population. Clin Cardiol 13:323, 1990.

49. Pitts WR, Vongpatanasin W, Cigarroa JE, et al: Effects of the intracoronary infusion of cocaine on left ventricular systolic and diastolic function in humans. Circulation 97:1270, 1998.
50. Bauman JL, DiDomenico RJ: Cocaine-induced channelopathies: Emerging evidence on the multiple mechanisms of sudden death. J Cardiovasc Pharmacol Ther 7:195, 2002.
51. Brickner ME, Willard JE, Eichhorn EJ, et al: Left ventricular hypertrophy associated with chronic cocaine abuse. Circulation 84:1130, 1991.
52. Chambers HF, Morris DL, Tauber MG, et al: Cocaine use and the risk for endocarditis in intravenous drug users. Ann Intern Med 106:833, 1987.
53. Hsue PY, Salinas CL, Bolger AF, et al: Acute aortic dissection related to crack cocaine. Circulation 105:1592, 2002.

Amphetamines

54. Waksman J, Taylor RN Jr, Bodor GS, et al: Acute myocardial infarction associated with amphetamine use. Mayo Clin Proc 76:323, 2001.
55. Costa GM, Pizzi C, Bresciani B, et al: Acute myocardial infarction caused by amphetamines: A case report and review of the literature. Ital Heart J 2:478, 2001.
56. Raper R, Fisher M, Bihari D: Profound, reversible, myocardial depression in acute asthma treated with high-dose catecholamines. Crit Care Med 20:710, 1992.
57. Akashi YJ, Nakazawa K, Sakakibara M, et al: Reversible left ventricular dysfunction "takotsubo" cardiomyopathy related to catecholamine cardiotoxicity. J Electrocardiol 35:351, 2002.

Inhalants

58. Carder JR, Fuerst RS: Myocardial infarction after toluene inhalation. Pediatr Emerg Care 13:117, 1997.
59. Shepherd RT: Mechanism of sudden death associated with volatile substance abuse. Hum Toxicol 8:287, 1989.
60. Brady WJ Jr, Stremski E, Eljaiek L, et al: Freon inhalational abuse presenting with ventricular fibrillation. Am J Emerg Med 12:533, 1994.

Antiretroviral Agents

61. Koppel K, Bratt G, Eriksson M, et al: Serum lipid levels associated with increased risk for cardiovascular disease is associated with highly active antiretroviral therapy (HAART) in HIV-1 infection. Int J STD AIDS 11:451, 2000.
62. Tabib A, Leroux C, Mornex JF, et al: Accelerated coronary atherosclerosis and arteriosclerosis in young human immunodeficiency virus–positive patients. Coron Artery Dis 11:41, 2000.
63. Domanski MJ, Sloas MM, Follmann DA, et al: Effect of zidovudine and didanosine treatment on heart function in children infected with human immunodeficiency virus. J Pediatr 127:137, 1995.
64. Herskowitz A, Willoughby SB, Baughman KL, et al: Cardiomyopathy associated with antiretroviral therapy in patients with HIV infection: A report of six cases. Ann Intern Med 116:311, 1992.
65. Lewis W, Grupp IL, Grupp G, et al: Cardiac dysfunction occurs in the HIV-1 transgenic mouse treated with zidovudine. Lab Invest 80:187, 2000.

Ergotamine and Serotonin Agonists

66. Klein LS, Simpson RJ Jr, Stern R, et al: Myocardial infarction following administration of sublingual ergotamine. Chest 82:375, 1982.
67. Mueller L, Gallagher RM, Ciervo CA: Vasospasm-induced myocardial infarction with sumatriptan. Headache 36:329, 1996.
68. Main ML, Ramaswamy K, Andrews TC: Cardiac arrest and myocardial infarction immediately after sumatriptan injection. Ann Intern Med 128:874., 1998.

Appetite Suppressants

69. Connolly HM, Crary JL, McGoon MD, et al: Valvular heart disease associated with fenfluramine-phentermine. N Engl J Med 337:581, 1997.
70. Mast ST, Gersing KR, Anstrom KJ, et al: Association between selective serotonin reuptake inhibitor therapy and heart valve regurgitation. Am J Cardiol 87:989, 2001.
71. Khan MA, Herzog CA, St Peter JV, et al: The prevalence of cardiac valvular insufficiency assessed by transthoracic echocardiography in obese patients treated with appetite-suppressant drugs. N Engl J Med 339:713, 1998.
72. Jick H, Vasilakis C, Weinrauch LA, et al: A population-based study of appetite-suppressant drugs and the risk of cardiac-valve regurgitation. N Engl J Med 339:719, 1998.
73. Weissman NJ, Tighe JF Jr, Gottdiener JS, et al: An assessment of heart-valve abnormalities in obese patients taking dexfenfluramine, sustained-release dexfenfluramine, or placebo. Sustained-Release Dexfenfluramine Study Group. N Engl J Med 339:725, 1998.
74. Weissman NJ, Panza JA, Tighe JF, et al: Natural history of valvular regurgitation 1 year after discontinuation of dexfenfluramine therapy: A randomized, double-blind, placebo-controlled trial. Ann Intern Med 134:267, 2001.

Paclitaxel and Other Chemotherapeutic Drugs

75. Arbuck SG, Strauss H, Rowinsky E, et al: A reassessment of cardiac toxicity associated with Taxol. J Natl Cancer Inst Monogr 117, 1993.
76. Keefe DL: Trastuzumab-associated cardiotoxicity. Cancer 95:1592, 2002.
77. Kuropkat C, Griem K, Clark J, et al: Severe cardiotoxicity during 5-fluorouracil chemotherapy: A case and literature report. Am J Clin Oncol 22:466, 1999.
78. Kleiman NS, Lehane DE, Geyer CE Jr, et al: Prinzmetal's angina during 5-fluorouracil chemotherapy. Am J Med 82:566, 1987.

Environmental Exposures

79. Alexander CS: Cobalt-beer cardiomyopathy: A clinical and pathologic study of twenty-eight cases. Am J Med 53:395, 1972.
80. Jarvis JQ, Hammond E, Meier R, et al: Cobalt cardiomyopathy: A report of two cases from mineral assay laboratories and a review of the literature. J Occup Med 34:620, 1992.
81. Kopp SJ, Barron JT, Tow JP: Cardiovascular actions of lead and relationship to hypertension: A review. Environ Health Perspect 78:91, 1988.
82. Marek K, Zajac-Nedza M, Rola E, et al: [Examination of health effects after exposure to metallic mercury vapors in workers engaged in production of chlorine and acetic aldehyde: I. Evaluation of general health status]. Med Pr 46:101, 1995.
83. Guallar E, Sanz-Gallardo MI, van't Veer P, et al: Mercury, fish oils, and the risk of myocardial infarction. N Engl J Med 347:1747, 2002.
84. Salonen JT, Seppanen K, Nyyssonen K, et al: Intake of mercury from fish, lipid peroxidation, and the risk of myocardial infarction and coronary, cardiovascular, and any death in eastern Finnish men. Circulation 91:645, 1995.
85. Yoshizawa K, Rimm EB, Morris JS, et al: Mercury and the risk of coronary heart disease in men. N Engl J Med 347:1755, 2002.
86. Chulay JD, Spencer HC, Mugambi M: Electrocardiographic changes during treatment of leishmaniasis with pentavalent antimony (sodium stibogluconate). Am J Trop Med Hyg 34:702, 1985.
87. Hall JC, Harruff R: Fatal cardiac arrhythmia in a patient with interstitial myocarditis related to chronic arsenic poisoning. South Med J 82:1557, 1989.
88. Allred EN, Bleecker ER, Chaitman BR, et al: Acute effects of carbon monoxide exposure on individuals with coronary artery disease. Res Rep Health Eff Inst 1, 1989.
89. Allred EN, Bleecker ER, Chaitman BR, et al: Effects of carbon monoxide on myocardial ischemia. Environ Health Perspect 91:89, 1991.
90. Fiorista F, Casazza F, Comolatti G: [Silent myocardial infarction caused by acute carbon monoxide poisoning]. G Ital Cardiol 23:583, 1993.
91. Marius-Nunez AL: Myocardial infarction with normal coronary arteries after acute exposure to carbon monoxide. Chest 97:491, 1990.
92. Ebisuno S, Yasuno M, Yamada Y, et al: Myocardial infarction after acute carbon monoxide poisoning: Case report. Angiology 37:621, 1986.

CHAPTER 63

Primary Tumors of the Heart

Marc S. Sabatine • Wilson S. Colucci • Frederick J. Schoen

With an incidence of approximately 0.02 percent in autopsy series,[1,2] primary tumors of the heart* are far less common than metastatic tumors to the heart. Nonetheless they may cause a wide variety of clinical signs and symptoms that often masquerade as many other more common cardiovascular and systemic diseases. Cardiac tumors have been misdiagnosed as other cardiac conditions (including rheumatic valvular disease, endocarditis, myocarditis, pericarditis, cardiomyopathies, and congenital heart disease), pulmonary conditions (including pulmonary emboli, pulmonary hypertension, and interstitial lung disease), cerebrovascular disease, and vasculitis. Advances in noninvasive cardiovascular imaging techniques—especially echocardiography, computed tomography (CT), and magnetic resonance imaging (MRI)—have greatly facilitated the diagnostic evaluation and permit the rapid identification of intracardiac masses (Table 63–1). Nevertheless, a high index of suspicion remains the most important element in diagnosing a cardiac tumor because the time from onset of symptoms to diagnosis can be months or even years.

Clinical Presentation

Cardiac tumors usually present with some combination of heart failure, arrhythmias, or embolic phenomena. Intracavitary tumors are more likely to cause heart failure or embolic phenomena, whereas intramural tumors are more likely to cause arrhythmias. However, all intracavitary tumors have some point of attachment and thus may be arrhythmogenic, and, if large enough, intramural tumors may bulge and partially obliterate a cardiac chamber or interfere with a ventricle's mechanical performance and thus cause heart failure. Therefore, the specific signs and symptoms produced by tumors are more closely related to their precise anatomical location, size, and effect on the surrounding structures than to their histological types.[3]

Heart Failure

Cardiac tumors may cause signs and symptoms of either backward, congestive heart failure or forward, low-output heart failure, or both. Mechanistically, these manifestations may arise from intracavitary obstruction of either filling or outflow or from intramural interference with function. Obstruction of filling or outflow can be due to cavitary obliteration as well as valvular dysfunction. Myocardial dysfunction can include both systolic dysfunction due to impaired contractility and diastolic dysfunction due to restrictive physiology.

LEFT ATRIAL TUMORS. In adults, 80 to 90 percent of primary cardiac tumors seen in the left atrium are benign myxomas. Typically intracavitary, mobile, and pedunculated, myxomas may prolapse to various degrees into the mitral valve orifice, resulting in obstruction of blood flow from the left atrium to the left ventricle as well as mitral regurgitation. The resultant signs and symptoms often mimic those of mitral valve disease, especially mitral stenosis, and include dyspnea, orthopnea, and paroxysmal nocturnal dyspnea. However, weight loss, syncope, and sudden death—manifestations that are uncommon with mitral valve disease—also occur. Furthermore, atrial fibrillation, common in advanced, symptomatic mitral stenosis, is rare in patients with atrial myxomas, presumably because atrial enlargement is uncommon. It is not unusual for the symptoms to be sudden in onset, intermittent, and related to body position.[3] Thus, although most of the symptoms produced by left atrial tumors are nonspecific, the occurrence of paroxysmal symptoms that arise characteristically in a particular body position and are out of proportion to the clinical findings should raise suspicion for a left atrial tumor.

Physical Examination. This may disclose signs of pulmonary congestion; a loud S_1, which is often widely split; an S_4, a sound rarely audible in mitral stenosis; a holosystolic murmur that is loudest at the apex and resembles mitral regurgitation; and a diastolic murmur resulting from obstruction to flow through the mitral orifice due to the tumor. The loud S_1 that occurs in patients with left atrial myxoma may be caused by the late onset of mitral valve closure resulting from either increased left atrial pressure or prolapse of the tumor through the mitral valve orifice. In some cases, an early diastolic sound (~100 msec after S_2), termed a *tumor plop,* can be identified. It is thought to be produced as the tumor strikes the endocardial wall or as its excursion is abruptly halted and its stalk tenses. Although in most cases the tumor plop occurs later than the opening snap of the mitral valve and earlier than an S_3, it is not surprising that this sound is frequently confused with either of those findings.

RIGHT ATRIAL TUMORS. Right atrial tumors frequently produce symptoms of right heart failure, including peripheral edema, ascites, and hepatomegaly.[3] As approximately half of right atrial tumors will turn out to be sarcomas, the development of right-sided heart failure may be rapidly progressive. Coincident with the development of heart failure, new systolic

*Tumors arising elsewhere in the body and metastasizing to the pericardium and heart are discussed in Chapters 64 and 83, respectively.

TABLE 63–1 Imaging Features of Cardiac Tumors

Cardiac Tumor	Echocardiography	CT	MRI
Myxoma	Mobile tumor Narrow stalk connected to fossa ovalis Heterogeneous with hypoechoic and hyperechoic foci	Narrow base of attachment Heterogeneous, low attenuation Occasionally with calcification	Heterogeneous Primarily isointense on T1, with areas of hypointensity and hyperintensity Hyperintense on T2 Heterogeneous enhancement
Papillary fibroelastoma	Mobile mass Short pedicle "Shimmering" edges	Difficult to see	Difficult to see
Lipomas	Intramural hyperechoic mass	Homogeneous Low (fat) attenuation	Hyperintense on T1 ↓ Signal with fat suppression No enhancement
Rhabdomyomas	Multiple small, lobulated hyperechoic intramural masses		Homogeneous Isointense on T1 Hyperintense on T2
Fibromas	Intramural large, solid mass Central hyperechoic foci	Homogeneous, low attenuation Calcification	Isointense on T1 Hypointense on T2 Minimal enhancement
Teratomas	Very heterogeneous Pericardial effusion	Very heterogeneous	Very heterogeneous
Hemangiomas	Hyperechoic	Heterogeneous Calcification Marked enhancement	Isointense on T1 Hyperintense on T2 Marked enhancement
Angiosarcoma	Mass protruding into right atrium Pericardial effusion	Low attenuation	Infiltrative Heterogeneous Nodular areas of hyperintensity on T1 Linear areas of enhancement
Other sarcomas	Left atrial mass Broad base of attachment to posterior atrial wall	Low attenuation ± Calcification	Infiltrative and heterogeneous Variable intensity on T1
Lymphoma	Hypoechoic masses Pericardial effusion	Low attenuation	Infiltrative Isointense to hypointense on T1 Heterogenous enhancement

Adapted from information in (1) Grebenc ML, Rosado de Christenson ML, Burke AP, et al: Primary cardiac and pericardial neoplasms: Radiologic-pathologic correlation. Radiographics 20:1073-1103, 2000; (2) Araoz PA, Mulvagh SL, Tazelaar HD, et al: CT and MR imaging of benign primary cardiac neoplasms with echocardiographic correlation. Radiographics 20:1303-1319, 2000; (3) Araoz PA, Eklund HE, Welch TJ, Breen JF: CT and MR imaging of primary cardiac malignancies. Radiographics 19:1421-1434, 1999; and (4) Frank H: Cardiac and paracardiac masses. *In* Manning WJ, Pennell DJ (eds): Cardiovascular Magnetic Resonance. New York, Churchill Livingstone, 2002, pp 342-354.

or diastolic murmurs or both may be appreciated. It is not surprising that right atrial tumors have been misdiagnosed as Ebstein's anomaly of the tricuspid valve, constrictive pericarditis, tricuspid stenosis, carcinoid syndrome, superior vena caval syndrome, and cardiomyopathy.

Physical Examination. This can reveal an elevated jugular venous pressure with prominent *a* waves and steep *y* descents, peripheral edema, evidence of superior vena cava obstruction, hepatomegaly, and ascites. An early diastolic rumbling murmur, due to obstruction to tricuspid flow, or a holosystolic murmur, secondary to tricuspid regurgitation, may demonstrate respiratory or positional variation. Because of the rarity of *isolated* rheumatic tricuspid valvular disease, the lack of other valvular findings should raise the question of a right atrial tumor. A protodiastolic tumor plop has been described and is thought to be similar in etiology to that produced by left atrial tumors.

VENTRICULAR TUMORS. Depending on which chamber is involved, intracavitary ventricular tumors may present with left- or right-sided heart failure as a result of obstruction to ventricular filling or outflow. The clinical manifestations are those typical for left- and right-sided heart failure and include dyspnea, pulmonary edema, and syncope and peripheral edema, hepatomegaly, and ascites, respectively. Systolic or diastolic murmurs and atrial or ventricular gallops may be heard and thus the cardiac findings often lead to an initial diagnosis of valvular heart disease or hypertrophic cardiomyopathy. However, whereas valvular disease is often slowly progressive, the symptoms due to cardiac tumors are often rapidly progressive. Ventricular tumors that are predominantly intramural may be asymptomatic; they can affect diastolic function mimicking a restrictive cardiomyopathy; or they can affect systolic function mimicking a dilated cardiomyopathy.

Arrhythmias

Cardiac tumors, especially those with significant intramural involvement, may cause disturbances of conduction or rhythm,[4] the precise nature of which is determined by the location of the tumor. Tumors with atrial involvement or attachment such as myxomas, sarcomas, and lipomatous hypertrophy of the septum may produce a wide variety of supraventricular tachyarrhythmias, including atrial fibrillation, atrial flutter, and ectopic atrial tachycardia. Tumors in the area of the atrioventricular (AV) node, typically angiomas and mesotheliomas, may produce AV conduction disturbances, including complete heart block, and asystole. Tumors located within the ventricular myocardium such as rhabdomyomas and fibromas can cause premature ventricular beats, ventricular tachycardia, ventricular fibrillation, and sudden cardiac death.

Embolic Phenomena

Embolization of tumor fragments or of thrombi from the surface of a tumor is a frequent and often dramatic clinical occurrence. Although myxomas are the source of most tumor emboli because of the combination of their friable consistency and intracavitary location, other types of cardiac tumors occasionally may embolize. The distribution of tumor emboli depends on the location of the tumor and the presence or absence of intracardiac shunts.

LEFT-SIDED EMBOLI. Left-sided tumors embolize to the systemic circulation, resulting in stroke, visceral infarction, peripheral limb ischemia, and peripheral vascular aneurysms. The neurological event may occasionally be the first or only clinical manifestation of a cardiac tumor. An embolic stroke in a young person without evidence of cerebrovascular disease, particularly in the presence of sinus rhythm, should raise the suspicion of intracardiac myxoma, as well as infective endocarditis. Multiple systemic emboli may mimic systemic vasculitis or infective endocarditis, especially when associated with other manifestations of a systemic illness such as fever, weight loss, arthralgias, and an elevated erythrocyte sedimentation rate (ESR). The finding at angiography of numerous vascular aneurysms secondary to tumor emboli in the cerebral, renal, femoral, and coronary arteries is not infrequent and may lead to the mistaken diagnosis of polyarteritis nodosa. Because the diagnosis of an intracardiac tumor may be made after histological examination of systemic embolic material, it is of critical importance to make every effort to recover and examine the entirety of the embolic material because what appears to be a thrombus may actually be a cardiac tumor embolism covered by thrombus.

RIGHT-SIDED EMBOLI. Right-sided cardiac tumors and left-sided cardiac tumors proximal to left-to-right intracardiac shunts may result in pulmonary emboli. Indeed, serious pulmonary hypertension and cor pulmonale due to chronic recurrent pulmonary emboli from right atrial tumors can occur.

Diagnostic Techniques

CHEST ROENTGENOGRAM. Cardiac tumors may display several findings on plain chest roentgenograms that may offer the first clue as to their presence. The cardiac contour may display generalized or specific chamber enlargement that mimics virtually any type of valvular heart disease, or may demonstrate a bizarre appearance. An enlarged cardiac contour may also be due to a pericardial effusion, which generally indicates invasion of the pericardial space by a malignant tumor. Calcification visible by roentgenographic methods may occur with several types of cardiac tumor, including rhabdomyomas, fibromas, teratomas, myxomas, hemangiomas, and osteosarcomas. However, many cardiac tumors may be entirely intracavitary, uncalcified, and not associated with any change in cardiac contour. Thus, when a cardiac tumor is suspected, a dedicated cardiac imaging study is required.

ANGIOGRAPHY. Cardiac catheterization and selective angiocardiography enabled the first antemortem diagnosis of a cardiac tumor but now are rarely necessary because echocardiography, CT, and MRI provide adequate preoperative information (see later). In several circumstances, however, the risk of cardiac catheterization is outweighed by the supplemental information it may provide. These include cases in which noninvasive evaluation has not been adequate in fully defining tumor location or attachment or when other cardiac conditions such as coronary artery disease, valvular heart disease, or pulmonary hypertension may coexist and possibly dictate a different surgical approach.

Intracavitary tumors are identified by injecting contrast material upstream to the tumor location and demonstrating a filling defect in the chamber of interest. For suspected left atrial tumors, contrast material may be injected into the pulmonary artery and then waiting for the levophase. Large intramural ventricular tumors may be identified by observing abnormalities in the typical chamber contours. Finally, highly vascular tumors may be detected on coronary angiography by seeing the characteristic tumor blush.

The major risk of angiography is peripheral embolization due to dislodgment of a fragment of tumor or of an associated thrombus. Therefore, thorough evaluation by noninvasive methods before catheterization is recommended for patients suspected of having cardiac tumors so that contrast material can be injected into the chamber proximal to the location of the tumor. Moreover, because cardiac tumors may be numerous and present in more than one chamber, all four chambers should be visualized noninvasively before cardiac catheterization whenever possible.

ECHOCARDIOGRAPHY. Echocardiography (see Chap. 11) has become the screening test of choice for cardiac tumors. In particular, two-dimensional echocardiography offers real-time, high spatial and temporal resolution imaging and thus can provide information about tumor size, attachment, and mobility (Fig. 63–1A). Continuous-mode Doppler ultrasonography may be useful for evaluating the hemodynamic consequences of valvular obstruction or incompetence caused by cardiac tumors. *Tissue harmonic imaging,* which relies on the gradual generation of harmonics as ultrasound waves propagate through tissue, results in reduced near-field and side-lobe artifacts and thus offers improved image

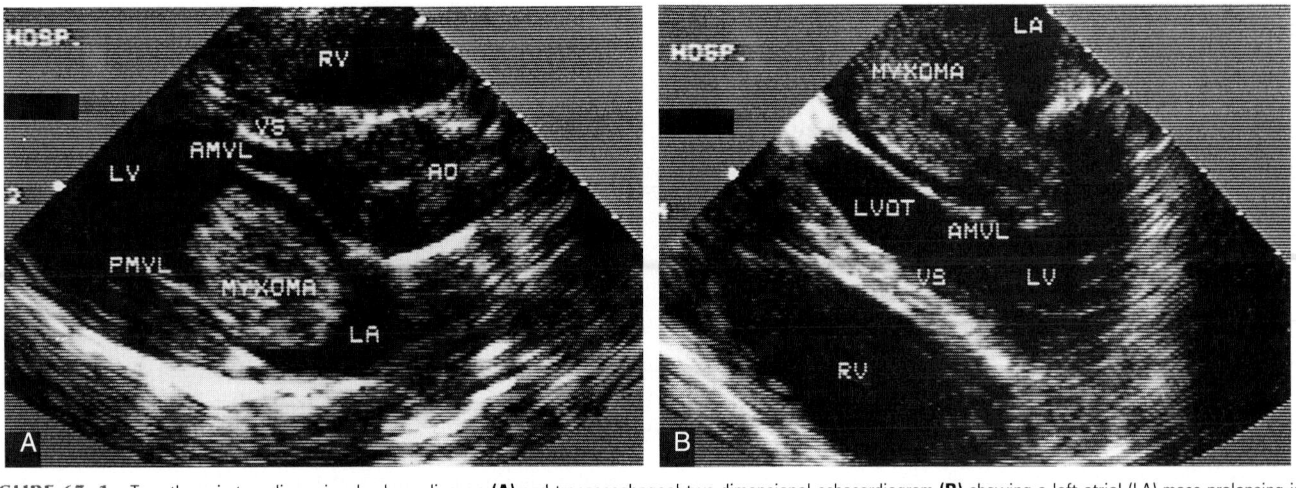

FIGURE 63–1 Transthoracic two-dimensional echocardiogram **(A)** and transesophageal two-dimensional echocardiogram **(B)** showing a left atrial (LA) mass prolapsing into and obstructing the mitral valve orifice. Note the superior resolution of the transesophageal echocardiogram. Although not visible here, the myxoma was attached to the midportion of the atrial septum. AO = aorta; AMVL = anterior mitral valve leaflet; PMVL = posterior mitral valve leaflet; LV = left ventricle; LVOT = left ventricular outflow tract; VS = ventricular septum. (From Allard MF, Taylor GP, Wilson JE, McManus BM: Primary cardiac tumors. *In* Goldhaber SZ, Braunwald E [eds]: Cardiopulmonary Diseases and Cardiac Tumors. Atlas of Heart Diseases. Vol 3. Philadelphia, Current Medicine, 1995, pp 15.1-15.22.)

quality. *Contrast echocardiography* uses microbubbles that are capable of transversing the pulmonary vascular bed and opacifying the left heart. This technique can be used to enhance endocardial border definition and thereby more clearly demonstrate filling defects caused by intracavitary tumors. *Myocardial contrast echocardiography*, in which the microbubbles are imaged within the myocardial capillary vascular bed, has already been used to demonstrate intracardiac mass perfusion,[5] thereby helping distinguish tumor from thrombus, and may someday be used to define the extent of intramural tumors.

Transesophageal Echocardiography. This appears to be superior to transthoracic echocardiography in many patients (see Fig. 63–1B). The potential advantages of transesophageal echocardiography include improved resolution of the tumor and its attachment, the ability to detect some masses not visualized by transthoracic echocardiography, and improved visualization of right atrial tumors.[6] Although transesophageal echocardiography does not appear warranted on a routine basis, it should be considered when the transthoracic study is suboptimal, and it is frequently used for intraoperative monitoring. *Three-dimensional transesophageal echocardiography* is a relatively new technique in which multiple cross-section images at slightly different angles are acquired by rotating a multiplane probe and using cardiac and respiratory gating.[7] The resulting volumetric data set is processed offline, and image reconstruction software is used to create a three-dimensional image that simulates intraoperative visualization.

COMPUTED TOMOGRAPHY. Recent advances in CT (see Chap. 15), including spiral, multislice spiral, and electron-beam CT (EBCT), have greatly improved its applicability to cardiac imaging.[8] A breath-hold technique is used to minimize respiratory motion artifact, and image resolution is further improved by gating the CT acquisition to the cardiac cycle. Electrocardiographic gating also allows cine-mode data to be obtained, thereby allowing assessment of mobility. Of note, data acquisition is sufficiently rapid (50 to 100 msec) for EBCT that cardiac gating is not absolutely necessary, permitting adequate imaging in patients with irregular rhythms. New rendering software has the ability to construct images in any plane and even create three-dimensional images.

CT provides a high degree of soft tissue discrimination, which is helpful in defining the degree of myocardial infiltration. CT can also be used to assess for calcification, which may be useful in the diagnosis of rhabdomyomas, fibromas, teratomas, myxomas, hemangiomas, and osteosarcomas. The administration of a contrast agent may clarify further the degree of intramural invasion (Fig. 63–2) and help differentiate a vascular tumor from an avascular thrombus. CT also allows for evaluation of the extracardiac structures. Thus, CT currently appears to be most useful in the evaluation of suspected tumors of the heart either to provide additional information when the echocardiographic data are equivocal or to determine the degree of myocardial invasion and the involvement of pericardial and extracardiac structures in lesions consistent with a malignant process.[9-11]

MAGNETIC RESONANCE IMAGING. MRI offers unsurpassed soft tissue characterization and the use of multiple, different pulse sequences presents clinicians with complementary information (see Chap. 14).[12] T1-weighted and T2-weighted dual-inversion recovery fast spin-echo sequences offer detailed morphological information, with T1-weighted images providing excellent soft tissue characterization and T2-weighted images providing superior tissue contrast and demonstration of fluid components. For complex, heterogeneous tumors such as myxomas and teratomas, studies have demonstrated excellent correlation between the MRI and pathological findings.[13] A short inversion recovery sequence permits suppression of fat signals and therefore is useful in detecting lipid-containing masses such as lipomas. Contrast enhancement with gadolinium provides information on the vascularity of the mass, often allows for better delineation of the degree of tumor infiltration within the myocardium, and assists in the differentiation of thrombus from tumor. Additionally, MRI allows for simultaneous assessment of all cardiac chambers, the pericardium, and surrounding structures. Multislice imaging can be performed in the standard cardiac axes as well as any modified axis as needed, thereby providing precise three-dimensional information (Fig. 63–3).

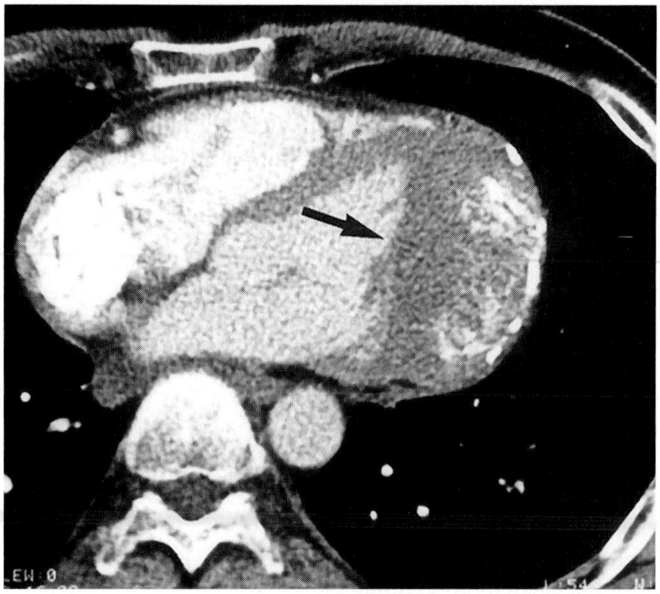

FIGURE 63–2 Contrast-enhanced electron-beam CT scan of a left ventricular fibroma. Note the coarse calcifications in the lateral wall (arrow). (From Araoz PA, Mulvagh SL, Tazelaar HD, et al: CT and MR imaging of benign primary cardiac neoplasms with echocardiographic correlation. Radiographics 20:1303-1319, 2000.)

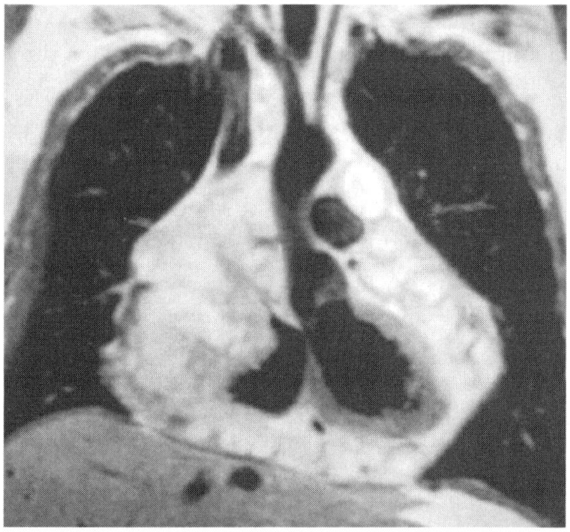

FIGURE 63–3 Coronal T2-weighted MRI of angiosarcoma demonstrating extensive circumferential cardiac involvement by the nodular, heterogeneous, hyperintense tumor, which invades the right atrium and encases the heart. (From Grebenc ML, Rosado de Christenson ML, Burke AP, et al: Primary cardiac and pericardial neoplasms: Radiologic-pathologic correlation. Radiographics 20:1073-1103, 2000.)

For evaluation of cardiac function and tumor mobility, gradient-echo sequences are used. These sequences have faster acquisition times, allowing for cine MRI. Recently developed steady-state free precession (SSFP) sequences offer even better contrast between blood and soft tissue and therefore can delineate the contour of tumors even in areas of slow blood flow. With up to 50 frames per second, SSFP cine acquisitions provide excellent three-dimensional visualization of cardiac function; valve motion; and the structure, size, attachment to adjacent structures, and mobility of cardiac masses. Thus, although the current limited availability and complex interpretation of cardiac MRI may prevent it from being adopted as a universal screening tool, MRI is emerging as the imaging modality of choice for complex cardiac masses.[9-11,14]

NUCLEAR IMAGING. Because tumors are typically in a relatively hypermetabolic state, positron-emission tomography imaging using a metabolic tracer such as 2-[fluorine 18]fluoro-2-deoxy-D-glucose (FDG) has proven useful in detecting malignant tumors. A few case reports have documented its usefulness in detecting primary cardiac tumors and in differentiating tumor from thrombus.[15] Malignant tumors also typically have a high apoptotic index. In one case report, imaging with ^{99m}Tc-p-annexin-V, a marker of apoptosis, demonstrated enhancement in an area containing a known cardiac mass. Subsequent resection revealed a sarcoma that, on immunohistochemistry, stained positive for annexin V.[16]

BIOPSY. Preoperative, catheter-based biopsy is rarely done. With a few exceptions, the treatment of choice for cardiac tumors is surgical excision. Therefore, once a tumor is identified, a definitive open surgical procedure is usually planned. Thrombus, the other major diagnostic possibility when faced with an intracardiac mass, can usually be differentiated from tumor by a combination of the clinical history and imaging data. Moreover, for left-sided intracavitary lesions, the risk of an embolic complication usually precludes consideration of biopsy, and for intramural masses endomyocardial biopsy may not yield an adequate sample.

However, there are several situations in which transvenous, catheter-based biopsy is indicated.[17] In children, certain types of tumors, such as rhabdomyomas, may spontaneously regress. Therefore, biopsy of (ideally) a right-sided mass may permit a histological diagnosis to be made that would then allow surgery to be deferred. In adults, biopsy of a lesion suspicious for malignancy may be necessary to define the specific histology, particularly if the anatomical extent of the lesion is such that there would be no role for attempted surgical resection. In these cases, the biopsy data can be used to optimize chemotherapy. Transesophageal echocardiography can be used to direct the biotome.[18] Intracardiac tumors have also been sampled by fine-needle aspiration.

Treatment Options and Prognosis

Benign Tumors

In 1952, the first antemortem diagnosis of a cardiac myxoma was made,[19] raising the possibility of surgical treatment for cardiac tumors. Two years later, on July 16, 1954, Clarence Crafoord performed the first successful surgical removal of a myxoma.[20] In adults, operative excision under direct vision using cardiopulmonary bypass has now become the treatment of choice for most benign cardiac tumors and in many cases results in a complete cure. Even benign cardiac tumors are potentially lethal as a result of intracavitary or valvular obstruction, peripheral embolization, and disturbances of rhythm or conduction, and, unfortunately, it is not unusual for patients to die or experience a major complication while awaiting operation. Therefore, it is mandatory to carry out the operation promptly after the diagnosis has been established.

In rare cases, the size of a tumor and the complexity of its sites of attachment or degree of infiltration have necessitated orthotopic heart transplantation. For benign tumors, this approach carries a good prognosis with a very low recurrence rate but the usual risks of transplantation.[21] In rare cases, rather than an allogeneic transplant, autotransplantation is performed, with complete removal of the heart, ex vivo repair, and then reimplantation of the patient's excised heart.[22]

The guidelines for myxoma removal outlined by Schaff and Mullany[23] can be generalized to cover the surgical approach to most benign cardiac tumors. These include the following:

1. Minimize manipulation of the heart before cardiopulmonary bypass.
2. Examine the other cardiac chambers for additional tumors not appreciated on preoperative imaging studies. Previously this meant direct visualization, but now intraoperative transesophageal echocardiography may suffice.
3. When technically feasible, attempt to excise the entire tumor to prevent residual tumor leading to a recurrence. However, for tumors with a substantial intramural component, this may not be possible without sacrificing ventricular contractile ability, proper AV valve function, and the preservation of the conduction system. In these situations, the type of tumor and its natural history must be weighed against the risks of total excision.
4. Carefully search for any dislodged tumor fragments that could lead to the generation of peripheral emboli and dispersion of micrometastases. To reduce this risk, the tumor should be removed en bloc when possible and the chamber then irrigated well with saline.
5. Carefully inspect any cardiac valves that may have had contact with any intracavitary component of the tumor to assess for traumatic damage and the need for repair.

Malignant Tumors

Operation is not an effective treatment for most primary malignant tumors of the heart because of the large mass of cardiac tissue involved or the presence of metastases. The major role for surgery in such cases is to establish a definitive diagnosis to preclude the possibility of a curable benign tumor. Left untreated, patients with primary malignant tumors of the heart generally have a life expectancy measured in months. In some cases, palliation of hemodynamics and/or constitutional symptoms and extension of life can be achieved by aggressive therapy. To that end, disease-free survival for more than 2 years has been reported after partial resection, chemotherapy, radiation therapy, orthotopic cardiac transplantation, or various combinations of these modalities.[24] Unfortunately, most case series indicate a failure to fundamentally alter the course of primary malignant tumors of the heart, and despite maximal therapy, median survival is no better than 1 year.

Specific Cardiac Tumors

Approximately 75 percent of all cardiac tumors are benign histologically and the remainder are malignant.[25] Most benign cardiac tumors are myxomas, followed in frequency by a wide variety of other tumors (Table 63–2 and Fig. 63–4). Almost all malignant cardiac tumors are sarcomas, and of these the angiosarcoma is the most common form (Table 63–3). Some tumors are associated with systemic syndromes (Table 63–4).[26]

Myxomas

Cardiac myxomas comprise approximately 50 percent of the total in most adult clinical case series and up to 90 percent in surgical case series. The histogenesis of cardiac myxomas is uncertain, but the weight of evidence favors benign neoplasia, with the tumor probably originating from subendocardial nests of primitive mesenchymal cells that may differentiate into several cell types, including endothelial and lipidic cells. Cytogenetic analyses demonstrating clonal chromosomal abnormalities provide the best support for this concept.[27]

The mean age at the time of presentation in patients with sporadic myxoma is 50 years.[28] However, there is a wide range—the youngest reported patient was a stillborn infant

TABLE 63–2 Relative Incidence of Benign Tumors of the Heart*

	Percentage of Group		
Benign Tumors	***Adults***	***Children***	***Infants***
Myxoma	52	17	0
Papillary fibroelastoma	16	0	0
Lipoma	16	0	0
Rhabdomyoma	1	42	62
Fibroma	3	18	17
Teratoma	1	12	12
Hemangioma	6	5	4
Other tumors†	5	4	4

Sources for the data include (1) McAllister HA, Fenoglio JJ: Tumors of the cardiovascular system. *In* Hartmann WH, Cowan WR (eds): Atlas of Tumor Pathology. Second Series, Fascicle 15. Washington, DC, Armed Forces Institute of Pathology, 1978, pp 1-3; (2) Nadas AS, Ellison RC: Cardiac tumors in infancy. Am J Cardiol 21:363-366, 1968; (3) Fine G: Neoplasms of the pericardium and heart. *In* Gould SE (ed): Pathology of the Heart and Blood Vessels. 3rd ed. Springfield, Charles C Thomas, 1968, pp 851-883; (4) Lam KY, Dickens P, Chan AC: Tumors of the heart: A 20-year experience with a review of 12,485 consecutive autopsies. Arch Pathol Lab Med 117:1027-1031, 1993; and (5) Virmani R, Burke A, Farb A, Atkinson JB: Cardiovascular Pathology. Major Problems in Pathology. Vol 40. 2nd ed. Philadelphia, WB Saunders, 2001.

*Data represent collective experience of multiple investigators with a total of 447, 92, and 82 benign tumors found in adults (age > 16 years), children (age 1-16 years), and infants (age < 1 year). Lipoma includes true lipomas and lipomatous hypertrophy of the septum.

†Other tumors include cystic tumors of the atrioventricular node, endocrine tumors, and histiocytoid tumors.

TABLE 63–3 Relative Incidence of Primary Malignant Tumors of the Heart*

	Percentage of Group		
Malignant Tumors	***Adults***	***Children***	***Infants***
Angiosarcoma	28	6	0
Rhabdomyosarcoma	11	41	50
Fibrosarcoma	8	18	17
Malignant fibrous histiocytoma	6	6	0
Osteosarcoma	7	0	0
Leiomyosarcoma	5	0	17
Myxosarcoma	3	6	0
Other sarcomas†	14	12	0
Undifferentiated sarcoma	12	12	17
Lymphoma	6	0	0

See Table 63–2 footnote for sources of the data.

*Data representing collective experience of multiple investigators with a total of 250, 17, and 6 malignant tumors found in adults (age > 16 years), children (age 1-16 years), and infants (age < 1 year).

†Other sarcomas included liposarcomas, synovial, and neurogenic sarcomas.

and the oldest was a 95-year-old woman. Two-thirds of patients are female. Approximately 75 percent of myxomas occur in the left atrium, where the site of attachment is almost always in the region of the limbus of the fossa ovalis. Although myxomas may occasionally be found on the posterior left atrial wall, tumors presenting in this location should raise the suspicion of malignancy. Myxomas also may occur in the right atrium (15 to 20 percent) and, less often, in the right or left ventricle. Myxomas of the AV valves have been

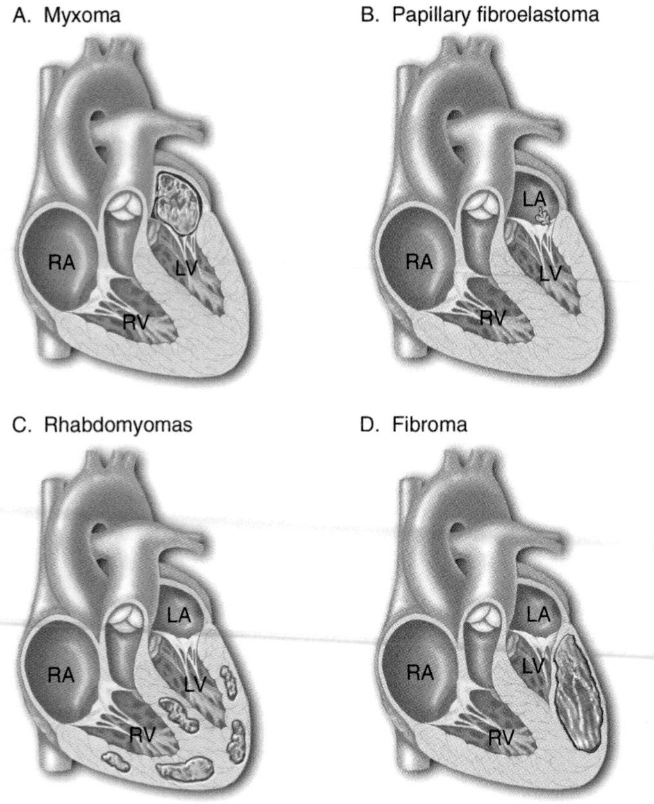

FIGURE 63–4 Characteristic appearance of the four most common benign primary cardiac tumors. **A,** Myxomas are typically a 5- to 6-cm globular mass, attached to the fossa ovalis in the left atrium, and can prolapse through the mitral valve. **B,** Papillary fibroelastomas are smaller than 1-cm, frond-like masses attached to the mitral or aortic valve. **C,** Rhabdomyomas usually present as multiple, rounded, smaller than 2-cm masses throughout the left and right ventricular myocardium. **D,** Fibromas are large, singular, 3- to 10-cm dense masses, typically found in the anterior free wall of the left ventricle.

reported. More than 90 percent of myxomas are solitary, but several myxomas within one atrium, as well as biatrial (usually extending through the foramen ovale), combined atrial and ventricular, and biventricular myxomas all have been reported. However, multiple tumors or atypical locations are more commonly seen in patients with familial myxomas (see later). The tumors average 5 to 6 cm in diameter but range from less than 1 to 15 cm or greater.[29]

CLINICAL MANIFESTATIONS. Myxomas present with one or more of the triad of intracardiac obstruction, systemic embolization, and constitutional symptoms (Table 63–5). Nearly 70 percent of patients with left atrial myxomas have cardiac symptoms, predominantly heart failure and syncope.[29] The pedunculated nature of myxomas and their predilection for the left atrium allow them to prolapse to various degrees into the mitral valve orifice, resulting in obstruction to left ventricular inflow as well as mitral regurgitation. Moreover, the recurrent collision between a left atrial myxoma and the mitral valve may cause permanent valvular damage, the so-called wrecking ball effect. In contrast to fixed mitral valve disease, the mobility of myxomas typically leads to paroxysmal symptoms of shortness of breath or syncope that may depend on body position. Large myxomas (>5 cm) are more likely to cause cardiac symptoms than their smaller counterparts.

Embolic events occur in 30 percent of patients. Of these patients, two-thirds have cerebral emboli causing transient ischemic attacks, strokes, or seizures, and half have peripheral limb emboli.[29] Cases of cardiac myxoma embolizing to coronary arteries, kidney, liver, spleen, eye, and skin have

TABLE 63–4 Syndromes Associated with Cardiac Tumors

Tumor	Syndrome	Gene	Prevalence (%) *Of Syndrome Among Patients with Tumor*	Prevalence (%) *Of Cardiac Tumor Among Patients with Syndrome*	Additional Features
Myxoma	Carney complex	*PRKAR1α*	<10	50-67	Spotty skin pigmentation, endocrine overactivity
Rhabdomyoma	Tuberous sclerosis	*TSC-1* *TSC-2*	80	50	Hamartomas, epilepsy, mental deficiency, adenoma sebaceum
Fibroma	Gorlin syndrome	*PTC*	5	<14	Nevoid basal cell carcinoma, medulloblastomas, odontogenic keratocysts, bifid ribs

TABLE 63–5 Symptoms and Signs of Cardiac Myxoma*

Variable	
Symptoms	**Incidence (%)**
Dyspnea	~70
Paroxysmal dyspnea	~25
Syncope	~20
Palpitations	~20
Chest pain	~10
Embolic event	~30
Fever	~20
Weight loss	~15
Signs	
Mitral systolic murmur	~50
Mitral diastolic murmur	~40
Loud S_1	~40
Tumor plop	~15
Laboratory Data	
Elevated ESR	~30
Anemia	~30
LA enlargement on CXR	~10

ESR = erythrocyte sedimentation rate; LA = left atrium; CXR = chest radiograph.

Sources for the data include (1) St John Sutton MG, Mercier LA, Giuliani ER, Lie JT: Atrial myxomas: A review of clinical experience in 40 patients. Mayo Clin Proc 55:371-376, 1980; (2) Burke AP, Virmani R: Cardiac myxoma: A clinicopathologic study. Am J Clin Pathol 100:671-680, 1993; (3) Bjessmo S, Ivert T: Cardiac myxoma: 40 years' experience in 63 patients. Ann Thorac Surg 63:697-700, 1997; (4) Pucci A, Gagliardotto P, Zanini C, et al: Histopathologic and clinical characterization of cardiac myxoma: Review of 53 cases from a single institution. Am Heart J 140:134-138, 2000; and (5) Pinede L, Duhaut P, Loire R: Clinical presentation of left atrial cardiac myxoma: A series of 112 consecutive cases. Medicine (Baltimore) 80:159-172, 2001.

*Summary of data representing collective experience of multiple investigators with a total of 284 cardiac myxomas.

been recorded.[30] One-fourth of patients with emboli have evidence of multiple embolic events. Compared to round and smooth tumors, polypoid, friable, and villous tumors are more than twice as likely to embolize.[29]

The third arm of the myxoma triad, constitutional symptoms, is unique among cardiac tumors. Although stated to occur in only 30 to 40 percent of patients, some investigators suggest that if searched for, they are found in up to 90 percent of patients. Symptoms include myalgias, muscle weakness, arthralgias, rash, fever, weight loss, and fatigue. Raynaud phenomenon and clubbing can be seen on physical examination. Laboratory evaluation may reveal an elevated ESR, anemia, leukocytosis, thrombocytopenia or thrombocytosis, and hypergammaglobulinemia. One can easily appreciate how a myxoma with prominent constitutional symptoms such as fever, arthralgias, Raynaud phenomenon, and an elevated ESR might initially be mistaken for collagen-vascular disease or how the combination of embolic events and fever might lead to the diagnosis of endocarditis. Rarely, myxomas are actually infected.[31]

Role of Interleukin 6. The association of constitutional symptoms with cardiac myxoma is likely due to the tumor's constitutive synthesis and secretion of interleukin (IL)-6, a cytokine that induces the acute-phase response. Increased levels of IL-6 and IL-6 messenger RNA have been found in myxoma tissue, and cultured myxoma cells have been shown to produce IL-6.[32] Patients with constitutional symptoms are more likely to have elevated levels of circulating IL-6, and in virtually all cases, serum IL-6 levels become undetectable and the autoimmune-like constitutional symptoms resolve on removal of the tumor.[33] Several cases of multiple myeloma developing in patients with cardiac myxoma have been reported, which is not unexpected given the important role IL-6 plays in promoting myeloma cell growth.

FAMILIAL MYXOMAS. These constitute 10 percent or less of all myxomas. Patients tend to present earlier (median age 20 years), are more likely to have myxomas in atypical locations, sometimes have multiple tumors, are more likely to develop recurrent tumors, and have associated dermatological and endocrine abnormalities. These observations were codified in 1985 by J. Aidan Carney, who described the "Carney complex" of myxomas, spotty skin pigmentation, and endocrine overactivity.[34] Patients with cardiac myxomas and pigmentary abnormalities had been previously described as having the NAME syndrome (*n*evi, *a*trial myxoma, *m*yxoid neurofibroma, *e*phelides)[35] or the LAMB syndrome (*l*entigines, *a*trial *m*yxoma, and *b*lue nevi).[36] However, it is now thought that these patients likely had unrecognized, subclinical endocrine abnormalities and thus had the Carney complex, which may be thought of as a form of multiple endocrine neoplasia.

Carney Complex. The diagnostic criteria for the Carney complex include having 2 of 12 recognized clinical manifestations (Table 63–6) or 1 clinical manifestation plus evidence of genetic transmission (affected first-degree relative or mutation in one of the genes linked to the Carney complex).[37] The possible clinical manifestations may be grouped into three categories: myxomas, pigmented skin lesions, and endocrine neoplasia. Cardiac myxomas are seen in half to two-thirds of patients at presentation. Although the left atrium is still the most common location for cardiac myxomas in Carney complex (~50 percent), atypical locations (right atrium ~40 percent, ventricles ~10 percent), multicentric foci (~50 percent), and recurrent tumors (10-22 percent) are far more common than in patients with nonsyndromic, isolated myxoma. In addition, one-third of patients have *mucocutaneous* myxomas at presentation, with classic sites being the eyelid, external ear canal, breast, and oropharynx. Pigmented skin lesions are the most common clinical manifestation,

TABLE 63–6 Diagnostic Criteria for Carney Complex*

Clinical Criteria

1. Spotty skin pigmentation with typical distribution (lips, conjunctiva and inner or outer canthi, vaginal and penile mucosa)
2. Myxoma (cutaneous and mucosal)
3. Cardiac myxoma
4. Breast myxomatosis or fat-suppressed MRI findings suggestive of this diagnosis
5. Primary pigmented nodular adrenocortical disease or paradoxical positive response of urinary glucocorticosteroids to dexamethasone administration during Liddle's test
6. Acromegaly due to growth hormone–producing adenoma
7. Large cell calcifying Sertoli cell tumors or characteristic calcification on testicular ultrasonography
8. Thyroid carcinoma or multiple, hyperechoic nodules on thyroid ultrasonography, in a young patient
9. Psammomatous melanotic schwannoma
10. Bule nevus, epithelioid blue nevus (multiple)
11. Breast ductal adenoma (multiple)
12. Osteochondromyxoma

Supplemental Genetic Criteria

1. Affected first-degree relative
2. Inactivating mutation of the *PRKAR1α* gene

From Stratakis CA, Kirschner LS, Carney JA: Clinical and molecular features of the Carney complex: Diagnostic criteria and recommendations for patient evaluation. J Clin Endocrinol Metab 86:4041-4046, 2001.

*A diagnosis of Carney complex requires that a patient have either 2 of the 12 clinical criteria (with histological confirmation of any suspected tumors or characteristic imaging or laboratory data) *or* 1 of the clinical criteria and 1 of the supplemental genetic criteria.

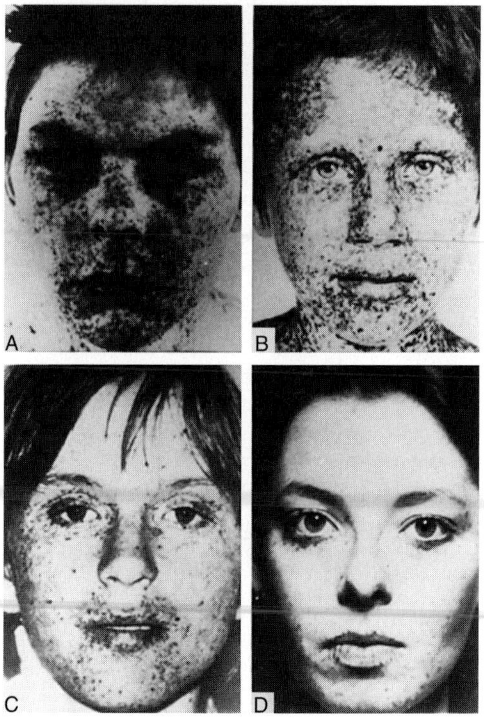

FIGURE 63–5 **A** to **D,** Four patients with extensive facial freckling, a finding associated with syndrome myxoma. Patients with this syndrome tend to be younger than patients with sporadic myxoma and have a substantially higher incidence of ventricular, multiple, biatrial, recurrent, and familial myxomas of the heart. In addition, these patients, in contrast with patients with sporadic myxoma, may have noncardiac myxomas and endocrine neoplasms. (From Vidaillet HJ Jr, Seward JB, Fyke FE, et al: "Syndrome myxoma": A subset of patients with cardiac myxoma associated with pigmented skin lesions and peripheral and endocrine neoplasms. Br Heart J 57:247, 1987.)

occurring in more than three-fourths of patients (Fig. 63–5). Blue nevi, café au lait spots, and depigmented lesions may be present at birth, but more commonly they develop in early childhood and may fade over time. Lentigines (macular melanoses) usually develop during the peripubertal period and typically involve the lips, conjunctiva, inner and outer canthi, and vaginal and penile mucosa. Endocrine abnormalities include primary pigmented nodular adrenocortical disease, growth hormone- and prolactin-producing pituitary adenomas, large cell calcifying Sertoli cell tumors, and thyroid adenoma or carcinoma. These neoplasms are identified in less than one-third of patients but are likely significantly underreported due to subclinical disease.

The Carney complex usually demonstrates autosomal dominant transmission, although such transmission may not be obvious due to incomplete penetrance and phenotypic variability even within the same family. Linkage studies have revealed two genetic loci: 2p16 and 17q22-24.[38,39] Among the families mapping to 17q, mutations in the gene encoding the protein kinase A regulatory subunit 1-α (*PRKAR1α*) have recently been identified,[40] but the cellular mechanism by which this genetic abnormality causes myxomas remains uncertain. Sporadic cardiac myxomas do not have these genetic alterations.[41]

In patients with established Carney complex, rigorous screening for the other aspects of the syndrome should be undertaken (e.g., measurement of urinary free cortisol, testicular ultrasound). Preoperatively, before resection of their cardiac myxoma, a careful search should be made in these patients for cardiac myxomas in other locations. Postoperatively, these patients should be observed closely for recurrence of myxomas. This occurs in 12 to 22 percent of such patients, and cardiac complications account for more than half the deaths in patients with Carney complex.[37] Routine echocardiographic screening of first-degree relatives of patients with familial myxomas is appropriate and should also be considered in patients with apparent sporadic myxomas but who are young or have multiple tumors.

DIAGNOSIS. On chest radiography, approximately half of patients with left atrial myxomas have evidence of left atrial enlargement or pulmonary venous hypertension, and half of patients with right atrial myxomas have evidence of calcification; however, one-third of patients have a completely normal radiograph.[42] Two-dimensional echocardiography is the imaging modality of choice, classically revealing a mobile, distensible tumor connected to the interatrial septum by a narrow stalk. Both hypoechoic and hyperechoic foci may be seen, reflecting areas of hemorrhage and calcification, respectively. Transthoracic echocardiography is usually sufficient to make the diagnosis, but if the results are suboptimal, transesophageal echocardiography should be employed. CT typically reveals a lobular, heterogeneous, low-attenuation mass with a narrow base of attachment (the stalk is usually too narrow to be visualized), and, in 14 percent of cases, punctate calcification. MRI often reveals a spherical, heterogeneous mass that is primarily isointense on T1-weighted images, with areas of hypointensity and hyperintensity, is hyperintense on T2-weighted images, and shows heterogeneous enhancement with administration of gadolinium.[42] Gradient echo-cine MRI can be used to demonstrate tumor mobility.

PATHOLOGY. On gross inspection, myxomas are gelatinous (often termed *myxoid*), smooth, and round, with a glistening surface, or they may be variably friable and either irregular or polypoid (Fig. 63–6). Areas of hemorrhage, calcification, and necrosis may be seen. The diagnosis of myxoma is now made by the observation of cords, rings, or florets of cells (often called *lipidic cells*) embedded in a myxoid stroma rich in glycosaminoglycans (Fig. 63–7).[43] Myxoma cells have a round, elongated, or polyhedral shape; scant pink cytoplasm; and an ovoid nucleus with an open chromatin pattern.

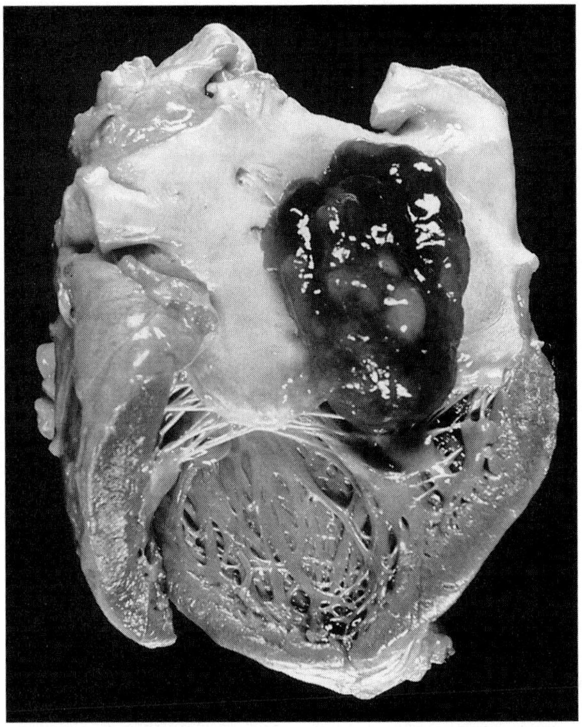

FIGURE 63–6 Photograph of the most frequent gross appearance of cardiac myxomas: a polypoid, smooth, round, hemorrhagic left atrial mass. The tumor mass nearly fills the left atrium and extends into the mitral valve orifice. (From Cotran RS, Kumar V, Robbins SL: Robbins Pathologic Basis of Disease. 5th ed. Philadelphia, WB Saunders, 1994.)

They are occasionally multinuclear. Myxoma cells have abundant fine cytoplasmic filaments similar to those of smooth muscle cells. The pathological characteristics of myxomas are well described and are independent of location or whether they are syndromic or nonsyndromic.

The cells most resemble embryonic mesenchymal cells with multipotential capabilities for cellular differentiation, including vasoformative activity and expression of vascular endothelial growth factor,[44] which can be found in the serum of patients with myxoma and resolves after excision of the tumor.[45] Myxoma cells are especially similar to embryonic endocardial cushion tissue, supporting the notion that myxomas arise from embryonic rests remaining from when the heart underwent septations. Immunohistochemical studies demonstrate positivity for vimentin, indicative of the mesenchymal derivation of the cells, as well as several neuroendocrine markers, including S-100 (89 percent of cases), protein gene product 9.5 (94 percent of cases), and calretinin (100 percent of cases).[46,47] Recent studies also demonstrate the presence of cardiomyocyte-specific transcription factors, supporting the idea that myxomas derive from mesenchymal cardiomyogenic precursor cells.[48]

Many of the morphological features of organizing mural thrombi resemble those of myxoma, including abundant loose amorphous extracellular matrix, connective tissue cells, and small vascular channels. It is difficult to distinguish between some myxomas and mural thrombi in various stages of organization; indeed, cellular intracardiac thrombi and peripheral thromboemboli occasionally receive an erroneous diagnosis of myxoma. The recent demonstration of calretinin expression in cardiac myxomas but not mural thrombi may lead to a useful tool for distinguishing myxomas from thrombi.[47] Cardiac myxomas also may be mistaken for cardiac sarcomas because a myxoid background rich in proteoglycans may be seen in both tumors. However, myxomas consist of polygonal myxoma cells that form syncytia and express S-100 protein, whereas sarcomas consist of spindle-shaped cells that show signs of nuclear atypia and mitoses and do not express S-100.

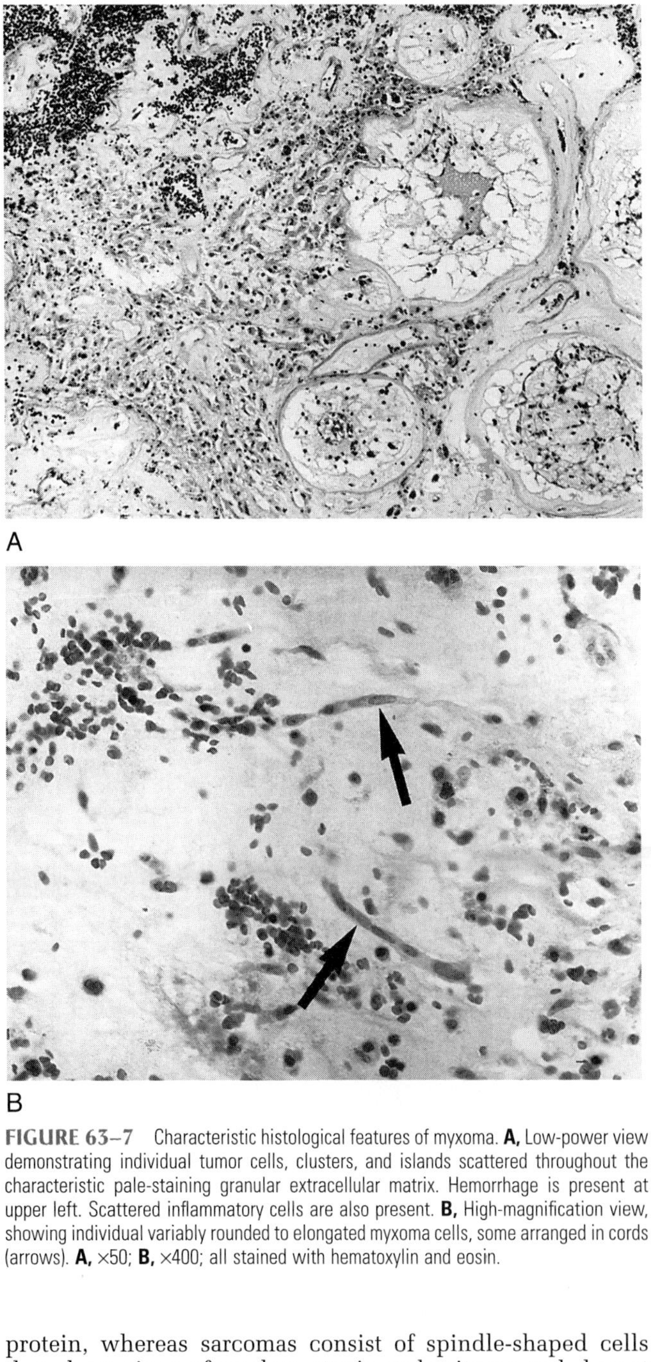

A

B

FIGURE 63–7 Characteristic histological features of myxoma. **A,** Low-power view demonstrating individual tumor cells, clusters, and islands scattered throughout the characteristic pale-staining granular extracellular matrix. Hemorrhage is present at upper left. Scattered inflammatory cells are also present. **B,** High-magnification view, showing individual variably rounded to elongated myxoma cells, some arranged in cords (arrows). **A,** ×50; **B,** ×400; all stained with hematoxylin and eosin.

TREATMENT. The usual surgical approach to a typical left-sided myxoma is through the right atrium and across the interatrial septum at the fossa ovalis with en bloc resection including a rim of septum around the base. In recent case series using such techniques, operative mortality approaches 1 percent.[23] In about 1 to 5 percent of cases, a recurrence or second cardiac myxoma has been reported after resection of the initial myxoma. Possible causes of the second tumor include incomplete excision of the original tumor with regrowth; growth from a second "pretumorous" focus (i.e., a metasynchronous tumor); or intracardiac implantation from the original tumor.[49] Because of the first two possibilities, some surgeons have advocated excision of the entire region of the fossa ovalis and repair of the resultant atrial septal defect to remove presumably high concentrations of pretumorous cells thought to be located in that region. Other surgeons have reported equally successful long-term recurrence-free periods with simple excision of the tumor and a small rim at the base. More recently, minimally invasive approaches via a minithoracotomy, with and without video-assisted endoscopy, have been reported.[50] Although short-term results appear excellent, long-term data on recurrence rates are lacking.

In patients with the Carney complex, the risk of a second tumor occurring in the future is in the range of 12 to 22 percent,[37] as compared with approximately 1 percent for patients with sporadic atrial myxoma.[23,29] It is believed that tumor recurrence in these cases is from a second pretumorous focus of cells. In these high-risk patients, a careful search for additional tumors preoperatively and more extensive resection of the underlying endocardium, atrial septum, or both is recommended. Careful echocardiographic follow-up for detection of metasynchronous tumors is recommended for all patients after resection of a myxoma.

Papillary Fibroelastomas

The most common tumors of the cardiac valves, papillary fibroelastomas are benign papillomas of the endocardium. Because they are easily overlooked at autopsy, the widespread use of echocardiography has led to increased preoperative and premortem recognition, and recent series suggest they are the second most common benign tumor of the adult heart.[25] The average age at detection is 60 years, although papillary fibroelastomas have been detected in neonates as well as in patients as old as 92 years.[51,52] The incidence in men and women appears to be similar. Most patients have concomitant valvular disease, suggesting that endocardial damage from infection, inflammation, radiation, or even prior invasive cardiac procedures may predispose to papilloma formation. More than 90 percent of the time papillary fibroelastomas are single. The median diameter is 8 mm; the largest reported tumor is 40 mm. Papillary fibroelastomas can occur on any valve or, far less commonly, on papillary muscle, chordae tendineae, or in the atria. The aortic and mitral valves are most commonly involved in adults. Most often, the arterial side of semilunar valves and the atrial surface of AV valves are affected. A short pedicle is seen approximately half of the time, typically in tumors arising from the endocardium of a cardiac chamber. Whether papillary fibroelastomas are truly neoplastic, as well as their relationship to cardiac mural thrombi and endocardial injury, remains uncertain.

CLINICAL MANIFESTATIONS. Although many are clinically insignificant, papillary fibroelastomas have the potential to embolize to vital structures.[51] These tumors may mimic infective endocarditis with the combination of embolic events and an abnormal appearing valve. Despite their valvular attachment, valvular dysfunction is distinctly uncommon.[51,52] However, tumors on the aortic valve can partially obstruct a coronary arterial orifice and lead to myocardial ischemia or infarction.[53] Transthoracic echocardiography has a sensitivity of 62 percent and transesophageal echocardiography a sensitivity of 77 percent.[52] The rates approach 90 percent when tumors smaller than 2 mm are excluded. A characteristic shimmer or vibration at the tumor-blood interface, ascribed to the finger-like projections of the tumor, has been described and is best appreciated on transesophageal echocardiography.[51] Typically these tumors are too small to be seen well on CT or MRI.

PATHOLOGY. On gross inspection, papillary fibroelastomas have a characteristic frond-like appearance resembling a sea anemone (Fig. 63–8). Histologically, the tumor is covered by endothelium that surrounds an avascular core of loose connective tissue rich in glycosaminoglycans, collagen, and elastic fibers and containing smooth muscle cells (often as a fine meshwork surrounding a central collagen or dense elastic fiber core).[54] Papillary fibroelastomas may be distinguished from Lambl's excrescences, which are acellular deposits of variably organized thrombus and connective tissue covered by a single layer of endothelium that are found on heart valves at the site of endothelial damage in many adults, particularly along the closure margins of the aortic valve cusps. In contrast, papillary fibroelastomas are not usually found at valvular contact areas. However, others have argued that neither gross nor microscopic criteria can reliably distinguish the two entities and suggest that the term *papillary fibroelastoma* be used when the papilloma is large, symptomatic, or atypically situated.

TREATMENT. Most investigators recommend complete resection of papillary fibroelastomas, especially for left-sided lesions.[55] Although these tumors are small, their frond-like structure results in a relatively large and irregular surface area. The risk of embolic events may be as high as 25 percent over 3 years, and even 6 percent in asymptomatic patients in whom papillary fibroelastoma was an incidental finding.[51] Anticoagulation does not appear to protect against embolic events.[56]

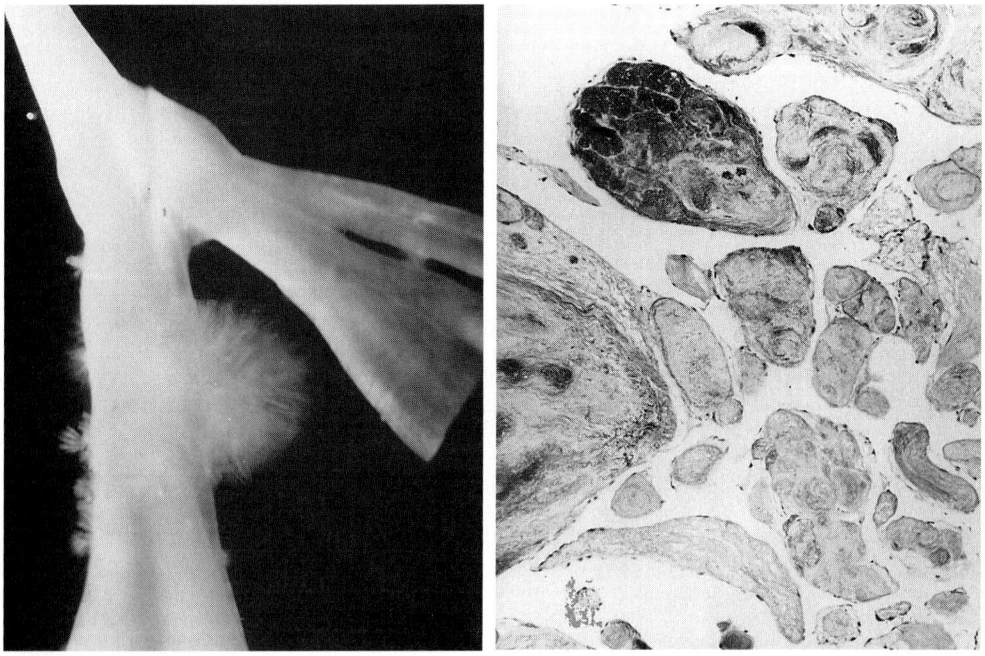
A B

FIGURE 63–8 Papillary fibroelastoma. **A,** Gross photograph demonstrating resemblance of this lesion to a sea anemone, with myriad papillary fronds, arising from the chordae tendineae near the mitral leaflet. In this case, many lesions were present, all associated with the mitral valve apparatus. **B,** Histological appearance of papillary fibroelastoma, demonstrating the numerous papillary fronds consisting of a collagen core surrounded by elastic fibers and loose connective tissue, all covered by endocardial endothelium. ×100; stained with elastica van Gieson stain (elastin black).

More than 90 percent of tumors can be resected using a conservative, valve-sparing approach with stalk excision or quadrangular resection and valve repair using a pericardial patch.[51] Recurrences have not been reported.

LIPOMAS AND LIPOMATOUS HYPERTROPHY

True lipomas are rare and can occur at any age and with equal frequency in both sexes. They range in diameter from 1 to 15 cm, although some very large lipomas weighing up to 4.8 kg have been reported. Most tumors are sessile or polypoid and occur in the subendocardium or subpericardium, although about one-fourth are completely intramuscular.

CLINICAL MANIFESTATIONS. The most common chambers affected are the left ventricle, right atrium, and interatrial septum. Many tumors are clinically silent, however, and are found only at autopsy. Echocardiography typically reveals a homogeneous, hyperechoic mass, but these findings are not diagnostic. On CT, lipomas appear as homogeneous masses with the same attenuation as fat. The best imaging modality is MRI, on which lipoma's signal intensity strikingly decreases during fat-saturated sequences.

PATHOLOGY. Microscopically, the lesions are usually well encapsulated and composed of typical mature fat cells; they occasionally contain fibrous connective tissue (fibrolipoma), muscular tissue (myolipoma), or vacuolated brown (fetal) fat, resembling a hibernoma.

LIPOMATOUS HYPERTROPHY OF THE INTERATRIAL SEPTUM. Whereas lipomas are true neoplasms, a more common cardiac lipomatous condition termed *lipomatous hypertrophy of the interatrial septum* represents a hamartoma consisting of fatty deposition in the interatrial septum. These lesions most commonly occur in obese, elderly, female patients.[57] Lipomatous hypertrophy classically involves the anterior or superior portion of the interatrial septum, spares the fossa ovalis, and protrudes into the right atrium. On average, the septum is thickened up to 2.5 cm (the septum is usually < 1 cm thick and the upper limit of normal is generally considered to be 2 cm); however, tumors up to 10 cm in diameter have been described.[25] The thickness of the septum correlates with body weight and the thickness of adipose tissue surrounding the heart.[57]

Clinically, lipomatous hypertrophy is associated with a high incidence of atrial arrhythmias that is correlated with the degree of hypertrophy. Massive lipomatous hypertrophy can cause obstruction of the superior vena cava. Pathologically, in contrast to true lipomas, lipomatous hypertrophy consists of a *nonencapsulated* accumulation of mature and fetal adipose tissue and atypical cardiac myocytes within the interatrial septum.[58] The term *hypertrophy* is therefore a misnomer because the lesion is due to an increased number rather than increased size of adipocytes and thus represents *hyperplasia*. Lipomatous hypertrophy is easily seen on transthoracic and transesophageal echocardiography as a highly echogenic, bilobed septal mass that spares the fossa ovalis and displays the tissue signal characteristics similar to subcutaneous fat on CT and MRI.[59]

TREATMENT. Because of their progressive growth, true lipomas usually require surgical intervention with complete excision. In contrast, surgical resection of lipomatous hypertrophy of the septum is usually performed only in the setting of superior vena cava obstruction or clinically significant arrhythmias.[60] The nonneoplastic nature of these lesions permits incomplete resections that restore normal hemodynamics to be performed.[61]

RHABDOMYOMAS

These are the most common cardiac tumors of infants and children; approximately three-fourths occur in patients younger than 1 year.[62] Evidence suggests that rhabdomyomas are actually myocardial hamartomas or malformations that are composed of myocytes that resemble fetal cardiac myocytes rather than true neoplasms. They occur with equal frequency in the left and right ventricular and septal myocardium; nearly all are multiple. Approximately one-third also involve either one or both atria. They are usually small and lobulated, with diameters in the range of 2 mm to 2 cm.[63]

CLINICAL MANIFESTATIONS. The type and severity of symptoms depend on the location and size of the tumors. Tumors close to the conduction system may result in arrhythmias. Heart block is the most common manifestation, but paroxysmal supraventricular tachycardia, ventricular tachycardia, and sudden cardiac death have also been reported and may be due to reentrant circuits created by the tumor. Intracavitary tumors may lead to signs and symptoms of congestive heart failure due to obstruction of blood flow, including death in utero and a hydropic infant. Echocardiography is usually adequate for diagnosis and typically reveals multiple small, lobulated, homogeneous, hyperechoic intramural tumors.[64] On MRI, rhabdomyomas are usually isointense on T1-weighted images and hyperintense on T2-weighted images.[65]

ASSOCIATION WITH TUBEROUS SCLEROSIS. Rhabdomyomas are strongly associated with tuberous sclerosis, which is an autosomal dominant hamartoma syndrome whose causative genes (*TSC-1* and *TSC-2*) are tumor suppressor genes that encode a protein complex that regulates cell size.[66] The syndrome is characterized by hamartomas in several organs, epilepsy, mental deficiency, and adenoma sebaceum. Several studies show that at least 80 percent of patients with cardiac rhabdomyomas have tuberous sclerosis,[63] and approximately 50 percent of patients younger than 18 years of age with tuberous sclerosis have cardiac rhabdomyomas.[67]

PATHOLOGY. Rhabdomyomas are yellowish gray and range from 1 mm to several centimeters in diameter (Fig 63–9). They are circumscribed but not encapsulated; microscopically, they are easily distinguished from the surrounding myocardium as clusters of abnormal cells. The microscopic hallmark, termed the *spider cell,* is a large (≤80-μm diameter) cell containing a central cytoplasmic mass that is suspended by fine myofibrillar processes radiating to the periphery, thus giving the appearance of a spider hanging in a net.

TREATMENT. Fifty percent or more of rhabdomyomas regress spontaneously after infancy.[63,67,68] Thus, in the absence of symptoms, surgery is not indicated.[69] This is fortunate because multiple nodular rhabdomyomas, the type associated with tuberous sclerosis, are difficult to resect. In contrast, intracavitary rhabdomyomas, which may cause heart failure, tend to be sporadic tumors not associated with tuberous sclerosis and are more amenable to surgical resection.[68] If the diagnosis is in question in an asymptomatic patient, a small, isolated tumor may be resected as part of the biopsy. For larger or multiple tumors, biopsy alone should be sufficient to yield the diagnosis and, if rhabdomyoma is confirmed, allow for observation with periodic echocardiograms rather than more involved surgery.

FIBROMAS

Fibromas are benign connective tissue tumors derived from fibroblasts that occur predominantly in children and constitute the second most common type of primary cardiac tumor occurring in the pediatric age

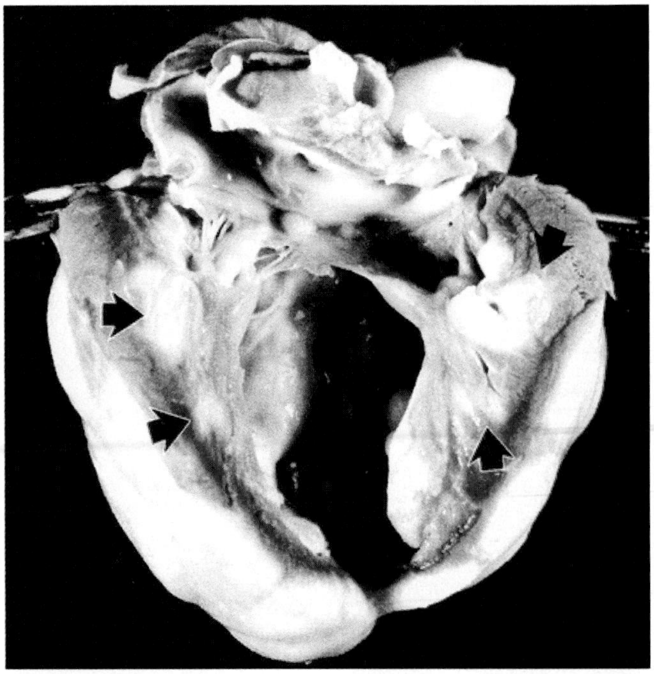

FIGURE 63–9 Photograph of a cut autopsy specimen from a 3-month-old boy with rhabdomyoma. Multiple, firm, white nodules can be seen distributed throughout the left ventricular myocardium (arrows). (From Grebenc ML, Rosado de Christenson ML, Burke AP, et al: Primary cardiac and pericardial neoplasms: Radiologic-pathologic correlation. Radiographics 20:1073-1103, 2000.)

group.[63] Most are detected in children younger than 10 years, and about one-third are diagnosed in infants younger than 1 year. Males and females appear to be equally affected. Cardiac fibromas typically are large tumors, ranging from 3 to 10 cm in diameter. They usually occur within the ventricular myocardium and much more frequently within the anterior free wall of the left ventricle or the interventricular septum than in the posterior left ventricular wall or right ventricle.[70]

CLINICAL MANIFESTATIONS. Approximately 70 percent of fibromas are symptomatic, causing mechanical interference with intracardiac flow (usually with bulky intracavitary left ventricular or right ventricular tumors), ventricular systolic function (usually with large intramyocardial left ventricular tumors), or conduction disturbances (usually with tumors arising in the interventricular septum). The most common clinical manifestations are congestive heart failure (21 percent), ventricular tachyarrhythmias (13 percent), and atypical chest pain (3.5 percent).[71] Sudden cardiac death occurs in 14 percent of patients with fibromas, typically in infants. Most symptomatic patients have cardiomegaly on their chest radiograph, with tumor calcification seen in 25 percent of cases.

Imaging. Echocardiography typically reveals an intramural, homogenous, echogenic mass. CT scanning often shows a homogeneous mass with calcification. On MRI, fibromas are usually homogeneous and isointense to hyperintense on T1-weighted images, and, owing to their dense fibrous nature, are hypointense on T2-weighted images and manifest minimal enhancement with gadolinium, although the latter finding is variable.[70]

GORLIN SYNDROME. The nevoid basal cell carcinoma, or Gorlin syndrome, is an autosomal dominant disorder characterized by multiple nevoid basal cell carcinomas, medulloblastomas, cardiac fibromas and fibrous histiocytomas and other tumors, as well as nonneoplastic features including odontogenic keratocysts, dyskeratotic pitting of the hands and feet, and a variety of skeletal abnormalities including bifid ribs.[72] In a small series of fibromas, Gorlin syndrome was identified in approximately 5 percent of patients, but many of these patients were infants in whom the other features of Gorlin syndrome might not have been apparent yet.[70] Fewer than 14 percent of patients with Gorlin syndrome have fibromas. The gene for this syndrome (*PTC*) was mapped to chromosome 9q22-31 and found to be a homolog of the *Drosophila* segment polarity gene *patched*.[73]

PATHOLOGY. Fibromas are gray, firm, circumscribed but not encapsulated, and exhibit a whorled appearance on cut sections (Fig. 63–10). Microscopically, cardiac fibromas consist of elongated fibroblasts admixed with fibrous tissue consisting mostly of collagen. Their cellularity is variable and appears to decrease with age; mitotic figures are rarely, if ever, seen.[70] Fibrous tissue is intermingled with adjacent myocardial fibers at the margins of the lesion. In older patients, fibromas may histologically resemble a scar from a healed infarct, but, unlike healed infarcts, fibromas appear as thickened or bulging masses on gross inspection. Calcification and islands of bone formation may be seen microscopically and occasionally radiographically.

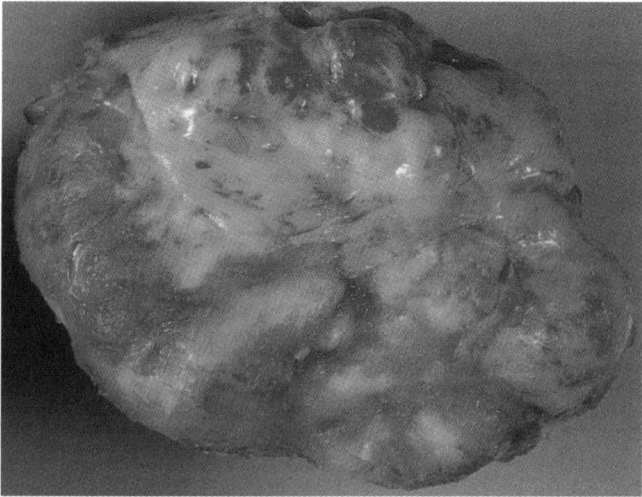

FIGURE 63–10 Photograph of an excised fibroma showing gross appearance. (From Allard MF, Taylor GP, Wilson JE, McManus BM: Primary cardiac tumors. *In* Goldhaber SZ, Braunwald E [eds]: Cardiopulmonary Diseases and Cardiac Tumors. Atlas of Heart Diseases. Vol 3. Philadelphia, Current Medicine, 1995, pp 15.1-15.22.)

TREATMENT. Surgical excision of cardiac fibromas is challenging but possible. Although these tumors lack capsules and may have extensions or satellites, it is usually possible to differentiate them from surrounding normal myocardium. Moreover, as fibromas displace rather than infiltrate the normal myocardium, reapproximation of the remaining myocardium post excision is often feasible.[71] Sometimes, though, the intramyocardial location of these tumors may preclude complete resection. Given the risk of fatal arrhythmias, resection is usually recommended even in asymptomatic cases. However, fibromas typically do not demonstrate continued growth after 1 or 2 years of age and cases of spontaneous regression have rarely been reported. Thus, patients who are able to undergo only partial resection may still do well postoperatively, and complete resection may be deferred if it will endanger the patient.

TERATOMAS

These tumors, which contain elements of all three germ cell layers, occur within the heart less frequently than they do in the anterior mediastinum.[74] Teratomas are generally observed in children and occur in the pericardium, attached to the root of the aorta or the pulmonary trunk. When located within the heart, they occur predominantly within the right atrium, right ventricle, or the interatrial or interventricular septum. Imaging studies typically reveal a heterogeneous mass with solid and cystic components.[75] They range from 0.5 to 9 cm in greatest diameter and tend to be lobulated with multiple cystic cavities containing clear, yellow, or brownish fluid.[74] On CT and MRI teratomas are very heterogeneous with areas of fat, cysts, soft tissue, calcification, and so forth.

HEMANGIOMAS

Composed of benign proliferations of endothelial cells, hemangiomas and lymphangiomas are extremely rare, with only 75 or so cases documented in the literature. Anatomically, they may occur in any part of the heart but more commonly are found in the lateral wall of the left ventricle (21 percent), the anterior wall of the right ventricle (21 percent), or the interventricular septum (17 percent).[76] Usually they are intramural, and, if in the interventricular septum or AV node, may cause complete heart block and sudden death. They may also protrude intraluminally and cause obstruction of the right ventricular outflow tract.

Hemangiomas are red, hemorrhagic, generally sessile or polypoid subendocardial nodules, ranging from 2 to 4 cm in diameter. Histologically, the tumors consist of endothelium-lined spaces that may contain blood, lymph, thrombi, or calcification; they are classified according to the predominant type of proliferating vascular channel. The natural history of these tumors is quite variable: some tumors involute, others stop growing after a certain time, and some continue to proliferate. Because there is no way to predict which course the tumor will take, resection is usually the treatment of choice. Radiation therapy has been used in instances when resection is not possible or complete,[77] and corticosteroids and interferon-alpha therapy may be considered.[78]

MISCELLANEOUS TUMORS

CYSTIC TUMOR ("MESOTHELIOMA") OF THE ATRIOVENTRICULAR NODE. Of controversial histogenesis, these small tumors (usually <15 mm in largest dimension) frequently cause death by complete heart block or ventricular fibrillation.[79] More common in women than in men, they occur at virtually any age and as poorly circumscribed, often multicystic nodules in the atrial septum, immediately cephalad to the commissure of the septal and anterior leaflets of the tricuspid valve, in the region of the AV node. These lesions are characterized by tubules and cysts lined by flat or cuboidal cells that are devoid of mitotic activity but may have secretory function.

ENDOCRINE TUMORS OF THE HEART. Approximately 2 percent of *paragangliomas* are intrathoracic, and of these, most are located in the posterior mediastinum. However, these tumors can also occur in close association with the left atrial or left ventricular epicardium, where they are thought to have arisen from sympathetic fibers to the heart or from ectopic chromaffin cells. More rarely still, paragangliomas may arise within the interatrial septum. Tumors in any of these locations may secrete catecholamines and therefore can be associated with signs and symptoms characteristic of pheochromocytoma.[80]

HISTIOCYTOID TUMORS. *Histiocytoid cardiomyopathy* (or *Purkinje cell hamartoma*) refers to a congenital collection of modified myocytes with few contractile elements. These tumors typically present as incessant ventricular tachycardia or sudden death in female infants and children.[81] *Benign fibrous histiocytomas* resemble fibromas, but with a greater number of histiocytic cells. In contrast to their malignant counterparts, mitotic figures are not seen and long-term prognosis is good.

Malignant Cardiac Tumors

About one-fourth of all cardiac tumors exhibit malignant histological characteristics and invasive or metastatic behavior. Nearly all (95 percent) of these are sarcomas, thus making these tumors second only to myxomas in overall frequency. Lymphomas account for the remaining 5 percent of primary malignant cardiac tumors.

Sarcomas

Sarcomas derive from mesenchyme and therefore may display a wide variety of morphological types, including angiosarcoma, rhabdomyosarcoma, fibrosarcoma and malignant fibrous histiocytomas, myxoid sarcomas, osteosarcoma, and others.[82] In a small case series, mutations in K-*ras* were seen in most primary cardiac sarcomas.[83] Sarcomas may occur at any age but are most common between the third and fifth decades. Except for rhabdomyosarcomas and fibrosarcomas, sarcomas are distinctly unusual in infants and children.

CLINICAL MANIFESTATIONS. The cardiac findings are determined primarily by the location of the tumor and by the extent of intracavitary obstruction.[82] Most patients present with progressive, unexplained dyspnea with evidence of heart failure, particularly of the right side. Precordial pain, uncommon in benign cardiac tumors, occurs in one-fourth of patients with sarcomas. Because of the rapid growth potential of sarcomas, they commonly extend into the pericardial space, and pericardial effusions, typically hemorrhagic and with or without tamponade physiology, are seen in one-fourth of patients. Obstruction of the superior vena cava (resulting in swelling of the face and upper extremities) and obstruction of the inferior vena cava (resulting in visceral congestion) have also been observed. In primarily intramural tumors, arrhythmias, conduction disturbances, and sudden death can occur. In older series, 75 percent of patients with cardiac sarcomas had evidence of distant metastases at the time of death; in more modern series, with superior noninvasive imaging facilitating earlier diagnosis, only 25 to 50 percent of patients have metastatic disease at the time of diagnosis. The most frequent sites are the lungs, thoracic lymph nodes, mediastinum, and vertebral column; the liver, kidneys, adrenals, pancreas, bone, spleen, and bowel are less often involved.

DIAGNOSIS. Although transthoracic echocardiography is a reasonable initial screening tool, transesophageal echocardiography may offer important clues as to the malignant nature of the lesion by showing intramyocardial and, for right atrial masses, vena caval invasion.[84] The superior soft tissue characterization possible with CT and especially MRI also allows them to determine the degree of tumor infiltration. However, there are no pathognomonic imaging signs, with most sarcomas showing heterogeneous signal intensity due to focal areas of hemorrhage and necrosis. Although pericardial involvement is common, even in those cases, pericardiocentesis may not yield malignant cells and endomyocardial or open biopsy may be needed.[85]

TREATMENT. Sarcomas proliferate rapidly and characteristically display a swift downhill course. Death is due to widespread infiltration of the myocardium, obstruction of flow within the heart, or distant metastases and most often occurs from a few weeks to 2 years after the onset of symptoms, with the median survival being 6 to 12 months. Undifferentiated tumors and those with a high mitotic rate and areas of necrosis have an especially poor prognosis.[82] Surgical excision should be considered to achieve local control and relieve symptoms. Patients who are able to undergo complete excision have a better prognosis (median survival 12 to 24 months) than those who only undergo incomplete resection (3 to 10 months).[82] Unfortunately, complete excision is possible in fewer than half of patients. Autotransplantation (i.e., cardiac explantation, ex vivo tumor resection, cardiac reconstruction and reimplantation) has been used in unusual cases to facilitate resection.[86] The benefits of chemotherapy are unclear, but based on data supporting anthracycline-based regimens in soft tissue sarcomas, adjuvant chemotherapy and/or radiation therapy is usually recommended.[87] Although orthotopic heart transplantation is a theoretical option for patients with locally unresectable disease but without evidence of metastasis, case series demonstrate that two-thirds of patients so treated will still die within 1 year, either of locally recurrent or metastatic disease.[21]

ANGIOSARCOMAS. Angiosarcomas, including Kaposi sarcomas, account for close to 30 percent of primary cardiac sarcomas.[25,82] In distinction to most other cardiac sarcomas, in which the sex distribution is equal, there appears to be a 3:1 male-to-female ratio among patients with angiosarcomas. These tumors have a striking predilection for the right atrium and may be either intracavitary and polypoid or diffuse and infiltrative, with sheet-like involvement of the pericardium occurring in the latter forms. Patients usually present with right-sided heart failure or tamponade as well as systemic signs such as fever and weight loss. Because these tumors are well vascularized and frequently have areas of hemorrhage and necrosis, MRI may reveal heterogeneous, nodular areas of hyperintensity, described as a "cauliflower" appearance, as well as linear areas of enhancement with gadolinium, described as a "sunray" appearance. Microscopically, angiosarcomas are characterized by ill-defined but variable anastomotic vascular channels lined with atypical, often heaped-up, endothelial cells. Approximately 25 percent of angiosarcomas contain spindled cells and the appearance of intracytoplasmic lumina containing red blood cells is a helpful diagnostic clue.[25] By electron microscopy, immature endothelial cells, primitive pericytes, and undifferentiated mesenchymal cells may be identified. Because these tumors are right sided, they tend to be discovered late and therefore have grown quite large and/or metastasized at the time of discovery. Thus they are often not amenable to complete resection and hence have a very poor prognosis even among the sarcomas.[87]

Kaposi sarcoma is a type of angiosarcoma seen in immunocompromised patients and whose pathogenesis is related to infection with human herpes virus 8. It is seen in less than 5 percent of patients with acquired immunodeficiency syndrome (AIDS) and in solid organ transplant recipients. Among those with visceral Kaposi sarcoma, rare cases of cardiac involvement have been reported, typically epicardial or pericardial, but occasionally myocardial.[88]

RHABDOMYOSARCOMAS. Embryonal rhabdomyosarcomas are the most common cardiac malignancy in infants and children and account for 10 percent of all primary cardiac sarcomas. These tumors of striated muscle often diffusely infiltrate the ventricular myocardium but may also occasionally form a polypoid extension into the cardiac chambers and therefore have been clinically mistaken for myxoma. There are usually multiple foci with occasional nodular involvement of the pericardium.[89] Rhabdomyoblasts are the histological hallmark of this tumor.

FIBROSARCOMAS. Fibrosarcomas of the heart account for 5 to 10 percent of cardiac sarcomas and have a whitish, soft "fish flesh" consistency. Fibroblastic in differentiation, they are composed of spindle-shaped cells with elongated, blunt-ended nuclei and frequent mitoses. They may contain areas of hemorrhage and necrosis and extensively infiltrate the heart, often involving more than one cardiac chamber and spreading to the pericardium.[90]

OSTEOSARCOMAS. Primary cardiac osteosarcomas comprise 5 to 10 percent of cardiac sarcomas. They almost always occur in adults and in the left atrium. Unlike myxomas, they have a broad base of attachment, typically to the posterior atrial wall. On CT, the tumors often but not invariably present as a low-attenuation mass with areas of dense calcification. Grossly, osteosarcomas are stone hard and heavily calcified.[91] Histologically, they resemble osteosarcomas of bone and may contain areas of chondrosarcoma or fibrosarcoma.

MALIGNANT FIBROUS HISTIOCYTOMAS. Previously classified as fibrosarcomas or undifferentiated sarcomas, malignant fibrous histiocytomas have a "storiform" appearance with a mix of malignant fibroblasts and histiocytes and may contain myxoid areas.[92] In modern series malignant fibrous histiocytomas account for 5 to 10 percent of sarcomas.[25] They typically involve the left atrium and can be confused with myxomas.

LEIOMYOSARCOMAS. Derived from smooth muscle cells, leiomyosarcomas account for 10 percent of cardiac sarcomas and most are located in the left atrium. Some of these tumors may actually originate in the smooth muscle lining the pulmonary veins. Patients typically present in their 30s, a decade younger than with other types of sarcoma. On CT, these tumors appear as low-attenuation masses in the left atrium. Although sessile and gelatinous, unlike myxomas these tumors usually originate from the posterior wall and may involve the pulmonary veins and mitral valve. Histologically, these tumors demonstrate fascicular growth of spindle cells that contain intracytoplasmic glycogen.

MYXOID SARCOMAS (MYXOSARCOMAS). These tumors comprise less than 5 percent of cardiac sarcomas and are usually found in the left atrium and contain extensive myxoid areas; thus, they can be confused with myxomas or thought to represent malignant transformation of a myxoma. However, the data that myxomas can undergo malignant transformation are lacking. Histologically, myxoid sarcomas are composed of spindled mesenchymal cells and lack the calcification, thrombus, and hemosiderin seen in benign myxomas.

UNDIFFERENTIATED SARCOMAS. Undifferentiated sarcomas lack specific histological features. Using strict morphological criteria and using modern immunohistochemistry, up to 25 percent of sarcomas remain unclassified.[93] These tumors are most commonly found in the left atrium.[25]

PRIMARY CARDIAC LYMPHOMAS

Primary lymphoma involving only the heart or pericardium is rare, although recently the incidence has increased due to an increased incidence of immunosuppression from AIDS and solid organ transplant. In immunocompetent patients,[94] the median age of presentation is 64 years and the male-to-female ratio is 3:1. Patients present with intractable, typically right-sided, heart failure (52 percent), precordial chest pain (17 percent), constitutional symptoms (17 percent), arrhythmias (12 percent), or tamponade (12 percent).The lymphoma usually arises from the right side of the heart (most commonly the right atrium) and half of patients have pericardial effusions, typically large.

Establishing the diagnosis of primary cardiac lymphoma is challenging.[94] Transthoracic echocardiography has only moderate sensitivity and therefore transesophageal echocardiography should be used if cardiac lymphoma is suspected. CT and MRI findings are not specific, but MRI appears to be the most sensitive diagnostic modality.A gallium-67 scan that shows marked uptake in the heart is suggestive but nonspecific.[95] Cytological analysis of pericardial fluid has reported sensitivities ranging from 14 to 67 percent.[94,96] Transvenous endomyocardial biopsy has a sensitivity of only 50 percent; open biopsy is the gold standard. On pathology, cardiac lymphoma appears as a firm, white, infiltrative process, occasionally with nodular foci that range from 3 to 12 cm in diameter. These tumors are almost universally aggressive diffuse, large B-cell lymphomas.[94]

Without treatment, the median survival of patients with cardiac lymphomas is less than 1 month. Patients treated with chemotherapy and/or radiation have median survivals on the order of 1 year.[94] Immediately after initiation of therapy patients may deteriorate due to rapid intramural tumor lysis causing heart failure,[97] arrhythmias,[98] and even cardiac rupture.[99] The long-term prognosis is almost universally dismal, although isolated cases of complete remissions after autologous stem cell transplant have been reported.[100]

REFERENCES

Clinical Presentation

1. McAllister HA, Fenoglio JJ: Tumors of the cardiovascular system. *In* Hartmann WH, Cowan WR (eds): Atlas of Tumor Pathology. Vol. Second Series, Fascicle 15. Washington, DC, Armed Forces Institute of Pathology, 1978, pp 1-3.
2. Reynen K: Frequency of primary tumors of the heart. Am J Cardiol 77:107, 1996.
3. Harvey WP: Clinical aspects of cardiac tumors. Am J Cardiol 21:328-343, 1968.
4. Kusano KF, Ohe T: Cardiac tumors that cause arrhythmias. Card Electrophysiol Rev 6:174-177, 2002.

Diagnostic Techniques

5. Tousek P, Orban M, Schomig A, Firschke C: Images in cardiovascular medicine: Real-time perfusion echocardiography of an intracardiac mass. Circulation 107:2390, 2003.
6. Shyu KG, Chen JJ, Cheng JJ, et al: Comparison of transthoracic and transesophageal echocardiography in the diagnosis of intracardiac tumors in adults. J Clin Ultrasound 22:381-389, 1994.
7. Espinola-Zavaleta N, Morales GH, Vargas-Barron J, et al: Three-dimensional transesophageal echocardiography in tumors of the heart. J Am Soc Echocardiogr 15:972-979, 2002.
8. Gerber TC, Kuzo RS, Karstaedt N, et al: Current results and new developments of coronary angiography with use of contrast-enhanced computed tomography of the heart. Mayo Clin Proc 77:55-71, 2002.
9. Grebenc ML, Rosado de Christenson ML, Burke AP, et al: Primary cardiac and pericardial neoplasms: Radiologic-pathologic correlation. Radiographics 20:1073-1103, 2000.
10. Araoz PA, Mulvagh SL, Tazelaar HD, et al: CT and MR imaging of benign primary cardiac neoplasms with echocardiographic correlation. Radiographics 20:1303-1319, 2000.
11. Araoz PA, Eklund HE, Welch TJ, Breen JF: CT and MR imaging of primary cardiac malignancies. Radiographics 19:1421-1434, 1999.
12. Hoffmann U, Globits S, Frank H: Cardiac and paracardiac masses: Current opinion on diagnostic evaluation by magnetic resonance imaging. Eur Heart J 19:553-563, 1998.
13. Masui T, Takahashi M, Miura K, et al: Cardiac myxoma: Identification of intratumoral hemorrhage and calcification on MR images. AJR Am J Roentgenol 164:850-852, 1995.
14. Frank H: Cardiac and paracardiac masses. In Manning WJ, Pennell DJ (eds): Cardiovascular Magnetic Resonance. New York, Churchill Livingstone, 2002, pp 342-354.
15. Plutchok JJ, Boxt LM, Weinberger J, et al: Differentiation of cardiac tumor from thrombus by combined MRI and F-18 FDG PET imaging. Clin Nucl Med 23:324-325, 1998.
16. Hofstra L, Dumont EA, Thimister PW, et al: In vivo detection of apoptosis in an intracardiac tumor. JAMA 285:1841-1842, 2001.
17. Veinot JP: Diagnostic endomyocardial biopsy pathology: Secondary myocardial diseases and other clinical indications—a review. Can J Cardiol 18:287-296, 2002.
18. Kang SM, Rim SJ, Chang HJ, et al: Primary cardiac lymphoma diagnosed by transvenous biopsy under transesophageal echocardiographic guidance and treated with systemic chemotherapy. Echocardiography 20:101-103, 2003.

Treatment Options and Prognosis

19. Goldberg HP, Glenn F, Dotter CT, Steinberg I: Myxoma of the left atrium: Diagnosis made during life with operative and post-mortem findings. Circulation 6:762-767, 1952.
20. Crafoord C: Discussion of Glover RP: Late results of mitral commissurotomy. *In* Lam CR (ed): Henry Ford Hospital International Symposium on Cardiovascular Surgery. Philadelphia, WB Saunders, 1955, pp 202-211.
21. Gowdamarajan A, Michler RE: Therapy for primary cardiac tumors: Is there a role for heart transplantation? Curr Opin Cardiol 15:121-125, 2000.
22. Scheld HH, Nestle HW, Kling D, et al: Resection of a heart tumor using autotransplantation. Thorac Cardiovasc Surg 36:40-43, 1988.
23. Schaff HV, Mullany CJ: Surgery for cardiac myxomas. Semin Thorac Cardiovasc Surg 12:77-88, 2000.
24. Mery GM, Reardon MJ, Haas J, et al: A combined modality approach to recurrent cardiac sarcoma resulting in a prolonged remission: A case report. Chest 123:1766-1768, 2003.

Specific Cardiac Tumors

25. Virmani R, Burke A, Farb A, Atkinson JB: Cardiovascular Pathology. Major Problems in Pathology. Vol. 40. Philadelphia, WB Saunders, 2001.
26. Vaughan CJ, Veugelers M, Basson CT: Tumors and the heart: Molecular genetic advances. Curr Opin Cardiol 16:195-200, 2001.
27. Dijkhuizen T, van den Berg E, Molenaar WM, et al: Rearrangements involving 12p12 in two cases of cardiac myxoma. Cancer Genet Cytogenet 82:161-162, 1995.
28. Yoon DH, Roberts W: Sex distribution in cardiac myxomas. Am J Cardiol 90:563-565, 2002.
29. Pinede L, Duhaut P, Loire R: Clinical presentation of left atrial cardiac myxoma: A series of 112 consecutive cases. Medicine (Baltimore) 80:159-172, 2001.
30. Reynen K: Cardiac myxomas. N Engl J Med 333:1610-1617, 1995.
31. Revankar SG, Clark RA: Infected cardiac myxoma: Case report and literature review. Medicine (Baltimore) 77:337-344, 1998.
32. Suzuki J, Takayama K, Mitsui F, et al: In situ interleukin-6 transcription in embryonic nonmuscle myosin heavy chain expressing immature mesenchyme cells of cardiac myxoma. Cardiovasc Pathol 9:33-37, 2000.
33. Parissis JT, Mentzikof D, Georgopoulou M, et al: Correlation of interleukin-6 gene expression to immunologic features in patients with cardiac myxomas. J Interferon Cytokine Res 16:589-593, 1996.
34. Carney JA, Gordon H, Carpenter PC, et al: The complex of myxomas, spotty pigmentation, and endocrine overactivity. Medicine (Baltimore) 64:270-283, 1985.

35. Atherton DJ, Pitcher DW, Wells RS, MacDonald DM: A syndrome of various cutaneous pigmented lesions, myxoid neurofibromata, and atrial myxoma: The NAME syndrome. Br J Dermatol 103:421-429, 1980.
36. Rhodes AR, Silverman RA, Harrist TJ, Perez-Atayde AR: Mucocutaneous lentigines, cardiomucocutaneous myxomas, and multiple blue nevi: The "LAMB" syndrome. J Am Acad Dermatol 10:72-82, 1984.
37. Stratakis CA, Kirschner LS, Carney JA: Clinical and molecular features of the Carney complex: Diagnostic criteria and recommendations for patient evaluation. J Clin Endocrinol Metab 86:4041-4046, 2001.
38. Stratakis CA, Carney JA, Lin JP, et al: Carney complex, a familial multiple neoplasia and lentiginosis syndrome: Analysis of 11 kindreds and linkage to the short arm of chromosome 2. J Clin Invest 97:699-705, 1996.
39. Casey M, Mah C, Merliss AD, et al: Identification of a novel genetic locus for familial cardiac myxomas and Carney complex. Circulation 98:2560-2566, 1998.
40. Kirschner LS, Carney JA, Pack SD, et al: Mutations of the gene encoding the protein kinase A type I-alpha regulatory subunit in patients with the Carney complex. Nat Genet 26:89-92, 2000.
41. Fogt F, Zimmerman RL, Hartmann CJ, et al: Genetic alterations of Carney complex are not present in sporadic cardiac myxomas. Int J Mol Med 9:59-60, 2002.
42. Grebenc ML, Rosado-de-Christenson ML, Green CE, et al: Cardiac myxoma: Imaging features in 83 patients. Radiographics 22:673-689, 2002.
43. Burke AP, Virmani R: Cardiac myxoma: A clinicopathologic study. Am J Clin Pathol 100:671-680, 1993.
44. Kono T, Koide N, Hama Y, et al: Expression of vascular endothelial growth factor and angiogenesis in cardiac myxoma: A study of fifteen patients. J Thorac Cardiovasc Surg 119:101-107, 2000.
45. Bennett KR, Gu JW, Adair TH, Heath BJ: Elevated plasma concentration of vascular endothelial growth factor in cardiac myxoma. J Thorac Cardiovasc Surg 122:193-194, 2001.
46. Pucci A, Gagliardotto P, Zanini C, et al: Histopathologic and clinical characterization of cardiac myxoma: Review of 53 cases from a single institution. Am Heart J 140:134-138, 2000.
47. Terracciano LM, Mhawech P, Suess K, et al: Calretinin as a marker for cardiac myxoma: Diagnostic and histogenetic considerations. Am J Clin Pathol 114:754-759, 2000.
48. Kodama H, Hirotani T, Suzuki Y, et al: Cardiomyogenic differentiation in cardiac myxoma expressing lineage-specific transcription factors. Am J Pathol 161:381-389, 2002.
49. Shinfeld A, Katsumata T, Westaby S: Recurrent cardiac myxoma: Seeding or multifocal disease? Ann Thorac Surg 66:285-288, 1998.
50. Ravikumar E, Pawar N, Gnanamuthu R, et al: Minimal access approach for surgical management of cardiac tumors. Ann Thorac Surg 70:1077-1079, 2000.
51. Klarich KW, Enriquez-Sarano M, Gura GM, et al: Papillary fibroelastoma: Echocardiographic characteristics for diagnosis and pathologic correlation. J Am Coll Cardiol 30:784-790, 1997.
52. Sun JP, Asher CR, Yang XS, et al: Clinical and echocardiographic characteristics of papillary fibroelastomas: A retrospective and prospective study in 162 patients. Circulation 103:2687-2693, 2001.
53. Israel DH, Sherman W, Ambrose JA, et al: Dynamic coronary ostial obstruction due to papillary fibroelastoma leading to myocardial ischemia and infarction. Am J Cardiol 67:104-105, 1991.
54. Fishbein MC, Ferrans VJ, Roberts WC: Endocardial papillary elastofibromas: Histologic, histochemical, and electron microscopical findings. Arch Pathol 99:335-341, 1975.
55. Shahian DM: Papillary fibroelastomas. Semin Thorac Cardiovasc Surg 12:101-110, 2000.
56. Nighoghossian N, Derex L, Loire R, et al: Giant lambl excrescences: An unusual source of cerebral embolism. Arch Neurol 54:41-44, 1997.
57. Shirani J, Roberts WC: Clinical, electrocardiographic and morphologic features of massive fatty deposits ("lipomatous hypertrophy") in the atrial septum. J Am Coll Cardiol 22:226-238, 1993.
58. Prior JT: Lipomatous hypertrophy of the cardiac interatrial septum: A lesion resembling hibernoma, lipo-blastomatosis and infiltrating lipoma. Arch Pathol 78:11-15, 1964.
59. Pochis WT, Saeian K, Sagar KB: Usefulness of transesophageal echocardiography in diagnosing lipomatous hypertrophy of the atrial septum with comparison to transthoracic echocardiography. Am J Cardiol 70:396-398, 1992.
60. Zeebregts CJ, Hensens AG, Timmermans J, et al: Lipomatous hypertrophy of the interatrial septum: Indication for surgery? Eur J Cardiothorac Surg 11:785-787, 1997.
61. Breuer M, Wippermann J, Franke U, Wahlers T: Lipomatous hypertrophy of the interatrial septum and upper right atrial inflow obstruction. Eur J Cardiothorac Surg 22:1023-1025, 2002.
62. Burke AP, Virmani R: Cardiac rhabdomyoma: A clinicopathologic study. Mod Pathol 4:70-74, 1991.
63. Beghetti M, Gow RM, Haney I, et al: Pediatric primary benign cardiac tumors: A 15-year review. Am Heart J 134:1107-1114, 1997.
64. Holley DG, Martin GR, Brenner JI, et al: Diagnosis and management of fetal cardiac tumors: A multicenter experience and review of published reports. J Am Coll Cardiol 26:516-520, 1995.
65. Berkenblit R, Spindola-Franco H, Frater RW, et al: MRI in the evaluation and management of a newborn infant with cardiac rhabdomyoma. Ann Thorac Surg 63:1475-1477, 1997.
66. Kwiatkowski DJ: Tuberous sclerosis: From tubers to mTOR. Ann Hum Genet 67:87-96, 2003.
67. Nir A, Tajik AJ, Freeman WK, et al: Tuberous sclerosis and cardiac rhabdomyoma. Am J Cardiol 76:419-421, 1995.
68. Bosi G, Lintermans JP, Pellegrino PA, et al: The natural history of cardiac rhabdomyoma with and without tuberous sclerosis. Acta Paediatr 85:928-931, 1996.
69. Stiller B, Hetzer R, Meyer R, et al: Primary cardiac tumours: When is surgery necessary? Eur J Cardiothorac Surg 20:1002-1006, 2001.
70. Burke AP, Rosado-de-Christenson M, Templeton PA, Virmani R: Cardiac fibroma: Clinicopathologic correlates and surgical treatment. J Thorac Cardiovasc Surg 108:862-870, 1994.
71. Parmley LF, Salley RK, Williams JP, Head GB III: The clinical spectrum of cardiac fibroma with diagnostic and surgical considerations: Noninvasive imaging enhances management. Ann Thorac Surg 45:455-465, 1988.
72. Gorlin RJ: Nevoid basal cell carcinoma syndrome. Medicine (Baltimore) 66:98-113, 1987.
73. Hahn H, Wicking C, Zaphiropoulous PG, et al: Mutations of the human homolog of *Drosophila* patched in the nevoid basal cell carcinoma syndrome. Cell 85:841-851, 1996.
74. Cox JN, Friedli B, Mechmeche R, et al: Teratoma of the heart: A case report and review of the literature. Virchows Arch A Pathol Anat Histopathol 402:163-174, 1983.
75. de Bustamante TD, Azpeitia J, Miralles M, et al: Prenatal sonographic detection of pericardial teratoma. J Clin Ultrasound 28:194-198, 2000.
76. Brizard C, Latremouille C, Jebara VA, et al: Cardiac hemangiomas. Ann Thorac Surg 56:390-394, 1993.
77. Tabry IF, Nassar VH, Rizk G, et al: Cavernous hemangioma of the heart: Case report and review of the literature. J Thorac Cardiovasc Surg 69:415-420, 1975.
78. Drolet BA, Esterly NB, Frieden IJ: Hemangiomas in children. N Engl J Med 341:173-181, 1999.
79. Cina SJ, Smialek JE, Burke AP, et al: Primary cardiac tumors causing sudden death: A review of the literature. Am J Forensic Med Pathol 17:271-281, 1996.
80. David TE, Lenkei SC, Marquez-Julio A, et al: Pheochromocytoma of the heart. Ann Thorac Surg 41:98-100, 1986.
81. Malhotra V, Ferrans VJ, Virmani R: Infantile histiocytoid cardiomyopathy: Three cases and literature review. Am Heart J 128:1009-1021, 1994.
82. Burke AP, Cowan D, Virmani R: Primary sarcomas of the heart. Cancer 69:387-395, 1992.
83. Garcia JM, Gonzalez R, Silva JM, et al: Mutational status of *K-ras* and *TP53* genes in primary sarcomas of the heart. Br J Cancer 82:1183-1185, 2000.
84. Hsieh PL, Lee D, Chiou KR, et al: Echocardiographic features of primary cardiac sarcoma. Echocardiography 19:215-220, 2002.
85. Hammoudeh AJ, Chaaban F, Watson RM, Millman A: Transesophageal echocardiography-guided transvenous endomyocardial biopsy used to diagnose primary cardiac angiosarcoma. Cathet Cardiovasc Diagn 37:347-349, 1996.
86. Conklin LD, Reardon MJ: Autotransplantation of the heart for primary cardiac malignancy: Development and surgical technique. Tex Heart Inst J 29:105-108, 2002.
87. Llombart-Cussac A, Pivot X, Contesso G, et al: Adjuvant chemotherapy for primary cardiac sarcomas: The IGR experience. Br J Cancer 78:1624-1628, 1998.
88. Burgert SJ, Strickman NE, Carrol CL, Falcone M: Cardiac Kaposi's sarcoma following heart transplantation. Catheter Cardiovasc Interv 49:208-212, 2000.
89. Raaf HN, Raaf JH: Sarcomas related to the heart and vasculature. Semin Surg Oncol 10:374-382, 1994.
90. Knobel B, Rosman P, Kishon Y, Husar M: Intracardiac primary fibrosarcoma: Case report and literature review. Thorac Cardiovasc Surg 40:227-230, 1992.
91. Reynard JS Jr, Gregoratos G, Gordon MJ, Bloor CM: Primary osteosarcoma of the heart. Am Heart J 109:598-600, 1985.
92. Laya MB, Mailliard JA, Bewtra C, Levin HS: Malignant fibrous histiocytoma of the heart: A case report and review of the literature. Cancer 59:1026-1031, 1987.
93. Donsbeck AV, Ranchere D, Coindre JM, et al: Primary cardiac sarcomas: An immunohistochemical and grading study with long-term follow-up of 24 cases. Histopathology 34:295-304, 1999.
94. Ceresoli GL, Ferreri AJ, Bucci E, et al: Primary cardiac lymphoma in immunocompetent patients: Diagnostic and therapeutic management. Cancer 80:1497-1506, 1997.
95. Hamada S, Nishimura T, Hayashida K, Uehara T: Intracardiac malignant lymphoma detected by gallium-67 citrate and thallium-201 chloride. J Nucl Med 29:1868-1870, 1988.
96. Chalabreysse L, Berger F, Loire R, et al: Primary cardiac lymphoma in immunocompetent patients: A report of three cases and review of the literature. Virchows Arch 441:456-461, 2002.
97. Chim CS, Chan AC, Kwong YL, Liang R: Primary cardiac lymphoma. Am J Hematol 54:79-83, 1997.
98. Rolla G, Bertero MT, Pastena G, et al: Primary lymphoma of the heart: A case report and review of the literature. Leuk Res 26:117-120, 2002.
99. Beckwith C, Butera J, Sadaniantz A, et al: Diagnosis in oncology. Case 1: Primary transmural cardiac lymphoma. J Clin Oncol 18:1996-1997, 2000.
100. Porcar Ramells C, Clemente Gonzalez C, Garcia Pares D, et al: [Primary cardiac lymphoma: Cytological diagnosis and treatment with response to polychemotherapy and hematopoietic precursor autotransplant. Presentation of a case a review of the literature]. An Med Interna 19:305-309, 2002.

CHAPTER 64

Pericardial Diseases

Martin M. LeWinter • Samer Kabbani

Anatomy and Physiology of the Pericardium

VISCERAL AND PARIETAL PERICARDIUM. The pericardium is composed of two layers.[1] The *visceral* pericardium is a serous membrane composed of a single layer of mesothelial cells adherent to the epicardial surface of the heart. The *parietal* pericardium is fibrous, is about 2 mm thick when measured post mortem in humans without pericardial disease, and surrounds most of the heart. The parietal pericardium is largely acellular and contains both collagen and elastin fibers. Collagen is probably the major structural component and appears as wavy bundles when the pericardium is at low levels of stretch. When it is stretched further, the bundles straighten, resulting in increased stiffness of the tissue. The visceral pericardium reflects back near the origins of the great vessels, becoming continuous with and forming the inner layer of the parietal pericardium. The pericardial space lies between these two layers. It normally contains up to about 50 ml of serous fluid. (The term pericardial *sac* refers to the parietal pericardium with its inner visceral layer.) The reflection of the visceral pericardium is a few centimeters proximal to the junctions of each of the caval vessels with the right atrium. Thus, portions of these vessels lie within the pericardial sac (Fig. 64–1). Posterior to the left atrium, the reflection occurs at the oblique sinus of the pericardium. As a result, the left atrium is largely extrapericardial.

The parietal pericardium has ligamentous attachments to the diaphragm, sternum, and other structures in the anterior mediastinum. These ensure that the heart occupies a relatively fixed position within the thoracic cavity regardless of phase of respiration and body position. The only noncardiovascular macrostructures associated with the pericardium are the phrenic nerves, which are enveloped by the parietal pericardium.

Although pericardiectomy does not result in any obvious negative consequences, the normal pericardium does have functions. As noted, it maintains the position of the heart relatively constant within the thoracic cavity. It may also function as a barrier to infection and provides lubrication between the visceral and parietal layers. The pericardium is remarkably well innervated, including mechano- and chemoreceptors and phrenic afferents.[2] The normal functions of these receptors are incompletely understood, but they probably participate in reflexes thought to result from irritation of pericardium or epicardium, or both (e.g., the Bezold-Jarisch reflex) as well as transmission of pericardial pain. The pericardium also secretes prostaglandins and related substances that may modulate epicardial-pericardial neural traffic and coronary tone by effects on coronary receptors.[3]

The best-characterized mechanical function of the normal pericardium is its *restraining* effect on cardiac volume.[4,5] This function reflects the mechanical properties of the pericardial tissue.[6] The parietal pericardium has a tensile strength similar to that of rubber. At low applied stresses approximating those at physiological or subphysiological cardiac volumes, the tissue is quite elastic (Fig. 64-2, top); i.e., small forces result in large amounts of stretch. As stretch increases, the pericardial tissue fairly abruptly becomes quite stiff and resistant to further stretch. The point on the pericardial stress-strain relationship (see Fig. 64-2, top) where this transition occurs probably corresponds to stresses present at the upper range and slightly above physiological cardiac volumes and is probably caused by straightening of the collagen bundles.

Pressure-Volume Relationship. The *pressure-volume relationship* of the pericardial sac parallels the properties of the isolated tissue[7] (see Fig. 64-2, bottom, left curve), i.e., a relatively flat, compliant segment changing relatively abruptly to a noncompliant segment, with the transition occurring in the range of the upper limit of normal total cardiac volume (in this case, for the dog). Thus, the pericardial sac has a relatively small reserve volume. As the reserve volume is exceeded, the pressure within the sac operating on the surface of the heart increases rapidly and is transmitted to the inside of the cardiac chambers. The shape of the pericardial pressure-volume relationship accounts for the fact that when a critical level of effusion is reached, relatively small amounts of additional fluid cause large increases in intrapericardial pressure and have marked effects on cardiac function; conversely, removal of small amounts of fluid in patients with tamponade can result in striking improvement.

The shape of the pericardial pressure-volume relationship suggests that the normal pericardium can restrain cardiac volume; i.e., the force exerted on the surface of the heart by the pericardium can significantly limit filling, with a component of intracavitary filling pressure representing transmission of the pericardial pressure. This relationship has been examined by directly measuring the pressure in the pericardial sac as cardiac volume is varied using devices specifically designed to measure a contact pressure between two surfaces.[8,9] These studies demonstrate a substantial contact pressure, especially when the upper limit of normal cardiac volume is exceeded. The contact pressure is proportionally more important for the right side of the heart, whose filling pressures are normally lower than those on the left. In some of these studies[9] pericardial pressure was actually found to be virtually identical to right-heart filling pressure, whereas

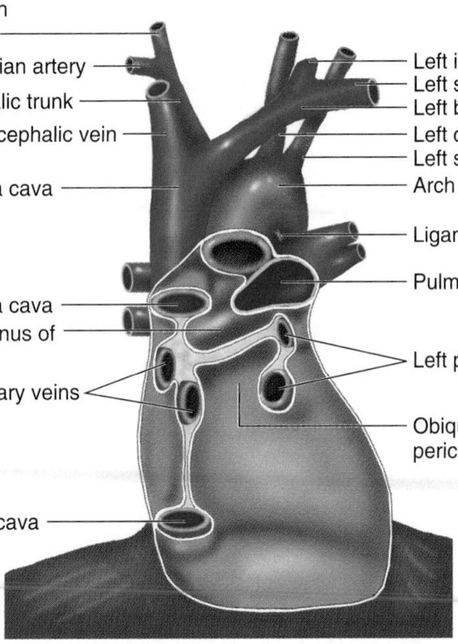

FIGURE 64–1 The pericardial reflections near the origins of the great vessels shown after removal of the heart. Note that portions of the caval vessels are within the pericardial space. (From Gabella G [sect ed]: The pericardium. *In* Gray H, Williams PL, Bannister LH [eds]: Gray's Anatomy: The Anatomical Basis of Medicine and Surgery. New York, Churchill-Livingstone, 1995, p 1471.)

in others[8] it was not as high but once again quite significant in relation to the right-heart pressure.

The pericardial contact pressure has also been estimated by quantifying the change in the right and left ventricular or right- and left-heart diastolic pressure-volume relationship before and after pericardiectomy.[4,5] Any decrease in pressure at a specified volume is the effective pericardial pressure at that volume. This method has the advantage of avoiding potential artifacts in direct pressure measurement. Studies in canine hearts using this approach[4] indicated negligible pericardial restraint at low normal filling volumes, with contact pressures in the range of 2 to 4 mm Hg at the upper end of the normal range. Contact pressure rapidly increases as filling is further augmented. With left-sided filling pressure about 25 mm Hg, estimated contact pressure is about 10 mm Hg, which accounts for a majority of the right-heart pressure at this level of filling.

Thus, it is clear that the normal pericardium can acutely restrain cardiac volume and influences measured intracavitary filling pressure. Moreover, patients undergoing pericardiotomy in conjunction with heart surgery with normal preoperative cardiac volumes were shown to have mild postoperative increases in cardiac mass and volume (as occurs with volume overload), consistent with relief of underlying, normally occurring restraint to filling by the pericardium.[10]

The normal pericardium also contributes to diastolic interaction[11] or the transmission of intracavitary filling pressure to adjoining chambers. For example, a portion of right ventricular diastolic pressure is transmitted to the left ventricle across the interventricular septum and contributes to left ventricular diastolic pressure. Because its presence increases right ventricular intracavitary pressure, the normal pericardium amplifies diastolic interaction. Thus, as cardiac volume increases above the physiological range the pericardium contributes increasingly to intracavitary filling pressures, directly because of the external contact pressure and indirectly because of increased diastolic interaction.

Passive Role of the Normal Pericardium in Heart Disease

When the cardiac chambers dilate rapidly, the restraining effect of the pericardium as well as its contribution to diastolic interaction can become markedly augmented, resulting in a hemodynamic picture with similarities to both cardiac tamponade and constrictive pericarditis. The most common example is acute right ventricular myocardial infarction (MI),[12] usually in conjunction with inferior left ventricular MI. In this situation, the right side of the heart dilates rapidly such that total heart volume exceeds the reserve volume of the pericardium. As a result of increased pericardial constraint and augmented interaction, left- and right-sided filling pressures equilibrate at elevated levels and a paradoxical pulse and inspiratory increase in systemic venous pressure (Kussmaul sign) can be observed. Other conditions in which similar hemodynamic effects are seen include acute pulmonary embolus and subacute mitral regurgitation. It is of note that these sorts of hemodynamic changes are not seen with purely left ventricular MI because of the largely extrapericardial location of the left atrium and the fact that the thicker walled left ventricle does not dilate acutely as much as the right ventricle.

Chronic cardiac dilation, as in dilated cardiomyopathy or regurgitant valvular disease, can result in cardiac volumes well in excess of the reserve volume of the normal pericardium. Despite this, exaggerated restraining effects are not ordinarily encountered. This observation implies that the pericardium undergoes chronic adaptation to accommodate marked increases in cardiac volume. In experimental chronic volume overload, the pericardial pressure-volume relationship shifts to the right and its slope decreases (see Fig. 64–2, bottom, right curve), i.e., it becomes more compliant, in association with increased pericardial area and mass and a decreased effect on the left ventricular diastolic pressure-volume relationship.[7,13] Thus, apparent growth of pericardial tissue occurs in response to chronic stretch. Presumably, a similar effect occurs with large, slowly accumulating pericardial effusions, which typically do not cause tamponade.

Acute Pericarditis

Etiology, Epidemiology, and Pathophysiology

Table 64–1 lists categories of diseases and specific conditions that can involve the pericardium. Acute pericarditis, defined as symptoms or signs resulting from pericardial inflammation of no more than 1 to 2 weeks duration, can occur in a wide variety of diseases (denoted by asterisks in Table 64–1). However, the majority of cases are idiopathic.[14,15] The term idiopathic is used to denote pericarditis for which no specific etiology can be found with routine diagnostic testing as outlined subsequently. Most such cases are presumed to be viral in etiology, but assessment of viral titers is not part of routine evaluation of sporadic cases because of cost and the fact that this knowledge does not usually alter management.

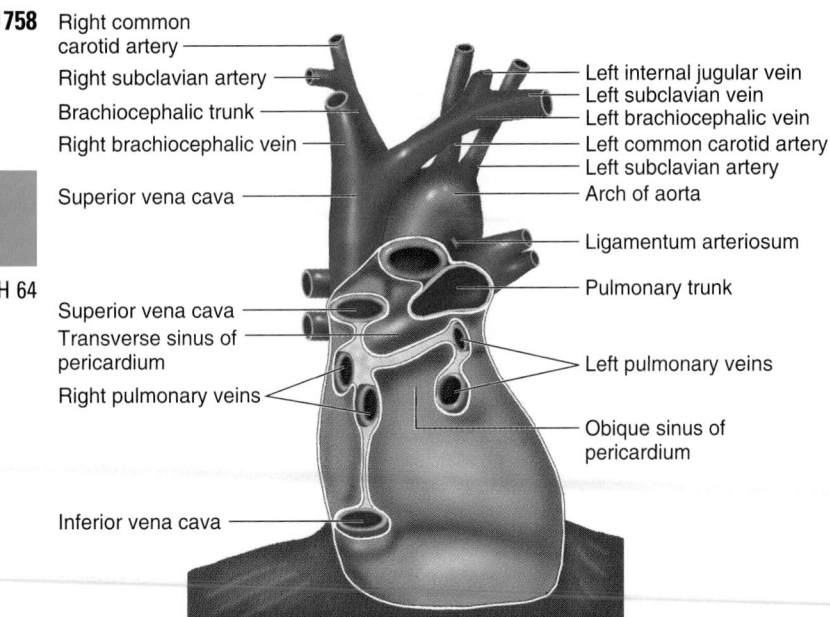

The overall incidence of acute pericarditis is impossible to define because there are undoubtedly a large number of undiagnosed cases. It is a relatively common diagnosis in the emergency department, but there are no large, modern series delineating its frequency in that setting. In one study,[16] it accounted for 1 percent of emergency department cases presenting with electrocardiographic (ECG) ST elevation, but this single criterion misses many cases. The fraction of all acute cases accounted for by idiopathic pericarditis is also uncertain and is influenced by population demographics and regional and seasonal variation in the prevalence of viral infections. However, 80 to 90 percent seems to be a reason-

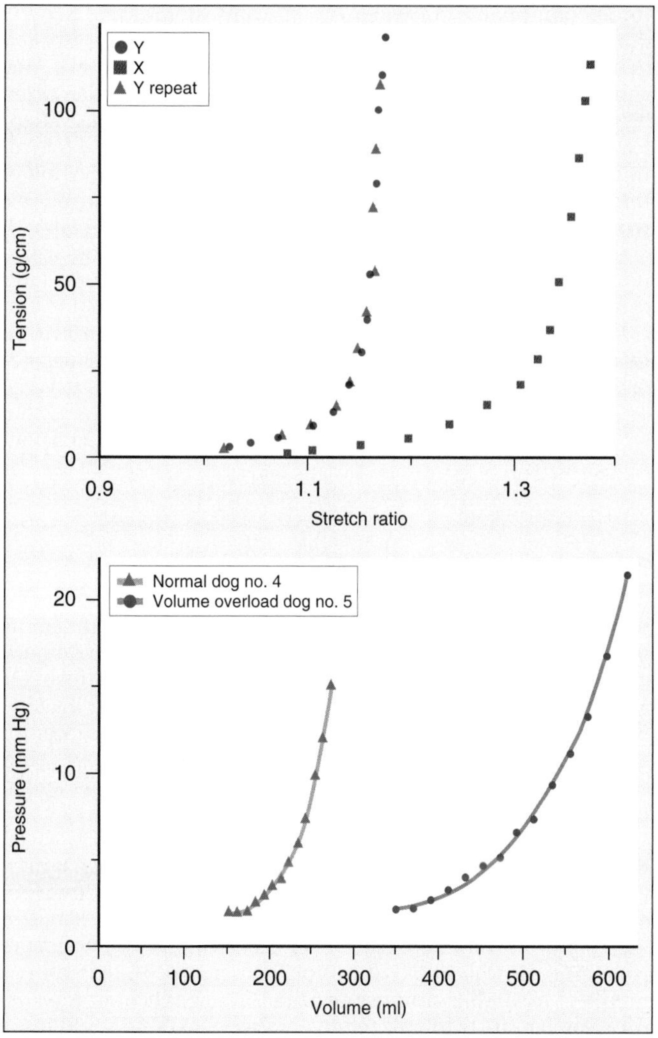

FIGURE 64–2 **Top,** Relationship between stretch and tension in vitro in normal human pericardial tissue. The tissue has been stretched in two, mutually orthogonal directions (X, Y). Note the relatively abrupt transition from a relatively flat to a steep, inelastic relationship. In addition, the tissue is anisotropic; i.e., the relation between tension and stretch depends on the direction of stretch. **Bottom,** Pressure-volume relationship of the normal canine pericardium (left) and after 4 weeks of cardiac dilation caused by volume overload (right). Note the relatively abrupt transition to a steep relationship in normal pericardium and marked shift to the right and flattening after chronic volume overload. (**Top,** From Lee M-C, Fung YC, Shabetai R, LeWinter MM: Biaxial mechanical properties of the human pericardium and canine comparisons. Am J Physiol 22:H75, 1987; **Bottom,** From Freeman G, LeWinter M: Pericardial adaptations during chronic cardiac dilation in dogs. Circ Res 54:294, 1984.)

able estimate.[14,15] The percentage is lower in patients with pericarditis who require hospitalization and higher in young, previously healthy patients. Tuberculous pericarditis is included in Table 64–1 as a cause of acute pericarditis but usually arises with more chronic symptoms. Bacterial pericarditis is also included because it can present with signs and symptoms of acute pericardial inflammation, but these patients are usually very sick and other components of their illness, including pericardial effusions, sepsis, and pneumonias, typically dominate the picture.

Pericarditis occurring 24 to 72 hours after transmural MI caused by local inflammation at the epicardial MI border and the delayed pericarditis of Dressler syndrome used to be common (see Chap. 46). The incidence has declined since the advent of thrombolytics and myocardial revascularization. With these exceptions, the distribution of etiologic diagnoses for acute pericarditis has changed little over time. In contrast,

TABLE 64–1 Categories of Pericardial Disease and Selected Specific Etiologies

Idiopathic*
Infectious
Viral* (echovirus, coxsackievirus, adenovirus, cytomegalovirus, hepatitis B, infectious mononucleosis, HIV/AIDs)
Bacterial* (*Pneumococcus, Staphylococcus, Streptococcus, Mycoplasma*, Lyme disease, *Hemophilus influenzae, Neisseria meningitidis*)
Mycobacteria*(*Mycobacterium tuberculosis, Mycobacterium avium-intracellulare*)
Fungal (histoplasmosis, coccidioidomyocosis)
Protozoal
Immune-inflammatory
Connective tissue disease* (systemic lupus erythematosus, rheumatoid arthritis, scleroderma, mixed)
Arteritis (polyarteritis nodosa, temporal arteritis)
Early post-myocardial infarction
Late post-myocardial infarction (Dressler syndrome),* late post-cardiotomy/thoracotomy*, late post-trauma*
Drug induced* (e.g., procainamide, hydralazine, isoniazid, cyclosporine)
Neoplastic disease
Primary: mesothelioma, fibrosarcoma, lipoma, and so on
Secondary*: breast and lung carcinoma, lymphomas, leukemias
Radiation induced*
Early post-cardiac surgery
Device and procedure related
Coronary angioplasty, implantable defibrillators, pacemakers
Trauma
Blunt and penetrating,* post-cardiopulmonary resuscitation*
Congenital
Cysts, congenital absence
Miscellaneous
Chronic renal failure, dialysis related
Hypothyroidism
Amyloidosis
Aortic dissection

AIDs = acquired immunodeficiency syndrome; HIV = human immunodeficiency virus.
*Etiologies that are manifest as acute pericarditis.

the epidemiology of pericardial effusion and constriction has changed considerably.

The pathophysiology of uncomplicated acute pericarditis is straightforward; all of the symptoms and signs result from inflammation of pericardial tissue. A minority of cases are complicated, as discussed later. In addition, some cases are associated with myocarditis.[17,18] Coexistent myocarditis is usually manifest only by release of biomarkers (creatine kinase, troponin I) (see Chap. 60). Occasionally, however, significant myocardial dysfunction occurs in conjunction with clinically manifest pericarditis.

History and Differential Diagnosis

Acute pericarditis almost always arises with chest pain as the chief complaint. A few cases without chest pain are diagnosed during evaluation of associated symptoms such as dyspnea or fever or incidentally in conjunction with noncardiac manifestations of systemic diseases such as rheumatoid arthritis or systemic lupus erythematosus (SLE).

The pain of pericarditis can be quite severe. It is variable in quality but often sharp and almost always pleuritic. It usually does not have the characteristic vise-like, constricting or oppressive features of ischemic discomfort. Pericardial pain typically has a relatively rapid onset and sometimes begins remarkably abruptly. It is most commonly substernal in location but can also be centered in the left anterior chest or the epigastrium. Radiation to the left arm is not unusual and can lead to confusion with myocardial ischemia. The most characteristic radiation is to the trapezius ridge, which is highly specific for pericarditis. Pericardial pain is almost always relieved by sitting forward and worsened by lying down. Associated symptoms can include dyspnea (often difficult to sort out with coexistent pleuritic pain), cough, and occasionally hiccoughs.

An antecedent history of fever or symptoms suggesting a viral syndrome are common. It is important to review the past medical history carefully for clues to specific etiologic diagnoses. Thus, a history of cancer or an autoimmune disorder, high fevers with shaking chills, skin rash, or weight loss should alert the physician to specific diseases that can cause pericarditis.

DIFFERENTIAL DIAGNOSIS. The differential diagnosis of chest pain is extensive (see Chap. 7). Diagnoses most easily confused with pericarditis include pneumonia or pneumonitis with pleurisy (which may coexist with pericarditis), pulmonary embolus or infarction, costochondritis, and gastroesophageal reflux disease. Myocardial ischemia and infarction are a major diagnostic concern. Acute pericarditis is usually relatively easily distinguished from ischemia on clinical and other grounds, but there are cases in which coronary angiography is required to resolve this issue. Other considerations include aortic dissection, intraabdominal processes, pneumothorax, and herpes zoster pain before skin lesions appear. Finally, acute pericarditis is occasionally the presenting manifestation of a preceding, clinically silent MI.

Physical Examination

Patients with uncomplicated acute pericarditis often appear quite uncomfortable and anxious and may have low-grade fever and sinus tachycardia. Other than this, the only abnormal physical finding is the pericardial friction rub, caused by contact between visceral and parietal pericardium. The classic rub is a distinctive and easily recognized auscultatory finding that is pathognomonic of pericarditis. It consists of three components corresponding to ventricular systole, early diastolic filling, and atrial contraction and has been likened to the sound made when walking on crunchy snow. The rub is usually loudest at the lower left sternal border, often extends to the cardiac apex, and is best heard with the patient leaning forward. It is often dynamic, disappearing and returning over short periods of time. Thus, it is often rewarding to listen frequently to a patient who has suspected pericarditis without an initially audible rub. Sometimes what is considered a pericardial rub in fact has only two or even one component. Labeling such findings rubs should be done with caution because the sound may actually represent a murmur.

It is important to perform a complete physical examination in a patient with acute pericarditis and look carefully for clues to specific etiologic diagnoses. The examiner must also be alert to findings indicating significant pericardial effusion, as discussed subsequently, and the presence of coexistent myocarditis.

Laboratory Testing

ELECTROCARDIOGRAM. The electrocardiogram is the most important laboratory test in the diagnosis of acute pericarditis (see Chap. 9). The classic finding is diffuse ST segment elevation (Fig. 64–3). The ST segment vector in acute pericarditis typically points leftward, anterior, and inferior. The result is ST segment elevation in all leads except aV_r and often V_1. Thus, the term "diffuse" is a slight misnomer. Usually, the ST segment is coved upward and resembles the current of injury of acute, transmural ischemia. However, the distinction between acute pericarditis and transmural ischemia is usually not difficult because of the more extensive lead involvement in pericarditis and the presence of much more prominent reciprocal ST segment depression in ischemia. However, ST elevation in pericarditis sometimes involves a smaller number of leads, in which case the distinction is more difficult. In other cases, the ST segment more closely resembles early repolarization. Here again, pericarditis usually involves more leads than typical early repolarization. As with the rub, ECG changes of acute pericarditis can be dynamic. Frequent recordings often yield a diagnosis in patients with suspected pericarditis who present initially with neither rub nor ST elevation.

PR segment depression is another common finding in acute pericarditis (see Fig. 64–3). In some cases, PR depression occurs in the absence of ST elevation and can be the initial ECG manifestation of acute pericarditis.[19] Thus, the finding is diagnostically useful in patients with neither rub nor ST elevation. In one study,[20] PR segment depression was a marker for clinically silent pericardial effusion in a series of patients referred for echocardiography, but this does not necessarily apply to those presenting with acute pericarditis.

ECG abnormalities other than ST elevation and PR depression are unusual in patients presenting soon after the onset of symptoms

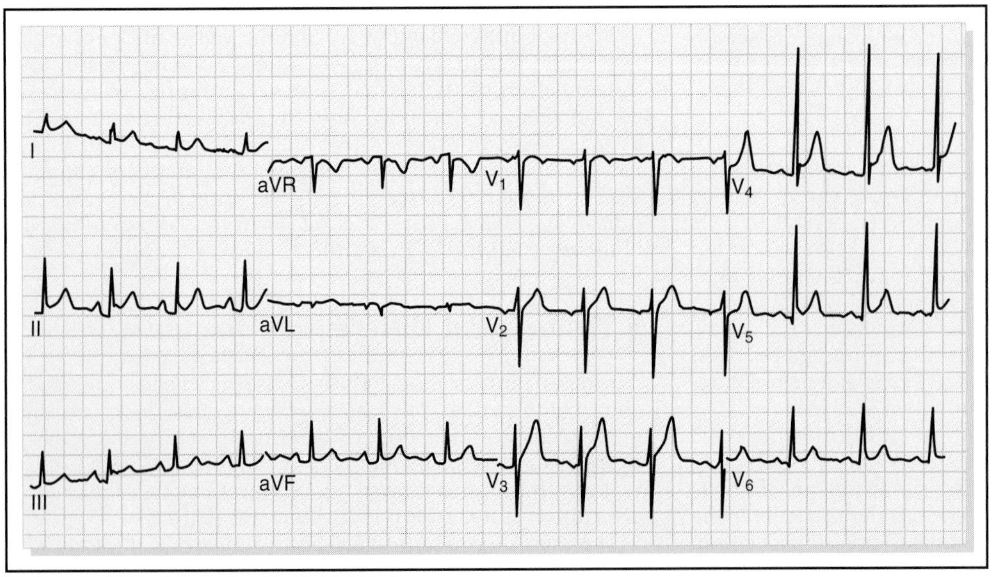

FIGURE 64–3 The electrocardiogram in acute pericarditis. Note both diffuse ST segment elevation and PR segment depression.

of acute pericarditis. Subsequent ECG changes are quite variable.[15] In some, the electrocardiogram simply reverts to normal over days or weeks. In others, the elevated ST segment passes through the isoelectric point and progresses to ST segment depression and T wave inversions in leads with upright QRS complexes. The latter changes can persist for weeks and months. They have no known significance in patients who have otherwise recovered. In patients presenting late after the onset of symptoms, these ECG changes can be difficult to distinguish from those of myocardial ischemia.

When present, ECG abnormalities other than the preceding ones should be considered carefully because they suggest diagnoses other than idiopathic pericarditis or complications. As examples, atrioventricular block may indicate Lyme disease, pathological Q waves can signify a previously silent MI with pericardial pain as its first manifestation, and low voltage or electrical alternans points toward significant effusion.

HEMOGRAM. Modest elevations of the white blood cell count, typically in the range 11,000 to 13,000/ml^3 with a mild lymphocytosis, are common in acute idiopathic pericarditis. Significantly higher counts are an alert for the presence of other etiologies. The red blood cell count should be normal. Anemia is also an alert for other etiologies. The erythrocyte sedimentation rate (ESR) should be no more than modestly elevated in acute idiopathic pericarditis. The ESR is a reasonable screening test in acute pericarditis because unusually high values may be a clue to etiologies such as autoimmune diseases or tuberculosis.

CARDIAC ENZYMES AND TROPONIN MEASUREMENTS. Several reports indicate that surprisingly large numbers of patients with a diagnosis of acute pericarditis without other evidence of myocarditis (see Chap. 60) or MI (see Chap. 46) have elevated cardiac enzymes (total creatine kinase or muscle-brain [MB] fraction) and troponin I.[17,18] These reports suggest a high incidence of concomitant, otherwise silent myocarditis. Patients with pericarditis with elevated biomarkers of myocardial injury appear to almost always have ST segment elevation. In our experience, evidence of myocardial injury in association with acute pericarditis, although it is certainly encountered, may not be as common as the relatively small studies in the literature[17,18] would suggest. Another concern in patients with elevated biomarkers is silent MI arising with subsequent pericarditis. Post-MI pericarditis usually (but not always) occurs after infarcts with pathological Q waves.

CHEST RADIOGRAPH (see Chap. 12). The chest radiograph, including the cardiac silhouette, is usually normal in uncomplicated cases of acute idiopathic pericarditis. Occasionally, small pulmonary infiltrates or pleural effusions are present, presumably related to viral or possibly mycoplasma infections. Other than this, pulmonary parenchymal or other abnormalities suggest diagnoses other than idiopathic pericarditis. Thus, bacterial pericarditis often occurs in conjunction with severe pneumonia. Tuberculous pericarditis can occur with or without associated pulmonary infiltrates. Mass lesions and enlarged lymph nodes suggestive of neoplastic disease also have great significance. Pulmonary vascular congestion may signal the presence of coexistent, severe myocarditis. Small to even moderate effusions may not cause an abnormal cardiac silhouette; thus, even modest enlargement is a cause for concern that a significant effusion is present.

ECHOCARDIOGRAPHY. The echocardiogram is normal in most patients presenting with acute idiopathic pericarditis (see Chap. 11). The main reason for performing echocardiography is to exclude an otherwise silent effusion. There are no modern data delineating the incidence of effusions in such patients. In our experience, most do not have effusions, but small ones are fairly common and not a cause for concern. Moderate or larger effusions are unusual and may signal a diagnosis other than idiopathic pericarditis. In addition to detecting effusions, echocardiography is useful in delineating whether associated myocarditis is severe enough to alter ventricular function as well as in detection of MI.

Natural History and Management

Because there have been no large, modern therapeutic trials, there are no established guidelines for management of acute pericarditis. Initial management should be focused on screening for specific etiologies that would alter management, detection of effusion and other echocardiographic abnormalities, symptomatic treatment, and appropriate treatment if a specific etiology is discovered. As initial evaluation, we recommend obtaining the laboratory data discussed previously, i.e., ECG, hemogram with ESR, chest radiograph, cardiac enzymes and troponin I, and echocardiography. In young women, it is not unreasonable to test for SLE as part of the initial evaluation.

Acute idiopathic pericarditis is a self-limited disease without significant complications or recurrence in about 70 to 90 percent of patients.[14,15] Accordingly, if the laboratory data support the diagnosis, symptomatic treatment with nonsteroidal antiinflammatory drugs (NSAIDs) should be initiated. Although indomethacin has frequently been used, ibuprofen is preferred because of its better side effect profile. The drug is administered in doses of 600 to 800 mg three times daily for 2 weeks and discontinued if pain is no longer present. Many patients have gratifying responses to the first dose or two of an NSAID. The majority respond fully to this regimen and need no additional treatment. Reliable patients with no more than small effusions who respond well to NSAIDs need not be admitted to hospital. Patients who do not respond well initially, have larger effusions, or have indications of an etiology other than idiopathic pericarditis should be hospitalized for additional observation, diagnostic testing and treatment as necessary.

Patients who respond slowly or inadequately to NSAIDs may require supplementary narcotic analgesics to allow time for a full response or a brief course of a corticosteroid, or both. For the latter, prednisone 60 mg by mouth is administered daily for 2 days with tapering to zero over a week. It is unusual not to achieve a satisfactory response to NSAIDs with narcotic analgesics or prednisone backup as necessary. Oral colchicine (1 mg daily with or without a 2- to 3-mg loading dose) can be an effective alternative to corticosteroids in patients who do not respond satisfactorily to NSAIDs. Colchicine has also been suggested as an alternative to NSAIDs for initial treatment.[21]

Complications of acute pericarditis include effusion and tamponade and constrictive pericarditis. It is not known how many patients presenting with acute pericarditis have moderate or larger effusions, but it is almost certainly less than 5 percent. As discussed earlier, a significant effusion increases the chance that a specific etiology is present. Management of effusion is discussed subsequently. The chance of developing constrictive pericarditis after a bout of acute pericarditis is also unknown but is undoubtedly extremely low. Strictly speaking, myocarditis is not a complication of pericarditis but an associated condition.

Relapsing and Recurrent Pericarditis

Perhaps 15 to 30 percent of patients with acute, apparently idiopathic pericarditis who respond satisfactorily to treatment as outlined previously suffer a relapse after completion of initial therapy.[14,15] A minority of these develop recurrent bouts of pericardial pain, which can sometimes be chronic and debilitating.[15] Recurrent pain is not necessarily associated with objective signs of pericardial inflammation. Some patients with what is initially thought to be idiopathic pericarditis manifest evidence of a specific etiology as they experience recurrences. Accordingly, a repeated evaluation for specific causes, especially autoimmune disorders, is appropriate. A pericardial biopsy to look for specific etiologic diagnoses in patients with recurrent pain without effusion is rarely if ever indicated because it is unlikely that a diagnosis would actually result or the information so obtained would alter management.

Treatment of recurrent pain is empirical. For an initial relapse, a second 2-week course of an NSAID is often effective. A course of colchicine may be at least as effective, although the optimal duration of treatment is uncertain. For bouts of recurrent pericardial pain beyond an initial relapse, we favor colchicine prophylaxis. There is now a fairly substantial favorable experience with chronic colchicine therapy as prophylaxis for recurrent pericardial pain, including that related to idiopathic pericarditis and other etiologies (e.g., postthoracotomy, SLE).[21] This experience strongly suggests that colchicine is at least as effective as chronic corticosteroid therapy, and it has a much more favorable side effect profile. The usual dose is 1 mg by mouth daily. Some recommend a 2- to 3-mg loading dose.[21] Initiation of prophylactic therapy does not preclude simultaneous use of NSAIDs or corticosteroids, although as discussed previously colchicine alone is often effective for acute episodes. The most common difficulty in using colchicine is nausea or diarrhea, or both, which in one study[21] required dose reduction or termination in 14 percent of patients.

Patients with recurrent pericardial pain despite NSAIDs and colchicine (or who cannot tolerate colchicine) are a challenging management problem. One option is a short course of prednisone as outlined earlier whenever symptoms first appear. Maintenance corticosteroid therapy should be avoided if at all possible. Nonsteroidal immunosuppressive therapy with drugs such as azathioprine and cyclophosphamide is an alternative to corticosteroids,[22] but published experience is extremely limited. In very difficult cases, low-dose maintenance therapy with these drugs may reduce the need for intermittent or maintenance corticosteroids and do so with less side effects. Pericardiectomy has occasionally been employed for recurrent pericarditis but appears to be effective in a small minority of patients at best.[23]

Pericardial Effusion and Tamponade

Etiology

Idiopathic pericarditis and any infection, neoplasm, or autoimmune or inflammatory process (including postradiation and drug induced) that can cause pericarditis can cause pericardial effusion (see Table 64–1). Effusions are common early after cardiac surgery,[24] but it is unusual for them to cause tamponade and they almost always resolve within several weeks. In addition, noninflammatory diseases, including hypothyroidism and amyloidosis, can cause effusion. Occasionally, patients with severe circulatory congestion have small to moderate transudative effusions. Bleeding into the pericardial sac occurs after blunt and penetrating trauma and as a consequence of post-MI rupture of the free wall of the left ventricle. Retrograde bleeding is an important cause of death related to dissecting aortic aneurysm (see Chap. 53). Last, occasional patients are encountered with large, silent pericardial effusions and no evidence of pericarditis.[25] Effusions in these patients are generally stable, but there is a significant incidence of tamponade over time.

Of the conditions that can cause effusion, those with a high incidence of progression to tamponade are bacterial (including mycobacteria), fungal, and human immunodeficiency virus (HIV)-associated infections (see Chap. 61), neoplastic involvement, and, of course, any form of bleeding into the pericardial space. Although large effusions related to acute idiopathic pericarditis are unusual, because of its high frequency this form of pericarditis accounts for a significant percentage of tamponade cases. Additional details of pericardial effusion pertinent to specific disease entities are discussed later in this chapter.

Pathophysiology and Hemodynamics

Formation of an effusion is simply a component of the response to inflammation when there is an inflammatory or infectious process affecting the pericardium. The latter is also probably the case with pericardial tumor implants (see Chap. 63). However, lymphomas occasionally cause effusion in association with enlarged mediastinal lymph nodes by obstructing pericardial lymph drainage. The pathophysiology of effusions in situations in which there is no obvious inflammation, for example, uremia and hypothyroidism, is poorly understood.

Cardiac tamponade is characterized by a continuum of hemodynamic events, from an effusion causing minimally detectable effects to the full-blown picture of circulatory collapse.[26a] Clinically, the most critical point occurs when an effusion reduces the volume of the cardiac chambers such that the cardiac output begins to decline. The key determinants of the hemodynamic consequences of a pericardial effusion are the level of pressure in the pericardial sac and the ability of the heart to compensate for the elevated pressure. The pressure, in turn, depends on the amount of fluid and the pericardial pressure-volume relationship. As discussed earlier, the pericardium normally has little reserve volume. As a result, relatively modest amounts of rapidly accumulating fluid can have major effects on cardiac function. Large, slowly accumulating effusions are often well tolerated, however, presumably because of chronic changes in the pericardial pressure-volume relationship as described earlier.

Compensatory Response. The compensatory response to a significant pericardial effusion includes increased adrenergic stimulation and parasympathetic withdrawal, which cause tachycardia and increased contractility.[26] Patients who cannot mount a normal adrenergic response, for example, those receiving beta-adrenergic blocking drugs, are more susceptible to the effects of a pericardial effusion. In the very late stages of tamponade, a depressor reflex with paradoxical bradycardia may supervene.[27]

Hemodynamic Consequences. The hemodynamic consequences of pericardial effusion have fascinated physiologists and physicians for many years.[26a,28,29] Non-steady-state responses to an abrupt increase in pericardial pressure provide insights into the mechanisms of the hemodynamic derangements of cardiac tamponade. Figure 64–4 shows an experiment performed in an open-chest dog in which aortic and pulmonary arterial flows (stroke volume) were measured on a beat-to-beat basis before and after a large amount of fluid was rapidly introduced into the pericardial sac over one to two cardiac cycles, indicated by the arrow. There was an immediate decrease in pulmonary arterial stroke volume but no change in aortic stroke volume. Two beats later, aortic stroke volume decreased and eventually a new steady state was achieved with equivalent decreases in aortic and pulmonary arterial stroke volume. During the time required to achieve a new steady state, pulmonary arterial stroke volume was less than aortic stroke volume. The transient inequality in left- and right-heart output resulted in net transfer of blood out of the pulmonary and into the systemic circulation and may explain the decrease in pulmonary vascularity on chest radiography in tamponade. In studies parallel to those in Figure 64–4, right-heart volume was

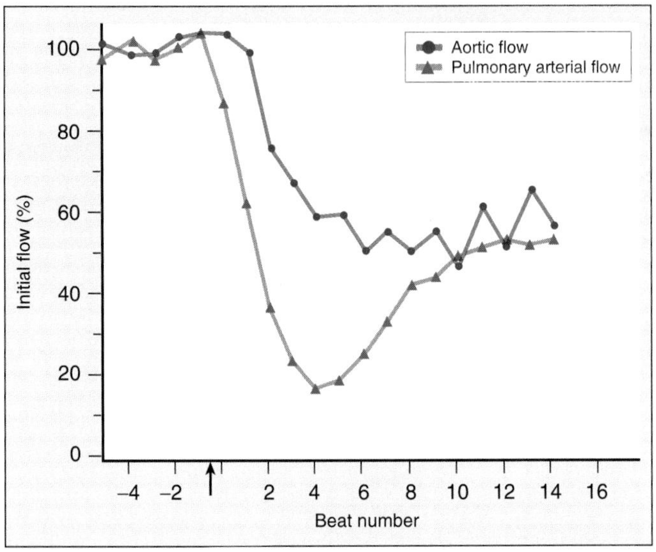

FIGURE 64–4 Beat-to-beat changes in pulmonary arterial and aortic stroke volume (as percentage of control) following abrupt production of cardiac tamponade (at arrow). Note that pulmonary arterial stroke volume decreases immediately, but there is a brief lag before aortic stroke volume decreases. Pulmonary arterial stroke volume is lower than aortic stroke volume until a new steady state is reached. (From Ditchey R, Engler R, LeWinter M, et al: The role of the right heart in acute cardiac tamponade in dogs. Circ Res 48:701, 1981.)

shown to decrease more than left-heart volume in response to a given increase in pericardial pressure. These results show that high pericardial pressure exerts its main effect by impeding filling of the right side of the heart, with much of the effect on the left side being secondary and due to underfilling. In studies employing regional tamponade[30] the greater importance of right-heart compression was confirmed and it was also shown that compressions of the right atrium and segments of the caval vessels within the pericardial sac are independent components of the response to a pericardial effusion. These observations also provide a mechanism for the observations that atrial and ventricular diastolic collapse detected in tamponade are usually confined to the right side of the heart.[15,31]

As fluid accumulates in the pericardial sac, left- and right-sided atrial and ventricular diastolic pressures gradually rise and in severe tamponade eventually equalize at a pressure similar to that in the pericardial sac, typically 15 to 20 mm Hg (Fig. 64-5). Equalization is closest during inspiration. Thus, the pressure in the pericardial sac dictates the intracavitary filling pressure and the *transmural* filling pressures of the cardiac chambers are very low. Correspondingly, cardiac volumes progressively decline until they are very small. The small end-diastolic ventricular volume (decreased preload) accounts for the small stroke volume. Because of compensatory increases in contractility, end-systolic volume also decreases, but not enough to normalize stroke volume (hence, the importance of tachycardia in maintaining cardiac output). Under normal conditions, transmural right-heart filling pressure is lower then left-heart filling pressure (upper limit of right atrial pressure ~7 mm Hg, left atrial pressure ~12 mm Hg). It follows that as fluid accumulates, filling pressure increases more rapidly in the right than the left side of the heart until equalization is achieved.

***x* AND *y* DESCENTS.** In addition to elevated and equal intracavitary filling pressures, markedly reduced transmural filling pressures, and small cardiac volumes, two other hemodynamic abnormalities are characteristic of tamponade. One is loss of the *y* descent of the right atrial or jugular venous pressure (see Fig. 64-5). The *x* and *y* descents of the venous pressure waveform correspond to periods when venous return is increasing (in veins, pressure is the mirror image of flow). Loss of the *y* descent has been explained on the basis of the concept that total heart volume is fixed in severe tamponade.[15,32] In consequence, blood can enter the heart only when blood is simultaneously leaving. The right atrial *y* descent begins when the tricuspid valve opens, i.e., when blood is not leaving the heart. Thus, no blood can enter the heart and the *y* descent is lost. In contrast, the *x* descent occurs during ventricular ejection. Because blood is leaving the heart at this time, venous inflow can increase normally and the *x* descent is retained. Although loss of the *y* descent can

TABLE 64–2 Hemodynamics in Cardiac Tamponade and Constrictive Pericarditis

Finding	Tamponade	Constriction
Paradoxical pulse	Usually present	Present in ~1/3
Equal left-right filling pressures	Present	Present
Systemic venous wave morphology	Absent *y* descent	Prominent *y* descent (M or W shape)
Inspiratory change in systemic venous pressure	Decrease (normal)	Increase or no change (Kussmaul sign)
"Square root" sign in ventricular pressure	Absent	Present

be difficult to discern at the bedside, especially in sick patients with tachycardia, it can easily be appreciated in recordings of systemic venous or right atrial pressure and provides a useful clue to the presence of significant tamponade.

PARADOXICAL PULSE. The second characteristic hemodynamic finding is the paradoxical pulse (Fig. 64-6), an abnormally large decline in systemic arterial pressure during inspiration (usually defined as a >10 mm Hg drop in systolic pressure). Other causes of *pulsus paradoxus* include constrictive pericarditis, pulmonary embolus, and pulmonary disease (asthma, emphysema) with large variation in intrathoracic pressure. In severe cardiac tamponade, the arterial pulse is impalpable during inspiration. The mechanism of the paradoxical pulse is multifactorial, but respiratory changes in systemic venous return are certainly important.[15,32,33] In tamponade, in contrast to constrictive pericarditis, the normal inspiratory *increase* in systemic venous return is retained. Therefore, the normal *decline* in systemic venous pressure on inspiration is present (Kussmaul sign is absent). The increase in right-heart filling occurs, once again, under conditions in which total heart volume is fixed and left-heart volume markedly reduced to start. The interventricular septum shifts to the left in exaggerated fashion on inspiration, encroaching on the left ventricle such that its stroke volume and pressure generation are abnormally reduced (see Fig. 64-6). Although the inspiratory increase in right-heart volume (preload) causes an increase in right ventricular stroke volume, it requires several cardiac cycles to increase left ventricular filling and stroke volume and counteract the septal shift effect. Other factors that may contribute to the paradoxical pulse include increased afterload caused by transmission of negative intrathoracic pressure to the aorta and traction on the pericardium caused by the descent of the diaphragm, which increases the pericardial pressure. Associated with these complex mechanisms are the striking findings that left- and right-heart pressures and stroke volume variations are exaggerated and 180 degrees out of phase (see Fig. 64-6). Table 64-2 lists the major hemodynamic findings in cardiac tamponade and compares them with those in constrictive pericarditis.

When there are preexisting elevations in diastolic pressures or volume, or both, tamponade can occur without a paradoxical pulse. Examples are patients with left ventricular dysfunction, aortic regurgitation, and atrial septal defect.[34,35] Retrograde bleeding into the pericardial sac is a common cause of death in type I dissecting aortic aneurysms. Tamponade may occur without a paradoxical pulse because of simultaneous aortic regurgitation related to valvular disruption.

Low-Pressure Tamponade. Although left- and right-sided filling pressures are characteristically 15 to 20 mm Hg in severe tamponade, tamponade can occur at lower levels of intracavitary filling pressure, a phenomenon termed *low-pressure tamponade*.[15] Low-pressure tamponade occurs when there is a decrease in blood volume in the setting of a preexisting effusion that did not previously have significant consequences. In these conditions, a relatively modestly elevated pericardial pressure can lower transmural filling pressure to levels at which stroke volume is compromised. Because the venous pressure is only modestly elevated or even normal, the diagnosis may not be suspected. Low-pressure tamponade is typically observed during hemodialysis, where it is signaled by hypotension during a dialysis run, and in patients with blood loss and dehydration. It may also be seen when diuretics are administered to patients with effusions.

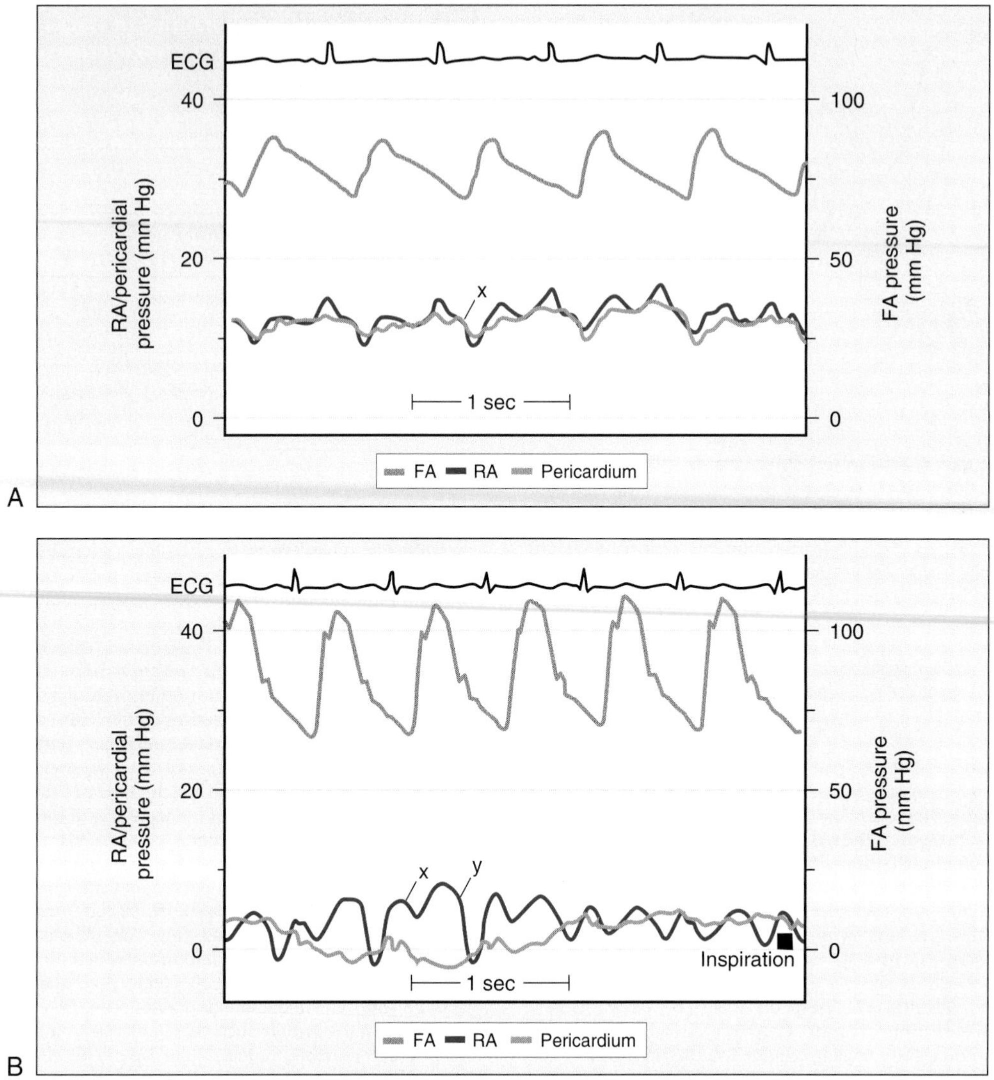

FIGURE 64–5 Femoral arterial (FA), right atrial (RA), and pericardial pressure before **(A)** and after **(B)** pericardiocentesis in a patient with cardiac tamponade. Both RA and pericardial pressure are about 15 mm Hg before pericardiocentesis. In this case there was a negligible paradoxical pulse. Note presence of *x* descent but absence of *y* descent before pericardiocentesis. Pericardiocentesis results in a marked increase in FA pressure and marked decrease in RA pressure. During inspiration, pericardial pressure becomes negative, there is clear separation between RA and pericardial pressure, and *y* descent is now evident and prominent, suggesting the possibility of an effusive-constrictive picture. (Adapted from Lorell BH, Grossman W: Profiles in constrictive pericarditis, restrictive cardiomyopathy and cardiac tamponade. *In* Baim DS, Grossman W [eds]: Grossman's Cardiac Catheterization, Angiography, and Intervention. Philadelphia, Lippincott Williams & Wilkins, 2000, p 840.)

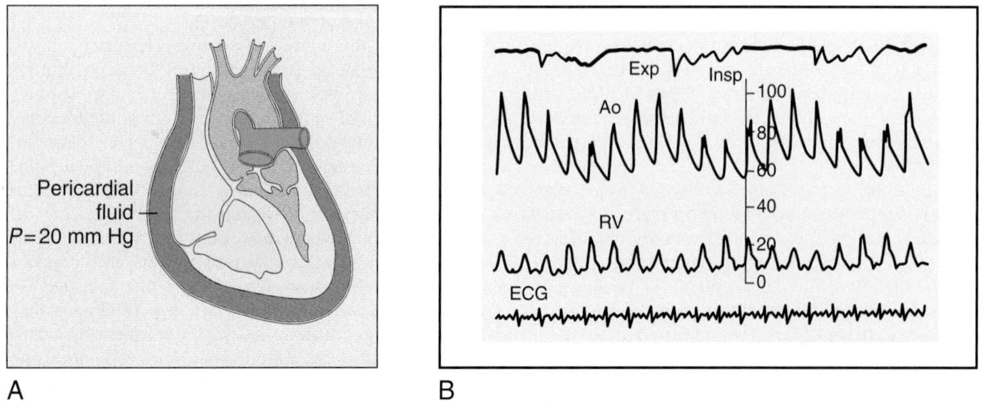

FIGURE 64–6 **A,** Schematic illustration of leftward septal shift with encroachment of left ventricular volume during inspiration in cardiac tamponade. **B,** Respiration marker and aortic and right ventricular pressure tracings in cardiac tamponade. Note paradoxical pulse and marked, 180 degrees out of phase respiratory variation in right- and left-sided pressures. Ao = aortic pressure; ECG = electrocardiogram; Exp = expiration; Insp = inspiration; RV = right ventricular pressure. (From Shabetai R: The Pericardium. New York, Grune & Stratton, 1981, p 266.)

Pericardial effusions can be loculated or localized, resulting in regional tamponade, as commonly encountered after cardiac surgery.[24,36] Regional tamponade can cause atypical hemodynamic abnormalities that can simulate heart failure, i.e., reduced cardiac output with unilateral filling pressure elevation. However, reports of the hemodynamics of regional tamponade are scarce and it is therefore difficult to generalize about this entity. Regional tamponade should be suspected whenever there are hemodynamic abnormalities in a setting in which a regional or loculated effusion is present.

Clinical Presentation

In any patient with effusion, a history pertinent to specific etiologies may be present and should be carefully sought. Occasionally, very large, asymptomatic chronic effusions are discovered when a chest radiograph is obtained for some unrelated reason.[25] As discussed earlier, specific etiologies are usually not found in these cases. Many patients with effusions also have pericardial pain. However, effusions do not by themselves cause symptoms unless tamponade is present. Patients with tamponade may complain of true dyspnea, whose mechanism is poorly understood because there is no pulmonary congestion. However, this is difficult to distinguish from tachypnea reflecting shock and respiratory alkalosis. Other symptoms reflect the extent to which the cardiac output is reduced. Usually, pericardial pain or a nonspecific sense of discomfort or both dominate the clinical picture. In our experience, patients with tamponade are almost always more comfortable sitting forward, even if they do not have pericardial pain.

A careful general physical examination in patients with pericardial effusion is critical because it may provide clues to a specific etiology. In pericardial effusion without tamponade, the cardiovascular examination is normal except that, if the effusion is very large, the cardiac impulse may be difficult or impossible to palpate and the heart sounds muffled. In addition, tubular breath sounds may be heard in the left axilla or left base because of bronchial compression.

If tamponade is present, patients usually appear uncomfortable, with signs reflecting varying degrees of reduced cardiac output and shock, including tachypnea, diaphoresis, cool extremities, peripheral cyanosis, and depressed sensorium. Hypotension is usually present, although in early stages compensatory mechanisms allow maintenance of normal blood pressure. A paradoxical pulse is the rule, but it is important to be alert to situations in which it may not be present. The paradoxical pulse is quantified using cuff sphygmomanometry by noting the difference between the pressure at which Korotkoff sounds first appear and that at which they are present with each heartbeat. In severe tamponade, the inspiratory decrease in arterial pressure is palpable and most obvious in pulses that are distant from the heart. Tachycardia is the rule unless heart rate–lowering drugs have been administered, conduction system disease coexists, or a preterminal bradycardic reflex has supervened.

The jugular venous pressure is markedly elevated, except in low-pressure tamponade, and the *y* descent is absent (see Fig. 64–5), although once again the latter can be difficult to appreciate at the bedside. The normal decrease in venous pressure on inspiration is retained. As with any large effusion, examination of the heart usually but not invariably reveals a reduced or absent cardiac impulse and, of course, a friction rub can also be present.

The clinical presentation of cardiac tamponade can be confused with the presentation of anything that can cause hypotension, shock, and elevated jugular venous pressure, including severe myocardial failure, right-sided heart failure related to pulmonary embolism or other causes of pulmonary hypertension, and right ventricular MI.

Laboratory Testing

ELECTROCARDIOGRAM. The only ECG abnormalities characteristic of pericardial effusion and tamponade are reduced voltage and electrical alternans of the QRS complex (Fig. 64–7).[15] Reduced voltage is a nonspecific finding that can be caused by several other conditions, including emphysema, infiltrative myocardial disease, and pneumothorax. Electrical alternans is virtually specific but relatively insensitive for large pericardial effusion with tamponade. It is caused by anterior-posterior swinging of the heart with each heartbeat. Its mechanism is poorly understood. When pericarditis coexists, the usual ECG findings may be present.

CHEST RADIOGRAPH (see Chap. 12). The cardiac silhouette remains normal until pericardial effusions are at least moderate in size. With moderate and larger effusions, the anteroposterior cardiac silhouette assumes a rounded, flask-like appearance (Fig. 64–8). Lateral views may reveal the pericardial fat pad sign, a linear lucency between the chest wall and the anterior surface of the heart, representing separation of parietal pericardial fat from epicardium. The lungs characteristically appear oligemic.

ECHOCARDIOGRAPHY (see Chap. 11). Because of its convenience and ease of application in critically ill patients, M-mode and two-dimensional Doppler echocardiography is currently the standard noninvasive diagnostic method for detection of pericardial effusion and noninvasive assessment of tamponade. A pericardial effusion appears as a lucent separation between parietal and visceral pericardium (Fig. 64–9). Separations should be present for the entire cardiac cycle to be classified as effusions. Small effusions are first evident over the posterobasal left ventricle. As the fluid increases it spreads anteriorly, laterally, and behind the left atrium, where its limit is demarcated by the visceral pericardial reflection. Ultimately, the separation becomes circumferential. Ordinarily, tamponade does not occur without a circumferential effusion and the diagnosis should be viewed with skepticism if this is not the case. However, in some types of pericardial disease and after cardiac surgery, effusions can be regional or loculated, or both, and, as discussed earlier, cause localized tamponade. Computed tomography (CT) and magnetic resonance (MR) are more precise than echocardiography for imaging the pericardium itself. However, frond-like or shaggy-appearing structures in the pericardial space

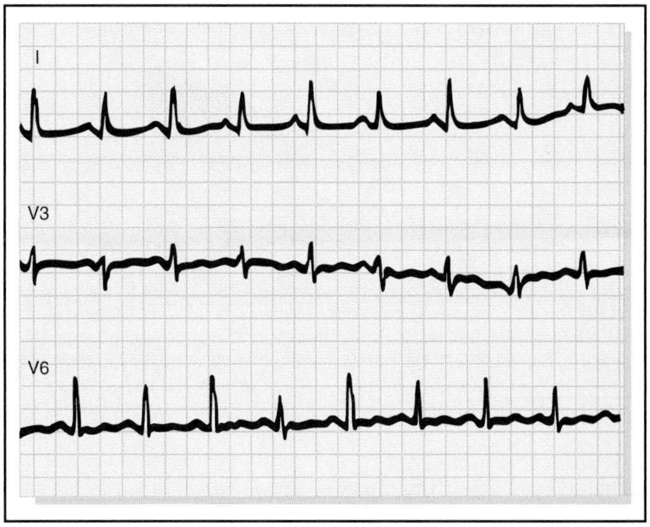

FIGURE 64–7 Electrocardiogram in cardiac tamponade showing alternans of the QRS complex. (From Shabetai R: The Pericardium. New York, Grune & Stratton, 1981, p 260.)

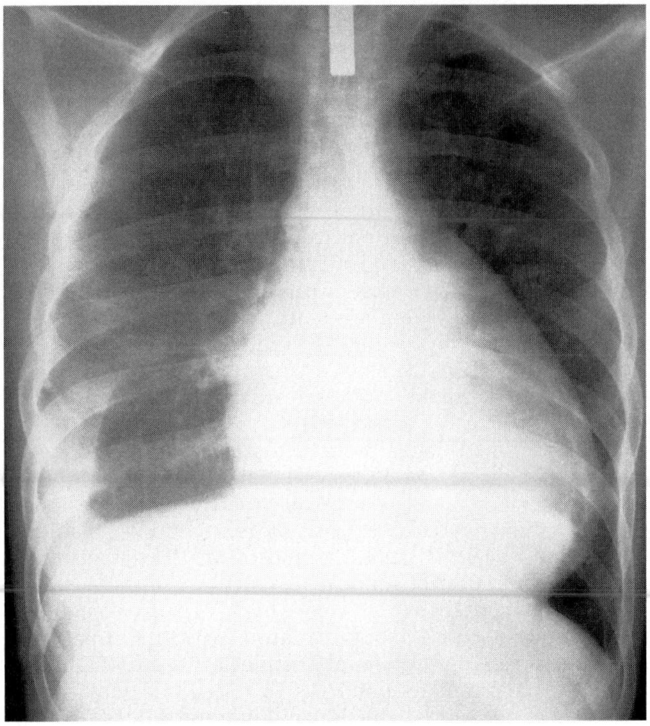

FIGURE 64–8 Anteroposterior chest radiograph of a patient with a large pericardial effusion (see text). (From Kabbani SS, LeWinter M: Cardiac constriction and restriction. *In* Crawford MH, DiMarco JP [eds]: Cardiology. St. Louis, Mosby, 2001, Sec. 5, Chap. 5, p 15.5.)

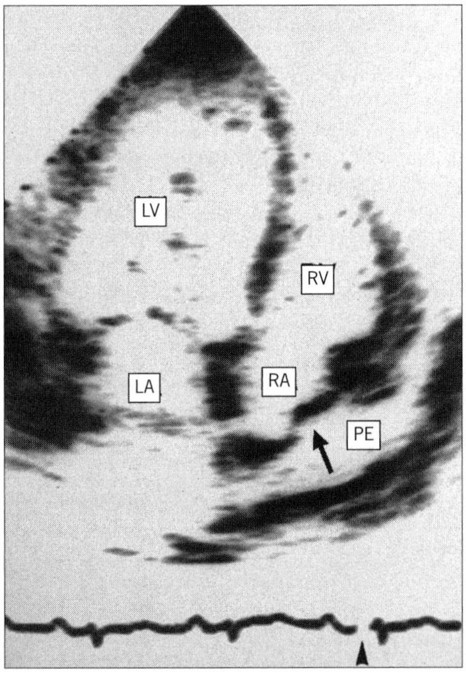

FIGURE 64–9 Two-dimensional echocardiogram of a large, circumferential pericardial effusion. LA = left atrium; LV = left ventricle; PE = pericardial effusion; RA = right atrium; RV = right ventricle. (From Kabbani SS, LeWinter M: Cardiac constriction and restriction. *In* Crawford MH, DiMarco JP [eds]: Cardiology. St. Louis, Mosby, 2001, Sec. 5, Chap. 5, p 15.5.)

detected by echocardiography suggest clots or chronic inflammatory or neoplastic pericardial processes.

As discussed previously, tamponade is best considered as a spectrum of severity of cardiac compression. Several findings indicate that tamponade is severe enough to cause some degree of hemodynamic compromise. Early diastolic collapse of the right ventricle (Fig. 64–10) and right atrium (which occurs during *ventricular* diastole) (Fig. 64–11) are sensitive and specific signs that appear relatively early during the course of tamponade.[15,30] Both occur because the pericardial pressure transiently exceeds the intracavitary pressure. A large *pleural* effusion can also elevate the pericardial pressure sufficiently to cause right ventricular collapse.[37] Left ventricular collapse[38] and left atrial collapse[39] have been reported with regional effusions after cardiac surgery but are distinctly unusual. The cardiac chambers are small and, as discussed earlier, in extreme cases the heart swings anteroposteriorly within the pericardial effusion. Distention of the caval vessels during their course outside the pericardial sac is useful as a sign of increased systemic venous pressure.

Reflecting the hemodynamic abnormalities discussed earlier, Doppler velocity recordings demonstrate exaggerated respiratory variation in right- and left-sided venous and valvular flow, with marked inspiratory increases on the right side and decreases on the left (Fig. 64–12).[28,31,35] As a result of reduced systemic venous inflow during early diastole with loss of the *y* descent, most caval and pulmonary venous inflow occurs during ventricular systole.[28,29] These changes in venous flow patterns are quite sensitive for tamponade.

In the vast majority of cases of pericardial effusion, transthoracic echocardiography provides sufficient diagnostic information to make informed management decisions. Transesophageal studies, although providing better quality images, are often impractical in sick patients. However, in intubated patients the transesophageal approach can easily be employed.

OTHER IMAGING MODALITIES. Pericardial effusion causes damping or abolition of cardiac pulsation. Accordingly, fluoroscopy is useful in the cardiac catheterization laboratory for detection of an acute effusion caused by perforations.

CT and MR imaging are useful adjuncts to echocardiography in the characterization of effusion and tamponade[15] (see Chaps. 14 and 15). Neither is ordinarily required or advisable in sick patients who require prompt management and treatment decisions. They can have an important ancillary role in situations in which hemodynamics are atypical and the presence and severity of tamponade less certain, and they are invaluable when echocardiography is technically inadequate for decision-making. Both CT and MR imaging provide more detailed quantitation and regional-spatial localization of pericardial effusion than echocardiography, and they are especially useful for loculated and regional effusions. Pericardial thickness can be measured with both, allowing indirect assessment of the severity and chronicity of inflammation. Electron beam CT is especially useful in this regard. Clues to the nature of the pericardial fluid (bloody, exudative, chylous) can also be gained, for example, from attenuation coefficients of CT images. Last, real-time CT or MR cine displays can provide information similar to that provided by echocardiography for assessment of tamponade, e.g., septal shifting, atrial and ventricular collapse.

Management of Pericardial Effusion and Tamponade

Management of pericardial effusion is dictated, first and foremost, by whether tamponade is present or has a high chance of developing in the near term. Situations in which tamponade should be considered a near-term threat include suspected bacterial or tuberculous pericarditis or bleeding into the pericardial space and any situation where there is a moderate to large effusion that is not thought to be chronic or is increasing in size, or both. When tamponade is present or threatened, clinical decision-making should be undertaken with great urgency and the threshold for pericardiocentesis should be low.

EFFUSIONS WITHOUT ACTUAL OR THREATENED TAMPONADE. In the absence of actual or threatened tamponade, management can be more leisurely. This cohort of patients includes several categories. Some have acute pericarditis with a small to moderate effusion detected as part of routine evaluation. Others undergo echocardiography because of diseases known to involve the pericardium. The remainder are asymptomatic and have effusions detected when diagnostic tests are performed for reasons other than suspected pericardial disease, for example, to evaluate an unexpectedly enlarged cardiac silhouette on chest radiography, when echocardiography is performed to assess possible cardiac disease, or when CT or MR is used to investigate thoracic pathology.

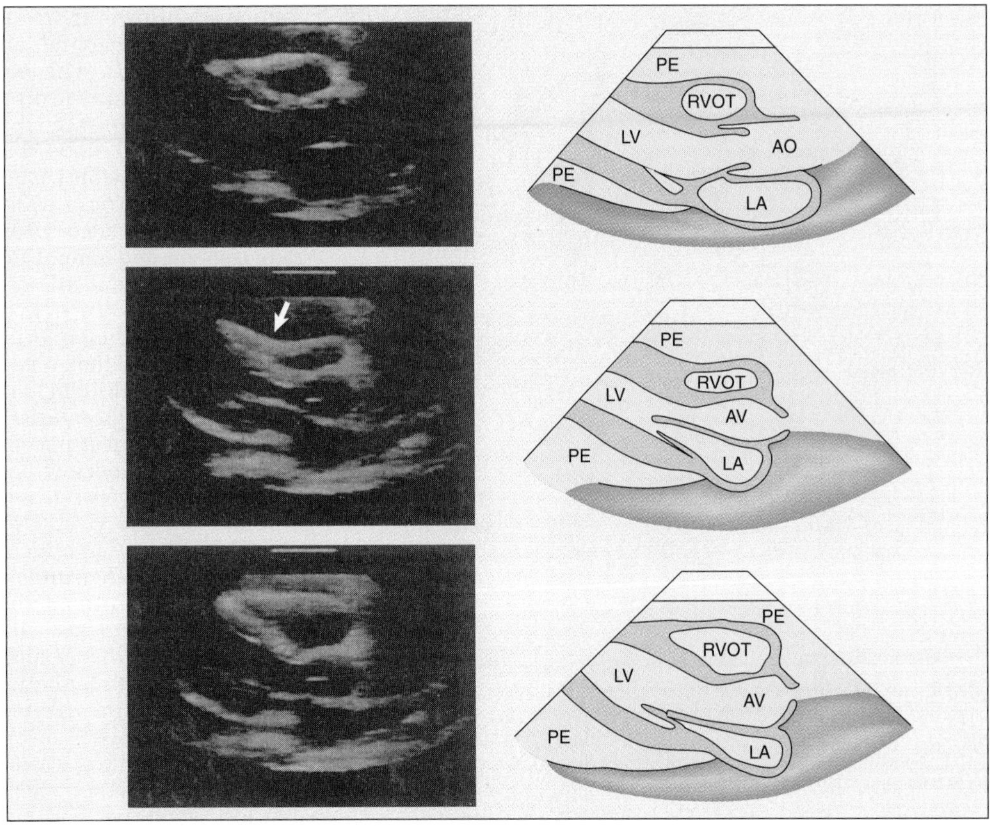

FIGURE 64–10 Two-dimensional echocardiogram illustrating diastolic collapse or indentation of the right ventricle in cardiac tamponade. **Top,** Systole; **middle,** early diastole with indentation indicated by arrow; **bottom,** late diastole with return of normal configuration. AV = aortic valve; LA = left atrium; LV = left ventricle; PE = pericardial effusion; RVOT = right ventricular outflow tract. (From Weyman AE: Principles and Practice of Echocardiography. Philadelphia, Lea & Febiger, 1994, p 1119.)

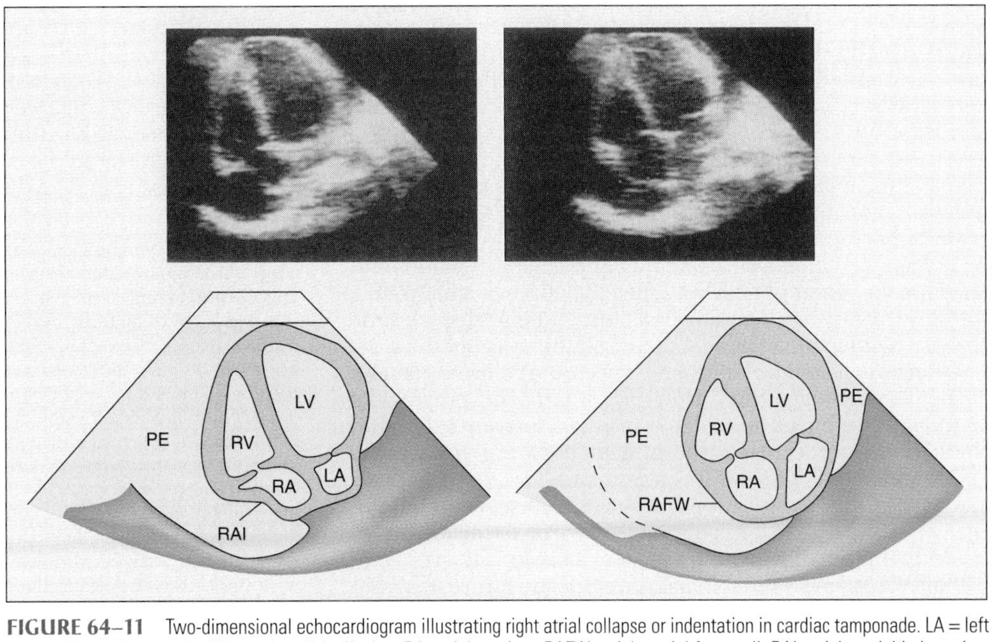

FIGURE 64–11 Two-dimensional echocardiogram illustrating right atrial collapse or indentation in cardiac tamponade. LA = left atrium; LV = left ventricle; PE = pericardial effusion; RA = right atrium; RAFW = right atrial free wall; RAI = right atrial indentation; RV = right ventricle. (From Gilliam LD: Hemodynamic compression of the right atrium: A new echocardiographic sign of cardiac tamponade. Circulation 68:294, 1983.)

In many cases of effusion in which tamponade is neither present nor threatened, an etiology is evident or strongly suggested on the basis of the history (e.g., known neoplastic or autoimmune disease, radiation therapy) or previously obtained diagnostic tests. When a diagnosis is not clear, an assessment of specific etiologies of pericardial disease should be undertaken. This assessment should in general include the diagnostic tests recommended for acute pericarditis, a careful medication review, and anything else dictated by the clinical picture. Thus, skin testing for tuberculosis and screening for neoplastic and autoimmune diseases and infections (e.g., Lyme disease) and hypothyroidism should be considered. At the same time, careful judgment should be exercised in the selection of tests for these patients. A patient with severe heart failure and circulatory congestion with a small, asymptomatic effusion does not need extensive testing. In contrast, patients with evidence of a systemic disease deserve careful attention. Serial titers of antibodies to viruses are usually not helpful or indicated in these cases because the results may be nonspecific or negative despite a viral etiology. However, situations occasionally arise in which evidence of a viral etiology, if present, is helpful in clarifying diagnostic dilemmas,

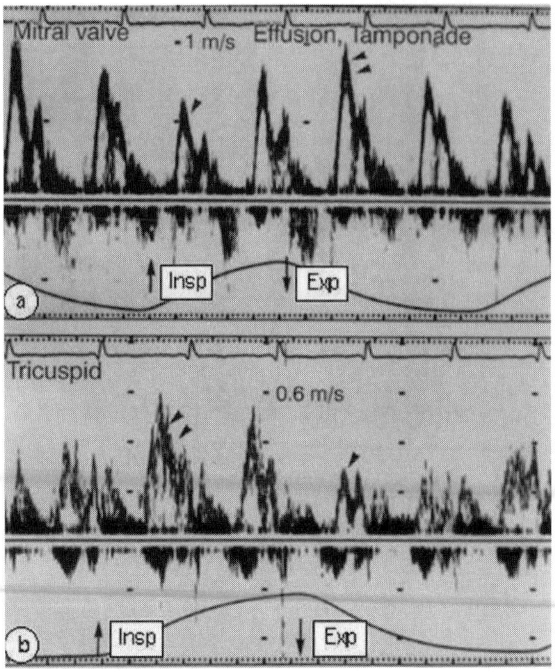

FIGURE 64–12 Transmitral and tricuspid Doppler velocity recordings in cardiac tamponade showing marked, 180 degrees out of phase respiratory variations. Exp = expiration; Insp = inspiration. (From Oh JK, Hatle LK, Mulvagh SL, Tajik AJ: Transient constrictive pericarditis: Diagnosis by two-dimensional Doppler echocardiography. Mayo Clin Proc 68:1158, 1993.)

providing reassurance, and avoiding unnecessary diagnostic testing or treatments. In these situations it is useful to save serum obtained at presentation should there be subsequent reasons for measurement of viral titers.

In this class of patients, pericardiocentesis (closed or open with biopsy) need be undertaken only for diagnostic purposes and is usually not indicated. As discussed earlier, in many cases a diagnosis either is obvious when the effusion is first noted or becomes evident as part of initial investigations. Moreover, in this setting analysis of pericardial fluid has a low yield for providing a specific diagnosis.[14,15,40] In occasional situations in which pericardiocentesis is thought to be necessary for diagnostic purposes, consideration should be given to open drainage with biopsy.

Occasional patients with large, asymptomatic effusions and no evidence of tamponade or a specific etiology constitute a special category.[25,40] The effusions are by definition chronic because tamponade would be present if this was not the case. They are in general stable, and specific etiologies usually do not emerge over time. However, a minority progress to tamponade in an unpredictable fashion. Interestingly, after closed pericardiocentesis the effusions do not necessarily reaccumulate.[25] Thus, there is a rationale for closed pericardiocentesis following routine evaluation for specific etiologies as outlined earlier. This decision can be made on an individual basis, however, because little is lost by conservative management in reliable patients who are aware of symptoms of tamponade. Before undertaking pericardiocentesis, however, a course of an NSAID, colchicine, or corticosteroids should be considered[21] as it will shrink some of these effusions.

EFFUSIONS WITH ACTUAL OR THREATENED TAMPONADE. These patients should be considered as having a true or potential medical emergency. With the exception of those who do not wish prolongation of life (mainly those with metastatic cancer), hospital admission and careful hemodynamic and echocardiographic monitoring are mandatory. Most patients require pericardiocentesis to treat or prevent tamponade. However, treatment should be carefully individualized and thoughtful clinical judgment is critical. For example, patients with acute, apparently idiopathic pericarditis or autoimmune diseases who have no more than mild tamponade can be treated with a course of prednisone and monitored in the hope that their effusions shrink rapidly. Patients with possible bacterial infections or bleeding into the pericardial sac *whose effusions are no more than moderate in size* may in some cases be suitable for initial conservative management and careful monitoring, especially because the risk of closed pericardiocentesis is increased with smaller effusions.

Hemodynamic monitoring with a balloon flotation pulmonary artery catheter is useful, especially in those with threatened or mild tamponade in whom a decision is made to defer pericardiocentesis. Hemodynamic monitoring is also helpful *after* pericardiocentesis to assess both reaccumulation and the presence of underlying constrictive disease (see Fig. 64–5), as discussed subsequently. However, insertion of a pulmonary artery catheter should not be allowed to delay definitive therapy in critically ill patients.

Intravenous Hydration. For most patients in this category, management should be directed toward urgent or emergent pericardiocentesis, with timing dependent on individual circumstances. When actual or threatened tamponade is diagnosed, intravenous hydration should be instituted, especially as some patients mistakenly receive diuretics because of an incorrect diagnosis of heart failure. In patients with tamponade who are critically ill, intravenous positive inotropes (dobutamine, dopamine) can be employed but are of limited efficacy. Hydration and positive inotropes are temporizing measures and should not be allowed to substitute for or delay pericardiocentesis.

Pericardiocentesis. In the vast majority of circumstances, closed pericardiocentesis is the initial treatment of choice. However, before proceeding it is important to be confident that there is indeed an effusion large enough to cause tamponade, especially if hemodynamics are atypical. Loculated effusions as well as effusions containing clots or fibrinous material are also of concern because the risk and difficulty of closed pericardiocentesis are increased. In these situations, if removal of pericardial fluid is thought to be necessary, an open approach should be considered for safety and to obtain pericardial tissue and create a pericardial window.

The most commonly employed approach to closed pericardiocentesis is subxiphoid needle insertion performed under echocardiographic guidance to minimize the risk of puncture of the myocardium and assess completeness of fluid removal.[41] When the needle has entered the pericardial space, a modest amount of fluid should be removed (perhaps 50 to 150 ml) in an effort to produce some degree of hemodynamic improvement. Then, a guidewire should be inserted and the needle replaced with a pigtail catheter. The catheter can then be manipulated with continuing echocardiographic guidance to maximize the amount of fluid removed. In a large, modern series from the Mayo Clinic,[41] the procedural success rate was 97 percent and the complication rate was 4.7 percent (major, 1.2 percent; minor, 3.5 percent). The procedure should be performed in the cardiac catheterization laboratory with experienced personnel in attendance unless the patient is too ill to be moved. If echocardiographic guidance is unavailable, the needle should be directed toward the right shoulder and then replaced with a catheter for subsequent fluid removal. CT fluoroscopy–guided drainage of effusions is an alternative when echocardiography cannot be used.[42]

If a pulmonary artery catheter has been inserted, right-heart, pulmonary capillary wedge, and systemic arterial pressures should be monitored before, during, and after and cardiac output measured before and after the procedure. Ideally, pressure should also be measured in the pericardial fluid. As discussed earlier, removal of relatively small amounts of fluid can result in substantial hemodynamic improvement. Hemodynamic monitoring before, during, and after pericardiocentesis is useful for several reasons. Initial measurements confirm and document the severity of tamponade. Assessment after completion establishes a baseline to assess reaccumulation, which is especially important if it is not possible to remove all fluid. As discussed in more detail subsequently, some patients presenting with tamponade have a coexisting component of constriction (i.e., effusive-constrictive pericarditis),[15] which is virtually impossible to detect when an effusion dominates the picture. Filling pressures that remain elevated after pericardiocentesis as well as the appearance of venous waveforms typical of constriction (rapid x and y descents) indicate coexistent constriction.

Following pericardiocentesis, continued hemodynamic monitoring and repeated echocardiography are recommended to check for reaccumulation. The length of continued monitoring is a matter of judgment but, typically, pulmonary artery catheter pressures are measured for about 24 hours and a follow-up echocardiogram is performed immediately before its removal. If hemodynamic changes indicating reaccumulation appear, echocardiography should be performed sooner. In most cases the intrapericardial catheter is left in place with heparinized saline in its lumen for 12 to 24 hours to facilitate repeated fluid removal. It also allows delivery of intrapericardial drugs to treat specific etiologies.

Open Pericardiocentesis. Open pericardiocentesis is occasionally preferred for the initial removal of pericardial fluid. Loculated effusions or effusions that are borderline in size are drained more safely in the operating room. Recurring effusions, especially those causing tamponade, are often initially drained using a closed approach because of logistical considerations. However, open pericardiocentesis, with biopsy and establishment of a pericardial window, is preferred for most recurrences when they are severe enough to cause tamponade. Creation of a window reliably eliminates future episodes of cardiac tamponade and provides pericardial tissue to assist in diagnosis. The surgeon should inspect the pericardium carefully and obtain multiple biopsies. Also, percutaneous balloon approaches have become available for drainage of effusions[43,44] as well as pericardioscopy and biopsy.[45] These methods appear to be quite safe and effective for producing pericardial windows, but at present they are available in only a few centers.

ANALYSIS OF PERICARDIAL FLUID (Table 64–3). Although analysis of pericardial fluid has a disappointing overall yield in identifying the etiology of pericardial disease, careful analysis can nonetheless be rewarding. *Assuming a diagnosis is not known before fluid removal,* routine pericardial fluid measurements should include specific gravity, white blood cell count and differential, hematocrit, and protein content.[14,15] Although most effusions are exudates, detection of a transudate reduces the diagnostic possibilities considerably. Blood in pericardial fluid is a nonspecific finding. Because pericardial blood usually undergoes rapid fibrinolysis, a low hematocrit does not exclude bleeding. Chylous effusions can occur after traumatic or surgical injury to the thoracic duct or obstruction by a neoplastic process. Occasionally they are idiopathic. Cholesterol-rich effusions occur in severe hypothyroidism. In certain circumstances, determination of bilirubin or cholesterol levels in pericardial fluid may be diagnostically useful.

Pericardial fluid should be routinely stained and cultured for detection of bacteria, including tuberculosis, and fungi. As much fluid as possible should be submitted for detection of malignant cells as there is a reasonably high yield for diagnosis of malignancy in patients with pericardial involvement. Elevated adenosine deaminase levels have high sensitivity and specificity for tuberculous pericardial disease.[46-48] Unless some other etiology is evident, adenosine deaminase should be a routine test because of the general difficulty of diagnosing tuberculous pericarditis and the delays involved in making a diagnosis by culture. Increased interferon-gamma in fluid also appears promising in the diagnosis of tuberculous pericarditis.[48] There may be a role for routine measurement of carcinoembryonic antigen as a general screen for malignant effusion and an adjunct to direct detection of malignant cells.[46,47]

TABLE 64–3 Routine Analysis of Pericardial Fluid

Specific gravity, white blood cell count and differential, hematocrit, protein content
Stain and culture for bacteria, including tuberculosis
Analysis for malignant cells
Adenosine deaminase
Consider: carcinoembryonic antigen, bilirubin, cholesterol

Constrictive Pericarditis

Etiology

Constrictive pericarditis represents the end stage of an inflammatory process involving the pericardium. Although virtually any of the inflammatory processes listed in Table 64–1 can cause constriction, in the industrialized world the etiology is most commonly infectious, postsurgical, or radiation injury (Table 64–4).[49] Tuberculosis was the most common cause of constrictive pericarditis in the developed world before the development of effective drug therapy. It is now much less prevalent. Although the constrictive process can follow an initial insult by as little as several months, constriction usually takes years to develop. The end result is dense fibrosis, often calcification, and adhesions of the parietal and visceral pericardium. Usually the scarring process is more or less symmetrical and impedes filling of all the heart chambers. The clinical presentation is dominated by signs and symptoms of right-sided heart failure.

Pathophysiology

The pathophysiological consequence of pericardial scarring is markedly restricted filling of all of the cardiac chambers This symmetrical effect results in elevation and equilibration of filling pressures in all chambers as well as the systemic and pulmonary veins. In early diastole the ventricles fill abnormally rapidly because of markedly elevated atrial pressures and accentuated early diastolic ventricular suction, the latter related to small end-systolic volumes. During early to mid-diastole, ventricular filling is abruptly halted when the intracardiac volume reaches the limit set by the noncompliant pericardium. As a result, almost all ventricular filling occurs very early in diastole. Systemic venous congestion results in hepatic congestion, peripheral edema, ascites, and sometimes anasarca and cardiac cirrhosis. Reduced cardiac index is also a consequence of impaired filling and results in fatigue, muscle wasting, and weight loss. In "pure" constriction, myocardial contractile function is preserved, although ejection fraction can be reduced as a consequence

TABLE 64–4 Causes of Constrictive Pericarditis

Idiopathic
Irradiation
Postsurgical
Infectious
Neoplastic
Autoimmune (connective tissue) disorders
Uremia
Posttraumatic
Sarcoid
Methysergide therapy
Implantable defibrillator patches

of reduced preload. However, the myocardium is occasionally involved in the chronic inflammation and fibrosis, leading to true contractile dysfunction that can at times be quite severe. The latter is also a predictor of a poor response to pericardiectomy.

An important contributor to the pathophysiology of constrictive pericarditis is failure of transmission of intrathoracic pressure changes during respiration to the cardiac chambers (Fig. 64–13). These changes continue to be transmitted to the pulmonary circulation. Thus, on inspiration the drop in intrathoracic pressure (and therefore pulmonary venous pressure) is not transmitted to the left side of the heart, including the left atrium. Consequently, on inspiration the small pulmonary vein to left atrial pressure gradient that normally drives left-heart filling is reduced, resulting in decreased left atrial inflow and transmitral filling. The inspiratory decrease in left ventricular filling allows an increase in right ventricular filling along with an interventricular septal shift to the left. The opposite sequence occurs with expiration.[15,50]

High systemic venous pressure and reduced cardiac output result in compensatory retention of sodium and water by the kidneys. Inhibition of atrial natriuretic peptide also contributes to renal sodium retention and further exacerbates increases in systemic venous and left-sided filling pressures.[51]

Clinical Presentation

The usual presentation consists of signs and symptoms of predominantly right-sided heart failure with normal or near-normal ventricular systolic function as assessed by echocardiography. At a relatively early stage these signs and symptoms include lower extremity edema, vague abdominal complaints, and some degree of passive hepatic congestion. As the disease becomes more severe, hepatic congestion worsens and can progress to frank jaundice, ascites or anasarca or both, and cardiac cirrhosis. Signs and symptoms ascribable to elevated pulmonary venous pressures such as exertional dyspnea, cough, and orthopnea may also appear with progressive disease. Atrial fibrillation and tricuspid regurgitation, which further exacerbates venous pressure elevation, may also appear at this stage. In the end stage of constrictive pericarditis, the effects of a chronically low cardiac output are prominent, including severe fatigue, muscle wasting, and weight loss. Rarely, initial symptoms include recurrent pleural effusions, transient ischemic attack and syncope. Clinically, severe end-stage constrictive pericarditis can be mistaken for any cause of severe right-sided heart failure as well as end-stage primary liver disease. Of course, the venous pressure is not elevated with primary liver disease.

Physical Examination

VENOUS PATTERN. Physical findings include marked elevation of jugular venous pressure with a prominent, rapidly collapsing *y* descent. This, combined with a normally prominent *x* descent, results in an M- or W-shaped venous pressure contour. At the bedside, this is best appreciated as two prominent descents with each cardiac cycle. In patients in atrial fibrillation the *x* descent is lost, leaving only the prominent *y* descent. The latter is difficult to distinguish from tricuspid regurgitation, which, as noted earlier, may itself occur as a consequence of constrictive pericarditis. The *Kussmaul sign*, an inspiratory increase in systemic venous pressure, is usually present.[15] Occasionally, the venous pressure simply fails to decrease on inspiration rather than actually increase. The Kussmaul sign reflects loss of the normal increase in right-heart venous return on inspiration even though tricuspid flow increases. These characteristic abnormalities of the venous waveform are in marked contrast to those observed in cardiac tamponade. A paradoxical pulse occurs in perhaps one-third of patients with constrictive pericarditis and is especially common when there is an effusive-constrictive picture. It is best explained by the aforementioned lack of transmission of decreased intrathoracic pressure to the left heart chambers.

PERICARDIAL KNOCK. In cases with extensive calcification and adhesion of the heart to adjacent structures, cardiac examination may reveal that the point of maximal impulse does not vary with changes in position. However, the most notable cardiac finding is the pericardial knock, which is an early diastolic sound best heard at the left sternal border or the cardiac apex, or both. It occurs slightly earlier and has a higher acoustic frequency than a third heart sound. The knock corresponds to the early, abrupt cessation of ventricular filling. Widening of second heart sound splitting may also be present. As noted previously, a significant number of patients with constrictive pericarditis have secondary tricuspid regurgitation with its characteristic systolic murmur.

Abdominal examination reveals hepatomegaly, often with palpable venous pulsations, with or without ascites. Other signs of chronic hepatic congestion may include jaundice,

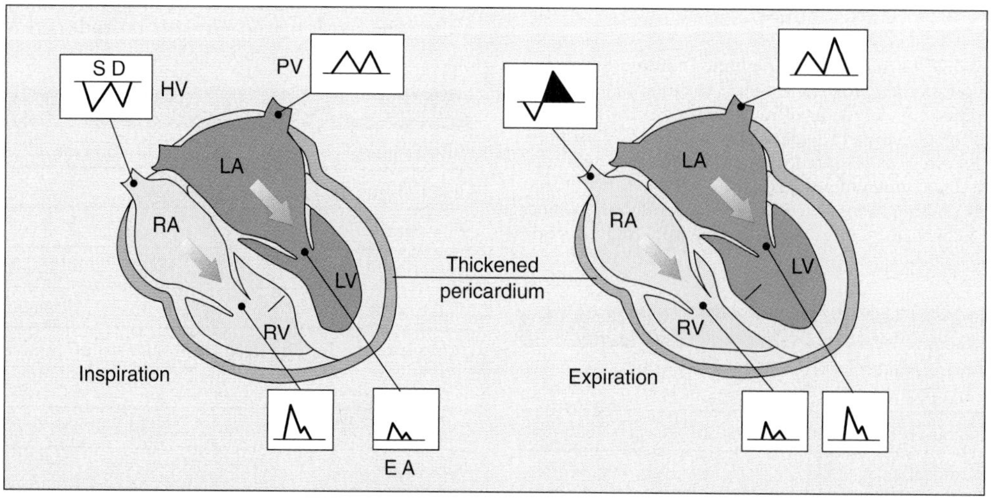

FIGURE 64–13 Schematic representation of transvalvular and central venous flow velocities in constrictive pericarditis. During inspiration the decrease in left ventricular filling results in a leftward septal shift allowing augmented flow into the right ventricle. The opposite occurs during expiration. D = diastolic venous flow; EA = mitral inflow; HV = hepatic vein; LA = left atrium; LV = left ventricle; PV = pulmonary venous flow; RA = right atrium; RV = right ventricle; S = systolic venous flow.

spider angiomata, and palmar erythema. Lower extremity edema is usually present and anasarca occurs in some cases. Patients with end-stage constrictive pericarditis may develop muscle wasting and cachexia with massive ascites and edema of the scrotum and lower extremities. The resemblance to end-stage, primary liver disease has already been noted.

Laboratory Testing

ELECTROCARDIOGRAM. There are no specific ECG findings. Nonspecific T wave abnormalities are often observed, as well as reduced voltage. Left atrial abnormality may also be present. Atrial fibrillation is present in a significant number of patients.

CHEST RADIOGRAPH (see Chap. 12). The chest radiograph frequently shows right atrial enlargement. The cardiac silhouette can be enlarged secondary to a coexisting pericardial effusion. Pericardial calcification is seen in a small number of patients and should raise suspicion of tuberculous pericarditis (Fig. 64–14). At the same time, calcification per se is by no means diagnostic of constrictive physiology. The lateral chest film is useful to detect pericardial calcification along the right heart border and in the atrioventricular groove. Isolated calcification of the left ventricular apex or posterior wall is typical of ventricular aneurysm rather than pericardial calcification. Pleural effusions are occasionally present and can be a presenting sign of constrictive pericarditis. When left-heart filling pressures are markedly elevated, pulmonary vascular congestion and redistribution can also be present.

ECHOCARDIOGRAM (see Chap. 11). M-mode and two-dimensional echocardiography findings include pericardial thickening and immobility, abrupt displacement of the interventricular septum during early diastole (septal "bounce"),[15] and signs of systemic venous congestion such as dilation of hepatic veins and distention of the inferior vena cava with blunted respiratory fluctuation. Premature pulmonic valve opening as a result of elevated right ventricular early diastolic pressure may also be observed. Exaggerated septal shifting during respiration is often present.

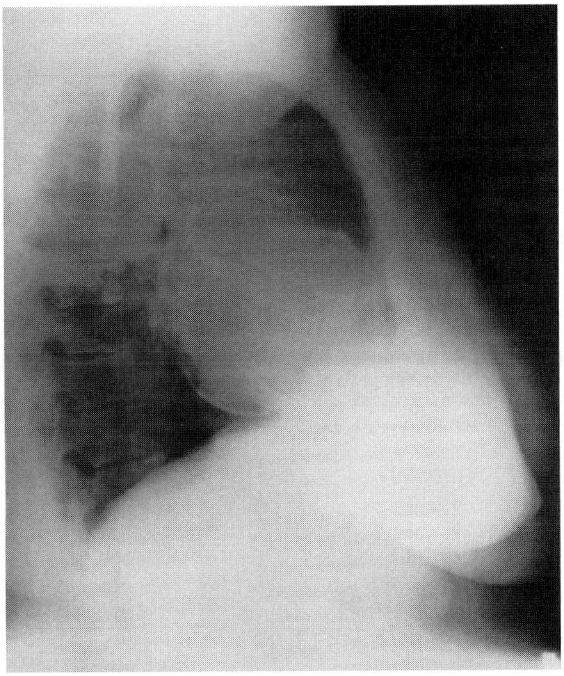

FIGURE 64–14 Chest radiograph showing marked pericardial calcifications in a patient with constrictive pericarditis.

Doppler Measurements. The role of lack of transmission of intrathoracic pressure to the cardiac chambers and resulting mitral and tricuspid inflow patterns in constrictive pericarditis has already been discussed. In accordance with these patterns, Doppler flow velocity measurements reveal exaggerated respiratory variation in both mitral inflow velocity and tricuspid-mitral inflow differences, with the latter being 180 degrees out of phase (see Fig. 64-13). Although there is some overlap with cardiac tamponade, these inflow patterns have good sensitivity and specificity for constrictive pericarditis and also help to distinguish between restrictive cardiomyopathy and constrictive pericarditis.[15,50,52] Typically, patients with pericardial constriction demonstrate an increase in mitral E velocity greater than or equal to 25 percent during expiration compared with inspiration and increased diastolic flow reversal with expiration in the hepatic veins. Mitral E wave deceleration time is usually but not always less than 160 msec. These Doppler echocardiographic findings have 88 percent sensitivity for the diagnosis of constrictive pericarditis. A subset of patients (up to 20 percent) with constriction do not exhibit typical respiratory changes, most likely because of markedly increased left atrial pressure or possibly a mixed constrictive-restrictive pattern related to myocardial involvement by the constrictive process. In patients without typical respiratory mitral-tricuspid flow velocity findings, examination after maneuvers that decrease preload (head-up tilt or sitting) can unmask the characteristic respiratory variation in mitral E velocity.[53]

A similar pattern of respiratory variation in mitral inflow velocity can be observed in chronic obstructive lung disease, right ventricular infarction, pulmonary embolism, and pleural effusion. Most of these conditions have other clinical and echocardiographic features that differentiate them from constrictive pericarditis. Superior vena caval flow velocities are particularly helpful in distinguishing between constrictive pericarditis and chronic obstructive pulmonary disease. Patients with pulmonary disease display a marked increase in inspiratory superior vena caval systolic forward flow velocity, which is not seen in constrictive pericarditis.

Transesophageal Echocardiography. Transesophageal echocardiography can be used as a valuable adjunct in assessing constrictive pericarditis. It is superior to transthoracic echocardiography for measuring pericardial thickness and has an excellent correlation with CT for this purpose.[54] Moreover, when mitral inflow velocities by transthoracic echocardiography are technically inadequate or equivocal, measurement of pulmonary venous Doppler velocities using the transesophageal approach demonstrates pronounced respiratory variation, even larger than that observed across the mitral valve.[55]

CARDIAC CATHETERIZATION AND ANGIOGRAPHY (see Chaps. 17 and 18). Right- and left-heart catheterization and coronary angiography in patients suspected of having constrictive pericarditis provide documentation of the hemodynamics of constrictive physiology and assist in the discrimination between constrictive pericarditis and restrictive cardiomyopathy.[56] Although there is limited need for contrast ventriculography in these patients, coronary angiography is used to detect occult coronary artery disease in those being considered for pericardiectomy. In addition, on rare occasions external pinching or compression of the coronary arteries or outflow tract regions by the constricting pericardium is detected.

Right- and left-heart pressures should be recorded simultaneously at equisensitive gains, with meticulous attention to calibration. Right atrial, right ventricular diastolic, pulmonary capillary wedge, and pre-a wave left ventricular diastolic pressure are elevated and equal, or nearly so, at around 20 mm Hg. Differences of more than 3 to 5 mm Hg between left- and right-heart filling pressures are rarely encountered. The right atrial pressure tracing shows a preserved x descent, a prominent y descent, and roughly equal a and v wave height, with the resultant M or W shape configuration. Both right and left ventricular pressures reveal an early, marked diastolic dip followed by a plateau ("dip and plateau" or "square root" sign) (Fig. 64-15). Pulmonary artery and right ventricular systolic pressures are usually modestly elevated, in the range 35 to 45 mm Hg. Pulmonary hypertension is not a feature of constrictive pericarditis and is indicative of coexisting cardiac or pulmonary disease. Hypovolemia, such as may occur secondary to diuretic therapy, can mask the typical hemodynamic findings. Rapid volume challenge with 1000 ml of normal saline over 6 to 8 minutes may unmask the hemodynamic features of constrictive pericarditis.[57]

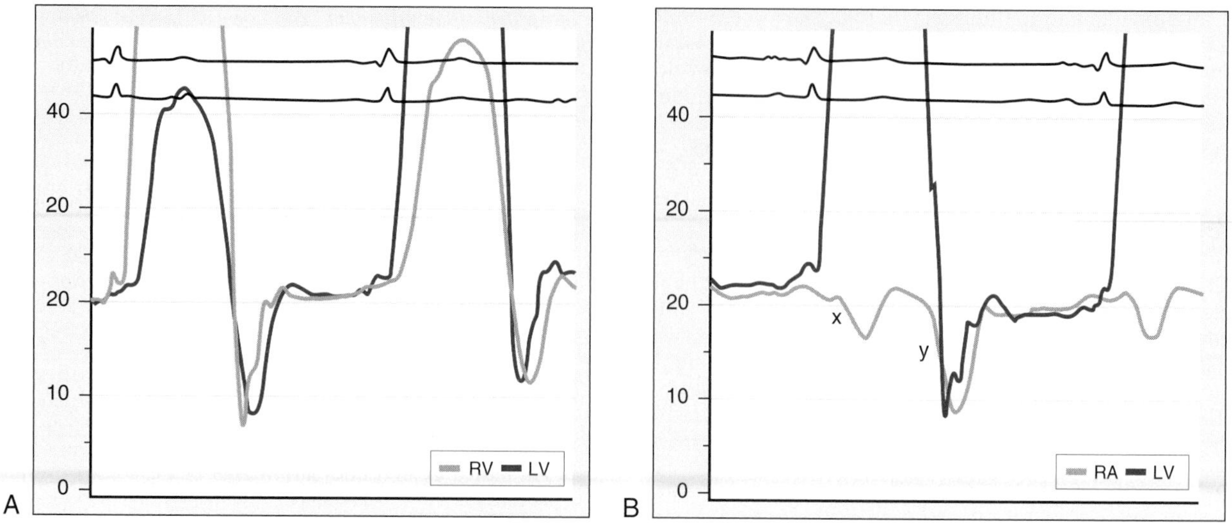

FIGURE 64–15 Pressure recordings in a patient with constrictive pericarditis. **A,** Simultaneous right ventricular (RV) and left ventricular (LV) pressure tracings with equalization of diastolic pressure as well as "dip and plateau" morphology. **B,** Simultaneous right atrial (RA) and LV pressure with equalization of RA and LV diastolic pressure. Note the prominent *y* descent. (From Vaitkus PT, Cooper KA, Shuman WP, Hardin NJ: Images in cardiovascular medicine: Constrictive pericarditis. Circulation 93:834, 1996.)

Stroke volume is almost always reduced but resting cardiac output can be preserved because of tachycardia. Depression of stroke volume is primarily related to reduced diastolic filling. In the absence of extensive coexisting myocardial involvement, left ventricular ejection fraction is normal or slightly reduced.

COMPUTED TOMOGRAPHY AND MAGNETIC RESONANCE IMAGING. CT provides detailed images of the pericardium and is especially helpful in detecting even minute amounts of pericardial calcification (Fig. 64–16). The major disadvantage of CT is the frequent need for administration of iodinated intravenous contrast material for best display of findings of pericardial pathology. The thickness of the normal pericardium measured by CT is less than 2 mm. MR imaging provides a detailed and comprehensive examination of the pericardium and heart without the need for iodinated contrast material or ionizing radiation. It is significantly less sensitive for detecting calcification than is CT. The "normal" pericardium visualized by MR imaging has been reported to be up to 4 mm in thickness. This measurement most likely reflects the entire pericardial "complex," with physiological fluid representing a significant component of the measured thickness.[58]

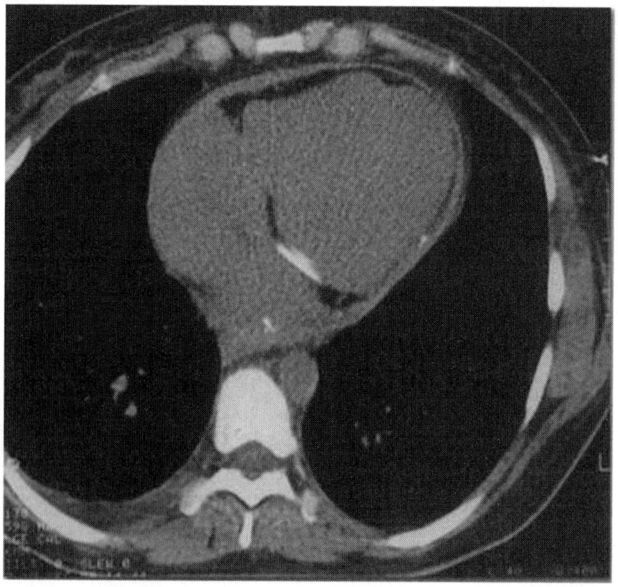

FIGURE 64–16 Computed tomographic scan showing increased pericardial thickness and mild calcification in a patient with constrictive pericarditis.

Demonstration of a thickened pericardium with or without calcification indicates acute or chronic pericarditis. If there is clinical evidence of impaired diastolic filling, pericardial thickening, especially if calcification is present, is virtually diagnostic of constriction. The absence of pericardial thickening argues against the diagnosis of constriction but does not completely rule it out. The pericardium can be globally thickened, but thickening is often focal. Localized compression of the heart caused by focal thickening is reported and occurs much more commonly on the right than the left side. In patients being considered for pericardiectomy, detailed descriptions of the location and severity of thickening and calcification aid the surgeon with respect to both risk stratification and planning of the operation. Additional CT and MR findings include distorted ventricular contours, hepatic venous congestion, ascites, pleural effusions, and occasionally pericardial effusion. Often there is dilation of the atria, coronary sinus, inferior vena cava, and hepatic veins. Cine acquisition (MR or electron beam CT) shows abnormal motion of the interventricular septum in early diastole.

Differentiating Constrictive Pericarditis from Restrictive Cardiomyopathy

Because their treatment is radically different, distinguishing constrictive pericarditis from restrictive cardiomyopathy is extremely important (Table 64–5). Their presentation and course overlap in many respects. An unequivocal pericardial knock points to constriction, but prominent third heart sounds in restrictive disease can confuse their bedside differentiation. ECG and chest radiographic findings are mostly nonspecific. However, a calcified pericardium indicates constrictive pericarditis and a low-voltage QRS suggests amyloidosis. There are some useful, albeit not invariably reliable, echocardiographic distinctions. Patients with restrictive cardiomyopathy usually have thick-walled ventricles because of infiltrative processes such as amyloidosis. Biatrial enlargement is also common in restriction. In constrictive pericarditis, the most distinctive finding is the ventricular septal bounce. As discussed earlier, the pericardium is usually thickened in constriction, but this may be difficult to assess

TABLE 64–5 Hemodynamic and Echocardiographic Features of Constrictive Pericarditis Compared with Restrictive Cardiomyopathy

Feature	Constriction	Restriction
Prominent *y* descent in venous pressure	Present	Variable
Paradoxical pulse	~1/3 of cases	Absent
Pericardial knock	Present	Absent
Equal right side–left side filling pressures	Present	Left at least 3–5 mm Hg > right
Filling pressures > 25 mm Hg	Rare	Common
Pulmonary artery systolic pressure > 60 mm Hg	No	Common
"Square root" sign	Present	Variable
Respiratory variation in left-right pressures or flows	Exaggerated	Normal
Ventricular wall thickness	Normal	Usually increased
Atrial size	Possible left atrial enlargement	Biatrial enlargement
Septal "bounce"	Present	Absent
Pericardial thickness	Increased	Normal

on transthoracic echocardiography. As noted, data indicate that transesophageal echocardiographic measurements of pericardial thickness correlate well with electron beam CT measurements.[54]

DOPPLER MEASUREMENTS. Doppler flow measurements are often useful in differentiating constrictive from restrictive physiology. Enhanced respiratory variation in mitral inflow velocity (>25 percent) is seen in constriction, whereas in restriction mitral inflow velocity varies by less than 10 percent (see Fig. 64–13). In restriction, pulmonary venous systolic flow is markedly blunted and diastolic flow is increased. This pattern is not observed in constriction. Hepatic veins demonstrate enhanced expiratory flow reversal with constriction, in contrast to increased inspiratory flow reversal in restriction.[15,59] Tissue Doppler echocardiography and color M-mode flow propagation have been shown to be complementary to mitral Doppler respiratory variation in distinguishing between constrictive pericarditis and restrictive cardiomyopathy.

HEMODYNAMICS. Hemodynamic differentiation between constrictive pericarditis and restrictive cardiomyopathy in the cardiac catheterization laboratory can be difficult. However, careful attention to the hemodynamic profile usually helps in making the distinction. In both conditions, right and left ventricular diastolic pressures are markedly elevated. In restrictive cardiomyopathy, however, diastolic pressure in the left ventricle is higher than in the right ventricle at rest or during exercise, usually by at least 3 to 5 mm Hg. As discussed earlier, in constrictive pericarditis left- and right-sided diastolic pressures are very close and demonstrate minimal change during exercise. Pulmonary hypertension is common with restrictive cardiomyopathy but rare in constrictive pericarditis. Marked elevation of right ventricular systolic pressure (>60 mm Hg) is usually indicative of restrictive cardiomyopathy. The absolute level of atrial or ventricular diastolic pressure elevation is also sometimes useful in distinguishing the two conditions, with extremely high pressures (>25 mm Hg) much more common in restrictive cardiomyopathy.[56]

COMPUTED TOMOGRAPHY AND MAGNETIC RESONANCE. CT (especially electron beam) and MR, because of their superior ability to provide detailed assessment of pericardial thickness and calcification, are very useful in differentiating constriction from restriction.[58] However, patients in whom constriction is present can rarely have normal pericardial thickness indicated by these imaging modalities.

Endomyocardial biopsy (or abdominal fat pad biopsy in amyloidosis) is often helpful in documenting the etiology of restrictive cardiomyopathy when an infiltrative process is involved. However, normal biopsy findings do not exclude restrictive cardiomyopathy.

The availability of the multiple diagnostic techniques that have been discussed has made it rare to have to resort to exploratory thoracotomy to distinguish between constriction and restriction. In difficult cases, however, it is often important to obtain as much diagnostic information as possible.

Management

Constrictive pericarditis is a progressive disease. Surgical pericardiectomy is the only definitive treatment. With the exception of patients with major comorbidities or severe debilitation who are considered to be at too high risk to withstand the surgery, the operation should not be delayed when the diagnosis is made. Medical management with diuretics and salt restriction is useful for symptomatic relief of fluid overload and peripheral edema, but patients ultimately become refractory. Sinus tachycardia is a compensatory mechanism. Thus, beta-adrenergic blockers and calcium antagonists that slow the heart rate should be avoided or used with great care. In patients with atrial fibrillation and a rapid ventricular response, digoxin is recommended as initial treatment to slow the ventricular rate before resorting to beta-adrenergic blockers or calcium antagonists. In general, the ventricular rate should not be allowed to drop below 80 to 90 beats/min.

PERICARDIECTOMY. Pericardiectomy is performed through a median sternotomy and involves radical excision of as much of the parietal pericardium as possible. After removal of the parietal pericardium, the visceral pericardium is inspected. Resection of the visceral pericardium should be considered if it is involved in the disease process. Most surgeons initially attempt to perform the operation without cardiopulmonary bypass. The latter should be available as back-up and is frequently required to facilitate access to the lateral and diaphragmatic surfaces of the left ventricle and allow safe removal of a maximal amount of pericardial tissue. Ultrasonic débridement is useful as an adjunct to conventional surgical débridement techniques.[60]

Hemodynamic and symptomatic improvement is achieved in some patients immediately after operation. However, in others symptomatic improvement may be delayed for weeks to months. Seventy to 80 percent of patients remain free from adverse cardiovascular outcomes at 5 years and 40 to 50 percent at 10 years after pericardiectomy.[49] Long-term results are worst in patients with radiation-induced disease. In an echocardiographic analysis, left ventricular diastolic function returned to normal in 40 percent of patients early and 57 percent late after pericardiectomy.[61] Persistence of abnormal diastolic filling was correlated with postoperative symptomatic status. Delayed or inadequate responses to pericardiectomy have been attributed to longstanding disease with myocardial atrophy or fibrosis, incomplete pericardial resection, and the development of recurrent cardiac compression by mediastinal inflammation and fibrosis. Lack of improvement after pericardiectomy may also be due to inadequate resection of visceral pericardium. Worsening of underlying tricuspid regurgitation can also cause hemodynamic deterioration after pericardiectomy.

Pericardiectomy is associated with 5 to 15 percent perioperative mortality in patients with constrictive pericarditis. Survival at 5 and 10 years is about 80 and 60 percent, respectively. Early mortality results primarily from low cardiac output, often in debilitated patients with prolonged cardiopulmonary bypass caused by difficult pericardial dissections. Sepsis, uncontrolled hemorrhage, and renal and respiratory insufficiency also contribute to early postoperative mortality.[15,61] The highest mortality occurs in patients with class III and IV preoperative symptoms. This observation supports the recommendation that pericardiectomy be performed early in the disease process, before marked clinical deterioration and myocardial damage occur.

Effusive-Constrictive Pericarditis

A significant number of patients with pericardial disease present with a syndrome that combines elements of effusion-tamponade and constriction, with a subacute or chronic course. It is common for an inflammatory effusion to dominate the picture initially, with constrictive findings prominent later. As noted earlier, these patients are sometimes identified when hemodynamics fail to normalize after pericardiocentesis. Etiologies are diverse, but the most common are probably malignancy, radiation, and tuberculosis. Physical, hemodynamic, and echocardiographic abnormalities are often mixtures of those associated with effusion and constriction and may vary considerably with time as the syndrome progresses. Diagnosis may require acquisition of pericardial fluid and biopsies if the etiology is not obvious. It is important to be cautious in performing closed pericardiocentesis in these patients when they do not have large effusions. Management is tailored to the specific etiology, if known. In our experience, it is usual for these patients to ultimately require pericardiectomy.

Specific Causes of Pericardial Disease

Bacterial Pericarditis

ETIOLOGY AND PATHOPHYSIOLOGY. Bacterial pericarditis is usually characterized by a purulent pericardial effusion. A wide variety of organisms can be causative.[15,62] Direct extension from pneumonia or empyema accounts for the majority of cases, with the most common agents being staphylococci, pneumococci, and streptococci. Hematogenous spread during bacteremia and contiguous spread after thoracic surgery or trauma are also important mechanisms of bacterial pericarditis. Hospital-acquired, penicillin-resistant staphylococcal pericarditis after thoracic surgery has increased during the past decade. There is increasing incidence of anaerobic organisms grown from pericardial fluid, the most common being *Prevotella* and *Peptostreptococcus* species and *Propionibacterium acnes*. Concomitant infection in the mediastinum or head and neck is most commonly associated with anaerobic isolates.[63,64]

Bacterial pericarditis can also result from rupture of perivalvular abscesses into the pericardial space in patients with endocarditis (see Chap. 58). Rarely, pericardial invasion spreads along fascial planes from the oral cavity, particularly periodontal and peritonsillar abscesses. The pericardium can become infected during meningococcal sepsis, producing primary meningococcal pericarditis. This can occur in the presence or absence of meningitis. In contrast to the usual purulent fluid, the *Neisseria* group can evoke a sterile effusion accompanied by systemic reactions such as arthritis, pleuritis, and ophthalmitis. This syndrome appears to have an immunological basis. It does not require antibiotic therapy and responds to antiinflammatory drugs.

CLINICAL FEATURES. The clinical presentation of bacterial pericarditis is usually high-grade fever with shaking chills and tachycardia, but one or more of these may be absent in debilitated patients. Patients may complain of dyspnea and chest pain. A pericardial friction rub is present in the majority of cases. Bacterial pericarditis can take a fulminant course with rapid development of cardiac tamponade. The disease may be unsuspected because underlying or associated illnesses such as severe pneumonia or mediastinitis after thoracic surgery dominate the clinical picture. Laboratory findings include leukocytosis with marked left shift. The pericardial fluid shows polymorphonuclear leukocytosis, low glucose, high protein, and elevated lactate dehydrogenase levels. Frank pus can occasionally be drained. The chest radiograph shows widening of the cardiac silhouette if the effusion is sufficiently large. With gas-producing organisms a lucent air-fluid interface may be observed. The electrocardiogram shows typical ST segment and T wave changes of acute pericarditis, along with low voltage if there is a large effusion. Two-dimensional echocardiography almost always demonstrates a significant pericardial effusion with or without adhesions. Cardiac tamponade is common and causes hemodynamic deterioration that can be confused with septic shock.

MANAGEMENT. Suspected or proven bacterial pericarditis should be considered a medical emergency and prompt closed pericardiocentesis or surgical drainage performed, with long-term catheter drainage if purulent fluid is obtained. Fluid should be submitted for Gram stain and cultured for aerobic and anaerobic bacteria with appropriate antibiotic sensitivity testing. Fungal and tuberculosis staining and cultures should also be performed on pericardial fluid. If not previously done, cultures of blood, sputum, urine, and recent surgical wounds should be obtained. Broad-spectrum antibiotics should be promptly started and then selected according to Gram stain and culture results. Anaerobic coverage is critical when pericardial infection secondary to head and neck infections is suspected.

Purulent pericardial effusions are likely to recur. Thus, surgical drainage with construction of a window is often needed. In patients with thick, purulent effusions and dense adhesions, extensive pericardiectomy may be required to achieve adequate drainage and prevent the development of constrictive pericarditis. *Early* surgical drainage may also help prevent late constriction. The prognosis for bacterial pericarditis is generally poor,[63,65,66] with survival in the range of 30 percent even in modern series. This poor prognosis probably reflects delays in diagnosis, disease severity, and comorbidities.[65,66]

Pericardial Disease and Human Immunodeficiency Virus (see Chap. 61)

ETIOLOGY AND PATHOPHYSIOLOGY A wide variety of pericardial disease etiologies have been reported in patients infected with HIV. It is estimated that 20 percent of patients infected with HIV have pericardial involvement. Pericardial disease is the most common cardiac manifestation of HIV disease, and the most common abnormality is a pericardial effusion.[67-69] The majority of effusions are small and asymptomatic. The effusion may be part of a generalized seroeffusive process also involving pleural and peritoneal surfaces. This "capillary leak" syndrome is probably related to enhanced cytokine expression in the later stages of HIV disease. Moderate to large effusions are more frequent in patients with more advanced stages of HIV infection. Congestive heart failure, Kaposi sarcoma, tuberculosis, and pulmonary infections are independently associated with moderate to large pericardial effusions in patients with HIV. Other forms of pericardial disease are less frequent and include involvement by various other neoplasms and classic pericarditis and myopericarditis. Constrictive pericarditis is rare in HIV patients. When present, it is usually secondary to *Mycobacterium tuberculosis*.[69]

CLINICAL FEATURES. Symptomatic patients with pericardial disease usually present with dyspnea or chest pain secondary to pericardial inflammation or a large effusion, or both. Large, symptomatic effusions are often caused by infection or a neoplasm. The most common infectious agents identified in symptomatic pericardial effusions are *M. tuberculosis* and *Mycobacterium avium-intracellulare*. However, a wide variety of organisms, often unusual, have been implicated, including *Cryptococcus neoformans*, cytomegalovirus, and *Mycobacterium kansasii*. Lymphomas and Kaposi sarcoma are the most common neoplasms associated with effusion.

MANAGEMENT. Asymptomatic patients with small to moderate pericardial effusions do not require pericardiocentesis. Most cases are idiopathic and usually remain asymptomatic or resolve spontaneously. Symptomatic, large effusions should be drained and an identifiable cause sought. One study demonstrated that pericardial effusion in HIV disease usually occurs in the context of full-blown acquired immunodeficiency syndrome and is strongly associated with a shortened survival independent of the CD4 count.[70] Mortality at 6 months for patients with pericardial effusion was ninefold greater than for patients without an effusion (Fig. 64–17).[70] The effects of highly active antiretroviral therapy on HIV-related pericardial disease have not yet been elucidated.

Tuberculous Pericarditis

ETIOLOGY AND PATHOPHYSIOLOGY. The incidence of pericardial tuberculosis has decreased markedly in the industrialized world in parallel with the deceased incidence of pulmonary tuberculosis. From 1 to 8 percent of patients with pulmonary tuberculosis develop pericardial involvement. Reflecting current epidemiology, in a modern series of cases of primary acute to subacute pericardial disease, tuberculosis was diagnosed in only 4 percent overall and in 7 percent of patients who developed cardiac tamponade. Similarly, tuberculous pericarditis was diagnosed in only 1 of 135 patients with constrictive pericarditis at the Mayo Clinic. However, pericardial tuberculosis remains a major problem in the immunocompromised host and the underdeveloped world, especially in southwest Africa. Moreover, the combination of HIV and pericardial tuberculosis is especially common in African populations. In a study of Tanzanian patients with large pericardial effusions, 14 of 14 HIV-positive patients had tuberculous pericarditis. Evidence of pericardial involvement in HIV-positive patients in African countries where both tuberculosis and HIV are endemic is usually sufficient to prompt antituberculous therapy.[71]

Pericardial involvement by tuberculosis is usually secondary to retrograde spread from peribronchial, peritracheal, or mediastinal lymph nodes or hematogenous spread from the primary focus. Less commonly, the pericardium is involved by the breakdown and contiguous spread of a necrotic lesion in the lung.

CLINICAL FEATURES. The clinical presentation of tuberculous pericarditis is usually subacute to chronic, with systemic symptoms of fever, malaise, and dyspnea in association with a pericardial effusion. Cough, night sweats, orthopnea, weight loss, and ankle edema are also common. The most common findings are radiographic cardiomegaly, pericardial rub, fever, and tachycardia. Findings related to large effusions such as paradoxical pulse, hepatomegaly, distended neck veins, pleural effusion, and distant heart sounds are common, as is severe hemodynamic compromise. Many patients are properly classified as having a subacute, effusive-constrictive syndrome, and a number develop late constrictive pericarditis despite antituberculous treatment.[72] Clinical evidence of pulmonary tuberculosis may be absent or subtle, which is one of the chief reasons the diagnosis is sometimes unsuspected.

Diagnosing tuberculous pericardial disease is notoriously difficult.[15,71,72] A definitive diagnosis is made by isolating the organism from pericardial fluid or a biopsy specimen. However, the yield for isolating the organism from pericardial fluid is relatively low. In a series of 41 patients with subacute tuberculous pericarditis, *M. tuberculosis* grew in only 4 of 13 cultures of pericardial fluid.[72] The probability of making a diagnosis is increased if both pericardial fluid and biopsy specimens are examined early in the effusive stage of the disease. Thus, there is a definite role for pericardial biopsy. Pericardial tissue reveals either granulomas or organisms in 80 to 90 percent of cases. The optimal diagnostic work-up (as well as management) of suspected tuberculous pericarditis includes a pericardial window with fluid and tissue sent for both culture and histopathological examination. The finding of granulomas without bacilli in biopsy tissue is helpful but not diagnostic of tuberculous pericarditis because granulomas can be found in rheumatoid and sarcoid pericardial disease.

A positive tuberculin skin test increases suspicion, but a negative skin test does not exclude the diagnosis and is often not useful in immunocompromised hosts. A positive skin test is also less helpful in populations with a high endemic incidence of tuberculosis. Measurement of adenosine deaminase, an enzyme produced by white blood cells in pericardial fluid, markedly improves diagnostic capabilities. Thus, in a prospective study of patients with pericardial effusion, an adenosine deaminase level greater than 40 units/liter had a sensitivity of 93 percent and a specificity of 97 percent for tuberculous pericarditis.[46] Adenosine deaminase should be routinely measured whenever tuberculous pericardial involvement is suspected. Measurement of interferon-gamma in pericardial fluid has been proposed as an additional marker for tuberculous involvement. Last, tuberculous pericarditis has also been presumptively diagnosed by polymerase chain reaction in pericardial biopsy specimens. This method offers the possibility of obtaining organism-specific results much more rapidly than do cultures.[73]

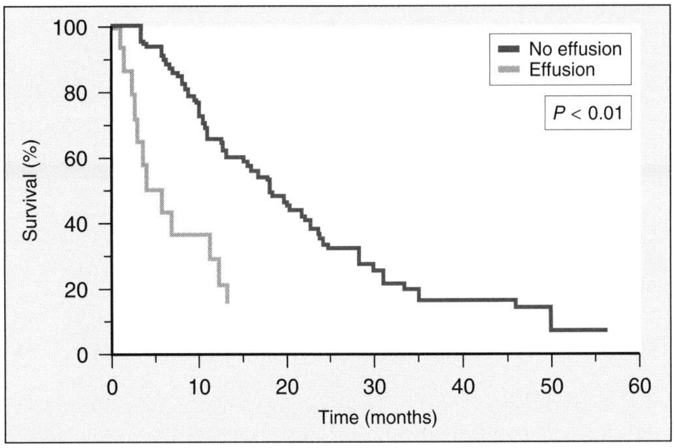

FIGURE 64–17 Kaplan-Meier survival curves in human immunodeficiency virus–positive patients with and without pericardial effusion. (From Heidenreich PA, Eisenberg MJ, Kee LL, et al: Pericardial effusion in AIDS. Incidence and survival. Circulation 92:3229, 1995.)

MANAGEMENT. The goals of therapy are to treat acute symptoms as well as tamponade, if present, and to prevent the progression to a constrictive stage. Antimycobacterial treatment has greatly decreased mortality. Effective multidrug therapy is mandatory. Two issues have arisen in the treatment of tuberculous pericarditis: the role of corticosteroids and the need for open surgical drainage versus closed pericardiocentesis. The most thorough study of closed pericardiocentesis versus open surgical drainage was performed in 240 South African patients with effusive tuberculous pericarditis.[74] After initial diagnostic evaluation, patients were randomly allocated to open pericardial biopsy and complete surgical drainage of fluid or percutaneous pericardiocentesis as needed. Patients were further randomly assigned to receive or not receive prednisolone. All patients were treated with isoniazid, streptomycin, rifampin, and pyrazinamide. The outcomes suggested that patients who undergo open drainage are less likely to require repeated pericardiocentesis, and there was a trend in the open drainage group toward reduced development of constriction. The role of corticosteroids was not fully elucidated. Their use did not influence the risk of death or progression to constriction but did speed the resolution of symptoms and decrease reaccumulation of fluid. There is no rationale for the use of corticosteroids when established constriction is present. No studies have addressed the use of corticosteroids in HIV-positive patients with tuberculous pericarditis. The optimal management of constrictive pericarditis related to tuberculosis is pericardiectomy.

FUNGAL PERICARDITIS

ETIOLOGY AND PATHOPHYSIOLOGY. Fungal infections are rare causes of pericarditis. They are mainly due to locally endemic organisms such as *Histoplasma* or *Coccidioides* or opportunistic fungi such as *Candida* and *Aspergillus*. Other fungi reported to cause pericardial disease include *Blastomyces*, *Cryptococcus*, and *Pneumocystis carinii*.

Histoplasmosis is the most common cause of fungal pericarditis. The organism is endemic in Ohio, the Mississippi River valley, and the western Appalachians; is acquired by inhalation; and can infect otherwise healthy patients living in the endemic areas.[75] Coccidioidomycosis is endemic in the American Southwest. The organism is acquired by inhalation of chlamydospores in an endemic area.[76] Immunocompromised patients, drug addicts, and those taking corticosteroids or potent broad-spectrum antibiotics are at increased risk for developing opportunistic fungal pericarditis.

CLINICAL FEATURES AND MANAGEMENT

Histoplasmosis. Pericardial histoplasmosis usually occurs in a previously healthy young patient. It is thought to be a noninfectious inflammatory process in response to infection confined to adjacent mediastinal lymph nodes. Accordingly, isolation of organisms from pericardial fluid is unusual. The fluid is serous, xanthochromic, or hemorrhagic. The clinical course usually begins with respiratory symptoms followed by pericardial pain. Effusion leading to cardiac tamponade occurs in almost half the cases. The diagnosis must be considered in endemic zones and is aided by rising complement fixation titers. Provided effusions are drained as needed, pericardial involvement eventually resolves with or without anti-inflammatory drugs. Antifungal agents are indicated only for disseminated histoplasmosis.

Coccidioidomycosis. Coccidioidomycosis pericarditis occurs as a complication of a progressive, disseminated form of infection. Patients are chronically ill and debilitated. Pericardial involvement does not occur in the self-limited influenza-like form of the infection. Physical findings suggestive of cardiac compression may be the first clues to the diagnosis of pericardial involvement. Treatment is directed at the disseminated fungal infection with intravenous amphotericin B. Pericardiocentesis is, of course, indicated when tamponade occurs.

Other Fungi. Pericarditis caused by opportunistic fungi such as *Candida* and *Aspergillus* usually occurs in patients who are immunosuppressed or receiving broad-spectrum antibiotics as well as patients recovering from complicated open-heart surgery. Pericardial involvement usually occurs in the setting of disseminated fungal infection. The prognosis is poor, and the diagnosis is often made at autopsy.

Uremic Pericarditis and Dialysis-Associated Pericardial Disease

(see Chap. 86)

ETIOLOGY AND PATHOPHYSIOLOGY. The incidence of classic uremic pericarditis has decreased markedly since the introduction of widespread dialysis. The pathophysiology of uremic pericarditis has never been fully elucidated, but it is clearly correlated with the levels of blood urea nitrogen (BUN) and creatinine in the blood. Toxic metabolites, hypercalcemia, hyperuricemia, and hemorrhagic, viral, and autoimmune mechanisms have been implicated.[15,77] However, there is no correlation between the development of uremic pericarditis and the level of catabolic metabolites. The acute or subacute phase is characterized by the appearance of shaggy, hemorrhagic, fibrinous exudates on both parietal and visceral surfaces with little in the way of inflammatory cellular reaction. Subacute or chronic constriction may develop with organization of the effusion and formation of thick adhesions within the pericardial space.

Dialysis-associated pericardial disease is now much more common than classic uremic pericarditis. It is characterized by de novo appearance of pericardial disease in patients undergoing chronic dialysis despite the fact that BUN and creatinine are normal or only mildly elevated. Its mechanism and relation to classic uremic pericarditis are unknown.

CLINICAL FEATURES. In modern populations of patients receiving chronic dialysis, the clinical presentation is sometimes that of acute pericarditis with chest pain, fever, leukocytosis, and pericardial friction rub. Alternatively, patients can present with an asymptomatic pericardial effusion that can cause hypotension during or after ultrafiltration (low-pressure tamponade). Although conventional cardiac tamponade with acute or subacute hemodynamic compromise can also occur, the extremely large, asymptomatic effusions typical of classic uremic pericarditis are rarely encountered today.

The electrocardiogram most often is not markedly affected and reflects a high incidence of associated abnormalities such as left ventricular hypertrophy, previous MI, or electrolyte abnormalities. The chest radiograph may demonstrate cardiac enlargement related to myocardial dysfunction and volume overload or pericardial effusion, or both. Asymptomatic effusions of small to moderate size are common in patients receiving chronic dialysis. Accordingly, the presence of typical pericardial pain or a friction rub, or both, is necessary for the diagnosis of pericarditis.

MANAGEMENT. The management of classic uremic pericarditis is intensive hemodialysis as well as drainage in patients with effusions that cause hemodynamic compromise. Patients with symptomatic pericarditis almost always respond to the initiation of intensification of dialysis. Heparin should be used cautiously during hemodialysis because of the possibility of causing hemorrhagic pericarditis with tamponade. Pericardial effusion without hemodynamic compromise resolves after several weeks of intensive hemodialysis in the majority of patients.[15]

Treatment of pericardial disease appearing de novo in patients receiving chronic dialysis is empirical. Cardiac tamponade, of course, requires drainage. In our experience, intensifying dialysis is marginally beneficial at best, presumably because these patients are already receiving most of the benefits of dialysis. Use of NSAIDs for pericardial pain is reasonable, but corticosteroids should be avoided if possible. There is no published experience with colchicine. A pericardial window may be required and is often the most effective approach in patients with recurring, hemodynamically significant effusions.

Early Post-Myocardial Infarction Pericarditis and Dressler Syndrome

(see Chap. 47)

ETIOLOGY AND PATHOPHYSIOLOGY. Early post-MI pericarditis occurs during the first 1 to 3 days and no more than a week after an MI and is due to transmural necrosis with inflammation affecting the adjacent visceral and parietal pericardium. Pericardial involvement is strongly associated with indices of infarct size. It is estimated from autopsy studies that about 40 percent of patients with large, Q wave MIs have pericardial inflammation.[78] Use of thrombolytic and mechanical revascularization therapy appears to have reduced the incidence of this form of pericarditis by at least 50 percent. On the basis of clinical criteria, the incidence in patients receiving thrombolytic therapy in the Gruppo Italiano per lo Studio della Sopravvivenza nell'Infarto Miocardico (GISSI) study was only 5 to 6 percent. Furthermore, the earlier the thrombolytic treatment is initiated, the lower the incidence of pericarditis.

Late pericarditis is characterized by pleuropericardial involvement with pericardial or pleural effusions, or both. This syndrome was initially described by Dressler and had an estimated incidence of 3 to 4 percent of MI patients in the past. However, there is a general impression that the incidence of Dressler syndrome has become markedly reduced during the reperfusion therapy era. Dressler syndrome is believed to have an autoimmune etiology because of sensitization to myocardial cells at the time of necrosis. Antimyocardial antibodies have been demonstrated in patients with the clinical syndrome,[15] although these antibodies are nonspecific. As noted previously, Dressler syndrome is a polyserositis involving the pleura and the pericardium. In contrast to that in early post-MI pericarditis, the inflammation in this syndrome is diffuse and not localized to the myocardial injury site.

CLINICAL FEATURES. Most commonly, early post-MI pericarditis is asymptomatic and identified by auscultation of a rub, usually within 1 to 3 days after presentation. Friction rubs in this setting are notoriously evanescent. Many are monophasic (usually systolic) and can be confused with a murmur of mitral regurgitation or ventricular septal defect. Acute post-MI pericarditis virtually never causes tamponade by itself. However, it can occur in association with left ventricular free wall rupture. Symptomatic patients develop pleuritic chest pain within the preceding time frame. It is important to distinguish pericardial pain from recurrent ischemic discomfort. Ordinarily, the distinction is not difficult on clinical grounds. However, the typical ECG changes of acute pericarditis are uncommon after MI. Pericardial inflammation is localized to the infarcted area; hence, the ECG changes usually involve subtle reelevation of the ST segment in the originally involved leads. An atypical T wave evolution has also been described that appears to be highly sensitive for acute post-MI pericarditis. It consists of persistent upright T waves or early normalization of inverted T waves following the MI. The presence of a pericardial effusion correlates with the presence of extensive MI but not with clinically evident pericarditis.

Dressler syndrome occurs as early as 1 week to a few months after an acute MI. Symptoms include fever and pleuritic chest pain. The physical examination may reveal pleural or pericardial friction rubs, or both. The chest radiograph may show a pleural effusion or enlargement of the cardiac silhouette, and the electrocardiogram often demonstrates ST elevation and T wave changes typical of acute pericarditis. Although pericardial effusions are common, tamponade is unusual.

MANAGEMENT. Although it is associated with relatively large, transmural MIs, early post-MI pericarditis per se is almost invariably a benign process that does not appear to affect in-hospital mortality independently. Treatment is entirely symptomatic. Augmentation of the usual low-dose aspirin administered to these patients (to 650 mg three or four times per day for 2 to 5 days) or acetaminophen can provide symptomatic relief. A brief course of prednisone may be useful in patients with unusually severe pain persisting more than 48 hours despite aspirin or acetaminophen. However, there is evidence that NSAIDs and corticosteroids interfere with the conversion of an MI into a scar, resulting in greater wall thinning and a higher incidence of post-MI rupture. Thus, these drugs should be avoided unless they are absolutely necessary. Because significant hemopericardium is extremely rare with early post-MI pericarditis and there is no evidence that heparin increases the risk, heparin administration should not be modified because of the presence of early post-MI pericarditis. However, coadministration of heparin and glycoprotein IIb/IIIa inhibitors should be done cautiously. There have been no reports of hemopericardium in patients with early post-MI pericarditis receiving dual oral antiplatelet therapy with aspirin and clopidogrel.

Although Dressler syndrome is ultimately a self-limited disorder, admission to the hospital for observation and monitoring should be considered if there is a substantial pericardial effusion or, as is often the case, other conditions, e.g., pulmonary infarction, are also being considered. Aspirin or NSAIDs are effective for symptomatic relief. A short course of prednisone, 40 to 60 mg/d with a 7- to 10-day taper, can be used in patients who do not respond to the preceding treatment or for recurrent symptoms.

POSTPERICARDIOTOMY AND POST-CARDIAC INJURY SYNDROME PERICARDITIS

Blunt or penetrating injury of the chest and heart with myocardial contusion can cause associated acute pericarditis (see Chap. 65). The pericarditis per se is rarely of clinical significance compared with other effects of the trauma. However, pericarditis can develop days to months after cardiac surgery, thoracotomy, or chest trauma. The pathogenesis of this syndrome is thought to involve production of antiheart antibodies in response to myocardial injury with resultant complement activation. A systemic inflammatory response occurs and is characterized by low-grade fever, elevated ESR, mild leukocytosis, and pleuropericardial inflammation with associated chest discomfort. The chest radiograph typically shows bilateral pleural effusions. A few patients demonstrate pulmonary infiltrates. The electrocardiogram reveals changes consistent with acute pericarditis in about 50 percent of patients. The echocardiogram usually shows a small to moderate-size pericardial effusion. Tamponade is rare. NSAIDs are first-line treatment, with an excellent response usually occurring within 48 hours of initiation. Treatment should be maintained for 2 to 3 weeks. Corticosteroid therapy is reserved for patients with unresponsive, severe, or recurrent symptoms.

RADIATION-INDUCED PERICARDITIS

Mediastinal and thoracic radiation is currently standard treatment for a variety of thoracic neoplasms. Hodgkin disease, non-Hodgkin lymphoma, and breast carcinoma are the most common neoplasms associated with radiation pericarditis (see Chaps. 63 and 83). Factors that influence the degree of injury to the pericardium include the total dose delivered, the amount of cardiac silhouette exposed, the nature of the radiation source, and the duration and fractionation of therapy. There is about a 2 percent incidence of clinically evident pericarditis in conjunction with modern techniques of radiation delivery.[79] However, the incidence can be as high as 20 percent when the entire pericardium is exposed.[15,79]

Radiation pericarditis takes one of two forms, an acute illness with chest pain and fever and a delayed form of pericardial injury that can occur years after treatment. Self-limited, asymptomatic effusions are common soon after radiation injury, but tamponade is unusual. Late manifestations of radiation injury occur from about a year to up to 20 years after exposure.[15,79] Patients can present with symptomatic pericarditis and effusion with or without cardiac compression or circulatory congestion related to constrictive pericarditis. Effusions can evolve into constriction, i.e., an effusive-constrictive syndrome.

Radiation-induced pericarditis and effusion can be confused with malignant effusions. Malignant effusions are usually associated with other evidence of disease recurrence and metastases. Hypothyroidism induced by mediastinal radiation can also contribute to pericardial effusion. Pericardiocentesis with fluid analysis for malignant cells and thyroid function tests help differentiate radiation-induced effusion from other etiologies. Large, symptomatic pericardial effusions may be drained either percutaneously or surgically. Recurrent pericardial effusions are usually best treated surgically with either a window or pericardiectomy. Pericardiectomy is, of course, the treatment of choice for patients with constrictive physiology. However, the perioperative mortality in this group of patients is higher than with idiopathic constrictive pericarditis.

METASTATIC PERICARDIAL DISEASE

Pericardial tumor implants are the usual cause of effusion in patients with known malignancies, although, as noted earlier, obstruction of lymphatic drainage by enlarged mediastinal lymph nodes is occasionally observed. The leading cause of cardiac tamponade in developed countries is malignancy. Lung (40 percent) and breast (22 percent) carcinoma and lymphomas (15 percent) are the most common causes of malignant effusion.[15] Gastrointestinal carcinoma, melanoma, and sarcomas are less common. With the advent of HIV infection, the incidence of Kaposi sarcoma and lymphomatous involvement of the pericardium have increased markedly.[69]

Pericardial tumor implants can cause pericardial pain. However, the dominant feature is usually an effusion. Effusions with elements of constriction are not unusual. An asymptomatic, incidentally discovered pericardial effusion can be the presenting sign of pericardial involvement in patients with malignant cancer. However, most patients present with symptomatic effusions or tamponade, or both. The electrocardiogram is variable but usually shows nonspecific T wave abnormalities with low-voltage QRS. ST segment elevation is somewhat unusual but can occur. In addition to echocardiography, CT and MR imaging are useful in evaluating the extent of metastatic disease to the pericardium and adjacent structures.

In most cancer patients with effusions or tamponade, it is important that metastatic involvement of the pericardium be confirmed by identification of malignant cells in pericardial fluid. Confirmation is important because of occasional cases of obstructed lymphatic drainage causing pericardial effusion, the possibility of confusion with radiation-induced disease, and the fact that other forms of pericardial disease can occur in patients who have or have had cancer. On the other hand, there are many exceptions in which clinical judgment dictates that this need not be done, especially when effusions are not large and specific treatment, e.g., instillation of drugs in the pericardial space, is not being contemplated.

It is important to evaluate the life expectancy of patients before performing pericardiocentesis and choosing treatment modalities. In terminally ill patients, drainage of effusions should be performed only to aid in relief of symptoms. However, patients with better prognoses deserve a more aggressive approach, which can be gratifying in a perhaps surprisingly large number. In a significant number of cases a single drainage provides prolonged relief as well as providing fluid for analysis. For this reason, drainage should be the initial step in the treatment of most patients, with careful attention to detection of reaccumulation. For recurrences, intrapericardial instillation of tetracycline or chemotherapeutic agents has been advocated to encourage pericardial sclerosis and has a reasonable record of success. External beam radiation therapy is an option in patients with radiation-sensitive tumors. A pericardial window or even complete surgical pericardiectomy should be considered in patients with recurrent effusions not responding to the preceding measures who continue to have a good prognosis otherwise.[80]

PRIMARY PERICARDIAL NEOPLASMS

A number of primary pericardial neoplasms have been reported. All are exceedingly rare. They include malignant mesotheliomas, fibrosarcomas, lymphangiomas, hemangiomas, teratomas, neurofibromas, and lipomas.[80,81] Because of their rarity, it is difficult to be precise about the clinical presentation and course of these neoplasms. In general, they are either locally invasive or compress cardiac structures or are detected from an abnormal cardiac silhouette on chest radiograph. Mesotheliomas and fibrosarcomas are quite lethal. Others such as lipomas are benign. CT and MR imaging are helpful in delineating the pathological anatomy of these tumors, but surgery is required for diagnosis and treatment.

AUTOIMMUNE AND DRUG-INDUCED PERICARDIAL DISEASE

Pericardial involvement can occur in almost any variety of autoimmune disease, but the great bulk of clinically recognized cases occur in rheumatoid arthritis, SLE, and progressive systemic sclerosis (scleroderma). In addition, a variety of drugs have been reported to cause pericarditis that is usually part of an autoimmune process.

RHEUMATOID ARTHRITIS. Pericardial involvement is common in rheumatoid arthritis (see Chap. 82). Older autopsy studies revealed pericardial inflammation in about 50 percent of patients. However, there are no systematic studies addressing the incidence of pericardial involvement in more contemporary patients. Clinically evident pericardial involvement is detected in up to 25 percent of patients with rheumatoid arthritis. Patients can present with chest pain, fever, and dyspnea related to acute pericarditis, which usually occurs in conjunction with exacerbation of the underlying disease. Asymptomatic large pericardial effusion or cardiac tamponade can also be the presenting manifestation of pericardial involvement in rheumatoid arthritis. The pericardial fluid is characterized by low glucose, neutrophilic leukocytosis, elevated titers of rheumatoid factor, and low complement levels. Constrictive pericarditis can also occur as the result of longstanding pericardial inflammation. In patients with joint disease exacerbation, the management of associated acute pericarditis or asymptomatic effusion is first and foremost the same as that employed to treat the exacerbation. Pericardial manifestations seem to respond well to high-dose aspirin or NSAIDs. Pericardial effusions causing cardiac tamponade should be drained, both to treat tamponade and to establish with confidence that there is no other etiology, e.g., infection, in patients who may be receiving immunosuppressive drugs. In general, the response to treatment of underlying disease exacerbations is too slow and uncertain to advocate a period of watchful waiting in the hope that effusions will shrink before drainage. Recurrent tamponade or large effusions are good indications for a pericardial window. Suppressive therapy with colchicine has also been shown to be effective for recurrent symptoms.[82]

SYSTEMIC LUPUS ERYTHEMATOSUS. Pericarditis is the most common cardiovascular manifestation of SLE,[15] and acute pericarditis can be the first manifestation of the disease. About 40 percent of patients with SLE develop pericarditis at some time, usually in conjunction with an overall flare and involvement of other serosal surfaces. Typical patients present with pleuritic chest pain, low-grade fever, and symptoms related to serosal inflammation elsewhere. The electrocardiogram often shows typical findings of acute pericarditis. The chest radiograph may show enlargement of the cardiac silhouette if pericardial effusion is present, along with pleural effusions and often parenchymal infiltrates. Pericardial effusions have high protein and low glucose contents and a white cell count below 10,000/ml. As with patients with rheumatoid arthritis, it is important to exclude purulent, fungal, or tuberculous pericarditis because the majority of these patients are being treated with immunosuppressive medications. Most patients respond to corticosteroids or immunosuppressive therapy used to treat the overall disease flare-up. Hemodynamic compromise secondary to cardiac tamponade is estimated to occur in 10 percent of patients with SLE. Accordingly, we recommend hospitalizing these patients to monitor for hemodynamic complications until clinical stability is achieved.

PROGRESSIVE SYSTEMIC SCLEROSIS (SCLERODERMA) (see Chap. 82). There is about a 10 percent incidence of acute pericarditis with chest pain and pericardial friction rub in progressive systemic sclerosis. However, pericardial involvement is found at autopsy in about 50 percent of patients. Pericardial effusion is detected by echocardiography in up to 40 percent of patients. Most effusions are small and asymptomatic, but there are occasional instances of large pericardial effusion. Late constrictive pericarditis has been described and carries a poor prognosis.[83] Treatment of acute pericarditis in patients with scleroderma is often unrewarding, with an unpredictable response to aspirin and NSAIDs. Although there is no published experience, colchicine should therefore be considered in these patients. It is important to perform right-heart catheterization in patients presenting with dyspnea or right-sided heart failure to evaluate pulmonary vascular disease, which is relatively common and can be confused with pericardial involvement.

DRUG-INDUCED PERICARDITIS

The great majority of cases of drug-induced pericardial disease occur as a component of drug-induced SLE syndromes. There have been no recent, systematic studies of the epidemiology or etiology of drug-induced SLE or drug-induced pericarditis. Therefore, it is difficult to generalize about current trends. Isoniazid and hydralazine are probably the most common current offenders. Procainamide used to be a major cause, but its use has decreased markedly in the last decade. Large effusions, tamponade, and even constriction have been reported but are rare in drug-induced SLE pericarditis. In addition to drug cessation, management is dictated by the specific elements of the SLE syndrome present as well as usual efforts aimed at detection and treatment of effusions. In rare cases, drug-induced pericarditis caused by agents such as penicillin and cromolyn has involved apparent hypersensitivity reactions with eosinophilia without an SLE picture.

PERICARDIAL DISEASE AND PERCUTANEOUS REVASCULARIZATION (see Chap. 48)

Cardiac tamponade is a rare but important complication of percutaneous revascularization. The incidence of cardiac tamponade ranges between 0.1 and 0.5 percent. The incidence has increased in the last 10 years, which is probably related to aggressive treatment of complex lesions and use of atherectomy devices and stiff or hydrophilic guidewires.

Cardiac tamponade during percutaneous revascularization is almost always a result of coronary artery perforation. Perforation can occur as a consequence of guidewire or balloon advancement. The clinical presentation is abrupt or rapidly progressive cardiac decompensation and severe hypotension. The diagnosis of perforation is made by the angiographic appearance of extravasation of dye from the coronary circulation into the pericardial space. Loss of cardiac pulsation on fluoroscopy indicates that a significant pericardial effusion is present. Management of pericardial tamponade requires sealing the coronary perforation, pericardiocentesis, and reversal of anticoagulation.[84] If the perforation cannot be managed percutaneously, emergency surgery is indicated.

HYPOTHYROID-ASSOCIATED PERICARDIAL DISEASE (see Chap. 79)

Patients with severe hypothyroidism develop pericardial effusions in perhaps 25 to 35 percent of cases.[15] These can become quite large but rarely, if ever, cause tamponade. Classically, they have high concentrations of cholesterol. The effusions gradually resolve with treatment of the thyroid condition.

CONGENITAL ANOMALIES OF THE PERICARDIUM

PERICARDIAL CYSTS. Pericardial cysts are rare, benign congenital malformations. They are usually fluid filled, located at the right costophrenic angle, and identified as an incidental finding on a chest radiograph. The diagnosis is usually confirmed by echocardiography. Patients should be managed conservatively.

CONGENITAL ABSENCE OF THE PERICARDIUM. Congenital absence of the pericardium is rare. Usually part or all of the left side of the parietal pericardium is absent, but partial absence of the right side has also been reported.[15] Partial absence of the left pericardium is often associated with other cardiac anomalies, including atrial septal defect, bicuspid aortic valve, or pulmonary malformations. It is often symptomatic and may even allow herniation of portions of the heart through the defect or torsion of the great vessels, with potentially life-threatening hemodynamic consequences. Recurrent pulmonary infections are occasionally seen. Patients can present with chest pain, syncope, or even sudden death. The electrocardiogram typically reveals an incomplete right bundle branch block. Absence of all or most of the left pericardium results in a characteristic chest radiograph, including a leftward shift of the cardiac silhouette, an elongated left heart border, and radiolucent bands between the aortic knob and the main pulmonary artery and between the left diaphragm and the base of the heart. Echocardiography reveals paradoxical septal motion and right ventricular enlargement. CT or MR imaging should be employed to establish a definitive diagnosis and elaborate the details of the defect. Appropriate surgical correction, i.e., pericardiectomy, should ordinarily be undertaken to ameliorate symptoms and eliminate the possibility of herniation.

REFERENCES

Anatomy and Physiology of the Pericardium

1. Gabella G (sect ed): The pericardium. *In* Gray H, Williams PL, Bannister LH (eds): Gray's Anatomy: The Anatomical Basis of Medicine and Surgery. New York, Churchill-Livingstone, 1995, pp 1471-1472.
2. Kostreva DR, Pontus SP: Pericardial mechanoreceptors with phrenic afferents. Am J Physiol 264:H1836, 1993.
3. Miyazaki T, Pride HP, Zipes DP: Prostaglandins in the pericardial fluid modulate neural regulation of cardiac electrophysiological properties. Circ Res 66:163, 1990.
4. Slinker BK, Bell S, Ditchey R, LeWinter MM: Pericardial pressure does not equal right heart pressure in the dog. Circulation 76:357, 1987.
5. Hamilton DR, Dani RS, Semlacher RA, et al: Right atrial and right ventricular transmural pressures in dogs and humans. Effects of the pericardium. Circulation 90:2492, 1994.
6. Lee MC, Fung YC, Shabetai R, LeWinter MM: Biaxial mechanical properties of the human pericardium and canine comparisons. Am J Physiol 22:H75, 1987.
7. Freeman G, LeWinter M: Pericardial adaptations during chronic cardiac dilation in dogs. Circ Res 54:294, 1984.
8. Freeman G, LeWinter M: Determinants of the intra-pericardial pressure in dogs. J Appl Physiol 60:758, 1986.
9. deVries G, Hamilton DR, Ter Keurs HE, et al: A novel technique for measurement of pericardial pressure. Am J Physiol 280:H2815, 2001.
10. Tischler M, Cooper K, LeWinter MM: Increased left ventricular volume and mass following coronary bypass surgery. A role for relief of pericardial constraint? Circulation 87:1921, 1993.
11. Baker AE, Dani R, Smith ER, et al: Quantitative assessment of independent contributions of pericardium and septum to direct ventricular interaction. Am J Physiol 275:H476, 1998.

Passive Role of the Normal Pericardium in Heart Disease

12. O'Rourke RA, Dell'Italia LJ: Right ventricular myocardial infarction. *In* Fuster V, Rorr R, Topol EJ (eds): Atherosclerosis and Coronary Artery Disease. Philadelphia, Lippincott-Raven, 1996, pp 1079-1096.
13. LeWinter M, Pavelec R: Influence of the pericardium on left ventricular end-diastolic pressure-segment length relations during early and late phases of experimental chronic volume overload in dogs. Circ Res 50:501, 1982.

Acute Pericarditis

14. Zayas R, Anguita M, Torres F, et al: Incidence of specific etiology and role of methods for specific etiologic diagnosis of primary acute pericarditis. Am J Cardiol 75:378, 1995.
15. Spodick DW: Pericardial diseases. *In* Braunwald E, Zipes D, Libby P (eds): Heart Disease. 6th ed. Philadelphia, WB Saunders, 2001, pp 1823-1876.
16. Brady WJ, Perron AD, Martin ML, et al: Cause of ST-segment abnormality in ED chest pain patients. Am J Emerg Med 19:25, 2001.
17. Bonnefoy E, Godon P, Kirkorian G, et al: Serum cardiac troponin I and ST-segment elevation in patients with acute pericarditis. Eur Heart J 21:798, 2000.
18. Brandt RR, Filzmaier K, Hanrath P: Circulating cardiac troponin I in acute pericarditis. Am J Cardiol 87:1326, 2001.
19. Baljepally R, Spodick DH: PR-segment depression as the initial electrocardiographic response in acute pericarditis. Am J Cardiol 81:1505, 1998.
20. Kudo Y, Yamasaki F, Doi Y, Sugiura T: Clinical correlates of PR-segment depression in asymptomatic patients with pericardial effusion. J Am Coll Cardiol 39:2000, 2002.
21. Adler Y, Finkelstein Y, Guindo J, et al: Colchicine treatment for recurrent pericarditis: A decade of experience. Circulation 97:2183, 1998.
22. Marcolongo R, Russo R, Laveder F, et al: Immunosuppressive therapy prevents recurrent pericarditis. J Am Coll Cardiol 26:1276, 1995.
23. Fowler NO, Harbin AD III: Recurrent acute pericarditis: Follow-up study of 31 patients. J Am Coll Cardiol 7:300, 1986.

Pericardial Effusion and Tamponade

24. Tsang TS, Barnes ME, Hayes SN, et al: Clinical and echocardiographic characteristics of significant pericardial effusions following cardiothoracic surgery and outcomes of echo-guided pericardiocentesis for management: Mayo Clinic experience, 1979-1998. Chest 116:322, 1999.
25. Goland S, Caspi A, Malnick S, et al: Idiopathic chronic pericardial effusion. N Engl J Med 342:1449, 2000.
26. Friedman HS, Lajam F, Zaman Q, et al: Effect of autonomic blockade on the hemodynamic findings in acute cardiac tamponade. Am J Physiol 232:H5, 1977.
26a. Spodick DH: Acute cardiac tamponade. N Engl J Med 349:684, 2003.
27. Friedman HS, Lajam F, Gomes JA, et al: Demonstration of a depressor reflex in acute cardiac tamponade. J Thorac Cardiovasc Surg 73:278, 1977.
28. Merce J, Sagrista-Sauleda J, Permanyer-Miralda G, et al: Correlation between clinical and Doppler echocardiographic findings in patients with moderate and large pericardial effusion: Implications for the diagnosis of cardiac tamponade. Am Heart J 138:759, 1999.
29. Hoit BD, Ramrakhyani K: Pulmonary venous flow in cardiac tamponade: Influence of left ventricular dysfunction and the relation to pulsus paradoxicus. J Am Soc Echocardiogr 4:559, 1991.
30. Fowler NO, Gabel M, Buncher CR: Cardiac tamponade: A comparison of right versus left heart compression. J Am Coll Cardiol 12:187, 1988.
31. Singh S, Wann LS, Schuchard GH, et al: Right ventricular and right atrial collapse in patients with cardiac tamponade—A combined echocardiographic and hemodynamic study. Circulation 70:966, 1984.
32. Shabetai R, Fowler NO, Guntheroth WG: The hemodynamics of cardiac tamponade and constrictive pericarditis. Am J Cardiol 26:480, 1970.
33. Shabetai R, Mangiardi L, Bhargava V, et al: The pericardium and cardiac function. Prog Cardiovasc Dis 22:107, 1979.
34. Winer HE, Kronzon I: Absence of paradoxical pulse in patients with cardiac tamponade and atrial septal defects. Am J Cardiol 44:378, 1979.
35. Hoit BD, Shaw D: The paradoxical pulse in tamponade: Mechanisms and echocardiographic correlates. Echocardiography 11:477, 1994.
36. Kuvin JT, Harati NA, Pandian NG, et al: Postoperative cardiac tamponade in the modern surgical era. Ann Thorac Surg 74:1148, 2002.
37. Vaska K, Wann LS, Sagar K, Klopfenstein HS: Pleural effusion as a cause of right ventricular diastolic collapse. Circulation 86:609, 1992.
38. Chuttani K, Pandian NG, Mohanty PK: Left ventricular diastolic collapse: An echocardiographic sign of regional cardiac tamponade. Circulation 83:1999, 1991.

39. Russo AM, O'Connor WH, Waxman HL: Atypical presentations and echocardiographic findings in patients with cardiac tamponade occurring early and late after cardiac surgery. Chest 104:71, 1993.
40. Merce J, Sagrista-Sauleda J, Permanyer-Miralda G, et al: Should pericardial drainage be performed routinely in patients who have a large pericardial effusion without tamponade? Am J Med 105:106, 1998.
41. Tsang TS, Enriquez-Sarano M, Freeman WK, et al: Consecutive 1127 therapeutic echocardiographically guided pericardiocenteses: Clinical profile, practice patterns, and outcomes spanning 21 years. Mayo Clin Proc 77:429, 2002.
42. Bruning R, Muehlstaedt M, Becker C, et al: Computed tomography–fluoroscopy guided drainage of pericardial effusions: Experience in 11 cases. Invest Radiol 37:328, 2002.
43. Wang HJ, Hsu KL, Chiang FT, et al: Technical and prognostic outcomes of double-balloon pericardiotomy for large malignancy-related pericardial effusions. Chest 122:893, 2002.
44. Del Barrio LG, Morales JH, Delgado C, et al: Percutaneous balloon window for patients with symptomatic pericardial effusion. Cardiovasc Intervent Radiol 25:360, 2002.
45. Maisch B, Ristic AD, Rupp H, Spodick DH: Pericardial access using the PerDUCER and flexible percutaneous pericardioscopy. Am J Cardiol 88:1323, 2001.
46. Koh KK, Kim EJ, Cho CH, et al: Adenosine deaminase and carcinoembryonic antigen in pericardial effusion diagnosis, especially in suspected tuberculous pericarditis. Circulation 89:2728, 1994.
47. Koh KK, In HH, Lee KH, et al: New scoring system using tumor markers in diagnosing patients with moderate pericardial effusions. Int J Cardiol 61:5, 1997.
48. Burgess LJ, Reuter H, Carstens ME, et al: The use of adenosine deaminase and interferon-gamma as diagnostic tools for tuberculous pericarditis. Chest 122:900, 2002.

Constrictive Pericarditis

49. Ling LH, Oh JK Schaff HV, et al: Constrictive pericarditis in the modern era: Evolving clinical spectrum and impact on outcome after pericardiectomy. Circulation 100:1380, 1999.
50. Oh JK, Hatle LK, Seward JB, et al: Diagnostic role of Doppler echocardiography in constrictive pericarditis. J Am Coll Cardiol 23:154, 1994.
51. Wolozin MW, Ortola FV, Spodick DH, Seifter JL: Release of atrial natriuretic factor after pericardiectomy for chronic constrictive pericarditis. Am J Cardiol 62:1323, 1988.
52. Klein AL, Cohen GI: Doppler echocardiographic assessment of constrictive pericarditis, cardiac amyloidosis, and cardiac tamponade. Cleve Clin J Med 59:278, 1992.
53. Oh JK, Tajik AJ, Appleton CP, et al: Preload reduction to unmask the characteristic Doppler features of constrictive pericarditis. A new observation. Circulation 96:3799, 1997.
54. Izumi C, Iga K, Sekiguchi K, et al: Usefulness of the transgastric view by transesophageal echocardiography in evaluating thickened pericardium in patients with constrictive pericarditis. J Am Soc Echocardiogr 15:1004, 2002.
55. Tabata T, Kabbani S, Murray RD, et al: Differences in the respiratory variation between pulmonary venous and mitral inflow Doppler velocities in patients with constrictive pericarditis with and without atrial fibrillation. J Am Coll Cardiol 37:1936, 2001.
56. Lorell BH, Grossman W: Profiles in constrictive pericarditis, restrictive cardiomyopathy, and cardiac tamponade. *In* Baim DS, Grossman W (eds): Cardiac Catheterization, Angiography and Intervention. Baltimore, Williams & Wilkins, 1996, pp 801-857.
57. Abdalla IA, Murray RD, Lee JC, et al: Does rapid volume loading during transesophageal echocardiography differentiate constrictive pericarditis from restrictive cardiomyopathy? Echocardiography 19:125, 2002.
58. Breen J: Imaging of the pericardium. J Thorac Imag 16:47, 2001.
59. Klein AL, Chen GI, Pietrolungo JF, et al: Differentiation of constrictive pericarditis from restrictive cardiomyopathy by Doppler transesophageal echocardiographic measurements of respiratory variation in pulmonary venous flow. J Am Coll Cardiol 22:1935, 1993.
60. Uchida T, Bando K, Minatoya K, et al: Pericardiectomy for constrictive pericarditis using the harmonic scalpel. Ann Thorac Surg 72:924, 2001.
61. Trotter MC, Chung KC, Ochsner JL, McFadden PM: Pericardiectomy for pericardial constriction. Am Surg 62:304, 1996.

Specific Causes of Pericardial Disease

62. Sagrista-Sauleda J, Barrabes JA, Permanyer-Miralda G, Soler-Soler J: Purulent pericarditis; review of a 20 year experience in a general hospital. J Am Coll Cardiol 22:1661, 1993.
63. Brook I, Frazier EH: Microbiology of acute purulent pericarditis. A 12-year experience in a military hospital. Arch Intern Med 156:1857, 1996.
64. Brook I: Pericarditis due to anaerobic bacteria. Cardiology 97:55, 2002.
65. Goodman LJ: Purulent pericarditis. Curr Treat Options Cardiovasc Med 2:343, 2000.
66. Keersmaekers T, Elshot SR, Sergeant PT: Primary bacterial pericarditis. Acta Cardiol 57:387, 2002.
67. Hakim JG, Matenga JA, Siziya S: Myocardial dysfunction in human immunodeficiency virus: An echocardiographic study of 157 patients in hospital in Zimbabwe. Heart 76:161, 1996.
68. Estok L, Wallach F: Cardiac tamponade in a patient with AIDS: A review of pericardial disease in patients with HIV infection. Mt Sinai J Med 65:33, 1998.
69. Silva-Cardoso J, Moura B, Martins L, et al: Pericardial involvement in human immunodeficiency virus infection. Chest 115:418, 1999.
70. Heidenreich P, Eisenberg M, Keel L, et al: Pericardial effusion in AIDS: Incidence and survival. Circulation 92:3229, 1995.
71. Sagrista-Sauleda J, Permanyer-Miralda G, Soler-Soler J: Tuberculous pericarditis: Ten year experience with a prospective protocol for diagnosis and treatment. J Am Coll Cardiol 11:724, 1988.
72. Barbara W, Trautner O, Rabih O: Tuberculous pericarditis: Optimal diagnosis and management. Clin Infect Dis 33:954, 2001.
73. Cegielski JP, Devlin BH, Morris AJ, et al: Comparison of PCR, culture, and histopathology for diagnosis of tuberculous pericarditis. J Clin Microbiol 35:3254, 1997.
74. Strang JI, Kakaza HHS, Gibson DG, et al: Controlled clinical trial of complete open surgical drainage and of prednisolone in treatment of tuberculous pericardial effusion in Transkei. Lancet 2:759, 1988.
75. Wheat L, Stein L, Corya BC, et al: Pericarditis as a manifestation of histoplasmosis during two large urban outbreaks. Medicine (Baltimore) 62:110, 1983.
76. Amundson DE: Perplexing pericarditis caused by coccidioidomycosis. South Med J 86:694, 1993.
77. Rostand SG, Rutsky EA: Pericarditis in end-stage renal disease. Cardiol Clin 8:701, 1998.
78. Oliva PB, Hammill SC, Talano JV: Effect of definition on incidence of postinfarction pericarditis. Is it time to redefine postinfarction pericarditis? Circulation 90:1537, 1994.
79. Tarbell N, Thompson L, Mauch P: Thoracic irradiation in Hodgkin's disease: Disease control and long-term complications. Int J Radiat Oncol Biol Phys 18:275, 1990.
80. Frankel KM: Treating malignancy-related effusions. Chest 123:1775, 2003.
81. Eren NT, Akar AR: Primary pericardial mesothelioma. Curr Treat Options Oncol 5:369, 2002.
82. Fernandez-Muixi J, Vidal F, Bardaji A: Recurrent pericarditis and cardiac tamponade in rheumatoid arthritis: Effectiveness of colchicine. Br J Rheumatol 33:596, 1994.
83. Armstrong GP, Whalley GA, Doughty RN, et al: Left ventricular function in scleroderma. Br J Rheumatol 35:983, 1996.
84. Ajuni SC, Glazier S, Blankenship L, et al: Perforation after percutaneous coronary interventions: Clinical, angiographic, and therapeutic observations. Cathet Cardiovasc Diagn 32:206, 1994.

CHAPTER 65

Traumatic Heart Disease

Kenneth L. Mattox • Anthony L. Estrera • Matthew J. Wall, Jr.

Incidence

In the United States, trauma currently is the fourth leading cause of death, and it is the leading cause of death in persons younger than 40 years of age. Thoracic trauma is responsible for 25 percent of the annual 50,000 deaths from vehicular accidents. As high a proportion as one-fourth of these deaths are due to traumatic cardiac injury. The actual incidence of cardiac injury from all of the diverse causes and classifications (including the confusing "cardiac contusion") is unknown. Cardiac injury may account for 10 percent of deaths from gunshot wounds.[1] Penetrating cardiac trauma is a highly lethal injury, with relatively few victims surviving long enough to reach the hospital. In a series of 1198 patients with penetrating cardiac injuries in South Africa, only 6 percent patients reached the hospital with any signs of life.[2] With improvements in organized emergency medical transport systems, up to 45 percent of those who sustain significant traumatic heart injury may reach the emergency department.

Blunt cardiac injuries have been reported less frequently than penetrating injuries. However, 10 to 70 percent of motor vehicle fatalities may have been the result of blunt cardiac rupture.

Etiology and Patterns of Cardiac Trauma

Categorization of traumatic heart disease is based on the mechanism of injury (i.e., penetrating, nonpenetrating [blunt], iatrogenic, metabolic, and other) (Table 65–1).

Penetrating Cardiac Trauma

Penetrating trauma is the most common cause of significant cardiac injury seen in the hospital setting, with the predominant injury being from guns and knives.[3-5] Other mechanisms, such as shotguns, ice picks, and fence impalement have also been reported.

The location of injury to the heart often correlates with the location of injury on the chest wall. Because of anterior location, the anatomical chambers at greatest risk for injury are the right and left ventricles. In a review of 711 patients with penetrating cardiac trauma, 54 percent sustained stab wounds and 42 percent had gunshot wounds. The right ventricle was injured in 40 percent of the cases, the left ventricle in 40 percent, the right atrium in 24 percent, and the left atrium in 3 percent. One-third of cardiac injuries involved multiple cardiac structures.[4] Significant intracardiac injuries involved the coronary arteries (n = 39), valvular apparatus (mitral) (n = 2), intracardiac fistulas (i.e., ventricular septal defects [VSD]) (n = 14), and unusual injuries (n = 10). Only 2 percent of patients surviving the initial injury and undergoing an operation required reoperation for a residual defect.[4]

Blunt Cardiac Trauma

Nonpenetrating or *blunt cardiac trauma* has replaced the term "cardiac contusion" and describes injury ranging from minor bruises of the myocardium to cardiac rupture. It can be caused by direct energy transferal to the heart or compression of the heart between the sternum and the vertebral column at the time of the accident, and even including cardiac contusion and cardiac rupture during external cardiac massage as a part of cardiopulmonary resuscitation (CPR). Within this spectrum, blunt cardiac injuries can manifest as free septal rupture, free wall rupture, coronary artery thrombosis, cardiac failure, complex arrhythmia, simple arrhythmia, and/or rupture of chordae tendineae or papillary muscles.[6] The incidence can be as high as three-fourths of the patients with severe bodily trauma. Causes include motor vehicle accidents, vehicular-pedestrian accidents, falls, crush injuries, blasts, assaults, CPR, and recreational events. Such injury is often associated with sternal or rib fractures. In one report, a fatal cardiac dysrhythmia occurred when the sternum was struck by a baseball,[7] which may be a form of commotio cordis (see Chap. 75).[8]

Cardiac rupture carries a significant risk of mortality. The biomechanics of cardiac rupture include[9] direct transmission of increased intrathoracic pressure to the chambers of the heart; hydraulic effect from a large force applied to the abdominal or extremity veins, causing force to be transmitted to the right atrium, resulting in rupture; decelerating force between fixed and mobile areas, which explains atriocaval tears; myocardial contusion, necrosis, and delayed rupture; and penetration from a broken rib or fractured sternum.

Blunt rupture of the cardiac septum occurs most frequently in late diastole or early systole near the apex of the heart. Multiple ruptures and disruption of the conduction system have been reported.[10] From autopsy data, blunt cardiac trauma with

TABLE 65–1 Etiology of Traumatic Heart Diseases

I. Penetrating	
	A. Stab wounds—knives, swords, ice picks, fence posts, wire, sporting
	B. Gunshot wounds—low-high caliber, handgun, rifles, nail guns, lawnmower projectiles
	C. Shotgun wounds—close range, distant
II. Nonpenetrating (Blunt)	
	A. Motor vehicle accident
	1. Seat belt
	2. Air bag
	B. Vehicular-pedestrian accident
	C. Falls from height
	D. Crushing—industrial accident
	E. Blasts—explosives, grenades
	F. Assault (aggravated)
	G. Sternal or rib fractures
	H. Recreational—sporting events (bull goring), baseball
III. Iatrogenic	
	A. Catheter induced
	B. Pericardiocentesis induced
IV. Metabolic	
	A. Traumatic response to injury
	B. "Stunning"
	C. Systemic inflammatory response syndrome (SIRS)
V. Others	
	A. Burn
	B. Electrical
	C. Factitious—needles, foreign bodies
	D. Embolic—missiles

ventricular rupture most often involves the left ventricle, followed by the right ventricle, and, least often, the left atrium. VSD can occur, with the most common tear involving both the membranous and the muscular portions of the septum. Injury to only the membranous portion of the septum is the least common blunt VSD. Traumatic rupture of the thoracic aorta is associated with lethal cardiac rupture in almost 25 percent of cases.

Blunt pericardial rupture results from pericardial tears secondary to increased intraabdominal pressure or lateral decelerative forces. Tears occur on the left side, most often parallel to the phrenic nerve, next most often to the diaphragmatic surface of the pericardium, then to the right of the pleuropericardium, and finally to the mediastinum. Cardiac herniation with cardiac dysfunction can occur in conjunction with these tears. The heart can be displaced into either pleural cavity or even into the peritoneum. In the instance of right pericardial rupture, the heart can become torsed, leading to the surprising discovery of an "empty" pericardial cavity at resuscitative left anterolateral thoracotomy. With a left-sided cardiac herniation through a pericardial tear, a distending heart prevents the heart from returning to the pericardium, and the term *incarcerated heart* has been applied. Venous filling is impaired, and unless the cardiac herniation is reduced, hypotension and cardiac arrest can occur.

Iatrogenic Cardiac Injury

Iatrogenic cardiac injury can occur with central venous line insertion, cardiac catheterization procedures, and pericardiocentesis. Cardiac injuries caused by central venous lines usually occur with placement from either the left subclavian or the left internal jugular vein.[11] Perforation causing tamponade has also been reported with a right internal jugular introducer sheath for transjugular intrahepatic portocaval shunts. Vigorous insertion of left-sided central lines, especially during dilation of the line tract, can lead to cardiac perforations. Even appropriate technique carries a discrete rate of iatrogenic injury secondary to central venous catheterization. Common sites of cardiac injury include the superior caval-atrial junction and the superior vena cava–innominate junction. These small perforations often lead to a compensated cardiac tamponade. Drainage by pericardiocentesis is often unsuccessful, and evacuation via subxiphoid pericardial window or full median sternotomy is required. Once access to the pericardial space is gained, the site of injury has often sealed and may be difficult to find.

Complications from coronary catheterization, including perforation of the coronary arteries, cardiac perforation, and aortic dissection can be catastrophic and require emergency surgical intervention. The incidence of coronary perforation with balloon angioplasty is estimated to be 0.1 to 0.2 percent, but with advanced interventional techniques (e.g., rotablation, directional atherectomy, coronary artery stenting, and laser ablation), the incidence may be as high as 3 percent.[12]

Other potential iatrogenic causes of cardiac injury include external and internal cardiac massage, right ventricular injury during pericardiocentesis, and intracardiac injections.[13]

Metabolic Cardiac Injury

Metabolic cardiac injury refers to cardiac dysfunction in response to traumatic injury and may be associated with injuries caused by burns, electrical injury, sepsis, the systemic inflammatory response syndrome, and multisystem trauma.[14-16] The exact mechanism responsible for this dysfunction is unclear, but responses to trauma induce a mediator storm, which is a release of cytokines that may have a direct affect on the myocardium. Endotoxin, tumor necrosis factor-alpha, tumor necrosis factor-beta, interleukin-1, interleukin-6, interleukin-10, catecholamines (epinephrine, norepinephrine), cell-adhesion molecules, and nitric oxide are all possible responsible mediators.[16-18]

Metabolic cardiac injury can manifest clinically as conduction disturbances or decreased contractility leading to decreased output. Myocardial depression can occur in response to the mediator storm and can alter calcium utilization and depression of the myocyte responsiveness to beta-adrenergic stimulation.[19,20] Myocytes have altered calcium utilization in patients with injuries from burns. The activation of constitutive nitric oxide synthase can modulate cardiac responsiveness to cholinergic and adrenergic stimulation, and production of inducible nitric oxide synthase can depress myocyte contractile responsiveness to beta-adrenergic agonists. The myocardial depressive effects appear to be reversible.[16]

Treatment of metabolic cardiac injury has been supportive, with correction of the initiating insults, but some practitioners have attempted to address the involved mediators using intravenous milrinone, corticosteroids, arginine, granulocyte-macrophage colony-stimulating factor, and glutamate.[20-22] Use of an intraaortic counterpulsation balloon pump can be considered to treat such myocardial depression, but controlled series do not exist to test this hypothesis.

Burns

Cardiac complications in the early postburn period are a major cause of death. The initial cardiovascular effect of burn injury is attributable to the profound reduction in cardiac output that can occur within minutes of the injury. The overall cardiac response has been described as an ebb and flow pattern, with the initial ebb phase lasting between 1 and 3 days and marked by hypovolemia and myocardial depression, and the flow phase characterized by a prolonged period of increased metabolic demand with increased cardiac output and peripheral blood flow. The reduction in cardiac output observed in the initial period of burn injury is the result of a dramatic and rapid decrease in intravascular volume due to a "capillary leak" and of a direct myocardial depression. Hypovolemia results from the capillary leak caused by endothelial injury and may be mediated by platelet-activating factor, complement, cytokines, arachidonic acid, or oxygen free radicals. Myocardial depression manifested by a decrease in myocardial contractility and abnormalities in ventricular compliance becomes apparent with a total body surface area burn of 20 to 25 percent. Myocardial-depressant factor, tumor necrosis factor, vasopressin, oxygen free radicals, and interleukins may be responsible for the depression.

Electrical Injury

Cardiac complications are most often the cause of death after electrical injury. An estimated 1100 to 1300 deaths occur annually in the United States from electrical injury (including lighting strikes). The cardiac complications after electrical injury include immediate cardiac arrest, acute myocardial necrosis with or without ventricular failure, pseudoinfarction, myocardial ischemia, dysrhythmias, conduction abnormalities, acute hypertension with peripheral vasospasm, and asymptomatic, nonspecific abnormalities evident on an electrocardiogram (ECG). Damage from electrical injury is due to direct effects on the excitable tissues, heat generated from the current, and accompanying associated injuries (e.g., falls, explosions, or fires).

Others

Intrapericardial and intracardiac foreign bodies can cause complications of acute suppurative pericarditis, chronic constrictive pericarditis, foreign body reaction, and hemopericardium.[23] Intrapericardial foreign bodies that have been reported to result in complications include bullets, hand grenades, shrapnel, knitting needles, and hypodermic needles. Needles and similar foreign bodies have been noted after deliberate insertion by patients, usually those with psychiatric diagnoses. A report by LeMaire and colleagues[23] advocated removal of those intrapericardial foreign bodies that are greater than 1 cm in size, that are contaminated, or that produce symptoms.

Intracardiac Missiles

Intracardiac missiles are foreign bodies that are embedded in the myocardium, retained in the trabeculations of the endocardial surface, or free in a cardiac chamber or in the pericardium. These are the result of direct penetrating thoracic injury or injury to a peripheral vascular structure with embolization to the heart. Location and other conditions determine the type of complications that can occur and the treatment required. Observation might be considered when the missile is (1) right sided, (2) embedded completely in the wall, (3) contained within a fibrous covering, (4) not contaminated, and (5) producing no symptoms. Right-sided missiles can embolize to the lung, at which point they can be removed, or, in rare cases, they embolize "paradoxically" through a patent foramen ovale or atrial septal defect.[24] Left-sided missiles can manifest as systemic embolization shortly after the initial injury. Diagnosis is determined with radiographs in two projections, fluoroscopy, echocardiography, or angiography. Treatment of retained missiles is individualized. Removal is recommended for missiles that are left-sided, larger than 1 to 2 cm, rough in shape, or produce symptoms.[24] Although direct approach, either with or without cardiopulmonary bypass, has been advocated in the past, a large percentage of right-sided foreign bodies can now be removed by interventional radiologists.

Clinical Presentation and Pathophysiology

Penetrating Cardiac Trauma

Wounds involving the precordial box, the anatomical area that includes the epigastrium and precordium within 3 cm of the sternum, carry a high incidence of cardiac injury. Stab wounds present a more predictable path of injury than gunshot wounds. Patients with cardiac injury can present with a clinical spectrum from full cardiac arrest with no vital signs, to asymptomatic with normal vital signs. Up to 80 percent of stab wounds eventually manifest tamponade (see Chap. 64). The weapon injures the pericardium and heart, but as the weapon is removed, the pericardium seals and may not allow blood to escape. Rapid bleeding into the pericardium favors clotting rather than defibrination.[25] As pericardial fluid accumulates, a decrease in ventricular filling occurs, leading to a decrease in stroke volume. A compensatory rise in catecholamines leads to tachycardia and increased right-sided heart filling pressures. The limits of distensibility are reached, and the septum shifts toward the left side, further compromising left ventricular function. If this cycle persists, ventricular function can continue to deteriorate, leading to irreversible shock. As little as 60 to 100 ml of blood in the pericardial sac can produce the clinical picture of tamponade.[25]

The rate of accumulation depends on the location of the wound. Because it has a thicker wall, wounds to the right ventricle seal themselves more readily than wounds to the right atrium. Patients with injuries to the coronary arteries present with rapid onset of tamponade combined with cardiac ischemia. With injuries to the left ventricle, the decompensated state can worsen, leading to cardiac arrest. The right side of the heart can compensate for injuries, and rapid deterioration may not occur; and patients with this sort of injury can benefit from early diagnosis and immediate intervention.

The classic finding of the Beck triad (muffled heart sounds, hypotension, and distended neck veins) is seen in only 10 percent of patients. Pulsus paradoxus (a substantial fall in systolic blood pressure during inspiration) and Kussmaul sign (increase in jugular venous distention on inspiration) may be present but are not reliable signs (see Chaps. 8 and 64).[26] A very valuable and reproducible sign of pericardial tamponade is a narrowing of the pulse pressure. An elevation of the central venous pressure often accompanies rapid and cyclic hyperresuscitation with crystalloid solutions, but in such instances, there is a widening of the pulse pressure. Elevation of the central venous pressure and narrowing of the pulse pressure represents a pericardial tamponade syndrome until proven otherwise.

In contrast to stab wounds, gunshot wounds to the heart are more frequently associated with hemorrhage than with tamponade. Twenty percent of gunshot wounds to the heart manifest as tamponade. With firearms, the kinetic energy is greater and the wounds to the heart and pericardium are frequently larger. Thus, these patients present in arrest more often due to hemorrhage.[26]

Nonpenetrating Cardiac Trauma

As in penetrating cardiac trauma, clinically severe blunt cardiac trauma (e.g., cardiac rupture) manifests as either tamponade or as hemorrhage, depending on the status of the pericardium. If the pericardium is intact, tamponade develops; if it is not intact, extrapericardial bleeding occurs and hypovolemic shock ensues. Tamponade is sometimes combined with hypovolemia, thus complicating the clinical presentation.

Blunt cardiac injury can be divided into clinically significant and clinically insignificant injuries. Clinically significant injuries include cardiac rupture (ventricular or atrial), septal rupture, valvular dysfunction, and coronary thrombosis. These injuries manifest as tamponade, hemorrhage, or severe cardiac dysfunction. Septal rupture and valvular dysfunction (leaflet tear, papillary muscle, or chordal rupture) can initially appear without symptoms but later demonstrate the delayed sequela of heart failure.[25]

Blunt cardiac injury can also appear as an arrythmia, most commonly premature ventricular contractions, the precise mechanism of which is unknown. Ventricular tachycardia can occur and degenerate into ventricular fibrillation. Supraventricular tachyarrhythmias can also occur. These symptoms commonly occur within the first 24 to 48 hours after injury (see Chap. 32).

Small isolated tears in the pericardium can lead to cardiac herniation. This is a rare complication of pericardial rupture and depends on the size of the pericardial tear. If large enough, cardiac herniation can occur, leading to acute cardiac dysfunction.[25]

Evaluation

Evaluation of suspected traumatic heart injury differs, depending on the whether the presenting patient is clinically stable or in extremis.

Initial Assessment

The diagnosis of traumatic heart injury requires a high index of suspicion (Fig. 65–1). On initial presentation to the emergency center, airway, breathing, and circulation (ABCs) under Advanced Trauma Life Support (ATLS) protocol are evaluated and established.[27] Two large-bore intravenous catheters are inserted, and blood is typed and cross-matched. The patient undergoes focused abdominal sonogram for trauma (FAST) and is examined for the Beck triad of muffled heart sounds, hypotension, and distended neck veins, as well as for pulsus paradoxus and Kussmaul sign. These findings suggest cardiac injury but are present in only 10 percent of patients with cardiac tamponade. If the FAST demonstrates pericardial fluid in the unstable patient (systemic blood pressure <90 mm Hg), immediate transfer to the operating room for definitive repair or damage control is required.

Patients in extremis require immediate surgical intervention and often require emergency thoracotomy for resuscitation. The clear indications for emergency department thoracotomy by surgical personnel include the following[28,29]:

1. Salvageable postinjury cardiac arrest (e.g., patients who have witnessed cardiac arrest with high likelihood of intrathoracic injury, especially penetrating cardiac wounds)
2. Severe postinjury hypotension (i.e., systolic blood pressure <60 mm Hg) due to cardiac tamponade, air embolism, or thoracic hemorrhage

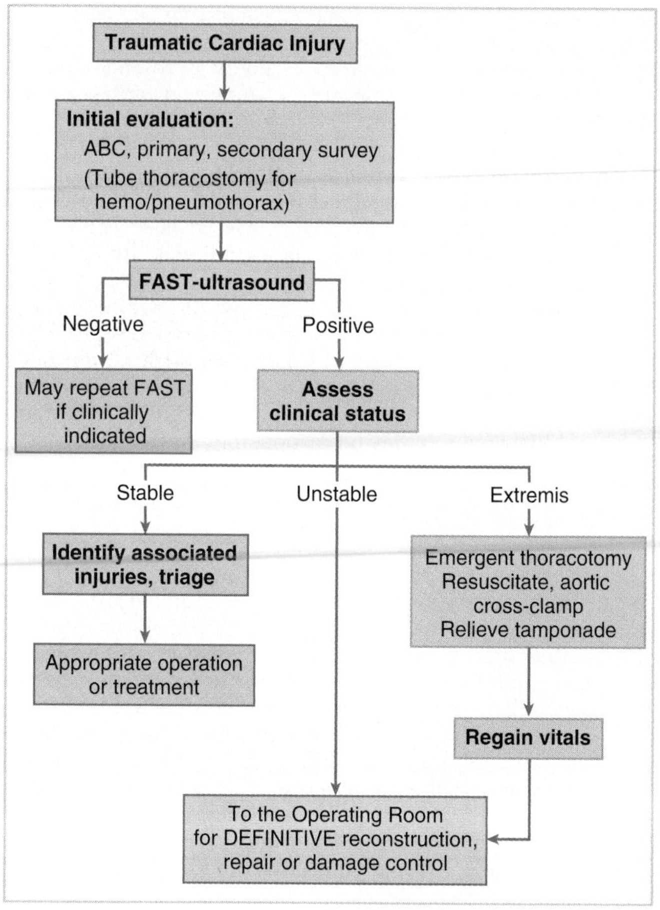

FIGURE 65–1 Algorithm for the initial assessment of traumatic cardiac injury. ABC = airway, breathing, and circulation; FAST = focused abdominal sonogram for trauma.

If, after resuscitative thoracotomy, vital signs are regained, the patient is transferred to the operating room for definitive repair. The patient with confirmed pericardial fluid by FAST, with normal vital signs (systemic blood pressure >90 mm Hg) may undergo a thorough evaluation to identify associated injuries. If other injuries are excluded, then open exploration may be required to exclude cardiac injury. In the absence of known causes of pericardial fluid (e.g., malignant pericardial effusion), a missed cardiac injury can lead to delayed bleeding, deterioration, or death.

Chest radiography is nonspecific, but it can identify hemothorax or pneumothorax and demonstrate an enlarged cardiac silhouette suggesting pericardial fluid. Other possibly indicated examinations include ultrasonography, central venous pressure measurements, subxiphoid pericardial window, thoracoscopy, laparoscopy, and pericardiocentesis.

ULTRASONOGRAPHY. Surgeons are increasingly performing ultrasonography for thoracic trauma, paralleling the use of ultrasonography for blunt abdominal trauma (see Chap. 11). The FAST evaluates four anatomical windows for the presence of intraabdominal or pericardial fluid (Fig. 65–2).[30] Ultrasonography in this setting is not intended to reach the precision of studies performed in the radiology suite but is merely intended to determine the presence of abnormal fluid collections, which aids in surgical decision making.[31] Ultrasonography is safe, portable, and expeditious and can be repeated as indicated.[31] If performed by a trained surgeon, the FAST examination has a sensitivity of nearly 100 percent and a specificity of 97.3 percent.[32]

To evaluate more subtle findings of blunt cardiac injury in the stable patient, transthoracic echocardiography (TTE) or

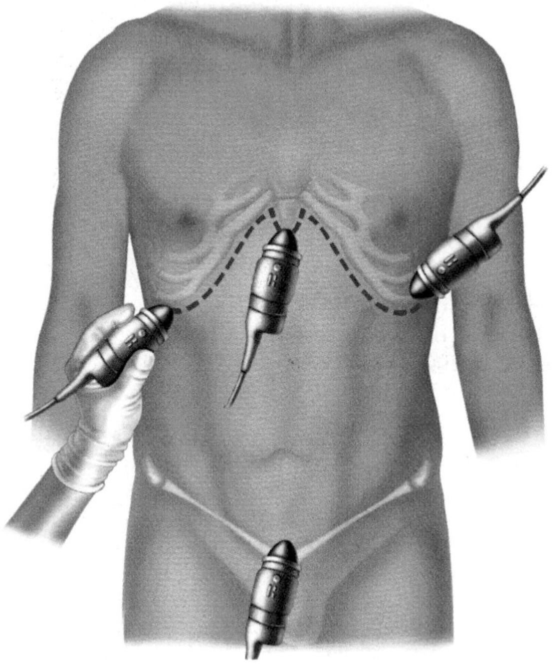

FIGURE 65–2 Focused Assessment for the Sonographic examination of the Trauma victim (FAST). (From Rozycki GS, Feliciano DV, Schmidt JA, et al: The role of surgeon performed ultrasound in patients with possible cardiac wounds. Ann Surg 223:737, 1996.)

transesophageal echocardiography (TEE) can be used. TEE is useful in identifying and characterizing valvular abnormalities and septal defects.

SUBXIPHOID PERICARDIAL WINDOW. Subxiphoid pericardial window has been performed both in the emergency department and in the operating room with the patient under either general or local anesthesia. Via a subxiphoid vertical incision, a small hole is made in the pericardium to determine the presence of blood. In a prospective study, Meyer and coworkers[33] compared the subxiphoid pericardial window with echocardiography in cases of penetrating heart injury and reported that the sensitivity and specificity of subxiphoid pericardial window were 100 percent and 92 percent, respectively, compared with 56 percent and 93 percent with echocardiography. They suggested the difference in sensitivity may have been due to the presence of hemothorax, which can confuse the pericardial and pleural space, or due to the fact that the blood had drained into the pleura.[33]

The disadvantage of a subxiphoid pericardial window is that it is an invasive procedure, and if a major injury is found, a second thoracic incision is required for definitive repair. Although there has been significant controversy in the past with regard to the indication for subxiphoid pericardial window, recent enthusiasm for ultrasonographic evaluation has almost eliminated the role of subxiphoid pericardial window in the evaluation of cardiac trauma.

PERICARDIOCENTESIS (see Chap. 64). Pericardiocentesis has had significant historical support, especially when the majority of penetrating cardiac wounds were produced by ice picks and the (surviving) patients arrived several hours and/or days after injury. In such instances, there was a natural triage of the more severe cardiac injuries and the intrapericardial blood had become defibrinated and was easy to remove. Currently, many trauma surgeons discourage pericardiocentesis for acute trauma. In general, pericardiocentesis has historically been used as a diagnostic or therapeutic maneuver to drain nonclotted pericardial fluid. In the setting of trauma, cardiac tamponade is acute and caused by hemorrhage. Clot forms quickly and is not amenable to needle drainage. Recurrence of tamponade and subsequent increase in mortality, as well as a significant incidence of false-negative results and potential for iatrogenic injury, makes pericardiocentesis a far less than optimal diagnostic tool.[13]

Indications for its use may apply in the case of iatrogenic injury caused by cardiac catheterization, at which time immediate decompression of the tamponade may be life saving, or in the trauma setting when a surgeon is not available.

Evaluation of Blunt Cardiac Injury

ELECTROCARDIOGRAPHY. In cases of blunt cardiac injury, conduction disturbances are common, and, thus, a screening 12-lead ECG could be helpful for evaluation (see Chap. 9). Sinus tachycardia is the most common rhythm disturbance seen. Other possible disturbances include T wave and ST segment changes (as seen with myocardial bruising), sinus bradycardia, first-degree atrioventricular block, right bundle branch block, right bundle branch block with hemiblock, third-degree block, atrial fibrillation, premature ventricular contractions, ventricular tachycardia, and ventricular fibrillation.

CARDIAC ENZYMES. Much has previously been written about the use of cardiac enzyme determinations in evaluating blunt cardiac injury. However, no correlation between serum assays (e.g., creatine phosphokinase myocardial band, cardiac troponin T, or cardiac troponin I) and identification and prognosis of injury has been demonstrated with blunt cardiac injury.[35-37] Therefore, cardiac enzyme assays should not be performed unless one is evaluating concomitant coronary artery disease.[32]

Treatment

Prehospital and Emergency Department

Only a small subset of patients with significant cardiac injury ever reaches the emergency department, and expeditious transport to a designated trauma facility is essential to survival. Transport times of less than 5 minutes and successful endotracheal intubation are positive factors for survival.

Definitive Treatment

Definitive treatment involves surgical exposure through a thoracotomy (Fig. 65–3A) or median sternotomy (Fig. 65–3B). The mainstays of treatment are relief of tamponade and correction of aberrant physiology, which involves correction of the acidosis and hypothermia and reestablishment of effective coronary perfusion (i.e., resuscitation of the heart).

Cardiorrhaphy should be performed by experienced surgeons (Fig. 65–4). Poor technique can result in enlargement of the lacerations or injury to the coronary arteries. If the initial treating physician is uncomfortable with the suturing technique, digital pressure can be applied until a more experienced surgeon arrives. Other techniques that have been described include the use of a Foley balloon catheter and a skin stapler (Fig. 65–5).[5]

Exposure to the heart is accomplished by a left anterolateral thoracotomy, which allows access to the pericardium and heart and exposure for aortic cross-clamping if necessary. This incision can be extended across the sternum to gain access to the right side of the chest and for better exposure of the right atrium or right ventricle. This usually requires ligation of both internal thoracic arteries. Manual access to the right hemithorax from the left side of the chest is achieved through the anterior mediastinum by blunt dissection. This maneuver allows rapid evaluation of the right side of the chest for major injuries without transecting the sternum. Once the left pleural space is entered, the lung is retracted to expose the descending thoracic aorta for cross-clamping of the pericardium for exposure. The amount of blood present in the left side of the chest indicates whether one is dealing with hemorrhage or tamponade. The pericardial sac anterior to the phrenopericardial vessels and phrenic nerve is opened, injuries are rapidly identified, and repair is performed.

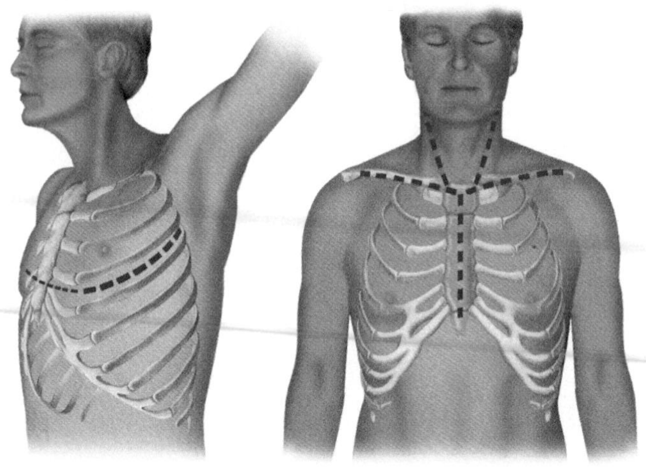

A B

FIGURE 65–3 Incisions for cardiac injury. **A,** Left anterior thoracotomy (extension across the sternum if required). **B,** Median sternotomy (extension to the neck can be performed for exposure of the great vessels).

In selected cases, particularly stab wounds to the precordium, median sternotomy can be used. This incision allows excellent exposure to the anterior structures of the heart, but difficulty with access to the posterior mediastinal structures and descending thoracic aorta for cross-clamping may be encountered.

Mechanical support is not often used in the acute setting.[5]

BLUNT CARDIAC INJURY. Much debate and discussion has occurred about the clinical relevance of "cardiac contusion." Most trauma surgeons conclude that this diagnosis should be eliminated because it does not affect how one treats these injuries. Thus, a normotensive patient with a normal initial ECG and suspected blunt cardiac injury is managed in emergency department or chest pain observation units, with no expected clinical significance. Patients with an abnormal ECG are admitted for monitoring and treated accordingly. Patients who present in cardiogenic shock are evaluated for a structural injury, which is then repaired.

Results

Factors determining survival in patients with traumatic cardiac injury are mechanism of injury, location of injury, associated injuries, coronary artery involvement, presence of tamponade, length of prehospital transport, requirement for resuscitative thoracotomy, and experience of the trauma team. The overall hospital survival rate for patients with penetrating heart injuries ranges from 30 to 90 percent.

The survival rate for patients with stab wounds is 70 to 80 percent, whereas survival after gunshot wounds is between 30 and 40 percent.[26] Cardiac rupture has a worse prognosis than penetrating injuries to the heart, with a survival rate of approximately 20 percent.

COMPLICATIONS. Primary injury-related cardiac complications include coronary artery injury, valvular apparatus injury (annulus, papillary muscles, and chordae tendineae), intracardiac fistulas, arrhythmias, and delayed tamponade. These delayed sequelae have been reported to have a broad range (4 to 56 percent), depending on the definition of complication.

Coronary artery injury is a rare complication, occurring in 5 to 9 percent of patients with cardiac injures, with a 69 percent rate of mortality.[4] A coronary artery injury is most often controlled by simple ligation, but bypass grafting using saphenous vein may be required for proximal left

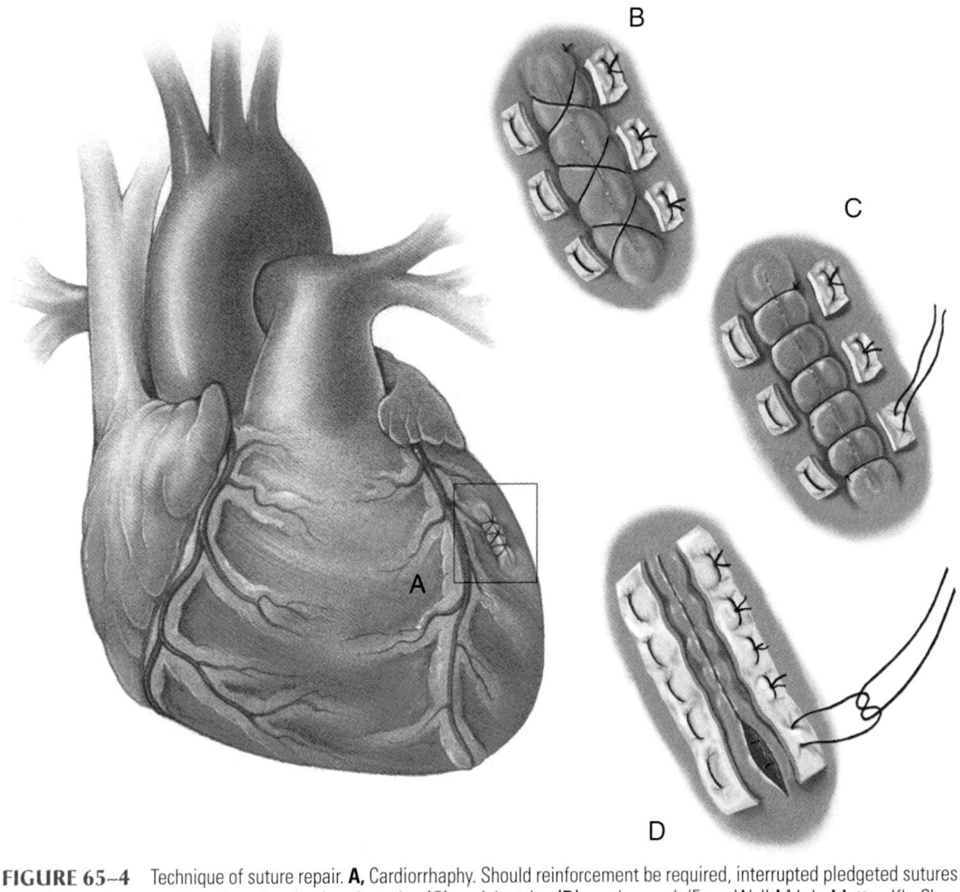

FIGURE 65–4 Technique of suture repair. **A,** Cardiorrhaphy. Should reinforcement be required, interrupted pledgeted sutures **(B)**, pledgeted sutures around previously placed staples **(C)**, or felt strips **(D)** can be used. (From Wall MJ Jr, Mattox KL, Chen CD, Baldwin JC: Acute management of complex cardiac injuries. J Trauma 42:905, 1997.)

anterior descending injuries (with total cardiopulmonary bypass).[4] With a resurrection of the old concept of coronary artery bypass grafting without cardiopulmonary bypass (off-pump bypass), this technique can theoretically be used for cases of these injuries in the highly unlikely event that the patient is hemodynamically stable.

Valvular apparatus dysfunction is rare (0.2 to 9 percent) and can occur with both blunt and penetrating trauma.[6] The aortic valve is most frequently injured, followed by the mitral and tricuspid valves. Often these injuries are identified after the initial cardiorrhaphy and resuscitation have been performed. Timing of repair depends on the patient's condition. If severe cardiac dysfunction exists at the time of the initial operation, immediate valve repair or replacement may be required; otherwise, delayed repair is advised.

Intracardiac fistulas include VSDs, atrial septal defects, and atrioventricular fistulas, with an incidence of 1.9 percent among cardiac injuries.[4] Management depends on symptoms and degree of cardiac dysfunction, with only a minority of these patients requiring repair.[12] These injuries are often identified after primary repair is accomplished, and they can be repaired after the patient has recovered from the original and associated injuries. Cardiac catheterization should be accomplished before repair so that specific anatomical sites of injury and incision planning can be accomplished.

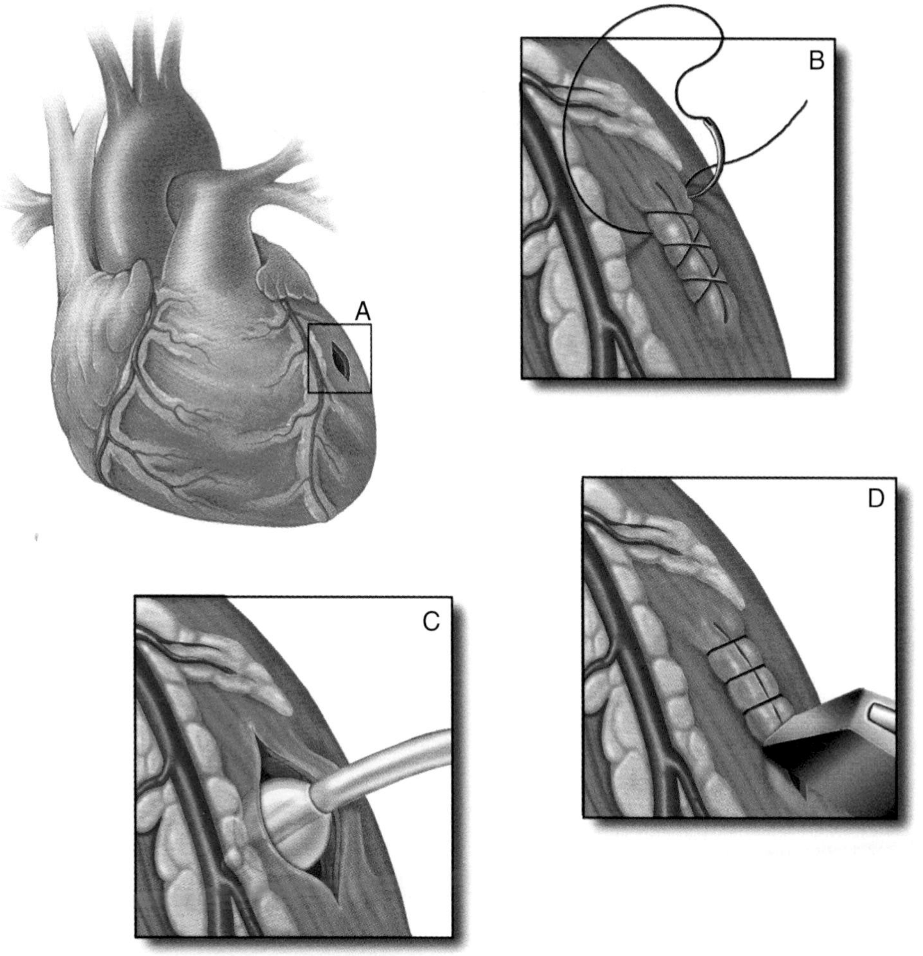

FIGURE 65–5 Temporary techniques to control bleeding. **A,** Stab wound to left ventricle. **B,** Initial management with interrupted or continuous 4-0 polypropylene sutures tied beneath the surgeon's finger. Additional techniques for complex injuries for temporary control include use of Foley balloon catheter **(C)** and skin stapler **(D)**. (From Wall MJ Jr, Mattox KL, Chen CD, Baldwin JC: Acute management of complex cardiac injuries. J Trauma 42:905, 1997.)

Arrhythmias can occur as a result of blunt injury, ischemia, or electrolyte abnormalities and are addressed according to the injury (Table 65–2) (see Chap. 32).

Delayed pericardial tamponade is very rare. It has been reported to occur as early as 1 hour after initial operation and as long as 76 days from the injury.[12]

Follow-Up

Secondary sequelae in survivors of cardiac trauma include valvular abnormalities and intracardiac fistulas.[33] These abnormalities can be identified intraoperatively by gross palpation of a thrill[15] or with the use of TEE. TEE may not be feasible, however, in the acutely injured patient. Early postoperative clinical examination and ECG findings are unreliable.[15] Thus, echocardiography is recommended during the initial hospitalization to identify occult injury and establish a baseline study. Because the incidence of late sequelae can be as high as 56 percent, follow-up echocardiography 3 to 4 weeks after injury has been recommended.[37]

In summary, the approach to the patient follows a well-defined plan. Patients with penetrating trauma arriving alive at a trauma center can have hemopericardium diagnosed by echocardiography. Urgent operation performed in the trauma resuscitation area or the operating room can result in

TABLE 65–2 Arrhythmias Associated with Cardiac Injury

Penetrating Injury
Sinus tachycardia
ST segment changes associated with ischemia
Supraventricular tachycardia
Ventricular tachycardia/fibrillation
Blunt Cardiac Injury
Sinus tachycardia
ST segment, T wave abnormalities
Atrioventricular blocks, bradycardia
Ventricular tachycardia/fibrillation
Electrical Injury
Sinus tachycardia
ST segment, T wave abnormalities
Bundle branch blocks
Axis deviation
Prolonged QT
Paroxysmal supraventricular tachycardia
Atrial fibrillation
Ventricular tachycardia, fibrillation (alternating current)
Asystole (lightnging strike)

survival. Blunt cardiac trauma can produce either minor ECG changes or frank rupture of the septum, free wall, or cardiac valves. Associated injuries are not uncommon. Stable patients can undergo evaluation in a cardiac evaluation unit, but unstable patients require rapid imaging and urgent operation. Late sequelae of fistula, coronary occlusion, and heart failure are rare and are most often detected by echocardiography within the first year after injury.

REFERENCES

1. Ivatury RR: Injury to the heart. *In* Feliciano DV, Moore EE, Mattox KL (eds): Trauma. 3rd ed. Stamford, CT, Appleton & Lange, 1996.
2. Campbell NC, Thomsen SR, Murkart DJ, et al: Review of 1198 cases of penetrating cardiac trauma. Br J Surg 84:1737, 1997.

Etiology and Patterns of Cardiac Trauma

3. Asensio JA, Berne JD, Demetriades D, et al: One hundred five penetrating cardiac injuries: A 2-year prospective evaluation. J Trauma 44:1073, 1998.
4. Wall MJ Jr, Mattox KL, Chen CD, Baldwin JC: Acute management of complex cardiac injuries. J Trauma 42:905, 1997.
5. Assencio JA, Soto SN, Forno W, et al: Penetrating cardiac injuries: A complex challenge. Injury 32:533, 2001.
6. Lin JC, Ott RA: Acute traumatic mitral valve insufficiency. J Trauma 47:165, 1999.
7. Amerongen RV, Rosen M, Winnik G, Horwitz J: Ventricular fibrillation following blunt chest trauma from a baseball. Pediatr Emerg Care 13:107, 1997.
8. Maron BJ, Link MS, Wang PJ, et al: Clinical profile of commotio cordis: An underappreciated cause of sudden death in young during sports and other activities. J Cardiovasc Electrophysiol 10:114, 1999.
9. Ivatury RR: Injury to the heart. *In* Mattox KL, Feliciano DV, Moore EE (eds): Trauma. 4th ed. New York, McGraw-Hill, 1999, pp 545-558.
10. Schaffer RB, Berdat PA, Seiler C, Carrel TP: Isolated rupture of the ventricular septum after blunt chest trauma. Ann Thorac Surg 67:853, 1999.
11. Baumgartner FJ, Rayhanabad J, Bongard FS, et al: Central venous injuries of the subclavian-jugular and innominate-caval confluences. Tex Heart Inst J 26:177, 1999.
12. Medizinische Klinik IV: Perforation und Ruptur Koronaryarterien. Herz 23:311, 1998.
13. Ivatury RR, Simon RJ, Rohman M: Cardiac complications. *In* Mattox KL (ed): Complications of Trauma. New York, Churchill Livingstone, 1994, pp 409-428.
14. Huang YS, Yang ZC, Tan BG, et al: Pathogenesis of early cardiac myocyte damage after sear burns. J Trauma 46:428, 1999.
15. Kirkpatrick AW, Chun R, Brown R, Simons RK: Hypothermia and the trauma patient. Can J Surg 42:333, 1999.
16. Sharkey SW, Shear W, Hodges M, Herzog CA: Reversible myocardial contraction abnormalities in patients with an acute non-cardiac illness. Chest 114:98, 1998.
17. Kumar A, Thota V, Dee L, et al: TNF-alpha and IL-1 are regulators for depression of in vitro myocardial cell contractility induced by serum from humans with septic shock. J Exp Med 183:949, 1996.
18. Meldrum DR, Shenkar R, Sheridan BC, et al: Hemorrhage activates myocardial NF-kappa and increases TNF-alpha in the heart. J Mol Cell Cardiol 29:2849, 1997.
19. Horton JW, Lin C, Maass D: Burn trauma and tumor necrosis factor alpha alter calcium handling by cardiomyocytes. Shock 10:270, 1998.
20. Horton JW, White J, Maass D, Sanders B: Arginine in burn injury improves cardiac performance and prevents bacterial translocation. J Appl Physiol 84:695, 1998.
21. Heinz G, Geppert A, Delle Karth G, et al: IV milrinone for cardiac output increase and maintenance: Comparison in nonhyperdynamic SIRS/sepsis and congestive heart failure. Intensive Care Med 25:620, 1999.
22. Flohe S, Borgermann J, Dominquez FE, et al: Influence of granulocyte-macrophage colony-stimulating factor (GM-CSF) on whole blood endotoxin responsiveness following trauma, cardiopulmonary bypass, and severe sepsis. Shock 12:17, 1999.
23. LeMaire SA, Wall MJ Jr, Mattox KL: Needle embolus causing cardiac puncture and chronic constrictive pericarditis. Ann Thorac Surg 65:1786, 1998.
24. Symbas PN, Symbas PJ: Missiles in the cardiovascular system. Surg Clin North Am 7:343, 1997.

Clinical Presentation and Pathophysiology

25. Ivatury RR: The injured heart. *In* Mattox KL, Moore EE, Feliciano DV (eds): Trauma. 4th ed. Stamford, CT, Appleton & Lange, 1999.
26. Brown J, Grover FL: Trauma to the heart. Chest Surg Clin North Am 7:325, 1997.

Evaluation

27. American College of Surgeons, Committee on Trauma: Advanced Trauma Life Support. Chicago, American College of Surgeons, 1997.
28. Read RA, Moore EE, Moore JB: Emergency department thoracotomy. *In* Feliciano DV, Moore EE, Mattox KL (eds): Trauma. 3rd ed. Stamford, CT, Appleton & Lange, 1996.
29. Working Group, Ad Hoc Subcommittee on Outcomes, American College of Surgeons-Committee on Trauma Practice Management Guidelines for Emergency Department Thoracotomy. J Am Coll Surg 193:303, 2001.
30. Rozycki GS, Feliciano DV, Schmidt JA, et al: The role of surgeon performed ultrasound in patients with possible cardiac wounds. Ann Surg 223:737, 1996.
31. Mattox KL, Wall MJ Jr: Newer diagnostic measures and emergency management. Chest Surg Clin North Am 7:214, 1997.
32. Rozycki GS, Schmidt JA, Oschner MG, et al: The role of surgeon-performed ultrasound in patients with possible penetrating wounds: A prospective multicenter study. J Trauma 45:190, 1998.
33. Meyer DM, Jessen ME, Grayburn PA: Use of echocardiography to detect occult cardiac injury after penetrating thoracic trauma: A prospective study. J Trauma 39:902, 1995.

Evaluation of Blunt Cardiac Injury

34. Feliciano DV, Rozycki GS: Advances in the diagnosis and treatment of thoracic trauma. Surg Clin North Am 79:1417, 1999.
35. Adams JE III, Davila-Roman VG, Bessey PQ, et al: Improved detection of cardiac contusion with cardiac troponin I. Am Heart J 131:308, 1996.
36. Ferjani M, Droc G, Dreux S, et al: Circulating cardiac troponin T in myocardial contusion. Chest 111:427, 1997.

Treatment

37. Bertinchant, JP, Polge A, Mohty D, et al: Evaluation of incidence, clinical significance and prognostic value of circulating cardiac troponin I and T elevation in hemodynamically stable patients with suspected myocardial contusion after blunt chest trauma. J Trauma 48:924, 2000.

CHAPTER 66

Pulmonary Embolism

Samuel Z. Goldhaber

Pulmonary embolism (PE) and deep venous thrombosis (DVT) account for hundreds of thousands of hospitalizations annually in the United States and afflict millions of individuals worldwide. The death rate among unselected patients is high, approximately 15 percent (Fig. 66–1).[1] Although D-dimer testing for exclusion of PE and chest computed tomography (CT) for imaging PE have revolutionized the diagnostic approach, PE and DVT nevertheless remain difficult to detect. More than 1,000,000 new cases of venous thromboembolism occur yearly in the United States, and most go unrecognized. Our understanding of the precipitants of PE has improved, especially the role of inherited hypercoagulable states and potentially modifiable risk factors such as long-haul air travel and obesity.

The most important therapeutic advance is among patients with idiopathic PE or DVT. They can now be treated safely over the long-term and at low cost to prevent most recurrent events with indefinite-duration warfarin anticoagulation. Cardiologists must provide expertise in the treatment of hemodynamically compromised patients with PE as well as those with right ventricular failure who maintain a stable blood pressure and heart rate. This requires accurate and rapid risk stratification, often with echocardiography or elevation of troponin or brain natriuretic peptide (BNP) levels, so that those patients with an adverse prognosis will be identified and treated with thrombolysis or embolectomy.

The selection of anticoagulant drugs has expanded beyond unfractionated heparin and warfarin. Low-molecular-weight heparins have improved therapeutic efficacy and can halve the rate of venous thromboembolism (VTE) in hospitalized medical patients, including those with congestive heart failure. A novel pentasaccharide drug, fondaparinux, has proved extremely effective in preventing VTE after orthopedic surgery. Oral direct thrombin inhibitors such as ximelagatran do not require serial blood testing and dose adjustment and may prove to be safer and more effective than warfarin.

Pathophysiology

Hypercoagulable States

In 1856, Rudolf Virchow postulated that a triad of factors leads to intravascular coagulation: (1) local trauma to the vessel wall, (2) hypercoagulability, and (3) stasis. Classically, the pathogenesis of PE was dichotomized as due to either unusual "inherited" (primary) or commonly "acquired" (secondary) risk factors. Now, however, it appears likely that many patients who develop PE are genetically predisposed with inherited procoagulant[2] and anticoagulant factors,[3] which often interact with a precipitating environmental stress to elicit overt thrombosis (Table 66–1).[4-13] There is also an association between atherosclerosis and the development of PE and DVT.[14]

PRIMARY HYPERCOAGULABLE STATES (see Chap. 80). Normally, a specified amount of activated protein C (aPC) can be added to plasma to prolong the activated partial thromboplastin time (PTT). Patients with "aPC resistance" have a blunted PTT prolongation and a predisposition to developing PE and DVT. The phenotype of aPC resistance is associated with a single point mutation, designated factor V Leiden, in the factor V gene.[5,6,8] Factor V Leiden triples the risk of developing VTE.[15] This genetic mutation is also a risk factor for recurrent pregnancy loss,[16] possibly due to placental vein thrombosis. Use of oral contraceptives by patients with factor V Leiden increases the risk of VTE by at least 10-fold.[17]

A single-point mutation in the 3′ untranslated region of the prothrombin gene (G-to-A transition at nucleotide position 20210) is associated with increased levels of prothrombin.[7] In the Physicians' Health Study, the prevalence of the prothrombin gene mutation was 3.9 percent, and this mutation doubled the risk of venous thrombosis.[18]

A careful family history remains the most rapid and cost-effective method of identifying a predisposition to venous thrombosis. Investigation with blood tests[19] can be misleading. For example, consumption coagulopathy due to venous thrombosis may be misdiagnosed as deficiency of antithrombin III, protein C, or protein S. Heparin administration can depress antithrombin III levels. Use of warfarin ordinarily causes a mild deficiency of protein C or S. Both oral contraceptives and pregnancy depress protein S levels.

ACQUIRED CONDITIONS THAT MAY PRECIPITATE VENOUS THROMBOSIS. Conditions that increase venous stasis or cause endothelial damage (Table 66–2) predispose to venous thrombosis, especially among patients who already have subclinical hypercoagulable states. Long-haul air travel[20] has captured the public's attention as a risk factor for PE (Fig. 66–2).

The stasis and immobilization associated with postoperative venous thrombosis may paradoxically increase after hospital discharge, because of the contemporary emphasis on minimizing the length of stay after surgery. Hospitalized patients with medical illnesses such as pneumonia or congestive heart failure are at high risk of developing VTE. There is a high prevalence of asymptomatic DVT at the time of admission of these patients.[21]

TABLE 66–1 Principal Hypercoagulable States Associated with Venous Thrombosis

Hypercoagulable State	Citation	Comments
Mutation in factor V gene (factor V Leiden)	Bertina et al[5]	Replaces arginine 506 with glutamine, rendering factor V resistant to inactivation by activated protein C
Resistance to activated protein C	Zöller et al[6]	Molecular background for resistance to activated protein C was found to be heterogeneous
Prothrombin gene mutation	Poort et al[7]	G20210A point mutation increases prothrombin levels
Mutation in protein C gene	Allaart et al[8]	Associated with protein C deficiency
Protein S deficiency	Gladson et al[9]	Protein S a cofactor for protein C
Antithrombin III deficiency	Bucciarelli et al[10]	Autosomal dominant inheritance; may cause resistance to heparin
Hyperhomocysteinemia	Langman et al[11] Ridker et al[12]	Triples risk[11]; potentiates risk from underlying factor V Leiden[12]
Antiphospholipid antibodies	Levine et al[13]	Encompasses anticardiolipin antibodies and lupus anticoagulant; associated with venous and arterial thrombosis

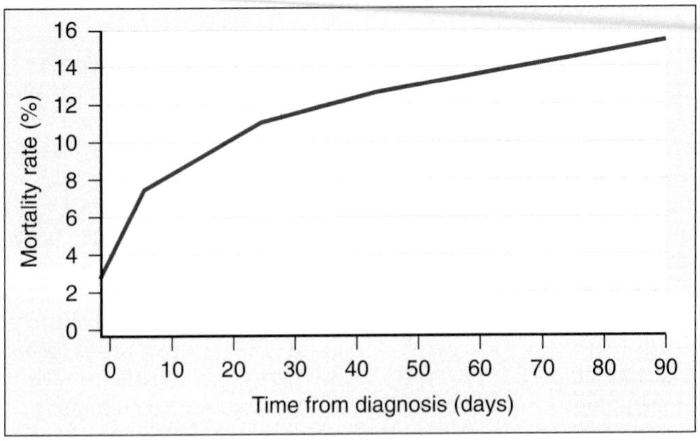

FIGURE 66–1 Overall cumulative mortality due to pulmonary embolism in the International Cooperative Pulmonary Embolism Registry (ICOPER) of 2454 patients was 11.4 percent at 2 weeks and 17.4 percent at 3 months. After exclusion of patients in whom pulmonary embolism was first discovered at autopsy, the mortality rate was 15.3 percent. (From Goldhaber SZ, Visani L, De Rosa M, for ICOPER: Acute pulmonary embolism: Clinical outcomes in the International Cooperative Pulmonary Embolism Registry [ICOPER]. Lancet 353:1386, 1999.)

Independent risk factors for PE and DVT include surgery, trauma, hospital or nursing home confinement, cancer, and cancer chemotherapy,[22] in addition to increasing age and diabetes mellitus. In the DVT FREE prospective registry of 5451 patients with ultrasonographically confirmed DVT, the five most common comorbidities were hypertension (50 percent), surgery within 3 months (38 percent), immobility within 30 days (34 percent), cancer (32 percent), and obesity (27 percent).[23]

With respect to oral contraceptives, the risk of fatal PE in a New Zealand case-control study was estimated to be 1 per 100,000 woman-years.[24] Hormone replacement therapy with estrogen plus progestin doubles the rate of PE and DVT. This finding was proven in the Women's Health Initiative, with 16,608 women randomized to hormone replacement therapy or placebo.[25] The risk of VTE also increases with raloxifene, a selective estrogen receptor modulator.[26]

The risk of newly diagnosed cancer after a first episode of PE or DVT is two- to threefold higher than expected for at least the following 2 years.[27] When cancer is detected, it is usually at an advanced stage with a poor prognosis.

Upper extremity DT is an increasingly important clinical entity because of more frequent placement of pacemakers and internal cardiac defibrillators, as well as more frequent use of chronic indwelling catheters for chemotherapy and nutrition. Patients with upper extremity DVT are at risk for PE, superior vena caval syndrome, and loss of vascular access.[28]

TABLE 66–2 Acquired Conditions that May Precipitate Venous Thrombosis

- Long-haul air travel
- Surgery/immobilization/trauma
- Hospitalization with medical illness such as pneumonia or congestive heart failure; stay in a medical or surgical intensive care unit
- Obesity
- Increasing age
- Cigarette smoking
- Systemic arterial hypertension
- Diabetes mellitus
- Use of oral contraceptives/pregnancy/postpartum state
- Cancer (sometimes occult adenocarcinoma) and cancer chemotherapy
- Stroke/spinal cord injury
- Indwelling central venous catheter, pacemakers, and internal cardiac defibrillators

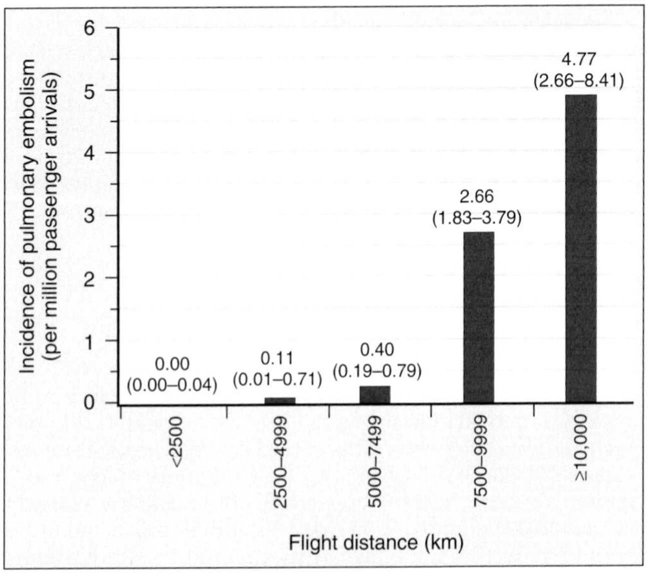

FIGURE 66–2 Incidence of pulmonary embolism increases as the distance traveled by air increases. Values shown above the bars are the number of cases per million passenger arrivals, with 95 percent confidence intervals. (From Lapostolle F, Surget V, Borron SW, et al: Severe pulmonary embolism associated with air travel. N Engl J Med 345:779, 2001.)

Relationship Between Deep Venous Thrombosis and Pulmonary Embolism

When venous thrombi detach from their sites of formation, they flow through the venous system toward the pulmonary arterial circulation. If an embolus is extremely large, it may lodge at the bifurcation of the pulmonary artery, forming a saddle embolus (Fig. 66–3, top). More commonly, a major pulmonary vessel is occluded (Fig. 66–3, bottom). Many patients with large PE do not have ultrasonographic evidence of DVT, probably because the clot has already embolized to the lungs.

RIGHT VENTRICULAR DYSFUNCTION. The extent of pulmonary vascular obstruction and the presence of underlying cardiopulmonary disease are probably the most important factors determining whether right ventricular dysfunction ensues. As obstruction increases, pulmonary artery pressure rises. The release of vasoconstricting compounds such as serotonin, reflex pulmonary artery vasoconstriction, and hypoxemia may further increase pulmonary vascular resistance and result in pulmonary hypertension.[29] The injured right ventricle releases biomarkers, including pro-brain natriuretic peptide,[30] brain natriuretic peptide,[31] and troponin,[32] all of which predict an increased likelihood of an adverse clinical outcome.

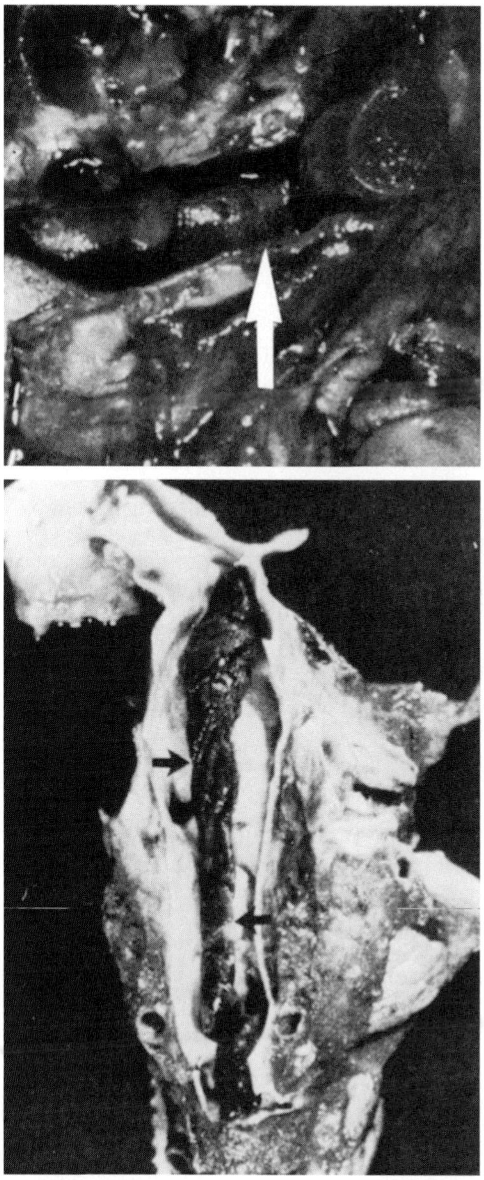

FIGURE 66–3 **Top,** Saddle embolus (arrow) at the bifurcation of the pulmonary artery. **Bottom,** Pulmonary embolus in left lower lobe pulmonary artery, with minimal attachment to the wall of the vessel. The embolus was dark red, typical of venous thrombi, and had indentations believed to represent impressions of the venous valves (arrows). (From Godleski JJ: Pathology of deep venous thrombosis and pulmonary embolism. *In* Goldhaber SZ [ed]: Pulmonary Embolism and Deep Venous Thrombosis. Philadelphia, WB Saunders, 1985, p 17.)

VENTRICULAR INTERDEPENDENCY. The sudden rise in pulmonary artery pressure reflects an abrupt increase in right ventricular afterload, with consequent elevation of right ventricular wall tension followed by right ventricular dilation and dysfunction (Fig. 66–4).[33] As the right ventricle dilates, the interventricular septum shifts toward the left, with resultant underfilling and decreased diastolic distensibility of this chamber. With underfilling of the left ventricle, systemic cardiac output and pressure both decline, potentially compromising coronary perfusion and producing myocardial ischemia.[34] Elevated right ventricular wall tension following massive PE reduces right coronary flow and increases right ventricular myocardial oxygen demand, which may result in ischemia and possibly cardiogenic shock. Perpetuation of this cycle can lead to right ventricular infarction, circulatory collapse, and death.

Summary of Pathophysiology

Pulmonary embolism can have the following pathophysiological effects: (1) increased pulmonary vascular resistance due to vascular obstruction, neurohumoral agents, or pulmonary artery baroreceptors; (2) impaired gas exchange due to increased alveolar dead space from vascular obstruction and hypoxemia from alveolar hypoventilation, low ventilation-perfusion units, and right-to-left shunting, as well as impaired carbon monoxide transfer due to loss of gas-exchange surface; (3) alveolar hyperventilation due to reflex stimulation of irritant receptors; (4) increased airway resistance due to bronchoconstriction; and (5) decreased pulmonary compliance due to lung edema, lung hemorrhage, and loss of surfactant.[35]

Diagnosis

Diagnosis of PE is more difficult than treatment or prevention. Fortunately, noninvasive diagnostic approaches have become increasingly reliable, particularly the plasma D-dimer enzyme-linked immunosorbent assay (ELISA), chest CT, and venous ultrasonography. The contemporary diagnostic strategy integrates clinical findings with various diagnostic techniques. Nevertheless, despite advances in diagnosis, major PE is missed antemortem in more than half the patients who have this condition at autopsy.[36]

CLINICAL PRESENTATION. Clinical suspicion of PE is of paramount importance in guiding diagnostic testing. Dyspnea is the most frequent symptom, and tachypnea is the most frequent sign of PE (Table 66–3). In general, severe dyspnea, syncope, or cyanosis portends a major life-threatening PE. However, pleuritic pain often signifies that the embolism is small and located in the distal pulmonary arterial system, near the pleural lining.

Pulmonary embolism should be suspected in hypotensive patients when (1) there is evidence of venous thrombosis or predisposing factors for it and (2) there is clinical evidence of acute cor pulmonale (acute right ventricular failure) such as distended neck veins, an S_3 gallop, a right ventricular heave, tachycardia, or tachypnea, especially if (3) there are echocardiographic findings of right ventricular dilation and hypokinesis or electrocardiographic (ECG) evidence of acute cor pulmonale manifested by a new S1Q3T3 pattern, new

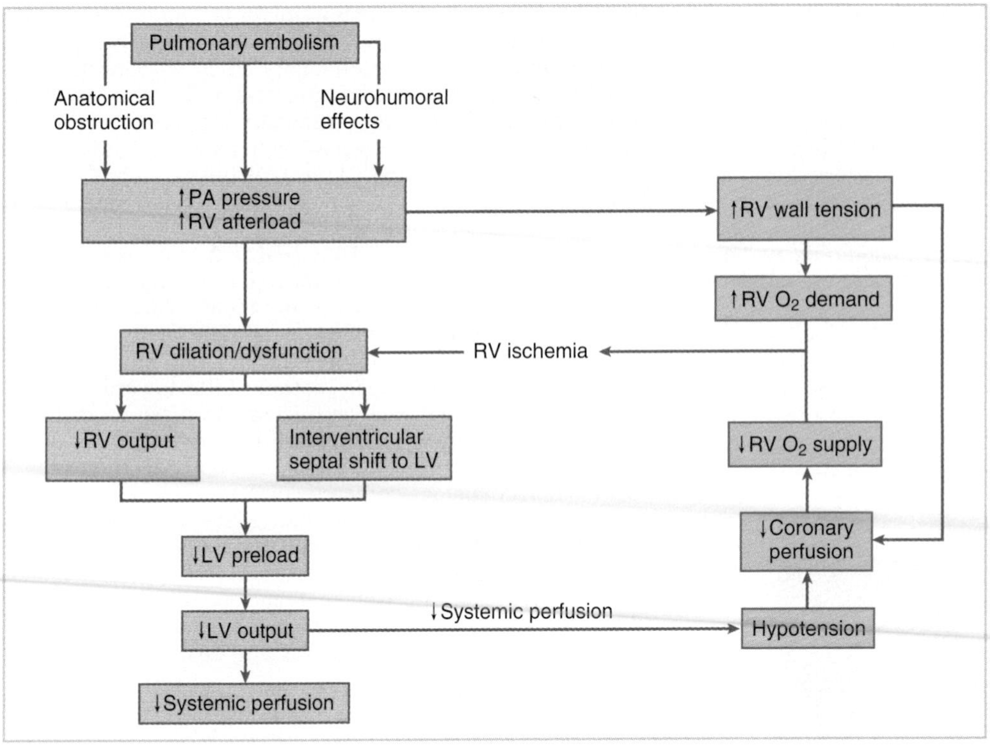

FIGURE 66–4 Pathophysiology of right ventricular dysfunction. LV = left ventricular; PA = pulmonary artery; RV = right ventricular.

incomplete right bundle branch block, or right ventricular ischemia (Fig. 66–5).

Wells and colleagues have developed a rapid seven-question bedside assessment (Table 66–4)[37] that is useful because with it almost half of their study patients could be categorized as "PE unlikely." They designated a score of 4.0 or lower as "PE unlikely." In this low-risk group, only about 5 percent of patients were subsequently diagnosed with PE.

DIFFERENTIAL DIAGNOSIS. The differential diagnosis of PE is broad and covers a spectrum from life-threatening disease such as acute myocardial infarction to innocuous anxiety states (Table 66–5). Some patients have concomitant PE and other illnesses. For example, if pneumonia or heart failure does not respond to appropriate therapy, the possibility of coexisting PE should be considered. Distinguishing between PE and primary pulmonary hypertension (see Chap. 67) warrants special vigilance. Some patients have a hybrid condition that is similar to primary pulmonary hypertension but that includes thrombi.[38] Among these patients, large central pulmonary artery thrombi can develop. It may be impossible to determine whether these thrombi formed in situ or whether they embolized to the pulmonary arteries from a separate site.

Clinical Syndromes of Pulmonary Embolism

Classification of PE into various syndromes (Table 66–6) is useful for prognostication and for deciding on subsequent clinical management.[39]

MASSIVE PULMONARY EMBOLISM. Patients with massive PE are at risk for cardiogenic shock. They have thrombosis often affecting at least half of the pulmonary arterial vasculature. Clot is almost always present bilaterally. Dyspnea is usually the most noticeable symptom, transient cyanosis is common, and systemic arterial hypotension requiring pressor support is the predominant sign. Often, these patients present without chest pain.

TABLE 66–3 Most Common Symptoms and Signs Among the 2454 Patients in the International Cooperative Pulmonary Embolism Registry (ICOPER)

Symptom or Sign	Percent
Dyspnea	82
Respiratory rate >20/min	60
Heart rate >100 beats/min	40
Chest pain	49
Cough	20
Syncope	14
Hemoptysis	7

Adapted from Goldhaber SZ, Visani L, De Rosa M, for ICOPER: Acute pulmonary embolism: Clinical outcomes in the International Cooperative Pulmonary Embolism Registry (ICOPER). Lancet 353:1386, 1999.

TABLE 66–4 Wells Clinical Bedside Scoring System for Suspected Pulmonary Embolism

Parameter	Points
Clinical signs and symptoms of DVT (minimum of leg swelling and pain with palpation of the deep veins)	3.0
An alternative diagnosis is less likely than PE	3.0
Heart rate greater than 100	1.5
Immobilization or surgery in the previous 4 weeks	1.5
Previous DVT/PE	1.5
Hemoptysis	1.0
Malignancy (on treatment, treated in the last 6 months, or palliative)	1.0

DVT = deep venous thrombosis; PE = pulmonary embolism.
Adapted from Wells PS, Anderson DR, Rodger M, et al: Derivation of a simple clinical model to categorize patients probability of pulmonary embolism: Increasing the models utility with the SimpliRED D-dimer. Thromb Haemost 83:416, 2000.

TABLE 66–5 Differential Diagnosis of Pulmonary Embolism

Myocardial infarction	Pericarditis
Pneumonia	Intrathoracic cancer
Congestive heart failure ("left-sided")	Rib fracture
Cardiomyopathy (global)	Pneumothorax
Primary pulmonary hypertension	Costochondritis
Asthma	"Musculoskeletal pain"
	Anxiety

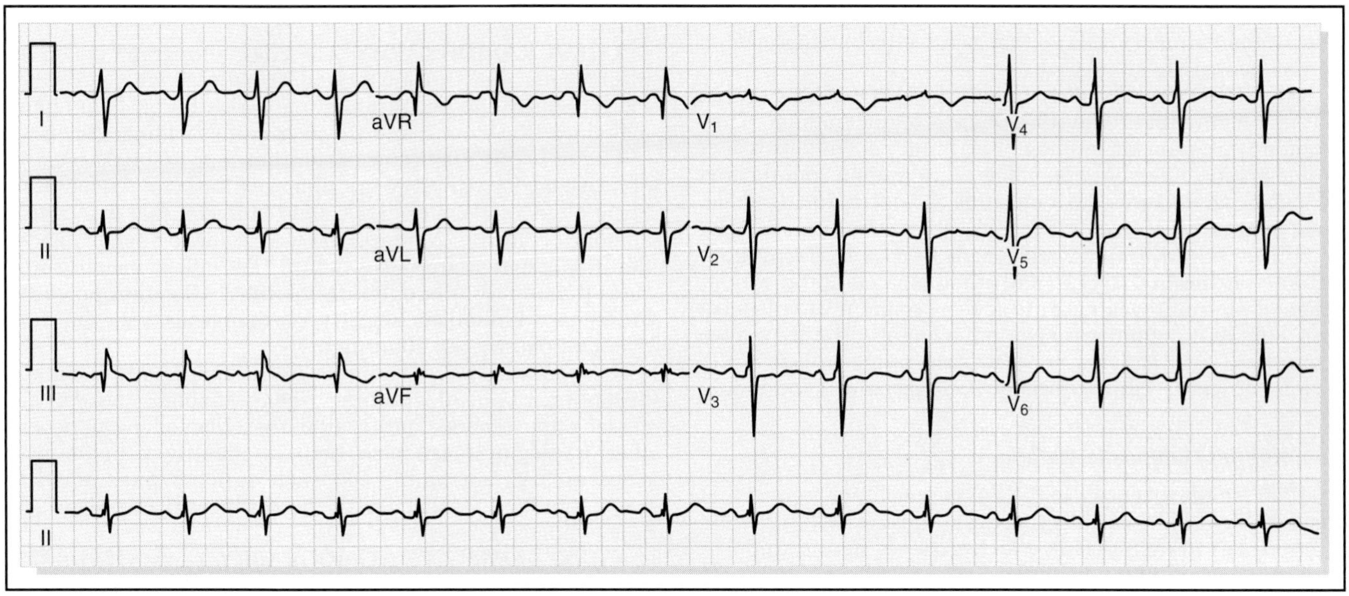

FIGURE 66–5 Electrocardiogram from a 33-year-old man who presented with a left main pulmonary artery embolism on chest computed tomographic scan. He was hemodynamically stable and had normal right ventricular function on echocardiogram. His troponin and brain natriuretic peptide levels were normal. He was managed with anticoagulation alone. On the initial electrocardiogram, he has a heart rate of 90 per minute, S1Q3T3, and incomplete right bundle branch block, with inverted or flattened T waves in Leads V1 through V4.

TABLE 66–6 Six Syndromes of Acute Pulmonary Embolism

Syndrome	Presentation	Right Ventricular Dysfunction	Therapy
Massive	Breathlessness, syncope, and cyanosis with persistent systemic arterial hypotension; typically >50 percent obstruction of pulmonary vasculature	Present	Heparin plus thrombolytic therapy or mechanical intervention
Moderate to large ("submassive")	Normal systemic arterial blood pressure; typically >30 percent perfusion defect on lung scan	Present	Heparin plus or minus thrombolytic therapy or mechanical intervention*
Small to moderate	Normal arterial blood pressure	Absent	Heparin
Pulmonary infarction	Pleuritic chest pain, hemoptysis, pleural rub, or evidence of lung consolidation; typically small peripheral emboli	Rare	Heparin and nonsteroidal antiinflammatory drugs
Paradoxical embolism	Sudden systemic embolic event such as stroke	Rare	Anticoagulation ± closure of right-to-left cardiac shunt
Nonthrombotic embolism	Most commonly air, fat, tumor fragments, or amniotic fluid	Rare	Supportive

*Therapy depends on degree of impairment of right ventricular function and presence or absence of contraindications to thrombolysis or heparin.
Adapted from Goldhaber SZ: Treatment of acute pulmonary embolism. *In* Goldhaber SZ (ed): Cardiopulmonary Diseases and Cardiac Tumors. *In* Braunwald E (series ed): Atlas of Heart Diseases. Vol 3. Philadelphia, Current Medicine, 1995, pp 7.1-7.12.

MODERATE TO LARGE ("SUBMASSIVE") PULMONARY EMBOLISM. Patients with this condition frequently have right ventricular hypokinesis, troponin or pro-BNP or BNP elevations, but normal systemic arterial pressure. Usually, one-third or more of the pulmonary artery vasculature is obstructed. These patients have various degrees of right ventricular hemodynamic instability masked by normal systemic arterial pressure. They are at risk for recurrent (and possibly fatal) PE, even with adequate anticoagulation. Most survive, but they may require escalation of therapy with pressor support or mechanical ventilation. Therefore, especially if right ventricular dysfunction persists, one should consider using thrombolytics or embolectomy.

SMALL TO MODERATE PULMONARY EMBOLISM. This syndrome is characterized by normal systemic arterial pressure, no troponin or pro-BNP release, and normal right ventricular function. Adequate anticoagulation results in an excellent clinical outcome.

PULMONARY INFARCTION. This syndrome is characterized by pleuritic chest pain that may be unremitting or may wax and wane. The pleurisy is occasionally accompanied by hemoptysis. The embolus usually lodges in the peripheral pulmonary arterial tree, near the pleura.[40] Tissue infarction usually occurs 3 to 7 days after embolism. The syndrome often includes fever, leukocytosis, an elevated erythrocyte sedimentation rate, and radiological evidence of infarction.

PARADOXICAL EMBOLISM. This syndrome often manifests with a sudden, devastating stroke and concomitant PE.[41] Although DVT is usually not detected in patients who suffer a paradoxical embolism in the presence of a patent foramen ovale, the DVT may embolize entirely to the pulmonary and systemic arteries, without residual leg or pelvic vein thrombosis. Contemporary management consists of closing the patent foramen ovale, either surgically but more often percutaneously.[42]

NONTHROMBOTIC PULMONARY EMBOLISM. Sources of embolism other than thrombus are uncommon. They include fat, tumor, air, and amniotic fluid. Fat embolism syndrome is most often observed after blunt trauma complicated by long-bone fractures.[43] Air embolus can occur during placement or removal of a central venous catheter.[44] Amniotic fluid embolism is catastrophic and characterized by respiratory failure, cardiogenic shock, and disseminated intravascular coagulation.[45] Intravenous drug abusers sometimes self-inject hair, talc, and cotton that contaminate the drug they have acquired. These patients are also susceptible to septic PE, which can cause endocarditis of the tricuspid or pulmonic valves.

Nonimaging Diagnostic Methods

To establish the diagnosis of PE, the astute clinician must first suspect this illness. Establishing the clinical probability of PE is important to help decide which patients should undergo further work-up. Many patients in whom PE is a theoretical possibility are exceedingly unlikely to have PE.

PLASMA D-DIMER ELISA. This blood-screening test relies on the principle that most patients with PE have ongoing endogenous fibrinolysis that is not effective enough to prevent PE but that does break down some of the fibrin clot to D-dimers. Although elevated plasma concentrations of D-dimers are sensitive for the presence of PE, they are not specific. Levels are elevated in patients for at least 1 week postoperatively and are also increased in patients with myocardial infarction, sepsis, cancer, or almost any other systemic illness. Therefore, the plasma D-dimer ELISA is ideally suited for outpatients or Emergency Department patients who have suspected PE but no coexisting acute systemic illness. This test is not useful for hospitalized inpatients.

At Brigham and Women's Hospital, we obtained D-dimer tests on consecutive Emergency Department patients suspected of acute PE.[46] After 1 year, 1106 assays were obtained: 559 patients had abnormally elevated D-dimer levels and 547 were within normal limits. Only 2 of the 547 patients had PE despite a normal D-dimer. Thus, the sensitivity of the D-dimer ELISA for acute PE was 96.4 percent and the negative predictive value was 99.6 percent. Similar findings have been observed in seven other urban Emergency Departments.[47] By ruling out PE with a normal D-dimer ELISA, fewer chest CT and lung scans will be required. A similar strategy works for excluding DVT, by combining a clinical risk assessment with a normal D-dimer ELISA.[48]

ARTERIAL BLOOD GASES. Among patients suspected of having PE in the Prospective Investigation of Pulmonary Embolism Diagnosis (PIOPED), there was no difference between the average PaO_2 (70 mm Hg) among those with and those without PE (72 mm Hg) at pulmonary angiography. In the subset with angiographically proven PE but no prior cardiopulmonary disease, 26 percent had a PaO_2 that was 80 mm Hg or greater.[49] Normal values of the alveolar-arterial oxygen gradient did not preclude the diagnosis of acute PE.[50] Therefore, arterial blood gas determinations should not be part of the diagnostic strategy when investigating suspected PE.

ELECTROCARDIOGRAM (see Chap. 9). The ECG helps exclude acute myocardial infarction and may raise suspicion or help confirm the diagnosis of PE among patients with ECG manifestations of right-heart strain. The converse is not true, however. Patients with massive PE may have sinus tachycardia, minor ST and T wave abnormalities, or even entirely normal ECGs. One of the most useful findings is negative T waves in precordial leads V1 through V4.[51] Other abnormalities include incomplete or complete right bundle branch block or an S1Q3T3 complex (see Fig. 66–5).[52]

Imaging Methods

CHEST RADIOGRAPHY. The chest radiograph is usually the first imaging study obtained in patients with suspected PE. Although one-fourth of patients with PE have an abnormal chest film examination, a near-normal radiograph in the setting of severe respiratory compromise is highly suggestive of massive PE. Chest x-ray abnormalities are uncommon. Focal oligemia (Westermark's sign) indicates massive central embolic occlusion. A peripheral wedge-shaped density above the diaphragm (Hampton's hump) (Fig. 66–6) usually indicates pulmonary infarction. In the International Cooperative Pulmonary Embolism Registry, cardiomegaly was the most common chest x-ray abnormality.[53]

One should always search for subtle abnormalities such as distention of the descending right pulmonary artery. The vessel often tapers rapidly after the enlarged portion. The chest radiograph can also help to identify patients with diseases that can mimic PE, such as lobar pneumonia or pneumothorax. Patients with these illnesses can also have concomitant PE.

CHEST COMPUTED TOMOGRAPHY. Chest CT has supplanted pulmonary radionuclide perfusion scintigraphy as the initial imaging test in most patients with suspected PE (Fig. 66–7).[53a] For patients with intrinsic lung disease and abnormal chest radiograph results, the chest CT scan can suggest an alternative or concomitant pulmonary disease to explain the clinical presentation. For the evaluation of suspected PE, the CT examination can include scanning of the venous system from the popliteal veins to the subsegmental pulmonary arteries. The CT examination can also provide valuable information about the size and function of the right ventricle relative to the left and can alert the clinician to the presence of right ventricular dysfunction. The latest generation of multidetector-row CT scanners permits image acquisition of the entire chest with 1 mm or submillimeter resolution with a breath-hold of less than 10 seconds.[54] With a properly performed CT scan on a multidetector row machine, it is likely that CT scanning supplants pulmonary angiography as the gold standard for PE imaging.

First-generation machines have poor resolution in the subsegmental pulmonary arteries. With first-generation machines, the sensitivity compared with pulmonary angiography is only 70 percent.[55] However, normal first-generation CT scans appear to predict a benign clinical course over the ensuing 3 months.[56]

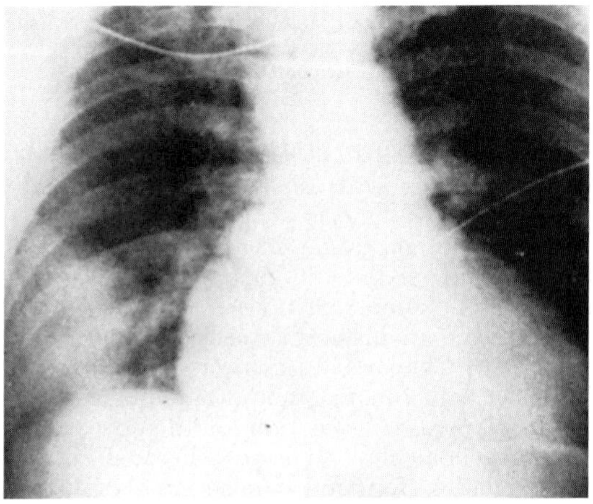

FIGURE 66–6 Posteroanterior chest film of a patient with pulmonary embolism shows a "Hampton's hump" in the right lower lung field, a homogeneous, wedge-shaped density in the peripheral field, convex to the hilum. (Courtesy of Dr. Jack L. Westcott, The New York Hospital and Cornell University Medical College.)

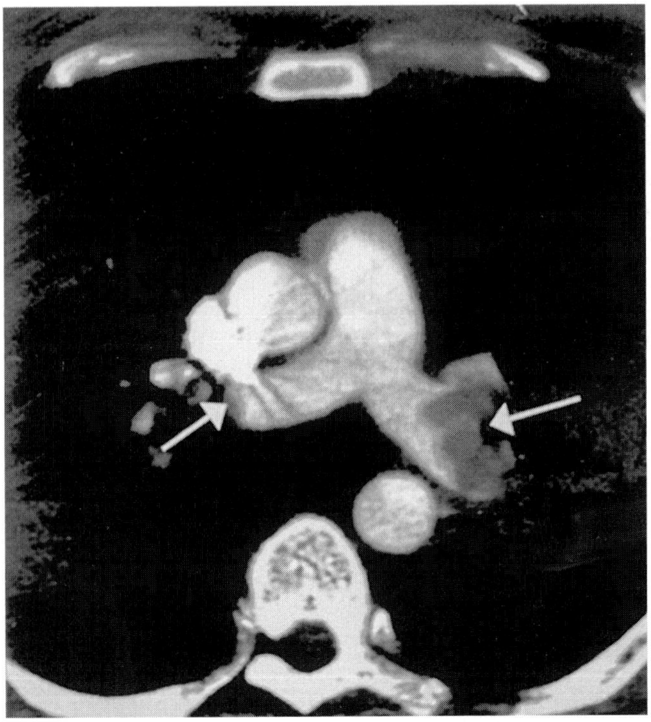

FIGURE 66–7 A 62-year-old physician suffered a massive pulmonary embolism 2 weeks after prostatectomy. Spiral chest computed tomography with contrast provided a definitive diagnosis, with a large thrombus burden apparent in the right and left main pulmonary arteries (arrows).

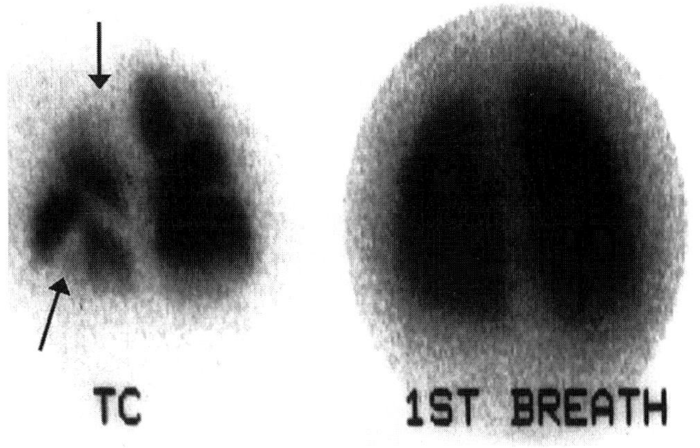

FIGURE 66–8 A 41-year-old woman presented with sudden onset of shortness of breath and retrosternal chest discomfort. Her heart rate was 168 beats/min, respiratory rate 32/min, oxygen saturation 86 percent, and blood pressure 112/70 mm Hg. She underwent a ventilation-perfusion (ventilation on the **left** and perfusion on the **right**) lung scan with xenon-133 gas (26 mCi) and technetium-99m macroaggregated albumin (3.2 mCi) in the left posterior oblique position. Numerous scattered segmental (arrows) and subsegmental perfusion defects with near normal ventilation were found. This ventilation-perfusion mismatch was interpreted as high probability for pulmonary embolism.

When ordering a CT scan, it is of paramount importance to know what generation of scanners are available. For patients suspected of massive PE, a first-generation scanner will suffice. For patients suspected of a small peripheral PE, the images should be acquired, if possible, on a newer machine with multirow detector capability. When CT scanning is preceded by D-dimer testing and venous ultrasonography of the legs, it is cost-effective in the work-up of suspected acute PE.[57]

LUNG SCANNING. Pulmonary radionuclide perfusion scintigraphy (lung scanning) is no longer the principal diagnostic imaging test when PE is suspected. Chest CT scanning with intravenous contrast has supplanted lung scanning because it provides direct and definitive results. Lung scanning is now a second-choice imaging test, usually reserved for patients with renal insufficiency, contrast allergy, or pregnancy (because of lower fetal radiation exposure than chest CT).

Perfusion scintigraphy uses radiolabeled aggregates of albumin or microspheres that are trapped in the pulmonary capillary bed. Six or eight standard views are obtained with a gamma camera. Patients with large PE may have many defects on the perfusion scan. If ventilation scanning is performed on a patient with PE but no intrinsic lung disease, a normal ventilation study result is expected, yielding a ventilation-perfusion mismatch (Fig. 66–8) and a lung scan interpreted as "high probability for PE." PE is very unlikely among patients with normal and near-normal scans. High-probability scans usually indicate acute PE, but no more than 25 percent of patients with suspected PE will have a high-probability scan.[58] Scans that fall between these extremes of the spectrum should be called "intermediate probability." Many patients with low-probability scans but high clinical suspicion for PE do, in fact, have PE at angiography.[59] Therefore, the term *low-probability* scan is a potentially lethal misnomer.[60]

TABLE 66–7	Echocardiographic Signs of Pulmonary Embolism
Direct visualization of thrombus (rare)	
Right ventricular dilation	
Right ventricular hypokinesis (with sparing of the apex)	
Abnormal interventricular septal motion	
Tricuspid valve regurgitation	
Pulmonary artery dilatation	
Lack of decreased inspiratory collapse of inferior vena cava	

MAGNETIC RESONANCE IMAGING. Gadolinium-enhanced magnetic resonance angiography (MRA) is a promising imaging test for suspected PE. When performed under ideal conditions with optimal imaging equipment, it appears to be sensitive and specific for segmental or larger PE.[61] Unlike chest CT or catheter-based pulmonary angiography, MRA does not require ionizing radiation or injection of iodinated contrast agent. Therefore, MRA can be performed safely in patients with poor renal function, at virtually no risk to the patient. Finally, magnetic resonance pulmonary angiography can include assessment of ventricular size and function, valuable in detecting patients at increased risk of an adverse clinical outcome. MRA also appears to be a promising tool for imaging leg vein thrombosis, including isolated calf vein thrombosis.[62]

ECHOCARDIOGRAPHY (see Chap. 11). Echocardiography is normal in about half of unselected patients with acute PE.[63] Therefore, echocardiography is not recommended as a routine diagnostic test for PE. However, it is a rapid, practical, and sensitive technique for detection of right ventricular overload among patients with established and large PE (Fig. 66-9). Moderate or severe right ventricular hypokinesis, persistent pulmonary hypertension, a patent foramen ovale, and free-floating thrombus in the right atrium or right ventricle help identify patients at high risk of death or recurrent thromboembolism. The frequency of echocardiographic signs of PE (Table 66-7) depends on the population being studied. For those patients in whom transthoracic imaging is unsatisfactory, transesophageal echocardiography can be carried out.[64]

Echocardiographic detection of right ventricular dysfunction at the time of presentation with PE is useful for risk stratification and prognostication.[65] Among patients with major PE, echocardiographic evidence of a patent foramen ovale signifies a high risk of death and paradoxical arterial thromboembolism.[66] Doppler echocardiography performed 6 weeks after the acute PE can identify patients with persistent pulmonary hypertension and right ventricular dysfunction. They are at high risk of developing chronic thromboembolic pulmonary hypertension.

PULMONARY ANGIOGRAPHY. Standard contrast pulmonary angiography was, for many years, considered the gold

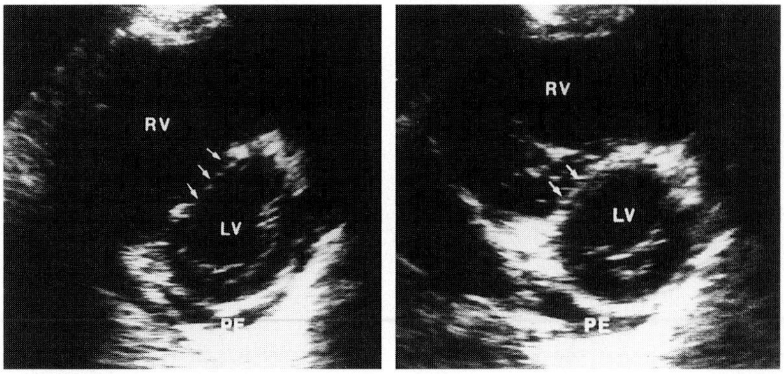

FIGURE 66–9 Parasternal short-axis views of the right ventricle (RV) and left ventricle (LV) in diastole **(left)** and systole **(right)**. Diastolic and systolic bowing of the interventricular septum (arrows) into the LV is compatible with RV volume and pressure overload, respectively. The RV is appreciably dilated and markedly hypokinetic, with little change in apparent RV area from diastole to systole. PE = small pericardial effusion. (From Come PC: Echocardiographic evaluation of pulmonary embolism and its response to therapeutic interventions. Chest 101:151S, 1992.)

standard for diagnosis but is now rarely performed because multiplanar chest CT scanning can solve most diagnostic dilemmas. However, pulmonary angiography is required when interventions are planned, such as suction catheter embolectomy, mechanical clot fragmentation, or catheter-directed thrombolysis.

The images from pulmonary angiographic evaluation can be displayed on conventional x-ray film or on a digital screen, with equivalent diagnostic accuracy.

In cases of chronic PE, CT scanning or pulmonary angiography will show arteries that appear pouched. The thrombus usually organizes with a concave edge (Fig. 66–10). Band-like defects called *webs* may be present, in addition to intimal irregularities and abrupt narrowing or occlusion of lobar vessels.

VENOUS ULTRASONOGRAPHY. The primary diagnostic criterion to establish the presence of DVT by ultrasonography is the loss of vein compressibility. Normally, the vein collapses completely when gentle pressure is applied to the skin overlying it. Upper extremity DVT can be more difficult to diagnose because the clavicle can hinder attempts to compress the subclavian vein. Venous ultrasonography is useful if it demonstrates DVT in patients with suspected PE. However, the majority of patients with PE have no imaging evidence of DVT.[67] *Therefore, if clinical suspicion of PE is high, patients without evidence of DVT should still be investigated for PE.*

CONTRAST PHLEBOGRAPHY. Although contrast phlebography was, for many years, the gold standard for DVT diagnosis, venograms are now rarely obtained. Venography is costly and invasive and occasionally results in contrast-induced renal failure, anaphylaxis, or phlebitis. Furthermore, there is considerable disagreement in the interpretation of contrast venograms among experienced readers. DVT is usually diagnosed with ultrasonography, which is widely available, convenient, and usually accurate. Alternative modes of diagnosis are contrast-enhanced CT and magnetic resonance imaging. Consequently, we reserve contrast phlebography for situations in which we anticipate an interventional procedure such as catheter-directed thrombolysis, suction embolectomy, angioplasty, stenting, or placement of an inferior vena caval filter.

Overall Strategy: An Integrated Diagnostic Approach

A wide array of diagnostic tests is available for the investigation of suspected PE. Familiarity with each test's strengths and weaknesses (Table 66–8) as well as knowledge of the availability and reliability of specific tests at one's hospital will facilitate a concise and streamlined work-up.

At Brigham and Women's Hospital (Fig. 66–11), the initial assessment includes the history, physical examination, and ECG, with special attention to the patient's clinical milieu and risk factors for venous thromboembolism. The Wells bedside assessment score is used to semiquantitate the clinical likelihood of PE. As part of the differential diagnostic work-up, we obtain an electrocardiogram and chest radiograph. To screen for PE in the Emergency Department, we obtain a rapid turn-around plasma D-dimer ELISA. If normal, then PE is exceedingly unlikely, and the diagnosis is ordinarily considered to have been excluded at that point. If elevated, we ordinarily pursue the diagnosis of PE with chest CT scanning. For the occasional equivocal result, we next

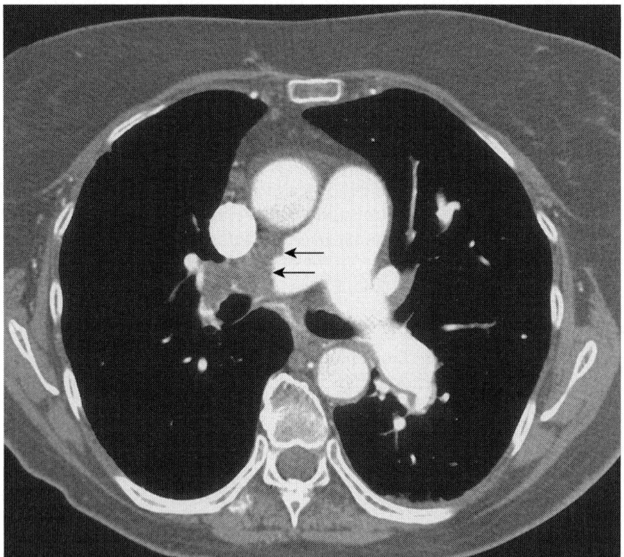

FIGURE 66–10 Chest computed tomography (CT) scan of a 59-year-old woman with chronic thromboembolic pulmonary hypertension. She has underlying antiphospholipid antibody syndrome. The chest CT scan demonstrates a large right pulmonary artery with an abrupt cut-off (arrows) in a jagged, irregular pattern due to chronic thromboembolism.

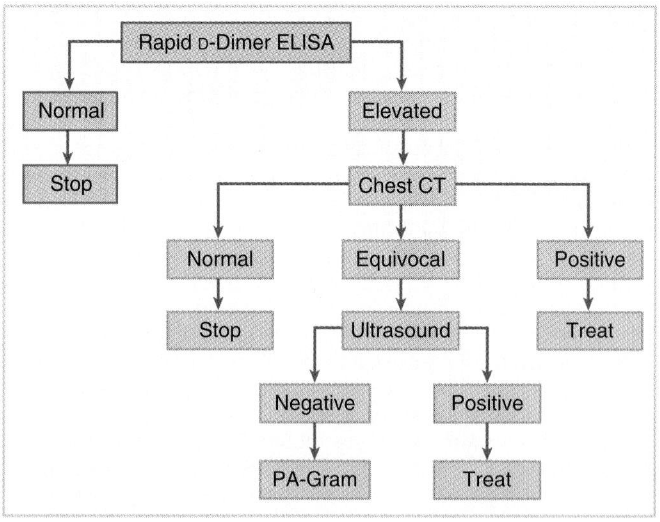

FIGURE 66–11 Emergency Department and outpatient pulmonary embolism diagnosis strategy: integrated diagnostic approach. CT = computed tomography; ELISA = enzyme-linked immunosorbent assay; PA-Gram = pulmonary arteriogram.

TABLE 66–8 Advantages and Disadvantages of Diagnostic Tests for Suspected Pulmonary Embolism

Diagnostic Test	Advantages	Disadvantages
Plasma D-dimer ELISA	A normal result in this rapid turnaround blood test makes PE exceedingly unlikely.	Level is elevated in patients with many systemic illnesses that mimic PE, such as pneumonia and myocardial infarction. Level is elevated in patients with sepsis, cancer, postoperative state, and pregnancy.
Electrocardiogram	Universally available; may indicate ominous acute cor pulmonale or benign pericarditis.	Acute cor pulmonale on electrocardiogram is not specific for PE; not a sensitive test.
Chest radiograph	Usually has minor abnormalities but occasionally pathognomonic; may indicate alternative diagnoses such as pneumothorax.	Not specific.
Chest computed tomography	New-generation scanners constitute the new gold standard for diagnosis.	Older generation scanners are insensitive for important but distal PE.
Lung scanning	High-probability scans are reliable for detecting PE; normal/near-normal scans are reliable for excluding PE.	Most scans are neither high probability nor normal/near-normal; lung scans are falling out of favor; most test results are equivocal.
Magnetic resonance imaging	Excellent for anatomy and cardiac function; the contrast agent does not cause renal failure.	In preliminary use; not widely available; experience very limited.
Echocardiography	Excellent for identifying right ventricular dilation and dysfunction that is not obvious clinically, thus providing an early warning of potentially adverse outcome.	Not specific; many patients with PE have normal echocardiograms; the test cannot reliably differentiate causes of right ventricular dysfunction.
Pulmonary angiography	Necessary for catheter-based interventions.	Invasive, costly, uncomfortable.
Venous ultrasonography	Excellent for detecting symptomatic proximal DVT; surrogate for PE.	Cannot image iliac vein thrombosis; imaging of calf is operator dependent; DVT may have embolized completely, resulting in a normal finding.
Contrast venography	Used to be gold standard; excellent for calf veins; necessary for catheter-based interventions.	Can cause chemical phlebitis; uncomfortable; costly; may fail to diagnose massive DVT because veins are filled with thrombus and cannot be opacified.

DVT = deep venous thrombosis; ELISA = enzyme-linked immunosorbent assay; PE = pulmonary embolism.

proceed to venous ultrasonography of the legs. If the ultrasonographic examination is normal and high clinical suspicion persists, a diagnostic pulmonary angiogram is obtained. An integrated diagnostic strategy that includes clinical probability assessment, chest CT, and venous ultrasonography will usually provide a noninvasive diagnosis or exclusion of PE. This approach is safe, is validated, and requires pulmonary angiography in at most 10 percent of patients.[68]

Management

Risk Stratification

Patients with PE present with a wide spectrum of illness that ranges from mild to severe. Therefore, rapid and accurate risk stratification is of paramount importance.[68a] Appropriate care can range from prevention of recurrent PE with anticoagulation alone in low-risk patients to clot dissolution or removal with thrombolysis or embolectomy in high-risk patients. High-risk patients may require intensive support with mechanical ventilation or pressors while the fundamental problem of PE is addressed with aggressive medical, interventional angiographic, or surgical therapy.

The three key components for risk stratification are (1) clinical evaluation, which can be undertaken systematically with the Geneva Prognostic Index,[69] (2) biomarkers such as troponin,[32] pro-BNP,[30] and BNP,[31] and (3) assessment of right ventricular function, usually accomplished with echocardiography.[34]

Clinical evaluation is straightforward if the patient feels perfectly well or, at the other end of the spectrum, is in cardiogenic shock. Most patients with PE, however, are

TABLE 66–9 The Geneva Point Score to Assess Pulmonary Embolism Prognosis

Variable	Point Score
Cancer	+2
Heart failure	+1
Prior DVT	+1
Hypotension	+2
Hypoxemia	+1
DVT on ultrasonogram	+1

DVT = deep venous thrombosis.

moderately ill. The traditional clinical assessment and prognostication has been done by *gestalt*. However, the Geneva Prognostic Index has quantified and validated a predictive model of clinical outcome, based on a bedside history and physical examination (Tables 66–9 and 66–10). This index was used to identify low-risk patients with PE who were managed successfully as outpatients, without hospitalization.[70]

Clinical evaluation should be supplemented by cardiac biomarkers that detect microinfarction or distention of the right ventricle.[70a] These tests should be readily available with rapid turn-around in Emergency Departments, thus providing the assessment with a quantitative estimate of risk.

Right ventricular dysfunction can be detected on physical examination, by noting distended jugular veins, a systolic murmur of tricuspid regurgitation, or an accentuated P2 (see Chap. 8). In practice, obese necks often make jugular vein

TABLE 66–10 The Geneva Adverse Outcome Score

Number of Points	Number of Patients	Cumulative Percentage	Percentage of Patients with Adverse Outcome (n)
0	52	19.4	0 (0)
1	79	48.9	2.5 (2)
2	49	67.2	4.1 (2)
3	56	88.1	17.8 (10)
4	22	96.3	27.3 (6)
5	7	98.9	57.1 (4)
6	3	100	100 (3)

From Wicki J, Perrier A, Perneger TV, et al: Predicting adverse outcome in patients with acute pulmonary embolism: A risk score. Thromb Haemost 84:548, 2000.

assessment difficult, and noisy Emergency Departments can obscure the subtle auscultatory findings of right ventricular dysfunction. The electrocardiogram may show a new right bundle branch block, but often, no comparison tracing is available. Therefore, the most commonly used tool for assessing right ventricular dysfunction is echocardiography (see Chap. 11).[34]

Adjunctive measures include provision of supplemental oxygen and adequate pain relief, usually most effective with nonsteroidal antiinflammatory medications. Patients who appear toxic and hypoxic should be considered for prompt temporary mechanical ventilation. Those with impending hypotension and/or poor organ perfusion require rapid institution of an inotropic agent such as dopamine (see Chap. 23). All patients find PE to be emotionally difficult to deal with. They and their families require constant reassurance that most patients have good outcomes once the diagnosis has been established.

Prevention of Recurrent Pulmonary Embolism or Deep Venous Thromboembolism

Heparin

UNFRACTIONATED HEPARIN (see Chap. 80). Standard unfractionated heparin (UFH) is a highly sulfated glycosaminoglycan that is partially purified from porcine intestinal mucosa. Its molecular weight ranges from 3000 to 30,000 and averages 15,000. Heparin acts primarily by binding to antithrombin III (AT III), an enzyme that inhibits the coagulation factors thrombin (factor IIa), Xa, IXa, XIa, and XIIa. Heparin subsequently promotes a conformational change in AT III that accelerates its activity approximately 100- to 1000-fold. This prevents additional thrombus formation and permits endogenous fibrinolytic mechanisms to lyse clot that has already formed. However, heparin does *not* directly dissolve thrombus that already exists. The efficacy of heparin is limited because clot-bound thrombin is protected from heparin-antithrombin III inhibition. Furthermore, heparin resistance can occur because UFH binds to plasma proteins.[71] The dose response to intravenous UFH is highly variable. Even when a therapeutic activated partial thromboplastin time between 55 to 85 seconds is achieved, and the dose maintained, subsequent measurements are usually not within the desired therapeutic range.[72]

An activated PTT that is at least one and one-half times greater than the control value should provide a minimum therapeutic level of unfractionated heparin. Commonly, the therapeutic range is 60 to 80 seconds. However, there are many different PTT reagent kits and virtually no standardization of PTT levels.

Initiation of heparin therapy is discussed later (see Initiating Heparin Therapy).

LOW-MOLECULAR-WEIGHT HEPARIN. Low-molecular-weight heparins (LMWHs) are fragments of UFH that exhibit less binding to plasma proteins and endothelial cells than UFH. Therefore, LMWHs have greater bioavailability, more predictable dose response, and longer half-life than UFH.[73] The introduction of LMWHs for treatment of venous thromboembolism is revolutionizing the management of DVT and PE, especially for the majority of patients who are hemodynamically stable (Table 66–11). Large randomized trials of patients with acute DVT have compared subcutaneously administered LMWH with continuous intravenous unfractionated heparin as a bridge to full and therapeutic anticoagulation.[74] LMWH was at least as effective and safe as continuous intravenous of unfractionated heparin.

A meta-analysis of randomized trials comparing 3674 patients with acute DVT receiving LMWH versus UFH demonstrated that LMWH reduced the mortality rate over 3 to 6 months of follow-up by 29 percent (Fig. 66–12).[75] The major bleeding complication rate was reduced by 43 percent. These data were used in a cost-effectiveness analysis that showed that LMWH is highly cost-effective compared with UFH for DVT management.[76] The excellent bioavailability and subcutaneous administration of LMWH permit a strategy of weight-based LMWH dosing (without laboratory tests for dose adjustment in most instances) coupled with the possibility of outpatient therapy or an abbreviated hospitalization. It appears that the majority of ambulatory patients who present with DVT can be treated as outpatients, as long as an infrastructure, such as an Anticoagulation Clinic, has been established to ensure meticulous follow-up.

TABLE 66–11 Low-Molecular-Weight Heparins

Name	Status	Molecular Weight (Daltons)	Anti-Xa/anti-Iia ratio	Treatment Dose
Enoxaparin	FDA approved for DVT treatment	4800	3.9	1.0 mg/kg twice daily, or 1.5 mg/kg once daily
Dalteparin	FDA approved, but not for DVT treatment	5000	2.2	100 U/kg twice daily, or 200 U/kg once daily
Nadroparin	Not available in the United States	4500	3.5	4100 U twice daily for patients weighing <50 kg, 6150 U twice daily for 50-70 kg, and 9200 U twice daily for >70 kg
Reviparin	Not available in the United States	3900	3.3	3500 U twice daily for patients weighing 35-45 kg, 4200 U twice daily for 46-60 kg and 6300 U twice daily for >60 kg
Tinzaparin	FDA approved for DVT treatment	4500	1.5	175 U/Kg once daily

DVT = deep venous thrombosis; FDA = Food and Drug Administration.

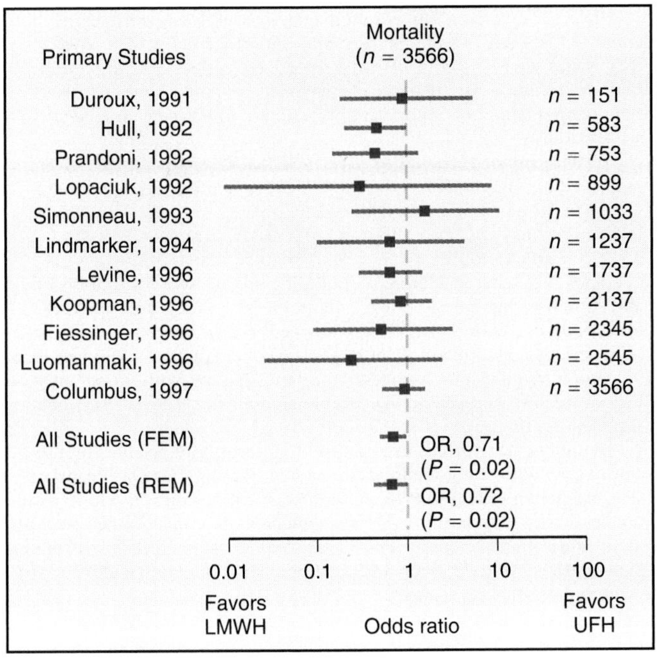

FIGURE 66–12 Meta-analysis for mortality rates comparing low-molecular-weight-heparin (LMWH) and unfractionated heparin (UFH). FEM = fixed-effects model; OR = odds ratio; REM = random-effects model. (Modified from Gould MK, Dembitzer AD, Doyle RL, et al: Low molecular weight heparins compared with unfractionated heparin for treatment of acute deep venous thrombosis: A meta-analysis of randomized, controlled trials. Ann Intern Med 130:800, 1999.)

In a randomized trial of 1137 DVT patients, the LMWH reviparin was more effective than UFH in causing thrombus regression, based on baseline and follow-up venography.[77] Reviparin reduced the recurrence rate by more than 50 percent compared with UFH. This reduction in recurrence rate correlated with successful thrombus regression on serial venography.

LMWH AS A "BRIDGE" TO WARFARIN. In patients with VTE and cancer, LMWH as monotherapy without oral anticoagulation may have advantages over traditional UFH as a "bridge" to warfarin. In one trial of 71 patients randomized to enoxaparin 1.5 mg/kg once daily versus UFH, the enoxaparin group experienced less bleeding.[78] In a larger trial of 672 patients with VTE and cancer, those randomized to dalteparin 200 U/kg once daily for 6 months had a much lower recurrence rate than patients receiving UFH: 8.8 percent versus 17.4 percent, respectively.[79]

In patients with symptomatic PE, LMWH appears at least as effective as intravenous UFH as a bridge to warfarin. Extended 3-month treatment with enoxaparin as monotherapy for symptomatic acute PE appears feasible and shortens the duration of hospitalization compared with patients receiving standard treatment.[80]

The Food and Drug Administration has approved outpatient treatment of DVT *without PE* using enoxaparin 1 mg/kg every 12 hours for a minimum of 5 days. Warfarin is usually begun on the first evening of therapy, and enoxaparin is continued until a stable and therapeutic INR of 2.0 to 3.0 is achieved. The dose of enoxaparin must be decreased in patients with renal insufficiency because LMWH is primarily renally excreted. The Food and Drug Administration approved the same enoxaparin dosing regimen for inpatient treatment of DVT *with or without PE*, as well as an alternative dosing regimen of 1.5 mg/kg once daily.

ANTI-Xa LEVELS. LMWH is usually dosed according to weight. However, if a quantitative assay is required to determine the anticoagulant effect, an anti-Xa level can be obtained. A therapeutic level for full anticoagulation is in the range of approximately 0.5 to 1.0 units/ml. Prophylactic doses of LMWH usually result in anti-Xa levels of 0.1 to 0.3 units/ml. The peak level is reached 3 to 6 hours after subcutaneous injection.

At Brigham and Women's Hospital, we assay the anti-Xa level with a HEPRN pack (Dupont) in the automated clinical analyzer used for other chemistry tests. This is a chromogenic assay based on the inhibition of factor Xa by heparin-activated antithrombin III. The plasma anti-Xa level is particularly useful in monitoring in five situations: (1) UFH anticoagulation with baseline elevated PTTs due to a lupus anticoagulant or anti-cardiolipin antibodies, (2) LMWH dosing in obese patients, (3) LMWH dosing in patients with renal dysfunction, (4) pregnancy,[81] and (5) determining the origin of an unexpected bleeding or clotting problem in patients who were receiving what appeared to be appropriate anticoagulant dosing.

INITIATING HEPARIN THERAPY. Heparin is the cornerstone of treatment for acute PE. Before heparin therapy is begun, risk factors for bleeding should be considered, such as a prior history of bleeding with anticoagulation, thrombocytopenia, vitamin K deficiency, increasing age, underlying diseases, and concomitant drug therapy. The most frequently overlooked portion of the physical examination is a rectal examination for occult blood.

Conventional anticoagulation for acute PE begins with a bolus of 5000 to 10,000 units of intravenous UFH, followed by a continuous intravenous infusion based on weight. Most patients require at least 30,000 units/24 hr. There are many nomograms, such as Raschke's,[82] to assist in adjusting the dose of continuous intravenous UFH, with guidelines provided by the patient's weight and PTT (Table 66–12). Unless a severe bleeding problem such as active gastrointestinal bleeding is detected, UFH can be started as soon as the diagnosis is suspected.

In patients with active bleeding, heparin therapy should be withheld, and nonpharmacological treatment (secondary prevention) with insertion of an inferior vena caval filter should be considered after confirmation of the diagnosis of PE. Although there is a trend toward the use of LMWH for patients who present with acute symptomatic PE, I prefer to initiate therapy with UFH if there is a possibility that the patient will require thrombolysis, catheter-based suction embolectomy, or open surgical embolectomy.

COMPLICATIONS. The most important adverse effect of heparin (UFH or LMWH) is hemorrhage. Major bleeding during anticoagulation may unmask a previously silent lesion, such as bladder or colon cancer. For most cases of moderate bleeding, cessation of heparin will suffice, and the PTT usually returns to normal within 6 hours. Resumption of heparin at a lower dose or implementing alternative therapy depends on the severity of the bleeding, the risk of recurrent thromboembolism, and the extent to which bleeding may have resulted from excessive anticoagulation.

In the event of life-threatening or intracranial hemorrhage, protamine sulfate can be administered at the time heparin is discontinued. Protamine, a strongly basic protein,

TABLE 66–12 Intravenous Unfractionated Heparin "Raschke Nomogram"

Variable	Action
Initial heparin bolus	80 U/kg bolus, then 18 U/kg/h
PTT <35 seconds (<1.2 × control)	80 U/kg bolus, then increase by 4 U/kg/h
PTT 35 to 45 seconds (1.2 to 1.5 × control)	40 U/kg bolus, then increase by 2 U/kg/h
PTT 46 to 70 seconds (1.5 to 2.3 × control)	No change
PTT 71 to 90 seconds (2.3 to 3 × control)	Decrease infusion rate by 2 U/kg/h
PTT >90 seconds (>3 × control)	Hold infusion 1 h, then decrease infusion rate by 3 U/kg/h

PTT = activated partial thromboplastin time.
From Raschke RA, Reilly BR, Guidry JR, et al: The weight-based heparin dosing nomogram compared with a "standard care" nomogram: A randomized controlled trial. Ann Intern Med 119:874, 1993.

immediately reverses anticoagulant activity by forming a stable complex with the acidic heparin. However, protamine only partially inhibits the anticoagulant activity of LMWH. For life-threatening hemorrhage, the usual dose is approximately 1 mg/100 units of heparin, administered slowly (e.g., 50 mg over 10 to 30 minutes). Protamine sulfate may cause allergic reactions, particularly in diabetic patients who have had prior exposure to protamine after using neutral protamine Hagedorn (NPH) insulin.

Heparin-induced thrombocytopenia and other complications of heparin therapy are discussed in Chapter 80.

Warfarin Sodium (see Chap. 80)

Warfarin is a vitamin K antagonist that prevents gamma carboxylation activation of coagulation factors II, VII, IX, and X. The full anticoagulant effect of warfarin may not be apparent for 5 days, even if the prothrombin time, used to monitor warfarin's effect, becomes elevated more rapidly. Elevation in the prothrombin time may initially reflect depletion of coagulation factor VII, which has a half-life of about 6 hours, whereas factor II has a half-life of about 5 days. Warfarin is a difficult drug to dose and monitor. Centralized anticoagulation clinics, staffed by nurses or pharmacists, have eased the administrative burden of prescribing warfarin and have assisted in safer and more effective anticoagulation.[83]

OVERLAP WITH HEPARIN. When warfarin therapy is initiated during an active thrombotic state, the levels of protein C and S decline, thus creating a thrombogenic potential. By overlapping heparin and warfarin for 5 days, the procoagulant effect of unopposed warfarin can be counteracted. In a Dutch study, patients with DVT were randomized to oral anticoagulation alone versus UFH plus oral anticoagulation. The recurrent DVT rate was three times higher in the group that received oral anticoagulation alone.[84]

MONITORING WARFARIN. The prothrombin time, used to adjust the dose of warfarin, should be reported according to the International Normalized Ratio (INR), not the prothrombin time ratio or the prothrombin time expressed in seconds. Not well appreciated is that warfarin can markedly increase the PTT. In a prospective cohort study, the PTT increased 16 seconds for each increase of 1.0 in the INR.[85] Unfortunately, INRs may not be a very reliable method for assessing anticoagulant effects. In a study of patients with similar INRs, there was substantial variability in tissue factor coagulation responses. This suggests that control of anticoagulation according to an INR target range may be less reliable than commonly thought.[86]

Nevertheless, from a practical viewpoint, we rely on the INR to dose warfarin. Under most circumstances, the initial dose should be 5 mg daily.[87] The dose should be reduced, however, for debilitated or elderly patients.[88] Some patients will have an extremely low warfarin requirement of 1.5 mg or less in the absence of liver dysfunction, drug interaction, or concomitant disease. They usually have CYP2CP variant alleles associated with impaired hydroxylation of S-warfarin. If not recognized when warfarin is initiated, these individuals are at a potentially high risk of bleeding complications.[89]

Warfarin is plagued by multiple drug-drug and drug-food interactions. Most antibiotics increase the INR. Even benign-sounding drugs such as acetaminophen increase the INR in a dose-dependent manner.[90] Green leafy vegetables have vitamin K and lower the INR.

COMPLICATIONS. Warfarin has a narrow therapeutic index, and the major toxic effect of warfarin is bleeding. At times, the dose response is unpredictable. The risk of bleeding increases as the INR increases. Risk factors for hemorrhage include severe hepatic or renal disease, alcoholism, drug interactions, trauma, malignant disease, and known previous bleeding sites in the gastrointestinal tract. The risk of major bleeding persists after hospital discharge and is greatest in the first 30 days following hospitalization.

Major life-threatening bleeding due to warfarin has traditionally required immediate treatment with enough cryoprecipitate or fresh frozen plasma to normalize the INR and achieve immediate hemostasis. An improved approach is to use recombinant human factor VIIa concentrate, which provides safe and rapid reversal of warfarin-induced excessive anticoagulation.[92]

Prior to "reversing" an elevated INR, it is useful to ensure that the abnormal laboratory value is "real" and not artifactual. An INR specimen that is not assayed promptly after blood collection can be spuriously high. In addition, "point of care" machines generally have higher INRs than central laboratories for patients who are intensively anticoagulated with warfarin.

To treat minor bleeding or a verified INR that exceeds 9.0 without any bleeding, vitamin K has traditionally been administered parenterally; a dose of 10 mg subcutaneously usually reverses the effects of warfarin in 6 to 12 hours. However, this approach makes patients relatively refractory to warfarin for up to 2 weeks, so that reinstitution of warfarin becomes problematic. Merely withholding one or two doses of warfarin and administering 2.5 mg of oral vitamin K is a reliable and safe method for rapidly correcting an INR that exceeds 5.0 in patients who do not have serious concomitant bleeding. Some patients with an INR less than 9.0 simply require interruption of warfarin therapy, without administration of fresh frozen plasma or vitamin K, until the INR has returned to the therapeutic range.

"Point-of-care" devices provide the INR result in 2 minutes by use of a drop of whole blood obtained from a fingertip puncture. Appropriately selected patients can self-manage their warfarin dosing at home. In a randomized trial comparing self-management with conventional management, the self-managed patients more frequently achieved their target INRs and reported an improved quality of life compared with the conventionally managed group.[93]

Optimal Duration and Intensity of Anticoagulation

There has been considerable debate about the optimal duration and intensity of anticoagulation for patients with idiopathic PE or DVT. During the past decade, a series of randomized trials[94-96a] has established that these patients benefit from either extended-duration or indefinite-duration anticoagulation.

The PREVENT Trial showed that anticoagulation can be administered safely and effectively for an indefinite period with a low-intensity target INR of 1.5 to 2.0. With this regimen, the incidence of PE and DVT was more than halved, and patients required INR testing only once every 8 weeks.[96] The benefit of low-intensity warfarin was not affected by whether the patient had factor V Leiden or the prothrombin gene mutation. Thus, the strategy of long-term, low-intensity warfarin was highly effective in preventing recurrence in all subgroups. In the ELATE study of 739 patients with idiopathic PE or DVT, indefinite-duration, full-intensity warfarin (target INR of 2.0-3.0) was more effective and as safe as indefinite-duration, low-intensity warfarin therapy (target INR of 1.5-2.0).[96a] At this time, there is no foolproof way to tell which patients with idiopathic PE or DVT are *unlikely* to require long-term anticoagulation. Therefore, we recommend 6 months of full-intensity anticoagulation (INR 2.0-3.0), followed by indefinite-duration anticoagulation for all suitable patients with idiopathic VTE (Fig. 66–13).

Inferior Vena Caval Interruption

The two major indications for placement of an IVC filter are (1) major hemorrhage that precludes anticoagulation, and (2) recurrent PE despite well-documented anticoagulation. An IVC filter prevents PE, not DVT.[97] Patients with filters after an initial PE are more than twice as likely as non-filter patients to require rehospitalization for DVT.[98] Therefore, when a filter is inserted, anticoagulation should also be used, whenever possible, to prevent further thrombosis. Some patients have an immediate contraindication to anticoagulation, but the duration of this contraindication is uncertain. Under these circumstances, placement of a nonpermanent filter may be appropriate. Temporary filters are attached to a guidewire or catheter. They can only be used for a few days because of concern for infection at the insertion site. Retrievable filters can be left in place for 10 to 14 days, or can remain perma-

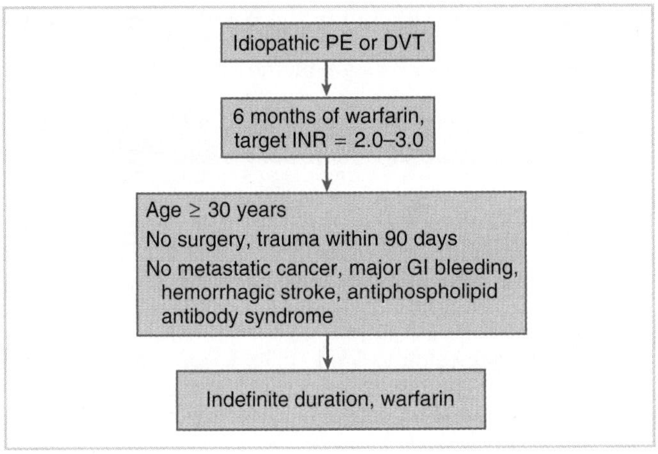

FIGURE 66–13 Optimal duration of anticoagulation for patients with idiopathic pulmonary embolism (PE) or deep venous thrombosis (DVT).

nently if necessary because of a trapped large clot or a persistent contraindication to anticoagulation.[99]

Thrombolysis

Thrombolysis is lifesaving in patients with cardiogenic shock due to massive PE (Fig. 66–14).[100] For patients with contraindications to thrombolysis, embolectomy in the Catheterization Laboratory or Operating Room can be substituted.

Thrombolysis may (1) prevent the downhill spiral of right-sided heart failure by physical dissolution of anatomically obstructing pulmonary arterial thrombus; (2) prevent the continued release of serotonin and other neurohumoral factors that might otherwise lead to worsening pulmonary hypertension; and (3) dissolve much of the source of the thrombus in the pelvic or deep leg veins, thereby decreasing the likelihood of recurrent large PE.

MAPPET-3, the largest randomized trial of thrombolytic therapy versus heparin alone, was carried out in patients with normal blood pressure but with right ventricular dysfunction or pulmonary hypertension. Tissue plasminogen activator minimized escalation of therapy—defined as the need for pressors, mechanical ventilation, cardiopulmonary resuscitation, or open-label thrombolysis—without an increase in major bleeding.[101]

The potential benefits of immediately reversing right heart failure and preventing recurrent PE must be balanced by the risk of hemorrhage. Contraindications to thrombolysis, such as intracranial disease, recent surgery, or trauma, preclude its use in some patients who can safely receive heparin alone. There is a 1 to 2 percent risk of intracranial hemorrhage.[102] Carefully screening patients for contraindications to thrombolysis is the best way to minimize bleeding risk (see Chap. 47).

At Brigham and Women's Hospital, we have coordinated five trials of PE thrombolysis. In a 101-patient trial of tissue plasminogen activator (t-PA; 100 mg as a continuous infusion over 2 hours) plus heparin versus heparin alone,[103] the initial systemic arterial systolic pressure was at least 90 mm Hg in every patient. Most importantly, no clinical episodes of PE recurred among patients receiving t-PA, but there were five (two fatal and three nonfatal) clinically suspected recurrent PEs within 14 days in patients randomized to heparin alone ($p < 0.06$). All five initially showed right ventricular hypokinesis on echocardiogram. This observation suggests that echocardiography may help identify a subgroup of patients with PE at high risk of adverse clinical outcomes if treated with heparin alone. Such patients in particular would appear to be excellent candidates for thrombolytic therapy in the absence of contraindications.

Qualitative assessment of right ventricular wall motion demonstrated that 39 percent of the t-PA recipients improved and 2.4 percent worsened, compared with 17 percent improvement and 17 percent worsening among those who received heparin alone ($p < 0.005$). Quantitative assessment showed that t-PA recipients had a significant decrease in right ventricular end-diastolic area during the 24 hours after randomization compared with none among those allocated to heparin alone ($p < 0.01$). Recipients of t-PA also had an absolute improvement in pulmonary perfusion of 14.6 percent at 24 hours, compared with 1.5 percent improvement among heparin-alone recipients ($p < 0.0001$).

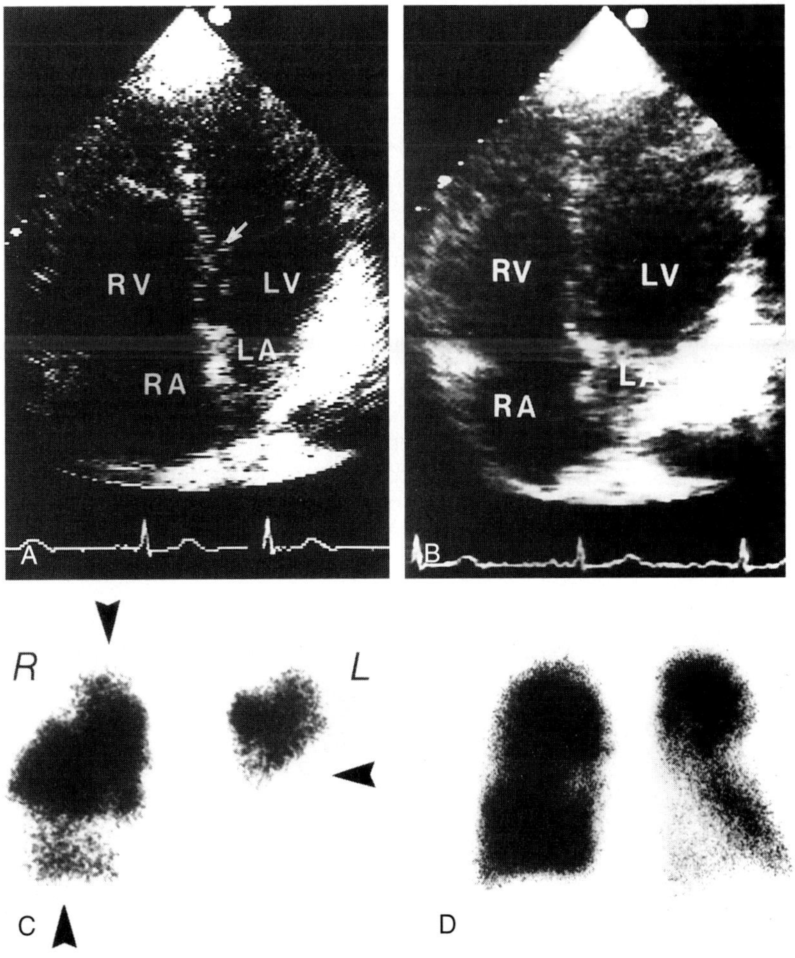

FIGURE 66–14 Echocardiograms (four-chamber view) and perfusion lung scans (anterior view) in a previously healthy 53-year-old man treated with tissue plasminogen activator (t-PA) for PE. **A,** Right ventricular (RV) enlargement before treatment. The RV end-diastolic area was 42.9 cm^2, and the interventricular septum (arrow) was displaced toward the left ventricle (LV). There was moderately severe RV hypokinesis. **B,** Three hours after initiation of t-PA therapy, the size of the RV normalized (with a planimetered area of 25.7 cm^2) and the interventricular septum resumed its normal configuration. RV wall motion normalized. **C,** The pretherapy lung scan shows absence of perfusion in the right middle lobe (lower arrowhead) and in most of the right upper lobe, particularly the apical segment of the right upper lobe (upper arrowhead). The left lung shows absence of perfusion in the lingula and anterior segment of the left upper lobe (horizontal arrowhead) and irregular perfusion in the apical-posterior segment of the left upper lobe. **D,** The posttherapy scan shows marked improvement in perfusion. LA = left atrium; RA = right atrium. (From Goldhaber SZ: Treatment of acute pulmonary embolism. *In* Goldhaber SZ [ed]: Cardiopulmonary Diseases and Cardiac Tumors. *In* Braunwald E [series ed]: Atlas of Heart Diseases. Vol 3. Philadelphia, Current Medicine, 1995, pp 3.1-3.25.)

Unlike patients receiving myocardial infarction thrombolysis, patients with PE have a wide "window" for effective use of thrombolysis. Specifically, patients who receive thrombolysis up to 14 days after new symptoms or signs maintain an effective response,[104] probably because of the bronchial collateral circulation. Therefore, patients suspected of having PE should be considered as potentially eligible for thrombolysis if they have had any new symptoms or signs within the 2 weeks before presentation.

DEEP VENOUS THROMBOSIS INTERVENTIONS

Indications for DVT thrombolysis include extensive iliofemoral or upper extremity venous thrombosis. Totally occlusive venous thrombosis usually does not lyse if the agent is administered through a peripheral vein. However, we often achieve a successful outcome with catheter-directed thrombolysis, catheter-directed suction embolectomy, venous angioplasty, venous stenting, or a combination of these interventional procedures.

VENOUS INSUFFICIENCY. Many patients with PE are plagued with chronic lower leg swelling and calf discomfort that can become problematic years after an episode of venous thromboembolism. This is known as *venous insufficiency* or *postthrombotic syndrome.*[105] In most situations, the pathophysiology is damage of venous valves from antecedent DVT. Under extreme circumstances, venous ulceration can occur, particularly in the medial malleolus. The condition is usually manageable with below-knee vascular compression stockings. However, the frequency of venous insufficiency can be halved by preventive use of sized-to-fit compression stockings of 20 to 40 mm Hg.[106]

Pulmonary Embolectomy

Emergency surgical embolectomy with cardiopulmonary bypass is reemerging as an effective and often successful strategy for managing patients with massive PE, or patients who have contraindications to thrombolysis with moderate size PE (Fig. 66–15), as well as those who require surgical excision of a right atrial thrombus or closure of a patent foramen ovale. The results of embolectomy can be optimized if patients are referred for this procedure before the onset of cardiogenic shock. At Brigham and Women's Hospital, 29 patients underwent surgical embolectomy in a 2-year period, with an 89 percent survival rate.[107] The procedure was performed without aortic cross-clamping, cardioplegic, or fibrillatory arrest on a warm, beating heart. It was imperative to avoid blind instrumentation of the fragile pulmonary arteries. Extraction was limited to directly visible clot, which was always possible throughout the segmental pulmonary arteries.

Catheter embolectomy occasionally results in extraction of massive pulmonary arterial thrombus (Fig. 66–16A). More often, multiple tiny clot fragments are suctioned through the catheter (Fig. 66–16B), with modest angiographic improvement, resulting nevertheless in rapid restoration of normal blood pressure with a decrease in hypoxemia. Interventional catheterization techniques include mechanical fragmentation of thrombus with a standard pulmonary artery catheter, clot pulverization with a rotating basket catheter, percutaneous rheolytic thrombectomy, and pigtail rotational catheter embolectomy.[108] Another approach is simultaneous mechanical clot fragmentation and pharmacological thrombolysis (Fig. 66–17).[109]

Management Approach for Acute Pulmonary Embolism

Therapy for PE should be tailored according to the patient's clinical status, the anatomical extent of the embolus, the presence of underlying cardiopulmonary disease, the presence of elevated cardiac biomarkers such as troponin, and the detection of right-sided-heart dysfunction by physical examination, electrocardiogram, and echocardiogram. High-risk patients warrant thrombolysis or embolectomy as primary therapy to dissolve or remove the thrombus, in addition to heparin anticoagulation to prevent recurrent venous thromboembolism. In low-risk patients, anticoagulation alone should suffice (Fig. 66–18).

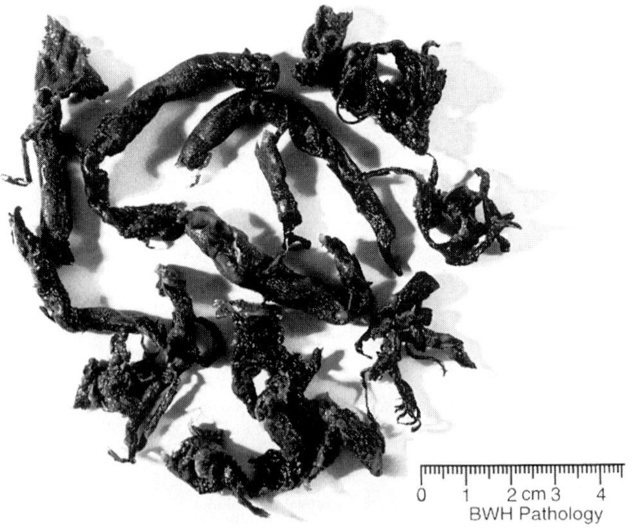

FIGURE 66–15 A 52-year-old woman was on the medical service to treat multiple sclerosis when she became short of breath and collapsed. Her echocardiogram showed a dilated right ventricle and collapsed left ventricle. Shortly thereafter, she suffered cardiac arrest and was immediately taken to the operating room with the presumptive diagnosis of pulmonary embolism. She was placed on cardiopulmonary bypass, and massive amounts of thrombus were removed from her pulmonary arteries. She subsequently recovered uneventfully.

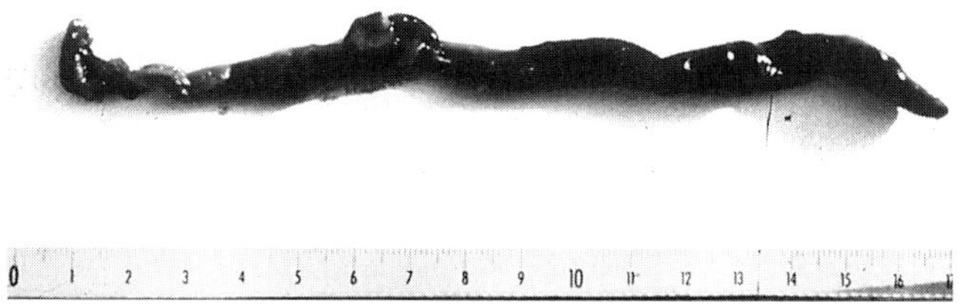

A

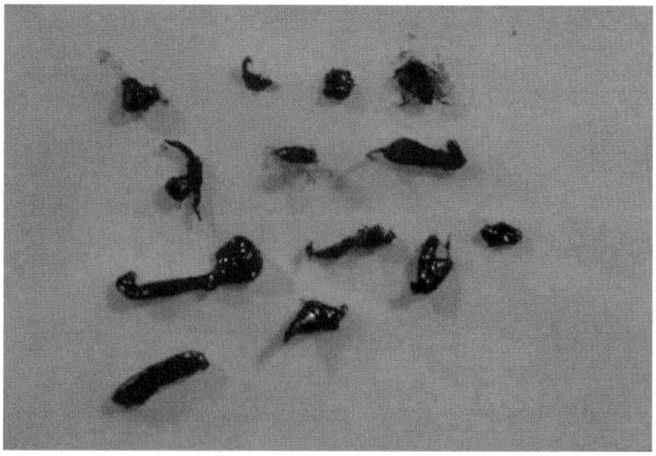

B

FIGURE 66–16 Philippe Reynaud, MD, at the Laennec Hospital in Paris, used a Greenfield embolectomy catheter to remove this 17-cm thrombus from a severely compromised patient with pulmonary embolism **(A)**. Rapid hemodynamic improvement ensued. (From Meyer G, Tamiser D, Reynaud P, Sors H: Acute pulmonary embolectomy. *In* Goldhaber SZ [ed]: Cardiopulmonary Diseases and Cardiac Tumors. *In* Braunwald E [series ed]: Atlas of Heart Diseases. Vol 3. Philadelphia, Current Medicine, 1995, pp 7.1-7.12.) Most of the time, however, suction catheter embolectomy removes multiple small clot fragments **(B)**. Despite modest angiographic improvement, marked clinical improvement often ensues.

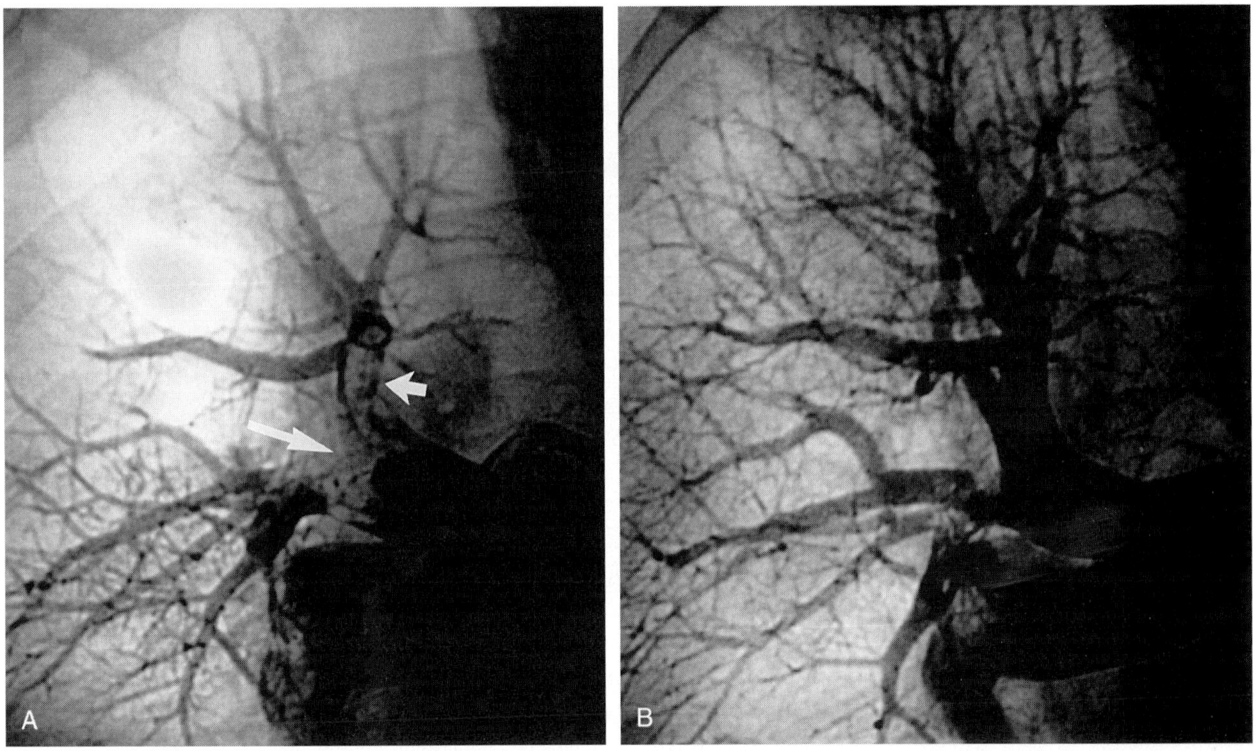

FIGURE 66–17 A 77-year-old woman had right-sided heart failure despite 3 days of full-dose heparin. Therefore, she underwent right heart catheterization and pulmonary angiography. Her pulmonary arterial pressure was 55/30 mm Hg. Seen on her baseline angiogram **(A)** were large right middle and right upper lobe pulmonary emboli (arrows). Because of relative contraindications to full-dose thrombolysis (systemic arterial hypertension and mild dementia), the patient underwent combined suction catheter embolectomy and catheter-directed thrombolysis with a bolus pulse spray of 8 mg of tissue plasminogen activator followed by an overnight infusion of 1 mg/hr. Her follow-up angiogram **(B)** shows marked improvement and reperfusion.

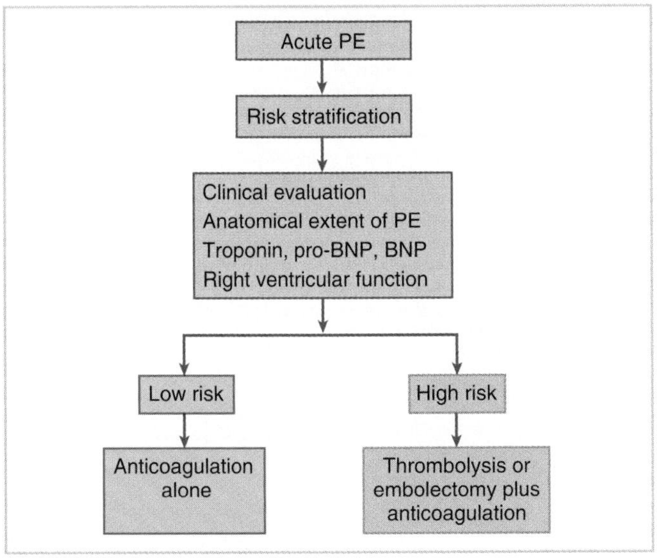

FIGURE 66–18 Management strategy for acute pulmonary embolism (PE), based on risk stratification. BNP = brain natriuretic peptide.

EMOTIONAL SUPPORT. Although PE can be as emotionally devastating as myocardial infarction, the psychological burden for patients with PE may be greater. The lay public is not familiar with PE, particularly in terms of the possibility of genetic predisposition, long-term disability, and recurrence of disease. There is a widespread lack of understanding of PE's pathophysiology[110] and treatment. By discussing the implications of PE with patients and their families, we can allay the emotional burden. For the past decade, one of my nurses and I have organized a Pulmonary Embolism Support Group for our patients. We meet at the hospital once every 3 weeks in the evening. Although these sessions have an educational component, the major emphasis is on discussing the anxieties and living difficulties that occur in the aftermath of PE.

Chronic Thromboembolic Pulmonary Hypertension (see Chap. 67; Figs 67–4 and 67–15)

Patients with chronic pulmonary hypertension due to previous PE[111] may be virtually bedridden with breathlessness due to high pulmonary arterial pressures. They should be considered for pulmonary thromboendarterectomy, which, if successful, can reduce and at times even cure pulmonary hypertension. The operation involves a median sternotomy, institution of cardiopulmonary bypass, and deep hypothermia with circulatory arrest periods. Incisions are made in both pulmonary arteries into the lower-lobe branches. Pulmonary thromboendarterectomy removes organized thrombus by establishing an endarterectomy plane in all involved vessels (Fig. 66–19).

At the University of California at San Diego, almost 2000 patients debilitated by chronic pulmonary hypertension due to PE have undergone pulmonary thromboendarterectomy with good results and at an acceptable risk. When surgery is not feasible, balloon pulmonary angioplasty can be considered. This procedure is associated with functional improvement and improved exercise tolerance.[112]

PREVENTION

Pulmonary embolism is difficult to diagnose, expensive to treat, and occasionally lethal despite therapy. Therefore, preventive measures are paramount. The concept of prophylaxis is gaining widespread acceptance, partly because of the medicolegal liability of physicians who omit prophylaxis among hospitalized patients with risk factors for venous thrombosis. Fortunately, numerous prophylaxis options are available for preventing PE and DVT in most patients (Table 66-13). The specific prophylaxis modality that is chosen is not nearly as important as upholding

TABLE 66–13 Specific Prevention Strategies for Pulmonary Embolism and Deep Venous Thrombosis

Indication	Prevention Strategy
Hospitalization with medical illness	Enoxaparin 40 mg daily or dalteparin 5000 U daily. GCS/IPC for patients with contraindications to anticoagulation. Combined LMWH or UHF *plus* GCS/IPC for patients at very high risk. Consider surveillance venous ultrasonography for medical intensive care unit patients.
General surgery	UFH 5000 U q8h, first dose 2 hr preoperatively, continued for 7 days or LMWH once daily.
Cancer surgery	Enoxaparin 40 mg daily, first dose 10-14 hr preoperatively, for 28 days.
Total hip replacement	Enoxaparin 40 mg daily, beginning preoperative evening, continuing out-of-hospital for 21-28 days. Enoxaparin 30 mg bid, first dose 12-24 hr postoperatively, until hospital discharge. Dalteparin 2500 U ≥4 hr postoperatively, then 5000 U daily until hospital discharge or for 35 days. Fondaparinux 2.5 mg 4-8 hr postoperatively, then ≥12 hr after first dose, then daily for 5-9 days. Warfarin daily, first dose 5 mg preoperative evening, adjusted to target INR of 2.0-3.0 and continued 4-6 weeks.
Total knee replacement	Enoxaparin 30 mg bid, beginning 12-24 hr postoperatively, continued for an average of 9 days. Fondaparinux 2.5 mg, first dose 4-8 hr postoperatively, second dose ≥12 hr after first dose, then daily for 5-9 days.
Hip fracture surgery	Fondaparinux 2.5 mg, first dose 4-8 hr postoperatively, second dose ≥12 hr after first dose, then daily for 5-9 days. However, if surgery is delayed >24-48 hr after admission, give first dose 10-14 hr preoperatively. Aspirin 160 mg daily for 35 days as adjunctive prophylaxis.

GCS = graduated compression stockings; IPC = intermittent pneumatic compression devices; LMWH = low-molecular-weight heparin; UFH = unfractionated heparin.

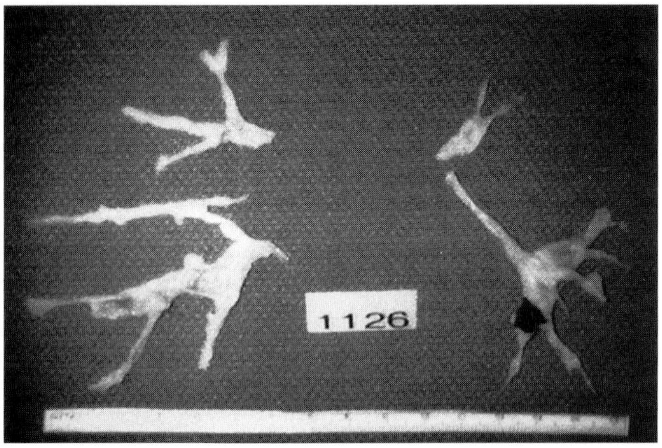

FIGURE 66–19 A 30-year-old man with chronic pulmonary embolism complained of exercise intolerance. His echocardiogram showed mild to moderate right ventricular dysfunction and enlargement. Lung scan, chest computed tomographic scan, and pulmonary angiogram showed numerous thrombi. The patient underwent pulmonary thromboendarterectomy after insertion of a prophylactic inferior vena caval filter. At surgery, a moderate amount of thromboembolic material was removed from both lungs. His pulmonary artery pressure decreased from a baseline of 35/10 mm Hg to 18/9 mm Hg before the pulmonary artery catheter was removed. He has enjoyed an excellent and uncomplicated recovery. (Courtesy of Dr. Kim M. Kerr.)

a standard that virtually all hospitalized patients receive some preventive measure appropriate to their level of risk.

American[113] and European[114] consensus conferences have provided detailed guidelines for prevention of venous thromboembolism with various mechanical measures and pharmacological agents. Computer-generated prompts increase the utilization of prophylactic measures.[115] However, even when implemented, prophylaxis may be inadequate.[116] Therefore, high-risk patients may warrant surveillance venous ultrasonography to detect "breakthrough" venous thrombi in high-risk settings.[117]

MECHANICAL MEASURES. Mechanical measures consist of graduated compression stockings and intermittent pneumatic compression devices, which enhance endogenous fibrinolysis[118] as well as increase venous blood flow. Mechanical measures are especially worthwhile among patients who have an absolute contraindication to anticoagulation.

PHARMACOLOGICAL AGENTS. Pharmacological prophylaxis options include unfractionated heparin[119] LMWH, fondaparinux,[120,121] and warfarin. Aspirin confers a slight benefit[122] but not enough to be considered a standard agent to prevent PE and DVT. For prophylaxis in the setting of total hip or knee replacement, the oral direct thrombin inhibitor ximelagatran appears promising when compared with warfarin[123] or with enoxaparin.[124] Postoperative PE often occurs several weeks after major surgery. Enoxaparin for 4 weeks postoperatively is superior to enoxaparin for 1 week postoperatively following surgery for cancer.[125] Extended-duration anticoagulation with LMWH is also worthwhile for patients undergoing total hip or knee replacement.[126]

PROPHYLAXIS STRATEGIES IN MEDICAL PATIENTS. Hospitalized medical patients are at risk for DVT and PE. The risk is greatest in intensive care units but it persists among less critically ill patients with diagnoses that include congestive heart failure, respiratory failure, pneumonia, or other serious infection. These venous thromboses can often be prevented with low, fixed, prophylactic doses of LMWH, such as enoxaparin 40 mg once daily[127] or dalteparin 5000 units once daily.[128] Nevertheless, in the DVT FREE Registry of 5451 DVT patients, 2295 of the 3894 patients (59 percent) who did not receive prophylaxis were medical patients.[23]

REFERENCES

1. Goldhaber SZ, Visani L, De Rosa M, for ICOPER: Acute pulmonary embolism: Clinical outcomes in the International Cooperative Pulmonary Embolism Registry (ICOPER). Lancet 353:1386, 1999.

Hypercoagulability

2. Ariens RA, de Lange M, Snieder H, et al: Activation markers of coagulation and fibrinolysis in twins: Heritability of the prethrombotic state. Lancet 359:667, 2002.
3. Rosendaal FR, Bovill EG: Heritability of clotting factors and the revival of the prothrombotic state. Lancet 359:638, 2002.
4. Seligsohn U, Lubetsky A: Genetic susceptibility to venous thrombosis. N Engl J Med 344:1222, 2001.
5. Bertina RM, Koeleman BPC, Koster T, et al: Mutation in blood coagulation factor V associated with resistance to activated protein C. Nature 369:64, 1994.
6. Zöller B, Dahlbäck B: Linkage between inherited resistance to activated protein C and factor V gene mutation in venous thrombosis. Lancet 343:1536, 1994.
7. Poort SR, Rosendaal FR, Reitsma PH, et al: A common genetic variation in the 3′-untranslated region of the prothrombin gene is associated with elevated plasma prothrombin levels and an increase in venous thrombosis. Blood 88:3698, 1996.
8. Allaart CF, Poort SR, Rosendaal FR, et al: Increased risk of venous thrombosis in carriers of hereditary protein C deficiency defect. Lancet 341:134, 1993.
9. Gladson CL, Scharrer I, Hach V, et al: The frequency of type heterozygous protein S and protein C deficiency in 141 unrelated young patients with venous thrombosis. Thromb Haemost 59:18, 1988.
10. Bucciarelli P, Rosendaal FR, Tripodi A, et al: Risk of venous thromboembolism and clinical manifestations in carriers of antithrombin, protein C, protein S deficiency, or activated protein C resistance: A multicenter collaborative family study. Arterioscler Thromb Vasc Biol 19:1026, 1999.
11. Langman LJ, Ray JG, Evrovski J, et al: Hyperhomocyst(e)inemia and the increased risk of venous thromboembolism: More evidence from a case-control study. Arch Intern Med 160:961, 2000.

12. Ridker PM, Hennekens CH, Selhub J, et al: Interrelation of hyperhomocyst(e)inemia, Factor V Leiden, and risk of future venous thromboembolism. Circulation 95:1777, 1997.
13. Levine JS, Branch DW, Rauch J: The antiphospholipid syndrome. N Engl J Med 346:752, 2002.
14. Prandoni P, Bilora F, Marchiori A, et al: An association between atherosclerosis and venous thromboembolism. N Engl J Med 348:1435, 2003.
15. Ridker PM, Hennekens CH, Lindpaintner K, et al: Mutation in the gene coding for coagulation factor V and risks of future myocardial infarction, stroke, and venous thrombosis in apparently healthy men. N Engl J Med 332:912, 1995.
16. Ridker PM, Miletich JP, Buring JE, et al: Factor V Leiden as a risk factor for recurrent pregnancy loss. Ann Intern Med 128:1000, 1998.
17. Vandenbroucke JP, Rosing J, Bloemenkamp KW, et al: Oral contraceptives and the risk of venous thrombosis. N Engl J Med 344:1527, 2001.
18. Ridker PM, Hennekens CH, Miletich JP: G20210A mutation in prothrombin gene and risk of myocardial infarction, stroke, and venous thrombosis in a large cohort of US men. Circulation 99:999, 1999.
19. Joffe HV, Goldhaber SZ. Laboratory thrombophilias and venous thromboembolism. Vasc Med 7:93, 2002.
20. Lapostolle F, Surget V, Borron SW, et al: Severe pulmonary embolism associated with air travel. N Engl J Med 345:779, 2001.
21. Oger E, Bressollette L, Nonent M, et al: High prevalence of asymptomatic deep vein thrombosis on admission in a medical unit among elderly patients. Thromb Haemost 88:592, 2002.
22. Heit JA, Silverstein MD, Mohr DN, et al: Risk factors for deep vein thrombosis and pulmonary embolism: A population-based case-control study. Arch Intern Med 160:809, 2000.
23. Goldhaber SZ, Tapson VF, for the DVT FREE Steering Committee: DVT FREE: A prospective registry of 5451 patients with ultrasound-confirmed deep vein thrombosis. Am J Cardiol 93:259, 2004.
24. Parkin L, Skegg DC, Wilson M, et al: Oral contraceptives and fatal pulmonary embolism. Lancet 355:2133, 2000.
25. Rossouw JE, Anderson GL, Prentice RL, et al: Risks and benefits of estrogen plus progestin in healthy postmenopausal women: Principal results From the Women's Health Initiative randomized controlled trial. JAMA 288:321, 2002.
26. Cummings SR, Eckert S, Krueger KA, et al: The effect of raloxifene on risk of breast cancer in postmenopausal women. Results from the MORE randomized trial. JAMA 281:2189, 1999.
27. Schulman S, Lindmarker P: Incidence of cancer after prophylaxis with warfarin against recurrent venous thromboembolism. Duration of Anticoagulation Trial. N Engl J Med 342:1953, 2000.

Pathophysiology

28. Joffe HV, Goldhaber SZ: Upper-extremity deep vein thrombosis. Circulation 106:1874, 2002.
29. Wood KE: Major pulmonary embolism: Review of a pathophysiologic approach to the golden hour of hemodynamically significant pulmonary embolism. Chest 121:877, 2002.
30. Kucher N, Printzen G, Doernhoefer T, et al: Low pro-brain natriuretic peptide levels predict benign clinical outcome in acute pulmonary embolism. Circulation 107:1576, 2003.
31. Kucher N, Printzen G, Goldhaber SZ: Prognostic role of BNP in acute pulmonary embolism. Circulation 107:2545, 2003.
32. Konstantinides S, Geibel A, Olschewski M, et al: Importance of cardiac troponins I and T in risk stratification of patients with acute pulmonary embolism. Circulation 106:1263, 2002.
33. Lualdi JC, Goldhaber SZ: Right ventricular dysfunction after acute pulmonary embolism: Pathophysiologic factors, detection, and therapeutic implications. Am Heart J 130:1276, 1995.
34. Goldhaber SZ: Echocardiography in the management of pulmonary embolism. Ann Intern Med 136:691, 2002.
35. Goldhaber SZ, Elliott, CE: Acute pulmonary embolism: Part I. Epidemiology, pathophysiology, and diagnosis. Circulation 108:2726, 2003.

Diagnosis

36. Pineda LA, Hathwar VS, Grant BJ: Clinical suspicion of fatal pulmonary embolism. Chest 120:791, 2001.
37. Wells PS, Anderson DR, Rodger M, et al: Derivation of a simple clinical model to categorize patients' probability of pulmonary embolism: Increasing the model's utility with the SimpliRED D-dimer. Thromb Haemost 83:416, 2000.
38. Moser KM, Fedullo PF, Finkbeiner WE, Golden J: Do patients with primary pulmonary hypertension develop extensive central thrombi? Circulation 91:741, 1995.
39. Goldhaber SZ: Treatment of acute pulmonary embolism. *In* Goldhaber SZ (ed): Cardiopulmonary diseases and cardiac tumors. *In* Braunwald E (series ed): Atlas of Heart Diseases. Vol 3. Philadelphia, Current Medicine 1995, p 3.1.
40. Dalen JE, Haffajee CI, Alpert JS, III, et al: Pulmonary embolism, pulmonary hemorrhage and pulmonary infarction. N Engl J Med 296:1431, 1977.
41. Goldhaber SZ, Polak JF: Deep vein thrombosis, pulmonary embolism, and primary pulmonary hypertension. *In* Creager MA (ed), Braunwald E (senior ed): Atlas of Vascular Disease. 2nd ed. Philadelphia, Current Medicine, 2003, pp 205-227.
42. Meier B, Lock JE: Contemporary management of patent foramen ovale. Circulation 107:5, 2003.
43. Fabian TC: Unraveling the fat embolism syndrome. N Engl J Med 329:961, 1993.
44. Muth CM, Shank ES: Gas embolism. N Engl J Med 342:476, 2000.
45. Baldisseri MR: Amniotic fluid embolism. UpToDate 2003.
46. Dunn KL, Wolf JP, Dorfman DM, et al: Normal D-dimer levels in emergency department patients suspected of acute pulmonary embolism. J Am Coll Cardiol 40:1475, 2002.
47. Kline JA, Nelson RD, Jackson RE, et al: Criteria for the safe use of D-dimer testing in emergency department patients with suspected pulmonary embolism: A multicenter US study. Ann Emerg Med 39:144, 2002.
48. Schutgens RE, Ackermark P, Haas FJ, et al: Combination of a normal D-dimer concentration and a non-high pretest clinical probability score is a safe strategy to exclude deep venous thrombosis. Circulation 107:593, 2003.
49. Stein PD, Terrin MI, Hales CA, et al: Clinical, laboratory, roentgenographic, and electrocardiographic findings in patients with acute pulmonary embolism and no preexisting cardiac or pulmonary disease. Chest 100:598, 1991.
50. Stein PD, Goldhaber SZ, Henry JW: Alveolar-arterial oxygen gradient in the assessment of acute pulmonary embolism. Chest 107:139, 1995.
51. Ferrari E, Imbert A, Chevalier T, et al: The ECG in pulmonary embolism. Predictive value of negative T waves in precordial leads—80 case reports. Chest 111:537, 1997.
52. Daniel KR, Courtney DM, Kline JA: Assessment of cardiac stress from massive pulmonary embolism with 12- lead ECG. Chest 120:474, 2001.
53. Elliott CG, Goldhaber SZ, Visani L, DeRosa M: Chest radiographs in acute pulmonary embolism. Results from the International Cooperative Pulmonary Embolism Registry. Chest 118:33, 2000.
53a. Schoepf UJ, Goldhaber SZ, Costello P: Spiral CT for acute pulmonary embolism. Circulation 109:2160, 2004.
54. Schoepf UJ, Holzknecht N, Helmberger TK, et al: Subsegmental pulmonary emboli: Improved detection with thin-collimation multi-detector row spiral CT. Radiology 222:483, 2002.
55. Perrier A, Howarth N, Didier D, et al: Performance of helical computed tomography in unselected outpatients with suspected pulmonary embolism. Ann Intern Med 135:88, 2001.
56. van Strijen MJ, de Monye W, Schiereck J, et al: Single-detector helical computed tomography as the primary diagnostic test in suspected pulmonary embolism: A multicenter clinical management study of 510 patients. Ann Intern Med 138:307, 2003.
57. Perrier A, Nendaz MR, Sarasin FP, et al: Cost-effectiveness analysis of diagnostic strategies for suspected pulmonary embolism including helical computed tomography. Am J Respir Crit Care Med 167:39, 2003.
58. Anonymous: Guidelines on diagnosis and management of acute pulmonary embolism. Task Force on Pulmonary Embolism, European Society of Cardiology. Eur Heart J 21:1301, 2000.
59. The PIOPED Investigators: Value of the ventilation/perfusion scan in acute pulmonary embolism: Results of the Prospective Investigation of Pulmonary Embolism Diagnosis (PIOPED). JAMA 263:2753, 1990.
60. Bone RC: The low-probability lung scan: A potentially lethal reading. Arch Intern Med 153:2621, 1993.
61. Oudkerk M, van Beek EJ, Wielopolski P, et al: Comparison of contrast-enhanced magnetic resonance angiography and conventional pulmonary angiography for the diagnosis of pulmonary embolism: A prospective study. Lancet 359:1643, 2002.
62. Fraser DG, Moody AR, Morgan PS, et al: Diagnosis of lower-limb deep venous thrombosis: A prospective blinded study of magnetic resonance direct thrombus imaging. Ann Intern Med 136:89, 2002.
63. Miniati M, Monti S, Pratali L, et al: Value of transthoracic echocardiography in the diagnosis of pulmonary embolism: Results of a prospective study in unselected patients. Am J Med 110:528, 2001.
64. Pruszczyk P, Torbicki A, Kuch-Wocial A, et al: Diagnostic value of transoesophageal echocardiography in suspected haemodynamically significant pulmonary embolism. Heart 85:628, 2001.
65. Grifoni S, Olivotto I, Cecchini P, et al: Short-term clinical outcome of patients with acute pulmonary embolism, normal blood pressure, and echocardiographic right ventricular dysfunction. Circulation 101:2817, 2000.
66. Konstantinides S, Geibel A, Kasper W, et al: Patent foramen ovale is an important predictor of adverse outcome in patients with major pulmonary embolism. Circulation 97:1946, 1998.
67. MacGillavry MR, Sanson BJ, Buller HR, Brandjes DP: Compression ultrasonography of the leg veins in patients with clinically suspected pulmonary embolism: Is a more extensive assessment of compressibility useful? Thromb Haemost 84:973, 2000.
68. Musset D, Parent F, Meyer G, et al: Diagnostic strategy for patients with suspected pulmonary embolism: A prospective multicentre outcome study. Lancet 360:1914, 2002.
68a. Goldhaber SZ, Elliott CG: Acute pulmonary embolism: Part II. Risk stratification, treatment, and prevention. Circulation 108:2834, 2003.

Management

69. Wicki J, Perrier A, Perneger TV, et al: Predicting adverse outcome in patients with acute pulmonary embolism: A risk score. Thromb Haemost 84:548, 2000.
70. Beer JH, Burger M, Gretener S, et al: Outpatient treatment of pulmonary embolism is feasible and safe in a substantial proportion of patients. J Thromb Haemost 1:186, 2003.
70a. Kucher N, Goldhaber SZ: Cardiac biomarkers for risk stratification of patients with acute pulmonary embolism. Circulation 108:2191, 2003.
71. Hirsh J, Anand SS, Halperin JL, Fuster V: Guide to anticoagulant therapy: Heparin: a statement for healthcare professionals from the American Heart Association. Circulation 103:2994, 2001.
72. Hylek EM, Regan S, Henault LE, et al: Challenges to the effective use of unfractionated heparin in the hospitalized management of acute thrombosis. Arch Intern Med 163:621, 2003.
73. Weitz JI: Low-molecular-weight heparins. N Engl J Med 337:688, 1997.
74. Merli G, Spiro TE, Olsson CG, et al: Subcutaneous enoxaparin once or twice daily compared with intravenous unfractionated heparin for treatment of venous thromboembolic disease. Ann Intern Med 134:191, 2001.
75. Gould MK, Dembitzer AD, Doyle RL, et al: Low-molecular-weight heparins compared with unfractionated heparin for treatment of acute deep venous thrombosis. A meta-analysis of randomized, controlled trials. Ann Intern Med 130:800, 1999.

76. Gould MK, Dembitzer AD, Sanders GD, Garber AM: Low-molecular-weight heparins compared with unfractionated heparin for treatment of acute deep venous thrombosis: A cost-effectiveness analysis. Ann Intern Med 130:789, 1999.
77. Breddin HK, Hach-Wunderle V, Nakov R, Kakkar VV: Effects of a low-molecular-weight heparin on thrombus regression and recurrent thromboembolism in patients with deep-vein thrombosis. N Engl J Med 344:626, 2001.
78. Meyer G, Marjanovic Z, Valcke J, et al: Comparison of low-molecular-weight heparin and warfarin for the secondary prevention of venous thromboembolism in patients with cancer: A randomized controlled study. Arch Intern Med 162:1729, 2002.
79. Lee AYY, Levine MN, Baker RI, et al: Low-molecular-weight heparin versus a coumarin for the prevention of recurrent venous thromboembolism in patients with cancer. N Engl J Med 349:146, 2003.
80. Beckman JA, Dunn K, Sasahara AA, Goldhaber SZ: Enoxaparin monotherapy without oral anticoagulation to treat acute symptomatic pulmonary embolism. Thromb Haemost 89:953, 2003.
81. Anticoagulation in Prosthetic Valves and Pregnancy Consensus Report Panel and Scientific Roundtable: Anticoagulation and enoxaparin use in patients with prosthetic heart valves and/or pregnancy. Clin Cardiol Consensus Rep 3: October 1, 2002.
82. Raschke RA, Reilly BR, Guidry JR, et al: The weight-based heparin dosing nomogram compared with a "standard care" nomogram: A randomized controlled trial. Ann Intern Med 119:874, 1993.
83. Grasso-Correnti N, Goldszer RC, Goldhaber SZ: The critical pathways of an anticoagulation service. Crit Pathways Cardiol 2:41, 2003.
84. Brandies DPM, Heijboer H, Buller HR, et al: Acenocoumarol and heparin compared with acenocoumarol alone in the initial treatment of proximal-vein thrombosis. N Engl J Med 327:1485, 1992.
85. Kearon C, Johnston M, Moffat K, et al: Effect of warfarin on activated partial thromboplastin time in patients receiving heparin. Arch Intern Med 158:1140, 1998.
86. Brummel KE, Paradis SG, Branda RF, Mann KG: Oral anticoagulation thresholds. Circulation 104:2311, 2001.
87. Harrison L, Johnston M, Massicotte MP, et al: Comparison of 5-mg and 10-mg loading doses in initiation of warfarin therapy. Ann Intern Med 126:133, 1997.
88. Joffe HV, Goldhaber SZ: Effectiveness and safety of long-term anticoagulation of patients ≥ 90 years of age with atrial fibrillation. Am J Cardiol 90:1397, 2002.
89. Higashi MK, Veenstra DL, Kondo LM, et al: Association between CYP2C9 genetic variants and anticoagulation-related outcomes during warfarin therapy. JAMA 287:1690, 2002.
90. Hylek EM, Heiman H, Skates SJ, et al: Acetaminophen and other risk factors for excessive warfarin anticoagulation. JAMA 279:657, 1998.
91. White RH, Beyth RJ, Zhou H, Romano PS: Major bleeding after hospitalization for deep-venous thrombosis. Am J Med 107:414, 1999.
92. Deveras RA, Kessler CM: Reversal of warfarin-induced excessive anticoagulation with recombinant human factor VIIa concentrate. Ann Intern Med 137:884, 2002.
93. Sawicki PT: A structured teaching and self-management program for patients receiving oral anticoagulation. JAMA 281:145, 1999.
94. Kearon C, Gent M, Hirsh J, et al: A comparison of three months of anticoagulation with extended anticoagulation for a first episode of idiopathic venous thromboembolism. N Engl J Med 340:901, 1999.
95. Agnelli G, Prandoni P, Santamaria MG, et al: Three months versus one year of oral anticoagulant therapy for idiopathic deep venous thrombosis. Warfarin Optimal Duration Italian Trial Investigators. N Engl J Med 345:165, 2001.
96. Ridker PM, Goldhaber SZ, Danielson E, et al: Long-term, low-intensity warfarin therapy for the prevention of recurrent venous thromboembolism. N Engl J Med 348:1425, 2003.
96a. Kearon C, Ginsberg JS, Kovacs MJ, et al: Comparison of low-intensity warfarin therapy with conventional-intensity warfarin therapy for long-term prevention of recurrent venous thromboembolism, N Engl J Med 349:631, 2003.
97. Decousus H, Leizorovicz A, Parent F, et al: A clinical trial of vena caval filters in the prevention of pulmonary embolism in patients with proximal deep-vein thrombosis. N Engl J Med 338:409, 1998.
98. White RH, Zhou H, Kim J, Romano PS: A population-based study of the effectiveness of inferior vena cava filter use among patients with venous thromboembolism. Arch Intern Med 160:2033, 2000.
99. Millward SF, Oliva VL, Bell SD, et al: Gunther Tulip Retrievable Vena Cava Filter: Results from the Registry of the Canadian Interventional Radiology Association. J Vasc Interv Radiol 12:1053, 2001.
100. Arcasoy SM, Kreit JW: Thrombolytic therapy of pulmonary embolism: A comprehensive review of current evidence. Chest 115:1695, 1999.
101. Konstantinides S, Geibel A, Heusel G, et al: Heparin plus alteplase compared with heparin alone in patients with submassive pulmonary embolism. N Engl J Med 347:1143, 2002.
102. Kanter DS, Mikkola KM, Patel SR, et al: Thrombolytic therapy for pulmonary embolism: Frequency of intracranial hemorrhage and associated risk factors. Chest 111:1241, 1997.
103. Goldhaber SZ, Haire WD, Feldstein ML, et al: Alteplase versus heparin in acute pulmonary embolism: Randomised trial assessing right-ventricular function and pulmonary perfusion. Lancet 341:507, 1993.
104. Daniels LB, Parker JA, Patel SR, et al: Relation of duration of symptoms with response to thrombolytic therapy in pulmonary embolism. Am J Cardiol 80:184, 1997.
105. Nicolaides AN: Investigation of chronic venous insufficiency: A consensus statement (France, March 5-9, 1997). Circulation 102:E126, 2000.
106. Brandjes DPM, Büller HR, Heijboer H, et al: Randomised trial of effect of compression stockings in patients with symptomatic proximal-vein thrombosis. Lancet 349:759, 1997.
107. Aklog L, Williams CS, Byrne JG, Goldhaber SZ: Acute pulmonary embolectomy: A contemporary approach. Circulation 105:1416, 2002.
108. Goldhaber SZ: Integration of catheter thrombectomy into our armamentarium to treat acute pulmonary embolism. Chest 114:1237, 1998.
109. Fava M, Loyola S, Flores P, Huete I: Mechanical fragmentation and pharmacologic thrombolysis in massive pulmonary embolism. J Vasc Interv Radiol 8:261, 1997.
110. Goldhaber SZ, Morrison RB: Pulmonary embolism and deep vein thrombosis. Circulation 106:1436, 2002.
111. Fedullo PF, Auger WR, Kerr KM, Rubin LJ: Chronic thromboembolic pulmonary hypertension. N Engl J Med 345:1465, 2001.
112. Feinstein JA, Goldhaber SZ, Lock JE, et al: Balloon pulmonary angioplasty for treatment of chronic thromboembolic pulmonary hypertension. Circulation 103:10, 2001.

Prevention

113. Geerts WH, Heit JA, Clagett GP, et al: Prevention of venous thromboembolism. Chest 119(1 Suppl):132S, 2001.
114. Prevention of venous thromboembolism: International Consensus Statement Guidelines compiled in accordance with the scientific evidence. International Angiology 20:1, 2001.
115. Durieux P, Nizard R, Ravaud P, et al: A clinical decision support system for prevention of venous thromboembolism: Effect on physician behavior. JAMA 283:2816, 2000.
116. Goldhaber SZ, Dunn K, MacDougall RC: New onset of venous thromboembolism among hospitalized patients at Brigham and Women's Hospital is caused more often by prophylaxis failure than by withholding treatment. Chest 118:1680, 2000.
117. Goldhaber SZ, Dunn K, Gerhard-Herman M, et al: Low rate of venous thromboembolism after craniotomy for brain tumor using multimodality prophylaxis. Chest 122:1933, 2002.
118. Comerota AJ, Chouhan V, Harada RN, et al: The fibrinolytic effects of intermittent pneumatic compression: Mechanism of enhanced fibrinolysis. Ann Surg 226:306, 1997.
119. Collins R, Scrimgeour A, Yusuf S, Peto R: Reduction in fatal pulmonary embolism and venous thrombosis by perioperative administration of subcutaneous heparin: Overview of results of randomized trials in general, orthopedic, and urologic surgery. N Engl J Med 318:1162, 1988.
120. Lassen MR, Bauer KA, Eriksson BI, Turpie AG: Postoperative fondaparinux versus preoperative enoxaparin for prevention of venous thromboembolism in elective hip-replacement surgery: A randomised double-blind comparison. Lancet 359:1715, 2002.
121. Bounameaux H, Perneger T: Fondaparinux: A new synthetic pentasaccharide for thrombosis prevention. Lancet 359:1710, 2002.
122. Antithrombotic Trialists' Collaboration: Collaborative meta-analysis of randomised trials of antiplatelet therapy for prevention of death, myocardial infarction, and stroke in high risk patients. BMJ 324:71, 2002.
123. Francis CW, Davidson BL, Berkowitz SD, et al: Ximelagatran versus warfarin for the prevention of venous thromboembolism after total knee arthroplasty: A randomized, double- blind trial. Ann Intern Med 137:648, 2002.
124. Eriksson BI, Agnelli G, Cohen AT, et al: Direct thrombin inhibitor melagatran followed by oral ximelagatran in comparison with enoxaparin for prevention of venous thromboembolism after total hip or knee replacement. Thromb Haemost 89:288, 2003.
125. Bergqvist D, Agnelli G, Cohen AT, et al: Duration of prophylaxis against venous thromboembolism with enoxaparin after surgery for cancer. N Engl J Med 346:975, 2002.
126. Eikelboom JW, Quinlan DJ, Douketis JD: Extended-duration prophylaxis against venous thromboembolism after total hip or knee replacement: A meta-analysis of the randomised trials. Lancet 358:9, 2001.
127. Samama MM, Cohen AT, Darmon J-Y, et al: A comparison of enoxaparin with placebo for the prevention of venous thromboembolism in acutely ill medical patients. N Engl J Med 341:793, 1999.
128. Leizorovicz A, Cohen AT, Turpie AG, et al: A randomized placebo controlled trial of dalteparin for the prevention of venous thromboembolism in acutely ill medical patients. Circulation 2004, submitted.

CHAPTER 67

Pulmonary Hypertension

Stuart Rich • Vallerie V. McLaughlin

Normal Pulmonary Circulation

Anatomy

The lung has a unique double arterial blood supply from the pulmonary and bronchial arteries, as well as double venous drainage into the pulmonary and azygos veins.[1] Inside the lung, each pulmonary artery accompanies the appropriate-generation bronchus and divides with it down to the level of the respiratory bronchiole. Additional supernumerary branches originate without relation to bronchial divisions and directly penetrate into the lung parenchyma. The diameter of the arteries decreases more rapidly than the diameter of the airways they accompany, so in the lung periphery, the diameters of the arteries are smaller than the diameters of the adjacent airways. Within the respiratory units, the pulmonary arteries and arterioles are centrally located and give rise to precapillary arterioles from which a network of capillaries radiate into the alveolar walls. The alveolar capillaries collect at the periphery of the acini and then drain into venules located within the interlobular and interlobar septa. During the passage of red blood cells through the lungs, hemoglobin is normally oxygenated to nearly full capacity and the blood is cleansed of much particulate matter and bacteria. The lungs, in addition to functioning as a blood oxygenator and filter, play a dominant role in achieving acid-base balance by excreting carbon dioxide, thereby helping to maintain optimal blood pH.

PULMONARY ARTERIES. The pulmonary arteries are classified as elastic or muscular based on the structure of the tunica media. The elastic arteries are conducting vessels, highly distensible at low transmural pressure. As the arteries decrease in size, the number of elastic laminae decreases and smooth muscle increases. Eventually, in vessels between 100 and 500 μm, elastic tissue is lost from the media and the arteries become muscular. The intima of the pulmonary arteries consists of a single layer of endothelial cells and their basement membrane. The adventitia is composed of dense connective tissue in direct continuity with the peribronchial connective tissue sheath. The muscular arteries are 500 μm in diameter or less and are characterized by a muscular media bounded by internal and external elastic laminae. In normal adults, the lumen is wide and the media is thin and represents less than 10 percent of the arterial cross-sectional area. Arterioles are precapillary arteries smaller than 100 μm in outer diameter and composed solely of a thin intima and single elastic lamina. The alveolar capillaries are lined with a continuous layer of endothelium resting on a continuous basement membrane and focally connected to scattered pericytes located beneath the basement membrane. The pulmonary circulation is characterized by high flow (the entire right ventricular output) and by low pressure and low resistance. Its wide and thin-walled vessels reflect these hemodynamic features. Thus, pulmonary vessels differ substantially from corresponding vessels in the systemic circulation (Table 67–1).

BRONCHIAL ARTERIES. These vessels ramify into a capillary network drained by bronchial veins; some empty into the pulmonary veins, and the remainder empty into the systemic venous bed. The bronchial circulation therefore constitutes a physiological "right-to-left" shunt. The function of the bronchial circulation is to provide nutrition to the airways. Normally, blood flow through this system is quite low and amounts to approximately 1 percent of the cardiac output; the resulting desaturation of left atrial blood is usually trivial. In some forms of pulmonary disease (e.g., severe bronchiectasis), however, and in the presence of many congenital cardiovascular malformations that cause cyanosis, blood flow through the bronchial circulation can increase to as much as 30 percent of left ventricular output and produce a significant right-to-left shunt.

Physiology

The normal pulmonary vascular bed offers less than one-tenth the resistance to flow offered by the systemic bed. Vascular resistance is generally quantified, by analogy to Ohm's law, as the ratio of pressure drop (ΔP in millimeters Hg) to mean flow (Q in liters

TABLE 67–1 Physiological Comparison of the Pulmonary and Systemic Circulations

	Pulmonary Circulation		Systemic Circulation	
Feature	*Range*	*Mean*	*Range*	*Mean*
Arterial pressure, mm Hg	25/10	15	120/80	90
Capillary pressure, mm Hg	6-9	7	10-30	17
Venous pressure, mm Hg	1-4	2	0-10	6
Arterial M/D ratio, %*	3-7	5	15-25	20
Venous M/D ratio, %*	2-5	3	3-6	5
Vascular resistance U^{m2}	1-4	3	10-25	15
Blood flow, liters/min	4-6	5	4-6	5

*M/D ratio = ratio of the medial thickness to the external diameter of the vessel.

per minute). The ratio is commonly multiplied by 79.9 (or 80 for simplification) to express the results in dynes-sec/cm^{-5}. This conversion to metric units can be avoided; that is, resistance can be expressed in millimeters Hg per liter per minute, which is sometimes referred to as hybrid units, PRU (peripheral resistance units), or Wood units (after the English cardiologist Paul Wood). The calculated pulmonary vascular resistance in normal adults is 67 ± 23 (SD) dyne-sec/cm^{-5} or 1 Wood unit.

Vascular resistance reflects a composite of variables that includes, but is not limited to, the cross-sectional area of small muscular arteries and arterioles. Other determinants are blood viscosity, the total mass of lung tissue (i.e., resistance is higher in infants and children than in adults), proximal vascular obstruction (e.g., pulmonary coarctation, pulmonary embolism, peripheral pulmonic stenosis), and extramural compression of vessels (perivascular edema).

Regulation of Vascular Tone

ADRENERGIC CONTROL. The pulmonary vasculature expresses both alpha and beta adrenoreceptors, which help regulate pulmonary vascular tone by producing vasoconstriction or vasodilation, respectively.[2] Alpha$_1$-adrenoreceptors in the pulmonary arteries have increased affinity and responsiveness to their agonists when compared with other vessels.[3] The downstream signaling events in alpha$_1$-adrenergic stimulation are an increase in ionic calcium levels and activation of protein kinase, which mediate vascular contractile and proliferative responses. The increased sensitivity of alpha$_1$-adrenoreceptors to norepinephrine in the pulmonary arteries may greatly facilitate local regulation of vascular tone in response to acute changes in oxygen concentrations, thereby adjusting regional perfusion. Stimulation of alpha$_1$-adrenoreceptors increases intracellular free calcium levels by at least two mechanisms: (1) coupling to specific G proteins on the cell membrane and (2) blockade of potassium ion channels.[4] Excessive stimulation of alpha$_1$-adrenergic receptors produces smooth muscle contraction, proliferation, and growth. Factors that produce an increase in alpha$_1$-adrenoreceptor gene synthesis, density, and activity greatly enhance pulmonary artery smooth muscle contractile and proliferative responses. Such factors include norepinephrine, appetite suppressants, and cocaine (Fig. 67–1).[5,6]

The alpha$_1$-adrenergic blocking agents phentolamine and tolazoline lower pulmonary vascular resistance, as does beta-adrenergic stimulation with isoproterenol. In contrast, beta-adrenergic blockade does not produce any change in pulmonary vascular resistance, which suggests that tonic activation of beta receptors is not necessary for maintenance of the normal low pulmonary vascular resistance. Acetylcholine is a potent relaxant of pulmonary arteries and arterioles and transiently lowers pulmonary vascular resistance in patients with elevated pulmonary vascular resistance with a major reversible component.

HYPOXIA. The hypoxic pulmonary vasoconstrictor response is an important adaptive mechanism in human physiology. Alveolar hypoxia results in local vasoconstriction so that blood flow is shunted away from hypoxic regions toward better ventilated areas of the lung, improving the ventilation-perfusion matching within the lung. Although the acute effects of this response are undoubtedly beneficial,

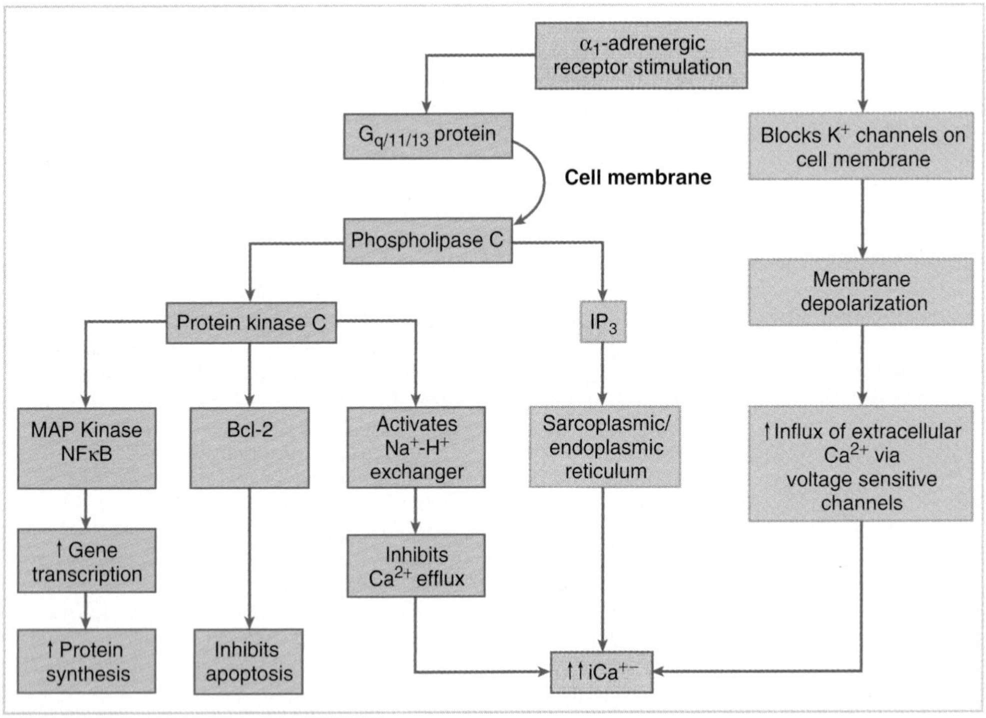

FIGURE 67–1 Signaling pathways of alpha$_1$-adrenergic receptors in smooth muscle cells that lead to pulmonary hypertension. Alpha$_1$-adrenergic receptors activate phospholipase C to produce inositol 1,4,5-triphosphate (IP_3), which mobilizes calcium from intracellular stores. Activation of protein kinase C also activates transcription factors such as mitogen-activated protein kinase (MAP kinase) and nuclear factor kappa-B (NFκB), which induce DNA synthesis and cell proliferation. By increasing levels of oncoprotein (Bcl-2) to inhibit apoptosis, the survival of vascular smooth muscle cells is promoted. Alpha$_1$-adrenergic receptors also couple to K^+ channels, which leads to entry of calcium from extracellular sources through voltage-sensitive channels. An increase in intracellular calcium is the major signal transduction mechanism responsible for producing smooth muscle contraction via the calcium calmodulin pathway, and protein kinase C activation is the major signal transduction pathway involved in the proliferation of pulmonary vascular smooth muscle cells. (From Salvi SS: α-1 Adrenergic hypothesis for pulmonary hypertension. Chest 115:1708, 1999.)

chronic hypoxemia can result in sustained elevation of pulmonary artery pressure, vascular remodeling, and the development of pulmonary hypertension.

Hypoxic pulmonary vasoconstriction can be observed in isolated pulmonary vascular smooth muscle cells.[7] The mechanism of hypoxic pulmonary vasoconstriction involves the inhibition of potassium currents and pulmonary vascular smooth muscle membrane depolarization as a result of changes in the membrane sulfhydryl redox status. Potassium, calcium, and chloride channels all play important roles in determining pulmonary vascular tone and are altered by changes in local oxygen tension in the pulmonary circulation.[8]

Increased calcium (Ca^{2+}) entry into the vascular smooth muscle cells appears to mediate hypoxic pulmonary vasoconstriction. The concentration of Ca^{2+} in the vicinity of the contractile machinery represents a balance between inflow and outflow across the cell membrane and intracellular release and uptake. Within the cell, Ca^{2+} can be mobilized from the sarcoplasmic reticulum and mitochondrial membrane, or the inner aspect of the cell membrane. Although most of the evidence favors an influx of Ca^{2+} from extracellular fluid, the relative contribution of differential mobilization from intracellular stores is unsettled. The mechanism responsible for intracellular mobilization of Ca^{2+} is also unclear.

THE ENDOTHELIUM. The vascular endothelium plays a central role as a mediator of hypoxia-induced pulmonary vasoconstriction. Balanced release of nitric oxide (NO) and endothelin by endothelial cells is a key factor in the regulation of tone in the pulmonary circulation. A reduction in NO production has been demonstrated in the chronically hypoxic piglet and rat, whereas prolonged inhalation of NO attenuates hypoxic pulmonary vasoconstriction and pulmonary vascular remodeling in rats.[9] Conversely, plasma levels of endothelin-1 are increased in association with hypoxemia in humans.[10] Endothelin receptor antagonists have been demonstrated to reduce hypoxic pulmonary vasoconstriction in animals.[11-14]

Pulmonary vascular remodeling in response to hypoxia is also meditated by a number of growth factors. Platelet-derived growth factor-A and platelet-derived growth factor-B levels are elevated in hypoxic rats, and vascular endothelial growth factor, which is an endothelial cell-specific mitogen, is upregulated during exposure to chronic hypoxia.[15,16] Vascular endothelial growth factor is likely involved in pulmonary vascular injury and endothelial cell proliferation in the setting of chronic hypoxic pulmonary vascular remodeling because of its permeability, angiogenesis, proinflammatory properties, and specificity for endothelial cells.

Hypoxia inducible factor 1[17] represents a vital link between oxygen sensing, gene transcription, and the physiological adaptation to chronic hypoxia in vivo. Hypoxia inducible factor 1 has been identified as a nuclear factor that is induced by hypoxia and bound to a site in the erythropoietin response element. Expression of hypoxia inducible factor 1 is tightly regulated by cellular oxygen tension. One of the classic adaptations to chronic hypoxia is an increased rate of erythropoiesis that is mediated by the glycoprotein growth hormone erythropoietin.

CHANGES IN ALVEOLAR OXYGENATION. These affect the oxygenation of small pulmonary arteries and arterioles by direct gaseous diffusion from the alveoli, respiratory bronchioles, and alveolar ducts in the pulmonary arterioles, even though the latter are "upstream" in relation to the alveoli. This fact, taken together with evidence for a reduction in pulmonary arterial blood volume during hypoxia, supports the view that the small pulmonary arteries and arterioles are the main sites of vasoconstriction and increased resistance in the pulmonary circulation during hypoxia. Although alveolar oxygen tension is a major physiological determinant of pulmonary arteriolar tone, a reduction in the oxygen tension in the mixed venous blood flowing through the small pulmonary arteries and arterioles may also contribute to pulmonary arterial vasoconstriction.

Acidosis significantly increases pulmonary vascular resistance and acts synergistically with hypoxia. In contrast, an increase in arterial $P\text{CO}_2$ seems to exert no direct effect but rather operates by way of the induced increase in hydrogen-ion concentration. Hypoxia and acidemia frequently coexist, and their interaction, which is clinically important, follows a predictable pattern.

Altitude. Life at high altitudes is associated with pulmonary hypertension of variable severity, reflecting the range of reactivities of different persons due to the pulmonary vasoconstrictive effect of chronic hypoxia. Altitude decreases the inspired partial pressure of oxygen ($P\text{O}_2$) because of a decrease in barometric pressure. At sea level, $P\text{O}_2$ is on average 150 mm Hg. At high altitudes (3000 to 5500 m), $P\text{O}_2$ decreases to 80 to 100 mm Hg, and at extreme altitudes (5500 to 8840 m), $P\text{O}_2$ decreases to 40 to 80 mm Hg. Corresponding alveolar $P\text{O}_2$ ($P\text{AO}_2$) and arterial $P\text{O}_2$ ($P\text{aO}_2$) depend on the hypoxic ventilatory response and associated respiratory alkalosis.[18] Mild pulmonary hypertension in adult natives at high altitude occurs at rest and may increase substantially with exercise. It is not immediately reversed by breathing of oxygen, does not seem to limit exercise capacity, and is rarely the cause of right ventricular failure.

Severe pulmonary hypertension may occur with high-altitude pulmonary edema, with infantile or adult forms of subacute mountain sickness, and with chronic mountain sickness. Subjects susceptible to high-altitude pulmonary edema often present with a slight increase in pulmonary vascular resistance at rest and exercise at sea level and with an enhanced pulmonary vascular reactivity to hypoxia. Transient right ventricular dysfunction has also been described with strenuous exercise at high altitude. In one study, 5 of 14 runners who completed an ultramarathon at high altitude developed marked right ventricular dilation and hypokinesis, paradoxical septal motion, and pulmonary hypertension. These echocardiographic abnormalities had all normalized at 1-day follow-up.[19]

FETAL AND NEONATAL CIRCULATION (see Chap. 56). In the fetus, oxygenated blood enters the heart from the inferior vena cava and streams across the foramen ovale to the left atrium, left ventricle, ascending aorta, and cranial vessels. Desaturated blood returns from the superior vena cava and passes through the tricuspid valve into the right ventricle and pulmonary artery. Because the resistance of the pulmonary vascular bed in the collapsed fetal lung is extremely high, only 10 to 30 percent of the total right ventricular output passes through the lungs, the remainder being shunted across the ductus arteriosus to the descending aorta and then back to the placenta.

An abrupt change in the pulmonary circulation occurs at birth. With the first breath, expansion of the lungs and the abrupt rise in $P\text{O}_2$ of blood lead to a reversal of pulmonary arteriolar vasoconstriction and stretching and dilation of muscular pulmonary arteries and arterioles, with a marked drop in vascular resistance. This decreased resistance facilitates a large increase in pulmonary blood flow and raises left atrial volume and pressure. The latter closes the flap valve of the foramen ovale, and interatrial right-to-left shunting ordinarily ceases within the first hour of life. Normally, the ductus arteriosus closes over the next 10 hours as a result of contraction of the thick smooth muscle bundles within its wall in response to rising arterial oxygen tension and a change in the prostaglandin milieu. Following the initial dramatic fall in pulmonary vascular resistance at birth, a continuous decline occurs over the first few months of life that is associated with thinning of the media of muscular pulmonary arteries and arterioles until the normal adult pattern is achieved.

AGING. In the elderly, the main pulmonary artery becomes mildly dilated, and a few shallow atheromas commonly develop in the elastic pulmonary arteries. Mild medial thickening and eccentric intimal fibrosis are commonly identified in muscular pulmonary arteries, capillaries become slightly thicker, and veins are frequently involved by intimal hyalinization with mild luminal narrowing. Pulmonary artery pressure and pulmonary vascular resistance increase with advanced age, similar to increases that occur in systemic vascular resistance. Reduced compliance of the pulmonary vascular bed secondary to intimal fibrosis and increased wall thickness in the muscular pulmonary arteries are factors. Changes in the pulmonary arteries are also affected by reduced compliance of left ventricular filling with age that is passively reflected back on the pulmonary vascular bed.

EXERCISE. With moderate exercise, a large increase in pulmonary blood flow is normally accompanied by only a small increase in pulmonary artery pressure. Exercise results in an increase in left atrial pressure that is progressive with exercise intensity and accounts for the majority of the increase in pulmonary arterial pressure that is observed. This marked effect of downstream pressure on upstream pressure is unique to the lung circulation inasmuch as systemic arterial pressure during exercise is largely independent of right atrial pressure. Because of the high vascular compliance in the normal lung microcirculation, an increase in left atrial pressure that results from the increased flow will act to distend the small vessels, thereby accounting for the fall in pulmonary vascular resistance during exercise.[20] Microcirculatory distention increases the surface area for diffusion and slows passage of red blood cells through the lung, which facilitates oxygen transfer.

Vascular Mediators

PROSTAGLANDINS. Lung tissue is particularly active in the synthesis, metabolism, and release of a number of prostaglandins, which may play a role in the regulation of pulmonary vascular resistance.[21] Prostaglandins I_2 (PGI_2) and E_1 (PGE_1) are active pulmonary vasodilators, whereas $PGF_{2\alpha}$ and PGA_2 are pulmonary vasoconstrictors. Counterregulatory actions have been ascribed to prostacyclin (PGI_2) and thromboxane within the pulmonary circulation.

Pulmonary endothelial cells have an abundance of prostacyclin synthase, whereas platelets are replete with thromboxane synthase. Both convert the cyclic endoperoxide precursors PGG_2 and PGH_2 into specific bioactive eicosanoids. Prostacyclin is a powerful vasodilator and inhibitor of platelet aggregation through activation of adenylate cyclase. Its metabolic half-life in the bloodstream is less than one circulation time, with its metabolite 6-keto-prostaglandin $F_{1\alpha}$ having little biological activity.

Physiologically, prostacyclin is a local hormone rather than a circulating one. Release of prostacyclin by endothelial cells causes relaxation of the underlying vascular smooth muscle and prevents platelet aggregation within the bloodstream. A variety of drugs with diverse mechanisms of action are reported to stimulate prostacyclin production and include calcium channel blockers, angiotensin-converting enzyme (ACE) inhibitors, diuretics, and nitrates.[17] Thromboxane is synthesized in platelets and macrophages. It also has a short half-life. Thromboxane is a potent agonist for platelet aggregation and vasoconstriction, and it may function as a growth factor for smooth muscles by acting via protein kinase C-linked pathways.[22]

NITRIC OXIDE. The biological action of NO is similar to that of prostacyclin in the way it relaxes vascular smooth muscle. It differs, however, in that its effects are mediated by rising levels of cyclic guanosine monophosphate.[23] Endothelial NO synthase is found in the vascular endothelium of the normal pulmonary vasculature, where it is responsible for generating NO to govern vascular tone. Release of NO occurs in response to a multitude of physiological stimuli, which include thrombin, bradykinin, and shear stress.[24] Besides its direct hemodynamic effects, NO inhibits platelet activation and confers an important antithrombotic property on the endothelial surface. NO also inhibits the growth of vascular smooth muscle cells and is probably involved in vascular remodeling in response to injury.[23] NO is also important in the signal transduction of angiogenesis inasmuch as vascular endothelial growth factor receptor activation results in increased NO production (Fig. 67–2).[25]

ENDOTHELIN. Endothelin is a potent mitogenic and vasoconstrictor peptide that plays an important role in the regulation of pulmonary vascular tone. ET-1 is the predominant isoform of endothelin in the cardiovascular system, generated through the cleavage of pre-pro ET-1 to big ET-1 and then to ET-1.[26] ET-1 is found in endothelial cells and released toward the vascular smooth muscle cell, consistent with a paracrine rule, but it is also produced by smooth muscle cells and cardiomyocytes. ET-1 has vasoconstrictive and mitogenic effects, simulates the production of growth factors such as vascular endothelial growth factor and basic fibroblast growth factor, and potentiates the effects of transforming growth factor (TGF)-β and platelet-derived growth factor.[27] In the lung, ET-1 is abundantly expressed in the pulmonary vasculature and appears to play an important role in the regulation of pulmonary vascular tone. ET-1 biosynthesis is regulated by physiochemical factors such as blood flow, pulsatile stretch, hypoxia, and thrombin. Endogenous inhibitors of ET-1 synthesis include nitric oxide and prostacyclin (Fig. 67–3).

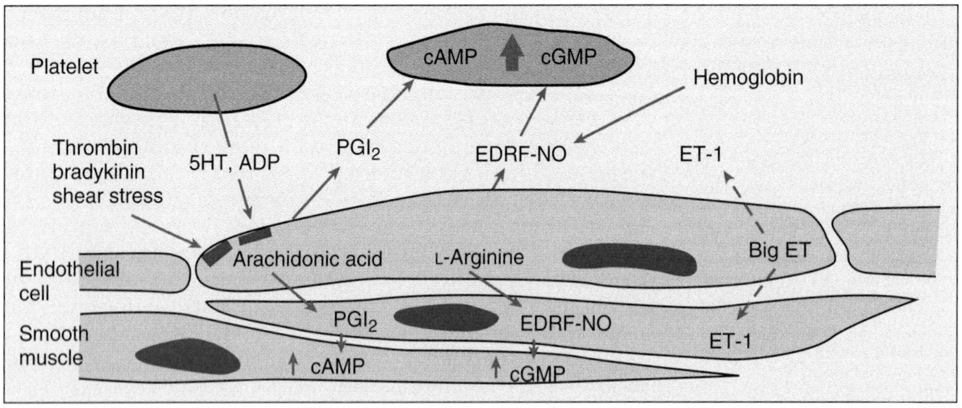

FIGURE 67–2 Generation of prostacyclin (PGI_2), endothelial-derived relaxing factor-nitric oxide (EDRF-NO), and endothelin-1 (ET-1) in endothelial cells. Stimulation of receptors on the cells by serotonin (5HT [5-hydroxytryptamine]) or adenosine diphosphate (ADP) released from platelets or by thrombin, bradykinin, or shear stress leads to the release of vasoactive mediators. PGI_2 relaxes vascular smooth muscle and inhibits platelet aggregation and adhesion by increasing levels of cyclic guanosine monophosphate (cGMP). The simultaneous increase in cyclic adenosine monophosphate (cAMP) and cGMP inhibits platelet aggregation. (From Vane JR, Anggard EE, Bolting RM: Regulatory functions of the vascular endothelium. N Engl J Med 323:27, 1990. Copyright 1990 Massachusetts Medical Society.)

ENDOTHELIN RECEPTORS. ET-1 exerts its major vascular effects through activation of two distinct G-protein-coupled ET_A and ET_B receptors. ET_A receptors are found in the medial smooth muscle layers of the blood vessels and atrial and ventricular myocardium. When stimulated, the ET_A receptors induce vasoconstriction and cellular proliferation by increasing intracellular calcium.[28] ET_B receptors are localized on endothelial cells and to some extent on smooth muscle cells and macrophages. The activation of ET_B receptors stimulates the release of nitric oxide and prostacyclin and prevents apoptosis.[29] Normally there is a balance between production and clearance, which is mediated by the ET_B receptor such that circulating endothelin is at a low level.

In pathological states, there is upregulation of the ET_B receptors located on the smooth muscle cells that function similar to ET_A receptors, which amplify the vasoconstrictive and mitogenic effects of ET-1. There is increasing evidence that pulmonary vascular smooth cells as well as endothelial cells synthesize and release ET-1 when stimulated by cytokines. A significant correlation between serum levels of ET-1 and pulmonary vascular resistance, right atrial pressure, and oxygen saturation in patients with pulmonary hypertension has been reported.[30] An increase in expression of ET-1 mRNA in pulmonary vascular endothelial cells of patients with pulmonary hypertension has also been described.[31]

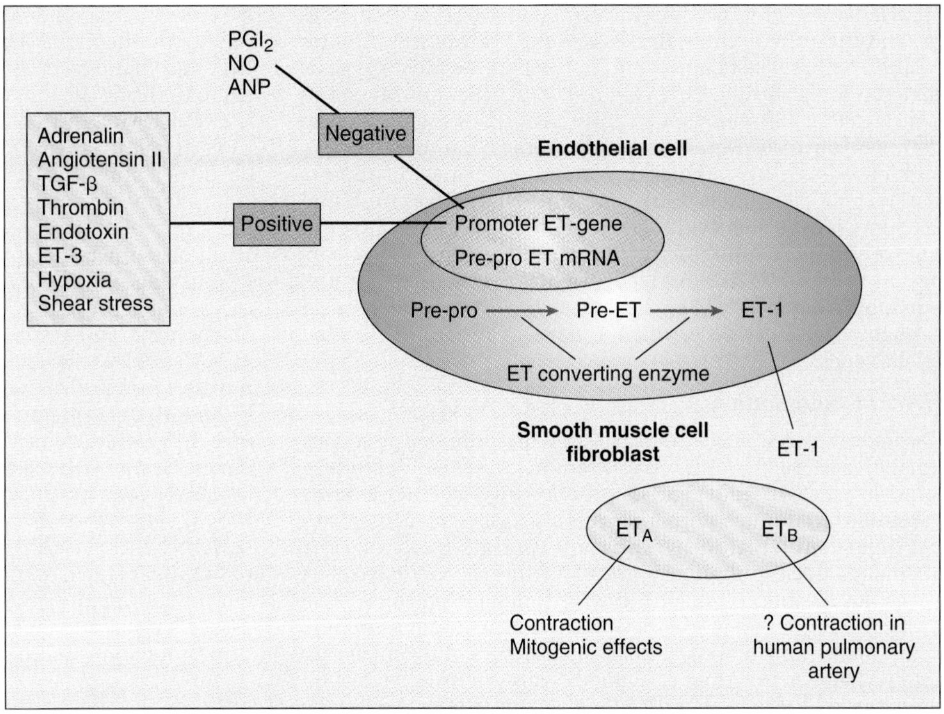

FIGURE 67–3 Regulation of the effects of endothelin (ET). ET may be active in the final stage of transduction of a number of pulmonary smooth muscle contractile and mitogenic factors. Nitric oxide (NO) and prostacyclin (PGI$_2$), together with atrial natriuretic peptide (ANP), inhibit expression of ET-1. ET$_A$ receptors are involved in contraction and in mitogenic effects on smooth muscle cells and fibroblasts. The small resistance arteries in humans appear to have contraction-inducing ET$_B$ receptors as well. TGF-β = transforming growth factor-beta. (From Higgenbottam TW, Laude EA: Endothelial dysfunction providing the basis for the treatment of pulmonary hypertension. Chest 114[Suppl]:72, 1998.)

SEROTONIN. Serotonin is an important constituent of platelet-dense granules and is released upon activation. Serotonin is a vasoconstrictor that promotes smooth muscle cell hypertrophy and hyperplasia. Normal endothelial cells respond to serotonin by enhancing the release of NO, thereby leading to vascular smooth muscle relaxation and vasodilation. In the setting of endothelial dysfunction, serotonin is unable to stimulate NO release and increases vascular smooth muscle tone, thereby leading to vasoconstriction.[32] In addition, serotonin can act as a growth factor and contribute to medial hypertrophy and promote vascular remodeling. Recently, hypoxia-dependent increased expression of the serotonin 5-hydroxytryptamine 2B receptor (5-HT 2BR) has been shown to be necessary for pulmonary hypertensive responses in mice.[33] It appears that active 5-HT 2BRs are necessary for pulmonary vascular proliferation and elastase and TGF-β dependent remodeling. Increased 5-HT receptor expression also occurs in cases of pulmonary hypertension in humans.[34]

ANGIOTENSIN II. This peptide is generated in the lung by means of enzymatic conversion of angiotensin I, a potent pulmonary vasoconstrictor. Angiotensin II stimulates cell proliferation, extracellular matrix proteins synthesis, and smooth muscle cell migration. The roles of ACE and angiotensin II in the pulmonary circulation are becoming more established. Local increases in right ventricular ACE activity and expression likely play an important role in the pathogenesis of right ventricular hypertrophy secondary to hypoxic pulmonary hypertension.[35] In chronically hypoxic rats, the development of pulmonary hypertension and right ventricular hypertrophy is associated with a significant increase in membrane-bound right ventricular ACE activity. ACE inhibitors attenuate the development of pulmonary hypertension in rats exposed to chronic hypoxia,[36] and acute hypoxic pulmonary vasoconstriction is attenuated by type 1 angiotensin II receptor blockade. Treatment of chronically hypoxic rats with ACE inhibitors also reduces right ventricular hypertrophy and fibrosis.[37]

Clinical Assessment of the Patient with Suspected Pulmonary Hypertension

History

A careful and detailed history of the patient with suspected pulmonary hypertension is often revealing. Since the earliest abnormalities in patients with pulmonary hypertension are manifest with exercise, it is characteristic that presenting symptoms are effort related. Because pulmonary hypertension can have an insidious onset, patients commonly experience dyspnea with effort that they attribute either to aging or to weight gain. With the onset of right ventricular failure, lower extremity edema from venous congestion is characteristic. Angina is also a common symptom, generally representing more advanced disease. It likely represents reduced coronary blood flow to a markedly hypertrophied right ventricle and has the typical qualities of angina from coronary artery disease. As the cardiac output becomes fixed and eventually falls, patients may have episodes of syncope or near syncope. Patients with pulmonary hypertension related to left ventricular diastolic dysfunction will characteristically have orthopnea and paroxysmal nocturnal dyspnea. Patients with underlying lung disease may also report frequent episodes of cough or wheezing. Hemoptysis is relatively uncommon in patients with pulmonary hypertension and may be associated with underlying thromboembolism and pulmonary infarction. Some patients with advanced mitral stenosis also present with hemoptysis.

Syncope is a characteristic symptom of pulmonary hypertension and is assumed to be due to a fixed cardiac output. A study on the systolic function and interactions of the left and right ventricles in patients with primary pulmonary hypertension (PPH) revealed an increased right ventricular end-diastolic volume and reduced right ventricular ejection fraction.[38] The mechanism for maintaining cardiac output with exercise was primarily through an increased heart rate inasmuch as stroke volume actually decreased. The right ventricular ejection fraction decreased with exercise, thus suggesting exercise-induced right ventricular failure. This result is expected because pulmonary artery pressure increases with exercise in patients with PPH. The left ventricular ejection fraction is maintained, but left ventricular end-diastolic volume decreases and left ventricular end-systolic volume becomes extremely small, which suggests that the left ventricle is shortening to its maximum extent. The fact that left ventricular end-diastolic and end-systolic volumes decreased whereas right ventricular end-systolic and end-diastolic volumes remained unchanged supports the concept that underfilling and not external compression accounts for the small left ventricular chamber size observed in patients with pulmonary hypertension. Syncope occurs because of exercise-induced right ventricular failure, whereby the heart rate becomes the only mechanism available to increase cardiac output, which has limited effectiveness.

Physical Examination

Cardiovascular findings consistent with pulmonary hypertension and right ventricular pressure overload include a large *a* wave in the jugular venous pulse; a low-volume carotid arterial pulse with a normal upstroke; a left parasternal (right ventricular) heave; a systolic pulsation produced by a dilated, tense pulmonary artery in the second left interspace; an ejection click and flow murmur in the same area; a closely split second heart sound with a loud pulmonic component; and a fourth heart sound of right ventricular origin. Late in the course, signs of right ventricular failure (hepatomegaly, peripheral edema, and ascites) may be present. Patients with severe pulmonary hypertension may also have prominent *v* waves in the jugular venous pulse as a result of tricuspid regurgitation, a third heart sound of right ventricular origin, a high-pitched early diastolic murmur of pulmonic regurgitation, and a holosystolic murmur of tricuspid regurgitation. Cyanosis is a late finding and usually attributable to a markedly reduced cardiac output with systemic vasoconstriction and ventilation-perfusion mismatch in the lung. Uncommonly, the left laryngeal nerve becomes paralyzed as a consequence of compression by a dilated pulmonary artery (Ortner syndrome).

CONCOMITANT ILLNESS. Patients whose pulmonary hypertension is associated with another illness often have clinical features of that disease. For example, patients with scleroderma typically report Raynaud phenomenon, dysphagia, sclerodactyly, and nonspecific arthritic symptoms. Patients with portal hypertension usually give a history of underlying chronic liver disease and may present with features that represent a blend of the high cardiac output state of cirrhosis and the low cardiac output state of pulmonary vascular disease. Many patients with congenital heart disease have a known history, but atrial septal defects in adults are frequently missed and patients may have symptoms manifest only later in life. These patients often have marked cyanosis that worsens with exercise. Patients with pulmonary venous hypertension, or pulmonary hypertension associated with lung disease, can also have extreme levels of hypoxemia. In patients with chronic obstructive pulmonary disease (COPD), the clinical signs are often obscured by hyperinflation of the chest. The jugular venous pressure may also be difficult to assess in patients with COPD because of large swings in intrathoracic pressure.

Diagnostic Tests

LABORATORY TESTS (Table 67–2). The results of these studies are usually normal in patients with pulmonary hypertension. If chronic arterial oxygen desaturation exists, polycythemia should be present. A number of investigators have reported hypercoagulable states, abnormal platelet function, defects in fibrinolysis, and other abnormalities of coagulation in patients with PPH.[39] Abnormal liver function test results

TABLE 67–2 Diagnostic Studies Useful for Elucidating Causes of Pulmonary Hypertension

Potential Cause	Diagnostic Studies
Pulmonary thromboembolic disease	Ventilation/perfusion scans, computed tomography of chest, pulmonary angiography
Pulmonary venous thrombosis or obstruction	Chest x-ray, angiography, computed tomography, magnetic resonance imaging
Congenital intracardiac shunts	Transesophageal echocardiography with contrast
Increased left atrial pressure secondary to mitral or aortic valve disease, left ventricular dysfunction, or systemic hypertension	Pulmonary artery wedge pressure, left atrial pressure (via patent foramen ovale), or LVEDP > 15 mm Hg
Pulmonary airway disease (e.g., chronic bronchitis and emphysema)	Respiratory function tests (FVC/FEV_1, chest x-ray)
Hypoxic pulmonary hypertension associated with (1) impaired ventilation, either central (CNS) or peripheral (chest wall problems or upper airway obstruction) and (2) residence at high altitude	Sleep apnea studies and respiratory function tests
Interstitial lung disease, pneumoconiosis, and fibrosis (e.g., silicosis, rheumatoid disease, and sarcoidosis)	Chest x-ray, spirometry and carbon monoxide diffusion, high-resolution chest computed tomography
Connective tissue disease (e.g., SLE, polyarteritis nodosa, scleroderma)	Serological and immunogenetic studies; skin, muscle, or other tissue biopsy: esophageal motility studies
Parasitic disease (schistosomiasis or filariasis)	Rectal biopsy, complement fixation, skin tests, blood smears
Cirrhosis with portal hypertension	Liver function tests, ultrasonography, computed tomography
Peripheral pulmonary artery stenosis (including Takayasu disease and fibrosing mediastinitis)	Selective pulmonary angiography or pressure gradient at catheterization
Sickle cell disease	Erythrocyte morphology, hemoglobin electrophoresis

CNS = central nervous system; FEV_1 = forced expiratory volume in 1 second; FVC = forced vital capacity; LVEDP = left ventricular end-diastolic pressure; SLE = systemic lupus erythematosus.

Modified from Weir EK: Diagnosis and management of primary pulmonary hypertension. *In* Weir EK, Reeves JT: Pulmonary Hypertension. Mt Kisco, NY, Futura, 1984, p 14.

can indicate right ventricular failure with resultant systemic venous hypertension.

B-type natriuretic peptide levels are elevated in patients with pulmonary hypertension and correlate positively with the pulmonary artery pressure.[40] B-type natriuretic peptide is secreted predominantly from cardiac ventricles through a constitutive pathway and is affected by the degree of myocardial stretch, damage, and ischemia in the ventricle.[41]

Uric acid levels are elevated in patients with pulmonary hypertension and correlate with hemodynamics.[42] Although the mechanism is uncertain, it may relate both to overproduction and to impaired uric acid excretion due to the low cardiac output and tissue hypoxia.

CHEST RADIOGRAPHY (see Chap. 12). Radiographic examination of the chest in patients with pulmonary hypertension shows enlargement of the main pulmonary artery and its major branches, with marked tapering of peripheral arteries. The right ventricle and atrium may also be enlarged. Fluoroscopic examination can disclose exaggerated pulsations of secondary pulmonary arterial branches reflecting an elevation in pulmonary arterial pulse pressure. However, in contrast to the plethoric peripheral lung fields in patients with left-to-right shunts, oligemia is noted in these lung regions in patients with pulmonary hypertension. The presence of pulmonary arterial hypertension in patients with COPD has been shown to be related to the width of the right descending pulmonary artery. A right descending pulmonary artery ranging from greater than 16 mm in its widest dimension to greater than 20 mm has been reported to identify patients with pulmonary arterial hypertension. In addition, a high value for the cardiothoracic ratio was 95 percent sensitive and 100 percent specific for the presence of pulmonary hypertension in patients with COPD. Dilation of the right ventricle gives the heart a globular appearance, but right ventricular hypertrophy or dilation is not easily discernible on a plain chest radiograph. Encroachment of the retrosternal air space on the lateral film may be a helpful sign to confirm that the enlarged silhouette is a result of right ventricular dilation.

ELECTROCARDIOGRAPHY (see Chap. 9). The detection of right ventricular hypertrophy by the electrocardiogram is highly specific but has a low sensitivity. The electrocardiogram in patients with PPH usually exhibits right atrial and right ventricular enlargement. A direct correlation between the amplitude of the R wave in V_1, the R/S ratio in V_2, and the level of pulmonary arterial pressure has been reported. These electrocardiographic abnormalities are usually less pronounced in patients with COPD than in patients with other forms of pulmonary hypertension because of the relatively modest degree of pulmonary hypertension that occurs and because of the effects of hyperinflation. Butler and coworkers suggested three criteria for right ventricular hypertrophy: (1) P wave amplitude less than 0.25 mV in II, III, aVF, and V_1 or V_2; (2) R wave amplitude equal to 0.2 mV in I; and (3) $A + R - PL = 0.7$ mV ($A = R$ or R' in V_1 or V_2; $R = S$ in I or V_6; $PL = S$ in V_2). A is the maximal amplitude of a positive waveform (R or R′) in leads V_1 or V_2, R is the maximal S amplitude in leads I or V_6, and PL is the S amplitude in V_1. These three criteria achieve 66 percent sensitivity in a group with right ventricular hypertrophy caused by mitral stenosis and 95 percent specificity in normal control subjects. When these criteria were evaluated in a population with pulmonary hypertension, their sensitivity was found to be even higher at 89 percent.[43]

ECHOCARDIOGRAPHY (see Chap. 11). Echocardiography usually demonstrates enlargement of the right atrium and ventricle, normal or small left ventricular dimensions, and a thickened interventricular septum.[44] Abnormal septal motion as a result of the right ventricular pressure overload is characteristic. Detection of right ventricular hypertrophy by echocardiography is limited by the ability to differentiate the right ventricular wall from its surrounding structures. Moreover, correlations between the thickness of the right ventricular wall and the right ventricular mass are poor, even when measured at autopsy. Right ventricular dysfunction is difficult to quantitate echocardiographically, but the position and curvature of the intraventricular septum gives an indication of right ventricular afterload. Echocardiographic findings that portend a poor prognosis include pericardial effusion, right atrial enlargement, and septal displacement.[45]

Doppler echocardiographic quantitation of right ventricular systolic hypertension can be obtained by measuring the velocity of the tricuspid regurgitant jet and using the Bernoulli formula (see Chap. 11). Doppler often overestimates the pulmonary artery pressure and may even suggest pulmonary hypertension in people who are normal.[46]

It is possible to estimate the pulmonary end-diastolic pressure noninvasively by summing the mean right atrial pressure and the end-diastolic gradient between the pulmonary artery and the right ventricular outflow track using the pulmonary regurgitation jet. When poor images make obtaining the estimates of peak tricuspid regurgitation velocities difficult, contrast enhancement with a saline medium should be used to improve the accuracy of the measurements. Doppler has also demonstrated left ventricular diastolic dysfunction with marked dependence on atrial contraction for ventricular filling.

RADIONUCLIDE VENTRICULOGRAPHY (see Chap. 13). Radionuclide ventriculography can provide useful information regarding right ventricular function, provided that adequate separation of the cardiac chambers can be accomplished.[47] Because radioactive counts are proportional to volume, variations in the geometric configuration of the ventricles are less important. Although pulmonary artery pressure cannot be estimated with this technique, there is an inverse relationship between pulmonary artery pressure and right ventricular ejection fraction.

LUNG SCINTIGRAPHY. A perfusion lung scan is an important test in making the correct diagnosis of pulmonary hypertension. Patients with PPH may reveal a relatively normal perfusion pattern or diffuse, patchy perfusion abnormalities. A perfusion lung scan will reliably distinguish patients with PPH from those who have pulmonary hypertension secondary to chronic pulmonary thromboembolism (Fig. 67–4).

PULMONARY FUNCTION TESTS. Although pulmonary function in patients with PPH is often completely normal, the vital capacity may be reduced to approximately 80 percent of predicted. A significant obstructive pattern is a rare finding, but hyperreactivity of the bronchial tree is common, which can lead to a misdiagnosis of asthma and could be a cause for delay in the diagnosis. In patients with PPH, the diffusing capacity for carbon monoxide (DLCO) is reduced to approximately 60 to 80 percent of predicted; there is no clear correlation between severity of the disease and the DLCO. The presence of arterial hypoxemia is due to ventilation-perfusion mismatch and/or reduced mixed venous oxygen saturations resulting from low cardiac output. The degree of arterial hypoxemia is often slight to moderate. A severe reduction of PaO_2 and SaO_2 can be due to right-to-left intra- or extracardiac shunts and/or intrapulmonary shunts. Consequently, PaO_2 and SaO_2 may vary markedly between patients with different constellations of associated abnormalities.

Approximately 20 percent of patients with systemic sclerosis have an isolated reduction in DLCO,[48] which, when severe (<55 percent of predicted) can be associated with the development of pulmonary arterial hypertension (PAH). In patients with limited systemic sclerosis, a fall in DLCO in the presence of normal lung volumes sometimes precedes PAH. A severe reduction in DLCO without changes in the pulmonary interstitium or the presence of a connective tissue

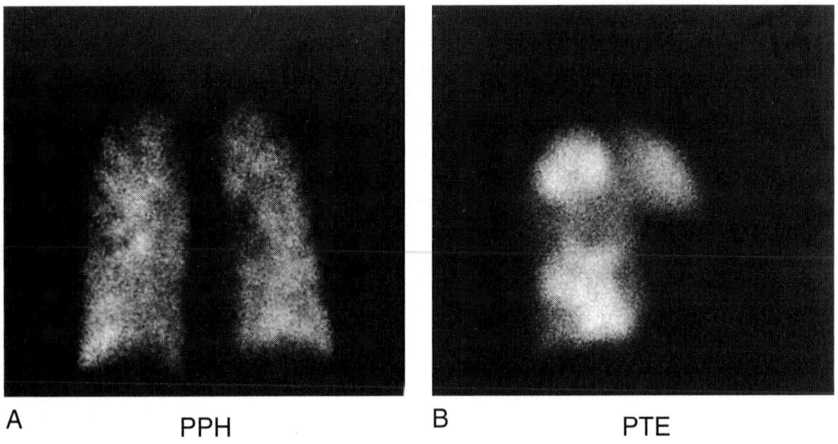

FIGURE 67–4 Perfusion lung scans in patients with pulmonary hypertension. **A,** Patient with primary pulmonary hypertension (PPH). **B,** Patient with pulmonary thromboembolism causing pulmonary hypertension (PTE). Both perfusion scans are abnormal. The scan from the patient with PPH shows a mottled distribution in a nonsegmental, nonanatomical manner. The scan from the patient with PTE reveals lobar, segmental, and subsegmental defects highly suggestive of an anatomical obstruction to pulmonary blood flow.

disease should alert the clinician to other diagnoses affecting the pulmonary vascular bed, such as pulmonary venoocclusive disease.

COMPUTED TOMOGRAPHY (see Chap. 15). Chest computed tomography (CT) scans have been used to determine the presence and severity of pulmonary hypertension based on the diameter of the main pulmonary arteries. Spiral chest CT scans have been used successfully in diagnosing chronic thromboembolic pulmonary hypertension (see Fig. 67–15). In addition to visualization of thrombi in the pulmonary vasculature with contrast enhancement, a mosaic pattern of variable attenuation compatible with irregular pulmonary perfusion can be determined in the unenhanced CT scan. Marked variation in the size of segmental vessels is also a specific feature of chronic thromboembolic disease. In some institutions, spiral CT scanning has replaced lung scintigraphy as a test to make this diagnosis.

A high-resolution CT scan of the chest is also the most accurate noninvasive means of detecting emphysema. The principal manifestation of emphysema is a hyperlucent region of lung tissue with no or only a very thin visible wall. Because CT has 10 times the density resolution of conventional radiography, it more readily distinguishes the emphysematous spaces from surrounding lung tissue. Other findings on high-resolution CT include ground-glass opacity, bullae, bronchial wall thickening, mucous plugging of bronchi and bronchioles, overinflation, air trapping (manifest as a lack of expected increase in lung opacity on exhalation scans), central arterial dilation reflecting pulmonary arterial hypertension, and modest mediastinal lymphadenopathy. CT can demonstrate emphysema in patients with little or no abnormality detected by pulmonary function tests. Because the aggregate cross-sectional area is so large, the respiratory bronchioles contribute only a small portion of the total resistance to air flow, which results in poor sensitivity of pulmonary function tests.

PULMONARY ANGIOGRAPHY. Pulmonary angiography establishes the correct diagnosis in patients with pulmonary hypertension in whom a perfusion lung scan suggests segmental or lobar defects. Typically, pulmonary angiography demonstrates large central pulmonary arteries with marked peripheral tapering. Postmortem arteriograms demonstrate the absence of "background haze" secondary to the loss of small, nonmuscular pulmonary arterioles. Although pulmonary angiography carries an increased risk in patients with pulmonary hypertension, it can be performed safely if adequate precautions are taken. Maintenance of adequate oxygenation by the administration of supplemental oxygen and the avoidance of vasovagal reactions (and rapid treatment of those that occur with intravenous atropine) should reduce the associated risk in this patient group. Placement of an arterial line for continuous arterial pressure monitoring is advised, and nonionic contrast agents appear to be better tolerated. Pulmonary wedge angiography with hand injection of small amounts of angiographic contrast material through the terminal lumen of a balloon flotation catheter is not a substitute for pulmonary angiography and may result in misleading findings.

EXERCISE TESTING (see Chap. 10). The use of a symptom-limited exercise test can be very helpful in the evaluation of patients with pulmonary hypertension.[49] Besides allowing objective assessment of the severity of symptoms, exercise testing has also been shown to be predictive of survival. The 6-minute walk test is commonly used in clinical trials as an endpoint for efficacy of therapy in patients with pulmonary hypertension. It has been correlated with workload, heart rate, oxygen saturation, and dyspnea response. In randomized clinical trials, a 6-minute walk has been shown to be an independent predictor of mortality.[50] Its drawbacks include the fact that the effort is often tester dependent and that anthropometric factors such as gait speed, age, weight, muscle mass, and length of stride can affect the test. Treadmill testing has also been used and compares with the 6-minute walk test in reflecting drug efficacy. The Naughton protocol uses a treadmill with increases in work of 1 metabolic equivalent (MET) increments at 2-minute stages to allow patients with very limited exercise tolerance to perform.[49]

Cardiopulmonary exercise testing using an upright bicycle and measurements of gas exchange has the potential to noninvasively grade the severity of exercise limitation in patients with pulmonary hypertension.[51] The breathlessness of patients with pulmonary hypertension during exercise can be related to the relative hypoperfusion of their lungs, which causes an increase in dead space ventilation manifest by a hyperbolic increase in minute ventilation. This can be exacerbated by lactic acidosis and hypoxemia as a result of their inability to increase cardiac output with exercise. Thus, dyspnea with pulmonary hypertension is attributable to worsening ventilation-perfusion mismatching, lactic acidosis, and arterial hypoxemia.[52]

CARDIAC CATHETERIZATION (see Chap. 17). Besides confirming the diagnosis and allowing the exclusion of other causes, cardiac catheterization also establishes the severity of disease and allows an assessment of prognosis. By definition, patients with PAH should have a low or normal pulmonary capillary wedge pressure. When a wedge pressure cannot be obtained, direct measurement of left ventricular end-diastolic pressure is advised. If the wedge pressure is increased, it should be correlated with left ventricular end-diastolic pressure and not attributed to a "falsely elevated" reading. It has been shown that left ventricular diastolic compliance becomes significantly impaired in patients with PAH and parallels the severity of the disease; thus, pulmonary capillary wedge pressure tends to rise slightly in the late stages of PAH, although it rarely exceed 16 mm Hg. Measurements of all right-sided pressures are properly made at end-expiration to avoid incorporating negative intrathoracic pressures.

It can be extremely difficult to pass a catheter into the pulmonary artery in patients with pulmonary hypertension because of the tricuspid regurgitation, dilated right atrium and ventricle, and low cardiac output. A specific flow-directed thermodilution balloon catheter has been developed for patients with pulmonary hypertension (American Edwards Laboratories, Irvine, CA); it has an extra port for the placement of a 0.32-inch guidewire to provide better stiffness to the catheter. The risk associated with cardiac catheterization in patients with pulmonary hypertension is extremely low in experienced hands, but deaths have been reported.

Acute Testing with Vasodilators (Table 67–3). Several vasodilators are of value in the assessment of pulmonary vasoreactivity in patients with PAH. Adenosine is an intermediate product in the metabolism of adenosine triphosphate that has potent vasodilator properties through its action on specific vascular receptors. It is believed to stimulate the endothelial cell and vascular smooth muscle receptors of the A_2 type, which induce vascular smooth muscle relaxation by increasing cyclic adenosine monophosphate. In patients with PAH, adenosine has been shown to be a potent vasodilator and predictive of the chronic effects of intravenous prostacyclin and oral calcium channel blockers.[53] Adenosine has an extremely short half-life (<5 sec), which provides a safety net by its rapid dissolution should any adverse side effects occur. It is administered intravenously as an infusion in doses of 50 μg/kg/min and titrated upward every 2 minutes until uncomfortable symptoms develop (such as chest tightness or dyspnea).

Epoprostenol has been used as an acute test of vasoreactivity in patients with PAH.[54] Like adenosine, its short half-life allows use of the drug to be discontinued if any acute adverse effects result. Also similar to adenosine, it is administered incrementally, at 2 ng/kg/min and increased every 15 to 30 minutes until systemic effects such as headache, flushing, or nausea occur, which limits the acute dose titration. Favorable acute effects from epoprostenol are predictive of a favorable response to oral calcium channel blockers.

Adenosine and epoprostenol possess potent inotropic properties, in addition to their ability to vasodilate the pulmonary vascular bed. When using these drugs for the acute testing of patients, one needs to pay particular attention to changes in cardiac output that occur in association with the changes in pulmonary arterial pressure. An increase in cardiac output with no change in pulmonary arterial pressure will result in a reduction in calculated pulmonary vascular resistance and may be erroneously interpreted as a vasodilator response.

Nitric oxide is also a useful drug to test pulmonary vasoreactivity.[55] Because it binds very rapidly to hemoglobin with high affinity and is thereby inactivated, inhalation of NO gas results in selective pulmonary vascular effects without influencing the systemic circulation.[56] Inhalation of NO by patients with PAH has been shown to produce a reduction in pulmonary vascular resistance acutely, similar to that achieved with intravenous adenosine, and to also predict the effectiveness of calcium channel blockers. NO differs importantly from adenosine and epoprostenol in that it has little effect on cardiac output. It is usually given via facemask at 20 to 40 ppm.

It must be emphasized that hemodynamic assessment of the entire circulatory system is essential when determining the influence of drugs in these patients. Small changes in pulmonary artery pressure are usually due to variability and are not related to direct drug influence. Changes in pulmonary vascular resistance cannot be directly measured but are computed by the change in pulmonary pressure and cardiac output simultaneously. Because thermodilution cardiac output—the method that is most commonly used in these patients—can be associated with large errors in reproducibility, particular care should be taken in the methodology of thermodilution used in these patients. In addition, when an underlying right-to-left shunt exists, the Fick determination of cardiac output is required.

Changes in pulmonary capillary wedge pressure can have important influences on the determination of pulmonary vascular resistance. A rising capillary wedge pressure secondary to increased cardiac output may be the first sign of impending left ventricular failure and an adverse effect of a drug, whereas the calculated pulmonary vascular resistance may become lower and suggest a beneficial effect. Right atrial pressure also reflects the filling characteristics of the right ventricle. A right atrial pressure increase in the face of rising cardiac output suggests right ventricular diastolic dysfunction. The resting heart rate is a physiological parameter of marked importance in patients with congestive heart failure, and treatments that cause an increased heart rate are likely to yield deleterious long-term results. Finally, the systemic arterial oxygen

TABLE 67–3 Hemodynamic Assessment of Vasodilators in Pulmonary Hypertension

Parameter Measured	Desired Acute Changes	Comments
Mean pulmonary artery pressure	>25% fall; ideally mean PAP below 30 mm Hg	Must not be any associated significant fall in systemic blood pressure
Pulmonary vascular resistance	>33% fall; ideally, PVR below 6 units	Should be associated with a fall in PAP *and* an increase in cardiac output. An increase in cardiac output alone may lead to future RV failure
Right atrial pressure	No change or fall	An increase in RA pressure signals impending RV failure
Pulmonary capillary wedge pressure	No change	An increase in wedge pressure suggests pulmonary venoocclusive disease or coexisting LV dysfunction
Systemic blood pressure	Minimal fall; mean arterial pressure should remain above 90 mm Hg	A significant hypotensive response makes chronic vasodilator therapy contraindicated
Cardiac output	Increase	The increase should be related to increased stroke volume and not solely due to increased heart rate
Heart rate	No significant change	A chronic increased heart rate will result in RV failure. Watch for bradycardia if high doses of diltiazem are used
Systemic arterial oxygen saturation	Increase if reduced on room air, little change if normal	A fall in systemic arterial oxygen saturation suggests lung disease or right-to-left shunting and prohibits chronic use
Pulmonary artery (mixed venous) oxygen saturation	Increase	Should reflect the increase in cardiac output and improved tissue oxygenation

LV = left ventricular; PAP = pulmonary artery pressure; PVR = pulmonary vascular resistance; RA = right atrial; RV = right ventricular.

From Rubin LJ, Rich S: Medical management. *In* Rubin LJ, Rich S (eds): Primary Pulmonary Hypertension. New York. Marcel Dekker, 1997, pp 271-286 by courtesy of Marcel Dekker, Inc.

content should be evaluated in patients with pulmonary hypertension. Effective vasodilator drugs can result in vasodilation of blood vessels supplying poorly ventilated areas of the lung and can worsen hypoxemia. This effect is particularly noticeable in patients with underlying chronic lung disease.

Classification of Pulmonary Hypertension

Pulmonary hypertension, in its simplest sense, refers to any elevation in the pulmonary arterial pressure above normal. The presence of pulmonary hypertension may reflect a serious underlying pulmonary vascular disease, which can be progressive and fatal, or simply an obligatory passive elevation in the pulmonary artery pressure in response to elevated pressures in the left heart. Consequently, an accurate diagnosis of the cause of pulmonary hypertension in a patient is essential to establish an effective treatment plan. In addition, therapies that may be beneficial in patients with some types of pulmonary hypertension may be harmful in patients with other types.

The diagnosis of pulmonary hypertension relies on establishing an elevation in pulmonary artery pressure above normal. Published norms have come from cardiac catheterizations performed in young subjects at rest without any evidence of cardiopulmonary disease. The upper limit of normal for pulmonary artery mean pressure is 19 mm Hg. However, this assumes that there are no abnormalities in downstream pressures of the left atrium or left ventricle, or an increased cardiac output. That is why a patient can have pulmonary hypertension from the standpoint of an elevated pulmonary artery pressure, but normal pulmonary vascular resistance. Recently, parameters for normal pulmonary arterial systolic pressure derived by echo-Doppler studies have been published that suggest that the upper limit of normal of pulmonary arterial systolic pressure in the general population may be higher than previously appreciated.[46]

There are patients whose resting hemodynamics are normal but in whom marked elevations in pulmonary pressure occur with exercise. It has been presumed that this represents an early stage of pulmonary vascular disease. However, because patients may have a hypertensive response to exercise with respect to the systemic vasculature, a similar type of response can occur in the pulmonary vascular disease, or reduced compliance of an otherwise normal pulmonary circulation can be difficult to ascertain.

In 1998, a new classification for pulmonary hypertension was developed at the World Symposium on Pulmonary Hypertension cosponsored by the World Health Organization. This classification catalogued clinical conditions based on common pathobiological features to serve as a guide in the clinical assessment and treatment of these patients. Recently, modifications to this classification have been proposed (Table 67–4). In addition, a functional classification patterned after the New York Heart Association functional classification for heart disease was developed to allow comparisons of patients with respect to the clinical severity of the disease process (Table 67–5).

Pulmonary arterial hypertension refers to pulmonary vascular disease affecting the arterioles, resulting in an elevation in pressure and vascular resistance. Although PPH is relatively rare, with an estimated incidence of 1 to 2 per million in the population, severe PAH associated with other conditions is more common (Table 67–6).[57] The most common etiology is associated with connective tissue disease states, primarily scleroderma, including the CREST syndrome (calcinosis cutis, Raynaud phenomenon, esophageal dysfunction, sclerodactyly, and telangiectasia), and mixed connective tissue disease. PAH is also relatively common in patients with congenital heart defects, especially those with ventricular septal defects or a patent ductus arteriosus.[58]

TABLE 67–4 Clinical Classification of Pulmonary Arterial Hypertension*

1. Pulmonary arterial hypertension
1.1 Primary pulmonary hypertension
(a) Familial
1.2 Associated with:
(a) Connective tissue disease
(b) Congenital heart disease
(c) Portal hypertension
(d) Human immunodeficiency virus infection
(e) Drugs/toxins
(1) Anorexigens
(2) Other
1.3 Persistent pulmonary hypertension of the newborn
1.4 Pulmonary veno-occlusive disease
1.5 Pulmonary capillary hemangiomatosis
2. Pulmonary venous hypertension
2.1 Left-sided atrial or ventricular heart disease
2.2 Left-sided valvular heart disease
2.3 Extrinsic compression of central pulmonary veins
(a) Fibrosing mediastinitis
(b) Adenopathy/tumors
2.4 Other
3. Pulmonary hypertension associated with disorders of the respiratory system and/or hypoxemia
3.1 Chronic obstructive pulmonary disease
3.2 Interstitial lung disease
3.3 Sleep-disordered breathing
3.4 Alveolar hypoventilation disorders
3.5 Chronic exposure to high altitude
3.6 Neonatal lung disease
3.7 Alveolar-capillary dysplasia
3.8 Other
4. Pulmonary hypertension due to chronic thrombotic and/or embolic disease
4.1 Thromboembolic obstruction of proximal pulmonary arteries
4.2 Thromboembolic obstruction of the distal pulmonary arteries
4.3 Pulmonary embolism (tumor, ova parasites, foreign material)
5. Pulmonary hypertension due to disorders directly affecting the pulmonary vasculature
5.1 Inflammatory
(a) Schistosomiasis
(b) Sarcoidosis
(c) Histiocytosis X
(d) Other

*Modified from Rich S (ed): Primary Pulmonary Hypertension: Executive Summary from the World Symposium—Primary Pulmonary Hypertension 1998. Available from the World Health Organization at http://www.who.int/ncd/cvd/pph.html.

Other comorbid conditions include cirrhosis with portal hypertension and human immunodeficiency virus (HIV) infection.

COR PULMONALE. This is defined as right ventricular hypertrophy and dilation secondary to pulmonary hypertension caused by diseases of the lung parenchyma and/or pulmonary vasculature, unrelated to the left side of the heart. Chronic cor pulmonale traditionally implies pulmonary hypertension related to either obstructive or restrictive lung disease, whereas acute cor pulmonale usually refers to the development of acute pulmonary hypertension from massive pulmonary embolism.

Primary Pulmonary Hypertension

Primary pulmonary hypertension is the diagnosis given to patients with pulmonary hypertension of unexplained etiol-

TABLE 67–5 World Health Organization Functional Classification of Pulmonary Hypertension*

A. Class I—Patients with pulmonary hypertension but without resulting limitation of physical activity. Ordinary physical activity does not cause undue dyspnea or fatigue, chest pain, or syncope.
B. Class II—Patients with pulmonary hypertension resulting in slight limitation of physical activity. They are comfortable at rest. Ordinary physical activity causes undue dyspnea or fatigue, chest pain, or near syncope.
C. Class III—Patients with pulmonary hypertension resulting in marked limitation of physical activity. They are comfortable at rest. Less than ordinary activity causes undue dyspnea or fatigue, chest pain, or near syncope.
D. Class IV—Patients with pulmonary hypertension with inability to carry out any physical activity without symptoms. Patients manifest signs of right heart failure. Dyspnea and/or fatigue may even be present at rest. Discomfort is increased by any physical activity.

*Modified from Rich S (ed): Primary Pulmonary Hypertension: Executive Summary from the World Symposium—Primary Pulmonary Hypertension 1998. Available from the World Health Organization at http://www.who.int/ncd/cvd/pph.html.

ogy. Although the name of the disease stems from its distinction from pulmonary hypertension secondary to known cardiac or pulmonary causes, PPH should not be considered as only pulmonary hypertension for which no cause is found. The clinical features, usual age of onset, progression of the disease, and autopsy findings make PPH a distinct clinical entity and distinguish it from other forms of pulmonary hypertension even though its diagnosis requires careful exclusion of secondary causes. The actual incidence of PPH appears to be approximately 2 cases per million population, thus qualifying it as an orphan disease.[59]

Etiology

By definition, the precise cause of PPH is unknown, but it probably represents the clinical expression of PAH as the final common pathway from multiple biological abnormalities within the pulmonary circulation. As understanding of vascular biology improves, many studies point to abnormalities in pulmonary endothelial cell function as causing or contributing to the development of pulmonary hypertension in humans.[60] It is now understood that the endothelial cell regulates pulmonary smooth muscle cell tone. Dysfunction of the counterregulatory systems within the pulmonary vascular bed seems to be common in cases of pulmonary hypertension. The normal pulmonary vascular endothelial cell maintains the vascular smooth muscle in a state of relaxation.[61] The finding of increased pulmonary vascular reactivity and vasoconstriction in patients with PPH suggests that a marked vasoconstrictive tendency underlies the development of PPH in predisposed individuals, possibly as a result of inappropriate smooth muscle hypertrophy.

Reduced expression of NO synthase in the endothelium of patients with pulmonary hypertension has been demonstrated and correlates inversely with the extent and severity of morphological lesions.[62] Although it is unsettled whether reduced NO synthase production is a cause or a result of the disease, it is consistent with endothelial dysfunction underlying PPH as part of the disease process. Endothelin may also play an important role in the elevated pulmonary vascular tone.[63] Because it has a long half-life, subtle disturbances in production or release could lead to sustained vasoconstriction. Elevations in endothelin levels within the pulmonary vasculature of patients with various forms of pulmonary hypertension have been documented.[64] This finding suggests that regardless of whether abnormal endothelial function is the underlying cause of PPH, progression of the disease is invariably accompanied by worsening of endothelial function, which itself can promote disease progression.

A striking feature of the pulmonary vasculature in patients with PPH is intimal proliferation, and in some vessels it causes virtually complete vascular occlusion (Fig. 67–5). Several growth factors have been implicated in the development of this type of vascular pathology, including basic fibroblast growth factor from the endothelium[65] and platelet-derived growth factor and TGF-β[66] from platelets. Enhanced growth factor release, activation, and intracellular signaling may lead to smooth muscle cell proliferation and migration, as well as extracellular matrix synthesis. Even advanced lesions show evidence of in situ activity of ongoing synthesis of connective tissue proteins such as elastin, collagen, and fibronectin.[60]

An equally important etiological feature of PPH is the widespread development of in situ thrombosis of the small pulmonary arteries with intraluminal thrombin deposition. Abnormalities in platelet activation and function and biochemical features of a procoagulant environment within the pulmonary vasculature support a role of thrombosis in disease initiation in some patients.[67,68] Interactions between growth factors, platelets, and the vessel wall suggest that thrombin may play a fundamental role in many of the pathobiological processes described in patients with PPH and in disease progression.[69] A prothrombotic state can arise as a consequence of fibrinolysis, enhanced coagulation, or increased platelet activation. Platelet activation not only promotes thrombosis but also leads to the release of granules that contain mitogenic agents and vasoconstrictive substances.[70]

LOCAL HEMODYNAMICS. Several studies suggest that local hemodynamics can influence pulmonary vascular remodeling.[71] A classic example is the pulmonary hypertension that occurs in congenital systemic-to-pulmonary shunts. It is believed that endothelial cells can release mediators that induce vascular smooth muscle cell growth in response to changes in pulmonary blood flow or pressure. Experimental data suggest that medial hypertrophy can be converted to a neointimal

TABLE 67–6 Advanced Pulmonary Hypertension by Disease Category

Disease	Prevalence	Percentage of Patients with PH	Estimated Number in North America and Europe
Systemic sclerosis	190/million	33	37,620
Congenital heart defects (ASD/VSD/PDA)	300/million	15-20	31,500
Cirrhosis	1600/million	0.6	5,760
HIV related	2500/million	0.5	7,500
Primary PH	7/million	100	4,200

ASD = atrial septal defect; HIV = human immunodeficiency virus; PDA = patent ductus arteriosus; PH = pulmonary hypertension; VSD = ventricular septal defect.

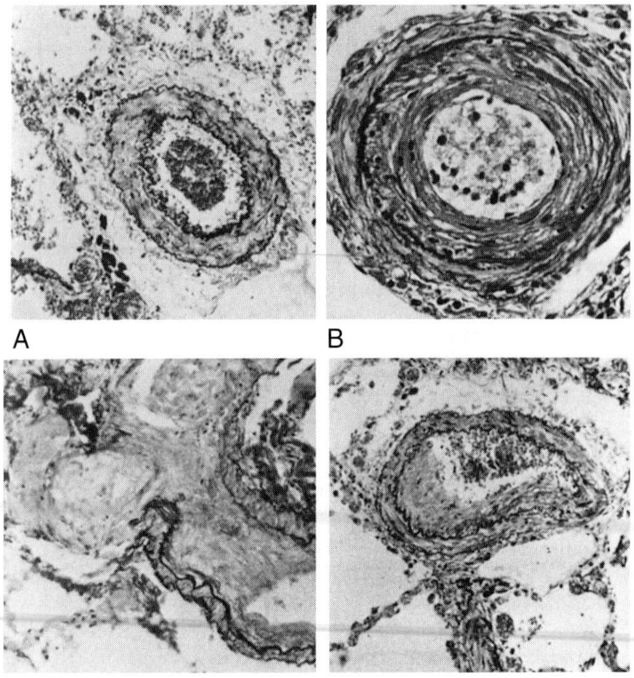

FIGURE 67–5 Photomicrographs of pulmonary arterial histological lesions seen in cases of clinically unexplained pulmonary hypertension. All slides were stained with Verhoeff-van Gieson stain. **A,** Medical hypertrophy (original magnification ×100). **B,** Concentric laminal intimal fibrosis, seen most often in association with plexiform lesions (original magnification ×200). **C,** Plexiform lesion demonstrating obstruction in the arterial lumen, aneurysmal dilation, and proliferation of anastomosing vascular channels (original magnification ×200). **D,** Eccentric intimal fibrosis, often seen in association with organized microthrombi but also present in many patients with plexiform lesions (original magnification ×100). (From Palevsky HI, Schloo BL, Pietra CC, et al: Primary pulmonary hypertension: Vascular structure, morphometry and responsiveness to vasodilator agents. Circulation 80:1207, 1989.)

pattern when pulmonary vascular injury is coupled with increased pulmonary blood flow. These neointimal lesions are composed of smooth muscle cells that are immunoreactive to anti-α smooth muscle actin antibody. It is now accepted that hemodynamic shear stress acts through the endothelium to regulate vessel tone and in the chronic restructuring of blood vessels.[71]

Endothelial denudation also results in platelet adherence to exposed tissue collagen, with release of platelet-derived smooth muscle mitogens that also have vasoconstrictor properties. This process in turn leads to an inflammatory response and thrombosis, thereby narrowing the lumen of pulmonary vessels. In a person who is susceptible—whether on a genetic or an acquired basis—intense vasoconstriction may lead to fibrinoid necrosis of the arteriolar wall and the development of plexiform lesions. Ultimately, the vessels are reduced in number, and the residua of these destroyed vessels can be seen histologically as "ghost vessels." Destruction of large numbers of pulmonary arterioles reduces the cross-sectional area of the pulmonary vascular bed, thereby producing a permanent increase in pulmonary vascular resistance and fixed pulmonary hypertension. The latter in turn damages other blood vessels and initiates a vicious circle, with progressively rising pulmonary arterial pressure.

ANGIOTENSIN-CONVERTING ENZYME. An essential role of ACE in the pathogenesis of pulmonary hypertension is strongly suggested by the presence of increased ACE immunoreactivity at sites of increased matrix gene expression in human hypertensive pulmonary arteries.[35] Further supporting a role for ACE in pulmonary vascular remodeling are observations that ACE protein and mRNA expression are focally increased in rat pulmonary arteries with medial hypertrophy from chronic hypoxia.[37]

INCREASED ACTIVITY OF ELASTOLYTIC ENZYMES. This appears to be important in the pathophysiology of pulmonary vascular disease.[72] High elastin turnover and neosynthesis of elastin have been attributed to degradation of elastin from the increased activity of serine elastase. A cause-and-effect relationship between elastase and pulmonary vascular disease was demonstrated when elastase inhibitors were shown to be effective in attenuating the development and retarding the progression of pulmonary hypertension in monocrotaline-injected hypoxic rats.[73] Progression of pulmonary hypertension may involve a series of switches in smooth muscle cell phenotype and proliferation to account for the medial hypertrophy and smooth muscle cell migration resulting in neointimal formation. Structural and functional alterations in the endothelial cell could result in loss of barrier function and allow leakage into the subendothelium of a serum factor normally excluded from this region. Enzymes released from precursor or mature smooth muscle cells could activate growth factors normally stored in the extracellular matrix, such as basic fibroblast growth factor and TGF-β, which are known to induce smooth muscle cell hypertrophy and proliferation and increase connective tissue protein synthesis. In muscular arteries, release of growth factors would result in hypertrophy of the vessel wall.

ION CHANNELS. Potassium channels are found throughout the pulmonary vascular bed.[74] They consist of voltage-dependent potassium channels and calcium-dependent potassium channels (see Chap. 27). The role of these channels has been studied primarily in the presence of acute hypoxia in animals. It is believed that potassium channels modulate adult pulmonary vascular tone. It is probable that calcium channels also serve a regulatory role in modulating vascular tone, particularly the L-type calcium channel. Inhibition of the voltage-regulated potassium channel by hypoxia or drugs can produce vasoconstriction and has been described in pulmonary artery smooth muscle cells harvested from patients with PPH. It has been suggested that defects in the potassium channel of pulmonary resistance smooth muscle cells are involved in the initiation or progression of pulmonary hypertension. A genetic defect related to potassium channels in the lungs of patients with PPH that leads to vasoconstriction may be one mechanism for the development of PPH in some patients (see Fig. 67–6).[74]

DYSFUNCTIONAL ENDOTHELIUM. The dysfunctional pulmonary hypertensive endothelial cell phenotype is characterized by uncontrolled proliferation, increased production of vasoconstrictor mediators such as endothelin, expression of 5-lipoxygenase, and decreased synthesis of prostacyclin. In patients with PPH, expression of prostacyclin synthase is reduced in pulmonary arteries ranging from 1 mm to less than 100 μm in diameter, which suggests that the reduction in prostacyclin synthesis in otherwise morphologically normal to minimally remodeled vessels may play a role in the early stages of pathogenesis. Alternatively, endothelial cells of pulmonary small arteries may become dysfunctional as the disease progresses and pulmonary artery pressure progressively rises. Loss of expression of prostacyclin synthase is one of the phenotypic alterations present in pulmonary endothelial cells in cases of severe pulmonary hypertension.[75]

SEROTONIN. This substance has also been implicated as being involved in PPH. Elevations in serotonin levels have been correlated with the pulmonary vascular pressure gradient in patients with acute respiratory distress syndrome. Children with congenital heart disease and pulmonary hypertension have increased turnover of serotonin.[76] PPH has been reported in a patient with familial platelet storage pool disease, which represents a defect in serotonin handling and release. One series reported increased serotonin in patients with pulmonary hypertension associated with the use of fenfluramine and with connective tissue disease.[77] Of interest is that after six of these patients underwent heart/lung transplantation, they had persistently elevated concentrations of plasma serotonin and decreased platelet serotonin concentrations, thus suggesting that the abnormality in platelet serotonin handling was a primary process in the evolution of their pulmonary hypertension.

Genetics

An important emerging concept in the development of PAH is that the disease develops in patients with an underlying genetic predisposition following exposure to specific stimuli, which serve as triggers. Predisposition to the development of pulmonary hypertension has been noted by the marked heterogeneity in responses of the pulmonary vasculature in a variety of disease states. Examples include the considerable variability among individuals to vasoconstrictive stimuli such as hypoxia or acidosis, which can produce marked pulmonary hypertension in one person and be essentially without effect in another. The pulmonary arterial pressure response to hypoxia is particularly great in individuals with blood group A. This variability in responsiveness of the pulmonary vascular bed undoubtedly accounts for the fact that

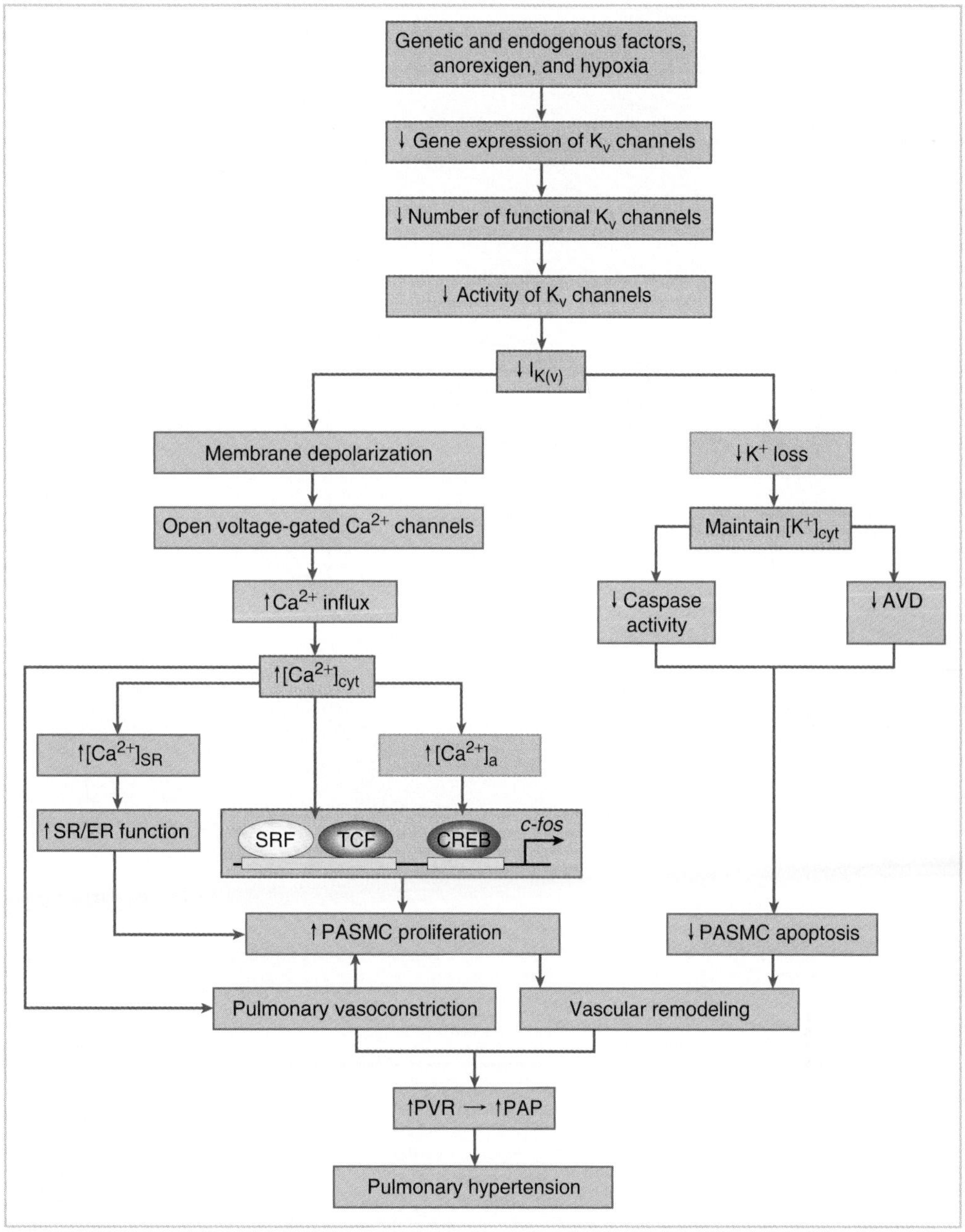

FIGURE 67–6 Schematic diagram depicting possible cellular mechanisms responsible for the development of pulmonary hypertension. The process is initiated by a series of endogenous and exogenous factors, which lead to abnormal gene transcription or expression of functional K_v channels and reduction in K_v channel activity. This leads to membrane depolarization and opening of voltage-gated Ca^{2+} channels, increasing $[Ca^{2+}]_{cyt}$. Because of the high ratio of Ca^{2+} in the SR ($[Ca^{2+}]_{SR}$) to $[Ca^{2+}]_{cyt}$ and the minimal resistance of the nuclear membrane to Ca^{2+}, a rise in $[Ca^{2+}]_{cyt}$ subsequently increases $[Ca^{2}]_{SR}$ and nuclear Ca^{2+} ($[Ca^{2+}]_n$). *c-fos* is a Ca^{2+}-responsive gene that has two Ca^{2+} elements in its promoter: the SRE (which binds with SRF), and the cyclic adenosine monophosphate response element (which binds to CREB). Activation of the early-responsive gene expression by increased $[Ca^{2+}]_{cyt}$, and $[Ca^{2+}]_n$, and the increased $[Ca^{2+}]_{SR}$ and SR/ER function stimulates pulmonary arterial smooth muscle cell (PASMC) proliferation. Increased $[Ca^{2+}]_{cyt}$ also causes increased vascular tone and vasoconstriction. Decreased IK_v, on the other hand, causes a decreased K^+ loss from the cell, maintaining sufficient K^+ in the cytosol ($[K^+]_{cyt}$). This in turn counteracts the apoptotic volume decrease (AVD) and decreases the activity of apoptotic mediators such as caspase and nucleases, leading to a reduced apoptosis of the SMCs. An increased cellular proliferation and decreased apoptosis cause vascular remodeling, ultimately leading to increased pulmonary vascular resistance (PVR), pulmonary artery pressure (PAP), and the development of pulmonary hypertension. CREB = cyclic AMP response element binding protein; SRF = serum response factor; TCF = ternary complex factor. (From Mandegar M, Yuan JX-J: Role of K^+ channels in pulmonary hypertension. Vasc Pharmacol 38:25, 2002.)

pulmonary edema develops in only a minority of individuals on exposure to high altitude. Also, the severity of pulmonary hypertension and the level of pulmonary vascular resistance vary considerably among individuals with congenital heart disease and comparably sized ventricular septal defects. Presumably, a genetic basis underlies these differences in pulmonary vascular reactivity, just as there appears to be a genetic basis for the increased reactivity of the systemic vascular bed in essential systemic hypertension.

FAMILIAL PPH. PPH has been diagnosed in families worldwide. The prevalence of familial PPH is uncertain, but it occurs in at least 6 percent of cases, and the incidence is probably higher. Many unique features are associated with the transmission and development of PPH in families.[78] The age of onset is variable and penetrance is incomplete. Many individuals in families with PPH inherit the gene and have progeny in whom PPH never develops. The observation that fewer males are born in PPH families than in the population at large suggests that the PPH gene might influence fertilization or cause male fetal wastage. Patients with familial PPH have a similar female-to-male ratio, age of onset, and natural history of the disease as those with sporadic PPH.

Documentation of familial PPH can be difficult, since remote common ancestry occurs in patients with apparently sporadic PPH and skip generations caused either by incomplete penetrance or by variable expression can mimic sporadic disease. Vertical transmission has been demonstrated in as many as five generations in one family and is probably indicative of a single dominant gene that is believed to be autosomal for PPH.[79] Genetic anticipation has been described in familial PPH since the early reports (Fig. 67–7). Because the clinical and pathological features of familial and sporadic PPH are virtually identical, it seems likely that the same genes are involved in both forms of the disease.

Familial PPH segregates as an autosomal dominant trait with markedly reduced penetrance. Using linkage analysis, the locus designated PPH-1 on chromosome 2q31-33 led to the discovery of the *PPH-1* gene.[80] *PPH-1* is the Human Genome Organization-approved designation DGB:1381541.[81] The low penetrance of this gene confers only about a 20 percent likelihood of development of the disease.

Bone Morphogenetic Protein Receptor Type 2 Gene. The gene (*BMPR-2*) coding for a receptor member of the TGF-β

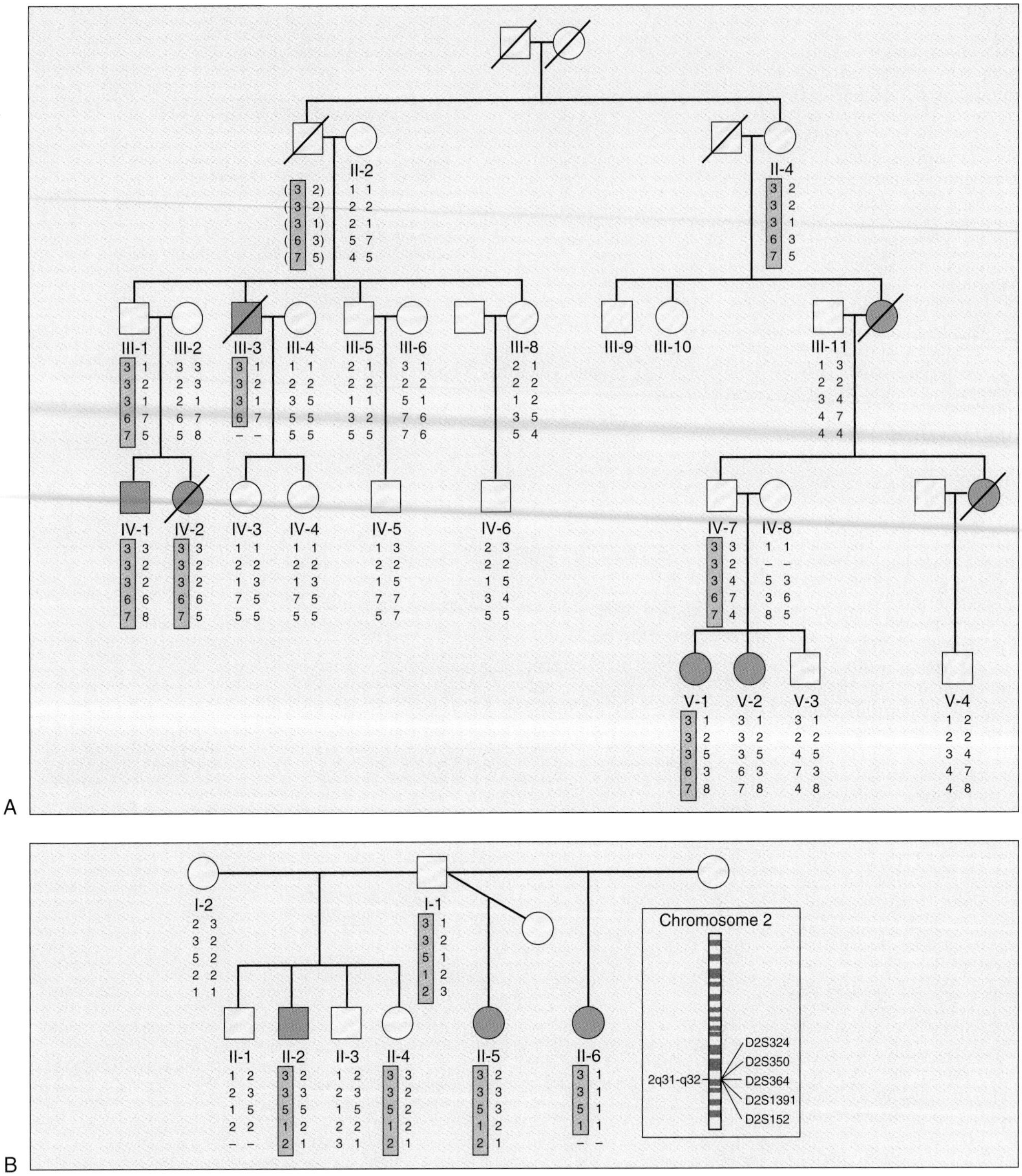

FIGURE 67–7 The pedigrees of two families (**A** and **B**) with familial primary pulmonary hypertension (PPH). Shaded symbols represent affected individuals. Genotyped individuals are indicated by the respective pedigree designations. The PPH-1 region on chromosome 2 (2q31-q32) contains a number of candidate genes. (From Morse JH, Jones AC, Barst RJ, et al: Mapping of familial primary pulmonary hypertension locus (*PPH-1*) to chromosome 2q31-32. Circulation 95:2603, 1997.)

family has been identified as causative of familial PPH.[82] The mutations ascribed to the locus interrupt the BMP-mediated signaling pathway, resulting in a predisposition to proliferation rather than apoptosis of cells within small pulmonary arteries. These molecular studies suggest that the target cells within the pulmonary arterial wall are sensitive to *BMPR-2* gene dosage and the TGF-β pathway mediated through *BMPR-2* is critical for the maintenance and/or normal response to injury of the pulmonary vasculature (Fig. 67–8).[83] It is clear, however, that additional factors, either environmental or genetic, are required in the pathogenesis of the disease. How defects in *BMPR-2* contribute to endothelial cell proliferation, smooth muscle cell hypertrophy, and fibroblast deposition in patients with PPH remains unknown. It is interesting to note that many patients with "sporadic" PPH actually have a kindred affected by familial PPH that can span many generations.[82] About one in four cases of sporadic PPH actually have germline mutations in the gene encoding the

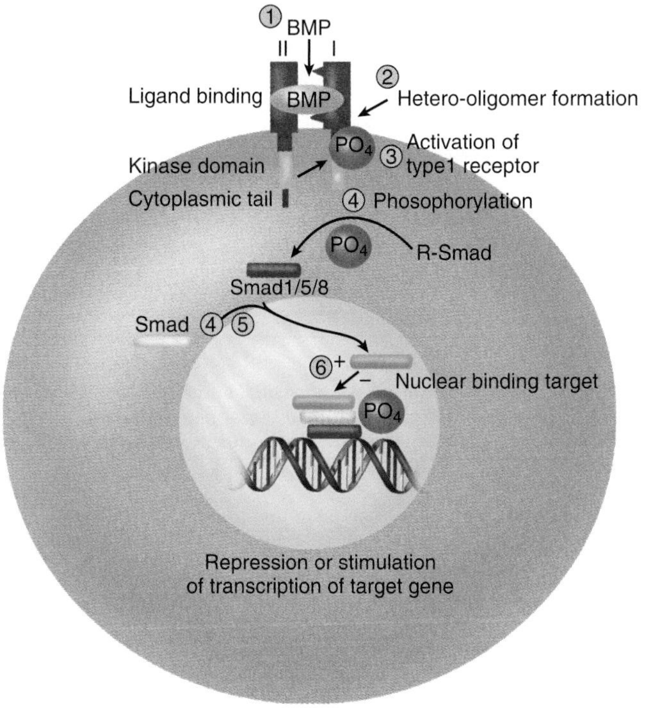

FIGURE 67–8 Bone morphogenetic protein (BMP) signaling pathway. **1** and **2,** BMPR1 and BMPR2 are present on most cell surfaces as homo-dimers or hetero-oligomers. With ligand binding, a complex of ligand, two type I receptors, and two type II receptors is formed. **3,** After ligand stimulation, the type II receptor phosphorylates the type I receptor in its juxtamembrane domain. **4,** The activated type I receptor then phosphorylates a receptor-regulated Smad (R-Smad); thus, the type I receptors determine the specificity of the signal. Smads 1, 5, and 8 are specific for BMP signaling pathway. **5,** Once activated by phosphorylation, the R-Smads interact with the common mediator Smad 4 to form hetero-oligomers that are translocated to the nucleus. **6,** In the nucleus, the Smad complex interacts with transcription factors and binds to DNA to induce or suppress transcription of target genes. Smads 6 and 7, inhibitory Smads (not shown), bind to activated type I receptors to prevent the phosphorylation of R-Smads. (From Runo JR, Loyd JE: Primary pulmonary hypertension. Lancet 361:1533, 2003.)

BMPR-2 receptor. Recent work suggesting that there are other causative genes supports the idea that there may be genetic determinants that modify the clinical expression of the disease. Endothelial cells and myofibroblast cells compose intimal lesions at the sites of pulmonary vascular expression of the *BMPR-2* receptor.[84]

Other Genetic Factors. Other factors suggested include ET-1, changes in potassium channels, sensitivity to prostacyclin, and serotonin. Adnot and colleagues demonstrated that there is overexpression of serotonin transporter (5-HTT) in pulmonary arteries and platelets from all the patients with PPH they studied and that increased activity of the 5-HTT is responsible for the associated smooth muscle hyperplasia.[85] In addition, they recently demonstrated that 5-HTT expression is elevated in cultured pulmonary artery smooth muscle cells from patients with PAH and that proliferation was also increased and related to 5-HTT expression and 5-HTT activity.[86] 5-HTT is encoded by a single gene on chromosome 17q11.2, and a variant in the upstream promotor region of the *5-HTT* gene has been described.[87] This polymorphism with long (L) and short (S) forms affects *5-HTT* expression and function, with the L-allele inducing a greater rate of *5-HTT* gene transcription than the S-allele. This L-allelic variant was found to be present in homozygous form in 65 percent of PPH patients but only in 27 percent of control subjects.[85] *5-HTT* gene polymorphism could also contribute to interindividual differences in hypoxia-induced *5-HTT* expression and potentially affects susceptibility to hypoxic PAH (Fig. 67–9).

Pathological Features

Morphological abnormalities in each cell line have been described in cases of PPH. The endothelium in particular displays marked heterogeneity in the pulmonary vascular bed. Although endothelial dysfunction has been clearly described in cases of PPH, discordance between phenotype and function is commonly noted.[88] It is not known at what stage during the evolution of PPH endothelial cell proliferation occurs. It has been proposed, however, that a somatic mutation rather than nonselective cell proliferation in response to injury accounts for the growth advantage of endothelial cells in patients with PPH.[89] Heterogeneity in the smooth muscle and fibroblast populations also contributes to discordance between phenotype and function. Interconversion between cell types (fibroblast to smooth muscle cell or endothelium to smooth muscle cell) in addition to neovascularization may occur.

Smooth muscle cell hypertrophy and increased connective tissue and extracellular matrix are found in the large muscular and elastic arteries.[72,73] In the subendothelial layer, increased thickness may be the result of recruitment and/or proliferation of smooth muscle-like cells. It is possible that precursor smooth muscle cells are in a continuous layer in the subendothelial layer along the entire pulmonary artery. These cells are similar to the pericytes that are responsible for the appearance of muscle in normally nonmuscular arteries and that contribute to intimal thickening in larger arteries. Alterations in the extracellular matrix secondary to proteolytic enzymes also play a role in the pathology of PPH. Matrix-degrading enzymes can release mitogenically active growth factors that stimulate smooth muscle cell proliferation. In addition, elastase and matrix metalloproteinases contribute to upregulation of proliferation. Degradation of elastin has also been shown to stimulate upregulation of the glycoprotein fibronectin, which in turn stimulates smooth muscle cell migration.[84]

HYPERTENSIVE PULMONARY ARTERIOPATHY. The most common vascular changes in PPH can best be characterized as a hypertensive pulmonary arteriopathy, which is present in 85 percent of cases (Table 67–7). These changes involve medial hypertrophy of the arteries and arterioles, often in conjunction with other vascular changes. Isolated medial hypertrophy is uncommon, and when present it has been assumed to represent an early stage of the disease. The intimal proliferation may be concentric laminar intimal fibrosis, eccentric intimal fibrosis, or concentric nonlaminar intimal fibrosis. The frequency of these findings differs from case to case and within regions of the same lung in the same patient. In addition, plexiform and dilation lesions, as well as a necrotizing arteritis, may be seen throughout the lungs. The fundamental nature of the plexiform lesion remains a mystery.[90] Morphologically, they represent a mass of disorganized vessels with proliferating endothelial cells, smooth muscle cells, myofibroblasts, and macrophages. Several studies have demonstrated the involvement of growth factors that have been implicated in angiogenesis.[91] Whether the plexiform lesion represents impaired proliferation or angiogenesis remains unclear.

THROMBOTIC PULMONARY ARTERIOPATHY. The other major pattern of vascular changes in PPH is that of a thrombotic pulmonary arteriopathy.[92] Typical features include medial hypertrophy of the arteries and arterioles with both eccentric and concentric nonlaminar intimal fibrosis. The presence of colander lesions, which represent recannalized thrombi, is also typical. These lesions are believed to arise as a result of primary in situ thrombosis of the small vascular arteries and not from recurrent pulmonary embolism.

On rare occasion, a diffuse pulmonary arteritis with secondary thrombosis has been reported in patients with PPH,

TABLE 67–7 Histopathological Classification of Hypertensive Pulmonary Vascular Disease

Classification	Characteristic Histopathological Features
Arteriopathy	
Isolated medial hypertrophy*	Medial hypertrophy: increase of medial muscle in muscular arteries, muscularization of nonmuscularized arterioles; no appreciable intimal or luminal obstructive lesions. No plexiform lesions.
Plexogenic pulmonary arteriopathy	Plexiform and dilation lesions. Medial hypertrophy; eccentric or concentric-laminar and nonlaminar intimal thickening; fibrinoid necrosis, arteritis, and thrombotic lesions.
Thrombotic pulmonary arteriopathy	Thrombi (fresh, organizing, or organized and colander lesions). Eccentric and concentric nonlaminar intimal thickening, varying degrees of medial hypertrophy. No plexiform lesions.
Isolated pulmonary arteritis	Active or healed arteritis. Limited to pulmonary arteries; varying degrees of medial hypertrophy, intimal fibrosis, and thrombotic lesions. No plexiform lesions. No systemic arteritis.
Venopathy	
Pulmonary venoocclusive disease	Eccentric intimal fibrosis and recanalized thrombi within pulmonary veins and venules; arterialized veins, capillary congestion, alveolar edema and siderophages, dilated lymphatics, pleural and septal edema, and arterial medial hypertrophy; intimal thickening and thrombotic lesions.
Microangiopathy	
Pulmonary capillary hemangiomatosis	Infiltrating thin-walled blood vessels throughout pulmonary parenchyma, pleura, bronchi, and walls of pulmonary veins and arteries. Medial hypertrophy and intimal thickening of muscular pulmonary arteries and arterioles.

From Pietra GG: Pathology of primary pulmonary hypertension. *In* Rubin LJ, Rich S (eds): Primary Pulmonary Hypertension. New York, Marcel Dekker, 1997, pp 19-61, by courtesy of Marcel Dekker, Inc.

*Medial hypertrophy includes muscularization of arterioles.

predominantly in children. Although the association has not been reported in patients with underlying connective tissue disease, it may reflect the vascular response to a specific but not clearly identified risk factor.

Clinical Features

NATURAL HISTORY AND SYMPTOMS. The most extensive study on the natural history of PPH was reported from the National Institutes of Health (NIH) Registry on Primary Pulmonary Hypertension from 1981 to 1987. The study included the long-term follow-up of 194 patients in whom PPH was diagnosed by established clinical and hemodynamic criteria. Sixty-three percent of the patients were female, and the mean age was 36 ± 15 years (range, 1 to 81 years) at the time of diagnosis. The mean interval from the onset of symptoms to diagnosis was 2 years, and the most common initial symptoms were dyspnea (80 percent), fatigue (19 percent), syncope or near syncope (13 percent), and Raynaud phenomenon (10 percent). No ethnic differentiation was observed, with 12.3 percent of patients being black and 2.3 percent being Hispanic.

HEMODYNAMIC CHANGES. Univariate analysis from the NIH Registry pointed to the mean right atrial pressure, mean pulmonary artery pressure, and cardiac index, as well as the diffusing capacity from carbon monoxide, as significantly related to mortality. The New York Heart Association (NYHA) classification was also strongly related to survival.

Right ventricular failure from pulmonary hypertension is a result of chronic pressure overload and associated volume overload with the development of tricuspid regurgitation. However, animal studies suggest that right ventricular ischemia may also be a common feature. The mechanism of right ventricular failure in patients with pulmonary hypertension is complex. The chronic pressure overload that induces right ventricular hypertrophy and reduced contractility has been shown to cause a reduction in coronary blood flow to the right ventricular myocardium, which can produce right ventricular ischemia, both acutely and chronically. Such right ventricular dysfunction appears to be a result of a reduction in right ventricular coronary artery driving pressure. In an interesting animal study by Vlahakes and colleagues, acute right ventricular failure secondary to right ventricular hypertension was overcome by increasing central aortic pressure, which resulted in an increase in right ventricular coronary driving pressure. Murray and Vatner reported that a moderate increase in aortic pressure was accompanied by a large increase in right ventricular myocardial perfusion only when the auto-

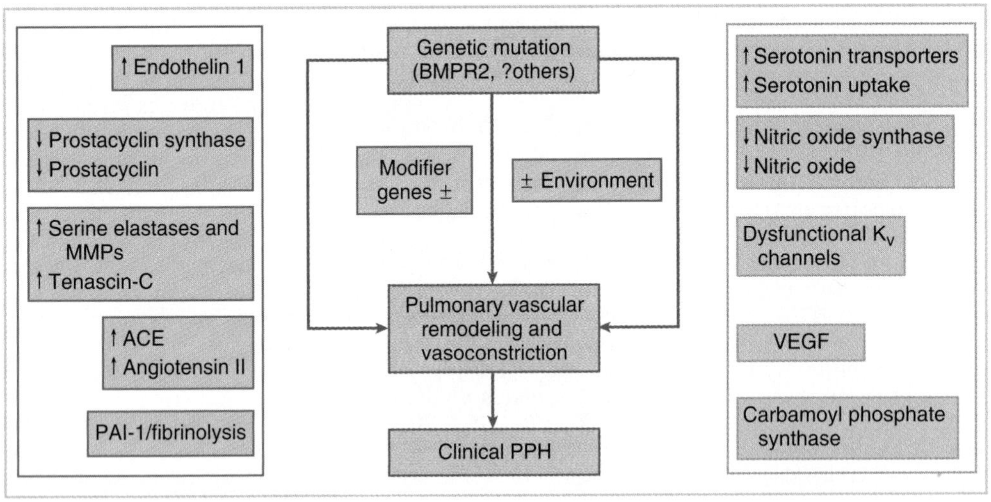

FIGURE 67–9 Proposed pathogenesis for the development of primary pulmonary hypertension (PPH). Genes implicated in the pathogenesis of PPH are bone morphogenetic protein receptor type 2 (BMPR2), prostacyclin synthase, serotonin transporters, nitric oxide synthase, serine elastases, and matrix metalloproteinases (MMPs), voltage-gated potassium (K) channels, angiotensin-converting enzyme (ACE), vascular endothelial growth factor (VEGF), carbamoyl phosphate synthase, and plasminogen activator inhibitor type 1 (PAI-1). Endothelin-1 production adds to the vasoconstriction in patients with PPH, but whether this is secondary to changes in the genes, a result of endothelial dysfunction, or a primary pathogenetic event is not clear. Pulmonary vascular remodeling results from the effects of genetics, modifying genes, and environment. (From Runo JR, Loyd JE: Primary pulmonary hypertension. Lancet 361:1533, 2003.)

nomic nervous system was blocked with an alpha blocker. Because the symptom of angina associated with PPH is characteristic of myocardial ischemia, it probably represents ongoing ischemia caused by this phenomenon.

LEFT VENTRICULAR FUNCTION. On occasion, patients with pulmonary hypertension have a reduced left ventricular ejection fraction and even regional wall motion abnormalities of the left ventricle.[93] In the past, these findings had been attributed to mechanisms related to interventricular dependence, which suggests that in some way a dysfunctional right ventricle can lead to a dysfunctional left ventricle. Clearly, the shared interventricular septum can affect the function of both ventricles. More recently, extrinsic compression of the left main coronary artery by the pulmonary artery in patients with chronic pulmonary hypertension has been described and may be associated with classic angina-like symptoms.[94,95] It is advisable to look for extrinsic compression of the left main coronary artery with coronary angiography in patients with long-standing pulmonary hypertension who have abnormal left ventricular function.

CAUSES OF DEATH. The most common cause of death in patients with PPH in the NIH Registry was progressive right-sided heart failure (47 percent). Sudden cardiac death was limited to patients who were NYHA class IV, suggesting that it is a manifestation of end-stage disease rather than a phenomenon that occurs early or unpredictably in the clinical course of the disease. The remainder of the patients died of some other medical complication, such as pneumonia or bleeding, which suggests that patients with PPH do not tolerate coexistent medical conditions well.

CLINICAL COURSE. The clinical course of patients with PPH can be highly variable. However, with the onset of overt right ventricular failure manifested by worsening symptoms and systemic venous congestion, patient survival is generally limited to approximately 6 months. Understanding the clinical course of patients with PPH is important, especially when considering major interventional therapy such as organ transplantation.

Management

LIFESTYLE CHANGES. The diagnosis of PPH does not necessarily imply total disability for the patient. However, physical activity can be associated with elevated pulmonary artery pressure inasmuch as marked hemodynamic changes have been documented to occur early in the onset of increased physical activity. For that reason, graded exercise activities, such as bike riding or swimming, in which patients can gradually increase their workload and easily limit the extent of their work, are thought to be safer than isometric activities. Isometric activities such as lifting weights or stair climbing can be associated with syncopal events and should be limited or avoided.

Pregnancy. The subject of pregnancy should also be discussed with women of childbearing age. The physiological changes that occur in pregnancy can potentially activate the disease and result in death of the mother and/or the child. Besides the increased circulating blood volume and oxygen consumption that will increase right ventricular work, circulating procoagulant factors and the risk of pulmonary embolism from deep vein thrombosis and amniotic fluid are serious concerns. Syncope and cardiac arrest have also been reported to occur during active labor and delivery, and a syndrome of postpartum circulatory collapse has been described.[96] For these reasons, surgical sterilization should be given strong consideration by women with PPH or their husbands.

DIGOXIN. Animal studies in right ventricular systolic overload show that prior administration of digoxin helps prevent the reduction in contractility of the right ventricle. Clinically, it has been shown that digoxin can exert a favorable hemodynamic effect when given acutely to patients with right ventricular failure from pulmonary hypertension.[97] An increase in resting cardiac output of approximately 10 percent was noted, which is similar to observations made in patients with left ventricular systolic failure. In addition, it was also observed that digoxin causes a significant reduction in circulating norepinephrine, which was markedly increased. Digitalis toxicity in patients with pulmonary hypertension and normal renal function is uncommon.

DIURETICS. These drugs appear to be of marked benefit in symptom relief of patients with PPH. Their traditional role has been limited to patients manifesting right ventricular failure and systemic venous congestion. However, patients with advanced PPH can have increased left ventricular filling pressures that contribute to the symptoms of dyspnea and orthopnea, which can be relieved with diuretics. Diuretics may also serve to reduce right ventricular wall stress in patients with concomitant tricuspid regurgitation and volume overload. The fear that diuretics will induce systemic hypotension is unfounded because the main factor limiting cardiac output is pulmonary vascular resistance and not pulmonary blood volume. Patients with severe venous congestion may require high doses of loop diuretics or the use of combined diuretics. In these instances, electrolytes need to be carefully watched to avoid hyponatremia and hypokalemia.

In humans, elevated plasma aldosterone concentrations are associated with endothelial dysfunction, left ventricular hypertrophy, and cardiac death. Spironolactone has been demonstrated to enhance the beneficial effect of ACE inhibition on mortality in patients with congestive heart failure.[98] Given the similarities between left and right heart failure on activation of the renin-angiotensin-aldosterone system, it seems reasonable to use aldosterone antagonists in patients with pulmonary hypertension.

SUPPLEMENTAL OXYGEN. Hypoxic pulmonary vasoconstriction can contribute to pulmonary vascular disease in patients with alveolar hypoxia from parenchymal lung disease. Supplemental low-flow oxygen alleviates arterial hypoxemia and attenuates the pulmonary hypertension in patients with these disorders. Although most patients with PPH do not exhibit resting hypoxemia, those who experience arterial oxygen desaturation with activity may benefit from ambulatory supplemental oxygen because increased oxygen extraction develops in the face of fixed oxygen delivery. Patients with severe right-sided heart failure and resting hypoxemia resulting from markedly increased oxygen extraction at rest should be treated with continuous oxygen therapy to maintain their arterial oxygen saturation above 90 percent. Patients with hypoxemia caused by a right-to-left shunt via a patent foramen ovale do not improve their level of oxygenation to an appreciable degree with supplemental oxygen.

ANTICOAGULANTS. Oral anticoagulant therapy is widely recommended for patients with PPH, although its clinical efficacy as a therapy is difficult to prove. A retrospective review of patients with PPH monitored over a 15-year period at the Mayo Clinic suggested that patients who received warfarin had improved survival over those who did not. The influence of warfarin therapy has been investigated in patients with PPH who failed to respond to high doses of calcium channel blockers.[99] Significant improvement in survival was observed in patients who received anticoagulation, with a 1-year survival rate of 91 percent and a 3-year survival rate of 47 percent as compared with 1- and 3-year rates of 62 and 31 percent, respectively, in patients who did not receive anticoagulants. The current recommendation is to use warfarin in relatively low doses, as has been recommended for prophylaxis of venous thromboembolism, with the international normalized ratio (INR) maintained at 2.0 to 3.0 times control. Given its inhibitory effects on smooth muscle proliferation, heparin might be a better anticoagulant in patients with PPH, although its use is more difficult. With the recent advent of low-molecular-weight heparins requiring once-a-day administration without the need for adjusting the dose to its antithrombotic effect, treatment with these agents is becoming a more viable alternative.

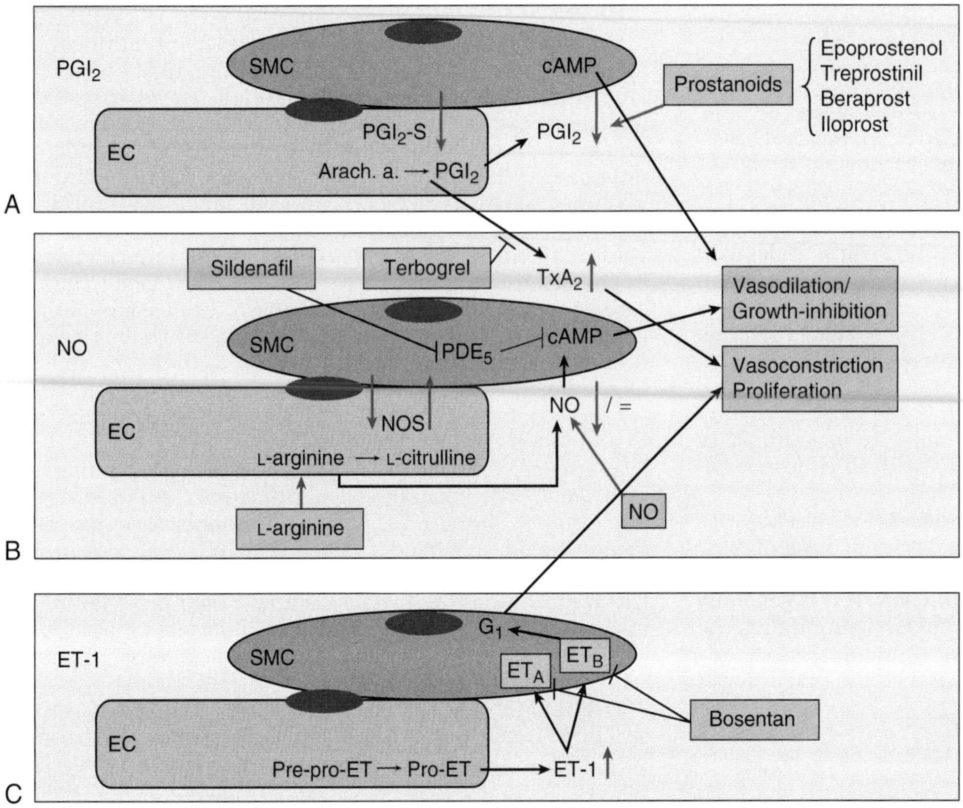

FIGURE 67–10 Endothelial dysfunction and its pharmacological correction in cases of pulmonary arterial hypertension. Arach. a. = arachidonic acid; cAMP = cyclic adenosine monophosphate; EC = endothelial cell; ET = endothelin; NO = nitric oxide; PDE = phosphodiesterase; PGI$_2$ = prostacyclin; S = synthase; SMC = smooth muscle cell; TxA$_2$ = thromboxane A$_2$. ↓ and ↑ denote pathobiological changes typical of pulmonary arterial hypertension. Boxes and arrows denote substances, sites, and modality of therapeutic interventions. (From Galie N, Manes A, Branzi A: Emerging medical therapies for pulmonary arterial hypertension. Prog Cardiovasc Dis 45:213, 2002.)

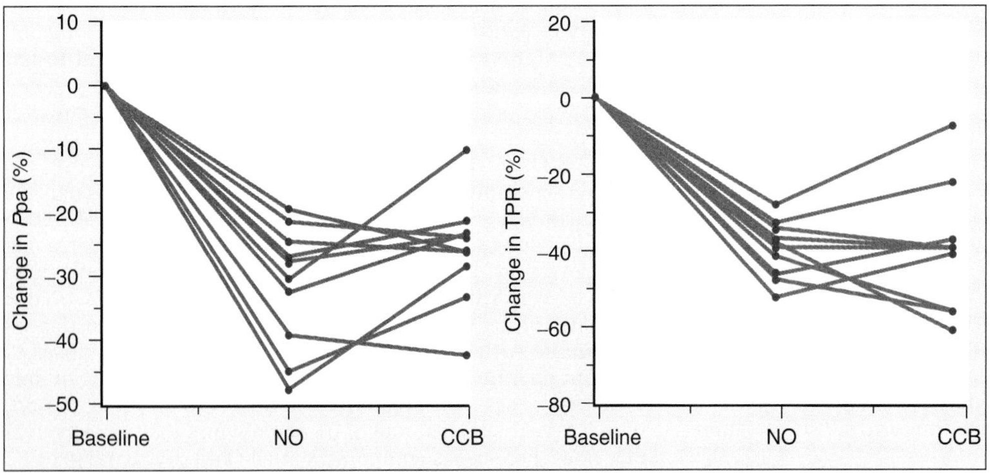

FIGURE 67–11 Comparison of individual pulmonary vasodilator response to inhaled nitric oxide (NO) and oral calcium-channel blockers (CCB) in patients with primary pulmonary hypertension (PPH). Inhalation of NO can predict acute and chronic response to oral calcium-channel blockers in PPH. P_{pa} = mean pulmonary artery pressure; TPR = total pulmonary resistance (P_{pa} divided by cardiac index). (From Sitbon O, Humbert M, Simonneau G: Primary pulmonary hypertension: Current therapy. Prog Cardiovasc Dis 45:115, 2002.)

Vasodilator Therapy

Because of early reports showing a reduction in pulmonary artery pressure following the acute administration of vasodilators, it has been presumed that vasodilators are the mainstay of treatment in patients with PPH. This presumption is not supported by the published literature, however. Vasodilators are effective in a subset of patients with PPH, but many complexities regarding vasodilator administration make their use in these patients very difficult.

The final common cellular pathway by which vasodilators work is through a reduction of intracellular calcium in the vascular smooth muscle cell. The same mechanism is also attributable to cellular growth inhibition. Indeed, most vasodilators have been shown to possess growth inhibitory properties of smooth muscle cells in culture. It is likely that the chronic effects of these agents in patients with pulmonary hypertension represent both mechanisms (Fig. 67–10).

CALCIUM CHANNEL BLOCKERS. Of the vasodilators prescribed for patients with PPH, calcium channel blockers appear to have the widest use (Fig. 67–11). Early studies using conventional doses failed to demonstrate a chronic sustained benefit. Moreover, calcium channel blockers have properties that could worsen the underlying pulmonary hypertension, including negative inotropic effects on right ventricular function and reflex sympathetic stimulation, which may increase the resting heart rate. It has been reported that 10 to 20 percent of patients with PPH who are challenged with very high doses of calcium channel blockers may manifest a dramatic reduction in pulmonary artery pressure and pulmonary vascular resistance, which upon serial catheterization has been maintained for more than 5 years.[99] Importantly, the patient's quality of life is restored with improved functional class, and survival (94 percent rate at 5 years) is improved when compared with nonresponders and historical control subjects (36 percent rate). This experience suggests that a select subset of patients with PPH have the ability to have their pulmonary hypertension reversed and their quality of life and length of survival enhanced.

It is unknown whether the response to calcium channel blockers identifies two subsets of patients with PPH, different stages of PPH, or a combination of both. However, it is essential to point out that patients who do not exhibit a dramatic hemodynamic response to calcium channel blockers do not appear to benefit from their long-term administration. Unfortunately, it is becoming common practice for physicians to prescribe calcium channel blockers at conventional doses to all patients with pulmonary hypertension, often without hemodynamic guidance. This unfortunate practice may result in quicker deterioration in these patients and should be strongly discouraged.

PROSTACYCLINS. Continuous-infusion epoprostenol has been shown in randomized clinical trials to improve quality of life and symptoms related to PPH, exercise tolerance, hemodynamics, and survival.[100-103] The initial enthusiasm for epoprostenol was based on the demonstration of pulmonary vasodilator effects when administered to experimental animals with acute pulmonary vasoconstriction. The long-term effects of epoprostenol in PPH include its vasodilator and antithrombotic effects, but its effects may also be importantly related to its ability to normalize cardiac output. Patients may have a reduction in pulmonary vascular resistance of greater than 50 percent even if no acute hemodynamic effects are noted.

Epoprostenol is administered through a central venous catheter that is surgically implanted and delivered by an ambulatory infusion system. The delivery system is complex and requires patients to learn the techniques of sterile drug preparation, operation of the pump, and care of the intravenous catheter. Most of the serious complications that have occurred with epoprostenol therapy have been attributable to the delivery system and include catheter-related infections and thrombosis and temporary interruption of the infusion because of pump malfunction. Anecdotal reports of rebound pulmonary hypertension occurring in patients in whom the infusion was interrupted suggest that great care must be taken to ensure that the infusion is never stopped.

Side effects related to epoprostenol include flushing, headache, nausea, diarrhea, and a unique type of jaw discomfort that occurs with eating. In most patients, these symptoms are minimal and well tolerated. Chronic foot pain and a poorly defined gastropathy with prolonged use develop in some patients. To date, epoprostenol has been given to patients with PPH for more than 10 years with continued favorable effectiveness. In some patients (NYHA class IV) who are critically ill, it serves as a bridge to lung transplantation by stabilizing the patient to a more favorable preoperative state. Patients who are less critically ill may do so well with epoprostenol therapy that they may delay the need to consider transplantation, perhaps indefinitely.

A high cardiac output state has been reported in a series of patients with PPH receiving chronic epoprostenol therapy and is consistent with the drug having positive inotropic effects.[104] Whether the effect is a direct one on the myocardium or indirect via neurohormonal activation has not been determined. Although most patients with PPH have reduced cardiac output on initial examination, the development of a chronic high-output state could have long-term detrimental effects on underlying cardiac function. The follow-up assessment of patients receiving intravenous epoprostenol is quite variable from medical center to medical center, but it does appear important to determine the cardiac output response to therapy periodically to optimize dosing.[105]

Long-Term Effects. The experience with epoprostenol in patients with PPH for more than 10 years has been reported by two large centers (Fig. 67–12). Survival rates over 5 years were markedly improved compared with survival in

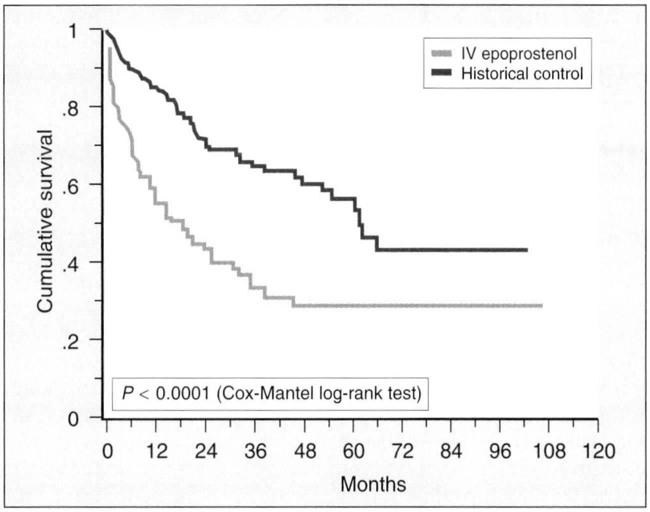

FIGURE 67–12 Kaplan-Meier survival estimates in 178 patients with primary pulmonary hypertension (PPH) from the initiation of epoprostenol therapy. For comparison, survival data are also shown for a historical group of 135 patients with PPH matched for New York Heart Association functional class and who never received epoprostenol therapy. In the population of patients treated with epoprostenol (blue line), overall survival rates at 1, 2, 3, and 5 years are 85, 75, 43, 33, and 28 percent in the historical control group (magenta line). (From Sitbon O, Humbert M, Simonneau G: Primary pulmonary hypertension: Current therapy. Prog Cardiovasc Dis 45:115, 2002.)

historical control subjects and the natural history predicted by the NIH Registry. Predictors of survival included NYHA functional class, exercise tolerance, and acute vasodilator responsiveness. Both studies provided important data for identifying patients who would do well over the long term, versus those in whom transplantation should be considered.[106,107]

Treprostinil. This is a stable prostacyclin analog, recently approved by the Food and Drug Administration, that has pharmacological actions similar to epoprostenol but differs in that it is chemically stable at room temperature and neutral pH and has a longer half-life (3-4 hours). In a large randomized clinical trial in patients with pulmonary arterial hypertension, treprostinil was effective in increasing distance walked in 6 minutes, symptoms of dyspnea associated with exercise, and hemodynamics.[108,109] Its pharmacological properties allow it to be administered through continuous subcutaneous infusion, thus eliminating the need for a central venous catheter and refrigeration during administrations. Infusion site pain was common.

Iloprost. This analog of prostacyclin has been utilized via inhalation. In randomized clinical trials, inhaled iloprost was shown to have an acute effect on hemodynamics similar to inhaled nitric oxide.[110,111] When iloprost was given chronically, patients reported an improvement in exercise, manifested by a 6-minute walk test, and in hemodynamics. Inhaled iloprost has advantages over intravenous epoprostenol in that it does not require a central venous catheter or infusion pump system or cause the attendant complications. Due to the short half-life of iloprost, however, it requires frequent (up to 12 per day) inhalations, which is very restrictive to patients on this therapy. Developments in the technology of nebulizers and the use of prostacyclin analogs with longer half-lives might allow for more widespread use of this treatment modality.

Beraprost. This is an orally active prostacyclin analog that has been evaluated in randomized double-blind placebo-controlled multicenter trials in patients with PPH. In one large European trial (the ALPHABET study), beraprost improved exercise capacity and symptoms over a 12-week period but had no significant effect on cardiopulmonary hemodynamics or functional class.[112] A similar trial conducted in the United States, however, failed to show long-term efficacy beyond 12 weeks.[113] Beraprost was associated with frequent side effects of headache, flushing, and diarrhea, which limited the ability to administer higher doses.

ENDOTHELIN RECEPTOR BLOCKERS. Bosentan is a nonselective endothelin receptor blocker that was recently approved as a treatment of pulmonary arterial hypertension. In a 12-week placebo-controlled trial of 32 patients with PAH, bosentan was superior to placebo in increasing 6-minute walk distance and hemodynamics.[114] In a large randomized clinical trial, bosentan showed a significant improvement in 6-minute walk distance after 16 weeks as compared with placebo.[115] It also was shown to lengthen the composite endpoint of time to clinical worsening, which included death, lung transplantation, hospitalization for pulmonary hypertension, lack of improvement, or worsening leading to discontinuation in need for epoprostenol therapy. Importantly, there was a dose-dependent increase in hepatic transaminases noted from the medication, with significant elevations in 14 percent of the patients randomized to the higher dose (250 mg twice a day). The Food and Drug Administration approved bosentan at the target dose of 125 mg twice a day for patients with pulmonary arterial hypertension who have World Health Organization (WHO) class III or IV disease. The investigational ET_A selective endothelin receptor antagonist, sitaxsentan, also improves exercise capacity in pulmonary arterial hypertension.[116] Further studies with this agent are ongoing (Fig. 67–13).

PHOSPHODIESTERASE-5 INHIBITORS. Sildenafil is a phosphodiesterase-5 (PDE5) inhibitor approved to treat erectile dysfunction. PDE5 inhibitors produce pulmonary vasodilation by promoting an enhanced and sustained level of cyclic guanosine monophosphate, an identical effect to inhaled NO. When tested as a single oral agent, sildenafil has been shown to be a potent and selective pulmonary vasodilator with equal efficacy to that of inhaled NO in lowering pulmonary artery pressure and pulmonary vascular resistance.[117] Sildenafil has a preferential effect on the pulmonary circulation because of the high expression of this isoform in the lung. Many anecdotal reports appear in the published medical literature on the success of sildenafil as an oral therapy for patients with primary pulmonary hypertension.[118-122] The safety and long-term effectiveness of sildenafil as a treatment of pulmonary arterial hypertension is currently under investigation and appears promising.

Invasive Techniques

ATRIAL SEPTOSTOMY. The rationale for the creation of an atrial septostomy in patients with PPH is based on experimental and clinical observations suggesting that an intra-atrial defect allowing right-to-left shunting in the setting of severe pulmonary hypertension might be of benefit. Although countless patients have undergone this procedure worldwide, it should still be considered investigational.[123] Indications for the procedure include recurrent syncope and/or right ventricular failure despite maximum medical therapy, as a bridge to transplantation if deterioration occurs in the face of maximum medical therapy, or when no other option exists. Because the disease process in PPH appears to be unaffected by the procedure, the long-term effects of atrial septostomy must be considered palliative.

The rate of procedure-related mortality with atrial septostomy in patients with PPH is high, and thus the procedure should be attempted only in institutions with an established track record in the treatment of advanced pulmonary hypertension and experience in performing atrial septostomy with a low rate of morbidity. It should not be performed in a patient with impending death and severe right ventricular failure or a patient receiving maximum cardiorespiratory support. Predictors of procedure-related failure or death have been identified and include a mean right atrial pressure of greater than 20 mm Hg, a pulmonary vascular resistance index of greater than 55 units/m^2, or a predicted 1-year survival rate of less than 40 percent.

The mechanisms responsible for the beneficial effects of atrial septostomy remain unclear. Possibilities include increased oxygen delivery at rest and/or with exercise,

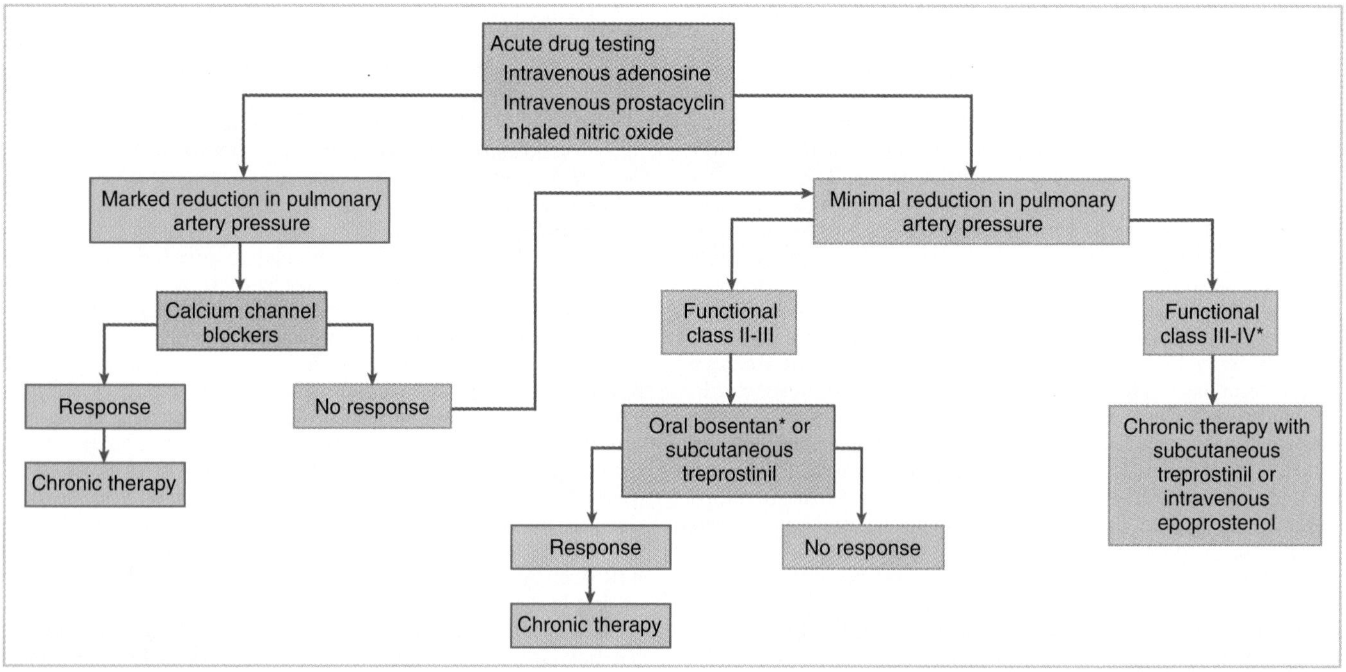

FIGURE 67–13 A treatment algorithm for pulmonary arterial hypertension (PAH) based on established clinical studies is presented. Although there is no consensus for the definition of a response to acute vasodilator testing, it appears that a reduction in mean pulmonary artery pressure below 40 mm Hg is necessary. A chronic response requires a documented improvement in resting hemodynamics, exercise tolerance, or preferably both. Patients who fail to respond chronically to epoprostenol should be considered for lung transplantation. *Bosentan is indicated for WHO functional class III and IV patients.

reduced right ventricular end-diastolic pressure or wall stress, improvement in right ventricular function by the Frank-Starling mechanism, or relief of ischemia.

HEART-LUNG AND LUNG TRANSPLANTATION (see Chap. 26). Heart-lung transplantation has been performed successfully in patients with PPH since 1981.[124] Because these patients have pulmonary vascular disease and severe right ventricular dysfunction, it was originally believed that heart-lung transplantation was the only transplantation option. Widespread application of heart-lung transplantation, however, has been limited by the number of centers with expertise to perform the procedure, the scarcity of suitable donor organs, and the very long waiting times required for patients with end-stage right-sided heart failure. Consequently, bilateral or double-lung transplantation and single-lung transplantation have been performed successfully in patients with PPH.[125] Hemodynamic studies have shown an immediate reduction in pulmonary artery pressure and pulmonary vascular resistance associated with improvement in right ventricular function.

The ages of recipients of heart-lung and lung transplantation for pulmonary hypertension have ranged from 2 months to 61 years.[126] The operative mortality rate ranges between 16 and 29 percent and is somewhat higher for recipients of a single-lung transplant. The 1-year survival rate is between 70 and 75 percent, the 2-year survival rate is between 55 and percent, and the 5-year survival rate is between 40 and 45 percent. Transplantation should be reserved for patients with pulmonary hypertension who have progressed in spite of optimal medical management (Table 67–8).[126]

Timing. In considering referral for evaluation for transplantation, the course of the disease and the waiting time must be taken into account, as well as other factors such as the anticipated waiting time before transplantation in the region and the expected survival after transplantation.[127] It is generally accepted that patients should be considered for transplantation when they have WHO functional class III or IV disease in spite of medical therapy or when treatment with prostacyclin is initiated. The major long-term complications in patients who survive the operation are the high incidence of bronchiolitis obliterans in the transplanted lungs, acute organ rejection, and opportunistic infection.[128] Although several studies have documented significant improvement in quality of life after heart-lung and lung transplantation for pulmonary hypertension, cost-effectiveness has not yet been addressed.

TABLE 67–8 General Guidelines for Selection of Lung Transplant Recipients

Indications
Advanced obstructive, fibrotic, or pulmonary vascular disease with a high risk of death within 2 to 3 yr
Lack of success or availability of alternative therapies
Severe functional limitation but preserved ability to walk
Age 55 yr or less for candidates for heart-lung transplantation, age 60 yr or less for candidates for bilateral lung transplantation, and age 65 yr or less for candidates for single-lung transplantation
Absolute Contraindications
Severe extrapulmonary organ dysfunction, including renal insufficiency with a creatinine clearance below 50 ml/min, hepatic dysfunction with coagulopathy or portal hypertension, and left ventricular dysfunction or severe coronary artery disease (consider heart-lung transplantation)
Acute, critical illness
Active cancer or recent history of cancer with substantial likelihood of recurrence (except for basal cell and squamous cell carcinoma of the skin)
Active extrapulmonary infection (including infection with human immunodeficiency virus, hepatitis B, hepatitis C)
Severe psychiatric illness, noncompliance with therapy, and drug or alcohol dependence
Active or recent (preceding 3 to 6 mo) cigarette smoking
Severe malnutrition (<70% of ideal body weight) or marked obesity (>130% of ideal body weight)
Inability to walk, with poor rehabilitation potential
Relative Contraindications
Chronic medical conditions that are poorly controlled or associated with target organ damage
Daily requirement for more than 20 mg of prednisone (or equivalent)
Mechanical ventilation (excluding noninvasive ventilation)
Extensive pleural thickening from prior thoracic surgery or infection
Active connective tissue disease
Preoperative colonization of the airways with pan-resistant bacteria (in patients with cystic fibrosis)

From Arcasoy SM, Kotlo RB: Lung transplantation. N Engl J Med 340:1081, 1999. Copyright © 1999 Massachusetts Medical Society.

Pulmonary Arterial Hypertension Associated with Congenital Heart Disease (see Chap. 56)

It has long been known that pulmonary hypertension can develop in adults with atrial septal defect. It is presumed that chronically increased pulmonary blood flow may have effects on pulmonary endothelium through mechanical means that cause perturbations in the integrity of the vascular wall and lead to the development of pulmonary vascular disease. Increased pulmonary blood flow from hyperthyroidism and beriberi have been reported to be associated with the development of unexplained pulmonary hypertension, which suggests that high pulmonary blood flow,[129] rather than mere coincidence, is the basis for the development of pulmonary hypertension in patients with pretricuspid shunts such as atrial septal defect or anomalous pulmonary venous drainage.

If a congenital cardiovascular defect causes pulmonary hypertension from the time of birth, the small, muscular arteries of the fetal lung may undergo delayed or only partial involution, with subsequent persistently high levels of pulmonary vascular resistance. This is especially true in lesions in which a left-to-right shunt enters the right ventricle or pulmonary artery directly (i.e., a post-tricuspid valve shunt, such as ventricular septal defect or patent ductus arteriosus): These patients experience a higher incidence of severe and irreversible pulmonary vascular damage than do those in whom the shunt is proximal to the tricuspid valve (pretricuspid shunts, as in atrial septal defect and partial anomalous pulmonary venous drainage). In the latter category, pulmonary hypertension may result from a large pretricuspid left-to-right shunt, which enhances the risk of pulmonary vascular damage.

Pathology

The extent of reversibility of pulmonary vascular obstructive disease in the presence of congenital heart disease varies. From an anatomical point of view, reversible conditions are those in which the decreased pulmonary arteriolar cross-sectional area is the result of medial hypertrophy and vasoconstriction; irreversibility is associated with the presence of necrotizing arteritis and plexiform lesions in these small vessels.

The classification by Heath and Edwards of six grades of structural change is widely used to assess the potential reversibility of pulmonary vascular disease and is summarized as follows: Grade I is characterized by hypertrophy of the media of small muscular pulmonary arteries and arterioles. In grade II, intimal cellular proliferation is added to the medial hypertrophy. Grade III is characterized by advanced medial thickening with hypertrophy and hyperplasia, together with progressive intimal proliferation and concentric fibrosis that result in obliteration of many arterioles and small arteries. In grade IV, dilation and so-called plexiform lesions of the muscular pulmonary arteries and arterioles are observed. The latter consist of a plexiform network of capillary-like channels within a dilated segment of a muscular pulmonary artery. The channels are separated by proliferating endothelial cells that often contain thrombi; indeed, the network of capillary channels may constitute recanalization of a thrombus. Grade V changes include complex plexiform, angiomatous, and cavernous lesions and hyalinization of intimal fibrosis. Finally, grade VI is characterized by the presence of necrotizing arteritis.

Clinical Considerations

EISENMENGER SYNDROME. This refers to any anomalous circulatory communication that leads to obliterative pulmonary vascular disease, including pretricuspid and posttricuspid shunts. Health-Edwards grade IV to VI changes are usual in these patients; occasionally, lesser anatomical changes predominate and may be reversible after successful corrective surgery. The long-term prognosis of patients with the Eisenmenger syndrome is substantially better than that of patients with other conditions associated with pulmonary hypertension.[130] Patients with the Eisenmenger syndrome have an 80 percent survival rate at 10 years, a 77 percent survival rate at 15 years, and a 42 percent survival rate at 25 years.[131,132] Survival is typically related to mean right atrial pressure and pulmonary vascular resistance.

When pulmonary vascular resistance has increased so that it equals or exceeds systemic resistance and the anatomical changes of the pulmonary vessels are predominantly those of grades IV to VI, surgical closure of the anomalous circulatory communication will be associated with a prohibitive immediate risk and, if the patient survives, will usually fail to relieve pulmonary hypertension. Surgery may in fact hasten death in most survivors who had either balanced shunts or predominant right-to-left shunts, because closure of the right-to-left communication merely increases the load on an already overburdened right ventricle. Structural changes in the pulmonary vascular bed are evident in pulmonary arteriograms, which reveal dilated central pulmonary arteries and narrowing of the peripheral branches. These changes can be evaluated by means of quantitative analysis of the pulmonary wedge angiogram.

TREATMENT. Intravenous epoprostenol therapy has been shown to improve exercise tolerance, quality of life, and hemodynamics in patients with congenital heart disease, irrespective of the severity or duration of the condition.[133,134] It is effective in patients who have had previous surgical repair of their defect and in those who have not. No increased incidence of systemic side effects has been noted in patients who have a persistent right-to-left shunt. In patients who have bidirectional shunts, the use of epoprostenol may be a therapeutic strategy to enable a patient who is considered inoperable to become eligible for surgery at a later date. Treprostinil has also been used effectively in patients with congenital heart disease.

Pulmonary Arterial Hypertension Associated with Connective Tissue Diseases (see Chap. 82)

Scleroderma, including the CREST syndrome, is the most common cause of pulmonary hypertension in connective tissue disease states.[57] Scleroderma is associated with pulmonary hypertension in as many as one-third of patients and CREST syndrome in as many as 50 percent. The high incidence suggests that periodic screening with echocardiography in these patients may be a reasonable practice. Although pulmonary hypertension may occur as a result of entrapment and obstruction of the pulmonary microvasculature by interstitial inflammation or fibrosis, patients initially seen with severe pulmonary hypertension usually do not have evidence of interstitial lung disease and have a pulmonary vasculature with histological features that resemble those of PPH.[135] Patients with systemic lupus erythematosus also have pulmonary hypertension, although less commonly than patients with scleroderma. Mixed connective tissue disease is a less common form of connective tissue disease, but pulmonary hypertension may occur in as many as two-thirds of these patients. Pulmonary hypertension has also been described in patients with polymyositis, dermatomyositis, and rheumatoid arthritis.

Because connective tissue diseases may have an insidious onset and slowly progressive course, early recognition of the symptoms of pulmonary hypertension may be difficult. Although easy fatigability may be a feature of the connective tissue disease, it may also be an initial symptom of pulmonary hypertension. Dyspnea is still the most common initial symptom and should not be attributed to advancing age. Syncope, presyncope, or peripheral edema represents advanced pulmonary hypertension and right-sided heart failure. Physical findings of an elevated jugular venous pressure and an increased pulmonic component of the second heart sound along with a right ventricular fourth heart sound are typical features of pulmonary hypertension and warrant an evaluation for pulmonary hypertension. A murmur of tricuspid regurgitation generally reflects more advanced disease. Arterial hypoxemia is characteristic and should also prompt an evaluation of possible pulmonary hypertension in these patients.

The prognosis of patients with connective tissue disease in whom pulmonary hypertension develops is very poor.[133] Conventional therapy with digitalis, diuretics, and supplemental oxygen is used, and anticoagulation has been recommended to provide a survival benefit similar to the practice in PPH. Although the use of oral vasodilators has been disappointing, intravenous epoprostenol has demonstrated therapeutic efficacy manifested by improved exercise tolerance, hemodynamics, and sense of well-being.[136] In patients with associated Raynaud phenomenon, it may provide relief of digital ischemia. Subcutaneous treprostinil and oral bosentan are also approved treatments of pulmonary hypertension associated with connective tissue diseases.

Pulmonary Arterial Hypertension Associated with Portal Hypertension

Pulmonary abnormalities have been commonly associated with the development of hepatic cirrhosis and portal hypertension[137] and include hypoxemia and intrapulmonary shunting, portal-pulmonary shunting, impaired hypoxic pulmonary vasoconstriction, and pulmonary hypertension. Although the relative risk associated with the development of pulmonary hypertension in patients with portal hypertension is unknown, a large postmortem study from the Johns Hopkins Hospital showed that the prevalence of unexplained or pulmonary hypertension in patients with cirrhosis was 5.6 times higher than that of PPH alone. A modest increase in pulmonary artery systolic pressure is not unusual in patients with cirrhosis and portal hypertension. The increase in pulmonary artery pressure is usually passive and relates to the increase in cardiac output and/or blood volume and is associated with near-normal pulmonary vascular resistance. Published studies indicate a strong association between portal hypertension and pulmonary hypertension regardless of whether liver disease is present.[138,139] Although the mechanisms are uncertain, several possibilities are consistent. Portal hypertension itself induces numerous modifications in the vascular media that may trigger a cascade of intracellular signals and/or cause activation or repression of various genes in endothelial and smooth muscle cells. Increased levels of several vasoactive mediators, cytokines, and growth factors have been demonstrated in patients with portal hypertension, including serotonin and interleukin-1.[139] Other angiogenic factors such as hepatocyte growth factor or vascular endothelial growth factor may be involved in pulmonary artery remodeling.

Patients in whom PPH develops in association with cirrhosis appear to be similar to patients without cirrhosis, with the sole exception that they tend to have higher cardiac output and consequently lower calculated systemic and pulmonary vascular resistance, which is characteristic of the cirrhotic state. Treatment of portal pulmonary hypertension generally follows the guidelines developed for treating patients with PPH. Although severe pulmonary hypertension is considered a contraindication to liver transplantation because of the risk of irreversible right-sided heart failure, successful liver transplantation has been reported in patients with very mild pulmonary hypertension treated successfully with intravenous epoprostenol.[140,141]

PULMONARY ARTERIAL HYPERTENSION ASSOCIATED WITH HUMAN IMMUNODEFICIENCY VIRUS INFECTION

Although well documented, it remains unclear how HIV infection results in an increased incidence of PPH in HIV-infected patients.[142,143] A direct pathogenic role of HIV seems unlikely inasmuch as no viral constituents have been detected in the vascular endothelium of these patients. On the other hand, reports of pulmonary arteriopathy with intimal proliferation in monkeys experimentally infected with the simian immunodeficiency virus and in a murine model of acquired immunodeficiency syndrome suggest a pathogenetic link between infection with an immunodeficiency virus and the development of PPH, possibly mediated by release of inflammatory mediators or by autoimmune mechanisms.[142] A large case-control study of HIV-associated PPH was recently conducted in the Swiss HIV Cohort Study.[143] The cumulative incidence was 0.6 percent within the entire HIV-infected population. PPH was diagnosed in patients in all stages of HIV infection and without an obvious relationship to immune deficiency. The clinical and hemodynamic features of these patients were similar to those of patients with PPH.

PULMONARY ARTERIAL HYPERTENSION RELATED TO ANOREXIGENS

Several anorexigenics have been demonstrated to cause pulmonary hypertension in humans. The first observation was made in 1967, when an epidemic of PPH was associated with the use of aminorex in Europe coincident with its introduction in the general population. The mechanism by which aminorex causes pulmonary hypertension remains uncertain, but it has similarities to both adrenaline and ephedrine in its chemical structure. The clinical features of pulmonary hypertension were identical to those attributed to PPH.

The association between the use of fenfluramine appetite suppressants and the development of PPH was established in the International Primary Pulmonary Hypertension Study (IPPHS), a case-control study conducted in Europe in 1992 to 1994.[59] The study resulted in severe restriction of the use of appetite suppressants in Europe, only to see their use popularized in the United States. Ultimately, the marked increase in the number of cases of PPH and cardiac valvulopathy ascribed to the use of fenfluramine drugs in the United States led to their withdrawal in 1997. Unfortunately, in the majority of patients, the development of pulmonary hypertension has been progressive despite withdrawal of the appetite suppressants.[144,145] Although the drugs mainly identified in the IPPHS were the fenfluramines, anorexigenics such as amphetamine were also implicated.

The mechanism by which the fenfluramines and aminorex produce pulmonary hypertension has been investigated. Experimental studies have demonstrated that these drugs can cause pulmonary vasoconstriction by inhibiting voltage-gated potassium channels in the smooth muscle cells of resistance-level pulmonary arteries.[146] Although the degree of pulmonary vasoconstriction noted was small, it increased dramatically when NO synthase was inhibited. One recent study compared NO production in patients with PPH and patients with pulmonary hypertension associated with the use of anorexigens.[147] It appears that the latter group had a deficiency in basal NO production when compared with patients with PPH, which suggests that NO may be a compensatory product of the pulmonary arterial endothelium that increases in pulmonary hypertension to counteract the effects of chronic vasoconstriction.

Because of the consistent association with anorexigenics and unexplained pulmonary hypertension, clinicians should be exceedingly careful in the use of these drugs in the future, especially in patients who may have increased susceptibility to the development of pulmonary hypertension. Although treatment is similar to that of PPH, prognosis may be worse.[148]

PERSISTENT PULMONARY HYPERTENSION OF THE NEWBORN

Three forms of persistent pulmonary hypertension of the newborn have been described. In the hypertrophic type, the muscular tissue of the pulmonary arteries is hypertrophied and extends peripherally to the acini. Medial hypertrophy causes narrowing of the arteries and an increase in pulmonary pressure and reduction in pulmonary blood flow. It is believed to be the result of sustained fetal hypertension from chronic vasoconstriction due to chronic fetal distress. In the hypoplastic type, the lungs including the pulmonary arteries are underdeveloped, usually as the result of a congenital diaphragmatic hernia or prolonged leakage of amniotic fluid.[149,150] The cross-sectional area of the pulmonary vascular bed is inadequate for normal neonatal pulmonary blood flow. In the reactive type, lung histology is presumably normal but vasoconstriction causes pulmonary hypertension. High levels of vasoconstrictive mediators such as thromboxane, norepinephrine, and leukotrienes may be responsible and may result in a streptococcal infection or acute asphyxia at birth.

Although persistent pulmonary hypertension of the newborn can vary in severity, severe cases are usually life threatening. It is usually associated with severe hypoxemia and the need for mechanical ventilation. Echocardiographic findings of severe pulmonary hypertension and right-to-left shunting at the level of the ductus arteriosus or foramen ovale are common. Inhaled nitric oxide has provided encouraging results through improvement in oxygenation in these patients (see Fig. 67-9). Intravenous epoprostenol has also been used and may even have additive effects to that of inhaled NO.[151] Alveolar capillary dysplasia is a very rare cause of persistent pulmonary hypertension of the newborn and is characterized by a developmental abnormality in the pulmonary vasculature. The antemortem diagnosis can be made only with open-lung biopsy. Despite aggressive treatment with NO, epoprostenol, and even extracorporeal membrane oxygenation, survival in the setting of alveolar capillary dysplasia is rare.[152]

PULMONARY VENOOCCLUSIVE DISEASE

Pulmonary venoocclusive disease is a rare form of PPH. The histopathological diagnosis is based on the presence of obstructive eccentric fibrous intimal pads within the pulmonary veins and venules. Arterialization of the pulmonary veins is often present and associated with alveolar capillary congestion. Other changes of chronic pulmonary hypertension such as medial hypertrophy and muscularization of the arterioles with eccentric intimal fibrosis may also be seen. The pulmonary venous obstruction explains the increased pulmonary capillary wedge pressure described in patients in the late stages of the disease and the increase in basilar bronchovascular markings described on the chest radiograph. These clinical findings, along with a perfusion lung scan showing diffuse, patchy nonsegmental abnormalities, is suggestive of the diagnosis on a clinical basis.[153] The chest CT scan may be very helpful, revealing smooth interlobular septal thickening, ground-glass opacities, and a mosaic attention pattern. The treatment of pulmonary venoocclusive disease is unsatisfactory. Anecdotal reports of success with calcium blockers or epoprostenol have been tempered by reports of these treatments producing fulminant pulmonary edema. Any therapy needs particularly close supervision, and early referral of the patient for lung transplantation should be considered.

PULMONARY CAPILLARY HEMANGIOMATOSIS

Pulmonary capillary hemangiomatosis was first described in 1978 as a very rare cause of pulmonary hypertension.[154] Because of the few reports in the medical literature, it is hard to characterize this abnormality. The typical chest radiographic appearance is a diffuse bilateral reticular nodular pattern associated with enlarged central pulmonary arteries.[155] Ventilation-perfusion scans are often abnormal and may show matched or unmatched defects. The most characteristic finding on high-resolution CT scan is diffuse bilateral thickening of the interlobular septa and small centrilobular, poorly circumscribed, nobular opacities.[156] Diffuse ground-glass opacities have also been described. Histological findings often include irregular small nodular foci of thin-walled capillary-sized vessels that diffusely invade the lung parenchyma, the bronchiolar walls, and the adventitia of large vessels. These nodular lesions are often associated with alveolar hemorrhage. Changes of hypertensive arteriopathy manifest by intimal fibrosis and medial hypertrophy are also common. Most patients appear to be young adults and present with dyspnea and/or hemoptysis. It is very difficult to distinguish pulmonary capillary hemangiomatosis from PPH clinically. A hereditary form with probable autosomal recessive transmission has been reported.

The clinical course of patients with this condition is usually one of progressive deterioration leading to severe pulmonary hypertension, right-sided heart failure, and death. Intravenous epoprostenol has been used, but it has been reported with the associated development of severe pulmonary edema.[157] The only definitive treatment for these patients is bilateral lung transplantation.

Pulmonary Venous Hypertension

PATHOPHYSIOLOGY. Increased resistance to pulmonary venous drainage is a mechanism common to several conditions of diverse causes in which pulmonary hypertension occurs. Altered resistance to pulmonary venous drainage may be the result of diseases affecting the left ventricle or pericardium, mitral or aortic valves, or rare entities such as cor triatriatum and left atrial myxoma.

The severity of pulmonary hypertension depends, in part, on the performance of the right ventricle. In response to an acute stress such as pulmonary embolism, the normal right ventricle of an adult living at sea level can achieve systolic pulmonary pressures of 45 to 50 mm Hg, above which right ventricular failure supervenes. Systolic pressures exceeding these levels can be generated only by a hypertrophied right ventricle. If right ventricular infarction or ischemia has occurred or if the right and left ventricles are both affected by a myopathic process, right ventricular failure occurs at lower pulmonary artery pressure and severe elevations in pulmonary artery pressure may not develop despite an increase in pulmonary vascular resistance.

In the presence of a normal right ventricle, an increase in left atrial pressure initially results in a fall in both pulmonary vascular resistance and the pressure gradient across the lungs. These reductions may reflect distention of a population of compliant small vessels, recruitment of additional vascular channels, or both. With further increases in left atrial pressure, pulmonary arterial pressure rises along with pulmonary venous pressure, so that at a constant pulmonary blood flow, the pressure gradient between the pulmonary artery and veins and pulmonary vascular resistance remains constant. When pulmonary venous pressure approaches or exceeds 25 mm Hg on a chronic basis, a disproportionate elevation in pulmonary artery pressure occurs, so that the pressure gradient between the pulmonary artery and veins rises while pulmonary blood flow remains constant or falls, which is indicative of an elevation in pulmonary vascular resistance that is due, in part, to pulmonary vasoconstriction. Such patients may have some of the pathological features of PPH (see later) and it may be this subgroup that benefits from therapy directed at pulmonary hypertension.

Pulmonary Arterial Vasoconstriction. Considerable variability in pulmonary arterial vasoconstriction occurs in response to pulmonary venous hypertension. Marked reactive pulmonary hypertension with pulmonary artery systolic pressures in excess of 80 mm Hg occurs in somewhat less than one-third of patients whose pulmonary venous pressures are elevated in excess of 25 mm Hg. The fact that severe reactive pulmonary hypertension develops in less than one-third of patients with severe mitral stenosis suggests a broad spectrum of pulmonary vascular reactivity to chronic increases in pulmonary venous pressure.

The mechanisms involved in elevating pulmonary vascular resistance are unclear. In addition to hypertrophy of the media of the vasculature, a neural component may be present. An elevation in pulmonary venous pressure may also narrow or close airways, which may diminish ventilation and lead to hypoxia and vasoconstriction, and interstitial pulmonary edema secondary to pulmonary venous hypertension may encroach on the vascular lumen.

PATHOLOGY. Structural changes in the pulmonary vascular bed develop in association with chronic pulmonary venous hypertension, irrespective of its origin. At the ultrastructural level, these changes include swelling of pulmonary capillary endothelial cells, thickening of their basal lamina, and wide separation of groups of connective tissue fibrils, indicative of interstitial edema. With persistence of the edema, reticular and elastic fibrils proliferate and the alveolar capillaries become embedded in dense connective tissue. The permeability of interendothelial junctions depends on pulmonary capillary pressure, with leakage of large molecules (40,000 to 60,000 daltons) occurring at capillary pressures in excess of approximately 30 mm Hg.

Light microscopic examination of the lungs of patients with pulmonary venous hypertension shows distention of pulmonary capillaries, thickening and rupture of the basement membranes of endothelial cells, and transudation of erythrocytes through these ruptured membranes into the alveolar spaces, which contain fragments of disintegrating erythrocytes. Pulmonary hemosiderosis is commonly observed and may progress to extensive fibrosis. In the late stages of pulmonary venous hypertension, areas of hemorrhage may be scattered throughout the lungs, edema fluid and coagulum may collect in the alveolar spaces, and widespread organization and fibrosis of pulmonary alveoli may be present. Occasionally, particularly in patients with chronic pulmonary venous hypertension caused by mitral valve disease, the alveolar spaces become ossified. Pulmonary lymphatics may become markedly distended and give the appearance of lymphangiectasis, particularly when pulmonary venous pressure chronically exceeds 30 mm Hg. Structural alterations in the small pulmonary arteries, arterioles, and venules include medial hypertrophy, intimal fibrosis, and rarely, necrotizing arteritis. However, plexiform lesions are not seen.

CAUSES. Pulmonary hypertension secondary to elevation of the pulmonary venous pressure occurs in left ventricular dysfunction (see Chaps. 21 and 22), mitral and aortic valve disease (see Chap. 57), cardiomyopathy (see Chap. 59), cor triatriatum (see Chap. 56), and pericardial disease (see Chap. 64).

Pulmonary Hypertension Associated with Disorders of the Respiratory System

Diseases of the lung parenchyma are a common cause of pulmonary hypertension. The pathogenic mechanisms that can lead to pulmonary hypertension in this setting are shown in Table 67–9.

Chronic Obstructive Pulmonary Disease

Chronic obstructive pulmonary disease is the fourth leading cause of death in the United States, affecting more than 16 million people. The incidence, morbidity rate, and mortality rate of COPD vary widely among countries and are rising. The variation is possibly related to differences in exposure to risk factors as well as to differences in individual susceptibility.

TABLE 67–9 Potential Pathogenetic Mechanisms Leading to Pulmonary Arterial Hypertension and Cor Pulmonale

Mechanisms	Example
Primary	
Anatomical decrease in cross-sectional area (vessel destruction; encroachment on lumen by hypertrophy) of the pulmonary resistance vessels	Interstitial fibrosis and granuloma
Vasoconstriction of pulmonary resistance vessels	Hypoxia and acidosis
Contributory	
Large increments in pulmonary blood flow	Exercise
Increased pressures on the left side of the heart and pulmonary veins	Left ventricular failure or pulmonary venoocclusive disease
Increased viscosity of the blood	Secondary polycythemia or chronic hypoxia
Unproved	
Compression of pulmonary resistance vessels by raised alveolar pressures in their vicinity	Asthmatic bronchitis
Bronchial arterial-pulmonary arterial anastomoses	Expanded bronchial circulation

From Fishman AP: Pulmonary hypertension and cor pulmonale. *In* Fishman AP: Pulmonary Diseases and Disorders. 2nd ed. New York, McGraw-Hill, 1988, p 1001.

Chronic obstructive pulmonary disease is a heterogeneous group of diseases that share a common feature: the airways are narrowed, which causes the inability to exhale completely. Although there are numerous disorders that fall under the heading of COPD, the two largest components are emphysema and chronic bronchitis. While clear-cut distinctions between these components can often be made, there is considerable overlap as to the dominant abnormality in the individual patient in whom features of both may be manifest. Chronic bronchitis is a condition associated with excessive tracheal bronchial mucus production sufficient to cause cough with expectoration for at least 3 months of the year for more than 2 consecutive years. Emphysema is defined as the permanent, abnormal distention of the air spaces distal to the terminal bronchi, with destruction of the alveolar septa. In lungs from patients with COPD studied at postmortem, the major site of air flow obstruction has been shown to be in the small airways.

Definitions of COPD have been prepared by expert panels of the American Thoracic Society,[158] the European Respiratory Society,[159] the British Thoracic Society,[160] and the Global Initiative for Chronic Obstructive Lung Disease (GOLD).[161] Despite some subtle differences, all four expert panels make essentially the same key points:

1. Irreversible air flow obstruction is a cardinal feature of COPD.
2. Although limited reversibility of airflow obstruction in response to bronchodilator drugs is common, absence of such reversibility does not preclude bronchodilator treatment.
3. Neither asthma with complete reversibility nor chronic airflow obstruction due to other diagnosable conditions such as cystic fibrosis, obliterative bronchiolitis, or panbronchiolitis are included in the definition of COPD.
4. Tobacco smoking is the major, but not the only, risk factor for COPD.
5. The cause of irreversible airflow obstruction in patients with COPD is the presence in the lungs of bronchiolitis or small airway disease and emphysema, which are present to a variable mix among patients.

Of all of these definitions, the GOLD definition has gained widespread acceptance because of its simplicity and emphasis on spirometry as the standard for the diagnosis of airflow obstruction.

RISK FACTORS. Cigarette smoking is the most commonly identified correlate with COPD and accounts for 80 to 90 percent of the risk of developing COPD.[162] It has been estimated that 15 percent of one-pack-per-day smokers and 25 percent of two-pack-per-day smokers develop COPD during their lifetime. Other potential environmental causes include air pollution, occupational exposures, and infection. It is likely that there are important interactions between environmental factors and a genetic predisposition to COPD. Individuals who are homozygous for alpha$_1$-antitrypsin deficiency develop severe emphysema in the third and fourth decades of life. Dusty occupational environments are well-established risks but probably not major factors in North America.

PATHOGENESIS. A chronic inflammatory process is involved in COPD that differs from that seen in asthma, with different inflammatory cells, mediators, inflammatory effects, and responses to treatment.[163] Most inflammation in cases of COPD occurs in the peripheral airways (bronchioles) and lung parenchyma. There is increased destruction of lung parenchyma and an increased number of macrophages and T-lymphocytes, which are predominantly CD8+ (cytotoxic) T cells.[164] Importantly, eosinophils are not prominent as they are in asthma, except during an exacerbation.[165] Other inflammatory mediators that are elevated in patients with COPD include leukotriene B_4, which is chemotactic for neutrophils, tumor necrosis factor (TNF)-alpha, and interleukin-8.[166] Macrophages also appear to play an important role, since the cells are five to 10 times more numerous, are activated, are localized to the sites of damage, and also have the capacity to produce the pathological changes of COPD.[167] Macrophages also appear to be activated by cigarette smoke and other irritants to release neutrophil-chemotactic factors such as leukotriene B_4 and interleukin-8. Neutrophils and macrophages also release multiple proteinases that break down connective tissue in the lung parenchyma, resulting in emphysema, and stimulate mucus secretion (Fig. 67–14).[168]

Protease-Antiprotease Imbalance. This likely contributes to the pathophysiology of COPD.[167] In this condition, the balance appears to be tipped in favor of increased proteolysis because of either an increase in proteases, including neutrophil elastase, cathepsins, and matrix metalloproteinases, or a deficiency of the antiproteases, which may include alpha$_1$-antitrypsin in the lung parenchyma and airways, epithelium-derived secreting leukoprotease inhibitor in the airways, or at least three tissue inhibitors of matrix metalloproteinases (called TIMP-1, TIMP-2, and TIMP-3).[168] There is accumulating evidence that oxidative stress may have an important role in COPD,[169] possibly exacerbating the condition through several mechanisms, including the activation of transcription factor nuclear factor-κB and oxidative damage of the antiproteases, thus enhancing inflammation and proteolytic injury.

Systemic Effects of COPD. These include increased circulating concentrations of interleukin-6 and of acute phase proteins such as C-reactive protein.[170,171] Weight loss in patients with COPD has been associated with increased circulating levels of TNF-α and soluble TNF receptors and with increased release of TNF-α from circulating cells. The subsequent elevation of circulating levels of leptin may lead to weight loss and skeletal muscle wasting in COPD patients.[172] The low-grade systemic inflammation that is present in patients with moderate to severe airflow obstruction is thought to play a role in the increased cardiovascular risk for COPD patients.[173]

PATHOPHYSIOLOGY OF PULMONARY HYPERTENSION. Most commonly, pulmonary hypertension in COPD patients is due to multiple factors, including pulmonary vasoconstriction caused by alveolar hypoxia, acidemia, and hypercarbia; the compression of pulmonary vessels by the high lung volume; the loss of small vessels in the vascular bed in regions of the emphysema and lung destruction; and

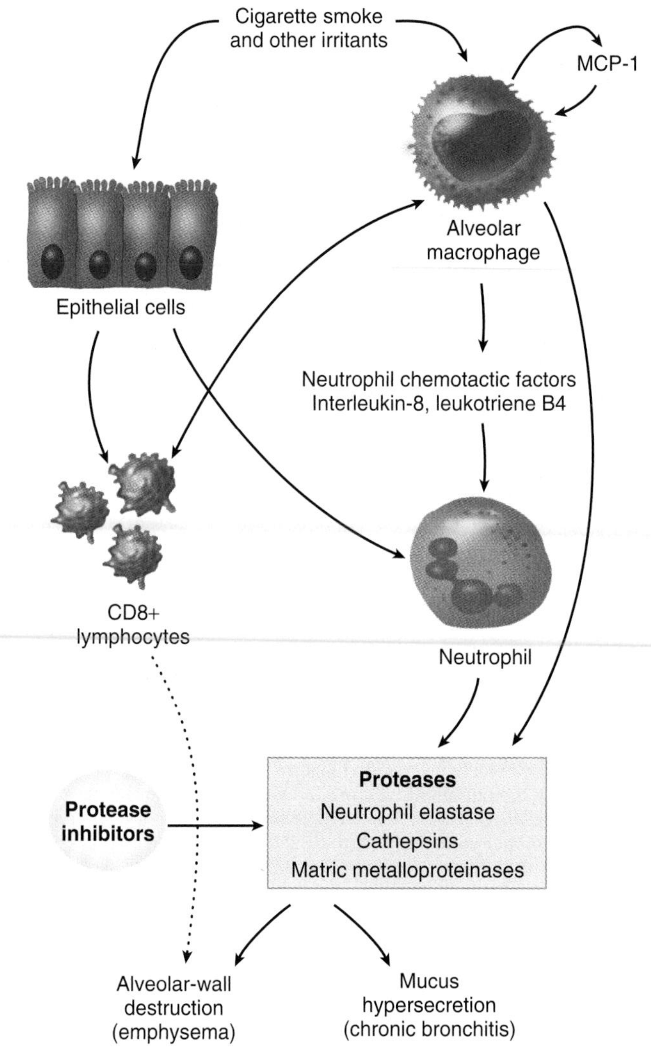

FIGURE 67–14 Inflammatory mechanisms in chronic obstructive pulmonary disease. Cigarette smoke and other irritants activate macrophages and airway epithelial cells in the respiratory tract, which release neutrophil chemotactic factors, including interleukin-8 and leukotriene B_4. Neutrophils and macrophages then release proteases that break down connective tissue in the lung parenchyma, resulting in emphysema, and also stimulate mucus hypersecretion. Proteases are normally counteracted by protease inhibitors, including alpha$_1$-antitrypsin, secretory leukoprotease inhibitor, and tissue inhibitors of matrix metalloproteinases. Cytotoxic T cells (CD8+ lymphocytes) may also be involved in the inflammatory cascade. MCP-1 denotes monocyte chemotactic protein 1, which is released by and affects macrophages. (From Barnes PJ: Chronic obstructive pulmonary disease. N Engl J Med 343:269, 2000.)

increased cardiac output and blood viscosity from polycythemia secondary to hypoxia. Of these, hypoxia is the most important factor and is associated with pathological changes that occur characteristically in the peripheral pulmonary arterial bed. The intima of small pulmonary arteries develop accumulations of vascular smooth muscle cells that are laid down longitudinally along the length of the vessels. Intimal thickening appears to be an early event that occurs in association with progressive air flow limitation. Medial hypertrophy in the muscular pulmonary arteries, and less commonly fibrinoid necrosis in these vessels, has also been reported in patients with COPD with chronic pulmonary arterial hypertension. Thus, structural change, rather than hypoxic vasoconstriction, is required for the development of sustained pulmonary hypertension in patients with COPD.

Changes in airway resistance may augment pulmonary vascular resistance in patients with COPD by increases in the alveolar pressure. The normal linear relationship between pressure and flow in the pulmonary circulation changes when alveolar pressure is elevated. The effect of airway resistance on pulmonary artery pressure may be particularly important when ventilation increases (such as in cases of acute exacerbation of COPD). In patients with COPD, even the small increases in flow that occur during mild exercise may increase pulmonary artery pressure significantly.

Alveolar hypoxia is a potent arterial constrictor in the pulmonary circulation that reduces perfusion with respect to ventilation in an attempt to restore PaO_2. In patients with COPD, there is a positive correlation between the $PaCO_2$ and the pulmonary artery pressure. Polycythemia, which may develop in response to chronic hypoxemia, increases the blood viscosity, which may also contribute to the severity of pulmonary arterial hypertension. Pulmonary arterial thrombosis may also occur in patients with COPD and may be a result of peripheral airway inflammation.

Evaluation of the Patient with Chronic Obstructive Pulmonary Disease

The diagnosis of COPD should be considered in patients with chronic cough, sputum production, dyspnea, or history of exposure to risk factors for the disease. Key indicators for considering a diagnosis of COPD are listed in Table 67–10. Although an important part of patient care, physical examination is relatively insensitive for diagnosing pulmonary hypertension and COPD. Clinical signs are often obscured by hyperinflation of the chest. Spirometry is the gold standard by which to diagnose and categorize COPD. Spirometry should measure the maximal volume of air forcibly exhaled from the point of maximal inhalation (FVC) and the volume of air exhaled during the first second of this maneuver (FEV_1). The

TABLE 67–10 Key Indicators for Considering a Diagnosis of Chronic Obstructive Pulmonary Disease (COPD)*

Stage	Characteristics
Chronic cough	Present intermittently or every day Often present throughout the day; seldom only nocturnal
Chronic sputum production	Any pattern of chronic sputum production may indicate COPD
Dyspnea that is:	Progressive (worsens over time) Persistent (present every day) Described by the patients as: "increased effort to breath," "heaviness," "air hunger," or "gasping" Worse on exercise Worse during respiratory infections
History of exposure to risk factors, especially:	Tobacco smoke Occupational dusts and chemicals Smoke from home cooking and heating fuels

Adapted from Pauwels RA, Buist AS, Calverley PM, et al: Global strategy for the diagnosis, management, and prevention of chronic obstructive pulmonary disease. Am J Respir Crit Care Med 163:1256, 2001.

*Consider COPD and performs spirometry if any of these indicators are present. These indicators are not diagnostic by themselves, but the presence of multiple key indicators increases the probability of a diagnosis of COPD. Spirometry is needed to establish a diagnosis of COPD.

ratio of these two components (FEV_1:FVC) should then be calculated. Patients with COPD typically show a decrease in both FEV_1 and FVC. An FEV_1:FVC ratio of less than 70 percent and a post-bronchodilator FEV_1 of less than 80 percent of predicted confirms the presence of airflow limitation that is not fully reversible. However, even patients who do not demonstrate reversibility with a short-acting bronchodilator can benefit symptomatically from long-term bronchodilator treatment.

ECHOCARDIOGRAPHY. Although echocardiography is an invaluable tool in the evaluation of most forms of pulmonary hypertension, its utility is more limited in cases of COPD because hyperinflation of the lungs and marked respiratory variations in intrathoracic pressures often result in suboptimal images. In a recent study, Doppler echocardiography was used to estimate systolic pulmonary artery pressure in a cohort of 374 lung transplantation candidates.[174] Of these patients, 68 percent had obstructive lung disease, 28 percent had interstitial lung disease, and 4 percent had pulmonary vascular disease. The prevalence of pulmonary hypertension was 18 percent among the COPD population, 59 percent among those with interstitial lung disease, and 100 percent among those with pulmonary vascular disease. Estimation of the systolic pulmonary artery pressure was possible in only 44 percent of the patients. Although the correlation between systolic pulmonary artery pressure estimated by echocardiography and that measured at the time of cardiac catheterization was good, 52 percent of the pressure measurements were found to be inaccurate, defined as a more than 10 mm Hg difference compared with the measured pressure at the time of cardiac catheterization. Furthermore, 48 percent of patients were misclassified as having pulmonary hypertension by echocardiography. Sensitivity, specificity, and positive and negative predictive values of systolic pulmonary artery pressure estimation by echocardiography for the diagnosis of pulmonary hypertension were 85, 55, 52, and 87 percent, respectively. Although the right ventricle was adequately visualized in nearly all of the patients, detection of right ventricular abnormalities did not enhance the poor positive predictive value of the Doppler echocardiogram. Given the inaccuracy of the echocardiogram in patients with pulmonary disease, an elevated estimated systolic pulmonary artery pressure obtained by echocardiogram must be interpreted with caution, because approximately half of the time it will represent a false-positive finding.

The largest hemodynamic characterization of patients with severe emphysema included 120 patients evaluated for participation in the National Emphysema Treatment Trial at 3 of the 17 participating centers.[175] These patients had severe airflow limitation with an FEV_1 of 27 percent of predicted, residual volume of 225 percent of predicted, and diffusing capacity of 27 percent of predicted. In 77.5 percent of the patients, pulmonary artery systolic pressure was between 30 and 45 mm Hg, whereas only 13.3 percent had a pulmonary artery systolic pressure of greater than 45 mm Hg. The mean pulmonary artery pressure was greater than 35 mm Hg in only 5 percent of patients.

In patients with mild COPD, right ventricular end-diastolic pressure and right ventricular stroke work, which were normal at rest, increased during exercise because of an increase in work against a higher pulmonary artery pressure.

Severe pulmonary arterial hypertension is uncommon in the presence of COPD. In a review of 500 patients with pulmonary hypertension, only 6 were found to have severe elevation in mean pulmonary artery pressure (>50 mm Hg), which was not related to the severity of their underlying lung disease.[176] This observation suggests that a different biological mechanism results in changes in the pulmonary vascular bed in susceptible patients and that severe pulmonary hypertension occurs in the presence of lung disease rather than as a result of the lung disease. Therefore, patients who present with severe pulmonary hypertension should be evaluated for another disease process that is responsible for the high pulmonary arterial pressures before it is attributed to the COPD.

Prognosis and Predictors of Survival

Chronic obstructive pulmonary disease is usually a progressive disease, and a patient's lung function can be expected to deteriorate over time, even with the best available care. Although pulmonary hypertension progresses slowly in patients with COPD, its presence confers a poor prognosis. For example, Weitzenblum and coworkers showed a 72 percent 4-year survival rate in patients with normal pulmonary artery pressure compared with a 49 percent survival rate in those with an elevated pulmonary artery pressure (mean >20 mm Hg).[177]

A study with a 10-year follow-up conducted on a cohort of 870 patients with severe COPD concluded that: (1) patients with COPD have a high mortality rate from acute respiratory failure, cor pulmonale, and lung cancer; (2) patients' age at the time of diagnosis influences the death risk; (3) patients who need long-term oxygen treatment have a higher death risk than those who do not; (4) the higher the FEV_1 or PaO_2 at the time of diagnosis, the lower the death risk; (5) patients who need and use long-term oxygen treatment have a lower death risk those who need it but do not use it properly; and (6) patients with a partial reversible airway obstruction who regularly attend the clinic for planned checkups have a lower death risk than those who have the same characteristics but do not show adherence to the care program.[178] In another study of 166 patients treated with long-term oxygen therapy, the overall survival rates were 78.3 and 67.1 percent at 2 and 3 years, respectively. A multivariate analysis showed an independent predictive power for right ventricular systolic pressure, age, and FEV_1.[179] Once endotracheal intubation is necessary, the prognosis is usually poor and the survival after 1 year is usually lower than 40 percent.[180] Pulmonary embolism is a common cause of death, with the frequency estimated to be approximately 11 percent.[181] Among patients with COPD in the intensive care unit, pulmonary embolism was the most frequent cause of death, at 40.6 percent.

Management

The overall approach to the management of stable COPD should revolve around a stepwise increase in treatment, depending on the severity of the disease. Disease severity is determined by the severity of symptoms and air flow limitation as well as other factors, including the frequency and severity of exacerbations, complications, respiratory failure, and comorbid factors, including cardiovascular disease and sleep-related disorders, in addition to the general health status of the patient. Patient education is paramount to effective treatment of COPD.

SMOKING CESSATION. The importance of smoking cessation cannot be overemphasized. The annual rate of decline of FEV_1 in smokers is approximately 80 ml per year, in contrast to 25 to 30 ml per year in nonsmokers. The Lung Health Study reported that patients who stopped smoking had a small improvement in FEV_1 (57 ml) after 1 year.[182] Thereafter, the rate of decline in lung function is similar to that of age-matched nonsmokers. The short-term success rates with smoking cessation are variable (18-77 percent), but success is more likely if the patient abstains from smoking within the first 2 weeks of entry into a program.

Numerous effective pharmacotherapies for smoking cessation now exist. They are generally recommended when counseling alone is not sufficient to help the patient to quit smoking. Numerous studies indicate that nicotine replacement therapy in any form (gum, inhaler, nasal spray, transdermal patch, sublingual tablets, or lozenges) reliably increases long-term smoking abstinence rates.[183] The antidepressants bupropion or nortriptyline have also been shown to increase long-term smoking cessation rates, although fewer data are available.[184]

PULMONARY REHABILITATION. The goals of pulmonary rehabilitation in COPD patients are to reduce symptoms, improve quality of life, and increase physical and emotional participation in everyday activities. Although a large study of 200 patients with disabling COPD demonstrated no difference in hospital admission among the patients randomized to receive rehabilitation versus the control patients, the rehabilitation group showed greater improvements in walking ability and general and disease-specific health status.[185]

PHARMACOLOGICAL TREATMENT. Pharmacological therapy is used to prevent and control symptoms, reduce the frequency and severity of exacerbations, improve health status, and improve exercise tolerance (Table 67–11). Although none of these medications has been demonstrated to modify the long-term decline in lung function, this should not preclude the use of these therapies to control symptoms.

Bronchodilators and Corticosteroids. Bronchodilators are central to the management of COPD and can be used either on an as-needed basis for relief of persistent or worsening symptoms or on a regular basis to help prevent and reduce symptoms. The choice of a beta-2 agonist, anticholinergic agent, theophylline, or combination therapy depends on the availability and individual response in terms of symptom relief and side effects. A combination of a short-acting beta-2 antagonist and an anticholinergic agent in stable COPD patients produces greater and more sustained improvements in FEV_1 than either agent alone and does not produce evidence of tachyphylaxis over 90 days of treatment.[186,187] Such combinations are commercially available. Prolonged treatment with corticosteroids does not modify the long-term decline in lung function in patients with COPD and should primarily be used in those who have a documented spirometric response to inhaled corticosteroids.[188]

Other Pharmacological Treatments. The use of vasodilators has been disappointing in the treatment of COPD patients, even those with pulmonary hypertension. No agent other than oxygen has been shown convincingly to vasodilate the pulmonary circulation in patients with COPD. Because of potential for worsening ventilation-perfusion mismatch, vasodilators may worsen hypoxemia. Data regarding the use of digoxin in COPD patients is insufficient to make recommendations, although short-term intravenous digoxin improved cardiac output and reduced circulating norepinephrine levels in patients with right ventricular dysfunction due to PPH.[97] Influenza and pneumococcal vaccines are recommended for prophylaxis..

OXYGEN. Hypoxemia is a common finding in patients with advanced COPD and is easily corrected with low-flow supplemental O_2. In key clinical trials, long-term O_2 therapy clearly improved the survival of hypoxemic patients with COPD.[189,190] The British study[191] compared the effect of treatment with oxygen for approximately 15 hours per day with the effects of no O_2 therapy, whereas the NIH study compared nocturnal O_2 therapy (about 12 hours per day) to "continuous" O_2 therapy (at least 19 hours per day).[189] In each study, the mean baseline PaO_2 when the patients were breathing ambient air was 51 mm Hg; the mean FEV_1 was 0.7 to 0.8 liters.

Oxygen therapy was beneficial in both studies. In the British study, 19 of 42 (45 percent) O_2-treated patients died within 5 years, whereas 30 of 45 (67 percent) untreated patients died. In the NIH study, the mortality rate after 1 year was 20.6 percent in the group receiving nocturnal O_2 and 11.9 percent in the group receiving continuous oxygen therapy; and after 2 years, mortality rates were 40.8 and 22.4 percent, respectively.[189] The relative risk of death for nocturnal O_2 therapy compared with continuous O_2 was 1.94. O_2 therapy is therefore effective, and continuous therapy is more effective than nocturnal therapy only.

HEMODYNAMIC EFFECTS OF OXYGEN. How oxygen therapy improves survival is unknown. Two major hypotheses have been proposed: (1) O_2 relieves pulmonary vasoconstriction, decreasing pulmonary vascular resistance and thus enabling the right ventricle to increase stroke volume; and (2) oxygen therapy improves arterial oxygen content, providing enhanced oxygen delivery to the heart, brain, and other vital organs. These two hypotheses are not mutually exclusive, and each one has supporting evidence. Oxygen therapy clearly alleviates the progressive pulmonary hypertension of untreated COPD. Patients who exhibit a significant decrease in pulmonary artery pressure (>5 mm Hg) after acute oxygen therapy (28 percent O_2 for 1 day) have better survival than patients who do not respond acutely when both groups of patients are subsequently treated with long-term continuous oxygen therapy.[190] Enhanced right ventricular performance during short-term oxygen therapy may also be the direct result of improved tissue (e.g., myocardial) oxygenation rather than decreased pulmonary vascular resistance.[191]

RECOMMENDATIONS FOR OXYGEN THERAPY. Criteria for chronic home oxygen therapy are shown in Table 67–12. Long-term oxygen therapy is warranted if the resting PaO_2 remains less than 55 mm Hg after a 3-week stabilization period on maximal medical therapy (e.g., bronchodilators, antimicrobial agents, diuretics). Patients with a PaO_2

TABLE 67–11 Therapy at Each Stage of Chronic Obstructive Pulmonary Disease (COPD)

Stage	Characteristics	Recommended Treatment
All		Avoidance of risk factors Influenza vaccination
0: At risk	Chronic symptoms (cough, sputum) Exposure to risk factors	
I: Mild COPD	$FEV_1/FVC < 70\%$ $FEV_1 \geq 80\%$ predicted With or without symptoms	Short-acting bronchodilator when needed
II: Moderate COPD	IIA $FEV_1/FVC < 70\%$ 50% < FEB1 < 80% predicted With or without symptoms	Regular treatment with one or more bronchodilators Inhaled glucocorticosteroids if significant symptoms and lung function response or if repeated exacerbations Rehabilitation
	IIB $FEV_1/FVC < 70\%$ $30\% \leq FEV_1 > 50\%$ predicted With or without symptoms	Regular treatment with one or more bronchodilators Inhaled glucocorticosteroids if significant symptoms and lung function response or if repeated exacerbations Rehabilitation
III: Severe COPD	$FEV_1/FVC < 70\%$ $FEV_1 < 30\%$ predicted or presence of respiratory failure or right heart failure	Regular treatment with one or more bronchodilators Inhaled glucocorticosteroids if significant symptoms and lung function response or if repeated exacerbations Treatment of complications Rehabilitation Long-term oxygen therapy if respiratory failure Consider surgical treatments

Adapted from Pauwels RA, Buist AS, Calverley PM, et al: Global strategy for the diagnosis, management, and prevention of chronic obstructive pulmonary disease. Am J Respir Crit Care Med 163:1256, 2001.

TABLE 67–12 Indications for Home Oxygen

Absolute
PaO_2 ≤55 mm Hg or SaO_2 ≤88%
PaO_2 55-59 mm Hg or SaO_2 = 89% in the presence of any of the following
Dependent edema suggesting congestive heart failure
P pulmonale on the ECG (P wave <3 mm in standard leads II, III, or aVF)
Erythrocytosis (hematocrit >56%)
Specific Situations
During exercise
PaO_2 <55 mm Hg or O_2 saturation <88% with low level of exertion
During sleep
PaO_2 <55 mm Hg or O_2 saturation <88% with associated complications, such as pulmonary hypertension, excessive daytime sleepiness, and cardiac arrhythmias

Adapted from ATS Statement: Comprehensive outpatient management of COPD. Am J Respir Crit Care Med 152(Suppl):S84, 1995.

above 55 mm Hg should be considered for oxygen therapy if they are polycythemic or have clinical evidence (e.g., electrocardiogram, physical examination) of pulmonary hypertension. Hypoxemia should be documented after the stabilization period to avoid the cost of long-term oxygen therapy in patients who do not require it. O_2 has been shown to delay the onset of fatigue in exercising muscles, thus improving ventilatory endurance and exercise capacity.[191] In addition, it decreases dyspnea and minute ventilation for a given workload.[192] Nocturnal oxygen therapy may be important in patients with sleep desaturation. Daily activities, such as walking, washing, and eating, are associated with transient oxygen desaturation in patients with moderate to severe COPD, even in the absence of resting hypoxemia[193]; this desaturation can be relieved with O_2.

NONINVASIVE VENTILATION. Noninvasive positive-pressure ventilation has been reported to improve gas exchange, sleep efficiency, quality of life, and functional status in patients with restrictive lung disease and chronic respiratory failure; however, its usefulness in patients with COPD is not as well established. Uncontrolled studies have demonstrated that noninvasive positive pressure ventilation used at home may improve oxygenation and reduce hospital admissions in patients with severe COPD and hypercapnia and improve long-term survival, although large controlled clinical trials are now needed.[194] The combination of noninvasive positive pressure ventilation and long-term O_2 therapy may be more effective,[195] but again large trials are needed before this approach can be recommended.

LUNG VOLUME REDUCTION SURGERY. Volume reduction surgery, which was originally described by Brantigan, has been advocated in selected patients with advanced emphysema. The surgical technique involves removing 20 to 30 percent of the volume of each lung by means of sternotomy, sequential thoracotomy, or thoracoscopy to reduce the severe hyperinflation commonly seen in patients with severe COPD.

A randomized trial comparing the results of lung volume reduction surgery with medical therapy for severe emphysema has been completed.[196] A total of 1218 patients with severe emphysema who underwent pulmonary rehabilitation were randomly assigned to undergo lung volume reduction surgery or to receive continued medical therapy. An interim analysis determined that patients with a FEV_1 of less than 20 percent of predicted and either homogeneous distribution of emphysema on CT scan or carbon monoxide diffusing capacity that was 20 percent or less of the predicted value were at high risk for death after lung volume reduction surgery with a low probability of functional benefit.[197] Such patients were subsequently excluded from entry into the trial. Overall, there was a death rate of 0.11 per person-year in both treatment groups, although it was determined that certain subgroups might benefit. Among patients with predominantly upper lobe emphysema and low exercise capacity, the mortality rate was lower in the surgery group than in the medical therapy group. Among patients with non-upper lobe emphysema and high exercise capacity, the mortality rate was higher in the surgery group than in the medical therapy group.

Exercise Capacity. Despite the lack of survival advantage, exercise capacity improved by more than 10 watts in 28, 22, and 15 percent of patients in the surgery group after 6, 12, and 24 months, respectively, as compared with 4, 5, and 3 percent of patients in the medical therapy group. Patients in the surgery group were also significantly more likely to have improvements in 6-minute walk distance, percentage of predicted value for FEV_1, general and health-related quality of life, and degree of dyspnea. Thus, patients with predominantly upper lobe emphysema and a low maximal workload have a lower mortality rate and a greater probability of improvement in exercise capacity with lung volume reduction surgery and should be considered for the procedure. In contrast, patients with predominantly non-upper lobe emphysema and high maximal workload had a higher mortality rate and little functional improvement, regardless of treatment received. These symptomatic improvements after lung volume reduction surgery appear to wane with time, and long-term data from the large National Emphysema Treatment Trial may be enlightening. Lung volume reduction is a palliative procedure that does not halt, but only slows, the rate of functional decline for COPD. The disease will still progress, and symptoms will likely worsen.

LUNG TRANSPLANTATION (see Chap. 26). COPD is the most common indication for lung transplantation worldwide. In 1995, approximately 60 percent of single lung and 30 percent of bilateral lung transplants were performed on patients with COPD.[198] Lung transplantation is a viable treatment option in patients with advanced pulmonary parenchymal or pulmonary vascular disease who have exhausted medical management. Both the number of patients waiting for lung transplantation and the waiting period have increased. Because of the scarcity of organ donors, the waiting time is now approximately 18 to 24 months in the United States. Patient selection and timing of referral for lung transplantation should take into account this waiting period. Selection criteria are outlined in Table 67–8. Both single-lung transplantation and bilateral lung transplantation result in significant improvement in postoperative lung function, exercise capacity, and quality of life.[199] The choice of the procedure needs to be individualized. In general, single-lung transplantation is used for emphysema because of the scarcity of organ donors, lower perioperative morbidity and mortality rates, and comparable improvement in exercise capacity compared with bilateral lung transplantation.[200] However, postoperative spirometry, single breath diffusing capacity, and arterial oxygen tension are all significantly higher in bilateral lung transplantation compared with single-lung transplantation, which may benefit young patients with emphysema because the higher pulmonary reserve will offset any decline in lung function due to infection or rejection. In most centers, bilateral lung transplantation is reserved for patients with suppurative lung disease or pulmonary vascular disease. The 1-year and 5-year survival rates for single and bilateral lung transplantation for emphysema are approximately 80 percent and 40 percent, respectively.

Interstitial Lung Diseases

Interstitial lung diseases represent a variety of conditions that involve the alveolar walls, perialveolar tissue, and other contiguous supporting structures.[201-203] Pulmonary hypertension occurs in patients with a variety of interstitial lung diseases and is often associated with obliteration of the pulmonary vascular bed by lung destruction and fibrosis. The mechanism for pulmonary hypertension may be related to hypoxemia, a loss of effective pulmonary vasculature from lung destruction, and/or by indirectly triggering a pulmonary vasculopathy. Interstitial lung disease may be due to environmental inhalant exposures, such as to asbestos, drugs, and chemotherapeutic agents, to radiation, and to recurring aspiration pneumonias. A large number of patients have interstitial lung disease of unknown origin, the most common being idiopathic pulmonary fibrosis and interstitial lung disease associated with connective tissue diseases.

Adult Cystic Fibrosis

Cystic fibrosis is the most common lethal genetic disease in white persons and occurs in approximately 1 of every 2000 live births. As the disease progresses, patients develop disabling lung disease and eventually respiratory failure, pulmonary hypertension, and cor pulmonale. The pathophysiology of pulmonary hypertension in cystic fibrosis is believed to be related to progressive destruction of the lung parenchyma and the pulmonary vasculature and to pulmonary vasoconstriction secondary to hypoxemia.[204] The development of pulmonary hypertension in patients with cystic fibrosis carries a grave prognosis. The mean survival time from the onset has been reported to be as short as 8 months. Typically, patients have severe hypoxemia, which may be a result of and a causative factor in the disease.

One study evaluated patients with cystic fibrosis and pulmonary hypertension in depth.[205] Right ventricular hypertrophy appears to be a precursor of right ventricular failure and an indicator of the onset of pulmonary hypertension. The severity of the pulmonary hypertension appeared to correlate significantly with declining pulmonary function, as well as with the degree of oxygen desaturation with exercise. In this study, patients who developed pulmonary hypertension had a much worse prognosis (average survival, 15 months) compared with those without pulmonary hypertension (average survival, 33 months). Once lung function is severely limited (FEV_1 <40 percent of predicted), the prevalence of pulmonary hypertension may be as a high as 40 percent. Because hypoxemia is universally found, supplemental oxygen is considered to be the mainstay of treatment in this group.

Sleep-Disordered Breathing (see Chap. 68)

PULMONARY HYPERTENSION. Observational studies have demonstrated a wide variation in the incidence of pulmonary hypertension as a complication of sleep apnea with a wide range of severity. The percentage has ranged from 17 to 73 percent, although these studies had variable entry criteria and some included patients with coexistent COPD.[206] The diagnosis of pulmonary hypertension in obstructive sleep apnea patients is also clouded by the coexistence of systemic hypertension, obesity, and diastolic dysfunction. Successful treatment with continuous positive airway pressure improves pulmonary hemodynamics in patients with obstructive sleep apnea,[207] supporting the relationship between these two disease entities. Acute pulmonary hemodynamic changes during obstructive apneas have been well defined; however, the extent to which these translate into persistent daytime pulmonary hypertension remains less certain.

ALVEOLAR HYPOVENTILATION DISORDERS

Alveolar hypoventilation disorders are characterized by hypoxemia and mechanical disorders of the ventilatory system which, in concert, may cause pulmonary hypertension.

CHEST WALL DISORDERS. Thoracovertebral deformities that can result in restrictive pulmonary syndromes, chronic alveolar hypoventilation, and pulmonary hypertension include idiopathic kyphoscoliosis, spinal tuberculosis, congenital spinal developmental abnormalities, spinal cord injury and other childhood myelopathies, ankylosing spondylitis, or other congenital and acquired muscular skeletal conditions, such as pectus excavatum. Kyphoscoliosis is a relatively common disorder of the spine and its articulations. When severe, it can have a profound impact on pulmonary function, characterized by a severe restrictive pattern on pulmonary function testing. In addition, there can be associated inspiratory muscle weakness that appears related to the increased elastic load from reduced lung and chest wall compliance. Scoliosis that appears before the age of 5 years has the worst respiratory prognosis. An angulation of greater than 100 degrees is considered very severe and is strongly associated with chronic alveolar hypoventilation.[208] Pulmonary compliance is often reduced by 50 percent or more as a result of lung underdevelopment and chronic lung hypoinflation. Patients can also have both central and obstructive apneas and hypopneas.

Pulmonary hypertension frequently occurs in patients with thoracovertibular deformities. Pulmonary hypertension is related to the reduction of the vascular bed because of hypoventilation and hypoxia. Symptoms are commonly slowly progressive. Hypoxemia can be seen from ventilation-perfusion mismatch or underlying atelectasis. In patients with advanced disease, intermittent positive-pressure breathing and noninvasive ventilation have been used successfully, as well as supplemental oxygen in patients who are hypoxemic.[209]

NEUROMUSCULAR DISEASE. The development of right-sided heart failure is an unusual manifestation of respiratory failure solely due to respiratory muscle weakness. It usually develops in response to the hypoxic and hypercapnic stimuli in patients with chronic forms of these disorders. Weakness of the respiratory muscles can be caused by either generalized muscle diseases, such as myopathic infiltrating diseases or muscular dystrophy (see Chap. 85), or more commonly by such neurological disorders as a cord lesion at or below the third cervical vertebra, amyotrophic lateral sclerosis, myasthenia gravis, poliomyelitis, and Guillain-Barré syndrome. The diagnosis of respiratory muscle weakness is confirmed by the finding of a restrictive ventilatory defect and a marked impairment of maximal respiratory pressures. Nocturnal ventilatory support, with either positive or negative pressure, has become established as effective therapy in appropriate cases, and its beneficial effects are well recognized.[210]

DIAPHRAGMATIC PARALYSIS. Bilateral diaphragmatic paralysis is an uncommon and rarely recognized cause of pulmonary hypertension. Diaphragmatic paralysis is a result of phrenic nerve injury, which can be traumatic or secondary to an underlying motor neuron disease. It may occur after cardiac surgery, as a manifestation of Lyme disease,[211] after radiation therapy,[212] or as a manifestation of other neurological disorders. When an affected patient is upright, ventilation may be normal or almost so, but when the patient is supine, gas exchange deteriorates. The diagnosis may be suspected in a patient with supine breathlessness, a disturbed sleep pattern, paradoxical motion of the abdomen on inspiration, and a low vital capacity in the upright position.

Patients with nontraumatic bilateral diaphragmatic paralysis may go unrecognized until they present either with respiratory failure or pulmonary hypertension. The diagnosis can be suspected when the vital capacity is reduced by more than 40 percent of predicted and paradoxic motion of the hemidiaphragms is noted on fluoroscopy.[213] Patients can also have unilateral paralysis of the diaphragm, which is more common but is associated with fewer symptoms and physiological abnormalities. The treatment should always be directed toward correcting the underlying chronic neuromuscular disease, if present, and addressing nocturnal hypoventilation with noninvasive ventilatory techniques. Intermittent positive airway pressure is an effective therapy.[214]

Pulmonary Hypertension due to Chronic Thrombotic or Embolic Obstruction of the Pulmonary Arteries (see Chap. 66)

Pulmonary thromboembolism, as a single event or as repeated events, rarely leads to the development of chronic pulmonary hypertension. In a subset of patients (believed to be less than 0.1 percent of all patients suffering from pulmonary embolism), however, the outcome is unusual. Rather than having inherent fibrinolytic resolution of the thromboembolism with restoration of vascular patency, the thromboemboli in these patients fail to resolve adequately. They undergo organization and incomplete recanalization and become incorporated into the vascular wall. Commonly, they are in the subsegmental, segmental, and lobar vessels, although it is believed that chronic thromboembolism tends to propagate retrograde, leading to slowly progressive vascular obstruction.

An identifiable hypercoagulable state is found in only a minority of patients. The lupus anticoagulant is present in 10 to 20 percent of patients with chronic thromboembolic pulmonary hypertension, whereas inherited deficiencies of protein C, protein S, and antithrombin III as a group can be identified in up to 5 percent of this population.[215] The development of a pulmonary hypertensive arteriopathy, similar to that seen in patients with other forms of pulmonary hypertension, has been documented in unobstructive lung regions as well as in vessels distal to partially or completely occluded proximal pulmonary arteries. These small vessel changes therefore appear to be a significant contributor to the hemodynamic progression seen in many patients. It appears that the vast majority of these patients have suffered one major thromboembolic event rather than multiple recurrences.

Chronic thromboembolic pulmonary hypertension involving the proximal pulmonary arteries is a well-characterized entity. The slowly progressive nature of the course of chronic thromboembolic pulmonary hypertension allows right ventricular hypertrophy to ensue and compensate for the increased pulmonary vascular resistance. However, owing to either progressive thrombosis or vascular changes in the "uninvolved" vascular bed,[216] the pulmonary hypertension becomes progressive and the patient manifests the clinical symptoms of dyspnea, fatigue, hypoxemia, and right-sided heart failure.

Patient Evaluation

The findings on clinical examination of patients with chronic thromboembolic pulmonary hypertension are similar to those of other patients with pulmonary hypertension, with the exception of the following features: These patients tend to have lower cardiac outputs than patients with PPH, which is often reflected in the reduced carotid arterial pulse volume. In addition, on occasion, bruits can be heard over areas of the lung that represent vessels with partial occlusions, but they must be carefully listened for.[217] It is important to make the diagnostic distinction between patients with chronic thromboembolic pulmonary hypertension and those with other forms of pulmonary hypertension, because the treatments are so different. For the former group, a potentially curative therapy through thromboendarterectomy is available, whereas for the latter group effective pharmacological regimens are now evolving. The symptoms and physical findings of chronic thromboembolic pulmonary hypertension are nonspecific and similar to those of patients with PPH.

PERFUSION LUNG SCAN. The perfusion lung scan is usually adequate to identify patients with this entity and is an important reason why lung scans are recommended for all patients who present with pulmonary hypertension (see Fig. 67–4). However, the lung scan typically underestimates the severity of the central pulmonary arterial obstruction.[218] Therefore, patients who present with one or more mismatched segmental or larger defects should undergo pulmonary angiography. This continues to be the gold standard for defining the pulmonary vascular anatomy and is performed to determine whether chronic thromboembolic obstruction is present, to determine its location and surgical accessibility, and to rule out other diagnostic possibilities. Maturation and organization of clot results in vessel retraction and partial recanalization, resulting in several angiographic patterns suggestive of chronic thromboembolic disease: pouch defect; pulmonary webs or bands; intimal irregularities; abrupt narrowing of major pulmonary vessels; and obstruction of main, lobar, or segmental pulmonary arteries, frequently at their point of origin.[219] Since chronic thromboembolic pulmonary hypertension is usually bilateral, the presence of unilateral central pulmonary artery obstruction should prompt consideration of other diagnoses, such as pulmonary vascular tumors or extravascular compression from a lung carcinoma, hilar or mediastinal adenopathy, or mediastinal fibrosis. Pulmonary angiography can be performed safely in these patients if careful attention is given to the hemodynamic state. Nonionic contrast medium has been demonstrated to cause no major hemodynamic effects, even in patients with severe chronic thromboembolic pulmonary hypertension,[220] and is preferred. Hypotension and/or bradycardia should be immediately treated with atropine.

COMPUTED TOMOGRAPHY. CT scanning can be a great aid in diagnosing chronic thromboembolic pulmonary hypertension (Fig. 67–15). Using high-resolution nonenhanced CT, areas of increased attenuation that do not obscure the vessels and that have a ground-glass appearance have been characterized as a mosaic pattern corresponding to hypoperfusion of the lung. Although this pattern is consistent with

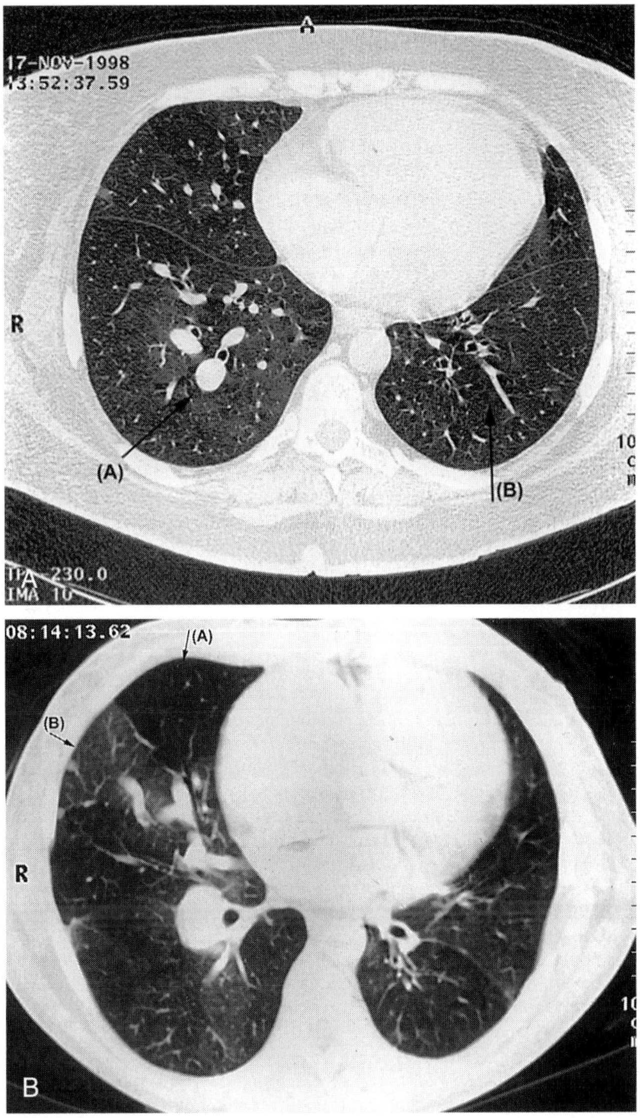

FIGURE 67–15 Chest computed tomographic scans in a patient with chronic thromboembolic pulmonary hypertension. **A,** Helical scan with contrast medium enhancement of the pulmonary vasculature shows a marked disparity in vessel size between the involved vessels (A), which are enlarged from thrombus, and the uninvolved vessels (B). **B,** Non-contrast-enhanced high-resolution scan illustrates a marked mosaic pattern manifest by differences in density of regions of the lung parenchyma reflecting the perfused areas (B) and the nonperfused areas (A), also consistent with underlying thromboembolic disease.

chronic thromboembolic pulmonary hypertension, it may also be seen in patients with cystic fibrosis, those with bronchiectasis, and lung transplant recipients, but it is virtually never seen in patients with PPH.[221] The contrast-enhanced CT features suggestive of chronic thromboembolic pulmonary hypertension include evidence of organized thrombus lining the pulmonary vessels in an eccentric or concentric fashion; enlargement of the right ventricle and central pulmonary arteries; variation in size of segmental arteries (relatively smaller in the affected segments compared to uninvolved segments); bronchial artery collaterals; and parenchymal changes to pulmonary infarcts. Marked variation in the size of the segmental vessels is more specific for chronic thromboembolic pulmonary hypertension and is believed to represent involvement of the segmental vessels due to thromboemboli. It has been reported that these findings might also be mimicked in patients with fibrosing mediastinitis.

CARDIAC CATHETERIZATION. Patients with chronic thromboembolic pulmonary hypertension tend to have higher right atrial pressures and lower cardiac outputs than comparable patients with PPH for the same level of pulmonary artery pressure. Because this is a disease that generally is progressive, the hemodynamic indications for surgical intervention are an elevation of pulmonary artery pressure and pulmonary vascular resistance for a period of more than 3 months despite adequate anticoagulation.

Treatment

Pulmonary thromboendarterectomy is considered in patients who are symptomatic and have evidence of hemodynamic or ventilatory impairment at rest or with exercise.[222] Operability is determined by the location and extent of proximal thromboemboli (see Fig. 66–19). Thrombi must involve the main, lobar, or proximal segmental arteries. It is important to evaluate whether the amount of surgically accessible thrombus is compatible with a degree of hemodynamic impairment. Failure to significantly reduce the pulmonary vascular resistance with endarterectomy, usually a result of the small vessel arteriopathy that may accompany this disease, is associated with a higher perioperative mortality rate and worse long-term outcome.[223]

Patients undergoing surgery usually have a preoperative pulmonary vascular resistance of greater than 4 Wood units and typically in the range of 10 to 12 Wood units. It is also important to assess the comorbid conditions preoperatively. Although severe left ventricular dysfunction is the only absolute contraindication to pulmonary thromboendarterectomy, advanced age, severe right ventricular dysfunction, and other significant comorbid illnesses increase the perioperative morbidity and mortality risks.[224] Right ventricular dysfunction is not considered a contraindication to surgery, because right ventricular function has been noted to improve once the obstruction of the pulmonary blood flow is removed. It is a true endarterectomy requiring establishment of a dissection plane at the level of the media. The procedure is performed on cardiopulmonary bypass and usually requires periods of complete circulatory arrest to allow for a bloodless field and define an adequate endarterectomy plane.

An operative classification of thromboembolic disease has recently been established and may be useful in terms of prognostication.[225] Among 202 patients who underwent pulmonary thromboendarterectomy, intraoperative classification of thromboembolism was defined as follows: type 1 (37.6 percent), thrombus in the main lobar pulmonary arteries; type 2 (40 percent), intimal thickening and fibrosis proximal to the segmental arteries; type 3 (18.8 percent), disease within distal segmental arteries only; and type 4 (3.4 percent), distal arteriolar vasculopathy without visible thromboembolic disease. Although all four patient groups were similar with respect to age, preoperative pulmonary artery pressures, and pulmonary vascular resistance, patients with proximal thromboembolic disease (groups 1 and 2) had a significantly greater improvement in pulmonary artery systolic pressure and pulmonary vascular resistance. There was also a greater increase in postoperative cardiac index and decrease in right ventricular systolic pressure in these patients as compared with those who had disease within the segmental or distal branches (groups 3 and 4). Although in previous series the operative mortality rate has been reported to be fairly high, the 1-month survival rate in patients who fell into groups 1 and 2 was 98.7 and 97.5 percent, respectively, whereas the 1-month survival rate in patients classified in groups 3 and 4 was 86.8 and 85.7 percent, respectively.

POSTOPERATIVE MANAGEMENT. Postoperative management can be extremely challenging. Patients in whom a large volume of central thrombus is removed, associated with back-bleeding from the distal vascular segments and an immediate fall in the pulmonary artery pressure, usually have an extremely good postoperative course and long-term follow-up. Patients in whom small amounts of thrombus can be removed, in whom the thrombus becomes fragmented at the time of thromboendarterectomy, or in whom there is no distal back-bleeding from the segment where the thrombus was removed usually have a difficult postoperative course. In addition, a lack of significant fall in pulmonary artery pressure and an increase in cardiac output portends a difficult postoperative recovery.

These patients may need mechanical ventilation and inotropic support for days to weeks during periods of slow recovery. Much of their mortality risk appears to be related to severe right ventricular dysfunction, which actually becomes initially worsened during the surgical procedure. Reperfusion injury, which is manifest by profound hypoxemia and pulmonary infiltrates corresponding to the segments where thrombus was removed, occurs in approximately 15 to 20 percent of patients and can be extensive. The only effective management of this complication is sustained assisted ventilation and oxygen supplementation. Attempts to reverse this with corticosteroids or other agents have not been successful. Other complications include atrial fibrillation, pneumonia, delirium, pneumothorax, pancreatitis, clostridium difficile, colitis, and gastrointestinal bleeding.

Those survivors who have a good result, with a significant reduction in postoperative pulmonary vascular resistance at 48 hours, can expect to realize an improvement in functional class and exercise tolerance.[226] Life-long anticoagulation with a goal INR ratio of 2.5 to 3.5 is indicated postoperatively.

PPH VERSUS CHRONIC THROMBOEMBOLIC PULMONARY HYPERTENSION. There are patients whose clinical presentation and evaluation findings are virtually identical to those of patients with PPH but who on autopsy have widespread thrombotic lesions throughout their pulmonary vasculature. It is unclear whether they represent PPH with an excessive tendency toward thrombosis or chronic thromboembolic pulmonary hypertension with persistent thromboemboli only at the arteriolar level. Often their lung scan will show a perfusion pattern characterized by a diffuse mottled abnormality. Because of the poor outcomes after surgery of patients with very distal thromboembolic disease, medical management has been attempted. Both the oral prostacyclin analog beraprost sodium and the phosphodiesterase inhibitor sildenafil have been reported in small case series to improve hemodynamics and exercise tolerance in patients with nonoperable chronic thromboembolic pulmonary hypertension.[227,228]

SICKLE CELL DISEASE

Cardiovascular abnormalities are prominent as part of the clinical spectrum of sickle cell disease. Evidence of right ventricular dysfunction, presumably resulting from pulmonary hypertension, is a poorly characterized complication. In one series of 60 consecutive patients undergoing echocardiography, the incidence of pulmonary hypertension in the setting of sickle cell disease was 20 percent. The mortality rate was also significantly greater in patients with pulmonary hypertension than in those without (42 vs. 8 percent; $p = 0.03$). One must always consider left ventricular dysfunction as a cause of pulmonary hypertension in patients with sickle cell disease because the elevation of pulmonary artery pressure is most often associated with elevation of the pulmonary capillary wedge pressure.[229] Patients with sickle cell disease can also have an increased risk of thromboembolism, and pulmonary thromboendarterectomy may be indicated in certain situations.[230] Sickle cell disease can rarely affect the lungs by causing embolization of bone marrow elements. Generally, the smaller pulmonary arteries, arterioles, and capillaries are affected. It can be associated with pulmonary infarction or local perivascular fibrosis.

Pulmonary Hypertension due to Disorders Directly Affecting the Pulmonary Vasculature

SCHISTOSOMIASIS

Although schistosomiasis is extremely rare in North America, hundreds of millions of people are affected worldwide, particularly in developing countries. The development of pulmonary hypertension almost always occurs in the setting of hepatosplenic disease and portal hypertension.[231] Clinical features appear when ova embolize to the lungs, where they induce formation of delayed hypersensitivity granulomas. In addition, deposition of fibrous tissue causes narrowing, thickening, and occlusion of the pulmonary arterioles. Histologically, focal changes related directly to the presence of schistosome ova may be located either within the alveolar tissue or within the pulmonary arteries, and plexiform or angiomatoid lesions may be found. Fibrosis surrounds most focal lesions. The clinical symptoms and radiographic findings in these patients who develop pulmonary hypertension are not distinctive. In developing countries, this condition can be confused with primary pulmonary hypertension.

The diagnosis of schistosomiasis-induced pulmonary hypertension is confirmed by finding the parasite ova in the urine or stools of persons with symptoms. However, the insidious onset of pulmonary vascular disease years after infection makes finding these parasite ova difficult. Active infections are treated with praziquantel, which kills the adult worms and stops further destruction of tissue by ova deposition.[232] Reversal of pathological lesions in the lungs after therapy has not been documented.

SARCOIDOSIS

Sarcoidosis is a multisystemic granulomatous disease of unknown origin characterized by an enhanced cellular immune response at the sites of involvement. Although any organ can be involved, sarcoidosis most commonly affects the lungs and intrathoracic lymph nodes.[233] The clinical manifestation and natural history of sarcoidosis vary greatly, but the lung is involved in more than 90 percent of patients. The most common presenting symptoms are cough and shortness of breath, which is of a progressive nature.[234] As the disease progresses in the lung parenchyma, extensive interstitial fibrosis is the result. In addition, obstructive airway disease, fibrocystic disease, bronchiectasis, endobronchial granulomas, and lobar atelectasis are common consequences of lung involvement.

Cardiac involvement from sarcoidosis appears to be more common than previously thought and may be present in up to one-third of the cases. Consequently, patients presenting with dyspnea should undergo a thorough cardiac evaluation for the possibility of cardiac involvement. Noncaseating granulomas may infiltrate the myocardium and leave fibrotic scars; and if enough of the myocardium is involved, the patients will develop clinical features of a restrictive cardiomyopathy. Patients with cardiac involvement from sarcoidosis also present with varying degrees of heart block, arrhythmias, and/or clinical features of biventricular diastolic heart failure. Sudden death can be a common manifestation of cardiac sarcoid, and it is one of the most feared sequelae. The prognosis of patients with cardiac involvement from sarcoidosis is variable but can be quite poor. Usually a trial of corticosteroids is given in the hope that it will alter the natural history of the disease.

The echocardiogram often demonstrates either diffuse or regional wall motion abnormalities in patients with cardiac involvement. It is not uncommon, however, to find the features of pulmonary hypertension. Pulmonary hypertension detected by echo-Doppler techniques may be the result of restrictive cardiomyopathy from sarcoid and needs to be clearly distinguished from pulmonary hypertension from direct pulmonary vascular involvement, because the clinical management of these two conditions differs dramatically.

Pulmonary hypertension is most commonly the result of chronic severe fibrocystic sarcoidosis.[235] Patients have chronic progressive dyspnea with effort, a chest radiograph demonstrating severe diffuse interstitial fibrotic lung disease, and pulmonary function tests that reflect severe restrictive physiology and hypoxemia. In these cases, the resulting pulmonary hypertension is usually mild to moderate and typical of patients presenting with restrictive lung disease of any cause.

MANAGEMENT. Management is generally focused on reversing any acute exacerbations of the lung disease and giving supplemental oxygen when indicated. Some patients with sarcoidosis, however, have mild to moderate restrictive lung disease with severe pulmonary hypertension, presumed from granulomatous vasculitis of the pulmonary vessels. It is critically important in the cardiopulmonary evaluation of the patient presenting with underlying sarcoidosis and dyspnea to distinguish whether the symptoms are from chronic interstitial lung disease, restrictive cardiomyopathy, or pulmonary vascular disease.[236] Although the traditional treatment of these patients has been unsatisfactory, it was recently demonstrated that some patients have a very favorable response to intravenous epoprostenol therapy.[133] Although interstitial lung involvement from sarcoidosis can result in mild pulmonary hypertension, a subset of patients present with severe pulmonary hypertension believed to be due to direct pulmonary vascular involvement. It appears that, as with other, secondary causes, these patients are predisposed to the development of pulmonary vascular disease that is triggered in some way by the sarcoid disease process. Although the use of intravenous epoprostenol chronically may reverse the right-sided heart failure and dramatically improve these patients' pulmonary hemodynamics, it will have no impact on any underlying fibrotic lung disease and/or hypoxemia, which still may render the patients symptomatic and dyspneic.

REFERENCES

Normal Pulmonary Circulation

1. Pietra G: The pathology of primary pulmonary hypertension. *In* Rubin LJ, Rich S (eds): Primary Pulmonary Hypertension. New York, Marcel Dekker, 1997, pp 19-61.
2. Salvi SS: Alpha1-adrenergic hypothesis for pulmonary hypertension. Chest 115:1708, 1999.
3. Bevan R: Influence of adrenergic innervation on vascular growth and mature characteristics. Am Rev Respir Dis 140:147, 1989.
4. Takizawa T, Hara Y, Saito T, et al: Alpha-1-adrenoceptor stimulation partially inhibits ATP-sensitive K^+ current in guinea pig ventricular cells: Attenuation of the action potential shortening induced by hypoxia and K^+ channel openers. J Cardiovasc Pharmacol 28:799, 1996.
5. Weir EK, Reeve HL, Huang JM, et al: Anorexic agents aminorex, fenfluramine, and dexfenfluramine inhibit potassium current in rat pulmonary vascular smooth muscle and cause pulmonary vasoconstriction. Circulation 94:2216, 1996.
6. Bento AC, de Moraes S: Effects of estrogen pretreatment of the spare α_1-adrenoceptors and the slow and fast components of the contractile response of the isolated female rat aorta. Gen Pharmacol 23:565, 1992.
7. Kourembanas S, Morita T, Christou H, et al: Hypoxic responses of vascular cells. Chest 114:25S, 1998.
8. Weir E, Reeve H, Peterson D, et al: Pulmonary vasoconstriction, oxygen sensing, and the role of ion channels. Chest 114:17, 1998.
9. Horstman D, Frank D, Rich G: Prolonged inhaled NO attenuates hypoxic, but not monocrotaline-induced, pulmonary vascular remodeling in rats. Anesth Analg 86:74, 1998.
10. Cargill R, Kiely D, Clark R, Lipworth B: Hypoxaemia and release of endothelin-1. Thorax 50:1308, 1995.
11. Peng W, Michael J, Hoidal J, et al: ET-1 modulates KCa-channel activity and arterial tension in normoxic and hypoxic human pulmonary vasculature. Am J Physiol 275:L729, 1998.
12. Bialecki R, Stinson-Fisher C, Murdoch W, et al: A novel orally active endothelin-A receptor antagonist, ZD1611, prevents chronic hypoxia-induced pulmonary hypertension in the rat. Chest 114:91S, 1998.
13. Haleen S, Schroeder R, Walker D, et al: Efficacy of CI-1020, an endothelin A receptor antagonist, in hypoxic pulmonary hypertension. J Cardiovas Pharmacol 31:S331, 1998.
14. Holm P, Liska J, Franco-Cereceda A: The ETA receptor antagonist, BMS-182874, reduces acute hypoxic pulmonary hypertension in pigs in vivo. Cardiovasc Res 37:765, 1998.
15. Christou H, Yoshida A, Arthur V, et al: Increased vascular endothelial growth factor production in the lungs of rats with hypoxia-induced pulmonary hypertension. Am J Respir Cell Mol Biol 18:768, 1998.
16. Partovian C, Adnot S, Eddahibi S, et al: Heart and lung VEGF mRNA expression in rats with monocrotaline- or hypoxia-induced pulmonary hypertension. Am J Physiol 275:H1948, 1998.
17. Semenza GL, Agani F, Iyer N, et al: Hypoxia-inducible factor 1: From molecular biology to cardiopulmonary physiology. Chest 114:40S, 1998.
18. Naeije R: Pulmonary circulation at high altitude. Respiration 64:429, 1997.
19. Davila-Roman VG, Guest TM, Tuteur PG, et al: Transient right but not left ventricular dysfunction after strenuous exercise at high altitude. J Am Coll Cardiol 30:468, 1997.
20. Cacciapuoti F, D'Avino M, Lama D, et al: Hemodynamic changes in pulmonary circulation induced by effort in the elderly. Am J Cardiol 71:1481, 1993.
21. Vane JR, Anggard EE, Botting RM: Regulatory functions of the vascular endothelium. N Engl J Med 323:27, 1990.
22. Murtha YM, Allen BM, Orr JA: The role of protein kinase C in thromboxane A2-induced pulmonary artery vasoconstriction. J Biomed Sci 6:293, 1999.
23. Cooper CJ, Landzberg MJ, Anderson TJ, et al: Role of nitric oxide in the local regulation of pulmonary vascular resistance in humans. Circulation 93:266, 1996.
24. Cooper CJ, Jevnikar FW, Walsh T, et al: The influence of basal nitric oxide activity on pulmonary vascular resistance in patients with congestive heart failure. Am J Cardiol 82:609, 1998.
25. Bouloumie A, Schini-Kerth VB, Busse R: Vascular endothelial growth factor upregulates nitric oxide synthase expression in endothelial cells. Cardiovasc Res 41:773, 1999.
26. Cacoub P, Dorent R, Nataf P, et al: Endothelin-1 in the lungs of patients with pulmonary hypertension. Cardiovasc Res 33:196, 1997.
27. Gray MO, Long CS, Kalinyak JE, et al: Angiotensin II stimulates cardiac myocyte hypertrophy via paracrine release of TGF-beta 1 and endothelin-1 from fibroblasts. Cardiovasc Res 40:352, 1998.
28. Wort S, Woods M, Warner T, et al: Endogenously released endothelin-1 from human pulmonary artery smooth muscle promotes cellular proliferation. Am J Respir Cell Mol Biol 25:104, 2001.
29. Dupuis J, Jasmin J, Prie S, Cernacek P: Importance of local production of endothelin-1 and of the ET_B receptor in the regulation of pulmonary vascular tone. Pulm Pharmacol Therap 13:135, 2000.
30. Rubens C, Ewert R, Halank M, et al: Big endothelin-1 and endothelin-1 plasma levels are correlated with the severity of primary pulmonary hypertension. Chest 120:1562, 2001.
31. Peifley K, Winkles J: Angiotensin II and endothelin-1 increase fibroblast growth factor-2 mRNA expression in vascular smooth muscle cells. Biochem Biophys Res Commun 242:202, 1998.
32. Fanburg B, Lee S:A new role for an old molecule: Serotonin as a mitogen. Am J Physiol 272:L795, 1997.
33. Eddahibi S, Hanoun N, Lanfumey L, et al: Attenuated hypoxic pulmonary hypertension in mice lacking the 5-hydroxytryptamine transporter gene. J Clin Invest 105:1555, 2000.
34. MacLean MR, Herve P, Eddahibi S, Adnot S: 5-hydroxytryptamine and the pulmonary circulation: Receptors, transporters and relevance to pulmonary arterial hypertension. Br J Pharmacol 131:161, 2000.
35. Schuster DP, Crouch EC, Parks WC, et al: Angiotensin converting enzyme expression in primary pulmonary hypertension. Am J Respir Crit Care Med 154:1087, 1996.
36. Okada K, Bernstein ML, Zhang W, et al: Angiotensin-converting enzyme inhibition delays pulmonary vascular neointimal formation. Am J Respir Crit Care Med 158:939, 1998.

37. Morrell NW, Atochina EN, Morris KG, et al: Angiotensin converting enzyme expression is increased in small pulmonary arteries of rats with hypoxia-induced pulmonary hypertension. J Clin Invest 96:1823, 1995.

Clinical Assessment of the Patient with Suspected Pulmonary Hypertension

38. Noutens M, Wolfkiel CJ, Chemka EV, et al: Understanding right and left ventricular systolic function and interactions at rest and with exercise in primary pulmonary hypertension. Am J Cardiol 73:379, 1995.
39. Wolf M, Boyer-Neumann C, Parent F, et al: Thrombotic risk factors in pulmonary hypertension. Eur Respir J 15:395, 2000.
40. Nagaya N, Nishikimi T, Okano Y, et al: Plasma brain natriuretic peptide levels increase in proportion to the extent of right ventricular dysfunction in pulmonary hypertension. J Am Coll Cardiol 31:202, 1998.
41. Wada A, Tsutamato T, Maeda Y, et al: Endogenous atrial natriuretic peptide inhibits endothelin-1 secretion in dogs with severe congestive heart failure. Am J Physiol 270:H1819, 1996.
42. Nagaya N, Uematsu M, Satoh T, et al: Serum uric acid levels correlate with the severity and the mortality of primary pulmonary hypertension. Am J Respir Crit Care Med 160:487, 1999.
43. Behar JV, Howe CM, Wagner NB, et al: Performance of new criteria for right ventricular hypertrophy and myocardial infarction in patients with pulmonary hypertension due to cor pulmonale and mitral stenosis. J Electrocardiol 24:231, 1991.
44. Zompatori M, Battaglia M, Rimondi M, et al: Hemodynamic estimation of chronic cor pulmonale by Doppler echocardiography. Clinical value and comparison with other noninvasive imaging techniques. Rays 22:73, 1997.
45. Raymond RJ, Hinderliter AL, Willis PW, et al: Echocardiographic predictors of adverse outcomes in primary pulmonary hypertension. J Am Coll Cardiol 39:1214, 2002.
46. McQuillan B, Picard M, Leavitt M, Weyman A: Clinical correlates and reference intervals for pulmonary artery systolic pressure among echocardiographically normal subjects. Circulation 104:2797, 2001.
47. Jain D, Zaret B: Assessment of right ventricular function: Role of nuclear imaging techniques. Cardiol Clin 10:23, 1992.
48. Steen VD, Graham G, Conte C, et al: Isolated diffusing capacity reduction in systemic sclerosis. Arthritis Rheum 35:765, 1992.
49. Butler J, Chomsky D, Wilson J: Pulmonary hypertension and exercise intolerance in patients with heart failure. J Am Coll Cardiol 34:1802, 1999.
50. Wax D, Garofano R, Barst R: Effects of long-term infusion of prostacyclin on exercise performance in patients with primary pulmonary hypertension. Chest 116:914, 1999.
51. Sun X-G, Hansen J, Oudiz R, Wasserman K: Exercise pathophysiology in patients with primary pulmonary hypertension. Circulation 104:429, 2001.
52. Myers J, Gullestad L, Vagelos R, et al: Clinical, hemodynamic, and cardiopulmonary exercise test determinants of survival in patients referred for evaluation of heart failure. Ann Intern Med 129:286, 1998.
53. Nootens M, Schrader B, Kaufmann E, et al: Comparative acute effects of adenosine and prostacyclin in primary pulmonary hypertension. Chest 107:54, 1995.
54. Raffy O, Azarian R, Brenot F, et al: Clinical significance of the pulmonary vasodilator response during short-term infusion of prostacyclin in primary pulmonary hypertension. Circulation 93:484, 1996.
55. Ricciardi MJ, Knight BP, Martinez FJ, Rubenfire M: Inhaled nitric oxide in primary pulmonary hypertension: A safe and effective agent for predicting response to nifedipine. J Am Coll Cardiol 32:1068, 1998.
56. Krasuski R, Warner J, Wang A, et al: Inhaled nitric oxide selectively dilates pulmonary vasculature in adult patients with pulmonary hypertension, irrespective of etiology. J Am Coll Cardiol 36:2204, 2000.
57. Mitchell H, Bolster MB, LeRoy EC: Scleroderma and related conditions. Med Clin North Am 81:129, 1997.

Primary Pulmonary Hypertension

58. Brickner M, Hillis L, Lange R: Congenital heart disease in adults: First of two parts. N Engl J Med 342:256, 2000.
59. Abenhaim L, Moride Y, Brenot F, et al: Appetite-suppressant drugs and the risk of primary pulmonary hypertension. N Engl J Med 335:609, 1996.
60. Botney MD, Liptay MJ, Kaiser LR, et al: Active collagen synthesis by pulmonary arteries in human primary pulmonary hypertension. Am J Pathol 143:121, 1993.
61. Higenbottam TW, Laude EA: Endothelial dysfunction providing the basis for the treatment of pulmonary hypertension. Chest 114(Suppl):72, 1998.
62. Giaid A, Saleh D: Reduced expression of endothelial nitric oxide synthase in the lungs of patients with pulmonary hypertension. N Engl J Med 333:214, 1995.
63. Giaid A: Nitric oxide and endothelin-1 in pulmonary hypertension. Chest 114(Suppl):208, 1998.
64. Stewart DJ, Levy RD, Cernacek P, Langleben D: Increased plasma endothelin-1 in pulmonary hypertension: Marker or mediator of disease? Ann Intern Med 114:464, 1991.
65. Lindner V, Lappi DA, Baird A, et al: Role of basic fibroblast growth factor in vascular lesion formation. Circ Res 68:106, 1991.
66. Botney MD, Bahadori L, Gold LI: Vascular remodeling in primary pulmonary hypertension. Potential role for transforming growth factor-beta. Am J Pathol 144:286, 1994.
67. Welsh CH, Hassell KL, Badesch DB, et al: Coagulation and fibrinolytic profiles in patients with severe pulmonary hypertension. Chest 110:710, 1996.
68. Morse JH, Barst RJ, Fotino M, et al: Primary pulmonary hypertension, tissue plasminogen activator antibodies, and HLA-DQ7. Am J Respir Crit Care Med 155:274, 1997.
69. Ware JA, Helstad DD: Platelet-endothelium interactions. N Engl J Med 328:628, 1993.
70. Nakonechnicov S, Gabbasov Z, Chazova I, et al: Platelet aggregation in patients with primary pulmonary hypertension. Blood Coagul Fibrinolysis 7:225, 1996.
71. Botney MD: Role of hemodynamics in pulmonary vascular remodeling: Implications for primary pulmonary hypertension. Am J Respir Crit Care Med 159:361, 1999.
72. Rabinovitch M: Insights into the pathogenesis if primary pulmonary hypertension from animal models. *In* Rubin LJ, Rich S (ed): Primary Pulmonary Hypertension. New York, Marcel Dekker, 1997, pp 63-82.
73. Rabinovitch M: Elastase and the pathobiology of unexplained pulmonary hypertension. Chest 114:213, 1998.
74. Yuan JX, Aldinger AM, Juhaszova M, et al: Dysfunctional voltage-gated K^+ channels in pulmonary artery smooth muscle cells of patients with primary pulmonary hypertension. Circulation 98:1400, 1998.
75. Tuder R, Cool C, Geraci M, et al: Prostacyclin synthase expression is decreased in lungs from patients with severe pulmonary hypertension. Am J Respir Crit Care Med 159:1925, 1999.
76. Breuer J, Georgaraki A, Sieverding L, et al: Increased turnover of serotonin in children with pulmonary hypertension secondary to congenital heart disease. Pediatr Cardiol 17:214, 1996.
77. Herve P, Launay JM, Scrobohaci ML, et al: Increased plasma serotonin in primary pulmonary hypertension. Am J Med 99:249, 1995.
78. Loyd JE, Newman JH: Familial primary pulmonary hypertension. *In* Rubin LJ, Rich S (ed). Primary Pulmonary Hypertension. New York, Marcel Dekker, 1997, pp 151-162.
79. Barst R, Loyd JE: Genetics and immunogenetic aspects of primary pulmonary hypertension. Chest 114(Suppl):231, 1998.
80. Deng Z, Haghighi F, Helleby L, et al: Fine mapping of *PPH1*, a gene for familial primary pulmonary hypertension, to a 3-cM region on chromosome 2q33. Am J Respir Crit Care Med 161:1055, 2000.
81. Morse JH, Jones AC, Barst RJ, et al: Mapping of familial primary pulmonary hypertension locus (*PPH1*) to chromosome 2q31-q32. Circulation 95:2603, 1997.
82. Newman J, Wheeler L, Lane K, et al: Mutation in the gene for bone morphogenetic protein receptor II as a cause of primary pulmonary hypertension in a large kindred. N Engl J Med 345:319, 2001.
83. Rudarakanchana N, Flanagan J, Chen H, et al: Functional analysis of bone morphogenetic protein type II receptor mutations underlying primary pulmonary hypertension. Hum Mol Genet 11:1517, 2002.
84. Atkinson C, Stewart S, Upton PD, et al: Primary pulmonary hypertension is associated with reduced pulmonary vascular expression of type II bone morphogenetic protein receptor. Circulation 105:1672, 2002.
85. Eddahibi S, Humbert M, Fadel E, et al: Serotonin transporter overexpression is responsible for pulmonary artery smooth muscle hyperplasia in primary pulmonary hypertension. J Clin Invest 108:1141, 2001.
86. Eddahibi S, Humbert M, Fadel E, et al: Hyperplasia of pulmonary artery smooth muscle in primary and secondary pulmonary hypertension is causally related to serotonin transporter overexpression. Am J Respir Crit Care Med 165:A97, 2002.
87. Lesch K-P, Engel D, Heils A, et al: Association of anxiety-related traits with a polymorphism in the serotonin transporter gene regulatory region. Science 274:1527, 1996.
88. Voelkel NF, Tuder RM, Weir EK: Pathophysiology of primary pulmonary hypertension: From physiology to molecular mechanisms. *In* Rubin LJ, Rich S (ed): Primary Pulmonary Hypertension. New York, Marcel Dekker, 1997, pp 83-129.
89. Lee SD, Shroyer KR, Markham NE, et al: Monoclonal endothelial cell proliferation is present in primary but not secondary pulmonary hypertension. J Clin Invest 101:927, 1998.
90. Tuder R: Plexiform lesions in primary pulmonary hypertension may represent an abnormal form of angiogenesis. Semin Respir Crit Care Med 15:207, 1994.
91. Tuder RM, Groves B, Badesch DB, Voelkel NF: Exuberant endothelial cell growth and elements of inflammation are present in plexiform lesions of pulmonary hypertension. Am J Pathol 144:275, 1994.
92. Wagenvoort CA, Mulder PG: Thrombotic lesions in primary plexogenic arteriopathy: Similar pathogenesis or complication? Chest 103:844, 1993.
93. Nagaya N, Satoh T, Ishida Y, et al: Impaired left ventricular myocardial metabolism in patients with pulmonary hypertension detected by radionuclide imaging. Nucl Med Commun 18:1171, 1997.
94. Patrat JF, Jondeau G, Dubourg O, et al: Left main coronary artery compression during primary pulmonary hypertension. Chest 112:842, 1997.
95. Kawut SM, Silvestry FE, Ferrari VA, et al: Extrinsic compression of the left main coronary artery by the pulmonary artery in patients with long-standing pulmonary hypertension. Am J Cardiol 83:984, A10, 1999.
96. Weiss BM, Zemp L, Seifert B, Hess OM: Outcome of pulmonary vascular disease in pregnancy: A systematic overview from 1978 through 1996. J Am Coll Cardiol 31:1650, 1998.
97. Rich S, Seidlitz M, Dodin E, et al: The short-term effects of digoxin in patients with right ventricular dysfunction from pulmonary hypertension. Chest 114:787, 1998.
98. Weber K: Aldosterone in congestive heart failure. N Engl J Med 345:1689, 2001.
99. Rich S, Kaufmann E, Levy PS: The effect of high doses of calcium-channel blockers on survival in primary pulmonary hypertension. N Engl J Med 327:76, 1992.
100. Barst RJ, Rubin LJ, Long WA, et al: A comparison of continuous intravenous epoprostenol (prostacyclin) with conventional therapy for primary pulmonary hypertension. The Primary Pulmonary Hypertension Study Group. N Engl J Med 334:296, 1996.
101. Barst RJ, Maislin G, Fishman AP: Vasodilator therapy for primary pulmonary hypertension in children. Circulation 99:1197, 1999.
102. Shapiro SM, Oudiz RJ, Cao T, et al: Primary pulmonary hypertension: Improved long-term effects and survival with continuous intravenous epoprostenol infusion. J Am Coll Cardiol 30:343, 1997.
103. McLaughlin VV, Genthner DE, Panella MM, Rich S: Reduction in pulmonary vascular resistance with long-term epoprostenol (prostacyclin) therapy in primary pulmonary hypertension. N Engl J Med 338:273, 1998.
104. Rich S, McLaughlin V: The effects of chronic prostacyclin therapy on cardiac output and symptoms in primary pulmonary hypertension. J Am Coll Cardiol 34:1184, 1999.

105. Robbins IM, Christman BW, Newman JH, et al: A survey of diagnostic practices and the use of epoprostenol in patients with primary pulmonary hypertension. Chest 114:1269, 1998.
106. Sitbon O, Humbert M, Nunes H, et al: Long-term intravenous epoprostenol infusion in primary pulmonary hypertension. J Am Coll Cardiol 40:780, 2002.
107. McLaughlin V, Shillington A, Rich S: Survival in primary pulmonary hypertension. The impact of epoprostenol therapy. Circulation 106:1477, 2002.
108. McLaughlin V, Gaine S, Barst R, et al: Efficacy and safety of treprostinil: An epoprostenol analog for primary pulmonary hypertension. J Cardiovasc Pharmacol 41:293, 2003.
109. Simonneau G, Barst RJ, Galie N, et al: Continuous subcutaneous infusion of treprostinil, a prostacyclin analogue, in patients with pulmonary arterial hypertension: A double-blind, randomized, placebo-controlled trial. Am J Respir Crit Care Med 165:800, 2002.
110. Hoeper M, Schwarze M, Ehlerding S, et al: Long-term treatment of primary pulmonary hypertension with aerosolized iloprost, a prostacyclin analogue. N Engl J Med 342:1866, 2000.
111. Olschewski H, Simonneau G, Galie N, et al: Inhaled iloprost for severe pulmonary hypertension. N Engl J Med 347:322, 2002.
112. Galie N, Humber M, Vachiery J-L, et al: Effects of beraprost sodium, an oral prostacyclin analogue, in patients with pulmonary arterial hypertension: A randomized, double-blind, placebo-controlled trial. J Am Coll Cardiol 39:1496, 2002.
113. Barst RJ, McGoon M, McLaughlin VV, et al: Beraprost therapy for pulmonary arterial hypertension. J Am Cell Cardiol 41:2119, 2003.
114. Channick R, Simonneau G, Sitbon O, et al: Effects of the dual endothelin-receptor antagonist bosentan in patients with pulmonary hypertension: A randomised placebo-controlled study. Lancet 358:1119, 2001.
115. Rubin L, Badesch D, Barst R, et al: Bosentan therapy for pulmonary arterial hypertension. N Engl J Med 346:896, 2002.
116. Barst RJ, Langleben D, Frost A, et al: Sitaxsentan therapy for pulmonary arterial hypertension. Am J Respir Crit Care Med 169:441, 2004.
117. Michelakis E, Tymchak W, Lien D, et al: Oral sildenafil is an effective and specific pulmonary vasodilator in patients with pulmonary arterial hypertension. Circulation 105:2398, 2002.
118. Ghofrani H, Wiedemann R, Rose F, et al: Sildenafil for treatment of lung fibrosis and pulmonary hypertension: A randomised controlled trial. Lancet 360:895, 2002.
119. Sitbon O, Humbert M, Simonneau G: Primary pulmonary hypertension: Current therapy. Prog Cardiovasc Dis 45:115, 2002.
120. Wilkens H, Guth A, Konig J, et al: Effect of inhaled iloprost plus oral sildenafil in patients with primary pulmonary hypertension. Circulation 104:1218, 2001.
121. Wensel R, Opitz C, Anker S, et al: Assessment of survival in patients with primary pulmonary hypertension. Circulation 106:319, 2002.
122. Ghofrani HA, Rose F, Schermuly RT, et al: Oral sildenafil as long-term adjunct therapy to inhaled iloprost in severe pulmonary arterial hypertension. J Am Coll Cardiol 42:158, 2003.
123. Rich S, Dodin E, McLaughlin VV: Usefulness of atrial septostomy as a treatment for primary pulmonary hypertension and guidelines for its application. Am J Cardiol 80:369, 1997.
124. Arcasoy SM, Kotloff RM: Lung transplantation. N Engl J Med 340:1081, 1999.
125. Trulock EP: Lung transplantation. Am J Respir Crit Care Med 155:789, 1997.
126. Maurer JR, Frost AE, Estenne M, et al: International guidelines for the selection of lung transplant candidates. Transplantation 66:951, 1998.
127. Rich S, McLaughlin VV: Lung transplantation for pulmonary hypertension: Patient selection and maintenance therapy while awaiting transplantation. Semin Thorac Cardiovasc Surg 10:135, 1998.

Pulmonary Arterial Hypertension with Associated Conditions

128. Sundaresan S: The impact of bronchiolitis obliterans on late morbidity and mortality after single and bilateral lung transplantation for pulmonary hypertension. Semin Thorac Cardiovasc Surg 10:152, 1998.
129. Okura H, Takatsu Y: High-output heart failure as a cause of pulmonary hypertension. Intern Med 33:363, 1994.
130. Clabby ML, Canter CE, Moller JH, Bridges ND: Hemodynamic data and survival in children with pulmonary hypertension. J Am Coll Cardiol 30:554, 1997.
131. Hopkins WE, Ochoa LL, Richardson GW, Trulock EP: Comparison of the hemodynamics and survival of adults with severe primary pulmonary hypertension or Eisenmenger syndrome. J Heart Lung Transplant 15:100, 1996.
132. Vongpatanasin W, Brickner ME, Hillis LD, Lange RA: The Eisenmenger syndrome in adults. Ann Intern Med 128:745, 1998.
133. McLaughlin VV, Genthner DE, Panella MM, et al: Compassionate use of continuous prostacyclin in the management of secondary pulmonary hypertension: A case series. Ann Intern Med 130:740, 1999.
134. Rosenzweig EB, Kerstein D, Barst RJ: Long-term prostacyclin for pulmonary hypertension with associated congenital heart defects. Circulation 99:1858, 1999.
135. Palevsky HI, Gurughagavatula I: Pulmonary hypertension in collagen vascular disease. Compr Ther 25:133, 1999.
136. Badesch DB, Tapson VF, McGoon MD, et al: Continuous intravenous epoprostenol for pulmonary hypertension due to the scleroderma spectrum of disease: A randomized controlled trial. Ann Intern Med 132:425, 2000.
137. Lange PA, Stoller JK: The hepatopulmonary syndrome. Ann Intern Med 122:521, 1995.
138. Kuo PC, Plotkin JS, Johnson LB, et al: Distinctive clinical features of portopulmonary hypertension. Chest 112:980, 1997.
139. Herve P, Lebrec D, Brenot F, et al: Pulmonary vascular disorders in portal hypertension. Eur Respir J 11:1153, 1998.
140. Kuo P: Pulmonary hypertension: Considerations in the liver transplant candidate. Transpl Int 9:141, 1996.
141. Schott R, Chaouat A, Launoy A, et al: Improvement of pulmonary hypertension after liver transplantation. Chest 115:1748, 1999.
142. Humbert M, Monti G, Fartoukh M, et al: Platelet-derived growth factor expression in primary pulmonary hypertension: Comparison of HIV seropositive and HIV seronegative patients. Eur Respir J 11:554, 1998.
143. Opravil M, Pechere M, Speich R, et al: HIV-associated primary pulmonary hypertension. A case control study. Swiss HIV Cohort Study. Am J Respir Crit Care Med 155:990, 1997.
144. Simonneau G, Fartoukh M, Sitbon O, et al: Primary pulmonary hypertension associated with the use of fenfluramine derivatives. Chest 114(Suppl):195, 1998 .
145. Rich S, Rubin L, Walker AM, et al: Anorexigens and pulmonary hypertension in the United States: Results from the surveillance of North American pulmonary hypertension. Chest 117:870, 2000.
146. Weir EK, Reeve HL, Huang JM, et al: Anorexic agents aminorex, fenfluramine, and dexfenfluramine inhibit potassium current in rat pulmonary vascular smooth muscle and cause pulmonary vasoconstriction. Circulation 94:2216, 1996.
147. Archer SL, Djaballah K, Humbert M, et al: Nitric oxide deficiency in fenfluramine- and dexfenfluramine-induced pulmonary hypertension. Am J Respir Crit Care Med 158:1061, 1998.
148. Rich S, Shillington A, McLaughlin V: Comparison of survival in patients with pulmonary hypertension associated with fenfluramine to patients with primary pulmonary hypertension. Am J Cardiol 92:1366, 2003.
149. Hulsmann AR, van den Anker JN: Evolution and natural history of chronic lung disease of prematurity. Monaldi Arch Chest Dis 52:272, 1997.
150. Langer JC: Congenital diaphragmatic hernia. Chest Surg Clin North Am 8:295, 1998.
151. Roberts JD Jr, Fineman JR, Morin FC III, et al: Inhaled nitric oxide and persistent pulmonary hypertension of the newborn. N Engl J Med 336:605, 1997.
152. Steinhorn RH, Cox PN, Fineman JR, et al: Inhaled nitric oxide enhances oxygenation but not survival in infants with alveolar capillary dysplasia. J Pediatr 130:417, 1997.
153. Valdes L, Gonzalez-Juanatey JR, Alvarez D, et al: Diagnosis of pulmonary veno-occlusive disease: New criteria for biopsy. Respir Med 92:979, 1998.
154. Masur Y, Remberger K, Hoefer M: Pulmonary capillary hemangiomatosis as a rare cause of pulmonary hypertension. Pathol Res Pract 192:290, discussion 296, 1996.
155. Lippert JL, White CS, Cameron EW, et al: Pulmonary capillary hemangiomatosis: Radiographic appearance. J Thorac Imaging 13:49, 1998.
156. Dufour B, Maitre S, Humbert M, et al: High-resolution CT of the chest in four patients with pulmonary capillary hemangiomatosis or pulmonary venoocclusive disease. AJR Am J Roentgenol 171:1321, 1998.
157. Humbert M, Maitre S, Capron F, et al: Pulmonary edema complicating continuous intravenous prostacyclin in pulmonary capillary hemangiomatosis. Am J Respir Crit Care Med 157:1681, 1998.

Pulmonary Hypertension Associated with Disorders of the Respiratory System

158. American Thoracic Society: Standards for the diagnosis and care of patients with chronic obstructive disease [official statement]. Am J Respir Crit Care Med 152:S77, 1995.
159. Siafakas NM, Vermeire P, Pride NB, et al: Optimal assessment and management of chronic obstructive pulmonary disease (COPD). European Respiratory Society Task Force. Eur Respir J 8:1398, 1995.
160. British Thoracic Society Group of the Standards of Care Committee: BTS guidelines for the management of chronic obstructive pulmonary disease. COPD Guidelines Group of the Standards of Care Committee of the BTS. Thorax 52:S1, 1997.
161. Pauwels RA, Buist AS, Calverley PM, et al: Global strategy for the diagnosis, management, and prevention of chronic obstructive pulmonary disease. NHLBI/WHO Global Initiative for Chronic Obstructive Lung Disease (GOLD) Workshop summary. Am J Respir Crit Care 163:1256, 2001.
162. Sherrill DL, Lebowitz MD, Burrows B: Epidemiology of chronic obstructive pulmonary disease. Clin Chest Med 11:375, 1990.
163. Barnes PJ: Mechanisms in COPD: Differences from asthma. Chest 117:10S, 2000.
164. Saetta M, Di Stefano A, Turato G, et al: CD8+ T-lymphocytes in peripheral airways of smokers with chronic obstructive pulmonary disease. Am J Respir Crit Care Med 157:822, 1998.
165. Saetta M, Di Stefano A, Maestrelli P, et al: Airway eosinophilia in chronic bronchitis during exacerbations. Am J Respir Crit Care Med 150:1646, 1994.
166. Keatings VM, Collins PD, Scott DM, et al: Differences in interleukin-8 and tumor necrosis factor-alpha in induced sputum from patients with chronic obstructive pulmonary disease or asthma. Am J Respir Crit Care Med 153:530, 1996.
167. Stockley RA: Neutrophils and protease/antiprotease imbalance. Am J Respir Crit Care Med 160:S49, 1999.
168. Shapiro SD, Senior RM: Matrix metalloproteinases: Matrix degradation and more. Am J Respir Cell Mol Biol 20:1100, 1999.
169. Repine JE, Bast A, Lankhorst I: Oxidative stress in chronic obstructive pulmonary disease. Oxidative Stress Study Group. Am J Respir Crit Care Med 156:341, 1997.
170. Di Francia M, Barbier D, Mege JL, et al: Tumor necrosis factor-alpha levels and weight loss in chronic obstructive pulmonary disease. Am J Respir Crit Care Med 150:1453, 1994.
171. Schols AM, Buurman WA, Staal van den Brekel AJ, et al: Evidence for a relation between metabolic derangements and increased levels of inflammatory mediators in a subgroup of patients with chronic obstructive pulmonary disease. Thorax 51:819, 1996.
172. Schols AM, Creutzberg EC, Buurman WA, et al: Plasma leptin is related to proinflammatory status and dietary intake in patients with chronic obstructive pulmonary disease. Am J Respir Crit Care Med 160:1220, 1999.
173. Sin DD, Man SF: Why are patients with chronic obstructive pulmonary disease at increased risk of cardiovascular diseases? The potential role of systemic inflammation in chronic obstructive pulmonary disease. Circulation 107:1514, 2003.

174. Arcasoy SM, Christie JD, Ferrari VA, et al: Echocardiographic assessment of pulmonary hypertension in patients with advanced lung disease. Am J Respir Crit Care Med 167:735, 2003.
175. Scharf SM, Iqbal M, Keller C, et al: Hemodynamic characterization of patients with severe emphysema. Am J Respir Crit Care Med 166:314, 2002.
176. Stevens D, Sharma K, Rich S, et al: Severe pulmonary hypertension associated with COPD. [abstract]. Am J Respir Crit Care Med 159:A155, 1999.
177. Weitzenblum E, Hirth C, Ducolone A, et al: Prognostic value of pulmonary artery pressure in chronic obstructive pulmonary disease. Thorax 36:752, 1981.
178. Piccioni P, Caria E, Bignamini E, et al: Predictors of survival in a group of patients with chronic airflow obstruction. J Clin Epidemiol 51:547, 1998.
179. Dallari R, Barozzi G, Pinelli GP, et al: Predictors of survival in subjects with chronic obstructive pulmonary disease treated with long-term oxygen therapy. Respiration 61:8, 1994.
180. Braghiroli A, Zaccaria S, Ioli F, et al: Pulmonary failure as a cause of death in COPD. Monaldi Arch Chest Dis 52:170, 1997.
181. Filipecki S, Kober J, Kaminski D, Tomowsi W: Pulmonary thromboembolism. Monaldi Arch Chest Dis 52:492, 1997.
182. Anthonisen N, Connett J, Kiley J, et al: Effects of smoking intervention and the use of an inhaled anticholinergic bronchodilator on the rate of decline of FEV_1: The Lung Health Study. JAMA 272:1497, 1994.
183. Lancaster T, Stead L, Silagy C, Sowden A: Effectiveness of interventions to help people stop smoking: Findings from the Cochrane Library. BMJ 321:355, 2000.
184. Jorenby DE, Leischow SJ, Nides MA, et al: A controlled trial of sustained-release bupropion, a nicotine patch, or both for smoking cessation. N Engl J Med 340:685, 1999.
185. Griffiths TL, Burr ML, Campbell IA, et al: Results at 1 year of outpatient multidisciplinary pulmonary rehabilitation: A randomised controlled trial. Lancet 355:362, 2000.
186. The COMBIVENT Inhalation Solution Study Group: Routine nebulized ipratropium and albuterol together are better than either alone in COPD. Chest 112:1514, 1997.
187. Gross N, Tashkin D, Miller R, et al: Inhalation by nebulization of albuterol-ipratropium combination (Dey combination) is superior to either agent alone in the treatment of chronic obstructive pulmonary disease. Dey Combination Solution Study Group. Respiration 65:354, 1998.
188. The Lung Health Study Research Group: Effect of inhaled triamcinolone on the decline in pulmonary function in chronic obstructive pulmonary disease. N Engl J Med 343:1902, 2000.
189. Nocturnal Oxygen Therapy Trial Group: Continuous or nocturnals oxygen therapy in hypoxemic chronic obstructive lung disease. Ann Intern Med 93:931, 1980.
190. Ashutosh K, Mead G, Dunsky M: Early effects of oxygen administration and prognosis in chronic obstructive pulmonary disease and cor pulmonale. Am Rev Respir Dis 127:399, 1983.
191. Dewan NA, Bell CW: Effect of low flow and high flow oxygen delivery on exercise tolerance and sensation of dyspnea: A study comparing the transtracheal catheter and nasal prongs. Chest 105:1061, 1994.
192. Meduri GU, Abou-Shala N, Fox RC, et al: Noninvasive face mask mechanical ventilation in patients with acute hypercapnic respiratory failure. Chest 100:445, 1991.
193. Soguel Schenkel N, Burdet L, de Muralt B, et al: Oxygen saturation during daily activities in chronic obstructive pulmonary disease. Eur Respir J 9:2584, 1996.
194. Antonelli M, Conti G, Rocco M, et al: A comparison of noninvasive positive-pressure ventilation and conventional mechanical ventilation in patients with acute respiratory failure. N Engl J Med 339:429, 1998.
195. Meecham Jones DJ, Paul EA, Jones PW, et al: Nasal pressure support ventilation plus oxygen compared with oxygen therapy alone in hypercapnic COPD. Am J Respir Crit Care Med 152:538, 1995.
196. National Emphysema Treatment Trial Research Group: A randomized trial comparing lung-volume-reduction surgery with medical therapy for severe emphysema. N Engl J Med 348:2059, 2003.
197. National Emphysema Treatment Trial Research Group: Patients at high risk of death after lung-volume-reduction surgery. N Engl J Med 345:1075, 2001.
198. Trulock EP, Edwards LB, Taylor DO, et al: The registry of the International Society for Heart and Lung Transplantation: Twentieth official adult lung and heart-lung transplant report-2003. J Heart Lung Transplant 22:625, 2003.
199. Lynch JP, Trulock EP: Lung transplantation in chronic airflow limitation. Med Clin North Am 80:657, 1996.
200. Low DE, Trulock EP, Kaiser LR, et al: Morbidity, mortality, and early results of single versus bilateral lung transplantation for emphysema. J Thorac Cardiovasc Surg 103:1119, 1992.
201. Katzenstein AL, Myers JL: Idiopathic pulmonary fibrosis: Clinical relevance of pathologic classification. Am J Respir Crit Care Med 157:1301, 1998.
202. Ryu JH, Colby TV, Hartman TE: Idiopathic pulmonary fibrosis: Current concepts. Mayo Clin Proc 73:1085, 1998.
203. Idiopathic pulmonary fibrosis: Diagnosis and treatment: International consensus statement. Am J Respir Crit Care Med 161:646, 2000.
204. Coffey MJ, FitzGerald MX, McNicholas WT: Comparison of oxygen desaturation during sleep and exercise in patients with cystic fibrosis. Chest 100:659, 1991.
205. Fraser KL, Tullis DE, Sasson Z, et al: Pulmonary hypertension and cardiac function in adult cystic fibrosis: Role of hypoxemia. Chest 115:1321, 1999.
206. Marrone O, Bonsignore MR: Pulmonary hemodynamics in obstructive sleep apnea. Sleep Med Rev 6:175, 2002.
207. Sajkov D, Wang T, Saunders NA, et al: Continuous positive airway pressure treatment improves pulmonary hemodynamics in patients with obstructive sleep apnea. Am J Resp Crit Care Med 165:152, 2002.
208. Leger P: Long-term noninvasive ventilation for patients with thoracic cage abnormalities. Respir Care Clin North Am 2:241, 1996.
209. Simonda A: Nasal intermittent positive pressure ventilation in neuromuscular and chest wall disease. Monaldi Arch Chest Dis 48:156, 1993.
210. Robert D, Gerard M, Leger P, et al: Domiciliary ventilation by tracheostomy for chronic respiratory failure. Rev Fr Mal Respir 11:923, 1983.
211. Faul JL, Ruoss S, Doyle RL, Kao PN: Diaphragmatic paralysis due to Lyme disease. Eur Respir J 13:700, 1999.
212. De Vito EL, Quadrelli SA, Montiel GC, Roncoroni AJ: Bilateral diaphragmatic paralysis after mediastinal radiotherapy. Respiration 63:187, 1996.
213. Gierada D, Slone R, Fleishman M: Imaging evaluation of the diaphragm. Chest Surg Clin North Am 8:237, 1998.
214. Lin MC, Liaw MY, Huang CC, et al: Bilateral diaphragmatic paralysis: A rare cause of acute respiratory failure managed with nasal mask bilevel positive airway pressure (BiPAP) ventilation. Eur Respir J 10:1922, 1997.

Pulmonary Hypertension due to Chronic Thrombotic or Embolic Obstruction of the Pulmonary Arteries

215. Wolf M, Boyer-Neumann C, Parent F, et al: Thrombotic risk factors in pulmonary hypertension. Eur Respir J 15:395, 2000.
216. Moser KM, Auger WR, Fedullo PF, Jamieson SW: Chronic thromboembolic pulmonary hypertension: Clinical picture and surgical treatment. Eur Respir J 5:334, 1992.
217. Auger WR, Moser KM: Pulmonary flow murmurs: A distinctive physical sign found in chronic pulmonary thromboembolic disease. Clin Res 37:145A, 1989.
218. Ryan KL, Fedullo PF, Davis GB, et al: Perfusion scan findings understate the severity of angiographic and hemodynamic compromise in chronic thromboembolic pulmonary hypertension. Chest 93:1180, 1988.
219. Auger WR, Fedullo PF, Moser KM, et al: Chronic major-vessel thromboembolic pulmonary artery obstruction: Appearance at angiography. Radiology 182:393, 1992.
220. Pitton MB, Duber C, Mayer E, Thelen M: Hemodynamic effects of nonionic contrast bolus injection and oxygen inhalation during pulmonary angiography in patients with chronic major-vessel thromboembolic pulmonary hypertension. Circulation 94:2485, 1996.
221. King M, Ysrael M, Bergin C: Chronic thromboembolic pulmonary hypertension: CT findings. AJR Am J Roentgenol 170:955, 1998.
222. Daily PO, Dembitsky WP, Iversen S, et al: Risk factors for pulmonary thromboendarterectomy. J Thorac Cardiovasc Surg 99:670, 1990.
223. Jamieson SW, Kapelanski DP: Pulmonary endarterectomy. Curr Probl Surg 37:165, 2000.
224. Thistlethwaite PA, Mo M, Madani MM, et al: Operative classification of thromboembolic disease determines outcome after pulmonary endarterectomy. J Thorac Cardiovasc Surg 124:1203, 2002.
225. Thistlethwaite PA, Mo M, Madani MM, et al: Operative classification of thromboembolic disease determines outcome after pulmonary endarterectomy. J Thorac Cardiovasc Surg 124:1203, 2002.
226. Mayer E, Dahm M, Hake U, et al: Mid-term results of pulmonary thromboendarterectomy for chronic thromboembolic pulmonary hypertension. Ann Thorac Surg 61:1788, 1996.
227. Ono F, Nagaya N, Okumura H, et al: Effect of orally active prostacyclin analogue on survival in patients with chronic thromboembolic pulmonary hypertension without major vessel obstruction. Chest 123:1583, 2003.
228. Ghofrani HA, Schermuly RT, Rose F, et al: Sildenafil for long-term treatment of nonoperable chronic thromboembolic pulmonary hypertension. Am J Respir Crit Care Med 167:1139, 2003.
229. Norris SL, Johnson C, Haywood LJ: Left ventricular filling pressure in sickle cell anemia. J Assoc Acad Minor Phys 3:20, 1992.

Pulmonary Hypertension due to Disorders Directly Affecting the Pulmonary Vasculature

230. Yung GL, Channick RN, Fedullo PF, et al: Successful pulmonary thromboendarterectomy in two patients with sickle cell disease. Am J Respir Crit Care Med 157:1690, 1998.
231. Morris W, Knauer CM: Cardiopulmonary manifestations of schistosomiasis. Semin Respir Infect 12:159, 1997.
232. Barbosa MM, Lamounier JA, Oliveira EC, et al: Pulmonary hypertension in schistosomiasis mansoni. Trans R Soc Trop Med Hyg 90:663, 1996.
233. Sheffield EA: Pathology of sarcoidosis. Clin Chest Med 18:741, 1997.
234. Nagai S, Shigematsu M, Hamada K, Izumi T: Clinical courses and prognoses of pulmonary sarcoidosis. Curr Opin Pulm Med 5:293, 1999.
235. Lynch JP 3rd, Kazerooni EA, Gay SE: Pulmonary sarcoidosis. Clin Chest Med 18:755, 1997.
236. Mana J, Badrinas F: Prognosis of sarcoidosis: An unresolved issue. Sarcoidosis 9:15, 1992.

CHAPTER 68

Sleep Disorders and Cardiovascular Disease

Meir H. Kryger

There is a complex interaction between the cardiovascular system and sleep. Sleep disorders, such as sleep apnea, can cause abnormal cardiovascular function and disease; cardiovascular disease, for example, congestive heart failure (see Chap. 21), can cause a sleep disorder. In addition, some cardiovascular disorders seem to be linked to a specific sleep state or time of day, such as coronary vasoconstriction (see Chap. 17) occurring during rapid eye movement sleep, and sudden death (see Chap. 33) occurring in the early morning hours during awakening. In this chapter, the most common sleep problems likely to be encountered by a cardiologist in clinical practice are reviewed, including obstructive sleep apnea syndrome and Cheyne-Stokes respiration. Cardiac physiology and pathophysiology during sleep and less common cardiovascular problems that are impacted by sleep and its disorders are reviewed elsewhere.[1]

Sleep Physiology

Using neurophysiological monitoring, sleep is divided into two types: (1) rapid eye movement (REM) sleep, which makes up about one-fourth of the night in young adults and (2) non-rapid eye movement (NREM) sleep, which makes up the remaining three-fourths.[2] During REM sleep, which is the time of the most intense dreaming, monitoring reveals that people are not moving and there are at times marked increases in activity in certain parts of the brain and brain stem. When the increased activity is in the region of the oculomotor nuclei, then the REMs occur. Because there are more abnormal cardiovascular events in REM than NREM sleep, it is possible that when the increased activity passes through the parts of the nervous system that control the cardiovascular system, instability in cardiovascular function might occur. NREM sleep is subdivided, again based on neurophysiological criteria, into stage 1 sleep, a transition between wakefulness and deeper sleep, which makes up in normal subjects roughly 5 percent of the night; stage 2 sleep, determined by the presence of characteristic waves (spindles and K complexes), which makes up half of the night; and stages 3 and 4, that together are often called *slow-wave sleep*, or *delta sleep*, which make up roughly a quarter of the night. During NREM sleep, most physiological functions appear to be normally controlled except for a dip in blood pressure that can occur with a transition from wakefulness to sleep. Thereafter, blood pressure and heart rate and rhythm do not vary a great deal unless an arousal (a brief awakening) occurs.

In contrast to the tight regulation in NREM sleep, during REM sleep, control of many physiological control systems, for example cardiovascular regulation and thermoregulation, may be more erratic (e.g., variability in heart rate and blood pressure), or virtually absent (e.g., thermoregulation). Superimposed on the change in physiology directly related to the sleep state are time-related changes in physiological systems, whether the person is awake or asleep. These are the circadian influences. For example, there appear to be circadian influences on myocardial ischemic threshold that are present even during the awake state (see Chap. 44). This circadian effect may explain the increased propensity to develop adverse cardiovascular events at certain times of the day. For example, even though one would expect the reduction in demands on the cardiovascular system during sleep to markedly reduce cardiovascular events, 20 percent of myocardial infarctions (see Chap. 46), 15 percent of sudden deaths (see Chap. 33), and 29 percent of episodes of atrial fibrillation (see Chap. 32) occur between midnight and 6:00 AM. Over the 24-hour period new onset of myocardial infarction, sudden cardiac death, and thrombotic stroke are most likely to occur between early and mid-morning.[3] Thus, abnormal cardiovascular physiology can be impacted by sleep state, circadian rhythm, and sleep pathology.

Types of Sleep Apnea

Sleep apnea refers to the cessation of breathing during sleep. In one type of apnea, *obstructive apnea*, the cessation is caused by obstruction in the upper airway. In *central apnea*, the cessation of breathing is caused by a reduction of impulses from the central nervous system to the muscles of respiration. Some patients have features of both. Cardiologists are likely to encounter many patients with sleep apnea in their practice. Obstructive sleep apnea is a common condition that causes cardiovascular morbidity. Cheyne-Stokes respiration, a form of central sleep apnea, is found in about 40 percent of cases of heart failure.

Obstructive Sleep Apnea Syndrome

Obstructive sleep apnea syndrome is characterized by repetitive upper airway obstruction during sleep, resulting in profound effects on cardiovascular function, gas exchange, and continuity of sleep. These in turn result in important clinical consequences that affect several organ systems (especially the cardiovascular system) and create a poor quality of life.

Epidemiology and Risk Factors

Obstructive sleep apnea occurs in all age groups and both genders.[4,5] Although it was previously believed that sleep apnea was rare in women, it is now thought to be much more common in that group. It has been estimated that 4 percent of adult men and 2 percent of adult women have obstructive sleep apnea syndrome. It has been estimated that 1 to 3 percent of children have sleep apnea, with the most common etiology being adenotonsillar hypertrophy. The mean age of presentation in adults in most series is between 48 and 51 years. Any disorder that can compromise the upper airway, including obesity, retrognathia (mandible too far posterior), micrognathia (small mandible), mass lesions in the airway, or nasal obstruction, can lead to obstructive sleep apnea syndrome. About 70 to 80 percent of adults with obstructive sleep apnea syndrome have obesity as the main cause of their problem.

Physiological Changes during Sleep in Obstructive Sleep Apnea

When patients with obstructive sleep apnea stop breathing during sleep, a reduction in arterial oxygen saturation (SaO_2) occurs, along with activation of the sympathetic and parasympathetic nervous systems. The episodes of sleep apnea by definition exceed 10 seconds in duration and, in our laboratory, average about 25 seconds in NREM sleep and about 35 seconds in REM sleep. On the average, patients spend 20 percent of sleep time with an SaO_2 of less than 90 percent.

CARDIAC RHYTHM. The changes in autonomic nervous system activity result in a slowing of the heart rate during the episodes of apnea and a speeding up of the heart rate once breathing resumes. Cardiac arrhythmias (see Chap. 32) are much more common in those patients who have more severe sleep apnea as measured by the apnea/hypopnea index, which is the number of abnormal breathing events per hour of sleep. The most common arrhythmias seen are bradyarrhythmias and ventricular extrasystoles.[6,7] In one series, almost 80 percent of cases had some rhythm abnormality, and 18 percent had a clinically significant abnormal rhythm including recurrent sinus pauses, asystolic periods lasting 6 seconds or longer, or ventricular extrasystoles.[7] The ventricular arrhythmias are not usually related to bradycardia and may be most frequent during the most severe hypoxemia. The bradyarrhythmias are likely related to increased vagal tone since they have been reported to be reversed by atropine and are more common during REM sleep.[6] Patients with the rhythms just mentioned, in whom the diagnosis of sleep apnea–induced bradyarrhythmia is not apparent, may end up having unnecessary cardiac pacemakers inserted and are best treated with continuous positive airway pressure (CPAP).[8] In cardiac disease patients who are at high risk for arrhythmias and have a low left ventricular ejection fraction (LVEF) (see later), coexistent sleep apnea increases the risk of ventricular arrhythmias.[9]

BLOOD PRESSURE. Systemic blood pressure increases during the apneic episodes, although in elderly patients the blood pressure may fall.[10] Pulmonary artery pressure can also increase in the presence of severe hypoxemia and some patients can develop cor pulmonale (see Chap. 67).[11-13]

VENTILATION. In the most severe cases, the abnormalities in ventilation during sleep can partially persist into the wakefulness period and patients can develop awake-hypoventilation documented by an elevated $P{CO_2}$. The combination of awake-respiratory failure, cor pulmonale, and obesity is the hallmark of the obesity-hypoventilation syndrome previously called *Pickwickian syndrome* (see Chap. 67).[13] Obesity does not have to be present for hypoventilation to occur in people with upper airway obstruction; hypoventilation causing right-sided cardiac failure has been described, for example, in children with enlarged tonsils. Some patients with obesity-hypoventilation syndrome do not actually develop apnea during sleep but instead have continuous hypoventilation with severe hypoxemia during wakefulness and sleep.[13]

AROUSALS. To resume unobstructed breathing, patients have a neurological arousal (a brief awakening), which results in an increase in the tone of the upper airway dilating muscles; this has the effect of opening the obstructed or occluded airway. These arousals result in markedly abnormal sleep structure; in particular, most patients have a decrease or absence of slow wave sleep and a reduction in REM sleep, which lead to the most common symptom—excessive daytime sleepiness.

Daytime Clinical Consequences of Sleep Apnea

Sleep apnea has its major clinical effects on the neurological and cardiovascular systems. The abnormal sleep causes severe daytime sleepiness and, in some patients, impaired daytime cognitive function. The latter may be responsible for an increased automobile accident rate.[14-16] Sleep apnea is associated with systemic hypertension (see Chap. 37), pulmonary hypertension (see Chap. 67), ischemic heart disease (see Chap. 46), and heart failure and stroke.[17-20] There is now no doubt that sleep apnea is a risk factor for systemic hypertension independent of age, gender, and body mass index.[20,21] Patients with sleep apnea are two or three times more likely than control groups to have arterial hypertension and are two or three times more likely to be treated with antihypertensive medications.[19,22] Patients with "idiopathic" hypertension are highly likely to include a substantial proportion of patients with obstructive sleep apnea, and this is particularly true in patients whose hypertension is resistant to therapy or difficult to control.[23] *Therefore, the clinical cardiologist should consider sleep apnea in the evaluation of hypertensive patients.*

Clinical Features

The most common presenting symptoms found in patients with obstructive sleep apnea include excessive daytime sleepiness, snoring, and the observation by others that the patient stops breathing during sleep. In most patients the snoring and observed apneas are present most nights. Other common symptoms in these patients include awakening with headache, sensation of choking, poor memory and concentration, and poor performance at work. There is frequently an associated history of arterial hypertension, and a previous history of depression and hypothyroidism are common, especially in women.[24]

Diagnosis

Patients with suspected obstructive sleep apnea syndrome should receive an overnight sleep study that has sufficient channels to be able to confirm the presence and type (central versus obstructive) of apnea, oxygenation, and sleep structure (Fig. 68–1). The latter measurement is particularly important because some patients, particularly women, can have a mild variant of obstructive sleep apnea called *upper airway resistance syndrome* in which the obstructions to inspiration are not sufficiently severe or long to be classed as an apnea (by definition 10 seconds), but would be sufficiently severe to disrupt sleep quality and result in many of the earlier mentioned pathophysiology and symptoms.

As part of the sleep evaluation, if a sleep breathing disorder is confirmed, the patient will also be studied using a ventilatory assist device, either CPAP or bilevel positive airway pressure (BiPAP) to determine the optimal settings for the equipment. These devices can stent the airway open and thus prevent the episodes of obstruction.

Indications for Treatment

It is recommended that all patients with polysomnographically proven obstructive sleep apnea with an apnea/hypopnea index exceeding 20 be treated, since that level of apnea has been associated with an increased death rate without treatment. Because hypertension has been associated with an apnea/hypopnea index higher than 15, some have recommended that patients be treated if the apnea/hypopnea index exceeds this level. Many authorities also recommend treating patients who have a proven apnea/hypopnea index higher than 5, if in addition they have known complications attributable to sleep apnea, including excessive daytime sleepiness and cardiovascular disease (Table 68–1). U.S. government guidelines for reimbursement for CPAP by Medicare and Medicaid Services in the United States have recently changed to reflect this latter indication.[25]

THERAPY. The principles of treatment of obstructive sleep apnea are first to reduce the risk factors, and then if a specific anatomic cause of the apnea is found, to treat that abnormality if possible and, if no abnormality is found, to use a ventilatory assistance device to reverse the obstruction (Fig. 68–2).

General Measures. Since 70 to 80 percent of obstructive sleep apnea patients are obese, weight loss is a critical component of any treatment plan for the obese patient. Because many of the patients also have hypertension and diabetes (see Chap. 40), this approach should help those conditions as well. Patients do not have to achieve their ideal weight for the apnea to resolve most of the time. It seems as though for many patients there is a threshold, and once the threshold is reached, the apnea improves dramatically even though they may continue to still snore and to be overweight.

Avoidance of Alcohol and Sedatives. Because alcohol can make a patient much more sleepy and dramatically worsen the episodes of apnea, patients should be encouraged to avoid drinking alcohol. The same advice can be given about the use of hypnotic or sedative drugs.

Specific Anatomical Treatment. If nasal obstruction or anatomical obstruction of the pharyngeal airway caused by lesions such as enlarged tonsils are present, the patient should be referred to a specialist to assess them to see whether they are candidates for surgical treatment. If the patient has significant retrognathia or micrognathia, the patient may benefit from the use of an oral appliance worn at night, which brings the lower jaw upward and forward. Sometimes the patient can benefit from reconstructive surgery of the mandible.

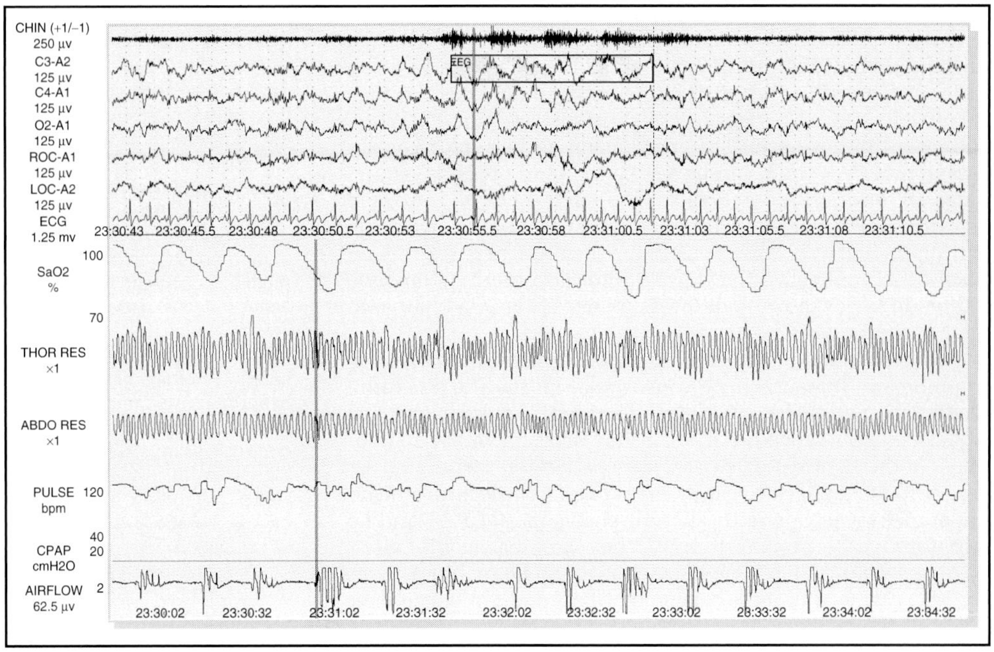

FIGURE 68–1 This is a fragment of an overnight sleep study from a patient with severe obstructive sleep apnea syndrome. The top seven channels represent about 30 seconds of data and show the information used to stage sleep and the electrocardiogram (ECG). The top channel is the chin electromyogram; the next three are used for the electroencephalogram (EEG), the next two for eye movements, followed by the ECG. The bottom six channels represent about 5 minutes of data and show the information used to document apnea type. The channels from top to bottom are oxyhemoglobin saturation (Sao_2), thoracic movement (THOR RES), abdominal movement (ABDO RES), pulse rate (bpm), continuous positive airway pressure (CPAP), and nasal airflow. There are 14 apneic episodes in this segment. The episodes are associated with efforts to breathe seen in the chest wall and abdomen, but notice the intermittent cessation of airflow in the bottom channel. The vertical blue line in each segment corresponds to an identical moment in time. Notice that resumption of breathing occurs right after an arousal on EEG (the yellow box). Also note the marked variability in pulse rate.

TABLE 68–1 Indications for CPAP Treatment

Treatment is indicated if either of the following criteria* is met:

AHI ≥ 15 events per hr

or

AHI ≥ 5 and ≤14 events per hr with documented symptoms of excessive daytime sleepiness, impaired cognition, mood disorders or insomnia, or documented hypertension, ischemic heart disease, or history of stroke

AHI = apnea/hypopnea index; CPAP = continuous positive airway pressure.

*If these criteria are met, CPAP therapy will be covered under Medicare in adult patients with obstructive sleep apnea. See http://cms.hhs.gov/mcd/index_list.asp?list_type=ncd for complete description at medicare coverage in the List of National Coverage Determinations.

Ventilatory Assist Devices. CPAP and BiPAP are the most widely used treatments and the treatment of first choice in patients with obstructive sleep apnea syndrome. The principle of these devices is that the positive pressure splints the pharyngeal airway open, counteracting its tendency to collapse during inspiration. The treatment is usually highly effective, although compliance appears to be between 50 and 70 percent, which is probably comparable to that of many other medical treatments. Treatment with nasal CPAP has been shown to improve quality of life, cognitive function, and arterial hypertension.[26-29]

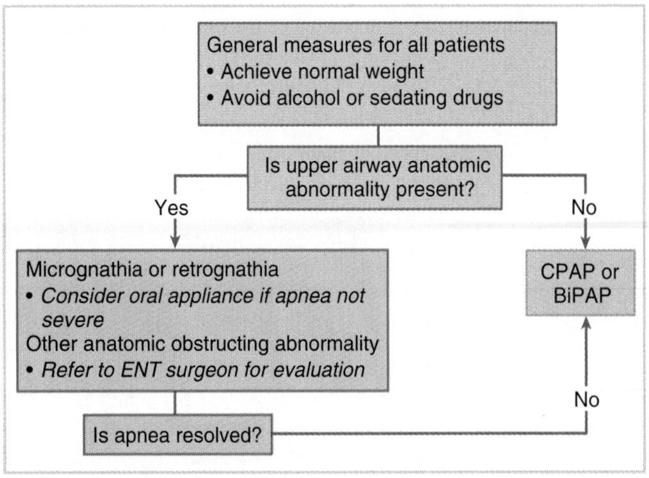

FIGURE 68–2 Approach to treatment of typical obstructive sleep apnea syndrome. ENT = ear, nose, throat; CPAP = continuous positive airway pressure; BiPAP = bilevel positive airway pressure.

Additional Issues of Particular Interest to Cardiologists. Arrhythmias and arterial hypertension were mentioned earlier. Difficult-to-control hypertension can be due to sleep apnea.[30] Thus it is appropriate to ask about sleep apnea symptoms in newly diagnosed hypertensive patients. When patients who have arterial hypertension and sleep apnea are started on CPAP, there can be a drop in blood pressure, sometimes to normotensive levels. Clinicians should routinely measure blood pressure in hypertensive patients receiving antihypertensive medication when they are first started on nasal CPAP to ensure that they do not become hypotensive. If they do lower their blood pressure excessively, a change in their antihypertensive drugs may be needed.

Anesthesia and Surgery. Because sleep apnea is so common and it results in cardiovascular morbidity, it is quite likely that patients with sleep apnea will undergo cardiac catheterization procedures or cardiac surgery. In both situations, in the established sleep apnea patient on treatment, the use of opiate analgesia results in an even more compromised upper airway and patients should receive nasal CPAP and be monitored with oximetry until they are reasonably alert. Some patients not on CPAP can develop heart block after surgery, which should be treated by CPAP and not pacemaker insertion.[31]

Patients who have had coronary artery bypass grafting (see Chap. 50) or other surgical procedures involving the chest can have a great deal of pain at the incision site when continued on nasal CPAP in the postoperative period. Such patients may benefit from switching (at least temporarily) from a CPAP to a BiPAP system. With the latter modality of airway support, in which the pressure during inspiration is higher than during expiration, patients find the application of pressure less painful, in our experience.

Sleep Abnormalities in Patients with Left Ventricular Cardiac Failure (Central Sleep Apnea)

In 1818, Cheyne first described repetitive cycles of apneas followed by hyperpneas in what is now called *Cheyne-Stokes respiration*.[32] Although this form of central apnea, characterized by a waxing and waning of ventilation, occurs in other conditions, such as after some cerebrovascular accidents, renal disease, and exposure to high altitude, it is generally most often linked to left ventricular cardiac failure (see Chap. 21). Cheyne-Stokes respiration in heart failure can cause sleep-onset insomnia and paroxysmal nocturnal dyspnea and treatment of the heart failure can ameliorate the breathing pattern.[33] More recent studies have shown that although Cheyne-Stokes respiration is by far the most common abnormal breathing pattern in heart failure, a significant number of patients have obstructive sleep apnea as their primary sleep breathing problem. In this section we focus primarily on Cheyne-Stokes respiration.

EPIDEMIOLOGY. About 40 percent of all the heart failure patients with an LVEF less than 0.45 have been reported to have Cheyne-Stokes respiration, whereas 10 percent have obstructive sleep apnea.[34] Those with obstructive sleep apnea were more obese and were more likely to have a snoring history. The consequences (apnea/hypopnea index, number of arousals per hour of sleep, and degree of hypoxemia) were similar in those with central or obstructive sleep apnea. Risk factors for Cheyne-Stokes respiration in heart failure include male gender, age older than 60 years, the presence of atrial fibrillation, and hypocapnia.[35] The presence of Cheyne-Stokes respiration is an indicator of poor prognosis.[36]

PATHOPHYSIOLOGY. Many theories and models have been proposed to explain the mechanisms that start and maintain the Cheyne-Stokes respiration pattern in left ventricular failure.[37] These mechanisms include heightened ventilatory response to carbon dioxide, alkalemia, prolonged circulation time, and effect of sleep state, all of which alone or in combination can be used to explain a periodic breathing pattern. Cheyne-Stokes respiration decreases during REM sleep, the time when chemical control of breathing is the most blunted, suggesting that chemical drives are necessary to perpetuate the abnormal breathing pattern. Sleep is not a necessary condition for Cheyne-Stokes respiration since it can occur during wakefulness.

The breathing pattern in Cheyne-Stokes respiration can be almost monotonously repetitive over long periods of time. Cheyne-Stokes respiration is present in the average patient with left-sided heart failure about half the night and might even be present while the patient is awake. Some trigger starts and another stops this breathing pattern. What seems to trigger Cheyne-Stokes respiration is an event that initially destabilizes breathing, perhaps a sigh, a deep breath, or an arousal. One can hypothesize that in response to the event, a temporary hyperventilation results in hypocapnia, which is sensed by the chemical ventilatory control system, which results in a reduction in output to the respiratory muscles, which then results in hypoventilation or apnea. Once Cheyne-Stokes respiration starts, it is perpetuated by the chemical ventilatory control systems that lead to repetitive overshooting and undershooting of ventilation.

The cycle time of the Cheyne-Stokes breathing pattern seems related to the circulation time. It has been predicted in models and shown in experiments that cycle time (the time between peaks of hyperpnea) is roughly four times the circulation time and therefore people with severe heart failure and a long circulation time will have a long cycle time. Thus, it is as though the breathing pattern goes on "autopilot." The breathing pattern normalizes when the main perpetuating factor, the ventilatory control of breathing, becomes blunted, as occurs during REM sleep.

One would expect that all patients with very low LVEF would have Cheyne-Stokes respiration, but this is not the case. Some patients with very low LVEFs do not have Cheyne-Stokes respiration, whereas some with LVEFs higher than 0.40 might have Cheyne-Stokes respiration. Thus, it is not the ejection fraction *per se* that determines whether Cheyne-Stokes respiration will be present but rather an interaction of the pathogenic mechanisms mentioned earlier.

PHYSIOLOGICAL CONSEQUENCES OF CHEYNE-STOKES RESPIRATION

Arousals. When Cheyne-Stokes respiration occurs at sleep onset, the episodes of decreased ventilation or apnea can cause an arousal. Thus, patients with Cheyne-Stokes respiration frequently complain of insomnia and have difficulty falling asleep.

Arousals from sleep are common with Cheyne-Stokes respiration. The arousals typically occur not at the end of apnea, which is the situation in patients with obstructive sleep apnea, but instead during the peak of hyperpnea. Not all episodes of Cheyne-Stokes breathing are associated with an arousal, however. The arousals are believed to be related to the increased work of breathing during the peak of hyperpnea.

Hypoxemia. Hypoxemia commonly occurs with Cheyne-Stokes respiration, and the lowest oxygen saturation occurring in a cycle usually coincides with the peak of hyperpnea. This is quite different from the situation in obstructive sleep apnea during which the lowest oxygen saturations are found immediately before breathing resumes. The reason why oxygen saturation is lowest when the patient is breathing the most, rather than at the end of the apneic episodes, is because patients with heart failure usually have a prolonged circulation time, and once breathing resumes, it takes longer for oxygenated blood to go from the lungs to peripheral tissues.

Additional Physiological Changes. There can be a substantial oscillation in systemic blood pressure[38] in association with Cheyne-Stokes respiration. The hypoxemia, and the increased systemic blood pressure, likely place an important burden on an already compromised cardiovascular system, whereas the changes in the central nervous system can lead to cognitive impairment.

CLINICAL FEATURES. The most common symptom of patients with Cheyne-Stokes respiration, besides the symptoms of the underlying cardiovascular disease, is severe insomnia, which can be of the sleep-onset type (i.e., an inability to fall asleep) as well as the sleep maintenance type (i.e., difficulty staying asleep). The insomnia can be particularly stressing for the patient because they can, in addition, have severe sleepiness. Thus, they can have the combination of being quite sleepy yet being unable to fall or stay asleep.

When patients with Cheyne-Stokes respiration awaken during the night, sometimes at the end of a long apneic episode, they can have severe shortness of breath consistent with paroxysmal nocturnal dyspnea (see Chap. 22). Severe cough and unpleasant dreams can precede these episodes of nocturnal dyspnea.[39] Some patients are short of breath when lying flat, and the shortness of breath can be relieved somewhat on sitting up or using several pillows (orthopnea). Some patients complain of symptoms consistent with angina pectoris that might awaken them.

Some patients also have a movement disorder that can lead to the symptoms of restless legs syndrome and periodic contractions of some muscle groups during sleep. This can also contribute to the sleeplessness of some of the patients. During the daytime the patients may complain of severe daytime sleepiness and may have markedly impaired cognitive function.

CLINICAL ASSESSMENT. All patients with heart disease should be asked about symptoms of sleep disorders. These questions should include how long it takes the patients to fall asleep, how often they wake up during sleep, have they been observed to snore, have they been observed to stop breathing during sleep, and do they have symptoms of paroxysmal nocturnal dyspnea, orthopnea, or angina. We have found, in our own practice, that some patients who do not normally have nocturia can have significant nocturia on nights in which they develop an arrhythmia (e.g., sustained atrial fibrillation). Some patients have palpitations that awaken them.

MANAGEMENT OF HEART FAILURE. With improvement in heart failure, Cheyne-Stokes respiration can resolve.[33] The cornerstone of management is the treatment of the heart failure (see Chap. 23); nocturnal symptoms can be a marker that the heart failure may not be under optimal control.

If, with what is considered to be optimal heart failure control, the patient still has symptoms of disturbed sleep (sleep-onset or sleep-maintenance insomnia), the patient should have a comprehensive overnight sleep study—polysomnography.

DIAGNOSIS. Polysomnography can be extremely helpful in deciding on treatment (Fig. 68–3). The sleep study should confirm that an abnormal breathing pattern is present and should be able to distinguish the reduced respiratory efforts in Cheyne-Stokes respiration from the findings seen in obstructive apnea. About 80 percent of heart failure patients with a sleep breathing problem have the findings of Cheyne-Stokes respiration, whereas 20 percent have the obstructive type. Many such patients also have periodic movements in sleep, which may also be a factor in disrupting sleep. The sleep study should also be able to yield information about the severity of hypoxemia, whether cardiac arrhythmias are present, and the extent of sleep disruption.

Our practice is to perform a split-night study in which patients have a baseline assessment for 3 to 4 hours so the diagnosis can be documented, followed by application of treatment for the remainder of the night. If Cheyne-Stokes respiration is confirmed, we first start the patient on oxygen at roughly 2 to 3 liters/min to assess its impact on the breathing pattern. If the patient has an element of obstructive sleep apnea, we would instead assess the patient using nasal CPAP or BiPAP.

Studying a patient who is still recovering from a bout of heart failure may not help in determining optimal treatment. The sleep evaluation should occur when the patient is on optimal treatment and stable. We do not recommend screening studies in this situation. Oximetry alone or many screening systems cannot differentiate apnea type (central or obstructive) and cannot determine whether a patient is actually sleeping, and they do not store the electrocardiogram.

TREATMENT OF ABNORMAL SLEEP BREATHING PATTERN. Treatment of sleep breathing abnormalities in heart failure (Fig. 68–4) is an area of great current research interest. If the patient is found to have obstructive sleep apnea (which is present in about 10 percent of heart failure patients), then CPAP treatment as outlined earlier should be instituted.

Administration of nocturnal oxygen,[40,41] nasal CPAP or BiPAP,[42-45] or more complex ventilatory assist modes[46] have

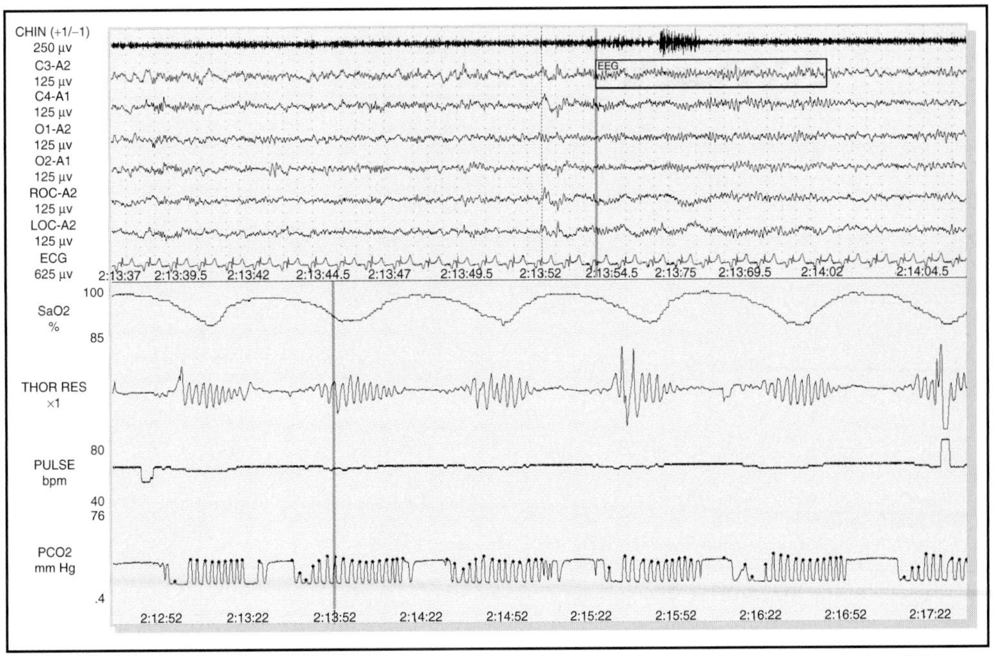

FIGURE 68–3 This is a fragment of an overnight sleep study from a patient with severe left ventricular failure who eventually had a heart transplant. The top eight channels represent about 30 seconds of data and show the information used to stage sleep and the electrocardiogram. The top channel is the chin electromyogram; the next four are used for the electroencephalogram (EEG), the next two for eye movements, followed by the electrocardiogram. The bottom four channels represent about 5 minutes of data and show the information used to document apnea type. The channels from top to bottom are oxyhemoglobin saturation, thoracic movement, pulse rate, and oronasal P_{CO_2} (see the Fig. 68–1 legend for abbreviations). There are six apneic episodes in this segment of Cheyne-Stokes respiration. Note the hyperpneas following each apnea. The apneic episodes are associated with decreased or absent efforts to breathe seen in the chest wall, and notice the intermittent cessation of airflow in the bottom channel. The vertical blue line in each segment corresponds to an identical moment in time. Notice that resumption of breathing occurs before an arousal on EEG (the yellow box), and that the nadir of Sa_{O_2} occurs during the peak of hyperpnea. Also note the lack of variability in pulse rate.

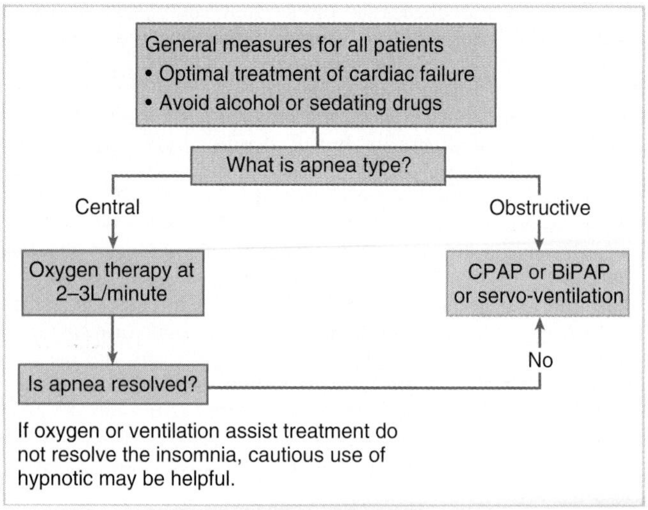
General measures for all patients
• Optimal treatment of cardiac failure
• Avoid alcohol or sedating drugs
What is apnea type?
Central
Obstructive
Oxygen therapy at 2–3L/minute
CPAP or BiPAP or servo-ventilation
No
Is apnea resolved?
If oxygen or ventilation assist treatment do not resolve the insomnia, cautious use of hypnotic may be helpful.

FIGURE 68–4 Approach to treatment of sleep disorders in left ventricular failure. CPAP = continuous positive airway pressure; BiPAP = bilevel positive airway pressure.

been suggested, and positive short-term results have been reported with them. In those patients who have obstructive sleep apnea, CPAP reduces daytime systolic blood pressure, heart rate, and the left ventricular end-systolic dimension and improves the LVEF.[42] In patients with heart failure and central apnea, CPAP and BiPAP may improve cardiac function by reducing afterload, and ongoing clinical trials will help determine the role of these treatments in the treatment of heart failure. Until long-term outcome trials are developed, the clinician must weigh the following factors in determining treatment choices: patient comfort and acceptance of treatment, response to treatment, and what is available in the local medical community.

If drug therapy with hypnotic agents is contemplated, published studies to date suggest that there is little risk of hypoventilation in patients with Cheyne-Stokes respiration who do not have an element of upper airway obstruction. Benzodiazepines such as temazepam may improve sleep in these patients. However, if the patient does have upper airway obstruction, using hypnotics may worsen the obstruction.

Acknowledgment

Dr. Kryger's work on this chapter was supported in part by NIH Grant R01 HL63342-01A1.

REFERENCES

1. Kryger M, Roth T, Dement WC: Principles and Practice of Sleep Medicine. 4th ed. Philadelphia, WB Saunders, 2004.
2. Carskadon MA, Dement WC: Normal human sleep: An overview. *In* Kryger M, Roth T, Dement WC: Principles and Practice of Sleep Medicine. 4th ed. Philadelphia, WB Saunders, 2004 (in press).
3. Verrier R: Sleep-related cardiovascular risk. *In* Kryger M, Roth T, Dement WC: Principles and Practice of Sleep Medicine. 4th ed. Philadelphia, WB Saunders, 2004 (in press).
4. Young T, Peppard PE, Gottlieb DJ: Epidemiology of obstructive sleep apnea: A population health perspective. Am J Respir Crit Care Med 165:1217-1239, 2002.
5. Kapsimalis F, Kryger MH: Gender and obstructive sleep apnea syndrome: I. Clinical features. Sleep 25:412-419, 2002.
6. Koehler U, Becker HF, Grimm W, et al: Relations among hypoxemia, sleep stage, and bradyarrhythmia during obstructive sleep apnea. Am Heart J 139:142-148, 2000.
7. Harbison J, O'Reilly P, McNicholas WT: Cardiac rhythm disturbances in the obstructive sleep apnea syndrome. Chest 118:591-595, 2000.
8. Stegman SS, Burroughs JM, Henthorn RW: Asymptomatic bradyarrhythmias as a marker of sleep apnea: Appropriate recognition and treatment may reduce the need for pacemaker therapy. Pacing Clin Electrophysiol 19:899-904, 1996.
9. Fichter J, Bauer D, Arampatzis S, et al: Sleep-related breathing disorders are associated with ventricular arrhythmias in patients with an implantable cardioverter-defibrillator. Chest 122:558-561, 2002.
10. Weiss JW, Launois SH, Anand A, Garpestad E: Cardiovascular morbidity in obstructive sleep apnea. Prog Cardiovasc Dis 41:367-376, 1999.
11. Sajkov D, Wang T, Saunders NA, et al: Continuous positive airway pressure treatment improves pulmonary hemodynamics in patients with obstructive sleep apnea. Am J Respir Crit Care Med 165:152-158, 2002.
12. Kessler R, Chaouat A, Weitzenblum E, et al: Pulmonary hypertension in the obstructive sleep apnea syndrome: Prevalence, causes, and therapeutic consequences. Eur Respir J 9:787-794, 1996.
13. Kessler R, Chaouat A, Schinkewitch P, et al: The obesity-hypoventilation syndrome revisited: A prospective study of 34 consecutive cases. Chest 120:369-376, 2001.
14. Roth T, Roehrs TA: Etiologies and sequelae of excessive daytime sleepiness. Clin Ther 18:562-576, 1996.
15. Naegele B, Pepin J-L, Levy P, et al: Cognitive executive dysfunction in patients with obstructive sleep apnea syndrome (OSAS) after CPAP treatment. Sleep 21:392-397, 1998.
16. George CF, Smiley A: Sleep apnea and automobile crashes. Sleep 22:790-795, 1999.
17. Smith R, Ronald J, Delaive K, et al: What are obstructive sleep apnea patients being treated for prior to this diagnosis? Chest 121:164-172, 2002.
18. Shamsuzzaman AB, Somers VK: Fibrinogen, stroke and obstructive sleep apnea: An evolving paradigm of cardiovascular risk. Am J Respir Crit Care Med 162:2018-2020, 2000.
19. D'Alessandro R, Magelli C, Gamberini G, et al: Snoring every night as a risk factor for myocardial infarction: A case control study. BMJ 300:1557-1558, 1990.
20. Nieto FJ, Young TB, Lind BK, et al: Association of sleep disordered breathing, sleep apnea, and hypertension in a large community-based study: Sleep Heart Health Study. JAMA 283:1829-1836, 2000.
21. Peppard PE, Young T, Palta M, Skatrud J: Prospective study of the association between sleep-disordered breathing and hypertension. N Engl J Med 342:1378-1384, 2000.
22. Otake K, Delaive K, Walld R, et al: Cardiovascular medication use in patients with undiagnosed obstructive sleep apnoea. Thorax 57:417-422, 2002.
23. Logan AG, Perlikowski SM, Mente A, et al: High prevalence of unrecognized sleep apnoea in drug-resistant hypertension. J Hypertens 19:2271-2277, 2001.
24. Shepertycki M, Kryger M: Effect of gender on clinical features of OSAS. Sleep 26:A221, 2004.
25. Web site for the List of National Coverage Determinations [NCDs] in the Indexes for the Medicare Coverage Databases. On the site, scroll down to "continuous positive airway pressure" (http://cms.hhs.gov/mcd/index_list.asp?list_type=ncd).
26. Engleman HM, Kingshott RN, Wraith PK, et al: Randomized placebo-controlled crossover trial of continuous positive airway pressure for mild sleep apnea/hypopnea syndrome. Am J Respir Crit Care Med 159:461-467, 1999.
27. Redline S, Adams N, Strauss ME, et al: Improvement of mild sleep-disordered breathing with CPAP compared with conservative therapy. Am J Respir Crit Care Med 157:858-865, 1998.
28. Faccenda JF, Mackay TW, Boon NA, Douglas NJ: Randomized placebo-controlled trial of continuous positive airway pressure on blood pressure in the sleep apnea-hypopnea syndrome. Am J Respir Crit Care Med 163:344-348, 2001.
29. White J, Cates C, Wright J: Continuous positive airways pressure for obstructive sleep apnoea. Cochrane Database Syst Rev CD001106, 2002.
30. Grote L, Hedner J, Peter JH: Sleep-related breathing disorder is an independent risk factor for uncontrolled hypertension. J Hypertens 18:679-685, 2000.
31. Block M, Jacobson LB, Rabkin RA: Heart block in patients after bariatric surgery accompanying sleep apnea. Obes Surg 11:627-630, 2001.
32. Cheyne J: A case of apoplexy in which the fleshy part of the heart was converted into fat. Dublin Hosp Rep 2:216-223, 1818.
33. Harrison TR, King CE, Calhoun JA, Harrison WG Jr: Congestive heart failure: XX. Cheyne-Stokes respiration as the cause of paroxysmal dyspnea at the onset of sleep. Arch Intern Med 53:891-910, 1934.
34. Javaheri S, Parker TJ, Liming JD, et al: Sleep apnea in 81 ambulatory male patients with stable heart failure: Types and their prevalences, consequences, and presentations. Circulation 97:2154-2159, 1998.
35. Sin DD, Fitzgerald F, Parker JD, et al: Risk factors for central and obstructive sleep apnea in 450 men and women with congestive heart failure. Am J Respir Crit Care Med 160:1101-1106, 1999.
36. Lanfranchi PA, Braghiroli A, Bosimini E, et al: Prognostic value of nocturnal Cheyne-Stokes respiration in chronic heart failure. Circulation 99:1435-1440, 1999.
37. Javaheri S: A mechanism of central sleep apnea in patients with heart failure. N Engl J Med 341:949-954, 1999.
38. Trinder J, Merson R, Rosenberg JI, et al: Pathophysiological interactions of ventilation, arousals, and blood pressure oscillations during Cheyne-Stokes respiration in patients with heart failure. Am J Respir Crit Care Med 162:808-813, 2000.
39. Harrison TR, King CE, Calhoun JA, Harrison WG Jr: Congestive heart failure: XVIII. Clinical types of nocturnal dyspnea. Arch Intern Med 53:561-573, 1934.
40. Javaheri S, Ahmed M, Parker TJ, Brown CR: Effects of nasal O_2 on sleep-related disordered breathing in ambulatory patients with stable heart failure. Sleep 22:1101-1106, 1999.
41. Franklin KA, Eriksson P, Sahlin C, Lundgren R: Reversal of central sleep apnea with oxygen. Chest 111:163-169, 1997.
42. Kaneko Y, Floras JS, Usui K, et al: Cardiovascular effects of continuous positive airway pressure in patients with heart failure and obstructive sleep apnea. N Engl J Med 348:1233-1241, 2003.
43. Kohnlein T, Welte T, Tan LB, Elliott MW: Assisted ventilation for heart failure patients with Cheyne-Stokes respiration. Eur Respir J 20:934-941, 2002.
44. Krachman SL, D'Alonzo GE, Berger TJ, Eisen HJ: Comparison of oxygen therapy with nasal continuous positive airway pressure on Cheyne-Stokes respiration during sleep in congestive heart failure. Chest 116:1550-1557, 1999.
45. Mansfield DR, Gollogly NC, Kaye DM, et al: Controlled trial of continuous airway pressure in obstructive sleep apnea and heart failure. Am J Respir Crit Care Med 169:329-331, 2004.
46. Pepperell JC, Maskell NA, Jones DR, et al: A randomized controlled trial of adaptive ventilation for Cheyne-Stokes breathing in heart failure. Am J Respir Crit Care Med 168:1109-1114, 2003.

PART VIII

Molecular Biology and Genetics

CHAPTER 69

Principles of Cardiovascular Molecular Biology and Genetics

Elizabeth G. Nabel

Molecular biology and genetics now form the solid foundation of cardiovascular science and medicine. In the past two decades, the concepts of molecular biology and genetics have permeated all aspects of medicine. The principles of these disciplines are a cornerstone of medical school curricula. Molecular genetic approaches are routinely used in physician-scientists' laboratories to test hypotheses about cardiovascular disease. Physicians have access to an array of molecular and genetic tools to guide the diagnosis and treatment of patients. Many therapeutic agents are now produced using recombinant DNA technology.

The breakthroughs in our understanding of the genetic basis of cardiovascular disease have been equally impressive. Our appreciation of the mechanism by which single genes cause disease, even when the diseases are uncommon, has led to an understanding of the pathogenesis of more common cardiovascular diseases. With completion of sequencing of the Human Genome Project, genomic discoveries in cardiovascular diseases now occur at a rapid pace. How these discoveries will be translated to the care of patients with cardiovascular disease is currently difficult to predict.

This chapter highlights the basic principles of molecular biology and genetics. It is designed as a brief review and reference source, intended to prepare the reader for discussions of specific cardiovascular applications in other chapters throughout the text. References are provided for a general coverage on a topic as well as an in-depth coverage of each subject.

Principles of Cell Biology and the Cell Cycle

All living organisms are composed of cells, and all cells arise from preexisting cells.[1,2] Cells are organized into compartments. Prokaryotes, such as bacteria, contain a single cell compartment bounded by a membrane or membranes. Eukaryotes, such as mammals, are defined by the division of each cell into a nucleus that contains the genetic material, surrounded by a cytoplasm, which in turn is bounded by the plasma membrane that marks the periphery of the cell. The cytoplasm also contains other discrete compartments, also bounded by membranes. To define the execution of genetic instructions in a cell, we must consider the nature of the various compartments and how they function to create regions with different properties.

The mammalian cell is a highly compartmentalized structure (Fig. 69–1). The outer membrane, called the *plasma membrane*, is a lipid bilayer intended to exclude an aqueous environment, such as extracellular fluid.[3] The plasma membrane is studded with a class of transmembrane proteins called *receptors*. A receptor has a binding site that recognizes some ligand on the exterior side of the membrane. Binding of the ligand usually triggers a change in the protein, which is transmitted to the

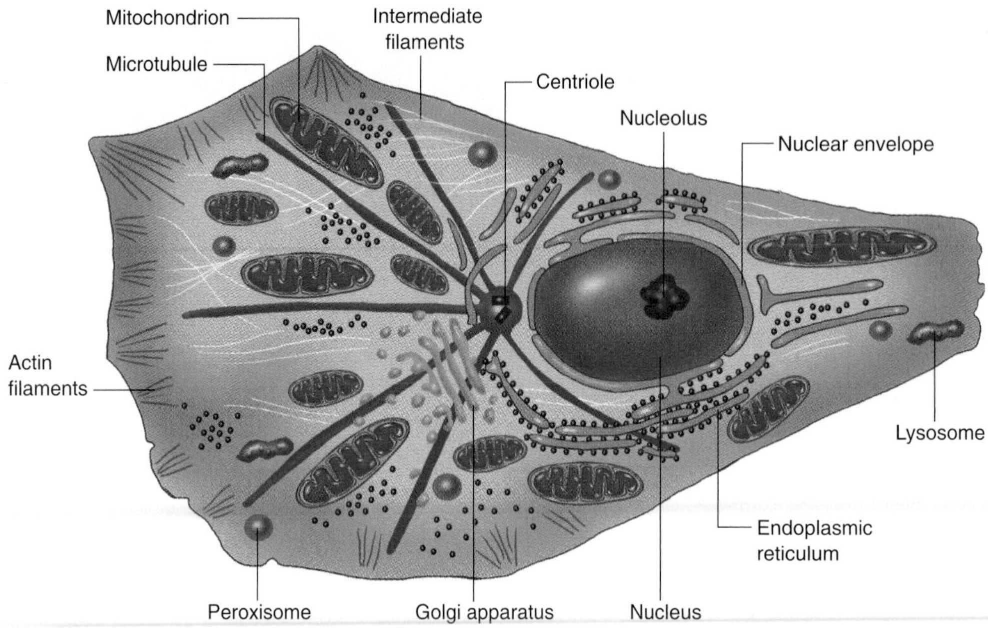

FIGURE 69–1 Structure of a mammalian cell. Schematic illustration of a cell, demonstrating structures common to most cells.

cytoplasmic face by a conformational change in the receptor protein, or as movement of the whole protein into the interior. This change, in turn, triggers other changes within the cell, and thus provides a means for responding to the environment. This type of relationship is called *signal transduction*.[4]

The cytoplasm contains networks of membranes. Membrane sheets make up the endoplasmic reticulum (ER) and the Golgi apparatus.[5] ER consists of a continuous sheet of highly folded membranes extending from the outer nuclear membrane. ER can be divided into two types, which are part of the same membrane sheet. Rough ER has ribosomes, the small particles concerned with the synthesis of proteins, on its surface, whereas smooth ER does not. The Golgi apparatus consists of stacks of separate cisternae. Proteins that have been modified in ER enter the Golgi apparatus, undergo further modifications, and then exit. A major function of the ER and Golgi apparatus is to sort proteins according to destination, using signals inherent in the protein sequence. This process of directing proteins to their final destination is called *protein sorting* or *trafficking*.[6] Mitochondria are specialized organelles in the cytoplasm that generate energy stored in the form of adenosine triphosphate from the oxidation of carbon-containing compounds such as sugars or fats. Lysosomes are membrane-enclosed bodies that contain hydrolytic enzymes, which further process proteins within the cell. Cell shape is determined by the cytoskeleton, which contains networks of protein fibers extending across and around the cell. The three classes of fibers are actin filaments, microtubules, and intermediate filaments.

The most important feature of the nucleus is the genetic material. It has a granular appearance, due to chromatin, that is easily recognized with certain stains. Between cell divisions, chromatin forms a single dense mass. When a cell divides, its chromatin can be seen to consist of a discrete number of thread-like particles, called chromosomes.[7] A common feature of cells, except those that have reached a final, specialized state of development (*terminal differentiation*), is their ability to divide. Many structural changes occur within a cell during division. There is extensive reorganization of membranes and the cytoskeleton. The cell is organized by a new structure, called the *spindle*, the function of which is to allow the distribution of chromosomes to daughter cells. The result of these changes is that many of the former activities of the cell—gene expression, protein synthesis and secretion, cell motility—come to a halt.[8]

The cell cycle, the period between the release of a newly formed cell as a progeny of a division and its own subsequent division into two daughter cells, consists of two parts.[9] Interphase, a relatively long period, represents the time during which the cell engages in its synthetic activities and reproduces its subcellular components. During interphase, the cell has a discrete nuclear compartment, containing a compact mass of chromatin. Mitosis is a short period of time during which the actual division into two daughter cells is accomplished. During mitosis, the internal organization of the cell is replaced by the spindle, and individual chromosomes are apparent. The products of the series of mitotic divisions that generate the organism are called the *somatic cells*. During embryonic development, many or most of the somatic cells proceed through the cell cycle. In the adult organism, many cells are terminally differentiated and no longer divide. They remain in a stationary phase in which there is no DNA synthesis, equivalent to a perpetual interphase.

Mitosis recapitulates the chromosome constitution of the cell. Each daughter cell starts its life with two copies of each chromosome. These copies are called *homologues*. The total number of chromosomes is called the *diploid set* and has 2n members (see Chap. 70). During interphase, a growing cell duplicates its chromosomal material. At the beginning of mitosis, each chromosome appears to split longitudinally to generate two copies, called *sister chromatids*. The cell now contains 4n chromosomes, organized as 2n pairs of sister chromatids. The process of mitosis consists of four phases: prophase, metaphase, anaphase, and telophase, ending in cytokinesis, in which the cell divides and each daughter has the same complete set of chromosomes, one member of each pair derived from each parent (Fig. 69–2). Each phase consists of distinct movements of the centromere, the central, constriction region of the chromosome. These movements are essential to separation of the pairs of chromosomes into each daughter cell and completion of cell division.

Just before mitosis, double-stranded chromosomal breaks or other DNA damage is repaired by a series of cell cycle checkpoints.[10] Under normal conditions, cellular DNA is repaired, and the cell completes mitosis. Cells in which DNA is not repaired undergo apoptosis, or programmed cell death.[11] This mechanism allows the perpetuation of cell division in which chromosomal DNA is intact. Carcinogenesis results when cell division escapes checkpoint control, and cells with double-stranded DNA break or other forms of damaged DNA divide uncontrollably and metastasize to other sites in the organism.

The essential proteins in cell cycle checkpoint control are the cyclins and the cyclin-dependent kinases (CDKs) (Fig. 69–3). The CDKs are holoenzyme complexes that contain cyclin regulatory subunits and CDK catalytic subunits.[12] Four distinct phases of the cell cycle are regulated by cyclin-CDK complexes: Gap 1 or G1 phase, DNA replication or S phase, Gap 2 or G2 phase, and mitosis or M phase. Restriction point control in G1 phase is mediated by two CDKs, the cyclin D- and cyclin E-dependent kinases. The D-type cyclins (D1, D2, and D3) interact combinatorially with two catalytic partners, CDK4 and CDK6, early in G_1 to yield at least six holoenzymes expressed in tissue-specific patterns.[13] Cyclin E enters into a complex with its catalytic partner CDK2 and collaborates with the cyclin D-dependent kinases to complete phosphorylation of the retinoblastoma tumor-suppressor protein (Rb) late in G1, which results in transit through the G1-S checkpoint into S phase.[14]

Endogenous inhibitors of the cyclins-CDKs, termed the *cyclin-dependent kinase inhibitors* or CKIs, are expressed throughout G1 to inhibit phosphorylation and activation of cyclin-CDK complexes, resulting in G1 arrest.[15] The CKIs function to prevent transition through the G1 checkpoint and inhibit mitosis, leading to growth arrest of cells. CKIs are classified into two families on the basis of their structures and CDK targets. The CIP/KIP proteins are broadly acting inhibitors that alter the activities of cyclin-D, cyclin E- and cyclin A-dependent kinases. This family includes p21(Cip1), p27(Kip1), and p57(Kip2). All three contain characteristic motifs in their amino-terminal regions that bind cyclin and CDK substrates. p21(Cip1) functions as a downstream effector of the transcription factor and tumor suppressor gene, p53, to cause DNA damage repair and/or promote apoptosis. p27(Kip1) is a potent inhibitor of cell proliferation in normal and diseased tissues and is a critical mediator in tissue injury, inflammation, and wound repair.[16] The INK4 (*in*hibitor of CD*K4*) family of proteins consists of INK4A (p16), INK4B (p15), INK4C (p18), and INK4D (p19).[17] These CKIs contain multiple ankyrin repeats, bind only to CDK4 and CDK6 and not to other CDKs, and specifically inhibit the catalytic subunits of CDK4 and CDK6. The INK proteins are important regulators of tumor growth and in developmental biology, but they play a lesser role in cardiovascular diseases.

Injury to the heart or blood vessels leads to a remodeling process that is adaptive under normal conditions or maladaptive in conditions of disease pathophysiology (see Chaps. 35 and 71). In response to physiological stimuli, vascular smooth muscle cells (VSMCs) within the media proliferate and migrate into the intima to form a multilayered vascular wound or *neointima*. Normally, this is a self-limited process that results in a well-healed vascular wound and preservation of luminal blood flow. In certain vascular diseases, however, VSMC proliferation becomes excessive, leading to a pathological lesion in the blood vessel, which in turn produces clinical symptoms. These diseases are often characterized by systemic or local inflammation, which exacerbates the VSMC proliferative response. The CIP/KIP CKIs are important regulators of tissue remodeling in the vasculature.[18] p27(Kip1) is constitutively expressed in VSMCs and endothelial cells of arteries and is downregulated after vascular injury or exposure of VSMCs and endothelial cells to mitogens. After a proliferative burst, VSMCs synthesize and secrete extracellular matrix molecules, which signal to VSMCs and endothelial cells, leading to induction of p27(Kip1) and p21(Cip1), and suppression of cyclin E-CDK2. Expression of the CIP/KIP CKIs leads to cell cycle arrest and inhibition of cell division.[19] p27(Kip1) is also an important regulator of tissue inflammation through its effects on T-lymphocyte proliferation. In the vasculature, p27(Kip1) mediates vascular repair through its regulation of proliferation, inflammation, and bone marrow progenitor cells. Genetic deletion of p27(Kip1) in mice results in a benign hyperplasia of epithelial and mesodermal cells in multiple organs, including the heart and vasculature.

p21(Cip1) is required for growth and differentiation in the heart, bone, skin, and kidney, and it confers susceptibility to apoptosis.[20] This CKI functions in a p53-dependent and p53-

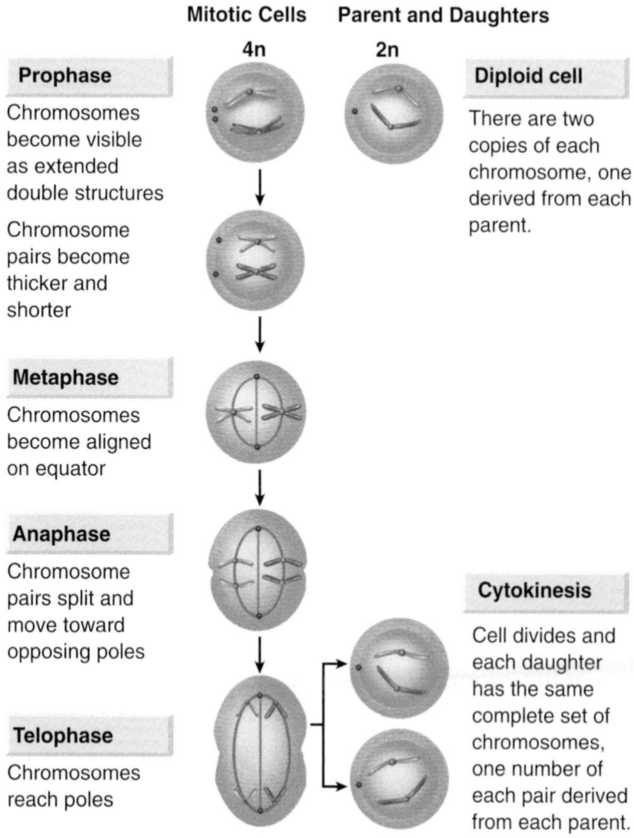

FIGURE 69–2 Process of mitosis in a mammalian cell in which the genetic material is duplicated and distributed during cell division (see text).

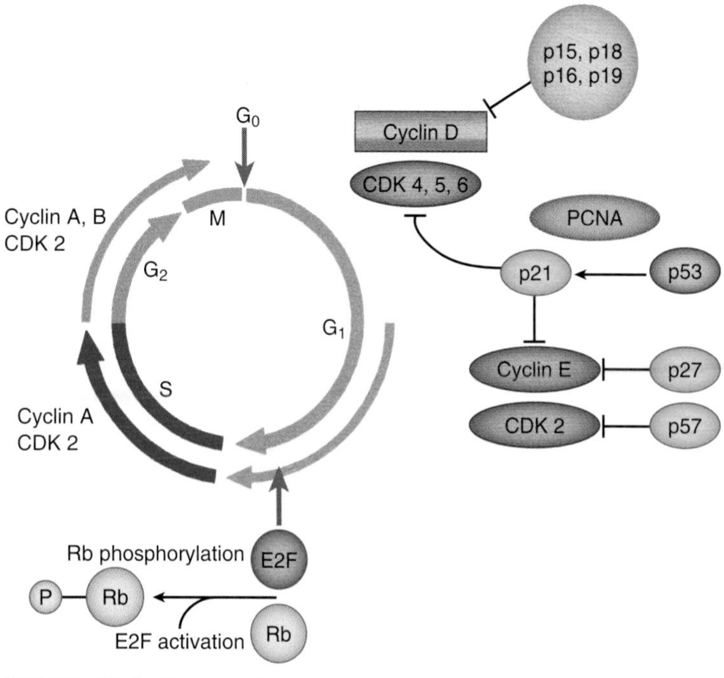

FIGURE 69–3 The mammalian cell cycle. The cyclins, cyclin-dependent kinases, and cyclin-dependent kinase inhibitors active in each phase are shown (see text for explanation and abbreviations).

independent manner. In the heart, p21(Cip1) is expressed independent of p53 in cardiac myocytes; overexpression of p21(Cip1) within myocytes leads to hypertrophy.

Most human cancer cells sustain mutations that alter the functions of p53 or Rb by direct mutation of gene sequences or by targeting genes that act epistatically to prevent their normal function. Rb limits cell proliferation by preventing entry into S phase. The mechanism is blockage of E2F transcription factors from activating genes required for DNA replication and nucleotide metabolism. p53 is mutated in more than 50 percent of human cancers. The protein accumulates in response to cellular stress from DNA damage, hypoxia, and oncogene activation. p53 initiates a transcriptional program that triggers cell cycle arrest or apoptosis.[21] When activated by p53, p21(Cip1) induces apoptosis in tumor and other cells.

The cell cycle functions as the major regulator of cell division. DNA replication and cytokinesis depend on normal functioning of the cell cycle. The cyclins, CDKS, and CKIs are, secondarily, important mediators of carcinogenesis, tissue inflammation, and wound repair.

The Genetic Code: DNA, RNA, and Protein

DNA

Deoxyribonucleic acid (DNA) is the building block of human life (Fig. 69–4). Its double helical structure is deceptively simple, yet the rules encoded within this structure specify the form and function of all cells within an organism. DNA consists of two long strands of polynucleotides that twist around each other clockwise to form an unbroken double helix. Alternating deoxyribose-phosphate groups form the backbone of the helix, with the phosphate group making a 5′-3′ phosphodiester bond between the fifth carbon of one pentose ring and the third carbon of the next pentose ring (Fig. 69–5). Nucleic acid bases attached to the sugar groups of each strand face each other within the helix, perpendicular to the strand axis. The order of the nucleic acids specifies the eventual sequence of the protein product of the gene. There are only four bases: the purines adenine and guanine (A and G) and the pyrimidines cytosine and thymine (C and T). During assembly of the double helix, a purine can pair only with a pyrimidine, and a pyrimidine with a purine. Each base pair (bp) forms one of the rungs in the twisted ladder of the DNA molecule, which can be millions of bases long. The two strands of DNA, which are held together by hydrogen bonds between complementary base pairs, have opposite chemical polarities. One strand is oriented in a 5′ to 3′ direction, while the other is in a 3′ to 5′ direction. Enzymes that recognize specific DNA sequences also recognize the polarity of the strand. An enzyme "reads" the nucleotide sequences on the two strands in opposite directions. Because the structure of the helical backbone is invariant, enzymes responsible for DNA copying, cleavage, and repairing strand breaks can act anywhere along the length of the DNA strand.

An important consequence of the A-T and G-C pairing is that the sequence of nucleotides on one strand of the double helix determines the sequence on the complementary strand. This base pairing rule is critical for the storage, retrieval, and

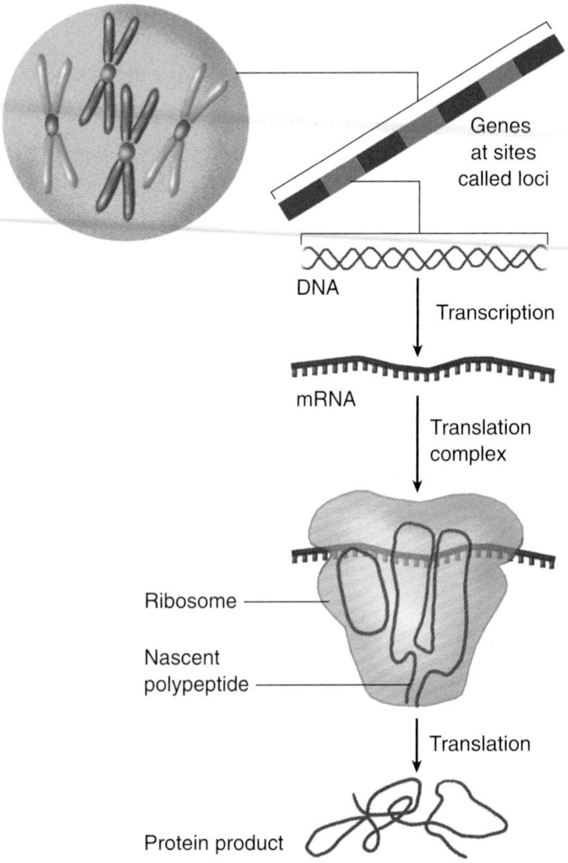

FIGURE 69–4 Depiction of the storage of genetic information in homologous chromosomes, which contain genes made up of DNA and genetic expression involving transcription of DNA into RNA, which is translated on a ribosome into protein.

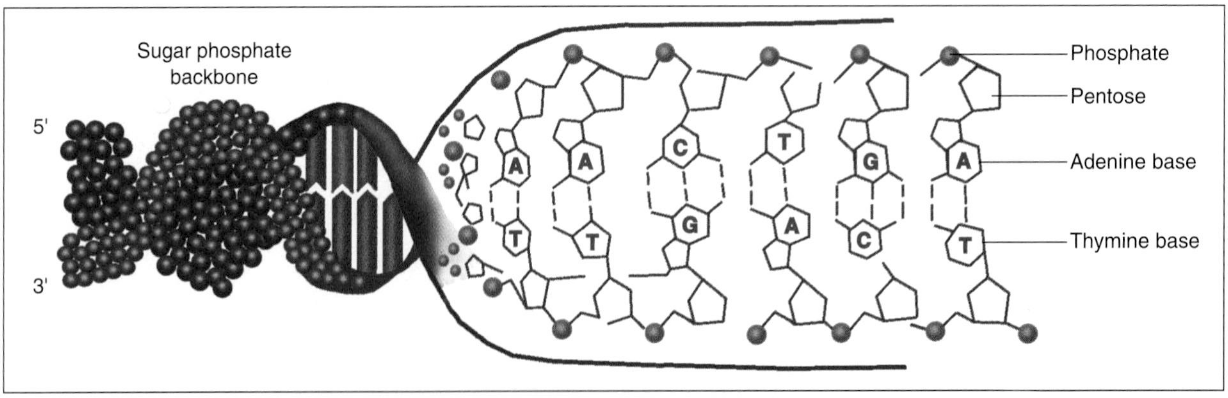

FIGURE 69–5 Schematic representation of the DNA double helix. The specificity of genetic information is carried in the four bases—guanine, adenine, thymine, and cytosine—that extend inward from a sugar-phosphate background and form pairs with complementary bases on the opposing strand.

transfer of genetic material, whether it be for duplication of DNA into a daughter cell, repair of a damaged DNA strand, or reading as a template for RNA transcription.

Chromosomes are long double helical strands of DNA tightly coiled into compacted, discrete lengths by nuclear proteins. Each chromosome varies in length and base pair composition. In human cells, the nucleus contains 23 different pairs of chromosomes, each with a specific length and base pair sequence. The combined DNA sequences (approximately 3×10^9) on all the chromosomes within a cell comprise the genome.[22,23] The information carried within the genome is identical in all cells of an organism and varies little between members of a species. Indeed, the genome of humans, *Homo sapiens*, is approximately 99 percent identical.[24]

During cell division, enzymes called *polymerases* unwind the DNA helix in each chromosome and copy each of the two strands separately along their entire length. Each daughter cell, then, inherits a double-stranded DNA molecule containing one old and one new strand. Each of these strands can in turn generate a new strand that faithfully reproduces the original template. This fidelity of DNA replication is essential for accurate transfer of genetic information. Errors in this process are a common source of gene mutations, which are inherited in successive rounds of cell division.

A gene is a section of base sequences used as a template for the copying process of transcription and, therefore, is the fundamental unit of inherited DNA information. Genes comprise only a small fraction of all the DNA carried on a chromosome. Only 1 to 2 percent of its bases encode proteins, and the full complement of protein-coding sequences still remains to be established. The human genome contains an estimated 30,000 distinct genes.[22,23] The protein coding information contained within a single gene is not continuous but instead is encoded in multiple discontinuous packets called *exons*. Between these exons are variably sized stretches of DNA called *introns*. The function of these introns is not known. They probably contain the bulk of the regulatory information controlling the expression of the approximately 30,000 protein-coding genes, and myriad other functional elements, such as non-protein-coding genes and the sequence determinants of chromosome dynamics. Even less is known about the function of the roughly half of the genome that consists of highly repetitive sequences or of the remaining noncoding, nonrepetitive DNA.

RNA

The first step in the expression of genetic information is transcription, which serves to carry the genetic information out of the nucleus into the cytoplasm where the synthesis of proteins occurs. In this process, transcription of DNA to RNA requires the expression of a gene template called messenger RNA (mRNA) in the nucleus (Fig. 69–6). A specialized enzyme, RNA polymerase, copies one of the two DNA strands (the antisense strand), creating a complementary stretch of sequence that is an exact copy of the sense strand. RNA structure differs slightly from DNA. One of the RNA bases, uracil, replaces the DNA base thymine, and the RNA sugar phosphate component ribose replaces DNA deoxyribose. Ribose renders the RNA molecule much more susceptible to degradation than the more stable deoxyribose. This allows RNAs to respond more rapidly to shifts in cellular signaling and move quickly to the cytoplasm for protein production.

From Genes to Proteins

The process of converting a gene to a protein involves two major steps: transcription of the DNA by RNA in the nucleus and translation of the RNA into protein in the cytoplasm.

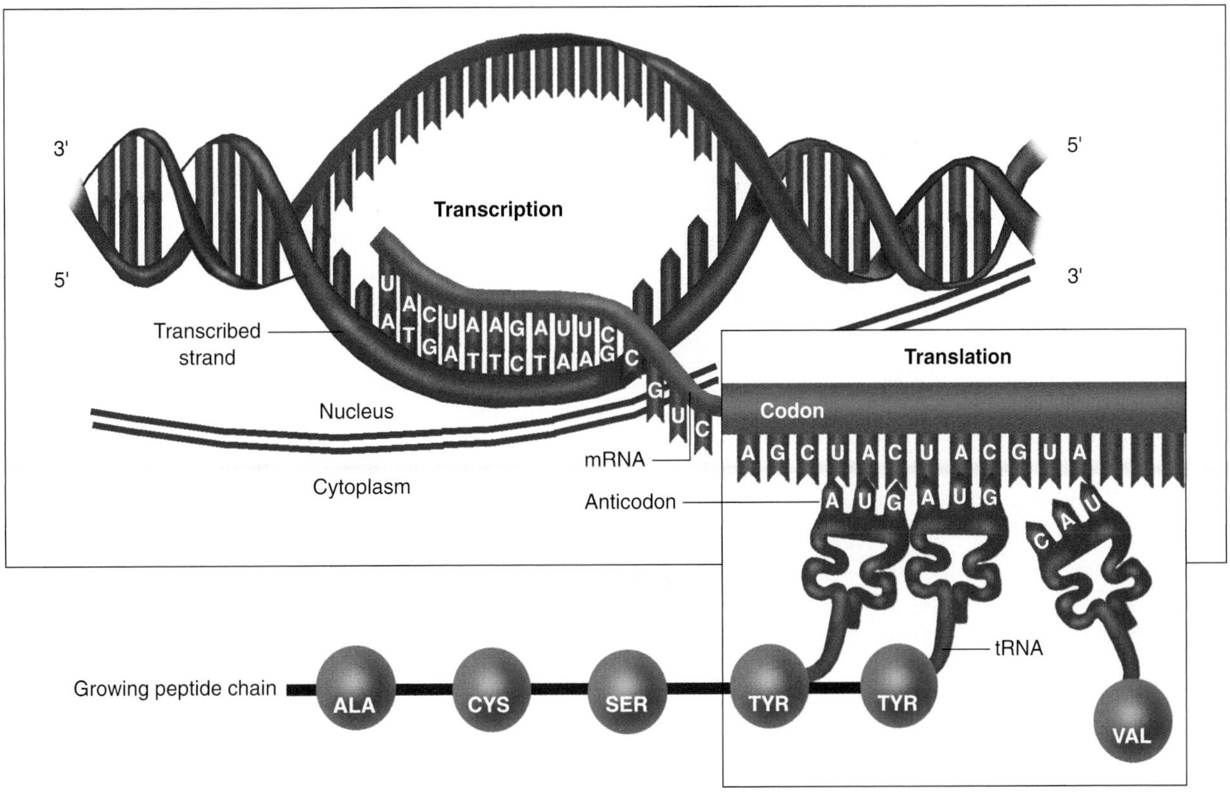

FIGURE 69–6 The flow of genetic information. Transcription in the nucleus creates a complementary ribonucleic acid copy from one of the DNA strands in the double helix. mRNA is transported into the cytoplasm, where it is translated into protein.

This is a complex and highly regulated process. Transcription begins in the nucleus by copying of the DNA sequence of the gene into mRNA (see Fig. 69–6). The single-stranded RNA is modified at both ends. At the 5′ end, a nucleotide structure called a *cap* is added to increase translation efficiency by allowing ribosomes to bind to RNA. At the 3′ end, a nucleotide recognizes an A/T rich sequence in a noncoding region and trims the transcript downstream by about 20 bp. An enzyme that adds a stretch of adenosine to form a polyA tail, which stabilizes the transcript, modifies the newly cleaved 3′ end. The transcript then undergoes splicing to remove intronic sequences. This is a highly regulated process, since unspliced transcripts are highly unstable and are cleared rapidly from the cell. Splicing is an important control point in gene expression. It must be absolutely precise, since the deletion or addition of a single nucleotide at the splice junction would throw out of frame the subsequent three-base codon translation of the RNA. The full significance of RNA splicing is not completely understood, but it must represent a critical point in the regulation of gene expression due to the large expanses of intron sequences and the inability of transcripts to leave the nucleus until their introns are removed.

Once in the cytoplasm, mRNA provides a template for translation or protein synthesis. Translation occurs on a macromolecular complex, like an assembly line, called *ribosomes*. The ribosomes read and translate the nucleotide sequence in mRNA into an amino acid sequence; that is, the four base mRNA code is translated into the 20 amino acid alphabet of proteins. This genetic code is remarkably simple and has been conserved in most organisms. Every three RNA nucleotides encodes for a single amino acid; therefore, the codon is a triplet of bases (Fig. 69–7). Permutations of the four RNA nucleotides results in 64 different triplets (4 × 4 × 4), so that any one of the 20 amino acids can be specified by more than one codon. One of the triplets, AUG, specifies methionine, which is the amino acid that starts each protein. Three other triplets, UAA, UGA, and UAG, program the ribosome to end translation and are therefore called *stop codons*.

The conversion of a codon into an amino acid requires an adapter molecule, called *transfer RNA* (tRNA), to decode mRNA. Each tRNA uses a unique three-base sequence or anticodon to line up with the complementary codon in mRNA (see Fig. 69–6). Ribosomal enzymes link adjoining amino acids, which frees them from the tRNA adapters and adds them to the growing amino acid chain. The order of the amino acids is specified by the order of the codons on the corresponding mRNA template. Translation then completes the transfer of information from DNA in the nucleus to a unique protein structure.

Since the genetic code is preserved across species, human genetic sequences can be transferred into bacteria, yeast, or insect cells, where the sequences will be faithfully replicated and decoded into RNA and protein. This principle constitutes the basis of recombinant DNA technology, which is used to produce recombinant proteins for research and therapeutic purposes (tissue plasminogen activator is an example).

The process of gene expression requires controlled and precise regulation at multiple steps. Only a small number of genes are expressed within a cell at a given time. One set of genes is constitutively expressed in most cells and are referred to colloquially as "housekeeping genes." These genes are necessary for cell replication, energy generation, and survival functions. A second set of genes are expressed in a lineage-specific manner, i.e., within certain cells. These genes are required for cell-specific functions, such as contractility. The precise regulation of lineage-specific genes determines the unique identity and function of a particular cell. Another set of genes is expressed in response to environmental stimuli. These sets of controls are required to produce the complex and dynamic patterns of gene expression, which allow an organism to respond to internal and external signals.

		Second Base			
First Base		U	C	A	G
	U	UUU, UUC Phe UUA, UUG Leu	UCU, UCC, UCA, UCG Ser	UAU, UAC Tyr UAA, UAG TERM	UGU, UGC Cys UGA TERM UGG Trp
	C	CUU, CUC, CUA, CUG Leu	CCU, CCC, CCA, CCG Pro	CAU, CAC His CAA, CAG Gin	CGU, CGC, CGA, CGG Arg
	A	AUU, AUC, AUA Ile AUG Met	ACU, ACC, ACA, ACG Thr	AAU, AAC Asn AAA, AAG Lys	AGU, AGC Ser AGA, AGG Arg
	G	GUU, GUC, GUA, GUG Val	GCU, GCC, GCA, GCG Ala	GAU, GAC Asp GAA, GAG Glu	GGU, GGC, GGA, GGG Gly

FIGURE 69–7 The genetic code. The amino acids corresponding to each nucleotide triplet in the mRNA are shown. There is a single start codon (AUG) and three stop codons (UAG, UAA, UGA).

Principles and Techniques of Molecular Biology

Recombinant DNA technologies developed in the 1970s as a response to the need for sufficient quantities of DNA for biochemical analysis. The method refers to the clipping of a segment out of surrounding DNA using sequence-specific endonucleases known as *restriction enzymes*. The segment then can be inserted at will into a vector that permits copying it millions of times (see later). The success of recombinant DNA techniques fueled most of the advances in molecular biology over the past 30 years. Many of these techniques are now commonplace in research laboratories. These approaches are routinely used for analysis of gene structure, expression, and organization; regulatory pathways by which cells control gene expression; and discovery of novel genes and therapeutics. These advances have changed the face of medical research. Genetic engineering in which an organism is modified to include new genes designed with desired characteristics is in routine practice in many research laboratories. Recombinant DNA technologies are used to mass-produce therapeutic proteins, such as recombinant tissue plasminogen activator. The ability to manipulate the human genome has opened up new possibilities for the development of diagnostic tests and new therapies. Yet, the techniques of molecular biology, like the structure of DNA itself, are surprisingly simple. The basic approaches are described here; the reader is guided to in-depth reviews for a primer on how to perform the techniques.[25]

Cloning DNA

Molecular cloning provides a means to produce millions of copies of a DNA sequence or gene within bacterial cells. A DNA fragment is first inserted into a cloning vector. The most commonly used vectors are small circular DNA molecules called *plasmids* or bacterial viruses called *phage*. The vectors also contain genetic information that allows the bacterial cell to replicate the DNA sequence. After insertion of a DNA sequence, the plasmid or phage vector is introduced into a bacterial cell. The growing bacterial culture replicates the vector containing the DNA sequence in hundreds of copies per cell, yielding multiple identical clones of the original DNA sequence. The vectors are then harvested from the bacterial culture using the same restriction enzymes used to insert the DNA sequence into the vector.

The molecular biologist uses restriction endonucleases derived from bacteria as molecular scissors that cut DNA motifs at predictable sequences. Each restriction enzyme recognizes a specific nucleotide sequence. These recognition sites occur randomly along the DNA of any organism and consist of a short symmetric sequence motif called a *palindrome*, which is repeated in opposing orientation on both strands of the double helix DNA. For example, the enzyme EcoRI from the bacteria *Escherichia coli* recognizes and cuts the sequence GAATTC in double-strand DNA at GA and AG junctions. Most restriction enzymes cleave their palindromic sequence asymmetrically, leaving a single-stranded overhang on each end of the cut. These "sticky" ends have unique and complementary sequences that can be used to connect a fragment of human DNA with complementary ends of DNA from another source. An enzymatic reaction connects the continuous double-stranded DNA to form a smooth splice. These principles are used to construct various DNA rearrangements for multiple purposes, such as gene cloning, generating knock-out mice, or constructing recombinant DNA therapies.

Blotting Techniques

Blotting is a tool that permits identification of DNA, RNA, or protein by its molecular size. Analysis of DNA is referred to as a Southern blot; RNA identification is a Northern blot; and protein isolation is a Western blot. The principles of blotting techniques are straightforward.[25] A mixture of molecules to be analyzed is subjected to gel electrophoresis, which separates different species according to size and/or electrical charge (Fig. 69–8). An agarose gel is used in which the molecules are loaded into wells at one end. The gel is submerged into buffer and subjected to an electrical current. The molecules migrate across the electrical field. Since DNA and RNA are acids that carry a negative charge, they migrate toward the positive pole of the gel. The agarose matrix hinders the migration of larger molecules, so that the molecules also separate by size. When the electrophoresis is completed, the gel is removed from the buffer, and a nylon filter and dry absorbent material are placed on top. The buffer from the gel is blotted into the absorbent material carrying with it the separated molecules, which remain on the nylon filter. The filter is treated to permanently fix the molecules on its surface, creating a mirror image of the original gel. The filter is then bathed with a tagged molecule that recognizes (hybridizes to) the molecule of interest (the probe) and washed to remove the unbound probe. For Southern (DNA) and Northern (RNA) blots, the probe is a small fragment of nucleic acid that carries a complementary sequence to the molecule being investigated. The nucleic acid is tagged with a radioactive element detectable by exposure to x-ray film or other techniques.

The position of the hybridized probe, which appears as a band, provides an estimate of the size of DNA or RNA segment. By running parallel lanes of molecular markers of known size, the precise size of the DNA or RNA element is determined. For protein identification (Western blot), the probe consists of a tagged antibody that recognizes the target protein. Size markers are also run in the gel to identify the size of the protein.

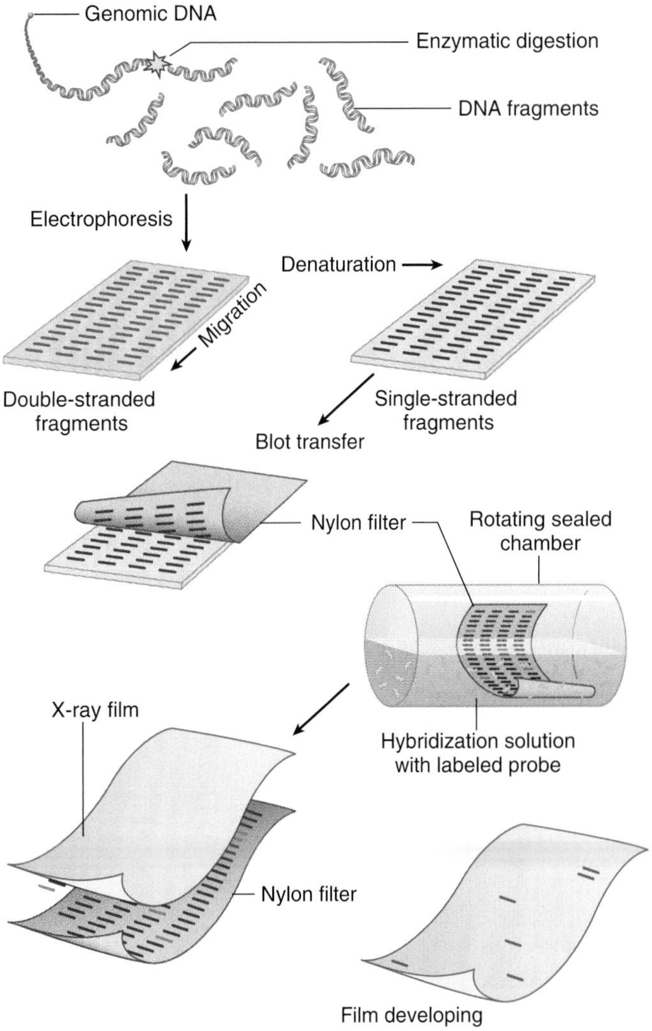

FIGURE 69–8 Blotting DNA. The process of Southern blotting to identify genomic DNA is shown.

Blotting techniques are also used for other purposes, including to map the position of restriction sites in a specific gene following restriction enzyme digestion, and in cytogenetic analysis to compare restriction sites in genomic DNA from a test and reference sample.

Polymerase Chain Reaction

Polymerase chain reaction (PCR) is an amplification procedure that takes place within a test tube (Fig. 69–9). The segment of DNA or RNA to be amplified is combined in a test tube with two short oligonucleotide primers (chemically synthesized single-stranded DNA fragments). The primers initiate the amplification, which then proceeds in a series of cycles in which the original DNA, called the *template*, is separated into single strands. The separation of the strands allows the primers to bind or anneal to the respective complementary sequences at each end of the single strands. A heat-stable DNA polymerase enzyme adds nucleotide bases at the ends of each primer, reading across the single DNA strand, generating a complementary copy of the single strand. By the time the polymerase has reached the end of the single

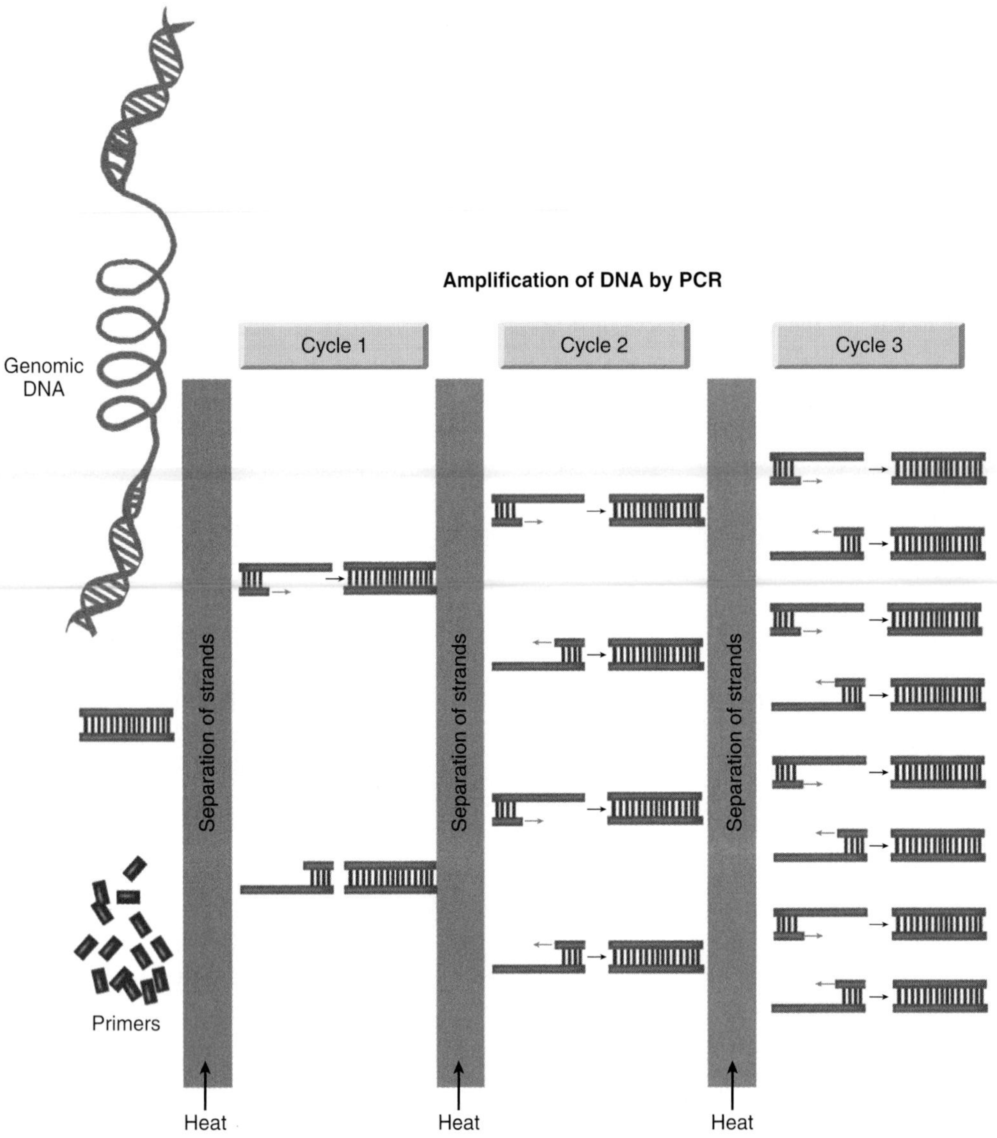

FIGURE 69–9 DNA amplification with the polymerase chain reaction (PCR). Synthetic primers corresponding to the 5′ and 3′ ends of the DNA sequence are chemically synthesized. The double-stranded DNA is melted by heating to 92°C, followed by cooling to 72°C to anneal the primers. A heat-stable DNA polymerase amplifies each strand of the target sequence, producing two copies of the DNA sequence. The process is repeated multiple times to achieve amplification of the target sequence.

strand, a new double-stranded sequence has been generated. The cycle begins again, heating and separating the double strand, followed by the generation of a new strand by the primer and polymerase. Each round of PCR amplification doubles the number of DNA templates. It is possible to create millions of copies of a DNA segment in several hours by PCR, even when the starting material is a single copy of DNA. The entire amplification is carried out in a sealed test tube or well in a specially designed machine that can be programmed to automatically heat and cool the sample. PCR has now become a commonplace tool to generate a sufficient quantity of identical genetic material for analysis.

Principles of Molecular Genetics

Genotype and the Identification of Disease-Causing Genes

The discovery of the structure and function of DNA in 1953 laid the foundation for molecular genetics.[26] The completion of sequencing of the human genome has added considerably to this foundation.[22,23] Clinicians now have at hand the tools of molecular genetics with which they can pursue diagnoses and treatments. In this regard, three concepts prove particularly useful in cardiovascular genetics: genotype, genomics, and proteomics. Genotype is the composite of DNA sequences within an individual's set of genes, or the complete sequence of an individual's DNA on all 23 pairs of chromosomes. Genomics is the expression of gene sequences as RNA. The focus of genomics is "Which genes are expressed?" Proteomics is the study of proteins expressed within a cell or organism and seeks to understand the networks of protein-protein interactions.

Historically, the field of genetics focused on monogenic disorders, i.e., diseases caused by a single gene deletion or mutation (see Chap. 70). With the newer tools of genomics and proteomics, attention has turned to the evaluation of the genetic susceptibility to complex disease traits, such as coronary artery disease and hyperlipidemias. Understanding the genetic basis of complex diseases requires knowledge of gene sequences, the proteins encoded by the genes, and the functions of the proteins. However, it is becoming increasingly clear that complex cardiovascular problems will not be resolved by deriving the nucleotide sequence of the human genome or from unraveling the approximately 30,000 loci that encode the corresponding proteins or regulate other genes. Considerable work is required to define precisely the molecular mechanisms by which changes in an individual gene or set of genes specify or confer risk for a specific disease phenotype.

Monogenic Disorders

Medical genetics has classically focused on single gene or monogenic diseases, where the cause of the disease is traced to a missing or mutated gene. Approximately 1000 disease-causing genes have been identified.[27] Monogenic disorders are rare and typically are inherited in a mendelian or autosomal manner. Interestingly, our understanding of the mechanism by which single genes cause disease, even though these mechanisms are uncommon, has led to an understanding of the pathogenesis of more common cardiovascular diseases.

Our current understanding of genetic factors in cardiovascular disease is reviewed in more detail elsewhere (see Chap. 70).[28] Briefly, each gene exists in two copies, known as *alleles*. An individual is homozygous at a given locus if the two alleles are identical, or heterozygous if the alleles are different. The specific alleles present at a given loci represent the genotype for those genes. Viewed more broadly, a genotype is a composite of the genetic factors responsible for creating a phenotype. A phenotype, in turn, is the visible or measurable properties resulting from a genotype, such as coronary artery disease or obesity. Phenotype can also be defined as the effect of gene action, whether due to a single gene or the entire genotype.

Differences in nucleotide sequences, either between two individuals or among all individuals within a population, constitutes genetic *variation*. Differences that arise in nucleotide sequences and lead to a structural change in the proteins they encode are called *mutations*. A mutation is defined as occurring in less than 1 percent of a given population.[29] Approximately 16,000 mutations in single-gene disorders have been identified.[27] Examples of mutations include missense, nonsense, frame shift, deletion, and insertion (Fig. 69–10). Missense mutations result from substitutions of one or more nucleotides in such a way as to change the primary sequence of the encoded protein. These missense mutations alter the function of the protein by changing its primary structure. A nonsense mutation introduces a premature stop codon into a gene, resulting in a truncated gene product that can display alterations in function and can be unstable. Insertions or deletions of nucleotides add or subtract amino acids from the resulting proteins, if the nucleotide changes lead to an addition or deletion of a triplet. Frame-shift mutations occur when codons of a gene are read in the wrong reading frame. These mutations typically cause abnormal protein structure due to the introduction of out-of-frame termination codons, which lead to premature termination of proteins. Mutations in introns and exons cause splicing errors that also lead to alterations in protein structure or premature termination. Finally, mutations in the promoters or enhancers of genes can lead to alterations in the levels of expression of a protein, or the temporal or spatial patterns of gene expression of a protein.

Wild-type Sequence							
... AUG	GCC	TAC	GTT	CGA	CCC ...		
... Met	Ala	Tyr	Val	Arg	Pro ...		
Missense							
AUG	ACC	TAC	GTT	CGA	CCC		
Met	Thr	Tyr	Val	Arg	Pro		
Nonsense							
AUG	GCC	TAG	GTT	CGA	CCC		
Met	Ala	Stop					
Frameshift							
AUG	GCC	TAC	•TTC	CGA	CCC		
Met	Ala	Tyr	Phe	Asp	...		
Deletion							
AUG	GCC	TAC	GTT	...	CCC		
Met	Ala	Tyr	Val	–	Pro		
OR							
AUG	GCC	TA•	G	TT	CCC		
Met	Ala	Stop	⟶				
Insertion							
AUG	GCC	AAA	TAC	GTT	CGA	CCC	
Met	Ala	Lys	Tyr	Val	Arg	Pro	
OR							
AUG	GCC	ATA	CGT	TCG	ACC ...		
Met	Ala	Ile	Arg	Ser	Thr ...		

FIGURE 69–10 Different types of mutations that alter the structure and expression of human genes.

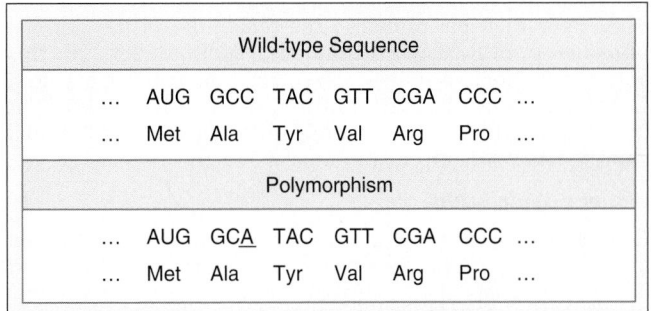

A variety of mutations have been found in monogenic cardiovascular diseases (see Chap. 70). For example, while the primary defect in familial hypercholesterolemia is a deficit of low-density lipoprotein receptors (LDLRs), more than 600 mutations in the LDLR gene have been identified in patients with this disorder.[30] Likewise, hypertrophic cardiomyopathy, an autosomal dominant disease, is caused by mutations in the genes encoding proteins of the myocardial-contractile apparatus. Multiple causative mutations in at least 10 different sarcomeric proteins have been identified, including cardiac beta-myosin heavy chain, cardiac myosin-binding protein, cardiac troponin T, cardiac troponin I, alpha-tropomyosin, essential and regulatory light chains, and cardiac actin.[31] Other monogenic cardiovascular disorders include familial long Q-T syndrome,[32] venous thrombosis due to factor V Leiden,[33] and inherited forms of hypertension.[34]

Complex Trait Analysis

Polymorphisms are common variations, defined as being present in more than 1 percent of the population. Single nucleotide polymorphisms (SNPs) are nucleotide substitutions that do not alter a protein structure (Fig. 69–11). SNPs are very useful markers to map genes to chromosomal loci.[35] An SNP may be a marker of disease susceptibility, i.e., it can associate with a disease due to either a direct effect of the SNP on the disease or linkage with a nearby susceptibility locus.[36] There are an estimated 1.4 million SNPs in the human genome.[37] Putative and confirmed SNPs are accessible through several public databases, such as dbSNP, a database maintained by the National Center for Biotechnology Information.[38]

A haplotype is a set of SNPs grouped by genetic regions and inherited en bloc within a given population. Haplotypes may have a true association with a disease or may only appear to be associated due to confounding factors.[39] If a SNP is associated with a disease, it is likely that the SNP is

Wild-type Sequence					
... AUG	GCC	TAC	GTT	CGA	CCC ...
... Met	Ala	Tyr	Val	Arg	Pro ...
Polymorphism					
... AUG	GCA	TAC	GTT	CGA	CCC ...
... Met	Ala	Tyr	Val	Arg	Pro ...

FIGURE 69–11 A polymorphism is a nucleotide substitution that does not alter the primary amino acid structure of the resulting protein.

inherited as part of a haplotype in which other SNPs are also statistically associated with the disease. This nonrandom association of alleles is called *linkage disequilibrium*. Linkage disequilibrium exists when alleles at two distinct locations in the genome are inherited together more frequently than expected. Since a SNP may simply be a marker of disease predisposition rather than a causal agent, demonstration of altered gene function must be shown in order to prove causality.

An international effort is underway to identify all SNPs on all 22 somatic chromosomes in 300 individuals from diverse backgrounds in Asia, Africa, Europe, and the Americas. This project, called the Haplotype Map or HapMap, was initiated in October 2002 to construct a genome-wide map of SNP clusters based on DNA samples from different human populations.[40] The HapMap will provide a SNP roadmap for performing linkage analysis, association studies, and evaluation of SNP partners for contribution to a disease. SNPs, then, provide insight into the genetic basis for disease for several reasons: direct causal agents of altered gene function; markers of disease, regardless of causality; and genome-wide markers for genetic studies due their presence at high density throughout the genome.[41,42]

Linkage Analysis and Association Studies

Two types of genetic studies examine inheritance: linkage analysis and association studies. Linkage studies are performed in families to study coinheritance of two traits passed down from parent to child.[43] Sets of polymorphic markers or SNPs are used to identify the location of the two alleles on a chromosomal locus. The genes encoding the two traits typically reside in close proximity to each other, and hence, the traits, or alleles, are linked. Linkage is determined by a LOD score, or the *l*ogarithm of the *od*ds that markers are linked at a particular distance, divided by the odds that they are linked at 50 percent coinheritance (not linked at all). Linkage analysis is commonly used to identify and study mendelian traits.[44] Allele-sharing methods are also used to compare similarity of alleles in closely affected individuals, such as affected sibling pairs.

Population-based association studies are useful for investigations of common disorders without clear mendelian inheritance.[45] Association studies often employ a case control approach in which an experimental and reference group are compared. Careful consideration of the most appropriate control population is necessary to draw valid conclusions and infer gene function from these studies. Case control studies should be sufficiently powered with a large enough sample size to achieve statistical significance. In this approach, known SNPs in candidate genes are investigated, using the alleles of a given SNP as variables, which are then associated with the presence or absence of disease or a particular outcome. If SNPs in a candidate gene are not known, then the gene is directly sequenced in a subset of the study and in control populations to determine which SNPs are differentially represented in the two populations. Confirmation of SNPs is then performed in the remainder of the population using PCR-based techniques. A limitation of this approach is the bias inherent in selection of candidate genes. Only those genes known or of interest are often chosen for investigation. In contrast, identification of genes by positional cloning has frequently led to unanticipated discoveries.

Genome-Wide Scans

Genome-wide scans of SNPs are newer techniques performed on high-throughput platforms and assay for several thousand SNPs simultaneously.[46-48] By taking advantage of the physical distribution of SNPs through the genome, chromosomal regions between SNPs are associated with a disease. With this technique, SNPs can be identified as biomarkers of disease. This approach will be an active area of research in the coming years.

Genomics

Genomics is the study of gene function through the parallel measurements of genomes, most commonly using the techniques of microarrays and serial analysis of gene expression (SAGE). Microarray usage in drug discovery is expanding, and its applications include basic research and target discovery, biomarker determination, pharmacology, toxicogenomics, target selectivity, development of prognostic tests, and disease-subclass determination.

The basic technique involves extraction of RNA from biological samples in either normal or test states (Fig. 69–12).[49] The RNA is copied, while incorporating either fluorescent nucleotides or a tag that is later stained with fluorescence. The labeled RNA is then hybridized to a microarray for a period of time, after which the excess is washed off and the microarray is scanned under laser light. The end result is 4000 to 5000 measurements of gene expression per biological sample. Because a complete experiment might involve any number up to hundreds of microarrays, the resultant RNA-expression data sets can vary greatly in size.

cDNA Microarrays

cDNA microarrays are created from probe cDNA libraries (500-5000 bases) by spotting a cDNA corresponding to an individual gene or probe at a precise location on a microscope slide. Each microarray measures two samples and provides a relative measurement level for each RNA molecule. Target RNAs labeled with a fluorescent dye are hybridized to the cDNA microarray surface, along with a control sample. The two RNA samples compete for binding to each probe. RNA that matches the cDNA sequence hybridizes to the cDNA spot on the microscope slide. The fluorescent labels are laser activated, and the signal intensities from fluorescent probes binding cDNA spots are compared. The comparison reflects the ratios of RNA abundance for each expressed gene. Normalization strategies that allow for standardization of interarray comparisons are applied, followed by analytical methods, as described previously.

Oligonucleotide Arrays

Oligonucleotide arrays are created by attachment of synthetic nucleotide probes (12-80-mer oligonucleotides) representa-

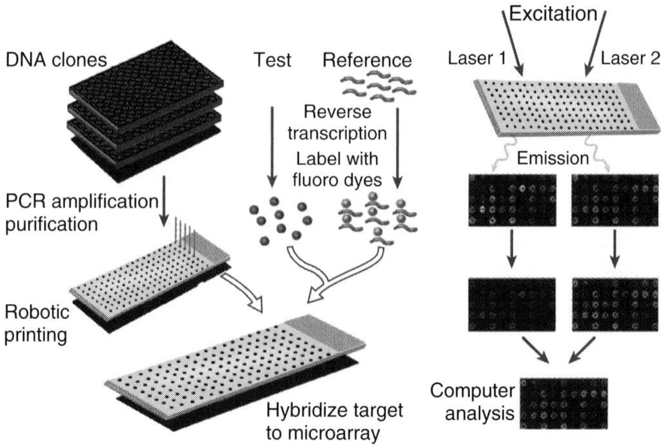

FIGURE 69–12 Detection of differential expression of mRNA from cells or tissues using gene expression profiling. After mRNA is isolated from cells or tissues, it is analyzed by hybridization to fluorescent-labeled cDNA clones imprinted onto a microscope slide. The fluorescent labels are laser activated, and the signal intensities from fluorescent probes binding cDNA spots are compared.

tive of unique portions of genes to an array surface. cDNA is synthesized from the experimental mRNA sample, followed by an in vitro transcription step to create biotin-labeled cRNA, which hybridizes to the microarray target. The microarray is treated with a fluorescent dye tagged to avidin (a protein that binds tightly to biotin) and subjected to laser activation. With oligonucleotide arrays, each microarray measures a single sample and provides an absolute measurement level of each RNA molecule. Signal intensities are measured as a reflection of expression level for each gene.

SAGE

SAGE is a technique for characterization of gene expression based on direct sequencing of transcripts. Its major strength is determination and analysis of transcripts when the sequence is unknown. SAGE requires approximately 10-fold larger quantities of mRNA for analysis and hence is much more labor intensive than some array platforms, even with automated sequencers, since the simplest two-sample comparison requires sequencing of approximately 1.5×10^6 bases. This factor alone poses difficulties when RNA abundance is low, whereas a major advantage is its higher sensitivity for changes in expression level.[50,51]

After acquisition of data by image processing, data are analyzed in three steps: normalization, filtering, and computation. Normalization accounts for technical factors, such as array manufacturing, differences in dye incorporation, and irregularities in probe distribution during hybridization, and is performed to allow meaningful comparisons between individual arrays. Filtering of data refers to the selection of those data likely to represent significant findings. Typical criteria for filtering include assessment of signal quality and fold-change in gene expression level. Differential gene expression in microarray analysis is often defined by a 1.5- to 2-fold difference in relative gene expression level.

Determination of similarity and dissimilarity is a critical component of the data analysis. Two general approaches are used: supervised and unsupervised. Supervised methods are employed for finding genes with expression levels that are significantly different between groups of samples, and finding genes that accurately predict a characteristic of the sample. Two commonly used supervised techniques include "nearest neighbors" and "support vector machines." Users of unsupervised methods try to find internal structure or relationships in a data set instead of trying to determine how best to predict a correct answer. Four commonly used unsupervised techniques include hierarchical clustering, self-organizing maps, relevance networks, and principal-component analysis. These analytical methods are described in detail elsewhere.[52] These computational approaches are then followed by a statistical analysis. Before any microarray data are taken at face value, significant findings should be validated with independent testing of RNA expression levels using quantitative reverse transcription PCR or conventional Northern blotting techniques.

Proteomics

Proteomics is the study of proteins expressed by the genome. Genomics and proteomics should be viewed as complementary components of the genetic spectrum, beginning with DNA and ending with modified proteins (Fig. 69–13). Proteins are the final product of the human genome and ultimately define human biology. Proteins are responsible for biological form and function. It is estimated that there are six to seven times as many proteins as genes (approximately 200,000) in humans, due to splicing, exchange of structural cassettes among genes during transcription, and posttranslational modifications. The field of proteomics seeks to understand the complex interactions of all proteins expressed within a tissue or organism under normal or perturbed conditions. Indeed, human proteomics is in its infancy.[53]

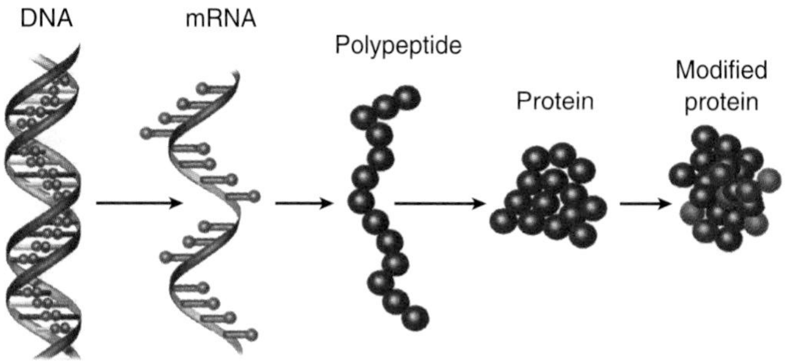

FIGURE 69–13 Relationship of the genome to the proteome. Examples of common posttranslational modifications include the addition to amino acids (blue balls) of sugars (glycosylation), phosphorylation, and prenylation depicted by the red and green balls.

The methods for proteome analysis are still under development and validation. However, there are five basic elements to any proteomic analysis: sample acquisition, protein extraction, protein separation, protein sequence determination, and sequence comparison to reference databases for protein identification.[54] Sample acquisition is straightforward, involving obtaining a tissue biopsy or a plasma sample from an individual (under informed consent). Protein extraction is generally performed by chemical methods, generally with methanol, to remove all DNA, RNA, carbohydrates, and lipids. Extracted proteins must be separated for identification, and this step has traditionally been performed by two-dimensional gel electrophoresis. In the first dimension, proteins are separated by mass, and in the second dimension, they are separated by isoelectric point or net charge. Because most spots on a two-dimensional gel contain multiple protein constituents, alternate methods for separating and identifying proteins have evolved, including liquid chromatography. Liquid chromatography utilizes solid- and liquid-phase media to separate proteins according to biochemical properties, including molecular mass, isoelectric point, or hydrophobicity. These liquid chromatography separations can be performed in series to improve resolution. Other types of chromatographic columns can be used to improve sensitivity and specificity, such as affinity chromatography in which a column contains antibodies specific to certain functions to achieve the desired separation. Following separation, the protein is identified, generally using some form of mass spectrometry (Fig. 69–14). Mass spectrometry converts proteins or peptides to charged species that can be separated on the basis of their mass-to-charge ratio. Several types of mass spectrometry ionization methods are in use, including electrospray ionization and matrix-assisted laser desorption ionization (MALDI). Peptide sequences identified with these methods must next be analyzed by comparison with known database sequences to determine the unequivocal identity of the protein. Once proteins in a given proteome have been identified, their relative abundance levels are determined to compare relative abundance of proteins in a normal or diseased state. Finally, a thorough analysis of a proteome should include some measure of function, whether it is in cultured cells or in animal models. This approach is similar to functional genomic analysis, in which it is critical to gauge the importance of a gene or mutation through determination of gene function.

Proteomic analysis is currently limited by sensitivity, specificity, and throughput. However, this field and its methodologies are developing rapidly. The application of proteomics to cardiovascular disease holds great promise for understanding the function of the cardiovascular system in all its complexity.

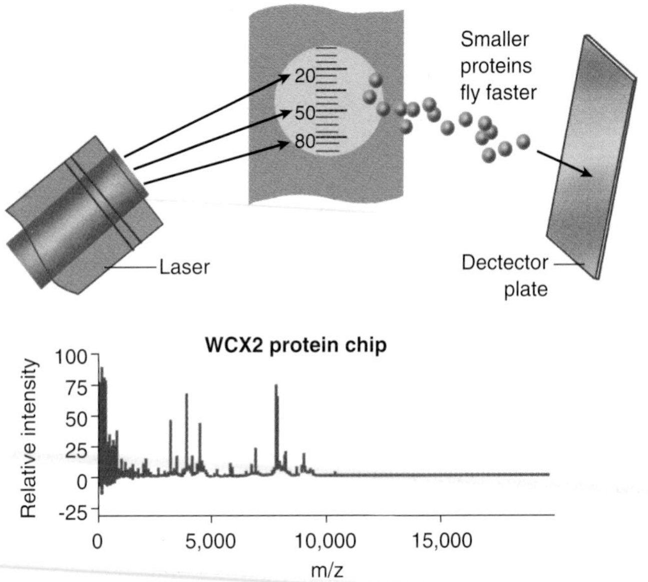

FIGURE 69–14 Mass spectrometry to identify separated proteins. A sample of serum or plasma is applied to the surface of a protein-binding chip, and the chip is irradiated with a laser where bound proteins are launched as ions. A time of flight to detection by an electrode is a measure of the mass-to-charge ratio (m/z) of the ion, which is displayed graphically.

Genetic Modification of Mice to Study Human Cardiovascular Disease

The techniques for generating genetically modified mice has had a tremendous impact on cardiovascular research. The mouse is a small animal with a short gestation period (21 days). Yet, there is remarkable conservation of the molecular pathways that control cardiovascular development and function between mice and humans. Similar genes and signaling pathways regulate the development of the heart and vasculature in both species.[55] With completion of sequencing of the mouse and human genome, comparative genetics is now possible.[56] For these reasons, genetically modified mice have become an essential animal model to study cardiovascular genetics, developmental biology, and physiology. Limitations of mouse models to study human cardiovascular disease are evident, but due to the simplicity of genetic manipulation in the mouse, it has become a standard starting place for hypothesis testing prior to evaluation in a larger animal. This section briefly describes the principles of four approaches to genetic modification in the mouse: transgenics, gene deletion or "knockout," conditional knockout, and studying mouse physiology. The reader is referred to other sources for in-depth reviews.[57]

Transgenic Mice

Creation of a transgenic mouse involves four steps: cloning of the gene of interest; fusion of the gene to transcriptional regulatory sequences that program its expression in all tissues of the mouse or in specific tissues; injection of the purified transgene into the male pronucleus of a fertilized one-cell mouse embryo; and reimplantation of the injected embryo into a foster mother. The injected transgene randomly integrates into a chromosome of the fertilized embryo, resulting in a founder mouse that expresses the injected transgene and that passes the transgene to 50 percent of its progeny. Comparative studies can then be performed between the transgenic mouse and nontransgenic littermate mouse as a control. Production of a founder transgenic mouse is now routinely performed in many laboratories and is accomplished generally in less than a month. Similar techniques have been used to create transgenic rabbits, rats, and pigs.

Refinements of these techniques have facilitated more sophisticated transgenic models. Cell-specific promoters program transgene expression exclusively in cardiomyocytes, endothelial cells, and vascular smooth muscle cells, creating a transgenic mouse with restricted expression in the cardiovascular system. While overexpression of a transgene results in a gain-of-function, it is also possible to eliminate the function of a single gene by overexpressing a dominant-negative mutant of that gene whose encoded protein interferes with the function of the wild-type protein. Expression of a transgene can also be turned on or off by administration of a simple drug like tetracycline using a tet operon system.[58] These mice allow precisely timed transgene expression as well as a comparison in the same animal of the phenotypes of transgene on and off states.

Gene Inactivation or Knockout Approaches

Gene deletion is a complementary approach to transgenesis for studying the role of a specific gene in mouse development and physiology (Fig. 69–15). In gene deletion studies, the expression of one or more genes is "knocked out" to produce a loss-of-function mutant mouse. The knockout approach involves the following steps: construction of a targeting vector containing the gene of interest with a deletion or nonsense mutation; transfection of a pluripotent mouse embryonic stem cell with the targeting vector; homologous recombination between the targeting construct and one copy of the endogenous gene, producing an embryonic stem cell with a homozygous deletion of the gene of interest; injection of the mutant embryonic stem cell into a fertilized mouse blastocyst; and implantation of the blastocyst into a foster mother. The resulting mouse pup is a chimera in which all tissues, including the gonads, are derived in part from the mutant embryonic stem cells and in part from the wild-type cells of the injected blastocysts. This chimeric animal is bred to a wild-type animal, and fertilization of a wild-type egg with a mutant sperm from the chimera produces a heterozygous knockout mouse in which one copy of the gene of interest in all cells is mutant and the other copy is wild-type. Heterozygous animals are then bred with each other to produce homozygous knockouts that have deletions of the gene of interest in all cells. The absence of the gene in the knockout animal produces a specific phenotype that reveals the direct function of the gene in development and normal and perturbed physiology. Creation of a knockout mouse is technically more challenging that transgenesis and often takes 9 to 12 months to complete.

Conditional Knockout Mice

Inactivation of important genes commonly results in early embryonic lethal phenotypes that are difficult to analyze and understand. As a result, methods have been developed to delete genes in a tissue-specific fashion and/or to inactivate genes at different times in development. In addition, it is often of interest to produce specific mutations of genes rather than to eliminate their expression completely. Homologous recombination is also used to introduce specific mutations into wild-type genes; the difference in technique is that these "knock-ins" utilize a targeting construct containing a mutant gene rather than a gene deletion. Other homologous recombination approaches permit introduction of a distinct or unrelated gene into a foreign genetic locus to regulate the new gene under the control of the promoter of the targeted locus.

Another approach to tissue-specific gene deletion is use of a bacterial phage recombination system called Cre-lox.[59] A P1

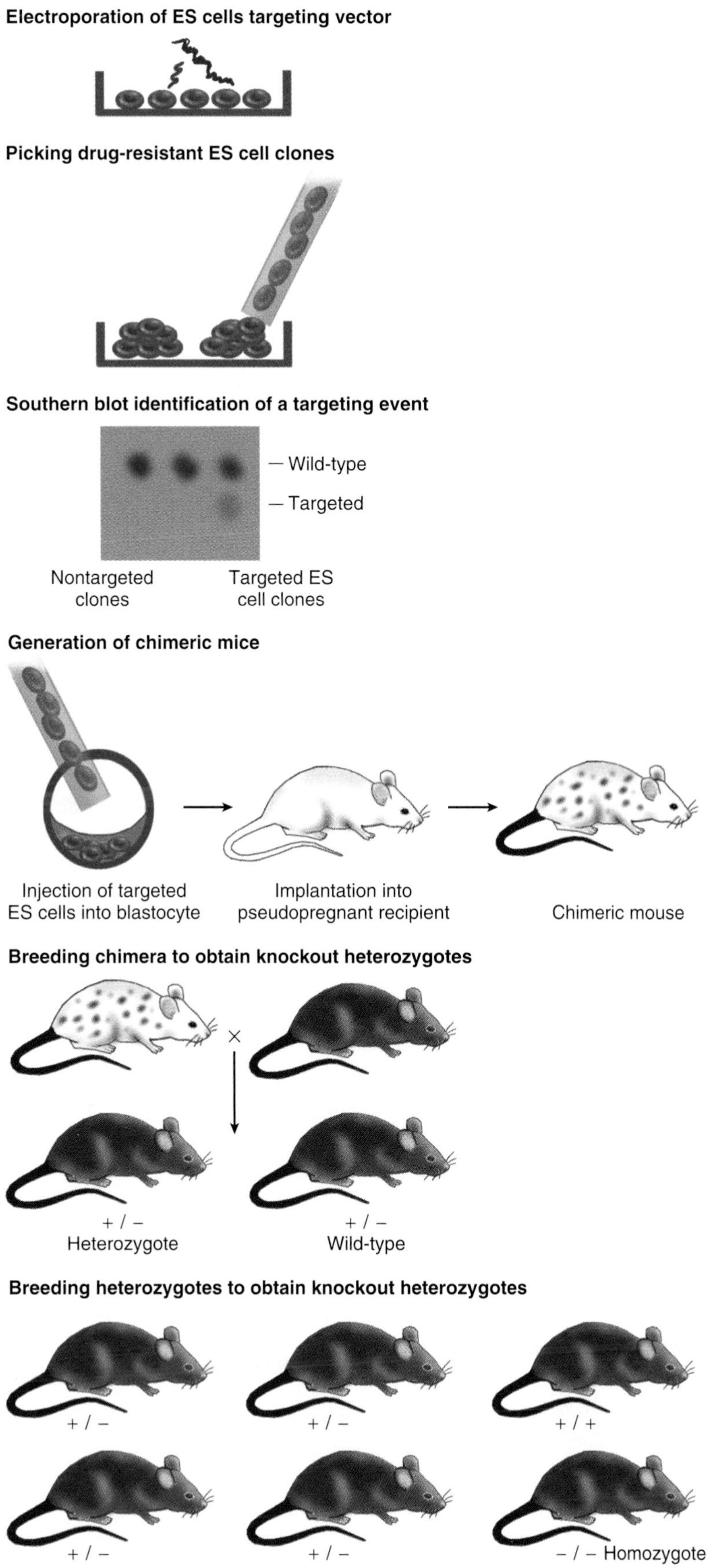

FIGURE 69–15 Scheme for generating heterozygous and homozygous gene knockout mice by homologous recombination in mouse embryonic stem (ES) cells.

bacteriophage encodes an enzyme called Cre that catalyzes recombination of DNA between two specific sequences (called loxP sites) that signal recombination. This system has been adapted in mice by producing a targeting construct in which the gene of interest is *flanked* by *lox*P sites (a "floxed allele"). Mice homozygous for the floxed allele are bred with transgenic mice that express the Cre recombinase in a tissue-specific manner (e.g., endothelial cells, vascular smooth muscle cells, cardiomyocytes). The resulting mice have a deletion of the gene of interest only in the tissue expressing the Cre recombinase. By placing the Cre transgene under the control of a tetracycline responsive promoter, gene deletion is programmed only following tetracycline feeding.

Studies of Mouse Physiology

Realizing the advantage of the potential of mouse genetics requires technologies that can characterize the phenotype of mutant mice. The mouse is technically challenging because the heart and blood vessels are very small in size and the resting mouse heart beat is greater than 500 beats/min. Miniaturized instrumentation and microsurgical techniques have helped solve these problems.[60,61] It is now possible to obtain a wide variety of physiological measurements in anesthetized and intubated mice, including aortic blood pressures, left ventricular pressure tracings, and cardiac hemodynamics before and after infusions of pharmacological agents, such as dobutamine or isoproterenol. Noninvasive imaging of the heart and vasculature has improved substantially, and two-dimensional echocardiograms are now routine in fetal and adult mice. Magnetic resonance imaging renders clear images of cardiac structure and function. These noninvasive techniques are used to measure end-systolic and end-diastolic left ventricular dimensions, left ventricular wall thickness and mass, and shortening fraction. Myocardial infarctions produced by coronary artery ligation, wire injuries to vessels that simulate angioplasty, and aortic banding to induce left ventricular hypertrophy are commonly performed in gene modified mice. Exercise testing, 24-hour electrocardiogram recordings on conscious mice using implanted transducers, and electrophysiological studies to detect inducible cardiac arrhythmias are also standard techniques. With the availability of techniques to study cardiovascular physiology, genetically modified mice now provide an accurate and convenient way to evaluate the function of specific genes in cardiovascular disease.

Gene- and Cell-Based Therapies

Gene transfer is the introduction and expression of recombinant genes in mammalian cells. Gene transfer aims to introduce recombinant genes into target cells to study the mechanisms and consequences of gene expression. Genes are transfected into cells using vectors. The recombinant gene undergoes transcription into RNA and translation into protein by host enzymes, culminating in the expression of the recombinant protein. The recombinant protein remains intracellular or is secreted into the extracellular space or circulation. Gene expression is transient or stable, depending on whether integration into chromosomes occurs. The efficiency of DNA uptake and gene expression, often referred to as *transfection efficiency*, depends on many factors, including delivery of DNA to the cell, uptake of DNA into the cytoplasm, degradation of DNA in endosomes, release of DNA from endosomes into the cytoplasm, transport to the nucleus, and persistence in the nucleus.

In vivo gene transfer is performed by cell-mediated or direct gene transfer methods. Cell-mediated or ex vivo gene transfer involves removing autologous cells from the host and transfecting the cells with the vector in vitro.[62] Genetically modified cells are reintroduced into the host by infusion or injection. Ex vivo gene transfer permits the introduction of recombinant genetic material into a specific cell—for example, endothelial or smooth muscle cells—and analysis of recombinant gene expression within that cell type.

In vivo gene transfer employs the direct introduction of recombinant genes into target cells and tissues.[63] Targeted gene transfer in the vasculature has been performed with cell-specific promoters to achieve gene expression within endothelial cells or smooth muscle cells.[64] Both ex vivo and in vivo gene transfer approaches have been employed in the development of animal models of vascular disease and in clinical trials of gene transfer to the cardiovascular system.

Vectors

Transfection of appropriate target cells represents the critical first step in gene transfer. As a result, development of gene transfer methods has represented a significant area of research in the field. Both viral and nonviral vectors have been employed in vascular gene transfer studies. A common feature of these methods is the efficient delivery of genes into cells. Vectors differ, however, in the processing of foreign DNA and the frequency of integration into chromosomal DNA. In the case of retroviral and lentiviral vectors, the transferred sequences are stably integrated into the chromosomal DNA of the target cell. These vectors have been considered most often for ex vivo gene therapy. Other methods of gene transfer result primarily in the introduction of foreign DNA into target cell nuclei in an unintegrated form. These methods result in high, but transient, gene expression. These vectors, including adenovirus, adeno-associated virus, and cationic liposomes, have been employed predominantly for in vivo gene transfer studies.

Retroviruses

Retroviruses were the first vectors employed in gene transfer studies, dating back to the 1980s. Initial interest in retroviruses as vectors arose from the observation that these vectors stably transduce nearly 100 percent of proliferating target cells in culture. Retroviral vectors were used initially in vascular gene transfer studies, primarily in ex vivo studies, but their use has been limited by low transfection efficiencies. Retroviral vectors have been used recently in clinical gene therapy studies for treatment of severe combined immune deficiency (SCID). Unfortunately, in one trial, two children experienced the complication of retroviral insertion into an oncogenic site of chromosome X, leading to leukemia.[65]

Adenovirus

Adenovirus type 2 and type 5 are the two serotypes used for vectors in cardiovascular gene transfer. The adenovirus genome is linear, double-stranded DNA, approximately 36 kb in length, which is divided into 100 map units, each of which is 360 base pairs in length. The DNA contains short inverted terminal repeats (ITRs) at the end of the genome that are required for viral DNA replication. The gene products are organized into early (E1-E4) and late (L1-L5) regions, based on expression before or after initiation of DNA replication. Adenoviruses have a lytic life cycle characterized by attachment to an adenoviral glycoprotein receptor on mammalian cells and entry into cells by receptor-mediated endocytosis. Adenoviral capsid proteins protect adenoviruses from lysosomal degradation, and viral DNA translocates to the nucleus. Expression of viral genes depends on cellular transcription factors and expression of the adenoviral E1 region, which encodes a transactivator of viral gene expression. During lytic infection, the viral genome replicates to several thousand copies per cell. The viral genome associates with core proteins and is packaged into capsids by self-assembling of major capsid proteins.

The adenovirus genome is rendered replication-deficient to generate a vector. Vectors are constructed by homologous recombination in a cell line known as 293 cells by cotransfection of (1) a bacterial plasmid containing the cDNA of interest and a small region of adenoviral genome deleted from E1A and E1B regions (these regions regulate adenoviral transcription and are required for viral replication), and (2) an incomplete adenoviral genome. Homologous recombination between the two DNAs generates a recombinant genome in which the foreign gene replaces the E1 region. Viral stock is further propagated in 293 cells to high titer, generally 10^9 to 10^{10} plaque-forming units (pfu) per milliliter.

Adenoviral vectors have several additional advantages, including efficient infection of mammalian cells and expression in nondividing cells in vitro and in vivo. These vectors are relatively stable and can be grown and concentrated to a high titer. Extrachromosomal replication of the vector greatly reduces the chance of mutation by random integration and dysregulation of host cellular genes. However, a number of shortcomings limit their use as gene transfer vectors. Gene expression in vascular and myocardial cells following adenoviral infection is short-lived, persisting for only several weeks.[66-68] Host immune response to adenoviral proteins is a major limitation to their in vivo use. Although low levels of neutralizing antibodies do not appear to have adverse clinical effects, it remains to be determined whether host immune responses to the adenovirus will preclude repeated administrations of the same serotype of adenovirus. First-generation recombinant adenoviral vectors (deletion of E1A and E1B genes and partial deletion of E3 genes) have been used clinically in gene therapy studies, even though in animal models these vectors are often associated with tissue inflammation, particularly in the liver and lung.[69] Direct exposure of diseased liver to high-titer adenoviral vectors is highly toxic, and in one case, unfortunately lethal.[70] Inactivation of the E2A gene has been associated with longer gene expression and less inflammation in lung and liver. In arterial gene transfer studies employing adenoviral vectors, mononuclear inflammatory cell infiltrates have been observed in the adventitia of peripheral[71] and pulmonary[68] arteries, but no necrosis or vasculitis was observed. Infection of pulmonary arteries with adenovirus was associated with mild degrees of perivascular inflammation; however, pulmonary arteries instilled with saline or liposomes also exhibited mild accumulation of perivascular mononuclear cells.[68] Despite the limitations of immune responses to adenoviral capsid proteins, adenoviral vectors are attractive vehicles for in vivo gene transfer in animal models because of the efficiency of transfection. Whether adenoviral vectors will be used clinically remains to be seen.

Adeno-Associated Virus

Adeno-associated virus (AAV) is a defective human parvovirus that has attractive features as a gene transfer vector. This viral vector is prepared at high titers, is not normally pathogenic in humans, and infects many cell types in vitro.[72] The AAV genome is a single-stranded, linear, 5 kb DNA molecule. The wild-type AAV integrates in a site-specific fashion into a single 7 kb region on human chromosome 19. The AAV genome is flanked by 145 base pair–inverted terminal repeats containing the sequences required for packaging, DNA replication, and integration. The coding region contains two open reading frames, which are deleted and replaced with one or more cDNAs plus transcriptional regulatory units during vector construction.[73] AAV vectors accept transgene cassettes of only 4 to 5 kb; this limits the types of transgenes that can be used. Propagation of AAV vectors requires complex packaging, including AAV Rep and Cap proteins and five adenoviral proteins (E1A, E1B, E2A, E4, and VA). These complex packaging requirements have precluded construction of a helper cell line for AAV. Currently, vectors are constructed by cotransfection of cells with the AAV vector and a non-packageable plasmid containing the AAV Rep and Cap proteins. This is followed by infection of the transfected cells with wild-type or mutant helper adenovirus. AAV is separated from contaminating adenovirus by heat treatment and equilibrium density gradation centrifugation. Protocols for constructing AAV vectors are described elsewhere.[72]

The AAV vectors infect multiple cell types in vitro, but their utility in vivo has not been established. Transduction of vascular endothelial and smooth muscle cells remains unknown.[74] Further limitations include a lack of packaging cell lines and a requirement for coinfection with adenovirus, making it difficult to prepare large quantities of pure AAV vectors. Deletion of viral genes during vector construction limits the ability of these vectors to integrate in a site-specific manner but does raise the possibility of insertional mutagenesis. AAV vectors are theoretically attractive, but considerable work is required before they can be implemented clinically.

Cationic Liposomes

Cationic lipids are preparations of positively charged lipids that spontaneously complex with negatively charged DNA to form DNA-lipid conjugates. The lipid component facilitates delivery of DNA to cells by fusion with plasmid membrane or with endosomal membranes after endocytosis. Following release from endosomes, plasmid DNA is maintained in an extrachromosomal form. Cationic liposomes have been employed in arterial gene transfer studies in many animal models, including rats, rabbits, dogs, and pigs. Advantages of cationic liposomes include a favorable safety profile, a lack of viral coding sequences, and no cDNA size constraints. Minimal biochemical, hemodynamic, or cardiac toxicity has been associated with their use in animals or humans.[75] These vectors are straightforward to prepare for experimental and clinical use. The limitations include a low transfection efficiency and short-term gene expression.

Polymers

Nucleic acids and drugs have been applied to polymer gels coated onto stents or balloons and directly applied to arteries. Hydrogel catheters were developed to transmit plasmid DNA to rabbit arteries in vivo and to humans in clinical gene therapy trials.[76] Over time, other polymers were developed associated with stenting of arteries, but many early polymers were associated with intense inflammatory reactions. Newer formulations have been successfully used in the development of drug-eluting stents.[77,78]

Animal Models

Gene transfer is a useful approach to introduce nucleic acids to somatic cells of an animal to define gene function, dissect disease pathophysiology, or achieve a therapeutic effect. Over the past decade, gene transfer has been employed in many animal models of cardiovascular disease.[79] Gene- and cell-based approaches have been used, including a recent interest in combining gene transfer with stem cell based therapies.[80,81] Gene transfer as a tool to induce vascular growth is an illustrative example.

Vascular growth proceeds through the stages of angiogenesis, arteriogenesis, and lymphangiogenesis. Angiogenesis is the sprouting of new blood vessels from preexisting vessels. Arteriogenesis is the enlargement of muscular collateral blood vessels from preexisting arteriolar anastomoses and is often referred to as "collateralization." Lymphangiogenesis is the generation of new lymphatic vessels from preexisting ones. It has been widely used in preclinical and clinical studies. Two splice variants of vascular endothelial growth factor (VEGF A), $VEGF_{165}$ and $VEGF_{121}$, have angiogenic properties in animal models[82] and have been evaluated in clinical trials.[83] Placental growth factor (PlGF) also has angiogenic activity in animals. PlGF binds to VEGFR-1 and has been implicated in angiogenesis under pathological conditions.[84] Interestingly, PlGF also promotes angiogenesis and arteriogenesis through mobilization of hematopoietic stem cells and endothelial progenitor cells from the bone marrow. The clinical relevance of VEGF, PlGF, and endothelial progenitor cells in the clinical treatment of ischemia remains undetermined, although there have been recent efforts at transducing stem cells with VEGF to enhance angiogenesis.[85,86] Other growth factors have been evaluated for their angiogenic properties in gene transfer models. Hypoxia-inducible transcription factor-1-alpha activates several angiogenic growth factors, including VEGF-A, VEGFR-2, insulin-like growth factor-2, and erythropoietin.[87] A leucine zipper transcription factor that activated VEGF transcription has also been recently described.[88]

The hypothesis that overexpression of growth factors will result in therapeutic vascular growth has been tested in several animal models of peripheral and myocardial ischemia, including ex vivo transduction of stem cells and endothelial progenitor cells.[82,86,89] Adenoviral-mediated VEGF and fibroblast growth factor delivery and vascular growth has been demonstrated in the myocardium and skeletal muscle by the proliferation and enlargement of capillaries, although cessation of therapy (or extinction of the transgene) leads to regression of most of the vessels. Expression of VEGF for more than 4 weeks leads to sufficient vascular remodeling that new vessel growth persists for several months after VEGF treatment is withdrawn.[90] In animal models, hemodynamic factors and persistence of blood flow are important for stabilization of the newly formed vessels. Furthermore, the predictive value of a preclinical animal model is inversely related to the animal size. Many applications and vectors work well in smaller animals, such as mice and rats, but scaling up to larger animals, such as pigs, dogs, and sheep, has proved difficult. Demonstration of efficacy in young, normal animals may not predict responses in older human patients with chronic diseases. Indeed, vascular growth is impaired in elderly and diabetic animals.[91] Many of the beneficial biological effects reported in animals may not be achievable in humans, given the limitations of current vectors.

Clinical Trials

Cardiovascular gene therapy trials have had a checkered course. Many phase I trials have been completed, but few have proceeded to phase II studies. Concerns have been raised about the use of adenoviral vectors, even for cardiac or vascular applications, as well as low transfection efficiencies in vivo. The majority of studies have focused on stimulation of angiogenesis and arteriogenesis to improve perfusion of myocardial or skeletal muscle. Three phases of therapeutic angiogenesis trials have been conducted to date. Initial phase I trials employed plasmid DNA[76,92,93] and adenoviruses[94,95] to induce angiogenesis for peripheral or myocardial ischemia. These trials evaluated the safety of vectors and catheter or direct injection delivery in small numbers of patients. Consistent findings were evident: no serious adverse events were encountered attributable to the gene vector or delivery device. With this demonstration of safety, phase I/II trials evaluated larger numbers of patients with soft efficacy endpoints.[96-104] No major adverse events were reported, and while positive efficacy findings were reported, many of these trials were not controlled. Collectively, however, the following clinical insights accrued. Placebo effects are common in treated patients, perhaps due to altered hemodynamics or improved clinical care. Meaningful clinical endpoints were not always predefined and hence cast doubt on efficacy data. The absence of controlled, randomized studies also did not help the field move forward. Recently, a third phase of clinical trials has been initiated with placebo-controlled studies, including larger numbers of patients and well-defined clinical endpoints.[105-114] Data from these phase III studies and long-term follow-up are essential in determining whether a gene therapy product will be approved by the Food and Drug Administration and clinically used to treat myocardial and/or peripheral ischemia. Improved understanding of the pharmacokinetics is essential.[115] Investigators must proceed with carefully conducted and evaluated trials.

Future Directions

Molecular and cellular biology are now part of mainstream cardiovascular research. These approaches have advanced our understanding of the pathogenesis of cardiovascular diseases, have led to the development of extremely useful animal models, and have provided the basic principles for molecular therapies. Cardiovascular research is now turning to molecular genetics as the next scientific arena in which major advances will occur. To date, we have begun to understand the mechanisms by which single genes cause cardiovascular disease. These mechanisms have provided great insight into the pathophysiology of complex common cardiovascular disorders. The next major challenge in the field of molecular genetics is to understand with greater clarity genetic susceptibility to common cardiovascular diseases. Genotyping, genomics, and proteomics are approaches with promise but are incompletely developed at this time. The information gleaned from these techniques will only be as good as the characterization of clinical phenotypes by thoughtful, observant physicians who detect unusual patterns of disease in their patients. While many investigators remain hopeful, we do not know the role that genetic or cell-based therapies will play in the practice of clinical cardiology. The efforts of many physician-scientists and clinical investigators are required to conduct careful, well-considered studies. Only then can the promise of molecular genetics be realized and applied to the care of cardiovascular patients.

REFERENCES

1. Alberts B, Johnson A, Lewis J, et al: Molecular Biology of the Cell. New York, Garland Science, 2002.
2. Lewin B. Genes VII. Oxford, Oxford University Press, 2000.
3. Edidin M: Lipids on the frontier: A century of cell-membrane bilayers. Nat Rev Mol Cell Biol 4:414, 2003.
4. Shi Y, Massague J: Mechanisms of TGF-beta signaling from cell membrane to the nucleus. Cell 113:685, 2003.
5. Weis K: Regulating access to the genome: Nucleocytoplasmic transport throughout the cell cycle. Cell 112:441, 2003.
6. Bonifacino JS, Lippincott-Schwartz J: Coat proteins: Shaping membrane transport. Nat Rev Mol Cell Biol 4:409, 2003.
7. Williams RR, Fisher AG: Chromosomes, positions please! Nat Cell Biol 5:388, 2003.
8. Eichler EE, Sankoff D: Structural dynamics of eukaryotic chromosome evolution. Science 301:793, 2003.
9. Page SL, Hawley RS: Chromosome choreography: The meiotic ballet. Science 301:785, 2003.
10. Cline SD, Hanawalt PC: Who's on first in the cellular response to DNA damage? Nat Rev Mol Cell Biol 4:361, 2003.
11. Lawen A: Apoptosis: An introduction. Bioessays 25:888, 2003.
12. Roberts JM: Evolving ideas about cyclins. Cell 98:129, 1999.
13. Sherr CJ: The Pezcoller lecture: Cancer cell cycles revisited. Cancer Res 60:3689, 2000.
14. Roberts JM, Sherr CJ: Bared essentials of CDK2 and cyclin E. Nat Genet 35:9, 2003.
15. Sherr CJ, Roberts JM: CDK inhibitors: Positive and negative regulators of G1-phase progression. Genes Dev 13:1501, 1999.

16. Conqueret O: New roles for p21 and p27 cell-cycle inhibitors: A function for each cell compartment? Trends Cell Biol 13:65, 2003.
17. Lowe SW, Sherr CJ: Tumor suppression by Ink4a-Arf: Progress and puzzles. Curr Opin Genet Dev 13:77, 2003.
18. Nabel EG: CDKs and CKIs: Molecular targets for tissue remodeling. Nat Rev Drug Discov 1:587, 2002.
19. Nabel EG, Boehm M, Akyurek LM, et at: Cell cycle signaling and cardiovascular disease. Cold Spring Harb Symp Quant Biol 67:163, 2002.
20. Gartel AL, Tyner AL: The role of the cyclin-dependent kinase inhibitor p21 in apoptosis. Mol Cancer Ther 1:639, 2002.
21. Vogelstein B, Lane D, Levine AJ: Surfing the p53 network. Nature Nov 408:307, 2000.
22. Lander ES, Linton LM, Birren B, et al: Initial sequencing and analysis of the human genome. Nature 409: 860, 2001.
23. Venter JC, Adams MD, Myers EW, et al: The sequence of the human genome. Science 291:1304, 2001.
24. Collins FS, Green ED, Guttmacher AE, et al: A vision for the future of genomics research. Nature 422:835, 2003.
25. Sambrook J, Russell DW: Molecular cloning: A laboratory manual. Cold Spring Harbor, Cold Spring Harbor Laboratory, 2001.
26. Watson JD, Crick FHC: Molecular structure of nucleic acids: A structure for deoxyribose nucleic acid. Nature 171:737, 1953.
27. NCBI: Online Mendelian Inheritance in Man. Available at: http://www.ncbi.nlm.nih.gov/omim
28. Nabel EG: Cardiovascular disease. N Engl J Med 349:60, 2003.
29. Wang DG, Fan JB, Siao CJ, et al: Large-scale identification, mapping, and genotyping of single-nucleotide polymorphisms in the human genome. Science 280:1077, 1998.
30. Goldstein JL, Hobbs HH, Brown MS: Familial hypercholesterolemia. *In* Scriver CR, Beaudet AL, Sly WS, et al (eds): The Metabolic & Molecular Bases of Inherited Disease. New York, McGraw-Hill, 2001.
31. Seidman JG, Seidman C: The genetic basis for cardiomyopathy: From mutation identification to mechanistic paradigms. Cell 104:557, 2001.
32. Keating MT, Sanguinetti MC: Molecular and cellular mechanisms of cardiac arrhythmias. Cell 104:569, 2001.
33. Ridker PM, Stampfer MJ: Assessment of genetic markers for coronary thrombosis: Promise and precaution. Lancet 353:687, 1999.
34. Lifton RP, Gharavi AG, Geller DS: Molecular mechanisms of human hypertension. Cell 104:545, 2001.
35. Riva A, Kohane IS: SNPper: Retrieval and analysis of human SNPs. Bioinformatics 18:1681-1685, 2002.
36. Cargill M, Altshuler D, Ireland J, et al: Characterization of single-nucleotide polymorphisms in coding regions of human genes. Nat Genetics 22:231, 1999.
37. Sachidanandam R, Weissman D, Schmidt SC, et al: A map of human genome sequence variation containing 1.42 million single nucleotide polymorphisms. Nature 409:928, 2002.
38. NCBI: Single Nucleotide Polymorphism. Available at: http://www.ncbi.nlm.nih.gov/SNP/
39. Sabeti PC, Reich DE, Higgins JM, et al: Detecting recent positive selection in the human genome from haplotype structure. Nature 419:832, 2002.
40. Couzin J: Human Genome. HapMap launched with pledges of $100 million. Science 298:941, 2002.
41. Syvänen A: Accessing genetic variation: Genotyping single nucleotide polymorphisms. Nat Rev Genet 2:930, 2001.
42. Wang DG, Fan J, Siao C, et al: Large-scale identification, mapping, and genotyping of single-nucleotide polymorphisms in the human genome. Science 280:1077, 1998.
43. Zwick ME, Cutler DJ, Chakravarti A: Patterns of genetic variation in Mendelian and complex traits. Annu Rev Genomics Hum Genet 1:387, 2000.
44. Glazier AM, Nadeu JH, Altman TJ: Finding genes that underlie complex traits. Science 298:2345, 2002.
45. Lohmueller KE, Pearce CL, Pike M, et al: Meta-analysis of genetic association studies supports a contribution of common variants to susceptibility to common disease. Nat Genet 33:177, 2003.
46. Mohike KL, Erdos MR, Scott LJ, et al: High-throughput screening for evidence of association by using mass spectrometry genotyping on DNA pools. PNAS 99:16928, 2002.
47. Storey JD, Tibshirani R: Statistical significance for genomewide studies. PNAS 100:9440, 2003.
48. Kennedy GC, Matsuzaki H, Dong S, et al: Large-scale genotyping of complex DNA. Nat Biotechnol 21:1233, 2003.
49. Butte A: The use and analysis of microarray DNA. Nat Rev Drug Disc 1:951, 2002.
50. Velculescu VE, Vogelstein B, Kinzler KW: Analysing uncharted transcriptomes with SAGE. Trends Genet 16:423, 2000.
51. Patino WD, Mian OY, Hwang PM: Serial analysis of gene expression: Technical considerations and applications to cardiovascular biology. Circ Res 91:565, 2002.
52. Lockhart DJ, Winzeler EA: Genomics, gene expression and DNA arrays. Nature 405:827, 2000.
53. Loscalzo J: Proteomics in cardiovascular biology and medicine. Circulation 108:380, 2003.
54. Arrell DK, Neverova I, Van Eyk JE: Cardiovascular proteomics: Evolution and potential. Circ Res 88:763, 2001.
55. Fishman MC, Olson EN, Chien KR: Molecular advances in cardiovascular development. *In* Chien KR, Braunwald E (eds): Molecular Basis of Cardiovascular Disease: A Companion to Braunwald's Heart Disease. Philadelphia, WB Saunders, 1999, pp 115-134.
56. Mouse Genome Sequencing Consortium: Initial sequencing and comparative analysis of the mouse genome. Nature 420:520, 2002.
57. Young SG, Lusis AJ, Hammer RE: Genetically modified animal models in cardiovascular research. *In* Chien KR, Braunwald E (eds): Molecular Basis of Cardiovascular Disease: A Companion to Braunwald's Heart Disease. Philadelphia, WB Saunders, 1999, pp 37-85.
58. Gossen M, Bujard H: Tight control of gene expression in mammalian cells by tetracycline-responsive promoters. Proc Natl Acad Sci U S A 89:5547, 1992.
59. Gu H, Marth JD, Orban PC, et al: Deletion of a DNA polymerase β gene segment in T cells using cell type-specific gene targeting. Science 265:103, 1994.
60. Chien KR: Cardiac muscle diseases in genetically engineered mice: Evolution of molecular physiology. Am J Physiol 269:h755, 1995.
61. Duckers HJ, Boehm M, True AL, et al: Heme oxygenase-1 protects against vascular constriction and proliferation. Nat Med 7:693, 2001.
62. Nabel EG, Plautz G, Boyce FM, et al: Recombinant gene expression in vivo within endothelial cells of the arterial wall. Science 244:1342, 1989.
63. Nabel EG, Plautz G, Nabel GJ: Site-specific gene expression in vivo by direct gene transfer into the arterial wall. Science 249:1285, 1990.
64. Akyürek LM, Yang Z-Y, Aoki K, et al: SM22 a promoter targets gene expression to vascular smooth muscle cells in vitro and in vivo. Mol Med 11:983, 2000.
65. Marshall E: Second child in French trial is found to have leukemia. Science 299:320, 2003.
66. Lemarchand P, Jones M, Yamada I, Crystal RG: In vivo gene transfer and expression in normal uninjured blood vessels using replication-deficient recombinant adenovirus vectors. Circ Res 72:1132, 1993.
67. Guzman RJ, Lemarchand P, Crystal RG, et al: Efficient gene transfer into myocardium by direct injection of adenovirus vectors. Circ Res 73:1202, 1993.
68. Muller DW, Gordon D, San H, et al: Catheter-mediated pulmonary vascular gene transfer and expression. Circ Res 75:1039, 1994.
69. Yang Y, Nunes FA, Berencsi K, et al: Cellular immunity to viral antigens limits E1-deleted adenoviruses for gene therapy. Proc Natl Acad Sci U S A 91:4407, 1994.
70. Somia N, Verma IM: Gene therapy: Trials and tribulations. Nat Rev Genet 1:91, 2002.
71. Ohno T, Gordon D, San H, et al: Gene therapy for vascular smooth muscle cell proliferation after arterial injury. Science 265:781, 1994.
72. Tal J: Adeno-associated virus-based vectors in gene therapy. J Biomed Sci 7:279, 2000.
73. Rolling F, Samulski RJ: AAV as a viral vector for human gene therapy. Generation of recombinant virus. Mol Biotechnol 3:9, 1995.
74. Lynch CM, Hara PS, Leonard JC, et al: Adeno-associated virus vectors for vascular gene delivery. Circ Res 80:497, 1997.
75. San H, Yang ZY, Pompili VJ, et al: Safety and short-term toxicity of a novel cationic lipid formulation for human gene therapy. Hum Gene Ther 4:781, 1993.
76. Isner JM, Pieczek A, Schainfeld R, et al: Clinical evidence of angiogenesis after arterial gene transfer of phVEGF165 in patient with ischaemic limb. Lancet 348:370, 1996.
77. Sousa JE, Serruys PW, Costa MA: New frontiers in cardiology: Drug-eluting stents: Part I. Circulation 107:2274, 2003.
78. Sousa JE, Serruys PW, Costa MA: New frontiers in cardiology: Drug-eluting stents: Part II. Circulation 107:2383, 2003.
79. Baskir R, Vale PR, Isner JM, Losordo DW: Angiogenic gene therapy: Pre-clinical studies and phase I clinical data. Kidney Int 61:110, 2002.
80. Mangi AA, Noiseux N, Kong D, et al: Mesenchymal stem cells modified with Akt prevent remodeling and restore performance of infarcted hearts. Nat Med 9:1195, 2003.
81. Hill JM, Dick AJ, Raman VK, et al: Serial cardiac magnetic resonance imaging of injected mesenchymal stem cells. Circulation 108:1009, 2003.
82. Isner JM: Myocardial gene therapy. Nature 415:234, 2002.
83. Yla-Herttuala S, Martin JF: Cardiovascular gene therapy. Lancet 355:213, 2000.
84. Lutun A, Tjwa M, Moons L, et al: Revascularization of ischemic tissues by PlGF treatment, and inhibition of tumor angiogenesis, arthritis and atherosclerosis by anti-Flt1. Nat Med 8:831, 2002.
85. Iwaguro H, Yamaguchi J, Kalka C, et al: Endothelial progenitor cell vascular endothelial growth factor gene transfer for vascular regeneration. Circulation 105:672, 2002.
86. Nabel EG: Stem cells combined with gene transfer for therapeutic vasculogenesis. Circulation 105:672, 2002.
87. Vincent KA, Shyu KG, Luo Y, et al: Angiogenesis is induced in a rabbit model of hindlimb ischemia by naked DNA encoding an HIF-1alpha/VP16 hybrid transcription factor. Circulation 102:2255, 2000.
88. Rebar EJ, Huang Y, Hickey R, et al: Induction of angiogenesis in a mouse model using engineered transcription factors. Nat Med 8:1427, 2002.
89. Yla-Herttuala S, Alitalo K: Gene transfer as a tool to induce therapeutic vascular growth. Nat Med 9:694, 2003.
90. Dor Y, Djonov V, Abramovitch R, et al: Conditional switching of VEGF provides new insights into adult neovascularization and pro-angiogenic therapy. EMBO J 21:1939, 2002.
91. Schratzberger P, Walter DH, Rittig K, et al: Reversal of experimental diabetic neuropathy by VEGF gene transfer. J Clin Invest 107:1083, 2001.
92. Baumgartner I, Pieczek A, Manor O, et al: Constitutive expression of phVEGF165 after intramuscular gene transfer promotes collateral vessel development in patients with critical limb ischemia. Circulation 97:1114, 1998.
93. Isner JM, Baumgartner I, Rauh G, et al: Treatment of thromboangiitis obliterans (Buerger's disease) by intramuscular gene transfer of vascular endothelial growth factor: Preliminary clinical results. J Vasc Surg 28:964, 1998.
94. Laitinen M, Makinen K, Manninen H, et al: Adenovirus-mediated gene transfer to lower limb artery of patients with chronic critical leg ischemia. Hum Gene Ther 9:1481, 1998.
95. Losordo DW, Vale PR, Symes JF, et al: Gene therapy for myocardial angiogenesis: Initial clinical results with direct myocardial injection of phVEGF165 as sole therapy for myocardial ischemia. Circulation 98:2800, 1998.
96. Symes JF, Losordo DW, Vale PR, et al: Gene therapy with vascular endothelial growth factor for inoperable coronary artery disease. Ann Thorac Surg 68:830, 1999.

97. Vale PR, Losordo DW, Milliken CE, et al: Left ventricular electromechanical mapping to assess efficacy of phVEGF(165) gene transfer for therapeutic angiogenesis in chronic myocardial ischemia. Circulation 102:965, 2000.
98. Laitinen M, Hartikainen J, Kiltunen MO, et al: Catheter-mediated vascular endothelial growth factor gene transfer to human coronary arteries after angioplasty. Hum Gene Ther 11:263, 2000.
99. Vale PR, Losordo DW, Milliken CE, et al: Randomized, single-blind, placebo-controlled pilot study of catheter-based myocardial gene transfer for therapeutic angiogenesis using left ventricular electromechanical mapping in patients with chronic myocardial ischemia. Circulation 103:2138, 2001.
100. Rajagopalan S, Shah M, Luciano A, et al: Adenovirus-mediated gene transfer of VEGF(121) improves lower-extremity endothelial function and flow reserve. Circulation 104:753, 2001.
101. Sarkar N, Ruck A, Kallner G, et al: Effects of intramyocardial injection of phVEGF-A165 as sole therapy in patients with refractory coronary artery disease—12-month follow-up: Angiogenic gene therapy. J Intern Med 250:373, 2001.
102. Comerota AJ, Throm RC, Miller KA, et al: Naked plasmid DNA encoding fibroblast growth factor type 1 for the treatment of end-stage unreconstructible lower extremity ischemia: Preliminary results of a phase I trial. J Vasc Surg 35:930, 2002.
103. Losordo DW, Vale PR, Hendel RC, et al: Phase 1/2 placebo-controlled, double-blind, dose-escalating trial of myocardial vascular endothelial growth factor 2 gene transfer by catheter delivery in patients with chronic myocardial ischemia. Circulation 105:2012, 2002.
104. Shyu KG, Chang H, Wang BW, Kuan P: Intramuscular vascular endothelial growth factor gene therapy in patients with chronic critical leg ischemia. Am J Med 114:85, 2003.
105. Henry TD, Annex BH, McKendall GR, et al: The VIVA trial: Vascular endothelial growth factor in ischemia for vascular angiogenesis. Circulation 107:1359, 2003.
106. Simons M, Annex BH, Laham RJ, et al: Pharmacological treatment of coronary artery fibroblast growth factor-2: Double-blind, randomized, controlled clinical trial. Circulation 105:788, 2002.
107. Lederman RJ, Mendelsohn FO, Anderson RD, et al: TRAFFIC Investigators. Therapeutic angiogenesis with recombinant fibroblast growth factor-2 for intermittent claudication (the TRAFFIC study): A randomized trial. Lancet 359:2058, 2002.
108. Seiler C, Pohl T, Wustmann K, et al: Promotion of collateral growth by granulocyte-macrophage colony-stimulating factor in patients with coronary artery disease: A randomized, double-blind, placebo-controlled study. Circulation 104:2012, 2001.
109. Grines CL, Watkins MW, Helmer G, et al: Angiogenic Gene Therapy (AGENT) trial in patients with stable angina pectoris. Circulation 105:1291, 2002.
110. Makinen K, Manninen H, Hedman M, et al: Increased vascularity detected by digital subtraction angiography after VEGF gene transfer to human lower limb artery: A randomized, placebo-controlled, double-blinded phase II study. Mol Ther 6:127, 2002.
111. Hedman M, Hartikainen J, Syvanne M, et al: Safety and feasibility of catheter-based local intracoronary vascular endothelial growth factor gene transfer in the prevention of postangioplasty and in-stent restenosis and in the treatment of chronic myocardial ischemia: Phase II results of the Kuopio Angiogenesis Trial (KAT). Circulation 107:2677, 2003.
112. Stewart DJ, et al: A phase 2, randomized, multicenter, 26-week study to assess the efficacy and safety of BIOBYPASS (AdGVVEGF121) delivered through minimally invasive surgery versus maximum medical treatment in patients with severe angina, advanced coronary artery disease, and no options for revascularizations. Circulation 106:23, 2002.
113. Rajagopalan S, Mohler E 3rd, Lederman RJ, et al: Regional Angiogenesis with Vascular Endothelial Growth Factor Trial. Regional angiogenesis with vascular endothelial growth factor (VEGF) in peripheral arterial disease: Design of the RAVE trial. Am Heart J 145:1114, 2003.
114. Kastrup J: Euroinject One trial. Late breaking clinical trials sessions, American College of Cardiology 2003, Chicago. J Am Coll Cardiol 41:1603, 2003.
115. Pislaru S, Janssens SP, Gersh BJ, Simari RD: Defining gene transfer before expecting gene therapy: Putting the horse before the cart. Circulation 106:631, 2002.

CHAPTER 70

Genetics and Cardiovascular Disease

Reed E. Pyeritz

Genetic Factors in Disease

Genes contribute to both the cause and the pathogenesis of virtually any abnormality of human physiology and behavior, including, of course, disorders of the heart and the vascular system. This statement carries two messages in addition to the obvious one. First, disease associated with even the most "environmental" of causes, such as trauma, malnutrition, and drug abuse, depends on the human body's response to the insult. How the stress of the initial insult is expressed (the *phenotype*) and how the patient suffers and perhaps recovers depend, to various and yet often poorly defined degrees, on the patient's *genotype*. This idea seems self-evident and verges on the trite, but it is frequently neglected. Some environmental insults, such as massive trauma or poisoning, are lethal to all, regardless of genotype. Nonetheless, as developments in fields such as pharmacogenetics and ecogenetics are defining genetic susceptibilities to human disease better and more simply, physicians must become increasingly attuned to the importance of the genotype.[1]

Second, the introductory statement emphasizes that genetic factors have roles in *both* cause and process; etiology and pathogenesis, although related, are conceptually distinct.[2] For example, the cause of sickle cell anemia is clearly a single mutant gene, but whether a patient homozygous for this mutation expresses all, some, or none of the manifestations of the disease depends on many other genetic and nongenetic factors. Conversely, the cause of pneumococcal pneumonia is equally evident, but the severity and resolution of the disease depend on the patient's immune competence (which in turn depends on genetic and nongenetic factors) as much as on treatment with an antibiotic.

The genotype, therefore, can be detrimental in at least two distinct ways. First, mutant genes can so upset embryology or physiology that a clinical abnormality occurs. Whereas the phenotype of any particular mutation depends on a host of factors, including which homeostatic systems are available to modulate the action of the defect, the genotype has the principal role in causing the disease. This class of mutations is usually referred to as *genetic diseases*. Second, a mutation can facilitate the action of an extrinsic cause in producing disease. Inherited susceptibilities are part of the pathogenesis of disease and are one reason for taking a patient's family history. Until recently, clinicians could do little to pursue tantalizing facts, such as several relatives' suffering myocardial infarction before age 50. The long-touted prospect of detecting a patient's inherited susceptibilities and intervening before irreversible clinical sequelae occur is becoming reality.

Two caveats are important. First, a considerable gap exists between identifying an apparently inherited susceptibility and prescribing an intervention of proven benefit. For example, several years ago a parental history of sudden death was found to identify middle-aged men at increased risk of sudden death, independent of myocardial infarction.[3] However, effective clinical use of this association will require understanding the pathological factors and conducting outcome studies of potential interventions. Second, the risk of "genetic determinism" remains ever-present. A recent study examined public perceptions of "a gene for heart disease"[4]; the concept was interpreted correctly by the majority of the sample, but an important minority thought in terms of an absolute risk that denoted inevitability.

Disorders Due to Microscopic Alterations in Chromosomes

The estimate of the total number of human genes has been revised downward, from 100,000 to about 35,000, as a result of the Human Genome Project. Two copies (termed *alleles*) of each gene are arrayed along 23 pairs of *chromosomes*. Twenty-two of the chromosomes are called *autosomes* (numbered 1 through 22), and the 23rd pair is the *sex chromosomes*, X and Y. Females have two X chromosomes and males have an X and a Y chromosome. Both autosomal alleles are potentially active in specifying RNA copies of their DNA sequences; whether a gene is active depends on the cell type, the developmental stage of the organism, and the regulatory molecules that interact with promoter and enhancer nucleotide sequences that control transcription of the gene. In cells with two X chromosomes (i.e., in all females, in persons with Klinefelter syndrome in which two Xs and one Y

TABLE 70–1 Genomic Disorders (Contiguous Gene Syndromes)

	Symbol	Genetic Defect	Cardiovascular Abnormalities
Syndromes with Cardiovascular Involvement			
Arteriohepatic dysplasia	AHD	del 20p11.23-p12.2	Peripheral pulmonic stenosis/hypoplasia
Cat-eye syndrome	CES	dup 22q11	Total anomalous pulmonary venous return
DiGeorge sequence	DGS	del 22q11	Truncus arteriosus, right aortic arch, TOF, PDA
Miller-Dieker syndrome	MDS	del 17p13	PDA ± complex anomalies
Prader-Willi syndrome	PWS/AS	del 15q12	Cor pulmonale (secondary to obesity and central apnea)
WAGR syndrome		del 11p13	Hypertension (secondary to Wilms tumor)
Syndromes without Frequent Cardiovascular Involvement			
Angelman syndrome	AS	del 15q12*	
Smith-Magenis syndrome	SMS	del 17p11.2	

*The deletion is often indistinguishable at the cytogenetic level from that of the Prader-Willi syndrome; genetic imprinting of locus *UBE3A* is thought to account in part for the phenotypic differences. In Prader-Willi syndrome, the deleted chromosome is always the chromosome 15 inherited from the father, whereas in Angelman syndrome, the deletion affects the maternal chromosome 15.

PDA = patent ductus arteriosus; TOF = tetralogy of Fallot; WAGR = Wilms tumor, aniridia, genitourinary, and retardation.

occur, and in persons with some other rare conditions), only one X is entirely active after early embryogenesis.

Human chromosomes can be examined by culturing cells capable of mitosis; T lymphocytes obtained from venous blood are the usual source, but fibroblasts, cells from chorionic villi, amniocytes, and leukocyte precursors present in bone marrow are also used clinically. Chromosomes are distinguished from one another by their size, shape (determined by the position of a constriction called the *centromere,* which functions as the attachment of the mitotic apparatus), and characteristic banding pattern as revealed by any of several staining techniques. The chromosomes are photographed, cut out, and arranged in pairs, from 1 through 22 and the sex chromosomes, in a display called the *karyotype.* This display and its interpretation are the end results of a clinical study of a patient's chromosomes. The chromosome constitution of a cell is designated by first specifying the number of chromosomes present (46 being normal in diploid cells), then specifying the sex chromosomes, and finally describing any abnormalities. For example, a normal male is designated 46,XY, and a female with an extra chromosome 21 is designated 46,XX,+21.

ANEUPLOIDY. Chromosome aberrations, especially too many or too few chromosomes (*aneuploidy*), are extremely common in human embryos; more than one-half of all conceptuses are spontaneously aborted in early pregnancy, and at least one-half of them are aneuploid. Among live-born infants, about 0.5 percent have a chromosome aberration.

Gain or loss of chromosomes generally happens by nondisjunction, or the failure of a homologous pair of chromosomes to separate. Absence of one chromosome is termed *monosomy;* all autosomal monosomies are embryonic lethals, as is presence of only a Y sex chromosome. The presence of three chromosomes is *trisomy,* and the presence of an entire extra set of chromosomes (for a total of 69) is *triploidy.* The most common autosomal aneuploidy, trisomy 21 associated with Down syndrome, and aneuploidy for sex chromosomes all are compatible with survival into adulthood.

CHROMOSOME REARRANGEMENTS. A chromosome can break and rejoin within itself, potentially giving rise to an *inversion* of genetic material. Often no apparent phenotypic effect occurs in people with an inversion, but because inversions can disrupt chromosome pairing during meiosis, their offspring may have more profound aberrations.

DELETIONS AND DUPLICATIONS. Just as their names imply, these aberrations are losses or gains of chromosomal material. Many clinical syndromes have been associated with aberrations of specific chromosome regions.[5] The smallest deletion detectable by light microscopy is associated with loss of considerable DNA, on the order of 1 million base pairs, so more than one gene is potentially disrupted or lost.

A number of conditions, each initially thought to be due to a mutation in a single locus, are associated with small interstitial chromosome aberrations affecting a cluster of genes (Table 70-1). So rather than pleiotropic manifestations of one mutation, these conditions are likely due to the effects of absences of several, and perhaps many, loci on one chromosome, and therefore are best thought of as *genomic disorders.* In the past, they were referred to as *contiguous gene syndromes.*[6] In the regions of the genome where these deletions occur, repetitive nucleotide sequences appear to predispose to aberrant recombination, and this accounts for their surprising incidence.[7] In addition, such defects are potentially heritable, and the occurrence of the disorder in a family behaves as a Mendelian dominant. Several interstitial deletions are both relatively common and important causes of congenital heart disease.

Disorders Due to Changes in Single Nuclear Genes (see Chap. 69)

Mutations of genes located on the 22 pairs of autosomes and the two sex chromosomes produce phenotypes inherited according to the two principal tenets of Mendel: alleles segregate and nonalleles assort. The first statement refers to gametes receiving only one of the two alleles at a given locus as a result of meiosis. The second statement describes the results of recombination, the meiotic process of rearranging DNA between the two chromosomes of the pair (*homologous chromosomes*); if two loci are widely spaced along a chromosome, their chances of being separated by recombination are 50-50, and they are said to be *unlinked.*

The Human Genome Project, begun in 1990, had goals to map all expressed genes, to create a physical map of overlapping pieces of DNA composing the entire genome, and finally, to sequence all 3.2 billion nucleotides in the haploid complement of human DNA. The project was completed well ahead of schedule, and more than 95 percent of the entire sequence now exists in public databases.[8] More than 12,000 individual loci have been identified, either on the basis of the phenotype that mutations in single genes produce, or through understanding the normal product or function of the gene.[9] The presumption of single-gene defects is based in most instances on the pattern of inheritance in families; segregation of the phenotype according to Mendelian principles is the central piece of evidence. For an increasing number of loci, however, molecular genetic techniques have mapped the phenotype to a narrow chromosome region or to a single gene, or even revealed the actual alteration in nucleotide sequence (see Chap. 69) (Table 70–2).[10] The range of known Mendelian variation in humans and information about gene mapping and molecular defects are routinely catalogued and available on-line.[11]

Of the more than 10,000 loci that have been clearly identified on the basis of either an abnormal phenotype or a normal product, 17.4 percent involve the heart.[11] Many others involve other parts of the cardiovascular system. Thousands

Text continued on p. 1873

TABLE 70–2 Mendelian Conditions that Involve the Cardiovascular System with Known Genetic Defects or Gene Mapping of the Phenotype

Phenotype	Gene Symbol	OMIM No.*	Gene Map Locus
Cardiomyopathies			
Adhalinopathy, primary	*SGCA*	600119	17q12-q21.33
Arrhythmogenic RV dysplasia-1	*ARVD1*	107970	14q23-q24
Arrhythmogenic RV dysplasia-2	*ARVD2*	600996	1q42-q43
Arrhythmogenic RV dysplasia-3	*ARVD3*	602086	14q12-q22
Arrhythmogenic RV dysplasia-4	*ARVD4*	602087	2q32.1-q32.3
Arrhythmogenic RV dysplasia-5	*ARVD5*	604400	3p23
Arrhythmogenic RV dysplasia-6	*ARVD6*	604401	10p12-p14
Becker and Duchenne muscular dystrophies	*DMD*	310200	Xp21.2
Emery-Dreifuss muscular dystrophy	*EMD*	310300	Xp28
Emery-Dreifuss muscular dystrophy	*LMNA*	150330	1q21.2-q21.3
Endocardial fibroelastosis-2	*TAZ*	302060	Xq28
FDC	*ACTC*	102540	15q14
FDC-1A	*CMD1A*	115200	1p11-q11
FDC-1B	*CMD1B*	600884	9q13
FDC-1C	*CMD1C*	601493	10q21-q23
FDC-1E	*CMD1E*	601154	3p25-p22
FDC-1F	*CMD1F*	602067	6q23
FDC-1G	*CMD1G*	604145	2q31
FDC-1H	*CMD1H*	604288	2q14-q22
FDC-2	*CMD1D*	601494	1q32
FDC, X-linked	*DMD*	310220	Xp21.2
FDC-3A	*TAZ*	302060	Xq28
FHC-1	*MYH7*	160760	14q12
FHC-2	*TNNT2*	191045	1q32
FHC-3	*TPM1*	191010	15q22.1
FHC-4	*MYBPC3*	600958	11p11.2
FHC	*TNNI3*	191044	19q13.4
FHC with WPW	*CMH6*	600858	7q3
FHC, mid-LV type	*MYL2*	160781	12q23-q24.3
FHC, mid-LV type	*MYL3*	160790	3p
Friedreich ataxia	*FRDA*	229300	9q13
Muscular dystrophy, Duchenne-like	*SGCA*	600119	17q12-q21.33
Myotonic dystrophy	*DMPK*	160900	19q13.2-q13.3
Myotonic dystrophy 2	*DM2*	602668	3q
Noncompaction of LV	*TAZ*	302060	Xq28
Developmental Disorders			
Alagille syndrome	*JAG1*	601920	20p12
Atrial septal defect, secundum	*ASDI*	108800	6p21.3
Atrial septal defect with AV conduction defects	*CSX*	600584	5q34
AV canal defect-1	*AVSD*	600309	1p31-p21
Bannayan-Zonana syndrome	*PTEN*	601728	10q23.3
Cardiac valve dysplasia-1	*CVD1*	314400	Xq28
Cat-eye syndrome	*CECR*	115470	22q11

Continued

TABLE 70–2 Mendelian Conditions that Involve the Cardiovascular System with Known Genetic Defects or Gene Mapping of the Phenotype—cont'd

Phenotype	Gene Symbol	OMIM No.*	Gene Map Locus
Conotruncal cardiac defects	*CTHM*	217095	22q11
DiGeorge sequence and velocardiofacial syndrome	*DGCR*	188400	del22q11
Down syndrome	*DCR*	190685	21q22.3
Ellis–van Creveld syndrome	*EVC*	225500	4p16
Goldenhar syndrome	*GHS*	141400	7p
Heterotaxy, X-lined visceral	*ZIC3*	306955	Xq26.2
Holt-Oram syndrome	*TBX5*	601620	12q24.1
Keutel syndrome	*MGP*	154870	12p13.1-p12.3
Left-right axis malformation	*TGFB4*	601877	1q42.1
Noonan syndrome	*NSI*	163950	12q24
Progeria	*LMNA*	176670	1q21.1
Total anomalous pulmonary venous return	*TAPVR1*	106700	4p13-q12
Turner syndrome	*RPS4X*	312760	Xq13.1
Werner syndrome	*WRN*	277700	8p12-p11.2
Williams syndrome	*ELN*	194050	del7q11
Wolf-Hirschhorn syndrome	*WHCR*	194190	4p16.3
Disorders of Blood Pressure			
Bartter syndrome	*SLC12A1*	600839	15q15-q21.1
Bartter syndrome with deafness	*BSND*	602522	1p31
Bartter syndrome, type 2	*KCNJ1*	600359	11q24
Bartter syndrome, type 3	*CLCNKB*	602023	1p36
Dysautonomia, familial	*DYS*	223900	9q31-q33
Hypertension, essential	*SAH*	145505	16p13.11
Hypertension, essential	*PNMT*	171190	17q21-q22
Hypertension, essential	*AGTR1*	106165	3q21-q25
Hypertension, essential	*GNB3*	139130	12p13
Hypertension, essential	*AGT*	106150	1q42-q43
Hypertension, low renin	*HSD11B2*	218030	16q22
Hypertension, salt resistant	*NPR3*	108962	5p14-p12
Hypertension, with brachydactyly	*HTNB*	112410	12p12.2-p11.2
Liddle syndrome	*SCNN1B*	600760	16p13-p12
Liddle syndrome	*SCNN1G*	600761	16p13-p12
Mineralocorticoid excess	*HSD11B2*	218030	16p22
Orthostatic hypotensive disorder	*OHDS*	143850	18q
Pheochromocytoma	*SDHB* *VHL* *RET* *SDHD*	185470 193300 164761 602690	1p36.1-p35 3p26-p25 10q11.2 11q23
Polycystic kidney disease, adult 1	*PKD1*	601313	16p13.3-p13.12
Polycystic kidney disease, adult 2	*PKD2*	173910	4q21-q23
Preeclampsia, susceptibility to	*NOS3*	163729	7q36
Preeclampsia, susceptibility to	*AGT*	106150	1q42-q43
Preeclampsia/eclampsia	*PEE*	189800	4q25-q34
Pulmonary hypertension, familial	*PPH1*	178600	2q31-q32

TABLE 70–2 Mendelian Conditions that Involve the Cardiovascular System with Known Genetic Defects or Gene Mapping of the Phenotype—cont'd

Phenotype	Gene Symbol	OMIM No.*	Gene Map Locus
Disorders of Coagulation and Thrombosis			
Antithrombin III deficiency	*AT3*	107300	1q23-q25
Antithrombin Pittsburgh defect	*PI*	107400	14q32.1
Coumarin resistance	*CYP2A6*	122720	19q13.2
Defective thromboxane A2 receptor	*TBXA2R*	188070	19p13.3
Dysfibrinogenemia, α type	*FGA*	134820	4q28
Dysfibrinogenemia, β type	*FGB*	134830	4q28
Dysfibrinogenemia, γ type	*FGG*	134850	4q28
Dysprothrombinemia	*F2*	176930	11p11-q12
Factor H deficiency	*HF1*	134370	1q32
Factor V deficiency	*F5*	227400	1q23
Factor VII deficiency	*F7*	227500	13q34
Factor X deficiency	*F10*	227600	13q34
Factor XI deficiency	*F11*	264900	4q35
Factor XII deficiency	*F12*	234000	5q33-qter
Factor XIIIA deficiency	*F13A1*	134570	6p25-p24
Factor XIIIB deficiency	*F13B*	134580	1q31-q32.1
Glanzmann thrombasthenia, type A	*ITGA2B*	273800	17q21.32
Glanzmann thrombasthenia, type B	*ITGB3*	173470	17q21.32
GNAQ deficiency	*GNAQ*	600998	9q21
Hemophilia A	*F8C*	306700	Xq28
Hemophilia B	*F9*	306900	Xq27.1-q27.2
PAI1 deficiency	*PAI1*	173360	7q21.3-q22
Plasmin inhibitor deficiency	*PLI*	262850	17pter-p12
Plasminogen activator deficiency	*PLAT*	173370	8p12
Plasminogen deficiency	*PLG*	173350	6q26
Platelet α/δ storage pool deficiency	*SELP*	173610	1q23-q25
Platelet disorder, familial with myeloid malignancy	*FPDMM*	601399	21q22.1-q22.2
Platelet glycoprotein IV deficiency	*CD36*	173510	7q11.2
Platelet-activating factor acetylhydrolase deficiency	*PAFAH*	601690	6p21.2-p12
Protein C inhibitor deficiency	*PCI*	601841	14q32.1
Protein S deficiency	*PROS1*	176880	3p11.1-q11.2
Thrombocythemia, essential	*THPO*	600044	3q26.3-q27
Thrombocytopenia, neonatal	*ITGA2B*	273800	17q21.32
Thrombocytopenia, Paris-Trousseau	*TCPT*	188025	11q23
Thrombocytopenia, X-linked	*WAS*	301000	Xp11.23-p11.22
Thrombophilia	*HRG*	142640	3q27
Thrombophilia	*PAI1*	173360	7q21.3-q22
Thrombophilia	*HCF2*	142360	22q11
Thrombophilia	*THBD*	188040	20p11.2
Thrombophilia	*PLG*	173350	6q26
Thromboxane synthase deficiency	*TBXAS1*	274180	7q34
Vitamin K–dependent coagulation defect	*GGCX*	137167	2p12
von Willebrand disease	*VWF*	193400	12p13.3
Warfarin sensitivity	*CYP2C9*	601130	10q24

Continued

TABLE 70–2 Mendelian Conditions that Involve the Cardiovascular System with Known Genetic Defects or Gene Mapping of the Phenotype—cont'd

Phenotype	Gene Symbol	OMIM No.*	Gene Map Locus
Disorders of Lipid Metabolism			
Abetalipoproteinemia	*MTP*	157147	4q22-q24
Abetalipoproteinemia	*APOB*	107730	2p24
Apo A-I and Apo C-III deficiency	*APOA1*	107680	11q23
Apo A-II deficiency	*APOA2*	107670	1q21-q23
Apo B-100 ligand defect	*APOB*	107730	2p24
Cerebrotendinous xanthomatosis	*CYP27A1*	213700	2q33-qter
Combined familial hyperlipidemia	*LPL*	238600	8p22
HMG-CoA synthetase-2 deficiency	*HMGCS2*	600234	1p13-p12
Hypercholesterolemia, familial	*LDLR*	143890	19p13.2-p13.1
Hypercholesterolemia, familial 3	*FH3*	603776	1p34.1-p32
Hypertriglyceridemia	*APOC3*	107720	11q23
Hypertriglyceridemia	*APOA1*	107680	11q23
Hypoalphalipoproteinemia	*APOA1*	107680	11q23
Hypobetalipoproteinemia	*APOB*	107730	2p24
Sitosterolemia	*STSL*	210250	2p21
Tangier disease	*HDLDT1*	205400	9q31
Wolman disease	*LIPA*	278000	10q24-q25
Metabolic Disorders with Primary Effects in the Cardiovascular System			
Carnitine acetyltransferase deficiency	*CRAT*	600184	9q34.1
Carnitine deficiency, systemic	*SLC22A5*	603377	5q33.1
Metabolic Disorders with Secondary Effects in the Cardiovascular System			
Amyloidosis	*APOA1*	107680	11q23
Amyloidosis, cerebroarterial	*APP*	104760	21q21.3-q22.05
Cerebral amyloid angiopathy	*CST3*	105150	20p11.2
Cerebrovascular disease, occlusive	*AACT*	107280	14q32.1
Coronary spasm, susceptibility to	*NOS3*	163729	7q36
Fabry disease	*GLA*	301500	Xq22
Gaucher disease with calcification	*GBA*	230800	1q21
Glycogen storage disease II (Pompe)	*GAA*	232300	17q25.2-q25.3
Hemochromatosis	*HFE*	235200	6p21.3
Homocystinuria	*CBS*	236200	21q22.3
Homocystinuria, MTHFR deficiency	*MTHFR*	236250	1p36.3
Menkes syndrome	*ATP7A*	300011	Xq12-q13
Mucopolysaccharidosis I	*IDUA*	252800	4p16.3
Mucopolysaccharidosis II	*IDS*	309900	Xq28
Mucopolysaccharidosis IVA	*GALNS*	253000	16q24.3
Mucopolysaccharidosis IVB	*GLB1*	230500	3p21.33
Mucopolysaccharidosis VI	*ARSB*	253200	5q11-q13
Mulibrey nanism	*MUL*	253250	17q22-q23
Pseudoxanthoma elasticum	*PXE*	264800	16p13.1
Neoplastic Disorders			
Carney (NAME) complex	*CNC*	160980	2p16
Paraganglioma, familial nonchromaffin 1	*PGL1*	168000	12q23

TABLE 70–2 Mendelian Conditions that Involve the Cardiovascular System with Known Genetic Defects or Gene Mapping of the Phenotype—cont'd

Phenotype	Gene Symbol	OMIM No.*	Gene Map Locus
Paraganglioma, familial nonchromaffin 2	*PGL2*	601650	11q13.1
von Hippel–Lindau syndrome	*VHL*	193300	3p26-p25
Primary Disorders of Rhythm and Conduction			
Heart block, progressive familial-1	*HB1*	113900	19q13.2-q13.3
Jervell and Lange-Nielsen syndrome	*KCNQ1*	192500	11p15.5
Jervell and Lange-Nielsen syndrome	*KCNE1*	176261	21q22.1-q22.2
Long-QT syndrome-1	*KCNQ1*	192500	11p15.5
Long-QT syndrome-2	*KCNH2*	152427	7q35-q36
Long-QT syndrome-3 and ventricular fibrillation, idiopathic	*SCN5A*	600163	3p24-p21
Long-QT syndrome-4	*LQT4*	600919	4q25-q27
Long-QT syndrome-5	*KCNE2*	603796	21q22.1
Ventricular tachycardia, idiopathic	*GNAI2*	139360	3p21
Primary Disorders of Vasculature			
Aneurysm, familial and Ehlers-Danlos, vascular type	*COL3A1*	120180	2q31
Arterial calcification of infancy	*ENPP1*	208000	6q22-q23
Cerebral arteriopathy with subcortical infarcts and leukoencephalopathy	*NOTCH3*	600276	19p13.2-p13.1
Cerebral cavernous malformations-1	*CCM1*	116860	7q11.2-q21
Cerebral cavernous malformations-2	*CCM2*	603284	7p15-p13
Cerebral cavernous malformations-3	*CCM3*	603285	3q25.2-q27
Fibromuscular dysplasia of arteries	*COL3A1*	120180	2q31
Hemangioma, capillary infantile	*HC1*	602089	5q31-q33
Hemiplegic migraine, familial	*CACNA1A*	601011	19p13
Hemiplegic migraine, familial 2	*MHP2*	602481	1q21-q23
Hemiplegic migraine, familial, susceptibility to	*MFTS*	300125	Xq
Hereditary hemorrhagic telangiectasia-1	*ENG*	131195	9q34.1
Hereditary hemorrhagic telangiectasia-2	*ALK1*	601284	12q11-q14
Lymphedema, hereditary	*FLT4*	136352	5q35.3
Marfan syndrome	*FBN1*	134797	15q21.1
Moyamoya disease	*MYMY*	252350	3p26-p24.2
Supravalvular aortic stenosis	*ELN*	130160	7q11.2
Venous malformations, multiple	*TEK*	600221	9p21

*Refers to the entry for the locus in http://www.ncbi.nlm.nih.gov/Omim/.
AV = atrioventricular; FDC = familial dilated cardiomyopathy; FHC = familial hypertrophic cardiomyopathy; LV = left ventricle; RV = right ventricle.
Disorders may have been mapped by the phenotype, by the gene, or both. The annotations p and q refer to band patterns in chromosomes detected cytochemically that mark specific regions.

of loci have been mapped to a specific region of the genome. Many of these loci, when mutated, cause Mendelian disorders, and the genetic map of these loci represents the "morbid anatomy of the human genome." Some of the cardiovascular and hemostatic disorders that were mapped by mid-2003 are shown in Figure 70–1. Knowledge of the molecular etiology of the monogenic disorders, most of which are relatively rare, will undoubtedly lead to improved understanding of the cause, pathogenesis, and treatment of more common conditions.[10,12]

Another product of the Human Genome Project is the identification and cataloging of tens of thousands of single nucleotide polymorphisms (SNPs), nonpathological alterations in 1 nucleotide that occur in all humans at a prevalence of about 1 per 1100 nucleotides. Two types of genetic analyses can be performed using SNPs: linkage and association. Association analyses have been especially common in studies of common cardiovascular disease; however, most investigations of individual phenotypes, such as myocardial infarction, have produced conflicting results.[13] Improved precision will require both larger numbers of subjects and careful attention to control populations, since the frequency and distribution of SNPs depend highly on ethnicity. Increasingly, studies of common conditions are melding large

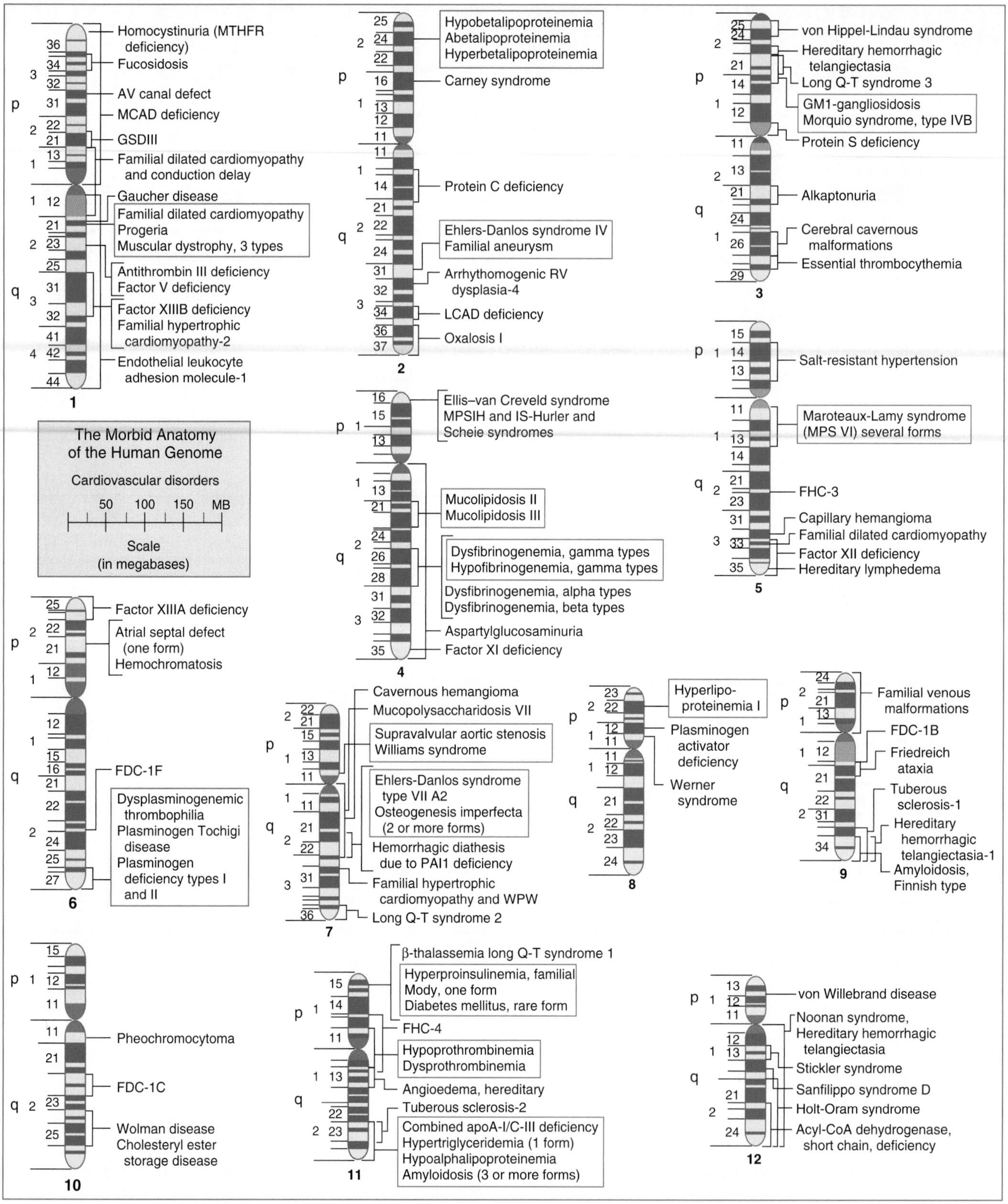

FIGURE 70–1 Chromosomal location of human genes associated with some disorders of the cardiovascular system. These genes affect the structure, function, and metabolism of the heart and blood vessels and hemostasis and have been identified by the deleterious effects of mutations. Numerous additional genes that encode structural proteins important to the cardiovascular system have been identified but not yet associated with disease. In the figure, brackets next to the chromosome show the regional localization of the gene causing a particular disorder. Brackets next to two or more disorders indicate that all of the genes causing the disorders map to the same region. Disorders surrounded by boxes are caused by different mutations at the same gene.

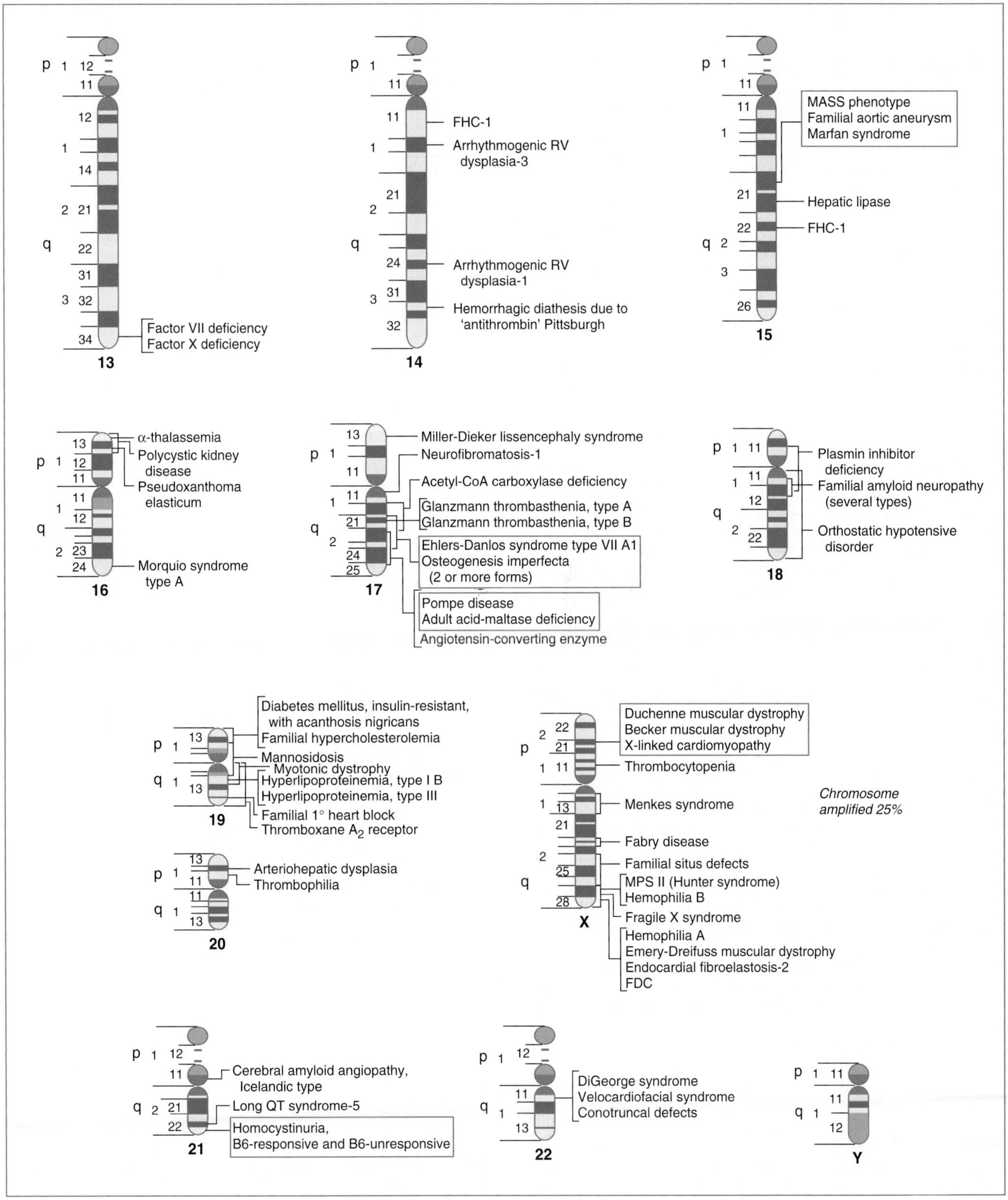

FIGURE 70–1, cont'd

databases of medical history, genealogy, and genotypes based on SNPs.[9,14]

Dominance and Recessiveness

The related concepts of dominance and recessiveness are characteristics of the phenotype, *not of the gene.* A phenotype is dominant when the patient is *heterozygous* for a mutation, i.e., when one copy of the mutant allele and one copy of the normal allele are present. This holds for genes on both autosomes and the X chromosome. A phenotype is recessive when the patient has two mutant alleles at the locus causing the condition. If the mutant alleles are identical, the patient is *homozygous* at that locus, a situation usually present either when the allele is identical by descent through both parents (i.e., the parents had a common ancestor and are *consanguineous*) or when the mutant allele is common in the population (e.g., the most prevalent mutation for cystic fibrosis and the mutation for sickle cell anemia). Biochemical and molecular genetic assessment of mutant alleles has shown that the majority of recessive phenotypes are due to two distinct mutant alleles, a situation termed a *genetic compound,* indicative of the widespread heterogeneity in mutations at each locus. Males have but one X chromosome, and each locus is therefore *hemizygous;* a mutant locus is always expressed in the phenotype of a male. Dominance and recessiveness for X-linked traits refer to expression in heterozygous and homozygous women, respectively.

Whether a disorder is called dominant or recessive depends on how carefully the phenotype is assessed and how it is defined. For example, familial hypercholesterolemia is a relatively common hereditary disorder caused by defects in the receptor for low-density lipoprotein (LDL; see Chap. 39). The vast majority of patients are heterozygous for a mutant allele at the *LDLR* locus on chromosome 19, and the disease is inherited as a Mendelian dominant trait. However, if a man and a woman, each heterozygous for an *LDLR* mutation, produce a child, that child has a 25 percent risk of inheriting both of the mutant alleles and thereby is either homozygous or a genetic compound for *LDLR.* Such a child has a much more severe form of familial hypercholesterolemia that is inherited as a Mendelian recessive trait. Similarly, homozygosity for the sickle hemoglobin mutation at the β-globin locus on chromosome 11 produces the familiar autosomal recessive disease sickle cell anemia. However, heterozygosity for the same mutation rarely produces disease but rather sickling of erythrocytes if they are examined under conditions of low oxygen tension; this phenotype is transmitted as a dominant trait.

AUTOSOMAL RECESSIVE INHERITANCE. Nearly all deficiencies of enzymatic activity—the classic inborn errors of metabolism first defined by Archibald Garrod in 1903—cause recessive phenotypes. Most homeostatic systems, which include all metabolic pathways, have sufficient flexibility to function well if one of the enzymatic steps functions at half-normal efficiency, as would occur in the case of heterozygosity for a mutant allele at a structural gene for an enzyme. However, homeostasis cannot cope if two mutant alleles cause a reduction in enzymatic activity to a few percent or less of normal activity. The characteristics of autosomal recessive inheritance, features common to such phenotypes, and a typical pedigree are shown in Figure 70–2.

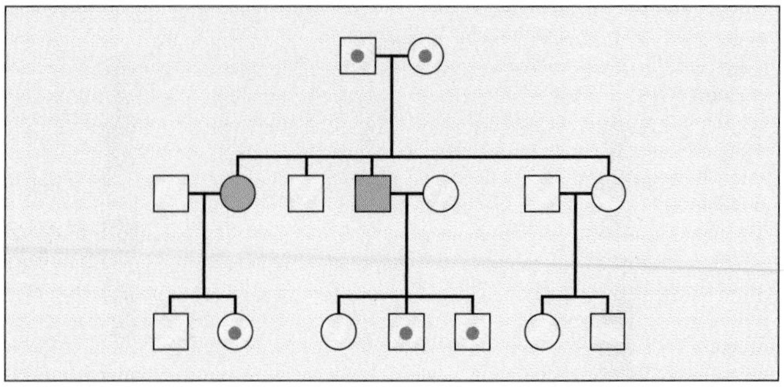

FIGURE 70–2 *Characteristics of autosomal recessive inheritance:*
A single generation is affected.
Both sexes are affected equally frequently.
Each parent is heterozygous (a carrier).
Each offspring of two carriers has a 25 percent chance of being affected, a 50 percent chance of being a carrier, and a 25 percent chance of inheriting neither mutant allele.
Two-thirds of clinically normal offspring are carriers.
The rarer the phenotype, the greater is the likelihood of consanguinity.
Characteristics of autosomal recessive phenotypes:
Often due to enzyme deficiencies.
Often more severe than dominant disorders.
Often early age of onset.

AUTOSOMAL DOMINANT INHERITANCE. Only a few enzyme deficiencies but many disorders of development and structure are inherited as dominant traits. The reasons for this are several. One possibility is that developmental homeostasis has a limited repertoire of responses to stress, and when a structural or regulatory macromolecule is reduced to only one-half normal amount, the system cannot cope. Another possibility, illustrated by mutations in procollagen molecules, pertains to gene products that must interact before becoming functional; an aberrant protein combined with a normal one would be a defective multimer, and the effect of being heterozygous for a mutation would be magnified—a *dominant-negative effect.*[2,15] The characteristics of autosomal dominant inheritance, features common to many such phenotypes, and a typical pedigree are shown in Figure 70–3.

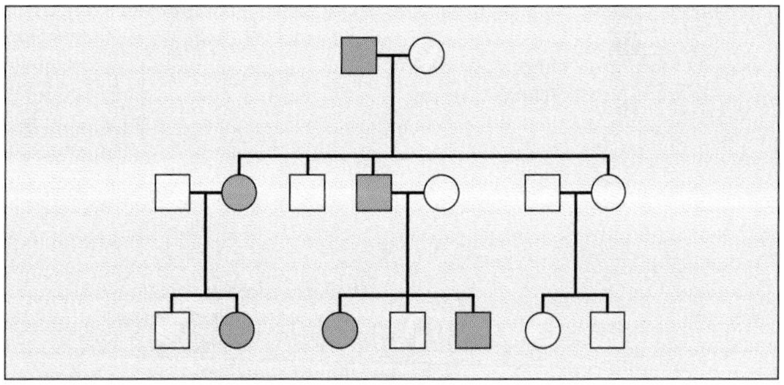

FIGURE 70–3 *Characteristics of autosomal dominant inheritance:*
Several generations are affected.
Both sexes are affected equally frequently.
In familial cases, only one parent need be affected.
Male-to-male transmission occurs.
Offspring of an affected parent has a 50 percent chance of being affected.
The frequency of sporadic cases is higher, the more severe the condition.
Paternal age has an effect in sporadic cases.
Characteristics of autosomal dominant phenotypes:
Often associated with malformations.
Often pleiotropic.
Usually variable.
Often age dependent.

Most human dominant traits are *incomplete,* because the heterozygote is less severely affected than the homozygote. Defects of *LDLR* are illustrative: the heterozygote has classic type IIa hyperlipidemia whereas the homozygote has a quantitatively worse form of the same disease. It may well be that homozygosity for most alleles that cause dominant disorders is incompatible with life.

X-LINKED INHERITANCE. The characteristics of X-linked inheritance, features common to such phenotypes, and a typical pedigree are shown in Figure 70–4. Whereas virtually

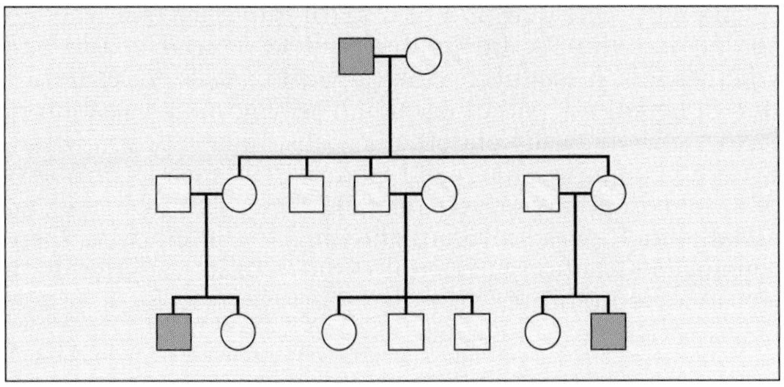

FIGURE 70–4 *Characteristics of X-linked inheritance:*
No male-to-male transmission.
All daughters of affected males are carriers.
Sons of a carrier mother have a 50 percent chance of being affected; daughters have a 50 percent chance of being carriers.
Some mothers of an affected male are not heterozygotes in all cells of their body, but they may have more affected sons if germinal mosaicism is present.
Characteristics of X-linked phenotypes:
More severe in males.
Heterozygous females may be unaffected.
Variable, especially in females.

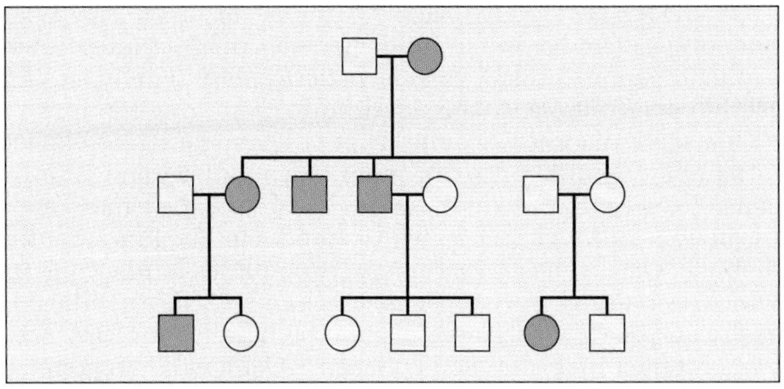

FIGURE 70–5 *Characteristics of disorders due to a mutation of the mitochondrial chromosome:*
Both sexes are equally frequently and severely affected.
Transmission is only through women; offspring of affected men are unaffected.
All offspring of an affected woman may be affected.
Variability of expression can be extreme in a family, including apparent nonpenetrance.
Phenotypes may be age dependent.

TABLE 70–3 Causes of Variability of Gene Expression

Genetic background	Physiological rearrangements
Age dependence	Variation in X inactivation*
Sex influence	Endogenous complementation*
Sex limitation	Maternal factors
Modifying loci:	Effects of mitochondrial genome
Hypostasis and epistasis	Intrauterine environment
Gene alteration	Imprinting
Somatic mutation	Exogenous and ecological factors
Somatic amplification	Ecology—temperature, diet
Transpositions and rearrangements	Teratogens
Mutations	Medical intervention
	Chance

*Pertains to female heterozygotes for X-linked disorders.

all diseases due to mutations on the X chromosome are more severe in hemizygous males, women heterozygous for the same mutations often show some manifestations, albeit less severe and of later age of onset. For example, most women carriers of alpha-galactosidase A deficiency (Fabry disease) eventually develop cerebrovascular disease or renal failure because of the accumulation of glycosphingolipid.

MITOCHONDRIAL INHERITANCE. Energy generation through oxidative phosphorylation occurs in mitochondria in the cytoplasm of most cell types. Numerous mitochondria, each containing a single chromosome, exist in each cell. Some of the enzymes of oxidative phosphorylation are encoded by genes on the nuclear chromosomes and the proteins transported into the mitochondrion; the rest of the proteins are encoded by genes on the mitochondrial chromosome. Thus, genetic defects of oxidative phosphorylation can be due to mutations of genes on the autosomes or the X chromosome, and the resulting diseases behave as Mendelian recessive traits, or they can be due to mutations of genes on the mitochondrial chromosome, in which case the resulting diseases do not behave as Mendelian traits.[16] The differences are explicable by the events of conception. The spermatocyte contributes few if any mitochondria to the zygote, and the effective complement of mitochondria that will ever be present in the fetus is derived from the mitochondria already present in the cytoplasm of the oocyte. Thus, phenotypes due to mutations of the mitochondrial chromosome show *maternal inheritance,* the characteristics of which are shown in Figure 70–5.

Principles of Clinical Genetics

PLEIOTROPY. Most mutant alleles have effects on more than one organ system, and a Mendelian phenotype frequently displays numerous, often diverse manifestations. For example, Marfan syndrome is defined by abnormalities in the eye, skeleton, skin, heart, and aorta, and until the recognition of a defect in extracellular microfibrils, the findings could not be linked either etiologically or pathogenetically.

VARIABILITY. The effects of the same mutant allele on phenotype can be different among people heterozygous (for dominant traits), homozygous (for autosomal recessive traits), or hemizygous (for X-linked traits) for the allele. Variability can be described in terms of the frequency of a particular pleiotropic manifestation among patients with the mutation; the severity of the phenotype; and the age of onset of manifestations. If a person has the mutant allele or alleles but shows no phenotypic effect, the trait is called *nonpenetrant.* To an important degree, whether a clinical phenotype is called nonpenetrant depends on the sensitivity of the techniques used for detection. For example, two decades ago, based on bedside examination, cardiovascular abnormalities were thought to affect about half of people with Marfan syndrome; echocardiography now reveals aortic dilation in more than 90 percent. The term *incomplete penetrance* should not be used with reference to individuals but rather to indicate that prevalence of the phenotype is less than 100 percent of people known to carry the mutation. The Holt-Oram syndrome (see Chap. 56) is an instructive example. In this autosomal dominant syndrome of reduction anomalies of the upper limb and congenital heart defect, patients in the same family can have only arm anomalies, only a heart defect, or both. Moreover, the severity of the reduction defect varies widely, from a proximally placed thumb to near total absence of the arm. The cardiac feature is incompletely penetrant because only about 50 percent of patients have it, but in any individual with the Holt-Oram allele, the heart is either structurally normal or not.

Numerous genetic and environmental factors can affect expression of a gene (Table 70–3), and it is often impossible to determine which of these factors are most important in a specific patient or particular disease. However, the pervasiveness of variable expression emphasizes that phenotypes determined by single genes are to some extent really "multifactorial."

GENETIC HETEROGENEITY. Similar or even identical phenotypes can be due to fundamentally distinct mutations, a phenomenon termed *genetic heterogeneity.* For example, Marfan syndrome and homocystinuria were long thought to be the same disorder, despite what now appear in retrospect to be obvious differences in inheritance pattern and intelligence.[17] As in the case of these two disorders, the causes may lie in two different genes whose products are functionally distinct. Osteogenesis imperfecta exemplifies a disorder in which mutations in two genes, α1(I) and α2(I) procollagen, each can produce the same phenotype because the two proteins interact to form type I collagen.[18] Genetic heterogeneity is pervasive at the intragenic level of analysis; except for sickle cell anemia, hemochromatosis, and achondroplasia, virtually all single-gene disorders are due to a wide variety of mutations at a given locus.

Nonpathological Variation in the Cardiovascular System

CARDIAC STRUCTURE AND PHYSIOLOGY. All aspects of the ontogeny of the cardiovascular system are dictated by the genome. If, as seems most credible, few genes have a large effect and many have small contributions, any specific aspect of "normal" cardiovascular phenotype—size, shape, function—exhibits multifactorial inheritance. In other words, to the extent that any given phenotype can be quantified, it shows a normal distribution within the population, and near-relatives are more similar to each other than they are to distant relatives and the rest of the population. The twin method should demonstrate a higher concordance of the trait in monozygotic than dizygotic twins. However, surprisingly few phenotypes have been examined.

Preliminary data on left ventricular dimensions measured echocardiographically showed higher correlations between parent and child than between matched control subjects, suggesting a genetic contribution; however, as in many such studies, the effect of shared environment was not estimated. In an attempt to minimize environmental contributions, left ventricular sizes of twins who were not exercise-trained were compared; the mean intrapair differences in echocardiographic dimensions were less in the monozygotic than in the dizygotic twins and nontwin siblings. The caliber and branch geometry of coronary arteries show familial resemblance, and both parameters are much more similar in monozygotic twins than in other relatives. Further support for the importance of genetic factors in normal development derives from studies that demonstrate ethnic differences in structure. For example, the thickness of the intima and the media of coronary arteries of children who died of noncardiovascular causes varied significantly with the ethnicity of the child.

Measures of cardiac electrophysiology show familial resemblance. Studies of both nuclear families[19] and twins suggest a genetic contribution to resting heart rate, conduction times, and repolarization time. Polymorphic variation in the beta-1 adrenergic receptor is associated with resting heart rate.[20] Genetic control of normal cardiovascular function has been especially difficult to study because of the multitude of environmental (training, diet), stochastic (age), and clinical (subtle, unrecognized pathological condition) issues that confound comparisons of relatives and control subjects. Thus far, no strong genetic contribution to an individual's response to physical conditioning has emerged.

VASCULAR SYSTEM. All members of certain inbred animal strains show little variation in arterial anatomy, especially branch angles, and considerable variation with other strains of the same species. Except for the studies of coronary arterial anatomy already noted, similar studies of humans have not been reported.

One intriguing question of clinical importance is whether certain individuals are predisposed to arterial spasm and whether this susceptibility has a genetic basis. An examination of hereditary pathological and polymorphic variation in factors elaborated by endothelial cells, platelets, and leukocytes to maintain patency of blood vessels, such as prostacyclin, endothelium-derived relaxing factor (nitric oxide), or endothelin-1, may prove enlightening.[21,22] Similarly, is there genetic contribution to arterial stiffness or its variation with age and conditioning?[23]

Cardiovascular Disorders Associated with Chromosome Aberrations

Chromosome aberrations occur in 0.5 percent of the population at birth and are common findings in tumors. Visible alterations of the amount of chromosomal material cause primarily structural defects of the cardiovascular system that are evident in the newborn. The frequency of chromosome aberrations among live-born children with congenital heart defects has been found to range from 5 to 13 percent. Upward of 40 percent of all fetuses with heart defects detected by ultrasonography at 18 to 20 weeks' gestation have chromosome aberrations; most are spontaneously aborted. Most forms of aneuploidy and most duplications and deletions of more than a chromosome band are associated with defects of the cardiovascular system (see Tables 70–1 and 70–4).[24] Exceptions are 47,XXX, 47,XYY, and 47,XXY (Klinefelter syndrome), in which the incidence of congenital heart disease is probably not elevated over the population baseline.

ANEUPLOIDY. How the abnormal phenotypes caused by autosomal aneuploidy develop remains controversial. One view holds that disturbance of the dosage of the genes present on the specific aneuploid chromosome segments is the central issue. The other view is that any aneuploid state disturbs developmental homeostasis in a nonspecific manner. The former theory predicts some distinctiveness of phenotype among the trisomy syndromes that occur in live-born children, whereas the latter predicts shared manifestations. At a coarse level, the clinical pictures are similar, with grave problems of the craniofacies, central nervous system, genitalia, distal limbs, and heart usually present. However when a more refined examination of the phenotypes is obtained, considerable distinctiveness emerges.

The three most common autosomal trisomies—13, 18, and 21—can be distinguished readily at the bedside. In all three, membranous ventricular and atrial septal defects are common. However, the detailed accounting of cardiovascular lesions among large numbers of patients with these trisomies reveals important differences that suggest aneuploidy exerts more than a global effect on development. In this and most other analyses of congenital heart defects, the system of classification based on the presumed pathogenetic mechanisms proves most instructive and is a useful approach to comparing different causative factors (Table 70–4).

About one-quarter of the defects in trisomies 13 and 18 are due to cell migration abnormalities, and two-thirds are flow lesions; when combined, these two mechanisms account for considerably more of these classes of defects than in the general population with congenital heart disease. By contrast, in trisomy 21, left-sided flow lesions are much less common, whereas abnormal closure of endocardial cushions is strikingly frequent. Indeed, in contrast to endocardial cushion defects without a chromosome 21 anomaly, left-sided flow lesions rarely occur in patients with Down syndrome and endocardial cushion defects. Furthermore, the high incidence of endocardial cushion defects and low incidence of

TABLE 70–4 Cardiovascular Manifestations Associated with Chromosome Aberrations

Chromosome Aberration	Eponym	Cardiovascular Manifestations
Triploidy		
69,XXX (or XXY or XYY)		>50% have CHD: ASD and VSD
Aneuploidy		
+13	Patau	~80% have CHD; 75% of CHD is complex: PDA, VSD, ASD, PS, AS, dextrocardia, CoA
+18	Edwards	~90% have CHD: most CHD is complex: VSD, PDA, ASD, bicuspid PV and AV, CoA
+21	Down	~40% have CHD: ECD, TOF; MVP in ~20%; AR
+8 mosaicism		~25% have CHD, most of little clinical consequence: VSD, PDA, CoA, PS
+9 mosaicism		~70% have CHD, usually complex: VSD, PDA, PLSVC
45,X	Turner	~10% have clinically important CHD: 50% of these have CoA; mild CoA is likely much more common; also AS, ARD, VSD, ASD, dextrocardia
47,XXX		CHD not increased
47,XXY	Klinefelter	CHD possibly slightly increased; ? mild conduction changes; venous thromboembolic disease
47,XYY		CHD not increased; ? mild conduction changes
Deletions		
4p–	Wolf-Hirschhorn	~50% have CHD, usually complex: VSD, ASD, PDA, PS
5p–	Cri du chat	~20% have CHD, usually single: VSD, PDA, ASD, PS
7q–		~20% have CHD, various, often complex
13q–		CHD common, often severe, but depends on region deleted
18p–		CHD uncommon
18q–		~25% have CHD, usually single, of little consequence: VSD, PDA, ASD, PS
ring 18		~20% have CHD: CoA, PA hypoplasia, HLH, PLSVC
Duplications		
4p trisomy		~10% have CHD, usually single: no defect predominates
9p trisomy		>10% have CHD: VSD, ASD, AS, PS
10p trisomy		~30% have CHD, usually single: no defect predominates
10q24-qter trisomy		~50% have CHD, usually complex: ECD, VSD, TOF
22pter-q11 trisomy or tetrasomy	Cat eye	~50% have CHD, usually complex: TAPVR, VSD, TOF
Other Aberrations		
Marker Xq27.3	Fragile X syndrome	~50% have aortic root dilatation, MVP, or both

AR = aortic regurgitation; ARD = aortic root dilation; AS = aortic stenosis; ASD = atrial septal defect; AV = aortic valve; CHD = congenital heart defect(s); CoA = coarctation of aorta; ECD = endocardial cushion defect; HLH = hypoplastic left heart; MVP = mitral valve prolapse; PA = pulmonary artery; PDA = patent ductus arteriosus; PLSVC = persistence of left superior vena cava; PS = valvular pulmonic stenosis; PV = pulmonic valve; TAPVR = total anomalous pulmonary venous return; TOF = tetralogy of Fallot; VSD = ventricular septal defect.

conotruncal and distal aortic anomalies have suggested a distinct pathogenetic mechanism in trisomy 21, potentially involving cell adhesiveness and the extracellular matrix.

TRISOMY 21–DOWN SYNDROME. This most common phenotype due to a human chromosome aberration occurs about once in every 600 births. Most patients have trisomy 21, and the risk of this aberration is exponentially related to maternal age: the risk is lowest for young women and rises steeply after age 35, reaching 4 percent for women older than 45. A small minority (3 percent) of cases of Down syndrome result from an extra copy of all or part of the long arm of chromosome 21 translocated to another chromosome. This situation is relatively more common in mothers younger than 30 years. The phenotypes of the two forms of Down syndrome do not differ. The phenotype tends to be less severe if the trisomy is mosaic (3 percent of Down syndrome) as a result of a mitotic nondisjunctional error in the embryo.

The most common causes of morbidity and mortality in patients with Down syndrome are congenital heart defects (present in 40 to 50 percent of cases),[25] hematological malignant disease, and duodenal atresia. If patients either escape or survive these problems, survival into the fifth decade and beyond is likely but is complicated by progressive dementia of the Alzheimer type. Premature aging may also affect the vasculature, although definitive studies are lacking.

The most characteristic cardiac anomaly in patients with Down syndrome is a defect of closure of the endocardial cushions (see Chap. 56). Complicating the clinical problems in such patients and those with simple septal defects is a seeming predisposition to pulmonary hypertension in the presence of elevated pulmonary blood flow. About one-third of congenital heart defects are complex, and affected individuals tend, not surprisingly, to be the most ill patients. Mitral valve prolapse (MVP) is found with a frequency exceeding that in age- and gender-matched control subjects. The aortic and pulmonary valve cusps seem predisposed to fenestrations in adulthood. In the neonate with Down syndrome, the physical examination has a sensitivity of 80 percent for detecting cardiovascular anomalies; echocardiography detects some additional infants who have normal physical examination findings but who will later require cardiac surgery.[26]

Through the study of individuals trisomic for only a portion of the long arm of chromosome 21, the region crucial to the development of heart defects has been narrowed to 5.5 megabases (mb) of DNA in band 21q22.3; a locus in this region, *DSCAM*, that encodes a cell adhesion molecule is a leading candidate gene for this aspect of the Down syndrome phenotype.[27]

Medical treatment of patients with Down syndrome has undergone evolution to more aggressive measures in recent years. Objections and hesitations on medical, societal, and ethical grounds to operative repair of heart defects in Down syndrome have been mollified substantially.[28] More follow-up data are becoming available, and early and late postoperative survival in patients with Down syndrome appears to be comparable to that in other patients with similar defects.

TRISOMY 18. Edwards syndrome is the second most common autosomal trisomy. Most cases are due to meiotic disjunction, and there is a strong relationship to maternal age. Routine prenatal diagnostic testing of women older than 34 years would detect all aneuploid fetuses in them, but this would represent only one-third of all autosomal trisomies; in the United States, less than one-half of all women of this advanced age undergo definitive testing. Prenatal detection of trisomies followed by termination of pregnancy is currently having a small but measurable impact on decreasing the incidence of Down, Edwards, and Patau syndromes.

Although the severity of the phenotype rarely enables survival beyond a few months, 5 to 10 percent of patients live to 1 year and a few survive to adulthood, perhaps because of undetected mosaicism for a chromosomally normal cell line.[29,30] However, central nervous system function is far less than in patients with Down syndrome and leads to complex medical management and supportive care for long-term survivors.[28]

Cardiovascular defects occur in at least 90 percent of cases and contribute to death. Complex lesions, usually involving septal defects, dysplastic valves that are rarely hemodynamically important, patent ductus arteriosus (PDA), and persistence of the left superior vena cava are common. Right ventricular enlargement is common and may indicate not only shunting from left to right but pulmonary hypertension due to anomalies of the pulmonary vasculature. As in Down syndrome, transposition of the great arteries is virtually unknown in patients with trisomy 18. Invasive diagnostic procedures or aggressive supportive measures should be undertaken only rarely in patients with Edwards syndrome.

TRISOMY 13. Patau syndrome occurs in about 0.01 percent of live births and in progressively higher frequencies in stillbirths and spontaneous abortions. The external phenotype is usually severe but occasionally not as characteristic as that of other trisomies; survival beyond a few weeks is rare, and the causes of death involve several organ systems, especially the heart. Cardiovascular anomalies occur a bit less frequently than in trisomy 18 and have a slightly different spectrum.[28] Septal defects are the most common isolated lesions, dextrocardia and bicuspid semilunar valves occur in association with other anomalies, and accessory papillary muscles occur in 30 percent of fetuses with trisomy 13.[31]

Median survival is about 10 days, but 5 to 10 percent survive to 1 year, and a very few live beyond one decade.[30,32] Patients who survive beyond 1 month often are mosaic for a chromosomally normal cell line; thus, prognosis is fraught with uncertainty until detailed analysis is completed. Whether invasive cardiological studies are performed or aggressive management is undertaken can be determined by the severity of involvement of other organ systems, especially the brain, pending cytogenetic investigation.

TURNER SYNDROME. About 1 in every 2500 females lacks an X chromosome and has a 45,X karyotype, which is by far the most common cause of Turner syndrome. The frequency of a nonmosaic 45,X karyotype is much higher in spontaneous abortuses than in live-borns, and probably less than 2 percent of such conceptuses come to term. The clinical phenotype is variable and often mild; typically, the diagnosis is not suspected until a child's short stature is evaluated or a woman complains of amenorrhea. Many cases are mosaic for cell lines with 46,XX or 46,XY constitutions. Various structural aberrations involving the X chromosome can cause partial or complete Turner syndrome.

Among patients with the 45,X karyotype, reported frequencies of congenital cardiovascular defects vary from 20 to 50 percent, depending on how patients were ascertained. Fifty to 70 percent of those with cardiovascular defects have clinically important aortic coarctation, usually of the postductal form. As noninvasive imaging studies of asymptomatic patients become routine, the frequency of coarctation may increase. Various other cardiac malformations may occur, either singly or combined with coarctation. However, there is strong support for left-sided flow abnormalities as a major pathogenetic mechanism. Bicuspid aortic valve, dilation of the ascending aorta (with a risk of dissection and histopathologic examination showing elastic fiber disruption), or both occur even in the absence of coarctation,[33] and hypoplastic left heart has been reported. Partial anomalous pulmonary venous drainage without an atrial septal defect is fairly common and should be suspected when echocardiography detects right ventricular overload.

Postmortem examination of midtrimester abortuses with 45,X showed a higher incidence of left-sided flow lesions than found at birth, suggesting an association between the pathogenesis of the cardiovascular anomalies and the uniform presence of lymphatic obstruction at the base of the heart. In fetuses with Turner phenotype that do not survive, the size of the heart is reduced, perhaps representing a mild but generalized form of hypoplastic left heart, the most severe form of left-sided flow defects.[34] The fetal hydrops common in cases of severe, fetal Turner syndrome could be due to inadequate cardiac function, rather than its cause. Blood pressure elevation is common, even without coarctation or after its repair; a high frequency of renal anomalies is one likely cause but not the sole explanation for the prevalence of hypertension. Elevated blood pressure is strongly associated with dilation of the ascending aorta, so aggressive treatment is warranted on several accounts.[33]

In about two-thirds of cases, the retained X chromosome derives from the oocyte (maternal X). Because entire chromosomes or regions of a chromosome may be differentially regulated (imprinted)[35] by passage through oogenesis versus spermatogenesis, could some of the variability in phenotype among patients with Turner syndrome be due to the origin of the retained X or the origin of the lost X? In a study of 63 patients, 10 had severe cardiovascular features, and 9 of them had retained the maternal X.[36] This is an idea worthy of further investigation. Women with mosaic karyotypes are less likely to have cardiovascular defects. Some studies also suggest a "critical region" of the X chromosome, which, when deleted, results in most of the features of Turner syndrome.[37]

Management of both children[38] and adults[39] with Turner syndrome requires careful and routine attention to the cardiovascular system. Chronic treatment of children with human growth hormone to increase mature height has no apparent deleterious effect on cardiac performance.[40]

Congenital Heart Disease (see Chap. 56)

In the past few decades, the reported incidence of structural heart defects in newborns has increased from 5 to 7 per 1000 in live births, probably as the result of increased diagnostic sensitivity (especially cross-sectional and Doppler echocardiography and magnetic resonance imaging), including prenatally.[40-42] Supporting this explanation is the lack of change over the same period in the incidence of critical defects diagnosed neonatally at 3.1 to 3.5 per 1000.[40,43] This enhanced resolving power of noninvasive methods should prove particularly useful in the study of familial structural defects, because apparently unaffected relatives can be evaluated for subclinical evidence of anomalies. Few investigations to date have capitalized on this approach.[44]

As is evident from the previous section, gross aberrations of chromosomes produce an extensive and varied array of structural heart disease, an observation as true for spontaneous abortuses as for live-born children. Unfortunately, cytogenetic aberrations have provided few clues about etiology and pathogenesis of congenital malformations.[45,46] Better understanding comes from investigating the other two mechanisms by which genes cause congenital heart defects: multifactorial processes and mutations of single genes. In addition to the Mendelian syndromes discussed later, evidence for the involvement of genes of large effect derives, in part, from studies of incidence of congenital heart disease in populations with a high rate of inbreeding. The increased occurrence of defects in offspring of consanguineous matings suggests that mutations in one or more genes, when homozygous, strongly predispose to abnormal cardiovascular development.

MULTIFACTORIAL PROCESSES. The empirical risks of recurrence of congenital heart defects have increased in recent years,[47] in keeping with the overall higher incidence noted earlier. However, this conclusion has been criticized because the studies focused on the offspring of women probands, in whom the recurrence risk appears higher than in men with congenital heart defects.[48] In addition to this unexplained maternal influence, other factors may be at work. For example, improved detection of subtle lesions, more faithful reporting of patients, and the assiduousness of epidemiologists may have shown a systematic variation. More patients with cardiovascular problems now survive[48] to bear children due to improved medical and surgical care; their offspring might be at increased risk because of the severity of the parents' problems, but some evidence refutes this idea.

The familial aggregation of congenital heart defects supports many of the predictions of the threshold liability model of multifactorial inheritance.[43,49] In most studies, whether focused on populations or families, defects were classified by their pathological findings; for example, all ventricular septal defects were considered as one group. There has been bias in reporting families in which one type of defect aggregates, leading to many reports of "familial atrial septal defect," "familial cardiomyopathy," and so on, although not all septal

TABLE 70–5 Classification of Congenital Heart Defects Based on Pathogenetic Mechanisms

Pathogenetic Mechanism	Examples of Defects
Embryonic blood flow defects	
Left-sided lesions	HLH; bicuspid aortic valve; IAA type A; CoA; PDA
Right-sided lesions	Secundum ASD; PS
Mesenchymal tissue migration defects	TOF; D-TGA
Extracellular matrix defects	ECD
Abnormal cellular death	Ebstein anomaly; muscular VSD
Defects of looping and situs	L-TGA
Abnormalities of targeted growth	TAPVR

ASD = atrial septal defect; CoA = coarctation of aorta; ECD = endocardial cushion defect; HLH = hypoplastic left heart; IAA = interrupted aortic arch; PDA = patent ductus arteriosus; PS = valvular pulmonic stenosis; TAPVR = total anomalous pulmonary venous return; TGA = transposition of great arteries; TOF = tetralogy of Fallot; VSD = ventricular septal defect.

defects or cardiopathies have the same structure on careful scrutiny, let alone the same cause.[50,51]

A major advance has been the movement to examine familial aggregation of defects based on presumed pathogenesis.[41] The scheme developed by Clark[52] and since modified and expanded (Table 70–5), has become widely used. Under this approach, some anatomically distinct lesions are related by common pathogenesis; if the pathogenetic mechanism has substantial genetic control, then the occurrence of distinct defects in the same family would still be consistent with a genetic model. Alternatively, defects unrelated by pathogenesis would require a different interpretation. This model rationalizes examination of apparently unaffected relatives, which increases the chances of detecting subtle manifestations of defective development of cardiovascular structures. Such investigation, in addition to targeted testing for single-gene mutations or chromosomal microdeletions, is now fundamental to genetic counseling for all congenital heart disease.[53]

ERRORS IN MESENCHYMAL TISSUE MIGRATION. Included in this category is a wide range of anomalies of the outflow tract, some due to failure of fusion and others due to failure of septation. Relatives of probands with interruption of the aortic arch type B or truncus arteriosus, both uncommon conotruncal malformations, had 2.5 percent and 6.6 percent incidences, respectively, of congenital heart defects. Both recurrence rates were higher than expected. The frequency of congenital malformations was much lower in relatives of patients with other forms of interrupted aortic arch. Moreover, relatives of probands with truncus arteriosus and other defects had a recurrence rate of 13 percent, the majority in the spectrum of conotruncal lesions. Here is an instance in which refined empirical risk data should improve the accuracy of genetic counseling.

Categorizing anatomical defects by presumed pathogenesis emphasizes that all ventricular septal defects are not alike. However, even within an embryologically circumscribed category, the situation is complex. Many perimembranous ventricular septal defects and tetralogy of Fallot can be considered errors in mesenchymal tissue migration. Evidence exists for the effects of major genes (e.g., as yet unidentified ones in the 22q11 region,[54] *JAG1*,[55,56] the gene that when mutated also causes Alagille syndrome[57,58] and *NKX2.5*[59,60]), and for multifactorial effects.[61]

CONOTRUNCAL DEVELOPMENT. Considerable progress has been made during the past few years in identifying a region of chromosome 22 that has a major role in development of the conotruncus, the branchial arches, and the face. Interest was first stimulated by detection of small deletions involving 22q11 in patients with DiGeorge sequence. This condition includes developmental anomalies of the fourth branchial arch and derivatives of the third and fourth pharyngeal pouches. Hypoplasia of the thymus and parathyroids causes immune deficiency and hypocalcemia. The cardiac defects range from tetralogy of Fallot to ventricular septal defect, truncus arteriosus, interrupted aorta type B, and right aortic arch, and are often lethal. Deletion of 22q11 accounts for about 90 percent of instances of DiGeorge sequence.[53]

Subsequently, patients with velocardiofacial syndrome (VCF, also called Shprintzen-Goldberg syndrome) and what has been called in Japan the *conotruncal anomaly face syndrome* were found to have deletions in the same region, albeit generally smaller ones than in patients with DiGeorge syndrome. Because the deletion is often too small to be detected by routine cytogenetics, fluorescent in situ hybridization (FISH) with a DNA probe for the region is the assay of choice. The VCF syndrome is unlike DiGeorge syndrome and includes an abnormal but characteristic facies, cleft palate, pharyngeal insufficiency, and conotruncal cardiac defects.

This same region of chromosome 22 has been examined in patients with familial occurrence of various congenital cardiac defects and in patients with nonfamilial occurrence, nonsyndromic conotruncal defects; an important fraction of patients in both categories have submicroscopic deletions of 22q11.[54,62-64] Thus, a gene or genes in this region account for much of the recurrence risk of defects due to mesenchymal tissue migration abnormalities. Further, accurate counseling about recurrence risks for this broad range of defects necessitates FISH or molecular analysis for the presence of a deletion in the proband and, if present, in both parents. Deletion of 22q11 occurs in about 13 per 100,000 live births and is, after trisomy 21, the second most common genetic cause of congenital heart disease.[65]

Investigation of a strain of Keeshond dogs prone to conotruncal defects has shown that a single gene can be responsible for pathogenetically related defects of widely varying severity.

FLOW DEFECTS. Left-sided flow lesions comprise a spectrum that includes hypoplastic left heart, congenital aortic stenosis, bicuspid aortic valve, interrupted aortic arch type A, and aortic coarctation. Various components of this spectrum can be present in the same patient. Data from the Baltimore-Washington Infant Study,[41] a population-based case-control study of congenital cardiovascular malformations, were used to show that in first-degree relatives of probands with isolated hypoplastic left heart, the incidence of bicuspid aortic valve was 12 percent; most of the cases were asymptomatic and unrecognized before they were detected by echocardiography as part of this investigation. In an exceptional family, four instances of aortic coarctation occurred in four generations. Coarctation, even when repaired, poses an important risk factor for a woman during pregnancy.[66]

The association of coarctation of the aorta, bicuspid aortic valve, and dilation of the ascending aorta, which may occur as part of Turner syndrome (see earlier discussion), is well known in the general population. Several intriguing questions about the genetics and pathogenesis of this association need to be addressed. To what extent is the ascending aorta intrinsically abnormal and hence predisposed to dilate, and to what extent is the dilation simply a result of abnormal turbulence created by a bicuspid aortic valve? Some patients with this association also have subtle evidence of a systemic connective tissue abnormality, reminiscent of Marfan syndrome, in support of the former hypothesis. Furthermore, some people with a bicuspid aortic valve and neither stenosis nor regurgitation develop aneurysms. It will be of interest to extend the study of left-sided flow lesions to include probands with coarctation or congenital aortic stenosis and to evaluate close relatives with techniques capable of detecting the entire range of flow defects.

EXTRACELLULAR MATRIX ABNORMALITIES. Enough is known about the biochemistry and cell biology of cardiac embryology to state with some confidence that the extracellular matrix ("connective tissue") has an important role. The endocardial cushions have received the most attention as an area where defects in the extracellular matrix might produce malformations.[52] The high frequency of endocardial cushion defects and atrioventricular septal defects in patients with Down syndrome has been noted. Of interest is the finding of increased adhesiveness of fibroblasts from patients with trisomy 21, a phenomenon that could reflect interaction with the extracellular matrix. The distinctiveness of endocardial cushion defects in patients with normal chromosomes and in those with trisomy 21 has been suggested because of differences in associated cardiovascular malformations.[50] However, of six families in which the proband had an endocardial cushion defect, three had recurrence of the same type of defect in a relative, including two with trisomy 21. Atrioventricular septal defects (AVSD) are also seen in patients with a number of other conditions, including deletions of the short arm of chromosome 3 (3p–). A gene in this region, *CRELD1*, has been found to be mutated in some families with AVSD in multiple generations.[67]

SITUS AND LOOPING DEFECTS. This is an area fraught with difficulties of nomenclature, diagnosis, and heterogeneity of both etiology and pathogenesis.[68] In analysis of clinical data, the most informative approach but clearly arduous because of the large amount of data required, would be to categorize probands and their relatives by the type of situs (solitus, inversus, dextroversion, or levoversion; see Chap. 56) and each of those by the presence or absence of other cardiac and visceral defects. This has not been done on epidemiological cohorts, and relatives in family studies have rarely been subjected to evaluations sufficient to characterize their phenotypes in detail. However, when careful family studies are performed, evidence for genetic contribution to specific defects may emerge, e.g., in cases of complete transposition of the great arteries.[69]

Many variable phenotypes are grouped in a category, *heterotaxy*, that accounts for 3 to 4 percent of all congenital heart defects. Several Mendelian phenotypes point to single genes that have a major effect on determining laterality. In the autosomal recessive Kartagener syndrome, a randomization of lateralization of the heart (situs solitus and situs inversus are equally likely in homozygotes) coexists with a defect in ciliary motility, which leads to sinusitis, bronchiectasis, and sperm immotility.[70]

Heterotaxy with splenic and other cardiac defects, particularly of the position of the great vessels, can be inherited as autosomal recessive, autosomal dominant, and X-linked recessive traits.[11] Some of the families with these apparently single-gene disorders have concordance of phenotype, but many do not, suggesting that in some cases various types of situs defects, polysplenia, and asplenia are different manifestations of the same mutation.

In recent years, investigation of molecular embryology has shed increasing light on cardiovascular development and maldevelopment.[71] The determination of laterality and defects involving heterotaxy have been especially revealing in both mice and humans.[72,73] In mice, the *inv* locus has long been associated with left/right asymmetry, and the gene was recently cloned.[74] In humans, mutations of two genes thus far, one encoding the activin receptor type IIB[75] and one encoding the connexin43 gap junction protein, have been associated with defects of laterality.

Few data define the recurrence risks of defects in the *cell death* (e.g., Ebstein anomaly) and *abnormal targeted growth* (e.g., anomalous pulmonary venous return) categories. Data from the Baltimore-Washington Infant Study do not show an increased risk of any cardiovascular defect in the relatives of a proband with a defect in either of these categories.[41]

DISORDERS OF UNCLEAR CAUSE. A number of disorders include an important likelihood of malformation of the cardiovascular system but are of unclear cause (Table 70–6). Familial recurrence is low enough to be incompatible with multifactorial inheritance. Several of these disorders deserve comment.

Certain congenital cardiac defects and other malformations occur together more frequently than expected by chance; this *association* of defects suggests a common cause, pathogenesis, or both, but the following disorders and those in Table 70–7 remain enigmatic on most of these counts. Designation as a *sequence* implies that some evidence exists for a common developmental problem to account for the features.

CHARGE Association (see Table 70-6). Patients with this condition by definition have congenital heart defects. The spectrum of cardiovascular malformations suggests not so much a common pathogenetic scheme as a common time of abnormal development. During gestational days 32 to 45, cardiac septation, fusion of the endocardial cushions and membranous ventricular septum, and formation of the outflow tracts and valves occur. An environmental insult or a breakdown in developmental homeostasis during this period could result in the malformation spectrum of this disorder. The defects in other systems could also arise during this embryological window and would be consistent with either environmental or intrinsic factors.

VACTERL Association (see Table 70-6). This condition has expanded over the years to include *v*ertebral, *v*entricular septal, *a*nal, cardiac, *t*racheoesophageal, *r*enal, and *l*imb defects. Omitted from the mnemonic is the single umbilical artery often present. Cardiac defects are present in about one-half of patients with more than two components of this association but usually are not life-threatening. VACTERL

TABLE 70–6 Disorders of Uncertain Cause and Inheritance that are Associated with a High Incidence of Cardiovascular Abnormalities

Disorder and Phenotype	OMIM No.*	Cardiovascular Abnormalities†
Aase syndrome (congenital anemia, triphalangeal thumbs)	205600	VSD
Bilateral left-sidedness sequence (polysplenia syndrome)	208530	ASD
Bilateral right-sidedness sequence (asplenia syndrome; Ivemark syndrome)	208530	Situs inversus, ECD, VSD
CHARGE association (*c*oloboma, *h*eart anomaly, choanal *a*tresia, *r*etardation, *g*enital, and *e*ar anomalies)	214800	TOF, PDA, ECD, VSD
Cornelia de Lange syndrome (short stature, retardation, synophrys, hypertrichosis, micromelia, genital anomalies)	122470	~20% Have CHD: VSD, PDA, ASD, PLSVC, TOF
DiGeorge sequence‡ (abnormalities of derivatives of third and fourth pharyngeal pouches and fourth branchial arch: hypoplastic thymus with cellular immune deficiency, hyoplastic parathyroids with hypocalcemia)	188400	CHD in ~100%: aortic arch anomalies (especially IAA type B and right-sided aortic arch); PDA, TOF
Goldenhar syndrome (abnormalities of derivatives of first and second branchial arches: hemifacial microsomia, microtia, vertebral anomalies)	141400, 164210, 257700	~50% have CHD: VSD, TOF, PDA, CoA, right-sided aortic arch, PLSVC
Klippel-Feil sequence (short neck, limited rotation of the head, cervical anomalies)	118100 148900, 214300	Variable estimates (5%-70%) of CHD: VSD, dextrocardia
Kabuki make-up syndrome (dwarfism, peculiar facies, scoliosis, mental retardation)	147920	30% have CHD: ASD, VSD, TOF, CoA, PDA
Pallister-Hall syndrome (hypothalamic hamartoblastoma, hypopituitarism, imperforate anus, postaxial polydactyly)	146510	ECD
Poland sequence (unilateral absence of sternocostal pectoralis major, ipsilateral synbrachydactyly)	173800	~10% have dextrocardia or dextroversion
Rubinstein-Taybi syndrome (short stature, retardation, microcephaly, characteristic facies, broad thumbs)	180849	~20% have CHD: ECD, ASD, TOF, PDA, VSD
VATER association (*v*ertebral defects, *a*nal atresia, *t*racheo *e*sophageal fistula, *r*adial dysplasia, renal anomaly)	192350	VSD

*None of these disorders is evidently due to a mutation in a single gene; however, most are listed in Online Mendelian Inheritance in Man (www.ncbi.nlm.nih.gov/omim)[8] and the OMIM no. is provided as a ready source to the literature.

†Listed in approximate order of decreasing frequency.

‡90% of cases associated with del(22q11); likely a contiguous gene deletion defect.

ASD = atrial septal defect; CHD = congenital heart defect(s); CoA = coarctation of aorta; ECD = endocardial cushion defect; IAA = interrupted aortic arch; PDA = patent ductus arteriosus; PLSVC = persistence of left superior vena cava; TOF = tetralogy of Fallot; VSD = ventricular septal defect.

TABLE 70–7 Congenital Heart Defects Occasionally Showing Familial Aggregation Consistent with Mendelian Inheritance

Defect	OMIM No.*
Aneurysm, intracranial berry	105800
Aneurysm, abdominal aortic	100070
Angioma	106050, 106070, 206570
ASD, ostium primum	209400
ASD, ostium secundum	108800, 108900, 178650
Bicuspid aortic valve	109730
Conotruncal defect	231060
Dextrocardia	244400, 304750
Ebstein anomaly	224700
Endocardial fibroelastosis	226000, 227280, 305300
Hemangioma	106070, 140800, 140900, 234800
Hemangioma, cavernous	116860, 140850
Hypoplastic left heart	140500, 241550
Hypoplastic right heart	277200
Lymphedema, congenital	153000, 153100, 153400, 214900, 247440
Mitral valve prolapse	157700
Patent ductus arteriosus	169100
Pulmonary venous return, anomalous	106700
Pulmonic stenosis	126190, 178650, 193520, 265500, 265600, 270460
Subaortic stenosis	271950, 271960
Tetralogy of Fallot	187500
Ventricle, single	234750

*Data from Online Mendelian Inheritance in Man (www.ncbi.nlm.nih.gov/omim).
ASD = atrial septal defect.

association occasionally occurs in relatives.[76] Although infants with this condition often fail to thrive initially, the long-term prognosis for health and mental function is good, so aggressive management of the multiple malformations is warranted. It is important to separate as soon as possible those patients who have the features of trisomy 18 or 13q chromosome aberrations, as prognosis in these cases is distinctly unfavorable.

Mendelian Disorders

Some congenital cardiovascular defects segregate in occasional families as predicted of a Mendelian phenotype. Strong bias favors reporting such occurrences, and equally strong is a temptation to conclude that, at least in some cases, the defect is caused by mutation in a single gene. However, rarely and by chance alone, a multifactorial trait recurs in a family in a pattern mimicking Mendelian segregation. This potential confusion and the resultant uncertainty in counseling patients and families pertains equally well to disturbances of conduction and rhythm, various cardiomyopathies, vascular anomalies, and hypertension, all discussed subsequently. The true cause of the cardiovascular diseases in such families may not become clarified until each is investigated in detail, in concert with efforts to map and sequence the entire human genome.

The subject of this section can therefore be parsed into three broad classes of conditions: congenital cardiac defects that occasionally seem to be inherited as Mendelian traits (see Table 70–7), pleiotropic Mendelian syndromes that always or frequently affect the structure of the cardiovascular system (Table 70–8), and Mendelian syndromes that occasionally affect the cardiovascular system (Table 70–9).

PATENT DUCTUS ARTERIOSUS. Most instances of PDA are sporadic occurrences, and a strong association with prematurity and all of its antecedents is noted. However, in a number of families that have been described, PDA occurs as an autosomal dominant trait. In some pedigrees, mild facial dysmorphism segregates with PDA; because the facial features differ among families, the number of syndromes remains unclear.[77] Some families with autosomal dominant PDA are predisposed to aortic dissection.[78] In other families, PDA occurs as a recessive trait, and a locus at 12q24 has been implicated.[79]

FAMILIAL ATRIAL SEPTAL DEFECT. Two Mendelian forms of atrial septal defect exist as autosomal dominant traits.[80] One has no associated problems and has been described in few pedigrees. Mutations in *GATA4* have been described recently in several families.[81]

The second, more common condition is associated with atrioventricular conduction delay.[82] The defect is of the secundum type, and relatives do not seem to be at increased risk of other cardiac malformations. The severity of heart block rarely progresses to third degree. The electrocardiographic abnormality in a patient with apparently sporadic atrial septal defect should prompt a detailed family history and evaluation of close relatives. Attention should be directed to the upper limbs, particularly the thumbs, to rule out the Holt-Oram syndrome; radiographic examination of the upper limbs of the proband is helpful on this account.

In patients with atrial septal defect due to aneuploidy (a syndrome with extracardiac features), when one of the autosomal dominant forms is excluded, the recurrence risk of secundum atrial septal defect is about 3 percent, a value that conforms closely to the multifactorial threshold model. Several pleiotropic Mendelian conditions have defects of the atrial septum as frequent manifestations.

HOLT-ORAM SYNDROME. This autosomal dominant condition, first elaborated in 1960, shows marked variability within a pedigree. The cardinal manifestations are dysplasia of the upper limbs and atrial septal defect. In heterozygotes for the mutation, arm deformity ranges from undetectable through distally placed thumbs and hypoplastic thenar eminences, triphalangeal thumbs, anomalies of the carpus, and radial aplasia, to phocomelia and hypoplasia of the clavicles and shoulders. Upper-extremity deformity is usually bilateral but may be asymmetrical in severity, with the left side more affected. Similarly, the atrial involvement ranges from none to a large secundum defect with early, severe hemodynamic compromise. Other cardiac malformations have been reported, with ventricular septal defects and PDA the most frequent. The skeletal and cardiac manifestations are not correlated in individuals, and how a parent is affected is not a reliable predictor of effects on offspring. Prenatal diagnosis by ultrasonography was reported in a fetus with severe limb abnormalities; a large septal defect could presumably be detected as well. Other manifestations include dermatoglyphic abnormalities, pectus excavatum, hypoplastic peripheral arteries, and cardiac conduction disturbance, the last usually involving the atrioventricular node and present in patients with septal defects. Although the Holt-Oram syndrome bears some resemblance to the VACTERL association, the clear Mendelian nature and lack of more extensive organ system involvement of the former indicate that the two conditions do not represent a pathogenetic spectrum.

TABLE 70–8 Mendelian Disorders with Congenital Defects of Cardiovascular Structure as Frequent Manifestations

Descriptive Name	Eponym	OMIM No.*	Cardiovascular Abnormalities
Adult polycystic kidney disease		173900	MVP, dilated aortic root, intracranial berry aneurysm
Arteriohepatic dysplasia	Alagille syndrome	118450	PPS
Cataract and cardiomyopathy		212350	HCM
Chondroectodermal dysplasia	Ellis–van Creveld syndrome	225500	ASD (ostium primum), common atrium
Deafness, mitral regurgitation, and short stature	Forney syndrome	157800	MR
Familial collagenoma syndrome		115250	DCM
Heart-hand syndrome	Holt-Oram syndrome	142900	ASD (ostium secundum), VSD, MVP, HLH
Keratosis palmoplantaris	Mal de Meleda syndrome	248300	DCM, dysrhythmia
Malignant hyperthermia and skeletal defects	King syndrome	145600	Malignant hyperthermia→cardiac arrest
Noonan syndrome		163950	PS, HCM
Pulmonic stenosis and deafness		178651	PS
Smith-Lemli-Opitz syndrome		270400	PDA, ASD, VSD, TOF, ECD, CoA
Velocardiofacial syndrome	Shprintzen syndrome	192430	TOF, tortuous retinal vasculature

*Data from Online Mendelian Inheritance in Man (www.ncbi.nlm.nih.gov/omim).

ASD = atrial septal defect; CoA = coarctation of aorta; DCM = dilated cardiomyopathy; ECD = endocardial cushion defect; HCM = hypertrophic cardiomyopathy; HLH = hypoplastic left heart; MR = mitral regurgitation; MVP = mitral valve prolapse; PDA = patent ductus arteriosus; PPS = peripheral pulmonic stenosis; PS = valvular pulmonic stenosis; TOF = tetralogy of Fallot; VSD = ventricular septal defect.

TABLE 70–9 Mendelian Disorders with Cardiovascular Abnormalities as Occasional Manifestations

Syndrome	Eponym	OMIM No.*	Cardiovascular Abnormalities
Acrocephalosyndactyly type I	Apert syndrome	101200	PS, PPS, VSD, EFE
Acrocephalopolysyndactyly type II	Carpenter syndrome	201000	PDA, VSD, PS, TGA
Hereditary angioedema		106100	Coronary arteritis
Imperforate anus with hand, foot, and ear anomalies	Townes-Brocks syndrome	107480	Sporadic cases have CHD: VSD, ASD
Mandibulofacial dysostosis	Treacher Collins syndrome	154500, 248390	10% have CHD: variable
Neuronal ceroid lipofuscinosis	Batten disease	204200	HCM
Orofacial digital syndrome type II	Mohr syndrome	252100	Variable
Short rib–polydactyly syndrome	Saldino-Noonan syndrome	263530	TGA, ECD, hypoplastic right heart
Thrombocytopenia–absent radius syndrome	TAR syndrome	274000	TOF

*Data from Online Mendelian Inheritance in Man (www.ncbi.nlm.nih.gov/omim).

ASD = atrial septal defect; CHD = congenital heart defect(s); ECD = endocardial cushion defect; EFE = endocardial fibroelastosis; HCM = hypertrophic cardiomyopathy; PDA = patent ductus arteriosus; PS = valvular pulmonic stenosis; PPS = peripheral pulmonic stenosis; TGA = transposition of great arteries; TOF = tetralogy of Fallot; VSD = ventricular septal defect.

The diagnosis of Holt-Oram syndrome is most likely to be missed in a patient with an unknown or unremarkable family history, a secundum septal defect, and minimal or no thumb anomaly. In any "sporadic" case of an atrial septal defect, the patient and the parents should be carefully examined for limb malformations and the family history studied in detail. Detection of a subtle limb defect alters the recurrence risk in offspring of the proband from the empirical risk of an isolated septal defect of 3 percent to the 50 percent of an autosomal dominant trait.

Mutations in the *TBX5* gene, a transcriptional regulator, cause one form of Holt-Oram syndrome.[83] The effect of different mutations on expression of the transcription factor does not appear to correlate with the marked differences seen in limb and cardiac development in different families.[84] Not all families with Holt-Oram syndrome are linked to this locus at 12q2, so at least one additional gene can cause this spectrum of defects.

ELLIS–VAN CREVELD SYNDROME (Fig. 70–6). This rare autosomal recessive chondrodysplasia is found among the old-order Amish because of a founder effect and consanguinity. Short stature, metaphyseal dysplasia, dysplastic nails and teeth, and postaxial polydactyly are the pleiotropic manifestations, in addition to congenital heart disease. Congenital heart disease is present in more than one-half of homozygotes, and most of the defects affect the atrial septum. The majority are defects of endocardial cushion closure, including ostium primum defects of widely varying size up to

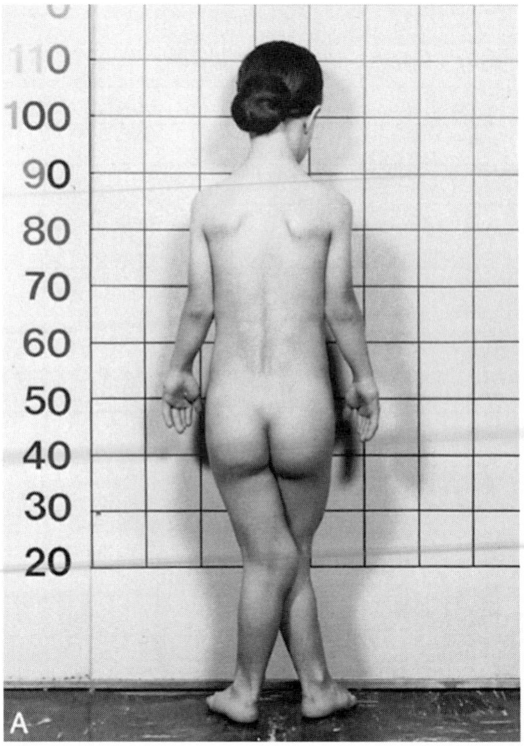

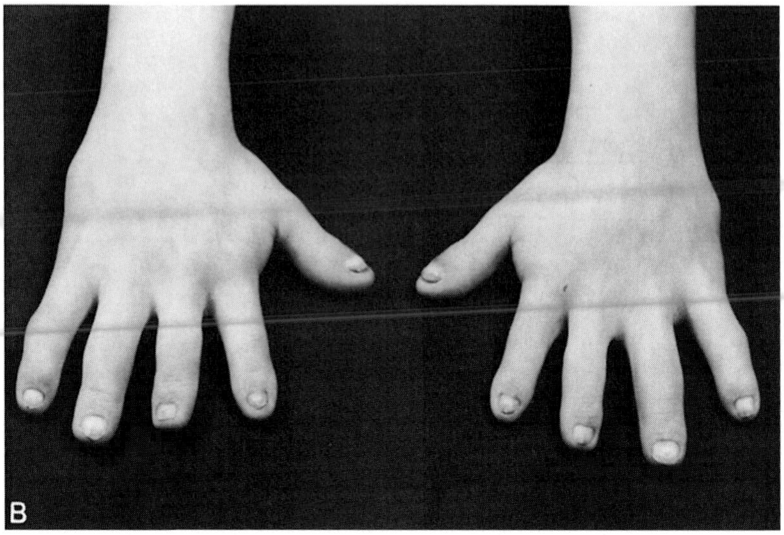

FIGURE 70–6 Ellis–van Creveld syndrome in a young woman. **A,** Note short stature, joint contractures at the elbows, and marked genu valgum. **B,** The fingers are short and the nails dysplastic. Note the protuberances along the ulnar edges of the hands where sixth digits were amputated.

a single atrium. This disorder has long been thought to be due to a yet unknown defect in the extracellular matrix, which would fit with the high frequency of endocardial cushion lesions. However, defects thought to be due to abnormal embryonic flow (coarctation, hypoplastic left heart, and patent ductus arteriosus) occur in about 20 percent of cases. The gene maps to 4p16 in patients of all ethnic derivations. A gene of unknown function within this locus, termed *EVC,* is mutated in some, but not all, patients.[85] A second gene in this chromosomal region, called *EVC2,* is mutated in patients of Ashkenazi ethnicity.[86] The finding that two closely linked genes cause the same condition is distinctly unusual. Ellis–van Creveld syndrome can be diagnosed prenatally by detection of polydactyly by ultrasonography.

FAMILIAL ATRIOVENTRICULAR CANAL DEFECTS. This spectrum of defects occasionally occurs in an autosomal dominant pattern in families and is unassociated with features in other systems. Because the cardiac defect is suggestive of that in Down syndrome, linkage to chromosome 21 markers was pursued, to no avail. In a large kindred that showed variable expression of nonsyndromic atrioventricular canal defects, analysis of shared markers among persons clearly affected identified a region on chromosome 1 (1p31-p21) that must harbor a gene that effects susceptibility to failure of closure of the endocardial cushions.[87]

VENTRICULAR SEPTAL DEFECT. This malformation does not seem to be inherited as an isolated Mendelian malformation, and no syndromes include it as a common, isolated manifestation.[80]

SUPRAVALVULAR AORTIC STENOSIS. This congenital lesion, which can be asymptomatic and detected long after birth because of an ejection murmur, occurs in at least three settings. It can be a sporadic anomaly, a component of Williams syndrome, or an autosomal dominant trait associated with peripheral pulmonic stenoses and a diffuse arteriopathy.

Williams syndrome is usually sporadic but, in more instances than previously recognized, is a highly variable autosomal dominant condition. The full spectrum includes infantile hypercalcemia, abnormal (elfin) facies (see Fig. 56–33), mental deficiency, short stature, numerous peripheral pulmonic stenoses, and supravalvular aortic stenosis. Although patients usually survive the problems of infancy and show catch-up growth, progressive problems of joint contractures, genitourinary and gastrointestinal dysfunction, hypertension, and psychosocial adjustment define the long-term prognosis.[88]

Supravalvular aortic stenosis (SVAS) is due to heterozygosity for a mutation in tropoelastin (discussed later). Because elastic fibers are intrinsic to the media of elastic and muscular arteries, a diffuse, progressive arteriopathy develops, with thickening of the wall and reduction of the lumen. The natural history of the arterial disease is just emerging as patients with Williams syndrome live longer and are monitored prospectively. A predisposition to cerebrovascular disease seems certain. Virtually all tested patients with Williams syndrome have a deletion of the long arm of chromosome 7.[89,90] Those with SVAS have a deletion involving the tropoelastin locus.[91] The crucial gene or genes involved in the rest of the Williams phenotype lie telomeric to the tropoelastin locus; considerable effort is currently directed at identifying the genes that have a role in development of the face, in calcium metabolism, and in development of personality and cognitive capability. Cultured cells from patients with either Williams syndrome or SVAS make less elastin than normal, but the cells have a higher than normal rate of proliferation, a finding that may explain the thickening of the arterial media seen in both conditions.[92]

Autosomal dominant SVAS is an entity distinct from Williams syndrome, although some patients have subtle defects in personality and intelligence. Peripheral pulmonary artery stenoses may be present but rarely cause hemodynamic problems. The aortic lesion requires surgery in less than half of patients.

MITRAL VALVE PROLAPSE (see Chap. 57). This trait is of heterogeneous cause and pathogenesis, although it has been called the most common abnormality of human heart valves. MVP is, equally clearly, not always an abnormality.[93,94] The heritable forms of MVP can be classified into three groups. The first is a familial form with minimal extracardiac involvement. The second is clinically variable, an autosomal dominant condition that merges at one end of its spectrum with Marfan syndrome; it could just as well be discussed as a heritable disorder of connective tissue. The third category is composed of the various Mendelian syndromes that include MVP as a pleiotropic manifestation. In all of these categories, prolapse of the tricuspid valve is a frequent accompaniment.

The first category, which some have called MVP syndrome or familial MVP, includes a condition centered on the mitral valve. The development of actual prolapse shows the age- and gender-dependent behavior characteristic of the idiopathic form. Formal genetic studies in most families confirm autosomal dominance with variable expression. This category has been partitioned into those patients with billowing of the mitral leaflets and those with excessive systolic mitral annular expansion; because this phenotype breeds relatively true, two distinct autosomal dominant forms may exist. The cause, or causes, of these entities is unknown. Moreover, when and how the phenotype of this condition can be distinguished from the sporadic cases of MVP and the cases with obvious evidence of a systemic disorder of connective tissue are unclear. The only consistent extracardiac manifestations are excessive arm span in women and relatively low body weight and systolic pressure. Recently, MVP has been mapped to three genetic loci; none of the genes has been identified. Two are autosomal loci, 11p15.4 and 16p11.2-p12.1.[95,96] Susceptibility to myxomatous degeneration of all cardiac valves can be inherited as an X-linked trait that maps to Xq28.[97]

Many clinical geneticists and cardiologists have referred patients with a suspicion of Marfan syndrome or Ehlers-Danlos syndrome. Some of these patients do not meet minimal diagnostic criteria for a recognized connective tissue disorder[98] but clearly have extracardiac features consistent with a defect of the extracellular matrix described later. MVP is commonly but not always present; when it is present and when evidence of a systemic abnormality of connective tissue is lacking, the patient should be considered to have *primary MVP* (see above). The clinical spectrum of the patients with syndromic MVP includes abnormal striae atrophicae, excessive arm span and leg length, joint hypermobility, pectus excavatum, scoliosis, reduction in thoracic kyphosis ("straight back"), myopia, and mild aortic root dilation.[99] Aortic dilation beyond 3 SD above the mean for body surface area, aortic dissection, ectopia lentis, or a family history of any of these three features *removes* a patient from this category. For the remainder of patients, the acronym MASS phenotype (*m*itral valve, *a*orta, *s*kin, and *s*keletal) describes what certainly is a heterogeneous grouping of patients and families. The aorta is mentioned specifically because of the appropriate concern that progressive dilation and dissection will occur; in fact, neither has been the case, although prospective evaluation has been unsystematic. Many of the associations between MVP and deformity of the thoracic cage and spontaneous pneumothorax are explained by the MASS phenotype.

Finally, MVP frequently accompanies Marfan syndrome, several of the Ehlers-Danlos syndromes, and cutis laxa and occurs more often than expected in patients with osteogenesis imperfecta, Larsen syndrome, pseudoxanthoma elasticum, and other Mendelian syndromes (see Table 70–13). In addition, occasional families with otherwise unclassified heritable disorders of connective tissue have prominent involvement of the mitral apparatus, with myxomatous deterioration, calcification, or both.[100]

NOONAN SYNDROME. Among the pleiotropic Mendelian syndromes with frequent cardiovascular involvement, Noonan syndrome is important because of its relatively high prevalence and clinical variability. This autosomal dominant condition has been called the male Turner syndrome in the past because of the short stature, cubitus valgus, neck webbing, congenital lymphedema, and congenital heart defects that coexist in the 45,X Turner syndrome. However, Noonan syndrome is distinct, but not simply because both men and women are affected. Patients with Noonan syndrome often have an unusual deformity of the sternum, mental dullness, hypertelorism, ptosis, and cryptorchidism. The cardiovascular defects, although widely varied, do not include an increased incidence of coarctation of the aorta. Due to the dysmorphism of the facies and the cardiac involvement, Noonan syndrome is often classified, along with William, LEOPARD, King, and Watson syndromes, as a cardiofacial syndrome.

The entire phenotype of Noonan syndrome is highly variable, and affected persons can escape clinical problems (or accurate diagnosis) even if they have obvious manifestations. Similarly, a wide range of cardiovascular involvement can occur. *Valvular pulmonic stenosis* was the first defect identified, and Noonan syndrome should always be considered in a patient with this lesion. The valve cusps are thickened and dysplastic, even in the absence of hemodynamic compromise. Obstruction to right-sided flow can also occur in patients with Noonan syndrome because of pulmonary artery hypoplasia or infundibular subvalvular changes. The latter finding reflects a generalized predisposition to hypertrophic cardiomyopathy, often asymmetrical, that can affect either ventricle. *Atrial septal defect* occurs in about one-third of patients, usually in association with pulmonic stenosis. *Ventricular septal defects* and *patent ductus arteriosus* each occur in about 10 percent. Congenital anomalies of coronary arteries are found occasionally and unexpectedly during evaluation of more obvious defects. The electrocardiogram often shows left anterior hemiblock and a deep precordial S wave, a pattern not common in pulmonic stenosis of other causes.

Lymphatic dysplasia, especially of the lower limbs, is common but causes clinical difficulties in less than 20 percent of cases. Although evidence of lymphedema often disappears during childhood, chylothorax and a protein-losing enteropathy represent the severe end of the spectrum.

Noonan syndrome shares features with other cardiofacial syndromes, and in sporadic cases (which account for 50 percent of Noonan syndrome), diagnosis can be difficult. All are autosomal dominant, so genetic counseling is somewhat easier. Affected males have reduced reproductive capabilities because of testicular abnormalities. Susceptibility to malignant hyperthermia can be detected by family history, elevated skeletal muscle creatine kinase levels, or muscle biopsy. Noonan syndrome occurs with a relatively high frequency, estimated to be as great as 1 per 1000. Mutations in the gene *PTPN11*, mapped to 12q24.2-q24.31, causes Noonan syndrome in about one-half of instances, so interlocus genetic heterogeneity is likely.[101] Intriguing issues that may shed light on both cause and pathogenesis are the overlap in phenotype with type I neurofibromatosis (the gene for which is on chromosome 17), and the frequent coexistence of Noonan syndrome and deficiency of coagulation factor XI.

Teratogenic Effects

A teratogen is any agent that adversely affects embryonic or fetal development, such as infectious vectors, radiation, drugs, and other chemicals (Table 70–10).[102,103] Teratogenic effects on the cardiovascular system are considered in this chapter for several reasons. First, the phenotypes are often reminiscent of those caused by chromosomal aberrations and single-gene mutations. Second, clinical geneticists and dysmorphologists are involved in diagnosing, managing, and investigating both teratogenic and genetic syndromes. Finally, an organism's response to an encounter with a potential teratogen is largely determined by its genome. The entire field of ecogenetics and part of pharmacogenetics are concerned with these issues.

TABLE 70–10 Cardiovascular Defects Associated with Prenatal Exposure to Teratogens

Teratogen	Cardiovascular Abnormalities*
Ethanol	~50% have CHD: VSD (~50% close spontaneously), TOF, ASD, ECD, absence of a pulmonary artery
Hydantoin	~10% have CHD: VSD, ASD, PS
Lithium	<3% have Ebstein anomaly
Phenylalanine	~20% have CHD: TOF
Retinoic acid	>50% have CHD: TGA, TOF, VSD, IAA
Rubella	>50% have CHD: PDA with or without ASD, VSD, PPS, IAA
Trimethadione	~50% have CHD: complex combinations most frequent (involving VSD, ASD, PDA, AS, PS), VSD, TOF
Valproic acid	>50% have CHD: left- and right-sided flow lesions: CoA, HLH, ASD, VSD, pulmonary atresia
Vitamin D	Supravalvular aortic stenosis is the cardinal manifestation; PPS
Warfarin	~10% have CHD: PDA, PS; rarely, intracranial hemorrhage.

*Among patients with the full clinical spectrum associated with each teratogen; cardiovascular defects listed in decreasing order of prevalence.

AS = aortic stenosis; ASD = atrial septal defect; CHD = congenital heart defect(s); CoA = coarctation of aorta; ECD = endocardial cushion defect; HLH = hypoplastic left heart; IAA = interrupted aortic arch; PDA = patent ductus arteriosus; PPS = peripheral pulmonic stenosis; PS = valvular pulmonic stenosis; TGA = transposition of great arteries; TOF = tetralogy of Fallot; VSD = ventricular septal defect.

The abilities to resist disruption of normal human embryogenesis and development involve systems quite distinct from physiological homeostasis and related only in part with developmental homeostasis. Genetic susceptibilities to teratogens can be illustrated by diverse mechanisms: reduced or inaccurate repair of radiation-induced DNA damage; enhanced receptiveness to viral entry or replication; immune deficiencies that prevent inactivation of infectious vectors or maintenance of immunity; slow inactivation of a compound that exerts a direct deleterious effect; or rapid conversion of an inoffensive drug to a teratogenic metabolite. These types of hereditary variation can be determined by single genes, with susceptibility inherited as a Mendelian trait, or by many genes, each of small effect. Either situation can account for the well-known fact that only a fraction of pregnancies exposed to a given agent are affected adversely. Variation in dose and timing of exposure also confound interpretation of epidemiological and family data. It is not surprising, then, that the actual appearance of the abnormal phenotype is not amenable to traditional pedigree analysis. Rather, examination of the biochemical susceptibilities have proved, and will continue to prove, more enlightening.

Some teratogens, such as warfarin, have a clear action that explains how the pleiotropic manifestations emerge. The action of other teratogens, such as alcohol, is obscure. Finally, in some teratogenic syndromes, such as that in offspring of women with diabetes mellitus, the actual offensive agent is unclear, and numerous pathogenetic mechanisms seem to pertain. Regardless of cause and pathogenetic mechanism, the phenotypes of many teratogens often share manifestations, especially prenatal growth retardation, abnormalities of the craniofacies, and mental retardation.[91] The following syndromes have prominent consequences on the cardiovascular system.

FETAL ALCOHOL SYNDROME. Ethanol is the most common teratogen to which the human embryo and fetus are exposed. The period of greatest vulnerability is the first trimester, and the risks are related clearly to the amount of alcohol consumed; the risk that fetal alcohol syndrome will occur in an offspring of a chronic alcoholic woman is 30 to 50 percent. The features are highly variable and include growth retardation, mild to moderate mental retardation, hyperactivity, short palpebral fissures, a smooth philtrum with a thin upper lip, and small distal phalanges.[104] Congenital heart defects occur in more than one-half of children with the full spectrum of the phenotype; ventricular septal defects are most common and often insignificant, but atrial septal defects, tetralogy of Fallot, and aortic coarctation can occur.

FETAL HYDANTOIN SYNDROME. Virtually all antiseizure medications can affect the fetus. Hydantoin was the first to be identified as a teratogen. The risk to the fetus depends in part on the genotype of the fetus; defects in arene oxidase predispose to the full syndrome. The features include prenatal and postnatal growth retardation, mild mental retardation, a broad face with a short nose, short distal phalanges with small nails, and hip dislocation. Cardiovascular defects, which are an inconstant part of the syndrome, include septal defects, right- and left-sided flow defects, and a single umbilical artery.

RETINOIC ACID EMBRYOPATHY. Isotretinoin was not recognized as a teratogen until after it was licensed for the treatment of acne. The vulnerable period extends from the first week through the fourth month of gestation. Isotretinoin increases the risks of miscarriage and stillbirth. The phenotype includes anomalies of the craniofacies and gross neuroanatomical disruption. Cardiovascular defects are common and emphasize various conotruncal malformations. Live-born infants often succumb to the cardiac and brain anomalies. Although the mechanism of action is not certain, vitamin A derivatives such as retinoic acid function as morphogens during embryogenesis, serving as signals for cell migration. The fact that the cardiovascular defects are primarily those of rotation and folding suggests disruption of a normal developmental homeostatic system.

WARFARIN EMBRYOPATHY. Coumarin-related vitamin K antagonists are usually prescribed for various cardiovascular problems in women of childbearing age and can cause diverse cardiovascular and other organ damage to the fetus. Coumarin interferes with embryogenesis directly when administered during gestational weeks 6 through 9. The most pronounced effects are on cartilage because of inhibition of enzymes of extracellular matrix metabolism. Congenital cardiac defects perhaps increase in frequency but fit no specific pathogenetic mechanism. The second pattern of coumarin effects involves exposure during the second and third trimesters and includes spontaneous abortion, stillbirth, and various central nervous system defects. The last are not due simply to intracranial hemorrhage as was once assumed.

What predisposes to the adverse fetal effects of coumarin remains undetermined. First, more than 75 percent of women who take coumarin derivatives throughout pregnancy have normal offspring; reassuring most women while identifying those at risk for adverse effects has obvious advantages. Second, placing all pregnant women on a regimen of heparin is not an acceptable solution, because heparin can cause stillbirth or premature fetal loss in about 20 percent of exposures, is not as effective as coumarin in some indications for anticoagulation, and is more difficult to administer and regulate.

MATERNAL PHENYLKETONURIA. The inborn error of metabolism phenylketonuria (PKU) produces severe mental retardation unless the phenylalanine content of the diet is markedly reduced soon after birth.[105] Deficiency of phenylalanine hydroxylase in the fetus produces no harm because fetal blood levels of phenylalanine are regulated by the heterozygous mother's enzyme. Because neonatal screening for this disease is now routine in all states, virtually all patients receive treatment and grow to adulthood with average intelligence. Many patients discontinue the rigorous dietary therapy during adolescence, when the elevated phenylalanine levels have far less deleterious effects. The embryopathy occurs when a woman with homozygous deficiency for phenylalanine hydroxylase becomes pregnant and her fetus is exposed to high levels of the amino acid, which overwhelm its ability to metabolize. The result is highly predictable if the mother does not restart dietary restriction of phenylalanine for the entire gestation: moderate to severe mental retardation, prenatal and postnatal growth retardation, microcephaly, and various cardiovascular defects in 15 to 20 percent of cases. This condition can largely be prevented by effective counseling of female patients with PKU.

FETAL RUBELLA EFFECTS (see Chap. 56). About 50 percent of fetuses become infected with the rubella virus when the mother is infected during the first trimester. An infected fetus not only suffers varied and severe interference with development and organogenesis but also acquires a chronic viral illness that can persist for years. The most common features of the embryopathy are mental deficiency, deafness, cataract, and cardiovascular defects. PDA is common, as are septal defects. Peripheral pulmonary stenosis and fibromuscular proliferation of medium and small arteries often improve postnatally.

Cardiomyopathies (see Chap. 59)

Each of the three clinical categories of primary cardiomyopathy—hypertrophic, dilated, and restrictive—can be caused by mutations in single genes as judged by Mendelian inheritance of a consistent phenotype in numerous families. Many other Mendelian and mitochondrial disorders also cause cardiomyopathies as a secondary consequence of their basic metabolic disturbance.

Hypertrophic Cardiomyopathy

In more than four decades since the recognition of hypertrophic cardiomyopathy as a clinical entity, many aspects of its natural history, pathology, and management have been clarified substantially.[106-111] The phenotype is most clearly defined anatomically and histologically and consists of myocardial hypertrophy without secondary cause; cellular and myofiber disarray; myocardial fibrosis; and mediointimal proliferation of small coronary arteries. None of these features is pathognomonic; for example, myofiber disorganization is present in the normal human heart during embryogenesis and in congenital heart defects that place strain on the right-sided circulation.

About half of probands with idiopathic hypertrophic cardiomyopathy of any segment of the left ventricle have affected first-degree relatives, and the phenotype in those families is inherited as an autosomal dominant, familial hypertrophic cardiomyopathy (FHC). There is wide variability of expression within a family, in part due to the age dependence of the trait.[107] Later generations of relatives in adolescence and childhood may not have developed echocardiographic evidence of hypertrophy. Hence, pedigree screening by phenotype for clinical, counseling, or investigative purposes should not be considered complete until the following criteria are satisfied: two-dimensional echocardiography is used to ensure that segmental hypertrophy is detected; a person at risk has normal echocardiographic findings and no evidence of electrocardiographic abnormality or important dysrhythmia after about age 20; and a person of any age has left ventricular hypertrophy without any other explanation, such as hypertension or aortic stenosis.

Familial hypertrophic cardiomyopathy is a disease of the sarcomere, with primary defects of thick and thin filaments now defined. Mutations of at least 10 and perhaps more loci cause FHC (see Table 70–2).[112] The first gene identified was the cardiac beta-myosin heavy chain gene (*MYH7*). Depending on the population studied, about 50 percent of all FHC mutations occur in *MYH7,* and many mutations have been described.[113,114] Patients with neither parent affected may also have *MYH7* mutations, suggesting that the genetic alteration occurred in the egg or sperm of a parent. The likelihood of germline mosaicism is suggested strongly by two siblings with FHC and the same mutation in *MHY7*, even though neither parent shows the mutation in leukocyte DNA.[115] Mutations that alter the charge of the beta-myosin heavy chain generally carry a worse prognosis in terms of age of detection, electrocardiographic abnormalities, and sudden death.[116-118] Thus, defining the specific gene involved, followed by the specific mutation, likely has clinical importance.[119] However, because of the substantial technical challenges and expense of identifying the specific mutation in any given patient with FHC, genetic testing is not yet routine.[120] A recent survey of families with FHC found that in 82 percent, a mutation in either *MYH7* or *MYBPC3* was responsible, a finding that should facilitate a systematic approach to molecular testing.[112] How the mutant protein interacts with other components of the sarcomere of both cardiac and skeletal muscle to produce the phenotype is another area of active research,[121] as is the generation and characterization of animal models of FHC. Both approaches suggest that abnormal signaling by calcium ions in the sarcomere and diminished myocardial energetics and contractile reserve represent common pathways to aberrant myocyte growth and myocardial remodeling.[122,123] The importance of presymptomatic and even prehypertrophy diagnosis through mutation analysis in families will become more important as improved methods of therapy evolve.[124] Apparent cases of sporadic noncompaction of the left ventricle may represent the first recognizable instance of FHC in a family.[125]

Although intergenic and intragenic heterogeneity account for much of the interfamilial variability in the FHC phenotype, considerable variation remains among relatives who share the same mutation. Both environmental and genetic factors have impacts. A possible example of the latter is the angiotensin I–converting enzyme (ACE) genotype, with different polymorphic variants of ACE associated with more or less hypertrophy. Prognosis also depends on the degree of involvement of the cardiac microvasculature; patients unable to increase blood flow in response to dipyridamole were more likely to have an unfavorable outcome.[126]

Dilated Cardiomyopathy

The prevalence of idiopathic dilated cardiomyopathy (DCM) is about double that of the hypertrophic form, or about 2 to 8 per 100,000. Approximately one-half of patients who are evaluated for unexplained DCM are left with the "idiopathic" designation.[127] Although numerous occurrences of familial dilated cardiomyopathy (FDC) are reported, few investigations have been conducted of an unselected series of probands for clinical and subclinical evidence of cardiac disease. Thus, it is unclear what fraction of patients with idiopathic DCM have a Mendelian disease, how many have a new mutation for a Mendelian disease, and how many have phenocopies of nongenetic causes. Estimates of a positive family history, which could suggest a Mendelian condition or a shared environmental cause, range from 7 to 30 percent.[113]

Because of the risk of severe dysrhythmia in patients with DCM, early detection of individuals with the disorder can be life saving. Echocardiography sensitively detects affected relatives with subclinical disease. Individuals who have equivocal left ventricular enlargement or dysfunction can have ambulatory electrocardiographic monitoring and, if the diagnosis is still uncertain, can have serial examinations. Certainly every patient with idiopathic DCM should have a detailed family history taken; about 20 percent reveal an affected relative.[128] If any close relative has a history consistent with cardiomyopathy, dysrhythmia, or sudden death at a relatively young age, counseling about the risk of a familial disease and the potential benefits of pedigree screening should be offered. The majority of instances of FDC fit autosomal dominant inheritance, but X-linked, autosomal recessive, and mitochondrial forms exist.[107,129-131] Clinical variability characterizes virtually all pedigrees; variation in severity, clinical phenotype, and age of onset is typical.

Considerable progress has been made in the past few years in defining the causes of many of the autosomal dominant forms of FDC. Mutations that affect either force generation or force transmission can result in the DCM phenotype. Histological examination of myocardium generally shows nonspecific hypertrophy and fibrosis. By electron microscopy, however, mitochondria are distinctly abnormal, a finding not seen in cases of congestive heart failure due to other causes. Although various mutations of the mitochondrial chromosome can cause dilated cardiomyopathy, including childhood onset, the inheritance pattern in most cases does not suggest maternal transmission.[131]

Some pedigrees show convincing evidence of X-linkage of dilated cardiomyopathy. At least three loci have been identified. In Barth syndrome, cardiac involvement is associated with skeletal myopathy, proportionate short stature, and neutropenia. The cause is mutation of the (*TAZ*) gene at Xq28. Mutations of this gene can also cause isolated FDC and noncompaction of the left ventricle.[107,132]

Many males with Duchenne and some with Becker muscular dystrophy develop myocardial dysfunction.[133] In the Becker form, right ventricular involvement may be unassociated with left ventricular dysfunction. Deletion of exon 49 of the dystrophin gene predisposes to cardiomyopathy. This pleiotropic feature in a disease that manifests as a skeletal myopathy prompted evaluation of the dystrophin locus in pedigrees with apparently isolated cardiomyopathy. Mutations in the 5′ end of the dystrophin gene have been found to account for some instances of X-linked dilated cardiomyopathy. Why some dystrophin mutations are selectively expressed in cardiac muscle (and others in brain) is unclear.

Emery-Dreifuss muscular dystrophy is distinguishable clinically from the Duchenne and Becker forms by absence of pseudohypertrophy of skeletal muscle, early involvement of the arms with elbow contractures, and early onset of cardiac conduction abnormalities and atrial dysrhythmia.[133,134] Autosomal dominant and X-linked recessive forms occur. In the latter, female heterozygotes are also commonly affected, albeit more mildly than males. The disease was mapped to the distal region of Xq28, and a previously unknown gene, called *emerin*, was found to be mutated. Hearts show replacement of myocardium, especially in the atria, with fat and fibrosis. Even though the conduction system is not primarily affected histologically, sudden death is common in both hemizygous men and heterozygous women; thus, carrier detection can be life saving.

The dominant form of Emery-Dreifuss muscular dystrophy is caused by mutations in the lamin A/C gene.[135] Both emerin and lamin A/C are expressed in the nuclear membrane of skeletal and heart muscle. Mutations in lamin A/C cause a number of diverse syndromes, including Hutchinson-Gilford progeria.[136]

Autosomal recessive forms of limb-girdle muscular dystrophy with DCM have been found to be due to mutations in the genes encoding β- and δ-sarcoglycan, and mutations in the same genes, when heterozygous, cause autosomal dominant FDC.[137,138]

The arrhythmogenic right ventricular dysplasias are distinct from idiopathic DCM but share some features with most of the FDCs in that they are generally autosomal dominant, and conduction defects, dysrhythmia, and sudden death can precede the appearance of overt heart failure.[139,140]

TABLE 70–11 Disorders Associated with Restrictive Cardiomyopathy

Phenotype	OMIM No.*
Primary endocardial fibroelastosis	
Familial endocardial fibroelastosis	226000, 305300
Faciocardiorenal syndrome	227280
Secondary endocardial fibroelastosis	
As a Relatively Common Manifestation	
Maternal lupus erythematosus	
Pseudoxanthoma elasticum	177850, 264800
Systemic carnitine deficiency	212140
Trisomy 18	
As a Relatively Infrequent Manifestation	
Cornelia de Lange syndrome	122470
Rubinstein-Taybi syndrome	268600
Secondary Infiltrative Cardiomyopathy	
Familial amyloidoses I and III	176300
Fabry disease	301500
Gaucher disease type I	230800
Glycogen storage disorder II	232300
Glycogen storage disorder III	232400
Hemochromatosis	235200
Mucopolysaccharidosis IH	252800
Mucopolysaccharidosis II	309900

*Data from Online Mendelian Inheritance in Man (www.ncbi.nlm.nih.gov/omim).

Restrictive Cardiomyopathy

Restrictive cardiomyopathy is primarily a defect of diastolic function.[141] The pathogenesis of the majority of cases of restrictive cardiomyopathy involves infiltration or replacement of the myocardium or both. The causes are varied and can be nongenetic or genetic; the latter are mostly metabolic diseases with secondary effects on the heart and are summarized in Table 70–11; some are reviewed subsequently. One form of restrictive cardiomyopathy that has primary genetic forms among many other causes is endocardial fibroelastosis. Other mutations produce restriction through pericardial constriction. Isolated pedigrees of primary myocardial fibrosis without secondary cause and leading to restrictive hemodynamics are not classifiable.

Endocardial Fibroelastosis

This abnormality is characterized by thickening of the endocardium, which leads to decreased compliance and impaired diastolic function. Primary forms, discussed here, are unassociated with other cardiac anomalies (see Table 70–9). In infants, there is often an indolent course of failure to thrive, tachypnea, and tachycardia, until a precipitant such as an upper respiratory infection leads to rapid cardiac decompensation. Treatment of children with primary endocardial fibroelastosis is ineffective; cardiac transplantation now offers some hope. Autopsy shows enlargement of the left ventricle and perhaps other chambers, no abnormality of lung vessels, and collapse of the left lower lobe. Histopathological study reveals extensive deposition of extracellular matrix, primarily collagen and elastic fibers, in the endocardium.

X-linked recessive inheritance is the most firmly established of the single-gene causes. Some pedigrees show mainly small, contracted cardiac chambers, whereas others have chamber dilation; both are compatible with the functional pathophysiology described by the term *restrictive*. Males are affected earlier and more severely by both forms, and death in infancy is not unusual. The condition must be distinguished from X-linked dilated cardiomyopathy and Barth syndrome. Morphological abnormalities of mitochondria occur on ultrastructural studies of heart and leukocytes. Insufficient longitudinal experience is recorded to know whether females heterozygous for this mutation develop a dilated or restrictive cardiomyopathy later in life.

Several pedigrees suggestive of autosomal recessive inheritance of primary endocardial fibroelastosis were reported before the routine availability of laboratory methods to diagnose metabolic derangements, especially defects in fatty acid catabolism. The occurrence of hydrocephalus, endocardial fibroelastosis, and neonatal cataracts may be due to a single gene mutation but could represent sequelae of a viral infection. Endocardial fibroelastosis can be a prominent finding at autopsy in patients with autosomal dominant dilated cardiomyopathy; whether the endocardial changes are primary, representing yet another Mendelian form of this disorder, or secondary remains unclear.

Restrictive cardiomyopathy often occurs with both hemodynamic evidence of impaired diastolic filling and wall thickening; any of the conditions causing pseudohypertrophy of the myocardium can eventually exhibit restrictive pathophysiology. Hemochromatosis and the amyloidoses, both hereditary and acquired forms, are especially likely to present in this manner. Connective tissue replaces myocytes or infiltrates the interstitium in a number of conditions. Fibrosis of the myocardium may cause pseudohypertrophy, but the clinical consequences are more those of restriction. Restrictive pathophysiology often accompanies fibrosis of the myocardium, at least in the early stages. Replacement of myocytes or infiltration of the interstitium by collagen and proteoglycan occurs in various conditions, such as muscular dystrophies and disorders that predispose to ischemia due to coronary artery occlusion, such as diabetes mellitus, hemoglobinopathies associated with sickling, Fabry disease, and the mucopolysaccharidoses. Severe fibrosis may produce considerable thickening of the myocardium, or pseudohypertrophy. Finally, a number of hereditary conditions associate with endocardial fibroelastosis (see Table 70-11).

CONSTRICTIVE PERICARDITIS (see Chap. 64). Two rare autosomal recessive disorders include fibrous thickening of the pericardium as a manifestation. In both, signs and symptoms of constrictive pericarditis develop insidiously, and treatment by pericardiotomy is life saving. One condition was first described in Finland and given the name *MULIBREY nanism,* a combination of a mnemonic for *mu*scle, *li*ver, *br*ain, and *ey*e and an archaic word for dwarfism (nanism). Growth failure from an early age is common, and growth does not improve once pericardial constriction is abated. Subsequently, more than a dozen patients, generally with consanguineous parents, have been reported from around the world.[142] The gene in which mutations occur maps to 17q22-q23 and encodes an apparent zinc-finger transcription factor of unclear function.[143]

The arthropathy-camptodactyly syndrome previously had been reported because of the skeletal and rheumatological manifestations before pericardial effusion and fibrous thickening of the pericardium were recognized as manifestations. The disease locus was mapped in consanguineous kindreds by homozygosity by descent to 1q25-q31, and mutations occur in the gene, *CACP,* that encodes a secreted proteoglycan.[144,145]

Cardiomyopathies Secondary to Other Causes

INBORN ERRORS OF METABOLISM. These can affect the left ventricle by various mechanisms (Table 70–12) and produce diverse anatomical, histological, and functional disturbances. The most common anatomical result is an apparent hypertrophic cardiomyopathy, which is actually pseudohypertrophic because the thickened walls are not due to myocardial cell hypertrophy but to cellular or interstitial infiltration by metabolites. Abnormalities of both systolic and diastolic function result, outflow obstruction may occur, and in some cases the hemodynamic characteristics resemble a restrictive cardiomyopathy. The offending metabolite may be an incompletely degraded macromolecule such as glycogen (glycogen storage disorder II [Pompe disease] and glycogen storage disorder III), proteoglycan and glycosaminoglycan (mucopolysaccharidoses I, III, IV, VI, and VII),[146] sphingolipid (Fabry disease,[147] Tay-Sachs disease, Farber disease, Refsum disease, and Gaucher disease), glycoprotein (fucosidosis and mannosidosis), and amyloid (familial amyloidoses I and III) or a small molecule such as iron in hemochromatosis. Some of these disorders are discussed later. True myocardial hypertrophy occurs as a part of Mendelian syndromes, such as Noonan syndrome, von Recklinghausen neurofibromatosis, Costello syndrome[148] and LEOPARD syndrome,[149] and monogenic errors of metabolism, notably those producing hyperthyroidism and pheochromocytoma. Any of the Mendelian disorders that cause hypertension may, over time, produce true myocardial hypertrophy.

Dilated cardiomyopathy often results from inborn errors of energy production, especially fatty acid metabolism. Various disorders associated with carnitine deficiency, mitochondrial and peroxisomal dysfunction, and muscle dysfunction can manifest with symptoms of congestive heart failure or dysrhythmia.

Primary Disorders of Rhythm and Conduction

See Chapter 28.

Disorders of Connective Tissue

The two broad classes of connective tissue disorders are those due to mutations in single genes that determine or somehow affect components of the extracellular matrix and those due to extrinsic factors affecting the extracellular matrix, such as rheumatoid arthritis and systemic lupus erythematosus. The former category includes many disorders that affect the cardiovascular system. Susceptibility to so-called acquired disorders of connective tissue is, in part, determined by genes, and this specific aspect is reviewed below.

Mendelian Disorders of the Extracellular Matrix

Close to 200 distinct phenotypes now make up this category, which was first defined less than four decades ago with fewer than 10 disorders. Several reviews and textbooks describe the phenotypes, genetics, and causes of many of the conditions (Table 70–13).[18,150,151]

Marfan Syndrome

This autosomal dominant disorder is relatively frequent (2-3 per 10,000) and occurs in all races and ethnic groups.[15,151] Even with the discovery of the genetic and biochemical bases of the condition, the diagnosis of Marfan syndrome outside families with the classic phenotype remains entirely clinical. Current criteria (Table 70–14) depend on the manifestations in the cardinal organ systems—the eye, the skeleton, the heart, and the aorta—and other systems as well as the family history (Fig. 70–7).[98,151] The presence of manifestations more specific for Marfan syndrome, such as aortic dilation, aortic dissection in a nonhypertensive young person, ectopia lentis, and dural ectasia, clearly is more important diagnostically

TABLE 70–12 Mendelian Errors of Metabolism with Manifestations in the Cardiovascular System

Disorder	Eponym or Common Name	OMIM No.*	Pathogenesis
Aminoacidopathies			
Alkaptonuria	Ochronosis	203500	Deposition of homogentisic acid in connective tissue
Cystinosis, nephropathic type		219800	Lysosomal storage
Homocystinuria		236200	Unknown
Oxalosis I	Hyperoxaluria	259900	Vascular and tissue accumulation of oxalate
Defects in Fatty Acid Metabolism			
Carnitine transport defect	Primary carnitine deficiency	212140	Lipid myopathy; defective energy generation
MCAD deficiency		201450	Lipid myopathy; defective energy generation
LCAD deficiency		201460	Lipid myopathy; defective energy generation
Glycogen Storage Disorders			
GSD II	Pompe	232300	Lysosomal storage
GSD II	Adult acid maltase deficiency	232300	Lysosomal storage
GSD III	Forbes; debrancher deficiency	232400	Intracellular glycogen accumulation; fibrosis
GSD VIII	GSD of the heart	306000	
Glycoproteinoses			
Fucosidosis, severe		230000	Lysosomal storage
Fucosidosis, mild		230000	Lysosomal storage
Mannosidosis		248500	Lysosomal storage
Aspartylglycosaminuria		208400	Lysosomal storage
Mucolipidoses			
ML II	I-cell	252500	Lysosomal storage
ML III	Pseudo-Hurler polydystrophy	252500	Lysosomal storage
Mucopolysaccharidoses			
MPS IH	Hurler	252800	Lysosomal storage
MPS IS	Scheie	252800	Lysosomal storage
MPS IH/S	Hurler-Scheie	252800	Lysosomal storage
MPS II	Hunter	209900	Lysosomal storage
MPS III A	Sanfilippo A	252900	Lysosomal storage
MPS III B	Sanfilippo B	252920	Lysosomal storage
MPS III C	Sanfilippo C	252930	Lysosomal storage
MPS III D	Sanfilippo D	252940	Lysosomal storage
MPS IV A	Morquio A	253000	Lysosomal storage
MPS IV B	Morquio B	253010	Lysosomal storage
MPS VI	Maroteaux-Lamy	253200	Lysosomal storage
MPS VII	Sly	253220	Lysosomal storage
Sphingolipidoses			
Fabry		301500	Cellular accumulation of trihexosyl ceramide, especially in endothelium
Farber		228000	Histiocytic infiltration
Gaucher, adult form		230800	Cellular accumulation of glucocerebroside
Miscellaneous Disorders			
Acid lipase deficiency	Wolman	278000	↑ Cholesterol; foam cell infiltration
Cholesterol ester storage disease		278000	↑ Cholesterol; foam cell infiltration
Geleophysic dysplasia		231050	Lysosomal storage
Hereditary angioedema		106100	Complement and kinin activation

*Data from Online Mendelian Inheritance in Man (www.ncbi.nlm.nih.gov/omim).
†Gene symbol; for chromosomal locus see Table 70–2.
‡Naturally occurring mutants; does not include transgenic and knockout rodent models.

Cardiovascular Involvement	Biochemical Defect	Gene Locus[†]	Animal Model[‡]
AS; atherosclerosis	Homogentisate oxidase	*HGD*	
Hypertension from renal failure, vascular wall thickening	Cystinosin	*CTNS*	
Early CAD; venous thrombosis; pulmonary embolism	Cystathionine β-synthase	*CBS*	
Conduction defect; vascular occlusions; Raynaud phenomenon	Peroxisomal alanine-glyoxylate aminotransferase	*AGT*	
DCM: ECF	Solute carrier 22	*OCTN2*	Syrian hamster
DCM	Medium-chain acyl-CoA dehydrogenase	*ACADM*	
DCM	Long-chain acyl-CoA dehydrogenase	*ACADL*	
Pseudohypertrophic CM; short PR interval; ECF	α-1,4-glucosidase	*GAA*	Canine and bovine
Primarily skeletal muscle; respiratory insufficiency; cor pulmonale	α-1,4-glucosidase	*GAA*	
Pseudohypertrophic CM	Amylo-1,6-glucosidase	*AGL*	
DCM	Phosphorylase kinase	*PHKA2*	
Myocardial thickening	α-Fucosidase	*FUCA1*	
Angiokeratoma	α-Fucosidase	*FUCA1*	
Myocardial thickening; valvular thickening; conduction disturbance	α-Mannosidase	*MANB*	
Valvular thickening	Aspartylglycosylamine aminohydrolase	*AGA*	
Same as MPS IH	Acetylglucosamine-1-phosphotransferase	*GNPTA*	
Valvular thickening and dysfunction, especially AS, AR	Acetylglucosamine-1-phosphotransferase	*GNPTA*	
Early CAD; PH and OAD→CP; valvular dysfunction, especially MR, AR; pseudohypertrophic CM	α-L-Iduronidase	*IDUA*	Canine and feline
Valvular dysfunction, especially AS	α-L-Iduronidase	*IDUA*	
Same as MPS IH	α-L-Iduronidase	*IDUA*	
Same as MPS IH; less severe in mild MPS II variant	Sulfoiduronate sulfatase	*IDS*	
Valvular thickening and occasional dysfunction	Heparan sulfate sulfatase	*SGSH*	
Valvular thickening and occasional dysfunction	*N*-Acetyl-α-D-glucosaminidase	*NAGLU*	
Valvular thickening and occasional dysfunction	Acetyl-CoA; α-glucosaminidase *N*-acetyltransferase	*MPS3C*	
Valvular thickening and occasional dysfunction	*N*-Acetylglucosamine-6-sulfatase	*GNS*	
Valvular dysfunction, especially AR	Galactosamine-6-sulfatase	*GALNS*	
Milder than MPS IV A	β-Galactosidase	*GLBI*	
Same as MPS IH	Arylsulfatase B	*ARSB*	Feline
Valvular thickening	β-Glucuronidase	*GUSB*	Murine and canine
Early CAD, valvular thickening and dysfunction; pseudohypertrophic CM; short PR interval; arteriolar occlusion; angiokeratoma	α-Galactosidase A	*GLA*	
Nodular thickening of valves	Ceramidase	*ASAH*	
PH→CP; interstitial infiltration of myocytes by Gaucher cells; constrictive pericarditis	β-Glucocerebroside	*GBA*	
Atherosclerosis	Lysosomal acid lipase	*LIPA*	
Atherosclerosis; PH	Lysosomal acid lipase	*LIPA*	
Valvular dysfunction	?		
Angioedema	C1 esterase inhibitor	*CINH*	

AR = aortic regurgitation; AS = aortic stenosis; CAD = coronary artery disease; CM = cardiomyopathy; CP = cor pulmonale; DCM = dilated cardiomyopathy; ECF = endocardial fibroelastosis; GSD = glycogen storage disease; MPS = mucopolysaccharoidoses; MR = mitral regurgitation; OAD = obstructive airway disease; PH = pulmonary hypertension.

TABLE 70–13 Cardiovascular Manifestations of Heritable Disorders of Connective Tissue

Disorder	OMIM No.*	Cardiovascular Manifestations
Cutis laxa	219100 123700	PS, PPS, CP MVP
Ehlers-Danlos, classic form	130000, 130010	MVP, occasional aortic root dilatation
Ehlers-Danlos, hypermobile form	130020	MVP
Ehlers-Danlos, vascular form	130050	Arterial rupture, MVP, occasionally aortic dissection and arterial aneurysms, easy bruising
Ehlers-Danlos, ocular-scoliotic form	225400	MVP
Ehlers-Danlos, tenascin-X deficiency[151a]	606408	MVP, easy bruising
Osteogenesis imperfecta I	166200	MVP, mild aortic root dilatation
Osteogenesis imperfecta II	166210	CP, arterial calcification
Osteogenesis imperfecta III	259420	MVP
Osteogenesis imperfecta IV	166220	Aortic root dilatation
Marfan syndrome	154700	MVP, aortic root dilatation, aortic dissection
MASS phenotype	157700	MVP, mild aortic root dilatation
Pseudoxanthoma elasticum	177850	Arteriolar sclerosis, claudication, myocardial infarction, endocardial fibroelastosis

CP = cor pulmonale; MVP = mitral valve prolapse; PPS = peripheral pulmonic stenosis; PS = valvular pulmonic stenosis.
*Data from Online Mendelian Inheritance in Man (www.ncbi.nlm.nih.gov/omim).

TABLE 70–14 Diagnostic Criteria for Marfan Syndrome

Phenotypic Manifestations*	
Skeleton	Joint hypermobility, tall stature, pectus excavatum, reduced thoracic kyphosis, scoliosis, arachnodactyly, dolichostenomelia, pectus carinatum, erosion of the lumbosacral vertebrae from dural ectasia[d]
Eye	Myopia, retinal detachment, elongated globe, precocious cataracts, ectopia lentis[d]
Cardiovascular	Mitral valve prolapse, endocarditis, dysrhythmia, dilated mitral annulus, mitral regurgitation, tricuspid valve prolapse, aortic regurgitation, aortic dissection,[d] dilation of the aortic root[d]
Pulmonary	Apical blebs, spontaneous pneumothorax
Skin and integument	Inguinal hernias, incisional hernias, striae atrophicae
Central nervous system	Attention deficit disorder, hyperactivity, verbal-performance discrepancy, dural ectasia,[d] anterior pelvic meningocele[d]
Family history	*If the family history is positive* for a close relative clearly affected by Marfan syndrome, to make the diagnosis in the patient, a major criterion should be present as well as findings in one other system. *If the family history is negative or unknown*, to make the diagnosis, the patient should have one major criterion and manifestations in two other systems.

*Manifestations are listed within each organ system in increasing specificity for Marfan syndrome, although none is completely specific; those indicated by[d] are the most specific and constitute major criteria.[141]

than features common in other connective tissue disorders and in the general population, such as scoliosis, joint hypermobility, myopia, and MVP.

The most common cardiovascular features are MVP and dilation of the sinuses of Valsalva.[151] Associated clinical problems of mitral regurgitation, aortic regurgitation, and aortic dissection account, if untreated, for most of the early mortality that results in an average age of death in the fourth and fifth decades of life.[152] Children tend to be more severely affected by mitral valve disease, whereas aortic problems are progressive and more likely in adolescence and beyond.

MITRAL VALVE INVOLVEMENT. MVP (see Chap. 57) is age dependent and more common in women with Marfan syndrome. The incidence reaches 60 to 80 percent when patients are studied by two-dimensional echocardiography, and the valve leaflets generally have an elongated and redundant appearance. Progression of severity, as judged by the appearance or worsening of mitral regurgitation by clinical and echocardiographic criteria, occurs in at least one-quarter of patients, a much higher rate than in MVP found in the general population. The mitral annulus dilates and contributes to the regurgitation, as do stretching and occasional rupture of chordae. About 10 percent of patients with marked prolapse have calcification of the mitral annulus. Standard treatment for chronic mitral regurgitation is indicated, but coexistent aortic root dilation usually requires that increasing inotropy be avoided. When mitral regurgitation becomes severe enough to warrant surgical intervention, two considerations must be added to the balance: (1) repair of the mitral apparatus is often successful and durable in patients with Marfan syndrome.[153] Repair is less easily accomplished when the cusps are extremely redundant, there is marked chordal damage, or the annulus is heavily calcified; (2) the aorta may be enlarged enough to permit concomitant repair. With Marfan syndrome, as with virtually all of the heritable disorders of connective tissue, there is an increased susceptibility to dehiscence of prosthetic mitral valves, regardless of the care taken in placing them.

AORTIC ROOT INVOLVEMENT (see Chap. 53). The sinuses of Valsalva are often dilated at birth, and the rate of progression varies widely among patients in general and also among relatives (Fig. 70–8). Thus, predicting long-term risks of developing aortic regurgitation (which clearly is positively associated with aortic root diameter), suffering aortic dissection (which is less clearly associated with diameter), or requiring aortic surgery is fraught with uncertainty.[154] Transthoracic echocardiography is sufficient for detecting and monitoring changes in diameter, because in the absence of dissection, dilation is limited to the proximal ascending aorta, and the rate of change is slow, measured in millimeters per year. Rare exceptions of principal dilation of the thoracic aorta can be monitored with transesophageal echocardiography or magnetic resonance imaging. Patients with dilation less than 1.5 times the mean diameter predicted for their body size can be observed annually; as the diameter increases, more frequent evaluation is necessary. Aortic regurgitation often appears in adults at a diameter of 50 mm but may be absent at diameters of more than 60 mm. The risk of dissection increases with the size of the aorta and fortunately occurs infrequently below a diameter of 55 mm in the adult. Many physicians have adopted the criterion of a 50 to 55 mm maximal aortic root dimension for performing elective surgery in adult patients with Marfan syndrome, regardless of the severity of the aortic regurgitation,[153] although patients with a family history of aortic dissection should have surgery at the lower end of this range. The perioperative results of both elective and emergency repair of the aortic root have been excellent and a marked improvement from the pre-composite graft era that ended in the mid-1970s. Long-term results of operation are limited by the problems of endocarditis and anticoagulation common to all prosthetic valves, but in the absence of chronic aortic dissection appear favorable for patients with Marfan syndrome.[153,155]

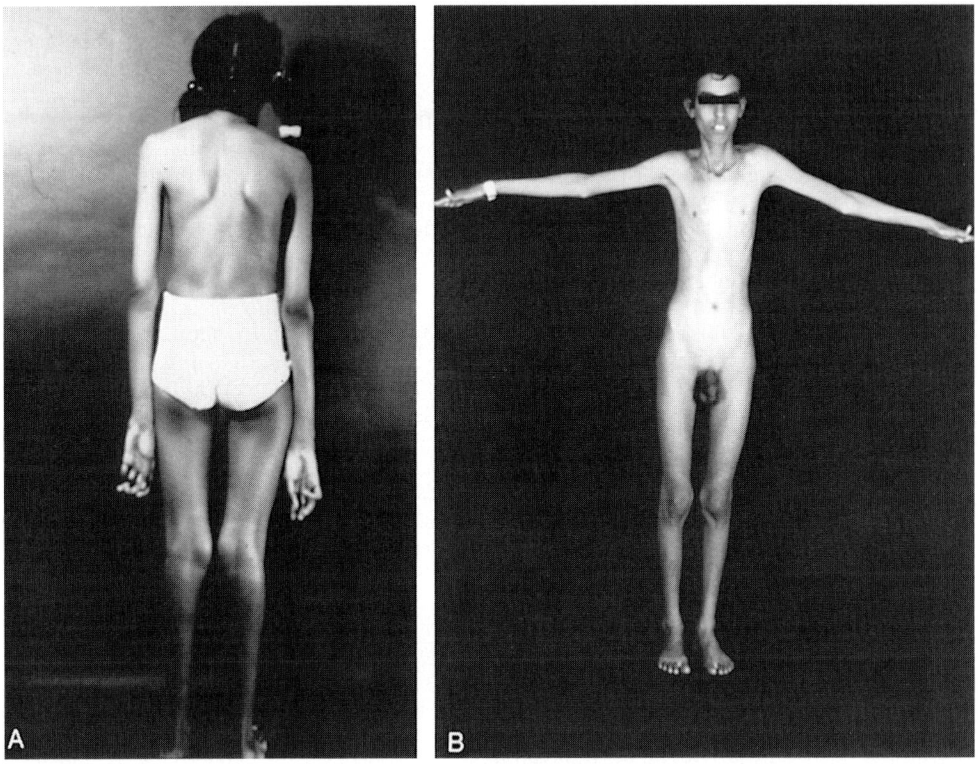

FIGURE 70–7 External phenotype of patients with Marfan syndrome, showing long extremities and digits, tall stature, and pectus carinatum.

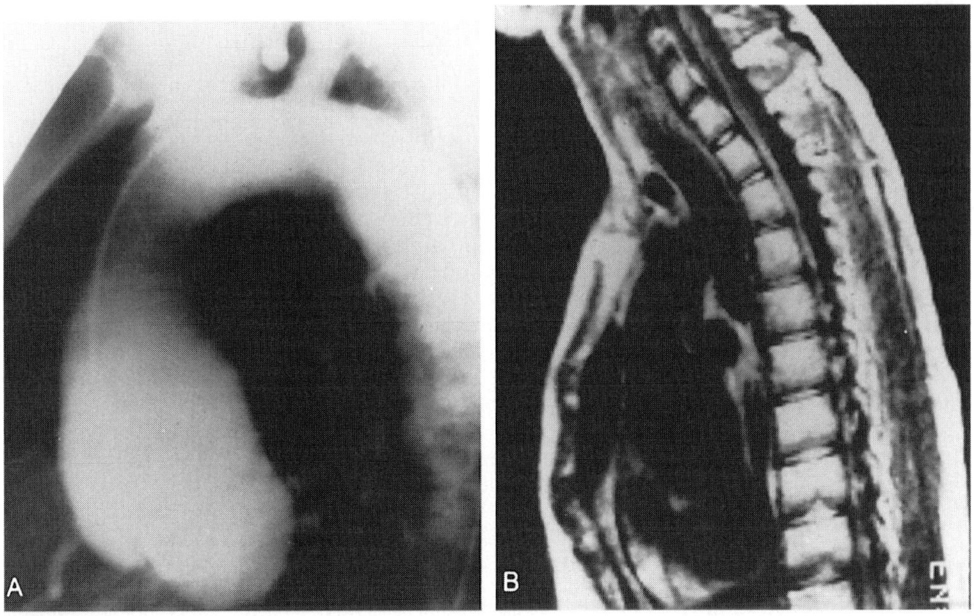

FIGURE 70–8 Dilation of the aortic root in Marfan syndrome. **A,** Lateral angiogram of the ascending aorta showing dilation of the sinuses of Valsalva and proximal ascending aorta and relatively normal caliber of the ascending aorta. **B,** Lateral magnetic resonance imaging scan of the same patient.

Several approaches to repairing the dilated or dissected aortic root while preserving the native aortic valve have been developed.[156] Findings at both short- and, now, long-term follow-up of patients with Marfan syndrome who have undergone this repair have been quite favorable.[153,157] The operation must be performed before the root is widely dilated and the valve commissures and cusps markedly stretched. This approach is increasingly being taken in all patients when the maximal root dimension reaches 50 mm, and it is an especially suitable procedure for women of childbearing age who want to consider pregnancy, as well as for all others in whom anticoagulation is contraindicated.

THORACIC ABNORMALITIES. Severe *pectus excavatum* can complicate cardiovascular surgery by hampering exposure of the heart by median sternotomy. For elective cardiovascular surgery, repair of the sternal deformity some months in advance permits sufficient healing of the costochondral junctions that a stable and functionally and cosmetically improved thoracic cage will facilitate further surgery and postoperative recovery. Simultaneous repair of cardiac and sternal defects, although possible, is a long procedure, and intraoperative bleeding from bone can be considerable due to the anticoagulation associated with cardiopulmonary bypass.

AORTIC DISSECTION (see Chap. 53). This complication usually begins just above the coronary ostia (type A in the Stanford scheme) and extends the entire length of the aorta (type I in DeBakey scheme). About 10 percent of dissections begin distal to the left subclavian artery (type B or III), but dissection rarely is limited to the abdominal aorta. Angiography, magnetic resonance imaging, and transesophageal echocardiography all have a role in the diagnosis of acute dissection in patients with Marfan syndrome; the capabilities and experience of the medical center and the stability of the patient are important determinants of the approach. Because many acute dissections of the ascending aorta in patients with Marfan syndrome have a stuttering course that culminates in death due to rupture or hemopericardium, rapid transfer to a facility prepared to perform immediate repair is essential.

Not all acute dissections in patients with Marfan syndrome involve severe, tearing chest pain that radiates to the back; indeed, some extensive dissections have been occult. This experience reinforces the need for a high index of suspicion by physicians whenever a tall, nearsighted young person with a thoracic cage deformity arrives at an emergency department with vague complaints of lightheadedness, chest or abdominal discomfort, or a murmur of aortic regurgitation. Similarly, patients known to have Marfan syndrome and their close relatives need education about the signs and symptoms of aortic dissection. In general, the management of acute and chronic dissection in patients with Marfan syndrome follows standard practice, with several departures. First, all dissections of the ascending aorta should be repaired promptly, preferably with a composite graft. Second, regular evaluation with magnetic resonance imaging is important, as the diameter of any region of dissected aorta is likely to expand over time. Third, reduction of systolic blood pressure and administration of negative-inotropic doses of beta-adrenergic blockers should be even more strictly adhered to than in dissections without a connective tissue abnormality. In most instances, any region of the aorta should be repaired when complications of further dissection, branch vessel occlusion, or dilation beyond about 50 mm occur. A staged approach to total replacement of the Marfan aorta is now both feasible and successful.

DYSRHYTHMIAS. Some patients develop serious ventricular or supraventricular dysrhythmia.[152] The latter often accompanies chronic mitral regurgitation, but the former may be of high grade and difficult to suppress when only MVP is present. Some patients have the syndrome of autonomic dysfunction, atypical chest pain, and palpitations seen in some patients with MVP unassociated with a flagrant connective tissue abnormality.

VENTRICULAR FUNCTION. Occasional patients with Marfan syndrome who have no clinically important valvular abnormalities develop moderate-to-severe left ventricular dysfunction. While this could represent the unlikely coincidence of Marfan syndrome and idiopathic dilated cardiomyopathy, we have speculated that certain fibrillin mutations could have a detrimental effect on myocardial function.[151] Evidence for and against this hypothesis has recently been produced.[158,159] Further study appears warranted.

MANAGEMENT. Routine cardiological management of Marfan syndrome is multifaceted: regular clinical and echocardiographic examinations; routine endocarditis prophylaxis for dental and other procedures; restriction of activity from heavy weightlifting, contact sports, and any exertion at maximal capacity; and long-term beta-adrenergic blocking agent therapy form the basic approach, with individual variation often appropriate. Support for the role of beta-adrenergic antagonists comes from several prospective studies that show a reduction in the rate of aortic dilation and the risk of aortic dissection in patients treated with negatively inotropic doses of propranolol or atenolol.[160] However, short-term administration of propranolol to patients with large sinus of Valsalva aneurysms, although reducing heart rate and peak systolic pressure, did not improve the impedance characteristics recorded in the ascending aorta. However, given studies that emphasize the importance of central pulse pressure to aortic dilation,[161] use of beta-adrenergic blocking agents seems warranted.

A woman with Marfan syndrome has two concerns about pregnancy (see Chap. 74). The first is the 50:50 risk that any child will inherit the condition; prenatal diagnosis can currently be attempted in selected situations. The second is the risk of dissection that the hemodynamic stresses of pregnancy place on the aorta. Several dozen case reports attest to the heightened incidence of dissection during the third trimester, parturition, and the first month postpartum. However, serious aortic dilation was present in the majority of instances. Prospective evaluation of 21 women through 45 pregnancies confirmed our earlier recommendation that the cardiovascular risks are relatively low if the aortic diameter does not exceed 40 mm and cardiac function is not compromised, a view shared by other investigators.[162]

ETIOLOGY. Marfan syndrome is caused by mutations in the gene that encodes fibrillin-1 (*FBN1*), the major constituent of microfibrils, which are components of the extracellular matrix that are widely dispersed and perform numerous functions.[151] Microfibrils and tropoelastin form elastic fibers. Fragmentation and disorganization of elastic fibers in the aortic media have long been a histological marker (inappropriately called *cystic medial necrosis*) of Marfan syndrome, although similar microscopic pathological lesions occur in familial aortic aneurysms and aging aortas of the normal population. A defect in microfibrils explains all of the pleiotropic manifestations of Marfan syndrome.

Several hundred distinct mutations in *FBN1,* the gene that encodes fibrillin-1, occur in different families, and only a few have emerged, by chance, in unrelated patients.[163,164] Because *FBN1* is such a large gene (approximately 9000 nucleotides in the mRNA, dispersed in 65 exons over 240kb of chromosome 15q21.1), finding a mutation is still not a simple matter.[165,166] Once the mutation is identified, diagnosis in that family is straightforward. In families with several alive and cooperative affected members, linkage analysis can be used for presymptomatic and prenatal diagnosis. The use of molecular testing is confounded, however, by the discovery that autosomal dominant ectopia lentis, familial tall stature, MASS phenotype, and familial aortic aneurysm all are phenotypes caused by mutations in *FBN1* and are exactly the conditions clinicians are interested in excluding in their patients of questionable diagnosis.[163]

Mutations in *FBN1* have distinct effects on microfibril formation: some affect synthesis, others secretion, and yet others incorporation of fibrillin-1 monomers into the extracellular matrix. Studies in mice deficient in fibrillin-1 suggest that microfibrils have an important role in embryological development through interaction with transforming growth factor-beta (TGF-β). Mutations in fibrillin may result in inappropriate or excessive activation of TGF-β signaling.[167]

MITRAL VALVE PROLAPSE AND THE MASS PHENOTYPE. This heterogeneous group of conditions, described earlier, likely contains large numbers of patients and families who have a defect of the extracellular matrix underlying the phenotypes. Some, but not all, have mutations in *FBN1*.[151,163]

Ehlers-Danlos Syndrome

Ehlers-Danlos syndrome is a group of heterogeneous conditions linked by variable involvement of the skin and the joints, with hyperelasticity and fragility of the former occurring with hypermobility of the latter (Fig. 70–9).[168] Mitral valve prolapse is clearly increased in frequency in most of the clinical types, but the occurrence of aortic root dilation is controversial. A recent study found that 25 to 30 percent of patients with the classic and hypermobile forms of Ehlers-Danlos syndrome had mild dilation of the aortic root,[169] a finding counter to what a previous survey had shown.[170]

The most serious cardiovascular problems occur in patients with the vascular form of Ehlers-Danlos syndrome with spontaneous rupture of large- and medium-caliber arteries.[171] Various defects of type III collagen caused the phenotype in virtually all patients studied.[172] Analysis of collagen production by cultured skin fibroblasts should be used to confirm the diagnosis.[18] True aneurysms form rarely; rather, a rupture without dissection usually occurs as a catastrophic event. Most prone are the abdominal aorta and its branches, the great vessels of the aortic arch, and the large arteries of the limbs. False aneurysms and fistulas may be one result in those patients who do not die of the initial rupture. Vascular surgery is difficult, as the normal-appearing vessels around the rent fail to hold sutures. As a consequence, elective surgery to repair vascular anomalies, such as false aneurysms, that are causing no immediate problem is contraindicated in most cases. The vascular form of Ehlers-Danlos syndrome is often sporadic but, when familial, is usually autosomal dominant.[173] Prenatal diagnosis is possible by examining collagen production in amniocytes. However, pregnancy is particularly hazardous to women with this condition because of vascular rupture, although some mutations may not be as dangerous.[172,174]

Pseudoxanthoma Elasticum

Pseudoxanthoma elasticum (PXE) is a clinically variable and genetically heterogeneous disorder caused by mutations in the gene *ABCC6*, which encodes a membrane protein of unclear function. Histopathological examination of affected tissues shows fragmentation and calcification of elastic fibers. The skin, eyes, gastrointestinal system, and cardiovascular system are the organs most severely affected.[175] The skin shows highly characteristic raised yellowish papules (pseudoxanthoma) overlying areas of flexural stress, such as the neck, cubital and popliteal fossae, and groin (Fig. 70–10). Breaks in the elastic lamella, Bruch membrane of the choroid, produce the fundoscopic finding of angioid streaks. Gastrointestinal hemorrhage is common and potentially fatal; mucosal arterioles bleed, and because the calcified elastic fibers prevent effective vessel retraction, hemostasis is difficult. Selective arterial embolization was life saving in one instance. The heart is affected in a number of ways. Endocardial fibroelastosis is common, but because primarily the atria are involved, a restrictive cardiomyopathy is uncommon. One patient with marked endocardial fibroelastosis was helped by resection of calcified elastic bands within the left ventricle. Mitral valve prolapse may be increased in frequency but is rarely a clinical problem. Coronary artery disease with myocardial ischemia and infarction is a common cause of early death.

Elastic and muscular arteries, including the coronaries, develop a type of arteriosclerosis similar to Mönckeberg; progressive luminal narrowing occurs and can produce complete occlusion. This is initially most evident at the radial and ulnar arteries, where absence of pulses and a positive Allen test result are noted early in the course. Interestingly, carotid-femoral pulse wave velocity was not increased in patients with PXE, and radial artery stiffness was reduced in female patients.[176] Because narrowing progresses slowly, collateral arteries form, and peripheral ischemia is a late complication. Because the arterial stenoses tend to be

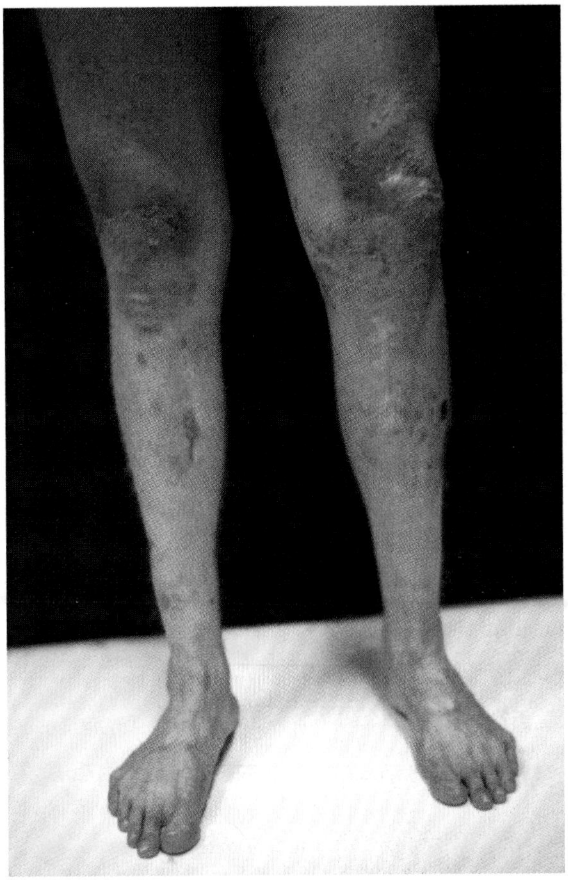

FIGURE 70–9 Legs of a patient with Ehlers-Danlos syndrome type IV who died of rupture of the subclavian artery. Note the mild joint hypermobility and the striking dermal abnormalities—elastosis perforans serpiginosa and thin, atrophic scars over areas of recurrent trauma.

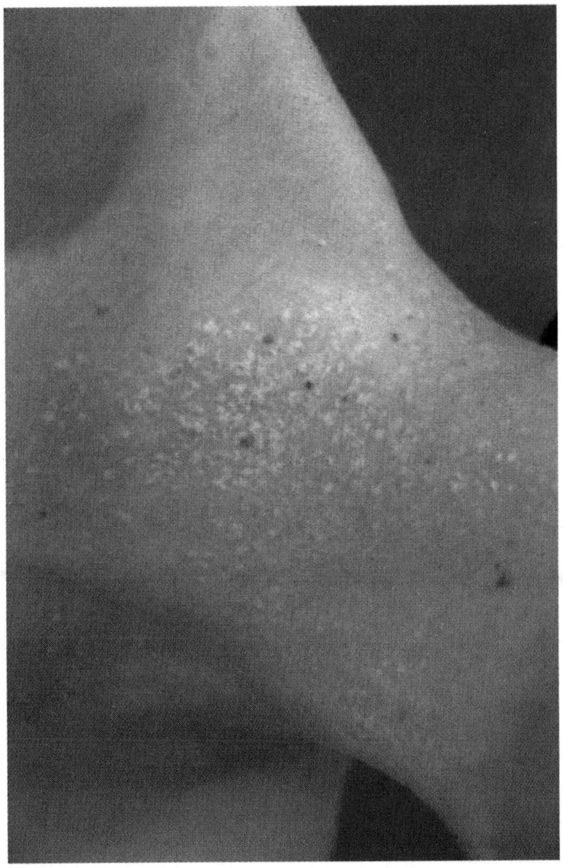

FIGURE 70–10 Skin of a young man with pseudoxanthoma elasticum. The neck is a typical location to notice the raised, yellowish papules from which the name of the condition derives.

diffuse, bypassing them often involves extensive surgery. Hypertension and all risk factors for atherosclerosis should be aggressively controlled.

Genetic Susceptibility to Acquired Disorders of Connective Tissue

Genetic factors are clearly implicated in the susceptibility to many of the rheumatic disorders and to specific complications of specific conditions. The cardiovascular manifestations of these disorders are particularly interesting in this regard. For example, study of HLA-DR antigen frequencies suggests that immune-response factors are involved in the pathogenesis of chronic rheumatic heart disease in black patients.

Inborn Errors of Metabolism that Affect the Cardiovascular System

Hundreds of biochemical defects that affect human metabolism have direct or secondary impact on the cardiovascular system (see Table 70–12).[177] Several examples are reviewed, selected for their relevance to clinical practice or their instructive lessons about pathophysiology.

Aminoacidopathies

Inborn errors of amino acid metabolism result in the accumulation of precursors and a deficit of end products, either or both of which can be detrimental.

ALKAPTONURIA. An intermediate of tyrosine catabolism polymerizes to homogentisic acid, which readily accumulates in the extracellular matrix.[178] Over many years, connective tissue of cartilage, heart valves, and arteries becomes increasingly abnormal. Aortic stenosis and arteriosclerosis are the cardiological sequelae.

HOMOCYSTINURIA. This condition is caused by a deficiency of cystathionine beta-synthase; the pathogenesis of the pleiotropic manifestations is largely unknown.[17,179,180] Perhaps the amino acid sulfhydryl groups bind to collagen, fibrillin, and other macromolecules and interfere with cross-linking. The clinical features, once confused with Marfan syndrome, include tall stature, skeletal deformity, ectopia lentis, mental retardation, psychiatric disturbances, and a predilection for venous and arterial thromboses. Those patients with mutations that render the enzyme activity able to be increased by pharmacological doses of pyridoxine are less severely affected; early treatment can prevent most aspects of the phenotype.[181] Patients unresponsive to pyridoxine can be helped by a low-protein diet to reduce intake of methionine and by oral betaine, a cofactor essential for remethylation of homocysteine.

Myocardial infarction, pulmonary embolism, and stroke are the most common causes of death. The pathogenesis of the vascular complications was once thought to involve abnormal platelet function, but platelet survival in untreated patients is normal. Growing evidence supports a susceptibility of heterozygotes, who have none of the external phenotype of the disease, to atherosclerosis.[182] Various actions of homocysteine on endothelial receptors, stimulation of smooth muscle growth, and production of extracellular matrix components are being explored for clinical relevance.[183] Current therapeutic approaches are focused on maintaining physiological levels of the cofactors involved in metabolism of sulfurated amino acids, folate and vitamins B_6 and B_{12}.

Disorders of Fatty Acid Metabolism

Although most organs can metabolize fatty acids when faced with hypoglycemia, only the heart depends on fatty acids as the primary source of energy generation. Thus, it is not surprising that virtually all genetic defects in fatty acid metabolism, including generalized defects in mitochondria and peroxisomes, are associated with myocardial dysfunction.[184] Other substrates—glucose, lactate, and oxaloacetate—also generate energy in myocardial cells by entry into mitochondria and the tricarboxylic acid (Krebs) cycle. Thus, defects in conversion of pyruvate to acetyl coenzyme A and in any point along the tricarboxylic acid cycle and the respiratory chain have a major impact on myocardial energy generation. Quite likely, some sporadic and familial instances of idiopathic cardiomyopathy represent undiagnosed or undefined metabolic disorders.

CARNITINE DEFICIENCIES. Carnitine is a required cofactor for entry of long-chain fatty acids into mitochondria and is both synthesized endogenously and available from dietary sources.[185] Deficiency of carnitine effectively blocks metabolism of long-chain fatty acids throughout the body and hepatic metabolism of ketones. Because of their relative dependence on fatty acids, muscle cells, including myocytes, suffer out of proportion to other tissue when carnitine levels are low for any reason. Cytoplasmic inclusions of lipid are characteristic findings in myocytes and hepatocytes.

Several Mendelian defects produce primary or secondary carnitine deficiency. An autosomal recessive defect in carnitine palmitoyltransferase I leads to increased plasma carnitine and a skeletal muscle myopathy with little effect on the heart.[185] So-called systemic carnitine deficiency can have various causes: primary deficiency of intake, synthesis, or function, and secondary deficiency, the majority now known to be a result of defects in fatty acid metabolism. The latter group of conditions usually does not respond to pharmacological doses of carnitine.[185]

Primary carnitine deficiency usually manifests in infancy with hypoglycemia, coma, and congestive heart failure due to dilated cardiomyopathy. In the few cases reported, problems largely resolve with carnitine treatment; they can be prevented from recurring by oral supplementation with L-carnitine. Primary systemic carnitine deficiency is due to a defect in carnitine transport, which leads to excessive urinary loss and affects muscle but not liver.[186] Thus, muscle cells still may be relatively deficient in carnitine, despite supplementation, and long-term prognosis is uncertain.

DEFECTS OF BETA-OXIDATION. At least 20 steps are involved when a molecule of free fatty acid leaves the plasma, enters beta-oxidation in the mitochondrion, and generates electrons and acetyl-CoA[185] At each turn of the oxidation spiral, two carbons are removed from the fatty acid, and the enzymes involved in this step are specific for substrates of only certain chain length: long-chain, medium-chain, and short-chain acetyl-CoA dehydrogenases, or LCAD, MCAD, and SCAD. Thus far, patients with defects in nine of the steps have been characterized.

Patients homozygous for these generally autosomal recessive disorders develop episodic hypoketotic hypoglycemia, usually associated with fasting or intercurrent illness. Deficiency of MCAD is the most common cause and occurs in about 1 of every 7000 newborns in the United States. Hypoglycemic crises can rapidly progress to coma and death, and 50 to 60 percent of affected infants die in the first 2 years of life.[186] Because infants between episodes or before a fatal crisis appear normal, MCAD deficiency accounts for a proportion of so-called sudden infant deaths.[180] Histopathological examination shows microvesicular accumulation of fat in cardiac and skeletal muscle. One mutation in MCAD (A985G) accounts for a large percentage of all alleles that predispose to this lethal disorder, and various approaches to newborn screening are being investigated.

MITOCHONDRIAL MYOPATHIES. All of the enzymes of fatty acid oxidation are encoded by genes located on nuclear chromosomes, but the components of the electron transport chain are encoded by both nuclear and mitochondrial genes. Several syndromes involving various types of myopathies have been shown to be due to mutations in the mitochondrial chromosome.[16] The *Kearns-Sayre* syndrome includes pigmentary degeneration of the retina, ophthalmoplegia, and cardiomyopathy as its most prominent manifestations; all of the affected tissues rely nearly exclusively on oxidative phosphorylation for energy generation.

The MELAS syndrome (*m*yopathy, *e*ncephalopathy, *l*actic *a*cidosis, and *s*troke-like episodes) is due to mutations in mitochondrial transfer RNA genes. In addition to the features that define the acronym, hypertrophic cardiomyopathy and diffuse coronary angiopathy are common. Various other mtDNA mutations are associated with hypertrophic or dilated cardiomyopathy.[131]

Variations in both the actual mutations and the fraction of abnormal mitochondria in the cells of the different organs (heteroplasmy) account for many of the clinical differences in phenotype, severity, and age of onset among patients with this disorder. Inheritance is maternal for patients with mitochondrial mutations; apparent autosomal recessive and dominant inheritance may indicate that mutations of nuclear genes can impair electron transport similarly to mitochondrial mutations. Some patients have been treated with moderate success over the short term with coenzyme Q and with cardiac transplantation in one case.

Glycogenoses

Several of the glycogen storage disorders affect cardiac muscle.

GLYCOGEN STORAGE DISEASE II. This autosomal recessive condition is due to deficiency of the lysosomal enzyme α-1,4-glucosidase and results in the lysosomal accumulation of glycogen in most tissues. Several allelic variants occur.[187] The condition with infantile onset is called *Pompe disease,* and cardiac involvement is profound.[185] Infants with Pompe disease appear well initially but soon fail to thrive and develop hypotonia, tachypnea, and tachycardia; the disease progresses during the first year to irreversible congestive heart failure and death due to pneumonia or cardiopulmonary failure. Auscultation typically reveals no murmurs until late in the course when obstruction develops, and hypoglycemia does not appear because the nonlysosomal pathway of glycogen catabolism is intact. The diagnosis is suggested by massive cardiomegaly on examination and chest radiography and by characteristic echocardiographic abnormalities of a short PR interval and markedly increased QRS voltage. Echocardiography shows tremendously thickened (pseudohypertrophic) ventricles, and Doppler interrogation or catheterization may reveal subaortic and subpulmonic pressure gradients characteristic of obstructive cardiomyopathy.

Reduced diastolic function of a restrictive cardiomyopathy develops eventually, and endocardial fibroelastosis is common. With these findings, the diagnosis of Pompe disease is virtually certain, but it can be confirmed by analysis of α-1,4-glucosidase activity in cultured fibroblasts. Prenatal diagnosis is possible by enzymatic assay of amniocytes. Treatment is supportive, but cardiac transplantation could correct the cardiac problem; unfortunately, involvement of other organs, including the lungs, liver, and skeletal muscle, might eventually prove just as serious as the cardiomyopathy. Bone marrow transplantation might be a solution if performed early in the course. An animal model of α-1,4-glucosidase deficiency exists in cattle and develops cardiac pathology typical of human Pompe disease.

Cardiomyopathy may develop in the juvenile-onset form of α-1,4-glucosidase deficiency, but it is not invariable because of allelic heterogeneity. In one sibship without cardiac involvement, three brothers had extensive hepatic, skeletal muscle, and arterial smooth muscle accumulation of glycogen, and each died of rupture of a basilar artery aneurysm. The adult-onset form usually presents with insidious onset of respiratory insufficiency, and clinically important cardiac disease is rare.

GLYCOGEN STORAGE DISEASE III. The striking clinical variability in phenotype associated with deficiency of α-1,4-glucosidase is due in large part to the extensive array of mutations that occur at the *GAA* locus. This autosomal recessive deficiency of amylo-1,6-glucosidase results in infantile- and juvenile-onset syndromes of muscle weakness, wasting, and hepatomegaly. Clinical cardiac disease is not common, although both cytoplasmic (nonlysosomal) and intermyofibril glycogen is routinely present in the heart and causes pseudohypertrophy and increased voltage on electrocardiography. The diagnosis has been established by enzymatic assay of an endomyocardial biopsy specimen.

GLYCOGEN STORAGE DISEASE IV. This is caused by deficiency of α-1,4-glucan: α-1,4-glucan 6-glycosyl transferase. It usually causes a fatal disorder of early childhood characterized by hepatic failure; although extensive deposition of polysaccharide occurs in the heart, death intervenes before cardiac symptoms appear. In the most severe form, the fetus has hydrops and generalized muscle degeneration.[188] As with all of the glycogen storage diseases, extensive allelic heterogeneity results in milder forms of the classic disorders. Patients with diagnosis later in adolescence tend to have more severe cardiomyopathy. Liver transplantation has been life saving in some cases and has, somewhat surprisingly, resulted in a reduction of glycogen deposits in the heart and skeletal muscles.

AMP-ACTIVATED PROTEIN KINASE DEFICIENCY. Mutations in the gene *PRKAG2,* which encodes the γ-2 regulatory subunit of the enzyme that controls the uptake of glucose by various cells, are associated with potentially severe cardiovascular manifestations.[189] Cardiac hypertrophy is an inconstant finding, but conduction defects and dysrhythmia, especially preexcitation, are common. Myocardial histopathology shows accumulation of glycogen in myocyte vacuoles and interstitial fibrosis.

CARDIAC PHOSPHORYLASE KINASE DEFICIENCY. Few cases of this enzyme deficiency have been reported: deposition of glycogen is confined to the heart, which may be massively thickened and enlarged, and leads to early death.

GLYCOPROTEINOSES. This group of disorders results in the lysosomal accumulation of various compounds that cannot be catabolized further because of the specific enzyme deficiency (see Table 70–12). Some have prominent cardiac pathological findings, generally of pseudohypertrophy and valvular thickening, which manifest with congestive failure, valvular dysfunction, conduction defects, or dysrhythmia.[190]

Hematological Disorders

HEMOCHROMATOSIS. This autosomal recessive disorder of unknown cause results in iron deposition in many tissues, including the myocardium. The manifestations include diabetes mellitus, skin hyperpigmentation, hypogonadism, hepatic failure with cirrhosis, hepatoma, and congestive heart failure; severity is less and age of onset later in women due to the autophlebotomy provided by menstruation.[191] The cause of the most common form of hereditary hemochromatosis is a gene, *HFE,* closely linked to the major histocompatibility locus on chromosome 6. One specific mutation accounts for a large proportion of the mutant alleles among white patients.[192] Fully 10 percent of the population is heterozygous for a hemochromatosis mutation. On the one hand, this allele prevalence might suggest that, at an incidence of 2 to 3 per 1000, hemochromatosis is underdiagnosed. On the other hand, a large population survey suggests that homozygosity for the mutation has markedly reduced penetrance.[193] The allele frequency has given rise to interest in population screening by molecular genetic techniques, but for now traditional clinical laboratory approaches are appropriate.[194] Diagnosis depends on finding increased serum iron, ferritin, and, especially, transferrin saturation in the absence of any obvious cause of excessive iron intake.

Cardiac involvement often appears first as dysrhythmia or congestive heart failure. Dysrhythmia, conduction abnormalities, and low QRS voltage are typical electrocardiographic findings; cardiomegaly is seen on chest radiography, and a dilated cardiomyopathy with reduced systolic function can be documented on echocardiography. Occasional patients have a restrictive pattern on cardiac catheterization. Treatment by repeated phlebotomy is most effective if begun before organ damage is irreversible. If a patient with congestive heart failure has not yet developed serious compromise in other organs, cardiac transplantation can be contemplated, as can combined heart-liver replacement.

HEMOGLOBINOPATHIES. Sickle cell disease and other hemoglobinopathies associated with sickling can produce ischemia and infarction in numerous organs by occlusion of small vessels; however, the heart is relatively resistant.[195] Nonetheless, the combination of chronic hypoxemia and anemia produces a sustained high-output state that leads to congestive heart failure in many adults. The cardiovascular system can also be compromised by systemic hypertension due to renal infarction, pulmonary embolism and infarction (the chest pain of which often causes concern about myocardial ischemia), pulmonary hypertension, stroke, and hemosiderosis from chronic transfusions.

In addition to a hyperdynamic congestive failure, iron overload is the principal risk to the myocardium in cases of decreased erythrocyte production of other causes (thalassemias) and increased erythrocyte consumption (hemolytic anemias) requiring repeated transfusions. Treatment with daily injections of deferoxamine can, if begun early, prevent the development of severe cardiac and hepatic disease. Development of an oral iron chelator would greatly improve compliance and efficacy. In patients with beta-thalassemia, heart failure can occur from an autoimmune mechanism, the risks for which depend on the patient's immunogenetic profile.[196] Various approaches to management of sickle cell disease, including hydroxyurea, show promise.[197] Combined heart-liver transplantation has been used in a case of end-stage organ failure with homozygous beta-thalassemia. Both sickle cell disease and thalassemias are associated with diffuse defects in elastic tissue, manifest in the skin and arteries, among other organs.[198,199]

Mucopolysaccharidoses and Disorders of Targeting Lysosomal Enzymes

Many of the specific disorders included in the groupings *mucopolysaccharidoses* and *disorders of targeting lysosomal enzymes* share phenotypic manifestations and are caused by various defects in the ability of lysosomes to catabolize proteoglycan and glycosaminoglycan. Short stature, progressive coarsening of facial features, a skeletal dysplasia termed *dysostosis multiplex*, corneal clouding, and protean effects on the cardiovascular system are common (Fig. 70–11).[200] Only MPS IS (Scheie syndrome), the mild form of MPS IH (mild Hunter syndrome), MPS IV (Morquio syndrome), and MPS VI (Maroteaux-Lamy syndrome) carry minimal or no mental impairment.

CARDIOVASCULAR MANIFESTATIONS. The cardiovascular complications of these disorders (see Table 70–12), which are all progressive and usually insidious, arise from engorgement of cells and tissues with macromolecular storage material. First, the ventricular walls become pseudohypertrophic, and systolic function gradually deteriorates. The electrocardiogram shows reduced QRS voltages; rarely is any conduction disturbance present. Second, coronary arteries narrow because of intimal and medial thickening. Myocardial infarction is common in MPS IH and the severe form of MPS II, although the patients are usually too impaired mentally to report classic symptoms, and the diagnosis is made postmortem. Third, valve leaflets thicken and cause progressive dysfunction oddly specific for individual disorders. For example, aortic stenosis is common in patients with MPS IS, and mitral regurgitation is frequently found in patients with MPS IH and MPS IV. Finally, narrowing of the upper and middle airways causes obstructive apnea, chronic hypoxemia and hypercarbia, pulmonary hypertension, and eventually cor pulmonale.[201]

MANAGEMENT. Treatment of children with those conditions that cause mental retardation has in the past been supportive. Increasing experience with bone marrow transplantation in many of the conditions shows that in the survivors of the transplant, somatic accumulation of mucopolysaccharide can be reduced, with clinical improvement in cardiopulmonary function.[200] However, improvement of central nervous system function has been marginal or absent. Nonetheless, bone marrow transplantation may have a role, especially in cases of MPS IV and MPS VI, in which cardiopulmonary compromise can greatly shorten otherwise productive lives. Attempts at cardiovascular surgery, indeed of any procedure requiring general anesthesia, are fraught with risks of difficult intubation, hyperextension of the neck with cervical cord damage (the odontoid process is often hypoplastic), and prolonged efforts to wean from mechanical ventilation.[201] Enzyme replacement therapy is being developed for most of the MPS disorders and received Food and Drug Administration (FDA) approval for MPS I in 1993. However, the enzyme does not cross the blood-brain barrier, and therapy is indicated only for the somatic manifestations.[202]

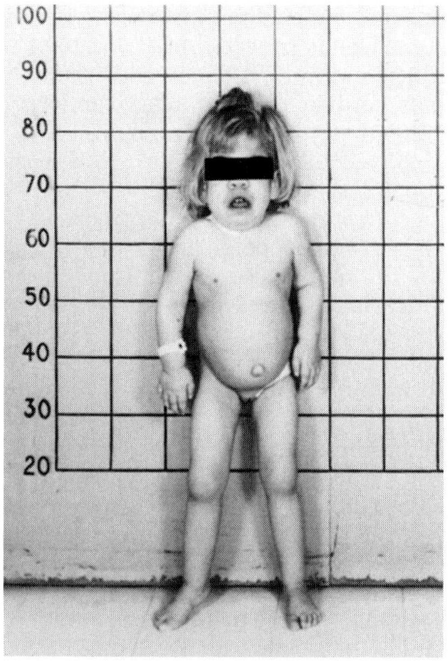

FIGURE 70–11 Hurler syndrome in a 4-year-old girl. Note the short stature and coarse facial features.

Sphingolipidoses

FABRY DISEASE. This X-linked condition deserves comment because the diagnosis is often not made until adulthood, when serious end-organ damage has occurred.[203,204] As a result of deficiency of alpha-galactosidase A, ceramide trihexoside and other glycosphingolipids accumulate in lysosomes of many cells and organs, especially endothelial cells, glomerular and tubular cells of the kidneys, and the heart. Microangiopathy causes the characteristic skin lesion, angiokeratoma, and may contribute, along with primary nerve involvement, to acroparesthesias and painful crises. Proteinuria and hypertension precede renal failure, which often has led to death in male subjects and often requires long-term dialysis or renal transplantation by the fourth decade. A successful kidney allograft does not correct the systemic metabolic defect, and the disease usually progresses in other organs. Infusion of purified human α-galactosidase A, which received FDA approval in 2003, reduces tissue storage of glycosphingolipid.[205,206]

CARDIAC MANIFESTATIONS. Structural and functional cardiac involvement is qualitatively similar to that in the mucopolysaccharidoses. Thickening of the myocardium is pseudohypertrophy due to deposition of glycosphingolipid in lysosomes; the diagnosis has been made by endocardial biopsy during the evaluation of unexplained ventricular hypertrophy or frank obstructive cardiomyopathy. Chronic hypertension can exaggerate left ventricular dysfunction, as can ischemia and infarction due to diffuse luminal narrowing of the coronary arteries. Echocardiography is useful for serial documentation of myocardial function. Although valvular thickening and MVP are common, hemodynamically important mitral regurgitation is not. The pulmonary vasculature becomes narrowed and right-sided pressures rise, but cor pulmonale is rarely a problem. The electrocardiogram often shows a shortened PR interval, increased left ventricular voltages, and dysrhythmia. Medium-sized arteries throughout the body develop luminal narrowing, with cerebrovascular disease the most common cause of death after renal failure.

Heterozygous females generally show some clinical manifestations, especially in the eyes, and at much later ages than hemizygous males develop renal, cerebrovascular, and cardiac disease.[204] Prenatal diagnosis is possible, and a detailed family history and genetic counseling are essential whenever the disease is found. Various mutations occur in the gene for alpha-galactosidase A and account for much of the clinical variability.

Familial Amyloidoses (see Chap. 59)

Various disorders, defined initially by clinical phenotype and due to progressive accumulation of amyloid in organs and tissues, are beginning to be categorized by the underlying biochemical and genetic defects.[207] The several conditions termed *familial amyloidosis with polyneuropathy* and originally classified as separate autosomal dominant disorders are now known to be due to different mutations in the same gene encoding transthyretin, a thyroxine- and retinol-binding protein also called *prealbumin.* Amyloidosis that occurs in the absence of a positive family history is often the first diagnosable case of familial amyloidosis.[208] Although polyneuropathy dominates the early course during young adulthood, renal failure and restrictive cardiomyopathy supervene later and cause death in most cases. Pulmonary hypertension can be a late complication.[209] The age of onset, severity, and predilection for kidney and cardiac involvement are determined by the type of mutation, with male subjects affected earlier and more severely. Autonomic dysfunction is common, reflected in reduced heart rate variability.[210]

Liver transplantation can prevent progression of the disease and potentially reverse some tissue accumulation but may not prevent progression of cardiomyopathy.[211] When the myocardium is severely infiltrated, combined liver-heart transplant offers the only hope.

Neuromuscular Disorders

See Chapter 85.

Cardiac Tumors (see Chap. 63)

The three most common tumors that originate in the heart are myxomas, fibromas, and rhabdomyomas. All occur as part of hereditary syndromes and as sporadic events. The new occurrence of any of these tumors, especially in a child, may represent the first manifestation of a systemic condition, so a detailed general examination and family history are always indicated.[212,213] For example, 51 to 86 percent of cardiac rhabdomyomas occur because of tuberous sclerosis.[214] Tumors due to hereditary disorders tend to be multiple and to recur after resection. An example is the NAME syndrome (for *n*evi, *a*trial myxoma, *m*yxoid neurofibromata, and *e*phelides; the acronym ignores the numerous endocrine tumors), also called *Carney complex*, in which many myxomas can occur throughout the myocardium.[215-217]

Inherited Disorders of the Circulation

Hereditary Hemorrhagic Telangiectasia

Hereditary hemorrhagic telangiectasia (HHT), an autosomal dominant condition often called *Osler-Rendu-Weber disease*, is more common than is appreciated. Because of marked intrafamilial and interfamilial variability, the condition can remain undiagnosed in affected patients for years despite mild manifestations.[218,219] Mucocutaneous telangiectases, 0.5 to 3 mm in diameter, occur on the tongue, lips, and fingertips most commonly. Small and moderate-sized arteriovenous fistulas occur in the nose, leading to recurrent epistaxis, in the gastrointestinal system, where they cause recurrent bleeding and occult anemia, and in the lungs, resulting in hypoxemia, hemoptysis, polycythemia, clubbing, paradoxical embolization through the right-to-left shunt, and a hyperdynamic circulation. Less common sites of vascular malformations are the brain,[220] liver, and kidneys. Diffuse ectasia of the coronary arteries was noted in one patient, and hemorrhagic pericarditis with tamponade in another.[221] Bleeding is facilitated, even in the presence of normal platelet function and clotting function, because of the lack of resistance channels in the telangiectatic lesions.

Patients with HHT and their close relatives should be screened for pulmonary arteriovenous malformations (PAVM) with a contrast echocardiogram.[222] Appearance of "bubbles" in the left atrium after 4 to 10 cardiac cycles is virtually pathognomonic of a shunt in the lung. A positive contrast echocardiogram should be followed by spiral computed tomography to document the number, size, and location of PAVMs. A low oxygen saturation should prompt angiography and therapeutic balloon occlusion of the feeding arteries of any sizable malformation to prevent systemic embolization, especially to the brain.[223] In a few patients, epistaxis and gastrointestinal blood loss have been reduced by antifibrinolytic therapy with danazol or aminocaproic acid.[224] Controlled trials of various approaches to chronic management, taking into account clinical and genetic variables, are sorely needed. Whether to screen all patients with HHT for cerebral vascular malformations and, if so, at what age screening should be started are both unclear.[225]

At least three genes are capable of causing HHT, and two have been mapped to 9q33-q34 and to 3p22. The former locus, *ENG*, encodes a TGF-β-binding protein called endoglin, and various mutations segregate with HHT in different families. The other locus, *ALK1*, encodes an activin receptor–like kinase, which is a member of the serine-threonine kinase receptor family, expressed in endothelial cells. This suggests that defects in this gene might affect development or repair of vessels.[226] Not all families link to these two genes, so a third locus is being sought. Thus, by mutation detection or linkage analysis, presymptomatic and prenatal diagnosis are available to a large number of patients with a potentially life-threatening disorder.

von Hippel–Lindau Syndrome

The features of this autosomal dominant condition involve malformations and abnormal growth of small blood vessels. Retinal angioma, hemangioblastoma of the cerebellum, and hemangioma of the spinal cord occur in association with renal cell carcinoma, pancreatic and epididymal cystadenomas, and pheochromocytoma. Secondary hypertension due to renal disease and pheochromocytoma, which is often bilateral, occurs and predisposes to subarachnoid hemorrhage. The cause is a tumor suppressor gene, *VHL*, at 3p26-p25. Patients inherit a germline mutation (and there is great diversity among families in the actual mutations) that is present in all cells. When a somatic mutation in the normal allele occurs in a susceptible cell, such as in the renal parenchyma or adrenal medulla, the cell becomes functionally homozygous for a lack of the gene product, and the cascade toward neoplasia is initiated.[227] How this gene product stimulates or permits angiomatous malformations is unclear.

Disorders Primarily Affecting Arteries

Mendelian disorders are associated with a diverse array of arterial pathological findings, and some were described or catalogued earlier in this chapter. This section deals with two categories of disorders caused by a single mutant gene: pleiotropic syndromes better known for affecting organ systems other than the vasculature, and primary abnormalities of arteries.

ADULT POLYCYSTIC KIDNEY DISEASE. Adult polycystic kidney disease (APKD) is a relatively common autosomal dominant disease that affects 0.5 million people and accounts for 8 to 10 percent of all long-term hemodialysis in the United States. Development of renal cysts is age-dependent, and presymptomatic detection of heterozygotes, even by ultrasonography, can be uncertain into adulthood. About one-half of patients are hypertensive, one-half have hepatic cysts, one-half eventually develop severe renal failure, and an unknown (but probably high) fraction have colonic diverticula. Elevated plasma renin levels contribute to hypertension long before renal failure occurs. The cardiovascular manifestations include MVP in one-quarter, mild dilation of the aortic root, occasional thoracic and abdominal aneurysms, and a predisposition to regurgitation of the aortic, mitral, and tricuspid valves. The association of diverticula, organ cysts, and cardiovascular lesions reminiscent of, but milder than, Marfan syndrome suggests some involvement of the extracellular matrix.

The most serious vascular problem is typical berry aneurysms of the cerebral circulation that occur in about 10 percent of heterozygotes but may remain asymptomatic throughout life. Hypertension predisposes to subarachnoid hemorrhage. How to screen for and treat intracranial aneurysms in patients without neurological symptoms remains controversial. Cerebral angiography carries higher risks in patients with APKD because of dissection and heightened vascular reactivity. Magnetic resonance imaging detects most saccular aneurysms down to 2 to 3 mm in diameter. Whether to attempt prophylactic repair when a small aneurysm is detected has not been investigated systematically. Without question, aggressive blood pressure control is indicated in any patient with APKD.

At least three genes cause APKD. The greatest portion of cases are due to mutations in a gene called *PBP* at the *PKD1* locus (16p13.3).[228] In most of the remaining families, the disease maps to the *PKD2* locus in the region 4q23-q23. Families affected by mutations in *PKD2* tend to develop renal failure later and have a milder course.[229] In both *PKD1* and *PKD2* cases, the multiorgan cysts develop when a somatic mutation occurs in the normal allele at the respective mutant locus, analogous to the two-hit model so familiar with tumorigenesis.[230] A French Canadian family with disease typical of *PKD1* is unlinked to either locus, indicating that a *PKD3* gene exists. Patients with mutations in *PKD1* and *PKD2* show marked intrafamilial variability. Discovering some of the factors that affect this variability could suggest novel approaches to modifying disease progression.[231]

ARTERIOHEPATIC DYSPLASIA. An autosomal dominant disorder of marked variability, *Alagille syndrome* causes neonatal jaundice due to aplasia of intrahepatic bile ducts and congestive heart failure in the most severely affected infants but may be asymptomatic in heterozygous relatives.[58,232] The cardiovascular findings include peripheral pulmonic and systemic arterial stenoses in the majority, occasionally associated with septal defects or PDA.[233-235] A diffuse vasculopathy is present in some patients.[56] Renal disease can produce hypertension. The locus was initially mapped by studying chromosomes and finding in some patients that part or all of band 20p12 was missing (an interstitial deletion). The *Jagged1* gene, which mapped to this exact region, was then identified as the cause.

ARTERIAL ANEURYSM, ECTASIA, OR DISSECTION (see Chap. 53). Pedigrees abound in which dilation of the aortic root, aneurysm of the abdominal aorta, aortic dissection without dilation, or a combination of these problems occurs in an autosomal dominant pattern without evidence of a recognized heritable disorder of connective tissue.[236,237] Because of the variable presentation and natural history of the aortic disease, presymptomatic detection of presumed heterozygotes is uncertain, as is reassurance of relatives at risk who are of childbearing age and would prefer not to pass this condition to offspring.

The association of dissection of the ascending aorta with bicuspid aortic valve and aortic coarctation is well known, although the cause and pathogenesis remain unclear. In such cases, the aortic wall shows abnormalities of elastic fibers. A person with a congenitally bicuspid aortic valve or aortic coarctation should be screened for dilation of the aortic root, and first-degree relatives should be screened for both lesions. This recommendation is based, in part, on the bicuspid aortic valve being a congenital heart defect of the left-sided flow category, with a relatively high recurrence risk.

In two families with autosomal dominant transmission of arterial aneurysms and mildly increased skin fragility and bruisability, different mutations in the gene encoding type III procollagen occurred. Thus, depending on the mutation, deficiency of type III collagen can cause the vascular form of Ehlers-Danlos syndrome or a form of the much subtler but just as deadly syndrome, familial arterial rupture. For these families in which the mutations have been defined, reliable presymptomatic and prenatal diagnoses are at hand. However, suggestions that mutations in type III collagen would account for the majority of aortic aneurysms, including abdominal aneurysms in the elderly, have proved unfounded.

Families with aneurysm, dissection, or both of the thoracic aorta have been studied extensively in the past few years. Linkage to three loci, 3p25-p24.2, 5q13-q14, and 11q23.2-q24, has been reported.[238-240] A predisposition to cervical arterial dissection in young people was found to be associated with diffuse lentiginosis in several families, with a suggestion of autosomal recessive inheritance. An association is also noted between cervical dissection and intracranial hemorrhage, which is increased when congenital cardiovascular defects are present, especially bicuspid aortic valve or aortic coarctation. Formal genetic analysis of 91 families ascertained through a proband with abdominal aortic aneurysm suggests that an autosomal recessive predisposition exists for late-onset aneurysms. This study and others[241] provide a rationale for offering ultrasonographic screening to siblings of patients with abdominal aortic dilation.

FAMILIAL ARTERIAL TORTUOSITY. This is a rare, possibly autosomal recessive condition of unknown cause. Paradoxically, diffuse ectasia of all systemic arteries occurs with peripheral pulmonic stenoses.[242]

FAMILIAL INTRACRANIAL HEMORRHAGE. In addition to APKD, three syndromes predispose to subarachnoid or cerebral hemorrhage. Berry aneurysms without pleiotropic manifestations in other organs are a rare but well-documented autosomal dominant trait. How aggressively near relatives should be screened for intracranial aneurysms remains controversial because of the relatively low risk of hemorrhage compared with the morbidity and mortality of current surgical techniques for repairing defects.[243-245] A defect in type III collagen was suggested by linkage analysis, but sequence analysis of the gene in 55 unrelated patients found no mutations.

The cerebral arterial type of familial amyloidosis (type VI) is an autosomal dominant condition caused by a defect in the proteinase inhibitor cystatin O. This disease is rare outside Iceland and Holland. The walls of cerebral arteries are thickened by a material resembling amyloid, and the vessels become tortuous and fragile. Recurrent cerebral hemorrhage is common in the fifth and sixth decades of life.

Familial hemangiomas have been reported infrequently to occur as an autosomal dominant condition. The brain and retina are the principal sites of vascular malformation, although cutaneous lesions occur in some pedigrees. The intracranial hemangioma can be large and the patient can present with varied neurological symptoms, including hemorrhage. A more benign familial disorder of primarily isolated cutaneous hemangiomas also exists.[246]

FAMILIAL ARTERIAL OCCLUSIVE DISEASES.[247] Fibromuscular dysplasia of the renal and other arteries occurs in cases of von Recklinghausen neurofibromatosis and, along with pheochromocytoma, can be a cause of hypertension. Severe deficiency of alpha 1-antiprotease is another cause of fibromuscular dysplasia. The arterial lesion can occur by itself in families and produce stroke, myocardial infarction, intermittent claudication, and hypertension as early as childhood. Inheritance is most consistent with autosomal dominance.

Familial hypoplasia of the carotid arteries, familial arteriopathy caused by concentric thickening of systemic and pulmonic arteries, familial moyamoya disease (which has been mapped to 3p24.2-p26),[248] and generalized arterial calcification of infancy all are rare, possibly Mendelian, syndromes of unknown cause.

Cerebral autosomal dominant arteriopathy with subcortical infarcts and leukoencephalopathy (CADASIL) is due to mutations in the *NOTCH3* gene.[249] Characteristic inclusions occur in vascular smooth muscle cells, and the deep, perforating cerebral arterioles develop occlusions that produce insidious onset of symptoms and transient ischemic attacks.

FAMILIAL HEMIPLEGIC MIGRAINE. The migraine syndrome is commonly familial and occurs in many generations. A severe form, associated with recurrent hemiplegia, is inherited as an autosomal dominant trait and is due to mutations in a sodium channel gene.[250] However, some families with hemiplegic migraine and others with simple migraine are unlinked to this locus. In the same region of 19p is a locus causing autosomal dominant cerebral arteriopathy with subcortical infarcts. Whether the two conditions are related through allelism is unclear.

FAMILIAL PULMONARY HYPERTENSION (see Chap. 67). Primary pulmonary hypertension (PPH) is occasionally familial. Inheritance is most consistent with an autosomal dominant predisposition with sex influence favoring expression in females.[251,252] Mutations in the *BMPR2* gene at 2q33 cause the disease in many of the families.[253]

Pulmonary hypertension can occur in patients with neurofibromatosis due to pulmonary fibrosis, and in patients with hereditary hemorrhagic telangiectasia caused by mutations in *ALK1*.

Disorders Primarily Affecting Veins

VARICOSE VEINS. Although a familial susceptibility to varicosities of the lower extremities clearly exists and favors women in a ratio of 2 : 1, Mendelian inheritance has not been confirmed. Marfan syndrome, various Ehlers-Danlos syndromes, and an autosomal recessive condition featuring distichiasis (a double row of eyelashes) predispose to varicose veins.

ATRETIC VEINS. Some patients with the Klippel-Trénaunay syndrome of cutaneous hemangioma and hemihypertrophy have atresia of the deep venous system. The concomitant superficial varicosities should not be stripped, lest the remaining venous drainage of the lower extremity be removed. This is a confusing syndrome that overlaps with several others; Mendelian inheritance is uncertain.[254] Renal arterial aneurysm and hemangioma occurred in one patient.

CAVERNOUS ANGIOMAS. Cavernous angiomas represent at least 15 percent of vascular malformations of the central nervous system, and familial occurrence is common. These are not arteriovenous malformations but primarily a tortuous collection of veins. Seizure is the most common presenting feature, followed by headache, stroke, and progressive neurological deficit. Magnetic resonance (T2-weighted) imaging is the procedure of choice because it is sensitive; arteriography is not likely to detect the venous malformation. In some families, hepatic angiomas are an important feature. Three genetic loci have been mapped to 7q, 7p and 3q; the locus on 7q is *KRIT1*, of unclear function.[255-257]

ARTERIOVENOUS MALFORMATIONS. The most common Mendelian causes of arteriovenous malformations (AVMs) are the various forms of hereditary hemorrhagic telangiectasia. However, AVMs, especially of the brain, are relatively common findings,[258] and other genetic susceptibilities exist, such as the Parkes Weber syndrome.[254]

Disorders Primarily Affecting Lymphatics

Several forms of hereditary lymphedema exist,[259,260] with the best studied inherited as autosomal dominant conditions. An early-onset form bears the eponym *Nonne-Milroy lymphedema* and can cause a protein-losing enteropathy and pleural effusion. A form called *Meige lymphedema* does not appear until about the time of puberty and is most severe in the legs, although one family with late-onset edema had involvement of the arms and face. Considerable intrafamilial variability in age of onset is noted, however, and whether two or more distinct conditions exist remains unclear. Mutations in one of the receptors for vascular endothelial growth factor, *VEGFR3*, have been found in some families.[261,262] Lymphedema associated with distichiasis is due to mutations in *FOXC2*, which encodes a transcription factor, and hypotrichosis-lymphedema-telangiectasia syndrome is caused by mutations in another transcription factor gene, *SOX18*.[263]

Genetic Factors Predisposing to Atherosclerosis (see Chaps. 36 and 39)

Various genetic factors, in addition to the well-studied errors of lipid metabolism, clearly predispose to atherosclerosis.[264] A few genes aside from those involved in lipid metabolism have such a prominent impact as to be identifiable from the family history. Two genes recently found to predispose to coronary artery disease are *ABCC6*, the gene that also causes pseudoxanthoma elasticum,[265] and *KLOTHO*, a gene of unclear function.[266] However, genes that predispose to hypertension and diabetes mellitus; control arterial diameter, reactivity, and branching angles; affect platelet adhesiveness, thrombosis, and fibrinolysis; and regulate endothelial and smooth muscle function all can be considered candidate genes for study in families predisposed to atherosclerosis. Screening numerous genes for common mutations and polymorphisms that convey risk information will be increasingly possible.[267-269]

Abnormal Regulation of Blood Pressure (see Chap. 37)

Blood pressure is a quantifiable trait that shows continuous variation within the population. Although many genes and environmental factors undoubtedly affect a person's blood pressure, familial transmission of some arbitrarily defined disease "hypertension" follows neither Mendelian nor multifactorial inheritance.[270,271] Various cybernetic systems operate to maintain the blood pressure within tolerable limits. When this physiological homeostasis goes awry or its limits are too lax, pathological and clinical consequences occur.[272] For example, sensitivity of the baroreflex was impaired in patients who had untreated essential hypertension and a positive family history of hypertension compared with hypertensive patients with no family history and to nonhypertensive control subjects. The complexities of such systems are considerable, and two approaches have been taken in recent years to focus the analysis.[271,272] One involves a candidate-gene approach in humans, based on loci known to be involved in physiological pathways; the second involves naturally occurring and experimentally created strains of animals.

STUDIES OF HUMANS. All the classic approaches to detecting genetic influences in diseases—twin studies, familial aggregation, adoption—confirm that genes have a role, but less than 5 percent of patients with hypertension have a defined genetic cause.[273]

Occasional families show striking Mendelian segregation of hypertension without being associated with one of the identifiable syndromes listed in Table 70–15. One example, in which early, severe hypertension is inherited as an autosomal dominant trait, is Liddle syndrome. Because of hypokalemia, aldosteronism was suspected, but both aldosterone and renin levels were low. Attention then focused on sodium resorption in the distal nephron and its regulation. Mutations discovered in the beta subunit of the epithelial sodium channel render the channel insensitive to the usual regulators.

Another example of successful application of the candidate gene approach is investigation of glucocorticoid-remediable

TABLE 70–15 Mendelian Disorders Associated with Abnormal Blood Pressure

Disorder	OMIM No.*	Pathogenesis
Primarily Elevated Blood Pressure		
Adrenal hyperplasia IV	202010	11-β-hydroxylase deficiency→ ↑ 11-deoxycorticosterone
Adrenal hyperplasia V	202110	17-α-hydroxylase deficiency→ ↑ 11-deoxycorticosterone
Aldosteronism	103900	↑ Aldosterone
Alport syndrome	104200 301050	Renal failure
Amyloidosis, familial visceral (amyloidosis VIII)	105200	Nephropathy
Arterial calcification of infancy	208000	Arteriosclerosis
Arterial fibromuscular dysplasia	135580	Renal artery stenosis→ ↑ renin
Arteriohepatic dysplasia	118450	Renal dysplasia; renal arterial stenosis
Bartter syndrome	241200	Secondary to hyperaldosteronism
Fabry disease	301500	Renal failure; renal arterial stenosis; arteriolar stenosis→ ↑ peripheral resistance
Liddle syndrome	177200	Defective epithelial sodium channel→ ↓ K^+ ↓ aldosterone, ↓ renin, ↓ angiotensin
Multiple endocrine neoplasia I	131100	Adrenocortical adenoma→ ↑ Cushing syndrome
Multiple endocrine neoplasia II	171400	Pheochromocytoma→ ↑ catecholamines
Nail-patella syndrome	161200	Nephropathy
Neurofibromatosis type I	162200	Pheochromocytoma→ ↑ catecholamines; renal arterial fibromuscular dysplasia
Paraganglioma	168000	↑ Catecholamines
Pheochromocytoma, familial	171300	↑ Catecholamines
Polycystic kidney disease, adult	173900, 173910	↑ Renin; renal failure
Porphyria, acute intermittent	176000	?, but only during acute attacks
Pseudohypoaldosteronism, type I	264350	Aldosterone receptor deficiency
Pseudohypoaldosteronism, type II	145260	Defective renal secretion of potassium
Pseudoxanthoma elasticum	177850, 264800	Arteriosclerosis
Riley-Day syndrome	223900	Dysautonomia
von Hippel–Lindau syndrome	193300	Pheochromocytoma→ ↑ catecholamines
Wilms tumor	194070, 194071, 194090	?
Primarily Low Blood Pressure†		
Dopamine β-hydroxylase deficiency	223360	↑ Synthesis of epinephrine
Fabry disease	301500	↓ Peripheral vascular tone
Hyperbradykininism	143850	↑ Bradykinin
Pelizaeus-Merzbacher, late-onset	169500	?
Peripheral motor neuropathy and dysautonomia	252320	?
Pheochromocytoma, familial	171300	↑ Catecholamines (epinephrine)
Shy-Drager syndrome	146500	Primary autonomic insufficiency

*Data from Online Mendelian Inheritance in Man (www.ncbi.nlm.nih.gov/omim).

†Does not include hypovolemia, obstruction of blood flow, and cardiogenic causes of hypotension, each of which subsumes numerous hereditary disorders as primary causes.

aldosteronism. The phenotype was mapped to chromosome 8q21, a region already known to contain two candidate genes, aldosterone synthase and 11β-hydroxylase. By honing in on these loci, mutations creating a chimeric gene by unequal recombination were found to be the cause. As a result of the fusion, aldosterone synthase comes under regulation of adrenocorticotropic hormone. The actual frequency of such mutational events is considerably higher than suspected in the population, and the molecular means are now available to assess the epidemiology of what will likely be a common cause of early hypertension.

Angiotensinogen, the gene for which is in the region 1q42-q43, is a logical candidate gene to investigate because of the central role of its product in blood pressure regulation. Several polymorphic variants involving single amino acid substitutions occur; at positions 174 and 235, either methionine (M) or threonine (T) can exist. The special effects of these polymorphisms on activity, if any, are unclear, but persons homozygous for the 235T allele have plasma angiotensinogen levels 20 percent higher than those with the 235M alleles. Some but not all studies have found an association between the 174M and 235T alleles and hypertension. The importance of these polymorphisms seems to depend on the subject's ethnic background.[274]

The ACE gene, at 17q23, contains a common insertion/deletion polymorphism termed I and D, respectively, that permits both association and linkage studies. The three possible genotypes are DD, ID, and II, and the plasma level of ACE is highest, for unclear reasons, in persons who are DD and lowest in those who are II. The DD genotype has been associated with predisposition to coronary artery disease and myocardial infarction, which may account for a relative decrease of hypertensive patients with the DD genotype at older ages.

Pregnancy is a clear risk factor for hypertension. A susceptibility locus for preeclampsia has been identified.[275,276]

The opposite of hypertension, inappropriate control of pressure on the low side, also has numerous genetic bases (see Table 70–15).[277,278] A number of Mendelian conditions, most of which are rare, cause major deviations of blood pressure from an appropriate physiological range (see Table 70–15). These disorders are likely to be underdiagnosed.

REFERENCES

1. Childs B: Genetic Medicine: A Logic of Disease. Baltimore, Johns Hopkins University Press, 1999.
2. Murphy EA, Pyeritz RE: Pathogenetics. *In* Rimoin DL, Connor JM, Pyeritz RE, Korf BR (eds): Principles and Practice of Medical Genetics. 4th ed. New York, Churchill Livingstone, 2002, pp 439-455.
3. Jouven X, Desnos M, Guerot C, et al: Predicting sudden death in the population. The Paris prospective study I. Circulation 99:1978, 1999.
4. Bates BR, Templeton A, Achter PJ, et al: What does "A gene for heart disease" mean? A focus group study of public understandings of genetic risk factors. Am J Med Genet 119A:156, 2003.
5. Pai GS, Lewandowski RC Jr, Borgaonkar D: Handbook of Chromosomal Syndromes. New York, John Wiley & Sons, 2002.
6. Shaffer LG, Ledbetter DH, Lupski JR: Molecular cytogenetics of contiguous gene syndromes: Mechanisms and consequences of gene dosage imbalance. *In* Scriver CR, Beaudet AL, Sly WA, Valle D (eds): The Metabolic and Molecular Bases of Inherited Disease. 8th ed. New York, McGraw-Hill, 2001, pp 1291-1326.
7. Bayés M, Magano LF, Rivera N, et al: Mutational mechanisms of Williams-Beuren syndrome deletions. Am J Hum Genet 73:131, 2003.
8. The International Human Genome Sequencing Consortium: Initial sequencing and analysis of the human genome. Nature 409:860, 2001.
9. Collins FS, Green ED, Guttmacher AE, et al: A vision for the future of genomics research. Nature 422:835, 2003.
10. Pyeritz RE: Genetic approaches to cardiovascular disease. *In* Chien KR, Breslow JL, Leiden JM, et al (eds): Molecular Basis of Cardiovascular Disease. Philadelphia, WB Saunders, 1999, pp 19-36.
11. Online Mendelian Inheritance in Man. Available at www.ncbi.nlm.nih.gov/omim
12. Epstein JA, Rader DJ, Parmacek MS: Perspective: Cardiovascular disease in the postgenomic era—lessons learned and challenges ahead. Endocrinology 143:2045, 2002.
13. Hirschhorn JN, Lohmueller K, Byrne E, et al: A comprehensive review of genetic association studies. Genet Med 4:45, 2002.
14. Lachmeijer AMA, Arngrímsson R, Bastiaans EJ, et al: A genome-wide scan for preeclampsia in the Netherlands. Eur J Hum Genet 9:758, 2001.
15. Pyeritz RE: Marfan syndrome and related disorders of connective tissue. Annu Rev Med 51:481, 2000.
16. Wallace DC, Lott MT: Mitochondrial genetics. *In* Rimoin DL, Connor JM, Pyeritz RE, Korf BR (eds): Principles and Practice of Medical Genetics. 4th ed. New York, Churchill Livingstone, 2002, pp 299-409.
17. Pyeritz RE: Homocystinuria. *In* Beighton P (ed): McKusick's Heritable Disorders of Connective Tissue. 5th ed. St. Louis, CV Mosby, 1993, p 137.
18. Byers PH: Disorders of collagen biosynthesis and structure. *In* Scriver CR, Beaudet AL, Sly WA, Valle D (eds): The Metabolic and Molecular Bases of Inherited Disease. 8th ed. New York, McGraw-Hill, 2001, pp 5241-5286.
19. Friedlander Y, Lapidos T, Sinnreich R, Kark JD: Genetic and environmental sources of QT interval variability in Israeli families: The kibbutz settlements family study. Clin Genet 56:200, 1999.
20. Ranade K, Jorgenson E, Sheu WH-H, et al: A polymorphism in the β1 adrenergic receptor is associated with resting heart rate. Am J Hum Genet 70:935, 2002.
21. Wang XL, Mahaney MC, Sim AS, et at: Genetic contribution of the endothelial constitutive nitric oxide synthase gene to plasma nitric oxide levels. Arterioscler Thromb Vasc Biol 17:3147, 1997.
22. Rudic RD, Sessa WC: Human Genetics '99: The cardiovascular system: Nitric oxide in endothelial dysfunction and vascular remodeling: Clinical correlates and experimental links. Am J Hum Genet 64:673, 1999.
23. Zannad F, Visvikis S, Gueguen R, et al: Genetics strongly determines the wall thickness of the left and right carotid arteries. Hum Genet 103:183, 1998.

Cardiovascular Disorders Associated with Chromosome Aberrations

24. van Karnebeek CDM, Hennekam RCM: Associations between chromosomal anomalies and congenital heart defects: A database search. Am J Med Genet 84:158, 1999.
25. Freeman SB, Taft LF, Dooley KJ, et al: Population-based study of congenital heart defects in Down syndrome. Am J Med Genet 80:213, 1998.
26. McElhinney DB, Straka M, Goldmuntz E, et al: Correlation between abnormal cardiac physical examination and echocardiographic findings in neonates with Down syndrome. Am J Med Genet 113:238, 2002.
27. Barlow GM, Chen X-N, Shi ZY, et al: Down syndrome congenital heart disease: A narrowed region and a candidate gene. Genet Med 3:91, 2001.
28. Tolmie JL: Down syndrome and other autosomal trisomies. *In* Rimoin DL, Connor JM, Pyeritz RE, Korf BR (eds): Principles and Practice of Medical Genetics. 4th ed. New York, Churchill Livingstone, 2002, pp 1129-1183.
29. Kelly M, Robinson BW, Moore JW: Trisomy 18 in a 20-year-old woman. Am J Med Genet 112:397, 2002.
30. Rasmussen SA, Wong LY, Yang Q, et al: Population-based analyses of mortality in trisomy 13 and trisomy 18. Pediatrics 111:777, 2003.
31. Wax JR, Pinette MG, Blackstone J, et al: Isolated multiple bilateral echogenic papillary muscles: A unique sonographic feature of trisomy 13. Obstet Gynecol 99:902, 2002.
32. Tunca Y, Kadandale JS, Pivnick EK: Long-term survival in Patau syndrome. Clin Dysmorphol 10:149, 2001.
33. Elsheikh M, Casadei B, Conway GS, et al: Hypertension is a major risk factor for aortic root dilatation in women with Turner's syndrome. Clin Endocrinol 54:69, 2001.
34. Lin AE: The heart of Turner syndrome: Small matters. Teratology 66:63, 2002.
35. Gravholt CH: Medical problems of adult Turner's syndrome. Horm Res 56(suppl 1):44, 2001.
36. Sapienza C, Hall JG: Genome imprinting in human disease. *In* Scriver CR, Beaudet AL, Sly WA, Valle D (eds): The Metabolic and Molecular Bases of Inherited Disease. 8th ed. New York, McGraw-Hill, 2001, pp 417-432.
37. Jacobs P, Dalton P, James R, et al: Turner syndrome: A cytogenetic and molecular study. Ann Hum Genet 61:471, 1997.
38. Zinn AR, Tonk VS, Chen Z, et al: Evidence for a Turner syndrome locus or loci at Xp11.2-p22.1. Am J Hum Genet 63:1757, 1998.
39. Frías JL, Davenport ML, et al: Health supervision for children with Turner syndrome. Pediatrics 111:692, 2003.
40. Radetti G, Crepaz R, Milanesi O, et al: Cardiac performance in Turner's syndrome patients on growth hormone therapy. Horm Res 55:240, 2001.

Congenital Heart Disease

41. Ferencz C, Loffredo CA, Correa-Villaseñor A, Wilson P: Genetic and Environmental Risk Factors of Major Cardiovascular Malformations: The Baltimore-Washington Infant Study 1981-1989. Armonk, NY, Futura, 1997.
42. Wong SF, Chan FY, Cincotta RB, et al: Factors influencing the prenatal detection of structural congenital heart diseases. Ultrasound Obstet Gynecol 21:19, 2003.
43. Lin AE, Herring AH, Scharenberg K, et al: Cardiovascular malformations: Changes in prevalence and birth status, 1972-1990. Am J Med Genet 84:102, 1999.
44. Pyeritz RE, Murphy EA: The genetics of congenital heart disease: Perspectives and prospects. J Am Coll Cardiol 13:1458, 1989.
45. Devriendt K, Matthijs G, Dael RV, et al: Delineation of the critical deletion region for congenital heart defects on chromosome 8p23.1. Am J Hum Genet 64:1119, 1999.
46. Clayton-Smith J, Donnai D: Human malformations. *In* Rimoin DL, Connor JM, Pyeritz RE, Korf BR (eds): Principles and Practice of Medical Genetics. 4th ed. New York, Churchill Livingstone, 2002, pp 488-500.
47. Siu SC, Colman JM, Sorensen S, et al: Adverse neonatal and cardiac outcomes are more common in pregnant women with cardiac disease. Circulation 105:2179, 2002.

48. Romano-Zelekha O, Hirsh R, Blieden L, et al: The risk for congenital heart defects in offspring of individuals with congenital heart defects. Clin Genet 59:325, 2001.
49. Anderson NH, Dominiczak AF: Genetic analysis of complex traits. *In* Rimoin DL, Connor JM, Pyeritz RE, Korf BR (eds): Principles and Practice of Medical Genetics. 4th ed. New York, Churchill Livingstone, 2002, pp 410-424.
50. Digilio MC, Marino B, Toscanno A, et al: Atrioventricular canal defect without Down syndrome: A heterogeneous malformation. Am J Med Genet 85:140, 1999.
51. Marino B, Digilio MC: Inlet ventricular septal defect is not a partial atrioventricular septal defect. Am J Med Genet 87:195, 1999.
52. Clark EB: Mechanisms in the pathogenesis of congenital cardiac malformations. *In* Pierpont MEM, Moller JH (eds): Genetics of Cardiovascular Disease. Boston, Martinus Nihjoff, 1986, p 3.
53. Hoess K, Goldmuntz E, Pyeritz RE: Genetic counseling for congenital heart disease: New approaches for a new decade. Curr Cardiol Rep 4:68, 2002.
54. Goldmuntz E, Clark BJ, Mitchell LE, et al: Frequency of 22q11 deletions in patients with conotruncal defects. J Am Coll Cardiol 32:492, 1998.
55. Eldadah ZA, Hamosh A, Biery NJ, et al: Familial tetralogy of Fallot caused by mutation in the jagged-1 gene. Hum Molec Genet 10:163, 2001.
56. McElhinney DB, Krantz ID, Bason L, et al: Analysis of cardiovascular phenotype and genotype-phenotype correlation in individuals with a *JAG1* mutation and/or Alagille syndrome. Circulation 106:2567, 2002.
57. Krantz ID, Smith R, Colliton RP, et al: *Jagged1* mutations in patients ascertained with isolated congenital heart defects. Am J Med Genet 84:56, 1999.
58. Krantz ID: Alagille syndrome: Chipping away at the tip of the iceberg. Am J Med Genet 112:160, 2002.
59. Benson DW, Silberbach GM, Kavanaugh-McHugh A, et al: Mutations in the cardiac transcription factor *NKX2.5* affect diverse cardiac developmental pathways. J Clin Invest 104:1567, 1999.
60. Kasahara H, Lee B, Schott J-J, et al: Loss of function and inhibitory effects of human CSX/NKX2.5 homeoprotein mutations associated with congenital heart disease. J Clin Invest 106:299, 2000.
61. Ewing CK, Loffredo CA, Beaty TH: Paternal risk factors for isolated membranous ventricular septal defects. Am J Med Genet 71:42, 1997.
62. Funke B, Puech A, Saint-Jore B, et al: Isolation and characterization of a human gene containing a nuclear localization signal from the critical region for velo-cardiofacial syndrome on 22q11. Genomics 53:146, 1998.
63. Hokanson JS, Pierpont ME, Hirsch B, et al: 22q11.2 microdeletions in adults with familial tetralogy of Fallot. Genet Med 3:61, 2001.
64. Maeda J, Yamagashi H, Matsuoka R, et al: Frequent association of 22q11.2 deletion with tetralogy of Fallot. Am J Med Genet 92:269, 2000.
65. Goodship J, Cross I, LiLing J, Wren C: A populations study of chromosome 22q11 deletions in infancy. Arch Dis Child 79:348, 1998.
66. Beauchesne LM, Connolly HM, Ammash NM, et al: Coarctation of the aorta: Outcome of pregnancy. J Am Coll Cardiology 38:1728, 2001.
67. Robinson SW, Morris CD, Goldmuntz E, et al: Missense mutations in *CRELD1* are associated with cardiac atrioventricular septal defects. Am J Hum Genet 72:1047, 2003.
68. Kathiriya IS, Srivastava D: Left-right asymmetry and cardiac looping: Implications for cardiac development and congenital heart disease. Am J Med Genet 97:271, 2000.
69. Digilio MC, Casey B, Toscano A, et al: Complete transposition of the great arteries: Patterns of congenital heart disease in familial precurrence. Circulation 104:2809, 2001.
70. Afzelius BA, Mossberg B, Bergström SE: Immotile-cilia syndrome (primary ciliary dyskinesia), including Kartagener syndrome. *In* Scriver CR, Beaudet AL, Sly WA, Valle D (eds): The Metabolic and Molecular Bases of Inherited Disease. 8th ed. New York, McGraw-Hill, 2001, pp 4817-4828.
71. Solloway MJ, Harvey RP: Molecular pathways in myocardial development: A stem cell perspective. Cardiovasc Res 58:265, 2003.
72. Casey B: Two rights make a wrong: Human left-right malformations. Hum Mol Genet 7:1565, 1998.
73. Towbin JA, Casey B, Belmont J: Human Genetics ‘99: The cardiovascular system: The molecular basis of vascular disorders. Am J Hum Genet 64:678, 1999.
74. Mochizuki T, Saijoh U, Tsuchiya K, et al: Cloning of *inv*, a gene that controls left/right asymmetry and kidney development. Nature Genet 395:177, 1998.
75. Kosaki R, Gebbia M, Kosaki K, et al: Left-right axis malformations associated with mutations in *ACVR2B*, the gene for human activin receptor type IIB. Am J Med Genet 82:70, 1999.
76. Nezarati MM, McLeod DR: VACTERL manifestations in two generations of a family. Am J Med Genet 82:40, 1999.
77. Slavotinek A, Clayton-Smith J, Super M: Familial patent ductus arteriosus: A further case of CHAR syndrome. Am J Med Genet 71:229, 1997.
78. Glancy DL, Wegmann M, Dhurandhar RW: Aortic dissection and patent ductus arteriosus in three generations. Am J Cardiol 87:813, 2001.
79. Mani A, Meraji S-M, Houshyar R, et al: Finding genetic contributions to sporadic disease: A recessive locus at 12q24 commonly contributes to patent ductus arteriosus. Proc Natl Acad Sci U S A 99:15054, 2002.
80. Vaughan CJ, Basson CT: Molecular determinants of atrial and ventricular septal defects and patent ductus arteriosus. Am J Med Genet 97:304, 2001.
81. Garg V, Kathiriya IS, Barnes R, et al: GATA4 mutations cause human congenital heart defects and reveal an interaction with TBX5. Nature 424:443, 2003.
82. Schott J-J, Benson DW, Basson CT, et al: Congenital heart disease caused by mutations in the transcription factor NKX2-5. Science 281:108, 1998.
83. Basson CT, Huang T, Lin RC, et al: Different TBX5 interactions in heart and limb defined by Holt-Oram syndrome mutations. Proc Natl Acad Sci U S A 96:2919, 1999.
84. Brassington A-ME, Sung SS, Toydemir RM, et al: Expressivity of Holt-Oram syndrome is not predicted by *TBX5* genotype. Am J Hum Genet 73:74, 2003.
85. Ruiz-Perez VL, Ide SE, Strom TM, et al: Mutations in a new gene in Ellis-van Creveld syndrome and Weyers acrodental dysostosis. Nature Genet 24:283, 2000.
86. Galdzicka M, Patnala S, Hirshman MG, et al: A new gene, *EVC2*, is mutated in Ellis-van Creveld syndrome. Molec Genet Metabolism 77:291, 2002.
87. Sheffield VC, Pierpont ME, Nishimura D, et al: Identification of a complex congenital heart defect susceptibility locus by using DNA pooling and shared segment analysis. Hum Molec Genet 6:117, 1997.
88. Broder K, Reinhardt E, Ahern J, et al: Elevated ambulatory blood pressure in 20 subjects with Williams syndrome. Am J Med Genet 83:356, 1999.
89. Tassabehji M, Metcalfe K, Karmiloff-Smith A, et al: Williams syndrome: Use of chromosomal microdeletions as a tool to dissect cognitive and physical phenotypes. Am J Hum Genet 64:118, 1999.
90. Francke U: Williams-Beuren syndrome: Genes and mechanisms. Hum Molec Genet 8:1947, 1999.
91. Metcalfe K, Rucka AK, Smoot L, et al: Elastin: Mutational spectrum in supravalvular aortic stenosis. Eur J Hum Genet 8:955, 2000.
92. Urbán Z, Riazi S, Seidl TL, et al: Connection between elastin haploinsfficiency and increased cell proliferation in patients with supravalvular aortic stenosis and Williams-Beuren syndrome. Am J Hum Genet 71:30, 2002.
93. Nishimura RA, McGoon MD: Perspectives on mitral-valve prolapse. N Engl J Med 341:48, 1999.
94. Freed LA, Levy D, Levine RA, et al: Prevalence and clinical outcome of mitral-valve prolapse. N Engl J Med 341:1, 1999.
95. Freed LA, Acierno JS Jr, Dai D, et al: A locus for autosomal dominant mitral valve prolapse on chromosome 11p15.4. Am J Hum Genet 72:1551, 2003.
96. Disse S, Abergel E, Berrebi A, et al: Mapping of a first locus for autosomal dominant myxomatous mitral-valve prolapse to chromosome 16p11.2-p12.1. Am J Hum Genet 65:1242, 1999.
97. Kyndt F, Schott JJ, Trochu JN, et al: Mapping of X-linked myxomatous valvular dystrophy to chromosome Xq28. Am J Hum Genet 62:627, 1998.
98. DePaepe A, Deitz HC, Devereux RB, et al: Revised diagnostic criteria for the Marfan syndrome. Am J Med Genet 62:417, 1996.
99. Glesby MJ, Pyeritz RE: Association of mitral valve prolapse and systemic abnormalities of connective tissue: A phenotypic continuum. JAMA 262:523, 1989.
100. James PA, Aftimos S, Skinner JR: Familial mitral valve prolapse associated with short stature, characteristic face, and sudden death. Am J Med Genet 119A:32, 2003.
101. Musante L, Kehl HG, Majewski F, et al: Spectrum of mutations in *PTPN11* and genotype-phenotype correlation in 96 patients with Noonan syndrome and five patients with cardio-facio-cutaneous syndrome. Eur J Hum Genet 11:201, 2003.
102. Friedman JM, Hanson JW: Clinical teratology. *In* Rimoin DL, Connor JM, Pyeritz RE, Korf BR (eds): Principles and Practice of Medical Genetics. 4th ed. New York, Churchill Livingstone, 2002, pp 1011-1045.
103. Shepard TH: Catalog of Teratogenic Agents. 10th ed. Baltimore, Johns Hopkins Press, 2001.
104. Bagheri MM, Burd L, Martsolf JT, Klug MG: Fetal alcohol syndrome. J Perinat Med 26:263, 1998.
105. Scriver CR, Kaufman S: Hyperphenylalaninemia: Phenylalanine hydroxylase deficiency. *In* Scriver CR, Beaudet AL, Sly WA, Valle D (eds): The Metabolic and Molecular Bases of Inherited Disease. 8th ed. New York, McGraw-Hill, 2001, pp 1667-1724.
106. Seidman JG, Seidman C: The genetic basis for cardiomyopathy: From mutation identification to mechanistic paradigms. Cell 104:557, 2001.
107. Vosberg H-P, McKenna WJ. Cardiomyopathies. *In* Rimoin DL, Connor JM, Pyeritz RE, Korf BR (eds): Principles and Practice of Medical Genetics. 4th ed. New York, Churchill Livingstone, 2002, pp 1342-1416.
108. Maron, BJ, Casey SA, Poliac LC, et al: Clinical course of hypertrophic cardiomyopathy in a regional United States cohort. JAMA 281:650, 1999.
109. Maron BJ: Hypertrophic cardiomyopathy. JAMA 287:1308, 2002.
110. McKenna W, Behr ER: Hypertrophic cardiomyopathy: Management, risk stratification, and prevention of sudden death. Heart 87:169, 2002.
111. Braunwald E, Seidman CE, Sigwart U: Contemporary evaluation and management of hypertrophic cardiomyopathy. Circulation 106:1312, 2002.
112. Richard P, Charron P, Carrier L, et al: Hypertrophic cardiomyopathy: Distribution of disease genes, spectrum of mutations, and implications for a molecular diagnosis strategy. Circulation 107:2227, 2003.

Cardiomyopathies

113. Semsarian C, Seidman J, Seidman CE: Molecular genetics of inherited cardiomyopathies. *In* Chien KR (ed): Molecular Basis of Cardiovascular Disease. 2nd ed. Philadelphia, Saunders, 2004, pp 293-305.
114. Fung DCY, Yu B, Littlejohn T, et al: An online locus-specific mutation database for familial hypertrophic cardiomyopathy. Hum Mutat 14:326, 1999.
115. Forissier J-F, Richard P, Briault S, et al: First description of germline mosaicism in familial hypertrophic cardiomyopathy. J Med Genet 37:132, 2000.
116. Jeschke B, Uhl K, Weist B, et al: A high risk phenotype of hypertrophic cardiomyopathy associated with a compound genotype of two mutated β-myosin heavy chain genes. Hum Genet 102:299, 1998.
117. Tesson F, Richard P, Charron P, et al: Genotype-phenotype analysis in four families with mutations in β-myosin heavy chain gene responsible for familial hypertrophic cardiomyopathy. Hum Mutat 12:385, 1998.
118. Richard P, Isnard R, Carrier L, et al: Double heterozygosity for mutations in the β-myosin heavy chain and in the cardiac myosin binding protein C genes in a family with hypertrophic cardiomyopathy. J Med Genet 36:542, 1999.

119. Yu B, French JA, Jeremy RW, et al: Counseling issues in familial hypertrophic cardiomyopathy. J Med Genet 35:183, 1998.
120. Maron BJ, Moller JH, Seidman CE, et al: Impact of laboratory molecular diagnosis on contemporary diagnostic criteria for genetically transmitted cardiovascular diseases: Hypertrophic cardiomyopathy, long-QT syndrome, and Marfan syndrome. Circulation 98:1460, 1998.
121. Lim D-S, Roberts R, Marian AJ: Expression profiling of cardiac genes in human hypertrophic cardiomyopathy: Insight into the pathogenesis of phenotypes. J Am Coll Cardiol 38:1175, 2001.
122. Fatkin D, McConnell BK, Mudd JO, et al: An abnormal Ca^{2+} response in mutant sarcomere protein-mediated familial hypertrophic cardiomyopathy. J Clin Invest 106:1351, 2000.
123. Javadpour MM, Tardiff JC, Pinz K, Ingwall JS: Decreased energetics in murine hearts bearing the R92Q mutation in cardiac troponin T. J Clin Invest 112:768, 2003.
124. Maron BJ, Shen W-K, Link MS, et al: Efficacy of implantable cardioverter-defibrillators for the prevention of sudden death in patients with hypertrophic cardiomyopathy. N Engl J Med 342:365, 2000.
125. Sasse-Klaassen S, Gerull B, Oechslin E, et al: Isolated noncompaction of the left ventricular myocardium in the adult is an autosomal dominant disorder in the majority of patients. Am J Med Genet 119A:162, 2003.
126. Cecchi F, Olivotto I, Gistri R, et al: Coronary microvascular dysfunction and prognosis in hypertrophic cardiomyopathy. N Engl J Med 349:1027, 2003.
127. Felker GM, Thompson RE, Hare JM, et al: Underlying causes and long-term survival in patients with initially unexplained cardiomyopathy. N Engl J Med 342:1077, 2000.
128. Legius E, Schollen E, Matthijs G, Fryns J-P: Fine mapping of Noonan/cardiofacio-cutaneous syndrome in a large family. Eur J Hum Genet 6:32, 1998.
129. Maeda M, Holder E, Lowes B, et al: Dilated cardiomyopathy associated with deficiency of the cytoskeletal protein metavinculin. Circulation 95:17, 1997.
130. Jung M, Poepping I, Perrot A, et al: Investigation of a family with autosomal dominant dilated cardiomyopathy defines a novel locus on chromosome 2q14-q22. Am J Hum Genet 65:1068, 1997.
131. Vilarinho L, Santorelli FM, Rosas MJ, et al: The mitochondrial A3243G mutation presenting as severe cardiomyopathy. J Med Genet 34:607, 1997.
132. Digilio MC, Marino B, Bevilacqua M, et al: Genetic heterogeneity of isolated noncompaction of the left ventricular myocardium. Am J Med Genet 85:90, 1999.
133. Emery AEH: Duchenne and other X-linked muscular dystrophies. *In* Rimoin DL, Connor JM, Pyeritz RE, Korf BR (eds): Principles and Practice of Medical Genetics. 4th ed. New York, Churchill Livingstone, 2002, pp 3266-3284.
134. Bushby KMD: Autosomally inherited muscular dystrophies. *In* Rimoin DL, Connor JM, Pyeritz RE, Korf BR (eds): Principles and Practice of Medical Genetics. 4th ed. New York, Churchill Livingstone, 2002, pp 3285-3302.
135. Morris GE, Manilal S: Heart to heart: From nuclear proteins to Emery-Dreifuss muscular dystrophy. Hum Molec Genet 8:1847, 1999.
136. De Sandre-Giovannoli A, Bernard R, Cau P, et al: Lamin A truncation in Hutchinson-Gilford Progeria. Science 300:2055, 2003.
137. Barresi R, Di Blasi C, Negri T, et al: Disruption of heart sarcoglycan complex and severe cardiomyopathy caused by β sarcoglycan mutations. J Med Genet 37:102, 2000.
138. Sylvius N, Duboscq-Bidot L, Bouchier C, et al: Mutational analysis of the β- and δ-sarcoglycan genes in a large number of patients with familial and sporadic dilated cardiomyopathy. Am J Med Genet 120A:8, 2003.
139. Tiso N, Stephan DA, Nava A, et al: Identification of mutations in the cardiac ryanodine receptor gene in families affected with arrhythmogenic right ventricular cardiomyopathy type 2 (ARVD2). Hum Molec Genet 10:189, 2001.
140. Rampazzo A, Beffagna G, Nava A, et al: Arrhythmogenic right ventricular cardiomyopathy type 1 (ARVD1): Confirmation of locus assignment and mutation screening of four candidate genes. Eur J Hum Genet 11:69, 2003.
141. Ammash NM, Seward JB, Bailey KR, et al: Clinical profile and outcome of idiopathic restrictive cardiomyopathy. Circulation 101:2490, 2000.
142. Lipsanen-Nyman M, Perheentupa J, Rapola J, et al: Mulibrey heart disease. Clinical manifestations, long-term course, and results of pericardiectomy in a series of 49 patients born before 1985. Circulation 107:2810, 2003.
143. Avela K, Lipsanen-Nyman M, Idanheimo N, et al: Gene encoding a new RING-B-box-Coiled-coil protein is mutated in mulibrey nanism. Nature Genet 25:298, 2000.
144. Bahabri SA, Suwairi WM, Laxer RM, et al: The camptodactyly-arthropathy-coxa vara-pericarditis syndrome: Clinical features and genetic mapping to human chromosome 1. Arthritis Rheum 41:730, 1998.
145. Marcelino J, Carpten JD, Suwairi WM, et al: CACP, encoding a secreted proteoglycan, is mutated in camptodactyly-arthropathy-coxa vara-pericarditis syndrome. Nature Genet 23:319, 1999.
146. Van Hove JLK, Wevers RA, Van Cleemput J, et al: Late-onset visceral presentation with cardiomyopathy and without neurological symptoms of adult Sanfilippo A syndrome. Am J Med Genet 118:282, 2003.
147. Kampmann C, Baehner F, Ries M, et al: Cardiac involvement in Anderson-Fabry disease. J Am Soc Nephrol 13:S147, 2002.
148. Lin AE, Grossfeld PD, Hamilton RM, et al: Further delineation of cardiac abnormalities in Costello syndrome. Am J Med Genet 111:115, 2002.
149. Coppin BD, Temple IK: Multiple lentigines syndrome (LEOPARD) syndrome or progressive cardiomyopathic lentiginosis. J Med Genet 24:582, 1997.

Disorders of Connective Tissue

150. Royce PM, Steinmann B (eds): Connective Tissue and Its Heritable Disorders: Molecular, Genetic and Medical Aspects. 2nd ed. New York, Wiley-Liss, 2002.
151. Pyeritz RE: Disorders of fibrillins and microfibrilogenesis: Marfan syndrome, MASS phenotype, contractural arachnodactyly and related conditions. *In* Rimoin DL, Connor JM, Pyeritz RE, Korf BR (eds): Principles and Practice of Medical Genetics. 4th ed. New York, Churchill Livingstone, 2002, pp 3977-4020.
151a. Schalkwijk J, Zweers MC, Steijlen PM, et al: A recessive form of the Ehlers-Danlos syndrome caused by tenascin-X deficiency. N Engl J Med 345:1167, 2001.
152. Yetman AT, Bornemeier RA, McCrindle BW: Long-term outcome in patients with Marfan syndrome: Is aortic dissection the only cause of sudden death? J Am Coll Cardiol 41:329, 2003.
153. Gott VL, Greene PS, Alejo DE, et al: Surgery for ascending aortic disease in Marfan patients: A multi-center study. N Engl J Med 340:1307, 1999.
154. van Karnebeek CDM, Naeff MSJ, Mulder BJM, et al: Natural history of cardiovascular manifestations in Marfan syndrome. Arch Dis Child 84:129, 2001.
155. Lepore V, Jeppsson A, Radberg G, et al: Aortic surgery in patients with Marfan syndrome: Long-term survival, morbidity and function. J Heart Valve Dis 10:25, 2001.
156. De Oliveira NC, David TE, Ivanov J, et al: Results of surgery for aortic root aneurysm in patients with Marfan syndrome. J Thorac Cardiovasc Surg 125:789, 2003.
157. Miller DC: Valve-sparing aortic root replacement in patients with the Marfan syndrome. J Thorac Cardiovasc Surg 125:773, 2003.
158. Porciani MC, Giurlani L, Chelucci A, et al: Diastolic subclinical primary alterations in Marfan syndrome and Marfan-related disorders. Clin Cardiol 25:416, 2002.
159. Chatrath R, Beauchesne LM, Connolly HM, et al: Left ventricular function in the Marfan syndrome without significant valvular regurgitation. Am J Cardiol 91:914, 2003.
160. Shores J, Borger KR, Murphy EA, et al: Chronic β-adrenergic blockade protects the aorta in the Marfan syndrome: A prospective, randomized trial of propranolol. N Engl J Med 330:1335, 1994.
161. Jondeau G, Boutouyrie P, Lacolley P, et al: Central pulse pressure is a major determinant of ascending aorta dilatation in Marfan syndrome. Circulation 99:2677, 1999.
162. Lipscomb KJ, Clayton-Smith J, Clarke B, et al: Outcome of pregnancy in women with Marfan's syndrome. Br J Obstet Gynaecol 104:210, 1997.
163. Pyeritz RE, Dietz HC: The Marfan syndrome and other fibrillinopathies. *In* Royce PM, Steinmann B (eds): Connective Tissue and Its Heritable Disorders: Molecular, Genetic and Medical Aspects. 2nd ed. New York, Wiley-Liss, 2002, pp 585-626.
164. Collod-Beroud G, Beroud C, Ades L: Marfan Database (3rd ed): New mutations and new routines for the software. Nucl Acids Res 26:229, 1998.
165. Yuan B, Thomas JP, von Kodolitsch Y, Pyeritz RE: Comparison of heteroduplex analysis, direct sequencing and enzyme mismatch cleavage for detecting mutations in a large gene, FBN1. Hum Mutat 14:440, 1999.
166. Korkko J, Kaitila I, Lonnqvist L, et al: Sensitivity of conformation sensitive gel electrophoresis in detecting mutations in Marfan syndrome and related conditions. J Med Genet 39:34, 2002.
167. Neptune ER, Frischmeyer PA, Arking DE, et al: Dysregulation of TGF-α activation contributes to pathogenesis in Marfan syndrome. Nature Genet 33:407, 2003.
168. Beighton P, De Paepe A, Steinmann B, et al: Ehlers-Danlos syndromes: Revised nosology, Villefranche, 1997. Am J Med Genet 77:31, 1998.
169. Wenstrup RJ, Meyer RA, Lyle JS, et al: Prevalence of aortic root dilation in the Ehlers-Danlos syndrome. Genet Med 4:112, 2002.
170. Dolan AL, Mishra MB, Chambers JB, et al: Clinical and echocardiographic survey of the Ehlers-Danlos syndrome. Br J Rheumatol 36:459, 1997.
171. Pyeritz RE: Ehlers-Danlos syndrome. N Engl J Med 342:730, 2000.
172. Gilchrist D, Schwarze U, Shields K, et al: Large kindred with Ehlers-Danlos syndrome type IV due to a point mutation (G571S) in the *COL3A1* gene of type III procollagen: Low risk of pregnancy complications and unexpected longevity in some affected relatives. Am J Med Genet 82:305, 1999.
173. Pepin M, Schwarze U, Superti-Furga A, Byers PH: Clinical and genetic features of Ehlers-Danlos syndrome type IV, the vascular type. N Engl J Med 342:673, 2000.
174. Lind J, Wallenburg HCS: Pregnancy and the Ehler-Danlos syndrome: A retrospective study in a Dutch population. Acta Obstet Gynecol Scand 81:293, 2002.
175. Uitto J, Pulkkinen L: Heritable disorders of elastic tissue: Cutis laxa, pseudoxanthoma elasticum and related disorders. *In* Rimoin DL, Connor JM, Pyeritz RE, Korf BR (eds): Principles and Practice of Medical Genetics. 4th ed. New York, Churchill Livingstone, 2002, pp 4044-4070.
176. Germain DP, Boutouyrie P, Laloux B, et al: Arterial remodeling and stiffness in patients with pseudoxanthoma elasticum. Arterioscler Thromb Vasc Biol 23:836, 2003.

Inborn Errors of Metabolism that Affect the Cardiovascular System

177. Wilcken DEL: Overview of inherited metabolic disorders causing cardiovascular disease. J Inherit Metab Dis 26:245, 2003.
178. La Du BN: Alkaptonuria: *In* Scriver CR, Beaudet AL, Sly WA, Valle D (eds): The Metabolic and Molecular Bases of Inherited Disease. 8th ed. New York, McGraw-Hill, 2001, pp 2109-2124.
179. Mudd SH, Levy HL, Skovby F: Disorders of transsulfuration. *In* Scriver CR, Beaudet AL, Sly WA, Valle D (eds): The Metabolic and Molecular Bases of Inherited Disease. 8th ed. New York, McGraw-Hill, 2001, pp 2007-2056.
180. Kraus JP, Janosik M, Kozich V, et al: Cystathionine β-synthase mutations in homocystinuria. Hum Mutat 13:362, 1999.
181. Wilcken DEL, Wilcken B: The natural history of vascular disease in homocystinuria and the effects of treatment. J Inher Metab Dis 20:295, 1997.
182. Eikelboom JW, Lonn E, Genest J Jr, et al: Homocyst(e)ine and cardiovascular disease: A critical review of the epidemiologic evidence. Ann Intern Med 131:363, 1999.
183. Majors A, Ehrhart LA, Pezacka EH: Homocysteine as a risk factor for vascular disease. Enhanced collagen production and accumulation by smooth muscle cells. Arterioscler Thromb Vasc Biol 17:2074, 1997.

184. Darras BT, Friedman NR: Metabolic myopathies: A clinical approach; Part II. Pediatr Neurol 22:171, 2000.
185. Roe CR, Ding J: Mitochondrial fatty acid oxidation disorders. *In* Scriver CR, Beaudet AL, Sly WA, Valle D (eds): The Metabolic and Molecular Bases of Inherited Disease. 8th ed. New York, McGraw-Hill, 2001, pp 2297-2326.
186. Goodman SI: Organic acidemias and disorders of fatty acid oxidation. *In* Rimoin DL, Connor JM, Pyeritz RE, Korf BR (eds): Principles and Practice of Medical Genetics. 4th ed. New York, Churchill Livingstone, 2002, pp 2550-2565.
187. Chen Y-T: Glycogen storage diseases. *In* Scriver CR, Beaudet AL, Sly WA, Valle D (eds): The Metabolic and Molecular Bases of Inherited Disease. 8th ed. New York, McGraw-Hill, 2001, pp 1521-1552.
188. Cox PM, Brueton LA, Murphy KW, et al: Early-onset fetal hydrops and muscle degeneration in siblings due to a novel variant of type IV glycogenosis. Am J Med Genet 86:187, 1999.
189. Arad M, Benson DW, Perez-Atayde AR, et al: Constitutively active AMP kinase mutations cause glycogen storage disease mimicking hypertrophic cardiomyopathy. J Clin Invest 109:357, 2002.
190. Leroy JG: Oligosaccharidoses and allied disorders. *In* Rimoin DL, Connor JM, Pyeritz RE, Korf BR (eds): Principles and Practice of Medical Genetics. 4th ed. New York, Churchill Livingstone, 2002, pp 2677-2711.
191. Beutler E, Bothwell TH, Charlton RW, Motulsky AG: Hereditary hemochromatosis. *In* Scriver CR, Beaudet AL, Sly WA, Valle D (eds): The Metabolic and Molecular Bases of Inherited Disease. 8th ed. New York, McGraw-Hill, 2001, pp 3127-3162.
192. Olynyk JK, Cullen DJ, Aquilia S, et al: A population-based study of the clinical expression of the hemochromatosis gene. N Engl J Med 341:718, 1999.
193. Beutler E, Felitti VJ, Koziol JA, et al: Penetrance of 845G → A(C282Y) *HFE* hereditary haemochromatosis mutation in the USA. Lancet 359:211, 2002.
194. Burke W, Thomson E, Khoury MJ, et al: Hereditary hemochromatosis: Gene discovery and its implications for population-based screening. JAMA 280:172, 1998.
195. Weatherall DJ, Clegg JB, Higgs DR, et al: The hemoglobinopathies. *In* Scriver CR, Beaudet AL, Sly WA, Valley D (eds): The Metabolic and Molecular Bases of Inherited Disease. 8th ed. New York, McGraw-Hill, 2001, pp 4571-636.
196. Kremastinos DT, Flevari P, Spyropoulou M, et al: Association of heart failure in homozygous β-thalassemia with the major histocompatibility complex. Circulation 100:2074, 1999.
197. Steinberg MH: Management of sickle cell disease. N Engl J Med 340:1021, 1999.
198. Tsomi K, Karagiorga-Lagana M, Karabatsos F, et al: Arterial elastorrhexis in β-thalassaemia intermedia, sickle cell thalassaemia and hereditary sperocytosis. Eur J Haematol 67:135, 2001.
199. Aessopos A, Farmakis D, Loukopoulos D: Elastic tissue abnormalities resembling pseudoxanthoma elasticum in β thalassemia and the sickling syndromes. Blood 99:30, 2002.
200. Spranger J: Mucopolysaccharidoses. *In* Rimoin DL, Connor JM, Pyeritz RE, Korf BR (eds): Principles and Practice of Medical Genetics. 4th ed. New York, Churchill Livingstone, 2002, pp 2666-2676.
201. Semenza GL, Pyeritz RE: Respiratory complications of the mucopolysaccharide storage disorders. Medicine 67:209, 1988.
202. Kakkis ED, Muenzer J, Tiller GE, et at: Enzyme-replacement therapy in mucopolysaccharidosis I. New Engl J Med 344:182, 2001.
203. Percy AK: Gangliosidoses and related lipid storage diseases. *In* Rimoin DL, Connor JM, Pyeritz RE, Korf BR (eds): Principles and Practice of Medical Genetics. 4th ed. New York, Churchill Livingstone, 2002, pp 2712-2751.
204. Desnick RJ, Brady R, Barranger J, et al: Fabry disease, an under-recognized multisystemic disorder: Expert recommendations for diagnosis, management, and enzyme replacement therapy. Ann Intern Med 138:338, 2003.
205. Schiffmann R, Murray GJ, Treco D, et al: Infusion of α-galactosidase A reduces tissue globotriaosylceramide storage in patients with Fabry disease. Proc Natl Acad Sci U S A 97:365, 2000.
206. Hopkin RJ, Bissler J, Grabowski, GA: Comparative evaluation of α-galactosidase A infusions for treatment of Fabry disease. Genet Med 5:144-53, 2003.
207. Boerkoel CN III, Lupski JR: Hereditary motor and sensory neuropathies. *In* Rimoin DL, Connor JM, Pyeritz RE, Korf BR (eds): Principles and Practice of Medical Genetics. 4th ed. New York, Churchill Livingstone, 2002, pp 3303-3320.
208. Lachmann HJ, Booth DR, Booth SE, et al: Misdiagnosis of hereditary amyloidosis as AL (primary) amyloidosis. N Engl J Med 346:1786, 2002.
209. Dingli D, Utz JP, Gertz MA: Pulmonary hypertension in patients with amyloidosis. Chest 120:1735, 2001.
210. Morelli S, Carmenini E, Sgreccia A, et al: Heart rate variability and familial amyloidosis. Inter J Cardiol 83:295, 2002.
211. Olofsson BO, Backman C, Karp K, et al: Progression of cardiomyopathy after liver transplantation in patients with familial amyloidotic polyneuropathy, Portuguese type. Transplantation 73:745, 2002.
212. Roach ES, DiMario FJ, Kandt RS, Northrup H: Tuberous sclerosis complex consensus conference: Recommendations for diagnostic evaluation. J Child Neurol 14:401, 1999.
213. Sperling D, Smith M: Novel 23-base-pair duplication mutation in TSC1 exon 15 in an infant presenting with cardiac rhabdomyomas. Am J Med Genet 84:346, 1999.
214. Astrinidis A, Khare L, Carsillo T, et al: Mutational analysis of the tuberous sclerosis gene *TSC2* in patients with pulmonary lymphangioleiomyomatosis. J Med Genet 37:55, 2000.
215. Harris NL, McNeely WF, Shepard JO, et al: Presentation of case 11-2002, MGH. N Engl J Med 346:1152, 2002.
216. Basson CT, MacRae CA, Korf B, Merliss A: Genetic heterogeneity of familial atrial myxoma syndromes (Carney complex). Am J Cardiol 79:994, 1997.
217. Groussin L, Kirschner LS, Vincent-Dejean C, et al: Molecular analysis of the cyclic AMP-dependent protein kinase A (PKA) regulatory subunit 1A (*PRKAR1A*) gene in patients with Carney complex and primary pigmented nodular adrenocortical disease (PPNAD) reveals novel mutations and clues for pathophysiology: Augmented PKA signaling is associated with adrenal tumorigenesis in PPNAD. Am J Hum Genet 71:1433, 2002.

Inherited Disorders of the Circulation

218. Shovlin CL, Guttmacher AE, Buscarini E, et al: Diagnostic criteria for hereditary hemorrhagic telangiectasia (Rendu-Osler-Weber syndrome). Am J Med Genet 91:66, 2000.
219. McDonald JE, Miller FJ, Hallam SE, et al: Clinical manifestations in a large hereditary hemorrhagic telangiectasia (HHT) type 2 kindred. Am J Med Genet. 93:320, 2000.
220. Fulbright RK, Chaloupka JC, Putman CM, et al: MR of hereditary hemorrhagic telangiectasia: Prevalence and spectrum of cerebrovascular malformations. Am J Neuroradiol 19:477, 1998.
221. Kopel L, Lage SG: Cardiac tamponade in hereditary hemorrhagic telangiectasia. Am J Med 105:252, 1998.
222. Lee WL, Graham AF, Pugash RA, et al: Contrast echocardiography remains positive after treatment of pulmonary arteriovenous malformations. Chest 123:351, 2003.
223. Lee DW, White RI Jr, Egglin TK, et al: Embolotherapy of large pulmonary arteriovenous malformations: Long-term results. Ann Thorac Surg 64:930, 1997.
224. Longacre AV, Gross CP, Gallitelli M, et al: Diagnosis and management of gastrointestinal bleeding in patients with hereditary hemorrhagic telangiectasia. Am J Gastroenterol 98:59, 2003.
225. Easey AJ, Wallace GM, Hughes JM, et al: Should asymptomatic patients with hereditary haemorrhagic telangiectasia (HHT) be screened for cerebral vascular malformations? J Neurol Neurosurg Psychiatry 74:743, 2003.
226. Marchuk DA, Srinivasan S, Squire TL, et al: Vascular morphogenesis: Tales of two syndromes. Hum Molec Genet 12:R97, 2003.
227. Prowse AH, Webster AR, Richards FM, et al: Somatic inactivation of the VHL gene in Von Hippel-Lindau disease tumors. Am J Hum Genet 60:765, 1997.
228. Watnick T, Phakdeekitcharoen B, Johnson A, et al: Mutation detection of *PKD1* identifies a novel mutation common to three families with aneurysms and/or very-early-onset disease. Am J Hum Genet 65:1561, 1999.
229. Hateboer N, van Dijk MA, Bogdanova N, et al: Comparison of phenotypes of polycystic kidney disease types 1 and 2. Lancet 353:103, 1999.
230. Koptides M, Hadjimichael C. Koupepidou P, et al: Germinal and somatic mutations in the PKD2 gene of renal cysts in autosomal dominant polycystic kidney disease. Hum Molec Genet 8:509, 1999.
231. Peters DJM, Breuning MH: Autosomal dominant polycystic kidney disease: Modification of disease progression. Lancet 358:1439, 2001.
232. Piccoli DA, Spinner NB: Alagille syndrome and the Jagged1 gene. Sem Liver Dis 21:525, 2001.
233. Woolfenden AR, Albers GW, Steinberg GK, et al: Moyamoya syndrome in children with Alagille syndrome: Additional evidence of a vasculopathy. Pediatrics 103:505, 1999.
234. Yuan Z-R, Kohsak T, Ikegaya T, et al: Mutational analysis of the Jagged 1 gene in Alagille syndrome families. Hum Molec Genet 7:1363, 1998.
235. Li L, Krantz ID, Deng Y, et al: Alagille syndrome is caused by mutations in human Jagged1, which encodes a ligand for Notch1. Nature Genet 16:243, 1997.
236. Biddinger A, Rocklin M, Coselli J, Milewicz DM: Familial thoracic aortic dilatations and dissections: A case control study. J Vasc Surg 25:506, 1997.
237. Milewicz DM, Chen H, Park E-S, et al: Reduced penetrance and variable expressivity of familial thoracic aortic aneurysms/dissections. Am J Cardiol 82:474, 1998.
238. Guo D, Hasham S, Kuang SQ, et al: Familial thoracic aortic aneurysms and dissections: Genetic heterogeneity with a major locus mapping to 5q13-14. Circulation 103:2461, 2001.
239. Vaughan CJ, Casey M, He J, et al: Identification of a chromosome 11q23-2-q24 locus for familial aortic aneurysm disease, a genetically heterogeneous disorder. Circulation 103:2469, 2001.
240. Hasham SN, Willing MC, Guo DC, et al: Mapping a locus for familial thoracic aortic aneurysms and dissections. Circulation 107:3184, 2003.
241. Multicentre Aneurysm Screening Study Group: Multicentre aneurysm screening study (MASS): Cost effectiveness analysis of screening for abdominal aortic aneurysms based on four year results from randomized controlled trial. BMJ 325:1135, 2002.
242. Franceschini P, Guala A, Licata D, et al: Arterial Tortuosity syndrome. Am J Med Genet 91:141, 2000.
243. Caplan LR: Should intracranial aneurysms be treated before they rupture? N Engl J Med 339:1774, 1998.
244. Magnetic Resonance Angiography Study Group: Risks and benefits of screening for intracranial aneurysms in first-degree relatives of patients with sporadic subarachnoid hemorrhage. N Engl J Med 241:1344, 1999.
245. Gaist D, Væth M, Tsiropoulos I, et al: Risk of subarachnoid haemorrhage in first degree relatives of patients with subarachnoid haemorrhage: Follow up study based on national registries in Denmark. BMJ 320:141, 2000.
246. Walter JW, Blei F, Anderson JL, et al: Genetic mapping of a novel familial form of infantile hemangioma. Am J Med Genet 82:77, 1999.
247. Iadecola C: Genetics of cerebrovascular disease. N Engl J Med 339:216, 1998.
248. Ikeda H, Sasaki T, Yoshimoto T, et al: Mapping of a familial Moyamoya disease gene to chromosome 3p24.2-p26. Am J Hum Genet 64:533, 1999.
249. De Lange RPJ, Bolt J, Reid E, et al: Screening British CADASIL families for mutations in the *NOTCH3* gene. J Med Genet 37:224, 2000.
250. Ducros A, Denier C, Joutel A, et al: Recurrence of the T666M calcium channel *CACNA1A* gene mutation in familial hemiplegic migraine with progressive cerebellar ataxia. Am J Hum Genet 64:89, 1999.
251. Trembath RC, Harrison R: Insights into the genetic and molecular basis of primary pulmonary hypertension. Pediatr Res 53:883, 2003.
252. Runo JR, Loyd JE: Primary pulmonary hypertension. Lancet 361:1533, 2003.

253. Deng Z, Morse JH, Slager SL, et al: Familial primary pulmonary hypertension (gene PPH1) is caused by mutations in the bone morphogenetic protein receptor-II gene. Am J Hum Genet 67:737, 2000.
254. Cohen MM Jr: Klippel-Trenaunay syndrome. Am J Med Genet 93:171, 2000.
255. Craig HD, Gunel M, Cepeda O, et al: Multilocus linkage identifies two new loci for a Mendelian form of stroke, cerebral cavernous malformation, at 7p15-13 and 3q25.2-27. Hum Molec Genet 7:1851, 1998.
256. Zhang J, Clatterbuck RE, Rigamonti D, et al: Mutations in KRIT1 in familial cerebral cavernous malformations. Neurosurgery 46:1272, 2000.
257. Cavé-Riant F, Denier C, Labauge P, et al: Spectrum and expression analysis of *KRIT1* mutations in 121 consecutive and unrelated patients with cerebral cavernous malformations. Eur J Hum Genet 10:733, 2002.
258. Arteriovenous Malformation Study Group: Arteriovenous malformations of the brain in adults. N Engl J Med 340:1812-1818, 1999.
259. Ferrell RE, Pyeritz RE: Hereditary disorders of the lymphatic and venous systems. *In* Rimoin DL, Conner JM, Pyeritz RE, Korf B (eds): Principles and Practice of Medical Genetics, 4th ed. Edinburgh: Churchill Livingstone, 2002, pp 1546-1560.
260. Van Balkom IDC, Alders M, Allanson J, et al: Lymphedema-lymphangiectasia-mental retardation (Hennekam) syndrome: A review. Am J Med Genet 112:412, 2002.
261. Ferrell RE, Levinson KL, Esman JH, et al: Hereditary lymphedema: Evidence for linkage and genetic heterogeneity. Hum Molec Genet 7:2073, 1998.
262. Evans AL, Brice G, Sotirova V, et al: Mapping of primary congenital lymphedema to the 5q35.3 region. Am J Hum Genet 64:547, 1999.
263. Irrthum A, Devriendt K, Chitayat D, et al: Mutations in the transcription factor gene *SOX18* underlie recessive and dominant forms of hypotrichosis-lymphedema-telangiectasia. Am J Hum Genet 72:1470, 2003.
264. Asad R, Thompson PD, Pyeritz RE: Genetic factors in occlusive arterial disease. *In* Rimoin DL, Conner JM, Pyeritz RE, Korf B (eds): Principles and Practice of Medical Genetics, 4th ed. New York, Churchill Livingstone, 2002, pp 1519-1545.
265. Trip MD, Smulders YM, Wegman JJ, et al: Frequent mutation in the ABCC6 gene (*R1141X*) is associated with a strong increase in the prevalence of coronary artery disease. Circulation 106:773, 2002.
266. Arking DE, Becker DM, Yanek LR, et al: KLOTHO allele status and the risk of early-onset occult coronary artery disease. Am J Hum Genet 72:1154, 2003.
267. von Kodolitsch Y, Pyeritz RE, Rogan PK: Splice site mutations in atherosclerosis candidate genes: Relating individual information to phenotype. Circulation 100:693, 1999.
268. Hacia JG, Collins FS: Mutational analysis using oligonucleotide microarrays. J Med Genet 36:730, 1999.
269. Elston RC: Linkage and association. Genet Epidemiol 15:565, 1998.
270. Hunt SC, Hopkins PN, Lalouel J-M: Hypertension. *In* King RA, Rotter JI, Motulsky AG (eds): The Genetic Basis of Common Diseases. 2nd ed. New York, Oxford University Press, 2002, pp 127-154.
271. Jeunemaitre X, Gimenez-Roqueplo A-P, Disse-Nicodeme S, Corvol P: Molecular basis of human hypertension. *In* Rimoin DL, Connor JM, Pyeritz RE, Korf BR (eds): Principles and Practice of Medical Genetics. 4th ed. New York, Churchill Livingstone, 2002, pp 1475-1479.
272. Halushka MK, Fan JB, Bentley K, et al: Patterns of single-nucleotide polymorphisms in candidate genes for blood-pressure homeostasis. Nature Genet 22:239, 1999.
273. Lifton RP, Gharavi AG, Geller DS: Molecular mechanisms of human hypertension. Cell 104:545, 2001.
274. Niu T, Xu X, Rogus J, et al: Angiotensinogen gene and hypertension in Chinese. J Clin Invest 101:188, 1998.
275. Arngrimsson R, Hayward C, Nadaud S, et al: Evidence for a familial pregnancy-induced hypertension locus in the eNOS-gene region. Am J Hum Genet 61:354, 1997.
276. Arngrimsson R, Siguroardottir S, Frigge ML, et al: A genome-wide scan reveals a maternal susceptibility locus for pre-eclampsia on chromosome 2p13. Hum Molec Genet 8:1799, 1999.
277. DeStefano AL, Baldwin CT, Burzstyn M, et al: Autosomal dominant orthostatic hypotensive disorder maps to chromosome 18q. Am J Hum Genet 63:1425, 1998.
278. Schwartz F, Baldwin CT, Baima J, Gavras H: Mitochondrial DNA mutations in patients with orthostatic hypotension. Am J Med Genet 86:145, 1999.

CHAPTER 71

Myocardial Regeneration

Piero Anversa • Annarosa Leri

Two distinct forms of myocardial regeneration occur in the adult heart after injury. The first is restricted to the unaffected portion of the myocardium and uses the growth reserve of the viable tissue. The process of generating new myocardial mass involves hypertrophy of terminally differentiated myocytes and replication of myocytes that have retained the ability to reenter the cell cycle and divide.[1] The second requires the repair of necrotic lost myocardium that can be accomplished only by cellular therapy. This novel procedure has been performed recently using exogenous primitive cells of various sources (Fig. 71–1). The expansion of the surviving myocardium by replication of parenchymal cells imposes a different view of the growth of the heart, whereas tissue reconstitution from nonresident cells demands that these cells be capable of developing myocytes and coronary vessels in an orderly manner to rebuild functionally competent new myocardium.[2]

Growth Reserve of the Heart

If the adult heart were a static organ, its biology would be rather simple. Shortly after birth, myocytes would cease to divide and would acquire a state of terminal differentiation.[3] The total number of parenchymal cells would become established at this time, and this cell population would remain constant throughout life. According to this paradigm, the myocardium would constitute a steady-state tissue because its most distinctive cellular compartment would persist intact until death of the individual. Although nature continuously teaches us the simplicity of natural events, the biological model of the postnatal heart as a lethargic organ is unrealistic. The evidence that has accumulated on the dynamic state of the cellular population of the heart[1,2,4] has forced us to deal with complexity.

As the basic components of a tissue, cells represent autonomous agents that are driven by built-in programs and also sense the chemical and mechanical signals dictated by the surrounding microenvironment. The integration of intrinsic and extrinsic cues regulates cell migration, growth, differentiation, and death, which constitute the basic processes of organ homeostasis. These notions, valid for any organ or tissue in the organism, have only recently been applied to the heart. Therefore, the new concept of cardiac development, maturation, aging, and disease must include these fundamental biological principles of myocardial homeostasis. These principles are critical for the identification of novel therapeutic strategies for the repair of the injured heart.

Aging, cardiac diseases, and, most apparently, ischemic injury and myocardial infarction are characterized by scattered or segmental loss of myocytes by apoptotic and necrotic death.[1,4] The lack of restoration of the myocyte compartment has been cited as unequivocal proof of the postmitotic condition of the old and damaged heart. This phenomenon is actually common to other organs, including highly proliferating tissues. A decline in the number of parenchymal cells as a function of age and pathological damage occurs in the bone marrow, immune system, testis, retinal epithelium, cochlea, liver, brain, and peripheral nervous system. Similarly, infarcts of the intestine, brain, skin, kidney, and liver evolve in a manner identical to the heart.[5] Additionally, as in the heart, other organs respond to stress by an increase in cell-replicative growth. However, this reaction is often unsuccessful and does not reestablish tissue homeostasis.[6] Cell death may exceed cell division, and cell regeneration may occur preferentially in the unaffected region of all organs, precluding effective repair.

The behavior of the heart, therefore, fits into a common model of organ growth. During development and physiological turnover of a tissue, cells divide for a defined number of rounds, ultimately reaching terminal differentiation. The process of commitment of primitive cells into more specialized units involves an increased restriction in their proliferative potential that culminates in cell cycle withdrawal. A precise coordination between cells entering a quiescent nondividing state and cells reaching terminal differentiation and functional competence is required to ensure proper performance of any organ, including the heart. Moreover, maintenance of cell cycle arrest in fully mature cells is crucial for tissue architecture and function. The preservation of the differentiated state of myocytes must be tightly regulated. In fact, the heart would fail if most of its parenchymal cells were involved not in contractile activity but in cell replication. Mitotic division is restricted to small amplifying myocytes that possess a minimal amount of myofibrils distributed at the periphery of the cell in the subsarcolemmal region (Fig. 71–2). This observation illustrates the new paradigm.

The old paradigm is strongly engrained among cardiologists and cardiovascular scientists who accept the principles that the heart can survive and exert its pump function throughout life with the same cells present at birth.[3] Because of this misconception, research in the past 50 years has focused on understanding the molecular control of myocyte hypertrophy,[7] with acrimonious objections to information supporting the replicative capacity of the adult heart.[8] The demonstration of myocyte cytokinesis during development was considered a biological curiosity rather than a relevant component of the physiological turnover of the normal heart. Concurrently, the identification of myocyte division in the overloaded ventricle was not recognized as

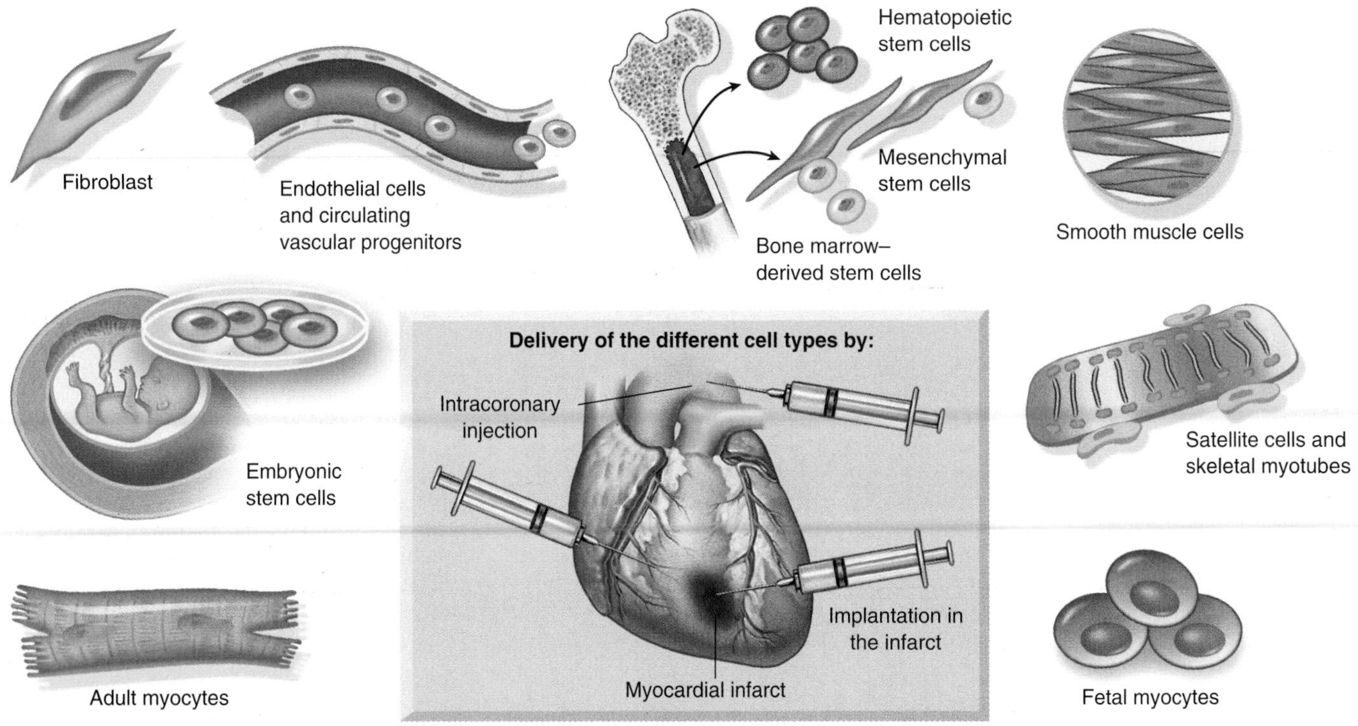

FIGURE 71–1 Myocardial repair. A variety of cell types from different origins have been employed in an attempt to repair and improve the function of the infarcted heart. The various cell populations used for this purpose are depicted here.

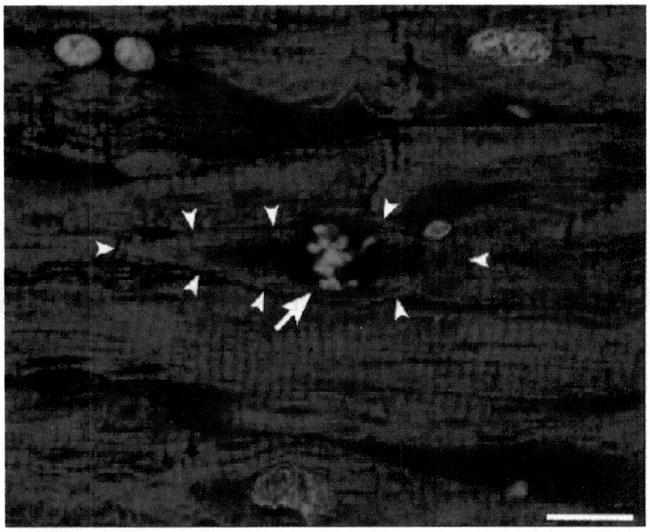

FIGURE 71–2 Dividing myocyte. In a small myocyte (alpha-sarcomeric actin = red), there is a nucleus in mitosis (propidium iodide [PI] = green; arrow) characterized by a cluster of metaphase chromosomes. The mitotic myocyte shows myofibrillar structures located at the periphery of the cell (arrowheads). This section derives from the heart of a patient affected by end-stage ischemic myopathy. Confocal microscopy, bar = 10 μm.

an important growth mechanism dramatically affecting the remodeling of the pathological heart. According to the established view, new cells cannot replace dead myocytes. This belief has delayed the understanding of the cellular response of the diseased heart. The answer to this conundrum has been provided by a series of findings that urge a reinterpretation of the biology of the heart, perennially viewed as a postmitotic organ.[3]

Identification of Myocyte Proliferation in the Damaged Heart

Cardiac regeneration by myocyte multiplication cannot be restricted to the detection of karyokinesis and cytokinesis, which are rapid events difficult to capture. The analysis of duplicating cells includes identification of cells and their nuclei in various phases of the cell cycle. Probes are available, and an accurate evaluation of the number of cycling myocytes can be obtained. This involves the identification of myocytes that express cyclins and cyclin-dependent kinases, replicate DNA, traverse the cell cycle, and divide. These approaches have provided information on the dynamic state of cell regeneration in the normal and pathological heart.[9,10] (For an extended discussion and pictorial representation of the cell cycle, see Chap. 69.)

The presence of myofibrils in cycling myocytes indicates that a subpopulation of partially differentiated parenchymal cells can divide in the adult organ. The basic cell cycle machinery of myocytes has its core in the cyclins and cyclin-dependent kinases. Key regulators of G_1 progression are the group of D cyclins that are synthesized during the G_0-G_1 transition. However, kinase activity becomes apparent only in mid-G_1. The increase in cyclin D_2 and cyclin D_2-associated kinase in myocytes demonstrates that these cells have left the quiescent state and have reentered the cell cycle.[11] The enhanced expression of cyclin A and cdk2 activity is followed by activation of cyclin B and cdc2, which promote the progression of myocytes in S phase and G_2-M before cytokinesis.[11]

Markers capable of recognizing different phases of the cell cycle or present during the entire cell cycle have been identified. DNA synthesis can be detected by modified nucleotides, including bromodeoxyuridine (BrdU). Immunofluorescence can visualize the incorporation of BrdU in the DNA; this technique has been used to assess cell proliferation (Fig.

71-3). This methodology visualizes cells undergoing DNA synthesis. Therefore, cells in S phase or in which DNA damage is repaired show BrdU labeling.[12] An obvious limitation of this procedure is that the chances that a cycling cell will incorporate the nucleotide are restricted to the period of exposure to the marker. Additionally, cells at the G_1-S boundary are not labeled and the G_1 phase may be particularly long, resulting in an underestimation of the actual number of cycling cells.

Expression of the proliferating cell nuclear antigen (PCNA) is associated with cell proliferation, being low in quiescent cells and high in cycling cells.[13] An increase in PCNA is observed in late G_1, and a further increase occurs in S phase. G_2-M cells show a markedly reduced level of PCNA immunofluorescence. PCNA acts as a sliding clamp that allows DNA polymerase δ and ε to move quickly along the DNA while remaining tightly bound.[13] Moreover, PCNA is an integral component of DNA repair,[13] limiting its utilization as a marker of cell proliferation in many pathological conditions where cell multiplication is coupled with cell death and DNA damage. In the myocardium, increased PCNA transcription has been linked to DNA synthesis, DNA repair, and myocyte proliferation. In the presence of ventricular failure following acute myocardial infarction or in conditions of global ischemia, PCNA and histone-H_3 messenger RNA levels are upregulated in myocytes, and the distribution of PCNA protein in the cells correlates closely with the regional variations in diastolic wall stress in the injured ventricle. PCNA labeling of myocytes occurs in the human heart affected by terminal failure in combination with the appearance of myocyte nuclear and cell division.[14]

Ki67 is a nuclear protein present only in proliferating cells (see Fig. 71-3). This antigen is expressed during late G_1, S, G_2, prophase, and metaphase, declining progressively in anaphase and telophase.[15] Of relevance, Ki67 is absent in quiescent cells and is not involved in DNA repair. The function of this protein is largely unknown. The localization of Ki67 in the outer dense compartment of the nucleolus suggests a participation in ribosome biogenesis, required only when a rapid production of these organelles is necessary, such as during the cell cycle. Additionally, the C-terminal domain of Ki67 has the ability to bind DNA sequences rich in adenine and thymine, and may work as a transcription factor. A certain similarity with the consensus sequences of p53, an inhibitor of the cell cycle, and the stretches of nucleotides that Ki67 binds in vitro has been reported.[16] These findings have favored intriguing speculations concerning the potential opposite role that these two proteins may play in the cell cycle. In contrast to markers of S phase, Ki67 protein expression reflects a physiological state of the cell and is closely coupled with cell proliferation. The evaluation of Ki67 labeling of nuclei offers a sensitive approach for the analysis of the degree of cell multiplication. This nuclear protein recognizes cells in all the active phases of the cell cycle. Additionally, there is not a single example of a Ki67-positive cell that cannot divide.[15]

More recently, Cdc6 and the minichromosome maintenance (MCM) family of proteins have been employed as novel markers of cell multiplication (see Fig. 71-3). Eukaryotic cells possess control mechanisms to restrict DNA replication to one in the entire cell cycle. At the level of DNA, the origin recognition complex (ORC) determines where replication can initiate, and this allows Cdc6 to recruit MCM proteins. At this stage, the DNA is licensed to replicate.[17] During M-G_1 transition, a multiprotein complex is assembled at the ORC and awaits a signal to initiate DNA synthesis. As cells progress from the G_1 to S, this complex is activated. In late S phase, the dissociation of Cdc6 and MCM from chromatin ensures that DNA is replicated only once during a single division cycle. Despite the restriction of DNA replication to S phase, changes in the proteins associated with ORC occur throughout the cell cycle. Thus, Cdc6 and MCM recognize cells throughout G_1, S, and late mitosis, including anaphase and telophase.[17] Both Cdc6 and MCM are downregulated in terminally differentiated and quiescent cells.

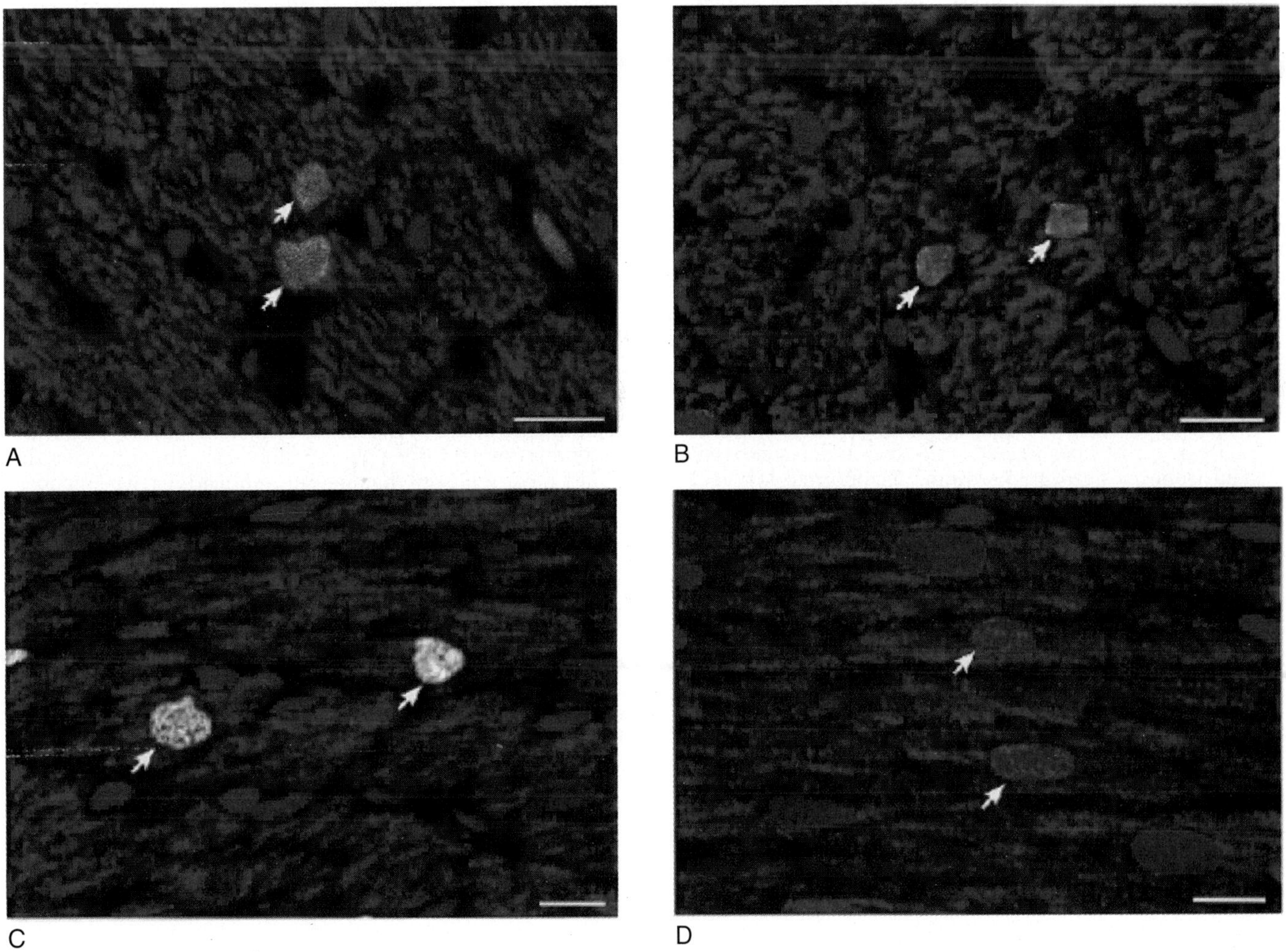

FIGURE 71–3 Markers of replicating myocytes. In each panel, two myocyte nuclei are positive for BrdU (**A,** yellow), Ki67 (**B,** green), MCM5 (**C,** white), and Cdc6 (**D,** magenta). Arrows point to cycling myocytes. Myocyte cytoplasm is recognized by alpha-sarcomeric actin (red) and nuclei by propidium iodide (blue). These sections derive from the ventricle of a Fischer rat. Confocal microscopy, bar = 10 μm.

On the basis of the earlier discussion, identification and quantification of the replicating pool in a given tissue or cell population require utilization of specific markers able to recognize molecules expressed only during the cell cycle and absent during quiescence. Colabeling with antibodies against contractile proteins recognizes dividing myocytes by high-resolution confocal microscopy.[9,10] Mitosis, the most impressive event within the cell cycle, is characterized by the formation of the mitotic spindle, with the bipolar shooting out of chromosomes, and the identification of the actomyosin contractile ring, which constricts and pinches off the membrane to form two daughter cells. These findings have shown unequivocally that adult cardiac myocytes undergo karyokinesis and cytokinesis. All stages of mitosis have been identified in myocytes and, thereby, mitotic indices have been computed by examining large areas of myocardium by confocal microscopy.

Magnitude of Myocyte Regeneration in the Damaged Heart

Evaluation of a myocyte mitotic index provides an important gauge of the rapidity and intensity of the response of the growth reserve of the heart to stressful conditions. The interpretation of the myocyte mitotic index is influenced by variables that are difficult to predict. For example, the time required for the completion of karyokinesis and cytokinesis of myocytes in vivo is unknown. Similarly, whether aging, ventricular loading, or disease states influence the duration of this nuclear or cellular event remains to be established. These determinants could attenuate or enhance myocardial growth and play a critical role in the adaptation of the heart to acute and chronic changes in wall stress. On this basis, the degree of myocyte division has been evaluated separately in acute and chronic heart failure of ischemic origin.

A myocyte mitotic index has been measured in myocyte nuclei of control and acutely infarcted human hearts by confocal microscopy. A value of $11/10^6$ myocytes was determined in control intact left ventricles, while a 47-fold higher value of $520/10^6$ myocytes was detected in the infarcted ventricles ($775/10^6$ in the border zone and $264/10^6$ in the remote myocardium). The expression of Ki67 was also measured. In comparison with $489/10^6$ myocytes in normal hearts, myocardial infarcts resulted in an 84-fold, $40{,}997/10^6$, and 28-fold, $13{,}799/10^6$, increase in the number of myocyte nuclei labeled by Ki67 in the region bordering and remote from infarction, respectively. Thus, the number of Ki67-positive myocyte nuclei was three times higher in the region adjacent to than distant from the dead myocardium.[9] The normal left ventricle contains 5.5×10^9 myocytes, and this value decreases to 3.8×10^9 myocytes after a 30 percent infarct. The fraction of mitotic myocytes implies that 60,500 myocytes are in mitosis in the normal left ventricle and 1,976,000 in the infarcted left ventricle. Since mitosis lasts approximately 30 minutes, a 30 percent infarct would be replaced in less than 3 weeks if this level of myocyte regeneration persisted with time.[9]

The degree of cell division detected acutely after infarction suggests that, in the absence of a change in the rate of cell regeneration, 17×10^9 myocytes would be formed over a period of 6 months. Essentially, all left ventricular myocytes would be replaced three times in half a year. A relationship exists between the number of myocyte nuclei expressing Ki67 and the number of myocyte nuclei in mitoses. The number of cycling myocytes measured by Ki67 labeling is 50 times as high as the number of mitotic myocytes. On the assumption that mitosis is completed in 30 minutes, the duration of the myocyte cell cycle in vivo should be approximately 25 hours. When MCM5 labeling of myocyte nuclei and the myocyte mitotic index are considered (our unpublished results), the computed length of the cell cycle is nearly 45 hours. This is because Ki67 is expressed only late in G_1 and MCM5 is expressed during the entire G_1 phase.[15,17]

A mitotic index of $150/10^6$ myocytes has been found in the left ventricle of postinfarcted hearts in end-stage cardiac failure.[18] In the presence of 3.8×10^9 left ventricular myocytes, a mitotic index of $150/10^6$ implies that 570,000 cells are in mitosis and 4.9×10^9 myocytes are formed in 6 months. Similar results have been obtained in patients with end-stage dilated cardiomyopathy.[18] Therefore, myocyte regeneration is attenuated in chronically decompensated hearts, suggesting that the duration of the disease and the persistence of a high loading state lead to a progressive utilization of the proliferative cell reserve of the myocardium, and this phenomenon may promote terminal failure.

In spite of these various approaches that provide relevant indices of myocyte multiplication, by definition, myocyte proliferation corresponds to an absolute increase in the number of parenchymal cells in the ventricle or the heart. However, myocyte loss, an event common to aging and cardiac diseases, complicates the estimation of the real number of newly formed myocytes. Myocyte loss results in an underestimation of myocyte hyperplasia, and myocyte hyperplasia leads to an underestimation of the magnitude of myocyte death in the heart. Thus, myocyte proliferation may be obscured by myocyte loss, and the measurement of cell number may not give unequivocal evidence of cell regeneration. This consideration pertains to several forms of heart failure, particularly of ischemic origin. Thus, the quantitative estimation of the actual number of newly generated myocytes presents a difficult challenge whether it concerns physiological or pathological conditions of the adult heart.[19]

Quantitative measurements of myocyte proliferation in the overloaded heart in animal models have documented increases in the number of myocytes that varied from 20 to 45 percent.[4] These values are significantly lower than those obtained in the decompensated human heart in which myocyte number is more than doubled in conditions of extreme hypertrophy with a heart weight of nearly 2 pounds.[19] In human hearts weighing more than 500 gm, myocyte proliferation has been identified as the prevailing mechanism of increased muscle mass.[19] Because of the contribution of myocyte death in heart failure, these levels of cell regeneration can be interpreted only as minimal indices of the actual magnitude of myocyte proliferation in the pathological heart. The remarkable degrees of myocyte reconstitution in the diseased heart emphasize the importance of defining the origin of the newly formed myocytes. This information is critical for the potentiation of a cellular process that could have relevant therapeutic implications for "mending the broken heart." Myocardial regeneration is the most promising form of remedy for the damaged failing heart.

The challenging results discussed earlier indicate that the old paradigm concerning the growth property of adult myocytes should be changed to the new paradigm that recognizes that myocytes can undergo cellular hypertrophy and cell division. This new view raises questions about the factors conditioning distinct growth reactions of the myocyte compartment. The critical issue is myocyte replication since myocyte hypertrophy can be interpreted as a terminally differentiated cell that has exercised the ability only to expand the myofibrillar and nonmyofibrillar components of the cytoplasm. Conversely, several feasible mechanisms of myocyte regeneration can be proposed, as follows:

1. The adult heart contains a subpopulation of partially differentiated myocytes, which can engage in a limited number of doublings before they acquire a mitotic block.
2. Resident primitive cells cluster in specific regions of the heart and, following activation, migrate to sites of cell turnover, where they replicate and differentiate, or

they undergo proliferation and differentiation.

translocate to the proximity of areas of damage, where they undergo proliferation and differentiation.

3. Circulating progenitor cells mobilized from the bone marrow might reach the myocardium through the systemic circulation and, after homing, are conditioned by the local microenvironment to commit themselves to cardiac cell lineages, replacing myocytes and vascular structures (Fig. 71–4).
4. These three pathways could conceivably operate in combination.

Recent observations favor the possibility that primitive cells reside in the heart and possess the ability to differentiate and generate myocytes and coronary vessels.[1,2,20,21] However, this is still an issue of great controversy and intense study. The available data do not allow an indisputable answer to this important question.

Attenuation of Myocyte Replication

The mechanisms that cause the progressive decrease in myocyte proliferation in the diseased heart are unknown but point to a critical reduction in telomeric length possibly mediated by a chronic decline in telomerase activity. During the S phase of the cell cycle, the semiconservative model of DNA replication encounters an intrinsic obstacle consisting of the inability of conventional DNA polymerase to complete the synthesis of the lagging strand of the replication fork of the DNA double helix. This end-replication problem would cause progressive loss of genetic material and DNA shortening.[22] In eukaryotic cells a specialized DNA polymerase and protective caps called *telomeres* preserve the integrity of chromosomes. Telomeres are chromatin structures bound to an array of proteins localized at the ends of chromosomes. Telomerase is a ribonucleoprotein that acts as a reverse transcriptase extending the 3′ chromosomal ends by using its own RNA as a template.[22] Synthesis of telomeric repeats by telomerase prevents loss of DNA and allows complete duplication of DNA (Fig. 71–5).

Telomerase activity is a property of dividing cells. In germ cells, this protein ensures telomere length and unlimited proliferative potential. Somatic cells, with stem cell–like characteristics such as hematopoietic and basal epithelial cells, are telomerase competent.[23] Telomerase does not operate in somatic replicating cells. The telomeric DNA, which is lost in each cell cycle, exceeds that synthesized.[24] However, telomeres are essential for chromosomal stability and, thereby, cell viability.[22,24] Telomere shortening coupled with cell division in the absence of telomerase activity is one of the major causes of telomere dysfunction in human cells.[24] Telomerase activity, however, does not necessarily prevent telomere erosion, which is also influenced by the telomeric proteins TRF1 and TRF2. Loss of these proteins leads to telomere instability, which is as critical as telomeric shortening in determining the destiny of a cell.[25] Telomere erosion to a critically short length results in end-to-end fusions or chromatin anaphase bridges and triggers cell arrest and/or apoptosis. This phenomenon can occur in cardiomyocytes (see Fig. 71–5). Average telomeric length varies between 9 and 10 kilobase pairs[26] in both dogs and humans,[27] and is approximately 30 to 40 kilobase pairs in mice, and undetermined as yet in rats.[24]

The proliferative history of a cell is written on telomeres: telomere erosion tells us the number of past divisions experienced by a somatic cell and, most important, its residual proliferative potential. However, average telomeric length provides only an approximate indication of the actual length of individual telomeres. This is because loss of DNA and telomeric shortening do not affect all telomeres homogeneously. Shortening preferentially occurs in a fraction of telomeres, and the shortest telomere present in a cell is critical for cell viability and chromosome integrity.[24] The identification in myocytes of specific chromosomes with shortest telomeres may clarify issues related to myocyte growth and death; the fate of a myocyte may be determined by its shortest telomere. Telomeric shortening has been detected in a subpopulation of myocytes in the old rat heart affected by chronic cardiac failure[28] in combination with an age-dependent decrease in telomerase activity.[29] Conversely, this enzyme activity is increased in acute cardiac failure in dogs preserving telomeric length in myocytes.[27]

Thus, cardiomyocyte hypertrophy and regeneration constitute the growth reserve mechanisms of the heart during aging and cardiac diseases. Cellular growth, however, is controlled by telomeric length and telomerase activity. The relative impact of these factors on myocyte growth can be better characterized when telomerase function is repressed. Knockout mice in which the RNA component of telomerase has been deleted have a severe attenuation in myocyte regeneration.[30] Because of the complete lack of telomerase activity, these mice exhibit shortening of telomeres at a rate of 3 to 5 kilobase pairs per cell cycle. This mutation severely affects cell death and markedly enhances cardiomyocyte renewal. The expression of the tumor suppressor p53 with activation of myocyte apoptosis becomes apparent when the mean length of telomeres is reduced by 55 to 65 percent to nearly 14 kilobase pairs. These phenomena result in pathological cardiac remodeling and ventricular decompensation at 6 to 8 months after birth, underlining the importance of the absence

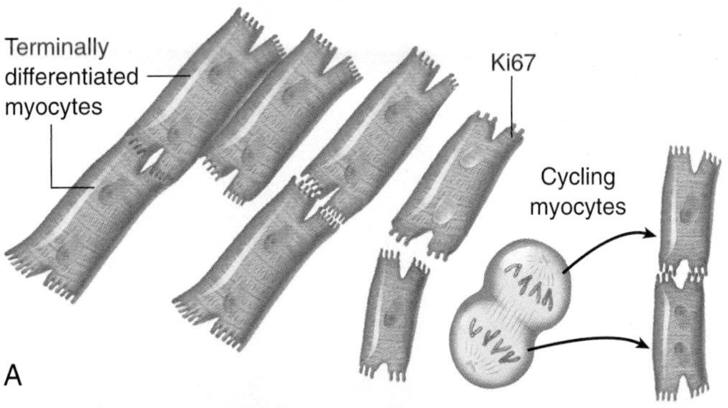

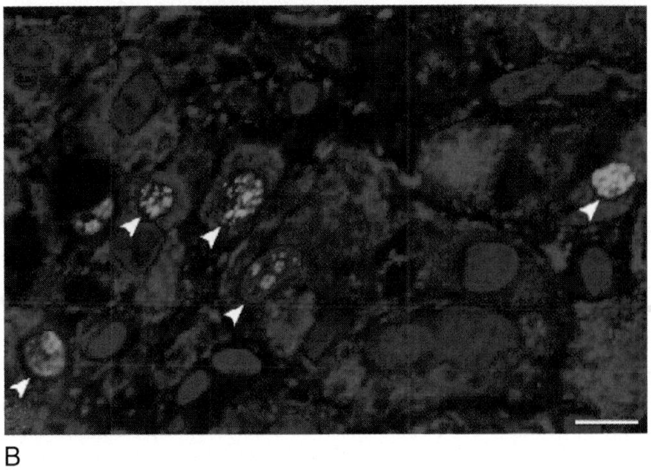

FIGURE 71–4 Mechanisms of myocardial regeneration. Several potential mechanisms of myocardial reconstitution are shown in schematic forms in **A, C,** and **E** and by confocal microscopy of tissue sections in **B, D,** and **F**. **A** schematically illustrates terminally differentiated myocytes and dividing or cycling myocytes. **B** shows a group of small developing myocytes expressing the cell cycle marker, Ki67 (green, arrowheads) in their nuclei. The myocyte cytoplasm is recognized by alpha-sarcomeric actin (red) and nuclei by propidium iodide (PI) (blue). This image corresponds to a human heart in end-stage failure. Confocal microscopy, bar = 10 μm. *Continued*

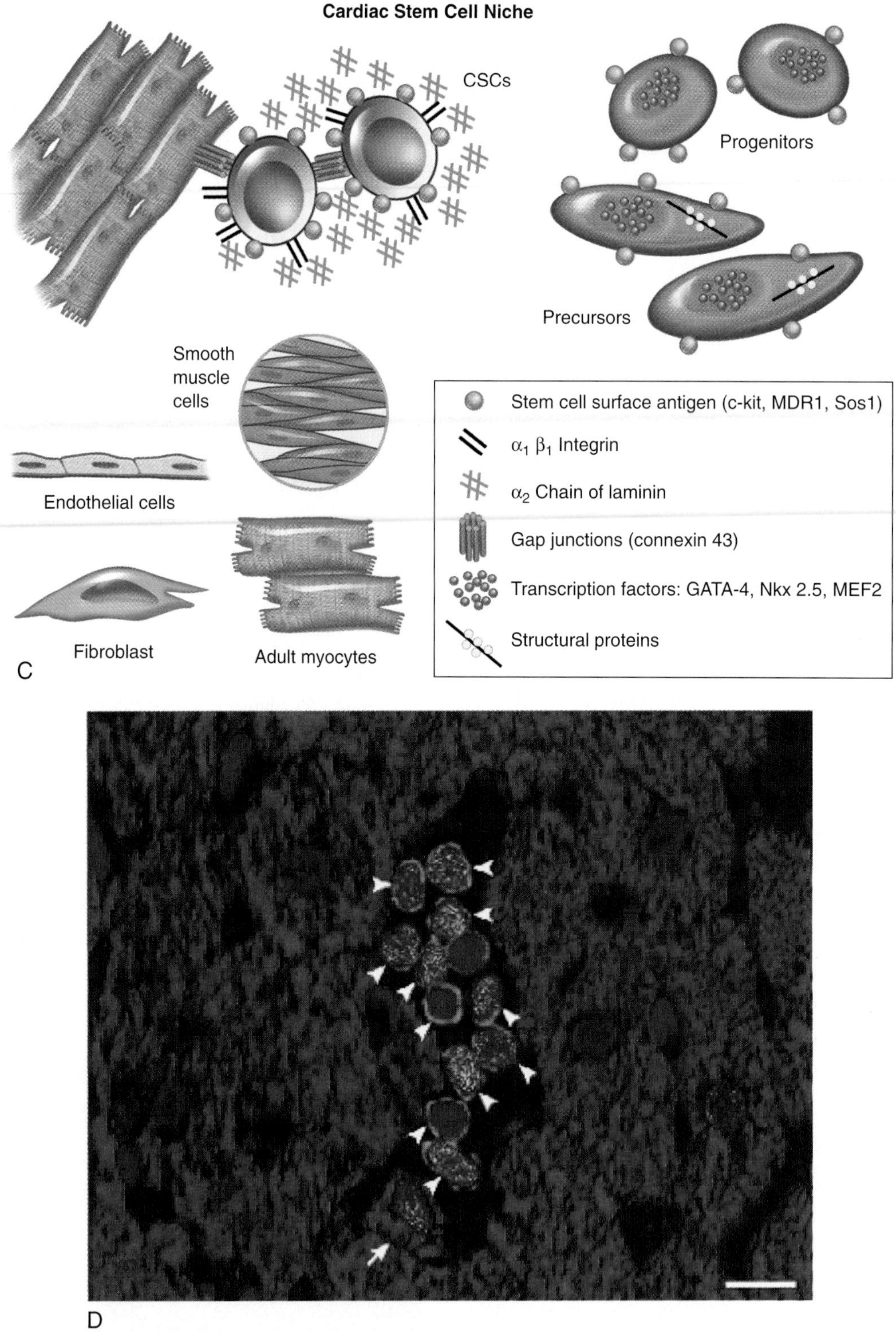

FIGURE 71–4, cont'd **C** illustrates schematically a cardiac stem cell (CSC) niche containing primitive cells, progenitors, and precursors. Primitive cells express stem cell surface antigens and integrin receptors. Progenitors are similar to primitive cells but also express cardiac or myocyte transcription factors. Precursor cells are similar to primitive and progenitor cells but contain in their cytoplasm structural proteins such as alpha-sarcomeric actin and cardiac myosin heavy chain. These cells lose the surface antigens and progressively become fully differentiated myocytes. A similar pattern of growth occurs in endothelial cells, smooth muscle cells, and fibroblasts. **D** demonstrates some of the aspects of cell differentiation illustrated in C. A cluster of primitive cells expressing the stem cell surface antigen c-kit (green) is documented within the ventricular myocardium. Nine (arrowheads) of the 12 c-kit positive cells express GATA-4 (white) in their nuclei. The nucleus of a small maturing myocyte is positive for GATA-4 (arrow). The myocyte cytoplasm is recognized by alpha-sarcomeric actin (red) and nuclei by PI (blue). This section corresponds to the ventricle of a Fischer rat. Confocal microscopy, bar = 10 μm.

of myocyte division in the development of heart failure.[30] This observation demonstrates the pivotal role of myocyte regeneration in the preservation of the performance of the heart under physiological conditions. Any imposition of an abnormal load might potentiate this impaired adaptation of the "nonmitotic heart" and favor precocious cardiac failure and death of the organism.

In summary, efforts have been made in the past 10 years to identify the mechanisms of myocyte growth in the pathological heart. Myocyte hypertrophy and proliferation in

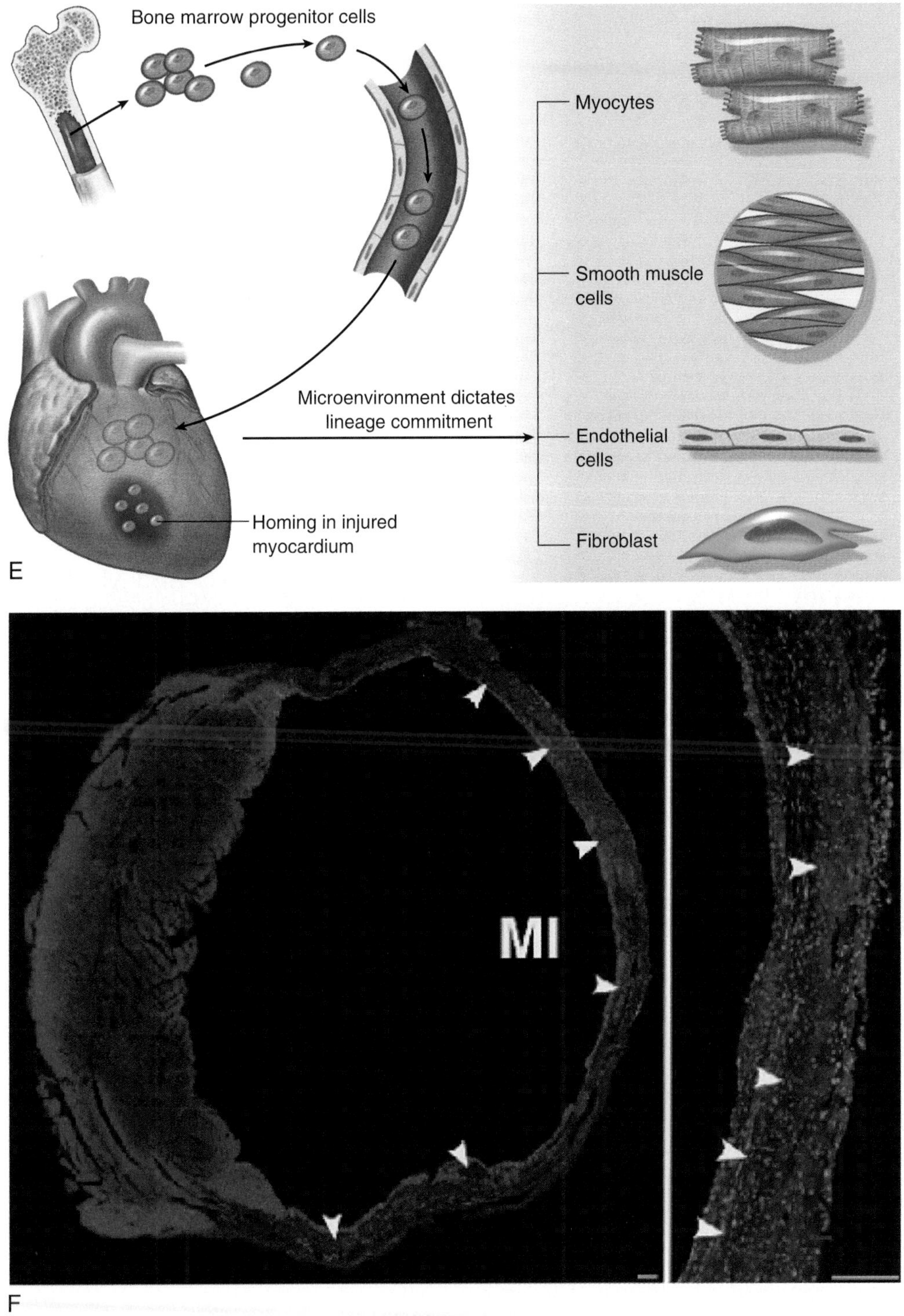

FIGURE 71–4, cont'd **E** presents in a schematic form the repair of infarcted myocardium by circulating and bone marrow–mobilized progenitor cells. **F** demonstrates the actual regeneration of infarcted myocardium 27 days after the increase in circulating progenitor cells mediated by the systemic administration of cytokines in mice. The regenerating band indicated by arrowheads in the large transverse section is shown at higher magnification in the adjacent panel. New myocytes are identified by the red fluorescence of cardiac myosin. Green-yellow fluorescence reflects PI labeling of nuclei. Confocal microscopy, bar = 200 μm. (**A** to **F**, From Orlic D, Kajstura J, Chimenti S, et al: Mobilized bone marrow cells repair the infarcted heart, improving function and survival. Proc Natl Acad Sci U S A 98:10344-10349, 2001.)

combination with myocyte death, apoptotic and necrotic in nature, constitute the fundamental elements of cardiac remodeling. Improvement in methodology enabled experiments that have disproved the dogma introduced more than 60 years ago that all myocytes are terminally differentiated. There is a group of myocytes that expresses the molecular components required for entry into the cell cycle and the regulation of their progression through S, G_2, karyokinesis, and cytokinesis. The recognition that myocyte hypertrophy and regeneration, and myocyte necrosis and apoptosis, occur in the diseased heart has significantly enhanced our understanding of the plasticity of the myocardium and the critical role played by cell death and cell division in the complex transition from cardiac hypertrophy to heart failure.

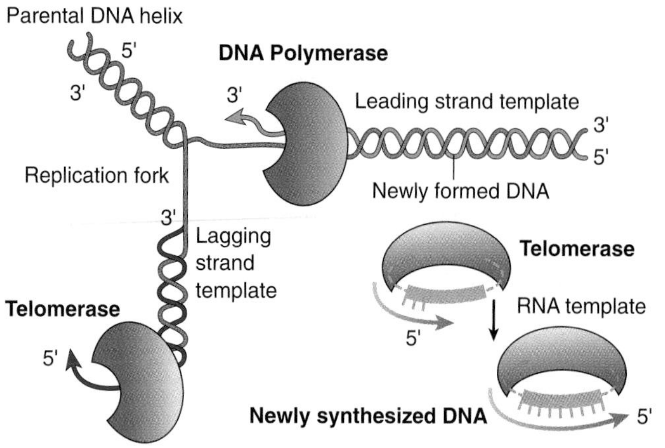

FIGURE 71–5 The end-replication problem. During cell division, conventional DNA polymerase cannot complete the synthesis of the lagging strand of the replication fork of the DNA double helix. This end-replication problem would cause progressive shortening of the DNA. However, telomerase, which is a reverse transcriptase, extends the 3′ chromosomal ends using its own RNA as a template. Synthesis of telomeric repeats by telomerase protects from loss of nucleic acid, allowing complete replication of DNA.

Myocardial Repair

Repair of damaged tissues and organs implies two distinct but interconnected processes: dead cells must be replaced by newly generated ones, and the newborn cells have to differentiate and become organized in a complex pattern that, ideally, restores the original structure of the injured tissue. However, this dual process usually occurs only during physiological cell turnover, in the absence of damage. For example, the bone marrow replenishes the blood with terminally differentiated cells, and the cells nested in the bulge of the hair follicle replace dead keratinocytes in the epidermis. Conversely, ischemic injury results in scar formation in all tissues, whether parenchymal cells are highly proliferating, slow cycling, or terminally differentiated. In the skin, which is an organ characterized by elevated levels of cell proliferation, wound healing leads to substitution of the damaged area with fibrotic tissue. The scarred portion of the skin does not possess the properties of the unaffected skin in terms of cellular composition, architecture, and biochemical and physical function. It is unknown why lesions of various etiologies cannot be repaired with complete *restitutio ad integrum*. Whether this depends on the accumulation of transforming growth factor-beta–like molecules (chalones) with massive inhibition of cell proliferation, chemorepellents of migrating cells (which could initiate the actual reconstitution of the damaged region), or inflammatory cytokines promoting leukocytes and fibroblast infiltration has not been identified. The need to overcome this biological obstacle of high clinical importance has stimulated the search for novel approaches to the replacement of dead cells with new functionally competent cells.

Several interventions have been used in the attempt to induce regeneration of damaged ventricular myocardium after infarction or cryoinjury in animal models. These therapeutic strategies have used a variety of cell types, including fetal cardiomyocytes and tissues, skeletal myoblasts, embryo-derived endothelial cells, bone marrow–derived immature myocytes, fibroblasts, smooth muscle cells, and bone marrow c-kit positive and negative primitive cells.[1,2,5,31,32] Promising results have been obtained with several of these cell types. Positive effects, including the successful survival of the implanted cells that occasionally integrated structurally and functionally with the host myocardium, have been reported. At times an improvement in cardiac performance has been found. Currently, however, there is no consensus but rather a vigorous debate on the most promising form of cellular therapy for myocardial injury.

Several problems confound the interpretation of attempts to ameliorate cardiac anatomy, function, or loading conditions with interventions involving fibroblasts, smooth muscle cells, and the other cell types indicated earlier. With the exception of bone marrow cells (BMCs) and neonatal myocytes, which generate cardiomyocytes and vascular structures,[33-35] it remains an open question how cell populations with no or minimal angiogenic properties furnish novel therapeutic tools of the decompensated heart of ischemic and nonischemic origin. Most important, the question concerning the reconstitution of scarred tissue into contracting myocardium has been addressed only peripherally. The ultimate form of cell therapy has to include an approach that can interfere and substitute acutely dead myocardium and areas of nonmechanically active scarred postischemic myocardium. Some specific therapeutic strategies are discussed in some detail because of their popularity and recent application to humans.[36-42] Questions are also raised in terms of the feasibility of these initial clinical trials in view of the data available from animal work.

Skeletal Myoblasts and Myocardial Repair

The first attempt to enwrap infarcted myocardium with a patch of skeletal muscle in humans was performed in the 1930s. Fifty years passed before large sheets of skeletal muscle tissue were positioned on the epicardial surface of the ischemic area and stimulated by a pacemaker. This surgical procedure, known as *dynamic cardiomyoplasty*, has prompted investigators to experimentally use individual myogenic cells instead of whole pieces of tissue. The new approach has been called *cellular cardiomyoplasty*. Isolated skeletal myoblasts or satellite cells have been directly injected into the ischemic zone or delivered through the coronary circulation.[43-46] Myogenic cells were obtained from the musculature of the limbs or abdomen of animals, which were subsequently exposed to ligation of the main left coronary artery or cryoinjury. The myogenic cells expanded in vitro were then injected in the infarcted or damaged portion of the ventricle to restore contractile function (Fig. 71–6). The autologous origin of the cells to be implanted constituted an obvious advantage compared with approaches of cardiac repair. The need for immunosuppressive therapy and the risk of immune rejection were circumvented. Moreover, skeletal myoblasts resist ischemia better than cardiomyocytes,[42] enhancing their survival in a region of the ventricle supplied by an occluded vessel. For these reasons, clinical trials of skeletal myoblast implantation have begun in patients with acute myocardial infarction injection of skeletal myoblasts during surgical revascularization.[42] Thus, two forms of treatment are applied simultaneously.

This intervention usually enhances cardiac function. However, it is difficult to establish whether the implanted cells constitute an active graft, which dynamically contributes to myocardial contractility, or a passive graft, which reduces negative remodeling by decreasing the stiffness of the scarred portion of the wall. Findings from different groups of investigators reflect these two possibilities. Hagège and collaborators report an improvement of systolic function in humans,[42] whereas Taylor and colleagues observe an amelioration of diastolic performance in animals.[45] Engraftment of other cell types, such as fibroblasts and embryonic cardiomyocytes, also improved diastolic function,[31,32] independent of their different origins. The elastic properties of the implanted myoblasts could, therefore, account for much of the improvement in ventricular hemodynamics. The lack of integration of skeletal myoblasts with surrounding viable

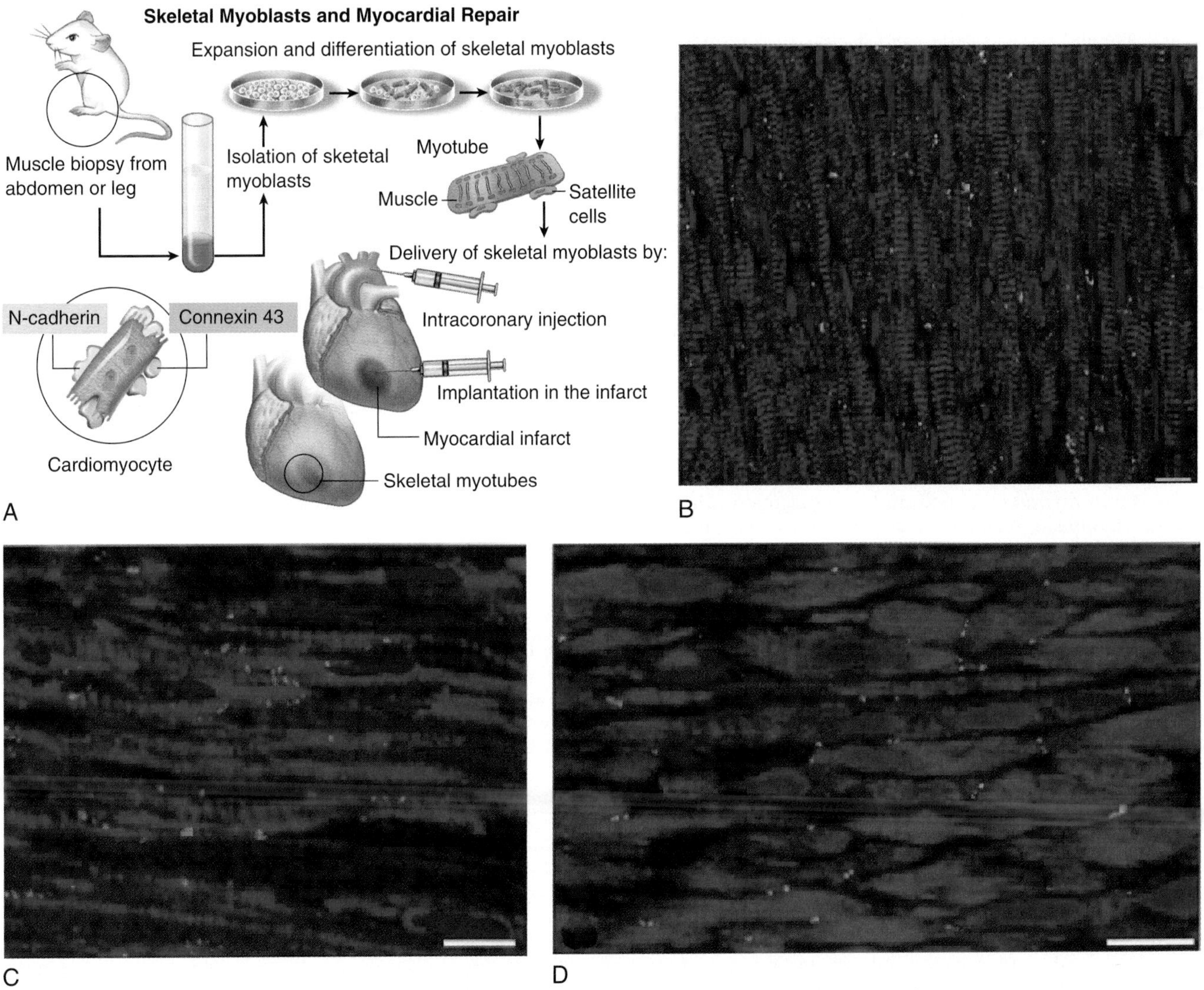

FIGURE 71–6 Skeletal myoblasts and myocardial injury. Schematic illustration of the different steps implicated in the preparation of skeletal myoblasts prior to injection **(A)**. The consequences of this form of intervention are also shown. Two critical proteins, connexin 43 and N-cadherin, are not expressed in implanted myoblasts. This deficiency does not allow electrical and mechanical coupling between injected skeletal myoblasts and between skeletal myoblasts and surrounding cardiomyocytes. **B** to **D,** Distribution of connexin 43 (green) is shown in adult mouse heart **(B)** and in regenerating tissue after infarction (**C,** green). Similarly, myocytes in the reconstituting myocardium possess N-cadherin (**D,** green). The myocyte cytoplasm is recognized by cardiac myosin antibody labeling (red) and nuclei are stained by propidium iodide (blue). Confocal microscopy, bar = 10 μm. (**C,** From Orlic D, Kajstura J, Chimenti S, et al: Mobilized bone marrow cells repair the infarcted heart, improving function and survival. Proc Natl Acad Sci U S A 98:10344-10349, 2001.)

tissue supports the likelihood of a passive graft. The absence of functional interaction between the graft and the spared myocardium represents a serious concern and limitation in the use of skeletal myoblasts for the repair of a dead region of the heart. Analysis of the graft-host organ interface has failed to provide evidence of mechanical or electrical coupling between skeletal myoblasts and resident cardiac myocytes. The microenvironment of the heart has apparently not permitted the desired effect of changing the biology of skeletal muscle cells into cardiomyocytes.

To appreciate the inherent problems with the therapeutic efficacy of skeletal myoblasts, a few comments on the role of the plasma membrane of cardiomyocytes in myocardial contractility may be helpful. Nexuses and fasciae adherentes of the intercalated discs constitute the intercellular junctions responsible, respectively, for electrical and mechanical coupling of myocytes (see Fig. 71–6). Nexuses or gap junctions are composed of clusters of intercellular channels at the interface of the cells.[47] By regulating the direct exchange of ions and small molecules between cells, these channels participate in various cellular processes, including differentiation, development, metabolic homeostasis, and electrical connection.[48] The connexins, a protein family with 15 distinct isoforms, form gap junctions. The rodent heart expresses at least three connexin proteins. Connexin 43 is the most abundant and localizes in both atrial and ventricular myocardium but not in pacemaker cells and the conduction system.[48] The fascia adherens or intermediate junction is a specialized region that provides strong cell-to-cell adhesion mediated by the cadherin/catenin complex through linkage to the actin cytoskeleton. This structure constitutes the site of attachment of myofibrils and aids the transmission of contraction across the plasma membrane of neighboring cells.[49] N-cadherin, a member of the Ca^{2+}-dependent cell-to-cell adhesion molecule family, is one of the distinctive components of the fascia adherens in the heart.[50] Cadherins act as adhesion-activated cell receptors.[50] The inhibition of N-cadherin causes myocytes to lose contact with adjacent cells, disrupting the organization of myofibrils. The integrity of the intercalated disc is, therefore, essential for the myocardium to function as a syncytium and to guarantee a synchronous contraction of its parenchymal cells.

Connexin 43 and N-cadherin are consistently absent in grafted skeletal muscle cells from 3 days to 3 months after surgery in both animal models and treated patients.[42] Thus, the grafts are unable to establish persistent electrical and mechanical interactions with the spared myocardium in vivo. A layer of dense, scarred tissue often separates the cardiomyocytes from the implanted skeletal muscle cells opposing the integration of these two cell populations in the infarcted heart. To evaluate whether the presence of this physical obstacle prevented the graft from making structural association with myocytes, skeletal myoblasts were injected in normal hearts. Although cardiac and skeletal muscle cells were nested together and there was a minimal amount of scarring, connexin 43 and N-cadherin did not develop in myoblasts and no direct communication was created with myocytes. Murry and collaborators[44] detected structures resembling adherens junctions and tight junctions exclusively in skeletal muscle cells. Unfortunately, in spite of an initial excitement, these structures correspond to low-resistance junctions, which commonly occur during fusion of myoblasts in myotubes in culture.[51] In vitro manipulation of skeletal myoblasts to force overexpression of connexin 43, has led to the appearance of gap junctions on the surface of cultured cells.[52] However, the efficacy of this approach remains to be shown in vivo. The absence of synchronous contraction may be one of the factors responsible for the episodes of arrhythmia in infarcted patients treated with skeletal myoblasts.[42]

Before skeletal myoblasts are employed for treatment, the cell population is expanded for 2 to 3 weeks in vitro. This necessity prevents the immediate clinical application of this form of therapy, and the delay may be critical in determining the number of surviving cells after implantation. The heart tissue shows extensive inflammation at this time, and the environment may be hostile for homing of skeletal myoblasts. Moreover, adult human myoblasts divide only 20 to 25 times before reaching senescence,[53] and the success of skeletal myoblast implantation is related to the number of donor cells. For this reason, the improvement in function in end-stage failure is delayed and detected only when large numbers of cells are administrated. A similar outcome has been found in patients with Duchenne myopathy. The need for a large quantity of cells has been attributed to acute and extensive cell death during the first week of engraftment.

During in vitro expansion and following introduction in the heart, myoblasts parallel the normal developmental process characterized by cell cycle withdrawal and myogenic differentiation with formation of myotubes.[44] The state of terminal differentiation rapidly acquired by skeletal myoblasts limits any possible proliferation of the implanted cells. The absence of cell turnover has a negative impact on the long-term efficacy of this kind of cellular cardiomyoplasty. Damaged cells within the graft cannot be replaced, impairing the mechanical and elastic properties of the graft and, ultimately, cardiac function. High-proliferative potential could be achieved with the implantation of immortalized myogenic cell lines. However, the risk of tumor formation precludes any clinical application.

Although this pioneer work with skeletal myoblasts has highlighted the need and importance of cellular therapy for ischemic heart disease, cardiac repair demands that the injured portion of the ventricular wall be replaced by tissue that has the same structural and functional properties of the lost myocardium. Complex manipulations of skeletal myoblasts have to be developed before these cells acquire the capability of reconstituting healthy functioning myocardium. The target of regenerative medicine must be the restoration of a tissue composed of parenchymal cells and vessels organized in an orderly manner, which resembles the native organ. In the cardiac microenvironment, the plasticity of skeletal muscle cells is quite limited. The only modification consists of a switch from fast-twitch muscle to slow-twitch muscle.[42] This phenotypic change is characterized by the expression of slow-twitch myosin isoforms,[44] suggesting that the cardiac milieu alters in part the developmental program of the implanted cells. However, transdifferentiation of skeletal myoblast in cardiac myocytes has never been observed. Conversely, the myocardial environment is permissive for a normal maturation of myogenic cells into skeletal myotubes.

Mesenchymal Stem Cells and Cardiac Repair

The bone marrow contains several cell types. In addition to differentiated cells, such as stroma, vascular cells, adipocytes, osteoblasts, and osteoclasts, a pool of primitive immature cells reside in the bone marrow. This class of cells has stem cell properties and is rather heterogeneous; it is composed of hematopoietic stem cells (HSCs) and mesenchymal stem cells[54] (MSCs). The bone marrow, followed by the peripheral and cord blood, constitutes the main source of MSCs in adulthood. However, MSCs or mesenchymal progenitor cells, which possess a more restricted lineage developmental potential, have been identified in tissues distant from the bone marrow. The oval cells of the liver, prostatic stem cells, metanephric mesenchymal cells, precursors of the Leydig cells in the testis, primitive osteoprogenitors, and satellite cells of the skeletal muscle have been classified as MSCs.[54] Not all studies agree that MSCs actually reside in these mesenchymal tissues. A "long-distance" traffic of MSCs may operate from the bone marrow through the blood stream.[54] Alternatively, embryonic primordia may be stored in a quiescent state in organs of mesodermal origin and participate in tissue repair in response to injury. We focus on MSCs of bone marrow origin, which have been used for cardiac repair.

Human and murine MSCs have been extensively characterized in vitro. MSCs are isolated from bone marrow aspirates and density gradient. These cells adhere quickly to the culture dish and grow as fibroblast-like cells, forming colonies that become visible 1 week after plating.[55] Following removal of HSCs and nonadherent cells, only a small percentage of the initial BMC population consists of MSCs, ranging from 0.001 to 0.01 percent. MSCs undergo a relatively few population doublings, from 4 to 20, maintaining the original normal karyotype and a constant level of telomerase activity.[54,55] Telomeric shortening does not occur in MSCs in culture. During the in vitro phase of amplification, MSCs usually do not differentiate spontaneously. However, by culturing them in distinct media containing different cytokines and growth factors, MSCs differentiate into multiple mesenchymal phenotypes, such as adipocytes, chondrocytes, and osteocytes.[54,55] The immunophenotype of MSCs has partially been defined. MSCs express adhesion receptors,[54,55] including CD29, CD44, CD71, CD90, CD106, CD120a, and CD124, and surface antigens[54] that are not present in HSCs, stromal hybridoma 2 (SH2), SH3, and SH4. These surface antigens have been identified in SH cell lines. They constitute early markers of undifferentiated MSCs and disappear with lineage commitment.[54] MSCs, however, are negative for markers of the hematopoietic lineage, including CD34 and the common leukocyte antigen CD45.[55]

This population of BMCs differentiates in cardiomyocytes in vitro. By dilution technique, clones of MSCs have been obtained.[56] Clonogenic cells have a fibroblast-like shape, but after stimulation with 5-aza-cytidine, which is a DNA demethylating agent that promotes the reactivation of gene expression, the morphology of nearly 30 percent of the cells changes from a spindle shape to a ball-like form and, with time, to a rod shape. Subsequently, the differentiating cells fuse together in a syncytium that resembles a myotube.[57] In spite of this characteristic that mimics the organization of skeletal muscle, MSC-derived cardiomyogenic cells exhibit markers of fetal cardiac myocytes.[57] The beta isoform of myosin heavy chain is expressed much more than the alpha isoform. Similarly, alpha skeletal actin predominates with respect to alpha cardiac actin. Myosin light chain-2v is also present. Specific transcription factors of the cardiac and myocyte lineage can be detected; they include GATA-4, Nkx2.5, and HAND1/2.[58] Alternative splicing forms of the *MEF2* gene are observed. From early to late passages, MEF2A and MEF2B are replaced by MEF2C and MEF2D.[57,58] The differentiation of this cardiomyogenic cell line seems to recapitulate the developmental program of gene expression during prenatal life, which is tightly regulated by the turning on and off of multiple genes. Finally, these cells express functionally competent alpha- and beta-adrenergic and muscarinic receptors on the membrane.[59] Cells beat spontaneously and synchronously in vitro, and the rate of contraction increases after exposure to isoproterenol, whereas the addition of a selective $beta_1$ blocker inhibits contractile activity.[59] The synchrony of contraction is most likely due to the formation of intercalated discs. The same phenomenon is observed when cardiomyogenic cells derived from MSCs are cocultured with neonatal myocytes.[60] Mechanical and electrical coupling between the two cell types has been observed in vitro. Intercalated discs have been identified in functionally competent myocytes by electron microscopy.

MSC-derived cardiomyogenic cells have been used for cardiac repair after experimental myocardial infarction. Four weeks after coronary artery occlusion in pigs, 100×10^6 autologous bone marrow stromal cells, which had been expanded and induced to differentiate in vitro, were injected in the infarcted region of the ventricular wall.[61] One month later, islands of cardiac-like tissue and new capillaries were found within the scarred tissue. Wall motion reappeared in the infarcted myocardium, suggesting that cell implantation led to partial reconstitution of dead myocardium that had positive consequences on the hemodynamics and anatomy of the damaged heart. Myocardial regeneration reduced cavitary volume, increased the thickness of the infarcted wall, and improved the contractile performance.[61] Similar results have been obtained in a model of ischemia reperfusion injury in pigs.[62] Two weeks after a 60-minute occlusion of the left anterior descending coronary artery, 6×10^7 labeled MSCs were directly injected in the infarcted area. By placing ultrasonic crystals within the ischemic region, the recovery of contractile activity could be followed during the entire period of observation. Systolic and diastolic function ameliorated and wall thinning was markedly reduced after 1 month. Cotransplantation of human MSCs and human fetal cardiomyocytes in infarcted pigs resulted in a greater improvement in cardiac function than with MSCs alone.[63]

Before discussing other results obtained with the injection of MSCs after infarction, it might be relevant to compare the efficacy of skeletal myoblasts and MSCs as distinct forms of therapy for the infarcted heart. In both cases, cells must be collected and expanded before utilization. The time factor can influence the engraftment of MSCs in the damaged area and how the changes in the microenvironment of the infarcted tissue interfere with cell growth and differentiation. However, MSCs possess the ability to generate myocytes and coronary vessels and, thereby, new myocardium.[61,63] MSCs should therefore have a greater therapeutic impact on cardiac repair than skeletal myoblasts. The latter does not differentiate into myocytes, and the creation of vascular structures by implantation of skeletal myoblasts remains to be demonstrated.

A number of other experiments have been performed in rats, utilizing MSC transplantation following cryoinjury of the myocardium.[64] BrdU-labeled cells were injected in the scar, which, 5 weeks later, contained muscle cells positive for troponin I, confirming their myocyte commitment. Additionally, large vascular structures and capillary profiles were detected in the area of damage.[64] The growing myocardium reduced the dimension of the scar in association with an improvement in peak systolic pressure and developed pressure of the treated infarcted rats. An alternative route of administration of MSCs has been attempted with the expectation that, if successful, the new procedure would have greater clinical relevance. Bone marrow stromal cells have been delivered directly through the coronary circulation.[65] However, MSCs differentiated into fibroblasts in the region of the scar and into cardiomyocytes in the surviving myocardium. This study emphasizes the importance of the microenvironment in guiding the developmental pathway of MSCs in vivo. These observations agree with in vitro reports of the medium-dependent specific lineage commitment engaged by MSCs.[54]

A lower degree of engraftment of MSCs has been found in the normal heart. In the study by Wang and collaborators,[66] MSCs implanted within the healthy rat ventricular myocardium were identified only at the site of injection. Conversely, in the paper by Toma and colleagues,[67] implanted cells were scattered throughout the myocardium, but they failed to accumulate in clusters. Only individual cells randomly distributed were detected up to 60 days after the intervention. Thus, in the absence of injury MSCs appear to remain in a viable partially quiescent state. In fact, they participate minimally in the physiological turnover of myocytes. In this regard, a relevant unexpected finding was that MSCs expressed connexin 43, forming gap junctions between engrafted cells and resident myocytes within the host myocardium.[66] A systemic infusion of MSCs was performed in lethally irradiated and nonconditioned adult baboons.[68] Transplantation was significantly more successful in animals exposed to irradiation. A broad distribution of MSCs was detected with a preferential engraftment in the gastrointestinal tract, kidney, lung, liver, thymus, and skin. Unfortunately, the heart was not harvested; therefore, no information is available regarding colonization of MSCs to the myocardium in nonhuman primates.

Recent work has identified a rare cell population within the MSC compartment of the bone marrow in mice.[55] These cells have been classified as multipotent adult progenitor cells (MAPCs). MAPCs can undergo more than 120 population doublings without modification of morphology or immunophenotype. Membrane antigens on MAPCs are not specific for a previously known progenitor cell. They share some characteristic with HSCs and some others with MSCs. MAPCs express low levels of Flk-1, Sca-1 and Thy-1, and higher levels of CD13 and stage-specific antigen I. In a manner similar to MSCs, MAPCs lack CD34, CD44, CD45, and the major histocompatibility complex classes I and II.[55] The surface antigen c-kit is typically present in HSCs and MSCs, although its level is lower in the latter group of stem cells.[54] A unique property of MAPCs is that c-kit is absent in this highly purified progenitor cell population. Whether this difference helps or hinders growth and commitment of MAPCs has not yet been determined.

In this regard, during embryogenesis in the blastocyst, MAPCs give rise to essentially all somatic tissues in the organism, including the myocardium. However, MAPCs only partly maintained this property following in vivo injection in the systemic circulation. The ability to differentiate into cardiac and skeletal muscle, kidney, skin, and brain tissues is lost, raising questions whether the therapeutic applications of these progenitor cells as a source of repair of several important vital organs. This limitation is particularly significant because similar results were obtained in intact and irradiated injured animals.

In summary, it is currently difficult to reach definitive conclusions concerning the use of MSCs and MAPCs for myocardial regeneration. The observations made so far require confirmation, and specific experimental protocols aiming at target organs have to be developed and tested. The actual potential of MSCs and progenitor cells in tissue reconstitution remains an open, important question.

Bone Marrow Cells and Myocardial Repair

In addition to MSCs, the bone marrow possesses a blood-forming stem cell. This is a rare cell population that corresponds to true HSCs, which are responsible for the permanent long-term reconstitution of hematopoiesis. These cells are few and their phenotype is well established.[69] HSCs are lineage negative, Sca-1-positive, c-kit-positive, and Thy1.1-low. The plasticity of HSCs defined by their ability to generate tissues different from the organ of origin has recently been challenged.[70] A major problem in tissue regeneration including the myocardium is the lack of purity of bone marrow donor cells. This heterogeneity raises questions regarding the type of BMC that actually promotes the repair of an injured portion of an organ. Moreover, the use of enriched cell preparations and the difficulty of obtaining an actually pure and uniform cell population have cast doubts on the actual plasticity of HSCs. Alternative explanations have been offered, varying from the possibility of in vivo cell fusion to models based on the notion of preexisting heterogeneity of primitive cells within the bone marrow. In the first case, the replacement of damaged tissue in the liver and intestinal epithelia in vivo has been shown to be the consequence of fusion of BMCs with the existing cells, which then reacquire primitive properties.[71-73] This sequence, however, does not seem to operate in the heart.[1] In the second case, the bone marrow is viewed as a reservoir that contains progenitor cells in an early stage of commitment to multiple cell lineages.[74] Physiological turnover or discrete areas of injury may transmit signals to these poorly differentiated cells, which migrate from the bone marrow to these sites where they become activated and substitute for the old cell or repair the damage.

In spite of uncertainty about the mechanisms of cardiac repair, the use of BMCs in the management of myocardial infarction has advantages over other approaches employed in animals and humans. As discussed, at least in part, in the previous sections, efforts have been made to restore function in the infarcted myocardium by transplanting cultured fetal myocytes or tissue, adult myocytes, skeletal myoblasts, and bone marrow–derived immature cardiomyocytes. When incorporation of the engrafted cells or tissue was successful, some improvement in ventricular performance occurred. However, these approaches failed to reconstitute healthy myocardium, integrated structurally and functionally with the spared portion of the wall. This limitation was particularly evident with skeletal myoblasts. Moreover, the formation of vessels in the implants remained an unresolved problem. With the exception of skeletal myoblasts obtained from the recipient, the use of cyclosporine was required to prevent rejection. These issues have tempered the enthusiasm for this pioneering work and stimulated the search for new therapeutic strategies for the regeneration of dead myocardium.

The growth potential of adult HSCs or less purified BMCs injected in the circulation or locally delivered in areas of injury[33,75,76] raises the possibility that these primitive cells sense signals from lesions, migrate to regions of damage, and ultimately result in the reconstitution of the damaged tissue.[33,75,76] On this basis, an enriched population of lineage-negative, c-kit–positive BMCs were implanted into the viable myocardium in the proximity of an acute infarct in mice.[33] In less than 2 weeks, numerous small cardiomyocytes and vascular structures developed within the infarcted zone and replaced a large fraction of the dead myocardium. Myocytes expressed connexin 43, and the newly formed arterioles and capillaries were connected with the primary coronary circulation and were uniformly distributed within the regenerated portion of the ventricular wall. BMCs developed functioning myocardium, reduced infarct size, and ameliorated cardiac performance.[33]

Cytokines and growth factors appear to participate in the mobilization of stem cells and their translocation to damaged organs. This issue is highly relevant clinically because it might permit the application of strategies that do not require local implantation of exogenous stem cells or their preventive storage from the recipient. It is well established that SCF and granulocyte colony–stimulating factor induce a marked increase in the total number of circulating HSCs.[75] Mobilization by cytokines of HSCs into the circulation results in their localization to the infarcted portion of the ventricle, promoting regeneration of parenchymal cells and vascular structures and de novo reconstitution of viable myocardium (see Fig. 71–4). Therefore, two independent approaches have been identified for the regeneration of infarcted myocardium. A partial recovery was accomplished by autologous BMC implantation in dogs with chronic infarcts[77] and following the intravenous injection of CD34-positive BMCs in rats with acute myocardial injury.[78] The number of microvessels increased in both cases, mostly in the border zone. Angiogenesis and wall thickening improve cardiac performance.

On the basis of these few initial studies of myocardial regeneration and before the long-term consequences of BMC implantation could be established in animals, this procedure was translated to humans. Patients with acute myocardial infarcts have been treated with intracoronary delivery of BMCs at the time of reperfusion of the occluded vessel.[38,40,41,79] The immunophenotype of the administered cells in infarcted heart was established only in one case, in which the cells employed were AC133 positive.[40] AC133-positive bone marrow–derived cells are CD34 negative and have a high potential for angiogenesis.[40] In all trials, echocardiography showed a marked increase in ejection fraction and coronary blood flow. In some patients, wall motion recovered in the previously akinetic region and signs of myocardial viability were detected by fluorodeoxyglucose-positron emission tomography. Patients have been followed up to 6 months or 1 year after surgery. Malignant neoplasms have not been detected. In contrast to coronary infusion, six patients with acute infarcts were treated with local myocardial implantation of BMCs. Early after the intervention, ventricular arrhythmia developed in two cases and pericardial effusion in two others. At 16 months, the six patients were alive and reported a noticeable improvement in exercise capacity.[40] Finally, eight patients with refractory stable angina received an injection of BMCs through a catheter, which was guided to the ischemic areas by nonfluoroscopic left ventricular electromechanical mapping. The cells were a mixed population of primitive and early committed cells: about 8 percent exhibited only CD34, and the remaining were CD3-positive T cells, CD11b-positive/D15-positive granulocyte precursors, and granulocyte colony–forming units. The episodes of angina were reduced and the thickness of the target wall was improved.[41] With the exception of this study, the major limitation of these small clinical trials is that the delivery of bone marrow–derived cells is done simultaneously with revascularization of the ischemic region, complicating interpretation of the results. Therefore, the success of BMC therapy as a novel treatment of the ischemic myopathy is unresolved.

REFERENCES

1. Nadal-Ginard B, Kajstura J, Leri A, et al: Myocyte death, growth and regeneration in cardiac hypertrophy and failure. Circ Res 92:139-150, 2003.
2. Anversa P, Nadal-Ginard B: Myocyte renewal and ventricular remodeling. Nature 415:240-243, 2002.
3. Chien KR, Olson EN: Converging pathways and principles in heart development and disease. Cell 110:153-162, 2002.
4. Anversa P, Kajstura J: Ventricular myocytes are not terminally differentiated in the adult mammalian heart. Circ Res 83:1-14, 1998.
5. Anversa P, Leri A, Kajstura J, et al: Myocyte growth and cardiac repair. J Mol Cell Cardiol 34:91-105, 2002.
6. Conlon I, Raff M: Size control in animal development. Cell 96:235-244, 1999.
7. Molkentin JD, Dorn GW II: Cytoplasmic signaling pathways that regulate cardiac hypertrophy. Annu Rev Physiol 63:391-426, 2001.
8. Taylor DA, Hruban R, Rodriguez ER, et al: Cardiac chimerism as a mechanism for self-repair: Does it happen and if so to what degree? Circulation 106:2-4, 2002.
9. Beltrami AP, Urbanek K, Kajstura J, et al: Evidence that human cardiac myocytes divide after myocardial infarction. N Engl J Med 344:1750-1757, 2001.
10. Quaini F, Urbanek K, Beltrami AP, et al: Chimerism of the transplanted heart. N Engl J Med 346:5-15, 2002.
11. Setoguchi M, Leri A, Wang S, et al: Activation of cyclins and cyclin-dependent kinases, DNA synthesis, and myocyte mitotic division in pacing-induced heart failure in dogs. Lab Invest 79:1545-1558, 1999.
12. Dolbeare F: Bromodeoxyuridine: A diagnostic tool in biology and medicine: III. Proliferation in normal, injured and diseased tissue, growth factors, differentiation, DNA replication sites and in situ hybridization. Histochem J 28:531-575, 1996.
13. Larsen JK, Landberg G, Roos G: Detection of proliferating cell nuclear antigen. Methods Cell Biol 63:419-431, 2001.
14. Quaini F, Cigola E, Lagrasta C, et al: End-stage cardiac failure in humans is coupled with the induction of PCNA and nuclear mitotic division in myocytes. Circ Res 75:1050-1063, 1994.
15. Scholzen T, Gerdes J: The Ki-67 protein: from the known to the unknown. J Cell Physiol 182:311-322, 2000.
16. MacCallum DE, Hall PA: The biochemical characterization of the DNA binding activity of pKi67. J Pathol 191:286-298, 2000.
17. Stoeber K, Tlsty TD, Happerfield L, et al: DNA replication licensing and human cell proliferation. J Cell Sci 114:2027-2041, 2001.
18. Kajstura J, Leri A, Finato N, et al: Myocyte proliferation in end-stage cardiac failure in humans. Proc Natl Acad Sci U S A 95:8801-8805, 1998.

19. Anversa P, Olivetti G: Cellular basis of physiological and pathological myocardial growth. *In* Page E, Fozzard HA, Solaro RJ (eds): Handbook of Physiology. Chicago, Oxford University Press, 2002, pp 75-144.
20. Anversa P, Kajstura J, Nadal-Ginard B, et al: Primitive cells and tissue regeneration. Circ Res 92:579-582, 2003.
21. Nadal-Ginard B, Kajstura J, Anversa P, et al: A matter of life and death. J Clin Invest 111:1457-1459, 2003.
22. Cong YS, Wright WE, Shay JW: Human telomerase and its regulation. Microbiol Mol Biol Rev 66:407-425, 2002.
23. Allsopp RC, Morin GB, DePinho R, et al: Telomerase is required to slow telomere shortening and extend replicative lifespan of HSC during serial transplantation. Blood 102:517-520, 2003.
24. Hande MP, Samper E, Lansdorp P, et al: Telomere length dynamics and chromosomal instability in cells derived from telomerase null mice. J Cell Biol 144:589-601, 1999.
25. Smogorzewska A, van Steensel B, Bianchi A, et al: Control of human telomere length by TRF1 and TRF2. Mol Cell Biol 20:1659-1668, 2000.
26. Nakamura K, Izumiyama-Shimomura N, Sawabe M, et al: Comparative analysis of telomere lengths and erosion with age in human epidermis and lingual epithelium. J Invest Dermatol 119:1014-1019, 2002.
27. Leri A, Barlucchi L, Limana F, et al: Telomerase expression and activity are coupled with myocyte proliferation and preservation of telomeric length in the failing heart. Proc Natl Acad Sci U S A 98:8626-8631, 2001.
28. Kajstura J, Pertoldi B, Leri A, et al: Telomere shortening is an in vivo marker of myocyte replication and aging. Am J Pathol 156:813-819, 2000.
29. Leri A, Malhotra A, Liew CC, et al: Telomerase activity in rat cardiac myocytes is age and gender dependent. J Mol Cell Cardiol 32:385-390, 2000.
30. Leri A, Franco S, Zacheo A, et al: Ablation of telomerase and telomere loss leads to cardiac dilatation and heart failure associated with p53 upregulation. EMBO J 22:131-139, 2003.
31. Gepstein L: Derivation and potential applications of human embryonic stem cells. Circ Res 91:866-876, 2002.
32. El Oakley RM, Ooi OC, Bongso A, et al: Myocyte transplantation for myocardial repair: A few good cells can mend a broken heart. Ann Thorac Surg 71:1724-1733, 2001.
33. Orlic D, Kajstura J, Chimenti S, et al: Bone marrow cells regenerate infarcted myocardium. Nature 410:701-705, 2001.
34. Hirschi KK, Goodell MA: Hematopoietic vascular and cardiac fates of bone marrow–derived stem cells. Gene Therapy 9:648-652, 2002.
35. Reffelmann T, Dow JS, Dai W, et al: Transplantation of neonatal cardiomyocytes after permanent coronary artery occlusion increases regional blood flow of infarcted myocardium. J Mol Cell Cardiol 35:607-613, 2003.
36. Hamano K, Mishida M, Hirata K, et al: Local implantation of autologous bone marrow cells for therapeutic angiogenesis in patients with ischemic heart disease: Clinical trial and preliminary results. Jpn Circ J 65:845-847, 2001.
37. Assmus B, Schachinger V, Teupe C, et al: Transplantation of progenitor cells and regeneration enhancement in acute myocardial infarction (TOPCARE-AMI). Circulation 106:3009-3017, 2002.
38. Strauer BE, Brehm M, Zeus T, et al: Repair of infarcted myocardium by autologous intracoronary mononuclear bone marrow cell transplantation in humans. Circulation 106:1913-1918, 2002.
39. Beran G: Autologous stem cells injection in a patient after acute myocardial infarction. Heart Surg Forum 6:9, 2002.
40. Stamm C, Westphal B, Kleine HD, et al: Autologous bone-marrow stem-cell transplantation for myocardial regeneration. Lancet 361:45-46, 2003.
41. Tse HF, Kwong YL, Chan JKF, et al: Angiogenesis in ischaemic myocardium by intramyocardial autologous bone marrow mononuclear cell implantation. Lancet 361:47-49, 2003.
42. Hagège AA, Carrion C, Menasché P, et al: Viability and differentiation of autologous skeletal myoblast grafts in ischaemic cardiomyopathy. Lancet 361:491-492, 2003.
43. Koh GY, Klug MG, Soonpaa MH, et al: Differentiation and long-term survival of C2C12 myoblast grafts in heart. J Clin Invest 92:1548-1554, 1993.
44. Murry CE, Wiseman RW, Schwartz SM, Hauschka SD: Skeletal myoblast transplantation for repair of myocardial necrosis. J Clin Invest 98:2512-2523, 1996.
45. Taylor DA, Atkins BZ, Hungspreugs P, et al: Regenerating functional myocardium: Improved performance after skeletal myoblast transplantation. Nat Med 4:929-933, 1998.
46. Suzuki K, Murtuza B, Suzuki N, et al: Intracoronary infusion of skeletal myoblasts improves cardiac function in doxorubicin-induced heart failure. Circulation 104:I213-I217, 2001.
47. Kumar NM, Gilula NB: The gap junction communication channel. Cell 84:381-388, 1996.
48. Spray DC, Suadicani SO, Srinivas M, et al: Gap junctions in the cardiovascular system. *In* Page E, Fozzard HA, Solaro RJ (eds): Handbook of Physiology. Chicago, Oxford University Press, 2002, pp 169-212.
49. Luo Y, Radice GL: Cadherin-mediated adhesion is essential for myofibril continuity across the plasma membrane but not for assembly of the contractile apparatus. J Cell Sci 116:1471-1479, 2003.
50. Yap AS, Kovacs EM: Direct cadherin-activated cell signaling: A view from the plasma membrane. J Cell Biol 160:11-16, 2003.
51. Bonincontro A, Cametti C, Hausman RE, et al: Changes in myoblast membrane electrical properties during cell-cell adhesion and fusion in vitro. Biochim Biophys Acta 903:89-95, 1987.
52. Suzuki K, Brand NJ, Allen S, et al: Overexpression of connexin 43 in skeletal myoblasts: Relevance to cell transplantation to the heart. J Thorac Cardiovasc Surg 122:759-766, 2001.
53. Decary S, Mouly V, Hamida CB, et al: Replicative potential and telomere length in human skeletal muscle: Implications for satellite cell–mediated gene therapy. Hum Gene Ther 8:1429-1438, 1997.
54. Minguell JJ, Erices A, Conget P: Mesenchymal stem cells. Exp Biol Med 226:507-520, 2001.
55. Jiang Y, Jahagirdar BN, Reinhardt RL, et al: Pluripotency of mesenchymal stem cells derived from adult marrow. Nature 418:41-49, 2002.
56. Colter DC, Sekiya I, Prockop DJ: Identification of a subpopulation of rapidly self-renewing and multipotential adult stem cells in colonies of human marrow stromal cells. Proc Natl Acad Sci U S A 98:7841-7845, 2001.
57. Makino S, Fukuda K, Miyoshi S, et al: Cardiomyocytes can be generated from marrow stromal cells in vitro. J Clin Invest 103:697-705, 1999.
58. Fukuda K: Development of regenerative cardiomyocytes from mesenchymal stem cells for cardiovascular tissue engineering. Artif Organs 25:187-193, 2001.
59. Hakuno D, Fukuda K, Makino S, et al: Bone marrow–derived regenerated cardiomyocytes (CMG cells) express functional adrenergic and muscarinic receptors. Circulation 105:380-386, 2002.
60. Tomita S, Nakatani T, Fukuhara S, et al: Bone marrow stromal cells contract synchronously with cardiomyocytes in a coculture system. Jpn J Thorac Cardiovasc Surg 50:321-324, 2002.
61. Tomita S, Mickle DA, Weisel RD, et al: Improved heart function with myogenesis and angiogenesis after autologous porcine bone marrow stromal cell transplantation. J Thorac Cardiovasc Surg 123:1132-1140, 2002.
62. Shake JG, Gruber PJ, Baumgartner WA, et al: Mesenchymal stem cell implantation in a swine myocardial infarct model: Engraftment and functional effects. Ann Thorac Surg 73:1919-1925, 2002.
63. Min JY, Sullivan MF, Yang Y, et al: Significant improvement of heart function by cotransplantation of human mesenchymal stem cells and fetal cardiomyocytes in postinfarcted pigs. Ann Thorac Surg 74:1568-1575, 2002.
64. Tomita S, Li RK, Weisel RD, et al: Autologous transplantation of bone marrow cells improves damaged heart function. Circulation 100:II247-II256, 1999.
65. Wang JS, Shum-Tim D, Chedrawy E, Chiu RC: The coronary delivery of marrow stromal cells for myocardial regeneration: Pathophysiologic and therapeutic implications. J Thorac Cardiovasc Surg 122:699-705, 2001.
66. Wang JS, Shum-Tim D, Galipeau J, et al: Marrow stromal cells for cellular cardiomyoplasty: Feasibility and potential clinical advantages. J Thorac Cardiovasc Surg 120:999-1005, 2000.
67. Toma C, Pittenger MF, Cahill KS, et al: Human mesenchymal stem cells differentiate to a cardiomyocyte phenotype in the adult murine heart. Circulation 105:93-98, 2002.
68. Devine SM, Cobbs C, Jennings M, et al: Mesenchymal stem cells distribute to a wide range of tissues following systematic infusion into non-human primates. Blood 101:2999-3001, 2003.
69. Kondo M, Wagers AJ, Manz MG, et al: Biology of hematopoietic stem cells and progenitors: Implications for clinical applications. Annu Rev Immunol 21:759-806, 2003.
70. Wagers AJ, Sherwood RI, Christensen JL, et al: Little evidence for developmental plasticity of adult hematopoietic stem cells. Science 297:2256-2259, 2002.
71. Spees JL, Olson SD, Ylostalo J, et al: Differentiation, cell fusion, and nuclear fusion during ex vivo repair of epithelium by human adult stem cells from bone marrow stroma. Proc Natl Acad Sci U S A 100:2397-2402, 2003.
72. Vassilopoulos G, Wang PR, Russell DW: Transplanted bone marrow regenerates liver by cell fusion. Nature 422:901-904, 2003.
73. Wang X, Willenbring H, Akkari Y, et al: Cell fusion is the principal source of bone marrow–derived hepatocytes. Nature 422:897-901, 2003.
74. Orkin SH, Zon LI: Hematopoiesis and stem cells: Plasticity versus developmental heterogeneity. Nat Immunol 3:323-328, 2002.
75. Orlic D, Kajstura J, Chimenti S, et al: Mobilized bone marrow cells repair the infarcted heart, improving function and survival. Proc Natl Acad Sci U S A 98:10344-10349, 2001.
76. Jackson KA, Majka SM, Wang H, et al: Regeneration of ischemic cardiac muscle and vascular endothelium by adult stem cells. J Clin Invest 107:1395-1402, 2001.
77. Hassink RJ, Brutel de la Riviere A, Mummery CL, et al: Transplantation of cells for cardiac repair. J Am Coll Cardiol 41:711-717, 2003.
78. Kawamoto A, Tkebuchava T, Yamaguchi J, et al: Intramyocardial transplantation of autologous endothelial progenitor cells for the therapeutic neovascularization of myocardial ischemia. Circulation 107:461-468, 2003.
79. Strauer BE, Brehm M, Zeus T, et al: Repair of infarcted myocardium by autologous intracoronary mononuclear bone marrow cell transplantation in humans. Circulation 106:1913-1918, 2002.

PART IX

Cardiovascular Disease in Special Populations

CHAPTER 72

Cardiovascular Disease in the Elderly

Janice B. Schwartz • Douglas P. Zipes

Demographics and Epidemiology[1]

The proportion of people aged 65 years and older in the United States is projected to increase from 12.4 percent (35 million) of the population in 2000 to 19.6 percent in 2030 (71 million) and to 82 million in 2050. The number of people older than 80 years is projected to double from 9.3 million in 2000 to 19.5 million in 2030 and to more than triple by 2050. Women represented 59 percent of persons older than 65 years in 2000 and are estimated to make up 56 percent of the older population in 2030 (Fig. 72-1). If current projections hold, there will be increases in the percentage of racial minorities. From 2000 to 2030, the proportion of persons older than 65 years who are members of racial minority groups (i.e., black, Native American–Alaska Native, Asian–Pacific Islander) is expected to increase from 11.3 to 16.5 percent and the proportion of Hispanic people is expected to increase from 5.6 to 10.9 percent. Almost half of people older than 65 years in the United States in 2000 had after-tax incomes at the poverty level (41 percent of 65- to 74-year-olds and 56 percent of those older than 75 years); and this trend is likely to continue.[2] Global trends are similar, with the worldwide population older than 65 years projected to increase to 973 million or 12.0 percent in 2030 and make up about 20 percent of the population in 2050. Increases will be greatest in undeveloped nations. Estimates are for twice as many women as men older than 80 years and three times as many women as men older than 90.

Cardiovascular disease is the most frequent diagnosis in elderly people and is the leading cause of death in both men and women older than 65 years. Hypertension occurs in one-half to two-thirds of people older than 65 years, and heart failure (HF) is the most frequent hospital discharge diagnosis among older Americans. The profile of these common cardiovascular diseases in older patients differs from that in younger patients. Systolic, but not diastolic, blood pressure increases with aging, and systolic hypertension becomes a stronger predictor of cardiovascular events, especially in women. HF with preserved systolic function becomes more common at older ages and is more common in women than men. Coronary artery disease (CAD) is more likely to involve multiple vessels and left main artery disease and is equally likely in women and men older than 65 years. Equal numbers of older men and women present with acute myocardial infarction (AMI) until age 80, after which more women present. More than 80 percent of all deaths attributable to cardiovascular disease occur in people older than 65 years, with approximately 60 percent of deaths in patients older than 75 years.

Furthermore, cardiovascular disease in older people is not seen in isolation. Eighty percent of older Americans have at least one chronic medical condition and half have at least two. Arthritis affects about 60 percent of persons older than 65 years, and diabetes affects about 20 percent (Fig. 72–2). Ear, nose, and throat problems, vision disorders, and orthopedic problems are also common. As U.S. adults live longer, the prevalence and incidence of dementia that impairs memory, decision-making capability, orientation to physical surroundings, and language also increase. The prevalence of Alzheimer's disease is estimated as 10 percent in community-dwelling whites older than 65 years and is higher in black and Hispanic populations. By age 80, approximately 40 percent of people may be affected.[3] One-third of Medicare

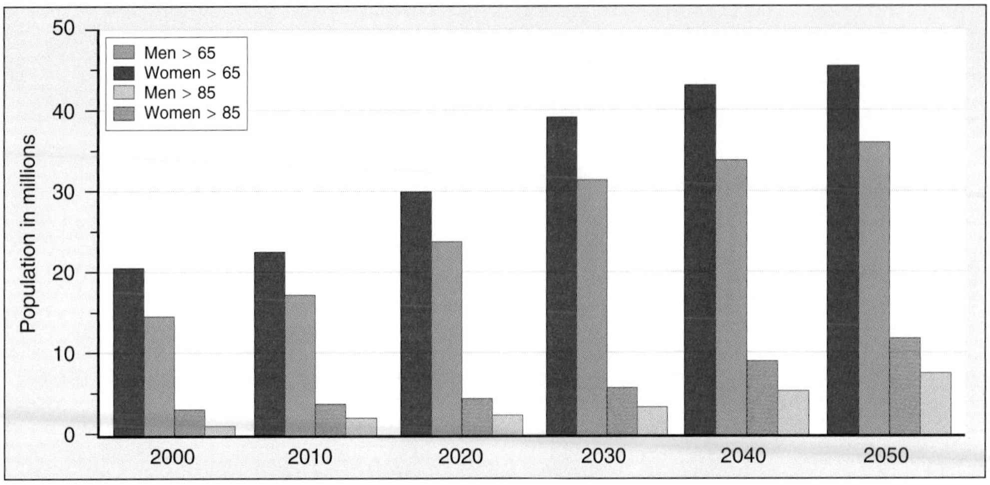

FIGURE 72–1 U.S. population estimates projected from 2000 to 2050. Dark pink bars represent numbers of women older than 65 years, dark blue bars represent numbers of men older than 65 years, light pink bars represent numbers of women older than 85 years, and light blue bars represent numbers of men older than 85 years, in millions of people. (From the U.S. Census Bureau.)

beneficiaries with Alzheimer's disease have CAD, one-quarter have had a stroke, and 22 percent have diabetes.[4]

The high morbidity and mortality from cardiovascular disease in elderly persons warrant aggressive approaches to treatment that have been shown to be effective in older patients. Compelling data demonstrate reduced morbidity and mortality rates for the treatment of hypertension, HF, atrial fibrillation, and lipid abnormalities in older patients 60 to 74 years of age, although data on minorities and women are limited.[5] Few trials of cardiovascular therapies have enrolled significant numbers of men or women older than 75 years, elderly patients with multisystem disease, or elderly patients with cognitive impairment, and none have addressed cardiovascular therapies in the nursing home population. The projected increase in numbers of older people from previously understudied and undertreated groups presents both medical and economic challenges for cardiovascular disease treatment.

PATHOPHYSIOLOGY

No universal definition of "elderly" and no accurate biomarker for aging exist. Although physiological changes associated with aging do not appear at a specific age and do not proceed at the same pace in all individuals, most definitions of elderly are based on chronological age. The World Health Organization uses 60 years of age to define "elderly," and most U.S. classifications use the age of 65 years. Gerontologists subclassify older age groups into young old (60 to 74 years), old old (75 to 85 years), and very old (over 85 years of age). Clinicians often separate older patients into two subgroups—those 65 to 80 years of age and those older than 80 years—to highlight the frailty, reduced capacity (physical and mental), and presence of multiple disorders that are more common after 80 years of age.

Hallmarks of cardiovascular aging in humans[6-8] include progressive increases in systolic blood pressure, pulse pressure (Fig. 72–3), pulse wave velocity, and left ventricular mass and increased incidence of CAD and atrial fibrillation. Reproducible age-related decreases are seen in rates of early left ventricular diastolic filling, maximal heart rates (Fig. 72–4), maximal cardiac output (see Fig. 72–4), maximal aerobic capacity or maximal oxygen consumption (VO_{2max}), exercise-induced augmentation of ejection fraction, reflex responses of heart rate, heart rate variability, and vasodilation in response to beta-adrenergic stimuli or endothelium-mediated vasodilator compounds (Fig. 72–5).

Cellular, enzymatic, and molecular alterations in the arterial vessel wall include migration of activated vascular smooth muscle cells into the intima, with increased matrix production related to altered activity of matrix metalloproteinases, angiotensin II, transforming growth factor beta, intercellular cell adhesion molecules, and production of collagen and collagen cross-linking. Loss of elastic fibers, increases in fibronectin, and calcification are also observed. These processes lead to arterial dilation and increased intimal thickness resulting in increased vascular stiffness. Increased arterial stiffness is manifested by increases in pulse wave velocity away from the heart and increased and earlier pulse wave reflections back toward the heart (often estimated as the aortic augmentation index). In both animal and human models of aging, endothelial cell production of nitric oxide (NO) decreases with age; there is decreased endothelial cell mass associated with increased cell senescence and apoptosis and increased NO consumption because of an age-dependent increase in vascular superoxide anion production. These changes contribute to reduced endothelial cell NO-mediated vasodilatory responses of the peripheral and coronary vasculature. Vascular responses to beta-adrenergic agonists and alpha-adrenergic blockade are also reduced with aging. In contrast, responses to non-endothelium-derived compounds such as nitrates or nitroprusside are preserved with aging but may vary by vascular bed or be altered by diseases such as hypertension or diabetes.

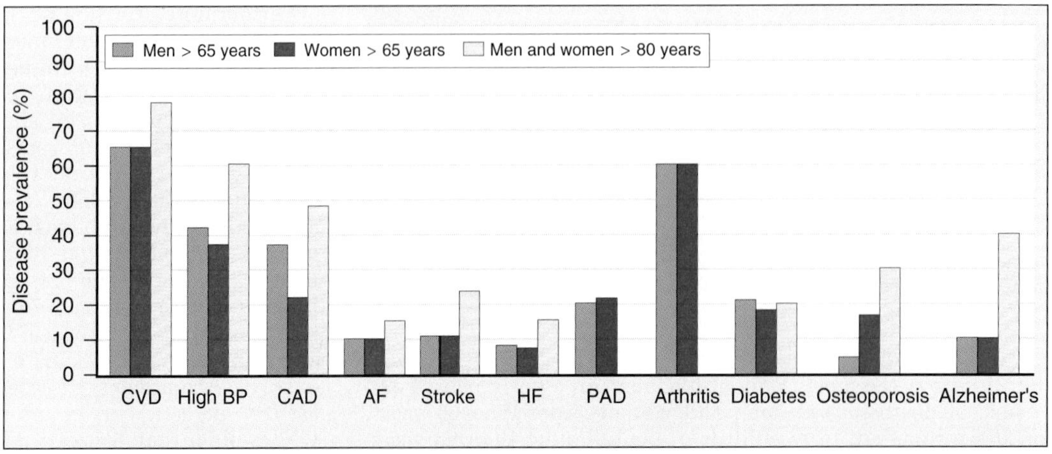

FIGURE 72–2 Prevalence of cardiovascular and other common chronic medical illnesses in older persons in the United States. Data are percentages. AF = atrial fibrillation; CAD = coronary artery disease; CVD = cardiovascular disease; HF = heart failure; High BP = hypertension (all forms); PAD = peripheral artery disease. Blue bars represent data for men older than 65 years, pink bars represent women older than 65 years, and yellow bars represent men and women older than 80 years.

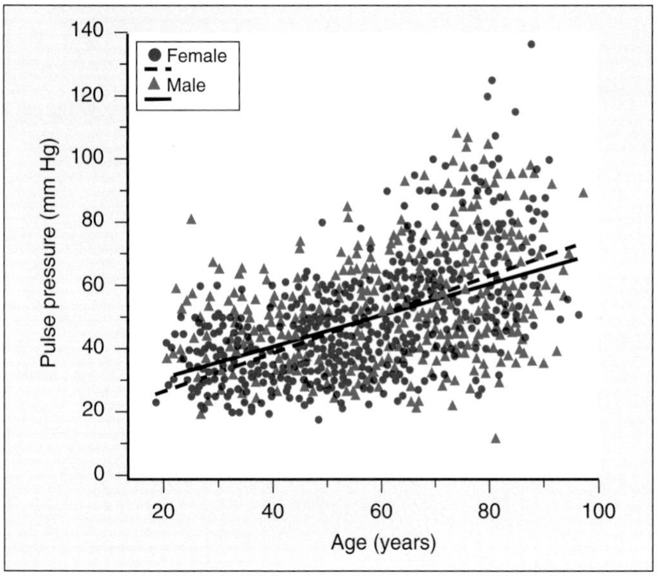

FIGURE 72–3 Pulse pressure (systolic minus diastolic pressure) with aging in apparently healthy subjects enrolled in the Baltimore Longitudinal Study of Aging . (From Pearson JD, Morrell CH, Brant LJ, et al: Age-associated changes in blood pressure in a longitudinal study of healthy men and women. J Gerontol Med Sci 53:M177, 1997.)

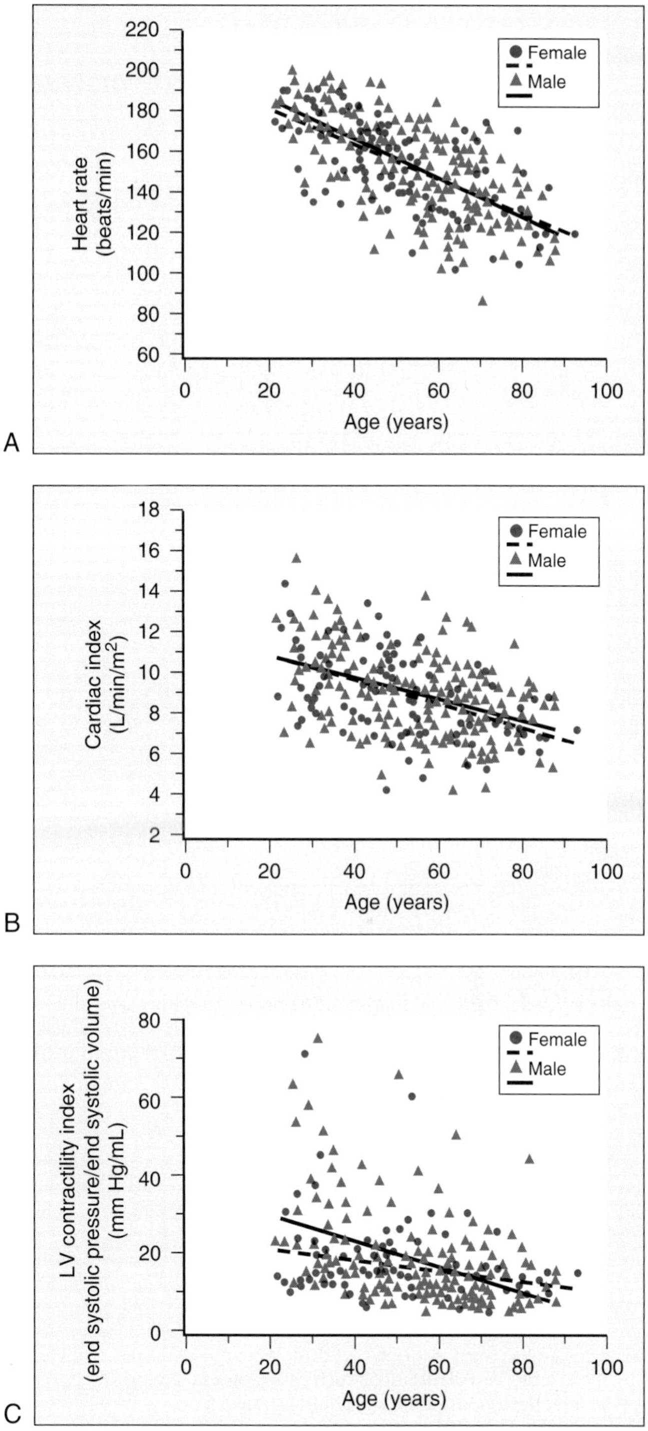

FIGURE 72–4 Maximum exercise heart rate **(A)**, cardiac index **(B)**, and left ventricular (LV) contractility index **(C)** in men and women in the Baltimore Longitudinal Study of Aging who had been prescreened to exclude clinical and occult cardiovascular disease. (From Fleg JL, O'Connor FC, Gerstenblith G, et al: Impact of age on the cardiovascular response to dynamic upright exercise in healthy men and women. J Appl Physiol 78:890, 1995.)

Changes in the extracellular matrix of the myocardium parallel those in the vasculature with increased collagen, increased fibril diameter and collagen cross-linking, an increase in the ratio of type I to type III collagen, decreased elastin content, and an increase in fibronectin. There may also be a shift in the balance between matrix metalloproteinases and tissue inhibitors of matrix metalloproteinases that favors increased production of extracellular matrix. Fibroblast proliferation is induced by growth factors, in particular angiotensin, transforming growth factors, tumor necrosis factor-alpha, and platelet-derived growth factor. These changes are accompanied by cell loss and altered cellular function.[9,10] In the atria, decreased sinus node cells and extracellular matrix changes contribute to sinus node dysfunction and atrial fibrillation. Collagen, elastic tissue, and calcification changes in or near the central fibrous body and the atrioventricular (AV) node or proximal bundle branches contribute to conduction abnormalities and annular valvular calcification. In the ventricle, collagen deposition and extracellular matrix changes contribute to loss of cells, hypertrophy of myocytes with changes in myosin subforms, and altered myocardial calcium handling.[11] Changes in myocardial calcium handling include reduced or delayed inactivation of L-type transmembrane calcium current, decreased and delayed intracellular ionized calcium uptake by cardiac myocyte sarcoplasmic reticulum (in part due to reduced sarcoendoplasmic reticulum calcium adenosine triphosphatase [SERCA2] activity), and reduced and delayed outwardly directed potassium rectifier current activation. The result is prolongation of the membrane action potential and inward calcium current with prolongation of both contraction and relaxation.[9,11,12]

Age-related changes are also seen in the intravascular environment. Increases in fibrinogen; coagulation factors V, VIII, and IX; and other coagulation proteins are seen without countering increases in anticoagulant factors. Platelet phospholipid content is altered and platelet activity is increased with increased binding of platelet-derived growth factor to the arterial wall in older individuals compared with younger individuals. Increased levels of plasminogen activator inhibitor 1 (PAI-1) are seen with aging, especially during stress, resulting in impaired fibrinolysis. Circulating prothrombotic inflammatory cytokines, especially interleukin-6, also increase with age and may play a role in the pathogenesis of acute coronary syndromes. Adipose cells associated with obesity are also sources of PAI-1 and inflammatory cytokines. All these changes also potentiate development of atherosclerosis.[9,13,14]

Consistent changes in the autonomic nervous system (see Chap. 87) accompany aging and influence cardiovascular function. For the beta-adrenergic system, age-related changes include decreased receptor numbers, altered G protein coupling, and altered G protein–mediated signal transduction. Age-related decreases in alpha-adrenergic platelet receptors and decreased alpha-adrenergic–mediated arterial vasoreactivity of forearm blood vessels occur, but alpha-adrenergic–mediated changes in human hand veins appear to be preserved. Dopaminergic receptor content and dopaminergic transporters decrease and cardiac contractile responses to dopaminergic stimulation may be blunted with aging. Decreased sensitivity and responses to parasympathetic stimulation are seen in cardiac and vascular tissues, but increased central nervous system effects are frequently seen in models of aging. The combined age-related autonomic changes lead to decreased baroreflex function and responses to physiological stressors with increased sensitivity to parasympathetic stimulation of the central nervous system.[6,7,9,15-20]

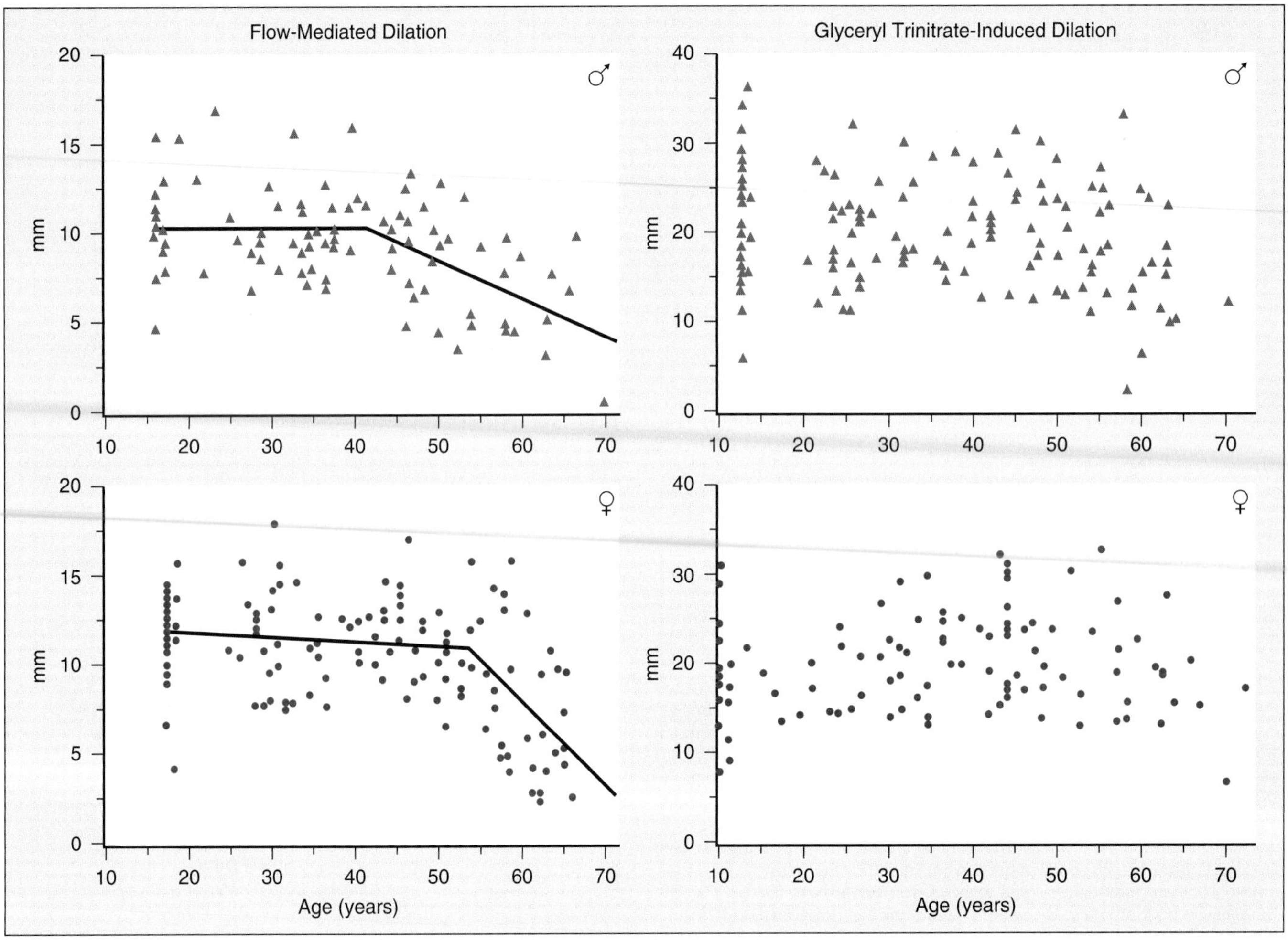

FIGURE 72–5 Endothelial (flow)-mediated and nonendothelial (glyceryl trinitrate)-induced arterial dilation in apparently healthy men and women. Age-associated declines are seen in flow-mediated dilation but not in glyceryl trinitrate–induced dilation. Age-related changes occur earlier in men than women. (From Celermajer DS, Sorensen KE, Spiegelhalter DJ, et al: Aging is associated with endothelial dysfunction in healthy men years before the age-related decline in women. J Am Coll Cardiol 24:471, 1994.)

Several unifying hypotheses for age-related changes throughout the body have been proposed and include cumulative oxidative damage, inflammatory responses to cellular stress or infection, and programmed cell death. Some of the age-related cardiovascular changes can be partially, if not totally, reversed. Exercise improves endothelial function, measures of arterial stiffness, and baroreceptor function in older people. Pharmacological approaches with antiinflammatory and antioxidant vitamin administration have not been successful, although dietary antioxidant intake has been associated with slowing of age-related changes in the vasculature, and medications such as angiotensin-converting enzyme (ACE) inhibitors, aldosterone antagonists, or beta blockers may influence the vascular and cardiac remodeling associated with hypertension, atherosclerosis, or HF.[21-29] Agents that directly target collagen cross-linking and inflammation are being evaluated.

Age-related changes create a cardiovascular system faced with increased pulsatile load and one that is less able to increase output in response to stress. Age-related changes also limit maximal capacity and decrease reserve capacity, contributing to lower thresholds for symptoms in the presence of cardiovascular diseases that become more common with increasing age. Table 72-1 summarizes age-related cardiovascular changes contrasted with cardiovascular disease.

Medication Modifications

The vast majority of therapeutic interventions for elderly people are pharmacological, making appropriate drug selection and modification of dosing regimens for the older patient important (see Chap. 5).

LOADING DOSES OF MEDICATIONS. On average, body size decreases with aging and body composition changes, resulting in decreased total body water, intravascular volume, and muscle mass. Age-related changes are continuous but most pronounced after 75 to 80 years. Women tend to weigh less and have smaller body and intravascular volumes and muscle mass than men at all ages. Higher serum concentrations of medications are found in older patients, and especially older women, if initial doses are the same as those in younger patients. Weight adjustments for loading doses of the cardiovascular drugs digoxin, lidocaine, and other type I antiarrhythmic drugs, and type III antiarrhythmic drugs; aminoglycoside antibiotics; chemotherapy regimens; and unfractionated heparin are standard. When fibrinolytic drugs have been administered without weight-based dosage adjustments, increased risk of intracranial hemorrhage (ICH) resulted with older age, smaller body weight, and female sex (in addition to hypertension and prior cerebrovascular disease).[30,31] Increased risk of bleeding in older patients is also seen after administration of "standard" doses of low-molecular-weight heparins in combination with other lytic agents. In contrast, increased risk of intracranial bleeding in older patients was not seen in trials using weight-based dosing.[32]

Routine dosage-weight adjustments should be made in loading doses of medications, especially those with low therapeutic-to-toxicity ratios, resulting in doses that are usually lower in older patients, especially older women.

TABLE 72–1 Differentiation Between Age-Associated Changes and Cardiovascular Disease in Older People

Organ	Age-Associated Changes	Cardiovascular Disease
Vasculature	Increased intimal thickness Arterial stiffening Increased pulse pressure Increased pulse wave velocity Early central wave reflections Decreased endothelium-mediated vasodilation	Systolic hypertension Coronary artery obstruction Peripheral artery obstruction Carotid artery obstruction
Atria	Increased left atrial size Atrial premature complexes	Atrial fibrillation
Sinus node	Decreased maximal heart rate Decreased heart rate variability	Sinus node dysfunction, sick sinus syndrome
Atrioventricular node	Increased conduction time	Type II block, third-degree block
Valves	Sclerosis, calcification	Stenosis, regurgitation
Ventricle	Increased left ventricular wall tension Prolonged myocardial contraction Prolonged early diastolic filling rate Decreased maximal cardiac output Right bundle branch block Ventricular premature complexes	Left ventricular hypertrophy Heart failure (with or without preserved systolic function) Ventricular tachycardia, fibrillation

CHRONIC MEDICATION ADMINISTRATION

RENAL CLEARANCE. Renal clearance by all routes (glomerular filtration, renal tubular reabsorption, and secretion) decreases with age and is lower in women than in men at all ages. There is considerable intersubject variability, but a general estimate is a 10 percent decline in glomerular filtration per decade with 15 to 25 percent lower rates in women than in men. Algorithms to estimate creatinine clearance or glomerular filtration often include age, sex, weight, serum creatinine concentrations, and, more recently, race as variables.[33] Two useful formulas to estimate glomerular filtration or creatinine clearance in people during stable conditions are:

$$\text{Creatinine clearance} = (140 - \text{age [yr]} \times \text{weight [kg]})/(\text{creatinine} \times 72)$$

multiplied by 0.85 for women[34]

$$\text{Glomerular filtration} = 186.3 \times (\text{creatinine})^{-1.154} \times (\text{age})^{-0.203} \times 1.212 \text{ (if black)} \times 0.742 \text{ (if female)}$$[35]

Significant decreases in renal elimination can be present in older patients in the presence of normal serum creatinine measurements. The algorithms predict that most women older than 70 have stage 3 renal function or moderate renal failure (National Kidney Foundation 2001 guidelines, available at http://www.kidney.org). With elevations of serum creatinine, severe renal impairment is likely to be present. Estimates of renal clearance are recommended before prescribing renally cleared medications, in determining risks for procedures, and before administration of contrast agents or other potentially nephrotoxic agents in older patients. They are not, however, accurate if the patient is clinically unstable.

HEPATIC (AND INTESTINAL) CLEARANCE. Most studies show decreases in oxidative drug metabolism or clearance by the cytochrome P450 (CYP) system with aging, suggesting that lower amounts of drug per unit time (or day) should be given to older patients compared with younger patients. Cardiovascular drugs showing such age-related changes in hepatic clearance include alpha blockers (doxazosin, prazosin, terazosin), some beta blockers (metoprolol, propranolol, timolol), calcium channel blockers (dihydropyridines, diltiazem, verapamil), several 3-hydroxy-3-methylglutaryl coenzyme A (HMG CoA) reductase inhibitors (atorvastatin, fluvastatin), and the benzodiazepine midazolam. Variability in age-related changes is marked, however, and the effects of disease states, gender, race, and medication interactions are usually greater than those of age in populations of patients.[36,37] CYP drug clearance is usually faster in men than women, even after correction for weight, suggesting that women should receive lower dosages per unit time and weight than men. The exceptions are CYP3A substrates such as midazolam and nifedipine that are cleared more rapidly in women. Additional information on sex-specific medication adjustments has been reviewed.[38,39]

Genetic variation in drug metabolism exists, and allelic variants for most of the CYP pathways have been described that affect drug clearance as well as responses.[40,41] Encainide, metoprolol, and warfarin are metabolized by the polymorphic CYP2D6 enzyme that can produce distinct phenotypes of ultrarapid, rapid, slow, and ultraslow drug clearance. Pharmacogenetic variants can also explain some of the variability in metabolism and toxicity with the HMG CoA reductase inhibitor simvastatin.[42] It is currently difficult to estimate the clinical impact of genetic polymorphisms of drug-metabolizing enzymes (or receptors or transcription-regulating elements), and routine pharmacogenomic screening is not recommended at present.[43] Further information can be found at the National Institutes of Health–sponsored Pharmacogenetics Research Network (www.pharmgkb.org or www.imm.ki.se/CYPalleles/). Data on CYP pathways of human metabolism have been reviewed,[44] and updates are available in a searchable data base (www.gentest.com).

Drugs metabolized by the conjugative reactions of glucuronidation (morphine, diazepam), sulfation (methyldopa), or acetylation (procainamide) do not appear to be affected by aging but show disease-related effects, and clearance is consistently lower in women than in men.

ELIMINATION HALF-LIVES. In general, elimination half-lives of drugs increase with age, so that the time between dosage adjustments needs to be increased in older patients before the full effect of a given dose can be assessed. Conversely, increased time is needed for complete drug elimination from the body and dissipation of the drug effects.

Age-related changes in protein binding of drugs are not usually found. Changes in free drug concentrations related to drugs competing for binding sites can occur, although these changes are predicted to be transitory.[45] Clinically significant examples involve warfarin and changes in anticoagulation when additional drugs are added to therapy. For example, markedly increased prolongation of coagulation times can occur when amiodarone is added to warfarin therapy (see Chap. 30). Drug interactions must be considered whenever an agent is added to warfarin therapy. Table 72–2 summarizes general guidelines for drug dosing in older patients.

ADVERSE DRUG EVENTS AND DRUG INTERACTIONS.

Adverse drug events are estimated to affect millions of people per year and account for up to 5 percent of hospital admissions.[46] Cardiovascular medications such digoxin, warfarin, diuretics, and calcium channel blockers are among those most frequently cited as responsible for "preventable" adverse drug events in community-dwelling elderly people and hospitalized elderly patients.[47,48] The odds ratio of severe adverse drug events with cardiovascular medications has been reported to be 2.4 times that of other medications in hospitalized patients.[49] In adult patients in ambulatory primary care settings, selective serotonin reuptake inhibitors (SSRIs), beta blockers, ACE inhibitors, and nonsteroidal anti-inflammatory drugs (NSAIDs) have been identified in adverse

TABLE 72–2 Guidelines for Drug Dosing in Older Patients

In general, loading doses should be reduced—weight (or body surface area) can be used to estimate loading dose requirements; doses in women are usually less than those in men.
Base doses of renally cleared drugs on estimates of glomerular filtration or creatinine clearance (or, if not possible, initiate with lower doses than in younger patient); reduce doses of hepatically cleared drugs.
Time between dosage adjustments and evaluation of dosing changes should be longer in older patients than in younger patients.
Routine use of strategies to avoid drug interactions is essential.
Assessment of adherence and attention to factors contributing to nonadherence should be part of the prescription process.

drug events.[50] In nursing home patients, drugs associated with adverse drug events are more frequently antibiotics, anticoagulants, antipsychotic drugs, antidepressants, antiseizure medications, or opioids.[51] Adverse drug effects may arise with "atypical" symptoms in the older patient, such as mental status changes and impaired cognition with digitalis excess.

The strongest risk factor for adverse drug-related events is the number of drugs prescribed, independent of age. Chronic administration of four drugs is associated with a risk of adverse effects of 50 to 60 percent; administration of eight or nine drugs increases the risk to almost 100 percent (Fig. 72–6). Although the goal is to prescribe as few drugs as possible for elderly patients, the presence of multiple diseases and multidrug regimens for common cardiovascular diseases often results in polypharmacy. A national survey of noninstitutionalized people older than 65 years found that over 40 percent used 5 or more different medications each week and 12 percent used 10 or more different medications per week.[52] American College of Cardiology/American Heart Association (ACC/AHA) guidelines for the pharmacological treatment of patients after uncomplicated myocardial infarction and for the management of chronic HF recommend use of four or five drugs.[53,54] Strategies that minimize the chance of drug interactions and adverse drug effects are thus essential.

PHARMACOKINETIC INTERACTIONS. Pharmacokinetic interactions that alter the concentration of concomitantly administered medications are more likely if drugs that are metabolized by or inhibit the same pathway are coadministered. Table 72-3 lists some examples of cardiovascular drugs by metabolic pathway with examples of inducers and inhibitors (see also Table 5-1, Chap. 5). The most potent inhibitors of the CYP oxidative enzymes are amiodarone (all CYP isoforms), the azole antifungal drugs itraconazole and ketoconazole (CYP3A), and protease inhibitors (CYP3A), followed by erythromycin (CYP3A) and terfenadine (CYP3A). Oral hypoglycemic agents are commonly prescribed drugs for elderly patients, and coadministration of sulfonamide antibiotics with sulfonylureas can lead to hypoglycemia, in part because of CYP2C9 inhibition. Some drugs are administered as prodrugs and metabolized to active agents (cardiovascular examples include many ACE inhibitors and clopidogrel). Inhibition of the antiplatelet effects of clopidogrel by coadministration of atorvastatin, which decreases clopidogrel activation (CYP3A), has been reported,[55] although the clinical significance is not entirely clear.[55a]

Inducibility of hepatic enzyme activity can lower concentrations of medications and lead to ineffective therapy. The antituberculous drug rifampin is the most potent inducer of CYP1A and CYP3A. With mandatory screening of nursing home residents for tuberculosis, treatment with rifampin may be initiated. Dosages of coadministered drugs cleared by CYP1A and CYP3A may need to be increased during rifampin administration and decreased upon discontinuation of rifampin. The clinical importance of this interaction was recognized with markedly decreased cyclosporine levels during rifampin coadministration. Reduced clopidogrel inhibition of platelet aggregation by atorvastatin has also been reported after rifampin administration.[55] Other significant hepatic enzyme inducers include dexamethasone and phenytoin (CYP2C); caffeine, cigarette smoke, lansoprazole, and omeprazole (CYP1A); and St. John's wort (CYP3A). Diet-drug and herb-drug interactions also occur.[56,57]

Despite the predictability of some of these interactions, many hospital admissions of elderly patients for drug toxicity involve administration of drugs known to interact.[58] Because of the multiplicity of potential interactions, release of new medications, and discovery of new interactions, use of pharmacy or computerized and on-line tools that provide comprehensive up-to-date information and guidelines for avoiding drug interactions is highly recommended. Available tools include the *Physician's Desk Reference* (PDR; traditional, pocket, or on-line versions), PDR handbook of drug interactions (traditional, computer version, or handheld computer version available free of charge at www.PDR.net), the Clinical Pharmacology modules (computer-based), the Medical Letter and the Medical Letter Drug Interactions Program (computer-based), Epocrates for the handheld computer (available free of charge at <www.epocrates.com>), and online pharmacology texts or data bases (the Food and Drug Administration: www.fda.gov/cder, drug reactions section; or www.druginteractions.org), among others. Many individual hospitals or health care systems and pharmacies provide internal reference sources. Information organized by CYP pathways is accessible in a searchable human P450 metabolism data base (www.gentest.com). Specialized clinics, use of specific algorithms, and computer-based dosage programs to monitor oral anticoagulant therapy in outpatients, especially, have been shown to reduce bleeding-related complications.[59]

Other approaches that have been shown to reduce adverse drug reactions in older patients include involvement of pharmacy-trained individuals to assess the appropriateness of doses and medication counseling using

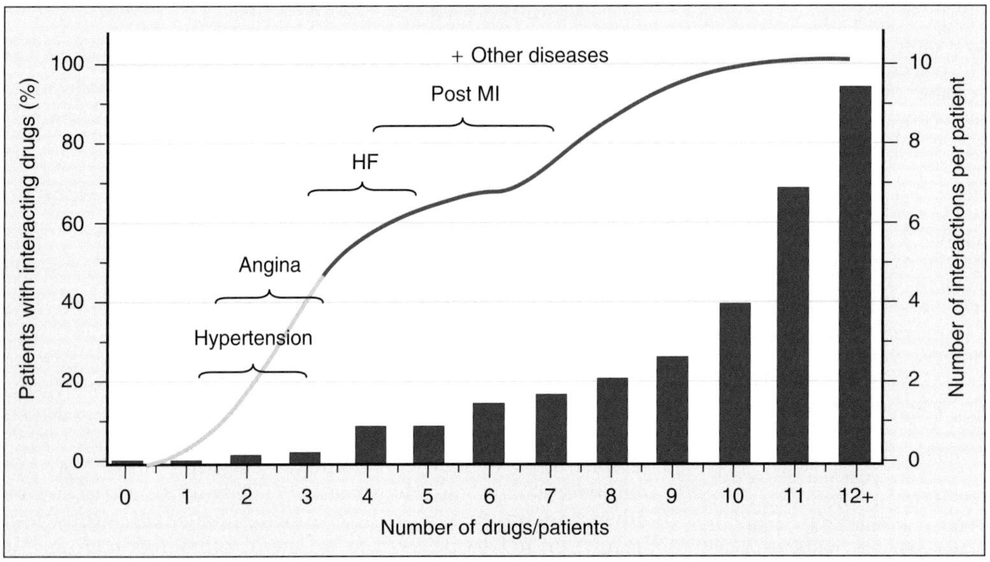

FIGURE 72–6 Relationship between the number of drugs consumed and drug interactions. Current guidelines for the pharmacological management of patients with heart failure (HF) or myocardial infarction (post MI) place them at higher risk for drug interactions (≥4 drugs). (From Schwartz JB: Clinical Pharmacology, American College of Cardiology Self-Assessment Program V, 2003 as modified from Nolan and O'Malley, Age Aging, 1989, and Denham, Br Med Bull, 1990.)

TABLE 72–3 Major Routes of Cytochrome P450 (CYP) Metabolism of Cardiovascular and Commonly Administered Drugs in Elderly People*

Enzyme Isoform	Cardiovascular	Other Substrates	Inducers†	Inhibitors†
CYP1A2	Carvedilol Fluvastatin Guanabenz Mexiletine Pimobendan Propranolol	Acetaminophen Caffeine Imipramine Mirtazapine Nicotine Tacrine Testosterone Theophylline	Rifampin Omeprazole Cigarette smoke Charbroiled, pan-fried meat Lansoprazole	Cimetidine Grapefruit juice Irbesartan, losartan Fluoroquinolones Fluvoxamine Mexiletine Omeprazole Ticlodipine Cholecalciferol
CYP2C 2C8/9 (Polymorphic)	ARB's (irbesartan, losartan) Fluvastatin Torsemide Warfarin	Acenocoumarol Celecoxib Fluoxetine Glipizide NSAIDs (diclofenac, flurbiprofen ibuprofen, meloxicam, naproxen, piroxicam) Phenytoin Tamoxifen Tolbutamide	Dexamethasone Phenobarbital Phenytoin Rifampin Secobarbital	Azole antifungals Amiodarone Cimetidine Fluconazole Isoniazid Sulfaphenazole Ticlodipine
2C19 (Polymorphic)		Cyclophosphamide Diazepam Lansoprazole Omeprazole, pantoprazole Phenytoin Progesterone Selegiline Sulfamethoxazole Tricyclic antidepressants (amitriptyline, clomipramine) Venlafaxine	Rifampin Phenobarbital	Ketoconazole Fluoxetine Fluvoxamine Fluconazole Lansoprazole Omeprazole Ticlodipine
CYP2D6 (Polymorphic)	Beta blockers (carvedilol, metoprolol, propranolol, timolol) Flecainide Metoprolol Mexiletine Pindolol Procainamide Propafenone	Amitriptyline Codeine Dextromethorphan DHEA Haloperidol Omeprazole Ondansetron Paroxetine Risperidone SSRI antidepressants Tamoxifen Tolterodine Tramadol Tricyclic antidepressants (desipramine, imipramine) Venlafaxine	Haloperidol	Amiodarone Ticlodipine Quinidine Chlorpheniramine Cimetidine Clomipramine Desipramine Flecainide Fluoxetine Haloperidol Lansoprazole Methadone Paroxetine
CYP3A4	Beta blockers (bisoprolol, metoprolol) Cilostazol Clopidogrel Dihydropyridines (nifedipine, amlodipine, felodipine, isradipine, nicardipine, nisoldipine) Diltiazem Eplerenone Fenofibrate Flosequinan HMG CoA reductase Inhibitors (atorvastatin, lovastatin, pravastatin, simvastatin) Gemfibrozil Lidocaine Losartan Propafenone	Alprazolam Astemizole Carbamazepine Cisapride Colchicine Clozapine Cyclosporine Diazepam Diclofenac Erythromycin Estradiol, ethinylestradiol Fentanyl Itraconazole Ketoconazole Medroxyprogesterone Midazolam Mirtazapine Nefazodone Paclitaxel	Rifampin Bosentan Nitric oxide St. John's wort	Ketoconazole Itraconazole Protease inhibitors Amiodarone Nefazodone Mibefradil Fluvoxamine Cimetidine Grapefruit juice Cyclosporine Erythromycin Verapamil Diltiazem Doxorubicin Losartan Quinidine Antibiotics (fluroquinolones, e.g.,

Continued

TABLE 72–3 Major Routes of Cytochrome P450 (CYP) Metabolism of Cardiovascular and Commonly Administered Drugs in Elderly People*—cont'd

Enzyme Isoform	Cardiovascular	Other Substrates	Inducers†	Inhibitors†
	Quinidine Verapamil Vesnarinone	Protease inhibitors Rifampin Salmeterol Sildenafil Sulfinpyrazone Tamoxifen Terfenadine Theophylline Triazolam Troglitazone Zolpidem		ciprofloxacin; macrolides, e.g., clarithromycin, troleandomycin)

ARB = angiotensin receptor blocker; DHEA = dehydroepiandrosterone; HMG CoA = 3-hydroxy-3-methylglutaryl coenzyme A; NSAID = nonsteroidal antiinflammatory drug; SSRI = selective serotonin reuptake inhibitor.

*Examples cite major pathway only for drugs that are substrates of multiple CYP pathways.

†In approximate order of potency.

multidisciplinary care team members. A major limitation to the success of all of these approaches is the frequent lack of complete and readily accessible information on medication consumption and disease state information, especially for the older patient with multiple diseases and physicians. Integrated medical record and pharmacy information and interactive data bases have been recommended by numerous panels investigating strategies to reduce adverse drug events and improve medication therapy but are not widely available.[60,61]

ADVERSE PHARMACODYNAMIC EFFECTS. Age-related changes in cardiovascular physiology and dynamics affect pharmacodynamics (see Table 72–1).[6,7,62] Greater age-related sensitivity to parasympathetic stimulation may explain the increased frequency of adverse effects such as urinary retention, constipation, and fecal impaction in older patients who receive drugs with anticholinergic properties (e.g., disopyramide). Gastrointestinal transit time is generally increased in elderly people, and constipation is a frequent complaint of hospitalized, less active, and institutionalized elderly persons. Drug-induced constipation and bowel obstruction can occur in older patients receiving bile acid sequestrants, anticholinergic medications, opiates, and verapamil.

Pharmacodynamic drug interactions are most likely to occur between drugs acting on the same system. A classical example of additive effects that can produce hypotension and postural hypotension in elderly people is the coadministration of direct vasodilators or nitrates combined with alpha blockers, beta blockers, calcium channel blockers, ACE inhibitors, diuretics, or sildenafil. Additional examples are combinations of amiodarone, beta-adrenergic blocking drugs, digoxin, diltiazem, or verapamil producing bradycardia and bleeding caused by increased inhibition of platelet and clotting factors with combinations of aspirin, NSAIDs (including cyclooxygenase 2 [COX-2] selective inhibitors), warfarin, or clopidogrel. Increased potassium concentrations caused by combined administration of ACE inhibitors and potassium-sparing diuretics in older patients are cited as causes of serious adverse drug reactions.[63] Combinations of NSAIDs, including selective COX-2 inhibitors, with ACE inhibitors can also decrease potassium excretion and cause hyperkalemia in the older patient or can cause a decrease in renal function.[64]

Examples of pharmacodynamic interactions with antagonistic effects include increased angina when a beta-agonist or theophylline is given to patients with CAD receiving beta blockers or nondihydropyridine calcium channel antagonists and loss of hypertension control when a drug such as fludrocortisone acetate is given for postural hypotension.

INAPPROPRIATE PRESCRIBING IN ELDERLY PATIENTS. Long-acting benzodiazepines, sedative and hypnotic agents, long-acting oral hypoglycemic agents, selected analgesics, antiemetics, and gastrointestinal antispasmodics are usually considered inappropriate in elderly patients on the basis of an unfavorable risk-to-benefit ratio.[65,66] Although most cardiovascular medications are not considered inappropriate for the older patient, more recent definitions of inappropriate drug use include failure to consider drug-disease interactions and failure to adjust drug dosages for age-related changes, drug duplication, drug-drug interactions, and duration of use. Using these criteria, most drug utilization review studies conclude that inappropriate drug prescribing occurs in a significant fraction of older patients. Explicit criteria for appropriate prescribing of digoxin, calcium channel blockers, and ACE inhibitors in older patients have been developed by expert consensus panels[67] and are accessible at www.ahrqpubs@ahrq.gov. It is pertinent that initial drug dose recommendations from resources such as the PDR may not be the minimally effective dose established by studies done after drug marketing approval or in guideline statements.[68]

ADHERENCE. Adherence taking medications is commonly thought to be lower in older patients than younger patients. In one report, hospitalization for decompensated congestive HF was attributed to medication noncompliance in 42 percent of elderly patients.[69] Contributing factors include the cost of medications; difficulty with understanding directions because of either small print of written directions, hearing impairment, or impaired memory; inadequate instructions; complex dosing regimens; difficulties with packaging materials; and insufficient eduction of the patient, family, or caregiver on medication use. Of these, the most limiting are thought to be the cost of medications, poor education of the patient regarding medications, and cognitive impairment in elderly patients, especially those living alone.[70] In a study of Medicare beneficiaries with CAD, use of HMG CoA reductase inhibitors was directly related to drug payment coverage.[71] It is of note that physicians routinely overestimate patients' adherence taking medications.[72] Assessment of adherence should be part of care and issues related to potential contributors to medication nonadherence should be addressed by prescribing health care professionals. Unfortunately, there are few trials of interventions to improve medication adherence with resources usually available in clinical settings.[73] Strategies to overcome these obstacles include programs for low-income seniors, visual or memory aids, medication dispensing tools, use of geriatric-friendly packaging, assessment of cognitive status and patients' understanding, and inclusion of caregivers or family members in discussion regarding medications.

Vascular Disease

HYPERTENSION (see Chaps. 37 and 38)

Prevalence and Incidence. Diastolic (>90 mm Hg) or systolic (>140 mm Hg) hypertension, or both, occurs in one-half to two-thirds of people older than 65 years. The prevalence varies by race (or genetics) and is slightly higher in black and Hispanic people than in non-Hispanic whites.[74] The profile of hypertension is altered by aging.[75] Systolic hypertension becomes more prevalent with aging, whereas diastolic blood pressure is relatively constant from 50 to 80 years of age with average diastolic pressures higher in men than women from ages 50 to 80 years. Systolic blood pressure rises with aging in both men and women but rises more steeply in women. Systolic blood pressure is lower in women than in men until about age 50 (average age of menopause) but rises to levels equal to those of men by age 65 years. "Isolated" systolic hypertension, without elevation of diastolic blood pressure, is present in about 8 percent of sexagenarians and more than 25 percent of the population older than 80 years. A large percentage of people are unaware that they have hypertension, and hypertension is not controlled in many older patients.[76]

Treatment. The cardiovascular benefits of treatment of systolic as well as diastolic hypertension in older patients have been well established in randomized clinical trials (Table 72–4). The Systolic Hypertension in the Elderly (SHEP) trial[77] also reported reduced rates of dementia in the open blind extended follow-up phase.[78] A comprehensive profile of older patients and responses to antihypertensive strategies, however, is still being elucidated. Most available data suggest that thiazide diuretics are as efficacious as any drug for first-line treatment of hypertension in elderly people[79] and offer advantages of use that include health outcomes and price as well as preservation of bone mineral density in older adults.[80,81] There may also be a role for ACE inhibitors compared with diuretics as first-line therapy in some older white men.[82] Neither the alpha blocker doxazosin nor dihydropyridine calcium channel blockers compare favorably with other first-line strategies for older patients with HF; and blacks may benefit less from ACE inhibitors (see Chaps. 37 and 38 for further discussion of hypertensive subgroups). Because most older patients require second (or third) medications to reach target blood pressures, treatment decisions for elderly patients with hypertension should focus on control of blood pressure and extend beyond first-line therapy.

Consideration of conditions that are highly prevalent in elderly people in the choice of antihypertensive therapy can optimize effects; minimize adverse effects, cost, and the number of medications; and increase adherence. In addition to recommendations based on concomitant cardiovascular diseases recognized in hypertension treatment guidelines (Table 72–5),[83,84] other conditions in elderly people warrant consideration. In older people, arthritis is second in prevalence to cardiovascular disease and NSAIDs are among the most frequently consumed drugs (prescription and over the counter). In addition to the potential for adverse renal effects or hyperkalemia when NSAIDs are given in combination with ACE inhibitors, angiotensin receptor blockers, or aldosterone antagonists, loss of blood pressure control and HF have been precipitated by nonselective NSAIDs as well as COX-2-selective NSAIDs. Age-related bone loss is accelerated in older men and women and is the major contributing cause of

TABLE 72–4 Trials of Blood Pressure Reduction in Elderly People

				Risk Reduction (%)			
Trial	***N***	**Age (yr)**	**Type**	***Stroke***	***CAD***	***HF***	***All CVD***
HDFP	2374	60-69	D	44	15	NR	16
Australian	582	60-69	D	33	18	NR	31
EWPHE	840	>60	D (+S)	36	20	22	29
Coope	884	60-79	D (+S)	42	−3	32	24
STOP-HTN	1627	70-84	D (+S)	47	13	51	40
MRC	4396	65-74	D (+S)	25	19	NR	17
SHEP	4736	≥60	S	33	27	55	32
Syst-Eur	4695	≥60	S	42	26	36	31
STONE	1632	60-79	S	57	6	68	60
Syst-China	2394	≥60	S	38	33	38	37

Age = age at study entry; CAD = coronary artery disease; all CVD = all cardiovascular disease composite endpoint; D = diastolic; EWPHE = European Working Party on High Blood Pressure in the Elderly; HDFP = Hypertension Detection and Follow-up Program; HF = heart failure; MRC = Medical Research Council; NR = not reported; S = systolic; SHEP = Systolic Hypertension in the Elderly Program; STONE = Shanghai Trial of Hypertension in the Elderly; Syst-China = Systolic Hypertension in China; Syst-Eur = Systolic Hypertension in Europe; type = type of hypertension.

References: randomized trials of pharmacological blood pressure reduction in the elderly: (1) HDFP: Five-year findings of the hypertension detection and follow up program: I. Reduction in mortality of persons with high blood pressure, including mild hypertension. JAMA 242:2562, 1979. Five-year findings of the hypertension detection and follow-up program: II. Mortality by race, sex and age. Hypertension detection and follow-up program cooperative. JAMA 242:2572, 1979. (2) Treatment of mild hypertension in the elderly: A study initiated and administered by the National Heart Foundation of Australia. Med J Austr 2:398, 1981. (3) Amery A, Birkenhäger W, Brixko P, et al: Mortality and morbidity results from the European Working Party on High Blood Pressure in the Elderly trial. Lancet 1:1349, 1985. (4) Coope J, Warrender TS: Randomised trial of treatment of hypertension in elderly patients in primary care. BMJ 293:1145, 1986. (5) Dahlöf B, Lindholm LH, Hansson L, et al: Morbidity and mortality in the Swedish Trial in Old Patients with Hypertension (STOP-hypertension). Lancet 338:1281, 1991. (6) MRC Working Party: Medical Research Council trial of treatment of hypertension in older adults: Principal results. BMJ 304:405, 1992. (7) SHEP Cooperative Research Group: Prevention of stroke by antihypertensive drug treatment in older persons with isolated systolic hypertension: Final results of the Systolic Hypertension in the Elderly Program (SHEP). JAMA 265:3255, 1991. (8) Syst-Eur: Staessen J, Fagard R, Thijs L, et al: Randomised double-blind comparison of placebo and active treatment for older patients with isolated systolic hypertension. Lancet 350:757, 1997. (9) Gong L, Zwang W, Zhu Y: Shanghai Trial of Nifedipine in the Elderly. Seventh European Meeting on Hypertension; June 9-12 1995; Milan. (10) Liu L, Wang JG, Gong L, et al for the Systolic Hypertension in China (Syst-China) Collaborative Group: Comparison of active treatment and placebo for older patients with isolated systolic hypertension. J Hypertens 16:1823, 1998.

TABLE 72–5 Considerations for Pharmacologic Therapy of Older Patients with Hypertension and Other Disorders

Hypertension Plus	Efficacy Considerations	Toxicity and Adverse Effect Considerations
Arthritis	—	ACE, ARB, aldosterone antagonist interactions with NSAIDs
Atrial fibrillation	Beta blocker,* calcium channel blocker (non-DHP),* amiodarone	Interactions with warfarin
Atrioventricular block	—	Beta blockers, non-DHP calcium channel blockers
Carotid disease or stroke	Calcium channel blocker,* ACE†	
Constipation	—	Verapamil
Coronary artery disease	Beta blocker,*,† calcium channel blocker*,†	Nitrates and postural hypotension
Dementia	Clonidine‡	
Diabetes	ACE,*,† ARB,*,† calcium channel blocker (non-DHP),† beta blocker†	
Gout		Diuretics
Heart failure	ACE,*,† ARB*,† + loop diuretic,*,† ± beta blocker,*,† ± aldosterone antagonist*,†,§	Calcium channel blockers (possible) ACE, ARB, aldosterone antagonist, and hyperkalemia
Hyponatremia	—	Diuretic (especially with SSRI)
Incontinence	—	Diuretic
Myocardial infarction	Beta blocker,*,† ± ACE,*,† ± aldosterone antagonist†	ACE, ARB, aldosterone antagonist, and hyperkalemia
Osteoporosis	Thiazides and bone density preservation	—
Peripheral artery disease	Calcium channel blocker (DHP)*	Beta blocker (if severe)
Postural hypotension	Thiazide‖	Alpha blocker, calcium channel blockers (DHP)
Prostatic hypertrophy	Alpha blocker*	
Renal failure	ACE,*,† ARB,*,† ACE + ARB; loop diuretic*	Aldosterone antagonists
Ventricular arrhythmias	Beta blocker*	Thiazide, loop diuretics, and hypokalemia

*Recommendations for first-line therapy from the European Society of Cardiology guidelines for the management of arterial hypertension.[84]

†Recommendations for second-line agents usually added to thiazide diuretics from the Seventh Report of the Joint National Committee on Prevention, Detection, Evaluation, and Treatment of High Blood Pressure.[83]

‡Only available transdermal formulation for patients unable to swallow or who refuse oral medications.

§Systolic heart failure only.

‖Nursing home patients.

ACE = angiotensin-converting enzyme inhibitor; ARB = angiotensin receptor blocking inhibitor; DHP = dihydropyridine; NSAID = nonsteroidal antiinflammatory drug; SSRI = selective serotonin reuptake inhibitor.

osteoporosis. Osteoporosis is a major risk factor for fractures in older people, and the lifetime risk of osteoporotic fracture in Americans is estimated as 40 percent for women and 13 percent for men. Thiazide administration has been associated with higher bone mineral density and a reduction in risk of hip fractures in epidemiological studies and preservation of bone mineral density compared with placebo in older adults.[81]

Effects of thiazides plus other agents have been evaluated in hypertension trials involving elderly patients. The Losartan Intervention for Endpoint reduction in hypertension study (LIFE) involving primarily whites with systolic hypertension and left ventricular hypertrophy found similar myocardial event and death rates with thiazides plus losartan compared with thiazides plus beta blockers, with more strokes and new-onset diabetes in the beta blocker arm.[85] The Study on Cognition and Prognosis in the Elderly (SCOPE) compared effects of low-dose diuretic therapy combined with either candesartan or placebo.[86] The combined incidence of cardiovascular death, nonfatal myocardial infarction, and nonfatal stroke did not differ; but candesartan plus thiazide was associated with a reduction in stroke risk compared with the thiazide plus placebo group. No difference in the rate of cognitive decline was seen between groups.

The older patients for whom thiazide diuretics may not be the best choice include patients with urinary frequency problems—stress incontinence, urinary frequency with or without incontinence related to prostatic hypertrophy, overactive bladders—and patients needing assistance with toileting. These patients may be more compliant with drugs that do not increase urinary frequency. Table 72–5 presents suggested antihypertensive regimens in older patients based on the presence of hypertension and concomitant diseases. Additional data on frequent geriatric problems and medications to use or avoid are available at www.geriatricsatyourfingertips.com.

Additional Considerations. Both the Seventh Report of the Joint National Committee on Prevention, Detection, Evaluation, and Treatment of High Blood Pressure (JNC 7)[83] and the European Guidelines for the Management of Arterial Hypertension[84] recommend lower initial drug dosages and slower medication titration in older patients and point out the need to monitor for postural hypotension.

A decrease in standing systolic blood pressure is estimated to be present in 15 percent of 70- to 74-year-old community-dwelling men or women and up to 30 percent of patients with systolic hypertension.[87] Postural hypotension of greater than 20 mm Hg or 20 percent of systolic pressure is a risk factor for falls and fractures that are associated with significant morbidity and mortality.[88] Antihypertensive medications add to the risk of postural hypotension, as do many antiparkinsonian agents, antipsychotic agents, or tricyclic antidepressant drugs. Postural blood pressure changes should be assessed (after more than 5 minutes supine, immediately after standing, and 2 minutes after standing) in older patients and volume depletion avoided.

Postprandial falls in both systolic and diastolic blood pressure occur in hospitalized, institutionalized,[89] and community-dwelling elderly persons.[90] The greatest fall occurs about 1 hour after eating, and the blood pressure returns to fasting levels 3 to 4 hours after eating. Blood pressure should be measured at least 4 hours after meals, and vasoactive medications with rapid absorption and peaks should not be administered with meals.

Smaller trials have shown weight loss and sodium restriction to be effective in patients from 65 to 75 years of age.[91] Manipulation of dietary calcium can also reverse some of the age-related change in blood pressure.[92]

The optimal blood pressure target is not known for the very old. Patients older than 80 years are a heterogeneous group. Meta-analyses of randomized trial data have concluded that there are cardiovascular morbidity benefits without mortality benefit for treatment of hypertension in patients older than 80 years[93] but have also reported a slightly higher overall risk of death in treated hypertensives older than 80 years compared with reduced deaths in patients aged 60 to 80 years.[94]

The frailest and oldest people may reside in long-term care facilities. It is estimated that 30 to 70 percent are hypertensive and 30 percent have postural hypotension. Diuretic therapy appears to be effective in controlling systolic blood pressure in these patients and may also decrease postural hypotension.[95]

Table 72-6 summarizes the approach to hypertension in older patients.

CORONARY ARTERY DISEASE (see Chaps. 47 to 50)

Prevalence and Incidence. Both the prevalence and severity of atherosclerotic CAD increase with age in men and women. Autopsy studies show that more than half of people older than 60 years have significant CAD with increasing prevalence of left main or triple-vessel CAD with older age. Using electrocardiographic (ECG) evidence of myocardial infarction, abnormal echocardiogram, carotid intimal thickness, or abnormal ankle-brachial index as measures of subclinical vascular disease in community-dwelling elderly people in the Cardiovascular Health Study, abnormalities were detected in 22 percent of women and 33 percent of men aged 65 to 70 years and 43 percent of women and 45 percent of men older than 85 years.[96-98] The lifetime risk of developing symptomatic CAD is estimated as 1 in 3 for men and 1 in 4 for women, with onset of symptoms about 10 years earlier in men than women and with hypertension, diabetes, and lipid abnormalities influencing individual risk.[99] By 80 years of age, similar frequencies of symptomatic CAD of about 20 to 30 percent are seen in men and women. Because of the increasing proportion of women at older ages, however, population studies show more absolute numbers of women with angina compared with men in the community.

TABLE 72–6 Approach to Hypertension in Older Patients

Systolic as well as diastolic hypertension should be treated • Diastolic target is <90 mm Hg • Systolic target is <140 mm Hg • Individualization is needed for patients older than 80 years
Initial therapy is often a low dose of a thiazide diuretic or is based on concomitant diseases (cardiac and noncardiac)
Drug dosing regimens should be reduced for age- and disease-related changes in drug metabolism and for drug-drug interactions
Patients should be monitored for postural hypotension • Blood pressure should be measured at least 4 hr from meals
Patients should be monitored for adverse effects and drug interactions, especially • Hypovolemia with diuretics • Hyperkalemia with angiotensin-converting enzyme, angiotensin receptor blocker, aldosterone antagonists • Renal function

Diagnosis

HISTORY. Angina symptoms are more likely to be absent or ischemia silent in older patients compared with young patients. Symptoms are also more likely to be termed "atypical" in older patients because the description differs from the classical description of substernal pressure with exertion. Symptoms may be described primarily as dyspnea, shoulder or back pain, weakness, fatigue (in women), or epigastric discomfort and may be precipitated by concurrent illnesses. Some older patients describe symptoms with effort but others may not because of limited physical exertion or altered manifestations of pain related to concomitant diabetes or possible age-related changes. Symptoms in these patients may occur at rest or during mental stress. Memory impairment may also limit the accuracy of the history. Lack of symptoms during evidence of myocardial ischemia on electrocardiography (silent ischemia) has been reported in 20 to 50 percent of patients 65 years of age or older.

TESTING FOR ISCHEMIA (see Chap. 50). The high prevalence of resting ST-T abnormalities in older people results in a modest age-associated reduction in specificity of exercise electrocardiography. Treadmill exercise testing can provide prognostic information in patients able to exercise sufficiently and can also provide information regarding functional capacity and exercise tolerance. Exercise results can be enhanced by the use of modified protocols beginning with low-intensity exercise. The ACC/AHA Guidelines on Exercise Testing estimate a slightly higher sensitivity (84 percent) and lower specificity (70 percent) in patients older than 75 years than in younger patients.[100] Echocardiography and nuclear testing can be used to overcome some of the limitations of ECG interpretation. In older patients unable to exercise, pharmacological agents such as dipyridamole or adenosine can be used with nuclear scintigraphy to assess myocardial perfusion at rest and after vasodilation; or agents such as dobutamine can be combined with echocardiography to assess ventricular function at rest and during increased myocardial demand.[101] Because of the high prevalence of coronary calcification with or without coronary flow decrease in the older population, electron beam cinetomography has little prognostic role in the older patient.

Treatment. Therapeutic goals and management goals that have been established for chronic stable angina are targeted primarily at risk reduction and symptom relief without modification for older patients[102] (see Chap. 50). No age restriction is considered for treatment of patients with CAD unless life expectancy is less than 2 years. Most data on lipid lowering for elderly people come from trials of HMG CoA reductase inhibitors (Table 72–7), with only the Heart Protection Study enrolling significant numbers of women and including patients older than 73.[103] The Heart Protection Study of low-density lipoprotein (LDL) cholesterol lowering with the HMG CoA reductase inhibitor simvastatin in patients with CAD from 40 to 80 years of age with concomitant disease demonstrated decreased total mortality in prespecified subgroups of women, patients older than 75, diabetics, and patients without elevated LDL cholesterol levels. Of the two large primary prevention trials of lipid lowering with HMG CoA reductase inhibitors, one enrolled only men up to age 64 and the other had an upper age cutoff of 73 years.[104,105] Thus, there are no published data about the use of cholesterol-lowering drugs for primary prevention in patients older than 75, especially women.

The incidence of rhabdomyolysis is low with HMG CoA reductase inhibitors, but risk factors for statin-induced myopathy include older age (>80 and women more than men), smaller body frame and frailty, multisystem disease (including chronic renal insufficiency, especially related to diabetes), the perioperative period, coadministration of certain medications (fibrates, nicotinic acid, cyclosporine,

TABLE 72–7 Secondary Prevention Trials of Lipid-Lowering Therapy with Elderly Participants

Study	Patients	N	% Older than 65 (n) (%, Women, n)	Drug (Dose)	Major Results
Scandinavian Simvastatin Survival Study (4S) Trial	CAD	4444	23% (1021) (19%, 827)	Simvastatin (20-40 mg/d)	Reduced all-cause and CAD mortality, CAD events, coronary revascularization, and stroke
Cholesterol and Recurrent Events (CARE) Trial	Post-MI	4159	31% (1283) (14%, 576)	Pravastatin (40 mg/d)	Reduced CAD mortality, death or events, coronary revascularization, and stroke
Long-Term Intervention with Pravastatin in Ischaemic Disease (LIPID) Study	Post-MI or unstable angina	9014	39% (3514) (17%, 1516)	Pravastatin (40 mg/d)	Reduced all-cause mortality, CAD death or events, coronary revascularization, and stroke
Veterans Affairs Cooperative Studies Program High-Density Lipoprotein Cholesterol Intervention Trial (VA-HIT)	CAD + high cholesterol and low HDL	2531	76%*(1936) (0, 0)	Gemfibrozil (1200 mg/d)	Reduced death from cardiovascular cause, no difference in coronary revascularization rates
Heart Protection Study (HPS)	CAD + other vascular disease, diabetes or hypertension	>20,000	28%† (5806) (33%, 5082)	Simvastatin (40 mg/d)	Reduced all-cause mortality, reduced cardiovascular events, reduced coronary revascularizations, and reduced stroke

*Age older than 60.
†Age older than 70.
CAD = coronary artery disease; MI = myocardial infarction.
References: Randomised trial of cholesterol lowering in 4444 patients with coronary heart disease: The Scandinavian Simvastatin Survival Study (4S). Lancet 344:1383, 1994. Miettinen T, Pyorala K, Olsson A, et al: Cholesterol-lowering therapy in women and elderly patients with myocardial infarction or angina pectoris. Findings from the Scandinavian Simvastatin Survival Study (4S). Circulation 96:4211, 1997. Sacks F, Pfeffer M, Moye L, et al: The effect of pravastatin on coronary events after myocardial infarction in patients with average cholesterol levels. Cholesterol and Recurrent Events Trial investigators. N Engl J Med 335:1001, 1996. Lewis S, Moye L, Sacks F, et al: Effect of pravastatin on cardiovascular events in older patients with myocardial infarction and cholesterol levels in the average range. Results of the Cholesterol and Recurrent Events (CARE) Trial. Ann Intern Med 129:681, 1998. The Long-Term Intervention with Pravastatin in Ischaemic Disease (LIPID) Study Group: Prevention of cardiovascular events and death with pravastatin in patients with coronary heart disease and a broad range of initial cholesterol levels. N Engl J Med 339:1349, 1998. Rubins H, Robins S, Collins D, et al for the Veterans Affairs High-density Lipoprotein Cholesterol Intervention Trial Study Group: Gemfibrozil for the secondary prevention of coronary heart disease in men with low levels of high-density lipoprotein cholesterol. N Engl J Med 341:410, 1999. Heart Protection Study Collaborative Group: MRC/BHF Heart Protection Study of cholesterol lowering with simvastatin in 20,536 high-risk individuals: A randomised placebo-controlled trial. Lancet 360:7, 2002.

azole antifungals, macrolide antibiotics, erythromycin, clarithromycin, nefazodone, verapamil, amiodarone), and alcohol abuse. Symptoms of myopathy may be difficult to differentiate from other types of pain in the older patient, and myopathy may not be recognized because of cognitive impairment or the presence of other musculoskeletal disorders. The smallest effective dose should be used and signs and symptoms monitored, and there should be a low threshold for laboratory tests. Muscle strength testing may be helpful in evaluating symptoms in older patients, including simple assessments of the ability to rise from a chair or climb stairs.

SPECIAL CONSIDERATIONS. Marked vasodilation related to rapid absorption or higher peak effects of isosorbide dinitrates can exacerbate postural hypotension, and agents with smooth concentration versus time profiles such as mononitrates or transdermal formulations may be preferred for daily administration, although cost may be prohibitive. Beta blockers have not been shown to increase the occurrence of depression in randomized trials, but beta blockers that are not lipophilic (e.g., atenolol, nadolol) may produce fewer central nervous system effects. Calcium channel blockers, especially the dihydropyridines, can produce pedal edema more frequently in the older patient. Shorter acting formulations can produce or exacerbate postural hypotension and should be avoided. Verapamil can exacerbate constipation, especially in inactive elderly persons. Beta blockers and nondihydropyridine calcium channel blockers both should be avoided in the presence of sinus node disease.

REVASCULARIZATION. There is increasing experience with both percutaneous coronary intervention (PCI) and coronary artery bypass grafting (CABG) in older patients. Half of all PCI and CABG procedures are performed in patients older than 65 years, with one-third of coronary artery revascularization procedures performed in patients older than 70 years. Randomized trials have demonstrated efficacy and successful outcomes in patients, including limited numbers of older patients (Table 72–8) (see Chap. 48). The largest enrollment of patients older than 75 years to date (109 patients) was in the Bypass Angioplasty Revascularization Investigation (BARI) trial involving patients with multivessel disease. Patients aged 65 to 80 had higher early morbidity and mortality after CABG compared with PCI but greater angina relief and fewer repeated procedures after CABG. Stroke was more common after CABG than after percutaneous transluminal coronary angioplasty (PTCA; 1.7 versus 0.2 percent), and HF and pulmonary edema were more common after PTCA (4.0 versus 1.3 percent). The 5-year survival rate was over 80 percent for both procedures (86 percent after CABG and 81.4 percent after PTCA) in these highly selected patients.[106] Women and minorities were underrepresented. Reports from the National Cardiovascular Revascularization Network also show increased early mortality rates after revascularization procedures in older patients, with a more rapid rise in the mortality risk in patients older than 75 years (Fig. 72–7).[107,108] Registry data suggest an in-hospital mortality risk of PCI of less than 1 percent in patients younger than 60 years that

TABLE 72–8 Representation of Elderly Patients with Coronary Artery Disease in Trials of Revascularization

Trial Name	Enrollment Year(s)	Treatment Comparisons	Number Enrolled	Age Inclusion	Number Enrolled ≥75 yr of Age
CASS	1970s	CABG vs. medical	780	Age ≤65 yr	0
VA	1970s	CABG vs. medical	686	None	0
European	1970s	CABG vs. medical	767	Age <65 yr	0
RITA	1980s-1990s	CABG vs. PCI	1011	None	22
EAST	1980s-1990	CABG vs. PCI	392	None	36
GABI	1986-1991	CABG vs. PCI	359	Age <75 yr	0
CABRI	1980s-1990s	CABG vs. PCI	1054	Age ≤75 yr	0
BARI	Late 1980s-1990s	CABG vs. PCI	1829	Age <80 yr	109
ERACI	1980s	CABG vs. PCI	127	Age <76	N/A (few)
ACME	Late 1980s	PCI vs. medical	328	N/A (mean = 60)	N/A
ARTS	1997-1998	PCI + stent vs. CABG	1205	Age ≤83 yr	70†
TIME	1996-2000	PCI or CABG vs. medical	282	>75 yr	282

ACME = Angioplasty Compared to Medicine Study (VA study); ARTS = Arterial Revascularization Therapy Study Trial; BARI = Bypass Angioplasty Revascularization Investigation; CABG = coronary artery bypass graft; N/A = not available; CABRI = Coronary Artery versus Bypass Revascularization Investigation; CASS = Coronary Artery Surgery Study; EAST = Emory Angioplasty versus Surgery Trial; ERACI = Argentine Randomized Trial of Percutaneous Transluminal Coronary Angioplasty versus Coronary Artery Bypass Surgery in Multivessel Disease; European = European Coronary Surgery Study; GABI = German Angioplasty versus Bypass Surgery Trial; PCI = percutaneous coronary intervention; RITA = Randomized Intervention Treatment of Angina; TIME = Trial of Invasive versus Medical Therapy in Elderly patients; VA = VA Cooperative Study of Coronary Artery Bypass for Stable Angina.

†Personal communication.

increases to about 4 percent in patients older than 75 years. Data for small numbers of patients older than 90 years suggest limited clinical benefit despite procedural success. Early CABG mortality rates increase from less than 2 percent in patients younger than 60 years to between 6 and 8 percent in patients older than 75 years; rates approaching 10 percent have been reported in patients older than 80 years. Elderly women are at highest risk, in part because of comorbid conditions.

Nonfatal complications with procedures also increase with age. PCI is associated with a slightly less than 1 percent risk of permanent stroke or coma and CABG is associated with a 3 to 6 percent incidence of permanent stroke or coma in patients older than 75 years. In the immediate postoperative period, longer durations of ventilatory support, greater need for inotropic support and intraaortic balloon placement, greater incidence of bleeding, delirium, renal failure, perioperative infarction, and infection are seen in older patients compared with younger patients. The highest rates of complications are usually seen in older women and in patients undergoing emergency procedures.

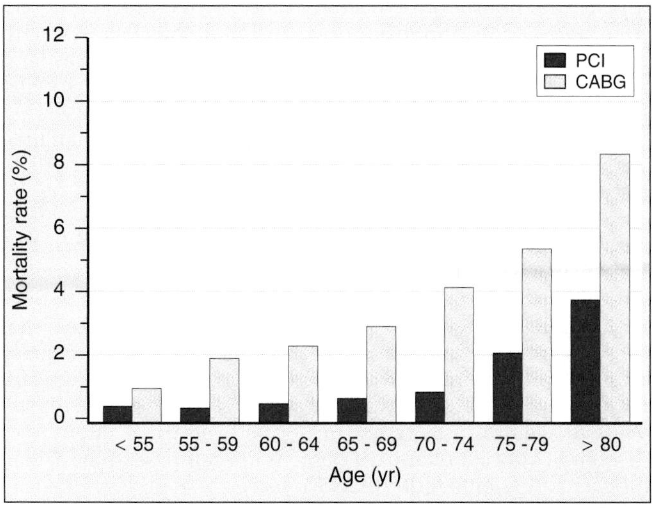

FIGURE 72–7 In-hospital mortality rates reported for revascularization procedures by age group. CABG = coronary artery bypass graft surgery; PCI = percutaneous intervention of all types. (Data from the National Cardiovascular Revascularization Network as reported by Alexander K, Anstrom K, Muhlbaier L, et al: Outcomes of cardiac surgery in patients ≥ 80 years: Results from the National Cardiovascular Network. J Am Coll Cardiol 35:731, 2000 and available at www.sgcard.org.)

In addition to the increased immediate mortality and morbidity associated with revascularization in older patients, the duration of disability and rehabilitation after procedures is usually longer for older persons. Preoperative considerations for older patients should address the potential need for in-home assistance or extended-care hospitalization. Postoperative considerations should also include evaluation for depression (see later). A current unknown is the precise risk of postoperative cognitive impairment in older patients, although neuropsychological testing detects impairment in significant numbers of patients after CABG.[109]

The Trial of Invasive versus Medical Therapy in Elderly patients (TIME) study compared invasive (PCI or CABG) versus optimized medical therapy in CAD patients older than 75 years with angina refractory to standard therapy.[110] Although the initial analysis at 6 months showed an advantage for revascularization, the advantage was no longer present at 1 year. Revascularization presented an early risk of death and complications and optimized medical therapy carried a chance of later events (hospitalization and revascularization) without a clear advantage of either strategy. This is the only revascularization study to enroll significant numbers of patients older than 75 years (see Table 72-8) and enroll significant numbers of women (40 percent). Data remain limited on comparisons involving stents, drug-eluting stents, and off-pump surgery in older groups.

Special Considerations. The ACC/AHA coronary bypass surgery and PCI guidelines conclude that age alone should not be used as the sole criterion when considering revascularization procedures (see www.acc.org or www.americanheart.org).[111] There is a clear role for individualized prognostic information based on multiple clinical factors and respect for patients' preferences in the decision-making process.[107-109,112] The possibility of disability or prolonged hospitalization after interventions must be considered. Recurrent angina or myocardial infarction may not be viewed as having the same negative impact as a stroke by many older patients. For the patient unable to make decisions, involvement of family members or agents is key to choices reflecting the prior wishes of the patient.

Acute Myocardial Infarction (see Chaps. 46 and 47). About 60 percent of hospital admissions for AMI are of people older than 65 years. With increasing age, the gender composition of patients presenting with AMI changes from predominantly men presenting in middle age, to equal number of men and women presenting between the ages of 75 to 84, to the majority of patients with AMI being women at ages older than 80 years. A review of the national Cooperative Cardiovascular Project (CCP) cohort of Medicare beneficiaries further characterized elderly patients presenting with AMI.[113] As age increases past 65 years, there are more patients with functional limitation, HF, prior coronary disease, and renal insufficiency; more women; and lower proportions of diabetics, smokers, or patients with prior revascularization. As age increased from 65 to more than 85 years, the proportion presenting with chest pain and ST elevation on electrocardiography within 6 hours of symptom onset also decreased. Mortality is at least threefold higher in patients older than 85 years than in patients younger than 65 years. Thus, the older old patient with AMI differs from both middle-aged and younger elderly patients.[114]

DIAGNOSIS. Chest pain or discomfort is the most common complaint in older as well as younger patients, but older patients may also present with sudden pulmonary edema or neurological symptoms such as syncope, stroke, or confusion. The electrocardiogram is also more likely to be nondiagnostic (because of baseline abnormalities of ventricular hypertrophy, intraventricular conduction, or pacing). The combination of atypical symptoms and nondiagnostic ECG findings increases the importance of rapid laboratory testing for circulating markers of myocardial damage such as troponin.

TREATMENT

THROMBOLYSIS. Randomized clinical trials of the effects of thrombolysis enrolled few patients older than 75 to 80 years. For patients up to the age of 75 years, most trials showed that fibrinolytic therapy is associated with a survival advantage similar to or greater than that seen in younger patients with ST elevation myocardial infarction. Population-based studies have suggested that community-dwelling elderly patients older than 75 years treated with thrombolytics, however, have an increased risk of ICH of approximately 1.4 percent[115] and some subgroups may not have an overall benefit.[116,117] Those with a high risk for ICH include patients older than 75 years, women, blacks, small patients (<65 kg in women and <80 kg for men), those with prior stroke, patients with systolic blood pressure greater than 160 mm Hg, and patients administered tissue plasminogen activator as compared with other agents. Cardiac rupture risk with thrombolysis is also increased in patients older than 70 years and in women, with an incidence of 0.5 to 2 percent.[32,118,119] The risk of cardiac rupture does not appear to be related to the intensity of anticoagulation. Complication rates of minor and major bleeding are also higher in older patients than younger patients. The ACC/AHA guidelines for management of myocardial infarction published in 1999 recommended thrombolytic administration in patients younger than 75 years with acute ischemic symptoms associated with ST elevation or left bundle branch block who present within 12 hours of symptom onset but acknowledged disagreement on recommendations for patients with this presentation who are older than 75 years[54] (accessible at www.acc.org; www.americanheart.org).

Fibrinolytic agents, especially fibrin-specific agents, are also associated with increased stroke risk related to ICH in the over 75 to 80 age group. Most agents are administered in combination with low-molecular-weight heparin, and dosage adjustments for weight may decrease risks of bleeding.

ANTIPLATELET AGENTS. Trial data show that aspirin reduces mortality in patients older than 70 years and aspirin is recommended for routine administration to older patients with AMI, although older patients have been less likely to receive aspirin than younger patients. The addition of clopidogrel to aspirin after non-ST-segment elevation myocardial infarction reduced major event rates by 20 percent, with similar absolute reductions in patients younger and older than 65 years; there are no significant data on patients older than 75 years. Newer glycoprotein (GP) IIb/IIIa inhibitors appear efficacious in patients older than 70 years, although net benefit may decline with increasing age. In clinical trials, bleeding risk was increased about twofold with GP IIb/IIIa inhibitors, with the risk being about 2 percent. Registry data estimate the increased risk of bleeding to be similar, with about a twofold greater (or 2 percent) risk in patients undergoing PCI who receive GP IIb/IIIa inhibitors compared with patients who do not.[120] A review of the Food and Drug Administration adverse event reports related to GP IIb/IIIa inhibitor administration found deaths in patients with a mean age of 69 to be associated with excessive bleeding, with intracranial bleeding the most common site.[121] It appears that older age is associated with an increased bleeding risk with GP IIb/IIIa inhibitors as well as aspirin and thrombolytics.

INVASIVE STRATEGIES. Results from several studies and data base reviews suggest that primary angioplasty in experienced centers is associated with improved outcomes compared with thrombolytic strategies in elderly patients with ST elevation AMI.[122,123] Primary angioplasty is associated with increased bleeding at the access site as well as increased transfusion requirements in the elderly. PCI procedures are also associated with an increased risk for contrast agent–mediated renal dysfunction in older patients that is an important predictor of adverse outcomes. The benefits of angioplasty compared with those of fibrinolysis have not been convincingly demonstrated in very elderly patients but are being investigated. Reperfusion strategies in elderly patients with acute coronary syndromes are under investigation by the Primary Angioplasty in Myocardial Infarction (PAMI) group.[124]

BETA BLOCKERS. Beta blocker administration is recommended for all patients with AMI regardless of age in the absence of contraindications. Age-related dosage adjustments are appropriate.

ANGIOTENSIN-CONVERTING ENZYME INHIBITORS. In the presence of left ventricular systolic dysfunction or anterior wall myocardial infarction, ACE inhibitors are recommended within the first 24 hours of onset of AMI. ACE inhibitors are recommended after 24 hours for all other patients with myocardial infarction, especially those with reduced left ventricular ejection and prior myocardial infarction. As with other agents in elderly people, smaller initial doses and slower titration are indicated, as is close monitoring of renal function.

Mortality rates are usually higher in older women than men with AMI, as are adverse outcomes with thrombolytics, fibrinolytics, and GP IIb/IIIa inhibitors.[114]

Post-Myocardial Infarction. Recommendations for administration of aspirin, beta blockers, ACE inhibitors, and lipid-lowering drugs for the post-myocardial infarction patient are based on clinical trial data showing benefit in populations that have included elderly patients. Data suggest that these agents are underutilized in older patients, especially women and minorities. Analyses of care delivery to Medicare recipients estimate that 24 percent of eligible patients 65 years of age or older are not prescribed aspirin at the time of discharge after AMI, and 50 percent are not prescribed a beta blocker.[125] Patients older than 75 years are even less likely to receive these therapies than patients 65 to 74 years of age. In contrast, calcium antagonist drugs may be more frequently prescribed in older than younger post-myocardial infarction patients. There is no role for routine administration of antiarrhythmic agents after myocardial infarction (with the exception of beta blockers).

ANTIDEPRESSANTS. Depression is considered relatively common in elderly persons, affecting 10 percent of community-dwelling older people. The prevalence of depression in patients after myocardial infarction is estimated at 20 percent for major depression to 27 percent for minor depression. Studies have shown associations between depression, low perceived social support, and increased cardiac morbidity and mortality in post-myocardial infarction patients[126] and patients undergoing CABG.[127,128] Individual trials of counseling interventions in patients with depression have not shown cardiac benefit, but meta-analyses suggest benefit.[129] Trials have addressed the efficacy and safety of SSRI antidepressant therapy in patients with depression after acute coronary syndromes or myocardial infarction. The Sertraline Antidepressant Heart Attack Randomized Trial (SADHART) involving depressed patients with unstable angina or myocardial infarction compared placebo with sertraline.[130] A small benefit was seen with sertraline that reached significance for patients with recurrent depression. A larger randomized trial, the Enhancing Recovery in Coronary Heart Disease Patients (ENRICHD) trial, compared interventions of cognitive therapy or cognitive therapy combined with an SSRI (sertraline) with "usual" care in patients diagnosed with depression early after myocardial infarction.[131] The intervention group showed increased quality of life and overall function without reduction in cardiac events or mortality after 2 years of treatment. Many patients assigned to usual care also received antidepressants (20.6 percent in the usual care group versus 28 percent in the intervention group). A post hoc analysis of all participants found SSRI use associated with reduced rates of death (hazard ratio = 0.58) and the combined endpoint of death or nonfatal myocardial infarction (hazard ratio = 0.57) without evidence of improvement of depression. General recommendations for all older patients with chronic medical diseases include screening for depression. Initial screening can take the form of a simple two-question test or the geriatric depression screen for older patients followed by additional evaluation for patients with answers suggesting the presence of depression.[132]

MODIFICATIONS IN THERAPY. Analyses showed that older post-myocardial infarction patients who were prescribed beta blockers had a greater risk of rehospitalization with HF if given high doses compared with low doses.[133] It is possible that higher use of beta blockers in the post-myocardial infarction regimen of older patients might be reached if recommendations were for lower and better tolerated doses of these drugs.

HORMONE REPLACEMENT THERAPY. Randomized trials comparing administration of hormone replacement therapy in the form of combined estrogen and progesterone or estrogen alone have shown overall lack of cardiovascular morbidity or mortality benefit and potential harm for both secondary and primary prevention in postmenopausal women.[134-135b] Estrogen with progesterone also increases both the risk of breast cancer and the invasiveness of tumors. Unopposed estrogen therapy has been associated with an increased risk of uterine cancer. The role of selective estrogen receptor modulators in prevention or treatment of vascular disease is under evaluation.

REHABILITATION PROGRAMS (see Chap. 43). The feasibility of and improvement with intensive exercise interventions have been shown for the frailest elderly people residing in the community as well as the nursing home.[136,137] The Cardiac Rehabilitation in Advanced Age (CR-AGE) trial compared hospital-based with home-based cardiac rehabilitation in cognitively intact patients from age 46 to 86 with recent myocardial infarction.[138] Similar improvement in total work capacity and health-related quality of life was seen with home-based rehabilitation compared with hospital-based rehabilitation in all age groups without improvement in the control group. The improvement, however, was somewhat smaller in those older than 75. Benefits decreased over time after hospital rehabilitation but were maintained with home cardiac rehabilitation. Complications were similar across groups; costs, however, were lower in the home rehabilitation group.

Table 72–9 summarizes the approach to the older patient with CAD.

TABLE 72–9 Approach to the Older Patient with Coronary Artery Disease

Morbidity and mortality from CAD and CAD treated medically or with revascularization increases with age and more steeply at ages older than 75 years. After age 70 to 75 years, there are few data to suggest clear advantages of one method of treatment of CAD over another.
Anticipated procedural complication rates should reflect the age and health status of the patient, not complication rates from series of younger patients.
Decisions regarding medical therapy versus revascularization or for PCI versus CABG should be based on the role of CAD in the context of the individual older patient's overall health, life style, projected life span, and preferences.

CABG = coronary artery bypass graft; CAD = coronary artery disease; PCI = percutaneous coronary intervention.

CAROTID ARTERY DISEASE AND STROKE

Prevalence and Incidence. Stroke is the third leading cause of death and leading cause of disability in the United States. The risk of stroke increases with age. Data from the Framingham Study estimate the 10-year probability of stroke as 11 percent in men at age 65 years and 7 percent in women at age 65. At age 80, the probability increases to 22 and 24 percent for men and women, respectively. One in 15 people older than 65 years reports a history of transient ischemic attacks (TIAs). Fifteen percent of patients with stroke report a prior TIA. The short-term risk of stroke after TIA appears to be higher than the risk after a completed stroke. Age older than 60, diabetes, longer duration of TIAs, and TIAs accompanied by weakness increase the risk of stroke after TIA. Carotid stenosis is responsible for about 25 percent of strokes. Risk factors for stroke and TIAs are the same as for other atherosclerotic diseases.

Diagnosis. The diagnosis of TIA is made following a spell of neurological impairment lasting less than 24 hours that is produced by ischemia in a discrete vascular territory in the brain, and the diagnosis is usually based on clinical history alone. Neurological deficits are not present unless there has been prior stroke or disease. Diagnosis of significant carotid disease is usually made in the presence of a stenosis greater than 70 to 80 percent defined by noninvasive imaging with Doppler ultrasonography or magnetic resonance angiography or less frequently with computed tomographic angiography (see Chap. 15). Carotid bruits may or may not be present and carotid disease may be asymptomatic.

Treatment. Preventive and secondary treatment is targeted at modifiable risk factors.[139] Increasing attention has been directed at antiplatelet or anticoagulant therapy in high-risk patients such as those with TIAs, prior stroke, or atrial fibrillation (see Chap. 30) and after myocardial infarction as well as carotid artery interventions for patients with severe lesions or symptomatic disease.[140-142]

STROKE PREVENTION

ANTIPLATELET DRUGS. Aspirin reduces the long-term risk of stroke, as well as cardiovascular events, after stroke or TIA and is considered standard therapy after a stroke regardless of the patient's age. The role of other agents such as the thienopyridine drugs ticlopidine and clopidogrel that inhibit platelet aggregation by blocking platelet adenosine diphosphate receptors is less clear. Ticlopidine-induced hematological side effects have limited its clinical use. Clopidogrel has substantially lower rates of hematological side effects than ticlopidine but is considerably more expensive than aspirin. Secondary prevention trials with clopidogrel that enrolled stroke patients found reductions in composite endpoints that included stroke, but the effect was not as great as the reduction in peripheral artery disease events.[143] Combined aspirin and extended-release dipyridamole has been reported to prevent more strokes than placebo or either aspirin or dipyridamole alone but was associated with greater gastrointestinal intolerance, headache, cost, and drug discontinuation.[144] A comparison of warfarin and aspirin did not find significant differences in the prevention of recurrent ischemic stroke or death or occurrence of serious adverse events.[145]

In most reports, bleeding complications with antiplatelet drugs are more frequent in older than in younger patients. No dose-response relationship was observed for the protective effects of aspirin from 50 to 1500 mg/d, but larger doses increased the risk of gastrointestinal bleeding.[146,147] Although the minimally effective dose for aspirin has not been determined, lower doses are recommended for older patients in particular.

WARFARIN. Antithrombotic prophylaxis should be determined individually on the basis of the estimated risk for stroke during aspirin therapy and the risk for bleeding during anticoagulation. For older patients at moderate and higher risk for stroke, anticoagulation with warfarin is appropriate, unless contraindicated. The target International Normalized Ratio (INR) is 2 to 3. Both initial and maintenance warfarin doses are usually lower in older adults than middle-aged patients, with initiation of warfarin at the estimated maintenance dosage (usually less than 5 mg/d in elderly persons) recommended, followed by frequent monitoring (www.americangeriatrics.org). See Table 72–10 for a summary of the approach to anticoagulation in the older patient.

ACUTE STROKE MANAGEMENT. Data support administration of aspirin in the acute stroke setting but do not support use of unfractionated or low-molecular-weight heparin, heparinoids, streptokinase, or recombinant urokinase. The overall benefit of recombinant tissue plasminogen activator may outweigh the bleeding risk in highly selected patients. Blood pressure management in the setting of acute stroke remains controversial, with aggressive reduction in pressure not generally recommended.[142]

SURGICAL AND ENDOVASCULAR APPROACHES. Several clinical trials have demonstrated that carotid endarterectomy in symptomatic patients with 70 to 99 percent internal carotid artery stenosis who have had a stroke or TIA attributable to the stenosis is safe and effective in reducing the risk of ipsilateral carotid ischemia. Surgery has performed better than medical treatment in preventing disabling ipsilateral stroke (Fig. 72–8).[148] Its benefit is less certain in patients with stenosis of 50 to 69 percent. In asymptomatic patients with carotid stenoses, carotid endarterectomy is less likely to benefit the patient. To achieve a net beneficial effect of carotid endarterectomy versus medical therapy alone, the combined mortality and morbidity rate should be less than 3 percent for asymptomatic patients and less than 6 to 7 percent for symptomatic patients. Increased risk of perioperative stroke or death is associated with surgery for completed stroke (versus TIA), female sex, age older than 75 years, systolic blood pressure higher than 180 mm Hg, and a history of peripheral vascular disease.[149] Intracranial vascular disease and bilateral carotid disease also increase the risk of stroke or death.

During the past few years, carotid angioplasty and stenting have evolved as an alternative to carotid endarterectomy, particularly in patients who are known to have a higher operative complication rate or technical contraindications to surgery such as previous neck surgeries, radiation, or restenosis after endarterectomy.[150]

Table 72–11 summarizes the general approach to the older patient with stroke.

TABLE 72–10 Approach to Anticoagulation in Older Patients

- Obtain complete medication and nutraceutical intake data to anticipate warfarin requirements, interactions, contraindications, and necessary adjustment
- Educate patient, family, and/or caregivers on diet, alcohol effects, and drug interactions and need for monitoring and communication
- Initiate at low doses—often at 2 mg/d, not to exceed 5 mg/d
- Monitor closely and titrate slowly; consider use of
  - anticoagulation clinics and/or
  - fingerstick self-testing programs (patient, family, or caregiver)
- Consider warfarin effects of all medication, supplement, and diet changes
- Use preventive measures for osteoporosis

PERIPHERAL ARTERY DISEASE

Prevalence and Incidence. Lower extremity peripheral arterial disease (PAD) is common among older men and women (see Chap. 54). The frequency of intermittent claudication increases with age from 0 to 6 percent of people aged 45 to 54 years to about 9 percent of patients aged 65 to 74 years. When an ankle brachial index of 0.9 is used to

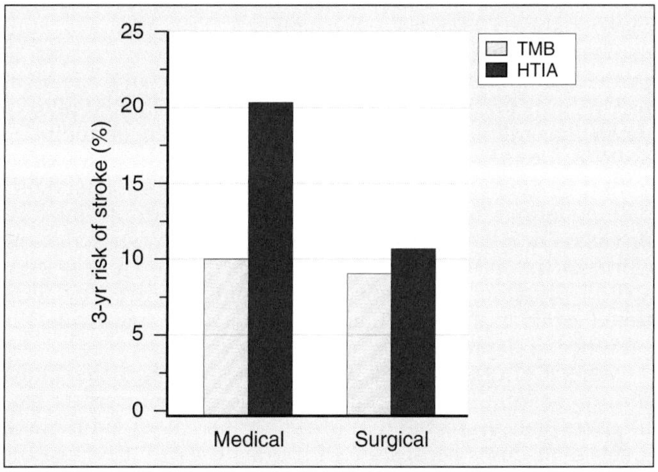

FIGURE 72–8 Three-year risk of ipsilateral stroke in patients with at least 50 percent stenosis and transient monocular blindness (TMB) or hemispheric transient ischemic attack (HTIA) in the North American Symptomatic Carotid Endarterectomy Trial (NASCET). (Data from Benevente O, Eliasziw M, Streifler J, et al: Prognosis after transient monocular blindness associated with carotid stenosis. N Engl J Med 345:1084, 2000.)

TABLE 72–11 Approach to the Older Patient with Stroke

- Modifiable risk factors of hypertension, elevated lipids, smoking, physical inactivity, and obesity should be treated; older patients with atrial fibrillation should have anticoagulation (in the absence of contraindications).
- Aspirin should be administered in the acute stroke setting and for secondary prevention with lower doses recommended for the older patient.
- Warfarin should be considered for patients with strokes while receiving aspirin in the absence of contraindications and with moderate to high likelihood of recurrent stroke.
- Anticoagulation with unfractionated or low-molecular-weight heparin, heparinoids, streptokinase, or urokinase is not recommended for acute stroke. Recombinant tissue plasminogen activator may have a role in selected patients.
- Carotid endarterectomy benefits symptomatic patients with 70-99% internal carotid artery stenosis who have had a stroke or transient ischemic attack attributable to the stenosis. Definitive conclusions regarding carotid angioplasty cannot be made at this time.

identify PAD, significant PAD is diagnosed in 17 to 20 percent of men and 21 percent of women older than 55, with somewhat higher rates in blacks compared with whites. Individuals with PAD have approximately the same relative risk of death from cardiovascular causes as patients with coronary or cerebrovascular disease.[96,151]

Diagnosis. Intermittent claudication is the earliest and most frequent presenting symptom in about one-third of patients with PAD. More than half of patients with abnormal ankle brachial index measurements indicating PAD have "atypical" leg discomfort.[152] About 20 percent of patients with PAD are asymptomatic. PAD is about equally prevalent in older men and women. Screening for PAD with the ankle brachial index is recommended in all patients older than 70 years, patients 50 to 69 years of age who smoke or have diabetes, patients with leg pain with exertion, those with abnormal results on vascular examinations of the leg, and patients with coronary, carotid, or renal arterial disease.

Treatment. Therapy in PAD should be directed at reduction of cardiovascular risk factors, exercise, and weight loss in overweight patients and improvement of symptoms and walking impairment with pharmacological or surgical intervention, if necessary (see Chap. 54). There are no age restrictions to therapeutic approaches.[153-156] Surgical recovery times, however, are longer in older patients. Table 72–12 presents the general approach to the older patient with PAD.

Heart Failure

Prevalence and Incidence. HF has become primarily a disorder of the elderly. HF contributes to at least 20 percent of hospital admissions of patients older than 65 years, with approximately three-quarters of hospitalizations for HF occurring in older patients. HF was reported as one of their medical conditions by 0.1 percent of people at ages 18 to 39 years, by about 4 percent aged 65 to 74 years, and by about 6 percent at ages 75 to 105 years in a national health interview survey.[157] In the Cardiovascular Health Study of independent community-dwelling subjects aged 66 to 103 years (n = 4842), HF defined by physician report and medical record review developed at a rate of 19.3 per 1000 patient-years. The incidence increased from 10.6 per 1000 person-years in participants 65 to 69 years of age at the initial evaluation to 42.5 per 1000 person-years in those older than 80 years[158] (Fig. 72–9). Asymptomatic left ventricular systolic dysfunction is estimated to occur in another 3 to 5 percent of the community with higher prevalences at older ages.[159]

HF of any type is associated with a reduction in life span as well as decreased quality of life and recurrent hospitalizations. Although HF treatments are improving, average 5-year mortality is approximately 50 percent for HF patients with systolic dysfunction and approximately 25 percent for HF patients with preserved systolic function.[160,161] In general, prognosis is worse in patients older than 65 years (Fig. 72–10).[162]

Age-Related Changes in Ventricular Function (see Chap. 19). In contrast to the etiology in middle-aged patients with HF, factors other than systolic function contribute to HF in the elderly population. Signs and symptoms of HF in older

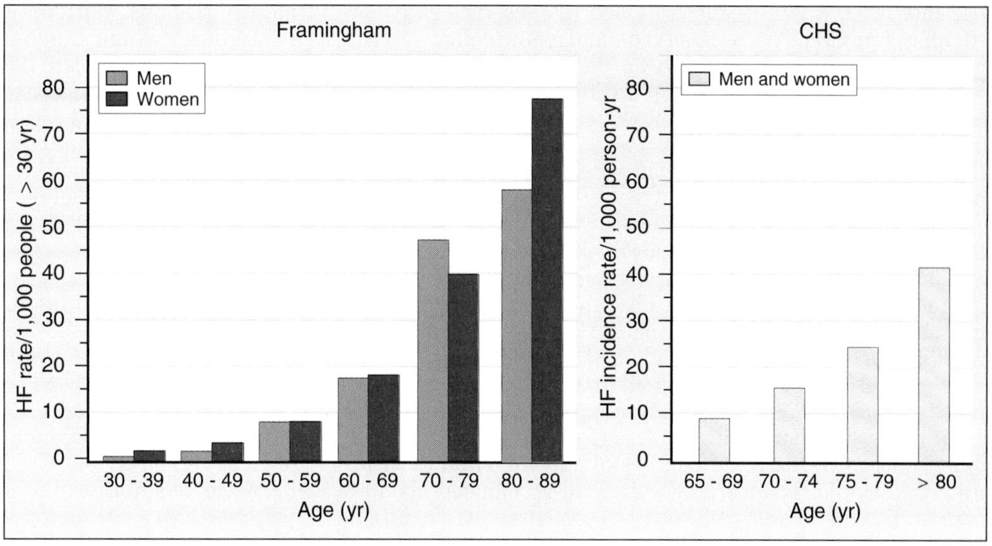

FIGURE 72–9 Prevalence and incidence rates of heart failure (HF) with aging in longitudinal studies. Prevalence rates of HF by age for men (blue) and women (pink) in the Framingham Study are shown in the **left panel** and incidence rates of congestive heart failure by age, from the Cardiovascular Health Study (CHS) are shown in the **right panel.** (Framingham data from Ho K, Pinsky J, Kannel W, Levy D: The epidemiology of heart failure: Framingham Study. J Am Coll Cardiol 22(Suppl A):6A, 1993; CHS data from Gottdiener J, Arnold A, Aurigemma G, et al: Predictors of congestive heart failure in the elderly: The Cardiovascular Health Study. J Am Coll Cardiol 35:1628, 2000.)

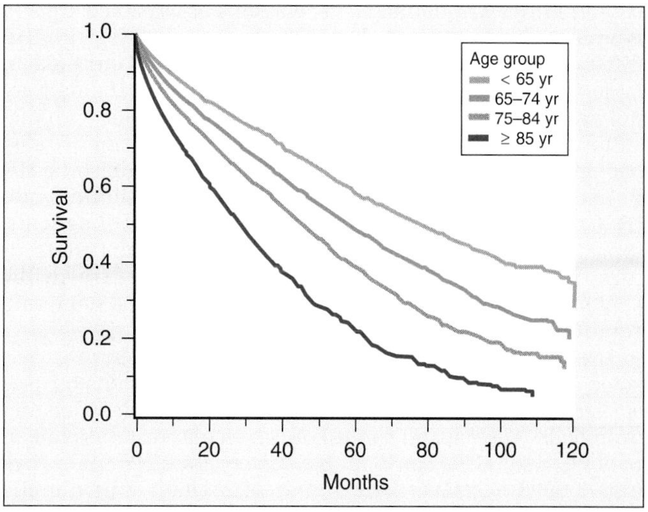

FIGURE 72–10 Age-stratified mortality (adjusted for gender and race) for patients with a diagnosis of heart failure in the Resource Utilization Among Congestive Heart Failure (REACH) study of 29,686 health care recipients during the years 1989 to 1999. (From McCullough P, Philbin E, Spertus J, et al: Confirmation of a heart failure epidemic: Findings from the Resource Utilization Among Congestive Heart Failure [REACH] study. J Am Coll Cardiol 39:60, 2002.)

TABLE 72–12 Approach to the Older Patient with Peripheral Artery Disease

Treatment of cardiovascular risk factors, aspirin, and supervised walking-based exercise programs are first-line therapy.
Medications can improve symptoms (cilostazol > clopidogrel > pentoxifylline; cilostazol should not be used in patients with heart failure).
Estrogen and progesterone should be avoided in women with PAD.
Revascularization options include percutaneous interventions for iliac disease but long-term efficacy requires surgical approaches at the femoropopliteal and infrapopliteal level.
Surgical morbidity and mortality increase with age and postoperative recovery times can be prolonged. All are highest in the setting of surgery for critical ischemia or limb salvage.

PAD = peripheral artery disease.

patients often occur in the presence of preserved left ventricular function.[163-165] Preserved left ventricular systolic function may be seen in 40 to 80 percent of older patients with HF and is almost twice as frequent in women as men.[166,167] Although HF with preserved systolic function has a slightly better prognosis than HF with abnormal function, there is a fourfold higher mortality risk compared with that of subjects free of HF.[168]

Diagnosis. Exercise intolerance is the primary symptom in chronic HF of either systolic or diastolic etiology. Dyspnea and fatigue are prominent symptoms in patients with HF, but fatigue also accompanies many chronic illnesses such as pulmonary disease, thyroid abnormality, anemia, or depression. Complaints of shortness of breath, orthopnea or development of nocturnal cough, or paroxysmal nocturnal dyspnea suggest the presence of HF. Despite these possible symptoms and complaints associated with HF, less than half of patients with moderate or severe diastolic or systolic dysfunction as measured by Doppler echocardiography had recognized HF in a community-based study.[164] Potential explanations for unrecognized HF in older patients include the nonspecificity of complaints of fatigue, with symptoms ascribed to aging, reduction in activities to avoid symptoms, and memory impairment leading to poor historical information. Physical examination may not be as definitive as in younger individuals. Peripheral edema can be due to age-related changes in venous tone, decreased skin turgor, or prolonged sedentary states. Evaluation of volume status on the basis of neck veins may also be difficult in the older patient. Rales and a third heart sound may be present only during episodes of acute decompensation, and differentiation of HF from pneumonia may be difficult in older patients, who are less likely to present with temperature elevations. With diastolic HF, fourth heart sounds may be present but third heart sounds are seldom present. Chest radiography shows pulmonary congestion during acute exacerbations and for some time after an episode; cardiomegaly is present in systolic HF but may or may not be present in diastolic HF. Because of the difficulties with diagnosing HF in the older patient by physician examination or by conventional radiography, use of echocardiography and serum markers of HF takes on greater diagnostic importance.[169]

Treatment. Most data regarding therapy for CHF are from studies of younger middle-aged men with systolic dysfunction resulting from ischemic CAD and few major medical comorbidities. Guidelines[53] are available at www.acc.org and www.americanheart.org. The elderly population with HF differs markedly from patients who have been enrolled in large trials of systolic HF treatment, and clinical trial data are not available to guide treatment of the older patient with diastolic HF. Conceptually, strategies that have demonstrated benefit for systolic HF may benefit patients with diastolic HF. Because the direct applicability of clinical trial findings and HF treatment guidelines to the majority of older HF patients, especially women and those residing in long-term care facilities, is unknown, it is important to consider care in the context of the individual patients and their goals, comorbid conditions, and estimated life expectancy.

SYSTOLIC HEART FAILURE. Pharmacological therapy is targeted at control of systolic and diastolic hypertension (see earlier), use of diuretics to control pulmonary congestion and pulmonary edema, and control of ventricular response rate in patients with atrial fibrillation. Most systolic HF trials have tested therapies on a background of digitalis and diuretic administration. Efficacy of the addition of ACE and angiotensin receptor blockers has been demonstrated in trials that have included elderly patients, and these agents have additional efficacy in diabetes, which is present in at least 10 percent of the older population.[85,170-172] Caution and close monitoring are necessary with use of ACE inhibitors in elderly persons, especially when given at "full doses" used in studies of younger patients. Beta blockers are usually considered next and can be instituted at low doses during periods of clinical stability. Direct vasodilators are efficacious but may have less of a role in older patients with increased likelihood of orthostatic hypotension. Studies of aldosterone antagonists and selective aldosterone blockers have enrolled limited numbers of older patients, especially minorities or women. Benefit may be seen with these drugs used at lower doses in patients with severe HF,[173] but age-related decreases in renal function increase the risk for hyperkalemia.[174] Data for natriuretic peptides in older patients are also lacking. Sex differences in HF etiology and prognosis have been suggested, but there are no sex-specific therapeutic recommendations to date.[175-177]

NONPHARMACOLOGICAL STRATEGIES. Dietary sodium restriction is advised and moderate physical activity should be encouraged if feasible. Cardiac resynchronization therapy can decrease hospitalizations and reduce mortality in selected patients with symptomatic systolic HF and prolonged cardiac repolarization or QRS intervals on the electrocardiogram (see Chap. 31).[178] Revascularization therapies are considered in the setting of ischemia. The few highly selected patients older than 65 years who have received cardiac transplantation appear to have survival times similar to those of younger patients, with slightly more morbidity and mortality related to the surgical procedure but lower rates of rejection than younger patients (see Chap. 26).

DIASTOLIC HEART FAILURE. Diuretics are advised for therapy of diastolic HF in the ACC/AHA guidelines for the evaluation and management of heart failure.[53] Digoxin was associated with symptomatic improvement and decreased hospitalizations (without mortality benefit) in the Digitalis Investigation Group study in patients with diastolic as well as systolic HF,[179] although its risk/benefit ratio in women has been questioned.[177] Small studies of HF in elderly persons with preserved left ventricular function suggest that ACE inhibitors or angiotensin receptor blockers may improve functional class, exercise duration, ejection fraction, diastolic filling, and left ventricular hypertrophy. Although calcium channel antagonists are often proposed for diastolic HF, supportive data are limited. Data are also lacking on nitrates, but some clinicians find them helpful in reducing orthopnea if given at bedtime. Finally, spironolactone and other aldosterone antagonists have not been tested in patients with diastolic HF. Studies of angiotensin II antagonists are ongoing (for a comprehensive review see reference 180).

ADDITIONAL CONSIDERATIONS. Education and involvement of the patient, family members, or caregivers is key to the management of older patients with HF. Recognition of warning signs of worsening failure, understanding of medication regimens, diet adjustments, and the role of regular moderate physical activity should be emphasized. Reliance cannot be on classical symptoms of HF, and weight should be measured daily with a mechanism for rapid communication of information and timely adjustment of diuretic dosages in order to prevent exacerbations of HF. Multidisciplinary team approaches with contacts with the patient between office visits can be highly beneficial, and use of primary care preventive strategies such as influenza vaccination can reduce hospitalizations for HF in older people.[181]

For very old patients or those with progressive symptoms of severe HF, goals of improving symptoms and quality of life and preventing acute exacerbations and hospitalization rather than prolongation of life become the emphasis. Hospice programs may have special expertise in the management of symptoms such as dyspnea with opiates and in providing support for family and caregivers as well as the patient with advanced HF (see Table 72–13 for the approach to the older patient with HF).

TABLE 72–13 Approach to the Older Patient with Heart Failure

Symptoms may be relatively nonspecific in the older patient.
Diagnosis may be facilitated by use of echocardiography or serum markers of heart failure.
Recognize that heart failure may be present in the older patient with preserved systolic function, especially older women.
Treat symptoms with a goal of improving quality of life as well as morbidity.
- Control blood pressure—systolic and diastolic.
- Control atrial fibrillation rate.
- Promote physical activity.
- Adjust medications for age- and disease-related changes in kinetics and dynamics.

Educate and involve patients, family members, or caregivers in management of heart failure.
- Monitor weight.
- Consider use of multidisciplinary team approaches.

Arrhythmias

PATHOPHYSIOLOGY AND AGE-RELATED ELECTROCARDIOGRAPHIC CHANGES. Cell loss and collagen infiltration occur in the area of the sinus node and throughout the atria, the central fibrous body, and cytoskeleton of the heart with increasing age. Changes are most marked in the area of the sinus node with destruction of as many as 90 percent of cells by age 75 years. The correlation between pathology and sinus node function, however, is poor, and sinus node function is preserved in most elderly patients although sinoatrial conduction is decreased. Collagen infiltration and fibrosis are of lesser magnitude in the area of the AV node and more marked in the left and right bundle branches. Conduction times through the AV node increase with aging with the site of delay above the His bundle. Despite age-related collagen infiltration, His-Purkinje conduction times are not usually increased by aging alone.

Resting heart rate is not altered by age, but maximal heart rate (see Fig. 72–4) and beat-to-beat variability in heart rate decrease with age because of age-related decreases in sinus node responses to beta-adrenergic and parasympathetic stimulation (see Chap. 87). On the surface electrocardiogram, the PR interval increases and the R, S, and T wave amplitude decrease. The QRS axis shifts leftward. This shift may reflect increased left ventricular mass or interstitial fibrosis of the anterior fascicular radiation. Right bundle branch block is found in 3 percent of healthy people older than 85 years and up to 20 percent of centenarians; it is found in 8 to 10 percent of older patients with heart disease but is not associated with cardiac morbidity or mortality. The presence of left bundle branch block increases with age and is more likely to be associated with cardiovascular disease. Similarly, nonspecific intraventricular conduction delays become more frequent with increasing age and are usually related to underlying myocardial disease. Repolarization times throughout the myocardium increase with age, and surface ECG QT intervals increase.

Atrial ectopy has been found on ECG recordings in 10 percent of community-dwelling elderly people without known cardiac disease and up to 80 percent during 24-hour ambulatory ECG recordings. Brief episodes of atrial tachyarrhythmias were seen in up to 50 percent of 24-hour ambulatory electrocardiograms of community-dwelling elderly people. Premature ventricular complexes also increase in prevalence and frequency with age. Ventricular ectopic beats are seen on ECG recordings in 6 to 11 percent of elderly people without known cardiovascular disease and as many as 76 percent on 24-hour ambulatory ECG recordings. In the absence of cardiac disease, these age-related changes have not been associated with subsequent cardiovascular events (see Table 72–1).

SINUS NODE DYSFUNCTION. Bradycardia related to sinus node dysfunction or AV conduction disease, or both, is more common as age increases. The mean age of patients undergoing permanent pacemaker implantation is about 74 years, with 70 percent of new pacemaker recipients being older than 70 years, and in the United States 85 percent of pacemaker implantations are in patients older than 65 years. The most common indication is for sinus node dysfunction.

ATRIOVENTRICULAR CONDUCTION DISEASE. First-degree AV block is diagnosed in 6 to 10 percent of healthy elderly people. Higher degree AV block is less common. Transient type II AV block occurs on 0.4 to 0.8 percent of 24-hour ambulatory ECG recordings of community-dwelling elderly people and transient third-degree AV block in less than 0.2 percent. These arrhythmias usually represent advanced conduction system disease requiring pacemaker implantation (see Chaps. 29 and 30).

ATRIAL ARRHYTHMIAS

Atrial Fibrillation. Atrial fibrillation is seen on 24-hour ambulatory recordings in 10 percent of community-dwelling older patients. The incidence of atrial fibrillation doubles with each decade beginning at age 60, so that by ages 80 to 89 years the incidence of atrial fibrillation is currently estimated to be 8 to 10 percent. Approximately one-half of patients with atrial fibrillation in the United States are older than 75 years. Atrial fibrillation in the population is increasing, however, and a 2.5-fold increase in the prevalence of atrial fibrillation over the next 50 years has been predicted (see Chap. 32).[182]

The focus of therapy in the older patient should be on anticoagulation to prevent stroke and recurrent stroke and rate control to improve symptoms. Rarely, rhythm control is needed to provide symptom relief. Patients should receive anticoagulation with warfarin in the absence of contraindications (see Table 72–10). The target INR is 2 to 2.5 in older patients in whom close monitoring of INRs can be performed. Low fixed warfarin doses of 1 mg/d are not efficacious. Patients older than 75 may require less than half the dose of middle-aged patients for equivalent anticoagulation. Warfarin dosing guidelines for elderly patients recommend initiation of warfarin at the estimated maintenance dosage of warfarin, usually less than 5 mg/d (www.americangeriatrics.org). Drug interaction information should be consulted whenever warfarin is being initiated or a drug is added to or deleted from a patient's medication regimen.

Chronic warfarin administration may contribute to osteoporosis. Vitamin K plays a role in bone metabolism, and oral anticoagulation with warfarin antagonizes vitamin K. In analyses of women receiving chronic oral anticoagulation compared with nonanticoagulated cohorts, increased risk of osteoporosis and higher rates of vertebral and rib fractures were associated with oral anticoagulation for more than 12 months.[183] Measures to prevent osteoporosis should accompany long-term anticoagulation with warfarin (calcium and vitamin D in most; bisphosphonates, calcitonin if needed) (Table 72–14).

TABLE 72–14 Approach to the Older Patient with Atrial Fibrillation

Atrial fibrillation is frequent in elderly people and confers a risk of stroke but the patient may be unaware of its presence, suggesting that routine examinations or electrocardiographic evaluations be targeted toward detection of atrial fibrillation.
Anticoagulation is the chief weapon against stroke.
- Both greater potential benefit and risk for fatal intracranial bleeding are present at ages older than 75 years, especially in women.
- Careful attention to anticoagulation monitoring is needed.
- Aspirin does not usually provide stroke risk reduction in older patients because of higher likelihood of the presence of cardiovascular diseases but has overall bleeding complication rates similar to those with warfarin.

Rate control produces equivalent benefits with lower costs than attempts at rhythm control.
- Useful agents for elderly patients include digoxin (rest control), beta blockers, nondihydropyridine calcium channel blockers, and amiodarone with dose adjustments for age, weight, and concomitant diseases.

VENTRICULAR ARRHYTHMIAS. Treatment of premature ventricular contractions with most type 1 antiarrhythmic agents either has been of no benefit or has decreased survival. If patients have symptoms, administration of a beta blocker may be helpful. Sustained ventricular tachycardia and ventricular fibrillation require treatment in patients of any age (see Chap. 30).

Valvular Disease (see also Chap. 57)

PATHOPHYSIOLOGY AND AGE-RELATED CHANGES. Age-related changes in the fibromuscular skeleton of the heart include myxomatous degeneration and collagen infiltration termed sclerosis. Sclerosis of the aortic valve is present in as many as 30 percent of elderly persons,[184] with the prevalence of sclerosis detected on echocardiography increasing as age increased from 65 to more than 85 years in the Cardiovascular Health Study.[185] Further age-related changes include calcification of the aortic valve leaflets, aortic annulus, base of the semilunar cusps, and the mitral annulus. Aortic valve calcium detected by electron beam computed tomography increases over time[186] with progression from valvular sclerosis to stenosis with a transvalvular pressure gradient in a significant percentage of patients (Table 72–15).[187] Aortic sclerosis appears to parallel atherosclerotic progression in other vessels.[188-190] This may explain the increased risk of myocardial infarction and death from cardiovascular causes in patients with aortic sclerosis without evidence of stenosis.[184] Risk factors identified for progression include hypertension, hyperlipidemia, smoking, end-stage renal disease, congenital bicuspid valves, and, in some series, diabetes, shorter stature, and male sex. In older patients, fibrosis with valve calcification is now the most common etiology of valvular stenoses, especially at the aortic position. Ischemic or hypertensive disease has become the most common etiology of valvular regurgitation, especially at the mitral valve. Similarly, pulmonary or tricuspid regurgitation in elderly persons is usually secondary to pulmonary hypertension and dilation of the right ventricle resulting from left ventricular ischemia, HF, or pulmonary disease. Less common etiologies of mild to moderate mitral or aortic regurgitation are ruptured chordae, endocarditis, trauma, aortic dissection, and rheumatic heart disease.

Infective endocarditis is seen with about equal frequency in younger and older patients but is more likely to be associated with nosocomial infections with the use of intravascular catheters or other devices, the presence of prosthetic implants, pacemaker leads, atheromas, or mitral annular calcification in older patients. Polymicrobial infections are uncommon in elderly people, and the most frequent pathogens are group D streptococci and enterococcus, *Staphylococcus epidermidis*, and *Streptococcus viridans* (see Chap. 58).

Treatment for symptomatic valvular disease relies on surgical approaches. Surgery in patients 70 to 80 years of age is increasingly common, but experience with those older than 90 years is limited and there is a high surgical mortality rate.

AORTIC STENOSIS. The prevalence of aortic stenosis in patients older than 65 years is estimated as 2 percent for severe stenosis, 5 percent for moderate stenosis, and 9 percent for mild stenosis. Aortic stenosis in more than 90 percent of older patients involves calcification of the aortic annulus and semilunar cusps of trileaflet valves without commissural fusion. The pathophysiological consequences of aortic stenosis are independent of etiology and include left ventricular hypertrophy, elevated left ventricular diastolic pressures, and decreased stroke volume in patients of all ages. For any given degree of aortic stenosis, left ventricular hypertrophy and decreased left ventricular compliance are greater in patients older than 65 than in younger patients. Approximately 50 percent of patients with severe aortic stenosis have significant CAD, further influencing left ventricular function, symptoms, and morbidity.

Diagnosis. Symptoms can be exertional angina, syncope, or HF and may be precipitated by atrial arrhythmias such as atrial fibrillation. Symptoms may be absent in inactive older patients or may not be elicited from patients with memory impairment. Physical findings of calcific aortic valve stenosis in older patients differ from those seen with rheumatic aortic stenosis and do not accurately reflect the degree of stenosis. The age-related arterial changes of decreased compliance and increased stiffness mask carotid artery findings associated with rheumatic aortic stenosis in younger individuals (see Chap. 8). The carotid artery upstroke and peak may appear normal and carotid amplitude may be unaltered or increased even in the presence of severe calcific stenosis. The presence of decreased carotid upstroke and volume (in the absence of carotid disease) usually indicates severe stenosis. Aortic sclerosis and aortic stenosis both produce systolic ejection murmurs. The volume of the murmur depends on flow as well as the pressure gradient and does not reflect the severity of stenosis. It may be absent in low-output states reflecting severe aortic valve obstruction. The murmur may be high pitched and musical as opposed to harsh and low in frequency. The loudness of the second heart sound may be preserved. Hypertension is common in elderly people, making left ventricular hypertrophy on electrocardiography or ventricular enlargement on chest radiography similarly of

TABLE 72–15 Prevalence of Aortic Valve Abnormalities Detected by Echocardiography in the Cross-Sectional Cardiovascular Health Study of 5201 Medicare Subjects Older than 65 Years

	Aortic Valve Abnormality*			
Subjects	***None***	***Sclerosis***	***Stenosis***	***Valve Replacement***
All subjects	3736 (72%)	1329 (26%)	88 (2%)	23 (0.4%)
Women	2249 (76%)	641 (22%)	43 (1.5%)	12 (0.4%)
Men	1487 (67%)	688 (31%)	45 (2%)	11 (0.5%)
65-74 yr old	2684 (78%)	697 (20%)	43 (1.3%)	16 (0.5%)
Women	1654 (82%)	344 (17%)	20 (1.0%)	9 (0.4%)
Men	1030 (73%)	353 (25%)	23 (1.6%)	7 (0.5%)
75-84 yr old	962 (62%)	542 (35%)	37 (2.4%)	7 (0.5%)
Women	546 (66%)	259 (31%)	22 (2.7%)	3 (0.4%)
Men	416 (58%)	283 (39%)	15 (2.1%)	4 (0.6%)
85+ yr old	90 (48%)	90 (48%)	8 (4%)	0 (0%)
Women	49 (56%)	38 (43%)	1 (1%)	0
Men	41 (41%)	52 (52%)	7 (7%)	0

From Stewart BF, Siscovick D, Lind BK, et al: Clinical factors associated with calcific aortic valve disease. Cardiovascular Health Study. J Am Coll Cardiol 29:630, 1997.

*Data are expressed as number (%) of subjects.

TABLE 72–16 Approach to the Older Patient with Suspected Valvular Disease

Physical examination cannot reliably assess the severity of valvular lesions in most older patients.
Doppler echocardiography is the clinical standard for diagnosis and evaluation of the severity of valve lesions.
- Differentiates sclerosis from stenosis
- Quantitates regurgitation
- Assesses calcification of valves and supporting structures

Age is a predictor of worse outcomes for the natural history of valvular lesions as well as surgical approaches.
Surgery is definitive therapy for valvular lesions with age, coronary artery disease, additional diseases, projected life span, and desired life style as factors in evaluating surgical options.

little diagnostic help. Thus, Doppler echocardiography has become the clinical standard for diagnosis of aortic stenosis in elderly patients. In the setting of low cardiac output, maneuvers (vasodilators, inotropes) to increase output may be helpful in quantifying stenosis. Catheterization is less commonly used to make the diagnosis, but coronary angiography is usually performed to evaluate CAD in older patients before surgical interventions.

Management. Management (Table 72–16) is similar to that of younger patients, with recognition of the increased likelihood of concomitant coronary disease and diseases of other organs (see Chap. 57).[191] Antibiotic prophylaxis should be used to prevent bacterial endocarditis. Risk factors should be treated, and current concepts support aggressive lipid lowering in patients with calcific aortic sclerosis and stenosis.[186,192,193]

Surgical morbidity and mortality are related to the severity and duration of aortic stenosis, presence or absence of HF or CAD, concomitant diseases (especially renal), urgency of the procedure, and complexity of the procedure. Combined valve replacement and CABG is associated with higher perioperative morbidity and mortality than isolated valve replacement. Estimates of operative mortality are in the range of 5 to 10 percent for selected older patients who have undergone valve replacement with or without CABG. Perioperative renal failure, pulmonary insufficiency, stroke, late cognitive impairment, and late death rates are higher than in younger individuals. Postoperative hospitalization and rehabilitation times are usually longer for older patients. Appropriate selection of patients includes assessment of the burden of disease in addition to that of valve disease, anticipated life span independent of valve disease, and symptom status. The frailer the patient and the more comorbidities, the more likely that the risk of perioperative mortality will outweigh the potential of benefit. Biological tissue valves are frequently implanted in elderly patients on the basis of a number of factors including shorter anticipated life expectancy, longer bioprosthesis durability with older age, and avoidance of chronic anticoagulation.[194,195] Estimated structural failure rates of current bioprosthetic valves are about 1 percent per patient-year in patients older than 65 years, and mechanical valves should be considered for younger old patients or those with longer estimated lifespans.[195]

Aortic balloon valvuloplasty has been used in symptomatic patients who were not surgical candidates. No studies have directly compared surgery with balloon valvuloplasty, but observed mortality rates for patients after aortic valvuloplasty are similar to those for patients with severe symptomatic aortic stenosis who do not undergo surgery. Valvuloplasty may improve hemodynamics and symptoms initially but is associated with high procedural morbidity and mortality, with rapid restenosis and recurrence of symptoms within months in most series. It may serve as a bridge to valve surgery in hemodynamically unstable patients (cardiogenic shock), patients undergoing emergent noncardiac surgery, and patients with severe comorbidities who are too ill to undergo cardiac surgery.[196]

Asymptomatic patients with aortic stenosis should be educated concerning signs and symptoms related to aortic stenosis and observed regularly for development of symptoms. Risk of sudden death in asymptomatic patients with aortic stenosis is estimated as 3 to 5 percent. Operative mortality in older patients exceeds this rate; thus, asymptomatic patients with severe aortic stenosis are not usually recommended for surgical interventions.

AORTIC REGURGITATION. The prevalence of aortic regurgitation also increases with age. Mild aortic regurgitation was detected by Doppler echocardiography in 13 percent of patients older than 80 years and moderate or severe regurgitation in 16 percent in one series.[197] Causes of aortic regurgitation in older patients include primary valvular disease (myxomatous or infective) or aortic root disease and dilation secondary to hypertension or dissection. Significant aortic regurgitation in older patients is usually seen in combination with aortic stenosis. When infective aortic regurgitation occurs in elderly patients, the clinical manifestations may be insidious and nonspecific and symptoms fewer than in younger patients with endocarditis. Central nervous system symptoms are common and may predict a less favorable clinical outcome. Patients who have acute HF and pulmonary congestion as the manifestation of aortic valve endocarditis have a mortality rate of 50 to 80 percent. Age is a predictor of worse outcome for the natural history of aortic regurgitation. The estimated life span of older patients with chronic severe aortic regurgitation who do not undergo valve replacement was estimated as 2 years after the onset of HF in earlier observational studies.

Aortic regurgitation can be diagnosed by the presence of the classic diastolic murmur on physical examination. The finding of a widened pulse pressure usually associated with aortic regurgitation in younger patients is of limited diagnostic value in the older patient because age-related changes in the vasculature usually produce a widened pulse pressure in older people. Doppler echocardiography is the usual method of quantitation of the regurgitation and assessment of ventricular function.

MITRAL ANNULAR CALCIFICATION. Mitral annular calcification is an age-related chronic degenerative process that is seen more commonly in women than men and in people older than 70 years. An increased prevalence of mitral annular calcification is seen in patients with systemic hypertension, increased mitral valve stress, mitral valve prolapse, raised left ventricular systolic pressure, aortic valve stenosis, chronic renal failure, secondary hyperparathyroidism, atrial fibrillation, and aortic atherosclerosis. As with aortic calcific processes, mitral annular calcification is associated with risk factors for the development of coronary atherosclerosis and may reflect generalized atherosclerosis.[189,190] Mitral annular calcification may produce mitral stenosis, mitral regurgitation, infective endocarditis, atrial arrhythmias, or heart block. It is an independent risk factor for systemic embolism and stroke, with the risk of stroke directly related to the degree of mitral annular calcification.

MITRAL STENOSIS. Symptoms and presentation are the same as in younger patients and include exertional dyspnea, orthopnea, paroxysmal nocturnal dyspnea, and pulmonary edema or right-sided HF. Physical findings of calcific mitral stenosis differ from those of rheumatic mitral stenosis, and neither a loud first heart sound nor an opening snap is usually heard. The characteristic diastolic rumbling murmur is usually present. Quantification of stenosis is usually accomplished by Doppler echocardiography.

MITRAL REGURGITATION. Myxomatous degenerative and ischemic papillary muscle dysfunction or rupture related to CAD and myocardial infarction as etiologies of mitral regurgitation (MR) in the older patient are increasing. Rheumatic mitral disease is declining, and endocarditis etiology is unchanged. MR may also be seen in the setting of left ventricular dilation related to HF.

Patients with acute MR present with HF and pulmonary edema, but this may also be the initial presentation for medical care of the older patient with chronic MR. Chronic MR may be asymptomatic, especially in the sedentary patient. In symptomatic patients, initial complaints are usually easy fatigability and decreasing exercise tolerance because of low forward cardiac output followed by dyspnea on exertion, orthopnea, paroxysmal nocturnal dyspnea, and dyspnea at rest as left ventricular function fails. Right-sided HF may also occur. Findings on examination are not altered by age, and a holosystolic murmur is usually present. Doppler echocardiography can quantitate the MR. Increasingly, transesophageal echocardiography plays a role in defining the structure of the mitral valve apparatus and evaluation of endocarditis.

Medical treatment is age independent and includes afterload reduction, diuretics as needed for HF, management of atrial fibrillation, and antibiotic prophylaxis. When symptoms cannot be controlled, surgical options are based on left ventricular function and the extent of comorbid diseases. Age older than 65 has been reported to be a predictor of hospital mortality with isolated mitral valve surgery. The presence of CAD and need for combined valve replacement and CABG also increase surgical morbidity and mortality. Survival at 5 years may be as low as 50 percent. Mitral valve repair is preferred to mitral valve replacement when possible in the older patient. Series reporting results of mitral valve repair (alone and with CABG) estimate early death rates in patients older than 70 of 9 percent.[198]

Additional Considerations. Drug-induced valve disease is uncommon, but there are case reports of fibroproliferative lesions producing valvular insufficiency or regurgitation in older patients receiving chronic treatment with the antiparkinsonian dopamine receptor agonist pergolide.[199,200]

REFERENCES

Demographics and Epidemiology

1. Trends in aging—United States and worldwide. MMWR Morb Mortal Wkly Rep 52(6):101, 2003.
2. U.S. Census Bureau: Income 2001 (http://www.census.gov/hhes/income ed).
3. Clark C, Karlawish J: Alzheimer disease: Current concepts and emerging diagnostic and therapeutic strategies. Ann Intern Med 138:400, 2003.
4. Alzheimer's Disease and Dementia. A Growing Challenge. Washington, DC, National Academy on an Aging Society; September 2000.
5. Harris D, Douglas P: Enrollment of women in cardiovascular clinical trials funded by the National Heart, Lung, and Blood Institute. N Engl J Med 343:475, 2000.

Pathophysiology

6. Lakatta E, Levy D: Arterial and cardiac aging: Major shareholders in cardiovascular disease enterprises: Part II: The aging heart in health: Links to heart disease. Circulation 107:346, 2003.
7. Lakatta E, Levy D: Arterial and cardiac aging: Major shareholders in cardiovascular disease enterprises: Part I: Aging arteries a "set up" for vascular disease. Circulation 107:139, 2003.
8. Kass D: Age-related changes in ventricular-arterial coupling: Pathophysiologic implications. Heart Fail Rev 7:51, 2002.
9. Lakatta E: Arterial and cardiac aging: Major shareholders in cardiovascular disease enterprises: Part III: Cellular and molecular clues to heart and arterial aging. Circulation 107:490, 2003.
10. Anversa P, Nadal-Ginard B: Myocyte renewal and ventricular remodelling. Nature 415:240, 2002.
11. Lakatta E, Sollott S: Perspectives on mammalian cardiovascular aging: Humans to molecules. Comp Biochem Physiol A Mol Integr Physiol 132:699, 2002.
12. Zhou Y, Lakatta E, Xiao R: Age-associated alterations in calcium current and its modulation in cardiac myocytes. Drugs Aging 13:159, 1998.
13. Wilkerson W, Sane D: Aging and thrombosis. Semin Thromb Hemost 28:555, 2002.
14. Willerson J: Systemic and local inflammation in patients with unstable atherosclerotic plaques. Prog Cardiovasc Dis 44:469, 2002.
15. Schwartz J: Dopaminergic responses in the Fischer 344 rat heart: Preserved chronotropic and dromotropic responses with aging. J Gerontol Med Sci 52:M36, 1997.
16. Supiano M, Hogikyan R, Sidani M, et al: Sympathetic nervous system activity and α-adrenergic responsiveness in older hypertensive humans. Am J Physiol 276:E519, 1999.
17. Seals D, Esler M: Human ageing and the sympathoadrenal system. J Physiol 528:407, 2000.
18. Rehman H, Masson E: Neuroendocrinology of ageing. Age Ageing 30:279, 2001.
19. Kaasinen V, Rinne J: Functional imaging studies of dopamine system and cognition in normal aging and Parkinson's disease. Neurosci Biobehav Rev 26:785, 2002.
20. Jones P, Christou D, Jordan J, Seals D: Baroreflex buffering is reduced with age in healthy men. Circulation 107:1770, 2003.
21. The ATBC Study Group: Incidence of cancer and mortality following alpha-tocopherol and beta-carotene supplementation. JAMA 290:476, 2003.
22. Liem A, Reynierse-Buitenwerf R, Zwinderman A, et al: Secondary prevention with folic acid: Effects on clinical outcomes. J Am Coll Cardiol 41:2105, 2003.
23. Salonen J: Clinical trials testing cardiovascular benefits of antioxidant supplementation. Free Radic Res 36:1299, 2002.
24. Waters D, Alderman E, Hsia J, et al: Effects of hormone replacement therapy and antioxidant vitamin supplements on coronary atherosclerosis in postmenopausal women. A randomized controlled trial. JAMA 288:2432, 2002.
25. Gruppo Italiano per lo Studio della Sopravivenza nell'Infarto miocardico (GISSI)-Prevenzione Investigators: Dietary supplementation with n-3 polyunsaturated fatty acids and vitamin E after myocardial infarction: Results of the GISSI-Prevenzione trial. Lancet 354:447, 1999.
26. Gale C, Ashurst H, Powers H, Martyn C: Antioxidant vitamin status and carotid atherosclerosis in the elderly. Am J Clin Nutr 74:402, 2001.
27. Miquel J: Can antioxidant diet supplementation protect against age-related mitochondrial damage? Ann NY Acad Sci 959:508, 2002.
28. Remme W: Aldosterone and myocardial infarction—Are aldosterone antagonists needed to prevent remodelling or does ACE inhibition suffice? Cardiovasc Drugs Ther 15:297, 2001.
29. Hansson L: ACE inhibition and left ventricular remodelling. Eur Heart J 18:1203, 1997.

Medication Modifications

30. Gurwitz J, Gore J, Goldberg R, et al: Risk for intracranial hemorrhage after tissue plasminogen activator treatment for acute myocardial infarction. Participants in the National Registry of Myocardial Infarction 2. Ann Intern Med 129:597, 1998.
31. Van de Werf F, Barron H, Armstrong P, et al: Incidence and predictors of bleeding events after fibrinolytic therapy with fibrin-specific agents. Eur Heart J 22:2253, 2001.
32. Van de Werf F: ASSENT-3: Implications for future trial design and clinical practice. Eur Heart J 23:911, 2002.
33. Levey A, Bosch J, Lewis J, et al: A more accurate method to estimate glomerular filtration rate from serum creatinine: A new prediction equation. Ann Intern Med 130:461, 1999.
34. Cockcroft DW, Gault MH: Prediction of creatinine clearance from serum creatinine. Nephron 16:31, 1976.
35. Manjunath G, Sarnak M, Levey A: Prediction equations to estimate glomerular filtration rate: An update. Curr Opin Nephrol Hypertens 10:785, 2001.
36. Kang D, Verotta D, Krecic-Shepard M, et al: Population analyses of sustained release verapamil in patients: Age, race, and sex effects. Clin Pharmacol Ther 73:31, 2003.
37. Krecic-Shepard M, Park K, Barnas C, et al: Race and sex influence clearance of nifedipine: Results of a population study. Clin Pharmacol Ther 68:130, 2000.
38. Schwartz J: Gender-specific implications for cardiovascular medication use in the elderly: Optimizing therapy for older women. Cardiol Rev 11:275, 2003.
39. Schwartz J: The influence of sex on pharmacokinetics. Clin Pharmacokinet 42:107, 2003.
40. Evans W, Relling M: Pharmacogenomics: Translating functional genomics into rational therapeutics. Science 286:487, 1999.
41. Weinshilboum R: Inheritance and drug response. N Engl J Med 348:529, 2003.
42. Mulder A, van Lijf H, Bon M, et al: Association of polymorphism in the cytochrome CYPD6 and the efficacy and tolerability of simvastatin. Clin Pharmacol Ther 70:546, 2001.
43. Roden DM, Brown NJ:. Preprescription genotyping: Not yet ready for prime time, but getting there. Circulation 103:1608, 2001.
44. Rendic S: Summary of information on human CYP enzymes: Human P450 metabolism data. Drug Metab Rev 34:83, 2002.
45. Benet L, Hoener B: Changes in plasma protein binding have little clinical relevance. Clin Pharmacol Ther 71:115, 2002.
46. Kohn LT, Corrigan JM, Donaldson MS (eds): To Err Is Human: Building a Safer Health System. Washington, DC, National Academies Press, 2000.
47. Onder G, Padone C, Landi F, et al: Adverse drug reactions as cause of hospital admission: Results from the Italian Group of Pharmacoepidemiology in the Elderly (GIFA). J Am Geriatr Soc 50:1962, 2002.
48. Gurwitz JH, Field TS, Harrold LR, et al: Incidence and preventability of adverse drug events among older persons in the ambulatory setting. JAMA 289:1107, 2003.
49. Bates D, Miller E, Cullen D, et al for the ADE Prevention Study Group: Patient risk factors for adverse drug events in hospitalized patients. Arch Intern Med 159:2553, 1999.
50. Gandhi TK, Weingart SN, Borus J, et al: Adverse drug events in ambulatory care. N Engl J Med 348:1556, 2003.
51. Field TS, Gurwitz JH, Avom J, et al: Risk factors for adverse drug events among nursing home residents. Arch Intern Med 161:1629, 2001.
52. Kaufman D, Kelly JP, Rosenberg L, et al: Recent patterns of medication use in the ambulatory adult population of the United States. The Slone survey. JAMA 287:337, 2002.
53. Hunt SA, Baker DW, Chin MH, et al: ACC/AHA guidelines for the evaluation and management of chronic heart failure in the adult: Executive summary: A report of the

American College of Cardiology/American Heart Association Task Force on Practice Guidelines (Committee to revise the 1995 Guidelines for the Evaluation and Management of Heart Failure). J Am Coll Cardiol 38:2101, 2001.
54. Ryan TJ, Antman EM, Brooks NH, et al: 1999 update: ACC/AHA Guidelines for the Management of Patients with Acute Myocardial Infarction: Executive Summary and Recommendations. A report of the American College of Cardiology/American Heart Association Task Force on Practice Guidelines (Committee on Management of Acute Myocardial Infarction). Circulation 100:1016, 1999.
55. Lau WC, Waskell LA, Watkins PB, et al: Atorvastatin reduces the ability of clopidogrel to inhibit platelet aggregation: A new drug-drug interaction. Circulation 107:32, 2003.
55a. Saw J, Steinhubl SR, Berger PB, et al: Lack of adverse clopidogrel-atorvastatin clinical interaction from secondary analysis of a randomized, placebo-controlled clopidogrel trial. Circulation 108:921, 2003.
56. De Smet P: Herbal remedies. N Engl J Med 347:2046, 2002.
57. Ioannides C: Pharmacokinetic interactions between herbal remedies and medicinal drugs. Xenobiotica 32:451, 2002.
58. Juurlink DN, Mamdani M, Kopp A, et al: Drug-drug interactions among elderly patients hospitalized for drug toxicity. JAMA 289:1652, 2003.
59. Schulman S. Care of patients receiving long-term anticoagulant therapy. N Engl J Med 349:675, 2003.
60. Institute of Medicine: Workshop on Pharmacokinetics and Drug Interactions in the Elderly and Special Issues in Elderly African-American Populations. Washington, DC, National Academy of Sciences, 1997.
61. Re-engineering the medication-use system. Am J Health Syst Pharm 57:537, 2000.
62. Pugh K, Wei J: Clinical implications of physiological changes in the aging heart. Drugs Aging 18:263, 2001.
63. Juurlink D, Mamdani M, Kopp A, et al: Drug-drug interactions among elderly patients hospitalized for drug toxicity. JAMA 289:1652, 2003.
64. Brater D: Anti-inflammatory agents and renal function. Semin Arthritis Rheum 32(3 Suppl 1):33, 2002.
65. Beers M: Explicit criteria for determining potentially inappropriate medication by the elderly. Arch Intern Med 157:1531, 1997.
66. Hanlon JT, Schmader KE, Boult C, et al: Use of inappropriate prescription drugs by older people. J Am Geriatr Soc 50:26, 2002.
67. Zhan C, Sangl J, Bierman AS, et al: Potentially inappropriate medication use in the community-dwelling elderly: Findings from the 1996 Medical Expenditure Panel Survey. JAMA 286:2866, 2001.
68. Cohn J: Adverse drug effects, compliance, and initial doses of antihypertensive drugs recommended by the Joint National Committee vs. the Physician's Desk Reference. Arch Intern Med 161:880, 2001.
69. Michalsen A, Konig G, Thimme W: Preventable causative factors leading to hospital admission with decompensated heart failure. Heart 80:437, 1998.
70. Salas M, Int'Veld BA, van der Linden PD, et al: Impaired cognitive function and compliance with antihypertensive drugs in elderly: The Rotterdam Study. Clin Pharmacol Ther 70:561, 2001.
71. Federman AD, Adams AS, Ross-Degnan D, et al: Supplemental insurance and use of effective cardiovascular drugs among elderly medicare beneficiaries with coronary heart disease JAMA 286:1732, 2001.
72. Barat I, Andreasen F, Damsgaard EMS: Drug therapy in the elderly: What doctors believe and patients actually do. Br J Clin Pharmacol 51:615, 2001.
73. McDonald HP, Garg AX, Haynes RB: Interventions to enhance patient adherence to medication prescriptions: Scientific review. JAMA 288:2868, 2002.

Vascular Disease

74. Hajjar I, Kotchen T: Trends in prevalence, awareness, treatment, and control of hypertension in the United States, 1988-2000. JAMA 290:199, 2003.
75. Franklin S, Gustin WT, Wong N, et al: Hemodynamic patterns of age-related changes in blood pressure. The Framingham Heart Study. Circulation 96:308, 1997.
76. Hyman D, Pavlik V: Characteristics of patients with uncontrolled hypertension in the United States. N Engl J Med 345:479, 2001.
77. Staessen J, Fagard R, Thijs L, et al: Randomised double-blind comparison of placebo and active treatment for older patients with isolated systolic hypertension. The Systolic Hypertension in Europe (Syst-Eur) Trial Investigators. Lancet 350:757, 1997.
78. Forette F, Seux ML, Staessen JA, et al for the Syst-Eur Investigators: The prevention of dementia with antihypertensive treatment. Arch Intern Med 162:2046, 2002.
79. The ALLHAT Collaborative Group: Major outcomes in high-risk hypertensive patients randomized to angiotensin-converting enzyme inhibitor or calcium channel blocker vs diuretic: The Antihypertensive and Lipid-Lowering Treatment to Prevent Heart Attack Trial (ALLHAT). JAMA 288:2981, 2002.
80. Psaty B, Lumley T, Furberg C, et al: Health outcomes associated with various antihypertensive therapies used as first-line agents. A network meta-analysis. JAMA 289:2534, 2003.
81. Lacroix A, Ott S, Ichikawa L, et al: Low-dose hydrochlorothiazide and preservation of bone mineral density in older adults. A randomized double-blind, placebo-controlled trial. Ann Intern Med 133:516, 2000.
82. Wing LM, Reld CM, Ryan P, et al for the Second Australian National Blood Pressure Study Group: A comparison of outcomes with angiotensin-converting-enzyme inhibitors and diuretics for hypertension in the elderly. N Engl J Med 348:583, 2003.
83. Chobanian AV, Bakris GL, Black HR, et al and the National High Blood Pressure Education Program Coordinating Committee: The Seventh Report of the Joint National Committee on Prevention, Detection, Evaluation, and Treatment of High Blood Pressure. The JNC 7 report. JAMA 289:2560, 2003.
84. Guidelines Committee: 2003 European Society of Hypertension–European Society of Cardiology guidelines for the management of arterial hypertension. J Hypertens 21:1011, 2003 (available on line at http://www.eshonline.org/documents/2003_guidelines.pdf).
85. Dahlof B, Devereux RB, Kjeldsen SE, et al: Cardiovascular morbidity and mortality in the Losartan Intervention For Endpoint reduction in hypertension study (LIFE): A randomised trial against atenolol. Lancet 359:995, 2002.
86. Lithell H, Hansson L, Skoog I, et al for the SCOPE Study Group: The Study on Cognition and Prognosis in the Elderly (SCOPE): Principal results of a randomized double-blind intervention trial. J Hypertens 21:875, 2003.
87. Fagard R: Epidemiology of hypertension in the elderly. Am J Geriatr Cardiol 11:23, 2002.
88. Tinetti M: Preventing falls in elderly persons. N Engl J Med 348:42, 2003.
89. Kohara K, Uemura K, Takata Y, et al: Postprandial hypotension: Evaluation by ambulatory blood pressure monitoring. Am J Hypertens 11:1358, 1998.
90. Smith N, Psaty B, Rutan G, et al: The association between time since last meal and blood pressure in older adults: The Cardiovascular Health Study. J Am Geriatr Soc 51:824, 2003.
91. Whelton P, Appel L, Espeland M, et al: Sodium reduction and weight loss in the treatment of hypertension in older persons: A randomized controlled trial of nonpharmacologic interventions in the elderly (TONE). JAMA 279:878, 1998.
92. Hajjar I, Grim C, Kotchen T: Dietary calcium lowers the age-related rise in blood pressure in the United States: The NHANES III Survey. J Clin Hypertens 5:122, 2003.
93. Gueyffler F, Bulpitt C, Boissel J-P, et al: Antihypertensive drugs in very old people: A subgroup meta-analysis of randomised controlled trials. INDANA Group. Lancet 353:793, 1999.
94. Goodwin J: Embracing complexity: A consideration of hypertension in the very old. J Gerontol Med Sci 58A:653, 2003.
95. Auseon A, Ooi W, Hossain M, Lipsitz L: Blood pressure behavior in the nursing home: Implications for diagnosis and treatment of hypertension. J Am Geriatr Soc 47:2377, 1999.
96. Kuller L, Fisher L, McClelland R, et al: Differences in prevalence of and risk factors for subclinical vascular disease among black and white participants in the Cardiovascular Health Study. Arterioscler Thromb Vasc Biol 18:283, 1998.
97. Newman AB, Shemanski L, Manolio TA, et al: Ankle-arm index as a predictor of cardiovascular disease and mortality in the Cardiovascular Health Study. Arterioscler Thromb Vasc Biol 19:538, 1999.
98. Kuller L, Borhani N, Furberg C, et al: Prevalence of subclinical atherosclerosis and cardiovascular disease and association with risk factors in the Cardiovascular Health Study. Am J Epidemiol 139:1164, 1994.
99. Wilson P, D'Agostino R, Levy D, et al: Prediction of coronary heart disease using risk factor categories. Circulation 97:1837, 1998.
100. Gibbons R, Balady G, Bricker J, et al: ACC/AHA 2002 Guideline Update for Exercise Testing: A Report of the American College of Cardiology/American Heart Association Task Force on Practice Guidelines (Committee on Exercise Testing). Available on the Web sites of the American College of Cardiology (www.acc.org) and the American Heart Association(www.americanheart.org), 2002.
101. Fleg J: Stress testing in the elderly. Am J Geriatr Cardiol 10:308, 2001.
102. Gibbons R, Abrams J, Chatterjee K, et al: ACC/AHA 2002 guideline update for the management of patients with chronic stable angina—Summary article: A report of the American College of Cardiology/American Heart Association Task Force on Practice Guidelines (Committee on the Management of Patients with Chronic Stable Angina). Circulation 107:149, 2003.
103. Heart Protection Study Collaborative Group: MRC/BHF Heart Protection Study of cholesterol lowering with simvastatin in 20,536 high-risk individuals: A randomised placebo-controlled trial. Lancet:7, 2002.
104. Downs J, Clearfield M, Weis S, et al: Primary prevention of acute coronary events with lovastatin in men and women with average cholesterol levels. Results of AFCAPS/TexCAPS. JAMA 279:1615, 1998.
105. Shepherd J, Cobbe S, Ford I, et al: Prevention of coronary heart disease with pravastatin in men with hypercholesterolemia. N Engl J Med 333:1301, 1995.
106. Mullany C, Mock M, Brooks M, et al: Effect of age in the Bypass Angioplasty Revascularization Investigation (BARI) randomized trial. Ann Thorac Surg 67:396, 1999.
107. Alexander K, Galanos A, Jollis J, et al: Post-myocardial infarction risk stratification in elderly patients. Am Heart J 142:37, 2001.
108. Batchelor W, Anstrom K, Muhlbaier L, et al: Contemporary outcome trends in the elderly undergoing percutaneous coronary interventions: Results in 7,472 octogenarians. National Cardiovascular Network Collaboration. J Am Coll Cardiol 36:723, 2000.
109. Newman MF, Kirchner J, Phillips-Bute B, et al: Neurological Outcome Research Group and the Cardiothoracic Anesthesiology Research Endeavors Investigators. Longitudinal assessment of neurocognitive function after coronary-artery bypass surgery. N Engl J Med 344:395, 2001.
110. Pfisterer M, Buser P, Osswald S, et al for the Trial of Invasive versus Medical Therapy in Elderly patients (TIME) Investigators: Outcome of elderly patients with chronic symptomatic coronary artery disease with an invasive vs. optimized medical treatment strategy. One-year results of the randomized TIME trial. JAMA 289:1117, 2003.
111. Eagle K, Guyton R, Davidoff R, et al: ACC/AHA Guidelines for Coronary Artery Bypass Graft Surgery: Executive Summary and Recommendations. A Report of the American College of Cardiology/American Heart Association Task Force on Practice Guidelines (Committee to Revise the 1991 Guidelines for Coronary Artery Bypass Graft Surgery). Circulation 100:1464, 1999.
112. Vaccarino V, Lin Z, Kasl S, et al: Gender differences in recovery after coronary artery bypass surgery. J Am Coll Cardiol 41:307, 2003.
113. Mehta R, Rathore S, Radford M, et al: Acute myocardial infarction in the elderly: Differences by age. J Am Coll Cardiol 38:736, 2001.
114. Rich MW, PRICE-2 Organizing Committee, PRICE-2 Investigators: Executive summary: Second Pivotal Research in Cardiovascular Syndromes in the Elderly (PRICE-II) Symposium. Acute coronary syndromes in the elderly: Mechanisms and management. Am J Geriatr Cardiol 12:307, 2003.

115. Brass LM, Lichtman JH, Wang Y, et al: Intracranial hemorrhage associated with thrombolytic therapy for elderly patients with acute myocardial infarction: Results from the Cooperative Cardiovascular Project. Stroke 31:1802, 2000.
116. Berger A, Radford M, Wang Y, et al: Thrombolytic therapy in older patients. J Am Coll Cardiol 36:366, 2000.
117. Thiemann D, Coresh J, Schulman S, et al: Lack of benefit for intravenous thrombolysis in patients with myocardial infarction who are older than 75 years. Circulation 101:2239, 2000.
118. Becker RC, Hochman JS, Cannon CP, et al: Fatal cardiac rupture among patients treated with thrombolytic agents and adjunctive thrombin antagonists: Observations from the Thrombolysis and Thrombin Inhibition in Myocardial Infarction 9 Study. J Am Coll Cardiol 33:479, 1999.
119. Angeja B, Rundle A, Gurwitz J, et al: Death or nonfatal stroke in patients with acute myocardial infarction treated with tissue plasminogen activator. Am J Cardiol 87:627, 2001.
120. Horwitz P, Berlin J, Sauer W, et al: Registry Committee of the Society for Cardiac Angiography Interventions. Bleeding risk of platelet glycoprotein IIb/IIIa receptor antagonists in broad-based practice (results from the Society for Cardiac Angiography and Interventions Registry). Am J Cardiol 91:803, 2003.
121. Brown D: Deaths associated with platelet glycoprotein IIb/IIIa inhibitor treatment. Heart 89:535, 2003.
122. Weaver W, Simes R, Betriu A, et al: Comparison of primary coronary angioplasty and intravenous thrombolytic therapy for acute myocardial infarction: A quantitative review. JAMA 278:2093, 1997.
123. Berger A, Schulman K, Gersh B, et al: Primary coronary angioplasty vs thrombolysis for the management of acute myocardial infarction in elderly patients. JAMA 282:341, 1999.
124. Rich MW: Executive summary: Second Pivotal Research in Cardiovascular syndromes in the Elderly (PRICE-2) symposium. Acute coronary syndromes in the elderly: Mechanisms and management. Am J Geriatr Cardiol 12:305, 2003.
125. Berwen D, Galusha D, Lewis J, et al: National and state trends in quality of care for acute myocardial infarction between 1994-1995 and 1998-1999. Arch Intern Med 163:1430, 2003.
126. Bush D, Ziegelstein R, Tayback M, et al: Even minimal symptoms of depression increase mortality risk after acute myocardial infarction. Am J Cardiol 88:337, 2001.
127. Scheir M, Matthews K, Owens J, et al: Optimism and rehospitalization after coronary artery bypass graft surgery. Arch Intern Med 159:829, 1999.
128. Connerney I, Shapiro P, McLaughlin J, et al: Relation between depression after coronary artery bypass surgery and 12-month outcome: A prospective study. Lancet 358:1766, 2001.
129. Dusseldorp E, van Elderen T, Maes S, et al: A meta-analysis of psychoeducational programs for coronary heart disease patients. Health Psychol 18:506, 1999.
130. Glassman A, O'Connor C, Califf R, et al: Sertraline treatment of major depression in patients with acute MI or unstable angina. JAMA 288:701, 2002.
131. Berkman LF, Blumenthal J, Burg M, et al: Effects of treating depression and low perceived social support on clinical events after myocardial infarction. The Enhancing Recovery in Coronary Heart Disease Patients (ENRICHD) Randomized Trial. JAMA 289:3106, 2003.
132. Whooley M, Avins A, Miranda J, Browner W: Case-finding instruments for depression: Two questions are as good as many. J Gen Intern Med 12:439, 1997.
133. Rochon P, Tu J, Anderson G, et al: Rate of heart failure and 1-year survival for older people receiving low-dose beta-blocker therapy after myocardial infarction. Lancet 356:639, 2000.
134. Grady D, Herrington D, Vittner V, et al: Cardiovascular disease outcomes during 6.8 years of hormone therapy. Heart and Estrogen/Progestin Replacement Study Follow-up (HERS II). JAMA 288:49, 2002.
135. Risks and Benefits of Estrogen Plus Progestin in Healthy Postmenopausal Women: Principal results from the Women's Health Initiative Randomized Controlled Trial. JAMA 288:321, 2002.
135a. Tanne JH: Oestrogen only arm of women's health initiative trial is stopped. BMJ 328:602, 2004.
135b. National Institutes of Health: NIH News. www.nhlbi.nih.gov/new/press/04-03-02.htm.
136. Binder F, Schechtman K, Ehsani A, et al: Effects of exercise training on frailty in community-dwelling older adults: Results of a randomized, controlled trial. J Am Geriatr Soc 50:2089, 2002.
137. Baum E, Jarjoura D, Polen A, et al: Effectiveness of a group exercise program in a long-term care facility: A randomized pilot trial. J Am Med Dir Assoc 4:74, 2003.
138. Marchionni N, Fattirolli F, Fumagalli S, et al: Improved exercise tolerance and quality of life with cardiac rehabilitation of older patients after myocardial infarction. Results of a randomized, controlled trial. Circulation 107:2201, 2003.
139. Straus S, Majumdar S, McAlister F: New evidence for stroke prevention. Scientific review. JAMA 288:1388, 2002.
140. Albers G, Hart R, Lutsep H, et al: AHA Scientific Statement. Supplement to the guidelines for the management of transient ischemic attacks. A statement from the Ad Hoc Committee on Guidelines for the Management of Transient Ischemic Attacks, Stroke Council, American Heart Association. Stroke 30:2502, 1999.
141. Johnston S: Transient ischemic attack. N Engl J Med 347:1687, 2002.
142. Adams HJ, Adams R, Brott T, et al: Stroke Council of the American Stroke Association. Guidelines for the early management of patients with ischemic stroke: A scientific statement from the Stroke Council of the American Stroke Association. Stroke 34:1056, 2003.
143. Committee CS: A randomized, blinded, trial of clopidogrel vs. aspirin in patients at risk of ischemic events (CAPRIE). Lancet 348:1329, 1996.
144. Diener H, Cunha L, Forbes C, et al: European Stroke Prevention Study-2. Dipyridamole and acetylsalicylic acid in the secondary prevention of stroke. J Neurol Sci 143:1, 1996.
145. Mohr J, Thompson J, Lazar R, et al: A comparison of warfarin and aspirin for the prevention of recurrent ischemic stroke. N Engl J Med 345:1444, 2001.
146. Antiplatelet Trialists' Collaboration: Collaborative meta-analysis of randomised trials of antiplatelet therapy for prevention of death, myocardial infarction and stroke in high risk patients. BMJ 324:71, 2002.
147. Johnson E, Lanes S, Wentwork CI, et al: A metaregression analysis of the dose-response effect of ASA on stroke. Arch Intern Med 159:1284, 1999.
148. Barnett H, Meldrum H, Eliasziw M: North American Symptomatic Carotid Endarterectomy Trial (NASCET) collaborators. The appropriate use of carotid endarterectomy. CMAJ 166:1169, 2002.
149. Rothwell P, Slatttery J, Warlow C: Clinical and angiographic predictors of stroke and death from carotid endarterectomy: Systematic review. BMJ 315:1571, 1997.
150. Hanel R, Xavier A, Kirmani J, et al: Management of carotid artery stenosis: Comparing endarterectomy and stenting. Curr Cardiol Rep 5:153, 2003.
151. Ouriel K: Peripheral arterial disease. Lancet 358:1257, 2001.
152. McDermott M, Greenland P, Liu K, et al: Leg symptoms in peripheral arterial disease. Associated clinical characteristics and functional impairment. JAMA 286:1599, 2001.
153. Dormandy J, Rutherford R: Management of peripheral arterial disease (PAD). J Vasc Surg 31:S1, 2000.
154. Hiatt W: Medical treatment of peripheral arterial disease and claudication. N Engl J Med 344:1608, 2001.
155. Trans Atlantic Inter-Society Consensus (TASC): Management of peripheral arterial disease (PAD). Eur J Vasc Endovasc Surg Suppl A(Sec A-D):S1, 2000.
156. Trans Atlantic Inter-Society Consensus (TASC): Management of peripheral arterial disease (PAD). Int Angiol 19(Suppl 1):1, 2000.

Heart Failure

157. Ni H: Prevalence of self-reported heart failure among US adults: Results from the 1999 National Health Interview Survey. Am Heart J 146:1, 2003.
158. Gottdiener J, Arnold A, Aurigemma G, et al: Predictors of congestive heart failure in the elderly: The Cardiovascular Health Study. J Am Coll Cardiol 35:1628, 2000.
159. Wang T, Levy D, Benjamin E, Vasan R: The epidemiology of "asymptomatic" left ventricular systolic dysfunction: Implications for screening. Ann Intern Med 138:907, 2003.
160. Gottdiener J, McClellan R, Marshall R, et al: Outcome of congestive heart failure in elderly persons: Influence of left ventricular systolic function. The Cardiovascular Health Study. Ann Intern Med 137:631, 2002.
161. MacCarthy P, Kearney M, Nolan J, et al: Prognosis in heart failure with preserved left ventricular systolic function: Prospective cohort study. Br Med J 327:78, 2003.
162. Croft J, Giles W, Pollard R, et al: Heart failure survival among older adults in the United States: A poor prognosis for an emerging epidemic in the Medicare population. Arch Intern Med 159:505, 1999.
163. Vasan R, Larson M, Benjamin E, et al: Congestive heart failure in subjects with normal versus reduced let ventricular ejection fraction: Prevalence and mortality in a population-based cohort. J Am Coll Cardiol 33:1948, 1999.
164. Redfield M, Jacobsen S, Burnett J, et al: Burden of systolic and diastolic ventricular dysfunction in the community. Appreciating the scope of the heart failure epidemic. JAMA 289:194, 2003.
165. Senni M, Tribouilloy C, Rodeheffer R, et al: Congestive heart failure in the community. Circulation 98:2282, 1998.
166. Kitzman DW, Gardin JM, Gottdiener JS, et al, Cardiovascular Health Study Research Group: Importance of heart failure with preserved systolic function in the elderly. CHS Research Group. Am J Cardiol 87:413, 2001.
167. Masoudi F, Havranek E, Smith G, et al: Gender, age, and heart failure with preserved left ventricular systolic function. J Am Coll Cardiol 41:217, 2003.
168. Philbin E, Erb T, Jenkins P: The natural history of heart failure with preserved left ventricular systolic function. J Am Coll Cardiol 29(2 Suppl A):245, 1997.
169. European Study Group on Diastolic Heart Failure: How to diagnose diastolic heart failure. Eur Heart J 19:990, 1998.
170. Garg R, Yusuf S, Trials C, GoAI: Overview of randomized trials of angiotensin converting enzyme inhibitors on mortality and morbidity in heart failure. JAMA 273:1450, 1995.
171. Flather M, Yusuf S, Kober L, et al for the ACE-Inhibitor Myocardial Infarction Collaborative Group: Long-term ACE-inhibitor therapy in patients with heart failure or left-ventricular dysfunction: A systematic overview of data from individual patients. Lancet 355:1575, 2000.
172. MacMahon S: The Blood Pressure Lowering Treatment Trialists' Collaboration: Second cycle of analyses. Program and abstracts of the 13th European Meeting on Hypertension, June 13-17, 2003, Milan, Italy.
173. Pitt B, Zannad F, Remme W, et al: The effect of spironolactone on morbidity and mortality in patients with severe heart failure. N Engl J Med 341:709, 1999.
174. Shlipak M: Pharmacotherapy for heart failure in patients with renal insufficiency. Ann Intern Med 139:917, 2003.
175. Petrie M, Dawson N, Murdoch D, et al: Failure of women's hearts. Circulation 99:2334, 1999.
176. Simon T, Mary-Krause M, Funck-Brentano C, Jaillon P: Sex differences in the prognosis of congestive heart failure. Results from the Cardiac Insufficiency Bisoprolol Study (CIBIS II). Circulation 103:375, 2001.
177. Rathore S, Wang Y, Krumholz H: Sex-based differences in the effect of digoxin for the treatment of heart failure. N Engl J Med 347:1403, 2002.
178. Bradley E, Baughman K, Berger R, et al: Cardiac resynchronization and death from progressive heart failure. A meta-analysis of randomized controlled trials. JAMA 289:730, 2003.
179. The effect of digoxin on mortality and morbidity in patients with heart failure. The Digitalis Investigation Group. N Engl J Med 336:525, 1997.
180. Kitzman D: Diastolic heart failure in the elderly. Heart Fail Rev 7:17, 2002.
181. Nichol K, Nordin J, Mullooly J, et al: Influenza vaccination and reduction in hospitalizations for cardiac disease and stroke among the elderly. N Engl J Med 348:1322, 2003.

Arrhythmias

182. Tsang T, Petty G, Barnes M, et al: The prevalence of atrial fibrillation in incident stroke cases and matched population controls in Rochester, Minnesota. Changes over three decades. J Am Coll Cardiol 42:93, 2003.
183. Caraballo P, Heit J, Atkinson E, et al: Long-term use of oral anticoagulants and the risk of fracture. Arch Intern Med 159:1750, 1999.

Valvular Disease

184. Otto C, Lind B, Kitzman D, et al: Association of aortic-valve sclerosis with cardiovascular mortality and morbidity in the elderly. N Engl J Med 341:142, 1999.
185. Stewart BF, Siscovick D, Lind BK, et al: Clinical factors associated with calcific aortic valve disease. Cardiovascular Health Study. J Am Coll Cardiol 29:630, 1997.
186. Shavelle D, Takasu J, Budoff M, et al: HMG CoA reductase inhibitor (statin) and aortic valve calcium. Lancet 359:1125, 2002.
187. Faggiano P, Antonini-Canterin F, Erlicher A, et al: Progression of aortic valve sclerosis to aortic stenosis. Am J Cardiol 91:99, 2003.
188. Pohle K, Maffert R, Ropers D, et al: Progression of aortic valve calcification. Association with coronary atherosclerosis and cardiovascular risk factors. Circulation 104:1927, 2001.
189. Atar S, Jeon D, Luo H, Siegel R: Mitral annular calcification: A marker of severe coronary artery disease in patients under 65 years old. Heart 89:161, 2003.
190. Adler Y, Herz I, Vaturi M, et al: Mitral annular calcium detected by transthoracic echocardiography is a marker for high prevalence and severity of coronary artery disease in patients undergoing coronary angiography. Am J Cardiol 81:784, 1998.
191. ACC/AHA guidelines for the management of patients with valvular heart disease. A Report of the American College of Cardiology/American Heart Association Task Force on Practice Guidelines (Committee on Management of Patients With Valvular Heart Disease). J Am Coll Cardiol 32:1486, 1998.
192. Peltier M, Trojette F, Enriquez-Sarano M, et al: Relation between cardiovascular risk factors and nonrheumatic severe calcific aortic stenosis among patients with a three-cuspid aortic valve. Am J Cardiol 91:97, 2003.
193. Bellamy M, Pellikka P, Klarich K, et al: Association of cholesterol levels, hydroxymethylglutaryl coenzyme-A reductase inhibitor treatment, and progression of aortic stenosis in the community. J Am Coll Cardiol 40:1723, 2002.
194. Cohen G, David T, Ivanov J, et al: The impact of age, coronary artery disease, and cardiac comorbidity on late survival after bioprosthetic aortic valve replacement. J Thorac Cardiovasc Surg 117:273, 1999.
195. Helft G, Tabone X, Georges J, et al: Late results with bioprosthetic valves in the elderly. J Card Surg 14:252, 1999.
196. Kauterman K, Michaels A, Ports T: Is there any indication for aortic valvuloplasty in the elderly? Am J Geriatr Cardiol 12:190, 2003.
197. Aronow W, Ahn C, Kronzon I: Comparison of echocardiographic abnormalities in African-American, Hispanic, and white men and women aged > 60 years. Am J Cardiol 87:1131, 2001.
198. Lee R, Sundt TI, Moon M, et al: Mitral valve repair in the elderly: Operative risk for patients over 70 years of age is acceptable. J Cardiovasc Surg 44:157, 2003.
199. Pritchett A, Morrison J, Edwards WD, et al: Valvular heart disease in patients taking pergolide. Mayo Clin Proc 77:1280, 2002.
200. Flowers C, Racoosin J, Lu S, Beitz J: The US Food and Drug Administration's registry of patients with pergolide-associated valvular heart disease. Mayo Clin Proc 78:730, 2003.

CHAPTER 73

Cardiovascular Disease in Women

Nancy K. Sweitzer • Pamela S. Douglas

More women die every year from cardiovascular disease than from any other cause (Fig. 73–1), yet women worry more about breast cancer than heart disease.[1,2] Women with heart disease may present differently than men, have unique underlying pathophysiologies, and have distinctive risk-benefit profiles with commonly accepted therapies. Heart disease is far more age dependent in women than in men; women with cardiovascular disease are older and have more comorbidities. This fact, in turn, makes diagnostic and treatment procedures more problematic in women. In addition, many effective pharmacological strategies are underutilized, and there is a lack of gender-specific data on numerous therapies. The fact that heart disease is on the decline in men but not women highlights our failure to treat this large segment of the population optimally (Fig. 73–2).

Gender and Mechanisms of Cardiovascular Disease

Genes and Hormones

Although men and women differ by only 1 chromosome out of 46, the impact on health and disease is large. Outside the reproductive systems, the heart and circulation are perhaps most affected. Clinicians have long known of the apparent "protection" of younger, premenopausal women from ischemic heart disease, and this protection has been attributed to estrogen.[3,4] The biological plausibility of this connection is indisputable—gonadal hormones do alter many pathophysiological processes thought to be fundamental to the development of atherosclerosis,[5] including thrombosis and inflammation.[6] Further, nuclear estrogen receptors are present in cardiac myocytes of both males and females, a potential explanation for gender differences in gene regulation.[7] However, these physiological differences have failed to translate into a useful pharmacopoeia. A series of experimental trials have failed to demonstrate any utility of estrogen therapy for either the primary or secondary prevention of vascular disease in men or women.[8-10] Many questions shade these results, and it may well be that in the future we will learn how to better harness the power of estrogens, through use of altered compounds, new delivery routes, and even pharmacogenomics, but for now, estrogens are not indicated in the treatment or prevention of atherosclerosis.

Gender, Genomics, and the Vulnerable Plaque

The differences between men and women in atherosclerosis are not limited to gonadal hormones. Research has shown some fundamental variation in the underlying mechanisms of disease. A Japanese study assayed a large population of myocardial infarction survivors for the presence of 71 single-nucleotide polymorphisms in candidate genes known to be relevant to the pathophysiology of atherosclerosis. Two were found to be significantly more prevalent in men—connexin37 and $p22^{phox}$—and two different genes were relevant in women—plasminogen activator inhibitor 1 (PAI-1) and stromelysin-1—suggesting that the genetic basis underlying coronary heart disease (CHD) varies by gender.[11]

Such genetic differences are manifest in the physiology of atherosclerosis, including plaque components (more cellular and fibrous tissue in women),[12] endothelial function (estrogen-induced coronary vasodilation),[13,14] and hemostasis (higher fibrinogen and factor VII levels in women).[15] Although coronary thrombosis is overwhelmingly the most likely cause of myocardial infarction in both genders (only rarely are infarctions due to spasm or syndrome X), women are twice as likely to have plaque erosion (37 percent in women versus 18 percent in men), whereas men have plaque rupture as the underlying cause of the infarction (82 percent in men versus 63 percent in women).[16]

Gender Differences in Ventricular Remodeling

Even after the onset of established clinical disease, compensation differs between men and women. In pressure overload syndromes (hypertension and aortic stenosis), female rats express different cardiac genes.[7] Women with aortic stenosis or hypertension tend to have more vigorous hypertrophy, with greater left ventricular mass, and better preserved systolic function and contractile reserve than men. In ischemic syndromes, animal studies suggest that females show less hypertrophy but also less pathological remodeling and dilation.[17] Apoptosis and

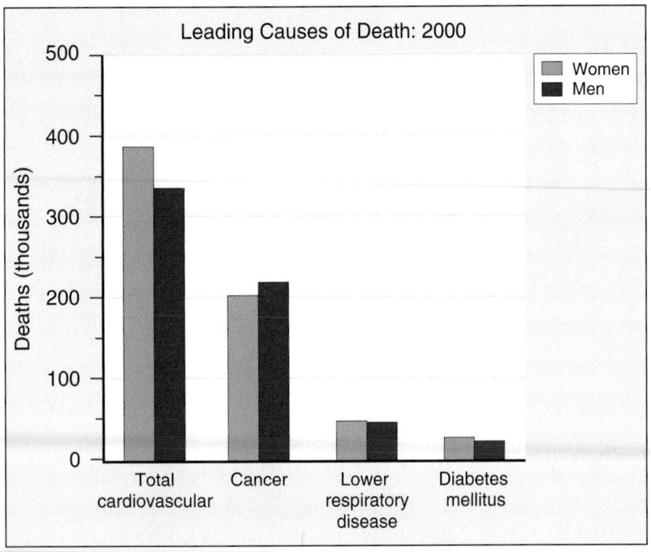

FIGURE 73–1 Number of deaths related to four leading causes of death in women and men in the United States in 2000, ranked in order for women. (Modified from the American Heart Association Heart Disease and Stroke Statistics—2003 Update; 2002. Available at http://www.americanheart.org/downloadable/heart/1059017971148 2003HDSStatsBookREV7-03.pdf. Accessed August 15, 2003.)

myocyte necrosis in response to aging, injury, or stress are more pronounced in males than in females.[18]

Gender Roles and Psychosocial Aspects of Cardiovascular Disease

It is important to recognize that, as patients, there are differences between the genders.[19] Because women are older and have a greater burden of risk factors and concomitant disease, they are more frail and less likely to recover fully from cardiovascular events. Women's greater longevity and our society's gender roles combine to make women caregivers to men with atherosclerotic disease but often leave the same women without social, emotional, or financial support at the time of their own illness.[20] Women, as well as their caregivers, may underestimate the importance of atherosclerotic disease and fail to implement preventive strategies fully or even recognize and act on symptoms appropriately. These factors have a significant, negative impact on optimal care delivery for women.[21]

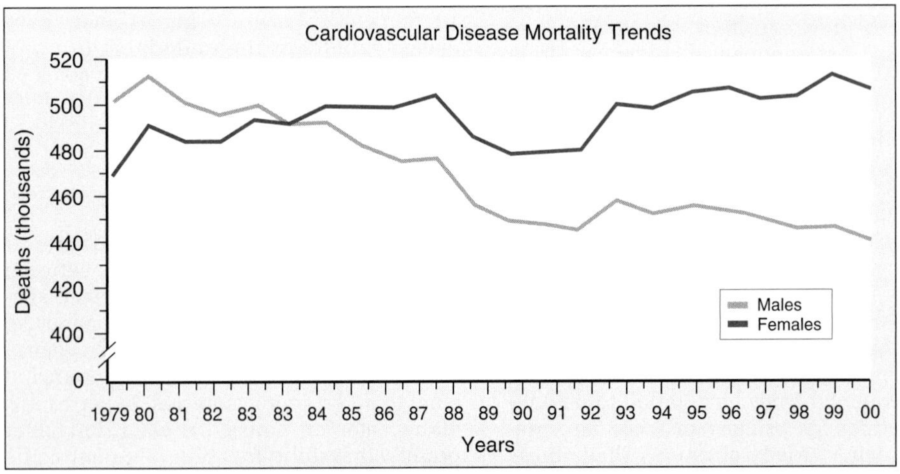

FIGURE 73–2 Trends in cardiovascular disease mortality in males and females in the United States from 1979 to 2000. (From the American Heart Association Heart Disease and Stroke Statistics—2003 Update; 2002. Available at http://www.americanheart.org/downloadable/heart/10590179711482003HDSStatsBookREV7-03.pdf. Accessed August 15, 2003.)

Atherosclerotic Vascular Disease

Risk Factors for Coronary Heart Disease in Women and Their Modification

Diabetes Mellitus and Metabolic Syndrome

Diabetes is associated with a greater incremental risk in women, completely eliminating the "female advantage."[22] The American Heart Association awards double weight to diabetes in women when calculating CHD risk,[23] similar to the weight given a systolic blood pressure of 173 mm Hg or above or a cholesterol level of 316 mg/dl or above. More than in men, diabetes dramatically increases the mortality of myocardial infarction in women (Fig. 73–3). Type 2 diabetes is associated with obesity, abdominal body fat distribution, hypertension, atherogenic dyslipidemia, and insulin resistance, all of which have been associated with higher CHD risk.[22] This complex of abnormalities, termed "metabolic syndrome," alters hepatic metabolism, lipoprotein levels, and circulating insulin levels.[24] More so than in men, obesity and body fat distribution appear to be independent coronary artery disease risk factors in women.[22] Diabetes is also linked with endothelial dysfunction and a variety of platelet abnormalities. Data from the Diabetes Control and Complications Trial suggest that intensive diabetes therapy reduces cardiovascular complications in men and women younger than 40 years.[25]

Hypertension

More than 25 million American women have high blood pressure, and cardiovascular risk related to hypertension rises steeply with age in females.[26] Further, although women have fewer cardiovascular events, the population risk attributable to hypertension is higher for women than men because of the increased incidence with age and the longevity of women.[27] Nonpharmacological interventions effectively decrease blood pressure in women, including a low-salt diet, physical activity, and weight loss. However, compliance with such changes is low (~10 percent)[28] and blood pressure increases again when physical activity decreases or weight is regained. Most trials have shown equal efficacy of blood pressure lowering to prevent cardiovascular events in men and women. The Seventh Joint National Committee on Prevention, Detection, Evaluation, and Treatment of High Blood Pressure includes a single set of guidelines for both men and women, stating that "large, long-term clinical trials of antihypertensive treatment have not demonstrated clinically significant gender differences in blood pressure response and outcomes."[29] Although it is clear that hypertension in women should be treated as aggressively as in men, it is possible that the optimal choice of antihypertensive agent may differ. The Antihypertensive and Lipid-Lowering Treatment to Prevent Heart Attack Trial (ALLHAT) demonstrated superiority of diuretic therapy in the prespecified female cohort, as in the trial as a whole.[30] The Second

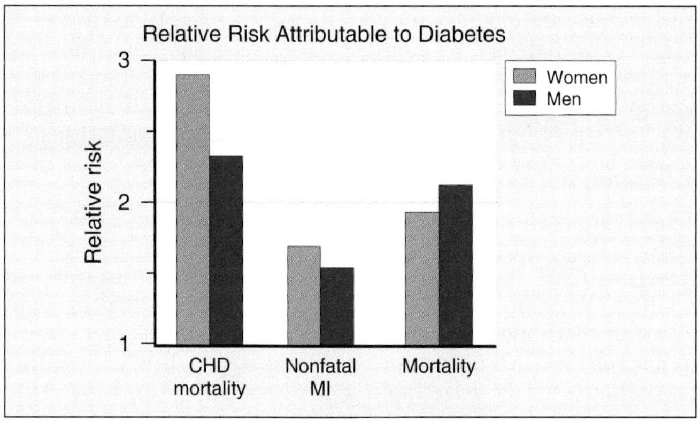

FIGURE 73–3 Relative risks of coronary heart disease (CHD) mortality, nonfatal myocardial infarction (MI), and total mortality attributable to diabetes in women compared with men. (Modified from Grady D, Chaput L, Kristof M: Diagnosis and Treatment of Coronary Heart Disease in Women: Systematic Reviews of Evidence on Selected Topics. Evidence Report/Technology Assessment No. 81. AHRQ Publication No. 03-0037. Rockville, Md, Agency for Healthcare Research and Quality, May 2003.)

Australian National Blood Pressure Study Group found that angiotensin-converting enzyme (ACE) inhibitor therapy decreased cardiovascular endpoints relative to hydrochlorothiazide in men but not in women.[31] The numbers of women included in trials are often too small to draw conclusions.

Smoking

Tobacco contributes to 17 percent of all female deaths in the United States and results in more deaths from CHD and stroke than any other cause.[32] The combination of accelerated atherosclerosis and propensity to vascular thrombosis induced by cigarette smoking is responsible for a six- to ninefold increased risk of myocardial infarction among female smokers compared with nonsmokers. There is a similar increase in stroke risk. The combination of cigarette smoking and oral contraceptive use appears to be particularly potent at increasing the risk of arterial thrombosis. Cigarettes have an antiestrogenic effect and induce an unfavorable lipid profile, leading women to lose their "natural" protection against atherosclerotic vascular disease. Currently available methods to assist with quitting may be less effective in women, perhaps because of a greater behavioral component and less nicotine addiction in women smokers.[33] Environmental exposure to tobacco smoke increases the risk of cardiovascular disease in women, and assessment of environmental exposure is an important part of risk assessment.[34]

Lipids

The average lipid profile in women is affected by hormonal status and changes throughout life. Young women have lower low-density lipoprotein (LDL) cholesterol levels and higher high-density lipoprotein (HDL) cholesterol levels than men of the same age.[35,36] As women age, LDL cholesterol increases, HDL cholesterol decreases, and the risk of CHD climbs.[37] Elevated total cholesterol and LDL levels are only weakly associated with CHD in women and only in women 65 years old or younger. Instead, HDL cholesterol is closely and inversely associated with CHD risk. Triglycerides are an independent predictor of CHD, particularly in older women. Lipoprotein(a), a composite of LDL, apolipoprotein B-100, and apolipoprotein(a), is also associated with higher cardiac risk in women.[35] Initial modification of a high-risk lipoprotein profile is generally accomplished by the same life-style changes and medications in men and women, although dietary interventions may be less effective in women.[38]

Multiple trials have demonstrated efficacy of 3-hydroxy-3-methylglutaryl coenzyme A (HMG CoA) reductase inhibitors, or statins, in both primary and secondary prevention of coronary events and death in women with both elevated and normal cholesterol, supporting the persistent theory that there are benefits of these agents independent of LDL-lowering effects (Fig. 73–4).[39] Women have generally not been included in trials of other classes of lipid-lowering agents, such as the bile acid sequestrant cholestyramine and the fibrate gemfibrozil. In addition, there are no data from large trials on the efficacy of lipid-lowering agents targeted more specifically at altering the HDL and triglyceride lipid subfractions, which appear more important in women. It seems reasonable to apply strategies shown to be successful in men, recognizing that optimal care of women with dyslipidemia may eventually be different from that of men.

Estrogen

The presence of estrogen in the premenopausal female population, the obvious protection this group enjoys against cardiovascular events, and documentation of estrogen receptors in cardiomyocytes and vascular tissues in both men and women led to tremendous enthusiasm for use of postmenopausal hormone replacement therapy as a preventive measure against atherosclerotic heart disease. This enthusiasm was bolstered by multiple observational studies suggesting improved longevity and decreased cardiac events in postmenopausal women receiving hormone replacement therapy as well as mechanistic data supporting biological plausibility.[40,41] Multiple randomized controlled trials in the past 3 years have refuted this hypothesis and provided strong evidence of an increase in cardiovascular risk (Fig. 73–5), particularly in the first year after beginning therapy, combined with increased risk of breast cancer, thromboembolic disease, and stroke, resulting in a withdrawal of prior recommendations.[8,9,42] In the Women's Health Initiative Study, use of estrogen alone, without a progestin, neither caused nor prevented cardiac events, although it did increase the risk of stroke and decrease the risk of hip fracture.[42a] Other studies documenting progression of atherosclerosis during hormone replacement therapy have confirmed the lack of benefit. Hormone replacement therapy has no place in prevention of heart disease in women at present.

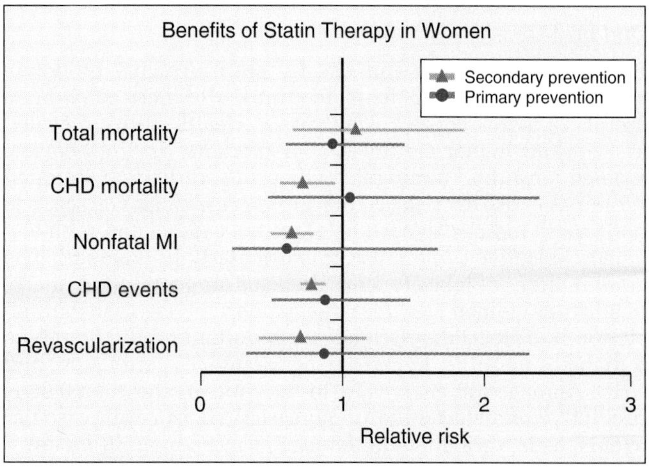

FIGURE 73–4 Risk reduction in multiple cardiovascular endpoints attributable to lipid-lowering therapy with statins in women with and without preexisting atherosclerotic disease. Summary odds ratios with 95 percent confidence intervals are presented. CHD = coronary heart disease; MI = myocardial infarction. (Modified from Grady D, Chaput L, Kristof M. Diagnosis and Treatment of Coronary Heart Disease in Women: Systematic Reviews of Evidence on Selected Topics. Evidence Report/Technology Assessment No. 81. AHRQ Publication No. 03-0037. Rockville, Md, Agency for Healthcare Research and Quality, May 2003.)

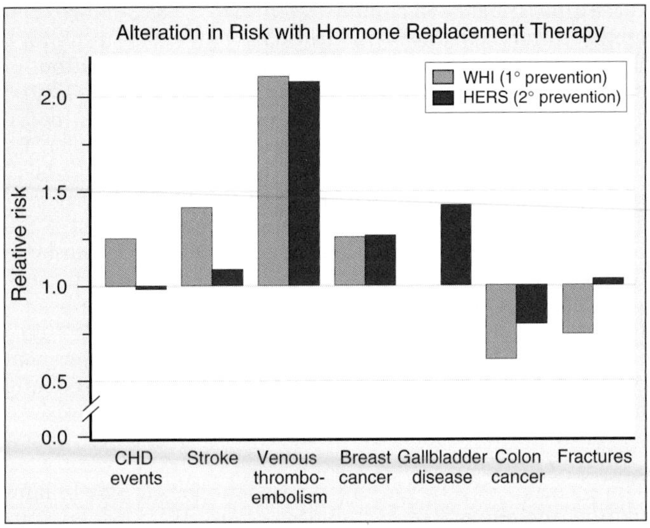

FIGURE 73–5 Relative risks of significant medical endpoints in large randomized controlled trials of postmenopausal hormone replacement therapy. CHD = coronary heart disease; WHI = Women's Health Initiative. (Modified from Grady D, Herrington D, Bittner V, et al: Cardiovascular disease outcomes during 6.8 years of hormone therapy: Heart and Estrogen/progestin Replacement Study follow-up [HERS II]. JAMA 288:49, 2002; and Rossouw JE, Anderson GL, Prentice RL, et al: Risks and benefits of estrogen plus progestin in healthy postmenopausal women: Principal results from the Women's Health Initiative randomized controlled trial. JAMA 288:321, 2002.)

Many questions about estrogen remain unanswered. Would alternative formulations of either estrogen or progesterone be of benefit? Does starting therapy immediately at menopause eliminate risk? Can genotype predict the risk-benefit profile of estrogen therapy? In addition, if the estrogen hypothesis is indeed a fallacy, what does afford the protection in the premenopausal female population? Several candidates have been suggested, although none have substantial scientific support: lower iron levels and higher oxytocin levels, for example.[3,43] Estrogen therapy is associated with impressive changes in so many risk factors, including lower LDL, higher HDL, improved glucose tolerance, and reductions in weight and waist circumference, that an understanding of the mechanism of increased risk is likely to revolutionize yet again our understanding of the atherosclerotic process.

Diet and Obesity

Excess caloric intake and obesity are a growing epidemic worldwide, and more than one-third of American women are classified as obese.[22] The Nurses' Health Study revealed a sevenfold higher cardiovascular mortality in the heaviest women, and the Framingham Offspring study demonstrated a dramatic rise in risk factors for cardiovascular disease at body mass indices above 20.[44] Obesity is associated with elevated C-reactive protein (CRP), particularly in women.[45] The combination of obesity and diabetes appears particularly deadly in women, as does the pattern of fat distribution. Abdominal fat accumulation is an important predictor of type 2 diabetes mellitus, hypertriglyceridemia, hypertension, and CHD. Among women, a waist-to-hip ratio greater than 0.88 is predictive of a substantially increased risk of cardiovascular events, as is a waist circumference of more than 38 inches.[46]

Physical Activity

Physical inactivity is more prevalent among women than men.[47] There is a strong inverse association between physical activity and coronary events in women.[48] Physical activity also has a salutary effect on other cardiovascular risk factors, including hypertension, obesity, and diabetes mellitus. The effect of regular exercise to increase HDL cholesterol and induce weight loss may be less in women than in men.[49] Significant barriers to regular exercise exist for American women, particularly older women. Caregiving duties, low energy, and lack of peers seen exercising are cited as impeding women's compliance with exercise recommendations.[50]

Inflammation

The close relationship between inflammation and cardiovascular risk is discussed in depth elsewhere (see Chap. 36). Baseline CRP levels predict future cardiovascular risk in healthy women, particularly those with metabolic syndrome.[51] Although we currently lack clinical trial evidence in support of CRP as a target of therapy, the ability of statins to reduce CRP is associated with benefit in lipid-lowering trials[52] and the ability of oral estrogen to raise CRP is associated with harm.[9,10]

Psychosocial Factors (see also Chap. 84)

The interaction of psychosocial and behavioral factors and heart disease is complex and has not been rigorously studied. Several cardiovascular risk factors are related to behavior (obesity, smoking, exercise), yet modification may be more difficult for women than for men, with caregiving roles often blamed for this failure. Perceived stress and lack of situational control have been found to increase CHD risk in both genders.[20,53] Social networks and support influence CHD outcome both independently and through the likelihood of compliance with therapeutic strategies (e.g., cardiac rehabilitation), and their impact may be greater in women, who are more likely to live alone. Although depression increases cardiac risk in both women and men, a causal relationship is unclear, as is the impact of treatment.[54]

Emerging Risk Factors

Many newer markers of increased cardiovascular risk apply equally to men and women, including abnormal endothelial reactivity, increased pulse pressure (thought to be a surrogate for increased vascular stiffness), factor V Leiden mutation, hyperhomocysteinemia, and elevated fibrinogen.[55,56] Estrogen increases fibrinogen levels, explaining the increased risk of vascular thrombosis associated with exogenous estrogen therapy. Although several members of the coagulation and fibrinolysis cascade have been proposed as possible risk factors, most recently through genetic polymorphisms,[56] current data support a role for these factors as modifiers of risk rather than causal. Whether targeting any of these emerging risk factors for intervention produces a reduction in cardiovascular events is unknown.

Strategies for Primary Prevention

Improvement in prevention of coronary artery disease in women requires earlier awareness and identification of risk. An overwhelming majority of women are unaware of their cardiovascular risk, and physicians do little to educate them.[1,21] Health care providers neglect to perform a formal assessment of cardiovascular risk with simultaneous education of the patient at risk about the real chance that she will experience cardiac disease and her role in altering modifiable risk factors. Identification of clustered risk factors, with aggressive treatment of hypertension and dyslipidemia, is imperative. Smoking cessation should be advised for every woman, regardless of overall risk profile. Early identification of glucose intolerance, abdominal adiposity, and metabolic syndrome, with aggressive behavior modification aimed at weight loss, is increasingly recognized as important. The role of aspirin is controversial in primary prevention in women, as most trials included only men. In the absence of compelling data, it is recommended that low-dose aspirin be considered as therapy only in women with a high estimated risk (>10 percent in 10 years).[23] The importance of encouraging life-style modification at each encounter with young women so that they may approach menopause with heart healthy behaviors in place is underscored by Nurses' Health Study data, which predict an 86 percent risk reduction in women who adopt healthy life styles including smoking cessation, achievement of ideal body weight, regular physical exercise, and a low-fat diet.[57]

Evaluation of Chest Pain

Clinical Syndromes and Natural History

Differences in presentation and disease manifestations between men and women exist and should be considered in the evaluation of chest pain. Women are on average 5 to 10 years older and have more comorbidities at the time of their first presentation with CHD. Angina is the most common first symptom of CHD in women, who are less likely than men to present initially with a concrete event such as myocardial infarction or sudden cardiac death (Fig. 73–6A).[2] Perhaps even more than in men, the prevalence of angiographic coronary disease varies dramatically according to the nature of the chest pain, age, and coronary risk factors. As illustrated in Figure 73–6B, typical or classic angina (defined as exertional substernal discomfort relieved rapidly by rest or nitroglycerin) is commonly due to atherosclerosis in women, particularly older women. Atypical chest pain (exertional substernal discomfort with atypical radiation or not relieved rapidly by rest or nitroglycerin) is less likely to be associated with angiographic coronary disease in women, particularly younger women, than in men.[53,58] Although equally likely to have effort angina, women with CHD are more likely than men to experience atypical symptoms, such as pain at rest, during sleep, or with mental stress. These differences make a gender-based approach essential in the recognition and assessment of acute and chronic ischemic syndromes.

The reasons for these differences are unclear. Although most women have typical angiographic findings of atherosclerosis, women have higher prevalences of vasospastic angina, microvascular angina, and abnormal coronary vasodilator reserve (syndrome X). These syndromes are associated with atypical chest pain patterns, have distinct treatments, and have a more favorable prognosis than epicardial coronary disease.[19,53] Finally, noncoronary chest pain syndromes are more common in women, further complicating clinical assessment of chest pain in females.

Women with undiagnosed chest pain have a better prognosis than men with chest pain because of a lower prevalence of atherosclerosis in women with chest pain. However, when a diagnosis of atherosclerotic disease is made conclusively (e.g., by a history of myocardial infarction), women are at equal and perhaps greater risk for adverse outcomes (Fig. 73–7). In subjects older than 65 with exertional chest pain, women and men have the same relative risks of CHD death (2.7 versus 2.4). Mortality after myocardial infarction is worse in women younger than 60 than that in men, reinforcing the fact that once an atherosclerotic etiology for the chest pain syndrome is identified, the prognosis is no different between the genders. The presence of elevated troponin in a woman with unstable angina predicts a worse outcome (Fig. 73–8), with a positive serum troponin predicting a greater increase in risk of death or myocardial infarction in women than in men.[59]

Noninvasive Diagnostic Testing

The general principles underlying noninvasive diagnostic testing do not differ in men and women.[60] Resting electrocardiography reveals a higher prevalence of repolarization (ST-T wave) abnormalities in women with suspected coronary disease than in men (32 versus 23 percent). Treadmill exercise testing is associated with a higher false-positive rate and a lower false-negative rate than in men (12 versus 40 percent), suggesting that routine testing reliably excludes the presence of CHD in women with negative tests. Variables that may alter test accuracy are resting ST-T wave abnormalities,

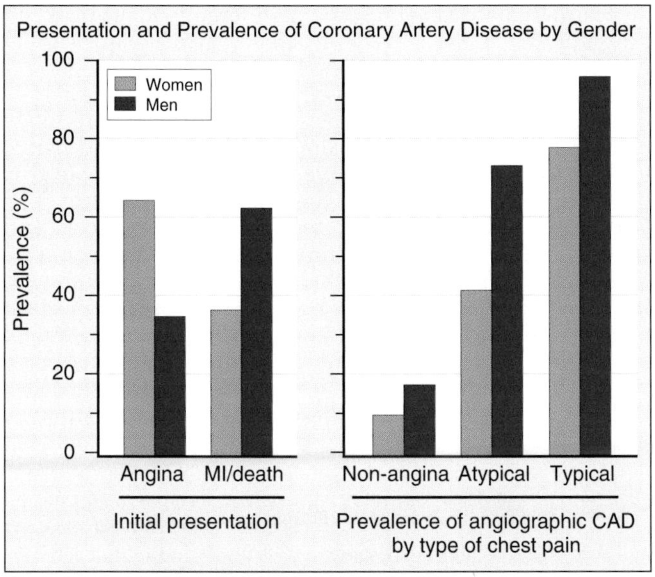

FIGURE 73–6 **A,** Differences in presenting symptom of coronary artery disease by sex. **B,** Prevalence of angiographically documented coronary artery disease (CAD) according to chest pain syndrome. Typical angina was defined as exertional substernal discomfort relieved rapidly by rest or nitroglycerin (NTG). Probable angina was similar to typical angina but varied in an important respect (atypical radiation, not relieved by NTG or rest). Nonanginal pain did not fit the preceding descriptions. MI = myocardial infarction. (Data from Kannel WB, Feinleib M: Natural history of angina pectoris in the Framingham study. Prognosis and survival. Am J Cardiol 29:154, 1972; and Chaitman BR, Bourassa MG, Davis K, et al: Angiographic prevalence of high-risk coronary artery disease in patient subsets [CASS]. Circulation 64:360, 1981.)

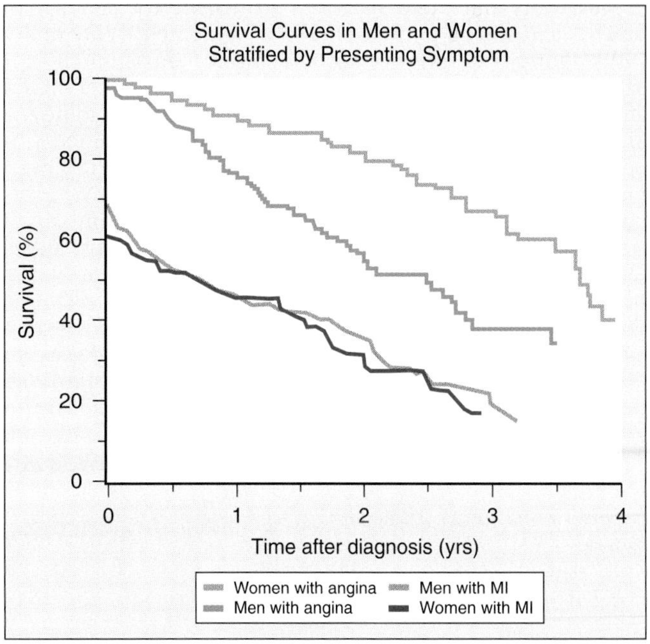

FIGURE 73–7 Survival curves of men and women 60 to 69 years of age presenting with angina, contrasted with those of men and women with documented coronary artery disease. The population of women with angina is more heterogeneous and includes more patients without an atherosclerotic etiology. MI = myocardial infarction. (From Hayes SN, Gersh BJ: *In* Douglas PS [ed]: Cardiovascular Health and Disease in Women. 2nd ed. Philadelphia, WB Saunders, 2002. Redrawn from Orencia A, Bailey K, Yawn BP, Kottke TE: Effect of gender on long-term outcome of angina pectoris and myocardial infarction/sudden unexpected death. JAMA 269:2392, 1993.)

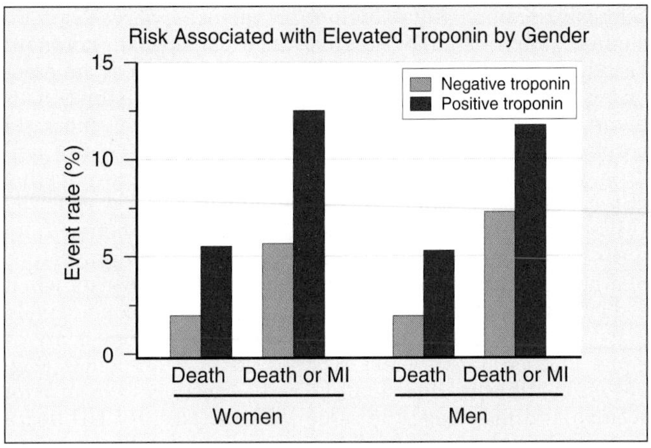

FIGURE 73–8 Impact of serum troponin level on risk of death and myocardial infarction (MI) in both men and women presenting with acute coronary syndromes. (Modified from Grady D, Chaput L, Kristof M: Diagnosis and Treatment of Coronary Heart Disease in Women: Systematic Reviews of Evidence on Selected Topics. Evidence Report/Technology Assessment No. 81. AHRQ Publication No. 03-0037. Rockville, Md, Agency for Healthcare Research and Quality. May 2003.)

peak exercise heart rate, number of diseased vessels, age, drug use (digitalis, diazepam), hyperventilation, conduction abnormalities, left ventricular hypertrophy, mitral valve prolapse, vasospasm, and hormonal influences. False-negative studies may be the result of gender-specific characteristics, including reduced exercise tolerance and the higher prevalence of single-vessel disease in women. The exercise component also provides useful prognostic information in women.[61]

The addition of imaging to electrocardiographic stress testing markedly improves its accuracy in women, as noted by meta-analyses[62,63] and reviews (see also Chaps. 10 and 13). Planar thallium scans during treadmill exercise testing suggest only moderate increases in sensitivity and specificity,[62] and single-photon emission computed tomography (SPECT) may not improve accuracy in women as much as it does in men.[64] Breast attenuation is reduced by use of higher energy isotopes such as technetium 99m sestamibi and newer algorithms for attenuation correction.[65] Exercise echocardiography improves diagnostic accuracy in women,[62] even more so than in men.[63] Meta-analyses[62,63] have shown exercise echocardiography to have similar sensitivity and superior specificity compared with nuclear perfusion studies (Table 73–1), with the accuracy of exercise electrocardiography and exercise nuclear studies, but not exercise echocardiography, showing gender dependence. Several formal cost-effectiveness models show stress echocardiography to dominate over nuclear techniques,[66,67] suggesting that diagnostic testing strategies employing exercise echocardiography as the first test might be superior (see also Chap. 15).

Coronary Angiography

Women are more likely than men to experience vascular and renal complications from diagnostic angiography, possibly because of more advanced age, higher prevalence of diabetes, and smaller body size. The incidences of myocardial infarction, stroke, and death complicating coronary angiography are similar in men and women.[68]

Gender Bias in the Diagnosis of Ischemic Heart Disease

A study in 1987 reporting that men with positive nuclear exercise tests were 6.3 times more likely to be referred to cardiac catheterization than women gave rise to concerns that female patients were receiving inadequate or inappropriate care, a conclusion that has been both substantiated and refuted by subsequent studies. Although awareness of the importance of CHD in women is growing, discrepancies still exist, and both gender and race influence management of chest pain.[69]

Less aggressive treatment strategies in women do not represent optimal care, nor can they be attributed solely to the difficulties in diagnosing coronary disease in women. In one study, subsequent CHD event rates after diagnostic testing were higher in women, whether they had a normal initial test (1.6 percent/yr death or myocardial infarction versus 0.8 percent in men) or an abnormal one (14.3 percent/yr versus 6.0 percent/yr). Revascularization was protective in both male and female patients, and untreated women had a worse prognosis. These data demonstrate not only a gender-based difference in clinical practice but also a worse outcome in women treated less aggressively.

Management of Symptomatic Coronary Heart Disease in Women

Acute Coronary Syndromes

Women have a different clinical presentation and hospital course following acute coronary syndromes and acute myocardial infarction and respond differently to medical and procedural therapies. Gender differences in acute myocardial infarction have been reviewed.[70-72]

Women suffering from an acute coronary syndrome or myocardial infarction are likely to be older; are more likely to have a history of hypertension, diabetes, unstable angina, hyperlipidemia, and congestive heart failure; and are less likely to be smokers than their male counterparts.[70,72,73] Women are also more likely to experience jaw, neck, and shoulder pain; abdominal pain; nausea; vomiting; palpitations; fatigue; and dyspnea in addition to chest pain and are less likely to report diaphoresis than men. Although chest pain is the single most common presenting symptom of myocardial infarction in women,[70] women seem more susceptible to "silent" infarction, particularly elderly women.[74] Perhaps in part because of these more atypical symptoms,

TABLE 73–1 Predictive Value of Noninvasive Testing in Women with Coronary Artery Disease*

Type of Study	Sensitivity	Specificity	Likelihood Ratio for Positive Test	Likelihood Ratio for Negative Test
Myocardial perfusion imaging	0.77 (0.69-0.81)	0.71 (0.69-0.78)	2.54 (1.95-3.32)	0.36 (0.28-0.46)
Exercise echocardiography	0.82 (0.73-0.89)	0.60 (0.48-0.71)	2.06 (1.53-2.77)	0.29 (0.18-0.47)

*Summary of data from good-quality clinical trials to determine clinical utility of noninvasive diagnostic testing in detection of coronary artery disease in women presenting with chest pain syndromes. Estimates with 95% confidence intervals are presented.

Modified from Grady D, Chaput L, Kristof M: Diagnosis and Treatment of Coronary Heart Disease in Women: Systematic Reviews of Evidence on Selected Topics. Evidence Report/Technology Assessment No. 81. AHRQ Publication No. 03-0037. Rockville, Md, Agency for Healthcare Research and Quality, May 2003.

women seek medical attention more slowly and even after hospital arrival may experience greater delays in receiving care. Physician uncertainty about the true clinical diagnosis is more common for women than men with acute myocardial infarction, and misdiagnosis is more likely.[75]

Women with infarction have higher risk initial presentations, with greater prevalences of tachycardia, rales, heart block, and a higher Killip class.[73] Women are less likely to be admitted to a coronary care unit or to be hospitalized in an institution in which catheterization is available. Most studies, but not all, find that women with acute infarction are less likely to undergo diagnostic catheterization during their hospital stay, even after controlling for age and a variety of clinical characteristics. Whether this distinction exists only for patients with equivocal indications for catheterization and whether it extends to lower rates of angioplasty and bypass surgery among catheterized patients are unclear. Women have higher rates of in-hospital complications from infarction, including bleeding, stroke, shock, myocardial rupture, and recurrent chest pain, than do men, although most of these differences appear attributable to age and comorbidities.

Mortality

Mortality in non-Q-wave myocardial infarction appears to be similar to that in men, but women with unstable angina are less likely to have angiographic CHD, reinfarction, or death.[76] In acute ST elevation myocardial infarction, early or in-hospital mortality in women is greater than in men, and adjustment for age or clinical characteristics, or both, reduces but does not eliminate this difference. In part, this gap may be due to a higher rate of prehospital sudden death in men, but this cannot explain the twofold greater mortality in women younger than 50 years compared with similarly aged men. Mortality 1 to 3 years after hospital discharge is also increased in younger women, although it is similar in postmenopausal women and men.[77]

Thrombolysis and Acute Medical Treatment

Because men and women show similar rates of intracoronary thrombosis on pretreatment angiography, it is not surprising that the efficacy of thrombolysis is equivalent with similar infarct-related artery patency and preservation of left ventricular function. However, whereas mortality is similar, complication rates, particularly hemorrhagic stroke and recurrent myocardial infarction, appear to be higher in women. In contrast to older studies, eligible women now seem to receive thrombolytic therapy at rates equal to those of men, but women more frequently have contraindications to thrombolysis.[78] Primary angioplasty is equally, if not more, effective in women, in part because of the greater reduction in hemorrhagic stroke. Despite a greater risk profile in women, percutaneous revascularization is as safe and effective in women as it is in men.[79]

Although there are physiological reasons to suspect that women may benefit from use of low-molecular-weight heparin and clopidogrel, adequate trial data assessing efficacy in women are unavailable. Use of glycoprotein IIb/IIIa inhibitors confers benefit in addition to that of aspirin in unstable coronary syndromes in women but not in men, provided there is evidence of injury (elevated troponin). Women do not appear to benefit in the absence of positive biomarkers. This finding suggests that, in women, platelets may play a more important role or may require more aggressive inhibition. Several studies, including Treat Angina with Aggrastat and determine Cost of Therapy with an Invasive or Conservative Strategy–Thrombolysis in Myocardial Infarction 18 (TACTICS-TIMI 18),[80] demonstrated equivalent benefit in men and women of an early invasive strategy over aggressive medical therapy alone even though women have a higher likelihood of no angiographic stenoses (17 versus 9 percent) and a lower likelihood of left main coronary disease. Other studies have suggested that the benefit in women is dependent upon the invasive strategy—women do not benefit when coronary artery bypass graft (CABG) surgery is used.[81]

Percutaneous Revascularization

Data show the efficacy of coronary artery stenting to be similar in men and women in both the short and long term.[82] The likelihood of angiographic success is similar in men and women in newer series, with lower success rates in women reported in older studies. However, the proportional risk of death from procedural complications remains greater in women, with higher complication and mortality rates, including groin complications, acute vessel closure, hemorrhagic complications, and death.[83] The difference in outcome has been variously attributed to women's older age, smaller body size, greater severity of angina, more fragile vessels, and greater burden of comorbidity. Care must be taken in the dosing of antiplatelet and anticoagulant therapies in women to minimize the incidence of hemorrhagic side effects.[72]

Surgical Therapies

In 2000, nearly 150,000 women had CABG in the United States, approximately 30 percent of the total number of CABG surgeries performed. Gender differences in outcome following CABG are well established and, although decreasing over time, persist in the new millennium.[84] In-hospital mortality is 1.4 to 4.4 times higher, particularly for younger women (<60 years) and low- and medium-risk patients, with no difference in highest risk patients, suggesting nonanatomical factors as the proximate cause.[85] Women are less likely to receive internal mammary grafts or undergo complete revascularization and are more likely to experience the complications of heart failure, perioperative infarction, and hemorrhage. Neurological complications of CABG, including stroke, transient ischemic attack, and coma, are more frequent in women.[86] Rehospitalization rates for women are two times those for men in the first 2 months after CABG.[84]

The causes of higher operative mortality and morbidity appear to be multiple, including technical factors such as smaller body size and coronary diameter, advanced age, comorbidities such as diabetes and hypertension, and clinical factors such as the urgency of the procedure. However, controlling for these eliminates only a small portion of the excess risk, with about 70 percent of the risk unaccounted for in well-controlled multivariate analyses.[85] Disease-related factors such as the extent and severity of angiographic stenoses and left ventricular dysfunction are consistently more favorable in women. Current data on "off-pump" CABG (OPCAB) appear to demonstrate a clear reduction in neurological events in both men and women compared with those associated with traditional coronary bypass techniques,[87] but the marked reduction in length of stay for men undergoing OPCAB may not be seen in women.[88]

After CABG, women have a lower likelihood of being free of angina than do men and experience greater physical disability and less return to work.[89,90] Rates of long-term survival, infarction, and reoperation are similar. Quality of life is worse for women, even when measures are adjusted for premorbid level of function.[84] The worse outcomes following CABG in women are related to more depression, slower recovery of normal physical function, greater physical symptoms, and a higher perceived degree of functional impairment. Much of this gap appears to be related to societal roles of women. Women undergoing CABG are more likely than men to be single and of lower socioeconomic class and thus lack adequate social support. In addition, women who have served as household managers return to this function rapidly after surgery and do not enjoy as extensive a recovery period free from obligations.

Adjunctive Medical Treatment and Secondary Prevention

Women with acute infarction are more likely than men to be treated with nitrates, digoxin, and diuretics and less likely to receive thrombolytics, antiarrhythmics, antiplatelet agents, ACE inhibitors, and beta blockers despite evidence for similar benefit in women.[73] Calcium channel blockade was not effective in either men or women. Although the Coronary Artery Surgery Study (CASS) showed that women treated medically had better 12-year survival with angiographically documented zero-, one-, or two-vessel disease than men with similar anatomy, other studies suggest that undertreatment of women is related to a worse outcome.[91]

Data from the Heart and Estrogen/progestin Replacement Study (HERS) provide the most extensive and distressing snapshot of the current state of secondary prevention in women with known CHD.[92] At the start of the study, only 33 percent of patients were receiving beta blockers, 53 percent were receiving lipid-lowering drugs, and 83 percent were receiving aspirin or other antiplatelet agents. Women at greatest risk were less likely to be taking aspirin ($p < 0.001$) or lipid-lowering drugs ($p = 0.006$). During the study period, the rate of aspirin use by participants actually fell. Current data on secondary prevention of coronary artery disease in women are summarized in Table 73–2.

Lipid lowering is efficacious in women with atherosclerotic disease, with several statin trials showing reductions in cardiac events and death.[39,93] Newer observational studies suggest benefit of aspirin in secondary prevention but still await confirmation by a randomized clinical trial. Diabetic, elderly, and symptomatic women appeared to benefit most, as did women with prior myocardial infarctions. Aspirin and other antiplatelet agents also reduced vascular events in women. Two studies suggest that men may experience more benefit than women when treated with ACE inhibitors after infarction. In contrast, administration of a beta-blocking agent clearly provides substantial improvement in postinfarction survival in women equal to, if not greater than, that in men.

After hospital discharge, women are less likely to be scheduled for exercise tests or referred for cardiac rehabilitation, and recovery from infarction appears delayed with slower return to work and full resumption of all activities and more sleep disturbance and psychiatric and psychosomatic complaints.[84]

Peripheral Arterial Disease

Peripheral arterial disease (PAD) is understudied from a gender-specific perspective. Although men have a higher reported prevalence of PAD, there is widespread failure to recognize PAD in women with documented reduction in ankle brachial index (ABI).[94,95] With noninvasive testing, the incidence of clinically significant PAD is equal in women and men at risk. Women with PAD have a higher incidence of confounding comorbidities, including osteoarthritis and spinal stenosis, and more often present with symptoms other than classical claudication or no symptoms.[94,96] They also have substantially increased mortality compared with age-matched healthy women, often because of myocardial ischemia.[95] Although all elderly women should receive a careful examination of peripheral pulses, ABI screening is recommended in women older than 60 at risk for PAD, including those with known atherosclerotic disease elsewhere, current smokers, and diabetics.

The risk factors for PAD are similar to those for CHD; however, diabetes and cigarette smoking have particularly strong associations with PAD. There are few data comparing evaluation or treatment between women and men, although women are less likely to be actively exercising or treated with aspirin or lipid-lowering agents, at least in part because of failure to recognize the disease.

Women with reduced ABI are less likely than men to have had prior revascularization. About a third of lower extremity revascularization procedures and amputations are performed in women. The rates of graft patency and long-term survival are significantly lower in women than in men.[97]

Hemostasis, Thrombosis, and Stroke

Gender and Hemostasis

The clotting and fibrinolysis systems are complex and intensively regulated (see also Chap. 80). Although genetic polymorphisms for many of the proteins involved in these

TABLE 73–2 Secondary Prevention of Coronary Artery Disease in Women*

Strategy	Level of Evidence	Reduction in Endpoints (%)	Underuse?
Lipid lowering	A	30-50	Y
Aspirin	A	20-25	Y
Beta blockers			
After MI	A	20-30	Y
With LV dysfunction	A	10-40	Y
ACE inhibitors			
After MI	A	5-10†	Y
With LV dysfunction	A	25-30†	Y
Smoking cessation	B	65	Y
Hypertension	C	?	?
Cardiac rehabilitation	C	?	Y
Hormone replacement therapy	A	Increase	N/A

*Summary of current data on secondary prevention of coronary artery disease in women, including level of evidence by American Heart Association criteria, reduction in endpoints noted in trials, and level of adoption by the medical community.

†Although the effect is probably positive, the 95% confidence interval crosses 1.0.

ACE = angiotensin-converting enzyme; LV = left ventricular; MI = myocardial infarction.

Modified from Grady D, Chaput L, Kristof M: Diagnosis and Treatment of Coronary Heart Disease in Women: Systematic Reviews of Evidence on Selected Topics. Evidence Report/Technology Assessment No. 81. AHRQ Publication No. 03-0037. Rockville, Md, Agency for Healthcare Research and Quality, May 2003.

cascades have been described, all identified to date are autosomal rather than gender linked. There are no identifiable differences in platelet function between the genders, although platelet levels in women fluctuate during the menstrual cycle.[15] Levels and function of several of the proteins involved in hemostasis do appear to be hormonally regulated. Fibrinogen and factor VII are slightly higher in women, and fibrinogen levels in women increase with age. Young women have higher plasma tissue plasminogen activator levels and lower PAI-1 levels than men, and levels of both increase with age in women. Changes in levels and activity of these and other factors are well described with alterations in the hormonal milieu seen with pregnancy, use of birth control pills and other exogenous estrogens, and hormonal cancer chemotherapy. On balance, the hemostatic profile in women appears slightly more thrombogenic, perhaps to protect against fetal hemorrhage, and is probably responsible for the increased rate of venous thromboembolism seen in women.[15]

Risk Factors and Their Modification

Hypertension and smoking are the most significant risk factors for stroke in women, although hyperlipidemia, diabetes, and obesity are also important predictors of stroke risk.[47,96] Nontraditional risk factors are increasingly being implicated in stroke risk, including homocysteine and, in young women, antiphospholipid antibody syndrome.[98] Single-gender studies in the last several years have shown that physical activity, a diet rich in omega-3 fatty acids, and intake of whole grains (but not processed grains) protect against ischemic stroke in women. Elevated serum levels of CRP in patients with an otherwise benign risk profile predict future stroke risk in both men and women. Abdominal obesity is also a predictor of stroke and is associated with elevated CRP levels. Aggressive treatment of hypertension with multiple agents has been shown to reduce the risk of first stroke, and treatment with angiotensin II receptor antagonists and diuretics reduces the risk of recurrent stroke even in patients without significant blood pressure elevation.[99] The Heart Outcomes Prevention Evaluation Study (HOPE) demonstrated a significant reduction in stroke risk with ramipril in both men and women with high risk for vascular disease, independent of blood pressure lowering effects.[100] In both trials, nearly 50 percent of treated patients were female.

In contrast to its effect in men, aspirin use does not appear to prevent first stroke in women,[101,102] but it may reduce the risk of recurrent stroke by approximately 25 percent. In patients with cardioembolic stroke, the risk reduction associated with aspirin therapy is 20 percent and that of warfarin is 60 percent for recurrent events. Elderly women in atrial fibrillation are less likely to be prescribed warfarin than men of the same age and more likely to receive aspirin therapy.[103] Multiple studies have demonstrated that physicians overestimate the risks associated with warfarin therapy, especially in elderly women.[104] Lipid-lowering therapy with HMG CoA reductase inhibitors is effective in both primary and secondary prevention of stroke.[39] Although experimental data suggest that estrogen is neuroprotective, estrogen as secondary prevention had no effect on stroke rate[8,10] and in the Women's Health Initiative trial of primary prevention there was a small increase in stroke risk among estrogen and progesterone users.

Clinical Syndromes, Natural History, and Treatment

Stroke incidence is approximately equal in both genders; however, 61 percent of all deaths associated with stroke occur in women.[47] Atherothrombotic stroke, which is strongly related to atherosclerotic disease, is the most common type of stroke in men, whereas the predominant stroke type in women is cardioembolic, typically related to atrial fibrillation. Significant carotid stenosis is found more frequently in men.[97] Hemorrhagic stroke occurs at roughly equal rates in men and women and accounts for 15 percent of all strokes. Subarachnoid hemorrhages are much more common in premenopausal women than in any other age group and are more often fatal in women than in men.[47,96]

Women are older when they have their first stroke and have more comorbidities. Stroke in women is more often complicated by congestive heart failure, typically in the presence of preserved systolic function. Treatment of acute ischemic stroke with thrombolytic therapy has apparently equal efficacy in both genders, although there is an increased risk of hemorrhage in women.[105]

Approximately one-third of carotid endarterectomies are performed in women.[97] The postoperative stroke rate is higher in women, perhaps because of smaller vessel size. Long-term outcome after carotid endarterectomy has not been extensively studied, but 5-year survival was higher in women than men in one study.[106] Women are more likely to develop recurrent carotid stenosis but have no increase in late stroke.[97] Following all types of stroke, women have more prolonged recovery, less often have adequate family support, and, as a result, account for a substantial portion of stroke victims requiring some type of long-term care.[107]

Arrhythmias

Gender and Cardiac Electrophysiology

(see also Chaps. 27 and 30)

Bazett first recognized a gender difference in the electrocardiogram between men and women in 1920, reporting higher heart rates and longer corrected QT intervals in women. Both gender and estrogen status affect the electrocardiogram in women. At birth and throughout life, the heart rate of a female is higher than that of a male. This difference has been ascribed variously to higher intrinsic parasympathetic tone in females, training effects related to higher fitness levels in men, intrinsic differences in quantities or kinetics, or both, of cardiac ion channels, and differences in cell coupling.[108] Estrogen modulates cardiac electrophysiology both in vitro and in vivo. Estrogen, but not dihydrotestosterone, prolongs action potential duration in ventricular myocytes. There is a direct effect of estrogen on both the rapidly and slowly activating inward-rectifying potassium channels (IK_r, IK_s). This gender difference in potassium channels has been tied to the higher incidence of drug-induced torsades de pointes among women. Estradiol-17β also reduces L-type calcium channel current rapidly through nongenomic mechanisms. Females with congenital long-QT syndrome have a different distribution of disease than men, with a larger number of women exhibiting the LQT2 subtype. Presentation of congenital long-QT syndrome in women commonly occurs during puberty or pregnancy. The postpartum period is a time of particular risk for women with this disorder, demonstrating the profound impact that fluctuating levels of sex steroids can have on channel biology and electrophysiology.[109]

Syncope (see also Chap. 34)

Women with syncope are older than men, less likely to have left ventricular dysfunction, and more often have a noncardiac etiology of the syncope identified.[110] Women with syncope have significantly higher cardiac event–free survival rates, with a cardiac event rate of 6 percent in more than 9 months of follow-up in one study compared to 21 percent in men.[110] Neurocardiogenic syncope is the most commonly identified type of syncope in women. Contrary to the usual teaching, this type of syncope is common among elderly patients, with a positive tilt-table test in approximately 30 percent of patients with unexplained syncope.[111] Older subjects with positive tilt-table tests are more likely to have a pure vasodepressor response without bradycardia, and midodrine has been proposed as the therapy of choice. Women have higher anxiety scores than men with neurocardiogenic syncope and also higher scores than women without positive tilt-table tests.[112] It is important to assess a woman with syncope fully before attributing the event to an underlying psychiatric disorder, as anxiety commonly coexists with electrophysiological abnormalities in women.

Atrial Arrhythmias

Palpitations are a common complaint with a large differential diagnosis. It is often difficult, particularly in women, to distinguish treatable atrial arrhythmias from other causes of palpitations. Inappropriate sinus tachycardia may arise as palpitations and an exaggerated heart rate response to mild exercise and has an almost 90 percent female prevalence.[113] Gender-specific dysregulation of the autonomic input to the sinus node is thought to be the etiology. Beta blockers are often poorly tolerated; selective sinus node ablation may be curative.

Among paroxysmal supraventricular tachycardias (PSVTs), electrocardiographic findings of Wolff-Parkinson-White syndrome are approximately 3.5 times more common in males than in females, whereas concealed bypass tracts occur with similar frequency in both genders. Two-thirds of patients with atrioventricular nodal tachycardia are female. Atrial fibrillation is 1.5 times more common in men than in women. In patients without overt heart disease, the incidence of atrial fibrillation increases with age in the male but not the female population. The incidence of paroxysms of atrial arrhythmias shows a distinct variance with phase of the menstrual cycle in women, again providing evidence for significant hormonal effects.[114]

Inappropriate and missed diagnoses among women with atrial arrhythmias are common. In 107 patients with documented PSVT, the disorder was unrecognized after initial evaluation in 59 patients (55 percent), including 68 percent of women.[115] In these patients the median time to diagnosis after presentation was 3.3 years, with symptoms attributed to panic, anxiety, or stress more often among women than men (65 versus 32 percent; $p < 0.04$). These investigators also looked at the prevalence of panic disorder according to the *Diagnostic and Statistical Manual of Mental Disorders*, fourth edition (DSM-IV), among patients with documented PSVT and found that 88 percent of patients had four or more symptoms of panic attack and 67 percent met DSM-IV criteria for panic disorder. Clearly, a history of palpitations must be thoroughly investigated before ascribing the complaint to an anxiety disorder, particularly in women. Among women with documented PSVT, multiple episodes of palpitations occurring frequently are the rule, with 75 percent of patients experiencing episodes at least monthly, making diagnosis less difficult if the proper level of suspicion is maintained. There is no evidence that the response of women to accepted therapy differs from that of men. However, few therapies have been tested in significant populations of women.

Ventricular Arrhythmias and Sudden Cardiac Death (see also Chap. 33)

Ventricular arrhythmias and sudden cardiac death are less common in women than in men. Approximately one in five sudden deaths occurs in women, and the etiology of sudden death more commonly is noncardiac among women, including a higher percentage of drug-related causes.[108] Among survivors of cardiac arrest, 80 percent of men are found to have coronary artery disease compared with 45 percent of women.

Women account for 70 percent of cases of torsades de pointes, probably because of their longer baseline QT interval. In addition, women have a higher risk of significant QT prolongation when exposed to drugs known to delay myocardial repolarization (Table 73–3) (see also Chap. 5). Despite this marker of increased risk, men die of sudden cardiac death at a much higher rate. This difference has been postulated to be the result of increased QT dispersion in men compared with women. It is possible that the combination of ischemia and increased QT dispersion is particularly lethal.[114]

When clinically significant ventricular arrhythmias have been documented, gender does not affect the subsequent clinical course. Mortality, defibrillator discharges, and arrhythmia-free survival are comparable among female and male survivors of sudden death. Nevertheless, risk stratification of women for ventricular arrhythmia is even more difficult than that of men because ventricular premature beats and nonsustained ventricular tachycardia do not carry the same negative prognostic implications, even after myocardial infarction. The optimal method of risk stratification is

TABLE 73–3 Drugs and Conditions Associated with QT Prolongation and Polymorphic Ventricular Tachycardia, Particularly in Women

Pharmaceutical Agents	Dofetilide
	Adenosine[†]
Antibiotics	
Erythromycin	**Other Agents**
Clarithromycin	Astemizole
Azithromycin	Terfenadine
Trimethoprim	Cisapride
Clindamycin	Famotidine
Ketoconazole*	Salmeterol
Pentamidine	Indapamide
Halofantrine	Nicardipine
Amantadine	Isradipine
Foscarnet	Moexipril/hydrochlorothiazide
Moxifloxacin	Bepridil
Gatifloxacin	Probucol
Psychiatric Drugs	Chloral hydrate
Thioridazine	Sumatriptan
Chlorpromazine	Dolasetron
Prochlorperazine	Felbamate
Quetiapine	Droperidol
Mesoridazine	Methadone
Pimozide	**Toxins**
Risperidone	Taxine (yew)
Haloperidol	Arsenic
Tricyclic antidepressants	Organophosphorus insecticides
Fluoxetine	
Paroxetine	**Physiological Conditions**
Citalopram	Intracranial hemorrhage
Sertraline	Liquid protein diets
Venlafaxine	Complete atrioventricular block
Antiarrhythmic Agents	Pacemaker malfunction
Quinidine	Hypokalemia
Procainamide	Hypocalcemia
Disopyramide	Hypomagnesemia
N-Acetyl-procainamide	Hypothyroidism
Sotalol	Acute myocardial infarction
Ibutilide	Human immunodeficiency virus infection
Amiodarone	

*Particularly in combination with terfenadine.
[†]In the setting of long-QT syndrome.

unclear.[114] Women survivors of sudden death have higher ejection fractions than men and are less often inducible at electrophysiological study. The Multicenter Unsustained Tachycardia Trial (MUSST), Multicenter Automatic Defibrillator Implantation Trials (MADIT I and MADIT II), and Amiodarone Versus Implantable Defibrillators (AVID) trial together enrolled less than 500 women, making gender-specific analysis impossible because of small numbers.[108]

Valvular Heart Disease

The epidemiology of several types of valvular heart disease demonstrates clear gender differences, but no data are available about variability in response to medical or surgical treatment (see also Chap. 57).

Mitral Valve Prolapse

Mitral valve prolapse is thought to be a genetic disorder with gender, body size, mean blood pressure, and thoracic geometry influencing the phenotype. Although clinically recognizable disease has a female predominance as high as 70 percent, major complications, most notably infective endocarditis and severe mitral regurgitation, have a strong male predominance.[116] The associations between mitral valve prolapse and chest pain, dyspnea at rest, anxiety, and panic attacks are related to a higher prevalence of these conditions in the female population rather than to the disease. There are, however, clear associations between mitral valve prolapse and midsystolic clicks, mitral systolic murmurs, thoracic bone abnormalities, low body weight, low systolic blood pressure, and palpitations. The majority of women with echocardiographic evidence of mitral valve prolapse have a benign natural history. The presence of a significant mitral valve murmur should prompt further diagnostic evaluation, including a prescription for antibiotic prophylaxis at the time of dental or other high-risk procedures (see also Chap. 58).

Rheumatic Valvular Disease

Development of mitral stenosis with a classic rheumatic deformity is more common in women than in men, although aortic disease is less common.[116] Women with rheumatic mitral stenosis often present during pregnancy, as the narrowed mitral orifice becomes limiting in the setting of increased cardiac output and relative tachycardia. Hemoptysis is a more common presenting feature of mitral stenosis in women than in men. There is no evidence that response to percutaneous balloon valvotomy or surgical valve replacement varies by gender, although the issue has not been closely studied.

Nonrheumatic Aortic Valve Disease

Bicuspid aortic valves have a nearly 3:1 male predominance, and aortic valve surgery among patients younger than 65 occurs predominantly in men. There is some evidence that women with bicuspid valves have less propensity to progression to stenosis or regurgitation and require surgical intervention less frequently.[116] In patients 65 or older, there is a twofold higher prevalence of calcific aortic valve disease in men than in women.[117]

Marfan Syndrome

Because Marfan syndrome is an autosomal dominant disorder, incidence, therapy, and outcome do not differ by gender. However, pregnancy increases the risk of aortic dissection, particularly in the presence of any abnormality of the aortic root.[116]

Heart Failure

Clinical Syndromes and Natural History

Given that the genetic and physiological responses to myocardial stress or injury clearly differ between men and women (see earlier), it is not surprising that the clinical spectrum and epidemiology of heart failure also differ. Women develop heart failure at a later age, are less likely to have had a prior myocardial infarction, and are more likely to have hypertension, diabetes, and obesity. In the Medicare population, 80 percent of patients with heart failure and preserved systolic function are women.[118] Alcoholic cardiomyopathy is encountered less frequently in women than in men, but this may be due to the lower prevalence of alcoholism among women because data suggest that alcohol may be more toxic to the myocardium in women, with a lower total dose required to produce cardiomyopathy.[119]

Diagnosis of heart failure may be more difficult in women than in men, in part because of higher prevalences of fluid retention and shortness of breath of noncardiac origin. Women prescribed diuretic therapy meet diagnostic criteria for heart failure less often than men. This difference seems to be related to higher rates of obesity in women and is not explained purely by the presence of diastolic abnormalities.[120] Following a diagnosis of heart failure, men more frequently undergo echocardiographic study, stress testing, and catheterization and are more likely to be referred to specialists.[120]

The prognosis in women with heart failure differs from that in men. Heart failure with preserved systolic function has been thought to have a better prognosis than that associated with systolic dysfunction, although the mortality in patients with preserved systolic function is four times that of age-matched patients without heart failure[121] and has been suggested to be equal to that of patients with systolic dysfunction in the modern era.[122] Because of this, general population studies show an improved prognosis for women with heart failure. However, women enrolled in the Studies of Left Ventricular Dysfunction (SOLVD) trial, all of whom had significant systolic dysfunction, had a distinctly worse prognosis than the men. The heterogeneity of populations and underlying disease in various studies probably explains discrepancies in the literature.

Medical Therapy

There is a disturbing uncertainty about the efficacy of many established therapies in women with heart failure. Clinical trials have focused almost exclusively on patients with systolic dysfunction and typically enrolled younger patients and patients with an ischemic etiology disproportionately, thus having a heavy predominance of male subjects and failing to address treatment of diastolic dysfunction.

Conclusive evidence for a reduction in mortality and morbidity with ACE inhibitor therapy in systolic dysfunction exists only for men because of the small numbers of women enrolled and the lack of prespecified analyses by gender. Adverse events are more common in women receiving ACE inhibitor therapy, perhaps in part because of the failure to account for body size when determining dosing regimens in the major clinical trials.[120] Meta-analyses have demonstrated improvement in outcomes in women treated with ACE inhibitors but suggested that the effect may be less than in men.[123] Beta-adrenergic blocking agent therapy appears equally effective for both genders with systolic dysfunction and symptoms of heart failure.[124]

A concerning report demonstrated an increased risk of death in women randomly assigned to digoxin therapy in the Digitalis Investigation Group (DIG) trial, with a smaller reduction in hospitalizations than was seen in men.[125] This may be due in part to higher serum digoxin levels in the physically smaller female population. However, there was an increase in the risk of both death from heart failure and death from other cardiovascular causes, which is difficult to explain solely on the basis of toxicity of the medication. Diuretic therapy has been associated with a greater risk of hypokalemia in women.[126] Combined with the longer basal QTc interval in women this raises the question of greater risk of iatrogenic arrhythmia. No studies have addressed this issue.

There are currently no gender-specific data on the use of newer therapies, such as aldosterone blockade, or therapies used in acutely decompensated patients, such as intravenous natriuretic peptides, inotropes, or inodilators, although the ongoing Acute Decompensated Heart Failure National Registry (ADHERE), collecting data on patients hospitalized with acutely decompensated heart failure, should provide some insight.

Surgical Therapies and Transplantation

Far fewer women than men have undergone cardiac transplantation, which is in part due to the older average age of women with heart failure as well as differences in patients' desires for transplantation.[127] There is no evidence of inherent bias against females in selection of candidates for transplantation, although age and body weight restrictions commonly employed reduce the numbers of eligible women. There are no gender-specific data on use or outcomes of high-risk surgical procedures or ventricular assist devices in women.

Issues of Death and Dying in Women

A growing body of literature suggests that women choose different paths from men when faced with chronic or terminal illness (see also Chap. 6).[128,129] Women are more concerned about comfort and have a greater fear of technology and associated suffering, avoiding therapies perceived as heroic or experimental. Women and men with heart failure and chronic disability both choose quality of life over longer life.[130] Although cardiology has justifiably focused on major life-saving advances, increasing attention is being paid to therapies that may improve but not necessarily lengthen life. Gender-specific aspects of palliative care and assisting the dying patient with cardiac disease remain relatively unexplored.

REFERENCES

1. Wenger NK: Coronary heart disease and women: magnitude of the problem. Cardiol Rev 10:211, 2002.
2. Kannel WB: The Framingham Study: Historical insight on the impact of cardiovascular risk factors in men versus women. J Gend Specif Med 5:27, 2002.

Gender and Mechanisms of Cardiovascular Disease

3. Sullivan JL: Are menstruating women protected from heart disease because of, or in spite of, estrogen? Relevance to the iron hypothesis. Am Heart J 145:190, 2003.
4. Mikkola TS, Clarkson TB: Estrogen replacement therapy, atherosclerosis, and vascular function. Cardiovasc Res 53:605, 2002.
5. Mendelsohn ME: Genomic and nongenomic effects of estrogen in the vasculature. Am J Cardiol 90:3F, 2002.
6. Zanger D, Yang BK, Ardans J, et al: Divergent effects of hormone therapy on serum markers of inflammation in postmenopausal women with coronary artery disease on appropriate medical management. J Am Coll Cardiol 36:1797, 2000.
7. Weinberg EO, Thienelt CD, Katz SE, et al: Gender differences in molecular remodeling in pressure overload hypertrophy. J Am Coll Cardiol 34:264, 1999.
8. Hulley S, Grady D, Bush T, et al: Randomized trial of estrogen plus progestin for secondary prevention of coronary heart disease in postmenopausal women. Heart and Estrogen/progestin Replacement Study (HERS) Research Group. JAMA 280:605, 1998.
9. Manson JE, Hsia J, Johnson KC, et al: Estrogen plus progestin and the risk of coronary heart disease. N Engl J Med 349:523, 2003.
10. Grady D, Herrington D, Bittner V, et al: Cardiovascular disease outcomes during 6.8 years of hormone therapy: Heart and Estrogen/progestin Replacement Study follow-up (HERS II). JAMA 288:49, 2002.
11. Yamada Y, Izawa H, Ichihara S, et al: Prediction of the risk of myocardial infarction from polymorphisms in candidate genes. N Engl J Med 347:1916, 2002.
12. Burke AP, Farb A, Malcom GT, et al: Effect of risk factors on the mechanism of acute thrombosis and sudden coronary death in women. Circulation 97:2110, 1998.
13. English JL, Jacobs LO, Green G, et al: Effect of the menstrual cycle on endothelium-dependent vasodilation of the brachial artery in normal young women. Am J Cardiol 82:256, 1998.
14. Sader MA, McCredie RJ, Griffiths KA, et al: Oestradiol improves arterial endothelial function in healthy men receiving testosterone. Clin Endocrinol (Oxf) 54:175, 2001.
15. Weksler B: Hemostasis and thrombosis. *In* Douglas PS (ed): Cardiovascular Health and Disease in Women. 2nd ed. Philadelphia, WB Saunders, 2002, pp 157-177.
16. Arbustini E, Dal Bello B, Morbini P, et al: Plaque erosion is a major substrate for coronary thrombosis in acute myocardial infarction. Heart 82:269, 1999.
17. Crabbe DL, Dipla K, Ambati S, et al: Gender differences in post-infarction hypertrophy in end-stage failing hearts. J Am Coll Cardiol 41:300, 2003.
18. Guerra S, Leri A, Wang X, et al: Myocyte death in the failing human heart is gender dependent. Circ Res 85:856, 1999.
19. Mosca L, Manson JE, Sutherland SE, et al: Cardiovascular disease in women: A statement for healthcare professionals from the American Heart Association. Writing Group. Circulation 96:2468, 1997.
20. Wenger NK: Social support and coronary heart disease in women: The challenge to learn more. Eur Heart J 19:1603, 1998.
21. Mosca L, Jones WK, King KB, et al: Awareness, perception, and knowledge of heart disease risk and prevention among women in the United States. American Heart Association Women's Heart Disease and Stroke Campaign Task Force. Arch Fam Med 9:506, 2000.

Atherosclerotic Vascular Disease

22. Skerrett PJ, Spelsberg A, Manson JE: Carbohydrate metabolism, obesity, and diabetes mellitus. *In* Douglas PS (ed): Cardiovascular Health and Disease in Women. 2nd ed. Philadelphia, WB Saunders, 2002, pp 39-70.
23. Pearson TA, Blair SN, Daniels SR, et al: AHA Guidelines for Primary Prevention of Cardiovascular Disease and Stroke: 2002 Update: Consensus Panel Guide to Comprehensive Risk Reduction for Adult Patients Without Coronary or Other Atherosclerotic Vascular Diseases. American Heart Association Science Advisory and Coordinating Committee. Circulation 106:388, 2002.
24. Wheatcroft SB, Williams IL, Shah AM, et al: Pathophysiological implications of insulin resistance on vascular endothelial function. Diabet Med 20:255, 2003.
25. Sowers JR: Diabetes mellitus and cardiovascular disease in women. Arch Intern Med 158:617, 1998.
26. Franklin SS: Definition and epidemiology of hypertensive cardiovascular disease in women: The size of the problem. J Hypertens 20(Suppl 2):S3, 2002.
27. Gueyffier F, Boutitie F, Boissel JP, et al: Effect of antihypertensive drug treatment on cardiovascular outcomes in women and men. A meta-analysis of individual patient data from randomized, controlled trials. The INDANA Investigators. Ann Intern Med 126:761, 1997.
28. Silaste ML, Junes R, Rantala AO, et al: Dietary and other non-pharmacological treatments in patients with drug-treated hypertension and control subjects. J Intern Med 247:318, 2000.
29. Chobanian AV, Bakris GL, Black HR, et al: The Seventh Report of the Joint National Committee on Prevention, Detection, Evaluation, and Treatment of High Blood Pressure: The JNC 7 report. JAMA 289:2560, 2003.
30. Major outcomes in high-risk hypertensive patients randomized to angiotensin-converting enzyme inhibitor or calcium channel blocker vs diuretic: The Antihypertensive and Lipid-Lowering Treatment to Prevent Heart Attack Trial (ALLHAT). JAMA 288:2981, 2002.
31. Wing LM, Reid CM, Ryan P, et al: A comparison of outcomes with angiotensin-converting-enzyme inhibitors and diuretics for hypertension in the elderly. N Engl J Med 348:583, 2003.
32. Bolego C, Poli A, Paoletti R: Smoking and gender. Cardiovasc Res 53:568, 2002.
33. Bohadana A, Nilsson F, Rasmussen T, et al: Gender differences in quit rates following smoking cessation with combination nicotine therapy: Influence of baseline smoking behavior. Nicotine Tob Res 5:111, 2003.
34. Steenland K, Thun M, Lally C, et al: Environmental tobacco smoke and coronary heart disease in the American Cancer Society CPS-II cohort. Circulation 94:622, 1996.
35. LaRosa JC: Lipids. *In* Douglas PS (ed): Cardiovascular Health and Disease in Women. 2nd ed. Philadelphia, WB Saunders 2002, pp 23-28.
36. Third Report of the National Cholesterol Education Program (NCEP) Expert Panel on Detection, Evaluation, and Treatment of High Blood Cholesterol in Adults (Adult Treatment Panel III) final report. Circulation 106:3143, 2002.
37. Bittner V: Lipoprotein abnormalities related to women's health. Am J Cardiol 90:77i, 2002.
38. Mosca LJ: Contemporary management of hyperlipidemia in women. J Womens Health Gend Based Med 11:423, 2002.
39. MRC/BHF Heart Protection Study of cholesterol lowering with simvastatin in 20,536 high-risk individuals: A randomised placebo-controlled trial. Lancet 360:7, 2002.
40. Mendelsohn ME, Karas RH: The protective effects of estrogen on the cardiovascular system. N Engl J Med 340:1801, 1999.

41. Manson JE, Martin KA: Clinical practice. Postmenopausal hormone-replacement therapy. N Engl J Med 345:34, 2001.
42. Rossouw JE, Anderson GL, Prentice RL, et al: Risks and benefits of estrogen plus progestin in healthy postmenopausal women: Principal results from the Women's Health Initiative randomized controlled trial. JAMA 288:321, 2002.
42a. Women's Health Initiative Study: Available at http://www.nhlbi.nih.gov/whi/
43. Pickering TG: Men are from Mars, women are from Venus: Stress, pets, and oxytocin. J Clin Hypertens (Greenwich) 5:86, 2003.
44. Manson JE, Willett WC, Stampfer MJ, et al: Body weight and mortality among women. N Engl J Med 333:677, 1995.
45. Visser M, Bouter LM, McQuillan GM, et al: Elevated C-reactive protein levels in overweight and obese adults. JAMA 282:2131, 1999.
46. Rexrode KM, Carey VJ, Hennekens CH, et al: Abdominal adiposity and coronary heart disease in women. JAMA 280:1843, 1998.
47. Heart Disease and Stroke Statistics—2003 Update. Dallas, American Heart Association, 2002 (http://www.americanheart.org/downloadable/heart/10590179711482003HDSStatsBookREV7-03.pdf).
48. Manson JE, Hu FB, Rich-Edwards JW, et al: A prospective study of walking as compared with vigorous exercise in the prevention of coronary heart disease in women. N Engl J Med 341:650, 1999.
49. Mensink GB, Ziese T, Kok FJ: Benefits of leisure-time physical activity on the cardiovascular risk profile at older age. Int J Epidemiol 28:659, 1999.
50. King AC, Castro C, Wilcox S, et al: Personal and environmental factors associated with physical inactivity among different racial-ethnic groups of U.S. middle-aged and older-aged women. Health Psychol 19:354, 2000.
51. Ridker PM, Buring JE, Cook NR, et al: C-reactive protein, the metabolic syndrome, and risk of incident cardiovascular events: An 8-year follow-up of 14 719 initially healthy American women. Circulation 107:391, 2003.
52. Ridker PM, Rifai N, Clearfield M, et al: Measurement of C-reactive protein for the targeting of statin therapy in the primary prevention of acute coronary events. N Engl J Med 344:1959, 2001.
53. Hayes SN, Gersh BJ: Chronic stable angina. *In* Douglas PS (ed): Cardiovascular Health and Disease in Women. 2nd ed. Philadelphia, WB Saunders, 2002, pp 291-315.
54. Bankier B, Littman AB: Psychiatric disorders and coronary heart disease in women—A still neglected topic: Review of the literature from 1971 to 2000. Psychother Psychosom 71:133, 2002.
55. Nguyen VH, McLaughlin MA: Coronary artery disease in women: A review of emerging cardiovascular risk factors. Mt Sinai J Med 69:338, 2002.
56. Donati MB, Zito F, Castelnuovo AD, et al: Genes, coagulation and cardiovascular risk. J Hum Hypertens 14:369, 2000.
57. Stampfer MJ, Hu FB, Manson JE, et al: Primary prevention of coronary heart disease in women through diet and lifestyle. N Engl J Med 343:16, 2000.
58. Kyker KA, Limacher MC: Gender differences in the presentation and symptoms of coronary artery disease. Curr Womens Health Rep 2:115, 2002.
59. Grady D, Chaput L, Kristof M: Diagnosis and Treatment of Coronary Heart Disease in Women: Systematic Reviews of Evidence on Selected Topics. Evidence Report/Technology Assessment No. 81. (Prepared by the University of California, San Francisco-Stanford Evidence-based Practice Center under Contract No 290-97-0013.) AHRQ Publication No. 03-0037. Rockville, Md, Agency for Healthcare and Research and Quality, May 2003.
60. Lualdi JC, Douglas PS: Considerations in the selection of noninvasive testing for the diagnosis of coronary artery disease. Cardiol Rev 6:278, 1998.
61. Alexander KP, Shaw LJ, Shaw LK, et al: Value of exercise treadmill testing in women. J Am Coll Cardiol 32:1657, 1998.
62. Kwok Y, Kim C, Grady D, et al: Meta-analysis of exercise testing to detect coronary artery disease in women. Am J Cardiol 83:660, 1999.
63. Fleischmann KE, Hunink MG, Kuntz KM, et al: Exercise echocardiography or exercise SPECT imaging? A meta-analysis of diagnostic test performance. JAMA 280:913, 1998.
64. Hansen CL, Kramer M, Rastogi A: Lower accuracy of TI-201 SPECT in women is not improved by size-based normal databases or Wiener filtering. J Nucl Cardiol 6:177, 1999.
65. Taillefer R, DePuey EG, Udelson JE, et al: Comparative diagnostic accuracy of Tl-201 and Tc-99m sestamibi SPECT imaging (perfusion and ECG-gated SPECT) in detecting coronary artery disease in women. J Am Coll Cardiol 29:69, 1997.
66. Kuntz KM, Fleischmann KE, Hunink MG, et al: Cost-effectiveness of diagnostic strategies for patients with chest pain. Ann Intern Med 130:709, 1999.
67. Kim C, Kwok YS, Saha S, et al: Diagnosis of suspected coronary artery disease in women: A cost-effectiveness analysis. Am Heart J 137:1019, 1999.
68. Steen MK, Jacobs AK, Freney D, et al: Gender related differences in complications during coronary angiography. Circulation 86:I-254, 1992.
69. Schulman KA, Berlin JA, Harless W, et al: The effect of race and gender on physicians' recommendations for cardiac catheterization. N Engl J Med 340:618, 1999.
70. Devon HA, Zerwic JJ: Symptoms of acute coronary syndromes: Are there gender differences? A review of the literature. Heart Lung 31:235, 2002.
71. Leopold JA, Jacobs AK: Catheter-based revascularization strategies for acute coronary syndromes in women. Rev Cardiovasc Med 2:181, 2001.
72. Hochman JS, Tamis-Holland JE: Acute coronary syndromes: Does gender matter? JAMA 288:3161, 2002.
73. Collins L, Douglas, PS: Acute coronary syndromes. *In* Douglas PS (ed): Cardiovascular Health and Disease in Women. 2nd ed. Philadelphia, WB Saunders, 2002, pp 316-342.
74. de Bruyne MC, Mosterd A, Hoes AW, et al: Prevalence, determinants, and misclassification of myocardial infarction in the elderly. Epidemiology 8:495, 1997.
75. Lundberg V, Wikstrom B, Bostrom S, et al: Exploring gender differences in case fatality in acute myocardial infarction or coronary death events in the northern Sweden MONICA Project. J Intern Med 251:235, 2002.
76. Hochman JS, Tamis JE, Thompson TD, et al: Gender, clinical presentation, and outcome in patients with acute coronary syndromes. Global Use of Strategies to Open Occluded Coronary Arteries in Acute Coronary Syndromes IIb Investigators. N Engl J Med 341:226, 1999.
77. Vaccarino V, Krumholz HM, Yarzebski J, et al: Gender differences in 2-year mortality after hospital discharge for myocardial infarction. Ann Intern Med 134:173, 2001.
78. Kaplan KL, Fitzpatrick P, Cox C, et al: Use of thrombolytic therapy for acute myocardial infarction: Effects of gender and age on treatment rates. J Thromb Thrombolysis 13:21, 2002.
79. Mehilli J, Kastrati A, Dirschinger J, et al: Gender-based analysis of outcome in patients with acute myocardial infarction treated predominantly with percutaneous coronary intervention. JAMA 287:210, 2002.
80. Cannon CP, Weintraub WS, Demopoulos LA, et al: Comparison of early invasive and conservative strategies in patients with unstable coronary syndromes treated with the glycoprotein IIb/IIIa inhibitor tirofiban. N Engl J Med 344:1879, 2001.
81. Wallentin L, Lagerqvist B, Husted S, et al: Outcome at 1 year after an invasive compared with a non-invasive strategy in unstable coronary-artery disease: The FRISC II invasive randomised trial. FRISC II Investigators. Fast Revascularisation during Instability in Coronary artery disease. Lancet 356:9, 2000.
82. Glaser R, Herrmann HC, Murphy SA, et al: Benefit of an early invasive management strategy in women with acute coronary syndromes. JAMA 288:3124, 2002.
83. Malenka DJ, O'Rourke D, Miller MA, et al: Cause of in-hospital death in 12,232 consecutive patients undergoing percutaneous transluminal coronary angioplasty. The Northern New England Cardiovascular Disease Study Group. Am Heart J 137:632, 1999.
84. Vaccarino V, Lin ZQ, Kasl SV, et al: Gender differences in recovery after coronary artery bypass surgery. J Am Coll Cardiol 41:307, 2003.
85. Vaccarino V, Abramson JL, Veledar E, et al: Gender differences in hospital mortality after coronary artery bypass surgery: Evidence for a higher mortality in younger women. Circulation 105:1176, 2002.
86. Hogue CW Jr, Barzilai B, Pieper KS, et al: Gender differences in neurological outcomes and mortality after cardiac surgery: A society of thoracic surgery national database report. Circulation 103:2133, 2001.
87. Stamou SC, Jablonski KA, Pfister AJ, et al: Stroke after conventional versus minimally invasive coronary artery bypass. Ann Thorac Surg 74:394, 2002.
88. Capdeville M, Chamogeogarkis T, Lee JH: Effect of gender on outcomes of beating heart operations. Ann Thorac Surg 72:S1022, 2001.
89. Jacobs AK: Coronary revascularization in women in 2003: Gender revisited. Circulation 107:375, 2003.
90. Ott RA, Gutfinger DE, Alimadadian H, et al: Conventional coronary artery bypass grafting: Why women take longer to recover. J Cardiovasc Surg (Torino) 42:311, 2001.
91. Schwartz LM, Fisher ES, Tosteson NA, et al: Treatment and health outcomes of women and men in a cohort with coronary artery disease. Arch Intern Med 157:1545, 1997.
92. Vittinghoff E, Shlipak MG, Varosy PD, et al: Risk factors and secondary prevention in women with heart disease: The Heart and Estrogen/progestin Replacement Study. Ann Intern Med 138:81, 2003.
93. Miettinen TA, Pyorala K, Olsson AG, et al: Cholesterol-lowering therapy in women and elderly patients with myocardial infarction or angina pectoris: Findings from the Scandinavian Simvastatin Survival Study (4S). Circulation 96:4211, 1997.
94. McDermott MM, Greenland P, Liu K, et al: Gender differences in peripheral arterial disease: Leg symptoms and physical functioning. J Am Geriatr Soc 51:222, 2003.
95. Higgins JP, Higgins JA: Epidemiology of peripheral arterial disease in women. J Epidemiol 13:1, 2003.
96. Langer RD, Criqui MH: Stroke and peripheral vascular disease in women. *In* Douglas PS (ed): Cardiovascular Health and Disease in Women. 2nd ed. Philadelphia, WB Saunders, 2002, pp 445-459.
97. Norman PE, Semmens JB, Lawrence-Brown M, et al: The influence of gender on outcome following peripheral vascular surgery: A review. Cardiovasc Surg 8:111, 2000.

Hemostasis, Thrombosis, and Stroke

98. Brey RL, Stallworth CL, McGlasson DL, et al: Antiphospholipid antibodies and stroke in young women. Stroke 33:2396, 2002.
99. Randomised trial of a perindopril-based blood-pressure-lowering regimen among 6,105 individuals with previous stroke or transient ischaemic attack. Lancet 358:1033, 2001.
100. Yusuf S, Sleight P, Pogue J, et al: Effects of an angiotensin-converting-enzyme inhibitor, ramipril, on cardiovascular events in high-risk patients. The Heart Outcomes Prevention Evaluation Study Investigators. N Engl J Med 342:145, 2000.
101. Hansson L, Zanchetti A, Carruthers SG, et al: Effects of intensive blood-pressure lowering and low-dose aspirin in patients with hypertension: Principal results of the Hypertension Optimal Treatment (HOT) randomised trial. HOT Study Group. Lancet 351:1755, 1998.
102. de Gaetano G: Low-dose aspirin and vitamin E in people at cardiovascular risk: A randomised trial in general practice. Collaborative Group of the Primary Prevention Project. Lancet 357:89, 2001.
103. Humphries KH, Kerr CR, Connolly SJ, et al: New-onset atrial fibrillation: Gender differences in presentation, treatment, and outcome. Circulation 103:2365, 2001.
104. Stafford RS, Singer DE: Recent national patterns of warfarin use in atrial fibrillation. Circulation 97:1231, 1998.
105. Kent DM, Ruthazer R, Selker HP: Are some patients likely to benefit from recombinant tissue-type plasminogen activator for acute ischemic stroke even beyond 3 hours from symptom onset? Stroke 34:464, 2003.
106. Schneider JR, Droste JS, Golan JF: Carotid endarterectomy in women versus men: Patient characteristics and outcomes. J Vasc Surg 25:890; discussion 897, 1997.
107. Holroyd-Leduc JM, Kapral MK, Austin PC, et al: Gender differences and similarities in the management and outcome of stroke patients. Stroke 31:1833, 2000.

108. Beauregard LA: Incidence and management of arrhythmias in women. J Gend Specif Med 5:38, 2002.
109. Rashba EJ, Zareba W, Moss AJ, et al: Influence of pregnancy on the risk for cardiac events in patients with hereditary long QT syndrome. LQTS Investigators. Circulation 97:451, 1998.
110. Freed LA, Eagle KA, Mahjoub ZA, et al: Gender differences in presentation, management, and cardiac event-free survival in patients with syncope. Am J Cardiol 80:1183, 1997.
111. McGavigan AD, Hood S: The influence of gender and age on response to head-up tilt-table testing in patients with recurrent syncope. Age Ageing 30:295, 2001.
112. Cohen TJ, Thayapran N, Ibrahim B, et al: An association between anxiety and neurocardiogenic syncope during head-up tilt table testing. Pacing Clin Electrophysiol 23:837, 2000.
113. Zimetbaum P, Josephson ME: Evaluation of patients with palpitations. N Engl J Med 338:1369, 1998.
114. Larsen JA, Kadish AH: Effects of gender on cardiac arrhythmias. J Cardiovasc Electrophysiol 9:655, 1998.
115. Lessmeier TJ, Gamperling D, Johnson-Liddon V, et al: Unrecognized paroxysmal supraventricular tachycardia. Potential for misdiagnosis as panic disorder. Arch Intern Med 157:537, 1997.

Valvular Heart Disease

116. Devereux RB: Valvular heart disease. *In* Douglas PS (ed): Cardiovascular Health and Disease in Women. 2nd ed. Philadelphia, WB Saunders, 2002, pp 405-425.
117. Stewart BF, Siscovick D, Lind BK, et al: Clinical factors associated with calcific aortic valve disease. Cardiovascular Health Study. J Am Coll Cardiol 29:630, 1997.

Heart Failure

118. Masoudi FA, Havranek EP, Smith G, et al: Gender, age, and heart failure with preserved left ventricular systolic function. J Am Coll Cardiol 41:217, 2003.
119. Fernandez-Sola J, Nicolas-Arfelis JM: Gender differences in alcoholic cardiomyopathy. J Gend Specif Med 5:41, 2002.
120. Petrie MC, Dawson NF, Murdoch DR, et al: Failure of women's hearts. Circulation 99:2334, 1999.
121. Vasan RS, Larson MG, Benjamin EJ, et al: Congestive heart failure in subjects with normal versus reduced left ventricular ejection fraction: Prevalence and mortality in a population-based cohort. J Am Coll Cardiol 33:1948, 1999.
122. Redfield MM, Jacobsen SJ, Burnett JC Jr, et al: Burden of systolic and diastolic ventricular dysfunction in the community: Appreciating the scope of the heart failure epidemic. JAMA 289:194, 2003.
123. Shekelle PG, Rich MW, Morton SC, et al: Efficacy of angiotensin-converting enzyme inhibitors and beta-blockers in the management of left ventricular systolic dysfunction according to race, gender, and diabetic status: A meta-analysis of major clinical trials. J Am Coll Cardiol 41:1529, 2003.
124. Ghali JK, Pina IL, Gottlieb SS, et al: Metoprolol CR/XL in female patients with heart failure: Analysis of the experience in Metoprolol Extended-Release Randomized Intervention Trial in Heart Failure (MERIT-HF). Circulation 105:1585, 2002.
125. Rathore SS, Wang Y, Krumholz HM: Gender-based differences in the effect of digoxin for the treatment of heart failure. N Engl J Med 347:1403, 2002.
126. Schwartz JB: Congestive heart failure medications: Is there a rationale for gender-specific therapy? J Gend Specif Med 3:17, 2000.
127. Aaronson KD, Schwartz JS, Goin JE, et al: Gender differences in patient acceptance of cardiac transplant candidacy. Circulation 91:2753, 1995.

Issues of Death and Dying in Women

128. Crawford BM, Meana M, Stewart D, et al: Treatment decision making in mature adults: Gender differences. Health Care Women Int 21:91, 2000.
129. Bookwala J, Coppola KM, Fagerlin A, et al: Gender differences in older adults' preferences for life-sustaining medical treatments and end-of-life values. Death Stud 25:127, 2001.
130. Lewis EF, Johnson PA, Johnson W, et al: Preferences for quality of life or survival expressed by patients with heart failure. J Heart Lung Transplant 20:1016, 2001.

CHAPTER 74

Pregnancy and Cardiovascular Disease

Uri Elkayam

Cardiovascular Physiology During Pregnancy and the Puerperium

Pregnancy and the peripartum period are associated with important cardiocirculatory changes[1] that can lead to marked clinical deterioration in the woman with heart disease. Hemodynamic changes occurring during pregnancy are summarized in Table 74–1.

BLOOD VOLUME. Blood volume increases substantially during pregnancy, starting as early as the sixth week and rising rapidly until midpregnancy, when the rise continues but at a much slower rate (Fig. 74-1).[1] The degree of maximum volume expansion varies considerably in the individual patient (20 to 100 percent) and averages 50 percent. This increase is reported to correlate with fetal weight, placental mass, weight of the products of conception, and maternal and neonatal weight.[1] A higher increment in blood volume is reported in multigravidas and in women with multiple pregnancies. Because increase in plasma volume is more rapid than increase in red blood cell mass (see Fig. 74-1), hemoglobin concentration falls during pregnancy gradually until week 30, causing the "physiological anemia of pregnancy" with hematocrit levels that can be as low as 33 to 38 percent, a condition that can be partially corrected with iron therapy. Changes in blood volume during pregnancy are attributable to estrogen-mediated stimulation of the renin-aldosterone system,[2] which results in sodium and water retention. Changes in other hormones, including deoxycorticosterone, prostaglandin, estrogen, prolactin, placental lactogen, growth hormone, and adrenocorticotropic hormone, may also be involved in water retention during pregnancy.

CARDIAC OUTPUT, STROKE VOLUME, AND HEART RATE. Cardiac output during pregnancy is estimated to increase by approximately 50 percent.[1] It begins to rise around the fifth week and increases rapidly until the 24th week, when it levels off or continues to rise slightly (Fig. 74-2; see Table 74-1).[1,3] During the third trimester, body position can substantially influence cardiac output, which increases in the lateral position and declines in the supine position owing to caval compression by the gravid uterus and decreased venous return to the heart. The increase in cardiac output early in pregnancy is predominantly due to augmentation in stroke volume, whereas in the third trimester it is largely due to an accelerated heart rate and stroke volume does not change or even declines as a result of caval compression (Fig. 74-3). Increase in cardiac output seems to be enhanced in subsequent pregnancies.[3]

Heart rate peaks during the third trimester with an average increase of 10 to 20 beats/min (see Fig. 74-2),[3,4] although on occasion it may be markedly faster. Pregnancy with multiple fetuses is associated with an even higher heart rate.

BLOOD PRESSURE AND SYSTEMIC VASCULAR RESISTANCE. Systemic arterial pressure begins to fall during the first trimester, reaches a nadir in midpregnancy, and returns toward pregestational levels before term (see Table 74-1).[3] Because diastolic blood pressure decreases substantially more than systolic pressure, the pulse pressure widens.[1] Reduction in blood pressure is caused by a decline in systemic vascular resistance related to reduced vascular tone,[5] probably mediated by (1) gestational hormonal activity, increased levels of circulating prostaglandins and atrial natriuretic peptides,[1] as well as endothelial nitric oxide; (2) increased heat production by the developing fetus; and (3) the creation of a low-resistance circulation in the pregnant uterus.

SUPINE HYPOTENSIVE SYNDROME OF PREGNANCY. The supine hypotensive or the uterocaval syndrome of pregnancy occurs with significant decreases in heart rate and blood pressure in up to 11 percent of pregnant women.[1] These hemodynamic changes are associated with weakness, lightheadedness, nausea, dizziness, and even syncope and are explained by acute occlusion of the inferior vena cava by the enlarged uterus. When the supine position is abandoned, these hemodynamic effects and symptoms are usually promptly relieved.

HEMODYNAMIC CHANGES DURING LABOR AND DELIVERY. Hemodynamics are altered substantially during labor and delivery secondary to anxiety, pain, and uterine contractions.[1] Oxygen consumption increases threefold; cardiac output rises progressively during labor because of increases in both stroke volume and heart rate, and it is higher in the lateral position. Both systolic and diastolic blood pressures increase markedly during contractions, with greater augmentation during the second stage.[1] The supine position is associated with a 20 percent reduction in stroke volume, cardiac output, and mean arterial pressure and a marked increase in systemic vascular resistance compared with the lateral position. Hemodynamic changes during labor and delivery are greatly influenced by the form of anesthesia and analgesia. Reduction of pain and apprehension by local, caudal, or epidural anesthesia may limit hemodynamic changes and the rise in oxygen consumption.

HEMODYNAMIC EFFECTS OF CESAREAN SECTION. To avoid the hemodynamic changes associated with vaginal delivery, cesarean section is frequently recommended for women with cardiovascular disease. However, this form of delivery can also be associated with considerable hemodynamic fluctuations related largely to intubation, drugs used for anesthesia and analgesia, larger extent of blood loss, the relief of caval compression, extubation, and postoperative awakening.[1]

HEMODYNAMIC CHANGES POST PARTUM. A temporary increase in venous return may occur immediately after delivery because of relief of caval compression and, in addition, blood shifting from the contracting uterus into the systemic circulation (autotransfusion). This change in effective blood volume occurs despite blood loss during delivery and can result in a substantial rise in ventricular

TABLE 74–1 Cardiocirculatory Changes During Normal Pregnancy

	Changes at Various Times (Weeks)					
Parameter	***5***	***12***	***20***	***24***	***32***	***38***
Heart rate	↑	↑↑↑	↑↑↑	↑↑↑	↑↑↑↑	↑↑↑↑
Systolic blood pressure	↔	↓	↓	↔	↑	↑↑
Diastolic blood pressure	↔	↓	↓↓	↓	↔	↑↑
Stroke volume	↑	↑↑↑↑↑	↑↑↑↑↑↑	↑↑↑↑↑↑	↑↑↑↑↑	↑↑↑↑↑
Cardiac output	↑↑	↑↑↑↑↑↑	↑↑↑↑↑↑↑	↑↑↑↑↑↑↑	↑↑↑↑↑↑↑	↑↑↑↑↑↑↑
Systemic vascular resistance	↓↓	↓↓↓↓↓	↓↓↓↓↓↓	↓↓↓↓↓↓	↓↓↓↓↓↓	↓↓↓↓↓
Left ventricular ejection fraction	↑	↑↑	↑↑	↑↑	↑	↑

↑, ≤5%; ↑↑, 6-10%; ↑↑↑, 11-15%; ↑↑↑↑, 16-20%; ↑↑↑↑↑, 21-30%; ↑↑↑↑↑↑, >30%; ↑↑↑↑↑↑↑, >40%.

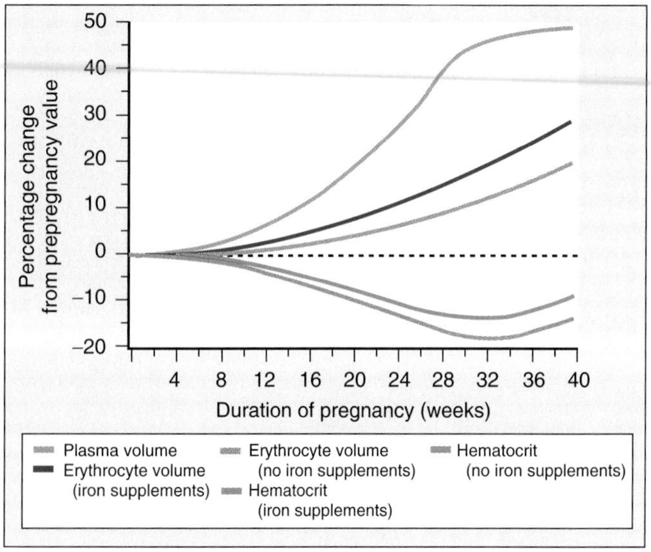

FIGURE 74–1 Changes in plasma volume, erythrocyte volume, and hematocrit during pregnancy. The increase in plasma volume is more rapid than the increase in erythrocyte volume, causing the "physiological anemia of pregnancy," which can be partially corrected with iron supplements. (From Pitkin RM: Nutritional support in obstetrics and gynecology. Clin Obstet Gynecol 19:489, 1976.)

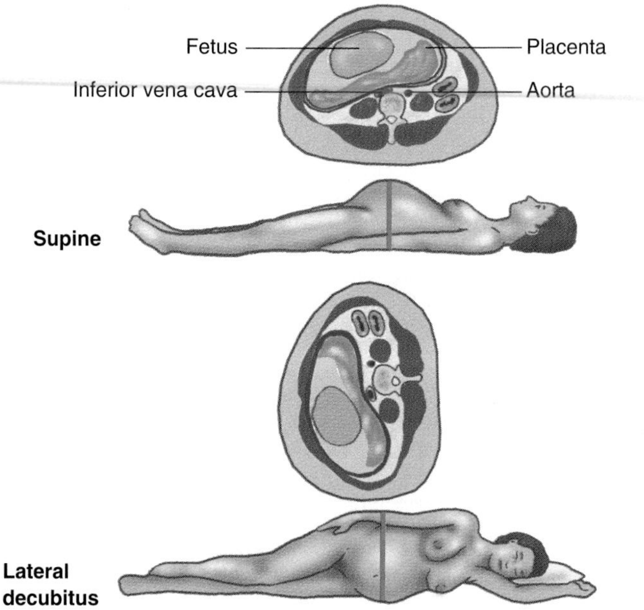

FIGURE 74–3 Venocaval compression of the inferior vena cava and abdominal aorta by the gravid uterus can lead to reduced venous return and thus to decreased cardiac output. (From Lee W, Shah PK, Amin DK, et al: Hemodynamic monitoring of cardiac patients during pregnancy. *In* Elkayam U, Gleicher N [eds]: Cardiac Problems in Pregnancy. 2nd ed. New York, Alan R. Liss, 1990, p 61.)

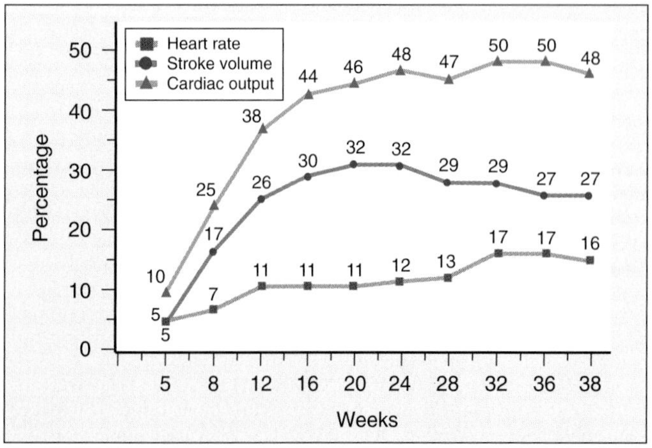

FIGURE 74–2 Percent changes of heart rate, stroke volume, and cardiac output measured in the lateral position throughout pregnancy compared with prepregnancy values. (Modified from Robson SC, Hunter S, Boys RJ, Dunlop W: Serial study of factors influencing changes in cardiac output during human pregnancy. Am J Physiol 256:H1060, 1989.)

filling pressure, stroke volume, and cardiac output and may lead to clinical deterioration.[6] Both heart rate and cardiac output return to prelabor values by 1 hour after delivery and mean blood pressure and stroke volume by 24 hours after delivery. Hemodynamic adaptation to pregnancy persists post partum and gradually returns to prepregnancy values within 12 to 24 weeks after delivery.[1]

Cardiovascular Evaluation During Pregnancy

History and Physical Examination

Normal pregnancy is often accompanied by symptoms of fatigue, decreased exercise capacity, hyperventilation, dyspnea, palpitations, lightheadedness, and even syncope (Table 74–2).[7] In addition, augmentation of jugular venous pulsation related to increased blood volume and leg edema (often observed in late pregnancy) could lead to an erroneous diagnosis of heart failure or overestimation of its severity.

TABLE 74–2 Cardiac Symptoms and Findings During Normal Pregnancy

Symptoms
Decreased exercise capacity
Tiredness
Dyspnea
Orthopnea
Palpitations
Lightheadedness
Syncope
Physical Findings
Inspection
Hyperventilation
Peripheral edema
Distended neck veins with prominent a and v waves and brisk *x* and *y* descents
Capillary pulsation
Precordial palpation
Brisk, diffuse, and displaced left ventricular impulse
Palpable right ventricular impulse
Palpable pulmonary trunk impulse
Auscultation
Pulmonary basilar rales
Increased first heart sound with exaggerated splitting
Exaggerated splitting of second heart sound
Midsystolic ejection-type murmurs at the lower left sternal edge and over the pulmonary area radiating to suprasternal notch and more to the left than right side of neck
Continuous murmurs (cervical venous hum, mammary souffle)
Diastolic murmurs (rare)

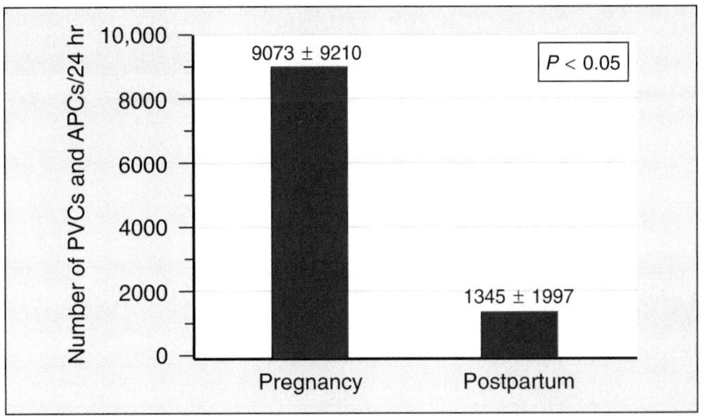

FIGURE 74–4 Total number of ventricular and atrial premature beats as recorded over 24 hours in nine healthy women with palpitations during pregnancy and in the postpartum period. APC = atrial premature complex; PVC = premature ventricular complex. (Modified from Shotan A, Ostrzega E, Mehra A, et al: Incidence of arrhythmias in normal pregnancy and relation to palpitations, dizziness, and syncope. Am J Cardiol 79:1061, 1997.)

TABLE 74–3 Electrocardiographic Findings During Normal Pregnancy

QRS axis deviation
Small Q wave and inverted P wave in lead III (abolished by inspiration)
ST segment and T wave changes (ritodrine tocolysis, cesarean section)
Frequent sinus tachycardia
Higher incidence of arrhythmias
Increased R/S ratio in leads V_2 and V_1

Systemic arterial pulses are full and collapsing and are similar to those palpated in patients with aortic regurgitation or hyperthyroidism. A left ventricular impulse is easily detected in most women in late pregnancy and is hyperactive and brisk. Right ventricular heave is usually present during the second and third trimesters, and the pulmonary trunk and pulmonic valve closure are often palpable. This group of findings may result in difficulty in assessing the presence or severity, or both, of pulmonary hypertension.

CARDIAC AUSCULTATION. Especially after the first trimester, auscultation often reveals an increased first heart sound (S_1) with exaggerated splitting that may be misinterpreted as a fourth heart sound (S_4) or as a systolic click.[7] The second heart sound (S_2) is often increased in late pregnancy and can exhibit persistent splitting when the patient is examined in the lateral position. These changes in S_2 may be interpreted as signs of pulmonary hypertension (loud P_2) or atrial septal defect (systolic murmur and splitting of S_2). Auscultation of the third and fourth heart sounds is uncommon in normal pregnancy.

Innocent Systolic Murmurs. These can be heard in most pregnant women and are the result of the hyperkinetic circulation of pregnancy. Murmurs are usually midsystolic and soft, are heard best at the lower left sternal edge and over the pulmonic area, and radiate to the suprasternal notch and more to the left than to the right side of the neck.[7] Not uncommonly, the benign murmur of pregnancy may be louder or longer and may sound like those associated with atrial septal defect or stenosis of one of the semilunar valves. In such cases an echocardiographic and Doppler evaluation is warranted to rule out an abnormal cardiac condition. Two benign continuous murmurs that may be heard during gestation are the cervical venous hum and mammary souffle. The venous hum is usually heard maximally over the right supraclavicular fossa but can radiate to the contralateral area and sometimes to the area below the clavicle. The mammary souffle may be either systolic or continuous, is heard over the breast late in gestation or in the lactating period, and is caused by increased flow in the mammary arteries. Characteristically, the murmur decreases or vanishes when pressure is applied to the stethoscope or when the patient moves to the upright position. Diastolic murmurs may be heard in normal pregnant women because of increased blood flow through the atrioventricular valve. Such a finding, however, is infrequent in the healthy pregnant woman and therefore requires careful diagnostic work-up to rule out organic disease.

Laboratory Examinations

ELECTROCARDIOGRAPHY (see Chap. 9). In normal pregnancy, the QRS axis may shift to either the left or the right, but it usually stays within normal limits (Table 74–3).[7] A small Q wave and an inverted P wave in lead III that vary with respiration as well as a greater R wave amplitude in leads V_1 and V_2 and an inverted T wave in V_2 can be present. ST segment depression mimicking myocardial ischemia but not associated with wall motion abnormalities has been described between induction of anesthesia and the end of surgery in patients undergoing cesarean section. Increased susceptibility to arrhythmias during pregnancy is manifested by the frequent finding of sinus tachycardia and atrial or ventricular premature beats (Fig. 74–4),[8] and an increased incidence of paroxysmal supraventricular tachycardia during normal pregnancy and several cases of ventricular tachycardia have been reported in healthy women (see Chap. 32).

CHEST RADIOGRAPHY. Although the radiation dose associated with a routine chest radiograph is minimal, because of the potential for adverse biological effects from

TABLE 74–4 Chest Radiograph Findings During Normal Pregnancy

Straightening of the left upper cardiac border
Horizontal position of the heart
Increased lung markings
Small plural effusion in early postpartum period

TABLE 74–5 Doppler and Echocardiographic Findings During Normal Pregnancy

Slightly increased systolic and diastolic left ventricular dimensions (when patient examined in the lateral position)
Unchanged or slightly improved left ventricular systolic function
Moderate increase in size of right atrium, right ventricle, and left atrium
Progressive dilation of pulmonary, tricuspid, and mitral valve annuli
Functional pulmonary, tricuspid, and mitral regurgitation
Small pericardial effusion

any amount of radiation the pelvic area should be shielded by protective lead material.[9]

Changes seen on chest films in normal pregnancy can simulate those of cardiac disease and should be interpreted with caution (Table 74–4).[7] Straightening of the left upper cardiac border because of prominence of the pulmonary conus is often seen. The heart may seem enlarged because of its horizontal positioning secondary to the elevated diaphragm. In addition, an increase in lung markings can simulate a pattern of flow redistribution seen with increased pulmonary venous pressure. Pleural effusion can be found early post partum; it is usually small and is resorbed 1 to 2 weeks after delivery.

DOPPLER ECHOCARDIOGRAPHY (see Chap. 5) (Table 74–5). Gestational use of both maternal and fetal cardiac ultrasonography is considered safe.[10] Transesophageal echocardiography has been increasingly used in pregnancy and seems to be well tolerated by both mother and fetus. Pericardial effusion, usually small or minimal, has been noted in normal pregnant women late in pregnancy.[7] There is a progressive increase in all cardiac chamber dimensions with an approximately 20 percent increase in the size of the right atrium and the right ventricle, 12 percent increase in left atrial size, and 10 percent increase in left ventricular size. Post partum, these changes gradually return toward baseline but may remain different from prepregnancy values for several months.[3] In addition, there is early and progressive dilation of mitral, tricuspid, and pulmonary annuli, which is associated with an increase in valvular regurgitation.

STRESS TESTING. An exercise test using bicycle ergometry or a treadmill can be carried out during pregnancy to help establish the diagnosis of ischemic heart disease and to assess functional capacity and cardiac reserve.[7] Although maximal exercise has been reported to be safe by some investigators,[11] a low-level exercise protocol allowing heart rate to increase to 70 percent of the maximal predicted heart rate with fetal monitoring is preferred when stress testing is indicated.[7]

RADIATION. Exposure of the embryo to irradiation during the first 10 days after conception would most likely either have no effect or lead to resorption.[9] Irradiation during organ formation (days 10 to 50) may have a teratogenic effect, whereas after completion of organogenesis it may cause intrauterine growth retardation, central nervous system abnormalities, and possibly an increased incidence of childhood cancer or leukemia.

Routine chest radiography is associated with radiation of 20 millirads to the chest. Standard fluoroscopy can deliver 1 to 2 rads/min to the chest and high-level fluoroscopy or cine as much as 5 to 10 rads/min. The amount of radiation scattered to the uterus and absorbed by the embryo is less than 5 percent of radiation absorbed by the directly radiated tissue. Direct irradiation to the fetus should be avoided and can be prevented by covering the patient with a lead apron during radiographic procedures. The use of a lead apron, however, is of little help in reducing fetal irradiation associated with Compton-scattered photons.

Radiation to the fetus from nuclear medicine procedures is mainly due to distribution of radiopharmaceuticals to the bladder or the placenta or directly across the placental barrier. The expected radiation with thallium-201 or technetium-99m–labeled sestamibi diagnostic procedures is less than 1 rad per examination. Cardiac function studies with technetium-99m–labeled red blood cells are associated with fetal radiation of 1 to 2 rads, peripheral contrast radiographic venography with 0.5 rad or less, and pulmonary scintigraphy with technetium-macroaggregated albumin with 0.05 rad or less.

Current recommendations related to intrauterine radiation exposure are as follows[9]:

- Less than 5 rads—patient can be reassured of very low likelihood of risk.
- Five to 10 rads—patient should be counseled regarding low risk of problems.
- Ten to 15 rads during first 6 weeks—individual considerations for termination of pregnancy should be made.
- More than 15 rads—termination of pregnancy recommended.

MAGNETIC RESONANCE IMAGING. The technique has been used increasingly during pregnancy for the diagnosis of fetal anomalities.[12] Although magnetic resonance imaging poses no known risks to the fetus and its use for diagnosis of fetal disease has increased, its safety has not been fully established. Currently, the U.S. Food and Drug Administration recommends prudence in using magnetic resonance imaging during pregnancy.

PULMONARY ARTERY CATHETERIZATION. Hemodynamic monitoring with the aid of a pulmonary artery catheter can be of great help in managing patients at high risk during pregnancy, labor, delivery, and the postpartum period. The ability to insert and position the flotation catheter with pressure monitoring without the need for fluoroscopy makes it particularly attractive for use during pregnancy. Hemodynamic monitoring is recommended throughout labor and delivery for any patient with symptomatic cardiac disease during pregnancy or with the potential for deterioration because of valvular, myocardial, or ischemic heart disease. Because significant circulatory changes that may lead to hemodynamic deterioration occur in the early postpartum period,[1] hemodynamic monitoring should be continued for at least several hours after delivery to ensure stability.

CARDIAC CATHETERIZATION. Cardiac catheterization may be indicated in rare instances of cardiac decompensation when sufficient information cannot be obtained by noninvasive techniques, especially if cardiac surgery, percutaneous coronary intervention, or balloon valvuloplasty is being considered. Although this technique provides high-quality images, it is associated with a relatively high dose of radiation.[9] To minimize radiation to the pelvic and abdominal areas, the brachial rather than the femoral approach is preferred, fluoroscopy and cine time should be reduced to the minimum required, and direct irradiation to the fetus should be avoided.

Pregnancy in Women with Congenital Heart Disease

Because of increased survival of children with congenital heart disease (see Chap. 56), pregnancy has become more common in this population of patients.[13,14] Preconception evaluation should include careful history and assessment of risk for both the mother and the fetus.[15] The patient should be counseled regarding contraceptive alternatives,[16] potential maternal and fetal risks of pregnancy,[17-19] and, when appropriate, expected long-term maternal morbidity and survival as well as the risk of congenital malformations in the offspring.[20] In addition, guidance concerning anticoagulation and prophylactic antibiotics, if needed, should be provided.

MATERNAL AND FETAL OUTCOME. In general, a good maternal outcome can be expected in most cases with noncyanotic congenital heart disease. Maternal outcome is determined by the nature of the disease, surgical repair, presence and severity of cyanosis, increased pulmonary vascular resistance, maternal functional capacity, myocardial dysfunction, left ventricular obstruction, and history of arrhythmias or other prior cardiac events.[14,19] An unfavorable outcome, including development of congestive heart failure, arrhythmias, and hypertension, is commonly seen in patients with impaired functional status and those with cyanosis.[17] Other reported complications include angina, infective endocarditis, and thromboembolic phenomena.[13,19] Pregnant women with congenital heart disease have an increased risk for neonatal complications including fetal wastage, low birth weight for gestational age, prematurity, congenital heart disease, and respiratory distress syndrome.[19] The risk of fetal and neonatal complications is increased in patients with cyanotic heart disease.[13,21] Fetal wastage was reported in 45 percent of cyanotic mothers compared with 20 percent of acyanotic mothers with congenital heart disease.[21] In addition, low birth weight for gestational age and prematurity are common in cyanotic mothers and correlate with maternal hemoglobin and hematocrit values.[13,21] Risk of congenital heart disease is increased for the offspring of mothers with congenital heart disease with a reported incidence of 4 to 8 percent,[19] and there are many noncardiac congenital malformations as well as mental and physical impairments in children born to mothers with congenital heart disease.[19]

LABOR AND DELIVERY. Elective induction of labor when fetal maturity is confirmed may be used in high-risk patients for better planning, hemodynamic monitoring, and availability of expert personnel during labor and delivery.[13] Vaginal delivery is preferred for most patients, and cesarean section is indicated in the stable patients only for obstetric reasons. Oxygen should be given to hypoxemic mothers, and blood gas monitoring is recommended in most patients with impaired functional capacity, cardiac dysfunction, pulmonary hypertension, and cyanotic malformations. Hemodynamic monitoring should be considered in selected patients, and blood volume loss must be anticipated and treated promptly.

ANTIBIOTIC PROPHYLAXIS. Official recommendations by the American Heart Association suggest that antibiotic prophylaxis for an uncomplicated delivery is unnecessary except for cases with prosthetic heart valves or a surgically constructed systemic-to-pulmonary shunt.[22] Because of difficulties in predicting complicated deliveries and potential devastating consequences of endocarditis,[23] antibiotic prophylaxis for vaginal delivery in all patients with congenital heart disease (except those with an isolated secundum type of atrial septal defect and those 6 months or more after repair of septal defects or surgical ligation and division of patent ductus arteriosus) seems reasonable.

Specific Malformations

ATRIAL SEPTAL DEFECT AND PATENT FORAMEN OVALE. Atrial septal defect is usually well tolerated in pregnancy even in patients with large left-to-right shunts. A retrospective review of 163 pregnancies in 80 women with atrial septal defect reported higher incidences of miscarriage, preterm delivery, and cardiac symptoms in cases in which pregnancy occurred before surgical correction.[24] The development of pulmonary hypertension and atrial arrhythmias rarely occurs in women of childbearing age. Because endocarditis is rare, antibiotic prophylaxis is not indicated in patients with secundum-type atrial septal defect. Recommendations concerning pregnancy in patients with atrial septal defect should be made on an individual basis, considering accompanying lesions, functional status, and the level of pulmonary vascular resistance. Paradoxical embolism leading to stroke has been reported in patients with patent foramen ovale during pregnancy.[25,26] In one of the cases, percutaneous closure of the patent foramen ovale was performed during pregnancy guided by echocardiography.[26]

VENTRICULAR SEPTAL DEFECT. Women with isolated ventricular septal defect usually tolerate pregnancy well, although congestive heart failure and arrhythmias have been reported.[13,14,18] The risk posed by pregnancy after closure of an uncomplicated ventricular septal defect should not differ from that in patients without heart disease. The incidence of ventricular septal defect in offspring has been reported to be 4 to 11 percent.[17] Marked reduction in blood pressure during or after delivery as a result of blood loss or anesthesia can lead to shunt reversal in patients with pulmonary hypertension. The use of vasopressors and volume replacement to stabilize blood pressure should prevent further complications.

PATENT DUCTUS ARTERIOSUS. Maternal outcome in patients with patent ductus arteriosus with left-to-right shunt is usually favorable,[13,14,18] but clinical deterioration and congestive heart failure can occur in some patients. There were no maternal deaths among a large number of patients with patent ductus arteriosus.[17] The need for surgical intervention during pregnancy is rare. A fall in systemic vascular resistance during gestation and hypotension early post partum can lead to shunt reversal in women with pulmonary hypertension. Peripartum decreases in systemic blood pressure should be corrected by means of vasopressor agents. Postoperative pregnancy is well tolerated by the mother, and recurrence of patent ductus arteriosus in the fetus is rare (<1 percent).[27]

CONGENITAL AORTIC VALVE DISEASE. Most patients with mild aortic stenosis have a favorable outcome of pregnancy.[6,13,14] At the same time, however, moderate or severe aortic stenosis is likely to be associated with symptomatic deterioration during pregnancy, may lead to maternal morbidity and even mortality, and is associated with important effects on the fetus including intrauterine growth retardation, premature delivery, and reduced birth weight.[6]

Symptoms usually develop in the second or third trimester and most commonly arise as exertional dyspnea, but chest pain, lightheadedness, and syncope may also occur. An increased incidence of cardiac defects has been reported in liveborn infants of mothers with left ventricular outflow obstruction.[13] Because of the risk involved, patients with severe aortic stenosis (aortic valve area <1.0 cm^2) should consider undergoing valve replacement before becoming pregnant. Optional management strategies for a pregnant patient with severe aortic stenosis include (1) early abortion followed by valve replacement and repeated pregnancy and (2) continuation of pregnancy and planning for percutaneous balloon valvuloplasty or surgical intervention in patients who show clinical deterioration not controlled by medical therapy. Both replacement of the aortic valve and percutaneous balloon valvuloplasty have been performed successfully in pregnant women with aortic stenosis.[28] These procedures, however, are not free of complications. Although valvuloplasty obviates the general anesthesia and cardiopulmonary bypass required for surgery, it can be associated with prolonged radiation exposure and hemodynamic fluctuations that can lead to immediate and late fetal complications. Surgical replacement of the aortic valve during pregnancy can be associated with an increased incidence of maternal complications and fetal loss.[29] These procedures should therefore be considered only for symptomatic patients with severe disease not manageable by medical therapy and should be avoided when possible during the first trimester.

COARCTATION OF THE AORTA. Both maternal and fetal outcomes are usually favorable in cases with aortic coarctation.[30,31] At the same time, however, cases of severe hypertension, congestive heart failure, and aortic dissection have been reported.[13,30-32] Systemic hypertension is common during pregnancy in women with a significant coarctation gradient.[31] Congenital heart disease was reported in 3 to 4 percent of newborns born to women with corrected coarctation.[30,31] Because increased incidences of hypertension and infective endocarditis in the mother and of congenital heart disease in the fetus have been shown in cases with surgically uncorrected compared with corrected coarctation,[13] it seems advisable to correct aortic coarctation before pregnancy.

Measures to reduce the incidence of aortic dissection and rupture of cerebral aneurysms during pregnancy consist of limiting physical activity and controlling blood pressure. Because beta blockade may decrease the risk of these events by reduction of aortic wall tension, beta blockers should be the antihypertensive drugs of choice. Excessive blood pressure reduction, however, may compromise uteroplacental blood flow and should be avoided. Surgical correction of coarctation has been performed successfully during pregnancy[30] and may be indicated in patients with severe, uncontrollable systolic hypertension or heart failure. No information is available on pregnancy in women with aortic coarctation following percutaneous dilation.

PULMONIC STENOSIS. Isolated pulmonic stenosis is usually well tolerated during pregnancy.[6] When possible, however, severe stenosis should be corrected before conception. In the rare instance of progressive right ventricular failure or symptoms clearly related to the stenotic valve, or in a patient with an intracardiac shunt at either the atrial or ventricular level with cyanosis, percutaneous balloon valvotomy should be considered during pregnancy.

TETRALOGY OF FALLOT. Hemodynamic changes associated with pregnancy may cause clinical deterioration in women with surgically uncorrected or only partially corrected tetralogy of Fallot. Increase in blood volume and venous return to the right atrium raises right ventricular pressure, which, combined with a fall in systemic vascular resistance, can produce or exacerbate right-to-left shunt and cyanosis. Labor and delivery are particularly important because a fall in blood pressure can also increase right-to-left shunt and the degree of cyanosis. Maternal hematocrit above 60 percent, arterial oxygen saturation below 80 percent, right ventricular hypertension, and syncopal episodes are poor prognostic signs. Pregnancies in women with cyanosis are associated with high rates of spontaneous abortion, premature delivery, and fetal growth retardation.[13,14,21]

Close monitoring of systemic blood pressure and blood gases during labor and delivery is recommended for cyanotic or symptomatic patients. The incidence of cardiac defects reported in the infants ranges between 3 and 17 percent.[17]

The risk of pregnancy in patients with good surgical repair is similar to that in the general population. Patients who have undergone only palliative procedures and have residual problems, such as pulmonic regurgitation, right ventricular outflow obstruction, and right ventricular dilation and dysfunction, are still at higher risk for the development of heart failure and arrhythmias during pregnancy.[33] Patients who have undergone shunt procedures to improve cyanosis may develop pulmonary hypertension, which increases the risk of pregnancy.[34] Because maternal and fetal outcomes seem to be markedly improved after surgical repair, this procedure should be performed before conception.[13,35] Because revision of an incompletely repaired defect is recommended in patients with residual ventricular septal defect when the pulmonary/systemic flow ratio is greater than 1.5:1.0, in those with right ventricular outflow obstruction (right ventricular systolic pressure >60 mm Hg), and in those with right ventricular failure related to pulmonic regurgitation, such revision should be performed before conception in a woman who plans to conceive. To determine the risk of defects in the fetus, patients with tetralogy of Fallot should be tested with fluorescent in situ hybridization to rule out 22q11 deletion syndrome. Negative results of this test indicates a low risk of a defect in the fetus.[36]

EISENMENGER SYNDROME. This condition continues to be associated with a high risk of maternal morbidity and mortality. Two reviews involving 55 and 65 women, respectively, reported maternal mortality of approximately 40 percent.[13,37] The cause of maternal death is often unclear; it usually occurs between the first few days and the first few weeks after delivery and is preceded by desaturation and hemodynamic and clinical deterioration.[38-41] Diffuse fibrinoid necrosis of pulmonary arterioles has been found in some patients,[42] and pulmonary embolism has been reported at necropsy.[42] Eisenmenger syndrome is also associated with a poor fetal outcome, with a high incidence of fetal loss, prematurity, intrauterine growth retardation, and perinatal death.[13,34]

Because of the high risk of maternal mortality, patients with Eisenmenger syndrome should be advised against pregnancy. Sterilization may be considered prior to pregnancy, and early abortion should be recommended for patients who are already pregnant. Management of a pregnant patient who decides to proceed to term must include close follow-up for early detection of clinical deterioration. To prevent an increased incidence of peripartum thromboembolism, anticoagulant therapy seems indicated in the third trimester of gestation and for 4 weeks post partum. Because premature delivery is common, women with Eisenmenger syndrome should be hospitalized for any sign of premature uterine activity. For this reason and to ensure restriction of activity and close follow-up, early elective hospitalization is recommended. Spontaneous labor is preferred to induction and should lower the chance of prematurity or the need for cesarean section. Blood pressure, electrocardiographic, and blood gas monitoring are essential during labor and delivery to ensure early detection and correction of problems; high concentrations of oxygen may be helpful. Most patients in stable condition tolerate vaginal delivery; however, an attempt should be made to shorten the second stage of labor by the use of forceps or vacuum extraction. Because of the higher risk of fetal distress during vaginal delivery and potential need for emergency cesarean section, a planned cesarean section is often preferred. Insertion of a Swan-Ganz catheter may be difficult and associated with the development of arrhythmias, and its routine use is not recommended. Inhaled nitric oxide has been used successfully to reduce pulmonary pressure and improve oxygenation during labor and the early postpartum period in two patients with Eisenmenger syndrome.[38,39] Patients gave birth to live infants but died 2 and 21 days post partum.

EBSTEIN ANOMALY. Pregnancy in women with noncyanotic Ebstein anomaly is well tolerated. In cyanotic cases, pregnancy is associated with increased risks of maternal heart failure, prematurity, and fetal loss.[35] The approach to labor and delivery in symptomatic or cyanotic patients with Ebstein anomaly includes antibiotic prophylaxis, oxygen administration, hemodynamic and blood gas monitoring, and efforts to prevent a drop in systemic blood pressure in response to peripheral vasodilation or blood loss.

COMPLEX CYANOTIC CONGENITAL HEART DISEASE. The more widespread use of palliative and corrective surgical procedures for complex cyanotic congenital cardiac anomalies has allowed more women who are so affected to reach childbearing age.[13] Although successful pregnancies have been reported in patients with partially corrected and uncorrected cyanotic heart disease, pregnancy is associated with increased risk in these patients. A report of 96 pregnancies in 44 patients with cyanotic heart disease without pulmonary hypertension demonstrated cardiovascular complications in 32 percent of the patients.[21] These complications included heart failure, thromboembolic events, supraventricular tachycardia, and peripartum bacterial endocarditis resulting in postpartum maternal death in one patient. In addition, a high incidence of fetal wastage (57 percent), premature deliveries, small-for-gestational-age newborns, and both cardiac and noncardiac congenital malformations have been reported.

More than 100 pregnancies in women with intraatrial repair for transposition of the great arteries have been reported without maternal mortality.[43] Pregnancy seems to be well tolerated in asymptomatic patients or those with only mild symptoms (Class II) prior to pregnancy. Worsening of systemic ventricular function during pregnancy or shortly thereafter has been reported in 10 percent of cases.

A report describing the experience in 60 pregnancies in 22 women with congenitally corrected transposition of great arteries indicated a successful outcome in most cases.[44] The rate of fetal loss and maternal morbidity was, however, increased. Morbidity included congestive heart failure, worsening valve regurgitation, endocarditis, and myocardial infarction. Because of the small number of cases, the risk of congenital heart disease in the offspring of women with congenitally corrected transposition is uncertain.

A report by Canobbio and colleagues[45] on patients after the Fontan operation indicated that a good pregnancy outcome was possible with small babies. Other reports, however, described thromboembolic complications with right atrial thrombus leading to embolic obstruction of the connection and to death.[42]

Valvular Heart Disease (see Chap. 57)

MITRAL STENOSIS. This condition is the most common rheumatic valvular lesion in pregnancy.[46,47] A majority of patients with moderate to severe mitral stenosis (mitral valve area <1.5 cm^2) demonstrate worsening of one or two classes in New York Heart Association functional status during gestation (Fig. 74–5).[6,46] Although mitral stenosis is often accompanied by some degree of mitral regurgitation, hemodynamic problems are related predominantly to flow obstruction. The pressure gradient across the narrowed mitral valve may increase greatly secondary to the physiological increase in heart rate and blood volume of pregnancy. Increased left atrial pressure can result in atrial arrhythmias that may lead to an acceleration of ventricular rate and further elevation of left atrial pressure. In addition, decreased serum colloid osmotic pressure during pregnancy and excessive peripartum intravenous fluid administration can both predispose to pulmonary edema. Studies have demonstrated a high incidence of worsening of functional class and the development of heart failure which led to the need for hospitalizations and either starting or increasing the dose of cardiac medications in patients with moderate to severe mitral stenosis (Figs. 74–6 and 74–7).[6,48] In addition, there was a marked increase in the rate of prematurity, fetal growth retardation, and low neonatal birth weight in these cases. Despite a marked increase in maternal morbidity, mortality is rare and is mostly due to standard care.[6,49]

Treatment. The therapeutic approach to patients with significant mitral stenosis should aim to reduce the heart rate and decrease left atrial pressure. Both heart rate and symptoms can be controlled effectively by restricting physical activity and administering beta-adrenergic receptor blockers. In patients with atrial fibrillation, digoxin may also be useful for control of ventricular rate. Left atrial pressure can be reduced by a decrease in blood volume through restriction of salt intake and the use of oral diuretics; aggressive use of diuretic agents should, however, be avoided to prevent hypovolemia and reduction of uteroplacental perfusion.

Although careful medical therapy allows successful completion of pregnancy in the great majority of women,[46] repair or replacement of the valve during pregnancy may be indicated in some patients with severe symptoms in spite of adequate medical therapy. The use of percutaneous mitral balloon valvuloplasty during pregnancy has been reported in an increasing number of pregnant patients with mitral stenosis.[50-53] In the majority of cases, hemodynamic and symptomatic improvement has been achieved without apparent untoward maternal and fetal effects. Follow-up for several

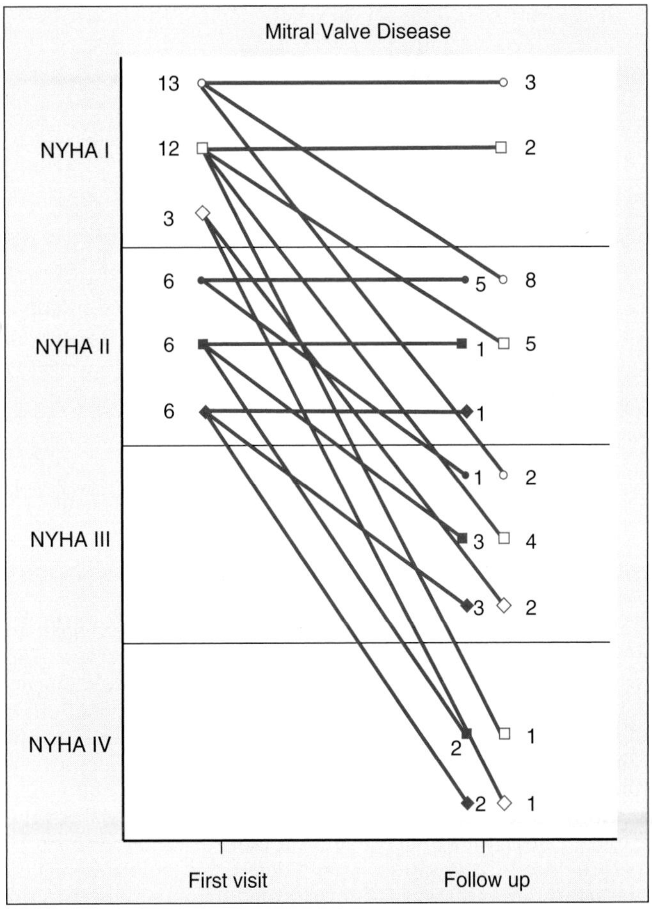

FIGURE 74–5 Change in New York Heart Association (NYHA) functional class between first visit and follow-up during pregnancy in patients with predominant mitral valve disease. Circles = mild mitral stenosis; squares = moderate mitral stenosis; diamonds = severe mitral stenosis; open symbols = NYHA functional Class I on presentation; closed symbols = NYHA functional Class II on presentation. (From Hameed A, Karaalp IS, Tummala PP, et al: The effect of valvular heart disease on maternal and fetal outcome of pregnancy. J Am Coll Cardiol 37:893, 2001.)

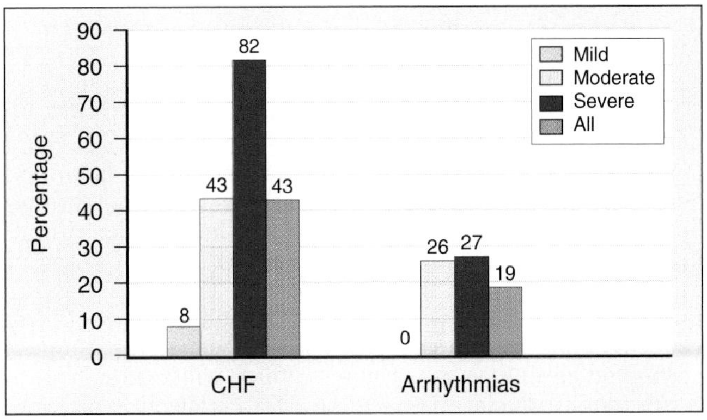

FIGURE 74–6 Percent development of symptoms of congestive heart failure (CHF) and arrhythmias during pregnancy in 46 patients with mitral stenosis. (From Hameed A, Karaalp IS, Tummala PP, et al: The effect of valvular heart disease on maternal and fetal outcome of pregnancy. J Am Coll Cardiol 37:893, 2001.)

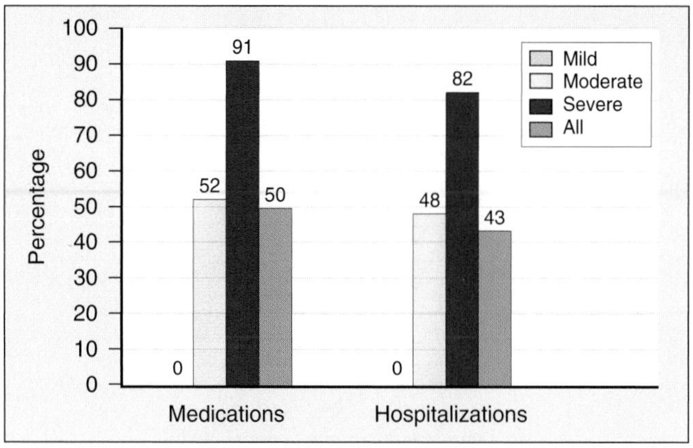

FIGURE 74–7 Percent usage of new cardiac medications or increase in their dose and hospitalizations during pregnancy in 46 patients with mitral stenosis. (From Hameed A, Karaalp IS, Tummala PP, et al: The effect of valvular heart disease on maternal and fetal outcome of pregnancy. J Am Coll Cardiol 37:893, 2001.)

years has shown normal development of children born to mothers who had mitral valve balloon valvuloplasty during pregnanacy.[52,53] At the same time, however, serious complications have occasionally been reported, including initiation of maternal arrhythmias leading to fetal distress, cardiac tamponade requiring surgical intervention, systemic embolization, uterine contraction, and even precipitous labor. In addition, this procedure is associated with some risk to the fetus secondary to unavoidable ionizing radiation. The procedure should, therefore, be avoided if possible during the first trimester and should be performed by experienced operators with adequate abdominal and pelvic shielding with minimum radiation exposure and under echocardiographic guidance, when possible.

Mitral valve repair or replacement should be considered during pregnancy only in cases with severe mitral stenosis (mitral valve area <1.0 cm^2) refractory to optimal medical therapy or when close follow-up during pregnancy, labor, and delivery is not possible. When valve replacement is indicated, selection of the type of prosthesis should be based on its hemodynamic profile and durability and the need for anticoagulation.

Vaginal delivery can be permitted in most patients with mitral stenosis.[6] In symptomatic patients and those with moderate or severe stenosis (mitral valve area <1.5 cm^2), hemodynamic monitoring is recommended during labor and delivery. Initiation of monitoring at onset of labor allows hemodynamic optimization by means of intravenous diuretics, digoxin (in case of atrial fibrillation), beta blockers, or nitroglycerin and prevention of a rise in left atrial pressure during labor and delivery. With delivery and thus relief of venocaval obstruction caused by the gravid uterus, there is an immediate increase in venous return, which may lead to a substantial increase in pulmonary artery wedge pressure and pulmonary edema.[1,6] For this reason, hemodynamic monitoring should be continued for at least several hours post partum.

Epidural anesthesia is the most appropriate form of analgesia in patients with mitral stenosis for both vaginal and abdominal delivery. This form of anesthesia is often associated with a significant fall in pulmonary arterial and left atrial pressures related to systemic vasodilation.[54] With this approach, the great majority of patients with mitral stenosis, even if it is severe, can be delivered with few complications.

MITRAL REGURGITATION. This condition is usually well tolerated in pregnancy, presumably because of left ventricular unloading secondary to the physiological fall in systemic vascular resistance.[1] In symptomatic patients, drug therapy with diuretics is indicated, and digoxin may be useful in those with impaired left ventricular systolic function. Hydralazine has been shown to be safe for use during pregnancy,[55] and it may be used for further reduction of left ventricular afterload and prevention of hemodynamic worsening associated with isometric exercise during labor. Because of risk of fetal loss, surgery should be avoided if possible during pregnancy and considered only in patients with severe heart failure and hemodynamic compromise in spite of adequate medical management.

AORTIC STENOSIS. Rheumatic aortic stenosis is rare during pregnancy and occurs in conjunction with mitral valve disease in approximately 5 percent of pregnant patients with rheumatic valvular disease.[46] Although most patients with aortic stenosis and valve area greater than 1.5 cm^2 tolerate pregnancy well, patients with more severe stenosis may demonstrate clinical deterioration with exertional dyspnea, near-syncope, or syncope and pulmonary edema.[6] Development of serious symptoms during pregnancy, especially if resistant to medical therapy, may require termination of pregnancy or repair of the valve either surgically (valve replacement) or by percutaneous balloon valvuloplasty.[56]

AORTIC REGURGITATION. Aortic regurgitation in young women may be due to a bicuspid aortic valve, rheumatic disease, previous endocarditis, or dilated aortic annulus. Like mitral regurgitation, aortic regurgitation is well tolerated during pregnancy, probably because of reduced systemic vascular resistance and increased heart rate, which results in shortening of diastole. In symptomatic patients, diuretics, digoxin, and hydralazine for left ventricular afterload reduction can be safely used.

Other Conditions Affecting the Valves, Aorta, and Myocardium

MITRAL VALVE PROLAPSE. The prevalence of mitral valve prolapse in the general population has been found to be 2.4 percent, and mitral valve prolapse was reported in approximately 1.2 percent of pregnant women.[57,58] Because of the high incidence of systolic functional murmurs and wide splitting of the first heart sound during pregnancy, mitral valve prolapse may be falsely diagnosed and needs to be confirmed by echocardiographic criteria.[57] At the same time, the incidence of prolapse-related auscultatory and echocardiographic findings may decrease during gestation as a result of an increase in left ventricular end-diastolic volume.[58]

For the few patients with mitral valve prolapse with chest pain or cardiac arrhythmias, the emphasis should be on reassurance and attempts to avoid the use of medications during pregnancy. Beta-adrenergic blocking agents are recommended when therapy is indicated for arrhythmias. Patients with mitral valve prolapse, especially those with a thickened mitral valve and mitral regurgitation, are at increased risk for infective endocarditis. Although antibiotic prophylaxis for uncomplicated vaginal delivery has not been uniformly recommended,[22] the development of bacteremia during vaginal delivery and cesarean section cannot always be predicted. For this reason, prophylaxis for labor and delivery in patients with mitral valve prolapse accompanied by valve thickening or regurgitation, or both, seems warranted.

MARFAN SYNDROME. Pregnancy in women with Marfan syndrome poses a twofold problem: (1) cardiovascular complications and (2) a high risk of having a child who inherits the condition.[59,60] Cardiovascular complications during pregnancy include dilation of the ascending aorta, which may lead to the development of aortic regurgitation and congestive heart failure, and proximal and distal dissections of the aorta with possible involvement of the iliac and coronary arteries. The risk of aortic dissection is significantly higher in patients with a dilated aorta or a history of previous dissection. Patients with Marfan syndrome who have only minor involvement of the cardiovascular system and aortic diameter less than 40 mm usually tolerate pregnancy well. The majority of complications are developed in the later phase of pregnancy. Marfan syndrome may also be responsible for obstetric complications including cervical incompetence, abnormal placental site, and postpartum hemorrhagic complications.[61]

The management of pregnancy in women with Marfan syndrome should include preconception counseling to discuss potential maternal and fetal risks.[59] Women with significant cardiac involvement—in particular, dilation of the aorta and previous history of aortic dissection—are at high risk for complications during gestation and should be advised against conception or, if they are already pregnant, advised to have an early abortion. In contrast, the risk in patients without cardiac complications and with a normal aortic diameter is significantly lower. Still, a favorable outcome is not guaranteed, and aortic dissection can occur, albeit infrequently, in patients with a normal-sized aorta.[59,60] Because of reported progressive dilation during gestation, preconception echocardiographic assessment of the aorta and periodic follow-up during pregnancy are highly recommended.[62] Because aneurysms and dissections of the aorta can occasionally involve the descending aorta, the use of transesophageal echocardiography seems preferred to transthoracic examination. During pregnancy, vigorous physical activity should be avoided. Beta blockers, which have been shown to reduce the rate of aortic dilation and the risk of complications in patients with Marfan syndrome, should be administered. In case of substantial dilation or dissection of the aorta during pregnancy, depending on the stage of pregnancy, therapeutic abortion, early delivery, or surgical intervention should be considered.[59,60,62,63] A number of patients have been reported to have successful full-term pregnancies without complications after an elective aortic root replacement.[64] In women with aortic dilation, aortic dissection, or other cardiac complications, abdominal delivery by cesarean section should be the preferred mode of delivery to minimize hemodynamic changes associated with vaginal delivery.[43,59,61]

Cardiomyopathies

HYPERTROPHIC CARDIOMYOPATHY. Reported experience in approximately 350 pregnancies in 200 women with hypertrophic cardiomyopathy (see Chap. 59) has suggested a favorable outcome in most cases but at the same time a potential for increased morbidity and even mortality.[65-67] Worsening of symptoms and increased shortness of breath and fatigue have been reported in approximately 15 to 20 percent of cases and are more common in women with symptoms prior to pregnancy[67]; chest pain, palpitations, dizzy spells, and syncope have also been reported. In addition, isolated cases of arrhythmias have been described, including poorly tolerated resistant supraventricular tachycardia with fetal distress,[65] atrial fibrillation leading to hemodynamic deterioration requiring electrical cardioversion, and ventricular fibrillation treated by electric shock. Pregnancy-related maternal mortality is low in patients with hypertrophic cardiomyopathy, but it is increased compared with that in the general population[67] and is due to ventricular arrhythmias.[65] Although fetal outcome is in general favorable, women with symptoms before pregnancy have an increased risk of fetal prematurity compared with healthy women.[67] The risk of inheriting the disease may be as high as 50 percent in familial cases and less in sporadic cases.[65]

The therapeutic approach to the pregnant patient with hypertrophic cardiomyopathy depends on the presence of symptoms and left ventricular outflow obstruction. In the symptomatic patient with obstructive hypertrophic cardiomyopathy, an attempt should be made to avoid blood loss and use of drugs that can lead to vasodilation or sympathetic stimulation during labor and delivery. Indications for drug therapy during gestation include arrhythmias and symptoms of heart failure. Symptoms associated with elevated left ventricular filling pressure should be treated with beta-adrenergic blocking agents, and diuretics and calcium antagonists may be added if beta blockers alone are not sufficient.[65] Because of the potential arrhythmogenic effect of pregnancy, implantation of an automatic defibrillator before pregnancy should be considered in patients with history of syncope, life-threatening arrhythmias, or a family history of death caused by the same condition.[65]

Vaginal delivery has been shown to be safe in women with hypertrophic cardiomyopathy.[65] In those with symptoms of outflow obstruction, the second stage of labor may be shortened by the use of forceps. The use of prostaglandins to induce uterine contractions may be risky in a patient with obstructive hypertrophic cardiomyopathy owing to their vasodilatory effect, whereas oxytocin should be well tolerated. Because tocolytic agents with beta-adrenergic receptor activity may worsen left ventricular outflow tract obstruction, other medications such as magnesium sulfate are preferred. Similarly, spinal and epidural anesthetics should be used with caution in obstructive hypertrophic cardiomyopathy because of their vasodilatory effect, and excessive blood loss should be avoided and if it occurs it should be replaced promptly with intravenous fluid or blood.[68]

Because the risk for infective endocarditis is increased in hypertrophic cardiomyopathy, especially the obstructive form, and in patients with mitral valve abnormalities, antibiotic prophylaxis should be considered for labor and delivery.

PERIPARTUM CARDIOMYOPATHY. Peripartum cardiomyopathy is a form of dilated cardiomyopathy with left ventricular systolic dysfunction that results in signs and symptoms of heart failure (see Chaps. 21 to 23).[69,70] The syndrome has been defined by the following four criteria: (1) the development of cardiac failure in the last month of pregnancy or within 5 months of delivery, (2) absence of an identifiable cause for the cardiac failure, (3) absence of recognizable heart disease prior to the last month of pregnancy, and (4) left ventricular systolic dysfunction demonstrated by classical echocardiographic criteria, such as depressed shortening fraction or ejection fraction.[70] However, there have been reports of an early presentation of peripartum cardiomyopathy during the second and third trimesters of pregnancy in a large minority of patients.[71] The incidence of the disease in the United States is not known and has been reported to range between 1 per 4000 and 1 per 15,000 deliveries; the incidence is higher in Haiti and in certain parts of Africa.[69,70,72]

Peripartum cardiomyopathy can occur at any age but is more common in women older than 30 years. In the United States, it involves women of various ethnic groups and it is related to first and second pregnancies in almost 60 percent of cases.[73] There is a strong relation between the development of peripartum cardiomyopathy, gestational hypertension, twin pregnancy, and the use of tocolytic therapy.[70,73]

Common symptoms and signs are shortness of breath, fatigue, chest pain, palpitations, weight gain, peripheral edema, peripheral or pulmonary embolization, and arrhythmias. Physical examination often reveals an enlarged heart, S_3, and murmurs of mitral and tricuspid regurgitation. The electrocardiogram may show tachycardia, ST-T wave changes, conduction abnormalities, and arrhythmias. Chest radiography usually shows cardiomegaly, pulmonary venous congestion with interstitial or alveolar edema, and occasionally pleural effusion. Doppler echocardiography commonly demonstrates enlargement of all four cardiac chambers, with marked reduction in left ventricular systolic function. Small to moderate pericardial effusion and mitral, tricuspid, and pulmonic regurgitation may be evident. The clinical presentation and hemodynamic changes are indistinguishable from those found in other forms of dilated cardiomyopathy.

The clinical course of peripartum cardiomyopathy varies, with 50 to 60 percent of patients showing complete or near-complete recovery of clinical status and cardiac function, usually within the first 6 months post partum[73]; the rest of the patients demonstrate either further clinical deterioration, leading to cardiac transplantation or premature death, or persistent left ventricular dysfunction and chronic heart failure.[69,70,74]

Management. Acute heart failure should be treated vigorously with oxygen, diuretics, digitalis, and vasodilator agents. The use of hydralazine as an afterload-reducing agent is safe during pregnancy.[55] The use of organic nitrates, dopamine, dobutamine, or milrinone has been reported in pregnancy in a limited number of cases, but the use of nesiritide during pregnancy has not been reported. Nitroprusside has been used successfully during pregnancy, but experiments in animals have shown a potential for fetal toxicity.[55] Angiotensin-converting enzyme inhibitors have a teratogenic effect, may cause fetal renal dysfunction, and should therefore not be used during pregnancy.[75] Because of the increased incidence of thromboembolic events, anticoagulant therapy is recommended.[76,77] Because the disease may be reversible, the temporary use of an intraaortic balloon pump or left ventricular assist device may help stabilize the patient's condition pending improvement. A small retrospective study of intravenous immune globulin showed a favorable effect on recovery of left ventricular dysfunction in patients with peripartum cardiomyopathy.[78] Similarly, the use of pentoxifylline in addition to standard care was reported to lead to a significant improvement in outcome in patients with peripartum cardiomyopathy.[79] Further evaluation of these therapies seems warranted. Because of continuous clinical deterioration, some patients with peripartum cardiomyopathy may need to undergo cardiac transplantation. Reports comparing results of cardiac transplantation in age-matched females with peripartum cardiomyopathy and idiopathic cardiomyopathy showed favorable and comparable long-term survival in both groups.[74] The rate of mortality in patients with peripartum cardiomyopathy was reported to be 10 and 32 percent in two reports.[80,81]

Subsequent pregnancies in women with peripartum cardiomyopathy are often associated with relapse, leading to left ventricular dysfunction, symptomatic deterioration, and even death (Fig. 74–8). Although the likelihood of such relapse is greater in patients with persistently abnormal cardiac function, it has also been reported in women in whom left ventricular function is restored after the first episode.[82] A survey on the risk of subsequent pregnancy in women with history of peripartum cardiomyopathy reported no mortality in patients with normal left ventricular ejection but 19 percent mortality in patients with a depressed left ventricular ejection fraction (25 percent in those who did not have an abortion [Fig. 74–8]). For these reasons, subsequent pregnancies should be discouraged in patients with peripartum cardiomyopathy who have persistent cardiac dysfunction; women with recovered cardiac function can also not be guaranteed an event-free pregnancy, and recurrence of the disease is possible. The risk of mortality in such cases, however, seems to be small.[82]

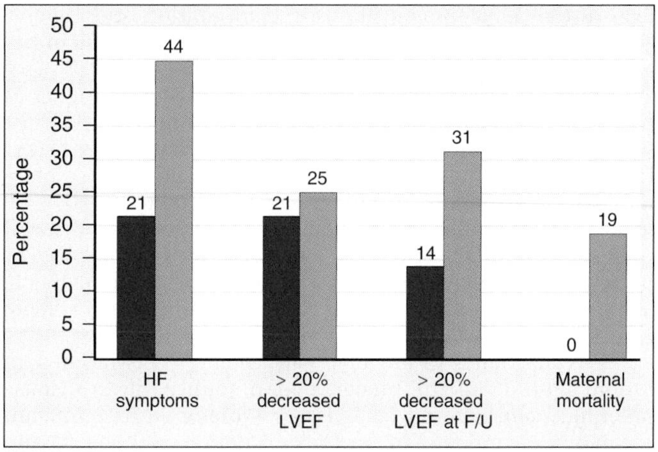

FIGURE 74–8 Maternal complications associated with subsequent pregnancy in women with a history of peripartum cardiomyopathy who did not have an abortion. F/U = follow-up; HF = heart failure; LVEF = left ventricular ejection fraction. (Modified from Elkayam U, Tummala PP, Rao K, et al: Maternal and fetal outcomes of subsequent pregnancies in women with peripartum cardiomyopathy. N Engl J Med 344:1567, 2001.)

Hypertension in Pregnancy (see Chap. 38)

Hypertensive disorders of pregnancy are a major cause of maternal and perinatal morbidity and mortality. Most adverse events are attributable to the preeclampsia syndrome, which is characterized by new-onset hypertension with proteinuria during pregnancy and is more common in women with chronic hypertension.[83,84] In general, hypertension in pregnancy is defined as blood pressure greater than 140 mm Hg systolic and 90 mm Hg diastolic on at least two occasions 6 hours apart. Hypertension complicates 8 to 10 percent of all pregnancies and is an important cause of maternal mortality and morbidity, including abruptio placentae, pulmonary edema, respiratory failure, disseminated intravascular coagulation, cerebral hemorrhage, hepatic failure, and acute renal failure. Fetal complications include prematurity, intrauterine growth retardation, stillbirth, and neonatal death.[83,84] Hypertensive disorders in pregnancy can be divided into three broad categories: chronic hypertension, gestational hypertension, and preeclampsia-eclampsia.[83-85]

CHRONIC HYPERTENSION. Chronic hypertension is defined as hypertension that precedes pregnancy. It can be assumed when elevated blood pressure is detected before the 20th gestational week, and it can also be diagnosed in retrospect when blood pressure fails to become normal 12 weeks after delivery.[86] It occurs in 1 to 5 percent of pregnancies and is associated with increased complications (15 percent), such as fetal growth retardation, premature delivery, abruptio placentae, acute renal failure, and hypertensive crisis; most of these complications occur in patients older than 30 years with a longer duration of hypertension or those who develop superimposed preeclampsia. Drug therapy is recommended for patients with high-risk characteristics of preeclampsia[87] (severe hypertension with evidence of end-organ involvement, a poor obstetric history, renal insufficiency, diabetes, or collagen-vascular disease) (Table 74–6). High-risk patients also require frequent monitoring of blood and urine chemistry and of fetal growth. In low-risk patients (blood pressure between 140 and 160 systolic and 90 and 110 diastolic, normal physical examination, normal electrocardiogram and echocardiogram, and no proteinuria), antihypertensive therapy has not been shown to prevent development of preeclampsia or affect fetal outcome.[64]

GESTATIONAL HYPERTENSION. Gestational hypertension is defined as hypertension induced by pregnancy

TABLE 74–6 Antihypertensive Drugs in Pregnancy

Class	Drug	Starting Dose	Maximum Dose
	Drugs for Long-Term Treatment of Hypertension		
Central $alpha_2$-agonist	Methyldopa Clonidine	250 mg tid 0.1-0.3 mg bid	4 g/d 1.2 mg/d
$Alpha_1$-adrenergic blocker	Prazosin	1 mg bid	20 mg/d
Calcium channel blocker	Nifedipine	10 mg qid	120 mg/d
Beta-adrenergic blocker	Atenolol	100 mg qd	100 mg/bid
Alpha/beta-adrenergic blocker	Labetalol	100 mg tid	2400 mg/d
Diuretics	Hydrochlorothiazide	25 mg qd	50 mg/d
Class	**Drug**	**Dose**	
	Drugs for Acute Treatment of Severe Hypertension		
Arterial dilator	Hydralazine Diazoxide	5-10 mg IV q 15-30 min 30-60 mg IV q 10-15 min	
Calcium channel blocker	Nifedipine	10-20 mg PO q 30 min	
Alpha/beta-adrenergic blocker	Labetalol	20-40-80 mg IV q 10-20 min (up to 300 mg)	
Arterial/venous dilator	Sodium nitroprusside	(50 mg/250 ml saline): 0.5-5.0 μg/kg/min	

beginning after 20 weeks of gestation and resolving by the sixth postpartum week.[86] Gestational hypertension is further classified as transient hypertension (hypertension without proteinuria) and preeclampsia (hypertension with proteinuria). Transient hypertension usually arises in the late third trimester with return of blood pressure to normal by the 10th postpartum day. It should be noted that the presence of proteinuria can occur late in the course of preeclampsia and the distinction between transient hypertension and preeclampsia can be difficult and can often be made only retrospectively. For this reason, in uncertain situations, preeclampsia should be considered and seizure prophylaxis should be instituted empirically in patients with blood pressure greater than 160/110 mm Hg. Pregnancy outcome is usually favorable in cases with transient hypertension, and use of antihypertensive therapy should be reserved for patients with blood pressure greater than 160/110 mm Hg.

PREECLAMPSIA-ECLAMPSIA. Preeclampsia is a pregnancy-specific syndrome that usually occurs after 20 weeks of gestation and is defined by the de novo appearance of hypertension (systolic blood pressure >140 mm Hg or diastolic blood pressure of ≥90 mm Hg) accompanied by new-onset proteinuria, defined as 300 mg or more per 24 hours. In the absence of proteinuria, the disease is highly suspect when increased blood pressure is accompanied by symptoms of headache, blurred vision, pulmonary edema, and abdominal pain or abnormal laboratory tests, specifically low platelet counts and abnormal liver enzymes. Preeclampsia is reversible and usually regresses within 24 to 48 hours post partum. In a minority of cases, postpartum eclampsia with hypertension, proteinuria, and convulsions occurs within 10 days after delivery. The maternal and fetal outcome for preeclampsia superimposed on existing hypertension is worse than that for de novo preeclampsia.

Management (see Table 74–6). The majority of women with chronic hypertension in pregnancy with a systolic blood pressure of 140 to 160 mm Hg or a diastolic blood pressure up to 110 mm Hg are at low risk for cardiovascular complications and are candidates for nondrug therapy. Most of the risk associated with chronic hypertension occurs in the setting of superimposed preeclampsia (25 percent of cases).

Indications for drug therapy include blood pressure exceeding 150 to 160 mm Hg systolic or 100 to 110 mm Hg diastolic or the presence of target organ damage, such as left ventricular hypertrophy or renal insufficiency. Methyldopa is the preferred therapy; alternatively, an effective prepregnancy regimen can be continued with the exception of converting enzyme inhibitors or angiotensin receptor antagonists.[75]

Delivery is the only definitive treatment for preeclampsia, and there is no evidence that any other therapy alters the underlying pathophysiology or improves perinatal outcome. All women with the diagnosis of preeclampsia should be considered for delivery at 40 weeks of gestation. Delivery may be indicated for women with mild disease and a favorable cervix for induction at 38 weeks of gestation and should be considered in women with severe preeclampsia beyond 32 to 34 weeks of gestation. Delivery is indicated even in women with fetal gestational age between 23 and 32 weeks if there are worsening maternal symptoms, laboratory evidence of end-organ dysfunction, or fetal deterioration.

Patients with stable, mild preeclampsia may be observed until fetal pulmonary maturity is verified or until after 37 weeks of gestation with cervical ripening.[86] There is no evidence of a need for or benefit from antihypertensive drug therapy in this subgroup of patients. Severe preeclampsia can be rapidly progressive, leading to sudden deterioration of the status of both mother and fetus. Patients with severe preeclampsia who are at or past 34 weeks of gestation should be delivered promptly. Patients with severe preeclampsia who are at 23 to 34 weeks of gestation should be treated with bed rest, intravenous magnesium sulfate for seizure prophylaxis, blood pressure control, fetal assessment, and corticosteroids for acceleration of fetal lung maturity. Indications for delivery include eclampsia; resistant, severe hypertension (refractory to maximum doses of three antihypertensive drugs); completion of 34 weeks of gestation; HELLP syndrome (hemolysis, elevated liver enzymes, and low platelet count); and abnormal fetal testing. Because of potential risks to the mother and fetus, conservative management of severe preeclampsia has been recommended only at tertiary perinatal centers under close maternal and fetal monitoring.

The primary goal of treatment is to prevent maternal cerebral complications. The recommended goal of therapy is reduction of mean blood pressure below 126 mm Hg but not less than 105 mm Hg and diastolic blood pressure between 90 and 105 mm Hg. Use of intravenous hydralazine is recommended as initial therapy; a 5-mg bolus is given intravenously over 1 to 2 minutes. After 20 minutes, subsequent doses are dictated by the initial response; when the desired effect is obtained, the drug is repeated as necessary. If this therapy is not effective or is associated with maternal side effect (tachycardia, headache, nausea), labetalol (given in divided doses [20 mg intravenonsly and, if needed, followed by 40 mg and 3 doses of 80 mg in intervals of 10 to 20 minutes] or continuous infusion of 1 to 2 mg/min as needed) or nifedipine should be given. In rare cases, intravenous nitroglycerin or nitroprusside may be needed after failure of hydralazine, labetalol, and nifedipine.

Pregnancy after Cardiac Transplantation (see Chap. 26)

A study conducted to determine the outcome of pregnancy in cardiac allograft recipients identified 47 pregnancies in 35 heart transplant recipients that resulted in 35 live births (74 percent).[88] Therapeutic abortion was performed in five cases owing to a short interval between transplantation and conception. Maternal hemodynamic changes during gestation seemed well tolerated, and rejection episodes were rare. At the same time, however, a higher incidence of maternal complications was reported, including chronic hypertension, preeclampsia, worsening kidney failure, premature rupture of membranes, and infections. Although fetal loss does not seem to be increased, an increased incidence of preterm deliveries and fetal growth retardation and cesarean sections has been reported. No maternal deaths were reported during pregnancy, but the incidence of late death was high compared with that in age-matched healthy women. None of the newborns was found to have congenital malformations, supporting a lack of teratogenic effect of immunosuppressive agents.[89] The limited available information suggests, therefore, that pregnancy in women after cardiac transplantation is not associated with increased maternal mortality; however, it results in increased maternal morbidity, preterm deliveries, and fetal growth retardation.

Coronary Artery Disease

(see Chaps. 46 to 50)

Pathogenesis

Although clinical manifestations of coronary artery diseases are expected to be encountered during pregnancy with increasing frequency because of increasing maternal age and fertility,[90,91] these are still rare among women of childbearing age, and the occurrence of peripartum acute myocardial infarction is anecdotal.[92]

Risk factors for coronary artery disease in women younger than 50 years include cigarette smoking, high levels of total plasma cholesterol, low levels of high-density lipoproteins, lipoprotein (a), diabetes mellitus, hypertension, a family history of coronary artery disease, toxemia of pregnancy, and the use of oral contraceptives.[91-93] The combination of heavy smoking or hypertension and concurrent use of oral contraceptives has been shown to be a powerful predictor of acute myocardial infarction. Women who have had very low birth weight babies or preterm delivery also seem to be at an increased risk for coronary artery disease.[94]

In the assessment of risk factors for coronary artery disease during pregnancy, it should be noted that total cholesterol, low-density lipoprotein cholesterol, and triglyceride levels are significantly increased during pregnancy.[95]

Acute Myocardial Infarction

Acute myocardial infarction has been reported at any stage of pregnancy and at ages between 16 and 45. The highest incidence, however, occurs in the third trimester and in women older than 33 years. In addition, acute myocardial infarction has been noted to occur more commonly in multigravidas and its location to be more commonly in the anterolateral wall. Most maternal deaths occurred either at the time of infarction or within 2 weeks.[92]

Although atherosclerotic disease seems to be the primary cause of acute myocardial infarction,[92] peripartum acute myocardial infarction is often associated with normal coronary angiograms and has been suggested to be due to a decrease in coronary perfusion caused by spasm or in situ thrombosis. A coronary atheroma with ruptured fibrous cap demonstrated by intravascular ultrasonography, in spite of a normal coronary vessel angiogram in a patient who experienced an acute myocardial infarction during cesarean section, may suggest plaque rupture as a cause of infarction in some of these patients.[96] Although the presence of spasm has not been documented and its cause is not clear, it has been suggested as a mechanism of myocardial infarction in some instances with pregnancy-induced hypertension and with the administration of ergot derivatives, bromocriptine, oxytocin, and prostaglandin[97] used to suppress lactation or uterine bleeding and in patients with pheochromocytoma. Coronary arterial dissection mostly in the immediate postpartum period has been commonly associated with peripartum acute myocardial infarction.[92,98] The dissection involves the left anterior descending artery in approximately 80 percent of cases and the right coronary artery in most other cases. Other potential causes of acute myocardial infarction during pregnancy have been collagen-vascular disease, Kawasaki disease (see Chap. 82), sickle cell anemia, and hemostatic abnormalities.[92]

DIAGNOSIS. The diagnostic approach to ischemic myocardial disease in pregnancy is influenced to some extent by whether a diagnostic procedure could harm the fetus and by normal changes seen during pregnancy that may mimic pathological changes. T wave inversion, Q wave in lead III, and increased R/S ratio in leads V_1 and V_2 are commonly seen in normal pregnancy. ST segment depressions, not associated with chest pain or echocardiographic wall motion abnormalities, have been described during elective cesarean section and can mimic myocardial ischemia.

Because fetal bradycardia has been reported during maximal exercise in normal women, a submaximal exercise protocol with fetal monitoring is recommended for the evaluation of ischemic myocardial disease during pregnancy.[7]

Radionuclide myocardial perfusion scans and radionuclide ventriculography expose the fetus to some radiation[9] and should be used only when the potential benefit seems to outweigh the risk. For similar reasons, cardiac catheterization involving fluoroscopy and cineangiography should be used only when relevant information cannot be obtained by other, noninvasive methods. The diagnosis of myocardial ischemia and infarction has been reported to be delayed during pregnancy because of the low level of suspicion.[92] Concentrations of myoglobin, creatine kinase, and creatine kinase with muscle and brain subunits (CK-MB) were found to be increased twofold 30 minutes after delivery, whereas the level of troponin I remained below the cutoff value for discriminating myocardial infarction. For this reason, troponin should be used to diagnose myocardial infarction after delivery.[99]

MANAGEMENT. Both maternal and fetal considerations should influence the therapeutic approach to ischemic heart disease during pregnancy. Morphine sulfate does not cause congenital defects. Because it crosses the placenta, it can cause neonatal respiratory depression when given shortly before delivery.[92] Available reports on the use of thrombolytic therapy during pregnancy do not support a teratogenic effect, and the majority of reported cases resulted in favorable maternal and fetal outcomes.[92] This therapy, however, is associated with risk of maternal hemorrhage, especially when given at the time of delivery. Because of their safety in pregnancy, beta blockers appear to be the drugs of choice. The use of organic nitrates and calcium antagonists in patients with acute myocardial ischemia or infarction has been described in a limited number of patients. These drugs should be given cautiously to prevent maternal hypotension and potential fetal distress. Use of high-dose aspirin during pregnancy is debatable because it has been reported to cause fetal growth retardation and bleeding in the neonate and in the mother.[100] Although the use of low-dose aspirin is considered safe during pregnancy,[101,102] a large-scale randomized study demonstrated that prolonged use of 100 mg of aspirin started in the second trimester of pregnancy was associated with increased bleeding complications and lower birth weight compared with placebo.[102]

Coronary reperfusion by means of percutaneous transluminal coronary angioplasty or coronary artery bypass graft surgery[92,93] has been reported to be successful during pregnancy, although experience is still limited. Such procedures should be avoided during the first trimester, if possible, owing to the potential deleterious fetal effects related to ionizing radiation as well as cardiopulmonary bypass.

Risk stratification after acute myocardial infarction during pregnancy should be determined by noninvasive methods. Total cholesterol, low-density lipoprotein cholesterol, and triglyceride levels are significantly increased during pregnancy.[95] Coronary angiography should be done only in cases in which coronary angioplasty or bypass surgery seems indicated during pregnancy.

Management of the Pregnancy. Management should focus on reducing cardiovascular stress during pregnancy and the peripartum period.[92] Termination of pregnancy may be preferred in patients with severe ischemia or heart failure in the early phase of gestation. During labor, adequate analgesia and supplemental oxygen should be given, and, if desired, cardiac output can be increased by placing the patient in the left lateral decubitus position. Labor in the supine position, however, may decrease venous return and thus reduce right and left ventricular filling pressures. Low forceps can be used to shorten the second stage of labor. Pulmonary artery catheterization with hemodynamic monitoring can help in the early detection and correction of hemodynamic abnormalities during labor and delivery. Although elective cesarean section is not indicated in every case, it should be used in patients with active ischemia or hemodynamic instability despite adequate medical therapy. Continued hemodynamic monitoring is advisable for several hours post partum to detect hemodynamic worsening associated with the postpartum hemodynamic changes described earlier.

Arrhythmias

Pregnancy is associated with an increased incidence of arrhythmias in women both with and without structural heart disease (see Chaps. 29 to 32).[8,103,104] In healthy women, multiple and even frequent atrial and ventricular premature complexes may occur, usually without effect on either the mother or the fetus (see Fig. 74–4).[8] There is also a strong suggestion of an increased frequency of paroxysmal supraventricular tachycardia during pregnancy.[104]

Atrial flutter and fibrillation are rare during normal pregnancy and are usually associated with rheumatic mitral valve disease.[6,104,105] Reports have described atrial fibrillation during gestation accompanied by treatment with terbutaline and magnesium sulfate and in the presence of preexcitation.[103,104,106,107] Ventricular tachycardia is a rare occurrence in pregnancy and the puerperium. It has been reported in women with normal hearts,[104] but it is usually associated with structural heart disease, drugs, electrolyte abnormalities, or eclampsia.[106,108-110]

Although palpitations, dizziness, and even syncope are relatively common symptoms in normal pregnancy, they are rarely associated with cardiac arrhythmias.[8] Cardiac arrhythmias, however, when they occur, can be hemodynamically significant during gestation even in patients with a normal heart. Reduction in blood pressure occasionally associated with such arrhythmias can result in fetal bradycardia and the need for immediate treatment with antiarrhythmic drugs, electric cardioversion, or urgent cesarean section. The effect of pregnancy on women with the hereditary long-QT syndrome has been reported (see Chap. 28).[111] The postpartum interval was associated with a significant increase in the risk for cardiac events, including death, aborted cardiac arrest, and syncope. Treatment with beta-adrenergic blockers was independently associated with a decrease in the risk for cardiac events.

Complete heart block has been described during pregnancy and is usually congenital. Patients with complete heart block may remain asymptomatic during pregnancy and have uncomplicated labor and delivery without treatment. Symptomatic patients with conduction abnormalities, including bifascicular block, second-degree atrioventricular block, and complete heart block, have been treated during pregnancy with either temporary or permanent pacemakers; and numerous pregnancies have been reported in patients after pacemaker implantation.[104,112]

MANAGEMENT OF ARRHYTHMIAS. A complete evaluation is indicated in patients with arrhythmias during pregnancy to rule out a treatable cause such as electrolyte imbalance, thyroid disease, and arrhythmogenic effects of drugs, alcohol, caffeine, and cigarette smoking. An identified cause should be treated and antiarrhythmic drug therapy initiated only if the arrhythmia persists and is symptomatic, hemodynamically important, or life threatening. When drug therapy seems necessary, the smallest therapeutic dose of drugs known to be safe for the fetus should be used (Table 74–7). Therapeutic blood levels and the indication for continuous drug therapy should be reevaluated periodically. Because of the unpredictable exposure to ionizing radiation, electrophysiological evaluation and catheter ablation procedures are usually postponed until the postpartum period but have been reported during pregnancy.[113] If delay of such procedures is undesirable, an attempt should be made to minimize radiation and use echocardiographic guidance whenever possible. Synchronized electrical cardioversion has been performed safely during all stages of pregnancy[114,115] and can be used in patients with tachyarrhythmias unresponsive to drug therapy that are associated with hemodynamic decompensation. Insertion of an implantable cardioverter-defibrillator has not been reported during pregnancy; however, pregnancies in women with an implantable cardioverter-defibrillator have been reported to be uneventful.[116]

Other Cardiovascular Disorders

AORTIC DISSECTION (see Chap. 53). A predisposition for aortic dissection during gestation has been suggested.[117] Over the past 50 years, more than 200 cases of aortic dissection in association with pregnancy have been reported; most cases occur in women with Marfan syndrome,[59,60,118] and cases of aortic dissection in women with systemic hypertension, coarctation of the aorta, Turner syndrome, and the use of crack cocaine have been reported.[119-121] Pregnancy-related aortic dissection may be due to increased hemodynamic stress and alterations in the structure of the vascular wall[117] and seems to occur most often in the third trimester and peripartum period.

Transesophageal echocardiography provides a powerful and safe tool for establishing the diagnosis of aortic dissection.[122] During pregnancy, this method is preferable to computed tomography, which involves radiation exposure, and to magnetic resonance imaging, whose safety during gestation has not been fully established.

The combination of intravenous nitroprusside and beta-adrenergic blocking agents is currently recommended to control hypertension in nonpregnant patients with aortic dissection[123] and has been used successfully during pregnancy. However, because nitroprusside can result in fetal toxicity, it should be used only post partum or in patients refractory

TABLE 74–7 Cardiovascular Drugs in Pregnancy

Drug	Use in Pregnancy	Potential Side Effects	Breast Feeding	Risk Factors
Adenosine	Maternal and fetal arrhythmias	No side effects reported; data on use during first trimester are limited.	Data NA	C
Amiodarone	Maternal arrhythmias	IUGR, prematurity, congenital goiter, hypothyroidism and hyperthyroidism, transient bradycardia, and prolonged QT in the newborn.	Not recommended	C
Angiotensin-converting enzyme inhibitors	Hypertension	Oligohydramnios, IUGR, prematurity, neonatal hypotension, renal failure, anemia, death, skull ossification defect, limb contractures, patent ductus arteriosus.	Compatible	C
Beta blockers	Hypertension, maternal arrhythmias, myocardial ischemia, mitral stenosis, hypertrophic cardiomyopathy, hyperthyroidism, Marfan syndrome	Fetal bradycardia, low placental weight, possible IUGR, hypoglycemia, no information on carvedilol.	Compatible, monitoring of infant's heart rate recommended	Acebutolol B Labetalol C Metoprolol C Propranolol C Atenolol D
Digoxin	Maternal and fetal arrhythmias, heart failure	No evidence for unfavorable effects on the fetus.	Compatible	C
Diltiazem	Myocardial ischemia, tocolysis	Limited data. Increased incidence of major birth defects.	Compatible	C
Disopyramide	Maternal arrhythmias	Limited data. May induce uterine contraction and premature delivery.	Compatible	C
Diuretics	Hypertension, congestive heart failure	Hypovolemia → reduced uteroplacental perfusion, fetal hypoglycemia, thrombocytopenia, hyponatremia, hypokalemia. Thiazide diuretics can inhibit labor and suppress lactation.	Compatible	C
Flecainide	Maternal and fetal arrhythmias	Limited data. Two cases of fetal death after successful treatment of fetal SVT reported, relation to flecainide uncertain.	Compatible	C
Lidocaine	Local anesthesia, maternal arrhythmias	No evidence for unfavorable fetal effects; high serum levels may cause central nervous depression at birth.	Compatible	C
Nifedipine	Hypertension, tocolysis	Fetal distress related to maternal hypotension reported.	Compatible	C
Nitrates	Myocardial infarction and ischemia, hypertension, pulmonary edema, tocolysis	Limited data. Use is generally safe, few cases of fetal heart rate deceleration and bradycardia have been reported.	Data NA	C
Procainamide	Maternal and fetal arrhythmias	Limited data. No fetal side effects reported.	Compatible	C
Propafenone	Fetal arrhythmias	Limited data. Fetal death reported after direct intrauterine administration in fetuses with fetal hydrops.	Data NA	C
Quinidine	Maternal and fetal arrhythmias	Minimal oxytoxic effect, high doses may cause premature labor or abortion. Transient neonatal thrombocytopenia and damage to eighth nerve reported.	Compatible	C
Sodium nitroprusside	Hypertension, aortic dissection	Limited data. Potential thiocyanate fetal toxicity, fetal mortality reported in animals.	Data NA	C
Sotalol	Maternal arrythmias, hypertension, fetal tachycardia	Limited data. Two cases of fetal death and two cases of significant neurological morbidity in newborns reported as well as bradycardia in newborns.	Compatible, monitoring of infant's heart rate recommended	B
Verapamil	Maternal and fetal arrhythmias, hypertension, tocolysis	Limited data. Other than a single case of fetal death of uncertain cause, no adverse fetal or newborn effects have been reported.	Compatible	C

IUGR = intrauterine growth retardation; NA = not available; SVT = supraventricular tachycardia.

to other drugs during pregnancy and can be substituted by hydralazine, nitroglycerin, or labetolol.[55] To avoid blood pressure elevation associated with labor and vaginal delivery in women with aortic dissection, cesarean section is recommended.[118]

TAKAYASU ARTERITIS (see Chap. 82)

Because Takayasu arteritis often occurs in young women, there is a high likelihood of pregnancy in patients with this condition.[123] Review of the literature revealed information on pregnancies in more than 60 women with Takayasu disease.[123,124] The majority of more recently published cases have had favorable maternal outcomes, although increase in blood pressure during pregnancy with or without superimposed preeclampsia, development of heart failure, and progression of renal insufficiency have been described.[124] Although a favorable fetal outcome has been reported in many cases, the incidence of fetal growth retardation, premature deliveries, and fetal loss is increased.[123,124] The mode of delivery in the majority of cases was vaginal, and forceps were often used to expedite the second stage of labor. Cesarean section delivery has been performed mainly for obstetrical indications or maternal hypertension and vascular disorders. In the great majority of patients, abdominal delivery has been performed under epidural anesthesia with favorable results.

PRIMARY PULMONARY HYPERTENSION (see Chap. 67)

Primary pulmonary hypertension is one of the few cardiovascular conditions that in pregnancy continues to be associated with high maternal mortality, estimated to be 30 to 40 percent.[125,126] Clinical deterioration or death during pregnancy cannot be predicted on the basis of the patient's preconceptual clinical status. Symptomatic deterioration usually occurs in the second or third trimester and may be manifested by fatigue, exertional dyspnea, syncope, chest pain, palpitations, nonproductive cough, hemoptysis, and leg edema. Worsening of symptoms during pregnancy led to early hospitalization in many reported cases.[125-129] Death often occurs a few hours to several days post partum, usually related to sudden death or progressive right ventricular failure.[130,131] Although the exact cause of death in patients with primary pulmonary hypertension is not clear, right ventricular ischemia and failure caused by an increase in pulmonary vascular resistance after delivery, cardiac arrhythmias, and pulmonary embolism are potential mechanisms. In addition to high maternal risk, primary pulmonary hypertension is associated with poor fetal outcome with high incidences of prematurity, fetal growth retardation, and fetal loss.[125]

Because of the high risk to both mothers with primary pulmonary hypertension and their fetuses, pregnancy should be discouraged in these patients and tubal ligation should be considered. In addition, early abortion should be considered in patients who become pregnant. The incidence of premature delivery is increased in patients with primary pulmonary hypertension, and should, therefore, be anticipated. Because of the beneficial effect of anticoagulation in patients with primary pulmonary hypertension[34] and the increased incidence of thromboembolism during pregnancy, such therapy is recommended throughout gestation or at least during the third trimester and early postpartum phase. Hemodynamic monitoring and blood gas measurements should be performed continuously during labor and delivery. Oxygen should be provided to prevent hypoxemia, and inhaled nitric oxide or prostaglandins administered either by inhalation or intravenously may be useful to lower pulmonary vascular resistance.[131-133]

Because of the high rate of early postpartum maternal death, close monitoring is recommended for several days post partum. Successful use of vasodilators including inhaled nitric oxide and intravenous and inhaled prostaglandins to lower pulmonary pressure during labor, delivery, and the early postpartum period has been reported.[131-133] In addition, a successful maternal and fetal outcome has been reported in one case treated with intravenous epoprostenol for 4 weeks prior to and then during cesarean section delivery; the drug was continued after the delivery.[128]

Cardiac Surgery During Pregnancy

Because heart disease that requires surgery is usually diagnosed and treated before pregnancy, cardiac surgery during gestation is uncommon.[29] The experience continues to be anecdotal and usually limited to urgent, life-threatening conditions in which surgery cannot be delayed and delivery is not desired, mostly because of fetal immaturity.[93,134,135] The effects of anesthesia and the surgical procedure, especially cardiopulmonary bypass, on the placental circulation and fetal outcome are still not well understood.[136] A review of the literature published between 1984 and 1996[137] identified 161 cases of various cardiovascular operations, 137 with and 24 without cardiopulmonary bypass. Surgery during pregnancy resulted in a high fetal-neonatal mortality of 30 percent. Week of gestation at time of surgery, surgery with cardiopulmonary bypass, longer duration, and temperature of cardiopulmonary bypass did not influence fetal-neonatal outcome. Operations performed during pregnancy resulted in a moderately high maternal mortality of 6 percent, and surgery performed immediately after delivery was associated with even higher mortality of 12 percent. Hospitalization after the 27th gestational week and emergency surgery were associated with poor maternal outcome. Nine percent maternal mortality was reported in cases that involved valvular surgery and 22 percent in cases of aortic or arterial dissection repairs and pulmonary embolectomies. Maternal risk associated with peripartum cardiovascular surgery therefore seems higher than the risk of similar surgery in nonpregnant patients.

Because of high incidence of fetal wastage and moderate increase in maternal risk, surgery should be recommended only for patients who do not respond to medical therapy and should be performed if possible after delivery.[138] To minimize the risk of teratogenicity, surgery should be avoided during the first trimester. Because heart surgery is indicated after failure of medical therapy, many of these patients are hemodynamically unstable and require hemodynamic evaluation and optimization before and monitoring during surgery. Anesthetic agents should be selected on the basis of their hemodynamic effects and fetal safety. When the patient is at or near term, abdominal delivery by cesarean section can be performed before cardiac surgery when fetal maturity has been confirmed.[138] Fetal heart monitoring should be performed continuously during surgery by experienced personnel.

Pregnancy in Patients with Prosthetic Heart Valves

VALVE SELECTION. The selection of a prosthetic heart valve for women of childbearing age remains difficult.[139-141] New-generation mechanical valves offer excellent durability, low risk of reoperation, and superior hemodynamic profile. However, the need for anticoagulation is associated with an increased risk of maternal bleeding and fetal loss.[142] Tissue valves have an inferior hemodynamic profile, especially with small valve sizes in the aortic position, and are associated with a high incidence of deterioration in young patients; deterioration may be further accelerated during pregnancy, with an expected rate of valve replacement as high as 30 to 50 percent within 10 years.[139,140] Although homograft valves and new pericardial valves appear to have better hemodynamics, information regarding pregnancy in women with these valves is limited.[141,143] In the nonpregnant population, homograft valves have been reported to have the same rate of deterioration as porcine, bioprosthetic valves.[144] An evaluation of long-term follow-up of young women with a prosthetic heart valve reported a substantially higher rate of reoperation in bioprosthetic valves compared with homografts in the aortic position (60 versus 30 percent).[145] Long-term follow-up of nonpregnant patients undergoing the Ross procedure also showed high rates of reoperation of 24 and 38 percent at 10 and 20 years, respectively, and mortality of 15 and 39 percent.[146]

Risks associated with pregnancy in women with prosthetic valves are related mainly to the increased hemodynamic burden and incidence of thromboembolic events as well as to untoward fetal effects caused by cardiovascular drugs and anticoagulation. Experience in more than 1000 pregnancies indicates that most patients who are asymptomatic or mildly symptomatic before gestation tolerate the hemodynamic burden of pregnancy, although decreased functional capacity and need to start or increase drug therapy are not uncommon.[140]

Increased thromboembolic events have been reported during pregnancy in women with mechanical prosthetic heart valves, with incidences as high as 10 to 15 percent (Fig. 74–9). Approximately two-thirds of these patients presented with valve thrombosis, which led to death in 40 percent of them.[139] Thromboembolism, however, has been reported mostly with older generation mechanical prostheses in the mitral position.[139] Heparin has been considered the anticoagulant of choice during pregnancy because of its proven safety for both the patient and the fetus.[147] Reports of an increased incidence of mechanical valve thrombosis during use of subcutaneous heparin in pregnancy[139] have raised concern regarding the effectiveness of heparin in pregnant women with mechanical heart valves.

ANTICOAGULATION. Thromboembolic prophylaxis for women at higher risk (old-generation prosthetic heart valve in the mitral position, atrial fibrillation, history of thromboembolic event despite adequate anticoagulation level) seems to be best achieved with oral anticoagulation (International Normalized Ratio of 3.0 to 4.5) for the first 35 weeks. An alternative therapy for patients electing to avoid warfarin in the first gestational trimester is unfractionated or low-molecular-weight heparin with close monitoring and appropriate dose adjustment for the first trimester, followed by warfarin between 13 and 36 weeks and then heparin until delivery. A high heparin intensity should be used in patients at high risk. Because peak levels cannot always predict trough levels, anticoagulation should aim at predose antifactor Xa levels higher than 0.55 units/ml or a midinterval activated partial thromboplastin time of 2.5 to 3.5 seconds (predose = 2.0 seconds) with unfractionated heparin and higher than 0.7 units/ml with low-molecular-weight heparin.

Oral anticoagulants cross the placenta and can be harmful to the fetus. Exposure during the first 8 to 12 weeks can be associated with a teratogenic effect leading to warfarin embryopathy (depressed nasal bridge, nasal hypoplasia, small nasal bones, hypoplastic alae nasi, telecanthus, upper airway obstruction related to choanal stenosis, and punctate epiphyseal dysplasia of the long bones and the cervical and lumbar vertebrae plates). Use of warfarin during pregnancy can also lead to fetal intracranial bleeding and is associated with a high rate of fetal loss, mostly because of spontaneous abortion.[142,147] One study suggested a relationship between fetal complications and warfarin dose with most of the fetal adverse effects occurring in women treated with warfarin at doses higher than 5 mg/d.[149] This relationship, however, has not been confirmed by other studies.[150,151]

A review of the literature showed the occurrence of warfarin embryopathy in 6.4 percent of women with prosthetic heart valves treated with warfarin throughout pregnancy.[142] The risk of embryopathy was eliminated by substitution of warfarin with heparin started at or prior to 6 weeks and continued until 12 weeks of gestation. The use of warfarin was also associated with a high frequency of spontaneous abortions (25 percent), congenital fetal anomalies (6 percent), and fetal wastage (34 percent) (Fig. 74–10).

Low-molecular-weight heparins have several potential advantages over unfractionated heparin, including a lower frequency of heparin-induced thrombocytopenia and osteoporosis, superior absorption from the subcutaneous injection site and bioavailability, and a two- to fourfold greater half-life and, therefore, a more predictable and sustained anticoagulant effect.[143]

There is substantial experience with the use of low-molecular-weight heparins in pregnancy, mostly for venous thromboembolism prophylaxis.[152,153] Limited information, however, is available regarding the use of low-molecular-weight heparin in pregnant patients with mechanical prosthetic heart valves, and several of the reports have described pregnancies complicated by valve thrombosis[154-158]; most of these cases, however, were associated with inadequate doses or subtherapeutic anti-Xa levels, or both.[159]

The latest recommendations as published by the American College of Chest Physicians for anticoagulation in pregnant patients with prosthetic heart valves[160] are as follows:

- Aggressive adjusted dose of unfractionated heparin, given every 12 hours subcutaneously throughout pregnancy; midinterval activated partial thromboplastin time maintained at two times control levels, or anti-Xa heparin level maintained at 0.35 to 0.70 IU/ml.
- Low-molecular-weight heparin throughout pregnancy, in doses adjusted according to weight, or as necessary to maintain a 4-hour postinjection anti-Xa heparin level of about 1.0 IU/ml.
- Unfractionated or low-molecular-weight heparin, as above, until the 13th week; change to warfarin until the middle of the third trimester, then restart heparin therapy until delivery.

Our recommendations are similar but further emphasize the need for frequent and careful monitoring of the predose level

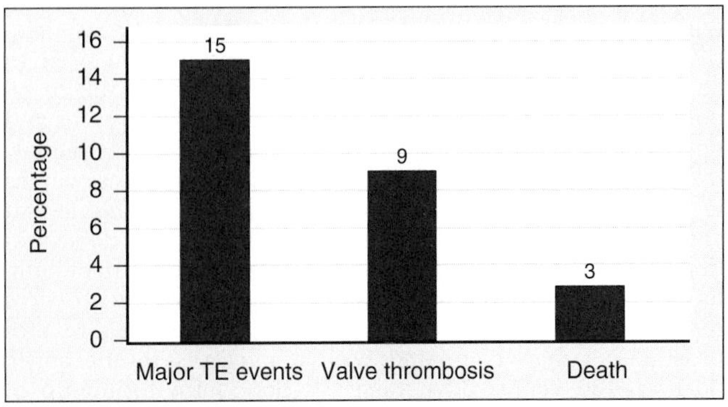

FIGURE 74–9 Incidence of major thromboembolic (TE) events during pregnancy in 326 pregnancies of women with mechanical prosthetic heart valves. (Modified from Elkayam U: Pregnancy through a prosthetic heart valve. J Am Coll Cardiol 33:1642, 1999.)

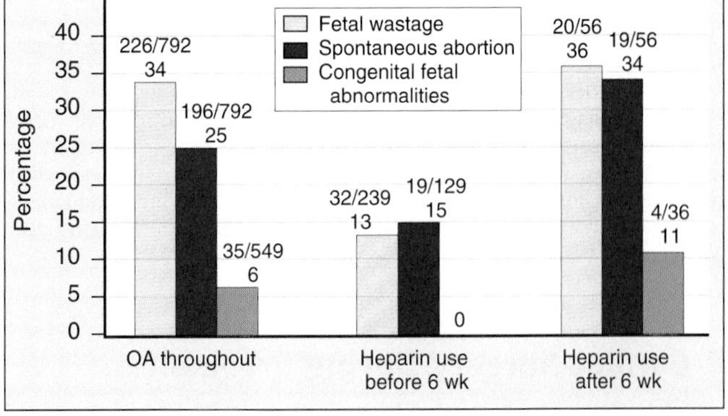

FIGURE 74–10 Frequency of fetal complications reported with various anticoagulation regimens. OA = oral anticoagulation. (Modified from Chan WS, Anand S, Ginsberg JS: Anticoagulation of pregnant women with mechanical heart valves: A systematic review of the literature. Arch Intern Med 160:191, 2000.)

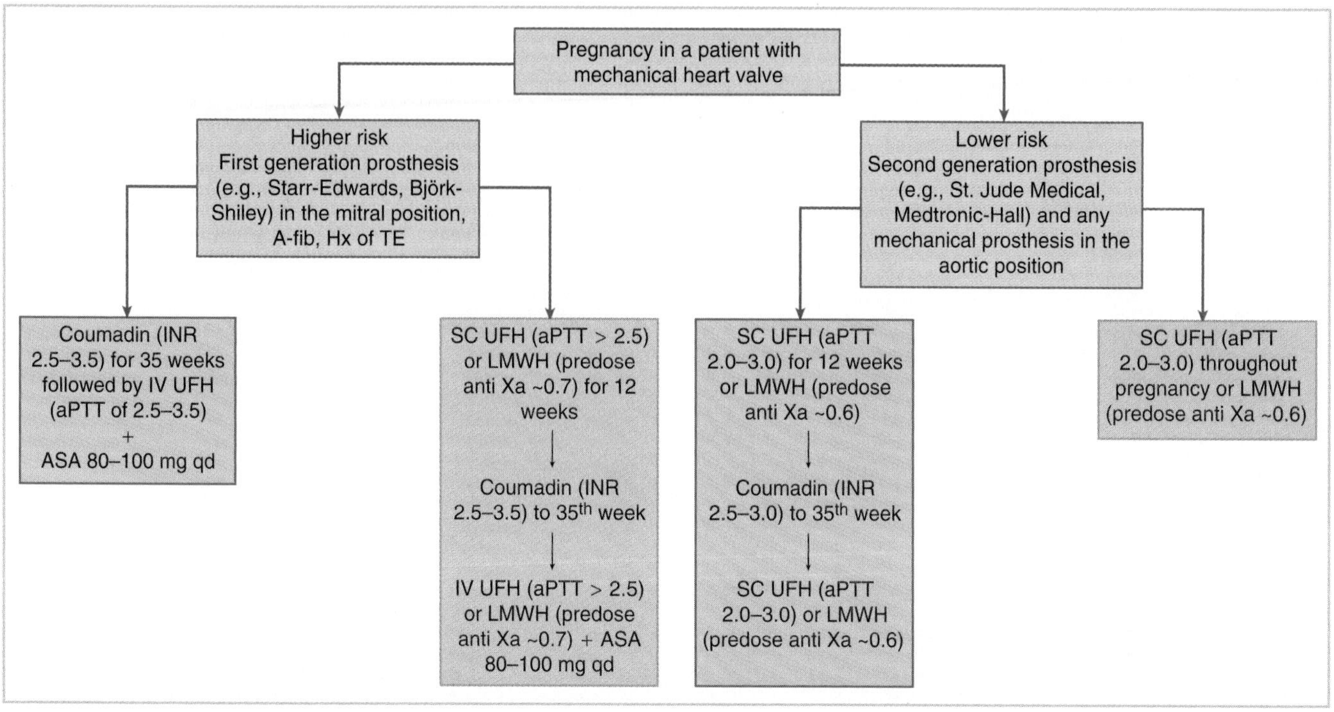

FIGURE 74–11 Recommended approach for anticoagulation prophylaxis in women with mechanical prosthetic heart valves during pregnancy. A-fib = atrial fibrillation; aPTT = activated partial thromboplastin time; ASA = acetylsalicylic acid; Hx =history; INR = International Normalized Ratio; LMWH = low-molecular-weight heparin; SC = subcutaneous; TE = thromboembolism; UFH = unfractionated heparin. (Elkayam U, Singh H, Irani A: Anticoagulation in pregnant women with prosthetic heart valves. Submitted for publication.)

of anticoagulation to ensure persistent thromboembolic prophylaxis in this high-risk group of patients (Fig. 74–11).[148,159]

Because of a high incidence of premature labor in patients with prosthetic heart valves, warfarin should be substituted for heparin at the 35th or 36th week to avoid onset of labor during warfarin therapy. The switch from warfarin to heparin should be performed in the hospital. In lower risk patients, including those with an aortic prosthetic valve and second-generation prosthesis in the mitral position, subcutaneous heparin therapy may be used throughout pregnancy (activated partial thromboplastin time of 2.0 to 3.0 seconds). A change from subcutaneous injections of heparin to an intravenous drip prior to elective delivery may be advisable because it allows discontinuation of therapy 4 hours before expected delivery. A higher level of anticoagulation seems justified in patients with mechanical prostheses in the mitral position, in patients with more than one mechanical prosthesis, in patients with atrial fibrillation, and in patients with a history of systemic embolization. The intensity of anticoagulation should be monitored frequently and immediately corrected if needed. Because a small dose of aspirin is safe during pregnancy[101] and can reduce the incidence of systemic embolization or death when added to oral anticoagulation, 80 mg of aspirin may be added to maximize the antithrombotic effect.

REFERENCES

Cardiovascular Physiology During Pregnancy and the Puerperium

1. Elkayam U, Gleicher N: Hemodynamic and cardiac function during normal pregnancy and the puerperium. *In* Elkayam U, Gleicher N (eds): Cardiac Problems in Pregnancy. 3rd ed. New York, Wiley-Liss, 1998, pp 3-20.
2. Brown MA, Gallery ED: Volume homeostasis in normal pregnancy and preeclampsia: Physiology and clinical implications. Baillieres Clin Obstet Gynecol 8:287, 1994.
3. Clapp JF III, Capeless E: Cardiovascular function before, during and after the first and subsequent pregnancies. Am J Cardiol 80:1469, 1997.
4. Mesa A, Jessurun C, Hernandez A, et al: Left ventricular diastolic function in normal human pregnancy. Circulation 99:511, 1999.
5. Poppas A, Shroff SG, Korcarz CE, et al: Serial assessment of the cardiovascular system in normal pregnancy. Circulation 95:2407, 1997.
6. Hameed AB, Karaalp IS, Tummala PP, et al: The effect of valvular heart disease on maternal and fetal outcome in pregnancy. J Am Coll Cardiol 37:893, 2001.

Cardiovascular Evaluation During Pregnancy

7. Elkayam U, Gleicher N: Cardiac evaluation during pregnancy. *In* Elkayam U, Gleicher N (eds): Cardiac Problems in Pregnancy. 3rd ed. New York, Wiley-Liss, 1998, pp 23-32.
8. Shotan A, Ostrzega E, Mehra A, et al: Incidence of arrhythmias in normal pregnancy and relation to palpitations, dizziness and syncope. Am J Cardiol 79:1061, 1997.
9. Colletti PM, Lee K: Cardiovascular imaging in the pregnant patient. *In* Elkayam U, Gleicher N (eds): Cardiac Problems in Pregnancy. 3rd ed. New York, Wiley-Liss, 1998, pp 33-36.
10. Allan L: Antenatal diagnosis of heart disease. Heart 83:367, 2000.
11. Veille JC, Kitzman D, Millsaps PD, et al: Left ventricular diastolic filling response to stationary bicycle exercise during pregnancy and the postpartum period. Am J Obstet Gynecol 185:822, 2001.
12. Colletti PM: Computer-assisted imaging of the fetus with magnetic resonance imaging. Comput Med Imaging Graph 20:491, 1996.

Pregnancy in Women with Congenital Heart Disease

13. Warnes CA, Elkayam U: Congenital heart disease and pregnancy. *In* Elkayam U, Gleicher N (eds): Cardiac Problems in Pregnancy. 3rd ed. New York, Wiley-Liss, 1998, pp 39-53.
14. Siu SC, Colman JM: Heart disease and pregnancy. Heart 85:710, 2001.
15. Swan L, Hillis WS, Cameron A: Family planning requirements of adults with congenital heart disease. Heart 78:9, 1997.
16. Kjos SL: Fertility control in the cardiac patient. *In* Elkayam U, Gleicher N (eds): Cardiac Problems in Pregnancy. 3rd ed. New York, Wiley-Liss, 1998, pp 451-456.
17. Sin SC, Sermer M, Harrison DA, et al: Risk and predictors for pregnancy-related complications in women with heart disease. Circulation 96:2789, 1997.
18. Zuber M, Gautschi N, Oechslin E, et al: Outcome of pregnancy in women with congenital shunt lesions. Heart 81:271, 1999.
19. Siu SC, Colman JM, Sorensen S, et al: Adverse neonatal and cardiac outcomes are more common in pregnant women with cardiac disease. Circulation 105:2179, 2002.
20. Ardinger RH Jr: Genetic counseling in congenital heart disease. Pediatr Ann 26:99, 1997.
21. Presbitero P, Somerville J, Stone S, et al: Pregnancy in cyanotic congenital heart disease: Outcome of mother and fetus. Circulation 89:2673, 1994.
22. Dajani AS, Taubert KA, Wilson W, et al: Prevention of bacterial endocarditis. Recommendations by the American Heart Association. JAMA 277:1794, 1997.
23. Ebrahimi R, Leung CY, Elkayam U, Reid CL: Infective endocarditis. *In* Elkayam U, Gleicher N (eds): Cardiac Problems in Pregnancy. 3rd ed. New York, Wiley-Liss, 1998, pp 191-198.
24. Actis Dato GM, Rinaudo P, Revelli A et al: Atrial septal defect and pregnancy: A retrospective analysis of obstetrical outcome before and after surgical correction. Minerva Cardioangiol 46:63, 1998.

25. Kozelj M, Novak-Antolic Z, Grad A, et al: Patent foramen ovale as a potential cause of paradoxical embolism in the post partum period. Eur J Obstet Gynecol Reprod Biol 84:55, 1999.
26. Daehnert I, Ewert P, Berger F, et al: Echocardiographically guided closure of a patent foramen ovale during pregnancy after recurrent strokes. J Interv Cardiol 14:191, 2001.
27. Actis Dato GM, Cavaglia M, Aidala E, et al: Patent ductus arteriosus. Follow up of 677 operated cases 40 years later. Minerva Cardioangiol 47:245,1999.
28. Bhargava B, Agarwal R, Yadav R, et al: Percutaneous balloon aortic valvuloplasty during pregnancy: Use of the Inoue balloon and the physiologic antegrade approach. Cathet Cardiovasc Diagn 45:422, 1998.
29. Cohen RG, Castro LJ: Cardiac surgery during pregnancy. *In* Elkayam U, Gleicher N (eds): Cardiac Problems in Pregnancy. 3rd ed. New York, Wiley-Liss, 1998, pp 277-284.
30. Saidi AS, Bezold LI, Altman CA, et al: Outcome of pregnancy following intervention for coarctation of the aorta. Am J Cardiol 82:786, 1998.
31. Beauchesne LM, Connolly HM, Ammash NM, et al: Coarctation of the aorta: Outcome of pregnancy. J Am Coll Cardiol 38:1728, 2001.
32. Plunkett MD, Bond LM, Geiss DM: Staged repair of acute type I aortic dissection and coarctation in pregnancy. Ann Thorac Surg 69:1945, 2000.
33. Therrian J, Marx GR, Gatzoulis MA: Late problems in tetralogy of Fallot—Recognition, management, and prevention. Cardiol Clin 20:395, 2002.
34. Weiss BM, Hess OM: Pulmonary vascular disease and pregnancy: Current controversies, management strategies, and perspectives. Eur Heart J 21:104, 2000.
35. Sawhney H, Suri V, Vasishta K, et al: Pregnancy and congenital heart disease—Maternal and fetal outcome. Aust NZ J Obstet Gyneol 38:266, 1998.
36. Burn J, Brennan P, Little J, et al: Recurrence risks in offspring of adults with major heart defects: Results from first cohort of British collaborative study. Lancet 351:311, 1998.
37. Branko WM, Otto H: Perioperative cardiovascular evaluation for noncardiac surgery: Congenital heart disease and heart disease in pregnancy deserve better guidelines. Circulation 95:530, 1997.
38. Goodwin TM, Gherman RB, Hameed A, Elkayam U: Favorable response of Eise menger's syndrome to inhaled nitric oxide during pregnancy. Am J Obstet Gynecol 180:64, 1999.
39. Lust KM, Boots RH, Dooris M, Wilson J: Management of labor in Eisenmenger syndrome with inhaled nitric oxide. Am J Obstet Gynecol 181:419, 1999.
40. Kansaria JJ, Salvi VS: Eisenmenger syndrome in pregnancy. J Postgrad Med 46:101, 2000.
41. Somerville J: The Denolin Lecture: The woman with congenital heart disease. Eur Heart J 19:1766, 1998.
42. Lao TT, Sermer M, Colman JM: Pregnancy after the Fontan procedure for tricuspid atresia: A case report. J Reprod Med 41:287, 1996.
43. Genomi M, Jenni R, Hoerstrup SP, et al: Pregnancy after atrial repair for transposition of the great arteries. Heart 81:276, 1999.
44. Connolly HM, Grogan M, Warnes CA: Pregnancy among women with congenitally corrected transposition of great arteries. J Am Coll Cardiol 33:1692, 1999.
45. Canobbio MM, Mair DD, van der Velde M, Koos BJ: Pregnancy outcome after the Fontan repair. J Am Coll Cardiol 28:763, 1996.

Valvular Heart Disease

46. Essop MR, Sareli P: Rheumatic valvular disease and pregnancy. *In* Elkayam U, Gleicher N (eds): Cardiac Problems in Pregnancy. 3rd ed. New York, Wiley-Liss, 1998, pp 55-60.
47. Reimold SC, Rutherford JD: Valvular heart disease in pregnancy. N Engl J Med 349:52, 2003.
48. Barbosa PJ, Lopes AA, Feitusa GS, et al: Prognostic factors of rheumatic mitral stenosis during pregnancy and puerperium. Arq Bras Cardiol 75:215, 2000.
49. Naidoo DP, Desai DK, Moodley J: Maternal death due to pre-existing cardiac disease. Cardiovasc J S Afr 13:17, 2002.
50. Birincioglu CL, Kucuker SA, Yapar EG, et al: Perinatal mitral valve interventions: A report of 10 cases. Ann Thorac Surg 67:1312, 1999.
51. de Souza JA, Martinez EE, Ambrosa JA, et al: Percutaneous balloon mitral valvuloplasty in comparison with open mitral valve commissurotomy for mitral stenosis during pregnancy. J Am Coll Cardiol 37:900, 2001.
52. Mangione JA, Lourenco RM, dos Santos ES, et al: Long-term follow-up of pregnant women after percutaneous mitral valvuloplasty. Catheter Cardiovasc Interv 50:413, 2000.
53. Kinsara AJ, Ismail O, Fawzi ME: Effect of balloon mitral valvuloplasty during pregnancy on childhood development. Cardiology 97:155, 2002.
54. Kubota N, Morimoto Y, Kemmotsu O: Anesthetic management for cesarean section in a patient with mitral stenosis and pulmonary hypertension. Masai Jpn J Anesthesiol 52:177, 2003.
55. Calvin SE: Use of vasodilators during pregnancy. *In* Elkayam U, Gleicher N (eds): Cardiac Problems in Pregnancy. 3rd ed. New York, Wiley-Liss, 1998, pp 391-398.
56. Bhargava B, Agarwal R, Yadar R, et al: Percutaneous balloon aortic valvuloplasty during pregnancy: Use of the Inoue balloon and the physiologic antegrade approach. Cathet Cardiovasc Diagn 45:422, 1998.

Other Conditions Affecting the Valves, Aorta, and Myocardium

57. Freed LA, Levy D, Levine RA, et al: Prevalence and clinical outcome of mitral-valve prolapse. N Engl J Med 341:1, 1999.
58. Rayburn WF: Mitral valve prolapse and pregnancy. *In* Elkayam U, Gleicher N (eds): Cardiac Problems in Pregnancy. 3rd ed. New York, Wiley-Liss, 1998, pp 175-182.
59. Elkayam U, Ostrzega E, Shotan A, Mehra A: Marfan syndrome and pregnancy. *In* Elkayam U, Gleicher N (eds): Cardiac Problems in Pregnancy. 3rd ed. New York, Wiley-Liss, 1998, pp 211-221.
60. Lind J, Wallenburg HC: The Marfan syndrome and pregnancy: A retrospective study in a Dutch population. Eur J Obstet Gynecol Reprod Biol 98:28, 2001.
61. Paternoster DM, Santarossa C, Vettore N, et al: Obstetric complications in Marfan's syndrome. Minerva Ginecol 50:441, 1998.
62. Uchida T, Ogino H, Ando M, et al: Aortic dissection in pregnant women with the Marfan syndrome. Jpn J Thorac Surg 55:693, 2001.
63. Gott VL, Greene PS, Alejo DE, et al: Replacement of the aortic root in patients with Marfan's syndrome. N Engl J Med 340:1307, 1999.
64. Oakley C, Child A, Jung B, et al: Expert consensus document on management of cardiovascular diseases during pregnancy. Eur Heart J 24:761, 2003.

Cardiomyopathies

65. Elkayam U, Dave R: Hypertrophic cardiomyopathy and pregnancy. *In* Elkayam U, Gleicher N (eds): Cardiac Problems in Pregnancy. 3rd ed. New York, Wiley-Liss, 1998, pp 211-221.
66. Probst V, Langlard JM, Desnos M, et al: Familial hypertrophic cardiomyopathy. French study of the duration and outcome of pregnancy. Arch Mal Coeur Vaiss 95:81, 2002.
67. Autore C, Conte MR, Piccinirino M, et al: Risk associated with pregnancy in hypertrophic cardiomyopathy. J Am Coll Cardiol 40:1864, 2002.
68. Autore C, Brauneis S, Fabrizio A, et al: Epidural anesthesia for cesarean section in patients with hypertrophic cardiomyopathy: A report of three cases. Anesthesiology 90:1205, 1999.
69. Lang RM, Lampert MB, Poppas A, et al: Peripartal cardiomyopathy. *In* Elkayam U, Gleicher N (eds): Cardiac Problems in Pregnancy. 3rd ed. New York, Wiley-Liss, 1998, pp 87-100.
70. Pearson GD, Veille JC, Rahimtoola S, et al: Peripartum cardiomyopathy: National Heart, Lung, and Blood Institute and Office of Rare Diseases (National Institutes of Health) workshop recommendations and review. JAMA 283:1183, 2000.
71. Akhter WM, Shotan A, Hameed A, et al: Pregnancy associated cardiomyopathy: Early versus late presentation. J Am Coll Cardiol 41:1039, 2003.
72. Fett JD: Peripartum cardiomyopathy. Insights from Haiti regarding a disease of unknown etiology. Minn Med 85:46, 2002.
73. Akhter WM, Shotan A, Hameed A, et al: Pregnancy associated cardiomyopathy: Clinical profile in 137 patients diagnosed in the U.S. J Am Coll Cardiol 41:1136, 2003.
74. Aziz TM, Burgess MI, Acladious NN, et al: Heart transplantation for peripartum cardiomyopathy: A report of three cases and a literature review. Cardiovasc Surg 7:565, 1999.
75. Shotan A, Widerhorn J, Hurst A, Elkayam U: Risks of angiotensin-converting enzyme inhibition during pregnancy: Experimental and clinical evidence, potential mechanisms, and recommendations for use. Am J Med 96:451, 1994.
76. Ford RF, Barton JR, O'Brien JM, et al: Demographics, management, and outcome of peripartum cardiomyopathy in a community hospital. Am J Obstet Gynecol 182:1036, 2000.
77. Carlson KM, Browning JE, Eggleston MK, et al: Peripartum cardiomyopathy presenting as lower extremity arterial thromboembolism; a case report. J Reprod Med 45:351, 2000.
78. Bozkurt B, Villaneuva FS, Halubkov R, et al: Intravenous immune globulin in the therapy of peripartum cardiomyopathy. J Am Coll Cardiol 34:177, 1999.
79. Sliwa K, Skudicky D, Candy G, et al: The addition of pentoxifylline to conventional therapy improves outcome in patients with peripartum cardiomyopathy. Eur J Heart Fail 4:305, 2002.
80. Sliwa K, Skudicky D, Bergemann A, et al: Peripartum cardiomyopathy: Analysis of clinical outcome, left ventricle function, plasma levels of cytokines and Fas/APO-O. J Am Coll Cardiol 35:701, 2000.
81. Felker GM, Thompson RE, Hare JM, et al: Underlying causes and long-term survival in patients with initially unexplained cardiomyopathy. N Engl J Med 342:1077, 2000.
82. Elkayam U, Tummala PP, Rao K, et al: Maternal and fetal outcomes of subsequent pregnancies in women with peripartum cardiomyopathy. N Engl J Med 344:1567, 2001.

Hypertension in Pregnancy

83. Roberts JM, Pearson G, Cutler J, et al: Summary of the NHLBI working group on research on hypertension during pregnancy. Hypertension 41:437, 2003.
84. Report of the national high blood pressure education program working group on high blood pressure in pregnancy. Am J Obstet Gynecol 183:S1, 2000.
85. Higgins JR, de Swiet M: Blood pressure measurement and classification in pregnancy. Lancet 357:131, 2001.
86. Chari RS, Frangieh AY, Sibai BM: Hypertension during pregnancy: Diagnosis, pathophysiology, and management. *In* Elkayam U, Gleicher N (eds): Cardiac Problems in Pregnancy. 3rd ed. New York, Wiley-Liss, 1998, pp 257-273.
87. Roberts JM, Cooper DW: Pathogenesis and genetics of pre-eclampsia. Lancet 357:53, 2001.
88. Branch KR, Wagoner LE, McGrory CH, et al: Risks of subsequent pregnancies on mother and newborn in female heart transplant recipient. J Heart Lung Transplant 17:698, 1998.
89. Alami WS, Young JB: Pregnancy after cardiac transplantation. *In* Elkayam U, Gleicher N (eds): Cardiac Problems in Pregnancy. 3rd ed. New York, Wiley-Liss, 1998, pp 327-337.

Coronary Artery Disease

90. Paulson RJ, Boostanfar R, Saadat P, et al: Pregnancy in the sixth decade of life. JAMA 288:2320, 2002.
91. Rutherford JD: Coronary artery disease in the childbearing age. *In* Elkayam U, Gleicher N (eds): Cardiac Problems in Pregnancy. 3rd ed. New York, Wiley-Liss, 1998, pp 121-130.
92. Roth A, Elkayam U: Acute myocardial infarction and pregnancy. *In* Elkayam U, Gleicher N (eds): Cardiac Problems in Pregnancy. 3rd ed. New York, Wiley-Liss, 1998, pp 131-151.
93. Hameed AB, Tummala PP, Godwin TM, et al: Unstable angina during pregnancy in two patients with premature coronary atherosclerosis and aortic stenosis in association with familial hypercholesterolemia. Am J Obstet Gynecol 182:1152, 2000.
94. Sattar N, Greer IA: Pregnancy complications and maternal cardiovascular risk: Opportunities for intervention and screening? BMJ 325:157, 2002.
95. Brizzi P, Tonalo G, Esposito F, et al: Lipoprotein metabolism during normal pregnancy. Am J Obstet Gynecol 181:430, 1999.
96. Kulka PJ, Scheu C, Tryba M, et al: Coronary artery plaque disruption as cause of acute myocardial infarction during cesarean section with spinal anesthesia. J Clin Anesth 12:335, 2000.
97. Chen FG, Koh KF, Chong YS: Cardiac arrest associated with sulprostone: Use during cesarean section. Anaesth Intensive Care 26:298, 1998.
98. Lerakis S, Manoukian S, Martin RP: Transesophageal echo detection of post partum coronary artery dissection. J Am Soc Echocardiogr 14:1132, 2001.

99. Shivvers SA, Wians FH Jr, Keffer JH, Ramin SM: Maternal cardiac troponin I levels during normal labor and delivery. Am J Obstet Gynecol 180:122, 1999.
100. Ginsberg JS, Hirsch J: Use of antithrombotic agents during pregnancy. Chest 114:524S, 1998.
101. Cartis S, Sibai B, Houth J, et al: Low-dose aspirin to prevent preeclampsia in women at high risk. National Institute of Child Health and Human Development, network of maternal-fetal medicine unit. N Engl J Med 338:701, 1998.
102. Subtil D, Goeusse P, Puech F, et al: Aspirin (100 mg) used for prevention of pre-eclampsia in nulliparous women: The Essai Regional Aspirine Mere-Enfant Study. Int J Obstet Gynecol 110:475, 2003.

Arrhythmias

103. Wolbrette D: Treatment of arrhythmias during pregnancy. Curr Womens Health Rep 3:135, 2003.
104. Leung CY, Brodsky MA: Cardiac arrhythmias and pregnancy. *In* Elkayam U, Gleicher N (eds): Cardiac Problems in Pregnancy. 3rd ed. New York, Wiley-Liss, 1998, pp 155-175.
105. Desai DK, Adanlawo M, Naidoo DP, et al: Mitral stenosis in pregnancy: A four year experience at King Edward VIII hospital, Durban, South Africa BJOG 107:953, 2000.
106. Braden GL, Von Oeyen PT, Germain MJ, et al: Ritodrine and terbutaline-induced hypokalemia in preterm labor: Mechanisms and consequences. Kidney Int 51:1867, 1997.
107. Carson MP, Fisher AJ, Scorza WE: Atrial fibrillation in pregnancy associated with oral terbutaline. Obstet Gynecol 100:1096, 2002.
108. Onagawa T, Ohkuchi A, Ohki R, et al: Woman with postpartum ventricular tachycardia and hypomagnesemia. J Obstet Gynecol Res 29:92, 2003.
109. Palma EC, Saxenberg V, Vijayaraman P, et al: Histopathological correlation of ablation lesions guided by noncontact mapping in a patient with peripartum cardiomyopathy and ventricular tachycardia. Pacing Clin Electrophysiol 24:1812, 2001.
110. Mela T, Galvin JM, McGovern BA: Magnesium deficiency during lactation as a precipitant of ventricular tachyarrhythmias. Pacing Clin Electrophysiol 25:231, 2002.
111. Rashba EJ, Zareba W, Moss AJ, et al: Influence of pregnancy on the risk for cardiac events in patients with hereditary long QT syndrome. Circulation 97:451, 1998.
112. Sharma JB, Malhotra M., Pundir P: Successful pregnancy outcome with cardiac pacemaker after complete heart block. Int J Gynaecol Obstet 68:145, 2000.
113. Dominguez A, Iterralde P, Hermosillo AG, et al: Successful radio frequency ablation of an accessory pathway during pregnancy. Pacing Clin Electrophysiol 22:131, 1999.
114. Brown O, Davidson, N, Palmer J: Cardioversion in the third trimester of pregnancy. Aust NZ J Obstet Gynecol 41:241, 2001.
115. Oktay C, Kesapli M, Altekin E: Wide-QRS complex tachycardia during pregnancy: Treatment with cardioversion and review. Am J Emerg Med 20:492, 2002.
116. Olufolabi AJ, Charlton GA, Allen SA, et al: Use of implantable cardioverter defibrillator and anti-arrhythmic agents in a parturient. Br J Anaesth 89:652, 2002.

Other Cardiovascular Disorders

117. Elkayam U, Hameed A: Vascular dissections and aneurysms during pregnancy. *In* Elkayam U, Gleicher N (eds): Cardiac Problems in Pregnancy. 3rd ed. New York, Wiley-Liss, 1998, p 201.
118. Brar HB: Anaesthetic management of a cesarean section in a patient with Marfan's syndrome and aortic dissection. Anaesth Intensive Care 29:67, 2001.
119. Plunkett MD, Bond LM, Geiss DM: Staged repair of acute type I aortic dissection and coagulation in pregnancy. Ann Thorac Surg 69:1945, 2000.
120. Garvey P, Elovitz M, Landsberger EJ: Aortic dissection and myocardial infarction in a pregnant patient with Turner syndrome. Obstet Gynecol 91:864, 1998.
121. Madu EC, Shala B, Baugh D: Crack-cocaine–associated aortic dissection in early pregnancy; a case report. Angiology 50:163, 1999.
122. Nienaberg CA, Eagle KA: Aortic dissection: New frontiers in diagnosis and management Part II: Therapeutic management and follow up. Circulation 108:772, 2003.
123. Elkayam U, Hameed A: Takayasu's arteritis and pregnancy. *In* Elkayam U, Gleicher N (eds): Cardiac Problems in Pregnancy. 3rd ed. New York, Wiley-Liss, 1998, p 237.
124. Sharma BK, Jain S, Vasishta K: Outcome of pregnancy in Takayasu arteritis. Int J Cardiol 75:S159, 2000.
125. Elkayam U, Dave R, Bokhari SWH: Primary pulmonary hypertension in pregnancy. *In* Elkayam U, Gleicher N (eds): Cardiac Problems in Pregnancy. 3rd ed. New York, Wiley-Liss, 1998, p 183.
126. Weiss BM. Zemp L. Seifert B, Hess OM: Outcome of pulmonary vascular disease in pregnancy: A systematic overview from 1978 through 1996. J Am Coll Cardiol 31:1650, 1998.
127. Satoh H, Masuda Y, Izuta S, et al: Pregnant patient with primary pulmonary hypertension: General anesthesia and extracorporeal membrane oxygenation support for termination of pregnancy. Anesthesiology 97:1638, 2002.
128. Stewart R, Tuazon D, Olson G, et al: Pregnancy and primary pulmonary hypertension; successful outcome with epoprostenol therapy. Chest 119:973, 2001.
129. Wong PS, Constantinides S, Kanellopoulos V, et al: Primary pulmonary hypertension in pregnancy. J R Soc Med 94:523, 2001.
130. Takeuchi K, Yokota H, Moriyama T, et al: Two cases of primary pulmonary hypertension diagnosed during pregnancy. J Perinat Med 26:248, 1998.
131. Monnery L, Nanson J, Charlton G: Primary pulmonary hypertension in pregnancy; a role for novel vasodilators. Br J Anaesth 87:295, 2001.
132. Decoene C, Bourzoufi K, Moreau D, et al: Use of inhaled nitric oxide for emergency cesarean section in a woman with unexpected primary pulmonary hypertension. Can J Anaesth 48:584, 2001.
133. Weiss BM, Maggiorini M, Jenni R, et al: Pregnant patient with primary pulmonary hypertension; inhaled pulmonary vasodilators and epidural anesthesia for cesarean delivery. Anesthesiology 92:1191, 2000.
134. Fabricius AM, Autschbach R, Doll N, et al: Acute aortic dissection during pregnancy. Thorac Cardiovasc Surg 49:56, 2001.
135. Ceresoli G, Passoni P, Benussi S, et al: Primary cardiac sarcoma in pregnancy: A case report and review of the literature. Am J Clin Oncol 22:460, 1999.
136. Mul TF, van Herwerden LA, Cohen-Overbeek TE, et al: Hypoxic-ischemic fetal insult resulting from maternal aortic root replacement, with normal fetal heart rate at term. Am J Obstet Gynecol 179:825, 1998.
137. Weiss BM, von Segesser LK, Alon E, et al: Outcome of cardiovascular surgery and pregnancy: A systematic review of the period 1984-1996. Am J Obstet Gynecol 179:1643, 1998.
138. Akashi H, Tayama K, Fujino T, et al: Surgical treatment for acute type A aortic dissection in pregnancy: A case of aortic root replacement just after cesarean section. Jpn Circ J 64:729, 2000.
139. Elkayam U: Pregnancy through a prosthetic heart valve. J Am Coll Cardiol 33:1642, 1999.
140. Elkayam U, Khan SS: Pregnancy in the patient with artificial heart valve. *In* Elkayam U, Gleicher N (eds): Cardiac Problems in Pregnancy. 3rd ed. New York, Wiley-Liss, 1998, pp 61-78.
141. Hung L, Rahimtoola SH: Prosthetic heart valves and pregnancy. Circulation 107:1240, 2003.
142. Chan WS, Ananad S, Ginsberg JS: Anticoagulation of pregnant women with mechanical heart valves: A systemic review of the literature. Arch Intern Med 160:191, 2000.
143. Dore A, Somerville J: Pregnancy in patients with pulmonary autograft valve replacement. Eur Heart J 18:1659, 1997.
144. Grunkemeir GL, Li HH, Naftel DC, et al: Long term performance of heart valve prosthesis. Curr Probl Cardiol 25:73, 2000.
145. North RA, Sadler L, Stewart AW, et al: Long-term survival and valve-related complications in young women with cardiac valve replacement. Circulation 99:2669, 1999.
146. Chambers JC, Somerville J, Stone S, et al: Pulmonary autograft procedure for aortic valve disease: Long-term results of the pioneer series. Circulation 96:2206, 1997.
147. McGehee W: Anticoagulation in pregnancy. *In* Elkayam U, Gleicher N (eds): Cardiac Problems in Pregnancy. 3rd ed. New York, Wiley-Liss, 1998, pp 407-417.
148. Elkayam U, Singh H, Irani A: Anticoagulation in pregnant women with prosthetic heart valves. Submitted for publication.
149. Vitale N, Defeo M, De Santo LS, et al: Dose-dependent fetal complications of warfarin in pregnant women with mechanical heart valves. J Am Coll Cardiol 33:1637, 1999.
150. Meschengieser SS, Fondevila CG, Santarelli MT, et al: Anticoagulation in pregnant women with mechanical valves prostheses. Heart 82:23, 1999.
151. Sadler L, McCowan L, White H, et al: Pregnancy outcomes and cardiac complications in women with mechanical bioprosthetic and homograft valves. Br J Obstet Gynaecol 17:245, 2000.
152. Laurent P, Dussarat GV, Bonal J, et al: Low molecular weight heparins: A guide to their optimum use in pregnancy. Drugs 62:463, 2002.
153. Ensom MH, Stephenson MD: Low molecular-weight heparins in pregnancy. Pharmacotherapy 19:1013, 1999.
154. Rowan JA, McCowan LM, Raudkivi PJ, et al: Enoxaparin treatment in women with mechanical heart valve during pregnancy. Am J Obstet Gynecol 185:633, 2001.
155. Arnaout MS, Kazma H, Khalil A, et al: Is there a safe anticoagulation protocol for pregnant women with prosthetic valves? Clin Exp Obstet Gynecol 25:101, 1998.
156. Berndt N, Khan I, Gallo R: A complication in anticoagulation using low-molecular weight heparin in a patient with a mechanical valve prosthesis. A case report. J Heart Valve Dis 9:844, 2000.
157. Saw J, Thompson E, Macdonald I: Mechanical valve thrombosis during pregnancy. Can J Cardiol 17:95, 2001.
158. Oles D, Berryessa R, Campbell K, et al: Emergency redo mitral valve replacement in a 27-year-old pregnant female with a clotted prosthetic mitral valve, preoperative fetal demise and postoperative ventricular assist device: A case report. Perfusion 16:159, 2001.
159. Sheshadi N, Goldhaber SZ, Elkayam U, et al: The clinical challenge of bridging anticoagulation in patients with mechanical prosthetic heart valves. Am Heart J (in press).
160. Ginsberg JS, Greer I, Hirsh J: Use of antithrombotic agents during pregnancy. Chest 119:122S, 2001.

GUIDELINES *Thomas H. Lee*

Pregnancy

Recommendations for management of heart disease in pregnancy are included in the 1998 American College of Cardiology/American Heart Association (ACC/AHA) guidelines on valvular disease[1] and in the 2003 ACC/AHA Scientific Statement on warfarin therapy.[2] These guidelines do not recommend routine antibiotic prophylaxis in patients with valvular heart disease undergoing uncomplicated vaginal delivery or cesarean section unless infection is suspected. For high-risk patients, such as those with prosthetic heart valves or prior histories of endocarditis, antibiotics are considered optional.

TABLE 74G–1 Guidelines for Anticoagulation During Pregnancy in Patients with Mechanical Prosthetic Valves

Indication	Class I	Class IIa	Class IIb	Class III
Anticoagulation during pregnancy in patients with mechanical prosthetic valves: Weeks 1 through 35	1. The decision whether to use heparin during the first trimester or to continue oral anticoagulation throughout pregnancy should be made after full discussion with the patient and her partner; if she chooses to change to heparin for the first trimester, she should be made aware that heparin is less safe for her, with a higher risk of both thrombosis and bleeding, and that any risk to the mother also jeopardizes the baby.[2] 2. High-risk women (a history of thromboembolism or an older generation mechanical prosthesis in the mitral position) who choose *not* to take warfarin during the first trimester should receive continuous unfractionated heparin intravenously in a dose to prolong the midinterval (6 hours after dosing) aPTT to two to three times the control value. Transition to warfarin can occur thereafter.	1. In patients receiving warfarin, INR should be maintained between 2.0 and 3.0 with the lowest possible dose of warfarin, and low-dose aspirin should be added.	1. Women at low risk (no history of thromboembolism, newer low-profile prosthesis) may be managed with adjusted-dose subcutaneous heparin (17,500 to 20,000 units b.i.d.) to prolong the midinterval (6 hours after dosing) aPTT to two to three times the control value.	
Anticoagulation during pregnancy in patients with mechanical prosthetic valves: After the 36th week		1. Warfarin should be stopped no later than week 36 and heparin substituted in anticipation of labor. 2. If labor begins during treatment with warfarin, a cesarian section should be performed. 3. In the absence of significant bleeding, heparin can be resumed 4 to 6 hours after delivery and warfarin begun orally.		

aPTT = activated partial thromboplastin time; INR = International Normalized Ratio.

Complex guidelines were offered in the 1998 ACC/AHA guidelines on valvular heart disease for management of anticoagulation in pregnant patients with mechanical prosthetic heart valves (Table 74G–1). These guidelines reflect high complication rates in pregnant women managed with subcutaneous heparin and support use of intravenous heparin during the first trimester. After the 36th week of pregnancy, transition from warfarin to heparin is recommended in anticipation of labor.

The 2003 Scientific Statement on anticoagulation notes a dilemma for physicians managing anticoagulation for pregnant patients. Three options are available:

1. Heparin or low-molecular-weight heparin throughout pregnancy,
2. Warfarin throughout pregnancy, changing to heparin or low-molecular-weight heparin at 38 weeks' gestation with planned labor induction at about 40 weeks, or
3. Heparin or low-molecular-weight heparin in the first trimester of pregnancy, switching to warfarin in the second trimester, continuing it until about 38 weeks' gestation, and then changing to heparin or low-molecular-weight heparin at 38 weeks with planned labor induction at about 40 weeks.

These strategies are complicated by the fact that low-molecular-weight heparin is not approved by the U.S. Food and Drug Administration (FDA) for use in any patients with mechanical prosthetic heart valves, and the FDA has issued an advisory warning against use of enoxaparin (Lovenox) in pregnant women with mechanical prosthetic heart valves. The guidelines note that some data indicate that low-molecular-weight heparin appears to be safe in nonpregnant patients with mechanical heart valves, but the expert panel could not recommend its use directly given the status of FDA-approved indications.

References

1. Bonow RO, Carabello B, de Leon AC Jr, et al: ACC/AHA guidelines for the management of patients with valvular heart disease: Executive summary: A report of the American College of Cardiology/American Heart Association Task Force on Practice Guidelines (Committee on Management of Patients With Valvular Heart Disease). Circulation 98:1949, 1998.
2. Hirsh J, Fuster V, Ansell J, Halperin JL: American Heart Association/American College of Cardiology Foundation guide to warfarin therapy. Circulation 107:1692, 2003.

CHAPTER 75

Cardiovascular Disease in Athletes

Barry J. Maron

Over the past several years interest has heightened considerably among medical practitioners and the lay public regarding the causes of sudden deaths in trained athletes, as well as the clinical significance of cardiac symptoms such as syncope and arrhythmias.[1-4] Catastrophic events in athletes are always unexpected, and although relatively uncommon, often achieve high visibility and convey a particularly devastating impact on the community.[2] Indeed, the possibility that young, highly trained high school, college, or even professional athletes may harbor potentially lethal heart disease[1-8] or are susceptible to sudden death under a variety of circumstances[1,2,9,10] may seem counterintuitive. Over the last several years, a large measure of clarification has resulted with regard to the causes of sudden death during sporting activities, as well as the most appropriate diagnostic and management strategies for this distinct subset of the population with a unique life style.

Causes of Sudden Death

Young Athletes (≤35 Years)

Although the overall athlete population is at low risk,[2] a number of largely congenital (usually unsuspected) cardiovascular diseases, each relatively uncommon in the general population, have been causally linked to exercise-related sudden death in young trained athletes or asymptomatic individuals with active sports-related life styles (Figs. 75–1 and 75–2).[1,2,6,7,11] Indeed, any cardiac disease capable of causing sudden death in young nonathletes can also be responsible for such events in athletes.

Based on autopsy surveys, about 80 percent of deaths in young athletes can be linked to structural cardiovascular disease.[1,2,6,7] In the United States, hypertrophic cardiomyopathy (HCM) has consistently been the single most common cause of such sudden deaths, accounting for about one-third of these events due to cardiovascular disease.[2] HCM is a relatively common genetic cardiac disease (1:500 in the general population) characterized by an asymmetrically hypertrophied and nondilated left ventricle with heterogeneous clinical, morphological, and genetic expression (see Chap. 59).[12,13] Indeed, HCM is the most common cause of sudden cardiac death in young individuals, frequently occurring with physical exertion. Sudden death due to ventricular tachyarrhythmias (see Chap. 32) probably emanates from an electrically unstable (and largely unpredictable) myocardial substrate,[1,2,6,7,11] evidenced by the histopathological markers of disorganized myocardial architecture and replacement scarring (a consequence of microvascular abnormalities and bursts of myocardial ischemia).[12] High-risk HCM patients are considered for primary prevention of sudden death with prophylactic implantation of cardioverter-defibrillators (see Chap. 31).[14]

In addition, not infrequently, hearts are encountered at autopsy with increased left ventricular mass (and wall thickness) and nondilated ventricular cavities, in which other objective morphological findings are suggestive of HCM, although not sufficient to permit definitive diagnosis.[1] In the absence of clinical data, it is uncertain whether such cases represent relatively mild morphological expressions of HCM or possibly unusual examples of marked physiological left ventricular hypertrophy associated with deleterious consequences.

The second most frequent causes of athletic field deaths, accounting for about 20 percent, are congenital coronary artery anomalies of wrong sinus origin (most commonly, left main coronary artery from right sinus of Valsalva) (Fig. 75–3); the mirror image malformation, anomalous right coronary from the left aortic sinus, has also been occasionally incriminated in such deaths (see Chap. 56).[1,2,15] These coronary anomalies may be more common than previously regarded, but diagnosis requires a high index of clinical suspicion, which is crucial given that surgical correction is possible.[15] Diagnosis of the coronary anomalies should be aroused in any young athlete with a history of chest pain or syncope, particularly if symptoms are triggered by exercise.[15,16] Suspicion may be raised with transthoracic echocardiography and identification possible with transesophageal echocardiography, multislice CT imaging, or magnetic resonance imaging (MRI) (see Chaps. 11, 14, and 15), ultimately with full confirmation achieved by coronary arteriography. Large, clinically identified patient cohorts with anomalous coronary artery and long-term follow-up (with or without surgery) are not presently available. Patients usually do not demonstrate abnormalities on 12-lead or exercise electrocardiogram (ECG) since myocardial ischemia is episodic,[15] thereby limiting the power for detection during preparticipation screening. Most likely mechanisms for myocardial ischemia include the acute-angled take-off and kinking at the origin of the left main coronary artery or compression, during exercise, of the anomalous artery between aorta and pulmonary trunk.

In addition, a diverse array of about 15 other congenital or acquired diseases account for only 5 percent or less of all athletic field deaths.[1,2] An unexpectedly high occurrence of premature atherosclerotic coronary artery disease has, however, been noted in some surveys of young athletes and is probably underrecognized in this population (see Chap. 46). Uncommon causes of sudden death include valvular heart disease (aortic stenosis or myxomatous mitral valve degeneration) (see Chap. 57), dilated cardiomyopathy (see Chap. 59), arrhythmogenic right ventricular cardiomyopathy (ARVC)

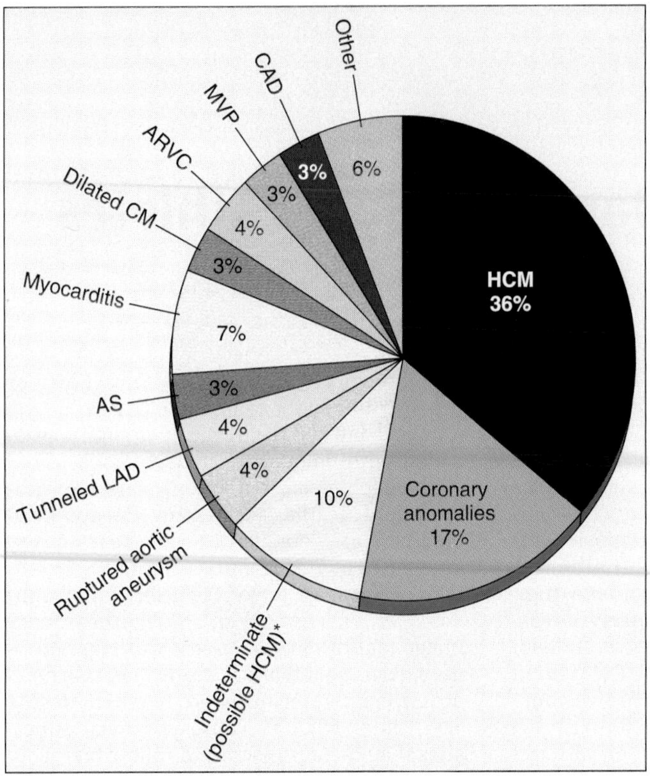

FIGURE 75–1 Causes of sudden cardiac death in young competitive athletes (median age, 17 years) based on systematic tracking in the U.S. Registry. In an additional 2 percent of the patients, no evidence of cardiovascular disease sufficient to explain death was identified at necropsy; *hearts with increased weight and some morphological features consistent with (but not diagnostic of) hypertrophic cardiomyopathy (HCM). LAD = left anterior descending coronary artery; AS = aortic stenosis; CM = cardiomyopathy; ARVC = arrhythmogenic right ventricular cardiomyopathy; MVP = mitral valve prolapse; CAD = coronary artery disease. (Adapted from Maron BJ, Thompson PD, Puffer JC, et al: Cardiovascular preparticipation screening of competitive athletes: A statement for health professionals from the Sudden Death Committee [Clinical Cardiology] and Congenital Cardiac Defects Committee [Cardiovascular Disease in the Young], American Heart Association. Circulation 94:850-856, 1996.)

(see Chap. 32), apparent coronary artery hypoplasia and other rare coronary anomalies, Marfan syndrome (see Chap. 56), and myocarditis (see Chap. 60).

Myocarditis is challenging to diagnose clinically (or at autopsy in the healed phase) and may be manifest only by ECG abnormalities, including heart block and ventricular arrhythmias, in the absence of symptoms. Although the inflammatory process of myocarditis is usually triggered by viral agents (most often enterovirus, but not uncommonly adenovirus), chronic cocaine ingestion can provoke a similar clinical and pathological profile (see Chap. 62).[2,9] Diagnosis is enhanced by testing endomyocardial biopsy specimens for viral genome by the polymerase chain reaction.

Athletes with Marfan syndrome can participate successfully in strenuous competitive sports for many years without experiencing a catastrophic event, presumably before aortic dilation becomes marked and the predisposition to dissection or rupture increases critically. Marfan syndrome may be underdiagnosed, particularly in populations of elite basketball players. ARVC is an uncommon familial cardiac disease, associated with ventricular or supraventricular tachyarrhythmias and sudden death, and characterized largely by diffuse or segmental right ventricular abnormalities with myocyte death, fibrous and adipose tissue replacement and myocarditis[7] resulting in chamber enlargement and systolic dysfunction, and T-wave inversion and epsilon waves in the right precordial ECG leads.[17] In athletes with heart disease, primary ventricular tachyarrhythmias are the predominant mechanism of sudden death, although in Marfan syndrome, demise is usually due to dissection and a ruptured aorta (associated with disruption of aortic media with decreased numbers of elastic fibers), or occasionally an arrhythmia.

Only about 2 percent of young athletes show normal cardiac structure without a definitive cause of death at autopsy.[1] Such deaths are probably due to conditions unassociated with gross or histological cardiac abnormalities, such as ion-channel disorders (long-QT and Brugada syndromes), Wolff-Parkinson-White syndrome, abnormalities of conducting system and microvasculature, catecholaminergic polymorphic ventricular tachycardia or right ventricular outflow tract tachycardia (see Chaps. 29 to 32), coronary vasospasm (see Chap. 46), and subtle morphological forms of HCM or ARVC.[2,7,18,19]

In addition, intramural tunneled coronary arteries (short segments of left anterior descending surrounded by myocardium) are occasionally the sole abnormality found at autopsy.[20] It remains unresolved as to whether these bridged coronary arteries are simply variants of normal or have pathophysiological significance in triggering myocardial ischemia and sudden death during exertion in otherwise healthy young individuals or patients with HCM. Sudden and unexpected arrhythmic death, nonfatal stroke, and acute myocardial infarction in trained athletes have also been attributed to illicit substance abuse with cocaine, anabolic steroids, or dietary and nutritional supplements (particularly ephedrine-containing compounds).[9,10]

Reports from the Veneto region of northeastern Italy provide an alternative profile for the causes of athletic field deaths, with ARVC the most common.[2,7] This unusual prevalence could possibly be due in part to genetic predisposition or, alternatively, the Italian national preparticipation athlete screening program, which probably identifies and disqualifies from competition disproportionately fewer athletes with ARVC than those with other diseases more readily identified during screening (e.g., HCM).[21]

Older Athletes (>35 Years)

Older athletes can also harbor occult cardiac disease and die suddenly and unexpectedly related to participation in athletic activities, usually road racing (including marathon), jogging, rugby, squash, and golf.[4,8] Unlike young athletes, the cause of death in most older conditioned athletes is atherosclerotic coronary artery disease (see Chaps. 47 and 50), with the remainder due to nonischemic diseases such as HCM or valvular heart disease. Many older athletes who have died of coronary heart disease had known risk factors, cardiovascular symptoms, or prior myocardial infarction (or coronary interventions) and severe atherosclerotic narrowing of two or three major extramural arteries with myocardial scarring. Although no strategies are in place for systematically screening older athletes in organized sports, it has been recommended that competitors in master's sports[8] with at least a moderate cardiovascular risk profile for coronary artery disease (≥1 independent risk factors) should undergo, in addition to history and physical examination, exercise (stress) testing before initiating training or competition.

There is overwhelming evidence that the cardiovascular benefits attributable to consistent exercise represent a primary prevention strategy for coronary artery disease in asymptomatic middle-aged and older persons. Although habitual exercise appears to mitigate the likelihood of sudden death in trained individuals (with unsuspected or known coronary artery disease), such events are triggered paradoxically with increased frequency when associated with vigorous exertion in untrained persons.[22] This supports the recommendation in sedentary persons for gradual entry into conditioning programs.[8]

COMMOTIO CORDIS

Virtually instantaneous cardiac arrest may result during sports activities from a relatively modest innocent-appearing and nonpenetrating blunt blow to the chest in the *absence* of underlying cardiovascular disease or structural injury to the chest wall or heart itself (i.e., commotio cordis).[5] Such occurrences are produced either by a projectile (most commonly a baseball, softball, or hockey puck) or by bodily contact with another athlete. The blow to the chest may be delivered with a wide range in velocities but is usually not perceived as particularly unusual for the sporting event nor of sufficient magnitude to result in death. A common scenario is that of a young baseball player struck in the chest (while batting) by a pitched ball thrown from a standard distance. However,

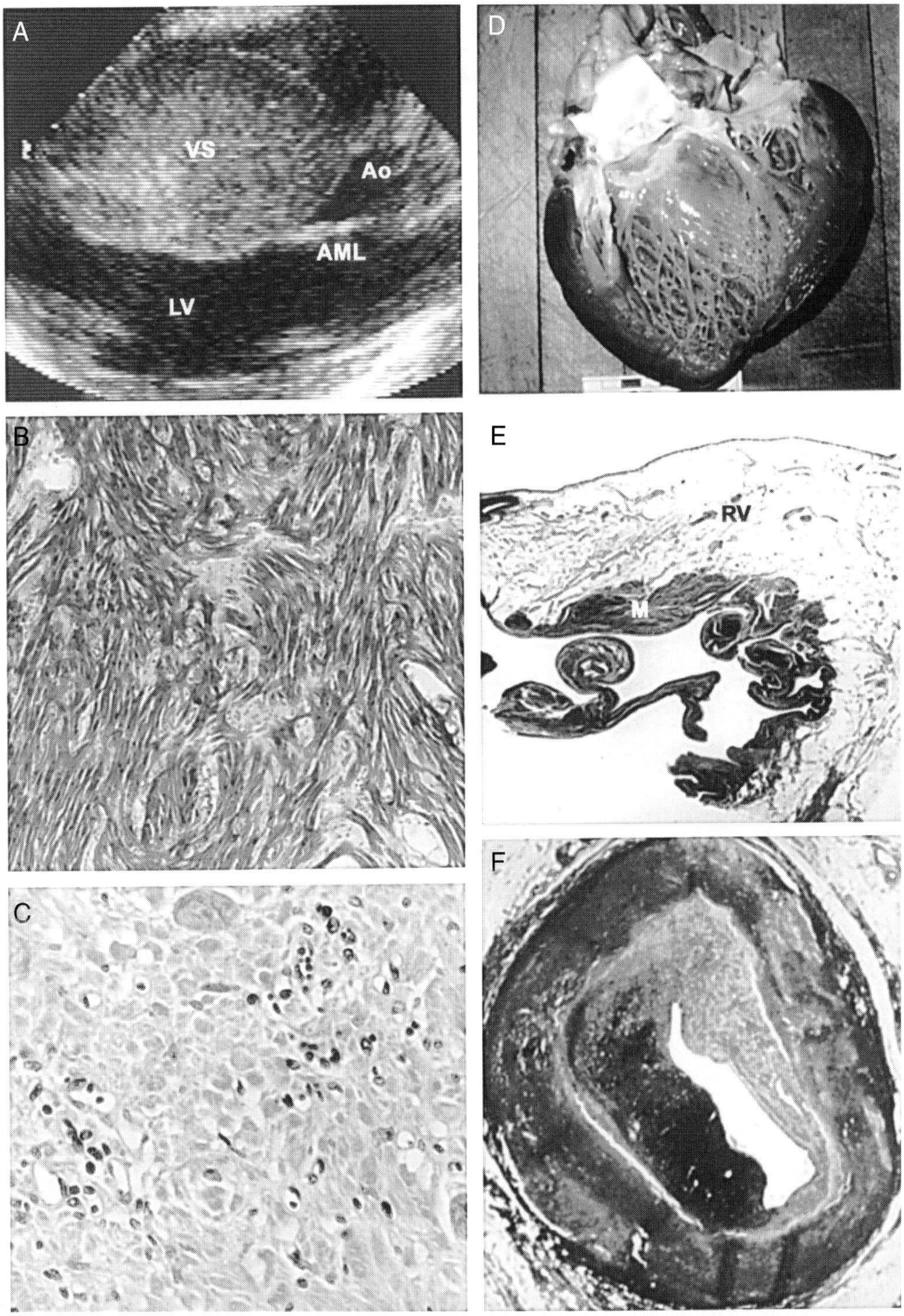

FIGURE 75–2 Causes of sudden cardiac death in young competitive athletes. **A,** Hypertrophic cardiomyopathy. Two-dimensional echocardiogram in parasternal long-axis view showing extreme asymmetrical thickening of the ventricular septum (VS) (i.e., 53 mm). LV = left ventricle; Ao = aorta; AML = anterior mitral leaflet. **B,** Hypertrophic cardiomyopathy. Histopathology showing the substrate of disorganized cardiac muscle cells and chaotic architectural pattern; hematoxylin and eosin stain. **C,** Myocarditis. Area of left ventricular myocardium with clusters of inflammatory mononuclear cells; hematoxylin and eosin stain, ×400. **D,** Idiopathic dilated cardiomyopathy, showing greatly enlarged left ventricular cavity. **E,** Arrhythmogenic right ventricular cardiomyopathy. Histological section of right ventricular (RV) wall showing extensive fatty replacement adjacent to a small area of residual myocytes (M); hematoxylin and eosin stain. **F,** Premature coronary artery disease. Portion of right coronary artery with atherosclerotic narrowing and ruptured plaque. (**A** to **F,** From Maron BJ: Sudden death in young athletes. N Engl J Med 349:1064-1075, 2003.)

many of these events occur in purely recreational situations at home or on the playground (some even unrelated to sports) with the fatal injuries often produced by family members.

Commotio cordis is most common in young children (mean age 13 years) with characteristically pliable chest walls that probably facilitate transmission of the chest impact energy to the myocardium.[5] There appear to be two other major determinants of a commotio cordis event: (1) the chest impact is located directly over the heart; and (2) the timing of the blow occurs precisely in a narrow 20-msec window during repolarization, just prior to the T wave peak, involving activation of the K^+-ATP channel.[23]

Certain measures aimed at prevention of commotio cordis during sports have been considered. Softer-than-normal ("safety") baseballs reduced the risk for ventricular fibrillation in an experimental model, suggesting that modification of athletic equipment could prevent sudden death; however, such projectiles do not provide absolute protection in

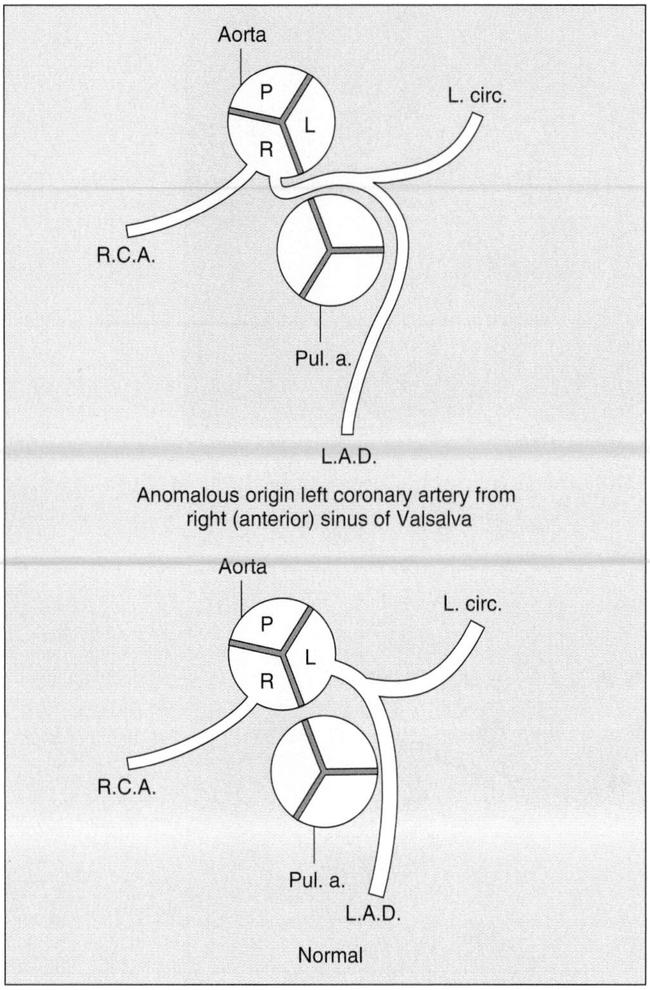

FIGURE 75–3 Congenital coronary artery anomaly of wrong aortic sinus origin, which may cause sudden death in young athletes. **Top,** Anomalous origin of the left main coronary artery arising from right (anterior) sinus of Valsalva. Note acute leftward bend of left main coronary artery at its origin and its posterior course between aorta and pulmonary artery trunk (Pul a.). **Bottom,** Normal coronary artery anatomy is shown for comparison. L.A.D. = left anterior descending; L. circ. = left circumflex; L = left sinus; R = right sinus; P = posterior sinus; R.C.A. = right coronary artery. (From Maron BJ, Epstein SE, Roberts WC: Causes of sudden death in competitive athletes. J Am Coll Cardiol 7:204-214, 1986.)

the field.[5] Greater use of chest barriers that effectively cover the precordium would theoretically protect against commotio cordis in young people competing in sports such as baseball, ice hockey, karate, and lacrosse. However, the infrequency of commotio cordis events remains an obstacle to documenting the effectiveness of any protective intervention.

Commotio cordis events are not uniformly fatal, with reported survival of 15 percent, usually associated with prompt cardiopulmonary resuscitation and defibrillation.[5] With enhanced public awareness of this syndrome and more widespread dissemination of automatic external defibrillators, effective emergency measures are likely to be implemented more rapidly on the athletic field, avoiding many future catastrophes.

Frequency and Demographics of Sudden Death in Athletes

Based largely on data assembled from U.S. populations, a profile of young competitive athletes with sudden death has emerged.[1,2,6] In young athletes, the frequency of sudden unexpected death due to cardiovascular disease during competitive sports appears to be low, occurring in about 1:200,000 individual student athletes per academic year and in about 1:70,000 over a 3-year high school career.[2] In comparison, older athletes have somewhat higher rates of exercise-related sudden death, reported to be from 1:15,000 to 1:50,000 per year.[2] Such estimates suggest that the intense and persistent public interest in these tragic events is disproportionate to their significance in numerical terms. However, such data are limited, and there is circumstantial evidence that the overall importance of this public health problem may have been underestimated. Regardless of prevalence, however, the social and emotional impact of an athlete dying suddenly (often fueled by the news media) is substantial, given the widely held perception that trained athletes epitomize the healthiest element of our society.[2]

Sudden death due to cardiovascular disease has been reported in a wide variety of sports, most commonly basketball and football in the United States[1,2] and soccer in Europe,[7,15,21] and is much more common in males (9:1), probably due to the overall lower participation rates of females and their absence from certain competitive sports (e.g., football). HCM is the most common cause of sudden cardiac death in previously undiagnosed young African American male athletes, contrasting sharply with the underrepresentation of African Americans in clinically identified HCM populations.[6] This suggests HCM is underdiagnosed in African Americans and that socioeconomic status and ethnicity may impact significantly on the access to cardiovascular diagnosis and ultimately the clinical identification of this disease.

The association of sudden death and unsuspected cardiovascular disease in young athletes does not appear coincidental.[24] Vigorous physical exertion in the context of competitive sports can act as a trigger for lethal ventricular arrhythmias and sudden death on the athletic field in certain susceptible athletes with underlying structural heart disease.[1-4,6,24] Indeed, most deaths in young athletes (i.e., 90 percent) occur on the athletic field during training or competition, predominantly in the late afternoon and early evening hours corresponding to the peak period of the day for intense physical activity, particularly with organized team sports.[1] Sudden cardiac death is not, however, limited to competitive athletes since similar tragedies can occur in young people during recreational or even sedentary activities.

Clinical Evaluation of Young Athletes

Young trained athletes present a unique challenge for cardiological assessment due to the many diverse alterations in cardiac physiology, structure, rhythm, and ECG pattern that can result from chronic conditioning and occasionally mimic pathological conditions.[2,4] Furthermore, despite the absence of cardiac symptoms, such highly conditioned individuals can in fact harbor unsuspected cardiovascular disease.[1,2,6,7]

Suspicion of cardiovascular disease in a trained athlete may arise by virtue of findings on preparticipation screening, onset of symptoms such as syncope, or fortuitously by recognition of a heart murmur on routine examination.[2,11] Thereafter, the preferred strategy should focus on systematically targeting with testing each of the heart diseases known to cause sudden death in young people until a cardiovascular abnormality is identified or each is effectively excluded (with priority afforded the most common). Since most of these causes of sudden death in young athletes are structural and functional abnormalities (e.g., HCM, coronary anomalies, valvular heart disease, ARVC, and myocarditis), tests such as echocardiography and possibly MRI become important implements in the differential diagnosis. Standard 12-lead

TABLE 76–1 Preoperative Laboratory Evaluation of Patients Undergoing Cardiac Surgery—cont'd

Preoperative Laboratory Test	Abnormal Finding	Comment
	3. Elevated pulmonary artery pressure (and pulmonary vascular resistance)	3. Fixed pulmonary vascular resistance should be suspected when the pulmonary artery diastolic pressure exceeds the mean pulmonary capillary wedge pressure. Vigorous oxygenation and pharmacological support with a pulmonary vasodilator (isoproterenol, prostaglandin E) are important in such cases. Patients with a pulmonary artery diastolic pressure equal to the pulmonary capillary wedge pressure usually have more rapid resolution of pulmonary hypertension postoperatively.
	4. LV mural thrombus	4. Increased risk of stroke perioperatively.
	5. Status of internal mammary arteries	5. Highly desirable arterial conduits for planned revascularization surgery.[40,41] Particular care is required during reoperation if patent internal mammary artery bypass is in place from previous surgery.
	6. Status of saphenous vein grafts	6. "Pseudoextravasation" of dye outside the lumen in a patent graft with slow flow probably represents thrombus-filled atherosclerotic aneurysm of the graft.
Vascular Doppler	1. Carotid stenosis	1. Suggests and increased risk of perioperative stroke. If symptomatic or if stenosis >80%, consideration for combined or staged carotid surgery.
	2. Aortic iliac disease	2. May contraindicate insertion of an intraaortic balloon pump and suggests increased risk of peripheral vascular complications.
	3. Absent or varicosed veins	3. In patients with severe varicosities or who have undergone venous stripping, alternative conduits such as bilateral internal mammary arteries or radial grafts must be considered.

BUN = blood urea nitrogen; FEV_1 = volume of air expired in 1 second; GI = gastrointestinal; Hct = hematocrit; LV = left ventricular; PT = prothrombin time; PTT = partial prothrombin time; RV = right ventricular; VC = vital capacity; WBC = white blood cell count.

TABLE 76–2 Risk Factors, Definitions, and Weights (Score)

Risk Factor	Definition	Score
Patient-Related Factors		
Age	Per 5 years or part thereof >60 yr)	1
Sex	Female	1
Chronic pulmonary disease	Long-term use of bronchodilators or steroids for lung disease	1
Extracardiac arteriopathy	Any one or more of the following: claudication, carotid occlusion or >50% stenosis, previous or planned intervention on the abdominal aorta, limb arteries, or carotid arteries	2
Neurological dysfunction	Disease severely affecting ambulation or day-to-day functioning	2
Previous cardiac surgery	Requiring opening of the pericardium	3
Serum creatinine	>200 μmol/liter preoperatively	2
Active endocarditis	Patient still receiving antibiotic treatment for endocarditis at the time of surgery	3
Critical preoperative state	Any one or more of the following: ventricular tachycardia or fibrillation or aborted sudden death, preoperative cardiac massage, preoperative ventilation before arrival in the operating room, preoperative inotropic support, intraaortic balloon counterpulsation, or preoperative acute renal failure (anuria or oliguria <10 ml/hr)	3
Cardiac-Related Factors		
Unstable angina	Rest angina requiring IV nitrates until arrival in the operating room	2
LV dysfunction	Moderate or LVEF 0.30-0.50 Poor or LVEF <0.30	1 3
Recent myocardial infarct	<90 days	2
Pulmonary hypertension	Systolic PA pressure >60 mm Hg	2
Operation-Related Factors		
Emergency	Carried out on referral before the beginning of the next working day	2
Other than isolated CABG	Major cardiac procedure other than or in addition to CABG	2
Surgery on thoracic aorta	For disorder of ascending, arch, or descending aorta	3
Postinfarct septal rupture		4

CABG = coronary artery bypass grafting; IV = intravenous; LV = left ventricular; LVEF = LV ejection fraction; PA = pulmonary artery.

severity scoring helps to identify patients at high risk for operative mortality (score > 6). By assembling and reviewing the data necessary for accurate assessment of a patient's operative risk, cardiologists can help with the appropriate clinical triage of patients, contain hospital costs, and facilitate consultations with other medical specialists (e.g., dialysis team) as needed. Patients at increased risk of mediastinal infection include the elderly and those with morbid obesity, diabetes mellitus, malnutrition, severe pulmonary disease that is likely to lead to prolonged postoperative ventilatory support, or macromastia in women.[52-54]

VENTRICULAR DYSFUNCTION. An especially important aspect of the preoperative evaluation of a cardiac surgical patient involves estimating the extent of underlying ventricular dysfunction. Un-revascularized viable myocardium after myocardial infarction likely serves as a substrate for recurrent ischemic events.[55-61] Also, patients with severe multivessel disease and akinetic myocardial zones who have chronic congestive heart failure as a result of hibernating myocardium (see Chap. 50) experience improved ventricular function after CABG.[55] Contemporary techniques that should be used for assessing myocardial viability in dysfunctional regions include imaging procedures that correlate perfusion with cell membrane integrity (thallium reperfusion), metabolic activity (positron-emission tomography), regional myocardial strain (magnetic resonance imaging), or contractile reserve (stress echocardiography) (see Chap. 16).[55-57,61] Clinicians should rely on imaging modalities with which they are most familiar and that are available at their institution. In addition to viability, the same imaging modalities can localize akinetic or dyskinetic segments. Patients with severe ventricular dysfunction as well as regional wall akinesia or dyskinesia may benefit from surgical ventricular restoration (Dor procedure) designed to restore mechanically the left ventricle to a more normal size and shape.[58]

The possibility of *right ventricular dysfunction* deserves careful consideration (see Table 76–1), particularly in patients with preoperatively elevated pulmonary artery systolic pressure (>60 mm Hg), a history of inferoposterior left ventricular infarction (which may be associated with right ventricular infarction), or longstanding tricuspid regurgitation. Patients with right ventricular dysfunction should receive an inotropic agent with vasodilating actions such as milrinone (0.5 μg/kg/min) or dobutamine (5 μg/kg/min) in addition to supplemental oxygen perioperatively in an attempt to lower pulmonary vascular resistance and improve right ventricular systolic performance. Intravenous nitrate infusions in the perioperative period have also been shown to reduce pulmonary hypertension and ameliorate right ventricular failure. Inhaled agents, including aerosolized prostacyclin and nitric oxide, can lower pulmonary vascular resistance and improve perioperative right ventricular performance.[62] Recombinant human B-type natriuretic peptide (BNP) is a promising new agent with pharmacological properties favorable for the treatment of right sided heart failure. Its ability to reduce markedly pulmonary vascular resistance and central venous pressure with mild systemic vasodilation may aid the management of selected patients.[63,64]

Patients with mitral regurgitation and severe heart failure should undergo preoperative afterload reduction with such agents as oral angiotensin-converting enzyme (ACE) inhibitors and intravenous sodium nitroprusside to a systolic pressure of about 90 to 100 mm Hg. Potential contraindications to such preoperative afterload reduction include concomitant severe aortic stenosis and hemodynamically significant cerebral or renal vascular disease. In these patients, early intervention with intraaortic balloon counterpulsation may be useful. This population may also benefit from preoperative tailored therapy with BNP in an ICU setting with pulmonary artery catheter monitoring to document lowering of pulmonary artery pressures and improved cardiac output. Intraaortic balloon support is also commonly used in the setting of severe decompensation from acute mitral regurgitation secondary to conditions such as papillary muscle rupture. Infarct-related ventricular septal defect may also require pharmacological and intraaortic balloon support in the perioperative period.

TABLE 76–3 Logistic Regression Model of EuroSCORE in the 1995 Pilot Study

Variables	Beta Coefficient
Age (continuous)	0.0666354
Female	0.3304052
Serum creatinine >200 μmol/liter	0.6521653
Extracardiac arteriopathy	0.6558917
Pulmonary disease	0.4931341
Neurological dysfunction	0.841626
Previous cardiac surgery	1.002625
Recent myocardial infarction	0.5460218
LVEF 0.30-0.50	0.4191643
LVEF <0.30	1.094443
Systolic pulmonary pressure >60 mm Hg	0.7676924
Active endocarditis	1.101265
Unstable angina	0.5677075
Emergency operation	0.7127953
Critical preoperative state	0.9058132
Ventricular septal rupture	1.462009
Other than isolated coronary surgery	0.5420364
Thoracic aortic surgery	1.159787
Constant (β_0)	−4.789594

LVEF = left ventricular ejection fraction. Full definitions of these variables are published and can be seen on-line (http://www.euroscore.org).

TABLE 76–4 Application of Scoring System

EuroSCORE	Patients	Died	95% Confidence Limits for Mortality: *Observed*	95% Confidence Limits for Mortality: *Expected*
0-2 (low risk)	4,529	36 (0.8%)	(0.56-1.10)	(1.27-1.29)
3-5 (medium risk)	5,977	182 (3.0%)	(2.62-3.51)	(2.90-2.94)
6 plus (high risk)	4,293	480 (11.2%)	(10.25-12.16)	(10.93-11.54)
Total	14,799	698 (4.7%)	(4.37-5.06)	(4.72-4.95)

TABLE 76–5 EuroSCORE Risk Profile: 66-year-old Female with COPD, Recent Myocardial Infarction for Isolated CABG

		Additive EuroSCORE	Logistic EuroSCORE *βi Xi*
Patient Factors			
Age	**66 yr**	**2**	**0.546775405**
Sex	☐ Female		
Chronic pulmonary disease	☑ Yes	**1**	**0.4931341**
Extracardiac arteriopathy	☐ Yes		
Neurological dysfunction	☐ Yes		
Previous cardiac surgery	☐ Yes		
Serum creatinine >200 μmol/liter	☐ Yes		
Active endocarditis	☐ Yes		
Critical preoperative state	☐ Yes		
Cardiac Factors			
Unstable angina	☐ Yes		
LV dysfunction moderate or LVEF 30-50%	☐ Moderate		
LV dysfunction poor or LVEF <30	☐ Poor		
Recent myocardial infarct	☑ Yes	**2**	**0.5460218**
Pulmonary hypertension	☐ Yes		
Operation Factors			
Emergency	☐ Yes		
Other than isolated CABG	☐ Yes		
Surgery on thoracic aorta	☐ Yes		
Postinfarct septal rupture	☐ Yes		
EuroSCORE		**5**	**3.90%**

Downloaded from http://euroscore.org.

CABG = coronary artery bypass grafting; COPD = chronic obstructive pulmonary disease; LV = left ventricular; LVEF = LV ejection fraction.

RISK OF MYOCARDIAL ISCHEMIA. Acute thrombolytic and interventional catheterization treatment regimens for acute myocardial infarction may not successfully restore coronary perfusion because of inadequate thrombolysis, reocclusion of the infarct-related artery following initially successful thrombolysis, or dissection/acute thrombosis of the target vessel during angioplasty.[65,66] Identification of patients for referral for emergency bypass surgery and decisions regarding the timing of such surgery remain a challenging clinical problem, particularly in view of the high perioperative mortality rate for patients who require surgery within 24 to 48 hours of thrombolysis.[66,67]

Potential indications for emergency bypass surgery following failed attempts at reperfusion in acute myocardial infarction include significant left main stenosis and inability to maintain patency of the infarct-related artery, severe multivessel coronary artery disease with anatomy unsuitable for angioplasty and ischemic dysfunction of the noninfarct zones, and inability to maintain patency of an infarct-related artery that places a large amount of myocardium in jeopardy (proximal left anterior descending) in patients with an infarct of less than 6 hours' duration. Although some clinical reports suggest that patients in cardiogenic shock who undergo urgent revascularization have improved survival in comparison to those who are not revascularized, these series suffer from potential selection bias, and definitive recommendations regarding the management of patients with cardiogenic shock and acute myocardial infarction must await the results of ongoing randomized trials.[65]

Patients who are referred for emergency revascularization surgery should be supported by an intraaortic balloon pump and, if technically feasible, an intracoronary perfusion catheter. Other methods for mechanical assistance of the failing circulation are described in Chapter 25. Because patients who undergo emergency bypass surgery within 6 to 12 hours of administration of a thrombolytic agent are at greater risk for intraoperative and postoperative hemorrhage, they should receive a hemostatic agent such as aprotinin (2 million kallikrein-inhibiting units [KIU] over a 20-minute period, followed by a continuous infusion of 500,000 KIU/hr).[68]

Patients with other manifestations of an acute coronary syndrome such as active, unstable angina may also be in tenuous hemodynamic balance as they proceed to the operating room, particularly if significant left main coronary artery stenosis or severe three-vessel coronary artery disease coexists with left ventricular dysfunction and/or mitral regurgitation. Delays while awaiting surgery and the time between the induction of anesthesia and the institution of cardiopulmonary bypass are high-risk periods during which a vicious spiral of myocardial ischemia and low-output syndrome can rapidly develop. Such patients should be protected by an intraaortic balloon pump inserted preoperatively and an infusion of nitroglycerin.

The risk of recurrent myocardial ischemia must be carefully weighed against the risk of early surgical intervention in patients sustaining a transmural myocardial infarction. Recent data suggest that the risk of coronary bypass surgery is high during the first several days following transmural injury, and a waiting period of 4 to 7 days should be sought unless patients are experiencing active, ongoing refractory myocardial ischemia or hemodynamic instability.[69,70] Preoperative intra-aortic balloon support may be extremely useful in stabilizing patients in the clinical setting of transmural injury.[71]

ANESTHESIA FOR CARDIAC SURGERY. The details of the practice of cardiac anesthesia are beyond the scope of this chapter and are available in other sources (see Chap. 77).[72,73] High-dose synthetic narcotics that do not cause vasodilation, such as fentanyl and sufentanil, have replaced morphine in many centers. Most cardiac units currently employ early extubation protocols for patients with low or moderate risk. Advantages of early extubation include a decrease in respiratory complications, ventilatory support, and length of stay in the ICU. To achieve early extubation within 6 hours of surgery, anesthetic techniques have included combinations of inhalational anesthetics, such as enflurane and isoflurane, together with low to moderate amounts of intravenous opioids, such as fentanyl and sufentanil, along with the intravenous anesthetic propofol. The newer, inhaled anesthetics that have replaced nitrous oxide still have the potential to cause vasodilation. Patients with critical aortic stenosis, critical mitral stenosis, and large right-to-left shunts may experience a dramatic reduction in cardiac output because ventricular stroke volume falls with a reduction in preload. Preoperative volume expansion and even administration of vasopressor agents may be necessary to avoid this problem.

Special attention in the perioperative setting should be focused on controlling heart rate and preventing intraoperative anemia or hypothermia to decrease the risk of myocardial injury and in-hospital mortality in patients undergoing CABG (Fig. 76–1).[74-76]

RHYTHM DEVICES AND CARDIAC SURGERY. Patients with high-grade (third-degree or type II second-degree) atrioventricular block and hemodynamic compromise (systolic pressure < 90 mm Hg) are at high risk during general anesthesia unless a temporary transvenous pacemaker wire or a flow-directed pacing system is inserted perioperatively. In a patient with a permanent pacemaker, its specifications (model, mode, and settings) and, if possible, a statement regarding the pacemaker dependency of the patient should be noted in the medical record (see Chap. 31). The possibility of postoperative malfunction in the permanent pacing system because of the effects of anesthesia, electrocautery, and surgical manipulation of the leads (e.g., during atrial cannulation) should be anticipated. Clinicians should have the appropriate pacemaker programming equipment available postoperatively because many problems (secondary to electromagnetic interference from the electrocautery apparatus) can be quickly resolved by interrogation of the generator and reprogramming in the recovery area. Patients with previously implanted cardioverter-defibrillator devices should have their unit disabled prior to surgery to minimize the risk of inappropriate shocks from sensing of electrocautery signals intraoperatively. Until the device is reactivated in the postoperative period, equipment for rapid external defibrillation should be available.

PERIOPERATIVE DRUG THERAPY. With the exception of oral anticoagulation with warfarin, most medications can and should be continued up to the time of surgery. Clinical trials of patients receiving saphenous vein bypass grafts demonstrated the importance of initiating antiplatelet therapy in the perioperative period. Because of the increased risk of postoperative bleeding, in the past some surgical groups discontinued aspirin use for several days preoperatively in elective

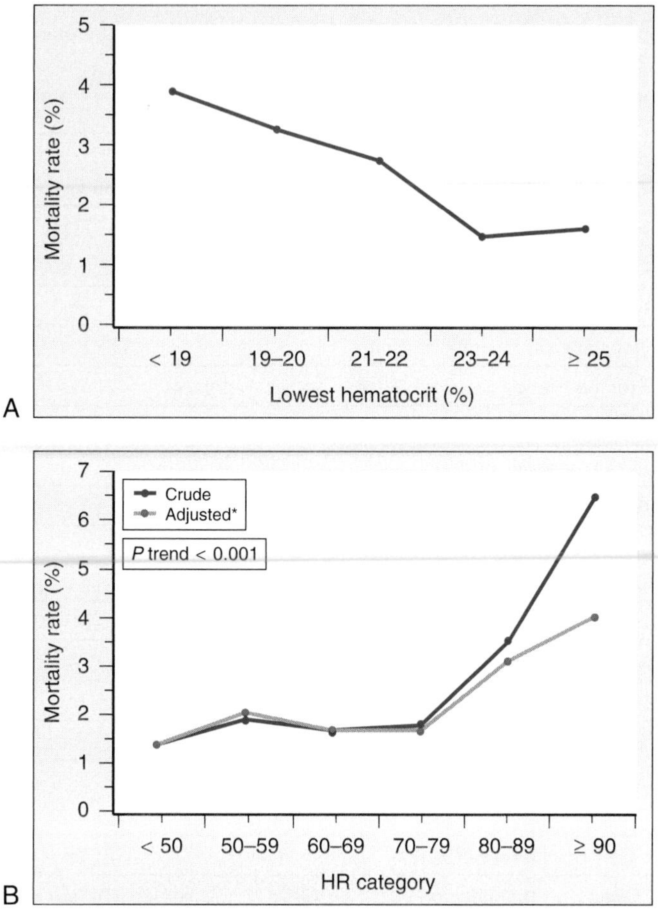

FIGURE 76–1 Intraoperative variables factors influencing mortality in coronary artery bypass patients. **A,** Adjusted mortality rates by lowest hematocrit on cardiopulmonary bypass. **B,** Preinduction heart rate (HR) and in-hospital mortality crude and adjusted rates. In both **A** and **B,** rates are adjusted for the following variables: age, sex, body surface area, comorbidity score, prior coronary artery bypass graft, ejection fraction, left ventricular end-diastolic pressure, and priority at surgery. (**A,** From DeFoe GR, Ross CS, Olmstead EM, et al: Lowest hematocrit on bypass and adverse outcomes associated with coronary artery bypass grafting. Ann Thorac Surg 71:769-776, 2001; and **B,** From Fillinger MP, Surgenor SD, Hartman GS, et al: The association between heart rate and in-hospital mortality after coronary artery bypass graft surgery. Anesth Analg 85:1483-1488, 2002.)

cases. Because of the risk of "breakthrough" episodes of ischemia if aspirin therapy is discontinued preoperatively, most cardiologists currently prefer to continue it up to the time of surgery and rely on preoperative donations of autologous red blood cells, cell-saver techniques, autotransfusion of shed blood intraoperatively, and antitibrinolytic drugs such as aprotinin to minimize the need for and potential hazards of homologous blood transfusion. If aspirin is withheld preoperatively, it should be restarted within 24 to 48 hours after surgery to reduce the risk of vein graft occlusion. Warfarin therapy should be stopped 2 to 3 days preoperatively and, if necessary, treatment with heparin or low-molecular-weight heparin initiated.

Although definitive data are not available, we usually continue both aspirin and clopidogrel up to the time of surgery in patients who have undergone implantation of a stent in the coronary circulation within the preceding 2 weeks to minimize the risk of stent thrombosis preoperatively. For patients who have had a stent implanted more than 2 weeks prior to surgery, we discontinue clopidogrel administration but continue aspirin up to the time of surgery. For patients receiving long-term clopidogrel as secondary prevention for vascular disease, we discontinue use of the drug 5 to 7 days preoperatively when feasible.

To minimize the risk of intraoperative bleeding, if patients are undergoing percutaneous intervention and have normal renal function and if cardiac surgery is likely to take place within the ensuing 24 to 48 hours, we prefer to use a short-acting intravenous glycoprotein IIb/IIIa inhibitor such as eptifibatide or tirofiban rather than a long-acting agent such as abciximab. Treatment with the short-acting agent is usually discontinued 6 to 12 hours preoperatively to permit platelet function to return toward normal. We prefer to use abciximab in patients with renal dysfunction since the small, short-acting inhibitors are cleared predominantly through renal elimination. When abciximab is used, we discontinue the infusion at least 12 hours prior to surgery.

For patients who have received an intravenous glycoprotein IIb/IIIa inhibitor and must proceed urgently to cardiac surgery, the antiplatelet effects of abciximab may be reversed by platelet transfusions.[77] In contrast, the high excess of free drug versus bound drug in the case of eptifibatide or tirofiban limits the ability of platelet transfusions to restore normal platelet function. In cases in which urgent removal of eptifibatide or tirofiban from the circulation is desired, hemodialysis may be necessary.

Calcium channel antagonists previously prescribed for control of ischemic heart disease should be continued up to the time of surgery to reduce the chance of myocardial ischemia from withdrawal of the drug. In the case of diltiazem and verapamil, the dose may need to be reduced because these agents may provoke bradycardia and a low-output syndrome postoperatively, especially if a beta-blocking agent or amiodarone is given concurrently or if the patient is elderly. Profound atropine- and isoproterenol-resistant bradyarrhythmias may occur postoperatively in patients treated with these calcium channel antagonists, particularly when the patient has not yet recovered from the hypothermia that is imposed intraoperatively; temporary dual-chamber pacing support should be available to manage such patients. Postoperative systemic hypotension is also common in patients receiving preoperative ACE inhibitors, and pharmacological strategies to increase systemic vascular resistance including vasopressin or norepinephrine maybe useful in selected patients.[78]

CONTINUATION OF ANTIARRHYTHMICS. With the exception of amiodarone, antiarrhythmic drugs that have been prescribed for hemodynamically compromising or life-threatening ventricular tachyarrhythmias should be continued up to the time of surgery because of the risk of breakthrough of a potentially lethal ventricular arrhythmia in the preoperative period.

Patients with a documented history of resuscitation from sudden cardiac death who are receiving amiodarone should continue to receive this drug up to the time of surgery. However, in cases in which amiodarone was prescribed for a less overtly life-threatening arrhythmia (e.g., atrial fibrillation), the maintenance dosage has been more than 200 mg/d, and the patient has a history of lung disease, we would consider omission of the drug for at least 3 months before subjecting the patient to elective cardiopulmonary bypass.

IMPLANTABLE CARDIOVERTER-DEFIBRILLATORS. Prophylactic implantation of cardioverter-defibrillators at the time of CABG in patients at high risk for ventricular arrhythmias (ejection fraction ≤ 0.35, abnormal signal-averaged electrocardiogram [ECG]) does not improve survival according to the results of the CABG-PATCH trial.[78a]

Intraoperative Management

Despite increased risks, particularly related to age and advanced disease, cardiac surgery patients today enjoy markedly improved outcomes when compared with patients operated on 10 years ago. Important intraoperative surgical advances that have contributed to this improved outcome include epiaortic echocardiographic scanning in patients with ascending aortic atherosclerosis (Fig. 76–2), transesophageal echocardiography, retrograde blood cardioplegia, carbon dioxide insufflation to prevent air embolization, vacuum-assisted venous drainage, and performance of all vascular anastomoses with a single aortic cross-clamp under cardioplegic arrest.[15] Emphasis on modern strategies to ensure blood conservation and minimize hemostatic complications has significantly decreased or eliminated homologous blood exposure for most patients undergoing cardiac surgery (Fig. 76–3).

Until the past decade, nearly all cardiac surgical procedures were performed via a standard median sternotomy with the use of cardiopulmonary bypass and cardiac arrest to provide a bloodless, motionless surgical field. Cardiac surgeons have now adopted less invasive approaches to coronary and valvu-

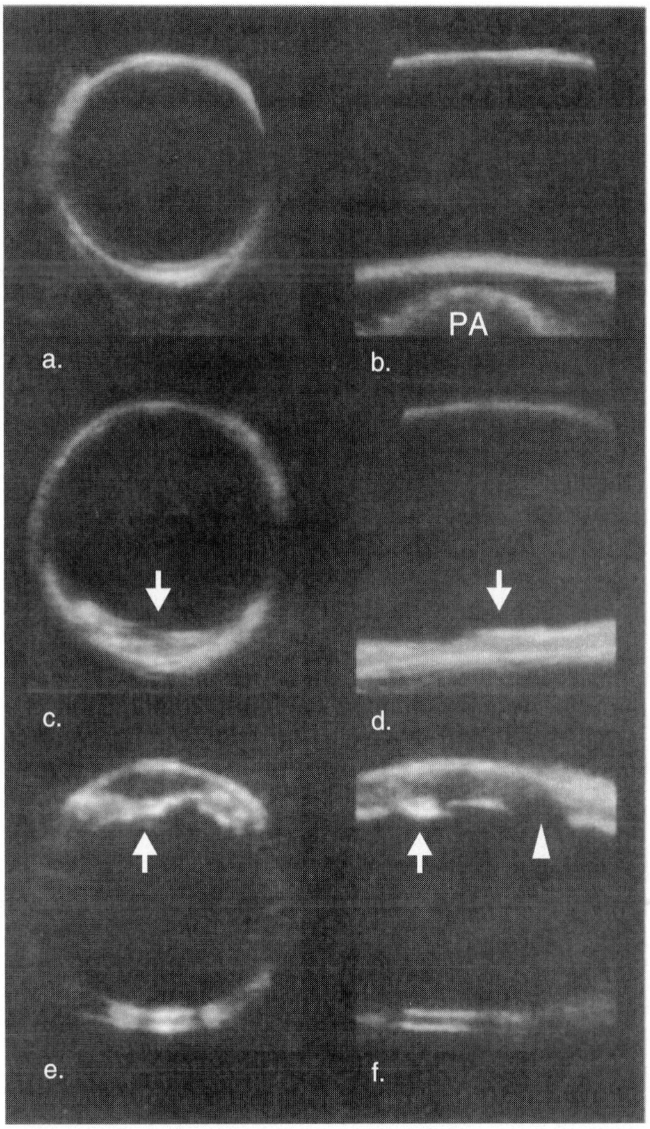

FIGURE 76–2 Ultrasonographic images of the ascending aorta, demonstrating transverse (a, c, and e) and longitudinal scans (b, d, and f). Panels a and b illustrate a normal patient. Panels c and d reveal a moderate arteriosclerosis (arrow). Panels e and f demonstrate typical severe arteriosclerosis (arrow) and ulcerated plaque (arrowhead) of the ascending aorta. PA = pulmonary artery. (From Goto T, Baba T, Matsuyama K, et al: Aortic atherosclerosis and postoperative neurological dysfunction in elderly coronary surgical patients. Ann Thorac Surg 75:1912-1918, 2003.)

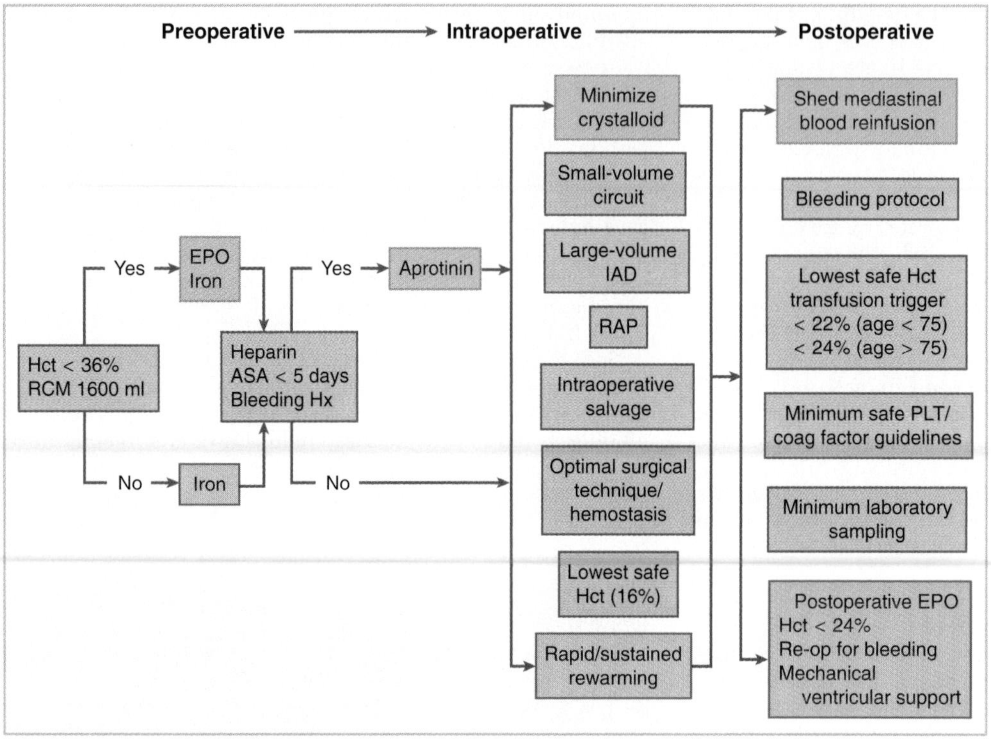

FIGURE 76–3 Multimodality algorithm designed to optimize blood conservation in cardiac surgical patients. Preoperative, intraoperative, and postoperative strategies all are important to eliminate the requirement for homologous blood transfusion. ASA = aspirin; coag = coagulation; EPO = erythropoietin; Hct = hematocrit; Hx = history; IAD = intraoperative autologous donation; PLT = platelet; RAP = retrograde autologous priming; RCM = red blood cell mass. (From Rosengart TK: Open heart surgery without transfusion in high-risk patients. Am J Cardiol 83:31B-37B, 1999.)

lar heart disease. The impetus for this change has been to decrease overall surgical trauma associated with full sternotomy and cardiopulmonary bypass without compromising the efficacy and safety of procedures. In valvular heart disease, cardiopulmonary bypass is essential, and therefore the focus has been on reducing trauma through a variety of less invasive incisions (Fig. 76–4). In coronary surgery, smaller incisions have also been used with or without cardiopulmonary bypass, particularly to perform single-vessel bypass to the left anterior descending artery. Recent technical advances in myocardial stabilization (Fig. 76–5) have now focused attention on off-pump multivessel coronary bypass through a full sternotomy.[79] This approach is particularly appealing in selected high-risk patients, including those with ascending aortic atherosclerosis, renal dysfunction, and severe pulmonary disease. Continued adoption of less invasive cardiac surgical techniques can be anticipated if ongoing clinical trials demonstrate medium- and long-term results comparable to those obtained with standard techniques.[79-86b]

Postoperative Management

Fluid, Electrolyte, and Acid-Base Balance

Extracorporeal circulation is associated with an increase in extracellular fluid and total exchangeable sodium, along with a decrease in exchangeable potassium. The cumulative experience in many centers has led to the following basic principles of management:

1. For the first 48 hours after surgery, free water is limited to about 1000 ml/d and intravenous fluids are administered in the form of dextrose (5%) in water. Sodium replacement varies with volume needs but is usually limited to 4 gm/liter.
2. Serum potassium levels can fluctuate dramatically; therefore, frequent measurement of serum potassium is indicated, especially in diabetic patients. We attempt to maintain serum potassium in the range of 4.5 ± 0.5 mEq/liter and magnesium at 2.0 mEq/liter or greater to minimize cardiac arrhythmias.
3. Serum glucose levels are frequently elevated (250 to 400 mg/dl), as a result of glucose-containing intravenous solutions and surgically induced increases in cortisol and catecholamine levels. Contemporary series have shown the importance of tight control of postoperative blood glucose levels to decrease morbidity following coronary bypass surgery. Protocols to maintain aggressively serum glucose levels to less than 150 mg/dl by continuous insulin infusion should be utilized in postoperative patients.[87-89]
4. Mild metabolic acidosis or metabolic alkalosis may be present for the first 24 hours postoperatively, particularly during rewarming. These acid-base abnormalities usually do not require correction in the absence of preoperative renal dysfunction or development of acute renal failure postoperatively. Significant metabolic acidosis (pH < 7.35) should be avoided during the rewarming phase, particularly if patients are dependent on an inotropic agent. Hyperventilation (P_{CO_2} < 35 mm Hg) and treatment with sodium bicarbonate should be instituted.
5. Serum total calcium, phosphorus, and magnesium levels are frequently depressed for about 24 to 48 hours in normally convalescing patients, partly because of the effects of hemodilution. Hypocalcemia and hypomagnesemia may predispose to the development of cardiac arrhythmias, and replacement therapy is generally warranted.

Respiratory Management

EFFECTS OF ANESTHESIA, STERNOTOMY, AND CARDIOPULMONARY BYPASS ON PULMONARY FUNCTION. To optimize respiratory management, four broad areas should be considered (Table 76–6). Most all patients experience alveolar dysfunction after open-heart surgery because of right-to-left intrapulmonary shunting of blood from various intrinsic alveolar abnormalities (e.g., atelectasis, edema, infection) and pulmonary vascular events (e.g., extravasation of fluid, inhibition of hypoxia-induced vasoconstriction).[90] Central respiratory drive and respiratory muscle function are depressed postoperatively because of a combination of pharmacological effects and mechanical derangements of thoracic function. Patients with preexisting pulmonary disease may experience more profound depression of respiratory function, necessitating vigorous pulmonary toilette.

EARLY EXTUBATION. Historically, most postoperative cardiac surgery patients received between 6 and 18 hours of ventilatory support. Early extubation protocols have now been widely adopted in cardiac ICUs, and stable patients are extubated within 4 hours (Table 76–7). Advantages of early extubation include improved patient mobility with early transition to step-down units.

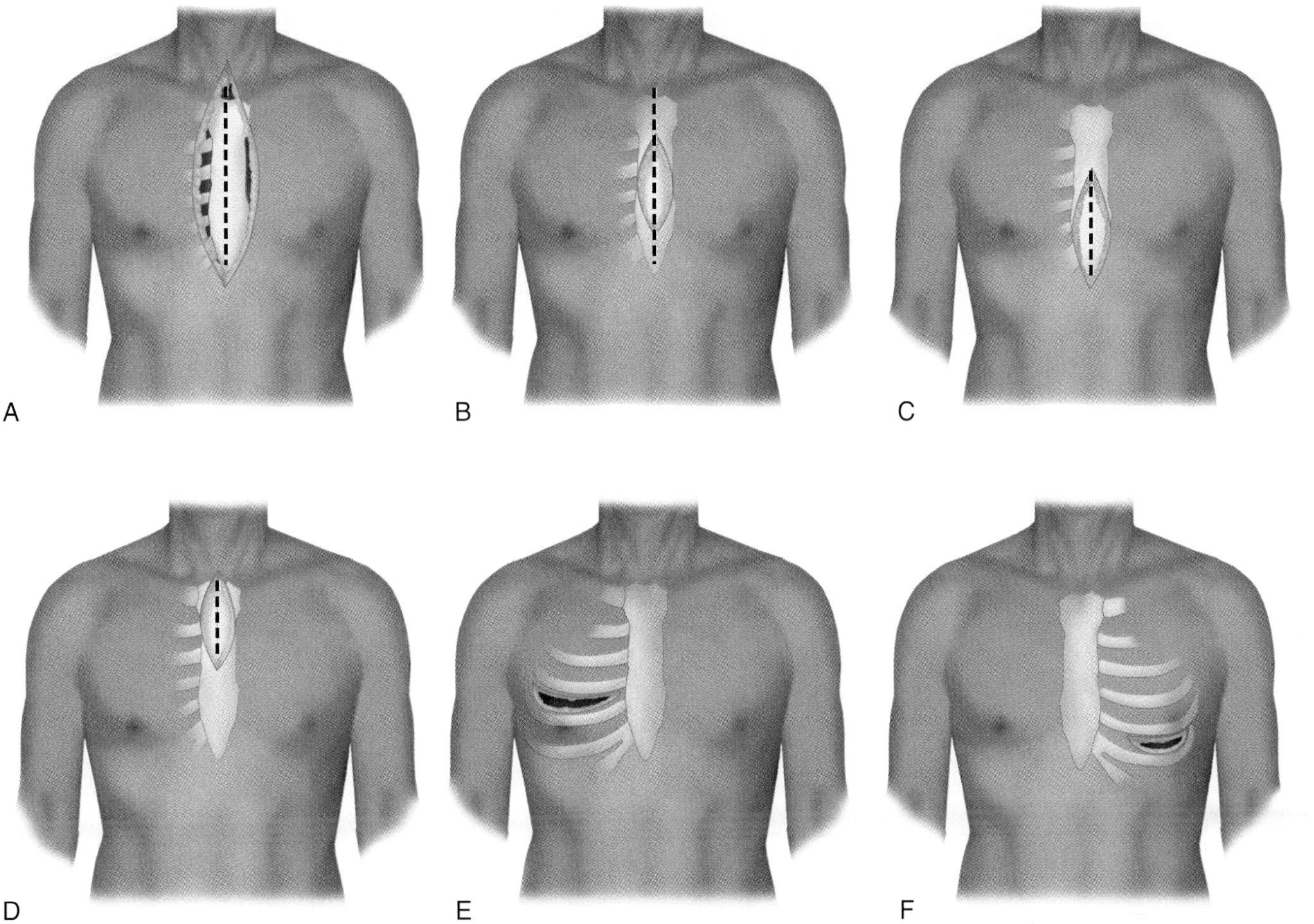

FIGURE 76–4 Schematic representation of traditional incision and sternotomy **(A)** compared with a variety of less invasive incisions (dotted lines represent chest wall incisions). Limited skin incision/full sternotomy **(B)** is gaining in popularity because of improved cosmetics and reduced trauma from the limited chest wall retraction. Partial lower or upper sternotomy **(C** and **D)** has been used predominantly in valve procedures. Limited right anterior thoracotomy **(E)** is a useful approach, particularly in mitral valve reoperations. Left anterior small thoracotomy **(F)** is currently used in robotic-assisted coronary bypass surgery.

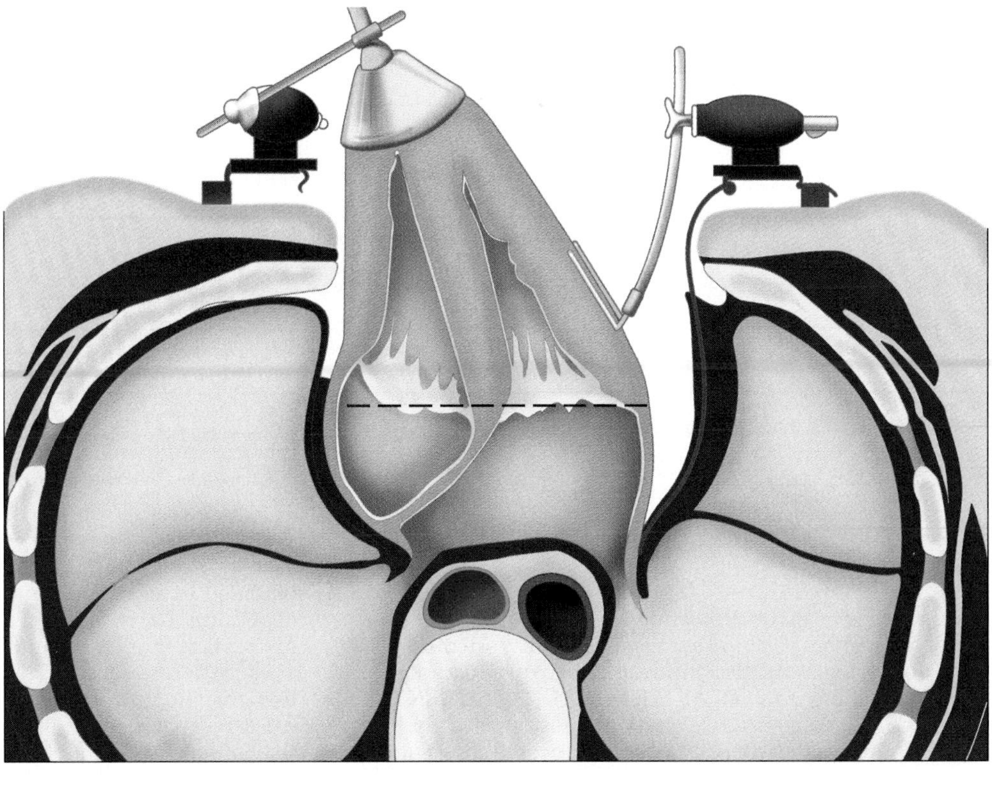

FIGURE 76–5 Off-pump coronary bypass surgery on the beating heart has been greatly facilitated by the development of positioning devices and platform stabilization systems. Positioning devices using apical suction cups **(left, top)** now allow optimal exposure of the posterolateral circulation while minimizing hemodynamic compromise. Platform stabilization systems **(right, top)** provide isolated immobilization during the performance of distal anastomoses.

TABLE 76–6 Abnormalities of Respiratory Function After Cardiac Surgery

Effects of Anesthesia, Thoracic Surgery, and Cardiopulmonary Bypass on Pulmonary Function	Potential Causes
Alveolar dysfunction (e.g., widened alveolar-arterial oxygen gradient because of right-to-left intrapulmonary shunting)	Scattered regions of atelectasis with preserved perfusion Pulmonary edema (e.g., cardiogenic, noncardiogenic "postpump" alveolar capillary leak) Pleural effusion Pneumothorax Infection Inhibition of hypoxic pulmonary vasoconstriction by anesthetic agents Exacerbation of ventilation/perfusion mismatch by vasodilating agents used postoperatively (e.g., nitroprusside)
Decreased central respiratory drive	General anesthetics Narcotic analgesics Cerebral insult in perioperative period
Decreased respiratory muscle function	Thoracic pain (incision, chest tubes) Persistent effects of muscle relaxants Age Obesity Depressed cardiac function Primary diaphragmatic dysfunction (e.g., phrenic nerve injury)
Exacerbation of underlying chronic pulmonary disease	Increase in airway resistance Increased secretions and worsening bronchitis Pneumonia Ventilatory management

TABLE 76–7 Cardiac Surgery Early Extubation Protocol

Definition	Extubation Within 4 hr after Surgery
Patient selection	
Inclusion criteria	All patients ≤80 yr old, LV ejection fraction >0.50
Excusion criteria	High inotropic requirement, postoperative bleeding or ischemia, severe pulmonary hypertension
Anesthetic management	
Intraoperative	Low-dose synthetic narcotics and inhalation agents
Postoperative	Muscle relaxant reversal Propofol 0.1 ml/kg/hr Minimize narcotic use
Ventilatory management	
Postoperative	SIMV mode Check ABGs and decrease ventilatory support every 20 min Always keep between pH 7.35 and 7.45 Always keep $pO_2 > 75$ mm Hg
Exubation guidelines	
Oxygenation	$pO_2 > 75$ mm Hg at an $FIO_2 \leq 0.50$
Respiratory drive	$pCO_2 < 45$ mm Hg and pH > 7.35 Spontaneously breathing
Mechanics	Respiratory rate < 25 breaths/min Negative inspiratory pressure > 20 cm H_2O Tidal volume > 8 ml/kg Vital capacity > 10 ml/kg
Airway protection	Alert with gag reflex Absence of heavy secretions
Cardiovascular	Cardiac index > 2.0 liter/min·m^{-2} MAP > 80 and < 120 mm Hg

ABG = arterial blood gas; LV = left ventricular; MAP = mean arterial pressure; SIMV = synchronized intermittent mandatory ventilation.

Special Problems

Failure to meet early extubation criteria may result from a variety of factors. Careful assessment usually identifies one or more etiologies resulting in respiratory dysfunction.

INCREASED ALVEOLAR-ARTERIAL GRADIENT. An increased alveolar-arterial gradient postoperatively is a serious problem that demands thorough evaluation. The ventilator settings should be checked and a chest radiograph obtained to ascertain the position of the tip of the endotracheal tube (to exclude, for example, intubation of the right main stem bronchus) and to rule out pneumothorax, lobar atelectasis or pneumonia, or a large pleural effusion. Hemodynamic monitoring by means of a pulmonary artery catheter can rarely cause pulmonary hemorrhage from overinflation of the balloon, and bronchoscopy may need to be performed to diagnose and manage the problem (e.g., occlusion of the bronchus draining the bleeding segment of the lung).

PULMONARY EDEMA. The most common cause of pulmonary edema postoperatively is elevated pulmonary venous pressure arising from left ventricular dysfunction. Patients with increased risk of pulmonary edema require aggressive diuresis, as well as vasodilator/inotropic and possibly intraaortic balloon support. Mechanical ventilation with positive end-expiratory pressure (PEEP) is used until the patient's ventricular function improves. A less common cause of postoperative respiratory failure is residual mitral regurgitation in a patient not undergoing concomitant mitral valve surgery at the time of other cardiac surgery. Repeat surgery may be needed if pulmonary edema persists despite attempts to control mitral regurgitation medically.[91,92]

In a few patients, pulmonary edema after cardiac surgery is due to adult respiratory distress syndrome. In its most extreme form, this disorder is associated with a generalized condition characterized by increased capillary permeability, interstitial edema, fever, leukocytosis, renal dysfunction, and occasionally hemodynamic collapse.

UNDERLYING CHRONIC LUNG DISEASE. General surgical preparation of patients with obstructive lung disease, including antibiotics, bronchodilators, and cessation of cigarette smoking, may help minimize the risk of respiratory failure from postoperative atelectasis and pneumonia. Inhaled bronchodilators should be continued postoperatively. Refractory patients may require a short course of corticosteroids (e.g., methylprednisolone 0.5 mg/kg every 6 hours for 3 days) to be weaned from the ventilator. Previous enthusiasm for intravenous methylxanthines has waned because of evidence of limited efficacy and the risk of agitation, arrhythmias, and grand mal seizures. Intravenous theophylline should therefore be reserved for extremely refractory cases and administered in a dose of 0.4 mg/kg/hr, with careful monitoring of plasma levels to maintain them in the range of 10 to 15 μg/ml.[93]

We have successfully operated on patients with severe respiratory compromise, including those with a forced expiratory volume in 1 second (FEV_1) of less than 0.8 liters who require home oxygen therapy. All patients with severe pulmonary dysfunction are considered for early extubation. It is important to maintain the arterial carbon dioxide tension close to the patient's baseline level to ensure an adequate respiratory drive.

DIAPHRAGMATIC FAILURE. Diaphragmatic dysfunction after cardiac surgical procedures usually occurs as a result of injury to the phrenic nerve. An elevated hemidiaphragm may be seen on postoperative radiographs in 25 percent of patients who undergo myocardial preservation, including topical ice slush and harvesting of an internal mammary artery.[94] A simple bedside test of diaphragmatic function is to ask the patient to protrude the umbilicus, a movement that requires diaphragmatic functional integrity. Of note, an elevated hemidiaphragm is not usually associated with increased postoperative morbidity or mortality.

Recovery of the hemidiaphragm to normal position occurs in 80 percent of patients at 1 year and nearly all patients by 2 years postoperatively. Clinically important diaphragmatic dysfunction caused by unilateral or bilateral phrenic nerve injury develops in less than 1 percent of patients after cardiac surgery.

Evidence of diaphragmatic failure includes an inability to wean the patient from the ventilator, vital capacity less than 500 ml, and paradoxical movement of the diaphragm on fluoroscopy (abnormal "sniff" test) or ultrasonography.

PROLONGED VENTILATORY INSUFFICIENCY. Patients who fail to be weaned from the ventilator within 48 hours require special attention. Because of the risk of stress-induced gastritis, H_2 receptor blockers (e.g., ranitidine 50 mg intravenously every 8 to 12 hours) or a mucosal cytoprotective agent (sucralfate 1 gm orally two to four times per day) is administered. Nutritional support is critical to provide metabolic needs and prevent the catabolism of respiratory muscles. Pressure support ventilation strategies are particularly useful for patients in need of prolonged ventilation. Barotrauma is minimized and patient comfort is improved while permitting incremental weaning in small steps.

High-compliance, low-pressure cuff (<20 mm Hg) endotracheal tubes have reduced the risk of mechanical complications (e.g., tracheal stenosis) and permit patients to remain intubated for several weeks. Nonetheless, we believe that patients requiring prolonged ventilatory support beyond 10 to 14 days benefit from a decision to proceed with early tracheostomy.[95] Tracheostomy provides improved patient comfort and greater pulmonary toilet and enhances weaning by minimizing pulmonary dead space. Percutaneous tracheostomy offers the advantage of bedside insertion with minimal surgical trauma and is particularly useful in patients with reasonable ventilatory mechanics but heavy secretions. Recent data suggest that early tracheostomy does not increase the risk of mediastinitis.

Hypertension

Postoperative hypertension has been defined variably in the literature,[96] but we consider it to be present if systolic pressure exceeds 140 mm Hg. The incidence of postoperative hypertension ranges from 40 to 60 percent. It occurs more commonly in patients with a preoperative history of hypertension, prior maintenance therapy with a beta-adrenergic antagonist, and well-preserved left ventricular function.[97] Postoperative hypertension is especially frequent after CABG and surgical relief of left ventricular outflow tract obstruction (e.g., aortic valve replacement, correction of coarctation of the aorta).

The mechanism of postoperative hypertension probably varies from patient to patient but usually includes (1) a "rebound" effect from withdrawal of beta-adrenergic antagonist administered preoperatively; (2) excessive sympathetic nervous system activity with elevated levels of circulating catecholamines (especially norepinephrine); (3) pressor reflexes originating in the heart, great vessels, or coronary arteries; and (4) a drop in aortic pressure proximal to the site of the corrected coarctation with resultant stimulation of aortic and carotid baroreceptors by apparent "hypotension." The renin-angiotensin system is stimulated and peripheral resistance is increased. Sudden exposure of vascular beds downstream from the coarctation to "undamped" aortic pressure can also cause mesenteric arteritis. Other frequent causes of transient hypertension in postoperative cardiac surgery patients include anxiety, pain, hypoxia, and pharyngeal manipulation. The adverse consequences of elevated systemic pressure include an increased risk of postoperative bleeding, suture line disruption, and aortic dissection; elevated left ventricular afterload and a consequent reduction in left ventricular output; and injury to aortocoronary bypass grafts, or postoperative stroke.

Management

Although a variety of agents may be used for treating acute postoperative hypertension, we prefer those that are rapidly acting and titratable and have a short half-life. Nitroglycerin is our first-choice agent, beginning at a dose of 25 μg/min and titrating up to a dose of 300 μg/min. Sodium nitroprusside (0.5 to 2 μg/kg/min) may be required in hypertension refractory to nitroglycerin therapy. Because of its prominent vasodilatory effects, sodium nitroprusside should be administered with caution for the first 3 to 4 hours after surgery since volume shifts may occur during the rewarming phase. Reflex tachycardia is a common side effect of sodium nitroprusside. The ultra-short-acting beta blocker esmolol (50 to 250 μg/kg/min) may be useful in patients with a hyperdynamic circulation. It is initially preferred over longer-acting beta blockers when evaluating patient tolerance to beta blockade (e.g., moderately severe left ventricular dysfunction). The need for transition to oral antihypertensive therapy is assessed on an individual basis; patients with a

TABLE 76–8 Diagnosis of Myocardial Infarction After Cardiac Surgery

Diagnostic Finding	Comment
Symptoms	
Early (<24 hr postop)	Not reliable because of residual effects of anesthesia and postoperative analgesics
Late (>24 hr postop)	Potentially reliable but may be confused with incisional pain and pleuritic pain from chest tubes, pericarditis
Electrocardiogram	
New, persistent Q waves	Most reliable diagnostic finding, but only if the Q waves persist on serial EGGs over several days
Evolutionary ST-T changes	Supportive data favoring the diagnosis or MI only if a typical evolutionary pattern is observed. Because of the effects of cardiopulmonary bypass, hypothermia, postoperative pericarditis, mediastinal chest tubes, and medications (e.g., digitalis), a variety of nonspecific ST-T wave abnormalities may be seen and should not be relied on for diagnosing perioperative MI
Myocardial-specific enzymes	
Total CK	Elevated total CK levels postoperatively may arise from multiple sources, including skeletal muscle in the thorax and calf, as well as myocardium
CK-MB	Myocardial-specific CK may be released from ischemia occurring during cardiopulmonary bypass, as well as myocardial and aortic incisions made intraoperatively (e.g., right atrium for cannulation of the cavae). Because of the nearly universal release of CK-MB, a diagnosis of MI should not be made unless CK-MB is significantly elevated (e.g., >30 units/liter)
Echocardiogram	A regional wall motion abnormality is a helpful finding, particularly if it can be shown to be a new finding by comparison with a peroperative study. Paradoxical motion of the high anterior portion of the interventricular septum is a common finding postoperatively in the absence of MI and should not be taken as the sole evidence of new perioperative myocardial necrosis

CK = creatine kinase; MI = myocardial infarction; ECG = electrocardiogram; postop = postoperative.

preoperative history of hypertension usually require chronic treatment.

Perioperative Myocardial Infarction (see Chap. 46)

Despite modern intraoperative myocardial protection and improvements in surgical technique, some degree of ischemia occurs nearly uniformly during CABG. Only a minority of patients (5 to 15 percent of patients undergoing CABG), however, actually experience a *perioperative myocardial infarction,* even in tertiary care centers currently operating on higher-risk patients, including those with failed percutaneous procedures.[98-100] Potential causes of myocardial ischemia and infarction in the perioperative period include incomplete revascularization; diffuse atherosclerotic disease of the distal coronary arteries; spasm, embolism, or thrombosis of the native coronary vessels or bypass grafts[101-103]; technical problems with graft anastomoses; inadequate myocardial preservation intraoperatively; increased myocardial oxygen needs, as in left ventricular hypertrophy; and hemodynamic derangements in the postoperative period (e.g., hypotension, hypertension, tachycardia). Although initially one might suspect that perioperative myocardial infarction results from occlusion of bypass grafts placed to circumvent diseased coronary arteries, autopsy studies have shown that bypass grafts are usually patent in patients dying of a perioperative myocardial infarction. This observation lends support to the concept that poor myocardial protection or a mismatch between myocardial oxygen supply and demand postoperatively accounts for much of the infarction noted.

DIAGNOSIS. The diagnosis of a myocardial infarction after cardiac surgery is more difficult than at other times because of the nonspecific ST-T wave abnormalities on ECG and nearly universal elevation of creatine kinase (CK) levels postoperatively. A number of diagnostic findings (Table 76–8) must be carefully interpreted and then integrated as shown in the algorithm displayed in Table 76–9. A 12-lead ECG should be obtained immediately on the patient's arrival in the ICU after surgery and no less frequently than once every 24 hours for the first few postoperative days. Measurements of total CK and CK-MB should be made every 8 hours for the first 24 to 36 hours if perioperative myocardial infarction is suspected.

Troponin. Experience with more sensitive serum markers of cardiac injury suggest that cardiac-specific troponin I and troponin T are elevated postoperatively in virtually all patients who undergo CABG.[104,105] Patients who experience a perioperative myocardial infarction release greater quantities of troponin such that serum measurements may remain 10- to 20-fold higher than the upper limit of the reference interval for at least 4 to 5 days postoperatively. Even in patients not experiencing perioperative myocardial infarctions by conventional diagnostic criteria, the relative increase in proteins such as cardiac troponin I over preoperative baseline values is greater than that of CK-MB, which suggests that troponin measurements can detect small amounts of myocardial tissue damage that are not detected by CK-MB.

Electrocardiography. The ECG is the most reliable tool for diagnosing a perioperative myocardial infarction. New and persistent Q waves accompanied by new, persistent, and evolutionary ST-T wave abnormalities are the most helpful criteria. Pathological Q waves resulting from perioperative myocardial infarction may appear with an earlier time course (i.e., immediately on arrival from the operating room) than in a nonrevascularized patient.

Echocardiography. Bedside echocardiograms (transthoracic and if necessary transesophageal) play an important role in establishing the diagnosis of a perioperative myocardial infarction by detecting new regional wall motion abnormalities in cases in which the ECG or serum marker measurements are unclear. It is especially helpful to compare new echocardiograms with the preoperative studies that are almost always available.

RISKS AND CONSEQUENCES OF PERIOPERATIVE INFARCTION. Variables that have been found to correlate with the development of perioperative myocardial infarction in patients undergoing CABG include emergency surgery, aortic cross-clamp time greater than 100 minutes, a recent myocardial infarction (within the prior week), intraoperative tachycardia, intraoperative anemia on cardiopulmonary bypass, left ventricular hypertrophy, and a history of previ-

TABLE 76–9 Algorithm for Diagnosis of Perioperative Myocardial Infarction After Cardiac Surgery

New Qs on ECG	CK-MB >30 IU/Liter	New RWMA On Echo*	Diagnosis	Comment
Yes	Yes	Yes	Definite MI	
Yes	Yes	No	Probable MI	New zone of necrosis not evident on Echo. The persistence of new Q waves and abnormally elevated CK-MB suggests that Q waves are not a "benign" postoperative finding
Yes	No	Yes	Definite MI	CK-MB peak probably missed because of infrequent sampling
Yes	No	No	Possible MI	New Q waves may be false-positive finding
No	Yes	Yes	Probable MI	Non-Q-wave MI
No	Yes	No	MI unlikely	Small non-Q-wave MI cannot be entirely excluded
No	No	Yes	MI unlikely	Removal of "restraining" effect of pericardium may result in new RWMAs, especially in high anterior septal area
No	No	No	No MI	Although small patchy areas of necrosis may be seen histologically, these abnormalities are probably not of clinical significance

Echo = echocardiography; MI = myocardial infarction; RWMA = regional wall motion abnormality; ECG = electrocardiogram.
*Perioperative echocardiography is not *required* for the diagnosis of a perioperative MI but can provide useful supportive data or aid in the diagnosis in unclear cases, especially if obtained acutely.

ous revascularization (either percutaneous transluminal coronary angioplasty or CABG).[100]

Patients with a perioperative myocardial infarction have increased hospital mortality (~10 to 15 percent) when compared with patients undergoing CABG who have not sustained a perioperative myocardial infarction (~1 percent).[100] Characteristics of patients who are especially at risk of increased short-term mortality after a perioperative myocardial infarction include age older than 65 years, unstable angina preoperatively, a myocardial infarction within 1 week before surgery, left ventricular aneurysm, intraventricular conduction disturbance (e.g., left bundle branch block), and the need for reoperation for bleeding. About two-thirds of the postoperative mortality is due to pump failure and one-third is due to malignant ventricular tachyarrhythmias. Perioperative myocardial infarction also adversely affects the long-term prognosis, particularly if associated with inadequate revascularization and depressed left ventricular function.[106]

MANAGEMENT OF MYOCARDIAL ISCHEMIA AFTER CABG. Patients with evidence of myocardial ischemia after coronary bypass surgery require an integrated assessment of clinical findings and laboratory tests on an individualized basis to define the appropriate management strategy. At the center of the decision pathway are the 12-lead ECG and hemodynamic observations (Fig. 76–6). Patients with ST elevations and a low cardiac index require intraaortic balloon pump support. Echocardiography may disclose new wall motion abnormalities that may necessitate coronary angiography and a percutaneous revascularization procedure or surgical reexploration in selected patients.

Low-Output Syndrome and Shock States

RECOGNITION. Sometimes, diagnosis of low-output syndrome and a shock state after cardiac surgery is difficult. Because cold extremities and mottled skin may result from hypothermia postoperatively, these observations lack sufficient specificity. Although reduced systolic pressure is the most striking manifestation of this disorder, low-output syndrome may be present even if the arterial systolic pressure exceeds 100 mm Hg because increased systemic vascular resistance (>1500 dyne-sec·cm^{-2}) may be supporting the peripheral perfusion pressure. It is important to recognize this syndrome because of the strong relationship between cardiac index in the early postoperative period and the probability of cardiac death after surgery. Common clinical features of the low-output syndrome and shock states after cardiac surgery include cold extremities, mottled skin, reduced systolic pressure (<90 mm Hg), decreased urine output (<30 ml/hr), low cardiac index (<2.0 liter/min·m^{-2}), low mixed venous oxygen saturation (<50 percent), and acidosis.

One should assess hemodynamic findings and integrate them with bedside echocardiographic recordings to confirm the diagnosis of low-output syndrome and attempt to segregate the findings into one of the patterns (*reduced preload, cardiogenic shock,* or *sepsis*) in Table 76–10. Although the hemodynamic findings among these patterns overlap and the coexistence of multiple disorders (e.g., bradycardia and hypovolemia) may blur the distinction between patterns, they offer a clinically useful approach to the evaluation of a patient with low-output syndrome. In addition to the specific treatment measures discussed later, a number of general measures are applicable to all patients who are in a shock-like condition after cardiac surgery, including prompt correction of any electrolyte and acid-base disturbances, transfusion to a hematocrit over 30 percent for improved oxygen-carrying capacity of the blood, and a "low threshold" for mechanical ventilatory support to minimize the work of breathing and thereby reduce total-body oxygen needs.

REDUCED PRELOAD

Hypovolemia. Low ventricular filling pressure, normal systemic vascular resistance, and a reduced cardiac index, coupled with echocardiographic demonstration of small ventricular volume with preserved systolic function, are indicative of *hypovolemia.* Possible causes include bleeding, excessive diuresis, the "leaky capillary state" associated with the postpump syndrome, and less frequently, inadequate vascular volume because of insufficient return of fluids at the conclusion of cardiopulmonary bypass. Rarely, adrenocortical insufficiency as a result of perioperative hemorrhage into the adrenal glands has been reported as a cause of hypovolemic hypotension after cardiac surgery.

Therapeutic maneuvers include the administration of intravenous fluids (normal saline solution, lactated Ringer solution), transfusion with packed red blood cells if the hemoglobin is less than 8 gm/dl, and administration of colloid-type volume expanders. It is also important to discontinue any vasodilators or antihypertensives that may have been prescribed during a period when the patient was hypertensive. While waiting for these measures to take effect, the patient may require transient infusion of a vasoconstrictor (usually phenylephrine) or an inotropic pressor (usually dopamine or epinephrine).

VASODILATION. Inhibition of sympathetic tone by the effects of anesthetic agents may cause peripheral vasodilation. In combination with the increased venous capacitance that may occur during rewarming, a low-output syndrome may develop as a result of markedly reduced systemic vascular resistance (<1000 dyne-sec·cm^{-5}). This situation is best treated by intravenous infusion of a vasoconstrictor such as norepinephrine in a dose of 1 to 10 μg/min until the systemic vascular resistance returns to a normal level. In patients not responsive to norepinephrine, commonly associated with preoperative ACE inhibition, the addition of intravenous vasopressin in a dose of 0.05 to 6 units per minute can restore normal systemic vascular resistance.

CARDIOGENIC SHOCK. When right ventricular and left ventricular filling pressures are in the normal range and systemic vascular resistance is not reduced, a frequent cause of a cardiac index less than 2 liter/min·m^{-2} is *bradycardia.* Because the cardiac index is the product of stroke volume and heart rate, this abnormality is easily corrected by atrial or atrioventricular pacing at 85 to 100 beats/min.

LEFT VENTRICULAR FAILURE. The pattern of predominant *left ventricular failure* in the early postoperative state is characterized by a disproportionately elevated pulmonary capillary wedge pressure in comparison to right atrial pressure, a low cardiac index, and normal or elevated systemic

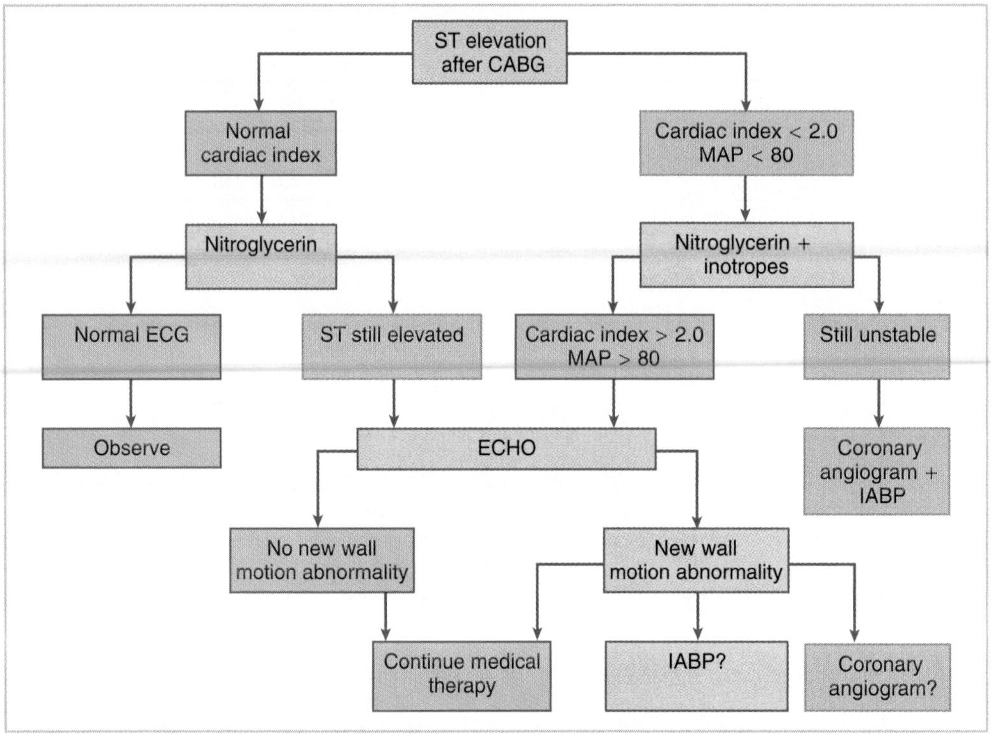

FIGURE 76–6 Myocardial ischemia after coronary bypass grafting occurs frequently. Hemodynamic assessment and ensuring of adequate coronary and systemic perfusion dictate early management strategies. Echocardiographic evaluation helps further tailor postoperative care. CABG = coronary artery bypass grafting; ECG = electrocardiogram; ECHO = echocardiography; IABP = intraaortic balloon pumping; MAP = mean arterial pressure.

TABLE 76–10 Hemodynamic Disturbances Following Cardiac Surgery

	Reduced Preload		
	Hypovolemia	***Vasodilation***	***Bradycardia (Inappropriately Slow HR Postoperatively)***
Hemodynamics			
RA	<8	<8	≤10
PCW	<15	<15	>15
CI	<2.0	<2.0	<2.0
SVR	<1200	<1000	>1200
Other			HR <60
Echocardiogram	Small ventricular chambers with vigorous systolic contraction unless LV dysfunction was present preoperatively	Small ventricular chambers with normal systolic contraction unless LV dysfunction was present preoperatively	Normal-sized ventricular chambers with vigorous systolic contraction, albeit at a slow rate
Management	IV fluids Transfusion if Hgb ≤ 10 Inotropes	Vasopressors	Cardiac pacing

CI = cardiac index; Hgb = hemoglobin; HR = heart rate; IV = intravenous; LV = left ventricular; PAD = pulmonary artery diastolic; PCW = pulmonary capillary wedge; RA = right arterial; RV = right ventricular; SVR = systemic vascular resistance; TR = tricuspid regurgitation.

vascular resistance. Echocardiography usually reveals a dilated, poorly contractile left ventricle, often exhibiting multiple regional wall motion abnormalities.

Diagnosis. The differential diagnosis of left ventricular failure after cardiac surgery includes the following conditions (which may coexist in the same patient): preoperative left ventricular dysfunction, inadequate surgical correction of the cardiac lesion (e.g., residual left ventricular outflow tract obstruction after repair of idiopathic hypertrophic subaortic stenosis, residual ventricular septal defect), complication of a surgical procedure (e.g., prosthetic valve leak or thrombosis, depression of stroke volume after correction of mitral regurgitation caused by elevation of afterload), dysrhythmia, depressant effect of a pharmacological agent (e.g., antiarrhythmic drug), acid-base or electrolyte disturbance, or myocardial ischemia and/or infarction. Bedside echocardiography can usually help identify mechanical disorders such as prosthetic valve dysfunction and dysrhythmias,[107] and metabolic abnormalities and toxic drug levels can be readily recognized by ECG and laboratory measurements.

Management. The objectives of hemodynamic management of patients with *left ventricular failure* postoperatively are to correct hypotension if present, increase forward left ventricular output, and return left and right ventricular filling pressures to the normal range. These variables are intimately related, and treatment may require careful titration of several intravenous agents for pharmacological support of the failing circulation. Boluses of calcium chloride (0.5 to 1 gm) increase myocardial contractility, but the effect is modest and short-lived. A continuous infusion of dopamine (5 to 10 μg/kg/min) or epinephrine (1 to 10 μg/min) is preferable if the primary goal is to increase systemic arterial pressure and cardiac output. Dobutamine (2 to 5 μg/kg/min), amrinone (bolus of 0.75 mg/kg and infusion of 5 to 10 μg/kg/min), or milrinone (bolus of 50 μg/kg/min and infusion of 0.375 to 0.75 μg/kg/min) also augment cardiac output and should be selected if a reduction in ventricular filling pressure is desired; systemic arterial pressure is usually unchanged or may even drop slightly because of the peripheral vasodilatory effects of these drugs. A commonly used combination is dopamine (2 μg/kg/min) to achieve greater renal perfusion in conjunction with dobutamine (2 to 5 μg/kg/min) for augmentation of cardiac output. If the mean arterial pressure is 90 mm Hg or higher, vasodilator therapy with nitroglycerin increases forward cardiac output and lowers pulmonary capillary wedge pressure further. When hypotension is profound (e.g., systolic pressure < 70 mm Hg), norepinephrine or epinephrine 1 to 10 μg/min or vasopressin 1 to 6 units per minute may be necessary to prevent coronary hypoperfusion.

We prefer to use an intraaortic balloon pump (see Chap. 25) for mechanical support of the circulation along with pharmacotherapy early in the course of management of postoperative left ventricular failure that does not respond to the initial pharmacological maneuvers already discussed. This protocol has the advantages of avoiding a continuous upward titration of the dose of sympathomimetic inotropic agents and vasoconstrictors associated with downregulation of beta-adrenergic antagonist receptors and diminished perfusion of the renal, mesenteric, and coronary vascular beds. Also, intraaortic balloon counterpulsation does not increase myocardial oxygen demand. The intraaortic balloon pump is contraindicated in the presence of severe aortic regurgitation and if an abdominal aortic aneurysm is present. In patients with severe peripheral vascular disease, balloon placement via the ascending aorta should be considered. Delayed sternal closure is another important adjunct in the management of cardiogenic shock following surgery (Fig. 76–7).[108,109] If the patient fails to improve despite a combination of intraaortic balloon pumping, open-chest management, and pharmacotherapy, a ventricular assist device may be inserted for temporary support or as a "bridge" to recovery or cardiac transplantation.[110-112] Serial evaluations of left ventricular function over time and under different loading conditions and supportive measures are best obtained with transesophageal echocardiograms.

Cardiogenic Shock			
LV Failure	***RV Failure***	***Cardiac Tamponade***	***Sepsis***
≥10 >20 <2.0 >1000	>10 ≤15 <2.0 >1000 PCW > 15 if LV failure is present	>15 >15 <2.0 >1000 RA = PCW = PAD (within 5 mm Hg) unless "asymmetrical" tamponade occurs because of pericardial clots	<10 <15 ≥2.0 <1000 Narrow A – VO_2 difference
Dilated LV with reduced systolic performance; regional wall motion abnormalities may reflect old or new myocardial ischemia and/or infarction	Dilated RA and RV with reduced RV systolic contraction TR often present on Doppler study IV contractile performance is variable	Small cardiac chambers with diastolic collapse of RA and RV Systolic contraction of RV and LV usually normal unless dysfunction was present preoperatively or coexistent LV or RV failure has occurred postoperatively	Small ventricular chambers with normal or slightly depressed contractile function (myocardial depressant factor)
Search for correctible lesion, offending agent, or laboratory abnormality Inotropes Vasopressors and vasodilators Mechanical assistance	Supplemental O_2 Pulmonary vasodilators Nitrous oxide Inotropes Mechanical assistance	Reexploration Supportive measures: IV fluids, inotropes	IV fluids Antibiotics Vasopressors Inotropes

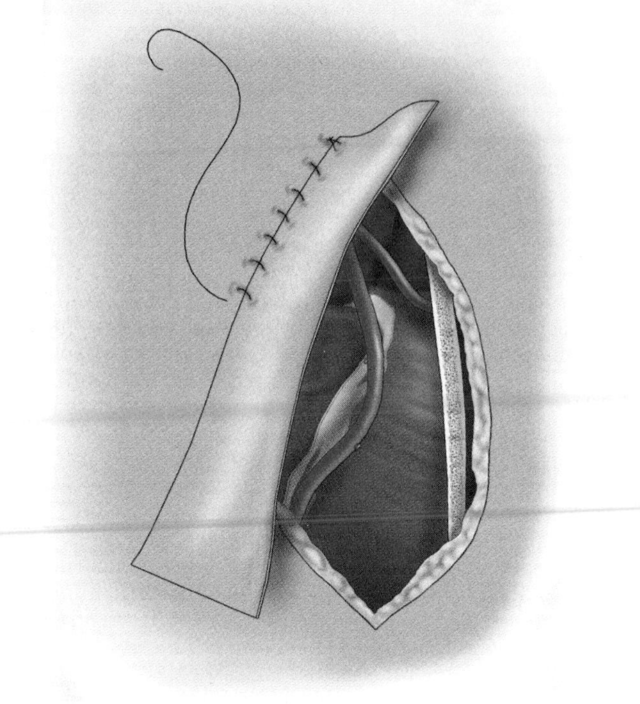

FIGURE 76–7 A patient in a low-output state may not tolerate immediate sternal closure, particularly in the setting of significant mediastinal and myocardial edema associated with prolonged cardiopulmonary bypass. Profuse coagulapathy represents an additional indication for open-chest management. After resolution of edema and recovery of myocardial function, the patient is returned to the operating room for a standard sternal closure.

RIGHT VENTRICULAR FAILURE. The pattern of predominant *right ventricular failure* is characterized by a disproportionate elevation in right atrial pressure in comparison to pulmonary capillary wedge pressure. In severe cases of postoperative right ventricular failure, right atrial pressure may exceed 20 mm Hg while pulmonary capillary wedge pressure remains equal to or less than 15 mm Hg. When left ventricular failure is present simultaneously, the difference between right atrial and pulmonary capillary wedge pressure lessens and differentiation from cardiac tamponade becomes difficult. Bedside echocardiography can aid the proper diagnosis (see Table 76–10).

Postoperatively, predominant right ventricular failure may be seen as a result of one or more of the following conditions: elevated pulmonary vascular resistance (persistently elevated from preoperative elevations in pulmonary artery pressure; postoperative hypoxia, pulmonary embolus, or pneumothorax), primary right ventricular ischemia/infarction,[113] or a mechanical lesion (tricuspid regurgitation, residual shunt flow, right ventriculotomy).

Massive pulmonary embolism occurs rarely after cardiac surgery (see Chap. 66). The diagnosis should be suspected when sudden deterioration in oxygenation occurs in association with confusion, systemic hypotension, tachycardia, ECG abnormalities (unexplained right axis deviation, right bundle branch block, a right ventricular strain pattern), and elevation of right atrial pressure. Angiographic confirmation of the diagnosis is not usually necessary. Expeditious noninvasive investigation by echocardiography is advisable in patients in whom the diagnosis remains uncertain.

Management. Hemodynamic management of predominant right ventricular failure should focus on improvement in right ventricular output to allow adequate filling of the left ventricle. Supplemental oxygen and hyperventilation to decrease P_{CO_2} levels help lower pulmonary artery pressure. Bradycardia (>60 beats/min) is corrected by atrial or atrioventricular pacing, isoproterenol (1 to 2 μg/min in an average adult) increases right ventricular contractility and also causes pulmonary vasodilation. Pulmonary hypertension may also be reduced by prostaglandin E_1 or intravenous nitroglycerin. In postoperative patients with massive pulmonary embolism and severe right ventricular dysfunction, emergency pulmonary embolectomy and placement of an inferior vena caval filter can be life-saving.

CARDIAC TAMPONADE (see Chap. 64). Postoperative echocardiography has shown that virtually all patients have pericardial effusion after cardiac surgery and that many such effusions are asymmetrical and loculated.[114] Even with mediastinal drains in place, cardiac tamponade can develop postoperatively; recognition of this condition requires a high index of suspicion and assessment of hemodynamics at the bedside.

Recognition. Important clinical features of tamponade, such as diminished heart sounds and pulsus paradoxus, may be obscured by mechanical ventilation. Asymmetrical, loculated accumulation of blood and clots in the mediastinum and pericardial space may cause isolated tamponade of one or two cardiac chambers and produce unusual elevations in diastolic pressure (e.g., right atrial tamponade with elevation of central venous pressure without an increase in right ventricular end-diastolic pressure or pulmonary capillary wedge pressure). Bedside transthoracic and transesophageal echocardiography is usually helpful for diagnosing pericardial effusions and assessing the hemodynamic significance of fluid collections.[115] Diastolic collapse of the right atrium and right ventricle is an indication of a hemodynamically significant external compressive force and should prompt urgent treatment.

Treatment. Although pericardiocentesis may be helpful in non-perioperative tamponade, it is unlikely to be successful in evacuating the organized pericardial and mediastinal material that develops after cardiac surgery; subxiphoid drainage and/or emergency resternotomy is preferred. Supportive measures that can be attempted in the interim include volume expansion with intravenous fluids (Plasmanate, whole blood) and inotropic agents (epinephrine).

SEPTIC SHOCK. Low ventricular filling pressure, markedly reduced systemic vascular resistance, and a normal or unexpectedly high cardiac index in the setting of hypotension and a shocklike state should raise suspicion of the early stages of *sepsis*. With progression of septic shock, a capillary leak syndrome develops (hypovolemia) and myocardial depression may occur and result in a somewhat reduced contractile pattern of the ventricles on echocardiography. Combined therapy with intravenous fluids, antibiotics, and inotropic agents is required to interrupt the vicious cycle of hypotension, acidosis, and diminished coronary perfusion. Most patients in a septic state during the first several days after cardiac surgery are infected with a skin organism (e.g., indwelling catheters) or from seeding the bloodstream from a pulmonary or urinary source. Broad antibiotic coverage (e.g., vancomycin plus ceftazidime) should be instituted. Because the offending organism is likely to be resistant to the prophylactic antibiotic given preoperatively, it is wise to not include it as one of the empirical antibiotics selected to treat sepsis.

Perioperative Arrhythmias (see Chaps. 30 and 32)

EVALUATION AND TREATMENT. There appear to be two peaks in the incidence of arrhythmias perioperatively: the first occurs in the operating room (most commonly during induction of anesthesia, weaning from cardiopulmonary bypass, or rewarming), and the second occurs in the ICU between the second and fifth postoperative days. The electrophysiological mechanisms underlying perioperative arrhythmias are incompletely understood, but they can probably be ascribed to a combination of the effects of circulating catecholamines, alterations in autonomic nervous system tone, transient electrolyte imbalance, myocardial ischemia or infarction, and mechanical irritation of the heart.

APPROACH TO THE PATIENT. Several factors may predispose to the development of arrhythmias, including ventilatory dysfunction, fever, electrolyte imbalance (hypokalemia, hypomagnesemia, hypocalcemia), anemia, myocardial ischemia or infarction, low cardiac output and reflex increase in sympathetic tone, hypertension, pericardial inflammation, and toxic effects of cardioactive medications (e.g., digitalis toxicity, bradycardia induced by diltiazem). *Every effort should be made to seek and eliminate any of the factors that may be provoking the arrhythmia.*

Although antiarrhythmic drug therapy and direct-current cardioversion are traditional methods for treating postoperative arrhythmias, cardiac pacing techniques have a number of advantages, including more rapid onset and offset of action, avoidance of potential drug toxicity (especially proarrhythmia), elimination of the need for anesthesia (required for cardioversion), reduced anxiety for the patient, greater safety in patients receiving digitalis, and perhaps most important, the ability to repeat the pacing protocol if the arrhythmia should recur, a not infrequent event. In addition to terminating arrhythmias, cardiac pacing can be used to suppress arrhythmias in many patients by atrial, atrioventricular sequential, or ventricular stimulation at a critical rate (e.g., 85 to 100 beats/min).

Surface Electrocardiogram. The value of a 12-lead ECG and simultaneously recorded multiple standard ECG lead rhythm strips cannot be overemphasized if one is attempting to analyze a wide-complex tachycardia. Unfortunately, a number of the criteria for differentiating supraventricular tachycardia with aberrant conduction from ventricular tachycardia (see Chap. 32) may not apply to postoperative patients because of previous or newly acquired infarction patterns, transient conduction defects (seen in 5 to 15 percent of patients in the early recovery period), and nonspecific repolarization patterns.

Epicardial Electrodes. It is desirable to place two wires on the free wall of the right atrium and a bipolar wire on the right ventricle intraoperatively to allow for bipolar atrial recording and pacing or dual-chamber pacing. The advantages of bipolar pacing include a smaller stimulus artifact, the ability to record a bipolar atrial electrogram during ventricular pacing, and a reduced likelihood of precipitating undesired atrial arrhythmias if an atrial wire is used as the indifferent electrode during unipolar ventricular pacing. Schematic diagrams showing the typical intrathoracic positioning of the atrial and ventricular wires are shown in Figure 76–8. In patients with severe heart failure, placement of biventricular pacing wires should be considered for postoperative support.[116,117]

Supraventricular Arrhythmias

ATRIAL PREMATURE DEPOLARIZATIONS. The hemodynamic consequences of atrial premature depolarizations are almost always minor, and one should resist the urge to suppress them with antiarrhythmic drugs. Instead, they should be considered a signal that the patient is possibly hypoxic or that an electrolyte or acid-base imbalance is present and a warning that the patient is at risk for more serious arrhythmia such as atrial fibrillation or atrial flutter. In the absence of such correctable abnormalities, one may want to administer a beta-adrenergic antagonist to inhibit the effects of circulating catecholamines and also to slow the ventricular rate if atrial fibrillation should develop.

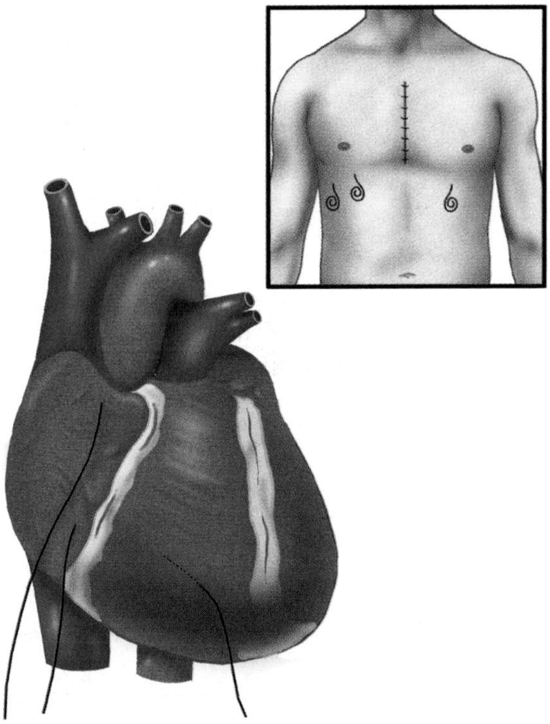

FIGURE 76–8 Epicardial electrodes in patients undergoing cardiac surgery. The precise number and location of pacing wires may vary among institutions and also according to the complexity of the operation (e.g., no atrial wires for routine coronary artery bypass surgery but both atrial and ventricular wires for valve surgery). In the example shown, the two atrial wires exit to the patient's right while the bipolar ventricular wire exits to the left.

ATRIAL FLUTTER. Control of the ventricular rate in atrial flutter is more difficult than in atrial fibrillation because of the limited number of ventricular responses to atrial activation (usually 2:1, 4:1, but rarely an odd-numbered multiple). Atrial flutter may be difficult to terminate with antiarrhythmic agents. Ibutilide 0.01 mg/kg up to 1 mg given intravenously over 10 minutes is useful as a first-line treatment of atrial flutter. Torsade de pointes can occur in up to 8 percent of cases, so patients post-ibultilide must be closely monitored during treatment with this drug. If ibultilide is unsuccessful, cardioversion with energy of 25 to 50 watt-seconds delivered as a single discharge can be expected to terminate atrial flutter in more than 90 percent of patients. Atrial flutter can also be terminated by rapid atrial pacing with the temporary epicardial atrial wires placed at the time of surgery (Fig. 76–9). The likelihood of success increases if one uses sufficiently rapid rates of pacing (up to 140 percent of the spontaneous atrial rate), a sufficient duration of pacing (10 to 30 seconds) with adequate strength (5 to 20 mA), and pretreatment of the patient with procainamide. To achieve the high drive rates required, a special stimulator is used.

ATRIAL FIBRILLATION. Although atrial fibrillation is an extremely common arrhythmia following cardiac surgery, etiology, predictors, and optimal management strategy remain elusive.[118-126] Even after prophylactic therapy with beta-adrenergic blockers, transient symptomatic atrial fibrillation occurs in at least 25 to 30 percent of patients after CABG and in 50 percent of patients following valvular surgery; atrial fibrillation appears with greatest incidence on the second or third postoperative day. Because of the hazards of postoperative atrial fibrillation, considerable effort has been devoted to identifying preoperative factors associated with an increased risk of postoperative arrhythmia.[118,121,123] Such factors include advanced age, male gender, hyperten-

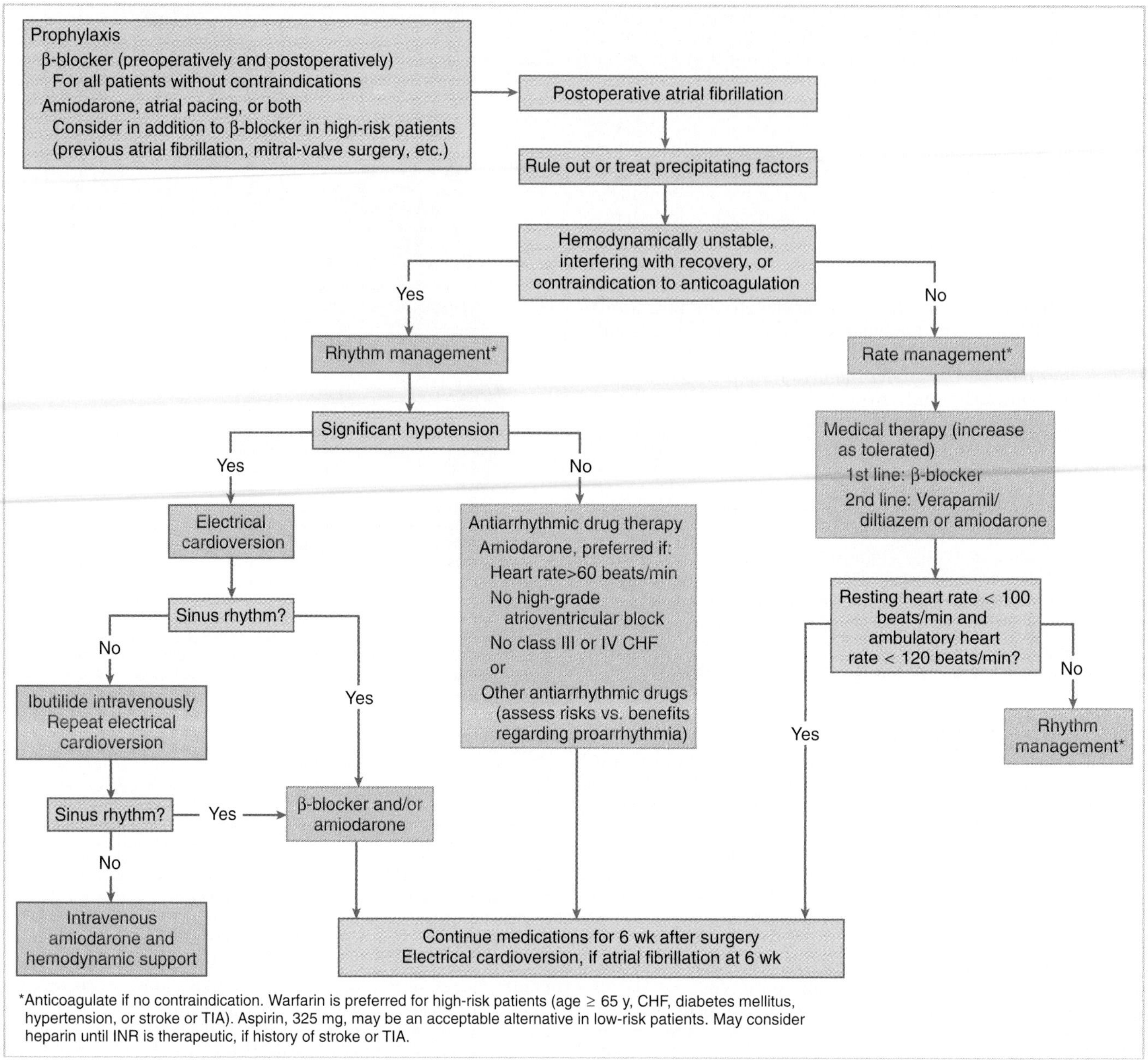

FIGURE 76–9 Algorithm for the prevention and management of atrial fibrillation after cardiac surgery. CHF = congestive heart failure; TIA = transient ischemic attack. (From Maisel WH, Rawn JD, Stevenson WG: Atrial fibrillation after cardiac surgery. Ann Intern Med 135:1061-1073, 2001.)

sion, intraaortic balloon pump, postoperative pneumonia, and mechanical ventilation for longer than 24 hours. A prolonged P wave duration recorded on a signal-averaged ECG and greater than 70 percent narrowing of the lumen of the right coronary artery may predict an increased risk of postoperative atrial fibrillation. However, for a substantial number of patients with postoperative atrial fibrillation, no apparent preoperative risk factor can be identified. Perhaps patients undergoing cardiac operations are vulnerable to postoperative atrial fibrillation because of mild nonuniformity in the distribution of their trial refractory periods. Intraoperative atrial ischemia associated with rapid rewarming of the atria during prolonged periods of cold cardioplegic arrest may increase the dispersion of refractoriness in the atria of such patients and thereby increase the risk of postoperative atrial fibrillation.

An algorithm for the prevention and management of atrial fibrillation after cardiac surgery is shown in Figure 76–9. Because of difficulties in reliably identifying patients at risk for atrial fibrillation preoperatively, it is common clinical practice to provide prophylactic therapy to most patients undergoing CABG. Beta-adrenergic blocking agents are most suitable for prophylaxis against atrial fibrillation. In the *absence* of an ejection fraction less than 30 percent, severe bronchospastic lung disease, or bradyarrhythmias, we advocate the use of prophylactic beta blockers in patients undergoing CABG. Conclusive data regarding the use of prophylactic antiarrhythmic therapy to prevent postoperative atrial fibrillation are lacking, although prophylactic amiodarone in selected patients has appeared promising in several clinical trials.[119,120,124] Unless hemodynamic collapse is present, in which case direct-current cardioversion should be performed, the initial treatment of choice in a postoperative patient is to slow the ventricular rate. Provided that the patient's ventricular function is adequate, acute intravenous administration of beta-adrenergic blocking agents (e.g., metoprolol 5 mg every 5 minutes for up to three doses), verapamil (5-mg bolus every 5 to 10 minutes for three or four doses), diltiazem (0.25- to 0.35-mg/kg bolus over a period of 2 minutes), or amiodarone (loading dose of 150-mg bolus, then 1 mg/min infusion for 6 hours, then 0.5 mg/min) is a more desirable option. Esmolol, an ultrashort-acting cardioselective beta blocker, when administered intravenously in a dose of 50 to 250 mg/kg/min, provides the option of rapid onset; in the event of hemodynamic deterioration, the effects of the drug are usually dissipated within 15 to 30 minutes after discontinuation of the infusion. In addition, the probability of conversion to sinus rhythm with esmolol appears to be better than with other agents such as verapamil.[127]

ANTICOAGULANTS. Epidemiological observations suggest that the development of postoperative atrial fibrillation is associated with a marked increase in the risk of stroke (odds ratio 3.0) and prolonged hospitalization. No consensus has been reached regarding anticoagulation recommendations in patients with postoperative atrial fibrillation. The risk of hemorrhage in the early postoperative period must be weighed against the risk of systemic thromboembolism. When atrial fibrillation develops beyond the second postoperative day, we generally advocate adherence to the guidelines established for nonsurgical patients and initiate anticoagulation (intravenous heparin followed by oral warfarin) in patients who have been in the arrhythmia for more than 48 hours, especially if the patient has a history of systemic embolism or if mitral valve disease or cardiomyopathy is present.

Beyond control of the ventricular rate acutely, the two treatment strategies for management of postoperative atrial fibrillation are similar to those for nonsurgical patients: chronic anticoagulation while administering rate-controlling agents versus restoration of sinus rhythm and attempts at suppression of recurrence of atrial fibrillation. Because large-scale clinical trial data are not available to guide decision making in this area, therapeutic approaches must be individualized. Ibutilide can acutely convert post-CABG atrial fibrillation when administered intravenously, albeit with a small risk (<2 percent) of torsades de pointes.[128] Procainamide is frequently used for the treatment of atrial fibrillation after open-heart surgery, although present evidence indicates that it has limited effectiveness in suppressing recurrence of atrial fibrillation.[129] Furthermore, any treatment decision formulated during hospitalization should be readdressed at the first postoperative visit (typically 4 to 6 weeks) to determine whether it is still a desirable course of action once the inflammation and metabolic alterations of the postoperative state have dissipated. Patients with depressed left ventricular function or striking ventricular hypertrophy who experience troublesome dyspnea and/or hypotension when in atrial fibrillation postoperatively are suitable candidates for a trial of restoration of sinus rhythm.

Patients with rheumatic heart disease and a preoperative history of atrial fibrillation often require permanent suppressive antiarrhythmic therapy despite successful aortic or mitral valve surgery even if sinus rhythm is present during the early postoperative period.

PAROXYSMAL SUPRAVENTRICULAR TACHYCARDIA. The reentrant forms of paroxysmal supraventricular tachycardia (PSVT)—atrioventricular nodal reentry tachycardia and atrioventricular reentry tachycardia—occur less frequently in postoperative patients than does atrial fibrillation or atrial flutter and, fortunately, retain their responsiveness to vagal maneuvers and pharmacotherapy designed to inhibit atrioventricular nodal conduction. The antiarrhythmic agent adenosine, an endogenous nucleoside, has a number of features that make it the drug of choice for treating PSVT in postoperative patients (see Chaps. 30 and 32). A rapid (2-second) intravenous bolus of 6 mg terminates about 60 percent of episodes of PSVT within 20 seconds; a subsequent bolus of 12 mg administered 1 to 2 minutes later terminates PSVT in virtually all patients who failed to respond to the lower dose. Because adenosine is rapidly transported into the cell or degraded enzymatically to inosine, the physiological effects of adenosine are dissipated in less than 5 minutes. Untoward reactions such as flushing, chest pain, or dyspnea, although common, are mild and short lived. PSVT may also be diagnosed by atrial recordings and terminated by burst atrial pacing or randomly delivered ventricular or atrial premature depolarizations that invade the reentrant circuit and interrupt the arrhythmia.

CARDIOVERSION. Direct-current cardioversion should be used in postsurgical patients with the following additional considerations. The recent cardiotomy with resultant pericardial and mediastinal inflammation, the presence of chest tubes and/or pleural effusions, and elevated catecholamine levels after surgery all may contribute to higher energy requirements for reversion of arrhythmias such as atrial fibrillation than are commonly required in patients who have not recently undergone cardiac surgery. To achieve the maximum transcardiac spread of current after median sternotomy, the anterior paddle should be placed to the *right* of the sternum between the third and sixth intercostal space, and the other paddle should be positioned in the fourth to sixth intercostal space as far in the left axilla as possible or in a posterior location under the tip of the left scapula. Firm pressure is applied to the paddles to maintain contact with the chest wall as the discharge buttons are depressed.

Ventricular Arrhythmias

VENTRICULAR PREMATURE DEPOLARIZATIONS. Isolated ventricular premature depolarizations (VPDs) commonly occur after cardiac surgery. An increase in the frequency of VPDs may be seen in patients with a preoperative history of VPDs, or they may appear de novo in patients with no history of ventricular arrhythmias. Although a fall in arterial pressure may be associated with isolated VPDs, this decreased pressure is usually extremely brief and of no significant hemodynamic consequence to the patient unless prolonged periods of bigeminy occur.

Management. We advocate a conservative approach focusing on prompt detection and correction of provocative factors (e.g. ischemia, hypoxia, metabolic derangement, or catheter initiation), liberal use of beta-adrenergic antagonists in patients with an ejection fraction greater than 0.30, and overdrive atrial or atrioventricular sequential pacing between 85 and 100 beats/min. We restrict suppressive antiarrhythmic therapy to patients with a preoperative history of serious ventricular tachyarrhythmias. If the decision is made to suppress VPDs in a patient without a history of symptomatic ventricular arrhythmias, the treatment period should be brief (6 to 24 hours) and the patient should not be automatically converted to treatment with an oral antiarrhythmic drug regimen without careful reconsideration of the indications for treatment.

VENTRICULAR TACHYCARDIA. Many of the same arguments cited earlier for isolated VPDs apply to paroxysms of nonsustained ventricular tachycardia. No definitive guidelines are available, but we believe that symptomatic episodes of nonsustained ventricular tachycardia in the absence of correctable factors and attempts at overdrive atrial or atrioventricular sequential pacing are indications for antiarrhythmic therapy, especially if the episodes are associated with hemodynamic compromise. *Sustained ventricular tachycardia* is a serious emergency that should be handled in an orderly approach. If the clinical situation permits, a 12-lead ECG should be obtained for future reference and confirmation of the diagnosis; simultaneous recording of surface ECG leads with electrograms from the epicardial wires may be helpful in establishing the mechanism of a wide-complex tachycardia.

Attempts at acute conversion of the tachycardia include the following maneuvers in the sequence listed: thumpversion, burst ventricular pacing, and boluses of antiarrhythmic agents (lidocaine 100 mg, procainamide up to 500 to 1000 mg over a period of 20 minutes, or amiodarone 75 to 150 mg infused over a 10-minute period). In urgent circumstances, synchronized direct-current cardioversion with a low-energy shock (25 to 50 watt-seconds) may be used. Unsynchronized shocks of 100 to 200 watt-seconds should be administered if the tachycardia rate is greater than 160 beats/min and/or has a sinusoidal waveform on ECG. After conversion, a search for correctable disorders should be undertaken, and if none is found, a continuous infusion of lidocaine (2 mg/min), procainamide (2 mg/min), or amiodarone (1 mg/min for 6 hours followed by a maintenance infusion of 0.5 mg/min).

VENTRICULAR FIBRILLATION. As in nonsurgical patients, ventricular fibrillation must be promptly treated with an unsynchronized direct-current shock. Ventricular fibrillation can often be reverted with shocks of 200 watt-seconds, provided that the intervention is performed promptly. It should be possible to defibrillate postoperative patients in the ICU expeditiously; therefore, the higher energies (360 to 400 watt-seconds) used in the "field" are probably unnecessary, at least initially. Because of the small number of patients experiencing unexpected sustained, hemodynamically compromising ventricular tachycardia or ventricular fibrillation, epidemiological data on provocative factors and the prognosis of these arrhythmias are difficult to evaluate. Unexplained ventricular tachycardia or ventricular fibrillation occurring within 24 hours after CABG is associated with very high in-hospital mortality, probably resulting from perioperative ischemia, infarction, and/or pump failure. Episodes of ventricular tachycardia or ventricular fibrillation occurring more than 24 hours after bypass surgery have a slightly less ominous prognosis and may be due to reperfusion of previously ischemic zones, early postoperative occlusion of coronary bypass grafts, or transmembrane shift of electrolytes during the process of recovery.[130]

Risk stratification of patients experiencing ventricular tachycardia or ventricular fibrillation postoperatively should include assessment of left ventricular function, coronary arteriography if ischemia/infarction is suspected, and consideration of an electrophysiological study to establish the most appropriate course of therapy. Because of the numerous metabolic fluxes taking place in the early postoperative period, electrophysiological study should, if possible, be postponed until at least 5 to 7 days following surgery. Serious consideration should be given to use of an implantable cardioverter-defibrillator in patients without an identifiable reversible cause of their arrhythmia, particularly those with a depressed ejection fraction (see Chap. 31).

ATRIOVENTRICULAR JUNCTIONAL RHYTHMS. Nonparoxysmal atrioventricular junctional rhythms (rate > 45 beats/min) can be seen after mitral or aortic valve surgery. Trauma and tissue swelling from surgical débridement and suture placement are believed to be the provocative mechanisms. Such rhythms are typically transient (≤48 hours) and easily treated with atrial or atrioventricular sequential pacing at a rate above that of the intrinsic junctional mechanism.

Bradyarrhythmias

Sinus bradycardia or sinus arrest with emergence of a slow atrioventricular junction escape rhythm can occur postoperatively when one or more of the following factors are present: advanced age, hypothermia, drug effects (diltiazem, beta blocker, digitalis, procainamide), preoperative sinus node dysfunction, intraoperative trauma to the sinus node, and postoperative elevation in vagal tone.[131] In addition to modifying the dose or discontinuing the use of offending drugs (such as those noted earlier), atrial pacing at 85 to 100 beats/min should be initiated to maintain adequate cardiac output and urine flow.

Although a new conduction defect may develop in up to 45 percent of patients following cardiac surgery, most are transient and related to myocardial hypothermia, perioperative electrolyte shifts, or surgical trauma during valve repair/replacement or closure of septal defects.[132] The risk of permanent, complete heart block postoperatively is increased in patients with preoperative conduction disturbances or multiple valve replacements and in those who have had previous valve surgery. However, implantation of a permanent epicardial pacing lead is rarely needed at the time of surgery because of the ease of implantation of a transvenous endocardial system postoperatively. An exception would be patients who are undergoing tricuspid valve replacement with a mechanical prosthesis, especially if they are simultaneously undergoing an aortic or mitral valve operation. Because of the contraindication to passing a transvenous lead through the mechanical tricuspid prosthesis, the surgical team should be alerted to the need for placement of permanent epicardial leads intraoperatively.

MANAGEMENT. The decision to insert a permanent pacemaker (see Chap. 31) after cardiac surgery should be based on the hemodynamic consequences of bradycardia in the individual patient rather than on a specific heart rate. Most new conduction defects resolve in the early postoperative period, but some persist for as long as 2 weeks. Few data are available to guide the decision about timing of implantation of a permanent pacemaker. We are willing to monitor a younger patient (<65 years) following CABG with a temporary pacing system postoperatively to see whether a conduction defect resolves. However, we have a low threshold for implanting a permanent pacemaker following aortic or mitral valve surgery or if antiarrhythmic therapy or beta-adrenergic blocker treatment is contemplated because these pharmacological measures might "stress" a diseased conduction system. We advocate early insertion of a permanent pacemaker in elderly patients with symptomatic bradycardia because the recuperative process is facilitated, the period of relative immobilization and ECG monitoring is minimized, and hospital stay is shortened. Finally, we are more aggressive about implantation of permanent pacemakers in patients with persistent advanced atrioventricular block than in those with isolated sinus bradycardia.

Hemostatic Disturbances (see Chap. 80)

EXCESSIVE BLEEDING. Multifactorial derangement of the hemostatic system develops in all patients who undergo cardiopulmonary bypass. These abnormalities are caused by exposure of the blood to artificial surfaces, hemodilution, and the effects of heparin (Table 76–11).[133] Platelet dysfunction is the most significant hemostatic abnormality that occurs after cardiopulmonary bypass, although diminution of coagulation factor levels may assume greater significance in patients with preoperative deficiencies in hemostasis. These abnormalities are increased in the setting of prolonged cardiopulmonary bypass times and the use of deep hypothermic circulatory arrest. Administration of the following drugs before surgery may predispose the patient to excessive bleeding: aspirin and other antiplatelet agents, nonsteroidal antiinflammatory agents, thrombolytic agents, certain antibiotics (carbenicillin, ticarcillin, moxalactam, cefamandole, third-generation cephalosporins), dextran, amrinone, quinidine, cytotoxic agents, gold, phenylbutazone, and fish oils. Other clinical conditions associated with increased postoperative hemorrhage include chronic renal failure, active endocarditis, and chronic hepatic congestion. The most obvious evidence of

TABLE 76–11 Hemostatic Disturbances Following Cardiopulmonary Bypass

Abnormality	Cause
Exposure of blood to artificial surfaces	
1. Platelet dysfunction A. Prolonged bleeding time B. Decreased adhesiveness	1. Depletion of platelet alpha granules, reduced response to wounds, and increased plasma levels of platelet factor 4 and beta-thromboglobulin
2. Inflammatory response	2. Activation of the complement, coagulation, fibrinolytic, and kallikrein cascades; activation of neutrophils with degranulation and protease enzyme release; oxygen free radical production; and synthesis of cytokines (tumor necrosis factor, IL-1, IL-6, IL-8)
Hemodilution	
1. Thrombocytopenia	1. Priming of extracorporeal bypass circuit with crystalloid solutions. Heparin-mediated immune thrombocylopenia may occur in about 5% of patients*
2. Coagulation factor depletion	2. Most coagulation factor levels are reduced by hemodilution by about 50%; factor V is reduced to 20-30% of normal and factor VIII is relatively unaffected. Factor levels usually return to normal within 12 hr after completion of cardiopulmonary bypass. Although plasminogen and fibrinogen levels are decreased by about 50%, fibrin degradation products usually do not appear in the plasma during bypass
Heparinization	Thrombus formation is inhibited and excessive bleeding is avoided intraoperatively by maintaining the activated clotting time between 400 and 480 sec

IL = interleukin.

*Reversal of heparin effects is accomplished with protamine sulfate. Vascular collapse has been reported in some patients during protamine treatment. To avoid the problem of heparin-induced thrombocytopenia and because heparin may not effectively inhibit all the thrombin generated during cardiopulmonary bypass ("heparin rebound"), novel antithrombins are being evaluated as alternatives to heparin during surgery.

bleeding in a postoperative cardiac surgical patient is by means of chest tube drainage. "Acceptable" rates of bleeding are usually less than 100 ml/hr. We advocate return to the operating room because of excessive bleeding include more than 500 ml/hr for 1 hour, more than 300 ml/hr for 3 hours, and 200 to 300 ml/hr for 4 hours. These criteria may be tempered by correctable extenuating circumstances, such as uncontrolled hypertension postoperatively, failure to achieve normothermia, or an abnormal coagulation status that is being corrected. In contrast, select patients undergoing minimally invasive surgery may be returned for exploration earlier if no explanation for excessive blood loss is obvious. Emergency medical maneuvers that can be attempted after sending coagulation studies to the laboratory include the use of PEEP up to 10 cm H_2O for mediastinal tamponade, empirical "correction" of putative platelet dysfunction with desmopressin acetate (DDAVP, a synthetic analog of arginine vasopressin that increases plasma levels of von Willebrand factor) 0.3 μg/kg infused over a period of 15 to 30 minutes, and empirical administration of a small dose of protamine sulfate 25 to 50 mg because heparin may be liberated from the patient's fat stores as rewarming occurs.

Once the coagulation profile returns, additional therapy in the form of platelet transfusions for a platelet count less than 100,000/mm^3 and fresh frozen plasma to correct an elevated prothrombin time can be prescribed. Aprotinin therapy (2×10^5 KIU loading bolus followed by infusion of 0.5×10^5 KIU/hr for 4 hours) is helpful in cases of excessive postoperative bleeding by virtue of its ability to inhibit fibrinolysis and preserve platelet glycoprotein Ib and von Willebrand factor activity.[134] When monitoring bleeding from a chest tube, it is important to be alert to sudden cessation of hemorrhage, which may indicate that the chest tubes have clotted and the fluid is now draining into the mediastinum or the pleural spaces. Serial chest radiographs may be helpful while observing a patient during a bleeding episode. With correct medical management, less than 2 percent of patients need to return to the operating room for control of bleeding, preferably within 3 to 4 hours of the original surgery, before hemodynamic destabilization occurs and large volumes of blood products are administered.

HYPERCOAGULABLE DISORDERS. Management of patients with hypercoagulable syndromes requiring cardiac surgery poses special challenges.[135-140] Common (factor V Leiden) and uncommon (antithrombin deficiency, proteins C and S deficiency) syndromes have different risk associations for venous thrombosis ranging between 2.5% (factor V Leiden) and 25% (antithrombin deficiency) (see Chap. 80). Surgery is a known trigger for thrombosis, and therefore aggressive prophylaxis with subcutaneous unfractionated heparin or low-molecular-weight heparin is warranted in the postoperative setting. If patients are on long-term anticoagulation, warfarin therapy should be switched to heparin therapy 3 to 5 days prior to surgery. As soon as adequate postoperative hemostasis is ensured, restarting heparin therapy within 2 days of surgery is recommended with simultaneous resumption of warfarin therapy. Patients with antiphospholipid antibody syndrome (lupus, anticoagulant/anticardiolipin antibodies, history of arterial or venous thrombosis, and/or recurrent fetal loss) can have associated valvular heart disease requiring surgery. Anticoagulation monitoring during cardiopulmonary bypass may be challenging, and preoperative in vitro testing to identify the most reliable assay for heparin monitoring may be warranted. In the postoperative setting aggressive anticoagulation is again recommended to prevent thromboembolic complications. In patients undergoing deep hypothermic circulatory arrest, particularly during aortic reconstructive surgery, cases of catastrophic circulatory thrombosis have been reported in patients with hypercoagulable states also receiving antifibrinolytics. We recommend factor V Leiden screening if circulatory arrest is planned, with avoidance of antifibrinolytics in patients who screen positive.[141]

HEPARIN-INDUCED THROMBOCYTOPENIA (see Chap. 80). Heparin-induced thrombocytopenia (HIT) is an immune-mediated, potentially life-threatening thrombotic complication that occurs in 3 percent of patients receiving heparin for 5 or more days.[142] HIT is a clinicopathological diagnosis that should be suspected in any patient who experiences a 50% or greater decrease in platelet count from baseline or a 30% or greater decrease in platelet count and associated thrombotic complication while on heparin for at least 5 days. Antibodies to heparin-platelet factor 4 cause platelet activation, aggregation and thrombin formation resulting often in deep venous thrombosis, pulmonary embolism, or cerebral sinus thrombosis. In general, thrombo-

TABLE 76–12 Anticoagulation Guidelines for Antithrombotic Therapy in Cardiac Surgery Patients

Surgery	Anticoagulant	INR*
Mitral mechanical valve	Warfarin	2.5-3.5
Aortic mechanical valve	Warfarin	2.0-3.0
Tricuspid mechanical valve	Warfarin	2.5-3.0
Atrial fibrillation	Warfarin	2.0-2.5
Mitral tissue valve	Warfarin	2.0-3.0 for 6 wk
Mitral valve repair	Warfarin	2.0-3.0 for 6 wk
Tricuspid tissue valve	Warfarin	2.0-3.0 for 6 wk
Tricuspid repair	Warfarin	2.0-3.0 for 6 wk
LV thrombus	Warfarin	2.0-3.0 for 6 mo
LV aneurysm repair	Warfarin	2.0-3.0 for 6 wk
Aortic tissue valve	ASA (80 mg/d)	
Coronary artery bypass	ASA 325 mg/d, 81 mg/d if taking warfarin	

ASA = acetylsalicylic acid (aspirin); LV = left ventricular.
*The target international normalized ratio (INR) is the midpoint of the range.

cytopenia resolves within 1 week of heparin discontinuation, but the prothrombotic state can persist for up to 1 month. Diagnostic tests for HIT are discussed in Chapter 80. In patients with suspicion of HIT, heparin should be stopped and, if a strong indication for anticoagulation persists, another antithrombotic agent (lepirudin, argatroban) should be initiated.[143-146] In patients with HIT, warfarin initiation should be done in the presence of lepirudin or argatroban due to warfarin's association with limb gangrene when used as the sole agent. HIT antibodies are usually undetectable 100 days after the cessation of heparin therapy, and if these antibodies are negative and the patient requires reoperative cardiac surgery, unfractioned heparin can be reused for cardiopulmonary bypass.

ANTITHROMBOTIC THERAPY IN CARDIAC SURGICAL PATIENTS. A wide spectrum of patients recovering from cardiac surgery may require either short- or long-term antithrombotic therapy (Table 76–12). Furthermore, the intensity of therapy is dictated by the estimated risk of thromboembolism. Variables that may have an impact on the risk of thromboembolism include insertion of a prosthetic valve (mechanical more than bioprosthetic), valve location (mitral more than aortic), the presence of atrial fibrillation, size of the left atrium, history of thromboembolism, left atrial thrombi visualized at surgery, and ventricular wall motion abnormalities associated with mural thrombi.

Neurological Complications

Neurological complications after cardiac surgery are quite common, particularly in the elderly, if one is attentive to the subtle cognitive (short-term memory loss, lack of concentration) and psychological (depression, increased sense of dependency) changes seen early after surgery.[29,147-149] A positive and supportive attitude on the part of the staff and enlistment of the aid of family members help minimize these problems. Although many patients return to their preoperative state by 4 to 6 weeks after surgery, about 10 percent continue to show deterioration in neuropsychological functioning over the next 6 months, especially if they are older than 65 years of age.[29,149] More serious neurological complications such as stroke occur in 1 to 5 percent of patients but may be seen in as many as 10 percent of patients older than 65.[29]

Symptomatic visual defects may be seen after cardiac surgery and result from retinal emboli, occipital lobe infarction, or anterior ischemic optic neuropathy. Risk factors for cerebrovascular accident or transient ischemic attack after cardiac surgery include preoperative carotid bruit, previous cerebrovascular accident or transient ischemic attack, postoperative atrial fibrillation, prolonged cardiopulmonary bypass (>2 hours), and preoperative left ventricular mural thrombus.[29]

Measures that decrease the risk of stroke in patients undergoing cardiac surgery include preoperative carotid scanning in high-risk patients, use of a soft-flow aortic cannula that minimizes disruption of aortic plaques, precise management of cardiopulmonary bypass with increased mean arterial pressure in elderly patients, and a strict strategy of minimal aortic manipulation if epiaortic ultrasound scanning reveals significant aortic atherothrombotic disease (see Fig. 76-3).[15]

Neuropathies in the upper extremities can occur after cardiac operations. A pattern of injury involving predominantly the ulnar nerve and medial antebrachial cutaneous nerve suggests that the lesion involves brachial plexus compression or a traction injury. The average duration of symptoms after such an injury is 2 months, but some patients show a slower time course of improvement extending over 6 to 12 months.

Infection

FEVER. Despite its nonspecific nature, fever is the most common initial clinical sign of a postoperative infection. It should be emphasized, however, that patients who experience a normal course of convalescence continue to show an elevated temperature for up to 6 days postoperatively. In the absence of infection, such early fevers probably result from alterations in blood components after cardiopulmonary bypass such as activation of polynuclear neutrophils and complement system. In addition to infectious causes, fevers that occur beyond 6 days may be due to drug reactions, phlebitis at the site of intravenous lines, atelectasis, pulmonary emboli, or the postpericardiotomy syndrome.

WOUND AND INCISION

Infections of the leg wound are typically manifested by fever, induration, pain, erythema, local warmth, and drainage from the suture line. The usual infectious agents include *Staphylococcus, Streptococcus,* and aerobic Gram-negative bacilli. Wound aspiration and Gram stain should be used to guide antibiotic treatment. More advanced cases require wound débridement and open drainage. Techniques of minimally invasive saphenous vein harvesting now make it possible to avoid a long leg incision, which decreases the risk of postoperative leg infection (Fig. 76-10).[150]

Recurrent bacterial cellulitis in the leg used for saphenous vein harvest may be a recalcitrant problem that appears months to years after surgery. Antibiotic courses directed against staphylococcal and streptococcal species for each individual occurrence may be insufficient, and a long-term course of antibiotic therapy may be needed. It is important to search for evidence of superficial fungal infections in the affected leg because persistent tinea pedis infection can cause recurrent lower extremity cellulitis. If a fungal infection is identified, treatment with topical miconazole or clotrimazole should be given in addition to antibacterial therapy.

Mediastinitis

Mediastinitis and sternal osteomyelitis are among the most serious complications of median sternotomy.[52,151,152] If one excludes operations that occur after thoracic trauma, it is estimated that mediastinitis occurs in about 2 percent of patients who undergo median sternotomy.

Most cases of mediastinitis occur within 2 weeks after sternotomy. Important diagnostic features of patients in whom mediastinitis develops early after cardiac surgery include persistent fever in excess of 101°F beyond the fourth postoperative day, a systemic toxic condition, leukocytosis, bacteremia, and a purulent discharge from the sternal wound. Recognition of mediastinitis requires a high index of suspicion

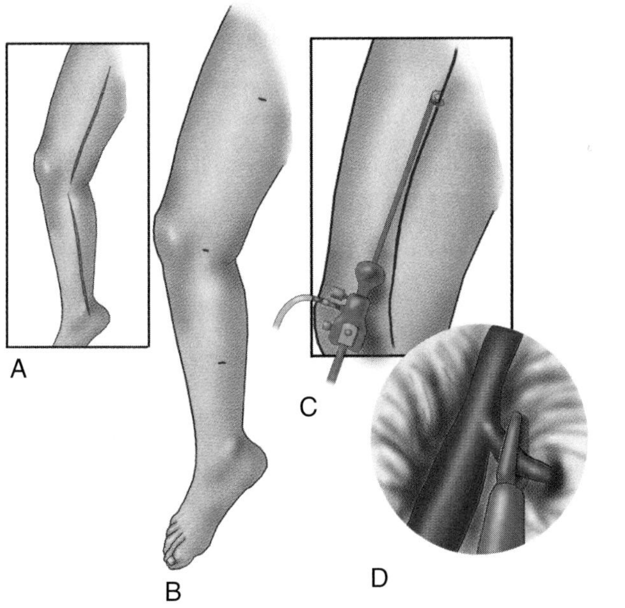

FIGURE 76–10 Minimally invasive approaches to saphenous vein harvesting have significantly reduced incisional morbidity. Traditional harvesting requires long leg incisions **(A)**, as compared with the less invasive videoscopic harvesting **(B)**. A dissection cannula is introduced through a small incision **(C)**, and branches are later divided **(D)** under videoscopic guidance.

and a vigorous, repetitive search for evidence of sternal wound drainage in patients who are persistently febrile late into the first week after surgery and who have no other obvious focus of infection, such as pneumonia or urinary tract infection. The diagnosis can be confirmed by needle aspiration from the subxiphoid approach followed by Gram stain and culture.

Risk Factors

Risk factors for the development of mediastinitis include prolonged cardiopulmonary bypass time, excessive postoperative bleeding with reexploration for control of hemorrhage, and diminished cardiac output in the postoperative period. The incidence of mediastinitis maybe increased when both internal mammary arteries are mobilized bilaterally for use as bypass conduits.[153] Therefore, many surgeons prefer to use only the left internal mammary artery, particularly in elderly diabetic patients, who may already be predisposed to delayed sternal wound healing. If both internal mammary arteries are utilized in this subgroup, they should be harvested without a large pedicle (skeletonized grafts) to preserve sternal vascularization.[35]

The spectrum of microorganisms that cause mediastinitis includes *Staphylococcus aureus* and *Staphylococcus epidermidis* in about 50 percent of patients and a variety of Gram-negative bacilli in about 40 percent of cases.[153,154] Mixed infections and fungal infections are rare. The organism isolated frequently is resistant to the prophylactic antibiotic used preoperatively, especially if the isolate includes a gram-negative bacillus or a beta-lactamase–producing *S. aureus.*

Diagnosis of Sternal Wound Infection

Definitive diagnosis requires exploration of the wound and culture of suspicious areas. In the past, closed (débridement, reclosure, and antibiotic irrigation) and open (débridement, packing, closure by secondary intent) approaches were commonly used. To facilitate functional recovery, we now favor early plastic surgical flap techniques to allow for immediate primary closure with vascularized tissue.[155] Regardless of the sternal closure strategy used, bacterial-specific intravenous antibiotics are typically administered for 6 weeks.

ANTIBIOTIC PROPHYLAXIS. Perioperative antibiotic prophylaxis benefits patients undergoing cardiac surgery.[156] Although the antibiotic regimen varies, in part related to local differences in microbiological flora and personal preference, it is directed against gram-positive cocci (the most frequent causative pathogens in infections after cardiac surgery) and usually contains a cephalosporin. A commonly used regimen consists of 1 gm of cefazolin intravenously 30 minutes before the skin incision and then repeated at 8-hour intervals for 48 hours after surgery.

PROSTHETIC VALVE ENDOCARDITIS (see Chaps. 57 and 58). Prosthetic valve endocarditis is a rare but extremely serious complication of cardiac surgery, frequently arising from nosocomial bacteremias.[33] It is estimated to occur in only 2 to 4 percent of patients; about half of the cases are classified as "early" (<60 days from the date of surgery) and half as "late" (>60 days from the date of surgery). Pooled data from several series indicate that the organism responsible for early prosthetic valve endocarditis includes a *Staphylococcus* species in about 50 percent of cases. The remainder of early cases of prosthetic valve endocarditis are caused by Gram-negative bacilli, dipthteroids, and fungi.[33,157]

Management. Features of prosthetic valve endocarditis that have been associated with increased mortality include invasive infection (i.e., extension into the myocardium); congestive heart failure resulting from dysfunction of the prosthesis; and the presence of antibiotic-resistant, virulent microorganisms or a fungal organism.[33,157] Appropriate antibiotic therapy for prosthetic valve endocarditis is discussed in Chapter 58, but practically all patients will require removal of the infected prosthesis.

VIRAL. Viral infections that occur after cardiac surgery are almost exclusively the result of infectious complications of transfusion therapy and, with the exception of human immunodeficiency virus, primarily result in hepatitis. The incidence of viral infections after cardiac operations is decreasing as a result of a reduction in the number of transfusions of blood bank products (e.g., cell-saver techniques and preoperative autologous blood donations) and improved screening techniques in contemporary blood bank practice. Cytomegalovirus infection is a febrile syndrome that typically occurs 1 month postoperatively. It is characterized by high-spiking fevers, abnormalities in liver function tests, and arthralgias. A self-limited illness, it is best treated with antipyretics and supportive fluid therapy.

FUNGAL. Fungal infections that involve the heart are rare. They are typically seen in cases of fungemia and are usually fatal. Although the problem of fungemia is well described in immunocompromised hosts (e.g., heart transplant recipient), in an autopsy study of 60 patients with fungal infections of the heart, 25 percent of cases occurred in association with conventional valvular surgery. About half of fungal infections of the heart are confined to the endocardium, and half involve both the endocardium and the myocardium. Extracardiac involvement is common, with spread of infection to the lungs, cerebrospinal fluid, urine, and skin. The most commonly encountered organisms, in descending order of frequency, are *Candida, Aspergillus,* and *Cryptococcus* species. Patients who appear to be at particular risk of fungal involvement of the heart are those who have received corticosteroids and long courses of antibiotic treatment postoperatively.

Peripheral Vascular Complications

Most adults who undergo cardiac surgery—especially coronary revascularization—have atherosclerosis of the peripheral arteries (e.g., iliofemoral system) and may experience lower extremity ischemia after surgery because of low flow in the perioperative period with in situ thrombosis, embolism from the heart or aorta, or vascular compromise from an intraaortic balloon pump catheter (see also Chaps. 54 and 55). Management consists of anticoagulation and removal of indwelling catheters, if clinically feasible. Thrombectomy and even revascularization surgery of the lower extremities (e.g., femorofemoral, femoropopliteal, or axillofemoral bypass) may be required to salvage threatened limbs.

Asymptomatic deep venous thrombosis of the calf can develop before hospital discharge in about one-third to one-half of patients who receive saphenous vein bypass grafts. Occasionally, these thrombi propagate to the proximal leg veins; only rarely do they cause massive pulmonary embolism. The best preventive strategy is rigorous perioperative prophylaxis against venous thromboembolism in all patients, including unfractionated or low-molecular-weight heparin.

Other Complications

PERICARDITIS (see Chap. 64). Pericardial friction rubs are commonly audible in the early postoperative period and probably result from local inflammation and mechanical irritation from the mediastinal chest tubes. The friction rubs usually subside by the second or third postoperative day and are asymptomatic because of the narcotic analgesics prescribed at that stage of recovery. Although pericardial rubs develop in some patients toward the end of the first postoperative week, they are usually benign, do not indicate a need for prolongation of hospitalization, and do not require treatment. A separate clinical syndrome that appears late in the first postoperative month is *postpericardiotomy syndrome.* The relationship between postpericardotomy syndrome and chronic constrictive pericarditis is not firmly established, but a number of patients with *postoperative constrictive pericarditis* have a history of postpericardiotomy syndrome.

RENAL FAILURE (see Chap. 86). All patients who undergo cardiac surgery experience a reduction in renal blood flow and the glomerular filtration rate as a consequence of both anesthesia and cardiopulmonary bypass. Risk factors for the development of persistent renal failure after cardiac surgery include a preoperative history of renal dysfunction or left ventricular dysfunction, prolonged bypass time (>180 minutes), prolonged aortic cross-clamping (>60 minutes), perioperative hypotension, advanced age (>70 years), and the development of medical complications postoperatively.[158,159]

Most cases of acute renal failure after cardiac surgery result from renal ischemia that lowers the glomerular filtration rate directly (prerenal disease) or, if severe or prolonged, can induce acute tubular necrosis. Possible additional contributory factors include sepsis, nephrotoxic drugs, radiocontrast material injection, embolization of cholesterol or other atheromatous debris in the renal circulation, increased urine free hemoglobin levels from hemolysis while undergoing cardiopulmonary bypass, and the effects of ACE inhibitors on glomerular capillary pressure. The detrimental effects of ACE inhibitors are most likely to occur when renal perfusion pressure is low because of renal artery stenosis or systemic hypotension caused by cardiac failure.

Urine output is variable in patients with postoperative acute renal failure. Anuria is uncommon and, if present, should raise the suspicion of urinary tract obstruction (e.g., occluded Foley catheter). More commonly, patients are either oliguric (<400 mg/d) or nonoliguric. Oliguric acute renal failure occurs less frequently than nonoliguric renal failure, usually reflects more severe renal injury, and is associated with a greater probability of requiring dialysis during the acute phase.

Differentiation Between Prerenal Azotemia and Acute Tubular Necrosis. Important diagnostic studies in all patients with acute renal failure include urinalysis and estimation of pulmonary capillary wedge pressure and cardiac output by means of pulmonary artery catheterization. Prerenal azotemia should be suspected if the urine sodium level is less than 20 mEq/liter, the fractional excretion of sodium is less than 1 percent, and urine osmolality is greater than 500 mOsm/liter. Acute tubular necrosis should be suspected if the urine sodium level is greater than 40 mEq/liter, fractional excretion of sodium is greater than 2 percent, and urine osmolality is less than 350 mOsm/liter.

Treatment. Essential elements of therapy for both prerenal azotemia and acute tubular necrosis include optimization of intravascular fluid volume and cardiac output. The latter is best accomplished with vasodilators and inotropic agents rather than vasoconstrictors to avoid further reductions in renal blood flow.

It is prudent to undertake a trial of furosemide and mannitol (only if the patient can tolerate the volume load of the latter) within the first 12 to 24 hours after the development of oliguria. The aim of such therapy is to increase urine output. Because of the renal-vasodilating effects of dopamine (2 to 3 µg/kg/min), patients with both oliguric and nonoliguric renal failure may experience an increase in urine output.

If oliguria persists beyond 12 hours, a number of supportive measures must be initiated, including careful attention to electrolyte balance, specifically avoiding hyperkalemia; avoidance of excessive free water administration, which might lead to hyponatremia; correction of acidosis (adding bicarbonate to daily fluids); and adjustment of medication dosages for delayed excretion if the drug is cleared by renal mechanisms. The care team should remain alert for pericarditis, refractory hyperkalemia, uremic encephalopathy, or colitis. Continuous arteriovenous hemofiltration can be used to remove excess fluid.

Cardiac Surgery in Patients with Chronic Renal Failure. Patients with chronic renal failure who undergo surgery have an increased risk of exacerbation of renal dysfunction perioperatively. Deterioration in renal function may require temporary or even permanent hemodialysis, and these eventualities should be addressed with the patient and the cardiac surgical team preoperatively. Surgery can be safely performed in patients who are already maintained by hemodialysis, but careful coordination of the surgical and dialysis schedules is essential to minimize postoperative problems with fluid and electrolyte management.[158]

GASTROINTESTINAL COMPLICATIONS. Serious gastrointestinal complications after cardiac surgery are rare (occurring in about 1 percent of patients) and can usually be handled by a conservative approach. Only about 0.5 percent of patients who undergo cardiac surgery require a general surgical operation for a gastrointestinal complication. Complications that may require intervention include upper or lower gastrointestinal bleeding, cholecystitis, and mesenteric ischemia. Patients with circulatory compromise on high-dose pressors and those who require intraaortic balloon pump support are more likely to have gastrointestinal complications. Despite their relative rarity, gastrointestinal complications are associated with significant mortality (approaching 40 percent in some series), thus highlighting the need for careful monitoring and repeated physical examination in high-risk patients. Most complications occur within 7 days of surgery.

Rehabilitation and Preparation for Discharge (see Chap. 43)

A coordinated, multidisciplinary cardiac exercise program is essential to overcome the physical deconditioning and psychosocial upheaval associated with cardiac surgery. Emphasis should be placed on early mobilization and progressively more patient self-care, including initiation of these measures in the ICU during the first 24 hours postoperatively. After transfer out of the ICU, the patient should be encouraged to engage in low-density (2 to 3 metabolic equivalent threshold) isotonic activities such as walking and range-of-motion exercises.[160] The nursing staff should monitor the patient's progress while being alert to any undue acceleration in heart rate (>120 beats/min) or hemodynamically compromising arrhythmias.

Patients should also participate in an education program focusing on instructions regarding postoperative medications and initiation of secondary measures targeted at preventing graft occlusion and progression of atherosclerosis.[161] Because of the overwhelming evidence indicating that platelet inhibition can prevent graft occlusion, all patients undergoing bypass surgery should receive long-term therapy with aspirin unless contraindicated. Clopidogrel may be useful in aspirin-intolerant patients, but there is no evidence of significant benefit from the routine use of either dipyridamole or sulfinpyrazone. Fast-track discharge protocols are now standard, and uncomplicated patients are typically discharged on the fifth postoperative day.[162,163]

REFERENCES

1. Braunwald E, Antman EM, Beasley JW, et al: ACC/AHA 2002 guideline update for the management of patients with unstable angina and non-ST-segment elevation myocardial infarction—summary article: A report of the American College of Cardiology/American Heart Association Task Force on Practice Guidelines (Committee on the Management of Patients With Unstable Angina). J Am Coll Cardiol 40:1366-1374, 2002.
2. Bech-Hanssen O, Caidahl K, Wall B, et al: Influence of aortic valve replacement, prosthesis type, and size on functional outcome and ventricular mass in patients with aortic stenosis. J Thorac Cardiovasc Surg 118:57-65, 1999.
3. Di Carli MF, Maddahi J, Rokhsar S, et al: Long-term survival of patients with coronary artery disease and left ventricular dysfunction: Implications for the role of myocardial viability assessment in management decisions. J Thorac Cardiovasc Surg 116:997-1004, 1998.

3a. Rahimatoola SH: The year in valvular heart disease. J Am Coll Cardiol 43:491, 2004.

3b. Schinkel AFL, Plodermans D, Vanoverschelde J-LL, et al: Incidence of recovery of contractile function following revascularization in patients with ischemic left ventricular dysfunction. Am J Cardiol 93:14, 2004.

4. Trachiotis GD, Weintraub WS, Johnston TS, et al: Coronary artery bypass grafting in patients with advanced left ventricular dysfunction. Ann Thorac Surg 66:1632-1639, 1998.
5. Bigger JT Jr: Prophylactic use of implanted cardiac defibrillators in patients at high risk for ventricular arrhythmias after coronary artery bypass graft surgery. Coronary Artery Bypass Graft (CABG) Patch Trial Investigators. N Engl J Med 337:1569-1575, 1997.
6. Aklog L, Adams DH, Couper GS, et al: Techniques and results of direct-access minimally invasive mitral valve surgery: A paradigm for the future. J Thorac Cardiovasc Surg 116:705-715, 1998.
7. Machler HE, Bergmann P, Anelli-Monti M, et al: Minimally invasive versus conventional aortic valve operations: A prospective study in 120 patients. Ann Thorac Surg 67:1001-1005, 1999.
8. Magovern JA, Benckart DH, Landreneau RJ, et al: Morbidity, cost, and six-month outcome of minimally invasive direct coronary artery bypass grafting. Ann Thorac Surg 66:1224-1229, 1998.
9. Allen KB, Griffith GL, Heimansohn DA, et al: Endoscopic versus traditional saphenous vein harvesting: A prospective, randomized trial. Ann Thorac Surg 66:26-32, 1998.
10. Filsoufi F, Aklog L, Adams DH: Minimally invasive CABG. Curr Opin Cardiol 16:306-309, 2001.
11. Byrne JG, Aklog L, Adams DH: Assessment and management of functional or ischaemic mitral regurgitation. Lancet 335:1743-1744, 2000.
12. Katz NM, Gersh BJ, Cox JL: Changing practice of coronary bypass surgery and its impact on early risk and long-term survival. Curr Opin Cardiol 13:465-475, 1998.
13. Aldea GS, Gaudiani JM, Shapira OM, et al: Effect of gender on postoperative outcomes and hospital stays after coronary artery bypass grafting. Ann Thorac Surg 67:1097-1103, 1999.
14. Mullany CJ, Mock MB, Brooks MM, et al: Effect of age in the Bypass Angioplasty Revascularization Investigation (BARI) randomized trial. Ann Thorac Surg 67:396-403, 1999.
15. Filsoufi F, Adams DH: Surgical approaches to coronary artery disease. Curr Treat Options Cardiovasc Med 4:55-63, 2002.
16. Blanche C, Khan SS, Chaux A, et al: Cardiac reoperations in octogenarians: Analysis of outcomes. Ann Thorac Surg 67:93-98, 1999.
17. Adams DH, Chen RH, Kadner A, et al: Impact of small prosthetic valve size on operative mortality in the elderly after aortic valve replacement for aortic stenosis: Does gender matter? J Thorac Cardiovasc Surg 118:815-822, 1999.
18. Jamieson WR, Edwards FH, Schwartz M, et al: Risk stratification for cardiac valve replacement. National Cardiac Surgery Database. Database Committee of The Society of Thoracic Surgeons. Ann Thorac Surg 67:943-951, 1999.
19. Lazar HL, Jacobs AK, Aldea GS, et al: Factors influencing mortality after emergency coronary artery bypass grafting for failed percutaneous transluminal coronary angioplasty. Ann Thorac Surg 64:1747-1752, 1997.
20. Gott JP, Thourani VH, Wright CE, et al: Risk neutralization in cardiac operations: Detection and treatment of associated carotid disease. Ann Thorac Surg 68:850-857, 1999.
21. Duarte IG, Murphy CO, Kosinski AS, et al: Late survival after valve operation in patients with left ventricular dysfunction. Ann Thorac Surg 64:1089-1095, 1997.
22. Couper GS, Dekkers RJ, Adams DH: The logistics and cost-effectiveness of circulatory support: Advantages of the ABIOMED BVS 5000. Ann Thorac Surg 68:646-649, 1999.
23. Erickson LC, Torchiana DF, Schneider EC, et al: The relationship between managed care insurance and use of lower-mortality hospitals for CABG surgery. JAMA 283:1976-1982, 2000.
24. Alexander KP, Anstrom KJ, Muhlbaier LH, et al: Outcomes of cardiac surgery in patients age ≥ 80 years: Results from the National Cardiovascular Network. J Am Coll Cardiol 35:731-738, 2000.
25. Byrne JG, Karavas AN, Filsoufi F, et al: Aortic valve surgery after previous CABG with functioning IMA grafts. Ann Thorac Surg 73:779-784, 2002.
26. Byrne JG, Karavas AN, Adams DH, et al: The preferred approach for mitral valve surgery after CABG: Right thoracotomy, hypothermia and avoidance of LIMA-LAD graft. J Heart Valve Dis 10:584-590, 2001.
27. Adams DH, Filsoufi F, Byrne JG, et al: Mitral valve repair in redo cardiac surgery. J Card Surg 17:40-45, 2002.

Preoperative Evaluation

28. Akins CW: Combined carotid endarterectomy and coronary revascularization operation. Ann Thorac Surg 66:1483-1484, 1998.
29. Scarborough JE, White W, Derilus FE, et al: Neurologic outcomes after coronary artery bypass grafting with and without cardiopulmonary bypass. Semin Thorac Cardiovasc Surg 15:52-62, 2003.
30. Levinson MM, Rodriguez DI: Endarterectomy for preventing stroke in symptomatic and asymptomatic carotid stenosis: Review of clinical trials and recommendations for surgical therapy. Heart Surg Forum 2:147-168, 1999.
31. Allie DE, Lirtzman M, Malik AP, et al: Rapid-staged strategy for concomitant critical carotid and left main coronary disease with left ventricular dysfunction: IABP use. Ann Thorac Surg 66:1230-1235, 1998.
32. Aranki SF, Adams DH, Rizzo RJ, et al: Determinants of early mortality and late survival in mitral valve endocarditis. Circulation 92(Suppl 2):143-149, 1995.
33. Filsoufi F, Adams DH: Surgical treatment of mitral valve endocarditis. *In* Cohn LH, Edmunds LH (eds): Cardiac Surgery in the Adult. 2nd ed. New York, McGraw-Hill, 2003, pp 987-997.
34. Leavitt BJ, O'Connor GT, Olmstead EM, et al: Use of the internal mammary artery graft and in-hospital mortality and other adverse outcomes associated with coronary artery bypass surgery. Circulation 103:507-512, 2001.
35. Uva MS, Braunberger E, Fisher M, et al: Does bilateral internal thoracic artery grafting increase surgical risk in diabetic patients? Ann Thorac Surg 66:2051-2055, 1998.
36. Engoren M, Buderer NF, Zacharias A, Habib RH: Variables predicting reintubation after cardiac surgical procedures. Ann Thorac Surg 67:661-665, 1999.
37. Milas BL, Jobes DR, Gorman RC: Management of bleeding and coagulopathy after heart surgery. Semin Thorac Cardiovasc Surg 12:326-336, 2000.
38. Meharwal ZS, Trehan N: Vascular complications of intra-aortic balloon insertion in patients undergoing coronary revascularization: Analysis of 911 cases. Eur J Cardiothorac Surg 21:741-747, 2002.
39. Rihal C, Eagle K, Mickel M, et al: Surgical therapy for coronary artery disease among patients with combined coronary artery and peripheral vascular disease. Circulation 91:46, 1995.
40. Higgins T, Estafanous F, Lloyd F, et al: Stratification of morbidity and mortality outcome by preoperative risk factors in coronary artery bypass patients: A clinical severity score. JAMA 207:2344, 1992.
41. Edwards FH, Carey JS, Grover FL, et al: Impact of gender on coronary bypass operative mortality. Ann Thorac Surg 66:125-131, 1998.
42. Athanasiou T, Al-Ruzzeh S, Del Stanbridge R, et al: Is the female gender an independent predictor of adverse outcome after off-pump coronary artery bypass grafting? Ann Thorac Surg 75:1153-1160, 2003.
43. Ferraris VA, Ferraris SP: Risk factors for postoperative morbidity. J Thorac Cardiovasc Surg 111:731-741, 1996.
44. Tu JV, Jaglal SB, Naylor CD, Steering Committee of the Provincial Adult Cardiac Care Network of Ontario: Multicenter validation of a risk index for mortality, intensive care unit stay, and overall hospital length of stay after cardiac surgery. Circulation 91:677, 1995.
45. Brooks MM, Jones RH, Bach RG, et al: Predictors of mortality and mortality from cardiac causes in the Bypass Angioplasty Revascularization Investigation (BARI) randomized trial and registry. Circulation 101:2682-2689, 2000.
46. Vogt A, Grube E, Glunz HG, et al: Determinants of mortality after cardiac surgery: Results of the Registry of the Arbeitsgemeinschaft Leitender Kardiologischer Krankenhausarzte (ALKK) on 10,525 patients. Eur Heart J 21:28-32, 2000.
47. Roques F, Nashef SA, Michel P, et al: Risk factors and outcome in European cardiac surgery: Analysis of the EuroSCORE multinational database of 19,030 patients. Eur J Cardiothorac Surg 15:816-822, 1999.
48. Nashef SA, Roques F, Michel P, et al: European system for cardiac operative risk evaluation (EuroSCORE). Eur J Cardiothorac Surg 16:9-13, 1999.
49. Geissler HJ, Hölzl P, Marohl S, et al: Risk stratification in heart surgery: Comparison of six score systems. Eur J Cardiothoracic Surg 17:400-406, 2000.
50. Nashef SA, Roques F, Hammill BG, et al: Validation of European system for cardiac operative risk evaluation (EuroSCORE) in North American cardiac surgery. Eur J Cardiothoracic Surg 22:101-105, 2002.
51. Roques F, Michel P, Goldstone AR, et al: The logistic EuroSCORE. Eur Heart J 24:881-882, 2003.
52. Borger MA, Rao V, Weisel RD, et al: Deep sternal wound infection: Risk factors and outcomes. Ann Thorac Surg 65:1050-1056, 1998.
53. Pevni D, Mohr R, Lev-Run O, et al: Influence of bilateral skeletonized harvesting on occurrence of deep sternal wound infection in 1,000 consecutive patients undergoing bilateral internal thoracic artery grafting. Ann Surg 237:277-280, 2003.

54. Braxton JH, Marrin CA, McGrath PD, et al: Mediastinitis and long-term survival after coronary artery bypass graft surgery. Ann Thorac Surg 70:2004-2007, 2000.
55. Pasquet A, Lauer MS, Williams MJ, et al: Prediction of global left ventricular function after bypass surgery in patients with severe left ventricular dysfunction: Impact of preoperative myocardial function, perfusion, and metabolism. Eur Heart J 21:125-136, 2000.
56. Reichek N: MRI myocardial tagging. J Magn Reson Imaging 10:609-616, 1999.
57. Bogaert J, Bosmans H, Maes A, et al: Remote myocardial dysfunction after acute anterior myocardial infarction—impact of left ventricular shape on regional function: A magnetic resonance myocardial tagging study. J Am Coll Cardiol 35:1525-1534, 2000.
58. Athanasuleas CL, Stanley AW, Buckberg GD, et al: Surgical anterior ventricular endocardial restoration (SAVER) for dilated ischemic cardiomyopathy. Semin Thorac Cardiovasc Surg 13:448-458, 2001.
59. Salati M, Lemma M, Di Mattia DG, et al: Myocardial revascularization in patients with ischemic cardiomyopathy: Functional observations. Ann Thorac Surg 64:1728-1734, 1997.
60. Bax JJ, Schinkel AFL, Boersma E, et al. Early versus delayed revascularization in patients with ischemic cardiomyopathy and substantial viability: Impact on outcome. Circulation 108:II39-II42, 2003.
61. Qin JX, Shiota T, McCarthy PM, et al. Importance of mitral valve repair associated with left ventricular reconstruction for patients with ischemic cardiomyopathy: A real-time three-dimensional echocardiography study. Circulation 108:II241-II246, 2003.
62. Fullerton DA, Jones SD, Jaggers J, et al: Effective control of pulmonary vascular resistance with inhaled nitric oxide after cardiac operation. J Thorac Cardiovasc Surg 111:753-762, 1996.
63. Moazami N, Damiano RJ, Bailey MS, et al: Nesiritide (BNP) in the management of postoperative cardiac patients. Ann Thorac Surg 75:1974-1976, 2003.
64. Young JB, Abraham WT, Stevenson LW, et al: Intravenous nesiritide vs nitroglycerin for treatment of decompensated congestive heart failure. JAMA 287:1531-1540, 2002.
65. Alvarez JM: Emergency coronary bypass grafting for failed percutaneous coronary artery stenting: Increased costs and platelet transfusion requirements after the use of abciximab. J Thorac Cardiovasc Surg 115:472-473, 1998.
66. Tardiff BE, Califf RM, Morris D, et al: Coronary revascularization surgery after myocardial infarction: Impact of bypass surgery on survival after thrombolysis. GUSTO Investigators. Global Utilization of Streptokinase and Tissue Plasminogen Activator for Occluded Coronary Arteries. J Am Coll Cardiol 29:240-249, 1997.
67. Braxton JH, Hammond GL, Letsou GV, et al: Optimal timing of coronary artery bypass graft surgery after acute myocardial infarction. Circulation 92:66, 1995.
68. Misfeld M, Dubbert S, Eleftheriadis S, et al: Fibrinolysis-adjusted perioperative low-dose aprotin reduces blood loss in bypass operations. Ann Thorac Surg 66:792-799, 1998.
69. Lee DC, Oz MC, Weinberg AD, et al: Optimal timing of revascularization: Transmural versus nontransmural acute myocardial infarction. Ann Thorac Surg 71:1197-1202, 2001.
70. Lee DC, Oz MC, Weinberg AD, et al: Appropriate timing of surgical intervention after transmural acute myocardial infarction. J Thorac Cardiovasc Surg 125:115-119, 2003.
71. Stone GW, Ohman EM, Miller MF, et al: Contemporary utilization and outcomes of intra-aortic balloon counterpulsation in acute myocardial infarction. J Am Coll Cardiol 41:1940-1945, 2003.
72. Kouchoukos NT, Blackstone EH, Doty DB, et al: Anesthesia for cardiovascular surgery. *In* Kirklin J, Barratt-Boyes B (eds): Cardiac Surgery. New York, Churchill Livingstone, 2003, p 163.
73. Savino JS, Floyd TE, Cheung AT: Cardiac anesthesia. *In* Cohn LH, Edmunds LH (eds): Cardiac Surgery in the Adult. New York, McGraw-Hill, 2003, p 249.
74. DeFoe GR, Ross CS, Olmstead EM, et al: Lowest hematocrit on bypass and adverse outcomes associated with coronary artery bypass grafting. Northern New England Cardiovascular Disease Study Group. Ann Thorac Surg 71:769-776, 2001.
75. Fillinger MP, Surgenor SD, Hartman GS, et al: The association between heart rate and in-hospital mortality after coronary artery bypass surgery. Anesth Analg 95:1483-1488, 2002.
76. DeFoe GR, Krumholz CF, DioDato CP, et al: Lowest core body temperature and adverse outcomes associated with coronary artery bypass surgery. Perfusion 18:127-133, 2003.
77. Lemmer JH Jr, Metzdorff MT, Krause AH Jr, et al: Emergency coronary artery bypass graft surgery in abciximab-treated patients. Ann Thorac Surg 66:90-95, 2000.
78. Morales DL, Garrido MJ, Madigan JD, et al: A double-blind randomized trial: prophylactic vasopressin reduces hypotension after cardiopulmonary bypass. Ann Thorac Surg 75:926-930, 2003.
78a. Bigger JT Jr, Whang W, Rottman JN, et al: Mechanisms of death in the CABG PATCH trial: A randomized trial of implantable cardiac defibrillator prophylaxis in patients with high risk of death after coronary bypass graft surgery. Circulation 99:1416, 1999.
79. Cartier R, Brann S, Dagenais F, et al: Systematic off-pump coronary artery revascularization in multivessel disease: Experience of three hundred cases. J Thorac Cardiovasc Surg 119:221-229, 2000.
80. Berger PB, Alderman EL, Nadel A, Schaff HV: Frequency of early occlusion and stenosis in a left internal mammary artery to left anterior descending artery bypass graft after surgery through a median sternotomy on conventional bypass: Benchmark for minimally invasive direct coronary artery bypass. Circulation 100:2353-2358, 1999.
81. Al-Ruzzeh S, Ambler G, Asimakopoulos, et al: Off-pump coronary artery bypass (OPCAB) surgery reduces risk-stratified morbidity and mortality: A United Kingdom multi-center comparative analysis of early outcome. Circulation 108:II1-II8, 2003.
82. Magee MJ, Coombs LP, Peterson ED, et al: Patient selection and current practice strategy for off-pump coronary artery bypass surgery. Circulation 108:II9-II14, 2003.
83. Sharony R, Bizekis CS, Kanchuger M, et al: Off-pump coronary artery bypass grafting reduces mortality and stroke in patients with atheromatous aortas: A case control study. Circulation 108:II15-II20, 2003.
84. Sharony R, Grossi EA, Saunders PC, et al: Minimally invasive aortic valve surgery in the elderly: A case-control study. Circulation 108:II43-II47, 2003.
85. Casselman FP, Slycke SV, Wellens F, et al: Mitral valve surgery can now routinely be performed endoscopically. Circulation 108:II48-II54, 2003.
86. Argenziano M, Oz MC, Kohmoto T, et al: Totally endoscopic atrial septal defect repair with robotic assistance. Circulation 108:II191-II194, 2003.
86a. Athanasion T, Al-Ruzzeh S, Kumar P, et al: Off-pump myocardial revascularization is associated with less incidence of stroke in elderly patients. Ann Thorac Surg 77:745, 2004.
86b. Khan NE, De Souza A, Mister R, et al: A randomized comparison of off-pump and on-pump multivessel coronary-artery bypass surgery. N Engl J Med 350:1, 2004.

Postoperative Management

87. Thourani VH, Weintraub WS, Stein B, et al: Influence of diabetes mellitus on early and late outcome after coronary artery bypass grafting. Ann Thorac Surg 67:1045-1052, 1999.
88. Fish LH, Weaver TW, Moore AL, et al: Value of postoperative blood glucose in predicting complications and length of stay after coronary artery bypass grafting. Am J Cardiol 92:74-76, 2003.
89. Furnary AP, Gao G, Grunkemeier GL, et al: Continuous insulin infusion reduces mortality in patients with diabetes undergoing coronary artery bypass grafting. J Thorac Cardiovasc Surg 125:1007-1021, 2003.
90. Canver CC, Chanda J: Intraoperative and postoperative risk factors for respiratory failure after coronary bypass. Ann Thorac Surg 75:853-857, 2003.
91. Adams DH, Filsoufi F, Aklog L: Surgical treatment of the ischemic mitral valve. J Heart Valve Dis Suppl 1:S21-S25, 2002.
92. Aklog L, Filsoufi F, Flores KQ, et al: Does coronary artery bypass grafting alone correct moderate ischemic mitral regurgitation? Circulation 104(Suppl 1):I68-I75, 2001.
93. ZuWallack RL, Mahler DA, Reilly D, et al: Salmeterol plus theophylline combination therapy in the treatment of COPD. Chest 119:1661-1670, 2001.
94. Katz MG, Katz R, Schachner A, Cohen AJ: Phrenic nerve injury after coronary artery bypass grafting: Will it go away? Ann Thorac Surg 65:32-35, 1998.
95. Stamenkovic SA, Morgan IS, Pontefract DR, Campanella C: Is early tracheostomy safe in cardiac patients with median sternotomy incisions? Ann Thorac Surg 69:1152-1154, 2000.
96. Vuylsteke A, Feneck RO, Jolin-Mellgard A, et al: Perioperative blood pressure control: A prospective survey of patient management in cardiac surgery. J Cardiothorac Vasc Anesth 14:269-273, 2000.
97. Cooper TJ, Clutton BTH, Jones SN, et al: Factors relating to the development of hypertension after cardiopulmonary bypass. Br Heart J 54:91, 1985.
98. Hamm CW, Reimers J, Ischinger T, et al: A randomized study of coronary angioplasty compared with bypass surgery in patients with symptomatic multivessel coronary disease. German Angioplasty Bypass Surgery Investigation (GABI). N Engl J Med 331:1037, 1994.
99. King SE, Lembo NJ, Weintraub WS, et al: A randomized trial comparing coronary angioplasty with coronary bypass surgery. Emory Angioplasty Versus Surgery Trial (EAST). N Engl J Med 331:1044, 1994.
100. Greaves S, Rutherford J, Aranki S, et al: Current incidence and determinants of perioperative myocardial infarction in coronary artery surgery. Am Heart J 132:572-573, 1996.
101. Myers MG, Fremes SE: Prevention of radial artery graft spasm: A survey of Canadian surgical centres. Can J Cardiol 19:677-681, 2003.
102. Muneretto C, Negri A, Manfredi J, et al: Safety and usefulness of composite grafts for total arterial myocardial revascularization: A prospective randomized evaluation. J Thorac Cardiovasc Surg 125:826-835, 2003.
103. Obarski TP, Loop FD, Cosgrove DM, et al: Frequency of acute myocardial infarction in valve repairs versus valve replacement for pure mitral regurgitation. Am J Cardiol 65:887, 1990.
104. Fransen EJ, Diris JH, Maessen JG, et al: Evaluation of "new" cardiac markers for ruling out myocardial infarction after coronary artery bypass grafting. Chest 122:1316-1321, 2002.
105. Kim LJ, Martinez EA, Faraday N, et al: Cardiac troponin I predicts short-term mortality in vascular surgery patients. Circulation 106:2366-2371, 2002.
106. Nalysnyk L, Fahrbach K, Reynolds MW, et al: Adverse events in coronary artery bypass graft (CABG) trials: A systematic review and analysis. Heart 89:767-772, 2003.
107. Joffe II, Jacobs LE, Lampert C, et al: Role of echocardiography in perioperative management of patients undergoing open heart surgery. Am Heart J 131:162, 1995.
108. Anderson CA, Filsoufi F, Aklog L, et al: Liberal use of delayed sternal closure for postcardiotomy hemodynamic instability. Ann Thorac Surg 73:1484-1488, 2002.
109. Shalabi RI, Amin M, Ayed AK, et al: Delayed sternal closure is a life-saving decision. Ann Thorac Cardiovasc Surg 4:220-223, 2002.
110. Frazier OH, Myers TJ, Westaby S, et al: Use of the Jarvik 2000 left ventricular assist system as a bridge to heart transplantation or as destination therapy for patients with chronic heart failure. Ann Surg 237:631-637, 2003.
111. Richenbacher WE, Naka Y, Raines EP, et al: Surgical management of patients in the REMATCH trial. Ann Thorac Surg 75:S86-S92, 2003.
112. Radovancevic B, Vrtovec B, Frazier OH: Left ventricular assist devices: An alternative to medical therapy for end-stage heart failure. Curr Opin Cardiol 18:210-214, 2003.
113. Costachescu T, Denault A, Guimond JG, et al: The hemodynamically unstable patient in the intensive care unit: Hemodynamic vs. transesophageal echocardiographic monitoring. Crit Care Med 30:1214-1223, 2002.
114. Kuvin JT, Harati NA, Pandian NG, et al: Postoperative cardiac tamponade in the modern surgical era. Ann Thorac Surg 74:1148-1153, 2002.
115. Schmidlin D, Schuepbach R, Bernard E, et al: Indications and impact of postoperative transesophageal echocardiography in cardiac surgical patients. Crit Care Med 29:2143-2148, 2001.
116. Mizuno T, Tanaka H, Makita S, et al: Biventricular pacing with coronary bypass and Dor's ventriculoplasty. Ann Thorac Surg 75:998-999, 2003.

117. DeRose JJ, Ashton RC, Belsley S, et al: Robotically assisted left ventricular epicardial lead implantation for biventricular pacing. J Am Coll Cardiol 41:1414-1419, 2003.
118. Aranki S, Shaw D, Adams D, et al: Predictors of atrial fibrillation following coronary artery surgery: Current trends and impact on hospital resources. Circulation 94:390-397, 1996.
119. Redle JD, Khurana S, Marzan R, et al: Prophylactic oral amiodarone compared with placebo for prevention of atrial fibrillation after coronary artery bypass surgery. Am Heart J 138:144-150, 1999.
120. Daoud EG, Strickberger SA, Man KC, et al: Preoperative amiodarone as prophylaxis against atrial fibrillation after heart surgery. N Engl J Med 337:1785-1791, 1997.
121. Ascione R, Caputo M, Calori G, et al: Predictors of atrial fibrillation after conventional and beating heart surgery: A prospective, randomized study. Circulation 102:1530-1535, 2000.
122. Creswell LL, Damiano RJ: Postoperative atrial fibrillation: An old problem crying for new solutions. J Thorac Cardiovasc Surg 121:638-641, 2003.
123. Maisel WH, Rawn JD, Stevenson WG: Atrial fibrillation after cardiac surgery. Ann Intern Med 135:1061-1073, 2001.
124. Crystal E, Kahn S, Roberts R, et al: Long-term amiodarone therapy and the risk of complications after cardiac surgery: Results from the Canadian Amiodarone Myocardial Infarction Arrhythmia Trial (CAMIAT). J Thorac Cardiovasc Surg 125:633-637, 2003.
125. Klein AL, Grimm RA, Murray RD, et al: Use of transesophageal echocardiography to guide cardioversion in patients with atrial fibrillation. N Engl J Med 344:1411-1420, 2001.
126. Gaita F, Riccardi R, Gallotti R: Surgical approaches to atrial fibrillation. Card Electrophysiol Rev 6:401-405, 2002.
127. Mooss AN, Wurdeman RL, Mohiuddin SM: Esmolol versus diltiazem in the treatment of postoperative atrial fibrillation/atrial flutter after open heart surgery. Am Heart J 140:176-180, 2000.
128. VanderLugt JT, Mattioni T, Denker S, et al: Efficacy and safety of ibutilide fumarate for the conversion of atrial arrhythmias after cardiac surgery. Circulation 100:369-375, 1999.
129. Raitt MH, Dolack GL, Kino K, et al: Procainamide has limited effectiveness for the treatment of atrial fibrillation after open heart surgery. Circulation 90(Supp 1):376, 1994.
130. Willems S, Weiss C, Meinertz T: Tachyarrhythmias following coronary artery bypass graft surgery: Epidemiology, mechanisms, and current therapeutic strategies. Thorac Cardiovasc Surg 45:232-237, 1997.
131. Koplan BA, Stevenson WG, Epstein LM, et al: Development and validation of a simple risk score to predict the need for permanent pacing after cardiac valve surgery. J Am Coll Cardiol 41:795-801, 2003.
132. Emlein G, Huang S, Pires L, et al: Prolonged bradyarrhythmias after isolated coronary artery bypass graft surgery. Am Heart J 126:1084, 1993.
133. Morse DS, Adams DH, Magnani B: Platelet and neutrophil activation during cardiac surgical procedures: Impact of cardiopulmonary bypass. Ann Thorac Surg 65:691-695, 1998.
134. Levi M, Cromheecke ME, de Jonge E, et al: Pharmacological strategies to decrease excessive blood loss in cardiac surgery: A meta-analysis of clinically relevant endpoints. Lancet 354:1940-1947, 2000.
135. Kearon C, Crowther M, Hirsh J: Management of patients with hereditary hypercoagulable disorders. Annu Rev Med 51:169-185, 2000.
136. Clagett GP, Anderson FA Jr, Geerts W, et al: Prevention of venous thromboembolism. Chest 114(5 Suppl):531S-560S, 1998.
137. Garcia-Torres R, Amigo MC, de la Rosa A, et al: Valvular heart disease in primary antiphospholipid syndrome (PAPS): Clinical and morphological findings. Lupus 5:56-61, 1996.
138. Brenner B, Blumenfeld Z, Markiewicz W, et al: Cardiac involvement in patients with primary antiphospholipid syndrome. J Am Coll Cardiol 18:931-936, 1991.
139. Levine JS, Branch DW, Rauch J: The antiphospholipid syndrome. N Engl J Med 346:752-763, 2002.
140. Hogan WJ, McBane RD, Santrach PJ, et al: Antiphospholipid syndrome and perioperative hemostatic management of cardiac valvular surgery. Mayo Clin Proc 75:971-976, 2000.
141. Fanashawe MP, Shore-Lesserson L, Reich DL: Two cases of fatal thrombosis after aminocaproic acid therapy and deep hypothermic circulatory arrest. Anesthesiology 95:1525-1527, 2001.
142. Ginsberg JA, Crowther MA, White RH, et al: Anticoagulation therapy. Hematology (Am Soc Hematol Educ Program) 339-357, 2001.
143. Greinacher A, Völpel H, Janssens U, et al: Recombinant hirudin (lepirudin) provides safe and effective anticoagulation in patients with heparin-induced thrombocytopenia: A prospective study. Circulation 99:73-80, 1999.
144. Sun Y, Greilich PE, Wilson SI, et al: The use of lepirudin for anticoagulation in patients with heparin-induced thrombocytopenia during major vascular surgery. Anesth Analg 92:344-346, 2001.
145. Verme-Gibboney CN, Hursting MJ: Argatroban dosing in patients with heparin-induced thrombocytopenia. Annu Pharmacother 37:970-975, 2003.
146. Koster A, Kuppe H, Hetzer R, et al: Emergent cardiopulmonary bypass in five patients with heparin-induced thrombocytopenia type II employing recombinant hirudin. Anesthesiology 89:777-780, 1998.
147. Taggart DP, Browne SM, Halligan PW, Wade DT: Is cardiopulmonary bypass still the cause of cognitive dysfunction after cardiac operations? J Thorac Cardiovasc Surg 118:414-420, 1999.
148. Puskas JD, Winston AD, Wright CE, et al: Stroke after coronary artery operation: Incidence, correlates, outcome, and cost. Ann Thorac Surg 69:1053-1056, 2000.
149. Newman MF, Kirchner JL, Phillips-Bute B, et al: Longitudinal assessment of neurocognitive function after coronary artery bypass surgery. N Engl J Med 344:395-402, 2001.
150. Carpino PA, Khabbaz KR, Bojar RM, et al: Clinical benefits of endoscopic vein harvesting in patients with risk factors for saphenectomy wound infections undergoing coronary artery bypass grafting. J Thorac Cardiovasc Surg 119:69-76, 2000.
151. The Parisian Mediastinitis Study Group: Risk factors for deep sternal wound infection after sternotomy: A prospective, multicenter study. J Thorac Cardiovasc Surg 111:1200-1207, 1996.
152. Braxton JH, Marrin CA, McGrath PD, et al: Mediastinitis and long-term survival after coronary artery bypass graft surgery. Ann Thorac Surg 70:2004-7, 2000.
153. He GW, Ryan WH, Acuff TE, et al: Risk factors for operative mortality and sternal wound infection in bilateral internal mammary artery grafting. J Thorac Cardiovasc Surg 107:196-202, 1994.
154. Milano CA, Georgiade G, Muhlbaier LH, et al: Comparison of omental and pectoralis flaps for poststernotomy mediastinitis. Ann Thorac Surg 67:377-381, 1999.
155. Rand RP, Cochran RP, Aziz S, et al: Prospective trial of catheter irrigation and muscle flaps for sternal wound infection. Ann Thorac Surg 65:1046-1049, 1998.
156. Hall J, Christiansen K, Carter M, et al: Antibiotic prophylaxis in cardiac operations. Ann Thorac Surg 56:916, 1993.
157. Niwaya K, Knott-Craig CJ, Santangelo K, et al: Advantage of autograft and homograft valve replacement for complex aortic valve endocarditis. Ann Thorac Surg 67:1603-1608, 1999.
158. Liu JY, Birkmeyer NJ, Sanders JH, et al: Risks of morbidity and mortality in dialysis patients undergoing coronary artery bypass surgery. Circulation 102:2973-2977, 2000.
159. Boldt J, Brenner T, Lehmann A, et al: Is kidney function altered by the duration of cardiopulmonary bypass? Ann Thorac Surg 75:906-912, 2003.

Rehabilitation and Preparation for Discharge

160. Fletcher G, Balady G, Froelicher V, et al: Exercise standards: A statement for healthcare professionals from the American Heart Association. Circulation 91:580, 1995.
161. Daida H, Yokoi H, Miyano H, et al: Relation of saphenous vein graft obstruction to serum cholesterol levels. J Am Coll Cardiol 25:193, 1995.
162. Walji S, Peterson RJ, Neis P, et al: Ultra-fast track hospital discharge using conventional cardiac surgical techniques. Ann Thorac Surg 67:363-370, 1999.
163. Ovrum E, Tangen G, Schiott C, et al: Rapid recovery protocol applied to 5,658 consecutive "on-pump" coronary bypass patients. Ann Thorac Surg 70:2008-2012, 2000.

CHAPTER 77

Anesthesia and Noncardiac Surgery in Patients with Heart Disease

Lee A. Fleisher • Kim A. Eagle

Cardiovascular morbidity and mortality represent a significant risk in the patient with known, or risk factors for, cardiovascular disease undergoing noncardiac surgery. Perioperative cardiovascular complications not only have implications in the immediate postoperative period but also may influence outcome over the subsequent 1 to 2 years. Over the past three decades there has been a steady progression of knowledge, from the identification of those at greatest risk, to randomized trials to identify strategies to reduce perioperative cardiovascular complications. However, much of the practice of management of the high-risk patient remains dependent on information from the nonsurgical arena. To disseminate best practices, guidelines have been developed to provide information for management of high-risk patients. This chapter attempts to distill this information, incorporating the available guidelines.

Assessment of Preoperative Risk for Noncardiac Surgery in Patients with Cardiovascular Disease

Ischemic Heart Disease

There are numerous care systems by which a patient may be evaluated prior to noncardiac surgery. The patient may be seen by his or her primary caregiver or a cardiologist. However, there are many patients who are evaluated only by the surgeon or anesthesiologist immediately before surgery. The stress of noncardiac surgery may raise heart rate and has been associated with a high incidence of symptomatic and asymptomatic myocardial ischemia. Therefore, the clinical evaluation of the patient may identify stable or unstable coronary artery disease (CAD). Patients with acute coronary syndromes, such as unstable angina or decompensated heart failure of ischemic origin, are at high risk for the development of further decompensation, myocardial necrosis, and death during the perioperative period. Such patients clearly warrant further evaluation and medical stabilization. If the noncardiac surgery is truly emergent, there are several case series utilizing intraaortic balloon bump counterpulsation as a means of providing short-term myocardial protection in addition to maximal medical therapy.

If the patient does not demonstrate unstable symptoms, the identification of known or symptomatic stable CAD or risk factors for CAD can guide the need for further diagnostic evaluation or changes in perioperative management. In determining the extent of the preoperative evaluation, it must be remembered that testing should not be performed unless the results would affect perioperative management. These management changes include cancellation of surgery because of prohibitive risk compared with benefit, delay of surgery for further medical management, coronary interventions before noncardiac surgery, utilization of an intensive care unit (ICU), and changes in monitoring.

Patients with stable angina represent a continuum from mild angina with extreme exertion to dyspnea with angina after walking up a few stairs. The patient who manifests angina only after strenuous exercise often does not demonstrate signs of left ventricular dysfunction and generally can be stabilized with adequate medical therapy, particularly treatment with beta-blocking agents. In contrast, a patient with dyspnea on mild exertion would be at high risk for perioperative ventricular dysfunction, myocardial ischemia, and possible myocardial infarction (MI). Such patients have a high probability of having extensive CAD, and additional monitoring or cardiovascular testing should be contemplated, depending upon the surgical procedure and institutional factors.

Traditionally, coronary risk assessment for noncardiac surgery in patients with a prior MI was based upon the time interval between the MI and surgery. Multiple studies demonstrated an increased incidence of reinfarction after noncardiac surgery if the prior MI was within 6 months of the operation. With improvements in perioperative care, this time interval has been shortened.[1] However, the intervening time interval is less relevant in the current era of thrombolytics, angioplasty, and routine coronary risk stratification after an acute MI. Although some patients with a recent MI may continue to have myocardium at risk for subsequent ischemia and infarction, most patients in the United

States have had their critical coronary stenosis evaluated and opened or bypassed or are receiving maximal medical therapy. The American Heart Association/American College of Cardiology Task Force on Perioperative Evaluation of the Cardiac Patient Undergoing Noncardiac Surgery has suggested that the highest risk cohort consists of patients within 6 weeks of their MI, a time period during which plaque and myocardial stabilization occur. After that period, risk stratification is based upon the presentation of disease (i.e., those with active ischemia are at highest risk).[2,3]

Hypertension

In the 1970s, a series of case studies changed the prevailing thought that antihypertensive agents should be discontinued before surgery, and suggested that poorly controlled hypertension was associated with untoward hemodynamic responses and that antihypertensive agents should be continued perioperatively. However, several large prospective studies did not establish mild to moderate hypertension as an independent predictor of postoperative cardiac complications such as cardiac death, postoperative MI, heart failure, or arrhythmias. Therefore, much of the approach to the patient with hypertension relies on management strategies from the nonsurgical literature.

More severe hypertension of a chronic nature, e.g., diastolic blood pressure higher than 110 mm Hg, should be controlled before any elective noncardiac surgery.[2] In contrast, a patient who is normally well controlled at home may demonstrate a markedly elevated blood pressure preoperatively because of anxiety. Although these patients are at increased risk for intraoperative hemodynamic lability, particularly with induction, most anesthesiologists proceed with surgery in the absence of other signs or symptoms of end-organ dysfunction.

A hypertensive crisis in the postoperative period, defined as a diastolic blood pressure higher than 120 mm Hg and clinical evidence of impending or actual end-organ damage, poses a definite risk of MI or cerebrovascular accident. Diagnostic criteria include papilledema or other evidence of increased intracranial pressure, myocardial ischemia, or acute renal failure. Several precipitants of hypertensive crises have been identified, including preeclampsia or eclampsia, pheochromocytomas, abrupt clonidine withdrawal prior to surgery, the use of chronic monoamine oxidase inhibitors with or without sympathomimetic drugs in combination, and inadvertent discontinuation of antihypertensive therapy.

Chronic hypertension may indirectly predispose patients to perioperative myocardial ischemia because CAD is more prevalent in these patients. Even in the absence of CAD, patients with chronic hypertension may have episodes of myocardial ischemia, perhaps related to impaired coronary vasodilator reserve and autoregulation such that higher arterial pressures are required to maintain adequate perfusion of vital organs. Because of vascular stiffness, hypertensive patients are also predisposed to hypotension and hence lower filling pressures. Thus, hypertensive patients with known peripheral and coronary vascular disease must have preoperative blood pressure levels monitored and maintained.

The Study of Perioperative Ischemia Research Group trial, in which patients had continuous perioperative electrocardiographic monitoring, showed that a history of hypertension was one of five independent predictors of postoperative ischemia and one of three independent predictors of increased postoperative mortality. Patients with a history of hypertension had almost twice the risk of postoperative myocardial ischemia and almost four times the risk of postoperative death compared with patients without hypertension in the first 48 hours postoperatively.

Thus, whether patients with mild to moderate hypertension should be considered at greater than average risk of perioperative myocardial ischemia remains uncertain due to often conflicting reports from the last 20 years. Surgery generally need not be postponed or canceled in the otherwise uncomplicated patient with mild to moderate hypertension.[2] Antihypertensive medications should be continued perioperatively,[2] and blood pressure should be maintained near preoperative levels to reduce the risk of myocardial ischemia. In patients with more severe hypertension, such as diastolic blood pressure higher than 110 mm Hg, the potential benefits of delaying surgery in order to optimize antihypertensive medications should be weighed against the risk of delaying the surgical procedure. With rapid-acting intravenous agents, blood pressure can usually be controlled within a matter of several hours. Weksler and colleagues studied 989 chronically treated hypertensive patients who presented for noncardiac surgery with diastolic blood pressure between 110 and 130 mm Hg and who had no previous MI, unstable or severe angina pectoris, renal failure, pregnancy-induced hypertension, left ventricular hypertrophy, previous coronary revascularization, aortic stenosis, preoperative dysrhythmias, conduction defects, or stroke.[4] The control group had their surgery postponed and remained in hospital for blood pressure control, and the study patients received 10 mg of nifedipine intranasally delivered. They observed no statistically significant differences in postoperative complications, suggesting that this subset of patients without significant cardiovascular comorbidities can proceed with surgery despite elevated blood pressure on the day of surgery.

Isolated systolic hypertension (systolic blood pressure greater than 160 mm Hg and diastolic blood pressure less than 90 mm Hg) has been identified as a risk factor for cardiovascular complications in the general population, and successful treatment reduces the future risk of stroke. However, only one study has directly assessed the relationship between cardiovascular disease and preoperative isolated systolic hypertension. In a multicenter study of patients undergoing coronary artery bypass grafting (CABG), isolated systolic hypertension was associated with a 30 percent increased incidence of cardiovascular complications compared with those in normotensive individuals.[5] Because it is unknown whether these findings can be generalized to noncardiac surgery and whether treatment will affect outcome, definition of the best approach requires further study. Treatment of systolic hypertension in elderly people is particularly challenging because the diastolic pressures are often low and unusually sensitive to hypovolemia.

Heart Failure

Heart failure has been associated in several studies with perioperative cardiac morbidity after noncardiac surgery.[6] Cohn and Goldman identified a third heart sound or other signs of heart failure as portending the most significant perioperative risks. For patients who present for noncardiac surgery with signs or symptoms of heart failure, its underpinnings need to be characterized before major noncardiac surgery. The goal of the preoperative evaluation should be identification of the underlying myocardial disease and assessment of the severity of systolic and diastolic dysfunction. Treatment of decompensated hypertrophic cardiomyopathy is very different from that of dilated cardiomyopathy, and the preoperative evaluation can influence perioperative management. In particular, this assessment may influence perioperative fluid and vasopressor management. Ischemic cardiomyopathy is of greatest concern because the patient has a substantial risk for developing further ischemia, leading to myocardial necrosis and potentially a downward spiral. In such patients, a pulmonary artery catheter or intraoperative transesophageal echocardiography could be indicated.

Obstructive hypertrophic cardiomyopathy was formerly regarded as a high-risk condition associated with high perioperative morbidity. A retrospective review of perioperative care in 35 patients concluded that the risk of general anesthesia and major noncardiac surgery is low in such patients. However, this study did suggest that spinal anesthesia may be relatively contraindicated in view of the sensitivity of cardiac output to hypovolemia in this condition. Haering and colleagues studied 77 patients with asymmetrical septal hypertrophy who were retrospectively identified from a large data base.[7] Forty percent of patients had one or more adverse perioperative cardiac events, including one patient who had an MI and ventricular tachycardia that required emergent cardioversion; the majority of the events were perioperative congestive heart failure. There were no perioperative deaths. Important independent risk factors for adverse outcome in all patients include major surgery and increasing duration of surgery. Unlike the findings in the original cohort of patients, the type of anesthesia was not an independent risk factor.

Valvular Heart Disease

The presence of critical aortic stenosis associates with a very high risk of cardiac decompensation in patients undergoing elective noncardiac surgery. The presence of any of the classical triad of angina, syncope, and heart failure in a patient with aortic stenosis should alert the clinician to the need for further evaluation and potential interventions, usually valve replacement. However, many patients with severe or critical aortic stenosis may be asymptomatic, and preoperative patients with aortic systolic murmurs warrant a careful history and physical examination and often further evaluation. There are several case series of patients with critical aortic stenosis demonstrating that, when necessary, noncardiac surgery can be performed with acceptable risk.[8] For the most part, these cases have included patients with few or no symptoms but a valve area less than 0.5 cm^2. Alternatively, aortic valvuloplasty represents an option for occasional patients. Although the long-term outcome of patients who undergo aortic balloon valvuloplasty is generally poor,[9] primarily because of restenosis, this procedure may be used for temporary benefit in noncardiac surgery in patients who cannot undergo valve replacement in the short term. The considerable procedure-related morbidity and mortality risk must be carefully considered before recommending this strategy as a means of trying to lower the risk of noncardiac surgery.

Mitral valve disease tends to cause less risk of perioperative complications than aortic stenosis. However, occult mitral stenosis from rheumatic heart disease is still encountered on occasion and can lead to severe left-sided heart failure in the presence of tachycardia or volume loading, or both. In contrast to aortic valvuloplasty, mitral valve balloon valvuloplasty often yields reasonable short- and long-term benefit, especially in younger patients with predominant mitral stenosis but without severe mitral valve leaflet thickening or significant subvalvular fibrosis and calcification.[10] In the perioperative patient with a functioning prosthetic heart valve, the major issues are antibiotic prophylaxis and anticoagulation. All patients with prosthetic valves who are undergoing procedures that can cause transient bacteremia should receive prophylaxis.[11,12]

In patients with prosthetic valves, the risk of increased bleeding during a procedure in a patient receiving antithrombotic therapy must be weighed against the increased risk of a thromboembolism caused by stopping the therapy. The common practice for patients with a mechanical prosthetic valve in place undergoing noncardiac surgery is the cessation of anticoagulants 3 days prior to surgery. This allows the International Normalized Ratio (INR) to fall to less than 1.5 times normal. The oral anticoagulants can then be resumed on postoperative day 1. Using a similar protocol, Katholi and colleagues observed no perioperative episodes of thromboembolism or hemorrhage in 25 patients. An alternative approach in patients at high risk for thromboembolism is conversion to heparin during the perioperative period. The heparin can be discontinued 4 to 6 hours prior to surgery and resumed shortly thereafter. Current prosthetic valves may involve a lower incidence, and the risk of heparin may outweigh the benefit in the perioperative setting. According to the American Heart Association/American College of Cardiology guidelines, heparin usually can be reserved for those who have had a recent thrombosis or embolus (arbitrarily within 1 year), those with demonstrated thrombotic problems when previously not receiving therapy, those with the Björk-Shiley valve, and those with more than three risk factors (atrial fibrillation, previous thromboembolism, hypercoagulable condition, and mechanical prosthesis).[13] A lower threshold for recommending heparin should be considered for patients with mechanical valves in the mitral position, in whom a single risk factor would be sufficient evidence of high risk. Subcutaneous low-molecular-weight heparin offers an alternative outpatient approach.[14] It is critical to have a discussion between the surgeon and cardiologist regarding the optimal perioperative management.

Congenital Heart Disease in Adults

(see also Chap. 56)

Congenital heart disease afflicts some 500,000 to 1 million adults in the United States alone. The nature of the underlying anatomy and any anatomical correction affect the perioperative plan and incidence of complications, including infection, bleeding, hypoxemia, hypotension, and paradoxical embolization. A major concern in the patient with congenital heart disease is the development of pulmonary hypertension and Eisenmenger syndrome. It has been thought traditionally that regional anesthesia should be avoided in these patients because of the potential for sympathetic blockade and worsening of the shunt. However, a review of the published literature incorporating 103 cases found that overall perioperative mortality was 14 percent; patients receiving regional anesthesia had a mortality of 5 percent, whereas those receiving general anesthesia had a mortality of 18 percent.[15] The authors concluded that most deaths probably occurred as a result of the surgical procedure and disease and not anesthesia. Although perioperative and peripartum mortalities were high, many anesthetic agents and techniques had been used with success. Patients with congenital heart disease are at risk for infective endocarditis and should receive antibiotic prophylaxis. A review discusses the anesthetic management of these patients in detail.[16]

Arrhythmias

Cardiac arrhythmias are common in the perioperative period, particularly in elderly patients or patients under-going thoracic surgery. Predisposing factors include pain (e.g., from hip fractures), severe anxiety, and other situations that heighten adrenergic tone. A prospective study of 4181 patients 50 years of age or older demonstrated supraventricular arrhythmia in 2 percent of patients during and 6.1 percent after surgery. Perioperative atrial fibrillation raises several concerns, including stroke.[17] Therefore, early treatment to restore sinus rhythm or control the ventricular response and anticoagulation is indicated. Amar and colleagues evaluated the prophylactic value of intravenous

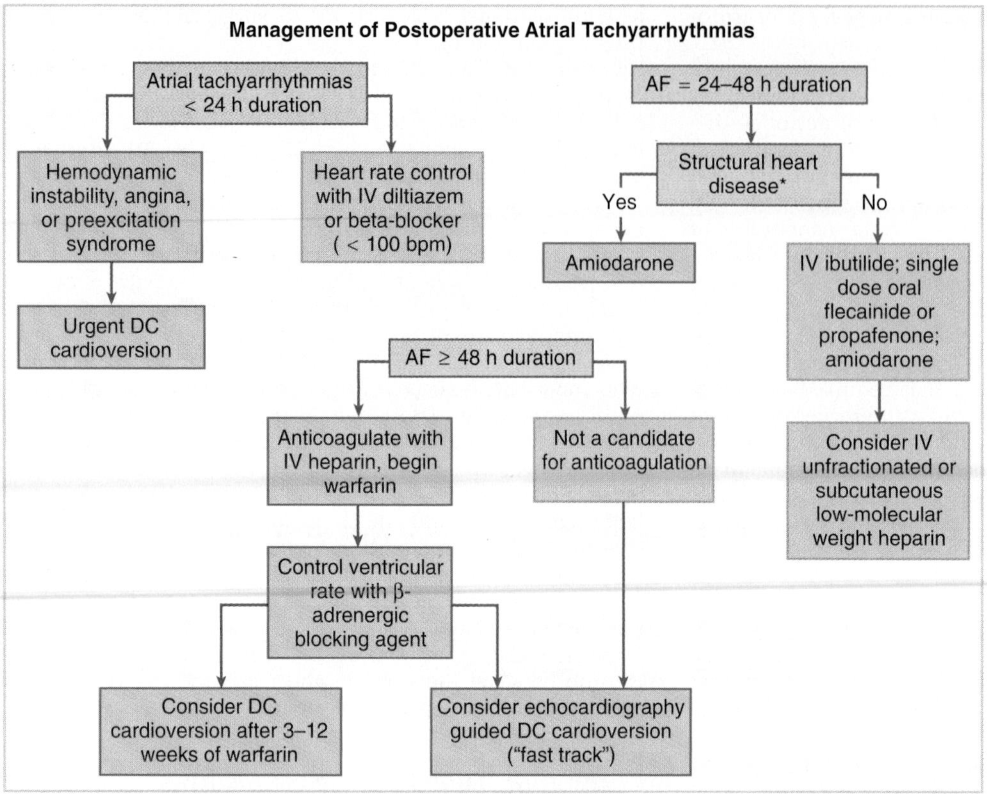

FIGURE 77–1 Proposed algorithm for the treatment of postoperative atrial tachyarrhythmias. AF = atrial fibrillation or flutter; bpm = beats/min; DC = direct current. *Structural heart disease is defined as the presence of one of the following: left ventricular hypertrophy with wall thickness greater than 1.4 cm, mitral valve disease, coronary artery disease, or heart failure. (From Amar D: Perioperative atrial tachyarrhythmias. Anesthesiology 97:1618, 2002.)

diltiazem in a randomized, placebo-controlled trial involving high-risk thoracic surgery and reported that prophylactic diltiazem reduced the incidence of clinically significant atrial arrhythmias.[18] Balser and colleagues studied 64 cases of postoperative supraventricular tachyarrhythmia.[19] After adenosine administration, patients who remained in supraventricular tachyarrhythmia were prospectively randomly assigned to receive either intravenous diltiazem or intravenous esmolol for ventricular rate control. The authors reported that intravenous esmolol produced a more rapid (2-hour) conversion to sinus rhythm than intravenous diltiazem. The literature has been reviewed and an algorithm for treatment produced (Fig. 77–1).[17]

Although ventricular arrhythmias were originally identified as a risk factor for perioperative morbidity, subsequent studies have not confirmed this finding. O'Kelly studied a consecutive sample of 230 male patients with known CAD or at high risk for CAD undergoing major noncardiac surgical procedures. Preoperative arrhythmias were associated with the occurrence of intraoperative and postoperative arrhythmias. However, nonfatal MI and cardiac death did not occur significantly more frequently in those with prior perioperative arrhythmias. Amar and colleagues studied 412 patients undergoing major thoracic surgery and determined that the incidence of nonsustained ventricular tachycardia is 15 percent but is not associated with poor outcome.[20] Despite this finding, the presence of an arrhythmia in the preoperative setting should provoke a search for underlying cardiopulmonary disease, ongoing myocardial ischemia or infarction, drug toxicity, or metabolic derangements.

Conduction abnormalities can increase perioperative risk and may require the placement of a temporary or permanent pacemaker. On the other hand, patients with intraventricular conduction delays, even in the presence of a left or right bundle branch block, and no history of advanced heart block or symptoms rarely progress to complete heart block perioperatively. Since transthoracic pacing units have become available, the need for temporary transvenous pacemakers has decreased.

Decision to Undergo Diagnostic Testing

The American College of Cardiology/American Heart Association Guidelines on Perioperative Cardiovascular Evaluation for Noncardiac Surgery proposed an algorithm based upon expert opinion, which has been reaffirmed in an update published in 2002.[2,3] A stepwise bayesian strategy that relies on assessment of clinical markers, prior coronary evaluation and treatment, functional capacity, and surgery-specific risk is outlined below. Successful use of the algorithm requires an appreciation for different levels of risk attributable to certain clinical circumstances, levels of functional capacity, and types of surgery.

Multiple studies have attempted to identify clinical risk markers for perioperative cardiovascular morbidity and mortality. As described earlier, patients with unstable coronary syndromes and severe valvular disease are at the highest risk. Patients with known, stable CAD are at intermediate risk. Through the use of large cohort studies and multivariate analyses, both diabetes and chronic renal insufficiency (creatinine >2.0 mg/dl) also have been associated with increased perioperative cardiovascular complications that place the patients at intermediate risk. Several clinical risk markers for cardiovascular disease, each associated with variable levels of perioperative risk, have been classified as "low risk factors." The classification of perioperative clinical risk markers for the purpose of assessing the need for further testing is shown in Table 77–1.

As described with regard to angina pattern, exercise tolerance is one of the strongest determinants of perioperative risk and the need for invasive monitoring.[21] In one study of outpatients referred for evaluation before major noncardiac procedures, patients were asked to estimate the number of blocks they could walk and flights of stairs they could climb without experiencing cardiac symptoms.[21] Patients who could not walk four blocks and climb two flights of stairs were considered to have poor exercise tolerance and were found to have twice as many perioperative cardiovascular complications as those with better functional status. The likelihood of a serious complication occurring was related inversely to the number of blocks that could be walked or flights of stairs that could be climbed. Several scales based upon activities of daily living have been proposed as a means of assessing exercise tolerance. One such scale (the Duke Activity Scale Index [DASI]) is advocated in the guidelines (Table 77–2).[2]

The type of surgical procedure itself has a significant impact on perioperative risks and the amount of preoperative preparation required for safe performance of anesthesia. For surgical procedures that are not associated with significant stress or a high incidence of perioperative myocardial ischemia or morbidity, the costs of the evaluation are often greater than any perceived benefits from the information gained by preoperative assessment. For example, outpatient procedures cause little morbidity and mortality. In such patients, perioperative management is rarely changed by the cardiovascular status unless the patient demonstrates unstable angina or overt congestive heart failure. In contrast, surgery for vascular disease is associated with a high risk of morbidity and ischemic potential. Intraabdominal, thoracic, and orthopedic procedures are considered to involve intermediate risk (Table 77–3).

In addition to the risk of the surgical procedure itself, risk is correlated with the surgical volume in a given center. Several studies have demonstrated differential mortality rates in both cancer and vascular surgery, with higher mortality seen in low-volume centers. Therefore, surgical mortality rates may be very institution specific, which may influence the decision to perform further perioperative evaluations and interventions.

The stepwise approach advocated in the American College of Cardiology/American Heart Association Task Force Guidelines on Perioperative Evaluation of the Cardiac Patient Undergoing Noncardiac Surgery is shown in Figure 77–2.[2,3]

TABLE 77–1 Clinical Predictors of Increased Perioperative Cardiovascular Risk (Myocardial Infarction, Congestive Heart Failure, Death)

Major
Unstable coronary syndromes
Recent myocardial infarction* with evidence of important ischemic risk by clinical symptoms or noninvasive study
Unstable or severe† angina (Canadian class III or IV)‡
Decompensated congestive heart failure
Significant arrhythmias
High-grade atrioventricular block
Symptomatic ventricular arrhythmias in the presence of underlying heart disease
Supraventricular arrhythmias with uncontrolled ventricular rate
Severe valvular disease
Intermediate
Mild angina pectoris (Canadian class I or II)
Prior myocardial infarction by history or pathological Q waves
Compensated or prior congestive heart failure
Diabetes mellitus
Chronic renal insufficiency
Minor
Advanced age
Abnormal electrocardiogram (left ventricular hypertrophy, left bundle branch block, ST-T abnormalities)
Rhythm other than sinus (e.g., atrial fibrillation)
Low functional capacity (e.g., inability to climb one flight of stairs with a bag of groceries)
History of stroke
Uncontrolled systemic hypertension

*The American College of Cardiology National Database Library defines recent myocardial infarction as greater than 7 days but less than or equal to 1 month (30 days).
†May include "stable" angina in patients who are unusually sedentary.
‡Campeau L: Grading of angina pectoris. Circulation 54:522, 1976.
From Eagle KA, Berger PB, Calkins H, et al: ACC/AHA guideline update for perioperative cardiovascular evaluation for noncardiac surgery: Executive summary: A report of the American College of Cardiology/American Heart Association Task Force on Practice Guidelines (Committee to Update the 1996 Guidelines on Perioperative Cardiovascular Evaluation for Noncardiac Surgery). J Am Coll Cardiol 39:542, 2002.

TABLE 77–3 Cardiac Risk* Stratification for Noncardiac Surgical Procedures

High (Reported Cardiac Risk Often >5%)
Emergent major operations, particularly in elderly people
Aortic and other major vascular
Peripheral vascular
Anticipated prolonged surgical procedures associated with large fluid shifts and/or blood loss
Intermediate (Reported Cardiac Risk Generally <5%)
Carotid endarterectomy
Head and neck
Intraperitoneal and intrathoracic
Orthopedic
Prostate
Low† (Reported Cardiac Risk Generally <1%)
Endoscopic procedures
Superficial procedure
Cataract
Breast

*Combined incidence of cardiac death and nonfatal myocardial infarction.
†Do not generally require further preoperative cardiac testing.
From Eagle KA, Berger PB, Calkins H, et al: ACC/AHA guideline update for perioperative cardiovascular evaluation for noncardiac surgery: Executive summary: A report of the American College of Cardiology/American Heart Association Task Force on Practice Guidelines (Committee to Update the 1996 Guidelines on Perioperative Cardiovascular Evaluation for Noncardiac Surgery). J Am Coll Cardiol 39:542, 2002.

TABLE 77–2 Estimated Energy Requirement for Various Activities*

1 MET ↓ 4 METs	Can you take care of yourself? Eat, dress, or use the toilet? Walk indoors around the house? Walk a block or two on level ground at 2-3 mph or 3.2-4.8 km/hr? Do light work around the house like dusting or washing dishes?	4 METs ↓	Climb a flight of stairs or walk up a hill? Walk on level ground at 4 mph or 6.4 km/hr? Run a short distance? Do heavy work around the house like scrubbing floors or lifting or moving heavy furniture? Participate in moderate recreational activities like golf, bowling, dancing, doubles tennis, or throwing a baseball or football?
		>10 METs	Participate in strenuous sports like swimming, singles tennis, football, basketball, or skiing?

*Adapted from the Duke Activity Status Index and AHA Exercise Standards.
MET = metabolic equivalent.
From Eagle KA, Berger PB, Calkins H, et al: ACC/AHA guideline update for perioperative cardiovascular evaluation for noncardiac surgery: Executive summary: A report of the American College of Cardiology/American Heart Association Task Force on Practice Guidelines (Committee to Update the 1996 Guidelines on Perioperative Cardiovascular Evaluation for Noncardiac Surgery). J Am Coll Cardiol 39:542, 2002.

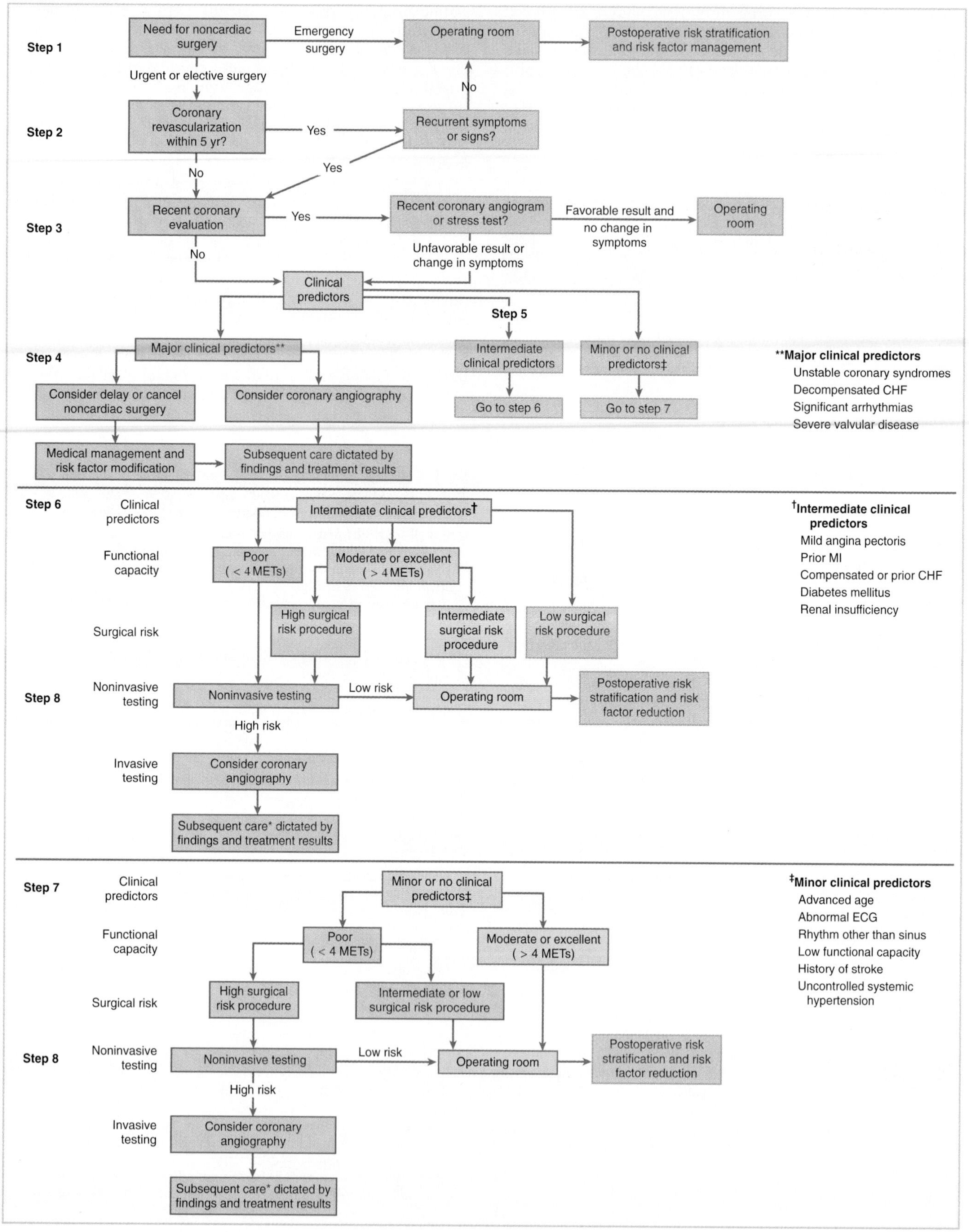

FIGURE 77–2 The American Heart Association/American College of Cardiology Task Force on Perioperative Evaluation of Cardiac Patients Undergoing Noncardiac Surgery has proposed an algorithm for decisions regarding the need for further evaluation. This represents one of multiple algorithms proposed in the literature. It is based upon expert opinion and incorporates eight steps. First, the clinician must evaluate the urgency of the surgery and the appropriateness of a formal preoperative assessment. Next, he or she must determine whether the patient has had a previous revascularization procedure or coronary evaluation. Patients with unstable coronary syndromes should be identified, and appropriate treatment should be instituted. The decision to have further testing depends on the interaction of the clinical risk factors, surgery-specific risk, and functional capacity. CHF = congestive heart failure; ECG = electrocardiogram; MET= metabolic equivalent; MI = myocardial infarction. (From Eagle KA, Berger PB, Calkins H, et al: ACC/AHA guideline update for perioperative cardiovascular evaluation for noncardiac surgery—Executive summary: A report of the American College of Cardiology/American Heart Association Task Force on Practice Guidelines [Committee to Update the 1996 Guidelines on Perioperative Cardiovascular Evaluation for Noncardiac Surgery]. J Am Coll Cardiol 39:542, 2002.)

First, the clinician must evaluate the urgency of the surgery and the appropriateness of a formal preoperative assessment. Next, the clinician must determine whether the patient has undergone a previous coronary revascularization procedure or coronary evaluation. Patients with unstable coronary syndromes should be identified and appropriate treatment instituted. Finally, the decision to undergo further testing depends upon the interaction of the clinical risk factors, surgery-specific risk, and functional capacity. High clinical risk markers include acute coronary syndromes and severe valvular disease. *Intermediate predictors* of increased risk are the factors that have been associated with higher perioperative risk in multiple studies. The guidelines currently consider mild angina pectoris, prior MI, compensated or prior congestive heart failure, chronic renal insufficiency, and diabetes mellitus as intermediate risk factors. *Minor predictors* of risk are those associated with CAD but whose relationship with perioperative cardiac complications is less well established. These include advanced age, an abnormal electrocardiogram, rhythm other than sinus, low functional capacity, history of stroke, and uncontrolled systemic hypertension; of these, low functional status is the most important. For patients at intermediate clinical risk, both exercise tolerance and the extent of the surgery are taken into account with regard to the need for further testing. No preoperative cardiovascular testing should be performed if the results would not change perioperative management.

Since the publication of the algorithm in 1996, several studies have suggested that this stepwise approach to the assessment of CAD is both effective and cost-effective.[22-24] Licker and colleagues compared data from two consecutive 4-year periods (1993 to 1996 [control period] versus 1997 to 2000 [intervention period]). Implementation of the American College of Cardiology/American Heart Association guidelines was associated with increased use of preoperative stress myocardial imaging (44.3 versus 20.6 percent; $p < 0.05$) and coronary revascularization (7.7 versus 0.8 percent; $p < 0.05$).[24] During the intervention period, there was a significant decrease in the incidence of cardiac complications (from 11.3 to 4.5 percent) and an increase in event-free survival at 1 year after surgery (from 91.3 to 98.2 percent). Froehlich and colleagues compared 102 historical control patients with 94 patients after guideline implementation and 104 patients later after guideline implementation.[23] Both resource utilization and costs were reduced after guideline implementation, and the effect was sustained for 2 years. We performed a small randomized trial involving 99 patients undergoing elective vascular surgery.[25] Patients at low or intermediate clinical risk were randomly assigned to testing or no testing, with no difference in perioperative or long-term outcome. The vast majority of these patients were highly functional and given perioperative beta blocker therapy, suggesting that exercise capacity can help determine the need for further diagnostic testing preoperatively.

Tests to Improve Identification and Definition of Cardiovascular Disease

Several noninvasive diagnostic methods have been proposed to evaluate the extent of coronary artery disease before noncardiac surgery. The exercise electrocardiogram has traditionally served to evaluate individuals for the presence of coronary artery disease. However, as outlined earlier, patients with excellent exercise tolerance in daily life rarely benefit from further testing. Patients with poor exercise capacity may not achieve heart rate and blood pressure adequate for diagnostic purposes on electrocardiographic stress tests. Such patients often require concomitant imaging.

A substantial number of high-risk patients either are unable to exercise or have contraindications to exercise. In surgical patients, this phenomenon is most evident in patients undergoing vascular surgery with claudication or an abdominal aortic aneurysm; both conditions associate with a high rate of perioperative cardiac morbidity. Therefore, pharmacological stress testing has become popular, particularly as a preoperative test in patients undergoing vascular surgery. Several authors have shown that the presence of a redistribution defect on dipyridamole or adenosine thallium or sestamibi imaging in patients undergoing peripheral vascular surgery predicts postoperative cardiac events. Pharmacological stress imaging is best employed in patients at moderate clinical risk. Several strategies may increase the predictive value of such tests. The redistribution defect can be quantitated, with larger areas of defect associated with increased risk. In addition, both increased lung uptake and left ventricular cavity dilation indicate ventricular dysfunction with ischemia. Several investigative groups have demonstrated that the delineation of "low-" and "high-" risk scintography (larger area of defect, increased lung uptake, and left ventricular cavity dilation) markedly improved the test's predictive value.[26] They demonstrated that patients with high-risk thallium scans had particularly increased risk for perioperative morbidity and long-term mortality.

Stress echocardiography has also been widely employed as a preoperative test.[27] One advantage of this test is that it assesses dynamically myocardial ischemia in response to increased inotropy and heart rate, such as may occur during the perioperative period. The presence of new wall motion abnormalities that occur at a low heart rate is the best predictor of increased perioperative risk, with large areas of defect being of secondary importance.[27]

Boersma and colleagues investigated the value of dobutamine stress echocardiography with respect to the extent of wall motion abnormalities and the ability of preoperative beta blocker treatment to attenuate risk in patients undergoing major aortic surgery. They assigned one point for each of the following characteristics: age older than 70 years, current angina, myocardial infarction, congestive heart failure, prior cerebrovascular disease, diabetes mellitus, and renal failure.[28] As the total of number of clinical risk factors increases, perioperative cardiac event rates also increase.

Which diagnostic test should be used (see also Chap. 16)? Several groups have published meta-analyses examining the various preoperative diagnostic tests. Mantha and colleagues demonstrated good predictive values of ambulatory electrocardiographic monitoring, radionuclide angiography, dipyridamole thallium imaging, and dobutamine stress echocardiography. Shaw and coworkers also demonstrated excellent predictive values for both dipyridamole thallium imaging and dobutamine stress echocardiography.[29] Although studies suggested the superior predictive value of dobutamine stress echocardiography, there was significant overlap of the confidence intervals with other tests. However, an important determinant with respect to the choice of preoperative testing is the expertise at the local institution. Another factor is whether assessment of valve function or myocardial thickness is of interest, in which case echocardiography may be preferred. Stress nuclear imaging may have slightly higher sensitivity, but stress echocardiography may be less likely to be falsely positive. The role in preoperative risk assessment of newer stress imaging modalities for preoperative assessment utilizing magnetic resonance imaging, 16-slice computed tomographic imaging, and position-emission tomography is rapidly evolving.

Overview of Anesthesia Used in Cardiac Patients Undergoing Noncardiac Surgery

There are three classes of anesthetics: general, regional, and local or sedation or monitored anesthetic care (MAC). General anesthesia can be defined best as a state including unconsciousness, amnesia, analgesia, immobility, and attenuation of autonomic responses to noxious stimulation. General anesthesia can be achieved with inhalational agents, intravenous agents, or a combination (frequently termed a balanced technique). In addition, general anesthesia can be achieved with or without an endotracheal tube. Laryngoscopy and intubation were traditionally thought to associate with the greatest stress and risk for myocardial ischemia, but extubation may involve greater risk. Alternative methods for delivering general anesthesia are through a mask or a laryngeal mask airway, a newer device that fits above the epiglottis and does not require laryngoscopy or intubation.

There are five currently approved inhalational anesthetic agents in the United States in addition to nitrous oxide, although enflurane and halothane are rarely utilized today. All inhalational agents have reversible myocardial depressant effects and lead to decreases in myocardial oxygen demand. The degree to which they depress cardiac output is a function of their concentration, effects on systemic vascular resistance, and effects on baroreceptor responsiveness. Therefore, they differ in their specific effects on heart rate and blood pressure.

Isoflurane causes negative inotropic effects, potent vascular smooth muscle relaxation, and minimal effects on baroreceptor function. Desflurane has the fastest onset and is used commonly in the outpatient setting. Sevoflurane's onset and offset of action are intermediate between those of isoflurane and desflurane. Its major advantage is that it is extremely pleasant smelling and therefore is used frequently as the agent of choice in children.

There have been several issues regarding the safety of the inhalational agents in patients with CAD. Isoflurane, because of its vasodilating properties, can cause a coronary artery steal leading to myocardial ischemia in an animal model. Several clinical cases have reported an association between myocardial ischemia and isoflurane, leading to an editorial suggesting that isoflurane should not be used in patients with CAD. However, several large-scale randomized and nonrandomized studies of the use of inhalational agents in patients undergoing CABG have not demonstrated any increased incidence of myocardial ischemia or infarction in patients receiving isoflurane compared with other inhalation agents or narcotic-based techniques. In a subsequent analysis of one of the randomized trials, the patients who were found to have steal-prone anatomy on coronary angiography did not have a higher incidence of myocardial ischemia. On the basis of the accumulated data from human studies, most anesthesiologists do not believe that isoflurane use presents a major threat of coronary steal, and it has become the most widely used anesthetic for patients, including those with CAD.

There are theoretical concerns regarding the safety of desflurane. Desflurane has been shown to be associated with airway irritability and led to tachycardia in volunteer studies. In a large-scale study comparing a narcotic-based anesthetic and a desflurane-based anesthetic, the desflurane group had a significantly higher incidence of myocardial infarction, although there was no difference in the incidence of MI. Including a narcotic with desflurane can prevent this tachycardia. Ongoing studies aim to determine the safety profile of desflurane in patients undergoing major vascular surgery. Sevoflurane has been studied in comparison with isoflurane in one randomized trial involving patients at high risk for cardiovascular disease. No difference in the incidence of myocardial ischemia was observed; however, the incidence of MI was too low to detect any difference. Overall, at this time no single inhalation anesthetic seems best for the patient with CAD.

There are theoretical advantages of the use of inhalational anesthetics in patients with CAD. Several investigative groups have demonstrated in vitro and in animal models that these agents have protective effects on the myocardium similar to those of ischemic preconditioning.[30,31] This favorable effect on myocardial oxygen demand would serve to offset the theoretical effects of coronary steal in patients with chronic coronary occlusion.

High-dose narcotic techniques offer the advantage of hemodynamic stability and lack of myocardial depression. In 1969, Lowenstein and colleagues proposed a high-dose narcotic technique for patients undergoing CABG. Narcotic-based anesthetics were frequently considered the "cardiac anesthesia" and advocated for use in all high-risk patients including those undergoing noncardiac surgery. The disadvantage of these traditional high-dose narcotic techniques is the requirement for postoperative ventilation. An ultra-short-acting narcotic (remifentanil) has been introduced into clinical practice, obviating the need for prolonged ventilation. It has been used in patients undergoing cardiac surgery and shown to facilitate early extubation.

Despite the theoretical advantages of a high-dose narcotic technique, several large-scale trials in patients undergoing CABG showed no difference in survival or major morbidity compared with the inhalation-based technique. This observation has led in part to the abandonment of high-dose narcotics in much of cardiac surgery and an emphasis on early extubation. Most anesthesiologists use a "balanced" technique that involves the administration of lower doses of narcotics with an inhalational agent. This approach allows the anesthesiologist to derive the benefits of each of these agents while minimizing the side effects.

An alternative mode of delivering general anesthesia is the intravenous agent propofol. Propofol is an alkyl phenol that can be used for both induction and maintenance of general anesthesia. It can result in profound hypotension because of reduced arterial tone with no change in heart rate. The major advantage of propofol is its rapid clearance with few residual effects on awakening; however, because it is quite expensive, its current use tends to be limited to operations of brief duration. Despite its hemodynamic effects, it has been used extensively to facilitate early extubation after coronary artery bypass surgery.

Current evidence indicates that there is no one best general anesthetic technique for patients with CAD undergoing noncardiac surgery and has led to the abandonment of the concept of a "cardiac anesthetic."

Spinal and Epidural Anesthesia

Regional anesthesia includes the techniques of spinal and epidural anesthesia as well as peripheral nerve blocks. Each technique has advantages and risks. Peripheral techniques, such as brachial plexus or Bier blocks, offer the advantage of having minimal or no hemodynamic effects. In contrast, spinal or epidural techniques can produce sympathetic blockade, which can reduce blood pressure and slow heart rate. Spinal anesthesia and lumbar or low thoracic epidural anesthesia can also evoke reflex sympathetic activation above the blockade, which might lead to myocardial ischemia.

The primary clinical difference between epidural and spinal anesthesia is the ability to provide continuous anesthesia or analgesia through placement of an epidural catheter as opposed to a single dose in spinal anesthesia, although some clinicians place a catheter in the intrathecal space. Although the speed of onset depends upon the local anesthetic agent used, spinal anesthesia and its associated autonomic effects occur sooner than the same agent administered epidurally. Because a catheter is usually left in place for epidural anesthesia, it can be more easily titrated. Epidural catheters can also be used postoperatively to provide analgesia.

A great deal of research has compared regional versus general anesthesia for patients with CAD, particularly patients undergoing infrainguinal bypass surgery. Overall mortality was reduced by about a third in patients allocated to neuraxial blockade, although the findings were controversial because most of the benefit was observed in older studies.[32] There were also reductions in MI and renal failure. Currently available evidence does not provide definitive data regarding one best anesthetic technique for patients undergoing high-risk noncardiac surgery.

Monitored Anesthesia Care

Monitored anesthesia care (MAC) encompasses local anesthesia administered by the surgeon with or without sedation. In a large-scale cohort study, MAC was associated with increased 30-day mortality in a univariate analysis compared with general anesthesia, although it did not remain significant in multivariate analysis when patients' comorbidity was taken into account.[33] The major issue with MAC is the ability to block the stress response adequately because inadequate analgesia associated with tachycardia may be worse than the potential hemodynamic effects of general or regional anesthesia. Since the introduction of the newer short-acting intravenous agents, general anesthesia essentially can now be administered without an endotracheal tube. This can allow the anesthesiologist to provide intense anesthesia for short or peripheral procedures without the potential effects of endotracheal intubation and extubation, blurring the distinction between general anesthesia and MAC.

Intraoperative Hemodynamics and Myocardial Ischemia

Over the past two decades, numerous studies have explored the relationship between hemodynamics, perioperative ischemia, and MI. Tachycardia is the strongest predictor of perioperative ischemia. Although traditionally heart rate higher than 100 beats/min has been defined as the lower limit for tachycardia, slower heart rates may result in myocardial ischemia. As described below, control of heart rate using beta blockers does decrease the incidence of myocardial ischemia and infarction.[34-37]

Although there has been concern about intraoperative hypotension in patients with CAD, there is no evidence to support such a contention. In CABG, the vast majority of episodes of intraoperative ischemia do not correlate with hemodynamic changes.[38] In the absence of tachycardia, hypotension has not been shown to be associated with myocardial ischemia.

Postoperative Management of Patients with Cardiac Disease after Noncardiac Surgery

Overview of the Postoperative Response to Surgery

To determine the best approach to preoperative testing, it is important to understand the pathophysiology of perioperative cardiac events. A full discussion of the pathophysiology of perioperative myocardial infarction has been published.[39]

All surgical procedures cause a stress response, although the extent of the response depends on the extent of the surgery and the use of anesthetics and analgesics to reduce the response. The stress response can lead to increases in heart rate and blood pressure, which can precipitate episodes of myocardial ischemia in areas distal to coronary artery stenoses. Prolonged myocardial ischemia (either prolonged individual episodes or cumulative duration of shorter episodes) has been associated with myocardial necrosis and perioperative MI and death.[39] Identification of patients with a high risk of coronary artery stenoses, through either history or cardiovascular testing, can lead to implementation of strategies to reduce morbidity from supply-demand mismatches.[40] As described previously, beta-blocking agents can reduce the increased demand and coronary revascularization may be of utility in improving supply-related issues in patients with critical stenoses.

A major mechanism of MI in the nonoperative setting is plaque rupture of a noncritical coronary stenosis with subsequent coronary thrombosis (see Chap. 35). Because the perioperative period is marked by tachycardia and a hypercoagulable state, plaque disruption and thrombosis may occur quite commonly. As the nidus for the thrombosis is a noncritical stenosis, preoperative cardiac evaluation may fail to identify such a patient before surgery, although control of heart rate may decrease the propensity of the plaque to rupture. The areas distal to the noncritical stenosis would not be expected to have collateral coronary flow, and therefore any acute thrombosis may have a greater detrimental effect than it would in a previously severely narrowed vessel. Preoperative cardiovascular testing clearly does not identify these patients. However, if the postoperative MI is due to a prolonged increase in myocardial oxygen demand in patients with one or more critical fixed stenoses, one would expect preoperative testing to identify such patients.

Some evidence supports both mechanisms. There have been several autopsy and postinfarction angiography studies after surgery. Ellis and colleagues demonstrated that one-third of all patients sustained events in areas distal to noncritical stenoses.[41] Dawood and colleagues demonstrated that fatal perioperative myocardial infarction occurs predominantly in patients with multivessel coronary disease, especially left main and three-vessel disease; however, the severity of preexisting underlying stenosis did not predict the resulting infarct territory.[42] This analysis suggests that fatal events occur primarily in patients with advanced fixed stenoses but that the infarct may be triggered by plaque rupture in a coexisting mild or only moderate stenosis of the area of diseased vessel.

Postoperative Intensive Care

Increasing evidence suggests that patients cared for in ICUs staffed by dedicated intensivists have improved outcomes. Pronovost and colleagues performed a systematic review of the literature on physician staffing patterns and clinical outcomes in critically ill patients.[43] They divided ICU physician staffing into low-intensity (no intensivist or elective intensivist consultation) and high-intensity (mandatory intensivist consultation or closed ICU [all care directed by intensivist]) groups. High-intensity staffing was associated with lower hospital mortality in 16 of 17 studies (94 percent) and with a pooled estimate of the relative risk for hospital mortality of 0.71 (95 percent confidence interval [CI], 0.62 to 0.82). High-intensity staffing was associated with lower ICU mortality in 14 of 15 studies (93 percent) and with a pooled estimate of the relative risk for ICU mortality of 0.61 (95 percent CI, 0.50 to 0.75). High-intensity staffing reduced hospital length of stay (LOS) in 10 of 13 studies and reduced ICU LOS in 14 of 18 studies without case-mix adjustment. High-intensity staffing was associated with reduced hospital LOS in two of four studies and ICU LOS in both studies that adjusted for case mix. No study found increased LOS with high-intensity staffing after case-mix adjustment. High-intensity versus low-intensity ICU physician staffing is associated with reduced hospital and ICU mortality and hospital and ICU LOS.

Postoperative Pain Management

There is interest in the value of postoperative analgesia regimens in reducing perioperative cardiac morbidity. The value of postoperative analgesia has been reviewed elsewhere.[44] Because postoperative tachycardia and catecholamine surges probably promote myocardial ischemia or coronary plaque rupture, or both, and postoperative pain is associated with tachycardia and increased catecholamines, effective postoperative analgesia may reduce cardiac complications. In addition, there is growing interest in the role of postoperative analgesia in reducing the hypercoagulable state. Epidural anesthesia may reduce platelet aggregability compared with general anesthesia. It is unclear whether this is related to intraoperative or postoperative management.

Future research will focus on how best to deliver postoperative analgesia to maximize the potential benefits in reducing complications.

Surveillance and Implications of Perioperative Cardiac Complications

The optimal and most cost-effective strategy for monitoring high-risk patients for major morbidity after noncardiac surgery is unknown. Myocardial ischemia and infarctions that occur postoperatively are usually silent, most likely because of the confounding effects of analgesics and postoperative surgical pain. Creatine kinase with muscle and brain subunits (CK-MB) is also less specific for myocardial necrosis postoperatively because this marker can rise during aortic surgery and after mesenteric ischemia. Further confounding the issue, most perioperative MIs are non-Q-wave in nature, and nonspecific ST-T wave changes are common after surgery with or without MI. Therefore, the diagnosis of a perioperative MI is particularly difficult using these traditional tests.

The approach to detection of perioperative MI has evolved with the use of troponins T and I. Adams and colleagues studied 108 patients undergoing high-risk surgery and obtained measures of CK-MB, total CK, and cardiac troponin I; daily electrocardiograms; and pre- and postoperative echocardiograms. Eight patients undergoing vascular surgery sustained a perioperative MI, as confirmed by the presence of new segmental-wall motion abnormalities. All eight patients had elevations of cardiac troponin I, and six patients had elevated CK-MB. Troponin I had a specificity of 99 percent and CK-MB a specificity of 81 percent. Lee and coworkers measured CK-MB and troponin T levels in 1175 patients undergoing noncardiac surgery and created receiver operating characteristic curves.[45] They found that troponin T had similar performance for diagnosing perioperative MI, but a significantly better correlation for major cardiac complications developing after an acute MI. Metzler and associates examined the sensitivity of troponin assay at variable cutoff levels—a value greater than 0.6 ng/ml demonstrated a positive predictive value of 87.5 percent and a negative predictive value of 98 percent.[46]

Traditionally, perioperative MI were associated with 30 to 50 percent short-term mortality. However, more recent series have reported a fatality rate associated with perioperative MIs as less than 20 percent.[39] This improvement may be due to more reliable detection of small nonfatal MIs. There also appears to be a shift in the timing of a perioperative MI. Studies from the 1980s suggested a peak incidence on the second and third postoperative days. Badner and colleagues, using troponin I as a marker for MI, suggested that the immediate and first postoperative days were the time of highest incidence.[47] This has been confirmed in other studies. Again, it is likely that this change is related to more robust surveillance methods, not a fundamental shift in how or when myocardial ischemia or infarction occurs.

Increasing evidence suggests that a perioperative MI or biomarker elevation predicts a worse long-term outcome. Lope-Jimenez and coworkers found that abnormal troponin T levels were associated with an increased incidence of cardiovascular complications within 6 months of surgery.[48] Kim and associates studied perioperative troponin I levels in 229 patients having aortic or infrainguinal vascular surgery or lower extremity amputation.[49] Twenty-eight patients (12 percent) had postoperative troponin I greater than 1.5 ng/mL, which was associated with a 6-fold increased risk of 6-month mortality and a 27-fold increased risk of MI. Furthermore, they observed a dose-response relation between troponin I concentration and mortality.

Strategies to Reduce Perioperative Cardiac Risk of Noncardiac Surgery

Coronary Artery Bypass Grafting

Coronary revascularization provides one means of reducing the perioperative risk of noncardiac surgery. There are currently no randomized trials of coronary revascularization, although there is an ongoing trial in the Veterans Affairs (VA) hospitals.[50] Some evidence exists that prior successful preoperative revascularization may decrease postoperative cardiac risk two- to fourfold in patients undergoing elective vascular surgery. The strongest evidence comes from the Coronary Artery Surgery Study (CASS) Registry, which enrolled patients from 1978 to 1981. The operative mortality for patients with CABG prior to noncardiac surgery was 0.9 percent but was significantly higher at 2.4 percent in patients without prior CABG. However, there was a 1.4 percent mortality rate associated with the CABG procedure itself.

Eagle and colleagues reported on a long-term analysis of patients entered into CASS.[51] They studied patients assigned for more than 10 years to medical or surgical therapy for CAD who underwent 3368 noncardiac operations in the years following assignment of coronary treatment. The reported rate of perioperative MI and death was stratified by type of surgical procedure. Specifically, low-risk surgeries such as skin, breast, urological, and minor orthopedic procedures were associated with a total morbidity and mortality less than 1 percent regardless of coronary treatment type, and prior revascularization did not affect outcome. Intermediate-risk surgery such as abdominal or thoracic surgery or carotid endarterectomy was associated with a combined morbidity and mortality of 1 to 5 percent with a small but significant improvement in outcome in patients who had undergone prior revascularization. The most significant improvement in outcome was in patients undergoing major vascular surgery such as abdominal or lower extremity revascularization. In this cohort, mortality after noncardiac surgery was reduced by two-thirds in patients who had had bypasses. However, this observational study did not randomly allocate patients and was undertaken in the 1970s and 1980s, before significant advances in medical, surgical, and percutaneous coronary strategies.[51]

The length of time between the coronary revascularization and noncardiac surgery most likely affects its protective effect. Back and colleagues studied 425 consecutive patients undergoing 481 elective major vascular operations at an academic VA Medical Center.[52] Coronary revascularization was classified as recent (CABG, <1 year; percutaneous transluminal coronary angioplasty [PTCA], <6 months) in 35 cases (7 percent), prior (1 year ≤ CABG < 5 year, 6 months ≤ PTCA < 2 year) in 45 cases (9 percent), and remote (CABG, ≥ 5 year; PTCA, ≥ 2 year) in 48 cases (10 percent). Outcomes in patients with previous PTCA were similar to those after CABG ($p = 0.7$). Significant differences in adverse cardiac events and mortality were found between patients with CABG within 5 years or PTCA within 2 years (6.3 and 1.3 percent, respectively), individuals with remote revascularization (10.4 and 6.3 percent), and nonrevascularized patients stratified as high risk (13.3 and 3.3 percent) or intermediate and low risk (2.8 and 0.9 percent). The authors concluded that previous coronary revascularization (CABG, <5 years; PTCA, <2 years) may provide only modest protection against adverse cardiac events and mortality following major arterial reconstruction.

An alternative approach to examining the optimal strategy for medical care in the absence of clinical trials is the construction of a decision analysis.[53] Such models assume that patients with significant CAD would undergo CABG prior to noncardiac surgery. The models found that the optimal decision was sensitive to local morbidity and mortality rates within the clinically observed range. These models suggest that preoperative testing for the purpose of coronary revascularization is not the optimal strategy if perioperative morbidity and mortality are low. If long-term survival is included in the models, coronary revascularization may lead to improved overall outcome and be a cost-effective intervention,[53] particularly in patients with significant left main or three-vessel coronary stenoses, or both.

Percutaneous Coronary Interventions

Several cohort studies have examined the benefit of percutaneous coronary intervention (PCI) before noncardiac surgery. Posner and colleagues utilized an administrative data set of patients who underwent PCI and noncardiac surgery in Washington State.[54] They matched patients with coronary disease undergoing noncardiac surgery with and without prior PCI and looked at cardiac complications. In this nonrandomized design, they noted a significantly lower rate of 30-day cardiac complications in patients who underwent PCI at least 90 days before the noncardiac surgery. PCI within 90 days of noncardiac surgery did not improve outcome. Although the explanation for these results is unknown, they may support the notion that PCI performed "to get the patient through surgery" may not improve perioperative outcome because cardiac complications may not occur in patients with stable or asymptomatic coronary stenosis and PCI may actually destabilize coronary plaques that become manifest in the days or weeks after noncardiac surgery. Hassan and colleagues evaluated the effect of multivessel angioplasty on subsequent noncardiac surgery in the Bypass Angioplasty Revascularization Investigation (BARI).[55] A total of 501 patients had noncardiac surgery a median of 29 months after the most recent revascularization procedure. Mortality and nonfatal MI occurred in 4 of the 250 surgery-assigned patients and 4 of the 251 angioplasty-assigned patients. Therefore, there does not appear to be an optimal choice of revascularization procedure for multivessel disease among patients who appear to be acceptable candidates for either strategy, although a larger scale study is necessary to confirm these findings.

PCI using coronary stenting poses several special issues. Kaluza and colleagues reported on the outcome in 40 patients who underwent prophylactic coronary stent placement less than 6 weeks before major noncardiac surgery requiring general anesthesia.[56] There were 7 MIs, 11 major bleeding episodes, and 8 deaths. All deaths and MIs, as well as 8 of 11 bleeding episodes, occurred in patients subjected to surgery fewer than 14 days after stenting. Four patients expired after undergoing surgery 1 day after stenting. The time between stenting and surgery appeared to be the main determinant of outcome, and the authors recommend that a minimum of 2 weeks, and preferably 4 weeks, elapse before elective surgery. Wilson and colleagues reported on 207 patients who underwent noncardiac surgery within 2 months of stent placement.[57] A total of 8 patients died or suffered an MI, all of whom were among the 168 patients undergoing surgery 6 weeks after stent placement. No events occurred in the 39 patients undergoing surgery 7 to 9 weeks after stent placement. These authors suggested that, whenever possible, noncardiac surgery should be delayed 6 weeks after stent placement has been performed, by which time stents are generally endothelialized, and a course of antiplatelet therapy to prevent stent thrombosis has been completed. For patients who must proceed to noncardiac surgery within the first 6 weeks of a PCI, balloon angioplasty without stent implantation may be the preferred strategy.

Pharmacological Interventions

Beta-Blocking Agents

Beta blockers are the best-studied medical treatment. They reduced perioperative cardiac morbidity, as shown in two well-designed randomized trials, and reduced surrogate endpoints of biomarker release and myocardial ischemia in other trials. Mangano and colleagues administered atenolol or placebo beginning the morning of surgery and continuing for 7 days postoperatively in a cohort of 200 patients with known coronary disease or risk factors for CAD undergoing high-risk noncardiac surgery.[34] They demonstrated a marked reduction in the incidence of perioperative myocardial ischemia but no differences in the rates of perioperative MI. There was a marked improvement in survival at 6 months in the atenolol group, which continued for at least 2 years.

The authors speculated that the lower incidence of myocardial ischemia was the result of less plaque destabilization with a resultant reduction in subsequent MI or death in the 6 months after noncardiac surgery. There were issues of randomization and uneven distribution of risk factors and treatment at baseline and upon discharge with beta blockers that may, at least in part, account for the findings. However, Poldermans and colleagues studied the perioperative use of bisoprolol versus routine care in elective major vascular surgery in the Dutch Echocardiographic Cardiac Risk Evaluation Applying Stress Echocardiography (DECREASE) trial.[37] This medication was started at least 7 days preoperatively, titrated to achieve a resting heart rate less than 60 beats/min, and continued postoperatively for 30 days. Of note, the study was confined to patients with at least one clinical marker of cardiac risk (prior MI, diabetes, angina pectoris, heart failure, age older than 70 years, or poor functional status) and evidence of inducible myocardial ischemia on a preoperative dobutamine stress echocardiogram. Patients with extensive regional wall abnormalities (large zones of myocardial ischemia) were excluded. Bisoprolol reduced perioperative MI or cardiac death by some 80 percent in this high-risk population. Because of the selection criteria, the efficacy of bisoprolol in the highest risk group, those who would be considered for coronary revascularization or modification or cancellation of the surgical procedure, cannot be determined from this trial. However, the event rate in the placebo group (nearly 40 percent) suggests that all but the highest risk patients were enrolled in the trial.

Boersma and colleagues reevaluated the use of dobutamine stress echocardiography with respect to the extent of wall motion abnormalities and use of beta blockers during surgery for the entire cohort of patients screened for the DECREASE trial.[28] They assigned one point for each of the following characteristics: age older than 70 years, current angina, MI, congestive heart failure, prior cerebrovascular disease, diabetes mellitus, and renal failure. As the total number of clinical risk factors increased, perioperative cardiac event rates also increased (Fig. 77–3). When the risk of death or MI was stratified by perioperative beta blocker usage, there was no significant improvement in those without any of the prior risk factors. In those with a risk factor score between 1 and 3, which represented more than half of all patients, the rate of cardiac events fell from 3 to 0.9 percent with effective beta blockade. Most important, in those with less than three risk factors, constituting 70 percent of the population, beta blocker therapy was very effective in reducing cardiac events in those with new wall motion abnormalities in one to four segments (33 versus 2.8 percent), having a smaller effect in those without new wall motion abnormalities (5.8 versus 2 percent). Beta blockers were not protective in patients with new wall motion abnormalities in more than five segments. The group with risk factors and extensive wall motion abnormalities on preoperative stress echocardiography may be the group to consider for prophylactic coronary revascularization.

On the basis of the accumulated evidence for the benefit of beta blockers in the perioperative period and that for the nonoperative benefit of beta blockers for CAD and heart failure, several groups have advocated prophylactic beta blockade in high-risk patients undergoing high-risk surgery. The American Heart Association/American College of Cardiology guidelines recommend treatment with a beta-blocking agent for patients previously receiving these agents and patients with positive stress tests undergoing major vascular surgery. They

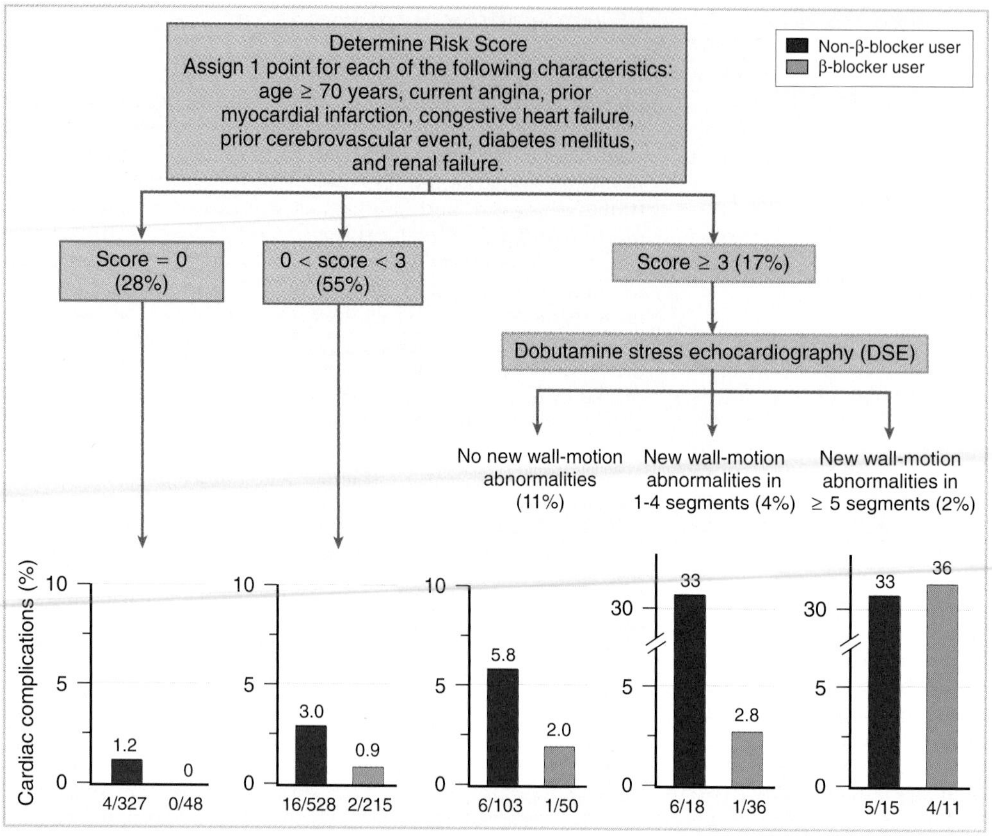

FIGURE 77–3 Perioperative cardiac risk and death in different populations of patients enrolled in the Dutch Echocardiographic Cardiac Risk Evaluation Applying Stress Echocardiography (DECREASE) trial. Risk is defined according to clinical risk and use of beta blockers in the randomized and nonrandomized cohorts of individuals. Patients with risk factors and a positive stress test demonstrating one to four areas of regional wall motion abnormality on dobutamine stress echocardiography were randomly assigned to perioperative bisoprolol titrated preoperatively to a heart rate less than 60 beats/min or to standard care. For all other patients who were not randomly assigned but were receiving preoperative beta blockers, the medication was switched to bisoprolol targeted to a heart rate less than 60 beats/min. (From Poldermans D, Boersma E, Bax JJ, et al: The effect of bisoprolol on perioperative mortality and myocardial infarction in high-risk patients undergoing vascular surgery. Dutch Echocardiographic Cardiac Risk Evaluation Applying Stress Echocardiography Study Group. N Engl J Med 341:1789, 1999.)

also recommend (level IIa evidence) prophylactic beta blocker administration in patients with known or major risk factors for CAD, although the strength of evidence is weaker and therefore the recommendation is based upon the general knowledge of beta blockers and cardiac disease. A report from the Agency for Healthcare Research and Quality has also suggested that prophylactic beta blocker treatment in patients with known risk factors for CAD is supported by the strongest forms of evidence.[58] Auerbach and Goldman have published recommendations regarding the use of beta-blocking drugs in the perioperative setting. These recommendations have led many institutions to develop protocols for implementation of perioperative beta-blocking agents.[59]

We have proposed an algorithm concerning beta blocker use (Fig. 77–4).[60] Several authors have demonstrated that the majority of patients presenting for noncardiac surgery and even for vascular surgery have not been started on beta blockers. One concern of the anesthesiologists is related to the acute administration of a beta-blocking agent on the morning of surgery. The combined effect of acute heart rate decrease coupled with the induction of anesthesia in a patient who had previously been beta blocker–naive has been associated anecdotally with marked bradycardia and hypotension. Treatment of these events could lead to wide swings in heart rate and blood pressure and less heart rate control than desired. The approach to the use of beta blockers depends on the preoperative status, the type of surgery, the cardiac risk factors, and any results of cardiac stress testing. If patients are receiving beta blockers preoperatively, it is important to continue perioperative beta blockers including intravenous administration in those unable to take the medication by mouth. If patients are undergoing vascular surgery and preoperative diagnostic imaging demonstrates areas at risk for myocardial ischemia, it would be important to initiate beta blocker therapy several days or more in advance and titrate to a heart rate of 60 to 70 beats/min.

Ideally, the beta blocker therapy should be initiated more than 7 days in advance, similar to the schedule in the Poldermans protocol, because there is a basal level of drug leading to modification of beta-adrenergic receptors. For a patient with a negative stress test and high clinical risk undergoing nonvascular surgery or vascular surgery, initiation of beta blockers several days in advance by the internist, cardiologist, or other primary care provider would be appropriate to ensure a stable beta blocker level on the day of surgery. If several days of beta blocker therapy cannot be achieved, the potential risks of new-onset beta blocker therapy during induction of general, epidural, or spinal anesthesia may outweigh the benefits of beginning drug therapy on the morning of surgery. Because the study by Mangano did not demonstrate any difference in outcome and the approach of Raby and colleagues[35] demonstrated similar efficacy with respect to perioperative ischemia, we suggest inducing general anesthesia or providing regional anesthesia prior to starting beta blocker therapy. If the induction is associated with tachycardia, administration of esmolol would be appropriate. After adequate anesthesia and analgesia are achieved, the heart rate should be controlled and maintained below 80 beats/min, as in the study by Poldermans, using short- and long-acting beta blocker therapy. If the patient is initially unstable, esmolol should be first-line therapy with eventual conversion to long-acting agents.

Alpha$_2$-Agonists

Several randomized trials have evaluated prophylactic alpha$_2$-agonists as a means of reducing perioperative cardiac morbidity. Wallace and colleagues published an abstract evaluating alpha$_2$-agonists compared with placebo in high-risk patients undergoing noncardiac surgery.[36] They reported results similar to those of Mangano and colleagues and demonstrated marked improvement in 2-year survival in the alpha$_2$-agonist group. Licker and colleagues reported on a cardioprotection protocol involving preoperative alpha$_2$-agonist administration and intra- and postoperative beta blocker administration compared with historical control studies that did not use preoperative testing or this pharmacological protocol. They reported markedly improved perioperative and long-term survival and reduced perioperative troponin levels in the more contemporary group employing the cardioprotection protocol. A meta-analysis of published studies demonstrated that perioperative clonidine reduced cardiac ischemic episodes in patients with known or at risk for coronary arterial disease without increasing the incidence of bradycardia, although the studies were underpowered to evaluate the efficacy for reduction of perioperative cardiac morbidity.[61]

Nitroglycerin

Only two randomized trials have evaluated the potential protective effect of prophylactic nitroglycerin in reducing perioperative cardiac complications after noncardiac surgery. In a small study by Coriat and colleagues involving patients undergoing carotid endarterectomy, high-dose (1 μg/kg/min) nitroglycerin was more effective than lower dose (0.5 μg/kg/min) nitroglycerin in reducing the incidence of myocardial ischemia, but MI did not occur in either group. The anesthetic used in this study was an oxygen-pancuronium-fentanyl anesthetic, and therefore inhalational agents, which may be cardioprotective and cause coronary vasodilation, were not administered. Dodds studied nitroglycerin versus placebo using a balanced anesthetic technique and reported no difference in the rates of myocardial ischemia or infarction. Taken together, the evidence suggests that prophylactic nitroglycerin does not reduce the incidence of perioperative cardiac morbidity, although neither trial was powered to detect a modest benefit of nitroglycerin. As these agents have considerable hemodynamic effects, it would seem prudent to avoid the prophylactic use of nitroglycerin, although there are clear indications for use as treatment when myocardial ischemia develops.

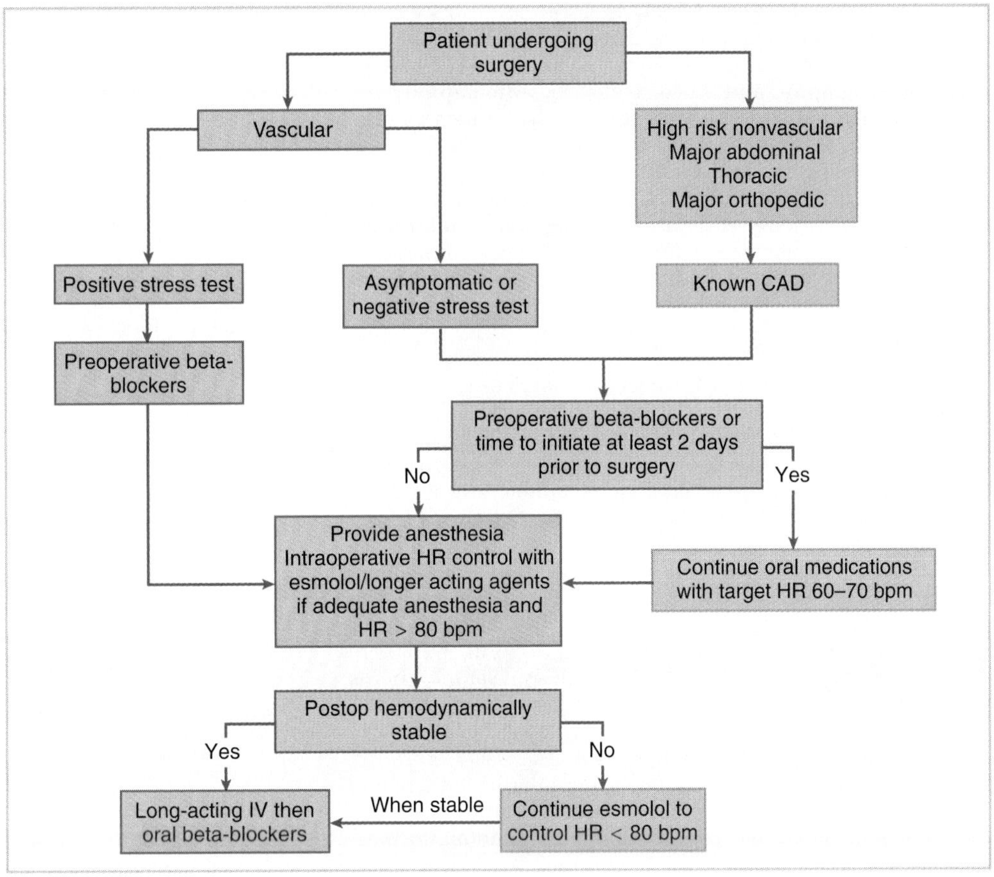

FIGURE 77–4 One proposed algorithm for the administration of beta blockers. CAD = coronary artery disease; HR = heart rate. (From Fleisher LA: Optimizing perioperative outcomes. International Anesthesia Research Society Refresher Course, Cleveland, Ohio, 2003.)

NONPHARMACOLOGICAL INTERVENTIONS

TEMPERATURE. Frank and colleagues completed a randomized trial of regional versus general anesthesia for lower extremity vascular bypass procedures and noted an association between hypothermia (temperature less than 35° C) and myocardial ischemia. They subsequently performed a randomized trial involving 300 high-risk patients undergoing a diverse group of intermediate- and high-risk procedures and randomly assigned patients to maintenance of normothermia or routine care. They observed a significantly reduced incidence of perioperative cardiac morbidity and mortality within 24 hours of surgery in the group that was kept normothermic.

Monitoring

Multiple studies have demonstrated the correlation between perioperative ST segment changes and major cardiac events, as described previously. Furthermore, the duration, either cumulative or continuous, of perioperative ST changes strongly predicts poor outcomes. Therefore, ST segment monitoring has become standard during the intraoperative and ICU periods for high-risk patients. However, patients at low to moderate risk may also develop ST segment changes. These changes may not reflect true myocardial ischemia, as suggested in one series.[62]

The period of greatest risk may be the time when the patient is in the ward and unmonitored. Many of the monitoring companies have developed ST segment telemetry monitors, but they have not been tested to any large degree in the perioperative period. This issue of whether early treatment of prolonged ST segment changes leads to improved outcome is not yet clarified. Until such studies are completed, the efficacy of such monitors remains debatable.

The value of pulmonary artery catheterization for noncardiac surgery has engendered controversy. Several small randomized trials did not demonstrate significant reductions in major cardiac morbidity and mortality in patients undergoing aortic surgery. A large-scale cohort study performed by Polanczyk and colleagues in which patients who had pulmonary catheters placed were matched with those who did not, using a propensity score, was also unable to demonstrate any significant benefit.[63] In fact, they observed an increased incidence of congestive heart failure and untoward noncardiac outcomes in the pulmonary artery catheter group. In a subsequent study, a total of 1994 patients were randomly assigned to goal-directed therapy guided by a pulmonary catheter or standard care without the use of a pulmonary catheter for patients undergoing urgent or elective major surgery.[64] There was no difference in survival, but there was a higher rate of pulmonary embolism in the catheter group compared with the standard care group. Therefore, current evidence does not support the routine use of pulmonary artery catheterization for high-risk patients undergoing major noncardiac surgery. Further work is required to understand whether these results can be generalized to the high-risk vascular surgical population and to determine the benefits of pulmonary artery catheters in specific clinical situations.

Transesophageal echocardiography (TEE) is another means of assessing intraoperative cardiac function. It is an extremely sensitive noninvasive tool for monitoring intraoperative wall motion abnormalities and fluid status. In patients undergoing aortic cross-clamping, TEE proved to have significantly better sensitivity for detecting intraoperative ischemia than electrocardiography. For noncardiac surgery, a study of TEE, 2-lead electrocardiography, and 12-lead electrocardiography demonstrated minimal additive value of TEE over 2-lead electrocardiography. Although TEE for routine monitoring of intraoperative ischemia in noncardiac surgery may have minimal additive value over ST segment recording for predicting which patients will sustain perioperative morbidity, TEE monitoring may be valuable to guide treatment in patients with unstable hemodynamics where filling status or myocardial function or both are uncertain.

Transfusion Threshold

There is a great deal of controversy regarding the optimal hemoglobin level at which to transfuse high-risk noncardiac surgical patients. No randomized trials have evaluated the optimal transfusion threshold, although there is a great deal of anecdotal evidence. Several small cohort studies have shown that hematocrits in the range 27 to 29 percent represent the point below which there is an increased incidence of myocardial ischemia and potentially MI. Data from a large-scale trial of transfusion triggers in the ICU were unable to document increased morbidity and mortality with a transfusion threshold of hemoglobin less than 7 gm/dl, but there were trends for increased morbidity in the subset of patients with ischemic heart disease. In the setting of acute MI, Wu demonstrated that lower hemoglobin levels, particularly below 10 gm/dl, are associated with increased mortality within 30 days. Therefore, there is accumulating evidence to suggest that patients with known ischemic heart disease who have not had revascularization should be maintained perioperatively with a hemoglobin greater than 9 gm/dl.

REFERENCES

Assessment of Preoperative Risk for Noncardiac Surgery in Patients with Cardiovascular Disease

1. Rivers SP, Scher LA, Gupta SK, et al: Safety of peripheral vascular surgery after recent acute myocardial infarction. J Vasc Surg 11:70, 1990.
2. Eagle KA, Brundage BH, Chaitman BR, et al: Guidelines for perioperative cardiovascular evaluation for noncardiac surgery. Report of the American College of Cardiology/American Heart Association Task Force on Practice Guidelines (Committee on Perioperative Cardiovascular Evaluation for Noncardiac Surgery). J Am Coll Cardiol 27:910, 1996.
3. Eagle KA, Berger PB, Calkins H, et al: ACC/AHA guideline update for perioperative cardiovascular evaluation for noncardiac surgery—Executive summary: A report of the American College of Cardiology/American Heart Association Task Force on Practice Guidelines (Committee to Update the 1996 Guidelines on Perioperative Cardiovascular Evaluation for Noncardiac Surgery). J Am Coll Cardiol 39:542, 2002.
4. Weksler N, Klein M, Szendro G, et al: The dilemma of immediate preoperative hypertension: To treat and operate, or to postpone surgery? J Clin Anesth 15:179, 2003.
5. Aronson S, Boisvert D, Lapp W: Isolated systolic hypertension is associated with adverse outcomes from coronary artery bypass grafting surgery. Anesth Analg 94:1079, 2002.
6. Cohn SL, Goldman L: Preoperative risk evaluation and perioperative management of patients with coronary artery disease. Med Clin North Am 87:111, 2003.
7. Haering JM, Comunale ME, Parker RA, et al: Cardiac risk of noncardiac surgery in patients with asymmetric septal hypertrophy. Anesthesiology 85:254, 1996.
8. Torsher LC, Shub C, Rettke SR, et al: Risk of patients with severe aortic stenosis undergoing noncardiac surgery. Am J Cardiol 81:448, 1998.
9. Otto C, Mickel M, Kennedy J, et al: Three-year outcome after balloon aortic valvuloplasty: Insights into prognosis of valvular aortic stenosis. Circulation 89:642, 1994.
10. Palacios I, Tuzcu M, Weyman A, et al: Clinical follow-up of patients undergoing percutaneous mitral balloon valvotomy. Circulation 91:671, 1995.
11. Dajani A, Taubert K, Wilson W, et al: Prevention of bacterial endocarditis. Recommendations by the American Heart Association. JAMA 277:1794, 1997.
12. Leport C, Horstkotte D, Burckhardt D: Antibiotic prophylaxis for infective endocarditis from an international group of experts towards a European consensus. Group of Experts of the International Society for Chemotherapy. Eur Heart J 16(Suppl B):126, 1995.
13. Bonow RO, Carabello B, de Leon AC Jr, et al: Guidelines for the management of patients with valvular heart disease: Executive summary. A report of the American College of Cardiology/American Heart Association Task Force on Practice Guidelines (Committee on Management of Patients with Valvular Heart Disease). Circulation 98:1949, 1998.
14. Ezekowitz MD: Anticoagulation management of valve replacement patients. J Heart Valve Dis 11(Suppl 1):S56, 2002.
15. Martin JT, Tautz TJ, Antognini JF: Safety of regional anesthesia in Eisenmenger's syndrome. Reg Anesth Pain Med 27:509, 2002.
16. Galli KK, Myers LB, Nicolson SC: Anesthesia for adult patients with congenital heart disease undergoing noncardiac surgery. Int Anesthesiol Clin 39:43, 2001.
17. Amar D: Perioperative atrial tachyarrhythmias. Anesthesiology 97:1618, 2002.
18. Amar D, Roistacher N, Rusch VW, et al: Effects of diltiazem prophylaxis on the incidence and clinical outcome of atrial arrhythmias after thoracic surgery. J Thorac Cardiovasc Surg 120:790, 2000.
19. Balser JR, Martinez EA, Winters BD, et al: Beta-adrenergic blockade accelerates conversion of postoperative supraventricular tachyarrhythmias. Anesthesiology 89:1052, 1998.
20. Amar D, Zhang H, Roistacher N: The incidence and outcome of ventricular arrhythmias after noncardiac thoracic surgery. Anesth Analg 95:537, 2002.
21. Reilly DF, McNeely MJ, Doerner D, et al: Self-reported exercise tolerance and the risk of serious perioperative complications. Arch Intern Med 159:2185, 1999.
22. Bartels C, Bechtel J, Hossmann V, et al: Cardiac risk stratification for high-risk vascular surgery. Circulation 95:2473, 1997.
23. Froehlich JB, Karavite D, Russman PL, et al: American College of Cardiology/American Heart Association preoperative assessment guidelines reduce resource utilization before aortic surgery. J Vasc Surg 36:758, 2002.
24. Licker M, Khatchatourian G, Schweizer A, et al: The impact of a cardioprotective protocol on the incidence of cardiac complications after aortic abdominal surgery. Anesth Analg 95:1525, 2002.
25. Falcone RA, Nass CM, Jermyn RM, et al: The value of preoperative pharmacological stress testing before vascular surgery using ACC/AHA guidelines: A prospective, randomized pilot trial. J Cardiothoracic Vasc Anesth 17: 694, 2003.
26. Fleisher LA, Rosenbaum SH, Nelson AH, et al: Preoperative dipyridamole thallium imaging and Holter monitoring as a predictor of perioperative cardiac events and long-term outcome. Anesthesiology 83:906, 1995.
27. Poldermans D, Arnese M, Fioretti PM, et al: Improved cardiac risk stratification in major vascular surgery with dobutamine-atropine stress echocardiography. J Am Coll Cardiol 26:648, 1995.
28. Boersma E, Poldermans D, Bax JJ, et al: Predictors of cardiac events after major vascular surgery: Role of clinical characteristics, dobutamine echocardiography, and beta-blocker therapy. JAMA 285:1865, 2001.
29. Shaw LJ, Eagle KA, Gersh BJ, et al: Meta-analysis of intravenous dipyridamole-thallium-201 imaging (1985 to 1994) and dobutamine echocardiography (1991 to 1994) for risk stratification before vascular surgery. J Am Coll Cardiol 27:787, 1996.

Overview of Anesthesia Used in Cardiac Patients Undergoing Noncardiac Surgery

30. Toller WG, Kersten JR, Pagel PS, et al: Sevoflurane reduces myocardial infarct size and decreases the time threshold for ischemic preconditioning in dogs. Anesthesiology 91:1437, 1999.
31. Chen Q, Camara AK, An J, et al: Sevoflurane preconditioning before moderate hypothermic ischemia protects against cytosolic [Ca^{2+}] loading and myocardial damage in part via mitochondrial K(ATP) channels. Anesthesiology 97:912, 2002.
32. Rodgers A, Walker N, Schug S, et al: Reduction of postoperative mortality and morbidity with epidural or spinal anaesthesia: Results from overview of randomised trials. BMJ 321:1493, 2000.
33. Cohen M, Duncan PG, Tate RB: Does anesthesia contribute to operative mortality? JAMA 260:2859, 1988.
34. Mangano DT, Layug EL, Wallace A, et al: Effect of atenolol on mortality and cardiovascular morbidity after noncardiac surgery. Multicenter Study of Perioperative Ischemia Research Group. N Engl J Med 335:1713, 1996.
35. Raby KE, Brull SJ, Timimi F, et al: The effect of heart rate control on myocardial ischemia among high-risk patients after vascular surgery. Anesth Analg 88:477, 1999.
36. Wallace A, Layug B, Tateo I, et al: Prophylactic atenolol reduces postoperative myocardial ischemia. McSPI Research Group. Anesthesiology 88:7, 1998.
37. Poldermans D, Boersma E, Bax JJ, et al: The effect of bisoprolol on perioperative mortality and myocardial infarction in high-risk patients undergoing vascular surgery. Dutch Echocardiographic Cardiac Risk Evaluation Applying Stress Echocardiography Study Group. N Engl J Med 341:1789, 1999.
38. Leung JM, O'Kelly BF, Mangano DT, et al: Relationship of regional wall motion abnormalities to hemodynamic indices of myocardial oxygen supply and demand in patients undergoing CABG surgery. Anesthesiology 73:802, 1990.

Postoperative Management of Patients with Cardiac Disease after Noncardiac Surgery

39. Landesberg G: The pathophysiology of perioperative myocardial infarction: Facts and perspectives. J Cardiothorac Vasc Anesth 17:90, 2003.
40. Fleisher LA, Eagle KA: Clinical practice. Lowering cardiac risk in noncardiac surgery. N Engl J Med 345:1677, 2001.
41. Ellis SG, Hertzer NR, Young JR, et al: Angiographic correlates of cardiac death and myocardial infarction complicating major nonthoracic vascular surgery. Am J Cardiol 77:1126, 1996.
42. Dawood MM, Gutpa DK, Southern J, et al: Pathology of fatal perioperative myocardial infarction: Implications regarding pathophysiology and prevention. Int J Cardiol 57:37, 1996.
43. Pronovost PJ, Angus DC, Dorman T, et al: Physician staffing patterns and clinical outcomes in critically ill patients: A systematic review. JAMA 288:2151, 2002.
44. Kehlet H, Holte K: Effect of postoperative analgesia on surgical outcome. Br J Anaesth 87:62, 2001.
45. Lee TH, Thomas EJ, Ludwig LE, et al: Troponin T as a marker for myocardial ischemia in patients undergoing major noncardiac surgery. Am J Cardiol 77:1031, 1996.
46. Metzler H, Gries M, Rehak P, et al: Perioperative myocardial cell injury: The role of troponins. Br J Anaesth 78:386, 1997.

47. Badner NH, Knill RL, Brown JE, et al: Myocardial infarction after noncardiac surgery. Anesthesiology 88:572, 1998.
48. Lopez-Jimenez F, Goldman L, Sacks DB, et al: Prognostic value of cardiac troponin T after noncardiac surgery: 6-month follow-up data. J Am Coll Cardiol 29:1241, 1997.
49. Kim LJ, Martinez EA, Faraday N, et al: Cardiac troponin I predicts short-term mortality in vascular surgery patients. Circulation 106:2366, 2002.

Strategies to Reduce Perioperative Cardiac Risk of Noncardiac Surgery

50. McFalls EO, Ward HB, Krupski WC, et al: Prophylactic coronary artery revascularization for elective vascular surgery: Study design. Veterans Affairs Cooperative Study Group on Coronary Artery Revascularization Prophylaxis for Elective Vascular Surgery. Control Clin Trials 20:297, 1999.
51. Eagle KA, Rihal CS, Mickel MC, et al: Cardiac risk of noncardiac surgery: Influence of coronary disease and type of surgery in 3368 operations. CASS Investigators and University of Michigan Heart Care Program. Coronary Artery Surgery Study. Circulation 96:1882, 1997.
52. Back MR, Stordahl N, Cuthbertson D, et al: Limitations in the cardiac risk reduction provided by coronary revascularization prior to elective vascular surgery. J Vasc Surg 36:526, 2002.
53. Glance LG: Selective preoperative cardiac screening improves five-year survival in patients undergoing major vascular surgery: A cost-effectiveness analysis. J Cardiothorac Vasc Anesth 13:265, 1999.
54. Posner KL, Van Norman GA, Chan V: Adverse cardiac outcomes after noncardiac surgery in patients with prior percutaneous transluminal coronary angioplasty. Anesth Analg 89:553, 1999.
55. Hassan SA, Hlatky MA, Boothroyd DB, et al: Outcomes of noncardiac surgery after coronary bypass surgery or coronary angioplasty in the Bypass Angioplasty Revascularization Investigation (BARI). Am J Med 110:260, 2001.
56. Kaluza GL, Joseph J, Lee JR, et al: Catastrophic outcomes of noncardiac surgery soon after coronary stenting. J Am Coll Cardiol 35:1288, 2000.
57. Wilson SH, Fasseas P, Orford JL, et al: Clinical outcome of patients undergoing noncardiac surgery in the two months following coronary stenting. J Am Coll Cardiol 42:234, 2003.

Perioperative Management in High-Risk Patients

58. Shojania KG, Duncan BW, McDonald KM, et al: Safe but sound: Patient safety meets evidence-based medicine. JAMA 288:508, 2002.
59. Auerbach AD, Goldman L: Beta-blockers and reduction of cardiac events in noncardiac surgery: Scientific review. JAMA 287:1435, 2002.
60. Fleisher LA: Optimizing perioperative outcomes. International Anesthesia Research Society Refresher Course, Cleveland, Ohio, 2003.
61. Nishina K, Mikawa K, Uesugi T, et al: Efficacy of clonidine for prevention of perioperative myocardial ischemia: A critical appraisal and meta-analysis of the literature. Anesthesiology 96:323, 2002.
62. Fleisher LA, Zielski MM, Schulman SP: Perioperative ST-segment depression is rare and may not indicate myocardial ischemia in moderate-risk patients undergoing noncardiac surgery. J Cardiothorac Vasc Anesth 11:155, 1997.
63. Polanczyk CA, Rohde LE, Goldman L, et al: Right heart catheterization and cardiac complications in patients undergoing noncardiac surgery: An observational study. JAMA 286:309, 2001.
64. Sandham JD, Hull RD, Brant RF, et al: A randomized, controlled trial of the use of pulmonary-artery catheters in high-risk surgical patients. N Engl J Med 348:5, 2003.

GUIDELINES *Thomas H. Lee*

Reducing Cardiac Risk with Noncardiac Surgery

Guidelines on the assessment and management of perioperative cardiovascular risk for patients undergoing noncardiac surgery were published by an American College of Cardiology/American Heart Association (ACC/AHA) task force in 1996 and updated in 2002.[1] Guidelines were also published by the American College of Physicians (ACP) in 1997,[2] but these guidelines preceded more recent research that has shifted the focus of management from noninvasive risk stratification to risk reduction through strategies such as use of perioperative beta blockade.[3]

Both ACC/AHA and ACP guidelines emphasize the importance of a directed history and physical examination, including assessment of patient functional capacity. Clinicians are urged to give attention to noncardiac comorbid conditions as well as cardiac issues. The ACC/AHA guidelines noted but did not endorse any single risk prediction decision aid; instead, these guidelines recommended a stepwise algorithm to identify patients most appropriate for noninvasive testing for further risk stratification (see Fig. 77–2).

The ACC/AHA guidelines also offer a simple alternative approach for clinicians to decide whether noninvasive cardiac testing is needed (Fig. 77G–1). The guidelines recommend noninvasive testing if any two of these three factors are present:

Intermediate clinical predictors are present (Canadian class 1 or 2 angina, prior myocardial infarction based on history or pathological Q waves, compensated or prior heart failure, or diabetes)
Poor functional capacity (less than 4 metabolic equivalents)
High surgical risk procedure (emergency major operations; aortic repair or peripheral vascular surgery; prolonged surgical procedures with large fluid shifts or blood loss)

Ancillary Testing

ACC/AHA recommendations for utilization of tests in patients undergoing noncardiac surgery are summarized in Table 77G–1. The routine 12-lead electrocardiogram (ECG) is supported for use in patients with high or intermediate clinical risk factors, including diabetes, or recent chest pain. The guidelines recommend restraint in the use of ECGs in asymptomatic patients undergoing low-risk procedures. Routine use of echocardiography to assess left ventricular function is discouraged unless patients have heart failure or dyspnea of unknown etiology. Similarly, routine use of exercise or pharmacological stress testing in asymptomatic patients without evidence of coronary artery disease is considered a class III indication (not supported by evidence).

The recommendations for use of coronary angiography (see Table 77G–1) reflect the goal of improving the patient's long-term cardiovascular prognosis and of minimizing the chances of the patient having an acute complication during the planned procedure. In general, the same indications that are used to determine whether a nonsurgical patient warrants coronary angiography should be used in the preoperative setting, but the threshold for performing angiography should decrease if the patient is to undergo a higher risk surgical procedure.

Risk Reduction Interventions

The guidelines emphasize that "It is almost never appropriate to recommend coronary bypass surgery or other invasive interventions such as coronary angioplasty in an effort to reduce the risk of noncardiac surgery when they would not otherwise be indicated." Thus, most of the attention of the guidelines is given to medical therapies and monitoring interventions for higher risk patients. Beta blockers receive strong support for patients with high cardiac risk who are undergoing vascular surgery. Evidence for use of alpha$_2$-agonists was considered less convincing.

Intraoperative nitroglycerin was supported for patients with acute ischemic syndromes who must undergo noncardiac procedures on a presumably urgent basis. The guidelines warn that prophylactic use of nitroglycerin must take into account the anesthetic plan and patient's hemodynamics and must recognize that vasodilation and hypovolemia can readily occur during anesthesia and surgery. The ACC/AHA task force did not find sufficient evidence to weight risks versus benefits of intraaortic balloon counterpulsation for patients with myocardial ischemic syndromes or routine use of transesophageal echocardiography.

The guidelines acknowledge data (primarily from observational studies) questioning the value of pulmonary artery catheterization for patients undergoing noncardiac surgery but note expert opinion that this procedure might provide valuable information in patients at highest risk for and from hemodynamic shifts with major procedures (Table 77G–2). These recommendations preceded a large randomized controlled trial that did not find benefit from pulmonary artery catheterization in elderly high-risk surgical patients.[4] There was some

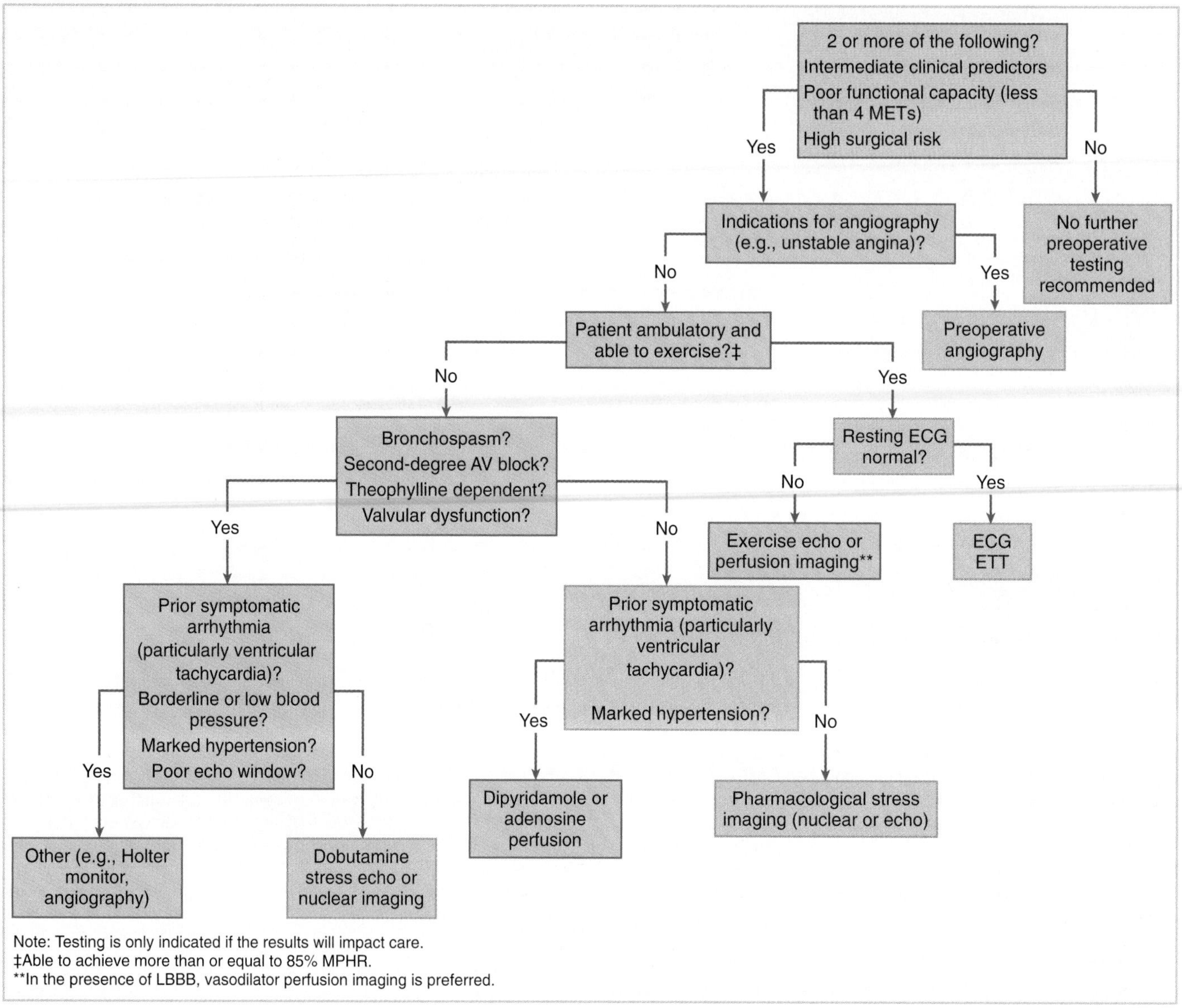

FIGURE 77G–1 Supplemental preoperative evaluation. AV = atrioventricular; ECG = electrocardiogram; ETT = exercise tolerance test; MET = metabolic equivalent. (From Eagle KA, Berger PB, Calkins H, et al: ACC/AHA guideline update for perioperative cardiovascular evaluation for noncardiac surgery: A report of the American College of Cardiology/American Heart Association Task Force on Practice Guidelines [Committee to Update the 1996 Guidelines on Perioperative Cardiovascular Evaluation for Noncardiac Surgery]. 2002. American College of Cardiology Web site. Available at: http://www.acc.org/clinical/guidelines/perio/dirIndex.htm.)

TABLE 77G–1 American College of Cardiology/American Heart Association Recommendations for Use of Ancillary Tests in Patients Undergoing Noncardiac Surgery

Indication	Class I (Indicated)	Class IIa (Good Supportive Evidence)	Class IIb (Weak Supportive Evidence)	Class III (Not Indicated)
Preoperative 12-lead rest ECG	1. Recent episode of chest pain or ischemic equivalent in clinically intermediate- or high-risk patients scheduled for an intermediate- or high-risk operative procedure.	1. Asymptomatic persons with diabetes mellitus.	1. Patients with prior coronary revascularization. 2. Asymptomatic male older than 45 yr or female older than 55 yr with two or more atherosclerotic risk factors. 3. Prior hospital admission for cardiac causes.	1. As a routine test in asymptomatic subjects undergoing low-risk operative procedures.
Preoperative noninvasive evaluation of left ventricular function	1. Patients with current or poorly controlled heart failure.	1. Patients with prior heart failure and patients with dyspnea of unknown origin.		1. As a routine test of left ventricular function in patients without prior heart failure.
Exercise or pharmacological stress testing	1. Diagnosis of adult patients with intermediate pretest probability of CAD. 2. Prognostic assessment of patients undergoing initial evaluation for suspected or proven CAD; evaluation of subjects with significant change in clinical status. 3. Demonstration of proof of myocardial ischemia before coronary revascularization. 4. Evaluation of adequacy of medical therapy; prognostic assessment after an acute coronary syndrome (if recent evaluation unavailable).	1. Evaluation of exercise capacity when subjective assessment is unreliable.	1. Diagnosis of CAD patients with high or low pretest probability; those with resting ST depression less than 1 mm, those undergoing digitalis therapy, and those with ECG criteria for left ventricular hypertrophy. 2. Detection of restenosis in high-risk asymptomatic subjects within the initial months after PCI.	1. For *exercise* stress testing, diagnosis of patients with resting ECG abnormalities that preclude adequate assessment, e.g., preexcitation syndrome, electronically paced ventricular rhythm, rest ST depression greater than 1 mm, or left bundle branch block. 2. Severe comorbidity likely to limit life expectancy or candidacy for revascularization. 3. Routine screening of asymptomatic men or women without evidence of CAD. 4. Investigation of isolated ectopic beats in young patients.
Coronary angiography in perioperative evaluation before (or after) noncardiac surgery	Patients with suspected or known CAD: 1. Evidence for high risk of adverse outcome based on noninvasive test results. 2. Angina unresponsive to adequate medical therapy. 3. Unstable angina, particularly when facing intermediate-risk* or high-risk* noncardiac surgery. 4. Equivocal noninvasive test results in patients at high clinical risk† undergoing high-risk* surgery.	1. Multiple markers of intermediate clinical risk† and planned vascular surgery (noninvasive testing should be considered first). 2. Moderate to large region of ischemia on noninvasive testing but without high-risk features and without lower LVEF. 3. Nondiagnostic noninvasive test results in patients of intermediate clinical risk† undergoing high-risk* noncardiac surgery. 4. Urgent noncardiac surgery while convalescing from acute MI.	1. Perioperative MI. 2. Medically stabilized class III or IV angina and planned low-risk or minor* surgery.	1. Low-risk* noncardiac surgery with known CAD and no high-risk results on noninvasive testing. 2. Asymptomatic after coronary revascularization with excellent exercise capacity (greater than or equal to 7 METs). 3. Mild stable angina with good left ventricular function and no high-risk noninvasive test results. 4. Noncandidate for coronary revascularization owing to concomitant medical illness, severe left ventricular dysfunction (e.g., LVEF less than 0.20), or refusal to consider revascularization. 5. Candidate for liver, lung, or renal transplantation older than 40 yr as part of evaluation for transplantation, unless noninvasive testing reveals high risk for adverse outcome.

CAD = coronary artery disease; ECG = electrocardiogram; HF = heart failure; LVEF = left ventricular ejection fraction; MET = metabolic equivalent; MI = myocardial infarction; PCI = percutaneous coronary intervention.

From Eagle KA, Berger PB, Calkins H, et al: ACC/AHA guideline update for perioperative cardiovascular evaluation for noncardiac surgery: A report of the American College of Cardiology/American Heart Association Task Force on Practice Guidelines (Committee to Update the 1996 Guidelines on Perioperative Cardiovascular Evaluation for Noncardiac Surgery). 2002. American College of Cardiology Web site. Available at: http://www.acc.org/clinical/guidelines/perio/dirIndex.htm.

*Cardiac risk according to type of noncardiac surgery. High risk: emergent major operations, aortic and major vascular surgery, peripheral vascular surgery, or anticipated prolonged surgical procedure associated with large fluid shifts and blood loss; intermediate risk: carotid endarterectomy, major head and neck surgery, intraperitoneal and intrathoracic surgery, orthopedic surgery, or prostate surgery; and low risk: endoscopic procedures, superficial procedures, cataract surgery, or breast surgery.

†Cardiac risk according to clinical predictors of perioperative death, MI, or HF. High clinical risk: unstable angina, acute or recent MI with evidence of important residual ischemic risk, decompensated HF, high degree of atrioventricular block, symptomatic ventricular arrhythmias with known structural heart disease, severe symptomatic valvular heart disease, or patient with multiple intermediate-risk markers such as prior MI, HF, and diabetes; intermediate clinical risk: Canadian Cardiovascular Society class I or II angina, prior MI by history or ECG, compensated or prior HF, diabetes mellitus, or renal insufficiency.

TABLE 77G–2 American College of Cardiology/American Heart Association Recommendations for Use of Interventions in Patients Undergoing Noncardiac Surgery

Indication	Class I (Indicated)	Class IIa (Good Supportive Evidence)	Class IIb (Weak Supportive Evidence)	Class III (Not Indicated)
Perioperative medical therapy	Beta blockers required in the recent past to control symptoms of angina or patients with symptomatic arrhythmias or hypertension. Beta blockers: patients at high cardiac risk owing to the finding of ischemia on preoperative testing who are undergoing vascular surgery.	Beta blockers: preoperative assessment identifies untreated hypertension, known coronary disease, or major risk factors for coronary disease.	Alpha$_2$-agonists: perioperative control of hypertension, or known CAD or major risk factors for CAD.	Beta blockers: contraindication to beta blockade. Alpha$_2$-agonists: contraindication to alpha$_2$-agonists.
Intraoperative nitroglycerin	High-risk patients previously taking nitroglycerin who have active signs of myocardial ischemia without hypotension.	As a prophylactic agent for high-risk patients to prevent myocardial ischemia and cardiac morbidity, particularly in those who have required nitrate therapy to control angina.		Patients with signs of hypovolemia or hypotension.
Intraoperative use of pulmonary artery catheters		Patients at risk for major hemodynamic disturbances that are most easily detected by a pulmonary artery catheter who are undergoing a procedure that is likely to cause these hemodynamic changes (e.g., suprarenal aortic aneurysm repair in a patient with angina) in a setting with experience in interpreting the results.	Either the patient's condition or the surgical procedure (but not both) places the patient at risk for hemodynamic disturbances (e.g., supraceliac aortic aneurysm repair in a patient with a negative stress test).	No risk of hemodynamic disturbances.
Perioperative ST segment monitoring		When available, proper use of computerized ST segment analysis in patients with known CAD or undergoing vascular surgery may provide increased sensitivity to detect myocardial ischemia during the perioperative period and may identify patients who would benefit from further postoperative and long-term interventions.	Patients with single or multiple risk factors for CAD.	Patients at low risk for CAD.

CAD = coronary artery disease.
From Eagle KA, Berger PB, Calkins H, et al: ACC/AHA guideline update for perioperative cardiovascular evaluation for noncardiac surgery: A report of the American College of Cardiology/American Heart Association Task Force on Practice Guidelines (Committee to Update the 1996 Guidelines on Perioperative Cardiovascular Evaluation for Noncardiac Surgery). 2002. American College of Cardiology Web site. Available at: http://www.acc.org/clinical/guidelines/perio/dirIndex.htm.

support for use of ST segment monitoring to detect perioperative ischemia, but the guidelines acknowledge that no studies have shown that this intervention improves outcome when therapy is based upon the resulting data.

Perioperative surveillance for acute coronary syndromes using routine ECGs and cardiac serum biomarkers was considered unnecessary in clinically low-risk patients undergoing low-risk operative procedures. In patients with high or intermediate clinical risk who have known or suspected coronary artery disease and who are undergoing high- or intermediate-risk surgical procedures, the guidelines recommend performance of ECGs at baseline, immediately after the surgical procedure, and daily on the first 2 days after surgery. For detection of myocardial injury, cardiac troponin measurements 24 hours postoperatively and on day 4 or hospital discharge (whichever comes first) were recommended.

References

1. Eagle KA, Berger PB, Calkins H, et al: ACC/AHA guideline update for perioperative cardiovascular evaluation for noncardiac surgery: A report of the American College of Cardiology/American Heart Association Task Force on Practice Guidelines (Committee to Update the 1996 Guidelines on Perioperative Cardiovascular Evaluation for Noncardiac Surgery). 2002. American College of Cardiology Web site (http://www.acc.org/clinical/guidelines/perio/dirIndex.htm).
2. American College of Physicians: Guidelines for assessing and managing the perioperative risk from coronary artery disease associated with major noncardiac surgery. Ann Intern Med 127:309, 1997.
3. Grayburn PA, Hillis LD: Cardiac events in patients undergoing noncardiac surgery: Shifting the paradigm from noninvasive risk stratification to therapy. Ann Intern Med 138:506, 2003.
4. Sandham JD, Hull RD, Brant RF, et al: A randomized, controlled trial of the use of pulmonary-artery catheters in high-risk surgical patients. N Engl J Med 348:5, 2003.

CHAPTER 78

Heart Disease in Varied Populations

Clyde W. Yancy

The Changing Demographics of the US Population

Cardiovascular disease remains the leading cause of death and disability in the United States, and its burden permeates the entirety of the US population. In the past, we have been comfortable extracting data from large epidemiological surveys, such as The Framingham Study, and from major clinical trials and applying those data to all persons at risk for heart disease. These databases have typically been overrepresented by predominantly white male study cohorts. Clinically naive assumptions have been made that the data discovered would be applicable to all persons, irrespective of gender, race, or ethnicity. However, current literature now strongly suggests that certain dissimilarities between cardiovascular disease in white populations and the other racial/ethnic populations in the United States do exist and that these differences are clinically relevant.

The need to focus on these dissimilarities has less to do with inclusiveness and more to do with the changing demographics of the United States. The United States is in the midst of a remarkable shift in population demographics. Currently, African Americans account for 14 percent of the US population and Hispanic Americans account for 13 percent. Asian Americans and Native Americans make up a smaller cohort of the US population, but together these four racial/ethnic or "varied" populations account for approximately 30 percent of the US population. The diversity of the American population is expected to increase over the next two to three decades. By 2050, the white non-Hispanic population may reach a nadir of 52.5 percent, compared to 75.7 percent in 1990, while Hispanic Americans may account for 22.5 percent and African Americans for 15.7 percent of the population. Asians and Pacific Islanders will account for 10.3 percent and American Indians and Alaska Natives will add 1.1 percent.[1] Thus, the epidemiology, pathophysiology, and treatment of heart disease in varied populations will have a major effect on the cardiovascular milieu in the United States.

DISTRIBUTION OF KNOWN RISK FACTORS FOR HEART DISEASE IN VARIED POPULATIONS

Hypertension. Within the varied populations, the incidence of known risk factors for cardiovascular disease is alarmingly high. The Third National Health and Nutrition Examination Survey (NHANES III) provides data on the distribution of hypertension among non-Hispanic white, non-Hispanic black, and Hispanic American groups. At least 33 million whites are hypertensive; nearly 6 million African Americans and 1.3 million Hispanic Americans are also affected with hypertension (see Chap. 37). Crude prevalence rates of hypertension for African Americans are 29.9 percent for men and 27.3 percent for women. For non-Hispanic whites, hypertension affects 25.6 percent of men and 23.8 percent of women, and for Hispanic Americans, it affects 14.6 percent of men and 14 percent of women. The higher prevalence of hypertension in African Americans is also accompanied by a worse disease severity. The prevalence of stage 3 hypertension (>180/110 mm Hg) is 8.5 percent for African Americans and 1 percent for whites. The mean systolic blood pressure and diastolic blood pressure for all African Americans is 125/75 mm Hg, which compares to a mean of 122/74 mm Hg for all whites. For hypertensive African Americans, the difference in blood pressure versus normotensive African Americans is 30/20 mm Hg, whereas for hypertensive whites, the difference is 23/15 mm Hg.[2]

Diabetes Mellitus. Diabetes is a deadly risk factor for cardiovascular disease and currently affects 17 million Americans (see Chap. 40). The incidence of the disease has increased 49 percent in the past decade; this is likely attributable to the alarming incidence of obesity. Among patients 40 to 74 years of age, the prevalence of diabetes is 11.2 percent for whites, 18.2 percent for African Americans, and 20.3 percent for Hispanic Americans. Despite the higher incidence of diabetes in Hispanic Americans, mortality rates due to diabetes are highest in African Americans, at 28.4 per 100,000 for men and 39.1 per 100,000 for women. This compares to 23.4 and 25.7 for white men and women, respectively.[3] Hypertension is concomitantly present in 75.4 percent of African American diabetic persons, 70.7 percent of Hispanic Americans with diabetes, and 64.5 percent of whites affected with diabetes.[4]

Metabolic Syndrome. Insulin resistance along with obesity, hypertension, and dyslipidemia constitutes the metabolic syndrome, which is associated with excessive cardiovascular disease (see Chap. 40). Using the NCEP ATP III criteria applied to the NHANES III database, the incidence of the metabolic syndrome is 22 percent overall for the US population over the age of 20 years but increases to more than 40 percent in elderly populations[5] and is highest in the varied populations. Hispanic Americans have the highest incidence of the metabolic syndrome, at 31.9 percent overall and 35 percent among Hispanic American women (Fig. 78-1). Of note, despite the high incidence of insulin resistance and the metabolic syndrome, Hispanic Americans have a lower prevalence of hypertension than African Americans. When the influence of obesity, body fat distribution, and insulin concentrations is followed prospectively in whites and Hispanic Americans, each factor is independently associated with the development of hypertension, with the greatest risk in subjects with the highest body mass index (BMI) (>30) and the highest insulin concentration (>95 pmol/liter). There does not appear to be an additional cardiovascular disease risk for Hispanic ethnicity versus white ethnicity, however.[6]

Obesity. The incidence of obesity (BMI > 25 is defined as overweight and BMI > 30 is defined as obese) in the US population is alarming, and the varied populations are disproportionately affected by this crisis (see Chap. 41). At the current rate of growth, the prevalence of obesity will be 40 percent by 2015.[7] The prevalence of both overweight and obesity is higher in African Americans and Hispanic Americans than in whites. The mean BMIs for African Americans, Hispanic Americans, and whites are 29.2, 28.6, and 26.3, respectively. African American women are on average 17 pounds heavier than white women of comparable age and socioeconomic status. Six of the 15 states with the highest prevalence of hypertension are in the

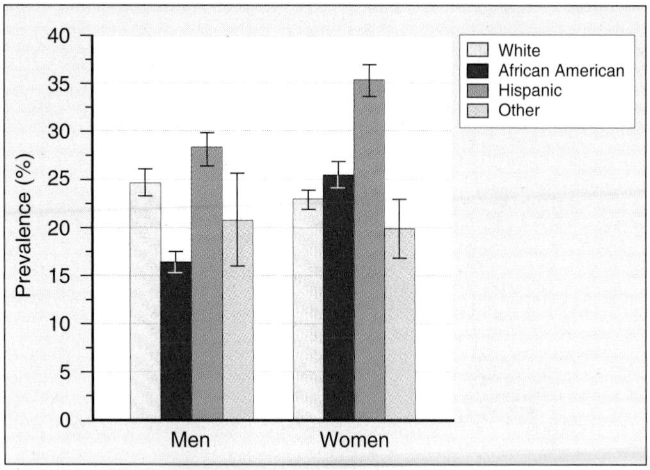

FIGURE 78–1 Age-adjusted prevalence of the metabolic syndrome among 8814 US adults aged at least 20 years, by sex and race or ethnicity, according to the National Health and Nutrition Examination Survey III, 1988-1994. Data are presented as percentage (shaded bars) and standard error (bracket). (From Ford ES, Giles WH, Dietz WH: Prevalence of the metabolic syndrome among US adults. JAMA 287:356, 2002.)

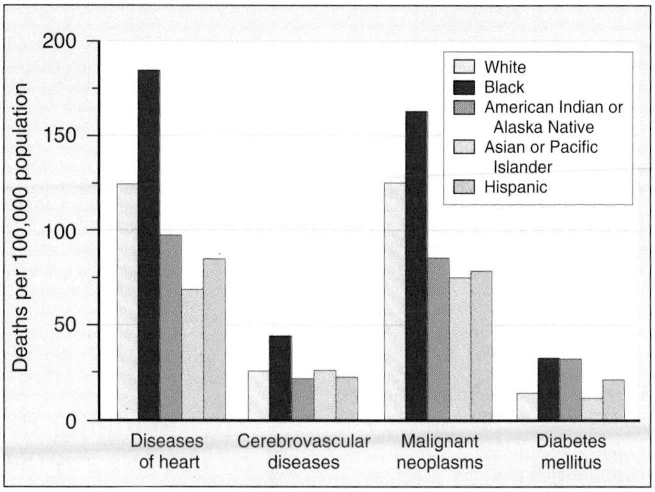

FIGURE 78–2 Age-adjusted death rates for selected causes of death by ethnicity, United States, 1950-1998. (From Smedley BD, Stith AY, Nelson AR [eds]: Unequal treatment: Confronting racial and ethnic disparities in health care. The Institute of Medicine. Washington, DC, National Academies Press, 2002, p 83.)

southeastern region of the United States (corresponding with the "stroke belt"). The highest prevalence of obesity is in African American women, at 44 percent, and in the Southeast, 71 percent of African American women are obese.[7,8]

The International Collaborative Study on Hypertension in Blacks (ICSHIB) demonstrated an important interaction of body mass index and hypertension across the course of the African Diaspora. Seven populations of West African origin were identified. A striking linear relationship was noted between BMI and the percentage of the respective population with hypertension, varying from less than 15 percent incidence of hypertension in Africans in Nigeria with a mean BMI of less than 24, to a hypertension incidence of nearly 35 percent in the Chicago area, where the mean BMI was 29.[9] Overall, 22 percent of the US population is physically inactive, but 40 percent of African American women are physically inactive. Data taken from the CARDIA study demonstrate that African American women have a higher BMI (by at least 2.7), higher energy intake, lower levels of physical activity, and lower overall physical fitness than white women.[10] Thus, the influence of obesity and physical inactivity on the development of hypertension and subsequent heart disease in African Americans is great.

Dyslipidemia is an important modifiable risk factor for heart disease in the United States, and correction of lipid disorders results in a decrease in the incidence of heart disease (see Chap. 39). Several reports have suggested that African Americans have lower low-density lipoprotein (LDL) cholesterol concentrations and less hypercholesterolemia. The Coronary Artery Risk Development in Young Adults study (CARDIA) identified the prevalence of LDL levels in young adults. An LDL cholesterol greater than 160 mg/dl was seen in 10 percent of young African American men and 5 percent of young African American women, which compared to 9 percent of young white men and 4 percent of young white women. High-density lipoprotein (HDL) levels were higher in African American men than in white men.[10]

Dietary Variations. In addition to greater energy intake, individuals in varied populations have several important dietary variations that are potentially associated with an increased incidence of cardiovascular disease. These dietary alterations include greater sodium consumption, less potassium consumption, and less calcium intake. The Treatment of Mild Hypertension Study (TOMHS) demonstrated dissimilar urinary Na^+ and Na^+:K^+ ratios for African Americans versus whites, especially at lower socioeconomic levels. This difference is related to dietary electrolyte intake, and the higher intake of dietary sodium is linked to the incidence of hypertension.[11] The recommended daily intake of sodium is quite low at 20 to 40 mmol. Currently, sodium consumption in the United States averages 140 to 150 mmol/day (8-10 gm/day) and is highest in African Americans and Hispanic Americans. Whereas there is a direct relationship between sodium intake and hypertension, there is an inverse relationship between potassium intake and hypertension.[12] African Americans consume a diet low in potassium. Low potassium consumption is typically associated with concurrent high sodium intake, caloric intake, and alcohol consumption; such diets are common in industrialized countries. African Americans also consume a diet low in calcium and perhaps lower in magnesium as well. The intake of calcium and magnesium is associated with lower blood pressures. The Dietary Approaches to Stop Hypertension Trial (DASH) tested the potential benefit of a diet rich in fruits, vegetables, and low-fat dairy products and low in saturated and total fats in control subjects and in patients with known hypertension. The diet led to an increase in potassium intake from 1700 mg/day to 4100 mg/day and a corresponding drop in sodium intake. The impact of the DASH diet was greatest in those subjects with the highest sodium intake, achieving a 12 mm Hg reduction in blood pressure in African Americans, which is equivalent to the results expected from pharmacological intervention with a single drug to control blood pressure.[13]

Left Ventricular Hypertrophy. In the setting of hypertension, the rates of left ventricular hypertrophy are highest in African Americans, at 31 percent versus 10 percent in whites, and the pattern of hypertrophy is more of the concentric type—a type known to be associated with increased cardiovascular events.[14] Left ventricular mass is correlated with systolic blood pressure and is a predictor of heart disease (see Chap. 37). The CARDIA study demonstrated a higher incidence of increased left ventricular mass in young adult African Americans and a close relationship between obesity, systolic blood pressure elevation, and left ventricular mass. Smoking rates are generally higher in African Americans and Hispanic Americans and may be increasing in teens and young adults.

Other risk factors for heart disease, such as hypertriglyceridemia, hyperuricemia, microalbuminuria, and elevated tissue plasminogen activator inhibitor-1 levels, may demonstrate subtle differences in these varied populations, but adequate data points are not available to make definitive comment.

Cardiovascular Mortality in Varied Populations

Heart disease is the leading cause of death for all cohorts of the US population, including the varied population. Of these groups, African Americans experience the highest rates of mortality from heart disease (Fig. 78–2). The mortality rate for African Americans is 1.6 times that of whites, a ratio that is identical to the black/white mortality ratio in 1950.[15] Hispanic Americans are twice as likely as all others to die from diabetes and Native Americans die disproportionately from diabetes as well. The average annual death rate due to heart disease expressed as deaths per 100,000 in the 45- to 64-year age range is 404 for African Americans, 219 for whites, 188 for Native Americans, 143 for Hispanic Americans, and 90 for Asian/Pacific Islanders. For the 65- to 74-year age range, the corresponding numbers are 1278 for African Americans,

871 for whites, 650 for Native Americans, 614 for Hispanic Americans, and 443 for Asian/Pacific Islanders. In women, cardiovascular disease is the leading cause of death, affecting 41 percent of white women, 41 percent of African American women, 33 percent of Hispanic American women, and 37 percent of Asian American women.[16,17]

The prevalence of coronary heart disease is higher in African Americans, with a prevalence of 7.1 percent and 9.0 percent, respectively, for men and women, as compared with 6.9 percent and 5.4 percent for white men and women. Death rates per 100,000 due to coronary heart disease are 272 and 193 for African American men and women, compared with 249 and 153 for white men and women.[16,17] In fact, death rates due to coronary heart disease in African Americans are the highest in the world.[18] Death rates from stroke are also higher in African Americans. Compared with whites, young African Americans have a threefold increased risk of ischemic stroke and a fourfold higher risk of stroke death. The death rate due to stroke is highest in the southeastern United States.[16] In addition, the five states with the highest rate of deaths due to congestive heart failure are also in the southeastern United States, and of the 15 states with the highest rates of end-stage renal disease (ESRD), 10 are in the Southeast.[8]

The prevalence of coronary heart disease in Mexican Americans is 7.2 percent for men and 6.8 percent for women, and the prevalence of myocardial infarction is 4.1 percent for men and 1.9 percent for women. This compares to 5.2 percent and 2.0 percent for white men and women and 4.3 percent and 3.3 percent for African American men and women. Death rates are similar for Hispanic Americans and whites (Table 78–1).[16]

Disparities in Cardiovascular Care and Outcomes in Varied Populations

The foregoing information clearly establishes important population differences regarding risk and outcomes for cardiovascular disease. The complete explanation for these differential outcomes is lacking but is likely to be a complex interplay of social, political, physiological, and genetic variances in these populations. These differences are best captured by an evaluation of the disparities in health care for the different racial and ethnic groups. *Disparities* in health care refers to differences in the quality of health care that are not due to access-related factors or clinical needs, preferences (patient choices), or appropriateness of the intervention (Fig. 78–3).[19] This is to be distinguished from *discrimination,* which implicates biases, prejudices, and stereotyping. Disparities may emanate from decisions made by the patient, provider, or health care system.

Members of ethnic minority groups have been found to refuse coronary artery bypass surgery (CABG) at a higher rate than others, but not sufficiently so to account for major differences in outcomes.[20] Greater issues are pertinent at the level of the health care delivery system. Language barriers are important obstacles for many patients. Nearly 14 million Americans are not proficient in English, and one in five Spanish-speaking persons report not seeking health care because of language issues. Nearly 8 million Hispanic Americans do not speak English well. One in 20 Native Americans does not speak English well, and among Asian Americans, the language barrier varies from 1 percent in persons of Hawaiian origin, to 15 percent for persons of Japanese origin and 55 percent for persons of Cambodian origin.[21] In addition to language barriers, lack of health insurance and geographic isolation both contribute further to disparities.

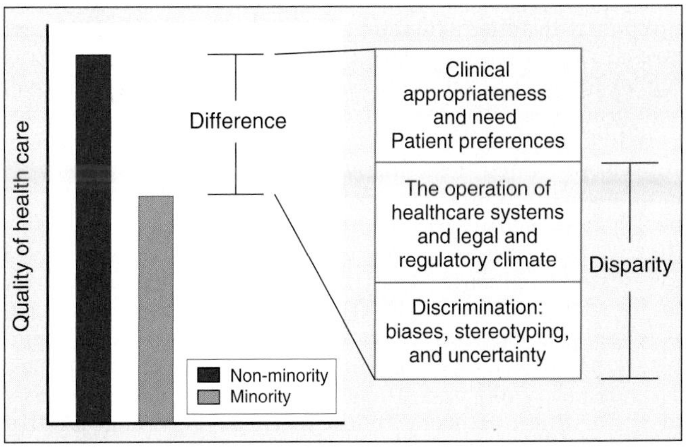

FIGURE 78–3 Differences, disparities, and discrimination: populations with equal access to health care. (From Gomes C, McGuire TG: Identifying the sources of racial and ethnic disparities in health care use. The Institute of Medicine Report. Washington, DC, National Academies Press, 2001.)

TABLE 78–1 Coronary Heart Disease and Angina Pectoris

Population Group	Prevalence CHD	Prevalence MI	Incidence CHD	Incidence MI	Mortality CHD	Mortality MI
Total population	12,900,000	7,600,000	1,100,000	540,000	515,204	192,898
Total males	6,300,000	4,700,000	660,000	330,000	260,574	100,306
Total females	6,600,000	2,900,000	440,000	210,000	254,630	92,585
White males	6.9%	5.2%	—	—	230,951	89,383
White females	5.4%	2.0%	—	—	224,449	81,201
Black males	7.1%	4.3%	68,200	—	24,625	9,045
Black females	9.0%	3.3%	47,700	—	26,640	10,067
Mexican-American males	7.2%	4.1%	—	—	—	—
Mexican-American females	6.8%	1.9%	—	—	—	—

CHD = coronary heart disease: includes heart attack angina pectoris (chest pain) or both; MI = myocardial infarction (heart attack).

Prevalence: NHANES III (1988-1994). CDC/NCHS: data for white and black males and females are for non-Hispanics. Total population data are for Americans age 20 and older: percentages for racial/ethnic groups are age-adjusted for age 20 and older. Incidence: ARIC (1987-1994). NHLBI. Mortality: CDC/NCHS: data for white and black males and females include Hispanics.

From American Heart Association: Heart Disease and Stroke Statistics—2003 Update. Dallas, American Heart Association, 2002.

Providers can contribute to disparities in health care as well through subconscious stereotyping, clinical uncertainty due to cultural ignorance, and delay in referral for indicated procedures. It has been demonstrated that physicians have lower rates of referrals for cardiac catheterization in African American women than in white men, white women, and African American men despite similar articulation of symptoms and reasonable indications for further evaluation.[22]

Because of the interdigitation of patient, system, and provider issues, Americans belonging to ethnic minority groups undergo cardiovascular procedures at a lower rate. In a survey of 4 million patients with acute myocardial infarction as indexed in the National Hospital Discharge Survey (NHDS), African American men and women have been demonstrated to undergo coronary angiography and CABG at much lower rates.[23] A separate Medicare survey suggested that there is a fourfold difference in the rate of CABG between whites and African Americans, even after adjusting for age and gender. These differences were most striking in the southeastern United States.[23] An analysis of Hispanic Americans and whites with a diagnosis of myocardial infarction revealed that Hispanic Americans were discharged on 38 percent fewer medications. Similarly, they were less likely to receive percutaneous coronary interventions.[24] Studies done at Veterans Administration hospitals are quite intriguing, as these facilities theoretically have removed any access to care issues. Nonetheless, referral for cardiac procedures was higher for whites. Of note, African Americans refused invasive procedures twice as often. Differences in rates of thrombolytic therapy and CABG were also observed, with African Americans much less likely to receive either strategy.[25] Patients with ESRD have access to Medicare funding for health care needs, which should theoretically reduce disparities. A longitudinal survey of health care disparities from Medicare beneficiaries with ESRD is quite compelling. Prior to the development of ESRD, white Americans were 300 percent more likely to undergo cardiac catheterization, angioplasty, or CABG after controlling for socioeconomic variables. This disparity fell to a 40 percent difference after the onset of ESRD and Medicare funding. These data suggest that similar health care funding could significantly diminish certain health care disparities in cardiovascular care.

The disproportionate risk for cardiovascular disease and apparent disparities in care are most evident in African American women. The Heart and Estrogen/Progestin Replacement Study (HERS) evaluated 2699 women, of whom 218 were African American. HERS evaluated women in a longitudinal study over 4 years to determine the health risks and benefits of hormone replacement therapy. Despite a definite twofold increase in cardiovascular event rates, African American women had less optimal control of hypertension and LDL cholesterol and lesser use of aspirin and statins.[26]

Hypertension in Varied Populations

No segment of the US population is devoid of excessive cardiovascular risk due to the consequences of hypertension (see Chap. 37). This risk is especially evident in the varied populations, however.

Hispanic Americans

A paradox exists in Hispanic Americans. Despite a higher incidence of diabetes and obesity, the prevalence of hypertension in Hispanic Americans is lower than in the general population. Hypertension among Hispanic Americans varies by gender and by the country of origin. Puerto Rican origin is associated with the highest incidence of hypertension, followed by Cuban origin and Mexican origin. When Hispanic Americans of Mexican origin are affected by hypertension, control of blood pressure can be more difficult.[27] The lower incidence of hypertension in Hispanic Americans of Mexican origin versus other Hispanic Americans is postulated to be due to a modernization phenomenon, implicating acclimatization to a Western lifestyle as a factor in the development of hypertension. In Puerto Rico, urban men with a high school education have a blood pressure 8 mm Hg higher than less educated men. This is not the same experience seen in other North American ethnic groups, in which education is associated with lower blood pressure measurements. For persons younger than 45 years, the prevalence of hypertension is twice the rate seen in the mainland United States. Death rates due to heart disease have increased by 72 percent over the last three decades while otherwise falling in the remainder of the United States. The incidence of ESRD is higher in Puerto Rico than in any other region of Latin America.[28]

Americans of South Asian Descent

Americans with ancestry from the Indian subcontinent have a major health problem with hypertension. Hypertension is a significant concern in the Indian subcontinent and is an important cardiovascular risk for South Asians worldwide. The World Health Organization has reported that Indian men in the age range of 40 to 55 years have the highest blood pressure among populations from 20 other developing countries. The prevalence of hypertension in Indian countries has increased from less than 2 percent in 1950 to nearly 20 percent currently. This increased risk is further exacerbated with emigration to North America and varies directly with the degree of urbanization. The Study of Health Assessment and Risk in Ethnic Groups (SHARE) done in Canada reported that South Asians had the highest self-reported incidence of hypertension.[29] Coincident with the hypertension risk is a growing risk of diabetes, dyslipidemia (perhaps related to a genetic predisposition to a low HDL level), and obesity. Tobacco consumption is likewise increasing in South Asians, and per capita fat consumption has increased. Taken together, the confluence of these risk factors contributes not only to the alarming rate of hypertension but also to the increasing rate of symptomatic coronary artery disease (CAD).[30]

African Americans

Hypertension in African Americans represents the most prolific variance in heart disease and cardiovascular disease risk factors in the varied populations. African Americans experience the highest prevalence of hypertension, perhaps in the world, with nearly 35 percent of all African Americans affected by hypertension.[31] It is estimated that 5.6 million African Americans have hypertension, a number that eclipses the total number of persons affected with congestive heart failure. The Hypertension and Detection Follow-up Program found that severe hypertension (diastolic blood pressure > 115 mm Hg) was five to seven times more likely to be present in African Americans than in white Americans.[31] The differential experience of hypertension is evident in childhood, with higher recorded blood pressures noted prior to the age of 10 years in black children as compared with white children.[32] The consequences of hypertension in African Americans are quite pathological, with a 50 percent higher frequency of heart failure,[33] a sixfold higher incidence of developing ESRD due to hypertension,[31] a 38 percent higher risk of stroke, and a higher risk of death due to stroke.[17] Overall, mortality due to hypertension and its consequences is four to five times more likely in African Americans than in whites.[31]

Hypertensive heart disease is manifest as left ventricular hypertrophy, which separately is a risk factor for sudden death and coronary events. The CARDIA study demonstrated that left ventricular mass is higher and independently correlated with systolic blood pressure in young African American males.[31,34] The Veterans Administration Cooperative Monotherapy Hypertension Trial determined that left ventricular hypertrophy diagnosed by electrocardiographic criteria is noted in 31 percent of African American hypertensive patients, as compared with 10 percent of white hypertensive patients.[35] The presence of increased left ventricular mass is associated with an increased rate of death and is thus a contributor to the excess rate of morbidity and mortality due to cardiovascular disease seen in African Americans. It is noted that CAD is the leading putative cause of heart failure in whites, but pooled data from published clinical trials suggest that hypertension may be the leading imputed cause of heart failure in blacks.[33]

Variances in the pathophysiology of stroke may also be extant. African Americans typically have more occlusive disease in the large and medium-sized intracranial arteries, whereas whites typically have more occlusive disease in the extracranial arteries. The incidence of hemorrhagic stroke is also higher. Similar observations have been made in the setting of ESRD. Hypertensive nephrosclerosis is the leading cause of ESRD for African Americans, and they disproportionately populate the hemodialysis cohort. For African Americans aged 20 to 44 years, hypertension-related ESRD is 20-fold higher than in whites. African Americans have been noted to lack the nocturnal dip in blood pressure and to have an earlier onset of proteinuria. Both of these findings are associated with a higher incidence of hypertension-induced nephrosclerosis.[36]

Several purported mechanisms may explain in part the excess burden of hypertension in African Americans. Peripheral vascular resistance may be higher in some African Americans with hypertension. Small studies have also demonstrated that vasodilatory responses are blunted in African Americans in a manner suggesting subtle differences in nitric oxide homeostasis.[37] Plasma renin activity is lower in African Americans than in age-matched white hypertensive patients,[38] urinary kallikrein excretion is lower, and insulin levels are higher.[33]

Much has been written about salt sensitivity in African Americans, including a theoretical assertion that Darwinian influences during the African Diaspora (active slave trading from West Africa to North America) led to selective pressure favoring genes that promote salt retention that now predispose to hypertension. This is an unproven but nevertheless prevalent theory.[39,40] Rates of hypertension in rural West Africa are the lowest in the world, but populations of West African origin in the Caribbean and in North America demonstrate dramatic rises in blood pressure that are linearly related to increases in body mass index (Fig. 78–4).[40] It is evident, however, that some African Americans do appear to be more salt sensitive than others. Salt restriction leads to a greater reduction in systolic blood pressure in African Americans (approximately 12 mm Hg) than in whites.[41] A genetic basis for sodium sensitivity may exist. The epithelial sodium channel is responsible for the final reabsorption of filtered sodium from the distal nephron and has now been found to have at least eight single nucleotide polymorphisms. One of these polymorphisms (T594M), is found only in people of West African descent and is four times more likely in hypertensive African Americans than in normotensive African Americans.[42] Unfortunately, variations in a single gene are not likely to be responsible for more than 2 to 4 percent of the difference in hypertension seen between ethnic groups.[40] Yet another very attractive candidate polymorphism related to the excess risk of hypertension-related cardiovascular disease in African Americans is noted within the inflammatory cytokines. Transforming growth factor beta-1 (TGF-β_1) is a proinflammatory cytokine associated with stimulation of fibrosis, extracellular matrix turnover, glomerular hyperplasia, and left ventricular hypertrophy. TGF-β_1 is overexpressed in African Americans, with higher circulating levels noted. A described polymorphism at codon 25 of the TGF-β_1 gene that involves the substitution of arginine for proline is associated with higher TGF-β_1 levels and is seen more frequently in African Americans.[43] Angiotensin-converting enzyme (ACE) inhibitors and angiotensin receptor blockers both reduce angiotensin-II-mediated stimulation of TGF-β_1, and this may be of clinical importance in the treatment of hypertension in African Americans. Beta blockers are reportedly less effective as monotherapy for hypertension in African Americans,[44] but data exist that suggest a strong correlation between visceral obesity in African American women and sympathetic nervous system activity.[45]

THERAPY FOR HYPERTENSION IN AFRICAN AMERICANS. The therapy for hypertension for all persons should be focused clearly on goal blood pressure reduction and the prevention of cardiovascular disease related to hypertension (see Chap. 38). The treatment of hypertension is similar for all demographic groups.[44] Within the African American group, the responsiveness to monotherapy with ACE inhibitors, angiotensin receptor blockers, and beta blockers may be less than the responsiveness to diuretics and calcium channel blockers, but these differences are corrected when diuretics are added to the neurohormonal antagonists. The African American Study of Kidney Disease and Hypertension (AASK) prospectively addressed the impact of three antihypertensive drug classes on decline of glomerular filtration rate in cases of hypertension. Diabetic patients were excluded. In patients with established hypertension-induced nephrosclerosis and reduced glomerular filtration rate (20-60 ml/min per 1.73 m^2), a clinical composite that included 50 percent reduction in glomerular filtration rate, ESRD, or death was most favorably affected by an ACE inhibitor as compared with either a beta blocker or a calcium channel blocker (Table 78–2). It was noted in this study that African American patients with hypertension uniformly required a multidrug regimen to achieve adequate blood pressure control.[46] An algorithm to guide ideal management of high blood pressure in African Americans is depicted in Figure 78–5[47] and its features are highlighted in Table 78–3. The reader is advised to note the lower goal blood pressure reduction.

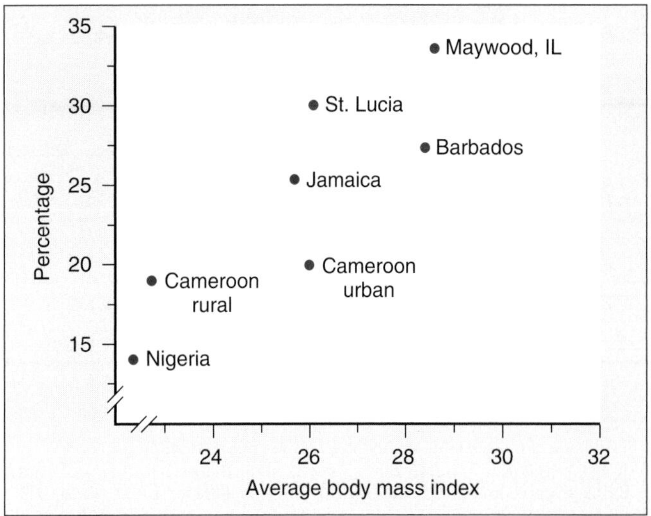

FIGURE 78–4 Hypertension prevalence across the African Diaspora. (From Cooper R, Rotimi C, Ataman S: The prevalence of hypertension in seven populations of West African origin. Am J Public Health 87:160, 1997.)

Ischemic Heart Disease in Varied Populations

All of the varied populations are experiencing increasing rates of ischemic heart disease related to the concurrent and often disproportionate presence of risk factors for CAD (see Chap. 36). Rates for CAD are increasing in Asian Americans, Hispanic Americans, Native Americans, and Americans of South Asian origin. It is important to note that the rates of CAD in these groups are approaching the rates seen in whites but do not exceed those rates. This is not the case, however, for African Americans.

African Americans have the highest rate of overall mortality due to CAD of any ethnic group in the United States. The risk for sudden cardiac death is higher and the onset of disease occurs approximately 5 years earlier. The usual presentation is more likely to be unstable angina or a non-ST segment elevation myocardial infarction rather than a typical ST segment elevation event.[48] Despite this increased incidence of disease, the presence of obstructive epicardial CAD on angiograms is less. Not infrequently, angiographic studies show normal epicardial vessels but autopsy studies demon-

TABLE 78–2 Analyses of Clinical Event Composite Outcomes

	Lower vs Usual Blood Pressure Goal Intervention		Drug Intervention: Ramipril vs Metoprolol		Drug Intervention: Metoprolol vs Amlodipine		Drug Intervention: Ramipril vs Amlodipine*	
Outcomes[‡]	% Risk Reduction (95% Confidence Interval)[†]	p Value	% Risk Reduction (95% Confidence Interval)[†]	p Value	% Risk Reduction (95% Confidence Interval)[†]	p Value	% Risk Reduction (95% Confidence Interval)[†]	p Value
GFR event, ESRD, or death	2 (−22 to 21)	0.85	22 (1 to 38)	0.04	20 (−10 to 41)	0.17	38 (14 to 56)	0.004
GFR event or ESRD	−2 (−31 to 20)	0.87	22 (−2 to 41)	0.07	24 (−9 to 47)	0.13	40 (14 to 59)	0.006
ESRD or death	12 (−13 to 32)	0.31	21 (−5 to 40)	0.11	42 (17 to 60)	0.003	49 (26 to 65)	<0.001
ESRD alone	6 (−29 to 31)	0.72	22 (−10 to 45)	0.16	59 (36 to 74)	<0.001	59 (36 to 74)	<0.001

ESRD = end-stage renal disease; GFR = glomerular filtration rate.
*Secondary comparison described in previous publication.
†All risk reductions adjusted for prespecified covariates: baseline proteinuria, mean arterial pressure, sex, history of heart disease, and age. Risk difference for ESRD or death composite and ESRD alone also adjusted for baseline GFR.
‡GFR event, ESRD, or death: main secondary composite clinical outcome with 340 events, including 179 declining GFR events, 84 additional participants with ESRD events, and 77 deaths; GFR event or ESRD: composite endpoint with 263 events, including 179 declining GFR events and 84 additional participants with ESRD events; ESRD, or death composite endpoint with 251 events, including 171 ESRD events and 80 deaths; and ESRD alone: endpoint with 171 events and deaths censored in this analysis.

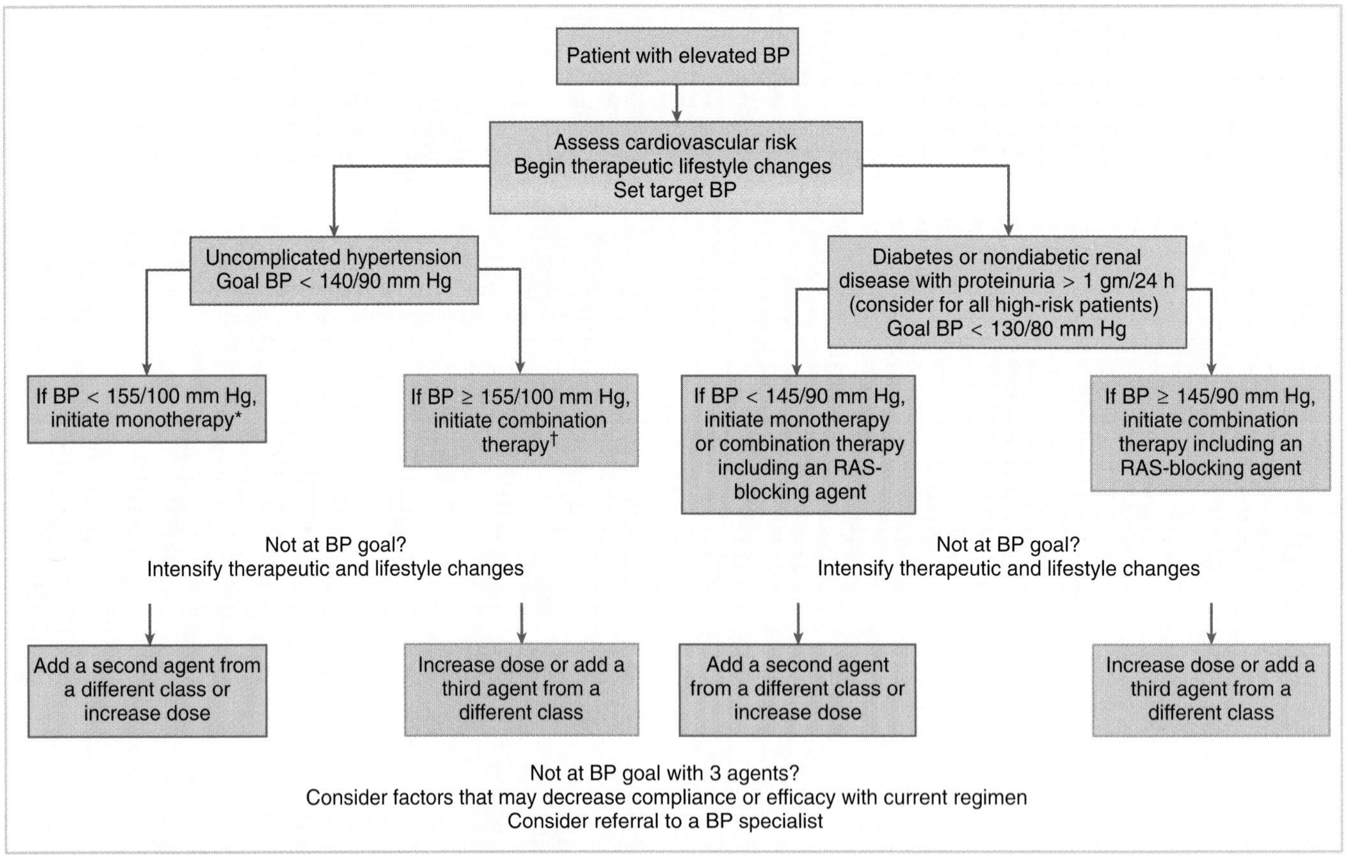

FIGURE 78–5 Clinical algorithm for achieving target blood pressure (BP) in African American patients with high BP. *Initiate monotherapy at the recommended starting dose with an agent from any of the following classes: diuretics, beta blockers, calcium channel blockers, angiotensin-converting enzyme inhibitors, or angiotensin II receptor blockers. †Initiate low-dose combination therapy with any of the following combinations: beta blocker/diuretic, angiotensin-converting enzyme inhibitor/diuretic, angiotensin-converting enzyme inhibitor/calcium channel blocker, or angiotensin II receptor blocker/diuretic. RAS = renin-angiotensin system.

strate a greater extent of atherosclerosis in African Americans despite a lesser degree of obstructive CAD.[49] As described earlier, interventions with thrombolytic therapy, percutaneous coronary interventions, and CABG are all less frequently administered.

The reason for the excess prevalence of CAD in African Americans is less likely related to pathophysiological variances, as suggested in the discussion on hypertension, and more likely due to the overabundance of cardiovascular risk factors. Obesity, left ventricular hypertrophy, type 2 diabetes, and physical inactivity are all more common in African Americans. Total cholesterol levels may be less in African Americans and HDL levels higher. Lipoprotein (a) levels are higher, by two- to threefold, in African Americans, but the

TABLE 78–3 Ideal Management of Hypertension in African Americans

Increase dietary potassium intake
Limit dietary sodium intake to <2.4 gm/day
Increase physical activity
Weight loss
All antihypertensive medications and combinations are effective
Multiple drug combinations may be required to achieve control
ACE inhibitors and beta blockers as monotherapy may be less effective but should be used when indicated (e.g., renal disease, heart failure, post-myocardial infarction)
Thiazide diuretics and calcium channel blockers may have greater blood pressure lowering efficacy
There is a higher incidence of angioedema when using ACE inhibitors

ACE = angiotensin-converting enzyme.

From Douglas JG, Bakris GL, Epstien M, et al: Management of high blood pressure in African Americans; consensus statement of the Hypertension in African Americans Working Group of the International Society of Hypertension in Blacks. Arch Intern Med 163:525, 2003.

TABLE 78–4 Polymorphisms Associated with Heart Failure

Genetic Polymorphism	Clinical Implications
Beta-1 adrenergic receptor; Gly-389	Subsensitive beta-1 receptor; decreased affinity for agonist and less cAMP generation
Beta-1 adrenergic receptor; ARG-389/alpha 2C Del322-325 receptor	Presence of both polymorphisms is associated with increased risk for heart failure in blacks; RR 10.11 when both are present
Enos	Subsensitive nitric oxide system
Aldosterone synthase	? Excessive fibrosis
Transforming growth factor beta-1	40% higher transforming growth factor beta-1 levels; higher endothelin levels?; more fibrosis
G Protein 825-T Allele	Marker of low renin hypertension, left ventricular hypertrophy, and stroke

From Yancy CW: Does race matter in heart failure? Am Heart J 146:203, 2003. See references 57-61.

relationship of lipoprotein (a) to coronary events remains unclear and may vary according to ethnicity. The relationship between total cholesterol, plaque formation, and coronary events may be weaker.[50]

The excess prevalence of left ventricular hypertrophy likely confounds the ischemic burden in the setting of CAD and may relate to excess mortality and sudden death. Mechanisms to support this theory are not yet clear. The increase in left ventricular mass with a disproportionately less robust vascular supply may lead to a lower threshold for arrhythmias and more damage due to ischemic events.[48] Endothelin-1 is a potent vasoconstrictor that has been demonstrated to be present in higher levels in African Americans.[51] Endothelin is stimulated by TGF-β_1, which, as described, is higher in hypertensive African Americans. The confluence of left ventricular hypertrophy and endothelial dysfunction may contribute to a greater risk of ischemia-related injury.

Importantly, there are no described differences in the presentation of acute coronary syndromes for any ethnic group, nor any described variations in treatment regimens or responses to standard medical and revascularization strategies. As such, no differences should be contemplated in the management of varied populations presenting with symptomatic CAD.

Heart Failure in Varied Populations

Heart failure has become one of the most pervasive cardiovascular illnesses in the United States (see Chap. 21). The prevalence of heart failure is increasing, as is the burden of excess mortality and morbidity—a burden that is once again borne in a disproportionate way by the demographics of varied populations. Although data for most ethnic groups are lacking in the realm of heart failure, data regarding African Americans are quite compelling and controversial.

Heart failure occurs in African Americans at a greater frequency, perhaps 50 percent higher overall and more than 100 percent higher in African American women than in whites. There are several striking differences in the natural history of heart disease in African Americans. The disease occurs at an earlier age; there is usually more profound left ventricular systolic dysfunction at the time of onset; and the clinical class is usually of more advanced severity.[33] The overall incidence of heart failure within the US population is 2 percent, but it occurs in 3 percent of the African American population. The issues regarding excess mortality and morbidity in African Americans with heart failure remain unresolved. The original data from the Studies of Left Ventricular Dysfunction (SOLVD) suggested a higher mortality rate,[52] but a reanalysis of African American and white cohorts matched for disease severity and left ventricular dysfunction demonstrated only an excess rate of hospitalization.[53] Data from the SOLVD prevention trial clearly demonstrated a higher incidence of heart failure, which is consistent with epidemiological surveys, but a similar responsiveness to ACE inhibitors.[54]

Based on the foregoing discussion, it is not surprising to discover that the leading putative cause of left ventricular dysfunction in African Americans with heart failure is hypertension. A survey of published clinical trials and registries suggests that the incidence of hypertension as the likely cause of heart failure in this population varies from approximately 30 percent to nearly 60 percent (Fig. 78–6).[33] True cause and effect is lacking, because few if any mechanistic data support the conversion from hypertensive heart disease to systolic dysfunction. Data from spontaneously hypertensive salt-sensitive animals suggest that the conversion from left ventricular hypertrophy to overt heart failure is associated with an increase in the progenitors of endothelin.[55] Although data do exist from the Systolic Hypertension in the Elderly Trial to justify therapy for hypertension as an effective means of preventing heart failure, these data are most pertinent for systolic hypertension of the elderly (which included 14 percent African Americans).[56] Similar inferences for the treatment of diastolic hypertension in African Americans are conjectural and not yet supported by definitive data.

A genomic basis to explain the differential epidemiology and natural history of heart failure in African Americans is under active investigation. Several candidate polymorphisms have emerged as plausible culprit genetic variations, but the relationship of these genes to the environment and the complex interplay of multiple physiological systems makes these discussions largely theoretical until additional data from large cohorts of the population are evaluated (Table 78–4).[57-61]

Data regarding the response to medical therapy for heart failure affecting African Americans emanate from post-hoc analyses of the African American subgroups in major clinical trials in heart failure. These analyses are all compromised by their retrospective nature, inconsistent sample sizes, and differences in disease expression between the African American and white cohorts. As such, the analyses yield provocative inferences and generate new hypotheses but do not alter current treatment recommendations (Table 78–5).[52-54,62-65]

Taken in aggregate, the data from Table 78–5 demonstrate that all approved therapeutic strategies for heart failure are effective and yield improved outcomes (see Chap. 23). There should be no reluctance to treat African Americans with

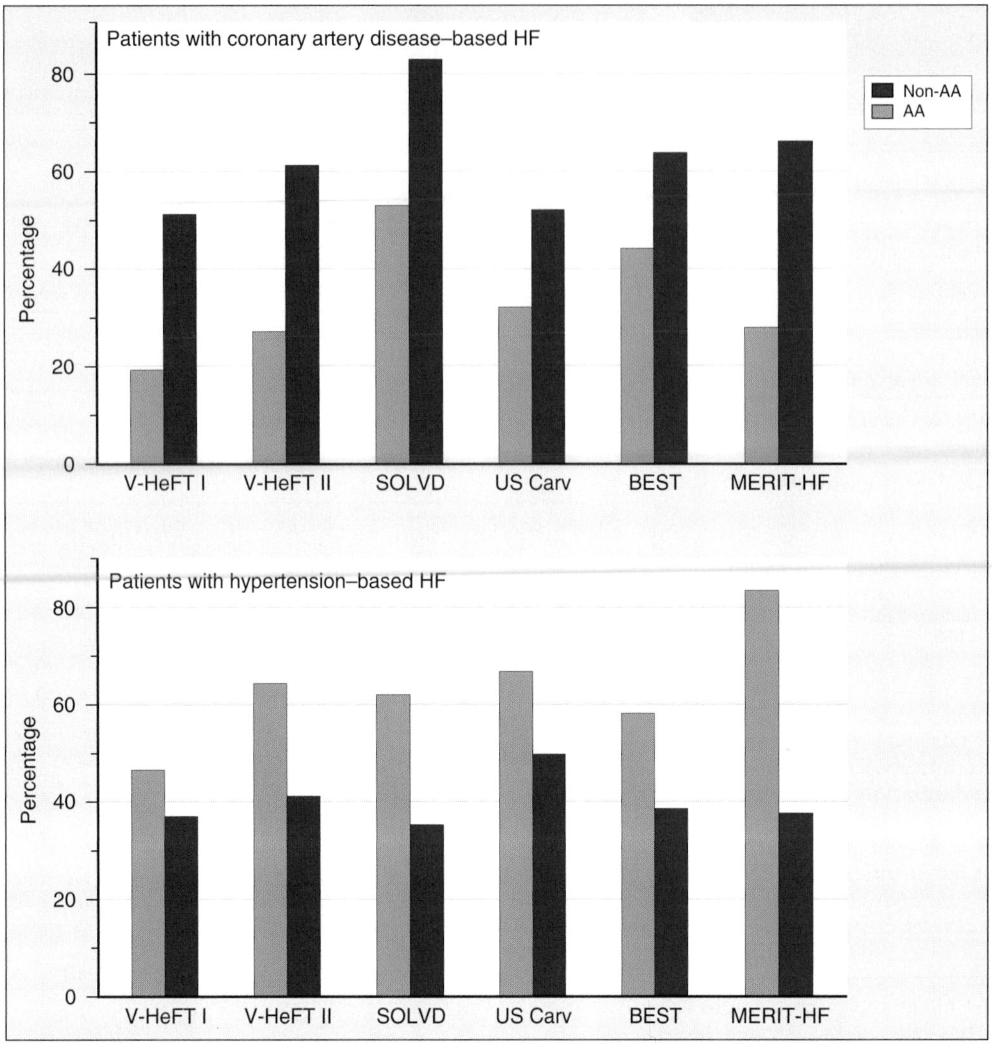

FIGURE 78–6 Etiology of heart failure (HF) in African Americans (AA). (Data from The BEST Investigators: N Engl J Med 344:1659, 2001 [BEST]; MERIT-HF Study Group: Lancet 353:2001, 1999 [MERIT]; The SOLVD Investigators: N Engl J Med 325:293, 1991 [SOLVD]; Packer M, et al: N Engl J Med 334:1349, 1996 [US Carv]; Cohn JN, et al: N Engl J Med 314:1547, 1986 [V-HeFT I]; Cohn JN, et al: N Engl J Med 325:303, 1991 [V-HeFT II].)

heart failure using any of the current treatment modalities. The data regarding beta blocker efficacy are least consistent. The analysis from the Beta Blocker Evaluation of Survival Trial was interpreted to mean that African American patients responded less well to beta blocker therapy and may have failed to benefit.[63] Given the presence of intrinsic sympathomimetic activity in this compound, it is more likely that these results are drug specific and not class specific. The number of African Americans exposed to extended release metoprolol in clinical trials has been insignificant, and subgroup analysis has been unrewarding.[64] However, the experience with carvedilol given in combination with ACE inhibitors to African Americans with all classes of heart failure are quite encouraging and are consistent with salutary outcomes. These data represent the strongest basis for recommended use of ACE inhibitors and beta blockers as primary therapy for heart failure in African Americans as in all other patients (Fig. 78–7).[65]

The African American Heart Failure Trial, A-HeFT, will prospectively identify the clinical benefit of therapy with a proprietary combination of isosorbide dinitrate and hydralazine as adjunctive therapy for heart failure in African Americans already receiving ACE inhibitors and beta blockers. A-HeFT will test the hypothesis that subtle differences in nitric oxide homeostasis are contributory to the excess cardiovascular risk seen in African Americans and that exogenous administration of a nitric oxide donor/antioxidant will overcome this perturbation. This first prospective trial in heart failure affecting African Americans will similarly address a number of additional questions regarding the natural history, epidemiology, and genetic profile of this disease.[66]

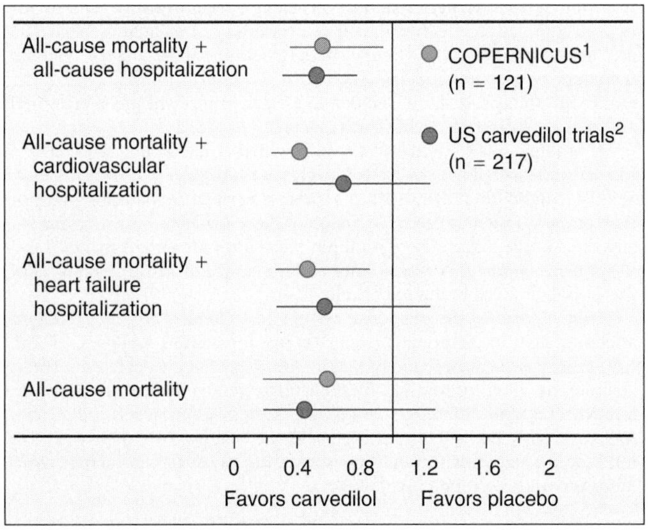

FIGURE 78–7 Effect of carvedilol in African American patients with heart failure. [1] Mean duration, 10.5 months. [2] Mean duration, 6.5 months. (Data from Packer M: Presentation at American Heart Association Scientific Sessions 2000 [COPERNICUS]; and Yancy CW: N Engl J Med 344:1358, 2001 [US Carvedilol Trials].)

The Construct of Race in Medicine

The inclusion of race or ethnicity in any discussion of medicine is problematic. Race is neither scientific nor physiological. The heterogeneity within race is similar to the heterogeneity between races,[67] and the very real requirements for the perpetuation of race, that is, intermarriage and similar environmental surroundings, are rapidly disappearing in the United States. Even the genomic debates are overshadowed by the observation that all persons share more than 99 percent of the same genetic code and that the variance between races is in approximately 0.1 percent of the code. Whether this one

44. Chobanian AV, Bakris GL, Black HR, et al: The Seventh Report of the Joint National Committee on Prevention, Detection, Evaluation and Treatment of High Blood Pressure. The JNC 7 report. JAMA 289:2560, 2003.
45. Nesbitt S, Victor RG: Pathogenesis of hypertension in African Americans. Congest Heart Fail 10:24, 2004.
46. Wright JT, Bakris G, Green T, et al: Effect of blood pressure lowering and antihypertensive drug class on progression of hypertensive kidney disease. Results from the AASK Trial. JAMA 19:2421, 2002.
47. Douglas JG, Bakris GL, Epstein M, et al: Management of high blood pressure in African Americans. Arch Intern Med 163:525, 2003.

Ischemic Heart Disease

48. Clark LT, Ferdinand KC, Flack JM, et al: Coronary heart disease in African Americans. Heart Dis 3:97, 2001.
49. Strong JP, Malcom GT, Oalmann MC, Wissler RW: The PDAY study: Natural history, risk factors, and pathobiology. Pathobiological Determinants of Atherosclerosis in Youth. Ann N Y Acad Sci 811:226, 1997.
50. Sorlie PD, Sharrett AR, Patsch W, et al: The relationship between lipids/lipoproteins and atherosclerosis in African Americans and whites: The Atherosclerosis Risk in Communities study. Ann Epidemiol 9:149, 1999.
51. Ergul S, Parish DC, Puett D, et al: Racial differences in plasma endothelin-1 concentrations in individuals with essential hypertension. Hypertension 28:652, 1996.

Heart Failure

52. Dries DL, Exner DV, Gersh BJ, et al: Racial differences in the outcome of left ventricular dysfunction. N Engl J Med 341:298, 1999.
53. Exner DV, Dries DL, Domanski MJ, et al: Lesser response to angiotensin-converting-enzyme inhibitor therapy in black as compared with white patients with left ventricular dysfunction. N Engl J Med 344:1351, 2001.
54. Dries DL, Strong MH, Cooper RS, Drazner M: Efficacy of angiotensin-converting enzyme inhibition in reducing progression from asymptomatic left ventricular dysfunction to symptomatic heart failure in black and white patients. J Am Coll Cardiol 40:311, 2002.
55. Iwanaga Y, Kihara Y, Hasegawa K, et al: Cardiac endothelin-1 plays a critical role in the functional deterioration of left ventricles during the transition from compensatory hypertrophy to congestive heart failure in salt-sensitive hypertensive rats. Circulation 98:2065, 1998.
56. Kostis JB, Davis BR, Cutler J, et al, for the SHEP Cooperative Research Group: Prevention of heart failure by antihypertensive drug treatment in older persons with isolated systolic hypertension. JAMA 278:212, 1997.
57. August P: TGF Beta-1 overexpressed in African American hypertensives. Proc Natl Acad Sci U S A 97:3479, 2000.
58. McNamara DM, Holubkov R, Janosko K, et al: Genetic Risk Assessment of Cardiac Events, GRACE, Circulation 103:1644, 2001.
59. Mason DA, Moore JD, Green SA, Liggett SB: A gain of function polymorphism in a G-protein coupling domain of the human beta-1 adrenergic receptor. J Biol Chem 274:12670, 1999.
60. Small KM, Wagoner LE, Levin AM, et al: Synergistic polymorphisms of beta 1 and alpha 2C adrenergic receptors and the risk of congestive heart failure. N Engl J Med 347:1135, 2002.
61. Turner ST, Schwartz GL, Chapman AB, Boperwinkle E: C825T polymorphism of the G protein beta-3 subunit and antihypertensive response to a thiazide diuretic. Hypertension 37:739, 2001.
62. Carson P, Ziesche S, Johnson G, et al: Racial differences in response to therapy for heart failure: Analysis of the vasodilator-heart failure trials. Vasodilator-Heart Failure Trial Study Group. J Card Fail 5:178, 1999.
63. The Beta-Blocker Evaluation of Survival Trial Investigators: A trial of the beta-blocker bucindolol in patients with advanced chronic heart failure. N Engl J Med 344:1659, 2001.
64. MERIT-HF Study Group: Effect of metoprolol CR/XL in chronic heart failure: Metoprolol CR/XL Randomised Intervention Trial in Congestive Heart Failure (MERIT-HF). Lancet 353:2001, 1999.
65. Yancy CW, Fowler MB, Colucci WS, et al: Race and the response to adrenergic blockade with carvedilol in patients with heart failure. N Engl J Med 344:1358, 2001.
66. Franciosa JA, Taylor AL, Cohn JN, et al, for the A-HeFT Investigators: African American Heart Failure Trial (A-HeFT): Rationale, design, and methodology. J Card Fail 8:128, 2002.

Race in Medicine

67. American Anthropological Association: American Anthropological Association statement on race, 1998. (http:/www.aaanet.org/stmts/racepp.htm)
68. Kaplan JB, Bennett T: Use of race and ethnicity in biomedical publication. JAMA 289:2709, 2003.

PART X

Cardiovascular Disease and Disorders of Other Organ Systems

CHAPTER 79

Endocrine Disorders and Cardiovascular Disease

Irwin Klein

Throughout medical science, there are very few areas where basic science investigation links as closely to clinical observations and therapy as in the field of cardiovascular endocrinology. As our knowledge of the cellular and molecular effects of various hormones evolves, we can better understand the clinical manifestations that arise from both excess hormone secretion and glandular failure leading to hormone deficiency states. More than 200 years ago, Caleb Hillier Parry described a woman with goiter and palpitations whose "each systole shook the whole thorax." He was the first to suggest that there was a connection between diseases of the heart and enlargement of the thyroid gland. The cardiovascular abnormalities associated with pathological changes of endocrine glands were recognized prior to the understanding of the specific hormones produced by these glands. This chapter reviews the broad spectrum of cardiac disease states that arise from changes in specific endocrine function. This approach allows us to explore the cellular mechanisms by which various hormones can produce changes in the cardiovascular system through actions on the cardiac myocyte, vascular smooth muscle cells, and other target cells and tissues.

Pituitary Gland

The pituitary gland is made up of two distinct anatomical portions. The anterior portion, or adenohypophysis, contains six different cell types, five of which produce polypeptide or glycoprotein hormones; the sixth classically has been referred to as nonsecretory chromophobic cells. Of these cell types, the somatotrophic cells, which secrete human growth hormone (hGH), and the corticotrophic cells, which produce adrenocorticotropic hormone (ACTH), have been linked to cardiac disease. The posterior pituitary, or neurohypophysis, is the anatomical location of the nerve terminals that secrete vasopressin (antidiuretic hormone) or oxytocin.

Growth Hormone

In adults, excessive growth hormone secretion before the fusion of the bone epiphysis leads to gigantism, whereas increased secretion of hGH after maturation of the long bones leads to acromegaly. The growth-promoting factor obtained from extracts of the pituitary gland was first identified by Evans and Long in the early 1920s. Almost 50 years later, the protein sequence and structure of hGH were first identified and its role as one member of a family of growth-promoting (somatic) factors emerged.

Growth hormone exerts its cellular effects through two major pathways. The first involves hormone binding to specific growth hormone receptors on target cells. These receptors have been identified in heart, skeletal muscle, fat, liver, and kidney and in many additional cell types throughout fetal development.[1] The second growth-promoting effect of hGH results from stimulation of synthesis of the insulin-like growth factor type 1

(IGF-1). This protein is produced primarily in the liver, but other cell types can produce IGF-1 under the influence of hGH.

Shortly after the identification of the IGF family, it was proposed that most actions of growth hormone were mediated through this second messenger. Clinical disease activity of patients with growth hormone excess (acromegaly) correlates better with serum levels of IGF-1 than with hGH. The ability to promote glucose uptake and cellular protein synthesis gave rise to the term insulin-like. IGF-1 binds to its cognate IGF-1 receptor, which is present in virtually all cell types. Transgenic experiments have demonstrated that the presence of IGF-1 receptors on cell types associates closely with the ability of those cells to divide. Ingenious studies in which the IGF-1 receptor was overexpressed in cardiac myocytes reportedly produced an increased myocyte number, mitotic rate, and the ability of the postdifferentiated myocytes to replicate.[2] The harnessing of this action holds potential benefit for genetic manipulation and repair of the diseased myocardium.

Acute changes in cardiovascular hemodynamics result from the infusion of both hGH and IGF-1. The acute increases in cardiac contractility and cardiac output may be due, at least in part, to a decrease in systemic vascular resistance and cardiac afterload.[3] Short-term administration of both hGH and IGF-1 does not increase blood pressure, implying that the increase in cardiac output is indeed a result of changes in systemic vascular resistance.[4-6]

Cardiovascular Manifestations of Acromegaly

Acromegaly is a relatively uncommon condition, and approximately 900 new cases are diagnosed each year in the United States. Acromegaly and pituitary-dependent human gigantism associate with markedly increased morbidity and mortality primarily resulting from cardiovascular disease. Untreated acromegaly, identified by its characteristic clinical signs and symptoms and by increased hGH secretion, markedly shortens life expectancy, with less than 20 percent of patients surviving beyond 60 years. Multiple studies implicate increased neoplasia arising from the gastrointestinal tract, colon polyps, colon cancer, and pulmonary disease in this increased mortality.[7] However, the cardiovascular and cerebral vascular changes including hypertension, cardiomegaly, congestive heart failure, and cerebral vascular accidents continue to be the major events that limit survival.[8] First recognized by Pierre Marie in 1886, cardiovascular involvement in acromegaly is a chronic insidious process.

The cardiovascular and hemodynamic effects of acromegaly are highly variable and differ among patients depending upon age, severity of disease, and disease duration.[9] In patients diagnosed with less than 5 years of disease activity, changes in systolic or diastolic blood pressure were not significant, but echocardiographic determination of left ventricular mass index increased almost 35 percent and cardiac index increased 24 percent. Measures of systolic function including stroke index increased significantly, and systemic vascular resistance increased by 20 percent.[10] Left ventricular diastolic function was normal. These studies stand in marked contrast to the reports that longer duration of acromegaly produces left ventricular dysfunction and cardiomyopathy.[8,9]

Known cardiac disease risk factors including hypertension, insulin resistance, diabetes mellitus, and hyperlipidemia frequently occur in patients with acromegaly. Although initial reports suggested that impairment of cardiac function in longstanding acromegaly was due to accelerated atherosclerosis, a postmortem study revealed significant coronary artery disease in only 11 percent of patients who died from disease-related causes. Angiography demonstrates the presence of either normal or dilated coronary arteries in most cases. Thallium stress testing is positive in less than 25 percent of patients and overall allows us to conclude that atherosclerosis and ischemic heart disease are unlikely to account for the marked degrees of biventricular cardiac hypertrophy, cardiac failure, and cardiovascular mortality associated with acromegaly.[11]

Rather specific functional and histological myocyte changes appear to arise in the setting of prolonged excess serum levels of hGH and IGF-1.[9,12] As many as two-thirds of acromegalic patients have echocardiographic criteria for left ventricular hypertrophy (LVH).[7,8] The right ventricle also increases in mass in acromegaly, indicating a more generalized process beyond systemic hypertension.[10] Asymmetrical septal hypertrophy, initially thought to be common in patients with acromegaly, is an unusual finding. There appears to be an increased prevalence of both aortic and mitral valve disease, which persists despite disease cure.[13] Individual patients with dilation of the aortic root and defects of the cardiac conduction system have been reported.[8,14]

Histological evaluation of acromegalic cardiac tissue reveals that there is an increase in myocyte size (hypertrophy) without an increase in cell number.[15] Acromegaly produces interstitial fibrosis and infiltration of a variety of inflammatory cells including mononuclear cells consistent with myocarditis.[8,11] The absence of cell necrosis in the presence of an inflammatory reaction has raised the question of whether part of these histological findings can be explained by IGF-1–promoted programmed cell death (apoptosis). A study of acromegalic patients with diastolic dysfunction indicated apoptotic cell death in endomyocardial biopsies.[16]

Given the breadth of pathological involvement of the heart in acromegaly, it is not surprising that there are associated functional changes.[10-12] Whereas approximately 10 percent of newly diagnosed patients have signs and symptoms of cardiac compromise, this percentage increases markedly with disease duration.[17] Some studies report a low incidence of overt left ventricular failure, suggesting that supervening factors including hypertension, type 2 diabetes, and hyperlipidemia are needed to impair function.[11] In acromegaly, LVH and congestive heart failure can occur in longstanding disease without hypertension, indicating that high levels of growth hormone or IGF-1, or both, can produce cardiac myopathic changes per se.[12,14] Successful therapy reverses many if not all of these findings.[18,19]

Electrocardiographic (ECG) abnormalities including left axis deviation, septal Q waves, ST-T wave depression, abnormal QT dispersion, and conduction system defects occur in as many as 50 percent of acromegalic patients. A variety of dysrhythmias including atrial and ventricular ectopic beats, sick sinus syndrome, and supraventricular and ventricular tachycardias have been described.[8,15] The finding in a signal average electrocardiogram of a fourfold increase in complex ventricular arrhythmias and late potentials, thought to be predictors of ventricular irritability, was also more common in patients with active acromegaly than in treated patients.[14] In contrast, exercise stress testing with ECG monitoring did not show inducible rhythm disturbances or evidence of ischemia, suggesting that left ventricular rhythm disturbances were not related to any underlying ischemia.

Secondary hypertension associated with acromegaly has been reported in 20 to 40 percent of patients.[7,8] Given the overall high prevalence rate of hypertension in the adult population and the insidious onset of acromegaly, it is difficult to determine whether the occurrence of hypertension is secondary or merely coincidental. The improvement with therapy, however, suggests that they are related.[19] Although epidemiological studies of survival in acromegaly initially suggested that hypertension was not an independent risk factor for mortality, a survey of patients who died of the disease demonstrated that mean blood pressures were higher than in those who survived.[7] The mechanism underlying hypertension in acromegaly is not clearly understood. Newly diagnosed patients with a short duration of disease had systolic and diastolic blood pressures no different from those of age- and sex-matched control subjects, but cardiac index was significantly increased. It does appear that the arterial intimal thickness is increased in patients with longstanding acromegaly, and these changes respond to hGH lowering.[8]

Growth hormone administration promotes sodium retention and volume expansion and appears to have a potent antinatriuretic effect independent of any effect on aldosterone.[20] Studies of the renin-angiotensin-aldosterone system show a failure to inhibit renin release optimally by volume expansion. When angiotensin II inhibitors are given to patients with acromegaly, there is a paradoxical increase in blood pressure.[11] The role of hyperinsulinemia in the hypertension of acromegaly has been questioned. Increased serum insulin can contribute to urinary sodium retention, impairment of endothelium-dependent vasodilation, and increased sympathetic activity.[21] There are rare associations of acromegaly with aldosterone-secreting adrenal adenomas and with pheochromocytoma.

Diagnosis

In 99 percent of cases, acromegaly arises from benign adenomas of the anterior pituitary gland.[7,19] At the time of diagnosis, the majority of these neoplasms are classified as macroadenomas (>10 mm), and patients have had clinical evidence of disease for more than 10 years. The diagnosis can be confirmed by demonstrating a serum growth hormone level greater than 5 ng/dl and a serum IGF-1 level greater than 300 μIU/ml measured 1 hour after a 100-gm glucose load. In the majority of patients, fasting growth hormone levels are higher than 10 ng/ml. Tumor localization can be established by magnetic resonance imaging dedicated to the pituitary gland. Rarely, growth hormone–releasing hormone can be secreted, causing diffuse hyperplasia of the pituitary. The existence of such changes must lead to the consideration of a neoplastic lesion residing in other parts of the endocrine system.

Therapy

Transsphenoidal surgery with resection of the adenoma is the procedure of choice for initial management. If hGH or IGF-1 or both remain elevated, radiotherapy in older patients, or dopamine or somatostatin receptor agonists in younger patients, can be used to restore serum growth hormone and IGF-1 levels to normal. Octreotide acetate, a pharmacological analog of somatostatin, is effective in the vast majority of patients in lowering hGH to less than 5 ng/ml. It may be primary therapy in selected cases. The cardiovascular complications of acromegaly including hypertension, LVH, and left ventricular dysfunction improve with treatment, and survival is significantly better in patients who achieve clinical and biochemical disease remission. A growth hormone receptor antagonist, pegvisomant, can normalize IGF-1 levels in long-term therapy and may play a role in somatostatin-resistant patients.[18,19]

Adrenocorticotropic Hormone and Cortisol

The adrenal corticotropic cells in the anterior pituitary synthesize a large protein (pro-opiomelanocortin) that is processed within the corticotropic cell into a family of smaller proteins that include alpha-melanocyte-stimulating hormone (αMSH), beta-endorphin, and ACTH. ACTH in turn binds to specific cells within the adrenal gland. The adrenal gland is anatomically divided into two major segments: the cortex and the medulla. The cortex zona glomerulosa produces aldosterone, the zona fasciculata produces primarily cortisol and some androgenic steroids, and the zona reticularis also produces cortisol and androgens. Synthesis of cortisol in the zona fasciculata and zona reticularis is primarily regulated by ACTH.[22] The zona glomerulosa shows a much lesser degree of ACTH responsiveness and responds primarily to angiotensin II by increased aldosterone secretion.

Cushing Disease

Excess cortisol secretion and its attendant clinical disease states can arise either from excess pituitary release of ACTH (Cushing disease) or through the adenomatous or rarely malignant neoplastic process arising in the adrenal gland itself (Cushing syndrome). Well-characterized conditions of both adrenal glucocorticoid and mineralocorticoid excess appear to result from the excessively high levels of (ectopic) ACTH produced by small cell carcinoma of the lung, carcinoid tumors, pancreatic islet cell tumors, medullary thyroid cancer, and other adenocarcinomas and hematological malignancies.[22]

Cortisol, a member of the glucocorticoid family of steroid hormones, binds to monomeric receptors located within the cytoplasm of many cell types (Fig. 79-1). The unliganded glucocorticoid receptors are bound to heat shock protein complexes. After binding cortisol, the receptors dissociate from these complexes, homodimerize or occasionally heterodimerize, translocate to the nucleus, and function as transcription factors. A variety of cardiac genes contain glucocorticoid response elements in their promoter regions that confer glucocorticoid responsiveness.[23] These genes include those that encode the voltage-gated potassium channel as well as protein kinases, which phosphorylate and regulate voltage-gated sodium channels. This expression may in turn be chamber specific.[24]

The cardiac effects of glucocorticoid excess in Cushing disease arise from both the direct effects of glucocorticoids on the heart and the effects of glucocorticoids on the liver, skeletal muscle, and fat tissue.[25] Accelerated atherosclerosis can result from abnormal glucose metabolism with hyperglycemia and hyperinsulinemia, hypertension, and altered clotting and platelet function. The mechanism for cortisol-mediated hypertension is multifactorial.[26] Studies have shown that, in contrast to the findings in aldosterone-induced hypertension, the central administration of glucocorticoids lowers blood pressure. Thus, cortisol-mediated hypertension appears not to result from activation of the mineralocorticoid receptor. In addition, antagonism of glucocorticoid effects through its cytosolic receptor can block cortisol-induced elevations of glucose and insulin but not those related to blood pressure.[27,28] Interestingly, one study suggested that inhibition of sodium retention is also insufficient to block the cortisol-mediated rise in blood pressure, pointing to the changes in vascular reactivity, systemic vascular resistance, and nitric oxide–mediated vasodilation as candidates for the hypertensive effect.[24,26]

The rise in serum glucose and the development of insulin resistance may give rise to activation of proinflammatory cytokines such as tumor necrosis factor-alpha and interleukin-6, which may underlie the accelerated atherosclerosis of insulin resistance found in other endocrine disease states.[27] Thus, while acting classically as an antiinflammatory hormone, cortisol excess can promote inflammation and accelerate atherosclerosis by producing insulin resistance, changes in corticosteroid-binding protein, and regulation of a variety of proinflammatory cytokines. The centripetal obesity characteristic of glucocorticoid excess resembles that seen in the insulin resistance syndromes. Excess androgen production resulting from increased ACTH stimulation of the adrenal cortex may also accelerate atherosclerosis in both men and women.[22]

The increased cardiovascular morbidity and mortality of Cushing syndrome can be explained in large part by cerebrovascular disease, peripheral vascular disease, coronary artery disease with myocardial infarction, and chronic congestive heart failure.[25,29] These are all changes that would be expected in the setting of accelerated atherosclerosis resulting from hypertension and hyperlipidemia.[30] Studies of left ventricular structure and function have shown hypertrophy and impaired contractility in 40 percent of patients.[31] In addition, the marked muscle weakness resulting from corticosteroid-induced skeletal myopathy contributes to impaired exercise tolerance.

Patients with Cushing disease can exhibit a variety of ECG changes. There appears to be a direct correlation between

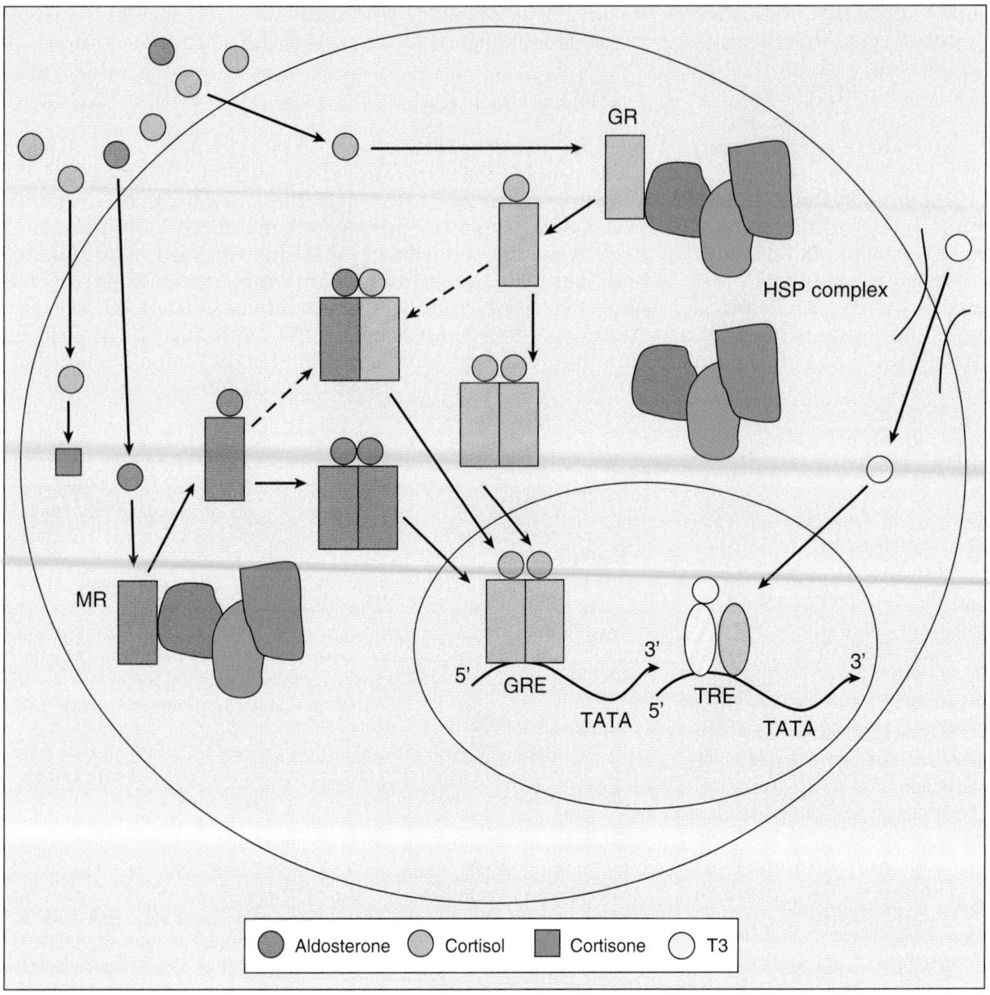

FIGURE 79–1 Scheme of a generalized nuclear hormone receptor mechanism of action. The mineralocorticoid receptor (MR) has similar affinities for aldosterone and cortisol. Circulating levels of cortisol are 100 to 1000 times greater than that of aldosterone. In MR-responsive cells, the enzyme 11beta-hydroxysteroid dehydrogenase metabolizes cortisol to cortisone, thereby allowing aldosterone to bind to MR. MR and the glucocorticoid receptor (GR) are cytoplasmic receptors that, after binding ligand, translocate to the nucleus and bind to glucocorticoid response elements (GREs) in the promoter regions of responsive genes. Triiodothyronine (T_3) enters the cell by facilitated diffusion and binds to thyroid hormone receptors (TRs), which are bound to thyroid hormone response elements (TREs) in the promoter regions of T_3-responsive genes. (Courtesy of Dr. S. Danzi.)

adrenal cortisol production rates and the duration of the PR interval. The underlying mechanism may be related to either the expression or the regulation of the voltage-gated sodium channel (SCN5A). Changes in electrocardiograms, specifically PR and QT intervals, may also arise as a result of the direct (nongenomic) effects of glucocorticoids on the voltage-gated potassium channel (Kv1.5) in a variety of excitable tissues.[24,25,32]

A particular complex of cardiac and adrenal lesions, referred to as the Carney complex, combines Cushing syndrome, cardiac myxoma, and a variety of pigmented dermal lesions (not café-au-lait).[33] This monogenic autosomal dominant trait maps to the q2 region of chromosome 17. Myxomas most commonly occur in the left atrium but can occur throughout the heart, at young ages, and be multicentric.

Diagnosis

Diagnosis of Cushing disease and syndrome requires demonstration of increased cortisol production, best accomplished by a 24-hour urinary free cortisol test.[22] ACTH measurements to determine whether the disease is pituitary, adrenal, or ectopically based and anatomical localization with magnetic resonance imaging of the suspected lesions confirm the laboratory tests.

Treatment

The treatment of excess cortisol production depends on the underlying mechanisms. In Cushing disease, transsphenoidal hypophysectomy can partially or completely reverse the increased ACTH production by the anterior pituitary. Cushing syndrome requires surgical removal of one (adrenal adenoma, adrenal carcinoma) or both (multiple nodular) adrenal glands. Immediately after surgery, it is necessary to replace both cortisol and mineralocorticoid (fludrocortisone) to prevent adrenal insufficiency. Treatment of the ectopic ACTH syndrome requires identification and treatment of the neoplastic process. Patients treated with exogenous steroids (e.g., prednisone, methylprednisolone) in doses above 10 mg/d for periods in excess of 1 month often develop clinical signs and symptoms of Cushing syndrome.[22] In nonsurgical patients, the adrenal enzyme inhibitor ketoconazole can reverse excess cortisol production. Even mild or subclinical degrees of Cushing syndrome (adrenal incidentaloma) appear to increase the risk for cardiovascular disease.[34]

Hyperaldosteronism

Aldosterone production by the zona glomerulosa is under the control of the renin-angiotensin system.[35] Renin secretion responds to changes in intravascular volume. Aldosterone synthesis and secretion are primarily regulated by angiotensin II, which binds to the angiotensin II type I receptor on the cells of the zona glomerulosa.[22,35]

The mechanism of action of aldosterone on target tissues resembles that reported for glucocorticoids (see Fig. 79–1).[36] Aldosterone is taken up into cells and binds to the mineralocorticoid receptor, which then translocates to the nucleus and promotes the expression of aldosterone-responsive genes.[28] In addition to kidney cells, where they control sodium transport, in vitro studies have demonstrated mineralocorticoid receptors in rat cardiac myocytes, which respond to stimulation with an increase in protein synthesis.[36-38] It is not clear whether these changes correspond to any relevant in vivo cardiac effects. Genetically engineered mice with an inactive mineralocorticoid receptor gene show classical features of mineralocorticoid deficiency and require sodium supplementation to survive. The aldosterone antagonists spironolactone and eplerenone compete for receptor binding in the cytosol (see Fig. 79–1).[39]

A variety of tissue-specific responses to aldosterone appear to be mediated at the level of the cell membrane and have been referred to as "nongenomic." Although these effects usually require a higher concentration of the hormone, they can change Na^+/H^+ transport and in vitro studies of cardiac myocytes have demonstrated a nongenomic effect on the Na^+/K^+ pump.[32]

Whereas the major cause of increased serum aldosterone is the physiological response to the activation of the renin-angiotensin system, there are well-recognized aldosterone-producing benign adrenal adenomas (Conn syndrome).[22,40] Primary hyperaldosteronism augments sodium retention, causes hypertension, increases renal loss of magnesium and potassium, decreases arterial compliance with a rise in systemic vascular resistance and resulting vascular damage, and alters the sympathetic and parasympathetic neural regulation. Many of the changes in the heart and cardiovascular system in hyperaldosteronism result from the associated hypertension. The degree of LVH, however, exceeds that expected from the hypertension alone, perhaps because of the increase in volume as well as pressure load resulting from increased aldosterone action.[41,42] The hyperaldosterone-mediated hypokalemia and much of the associated hypertension respond to the surgical removal of a unilateral (or occasionally bilateral) benign adrenal adenoma.

Addison Disease

Long before recognition that the glands situated just above the upper pole of each kidney (suprarenal) synthesize and secrete glucocorticoids and mineralocorticoids, Thomas Addison described the association of atrophy with loss of function of these structures with marked changes in the cardiovascular system. The hypovolemia, hypotension, and acute cardiovascular collapse resulting from renal sodium wasting, hyperkalemia, and loss of vascular tone are the hallmarks of acute Addisonian crisis, one of the most severe endocrine emergencies. Adrenal insufficiency most commonly arises from bilateral loss of adrenal function on an autoimmune basis; as a result of infection, hemorrhage, or metastatic malignancy; or in selected cases as a result of inborn errors of steroid hormone metabolism. In contrast, secondary adrenal insufficiency, which results from pituitary-dependent loss of ACTH secretion, leads to a fall in glucocorticoid production while mineralocorticoid production, including aldosterone production, remains at relatively normal levels. Studies have addressed the issue of relative hypothalamic-pituitary-adrenal insufficiency in acutely ill patients.[43] This issue has reopened the question of the need for stress dose cortisol treatment of patients with critical illness.

Addison disease can occur at any age. The noncardiac symptoms including increased pigmentation, abdominal pain with nausea and vomiting, and weight loss can be chronic, whereas the tachycardia, hypotension, and electrolyte abnormalities are harbingers of impending cardiovascular collapse and crisis.[44] Blood pressure measurements uniformly show low diastolic pressure (<60 mm Hg) with significant orthostatic changes reflecting volume loss. Laboratory findings of hyponatremia and hyperkalemia indicate loss of aldosterone production (renin levels are high). The hyperkalemia can alter the electrocardiogram producing low-amplitude P waves and peaked T waves.[45] In newly diagnosed, untreated patients with Addison disease, both left ventricular end-systolic and end-diastolic dimensions were reduced compared with control values. Cardiac atrophy is an unusual condition. It is seen in malnutrition related to anorexia, in astronauts after prolonged space flight, in populations with sodium-deficient diets, and characteristically with Addison disease (teardrop heart) (Fig. 79–2). This atrophic process is in response to decreases in cardiac workload because restoration of normal plasma volume with both mineralocorticoid and glucocorticoid replacement increases ventricular mass.[46]

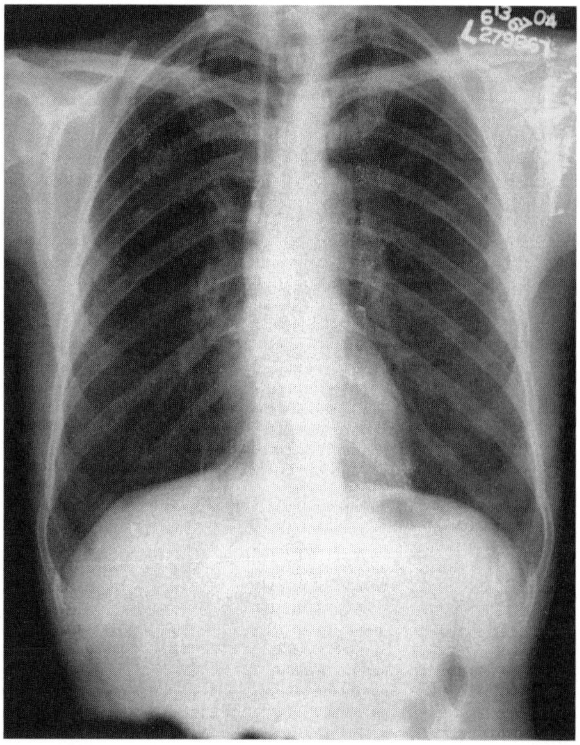

FIGURE 79–2 Routine chest radiograph of a patient with Addison disease related to tuberculosis. In addition to the small cardiac silhouette, there are calcified lymph nodes in the hilum of the right lung. (Courtesy of Dr. J. B. Naidich.)

Diagnosis

Acute adrenal insufficiency characteristically occurs in the setting of an acute stress, infection, or trauma in a patient with chronic adrenal insufficiency. It can also result from bilateral adrenal hemorrhage in patients with severe systemic infection or disseminated intravascular coagulation. Secondary adrenal insufficiency can occur in the setting of hypopituitarism, which in most situations is chronic; however, acute changes related to pituitary hemorrhage (apoplexy) or pituitary inflammation (lymphocytic hypophysitis) have been observed. Patients treated with long-term suppressive doses of corticosteroids (>10 mg of prednisone for more than 1 month) can develop acute adrenal insufficiency should such treatment be stopped precipitously.

The diagnosis is established when, in the morning or during severe stress, cortisol levels are low (<8 μg/dl) and fail to rise above 20 μg/dl 30 minutes after an intravenous injection of 0.25 mg of cosyntropin.

Treatment

Management of acute Addisonian crisis needs to address three major issues. The first is adequate hydrocortisone replacement, 100 mg given as an initial intravenous bolus and then 100 mg every 8 hours for the first 24 hours, tapering the dose for the next 72 to 96 hours. The second is restoration of the intravascular fluid deficit using large volumes of normal saline with 5 percent dextrose. Last is the need to identify and treat any underlying precipitating cause, including infection, acute cardiac or cerebral ischemia, or intraabdominal emergency. Chronic treatment is with oral corticosteroid and mineralocorticoid (fludrocortisone 0.1 mg/d) replacement.[22,46]

Parathyroid Disease

Diseases of the parathyroid glands can produce cardiovascular disease and alter cardiac function by two mechanisms. The first is through changes in the secretion of parathyroid hormone (PTH), a protein hormone that exerts effects on the heart, vascular smooth muscle cells, and endothelial cells.[47] The second is by way of changes in serum calcium. There is an exquisitely sensitive negative feedback mechanism by which serum ionized calcium regulates the synthesis and secretion of PTH.

PTH can bind to its cell surface receptor and alter the spontaneous beating rate of neonatal cardiac myocytes by an increase in intracellular cyclic adenosine monophosphate (AMP). PTH can also alter calcium influx and cardiac contractility in adult cardiac myocytes. In vascular smooth muscle cells, this alteration causes vasodilation. In addition to PTH, there is a parathyroid hormone–related peptide (PTHrP) that is structurally related to PTH and is synthesized and secreted in a variety of tissues including cardiac myocytes. PTHrP was first characterized as the humoral substance secreted by malignant tumors producing hypercalcemia. Interestingly, PTHrP can bind to the PTH receptor on cardiac cells and stimulate cyclic AMP accumulation and contractile activity and regulate L-type calcium currents. Thus, in a variety of paraneoplastic syndromes characterized by hypercalcemia, the direct effects of PTHrP on the heart and systemic vasculature can be manifested.[47]

HYPERPARATHYROIDISM

Classical primary hyperparathyroidism producing hypercalcemia most often arises as a result of the adenomatous enlargement of one of four parathyroid glands. The cardiovascular actions of hypercalcemia include an increase in cardiac contractility, a shortening of the ventricular action potential duration primarily through changes in phase 2, and blunting of the T wave and changes in the ST segment occasionally suggesting cardiac ischemia.[48] The QT interval is shortened, and occasionally accompanied by decreases in the PR interval as well. Treatment with digitalis glycosides appears to increase sensitivity of the heart to hypercalcemia.

Hypercalcemia has been linked to pathological changes in the heart including the myocardial interstitium, the conducting system, and calcific deposits in the valve cusps and annuli. Although initially observed in fairly longstanding and severe hypercalcemia, so-called metastatic calcifications can also occur in secondary parathyroid disease arising from chronic renal failure in which the serum calcium-phosphorus product constant is exceeded.[49]

Presumably as a result of the direct effect of calcium on vascular smooth muscle tone, patients with primary hyperparathyroidism have increased arterial pressure. Because PTH exerts a direct vasodilator effect and increased dietary calcium has been linked with a decrease in arterial pressure, the mechanisms that link PTH to blood pressure are complex.[47,48]

A simultaneous increase in serum immunoreactive PTH (best represented by the intact PTH assay) with an elevation of serum calcium establishes the diagnosis of primary hyperparathyroidism. Other causes include hypercalcemia of malignancy with an increased level of PTHrP or direct bone metastasis and neoplastic (lymphoma) or nonneoplastic (sarcoidosis) diseases leading to an increase in synthesis and release of 1,25-dihydroxyvitamin D_3. Treatment of hyperparathyroidism is the surgical removal of the parathyroid adenoma.

HYPOCALCEMIA

Low serum levels of total and ionized calcium directly alter myocyte function. Hypocalcemia prolongs phase 2 of the action potential duration and the QT interval. Severe hypocalcemia can potentially impair cardiac contractility and gives rise to a diffuse musculoskeletal syndrome including tetany and rhabdomyolysis. Primary hypoparathyroidism is a rare disease that can be seen after surgical removal of the parathyroid glands, in the setting of polyglandular dysfunction syndromes, as the result of glandular agenesis (DiGeorge) syndrome, and in the rare but interesting heritable disorder pseudohypoparathyroidism.

The most common cause of low serum calcium is chronic renal failure, and PTH levels are high (secondary hyperparathyroidism). In such patients it appears that the chronic effects of high levels of PTH on the heart and cardiovascular system predominate. Thus, the ability of PTH to stimulate G protein–coupled receptors may contribute to the LVH commonly observed in patients with chronic renal failure.[47] Systemic vascular resistance is often low, potentially reflecting the vasodilatory action of PTH. In patients with chronic renal failure, however, a variety of other important cardiovascular variables including anemia, accelerated atherosclerosis, hypertension, and changes in other vasoactive hormones contribute to the overall picture. Whether direct actions of the markedly elevated levels of PTH can produce alterations in myocyte physiology sufficient to cause further impairment of contractile function remains speculative.

Thyroid Gland

The thyroid gland and the heart share a close relationship arising in embryology. In ontogeny, the thyroid and heart Anlage migrate together. The close physiological relationship is affirmed by predictable changes in cardiovascular function across the entire range of thyroid disease states. In fact, cardiovascular manifestations are some of the most common and characteristic findings of hyperthyroidism.[50] To approach the diagnosis and management of thyroid hormone–mediated cardiac disease states, it is important to understand the cellular mechanisms of thyroid hormone action on the heart and vascular smooth muscle cells.[51]

CELLULAR MECHANISMS OF THYROID HORMONE ACTION ON THE HEART

Under the regulation of thyroid stimulating hormone (thyrotropin, TSH), the thyroid gland has the unique property of concentrating serum iodide and through a series of enzymatic steps synthesizes predominantly tetraiodothyronine (T_4, 85 percent) and a smaller percentage of triiodothyronine (T_3, 15 percent) (Fig. 79-3).[52] The major source of T_3 synthesis is conversion by 5′ monodeiodination primarily in the liver and to a lesser degree in the kidney.[53] A variety of studies have confirmed that T_3 is the active form of thyroid hormone and accounts for the vast majority of biological effects, including stimulation of tissue thermogenesis, alterations in the expression of various cellular proteins, and actions on the heart and vascular smooth muscle cells.[50,54] Serum free T_3 in turn is available to be taken up by a process of facilitated diffusion within cells, where it appears to pass without additional protein binding to the cell nucleus (Fig. 79-4). Most data indicate that the cardiac myocyte cannot metabolize T_4 to T_3 and therefore, all nuclear actions and changes observed in gene expression result from changes in blood levels of T_3. The cardiac myocyte expresses both the alpha and beta isoforms of the thyroid hormone receptors (TRs), which arise from two separate genes. These genes give rise to splice variants $TRalpha_1$ and $TRalpha_2$, of which only the former binds thyroid hormone, as well as $TRbeta_1$, $TRbeta_2$, and $TRbeta_3$[54] (see Fig. 79-1). It has been suggested, although direct confirmatory data are lacking, that $TRalpha_1$ is the predominant T_3 binding isoform in the heart and that isoform specificity may in turn determine myocyte-specific gene expression.[51,54] Similarly to the steroid and retinoic acid family of receptor proteins, the TRs act by binding as either homodimers or heterodimers to the thyroid hormone response elements in a promoter region of specific genes.[54] Binding to the promoter regions can either activate or repress gene expression.[55]

The cardiac proteins transcriptionally regulated by thyroid hormone are listed in Table 79-1. They include structural as well as regulatory proteins and also a variety of cardiac membrane ion channels and cell surface receptors, thus providing a molecular mechanism to explain many of the diverse effects of thyroid hormone on the heart. The first reported and the best studied to date have been the myosin heavy chain isoforms alpha and beta.[56] However, in the human ventricle, myosin isoform expression is primarily beta and there appears to be little if any alteration in isoform expression accompanying thyroid disease states.[57] There are changes in myosin heavy chain isoform expression in the human atria in a variety of disease states including congestive heart failure, and it remains to be determined whether these changes are thyroid hormone mediated.[58]

The sarcoplasmic reticulum calcium-activated adenosine triphosphatase (ATPase) is an important ion pump that determines the magnitude of myocyte calcium cycling (see also Chap. 19). The reuptake of calcium into the sarcoplasmic reticulum early in diastole in part determines the rate at which the left ventricle relaxes (isovolumetric relaxation time).[50] The activity of sarcoendoplasmic reticulum Ca^{2+}-ATPase (SERCA2), in turn, is regulated by the polymeric protein phospholamban, with its ability to inhibit SERCA activity further modified by the level of phosphorylation of the individual phospholamban monomers.[59] Inotropic agents that enhance cardiac contractility through increases in myocyte cyclic AMP do so by stimulating the phosphorylation of phospholamban. Thyroid hormone inhibits the genetic expression of phospholamban and increases phospholamban phosphorylation,[60] and genetically engineered animals deficient in phospholamban do not further increase cardiac contractility after exposure to excess thyroid hormone.[59] These data indicate that thyroid hormone exerts most of its direct effects on cardiac contractility by regulating calcium cycling through the SERCA-phospholamban system both transcriptionally and posttranscriptionally. Somewhat in conflict with these conclusions is the observation that patients with a homozygous deletion of phospholamban develop a dilated cardiomyopathy.[61] This molecular mechanism can explain why diastolic function varies inversely across the entire spectrum of thyroid disease states (Fig. 79-5).[50,62,63] In addition, beta-adrenergic blockade of the heart in hyperthyroidism does not decrease the rapid diastolic relaxation, further dissociating the thyroid hormone from the adrenergic effects of thyrotoxicosis.[50]

Changes in other myocyte genes, including Na^+, K^+-ATPase, account for the increase in basal oxygen consumption of the experimental hyperthyroid heart as well as explain the decrease in digitalis sensitivity of hyperthyroid patients. A variety of studies have shown that thyroid hormone can regulate the genetic expression of its own nuclear receptors within the cardiac myocyte (see Table 79-1).

In addition to the well-characterized nuclear effects of thyroid hormone, a growing body of cardiac responses to thyroid hormone appear to be mediated through nongenomic mechanisms,[64] as suggested by their relatively rapid onset of action (faster than can be accounted for by changes in gene expression and protein synthesis) and failure to be affected by inhibitors of gene transcription. The significance of these diverse actions remains to be established. They may alter the functional properties of membrane ion channels and pumps including the sodium channel and the inward-rectifying potassium current (I_k).

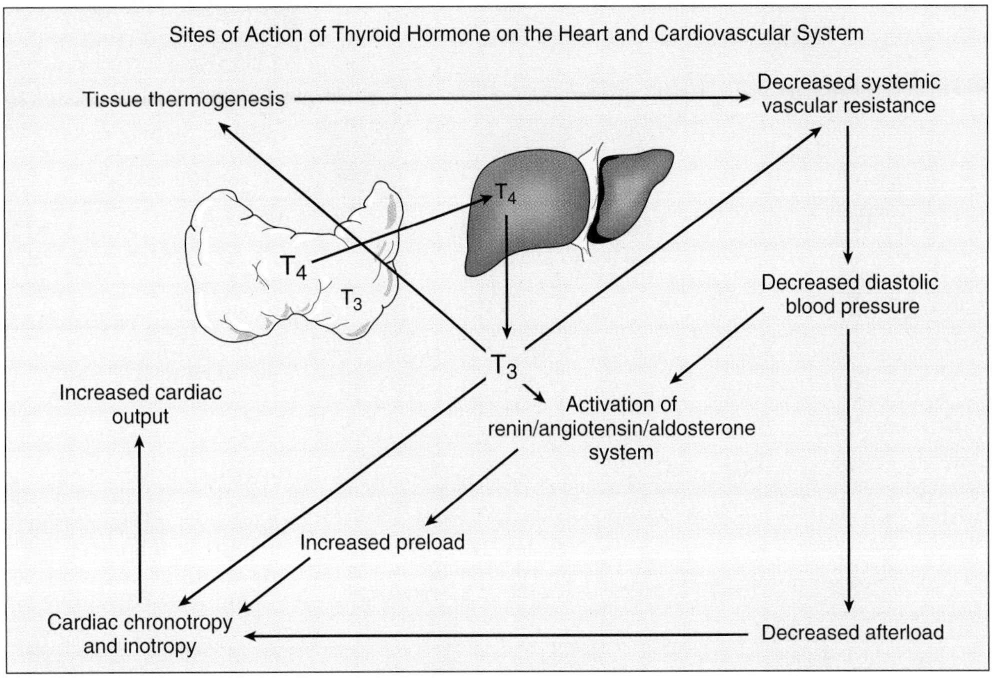

FIGURE 79–3 Schematic representation of thyroid hormone metabolism and the effects of triiodothyronine (T_3) on the heart and systemic vasculature.

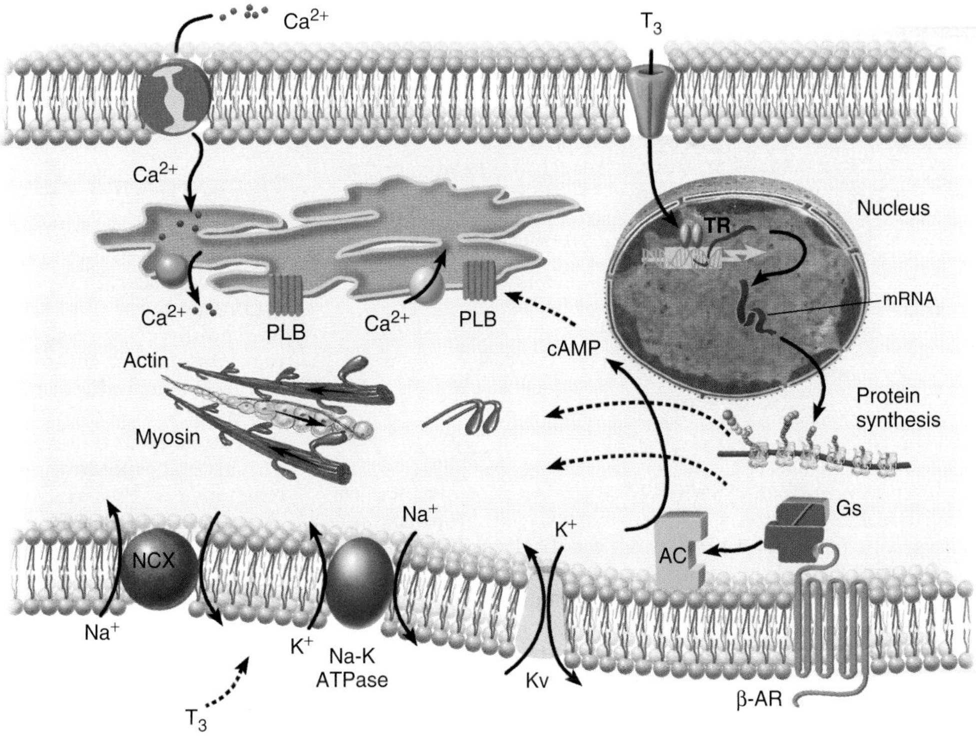

FIGURE 79–4 Triiodothyronine (T_3) enters the cell and binds to nuclear T_3 receptors. The complex then binds to thyroid hormone response elements (TREs) and regulates transcription of specific genes. Nonnuclear T_3 actions on ion channels for sodium (Na^+), potassium (K^+), and calcium (Ca^{2+}) ions are indicated. ATPase = adenosine triphosphatase; cAMP = cyclic adenosine monophosphate; mRNA = messenger RNA; TR = T_3 receptor protein; AC = adenylyl cyclase; β-AR = beta adrenergic receptor; Kv = voltage-gated potassium channel; NCX = sodium channel; PLB = phospholamban.

Thyroid Function Testing

A number of sensitive and specific laboratory tests can establish a diagnosis of thyroid disease with a high degree of precision. Serum TSH is the most widely used and most sensitive measure for the diagnosis of both hypothyroidism

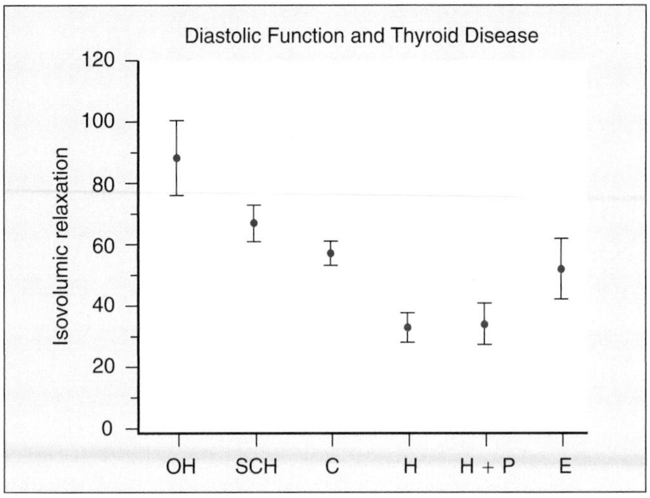

FIGURE 79–5 Diastolic function as measured by the isovolumic relaxation time varies over the entire range of thyroid disease including overt hypothyroidism (OH), subclinical hypothyroidism (SCH), control (C), hyperthyroidism (H), hyperthyroidism after beta-adrenergic blockade (H + P), and hyperthyroidism after treatment to restore normal thyroid function studies (E).

TABLE 79–1 Thyroid Hormone Regulation of Cardiac Gene Expression

Positively Regulated	Negatively Regulated
Alpha-myosin heavy chain	Beta-myosin heavy chain
Sarcoplasmic reticulum Ca^{2+}-ATPase	Phospholamban
Na^+, K^+-ATPase	Na^+/Ca^{2+} exchanger
Voltage-gated potassium channels (Kv1.5, Kv4.2, Kv4.3)	Thyroid hormone receptor alpha1
Atrial and brain natriuretic peptide	Adenylyl cyclase (AC) types V, VI
Malic enzyme	Guanine nucleotide–binding protein G_i
Beta-adrenergic receptor	
Guanine nucleotide–binding protein G_s	
Adenine nucleotide transporter 1	

ATPase = adenosine triphosphatase.

and hyperthyroidism.[65] Serum TSH levels uniformly increase (>5 μIU/mL) in patients with primary hypothyroidism and conversely, because of the normal feedback of excess levels of T_4 (and T_3) on the pituitary synthesis and secretion of TSH, the levels are low (<0.01 to 0.001 μIU/mL) in hyperthyroidism. Measures of free T_4 (and rarely free T_3) can be useful when coexistent hepatic, nutritional, or genetic disease may alter thyroxine-binding globulin content. Autoimmune thyroid diseases (Hashimoto and Graves) can be further diagnosed by the use of serological measures of antithyroid antibodies, most specifically antithyroid peroxidase or antithyroglobulin antibodies.

Thyroid Hormone–Catecholamine Interaction

Early observations of the heart in hyperthyroidism emphasize the similarity to that of hyperadrenergic states and moreover suggest enhanced sensitivity to catecholamines in this setting. This postulate forms the basis for the test described by Goetsch in 1918 in which hyperthyroidism could be diagnosed by demonstrating a marked cardioacceleration and blood pressure response to subcutaneous doses of epinephrine. Measurements of circulating catecholamine concentrations in hyperthyroid subjects revealed that despite the appearance of increased adrenergic signs and symptoms, levels of epinephrine and norepinephrine were decreased. This finding gave rise to the concept of enhanced catecholamine sensitivity, and molecular measures of increased beta$_1$-adrenergic receptors on cardiac myocytes in experimentally induced hyperthyroidism support this mechanism. A carefully controlled study of subhuman primates, however, has clearly demonstrated that there is no increase in sensitivity of the heart or cardiovascular system to catecholamines in experimental hyperthyroidism.[66] Accompanying the increased levels of beta$_1$-adrenergic receptors and guanosine triphosphate binding proteins, thyroid hormone decreases the genetic expression of cardiac-specific (V, VI) adenylyl cyclase catalytic subunit isoforms and thereby maintains cellular response to beta-adrenergic agonists within normal limits.[67]

TABLE 79–2 Cardiovascular Changes with Thyroid Disease

Parameter	Normal	Hyperthyroid	Hypothyroid
Systemic vascular resistance (dyne-cm) sec^{-5}	1500-1700	700-1200	2100-2700
Heart rate (beats/min)	72-84	88-130	60-80
Cardiac output (liter/min)	5.8	>7.0	<4.5
Blood volume (% of normal)	100	105.5	84.5

Hemodynamic Alterations in Thyroid Disease

Predictable changes in myocardial contractility and cardiovascular hemodynamics occur across the entire spectrum of thyroid disease (Table 79–2; see Fig. 79–5).[50] Multiple studies including those in experimental animals as well as invasive and noninvasive measurements in patients indicate that T_3 regulates cardiac inotropy and chronotropy through a variety of direct and indirect mechanisms.[50,68-70] Figure 79–3 shows the integrated schema by which T_3 acts on tissues throughout the body to increase tissue thermogenesis. Direct effects on vascular smooth muscle cells decrease systemic vascular resistance of the arterioles of the peripheral circulation.[68,71] There is a decrease in mean arterial pressure and activation of the renin-angiotensin-aldosterone system and an increase in renal sodium reabsorption. The increase in plasma volume coupled with an increase in erythropoietin leads to an increase in blood volume and a rise in cardiac preload.[70] Thus, a decrease in systemic vascular resistance (by as much as 50 percent), coupled with increases in venous return and preload, increases cardiac output. Cardiac output may more than double in hyperthyroidism and conversely may decrease by as much as 30 to 40 percent in hypothyroidism. Studies using positron-emission tomography (PET) measurements of acetate metabolism have demonstrated that the marked increase in cardiac output in hyperthyroidism is accomplished with no change in energy efficiency.[72]

T_3 appears to reduce systemic vascular resistance by both direct effects on vascular smooth muscle cells and changes in the vascular endothelium potentially involving the synthesis and secretion of nitric oxide.[68] The vasodilatory effect of T_3 can be observed within hours after administration of T_3 to patients undergoing coronary artery bypass grafting as well as patients with chronic congestive heart failure.[58,71] Arterial

TABLE 79–3 Cardiovascular Symptoms of Hyperthyroidism	
Palpitations	Anginal-like chest pain
Exercise intolerance	Peripheral edema
Dyspnea	Congestive heart failure

compliance also falls in hypothyroidism and may explain why mean arterial and diastolic pressures are low and peak systolic pressures increase.[69] Thus, the combination of increased cardiac output and decreased arterial compliance, which may be more pronounced in older patients with some degree of arterial vascular disease, leads to systolic hypertension in as many as 30 percent of patients.[69] In hypothyroidism, systemic vascular resistance may be increased by as much as 30 percent. Mean arterial pressure rises with as many as 20 percent of patients having significant diastolic hypertension.[69] Even mild hypothyroidism may decrease endothelium-derived relaxing factors.[73] The diastolic hypertension of hypothyroidism is frequently associated with a low renin level and a decrease in hepatic synthesis of renin substrate. This leads to a characteristically low level of salt sensitivity, again reinforcing the importance of an increase in systemic vascular resistance underlying the mechanism for diastolic hypertension.[74]

Hyperthyroidism

Cardiovascular symptoms are an integral and often the predominant clinical presentation of patients with hyperthyroidism (Table 79–3). Palpitations resulting from an increase in the rate and force of cardiac contractility are present in the majority of patients.[75] The increase in heart rate results from both an increase in sympathetic tone and a decrease in parasympathetic stimulation.[75] It is common to observe heart rates higher than 90 beats/min both at rest and during sleep; the normal diurnal variation in heart rate is blunted and the increase during exercise is exaggerated. Many hyperthyroid patients experience exercise intolerance and exertional dyspnea, in part because of weakness in skeletal and respiratory muscle.[76] In the setting of a low vascular resistance and increased preload, cardiac functional reserve is compromised and cannot rise further to accommodate the demands of submaximal or maximal exercise.[77]

A subset of thyrotoxic patients can experience angina-like chest pain. In older patients with known or suspected coronary artery disease, the increase in cardiac work associated with the increase in cardiac output and cardiac contractility of hyperthyroidism can produce myocardial ischemia, which can respond to beta-adrenergic blocking agents or the restoration of a euthyroid state. In rare patients, usually younger women, a syndrome of chest pain at rest associates with ischemic ECG changes. Cardiac catheterization has demonstrated that the majority of these patients have angiographically normal coronary arteries; however, coronary vasospasm has been reported similar to that found in variant angina. Myocardial infarction rarely develops, and these patients appear to respond to calcium channel blockers or nitroglycerin.

Atrial Fibrillation

The most common rhythm disturbance in patients with hyperthyroidism is sinus tachycardia.[75] Its clinical impact, however, is overshadowed by that of patients with atrial fibrillation resulting from thyrotoxicosis. The prevalence of atrial fibrillation and the less common forms of supraventricular tachycardia in this disease ranges between 2 and 20 percent.[78,79] When compared with a prevalence of atrial fibrillation of 2.3 percent in a control population with normal thyroid function, the prevalence of atrial fibrillation in overt hyperthyroidism was 13.8 percent.[79] It was reported that in more than 13,000 hyperthyroid patients the prevalence of atrial fibrillation was less than 2 percent, perhaps because of earlier recognition and disease treatment. When the same group of patients was analyzed for age distribution, it was seen that there was a stepwise increase in prevalence in each decade, peaking at about 15 percent in patients older than 70 years.[78] The latter study confirms essentially all reports that atrial fibrillation related to hyperthyroidism is more common with advancing age. In a study of unselected patients presenting with atrial fibrillation, less than 1 percent of cases were caused by overt hyperthyroidism.[80] Thus, the yield of abnormal thyroid function testing including a low serum TSH appears to be low in patients with new-onset atrial fibrillation. However, the ability to restore thyrotoxic patients to a euthyroid state and sinus rhythm justifies TSH testing in all patients with the recent onset of otherwise unexplained atrial fibrillation or other supraventricular arrhythmias.

Treatment of atrial fibrillation in the setting of hyperthyroidism includes beta-adrenergic blockade using one of a variety of beta$_1$-selective or nonselective agents to control the ventricular response. This symptomatic measure can be accomplished rapidly, but the treatments leading to a restoration of the euthyroid state require more time. Digitalis has been used to control the ventricular response in hyperthyroidism-associated atrial fibrillation; however, because of the increased rate of digitalis clearance as well as decreased sensitivity of the drug action resulting from high cellular levels of Na^+,K^+-ATPase and the presence of decreased parasympathetic tone, patients usually require higher doses of this medication. Anticoagulation in patients with hyperthyroidism and atrial fibrillation is controversial.[50,81] The potential for systemic or cerebral embolization must be weighed against the risk of bleeding and complications related to this therapy. Whether hyperthyroid patients are at increased risk for systemic embolization is not totally resolved. In a retrospective study of patients with hyperthyroidism, it was age rather than the presence of atrial fibrillation that was the main risk factor for embolization. Retrospective analysis of large series of patients did not demonstrate a prevalence of thromboembolic events greater than the reported risk of major bleeding from warfarin treatment.[81] Thus, in younger patients with hyperthyroidism and atrial fibrillation in the absence of other heart disease, hypertension, or other independent risk factors for embolization, the benefits of anticoagulation have not been proved and may well be outweighed by the risk. Aspirin provides an alternative for lowering risk for embolic events in young people and can be used safely.

Successful treatment of hyperthyroidism with either radioiodine or antithyroid drugs and restoration of normal serum levels of T_4 and T_3 associates with reversion to sinus rhythm in two-thirds of patients within 2 to 3 months.[78] In older patients or in the setting of atrial fibrillation of longer duration, the rate of reversion to sinus rhythm is lower and therefore electrical or pharmacological cardioversion should be attempted but only after the patient has been rendered euthyroid. The majority of patients (90 percent) can be restored to sinus rhythm by either electrical cardioversion or pharmacological measures, and many remain in sinus rhythm for periods up to 5 years or more. In a regimen in which disopyramide 300 mg/d was added for 3 months after successful cardioversion, patients were more likely to remain in sinus rhythm than those not treated.[81]

Heart Failure

The cardiovascular alterations in hyperthyroidism include increased resting cardiac output and enhanced cardiac contractility (Fig. 79–6; see Table 79–2). Despite this, a minority

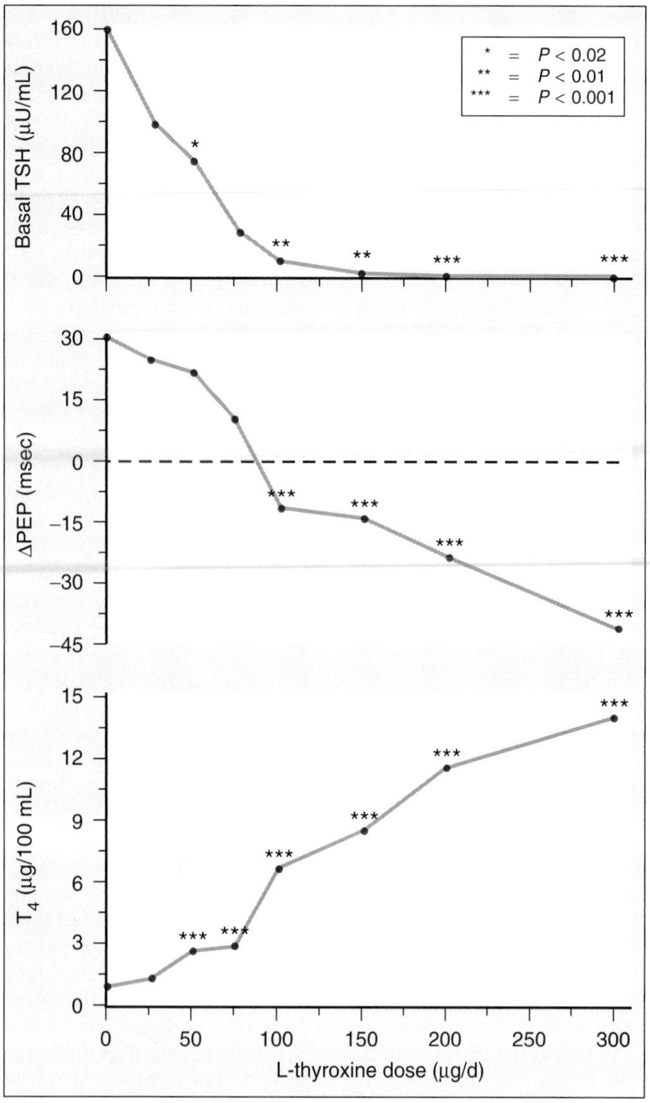

FIGURE 79–6 Response to stepwise L-thyroxine sodium treatment of hypothyroid patients as assessed by serum thyrotropin (TSH), serum tetraiodothyronine (T_4), and the improvement in left ventricular contractility as measured noninvasively by the preejection period (PEP). (From Crowley WF Jr, Ridgway EC, Bough EW, et al: Noninvasive evaluation of cardiac function in hypothyroidism. Response to gradual thyroxine replacement. N Engl J Med 296:1, 1977.)

of patients present with symptoms including dyspnea on exertion, orthopnea, and paroxysmal nocturnal dyspnea as well as signs demonstrating peripheral edema, neck vein distention, and an S_3 indicative of heart failure (see Table 79–3). This complex of findings coupled with a failure to increase the left ventricular ejection fraction with exercise has suggested the possibility of a hyperthyroid cardiomyopathy. The term often used in this setting, "high-output failure," is inappropriate; although resting cardiac output is as much as two to three times normal, the exercise intolerance appears to be a result not of cardiac failure but rather of skeletal muscle weakness.[50,76] High-output states, however, can increase renal sodium reabsorption, expand plasma volume, and cause development of peripheral edema, pleural effusions, and neck vein distention. Interestingly, although systemic vascular resistance falls with hyperthyroidism, the pulmonary vascular bed is not similarly affected and as a result of the increase in output to the pulmonary circulation, there is an increase in pulmonary artery pressures. This effect results in a rise in mean venous pressure, neck vein distention, hepatic congestion, and peripheral edema of the type associated with primary pulmonary hypertension or right-sided heart failure.[69]

Patients with longstanding hyperthyroidism and marked sinus tachycardia or atrial fibrillation can experience the development of low cardiac output, impaired cardiac contractility with a low ejection fraction, an S_3, and pulmonary congestion, all consistent with congestive heart failure.[50] Review of such cases suggests that impairment in left ventricular function is the result of a prolonged high heart rate and the development of rate-related heart failure. When the left ventricle becomes dilated, mitral regurgitation may also develop. Recognition of this entity is important because treatments aimed at slowing heart rate or controlling the ventricular response in atrial fibrillation appear to improve left ventricular function even before initiation of antithyroid therapy.[50] Because these patients are critically ill, they should be managed in an intensive care unit setting. Some patients with hyperthyroidism (similar to the overall congestive heart failure population) do not tolerate initiation of beta-adrenergic blocking drugs in full doses, and treatment can be started with lower doses of short-acting beta-blocking drugs in conjunction with classical forms of treatment of acute congestive heart failure, including diuresis.

The increase in rate pressure product and oxygen consumption that results from hyperthyroidism can impair cardiac function in older patients with known or suspected ischemic, hypertensive, or valvular heart disease. It is important to recognize promptly the cardiac manifestations of hyperthyroidism in older patients as they may have a higher risk for adverse cardiovascular and cerebral vascular outcomes.[82]

Treatment

Treatment of patients with thyrotoxic cardiac disease should include a beta-adrenergic antagonist to lower the heart rate to 10 or 15 percent above normal. This treatment causes the tachycardia-mediated component of ventricular dysfunction to improve, whereas the direct inotropic effects of thyroid hormone persist (see Fig. 79–4).[50] The rapid onset of action and the improvement in many of the signs and symptoms of hyperthyroidism indicate that most patients with overt symptoms should receive beta-blocking agents. Definitive therapy then can be accomplished safely with iodine-131 alone or in combination with an antithyroid drug.

Hypothyroidism

In contrast to the dramatic clinical signs and symptoms of hyperthyroidism, the cardiovascular findings of hypothyroidism are more subtle. Mild degrees of bradycardia, diastolic hypertension, a narrow pulse pressure and a relatively quiet precordium, and decreased intensity of the apical impulse are characteristic. Hemodynamic changes of hypothyroidism are diametrically opposite to those of hyperthyroidism (see Table 79–2) and explain many of the findings on physical examination. Despite the decrease in cardiac output and contractility of the hypothyroid myocardium, studies of myocardial metabolism using PET scan methodology have shown that the hypothyroid myocardium is energy inefficient. The oxygen cost of work increases primarily as a result of the increase in afterload.[83] Treatment of hypothyroid patients with restoration of a euthyroid state resolves these changes in parallel with a return of systemic vascular resistance to lower levels.

Hypothyroidism also produces increases in total and low-density lipoprotein (LDL) cholesterol as well as apolipoprotein B.[84] Although thyroid hormone can alter cholesterol metabolism through multiple mechanisms, including a decrease in biliary excretion, it appears that changes in LDL metabolism related to decreases in LDL receptor number are a primary mechanism. Thus, the finding of a direct relationship between the level of TSH as a measure of hypothyroidism and serum total cholesterol and LDL cholesterol is not surprising.[85]

Serum creatine kinase (CK) is elevated by 50 percent to 10-fold in as many as 30 percent of patients with hypothyroidism. Analysis of isoform specificity indicates that more than 96 percent is the muscle form (MM), consistent with a skeletal muscle origin of increased enzyme release.[86] In contrast to the half-life of CK after acute myocardial infarction (12 hours), the half-life in hypothyroidism after initiation of standard oral thyroid hormone replacement is approximately 10 to 14 days. Pericardial effusions can occur, consistent with observation that patients with hypothyroidism have an increase in volume of distribution of albumin and a decrease in lymphatic clearance function. Occasionally, the pericardial effusions are quite large, causing the appearance of cardiomegaly on routine chest radiographs. Echocardiography demonstrates small to moderate effusions in as many as 30 percent of overtly hypothyroid patients. The presence of pericardial fluid in hypothyroid patients does not compromise cardiac output, cardiac tamponade is exceedingly rare, and the effusion resolves over a period of weeks to months after initiation of thyroid hormone replacement.

As a result of changes in ion channel expression, the electrocardiogram in hypothyroidism is characterized by sinus bradycardia, low voltage, and prolongation of the action potential duration and the QT interval. The latter, in turn, predisposes patients to ventricular arrhythmias, and there are case reports of patients with acquired torsades de pointes that has improved or completely resolved with thyroid hormone replacement.[50]

As a result of increases in risk factors, including hypercholesterolemia, hypertension, and elevated levels of homocysteine, patients with hypothyroidism may have increased risk for atherosclerosis and coronary and systemic vascular disease.[87] Studies have shown increases in abdominal aortic atherosclerosis in patients with even mild hypothyroidism.[88] Small autopsy series have shown an increase in coronary artery disease, but only in patients with both hypertension and hypercholesterolemia. Whether patients with hypothyroidism have an increase in coronary artery disease is an important clinical issue. Noninvasive studies including thallium scanning have demonstrated abnormalities in perfusion suggestive of myocardial ischemia, but these defects appear to resolve with thyroid hormone treatment and may not reflect flow limitation related to fixed stenoses.

In patients younger than 50 years, it is possible to initiate full replacement doses of L-thyroxine (0.1 to 0.15 mg/d) without concern about untoward cardiac effects. In patients older than 50 with known or suspected coronary artery disease, the issue is more complicated. In patients with known coronary artery disease and a coexistent diagnosis of hypothyroidism, three major issues need to be addressed.

The first issue is whether coronary artery revascularization is required before initiating thyroid hormone replacement. If patients are not candidates for percutaneous intervention, coronary artery bypass grafting can be accomplished in patients with unstable angina, left main coronary artery disease, or three-vessel disease with impaired left ventricular function, even in the setting of overt hypothyroidism. Rarely, a patient is so profoundly hypothyroid that bleeding times and partial thromboplastin times are prolonged, requiring preoperative supplementation of clotting factors. Thyroid hormone replacement can be delayed until the postoperative period, when it can be administered in full dose either parenterally or orally.[71]

The second issue concerns patients with known stable cardiac disease in whom cardiac revascularization is not clinically indicated. Treatment of such patients should begin with low doses (12.5 μg) of L-thyroxine with doses increased stepwise (12.5 to 25 μg) every 6 to 8 weeks until serum TSH is normal. Thyroid hormone replacement in this setting and its ability to lower systemic vascular resistance and lower afterload as well as improve myocardial efficiency can actually decrease clinical signs of myocardial ischemia. Beta-adrenergic blocking agents are an ideal concomitant therapy to control heart rate.

The third issue concerns the group of patients who, although potentially at risk for coronary artery disease, exhibit no clinical signs or symptoms. In this group, thyroid hormone replacement can be started at low doses generally in the range of 25 to 50 μg/d and increased 25 μg every 6 to 8 weeks until serum TSH is normal. Should signs or symptoms of ischemic heart disease develop, the same recommendations apply as to patients with known underlying heart disease.

In all patients, thyroid hormone replacement should continue until serum TSH is normal and the patients are clinically euthyroid. The concept that these patients benefit from maintenance of "mild hypothyroidism" is not supported by the known effects of thyroid hormone on the heart and cardiovascular system. Thyroid hormone replacement should be accomplished with purified preparations of levothyroxine sodium. Preparations containing T_4 with T_3 (thyroid extract) or the existing purified preparations of T_3 do not offer benefit. The short half-life of T_3 and the inability to maintain serum levels within normal range in patients so treated can add to cardiac risk.[89]

Diagnosis

Hashimoto disease, radioiodine therapy for Graves disease, and iodine deficiency (in parts of the world where that remains a public health problem) are the leading causes of hypothyroidism and produce diagnostic elevations in serum TSH.[65] Thus, the finding of elevated TSH is sufficient to establish the diagnosis and form the basis for treatment. In routine practice, additional testing with a serum T_4 and T_3 resin uptake test is confirmatory. The prevalence of hypothyroidism is estimated as 3 to 4 percent for overt disease and 7 to 10 percent for the milder forms of disease. Thus, TSH screening can be advised for all adults and particularly patients demonstrating hypertension, hypercholesterolemia, hypertriglyceridemia, coronary or peripheral vascular disease, unexplained pericardial or pleural effusions, and a variety of musculoskeletal syndromes.[52]

Treatment

The response to treatment of hypothyroidism is predictable, especially from a cardiovascular perspective. Stepwise thyroid hormone replacement using levothyroxine sodium (Levoxyl, Synthroid) produces an incremental decrease in serum TSH, serum cholesterol, and serum CK and an improvement in left ventricular performance. Full replacement is accomplished when serum TSH is normal.[65] In the rare condition of myxedema coma, which is characterized by severe and longstanding hypothyroidism with the development of hypothermia, altered mental status, hypotension, bradycardia, and hypoventilation, the need for thyroid hormone replacement is more emergent and treatment can be accomplished with either T_4 at 100 μg/d or T_3 at 25 μg/d administered intravenously. These patients often require intensive care unit monitoring with volume repletion, gentle warming, and ventilatory support in the presence of CO_2 retention. Administration of hydrocortisone (100 mg every 8 hours) should be undertaken until results of serum cortisol testing are obtained. When patients are treated in this manner, hemodynamics including systemic vascular resistance, cardiac output, and heart rate improve within 24 to 48 hours.

SUBCLINICAL THYROID DISEASE

In contrast to overt symptomatic thyroid disease, subclinical thyroid disease implies the absence of classical hyper- or hypothyroidism-related symptoms in patients with thyroid dysfunction. The definition has been further refined to include the demonstration of an abnormal TSH level in the presence of normal serum levels of total T_4 and free T_4.[65] With the advent of widespread TSH screening, the magnitude of subclinical thyroid disease may exceed that of overt disease by three- to fourfold.[85]

Subclinical Hypothyroidism

Subclinical hypothyroidism, defined by a TSH level above the upper range of the reference population (usually >5 μIU/ml), is seen in as many as 9 percent of unselected populations and prevalence clearly increases with advancing age.[85] In contrast to younger patients, in whom there is a strong female predilection, this difference is lost in older populations. Studies of lipid metabolism, atherosclerosis, cardiac contractility, and systemic vascular resistance are altered in subclinical hypothyroidism. Cholesterol levels rise in parallel with increments in TSH elevations starting at 5 μIU/L. In a large study of women in Rotterdam, it was noted that atherosclerosis and myocardial infarction were increased with odds ratios of 1.7 and 2.3, respectively, in women with subclinical hypothyroidism. Interestingly, the presence of antithyroid antibodies indicated heightened risk.[88] Restoration of serum TSH to normal after thyroid hormone replacement improved lipid levels, lowered systemic vascular resistance, and improved cardiac contractility.[90] In patients with subclinical hypothyroidism, isovolumetric relaxation times are prolonged while systolic contractile function is unchanged (see Fig. 79–6). Replacement with L-thyroxine sodium at a mean dose of 68 μg/d (range 50 to 100 μg/d) restored isovolumetric relaxation times to normal, and compared with those in the same patients before therapy, systemic vascular resistance declined and systolic function was significantly improved.[91] A variety of studies have indicated that the changes in systemic vascular resistance may result from alterations in endothelium-dependent vasodilation.[73,87] Taking these findings together, it seems appropriate to recommend thyroid hormone replacement for all patients with subclinical hypothyroidism from a cardiovascular perspective. The lack of untoward cardiac effects observed when serum TSH levels have been restored to normal indicates that the potential benefits far outweigh the risks of treatment.[50]

Subclinical Hyperthyroidism

Subclinical hyperthyroidism is diagnosed when serum TSH is low (<0.1 μIU/ml) and both T_4 and T_3 are normal.[65] The significance of subclinical hyperthyroidism was conclusively established from a study of atrial fibrillation in patients 60 years of age or older in the Framingham cohort.[92] Prevalence of atrial fibrillation after 10 years was 28 percent in the patients with subclinical hyperthyroidism compared with 11 percent in patients with normal thyroid function with a relative risk of 3.1 (Fig. 79–7). A population-based study of more than 1000 individuals with subclinical hyperthyroidism not receiving L-thyroxine therapy or antithyroid medication demonstrated that a TSH level less than 0.5 was associated with twofold increased mortality with relative risk of 2.3 to 3.3 from all causes, which in turn was largely accounted for by increases in cardiovascular mortality.[93]

Whereas the cardiovascular changes are well established, the management of patients with subclinical hyperthyroidism is controversial. Therapy can be individualized with regard to three specific groups. The first group includes patients receiving thyroid hormone replacement for hypothyroidism in whom the low TSH is thought to be the result of excess medication and reduction of the dose is indicated. The second group includes patients with a prior diagnosis of thyroid cancer currently receiving L-thyroxine for the purpose of TSH suppression. In younger patients or those with more advanced disease (stage 3 or 4), beta-adrenergic blocking agents can reverse many if not all of the cardiovascular manifestations including heart rate control, LVH, and atrial ectopy. In older patients or patients with milder disease, the degree of TSH suppression can be relaxed by lowering the T_4 dosage.[94]

The third group includes patients in whom subclinical hyperthyroidism results from endogenous thyroid gland overactivity, including Graves disease, chronic thyroiditis, nodular goiter, or autonomously functioning adenoma. In this category, younger patients appear to have few or no untoward effects but older patients are potentially at risk from atrial fibrillation. In patients older than 60 years, antithyroid therapy (methimazole [Tapazole] 5 to 10 mg/d) can produce improvement, and in patients who do respond consideration should be given to the use of radioiodine for definitive treatment.[50]

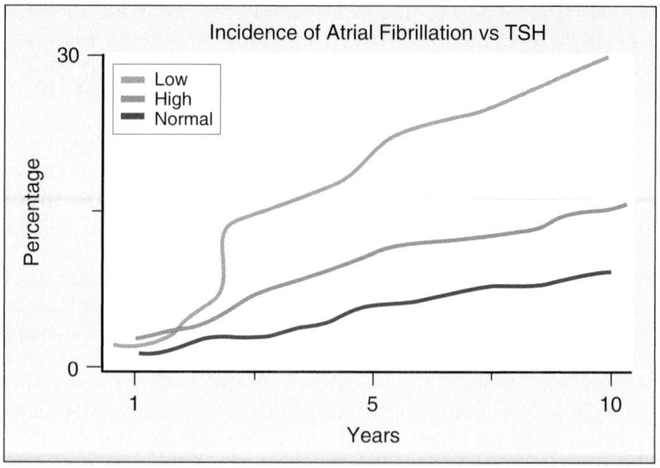

FIGURE 79–7 Atrial fibrillation in subclinical hyperthyroidism. Low thyrotropin (TSH) designates patients who have serum TSH less than 0.1 μIU/ml. (Adapted from Sawin CT: Subclinical hyperthyroidism and atrial fibrillation. Thyroid 12:501, 2002.)

Amiodarone and Thyroid Function

Amiodarone is an iodine-rich antiarrhythmic agent effective in the treatment of both ventricular and atrial tachyarrhythmias. It is currently used extensively in patients with a variety of cardiac diseases. As a result of the 30 percent by weight iodine content, this drug commonly causes abnormalities in thyroid function testing in patients treated for either short or long periods of time.[95] Similarly to other iodinated drugs, amiodarone inhibits the 5′ monodeiodination of T_4 in both the liver and the pituitary. Inhibition of T_4 metabolism in the liver decreases serum T_3 and increases serum T_4 while serum TSH levels initially remain normal. With more chronic treatment and as the total iodide content of the body rises, there is a potential for inhibition of T_4 synthesis and release from the thyroid gland, producing a rise in TSH. In patients with underlying goiter, autoimmune thyroid disease, or enzymatic defects in thyroid hormone biosynthesis and in some patients without any risk factors there is a progression to overt chemical and clinical hypothyroidism with a marked rise in serum TSH.[95] The overall prevalence of hypothyroidism in amiodarone-treated patients is reported to be between 15 and 20 percent. It is important to note that the symptoms of hypothyroidism in this setting can be quite subtle and significant hypothyroidism can occur even in their absence.

Thyroid function should be measured every 3 months in all patients receiving amiodarone. The effect on thyroid function does not depend on dose and can occur any time after initiating treatment and, because of the high lipid solubility and long half-life of the drug, for periods up to a year after discontinuation of therapy.[95]

Less common but perhaps more challenging is the development of amiodarone-induced thyrotoxicosis. Although it was initially not observed in the iodine-replete American population, the experience from Italy suggested that it occurred with a prevalence as high as 10 percent.[95] The onset was often sudden and could occur shortly after drug initiation, during chronic treatment, or up to 1 year after stopping therapy. Although the pathogenesis is multifactorial, early studies distinguished two forms of amiodarone-induced thyrotoxicosis. Type I occurs primarily in patients with preexisting thyroid disease and most commonly in iodine-deficient areas. These patients may rarely have an increase in 24-hour radioiodine uptake measures and frequently some measures of thyroid autoimmunity, including antithyroid antibodies. Color flow Doppler sonography of the thyroid gland has a "characteristic" appearance consistent with other forms of autoimmune thyroid disease. In contrast, type II disease was identified as a form of thyroiditis presumably mediated by a variety of proinflammatory cytokines including interleukin-6.[96] This disease is primarily a destructive process causing release of preformed thyroid hormone, which may continue for periods of weeks and months and is most often associated with low to absent radioiodine uptake. Further experience has shown that these two types have substantial overlap for many of the distinguishing parameters.

Because of the increased thyroidal and total body iodine content, use of iodine-131 is almost always ineffective. Similarly, treatment with antithyroid drugs has marginal effectiveness. Corticosteroids (prednisone 20 to 40 mg/d) have been recommended and proved to be of benefit, perhaps with increased utility in patients with type II disease in whom serum levels of interleukin-6 are high.[95] Alternatively, corticosteroids can be instituted in all patients; when they are effective, the response usually occurs within 1 week of initiating treatment. Treatment can then be tapered over 3 months leading to disease remission.[95] In patients unresponsive to glucocorticoids with evidence of hyperthyroidism including weight loss, tachycardia, palpitations, worsening angina, or other untoward cardiac effects, treatment with a combination of antithyroid therapy (methimazole 10 to 30 mg/d) and potassium perchlorate is variably effective.[97] Treatment can cause significant side effects including bone marrow toxicity resulting from the potassium perchlorate. A report confirms that total thyroidectomy can be performed safely and is an effective means of rapidly reversing the hyperthyroidism. Preoperative treatment with beta-adrenergic blocking drugs is indicated, and there have been no reported cases of resulting thyroid storm.[98]

An important issue is whether amiodarone-mediated thyroid dysfunction should mandate discontinuation of the drug. Because certain patients require amiodarone therapy to manage critical arrhythmias and the duration of drug retention in the body in lipid-soluble stores is in excess of 6 months, it seems prudent to continue amiodarone therapy while making separate management plans to deal with the thyroid dysfunction.

CHANGES IN THYROID HORMONE METABOLISM THAT ACCOMPANY CARDIAC DISEASE

In addition to the changes in thyroid function, which can result from classical thyroid disease, there are primary alterations in serum total and free T_3 and occasionally serum T_4 that accompany a variety of acute and chronic illnesses including sepsis, starvation, and cardiac disease.[99] In the absence of thyroid gland abnormality, changes in serum T_3 levels result from alterations in thyroid hormone metabolism. These cases have been referred to as "nonthyroidal illness." The mechanism for this decrease in serum T_3 is multifactorial and in part related to a decrease in 5′ monodeiodination in the liver.

A wide variety of acute and chronic cardiac diseases can alter thyroid hormone metabolism associated with marked declines in serum T_3. A population-based study of patients with cardiac disease has shown that a low serum T_3 level is a strong predictor of all-cause and cardiovascular mortality.[100] Following uncomplicated acute myocardial infarction, serum T_3 levels fall by about 20 percent and reach a nadir after approximately 96 hours. Experimental myocardial infarction in animal models produces a similar decrease in serum T_3, and replacement of T_3 levels to normal has been reported to increase left ventricular contractile function.[58]

Both children and adults undergoing cardiac surgery with cardiopulmonary bypass demonstrate a predictable fall in serum T_3 in the perioperative period.[101] Although treatment strategies using acute administration of intravenous T_3 to adults after coronary artery bypass grafting have resulted in an improvement in cardiac output and a fall in systemic vascular resistance, there was no alteration in overall mortality.[71] When the prevalence of atrial fibrillation was studied in this group of patients, however, it was shown to be decreased by as much as 50 percent compared with that in age-matched control subjects.[102] Pediatric cardiac patients, especially those undergoing surgery in the neonatal period, demonstrate an even greater decline in serum T_3 that can last for longer periods of time. The low postoperative T_3 level identifies patients at increased risk for morbidity and mortality.[103] A prospective randomized study has shown, especially in neonates, that the degree of therapeutic intervention and the need for postoperative inotropic agents are decreased by the administration of T_3 in doses sufficient to restore serum T_3 levels to normal.[104]

In patients with chronic congestive heart failure, the fall in serum T_3 is proportional to the severity of heart failure as assessed by the New York Heart Association classification.[58] As many as 30 percent of patients with heart failure have a low serum T_3, which occurs in both patients treated with amiodarone and those who are not.[58,100] In view of the deleterious effects of hypothyroidism on the myocardium, T_3 replacement may be of benefit. Human studies using a novel form of T_3 that is capable of restoring serum T_3 levels to normal and avoiding the peaks and valleys of drug levels associated with existing drug preparations are required to answer this question.[58]

Pheochromocytoma

Pheochromocytomas are primarily benign tumors arising from neuroectodermal chromaffin cells primarily within the adrenal medulla and abdomen, but they may arise anywhere within plexus of sympathetic adrenergic nerves. Although the prevalence is probably less than one per 2000 cases of diastolic hypertension, the importance of pheochromocytoma derives from the dramatic way in which symptoms can arise. Various autopsy studies have shown that in 75 percent of patients the diagnosis was not clinically suspected and in more than half it was thought to be a factor contributing to mortality.[105]

A variety of tumor characteristics have been established.[106] Most pheochromocytomas are 1 cm or greater in size, the vast majority arise as a unilateral adrenal lesion, and extraadrenal tumors are more common in children. Although most tumors are sporadic, approximately 10 percent are familial, and the latter are more often bilateral or occur in an extraadrenal location. When pheochromocytoma coexists with medullary thyroid carcinoma or occasionally with hyperparathyroidism, it is a designated multiple endocrine neoplasia (MEN) syndrome type II. These patients have a mutation in the RET proto-oncogene. In patients with MEN IIB, pheochromocytomas coexist with medullary thyroid cancer and mucosal neuromas are frequently seen on the lips and tongue. Pheochromocytoma may be present in up to 1 percent of patients with neurofibromatosis, and in von Hippel–Lindau disease pheochromocytoma develops in association with cerebellar or retinoangiomas.[107]

The clinical presentation of pheochromocytoma is characterized by headache, palpitations, excessive sweating, tremulousness, chest pain, weight loss, and a variety of other constitutional complaints. Hypertension may be episodic but is most commonly constant and is paradoxically associated with orthostatic hypotension upon arising in the morning. The paroxysmal attacks and classical symptoms result from episodic excess catecholamine secretion.[105]

The first onset of hypertension related to pheochromocytoma can be at the time of elective surgical intervention for an unrelated condition. As a result of norepinephrine release with an increase in systemic vascular resistance, cardiac output is increased minimally if at all despite increases in heart rate. The electrocardiogram can show LVH as well as the presence of inverted T waves, suggesting a left ventricular strain pattern. Although ventricular and atrial ectopy and episodes of supraventricular tachycardia can occur, there is little to distinguish the LVH from that of essential hypertension.[105]

There are reports of impaired left ventricular function and cardiomyopathy in patients with pheochromocytoma. The underlying mechanism is complex and includes increased left ventricular work and LVH from associated hypertension, potential adverse effects of excess catecholamines on myocyte structure and contractility, and changes in coronary arteries including thickening of the media presumably potentially impairing blood flow to the myocardium. Histological evidence of myocarditis is present post mortem in patients with previously diagnosed or undiagnosed disease.[105] The possibility of catecholamine-stimulated tachycardia in turn mediating left ventricular dysfunction should be addressed because treatments designed to slow the heart rate may rapidly improve left ventricular function.

Release of catecholamines from pheochromocytomas involves diffusion out of chromaffin cells as well as release from storage vessels, accounting for the demonstration of chromogranin A in the circulation. The primary catecholamine released is norepinephrine, but increases in epinephrine can also be measured. Demonstration of elevated serum dopamine implies the possibility of malignant transformation, which in turn suggests that the tumor may arise in an extraadrenal site. Rarely, pheochromocytoma can arise within the heart, presumably from chromaffin cells, which are part of the adrenergic autonomic paraganglia.[108]

Diagnosis

The diagnosis is established by demonstrating an increase in norepinephrine or epinephrine or its metabolites in serum or blood. Quantitative 24-hour urinary metanephrines are the most reliable for screening, and plasma catecholamines, when obtained under proper conditions, are also fairly sensitive.[108,109] A variety of provocative tests have been used to increase plasma catecholamines in patients with episodic disease. In contrast, the clonidine suppression test is safe and suppresses plasma norepinephrine by more than 50 percent in essential hypertensive patients but not in those with pheochromocytoma.[106] Imaging modalities include magnetic resonance imaging, which has a high degree of specificity, and computed tomographic scanning, which has a high degree of sensitivity because adrenal lesions are of sufficient size to be detected. Further studies with isotopic precursors of catecholamine biosynthesis, including [^{131}I]metaiodobenzylguanidine (MIBG), are useful for confirming that anatomical lesions are producing catecholamines.

Treatment

Definitive treatment of pheochromocytoma requires removal of the lesion. Accurate preoperative localization has reduced operative mortality and eliminates the need for exploratory laparotomy. Endoscopic procedures are now standard.[110] Preoperative pharmacological management includes 7 to 14 days of alpha-adrenergic blockade, usually with prazosin or phenoxybenzamine. Beta-adrenergic blocker therapy is considered contraindicated before establishing sufficient alpha blockade. If supraventricular arrhythmias or unremitting tachycardia is present, β_1-selective agents such as atenolol are preferred.[109] Operative intervention requires constant blood pressure monitoring, and the use of intravenous phentolamine or sodium nitroprusside may be required to treat episodic hypertension.[105,110] Postoperative management includes the use of large volumes of crystalloid-containing fluids to maintain blood volume and prevent hypotension. Glucose may be needed to replace depleted liver glycogen stores. In patients who are not candidates for surgical treatment, metyrosine can decrease catecholamine synthesis and improve the majority of cardiovascular signs and symptoms.[105,110]

REFERENCES

Pituitary Gland

1. Lu C, Schwartzbauer G, Sperling MA, et al: Demonstration of direct effects of growth hormone on neonatal cardiomyocytes. J Biol Chem 276:22892, 2001.
2. Reiss K, Cheng W, Ferber A, et al: Overexpression of insulin-like growth factor-1 in the heart is coupled with myocyte proliferation in transgenic mice. Proc Natl Acad Sci USA 93:8630, 1996.
3. Napoli R, Guardasole V, Angelini V, et al: Acute effects of growth hormone on vascular function in human subjects. J Clin Endocrinol Metab 88:2817, 2003.
4. Colao A, Marzullo P, Di Somma C, et al: Growth hormone and the heart. Clin Endocrinol (Oxf) 54:137, 2001.
5. Brevetti G, Marzullo P, Silvestro A, et al: Early vascular alterations in acromegaly. J Clin Endocrinol Metab 87:3174, 2002.
6. Chanson P, Megnien JL, del Pino M, et al: Decreased regional blood flow in patients with acromegaly. Clin Endocrinol (Oxf) 49:725, 1998.
7. Melmed S, Ho K, Klibanski A, et al: Clinical review 75: Recent advances in pathogenesis, diagnosis, and management of acromegaly. J Clin Endocrinol Metab 80:3395, 1995.
8. Clayton RN: Cardiovascular function in acromegaly. Endocr Rev 24:272, 2003.
9. Bruch C, Herrmann B, Schmermund A, et al: Impact of disease activity on left ventricular performance in patients with acromegaly. Am Heart J 144:538, 2002.
10. Colao A, Spinelli L, Cuocolo A, et al: Cardiovascular consequences of early-onset growth hormone excess. J Clin Endocrinol Metab 87:3097, 2002.
11. Lopez-Velasco R, Escobar-Morreale HF, Vega B, et al: Cardiac involvement in acromegaly: Specific myocardiopathy or consequence of systemic hypertension? J Clin Endocrinol Metab 82:1047, 1997.
12. Minniti G, Jafrain-Rea ML, Moroni C, et al: Echocardiographic evidence for a direct effect of GH/IGF-1 hypersecretion on cardiac mass and function in young acromegalics. Clin Endocrinol (Oxf) 49:101, 1998.
13. Colao A, Spinelli L, Marzullo P, et al: High prevalence of cardiac valve disease in acromegaly: An observational, analytical, case-control study. J Clin Endocrinol Metab 88:3196, 2003.
14. Herrmann BL, Bruch C, Saller B, et al: Acromegaly: Evidence for a direct relation between disease activity and cardiac dysfunction in patients without ventricular hypertrophy. Clin Endocrinol (Oxf) 56:595, 2002.
15. Ciulla M, Arosio M, Barelli MV, et al: Blood pressure–independent cardiac hypertrophy in acromegalic patients. J Hypertens 17:1965, 1999.
16. Frustaci A, Chimenti C, Setoguchi M, et al: Cell death in acromegalic cardiomyopathy. Circulation 99:1426, 1999.
17. Damjanovics SS, Neskovic AN, Petakov MS, et al: High output heart failure in patients with newly diagnosed acromegaly. Am J Med 112:610, 2002.
18. Trainer PJ, Drake WM, Katznelson L, et al: Treatment of acromegaly with the growth hormone-receptor antagonist pegvisomant. N Engl J Med 342:1171, 2000.
19. Melmed S, Casanueva FF, Cavagnini R, et al: CONSENSUS: Guidelines for acromegaly management. J Clin Endocrinol Metab 87:4054, 2002.
20. Fazio S, Cittadini A, Biondi B, et al: Cardiovascular effects of short-term growth hormone hypersecretion. J Clin Endocrinol Metab 85:179, 2000.
21. Maison P, Demolis P, Young J, et al: Vascular reactivity in acromegalic patients: Preliminary evidence for regional endothelial dysfunction and increased sympathetic vasoconstriction. Clin Endocrinol (Oxf) 53:445, 2000.
22. Orth DN, Kovacs WJ, DeBold CR: The adrenal cortex. *In* Wilson JD, Foster DW, Kronenberg HM, Larsen PR (eds): Williams Textbook of Endocrinology. Philadelphia, WB Saunders, 1998, pp 517-664.
23. Wallerath T, Witte K, Schafer SC, et al: Down-regulation of the expression of endothelial NO synthase is likely to contribute to glucocorticoid-mediated hypertension. Proc Natl Acad Sci USA 96:13357, 1999.
24. Whitworth JA, Mangos GJ, Kelly JJ: Cushing, cortisol, and cardiovascular disease. Hypertension 36:912, 2000.
25. Colao A, Pivonello R, Spiezia S, et al: Persistence of increased cardiovascular risk in patients with Cushing's disease after five years of successful cure. J Clin Endocrinol Metab 84:2664, 1999.
26. Kelly JJ, Mangos G, Williamson PM, et al: Cortisol and hypertension. Clin Exp Pharmacol Physiol 25(Suppl):S51, 1998.
27. Fernandez-Real J, Ricard W: Insulin resistance and chronic cardiovascular inflammatory syndrome. Endocr Rev 24:278, 2003.
28. Mortensen RM, Williams GH: Aldosterone action. *In* DeGroot L, Jameson L (eds): Endocrinology. Philadelphia, WB Saunders, 2001, p 1783.
29. Suzuki T, Shibata H, Ando T, et al: Risk factors associated with persistent postoperative hypertension in Cushing's syndrome. Endocr Res 26:791, 2000.
30. Faggiano A, Pivonello R, Spiezia S, et al: Cardiovascular risk factors and common carotid artery caliber and stiffness in patients with Cushing's disease during active disease and 1 year after disease remission. J Clin Endocrinol Metab 88:2527, 2003.
31. Muiesan ML, Lupia M, Salvetti M, et al: Left ventricular structural and functional characteristics in Cushing's syndrome. J Am Coll Cardiol 41:2275, 2003.
32. Norman WN, Wehling M (eds): Proceedings of the First International Meeting on Rapid Responses to Steroid Hormones. Steroids 64:3, 1999.
33. Basson CT: Case records of the Massachusetts General Hospital, case 11-2002. N Engl J Med 346:1152, 2002.
34. Ambrosi B, Sartorio A, Pizzocaro A, et al: Evaluation of haemostatic and fibrinolytic markers in patients with Cushing's syndrome and in patients with adrenal incidentaloma. Exp Clin Endocrinol Diabetes 108:294, 2000.
35. Carey RM, Siragy HM: Newly recognized components of the renin-angiotensin system: Potential roles in cardiovascular and renal regulation. Endocr Rev 24:261, 2003.
36. Young MJ, Funder JW: Mineralocorticoid receptors and pathophysiological roles for aldosterone in the cardiovascular system. J Hypertens 20:1465, 2002.
37. White PC: Aldosterone: Direct effects on and production by the heart. J Clin Endocrinol Metab 88:2376, 2003.
38. Mihailidou AS, Buhagiar KA, Rasmussen HH: Na^+ influx and Na^+-K^+ pump activation during short-term exposure of cardiac myocytes to aldosterone. Am J Physiol 274:C175, 1998.

39. Pitt B, Zannad F, Remme WJ, et al: The effect of spironolactone on morbidity and mortality in patients with severe heart failure. N Engl J Med 341:709, 1999.
40. Rossi GP, Sacchetto A, Pavan E, et al: Remodeling of the left ventricle in primary aldosteronism due to Conn's adenoma. Circulation 95:1471, 1997.
41. Pessina AC, Sacchetto A, Rossi GP: Left ventricular anatomy and function in primary aldosteronism and renovascular hypertension. Adv Exp Med Biol 432:63, 1997.
42. Shigematsu Y, Hamada M, Okayama H, et al: Left ventricular hypertrophy precedes other target-organ damage in primary aldosteronism. Hypertension 29:723, 1997.
43. Cooper MS, Stewart PM: Corticosteroid insufficiency in acutely ill patients. N Engl J Med 348:727, 2003.
44. Espinosa G, Santos E, Cervera R, et al: Adrenal involvement in the antiphospholipid syndrome: Clinical and immunologic characteristics of 86 patients. Medicine (Baltimore) 82:106, 2003.
45. Bhattacharyya A, Jagadeesan S, Wolstenholme RJ, et al: Acute adrenocortical crisis and an abnormal electrocardiogram. Hosp Med 60:908, 1999.
46. Fallo F, Betterle C, Budano S, et al: Regression of cardiac abnormalities after replacement therapy in Addison's disease. Eur J Endocrinol 140:425, 1999.

Parathyroid Disease

47. Schluter K, Piper HM: Cardiovascular actions of parathyroid hormone and parathyroid hormone–related peptide. Cardiovasc Res 37:34, 1998.
48. Stefenelli T, Abela C, Frank H, et al: Cardiac Abnormalities in patients with primary hyperparathyroidism: Implications for follow-up. J Clin Endocrinol Metab 82:106, 1997.
49. Stefenelli T, Mayr H, Bergler-Klein J, et al: Primary hyperparathyroidism: Incidence of cardiac abnormalities and partial reversibility after successful parathyroidectomy. Am J Med 95:197, 1993.

Thyroid Gland

50. Klein I, Ojamaa K: Thyroid hormone and the cardiovascular system. N Engl J Med 344:501, 2001.
51. Dillmann WH: Cellular action of thyroid hormone on the heart. Thyroid 12:447, 2002.
52. Levey GS, Klein I: Disorders of the thyroid. *In* Stein JH (ed): Internal Medicine. 5th ed. St. Louis, Mosby, 1998, pp 1323-1349.
53. Pachucki J, Hopkins J, Peeters R, et al: Type 2 iodothyronine deiodinase transgene expression in the mouse heart causes cardiac-specific thyrotoxicosis. Endocrinology 142:13, 2001.
54. Harvey CB, Williams GR: Mechanism of thyroid hormone action. Thyroid 12:441, 2002.
55. Danzi S, Klein I: Thyroid hormone–regulated cardiac gene expression and cardiovascular disease. Thyroid 12:467, 2002.
56. Morkin E: Control of cardiac myosin heavy chain gene expression. Microsc Res Tech 50:522, 2000.
57. Reiser PJ, Portman MA, Ning X, et al: Human cardiac myosin heavy chain isoforms in fetal and failing adult atria and ventricles. Am J Physiol 280:H1814, 2001.
58. Ojamaa K, Ascheim D, Hryniewicz K, et al: Thyroid hormone therapy of cardiovascular disease. Cardiovasc Rev Rep 23:20, 2002.
59. Carr AN, Kranias EG: Thyroid hormone regulation of calcium cycling proteins. Thyroid 12:453, 2002.
60. Ojamaa K, Kenessey A, Klein I: Thyroid hormone regulation of phospholamban phosphorylation in the rat heart. Endocrinology 141:2139, 2000.
61. Haghighi K, Kolokathis F, Pater L, et al: Human phospholamban null results in lethal dilated cardiomyopathy revealing a critical difference between mouse and human. J Clin Invest 111:869, 2003.
62. Biondi B, Palmieri EA, Lombardi G, et al: Subclinical hypothyroidism and cardiac function. Thyroid 12:505, 2002.
63. Virtanen VK, Saha HH, Groundstroem KW, et al: Thyroid hormone substitution therapy rapidly enhances left-ventricular diastolic function in hypothyroid patients. Cardiology 96:59, 2001.
64. Davis PJ, Davis FB: Nongenomic actions of thyroid hormone on the heart. Thyroid 12:459, 2002.
65. Demers LM, Spencer CA: Laboratory medicine practice guidelines, laboratory support for the diagnosis and monitoring of thyroid disease. Thyroid 13:3, 2003.
66. Hoit BD, Khoury SF, Shao Y, et al: Effects of thyroid hormone on cardiac beta-adrenergic responsiveness in conscious baboons. Circulation 96:592, 1997.
67. Ojamaa K, Klein I, Sabet A, et al: Changes in adenylyl cyclase isoforms as a mechanism for thyroid hormone modulation of cardiac beta-adrenergic receptor responsiveness. Metabolism 49:275, 2000.
68. Park KW, Kai HB, Ojamaa K, et al: The direct vasomotor effect of thyroid hormones on rat skeletal muscle resistance arteries. Anesth Analg 85:734, 1997.
69. Danzi S, Klein I: Thyroid hormone and blood pressure regulation. Curr Hypertens Rep 5:513, 2003.
70. Biondi B, Palmieri EA, Lombardi G, et al: Effects of thyroid hormone on cardiac function: The relative importance of heart rate, loading conditions, and myocardial contractility in the regulation of cardiac performance in human hyperthyroidism. J Clin Endocrinol Metab 87:968, 2002.
71. Klemperer JD, Klein I, Gomez M, et al: Thyroid hormone treatment after coronary-artery bypass surgery. N Engl J Med 333:1522, 1995.
72. Bengel FM, Lehnert J, Ibrahim T, et al: Cardiac oxidative metabolism, function, and metabolic performance in mild hyperthyroidism: A noninvasive study using positron emission tomography and magnetic resonance imaging. Thyroid 13:471, 2003.
73. Taddei S, Caraccio N, Virdis A, et al: Impaired endothelium-dependent vasodilatation in subclinical hypothyroidism: Beneficial effect of levothyroxine therapy. J Clin Endocrinol Metab 88:3731, 2003.
74. Marcisz C, Jonderko G, Kucharz EJ: Influence of short-time application of a low sodium diet on blood pressure in patients with hyperthyroidism or hypothyroidism during therapy. Am J Hypertens 14:995, 2001.
75. Cacciatori V, Bellavere F, Pessarossa A, et al: Power spectral analysis of heart rate in hyperthyroidism. J Clin Endocrinol Metab 81:2828, 1996.
76. Klein I, Levey GS: The cardiovascular system in thyrotoxicosis. *In* Braverman LE, Utiger RD (eds): Werner and Ingbar's the Thyroid: A Fundamental and Clinical Text. 8th ed. Philadelphia, Lippincott Williams & Wilkins, 2000, pp 596-604.
77. Kahaly GJ, Kampmann C, Mohr-Kahaly S: Cardiovascular hemodynamics and exercise tolerance in thyroid disease. Thyroid 12:473, 2002.
78. Shimizu T, Koide S, Noh JY, et al: Hyperthyroidism and the management of atrial fibrillation. Thyroid 12:489, 2002.
79. Auer J, Scheibner P, Mische T, et al: Subclinical hyperthyroidism as a risk factor for atrial fibrillation. Am Heart J 142:838, 2001.
80. Forfar JC: Atrial fibrillation and the pituitary-thyroid axis: A re-evaluation. Heart 77:3, 1997.
81. Nakazawa H, Lythall DA, Noh J, et al: Is there a place for the late cardioversion of atrial fibrillation? A long-term follow-up study of patients with post-thyrotoxic atrial fibrillation. Eur Heart J 21:327, 2000.
82. Franklyn JA, Maisonneuve P, Sheppard MC, et al: Mortality after the treatment of hyperthyroidism with radioactive iodine. N Engl J Med 338:712, 1998.
83. Bengel FM, Nekolla SC, Ibrahim T, et al: Effect of thyroid hormones on cardiac function, geometry, and oxidative metabolism assessed noninvasively by positron emission tomography and magnetic resonance imaging. J Clin Endocrinol Metab 85:1822, 2000.
84. Bakker S, ter Maaten JC, Popp-Snijders C, et al: The relationship between thyrotropin and low density lipoprotein cholesterol is modified by insulin sensitivity in healthy euthyroid subjects. J Clin Endocrinol Metab 86:1206, 2001.
85. Canaris GJ, Manowitz NR, Mayor G, et al: The Colorado thyroid disease prevalence study. Arch Intern Med 160:526, 2000.
86. Klein I, Ojamaa K: Thyroid (neuro) myopathy. Lancet 356:614, 2000.
87. Cappola AR, Ladenson PW: Hypothyroidism and atherosclerosis. J Clin Endocrinol Metab 88:2438, 2003.
88. Hak AE, Pols HAP, Visser TJ, et al: Subclinical hypothyroidism is an independent risk factor for atherosclerosis and myocardial infarction in elderly women: The Rotterdam Study. Ann Intern Med 132:270, 2000.
89. Danzi S, Ojamaa K, Klein I: Triiodothyronine-mediated myosin heavy chain gene transcription in the heart. Am J Physiol 284:H2255, 2003.
90. Monzani F, Di Bello V, Caraccio N, et al: Effect of levothyroxine on cardiac function and structure in subclinical hypothyroidism: A double blind, placebo-controlled study. J Clin Endocrinol Metab 86:1110, 2001.
91. Biondi B, Fazio S, Palmieri EA, et al: Left ventricular diastolic dysfunction in patients with subclinical hypothyroidism. J Clin Endocrinol Metab 84:2064, 1999.
92. Sawin CT: Subclinical hyperthyroidism and atrial fibrillation. Thyroid 12:501, 2002.
93. Parle, JV, Maisonneuve P, Sheppard MC, et al: Prediction of all-cause and cardiovascular mortality in elderly people from one low serum thyrotropin result: A 10-year cohort study. Lancet 358:861, 2001.
94. Burmeister LA, Flores A: Subclinical thyrotoxicosis and the heart. Thyroid 12:495, 2002.
95. Martino E, Bartalena L, Bogazzi F, et al: The effects of amiodarone on the thyroid. Endocr Rev 22:240, 2001.
96. Wiersinga WM: Amiodarone and the thyroid. *In* Weetman AP, Grossman A (eds): Pharmacotherapeutics of the Thyroid Gland. Berlin, Springer Verlag, 1997, pp 225-287.
97. Bogazzi F, Bartalena L, Cosci C, et al: Treatment of type II amiodarone-induced thyrotoxicosis by either iopanoic acid or glucocorticoids: A prospective, randomized study. J Clin Endocrinol Metab 88:1999, 2003.
98. Williams M, Lo Gerfo P: Thyroidectomy using local anesthesia in critically ill patients with amiodarone-induced thyrotoxicosis: A review and description of the technique. Thyroid 12:523, 2002.
99. DeGroot LJ: Dangerous dogmas in medicine: The nonthyroidal illness syndrome. J Clin Endocrinol Metab 84:151, 1999.
100. Iervasi G, Pingitore A, Landi P, et al: Low-T3 syndrome: A strong prognostic predictor of death in patients with heart disease. Circulation 107:708, 2003.
101. Portman MA, Fearneyhough C, Ning W, et al: Triiodothyronine repletion in infants during cardiopulmonary bypass for congenital heart disease. J Thorac Cardiovasc Surg 120:604, 2000.
102. Klemperer JD, Klein I, Ojamaa K, et al: Triiodothyronine therapy lowers the incidence of atrial fibrillation after cardiac operations. Ann Thorac Surg 61:1323, 1996.
103. Mainwaring RD, Capparelli E, Schell K, et al: Pharmacokinetic evaluation of triiodothyronine supplementation in children after modified Fontan procedure. Circulation 101:1423, 2000.
104. Chowdhury D, Parnell V, Ojamaa, K, et al: Usefulness of triiodothyronine (T3) treatment after surgery for complex congenital heart disease in infants and children. Am J Cardiol 84:1107, 1999.
105. Bravo EL: Pheochromocytoma. Cardiol Rev 10:44, 2002.
106. Manger WM, Gifford RW: Pheochromocytoma. J Clin Hypertens (Greenwich) 4:62, 2002.
107. Pacak K, Linehan WM, Eisenhofer G, et al: Recent advances in genetics, diagnosis, localization, and treatment of pheochromocytoma. Ann Intern Med 134:315, 2001.
108. Lenders JW, Pacak K, Eisenhofer G: New advances in the biochemical diagnosis of pheochromocytoma: Moving beyond catecholamines. Ann NY Acad Sci 970:29, 2002.
109. Schiff RL, Welsh GA: Perioperative evaluation and management of the patient with endocrine dysfunction. Med Clin North Am 87:175, 2003.
110. Eigelberger MS, Duh QY: Pheochromocytoma. Curr Treat Options Oncol 2:321, 2001.

CHAPTER 80

Hemostasis, Thrombosis, Fibrinolysis, and Cardiovascular Disease

Barbara A. Konkle • Andrew I. Schafer

Basic Mechanisms of Hemostasis and Thrombosis

The human hemostatic system has evolved as a remarkably orchestrated scheme of linked activities designed to preserve the integrity of blood circulation. Hemostasis is regulated to promote blood fluidity under normal circumstances. It is also prepared to clot blood with speed and precision to arrest blood flow and prevent exsanguination whenever and wherever the integrity of the circulation is disrupted. Finally, hemostasis has the capability to restore blood flow and perfusion upon subsequent healing of a damaged vessel. The major components of the hemostatic system are (1) the vessel wall itself, (2) plasma proteins (the coagulation and fibrinolytic factors), and (3) platelets (and probably other formed elements of blood, such as monocytes and red blood cells). These constituents function virtually inseparably (Fig. 80–1). Although this chapter discusses them individually, it is important to recognize the interdependence of the actions of the vessel wall, plasma clotting factors, and platelets.

Vascular Endothelium

Endothelial cells arise from hemangioblasts, which collect in blood islands, the precursors of blood vessels, in the yolk sac of the developing embryo.[1] Hemangioblasts differentiate into both primitive endothelial cells (angioblasts) and hematopoietic cells.[2] The endothelial cell progenitors that arise from hemangioblasts can form new blood vessels (a process termed *vasculogenesis*) under the influence of vascular endothelial growth factors and their tyrosine kinase receptors, as well as other tyrosine kinase receptors and their ligands. Endothelial cell precursors may actually circulate in adult human blood, and their numbers may increase as they participate in neovascularization (*angiogenesis*) of target tissues in response to ischemia, injury, tumor growth, and other pathological processes. Endothelial cell progenitors enter the adult circulation from bone marrow-derived angioblasts as well by shedding from the vessel wall.[3]

A monolayer of endothelial cells lines the intimal surface of the entire circulatory tree, thereby representing the only stationary cell type that components of blood ever come in contact with under normal circumstances. The endothelial surface of the adult human is enormous; it is composed of about 1 to 6×10^{13} cells, weighs approximately 1 kg, and covers a surface area equivalent to about six tennis courts.[4] Yet as recently as the first half of the 20th century, endothelial cells were viewed simply as barriers of blood flow, acting "merely in a negative manner," "similarly to a layer of paraffin or oil."[5] Today, we recognize that endothelium is a dynamic organ with complex metabolic capabilities, including the ability to control vascular permeability, the flow of biologically active molecules and nutrients, cell-cell and cell-matrix interactions within the vessel wall, blood flow and vascular tone, interactions of blood cells, the inflammatory response, and angiogenesis.

Endothelium is also an ideal regulator of hemostasis.[6] It possesses a remarkable repertoire of activities that permit it to transform rapidly from a potent antithrombotic to a prothrombotic surface wherever the need arises. Indeed, attempts to reproduce these properties clinically—for example, in cardiovascular prostheses, extracorporeal circuits, and bypass grafts—by pharmacological or even gene transfer methods have proved suboptimal.

Normal, quiescent endothelium constitutively displays a potent antithrombotic (thromboresistant) surface to blood (Fig. 80–2). It expresses anticoagulant, profibrinolytic, and platelet inhibitory properties. Whenever endothelium is activated or perturbed, however, it rapidly transforms to a prothrombotic surface that actually promotes coagulation, inhibits fibrinolysis, and activates platelets. These are not entirely uniform phenomena, however. Throughout the circulatory tree, even within a single organ, there is marked heterogeneity in the phenotype of endothelial cells. With respect to hemostasis, for example, endothelial cells from different tissues are heterogeneous in their expression of the various antithrombotic and prothrombotic mediators. Vascular bed–specific phenotypic characteristics of endothelium may account for the distinctively focal nature of thrombosis in the face of systemic abnormalities of hemostasis.[7,8] This endothelial heterogeneity depends on both genetic and environmental factors. Exposure to different microenvironmental stimuli, including variable hemodynamic forces, extracellular matrix composition, and cellular and humoral mediators, contributes significantly to the heterogeneity of endothelial phenotypes that develops throughout the circulation.

The specific antithrombotic and prothrombotic properties of endothelial cells

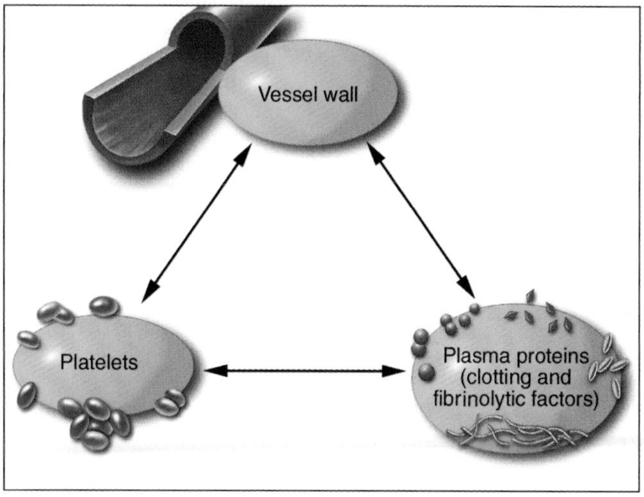

FIGURE 80–1 Interactions between the major components of the hemostatic system: the vessel wall, plasma proteins (clotting and fibrinolytic factors), and platelets.

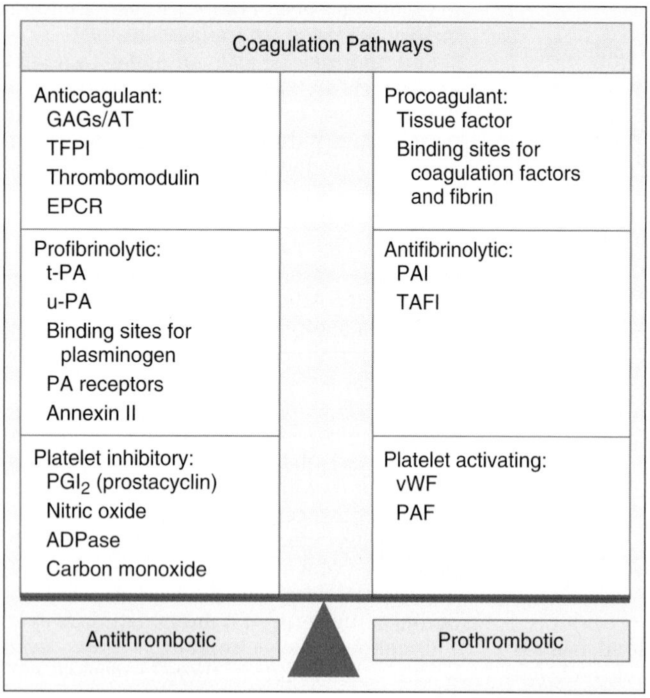

FIGURE 80–2 Balance of antithrombotic and prothrombotic properties of vascular endothelium. In general, antithrombotic properties dominate in quiescent endothelium under normal physiological conditions. In contrast, prothrombotic properties are expressed whenever endothelium is perturbed or activated. AT = antithrombin; EPCR = endothelial cell protein C receptor; GAGs = glycosaminoglycans; PAF = platelet-activating factor; PAI = plasminogen activator inhibitor; TAFI = thrombin-activatable fibrinolysis inhibitor; TFPI = tissue factor pathway inhibitor; t-PA = tissue-type plasminogen activator; u-PA = urokinase-type plasminogen activator; vWF = von Willebrand factor. (Modified from Rosendaal FR: Venous thrombosis: A multicausal disease. Lancet 353:1167, 1999.)

are described in more detail in the following sections (see Fig. 80–2). The hemostatic conversion of the vessel wall is triggered by mechanical damage or by perturbation and activation of the vascular cells by agents such as cytokines, bacterial endotoxin, hypoxia, and hemodynamic forces.

Similarly, a delicate balance exists in the capability of endothelial cells to modulate vascular tone (Fig. 80–3). An important physiological vasodilator released by endothelial cells is nitric oxide (NO), a gas synthesized from the terminal guanidino nitrogen atoms of L-arginine by the action of a group of enzymes known as nitric oxide synthases (NOSs). The major isoform of NOS present in endothelial cells, eNOS, is constitutively active and is further activated by stimuli that increase intracellular calcium, including several receptor-dependent agonists (e.g., thrombin) and hemodynamic forces (shear stress and cyclic stretch).[9] NO acts as a potent vasodilator as well as an inhibitor of platelet adhesion and platelet aggregation by stimulating soluble guanylate cyclase and thereby elevating intracellular levels of cyclic guanosine monophosphate in vascular smooth muscle cells and platelets. Prostaglandin I_2 (PGI_2, prostacyclin) is a major endothelium-derived oxygenation product of arachidonic acid, synthesized by the sequential actions of cyclooxygenase (COX) and prostacyclin synthase.[10,11] Prostacyclin, like NO, is both a vasodilator and an inhibitor of platelet aggregation (but not adhesion), exerting these actions by stimulating adenylate cyclase and thereby elevating intracellular cyclic adenosine monophosphate in target vascular smooth muscle and platelets. Endothelium-derived hyperpolarizing factor[12] and carbon monoxide, a byproduct of heme metabolism to biliverdin by heme oxygenases,[13] are also direct vasodilators elaborated by endothelial cells. Endothelial ecto-adenosine diphosphatase (ADPase), or CD39,[14] is a membrane-associated platelet inhibitor but may also indirectly promote vasodilation by generating adenosine. These vasodilator properties of endothelium are counterbalanced by endothelium-derived vasoconstrictors, including platelet-activating factor, endothelin-1, and thromboxane A_2 (TXA_2).[15,16]

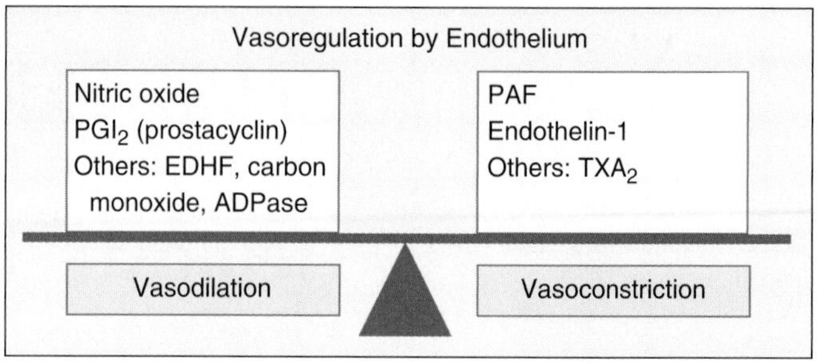

FIGURE 80–3 Regulation of vascular tone by the balance of endothelium-derived vasodilators and vasoconstrictors. ADPase = adenosine diphosphatase; EDHF = endothelium-derived hyperpolarizing factor; PAF = platelet-activating factor; TXA_2 = thromboxane A_2.

In many cases, endothelium-derived vasodilators also inhibit platelets and, conversely, endothelium-derived vasoconstrictors can also activate platelets. The net effect of vasodilation and inhibition of platelet function is to promote blood fluidity, whereas the net effect of vasoconstriction and platelet activation is to promote hemostasis. Thus, blood fluidity and hemostasis can be exquisitely regulated by the balance of antithrombotic/prothrombotic and vasodilatory/vasoconstrictor properties of endothelial cells, which are often coordinately modulated by their relative states of quiescence and activation (see Figs. 80–2 and 80–3).[6]

Coagulation

Plasma coagulation proteins ("clotting factors") normally circulate in plasma in their biologically inactive zymogen (or proenzyme) forms. When the thromboresistant nature of the vascular system is altered, by either mechanical injury or inflammatory and other systemic stimuli (e.g., coronary plaque rupture in patients who develop unstable angina), the coagulation system is activated. If the physiological antithrombotic defenses can be overwhelmed, the result will be the formation of hemostatic thrombi composed of platelets and fibrin. In cases in which focal vascular injury triggers

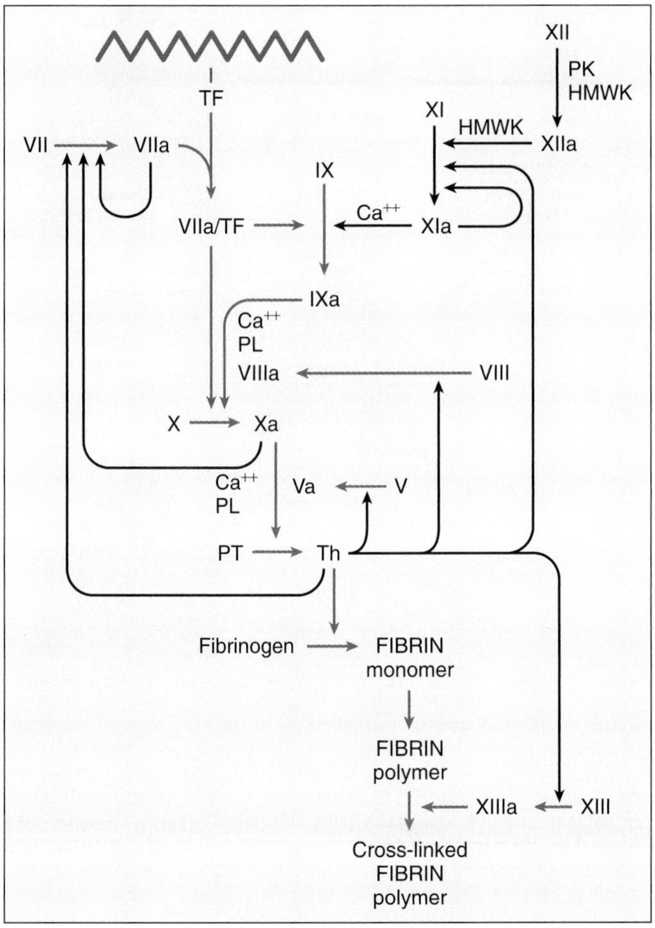

FIGURE 80–4 The coagulation cascade. This scheme emphasizes recent understanding of the importance of the tissue factor pathway in initiating clotting in vivo, the interactions between pathways, and the pivotal role of thrombin in sustaining the cascade by feedback activation of coagulation factors. HMWK = high-molecular-weight kininogen; PL = phospholipid; PT = prothrombin; TF = tissue factor; PK = prekallikrein; Th = thrombin. (Modified from Schafer AI: The primary and secondary hypercoagulable states. *In* Schafer AI [ed]: Molecular Mechanisms of Hypercoagulable States. Austin, TX, Landes Bioscience, 1997, pp 1-48.)

activation of the coagulation system, the occlusive hemostatic thrombus will be precisely localized at and limited to the site of damage.

The sequence of coagulation protein reactions that culminate in the formation of fibrin was originally described as a "waterfall" or a "cascade" (Fig. 80–4). The coagulation cascade is a highly coordinated and regulated series of linked enzymatic reactions that involves the sequential activation of plasma zymogens to serine proteases. Each protease then catalyzes the subsequent zymogen-protease transition by cleavage of peptide bonds. This creates a biochemical amplifier in which a small initiating stimulus rapidly generates high levels of the end-product fibrin. Our understanding of the coagulation cascade has been refined with the recognition that it actually involves a series of linked enzymatic multiprotein complexes, each consisting of a serine protease, one or more cofactor proteins, divalent cations, and a cellular surface (e.g., platelet membranes) on which these components can be assembled.[17,18]

Two pathways of blood coagulation have been recognized: the so-called extrinsic or tissue factor pathway and the so-called intrinsic or contact activation pathway. These two pathways of activation of the coagulation cascade converge to form a "common" pathway, which leads to the generation of the pivotal coagulation enzyme thrombin. Thrombin not only catalyzes the conversion of fibrinogen to fibrin but also serves an important role in sustaining the cascade by feedback activation of coagulation factors at several strategic sites (see Fig. 80–4).

EXTRINSIC PATHWAY. Coagulation in vivo is probably initiated through the extrinsic pathway. The immediate trigger is the injury-induced expression of tissue factor, an integral membrane glycoprotein on the surfaces of activated endothelial cells and circulating blood cells (particularly leukocytes), cells that normally do not express tissue factor activity on their surfaces.[18,19] Alternatively, vascular damage can expose blood to tissue factor expressed within the vessel wall, such as activated smooth muscle cells in atheromata, and constitutively by adventitial fibroblasts. The serine protease factor VIIa (activated factor VII) circulates in blood at trace levels but possesses very poor enzymatic activity in its free form. Exposure of blood to cell surface tissue factor activates coagulation by binding this free factor VIIa. The tissue factor/factor VIIa complex then acts as a bimolecular enzyme to accelerate the conversion of factor VII to VIIa, thereby generating more tissue factor/factor VIIa complexes and amplifying this initial hemostatic response.[20] Factor Xa and thrombin can also induce factor VII activation (see Fig. 80–4); in fact, these two enzymes may be kinetically preferred over the tissue factor/factor VIIa complex as physiological activators of factor VII. The final reaction in the extrinsic pathway is the activation of factor X to factor Xa. This can be catalyzed directly by the tissue factor/factor VIIa complex. Alternatively, this complex can activate factor X indirectly by initially converting factor IX to factor IXa (providing communication between the extrinsic and intrinsic pathways of coagulation), which then activates factor X. This indirect route of factor X activation is probably the one that is favored kinetically.

INTRINSIC PATHWAY. This pathway of coagulation is triggered by the autoactivation of factor XII to its active serine protease form (factor XIIa) on "negatively charged" surfaces, optimally in the presence of two other contact activation proteins, prekallikrein and high-molecular-weight kininogen.[21] A physiological negatively charged surface for contact activation of factor XII and the intrinsic pathway of coagulation has not been identified. However, this pathway is important in in vitro activation of coagulation, and knowledge of this pathway is necessary for interpretation of coagulation laboratory testing. In this pathway, factor XIIa converts the zymogen factor XI to its corresponding serine protease, factor XIa. Factor XIa, in turn, serves as an activator of factor IX to IXa. The final step in the intrinsic pathway is the activation of the plasma zymogen factor X to factor Xa by factor IXa, a reaction that requires the activated form of the plasma cofactor, factor VIIIa. Factor VIIIa is generated by thrombin-induced limited proteolysis of factor VIII.

The most compelling support that coagulation is not initiated by the intrinsic pathway is the clinical observation that individuals with inherited deficiencies of any of the contact activation factors (factor XII, prekallikrein, high-molecular-weight kininogen) do not have a bleeding tendency. Thus, it has been argued that this system has little to do with the initiation of hemostasis. In fact, these proteins may play important roles in other physiological systems, such as vasoregulation, and as antithrombotic and profibrinolytic agents.[22] In contrast, individuals with deficiencies of factors XI, IX, or VIII do have clinical bleeding tendencies and, therefore, these proteins in the intrinsic pathway do appear to play important roles in hemostasis. Therefore, the participation of factor XI in hemostasis probably does not depend on its activation by factor XIIa but rather on its positive feedback activation by thrombin. Thus, this positive feedback loop (see Fig. 80–4) would permit factor XIa to function in the propagation and amplification, rather than in the initiation, of the coagulation cascade.

COMMON PATHWAY. Factor Xa, which can be formed through the actions of either the tissue factor/factor VIIa complex or factor IXa (with factor VIIIa as a cofactor), initiates the common pathway of coagulation by converting the inactive plasma zymogen prothrombin to thrombin, the pivotal protease of the coagulation system. The essential cofactor for this reaction is factor Va, a plasma protein that shares about 30 percent sequence identity with the other plasma coagulation cofactor, factor VIIIa. Like the homologous factor VIIIa, factor Va is produced by thrombin-induced limited proteolysis of factor V. As noted earlier and further described later, thrombin is a multifunctional enzyme, but its major role in the common pathway is to convert soluble plasma fibrinogen to an insoluble fibrin matrix.[23] Fibrin polymerization involves an orderly process of intermolecular associations. Thrombin also activates factor XIII (fibrin-stabilizing factor) to factor XIIIa, a transglutaminase that covalently cross-links and thereby stabilizes the fibrin clot.

The coagulation cascade that culminates in fibrin formation would occur extremely inefficiently and slowly in fluid phase plasma. However, the assembly of these clotting factors on activated cell membrane surfaces greatly accelerates their reaction rates and also serves to localize blood clotting to sites of vascular injury.[18,24,25] In addition, proteases in the coagulation factor complexes assembled on cell surfaces are sequestered from inactivation by their physiological antithrombotic regulators (described later), further enhancing the efficiency of membrane-dependent reactions. The critical cell membrane components on which these coagulation reactions proceed are acidic phospholipids. These phospholipid species are not normally exposed on resting cell membrane surfaces. However, when platelets, monocytes, and endothelial cells are activated by vascular injury or inflammatory stimuli, the procoagulant head groups of the membrane anionic phospholipids translocate to the surfaces of these cells, making them available to support and promote the plasma coagulation reactions.[26]

PHOSPHOLIPID-ASSOCIATED ENZYME COMPLEXES. Major membrane phospholipid-associated enzyme complexes in the coagulation cascade include the "Xase" (or tenase) and "prothrombinase" complexes (Fig. 80–5). Each complex consists of a serine protease enzyme, its zymogen substrate, and its cofactor assembled in association with each other on the membrane surface. The extrinsic Xase complex consists of the tissue factor/factor VIIa enzyme complex and its zymogen substrates, factor IX and factor X. The intrinsic Xase complex consists of factor IXa as the enzyme, factor X as its substrate, and factor VIIIa as the cofactor. The prothrombinase complex consists of factor Xa as the enzyme, prothrombin (factor II) as its substrate, and factor Va as the cofactor. Factor IXa generated by the extrinsic Xase complex becomes the enzyme of the intrinsic Xase complex. Factor Xa generated by either the extrinsic Xase or the intrinsic Xase complex becomes the enzyme of the prothrombinase complex. These successive reaction complexes of coagulation most likely occur by diffusion of products along the same cell membrane surface.

The final enzyme product, thrombin, detaches from cell membranes and circulates in the blood to serve its multiple purposes. A major terminating reaction (see Fig. 80–5) involves membrane assembly of the protein Case complex in which free thrombin (factor IIa) binds to the integral membrane protein, thrombomodulin, which serves as the site for activation of protein C, a major antithrombotic protein discussed later in the chapter.

Anticoagulant (Antithrombotic) Mechanisms

Several physiological antithrombotic mechanisms act in concert to prevent clotting under normal circumstances.

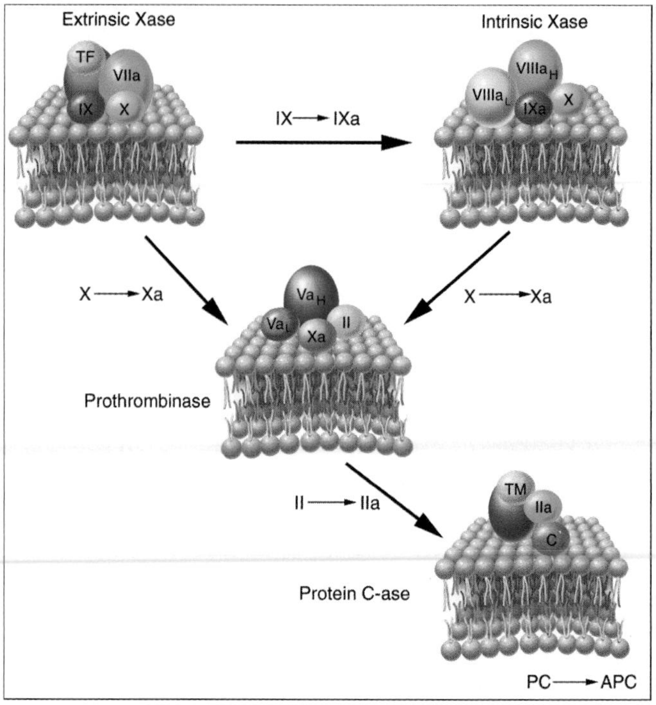

FIGURE 80–5 Schematic representation of the phospholipid membrane-associated enzyme complexes of coagulation. Each vitamin K–dependent serine protease (factors VIIa, IXa, and Xa and α-thrombin [IIa]) is shown in association with its cofactor protein (tissue factor [TF], factors VIIIa and Va, and thrombomodulin [TM]) and zymogen substrate(s) (factors IX and X, prothrombin [II] and protein C [C]) on the membrane surface. The cofactor proteins, factor VIIIa and factor Va, are characterized by a two-domain structure and consist of heavy (H) and light (L) chains that are bridged together by Ca^{2+} ions. Both domains are required for cofactor-membrane association and cofactor-protease binding. (Modified from Jenny NS, Mann KG: Coagulation cascade: An overview. *In* Loscalzo J, Schafer AI [eds]: Thrombosis and Hemorrhage. 2nd ed. Baltimore, Williams & Wilkins, 1998, pp 3-27.)

Optimal activity of each of the anticoagulant systems depends on the integrity of vascular endothelium. Thus, these physiological mechanisms operate to preserve blood fluidity in the intact circulation and also to limit blood clotting to specific focal sites of vascular injury.

Endothelial PGI_2, nitric oxide, ADPase, and carbon monoxide are physiological platelet-inhibitory mediators (see Fig. 80–2). Other anticoagulant systems are designed to limit fibrin accumulation. Several of these mechanisms, including antithrombin, the protein C/protein S/thrombomodulin system, and tissue factor pathway inhibitor (TFPI), act at different sites in the coagulation cascade to dampen fibrin accumulation. Fibrin that forms despite these anticoagulant defenses is then degraded by the fibrinolytic system. The sites of action of the major physiological antithrombotic pathways are shown in Figure 80–6.

ANTITHROMBIN. Antithrombin (or antithrombin III), the major plasma protease inhibitor of thrombin and the other clotting factors in the intrinsic and common pathways of coagulation, is a single-chain glycoprotein synthesized primarily in the liver and belonging to the serine protease inhibitor (*serpin*) family of proteins.[27,28] Antithrombin neutralizes thrombin and other activated coagulation factors by forming a complex between the active site of the enzyme and the reactive center (Arg393 and Ser394) of antithrombin. The rate of formation of these inactivating complexes increases by a factor of several thousand in the presence of heparin. This is the major anticoagulant mechanism of action of heparin (see later). Heparin and heparan sulfate proteoglycans are actually present as endogenous components of the vessel wall. Thus, antithrombin inactivation of thrombin and other

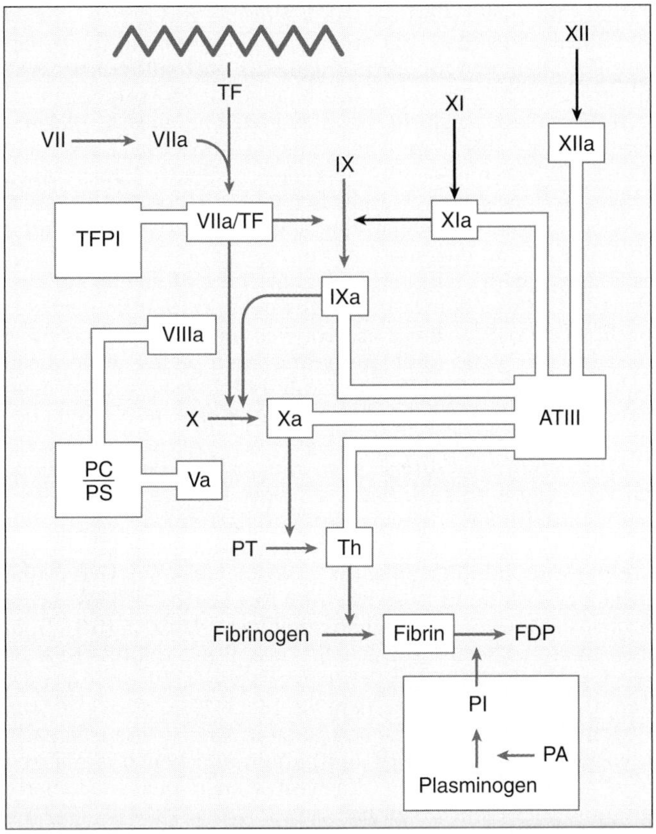

FIGURE 80–6 Sites of action of the four major physiological antithrombotic pathways: antithrombin (AT); protein C/protein S (PC/PS); tissue factor pathway inhibitor (TFPI); and the fibrinolytic system, consisting of plasminogen, plasminogen activator (PA), and plasmin (PI). (From Schafer AI: The primary and secondary hypercoagulable states. *In* Schafer AI [ed]: Molecular Mechanisms of Hypercoagulable States. Austin, TX, Landes Bioscience, 1997, pp 1-48.)

activated clotting factors probably occurs physiologically on vascular surfaces, where heparins are present to catalyze these reactions, rather than in fluid phase plasma. Inherited quantitative or qualitative deficiencies of antithrombin lead to a lifelong predisposition to venous thromboembolism.

PROTEIN Z. Protein Z–dependent protease inhibitor (ZPI) is a recently described, heparin-independent inhibitor of factor Xa.[29] Protein Z is a vitamin K–dependent protein that circulates in plasma in a complex with ZPI. Inhibition of factor Xa by ZPI, a member of the serpin superfamily of proteinase inhibitors, is enhanced 1000-fold by protein Z. The potential roles of protein Z and ZPI deficiency in thrombosis are under study.[29]

PROTEIN C/PROTEIN S/THROMBOMODULIN. Protein C is another plasma glycoprotein synthesized by the liver, which becomes an anticoagulant when it is activated by thrombin through cleavage of an Arg169-Leu170 bond in its heavy chain.[30] The thrombin-induced activation of protein C occurs physiologically on thrombomodulin, a transmembrane proteoglycan binding site for thrombin on endothelial cell surfaces.[31,32] Thrombomodulin thus serves an antithrombotic function both by binding and thereby removing thrombin from the circulation and by promoting the generation of anticoagulantly active protein C. The binding of protein C to its receptor on endothelial cells (endothelial cell protein C receptor) allows its concentration in proximity to the thrombin-thrombomodulin complex, therefore enhancing its efficiency of activation. Activated protein C acts as an anticoagulant by cleaving multiple bonds and thereby destroying the membrane-bound activated forms of coagulation factors V (Va) and VIII (VIIIa). This reaction is accelerated by a cofactor, protein S. Like protein C, protein S is a glycoprotein that undergoes vitamin K–dependent posttranslational carboxylations to form gamma-carboxyglutamic acid (Gla) residues that allow it to bind to negatively charged phospholipid surfaces. Protein S acts as a cofactor by increasing the affinity of activated protein C for phospholipids in the formation of the membrane-bound protein Case complex (see Fig. 80–5).[32] Quantitative or qualitative deficiencies of protein C or protein S, or resistance to the action of activated protein C by a specific mutation at its target cleavage site in factor Va (factor V Leiden), lead to hypercoagulable states.[28,33]

TISSUE FACTOR PATHWAY INHIBITOR. Tissue factor pathway inhibitor is a plasma protease inhibitor that regulates the tissue factor–induced extrinsic pathway of coagulation.[34] Unlike other coagulation inhibitors, which are members of the serpin family, TFPI is a multivalent Kunitz-type serine protease inhibitor. This structure permits TFPI to exert dual inhibitory actions against both tissue factor/factor VIIa (mediated by its Kunitz-1 domain binding to factor VIIa) and factor Xa (mediated by its Kunitz-2 binding to factor Xa) (see Fig. 80–6). Circulating plasma TFPI is bound to lipoproteins. TFPI can also be released by heparin from endothelial cells, where it is bound to glycosaminoglycans, and from platelets. The heparin-mediated release of TFPI may play a role in the anticoagulant effects of unfractionated and low-molecular-weight heparins.[35] Recent studies have demonstrated impairment of TFPI activity[36] and antibodies to TFPI in patients with antiphospholipid antibody syndrome.[37] Lipoprotein (a) [Lp(a)] has been shown to bind and inactivate TFPI, a novel mechanism by which Lp(a) may promote thrombosis.[38] Low levels of TFPI have also been recently reported to constitute a risk factor for venous thrombosis.[39]

THE FIBRINOLYTIC SYSTEM. Any thrombin that escapes the inhibitory effects of the physiological anticoagulant systems described earlier is available to convert fibrinogen to fibrin. In response, the endogenous fibrinolytic system is then activated to dispose of intravascular fibrin and thereby maintain or reestablish the patency of the circulation (Fig. 80–7). Just as thrombin is the key protease enzyme of the coagulation system, plasmin is the major protease enzyme of the fibrinolytic system, acting to digest fibrin to fibrin degradation products. Plasminogen, the inactive zymogen form of plasmin, is synthesized primarily in the liver and circulates in plasma in high (micromolar) concentrations. This single-chain glycoprotein has significant sequence homology with

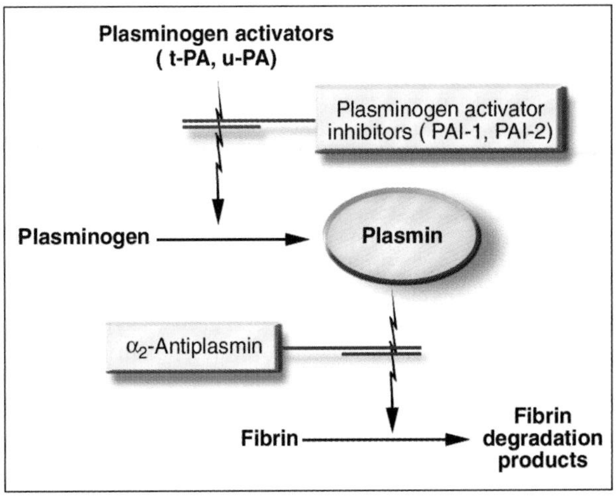

FIGURE 80–7 Scheme of the fibrinolytic system and its control. See text for explanation of abbreviations.

apolipoprotein A. Elevated plasma levels of lipoprotein A are associated with atherosclerotic cardiovascular risk (see Chap. 36).[40] Indeed, one possible atherogenic mechanism for Lp(a) might be to inhibit fibrinolysis by competing with plasminogen for plasmin generation.

Plasminogen Activators. Plasminogen activators cleave the Arg560-Val561 bond of plasminogen to generate the active enzyme plasmin, a two-chain molecule that derives its heavy chain (or A chain) from the amino-terminal region and its light chain (or B chain) from the carboxy-terminal region of plasminogen. The enzyme-active site of plasmin is localized in the B chain, whereas the A chain contains lysine-binding sites. The lysine-binding sites of plasmin (and plasminogen) permit it to bind to fibrin, so that physiological fibrinolysis is "fibrin specific."[17,41] Plasmin, a serine protease whose actions reach beyond fibrinolysis, plays important roles in tissue remodeling, wound healing, angiogenesis, and cell migration.[42]

The major physiological plasminogen activators that convert plasminogen to plasmin are tissue-type plasminogen activator (t-PA) and urokinase-type plasminogen activator (u-PA).[41] Both are serine proteases that are released by endothelial cells into plasma in trace concentrations. Plasmin can convert t-PA from its single-chain form to a two-chain molecule, in which the heavy and light chains are disulfide bonded. Both single-chain and two-chain forms of t-PA can convert plasminogen to plasmin. In contrast, single-chain u-PA (scu-PA) has little enzyme activity and must be converted to its disulfide bonded, two-chain active form by hydrolysis of a Lys158-Ile159 bond. t-PA and u-PA are released from endothelial cells by a variety of humoral factors (e.g., growth factors, hormones, and cytokines), as well as hemodynamic forces, but many of these stimuli also induce the release of plasminogen activator inhibitors.

Both plasminogen (through its lysine-binding sites) and t-PA possess specific affinity for fibrin and thereby bind selectively to clots. In the absence of fibrin, t-PA activates plasminogen to plasmin relatively slowly. Fibrin provides a surface for the sequential binding of t-PA and plasminogen. The assembly of a ternary complex, consisting of fibrin, plasminogen, and t-PA, promotes the localized interaction between plasminogen and t-PA and thereby greatly accelerates the rate of plasminogen activation to plasmin. Moreover, partial degradation of fibrin by plasmin exposes new plasminogen and t-PA binding sites in carboxy-terminus lysine residues of fibrin fragments, further enhancing these reactions. Thus, early fibrin digestion by plasmin further accelerates fibrinolysis, thereby amplifying the process. This creates a highly efficient mechanism to generate plasmin focally on the fibrin clot, which then becomes plasmin's substrate for digestion to fibrin degradation products. Thus, the fibrin surface itself is an important regulator of its own degradation by providing binding sites for fibrinolytic proteins.

In addition to its interactions with fibrin, components of the fibrinolytic system are also efficiently assembled on cell surfaces, similar to the coagulation system, to localize and kinetically optimize the generation of plasmin.[42,43] The surface of endothelial cells contain specific binding sites for plasminogen and t-PA, identified with annexin II, and other cell surfaces to catalyze plasminogen activation. u-PA receptors (u-PAR) also localize on endothelial cells and other cell types. The capacity of endothelial cells to synthesize and release plasminogen activators and then to bind these and other components of the fibrinolytic system provides a powerful paracrine mechanism to concentrate and activate fibrinolysis in proximity to intravascular thrombi contiguous to sites of endothelial damage. At the same time, receptors for the fibrinolytic proteins are also present on the surfaces of other cell types, including platelets and leukocytes that accumulate within thrombi.[42]

Plasmin cleaves fibrin at different rates at different sites of the fibrin molecule. This orderly process leads to the generation of characteristic fibrin fragments during the process of fibrinolysis. At the end of this sequential proteolysis, the D and E domains of fibrin are liberated. The sites of plasmin cleavage of fibrin are the same as those in fibrinogen. However, when plasmin acts on covalently cross-linked fibrin, D-dimers are released; hence, D-dimers can be measured in plasma as a relatively specific test of fibrin (rather than fibrinogen) degradation. Fibrin(ogen) degradation products may have potent anticoagulant and antiplatelet actions, thereby further contributing to the net antithrombotic effects of fibrinolysis. D-Dimer assays can be used as sensitive markers of blood clot formation, and some have been validated for clinical use to exclude the diagnosis of deep venous thrombosis and pulmonary embolism in selected populations (see Chap. 66).[44,45]

Fibrinolytic Inhibitors. Physiological regulation of fibrinolysis occurs primarily at two levels: (1) plasminogen activator inhibitors (PAIs), specifically PAI-1 and PAI-2, inhibit the physiological plasminogen activators, and (2) alpha$_2$-antiplasmin inhibits plasmin (see Fig. 80–7). PAI-1 is the primary inhibitor of t-PA and u-PA in plasma.[46,47] This serine protease inhibitor is a single-chain glycoprotein derived from endothelial cells and other cell types. PAI-1 inhibits t-PA by the formation of a complex between the active site of t-PA and the "bait" residues (Arg346-Met347) of PAI-1. PAI-2, which also belongs to the serpin superfamily, was originally identified in trophoblastic epithelium and hence is referred to as *placental-type PAI*.[48] Pregnant women have particularly elevated plasma levels of PAI-2.

Alpha$_2$-antiplasmin is a single-chain glycoprotein serpin that is synthesized predominantly by the liver. It is the main inhibitor of plasmin in human plasma, forming a 1:1 stoichiometric complex with plasmin that inactivates the enzyme.[41] Alpha$_2$-macroglobulin also inhibits plasmin, but at a much slower rate than alpha$_2$-antiplasmin; therefore, alpha$_2$-macroglobulin is of questionable importance in the physiological regulation of fibrinolysis.

Further regulation of fibrinolysis occurs by a unique feedback mechanism of thrombin generation via the thrombin-activatable fibrinolysis inhibitor (TAFI).[49] TAFI is activated by thrombin, a reaction that is increased more than 1000-fold in the presence of thrombomodulin. TAFI suppresses fibrinolysis through the removal of carboxy-terminal lysine residues on fibrin monomers, eliminating plasminogen and t-PA binding sites that normally serve to augment t-PA mediated conversion of plasminogen to plasmin. Elevated TAFI levels may constitute a mild risk factor for venous thrombosis.[50]

Platelets

Platelets, cytoplasmic fragments released into blood from bone marrow megakaryocytes, circulate with an average life span of 7 to 10 days.[51] These terminal cell fragments lack nuclei and therefore have limited capacity to synthesize new protein. The antithrombotic properties of intact vascular endothelium include potent platelet inhibitors (Figs. 80–2 and 80–8A). These inhibitors include PGI_2, NO, and carbon monoxide, which are labile molecules that are released by endothelial cells and act locally as autocoids, and ADPase, an ectonucleotidase of endothelial membranes that breaks down platelet-activating ADP.

PLATELET ADHESION. Vascular intimal injury diminishes locally the antiplatelet properties of endothelium, whereas previously cryptic, thrombogenic subendothelial substances (e.g., collagen) become exposed to flowing blood. Circulating platelets recognize sites of vascular disruption and adhere to the site of injury (Fig. 80–8B). Adhesion results

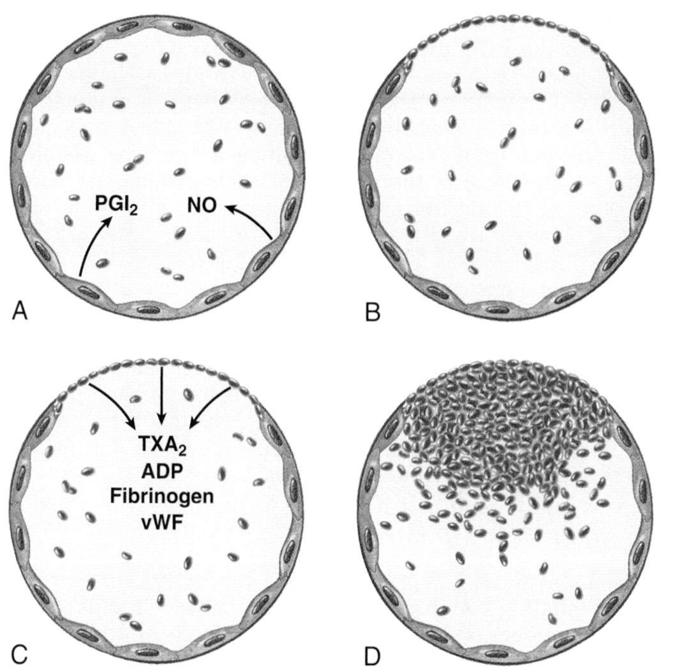

FIGURE 80–8 Sequence of events in platelet activation. **A,** Under normal conditions, a monolayer of endothelial cells lines the intimal surface of the circulatory tree, releasing platelet-inhibitory mediators such as PGI_2 (prostacyclin) and nitric oxide (NO). **B,** At a site of vascular injury (depicted from 11 o'clock to 1 o'clock), endothelium is lost and platelets undergo "adhesion" (platelet–vessel wall interactions) to subendothelial structures that are now exposed (e.g., collagen). **C,** Adherent platelets are activated and release granule constituents (e.g., ADP, fibrinogen, von Willebrand factor) and thromboxane A_2 (TXA_2). **D,** Substances released from activated platelets recruit additional platelets from the circulation to the site of injury and mediate the process of platelet "aggregation" (platelet-platelet interactions), resulting in the formation of an occlusive platelet plug.

in the formation of a monolayer of platelets that are attached to the denuded vascular intimal surface. Platelet adhesion (i.e., platelet–vessel wall interaction) is mediated primarily by von Willebrand factor (vWF), a multimeric protein consisting of a wide spectrum of polymerized subunits that create a mature protein with a molecular mass that ranges from about 550 to more than 10,000 Da, one of the largest soluble proteins in plasma.[52] vWF is synthesized by both endothelial cells and megakaryocytes, where it is stored in Weibel-Palade bodies and alpha granules, respectively, before its regulated secretion.[53] Released vWF is present in both plasma and in the extracellular matrix of the subendothelial vessel wall, to which the platelets are anchored. The large vWF multimers serve as the primary "molecular glue" to attach platelets to a damaged vessel wall with sufficient strength to withstand the high levels of shear stress that would tend to detach them with the flow of blood. The receptor for vWF on the platelet surface is localized in membrane glycoprotein (Gp) Ib, part of the platelet membrane Gp Ib/IX-V complex.[54] Higher levels of shear stress on the arterial side of the circulation promote the interaction between vWF and platelet membrane Gp Ib, probably through subtle shear-induced changes in the vWF molecule and/or its platelet receptor.[54,55] A Gp Ib–vWF dependent platelet adhesion to intact "activated" mesenteric venule endothelium under low-flow conditions has been described.[56] Platelet adhesion is also facilitated by direct binding to subendothelial collagen by means of specific platelet membrane collagen receptors, including $\alpha_2\beta_1$ integrin (also known as Gp Ia/IIa) and the immunoglobulin superfamily member Gp VI.[57,58] Under conditions of high shear stress in small arteries, Gp Ib and Gp VI may act in concert to rapidly tether platelets to the exposed extracellular matrix of the injured vessel wall through their respective ligands, vWF and collagen.[59] Subsequently, the generation of intracellular signals from Gp Ib and Gp VI leads to platelet activation (see next paragraph) and activation of integrin receptors to reinforce the initial adhesion.

PLATELET ACTIVATION. Adherent platelets then become activated (Fig. 80–8C). The platelet activation process results from the combined actions of several agonists that bind to their respective membrane receptors on adherent platelets and transmit platelet-activating intracellular signals.[60,61] These platelet stimuli include humoral mediators in plasma (e.g., epinephrine, thrombin), mediators released from activated cells (e.g., ADP, serotonin), and vessel wall extracellular matrix constituents that come in contact with adherent platelets (e.g., collagen, vWF). Several of these stimuli can activate platelets synergistically and may also act in concert with shear forces to which platelets are simultaneously exposed. Activated platelets undergo the release reaction, during which they secrete prepackaged constituents of their cytoplasmic granules: ADP, adenosine triphosphate, and serotonin from the dense granules; soluble adhesive proteins (fibrinogen, vWF, thrombospondin, fibronectin), growth factors (including platelet-derived growth factor, transforming growth factor-alpha, and transforming growth factor-beta), and procoagulants (platelet factor 4, factor V) from the alpha granules. Simultaneously, activated platelets synthesize de novo and release the potent platelet activator and vasoconstrictor TXA_2. TXA_2 is the major cyclooxygenase product of arachidonic acid metabolism in platelets. As described later in the section on antiplatelet agents, aspirin inhibits cyclooxygenase and thereby blocks TXA_2 synthesis in platelets. TXA_2 acts in concert with several of the substances released from granules to induce the activation of additional platelets in the microenvironment of the developing thrombus.[60,62]

AGGREGATION. The products of the platelet release reaction, including secreted granule constituents and TXA_2, mediate the final phase of platelet activation, the process of aggregation (Fig. 80–8D).[60,61] During platelet aggregation (platelet-platelet interaction), additional platelets are recruited from the circulation to the site of vascular injury, leading to the formation of an occlusive platelet thrombus. As discussed earlier, the platelet plug is anchored and stabilized by the fibrin mesh that develops simultaneously as the product of the coagulation cascade. At lower shear levels (e.g., in the venous circulation), the "molecular glue" that mediates aggregation is fibrinogen, which can be derived either from plasma or from the alpha-granule releasate of activated platelets. At higher shear levels (e.g., in arteries), vWF itself, which is also the ligand that mediates platelet adhesion, can substitute for fibrinogen as the ligand of aggregation. Fibrinogen or vWF binds to specific platelet membrane receptors that are located in the Gp IIb/IIIa integrin complex. Integrins are widely distributed on the surfaces of adherent eukaryotic cells. All receptors in the integrin superfamily contain an alpha and a beta subunit. Individual integrins can often bind to more than one ligand; thus, platelet Gp IIb/IIIa can recognize both fibrinogen and vWF, as well as some other adhesive proteins.

The Gp IIb/IIIa complex is the most abundant receptor on the platelet surface. Its alpha subunit (Gp IIb) is expressed specifically on platelets, but its $beta_3$ subunit (Gp IIIa) is shared by other integrins, including receptors on vascular cells. The heterodimeric, ligand-binding Gp IIb/IIIa complexes are not normally exposed in their active forms on the surfaces of quiescent circulating platelets. However, platelet activation converts Gp IIb/IIIa into competent receptors by means of specific signal transduction pathways,[63] enabling Gp IIb/IIIa to bind fibrinogen and vWF. The binding of these adhesive proteins requires that they contain the specific tripeptide sequence Arg-Gly-Asp (RGD). Recognition of

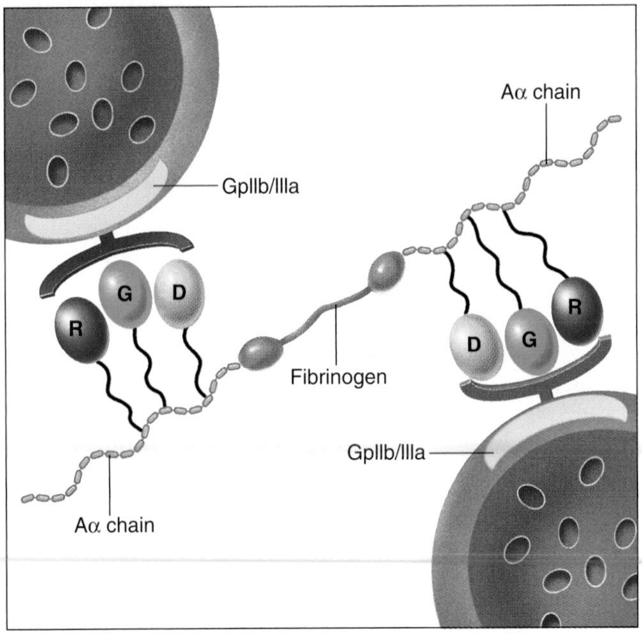

FIGURE 80–9 Linkage of two activated platelets by fibrinogen, which binds to its receptors in the platelet Gp IIb/IIIa complex by means of tripeptide RGD (arginine-glycine-aspartic acid) sequences located on the α chains of dimeric fibrinogen. The high density of Gp IIb/IIIa complexes on the surfaces of activated platelets permits the rapid formation of a network of fibrinogen bridges, leading to platelet aggregation at the site of vascular injury. (In regions of high shear stress, such as in diseased coronary arteries, von Willebrand factor may replace fibrinogen as the primary aggregating ligand. Like fibrinogen, the von Willebrand factor molecule has RGD sequences that mediate this process.) The result of platelet aggregation is the formation of an occlusive platelet thrombus. (From Schafer AI: Antiplatelet therapy with glycoprotein IIb/IIIa receptor inhibitors and other novel agents. Tex Heart Inst J 24:90, 1997.)

fibrinogen and other ligands by the active Gp IIb/IIIa complex involves the RGD tripeptide sequence (located at positions 95-97 and 572-574 of each of the two A-alpha chains of fibrinogen). When two activated platelets with functional Gp IIb/IIIa receptors each bind the same fibrinogen molecule, a fibrinogen bridge is created between the two platelets (Fig. 80–9). Because the surface of each platelet has about 50,000 Gp IIb/IIIa fibrinogen binding sites, numerous activated platelets recruited to the site of vascular injury can rapidly form an occlusive aggregate by means of a dense network of intercellular fibrinogen bridges.[64] In addition to its RGD sequences, the gamma chains of fibrinogen also contain a 12-amino acid residue (dodecapeptide HHLGGAKQAGDV) that also has the ability to bind to the platelet Gp IIb/IIIa receptor. These events of ligand binding to activated platelet membrane Gp IIb/IIIa receptors, which mediate the process of platelet aggregation, have served as targets for antiplatelet therapy with Gp IIb/IIIa antagonists.[65]

Central Role of Thrombin

Thrombin plays a pivotal role in coordinating, integrating, and regulating hemostasis. Depending on the circumstances, it can either promote or prevent blood clotting. This multifaceted effect of thrombin has been referred to as the *thrombin paradox*.[66] The balance of prothrombotic and antithrombotic activities of thrombin depends on at least three variables: (1) the concentration of free thrombin in blood, (2) the presence or absence of endothelial cells at thrombin's site of action, and, (3) the physiological state of the endothelium, if present.

When free thrombin is available in blood at high concentrations, particularly at a site of vascular injury where the antithrombotic influence of endothelium is lost, thrombin potently induces clotting (Fig. 80–10). This enzyme catalyzes several coagulation factor activation reactions that lead to fibrin formation, factor XIII activation to promote fibrin cross-linking, and activation and aggregation of platelets. In fact, under these procoagulant conditions, reciprocal, interdependent, and mutually self-amplifying interaction occurs between thrombin generation and platelet activation. Membranes of activated platelets facilitate thrombin generation by providing a surface for the assembly of coagulation factors and cofactors (Fig. 80–11; see earlier description). Conversely, thrombin is a potent activator of platelets, stimulating the availability of additional activated platelet surface for further thrombin generation. Thus, this reciprocal interaction between thrombin and platelets promotes and amplifies the formation of a tightly focused hemostatic plug composed of platelets and fibrin.

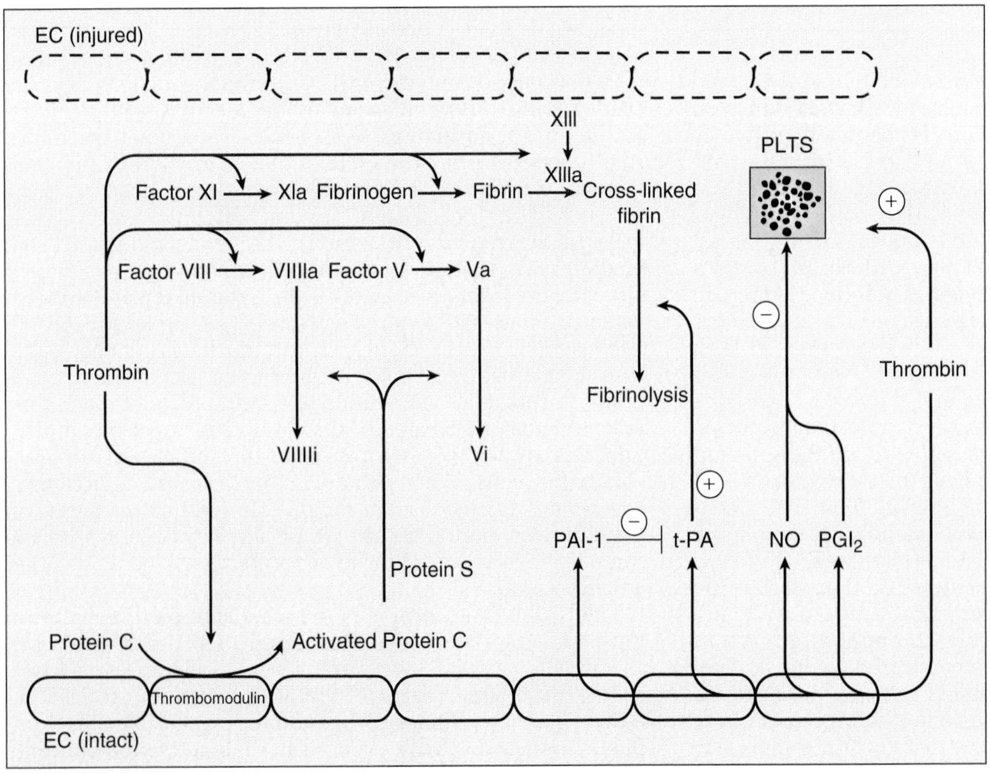

FIGURE 80–10 Central role of thrombin in modulating the state of blood coagulability, depending on the presence or absence of intact endothelial cells (EC) at its site of action. In the presence of intact EC (lower part of figure), free thrombin is removed from the circulation by EC thrombomodulin, and the antithrombotic effects of thrombin predominate: activation of protein C, release of tissue-type plasminogen activator (t-PA), and release of platelet-inhibitory nitric oxide (NO) and prostaglandin I_2 (PGI_2) by intact EC. In the absence of intact EC (upper part of figure), free thrombin is available in blood at higher concentrations and its prothrombotic effects predominate: activation of coagulation factors, fibrin formation and cross-linking, and activation of platelets (PLTS). PAI-1 = plasminogen activator inhibitor-1.

At lower concentrations of thrombin and in the presence of intact, "nonactivated," or

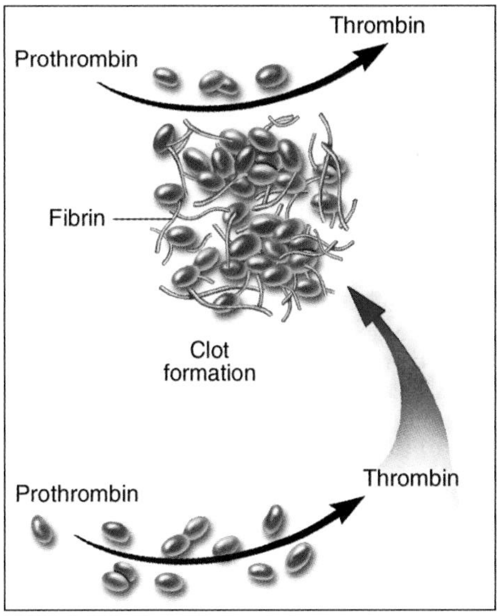

FIGURE 80–11 Reciprocal interaction between thrombin generation and platelet activation. The oval objects represent platelets. Membranes of activated platelets facilitate thrombin generation by providing a surface for assembly of coagulation factors. Conversely, thrombin is a potent activator of platelets, thus acting to promote and amplify activation of the coagulation system. This reciprocal interaction results in the accelerated and tightly focused formation of a hemostatic plug composed of platelets and fibrin. (From Schafer AI: The primary and secondary hypercoagulable states. *In* Schafer AI [ed]: Molecular Mechanisms of Hypercoagulable States. Austin, TX, Landes Bioscience, 1997, pp 1-48.)

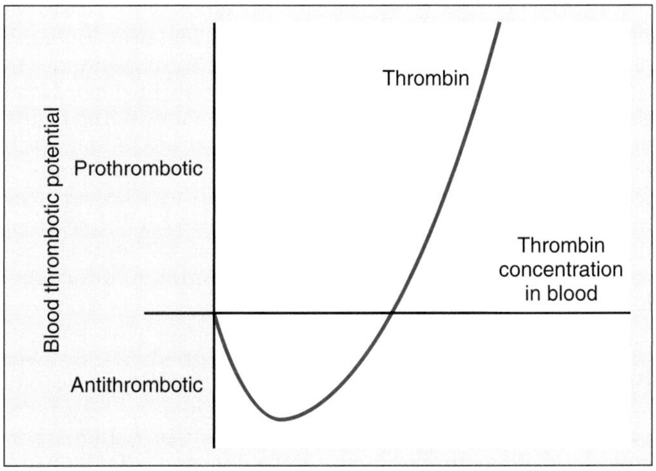

FIGURE 80–12 The thrombin paradox. At low concentrations of thrombin, protein C is activated, and elevated activated protein C exhibits antithrombotic activity. At increasingly higher levels of thrombin, the procoagulant properties of thrombin become dominant and prothrombotic potential is markedly increased. (Adapted from Griffin JH: The thrombin paradox. Nature 378:337, 1995.)

"noninflamed" endothelium, the antithrombotic effects of thrombin predominate (see Fig. 80–10). Low levels of thrombin stimulate increased levels of the endogenous circulating anticoagulant, activated protein C.[67,68] Accordingly, a J-shaped curve describes the relationship between the thrombotic potential of blood and free thrombin concentration (Fig. 80–12).[66] Furthermore, in the presence of normal endothelial cells in the intact circulation (see Fig. 80–10), endothelial thrombomodulin removes free thrombin from blood and low concentrations of thrombin stimulate t-PA release and the release of antiplatelet PGI_2 and NO from endothelial cells. Inflammation results in decreased endothelial thrombomodulin expression, diminishing its antithrombotic effect.[69] Thus, thrombin plays a central role in modulating the state

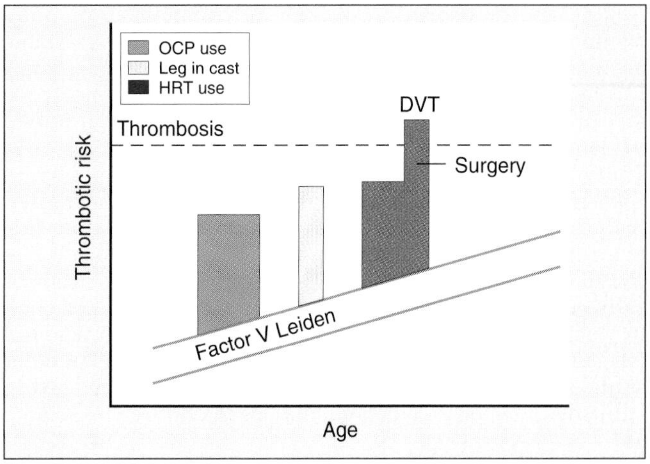

FIGURE 80–13 Thrombotic risk over time. Shown schematically is an individual's thrombotic risk over time. An underlying factor V Leiden mutation provides a "theoretically" constant increased risk. The thrombotic risk increases with age and, intermittently, oral contraceptive (OCP), hormone replacement (HRT) use, or other events increase that risk further. At some point, the cumulative risk may increase to the threshold for thrombosis and result in deep venous thrombosis (DVT). Note: The magnitude and duration of risk portrayed in the figure is meant for example only and may not precisely reflect the relative risk determined by clinical study. (Modified from Rosendaal FR: Venous thrombosis: A multicausal disease. Lancet 353:1167, 1999.)

of blood coagulability, depending on its free concentration in blood and the presence or absence of intact nonactivated endothelial cells at its site of action.

Thrombophilic Disorders

Pathological arterial or venous thromboembolism results from a complex interplay of inherited and acquired risk factors. An individual's likelihood of suffering a thrombotic event over his or her lifetime results from a combination of risk factors; an example is illustrated in Figure 80–13. Although an individual's risk at any given time cannot currently be completely defined, research is moving toward that goal. The major risk factor for arterial thrombosis in adults is atherosclerosis (see Chap. 35). This section focuses on inherited and acquired risk factors for venous or both venous and arterial thrombosis, as listed in Table 80–1.

Inherited Thrombophilia

FACTOR V LEIDEN. Factor V Leiden is the most common inherited thrombophilia, with a prevalence in whites of approximately 5 percent and as high as 20 to 40 percent in patients with venous thromboembolism (VTE), depending on selection criteria.[70,72] Factor V Leiden results from a single mutation (G1691A) in the factor V gene, which results in an arginine at amino acid 506 being replaced by a glutamine. This site is one of three activated protein C (APC) cleavage sites in factor V, by which APC, with free protein S as a cofactor, inactivates factor V and thus inhibits blood clot formation (see Fig. 80–6). Individuals heterozygous for this mutation have an approximately three- to eightfold increased risk of VTE, and those homozygous for the mutation have an approximately 50- to 80-fold increased risk of VTE. Interestingly, it appears to be a stronger risk factor for deep venous thrombosis (DVT) than for pulmonary embolism (see Chap. 66). Some investigators have speculated that a more adherent clot is formed in these individuals, which is therefore less likely to embolize. Although the mutation is most common in patients of European descent, and rare in sub-Saharan Africa and Asia, its prevalence in the United States in African Americans is approximately 1 percent, and among Asian

Americans 0.5 percent, which is as common as or more common than protein C, protein S, or AT deficiency (Table 80–2).[72-74]

Factor V Leiden does not appear to be a risk factor for myocardial infarction or ischemic stroke. This is supported by large cohort studies, including the Physician's Health Study, the Cardiovascular Health Study, and the Copenhagen City Heart Study. A meta-analysis evaluated 18 studies, including 4623 patients with myocardial infarction (7.4 percent with factor V Leiden) and 12,856 control subjects (7.4 percent with factor V Leiden).[75] One study found a statistically significant increased risk of early myocardial infarction in women who smoked cigarettes but not in women who did not smoke.[76] This finding has not been confirmed by other studies. The risk of ischemic stroke is also not increased in adults with factor V Leiden but may be in children (see Chap. 36).[72]

Women with the factor V Leiden mutation have an enhanced risk of thrombosis with hormonal therapy, including oral contraceptives and postmenopausal hormone replacement.[71,77-79] The risk of VTE with oral contraceptive use in women heterozygous for the mutation is increased 20- to 50-fold, compared to three- to fivefold in women without thrombophilia. A higher risk is seen in women using third-generation versus second-generation oral contraceptives, presumably due to the synthetic progestins used in the third-generation preparations. Since young women have a low underlying risk of DVT (approximately 1 in 10,000 per year), the number of women who will actually suffer a DVT, even when risk is increased significantly, is low in this age group. The risk of VTE in women receiving hormone replacement therapy is increased 13- to 14-fold, versus two- to fourfold in women without factor V Leiden or other identified underlying thrombophilia. Hormone-induced VTE in thrombophilic women occurs earlier after initiation of therapy than in women without an identified thrombophilia.

The factor V Leiden mutation accounts almost exclusively for the inherited form of the laboratory phenomenon of APC resistance. Rare cases of other factor V mutations affecting APC cleavage have been reported.[72] APC resistance was first described as impairment of APC-mediated prolongation of the aPTT in the plasma of selected thrombophilic patients.[80] In the absence of factor V Leiden, this abnormality has been associated with an increased risk of thrombosis, but the testing cannot be well standardized and the clinical utility of this finding is unclear. APC resistance is acquired in patients with many conditions, including hormone therapy, pregnancy, and antiphospholipid antibody syndrome, but its role in the pathogenesis of thrombosis in patients with these conditions has not been defined. Many laboratories use a factor V–specific APC resistance test that is highly sensitive and specific for the factor V Leiden mutation. Only other factor V mutations affecting APC cleavage and, rarely, lupus anticoagulants have been reported to produce false-positive results in this assay.

PROTHROMBIN GENE MUTATION. In 1996, a polymorphism in the 3′ untranslated region of the prothrombin gene (PT G20210A) was found to be associated with a two- to threefold increased risk of VTE.[28,81] This mutation is found predominantly in whites (1-6 percent), is uncommon in African Americans (0.2 percent) and is rare in other racial groups.[81,82] Although this mutation is not in the coding region of the prothrombin gene, it appears to result in increased prothrombin levels, probably by an increase in mRNA. Overall, studies do not show a greater risk of VTE recurrence in individuals heterozygous for either the factor V Leiden or the PT G20210A mutations. Thus, these states alone do not modify general recommendations for duration of anticoagulation after a single episode of VTE.

Like factor V Leiden, PT G20210A is associated with an increased risk of venous but not arterial thrombosis. Because PT G20210A is such a mild risk factor, thrombosis usually occurs in the setting of additional risk factors, either genetic or acquired. The risk of VTE is increased in patients heterozygous for both the factor V Leiden and PT G20210A mutations above that for either mutation alone. Since both are common in white populations, homozygous and compound heterozygous states are seen.

Hormonal therapy further increases the thrombotic risk in patients with PT G20210A. The VTE risk in patients heterozygous for this mutation who use OCP is increased 16-fold.[83] In addition, a markedly increased risk of cerebral

TABLE 80–1 Risk Factors for Thrombosis

Venous	Venous and Arterial
Inherited	Inherited
Factor V Leiden	Homocysteinuria
Prothrombin G20210A	Dysfibrinogenemia
Antithrombin deficiency	
Protein C deficiency	Mixed
Protein S deficiency	Hyperhomocysteinemia
Elevated factor VIII activity	
Acquired	Acquired
Age	Malignancy
Previous thrombosis	Antiphospholipid antibody syndrome
Immobilization	Hormonal therapy (oral contraceptives and hormone replacement therapy)
Major surgery	Polycythemia vera
Pregnancy and puerperium	Essential thrombocythemia
Hospitalization	Paroxysmal nocturnal hemoglobinuria
Activated protein C resistance, nongenetic	
Unknown*	
Elevated factor VII, IX, XI, von Willebrand factor	
Elevated levels of thrombin-activatable fibrinolysis inhibitor	
Low levels of tissue factor pathway inhibitor	

*Unknown whether risk factor is inherited or acquired.

TABLE 80–2 Ethnic Distribution of Inherited Thrombophilia in the United States (Prevalence %)

	Factor V Leiden	PT G20210A	↓Protein C*	↓Protein S*	↓AT*
White Americans	3-7	1-3	0.2-0.5	0.1-1	0.02-0.04
African Americans	~1	0-0.2			
Hispanic Americans	~2	†			
Asian Americans	~0.05	†			
Native Americans	~1	†			

*The prevalence of protein C, protein S, or AT deficiency is not known to vary by ethnic origin of the population tested.
†Unknown.

venous thrombosis, a rare clinical event, has been reported in women using oral contraceptives who are heterozygous for this mutation.[84]

ANTITHROMBIN DEFICIENCY. Antithrombin deficiency was the first described inherited risk factor for thrombosis.[27,28] Inherited antithrombin deficiency can be due to a quantitative (type I) or a qualitative (type II) abnormality, the latter manifest by decreased function with a normal protein level. Complete antithrombin deficiency has not been described and is likely incompatible with life. Patients with inherited type I deficiency carry the highest risk of thrombosis with a likelihood of thrombosis, based on small cohort studies, of up to 85 percent by the age of 50 years. Population studies do not support such a high risk. The discrepancy is likely due to a number of factors, including issues with testing, acquired antithrombin deficiency not carrying the same risk of thrombosis, and possible additional unrecognized genetic defects in the most affected families. In antithrombin-deficient individuals who present with thrombosis, anticoagulation is usually continued indefinitely.

While rare instances of arterial thrombosis have been reported, antithrombin deficiency is predominantly a risk for VTE. Venous thrombosis at unusual sites (including the portal and mesenteric veins) has been reported. Evaluation for antithrombin deficiency should not be done in patients with arterial thrombosis alone, except in unusual circumstances.

PROTEIN C AND S DEFICIENCIES. As described previously, free protein S serves as a cofactor for activated protein C in the inactivation of factor V and factor VIII (see Fig. 80–6). Homozygous deficiency of either protein C or S manifests in infancy as purpura fulminans. The risk of thrombosis in individuals heterozygous for these mutations is unclear, as reports vary, but is probably increased approximately 10-fold.[28,33,85] There appears to be substantial variability between affected families, which may be secondary to additional inherited factors. Factor V Leiden can be a significant cofactor in the increased thrombotic risk in families with protein C or protein S deficiency. Because factor V Leiden is so common, at least in white populations, a combination of these defects can occur and the combined effect may be enhanced by a "double-hit" of the same anticoagulant pathway. While rare cases of arterial thrombosis, particularly for protein S deficiency, have been reported, deficiencies of these proteins are predominantly, if not exclusively, risk factors for VTE. Therefore, determination of levels of protein C and protein S should not be included in an evaluation of adult patients with arterial thrombosis only.

Acquired deficiencies, not clearly associated with a thrombotic risk, and difficulties in laboratory testing, make diagnosis of these deficiencies challenging.[33,85] Ideally, an inherited deficiency is confirmed in family members. Proteins C and S are affected by vitamin K deficiency, warfarin ingestion, and liver disease, all of which tend to reduce their levels. Mildly decreased protein C levels can be an early marker of liver disease. Approaches to diagnosing protein C or protein S deficiency in patients on warfarin have been proposed by comparing values with other vitamin K–dependent factors. However, relationships between factor levels in patients on warfarin have significant interpatient variability, and this approach has not been validated.

Functional protein S assays are used as initial testing for protein S deficiency in many laboratories.[85] This test is known to have a significant false-positive rate and should not be used alone to diagnose protein S deficiency without further testing or family studies. Acquired protein S deficiency, particularly a low free protein S level, occurs in a number of settings, including pregnancy, inflammatory states, and hormone use. Although a decreased level of free protein S with a normal total protein S level is frequently an acquired

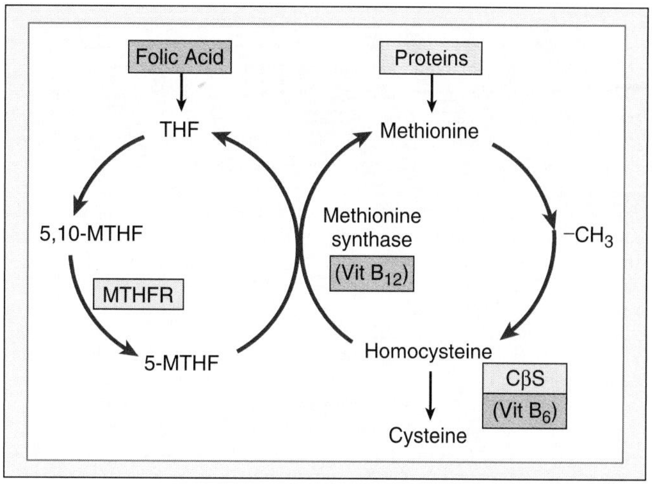

FIGURE 80–14 Homocysteine metabolism. Metabolism of homocysteine can occur through remethylation to methionine, a reaction that requires the enzyme methionine synthase and the cofactor, vitamin B12, or through transsulfuration to cysteine, via initial condensation with serine to form cystathionine, in a reaction catalyzed by cystathionine-β-synthase (CβS) followed by hydrolysis by the enzyme γ-cystathionase to cysteine and α-ketobutyrate. Both steps in the transsulfuration pathway require vitamin B6 as a cofactor. In the liver, remethylation also occurs with betaine as the methyl donor (not shown). Methyltetrahydrofolate is derived from the reduction of 5,10-methylene-tetrathydrofolate in a reaction catalyzed by methylene-tetrahydrofolate reductase (MTHFR). Enzymes in which mutations occur that may increase thrombotic risk are depicted in blue. Vitamins, supplementation with which is used for therapy, are depicted in red. MTHF = methylene-tetrahydrofolate; THF = tetrahydrofolate.

condition, individuals with inherited deficiency may have a similar picture (type III deficiency or type I in older individuals), making the distinction difficult. A diagnosis of protein S deficiency should be made with caution in individuals taking medications or in those with conditions known to affect protein S levels.

HOMOCYSTEINE. Homocysteine is a sulfhydryl amino acid formed from the demethylation of dietary methionine (Fig. 80–14).[86] Homocysteine can be remethylated to methionine by donation of a methyl group from (1) methyltetrahydrofolate (MTHF) in a reaction catalyzed by methionine synthase using vitamin B12 as an essential cofactor, or from (2) betaine. MTHF is derived from the reduction of 5-10, methylene tetrahydrofolate in a reaction catalyzed by MTHF reductase (MTHFR). Homocysteine is also condensed with serine to form cystathionine, a reaction catalyzed by cystathionine beta-synthase (CβS). Vitamin B6 is an essential cofactor in this reaction.

Patients with severe deficiencies in the enzymes methionine synthase, MTHFR, and, particularly, CβS can have marked elevations in plasma homocysteine (hyperhomocysteinemia) and suffer from premature atherosclerosis and arterial and venous thrombosis.[86] Homocysteinuria, due almost exclusively to homozygous CβS deficiency, is rare, with a frequency in the general population of 1 in 250,000, and is manifest by mental retardation, ectopic lenses, and skeletal abnormalities, as well as premature atherosclerosis and thrombosis. Approximately 25 percent of affected individuals will suffer a vascular occlusive event by 16 years of age and approximately 50 percent will do so by 29 years of age. In a review of reported cases, 51 percent were VTE, 32 percent were cerebrovascular accidents, 11 percent were peripheral vascular disease, and 4 percent were myocardial infarctions. Pathogenic effects of markedly elevated homocysteine levels are supported by in vitro studies and include induction of smooth muscle proliferation, accelerated oxidation of low-density lipoprotein cholesterol, direct endothelial toxicity, impairment of endothelial derived NO, decreased synthesis of heparan sulfate, proteoglycan synthesis, and induction of proinflammatory changes including increased tissue factor synthesis, decreased cell-surface expression of thrombomodulin, and increased expression of vascular adhesion molecule-1.[86,87]

The strong association of markedly elevated homocysteine levels with atherosclerotic and thrombotic disease prompted the evaluation of the effects of less marked elevations of homocysteine[88] (see Chap. 36). Mild (16-24 μmol/liter) or moderate (25-100 μmol/liter) hyperhomocysteinemia usually results from mutations in MTHFR and/or acquired dietary deficiencies of vitamin B12, folic acid, or vitamin B6, which are cofactors in homocysteine metabolism. The relationship of hyperhomocysteinemia to atherosclerotic vascular disease has been evaluated primarily by retrospective case-control studies but also by some prospective studies. One meta-analysis of 27 retrospective case-control studies demonstrated that for each 5 μmol/liter incremental rise in total plasma homocysteine, the odds ratios for coronary artery disease and cerebrovascular disease were 1.6 and 1.5, respectively. However, when studied prospectively, the relationship has not been found to be as strong, and a meta-analysis of prospective studies suggested at best a weak association.[86]

In assessing VTE risk, two meta-analyses found a 2.5 to 3 pooled odds ratio of VTE in individuals with an elevated fasting homoscysteine level.[86,89] While MTHFR mutations that can result in higher plasma homocysteine levels are common, it is the fasting plasma homocysteine levels, and not the presence of specific mutations, that correlate with increased thrombotic risk.[90] In a recent study evaluating genetic (five common functional polymorphisms in MTHFR) and nutritional factors contributing to hyperhomocysteinemia, the genetic contribution to the variance in homocysteine levels was estimated to be approximately 9 percent, compared with approximately 35 percent that could be attributed to low levels of folate and vitamin B12.[91] In evaluating patients for hyperhomocysteinemia, methionine loading to detect elevated plasma homocysteine not detected by fasting studies is probably not needed. Many small studies evaluating thrombophilic factors have reported that elevated homocysteine levels further increase the risk of thrombosis in individuals with other causes of thrombophilia.[92]

Elevated plasma homocysteine levels are usually responsive to vitamin supplementation, particularly folic acid supplementation. Implementation of folic acid fortification programs results in decreased rates of folic acid deficiency.[93] While vitamin supplementation can biochemically correct hyperhomocysteinemia, the clinical efficacy of such intervention in preventing thrombotic and vascular complications is currently under study. However, since oral supplementation with folic acid, vitamin B12, and vitamin B6 is an easily tolerated treatment, inclusion of fasting homocysteine levels in a thrombophilia evaluation and institution of treatment, if they are elevated, seems warranted.

OTHERS. Recent studies have provided data that increased levels of procoagulants may be associated with an increased risk of thrombosis.[94] The strongest association is with elevated factor VIII levels.[95] Persistently elevated factor VIII levels, remote from acute events, can be inherited, and in that setting have been found to increase the risk of VTE fivefold (individuals with factor VIII >150 U/dl versus those with factor VIII <100 U/dl). As a risk factor for thrombosis, factor VIII levels are independent of vWF levels. Elevated vWF levels were found to be a risk factor for VTE independent of factor VIII levels in one study,[96] but not in another.[97] Elevated factor VIII levels may increase the risk of VTE recurrence, with the highest levels imparting the greatest risk. One study found a 37 percent likelihood of recurrence at 2 years in individuals with factor VIII levels above the 90th percentile of the normal range.[98] Since factor VIII is an acute-phase reactant, it is important that if testing is performed, this be done remote from an acute event.

Elevated fibrinogen levels are associated with an increased risk of atherothrombotic disease, but not VTE. However, this likely reflects an inflammatory response, and inherited factors resulting in increased fibrinogen have not been clearly associated with an increased risk of thrombosis (see Chap. 36).[94,96] Also, lowering fibrinogen levels has not been shown to decrease risk. Increased prothrombin (factor II) levels not due to the prothrombin G20210A mutation has been associated with an increased risk of thrombosis, similar to that seen in individuals with the PT G20210A mutation.[83] Elevated factor IX, XI, or VII levels may be weakly associated with an increased risk of VTE.[94,96] Other than for factor VIII, there is no evidence that levels of these factors should alter management of VTE at this time. In the future, multiple levels may be assessed in a multifactorial approach to thrombotic risk. Until such an approach is validated in clinical study, testing these factors as part of a routine thrombophilia evaluation cannot be recommended.

Inherited heparin cofactor II deficiency is currently not considered a strong risk factor for thrombosis, although it may contribute to thrombotic risk when combined with other thrombophilias. Routine testing of patients with thromboembolic disease for heparin cofactor II deficiency is not recommended. Qualitative abnormalities of fibrinogen (dysfibrinogenemias) are usually associated with no clinical manifestations, although both mild bleeding symptoms and venous or arterial thrombosis have been reported. These are inherited in an autosomal dominant fashion. Because thrombosis-related dysfibrinogenemia is so rare, its inclusion in a thrombophilia evaluation is not routine.[99] Plasminogen deficiency, previously proposed as a thrombophilic condition, has not been substantiated in studies of deficient families.

Acquired Thrombophilia

Most instances of VTE are at least partially due to acquired conditions. Age itself is a strong risk factor for VTE, with the underlying risk in octogenarians (baseline risk of approximately 1 in 100 per year) 100-fold that of young children (baseline risk of approximately 1 in 100,000 per year).[71] Thrombotic risk in acquired situations as assessed in the Leiden Thrombophilia Study are shown in Table 80–3. Malignancy is strongly associated with thrombosis and should always be considered in adults who present with thrombosis, particularly if it is apparently "idiopathic" in individuals without a family history of thrombosis. Evaluations in these individuals beyond age-appropriate recommended cancer screening has not been shown to prolong survival.[100] Many individuals presenting with thrombosis and diagnosed with malignancy have abnormalities on physical examination or routine laboratory or radiological studies. A frequent laboratory finding in this setting is unexplained anemia. Individuals with myeloproliferative disorders, notably polycythemia vera and essential thrombocythemia, have an increased risk of venous and arterial thrombosis, and a complete blood cell count should be part of a thrombophilia evaluation. Although uncommon, essential thrombocythemia has been reported as a cause of myocardial infarction, particularly in young women.

HORMONAL THERAPY. Hormonal therapy carries an increased risk of VTE, and this risk may be increased significantly in thrombophilic women, as discussed earlier in this chapter (see also Chap. 73). Second-generation oral contraceptives and hormone replacement therapy increase the risk of thrombosis two- to fourfold.[79,101,102] Because middle-aged women have an underlying risk of VTE approximately 10-fold greater than that of young women, they are more likely to experience thrombosis when placed on hormonal therapy. Third-generation oral contraceptives, which contain less estrogen and a different progestin, are associated with a twofold increased risk of VTE compared to second-generation products. This surprising finding of increased risk, which has been confirmed in a number of large studies, is presumably due to the progestins in the third-generation preparations. Oral contraceptive use is associated with an increased risk of peripheral arterial disease[103] and a modest increase in myocardial infarction.[104] The pathogenesis of hormone-induced thrombosis is not clear. Estrogens have many differ-

TABLE 80–3 Thrombosis Risk in Acquired Situations: Data from the Leiden Thrombophilia Study

Risk Factor	Patients (n = 474), n (%)	Controls (n = 474), n (%)	Odds Ratio	95% Confidence Interval
Surgery	85 (18)	17 (3.6)	5.9	3.4-10.1
Hospitalization	59 (12)	6 (1.3)	11.1	4.7-25.9
Immobilization	17 (3.6)	2 (0.4)	8.9	2.0-38.2
Pregnancy	8 (5.0)	2 (1.3)	4.2	0.9-19.9
Puerperium	13 (8.2)	1 (0.6)	14.1	1.8-109
Oral contraceptives	109 (70)	65 (38)	3.8	2.4-6.0

From the Leiden Thrombophilia Study, a population based case-control study. Cases were unselected consecutive patients aged 18-70 years with a first objectively diagnosed deep vein thrombosis, and controls were acquaintances of cases or spouses of (other) cases. Controls were matched for age and sex and subjects with active malignancies were excluded. Time window for surgery, hospitalization (without surgery), and immobilization (not in the hospital, immobilized >13 days) was 1 year preceding the index date. For puerperium, it was delivery 30 days or less before the index date and for pregnancy and oral contraceptives it was at the index date. Data on pregnancy, puerperium, and oral contraceptive use refer to women of childbearing age only.

Adapted from Bauer KA, Rosendaal FR, Heit JA: Hypercoagulability: Too many tests, too much conflicting data. Hematology. Am Soc Hematol Edu Program Book 353, 2002.

ent effects on the coagulation system that include increases in procoagulant factors, reductions in free protein S and antithrombin, and acquired protein C resistance. Hormone-induced increases in fibrinolytic activity do not counterbalance this procoagulant effect.[101]

ANTIPHOSPHOLIPID ANTIBODY SYNDROME (APS). APS is defined by a characteristic constellation of clinical and laboratory abnormalities, including an increased risk of thrombosis.[105-107] Clinical findings can include unexplained venous or arterial thrombosis and pregnancy morbidity, including repeated miscarriages or fetal growth retardation. These are associated with persistent antibodies to certain phospholipid binding proteins. These antibodies, and particularly antibodies to the phospholipid cardiolipin (anticardiolipin antibodies, ACA), can be induced by infections or drugs, but in those settings they are not clearly associated with thrombosis. "True" APS likely results from an autoimmune reaction, either not associated with a defined autoimmune disorder, designated primary APS, or associated with an autoimmune disease, such as systemic lupus erythematosus, designated secondary APS.

In the 1990s, work from a number of laboratories clarified that the antibodies found in individuals with this syndrome were actually directed against phospholipid-binding proteins, not against the phospholipid itself. Actually, most positive ACA reactions require beta$_2$-glycoprotein 1 (β_2GP1) in the assay. β_2GP1 is an abundant protein in bovine and human plasma and thus is present in many assays without specifically being added. Antibodies against other phospholipid-binding proteins, most notably against prothrombin, but also against protein C, protein S, annexin V, and tissue factor pathway inhibitor, can also be found in patients with this syndrome. The role these autoantibodies play in the pathogenesis of APS has not been elucidated, although many studies are under way. Two mechanisms proposed whereby antiphospholipid antibodies promote thrombosis are as follows: (1) interfering with phospholipid-dependent anticoagulant pathways, including APC and TFPI functions, and (2) binding to cell surfaces and inducing cell activation.[107]

Patients with APS may have antibodies that react only in an immunoassay, as described, or that interfere with phospholipid dependent tests (termed *lupus anticoagulants*), or both. The presence of antibodies to β_2GP1 appear to be better predictors of thrombosis than antibodies to prothrombin, but testing for anti-β_2GP1 antibodies has not clearly been shown to improve the diagnosis of APS over the use of ACA determinations alone. Anti-prothrombin antibodies do not prevent conversion of prothrombin to thrombin but may result in prothrombin deficiency, which rarely is associated with bleeding, in contrast to the more characteristic thrombotic tendency of APS. A pattern of positive ACA and negative anti-β_2GP1 antibodies is seen in cases of infection, and in that setting it has not been associated with thrombosis.

A number of laboratory tests are used to diagnose lupus anticoagulants.[105,108] Many of these tests have been developed to detect lupus anticoagulants by modifications that make them more sensitive to interactions of the antibody with the phospholipid component of the assay. The aPTT can be prolonged, depending on the strength of the lupus anticoagulants and the aPTT reagent used. A widely used test, which when yielding positive results probably correlates best with an increased risk of thrombosis, is the dilute Russell viper venom test (dRVVT). Russell viper venom activates factor X directly, and results of the test are affected by underlying conditions or drugs that decrease common pathway factors. Prolongation of the dRVVT corrects with mixing with normal plasma if the prolongation is due to factor deficiency, which could be inherited, or it could be secondary to liver disease, vitamin K deficiency, or warfarin therapy. Heparin functions as an inhibitor and the finding does not correct when mixed with normal plasma, resulting in a false-positive test result. Many dRVVT assay procedures absorb out heparin, eliminating this problem; however, if positive values are found in a patient on heparin, the test should be repeated with the patient off heparin at a later date to confirm the finding. Laboratory confirmation of a lupus anticoagulant requires prolongation of a phospholipid-dependent test that does not correct with mixing but does correct with the addition of the correct phospholipid, usually a hexagonal phase phospholipid or platelet membranes (platelet neutralization procedure).

Antiphospholipid antibody syndrome can be manifest by arterial and/or venous thrombosis. Recurrence rates in patients with "true" APS have been reported to be as high as 70 percent, making this an indication for long-term anticoagulation. Patients with systemic lupus erythematosus or rheumatoid arthritis with persistently positive ACA or lupus anticoagulant have a higher rate of venous and arterial thrombosis than those without these laboratory findings. Recent studies have raised questions about the need for routine warfarin anticoagulation in these individuals above an international normalized ratio (INR) of 2 to 3, as previously proposed. However, there is a subset of patients who will develop recurrent arterial or venous thrombosis, even at higher levels of anticoagulation, who require alternative prophylactic approaches.

Diagnosis of APS based on laboratory findings, particularly ACA or anti-β_2GP1 antibody positivity alone, is problematic. The association of IgM ACA or anti-β_2GP1 antibodies or low titer IgG antibodies with thrombosis has not been documented by clinical study.[105-110] Many individuals without evidence of underlying disease have circulating ACA, including approximately 7 percent of normal blood donors. In data from the Physician's Health Study, there was no difference in the incidence of arterial or venous thrombosis in subjects testing positive versus those testing negative for ACA. In a recent meta-analysis of published studies (1988-2000), lupus anticoagulants and, less strongly, IgG ACA at medium or high titer, were associated with thrombosis.[110]

Most, but not all, patients who are positive for lupus anticoagulants also have ACA or anti-β_2GP1 antibodies. β_2GP1 has a weak affinity for binding to physiological procoagulant phospholipids. In the presence of such phospholipids, some anti-β_2GP1 antibodies can cross-link two phospholipid-bound β_2GP1 molecules, thereby attaching these with high affinity to the phospholipid surface.[107] It has been postulated that only anti-β_2GP1 antibodies with lupus anticoagulant activity can do this. If this mechanism were involved in the pathogenesis of APS, this would be consistent with the stronger association of thrombosis with lupus anticoagulant than with positive anti-β_2GP1 antibodies or ACA detected by immunoassay only.

Antithrombotic Drugs

Heparin and Related Drugs

Because its onset of action is practically immediate when administered parenterally, heparin is the anticoagulant of choice when rapid anticoagulation is required.[111] Commercial preparations of unfractionated heparin consist of a heterogeneous mixture of glycosaminoglycans, with molecular weights ranging from 3000 to 30,000.[35] However, only about one-third of the molecules in these products are anticoagulantly active. Heparin exerts its anticoagulant effect by interacting with antithrombin (Fig. 80–15). A specific pentasaccharide sequence in heparin accounts for its ability to bind with high affinity to lysine sites on antithrombin. In the absence of heparin, antithrombin binds to and neutralizes thrombin and other activated clotting factors (see earlier) slowly; however, heparin-bound antithrombin undergoes a conformational change that dramatically accelerates its ability to bind to and neutralize these factors. In these reactions, arginine reactive centers in antithrombin bind to the enzyme active center serines of thrombin and other serine protease coagulation factors, thereby inhibiting their activities. Heparin then dissociates from these complexes and can be reused to bind to other antithrombin molecules. Heparin thus acts as a true catalyst in accelerating the neutralization of thrombin and other activated clotting factors by antithrombin.[112] Fibrin-bound thrombin is relatively protected from inactivation by the heparin/ antithrombin complex.

Heparin is poorly absorbed from the gastrointestinal tract and therefore is administered parenterally. The complex pharmacokinetics of unfractionated heparin is due to its nonspecific binding to many plasma proteins (including some acute-phase reactants) and to vascular and blood cells. Provided that the doses used are adequate, the efficacy and safety of heparin are comparable when administered by continuous intravenous infusion or by subcutaneous injection.[112] Intermittent intravenous injections of heparin are associated with more bleeding complications than is continuous intravenous infusion.

UNFRACTIONATED HEPARIN MONITORING. Because of unfractionated heparin's often unpredictable pharmacokinetics and its narrow therapeutic range, therapy with this agent requires laboratory monitoring for proper dosing.[111] This is performed conventionally with the activated partial thromboplastin time (aPTT), a test sensitive to the inhibitory effects of heparin on thrombin, factor Xa, and factor IXa. For the treatment of DVT or pulmonary embolism, weight-based nomograms have been recommended because this approach results in more prompt anticoagulation without an increased risk of bleeding compared with other approaches. Treatment is initiated with an 80 U/kg bolus, followed by 18 U/kg/hr, with a target aPTT that has been standardized in the laboratory to reflect heparin levels measured by anti-Xa levels of 0.3 to 0.7 U/ml. The aPTT is sensitive over a heparin range of 0.1 to 1.0 U/ml. Because the aPTT becomes immeasurably prolonged at heparin concentrations of more than 1.0 U/ml, this test is unsuitable for monitoring heparin dosage during percutaneous coronary interventions (angioplasty and stenting) and during cardiac bypass surgery, in which patients require higher levels of anticoagulation with heparin. In these procedures, heparin can be monitored by the activated clotting time, because this test provides a graded response to heparin concentrations in the range of 1 to 5 U/ml. Low-dose subcutaneous unfractionated heparin has also been used to prevent (rather than treat) venous thromboembolism in high-risk patients. Doses of 5000 U every 8 or 12 hours generally

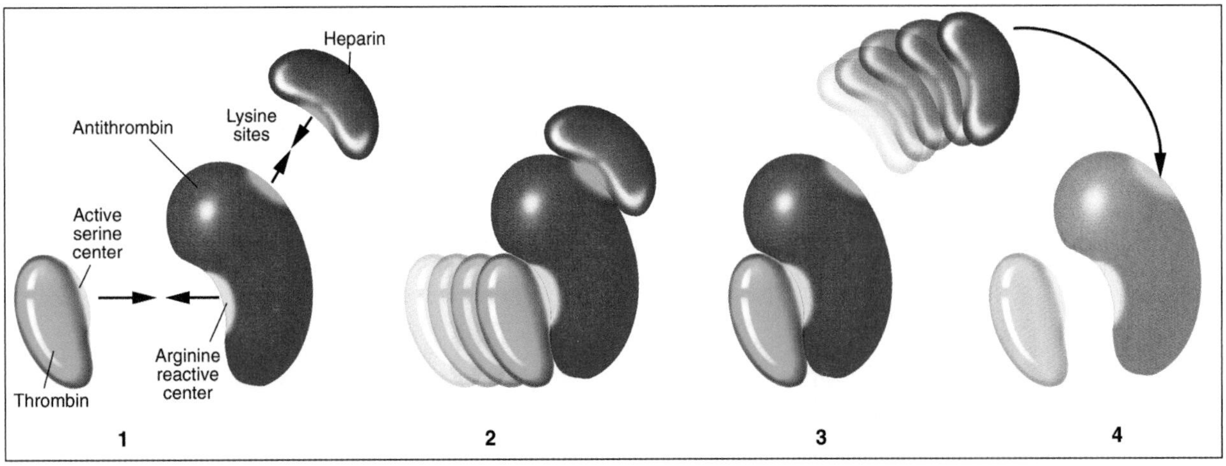

FIGURE 80–15 Mechanism of heparin action. See text for explanation. (Modified from Rosenberg RD: Hemorrhagic disorders: I. Protein interactions in the clotting mechanism. *In* Beck WS [ed]: Hematology. 5th ed. Cambridge, MIT Press, 1991, pp 507-542.)

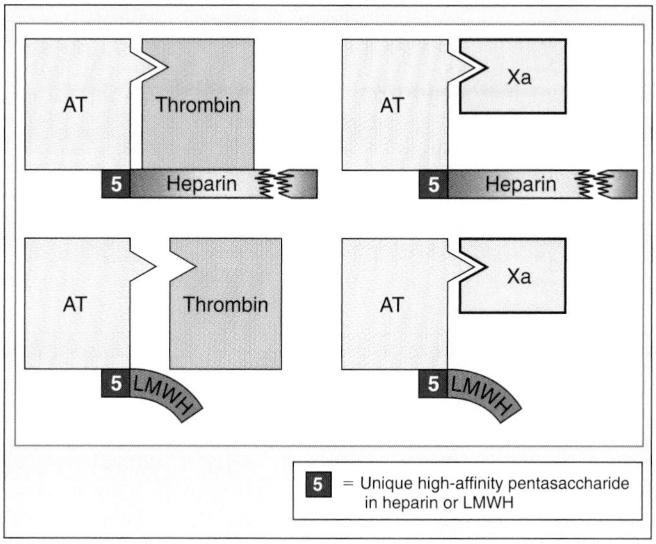

FIGURE 80–16 Mechanisms of inhibitory action of unfractionated heparin (heparin) and low-molecular-weight heparin (LMWH) on thrombin and factor Xa. Both unfractionated heparin and LMWH bind to antithrombin (AT) through a high-affinity pentasaccharide sequence (5) that both types of heparin contain. Inhibition of thrombin (left side of figure) requires formation of a ternary complex of heparin with both antithrombin and thrombin. Unfractionated heparins have sufficient length (≥18 saccharide residues, including the pentasaccharide sequence) to accomplish this, but LMWHs do not. In contrast, inhibition of factor Xa (right side of figure) requires that heparin bind only to antithrombin, which unfractionated heparin and LMWH can catalyze equally effectively through their common pentasaccharide sequences. Thus, LMWH (but not unfractionated heparin) inactivates factor Xa selectively relative to thrombin.

do not prolong the aPTT and therefore do not require monitoring in this setting.

LOW-MOLECULAR-WEIGHT HEPARINS. Low-molecular-weight heparins (LMWH) are manufactured from standard, unfractionated heparin by chemical or enzymatic depolymerization that yields fragments about one-third the size of unfractionated heparin.[35,111] Inhibition of thrombin requires that heparin bind to both antithrombin and thrombin, thereby forming a ternary complex (Fig. 80–16). Ternary complex formation requires that heparin contain at least 18 saccharide residues, including the high-affinity pentasaccharide sequence that binds to antithrombin. In contrast, inhibition of factor Xa requires that heparin bind only to antithrombin; hence, only the pentasaccharide sequence of heparin is needed for this simpler reaction. Most heparin chains in LMWH preparations have fewer than 18 saccharide units and therefore are of insufficient length to bind to both antithrombin and thrombin. However, the shorter heparin fragments in LMWH are able to catalyze the inhibition of factor Xa by antithrombin, provided that they contain the essential pentasaccharide sequence. Thus, the effects of LMWH in the coagulation cascade are restricted to relatively selective inactivation of factor Xa, whereas standard (unfractionated) heparin has equivalent inhibitory activity against factor Xa and thrombin.

Low-molecular-weight heparin has theoretical advantages over standard heparin for several additional reasons[113] First, unlike unfractionated heparin, it can inhibit platelet-bound factor Xa and therefore should be a more effective anticoagulant. Second, LMWH binds less readily to plasma proteins (including acute phase reactants) and vascular and blood cells, and LMWH is more resistant to neutralization by platelet factor 4; this produces a longer plasma half-life, more predictable bioavailability, and more favorable pharmacokinetics than standard heparin. Third, LMWH has less pronounced effects on platelet function and vascular integrity, properties that presumably contribute to its lower risk of bleeding complications than standard heparin. The longer plasma half-life and more predictable anticoagulant response of LMWH preparations allow their administration as fixed-dose, once-daily or twice-daily subcutaneous injections, without need for laboratory monitoring. The convenience of use of LMWH has been extended to outpatient management of patients with uncomplicated acute venous thromboembolism, a situation that previously required continuous intravenous heparin infusion in the hospital. Although several LMWH preparations have been approved for use in North America and Europe, they are prepared by different depolymerization methods and have somewhat different molecular compositions, pharmacological properties, and anticoagulant profiles.[114,115] Therefore, caution may need to be exercised in the interchangeability of these LMWH products.

COMPLICATIONS OF HEPARIN AND LMWH. The major complication of heparin is bleeding. Early studies suggested that treatment with LMWH caused significantly less bleeding than with unfractionated heparin; however, data from more recent and larger studies do not show as great a difference in bleeding risks between the two preparations (see Chap. 47). Factors that predispose to increased bleeding risk include advanced age, serious concurrent illness, heavy consumption of alcohol, concomitant use of aspirin, and renal failure.[35] LMWHs are cleared by renal excretion and should be used with caution in patients with renal insufficiency. In the TIMI 11A trial, a multicenter dose-ranging trial to evaluate the safety of enoxaparin in the treatment of patients with non-ST-segment elevation acute coronary syndrome, patients with a creatine clearance of less than 40 ml/min had higher trough and peak anti-Xa activity and were more likely to have major hemorrhagic events than subjects with normal renal function.[116]

Due to the relatively short half-life of unfractionated heparin, simple discontinuation is usually adequate to control bleeding complications. Protamine sulfate can be used in emergency situations with serious bleeding. Protamine, a strongly basic protein, practically instantaneously neutralizes heparin, which is highly negatively charged. Protamine is effective in neutralizing the antithrombin activity of LMWH but does not completely reverse its anti-factor X activity.

Two distinct types of thrombocytopenia are associated with heparin therapy.[117] The more common form, which may occur in up to 15 percent of patients receiving therapeutic doses of heparin, is a benign and self-limited side effect. This dose-dependent, non-immune-mediated type of thrombocytopenia rarely causes severe reductions in the platelet count or clinical complications and usually does not require discontinuation of heparin. In contrast, the immune form of heparin-induced thrombocytopenia (HIT) can, paradoxically, cause serious, limb- and life-threatening arterial as well as venous thrombosis (HITT). The mechanism in these cases is the interaction of antibody (usually IgG) with a complex of heparin and platelet factor 4 on the surfaces of platelets from which platelet factor 4 is released upon activation (Fig. 80–17A).[117,118] This complex results in the activation of platelets and monocytes through their FcγIIa receptors or on the surface of endothelial cells where released platelet factor 4 also binds (Fig. 80–17B).[119]

In HIT, patients develop absolute or relative (greater than 50 percent drop in platelet count) thrombocytopenia in a reproducible and diagnostic manner.[120] Thrombocytopenia begins at least 4 days after the initiation of heparin and rarely occurs more than 14 days after this time point. The exceptions are patients who received heparin within the recent past, usually within the past 3 months, and have circulating anti-heparin/platelet factor 4 antibodies. In those individuals, re-exposure to heparin can abruptly decrease platelet

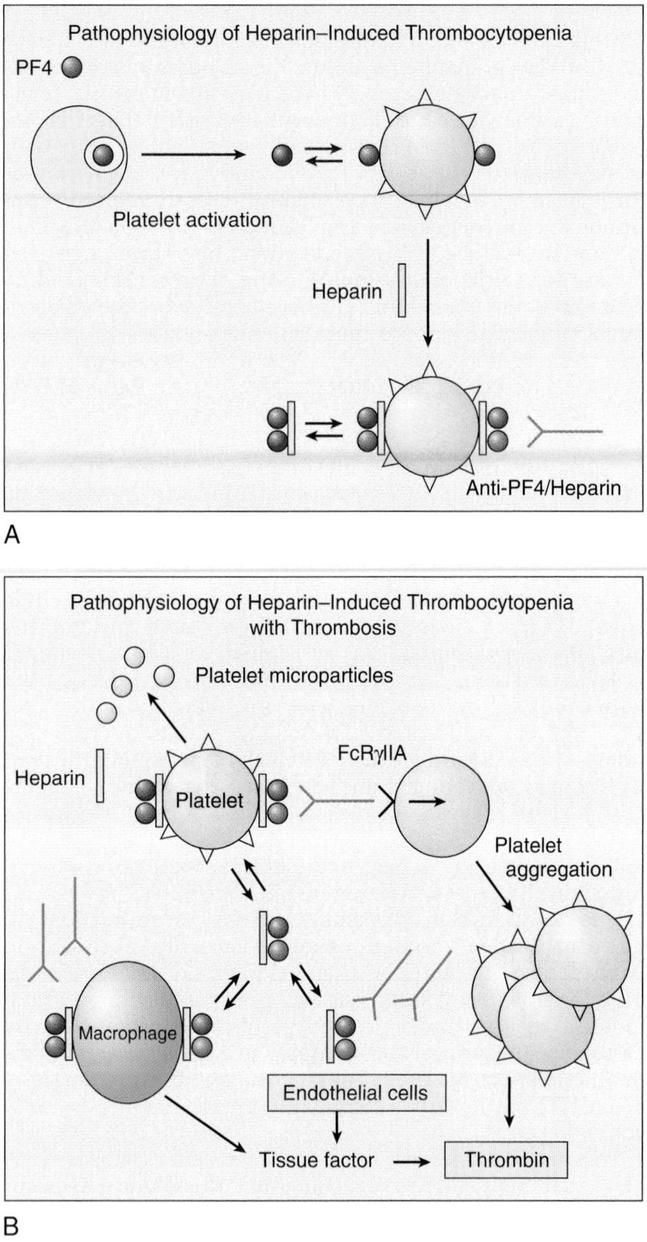

FIGURE 80–17 **A,** Pathophysiology of HIT. With platelet activation, platelet factor 4 (PF4) is released from the platelet α-granule and binds the surface of the activated platelet. PF4, a very basic protein, can complex with circulating negatively charged heparin, forming an antigenic complex. **B,** Pathophysiology of HITT. PF4/heparin antibodies can activate coagulation by a number of mechanisms, including (1) activation of platelets via the platelet FCRγIIa receptor resulting in platelet microparticle formation and the provision of a phospholipid surface for coagulation and (2) activation of endothelial cells and monocytes resulting in tissue factor expression, initiation of coagulation, and ultimately thrombin formation, which results in amplification of coagulation and further platelet activation. (Courtesy of D. Cines, University of Pennsylvania, Philadelphia, PA.)

count, and systemic reactions can occur. Except in this circumstance, prior exposure to heparin does not alter the time course of HIT. The decline in platelet count in HIT is usually moderate, with a typical nadir of 50,000 to 60,000/mm^3. However, HIT can cause severe thrombocytopenia even in the absence of thrombosis; and, conversely, heparin-induced thrombosis can actually occur with a normal platelet count. Immune-mediated HIT is not heparin dose-dependent and can develop with low-dose heparin or even with heparin flushes or the use of heparin-bonded catheters. Delayed-onset HIT has been described recently, a clinical scenario in which patients present a few weeks after heparin exposure with thrombosis and strongly positive testing for HIT, with or without thrombosis.[121,122] The pathogenesis of this variant is unclear but may result from ongoing antigenic stimulation, possibly from vascular wall bound complexes.

No single definitive laboratory test can ascertain the diagnosis of HIT, and HIT remains a clinical diagnosis supported by laboratory testing.[117] Laboratory testing for HIT can involve functional assays in which the heparin-induced activation of platelets in vitro is tested by aggregation, serotonin release, or platelet activation markers. Alternatively, enzyme immunoassays of antibody-heparin-platelet factor 4 complexes can be used to test for HIT. The latter have a high sensitivity but low specificity for HIT. Up to 70 percent of patients undergoing cardiopulmonary bypass surgery will develop anti-heparin/platelet factor 4 antibodies, whereas only 2 percent of those individuals will actually develop HIT.[123] Platelet activation assays, notably the serotonin-release assay, are more specific but less sensitive. In general, a negative immunoassay result excludes HIT, although false-negative results have been reported early in the presentation while the patient is still receiving heparin, presumably due to antigen to antibody excess. Therefore, if the initial test finding is negative in patients strongly suspected of HIT, treatment modifications should still be made and laboratory testing should be repeated a few days later.

When HIT is suspected, any source or route of heparin being administered to the patient must be discontinued immediately. LMWH therapy can result in HIT, although the incidence is approximately one-tenth that seen with unfractionated heparin. HIT is associated with a marked hypercoagulable state, and as many as 30 to 50 percent of individuals with HIT will develop thrombosis in the 30 days after diagnosis.[117] For this reason, patients with HIT should be assessed for thrombosis and, even in its absence, should be considered for anticoagulant therapy. Two direct thrombin inhibitors have been studied and have efficacy as anticoagulants in this setting: recombinant hirudin (lepirudin)[124] and argatroban,[125] a small-molecule synthetic antithrombin. LMWHs should not be substituted for heparin because they have strong cross-reactivity with HIT sera.

Other side effects of heparin include cumulative dose-dependent osteoporosis, skin necrosis, alopecia, hypersensitivity reactions, and hypoaldosteronism.[126] Heparin is the anticoagulant of choice during pregnancy; unlike warfarin, it does not cross the placenta and is not teratogenic. However, warfarin may be needed in women with mechanical heart valves who are at high risk of thromboembolism, at least in the periods of low risk of teratogenicity, because of the increased effectiveness of warfarin in this setting (see Chap. 57).[127]

OTHER GLYCOSAMINOGLYCAN-DERIVED DRUGS. Heparan sulfate, dermatan sulfate, and proteoglycans are endogenous heparin-like molecules with antithrombotic activity.[128] Several of these endogenous glycosaminoglycans have been developed as clinical anticoagulants.[128,129] Danaparoid (Orgaran), a mixture of low-molecular-weight anticoagulant glycosaminoglycans, predominantly heparan sulfate (84 percent) and dermatan sulfate (12 percent), was recently removed from the US market.[130] Dermatan sulfate, a naturally occurring glycosaminoglycan, promotes the inactivation of thrombin by heparin cofactor II. Like direct thrombin inhibitors (see later), and unlike standard and low-molecular-weight heparins, dermatan sulfate can inactivate fibrin-bound thrombin.[128] Heparins that can be absorbed orally are under development and some have entered clinical trials, although their efficacy has yet to be documented.

Fondaparinux, a chemically synthesized methoxy-derivative of the naturally occurring antithrombin-binding pentasaccharide, selectively catalyzes the inactivation of factor

Xa by antithrombin without inhibiting thrombin (see Fig. 80–15). Once-daily treatment with fondaparinux (2.5 mg subcutaneously) initiated in the early postoperative period is more effective than an LMWH preparation in preventing venous thromboembolism after hip or knee surgery, without increasing the risk of bleeding.[131,132] Fondaparinux is administered by subcutaneous injection, and its elimination half-life of 17 to 21 hours allows once-daily dosing. Unlike unfractionated heparin and LMWH, it does not bind platelets or platelet factor 4, nor does it result in release of TFPI. Since it does not bind platelet factor 4, an association with HIT would not be expected, and it may become a therapeutic option in this setting. There is no known antidote for reversal of the anticoagulant effect of fondaparinux. Even with a low bleeding risk, given its long half-life, this may become an issue in the clinical management of patients receiving this drug. In the completed studies, clinical situations requiring rapid reversal of the anticoagulant effect were not reported. Additional synthetic pentasaccharides for anticoagulation are under clinical study, including the drug idraparinux, which has a longer half-life than fondaparinux.

Warfarin

Warfarin (Coumadin) is the most frequently used oral anticoagulant.[133] Oral anticoagulants, which are derivatives of coumarins, exert their anticoagulant actions as vitamin K antagonists. The reduced form of vitamin K, vitamin KH_2, is normally required as a cofactor for the gamma-carboxylation of glutamic acid residues in coagulation factors II (prothrombin), VII, IX, and X[134] (Fig. 80–18). This post-translational modification of these clotting factors is necessary for them to function physiologically in the coagulation cascade by allowing them to bind to and form calcium-dependent complexes on cellular phospholipid surfaces. Oral anticoagulants block the reductase enzymes that are required to recycle vitamin K epoxide to vitamin KH_2 after the gamma-carboxylation reaction, thereby depleting the active vitamin K cofactor.

Warfarin is rapidly and almost completely absorbed from the gastrointestinal tract and circulates bound to albumin with a mean plasma half-life of approximately 40 hours. Metabolism is affected by inherited allelic variants of P450 CYP2C9, which catalyzes the conversion of S-warfarin to its inactive metabolite. Subjects homozygous for the least active alleles are more likely to require a low warfarin dose and to experience warfarin-related bleeding complications.[135] Numerous drugs alter the anticoagulant response to warfarin by pharmacokinetic or pharmacodynamic interactions. Drugs such as phenylbutazone, erythromycin, fluconazole, cimetidine, amiodarone, clofibrate, isoniazid, and propranolol increase warfarin levels, whereas drugs such as cholestyramine, barbiturates, rifampin, and sucralfate decrease warfarin levels. Dietary variations in vitamin K likewise alter warfarin's anticoagulant effects; high vitamin K intake in the diet (including nutritional supplements and vitamin preparations) reduces the anticoagulant response to warfarin. Conversely, liver disease, malabsorption, and hypermetabolic states enhance the anticoagulant effect of warfarin.

MONITORING. Oral anticoagulant therapy requires laboratory monitoring with the prothrombin time test. Commercially available thromboplastin reagents that are used in the prothrombin time assay vary considerably in their clotting ability. This problem previously created major variability in the prothrombin time values reported by different laboratories. To standardize prothrombin time reporting, the INR is now used. The INR corrects for differences in the thromboplastin reagents used by different laboratories. The optimal therapeutic range of warfarin for the prevention of venous thromboembolism and systemic embolism from atrial fibrillation and tissue heart valves targets an INR of 2.0 to 3.0. Higher intensity anticoagulation (INR, 2.5-3.5) is required in patients with mechanical prosthetic heart valves.

"Loading doses" of warfarin should not be employed in initiating oral anticoagulation. Although warfarin has a rapid onset of action, its optimal antithrombotic effect requires several days. The activity of all four of the vitamin K–dependent clotting factors must be inhibited to achieve clinically effective anticoagulation. The effects of warfarin require depletion of circulating clotting factors that are already gamma-carboxylated and hence biologically active when warfarin is started. The vitamin K–dependent clotting factors have different half-lives, with factor VII having the shortest. Therefore, the initial increase in the INR is predominantly due to a decrease in functional factor VII. A large "loading dose" of warfarin (i.e., 10 mg or more per day) will thus create a selective, severe factor VII deficiency state, while still failing to provide antithrombotic effect. In addition, a precipitous reduction in the plasma level of protein C, a vitamin

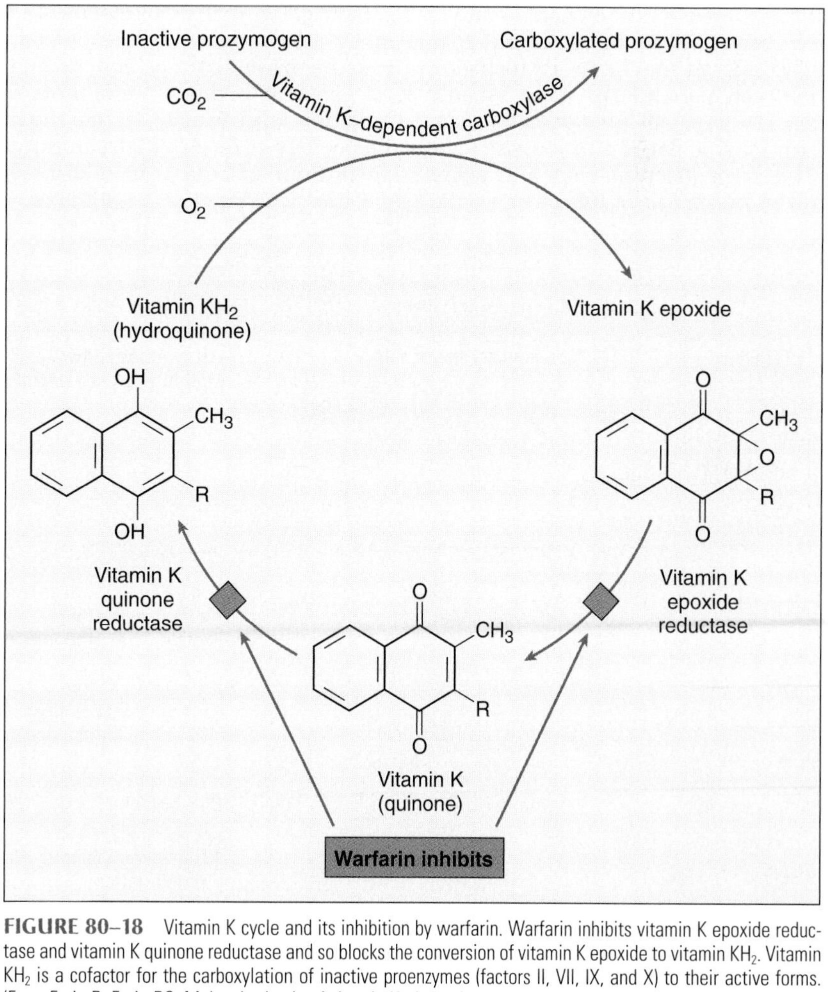

FIGURE 80–18 Vitamin K cycle and its inhibition by warfarin. Warfarin inhibits vitamin K epoxide reductase and vitamin K quinone reductase and so blocks the conversion of vitamin K epoxide to vitamin KH_2. Vitamin KH_2 is a cofactor for the carboxylation of inactive proenzymes (factors II, VII, IX, and X) to their active forms. (From Furie B, Furie BC: Molecular basis of vitamin K–dependent gamma-carboxylation. Blood 75:1753, 1990.)

K–dependent anticoagulant (rather than clotting) factor, which has the shortest half-life of all vitamin K–dependent proteins, can lead to a transient paradoxical hypercoagulable state during the first 36 hours of warfarin therapy (see later).[136,137] Therefore, the initial dose of warfarin should approximate the chronic maintenance dose that is anticipated, generally in the range of 4 to 6 mg/d in most adults.

COMPLICATIONS. Skin necrosis, a very rare complication that occurs within the first few days of starting warfarin therapy, tends to occur in patients with underlying inherited protein C or protein S deficiency. As noted earlier, it is likely related to the initial precipitous decrease in protein C levels (especially in individuals who may already have a congenitally low level of protein C). This leads to a transient prothrombotic imbalance, particularly with the use of large loading doses of warfarin. Warfarin should be avoided in pregnant patients, if possible, because of its potential to cause embryopathy and peripartum neonatal and maternal bleeding complications.

As with heparin, bleeding complications are the most frequent adverse effects of warfarin. For an individual patient, the cumulative risk of bleeding complications relates directly to the intensity and duration of anticoagulant therapy.[138] Major bleeding on warfarin occurs at a rate of 5 to 7 percent per year.[139] As noted earlier, the INR can vary despite a stable, chronic dose of warfarin as a function of changes in either medications or diet. When the INR exceeds the therapeutic range, discontinuing or reducing the dose of warfarin is usually sufficient; stopping warfarin generally normalizes the INR within about 3 days. If more rapid reversal of warfarin effect is required due to extreme elevations of the INR or clinical bleeding, vitamin K can be administered orally or parenterally. Vitamin K given orally has been shown to be superior to that given by subcutaneous injection, as the latter is ineffective in some patients.[140] However, particularly when vitamin K is given at higher doses, a transient resistance to re-anticoagulation with warfarin may be encountered subsequently. Emergency reversal of warfarin effect can be rapidly achieved by infusion of fresh frozen plasma (usually starting with 2 to 4 units). A single dose of recombinant factor VIIa reduced the prothrombin level in a small number of patients who had an elevated INR with serious bleeding (n = 4), required a procedure (n = 5), or were at high risk of bleeding and had an INR greater than 10 (n = 4).[141] Clinical efficacy was reported, although larger trials are needed to determine the efficacy and safety of this drug in this setting. Algorithms for the management of elevated INR with or without bleeding have been proposed.[136]

Thrombin Inhibitors and Other Specific Coagulation Inhibitors

Newly developed anticoagulants specifically target inactivation of thrombin, factor Xa, factor IXa, and the factor VIIa/tissue factor complex, as well as inactivation of factors VIIIa and Va by enhancement of the protein C anticoagulant pathway.[142-146] The sites of action of these anticoagulants are shown in Figure 80–19. Except for the direct thrombin inhibitors, most of these agents still await evaluation in phase 3 trials.

THROMBIN INHIBITORS. Direct thrombin inhibitors inactivate both free (fluid-phase) thrombin and fibrin-bound thrombin. In this respect, these agents differ from heparin and its low-molecular-weight derivatives, which require complex formation with antithrombin and thus are weak inhibitors of clot-bound thrombin.[142-144]

The thrombin molecule has distinct functional domains. The "active site" of thrombin is the catalytic site that possesses serine protease activity. "Exosite 1" of thrombin serves to dock substrates in the proper orientation and is the binding site for fibrin(ogen). Direct thrombin inhibitors interact with one or both of these sites. Hirudin and bivalirudin are more specific for thrombin than active-site inhibitors because they are bivalent, binding to thrombin at both the active site and exosite 1. In contrast, low-molecular-weight thrombin inhibitors such as argatroban and efegatran bind only to the active site of thrombin. Because the active site of thrombin is structurally similar to other serine proteases, these active-site inhibitors are less selective for thrombin than the bivalent inhibitors.

Hirudin, the prototype of the direct thrombin inhibitors, is a 65-amino acid polypeptide originally isolated from the saliva of *Hirudo medicinalis*, the medicinal leech. Hirudin is now produced by recombinant DNA technology (lepirudin). It binds tightly to thrombin, forming a slowly reversible, 1:1 stoichiometric complex. In this complex, the amino-terminus of hirudin binds to the active site and its carboxy-terminal binds to exosite 1 of thrombin.

Bivalirudin (formerly Hirulog) is a synthetic 20-amino acid polypeptide composed of a peptide sequence (D-Phe-Pro-Arg-Pro) that is directed at the active site of thrombin, linked to a dodecapeptide analog of the exosite 1–binding carboxy-terminal of hirudin. Thus, like hirudin, bivalirudin interacts bivalently with both the active

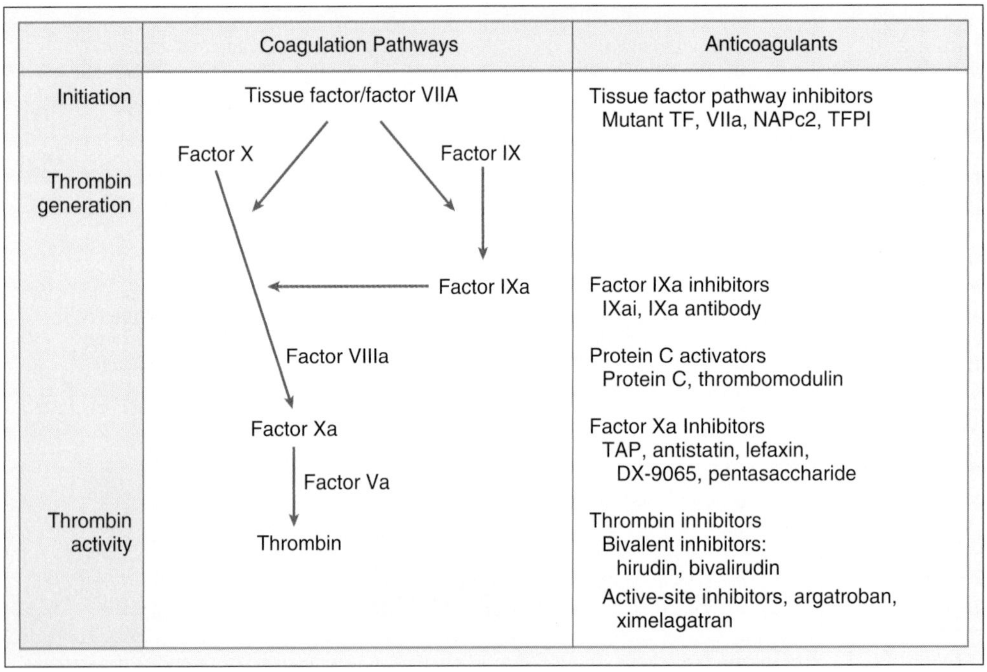

FIGURE 80–19 Activation and inhibitors of coagulation. New anticoagulants act by inhibiting the tissue factor pathway (initiation), thrombin generation, and thrombin activity. Ximelagatran is the product of the active thrombin inhibitor melagatran. (Modified from Hirsh J, Weitz JI: New antithrombotic agents. Lancet 353:1431, 1999.)

site and exosite 1 of thrombin, forming a 1:1 stoichiometric complex. However, once bound, thrombin cleaves the Arg-Pro bond and thereby removes the active site-binding part of bivalirudin, leaving only a low-affinity, weaker inhibitory interaction with thrombin. Consequently, the potent thrombin inhibitory effect of bivalirudin is short lived, conferring on it a potential safety advantage.

Several low-molecular-weight direct thrombin inhibitors have been developed. These less-specific agents target only the active site of thrombin. Argatroban is the prototype of the noncovalent class of these active site inhibitors, which also includes napsagatran, inogatran, and melagatran.

Direct thrombin inhibitors have theoretical advantages over heparin. First, as noted earlier, they can inactivate clot-bound thrombin. Second, unlike heparin, they do not bind to plasma proteins. Therefore, they have the pharmacokinetic advantage of a more predictable anticoagulant response. This may permit their administration without laboratory monitoring, which has not been true for the currently available parenterally administered agents due to their narrow therapeutic window and their use in combination with other anticoagulants, such as for coronary procedures.[144] However, laboratory monitoring may not be needed for the oral agents under development and in clinical study (see later). Clinical trial results and clinical experience suggest that the bleeding risk with the parenteral agents is greater than that seen with heparin. Because of their short half-lives, discontinuation of the drug is usually adequate to control bleeding symptoms.

Orally administered direct thrombin inhibitors have been developed and one, ximelagatran, is in phase 3 clinical trials. After oral administration, ximelagatran is rapidly absorbed and converted to its active metabolite melagatran, a small molecule direct thrombin inhibitor. In clinical trials, ximelagatran is given by twice-daily dosing and without laboratory monitoring. Efficacy in prevention of VTE after total knee arthroplasty has been reported, without increased bleeding risk as compared with warfarin.[146] Phase II trials showed promising results in the treatment of DVT,[147] and large international randomized controlled trials in thromboprophylaxis in atrial fibrillation and in the treatment of DVT were completed in 2003. Melagatran is excreted renally, and patients with significant renal impairment have not been included in clinical trials. Additional oral direct thrombin inhibitors are in clinical development.

OTHER SPECIFIC COAGULATION INHIBITORS. Inhibitors of factor Xa (see Fig. 80–19) include tick anticoagulant peptide (TAP), antistatin, and lefaxin.[145,148] The latter two are extracts of the salivary glands of two species of leeches. All are potent and specific factor Xa inhibitors that are available in recombinant forms. DX-9065 is a synthetic, low-molecular-weight, reversible factor Xa inhibitor that has oral bioavailability. Experimental agents that are inhibitors of factor IXa include a monoclonal antibody and active site-blocked-factor IXa.[149] Specific inhibitors of the tissue factor pathway under study include a soluble mutant form of tissue factor that has decreased cofactor function for factor VIIa-induced activation of factor X; active-site-blocked factor VIIa (VIIai), which competes with factor VII for tissue factor binding; NAPc2, a small, nematode-derived anticoagulant protein that binds to factor X and inhibits factor VIIa within the factor VII/tissue factor complex; and recombinant TFPI.[150] Protein C activators that have been studied as therapeutic anticoagulants include plasma and recombinant forms of protein C and recombinant soluble thrombomodulin. Recombinant human activated protein C, or drotrecogin alfa (activated), has antithrombotic, antiinflammatory, and profibrinolytic properties. A randomized, double-blind, placebo-controlled trial showed that this agent significantly reduced mortality in patients with severe sepsis, although with an increased risk of bleeding.[151]

Thrombolytic (Fibrinolytic) Drugs (see Chap. 47)

The common mechanism of action of currently available thrombolytic (fibrinolytic) agents, including streptokinase, urokinase, and alteplase (recombinant tissue-type plasminogen activator [rt-PA]), involves the conversion of the inactive plasma zymogen, plasminogen, to the active fibrinolytic enzyme, plasmin (see Fig. 80–7). Plasmin has relatively weak substrate specificity and can degrade not only fibrin but also any protein that has an arginyl-lysyl bond available for enzymatic attack, including fibrinogen. Indiscriminate plasmin lysis of both fibrin and fibrinogen can produce a systemic state of fibrin(ogen)olysis (or "systemic lytic state"), which might cause a serious systemic bleeding tendency, so attempts have been made to develop thrombolytic agents that generate plasmin preferentially at the fibrin surface in a preformed thrombus ("fibrin-specific agents"). Plasmin associated with fibrin is protected from rapid inhibition by $alpha_2$-antiplasmin (see earlier) and can thereby effectively degrade the fibrin of a clot. Thus, the biochemical strategy was to develop fibrinolytic agents that bind to fibrin and thereby produce only fibrin-bound plasmin from fibrin-bound plasminogen.

Streptokinase and urokinase induce a systemic lytic state, with extensive systemic activation of the fibrinolytic system, deplete $alpha_2$-antiplasmin, and degrade circulating fibrinogen. In contrast, the physiological plasminogen activators t-PA and scu-PA activate plasminogen preferentially at the fibrin surface. The promise of a marked reduction in the risk of hemorrhage with "second-generation" fibrin-specific agents has not been fulfilled in large clinical trials, however. This may be due to the inability of plasmin to discriminate between fibrin in pathological thrombi, which is the desired target, and fibrin in physiological hemostatic plugs, the lysis of which will induce bleeding.

STREPTOKINASE. Streptokinase is isolated from hemolytic streptococci and is produced from bacterial cultures. The mechanism of activation of plasminogen by streptokinase is unique among plasminogen activators in that streptokinase itself possesses no enzymatic activity.[152,153] Streptokinase forms a complex with plasminogen, and it is the streptokinase-plasminogen complex that actually possesses enzymatic activity toward plasminogen. The streptokinase-plasminogen complexes are thereby converted to streptokinase-plasmin complexes, and the enzyme active sites in the streptokinase-plasmin complexes are the same as those in plasmin. The streptokinase-plasmin(ogen) complexes activate circulating and fibrin-bound plasminogen relatively indiscriminately, producing a systemic lytic state.

Because of its bacterial source, streptokinase is antigenic. Most individuals have preexisting antibodies resulting from previous streptococcal infection. The administration of streptokinase stimulates the rapid formation of high titers of neutralizing antistreptokinase antibodies, which are sufficient to neutralize standard doses of streptokinase. Although antibody titers may return to near-baseline levels as early as 2 years after a single dose, once streptokinase has been used, subsequent thrombolytic treatment should be with an immunologically unrelated agent because of the uncertain efficacy of repeated treatment. Streptokinase causes transient hypotension in many patients and significant allergic reactions in some, including a serum sickness–type syndrome, fever, rash, and bronchospasm.

UROKINASE. Urokinase, or two-chain urokinase-type plasminogen activator (tcu-PA), is a trypsin-like serine protease composed of two polypeptide chains linked by a disulfide bridge.[152,153] Urokinase is produced from cultures of human fetal kidney cells. It directly activates plasminogen to plasmin, leading to relatively nonspecific degradation of fibrin, fibrinogen, and other plasma proteins, depletion of circulating alpha$_2$-antiplasmin, and a systemic lytic state. Urokinase is not antigenic and does not cause allergic reactions.

TISSUE-TYPE PLASMINOGEN ACTIVATOR. Tissue-type plasminogen activator is a naturally occurring molecule released from vascular endothelial cells. For therapeutic thrombolysis, it is produced commercially by recombinant DNA technology (rt-PA; alteplase) and, as a "second-generation" agent, it is relatively fibrin specific.[152,153]

Tissue-type plasminogen activator, a single-chain serine protease, activates plasminogen directly. Fibrin significantly enhances the efficiency of plasminogen activation by t-PA. The basis for the relative fibrin specificity of t-PA action is described previously in the section on the fibrinolytic system. Briefly, fibrin provides a surface for the sequential binding of enzyme (t-PA) and substrate (plasminogen). The assembly of this ternary complex thereby promotes the activation of plasminogen to plasmin that is efficiently localized to the fibrin clot; fibrin then becomes the substrate for lysis by the plasmin that is generated on its surface.

Tissue-type plasminogen activator is converted by plasmin to a disulfide-linked two-chain form by hydrolysis of the Arg 275-Ile276 bond; alteplase consists mainly of the single-chain form of t-PA. Both the single-chain and two-chain forms of t-PA are cleared from plasma according to a two-compartment model, with initial half-lives of 3 to 6 minutes and terminal half-lives of 40 to 50 minutes. The currently preferred dosage regimen of fibrin-selective alteplase for coronary thrombolysis consists of weight-adjusted, accelerated ("front-loaded") administration (see Chap. 47). The front-loaded administration of alteplase achieves a mean steady-state plasma concentration during the initial 30 minutes that is 45 percent higher than that achieved with standard infusion, although it does not alter the plasma half-life.

VARIANTS OF PLASMINOGEN ACTIVATORS. These thrombolytic agents have been engineered to favorably alter the pharmacokinetic and functional properties of currently used drugs. They are designed to have prolonged half-lives, improved enzymatic efficiency, enhanced local concentrations in the clot by altered binding to fibrin and stimulation by fibrin, and resistance to plasma protease inhibitors.[153]

Variants of u-PA have been developed and evaluated in clinical study.[153] Saruplase is an unglycosylated, single-chain recombinant u-PA. Clinical trials have demonstrated similar efficacy of this drug to other thrombolytics, but in some studies, increased bleeding complications occurred. M23 is a single-chain molecule composed of the kringle and protease domain of saruplase and the carboxy-terminal fragment of the direct thrombin inhibitor hirudin, providing both fibrinolytic and antithrombotic activity.

A number of t-PA mutants have been developed. These can be divided into those in which amino acid substitutions have been made (monteplase, tenecteplase) and deletion mutants (reteplase, lanoteplase, pamiteplase). In monteplase, there is a cysteine to serine substitution at position 84, resulting in an increased half-life of the drug compared to native t-PA. Tenecteplase contains amino acid substitutions at three sites: threonine at position 103 is replaced by asparagine; asparagine at position 117 is replaced by glutamine; and four amino acids, lysine, histidine, arginine, and arginine, are replaced by alanine-alanine-alanine-alanine at positions 296 through 299. Tenecteplase is characterized by a prolonged half-life, increased fibrin specificity, and increased resistance to inhibition by PAI-1.[154,155]

Reteplase (r-PA) is a single-chain nonglycosylated deletion variant of t-PA, containing only the kringle-2 and serine protease domains. This deletion mutant has a prolonged half-life and, therefore, can be administered by bolus injection. Another third-generation drug is lanoteplase (n-PA), which retains kringle-1, kringle-2, and protease domains and also has a glutamine substituted for asparagines at position 117. It has an even longer half-life (37 min) and can be administered by single-bolus, weight-adjusted injection.[155] Pamiteplase is a modified t-PA with deletion of the kringle-1 domain and a point substitution of glutamine for arginine at position 274. These modifications make the drug resistant to plasmin-mediated cleavage.

The t-PA of saliva from the vampire bat *Desmodus rotundus* (bat-PA) has potent and relatively fibrin-specific thrombolytic properties.[153,156] Different molecular forms of bat-PA have been purified, characterized, cloned, and expressed. These are being evaluated in preclinical ex vivo and animal studies.

Antibody targeting of thrombolytic agents is a potentially powerful approach to localizing the actions of these drugs to specific components of different types of thrombi (e.g., directed at platelet antigens in arterial thrombi, or thrombin in recently formed thrombi). This can be achieved by conjugating plasminogen activators with monoclonal antibodies that are specific, for example, for fibrin but do not cross-react with fibrinogen. These bifunctional molecules are engineered to contain both a highly specific antigen-binding site that concentrates the drug at the clot and an effector site that promotes thrombolysis.

Antiplatelet Agents

The sequence of events involved in the process of platelet activation is described in detail in the previous section on platelets (Figs. 80–8 and 80–20). Inhibition of platelet function can be targeted at any one of these activation steps.[157,158] Platelet blockade would be expected to be most effective if it is directed at either the initial (adhesion) (see Fig. 80–20A) or final (aggregation) (see Fig. 80–20D) points in the sequence. Antiplatelet agents targeted at any one of the intermediate events should be less potent, because platelet adhesion is followed by the binding of several specific agonists to their respective receptors and the activation of several simultaneous intracellular pathways (e.g., ADP release, TXA_2 synthesis) that act in concert to induce the final step of platelet aggregation. Therefore, pharmacological interruption of only one of these intermediate steps (e.g., with aspirin, antithrombins, clopidogrel) may permit platelet activation through alternative, uninhibited pathways. Agents that block the interaction of vWF with its platelet membrane Gp Ib receptor should inhibit adhesion (see Fig. 80–20A) as well as the subsequent downstream cascade of platelet activation events, including secretion of mitogens into the vessel wall and platelet aggregation. Therapeutic approaches to inhibit adhesion could involve anti-vWF or anti-Gp Ib monoclonal antibodies or agents that interfere with vWF-platelet Gp-Ib binding. These strategies have yet to be translated to clinical practice, however. In contrast, considerable clinical evidence has now validated powerful therapeutic strategies to block the final step of platelet aggregation that is mediated by the interaction of fibrinogen (or vWF) with its platelet Gp IIb/IIIa receptors (see Fig. 80–20D).

ASPIRIN. Aspirin (acetylsalicylic acid), known for more than 50 years to have antithrombotic efficacy, has stood the test of time as an effective, inexpensive, and relatively safe drug for the prevention of various thrombotic and vascular disorders, particularly in the arterial circulation where platelets are the predominant participants in the thrombotic process.[159] Until recently, aspirin has been essentially the only available, clinically effective antiplatelet drug. However, there are several clinical settings in which aspirin fails to provide full (or even partial) antithrombotic benefit.[160]

Aspirin is readily absorbed from the stomach and upper small intestine and is then hydrolyzed to release free acetyl groups. This moiety acetylates serine residues at position 529 of cyclooxygenase (COX; prostaglandin G/H synthase), which leads to irreversible inactivation of the enzyme (Fig. 80–21). Inactive, acetylated COX cannot function to catalyze the oxygenation of arachidonic acid to prostaglandin G_2. Aspirin thereby blocks the formation of TXA_2, a potent mediator of platelet aggregation and vasoconstrictor. Because anucleate platelets essentially are unable to synthesize new, unacetylated COX, aspirin blocks the function of platelets exposed to it for their remaining lifetime (normally 7 to 10 days) in the circulation. This accounts for the lengthy therapeutic effect of aspirin despite its plasma half-life of only 20 minutes.

The inhibitory effects of aspirin on platelet TXA_2 production and ex vivo aggregation are rapid, with maximal effects achieved within 15 to 30 minutes of oral administration of a dose as low as 81 mg. A single oral dose of 100 mg of aspirin almost completely suppresses platelet TXA_2 synthesis in both normal individuals and patients with cardiovascular disease. Daily administration of only 30 to 50 mg of aspirin exerts a cumulative effect and likewise results in almost complete inhibition of platelet TXA_2 production within 7 to 10 days. These aspirin effects on platelet TXA_2 formation generally correlate well with inhibition of ex vivo platelet aggregability and prolongation of the skin bleeding time. Although platelet function remains impaired for 4 to 7 days after a single dose of aspirin, reflecting the life span of irreversibly inhibited platelets, the prolonged bleeding time generally returns to normal within 24 to 48 hours of aspirin ingestion. This discrepancy is due to the release from bone marrow into the circulation of a sufficient cohort of uninhibited platelets after the elimination of aspirin from blood to restore normal in vivo hemostasis (bleeding time) even before complete normalization of ex vivo platelet function.

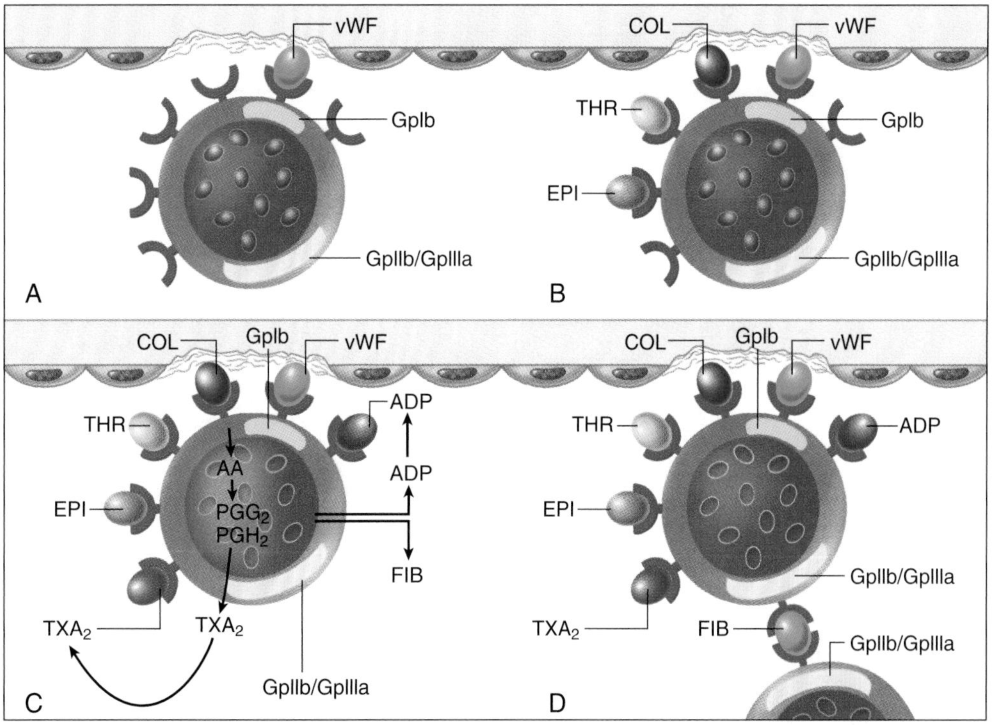

FIGURE 80–20 Sequence of events in platelet activation, with potential targets for antiplatelet therapy. **A,** Platelet adhesion to the injured vascular intimal surface is mediated by von Willebrand factor (vWF) binding to its receptor on platelet membrane Gp Ib. **B,** Adherent platelets are also anchored to the damaged vessel wall by binding of subendothelial collagen (COL) to its platelet surface COL receptors. Other platelet stimuli in blood, including thrombin (THR) and epinephrine (EPI), bind to their respective receptors. **C,** In response to these different stimuli, adherent platelets are activated and release thromboxane A_2 (TXA_2) and adenosine diphosphate (ADP), which bind to their own respective platelet receptors and amplify the activation process. **D,** Platelet aggregation is mediated by fibrinogen (FIB) binding to its receptors on adjoining platelets, forming fibrinogen bridges. The FIB receptor is formed by the complexing of Gp IIb/IIIa in the membrane of activated platelets. AA = arachidonic acid; PGG_2 and PGH_2 = labile prostaglandin endoperoxides. (Modified from Schafer AI: Antiplatelet therapy with glycoprotein IIb/IIIa receptor inhibitors and other novel agents. Tex Heart Inst J 24:90, 1997.)

Aspirin also inhibits COX in vascular endothelial cells, leading to suppression of platelet inhibitory and vasodilatory endothelium-derived PGI_2; this would be expected to offset the antiplatelet effects of aspirin. Attempts to design "platelet selective" aspirin regimens have not translated to clinical feasibility. Nevertheless, there is ample evidence that the antithrombotic effects of aspirin predominate in vivo, possibly due to mechanisms in addition to platelet TXA_2 inhibition.

Up to 50 percent of individuals exhibit a relative state of "aspirin resistance."[161] This phenomenon is defined as suboptimal inhibition of ex vivo platelet function or TXA_2 blockade in response to conventional doses of aspirin. "Aspirin resistance" has not yet been conclusively linked to aspirin "treatment failure," so its clinical relevance requires further study. Potential mechanisms may include pharmacodynamic interactions with other drugs (see next section), extraplatelet sources of TXA_2, or COX polymorphisms that lead to interindividual variability in response.[162]

NON-ASPIRIN NONSTEROIDAL ANTIINFLAMMATORY DRUGS (NSAIDS). Non-aspirin NSAIDs likewise inhibit COX. Unlike aspirin, however, these other NSAIDs inhibit the enzyme reversibly, and therefore their durations of TXA_2 and platelet inhibitory action depend on the clearance of the drugs from the circulation.[163] Thus, there is considerable variability in the extent and duration of the effects of various NSAIDs on ex vivo platelet aggregation and bleeding time prolongation. Non-aspirin NSAIDs reversibly inhibit COX by preventing its arachidonic acid substrate from gaining access to the active site of the enzyme.

COX-1, the constitutive isoform of COX, is present in platelets and produces TXA_2. Aspirin and the traditional NSAIDs are nonselective inhibitors of both COX-1 and COX-2. The newer COX-2-specific inhibitors are designed to maximize the antiinflammatory effects mediated by the COX-2 isoform, while minimizing the common side effects (e.g., bleeding) attributed to the COX-1 isoform. Therefore, the antiplatelet potency of the new COX-2 inhibitors is several orders of magnitude lower than that of aspirin and the standard NSAIDs, and generally cannot be assumed to afford antithrombotic protection. In fact, in clinical reports, COX-2 ingestion may promote, or at least not provide protection from, thromboembolism.[164] Concerns have been raised about the cardiovascular safety of long-term use of these agents because of their inhibition of COX-2-dependent PGI_2 production.[165]

Interaction of NSAIDs with COX may prevent acetylation of the enzyme by aspirin. This suggests that the concomitant administration of nonselective NSAIDs (e.g., ibuprofen), but not COX-2-selective NSAIDs, may actually antagonize the

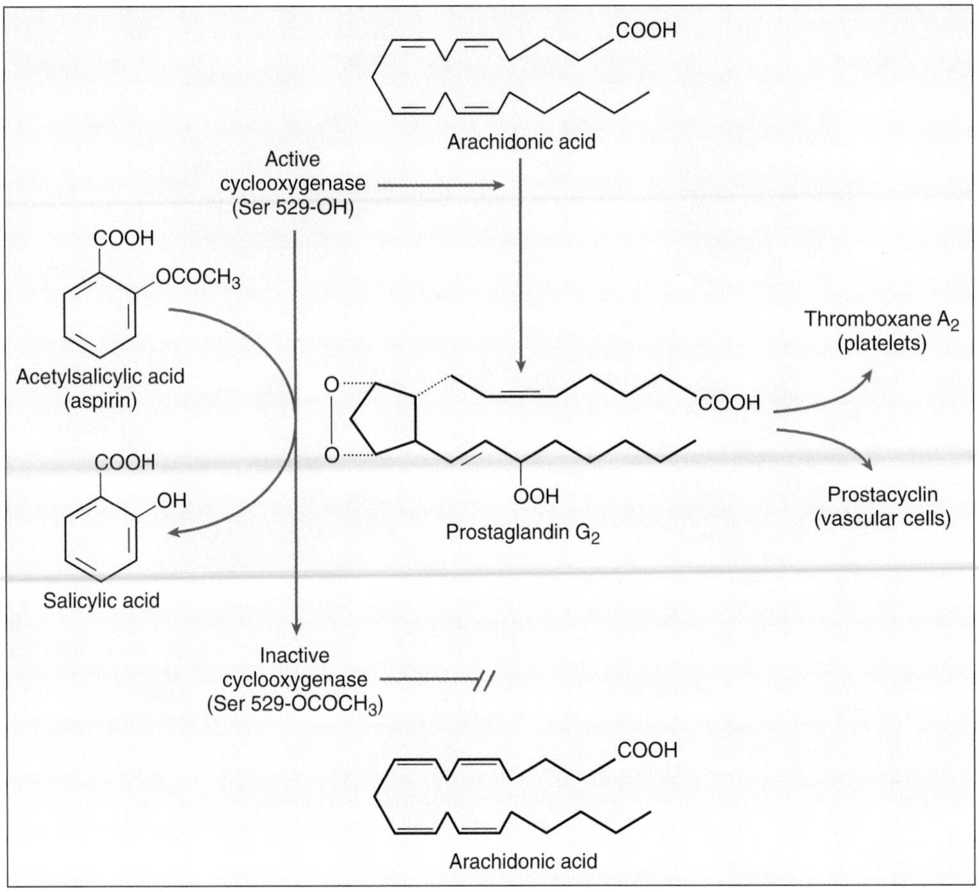

FIGURE 80–21 Aspirin (acetylsalicylic acid) inhibition of cyclooxygenase (prostaglandin-G/H synthase). Aspirin acetylates serine at position 529 of cyclooxygenase, rendering the enzyme inactive. Acetylated cyclooxygenase does not function to catalyze the oxygenation of arachidonic acid to prostaglandin G_2. Aspirin thereby blocks the formation of thromboxane A_2 (in platelets) and prostacyclin (in vascular cells). (From Loscalzo J, Schafer AI: Anticoagulants, antiplatelet agents, and fibrinolytics. *In* Loscalzo J, Creager MA, Dzau MV [eds]: Vascular Medicine: A Textbook of Vascular Biology and Diseases. Philadelphia: Lippincott Williams & Wilkins, 1996.)

effects of aspirin on COX by competitive interaction and consequently blunt aspirin's antiplatelet efficacy.[166] The mechanism of this pharmacodynamic interaction is competition between aspirin and NSAIDs for a common docking site within the COX channel, which aspirin binds to in platelets prior to irreversible acetylation of Ser529.[167]

OTHER THROMBOXANE INHIBITORS. Figure 80–20C illustrates other opportunities to interrupt platelet TXA_2 synthesis and/or action in addition to COX blockade. The reduced incidence of atherosclerotic cardiovascular disease in Greenland Eskimos has been attributed, at least in part, to their diets rich in fish oils containing omega-3 polyunsaturated fatty acids. A major omega-3 fatty acid in fish oils is eicosapentaenoic acid, which incorporates into phospholipids of cell membranes and competes with arachidonic acid as substrate for COX. The product of eicosapentaenoic acid oxygenation is TXA_3, an eicosanoid that is devoid of the potent platelet-activating and vasoconstrictor actions of arachidonic acid-derived TXA_2. Large and often unpalatable doses (>10 gm eicosapentaenoic acid daily) of medicinal fish oils are required to simulate changes in platelet membrane fatty acid content attained with Eskimo diets and thereby produce antiplatelet actions. Thromboxane synthase inhibitors (e.g., dazoxiben) and TXA_2 receptors antagonists (e.g., vapiprost), as well as dual thromboxane synthase/TXA_2 receptor inhibitors (e.g., ridogrel), have been developed but generally have not been found to be superior to aspirin in limited clinical trials.[158]

CLOPIDOGREL AND TICLOPIDINE. Clopidogrel (Plavix) and ticlopidine (Ticlid) are structurally related thienopyridine derivatives. Clopidogrel is largely replacing ticlopidine in clinical practice because of its more favorable side-effect profile and more rapid onset of action. These drugs produce their antiplatelet effects by inhibiting the ADP-dependent pathway of platelet activation.[158,168] After oral administration, both drugs require modification to active forms. They exert a permanent effect on a platelet protein, which is the ADP receptor itself or a platelet membrane component closely related to the ADP receptor. As ADP receptor blockers, these drugs inhibit ADP-induced platelet aggregation (see Fig. 80–20C).

Presumably because they must be converted to an active form in vivo, clopidogrel and ticlopidine have a relatively slow onset of antiplatelet action. On repeated daily dosing of 75 mg clopidogrel, partial inhibition of platelet aggregation occurs from the second day of treatment and reaches steady-state inhibition after 4 to 7 days. Ticlopidine has a slower onset of antiplatelet effect than clopidogrel. Using a larger loading dose of clopidogrel (300-400 mg) results in platelet inhibition within hours of adminstration.[169] The antiplatelet activity of clopidogrel and ticlopidine persists for 4 to 8 days after discontinuation of the drug, reflecting the circulating lifetime of platelets and consistent with an irreversible antiplatelet effect, as is the case with aspirin. Individual variability in platelet inhibition and the occurrence of "clopidogrel resistance" (similar to aspirin resistance) has been described, but the clinical relevance of these phenomena is as yet unclear.[162]

Ticlopidine can cause severe neutropenia, which is usually reversible with discontinuation of the drug, in up to 1 percent of patients.[158] The risk of this adverse effect is much lower (about 0.1 percent) with clopidogrel. In addition, thrombotic thrombocytopenic purpura, a serious and sometimes fatal disorder, is a rare complication of therapy with both ticlopidine and clopidogrel. Thrombotic thrombocytopenic purpura typically occurs within 2 to 8 weeks of initiation of the thienopyridine and was noted in 0.02 percent of patients receiving ticlopidine after coronary stenting.[170-172] Other side effects, including gastrointestinal symptoms, pruritus, urticaria, and bleeding, also appear to occur less often with clopidogrel than with ticlopidine.

PHOSPHODIESTERASE INHIBITORS

Dipyridamole. The mechanism of antiplatelet action of dipyridamole is unclear. Although this drug can stimulate PGI_2 synthesis, potentiate the platelet inhibitory effects of PGI_2, raise platelet cyclic adenosine monophosphate levels by inhibiting phosphodiesterase, and block uptake of adenosine into vascular and blood cells, these potential antiplatelet actions generally do not occur at therapeutically achievable drug concentrations.[158] Unlike aspirin, dipyridamole does not prolong the bleeding time or inhibit ex vivo platelet aggregation at therapeutic doses. Although numerous clinical trials have failed to demonstrate antithrombotic efficacy of dipyridamole when it is used alone in any clinical setting, it may enhance the effect of warfarin in preventing systemic embolization from mechanical heart valve prostheses and add to the beneficial effect of aspirin in preventing the progression of peripheral occlusive arterial disease or, when used in a sustained-release preparation, in the secondary prevention of ischemic stroke.[173]

Cilostazol. Cilostazol is a quinolone derivative that is a potent inhibitor of platelet phosphodiesterase-3 and has vasodilatory effects. It may be beneficial in the treatment of intermittent claudication due to peripheral vascular disease, an indication for which it has been approved by the Food and Drug Administration.[158]

GLYCOPROTEIN IIB/IIIA ANTAGONISTS. Regardless of the stimulus for their activation, the aggregation of platelets is finally regulated through their membrane binding sites for fibrinogen in the Gp IIb/IIIa receptor complex (see Fig. 80–20D). This provides the rationale for pharmacological intervention directed against the platelet Gp IIb/IIIa complex. The role of the platelet Gp IIb/IIIa complex in platelet activation is discussed in more detail earlier in the section on platelets. Because Gp IIb/IIIa antagonists do not block TXA_2 production by activated platelets, concomitant use of aspirin may enhance their antithrombotic efficacy.

Platelet Gp IIb/IIIa antagonists generally belong to one of the following classes: (1) monoclonal antibody against Gp IIb/IIIa; (2) peptide (peptidomimetic) antagonists, many of which contain the RGD sequence that can compete with fibrinogen for its Gp IIb/IIIa binding site; and (3) nonpeptide (nonpeptide-mimetic) antagonists of Gp IIb/IIIa. Three drugs currently available for coronary intervention or acute coronary syndromes represent the prototypes for these groups: abciximab (c7E3 Fab, ReoPro), a monoclonal antibody; eptifibatide (Integrilin), a peptide antagonist; and tirofiban (Aggrastat), a nonpeptide mimetic (see Chaps. 47, 48, and 52). These agents are approved for intravenous administration.[157,158,174] Although these agents have similar mechanisms of action (i.e., inhibition of ligand binding to the receptor), it should not be assumed that they react at the same site within the receptor or that the consequences of their binding to Gp IIb/IIIa are identical. Monoclonal antibody has a relatively extended duration of antiplatelet action, whereas the peptides and nonpeptide mimetics have a shorter elimination half-life.

Abciximab is the Fab fragment of a monoclonal antibody to Gp IIb/IIIa that has been humanized (mouse/human chimera) to reduce immunogenicity.[175] Abciximab is not specific to platelet Gp IIb/IIIa: it cross-reacts with the related integrin, alpha$_v$-beta$_3$, the vitronectin receptor that is present on vascular cells. This cross-reactivity was originally considered to be of potential therapeutic benefit in the prevention of coronary restenosis and inhibition of thrombin generation. Abciximab is currently administered as an intravenous bolus followed by infusion for 12 to 24 hours for coronary interventions. Because abciximab is derived from an antibody, concern has been raised about repeat administration. However, data indicate that readministration is safe and efficacious and that the same indications for first-time use can apply to subsequent readministration.[176]

Eptifibatide is a synthetic cyclic heptapeptide that contains a modified lysine-glycine-aspartic acid (KGD), rather than RGD, sequence that recognizes the binding site of platelet Gp IIb/IIIa (see Fig. 80–9). The rationale for eptifibatide is that the substitution of a single lysine (K) for arginine (R) makes this agent specific for the platelet Gp IIb/IIIa integrin. Whether this is an advantageous or a disadvantageous property (see earlier) has yet to be definitely determined. Eptifibatide is not immunogenic and is safe for repeated administration.[177]

Tirofiban (Aggrastat) is a nonpeptide mimetic. In contrast to the RGD (or KGD) peptidomimetics, which inhibit platelet aggregation by binding competitively to the RGD recognition site of Gp IIb/IIIa, the nonpeptides mimic the structural steric and charge characteristics of the RGD sequence.[158]

The clinical experience with oral Gp IIb/IIIa antagonists has been disappointing. The lack of clinical benefit for these agents as compared with the established efficacy with intravenous inhibitors may be in part due to inadequate in vivo platelet Gp IIb/IIIa blockade. Oral Gp IIb/IIIa antagonists may also cause paradoxical platelet activation. Ligand-mimetic Gp IIb/IIIa blockers can have intrinsic platelet-activating properties or can stimulate outside-inside signal transduction, leading to paradoxical platelet aggregation. These ligand-mimetic properties of Gp IIb/IIIa antagonists may also cause thrombocytopenia (see later).[178]

Complications. Bleeding complications with currently approved intravenous platelet Gp IIb/IIIa antagonists have primarily involved vascular access puncture sites in patients undergoing percutaneous intervention. Reduction and weight-adjustment in adjunctive heparin dosing in patients undergoing coronary interventions have reduced the incidence of these bleeding problems. No increase in intracerebral hemorrhage has been observed with the Gp IIb/IIIa antagonists. Therefore, the need for platelet transfusion to treat life-threatening bleeding is extremely rare, particularly with the short-acting agents such as eptifibatide and tirofiban. Severe thrombocytopenia (platelet count $<20{,}000/\mu l$) occurs in 0.1 to 0.5 percent of patients treated with the intravenous agents, and the incidence appears to be slightly higher with abciximab.[158] A precipitous decrease in platelet count may occur within 1 to 2 hours of initial exposure, or there may be a significant decline several days after initiation of therapy. Preexisting antibodies appear to play a role in some cases of thrombocytopenia induced by these agents, and in the future, pretreatment detection of these antibodies may select for patients at greater risk of thrombocytopenia.[179,180] Alterations in platelet Gp IIb/IIIa, similar to those induced by these drugs, may occur in some patients with intermittent platelet activation, such as from atherosclerosis, leading to neo-antigen and subsequent antibody formation.[181]

REFERENCES

Basic Mechanisms of Hemostasis and Thrombosis

1. Hajjar KA: The endothelium in thrombosis and hemorrhage. *In* Loscalzo J, Schafer AI (eds): Thrombosis and Hemorrhage, 3rd ed. , Lippincott Williams & Wilkins, 2003, pp 206-209.
2. Kubo H, Alitalo K: The bloody fate of endothelial stem cells. Genes Dev 17:322, 2003.
3. Carmeliet P: Angiogenesis in health and disease. Nature Med 9:653, 2003.
4. Cines DB, Pollak ES, Buck CA, et al: Endothelial cells in physiology and in the pathophysiology of vascular disorders. Blood 91:3527, 1998.
5. Schafer AI: Preface. *In* Schafer AI (ed): Molecular Mechanisms of Hypercoagulable States. Austin, Landes Bioscience, 1997.
6. Schafer AI: Vascular endothelium: In defense of blood fluidity. J Clin Invest 99:1143, 1997.
7. Rosenberg RD, Aird WC: Vascular-bed-specific hemostasis and hypercoagulable states. N Engl J Med 340:1555, 1999.
8. Edelberg JM, Christie PD, Rosenberg RD: Regulation of vascular bed–specific prothrombotic potential. Circ Res 89:117, 2001.
9. Cook JP: Flow, NO, and atherogenesis. Proc Natl Acad Sci U S A 100:1420, 2003.
10. Davidge ST: Prostaglandin H synthase and vascular function. Circ Res 89:650, 2001.
11. Smyth EM, FitzGerald GA: Human prostacyclin receptor. Vitam Horm 65:149, 2002.
12. Busse R, Edwards G, Feletou M, et al: EDHF: Bringing the concepts together. Trends Pharmacol Sci 23:374, 2002.
13. Durante W, Schafer AI: Carbon monoxide and vascular cell function. Int J Mol Med 2:255, 1998.

14. Marcus AJ, Broekman MJ, Drosopoulos JH, et al: Metabolic control of excessive extracellular nucleotide accumulation by CD39/ectonucleotidase-1: Implications for ischemic vascular diseases. J Pharmacol Exp Ther 305:9, 2003.
15. Busse R, Fleming I: Regulation of endothelium-derived vasoactive autacoid production by hemodynamic forces. Trends Pharmacol Sci 24:24, 2003.
16. Schiffrin EL: A critical review of the role of endothelial factors in the pathogenesis of hypertension. J Cardiovac Pharmacol 38(Suppl 2):S3, 2001.
17. Walsh PN, Ahmad SS: Proteases in blood clotting. Essays Biochem 38:95, 2002.
18. Mann KG, Butenas S, Brummel K: The dynamics of thrombin formation. Arterioscler Thromb Vasc Biol 23:17, 2003.
19. Morrissey JH: Tissue factor: An enzyme cofactor and a true receptor. Thromb Haemost 86:66, 2001.
20. Edgington TS, Dickinson CD, Ruf W: The structural basis of function of the TF VIIa complex in the cellular initiation of coagulation. Thromb Haemost 78:401, 1997.
21. Kitchens CS: The contact system. Arch Pathol Lab Med 126:1382, 2002.
22. Colman RW, Schmaier AH: Contact system: A vascular biology modulator with anticoagulant, profibrinolytic, antiadhesive, and proinflammatory attributes. Blood 90:3819, 1997.
23. Mosesson MW: Fibrinogen structure and fibrin clot assembly. Semin Thromb Hemost 24:169, 1998.
24. Schafer AI: The primary and secondary hypercoagulable states. *In* Schafer AI (ed): Molecular Mechanisms of Hypercoagulable States. Austin, Landes Bioscience, 1997, pp 1-48.
25. Walsh PN, London FS, Ahmad SS: The assembly of the factor X-activating complex on activated human platelets. J Thromb Haemost 1:48, 2003.
26. Zwaal RF, Comfurius P, Beevers EM: Lipid-protein interactions in blood coagulation. Biochim Biophys Acta 1376:433, 1998.
27. Kottke-Marchant K, Duncan A: Antithrombin deficiency. Arch Pathol Lab Med 126:1326, 2002.

28. Crowther, MA, Kelton JG: Congenital thrombophilic states associated with venous thrombosis: A qualitative overview and proposed classification system. Ann Intern Med 138:128, 2003.
29. Broze GJ Jr: Protein Z-dependent regulation of coagulation. Thromb Haemost 86:8, 2001.
30. Simmonds RE, Rance J, Lane DA: Regulation of coagulation. *In* Loscalzo J, Schafer AI (eds): Thrombosis and Hemorrhage, 3rd ed. Philadelphia, Lippincott Williams & Wilkins, 2003, pp 35-61.
31. Weiler H, Isermann BH: Thrombomodulin. J Thromb Haemost 1:1515, 2003.
32. Esmon CT: Regulation of blood coagulation. Biochim Biophys Acta 1477:349, 2000.
33. Kottke-Marchant K, Comp P: Laboratory issues in diagnosing abnormalities of protein C, thrombomodulin, and endothelial cell protein C receptor. Arch Pathol Lab Med 126:1337, 2002.
34. Bajaj MS, Birktoft JJ, Steer SA, Bajaj SP: Structure and biology of tissue factor pathway inhibitor. Thromb Haemost 86:959, 2001.
35. Morris TA: Heparin and low molecular weight heparin: Background and pharmacology. Clin Chest Med 24:39, 2003.
36. Adams MJ, Donohoe S, Mackie IJ, Machin SJ: Anti-tissue factor pathway inhibitor activity in patients with primary antiphospholipid syndrome. Br J Haematol 114:375, 2001.
37. Forastiero RR, Martinuzzo ME, Broze GJ Jr: High titers of autoantibodies to tissue factor pathway inhibitor are associated with the antiphospholipid syndrome. J Thromb Haemost 1:718, 2003.
38. Caplice NM, Panetta C, Peterson TE, et al: Lipoprotein(a) binds and inactivates tissue factor pathway inhibitor: A novel link between lipoproteins and thrombosis. Blood 98:2980, 2001.
39. Dahm A, van Hylekama Vlieg A, Bendz B, et al: Low levels of tissue factor pathway inhibitor (TFPI) increase the risk of venous thrombosis. Blood 101:4387, 2003.
40. Kostner KM, Kostner GM: Lipoprotein (a): Still an enigma? Curr Opin Lipidol 13:391, 2002.
41. Vaughan DE, Declerck PJ: Regulation of fibrinolysis. *In* Loscalzo J, Schafer AI (eds): Thrombosis and Hemorrhage, 3rd ed. Philadelphia, Lippincott Williams & Wilkins, 2003, pp 105-119.
42. Taubman MB: Interactions of coagulation and fibrinolytic proteins with the vessel wall. *In* Loscalzo J, Schafer AI (eds): Thrombosis and Hemorrhage. 3rd ed. Philadelphia, Lippincott Williams & Wilkins, 2003, pp 266-277.
43. Longstaff C: Plasminogen activation on the cell surface. Frontiers Biosci 7:244, 2002.
44. Oswald CT, Menon V, Stouffer GA: The use of D-dimer in emergency room patients with suspected deep vein thrombosis: A test whose time has come. J Thromb Haemost 1:635, 2003.
45. Schutgens REG, Haas FJLM, Gerritsen WBM, et al: The usefulness of five D-dimer assays in the exclusion of deep venous thrombosis. J Thromb Haemost 1:976, 2003.
46. Eitzman DT, Ginsberg D: Of mice and men: The function of plasminogen activator inhibitors (PAIs) in vivo. Adv Exp Med Biol 425:131, 1997.
47. Vaughn DE: Plasminogen activator inhibitor-1: A common denominator in cardiovascular disease. J Invest Med 46:370, 1998.
48. Astedt B, Lindoff C, Lecander I: Significance of the plasminogen activator inhibitor of placental type (PAI-2) in pregnancy. Semin Thromb Hemost 24:431, 1998.
49. Bouma BN, Meijers JCM: Thrombin activatable fibrinolysis inhibitor (TAFI, plasma procarboxypeptidase B, procarboxypeptidase R, procarboxypeptidase U). J Thromb Haemost 1:1566, 2003.
50. van Tiburg NH, Rosendaal FR, Bertina RM: Thrombin activatable fibrinolysis inhibitor and the risk for deep vein thrombosis. Blood. 95:2855, 2000.
51. Kaushansky K: Thrombopoietin. N Engl J Med 339:746, 1998.
52. Ruggeri ZM: Structure of von Willebrand factor and its function in platelet adhesion and thrombus formation. Baillieres Best Practice Clin Haematol 14:257, 2001.
53. de Wit TR, van Mourik JA: Biosynthesis, processing and secretion of von Willebrand factor: Biological implications. Baillieres Best Practice Clin Haematol 14:241, 2001.
54. Andrews RK, Shen Y, Gardiner EE, et al: The glycoprotein Ib-IX-V complex in platelet adhesion and signaling. Thromb Haemost 82:357, 1999.
55. McEver RP: Adhesive interaction of leukocytes, platelets, and the vessel wall during hemostasis and inflammation. Thromb Haemost 86:746, 2001.
56. Andre P, Denis CV, Ware J, et al: Platelets adhere to and translocate on von Willebrand factor presented by endothelium in stimulated veins. Blood 96:3322, 2000.
57. Savage B, Almus-Jacobs F, Ruggeri ZM: Specific synergy of multiple substrate receptor interactions in platelet thrombus formation under flow. Cell 94:657, 1998.
58. Nakamura T, Kambayashi J, Okuma M: Activation of the Gp IIb/IIIa complex induced by platelet adhesion to collagen is mediated by both alpha$_2$-beta$_1$ integrin and Gp VI. J Biol Chem 274:11897, 1999.
59. Nieswandt B, Watson SP: Platelet-collagen interactions: Is Gp VI the central receptor? Blood 102:449, 2003.
60. Ruggeri ZM: Platelets in atherothrombosis. Nature Med 8:1227, 2002.
61. Kroll MH, Resendiz JC: Mechanisms of platelet activation. *In* Loscalzo J, Schafer AI (eds): Thrombosis and Hemorrhage. 3rd ed. Philadelphia, Lippincott Williams & Wilkins, 2003, pp 187-205.
62. Thomas DW, Mannon RB, Mannon PJ, et al: Coagulation defects and altered hemodynamic responses in mice lacking receptors for thromboxane A_2. J Clin Invest 102:1994, 1998.
63. Jackson SP, Nesbitt WS, Kulkarni S: Signaling events underlying thrombus formation. J Thromb Haemost 1:1602, 2003.
64. Bennett JS: Platelet-fibrinogen interactions. Ann New York Acad Sci 936:340, 2001.
65. Schafer AI: Antiplatelet therapy with glycoprotein IIb/IIIa receptor inhibitors and other novel agents. Tex Heart Inst J 24:90, 1997.
66. Griffin JH: The thrombin paradox. Nature 378:337, 1995.
67. Hanson SR, Griffin JH, Harker LA, et al: Antithrombotic effects of thrombin-induced activation of endogenous protein C in primates. J Clin Invest 92:2003, 1993.
68. Mann KG, Butenas S, Brummel K: The dynamics of thrombin formation. Arterioscler Thromb Vasc Biol 23:17, 2003.
69. Esmon CT: Inflammation and thrombosis. J Thromb Haemost 1:1343, 2003.

Thrombophilic Disorders

70. Price DT, Ridker PM: Factor V Leiden mutation and the risks for thromboembolic disease: A clinical perspective. Ann Intern Med. 127:895, 1997.
71. Bauer KA, Rosendaal FR, Heit JA: Hypercoagulability: Too many tests, too much conflicting data. Hematology. Am Soc Hematol Educ Program Book 353-38168, 2002.
72. Press RD, Bauer KA, Kujovich JL, Heit JA: Clinical utility of factor V Leiden (R506Q) testing for the diagnosis and management of thromboembolic disorders. Arch Pathol Lab Med 126:1304, 2002.
73. Ridker PM, Miletich JP, Hennekens, Buring JE: Ethnic distribution of factor V Leiden in 4047 men and women. JAMA 277:1305, 1997.
74. Dowling NF, Austin H, Dilley A, et al: The epidemiology of venous thromboembolism in Caucasians and African-Americans: The GATE study. J Thromb Haemost 1:80, 2003.
75. Juul K, Tybjaerg-Hansen A, Steffensen R, et al: Factor V Leiden: The Copenhagen city heart study and 2 meta-analyses. Blood 100:3, 2002.
76. Rosendaal FR, Siscovick DS, Schwartz SM, et al: Factor V Leiden (resistance to activated protein C) increases the risk of myocardial infarction in young women. Blood 89:2817, 1997.
77. MacGillavry MR, Prins MH: Oral contraceptives and inherited thrombophilia: A gene-environment interaction with a risk of venous thrombosis. Sem Thromb Hemost 29:219, 2003.
78. Bauer KA: Hormone replacement therapy and the factor V Leiden mutation. Arterioscler Throm Vasc Biol 22:879, 2002.
79. Rosendaal FR, Van Hylckama Vlieg A, Tanis BC, Helmerhorst FM: Estrogens, progestogens and thrombosis. J Haemost Thromb 1:1371, 2003.
80. Dahlback B: The discovery of activated protein C resistance. J Thromb Haemost 1:3, 2003.
81. McGlennen RC, Key NS: Clinical and laboratory management of the prothrombin G20210A mutation. Arch Pathol Lab Med 126:1319, 2002.
82. Dilley A, Austin H, Hooper WC, et al: Prevalence of the prothrombin 20210 G-to-A variant in blacks: Infants, patients with venous thrombosis, patients with myocardial infarction, and control subjects. J Lab Clin Med 132:452, 1998.
83. Legnani C, Cosmi B, Valdre L, et al: Venous thromboembolism, oral contraceptives and high prothrombin levels. J Thromb Haemost 1:112, 2002.
84. Martinelli I, Sacchi E, Landi G, et al: High risk of cerebral-vein thrombosis in carriers of a prothrombin-gene mutation and in users of oral contraceptives. N Engl J Med 338:1793, 1998.
85. Goodwin AJ, Rosendaal FR, Kottke-Marchant K, Bovill EG: A review of the technical, diagnostic, and epidemiologic considerations for protein S assays. Arch Pathol Lab Med 126:1349, 2002.
86. Key NS, McGlennen RC: Hyperhomocyst(e)inemia and thrombophilia. Arch Pathol Lab Med 126:1367, 2002.
87. Langman LJ, Ray JG, Evrovski J, et al: Hyperhomocyst(e)inemia and the increased risk of venous thromboembolism: more evidence from a case-control study. Arch Intern Med 160:961, 2000.
88. Mangoni AA, Jackson SH: Homocysteine and cardiovascular disease: Current evidence and future prospects. Am J Med 112:556, 2002.
89. Ray JG: Meta-analysis of hyperhomocysteinemia as a risk factor for venous thromboembolic disease. Arch Intern Med 158:2101, 1998.
90. Ray JG, Shmorgun D, Chan WS: Common C677T polymorphism of the methylenetetrahydrofolate reductase gene and the risk of venous thromboembolism: Meta-analysis of 31 studies. Pathophys Haemost Thromb 32:51, 2002.

91. Kluijtmans LAJ, Young IS, Boreham CA, et al: Genetic and nutritional factors contributing to hyperhomocysteinemia in young adults. Blood 101:2483, 2003.
92. Keijzer MBAJ, den Heijer M, Blom HJ, et al: Interaction between hyperhomocysteinemia, mutated methylenetetrahydrofolate reductase (MTHFR) and inherited thrombophilic factor in recurrent venous thrombosis. Thromb Haemost 88:723, 2002.
93. Ray JG, Vermeulen MJ, Boss SC, Cole DE: Declining rate of folate insufficiency among adults following increased folic acid food fortification in Canada. Can J Public Health. Rev Can Sante Publique 93:249, 2002.
94. Chandler WL, Rodgers GM, Sprouse JT, Thompson AR: Elevated hemostatic factor levels as potential risk factor for thrombosis. Arch Pathol Lab Med 126:1405, 2002.
95. Kamphuisen PW, Eikenboom JCJ, Bertina RM: Elevated factor VIII levels and the risk of thrombosis. Arterioscler Thromb Vasc Biol 21:731, 2001.
96. Tsai AW, Cushman M, Rosamond WD, et al: Coagulation factors, inflammation markers, and venous thromboembolism: the longitudinal investigation of thromboembolism etiology (LITE). Am J Med 113:636, 2002.
97. Koster T, Blann AD, Briet E, et al: Role of clotting factor VIII in effect of von Willebrand factor on occurrence of deep-vein thrombosis. Lancet 345:152, 1995.
98. Kyrle PA, Minar E, Hirschl M, et al: High plasma levels of factor VIII and the risk of recurrent venous thromboembolism. N Engl J Med 343:457, 2000.
99. Haynes T: Dysfibrinogenemia and thrombosis. Arch Pathol Lab Med 126:1387, 2002.
100. Rickles FR, Levine MN: Hemostatic and thrombotic disorders of malignancy. *In* Kitchens CS, Alving BM, Kessler CM (eds): Consultative Hemostasis and Thrombosis. Philadelphia, WB Saunders, 2002, pp 325.
101. Stein S, Konkle BA: Thrombotic risk of oral contraceptives, postmenopausal hormone replacement, and selective estrogen receptor modulators (SERMs). *In* Kitchens CS, Alving BM, Kessler CM (eds): Consultative Hemostasis and Thrombosis. Philadelphia, WB Saunders, 2002, pp 427-436.
102. Vandenbroucke JP, Rosing J, Bloemenkamp K, et al: Oral contraceptives and the risk of venous thrombosis. N Engl J Med 344:1527, 2001.
103. van den Bosch MAAJ, Kemmeren JM, Tanis BC, et al: The RATIO study: Oral contraceptives and the risk of peripheral arterial disease in young women. J Thromb Haemost 1:439, 2002.
104. Tanis BC, van den Bosch MAAJ, Kemmeren JM, et al: Oral contraceptives and the risk of myocardial infarction. N Engl J Med 345:1787, 2001.
105. Levine JS, Branch DW, Rauch J: The antiphospholipid syndrome. N Engl J Med 346:752, 2002.
106. Galli M, Barbui T: Antiphospholipid syndrome: Definition and treatment. Semin Thromb Hemost 29:195, 2003.
107. Arnout J, Vermylen J: Current status and implications of autoimmune antiphospholipid antibodies in relation to thrombotic disease. J Thromb Haemost 1:931, 2002.
108. Triplett DA: Antiphospholipid antibodies. Arch Pathol Lab Med 126:1424, 2002.
109. Previtali S, Barbui T, Galli M: Anti-β2-glycoprotein 1 and anti-prothrombin antibodies in antiphospholipid-negative patients with thrombosis. Thromb Haemost 88:729, 2002.
110. Galli M, Luciani D, Bertolini G, Barbui T: Lupus anticoagulants are stronger risk factors for thrombosis than anticardiolipin antibodies in the antiphospholipid syndrome: A systematic review of the literature. Blood 101:1827, 2003.

Antithrombotic Drugs

111. Hirsh J, Warkentin TE, Shaughnessy S, et al: Heparin and low-molecular-weight heparin: Mechanisms of action, pharmacokinetics, dosing, monitoring, efficacy and safety. Chest 119:64S, 2001.
112. Ginsberg JS: Pharmacology of heparin-related compounds and coumarin derivatives. *In* Loscalzo J, Schafer AI (eds): Thrombosis and Hemorrhage. 3rd ed. Philadelphia, Lippincott Williams & Wilkins, 2003, pp 937-948.
113. Schafer AI: Low-molecular-weight heparin for venous thromboembolism. Hosp Pract 31:99, 1997.
114. Nenci GG: Low molecular weight heparins: Are they interchangeable? No. J Thromb Haemost 1:12, 2003.
115. Prandoni P: Low molecular weight heparins: Are they interchangable? Yes. J Thromb Haemost 1:10, 2003.
116. Becker RC, Spencer FA, Gibson M, et al: Influence of patient characteristics and renal function on factor Xa inhibition pharmacokinetics and pharmacodynamics after enoxaparin administration in non-ST-segment elevation acute coronary syndromes. Am Heart J 143:753, 2002.
117. McCrae KR, Cines DB: Drug-induced thrombocytopenias. *In* Loscalzo J, Schafer AI (eds): Thrombosis and Hemorrhage. 3rd ed. Philadelphia, Lippincott Williams & Wilkins, 2003, pp 457-475.
118. Aster RH: Heparin induced thrombocytopenia and thrombosis. N Engl J Med 332:1374, 1995.
119. Arepally GM, Poncz M, Cines DB: Immune vascular injury in heparin-induced thrombocytopenia. *In* Warkentin TE, Greinacher A (eds): Heparin-Induced Thrombocytopenia. 2nd ed. New York, Marcel Dekker, 2001, pp 215-230.
120. Warkentin TE, Kelton JG: Temporal aspects of heparin-induced thrombocytopenia. N Engl J Med 344:1286, 2001.
121. Warkentin TE, Kelton JG: Delayed-onset heparin-induced thrombocytopenia and thrombosis. Ann Intern Med 135:502, 2001.
122. Warkentin TE, Bernstein RA: Delayed-onset HIT and cerebral thrombosis after a single administration of unfractionated heparin. N Engl J Med 348:1067, 2003.
123. Warkentin TE, Sheppard JL, Horsewood P, et al: Impact of the patient population on the risk for heparin-induced thrombocytopenia. Blood 96:1703, 2000.
124. Greinacher A, Volpel H, Janssens U, et al: Recombinant hirudin (lepirudin) provides safe and effective anticoagulation in patients with heparin-induced thrombocytopenia: A prospective study. Circulation 99:73, 1999.
125. Lewis BE, Walenga JM, Wallis DE: Anticoagulation with Novastan (argatroban) in patients with heparin-induced thrombocytopenia and thrombosis syndrome. Semin Thromb Hemost 23:197, 1997.
126. Warkentin TE: Nonhemorrhagic complications of antithrombotic therapy. *In* Spandorfer J, Konkle B, Merli G (eds): Management and prevention of thrombosis in primary care. New York, Oxford University Press, 2001, pp 202-220.
127. Ginsberg J, Chan WS, Bates S, Kaatz S: Anticoagulation of pregnant women with mechanical heart valves. Arch Intern Med. 163:694, 2003.
128. Freedman JE, Loscalzo J: New antithrombotic strategies. *In* Loscalzo J, Schafer AI (eds): Thrombosis and Hemorrhage. 3rd ed. Philadelphia, Lippincott Williams & Wilkins, 2003, pp 978-995.
129. Bates SM, Weitz JI: The new heparins. Coron Artery Dis 9:65, 1998.
130. Ibbotson T, Perry CM: Danaparoid: A review of its use in thromboembolic and coagulation disorders. Drugs 62:2283, 2002.
131. Eriksson BI, Bauer KA, Lassen MR, et al: Fondaparinux compared with enoxaparin for the prevention of venous thromboembolism after hip-fracture. N Engl J Med 345:1298, 2001.
132. Bauer KA, Eriksson BI, Lassen MR, et al: Fondaparinux compared with enoxaparin for the prevention of venous thromboembolism after elective major knee surgery. N Engl J Med 345:1305, 2001.
133. Keller C, Matzdorff AC, Kemkes-Matthes B: Pharmacology of warfarin and clinical implications. Semin Thromb Hemost 25:13, 1999.
134. Furie B, Furie BC: Molecular basis of vitamin K-dependent gamma-carboxylation. Blood 75:1753, 1990.
135. Aithal GP, Day CP, Kesteven PJL, Daly AK: Association of polymorphisms in the cytochrome P450 CYP2C9 with warfarin dose requirement and risk of bleeding complications. Lancet 353:717, 1998.
136. Hirsh J, Dalen JE, Anderson D, et al: Oral anticoagulants: Mechanism of action, clinical effectiveness, and optimal therapeutic range. Chest 119(Suppl): 8S, 2001.
137. Harrison L, Johnston M, Massicotte MP, et al: Comparison of 5-mg and 10-mg loading doses in initiation of warfarin therapy. Ann Intern Med 126:133, 1997.
138. Levine MN, Raskob G, Landefeld S, et al: Hemorrhagic complications of anticoagulant treatment. Chest 119(Suppl):108S, 2001.
139. Schafer AI: Venous thrombosis as a chronic disease. N Engl J Med 340:955, 1999.
140. Crowther MA, Douketis JD, Schnurr T, et al: Oral vitamin K lowers the international normalized ratio more rapidly than subcutaneous vitamin K in the treatment of warfarin-associated coagulopathy: A randomized, controlled trial. Ann Intern Med 137:251, 2002.
141. Deveras RAE, Kessler CM: Reversal of warfarin-induced excessive anticoagulation with recombinant human factor VIIa concentrate. Ann Intern Med 137:884, 2002.
142. Heit JA: Mapping out the future in venous thromboembolism and acute coronary syndromes. Semin Thromb Hemost 28:33, 2002.
143. Hirsh J: New anticoagulants. Am Heart J 142(2 Suppl):S3, 2001.
144. Kaplan KL, Francis CW: Direct thrombin inhibitors. Semin Hematol 39:187, 2002.
145. Samama MM: Synthetic direct and indirect factor Xa inhibitors. Thromb Res106:V267, 2002.
146. Francis CW, Davidson BL, Berkowitz SD, et al: Ximalagatran versus warfarin for the prevention of venous thromboembolism after total knee arthroplasty. Ann Intern Med 137:648, 2002.
147. Eriksson H, Wahlander K, Gustafsson D, et al: A randomized, controlled, dose-guiding study of the oral direct thrombin inhibitor ximelagatran compared with standard therapy for the treatment of acute deep vein thrombosis. J Thromb Haemost 1:41, 2002.
148. Hauptmann J, Stürzebecher J: Synthetic inhibitors of thrombin and factor Xa: From bench to bedside. Thromb Res 93:203, 1999.
149. Bauer KA: Selective inhibition of coagulation factors: Advance in antithrombotic therapy. Semin Thromb Hemost 28:15, 2002.
150. Golino P: The inhibitors of the tissue factor: Factor VII pathway. Thromb Res 106:V257, 2002.
151. Bernard GR, Vincent J-L, Laterre P-F, et al: Efficacy and safety of recombinant human activated protein C for severe sepsis. N Engl J Med 344:699, 2001.
152. Collen D: Thrombolytic therapy. Thromb Haemost 78:742, 1997.
153. Leopold JA, Loscalzo J: Pharmacology of thrombolytic agents. *In* Loscalzo J, Schafer AI (eds): Thrombosis and Hemorrhage. 3rd ed. Philadelphia, Lippincott Williams & Wilkins, 2003, pp 949-977.
154. Tanswell P, Modi N, Combs D, Danays T: Pharmacokinetics and pharmacodynamics of tenecteplase in fibrinolytic therapy of acute myocardial infarction. Clin Pharmacokinet 45:1229, 2002.
155. Al-Shwafi KA, de Meester A, Pirenne B, Col JJ: Comparative fibrinolytic activity of front-loaded alteplase and the single-bolus mutants tenecteplase and lanoteplase during treatment of acute myocardial infarction. Am Heart J 145:127, 2003.
156. Toschi L, Bringmann P, Petri T, et al: Fibrin selectivity of the isolated protease domains of tissue-type and vampire bat salivary gland plasminogen activators. Eur J Biochem 252:108, 1998.
157. Bennett JS, Mousa S: Platelet function inhibitors in the year 2000. Thromb Haemost 85:395, 2001.
158. Bennett JS: Novel platelet inhibitors. Annu Rev Med 52:161, 2001.
159. Mehta P: Aspirin in the prophylaxis of coronary artery disease. Curr Opin Cardiol 17:552, 2002.
160. Folts JD, Schafer AI, Loscalzo J, et al: A perspective on the potential problems with aspirin as an antithrombotic agent: A comparison of studies in an animal model with clinical trials. J Am Coll Cardiol 33:295, 1999.
161. Patrono C: Aspirin resistance: Definition, mechanisms and clinical read-outs. J Thromb Haemost 1:1710, 2003.
162. Schafer AI: Genetic and acquired determinants of individual variability of response to antiplatelet drugs. Circulation 108:910, 2003.
163. Schafer AI: Effects of nonsteroidal anti-inflammatory therapy on platelets. Am J Med 106:25S, 1999.

164. McAdam B, Catella-Lawson F, Mardini L, et al: Systemic biosynthesis of prostacyclin by cyclooxygenase (COX)-2: The human pharmacology of a selective inhibitor of COX-2. Proc Natl Acad Sci U S A 96:272, 1999.
165. FitzGerald GA, Patrono C: The coxibs, selective inhibitors of cyclooxygenase-2. N Engl J Med 345:433, 2001.
166. Catella-Lawson F, Reilly MP, Kapoor SC, et al: Cyclooxygenase inhibitors and the antiplatelet effects of aspirin. N Engl Med 345:1809, 2001.
167. Patrono C, Coller B, Fitzgerald GA, et al: Platelet-active drugs: The relationship among dose, effectiveness, and side effects. Chest 119(1 Suppl):395, 2001.
168. Jneid H, Bhatt DL, Corti R, et al: Aspirin and clopidogrel in acute coronary syndromes. Arch Intern Med 163:1145, 2003.
169. Gurbel PA, Cummings CC, Bell CR, et al: Onset and extent of platelet inhibition by clopidogrel loading in patients undergoing elective coronary stenting: The plavix reduction of new thrombus occurrence (PRONTO) trial. Am Heart J 145:239, 2003.
170. Chen DK, Kim JS, Sutton DM: Thrombotic thrombocytopenic purpura associated with ticlopidine use: A report of 3 cases and review of the literature. Arch Intern Med 159:311, 1999.
171. Steinhubl SR, Tan WA, Foody JM, et al: Incidence and clinical course of thrombotic thrombocytopenia purpura due to ticlopidine following coronary stenting. EPISTENT Investigators. Evaluation of platelet IIb/IIIa inhibitor for stenting. JAMA 281:806, 1999.
172. Bennett CL, Connors JM, Carwile JM, et al: Thrombotic thrombocytopenic purpura associated with clopidogrel. N Engl J Med 342:1773, 2000.
173. De Schryver EL, Algra A, van Gijn J: Dipyridamole for preventing stroke and other vascular events in patients with vascular disease. Cochrane Database of Systematic Reviews CD001820, 2003.
174. Plow EF, Cierniewski CS, Xiao Z et al: Alpha IIbbeta3 and its antagonism at the new millennium. Thromb Haemost 86:34, 2001.
175. Bhatt DL, Lincoff AM: Abciximab. *In* Sasahara AA, Loscalzo J (eds): New Therapeutic Agents in Thrombosis and Thrombolysis. 2nd ed. New York, Marcel Dekker, 2003, pp 349-369.
176. Tcheng JE, Kereiakes DJ, Braden GA, et al: Readministration of abciximab: Interim report of the ReoPro Readministration Registry. Am Heart J 138:33, 1999.
177. Lorenz TJ, Macdonald F, Kitt MM: Nonimmunogenieity of eptifibatide, a cyclic heptapeptide inhibitor of platelet glycoprotein IIb-IIIa. Clin Ther 21:128, 1999.
178. Peter K, Bode C: Procoagulant activities of glycoprotein IIb/IIIa receptor blockers: *In* Sasahara AA, Loscalzo J (eds): New Therapeutic Agents in Thrombosis and Thrombolysis. 2nd ed. New York, Marcel Dekker, 2003, pp 401-411
179. Curtis BR, Swyers J, Divgi A, McFarland JG, Aster RH: Thrombocytopenia after second exposure to abciximab is caused by antibodies that recognize abciximab-coated platelets. Blood 99:2054, 2002.
180. Billheimer JT, Dicker IB, Wynn R, et al: Evidence that thrombocytopenia observed in humans treated with orally bioavailable glycoprotein IIb/IIIa antagonists is immune mediated. Blood 99:3540, 2002.
181. Abrams CS, Cines DB: Platelet glycoprotein IIb/IIIa inhibitors and thrombocytopenia: Possible link between platelet activation, autoimmunity and thrombosis. Thromb Haemost 88:888, 2002.

CHAPTER 81

Rheumatic Fever

Adnan S. Dajani

Rheumatic fever (RF) is generally classified as a connective tissue disease or collagen-vascular disease. Its anatomical hallmark is damage to collagen fibrils and to the ground substance of connective tissue. The rheumatic process is expressed as an inflammatory reaction that involves many organs, primarily the heart, the joints, and the central nervous system. The clinical manifestations of acute RF follow a group A streptococcal (group A strep) infection of the tonsillopharynx after a latent period of approximately 3 weeks. The major importance of acute RF is its ability to cause fibrosis of heart valves, leading to crippling hemodynamics of chronic heart disease.

RF is the most common cause of acquired heart disease in children and young adults worldwide. Although the incidence of RF declined sharply in many developed countries, the disease remains a major problem in many developing countries. The precise reasons for the fluctuations in the incidence of the disease remain only partly understood. Although RF has been studied extensively, the pathogenesis of the disease is not well defined.

EPIDEMIOLOGY

The incidence of RF and prevalence of rheumatic heart disease are markedly variable in different countries.[1,2] At the beginning of the 20th century, the incidence of RF in the United States exceeded 100 per 100,000 population; it ranged between 40 and 65 per 100,000 between 1935 and 1960 and is currently estimated as less than 2 per 100,000. Beginning in 1984, several outbreaks of acute RF were reported from a number of geographically distinct areas in the United States.[2] These focal outbreaks were not associated with a national increase in the incidence of RF. The decline in the incidence of RF in industrialized countries is in sharp contrast to the persistent high incidence of the disease in nonindustrialized countries.

In many developing countries, the incidence of acute RF approaches or exceeds 100 per 100,000.[1] In keeping with the falling incidence of RF in industrialized countries, the prevalence of rheumatic heart disease has declined. Table 81-1 compares the prevalence of rheumatic heart disease in school-age children in different regions of the world.

The decline in incidence of RF and prevalence of rheumatic heart disease has been attributed to several factors. Although the decline preceded the introduction of antimicrobial agents for the treatment of streptococcal pharyngitis, the use of these agents may have enhanced the rate of this decline. Improved economic standards, better housing conditions, decreased crowding in homes and schools, and access to medical care are often credited, at least in part, for the marked decline in RF.[1] Epidemiological observations show periodic shifts in the appearance and disappearance of specific M types in a particular geographical location. Such shifts may be another explanation for the decline and resurgence of RF in some parts of the world.

Because of the causal relationship between RF and group A strep pharyngitis, the epidemiologies of the two illnesses are very similar. Initial attacks of RF occur most commonly between the ages of 6 and 15 years, and RF rarely occurs before the age of 5 years. The risk of RF is increased in populations at high risk for streptococcal pharyngitis, such as military recruits, persons living in crowded conditions, and those in close contact with school-age children. The incidence of RF is equal in male and female patients. The seasonal incidence of RF also parallels that of streptococcal pharyngitis. The peak incidence of RF in Europe and the United States is in spring. Although RF used to be considered a disease of temperate climates, it is now more common in warm tropical climates, particularly in developing countries.

Pathogenesis

The evidence that group A streptococcus is the agent causing initial and recurrent attacks of RF is strong but indirect. It is based on clinical, epidemiological, and immunological observations. Factors that contribute to the pathogenesis of RF are related to both the putative causative agent and the host (Table 81–2).

THE ETIOLOGICAL AGENT. An untreated group A strep tonsillopharyngitis is the antecedent event that precipitates RF. RF does not follow streptococcal skin infection (impetigo). Proper antimicrobial treatment of streptococcal pharyngitis with eradication of the organism virtually eliminates the risk of RF. In situations conducive to epidemic streptococcal pharyngitis (such as the military population, crowding), as many as 3 percent of untreated acute streptococcal sore throats may be followed by RF. Endemic infections result in much lower attack rates. It has been well documented that about one-third of all cases of acute RF follow mild, almost asymptomatic pharyngitis. The lack of symptomatic pharyngitis was particularly striking in most of the more recent outbreaks of acute RF in which the majority of patients (58 percent) had no history of pharyngitis.[2] This is an alarming observation because primary prevention of acute RF relies on identification and proper treatment of streptococcal pharyngitis.

The major factors that are related to the risk of RF are the magnitude of the immune response to the antecedent streptococcal pharyngitis and persistence of the organism during convalescence. Variations in the rheumatogenicity of group A strep strains are a factor influencing the attack rate of RF.[3] The concept that RF is associated with infections with virulent encapsulated (mucoid) strains capable of inducing strong type-specific immune responses to M protein and other streptococcal antigens[4] has been strengthened by observations made during the outbreaks of acute RF in the mid-1980s. The streptococci isolated from patients with RF and their sibling contacts during these outbreaks were primarily strains belonging to M types 1, 3, 5, 6, and 18.[5] M proteins of rheumatogenic streptococci show distinct structural characteristics. They share a long terminal antigenic domain[6-8] and contain epitopes that are shared with human heart tissue, particularly sarcolemmal membrane proteins and cardiac myosin.

THE HOST. Although only a small proportion of individuals with untreated streptococcal pharyngitis may develop RF (3 percent), the incidence of the disease after

TABLE 81–1 Rheumatic Heart Disease in School-Age Children

Location	Prevalence Per 1000
United States	0.6
Japan	0.7
Asia (other)	0.4–21.0
Africa	0.3–15.0
South America	1.0–17.0

TABLE 81–2 Pathogenesis of Rheumatic Fever Group A Streptococcus

Tonsillopharyngeal infection, no other sites
Intensity of the infection Brisk antibody response Persistence of the organism
Rheumatogenic strains M types 1, 3, 5, 6, 14, 18, 19, 27, and 29 Distinct structural characteristics of M proteins Long terminal antigenic domain Epitopes shared with human heart tissue Heavily encapsulated, forming mucoid colonies Resistance to phagocytosis Does not produce opacity factor
Susceptible Host Genetic predisposition Presence of specific B-cell alloantigen
High incidence of class II HLA antigens

HLA = human leukocyte antigen.

streptococcal pharyngitis in patients who have had a previous episode of RF is substantially greater (about 50 percent). Numerous epidemiological studies also indicate familial predisposition to the disease. These observations and more recent studies strongly suggest a genetic basis for susceptibility to RF. A specific B-cell alloantigen, identified by monoclonal antibodies, has been described in almost all patients (99 percent) with RF but in only a small number (14 percent) of control subjects. Furthermore, susceptibility to RF has been linked with human leukocyte antigen (HLA) DR 1, 2, 3, and 4 haplotypes in various ethnic groups.

PATHOLOGY

The acute phase of RF is characterized by exudative and proliferative inflammatory reactions involving connective or collagen tissue. Although the disease process is diffuse, it affects primarily the heart, joints, brain, and cutaneous and subcutaneous tissues.

The basic structural change in collagen is fibrinoid degeneration. The interstitial connective tissue becomes edematous and eosinophilic, with fraying, fragmentation, and disintegration of collagen fibers. This change is associated with infiltration of mononuclear cells including large modified fibrohistiocytic cells (Aschoff cells). Some of the histiocytes are multinucleated and form Aschoff giant cells.

The Aschoff nodule in the proliferative stage is considered pathognomonic of rheumatic carditis. These nodules have been found almost invariably in the autopsies of patients who died of rheumatic carditis; however, more recent observations indicate that Aschoff nodules are observed in only 30 to 40 percent of biopsy specimens from patients with primary or recurrent episodes of RF.[9] Aschoff bodies may be seen in any area of the myocardium but not in other affected organs such as joints or brain. They are most often noted in the interventricular septum, the wall of the left ventricle, or the left atrial appendage. Aschoff nodules persist for many years after a rheumatic attack, even in patients with no evidence of recent or active inflammation.

TABLE 81–3 Guidelines for the Diagnosis of Initial Attacks of Rheumatic Fever (Jones Criteria, Updated 1992)

Major Manifestations	Minor Manifestations
Carditis	Clinical findings
Polyarthritis	Arthralgia
Chorea	Fever
Erythema marginatum	Laboratory findings
Subcutaneous nodules	Elevated acute phase reactants Erythrocyte sedimentation rate C-reactive protein Prolonged PR interval
Supporting Evidence of Antecedent A Streptococcal Infection Positive throat culture or rapid streptococcal antigen test Elevated or rising streptococcal antibody titer	

From Dajani AS, Ayoub EM, Bierman FZ, et al: Guidelines for the diagnosis of rheumatic fever: Jones criteria, updated 1992. JAMA 268:2069, 1992. Copyright 1992 American Medical Association.

Inflammation of valvular tissue accounts for the more commonly recognized clinical manifestations of rheumatic carditis. Initial inflammation leads to valvular insufficiency. The extravasation of lymphocytes through the valvular endothelium may initiate the pathological process.[10] The histological findings in endocarditis consist of edema and cellular infiltration of the valvular tissue and the chordae tendineae. Hyaline degeneration of the affected valve leads to the formation of verrucae at its edge, preventing total approximation of the leaflets. Fibrosis and calcification of the valve occur if inflammation persists. This process may eventually lead to valvular stenosis.

Diagnosis

No specific clinical, laboratory, or other test establishes the diagnosis of RF. In 1944, T. Duckett Jones formulated his criteria for the diagnosis of RF, which are still valuable. They have been modified, revised, edited, and updated by the Committee on Rheumatic Fever, Endocarditis, and Kawasaki Disease of the Council on Cardiovascular Disease in the Young (American Heart Association)[11] and, more recently, they have been reaffirmed.[12] The most recent guidelines (Table 81–3) emphasize the diagnosis of *initial attacks* of RF. Dividing clinical and laboratory findings into major and minor manifestations is based on the diagnostic importance of a particular finding. If supported by evidence of preceding group A strep infection, the presence of two major manifestations or of one major and two minor manifestations indicates a high probability of acute RF.

Major Clinical Manifestations

CARDITIS. Rheumatic carditis is a pancarditis affecting the endocardium, myocardium, and pericardium to various degrees. Clinically, rheumatic carditis is almost always associated with a murmur of valvulitis. The severity of carditis is variable. In its most severe form, death from cardiac failure may occur. More commonly, carditis is less intense, and the predominant effect is subsequent scarring of the heart valves. Evidence of carditis may be subtle; signs of valvular involvement may be mild and transient and may be easily missed on auscultation. Baseline studies, including electrocardiograms, echocardiograms, and Doppler studies,[12,13] should be obtained in patients in whom RF is suspected. The use of echocardiographic abnormalities in the recognition of carditis in patients without a heart murmur is controversial.[12,14]

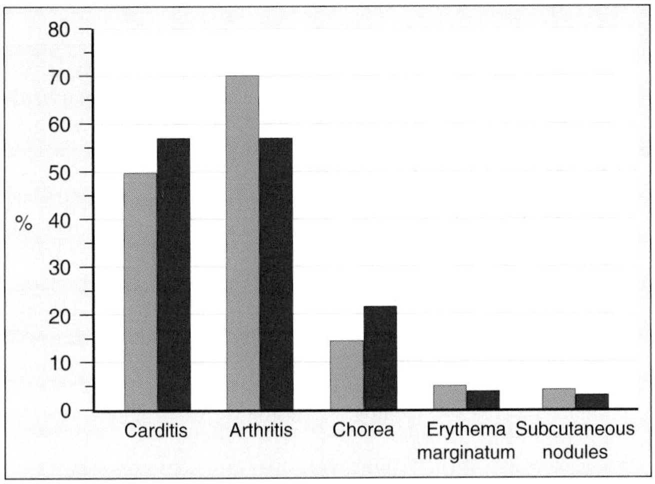

FIGURE 81–1 Relative frequency of major manifestations of rheumatic fever in earlier (blue) and more recent (purple) reports in the 1980s.

Patients who show no clear evidence of carditis on initial examination should be closely monitored for a few weeks to assess cardiac involvement.

Carditis is often regarded as the most specific manifestation of RF. It is noted in at least 50 percent of patients with acute RF (Fig. 81–1). More recent outbreaks in the United States suggested that the frequency of carditis was somewhat higher than traditionally reported, which may be due in part to more sophisticated diagnostic methods.[2] In one report, carditis was diagnosed in 72 percent of cases by auscultation and in 91 percent of cases by Doppler ultrasonography. The risk of overdiagnosing valvular incompetence by echocardiography should be emphasized, and overreliance on this tool in diagnosing rheumatic carditis should be avoided.

Valvulitis (endocarditis) involving mitral and aortic valves and the chordae of the mitral valve is the most characteristic component of rheumatic carditis. Mitral regurgitation is the hallmark of rheumatic carditis. Aortic regurgitation is less common and usually associated with mitral regurgitation. The pulmonic and tricuspid valves are rarely involved. Residual valvular damage is a major concern in patients with RF and may lead to intractable cardiac failure requiring surgical intervention. Valvular abnormalities, especially aortic and mitral regurgitation, rather than myocardial damage appear to be dominant in causing cardiac dysfunction.[12,14]

Myocarditis or pericarditis in the *absence* of valvulitis is *not* likely to be due to RF. Tachycardia is an early sign of myocarditis but may also be due to fever or cardiac failure. Transient arrhythmias may occur in patients with myocarditis. Severe myocarditis or valvular regurgitation may lead to cardiac failure. Cardiac enlargement occurs when severe hemodynamic changes result from valvular, myocardial, or pericardial disease.

ARTHRITIS. Polyarthritis is the most common major manifestation of RF (see Fig. 81–1) but the least specific. It is almost always asymmetrical and migratory and involves larger joints (knees, ankles, elbows, and wrists). Swelling, redness, heat, severe pain, limitation of motion, and tenderness to touch are characteristic. The arthritis of RF is benign and does not result in permanent joint deformity. Joint fluid shows findings characteristic of inflammation (not infection). In untreated cases, arthritis usually lasts 2 to 3 weeks. A striking feature of rheumatic arthritis is its dramatic response to salicylates.

Some patients may develop arthritis and other multisystem manifestations after acute streptococcal pharyngitis that do not fulfill the Jones criteria for the diagnosis of acute RF. This "syndrome" has been referred to as poststreptococcal reactive arthritis (PSRA). The arthritis of PSRA does not respond dramatically to antiinflammatory agents. Some patients with PSRA may have silent or delayed-onset carditis[15]; therefore, these patients should be carefully observed for several months for the subsequent development of carditis.

CHOREA. Sydenham chorea, St. Vitus dance, or chorea minor occurs in about 20 percent of patients with RF (see Fig. 81–1). The rheumatic inflammatory process in the central nervous system specifically involves the basal ganglia and caudate nuclei. Chorea is a *delayed* manifestation of RF, usually appearing 3 months or longer after the onset of the precipitating streptococcal infection. This period is in sharp contrast to the latent period of carditis or arthritis, which is usually 3 weeks. Thus, chorea is frequently the only manifestation of RF. Furthermore, evidence of a recent group A strep infection may be difficult to document, and other supporting historical, clinical, or laboratory findings to fulfill the Jones criteria may be lacking. The diagnosis of RF can be made in a patient with chorea without strictly adhering to the Jones criteria.

Sydenham chorea is characterized clinically by purposeless and involuntary movements, muscle incoordination and weakness, and emotional lability. The manifestations are more evident when a patient is awake and under stress and may disappear during sleep. All muscles, but primarily muscles of the face and extremities, may be involved. Speech may be affected, being explosive and halting. Handwriting deteriorates, and patients become uncoordinated and easily frustrated. The symptoms of Sydenham chorea must be distinguished from tics, athetosis, conversion reactions, hyperkinesis, and behavior problems. Symptoms usually resolve in 1 to 2 weeks, even without treatment. Patients with RF, and especially those with Sydenham chorea, are at higher risk for the development of neuropsychiatric disorders, including obsessive-compulsive and depressive disorders.[16]

ERYTHEMA MARGINATUM. This distinctive rash is a rare manifestation of RF, occurring in less than 5 percent of patients. It is an evanescent, erythematous, macular, nonpruritic rash with pale centers and rounded or serpiginous margins. Lesions vary greatly in size and occur mainly on the trunk and proximal extremities, not on the face. The rash may be induced by application of heat.

SUBCUTANEOUS NODULES. These are firm, painless, freely movable nodules that measure 0.5 to 2 cm. They are rarely seen in patients with RF (about 3 percent); when present, they are most often seen in patients with carditis. They are usually located over extensor surfaces of the joints (particularly elbows, knees, and wrists), in the occipital portion of the scalp, or over spinous processes. The overlying skin is freely movable, shows no discoloration, and is not inflamed.

Minor Manifestations

CLINICAL FINDINGS. Fever and arthralgia are nonspecific, common findings in patients with acute RF. Their diagnostic value is limited because they are encountered commonly in various other diseases. They are used to support the diagnosis of RF when only a single major manifestation is present. Fever is noted during the acute stages of the disease and has no characteristic pattern. Arthralgia is pain in one or more large joints without objective findings on examination and must not be considered a minor manifestation if arthritis is present. Epistaxis and abdominal pain may also occur but are not included as minor diagnostic criteria for RF.

LABORATORY FINDINGS. Elevated acute phase reactants offer objective but nonspecific indications of tissue inflammation. The erythrocyte sedimentation rate (ESR) and

C-reactive protein (CRP) level are almost always elevated during the acute stages of the disease in patients with carditis or polyarthritis but are usually normal in patients with chorea. The ESR is useful in monitoring the course of the disease; it usually returns to normal as the rheumatic activity subsides. The ESR may be elevated in patients with anemia and may be suppressed to normal levels in patients with congestive cardiac failure. Unlike the ESR, the CRP level is unaffected by anemia or cardiac failure.

A common finding in patients with acute RF is a prolonged PR interval for age and rate on electrocardiography. This finding alone is not diagnostic of carditis and does not correlate with the ultimate development of chronic rheumatic cardiac disease. Other findings on electrocardiography include tachycardia, atrioventricular block, and QRS-T changes suggestive of myocarditis; these changes are not considered minor manifestations.

Leukocytosis may be observed in the acute stages of RF, but the leukocyte count is variable and not dependable. Anemia is usually mild or moderate and normocytic normochromatic in morphology (anemia of chronic inflammation). Chest roentgenograms are useful in assessing cardiac size; however, normal findings on a chest roentgenogram do not preclude the presence of carditis. Pericarditis, pulmonary edema, and increased pulmonary vascularity are also detected by this examination. Echocardiography may be helpful in detecting endocardial, myocardial, and pericardial involvement. Antimyosin antibody imaging has been reported to be useful in the detection of rheumatic carditis.[17]

Antecedent Group A Streptococcal Infection

A number of illnesses mimic acute RF, and no laboratory test or tests establish a specific diagnosis of RF. It is therefore important to establish an antecedent streptococcal infection by demonstrating group A streptococcus in the tonsillopharynx or an elevated or rising streptococcal antibody titer. *Evidence of an antecedent streptococcal infection is required for confirmation of the initial diagnosis of acute RF.*

At the time of diagnosis of acute RF, only about 11 percent of patients have throat cultures positive for group A streptococcus.[2] The paucity of positive cultures is due, in part, to elimination of the organism by host defense mechanisms during the latent period between the onset of the infection and the subsequent development of RF. Several rapid group A strep antigen detection tests are commercially available. These tests vary in method. Most have a high degree of specificity but low sensitivity in a clinical setting. A negative test result does not preclude the presence of group A streptococcus in the pharynx. A positive throat culture result or rapid antigen test does not distinguish between a recent infection that can be associated with acute RF and chronic pharyngeal carriage of the organism.

Because the presence of group A streptococci in the pharynx may not represent active infection, elevated or rising antistreptococcal antibody titers provide more reliable evidence of a recent streptococcal infection than does a positive culture or a positive rapid antigen test result. The most commonly used antibody tests are the antistreptolysin O (ASO) and antideoxyribonuclease B (anti-DNase B) tests. The ASO test is usually performed first, and if results are not elevated, the anti-DNase B test is done. Elevated titers for both tests may persist for several weeks or months. ASO titers rise and fall more rapidly than anti-DNase B titers. A commercially available slide agglutination test measures antibodies to several streptococcal antigens. It is simple to perform, rapid, and widely available; however, the test is not well standardized and not very reproducible and is not recommended as a definitive test for evidence of a preceding group A strep infection.

Treatment

GENERAL. Whenever possible, patients should be admitted to a hospital for close observation and appropriate workup. Bed rest is generally considered important because it lessens joint pain. Ambulation may be attempted when fever abates and acute phase reactants return to normal. Patients should be allowed to return to a reasonably active life with normal physical activity. Strenuous physical exercise should be avoided, however, particularly if carditis was present. Although throat cultures are rarely positive for group A streptococcus at the time of onset of RF, patients should receive a 10-day course of penicillin therapy. Patients allergic to penicillin should be treated with erythromycin.

If heart failure intervenes, patients should receive diuretics, oxygen, and digitalis and have a restricted sodium diet. Digitalis preparations should be used cautiously because cardiac toxicity may occur with conventional dosages.

ANTIRHEUMATIC THERAPY. There is no specific treatment for the inflammatory reactions initiated by RF. Supportive therapy is aimed at reducing constitutional symptoms, controlling toxic manifestations, and improving cardiac function.

Patients with mild or no carditis usually respond well to salicylates. Salicylates are particularly effective in relieving joint pain; such pain usually abates within 24 hours of starting salicylates. Indeed, if joint pain persists after salicylate treatment, the diagnosis of RF may be questionable and patients should be re-evaluated. Because no specific diagnostic tests for RF exist, antiinflammatory therapy should be withheld until the clinical picture has become sufficiently clear to allow a diagnosis. Early administration of antiinflammatory agents may suppress clinical manifestations and prevent appropriate diagnosis. For optimal antiinflammatory effect, serum salicylate levels around 20 mg percent are required. Aspirin, at doses of 100 mg/kg/d, given four to five times daily, usually results in adequate serum levels to achieve a clinical response. Optimal salicylate therapy must be individualized, however, to ensure adequate response and avoid toxicity. Tinnitus, nausea, vomiting, and anorexia are common dose-related toxicities associated with salicylism. Side effects can subside after a few days of treatment despite continuation of the medication.

Patients with significant cardiac involvement—particularly those with pericarditis or congestive heart failure—respond more promptly to corticosteroids than to salicylates. Patients who do not respond to adequate doses of salicylates may occasionally benefit from a trial course of corticosteroids. Prednisone, 1 to 2 mg/kg/d, is the usual agent.

There is no evidence that salicylate, corticosteroids, or intravenous immunoglobulin therapy affects the course of carditis or diminishes the incidence of residual heart disease.[18-20] Therefore, the duration of therapy with antiinflammatory agents is arbitrarily based on an estimate of the severity of the episode and the promptness of the clinical response.

Mild attacks with little or no cardiac involvement can be treated with salicylates for about 1 month or until there is sufficient clinical and laboratory evidence of inflammatory inactivity. In more severe cases, therapy with corticosteroids may be continued for 2 to 3 months. The medication is then gradually reduced over the next 2 weeks. Even with prolonged therapy, some patients (approximately 5 percent) continue to demonstrate evidence of rheumatic activity for 6 months or more. A "rebound," manifested by reappearance of mild symptoms or of acute phase reactants, may occur in some patients after antiinflammatory medications have been discontinued, usually within 2 weeks. Modest symptoms usually subside without treatment; more severe symptoms may require treatment with salicylates. Some physicians recommend the use of salicylates (aspirin, 75 mg/kg/d) during the period when corticosteroids are being tapered and believe that such an approach may reduce the likelihood of a rebound.

Information about the use of salicylates other than aspirin is limited. In patients who cannot tolerate aspirin or who are allergic to it, a trial of other nonsteroidal agents may be warranted. Aspirin preparations that are coated or that contain alkali or buffers may also be tried; however, little evidence shows that such preparations are better tolerated, and some may have undesirable side effects.

Prevention

Primary Prevention

Prevention of primary attacks of RF depends on prompt recognition and proper treatment of group A strep tonsillopharyngitis. Eradication of group A streptococcus from the throat is essential. Although appropriate antimicrobial therapy started up to 9 days after the onset of acute streptococcal pharyngitis is effective in preventing primary attacks of RF, early therapy is advisable because it reduces both morbidity and the period of infectivity. In selecting a regimen for the treatment of group A strep pharyngitis, various factors should be considered, including bacteriological and clinical efficacy, ease of adherence to the recommended regimen (frequency of daily administration, duration of therapy, palatability), cost, spectrum of activity of the selected agent, and potential side effects.[21]

Penicillin is the antimicrobial agent of choice for the treatment of group A strep pharyngitis, except in patients with history of allergy to penicillin.[22] Penicillin has a narrow spectrum of activity, has longstanding proven efficacy, and is the least expensive regimen. Group A streptococcus resistant to penicillin has not been documented. Penicillin can be administered intramuscularly or orally (Table 81–4), depending on the patient's likely adherence to an oral regimen.

Intramuscular benzathine penicillin G is preferred, particularly for patients who are unlikely to complete a 10-day course of oral therapy and for patients with a personal or family history of RF or rheumatic heart disease. Benzathine penicillin G injections should be given as a single dose in a large muscle mass. This formulation is painful; injections that contain procaine penicillin in addition to benzathine penicillin G are less painful. Less discomfort is associated with intramuscular benzathine penicillin G if the medication is warmed to room temperature before administration.

The oral antibiotic of choice is penicillin V (phenoxymethyl penicillin). Patients should take oral penicillin regularly for an entire 10-day period, although they are likely to be asymptomatic after the first few days. Although the broader spectrum amoxicillin is often used for treatment of group A strep pharyngitis, it offers no microbiological advantage over penicillin.

Oral erythromycin is acceptable for patients allergic to penicillin. Treatment should also be prescribed for 10 days. Erythromycin estolate (20 to 40 mg/kg/d in two to four divided doses) or erythromycin ethyl succinate (40 mg/kg/d in two to four divided doses) is effective in treating streptococcal pharyngitis. The maximal dose of erythromycin is 1 gm/d. Although strains of group A streptococci resistant to erythromycin are prevalent in some areas of the world and have resulted in treatment failures, they are uncommon in most parts of the United States.

The macrolide azithromycin has susceptibility similar to that of erythromycin against group A streptococcus but may cause fewer gastrointestinal side effects. Azithromycin can be administered once daily and produces high tonsillar tissue concentrations. A 5-day course of azithromycin is acceptable as a second-line therapy for the treatment of patients with group A strep pharyngitis. The recommended dosage is 500 mg as a single dose on the first day followed by 250 mg once daily for 4 days.

A 10-day course of an oral cephalosporin is an acceptable alternative, particularly for penicillin-allergic patients. Narrower spectrum cephalosporins, such as cefadroxil or cephalexin, are probably preferable to the broader spectrum cephalosporins such as cefaclor, cefuroxime, cefixime, and cefpodoxime. Some penicillin-allergic persons (<15 percent) are also allergic to cephalosporins, and these agents should

TABLE 81–4 Prevention of Rheumatic Fever

Agent	Dose	Route	Duration
Primary Prevention			
Benzathine penicillin G	600,000 units for patients ≤27 kg 1,200,000 units for patients >27 kg *or*	IM	Once
Pencillin V	Children: 250 mg 2-3 times daily Adolescents and adults: 500 mg 2-3 times daily	PO	10 d
For patients allergic to penicillin:			
Erythromycin	40 mg/kg/d 2-4 times daily (maximum 1 gm/d)	PO	10 d
Secondary Prevention			
Benzathine penicillin G	1,200,00 units every 3-4 wk *or*	IM	See Table 81–5
Penicillin V	250 mg b.i.d. *or*	PO	See Table 81–5
Sulfadiazine	0.5 gm once daily for patients ≤27 kg (60 lb) 1.0 gm once daily for patients >27 kg (60 lb)	PO	See Table 81–5
For patients allergic to penicillin and sulfadiazine:			
Erythromycin	250 mg b.i.d.	PO	See Table 81–5

Modified from Dajani AS, Taubert K, Ferrieri P, et al: Treatment of streptococcal pharyngitis and prevention of rheumatic fever. Pediatrics 96:758, 1995, with permission.

not be used by patients with immediate (anaphylactic-type) hypersensitivity to penicillin.

A 10-day course with an oral cephalosporin is superior to 10 days of oral penicillin in eradicating group A streptococcus from the pharynx. Reports suggest that a 5-day course with selected oral cephalosporins is comparable to a 10-day course of oral penicillin in eradicating group A streptococcus from the pharynx.

Secondary Prevention

Patients who have suffered a previous attack of RF and who develop streptococcal pharyngitis are at high risk for a recurrent attack of RF. A group A strep infection need not be symptomatic to trigger a recurrence. Furthermore, RF can recur even when a symptomatic infection is optimally treated. For these reasons, prevention of recurrent RF requires continuous antimicrobial prophylaxis rather than recognition and treatment of acute episodes of streptococcal pharyngitis. Continuous prophylaxis is recommended for patients with a well-documented history of RF (including cases manifested solely by Sydenham chorea) and those with definite evidence of rheumatic heart disease. Such prophylaxis should be initiated as soon as acute RF or rheumatic heart disease is diagnosed. A full therapeutic course of penicillin (as outlined in Table 81–4) should first be given to patients with acute RF to eradicate residual group A streptococci even if a throat culture is negative at that time. Streptococcal infections occurring in family members of rheumatic patients should be treated promptly.

CONTINUOUS ANTIMICROBIAL PROPHYLAXIS. Continuous prophylaxis provides the most effective protection from RF recurrences. Risk of recurrence depends on several factors. Risk increases with several previous attacks, whereas the risk decreases as the interval since the most recent attack lengthens. The likelihood of acquiring a streptococcal upper respiratory tract infection is an important consideration. Patients with increased exposure to streptococcal infections include children and adolescents; parents of young children; teachers, physicians, nurses, and allied health personnel in contact with children; military recruits; and others in crowded housing. A higher risk of recurrences in economically disadvantaged populations has been demonstrated.

Physicians must consider each individual situation when determining the appropriate duration of prophylaxis. Patients who have had rheumatic carditis are at a relatively high risk for recurrences of carditis and are likely to sustain increasingly severe cardiac involvement with each recurrence. Therefore, patients who have had rheumatic carditis should receive long-term antibiotic prophylaxis, perhaps for life. Duration of prophylaxis depends on whether residual valvular disease is present or absent (Table 81–5). Prophylaxis should continue even after valve surgery, including prosthetic valve replacement. Patients who have had RF without carditis are at considerably less risk of cardiac involvement with a recurrence. Therefore, prophylaxis may be discontinued in these individuals after several years.[23] In general, prophylaxis should continue until 5 years have elapsed since the last RF attack or age 21 years, whichever is longer. The decision to discontinue prophylaxis or reinstate it should be made after discussion with the patient of potential risks and benefits and careful consideration of the epidemiological risk factors enumerated earlier.

An injection of 1,200,000 units of a long-acting penicillin preparation every 4 weeks is the recommended regimen for secondary prevention in most circumstances in the United States (see Table 81–4). In countries where the incidence of RF is particularly high, in special circumstances, or in certain high-risk individuals, such as patients with residual rheumatic carditis, the administration of benzathine penicillin G every 3 weeks is recommended.[24] Long-acting penicillin is of particular value in patients with a high risk of recurrence of RF. The advantages of benzathine penicillin G must be weighed against inconvenience to patients and pain of injection, which cause some patients to discontinue prophylaxis.

TABLE 81–5 Duration of Secondary Prophylaxis in Patients with Rheumatic Fever

Category	Duration
Rheumatic fever with carditis and residual valvular disease	At least 10 yr after last episode and at least until age 40 Sometimes lifelong prophylaxis
Rheumatic fever with carditis but no residual valvular disease	10 yr or well into adulthood, whichever is longer
Rheumatic fever without carditis	5 yr or until age 21, whichever is longer

From Dajani AS, Taubert K, Ferrieri P, et al: Treatment of streptococcal pharyngitis and prevention of rheumatic fever. Pediatrics 96:758, 1995, with permission.

Successful oral prophylaxis depends primarily on patients' adherence to prescribed regimens. Patients need careful and repeated instructions about the importance of continuing prophylaxis. Most failures of prophylaxis occur in nonadherent patients. Even with optimal adherence, risk of recurrence is higher in individuals receiving oral prophylaxis than in those receiving intramuscular benzathine penicillin G.[21] Oral agents are more appropriate for patients at lower risk for rheumatic recurrence. Accordingly, some physicians switch patients to oral prophylaxis when they have reached late adolescence or young adulthood and have remained free of rheumatic attacks for at least 5 years.

Penicillin V is the preferred oral agent (see Table 81–4). There are no published data about the use of other penicillins, macrolides, or cephalosporins for secondary prevention of RF. Although sulfonamides are not effective in eradication of group A streptococci, they do prevent infection. Sulfadiazine and sulfisoxazole appear to be equivalent; the use of sulfisoxazole is acceptable on the basis of extrapolation from data demonstrating that sulfadiazine has proven effectiveness in secondary prophylaxis. The recommended dose of sulfisoxazole is the same as that for sulfadiazine. Sulfonamide prophylaxis is contraindicated in late pregnancy because of transplacental passage of the drugs and potential competition with bilirubin for albumin binding sites. Erythromycin is recommended for patients who are allergic to penicillin and sulfisoxazole.

Infective Endocarditis Prophylaxis

(see also Chap. 58)

Patients with rheumatic valvular heart disease also require additional short-term antibiotic prophylaxis before certain surgical and dental procedures to prevent possible development of infective endocarditis. Patients with prosthetic valves or previous endocarditis are at particularly high risk. *Antibiotic regimens used to prevent recurrences of acute RF are inadequate for prevention of bacterial endocarditis.* The current recommendations of the American Heart Association concerning prevention of bacterial endocarditis should be followed.[25] Because alpha-hemolytic streptococci in the oropharynx may have developed resistance to oral penicillin being used for secondary prevention of RF, the agent selected to prevent endocarditis should not be a penicillin. Patients who have had RF but who do not have evidence of rheumatic heart disease do not need endocarditis prophylaxis.

GENERAL REFERENCES

Narula J, Virmanil R, Reddy KS, et al: Rheumatic Fever. American Registry of Pathology. Washington, DC, Armed Forces Institute of Pathology, 1999.
Jones TD: Diagnosis of rheumatic fever. JAMA 126:481, 1944.

REFERENCES

1. World Health Organization: Rheumatic fever and rheumatic heart disease. WHO Technical Report Series 764. Geneva, World Health Organization, 1998.
2. Dajani AS: Current status of nonsuppurative complications of group A streptococci. Pediatr Infect Dis J 10:S25, 1991.
3. Stollerman GH: Rheumatogenic group A streptococci and the return of rheumatic fever. Adv Intern Med 35:1, 1990.
4. Stollerman GH: Rheumatogenic streptococci and autoimmunity. Clin Immunol Immunopathol 61:131, 1991.
5. Kaplan EL, Johnson DR, Cleary PP: Group A streptococcal serotypes isolated from patients and sibling contacts during the resurgence of rheumatic fever in the United States in the mid-1980s. J Infect Dis 159:101, 1989.
6. Bessen D, Jones KF, Fischetti VA: Evidence for two distinct classes of streptococcal M protein and their relationship to rheumatic fever. J Exp Med 169:269, 1989.
7. Stollerman GH: Rheumatic fever in the 21st century. J Clin Infect Dis 33:806, 2001.
8. Smoot JC, Barbian KD, Van Gompel JJ, et al: Genome sequence and comparative microarray analysis of serotype M18 group A streptococcus strains associated with acute rheumatic fever outbreaks. Proc Natl Acad Sci USA 99:4668, 2002.
9. Narula J, Chopra P, Talwar KK, et al: Does endomyocardial biopsy aid in the diagnosis of active rheumatic carditis? Circulation 88:2198, 1993.
10. Roberts S, Kosanke S, Terrence Dunn S, et al: Pathogenic mechanisms in rheumatic carditis: Focus on valvular endothelium. J Infect Dis 183:507, 2001.
11. Dajani AS, Ayoub EM, Bierman FZ, et al: Guidelines for the diagnosis of rheumatic fever: Jones criteria, updated 1992. JAMA 268:2069, 1992.
12. Ferrieri P for the Jones Criteria Working Group: Proceedings of the Jones Criteria Workshop. Circulation 106:2521, 2002.
13. Veasy LG: Time to take soundings in acute rheumatic fever. Lancet 357:1994, 2001.
14. Gentles TL, Colan SD, Wilson NJ, et al: Left ventricular mechanics during and after acute rheumatic fever: Contractile dysfunction is closely related to valve regurgitation. J Am Coll Cardiol 37:201, 2001.
15. Schaffer FM, Agarwal R, Helm J, et al: Poststreptococcal reactive arthritis and silent carditis: A case report and review of the literature. Pediatrics 93:837, 1994.
16. Mercadente MT, Busatto GF, Lombroso PJ, et al: The psychiatric symptoms of rheumatic fever. Am J Psychiatry 157:2036, 2000.
17. Narula J: Usefulness of antimyosin antibody imaging for the detection of active rheumatic myocarditis. Am J Cardiol 84:946, 1999.
18. Cilliers AM, Manyemba J, Saloojee H: Anti-inflammatory treatment for carditis in acute rheumatic fever (Cochrane review). Cochrane Database Syst Rev 2:CD003176, 2003.
19. Voss LM, Wilson NJ, Neutze JM, et al: Intravenous immunoglobulin in acute rheumatic fever: A randomized controlled trial. Circulation 103:401, 2001.
20. Rullan E, Sigal LH: Rheumatic fever. Curr Rheumatol Rep 3:445, 2001.
21. Dajani AS: Adherence to physicians' instructions as a factor in managing streptococcal pharyngitis. Pediatrics 97:976, 1996.
22. Dajani AS, Taubert K, Ferrieri P, et al: Treatment of streptococcal pharyngitis and prevention of rheumatic fever. Pediatrics 96:758, 1995.
23. Berrios X, del Campo E, Guzman B, et al: Discontinuing rheumatic fever prophylaxis in selected adolescents and young adults. Ann Intern Med 118:401, 1993.
24. Lue HC, Wu MH, Wang JK, et al: Long-term outcome of patients with rheumatic fever receiving benzathine penicillin G prophylaxis every three weeks versus every four weeks. J Pediatr 125:812, 1994.
25. Dajani AS, Taubert KA, Wilson W, et al: Prevention of bacterial endocarditis: Recommendations by the American Heart Association. JAMA 277:1794, 1997.

CHAPTER 82

Rheumatic Diseases and the Cardiovascular System

Brian F. Mandell • Gary S. Hoffman

General Principles

Systemic rheumatological conditions often involve the cardiovascular system. They may first come to medical attention because of constitutional symptoms, muscle or joint pain, fever, regional or visceral ischemia, or organ failure. Rheumatological events that affect the heart and vessels vary from inapparent to catastrophic. Although cardiologists or cardiothoracic surgeons are usually not the initial source of care, in certain instances they may be the first to recognize that cardiovascular disease may have a primary immunological basis. Examples include patients with the vasculitides, who may present with claudication, aortic aneurysms, or ischemic heart disease (Takayasu or giant cell arteritis), and patients with systemic lupus erythematosus, who may first require medical attention for treatment of pericarditis.

Vasculitis

Discrimination between the various forms of rheumatic diseases and vasculitis begins with the concept of *primary* (i.e., the primary process is immune dysregulation without a known trigger) versus *secondary* (i.e., the cause is known and inflammation- or immune-mediated injury requires treatment or removal of the causative agent). Not knowing which group a patient fits into can lead to inappropriate use of immunosuppressive therapy that may have adverse or lethal consequences. Examples of secondary vasculitides include vasculitis secondary to sepsis, particularly endocarditis; drug toxicity and poisonings; malignancies; cardiac myxomas; and multifocal emboli from large-vessel aneurysms (Table 82–1). Each can mimic vasculitis or cause multifocal ischemia or infarction with accompanying vasculitis.

The greatest certainty in the diagnosis of primary vasculitis is in the setting of classic clinical and laboratory patterns, e.g., a 70-year-old woman with new-onset severe headache, temporal region pain, hip and shoulder girdle stiffness, visual aberration (amaurosis or blindness), and a high sedimentation rate. This picture would be so compatible with giant cell arteritis as not to require biopsy evidence of the diagnosis. Unfortunately, many patients with vasculitis do not present with such recognizable features. Instead, one may have to depend on combinations of less typical clues. A patient with ischemic digits, active urinary sediment, and peripheral neuropathy is likely to have vasculitis, especially if the previously noted secondary causes of vasculitis and its mimics have already been ruled out. The presence of a purpuric rash, particularly if it is palpable (Fig. 82–1), furthers the probability of this diagnosis, which can be confirmed by a simple skin biopsy. Such features occurring in the setting of an established autoimmune disease (e.g., rheumatoid arthritis, systemic lupus erythematosus, Sjögren syndrome, or relapsing polychondritis) enhance the likelihood of vasculitis being present. The physician must still distinguish primary from secondary causes.

Approach to Proving the Diagnosis of Vasculitis

Definitive proof of the diagnosis depends on visualizing vasculitic lesions in affected tissue. The greatest success in achieving a tissue diagnosis comes from biopsy of abnormal or symptomatic sites. In patients with proven vasculitis, the yield from biopsies of clinically normal sites is considerably less than 20 percent. Therefore, a biopsy of apparently normal tissue is not recommended. Biopsies of abnormal organs provide diagnostically useful information in more than 65 percent of cases. Biopsies of involved viscera have less than 100 percent yield because needle and organ-penetrating biopsies often do not directly visualize the affected tissue, and uniform involvement of vessels in affected viscera is uncommon.

A biopsy may not be practical in certain circumstances, such as systemic illness with symptoms of visceral ischemia, carotidynia, or findings of unequal pulses or blood pressures. Because biopsy of large vessels is usually impractical, angiography may be helpful. In this setting, vascular stenoses or aneurysms, or both, that cannot be explained on the basis of atherosclerosis may provide sufficient circumstantial evidence to proceed with treatment for primary systemic vasculitis.

Forms of Vasculitis Relevant to Cardiologists and Cardiovascular Surgeons

Takayasu Arteritis

Takayasu arteritis (TA) is an idiopathic large-vessel vasculitis of young individuals that affects the aorta and its major branches.

EPIDEMIOLOGY. Women are affected about 10 times more often than men. The median age at onset is 25 years. Although TA is best known to occur in Asia, the distribution of the disease is worldwide and it has been reported among people of all races

TABLE 82–1 Diagnosis of Vasculitis: Diseases That Can Mimic Primary Systemic Vasculitis

Sepsis, especially endocarditis
Drug toxicity or poisoning Cocaine Amphetamines Ephedra Phenylpropanolamine
Coagulopathy Anticardiolipin antibody syndrome Disseminated intravascular coagulation
Malignancy (solid organ or "liquid" tumors)
Cardiac myxoma
Multifocal emboli from large-vessel aneurysms (cholesterol, mycotic)
Ehlers-Danlos syndrome (vascular ectatic type)
Fibromuscular dysplasia

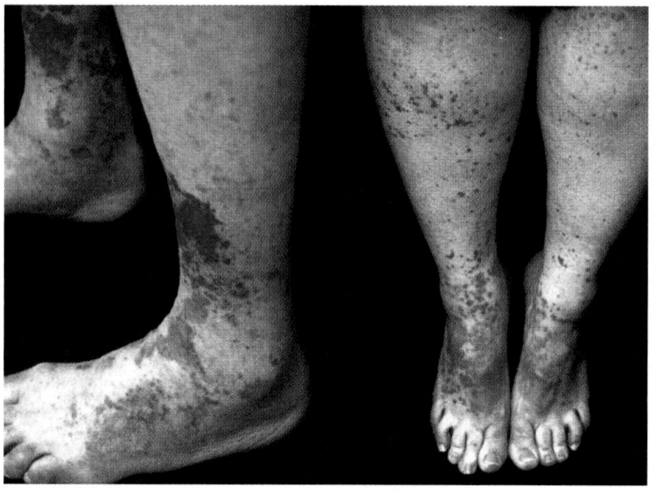

FIGURE 82–1 Palpable purpura. Vascular inflammation at the level of capillaries and venules leads to exudation of formed elements and the color and texture of lesions noted in these patients. The legs on the right are those of a young woman with Henoch-Schönlein vasculitis or purpura. The elderly man on the left has a similar lesion. However, in this case it was associated with hepatitis C virus (HCV), acquired in the course of transfusions for heart surgery. HCV infection led to cryoglobulinemia and *secondary* vasculitis. The treatment for each patient is quite different. The one with Henoch-Schönkin purpura, who does not have extracutaneous disease, requires only reassurance and monitoring for her usually self-limiting problem, whereas the patient with HCV and vasculitis requires antiviral therapy.

and ethnicities. The incidence of TA is estimated to be 2.6 per 1,000,000 persons in the United States and 1.26 per 1,000,000 in northern Europe.[1] Autopsy series from Japan point to a higher incidence, with 1 in every 3000 autopsies having features of TA.[2]

PATHOGENESIS. Although the cause of TA is unknown, studies of acute lesions reveal mononuclear cell infiltrates that appear to have reached the vessel wall through the vasa vasorum and subsequently migrate to the macroluminal intima (Fig. 82–2A, left). These cells are predominantly macrophages and T, gamma-delta, cytotoxic, and natural killer lymphocytes. There is also a small admixture of B lymphocytes. The presence of a variety of cytokines, including interleukin-6 (IL-6) and tumor necrosis factor (TNF), in these granulomatous lesions has suggested a variety of therapeutic approaches using biological agents. The finding of the mycobacterial heat shock protein, HSP-65, in the affected media and vasa vasorum of TA-affected vessels is intriguing. However, it is uncertain whether this is an epiphenomenon or a primary or intermediate step in TA pathogenesis.[3]

CLINICAL FEATURES. In TA, arterial stenoses occur three to four times more often than aneurysms. Claudication (>60 percent upper versus ~30 percent lower extremities) is the most common complaint, and bruits (~80 percent) and blood pressure and pulse asymmetries (60 to 80 percent) are the most common findings. Aneurysms are most common and clinically most significant in the aortic root, where they can lead to valvular regurgitation (~20 percent) (Fig. 82–2A, left, and B). Hypertension is most often due to renal artery stenosis but can also be associated with suprarenal aortic stenosis or a chronically damaged, rigid aorta. Cardiac, renal, and central nervous system vascular diseases are the principal causes of severe morbidity and mortality. Estimates of mortality range from a low of about 3 percent at 8 years[4] to about 35 percent at 5 years follow-up.[1,4]

Symptoms of large-vessel abnormalities or the finding of hypertension, especially in young patients, necessitates examination of extremity pulses and blood pressures for asymmetry and a search for bruits. Increasing extremity or visceral ischemia, malaise, myalgias, arthralgias, night sweats, and fever may indicate active disease. When such symptoms occur in the setting of an elevated erythrocyte sedimentation rate (ESR), active disease is assumed to be present. Yet, many patients may not have any constitutional or new vascular symptoms, and as many as 50 percent may have normal ESRs and still experience progressive disease.[1,4] The following findings indicate that active TA can occur in this setting:

1. New vascular abnormalities on sequential angiographic studies in patients who were thought to be in remission and
2. The presence of inflammatory changes in arterial biopsy specimens from patients in whom surgery was performed because of critical flow abnormalities in the setting of clinically "quiescent" disease.[1,4]

Until we are better able to judge the degree of disease activity in TA, outcomes will be compromised. Studies using refinements in magnetic resonance and positron-emission tomography imaging techniques may enable the clinician to detect qualitative abnormalities in the vessel wall that imply inflammatory change.[5] These abnormalities may then be followed sequentially to determine response to therapy.

The cardiac sequelae of TA are more often due to aortic regurgitation and inadequately treated hypertension than to arteritis affecting the coronary vessels.[1,4] When coronary artery vasculitis is detected (<5 percent), it is most frequent in the ostial regions. However, more distal involvement has also been reported and both types of lesions may occur in the same patient. These observations underscore the importance of considering vasculitis in the differential diagnosis for young patients with ischemic symptoms.

DIFFERENTIAL DIAGNOSIS. Certain congenital diseases cause abnormalities of tissue matrix and aortic regurgitation (e.g., Marfan syndrome, Ehlers-Danlos syndrome). However, these conditions are not associated with stenotic lesions in large vessels, the most common feature of TA. "Inborn" genetic errors that affect matrix structure are also not associated with systemic symptoms, abnormal acute phase reactants, anemia, or thrombocytosis, which may be present with large-vessel vasculitis. The young female predominance of TA distinguishes it from typical atherosclerosis, a disease much more likely to affect the lower extremity large vessels than the arms and the abdominal aorta than the aortic root. Infectious causes of large-vessel aneurysms (e.g., bacterial, syphilitic, mycobacterial, and fungal) must be considered in either gender and all age groups but usually are not associated with vascular stenoses affecting the arch vessels. Certain "autoimmune" diseases may be complicated by large-vessel vasculitis, but they are readily discerned by their associated characteristics (e.g., systemic lupus, Cogan syndrome, Behçet disease, spondyloarthropathies) and characteristic age preferences (e.g., Kawasaki disease and giant cell arteritis of the elderly). Sarcoidosis can closely mimic TA. Making the correct diagnosis depends on other characteristic features of sarcoidosis being present (e.g., proliferative synovitis, skin lesions, Bell palsy, hilar adenopathy).

There are no specific diagnostic tests for TA. The diagnosis is based on clinical features in conjunction with vascular imaging abnormalities. In patients who undergo vascular surgery, histopathological abnormalities may further support the diagnosis.

TREATMENT. Approximately 50 percent of patients with TA respond to corticosteroid therapy (e.g., prednisone 1 mg/kg/d), with subsequent resolution of symptoms and stabilization of abnormalities noted on arteriography. However, relapse can occur in more than 40 percent of patients with tapering of corticosteroid therapy. Corticosteroid-resistant patients or those with relapses may respond to the addition of daily therapy with cyclophosphamide (~2 mg/kg) or weekly therapy with methotrexate (~20 mg).[6] About 40 percent of patients who are treated with a cytotoxic agent and corticosteroid achieve remission, but in time about half of these patients also have relapses, leading to the need for chronic immunosuppressive therapy in at least 25 percent of all patients with TA.[1,4,6] Such unsatisfactory results have led to ongoing studies that seek to take advantage of new insights into pathogenesis. Preliminary studies have demonstrated that treatment designed to block TNF may dramatically benefit most patients (14 of 15) with TA who have had relapses during tapering of steroid therapy.[7]

A discussion of pharmacological therapy for TA addresses only one important aspect of care. Other important issues include treatment of the anatomical effects of vascular lesions. Patients with TA may have signs of clinical deterioration related to fixed critical stenoses or aneurysms. Hypertension affects about 40 to 90 percent of patients.[1,4] In Asia, India, and Mexico, TA is one of the most common causes of hypertension in adolescents and young adults. One of the most common errors in clinical management is related to the physician not knowing whether blood pressure recordings in an extremity are representative of aortic root pressure. Because more than 90 percent of patients have stenotic lesions and the most common sites of stenosis are the subclavian and innominate arteries, blood pressure in one or both arms may underestimate pressure in the aorta. Elevated aortic root pressure, when unrecognized and untreated, enhances the risks of hypertensive complications. This potential dilemma can best be appreciated when angiographic procedures include intravascular pressure recordings. These observations emphasize the importance of knowing the distribution and severity of all vascular lesions. In the setting of renal insufficiency, the potential of contrast agents to cause further renal impairment may limit exploration of the extent of all potential vascular lesions. However, if contraindications are not present, patients should have the entire aorta and its primary branches included in vascular imaging studies. Magnetic resonance angiography lacks the ability to measure intravascular pressures. If the clinical examination does not suggest that lesions affecting extremity-recorded blood pressures are present and extremity pressures are equal, a magnetic resonance study may be sufficient to delineate other vascular lesions without resorting to catheter-guided angiography.

Whenever feasible, anatomical correction of clinically significant lesions should be considered, especially in the setting of renal artery stenosis and hypertension. In about 20 percent of patients, aortic root involvement may lead to valvular insufficiency, angina, and congestive heart failure (Fig. 82–3).[1,4] Severe or progressive changes may require aortic surgery, with or without valve replacement. Although it is always preferable to operate on patients in remission, because judgment of TA activity may be difficult, *all* such surgeries should include obtaining vascular specimens for histopathological evaluation. Findings from surgical specimens should guide the need for postoperative immunosuppressive treatment.

The care of patients with TA requires a team approach that includes clinicians familiar with the proper use of immunosuppressive therapies, vascular imaging or intervention specialists, and, in the setting of critical stenoses or aneurysms, cardiovascular physicians and surgeons. For most patients, medical and surgical therapies provide important palliation.

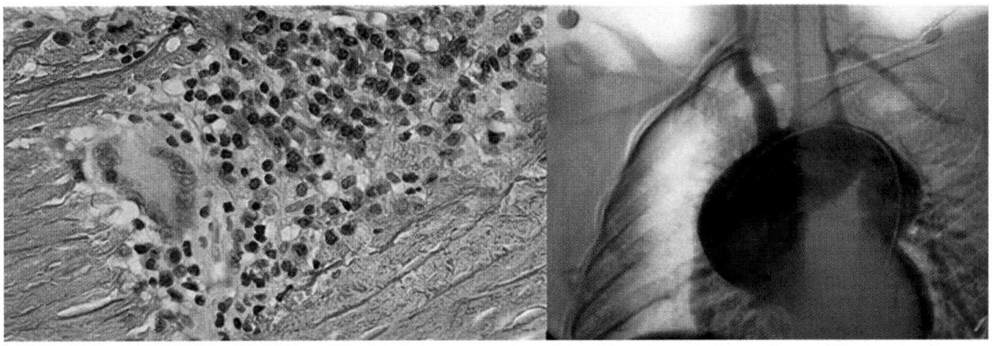

A

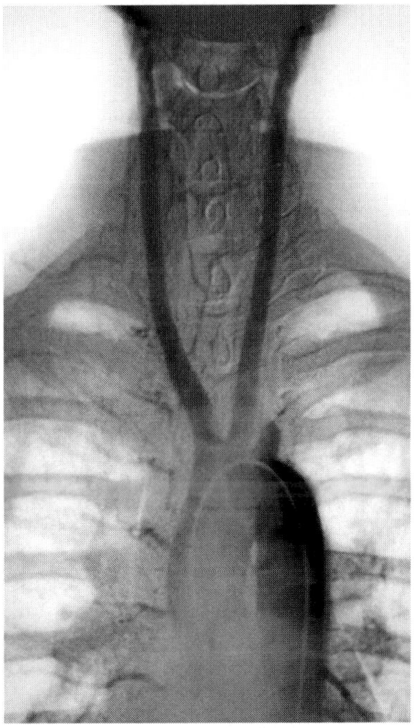

B

FIGURE 82–2 Takayasu arteritis. **A,** Granulomatous inflammation and medial destruction **(left)** have led to marked aortic root dilation **(right)** in a 17-year-old female high school student who developed symptoms of congestive heart failure and exertional angina. She also had diffuse narrowing of the left common carotid artery and irregular dilation of the innominate artery. **B,** Occlusion of both subclavian arteries has led to leg pressures being the only reliable measure of central aortic pressure.

Giant Cell Arteritis of the Elderly

Giant cell arteritis (GCA) and TA are the principal diseases associated with sterile granulomatous inflammation of large and medium-sized vessels.

EPIDEMIOLOGY. In the United States, GCA affects approximately 18 people per 100,000 population, and the affected people are older than 50 years (mean = 74 years). Although it is not understood, it is particularly interesting

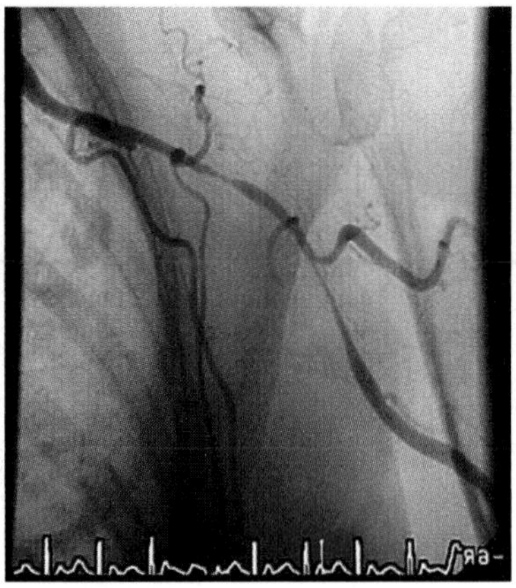

FIGURE 82–3 Giant cell arteritis. "Takayasu-like" lesions involving the subclavian and axillary arteries in a case of giant cell arteritis are shown.

that the incidence of GCA is much greater in northern latitudes. For example, in Iceland and Denmark, the incidence is 27 and 21 per 100,000, respectively, in the age group older than 50 years. Although women predominate in frequency of being affected (2 to 3:1), this predominance is not as striking as in TA (6 to 10:1). The demographic characteristics of patients with GCA are the same as those of patients with polymyalgia rheumatica, and in fact 30 to 50 percent of patients with GCA may concurrently have features of polymyalgia rheumatica.[8]

PATHOGENESIS. Although the cause of GCA remains unknown, much has been learned over the past 10 years about the inflammatory lesion. It begins in the adventitia, where the vasa vasorum are the conduit for the mononuclear cells (macrophages and Th1-type lymphocytes) that mediate vascular injury. Dendritic cells participate in the process by presenting to lymphocytes the putative antigen that is believed to "drive" GCA. This concept is supported by the finding of clonality of approximately 4 percent of T lymphocytes in the vessel wall. Clonality is not found in peripheral blood lymphocytes, enhancing the likelihood that a responsible antigen is presented in the adventitia or media. Vascular lesions are initially rich in proinflammatory cytokines such as IL-1, IL-6, TNF, and interferon-gamma. Intermediate lesions harbor mediators of matrix destruction (e.g., metalloproteinases, reactive oxygen and nitrogen species). In later stages, growth factors such as platelet-derived growth factor (PDGF) and fibroblast growth factor participate in stimulating myointimal proliferation, leading to vessel stenosis. Preliminary reports of improvement of GCA with anti-TNF treatment suggest that the cytokines play a pathogenetic role. The use of other anticytokine therapies that target the Th1 pathway merits evaluation in the future and may shed further light on the pathogenesis of GCA.[8]

CLINICAL FEATURES. The most characteristic features of GCA are new onset of atypical and often severe headaches, scalp and temporal artery tenderness, acute visual loss, polymyalgia rheumatica, and pain in the muscles of mastication (Table 82–2). Conjunction of such abnormalities with an increase in ESR supports a clinical diagnosis of GCA and treatment, even without temporal artery biopsy. The diagnosis is doubtful if dramatic improvement does not occur within 24 to 72 hours. In the instances in which typical features are not present but the diagnosis is suggested by vague systemic symptoms and atypical headache in the setting of a normal or elevated sedimentation rate, and all other reasonable diagnoses have been ruled out, the specific findings of a positive biopsy would be helpful in guiding treatment. The yield of positive temporal artery biopsies in patients clinically diagnosed with GCA has been estimated to be about 50 to 80 percent, depending in part on the size of the biopsy and whether bilateral samples have been obtained.[9]

TABLE 82–2 Giant Cell Arteritis: Clinical Profile

Abnormality	Frequency (%)
Atypical headache	60-90
Tender temporal artery	40-70
Systemic symptoms not attributable to other diseases	20-50
Fever	20-50
Polymyalgia rheumatica	30-50
Acute visual abnormalities	12-40
Transient ischemic attacks or stroke	5-10
Claudication	
"Jaw"	30-70
Extremities	5-15
Aortic aneurysm	15-20
Dramatic response to corticosteroid	~100
Positive temporal artery biopsy	~50-80

GCA may produce clinically apparent aortitis in at least 15 percent of cases and involve the primary branches of the aorta, especially the subclavian arteries, in a similar number of individuals.[10,11] Postmortem studies suggest that large-vessel involvement is far more common than clinically appreciated. Consequently, some patients with GCA may present with features that resemble those of TA. Among elderly people with inflammatory large-vessel disease, the same considerations and precautions must be applied in GCA as in TA: the need to identify an extremity that provides a reliable blood pressure that is equivalent to aortic root pressure and follow-up including careful observation for new bruits, pulse and blood pressure asymmetry, and the possible development of aortic aneurysms.

Studies have demonstrated that patients with GCA were more than 17 times more likely than age-matched control subjects to have thoracic aortic aneurysms and about 2.5 times more likely than age-matched control subjects to have abdominal aortic aneurysms[10,11] (see also Chap. 53). Fifty-five percent of patients with thoracic aortic aneurysms died as a result of those lesions. Because aneurysms were found either in the course of routine care or at postmortem examination, these may be conservative estimates. The finding of large-vessel disease, including aortic aneurysms, in elderly persons with GCA should not merely be assumed to be secondary to atheromatous disease. It is not surprising that about half of all patients with GCA have objective features of cardiac disease. However, it appears that myocardial infarction related to GCA is rare or rarely appreciated because histopathological findings in coronary arteries are infrequently sought in patients whose mean age is 74 years.

DIFFERENTIAL DIAGNOSIS. Mimics of GCA include other vasculitides that may cause musculoskeletal pain, headache, visual aberrations, fever, and malaise. These include Wegener granulomatosis (WG), Churg-Strauss vasculitis, and microscopic polyangiitis, and it is relatively simple to rule these out on the basis of more characteristic features of those illnesses (e.g., upper or lower airway disease, or both, and features of small-vessel vasculitis). Rarely, the GCA phenotype may be part of a paraneoplastic process. If polymyalgia rheumatica is the most compelling symptom of GCA, the differential also includes polymyositis and proximal-onset rheumatoid arthritis.

No precise serological test exists for GCA. Diagnosis is based on a clinically compatible presentation, concurrent highly abnormal acute phase reactants (>80 percent of cases), a positive temporal artery biopsy (50 to 80 percent of cases), or angiographic abnormalities of large vessels (see Fig. 82-3) that are compatible with GCA.

TREATMENT. Corticosteroids continue to be the most effective therapy for GCA. Prednisone (~0.7 to 1 mg/kg/d) reduces symptoms within 1 to 2 days and often eliminates symptoms within a week. About 2 to 4 weeks after clinical and laboratory parameters, particularly the ESR, have become normal, tapering of corticosteroid can begin. Unfortunately, the ESR does not always become normal even with disease control and should not be relied on as the only measure of disease activity. Occasional patients may either not achieve complete remission or not be able to have corticosteroid tapered. Cytotoxic or immunosuppressive agents have been recommended for such individuals by some authors, but the utility of these agents has not been proved in controlled comparative trials.[12]

Idiopathic Aortitis

Aortitis is a recognized feature of TA and GCA. It may also occur in diseases such as Behçet disease, Cogan syndrome, and in children as a complication of Kawasaki disease. Occasionally, it is an unanticipated finding in patients undergoing surgery for aortic valve regurgitation, aneurysm resection, or coarctation.[13] Little is known about the frequency and clinical characteristics of idiopathic aortitis. (Aortitis in the context of retroperitoneal fibrosis is a separate topic that is not discussed in this section.)

EPIDEMIOLOGY. A 20-year review of pathological specimens from consecutive aortic surgeries at the Cleveland Clinic Foundation revealed that 52 (4.3 percent) of 1204 specimens were classified as idiopathic aortitis. Sixty-seven percent of patients with idiopathic aortitis were women.[13]

PATHOGENESIS. Unless the patient with idiopathic aortitis had a past history of GCA or TA, the mechanisms of disease have remained unexplored.

CLINICAL FEATURES. In our series, 96 percent of cases with idiopathic aortitis had findings limited to the thoracic aorta. These data are similar to those from large postmortem series in which aortas have been examined in spite of the absence of overt aortic disease during life. In 96 percent of our cases, symptoms of systemic illness were not present at the time of surgery. In 69 percent of cases, idiopathic aortitis was not related to a current or past history of systemic disease. However, in 31 percent (16 of 52), aortitis was associated with a past history of GCA, TA, systemic lupus, WG, or a variety of other disorders. Thus, a past history of these illnesses and reports that they are presumably in remission become suspect in the setting of a newly recognized thoracic root aneurysm.

DIFFERENTIAL DIAGNOSIS. Patients with idiopathic aortitis vary in age from children to very elderly individuals. Consequently, differential diagnostic considerations might include Kawasaki disease, TA, GCA, systemic lupus, sarcoidosis, Cogan syndrome, Behçet disease, spondyloarthropathies, rheumatoid arthritis, rheumatic fever, and aortitis related to infectious agents (e.g., tuberculosis, syphilis, mycotic and bacterial agents). Symptoms or findings of these diseases may immediately allow prioritization of diagnostic choices. However, some processes may be clinically silent and diagnosis may be aided by ancillary laboratory studies (e.g., RPR, antinuclear antibody), skin tests (e.g., purified protein derivative), cultures, and special stains of surgical specimens. Because idiopathic aortitis is a syndrome that requires ruling out all causes of aortitis that may have specific therapies (e.g., antibiotics), it should be clear that no diagnostic tests for this entity exist apart from histopathological ones.

TREATMENT. In our experience with 36 patients, observed for a mean period of 42 months and analyzed retrospectively, new aneurysms were identified among 6 of 25 patients who were not treated with glucocorticosteroids and none of 11 patients who were treated with glucocorticosteroids. Although these results suggest that such therapy is indicated in this setting, there were marked variations of dose and duration of therapy that led to uncertainty about corticosteroid efficacy. Because only 17 percent of all patients subsequently developed new aneurysms over 3.5 years, we do not feel that all such patients require medical treatment.[13] These observations suggest that inflammatory disease may be isolated to the aortic root in most patients. To justify treatment, one would have to prove the existence of ongoing inflammatory disease. We approach this by routine history and physical examination, laboratory evaluation (complete blood count, ESR, C-reactive protein), and imaging studies (magnetic resonance angiography or imaging of the entire aorta and its primary branches). Because new lesions may occur over time, patients with idiopathic aortitis identified at the time of surgery should be periodically evaluated for recurrence. If proof of recurrent disease is present, treatment should be pursued, as recommended for TA and GCA. Although proof of the effectiveness of this approach is lacking, it can be defended on the basis of the similarities of these conditions and demonstrated efficacy in GCA and TA.

Kawasaki Disease

Kawasaki disease (KD) is an acute febrile systemic illness of childhood. It is the principal cause of acquired heart disease in children in Japan and the United States.

EPIDEMIOLOGY. KD was first described more than 35 years ago.[14] It occurs primarily in children younger than 4 to 5 years. Peak incidence is in children younger than 2 years. Boys are affected 1.5 times more often than girls. KD almost never occurs beyond age 8 years (mean age in Japan is 12 months and in the United States 2.8 years). Although all racial groups can be affected, Asian children have the highest incidence of KD (50 to 200 per 100,00 children younger than 5 years versus 6 to 15 per 100,000 in the United States). Asian Americans have a higher incidence of KD than blacks, in whom the incidence exceeds that of whites.[15] Although siblings of patients with KD are infrequently affected, KD does affect siblings more often than the general age-matched population (2.1 percent versus 0.19 percent). When siblings are affected, symptoms often occur shortly after their family member became ill. This finding raises questions about an infectious etiology in the setting of an immunological predisposition.[15-18]

PATHOGENESIS. Fever, rash, conjunctivitis, adenopathy, and geographical clustering suggest an infectious cause. However, no agent has yet been identified. The following scenarios remain possible:

1. An undiscovered pathogen is responsible for KD.
2. A known infectious agent plays a role in triggering an abnormal immune response, but the pathogen itself is cleared.
3. A pathogen triggers disease by molecular mimicry to normal host antigens.
4. A sequence of stochastic events leads to clinically apparent disease, but by the time the patient presents, the most critical early features of pathogenesis have disappeared.

The essential absence of disease in neonates invites speculation about protection related to maternal antibodies, and the rarity of KD in adults suggests that protection may occur through acquired immunity.[16,17]

The acute phase of illness is characterized by widespread evidence of immunoinflammatory activation. This evidence includes high levels of acute phase reactants, leukocytosis with a left shift, lymphocytosis with a predominance of polyclonal B cells, and thrombocytosis that frequently reaches 1,000,000/mm^3. Blood T lymphocytes, including CD4+ and CD8+ cells, increase in number and show signs of activation. In spite of these observations, children with acute KD are often anergic, indicating T-cell dysfunction. Increased blood levels of a broad range of cytokines and fragments of endothelial cell adhesion molecules indicate widespread immune activation. Cytokine-mediated endothelial cell activation and factors cytotoxic to endothelial cells may play an important early role in pathogenesis. Pathology specimens reveal vasculitis with endothelial cell edema, necrosis, desquamation, and a changing profile of leukocytes in the vessel wall (first neutrophils and later macrophages and T lymphocytes). After months, the inflammatory infiltrate diminishes, and as it fades, myointimal proliferation may produce stenoses or wall weakening may lead to aneurysm formation. In either case, the stage is set for subsequent thrombosis.[16,17]

CLINICAL FEATURES. The most prominent features are included in the case definition guidelines of the Centers for Disease Control and Prevention (Table 82–3). These guidelines lack any specific, single serological diagnostic test. The illness is usually self-limiting within 4 to 8 weeks, and mortality is 2 percent.

Cardiac abnormalities include pericardial effusions (~30 percent), myocarditis, mitral regurgitation (~30 percent), aortic regurgitation (infrequent), congestive heart failure, and atrial and ventricular arrythmias.[16,17] Electrocardiographic findings include decreased R wave voltage, ST segment depression, and T wave flattening or inversion. Slowed conduction may be seen with prolonged PR or QT prolongation. Deaths usually result from acute coronary artery thrombosis in aneurysms that form after vasculitis. Noninvasive techniques disclose coronary artery aneurysms in about 20 percent of patients, compared with 60 percent shown by angiography. Aneurysms usually appear 1 to 4 weeks after onset of fever. New aneurysms seldom form after 6 weeks. Aneurysms are more common in the proximal than distal coronary arteries. Although larger aneurysms (>8 mm) (Fig. 82–4) are among the most susceptible to later thrombosis and occlusion, leading to infarction and even sudden death, endothelial abnormalities and intimal proliferation in smaller lesions (<4 mm) may lead to cardiac ischemia as well. Myocardial infarction is most common in the first year after illness but can occur in young adults as well.[16,17]

Data from postmortem studies have also demonstrated vasculitis of the aorta and celiac, carotid, subclavian, and pulmonary arteries. Rare case reports of gut vasculitis in KD exist.[17,18] Gastrointestinal morbidity may depend more on small-vessel than large-vessel disease.

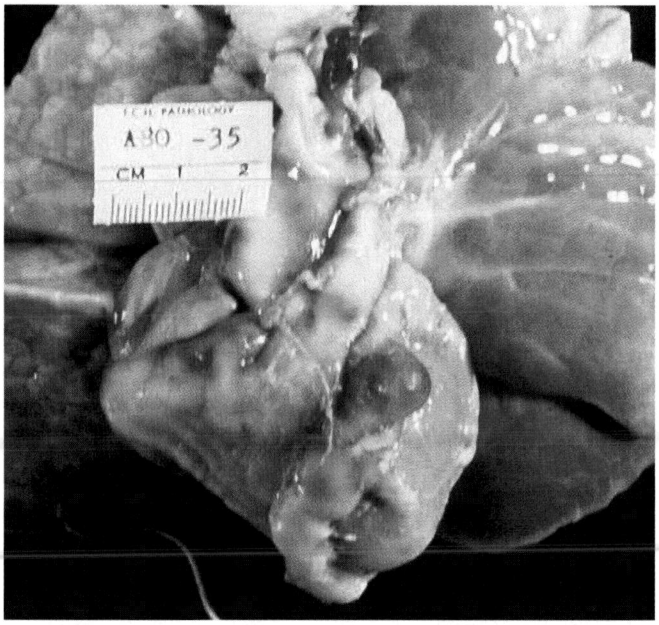

FIGURE 82–4 Giant coronary artery aneurysms related to Kawasaki disease. Note the bulbous protrusion from the left anterior descending coronary artery. (Courtesy of Dr. Karyl Barron.)

DIFFERENTIAL DIAGNOSIS. Given the resemblance of KD to infectious diseases, competing diagnoses include bacterial, spirochetal (e.g., leptospirosis), rickettsial (e.g., Rocky Mountain spotted fever), and viral illnesses. Drug reactions, poisonings (e.g., mercury), juvenile rheumatoid arthritis, systemic lupus, other vasculitides, and malignancies, especially lymphomas and leukemias, may also share aspects of KD.[17]

TREATMENT. Before the use of high doses of aspirin and intravenous gamma globulin, coronary artery aneurysms were relatively common. However, such treatment appears to have reduced the incidence of aneurysms to less than 10 percent.[16] The current standard of care consists of 2 gm/kg of intravenous gamma globulin as a single infusion. Treatment provided within the first 10 days of illness shows efficacy most convincingly. Aspirin (80 to 100 mg/kg/d until the patient is afebrile) has both antiinflammatory and antithrombotic effects. After fever subsides, the dose of aspirin is reduced (3 to 5 mg/kg/d) to achieve primarily antiplatelet effects. This treatment should continue until the platelet count and other inflammatory parameters return to normal (about 8 weeks). Long-term, low-dose aspirin is recommended in children with echocardiogram-demonstrated aneurysms, although the efficacy of such therapy has not been proved in controlled studies.

A small subset of patients with KD resist conventional therapy. They constitute a group that is most prone to aneurysm formation and long-term disease sequelae. The use of corticosteroids in this group and other patients remains controversial. The reported increased frequency of coronary artery aneurysms in an early report of corticosteroid-treated patients has not been seen by others.[16]

Recommendations for long-term follow-up by the American Heart Association include consideration of anticoagulation therapy in children with multiple giant aneurysms and known obstructive lesions and evaluation by stress testing during adolescence. Severe coronary artery lesions have been treated by bypass, but if disease is widespread and bypass is not possible, transplantation should be considered.[16]

TABLE 82–3 CDC Case Definition of Kawasaki Syndrome

Fever ≥5 days, without other explanation, plus at least four of the following: 1. Bilateral conjunctival injection 2. Mucous membrane changes: injected or fissured lips; injected pharynx or "strawberry" tongue 3. Extremity abnormality: erythema of palms/soles, edema of hands/feet or generalized, or peripheral desquamation (hands, feet) 4. Rash (polymorphous) 5. Cervical lymphadenopathy (usually a single node >1.5 cm)
Associated manifestations Irritability Sterile pyuria, meatitis Perineal erythema and desquamation Arthralgias, arthritis Abdominal pain, diarrhea Aseptic meningitis Hepatitis Obstrucive jaundice Hydrops of gallbladder Uveitis Sensorineural hearing loss Cardiovascular changes

Note: 80% of cases <4 years old; rare >8 years old.
CDC = Centers for Disease Control and Prevention.
Adapted from Barron KS: Kawasaki disease. *In* Hoffman GS, Weyand CM (eds): Inflammatory Disease of Blood Vessels. New York, Marcel Dekker, 2002, pp 305-319.

Vasculitis of Small or Medium-Sized Vessels That May Affect the Cardiovascular System

Churg-Strauss Syndrome (Allergic Angiitis and Granulomatosis)

Churg-Strauss syndrome (CSS) is a rare syndrome that typically includes a history of asthma, eosinophilia, pulmonary infiltrates, upper airway inflammation, and a variable frequency of renal, neurological, cutaneous, and cardiac involvement. Histopathological observations of involved lesions reveal eosinophilic, granulomatous infiltrates and vasculitis.

EPIDEMIOLOGY. The most generous estimate of the annual incidence of CSS is 2.4 cases per 1,000,000 persons per year. Those affected may be children or adults, with the peak age being 35 to 50 years. Significant gender bias does not exist.[19]

PATHOGENESIS. The cause of CSS remains unknown. Nonetheless, authorities have recommended withdrawal of any newly introduced drugs or treatments (e.g., desensitization) and avoidance of new environmental stimuli (e.g., farms, industry, if relevant to the medical history). A role for leukotriene antagonists, as used in the treatment of asthma, in precipitating CSS is a subject of controversy. Most would agree that if such an agent were introduced just before the emergence of CSS, it should be discontinued. Whether antineutrophil cytoplasmic antibodies (ANCAs) play a role in CSS is uncertain. ANCAs occur in 30 to 60 percent of cases, suggesting that if they play a role, it is not an essential one. Most often the immunofluorescent pattern for ANCAs in CSS is perinuclear (P pattern), but in a minority of cases it can be cytoplasmic (C). The specific antigen targeted by ANCA is usually myeloperoxidase, but in some cases it is proteinase 3 and the corresponding immunofluorescent pattern is C.

The granulomatous nature of CSS lesions suggests an involvement of Th1 lymphocytes and macrophages, whereas ANCA, if relevant, and eosinophils argue for a role of Th2-biased lymphocytes. The latter are a source of IL-5, which increases eosinophil production and release from the bone marrow.

CLINICAL FEATURES. By definition, the diagnosis requires a past or present history of asthma. Nonetheless, rare cases have been recognized with only a history of allergies and allergic rhinitis. Systemic symptoms are present in 70 to 100 percent of cases from different series. Chest imaging reveals infiltrates, usually multifocal, in 30 to 75 percent. Much less often, pulmonary nodules may be seen, as in WG; however, in CSS nodules are unlikely to cavitate, a finding that is common in WG. Cardiac disease in CSS is the most common cause of death. It is reported in 15 to 55 percent and may include pericarditis, myocarditis, and coronary arteritis. Congestive heart failure occurs in 15 to 30 percent of cases. Gastrointestinal ischemia (~5 percent) contributes significantly to morbidity and mortality. It may be manifest by frank blood from the rectum, melena, or bowel perforation. Many more patients have abdominal pain (30 to 60 percent) for which the ultimate cause is suspected to be CSS. The small intestine and colon are the sites more often affected. Peripheral neurological abnormalities (sensory or motor or both) affect more than two-thirds of patients. Although these features are not life-threatening, they can be a source of profound morbidity. Musculoskeletal symptoms and rashes may be seen in about one-half of all patients, and renal disease (glomerulonephritis) is seen in at least one-third.[19]

DIFFERENTIAL DIAGNOSIS. CSS may be confused with WG. However, patients who suffer from WG do not have an unusually high frequency of allergies and asthma and striking eosinophilia (although in some patients with WG eosinophils can be approximately 10 percent of the total white blood cell count). In WG, the most common ANCA pattern is C and antibody is usually directed to proteinase 3 (70 to 80 percent of ANCA-positive cases). Pulmonary nodules may cavitate in WG, an event that would be rare in CSS.

Other considerations in the differential are parasitic infections (especially helminths, larvae and adults, e.g., hookworm, ascaris, *Trichinella*, *Strongyloides*, filaria, flukes) that may produce chronic eosinophilia by stimulating IL-5 in affected organs. Because helminths may migrate through the lungs, infiltrates and bronchospasm may result, producing a picture of eosinophilic pneumonia and asthma. Idiopathic hypereosinophilic syndrome (HES) is a diagnosis to be considered only after all other causes of eosinophilia have been ruled out. In some cases it is part of a leukoproliferative syndrome and may be associated with splenomegaly, cytogenetic abnormalities, myelofibrosis, myelodysplasia, anemia, and abnormal red blood cell forms. When such findings are not present, the absence of vasculitis and asthma distinguishes HES from CSS. HES is of particular interest to cardiologists because of the risks of cardiac fibrosis, ventricular apical necrosis, and intraventricular thrombus formation. Emboli from the ventricles may lead to pulmonary infarction or systemic circulatory events, including stroke and peripheral occlusive lesions. Myocarditis and cardiac fibrosis may lead to a restrictive cardiomyopathy.

TREATMENT. Corticosteroids (most often prednisone, 1 mg/kg/d orally) usually produce dramatic improvement. In patients with critical organ system involvement (heart, brain, kidneys, gut) it may be prudent to provide "pulse" intravenous therapy (1 gm/d of methylprednisolone) for 1 to 3 days. Although recommended, this regimen has never been the subject of controlled clinical trials. Patients who are critically ill should also receive a second agent (most often cyclophosphamide). Cyclophosphamide is utilized daily in a dose of 2 mg/kg, assuming normal renal function. In the presence of renal impairment, the dose must be proportionately reduced to avoid severe bone marrow suppression. Long-term cyclophosphamide therapy carries many risks. Although once the standard of care, cyclophosphamide is now utilized to induce remission and then after 3 to 6 months, while corticosteroids are being tapered, if remission continues, cyclophosphamide is switched to maintenance therapy with either daily azathioprine or weekly methotrexate.

Polyarteritis Nodosa

Polyarteritis nodosa (PAN) is a nongranulomatous disease of only medium-sized arteries. The old literature on PAN has been a source of confusion to modern students of vasculitis. The older series included patients with both PAN and microscopic polyangiitis (MPA), a disease that can have features of PAN but is defined by the presence of small-vessel vasculitis (capillaries, venules, and arterioles). In modern parlance, cases of nongranulomatous vasculitis with glomerulonephritis (renal capillaritis) and pulmonary infiltrates (alveolitis or capillaritis) would be considered MPA and not PAN. The Chapel Hill Consensus Conference (CHCC) on Nomenclature set forth these guidelines.[20] The guidelines also stress that PAN and MPA are not immune complex mediated and not secondary forms of vasculitis, as might be due to infections, hepatitis viruses, or systemic lupus and other rheumatological diseases.

EPIDEMIOLOGY. Because not all authors adhere strictly to the CHCC guidelines, it is difficult to know the incidence of PAN. Even liberal application of these guidelines indicates that PAN is a rare disease, with an annual incidence of less than 1 per 100,000. Some authors include vasculitis related to hepatitis, mediated by immune complexes and cryoglobulins, in this figure. Men and women are equally affected. PAN may affect people of any age, but the incidence peaks between 40 and 60 years of age.

PATHOGENESIS. When one properly excludes cases associated with hepatitis, the etiology of medium-sized vessel vasculitis compatible with PAN is unknown. The histopathology of lesions varies and often evolves in time, at first having a predominance of neutrophils and later mononuclear cells. Granulomas and increased numbers of eosinophils *are not* present. Necrotizing changes may follow, with weakening of the vessel wall and aneurysm formation, or myointimal proliferation, causing stenosis and occlusion.

CLINICAL FEATURES. Systemic symptoms are present in at least 50 percent of all patients in different series. Any organ system can be involved. However, if one adheres to CHCC guidelines, several features should not be included because they reflect microvascular (capillary-venule) disease: palpable purpura, pulmonary infiltrates or hemorrhage, and glomerulonephritis. In contrast, these may be findings in MPA.

PAN would more typically include deep skin inflammatory changes that may produce painful nodules (similar to

extraskeletal B27-related complications without overt rheumatic disease. Most important, the HLA-B27 gene is *not* a diagnostic test.

Pericarditis, although reported, is not characteristic of the spondyloarthropathies. CAD does not occur at an increased rate, and coronary arteritis is not expected. Diastolic dysfunction has been reported[24] in patients who have HLA-B27 but is rarely of clinical significance. Cardiac conduction disease has been well described in patients with AS as well as Reiter syndrome. It has been estimated that up to one-third of patients with AS experience conduction disease. Atrioventricular conduction block may initially be intermittent but tends to progress. Conduction disease is more common in male patients, and as many as 20 percent of males with permanent pacemakers carry the HLA-B27 gene. Conduction disease may be the only abnormality associated with the HLA-B27 gene. Electrophysiological studies indicate that the level of block is usually at the atrioventricular node, not fascicular.[25] Atrial fibrillation may occur more commonly than expected in patients with the HLA-B27 gene.

Aortic root disease, with involvement of the aortic valve, has been reported in up to 100 percent of AS patients in autopsy series and 82 percent in a transesophageal echocardiographic study of patients with AS. Characteristic findings have included thickening of the aortic root with subsequent dilation. Aortic cusp nodularity with proximal thickening constitutes the "subaortic bump." The subaortic bump was found in 74 percent of 44 patients with AS[26] using transesophageal echocardiography. In this study, aortic regurgitation developed in 50 percent of patients, and 20 percent of patients had congestive heart failure, underwent valve replacement, had a stroke, or died compared with only 3 percent of age- and sex-matched volunteers. The aortic lesions progressed in 24 percent of patients and resolved in an additional 20 percent of patients over approximately a 2-year follow-up. The severity of aortic root disease was associated with the patients' age and duration of spondylitis. Dilation and stiffening of the aortic root may contribute to the aortic regurgitation. Hence, the regurgitant murmur, as in syphilitic aortitis, may be best heard along the right sternal border. There seems to be a unique B27-associated syndrome of aortic regurgitation and atrioventricular conduction block.

DIFFERENTIAL DIAGNOSIS. The B27-associated spondyloarthropathies are characterized by inflammation of the spine, with morning stiffness of the involved areas. Unlike that in RA, the peripheral arthritis is asymmetrical and usually involves large joints. The specific spondyloarthropathies are suggested by their associated extraarticular features (e.g., psoriasis, balanitis, urethritis, oral or genital ulcers or both). Cardiac involvement seems more linked to the presence of the HLA-B27 gene than to any specific rheumatic disorder.

TREATMENT. For years the spondyloarthropathies have been treated symptomatically, with marginal success, with NSAIDs and physical therapy. Modification of the disease course had not been expected from such therapy. The disease-modifying drugs used successfully in patients with RA (methotrexate, sulfasalazine) had minimal efficacy in relieving the symptoms and findings of spinal inflammation, although they were variably successful in treating peripheral arthritis. The B27 extraarticular manifestations were treated, as needed, with corticosteroids (uveitis) or surgery (aortic regurgitation or aortitis). The anti-TNF agents (etanercept, infliximab, adalimumab) have been found to have dramatic clinical efficacy in treating the symptoms of spondylitis; whether they will have a salubrious effect in treating or preventing the cardiovascular and ocular manifestations is currently unknown.

Systemic Lupus Erythematosus

Systemic lupus erythematosus (SLE) is a systemic autoimmune disease characterized by the presence of immune complexes and antinuclear antibodies (ANAs) and a constellation of clinical features, which may include serositis, arthritis, glomerulonephritis, central nervous system dysfunction, hemolytic anemia, thrombocytopenia, and leukopenia. Antiphospholipid antibodies (APLAs) are present in more than 20 percent of patients with lupus and may predispose the individual patient to arterial and venous thrombosis, pulmonary hypertension, or miscarriage (see also Chap. 80).

EPIDEMIOLOGY. SLE is more common in women and can occur at any age. Both idiopathic and drug-induced lupus have cardiac manifestations. Drug-induced lupus is well recognized following treatment with various cardiac medications including procainamide, quinidine, and hydralazine.

PATHOGENESIS. More than 90 percent of patients with SLE have ANAs; however, the presence of even high titers of ANA is *not* diagnostic of SLE. Antibodies to double-stranded DNA are present in approximately 50 to 70 percent of patients with idiopathic SLE and is more common in those with glomerulonephritis. SLE is an immune complex disorder, with immunoglobulin and complement deposition in involved organs, including the heart. The view of SLE as only an immune complex disorder is probably an oversimplification because (1) removal of complexes by apheresis has not been shown to alter the course of the disease, (2) immune deposits can be found in tissue (skin, heart) without resultant inflammation, and (3) T-cell hyperreactivity is an acknowledged component of SLE. Some lupus animal models have been associated with retroviral infections, but there are no consistently demonstrable viral agents in humans with SLE. Twin studies have suggested important roles for genetic factors.

CLINICAL FEATURES. Pericarditis is the most common cardiac problem in SLE.[27] Imaging and autopsy series demonstrate pericardial involvement in more than 60 percent of patients, and clinically significant pericarditis occurs in less than 30 percent. Unexplained chest pain is common in patients with SLE but is more likely due to etiologies other than pericarditis. Pericarditis may occur as the initial manifestation of SLE, appear at any point during the disease course, or occur as a complication of chronic renal disease. Pericardial fluid has generally demonstrated a neutrophil predominance, elevated protein, and a low or normal glucose level. Complement levels in pericardial fluid tend to be low, but this is not a characteristic unique to SLE. The fluid is indistinguishable from that obtained from patients with bacterial pericarditis, and thus infection must be excluded. Pericardial tamponade may occur at any point in the course of SLE, including the initial presentation. When effusions occur in the setting of chronic renal failure, it is difficult to distinguish uremic from lupus pericarditis. Pericarditis, as well as tamponade, can occur with drug-induced lupus. Constrictive pericarditis, presumably as a sequela of lupus pericarditis, has been reported.

Coronary arteritis, resulting in ischemic syndromes, rarely occurs in patients with SLE. The distinction between CAD and coronary arteritis may require sequential angiographic studies, with documentation of more rapid change in luminal images than is usually seen with CAD. Despite the young age of many patients with lupus, atherosclerosis remains the most common cause of ischemic cardiac disease. The prevalence of subclinical CAD is quite high, as determined by scintigraphy, electron beam computed tomography, and autopsy studies. Angina or myocardial infarction occurs in less than 20 percent of patients. As patients live longer with their disease, the prevalence of clinical cardiovascular events will increase. The most common cause of death in patients with longstanding SLE is cardiovascular disease. There are reports of young patients with SLE suffering myocardial infarction as the initial manifestation of their CAD. Middle-aged women with lupus are more than 50 times more likely to have a myocardial infarction[28] than age- and gender-matched control subjects. Risk factors include disease duration, period of time treated with corticosteroids, postmenopausal status, and hypercholesterolemia.

Additional causes of acute coronary syndromes in SLE include thrombosis, often related to the presence of APLA, and embolism from nonbacterial vegetative endocarditis (Libman-Sacks). The presence of APLA predisposes to thrombosis in some patients and has been associated in some echocardiographic studies with valve thickening and nonbacterial endocarditis. Antiendothelial cell antibodies may accelerate atherogenesis. The presence of APLA independently predicted CAD in a subset analysis of the Helsinki heart study.[29] Treatment of ischemic disease in patients with SLE is similar to that in patients with "routine" atherosclerotic disease, but because the mechanism for the increased risk of cardiovascular events is unknown and thus untreatable, an extremely aggressive approach to reducing known risk factors is warranted. The rare patient with coronary arteritis should be treated aggressively with high-dose corticosteroids, and patients with thrombotic disease related to APLA should receive long-term high-dose anticoagulation. Aspirin is *not* sufficient as an anticoagulant. Thrombocytopenia is common in patients with APLA and may complicate therapy.

Myocardial dysfunction in lupus is usually multifactorial and may result from immunological injury, ischemia, valvular disease, or coexistent problems such as hypertension. Acute myocarditis is infrequent but can be the initial presentation of SLE. Patients with peripheral skeletal myositis are reportedly at increased risk for myocarditis. Measurement of troponin I may be of value in documenting cardiac involvement, but the muscle-brain (MB) fraction of creatine kinase (CK) may be significantly elevated in the presence of skeletal myositis even in the absence of myocarditis. Noninvasive studies have demonstrated abnormal systolic and diastolic function in patients with active SLE. These changes are usually reversed with control of disease activity. Acute or chronic congestive heart failure related to SLE, in the absence of other confounding factors, is not common. Endomyocardial biopsy of the patient with cardiomyopathy and suspected lupus may not provide a specific diagnosis of lupus. The biopsy generally reveals patches of myocardial fibrosis, sparse interstitial mononuclear cell infiltrates, and occasional myocyte necrosis with some immune complex deposition even in areas devoid of inflammatory changes. If acute left ventricular failure occurs in patients with active SLE, in the absence of CAD or valve disease, a trial of corticosteroid therapy is indicated.

Tachyarrhythmias can occur in patients with SLE secondary to pericarditis or ischemia. Sinus tachycardia may be the earliest manifestation of myocarditis. A gallium scan may be abnormal in lupus myocarditis, but this has not been studied in adequate numbers of patients to be validated. Abnormal heart rate variability may be due to autonomic dysfunction or to occult myocarditis. Abnormal myocardial single-photon emission computed tomography scans have been noted, even among some patients with a normal resting echocardiogram.[30] Unexplained sinus tachycardia, which resolves with treatment of SLE, can occur in the presence of active lupus, even when evidence of cardiac dysfunction is absent. Occult pulmonary embolism should always be considered as a cause of tachycardia in patients with SLE, especially in the presence of APLA.

Babies born to mothers with SLE and other systemic autoimmune diseases have an increased incidence of congenital complete heart block. The pathogenic mechanism is the transmission of maternal anti-Ro and anti-La antibodies in utero causing myocardial inflammation and fibrosis of the conduction system.[31] The risk for development of complete heart block in infants born to mothers carrying the antibodies is low. However, women with systemic autoimmune diseases, known to be associated with these antibodies, should be screened before pregnancy for their presence. If the antibodies are present, the women should be observed throughout pregnancy with ultrasound studies to detect fetal complete heart block or hydrops. Heart block usually appears after the first trimester of pregnancy and is almost always irreversible. If it is recognized early, dexamethasone in utero *may* be successful in reversing myocarditis. Data to support this intervention are limited. Pacemaker placement is frequently necessary in the infant and may be required shortly after delivery.

Valvular involvement in SLE is common. Recognized 50 years ago as noninfectious vegetations (Libman-Sacks endocarditis), valvular abnormalities have been shown by transesophageal studies in more than 50 percent of patients with SLE.[32] Valvular thickening is the most common echo finding, followed by vegetations and valvular insufficiency. The vegetations are generally located on the atrial side of the mitral valve and the arterial side of the aortic valve. The vegetations are usually nonmobile. Over time, the lesions may resolve or worsen; fibrosis may cause retraction of the valve, resulting in insufficiency. Less commonly, the vegetations on the valve may occlude the orifice, causing stenosis. Valvulitis (Fig. 82–6), with valve fenestrations and rapidly progressing dysfunction, has been described. There are descriptions of mitral and aortic valve replacement in patients with SLE.[33] Valve repair has also been described.[34] Recurrence of valve disease, particularly thrombosis, may affect prosthetic valves. The nonbacterial vegetations rarely embolize and cause stroke syndromes. Several studies have demonstrated an increased prevalence of cardiac valve dysfunction in the presence of APLA with or without SLE. Because vegetations may occur in APLA-negative patients with SLE, there appear to be multiple mechanisms by which heart valves are affected in patients with lupus. Because of the high prevalence of valvular abnormalities in patients with SLE, it has been suggested that all patients with SLE receive antibiotic prophylaxis for endocarditis. Adequate studies do not exist to allow objective evaluation of this proposal.

On the basis of Doppler echocardiography, pulmonary artery hypertension is common in SLE.[35] Clinically significant pulmonary hypertension is less common. Etiologies for the development of pulmonary hypertension include thromboembolic disease related to APLA, intimal proliferation of the pulmonary artery, chronic vasospastic disease associated with peripheral Raynaud disease, and rarely arteritis of the pulmonary vessels. Successful heart-lung transplantation has been reported in a patient with SLE and progressive pulmonary hypertension. Aortitis can rarely occur in SLE.[36]

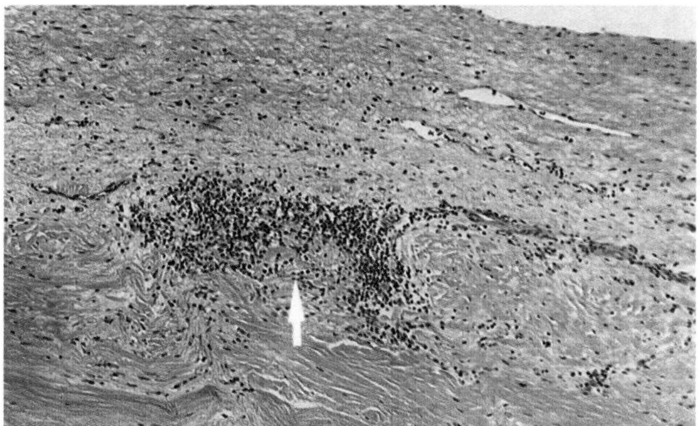

FIGURE 82–6 Valvulitis in systemic lupus erythematosus (SLE). Patients with SLE can experience valve dysfunction caused by bland vegetations (Libman-Sacks endocarditis), valve-associated thrombosis, and rarely true valvulitis. This photomicrograph illustrates aortic valve valvulitis that was discovered at the time of surgery for aortitis and aortic insufficiency (×400). The white arrow indicates a cluster of infiltrating leukocytes.

DIFFERENTIAL DIAGNOSIS. Among the most common features of SLE are ANAs (>90 percent), arthralgias and arthritis (60 to 90 percent), constitutional symptoms (50 to 75 percent), rash (50 to 80 percent), Raynaud vasospasm (30 to 60 percent), and glomerulonephritis (30 to 75 percent). More characteristic features that further enhance diagnostic likelihood include "butterfly" rash, sun-sensitive skin eruptions, discoid skin lesions, hemocytopenias (especially thrombocytopenia and leukopenia), antibodies to double-stranded DNA and Sm (anti-Smith), hypocomplementemia, and characteristic findings on biopsies of involved sites. Diseases that are occasionally confused with SLE include dermatomyositis, infections, lymphomas, thrombotic thrombocytopenic purpura (TTP), idiopathic thrombocytopenic purpura (ITP), Still disease, and sarcoidosis. The pattern of cardiac involvement in SLE is not diagnostic of this disorder.

TREATMENT. There is no single treatment for SLE per se. The specific manifestations are managed on an individual basis. Life-threatening organ involvement is controlled by high-dose corticosteroids, often with the addition of cyclophosphamide. Patients with mild pericarditis without threat of hemodynamic compromise are generally treated with NSAIDs unless there is a contraindication to such therapy, such as renal insufficiency. Corticosteroids are used for more severe disease. If prompt response to steroid therapy does not occur, large sterile pericardial effusions, particularly those accompanied by fever or hemodynamic compromise or both, are best treated with drainage and, if recurrent, consideration of a pericardial window. Arteritis and myocarditis are treated with high-dose corticosteroids with or without adjunctive cyclophosphamide or azathioprine. Corticosteroids may be used for acute valvulitis, and the indications for surgery are the same as for other causes of valvular dysfunction.

Antiphospholipid Antibody Syndrome

(see also Chap. 80)

APLA syndrome is defined as the presence of either APLA or a lupus anticoagulant *and* a history of otherwise unexplained recurrent venous or arterial thrombosis or frequent second- or third-trimester miscarriages. Mild thrombocytopenia, hemolytic anemia, and livedo reticularis are commonly present. APLAs are quite common (10 to 30 percent) in SLE, although not all of these patients exhibit the clinical syndrome. Low to moderate levels of APLA can also be found in association with a number of infectious and other autoimmune diseases, usually without clinical consequence. In the absence of an underlying systemic disease, APLA syndrome is termed primary.

EPIDEMIOLOGY. The true prevalence of the APLA syndrome is unknown. The presence of a lupus anticoagulant or APLA does not define the clinical syndrome, which requires a coincident clinical thrombotic or embolic event or events.

PATHOGENESIS. See Chapter 80.

CLINICAL FEATURES. Venous thromboembolic disease is the most common manifestation and most often occurs in the legs and lungs. Arterial thrombosis most often leads to stroke but can occur in a wide range of locations. Primary APLA syndrome is not associated with pericarditis, myocarditis, or conduction disease. Cardiac manifestations include thrombotic CAD, intracardiac thrombi, and nonbacterial endocarditis.[37] Heart valve abnormalities occur in approximately 30 percent of patients with primary APLA syndrome and include thrombotic masses extending from the valve ring or leaflets, vegetations, or thickening. The mitral valve is affected more frequently than the aortic valve, and regurgitation is far more common than stenosis (Fig. 82–7). Most valvular involvement is clinically silent. The first manifestation of valvular involvement with APLA syndrome may be a thromboembolic event such as stroke. The incidence of superimposed bacterial endocarditis is not known. Clinically significant valvular or intracardiac masses are treated by high-dose anticoagulation with warfarin,[38] with or without the addition of aspirin. Full-dose heparin therapy is probably also effective. Management of heparin dosing in the setting of a lupus anticoagulant, which prolongs the baseline partial thromboplastin time, may require consultation with the coagulation laboratory.[39] Vegetations may resolve with anticoagulation therapy over several months,[40] but spontaneous resolution has also been noted. Patients with APLA are at risk for myocardial infarction and reocclusion after angioplasty or bypass grafting. Aggressive prophylactic anticoagulation should be employed perioperatively in patients with APLA and previous thrombosis. Pulmonary hypertension can

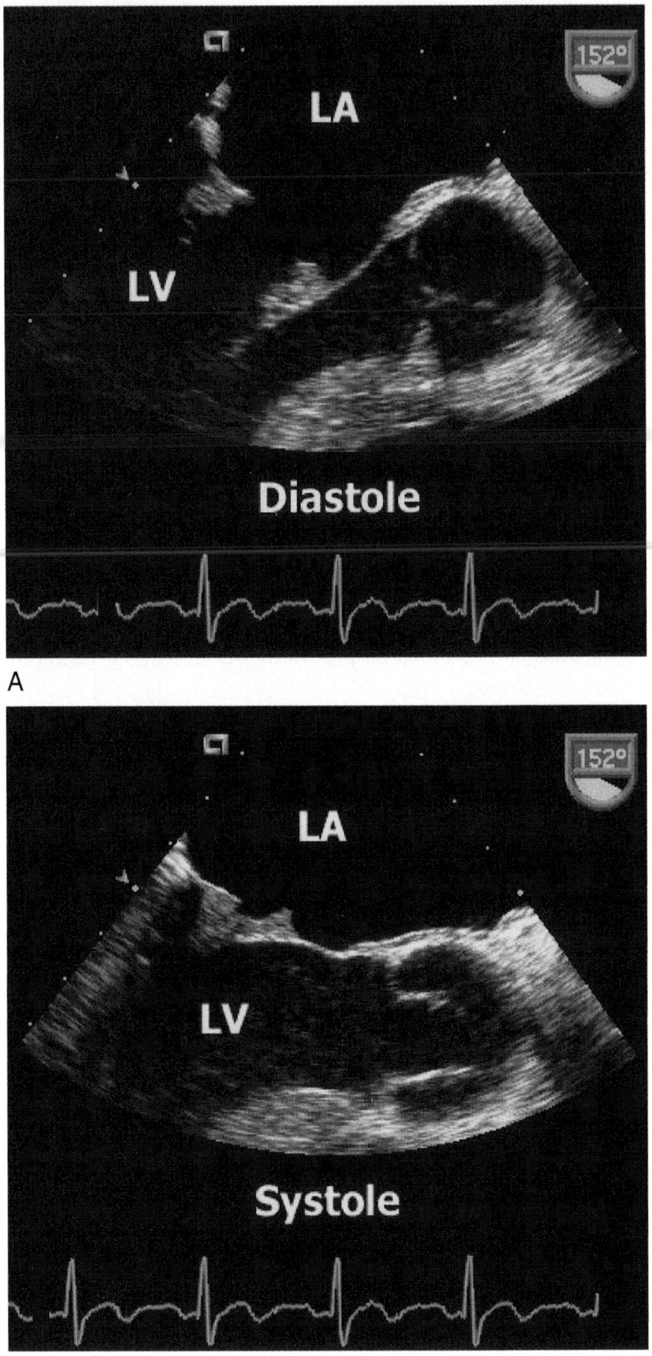

FIGURE 82–7 **A** and **B,** Transesophageal echocardiogram demonstrating large sterile vegetations in a 41-year-old man with a previous history of deep venous thrombosis, symptoms of dyspnea on exertion, and a holosystolic apical murmur. A transthoracic echocardiogram demonstrated severe mitral regurgitation. The presence of apposing lesions on both the anterior (right) and posterior (left) leaflets of the mitral valve, also known as "kissing" vegetations, is characteristic of the anticardiolipin antibody syndrome. LA = left atrium; LV = left ventricle. (Courtesy of Dr. Mario Carcia, Cleveland Clinic, Cleveland, OH.)

occur in patients with APLA secondary to chronic thromboembolic disease. It has also been proposed that APLA can directly stimulate pulmonary artery intimal proliferation.

DIFFERENTIAL DIAGNOSIS. The differential diagnosis of APLA syndrome includes SLE, TTP, ITP, and frequently occult neoplasia. SLE can involve the heart, as discussed earlier. TTP can cause coronary ischemia but not valvular disease, and occult neoplasia has been associated with nonbacterial thrombotic endocarditis.

TREATMENT. The primary therapy of APLA syndrome is anticoagulation, generally to a level similar to that used for patients with prosthetic valves. Monitoring of the anticoagulation level can be difficult in the presence of a prolonged partial thromboplastin time, but use of weight-based algorithms and low-molecular-weight heparin while waiting for a full warfarin effect makes it easier. There are no long-term controlled studies of the effect of chronic anticoagulation and valve disease. Valve replacement can be successfully accomplished in these patients; the indications for surgery are the same as in other patients. The consideration of the type of valve may be influenced by the need for lifelong anticoagulation in these patients, independent of the valve surgery.

Scleroderma (Progressive Systemic Sclerosis, CREST Syndrome)

Scleroderma and its variants are characterized by the presence of microvascular occlusive disease with vasospasm and intimal proliferation and various patterns of cutaneous and parenchymal fibrosis. Although early lesions are inflammatory, the most obvious clinical manifestations are due to enhanced extracellular matrix accumulation (fibrosis).

EPIDEMIOLOGY. Scleroderma, particularly progressive systemic sclerosis (PSS), is a rare disease that affects less than 1 to 19 per million persons per year. An increased prevalence occurs in certain populations such as the Choctaw Native Americans. The average age of onset is 45 to 65 years. Children are infrequently affected. Among younger individuals, there is a female bias (~7:1 versus 3:1 for entire scleroderma cohorts).

PATHOGENESIS. The cause of scleroderma is unknown. An increased frequency of autoimmune disorders and autoantibodies among relatives of patients suggests the importance of genetic factors. Nonetheless, the presence of scleroderma is extremely rare in both members of twin pairs, indicating that if inheritance plays a role, it is complex, almost certainly polygenic, and perhaps influenced by environmental factors. The influence of environmental factors is supported by the association of scleroderma-like conditions with exposures to "tainted" oils (rapeseed oil) and drugs (certain preparations of L-tryptophan).

The earliest lesions are mononuclear infiltrates, primarily T lymphocytes, surrounding terminal vessels. Endothelial injury and vascular leak probably account for the edema seen in the early stages of scleroderma in some patients. Immunocyte and endothelial cell activation is subsequently associated with release of cytokines (e.g., transforming growth factor-beta, PDGF, IL-4) that is linked to an increase in fibroblast production of extracellular matrix, especially types I and III collagen and glycosaminoglycans.

More than 90 percent of patients have ANA positivity in both PSS and the more limited CREST (*c*alcinosis, *R*aynaud phenomenon, *e*sophageal dysmotility, *s*clerodactyly, *t*elangiectasia) variant. This observation demonstrates a likely role for both T-cell and B-cell dysregulation.

CLINICAL FEATURES. Raynaud phenomenon usually precedes skin "hardening" and occurs in more than 90 percent of patients, again providing testimony to the initial and critical role of vascular dysfunction. Common features among patients with either limited (CREST) or generalized scleroderma are arthralgias (>90 percent), proximal weakness (>60 percent), esophageal dysmotility (>80 percent), telangiectasias (90 percent with CREST, ~60 percent with generalized disease), and pulmonary fibrosis (35 percent with CREST, 70 percent generalized). Renal crisis[41] is 20-fold more common in generalized disease than in CREST (20 percent versus 1 percent). Calcinosis may occur in both subtypes but is twice as common in the CREST variant (40 percent versus 20 percent). Generalized scleroderma (PSS) is distinguished by proximal cutaneous fibrosis. Thus, the term "limited" is not meant to indicate the absence of risk of visceral disease; it refers only to the distribution of skin lesions. The pattern of visceral involvement differs somewhat between CREST and PSS.

Pericardial involvement is common in PSS and includes fibrinous pericarditis in up to 70 percent of patients at autopsy.[42] Echocardiography demonstrates small pericardial effusions in less than 40 percent of patients. Acute pericarditis syndromes, including significant effusions, also occur.[43] The presence of moderate or large pericardial effusions is an independent risk factor for mortality. Pericarditis with effusions may require corticosteroid therapy, but there is concern about the risk of inducing scleroderma renal crisis with the use of corticosteroids

Necropsy and endomyocardial biopsies demonstrate the presence of patchy fibrosis, occasionally with contraction band necrosis. These findings may result from intermittent, intense ischemia produced by microvascular occlusion, perhaps related to vasospasm. The epicardial coronary arteries are generally angiographically normal. However, approximately 80 percent of PSS and 65 percent of CREST patients have fixed perfusion defects on scintigraphic imaging. Myocardial infarctions have been documented in PSS patients who have angiographically normal coronary arteries. Ventricular conduction abnormalities are common and, along with a septal pseudoinfarct pattern, correlate with reduced myocardial function with exercise. Electrical abnormalities can be found throughout the conduction system, and ventricular ectopy is present in more than 60 percent of patients. Patients with scleroderma, especially those with a history of palpitations or syncope, are susceptible to sudden death. The risk of sudden death is increased in patients with coexistent skeletal myositis. Primary valvular disease is not common. Renal crisis[41] may be associated with variable degree of hypertension, rapidly rising creatinine, microangiopathy, thrombocytopenia, and left ventricular failure. Treatment is with angiotensin-converting enzyme inhibitors, not corticosteroids.

Pulmonary hypertension occurs in both limited scleroderma and PSS and is a major clinical problem. It may be due to intrinsic pulmonary artery disease or secondary to interstitial fibrosis.[44] Patients with CREST, as well as PSS, should have periodic echocardiograms to screen for asymptomatic pulmonary hypertension.

DIFFERENTIAL DIAGNOSIS. Initially, prior to skin hardening or sclerodactyly, SLE, RA, or severe primary Raynaud disease can be confused with early scleroderma. Buerger disease does not lead to thick, tight skin and is more often seen in male smokers but can cause Raynaud phenomenon and digital necrosis (see also Chap. 54). Cryoglobulinemia and its primary causes (hepatitis, malignancy, other systemic autoimmune diseases) should be excluded in patients presenting with principally vascular symptoms and ischemic lesions. Eosinophilic fasciitis, carcinoid syndrome, and several paraneoplastic syndromes can rarely cause some diagnostic confusion. In time, the emergence of typical scleroderma features enables clarification of the diagnosis.

TREATMENT. At present, there is no proven effective treatment to limit the underlying mechanisms responsible for progression of PSS. Anecdotes and uncontrolled studies have suggested that cyclophosphamide may alter pulmonary progression and improve mortality. Controlled trials have been planned for the future.

Treatment of Raynaud vasospasm is symptomatic. Gastric reflux is often severe and can be improved by avoiding food and liquid intake before reclining, not assuming a fully horizontal position (wedged pillows for beds or raising the head of the bed), and aggressive antacid regimens with proton pump inhibitors. Renal crisis usually responds to aggressive control of blood pressure; angiotensin-converting enzyme inhibitors are the initial agents of choice. A few of the complications (myositis, alveolitis, and pericarditis) may respond to corticosteroids. Conduction disease and arrhythmias are treated as they would be in the absence of PSS. Pulmonary hypertension may respond to vasodilator therapy with endothelin antagonists or prostanoids.

Polymyositis and Dermatomyositis

Myositis with resultant weakness of proximal more than distal skeletal muscles characterizes polymyositis (PM) and dermatomyositis. CK is usually elevated. Respiratory muscles can be involved in severe cases. Both can be associated with fever and interstitial lung disease. Other visceral organ involvement is uncommon in adults. Dermatomyositis involves characteristic skin lesions, which include extensor surface erythema; Gottron papules overlying knuckles, elbows, and knees; edema of the eyelids; and a photosensitive diffuse papular eruption with scaling. Dermatomyositis, in a minority of older patients, may be a paraneoplastic syndrome.

EPIDEMIOLOGY. The incidence of inflammatory myositis is about 2 to 10 new cases per million population per year. People in all races and ethnic groups may have PM or dermatomyositis. There is an overall predilection that favors females, 2.5:1. In children there is less gender bias (1:1), and when myositis coexists with other autoimmune diseases (e.g., SLE, scleroderma—"overlap syndromes") gender bias is enhanced (10:1 females). When myositis coexists with malignancy in the adult population (mean age = 60), there is no gender bias.

Inflammatory myositis can affect patients of all ages. Juvenile dermatomyositis has no association with malignancy, but it may be associated with visceral arteritis that can cause bowel ischemia.

PATHOGENESIS. The cause of these disorders is unknown. Involved muscles are infiltrated with lymphocytes, and the lymphocyte subsets and histopathological pattern of inflammation differ between the two disorders. Autoantibodies are demonstrable, and certain antibody profiles may be associated with specific clinical patterns of presentation of PM and response to therapy; but at present these autoantibodies cannot be used reliably to dictate therapeutic decisions. The increased frequency of other autoimmune diseases in relatives, as in scleroderma and lupus, suggests at least some genetic component in the pathogenesis.

CLINICAL FEATURES. Both diseases affect skeletal muscle but can also affect the heart. Pericarditis is not common but can occur when PM is part of an overlap syndrome with other autoimmune diseases such as SLE or PSS. Coronary arteritis and ischemic CAD are rarely part of these overlap syndromes. Localized or generalized myocardial dysfunction is commonly found by echocardiographic assessment but infrequently causes clinical failure. The cardiomyopathy may be steroid responsive. Corticosteroid myopathy, a complication of treatment that can mimic PM although with a normal CK, generally affects skeletal but not respiratory or cardiac muscle. PM and dermatomyositis frequently affect the conduction system. In an electrocardiographic study of 77 patients, 23 percent had conduction block,[45] which can occur in the absence of cardiomyopathy and usually in the absence of symptoms. Pulmonary hypertension can occur but is usually secondary to interstitial lung disease.

DIFFERENTIAL DIAGNOSIS. PM is recognized by either the presence of chronically elevated CK or proximal weakness. Statin therapy can cause myopathy and occasionally elevated CK and thus can mimic PM. Myalgias are more common than in PM and weakness less common. Other drugs can also induce elevations in CK, and drug-induced myopathy should always be considered before proceeding with diagnostic tests for PM (electromyography, biopsy). Hypothyroidism can mimic PM and is easily ruled out by appropriate laboratory studies. Inclusion body myositis causes an elevated CK but is usually more indolent than PM and frequently involves the distal muscles. The distinction is important because it is less responsive to therapy. Polymyalgia rheumatica is not associated with an increase in muscle enzymes and may be associated with GCA. Dermatomyositis is recognized by one of several characteristic rashes, although SLE can closely mimic dermatomyositis in some patients.

TREATMENT. There are no controlled trials to guide treatment decisions. Nonetheless, initial therapy of inflammatory myositis when an underlying malignancy is not identified includes high doses of daily oral corticosteroids. In severe disease, i.e., in the setting of proximal dysphagia or myocarditis, a pulse regimen of several grams of methylprednisolone is often prescribed. Many clinicians frequently use a second agent (methotrexate, azathioprine, cyclosporine, tacrolimus) along with corticosteroids from the outset or if the patient demonstrates a chronic requirement for high-dose corticosteroid therapy. Long-term immunosuppressive therapy is frequently required. Refractory cases may respond to the addition of high-dose intravenous immunoglobulin therapy.

Sarcoidosis

Sarcoidosis is a granulomatous inflammatory disease of unknown etiology that primarily affects the lung parenchyma but can cause significant adenopathy, arthropathy, myositis, fever, and renal, liver, skin, eye, and cardiac disease.

EPIDEMIOLOGY. Sarcoidosis can affect men and women of all ages. The peak incidence is in the second to fourth decades. Few cases are diagnosed in childhood. The prevalence varies with the degree of vigilance applied to screening and the susceptibility of populations. In Sweden the prevalence is 64 per 100,000, and that in the United States has been variably reported as 10 to 40 per 100,000. The manifestations of the disease are seemingly different in different populations. Scandinavians seem more predisposed to acute sarcoid presentations. There appears to be a preponderance of cases with cardiac involvement reported from Japan. Blacks and Hispanic Americans are more susceptible to severe multisystem disease.

PATHOGENESIS. The etiology of sarcoidosis is unknown. A multicenter U.S study of sarcoidosis found limited evidence to support an environmental or occupational exposure etiology for sarcoidosis. In contrast, studies have linked infectious agents including mycobacterial and propionibacterial organisms with sarcoidosis. Evidence of polyclonal B-cell activation in the blood and several reports of transmission of sarcoidosis to recipients of organs donated by patients with sarcoidosis also support the presence of a transmissible agent, despite the general successful use of immunosuppressive therapy. Analysis of tissue involved with sarcoidosis reveals that T helper lymphocytes drive the granulomatous inflammatory response. There is evidence for a genetic predisposition to sarcoidosis, including familial clustering and shared HLA haplotypes in different populations.

CLINICAL PRESENTATION. Pericarditis has frequently been described, and necropsy studies have documented cardiac involvement in 27 percent of patients. Clinically significant pericarditis is uncommon. The granulomatous, infiltrative disease of the myocardium is often asymptomatic but can cause arrhythmias, conduction disease, and rarely otherwise unexplained congestive heart failure. Granulomatous infiltration may be patchy, and there is a predilection toward involvement of the left ventricle, particularly the upper septal area. This distribution influences the likelihood of obtaining a diagnostic right-sided endomyocardial biopsy. Gallium imaging may be helpful in determining the need for and duration of immunosuppressive therapy, but this has not been proved in any formal trial. Sarcoid dilated cardiomyopathy may be difficult to distinguish from idiopathic cardiomyopathy or occasionally from giant cell myocarditis. Conduction disease is more common than pump dysfunction in patients with sarcoidosis.[46] Biopsy may help to distinguish sarcoidosis from idiopathic or giant cell myocarditis, but the diagnostic yield of endomyocardial biopsy is low.[47] Sarcoidosis is, at least anecdotally, somewhat steroid responsive. Pulmonary artery hypertension and cor pulmonale can occur in sarcoidosis, generally as a result of pulmonary fibrosis. Systemic vasculitis is an uncommon complication of sarcoidosis. Its prevalence remains unknown. Sarcoid vasculitis can affect small- to large-caliber vessels, including the aorta. The latter presentation can easily be confused with Takayasu arteritis (Fig. 82–8). Black patients appear predisposed to large-vessel involvement.

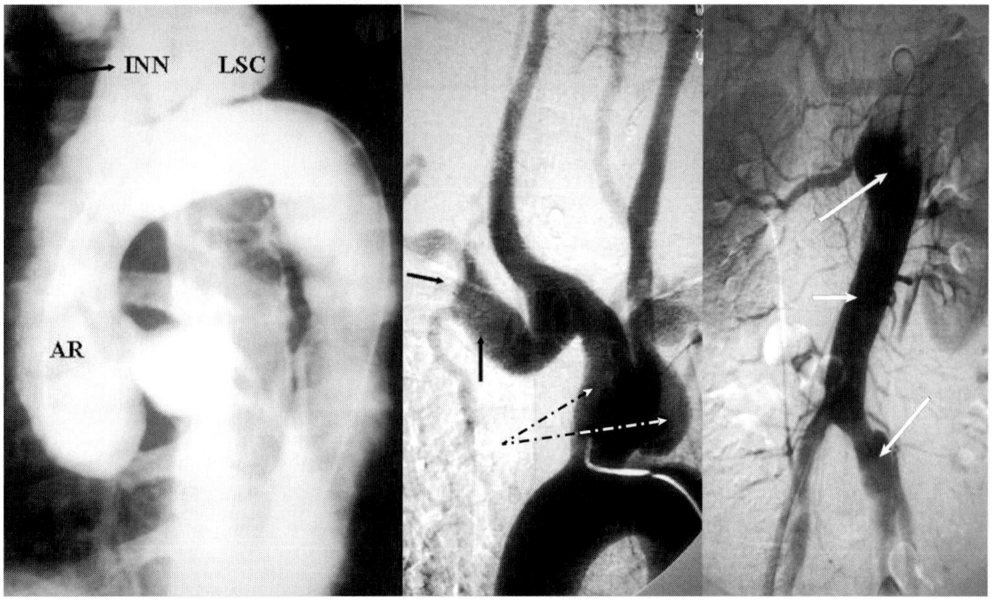

FIGURE 82–8 Sarcoid vasculitis. Aortogram of a 20-year-old black man who presented with chronic polyarthritis, uveitis, Bell palsy, and upper extremity claudication. The angiogram shows aneurysmal dilation of the innominate and proximal subclavian arteries (dotted arrows), the entire aortic root (AR, **left**), occlusion of both subclavian vessels (arrows) associated with arm claudication **(middle)**, and stenosis of the iliac vessels **(right)**. Note that sarcoid vasculitis can mimic Takayasu arteritis (TA). However, TA is associated with stenoses three to four times more often than aneurysms. Therefore, this angiographic picture should raise the differential diagnosis of TA. INN = innominate artery; LSC = left subclavian artery.

DIFFERENTIAL DIAGNOSIS. Clinically, there are many mimics of systemic sarcoidosis including chronic viral hepatitis, granulomatous hepatitis, SLE, Still disease, lymphoma, HIV infection, fungal infections, and Sjögren syndrome. When tissue specimens are available, special stains and cultures should be used to seek fungal and mycobacterial infection. Cardiac sarcoidosis is usually diagnosed by the presence of otherwise unexplained cardiomyopathy or conduction disease in the presence of documented pulmonary or hepatic sarcoidosis. Despite the inherent sampling errors, myocardial biopsy is desirable whenever reasonable.

TREATMENT. Although corticosteroid therapy may be palliative for all forms of sarcoidosis, including vasculitis, relapses of the disease are common and often preclude total withdrawal of treatment. Myocardial involvement is generally treated with long-term therapy, and frequently "steroid-sparing" therapies such as methotrexate are added. Morbidity from disease and treatment is common. There are no controlled trials of therapeutic interventions in cardiac sarcoid, and specifically there are no data to guide the duration of therapy. The serum angiotensin-converting enzyme level is an imperfect guide to therapy.

REFERENCES

Takayasu Arteritis

1. Kerr GS, Hallahan CW, Giordano J, et al: Takayasu's arteritis. Ann Intern Med 120:919, 1994.
2. Hashimoto Y, Tanaka M, Hata A, et al: Four years followup study in patients with Takayasu arteritis and severe aortic regurgitation; assessment by echocardiography. Int J Cardiol 54(S):173, 1997.
3. Seko Y, Sato O, Takagi A, et al: Restricted usage of T-cell receptor V alpha-V beta genes in infiltrating cells in aortic tissue of patients with Takayasu's arteritis. Circulation 93:1788, 1996.
4. Hoffman GS: Treatment of resistant Takayasu's arteritis. Rheum Dis Clin North Am 21:73, 1995.
5. Tso E, Flamm SD, White RD, et al: Takayasu's arteritis: Utility of magnetic resonance imaging in diagnosis and treatment. Arthritis Rheum 46:1634, 2002.
6. Hoffman GS, Leavitt RY, Kerr GS, et al: Treatment of Takayasu's with methotrexate. Arthritis Rheum 37:578, 1994.
7. Hoffman GS, Merkel PA, Tan-Ong M, et al: Anti-tumor necrosis factor therapy in patients with Takayasu's arteritis. Arthritis Rheum 2004 (in press).

Giant Cell Arteritis

8. Weyand CM, Goronzy JJ: Medium and large vessel vasculitis. N Engl J Med 349:160, 2003.
9. Rodriguez-Valverde V, Sarabia JM, Gonzalez-Gay MA, et al: Risk factors and predictive models of giant cell arteritis in polymyalgia rheumatica. Am J Med 102:331, 1997.
10. Evans J, Hunder GG: The implications of recognizing large-vessel involvement in elderly patients with giant cell arteritis. Curr Opin Rheumatol 9:37, 1997.
11. Evans JM, O'Fallon WM, Hunder GG: Increased incidence of aortic aneurysm and dissection in giant cell (temporal) arteritis. Ann Intern Med 122:502, 1995.
12. Hoffman GS, Cid MC, Hellmann DB, et al: A multicenter, randomized, double-blind, placebo-controlled trial of adjuvant methotrexate treatment for giant cell arteritis. Arthritis Rheum 46:1309, 2002.

Idiopathic Aortitis

13. Rojo-Leyva F, Ratliff N, Cosgrove DM, Hoffman GS: Study of 52 patients with idiopathic aortitis from a cohort of 1,204 surgical cases. Arthritis Rheum 43:901, 2000.

Kawasaki Disease

14. Kawasaki T: Acute febrile mucocutaneous lymph node syndrome with accompanying specific peeling of the fingers and the toes [in Japanese]. Allergy 16:178, 1967.
15. Davis RL, Waller PL, Mueller BA, et al: Kawasaki syndrome in Washington State: Race-specific incidence rates and residential proximity to water. Arch Pediatr Adolesc Med 149:66, 1995
16. Barron K: Kawasaki disease: Etiology, pathogenesis and treatment. Cleve Clin J Med 69(Suppl II):SII69, 2002.
17. Barron KS: Kawasaki disease. *In* Hoffman GS, Weyand CM (eds): Inflammatory Disease of Blood Vessels. 1st ed. New York, Marcel Dekker, 2002, pp 305-319.
18. Bell DM, Brink EW, Nitzkin JL, et al: Kawasaki's syndrome: Description of two outbreaks in the United States. N Engl J Med 304:1568, 1981.

Churg-Strauss Syndrome, Polyarteritis Nodosa

19. Guillevin L, Lhote F, Gayraud M, et al: Prognostic factors in polyarteritis nodosa and Churg-Strauss syndrome. Medicine (Baltimore) 75:17, 1996.
20. Jennette JC, Falk RJ, Andrassy K, et al: Nomenclature of systemic vasculitides: The proposal of an International Consensus Conference. Arthritis Rheum 37:187, 1994.

Rheumatoid Arthritis

21. Kitas G, Banks MJ, Bacon PB: Cardiac involvement in rheumatoid disease. Clin Med 1:18, 2001.
22. Van Doornum S, McColl G, Wicks IP: Accelerated atherosclerosis. An extraarticular feature of rheumatoid arthritis? Arthritis Rheum 46:862, 2002.
23. Levine AJ, Dimitri WR, Bonser RS: Aortic regurgitation in rheumatoid arthritis necessitating aortic valve replacement. Eur J Cardiothoracic Surg 15:213, 1999.

HLA-B27–Associated Spondyloarthropathies

24. Lautermann D, Braun J: Ankylosing spondylitis—Cardiac manifestations. Clin Exp Rheumatol 20:S11, 2002.
25. Bergfeldt L: HLA-B27-associated cardiac disease. Ann Intern Med 127:621, 1997.
26. Roldan CA, Chavez J, Wiest PW, et al: Aortic root disease associated with ankylosing spondylitis. J Am Coll Cardiol 32:1397, 1998.

Systemic Lupus Erythematosus

27. Moder KG, Miller TD, Tazelaar HD: Cardiac involvement in systemic lupus erythematosus. Mayo Clin Proc 74:275, 1999.

28. Manzi S, Meilahn EN, Rairie JE, et al: Age-specific incidence rates of myocardial infarction and angina in women with systemic lupus erythematosus: Comparison with the Framingham study. Am J Epidemiol 145:408, 1997.
29. Vaarala O, Manttari M, Manninen V, et al: Anti-cardiolipin antibodies and risk for myocardial infarction in a prospective cohort of middle-aged men. Circulation 91:23, 1995.
30. Laganà B, Schillaci O, Tubani L, et al: Lupus carditis: Evaluation with technetium-99m MIBI myocardial SPECT and heart rate variability. Angiology 50:143, 1999.
31. Finkelstein Y, Adler Y, Harel L, et al: Anti-Ro (SSA) and anti-La (SSB) antibodies and complete congenital heart block. Ann Med Interne (Paris) 148:204, 1997.
32. Roldan CA, Shively BK, Crawford MH: An echocardiographic study of valvular heart disease associated with systemic lupus erythematosus. N Engl J Med 335:1424, 1996.
33. Morin AM, Boyer A, Nataf P, Gandjbakhch I: Mitral insufficiency caused by systemic lupus erythematosus requiring valve replacement: Three case reports and a review of the literature. Thorac Cardiovasc Surg 44:313, 1996.
34. Kalangos A, Panos A, Sezerman O: Mitral valve repair in lupus valvulitis—Report of a case and review of the literature. J Heart Valve Dis 4:202, 1995.
35. Winslow TM, Ossipov MA, Fazio GP, et al: Five-year follow-up study of the prevalence and progression of pulmonary hypertension in systemic lupus erythematosus. Am Heart J 129:510, 1995.
36. Peguero A, Rabb H, Morgan M, et al: Lupus aortitis and aneurysm. Case report and review of the literature. J Clin Rheumatol 5:32, 1999.

Antiphospholipid Antibody Syndrome

37. Hojnik M, George J, Ziporen L, Shoenfeld Y: Heart valve involvement (Libman-Sacks endocarditis) in the antiphospholipid syndrome. Circulation 92:1579, 1996.
38. Khamashta MA, Buadrado MJ, Mujic F, et al: The management of thrombosis in the antiphospholipid-antibody syndrome. N Engl J Med 332:992, 1985.
39. Bartholomew J: Dosing of heparin in the presence of a lupus anticoagulant. J Clin Rheumatol 4:307, 1998.
40. Agirbasli MA, Hansen DE, Byrde BF: Resolution of vegetations with anticoagulation after myocardial infarction in primary antiphospholipid syndrome. Echocardiography 10:877, 1997.

Scleroderma

41. Steen VD: Scleroderma renal crisis. Rheum Dis Clin North Am 22:861, 1996.
42. Byers RJ, Marshall DAS, Freemont AJ: Pericardial involvement in systemic sclerosis. Ann Rheum Dis 45:393, 1997.
43. Deswal A, Follansbee WP: Cardiac involvement in scleroderma. Rheum Dis Clin North Am 22:841, 1996.
44. Koh ET, Lee P, Gladman DD, Abu-Shakra M: Pulmonary hypertension in systemic sclerosis: An analysis of 17 patients. Br J Rheumatol 35:989, 1996.

Polymyositis and Dermatomyositis

45. Stern R, Godblold J, Chess Q, Kagen L: ECG abnormalities in polymyositis. Arch Intern Med 144:2185, 1984.

Sarcoidosis

46. Yazaki Y, Isobe M, Hiramitsu S, et al: Comparison of clinical features and prognosis of cardiac sarcoidosis and idiopathic dilated cardiomyopathy. Am J Cardiol 82:537, 1998.
47. Uemura A, Morimoto SI, Hiramissu S, et al: Histologic diagnostic rate of cardiac sarcoidosis: Evaluation of endomyocardial biopsies. Am Heart J 138:299, 1999.

CHAPTER 83

The Patient with Cardiovascular Disease and Cancer

Karen Antman • Andrew R. Marks

Cardiovascular disease and cancer are both common; therefore, many patients with cardiovascular disease also have cancer. Because of overlapping risk factors such as obesity, hormone replacement therapy, and, particularly, smoking, heart disease patients are likely to have a higher risk of cancer than the general population.[1,2] Certainly cardiac transplant patients are at significant risk for squamous skin cancers[3–6] and Kaposi sarcoma.[7] Exercise, healthy body weight, and moderate wine intake may decrease the risk of both coronary heart disease and cancer.[8,9]

Cardiac complications of cancer such as pericardial tamponade or superior vena cava syndrome are frequent first manifestations of advanced neoplasia. Cancer treatments frequently compromise cardiac function. Radiation ports that include the heart for the treatment of lymphoma or lung or breast cancers can, rarely, produce late coronary artery disease or constrictive pericarditis. Oncolytic drugs, most frequently anthracyclines, paclitaxel, and trastuzumab, but also cyclophosphamide, 5-fluorouracil, and others, result in cardiotoxicity.

Although cardiac resuscitation is often attempted in patients with end-stage cancer, the chance of meaningful survival and even discharge in this setting is low. In one series, 22 percent of cancer patients with a sudden unanticipated cardiac arrest survived to be discharged from the hospital, but 0 of 171 patients with cardiac arrest from end-stage cancer survived.[10] Expert care of patients with both cancer and heart disease requires a basic knowledge of oncology.

Direct Complications of Neoplasia

Primary cardiac malignancies are rare[11-13] (see Chap. 63). Metastases to various cardiac structures are common. Tumor involvement can occur via hematogenous spread leading to multiple nodules involving all cardiac structures, possibly obstructing outflow tracts[14]; via direct invasions from primary lung or mediastinal tumors or metastases to mediastinal lymph nodes; or by direct intravascular spread up the inferior vena cava, most commonly from renal or uterine primary tumors.[15,16] Pericardial metastases occur in one third or more of dying patients, and metastases to the myocardium develop in about 10 percent, particularly in lung cancer patients with mediastinal lymph node involvement.

Cardiac Tamponade and Constrictive Pericarditis

A pericardial effusion with cardiac compression becomes a life-threatening medical emergency when it causes cardiac tamponade.[17–19] A thickened, fibrotic pericardium restricts diastolic filling and the diastolic volume of the heart in cases of constrictive pericarditis. Patients with large pericardial effusions from metastases may report dull chest pain, edema, fever, dyspnea, or cough. Distant heart sounds, pulsus paradoxus, jugular vein distention, and a narrow pulse pressure are characteristic on examination (see Chap. 64). The electrocardiogram (ECG) classically shows low voltage and perhaps electrical alternans. The chest radiograph often shows an enlarged cardiac silhouette. Echocardiography confirms the presence of a large pericardial effusion. Right atrial and ventricular collapse indicates tamponade.

The development of increased intrapericardial pressure depends on the rate of fluid accumulation and the volume of the effusate. Pericardiocentesis can be life saving, but pericardiectomy may be required to prevent rapid reaccumulation of fluid. Fluid should be sent for cytology even in the absence of a history of cancer.

ETIOLOGY. Cardiac tamponade can occur due to pericardial fluid accumulation that may be associated with pericarditis. Pericarditis can result from neoplasms, including metastases.[18,19] The differential diagnosis should include viral pericarditis, uremia, Dressler syndrome after myocardial infarction, iatrogenic cardiac perforation, bacterial infection, radiation therapy, aortic dissection, and others. The pericardium is frequently involved in metastatic lung cancer, breast cancer, leukemia, Hodgkin disease, and non-Hodgkin lymphoma, which account for the majority of cases of malignant pericarditis. Acute pericarditis can occur during radiation treatment of a mediastinal tumor adjacent to the pericardium due to inflammatory necrosis and usually does not cause chronic inflammation. Chronic constrictive pericarditis is becoming increasingly important in patients with breast cancer or lymphoma because of prolonged survival. Chemotherapeutic agents, including doxorubicin (Adriamycin), daunorubicin, cyclophosphamide, and others, may cause an acute form of pericarditis.

DIAGNOSIS. Patients with cancer can present with cardiac tamponade or constrictive pericarditis that is secondary either to a neoplastic process or to the therapy for a cancer. The diagnosis of malignant pericarditis depends on the documentation of pericardial inflammation and the clinical association with a neoplasm. Patients with pericarditis and neoplasm may have symptoms from radiation therapy. Many patients with advanced neoplastic disease are prone to infections that can cause pericarditis, and additional instrumentation with intravascular ports for chemotherapy substantially increases the risk of infections. Constrictive pericarditis should be suspected in patients with increased central venous pressure or unexplained pleural effusion, ascites, shortness of breath, and edema.

An important finding on physical examination is the Kussmaul sign, which is a paradoxical rise in the jugular venous pulse on inspiration. This finding is caused by increased pericardial fluid or a noncompliant pericardium. Normally, during inspiration, there is an increase in the "a" wave of the jugular venous pulse and a decrease in the mean jugular venous pressure as a result of the increased filling of the right-sided chambers associated with the decrease in intrathoracic pressure. The differential diagnosis for the Kussmaul sign includes cardiac tamponade, constrictive pericarditis, restrictive cardiomyopathy, severe right-sided heart failure, and right ventricular infarction.

TREATMENT. Cytological examination of pericardial fluid is diagnostic for malignant pericarditis in about 85 percent of cases.[19] Pericardial biopsy provides a histological diagnosis in up to 90 percent of cases. Removal of pericardial fluid can be therapeutic as well as diagnostic.[20] However, pericardial fluid often reaccumulates and may require insertion of a draining catheter, removal of the pericardium (pericardiectomy), or sclerosis with agents that induce scar formation, including tetracycline instilled into the pericardial space. Control often requires systemic treatment of the underlying malignancy with chemotherapy, although intrapericardial chemotherapy can be effective.[18] Radiotherapy can be helpful in patients with lymphoma or breast cancer but is limited in patients with less radiosensitive diseases by the radiation tolerance of normal cardiac structures.

Superior Vena Cava Obstruction

Superior vena cava syndrome (SVCS) occurs when obstruction of the thin-walled superior vena cava (SVC) interrupts venous return of blood from the head, upper extremities, and thorax to the right atrium. The SVC is encircled by lymph nodes that drain from the right thoracic cavity and the lower left thorax (Fig. 83–1). SVCS often manifests with slowly progressive symptoms worsening over weeks and recruitment of collateral circulation via the azygos, internal mammary, paraspinous, subcutaneous, or lateral thoracic veins and the esophageal venous complex. When symptoms occur abruptly, SVCS can constitute a medical emergency.[21]

SYMPTOMS. Obstruction of the SVC is a distressing manifestation of malignant or benign disease. Clinically, patients report the progressive development of shortness of breath (60 percent), facial swelling (50 percent), cough (24 percent), arm swelling (18 percent), chest pain (15 percent), and dysphagia (9 percent) as well as distorted vision, hoarseness, nausea, headache, and loss of consciousness. Physical findings include venous distention over the neck (66 percent) and chest wall (54 percent) (Fig. 83–2), facial edema (46 percent), plethora (19 percent), and cyanosis (19 percent) as well as dyspnea, orthopnea, stridor, and syncope. Symptoms may be exacerbated by lying in a supine position or bending forward. Patients with this syndrome can be uncomfortable or may develop life-threatening complications such as laryngeal or cerebral edema.

ETIOLOGY. Seventy-five to 85 percent of cases of SVCS result from neoplasia (Table 83–1), with lung cancer accounting for the majority of cases.[22,23] Of patients with lung cancer, 2 to 5 percent develop SVCS. However, 10 to 20 percent of patients with small cell lung cancer (SCLC), which constitutes only 20 percent of lung cancers, develop SVCS, accounting for almost 40 percent of patients with SVCS and lung cancer. Of patients with lung cancer–associated SVCS, 80 percent have right-sided primary lesions.

Lymphoma is the second most common cause of neoplasia associated with SVCS, comprising 2 to 21 percent of SVCS patients. Diffuse large cell lymphoma is the most common form (64 percent), followed by lymphoblastic lymphoma (33 percent). Similar to patients with lung

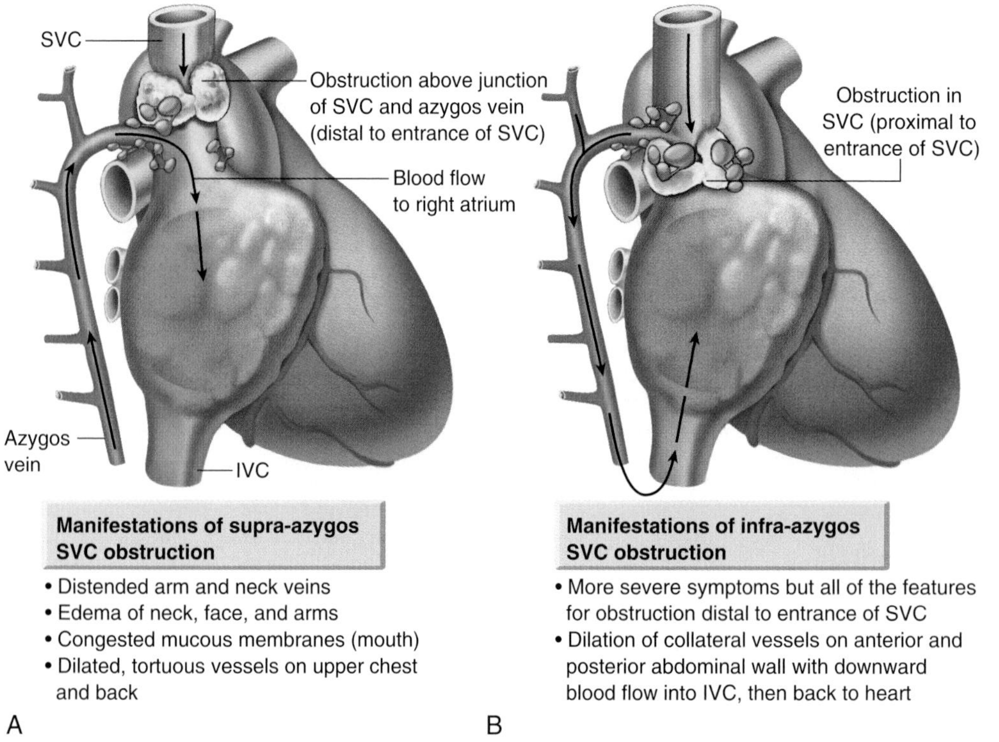
SVC
Obstruction above junction of SVC and azygos vein (distal to entrance of SVC)
Blood flow to right atrium
Azygos vein
IVC
Manifestations of supra-azygos SVC obstruction
• Distended arm and neck veins
• Edema of neck, face, and arms
• Congested mucous membranes (mouth)
• Dilated, tortuous vessels on upper chest and back
A
Obstruction in SVC (proximal to entrance of SVC)
Manifestations of infra-azygos SVC obstruction
• More severe symptoms but all of the features for obstruction distal to entrance of SVC
• Dilation of collateral vessels on anterior and posterior abdominal wall with downward blood flow into IVC, then back to heart
B

FIGURE 83–1 Anatomy of superior vena cava (SVC) syndrome. Lymph nodes may obstruct blood return above the entrance of the azygos vein **(A)**, resulting in edema of the face, neck, and arms and distended veins in the neck and arms and over the upper chest. Obstruction below the return of the azygos vein **(B)** results in retrograde flow through the azygos via collateral veins to the inferior vena cava (IVC), resulting in all the symptoms and signs in **A** plus dilation of the veins over the abdomen as well. (Modified from Skarin AT [ed]: Atlas of Diagnostic Oncology, 3rd ed. Philadelphia, Elsevier Science, 2003.)

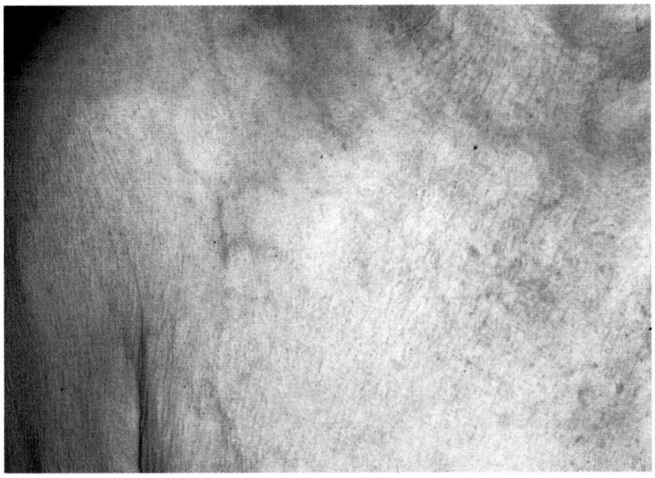

FIGURE 83–2 Distended veins in the skin over the chest wall of a patient with superior vena cava syndrome. (From Skarin AT [ed]: Atlas of Diagnostic Oncology, 3rd ed. Philadelphia, Elsevier Science, 2003.)

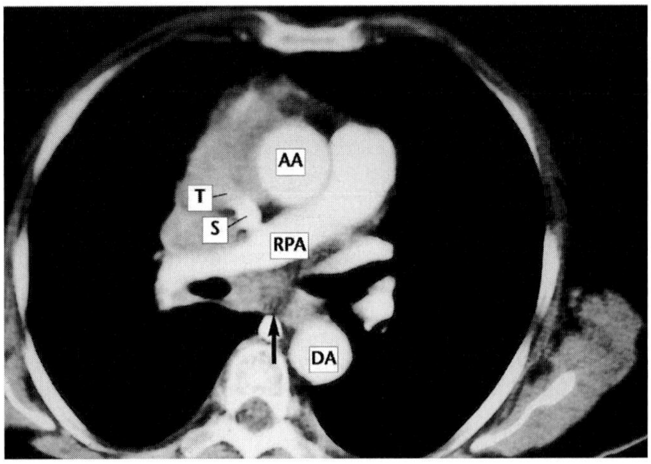

FIGURE 83–3 Superior vena cava syndrome in a case of diffuse large cell lymphoma. Computed tomography image with intravenous contrast at the level of the right pulmonary artery (RPA) showing tumor (T) infiltrating into the area of the superior vena cava (S), which is narrowed. Tumor is also present in the subcarinal space (arrow). AA = ascending aorta; DA = descending aorta. (From Skarin AT [ed]: Atlas of Diagnostic Oncology, 3rd ed. Philadelphia, Elsevier Science, 2003.)

TABLE 83–1 Malignancies Associated with Superior Vena Cava (SVC) Syndrome in Adults*

Neoplastic Diagnosis	Percentage of SVC	Percentage of Disease-Associated SVC
Lung cancer, stage 3B or 4:	48-81	
Small cell lung cancer		15-45
Squamous cell cancer		20-25
Adenocarcinoma		5-25
Large cell carcinoma		4-30
Lymphoma:	2-21	
Diffuse large cell lymphoma		64
Lymphoblastic lymphoma		33
Breast cancer	11	

*Include lung cancer, lymphomas, and metastases from other solid tumors. Seventy-five percent to 85% of patients with SVC have neoplastic disease.

cancer, only 1 to 5 percent of patients with lymphoma develop SVCS (21 percent of lymphoblastic lymphomas and 7 percent of diffuse large cell lymphomas). Of patients with primary mediastinal B-cell lymphoma with sclerosis, 57 percent developed SVCS. Although Hodgkin lymphoma often involves the mediastinum, SVCS rarely develops. Thymoma and germ cell tumors are other primary mediastinal malignancies that occasionally cause SVCS. The most common metastatic disease that causes SVCS is breast cancer, accounting for 11 percent of SVCS cases.

DIFFERENTIAL DIAGNOSIS. Benign causes of SVC obstruction not associated with neoplasia result from mediastinal fibrosis caused by radiotherapy or histoplasmosis, tuberculosis, collagen-vascular disease, arteriovenous shunts, or SVC thrombosis as a complication of central venous catheters, pacemaker leads, peritoneovenous shunts, Swan-Ganz catheters, or hyperalimentation catheters. Pacemakers and implantable cardioverter defibrillators result in up to 30 percent of local venous thrombosis, in some cases associated with infection; however, SVC obstruction is uncommon and relates to acute or previous lead infection or retention of a severed lead.[24]

In children with SVCS, up to 70 percent of cases are iatrogenic, developing after correction surgery for congenital heart disease, ventriculoatrial shunt to decompress hydrocephalus, and SVC catheterization for parenteral nutrition. Other benign causes include granulomas, congenital anomalies, and mediastinal fibrosis secondary to histoplasmosis. Neoplasia-associated SVCS in children results from lymphomas, acute lymphoblastic leukemia, rhabdomyosarcoma, neuroblastoma, and other solid tumors.[21]

DIAGNOSTIC PROCEDURES. In a patient with characteristic symptoms of SVC obstruction, physical evaluation is usually informative and raises a high level of suspicion. In patients with SVCS due to neoplasia, 60 percent lack a prior history of cancer. A mass is generally present on chest radiograph, with superior mediastinal widening and often pleural effusions. Computed tomography (CT) provides critical additional information (Fig. 83–3).

Imaging. Although the clinical picture usually makes diagnosis straightforward, patients with SVC obstruction frequently require imaging evaluation for assessment and therapy planning. Chest radiography in two planes reveals abnormal mediastinal widening suspicious of lymphoma or other mediastinal masses. Lesions in the lung fields or pleural effusions strongly suggest lung malignancy. Sonographic analysis is used to assess the extrathoracic systemic veins for thrombosis, and Doppler analysis may reveal the lack of transmitted right heart pulsations or dampened pulsations, which raises the suspicion of intrathoracic venous obstruction.

Most patients with suspected SVCS undergo contrast-enhanced CT when the modality is available. CT can document the presence of obstruction and establish the level, extent, and therapeutic options by mapping collateral and patent vasculature to aid interventional access and documenting any pulmonary emboli. Increased imaging of patients with neoplasm has identified many asymptomatic patients with "impending" SVC obstruction. The CT scan can illustrate the strategic relationship of growing tumor masses or the development of nonocclusive, early intraluminal thrombus. Magnetic resonance imaging can also perform this role effectively. If neoplasm was diagnosed previously, earlier radiation therapy may prevent SVCS. If CT is not an option, a venogram of the arms can provide additional information for therapeutic decisions.

The causes of SVCS include intraluminal, mural, and extraluminal obstruction. Intraluminal causes include bland and neoplastic thrombus as well as direct tumor extension. Bland thrombus is usually associated with intravenous lines or infected pacemaker leads, although it is an uncommon cause of complete occlusion. A paraneoplastic bland thrombus can also occur, and tumor vascularization can be used to differentiate a bland from a neoplastic thrombus. Mural causes include benign stenoses related to renal dialysis and strictures resulting from radiation therapy. Extraluminal causes are usually direct compression by bronchogenic tumors or malignant lymphadenopathy and represent the most common causes detected by imaging.

Oncological Intervention. Because the underlying cause will guide any therapeutic recommendations, obtaining tissue samples is essential to establishing the cause of SVCS. Sputum cytology can establish the diagnosis in almost half of patients. Biopsy of enlarged lymph nodes, when present, is frequently a relatively noninvasive method to obtain reliable tissue diagnosis. Thoracentesis can establish the diagnosis of malignancy in 70 percent of patients with pleural effusions. A diagnosis is made in most of the remaining cases with bronchoscopy, including brushing, washing, and biopsy samples. A marrow biopsy may be diagnostic of lymphoma or SCLC. If the diagnosis remains obscure, percutaneous transthoracic CT-guided fine-needle biopsy is a safe and effective method of diagnosis. When other methods have been unsuccessful, mediastinoscopy has a high diagnostic yield but at a somewhat higher risk of complications (5 percent).

MANAGEMENT. During medical evaluation and before institution of specific therapy, oxygen is administered to reduce the cardiac output and venous pressure, and head elevation, diuretics, and a low-salt diet are used to reduce edema. Dehydration increases the risk of further thrombosis, however. In patients with SVCS caused by malignant tumors, radiotherapy and chemotherapy are the most common first-line treatment options. Steroids can decrease inflammation or tumor-associated obstruction, but may obscure the diagnosis of lymphoma. Anticoagulation has not been proved to provide benefit in patients with neoplasia-associated SVCS and may interfere with diagnostic biopsies and interventions. Percutaneous transluminal angioplasty or stent insertion may relieve symptoms without obscuring the diagnosis.

Vascular Interventions. Endovascular stenting or angioplasty and thrombolysis can provide prompt relief of symptoms, particularly for patients with palliative treatment.[25] Balloon venoplasty and stenting, which may be augmented by catheter-applied thrombolysis, are prompt treatment options to decrease morbidity or to prevent impending SVC obstruction. Despite the historical concern that invasive diagnostic procedures in the setting of increased intrathoracic venous pressure would result in severe bleeding and complications of anesthesia, complication rates in experienced centers have proved acceptably low. Ideally, there is a remaining lumen for passage of a guidewire. Balloon angioplasty is undertaken and one or more stents are placed. The results of stent insertion are excellent, with a high percentage of technical success and rapid relief of symptoms. Adjuvant radiation therapy can be given. In the case of a preexisting paraneoplastic thrombus, the risk of stent thrombosis remains.

Surgical treatment involves the insertion of a bypass graft between the left innominate or jugular vein and the right atrial appendage, using an autologous or Dacron graft. However, this operation is very invasive and difficult. Therefore, it should be avoided if possible and, if necessary, performed only in patients with a relatively long life expectancy. In the chronic situation devoid of vascular interventions, patients may develop a network of chest wall and azygos/hemiazygos collateral vessels that effectively restore venous return to the right heart.[26]

Oncological Treatment of SVCS. The goal is to determine as rapidly as possible the histological type of the primary lesion and to institute curative therapy for lymphomas, germ cell tumors, and even SCLC and to provide palliation for advanced non-small-cell lung cancers and other metastatic solid tumors (Table 83–2). The prognosis of patients who present with SVCS depends greatly on the prognosis of the underlying neoplasm. Combination chemotherapy with or without radiation therapy relieves SVCS symptoms within 1 to 2 weeks in cases of newly diagnosed SCLC and lymphoma.

TABLE 83–2 Yields of Various Procedures for Diagnosis in Patients with Superior Vena Cava Syndrome

Procedure	% Diagnostic
Thoracotomy	98
Mediastinoscopy	90
Thoracentesis	71
Lymph node biopsy	67
Bronchoscopy	52
Sputum cytology	49

Treatment of SCLC with both chemotherapy and radiation significantly decreases the risk of SVCS recurrence over chemotherapy alone but may not improve survival. In some series of patients with SCLC, presentation with SVCS indicated a more favorable prognosis. SVCS secondary to lymphoma is rarely an emergency that requires treatment before histological diagnosis and complete staging. Chemotherapy provides both local and systemic therapy. Consolidation with radiation therapy may be appropriate for patients with large mediastinal masses (>10 cm). Dysphagia, hoarseness, and stridor are poor prognostic signs. Non-small-cell lung cancers and breast or other cancers metastatic to SVC lymph nodes are generally managed with radiation therapy or percutaneous transluminal angioplasty or stent insertion, or both.

Valvular Heart Disease in the Cancer Patient

Cardiac valves can be involved directly by primary or metastatic tumor, by bacterial or candidal infections, with nonbacterial thrombotic endocarditis, by trauma from semipermanent catheters inserted to facilitate treatment, and as a late effect of radiation therapy (see section on radiation complications).

Nonbacterial thrombotic endocarditis complicates the course of various malignancies, most commonly adenocarcinomas from the gastrointestinal tract and lung.[27] Morbidity and mortality mainly result from systemic embolism. Two hundred nonselected ambulatory patients with solid tumors evaluated for evidence of thromboembolic events and for plasma D-dimer levels were compared with a control group of 100 consecutive patients without overt heart disease referred to echocardiography for the detection of an occult arterial embolic source. Of 38 cancer patients with cardiac valvular vegetations from the group of 200, the valves affected were mitral (n = 19), aortic (n = 18), and tricuspid (n = 1). Primary lesions were lymphoma (n = 10), lung (n = 9), and pancreatic (n = 3). Thromboembolism to extremities was diagnosed in 4 patients, cerebrovascular accidents were diagnosed in 2, and 4 patients had silent segmental left ventricular wall motion abnormalities on echocardiography. Nine of 38 patients (24 percent) with vegetations developed thromboembolism, as compared with 13 of 162 patients without vegetations (8 percent; $p = 0.013$). D-Dimer levels were increased in 19 of 21 patients (90 percent) with thromboembolism and in 76 of 149 patients without thromboembolism

(51 percent; $p = 0.001$).[27] Treatment of cancer-associated nonbacterial thrombotic endocarditis remains difficult.

Ischemic Heart Disease and Malignancy

Cancer patients are at a higher risk for coronary artery disease due to prior radiation to the heart (see later), extrinsic compression by tumor of a coronary artery, or even tumor emboli within a coronary artery. Hypercoagulable states particularly associated with mucin-secreting adenocarcinomas also increase the risk of a coronary thrombosis.

Arrhythmias

Arrhythmias in cancer patients result from cardiomyopathies due to drugs or radiation (see later), electrolyte imbalance (particularly potassium wasting) from renal complications of antineoplastic and antibiotic drugs, and hypoxia from underlying chronic obstructive pulmonary disease,[28] pulmonary or pleural involvement with tumor, or infection with large pleural or pericardial effusions.[28] Rhythm disturbances, sinus tachycardia, ST segment and T wave changes, atrial fibrillation or flutter, and complete heart block can result. Cervical lymph node involvement can rarely lead to carotid sinus syncope.

Indirect Cardiovascular Complications of Cancer

Hyperviscosity

ERYTHROCYTOSIS. Elevated red blood cell mass can occur from a variety of stimuli. Polycythemia vera is a clonal chronic myeloproliferative disorder characterized by an increase in red blood cell mass with or without elevated leukocytes and platelets. Hyperviscosity is in part related to decreased red blood cell membrane fluidity and deformability.[29] An increased sensitivity of hematopoietic progenitor cells to regulatory factors such as erythropoietin; dysregulation of the *SHP1* gene, which encodes an intracellular phosphatase involved in cell signaling pathways; and mutations in the erythropoietin receptor gene are possible mechanisms for the development of polycythemia vera.

Patients with polycythemia vera have a 30 percent risk of thrombosis (extremity deep venous thrombosis, hepatic vein thrombosis [Budd-Chiari syndrome], pulmonary embolism, or coronary occlusions). Cerebrovascular occlusion and basilar artery insufficiency develop. Mitral valve thickening or nonbacterial vegetations also occur. Reduced cerebral blood flow caused by the erythrocytosis is associated with confusion and abnormal mental status, visual disturbances, dizziness, and headache.

Phlebotomy should maintain the hematocrit in the 40 to 45 percent range. Hydroxyurea is often used if phlebotomy alone is insufficient. Phlebotomy alone increases the risk of thrombosis, but hydroxyurea can, rarely, result in leukemia.

THROMBOCYTOSIS. Reactive thrombocytoses, which appropriately develop after surgery or in pregnancy, are not associated with an increased risk of thrombosis. However, essential thrombocytosis, a myeloproliferative disorder, increases the risk of both hemorrhage and thrombosis. Hydroxyurea, used to lower the platelet count, also reduces the risk of myocardial infarction.

LEUKOCYTOSIS. Although very high white blood cell counts associated with acute and chronic lymphoid leukemia generally do not cause significant hyperviscosity, leukemic white blood cell counts greater than 100,000/μl in patients with acute myeloid leukemia can cause leukostasis producing thrombosis and hemorrhages in microcapillaries of the brain (encephalopathy) and lung (pulmonary infiltrates and hypoxia). Hydroxyurea, definitive antileukemic chemotherapy, central nervous system radiation, and leukophoresis are used to limit complications. Patients with chronic myeloid leukemia often tolerate high white blood cell counts without leukostatic/thrombotic complications.

PLASMA PROTEINS. Multiple myeloma and Waldenström macroglobulinemia are clonal proliferations of plasma cells that elaborate a single immunoglobulin, the M-component. The immunoglobins produced are IgG and IgM, respectively. Congestive heart failure can result from anemia and expanded plasma volume as well as increased viscosity from circulating immunoglobulins. Hyperviscosity is more likely at any given IgM level compared to a similar IgG level. Most patients with Waldenström disease have elevated serum viscosity, but symptoms such as headache, dizziness, blurry vision, diplopia, and ataxia are uncommon (15 to 20 percent). Retinal examination can reveal distention of vessels with constrictions, especially of veins (a "sausage links" or "box car" effect) (Fig. 83–4). Symptoms can progress to confusion, stroke, or coma. Hyperviscosity syndrome, confirmed by measurements of serum viscosity, requires immediate reduc-

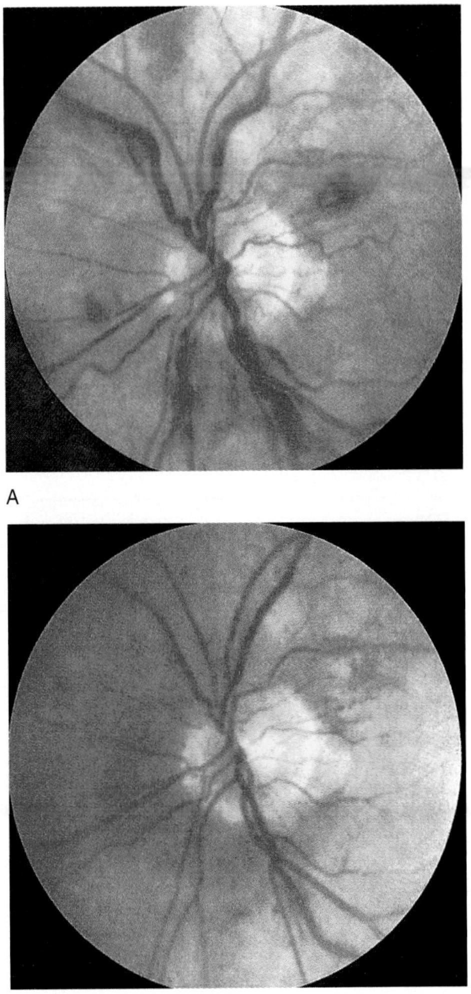

A

B

FIGURE 83–4 Waldenström macroglobulinemia (hyperviscosity syndrome). **A,** The retina of a patient who presented with blurred vision, headache, and dizziness exhibits gross distention of vessels, particularly the veins, which show bulging and constriction (the "linked sausage" effect), as well as areas of hemorrhage. **B,** After plasmapheresis, the vascular diameters are normal and the hemorrhagic areas have cleared. (From Skarin AT [ed]: Atlas of Diagnostic Oncology, 3rd ed. Philadelphia, Elsevier Science, 2003.)

tion in the M-component, generally with plasmapheresis and chemotherapy.

Cryoglobulins, immunoglobulins that aggregate at temperatures below 37°C, are associated with a variety of inflammatory conditions as well as with lymphoma and infections, particularly hepatitis C.[30] Severe hypertension from peripheral vasculitis can lead to renal failure, stroke, and cardiovascular events.

Cardiac Complications of Chemotherapy

Oncolytic drugs, most frequently anthracyclines, paclitaxel, and trastuzumab, but also cyclophosphamide, 5-fluorouracil, and others, result in cardiotoxicity.[31–34] Some hormone therapies are associated with increased risks of myocardial infarction and cardiomyopathies (Table 83–3).

Anthracycline Cardiotoxicity

ACUTE MANIFESTATIONS. Acute anthracycline toxicity includes arrhythmias, myocardial dysfunction, and pericardial effusions.

CHRONIC OR LATE CARDIOTOXICITY. Late cardiomyopathy was reported soon after anthracyclines were introduced—with congestive heart failure in up to 30 percent in patients who had received more than 500 mg/m^2 of doxorubicin (Adriamycin).[35] In randomized trials, congestive heart failure (CHF) developed significantly more often in the anthracycline arms of the studies, thus establishing cardiomyopathy due to anthracyclines. Endomyocardial biopsy studies documented a correlation between cumulative anthracycline dose and myocardial pathological condition.[36] Based on these studies, cumulative anthracycline doses are now generally kept lower than 450 mg/m^2, resulting in a risk of clinical symptoms of about 3 percent of cases. The risk is up to 26 percent for cumulative doses of 550 mg/m^2.[37] Measurably decreased function is found in asymptomatic patients (Fig. 83–5).

Although anthracycline-associated cardiomyopathy can develop as late as decades after the last anthracycline therapy, it classically produces congestive heart failure within a median of 3 months after the last anthracycline dose. Tachycardia and fatigue are followed by shortness of breath, pulmonary edema, and cardiac dilation. Associated arrhythmias include ventricular tachycardia or fibrillation, heart block, and occasional sudden death. Autopsy reveals fibrosis and hypertrophy of remaining myocytes. Cardiac function in patients who progress to this state but survive generally improves over a period of years.

In a retrospective study at M.D. Anderson Cancer Center, 682 consecutive women with metastatic breast cancer received doxorubicin by bolus infusion. Doxorubicin-associated CHF developed in 33 of 538 patients aged 50 to 64 years and in 13 of 144 aged 65 years and older after cumulative doses of 410 mg/m^2 (range, 150-550 mg/m^2) and 400 mg/m^2 (range, 100-570 mg/m^2), respectively, a median of 5 (range, <1-65 months) and 9 months (range, <1-28 months) after the last dose of doxorubicin. No risk factors could be identified. Thus, in this study, patients older than 65 years had no added risk of developing congestive heart failure.[38]

TABLE 83–3 Cardiotoxicity of Antineoplastic Agents

Implicated Agent	Comments
Anthracyclines	
Doxorubicin or daunorubicin	CHF at cumulative doses above 450 mg/m^2, arrhythmias
Mitoxantrone, idarubicin	CHF, decreases in left ventricular ejection fraction
Alkylating agents	
Cyclophosphamide	Produces a hemorrhagic myopericarditis 1-2 weeks after marrow transplant doses
Busulfan	Endocardial fibrosis
Cisplatin	Acute myocardial ischemia
Other cytotoxics	
Paclitaxel (Taxol)	Exacerbates anthracycline-associated CHF, bradycardia
5-Fluorouracil	Angina/myocardial infarction
Vincristine, vinblastine, vinorelbine (Navelbine)	Myocardial infarction
Biologics	
Trastuzumab (Herceptin)	Exacerbates anthracycline-associated CHF
Interferons	Exacerbates underlying cardiac disease
Interleukin-2	Acute myocardial injury, ventricular arrhythmias, hypotension
Hormones	
Megestrol (progestin)	Cardiomyopathy
Estramustine (androgen antagonist [Emcyt])	Myocardial infarction, CHF
Goserelin (gonadotropin-releasing hormone analog [Zoladex])	Myocardial infarction, CHF
Diethylstilbestrol (estrogen)	Myocardial infarction
Toremifene (antiestrogen [Fareston])	Myocardial infarction
Bicalutamide (antiandrogen [Casodex])	Angina, CHF, myocardial infarction
All-*trans*-retinoic acid	Myocardial dysfunction, heart failure, fever, shortness of breath, pleural and pericardial effusions, pulmonary infiltrates, and peripheral edema
Hematopoietic growth factors	
Granulocyte macrophage colony-stimulating factor (sargramostim [Leukine])	Capillary leak syndrome
Antiemetic	
Granisetron	Sinus bradycardia, atrioventricular block and increased PR interval or a Wenckebach block (Mobitz I).

CHF = congestive heart failure.

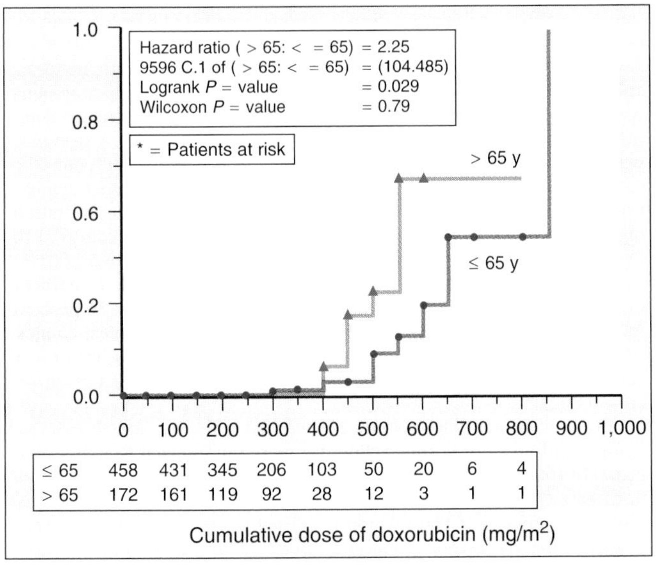

FIGURE 83–5 Risk of doxorubicin-associated congestive heart failure by patient age: Cumulative doxorubicin dose at onset of doxorubicin-associated congestive heart failure in 630 patients according to patient age older or younger than 65 years (y). (Redrawn from Swain SM, Whaley FS, Ewer MS: Congestive heart failure in patients treated with doxorubicin: A retrospective analysis of three trials. Cancer 97:2869, 2003.)

Children are at increased risk.[39,40] In a Roswell Park Cancer Institute study of 15-year survivors of childhood or adolescent cancer, cardiac mortality exceeded that expected, particularly for men after doxorubicin treatment. Risk was not ameliorated by treatment era (1960-1970 or 1971-1984).[41]

A Finnish group studied serum *N*-terminal atrial natriuretic peptide (NT-ANP) in 43 children during and in 48 children after chemotherapy for cancer. Cumulative anthracycline doses ranged between 0 and 600 mg/m^2 (median 225 mg/m^2). Cardiac evaluation included an ECG and echocardiographic assessment of systolic and diastolic left ventricular function. During chemotherapy, serum NT-ANP levels rose compared to controls but varied markedly in the same individuals. Serum NT-ANP levels were highest in patients after bone marrow transplantation or cardiac irradiation.[42]

In a Japanese study of 34 children (18 boys and 16 girls) who had received doxorubicin, plasma ANP and brain natriuretic peptide (BNP) were assayed at the first echocardiogram for cardiac function; 8 (23.5 percent) had left ventricular dysfunction. Both ANP and BNP were significantly elevated in comparison with healthy controls ($p < 0.01$) or patients with normal cardiac function ($p < 0.05$) and correlated significantly with systolic but not diastolic function. Plasma ANP and BNP levels may provide early markers for doxorubicin-induced cardiotoxicity in children.[43]

MECHANISMS. Despite many hypotheses, no mechanism underlying doxorubicin cardiotoxicity has proved definitive. Doxorubicin binds to cardiolipin in the inner mitochondrial membrane and interrupts synthesis of adenosine triphosphate (ATP). The doxorubicin-cardiolipin complex promotes transfer of electrons through doxorubicin-producing reactive oxygen species. Resulting peroxides lead to mitochondrial membrane damage. Glutathione peroxidase is depleted, which is particularly important in myocytes that lack catalase. The iron-doxorubicin complex disrupts the sarcoplasmic reticulum. Doxorubicinol also disturbs calcium transport.

PREVENTION. Limiting the cumulative dose of doxorubicin to less than 450 mg/m^2 provides the first line of defense against cardiotoxicity.[37] Anthracycline toxicity is also associated with peak dose per course. For tumors that require high doses of doxorubicin per course, the dose can be divided over several days or given by continuous infusion. Smaller weekly doses also provide an effective antitumor dose density but with lower peak doses. Liposome-encapsulated anthracycline decreases the risk of cardiac toxicity in clinical trials. Dexrazoxane (Zinecard or Cardioxane), an iron chelator, has been protective in randomized trials.[44,45] Other anthracycline analogs may have lower rates of cardiotoxicity for given level of efficacy, but this has been difficult to prove.

Patients are generally monitored for falling left ventricular ejection fractions with noninvasive techniques.[46] Troponin and natriuretic peptide levels as well as single-photon emission computed tomography scans have been monitored as well but are not established.[43,47,48]

MANAGEMENT. Management includes afterload reduction and angiotensin II converting enzyme inhibitors; selective beta-receptor blockers such as metoprolol may also be useful in patients with congestive heart failure. Malignant arrhythmias may also require treatment.

Trastuzumab (Herceptin) Cardiotoxicity

Amplification of the gene encoding the ErbB2 (Her2/neu) receptor tyrosine kinase, a coreceptor for neuroregulin signaling, promotes the progression of several forms of breast cancer.[49] Trastuzumab (Herceptin) is a humanized monoclonal antibody specific for the extracellular domain of ErbB2 and has been approved by the United States Food and Drug Administration to treat breast cancers that overexpress ErbB2. In a large-scale trial, treatment with trastuzumab led to marked improvement in survival.[50] However, 7 percent of patients receiving trastuzumab as a second-line therapy, following anthracycline treatment as a first-line therapy, develop cardiac dysfunction.[50,51] Such observations suggest an important role for ErbB2 signaling as a modifier of human heart failure. Trastuzumab-related cardiomyopathy likely results from downregulation of ErbB2 signaling, which appears to protect against the development of dilated cardiomyopathy.[52] Myocardial levels of ErbB2 receptors decrease during the transition from hypertrophy to decompensated heart failure.[53] Previous studies have shown that neuroregulins promote cardiomyocyte cell survival in vitro,[54] and ErbB2 signaling may prevent myocytic apoptosis and slow cardiac remodeling in cases of heart failure.[52]

In clinical trials, trastuzumab is effective as a single agent in the treatment of breast cancer but can also have additive or synergistic effects when used in combination with chemotherapeutic agents. Because the majority of patients with breast cancer receive anthracycline treatment, the incidence of cardiomyopathy in trastuzumab-treated patients in the absence of concurrent or prior anthracycline treatment remains uncertain. When trastuzumab is combined with anthracyclines, the incidence of cardiac dysfunction is 28 percent.[50,51,55] Trastuzumab appears to increase the sensitivity of heart muscle cells to anthracycline toxicity.[52] The essential role of ErbB2 signaling in the development of the embryonic heart and the slowing of cardiac myocyte cell death in heart failure models suggests that trastuzumab-related cardiac dysfunction is not mediated by immunological mechanisms or drug-drug interaction. Currently, the use of trastuzumab is restricted to treatment of metastatic breast cancer. Clinical trials are underway to test the effectiveness of trastuzumab in other forms of ErbB2-overexpressing cancers, such as breast cancer at earlier stages, as well as lung, prostate, and ovarian cancers.[51,56]

Cyclophosphamide at Conventional and Marrow Transplant Doses

The alkylating agents cyclophosphamide and ifosfamide can cause an acute myopericarditis, particularly in the setting of bone marrow transplantation.[47,57–60] Risk is associated with peak dose and thus can be decreased by dividing the transplant doses of cyclophosphamide over 2 to 4 days. Prior expo-

CONDUCTION SYSTEM AND PACEMAKERS. Electrical abnormalities include complete bundle branch block developing a decade after radiation doses due to fibrosis of the conduction system. Implanted pacemakers have been damaged by radiation as well, and pacemaker function requires careful monitoring.

CORONARY ARTERY DISEASE. Coronary artery disease has emerged as a late risk of cardiac radiation. Coronary spasm can also occur in patients with angiographically normal–appearing coronary arteries. Deaths have occurred in up to 1 percent of patients irradiated with curative intent for Hodgkin disease and after patients have been irradiated for breast cancer.

Risks of Radiation and Drug-Associated Cardiotoxicity

Cardiac function must be monitored when patients receive combinations of radiation and drugs known to cause dysfunction.[48,84] In a Duke University study of 20 patients with left-sided breast cancer who underwent cardiac perfusion imaging using single-photon emission computed tomography before doxorubicin chemotherapy (10 patients), before radiation, and 6 months after radiation, 60 percent of the patients had new perfusion defects 6 months after radiation. The defects were dose dependent, with minimal changes at 0 to 10 Gy but a 20 percent decrease in regional perfusion at 41 to 50 Gy. Two patients developed transient pericarditis, although none had myocardial infarction or clinical congestive heart failure. Follow-up was insufficient to determine whether these perfusion changes were transient, permanent, or associated with later clinical dysfunction.[48]

In a Dana-Farber Cancer Institute study, 299 women with breast cancer were randomized to 5 versus 10 cycles of adjuvant cyclophosphamide (500 mg/m^2) and doxorubicin (45 mg/m^2) intravenously every 21 days; 122 patients also received radiation. At a median follow-up of 6.0 years (range, 0.5 to 19.4 years), the rate of cardiac events per 100 patient-years was significantly higher for the patients who received 10 cycles than for those who received 5 cycles (1.7 [CI, 1.0-2.8] vs. 0.5 [CI, 0.1 to 1.2]; $p = 0.02$]. Cardiac risk in patients receiving 5 months of chemotherapy did not differ significantly from that of women in the Framingham Heart Study, irrespective of cardiac radiation dose-volume. In women receiving 10 chemotherapy cycles, however, cardiac events were significantly increased (relative risk, 3.6; $p < 0.00003$) compared with the Framingham population, particularly for women who also received moderate and high dose-volume cardiac radiation.[85]

In a retrospective analysis of 825 women entered in randomized adjuvant chemotherapy trials with or without doxorubicin (Adriamycin) at the Istituto Nazionale Tumori (Milan, Italy), 360 women (44 percent) also received breast irradiation. Congestive heart failure occurred in 4 women after doxorubicin-containing chemotherapy (2.6 percent of those who received both doxorubicin and radiation to the left breast) and was fatal in 2. Cardiac events were documented in 6.8 percent, more frequently in women who received left breast radiation and in those older than 55 years of age.[86]

Cardiac Neoplasm and Acquired Immunodeficiency Syndrome

(see also Chap. 61)

KAPOSI SARCOMA. In patients with acquired immunodeficiency syndrome (AIDS) and human immunodeficiency virus (HIV) infection, Kaposi sarcoma and malignant lymphoma have been described as malignant neoplasms that affect the heart. The incidence of Kaposi sarcoma involving the heart ranged from 12 to 28 percent in retrospective autopsy findings. During HIV infection, cardiac involvement with Kaposi sarcoma usually occurs as a part of disseminated Kaposi sarcoma. AIDS-related metastatic Kaposi sarcoma involves either the visceral layer of pericardium or the subepicardial fat, where it can involve the subepicardial adipose tissue adjacent to a major coronary artery with involvement of the adventitia of the ascending aorta or pulmonary trunk. Pericardial and myocardial involvement can also occur. Fatal cardiac tamponade and pericardial constriction can complicate cardiac Kaposi sarcoma.[87] Pericardiocentesis has no diagnostic role and is a high-risk procedure in this group of patients. In patients with AIDS in whom the clinician has a high index of suspicion of Kaposi sarcoma pericardial effusion, a transthoracoscopic pericardial window can provide decompression and establish the pathological diagnosis.[88] Kaposi sarcoma generally responds well to chemotherapy.[7]

LYMPHOMA. Intermediate- or high-grade lymphoma is among the diagnostic criteria for AIDS. Cardiac involvement with non-Hodgkin lymphoma, usually derived from B cells, is typically high grade and is often disseminated early in patients with AIDS. Involvement of the heart by disseminated lymphoma is more common than primary cardiac lymphoma.[89] Patients usually have nonspecific symptoms, but rapid progression of cardiac dysfunction can present as intractable congestive heart failure, pericardial effusion, cardiac arrhythmia, or cardiac tamponade. Masses commonly infiltrate the pericardium with or without extension into the myocardium in cases of aggressive HIV-related lymphomas. Patients with mechanical obstruction can benefit from surgical resection. The prognosis of patients with HIV-associated cardiac lymphoma is generally poor, although combination chemotherapy can produce clinical remission.[90]

Summary

Because cardiovascular disease and cancer are both common, the cardiologist will care for many patients with cancer or a history of cancer. Because of overlapping risk factors such as obesity, hormone therapy, and, in particular, smoking, patients with coronary artery disease also have an elevated risk of cancer.

Cardiac complications of cancer such as pericardial tamponade or superior vena cava syndrome are frequent first manifestations of advanced neoplasia. Cancer treatments frequently compromise cardiac function. Radiation ports that include the heart for the treatment of lymphoma or lung or breast cancers can rarely produce late coronary artery disease or constrictive pericarditis. Oncolytic drugs, most frequently anthracyclines, paclitaxel, and trastuzumab, but also cyclophosphamide, 5-fluorouracil, and others, result in cardiotoxicity. Conversely, cardiac transplant patients have significant risk for lymphoma, squamous skin cancers, and Kaposi sarcoma, likely related to immunosuppressive therapy. The dismal outcome of cardiac resuscitation in patients with end-stage cancer requires careful coordination of end-of-life planning between the patients and families and the cardiology and oncology teams. Increased monitoring and heightened awareness of the cardiovascular complications of cancer can improve quality of life and survival in many with oncologic diseases.

REFERENCES

1. Reicher-Reiss H, Jonas M, Goldbourt U, et al: Selectively increased risk of cancer in men with coronary heart disease. Am J Cardiol 87:459, A6, 2001.

2. Kuller LH, Matthews KA, Meilahn EN: Estrogens and women's health: Interrelation of coronary heart disease, breast cancer and osteoporosis. J Steroid Biochem Mol Biol 74:297, 2000.
3. Gjersvik P, Hansen S, Moller B, et al: Are heart transplant recipients more likely to develop skin cancer than kidney transplant recipients? Transpl Int 13(Suppl 1):S380, 2000.
4. Caforio AL, Fortina AB, Piaserico S, et al: Skin cancer in heart transplant recipients: Risk factor analysis and relevance of immunosuppressive therapy. Circulation 102:III222, 2000.
5. Jensen P, Moller B, Hansen S: Skin cancer in kidney and heart transplant recipients and different long-term immunosuppressive therapy regimens. J Am Acad Dermatol 42:307, 2000.
6. Fortina AB, Caforio AL, Piaserico S, et al: Skin cancer in heart transplant recipients: Frequency and risk factor analysis. J Heart Lung Transplant 19:249, 2000.
7. Antman K, Chang Y: Kaposi's sarcoma. N Engl J Med 342:1027, 2000.
8. Calle EE, Rodriguez C, Walker-Thurmond K, Thun MJ: Overweight, obesity, and mortality from cancer in a prospectively studied cohort of U.S. adults. N Engl J Med 348:1625, 2003.
9. Gronbaek M, Becker U, Johansen D, et al: Type of alcohol consumed and mortality from all causes, coronary heart disease, and cancer. Ann Intern Med 133:411, 2000.
10. Ewer MS, Kish SK, Martin CG, et al: Characteristics of cardiac arrest in cancer patients as a predictor of survival after cardiopulmonary resuscitation. Cancer 92:1905, 2001.

Direct Complications of Neoplasia

11. Veinot JP, Burns BF, Commons AS, Thomas J: Cardiac neoplasms at the Canadian Reference Centre for Cancer Pathology. Can J Cardiol 15:311, 1999.
12. Grebenc ML, Rosado de Christenson ML, Burke AP, et al: Primary cardiac and pericardial neoplasms: Radiologic-pathologic correlation. Radiographics 20:1073, quiz 1110, 2000.
13. Eren NT, Akar AR: Primary pericardial mesothelioma. Curr Treat Options Oncol 3:369, 2002.
14. Youn HJ, Jung SE, Chung WS, et al: Obstruction of right ventricular outflow tract by extended cardiac metastasis from esophageal cancer. J Am Soc Echocardiogr 15:1541, 2002.
15. Bissada NK, Yakout HH, Babanouri A, et al: Long-term experience with management of renal cell carcinoma involving the inferior vena cava. Urology 61:89, 2003.
16. Nam MS, Jeon MJ, Kim YT, et al: Pelvic leiomyomatosis with intracaval and intracardiac extension: A case report and review of the literature. Gynecol Oncol 89:175, 2003.

Cardiac Tamponade and Constrictive Pericarditis

17. Ortega-Carnicer J, Benezet J, Porras L: Lung cancer presenting as cardiac tamponade associated with transmural myocardial ischaemia. Resuscitation 51:317, 2001.
18. Bishiniotis TS, Antoniadou S, Katseas G, et al: Malignant cardiac tamponade in women with breast cancer treated by pericardiocentesis and intrapericardial administration of triethylenethiophosphoramide (thiotepa). Am J Cardiol 86:362, 2000.
19. Wang PC, Yang KY, Chao JY, et al: Prognostic role of pericardial fluid cytology in cardiac tamponade associated with non-small cell lung cancer. Chest 118:744, 2000.
20. Okamoto H, Shinkai T, Yamakido M, Saijo N: Cardiac tamponade caused by primary lung cancer and the management of pericardial effusion. Cancer 71:93, 1993.

Superior Vena Cava Obstruction

21. Case records of the Massachusetts General Hospital: Weekly clinicopathological exercises. Case 33-2000. A seven-year-old girl with the superior vena cava syndrome after treatment for a peripheral rhabdomyosarcoma. N Engl J Med 343:1249, 2000.
22. Wudel LJ Jr, Nesbitt JC: Superior vena cava syndrome. Curr Treat Options Oncol 2:77, 2001.
23. Kvale PA, Simoff M, Prakash UB: Lung cancer: Palliative care. Chest 123:284S, 2003.
24. Teo N, Sabharwal T, Rowland E, et al: Treatment of superior vena cava obstruction secondary to pacemaker wires with balloon venoplasty and insertion of metallic stents. Eur Heart J 23:1465, 2002.
25. Lanciego C, Chacon JL, Julian A, et al: Stenting as first option for endovascular treatment of malignant superior vena cava syndrome. AJR Am J Roentgenol 177:585, 2001.
26. Kovacs RG, Aguayo SM: Images in clinical medicine: Superior vena cava syndrome. N Engl J Med 329:1007, 1993.

Valvular Heart Disease in the Cancer Patient

27. Edoute Y, Haim N, Rinkevich D, et al: Cardiac valvular vegetations in cancer patients: A prospective echocardiographic study of 200 patients. Am J Med 102:252, 1997.

Arrhythmias

28. Sekine Y, Kesler KA, Behnia M, et al: COPD may increase the incidence of refractory supraventricular arrhythmias following pulmonary resection for non-small cell lung cancer. Chest 120:1783, 2001.

Indirect Cardiovascular Complications of Cancer

Hyperviscosity

29. Ambrus JL, Ambrus CM, Dembinsky W, et al: Thromboembolic disease susceptibility related to red cell membrane fluidity in patients with polycythemia vera and effect of phlebotomies. J Med 30:299, 1999.
30. Dammacco F, Sansonno D, Piccoli C, et al: The cryoglobulins: An overview. Eur J Clin Invest 31:628, 2001.

Cardiac Complications of Chemotherapy

Anthracycline Cardiotoxicity

31. Biganzoli L, Cufer T, Bruning P, et al: Doxorubicin-paclitaxel: A safe regimen in terms of cardiac toxicity in metastatic breast carcinoma patients. Results from a European Organization for Research and Treatment of Cancer multicenter trial. Cancer 97:40, 2003.
32. Giordano SH, Booser DJ, Murray JL, et al: A detailed evaluation of cardiac toxicity: A phase II study of doxorubicin and one- or three-hour-infusion paclitaxel in patients with metastatic breast cancer. Clin Cancer Res 8:3360, 2002.
33. Tham YL, Verani MS, Chang J: Reversible and irreversible cardiac dysfunction associated with trastuzumab in breast cancer. Breast Cancer Res Treat 74:131, 2002.
34. Keefe DL: Cardiovascular emergencies in the cancer patient. Semin Oncol 27:244, 2000.
35. Von Hoff DD, Layard MW, Basa P, et al: Risk factors for doxorubicin-induced congestive heart failure. Ann Intern Med 91:710, 1979.
36. Bristow MR, Mason JW, Billingham ME, Daniels JR: Doxorubicin cardiomyopathy: Evaluation by phonocardiography, endomyocardial biopsy, and cardiac catheterization. Ann Intern Med 88:168, 1978.
37. Swain SM, Whaley FS, Ewer MS: Congestive heart failure in patients treated with doxorubicin: A retrospective analysis of three trials. Cancer 97:2869, 2003.
38. Ibrahim NK, Hortobagyi GN, Ewer M, et al: Doxorubicin-induced congestive heart failure in elderly patients with metastatic breast cancer, with long-term follow-up: The M.D. Anderson experience. Cancer Chemother Pharmacol 43:471, 1999.
39. Li CK, Sung RY, Kwok KL, et al: A longitudinal study of cardiac function in children with cancer over 40 months. Pediatr Hematol Oncol 17:77, 2000.
40. Lanzarini L, Bossi G, Laudisa ML, et al: Lack of clinically significant cardiac dysfunction during intermediate dobutamine doses in long-term childhood cancer survivors exposed to anthracyclines. Am Heart J 140:315, 2000.
41. Green DM, Hyland A, Chung CS, et al: Cancer and cardiac mortality among 15-year survivors of cancer diagnosed during childhood or adolescence. J Clin Oncol 17:3207, 1999.
42. Tikanoja T, Riikonen P, Perkkio M, Helenius T: Serum N-terminal atrial natriuretic peptide (NT-ANP) in the cardiac follow-up in children with cancer. Med Pediatr Oncol 31:73, 1998.
43. Hayakawa H, Komada Y, Hirayama M, et al: Plasma levels of natriuretic peptides in relation to doxorubicin-induced cardiotoxicity and cardiac function in children with cancer. Med Pediatr Oncol 37:4, 2001.
44. Venturini M, Michelotti A, Del Mastro L, et al: Multicenter randomized controlled clinical trial to evaluate cardioprotection of dexrazoxane versus no cardioprotection in women receiving epirubicin chemotherapy for advanced breast cancer. J Clin Oncol 14:3112, 1996.
45. Lopez M, Vici P, Di Lauro K, et al: Randomized prospective clinical trial of high-dose epirubicin and dexrazoxane in patients with advanced breast cancer and soft tissue sarcomas. J Clin Oncol 16:86, 1998.
46. Mitani I, Jain D, Joska TM, et al: Doxorubicin cardiotoxicity: Prevention of congestive heart failure with serial cardiac function monitoring with equilibrium radionuclide angiocardiography in the current era. J Nucl Cardiol 10:132, 2003.
47. Morandi P, Ruffini PA, Benvenuto GM, et al: Serum cardiac troponin I levels and ECG/Echo monitoring in breast cancer patients undergoing high-dose ($7\ g/m^2$) cyclophosphamide. Bone Marrow Transplant 28:277, 2001.
48. Hardenbergh PH, Munley MT, Bentel GC, et al: Cardiac perfusion changes in patients treated for breast cancer with radiation therapy and doxorubicin: Preliminary results. Int J Radiat Oncol Biol Phys 49:1023, 2001.

Herceptin Cardiotoxicity

49. Klapper LN, Kirschbaum MH, Sela M, Yarden Y: Biochemical and clinical implications of the ErbB/HER signaling network of growth factor receptors. Adv Cancer Res 77:25, 2000.
50. Slamon DJ, Leyland-Jones B, Shak S, et al: Use of chemotherapy plus a monoclonal antibody against HER2 for metastatic breast cancer that overexpresses HER2. N Engl J Med 344:783, 2001.
51. Baselga J: Current and planned clinical trials with trastuzumab (Herceptin). Semin Oncol 27:27, 2000.
52. Crone SA, Zhao YY, Fan L, et al: ErbB2 is essential in the prevention of dilated cardiomyopathy. Nat Med 8:459, 2002.
53. Rohrbach S, Yan X, Weinberg EO, et al: Neuregulin in cardiac hypertrophy in rats with aortic stenosis: Differential expression of erbB2 and erbB4 receptors. Circulation 100:407, 1999.
54. Zhao YY, Sawyer DR, Baliga RR, et al: Neuregulins promote survival and growth of cardiac myocytes: Persistence of ErbB2 and ErbB4 expression in neonatal and adult ventricular myocytes. J Biol Chem 273:10261, 1998.
55. Sparano JA: Cardiac toxicity of trastuzumab (Herceptin): Implications for the design of adjuvant trials. Semin Oncol 28:20, 2001.
56. Agus DB, Bunn PA Jr, Franklin W, et al: HER-2/neu as a therapeutic target in non-small cell lung cancer, prostate cancer, and ovarian cancer. Semin Oncol 27:53, discussion 92, 2000.

Cyclophosphamide at Conventional and Marrow Transplant Doses

57. Gralow JR, Livingston RB: University of Washington high-dose cyclophosphamide, mitoxantrone, and etoposide experience in metastatic breast cancer: Unexpected cardiac toxicity. J Clin Oncol 19:3903, 2001.
58. Nieto Y, Cagnoni PJ, Bearman SI, et al: Cardiac toxicity following high-dose cyclophosphamide, cisplatin, and BCNU (STAMP-I) for breast cancer. Biol Blood Marrow Transplant 6:198, 2000.
59. Klein JL, Rey PM, Dansey RD, et al: Cardiac sequelae of doxorubicin and paclitaxel as induction chemotherapy prior to high-dose chemotherapy and peripheral blood progenitor cell transplantation in women with high-risk primary or metastatic breast cancer. Bone Marrow Transplant 25:1047, 2000.
60. Brockstein BE, Smiley C, Al-Sadir J, Williams SF: Cardiac and pulmonary toxicity in patients undergoing high-dose chemotherapy for lymphoma and breast cancer: Prognostic factors. Bone Marrow Transplant 25:885, 2000.

61. Sohn SK, Kim JG, Kim DH, Lee KB: Cardiac morbidity in advanced chronic myelogenous leukaemia patients treated by successive allogeneic stem cell transplantation with busulphan/cyclophosphamide conditioning after imatinib mesylate administration. Br J Haematol 121:469, 2003.
62. Ando M, Yokozawa T, Sawada J, et al: Cardiac conduction abnormalities in patients with breast cancer undergoing high-dose chemotherapy and stem cell transplantation. Bone Marrow Transplant 25:185, 2000.

Taxanes

63. Markman M, Kennedy A, Webster K, et al: Paclitaxel administration to gynecologic cancer patients with major cardiac risk factors. J Clin Oncol 16:3483, 1998.
64. Ekholm E, Rantanen V, Syvanen K, et al: Docetaxel does not impair cardiac autonomic function in breast cancer patients previously treated with anthracyclines. Anticancer Drugs 13:425, 2002.
65. Syvanen K, Ekholm E, Anttila K, Salminen E: Immediate effects of docetaxel alone or in combination with epirubicin on cardiac function in advanced breast cancer. Anticancer Res 23:1869, 2003.
66. Valero V, Perez E, Dieras V: Doxorubicin and taxane combination regimens for metastatic breast cancer: Focus on cardiac effects. Semin Oncol 28:15, 2001.

Doxorubicin and Paclitaxel Combinations

67. Gianni L, Munzone E, Capri G, et al: Paclitaxel by 3-hour infusion in combination with bolus doxorubicin in women with untreated metastatic breast cancer: High antitumor efficacy and cardiac effects in a dose-finding and sequence-finding study. J Clin Oncol 13:2688, 1995.
68. Gianni L, Dombernowsky P, Sledge G, et al: Cardiac function following combination therapy with paclitaxel and doxorubicin: An analysis of 657 women with advanced breast cancer. Ann Oncol 12:1067, 2001.

69. Hortobagyi GN, Willey J, Rahman Z, et al: Prospective assessment of cardiac toxicity during a randomized phase II trial of doxorubicin and paclitaxel in metastatic breast cancer. Semin Oncol 24:S17, 1997.
70. Perez EA: Doxorubicin and paclitaxel in the treatment of advanced breast cancer: Efficacy and cardiac considerations. Cancer Invest 19:155, 2001.
71. Doxorubicin/paclitaxel combination does not expose breast cancer patients to excessive cardiac risk. Oncology (Huntingt) 15:830, 2001.

All-Trans-Retinoic Acid Syndrome

72. Tallman MS, Andersen JW, Schiffer CA, et al: Clinical description of 44 patients with acute promyelocytic leukemia who developed the retinoic acid syndrome. Blood 95:90, 2000.

Other Agents

73. David JS, Gueugniaud PY, Hepp A, et al: Severe heart failure secondary to 5-fluorouracil and low-doses of folinic acid: Usefulness of an intra-aortic balloon pump. Crit Care Med 28:3558, 2000.
74. Reis SE, Costantino JP, Wickerham DL, et al: Cardiovascular effects of tamoxifen in women with and without heart disease: Breast cancer prevention trial. National Surgical Adjuvant Breast and Bowel Project Breast Cancer Prevention Trial Investigators. J Natl Cancer Inst 93:16, 2001.
75. Caorsi C, Quintana E, Valdes S, Munoz C: Continuous cardiac output and hemodynamic monitoring: High temporal correlation between plasma TNF-alpha and hemodynamic changes during a sepsis-like state in cancer immunotherapy. J Endotoxin Res 9:91, 2003.

Cardiac Complications of Radiation Therapy

76. Gustavsson A, Bendahl PO, Cwikiel M, et al: No serious late cardiac effects after adjuvant radiotherapy following mastectomy in premenopausal women with early breast cancer. Int J Radiat Oncol Biol Phys 43:745, 1999.
77. Gyenes G, Rutqvist LE, Liedberg A, Fornander T: Long-term cardiac morbidity and mortality in a randomized trial of pre- and postoperative radiation therapy versus surgery alone in primary breast cancer. Radiother Oncol 48:185, 1998.
78. Canney PA, Deehan C, Glegg M, Dickson J: Reducing cardiac dose in post-operative irradiation of breast cancer patients: The relative importance of patient positioning and CT scan planning. Br J Radiol 72:986, 1999.
79. Chen MH, Cash EP, Danias PG, et al: Respiratory maneuvers decrease irradiated cardiac volume in patients with left-sided breast cancer. J Cardiovasc Magn Reson 4:265, 2002.
80. Sixel KE, Aznar MC, Ung YC: Deep inspiration breath hold to reduce irradiated heart volume in breast cancer patients. Int J Radiat Oncol Biol Phys 49:199, 2001.
81. Gagliardi G, Lax I, Soderstrom S, et al: Prediction of excess risk of long-term cardiac mortality after radiotherapy of stage I breast cancer. Radiother Oncol 46:63, 1998.
82. Vallis KA, Pintilie M, Chong N, et al: Assessment of coronary heart disease morbidity and mortality after radiation therapy for early breast cancer. J Clin Oncol 20:1036, 2002.
83. Muren LP, Maurstad G, Hafslund R, et al: Cardiac and pulmonary doses and complication probabilities in standard and conformal tangential irradiation in conservative management of breast cancer. Radiother Oncol 62:173, 2002.

Risks of Radiation and Drug-Associated Cardiotoxicity

84. Zambetti M, Moliterni A, Materazzo C, et al: Long-term cardiac sequelae in operable breast cancer patients given adjuvant chemotherapy with or without doxorubicin and breast irradiation. J Clin Oncol 19:37, 2001.
85. Shapiro CL, Hardenbergh PH, Gelman R, et al: Cardiac effects of adjuvant doxorubicin and radiation therapy in breast cancer patients. J Clin Oncol 16:3493, 1998.
86. Valagussa P, Zambetti M, Biasi S, et al: Cardiac effects following adjuvant chemotherapy and breast irradiation in operable breast cancer. Ann Oncol 5:209, 1994.

Cardiac Neoplasm and AIDS

87. Chyu KY, Birnbaum Y, Naqvi T, et al: Echocardiographic detection of Kaposi's sarcoma causing cardiac tamponade in a patient with acquired immunodeficiency syndrome. Clin Cardiol 21:131, 1998.
88. Rerkpattanapipat P, Wongpraparut N, Jacobs LE, Kotler MN: Cardiac manifestations of acquired immunodeficiency syndrome. Arch Intern Med 160:602, 2000.
89. Roberts WC: Primary and secondary neoplasms of the heart. Am J Cardiol 80:671, 1997.
90. Duong M, Dubois C, Buisson M, et al: Non-Hodgkin's lymphoma of the heart in patients infected with human immunodeficiency virus. Clin Cardiol 20:497, 1997.

CHAPTER 84

Psychiatric and Behavioral Aspects of Cardiovascular Disease

Arthur J. Barsky

Daily life offers ample empirical evidence of an intimate relationship between the psyche and the heart. Intense emotions such as anxiety, anger, elation, and sexual arousal are accompanied by predictable increases in heart rate and blood pressure. Our everyday speech is filled with cardiac metaphors—the heart "races" with excitement, "pounds" in eager anticipation, "stands still" in dread, "aches" with grief. Many cultures have regarded the heart as the seat of emotion, the origin of love, the source of courage, or the abode of the soul. Generous people have "big hearts" and stingy people are "heartless." When you first met your first love, your heart "skipped a beat," and you were "broken hearted" when you parted ways soon thereafter. We attend funerals with a "heavy heart" and offer our "heartfelt" condolences. The interaction of heart and psyche is bidirectional. Emotions and stressful experiences affect the heart directly through the autonomic nervous system and indirectly via neuroendocrine pathways. Conversely, cardiac activity and function can reach conscious awareness and may be experienced as symptoms.

Psychiatric and Behavioral Aspects of Coronary Heart Disease

Type A Behavior Pattern and Anger

Clinicians have long observed that many patients with coronary heart disease (CHD) seem to be compulsive, driven overachievers who are unable to relax and are quick to feel angry and frustrated when things do not proceed as planned. These observations were reinforced in the 1960s by Friedman and Rosenman, who advanced the concept of type A behavior. Type A behavior is suffused with a sense of ambition, time urgency, and anger and hostility; type A people are excessively competitive and aggressive, with an extreme drive for achievement—impatient people leading fast-paced lives in continual and strenuous pursuit of a goal. This was contrasted with type B individuals, who are relaxed, unhurried, less aggressive, and who do not get as upset when thwarted. Large-scale, prospective studies in the 1970s and 1980s conducted on initially healthy individuals showed that those with type A behavior pattern, compared to type B individuals, had a significantly elevated rate of developing CHD and myocardial infarction at 5- to 8.5-year follow-up and had more extensive CHD at the time of angiography. Although some subsequent studies replicated these findings,[1] a number failed to support the association.

These contradictory findings led to a search for a specific component of type A behavior that might be more closely associated with CHD. This work suggested that anger and/or suppressed anger are the pathogenic components of type A personality. Anger, hostility, antagonistic interactions, cynicism, and mistrust have now been associated in long-term, prospective studies with the incidence of CHD, coronary events, and total mortality. For example, in a sample of 2890 middle-aged men followed prospectively for more than 8 years, suppressed anger was a significant predictor of a major cardiac event, and this relationship persisted after controlling for physiological, psychosocial, and behavioral risk factors.[2] In a prospective study of young adults, high levels of hostility were associated with subsequent coronary artery calcification,[3] and cross-sectional studies also report an association between the degree of hostility and the severity of CHD.[4] In large, prospective studies of initially healthy individuals, higher levels of anger were associated with a twofold to threefold increased incidence of developing CHD, after adjusting for other biological risk factors.[5]

Some studies, however, have failed to find an association between anger and CHD, and in general it appears that hostility and anger may predispose more to the initial cardiac event than adversely influencing the course of already established CHD. It is unclear to what degree hostility's effect may be mediated through its effect on other risk factors such as lack of social support, smoking, obesity, and alcohol use. The combination of both anger and low social support may be particularly hazardous.[6] Possible associations between anger and race, socioeconomic status, and gender also represent potential confounds. Although more research is necessary, it does appear that anger and hostility play some role in the development of CHD.

Depression and Anxiety

DEPRESSION. Depression is prevalent in CHD patients but is consistently underdiagnosed by their cardiologists and primary care physicians. Clinically significant depressive symptoms are found in 40 to 65 percent of patients following a myocardial infarction, and major depressive disorder is found in 15 to 25 percent of such patients.[7,8] In one study, 31.5 percent of patients with myocardial infarction experienced major depression while in the hospital or in the year following discharge.[9] The prevalence of depression is also elevated in patients with stable CHD who have not had a recent myocardial infarction and in patients who have undergone coronary artery bypass grafting (CABG).[10] Depression is often chronic: Three-fourths of the patients with major depression 2 weeks after a myocardial infarction remain depressed 3 months later. Although most subjects in these studies have been men, the risk of depression in women with CHD is twice as high as that of men.

Depression is important in itself because of the considerable suffering it imposes. In addition, depression exacerbates and amplifies cardiac symptoms. Depressed CHD patients have more severe cardiac symptoms than nondepressed CHD patients, even after controlling for the severity of cardiac disease[11]: They have more angina during exercise treadmill testing, terminate the treadmill test sooner, and have more persistent angina following myocardial infarction. Depression adversely affects compliance with medical therapy, and it is detrimental to cardiac rehabilitation. Depression also predicts a slower resumption of activities, poorer social readjustment, a lower likelihood of returning to work, and poorer quality of life following myocardial infarction.[12] In a 1-year, prospective study of patients who had undergone catheterization for documented CHD, physical functioning and interference with activities were better predicted by baseline depression and anxiety than by the number of stenosed vessels, even after controlling for medical comorbidity and treatment.[13]

Depression both worsens the prognosis of established CHD and constitutes a risk factor for the development of CHD in healthy individuals; that is, it confers an increased risk of cardiac mortality in both those with and without CHD at baseline.[14] In patients with documented CHD, depression predicts future cardiac events and is associated with significantly elevated rates of cardiac mortality (primarily as a result of sudden cardiac death [SCD]).[7] This risk is elevated for women as well as men and is not limited to major depressive disorder but also includes milder depressive symptoms. Thus, there is a continuous, linear relationship between the severity of depression and the risk of subsequent cardiac events.[15] Major depressive disorder at the time of cardiac catheterization is a significant predictor of subsequent myocardial infarction, angioplasty, CABG, and death in patients with evidence of CHD, and this effect is independent of disease severity, ejection fraction, and smoking. Depression prior to undergoing CABG surgery is an independent predictor of rehospitalization, continued surgical pain, and failure to resume previous activity.[16] Following myocardial infarction, depression increases the risk of reinfarction, cardiac arrest, and death, after adjusting for CHD severity.[7]

In an important longitudinal study of 222 patients, baseline depression was a significant predictor of cardiac mortality 6 and 18 months after myocardial infarction, and this association persisted after controlling statistically for the effects of baseline left ventricular dysfunction, Killip class, previous myocardial infarction, and frequency of premature ventricular complexes.[7] For longer follow-up periods, from 5 to 15 years, the relative risk of recurrent myocardial infarction or cardiac mortality associated with depression is between 1.5 and 6, after controlling for disease severity, smoking, diabetes, and age in multivariate analyses.[15] The degree of risk associated with depression is as great as that associated with traditional risk factors (e.g., cholesterol, smoking, hypertension) and is largely independent of them. In some studies, however, the association between depression and post-myocardial reinfarction is no longer significant when adjusted for all other predictors of cardiac mortality and for possible confounds (e.g., fatigue) that are common to both CHD and depression.[17] Much of the increased cardiac mortality associated with depression appears to be attributable to SCD due to arrhythmias. This suggests that the effect of depression may be more arrhythmogenic than atherogenic. An interaction effect may exist, in which the co-occurrence of depression with ventricular arrhythmias constitutes a particularly ominous prognostic factor. Conversely, optimism seems to have a positive influence on prognosis; optimism at the time of CABG is associated with a lower rate of rehospitalization for cardiac events over the subsequent 6 months, after controlling for sociodemographic differences and disease severity.[18]

Depression as a Risk Factor. Depression also appears to be a risk factor for the development of CHD in healthy individuals, though the evidence here is somewhat less conclusive. In prospective studies of initially healthy, community residents without a history of CHD, depression has been associated with an adjusted relative risk between 1.5 and 2 for the subsequent development of CHD, myocardial infarction, and cardiac death over periods from 6 to 40 years in men and in women, and this risk is largely independent of the more traditional risk factors.[19] A dose-response relationship seems to exist such that the more severely depressed the patient is, the greater the risk of developing CHD.

In *summary*, depression is a negative prognostic indicator for patients with established CHD and a risk factor for the development of CHD in healthy individuals. It is associated with increased morbidity, mortality, disability, and impaired quality of life. Both major depressive disorder and less severe depressive symptoms are significant in this regard. The degree of risk associated with major depression is comparable to that associated with other, established risk factors and is largely independent of them.

Several behavioral and physiological mechanisms may mediate the relationship between depression and CHD. Depression may operate through its influence on lifestyle and behavior[20]: Depressed individuals take poorer care of themselves; are less physically active; pay less attention to diet; drink more alcohol; smoke more and have worse quitting rates; have less motivation and energy to exercise regularly; and may be less likely to seek medical care. Depression is associated with poorer adherence to the medical regimen and to cardiac risk factor modification and rehabilitation, and depressed patients are more likely to drop out of exercise programs. For reasons that remain unclear, patients with a range of psychiatric disorders, including depression, undergo revascularization procedures (percutaneous transluminal coronary angioplasty and CABG) less frequently than those without psychiatric disorders, even after adjusting for disease severity.[21]

Pathophysiological Mechanisms. Several pathophysiological mechanisms may link depression and CHD.[22] First, depression results in autonomic arousal and hypothalamic-adrenocortical and sympathoadrenal hyperactivity. Depressed patients show hyperactivity of the hypothalamic-pituitary-adrenocortical axis and hypercortisolemia, and corticosteroids have atherogenic effects, including the induction of high blood pressure and increases in cholesterol and free fatty acids,[22] as well as possible effects on arterial endothelial function.[23] In addition, there is hypersecretion of norepinephrine in depression, and plasma catecholamines stimulate heart rate, blood pressure, and myocardial oxygen consumption. Catecholamines are also proarrhythmic, and an increased incidence of ventricular tachyarrhythmias has been found in depressed patients. (This observation is compatible with the finding that SCD accounts for a large share of the excess cardiac mortality found in depressed CHD patients.)[15,24] Second, depressed cardiac patients exhibit diminished heart rate variability,[25] resulting from a relative increase in sympathetic tone and/or a relative decrease in parasympathetic tone, which increases the risk of fatal arrhythmias. Third, depression may be accompanied by changes in platelet aggregability.[22,26] Serotonin plays a major role in depression, and it is also known to influence thrombogenesis and enhance platelet activation and responsiveness to other thrombogenic agents. Serotonin reuptake inhibitor antidepressants appear to normalize this platelet hyperactivity seen in depression.

ANXIETY. Chronically high levels of anxiety, panic disorder, and phobic anxiety appear to be both a risk factor for developing CHD and a negative prognostic influence on the course of established disease.[24] In the former instance, several prospective studies of initially healthy men and women reveal that those who are highly anxious at the outset are more likely to subsequently develop arteriosclerotic plaques, carotid artery intimal thickening, nonfatal myocardial infarction, and cardiac death.[27] Anxiety may also worsen the course of established CHD. Thus high levels of anxiety following myocardial infarction appear to confer a 2.5-fold to fivefold increased risk of recurrent ischemia, reinfarction, ventricular fibrillation, and SCD. In one study, for example, anxiety was an independent predictor of cardiac events following myocardial infarction, after adjusting for the influence of depression. In another study, higher levels of anxiety in patients hospitalized for myocardial infarction were independent predictors of more in-hospital ischemic and arrhythmic complications.[28] It remains unclear whether anxiety is more closely related to arrhythmias and SCD than to arteriosclerosis and infarction.

Possible mechanisms explaining these associations include sympathetic nervous system upregulation with increased catecholamine production and decreased vagal activity, microvascular angina, and idiopathic cardiomyopathy.

Psychosocial Factors

Psychosocial, cultural, and environmental factors increase the risk of CHD, either independently or in combination. These include social isolation and lack of social support, life stresses (such as job strain), and sociodemographic characteristics. These psychosocial risk factors tend to be associated with each other and often co-occur. For example, job strain and socioeconomic position may be inversely correlated, and depression is associated with social isolation. Furthermore, these psychosocial factors tend to be associated with unhealthy lifestyle behaviors. For example, life stress may be correlated with smoking, increased alcohol consumption, and body weight, and people with fewer social supports are less likely to stop smoking or adhere to the medical regimen.

SOCIAL ISOLATION, LACK OF SOCIAL SUPPORT, AND SOCIAL DISRUPTION. Population-based, cross-sectional surveys reveal that social integration (e.g., being married, having regular contact with friends, and belonging to organizations) is associated with lower levels of CHD. Conversely, social isolation and low social support (living alone, having few friends or family members, and not belonging to organizations, clubs, or churches) is associated with an increased incidence of CHD and a poorer outcome following first diagnosis of CHD.[29] In a recent prospective study of 430 CHD patients, those with fewer than four people in their social network had a 2.4 times greater risk of cardiac mortality after adjusting for differences in age, disease severity, psychological distress, smoking, and income.[30] Social support and depression seem to interact, such that high levels of social support blunt the impact of depression on cardiac mortality.[31]

Animal studies also suggest a protective role for social support against atherogenesis. When research personnel fondle laboratory rabbits placed on an atherogenic diet, the development of coronary atherosclerosis is retarded. Crowding and social disruption of animal colonies, as well as isolation of individual laboratory animals, increase the rates of atherogenesis.

Several mediating mechanisms have been proposed to explain this relationship between social integration and CHD. First, concerned and supportive others may encourage healthy behaviors and adherence to the medical regimen and provide a motivation for altering unhealthy behavioral risk factors; conversely, loneliness may foster unhealthy behaviors such as smoking and drinking. Second, social support, by providing comfort, encouragement, and consolation, may attenuate and buffer the individual's emotional and/or physiological response to environmental stress. Finally, significant others can provide practical assistance that mitigates the impact of stressful life events, for example, lending money, doing errands, and providing transportation.

LIFE STRESS AND JOB STRAIN. The relationship between life stress and CHD has long been of interest. Animal work is provocative in this regard. In studies ranging from mice to primates, stressful experimental paradigms that increase aggression and fear and that disturb stable social hierarchies and decrease social affiliation are associated with atherosclerosis. Thus, dominant male monkeys fed an atherogenic diet develop coronary atherosclerosis at a higher rate when repeatedly moved from one social group to another rather than when left in a single, stable group.

In humans, two different forms of stress have received particular attention: major life events that tax one's abilities to adapt (e.g., getting divorced, moving, encountering financial difficulties, or being involved in a lawsuit) and minor, recurrent irritants and frustrations. Some studies of individuals undergoing major, stressful life events have found an association with the incidence of myocardial infarction, the development of CHD, or cardiac mortality, but other prospective studies have not. At present, the evidence remains inconclusive.

When turning to recurrent daily stresses, job strain and work-related pressures have received considerable attention. *Job strain* is defined as the combination of high demands with little autonomy or control over one's working conditions, routine, or schedule. Job strain has been associated with an increased risk of CHD in previously healthy people,[32] but its impact on the progress of already established CHD is less clear. Cross-sectional studies in the United States and Europe disclose that both men and women workers with high job strain have a higher prevalence of CHD and higher incidence of myocardial infarction than do those with low job strain. Longitudinal studies also provide some support for this hypothesis.[33,33a] In a longitudinal study of 12,517 Swedish men over a 14-year period, low levels of control over one's work conditions were an independent risk factor for cardiovascular disease mortality.[34] After adjusting for age, smoking, exercise, and social class, workers with low levels of control over their jobs had a relative risk of 1.83 for cardiovascular mortality. Workers with both low control over their work and low levels of social support had a relative risk of 2.62 for cardiovascular mortality. Marital stress has been found to exert a negative prognostic influence on CHD in women and may be even more important than job stress for women.[35]

SOCIODEMOGRAPHIC CHARACTERISTICS. Lower socioeconomic status (whether assessed by education, occupation, or income) prospectively predisposes healthy people to an increased risk of CHD and CHD patients to a poorer prognosis. The decline in cardiovascular disease mortality over the past 30 years in the United States has been more pronounced among those of higher socioeconomic status, and the reasons for this are not clear. Because beneficial health habits (including not smoking and weight control) tend to be associated with socioeconomic status, they may play a role. Poorer nutrition and difficulty obtaining medical care may contribute, and hostility and depression may be weakly inversely correlated with social position. Stressful life events, greater job strain, lack of social support, and diminished sense of self-control may mediate the relationship between socioeconomic status and CHD. There are also complex racial and ethnic differences in cardiovascular disease that remain poorly understood. Because race and ethnicity tend to be confounded with differences in socioeconomic position, it has been difficult to isolate their effects.

Acute Mental Stress

Acute mental stress has negative cardiovascular consequences. Cardiovascular mortality rises in the month following the death of a loved one, and the incidence of cardiac events rises immediately after natural disasters and among civilians subjected to military attack. The direct cardiovascular effects of acute mental stress have been observed during daily life and with laboratory paradigms of experimental stress. Experimental stress (induced, for example, by public speaking or accomplishing difficult intellectual tasks under time pressure or in frustrating circumstances) reliably increases heart rate, blood pressure, and myocardial oxygen demands. The effect of acute mental stress on the heart already damaged by preexisting CHD has been studied with relatively sensitive measures of myocardial ischemia such as regional myocardial perfusion and wall motion abnormalities. Such stress precipitates myocardial ischemia in 30 to 60 percent of CHD patients.[36]

Mental stress-induced ischemia occurs at lower heart rates and at a lower levels of myocardial work than does exercise-induced ischemia, suggesting that decreases in myocardial perfusion may play a role in mental stress-induced ischemia. In a representative study, 59 percent of CHD patients (and 8 percent of controls) exhibited wall motion abnormalities during periods of experimentally induced stress. One third of the CHD patients had a decrease of at least 5 percent in ejection fraction. Mental stress–induced ischemia is more likely to be "silent," or asymptomatic, than is ischemia induced by exercise. In the study just referred to, 83 percent of mental stress-induced ischemic episodes were asymptomatic.

When CHD patients are monitored during daily life, mental challenges unaccompanied by strenuous physical exertion are frequently associated with transient myocardial ischemia. Such ischemia has been observed, for example, while driving and during public speaking. Although most ischemic episodes during daily life do not appear to be precipitated by psychological or mental stress, a sizable minority (perhaps as many as one fourth) are.

CHD patients who exhibit mental stress-induced ischemia appear to be at increased risk of subsequent fatal and nonfatal cardiac events.[37] This relationship persists after other risk factors (including age, left ventricular function, and prior myocardial infarction) have been taken into account.

Acute stress may promote ischemic heart disease in a number of ways. First, stress increases myocardial oxygen demands as a result of its hemodynamic effects. Second, vasospasm may reduce coronary blood flow, especially in more severely diseased vessels. Third, the stress response increases circulating cortisol and catecholamines, which activate platelets and promote platelet aggregation and which increase cholesterol and decrease high-density lipoproteins. The net result of these actions is to increase cardiac demand while at the same time decreasing coronary blood supply and to promote plaque rupture and thrombus formation.

Sudden Emotion

The work on anger, depression, and anxiety discussed earlier deals with the long-term consequences and sequelae of enduring, persistent emotions. There is also a body of work on the immediate and acute effects of sudden, intense, negative emotion. Because much of this work focuses on arrhythmias and SCD, it will be reviewed in the next section. However, mental activities leading to intense anger or frustration and, to a lesser degree, to anxiety and sadness can trigger myocardial ischemia.[38] The relative risk for myocardial infarction in the 1 to 2 hours following an episode in which the patients report feeling very angry is between 2.3 and 9.[39] Because these intense, negative emotional states involve sympathetic arousal, they may act by triggering coronary vasospasm, rupture of atherosclerotic plaques, and increased platelet aggregation. Anger and hostility in particular have been associated with increased platelet adhesion.[40] Hostility is also associated with decreased parasympathetic arousal during ambulatory monitoring. When anger is experimentally induced, patients scoring higher on hostility scales exhibit greater sympathetic nervous system–mediated cardiovascular responses than those who are less hostile.[41]

Arrhythmias and Sudden Cardiac Death

Increasing evidence links mentally stressful and emotionally powerful events with lethal arrhythmias and SCD. Intense, overwhelming emotions such as fear and anger have been associated with both benign and lethal arrhythmias, including ventricular premature complexes, ventricular tachycardia, and ventricular fibrillation. This effect is most evident in hearts that are already diseased, ischemic, or electrically unstable. There are at least three lines of investigation into the arrhythmogenic potential of stress and intense emotion: retrospective case series of psychological distress immediately preceding lethal arrhythmias or SCD; psychophysiological experiments demonstrating that arrhythmias immediately follow sudden, intense emotion or acute stress; and investigations of the neural control of cardiac rate and rhythm.

OBSERVATIONAL STUDIES. has long been suspected that acutely stressful events and sudden, intense emotion can precipitate fatal arrhythmias and SCD, and there are many anecdotal case reports of SCD following immediately after severe psychological stress and intense emotional arousal. Careful psychiatric interviews of patients hospitalized after ventricular tachycardia or ventricular fibrillation revealed that 21 percent had undergone a major emotional disturbance or psychological trigger in the preceding 24 hours. These included interpersonal conflicts, bereavement, public humiliation, marital separation, and business losses. Studies like these suffer from retrospective bias and selective recall, inadequate or absent control groups, and sampling bias. When taken together, however, they nonetheless suggest that acute stress (perhaps in conjunction with other factors such as preexisting CHD) has the power on occasion to precipitate lethal arrhythmias and contribute to SCD.

STRESS AND ARRHYTHMIAS. Other research has probed the link between emotionally provocative daily stresses and arrhythmias. Healthy subjects manifest ventricular ectopy during driving, public speaking, and stressful interviews. Among cardiac patients undergoing ambulatory monitoring, daily life stresses are associated with ectopy. Experimentally induced psychological stress has been shown to lower the ventricular vulnerable period and the threshold for ventricular fibrillation and to increase the frequency of ventricular ectopic beats in patients with preexisting ventricular arrhythmias. Thus it is clear that stressful experiences and events can produce rhythm changes in both normal subjects and CHD patients. The clinical importance of this remains to be established, but the combination of severe, acute mental distress and a myocardium made vulnerable by preexisting disease can result in lethal arrhythmias and SCD.

The link between stress and arrhythmias has been explored in experimental animal work. When dogs are subjected to aversive restraint and electric shock, there is a 49 to 66 percent decrease in the repetitive extrasystole threshold. If a coronary artery occlusion is first produced experimentally, then the same stressful paradigm induces spontaneous ventricular fibrillation. Similarly, when pigs with a coronary artery occlusion are placed in a stressful environment, there is a high incidence of spontaneous ventricular fibrillation.

Some psychiatric disorders, particularly anxiety and depressive disorders, may predispose to SCD. The empirical evidence, however, remains scanty. In one study, psychiatric distress after myocardial infarction predicted ventricular arrhythmias in the year following the infarct, although subsequent work failed to confirm these findings. Depressed patients with CHD have an increased incidence of significant ventricular arrhythmias.[24] Post-myocardial infarction depression in particular has been linked to SCD, and much of its negative influence on cardiac mortality in patients with CHD is mediated through SCD. However, a number of methodological problems make this work difficult to interpret, and on balance the evidence at this time must be considered equivocal.

Sociocultural and sociodemographic factors may also play a role in SCD. The inverse relationship between socioeconomic status and cardiac mortality in general is especially robust for SCD, although this may well be confounded by an association between social position and access to emergency medical care. Other work has disclosed that cardiac mortality is significantly higher immediately after, as compared with immediately before, an important religious holiday. There are also well-recognized, culture-specific syndromes in which sudden death follows highly ritualized events with a powerful, culture-specific significance, such as "voodoo death."

NEURAL INFLUENCES ON RATE AND RHYTHM. A number of pathways mediate the neural control of heart rate and rhythm. First, activation of the hypothalamic-adrenomedullary axis increases myocardial irritability and decreases the threshold for inducing ventricular fibrillation. Second, direct sympathetic innervation of the heart exerts a proarrhythmic effect, increasing ventricular ectopy and lowering the threshold for inducing ventricular arrhythmias, especially in the heart with preexisting ischemic damage or electrical instability. Animal work provides evidence of cortical and brain stem influence over cardiac rhythm: Pathways run from the frontal cortex and hypothalamus to the brain stem nuclei controlling cardiovascular function. Thus, stimulation of the lateral and posterior hypothalamus lowers the ventricular fibrillation threshold, and blockade of these corticofrontal pathways raise it. In humans, electrocardiographic (ECG) changes in rhythm and/or repolarization are seen in patients suffering cerebrovascular accidents involving the cortex. Finally, extreme stress and acute psychological trauma can cause myocardial necrosis. In animal models, large quantities of catecholamines, either exogenously administered or stress induced, can result in myofibrillar degeneration and myocardial necrosis. On pathological examination, widespread calcification is found, the result of peroxidation of myocardial lipid membranes and blockage of the calcium-channel pump. This same lesion has also been reported in humans who died suddenly at the peak of extreme psychic stress and trauma.

Implantable cardioverter-defibrillators are increasingly used in the treatment of potentially lethal arrhythmias (see Chap. 31). Although these devices are medically efficacious and generally meet with a high degree of patient acceptance, in a substantial minority of patients (probably between 25 and 50 percent) the implantation of the device results in significant emotional distress (anxiety, depression, anger, withdrawal).[42]

Psychiatric and Behavioral Aspects of Hypertension and Heart Failure

Hypertension (see Chap. 37)

Stress, conditioned learning, and autonomic arousal all can elevate blood pressure. Stimulation of brain sites with connections to the sympathetic nervous system have a pressor effect, and many of these sites are in turn connected with higher centers involved in the perception of the environment. However, the transient elevations of blood pressure seen in stressful and provocative situations may be unrelated to the persistent, sustained elevation that constitutes the disease of hypertension.

STRESS AND BLOOD PRESSURE. Stressful environments and challenging or aversive situations transiently increase the blood pressure both of normotensive and hypertensive individuals. This has been demonstrated in field studies using ambulatory monitoring of blood pressure during daily life and in laboratory studies assessing blood pressure reactivity to a discrete stimulus or specific experimental stressor. Some individuals exhibit greater cardiovascular reactivity than others, consistently responding to psychological stressors with greater increases in blood pressure and heart rate, more vasoconstriction and catecholamine secretion, and a more prolonged recovery phase. These individual differences in cardiovascular reactivity emerge early in life and are thought to be stable and enduring. Such hyperreactivity to stress has long been believed to predispose the individual to the eventual development of hypertension (and atherosclerosis), but the empirical evidence remains inconclusive. Several large epidemiological surveys of initially normotensive individuals have found that exaggerated blood pressure responses to psychological and physical stress predict the subsequent development of essential hypertension on long-term follow-up.[43] However, a number of questions remain about the hypothesis that an exaggerated stress response predisposes individuals to hypertension: cardiovascular reactivity may vary over time; it may vary within the same individual depending on the nature of the stress; and it is not yet clear that transient blood pressure increases in response to such stressors are the precursors of pathological, sustained hypertension.

In surveys examining the relationship between naturally occurring stress and blood pressure, stress has been associated with the onset or worsening of essential hypertension. Job strain in particular has been associated with an elevated prevalence and incidence of hypertension in men (this is less clear in women), and the blood pressures of people in more stressful occupations tend to be higher than those in less stressful jobs. However, it appears that such chronic stress requires the co-occurrence of other etiological factors (e.g., genetic endowment, dietary factors, or psychological characteristics) to cause sustained hypertension. This situation may be analogous to that emerging from animal work: Repeated exposure to stress can lead to sustained hypertension in animals that are predisposed to hypertension by genetic endowment or salt ingestion, but not in healthy animals free of such predisposing factors.

PSYCHOLOGICAL STATES. Anger and anxiety are accompanied by increases in peripheral vascular resistance and blood pressure, and anger has long been thought to contribute to the development of essential hypertension. Hostile individuals respond to provocation, conflict, and disagreement with larger increases in blood pressure than people who are less hostile,[44] and there have been reports of higher levels of anger and suppressed anger among hypertensive patients.[45] Other studies, however have failed to detect an association between anger or aggression and hypertension.[46] The relationship between anger and hypertension may be stronger in some minority groups than in non-minorities. In sum, the evidence linking anger and hypertension remains equivocal. Recent work has focused on the more-difficult-to-measure construct of repressed or *suppressed* emotion (particularly anger), and there are reports of an association between emotional inhibition and essential hypertension. Although one meta-analysis concluded that there appears to be an association between suppressed anger and resting blood pressure, overall, this literature must still be considered inconclusive.

Other work has examined the role of anxiety. There is some evidence that chronically anxious persons develop greater increases in systolic blood pressure over the ensuing years and may also be at increased risk of developing essential hypertension.[47] However, although several prospective studies confirmed this association, others have not.[16,48] Finally, the possible etiological role of depression has also been investigated. The prevalence of hypertension is reported to be higher in depressed community residents, depressed medical patients, and depressed psychiatric patients than in nondepressed comparison groups. In a recent, large, population-based study, the symptoms of depression and anxiety were significantly associated with the development of hypertension, even after adjusting for sociodemographic characteristics, smoking and alcohol use, and blood pressure at inception.[49]

Based on this work, relaxation training, meditation, and blood pressure and heart rate biofeedback have been employed to treat hypertension. Relaxation techniques and meditation apparently decrease blood pressure by lowering total vasoconstrictor tone and peripheral resistance, but it is unclear to what degree the treatment effect persists after the discontinuation of active treatment. Several expert groups and consensus panels have concluded that the benefits of such psychological treatments for hypertension have not yet been conclusively demonstrated.[50] On the other hand, several meta-analyses suggest that they are beneficial.[51] For example, a recent, small, controlled trial of individualized stress management reported statistically significant and clinically meaningful reductions of systolic and diastolic blood pressure at 6-month follow-up.[52] Some of the confusion is because the empirical findings seem to vary depending on the study design, methods, and measurements. Although these behavioral techniques may not be very effective when used alone, they may provide some incremental benefit when used to augment conventional antihypertensive therapy, perhaps enabling the physician to lower the doses of antihypertensives. This is important since nonadherence to the antihypertensive medication regimen is common and constitutes a major impediment to effective treatment. Relaxation training, meditation, and biofeedback may be most suitable for those patients who report a subjective sense of stress in their lives and for those who are attracted to the idea of psychological treatments for medical conditions.[52]

SOCIOCULTURAL FACTORS. Epidemiological and animal studies suggest a relationship between high blood pressure and sociocultural conditions. Individuals in more crowded and stressful living and working environments tend to show increased levels of catecholamines, increased cardiovascular reactivity, and higher blood pressures. Essential hypertension tends to be less prevalent in societies with stronger cultural traditions and more commonly shared value systems, and in those that are safer and more stable, than in societies with more disintegration, higher crime rates, and less stable social orders. In societies undergoing transition, conflict, or disintegration, blood pressures tend to rise over time, but many factors (e.g., changes in diet) may be contributing. Animal studies seem to corroborate these findings: Mice subjected to crowding or exposed to repeated threat from cats develop sustained high blood pressure.

Heart Failure (see Chap. 22)

The psychiatric and behavioral aspects of congestive heart failure (CHF) have only recently been subjected to study. CHF patients report high levels of psychological distress and diminished quality of life.[53] It appears that the same sorts of psychosocial factors that affect the course and outcome of CHD also influence CHF. Stress and emotional distress have been linked to the onset and exacerbation of CHF, perhaps by increasing heart rate and blood pressure and/or by provoking myocardial ischemia in patients with preexisting CHD. It has been suggested that left ventricular function is impaired during psychological stress,[54] and stress-induced heart failure has been described. In patients with idiopathic cardiomyopathy, experimental psychological stress (mental arithmetic) has been shown to induce changes in left ventricular diastolic function.

Depression has received particular attention in CHF patients because of its high prevalence in the elderly and because it appears to worsen the medical outcome. Approximately one-fourth of patients hospitalized for CHF have major depression.[55-57] Depression is an independent predictor of hospital admission and of increased medical care utilization in CHF.[56,58] It may also predict subsequent mortality.[55,56] Depression may also predispose to the development of CHF; in a prospective study of 2500 elderly community residents who were initially free of heart failure, depression at inception independently increased the risk of developing CHF in women, but not in men, over a 14-year follow-up period.[59] Research in this area is complicated by difficulty in differentiating the symptoms of CHF from those of depressive disorder. The anorexia, fatigue, weakness, and insomnia (resulting from orthopnea and paroxysmal nocturnal dyspnea) accompanying CHF can be confused with the symptoms of depression, and the cardiac cachexia of end-stage CHF may also suggest severe depression. When CHF is severe enough to cause cerebral ischemia, then cognitive dysfunction, confusion, and delirium with psychotic symptoms may result. This may at times be difficult to distinguish from anxiety disorder and panic.

Social support is an important moderator of the clinical course of CHF. Elderly women hospitalized with CHF who were without sources of emotional support had a more than threefold increase in the risk of cardiovascular events in the ensuing year than comparable patients with emotional support.[60] Elderly men without emotional support were not at increased risk. Social isolation was also found to be a significant predictor of mortality in CHF patients over a 2-year follow-up period, while controlling for depression, age, and disease severity.[60a]

Cardiac Symptoms: Chest Pain and Palpitations

Chest Pain (see Chaps. 7 and 45)

Chest pain, the classic symptom of CHD, is a nonspecific, insensitive, and unreliable indicator of ischemia. Pain does not bear a fixed, one-to-one relationship to demonstrable pathology; many patients with chest pain have no heart disease, and conversely, ischemia and infarction are often asymptomatic. Approximately one-fourth of myocardial infarctions are silent, and 70 to 80 percent of out-of-hospital, ischemic episodes in CHD patients are asymptomatic. Conversely, no cardiac cause can be found to explain most complaints of chest pain. Even in patients with documented CHD, two-thirds of chest pain episodes occur in the absence of ST segment depression indicative of ischemia, and approximately one-third of revascularized patients continue to have chest pain. Even among patients undergoing coronary angiography for chest pain, 10 to 30 percent have minimal or no angiographic evidence of CHD.

The absence of demonstrable heart disease does not mean that the patient's chest pain is either inconsequential or self-limited. Follow-up studies of chest pain patients with negative angiography and/or negative exercise stress testing reveal persistent distress and disability and a generally poor response to conventional antiischemic therapy. Although rates of myocardial infarction and of cardiac morbidity and mortality remain low, these patients continue to exhibit elevated levels of symptoms, disability, and medical care utilization. At least half continue to report recurrent chest pain, the persistent belief that they have serious heart disease, and impaired functioning (at work, socially, and in daily activities), at levels that are comparable to that of patients with CHD.

Psychological, psychiatric, and behavioral factors mediate some of this variance in symptoms among CHD patients. Thus, emotional distress is highly correlated with reports of chest pain in both those with and without CHD.[13] Mood and daily activities may account for as much of the variability in ambulatory patients' reports of chest pain as does ST depression indicative of ischemia.[61] Several psychological factors differentiate chest pain patients with and without demonstrable cardiac disease. Generalized psychological distress and body awareness is higher in patients with chest pain and normal coronary arteries than in chest pain patients with CHD. When those with normal angiography or normal stress tests are compared to those with positive tests, the former group is younger, more likely to be female, somatizes more, and has more psychological distress and a higher prevalence of diagnosable psychiatric disorder. Patients with medically unexplained chest pain, when compared to chest pain patients with abnormal angiographic findings have elevated rates of panic disorder (~35 to 50 percent vs. 5 percent) and of major depression (~35 to 40 percent vs. 5 to 8 percent). Of course, cardiac and psychiatric disorders are not mutually exclusive and therefore not infrequently co-occur. Thus, 5 to 23 percent of patients with angiographic evidence of CHD also have panic disorder. These cases of psychiatric and cardiac comorbidity pose especially difficult diagnostic dilemmas, and it is in these patients that panic disorder is most likely to be overlooked. The chest pain seen in panic disorder is more likely to be atypical in clinical character and to be accompanied by palpitations, dizziness, paresthesias, and multiple other somatic symptoms.

Palpitations (see Chap. 29)

Palpitations are among the most common symptoms encountered in medical practice, reported by 16 percent of primary care patients. Yet this subjective sensation corresponds poorly to demonstrable abnormalities of cardiac rate or rhythm. Most palpitations are not accompanied by arrhythmias, and most arrhythmias are not perceived and reported as palpitations. When patients complaining of palpitations undergo 24-hour, ambulatory ECG monitoring, 39 to 85 percent manifest a rhythm disturbance (most being benign and clinically insignificant). Approximately three-fourths of these patients with arrhythmias report at least one palpitation during 24 hours of monitoring, but in less than 15 percent of them are their symptoms coincident with the arrhythmia. Thus, accurate symptom reports occur in less than 10 percent of all patients being monitored.

A high proportion of patients with palpitations either have a psychiatric cause for their symptom or no etiology can be established. In a careful survey of 190 patients presenting with palpitations, 31 percent were judged to have a psychiatric basis for their presenting symptom and no etiology could be established in an additional 16 percent. The most common psychiatric cause of palpitations is panic disorder, found in more than one-fourth of ambulatory medical patients complaining of palpitations. In one study, 31 percent of 229 such patients had panic disorder or panic attacks, and in another study, 28 percent of patients complaining of palpitations had lifetime panic disorder and 19 percent had current panic disorder.

Palpitations that have no demonstrable cardiac basis may nonetheless be persistent and disturbing. In an observational 1-year follow-up study, 75 percent of palpitation patients reported recurrent symptoms, 19 percent reported impairment of their work performance, and 37 percent reported impairment in their role functioning at home. In another study, 84 percent of palpitation patients remained symptomatic 6 months after initially presenting and had an elevated rate of medical care utilization.

Panic attacks and arrhythmias may be difficult to distinguish clinically. Both may present as palpitations, shortness of breath, and light-headedness, and both not infrequently occur in those who are young and otherwise healthy. Frank syncope, however, is unusual in panic disorder, and if there have been multiple episodes, panic attacks are more stereotyped and more consistent from episode to episode. Recurrent panic attacks tend to lead to agoraphobia, in which the patient first becomes apprehensive about, and then avoids, being left alone, trapped in large crowds, and journeying far from home. Conversely, to make matters more difficult, the sympathetic arousal that may accompany an arrhythmia (and other acute cardiac events such as pulmonary emboli, acute valvular dysfunction, and myocardial ischemia as well) may be experienced and reported by the patient as acute anxiety or panic rather than as a cardiac event.

Delay and Denial of Cardiac Symptoms

Myocardial infarction patients commonly rationalize, ignore, or deny their symptoms, so that the average interval between the onset of symptoms and arrival in an emergency department is between 3 and 9 hours. Such delay poses a serious problem since a high proportion of myocardial infarction deaths occur soon after the event, and the newer therapies to preserve myocardial tissue require early intervention (see Chap. 47). Delay is greater in women and in the elderly[62] and (paradoxically) in those with a history of previous myocardial infarction.[63] A crucial determinant of the extent of delay is the length of time before the myocardial infarction sufferer informs another person of his or her symptoms; once the patient tells someone else, medical attention is usually obtained promptly.

Psychiatric Care of the Cardiac Patient

Acute Care of the Hospitalized Patient

ANXIETY. The onset or sudden progression of cardiac disease is terrifying. Pain and physical discomfort, the specter of sudden death or prolonged invalidism, and the knowledge that one has a chronic and potentially lethal disease all are profoundly distressing. The initial reaction is almost always one of anxiety. Fears of premature and sudden death loom, and worries about physical, sexual, social, and occupational incapacity materialize and plague patients. They may become terrified of any physical activity or strong emotion, fearing that these will trigger sudden death. As time passes, anxiety may be replaced with despondency and a heightened sense of physical vulnerability and of one's mortality. The individual may come to feel useless, damaged, or diminished. Patients may believe that their job performance and future livelihood have been irrevocably compromised, that they have become worn out and decrepit, and that they face a meager and empty future. They may feel guilty and blame themselves for falling ill, ascribing their plight to their failure to exercise enough, diet sufficiently, or maintain other "healthy" habits. All of this may presage a clinically significant, depressive episode.

Several psychiatric and behavioral problems commonly arise in patients while they are hospitalized for an acute cardiac event. The hospitalization itself (in particular, admission to the coronary care or intensive care unit) can be frightening and stressful. Patients suddenly find themselves in an unfamiliar, alien and frightening world, surrounded by fearsome machines with blinking lights and beeping alarms, subjected to painful procedures and tests about which they know little and understand less, while their lives seemingly hang in the balance from moment to moment. They are cut off from family, friends, neighbors, and all that is familiar. Sustained sleep is next to impossible, and many are afraid to fall asleep believing that the heart is in greater jeopardy during sleep. Their worst fears are substantiated if they witness the death or cardiac arrest of another patient.

Hospitalized patients should be kept well informed about what is transpiring, what is being done medically for them, and why. They should be told what to expect before procedures are carried out; the functions of equipment should be explained; and the effects and (especially) side effects of medications should be described in advance. The patient should be reassured that anxiety is a normal and entirely appropriate reaction. Early and frequent family visitation generally helps the patient to feel supported. Anxiolytics are often prescribed because anxiety is not only uncomfortable but its concomitant sympathetic arousal can be medically dangerous. Benzodiazepines are most commonly used for this purpose and should be prescribed on a regular, round-the-clock (rather than as-needed) basis. In the elderly and in those with compromised liver function, the shorter-acting benzodiazepines (e.g., oxazepam or lorazepam) are preferred, because they are cleared primarily by the kidney. The pharmacology of anxiolytics is discussed in the following section.

DELIRIUM AND COGNITIVE IMPAIRMENT. Delirium is frequent in hospitalized cardiac patients, especially following cardiac surgery. The delirious patient is confused, disoriented to time and place, has impaired memory and attention, has delusional ideas, and experiences perceptual disturbances such as illusions or hallucinations. The sleep-wake cycle is disrupted, and the level of consciousness and arousal is disturbed, so that the patient may be either stuporous and obtunded, or hyperalert and agitated. The onset of delirium may be insidious (e.g., insomnia, mild nocturnal confusion, and restlessness) and go unnoticed by the staff, or it may be dramatic and abrupt. The patient begins to misinterpret sensory information (e.g., mistaking a shadow for someone lurking in a corner of his or her room) and becomes suspicious and increasingly frightened. As confusion, fear, and excitement mount, frank paranoia sets in and the patient may become agitated, disruptive, belligerent, and out of control. This is a psychiatric emergency, because in their confusion and frenzy, delirious patients may harm themselves accidentally, fall, or pull out therapeutic life-lines, catheters, and implanted devices. The incidence of delirium after cardiac surgery is between 10 and 30 percent,[64] typically following a lucid interval of 3 to 5 days following surgery. The risk factors for postcardiotomy delirium are advanced age (>70 years of age); more extensive aortic atherosclerosis (large atheromas may be liberated by surgical manipulation of the aorta); a prior history of neurological disease, particularly preexisting cerebrovascular disease; a history of pulmonary disease, with the concomitant risks of poorer cerebral oxygenation and more hypoxia; and higher doses of narcotics and sedatives.[65]

Treatment of Delirium. This rests on rapid identification and correction of its underlying cause, medication for behavioral control if necessary, and supportive measures to provide comfort and safety. The etiological search is paramount. This means checking for cerebral hypoperfusion or hypoxia, acid-base disturbance, inadequate hydration, fluid and electrolyte imbalance, renal or hepatic failure, endocrine dysfunction, infection, and nutritional deficiency. Alcohol or drug withdrawal is a frequent cause, and the history must be searched carefully with this possibility in mind. Medications must be carefully reviewed because anticholinergics, narcotics, sedative-hypnotics, and H_2 blockers are common causes of delirium. Common offenders include cimetidine, digoxin, aminophylline, anticonvulsants, and all sedatives and hypnotics.

If the patient is agitated, disruptive, or confused enough to require behavioral control, high-potency antipsychotic drugs can be administered. Haloperidol has been widely used for this purpose and is safe and effective in critically ill patients, whether given orally or parenterally (including intravenously in emergency situations). Mild, delirious agitation is treated with 0.5 to 2 mg of haloperidol, moderate delirium with 5 to 10 mg; and the severely delirious patient can be given 10 or more mg of haloperidol. If the agitation persists unabated after 20 to 30 minutes, twice the original dose may be readministered. It has a minimal effect on heart rate, blood pressure, and respiration, and extrapyramidal effects are rare when it is administered intravenously. Parenteral droperidol is sometimes used. If excitement, hyperarousal, and motor agitation are especially prominent, the antipsychotic may be supplemented with a short-acting benzodiazepine such as lorazepam. The newer, "atypical" antipsychotics are increasingly used to treat delirium.[66] They appear to be safe and effective but have not yet been studied definitively. Antipsychotic agents are discussed in the following section.

Supportive measures should be undertaken to calm, orient, and comfort the delirious patient. He or she should be reoriented frequently by the staff, and a clock and calendar should be prominently displayed to aid in this process. It is helpful to preserve as much of a normal day-night cycle as is feasible considering the hospital routine. Family visitation should be encouraged because it is helpful in reassuring and calming the patient and in reducing paranoia. Familiar objects, such as family photographs, should be prominently displayed and plainly visible. Staff need to continually reintroduce themselves, educate the patient about what they are doing, and repeatedly explain the situation. Physical restraint should be employed whenever necessary to prevent self-harm or harm to the staff.

Longer-term cognitive changes also occur following cardiac surgery. These often involve memory, arithmetic skills, and the sequencing of complex actions. Neurocognitive testing of patients following CABG disclosed cognitive decline in 53 percent at discharge, 36 percent at 6 weeks, and in 24 percent of patients 6 months after discharge.[67] This study lacked a noncardiac surgery comparison group, however.

Convalescence and Recovery after Hospitalization

In the weeks and months after hospital discharge, depression is common. It is often self-limited, gradually diminishing as the patient resumes his or her old activities and as the specter of the acute episode and the hospitalization recede into the past. Frank discussion of the patient's concerns and specific information about common myths and fears are helpful. Lingering anxiety may lead patients to avoid activities or situations that they fear will provoke symptoms or even sudden death. Early, progressive mobilization is the best antidote. The patient may be dismayed by the degree of exhaustion resulting from even mild exertion, and although this easy fatigability is actually the result of deconditioning, it is mistakenly interpreted as evidence of permanent cardiac damage. As a result, exercise may be assiduously avoided, further exacerbating the problem.

Patients are often apprehensive about returning to work because of the stress it engenders. Many believe that strong emotions can be lethal and try to protect themselves by assiduously avoiding all situations or activities that arouse strong feelings, such as sexual activity or watching sports on television. Sexual activity in particular is diminished, and sexual dysfunction is common in both women and men with cardiac disease. Such concerns should be elicited by the physician and then discussed frankly and openly. Recommendations about proscribed and prescribed activities should be as specific as possible; simply saying "use your judgment" or "do it in moderation" is not helpful. Group meetings in which cardiac patients share common concerns, provide mutual support, obtain educational information, and guide the progressive resumption of activities are helpful.

TREATMENT. If depression lasts more than several weeks and meets diagnostic criteria for major depressive disorder, as happens in one-third or more of patients in the year after myocardial infarction,[9] pharmacotherapy is indicated. If left untreated, depression imposes a serious psychosocial burden, medical rehabilitation and recovery are impeded, and the depression itself is likely to become chronic. Because of this, and its negative effect on cardiac outcomes, increasing emphasis is being placed on the prompt detection and treatment of post-myocardial infarction depression. The Sertraline Antidepressant Heart Attack Randomized Trial (SADHART) was a double-blind, randomized, placebo-controlled trial of a selective serotonin reuptake inhibitor (SSRI) for major depressive disorder in patients hospitalized for myocardial infarction or unstable angina. At 6-month follow-up, when compared with placebo, the more severely depressed patients who received active drug were less depressed, although the less severely depressed patients did not show a treatment effect. There was a 20 percent reduction in life-threatening cardiac events (including nonfatal myocardial infarction and death) among those on active drug, but this difference in cardiac outcomes was not statistically significant due to the number of patients in the trial. In a case-controlled study of smokers hospitalized for myocardial infarction, SSRI administration was associated with a lowered risk of recurrent myocardial infarction, suggesting that treatment of depression may reduce its negative prognostic influence on cardiac outcomes.[68] Thus it remains to be definitively demonstrated that the treatment of depression following myocardial infarction significantly improves cardiac outcomes. The pharmacotherapy of depression is discussed in the following section.

Interest in psychosocial interventions for depression and/or social isolation has also been high. In one study of 435 post-myocardial infarction patients, a nursing-based psychosocial intervention reduced 1-year cardiac mortality, and the incidence of recurrent myocardial infarction was significantly lower at 7-year follow-up. However, two subsequent, large, randomized trials of multimodal interventions delivered by nurses or health visitors failed to improve depression or cardiac outcomes.[69] In the Montreal Heart Attack Readjustment Trial (M-HART), a supportive and educational home nursing intervention was provided to the most psychologically distressed post-myocardial infarction patients. This rather limited intervention was compared to usual care. At 1-year follow-up, the intervention had no effect on psychological distress and no overall effect on cardiac mortality, while it was actually associated with a *higher* mortality rate among women.[70] However, a subgroup analysis revealed that those patients whose psychological distress did improve with treatment did have more favorable long-term cardiac outcomes.[71] In the Enhancing Recovery in Coronary Heart Disease (ENRICHD), 2500 recent myocardial infarction patients with depression and/or low social support randomly received either cognitive behavior therapy (and SSRI antidepressants if indicated) or care as usual. Preliminary results suggest that there was no benefit in terms of cardiac outcomes or mortality, and outcomes appear worse for women. At the least, one can safely conclude from these studies that when the psychosocial treatment fails to improve depression (because the patient population is not sufficiently depressed or the treatment is not effective enough), then it does not improve cardiac outcomes. There is also a suggestion that women may benefit less from these psychosocial interventions in terms of cardiac outcomes than men.

Over the long term, some cardiac patients adopt a persistent coping style that is maladaptive and dysfunctional. They may ignore and deny their illness entirely, maintaining that nothing serious has happened at all. They may refuse to acknowledge any limitations or adhere to a therapeutic regimen and generally overdo things. Alternatively, they may capitulate completely to their illness and retreat into unwarranted invalidism, becoming "cardiac cripples" who are preoccupied with their health, terrified by every benign twinge or cramp, and living a life of psychological invalidism and disability. Each of these profoundly maladaptive coping patterns deserves psychotherapeutic attention.

Cardiac Rehabilitation Programs (see Chap. 43)

Cardiac rehabilitation programs seek to modify biobehavioral risk factors and retard the progression of the disease. These psychosocial, educational, and behavioral programs include various components. Almost all emphasize a formal program of graduated, progressive, aerobic exercise. Most assist patients in smoking cessation, curtailing alcohol abuse, lowering saturated fat intake, and controlling weight.

Most cardiac rehabilitation programs also include psychosocial interventions.[72] These involve the identification of psychosocial stressors and problems (depression, anxiety, anger, social isolation), individual or group counseling to deal with them, and instruction in stress reduction and stress management. The latter often entails relaxation training, which generally combines elements of progressive muscle relaxation, diaphragmatic breathing, and the use of calming mental imagery.

It is difficult to evaluate the effectiveness of these heterogeneous psychotherapeutic, psychosocial, and behavioral programs because they vary so widely in quality, content, design, and intensity. Many intervention trials are flawed by small sample size, high dropout rates, lack of randomization, insufficient long-term follow-up, and inadequate comparison or control groups. In addition, as standard cardiac care improves so substantially, it becomes more difficult to demonstrate the incremental benefit of these programs in terms of hard cardiac endpoints. Nonetheless, there are now a substantial number of intervention trials and several careful meta-analyses assessing the incremental benefit of adding a specific psychosocial component to cardiac rehabilitation programs. These studies generally indicate that, when compared to rehabilitation programs without such components, these programs further reduce psychological distress and anxiety and depressive symptoms, and improve coping skills and quality of life.[72] The empirical evidence also suggests that they lead to significantly lower rates of cardiac death and nonfatal, recurrent myocardial infarction.[73,74] When these psychological interventions have been found ineffective against cardiac endpoints, they have at the same time failed to lower psychosocial distress, depression, and anxiety.[74] The cardiac benefits of psychosocial treatment generally seem less clear for women and perhaps for older patients as well.

Psychopharmacology in the Cardiac Patient

Cardiovascular Aspects of Psychotropic Agents

ANTIDEPRESSANTS (Table 84–1)

Selective Serotonin Reuptake Inhibitors. The SSRIs have superseded the tricyclic antidepressants (TCAs) as the first-line agents for treating the cardiac patient with major depressive disorder. Their efficacy is comparable to that of the older TCAs; they are better tolerated, safer in overdose, and have less pharmacological action on the heart. The data thus far suggest that the SSRIs have minimal cardiovascular effects and a large margin of safety in treating patients with even very severe heart disease.[75] The SSRIs have little anticholinergic, antihistaminic, or noradrenergic activity and appear to inhibit platelet aggregation.

In healthy patients, the SSRIs have no adverse effects on cardiac contractility or conduction and there is no evidence of cardiotoxicity in overdose. In cardiac populations, they do not appear to cause significant ECG or blood pressure changes, although they can slow heart rate. Only rarely do they produce a clinically significant degree of sinus bradycardia. Because the SSRIs interfere with platelet aggregation, they can increase bleeding time. The SSRIs do have the potential to interact with a number of medications used in cardiac patients. They inhibit hepatic cytochrome P450 isoenzymes,[76] a series of isoenzymes involved in the oxidative metabolism of many drugs. These include lipophilic beta blockers (e.g., metoprolol and propranolol), calcium-channel blockers, type IC antiarrhythmics, angiotensin-converting enzyme (ACE) inhibitors, anticonvulsants, antihistamines, benzodiazepines, TCAs, codeine, and warfarin. The SSRIs therefore can raise the blood levels of these other agents when coadministered. Caution should be exercised when giving SSRIs to patients on these medications, and in particular the prothrombin time of patients receiving both warfarin and an SSRI should be monitored closely. Because the SSRIs are highly protein bound, they may displace other protein-bound drugs when coadministered, thereby increasing their bioavailability. This interaction can occur with warfarin and digitoxin, but it does not appear to be clinically significant in magnitude.

Tricyclic Antidepressants. TCAs were previously the mainstay of antidepressant pharmacotherapy and remain effective agents that are still widely employed. However, their multiple cardiovascular side effects and their potential lethality in overdose are disadvantages in patients with cardiac disease. TCAs act on adrenergic and serotoninergic neurons in the central nervous system and, in the periphery, have anticholinergic properties. They also have quinidine-like effects and produce alpha-adrenergic receptor blockade. They affect heart rate, rhythm, conduction, contractility, and blood pressure. Accordingly, these agents are not generally used in the presence of rhythm or conduction disturbances, severe CHF, or within 4 to 6 weeks of a myocardial infarction. Among the TCAs, the tertiary amines (e.g., imipramine and amitriptyline) are associated with more side effects, and the secondary amines (e.g., nortriptyline) have a preferable side effect profile in cardiac patients.[77]

The TCAs are type IA antiarrhythmic agents (see Chap. 30) and accordingly depress cardiac conduction, decrease ventricular irritability, and suppress ectopic activity. They slow atrial and ventricular depolarization; increase the QT, PR, and QRS intervals; and decrease T wave amplitude. In the absence of preexisting conduction abnormalities, this action is unlikely to be clinically significant at therapeutic doses. However, second-degree heart block, sick sinus syndrome, bundle branch block, a prolonged QT interval, and the concurrent administration of antiarrhythmic agents all are considered contraindications to their use. In contrast to this antiarrhythmic effect, the TCAs can on occasion be arrhythmogenic, probably by virtue of their prolongation of the QT interval and/or an increase in myocardial norepinephrine resulting from their peripheral inhibition of norepinephrine reuptake. Although the most common such arrhythmias are atrial and ventricular premature beats, these may give way to more malignant ventricular arrhythmias. These toxic, proarrhythmic effects are seen primarily in overdose, and are more likely in those with preexisting CHD, a prolonged QT interval, electrical instability, or a recent myocardial infarction. The TCAs also elevate heart rate 5 to 20 beats/min as a result of their anticholinergic blockade. Although this does not pose a problem in relatively healthy patients, it may be a consideration in those with heart disease.

TCAs produce postural hypotension in up to 20 percent of patients. In the elderly, in whom orthostatic hypotension can produce cerebral hypoperfusion and lead to falls and fractures, this side effect can be crucial. Blood pressure and pulse should be monitored for signs of orthostasis in patients treated with TCAs, especially when initiating treatment and when adjusting the dose. Elderly patients should be advised to stand up slowly after lying or sitting for prolonged periods. The magnitude of this effect is related to the magnitude of pretreatment orthostatic hypotension, and it is more likely to be clinically significant in patients with CHF, impaired left ventricular function, or volume depletion or who are taking antihypertensive medications. Caution is indicated when treating patients with poor ejection fractions because in animal studies TCAs exert a depressant effect on myocardial contractility, although in humans this effect is evident only at toxic doses and only rarely aggravates CHF.

Other Antidepressants. *Bupropion*, a non-TCA that acts on both the dopamine and norepinephrine systems, causes less hypotension than the TCAs; does not affect cardiac conduction or contractility; and is safely used in patients with cardiac disease. It does not exacerbate ventricular arrhythmias or conduction block in patients with these conditions. An additional benefit of bupropion in cardiac patients is that it is apparently effective in smoking cessation. An increased incidence of seizures is seen at higher doses, and bupropion may occasionally elevate blood pressure and heart rate, though rarely to a clinically significant degree. Because it inhibits the cytochrome P450 isoenzymes, bupropion can raise the levels of beta blockers and type 1C antiarrhythmics when administered concurrently.

Venlafaxine affects the reuptake of both serotonin and norepinephrine. It appears to have few cardiovascular actions and no effect on the ECG.[78] At higher doses venlafaxine has been associated with an elevation in blood pressure and pulse. Unlike the SSRIs, it does not inhibit cytochrome P450

TABLE 84–1 Antidepressants

Agent	Starting Dose	Maximum Dose	Side Effects	Cardiovascular Effects
Serotonin Reuptake Inhibitors				
Sertraline	12.5-25 mg/d	200 mg/d	Sexual dysfunction Nausea, diarrhea,headache, anxiety, agitation, insomnia, somnolence, sedation, tremor	Benign bradycardia
Fluoxetine	5-10 mg/d	80 mg/d		
Paroxetine	10 mg/d	50 mg/d		
Tricyclics			Dry mouth Blurry vision Constipation Urinary retention Postural hypotension Weight gain	Increased QT, PR, QRS intervals Decreased T wave amplitude Tachycardia Arrhythmias Postural hypotension
Amitriptyline	10-25 mg h.s.	300 mg/d	Sedation, somnolence	
Imipramine	10-25 mg h.s.	300 mg/d		
Nortriptyline	10 mg/d	150 mg/d	Anxiety, insomnia	
Desipramine	25 mg/d	300 mg/d		
Psychostimulants				
Methylphenidate	2.5 mg b.i.d.	20 mg b.i.d.	Anxiety, agitation Insomnia Anorexia Paranoia	Tachycardia (mild) Hypertension (mild)
Other Agents				
Bupropion	75 mg/d	150 mg t.i.d.	Anorexia, nausea Anxiety, agitation Insomnia Seizures	
Venlafaxine	25 mg b.i.d.	125 mg t.i.d.	Nausea Headache Sexual dysfunction Anxiety, insomnia Somnolence Dizziness	Hypertension (dose related) Tachycardia (dose related)
Trazodone	25 mg/d	300 mg b.i.d.	Sedation Nausea Headache Priapism (rare)	Postural hypotension
Mirtazapine	15 mg q.h.s.	45 mg q.h.s.	Sedation, somnolence Weight gain Dry mouth, anticholinergic effects Dizziness Agranulocytosis (rare)	Tachycardia (mild)

isoenzymes and is not highly protein bound; it may therefore be useful in patients on cardiac medications.

Trazodone, a triazolopyridine antidepressant, is often used in low doses as a hypnotic. Cardiovascular complications from trazodone are rare. It has few, if any, antiarrhythmic properties, although it has rarely been associated with heart block and ventricular arrhythmias. Because of its weak alpha-adrenergic blockade, it may also produce orthostatic hypotension. Nefazodone, a closely related drug, can also occasionally produce orthostatic hypotension and has significant P450 isoenzyme inhibition, and it can therefore increase the levels of concurrently administered calcium-channel blockers, quinidine, and lidocaine.

Mirtazapine is a tetracyclic antidepressant with a complex mechanism of action. It has not been studied in patients with cardiovascular disease, but in noncardiac populations it does not affect blood pressure or cardiac conduction. It has no anticholinergic activity, but it may increase heart rate slightly.[78a]

Psychostimulants such as dextroamphetamine and methylphenidate are used to treat depression in medically compromised and elderly patients. These agents tend to be used when depression is life threatening, when immediate treatment response is crucial (because they have a rapid onset of action), and in depressions with prominent anergia and apathy. Although there is considerable clinical support for their use, empirical evidence of their sustained efficacy over time is lacking. Serious cardiovascular side effects such as tachycardia, hypertension, and arrhythmias are relatively rare, but caution must be exercised when administering these medications to patients with significant hypertension, tachycardia, or ventricular ectopy, and blood pressure and heart rate should be monitored.

NEUROLEPTICS (Table 84–2). Neuroleptic or antipsychotic drugs are used in the treatment of schizophrenia, organic psychoses, and mood disorders that are refractory or have psychotic features. They are also widely used for agitation, confusion, excitement, and behavioral dyscontrol in geriatric patients. Neuroleptic drugs generally affect cardiac conduction and rhythm and produce hypotension. They have alpha-adrenergic blocking and quinidine-like properties, along with anticholinergic activity. They can produce prolongation of the PR and QT intervals, ST segment depression, T wave changes, ventricular arrhythmias, and heart block. Increasing attention has been devoted to their potential to increase the QT interval, leading in rare instances to torsades de pointes. *Thioridazine* is most frequently implicated in this

TABLE 84–2 Neuroleptic (Antipsychotic) Agents

Agent	Starting Dose	Maximum Dose	Side Effects	Cardiovascular Effects
Haloperidol	0.5 mg/d	>10 mg q.i.d.	Akathisia Dystonia Parkinsonism Tardive dyskinesia Neuroleptic malignant syndrome Rash Anticholinergic effects	Tachycardia QT interval prolongation Torsades de pointes
Clozapine	12.5 mg q.h.s. or b.i.d.	200-300 mg t.i.d.	Dizziness Somnolence Weight gain Hypersalivation Seizures Agranulocytosis Anticholinergic effects	Tachycardia Postural hypotension
Olanzapine	2.5-5 mg/d	20 mg/d	Sedation Constipation Weight gain Seizures Akathisia Extrapyramidal symptoms	Postural hypotension (mild) QT interval prolongation
Risperidone	0.25-0.5 mg/d	>6 mg/d	Somnolence Fatigue Nausea, diarrhea Weight gain Sexual dysfunction Nasal congestion Extrapyramidal symptoms	Hypotension QT interval prolongation Tachycardia

respect.[79] Although the quinidine-like effects of the neuroleptics are usually negligible, they can become significant in patients already taking type I antiarrhythmics or in those with hypokalemia or with clinically significant conduction delays. When administering a low-potency neuroleptic along with an antiarrhythmic, the ECG should be monitored for conduction delays. The lower potency neuroleptics produce more orthostatic hypotension (by means of alpha-adrenergic blockade) and tachycardia (by means of anticholinergic action), and this is of particular concern in the elderly and in the acute myocardial infarction patient.[80] Orthostasis is more likely to be a problem when these agents are combined with antihypertensives.

The higher potency neuroleptic agents, such as *haloperidol* and the piperazine phenothiazines, produce less of these effects and are therefore preferred in the presence of significant cardiac disease (especially conduction problems) and after cardiac surgery. Haloperidol in particular has been frequently used with safety and efficacy in severely ill cardiac patients. Oral haloperidol does not significantly affect the ECG, and intravenous haloperidol is used in acute emergencies such as agitated deliria. Administration can on rare occasions result in torsades de pointes and even SCD, and the QT interval should therefore be monitored during aggressive intravenous haloperidol therapy.

Experience with the newer "atypical" antipsychotics in cardiac patients is much more limited but suggests a generally similar profile. *Clozapine* can cause tachycardia and orthostatic hypotension and has significant anticholinergic activity (along with a risk of myelosuppression and agranulocytosis). There are reports of an infrequent association of clozapine with myocarditis and cardiomyopathy.[81] This risk is greatest in the first month of therapy.[82] *Olanzapine* produces mild orthostatic hypotension but has little effect on the ECG. *Risperidone* produces hypotension and has a quinidine-like effect, prolonging the QT interval, although this may not be of clinical significance. *Ziprasidone* has been associated with QT prolongation and is not recommended in patients with recent myocardial infarction, heart failure, QT prolongation, or arrhythmias. Thus it is clear that the new atypical neuroleptics, like the phenothiazines and haloperidol, can prolong QT interval.[79] However, the relationship to torsades de pointes and SCD is less clear since the tendency to prolong the QT interval is not closely associated with the tendency to cause torsades de pointes.[79] Recently, concern with atypical antipsychotics has focused on the incidence of new-onset diabetes and increased glucose levels in patients with preexisting diabetes, on hyperlipidemia, and on the weight gain seen in patients on these agents.

MOOD STABILIZERS (Table 84–3)

Lithium. Lithium exerts minimal cardiotoxicity at therapeutic doses in most patients and can be used safely in cardiac disease if initiated at a low dose, increased gradually, and monitored carefully. Clinically significant, cardiovascular side effects of lithium are rare; they may include sinus node dysfunction and increases in ventricular irritability. Benign, reversible T wave changes (including inversion and flattening) are common with lithium administration and are not clinically significant. The major toxic effects of lithium are neural (confusion, sedation), and the primary concern in cardiac patients is lithium toxicity resulting from decreased renal clearance or hypovolemia. This is of concern in patients with CHF, and it is exacerbated by their diuretics and restricted sodium intake. Sodium depletion decreases renal clearance of lithium. In the kidney, lithium is filtered out at the glomerulus and then reabsorbed in the proximal tubules. Sodium depletion, such as with diuretics, causes an increased proximal reabsorption of sodium, and lithium is reabsorbed more efficiently at the same time. A given lithium dose thus results in a higher blood level. Lithium may still be administered to the patient on diuretics, but levels must be monitored and dosage may need to be reduced. The elderly also require lower lithium doses because of a decline in the glomerular filtration rate. On rare occasion, lithium may worsen arrhythmias in patients with sinus node dysfunction.

TABLE 84–3 Mood Stabilizers

Agent	Staring Dose	Maximum Dose	Side Effects	Cardiovascular Effects
Lithium	300 mg b.i.d.	2100 mg/d (titrate against serum concentration)	Drowsiness, sedation Confusion Nausea, diarrhea Metallic taste Polyuria/polydipsia Tremor Hypothyroidism	T wave inversion or flattening Sinus node dysfunction Ventricular irritability
Carbamazepine	100 mg b.i.d.	1600 mg/d	Dizziness Drowsiness, sedation Ataxia Diplopia, blurred vision Rash Nausea Leukopenia Hyponatremia	Depressed cardiac conduction
Valproate	250 mg b.i.d.	3500 mg/d-4500 mg/d	Nausea, vomiting, anorexia Sedation Confusion Weight gain Tremor	

TABLE 84–4 Benzodiazepines

Agent	Starting Dose	Maximum Dose	Side Effects
Short-Acting Benzodiazepines			
Oxazepam	10 mg b.i.d.	120 mg/d	Sedation, drowsiness Slowed psychomotor function Exacerbation of underlying cognitive impairment Ataxia/falls in elderly Respiratory depression Tolerance/addiction Amnesia
Lorazepam	0.5 mg b.i.d.	10 mg/d	
Long-Acting Benzodiazepines			
Diazepam	2-5 mg q.d.	60 mg/d	
Chlordiazepoxide	5 mg q.d.	100 mg/d	
Clonazepam	0.25 mg/d	6 mg/d	
Alprazolam	0.25 mg b.i.d.	8 mg/d	

Anticonvulsants. These drugs are increasingly prescribed to stabilize the mood of patients with bipolar disorder (manic-depressive illness). Their use in cardiac patients has not yet been systematically studied. It is known that carbamazepine has quinidine-like effects and can aggravate heart block,[83] and it may also exacerbate CHF. *Carbamazepine* can also produce hyponatremia, and this effect is potentiated by other causes of hyponatremia, such as diuretics and CHF. *Valproate*, although not yet studied widely in cardiac populations, does not appear to have adverse cardiac effects. It can, however, lower the platelet count, decrease fibrinogen levels, and increase the prothrombin time. *Lamotrigine* is increasingly used in refractory depression and appears to have no significant cardiac effects nor impact on the cytochrome P450 system. *Topiramate* may have a role in the treatment of mania and anxiety. It is renally excreted, and care must be taken to ensure adequate hydration.

Benzodiazepines (Table 84–4). Benzodiazepines have anxiolytic, sedative, anticonvulsant, and muscle relaxant properties. Anxiety disorders, especially panic disorder and generalized anxiety disorder, are prevalent in patients with cardiac disease. Panic disorder is treated either with a benzodiazepine with antipanic efficacy (such as clonazepam, lorazepam, or alprazolam) or an antidepressant. Generalized anxiety disorder can also be treated with benzodiazepines, buspirone, or SSRIs. Hospitalized cardiac patients are acutely anxious and benzodiazepines are widely used in coronary care units. They can decrease respiratory drive in patients with chronic obstructive pulmonary disease and chronic hypercapnia but are free of cardiac side effects and are safe in seriously ill cardiac patients, even in the period immediately after myocardial infarction.

Benzodiazepines with longer half-lives and/or active metabolites (e.g., diazepam, flurazepam, clonazepam, chlordiazepoxide) accumulate in the body with repeated administration. A steady state is reached slowly, and clearance of the drug after discontinuation is prolonged. Thus the benzodiazepines with shorter half-lives and fewer active metabolites (lorazepam, oxazepam) are generally preferable, particularly in the elderly. Intramuscular absorption of these agents, other than lorazepam and midazolam, is erratic and unpredictable. The most prominent side effects are sedation, fatigue, memory complaints, and psychomotor impairment. In hospitalized patients and in the elderly, these effects can result in frank oversedation or delirium. Patients with preexisting cognitive impairment or organic brain syndromes often react to benzodiazepines with further confusion, increased memory loss, behavioral disinhibition, and belligerence. Ambulatory patients should be cautioned about driving and participating in activities requiring a high degree of alertness.

Psychiatric Side Effects of Cardiovascular Drugs

ANTIHYPERTENSIVES. Many antihypertensive agents have central nervous system side effects. Depression is not uncommon with methyldopa, clonidine, reserpine, and guanethidine. Therefore, calcium-channel blockers and ACE inhibitors may be preferable in the hypertensive patient with a history of depression. Abrupt discontinuation of antihypertensive agents can cause anxiety, agitation, and vivid dreams. *Methyldopa* is a relatively common cause of insomnia.

BETA-ADRENERGIC RECEPTOR ANTAGONISTS. There is a longstanding clinical impression that beta blockers can cause depression. Although there are reports that patients maintained on these agents have an elevated rate of concurrent antidepressant pharmacotherapy, other studies have failed to find an association between beta-blocker use and depression. Some of the confusion may stem from the fact that these agents cause sedation, lethargy, fatigue, and impotence, side effects that may be confused with depression. Depression may be more likely in those with a past history of depressive disorder, with the more lipophilic agents (e.g., propranolol, metoprolol), and when using higher doses. Beta blockers also occasionally cause vivid dreams and nightmares, hallucinations, and other psychotic symptoms, particularly in the elderly.

CALCIUM-CHANNEL BLOCKERS. In general, calcium-channel blockers do not have prominent psychiatric side effects. There are isolated case reports of depression associated with their administration, but this has not been demonstrated conclusively. Care should be taken when these agents are coadministered with the psychotropic drugs that inhibit the cytochrome P450 system, such as nefazodone and high doses of fluoxetine and paroxetine.

ANGIOTENSIN-CONVERTING ENZYME INHIBITORS. These inhibitors appear to have relatively few central nervous system side effects, although they may, on rare occasion, induce depression.

ANTIARRHYTHMICS. *Lidocaine* is a relatively common cause of anxiety, confusion, disorientation, hallucinations, and central nervous system excitement. Confusion, hallucinations, and delirium have also been reported with high doses of quinidine. Procainamide may cause depression, hallucinations, and other psychotic symptoms.

DIGITALIS. Anxiety, depression, visual illusions (e.g., yellow halos), and confusion may be the first signs of digitalis toxicity, but psychiatric symptoms may emerge at therapeutic levels as well.

DIURETICS. Diuretics can induce cognitive mental status changes by causing electrolyte imbalance (e.g., hyponatremia) or hypovolemia, and a secondary mood disorder may also occur, often characterized by anorexia, lethargy, and weakness.

Interactions of Psychotropic and Cardiac Drugs (Table 84–5)

Because many cardiac and psychotropic agents lower blood pressure, additive hypotensive effects are not uncommon, as for example between the TCAs and antihypertensives. Many psychotropic agents slow conduction and prolong the PR, QRS, and QT intervals, and synergistic effects can occur when they are used in conjunction with antiarrhythmic medications, resulting in heart block or the long-QT syndrome. Extreme caution is required if atypical neuroleptics are administered concomitantly with other drugs that increase

TABLE 84–5 Interactions of Psychotropic and Cardiac Drugs

Medication	Effect on Cardiac Agent
Interactions Involving Tricyclic Antidepressants	
Type IA antiarrhythmics	Potentiate delay in cardiac conduction; heart block
Antihypertensives: guanethidine, clonidine, reserpine	Antagonize antihypertensive effect; potentiate orthostatic hypotension
Sublingual nitrates	Oral absorption hindered by dry mouth
Alpha-adrenergic blocking agents	Potentiate antihypertensive effect
Interactions Involving Serotoninergic Antidepressants	
Lipophilic beta blockers	Increase blood levels due to decreased hepatic degradation
Calcium channel blockers	Increase blood levels due to decreased hepatic degradation
Type IC antiarrhythmics	Increase blood levels due to decreased hepatic degradation
Angiotensin-converting enzyme inhibitors	Increase blood levels due to decreased hepatic degradation
Warfarin	Increase blood levels due to decreased hepatic degradation
Digitoxin	Increase bioavailability due to displacement from protein-binding sites
Warfarin	Increase bioavailability due to displacement from protein-binding sites
Medication	**Effect on Psychotropic Agent**
Interactions Involving Lithium	
Diuretics that cause sodium loss	Increase blood lithium levels
Calcium channel blockers	Enhance lithium toxicity; bradycardia
Angiotensin-converting enzyme inhibitors	Enhance lithium toxicity
Methyldopa	Enhance lithium toxicity
Medication	**Effect on Psychotropic or Cardiac Agent**
Interactions Involving Carbamazepine	
Calcium channel blockers	Enhance carbamazepine toxicity
Antiarrhythmics	Potentiate delay in cardiac conduction

the QT interval such as *ketoconazole, quinidine,* and *cisapride*. There are several interactions between the TCAs and cardiac medications: The TCAs interfere with neuronal reuptake of clonidine and guanethidine and thus antagonize their antihypertensive action. They may potentiate the antihypertensive action of prazosin, and the dry mouth induced by TCAs may hinder the absorption of sublingual nitrates.

SSRIs are bound to plasma proteins and can displace other protein-bound drugs, thereby increasing the level of active drug and resulting in possible toxicity. This is particularly salient with *warfarin* and *digitoxin*, although the clinical significance of these interactions is not yet clear. As noted earlier, diuretics may raise *lithium* levels into the toxic range. This can generally be dealt with by reducing the lithium dose, although during acute diuresis the proper adjustment of lithium is difficult because of the massive shifts in sodium and fluid balance.

There are reports of idiosyncratic toxic reactions and of bradycardia when lithium is coadministered with the calcium-channel blockers *verapamil* and *diltiazem* and of lithium toxicity precipitated by the use of ACE inhibitors. *Methyldopa* seems to have a number of interactions with psychotropic agents, including possible toxicity when combined with lithium. The metabolic degradation of *carbamazepine* may be inhibited by calcium-channel blockers, thereby increasing the risk of carbamazepine toxicity. Carbamazepine and antiarrhythmics may have additive effects in slowing cardiac conduction.

REFERENCES

Psychiatric and Behavioral Aspects of Coronary Heart Disease

1. Kawachi I, Kubzansky LD, Spiro A, et al: Prospective study of a self-report type A scale and risk of coronary heart disease: Test of the MMPI-2 type A scale. Circulation 98:405-412, 1998.
2. Gallacher JE, Yarnell JW, Sweetnam PM, et al: Anger and incident heart disease in the Caerphilly study. Psychosom Med 61:446-454, 1999.
3. Iribarren C, Sidney S, Bild DE, et al: Association of hostility with coronary artery calcification in young adults: The Cardia Study. JAMA 283:2546-2551, 2000.
4. Siegman AW, Townsend ST, Civelek AC, et al: Antagonistic behavior, dominance, hostility, and coronary disease. Psychosom Med 62:248-257, 2000.
5. Chang PP, Ford DE, Meoni LA, et al: Anger in young men and subsequent premature cardiovascular disease: The precursors study. Arch Intern Med 162:901-906, 2002.
6. Angerer P, Siebert U, Kothny W, et al: Impact of social support, cynical hostility, and anger expression on progression of coronary atherosclerosis. J Am Coll Cardiol 36:1781-1788, 2000.
7. Frasure-Smith N, Lespérance F, Talajic M: Depression following myocardial infarction. Impact on 6-month survival. JAMA 270:1819-1825, 1993.
8. Glassman AH, O'Connor CM, Califf RM, et al: Sertaline treatment of major depression in patients with acute MI or unstable angina. JAMA 288:701-709, 2002.
9. Lespérance F, Frasure-Smith N, Talajic M: Major depression before and after myocardial infarction: Its nature and consequences. Psychosom Med 58:99-110, 1996.
10. McKhann GM, Borowicz LM, Goldsborough MA, et al: Depression and cognitive decline following coronary artery bypass grafting. Lancet 349:1282-1284, 1996.
11. Sullivan M, LaCroix A, Russo J, et al: Depression in coronary heart disease: What is the appropriate diagnostic threshold? Psychosomatics 40:285-292, 1999.
12. Carney RM, Jaffe AS: Treatment of depression following acute myocardial infarction. JAMA 288:750-751, 2002.
13. Sullivan MD, LaCroix AZ, Baum C, et al: Functional status in coronary artery disease: A one-year prospective study of the role of anxiety and depression. Am J Med 103:348-356, 1997.
14. Penninx BWJH, Beekman ATF, Honig A: Depression and cardiac mortality: Results from a community-based longitudinal study. Arch Gen Psychiatry 58:221-227, 2001.
15. Lespérance F, Frasure-Smith N, Talajic M, et al: Five-year risk of cardiac mortality in relation to initial severity and one-year changes in depression symptoms after myocardial infarction. Circulation 105:1049-1053, 2002.
16. Burg MM, Benedetto MC, Rosenberg R, et al: Presurgical depression predicts medical morbidity 6 months after coronary artery bypass graft surgery. Psychosom Med 65:111-118, 2003.
17. Ziegelstein RC: Depression in patients recovering from myocardial infarction. JAMA 286:1621-1627, 2001.
18. Scheier MF, Matthews KA, Owens JF, et al: Optimism and rehospitalization after coronary artery bypass surgery. Arch Intern Med 159:829-835, 1999.
19. Rugulies R: Depression as a predictor for coronary heart disease: A review and meta-analysis. Am J Prev Med 23:51-61, 2002.
20. Rutledge T, Reis SE, Olson M, et al: Psychosocial variables are associated with atherosclerosis risk factors among women with chest pain: The WISE Study. Psychosom Med 63:282-288, 2001.
21. Druss RG, Bradford DW, Rosenheck RA: Mental disorders and use of cardiovascular procedures after myocardial infarction. JAMA 283:506-511, 2000.
22. Musselman DL, Evans DL, Wemeroff CB: The relationship of depression to cardiovascular disease: Epidemiology, biology, and treatment. Arch Gen Psychiatry 55:580-592, 1998.
23. Broadley AJM, Korszun A, Jones CJH, et al: Arterial endothelial function is impaired in treated depression. Heart 88:521-524, 2002.
24. Januzzi JL, Stern TA, Pasternak RC, et al: The influence of anxiety and depression on outcomes of patients with coronary artery disease. Arch Intern Med 160:1913-1925, 2000.
25. Carney RM, Blumenthal JA, Stein PK, et al: Depression, heart rate variability, and acute myocardial infarction. Circulation 104:2024-2028, 2001.
26. Musselman DL, Marzec UM, Manatunga A: Platelet reactivity in depressed patients treated with paroxetine: Preliminary findings. Arch Gen Psychiatry 57:875-882, 2000.
27. Paterniti S, Zureik M, Ducimetière P, et al: Sustained anxiety and 4-year progression of carotid atherosclerosis. Arterioscler Thromb Vasc Biol 21:136-141, 2001.
28. Moser DK, Dracup K: Is anxiety early after myocardial infarction associated with subsequent ischemic and arrhythmic events? Psychosom Med 58:395-401, 1996.
29. King KB: Psychologic and social aspects of cardiovascular disease. Ann Behav Med 19:264-270, 1997.
30. Brummett BH, Barefoot JC, Siegler IC, et al: Characteristics of socially isolated patients with coronary artery disease who are at elevated risk for mortality. Psychosom Med 63:267-272, 2001.
31. Frasure-Smith N, Lespérance F, Gravel G, et al: Social support, depression, and mortality during the first year after myocardial infarction. Circulation 101:1919-1924, 2000.
32. Bosma H, Peter R, Siegrist J, et al: Two alternative job stress models and the risk of coronary heart disease. Am J Public Health 88:68-74, 1998.
33. Wamala SP, Mittleman MA, Schenck-Gustafsson K, et al: Potential explanations of the educational gradient in women: A population-based case-control study of Swedish women. Am J Public Health 89:315-321, 1999.

33a. Wamala SP, Mittleman MA, Horsten M, et al: Job stress and the occupational gradient in coronary heart disease risk in women. The Stockholm Female Coronary Risk Study. Soc Sci Med 51:481-489, 2000.

34. Johnson JV, Stewart W, Hall EM, et al: Long-term psychosocial work environment and cardiovascular mortality among Swedish males. Am J Public Health 86:324-331, 1996.
35. Orth-Gomér K, Wamala SP, Horsten M, et al: Marital stress worsens prognosis in women with coronary heart disease. JAMA 284:3008-3014, 2000.
36. Krantz DS, Kop WJ, Santiago HT, et al: Mental stress as a trigger of myocardial ischemia and infarction. Cardiol Clin 14:271-287, 1996.
37. Jiang W, Babyak M, Krantz DS, et al: Mental stress–induced myocardial ischemia and cardiac events. JAMA 21:1651-1656, 1996.
38. Gullette ECD, Blumenthal JA, Babyak M, et al: Effects of mental stress on myocardial ischemia during daily life. JAMA 277:1521-1526, 1997.
39. Möller J, Hallqvist J, Diderichsen F, et al: Do episodes of anger trigger myocardial infarction? A case-crossover analysis in the Stockholm Heart Epidemiology Program (SHEEP). Psychosom Med 61:842-849, 1999.
40. Markowitz JH: Hostility is associated with increased platelet activity in coronary heart disease. Psychosom Med 60:586-591, 1998.
41. Suarez EC, Kuhn CM, Schanberg SM, et al: Neuroendocrine, cardiovascular, and emotional responses of hostile men: The role of interpersonal challenge. Psychosom Med 60:78-88, 1998.
42. Heller SS, Ormont MA, Lidagoster L: Psychosocial outcome after ICD implantation: A current perspective. Pacing Clin Electrophysiol 21:1207-1215, 1998.

Psychiatric and Behavioral Aspects of Hypertension and Heart Failure

43. Weidner G, Kohlmann C, Horsten M, et al: Cardiovascular reactivity to mental stress in the Stockholm Female Coronary Risk Study. Psychosom Med 63:917-924, 2001.
44. Smith TW, Gallo LG: Hostility and cardiovascular reactivity during marital interaction. Psychosom Med 61:436-445, 1999.
45. Perini C, Muller FB, Rauchfliesch U, et al: Psychosomatic factors in borderline hypertensive subjects and offspring of hypertensive parents. Hypertension 16:627-634, 2002.
46. Friedman R, Schwartz JE, Schnall PL, et al: Psychological variables in hypertension: Relationship to casual or ambulatory blood pressure in men. Psychosom Med 63:19-31, 2001.
47. Jonas BS, Franks P, Ingram DD: Are symptoms of anxiety and depression risk factors for hypertension? Longitudinal evidence from the National Health and Nutrition Survey I Epidemiologic Follow-up Study. Arch Fam Med 6:43-49, 1997.
48. Shinn EH, Poston WSC, Kimball KT, et al: Blood pressure and symptoms of depression and anxiety: A prospective study. Am J Hypertens 14:660-664, 2001.
49. Jonas BS, Lando JF: Negative affect as a prospective risk factor for hypertension. Psychosom Med 62:188-196, 2000.
50. The Sixth Report of the Joint National Committee on Prevention, Detection, Evaluation, and Treatment of High Blood Pressure. Arch Intern Med 157:2413-2446, 1997 [published correction appears in Arch Intern Med 158:573, 1998.]
51. Linden W, Chambers LA: Clinical effectiveness of non-drug therapies for hypertension: A meta-analysis. Ann Behav Med 16:35-45, 1994.
52. Linden W, Lenz JW, Con AH: Individualized stress management for primary hypertension: A randomized trial. Arch Intern Med 161:1071-1080, 2001.
53. MacMahon K, Lip GYH: Psychological factors in heart failure: A review of the literature. Arch Intern Med 162:509-516, 2002.
54. Feenstra J, Grobee DE, Jonkman FAM, et al: Prevention of relapse in patients with congestive heart failure: The role of precipitating factors. Heart 80:432-436, 1998.
55. Koenig HG: Depression in hospitalized older patients with congestive heart failure. Gen Hosp Psychiatry 20:29-43, 1998.

56. Jiang W, Alexander J, Christopher E, et al: Relationship of depression to increased risk of mortality and rehospitalization in patients with congestive heart failure. Arch Intern Med 161:1849-1856, 2001.
57. Freedland KE, Rich MW, Skala JA, et al: Prevalence of depression in hospitalized patients with congestive heart failure. Psychosom Med 65:119-128, 2003.
58. Sullivan M, Simon G, Spertus J, et al: Depression-related costs in heart failure care. Arch Intern Med 162:1860-1866, 2002.
59. Williams SA, Kasl SV, Heiat A, et al: Depression and risk of heart failure among the elderly. Psychosom Med 64:6-12, 2002.
60. Krumholtz HM, Butler J, Miller J, et al: Prognostic impact of emotional support for elderly patients hospitalized with heart failure. Circulation 97:958-964, 1998.
60a. Murberg TA, Bru E: Social relationships and mortality in patients with congestive heart failure. J Psychosom Res 51:521-527, 2001.
61. Krantz DS, Hedges SM, Gabbay FH, et al: Triggers of angina and ST segment depression in ambulatory patients with coronary artery disease: Evidence for uncoupling of angina and ischemia. Am Heart J 128:703-712, 1994.
62. Leizorovicz A, Haugh MC, Mercier C, et al: Pre hospital and hospital time delays in thrombolytic treatment in patients with suspected myocardial infarction. Eur Heart J 18:248-253, 1997.
63. Meischke H, Larsen MP, Eisenberg MS: Gender differences in reported symptoms for acute myocardial infarction: Impact of prehospital delay time interval. Am J Emerg Med 16:363-366, 1998.

Psychiatric Care of the Cardiac Patient

64. Selnes OA, McKhann GM: Coronary-artery bypass surgery and the brain. N Engl J Med 344:451-452, 2001.
65. Roach GW, Kanchuger M, Mangano CM, et al: Adverse cerebral outcomes after coronary bypass surgery. N Engl J Med 335:1857-1863, 1996.
66. Schwartz TL, Masand PS: The role of atypical antipsychotics in the treatment of delirium. Psychosomatics 43:171-174, 2002.
67. Newman MF, Kirchner JL, Phillips-Bute B, et al: Longitudinal assessment of neurocognitive function after coronary-artery bypass surgery. N Engl J Med 344:395-402, 2001.
68. Sauer WH, Berlin JA, Kimmel SE: Selective serotonin reuptake inhibitors and myocardial infarction. Circulation 104:1894-1898, 2001.
69. Taylor CB, Miller NH, Smith PM, et al: The effect of a home-based, case-managed, multifactorial risk-reduction program on reducing psychological distress in patients with cardiovascular disease. J Cardiopulm Rehabil 17:157-162, 1997.
70. Frasure-Smith N, Lespérance F, Prince RH, et al: Randomized trial of home-based psychosocial nursing intervention for patients recovering from myocardial infarction. Lancet 350:473-479, 1997.
71. Cossette S, Frasure-Smith N, Lespérance F: Clinical implications of a reduction in psychological distress on cardiac prognosis in patients participating in a psychosocial intervention program. Psychosom Med 63:257-266, 2001.
72. Ades PA: Cardiac rehabilitation and secondary prevention of coronary heart disease. N Engl J Med 345:892-902, 2001.
73. Dusseldorp E, van Elderen T, Maes S, et al: A meta-analysis of psychoeducational programs for coronary heart disease patients. Health Psychol 18:506-519, 1999.
74. Linden W: Psychological treatments in cardiac rehabilitation: Review of rationales and outcomes. J Psychosom Res 48:443-454, 2000.

Psychopharmacology in the Cardiac Patient

75. Roose SP, Glassman AH, Attia E, et al: Cardiovascular effects of fluoxetine in depressed patients with heart disease. Am J Psychiatry 155:650-655, 1998.
76. Harvey AT, Preskorn SH: Cytochrome P450 enzymes: Interpretation of their interactions with selective srotonin reuptake inhibitors: I. J Clin Psychopharmacol 16:273-285, 1996.
77. Nelson JC, Kennedy JS, Pollock BG, et al: Treatment of major depression with nortriptyline and paroxetine in patients with ischemic heart disease. Am J Psychiatry 156:1024-1028, 1999.
78. Beliles K, Stoudemire A: Psychopharmacologic treatment of depression in the medically ill. Psychosomatics 39:S2-S19, 1998.
78a. Nelson JC: Safety and tolerability of the new antidepressants [review]. J Clin Psychiatry 58(Suppl 6):26-31, 1997.
79. Glassman AH, Bigger JT: Antipsychotic drugs: Prolonged QTc interval, torsade de pointes, and sudden death. Am J Psychiatry 158:1774-1782, 2001.
80. Stoudemire A, Moran MF: Psychopharmacology in the medically ill patient. *In* Schatzberg AF, Nemeroff CB (eds): Textbook of Psychopharmacology. Washington, DC, American Psychiatric Press, 1998, pp 931-959.
81. Killian JG, Kerr K, Lawrence C, et al: Myocarditis and cardiomyopathy associated with clozapine. Lancet 354:1841-1845, 1999.
82. Lieberman JA: Maximizing clozapine therapy: Managing side effects. J Clin Psychiatry 59(Suppl 3):38-43, 1998.
83. Benassi E, Bo GP, Cociot L, et al: Carbamazepine and cardiac conduction disturbances. Ann Neurol 22:280-281, 1999.

CHAPTER 85

Neurological Disorders and Cardiovascular Disease

William J. Groh • Douglas P. Zipes

Cardiovascular disease that occurs secondary to an underlying neurological disorder is related either to a direct involvement of the heart or to induced neurohormonal abnormalities that act on the heart. In several neurological disorders, the cardiovascular manifestations can be responsible for a greater risk of morbidity and mortality than the neurological manifestations. This chapter reviews those neurological disorders associated with important cardiovascular sequelae.

Muscular Dystrophies

The muscular dystrophies are a diffuse group of heritable disorders in which direct involvement of cardiac muscle and/or the cardiac conduction system is present to a variable degree. The muscular dystrophies can be classified into the following types:

1. X-linked—Duchenne and Becker muscular dystrophy
2. Myotonic muscular dystrophy
3. Emery-Dreifuss muscular dystrophy and associated disorders
4. Limb-girdle muscular dystrophy
5. Facioscapulohumeral muscular dystrophy

Duchenne and Becker Muscular Dystrophies

GENETICS. Both Duchenne and Becker muscular dystrophy are X-linked recessive disorders in which the genetic locus has been identified as an abnormality in the dystrophin gene. The dystrophin protein and dystrophin-associated glycoproteins provide a structural link between the myocyte cytoskeleton and extracellular matrix functioning to link contractile proteins to the cell membrane.[1] Dystrophin messenger RNA is expressed predominantly in skeletal, cardiac, and smooth muscle with lower levels in brain. Its absence can lead to membrane fragility resulting in myofibril necrosis and eventual loss of muscle fibers with fibrotic replacement. Abnormalities in dystrophin and in dystrophin-associated glycoproteins underlie the degeneration of cardiac and skeletal muscle in several inherited myopathies, including X-linked dilated cardiomyopathy.[2] Beyond the inherited disorders, the loss of dystrophin plays a role in myocyte failure in many cardiomyopathies including those associated with coronary artery disease.[3] In Duchenne muscular dystrophy, dystrophin is nearly absent, whereas in Becker muscular dystrophy, dystrophin is present but reduced in size or amount. This leads to the characteristic rapidly progressive skeletal muscle disease in Duchenne and the more benign course in Becker muscular dystrophy. The heart as a muscle is involved in both disorders.

CLINICAL PRESENTATION. Duchenne muscular dystrophy is the most common inherited neuromuscular disorder, with an incidence of 30 per 100,000 live male births. Patients typically become symptomatic before 5 years of age, presenting with skeletal muscle weakness that progresses such that the boy becomes wheelchair bound before 13 years of age (Fig. 85–1).[4] Death occurs commonly by age 20 to 25 years primarily from respiratory failure or cardiac arrest. Becker muscular dystrophy is less common (3 per 100,000 live male births) and has a more variable presentation of skeletal muscle weakness (Fig. 85–2) and a better prognosis, with most patients surviving to age 40 to 50 years.

In both Duchenne and Becker muscular dystrophy, elevated serum creatinine kinase activity is observed, over 10-fold and 5-fold normal values, respectively.

CARDIOVASCULAR MANIFESTATIONS. Virtually all patients with Duchenne muscular dystrophy develop a cardiomyopathy (see Chap. 59), but clinical recognition may be masked by severe skeletal muscle weakness. Preclinical cardiac involvement is present in one-fourth by 6 years of age, with the onset of clinically apparent cardiomyopathy after the age of 10 years being common. Predilection for involvement in the posterobasal and posterolateral left ventricle has been observed (Fig. 85–3). As with the skeletal muscle weakness, cardiac involvement in Becker muscular dystrophy is more variable than in Duchenne muscular dystrophy, ranging from none or subclinical to severe cardiomyopathy requiring transplant. Cardiac involvement in Becker muscular dystrophy is independent of the severity of skeletal muscle involvement, with some but not all investigators observing increased likelihood of cardiovascular disease in older individuals.[5] More than one-half of patients with subclinical or benign skeletal muscle disease were noted to have cardiac involvement if carefully evaluated.[6] In follow-up studies, progression in the severity of cardiac involvement is common. Cardiomyopathy can initially solely involve the right ventricle.

Thoracic deformities and a high diaphragm can alter the cardiovascular examination in Duchenne muscular dystrophy. A reduction in the anteroposterior chest dimension is commonly responsible for a systolic impulse displaced to the left sternal border, a grade 1–3/6 short midsystolic murmur in the second left interspace, and a loud pulmonary component of the second heart sound. In both Duchenne and Becker muscular dystrophy, mitral regurgitation is commonly observed. The presence of mitral regurgitation is related to posterior papillary muscle dysfunction in Duchenne

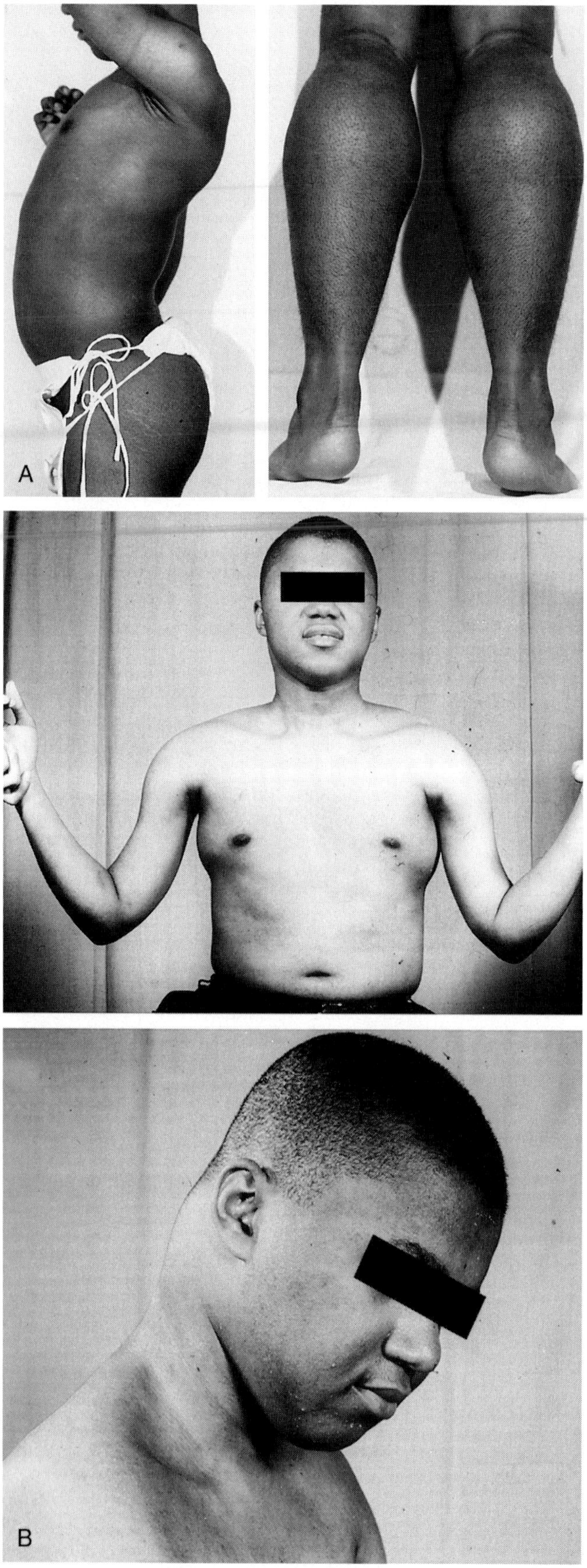

FIGURE 85–1 **A,** Classic X-linked muscular dystrophy. **Left,** Exaggerated lumbar lordosis. **Right,** Calf pseudohypertrophy and shortening of the Achilles tendons. **B,** Seventeen-year-old boy with Duchenne muscular dystrophy. There is striking enlargement (hypertrophy/pseudohypertrophy) of the deltoid and pectoralis major muscles **(upper panel)** and of the trapezius **(lower panel)**. There was also striking enlargement of both calves (not shown). (**A** and **B,** Courtesy of Joseph K. Perloff, MD.)

muscular dystrophy and to mitral annular dilation in Becker muscular dystrophy.[7]

Female carriers of Duchenne and Becker muscular dystrophy are at increased risk of dilated cardiomyopathy.[8]

ELECTROCARDIOGRAPHY. In patients with Duchenne muscular dystrophy the electrocardiogram (ECG) is abnormal in 90 percent, demonstrating a distinctive pattern of tall R waves and an increased RS amplitude in V_1 and deep narrow Q waves in the left precordial leads related to the characteristic posterolateral left ventricular involvement (Fig. 85–4). In patients with Becker muscular dystrophy, ECG abnormalities are present in up to 75 percent.[5] The ECG abnormalities observed include tall R waves and an increased RS amplitude in V_1, similar to that seen in Duchenne muscular dystrophy, but may also show frequent incomplete right bundle branch block. This may be related to early involvement of the right ventricle. In patients with congestive heart failure, left bundle branch block is common (Fig. 85–5).

ARRHYTHMIAS (see Chap. 32). In Duchenne muscular dystrophy, arrhythmias secondary to disturbances in both rhythm and conduction are observed. Persistent or labile sinus tachycardia is the most recognized abnormality. The pathogenesis of this tachycardia is unknown but does not appear related to abnormal autonomic function. Atrial arrhythmias including atrial fibrillation and atrial flutter occur commonly as a preterminal rhythm. Abnormalities in atrioventricular conduction have been observed. Up to 10 percent of individuals have PR intervals less than 120 milliseconds, while an additional 10 percent have prolonged PR intervals. Ventricular arrhythmias, primarily ventricular premature complexes, occur on monitoring in 30 percent. More complex ventricular arrhythmias have been reported, more commonly in individuals with severe muscle disease. Sudden death occurs in Duchenne muscular dystrophy, primarily in patients with severe skeletal muscle weakness. Whether the sudden death is primarily arrhythmic in nature is not clear. Several follow-up studies have shown a correlation between sudden death and complex ventricular arrhythmias.

Arrhythmic manifestations in Becker muscular dystrophy tend to correspond to the degree of the associated dilated cardiomyopathy but are not well characterized. Distal conduction system disease with complete heart block and bundle branch reentry ventricular tachycardia has been observed (see Chaps. 30 through 32).[9]

TREATMENT AND PROGNOSIS. Duchenne muscular dystrophy is a progressive disorder with respiratory or cardiac death common by age 20 to 25 years. Steroids and steroid derivatives have shown promise in delaying disease progression.[4] Gene replacement therapy holds future promise. A primary cardiac etiology for death occurs in about one-fourth of patients, with an equal distribution of death from progressive heart failure and sudden death. Intravenous verapamil used for preterminal atrial arrhythmias can lead to acute respiratory failure.

In Becker muscular dystrophy or female carriers of Duchenne muscular dystrophy, it is not known whether therapy to decrease myocardial wall stress is beneficial in preventing or delaying progression to cardiac failure. Once heart failure is established, conventional therapy is indicated. Cardiac transplantation has been reported.[10]

Myotonic Muscular Dystrophy

GENETICS. Myotonic muscular dystrophy (dystrophica myotonia, Steinert disease) is an autosomal dominant inherited disorder characterized by reflex and percussion myotonia, weakness and atrophy of distal skeletal muscles as well as systemic manifestations of early balding, gonadal atrophy, cataracts, mental retardation, and cardiac involvement (Fig. 85-6).[11] The genetic abnormality responsible is an amplified and unstable trinucleotide (cytosine-thymine-guanine [CTG]) repeat found on the long arm of chromosome 19 (myotonic dystrophy type 1). In individuals without myotonic dystrophy, between 5 and 37 copies of the CTG repeat are present. In individuals with myotonic dystrophy, 50 to several thousand CTG repeats are observed. A direct correlation exists between an increasing number of CTG repeats and earlier age of onset and increasing severity of neuromuscular involvement. Cardiac involvement, including conduction disease and arrhythmias, also correlates with the length of CTG repeat expansion.[12] The mechanism by which an amplified CTG repeat leads to the characteristic involvement in myotonic dystrophy is multifactorial.[13-15]

Proximal myotonic myopathy, or myotonic dystrophy type 2, is a disorder similar to myotonic dystrophy type 1 but with typically less severe muscular involvement.[16,17] Cardiac abnormalities including conduction disease have been reported in proximal myotonic myopathy but also appear much less common than in myotonic dystrophy type 1.[18] The differences in the reported prevalence of cardiac involvement in proximal myotonic myopathy are likely related to genetic heterogeneity in the clinical syndrome. A repeat expansion at a separate genetic loci (3q21) has been identified as being responsible for proximal myotonic myopathy in many but not all families.[19,20] The remainder of the section focuses on the more common myotonic dystrophy type 1, hereafter referred to as *myotonic dystrophy*.

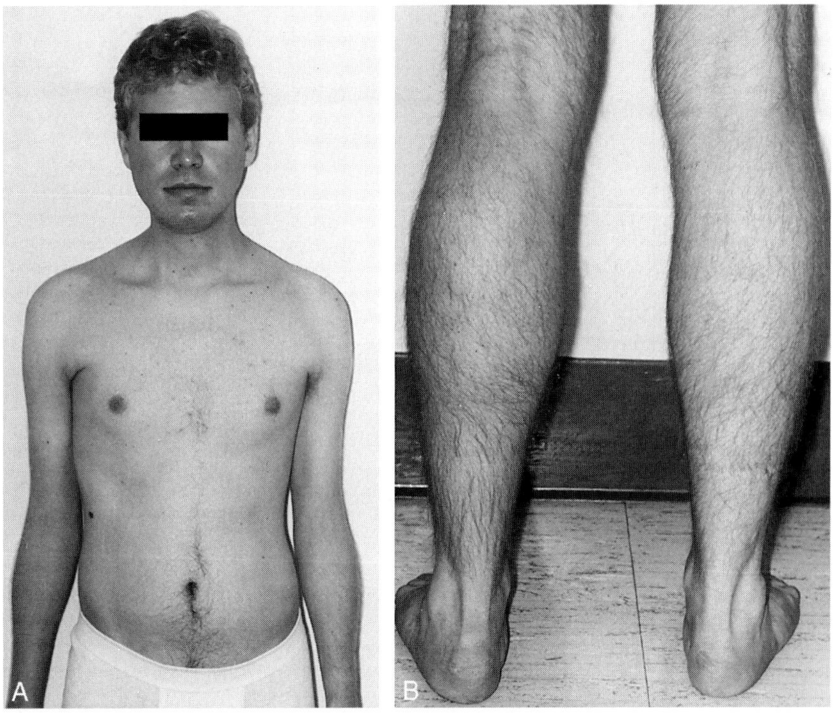

FIGURE 85–2 Late-onset, slowly progressive Becker muscular dystrophy in a 22-year-old man. **A,** There is dystrophy of the shoulder girdle, arms, and pelvic girdle (last not shown). **B,** Asymmetrical calf pseudohypertrophy, greater on the left than on the right. Dystrophy of proximal leg muscles is not shown. (**A** and **B,** Courtesy of Joseph K. Perloff, MD.)

CLINICAL PRESENTATION. Myotonic dystrophy is the most common inherited neuromuscular disorder in patients presenting as adults. The global incidence has been estimated to be 1 in 8000, although it is higher in certain populations, such as French Canadians and lower to nonexistent in other populations, such as African blacks. The age at onset of symptoms and diagnosis averages 20 to 25 years. Common early manifestations are weakness in the muscles of the face, neck, and distal extremities. On examination, myotonia (delayed muscle relaxation) can be demonstrated in the grip, thenar muscle group, and tongue (Fig. 85–7). Diagnosis when the individual is asymptomatic is possible using electromyography and genetic testing. Symptomatic myotonic dystrophy tends to present at an earlier age and with increasing severity in successive generations. This property is called *anticipation* and is related to the increasing amplification of CTG repeat length in successive generations. In general, cardiac symptoms occur after the onset of skeletal muscle weakness but can be the initial manifestation of the disease.

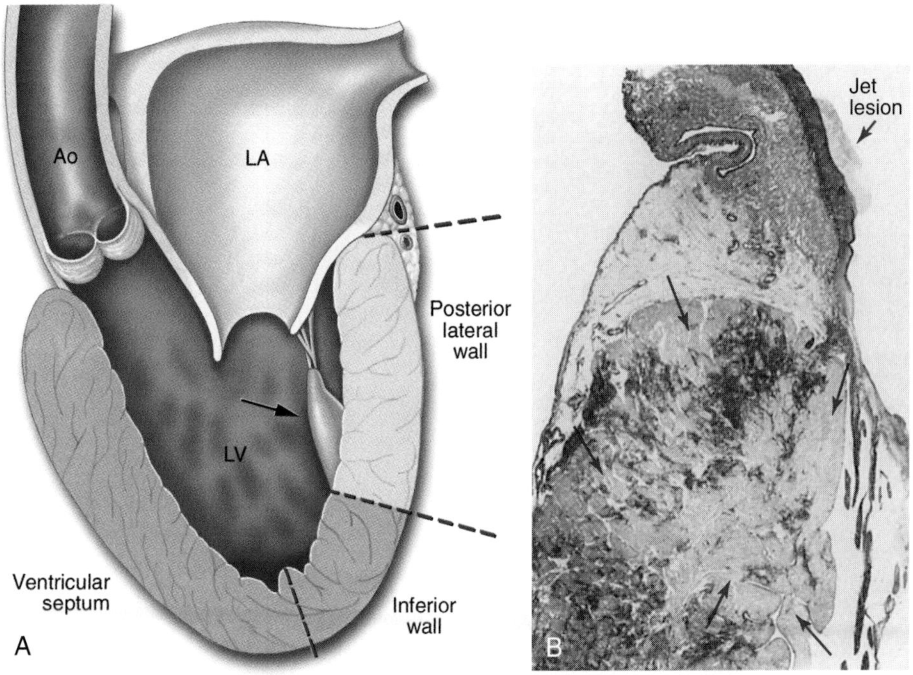

FIGURE 85–3 **A,** Schematic illustration showing the typical posterobasal myocardial involvement with lateral extension in classic Duchenne muscular dystrophy. The posterolateral papillary muscle is involved (arrow). **B,** Necropsy section showing posterobasal involvement (long arrows) of the left ventricle in a boy with classic Duchenne muscular dystrophy. The posterolateral papillary muscle was involved, resulting in mitral regurgitation and the jet lesion shown at upper right (arrow). LA = left atrium; LV = left ventricle; Ao = aorta. (**A** and **B,** Courtesy of Joseph K. Perloff, MD.)

CARDIOVASCULAR MANIFESTATIONS. Cardiac pathology is commonly seen in myotonic dystrophy primarily involving degeneration (fibrosis and fatty infiltration) of the specialized conduction tissue including the sinus node, atrioventricular node, and His-Purkinje system. Degenerative changes are observed in working atrial and ventricular tissue but only rarely progress to a symptomatic dilated cardiomyopathy (Fig. 85–8). It is not surprising, based on the preferential degeneration of conduction tissue, that the

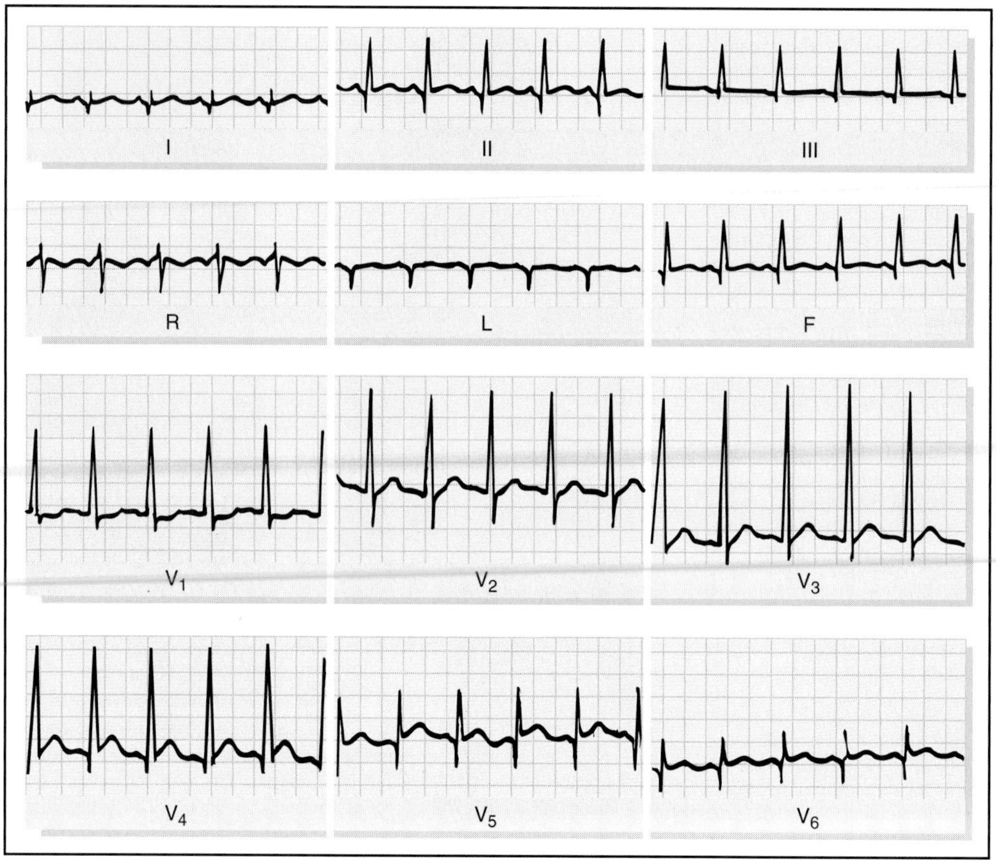

FIGURE 85–4 Electrocardiogram from a 12-year-old boy with classic Duchenne muscular dystrophy. Sinus tachycardia is observed. The QRS complex is typical of Duchenne dystrophy, showing tall R waves in lead V_1 and deep, narrow Q waves in leads I, aVL, and V_4 to V_6. (Courtesy of Charles Fisch, MD, Indiana University School of Medicine, Indianapolis, IN.)

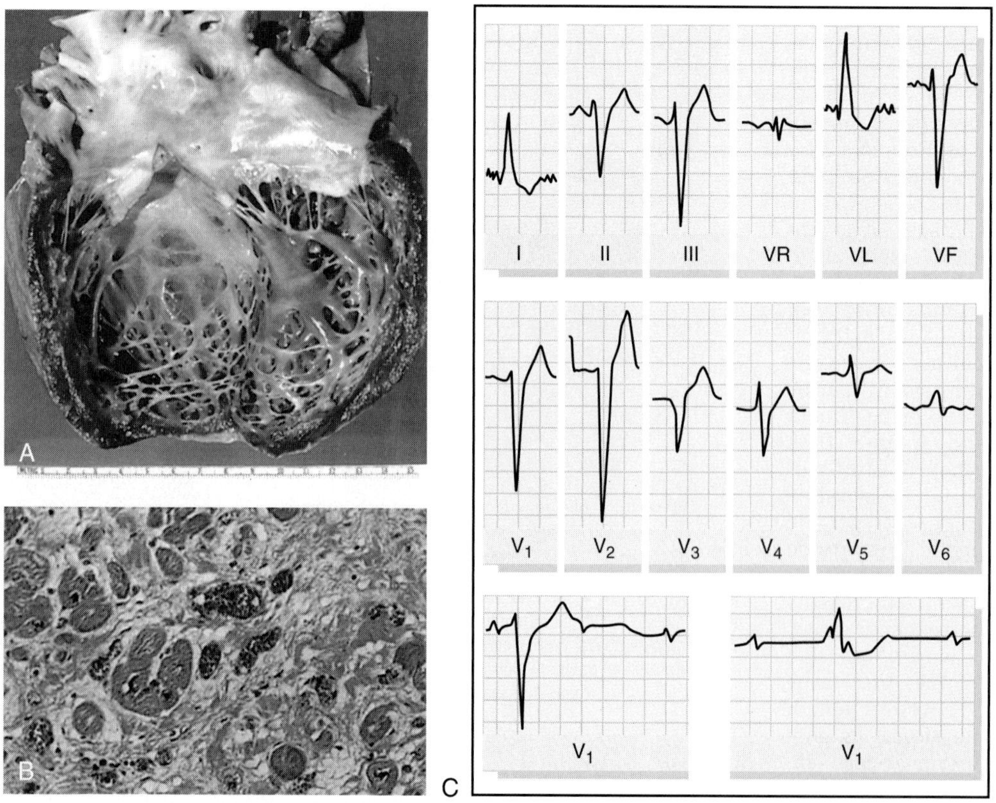

FIGURE 85–5 Gross and microscopic cardiac pathological specimens and the electrocardiogram from a 45-year-old man with late-onset, slowly progressive Becker muscular dystrophy. **A,** Dilated, flabby left ventricle with focal endocardial thickening. **B,** Microscopic section from the left ventricle shows marked confluent scarring with variations in fiber size; there was no significant coronary artery disease. **C,** Electrocardiogram recorded at age 40 years. The 12-lead tracing shows left axis deviation, a QRS of 0.14 second, small Q waves in leads I and aVL, and loss of R waves in leads V_2 and V_3. The lower tracings, taken 4 years later (a year before death), show complete heart block with a variable QRS configuration. (**A** to **C,** From Perloff JK, de Leon AC Jr, O'Doherty D: The cardiomyopathy of progressive muscular dystrophy. Circulation 33:625, 1966.)

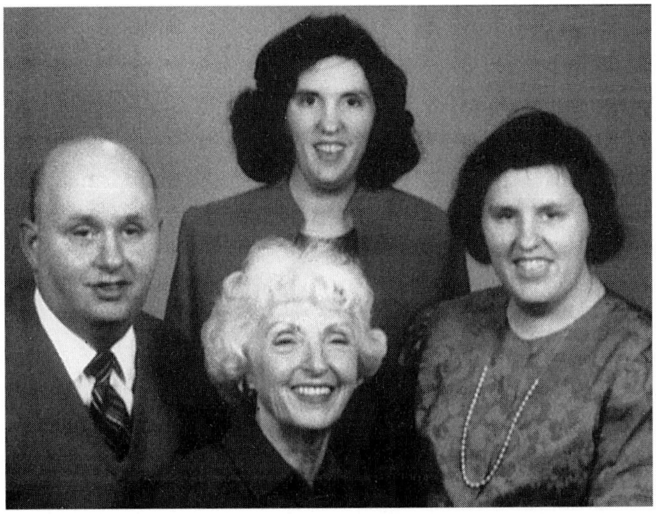

FIGURE 85–6 Myotonic muscular dystrophy in three siblings. Note the unaffected mother (front). Premature balding (left) and characteristic thin facies (rear) are demonstrated.

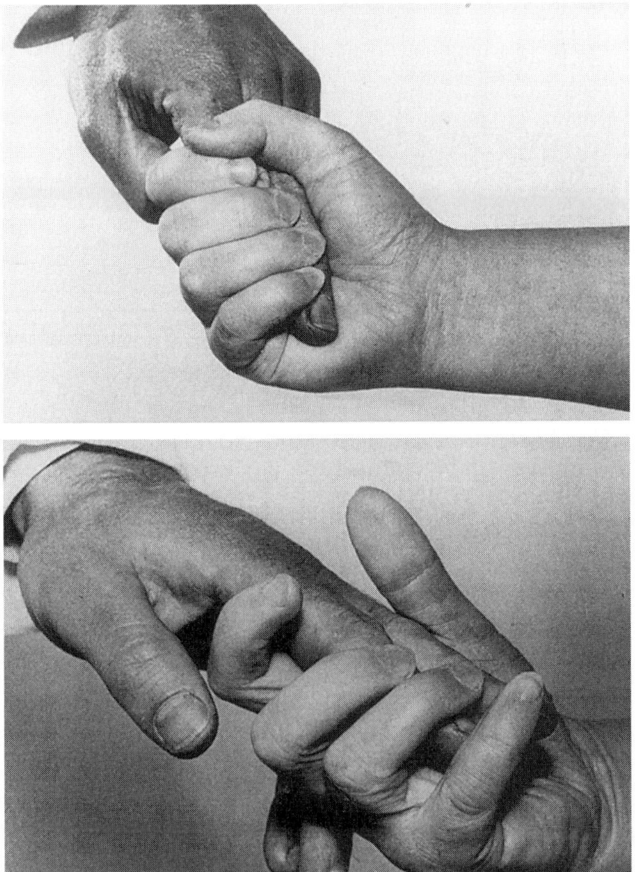

FIGURE 85–7 Grip myotonia in myotonic muscular dystrophy. Inability to release **(bottom)** after exerting grip **(top)**. (From Engel AG, Franzini-Armstrong C [eds]: Myology: Basic and Clinical. 2nd ed. Vol. II. New York, McGraw-Hill, 1994, p 1195.)

primary cardiac manifestations of myotonic dystrophy are arrhythmias.

Electrocardiography. The majority of adult patients with myotonic dystrophy have ECG abnormalities. In a large, unselected myotonic population followed in a U.S. neuromuscular clinic setting, 65 percent of patients had an abnormal ECG.[12] Abnormalities included first-degree atrioventricular

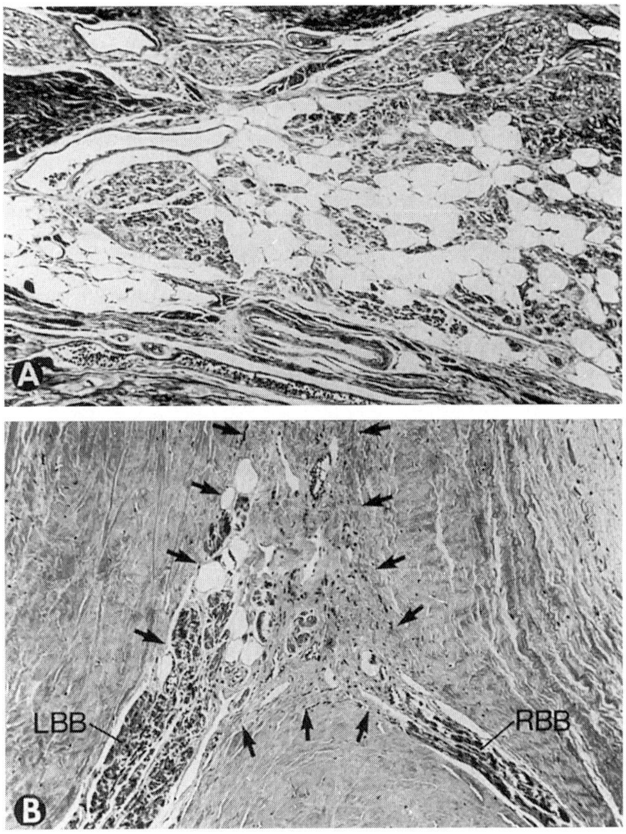

FIGURE 85–8 Histopathology of the atrioventricular bundle in myotonic dystrophy. **A,** Fatty infiltration in a 57-year-old man (Masson trichrome stain, ×90). **B,** Focal replacement fibrosis and atrophy in a 48-year-old woman. Arrows demarcate expected size and shape of the branching atrioventricular bundle (hematoxylin-eosin stain, ×90). LBB = left bundle branch; RBB = right bundle branch. (**A** and **B,** From Nguyen HH, Wolfe JT III, Holmes DR Jr, Edwards WD: Pathology of the cardiac conduction system in myotonic dystrophy: A study of 12 cases. J Am Coll Cardiol 11:662, 1988.)

block in 42 percent, right bundle branch block in 3 percent, left bundle branch block in 4 percent, and nonspecific intraventricular conduction delay in 12 percent. Q waves not associated with a known myocardial infarction are common. ECG abnormalities often progress over time (Fig. 85–9).

Echocardiography. Left ventricular systolic and diastolic dysfunction, left ventricular hypertrophy, and mitral valve prolapse have been reported in myotonic dystrophy patients at a higher prevalence than expected in an age-matched population.[21] The prevalence of symptomatic heart failure is estimated at 6 percent.

Arrhythmias. Patients with myotonic dystrophy demonstrate a wide range of arrhythmias. At cardiac electrophysiological study, the most common abnormality found is a prolonged His-ventricular interval, observed in 56 to 90 percent of selected patients.[22] Conduction system disease can progress to symptomatic atrioventricular block and necessitate pacemaker implantation. The prevalence of permanent cardiac pacing in patients with myotonic dystrophy varies widely between studies based on referral patterns and the indications used for implant. In a large, unselected myotonic population seen in a U.S. neuromuscular clinic setting, 3 percent had received a pacemaker.[12] In France, where early prophylactic pacemaker implantation in myotonic patients is practiced commonly, up to one-half of all myotonic patients receive a pacemaker.[22] Recent pacing guidelines have recognized that asymptomatic conduction abnormalities in neuromuscular diseases such as myotonic dystrophy may warrant special consideration for pacing.[23]

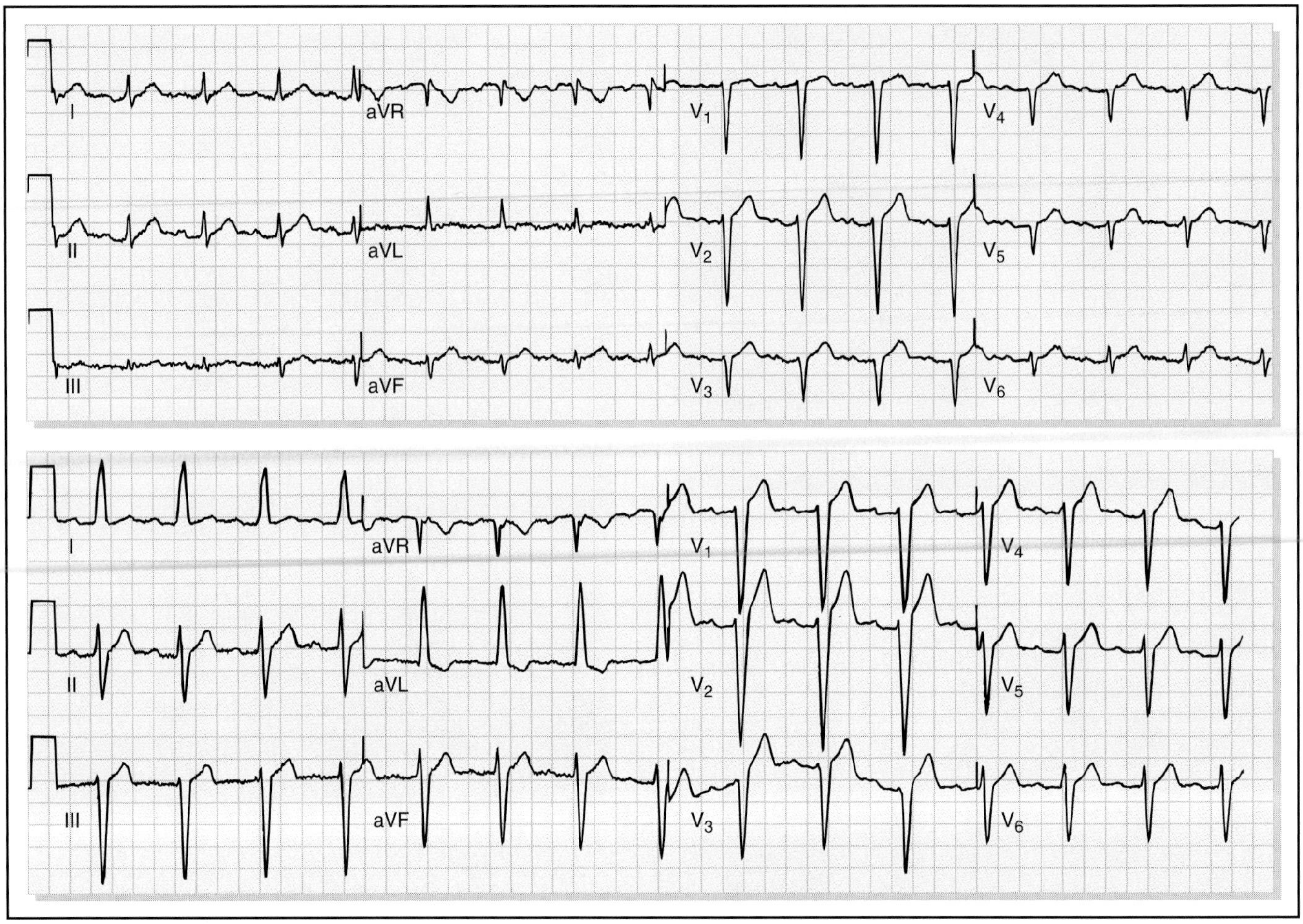

FIGURE 85–9 Electrocardiograms obtained 1 year apart in a 36-year-old man with myotonic dystrophy (the top set is older). Note the abnormal Q waves in the precordial leads. An increasing PR interval and QRS duration are observed consistent with increasing severity of conduction disease.

Atrial arrhythmias, primarily atrial fibrillation and atrial flutter, are the most common arrhythmias observed in myotonic dystrophy, being seen in approximately 4 percent of a general population.[12] Ventricular tachycardia can occur in patients with myotonic dystrophy. In at least two reports and a series of 6 patients, the ventricular tachycardia observed was related to reentry in the diseased distal conduction system, as characterized by bundle branch reentry and interfascicular reentry tachycardia (see Chaps. 27 and 32).[24] Therapy with right bundle branch and/or fascicular radiofrequency ablation resulted in absence of further inducible ventricular tachycardia.

The incidence of sudden death in patients with myotonic dystrophy is substantial and is believed to be primarily caused by arrhythmias. In a registry of 180 myotonic dystrophy patients from the Netherlands collected from 1950 to 1997, 29 percent of all deaths were classified as sudden presumably secondary to arrhythmias.[25] This was secondary only to pneumonia (31 percent) as a cause of death. In a 10-year study of mortality in a cohort of 367 patients from Quebec, 75 (20 percent) of patients died.[26] In these 75 deaths, 31 percent were characterized as secondary to cardiovascular causes, with 11 percent sudden. The mechanisms leading to sudden death in myotonic dystrophy are not clear. Distal conduction disease producing atrioventricular block can result in the lack of an appropriate escape rhythm and asystole or bradycardia-mediated ventricular fibrillation. Sudden death can occur in myotonic dystrophy despite previous permanent cardiac pacing, implicating the role of ventricular arrhythmias.

TREATMENT AND PROGNOSIS. Cardiac management in individuals with myotonic dystrophy is not well established. In the unusual patient in whom a dilated cardiomyopathy does develop, standard therapy including angiotensin-converting enzyme inhibitors and beta blockers has improved symptoms.[27] Patients presenting with symptoms indicative of arrhythmias such as syncope and palpitations should undergo an extensive evaluation, including cardiac electrophysiological study, to determine an etiology. A low threshold for permanent pacing is warranted. An appropriate level of screening for patients who do not manifest cardiac symptoms is unclear. Yearly ECGs and consideration for 24-hour ambulatory monitoring have been recommended. Whether significant or progressive ECG abnormalities require intervention such as prophylactic pacing or cardiac electrophysiological study is unclear. In one study, a combined arrhythmic endpoint was predicted by ECG markers indicative of conduction disease.[28] Trials encompassing more patients by using a multicenter approach have been recommended.[29] Certain families may be more prone to arrhythmic manifestations of myotonic dystrophy. Anesthesia in individuals with myotonic dystrophy can increase the risk of atrioventricular block and other arrhythmias. Careful monitoring during the perioperative period with a low threshold for prophylactic temporary pacing is recommended.

In patients presenting with wide complex tachycardia, cardiac electrophysiological study with particular evaluation for bundle branch reentry tachycardia should be done. The use of class I antiarrhythmic agents in suppressing ventricular tachycardia in myotonic dystrophy has had limited efficacy. Sotalol may be more effective. Implantable cardioverter-defibrillators are being used in myotonic patients.[30]

The course of neuromuscular abnormalities in myotonic dystrophy is highly variable. Death from progressive weakness and respiratory difficulty can occur in advanced skeletal muscle disease. Other individuals may be only minimally limited by weakness to ages of 60 to 70 years. Sudden death may significantly reduce survival in patients with myotonic dystrophy including those minimally symptomatic from a neuromuscular status. What evaluation and interventions are appropriate and the degree of effectiveness to decrease the risk of sudden death are unclear.

Emery-Dreifuss Muscular Dystrophy and Associated Disorders

GENETICS AND CARDIAC PATHOLOGY. Emery-Dreifuss muscular dystrophy is a rare familial disorder in which skeletal muscle symptoms are often mild but with cardiac involvement that is common and life threatening. The disease is classically inherited in an X-linked recessive fashion, but there is heterogeneity in that families have been reported that fit an autosomal dominant and recessive inheritance pattern. The gene responsible for the X-linked recessive Emery-Dreifuss muscular dystrophy, *STA*, encodes a nuclear membrane protein termed *emerin*.[31] The lack of emerin in skeletal and cardiac muscle is responsible for the disease phenotype.[32] Mutations in genes encoding two other nuclear membrane proteins, lamins A and C, have been identified as being responsible for a variety of other disorders with a phenotypic expression related to X-linked Emery-Dreifuss muscular dystrophy. The disorders include autosomal dominant and recessive Emery-Dreifuss muscular dystrophy, autosomal dominant dilated cardiomyopathy with conduction disease, autosomal dominant limb-girdle muscular dystrophy with conduction disease, and lipodystrophy with associated cardiac abnormalities.[33-37]

The mechanisms by which abnormalities in emerin and lamins A and C lead to cardiac involvement in Emery-Dreifuss muscular dystrophy and the associated disorders are not clear. The nuclear membrane proteins provide structural support for the nucleus as well as interact with the cell's cytoskeleton. One group of investigators have reported that emerin localizes to cardiac desmosomes and fasciae adherentes, possibly accounting for the predominance of conduction disease.[38] Localization of emerin in intercalated discs has not been observed by others.[39] Mutations in the tail regions of lamins A and C are responsible for most of the cases of autosomal dominant Emery-Dreifuss muscular dystrophy with a phenotype of both cardiac and skeletal muscle involvement.[33] Mutations in the rod domain of the lamins A and C gene primarily cause isolated cardiac disease including dilated cardiomyopathy, conduction system degeneration, and atrial and ventricular arrhythmias.[36] A rod domain deletion mutation has been reported as being responsible for a phenotype consistent with autosomal dominant Emery-Dreifuss muscular dystrophy.[40]

CLINICAL PRESENTATION. Emery-Dreifuss muscular dystrophy is characterized by a triad of (1) early contractures of the elbow, Achilles tendon, and posterior cervical muscles; (2) slowly progressing muscle weakness and atrophy primarily in humeroperoneal muscles; and (3) cardiac involvement. The disorder has been labeled *benign X-linked muscular dystrophy* to differentiate the slowly progressive muscular weakness from that of Duchenne muscular dystrophy. A definitive diagnosis can be made in Emery-Dreifuss muscular dystrophy and in carriers using antiemerin antibodies.[41]

In the autosomal dominant and recessive inheritance of Emery-Dreifuss muscular dystrophy, a more variable phenotypic expression and penetrance is typically observed.[34]

A mutation in the lamins A and C gene is also responsible for an autosomal dominantly–inherited familial partial lipodystrophy characterized by marked loss of subcutaneous fat, diabetes, hypertriglyceridemia, and cardiac abnormalities.[37]

CARDIOVASCULAR MANIFESTATIONS. Arrhythmias and dilated cardiomyopathy are the major manifestations of cardiac disease in Emery-Dreifuss muscular dystrophy and the associated disorders. In X-linked recessive Emery-Dreifuss muscular dystrophy, abnormalities in impulse generation and conduction are exceedingly frequent. ECGs are generally abnormal by age 20 to 30 years, commonly showing first-degree atrioventricular block. The atria appear to be involved earlier than the ventricles, with atrial fibrillation and atrial flutter, or more classically, permanent atrial standstill and junctional bradycardia, observed. Abnormalities in impulse generation or conduction are present in virtually all individuals by age 35 to 40 years, and pacing is often required. Ventricular arrhythmias, including sustained ventricular tachycardia and ventricular fibrillation, have been reported. Invasive cardiac electrophysiological study data are limited in this rare condition. Mild prolongation of the His-ventricular interval, atrial, atrioventricular nodal, and ventricular refractory periods have been observed. Sudden death (presumed cardiac) before 50 years of age is common. The incidence of sudden death may decrease with prophylactic pacing. Female carriers of X-linked recessive Emery-Dreifuss muscular dystrophy do not develop skeletal muscle disease, but late cardiac disease, including conduction abnormalities and sudden death, can occur.

Although arrhythmic disease is the most common presentation of cardiac involvement in X-linked recessive Emery-Dreifuss muscular dystrophy, a dilated cardiomyopathy can develop. The dilated cardiomyopathy is more common in patients in whom survival has been improved with pacemaker implantation. Both autopsy and endomyocardial biopsy have shown abnormal cardiac fibrosis.

Patients with disorders caused by lamins A and C mutations typically present at the ages of 20 to 40 years with cardiac conduction disease, atrial fibrillation, and dilated cardiomyopathy.[33-37] Skeletal muscle disease is typically subclinical or absent. Progression of a cardiomyopathy to an extent that heart transplant is required has been observed. Sudden death in those patients with a dilated cardiomyopathy is common. Permanent pacing is often required for symptomatic heart block.

TREATMENT AND PROGNOSIS. Affected patients should be monitored for development of ECG conduction abnormalities and other arrhythmias. Atrioventricular block can occur with anesthesia. In X-linked recessive Emery-Dreifuss muscular dystrophy, permanent pacing is recommended once conduction disease is evident, and it can be life saving. Whether similar pacing recommendations should be followed in patients with disorders caused by lamins A and C mutations is not clear. History, examination, and cardiac imaging for evaluation of left ventricular function is appropriate in all of the patients with Emery-Dreifuss muscular dystrophy and the associated disorders. Patients with left ventricular dysfunction should benefit from appropriate pharmacological therapy. These patients appear to benefit from heart transplant. Sudden death even in patients with pacemakers is common. Whether prophylactic implantable cardioverter-defibrillators should be considered in certain subgroups of patients is not clear. Female carriers of X-linked recessive Emery-Dreifuss muscular dystrophy develop conduction disease, and ECG monitoring on a routine basis is appropriate.

Limb-Girdle Muscular Dystrophy

GENETICS. Limb-girdle muscular dystrophy constitutes a group of disorders with a limb–pelvic girdle distribution of weakness but with otherwise heterogeneous inheritance and genetic etiology.[42] Inheritance is autosomal recessive (limb-girdle muscular dystrophy type 2), with many of the cases sporadic or autosomal dominant (limb-girdle muscular dystrophy type 1). At least 15 different gene abnormalities have been reported. The genes involved encode dystrophin-associated glycoproteins.[43]

CLINICAL PRESENTATION. The onset of muscle weakness is variable but usually occurs before 30 years of age. The recessive disorders tend to cause earlier weakness than the dominant disorders. Creatine kinase levels are typically moderately elevated. Patients commonly present with complaints of difficulty with walking or running secondary to pelvic girdle involvement. As the disease progresses, involvement of the shoulder muscles and then more distal muscles occurs, with sparing of facial involvement. Slow progression to severe disability and death can occur.

CARDIOVASCULAR MANIFESTATIONS. As with many of the features of limb-girdle muscular dystrophy, there is heterogeneity also observed in the presence and degree of cardiac involvement.

Limb-girdle muscular dystrophy types 2C to 2F are autosomal recessive disorders caused by mutations in a subunit of the sarcoglycan subcomplex.[42] These sarcoglyconopathy

disorders are associated with a dilated cardiomyopathy.[44-48] ECGs in these patients have shown abnormalities such as an increased R wave in V_1, consistent with a pattern of dystrophin-related cardiomyopathy, similar to that observed in Duchenne muscular dystrophy. With ECG or echocardiographic evaluations, cardiac abnormalities have been detected in up to 80 percent of patients. A smaller proportion of patients are symptomatic related to the cardiac involvement. A severe cardiomyopathy, including presentation with heart failure in childhood, may occur.[44,47,48] Sudden death associated with the cardiomyopathy has been reported. The mechanisms by which sarcoglycan abnormalities lead to a dilated cardiomyopathy are not clear. Recent studies support abnormalities in vascular supply to the myocardium rather than a direct myopathic effect.[49-51]

The autosomal dominant limb-girdle muscular dystrophy type 1B is caused by mutations in the gene encoding lamins A and C, similar to that observed in Emery-Dreifuss muscular dystrophy.[35] It is not surprising that the clinical phenotype is also similar to Emery-Dreifuss muscular dystrophy, with mild skeletal muscle symptoms and more severe cardiac involvement, primarily arrhythmic in nature.[52] Affected patients develop atrioventricular block by early middle age often necessitating pacing. Sudden death, believed to be cardiac, is common, including in those in whom pacing was previously instituted. A dilated cardiomyopathy can occur.

TREATMENT AND PROGNOSIS. Because of the heterogeneous nature of limb-girdle muscular dystrophy, specific recommendations for routine cardiac evaluation and therapy are difficult to formulate. Genetic testing can determine those with sarcoglyconopathies or lamins A and C mutations who are at the highest risk for cardiac involvement. In these patients (and families), cardiac evaluation for arrhythmias and ventricular dysfunction should be done. Whether standard heart failure therapy will decrease the progression of cardiomyopathy is unclear. Prophylactic pacing in those with lamins A and C mutations after conduction disease is observed should be considered. The high risk of sudden death in spite of pacing may point toward the implantable cardioverter-defibrillator as being a more appropriate electrical therapy.

Facioscapulohumeral Muscular Dystrophy

GENETICS. Facioscapulohumeral muscular dystrophy is the third most common type of muscular dystrophy after Duchenne and myotonic, with a prevalence of 1 per 20,000 persons.[53] It is an autosomal dominant disorder in which the genetic locus has been mapped to chromosome 4q35. Genetic heterogeneity has been reported. The diagnosis can be confirmed by a 4q35 *EcoRI* allele size of 38 kilobases or less.[54] Neither the definitive gene nor the gene product responsible for facioscapulohumeral muscular dystrophy has been identified.

CLINICAL PRESENTATION. Muscle weakness tends to follow a slowly progressive but variable course, presenting with facial and/or shoulder girdle muscle weakness and progressing to involve the pelvic musculature (Fig. 85–10). Major disability affecting walking eventually occurs in 20 percent of individuals.

CARDIOVASCULAR MANIFESTATIONS. Cardiac involvement in facioscapulohumeral muscular dystrophy is reported but does not constitute as significant of a problem in prevalence or severity as in other muscular dystrophies. In some series no evidence of cardiac abnormalities were found. Other series have reported a propensity toward arrhythmias, primarily atrial in origin, with atrioventricular conduction abnormalities less common.[55]

TREATMENT AND PROGNOSIS. Because significant clinical cardiac involvement is rare in facioscapulohumeral

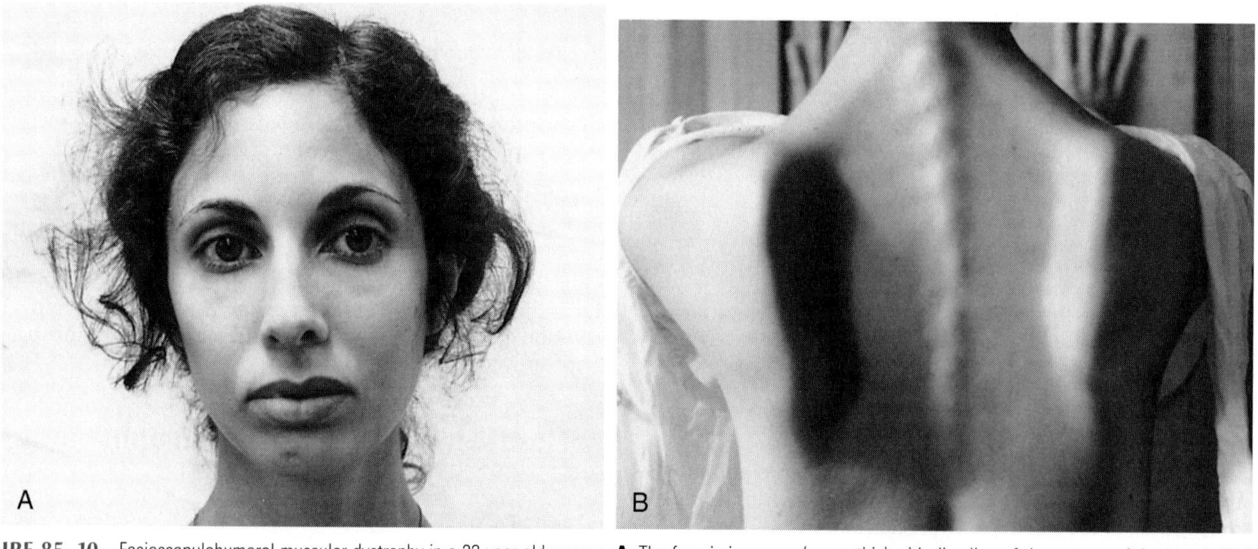

FIGURE 85–10 Facioscapulohumeral muscular dystrophy in a 32-year-old woman. **A,** The face is in repose (myopathic) with dimpling of the corners of the mouth. **B,** Typical winging of the scapulae. (**A** and **B,** Courtesy of Joseph K. Perloff, MD.)

muscular dystrophy, specific monitoring or treatment recommendations are not well defined. One group has recommended yearly ECGs.[55]

Friedreich Ataxia

GENETICS. Friedreich ataxia is an autosomal recessive spinocerebellar degenerative disease characterized clinically by ataxia of the limbs and trunk, dysarthria, loss of deep tendon reflexes, sensory abnormalities, skeletal deformities, diabetes mellitus, and cardiac involvement.[56] The disease is linked to chromosome 9, with the gene mutation affecting the encoding of a 210-amino acid protein, frataxin. Frataxin is a mitochondrial protein important in iron homeostasis and respiratory function. Messenger RNA for frataxin is highly expressed in the heart. The mutation responsible for Friedreich ataxia is an amplified trinucleotide (guanine-adenine-adenine [GAA]) repeat found in the first intron of the gene encoding frataxin. Whereas normal individuals have fewer than 33 repeats, patients with Friedreich ataxia have 66 to 1500 GAA repeats. In 95 percent of patients, both alleles of the gene have the expanded repeat. In 5 percent of patients, a point mutation occurs on one allele in association with an expanded repeat on the other. The GAA repeat disrupts transcription severely decreasing frataxin synthesis. The decrease in frataxin leads to mitochondrial dysfunction, poor cellular response to oxidative stress, and apoptosis.[57] Endomyocardial biopsies in patients with Friedreich ataxia have shown deficient function in mitochondrial respiratory complex subunits and in aconitase, an iron-sulfur protein involved in iron homeostasis.[58] Abnormal cardiac bioenergetics appear to result from the abnormalities in respiratory function and iron handling.[59] As the GAA triplet size increases an earlier age of symptom onset, increasing severity of neurological symptoms and worsening left ventricular hypertrophy by echocardiography are observed.[60]

CLINICAL PRESENTATION. The estimated prevalence of Friedreich ataxia is 1 in 50,000. Neurological symptoms usually manifest around puberty and almost always before age 25 years. Progressive loss of neuromuscular function, with the individual wheelchair bound 10 to 20 years after symptom onset, is the norm. Neurological symptoms precede cardiac symptoms in most but not all cases.

CARDIOVASCULAR MANIFESTATIONS. Friedreich ataxia is commonly associated with a concentric hypertrophic cardiomyopathy (see Chap. 59) (Fig. 85–11). Less commonly, asymmetrical septal hypertrophy is observed. The presence of a left ventricular outflow gradient associated with the septal hypertrophy has been reported. Presentation with a dilated cardiomyopathy is more rare but can occur (Fig. 85–12). The dilated cardiomyopathy appears to occur as a progressive transition from a hypertrophic cardiomyopathy. The prevalence of hypertrophy varies between studies but does increase in prevalence with a younger age at diagnosis and with increasing GAA trinucleotide repeat length.[60,61] Up to 95 percent of neurologically symptomatic patients have abnormalities on ECG and echocardiographic evaluations.

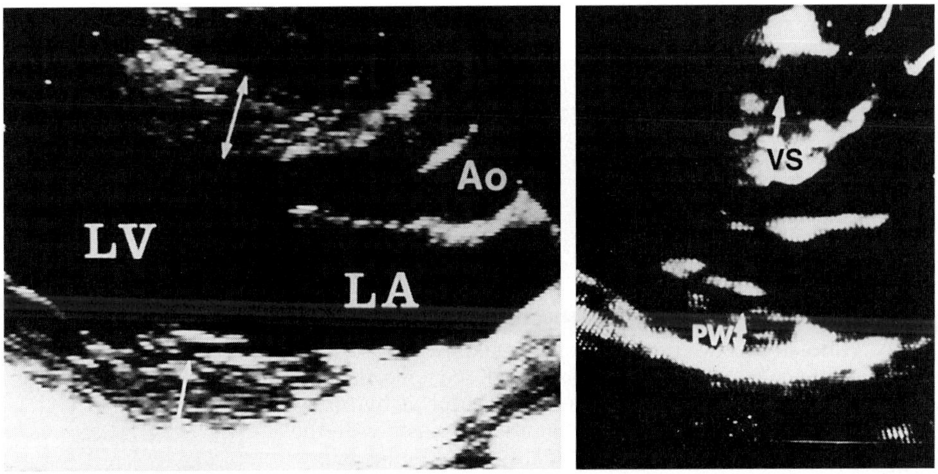

FIGURE 85–11 **A,** Two-dimensional echocardiogram (parasternal long axis diastolic frames) from a 14-year-old girl with Friedreich ataxia and concentric hypertrophy (arrows) of the LV. **B,** Two-dimensional echocardiogram (parasternal long axis) from a 17-year-old boy with Friedreich ataxia and hypertrophic cardiomyopathy characterized by disproportionate thickness (arrows) of the VS compared with the PW. LV = left ventricle; Ao = aorta; LA = left atrium; PW = posterior wall; VS = ventricular septum. (**A** and **B,** From Perloff JK: Cardiac manifestations of neuromuscular disease. *In* Abelmann WH [ed]: Cardiomyopathies, Myocarditis, and Pericardial Disease. *In* Braunwald E [series ed]: Atlas of Heart Diseases. Vol 2. Philadelphia, Current Medicine, 1995.)

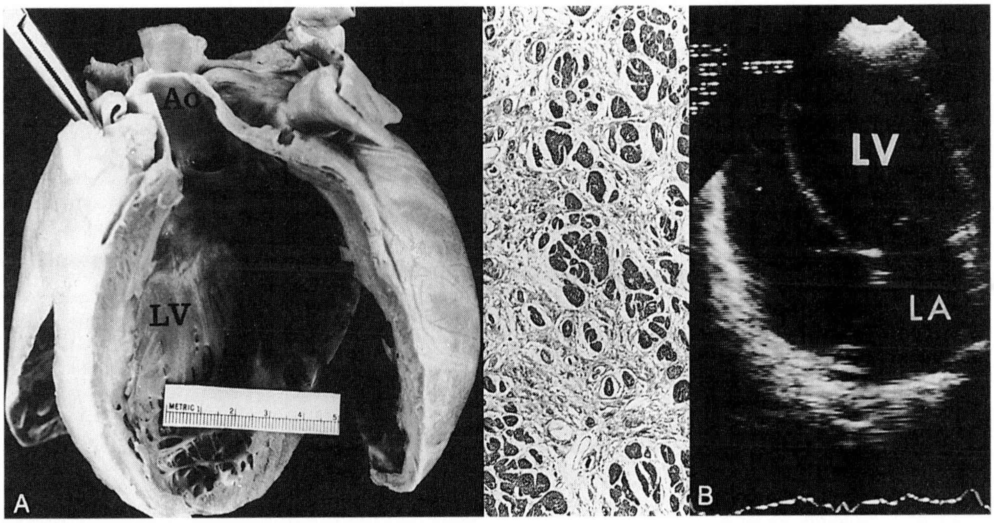

FIGURE 85–12 **A,** Gross and histological specimens from a 17-year-old boy with Friedreich ataxia whose echocardiogram progressed from normal at age 13 years to a minimally dilated, hypocontractile left ventricle 3 to 4 years later. The gross specimen shows a mildly dilated LV with normal wall thickness; the walls were flabby. The microscopic section from the LV free wall (middle panel) shows marked connective tissue replacement. Although specifically sought, small-vessel coronary artery disease was not identified. **B,** Two-dimensional echocardiogram (apical window) showing the mildly dilated, thin-walled LV. LA = left atrium; LV = left ventricle. (**A** and **B,** From Child JS, Perloff JK, Bach PM, et al: Cardiac involvement in Friedreich ataxia. J Am Coll Cardiol 7:1370, 1986.)

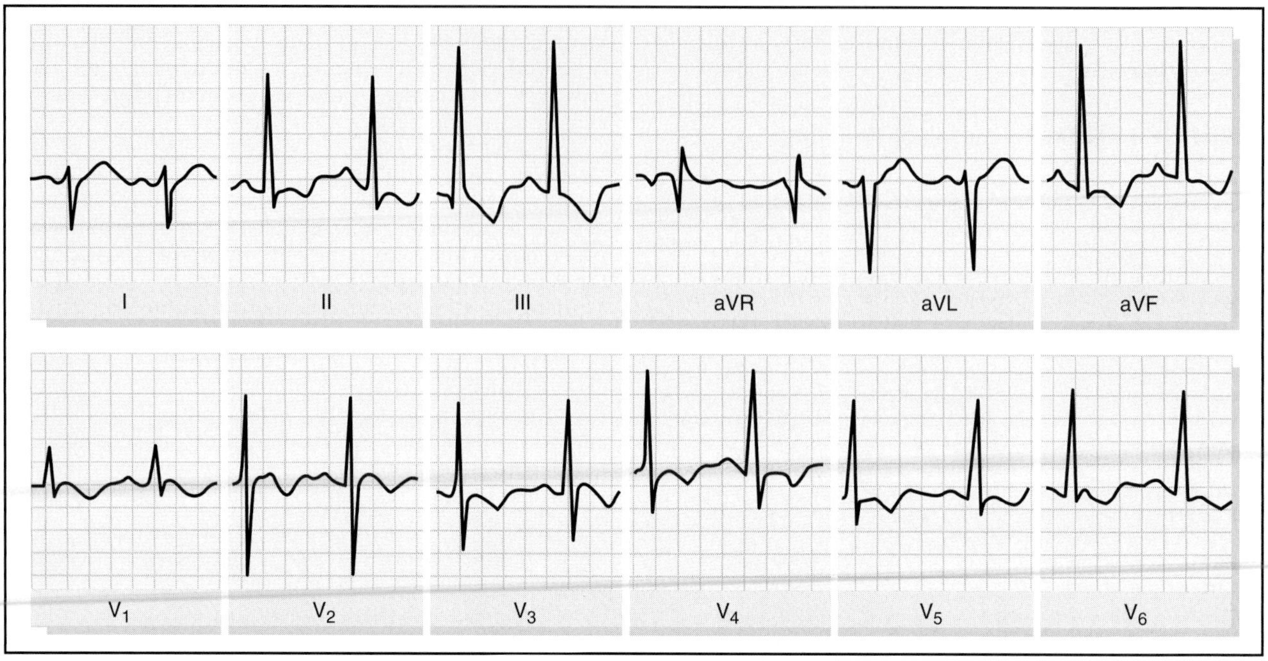

FIGURE 85–13 Electrocardiogram from a 34-year-old man with Friedreich ataxia. Widespread ST and T changes are observed. (Courtesy of Charles Fisch, MD, Indiana University School of Medicine, Indianapolis, IN.)

Findings are primarily consistent with ventricular hypertrophy. Left ventricular hypertrophy is not always present on ECGs despite echocardiographic evidence. Widespread T wave inversions are common (Fig. 85–13).

Arrhythmias occur in Friedreich ataxia but are less common than what might be expected, considering the high incidence of cardiac involvement. Atrial arrhythmias including atrial fibrillation and flutter are associated with the progression to a dilated cardiomyopathy. Ventricular tachycardia, again in the setting of a dilated cardiomyopathy, has been observed. The hypertrophic cardiomyopathy of Friedreich ataxia is not associated with serious ventricular arrhythmias as observed in the other types of heritable hypertrophic cardiomyopathies. Myocardial fiber disarray is not commonly observed in the hypertrophic cardiomyopathy of Friedreich ataxia. Sudden death has been reported, but a mechanism has not been well characterized.

Endomyocardial biopsies in Friedreich ataxia have demonstrated myocyte hypertrophy and interstitial fibrosis. Histopathological examination has revealed myocyte hypertrophy and degeneration, interstitial fibrosis, active muscle necrosis, bizarre pleomorphic nuclei, and periodic acid–Schiff-positive deposition in both large and small coronary arteries. Degeneration and fibrosis in cardiac nerves and ganglia and the conduction system have also been observed. Deposition of calcium salts and iron has been reported.

TREATMENT AND PROGNOSIS. Idebenone, a free radical scavenger, was reported to significantly decrease overall left ventricular mass in one-half of Friedreich ataxia patients treated in an unblinded, noncontrolled trial for 6 months.[62] No characteristics were found that separated responders from nonresponders. In patients with depressed left ventricular function at the initiation of idebenone therapy most showed improvement. Idebenone decreases markers of oxidative DNA damage in patients with Friedreich ataxia.[63] Whether an improvement in neurological outcome will result is unclear.

In general, progressive neurological dysfunction is the norm in Friedreich ataxia, with death from respiratory failure or infection in the fourth or fifth decades. Cardiac death occurs primarily in those developing a dilated cardiomyopathy. These patients tend do poorly, with rapid progression to end-stage congestive heart failure.

Less Common Neuromuscular Diseases Associated with Cardiac Manifestations

The Periodic Paralyses

GENETICS. The primary periodic paralyses are rare, nondystrophic, autosomal dominant disorders that result from abnormalities in ion channel genes. They can be classified into hypokalemic, hyperkalemic (potassium-sensitive), and normokalemic periodic paralyses, with several subclassifications in each.[64]

Hypokalemic periodic paralysis is characterized by episodic attacks of weakness in association with decreased serum potassium levels. Penetrance is complete in males and approximately 50 percent in females. Hypokalemic periodic paralysis has been mapped to chromosome 1q31-32 with subsequent identification of mutations in the alpha$_1$ subunit of the dihydropyridine-sensitive calcium channel. The disease may be genetically heterogeneous, as observed with the identification of a family with hypokalemic periodic paralysis and a mutation in the skeletal muscle sodium channel (SCN4A).[65]

Hyperkalemic periodic paralysis also manifests with episodic weakness but with symptoms worsening with potassium supplementation. Complete penetrance is observed. Potassium levels are usually high but may be normal during an attack. Hyperkalemic periodic paralysis is due primarily to mutations in the alpha subunit of SCN4A found on chromosome 17.[66] Multiple different mutations in this gene have been reported and result in a potassium-sensitive failure of inactivation in the sodium channel. Hyperkalemic periodic paralysis is genetically heterogeneous.

Andersen syndrome is a distinct potassium-sensitive periodic paralysis associated with dysmorphic features of low-set ears, micrognathia, and clinodactyly as well as a long-QT interval and ventricular arrhythmias (Fig. 85–14).[67] Andersen syndrome is linked to chromosome 17q23 with the mutation responsible in the *KCNJ2* gene encoding an inward rectifier potassium channel (Kir2.1).[68-70] Andersen syndrome has been given an alternate long-QT syndrome 7 nomenclature.

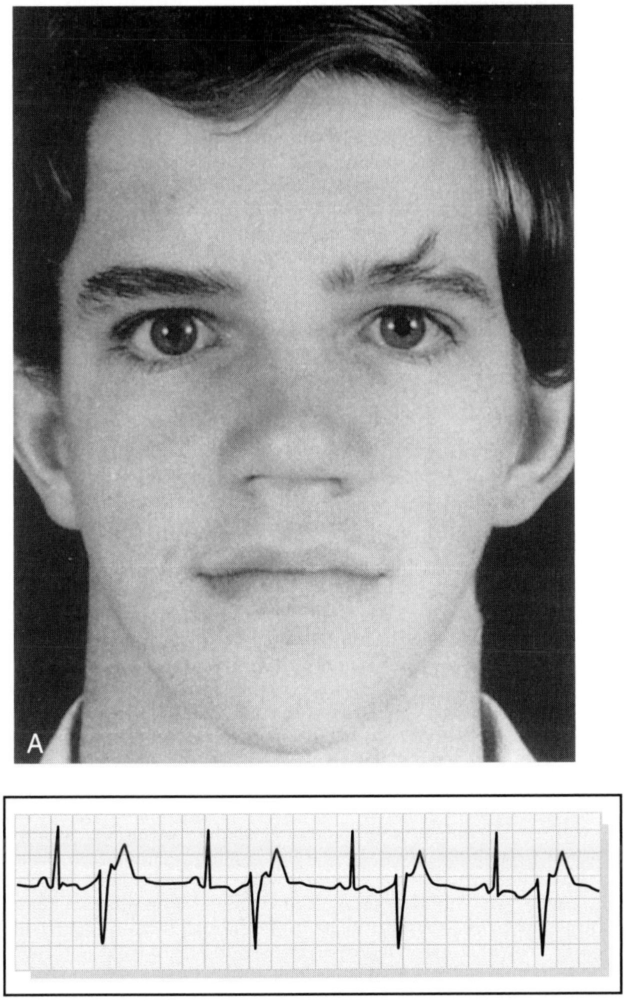

B

FIGURE 85–14 Andersen syndrome in a 22-year-old man. **A,** Characteristic low-set ears and hypoplastic mandible. **B,** Electrocardiographic recording revealing ventricular bigeminy. (**A** and **B,** From Tawil R, Ptacek LJ, Pavlakis SG, et al: Andersen's syndrome: Potassium-sensitive periodic paralysis, ventricular ectopy, and dysmorphic features. Ann Neurol 35:326, 1994.)

CLINICAL PRESENTATION. The primary manifestation of the periodic paralyses is episodic weakness. Attacks of weakness tend to be more severe and of longer duration with hypokalemic periodic paralysis than with hyperkalemic periodic paralysis. In both diseases, cold and rest after exercise can trigger an attack. Ingestion of carbohydrates can trigger an attack in hypokalemic periodic paralysis but may ameliorate an attack in hyperkalemic periodic paralysis.

CARDIOVASCULAR MANIFESTATIONS. The periodic paralyses are associated with ventricular arrhythmias. Arrhythmias occur primarily in hyperkalemic periodic paralysis and Andersen syndrome. Bidirectional ventricular tachycardia has been observed independent of digitalis intoxication. The episodes of bidirectional ventricular tachycardia are independent of attacks of muscle weakness, do not correlate with serum potassium levels, and can convert to sinus rhythm with exercise. Ventricular ectopy is common.

A prolonged QT interval can be observed. In some reports, this is episodic and associated with weakness, hypokalemia, or antiarrhythmic therapy. In other cases, a prolonged QT interval can be constant. Andersen syndrome is typically associated with a prolonged QT interval. Ventricular arrhythmias have been reported but are less likely in Andersen syndrome than other long-QT syndromes.

Sudden death has been reported in the periodic paralyses.

TREATMENT AND PROGNOSIS. The episodes of weakness typically respond to measures that work to normalize potassium levels. Weakness in hyperkalemic periodic paralysis can respond to mexiletine. Weakness in hypokalemic periodic paralysis can respond to acetazolamide. Treatment of electrolytes usually does not improve arrhythmias, or if it does, only transiently. Improvement in symptomatic nonsustained ventricular tachycardia associated with a prolonged QT interval has been reported with beta-blocker therapy. Class 1A antiarrhythmic agents can worsen muscle weakness and exacerbate arrhythmias associated with a prolonged QT interval. Bidirectional ventricular tachycardia, not associated with a prolonged QT interval, may not respond to beta-blocker therapy. Amiodarone has been observed to decrease episodes of sustained polymorphic ventricular tachycardia in Andersen syndrome.

MITOCHONDRIAL DISORDERS

GENETICS. The mitochondrial disorders are a heterogeneous group of diseases resulting from abnormalities in mitochondrial DNA and function.[71] The number of distinct disorders is extensive. Mitochondrial DNA is inherited maternally, and most of these disorders are thus transmitted from mother to children of both sexes. Some of the disorders occur sporadically or are inherited in an autosomal fashion. Disease severity can vary between patients and family members because both mutant and normal mitochondrial DNA can be present in tissue in a variable proportion. It is not surprising, based on the important metabolic function of mitochondria, that these disorders manifest with systemic pathology. Tissue with a high respiratory workload such as brain, skeletal muscle, and cardiac muscle are especially affected.

Mitochondrial disorders, which have cardiac manifestations, present as several clinical phenotypes, consisting of chronic progressive external ophthalmoplegia, which includes Kearns-Sayre syndrome; myoclonus epilepsy with red ragged fibers (MERRF); mitochondrial myopathy, encephalopathy, lactic acidosis, and stroke-like episodes (MELAS); and Leber hereditary optic neuropathy. Other, more rare mitochondrial point mutation disorders, present primarily with cardiac manifestations, typically a hypertrophic or dilated cardiomyopathy.[72] Chronic progressive external ophthalmoplegia is primarily a sporadic disease, whereas the others listed are maternally inherited.

CLINICAL PRESENTATION. *Kearns-Sayre syndrome* is characterized by the clinical triad of progressive external ophthalmoplegia, pigmentary retinopathy, and atrioventricular block (Fig. 85–15). Diabetes, deafness, and ataxia can also be associated. Clinical features of MERRF include myoclonus, seizures, ataxia, dementia, and skeletal muscle weakness. MELAS is the most common of the maternally inherited mitochondrial disorders and is characterized by encephalopathy, subacute stroke-like events, migraine-like headaches, recurrent emesis, extremity weakness, and short stature. *Leber hereditary optic neuropathy* manifests as a severe, subacute, painless loss of central vision, predominantly affecting young men.

CARDIOVASCULAR MANIFESTATIONS. In chronic, progressive external ophthalmoplegia, most commonly in Kearns-Sayre syndrome, cardiac involvement manifests primarily as conduction abnormalities.[73] A dilated cardiomyopathy has also been reported.[74] In Kearns-Sayre syndrome, atrioventricular block is common, usually presenting after eye involvement. The His-ventricular interval is prolonged, consistent with distal conduction disease. Pacing is often required before 20 years of age. An increased prevalence of preexcitation has also been reported.

Leber hereditary optic neuropathy can be associated with a short PR interval on the ECG and preexcitation. Supraventricular tachycardia has been reported.

In MERRF and MELAS, cardiac involvement manifesting as hypertrophic (symmetrical or asymmetrical) or dilated cardiomyopathy is observed. Other disorders caused by mitochondrial point mutations can present with a similar cardiac phenotype.[74] Patients can present with chest pain with ECG abnormalities and myocardial perfusion defects. Whether the dilated cardiomyopathy represents a progression from the hypertrophic cardiomyopathy or a separate syndrome is not clear. The dilated cardiomyopathy can result in heart failure and death.

Preexcitation has been described with MELAS.

TREATMENT AND PROGNOSIS. In Kearns-Sayre syndrome, the prophylactic implantation of a pacemaker has been advocated when distal conduction disease is evident. Pacing appears to improve survival.[73] The

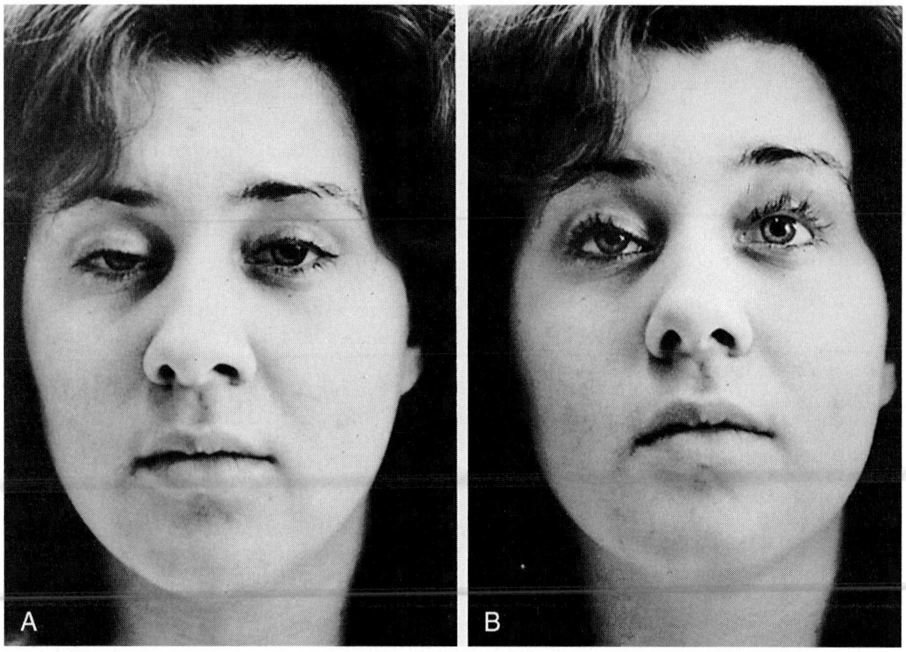

FIGURE 85–15 An 18-year-old girl with Kearns-Sayre syndrome and bilateral asymmetrical ptosis. Within 24 months, her electrocardiogram changed from normal to bifascicular block (complete right bundle branch block and left anterior fascicular block). **A,** Asymmetrical ptosis when the patient looks straight ahead. **B,** Ptosis of the right lid persists when the patient looks up. She also had typical pigmentary retinopathy. (**A** and **B,** Courtesy of Joseph K. Perloff, MD.)

degree of distal conduction disease that warrants prophylactic pacing is not clear. In Leber hereditary optic neuropathy, a baseline ECG may be prudent. In the other mitochondrial disorders, an understanding of the potential for cardiac involvement is necessary. Screening echocardiography has been recommended.[72] Whether other specific screening evaluations are warranted in these disorders is uncertain.

SPINAL MUSCULAR ATROPHY

GENETICS AND CLINICAL PRESENTATION. The spinal muscular atrophies are a group of lower motor neuron disorders presenting as progressive, symmetrical muscular weakness.[75,76] The disorders are inherited in an autosomal recessive fashion or are sporadic. The spinal muscular atrophies are classified clinically by the age of symptom onset and disease severity. *Type I (Werdnig-Hoffman disease)* and *type II* have early childhood onset with severe limitation of life span. *Type III (Kugelberg-Welander disease)* is characterized by later onset and slower progression, typically with survival to adulthood.

The spinal muscular atrophies link to chromosome 5q13. Mutations in two genes, *SMN* (survival of motor neuron) and *NAIP* (neuronal apoptosis inhibitory protein), are responsible for most cases.[77,78]

CARDIOVASCULAR MANIFESTATIONS. Cardiac involvement in spinal muscular atrophies includes coexisting complex congenital heart disease, cardiomyopathy, and arrhythmias. Congenital heart disease has been associated with types I and III spinal muscular atrophies. The most common abnormality is atrial septal defect, with other abnormalities reported. In spinal muscular atrophy type III, a dilated cardiomyopathy may occur with endomyocardial biopsies demonstrating fibrosis. Progression leading to a fatal outcome has been reported. Arrhythmic abnormalities including atrial standstill, atrial fibrillation, atrial flutter, and atrioventricular block may be the most common cardiac manifestation in these diseases. Permanent pacing for atrial standstill and atrioventricular block has been reported.

TREATMENT AND PROGNOSIS. The skeletal muscle involvement in spinal muscular atrophy types I and II limit life span to such a significant degree that treatment of associated cardiac abnormalities is often not indicated. In spinal muscular atrophy type III, awareness of the potential for associated cardiac abnormalities is necessary. Permanent pacing may be required.

GUILLAIN-BARRÉ SYNDROME

CLINICAL PRESENTATION. Guillain-Barré syndrome is an acute inflammatory demyelinating neuropathy characterized by peripheral, cranial, and autonomic nerve dysfunction.[77] It is the most common acquired demyelinating neuropathy, with an annual incidence of 1.7 per 100,000 population. In two-thirds of affected patients, an acute viral or bacterial illness, typically respiratory or gastrointestinal, precedes the onset of neurological symptoms by 5 days to 3 weeks. The disorder typically presents with symmetrical limb weakness that can progress to involve cranial and respiratory muscles. Approximately one-third of individuals require assisted ventilation.

CARDIOVASCULAR MANIFESTATIONS. Cardiac involvement in Guillain-Barré syndrome is related to accompanying autonomic nervous system dysfunction that manifests as hypertension, orthostatic hypotension, resting sinus tachycardia, loss of heart rate variability, ECG ST abnormalities, and both bradycardia and tachycardias. Significant autonomic nervous system dysfunction occurs primarily in severe cases of Guillain-Barré syndrome. Microneurographic recordings have shown increased sympathetic outflow during the acute illness that normalizes with recovery.

Life-threatening arrhythmias are common in severe cases of Guillain-Barré syndrome, primarily those requiring assisted ventilation. Arrhythmias observed include asystole, symptomatic bradycardia, rapid atrial fibrillation, and ventricular tachycardia/fibrillation. Deaths due to arrhythmias occur. Asystole was commonly associated with tracheal suctioning.

TREATMENT AND PROGNOSIS. In addition to supportive care, early plasmapheresis and intravenous immunoglobulin can improve recovery. In patients requiring ventilation, cardiac rhythm monitoring is mandatory. If serious bradycardia or asystole is observed, temporary or permanent pacing can improve survival. Atropine or isoproterenol during tracheal suctioning can be of benefit. The mortality rate in individuals hospitalized with Guillain-Barré syndrome is as high as 20 percent. In individuals who recover from Guillain-Barré syndrome, autonomic function also recovers and long-term arrhythmia risk has not been observed.

MYASTHENIA GRAVIS

CLINICAL PRESENTATION. Myasthenia gravis is a disorder of neuromuscular transmission resulting from production of antibody targeted against the nicotinic acetylcholine receptor. The primary symptom, fluctuating weakness, usually begins with the eye and facial muscles and later can involve the large muscles of the limbs. Patients can present at any age, typically at a younger age in women and an older age in men. Myasthenia gravis is usually associated with hyperplasia or a benign or malignant tumor (thymoma) of the thymus gland. The prevalence in the United States is 1 per 33,000 persons.

CARDIOVASCULAR MANIFESTATIONS. A myocarditis can be associated with myasthenia gravis, especially that occurring with thymoma. A cardiac muscle antibody is believed to be responsible. Up to 16 percent of patients with myasthenia gravis have cardiac manifestations not explained by another etiology. Presentation is typically with arrhythmic symptoms including atrial fibrillation, atrioventricular block, asystole, and unexplained sudden death. Autopsy findings were consistent with myocarditis.

TREATMENT AND PROGNOSIS. Myasthenia gravis is treated with anticholinesterase and immunosuppressive agents. Thymectomy is often indicated. Anticholinesterase agents may slow heart rate and cause hypotension. Whether immunosuppressive agents or thymectomy improve associated cardiac disease is unknown. Use of quinidine or propranolol in patients with myasthenia gravis may precipitate an acute exacerbation of weakness.

Acute Cerebrovascular Disease

CARDIOVASCULAR MANIFESTATIONS. Acute cerebrovascular diseases, including subarachnoid hemorrhage, other stroke syndromes and head injury, can be associated with severe cardiac manifestations.[78] The mechanism by which this occurs appears to be related to abnormal autonomic nervous system function, primarily a markedly increased sympathetic and parasympathetic output (see Chap. 87). Hypothalamic stimulation can reproduce the ECG changes observed in acute cerebrovascular disease. ECG changes associated with hypothalamic stimulation or blood in the subarachnoid space can be diminished with spinal cord transection, stellate ganglion blockade, vagolytics, and adrenergic blockers.

ECG abnormalities are observed in as high as 80 to 90 percent of individuals with subarachnoid hemorrhage. Abnormalities including ST elevation and depression, T wave inversion, and pathologic Q waves are observed.[79] Peaked inverted T waves and a prolonged QT interval can occur in 25 to 40 percent of patients (Fig. 85–16). Hypokalemia is observed in up to 50 percent of patients with subarachnoid hemorrhage, and this increases the likelihood of QT interval prolongation. Other stroke syndromes are often associated with abnormal ECGs but whether these are related to the stroke syndrome or to underlying intrinsic cardiac disease is often difficult to discern. A prolonged QT interval is more common in subarachnoid hemorrhage than other stroke syndromes. Closed-head trauma can cause similar ECG abnormalities as subarachnoid hemorrhage including a prolonged QT interval.

Myocardial damage with liberation of myocardial enzymes and subendocardial hemorrhage or fibrosis at autopsy can occur in the setting of acute cerebrovascular disease. Like the ECG changes, these abnormalities are believed to be related to local myocardial catecholamine excess.

Neurogenic pulmonary edema can accompany the acute neurological insult. The edema can have both a cardiogenic component, related to systemic hypertension, and a noncardiogenic (pulmonary capillary leak) component.

Life-threatening arrhythmias can occur in the setting of acute cerebrovascular disease. Ventricular tachycardia or fibrillation has been observed in patients with subarachnoid hemorrhage and head trauma. A torsades de pointes–type of ventricular tachycardia can occur (Fig. 85–17). Often this is observed in the setting of a prolonged QT interval and hypokalemia. Stroke syndromes, other than subarachnoid hemorrhage, appear to be only rarely associated with serious ventricular tachycardias. Atrial arrhythmias including atrial fibrillation and regular supraventricular tachycardia have been observed. Atrial fibrillation is most common in individuals presenting with what is believed to be an acute thromboembolic stroke. Separating an effect from the cause can be difficult. Bradycardias including sinoatrial block, sinus arrest, and atrioventricular block occur in up to 10 percent of individuals with subarachnoid hemorrhage.

TREATMENT AND PROGNOSIS. Beta-adrenergic blockers appear effective in decreasing myocardial damage and in controlling both supraventricular and ventricular arrhythmias associated with subarachnoid hemorrhage and head trauma. Beta-adrenergic blockers can increase the likelihood of bradycardia. Life-threatening arrhythmias occur primarily in the first day following the neurological event. Continuous ECG monitoring during this period is indicated. Careful monitoring of potassium levels especially in patients with subarachnoid hemorrhage is warranted. Refractory ventricular arrhythmias have been controlled effectively with stellate ganglion blockade. ECG abnormalities reflect adverse intracranial factors but do not appear to portend a poor cardiovascular outcome.

Head injury (blunt trauma or gunshot wound) and cerebrovascular accident are the leading causes of brain death in individuals being considered as heart donors. These donors can manifest ECG abnormalities, hemodynamic instability,

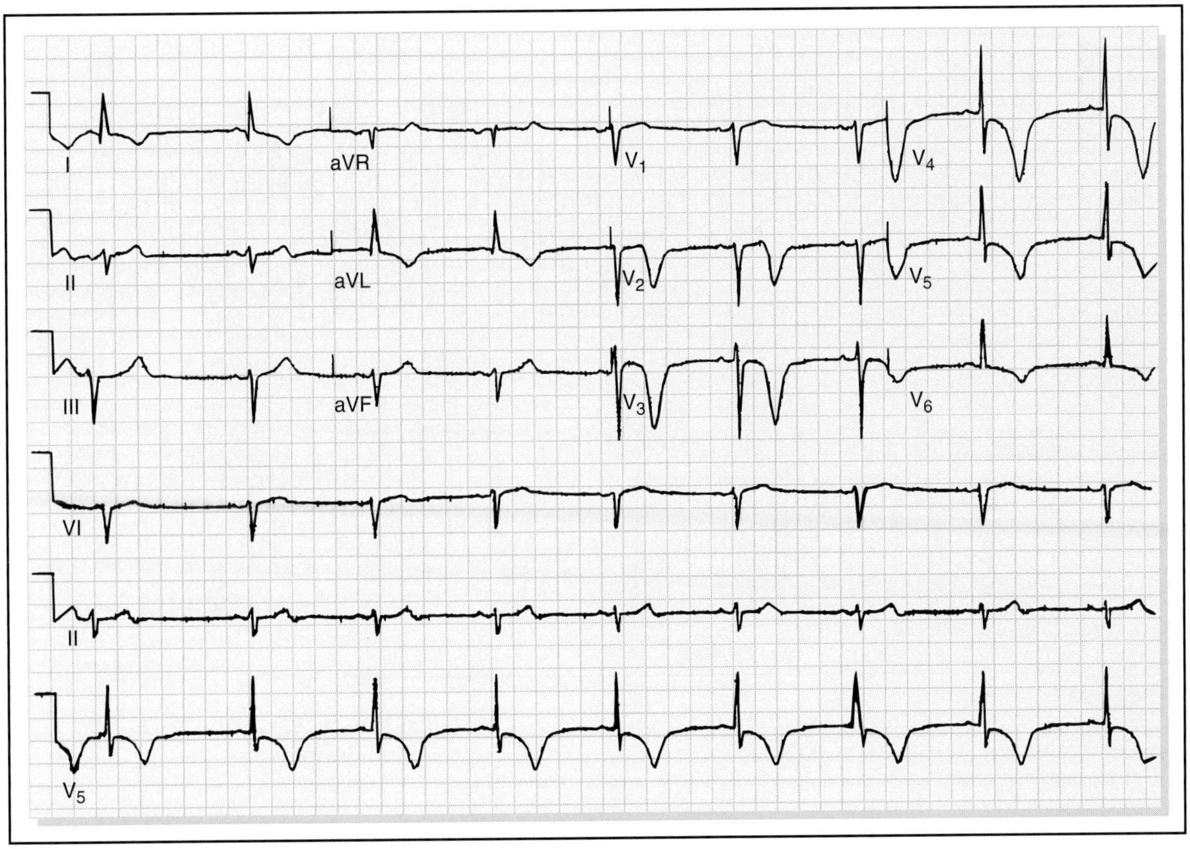

FIGURE 85–16 Electrocardiogram from a patient with cerebral hemorrhage. Deep and symmetrical T wave inversions are observed. (Courtesy of Charles Fisch, MD, Indiana University School of Medicine, Indianapolis, IN.)

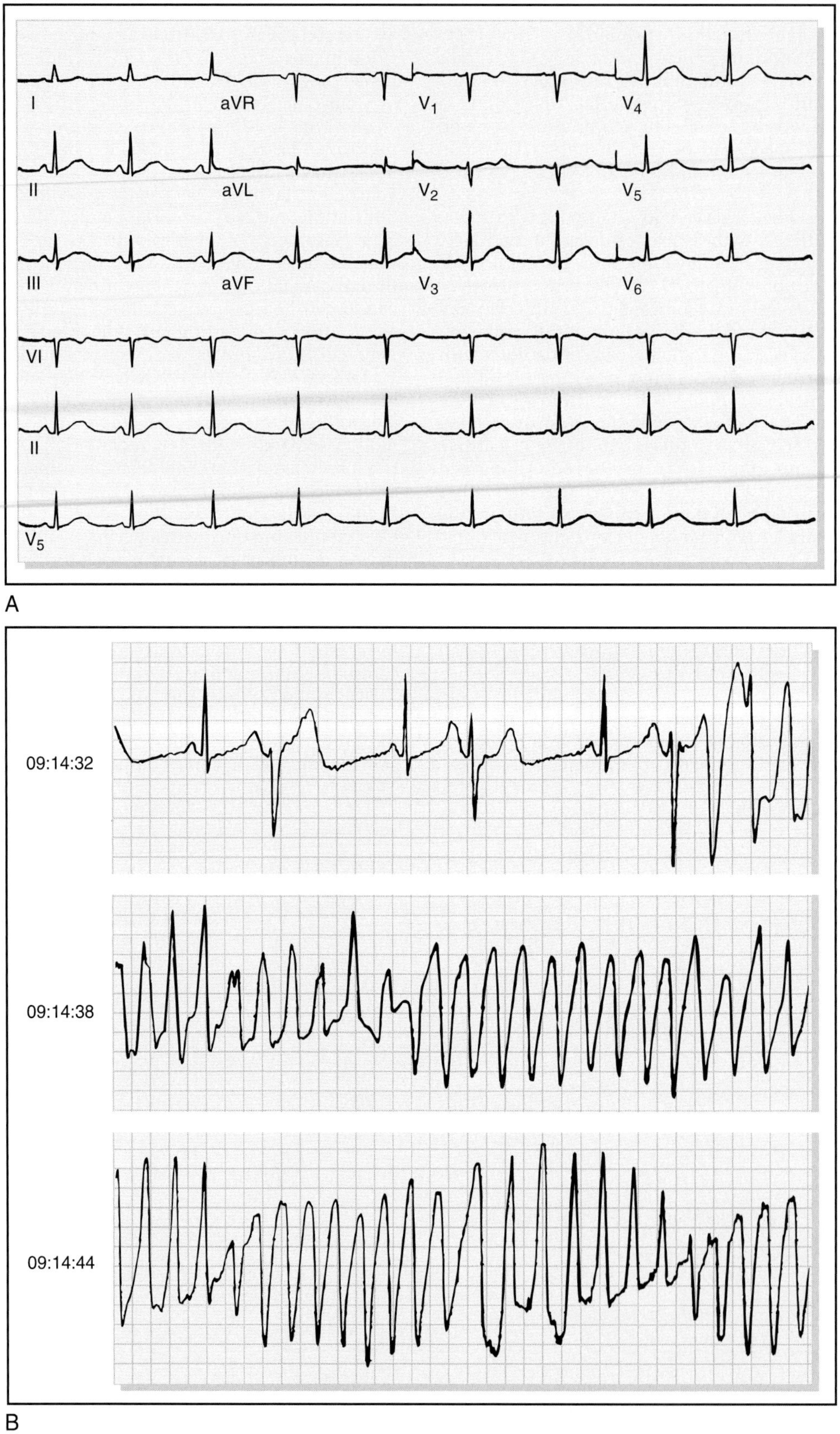

FIGURE 85–17 A 49-year-old patient with cerebral hemorrhage. **A,** Electrocardiogram recorded within 3 hours of admission and 4 hours after onset of symptoms. QT interval prolongation is observed. **B,** Electrocardiographic monitoring 6 hours after admission. Ventricular bigeminy precedes the onset of polymorphic ventricular tachycardia. Cardioversion was required. The patient was subsequently treated with a beta-adrenergic blocker without further ventricular tachycardia.

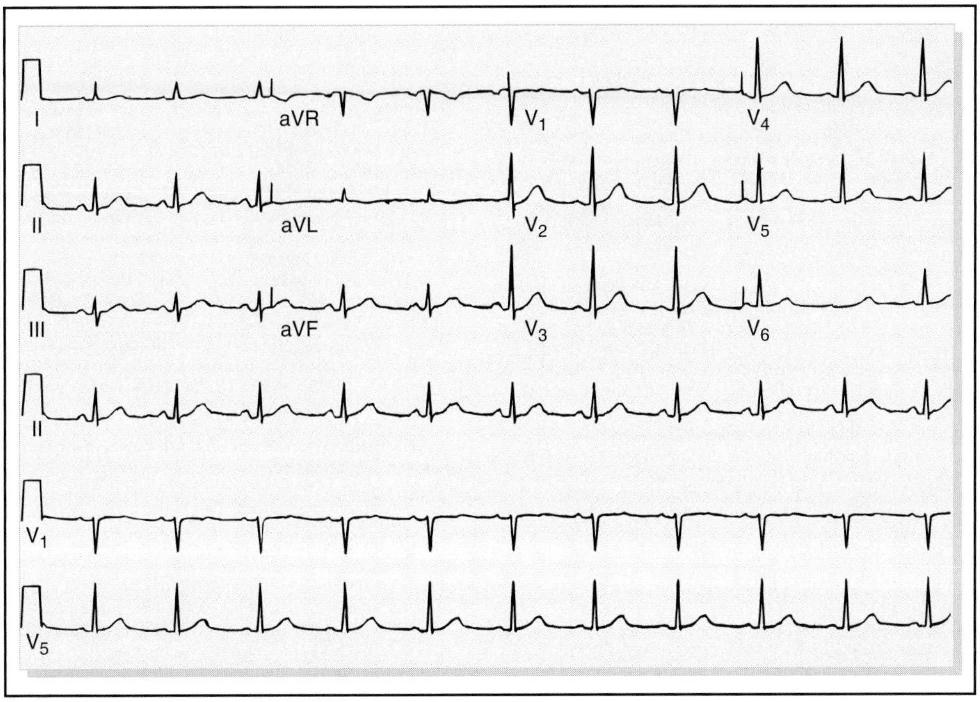

C

FIGURE 85–17, cont'd **C,** Electrocardiogram done 2 weeks after admission. The QT interval has normalized.

and myocardial dysfunction related primarily to adrenergic storm and not to intrinsic cardiac disease. Experimental studies on whether contractile performance recovers with transplantation are still controversial.[80] Optimization of volume status and inotropic support with careful echocardiographic evaluation and possibly left heart catheterization can allow the use of some donor hearts that would have otherwise been rejected.

REFERENCES

Duchenne and Becker Muscular Dystrophies

1. Towbin JA: The role of cytoskeletal proteins in cardiomyopathies. Curr Opin Cell Biol 10:131-9, 1998.
2. Ortiz-Lopez R, Li H, Su J, et al: Evidence for a dystrophin missense mutation as a cause of X-linked dilated cardiomyopathy. Circulation 95:2434-40, 1997.
3. Kaprielian RR, Stevenson S, Rothery SM, et al: Distinct patterns of dystrophin organization in myocyte sarcolemma and transverse tubules of normal and diseased human myocardium. Circulation 101:2586-94, 2000.
4. Biggar WD, Klamut HJ, Demacio PC, et al: Duchenne muscular dystrophy: Current knowledge, treatment, and future prospects. Clinical Orthop 88-106, 2002.
5. Hoogerwaard EM, de Voogt WG, Wilde AA, et al: Evolution of cardiac abnormalities in Becker muscular dystrophy over a 13-year period. J Neurol 244:657-63, 1997.
6. Melacini P, Fanin M, Danieli GA, et al: Myocardial involvement is very frequent among patients affected with subclinical Becker's muscular dystrophy. Circulation 94:3168-75, 1996.
7. Saito M, Kawai H, Akaike M, et al: Cardiac dysfunction with Becker muscular dystrophy. Am Heart J 132:642-7, 1996.
8. Hoogerwaard EM, Bakker E, Ippel PF, et al: Signs and symptoms of Duchenne muscular dystrophy and Becker muscular dystrophy among carriers in The Netherlands: A cohort study. Lancet 353:2116-9, 1999.
9. Negri SM, Cowan MD: Becker muscular dystrophy with bundle branch reentry ventricular tachycardia. J Cardiovasc Electrophysiol 9:652-4, 1998.
10. Case records of the Massachusetts General Hospital: Weekly clinicopathological exercises. Case 22-1998. A 22-year-old man with a cardiac transplant and creatine kinase elevation. N Engl J Med 339:182-90, 1998.

Myotonic Muscular Dystrophy

11. New nomenclature and DNA testing guidelines for myotonic dystrophy type 1 (DM1). The International Myotonic Dystrophy Consortium (IDMC). Neurology 54:1218-21, 2000.
12. Groh WJ, Lowe MR, Zipes DP: Severity of cardiac conduction involvement and arrhythmias in myotonic dystrophy type 1 correlates with age and CTG repeat length. J Cardiovasc Electrophysiol 13:444-8, 2002.
13. Tapscott SJ: Deconstructing myotonic dystrophy. Science 289:1701-2, 2000.
14. Tapscott SJ, Thornton CA: Biomedicine. Reconstructing myotonic dystrophy. Science 293:816-7, 2001.
15. Berul CI, Maguire CT, Aronovitz MJ, et al: DMPK dosage alterations result in atrioventricular conduction abnormalities in a mouse myotonic dystrophy model. J Clin Invest 103:R1-7, 1999.
16. Abbruzzese C, Krahe R, Liguori M, et al: Myotonic dystrophy phenotype without expansion of (CTG)n repeat: An entity distinct from proximal myotonic myopathy (PROMM)? J Neurol 243:715-21, 1996.
17. Meola G, Sansone V, Marinou K, et al: Proximal myotonic myopathy: A syndrome with a favourable prognosis? J Neurol Sci 193:89-96, 2002.
18. von zur Muhlen F, Klass C, Kreuzer H, et al: Cardiac involvement in proximal myotonic myopathy. Heart 79:619-21, 1998.
19. Ranum LP, Rasmussen PF, Benzow KA, et al: Genetic mapping of a second myotonic dystrophy locus. Nature Genet 19:196-8, 1998.
20. Liquori CL, Ricker K, Moseley ML, et al: Myotonic dystrophy type 2 caused by a CCTG expansion in intron 1 of ZNF9. Science 293:864-7, 2001.
21. Finsterer J, Gharehbaghi-Schnell E, Stollberger C, et al: Relation of cardiac abnormalities and CTG-repeat size in myotonic dystrophy. Clin Genet 59:350-5, 2001.
22. Lazarus A, Varin J, Ounnoughene Z, et al: Relationships among electrophysiological findings and clinical status, heart function, and extent of DNA mutation in myotonic dystrophy. Circulation 99:1041-6, 1999.
23. Gregoratos G, Abrams J, Epstein AE, et al: ACC/AHA/NASPE 2002 guideline update for implantation of cardiac pacemakers and antiarrhythmia devices. Circulation 106:2145-61, 2002.
24. Merino JL, Carmona JR, Fernandez-Lozano I, et al: Mechanisms of sustained ventricular tachycardia in myotonic dystrophy: Implications for catheter ablation. Circulation 98:541-546, 1998.
25. de Die-Smulders CE, Howeler CJ, Thijs C, et al: Age and causes of death in adult-onset myotonic dystrophy. Brain 121:1557-63, 1998.
26. Mathieu J, Allard P, Potvin L, et al: A 10-year study of mortality in a cohort of patients with myotonic dystrophy. Neurology 52:1658-62, 1999.
27. Stollberger C, Finsterer J, Keller H, et al: Progression of cardiac involvement in patients with myotonic dystrophy, Becker's muscular dystrophy and mitochondrial myopathy during a 2-year follow-up. Cardiology 90:173-9, 1998.
28. Colleran JA, Hawley RJ, Pinnow EE, et al: Value of the electrocardiogram in determining cardiac events and mortality in myotonic dystrophy. Am J Cardiol 80:1494-1497, 1997.
29. Phillips MF, Harper PS: Cardiac disease in myotonic dystrophy. Cardiovasc Res 33:13-22, 1997.
30. Hadian D, Lowe MR, Scott LR, et al: Use of an insertable loop recorder in a myotonic dystrophy patient. J Cardiovasc Electrophysiol 13:72-3, 2002.

Emery-Dreifuss Muscular Dystrophy and Associated Disorders

31. Nigro V, Bruni P, Ciccodicola A, et al: SSCP detection of novel mutations in patients with Emery-Dreifuss muscular dystrophy: Definition of a small C-terminal region required for emerin function. Hum Mol Genet 4:2003-4, 1995.
32. Nagano A, Koga R, Ogawa M, et al: Emerin deficiency at the nuclear membrane in patients with Emery-Dreifuss muscular dystrophy. Nature Genet 12:254-9, 1996.

33. Bonne G, Di Barletta MR, Varnous S, et al: Mutations in the gene encoding lamin A/C cause autosomal dominant Emery-Dreifuss muscular dystrophy. Nature Genet 21:285-8, 1999.
34. Di Barletta MR, Ricci E, Galluzzi G, et al: Different mutations in the LMNA gene cause autosomal dominant and autosomal recessive Emery-Dreifuss muscular dystrophy. Am J Hum Genet 66:1407-12, 2000.
35. Muchir A, Bonne G, van der Kooi AJ, et al: Identification of mutations in the gene encoding lamins A/C in autosomal dominant limb girdle muscular dystrophy with atrioventricular conduction disturbances (LGMD1B). Hum Mol Genet 9:1453-9, 2000.
36. Fatkin D, MacRae C, Sasaki T, et al: Missense mutations in the rod domain of the lamin A/C gene as causes of dilated cardiomyopathy and conduction-system disease. N Engl J Med 341:1715-24, 1999.
37. van der Kooi AJ, Bonne G, Eymard B, et al: Lamin A/C mutations with lipodystrophy, cardiac abnormalities, and muscular dystrophy. Neurology 59:620-3, 2002.
38. Cartegni L, di Barletta MR, Barresi R, et al: Heart-specific localization of emerin: New insights into Emery-Dreifuss muscular dystrophy. Hum Mol Genet 6:2257-64, 1997.
39. Manilal S, Sewry CA, Pereboev A, et al: Distribution of emerin and lamins in the heart and implications for Emery-Dreifuss muscular dystrophy. Hum Mol Genet 8:353-9, 1999.
40. Felice KJ, Schwartz RC, Brown CA, et al: Autosomal dominant Emery-Dreifuss dystrophy due to mutations in rod domain of the lamin A/C gene. Neurology 55:275-80, 2000.
41. Manilal S, Sewry CA, Man N, et al: Diagnosis of X-linked Emery-Dreifuss muscular dystrophy by protein analysis of leucocytes and skin with monoclonal antibodies. Neuromusc Disord 7:63-6, 1997.

Limb-Girdle Muscular Dystrophy

42. Mathews KD, Moore SA: Limb-girdle muscular dystrophy. Curr Neurol Neurosci Rep 3:78-85, 2003.
43. Beckmann JS, Brown RH, Muntoni F, et al: 66th/67th ENMC sponsored international workshop: The limb-girdle muscular dystrophies, 26-28 March 1999, Naarden, The Netherlands. Neuromusc Disord 9:436-45, 1999.
44. Fadic R, Sunada Y, Waclawik AJ, et al: Brief report: deficiency of a dystrophin-associated glycoprotein (adhalin) in a patient with muscular dystrophy and cardiomyopathy. N Engl J Med 334:362-6, 1996.
45. van der Kooi AJ, de Voogt WG, Barth PG, et al: The heart in limb girdle muscular dystrophy. Heart 79:73-7, 1998.
46. Melacini P, Fanin M, Duggan DJ, et al: Heart involvement in muscular dystrophies due to sarcoglycan gene mutations. Muscle Nerve 22:473-9, 1999.
47. Tsubata S, Bowles KR, Vatta M, et al: Mutations in the human delta-sarcoglycan gene in familial and sporadic dilated cardiomyopathy. J Clin Invest 106:655-62, 2000.
48. Barresi R, Di Blasi C, Negri T, et al: Disruption of heart sarcoglycan complex and severe cardiomyopathy caused by beta sarcoglycan mutations. J Med Genet 37:102-7, 2000.
49. Coral-Vazquez R, Cohn RD, Moore SA, et al: Disruption of the sarcoglycan-sarcospan complex in vascular smooth muscle: A novel mechanism for cardiomyopathy and muscular dystrophy. Cell 98:465-74, 1999.
50. Gnecchi-Ruscone T, Taylor J, Mercuri E, et al: Cardiomyopathy in Duchenne, Becker, and sarcoglycanopathies: A role for coronary dysfunction? Muscle Nerve 22:1549-56, 1999.
51. Cohn RD, Durbeej M, Moore SA, et al: Prevention of cardiomyopathy in mouse models lacking the smooth muscle sarcoglycan-sarcospan complex. J Clin Invest 107:R1-7, 2001.
52. van der Kooi AJ, Ledderhof TM, de Voogt WG, et al: A newly recognized autosomal dominant limb girdle muscular dystrophy with cardiac involvement. Ann Neurol 39:636-42, 1996.

Facioscapulohomeral Muscular Dystrophy

53. A prospective, quantitative study of the natural history of facioscapulohumeral muscular dystrophy (FSHD): Implications for therapeutic trials. The FSH-DY Group. Neurology 48:38-46, 1997.
54. Orrell RW, Tawil R, Forrester J, et al: Definitive molecular diagnosis of facioscapulohumeral dystrophy. Neurology 52:1822-6, 1999.
55. Laforet P, de Toma C, Eymard B, et al: Cardiac involvement in genetically confirmed facioscapulohumeral muscular dystrophy. Neurology 51:1454-6, 1998.

Friedreich Ataxia

56. Lynch DR, Farmer JM, Balcer LJ, et al: Friedreich ataxia: Effects of genetic understanding on clinical evaluation and therapy. Arch Neurol 59:743-7, 2002.
57. Wong A, Yang J, Cavadini P, et al: The Friedreich's ataxia mutation confers cellular sensitivity to oxidant stress which is rescued by chelators of iron and calcium and inhibitors of apoptosis. Hum Mol Genet 8:425-30, 1999.
58. Rotig A, de Lonlay P, Chretien D, et al: Aconitase and mitochondrial iron-sulphur protein deficiency in Friedreich ataxia. Nature Genet 17:215-7, 1997.
59. Lodi R, Rajagopalan B, Blamire AM, et al: Cardiac energetics are abnormal in Friedreich ataxia patients in the absence of cardiac dysfunction and hypertrophy: An in vivo 31P magnetic resonance spectroscopy study. Cardiovasc Res 52:111-9, 2001.
60. Isnard R, Kalotka H, Durr A, et al: Correlation between left ventricular hypertrophy and GAA trinucleotide repeat length in Friedreich's ataxia. Circulation 95:2247-9, 1997.
61. Maione S, Giunta A, Filla A, et al: May age onset be relevant in the occurrence of left ventricular hypertrophy in Friedreich's ataxia? Clin Cardiol 20:141-5, 1997.
62. Hausse AO, Aggoun Y, Bonnet D, et al: Idebenone and reduced cardiac hypertrophy in Friedreich's ataxia. Heart (British Cardiac Society) 87:346-9, 2002.
63. Schulz JB, Dehmer T, Schols L, et al: Oxidative stress in patients with Friedreich ataxia.[comment]. Neurology 55:1719-21, 2000.

Less Common Neuromuscular Diseases Associated with Cardiac Manifestations

64. Bulman DE: Phenotype variation and newcomers in ion channel disorders. Hum Mol Genet 6:1679-85, 1997.
65. Bulman DE, Scoggan KA, van Oene MD, et al: A novel sodium channel mutation in a family with hypokalemic periodic paralysis. Neurology 53:1932-6, 1999.
66. Ptacek LJ: Channelopathies: Ion channel disorders of muscle as a paradigm for paroxysmal disorders of the nervous system. Neuromusc Disord 7:250-5, 1997.
67. Sansone V, Griggs RC, Meola G, et al: Andersen's syndrome: A distinct periodic paralysis. Ann Neurol 42:305-12, 1997.
68. Plaster NM, Tawil R, Tristani-Firouzi M, et al: Mutations in Kir2.1 cause the developmental and episodic electrical phenotypes of Andersen's syndrome. Cell 105:511-9, 2001.
69. Ai T, Fujiwara Y, Tsuji K, et al: Novel KCNJ2 mutation in familial periodic paralysis with ventricular dysrhythmia. Circulation 105:2592-4, 2002.
70. Tristani-Firouzi M, Jensen JL, Donaldson MR, et al: Functional and clinical characterization of KCNJ2 mutations associated with LQT7 (Andersen syndrome). J Clin Invest 110:381-8, 2002.
71. Simon DK, Johns DR: Mitochondrial disorders: Clinical and genetic features. Ann Rev Med 50:111-27, 1999.
72. Santorelli FM, Tessa A, D'Amati G, et al: The emerging concept of mitochondrial cardiomyopathies. Am Heart J 141:E1, 2001.
73. Anan R, Nakagawa M, Miyata M, et al: Cardiac involvement in mitochondrial diseases. A study on 17 patients with documented mitochondrial DNA defects. Circulation 91:955-61, 1995.
74. Akaike M, Kawai H, Yokoi K, et al: Cardiac dysfunction in patients with chronic progressive external ophthalmoplegia. Clin Cardiol 20:239-43, 1997.
75. Stewart H, Wallace A, McGaughran J, et al: Molecular diagnosis of spinal muscular atrophy. Arch Dis Child 78:531-5, 1998.
76. Iannaccone ST, American Spinal Muscular Atrophy Randomized Trials G: Outcome measures for pediatric spinal muscular atrophy. Arch Neurol 59:1445-50, 2002.
77. Hahn AF: Guillain-Barre syndrome. Lancet 352:635-41, 1998.

Acute Cerebrovascular Disease

78. Sakr YL, Ghosn I, Vincent JL: Cardiac manifestations after subarachnoid hemorrhage: A systematic review of the literature. Prog Cardiovasc Dis 45:67-80, 2002.
79. Zaroff JG, Rordorf GA, Newell JB, et al: Cardiac outcome in patients with subarachnoid hemorrhage and electrocardiographic abnormalities. Neurosurg 44:34-9, 1999.
80. Szabo G, Sebening C, Hackert T, et al: Effects of brain death on myocardial function and ischemic tolerance of potential donor hearts. J Heart Lung Transplant 17:921-30, 1998.

CHAPTER 86

Interface Between Renal Disease and Cardiovascular Illness

Peter A. McCullough

The Cardiorenal Intersection

The heart and kidney are inextricably linked in terms of hemodynamic and regulatory functions. In a normal 70-kg man, each kidney weighs about 130 to 170 gm and receives blood flow of 400 ml/min per 100 gm, which is approximately 20 to 25 percent of the cardiac output, allowing the needed flow to maintain glomerular filtration. This flow is several times greater per unit weight of organ than the blood flow through most other organs. Although the oxygen extraction is low, the kidneys account for about 8 percent of the total oxygen consumption of the body. The kidney has a central role in electrolyte balance, volume, and blood pressure regulation. Communication between these two organs occurs at multiple levels, including the sympathetic nervous system, the renin-angiotensin-aldosterone system (RAAS) (Fig. 86–1), antidiuretic hormone, endothelin, and the natriuretic peptides (Fig. 86–2). With the understanding of these systems has come the development of key diagnostic and therapeutic targets in cardiovascular medicine.

The modern epidemics of obesity and hypertension (HTN) in the developed countries are central drivers of a secondary epidemic of type 2 diabetes with combined chronic kidney disease (CKD) and cardiovascular disease (CVD).[1] Among those with diabetes for 25 years or more, the prevalence of diabetic nephropathy in type 1 and type 2 diabetes is 57 and 48 percent, respectively.[2] Approximately half of all cases of end-stage renal disease (ESRD) are due to diabetic nephropathy. With the aging of the general population and cardiovascular care shifting toward the elderly population, an understanding of why decreasing levels of renal function act as a major adverse prognostic factor after a variety of cardiac events is imperative. Considerable evidence shows that CKD accelerates atherosclerosis, myocardial disease, and valvular disease and promotes an array of cardiac arrhythmias.[3]

Chronic Kidney Disease and Cardiovascular Risk

CKD is defined through a range of estimated glomerular filtration rate (eGFR) values by the National Kidney Foundation Kidney Disease Outcomes Quality Initiative (KDOQI) (Fig. 86–3).[4] A common definition for CKD stipulates an eGFR of less than 60 ml/min/1.73 m^2 or the presence of albuminuria, defined as an albumin-to-creatinine ratio greater than 30 mg/gm on a spot urine sample (Fig. 86–4). Although with normative aging (age 20 to 80), the eGFR declines from about 130 to 60 ml/min/1.73 m^2, a variety of pathobiological processes appear to begin when the eGFR drops below 60 ml/min/1.73 m^2. Most studies of cardiovascular outcomes have found that a break point for the development of contrast-induced nephropathy (CIN), restenosis after percutaneous coronary intervention (PCI), recurrent myocardial infarction (MI), diastolic/systolic congestive heart failure (CHF), arrhythmias, and cardiovascular death occurs below an eGFR of 60 ml/min/1.73 m^2, which roughly corresponds to a serum creatinine (Cr) greater than 1.5 mg/dl in the general population.[4-8] Because Cr is a crude indicator of renal function and often underestimates renal dysfunction in women and elderly people, calculated measures of eGFR or creatinine clearance (CrCl) using the Cockcroft-Gault equation or the Modification of Diet in Renal Disease (MDRD) equation are superior methods for the assessment of renal function.[4] The four-variable MDRD equation for CrCl is the preferred method because it does not rely on body weight.[4] This equation is

$$\text{CrCl} = 186.3\,(\text{serum creatinine}^{-1.154}) \times (\text{age}^{-.203})$$

and calculated values are multiplied by 0.742 for women and by 1.21 for blacks.

In addition, microalbuminuria at any level of eGFR is considered to represent CKD and has been thought to occur as the result of hyperfiltration in the kidneys because of diabetes and HTN-related changes in the glomeruli.[9] Several definitions have been proposed for microalbuminuria.[9] The most widely accepted is a random urine albumin/creatinine ratio (ACR) of 30 to 300 mg/gm. An ACR greater than 300 mg/gm is usually considered gross proteinuria. Microalbuminuria as an independent CVD risk factor is covered elsewhere in this text. The Seventh Report of the Joint National Committee on Prevention, Detection, Evaluation, and Treatment of High Blood Pressure (JNC 7) has recognized CKD as an independent cardiovascular risk state.[10] This risk state has a host

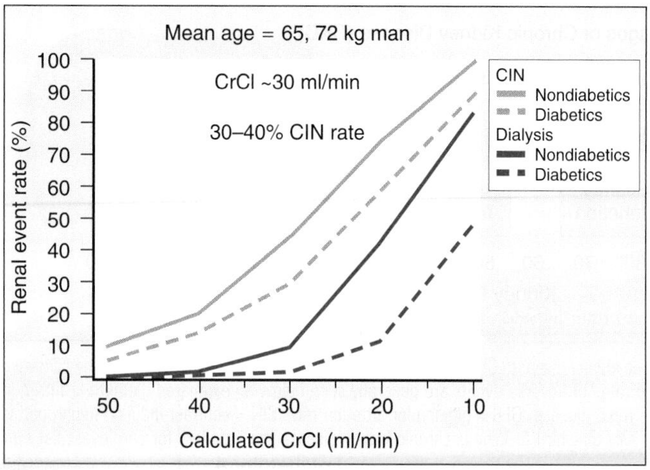

FIGURE 86–5 Validated risk of acute renal failure requiring dialysis after diagnostic angiography and ad hoc angioplasty, assuming a mean contrast dose of 250 ml and a mean age of 65. CrCl = creatinine clearance; CIN = contrast-induced nephropathy. (Data adapted from McCullough PA, Manley HJ: Prediction and prevention of contrast nephropathy. J Interv Cardiol 14:547, 2001.)

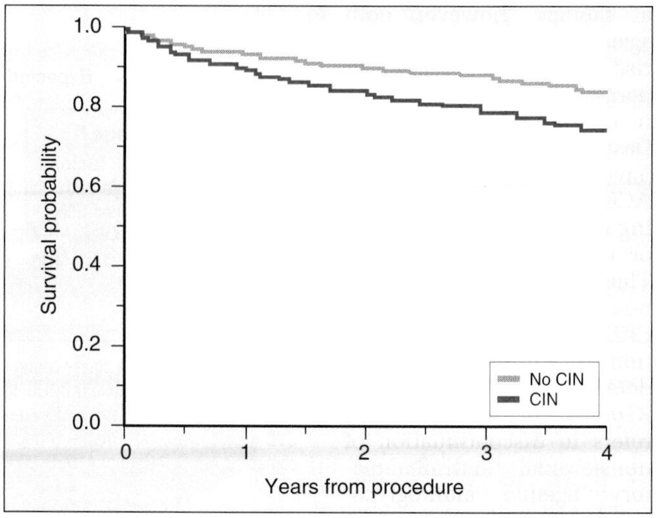

FIGURE 86–6 Adjusted, long-term outcomes in 7586 patients with and without contrast-induced nephropathy (CIN) after angioplasty, $p < 0.0001$. Contrast-induced nephropathy is defined as a 0.5 mg/dl rise in creatinine after percutaneous coronary intervention. (Adapted from Rihal CS, Textor SC, Grill DE, et al: Incidence and prognostic importance of acute renal failure after percutaneous coronary intervention. Circulation 105:2259, 2002.)

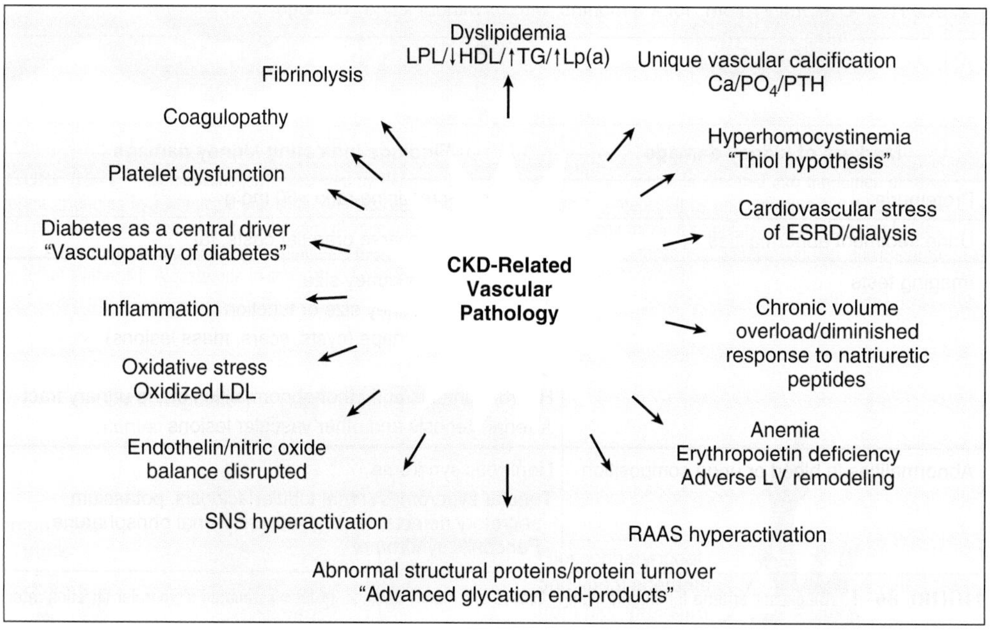

FIGURE 86–7 The pathobiology of the chronic kidney disease state and its effects on the cardiovascular system. Ca = calcium; CKD = chronic kidney disease; ESRD = end-stage renal disease; HDL = high-density lipoprotein; LDL-C = low-density lipoprotein cholesterol; Lp(a) = lipoprotein (a) ; LPL = lipoprotein lipase; LV = left ventricle; NO = nitric oxide; PO_4 = phosphate; PTH = parathyroid hormone; RAAS = renin-angiotensin-aldosterone system; SNS = sympathetic nervous system; TG = triglyceride. (Adapted from McCullough PA: Why is chronic kidney disease the "spoiler" for cardiovascular outcomes? J Am Coll Cardiol 41:725, 2003.)

provoke a vasodilation and an osmotic diuresis. However, when there is vascular disease, endothelial dysfunction, and glomerular injury, the contrast agent and the multifactorial insult of renal hypoxia provoke a vasoconstrictive response and mediate ischemic injury. The most important predictor of CIN is underlying renal dysfunction. The "remnant nephron" theory postulates that after sufficient chronic kidney damage has occurred and the eGFR is reduced to less than 60 ml/min/1.73 m^2, the remaining nephrons must assume the residual filtration load. The residual nephrons also have increased oxygen demands and are more susceptible to ischemic and oxidative injury.

Prevention of Contrast-Induced Nephropathy after Percutaneous Coronary Intervention

A prevention strategy for CIN should be employed for patients with diabetes as well as patients with preexisting CKD (baseline eGFR < 60 ml/min/1.73 m^2). In general, at an eGFR of 30 ml/min/1.73 m^2, the expected rate of contrast nephropathy is 30 to 40 percent and the rates of acute renal failure requiring dialysis are approximately 2 to 8 percent (see Fig. 86–4).[12] There are four basic concepts in contrast nephropathy prevention: (1) hydration, (2) choice and quantity of contrast material, (3) pre-, intra-, and postprocedural end-organ protection with pharmacotherapy, and (4) postprocedural monitoring and expectant care.

Hydration with intravenous normal or half-normal saline is reasonable, starting 3 to 12 hours prior to the procedure at a rate of 1 to 2 ml/kg/hr.[33-36] In those at risk, at least 300 to 500 ml of intravenous hydration should be received before the contrast material is administered. If there are particular concerns regarding volume overload or CHF in individuals in whom clinical assessment of volume status is difficult, a right-heart catheterization may aid management during and after the procedure. The postprocedure hydration target is a urine output of 150 ml/hr. If patients have a diuresis of more than a 150 ml/hr, they should have replacement of extra losses with more intravenous fluid. In general, this strategy calls for hydration orders of normal or half-normal saline at 150 ml/hr for at least 6 hours after the procedure. Achieving adequate urine flow rates in a clinical trial setting reduced the rate of contrast nephropathy by 50 percent.[35]

As discussed previously, two large-scale, double-blind randomized controlled trials indicated that the lower the ionicity and osmolality of the contrast agent, the less renal toxicity is expected; this has now been confirmed. In the Iohexol Cooperative Study, $n = 1196$, iohexol (Omnipaque) was found to be superior to a high-ionic contrast agent (diatrizoate meglumine [Hypaque-76]) in patients with diabetes and baseline CKD.[36] In the Nephrotoxicity in High-Risk Patients Study of Iso-Osmolar and Low-Osmolar Non-Ionic Contrast Media (NEPHRIC), iodixanol (Visipaque), a nonionic, isosmolar contrast agent, proved to be superior to iohexol with lower rates of contrast nephropathy observed.[37] Iodixanol was also demonstrated to be less thrombogenic than other contrast agents in the Contrast Media Utilization in High-Risk Percutaneous Transluminal Coronary Angioplasty (COURT) trial, with a 45 percent reduction in major adverse cardiac events compared with ioxaglate meglumine (Hexabrix); hence, iodixanol is the contrast agent of choice in patients at high renal risk undergoing intervention.[38] Although it is desirable to limit contrast to the smallest volume possible in any setting, there is disagreement about a "safe" contrast limit.[39] The lower the eGFR, the smaller the amount of contrast material needed to cause CIN.[39] In general, it is desirable to limit the contrast medium to less than 100 ml for any procedure.[12,13] If staged procedures are planned, it is advantageous to have more than 10 days between the first and second contrast exposures if contrast nephropathy has occurred with the first procedure.[40]

More than 35 randomized trials have tested various strategies in the prevention of CIN.[12] The majority of these trials were small, underpowered, and did not find the preventive strategy under investigation to be better than placebo. A few lessons have been learned from these trials: (1) diuretics in the form of loop diuretics or mannitol can worsen contrast nephropathy if there is inadequate volume replacement for the diuresis that follows; (2) low-dose or "renal dose" dopamine cannot be achieved despite its popularity in practice, given the counterbalancing forces of intrarenal vasodilation through the dopamine-1 receptor and the vasoconstricting forces of the dopamine-2, alpha, and beta receptors; and (3) renal toxic agents including nonsteroidal antiinflammatory agents, aminoglycosides, and cyclosporine should not be administered in the periprocedural period. There are currently no approved agents for the prevention of CIN.

The most popular strategy at the time of this writing is optimal hydration, iodixanol as the contrast agent of choice, and administration of oral or intravenous *N*-acetylcysteine (NAC), a cytoprotective agent against oxidative injury. In addition, one supportive, double-blind randomized trial of fenoldopam versus placebo demonstrated improved renal blood flow after contrast exposure.[41] However, a large confirmatory trial of fenoldopam failed to demonstrate a protective effect of this agent.[42] Ten trials regarding NAC have now been completed. Five were positive and five were neutral, with an overall edge in favor of NAC (Table 86–1).[43-52] Most operators believe—given the seriousness of CIN, the relative safety of the strategies used, and the evolution of clinical trials shaping our practice—that the combination of hydration, use of iodixanol, and NAC is a reasonable three-pronged approach to minimize CIN and the risk of acute renal failure requiring dialysis in patients at risk.

Postprocedural monitoring is critical in the current era of short stays and outpatient procedures. In general, high-risk patients in the hospital should have hydration started 12 hours before the procedure and continued at least 6 hours

TABLE 86–1 Randomized, Double-Blind, Placebo-Controlled Trials of *N*-Acetylcysteine in the Prevention of Contrast Nephropathy*

Author	Year	*N*	NAC Dose	Contrast Nephropathy Definition	NAC Contrast Nephropathy Rate	Placebo Contrast Nephropathy Rate	*p* Value
Tepel et al[43]	2000	83	600 mg PO b.i.d.	>0.5 mg/dl	1/41 (2.4)	9/42 (21.4)	0.01
Diaz-Sandoval et al[44]	2002	54	600 mg PO b.i.d. (one dose before PCI)	>0.5 mg/dl or >25% rise	2/26 (8.0)	12/28 (45.0)	0.005
Shyu et al[45]	2002	121	400 mg PO b.i.d.	>0.5 mg/dl	2/60 (3.3)	15/61 (24.6)	<0.0001
Kay et al[46]	2003	200	600 mg PO b.i.d.	>25%	4/102 (3.9)	12/98 (12.2)	0.03
Durham et al[47]	2002	79	1200 mg 1 hr before and 3 hr after PCI	>0.5 mg/dl	10/38 (26.3)	9/41 (22.0)	>0.05
Briguori et al[48]	2002	183	600 mg PO b.i.d.	>25%	6/92 (6.5)	10/91 (11.0)	0.22
Allaqaband et al[49]	2002	84	600 mg PO b.i.d.	>0.5 mg/dl	8/45 (17.7)	6/39 (15.3)	0.92
Loutrianakis et al[50]	2003	47	600 mg PO b.i.d.	>0.5 mg/dl >25% rise	6/24 (25.0) 8/24 (33.3)	3/23 (13.0) 2/23 (8.7)	0.20 0.04
RAPPID[51]	2003	80	150 mg/kg over 30 min before and 50 mg/kg over 4 hr after PCI	>0.5 mg/dl or >25% rise	2/41 (4.9)	8/39 (20.5)	0.05
Goldenberg et al[52]	2003	80	600 mg PO t.i.d.	0.5 mg/dl	4/41 (9.8)	3/39 (7.7)	0.52
Total weighted proportions		**1011**	**Various**	**Various**	**45/510 (8.8)**	**85/501 (17.0)**	**0.00001**

*Contrast nephropathy is defined as a rise in creatinine >25% from baseline or an absolute increase >0.5 mg/dl from baseline prior to contrast exposure.
NAC = *N*-acetylcysteine.

afterward. A serum Cr should be measured 24 hours after the procedure. For outpatients, particularly those with eGFR less than 60 ml/min/1.73 m^2, either an overnight stay or discharge to home with 48-hour follow-up and Cr measurement is advised. Individuals in whom severe CIN develops have a rise of Cr greater than 0.5 mg/dl in the first 24 hours after the procedure.[53] Thus, for those who do not have this degree of Cr elevation and an otherwise uneventful course, discharge to home may be considered. Table 86–2 summarizes a strategy for CIN risk assessment and prevention. It is important that CIN risks be discussed in the consent process. For those with eGFR less than 30 ml/min/1.73 m^2, the possibility of dialysis should be mentioned. Lastly, in those with eGFR less than 15 ml/min/1.73 m^2, nephrology consultation is advised with possible planning for dialysis after the procedure.

CKD is the most important factor in predicting adverse short- and long-term outcomes after PCI. The rationale for renal end-organ protection is based on chronic renal protection, avoidance of additive renal insults, and comprehensive CIN prophylaxis. The pathogenesis of CIN goes beyond serum Cr and involves a special vascular pathobiology that interrelates both renal and CVD outcomes.

TABLE 86–2 Ten-Step Checklist for Contrast Nephropathy Risk Stratification and Prevention for Patients at Risk Undergoing Percutaneous Coronary Intervention

Action
1. Calculate eGFR (creatinine clearance)—high risk if <60 ml/min/1.73 m^2
2. Check diabetic status—fivefold higher risk if diabetic
3. Discuss contrast nephropathy risk in informed consent process
4. Discontinue NSAIDs and other renal toxic drugs
5. Nephrology consultation for eGFR <15 ml/min for dialysis planning after PCI
6. Hydration with NS or 0.5 NS 150 ml/hr 3 hr before and 6 hr after procedure
7. Ensure urine flow rate >150 ml/hr after PCI
8. Iodixanol preferred contrast agent
9. Limit contrast volume to <100 ml
10. NAC 600 mg in 30 ml of ginger ale, two doses PO b.i.d. before and 2 doses PO b.i.d. after PCI

eGFR = estimated glomerular filtration rate; NAC = *N*-acetylcysteine; NS = normal saline; NSAID = nonsteroidal antiinflammatory drug; PCI = percutaneous coronary intervention.

Renal Disease and Hypertension

The kidney is a central regulator of blood pressure and controls intraglomerular pressure through autoregulation. When glomerular injury is present, a variety of pathways are activated resulting in increased systemic blood pressure (Fig. 86–8). This effect sets up a viscous circle of more glomerular and tubulointerstitial injury and worsened HTN (see Fig. 86–8). A cornerstone of management of combined CKD and CVD is strict blood pressure control (Fig. 86–9). An optimal blood pressure can be defined as less than 120/80 mm Hg, and most patients with CKD and HTN require three or more antihypertensive agents to achieve a goal blood pressure of less than 130/80 mm Hg.[10] Detection and treatment of HTN are outlined elsewhere in this text (see Chaps. 37 and 38). The key life-style issues with CKD and HTN include dietary changes with sodium restriction, weight reduction to a target body mass index less than 25 kg/m^2, and exercise for 60 minutes per day most days of the week. Pharmacological therapy aims for strict blood pressure control with an agent that antagonizes the RAAS often in combined action with a thiazide-type diuretic. Special diagnostic consideration should be given to the possibility of underlying bilateral renal artery stenosis from the clinical clues of poorly controlled blood pressure on more than three agents, abdominal bruits, smoking history, peripheral arterial disease, and a marked change in serum Cr with administration of ACEI.[54] Although renal artery stenosis accounts for less than 3 percent of ESRD cases, it represents a potentially treatable condition. Diagnostic approaches discussed elsewhere in this text should be considered (see Chap. 55).[55]

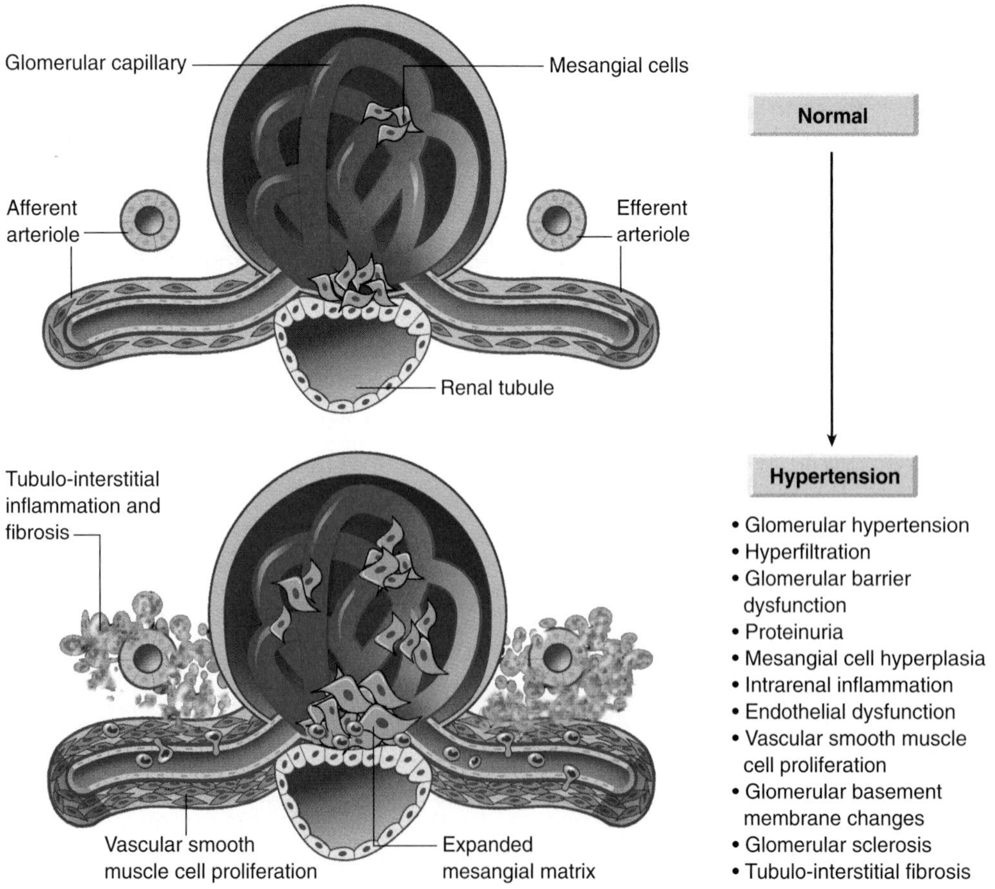

FIGURE 86–8 Pathological changes related to hypertension that occur within the kidney.

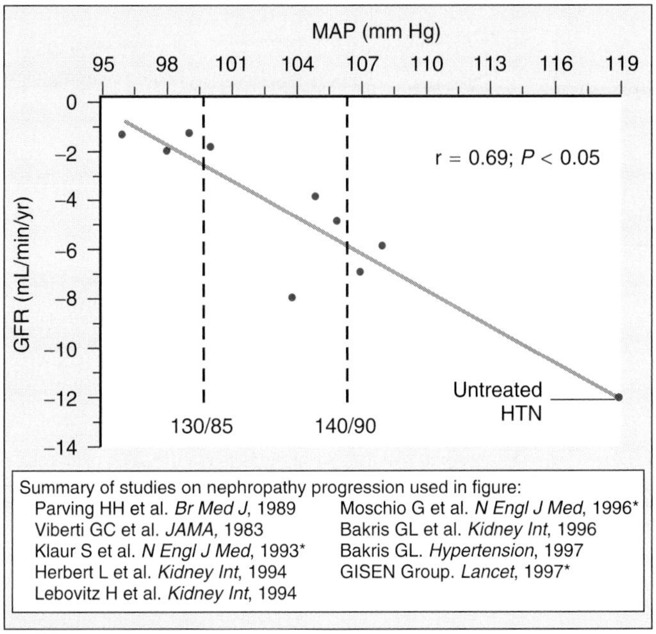

FIGURE 86–9 The influence of systemic blood pressure on the rate of decline in renal function. GFR = glomerular filtration rate; HTN = hypertension; MAP = mean arterial pressure. (Adapted from Bakris GL, Williams M, Dworkin L, et al: Preserving renal function in adults with hypertension and diabetes: A consensus approach. National Kidney Foundation Hypertension and Diabetes Executive Committees Working Group. Am J Kidney Dis 36:646, 2000.)

Diagnosis of Acute Coronary Syndromes in Patients with Chronic Kidney Disease

Multiple studies have found that elderly persons and those with diabetes have higher rates of silent ischemia.[56] Likewise, patients with CKD have shown higher rates of silent ischemia, which cluster with serious arrhythmias and other cardiac events.[57] Hemodialysis patients with ESRD bear considerable hemodynamic stress three times per week during dialysis sessions. Several studies have demonstrated a relationship between ST segment depression and release of cardiac biomarkers (primarily troponin T), before or during dialysis, and poor long-term survival.[57] From a practical perspective, it is important to realize that patients with CKD presenting to the hospital with chest discomfort represent a high-risk group, having a 40 percent cardiac event rate at 30 days.[58] In making the diagnosis of acute myocardial infarction (AMI) in patients with CKD or ESRD, troponin I is the preferred biomarker on the basis of its kinetic profile in patients with renal impairment.[59] The skeletal myopathy of renal disease can elevate creatine kinase, myoglobin, and some troponin T assays, making these tests less desirable. In addition to an elevated biomarker of cardiac injury, supporting evidence of the diagnosis of AMI could be characteristic chest pain, electrocardiographic changes (ST segment elevation or depression, new Q waves), or the identification of a culprit lesion on angiography. Because of the high event rate and prevalence of CVD among patients with CKD, it is advisable to consider admission to the hospital when the presenting symptom is chest discomfort and the eGFR is less than 60 ml/min/1.73 m^2 or the patient has ESRD and is receiving dialysis.[58]

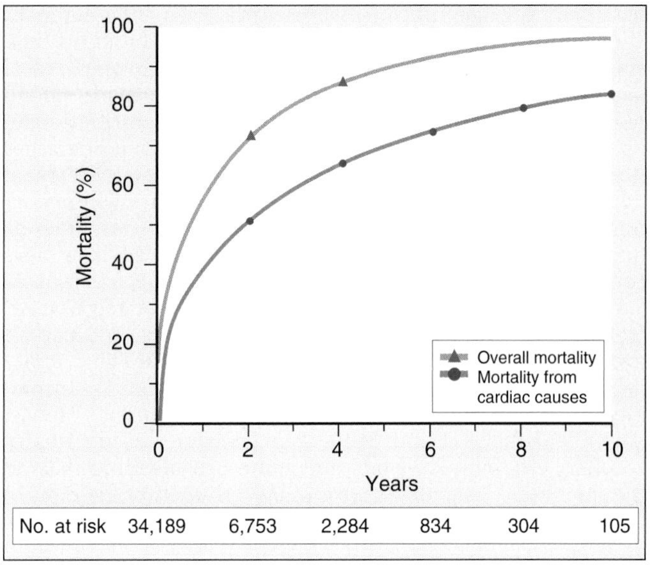

FIGURE 86–10 Cumulative mortality after myocardial infarction in patients with end-stage renal disease from the U.S. Renal Data System. (Adapted from Herzog CA, Ma JZ, Collins AJ: Poor long-term survival after acute myocardial infarction among patients on long-term dialysis. N Engl J Med 339:799, 1998.)

Renal Dysfunction as a Prognostic Factor in Acute Coronary Syndromes

In the last several decades, considerable advances have been made in the diagnosis and treatment of acute coronary syndromes (ACSs) in the general population. These advances include early paramedic response and defibrillation, coronary care units, and pharmacotherapy including antiplatelet agents, antithrombotics, beta receptor–blocking agents, ACEIs, and intravenous thrombolytic agents. Primary angioplasty for ST segment elevation myocardial infarction (STEMI) has become a well-accepted mode of treatment. These advances, however, have not been tested in patients with CKD or ESRD, primarily because these patients have been excluded from randomized treatment trials. Retrospective studies of patients in coronary care units have identified renal dysfunction as the most significant prognostic factor for long-term mortality when adjusting for other clinical factors, including age, gender, and comorbidities.[5-8] In addition, retrospective studies of patients with AMI consistently find renal dysfunction as an independent predictor of death, with a greater impact on mortality than baseline demographics or therapies received.[8] Patients with ESRD have the highest mortality after AMI of any large, chronic disease population (Fig. 86–10).[60]

Reasons for Poor Outcomes in Patients with Renal Dysfunction

Four reasons may explain why patients with renal dysfunction have poor cardiovascular outcomes in a variety of settings: (1) excess comorbidities associated with CKD and ESRD, in particular diabetes and heart failure; (2) therapeutic nihilism; (3) toxicity of therapies; and (4) special biological and pathophysiological factors in renal dysfunction that cause worsened outcomes.[11] In one study by Beattie and coworkers, the comorbidities of patients with STEMI and CKD (mean Cr = 2.7 mg/dl) included older age (mean 70.2 years), diabetes (38.1 percent), and prior heart failure (23.2 percent).[6] Those with ESRD had similar rates of comorbidities including age (mean 64.9 years), diabetes (40.4 percent), and prior heart failure (31.7 percent). This study found that, among the CKD and ESRD groups, there were lower rates of use of reperfusion therapy (thrombolysis or primary angioplasty) and beta blockers, suggesting some contribution to poor outcomes from underutilization of proven therapies (therapeutic nihilism). It is possible that patients with renal dysfunction may present later in their course, have more contraindications, or have other aspects about their presentations that prompt clinicians to use fewer therapies or take a more conservative approach.

Data on the toxicity of treatments for ACSs related to renal dysfunction are often unavailable, primarily because of exclusion of patients with CKD from these trials. The primary defects in thrombosis attributable to uremia are excess thrombin generation and decreased platelet aggregation.[61] Hence, patients with CKD and ESRD can have increased rates of coronary thrombotic events and increased bleeding risks at the same time. In patients with renal dysfunction the risks of bleeding increase with aspirin, unfractionated heparin, low-molecular-weight heparin, thrombolytics, glycoprotein IIb/IIIa receptor antagonists, and thienopyridine antiplatelet agents. The reason is primarily that uremia causes platelet dysfunction in a mechanism that is independent of and therefore additive to pharmacologically induced platelet antagonism or antithrombosis.[61] In patients with renal dysfunction, the best measure of bleeding risk is the bleeding time.[61] Unfortunately, the bleeding time is not a practical test for the ACS patient; consequently, clinicians cannot readily assess the a priori bleeding risk for any given CKD or ESRD patient. However, it is unlikely that bleeding complications account for the large differences seen in mortality between CKD and ESRD and those with preserved renal function with AMI.

The final and most important reason why patients with CKD and ESRD have poor outcomes after ACS is the enhanced vascular pathobiology induced by the chronic renal failure state.[24-26] The processes that contribute to accelerate atherosclerosis include a dyslipidemia characterized by decreased function of lipoprotein lipase, reductions in high-density lipoprotein cholesterol (HDL-C), elevated triglycerides, and normal low-density lipoprotein cholesterol (LDL-C) (see Fig. 86–7). In addition, accelerated vascular calcification is due in part to hypercalcemia, hyperphosphatemia, and elevated parathyroid hormone and is possibly worsened by chronic acidosis and mobilization of calcium from bone. Elevations in homocysteine and other thiols are present when the eGFR drops below 60 ml/min/1.73 m^2, enhancing oxidation of LDL-C and progression of atherosclerotic lesions. Renal dysfunction is a highly inflammatory state, associated with higher rates of plaque rupture and incident CVD events. Lastly, chronic hyperactivation of the sympathetic nervous system and an imbalance between endothelin, a powerful vasoconstrictor, and nitric oxide, a local paracrine vasodilator, may worsen HTN and may augment intravascular wall stress that could further contribute to incident CVD events.

Treatment of Acute Myocardial Infarction in Patients with Renal Dysfunction

The clinician must confront the high-risk populations, those with CKD and ESRD, with little evidence upon which to base treatment decisions in ACS. Therapies that benefit the general population often yield enhanced benefit in patients with CKD and ESRD.[62] A favorable benefit-to-risk ratio has now been demonstrated for aspirin, beta blockers, ACEI, aldosterone receptor antagonists, and statins and is expected for ARBs.[62] Therapies that require dose adjustment on the basis of CrCl include low-molecular-weight heparins and glycoprotein IIb/IIIa antagonists (Table 86–3). Given that the major inputs for bleeding risks include older age, low body weight, and renal dysfunction, Table 86–3 also lists agents that are approved in a weight-adjusted dose form and gives the currently recommended dose adjustments for commonly used antiplatelet and antithrombotic agents.[61] It is possible that greater utilization of such therapies, despite the heightened risk for complications, will attenuate the excess mortality reported in the CKD and ESRD populations. There have been no randomized trials of PCI or bypass surgery in patients with CKD or ESRD. However, in the Bypass Angioplasty Revascularization Investigation (BARI), whether PCI or surgery was used in the management of multivessel coronary disease, CKD and diabetes were associated with worsened long-term survival (Fig. 86–11).[8] Further research is needed into the particular pathogenic mechanisms in the renal failure state that promote plaque rupture, accelerate atherosclerosis, lead to ACS complications, and promote the development of heart failure and arrhythmias.

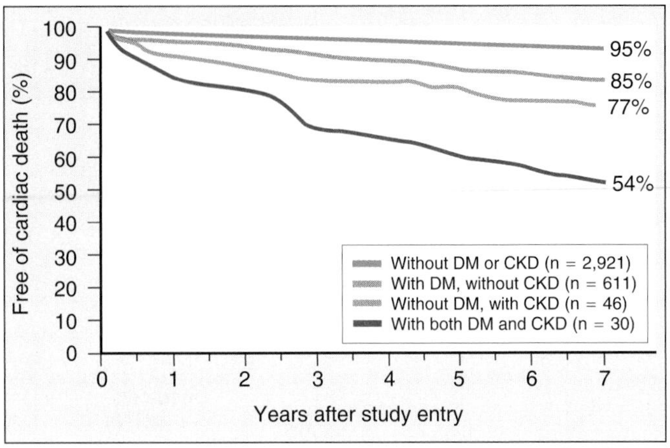

FIGURE 86–11 Freedom from cardiovascular death after angioplasty or bypass surgery in the Bypass Angioplasty Revascularization Investigation (BARI) Trial and Registry, $n = 3608$. CKD = chronic kidney disease; DM = diabetes mellitus. (Adapted from Szczech LA, Best PJ, Crowley E, for the Bypass Angioplasty Revascularization Investigation (BARI) Investigators: Outcomes of patients with chronic renal insufficiency in the bypass angioplasty revascularization investigation. Circulation 105:2253, 2002.)

Chronic Kidney Disease Complicating Congestive Heart Failure

The diagnosis of CHF with concomitant renal failure presents a particular challenge. Patients with CKD, and in particular ESRD, have three key mechanical contributors to CHF: pressure overload (related to HTN), volume overload, and cardiomyopathy. Approximately 20 percent of patients approaching hemodialysis have a diagnosis of CHF.[63] It is unclear how much of this diagnosis can be attributable purely to chronic volume overload from renal failure and how much is due to impaired systolic or diastolic function. Notably, CKD influences the levels of B-type natriuretic peptide (BNP), a diagnostic blood test for CHF. In general, when the eGFR is less than 60 ml/min/1.73 m^2, a higher BNP cut point of 200 pg/ml should be used in the diagnosis of CHF.[64] It is now well recognized that CKD, when it is present in patients with CHF, independently predicts poor outcomes.[65] Again, this excess risk seems to occur at a cut point in eGFR below 60 ml/min/1.73 m^2 (Fig. 86–12).[65] Estimated and actual GFRs clearly can be reduced by decreased renal blood flow related

TABLE 86–3 Recommended Dose Adjustment of Conventional Antithrombotics Used for Acute Coronary Syndromes in Patients with Chronic Kidney Disease and End-Stage Renal Disease

	eGFR (ml/min/1.73 m²)		Creatinine Clearance (ml/min)	
Agent	60–90 ml/min	30–60 ml/min	<30 ml/min	Dialysis Dependent
Aspirin	No adjustment needed	No adjustment needed	No adjustment needed	No adjustment needed
Clopidogrel	No adjustment needed	No adjustment needed	No adjustment needed	No adjustment needed
Ticlopidine	No adjustment needed	No adjustment needed	No adjustment needed	No adjustment needed
Heparin	No guidelines	No guidelines	No guidelines	No guidelines
LMWH	No guidelines	No guidelines	Reduced dose by 30%; factor Xa monitoring advocated	No guidelines
Lepirudin	No guidelines	CrCl 45-60 ml/min or SrCr 1.6–2 mg/dl: Reduce bolus to 0.2 mg/kg IV + decrease infusion rate by 50% (0.075 mg/kg/hr IV) CrCl 30-44 ml/min or SrCr 2.1-3 mg/dl: Reduce bolus to 0.2 mg/kg IV + decrease standard initial infusion rate by 70% (0.045 mg/kg/hr IV)	CrCl 15-29 ml/min or SrCr 3.1–6 mg/dl: Reduce bolus to 0.2 mg/kg IV + decrease infusion rate by 85% (0.0225 mg/kg/hr IV) CrCl <15 ml/min or SrCr >6 mg/dl: Reduce bolus to 0.2 mg/kg IV; No infusion	Reduce the bolus dose to 0.2 mg/kg IV; No infusion
Bivalirudin	No guidelines	Reduce infusion dose by 20%	Reduce infusion dose by 60%	Reduce infusion dose by 90%
Argatroban	No dose adjustment	No dose adjustment	No dose adjustment	
Abciximab	No guidelines Monitoring advocated	No guidelines Monitoring advocated	No guidelines Monitoring advocated	No guidelines Monitoring advocated
Eptifibatide	No guidelines	SrCr 2-4 mg/dl: 135 μg/kg IV bolus + 0.5 μg/kg/min IV infusion	SrCr >4.0 mg/dl Contraindicated	No clinical data In vitro data demonstrate clearance
Tirofiban	No dose adjustment	No dose adjustment	0.2 μg/kg/min IV for 30 min, followed by 0.05 μg/kg/min IV	No clinical data In vitro data demonstrate clearance

CrCl = creatinine clearance; eGFR = estimated glomerular filtration rate; LMWH = low-molecular-weight heparin; SrCr = serum creatinine.
Adapted from Sica D: The implications of renal impairment among patients undergoing percutaneous coronary intervention. J Invasive Cardiol 14(Suppl B):30B, 2002.

to low cardiac output. However, multiple studies of patients with class II and III CHF, in whom a low cardiac output state is not present, have shown decreased survival in a graded fashion related to renal impairment (see Fig. 86–12). A leading explanation for this observation is that the anemia that predictably develops when the eGFR drops below 60 ml/min/1.73 m², because of a functional deficiency of erythropoietin alpha, accelerates left ventricular hypertrophy and adverse cardiac remodeling. Small observational studies and randomized trials have suggested that treating patients with CHF, CKD, and anemia with exogenous epoetin alfa and supplemental iron improves symptoms, functional class, and peak oxygen consumption.[24,66] To date, there have been no completed mortality trials utilizing this strategy.

The combination of CHF and CKD presents a challenge to cardiologists with respect to proven treatment options. ACEI, if tolerated, or ARBs, if ACEI is not tolerated, beta blockers, aldosterone antagonists, and loop diuretics are all acceptable combination therapies.[67] Caveats in the use of ACEI and ARBs are the marked elevation in the serum Cr and acute renal failure that are more likely to occur when the patient is volume depleted or in the presence of occult bilateral renal artery stenosis or equivalent (unilateral renal artery stenosis present in a renal transplant recipient).[68] When initiating therapy to block the RAAS, it is advisable to have the systolic blood pressure stable and greater than 90 mm Hg, euvolemia, and a drug regimen without concurrent renal toxic agents. In general, an attempt should be made to use ACEI or ARB in patients down to an eGFR of 15 ml/min/1.73 m².

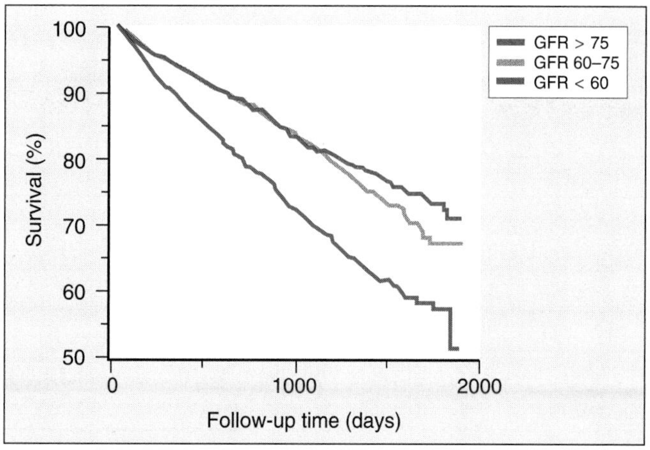

FIGURE 86–12 Kaplan-Meier survival analysis by level of glomerular filtration rate (GFR) as baseline from the Studies of LV Dysfunction (SOLVD) database, which includes patients with functional class I to III congestive heart failure, $n = 6630$. (Adapted from Al-Ahmad A, Rand WM, Manjunath G, et al: Reduced kidney function and anemia as risk factors for mortality in patients with left ventricular dysfunction. J Am Coll Cardiol 38:955, 2001.)

Below this level, case reports suggest a high rate of hyperkalemia and the concern of accelerating the course to ESRD and dialysis.

The management of the patient who is already receiving dialysis and in CHF requires particular care. In general, proven CHF therapies, provided they are tolerated, should be employed along with regular and ad hoc dialysis as needed to control volume overload. In a randomized trial, carvedilol did provide additional benefit in this scenario.[69] In addition, retrospective analysis supports the use of ACEI in patients with ESRD admitted with CHF.[70] Lastly, the acute management of decompensated CHF in patients with impaired eGFR poses a particularly difficult challenge. In fact, an elevated Cr is the single most common reason for the use of positive inotropes or inodilators in hospitalized patients with CHF.[71] There are no published reports of dobutamine leading to long-term favorable outcomes, and in the short term it increases arrhythmias and mortality. Likewise, milrinone has not been shown to reduce mortality, causes arrhythmias, and must be dose adjusted when the eGFR drops below 45 ml/min/1.73 m^2 (Table 86–4).[72] Another option is the use of intravenous BNP (nesiritide), which causes primarily venodilation and natriuresis.[73] Completed studies with nesiritide have evaluated the CKD subgroups and found benefit in CKD equal to that in those with preserved renal function, although the overall effect is modestly better than that with intravenous nitroglycerin.[74] Patients with advanced CHF have reduced renal blood flow, decreased glomerular filtration rate, enhanced proximal reabsorption of water, and an overall reduced capacity of the nephron to excrete water (Fig. 86–13). Furthermore, reduced effective arterial blood volume is a stimulus for antidiuretic hormone release, which plays a dominant role in worsening water retention (see Fig. 86–13). The clinical signs of this deterioration are an elevation in the serum Cr and blood urea nitrogen, hyponatremia, volume retention, and excessive thirst. Treatment efforts should be aimed at improving left ventricular systolic function, often in the hospitalized setting, with the intravenous therapies mentioned previously and discussed in detail elsewhere in this text.

In summary, CKD and CHF present a particularly challenging scenario for clinicians and patients. Frequent monitoring and the combined use of renal and cardioprotective strategies are critical. Future research is needed to confirm anemia correction with erythropoietin as an additional strategy in patients who have a CKD-related anemia. Dialysis patients, despite having volume reduction with mechanical

TABLE 86–4 Recommended Dose Adjustment of Selected Medical Therapy for Hypertension, Dyslipidemia, Heart Failure, and Arrhythmias in Patients with Chronic Kidney Disease and End-Stage Renal Disease

Drug	Elimination Route	eGFR (ml/min/1.73 m²) (CrCl ml/min) 90-60	60-30	<30	Dialysis Dependent
Central Adrenergic Blockers					
Clonidine	Renal				↓ Dose 50%
Methyldopa	Renal	q.i.d.	q.i.d.	↓ t.i.d.	↓ b.i.d. or qd
Angiotensin-Converting Enzyme Inhibitors (ACEIs)					
Captopril	Renal				↓ Dose 50%
Enalapril	Hepatic			↓ Dose 25%	↓ Dose 50%
Lisinopril	Renal			↓ Dose 25%	↓ Dose 50%
Ramipril	Renal/GI			↓ Dose 75%	↓ Dose 75%
Benazepril	Renal			↓ Dose 25%	↓ Dose 75%
Inotropic Agents					
Digoxin	Renal/nonrenal		↓ Dose 50%	↓ Dose 50%	↓ Dose 75%; change to q.o.d.
Milrinone	Renal		↓ Dose 25%	↓ Dose 50%	↓ Dose 75%
Antiarrhythmics					
Disopyramide	Renal/hepatic	b.i.d.	b.i.d.	↓ qd	↓ q.o.d.
Flecainide	Renal/hepatic				↓ Dose 25–50%
Mexiletine	Renal/hepatic				↓ Dose 50–75%
Procainamide	Renal/hepatic	q.i.d.	↓ t.i.d.	↓ b.i.d.	↓ b.i.d. or qd
Dofetilide	Renal/nonrenal		↓ Dose 50%	↓ Dose 75%	Contraindicated
Beta Blockers					
Atenolol	Renal			↓ Dose 50%	↓ Dose 75%; ↓ q.o.d.
Sotalol	Renal			↓ Dose 50%	↓ Dose 75%
Others					
Verapamil	Hepatic				↓ Dose 50–75%
Hydralazine		q.i.d.	↓ t.i.d	↓ t.i.d.	↓ b.i.d.
Gemfibrozil	Renal			↓ Dose 50%	↓ Dose 75%
Nicotinic acid	Renal/hepatic			↓ Dose 25%	↓ Dose 25%

CrCl = creatinine clearance; eGFR = estimated glomerular filtration rate; GI = gastrointestinal.

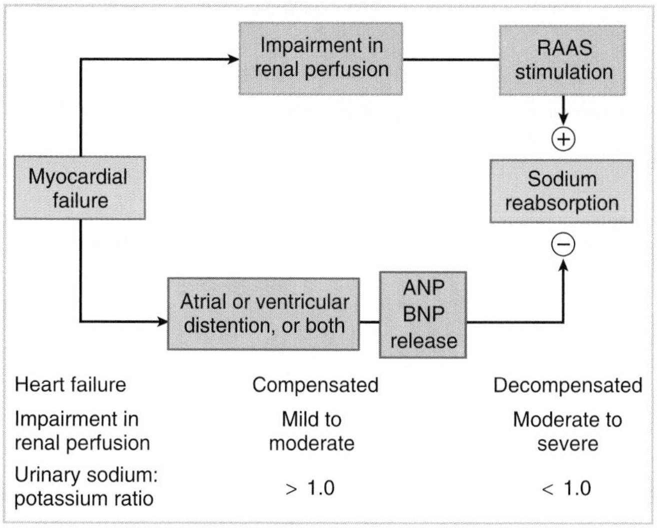

FIGURE 86–13 Pathophysiological processes in combined heart and kidney failure. ANP = A-type natriuretic peptide; BNP = B-type natriuretic peptide; RAAS = renin-angiotensin-aldosterone system. (From Weber KT: Aldosterone in congestive heart failure. N Engl J Med 345:1689, 2001.)

fluid removal, should have medical therapy with ACEIs or ARBs, beta blockers, and additional agents for blood pressure control if needed.

Chronic Kidney Disease and Valvular Heart Disease

Impaired renal function has been linked to mitral annular calcification and to aortic sclerosis. Advanced thickening of the cardiac valves and calcification have been observed in patients with ESRD.[75] Some 80 percent of patients with ESRD have the murmur of aortic sclerosis. Neither of these lesions usually progresses to the point where studies beyond echocardiography are needed. There are no published cases of renal dysfunction being isolated as the cause of valvular disease that required surgical intervention. However, CKD may accelerate degeneration of a tissue valvular prosthesis. Bacterial endocarditis may develop in patients with ESRD who have temporary dialysis access catheters.[76] Endocarditis with common pathogens including *Staphylococcus*, *Streptococcus*, and *Enterococcus*, in the aortic or mitral position, is associated with a mortality rate greater than 50 percent in this setting.[76] It becomes very difficult to treat given the continued need for dialysis access and the delay in surgical placement of permanent arteriovenous shunts or fistulas. Unfortunately, surgical mortality associated with valve replacement in ESRD related to endocarditis is quite high. Infection, and endocarditis in particular, is an increasingly common cause of death in patients with ESRD.

Renal Function and Arrhythmias

Uremia, hyperkalemia, and disorders of calcium-phosphorous balance have all been linked to higher rates of atrial and ventricular arrhythmias.[77] Given a concurrent substrate of left ventricular hypertrophy, left ventricular dilation, CHF, and valvular disease, it is not surprising that higher rates of virtually all arrhythmias have been reported in CKD, including bradyarrhythmias and heart block.[77] Caveats for practical management include dose adjustment for many antiarrhythmic medications including digoxin, sotalol, and procainamide (see Table 86–4). Of concern, CKD, and ESRD in particular, may cause elevated defibrillation thresholds and failure of implantable cardioverter-defibrillators (ICDs).[78] Until this association is better understood, patients receiving ICDs should have frequent surveillance and consideration for noninvasive programmed stimulation for appropriate antitachycardia and defibrillation therapy. Considering the high rates of sudden death in patients with ESRD, clinical trials of prophylactic ICDs in this population are under consideration.

Summary

Recognition has increased over the last decade that patients with CKD have a high risk for CVD. Frequent clinical scenarios in which renal function influences care include CIN, ACS, CHF, valvular disease, and arrhythmias. Results from retrospective studies and clinical trial subgroups form the basis of current recommendations, given the lack of prospective randomized trials in CKD and ESRD. Further study of the adverse metabolic milieu of chronic renal failure is likely to lead to generalizable diagnostic and therapeutic targets for the future management of renal patients with cardiovascular illness.

REFERENCES

Epidemiology and Outcomes

1. Lewis CE, Jacobs DR Jr, McCreath H, et al: Weight gain continues in the 1990s: 10-year trends in weight and overweight from the CARDIA study. Coronary Artery Risk Development in Young Adults. Am J Epidemiol 151:1172, 2000.
2. Bakris GL, Williams M, Dworkin L, et al: Preserving renal function in adults with hypertension and diabetes: A consensus approach. National Kidney Foundation Hypertension and Diabetes Executive Committees Working Group. Am J Kidney Dis 36:646, 2000.
3. McCullough PA: Cardiorenal risk: An important clinical intersection. Rev Cardiovasc Med 3:71, 2002.
4. National Kidney Foundation: Clinical practice guidelines for chronic kidney disease: Evaluation, classification, and stratification. Am J Kidney Dis 2(Suppl 1):S46, 2002.
5. McCullough PA, Soman SS, Shah SS, et al: Risks associated with renal dysfunction in patients in the coronary care unit. J Am Coll Cardiol 36:679, 2000.
6. Beattie JN, Soman SS, Sandberg KR, et al: Determinants of mortality after myocardial infarction in patients with advanced renal dysfunction. Am J Kidney Dis 37:1191, 2001.
7. Chertow GM, Lazarus JM, Christiansen CL, et al: Preoperative renal risk stratification. Circulation 95:878, 1997.
8. Szczech LA, Best PJ, Crowley E, for the Bypass Angioplasty Revascularization Investigation (BARI) Investigators: Outcomes of patients with chronic renal insufficiency in the bypass angioplasty revascularization investigation. Circulation 105:2253, 2002.
9. Keane WF, Eknoyan G: Proteinuria, albuminuria, risk, assessment, detection, elimination (PARADE): A position paper of the National Kidney Foundation. Am J Kidney Dis 33:1004, 1999.
10. Chobanian AV, Bakris GL, Black HR, for the National Heart, Lung, and Blood Institute Joint National Committee on Prevention, Detection, Evaluation, and Treatment of High Blood Pressure; National High Blood Pressure Education Program Coordinating Committee: The Seventh Report of the Joint National Committee on Prevention, Detection, Evaluation, and Treatment of High Blood Pressure: The JNC 7 report. JAMA 289:2560, 2003.
11. McCullough PA: Why is chronic kidney disease the "spoiler" for cardiovascular outcomes? J Am Coll Cardiol 41:725, 2003.
12. McCullough PA, Manley HJ: Prediction and prevention of contrast nephropathy. J Interv Cardiol 14:547, 2001.
13. McCullough PA, Wolyn R, Rocher LL, et al: Acute renal failure after coronary intervention: Incidence, risk factors, and relationship to mortality. Am J Med 103:368, 1997.
14. Mangano CM, Diamondstone LS, Ramsay JG, et al: Renal dysfunction after myocardial revascularization: Risk factors, adverse outcomes, and hospital resource utilization. The Multicenter Study of Perioperative Ischemia Research Group. Ann Intern Med 128:194, 1998.
15. Rihal CS, Textor SC, Grill DE, et al: Incidence and prognostic importance of acute renal failure after percutaneous coronary intervention. Circulation 105:2259, 2002.

Therapy

16. Pitt B, Segal R, Martinez FA, et al: Randomised trial of losartan versus captopril in patients over 65 with heart failure (Evaluation of Losartan in the Elderly Study, ELITE). Lancet 349:747, 1997.
17. Toto R: Angiotensin II subtype 1 receptor blockers and renal function. Arch Intern Med 161:1492, 2001.

18. Brenner BM, Cooper ME, de Zeeuw D, for the RENAAL Study Investigators: Effects of losartan on renal and cardiovascular outcomes in patients with type 2 diabetes and nephropathy. N Engl J Med 345:861, 2001.
19. Lewis EJ, Hunsicker LG, Clarke WR, for the Collaborative Study Group: Renoprotective effect of the angiotensin-receptor antagonist irbesartan in patients with nephropathy due to type 2 diabetes. N Engl J Med 345:851, 2001.
20. Parving HH, Lehnert H, Brochner-Mortensen J, for the Irbesartan in Patients with Type 2 Diabetes and Microalbuminuria Study Group: The effect of irbesartan on the development of diabetic nephropathy in patients with type 2 diabetes. N Engl J Med 345:870, 2001.
21. Dahlof B, Devereux RB, Kjeldsen SE, for the LIFE Study Group: Cardiovascular morbidity and mortality in the Losartan Intervention For Endpoint reduction in hypertension study (LIFE): A randomised trial against atenolol. Lancet 359:995, 2002.
22. Mann JF, Gerstein HC, Pogue J, et al: Renal insufficiency as a predictor of cardiovascular outcomes and the impact of ramipril: The HOPE randomized trial. Ann Intern Med 134:629, 2001.
23. Agodoa LY, Appel L, Bakris GL, for the African American Study of Kidney Disease and Hypertension (AASK) Study Group: Effect of ramipril vs amlodipine on renal outcomes in hypertensive nephrosclerosis: A randomized controlled trial. JAMA 285:2719, 2001.
24. Silverberg DS, Wexler D, Sheps D, et al: The effect of correction of mild anemia in severe, resistant congestive heart failure using subcutaneous erythropoietin and intravenous iron: A randomized controlled study. J Am Coll Cardiol 37:1775, 2001.
25. Friedman AN, Bostom AG, Selhub J, et al: The kidney and homocysteine metabolism. J Am Soc Nephrol 12:2181, 2001.
26. Chertow GM, Burke SK, Raggi P for the Treat to Goal Working Group: Sevelamer attenuates the progression of coronary and aortic calcification in hemodialysis patients. Kidney Int 62:245, 2002.

Percutaneous Coronary Interventions and Contrast-Induced Nephropathy

27. Andersen KJ, Christensen EI, Vik H: Effects of iodinated x-ray contrast media on renal epithelial cells in culture. Invest Radiol 29:955, 1994.
28. Keeley EC, Grines CL: Scraping of aortic debris by coronary guiding catheters: A prospective evaluation of 1,000 cases. J Am Coll Cardiol 32:1861, 1998.
29. Chertow GM, Lazarus JM, Christiansen CL, et al: Preoperative renal risk stratification. Circulation 95:878, 1997.
30. Denton KM, Shweta A, Anderson WP: Preglomerular and postglomerular resistance responses to different levels of sympathetic activation by hypoxia. J Am Soc Nephrol 13:27, 2002.
31. Uder M, Humke U, Pahl M, et al: Nonionic contrast media iohexol and iomeprol decrease renal arterial tone: Comparative studies on human and porcine isolated vascular segments. Invest Radiol 37:440, 2002.
32. Rauch D, Drescher P, Pereira FJ, et al: Comparison of iodinated contrast media–induced renal vasoconstriction in human, rabbit, dog, and pig arteries. Invest Radiol 32:315, 1997.
33. Mueller C, Buerkle G, Buettner HJ, et al: Prevention of contrast media–associated nephropathy: Randomized comparison of 2 hydration regimens in 1620 patients undergoing coronary angioplasty. Arch Intern Med 162:329, 2002.
34. Solomon R, Werner C, Mann D, et al: Effects of saline, mannitol, and furosemide to prevent acute decreases in renal function induced by radiocontrast agents. N Engl J Med 331:1416, 1994.
35. Stevens MA, McCullough PA, Tobin KJ, et al: A prospective randomized trial of prevention measures in patients at high risk for contrast nephropathy: Results of the P.R.I.N.C.E. Study. Prevention of Radiocontrast Induced Nephropathy Clinical Evaluation. J Am Coll Cardiol 33:403, 1999.
36. Rudnick MR, Goldfarb S, Wexler L, et al: Nephrotoxicity of ionic and nonionic contrast media in 1196 patients: A randomized trial. The Iohexol Cooperative Study. Kidney Int 47:254, 1995.
37. Aspelin P, Aubry P, Fransson SG, for the Nephrotoxicity in High-Risk Patients Study of Iso-Osmolar and Low-Osmolar Non-Ionic Contrast Media Study Investigators: Nephrotoxic effects in high-risk patients undergoing angiography. N Engl J Med 348:491, 2003.
38. Davidson CJ, Laskey WK, Hermiller JB, et al: Randomized trial of contrast media utilization in high-risk PTCA: The COURT trial. Circulation 101:2172, 2000.
39. Manske CL, Sprafka JM, Strony JT, Wang Y: Contrast nephropathy in azotemic diabetic patients undergoing coronary angiography. Am J Med 89:615, 1990.
40. Stone GW, Tumlin JA, Madyoon H, et al: Design and rationale of CONTRAST—A prospective, randomized, placebo-controlled trial of fenoldopam mesylate for the prevention of radiocontrast nephropathy. Rev Cardiovasc Med 2(Suppl 1):S31, 2001.
41. Tumlin JA, Wang A, Murray PT, Mathur VS: Fenoldopam mesylate blocks reductions in renal plasma flow after radiocontrast dye infusion: A pilot trial in the prevention of contrast nephropathy. Am Heart J 143:894, 2002.
42. Stone GW, McCullough PA, Tumlin J, et al: A prospective, randomized placebo-controlled multicenter trial evaluating fenoldopam mesylate for the prevention of contrast induced nephropathy: The CONTRAST Trial. J Am Coll Cardiol 41:83A, 2003.
43. Tepel M, van der Giet M, Schwarzfeld C, et al: Prevention of radiographic-contrast-agent-induced reductions in renal function by acetylcysteine. N Engl J Med 343:180, 2000.
44. Diaz-Sandoval LJ, Kosowsky BD, Losordo DW: Acetylcysteine to prevent angiography-related renal tissue injury (the APART trial). Am J Cardiol 89:356, 2002.
45. Shyu KG, Cheng JJ, Kuan P: Acetylcysteine protects against acute renal damage in patients with abnormal renal function undergoing a coronary procedure. J Am Coll Cardiol 40:1383, 2002.
46. Kay J, Chow WH, Chan TM, et al: Acetylcysteine for prevention of acute deterioration of renal function following elective coronary angiography and intervention: A randomized controlled trial. JAMA 289:553, 2003.
47. Durham JD, Caputo C, Dokko J, et al: A randomized controlled trial of *N*-acetylcysteine to prevent contrast nephropathy in cardiac angiography. Kidney Int 62:2202, 2002.
48. Briguori C, Manganelli F, Scarpato P, et al: Acetylcysteine and contrast agent–associated nephrotoxicity. J Am Coll Cardiol 40:298, 2002.
49. Allaqaband S, Tumuluri R, Malik AM, et al: Prospective randomized study of *N*-acetylcysteine, fenoldopam, and saline for prevention of radiocontrast-induced nephropathy. Catheter Cardiovasc Interv 57:279, 2002.
50. Loutrianakis E, Stella D, Hussain A, et al: Randomized comparison of fenoldopam and *N*-acetylcysteine to saline in the prevention of radiocontrast nephropathy. J Am Coll Cardiol 41:327A, 2003.
51. Baker CS, Wragg A, Kumar S, et al: A rapid protocol for the prevention of contrast-induced renal dysfunction (RAPPID Study). J Am Coll Cardiol 41:39A, 2003.
52. Goldenberg I, Jonas M, Matetzki S, et al: Contrast-associated nephropathy and clinical outcome of patients with chronic renal insufficiency undergoing cardiac catheterization: Lack of additive benefit of acetylcysteine to saline infusion. J Am Coll Cardiol 41:537A, 2003.
53. Guitterez N, Diaz A, Timmis GC, et al: Determinants of serum creatinine trajectory in acute contrast nephropathy. J Interv Cardiol 15:349, 2002.
54. Krijnen P, van Jaarsveld BC, Steyerberg EW, et al: A clinical prediction rule for renal artery stenosis. Ann Intern Med 129:705, 1998.

Ischemic Heart Diseases in Patients with Impaired Renal Function

55. Fatica RA, Port FK, Young EW: Incidence trends and mortality in end-stage renal disease attributed to renovascular disease in the United States. Am J Kidney Dis 37:1184, 2001.
56. Conti CR: Silent cardiac ischemia. Curr Opin Cardiol 17:537, 2002.
57. George SK, Singh AK: Current markers of myocardial ischemia and their validity in end-stage renal disease. Curr Opin Nephrol Hypertens 8:719, 1999.
58. McCullough PA, Nowak RM, Foreback C, et al: Emergency evaluation of chest pain in patients with advanced kidney disease. Arch Intern Med 162:2464, 2002.
59. McCullough PA, Nowak RM, Foreback C, et al: Performance of multiple cardiac biomarkers measured in the emergency department in patients with chronic kidney disease and chest pain. Acad Emerg Med 9:1389, 2002.
60. Herzog CA, Ma JZ, Collins AJ: Poor long-term survival after acute myocardial infarction among patients on long-term dialysis. N Engl J Med 339:799, 1998.
61. Sica D: The implications of renal impairment among patients undergoing percutaneous coronary intervention. J Invasive Cardiol 14(Suppl B):30B, 2002.
62. McCullough PA: Acute coronary syndromes in patients with renal failure. Curr Cardiol Rep 5:266, 2003.

Heart Failure in Patients with Kidney Disease

63. Schreiber BD: Congestive heart failure in patients with chronic kidney disease and on dialysis. Am J Med Sci 325:179, 2003.
64. McCullough PA, Duc P, Omland T, for the BNP Multinational Study Investigators: B-type natriuretic peptide and renal function in the diagnosis of heart failure: An analysis from the breathing not properly multinational study. Am J Kidney Dis 41:571, 2003.
65. Al-Ahmad A, Rand WM, Manjunath G, et al: Reduced kidney function and anemia as risk factors for mortality in patients with left ventricular dysfunction. J Am Coll Cardiol 38:955, 2001.
66. Mancini DM, Katz SD, Lang CC, et al: Effect of erythropoietin on exercise capacity in patients with moderate to severe chronic heart failure. Circulation 107:294, 2003.
67. Shlipak MG: Pharmacotherapy for heart failure in patients with renal insufficiency. Ann Intern Med 138:917, 2003.
68. Schoolwerth AC, Sica DA, Ballermann BJ, Wilcox CS for the Council on the Kidney in Cardiovascular Disease and the Council for High Blood Pressure Research of the American Heart Association: Renal considerations in angiotensin converting enzyme inhibitor therapy: A statement for healthcare professionals from the Council on the Kidney in Cardiovascular Disease and the Council for High Blood Pressure Research of the American Heart Association. Circulation 104:1985, 2001.
69. Cice G, Ferrara L, D'Andrea A, et al: Carvedilol increases two-year survival in dialysis patients with dilated cardiomyopathy: A prospective, placebo-controlled trial. J Am Coll Cardiol 41:1438, 2003.
70. McCullough PA, Sandberg KR, Yee J, Hudson MP: Mortality benefit of angiotensin-converting enzyme inhibitors after cardiac events in patients with end-stage renal disease. J Renin Angiotensin Aldosterone Syst 3:188, 2002.
71. Smith GL, Vaccarino V, Kosiborod M, et al: Worsening renal function: What is a clinically meaningful change in creatinine during hospitalization with heart failure? J Card Fail 9:13, 2003.
72. Jain P, Massie BM, Gattis WA, et al: Current medical treatment for the exacerbation of chronic heart failure resulting in hospitalization. Am Heart J 145(2 Suppl):S3, 2003.
73. Keating GM, Goa KL: Nesiritide: A review of its use in acute decompensated heart failure. Drugs 63:47, 2003.
74. Butler J, Emerson C, Peacock WF, et al: The efficacy and safety of B-type natriuretic peptide (nesiritide) in patients with renal insufficiency and acutely decompensated congestive heart failure. Nephrol Dial Transplant 19:391, 2004.

Valvular Heart Disease and Arrhythmias in Patients with Kidney Disease

75. Umana E, Ahmed W, Alpert MA: Valvular and perivalvular abnormalities in end-stage renal disease. Am J Med Sci 325:237, 2003.
76. Manian FA: Vascular and cardiac infections in end-stage renal disease. Am J Med Sci 325:243, 2003.
77. Soman SS, Sandberg KR, Borzak S, et al: The independent association of renal dysfunction and arrhythmias in critically ill patients. Chest 122:669, 2002.
78. Wase A, Basit A, Nazir R, et al: Does chronic renal insufficiency raise defibrillation threshold? [Abstract] Pacing Clin Electrophysiol 25(4, Pt II):594, 2002.

CHAPTER 87

Cardiovascular Manifestations of Autonomic Disorders

Rose Marie Robertson • David Robertson

General Principles

Autonomic control of the cardiovascular system provides second-to-second adjustments of blood pressure and heart rate, allowing humans great flexibility in posture and environment. Normally, autonomic integration of cardiovascular, renal, gastrointestinal, and temperature control adds to the metabolic control directed by the needs of each organ to maintain homeostasis for the entire organism and can even compensate for circumstances of stress or disease. Thus, when the autonomic nervous system fails and this finely tuned cardiovascular control is lost, significant impairment in function results.

Because most autonomic disorders are relatively uncommon, and because many clinicians are unfamiliar with these disorders and their presentation, consultation is usually sought. Since abnormalities in blood pressure, heart rate, or both are prominent features in these patients, and specialists in autonomic function are found in only a few centers, it is the cardiologist who is called upon to provide diagnostic and therapeutic information. In this chapter, we review the current understanding of abnormalities in autonomic cardiovascular control, as well as provide a guide for the consultant cardiologist in arriving at a diagnosis in these circumstances.

Several classification systems exist that can be applied to autonomic disorders, based on whether the disorder is acute or chronic, congenital or acquired, severe or mild, on the etiology (if known), and, in a few cases, on the specific underlying genetic abnormality.[1] Here, we use severity of autonomic impairment as the major feature differentiating these disorders and add the additional factor of the usual circumstances of presentation. This presents a simple approach to differential diagnosis. We also provide the initial approach to therapy for each disorder, recognizing that patients who do not respond adequately may require referral to a center specializing in autonomic dysfunction.

AUTONOMIC CARDIOVASCULAR CONTROL. The autonomic nervous system provides an integrated response by centrally coordinating physiological responses. It may be divided into sympathetic, parasympathetic, and enteric components. We focus on the first two. The effects of autonomic input to the cardiac conduction system,[2] the myocardium itself, and to the coronary and systemic vasculature are discussed in Chapters 19, 27, 37 and 44. Integrated control of blood pressure and heart rate and their modifications by disease are less familiar, and we delineate these in some detail, focusing first on the baroreflex.

BAROREFLEX. The maintenance of blood pressure with postural change in humans is accomplished by a group of reflexes referred to collectively as the *baroreflex*, provided by an integrated complex of neurons whose function reduces the lability of blood pressure. It includes the arterial baroreceptors, with sensory nerve endings within the aortic arch, at the origin of the right subclavian artery, and within the carotid sinuses, as well as the cardiopulmonary receptors (low-pressure receptors) in the walls of the atria and pulmonary artery. At baseline, the baroreflex tonically inhibits sympathetic activity and enhances parasympathetic activity. In the normal healthy human at rest, parasympathetic tone predominates. Additional complexities in the system (e.g., the presence of different populations of sympathetic neurons projecting from the paraventricular nucleus to the spinal cord, some participating in baroreflex-mediated responses, and others with a possible role in nonvasomotor sympathetic control[3]) allow further differentiation of response. However, we focus on the vasomotor aspects of autonomic function.

ARTERIAL BARORECEPTORS. Change in vascular pressure causes a change in the stretch applied to the arterial baroreceptors, and this in turn alters the frequency of discharge of the aortic depressor and carotid sinus nerves, whose first synapse lies within the nucleus tractus solitarii in the brain stem. Baroreceptor function is not the same in all individuals or even in the same individual at different times or in different experimental or disease states. For example, it has been demonstrated that adenoviral-mediated gene transfer of endothelial nitric oxide synthase to carotid sinus adventitia causes sustained, nitric oxide–dependent inhibition of baroreceptor activity and resetting of the baroreceptor function curve to higher pressures, suggesting that nitric oxide levels can modulate baroreceptor function.[4] When blood pressure is altered, afferent information from the baroreceptors is integrated on a beat-to-beat basis and determines efferent sympathetic and parasympathetic activity to minimize fluctuations in arterial pressure. This is accomplished via projections from the nucleus tractus solitarii to those hindbrain nuclei that govern efferent sympathetic activity (the caudal ventrolateral medulla, which projects to the rostral ventrolateral medulla and thus to the intermediolateral columns of the spinal cord) and parasympathetic activity (the nucleus ambiguus and the dorsal motor nucleus of the vagus). For example, when blood pressure rises, activation of the arterial baroreflex, producing an increase in the frequency of firing, leads to a decrease in sympathetic activity and an increase in parasympathetic activity, with the final integrated response being minimal change in blood pressure and heart rate.

In addition to the classic neurotransmitters such as norepinephrine and acetylcholine, cotransmitters such as neuropeptide Y may be released.[5] Studies of animals in which neuropeptide Y is overexpressed demonstrate that this peptide has sympatholytic and hypotensive effects and may have a role in blood pressure regulation. Although the effects of the classic neurotransmitters would seem to predominate, neuropeptide Y may buffer these effects, and in these studies, led to increased longevity.[5]

CARDIOPULMONARY RECEPTORS. Input from cardiopulmonary receptors in the heart and lungs, primarily in response to changes in volume, is also projected via vagal afferents to the nucleus tractus solitarii. These receptors are sensitive to chemical as well as mechanical activation and also provide input to the spinal cord via spinal sympathetic afferents. Stimulation of these receptors produces bradycardia, vasodilation, a resulting fall in blood pressure, and inhibition of vasopressin release. For example, the stimulation of cardiopulmonary receptors by an increase in intracardiac volume produces, via vasopressin and its effect on renal sympathetic nerve activity, an increase in salt and water excretion, an important regulatory mechanism directed at maintaining an optimal central blood volume. The components of the baroreflex are illustrated in Figure 87–1.

POSTURAL RESPONSES. With standing, the blood volume is subjected to gravitational forces that produce pooling of 500 to 800 ml of blood in the capacitance vessels of the lower extremities. Plasma moves to the interstitium (12 to 15 percent of the plasma volume over 20 to 40 minutes),[6] and there is a decrease in venous return and cardiac output.[7,8] This rapid fall in plasma volume with assumption of the upright posture in normal subjects was described in the 1930s by Youmans and associates.[9] The baroreceptor afferent nerves, both arterial and cardiopulmonary, detect reduced stretch and synapse in the nucleus tractus solitarii, and a decrease in parasympathetic tone and increase in sympathetic activity ensue, with the release of norepinephrine and an increase in peripheral resistance. Vasopressin release from the paraventricular nucleus and the supraoptic nucleus is also inhibited by the baroreflex, via the caudal ventrolateral medulla. When intact, this complex of autonomic reflex function protects blood pressure and cerebral perfusion.

Abnormalities of the integrated blood pressure and heart rate control provided by the baroreflex can be caused by dysfunction or failure of any of its separate components, from

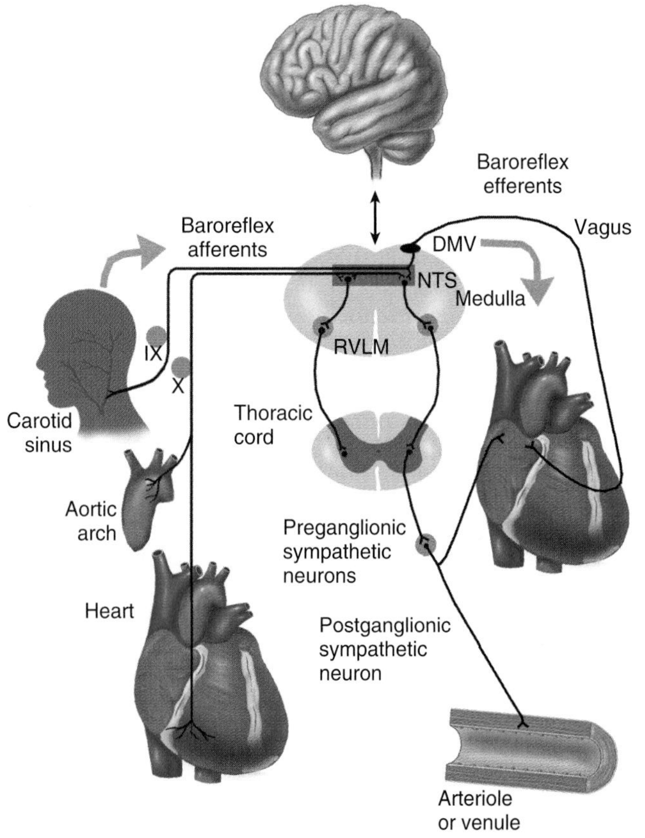

FIGURE 87–1 Components of the baroreflex. DMV = dorsal motor nucleus of the vagus; NTS = nucleus tractus solitarii; RVLM = rostroventrolateral medulla; NE = norepinephrine. (Courtesy of Dr. André Diedrich.)

sensory afferents, to areas of central integration in the brain stem, or efferent effector neurons. The clinical manifestations depend not only on the anatomic sites affected but also on the degree of dysfunction of the components affected. Although there is profound lability of blood pressure and heart rate in patients with complete baroreflex failure, there is a broad range of other disorders that can also produce abnormal blood pressure and heart rate responses.

Autonomic Disorders

Autonomic disorders, also referred to as *dysautonomias*, can be divided according to their effects on blood pressure in the upright posture. The first group includes those that are severe, always causing significant orthostatic hypotension (a fall in blood pressure with standing of more than 20/10 mm Hg, measured with the patient lying quietly and after 5 minutes of quiet standing, or as long as the patient can stand if symptoms limit the duration of standing.). Although these disorders are rare, some can significantly affect longevity, and all are serious.[7,8,10-13] The second group, the mild dysautonomias, are more common but less serious, and orthostatic hypotension is usually absent, though heart rate abnormalities are often prominent.[14-16] Animal models of a number of these disorders have been developed and are useful in studying pathophysiology and therapeutic options.[17] Table 87–1 provides a useful checklist to consider.

SETTINGS. It is also useful to consider the settings in which disorders present. Newly acquired autonomic dysfunction can appear in hospitalized patients and often prompts consultation, either because of new and profound hypotension or hypertension or an inability to discharge the patient due to marked orthostatic hypotension.. However, although patients with disorders that come on gradually over months to years may be referred for outpatient consultation, a subclinical autonomic disorder may also be noticed for the first time during a hospitalization for another disease, unmasked either by that disease or some aspect of its treatment. Chronic disorders often seem acute to the patient, especially if the first manifestation is dramatic, such as syncope, but careful review of the history usually reveals subtle premonitory symptoms. Table 87–2 lists some factors that are likely to worsen symptoms in patients with autonomic dysfunction and thus bring subclinical disorders to attention or, conversely, to improve orthostatic symptoms.[18-27]

TABLE 87–1 Autonomic Disorders Grouped by Severity
Severe dysautonomias—afferent/central dysfunction
Baroreflex failure
Glossopharyngeal neuralgia
Severe dysautonomias—efferent dysfunction
Acquired—symptoms beginning later in life
Multiple system atrophy
Pure autonomic failure
Autoimmune autonomic failure
Autonomic neuropathy (diabetes, amyloid, renal failure associated, vitamin B_{12} deficiency, paraneoplastic syndromes, idiopathic)
Guillain-Barré syndrome
Congenital—symptoms present from birth
Dopamine beta-hydroxylase deficiency
Mild dysautonomias
Postural tachycardia syndrome
Neurally mediated syncope
Norepinephrine transporter deficiency
Medications (norepinephrine transporter blockers)
Bed rest

TABLE 87–2 Factors Altering Blood Pressure in Patients with Autonomic Dysfunction		
Factor	**Raises Blood Pressure**	**Lowers Blood Pressure**
Intake	Water drinking	Food ingestion
Volume	Hypervolemia	Hypovolemia
Ventilation	Hypoventilation	Hyperventilation
Environment	Cold	Heat
Medications	Sympathomimetics	Vasodilators
Other	—	Infection (even subclinical)

AUTONOMIC TESTING AT THE BEDSIDE. Although there is a wide spectrum of autonomic tests that can be applied to differentiate autonomic disorders, evaluating the sympathetic adrenergic, sympathetic cholinergic, and parasympathetic branches of the autonomic nervous system, a few simple maneuvers at the bedside offer substantial information. Careful measurement of the blood pressure and heart rate in the supine posture should be followed by having the patient stand next to the bed, with support if necessary, with repeat determinations made as soon as the patient complains of symptoms or at 5 minutes. If the patient cannot continue standing for 5 minutes, blood pressure and heart rate should be obtained just prior to sitting. In most healthy individuals, the diastolic blood pressure rises slightly and the systolic pressure falls minimally, if at all. Orthostatic hypotension is defined as a fall of more than 20/10 mm Hg. Heart rate should increase no more than 20 beats/min.

If beat-to-beat heart rate can be obtained via continuous electrocardiographic (ECG) monitoring or an ECG machine set to record continuously for 30 seconds, it may be useful to add a Valsalva maneuver. During continuous recording, the patient blows into a closed system for 12 seconds at 40 mm Hg. A convenient system can be made by attaching the external tube of a 5-ml plastic syringe to the manometer of a sphygmomanometer. Divide the fastest heart rate during the Valsalva maneuver, when increased intrathoracic pressure impedes venous return and leads to a fall in blood pressure, by the slowest heart rate immediately afterward, during the rebound of blood pressure. A ratio of less than 1.4 suggests autonomic impairment. This is most useful if the patient is also instrumented for arterial pressure monitoring, so that the appropriate fall in blood pressure during the Valsalva maneuver can be documented.[28] Patients with congestive heart failure do not have the normal hemodynamic response to the Valsalva maneuver because they are less able to restrict the return of blood to the right atrium, so the maneuver is less helpful in this group. A normal Valsalva maneuver as well as the maneuver in a patient with pure autonomic failure is depicted in Figure 87–2.

Severe Dysautonomias

BAROREFLEX FAILURE. For many years, all patients with abnormalities of autonomic cardiovascular reflex control were considered to have baroreflex failure. And, in the broadest sense, autonomic efferents are a component of the baroreflex arc. However, there is a more specific syndrome of baroreflex failure involving a variety of disorders (surgery,[15] radiation,[29] cerebrovascular accident) affecting afferent neuronal input via the vagus and glossopharyngeal nerves, or damage to brain stem nuclei or interneurons, and we have elucidated its characteristics and distinguished it from the broader group of patients with other forms of

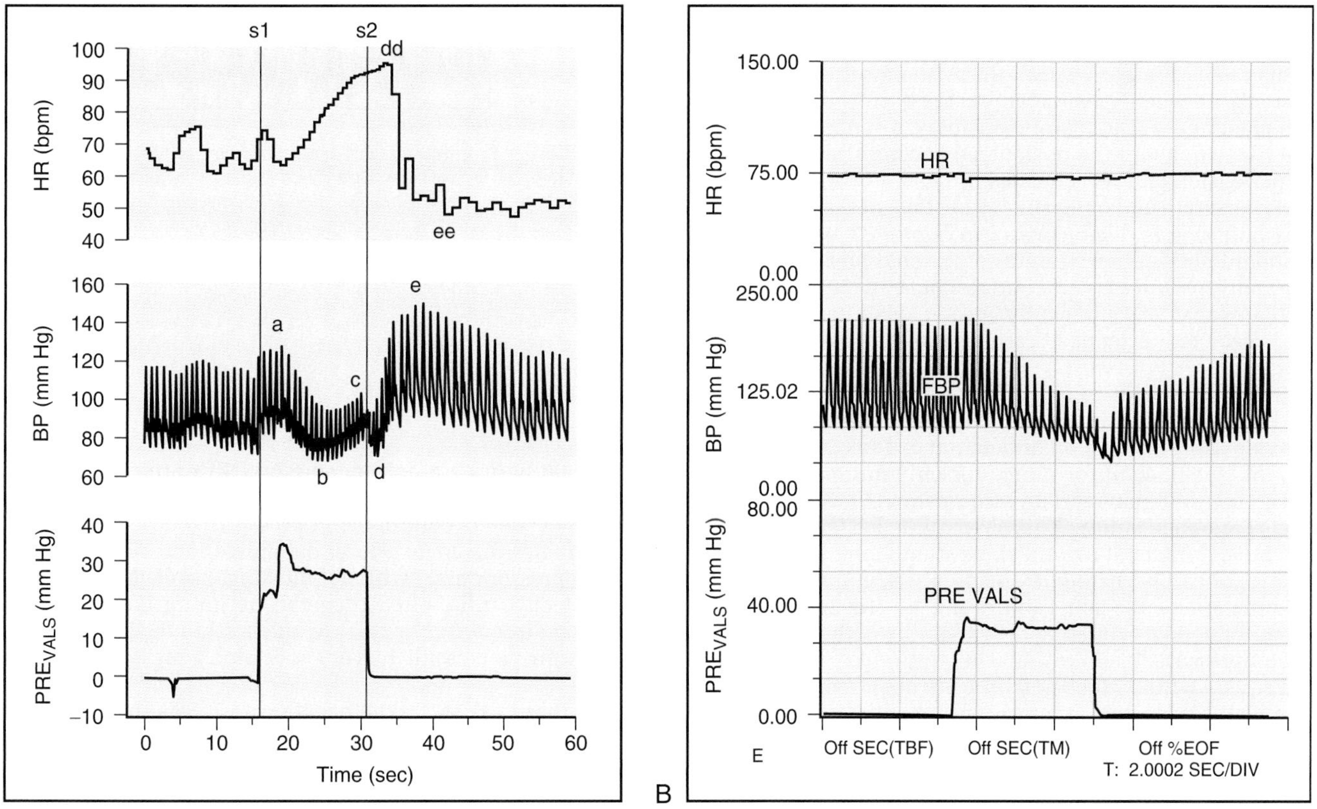

FIGURE 87–2 The Valsalva maneuver in a normal subject **(A)** and in a patient with pure autonomic failure **(B)**. a = increased intrathoracic pressure, beginning of phase 2; b = maximal fall in BP; HR = heart rate; BP = blood pressure; c = return of BP to within 20 mm Hg of baseline, due to sympathetically-mediated peripheral vasoconstriction; d = minimal BP after release of intrathoracic pressure, followed closely by maximal heart rate; e = increased BP as increased venous return is pumped into a vasoconstricted peripheral vascular bed; ee = slowed heart rate due to baroreflex response to the elevated pressure; PRE_{VALS} = pressure against which the subject is blowing with an open glottis; s1 = beginning of phase 1.

autonomic failure.[7] These patients have extremely labile blood pressure with alterations unbuffered by normal control mechanisms. The level of blood pressure at any given moment appears to be dependent on the sum of the input from higher centers on autonomic brain stem nuclei. Our ability to define this syndrome has greatly benefited from identification of a large kindred with an autosomal dominant disorder causing a high incidence of carotid body, glomus jugulare, and glomus vagale tumors, which can cause physical damage to adjacent nerves (glossopharyngeal and vagal).[15] Even if there is minimal impact of the tumors themselves, surgical resection may lead to unavoidable damage of underlying nervous structures, and baroreflex function can be studied in these patients before and after the procedure. This has allowed us to determine that the clinical presentation of baroreflex failure varies over time, with acute baroreflex dysfunction[30,31] appearing much more like pheochromocytoma, with extremely labile blood pressure and heart rate changing in concert (i.e., a rise in blood pressure does not lead to the expected baroreflex-mediated fall in heart rate, but rather heart rate and blood pressure rise and fall together), little or no orthostatic hypotension (presumably because the cortical arousal associated with taking the upright posture leads to increased sympathetic outflow, with its effects on the peripheral vasculature unbuffered), but with more orthostatic hypotension seen later in the course. Figure 87–3 demonstrates the loss of response to changes in carotid baroreceptor stimulation with baroreflex failure.

Some patients undergoing carotid endarterectomy, especially those who have previously had surgery on the other carotid, also develop baroreflex failure acutely, presenting in the postoperative period. Although the proportion is not clearly defined, 9 to 30 percent of carefully studied series of patients exhibit hypertension consistent with this problem,[32-34] and tens of thousands of these procedures are done yearly in the United States.[35] Both the hypertension and hypotension are often difficult to control with usual medical therapy. Although carotid angioplasty and stenting have been proposed as alternative procedures, their long-term outcomes are only now being evaluated. As these procedures also have the potential to affect carotid anatomy, it is not clear that they are likely to avoid the postoperative complications of severe hypertension and its sequelae.

An example of the physiological effect of the loss of baroreflex buffering is demonstrated in Figure 87–4, in which the standard nociceptive stimulus of the cold pressor test, which normally produces a pressor response of 20 to 40 mm Hg, not only has a significantly greater quantitative effect but also leads to a prolonged response in the absence of normal buffering.

In patients with only unilateral involvement, the extent of baroreflex impairment is variable. Although one might assume that preservation of function on the contralateral side would be sufficient for normal or only minimally abnormal baroreflex function, in fact some patients have nearly complete baroreflex failure. This observation led to studies of unilateral and bilateral carotid sinus stimulation, demonstrating that right carotid baroreflex loading was more effective than stimulation of the left carotid and as efficient as bilateral stimulation in modulating the variability of the heart rate and blood pressure.[36,37]

Patients with baroreflex failure are often seen acutely, after surgical intervention, trauma, or stroke (bilateral damage to the nucleus tractus solitarii), and in this setting the hypertension may sometimes be the highest one encounters in contemporary practice (systolic pressures of 200 to 320 mm Hg, with heart rates of 130 to 160 beats/min), with headaches of great severity. Apneic episodes also occur, possibly because of loss of neural afferents conveying information from vascular chemoreceptors. Plasma norepinephrine levels of 1000

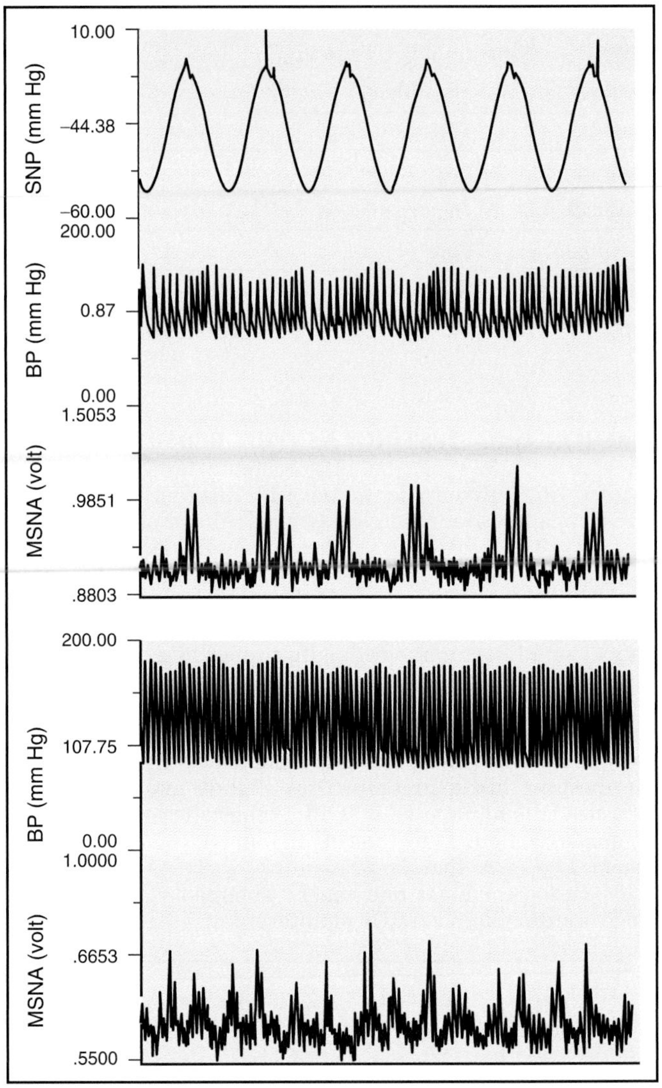

FIGURE 87–3 Effect of carotid sinus stimulation via neck suction in a healthy subject **(top)** and in a patient with chronic baroreflex failure **(bottom)**. **Top,** The effect of bilateral neck suction in a healthy volunteer for sinusoidal carotid sinus stimulation (SNP, period 10 sec) and the blood pressure response (middle trace) modulated by synchronized sympathetic nerve activity (lower trace). **Bottom,** Absent modulation of blood pressure (upper trace) and muscle sympathetic nerve activity (lower trace) by sinusoidal neck suction (period 10 sec) in a patient with baroreflex failure. The timing of carotid sinus stimulation is identical for both panels, although shown only in the top panel. BP = blood pressure; MSNA = muscle sympathetic nerve activity; SNP = sinusoidal neck pressure.

to 3000 pg/ml are not uncommon. Nitroprusside and a centrally acting alpha$_2$-agonist (clonidine) in combination are often needed to control blood pressure over the first 72 hours. Even after the acute phase, patients often continue to suffer from pressor crises, with hot flushing, headache, diaphoresis, and tachycardia, often triggered by minor cortical (anxiety, stress, discomfort, or fear) or other stimuli. Rest, sleep, and sedation may result in very low blood pressures and heart rates.

In these patients, whether the cause was the tumors mentioned earlier, surgery, radiation, trauma, or stroke, we found that the most helpful diagnostic criteria were the depressor response to a small (0.1 to 0.2 mg) dose of clonidine and the absence of heart rate responses to depressor or pressor drug infusions (at a time when stimuli and suppression of endogenous cortical activity, such as mental arithmetic and sedation, respectively, could raise and lower heart rate). These studies

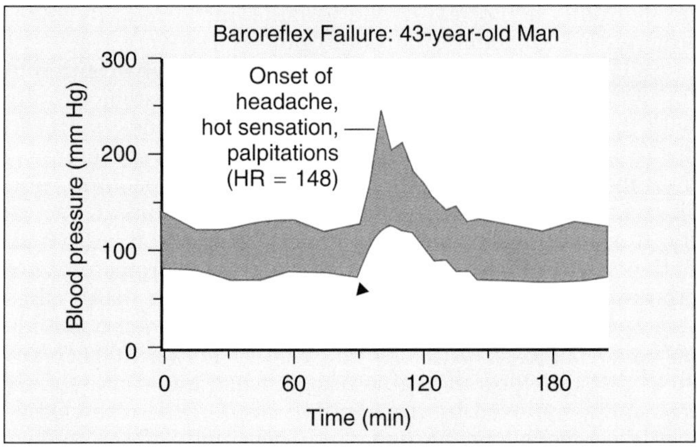

FIGURE 87–4 Response to cold pressor testing in baroreflex failure. The graph shows blood pressure monitoring in a 43-year-old man about 2 weeks after surgical removal of a second carotid body tumor. A 60-second cold pressor test (immersion of the hand in ice water; arrowhead) usually produces a 25- to 50-mm Hg pressor response that resolves within a few minutes. Here, the blood pressure continued to rise after the stimulus was removed and remained elevated above baseline for more than 45 minutes. HR = heart rate (beats/min). HR (trace not shown) peaked at 148, simultaneously with the peak of blood measure.

led to the use of clonidine and methyldopa in the chronic treatment of these patients, usually with good effect.

Chronically, the hallmark of baroreflex failure is labile hypertension and tachycardia, alternating with periods of hypotension and bradycardia. In many patients, low doses of a benzodiazepine aid in preventing cortically induced sympathetic surges, and in some cases, clonidine provides additional benefit in suppressing these surges.

GLOSSOPHARYNGEAL NEURALGIA. In patients who have had recent trauma in the area of the carotid sinus, secondary to causes such as surgery, tumor, or radiation, occasionally an intermittent activation of the glossopharyngeal nerve results. The patient experiences sudden, lancinating pain in the face, neck, or jaw on the affected side, and there is a sudden drop in both blood pressure and heart rate. This may be seen postoperatively and is an unexpected complication in what may be an otherwise benign course. Consultation is often sought for the episodes of hypotension, and the critical historical finding of pain may be overlooked in the focus on the hemodynamics. The episodes are usually self-limited, lasting for minutes, but the hypotension can be severe and symptomatic in itself, especially if the patient is upright. Treatment with yohimbine may ameliorate the episodes, but if all else fails, transection of the nerve may be necessary.[38,39]

MULTIPLE SYSTEM ATROPHY. Multiple system atrophy is a neurodegenerative disorder first described by Shy and Drager in 1960,[40] in which patchy central nervous system lesions are seen, consisting of oligodendroglial cells with cytoplasmic inclusions made up of multilayered fibrils of alpha-synuclein.[41,42] Although several other compounds, such as 14-3-3 proteins and tau, have been suggested to be involved,[43] careful study has shown that lesions can exist without the presence of either.[44] It appears that these inclusions eventually produce cellular degeneration. Patients gradually develop symptoms beginning in their 50s to 60s and exhibit both sympathetic and parasympathetic abnormalities. Autonomic symptoms and findings include impotence, lightheadedness due to orthostatic hypotension,[45] loss of sweating, abnormal pupillary responses,[46] urinary incontinence,[47-49] and respiratory abnormalities such as laryngeal stridor[50] and sleep apnea.[50,51] Urodynamic testing may be helpful in diagnosis in uncertain cases. At the bedside, significant orthostatic hypotension (the upright systolic pressure may fall by as much as 100 mm Hg, and may, in fact, be unobtainable) is accompanied by a minimal rise in heart rate. The fall in blood pressure can cause variable symptoms, with some patients reporting a headache involving the back of the neck,[52] blurring of vision, or a distancing of auditory sensation.

In addition, movement disorders of several forms can be seen in any posture. If there is rigidity, tremor, and bradykinesia, the patient may appear to have Parkinson's syndrome, but the movement generally does not improve with antiparkinsonian medications. A syndrome referred to as *atypical Parkinson's syndrome* has been described as a form of Parkinson's disease, with cell loss and Lewy bodies in autonomic regulatory regions, including the hypothalamus, sympathetic (intermediolateral nucleus of the thoracic cord and sympathetic ganglia), and parasympathetic (dorsal, vagal, and sacral parasympathetic nuclei) systems. Symptoms include orthostatic hypotension, gastrointestinal and urogenital dysfunction, pupillary abnormalities (pupillary control is dependent on both sympathetic and parasympathetic innervation), and disorders of sweating and regulation of temperature.[53] This syndrome may be clinically indistinguishable from multiple system atrophy.

In other patients with multiple system atrophy, the syndrome can be mistaken for spinocerebellar disease because of common symptoms of urinary incontinence and unsteadiness of gait.[54] The autonomic abnormalities, however, especially orthostatic hypotension, help determine that the patient has multiple system atrophy. Magnetic resonance imaging can also be helpful in defining the specific areas involved in multiple system atrophy.[54-56] Plasma catechols in multiple system atrophy show preservation of supine plasma norepinephrine, plasma dihydroxyphenolglycol, and urinary catecholamines.[57] But because the ability of the central nervous system to engage the periphery is impaired, the usual doubling with the upright posture is absent.

Although one might assume that the fall in blood pressure with upright posture is due to reduced arterial resistance, in fact, peripheral vascular resistance is increased in all postures in these patients, and it appears that increased venous compliance is a greater part of the problem.[58] Blood pressure while supine is markedly elevated in more than 50 percent of patients, with low renin levels.[59-62] Although the mechanism of supine hypertension is controversial,[63] studies in some patients suggest that it is due to inappropriately high constitutive catecholamine release.[12]

An additional symptom is a shift in urine production to the night, likely due to pressure diuresis as the low upright pressure during the day is replaced by the high blood pressure seen with the supine posture at night. This then leaves the patient relatively hypovolemic in the morning and worsens orthostatic hypotension.

THERAPEUTIC MANEUVERS. The first line of therapy in these patients is the timing of food and water. It has been demonstrated that food ingestion, particularly of carbohydrates, can lower blood pressure by 30 to 40 mm Hg,[42,60] and this may be helpful in reducing supine hypertension at night. During the day, however, the depressor effect of food ingestion produces an increased need for therapeutic maneuvers with a pressor effect for the periods immediately after meals. Caffeine ingestion of 100 to 250 mg with meals is helpful in some patients,[64] and somatostatin (which must be given by subcutaneous injection) is useful when the depressor effect is severe.[65,66] In contrast to food, drinking water has a significant, dose-dependent pressor effect in patients with autonomic dysfunction, with 16 ounces raising pressure by as much as 100 mm Hg in extreme cases, but routinely by 20 to 40 mm Hg.[21,67-69]

Second, physical maneuvers and exercise are helpful. Patients often have learned some maneuvers on their own to support blood pressure while upright, such as entwining the legs while constricting leg muscles, raising one foot to the seat of a chair, or squatting. Since patients are usually lightheaded with standing, they find it difficult to pursue their usual forms of exercise. Exercise in water is an excellent solution, because water pressure in effect provides compression of the lower extremities. Water temperatures that are excessively warm should be avoided, and care must be taken when emerging from the water. Analogous to standing in water is wearing waist-high garments providing 30 to 40 mm Hg graduated compression over the lower extremities. These should be removed when the patient is supine. Patients often need assistance in putting these garments on if they are tight enough to be effective. Open-crotch models are available. An additional maneuver is elevating the head of the bed 8 to 12 inches at night to reduce nocturia, thus leaving patients less volume depleted when they need to arise in the morning. Nocturia may also be treated with intranasal desmopressin.[67,70,71]

If these maneuvers are inadequate, pharmacological therapy should be instituted. Volume expansion via sodium retention can be produced by fludrocortisone, 0.05 to 0.2 mg orally twice a day. An addition of sodium to the diet is needed to see the full effect of fludrocortisone, and we encourage patients to eat a salty diet or to add 1 gm of salt to breakfast and lunch. A pressor agent is often also needed, and medications such as midodrine (2.5 to 10 mg orally two or three times a day) and yohimbine (5.4 mg orally two or three times a day) have a short enough duration of action to minimize worsening of supine hypertension at night. It is most effective to have patients keep water at the bedside and drink 16 ounces of water with their morning medications (fludrocortisone and a pressor agent) 20 to 30 minutes before arising. The combined pressor effects of the water and the pressor medication reduces the chance that marked orthostatic hypotension will cause a fall when the patient first arises. Anemia is common in patients with severe sympathetic failure, due at least in part to reduced sympathetically mediated erythropoietin release, and treatment with recombinant erythropoietin may be helpful.[72]

Unfortunately, although blood pressure control can be improved in patients with multiple system atrophy, there is currently no therapeutic approach to the overall degenerative neurologic process.[70] Nocturnal stridor is often troublesome in the later stages of the disorder but can be improved by continuous positive-pressure breathing.[73] Since difficulty with ambulation is often compromised more by loss of cell function in brain areas related to movement than by blood pressure, sustained improvement is unlikely. Multiple system atrophy does shorten life, and survival averages 9 years after diagnosis.[63,74] However, the course is variable, and some patients have survived for as long as 14 years. Since patients eventually become bedridden, careful planning with them and their caregivers for measures that maintain quality of life for as long as possible is essential.[59,60,75]

PURE AUTONOMIC FAILURE. In 1925, Bradbury and Eggleston described an "extensive and peculiar disturbance in the functional activity of the vegetative nervous system [accompanied by] idiopathic hypotension."[76] In these patients, with what was later referred to as *pure autonomic failure*, there is no central nervous system abnormality, but dysfunctional peripheral neurons prevent appropriate norepinephrine release. Norepinephrine levels are low in the supine posture and rise only minimally with standing. Autonomic symptoms and findings are as described earlier for multiple system atrophy but with the absence of any central nervous system lesions to produce a movement disorder. Longevity is normal, and control of orthostatic hypotension, using the same therapeutic maneuvers described for multiple system atrophy, is often sufficient to restore patients to most normal daily activities. At the bedside, orthostatic hypotension and an inadequate chronotropic response are seen.

ORTHOSTATIC ANGINA. In some patients, in addition to the symptoms described earlier for multiple system atrophy with the upright posture, or in place of them, chest pain can occur as the signal postural symptom. This symptom as described is indistinguishable from angina pectoris, and since it occurs when the patient stands to undertake an activity, it may appear to be precipitated by exertion. Although patients with pure autonomic failure are not protected from atherosclerosis and coronary artery disease, in many cases this apparent angina occurs in the absence of demonstrable coronary stenosis. With careful history taking, it becomes clear that this form of angina occurs when blood pressure is low and is relieved by the supine posture. It is also significantly worsened by nitroglycerin, especially if the patient remains upright, and appears to be due to severe orthostatic hypotension and inadequate coronary perfusion pressure. It is unclear why this occurs in some patients and not others, but it is important to recognize this pattern of orthostatic angina to provide the appropriate treatment. To determine whether conventional angina is present, supine exercise testing can be used.

AUTOIMMUNE AUTONOMIC FAILURE. In some patients, severe autonomic failure appears to result from immune damage to some aspect of neurons[77-81] and can be modeled by blockade of the N(N)-nicotinic receptor.[82] The findings of autonomic failure may appear suddenly, over days to weeks, or gradually over months to years.[79,83] In some of these patients, antibodies to ganglionic acetylcholine receptors have been demonstrated. When autoimmune autonomic failure appears gradually, it appears clinically indistinguishable from idiopathic pure autonomic failure. However, autoimmune autonomic failure may appear to occur overnight, often in a patient hospitalized for another illness, sometimes infectious in nature. The infection may seem to clear, but as the patient begins to ambulate, orthostatic hypotension can be so severe as to prevent discharge. Autonomic function testing shows postural vital signs with severe orthostatic hypotension and inadequate chronotropic response of heart rate for the degree of hypotension while upright. Autonomic abnormalities of bowel and bladder function are also common, and cholinergic dysfunction is more severe in those with higher antibody titers. Plasma catecholamines show very low norepinephrine levels, which rise only minimally with the upright posture. Although it has been suggested that intravenous gamma globulin may aid in reversing this syndrome,[84] it is not efficacious in all patients. Treatment is identical to that employed in patients with severe pure autonomic failure and multiple system atrophy.

SECONDARY AUTONOMIC NEUROPATHY (DIABETES, AMYLOID, RENAL FAILURE–ASSOCIATED, VITAMIN B_{12} DEFICIENCY, PARANEOPLASTIC SYNDROMES). Autonomic dysfunction is one of the frequent long-term complications of diabetes (see Chap. 51), and diabetes is one example of a number of disorders that lead to peripheral autonomic nerve dysfunction.[85] In patients with diabetes mellitus, both somatic and autonomic (both sympathetic and parasympathetic) neuropathy develop over time,[86,87] and abnormalities of autonomic cardiovascular control have been described both in animal models of diabetes[88,89] and in diabetic patients both with and without orthostatic hypotension.[86,87] In such patients, impairment of autonomic function has independent negative prognostic value,[90] although the underlying basis and extent of the abnormality remain unclear. Jensen-Urstad and associates[86] found a relationship between vascular stiffness, as determined by ultrasound of the carotid artery, and baroreflex sensitivity, suggesting that the abnormality may be caused by changes in the environment of the baroreceptor. Hoeldtke and colleagues[91] have recently demonstrated abnormal sudomotor responses in patients newly diagnosed with type 1 diabetes, especially in the upper body, and believed that this likely represented early sympathetic nerve injury. McDowell and coworkers[88,89] assessed baroreflex function at multiple levels in rabbits rendered diabetic with alloxan, finding normal control of renal sympathetic nerve activity but a selective deficit in baroreflex-mediated bradycardia; they suggested that the abnormal autonomic control seen in diabetics might be due primarily to defective activation of central parasympathetic pathways rather than of parasympathetic withdrawal.[88] This is consistent with studies in streptozotocin-diabetic rats. Gouty and associates[92] used the numbers of c-*Fos*-immunoreactive neurons in the nucleus of the solitary tract to assess function of the afferent limb of the baroreflex and found a reduction at 8 and 16 weeks. These studies strongly suggest that afferent as well as efferent neurons are involved. In humans, it has been clearly demonstrated that rigorous control of glucose provides protection against the microvascular complications of diabetes,[83] and the development of autonomic dysfunction appears to be improved.[83] Indeed, hypoglycemia itself can lead to autonomic dysfunction.[93]

When no obvious cause for peripheral autonomic dysfunction is present, an assessment of renal function and a fat pad biopsy for amyloid[20,94] are appropriate. Antibodies to various aspects of the peripheral autonomic nervous system can also be associated with neoplasms that may be clinically inapparent[81,95] but can still cause neuronal damage.[96] Since there have been reports of the autonomic disorder resolving after removal of the neoplasm, this diagnosis should be sought if antibodies can be demonstrated. In general, patients with this disorder and those with amyloid are poorly responsive to therapeutic measures that are quite effective in other forms of autonomic dysfunction.

GUILLAIN-BARRÉ SYNDROME. Although ascending motor abnormalities are prominent in this rare syndrome, they may be accompanied by autonomic dysfunction as well, which worsens the prognosis.[97,98] If this is the case, there are two aspects of treatment that are affected. While the patient is at bed rest, attention must be paid to potential hypersensitivity to sympathomimetic agents and to the effects of food and water on blood pressure. If autonomic dysfunction persists when the patient is able to assume the upright posture, the treatment of orthostatic hypotension, as in other patients with severe dysautonomias, must be included in the treatment regimen. For some patients, the only autonomic abnormality is orthostatic intolerance secondary to prolonged bed rest that resolves over a few days to weeks as ambulation is undertaken.

DOPAMINE BETA-HYDROXYLASE DEFICIENCY. Dopamine beta-hydroxylase deficiency is a congenital disorder and the first autonomic disorder in which a specific genetic abnormality was identified.[99] These patients lack a functional version of the enzyme that normally converts dopamine to norepinephrine in the vesicle within noradrenergic neurons. The sympathetic cholinergic and parasympathetic systems are normal. Figure 87–5 demonstrates the abnormality in the noradrenergic neuron.

Tyrosine hydroxylase, not dopamine beta-hydroxylase, is the rate-limiting enzyme in the generation of catecholamines. When norepinephrine is not made and cannot exert feedback control on tyrosine hydroxylase, the product just prior to the enzymatic block, in this case dopamine, is present in excess. These patients have two problems: First, they have no norepinephrine to release when sympathetic nerve activity increases, and thus, for example, cannot mount a vasoconstrictor response to upright posture. They have marked orthostatic hypotension (usually a fall in blood pressure to levels < 80 mm Hg systolic), with less heart rate rise than one would expect for this fall in blood pressure. Some heart rate rise is seen due to parasympathetic withdrawal. The patient is usually unable to stand quietly for even 60 seconds. Second, since these patients have constitutively higher levels of dopamine, and they release dopamine rather than norepinephrine with sympathetic stimuli, urinary sodium excretion is increased, and patients are slightly volume depleted. In addition, there is ptosis, nasal stuffiness, hyperextensibility of joints, and retrograde ejaculation in men.[100]

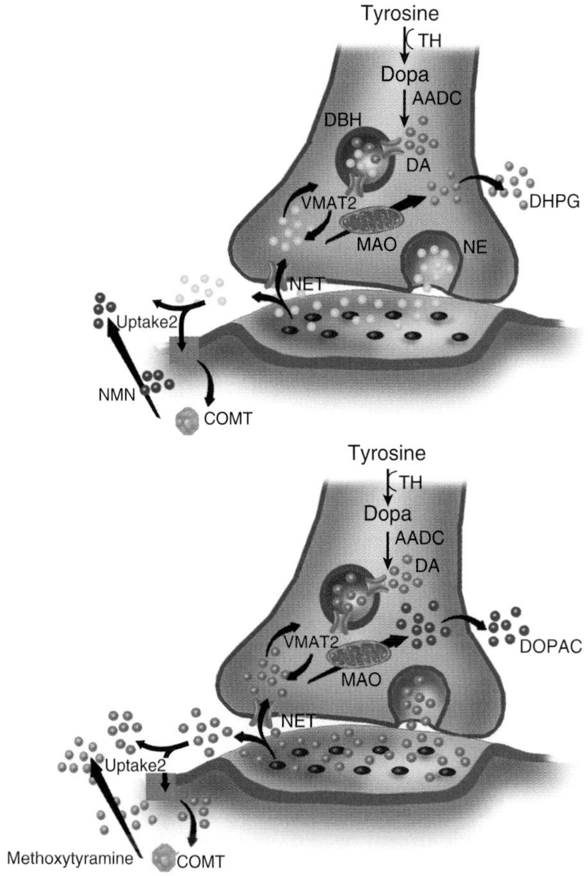

FIGURE 87–5 The enzymatic abnormality in dopamine beta-hydroxylase deficiency. TH = tyrosine hydroxylase; AADC = aromatic acid decarboxylase; DA = dopamine; Dopa = dihydroxyphenylalanine; DBH = dopamine beta-hydroxylase; VMAT2 = vesicular monoamine transporter 2; DHPG = dihydroxyphenylglycol; MAO = monoamine oxidase; NE = norepinephrine; NET = norepinephrine transporter; DOPAC = dihydroxyphenylacetic acid; NMN = normetanephrine; COMT = catechol *O*-methyltransferase. In the absence of functional dopamine beta-hydroxylase, the vesicles in noradrenergic neurons are filled with and release dopamine when the nerve is stimulated.

Since patients have normal levels of dopa decarboxylase, they are able to convert dihydroxyphenylserine to norepinephrine, and this drug has been used effectively to restore plasma norepinephrine levels and sympathetic responsiveness.[101] It has also been used with some benefit in patients with the more common forms of orthostatic hypotension due to autonomic failure.[102,103]

AUTONOMIC IMPAIRMENT IN CARDIAC DISEASE. Several forms of alteration in autonomic function have been demonstrated in patients with cardiovascular disease.[104-107] For example, increased neurohumoral tone in patients with heart failure has been associated with a worsened prognosis (see Chap. 22); this was the initial motivation for the expanded use of beta blockers in these patients. Of interest is a recent report of studies in a rabbit model of experimental heart failure that demonstrated a beneficial effect of simvastatin on plasma norepinephrine, renal sympathetic nerve activity, and baroreflex function.[108] Although many patients with heart failure are prescribed these agents because of other risk factors or known coronary disease, this suggests that they may have yet another non–lipid-lowering beneficial effect. Studies of autonomic effects in patients without conventional indications for 3-hydroxy-3-methylglutarylcoenzyme A (HMG-CoA) reductase inhibitors should be done.

A recent in vivo study in apolipoprotein E–/– mice, who are genetically dyslipidemic, showed increased blood pressure and heart rate, with decreased circadian rhythm, decreased heart rate variability, and increased blood pressure variability. When treated with rosuvastatin, they demonstrated an improvement in heart rate and blood pressure variability and decreased levels of caveolin 1, an inhibitor of aortic endothelial nitric oxide synthase.[109] It has also been demonstrated in a preliminary study that hypercholesterolemic patients with or without clinical coronary artery disease can improve heart rate variability after treatment with atorvastatin.[110] If confirmed in further studies in humans, this would suggest an additional beneficial effect of HMG-CoA reductase inhibitors in this population.

Mild Dysautonomias

POSTURAL TACHYCARDIA SYNDROME. In recent years, an increasing number of young to middle-aged patients have been recognized to have symptoms on standing, primarily tachycardia and weakness. Many demonstrate excessive sinus tachycardia on standing, according to the criteria of Streeten.[111] Most complain of orthostatic weakness, fatigue, chest discomfort, dizziness, anxiety, and occasionally presyncope or syncope after a period of standing.[112] These symptoms have also been used in the definition of postural tachycardia syndrome (POTS) by Low and coworkers,[112,113] but there is some variability in the inclusion criteria in studies by different investigators. The following criteria are now generally accepted in the clinical and laboratory definition of POTS:

- Orthostatic symptoms of sympathetic activation
- Orthostatic tachycardia (>30 beats/min)
- A fall in blood pressure of <20/10 mm Hg
- Elevated standing plasma norepinephrine (>600 pg/ml)

POTS is not a disease but indeed is a syndrome. Like "anemia" or "fever," this constellation of symptoms and findings represents the "final common pathway" of likely hundreds of genetic and acquired autonomic and cardiovascular entities. The disorder is not new. It has been recognized for many years and has been reported especially when large groups of young people were evaluated, often in times of war. Many different names have been applied, including *effort syndrome, hyperdynamic beta-adrenergic state, idiopathic hypovolemia, irritable heart, mitral valve prolapse syndrome, neurocirculatory asthenia, orthostatic tachycardia syndrome, soldier's heart, vasoregulatory asthenia*, as well as POTS.

In some cases, specific etiologies have been documented,[57,114-119] and several of these are listed in Table 87–3. We assessed baroreflex function in a group of patients with neuropathic orthostatic intolerance, demonstrating that there is not only alpha- and beta-receptor hypersensitivity but also a reduced baroreflex index (Fig. 87–6).[120]

Because it had been suggested that the tachycardia was an appropriate response to either an effective reduction in blood volume or a circulating vasodilator and that it might represent a healthy autonomic response appropriately maintaining blood pressure and cardiac output, blood flow in the middle cerebral artery has been assessed in these patients during head-up tilt. The more rapid than normal decline in blood velocity in these patients than in matched normal controls confirms that the compensatory response is hemodynamically inadequate.[37,121]

TABLE 87–3 Etiologies of Subsets of Orthostatic Tachycardia

Subset	Cause
Structural	Ehlers-Danlos syndrome
Hypovolemia (absolute)	Channelopathies
Hypovolemia (orthostatic)	Idiopathic
Autoimmune	Anti-NNA3 subunit
Neuropathic	Neuropathic postural tachycardia syndrome
Hyperadrenergic (increased release)	Hyperadrenergia
Hyperadrenergic (decreased clearance)	Norepinephrine transporter deficiency

NNA3 = $N_n\alpha_3$ = the α_3 subunit of the neural nicotinic receptor.

DYNAMIC PLASMA VOLUME CHANGES. Figure 87–7 demonstrates the abnormally increased dynamic plasma volume shifts in a patient with orthostatic intolerance, demonstrating coincident increases in plasma norepinephrine and heart rate and a more gradual rise in dihydroxyphenylglycol, the norepinephrine metabolite.

The magnitude of these changes has important consequences for the study of any orthostatic syndrome, but it has rarely been taken into account. These dynamic changes could either differentially activate cardiopulmonary receptors in patients with orthostatic intolerance or could be quantitatively distinct. Some patients with orthostatic intolerance seem to have both a chronically decreased blood volume (5 to 20 percent) and an excessive dynamic decrease as well.

Treatment is aimed at restoring normal plasma volume and preventing pooling of volume in the periphery, usually beginning with fludrocortisone and compression garments. Additional restraint of beta-mediated tachycardia with beta blockers may be helpful. Often only very low doses of medication are tolerated.

NOREPINEPHRINE TRANSPORTER DEFICIENCY. A rare specific etiology for POTS has been demonstrated to be a mutation in the norepinephrine transporter gene, leading to a higher than 98 percent reduction in the ability to transport released norepinephrine back into the sympathetic nerve ending.[122] The mutant form also exerts a dominant negative effect when it is co-transfected into a heterologous expression system, by causing a conformational disruption interfering with transporter biosynthetic progression and trafficking of not only the mutant transporter but also of the wild-type norepinephrine transporter.[117-119] This results in elevated synaptic levels of the neurotransmitter whenever norepinephrine release is triggered, with resultant excessive heart rate.

MEDICATIONS (NOREPINEPHRINE TRANSPORTER BLOCKERS). Medications such as tricyclic antidepressants produce a syndrome of orthostatic tachycardia and sometimes orthostatic hypotension.[123] Vasodilators may produce a similar effect. A review of the patient's medications for drugs with a potential hemodynamic effect should be a first consideration in evaluating patients with autonomic findings.

BED REST. Studies of normal subjects after a period of bed rest and studies of astronauts during exposure to microgravity have demonstrated the development of orthostatic tachycardia and, in some, an increased propensity to syncope with prolonged (30 minutes) quiet standing.[117,118,124] This resolves completely after normal ambulation is resumed, but symptoms may take several days to weeks to abate, especially if the period of bed rest is long. Gradually increasing periods

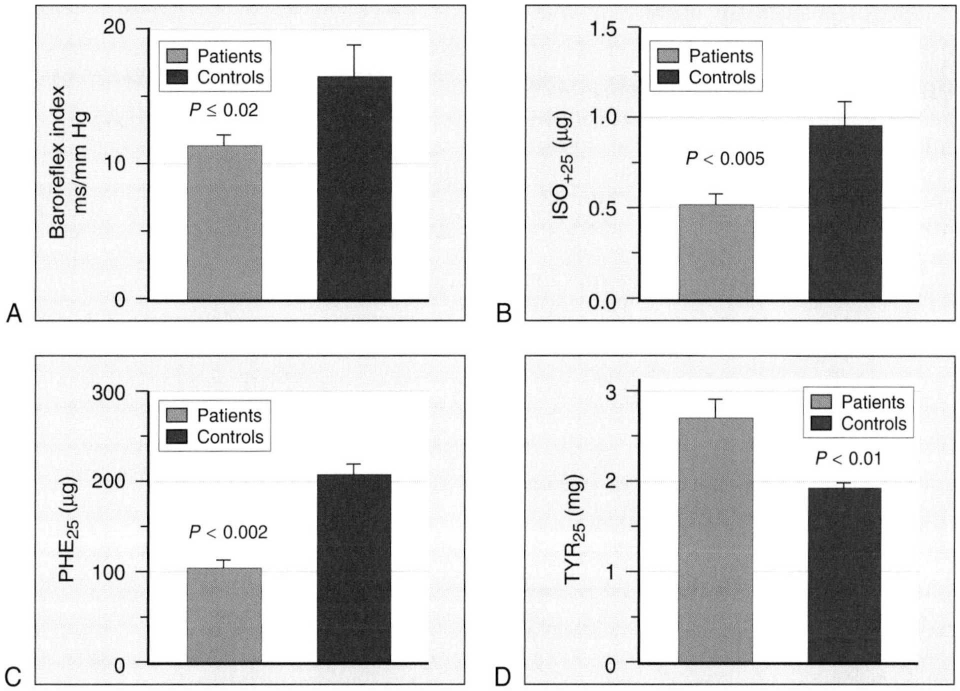

FIGURE 87–6 Pharmacological assessment of adrenergic receptor and baroreflex function in patients with orthostatic intolerance. For each agent (PHE = phenylephrine; ISO = isoproterenol; TYR = tyramine), the dose required to produce a pressor (PHE and TYR) or depressor (ISO) effect of 25 mm Hg is compared with the doses required in age-matched normal control subjects.

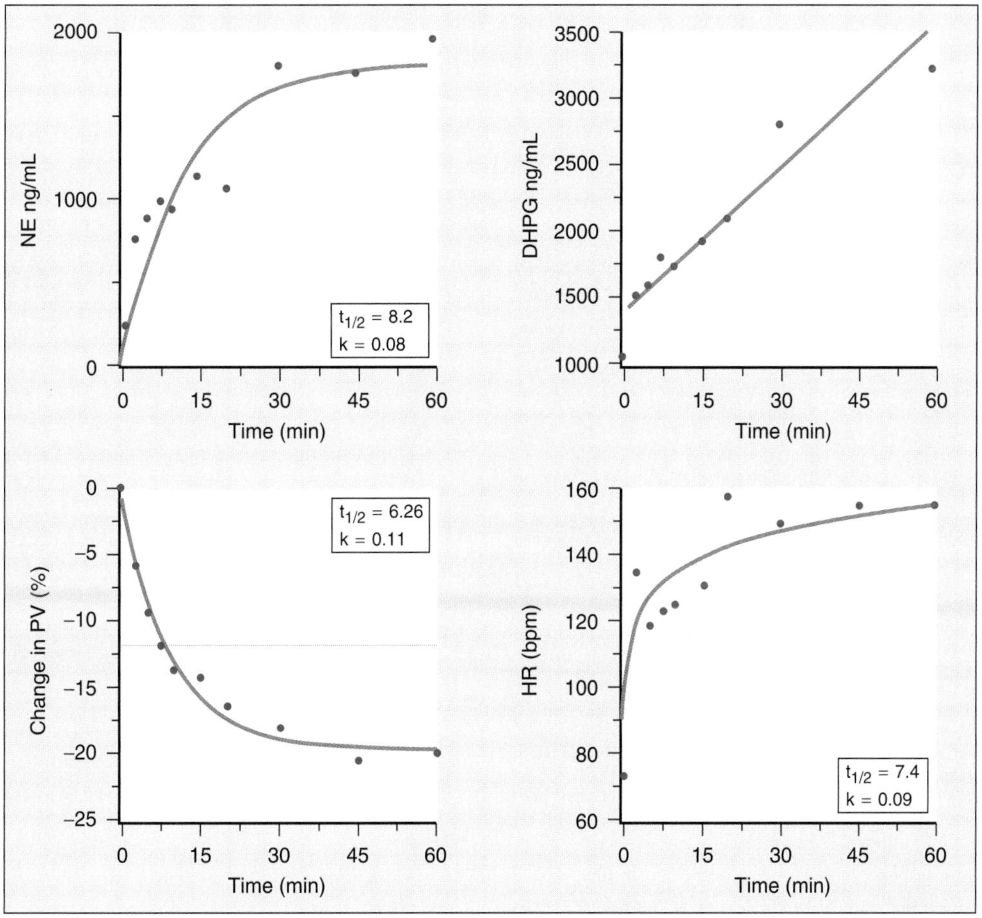

FIGURE 87–7 Effect of assuming the upright posture in a 39-year-old woman with orthostatic intolerance. From the bottom left, going counterclockwise, the PV decreases 20 percent over 45 minutes and is mirrored by an increase in HR. While the dihydroxyphenylglycol (DHPG) rises more gradually, the change in plasma norepinephrine (NE) parallels the change in heart rate.

of seated and then upright posture are usually all that is required, but compression garments may be helpful in situations where resolution is slow.

NEURALLY MEDIATED SYNCOPE. Most patients referred with syncope do not have either the orthostatic hypotension of the severe dysautonomias or the orthostatic tachycardia characteristic of orthostatic intolerance. In fact, between episodes of syncope, their autonomic function testing is entirely normal. After elimination of cardiac causes, most patients with neurally mediated syncope have a relatively benign prognosis, with risk related only to the circumstances in which they might have episodes of syncope. Their evaluation and treatment are covered in Chapter 34.

REFERENCES

General Principles

1. Diedrich, A, Jordan, J, Shannon, JR, et al: Modulation of QT interval during autonomic nervous system blockade in humans. Circulation 106:2238-2243, 2002.
2. Choy, AMJ, Lang, CC, Roden, DM, et al: Abnormalities of the QT interval in primary disorders of autonomic failure. Am Heart J 136:664-671, 1998.
3. Chen QH, Toney GM: Identification and characterization of two functionally distinct groups of spinal cord–projecting paraventricular nucleus neurons with sympathetic-related activity. Neuroscience 118:797-807, 2003.
4. Meyrelles, S, Sharma, R, Mao, H, et al: Modulation of baroreceptor activity by gene transfer of nitric oxide synthase to carotid sinus adventitia. Am J Physiol Regul Integr Comp Physiol 284: R1190-R1198, 2003.
5. Michalkiewicz M, Knestaut K, Bytchkova E, Michalkiewicz T: Hypotension and reduced catecholamines in neuropeptide Y transgenic rats. Hypertension 41:1056-1062, 2003.
6. Jacob G, Ertl AC, Shannon JR, et al: Effect of standing on neurohumoral responses and plasma volume in healthy subjects. J Appl Physiol 84:914-921, 1998.
7. Ketch T, Biaggioni I, Robertson R, Robertson D: Four faces of baroreflex failure: Hypertensive crisis, volatile hypertension, orthostatic tachycardia, and malignant vagotonia. Circulation 105:2518-2523, 2002.
8. Kim CH, Zabetian CP, Cubells JF, et al: Mutations in the dopamine beta-hydroxylase gene are associated with human norepinephrine deficiency. Am J Med Genet 108:140-147, 2002.
9. Youmans J, Akeroyd JJ, Frank H: Changes in the blood and circulation with changes in posture: The effect of exercise and vasodilatation. J Clin Invest 14:739-753, 1935.

Autonomic Disorders

10. Jordan J, Shannon JR, Black BK, et al: Malignant vagotonia due to selective baroreflex failure. Hypertension 30:1072-1077, 1997.
11. Parikh SM, Diedrich A, Biaggioni I, Robertson D: The nature of the autonomic dysfunction in multiple system atrophy. J Neurol Sci 200:1-10, 2002.
12. Shannon JR, Jordan J, Diedrich A, et al: Sympathetically mediated hypertension in autonomic failure. Circulation 101:2710-2715, 2000.
13. Takaya N, Sumiyoshi M, Nakata Y: Prolonged cardiac arrest caused by glossopharyngeal neuralgia. Heart 89:381, 2003.
14. Robertson D: The epidemic of orthostatic tachycardia and orthostatic intolerance. Am J Med Sci 317:75-77, 1999.
15. Shannon JR, Flattem NL, Jordan J, et al: Orthostatic intolerance and tachycardia associated with norepinephrine-transporter deficiency. N Engl J Med 342:541-549, 2000.
16. Mosqueda-Garcia R, Furlan R, Fernandez-Violante R, et al: Sympathetic and baroreceptor reflex function in neurally mediated syncope evoked by tilt. J Clin Invest 99:2736-2744, 1997.
17. Carson RP, Robertson D: Genetic manipulation of noradrenergic neurons. J Pharmacol Exp Ther 301:410-417, 2002.
18. Thomaides T, Bleasdale-Barr K, Chaudhuri KR, et al: Cardiovascular and hormonal responses to liquid food challenge in idiopathic Parkinson's disease, multiple system atrophy, and pure autonomic failure. Neurology 43:900-904, 1993.
19. Robertson D, Biaggioni I, Ertl AC, et al: Orthostatic intolerance: Emerging genetic and environmental etiologies. J Gravit Physio 6:151-154, 1999.
20. Carvalho MJ, van den Meiracker AH, Boomsma F, et al: Diurnal blood pressure variation in progressive autonomic failure. Hypertension 35:892-897, 2000.
21. Cariga P, Mathias CJ: Haemodynamics of the pressor effect of oral water in human sympathetic denervation due to autonomic failure. Clin Sci (Lond) 101:313-319, 2001.
22. Jordan J, Shannon JR, Grogan E, et al: The acute pressor effect of drinking water. J Hypertens 16:S32-S32, 1998.
23. Novak V, Spies JM, Novak P, et al: Hypocapnia and cerebral hypoperfusion in orthostatic intolerance. Stroke 29:1876-1881, 1998.
24. Jordan J, Shannon JR, Pohar B, et al: Contrasting effects of vasodilators on blood pressure and sodium balance in the hypertension of autonomic failure. J Am Soc Nephrol 10:35-42, 1999.
25. Shannon JR, Jordan J, Robertson D: Blood pressure in autonomic failure: Drinks, meals, and other ordeals. Clin Sci (Lond) 94:5, 1998.
26. Jordan J, Shannon JR, Diedrich A, et al: Interaction of carbon dioxide and sympathetic nervous system activity in the regulation of cerebral perfusion in humans. Hypertension 36:383-388, 2000.
27. Jordan J, Tank J, Shannon JR, et al: Baroreflex buffering and susceptibility to vasoactive drugs. Circulation 105:1459-1464, 2002.
28. Goldstein DS, Tack C: Noninvasive detection of sympathetic neurocirculatory failure. Clin Auton Res 10:285-291, 2000.

Severe Dysautonomias

29. Sharabi Y, Dendi R, Holmes C, Goldstein DS: Baroreflex failure as a late sequela of neck irradiation. Hypertension 42:110-116, 2003.
30. Robertson D, Hollister AS, Biaggioni I, et al: The diagnosis and treatment of baroreflex failure. N Engl J Med 329:1449-1455, 1993.
31. Robertson D, Jacob G, Ertl A, et al: Clinical models of cardiovascular regulation after weightlessness. Med Sci Sports Exerc 28(10 Suppl):S80-S84, 1996.
32. Dorman T, Thompson D, Breslow M, et al: Nicardipine versus nitroprusside for breakthrough hypertension following carotid endarterectomy. J Clin Anesth 13:16-19, 2001.
33. Dimakakos P, Antoniou A, Mourikis D, et al: Surgical outcome of carotid artery disease: Analysis of 367 carotid endarterectomies. Int Surg 83:350-354, 1998.
34. Landesberg G, Adam D, Berlatzky Y, Akselrod S: Step baroreflex response in awake patients undergoing carotid surgery: Time-and frequency-domain analysis. Am J Physiol 274:H1590-H1597, 1998.
35. Kresowik T, Bratzler D, Karp H, et al: Multistate utilization, processes, and outcomes of carotid endarterectomy. J Vasc Surg 32:227-234, 2001.
36. Furlan R, Diedrich A, Rimoldi A, et al: Effects of unilateral and bilateral carotid baroreflex stimulation on cardiac and neural sympathetic discharge oscillatory patterns. Circulation 108:717-723, 2003.
37. Jordan J, Shannon JR, Black BK, et al: Evidence for sympathetically-mediated cerebral vasoconstriction in idiopathic orthostatic intolerance. Circulation 98:827-827, 1998.
38. Moretti R, Torre P, Antonello RM, et al: Gabapentin treatment of glossopharyngeal neuralgia: A follow-up of four years of a single case. Eur J Pain 6:403-407, 2002.
39. Ozenci M, Karaoguz R, Conkbayir C, et al: Glossopharyngeal neuralgia with cardiac syncope treated by glossopharyngeal rhizotomy and microvascular decompression. Europace 5:149-152, 2003.
40. Shy G, Drager G: A neurological syndrome associated with orthostatic hypotension. Arch Neurol 2:511-527, 1960.
41. Benarroch EE: New findings on the neuropathology of multiple system atrophy. Auton Neurosci 96:59-62, 2002.
42. Robertson D, Shannon JR, Jordan J, et al: Multiple system atrophy: New developments in pathophysiology and therapy. Parkinsonism Relat Disord 7:257-260, 2001.
43. Abe H, Yagishita S, Amano N, et al: Argyrophilic glial intracytoplasmic inclusions in multiple system atrophy: Immunocytochemical and ultrastructural study. Acta Neuropathol (Berl) 84:273-277, 1992.
44. Giasson BI, Mabon ME, Duda JE, et al: Tau and 14-3-3 in glial cytoplasmic inclusions of multiple system atrophy. Acta Neuropathol (Berl) 106;243-250, 2003.
45. Austin MT, Davis TL, Robertson D, Charles PD: Multiple system atrophy: Clinical presentation and diagnosis. Tenn Med 92:55-57, 1999.
46. Micieli G, Tassorelli C, Martignoni E, et al: Further characterization of autonomic involvement in multiple system atrophy: A pupillometric study. Funct Neurol 10:273-280, 1995.
47. Oertel WH, Bandmann O: Multiple system atrophy. J Neural Transm 56:(Suppl):155-164, 1999.
48. Sakakibara R, Hattori T, Uchiyama T, et al: Urinary dysfunction and orthostatic hypotension in multiple system atrophy: Which is the more common and earlier manifestation? J Neurol Neurosurg Psychiatry 68:65-69, 2000.
49. Beck RO, Betts CD, Fowler CJ: Genitourinary dysfunction in multiple system atrophy: Clinical features and treatment in 62 cases. J Urol 151:1336-1341, 1994.
50. Yamaguchi M, Arai K, Asahina M, Hattori T: Laryngeal stridor in multiple system atrophy. Eur Neurol 49:154-159, 2003.
51. Asahina M, Yamaguchi M, Fukutake T, Hattori T: [Sleep apnea in multiple system atrophy]. Nippon Rinsho 58:1722-1727, 2000.
52. Bleasdale-Barr KM, Mathias CJ: Neck and other muscle pains in autonomic failure: Their association with orthostatic hypotension. J R Soc Med 91:355-359, 1998.
53. Micieli G, Tosi P, Marcheselli S, Cavallini A: Autonomic dysfunction in Parkinson's disease. Neurol Sci 24(Suppl 1):S32-S34, 2003.
54. Lee WY, Jin DK, Oh MR, et al: Frequency analysis and clinical characterization of spinocerebellar ataxia types 1, 2, 3, 6, and 7 in Korean patients. Arch Neurol 60:858-863, 2003.
55. Savoiardo M: Differential diagnosis of Parkinson's disease and atypical parkinsonian disorders by magnetic resonance imaging. Neurol Sci 24(Suppl 1):S35-S37, 2003.
56. Miwa H, Kajimoto Y, Nakanishi I, et al: T2-low signal intensity in the cortex in multiple system atrophy. J Neurol Sci 211:85-88, 2003.
57. Goldstein DS, Holmes C, Sharabi Y, et al: Plasma levels of catechols and metanephrines in neurogenic orthostatic hypotension. Neurology 60:1327-1332, 2003.
58. Smit AA, Halliwill JR, Low PA, Wieling W: Pathophysiological basis of orthostatic hypotension in autonomic failure. J Physiol 519:1-10, 1999.
59. Biaggioni I, Robertson RM: Hypertension in orthostatic hypotension and autonomic dysfunction. Cardiol Clin 20:291-301, 2002.
60. Colosimo C, Pezzella FR: The symptomatic treatment of multiple system atrophy. Eur J Neurol 9:195-199, 2002.
61. Jordan J, Biaggioni I: Diagnosis and treatment of supine hypertension in autonomic failure patients with orthostatic hypotension. J Clin Hypertens (Greenwich) 4:139-145, 2002.
62. Chandler MP, Mathias CJ: Haemodynamic responses during head-up tilt and tilt reversal in two groups with chronic autonomic failure: Pure autonomic failure and multiple system atrophy. J Neurol 249:542-548, 2002.
63. Goldstein DS, Pechnik S, Holmes C, et al: Association between supine hypertension and orthostatic hypotension in autonomic failure. Hypertension 42:136-142, 2003.
64. Onrot J, Goldberg MR, Biaggioni I, et al: Hemodynamic and humoral effects of caffeine in autonomic failure: Therapeutic implications for postprandial hypotension. N Engl J Med 313:549-554, 1985.

65. Hoeldtke RD, Dworkin GE, Gaspar SR, et al: Effect of the somatostatin analogue SMS-201-995 on the adrenergic response to glucose ingestion in patients with postprandial hypotension. Am J Med 86:673-677, 1989.
66. Lamarre-Cliche M, Cusson J: Octreotide for orthostatic hypotension. Can J Clin Pharmacol 213-215, 1999.
67. Mathias C, Young T: Plugging the leak—benefits of the vasopressin-2 agonist, desmopressin in autonomic failure. Clin Auton Res 13:85-87, 2003.
68. Shannon JR, Diedrich A, Biaggioni I, et al: Water drinking as a treatment for orthostatic syndromes. Am J Med 112:355-360, 2002.
69. Jordan J: Acute effect of water on blood pressure: What do we know? Clin Auton Res 12:250-255, 2002.
70. Riley DE: Orthostatic hypotension in multiple system atrophy. Curr Treat Options Neurol 2:225-230, 2000.
71. Sakakibara R, Matsuda S, Uchiyama T, et al: The effect of intranasal desmopressin on nocturnal waking in urination in multiple system atrophy patients with nocturnal polyuria. Clin Auton Res 13:106-108, 2003.
72. Winkler AS, Marsden J, Parton M, et al: Erythropoietin deficiency and anaemia in multiple system atrophy. Mov Disord 16:233-239, 2001.
73. Iranzo A, Santamaria J, Tolosa E: Continuous positive air pressure eliminates nocturnal stridor in multiple system atrophy. Barcelona Multiple System Atrophy Study Group. Lancet 356:1329-1330, 2000.
74. Wenning GK, Geser F: Multiple system atrophy. Rev Neurol (Paris) 159:3S31-3S38, 2003.
75. Gill CE, Khurana RK: Caregiver burden in Shy-Drager syndrome. J Nerv Ment Dis 188:47-50, 2000.
76. Bradbury S, Eggleston C: Postural hypotension: A report of three cases. Am Heart J 1:73-86, 1925.
77. Vernino S, Low PA, Fealey RD, et al: Autoantibodies to ganglionic acetylcholine receptors in autoimmune autonomic neuropathies. N Engl J Med 343:847-855, 2000.
78. Goldstein DS, Holmes C, Dendi R, et al Pandysautonomia associated with impaired ganglionic neurotransmission and circulating antibody to the neuronal nicotinic receptor. Clin Auton Res 12:281-285, 2002.
79. Klein CM, Vernino S, Lennon VA, et al: The spectrum of autoimmune autonomic neuropathies. Ann Neurol 53:752-758, 2003.
80. Low PA, Vernino S, Suarez G: Autonomic dysfunction in peripheral nerve disease. Muscle Nerve 27:646-661, 2003.
81. Vernino S, Adamski J, Kryzer TJ, et al: Neuronal nicotinic ACh receptor antibody in subacute autonomic neuropathy and cancer-related syndromes. Neurology 50:1806-1813, 1998.
82. Jordan J, Shannon JR, Black BK, et al: N(N)-nicotinic blockade as an acute human model of autonomic failure. Hypertension 31:1178-1184, 1998.
83. UK Prospective Study Group: Intensive blood-glucose control with sulphonylureas or insulin compared with conventional treatment and risk of complications in patients with type 2 diabetes (UKPDS 33). Lancet 352:837-853, 1998.
84. Smit AA, Vermeulen M, Koelman JH, Wieling W: Unusual recovery from acute panautonomic neuropathy after immunoglobulin therapy. Mayo Clin Proc 72:333-335, 1997.
85. Vinik AI, Erbas T: Recognizing and treating diabetic autonomic neuropathy. Cleve Clin J Med 68:928-944, 2001.
86. Jensen-Urstad K, Reichard P, Jensen-Urstad M: Decreased heart rate variability in patients with type 1 diabetes mellitus is related to arterial wall stiffness. J Intern Med 245:57-61, 1999.
87. Bernardi L: Clinical evaluation of arterial baroreflex activity in diabetes. Diabetes Nutr Metab 13:331-340, 2000.
88. McDowell T, Chapleau M, Hajduczok G, Abboud FM: Baroreflex dysfunction in diabetes mellitus: I. Selective impairment of parasympathetic control of heart rate. Am J Physiol 266:H235-H243, 1994.
89. McDowell T, Hajduczok G, Abboud F, Chapleau M: Baroreflex dysfunction in diabetes mellitus: II. Site of baroreflex impairment in diabetic rabbits. Am J Physiol 266:H244-H249, 2003.
90. Valensi P, Sachs RN, Harfouche B, et al: Predictive value of cardiac autonomic neuropathy in diabetic patients with or without silent myocardial ischemia. Diabetes Care 24:339-343, 2001.
91. Hoeldtke RD, Bryner KD, Horvath GG, et al: Redistribution of sudomotor responses is an early sign of sympathetic dysfunction in type 1 diabetes. Diabetes 436:436-443, 2001.
92. Gouty S, Regalia J, Helke C: Attenuation of the afferent limb of the baroreceptor reflex in streptozotocin-induced diabetic rats. Auton Neurosci 89:86-95, 2001.
93. Diedrich L, Sandoval D, Davis SN: Hypoglycemia-associated autonomic failure. Clin Auton Res 12:358-365, 2002.
94. Singer W, Opfer-Gehrking TL, McPhee BR, et al: Acetylcholinesterase inhibition: A novel approach in the treatment of neurogenic orthostatic hypotension. J Neurol Neurosurg Psychiatry 74:1294-1298, 2003.
95. Low PA: Autonomic neuropathies. Curr Opin Neurol 15:605-609, 2002.
96. Scaravilli F, An SF, Groves M, Thom M: The neuropathology of paraneoplastic syndromes. Brain Pathol 9:251-260, 1999.
97. Low PA: Autonomic neuropathies. Curr Opin Neurol 7:402-406, 1994.
98. Santiago S, Ferrer T, Espinosa ML: Neurophysiological studies of thin myelinated (A delta) and unmyelinated (C) fibers: Application to peripheral neuropathies. Neurophysiol Clin 30:27-42, 2000.
99. Robertson D, Goldberg MR, Onrot J, et al: Isolated failure of autonomic noradrenergic neurotransmission—evidence for impaired beta-hydroxylation of dopamine. N Engl J Med 314:1494-1497, 1986.
100. Biaggioni I, Goldstein DS, Atkinson T, Robertson D: Dopamine-beta-hydroxylase deficiency in humans. Neurology 40:370-373, 1990.
101. Vincent S, Robertson D: The broader view: Catecholamine abnormalities. Clin Auton Res 12(Suppl 1):I44-I49, 2002.
102. Freeman R, Landsberg L, Young J: The treatment of neurogenic orthostatic hypotension with 3,4-D,L-threo-dihydroxyphenylserine: A randomized, placebo-controlled, crossover trial. Neurology 53:2151-2157, 1999.
103. Kaufmann H, Saadia D, Voustianiouk A, et al: Norepinephrine precursor therapy in neurogenic orthostatic hypotension. Circulation 108:724-728, 2003.
104. Lanfranchi PA, Somers VK: Arterial baroreflex function and cardiovascular variability: Interactions and implications. Am J Physiol Regul Integr Comp Physiol 283:R815-R826, 2002.
105. Gerritsen J, Dekker JM, TenVoorde BJ, et al: Impaired autonomic function is associated with increased mortality, especially in subjects with diabetes, hypertension, or a history of cardiovascular disease: The Hoorn Study. Diabetes Care 24:1793-1798, 2001.
106. Stevens MJ: New imaging techniques for cardiovascular autonomic neuropathy: A window on the heart. Diabetes Technol Ther 3:9-22, 2001.
107. Sleight P: The importance of the autonomic nervous system in health and disease. Aust N Z J Med 27:467-473, 1997.
108. Pliquett R, Cornish K, Peuler J, Zucker I: Simvastatin normalizes autonomic neural control in experimental heart failure. Circulation 107:2493-2498, 2003.
109. Pelat M, Dessy C, Massion P, et al: Rosuvastatin decreases caveolin-1 and improves nitric oxide-dependent heart rate and blood pressure variability in apolipoprotein E-/- mice in vivo. Circulation 107:2480-2486, 2003.
110. Pehlivanidis AN, Athyros VG, Demitriadis DS, et al: Heart rate variability after long-term treatment with atorvastatin in hypercholesterolaemic patients with or without coronary artery disease. Atherosclerosis 157:463-469, 2001.

Mild Dysautonomias

111. Streeten DH: Orthostatic intolerance: A historical introduction to the pathophysiological mechanisms. Am J Med Sci 11:78-87, 1999.
112. Low PA, Schondorf R, Rummans TA: Why do patients have orthostatic symptoms in POTS? Clin Auton Res 11:223-224, 2001.
113. Novak V, Novak P, Opfer-Gehrking TL, et al: Clinical and laboratory indices that enhance the diagnosis of postural tachycardia syndrome. Mayo Clin Proc 73:1141-1150, 1998.
114. Rowe PC, Barron DF, Calkins H, et al: Orthostatic intolerance and chronic fatigue syndrome associated with Ehlers-Danlos syndrome. J Pediatr 135:494-499, 1999.
115. Kuchel O, Leveille J: Idiopathic hypovolemia: A self-perpetuating autonomic dysfunction? Clin Auton Res 8:341-346, 1998.
116. Jacob G, Costa F, Shannon JR, et al: The neuropathic postural tachycardia syndrome. N Engl J Med 343:1008-1014, 2000.
117. Ertl AC, Diedrich A, Biaggioni I: Baroreflex dysfunction induced by microgravity: Potential relevance to postflight orthostatic intolerance. Clin Auton Res 10:269-277, 2000.
118. Ertl AC, Diedrich A, Biaggioni I, et al: Human muscle sympathetic nerve activity and plasma noradrenaline kinetics in space. J Physiol 538:321-329, 2002.
119. Hahn MK, Robertson D, Blakely RD: A mutation in the human norepinephrine transporter gene (SLC6A2) associated with orthostatic intolerance disrupts surface expression of mutant and wild-type transporters. J Neurosci 23:4470-4478, 2003.
120. Jacob G, Shannon JR, Costa F, et al: Abnormal norepinephrine clearance and adrenergic receptor sensitivity in idiopathic orthostatic intolerance. Circulation 99:1706-1712, 1999.
121. Schondorf R, Benoit J, Stein R: Cerebral autoregulation in orthostatic intolerance. Ann N Y Acad Sci 940:514-526, 2001.
122. Robertson D, Flattem N, Tellioglu T, et al: Familial orthostatic tachycardia due to norepinephrine transporter deficiency. Ann N Y Acad Sci 940:527-543, 2001.
123. Schroeder C, Tank J, Boschmann M, et al: Selective norepinephrine reuptake inhibition as a human model of orthostatic intolerance. Circulation 105:347-353, 2002.
124. Convertino VA: G-factor as a tool in basic research: mechanisms of orthostatic tolerance. J Gravit Physiol 6:73-76, 1999.

DISCLOSURE INDEX

The following contributors have indicated that they have a relationship that, in the context of their participation in the writing of a chapter for the seventh edition of *Braunwald's Heart Disease,* could be perceived by some people as a real or apparent conflict of interest, but do not consider that it has influenced the writing of their chapter. Codes for the disclosure information (institution[s] and nature of relationship[s]) are provided below.

Relationship Codes

A—Stock options or bond holdings in a for-profit corporation or self-directed pension plan
B—Research grants
C—Employment (full or part-time)
D—Ownership or partnership
E—Consulting fees or other remuneration received by the contributor or immediate family
F—Nonremunerative positions, such as board member, trustee, or public spokesperson
G—Receipt of royalties
H—"Speaker's bureau"

Institution and Company Codes

001—ARCA Discovery, Inc.
002—Abbott Labs
003—Adelphi, Inc.
004—Aderis Pharmaceuticals, Inc.
005—Actelion
006—Ajinomoto Pharmaceuticals
007—Alexion Pharmaceuticals
008—Alliance Medical
009—Alza
010—American Association for Cancer Research
011—American Cancer Society
012—American College of Cardiology
013—American Heart Association
014—American Society of Echocardiography
015—Amersham Health
016—Amersham, Inc.
017—Arrow
018—Asahi Chemical Company
019—Astra Zeneca, Inc.
020—Avant Immunotherapeutics
021—Aventis
022—Avon Foundation
023—BASF
024—Baxter Pharmaceuticals
025—Bayer
026—Bayer Diagnostics
027—Berkeley Heart Lab
028—Berlex
029—Best Med
030—Beth Israel Deaconess Medical Center
031—Bioheart Scientific
032—Biomarin Pharmaceuticals
033—Biosite, Inc.
034—Blue Cross Blue Shield of Michigan
035—Boeringer Ingelheim
036—Boston Scientific Corporation
037—Bracco
038—Bristol Meyers Squibb, Co.
039—British Biotech
040—Burrill and Company
041—C2R
042—Cardiac Dimensions
043—Cardiofocus
044—Cardiovascular Biosciences
045—Cardiovascular Imaging Solutions
046—Cell Therapeutics
047—Centocor
048—Chiron
049—Churchill Livingstone
050—Columbia University
051—Cordis Corporation
052—Corvas BMS
053—Covalent
054—Cryocor
055—CTI, Inc.
056—Cubist Pharmaceuticals
057—Current Medicine LLC
058—Current Science
059—CV Therapeutics, Inc.
060—CVRx
061—Dade Behring
062—Denver Health Medical Center
063—Discovery East
064—Discovery, Inc.
065—Doris Duke Foundation
066—EBR systems
067—Eli Lilly and Company
068—Encysive
069—Esperion Therapeutics
070—Excerpta Medica
071—Exhale Therapeutics
072—eV3
073—Fondation Leducq (Paris)
074—Fujisawa
075—Genentech
076—Genvec
077—Genzyme
078—Glaxo Smith Kline
079—GMP Companies, Inc.
080—Goldant
081—GSK
082—GTC Therapeutics
083—Guerbet
084—Guidant Corporation
085—Interleukin Genetics
086—Intraluminal
087—Johnson and Johnson
088—Johnson and Johnson—Merck Consumer Pharmaceuticals
089—K-23 National Institute of Health
090—King Pharmaceuticals
091—KOS
092—Lancet International
093—Life Sentry
094—Lippincott
095—MC Communications
096—McGraw Hill
097—McNeil
098—Medical Decision Point
099—Medicines Company
100—Medreviews
101—Medtronic, Inc.
102—Merck & Co., Inc.
103—Merck Frosst/Schering Plough
104—Merck-Schering Plough Corp.
105—Michael Marcus and Associates Science Partners, LLC
106—Micromed
107—Millennium Pharmaceuticals
108—Mitsubishi
109—Molecular Insight Pharmaceuticals
110—Momenta Pharmaceuticals
111—Mylan
112—Myogen, Inc.
113—National Cancer Institute
114—National Heart, Lung and Blood Institute
115—NCME
116—New York University School of Medicine
117—NIH/NCRR Research Resource for Complex Physiologic Signals
118—Nitromed
119—Novartis, Inc.
120—Novonordisk Pharmaceuticals
121—Nuvelo
122—Octagon Corporation
123—Omnisonics
124—Ortho Biotech, Inc.
125—Ortho-Clinical Diagnostics
126—Ortho-McNeil
127—Otsuka
128—Pacific Mountain Affiliate
129—Paion
130—Pfizer, Inc.

131—Pharmacia Diagnostics
132—Pharmacia-Upjohn, Inc.
133—Philips
134—Philips Canada
135—Pierre Fabre
136—Point Biomedical
137—Procter and Gamble
138—Radiant Medical
139—Reliant Pharmaceuticals
140—Restore Medical
141—Rey Institute for Nonlinear Dynamics in Medicine
142—Roche Diagnostics
143—Sankyo
144—Sanofi-Synthelabo, Inc.
145—Sanyo
146—Scientific American Medicine Editorial Board
147—Scios, Inc.
148—Servier
149—Schering Plough Corp.
150—Siemens
151—SmithKline Beecham
152—St. Jude Medical
153—Stanford University
154—Sunol Molecular
155—Takeda
156—Terumo Cardiovascular Systems Corporation
157—Terumo Heart, Inc.
158—Thoratec
159—TJ Martel Foundation
160—Transneuronix
161—TYCO
162—United Therapeutics, Inc.
163—University of Colorado Health Sciences Center
164—University of Wisconsin, Medical School
165—Vasogen
166—Vasogenix
167—Vertex
168—Vicaron
169—Volcano Therapeutics
170—Women's Health Initiative
171—Wyeth
172—ZLB Behring

Contributors

Antman, Elliot, B-033, B-038, B-039, B-047, B-052, B-061, B-067, B-075, B-102, B107, B-142, B-154
Antman, Karen, A-055; B-011, B-022, B-113, B-159; E-019, E-065, E-110, E-146; F-010, F-011, F-092; G-094
Armstrong, William F., E-019, E-152; H-038
Baim, Donald S., E-036
Barsky, Arthur, B-130
Beckman, Joshua A., B-067, B-130; E-038; H-067, H-102, H-119
Beller, George A., B-038
Bonow, Robert O., B-114; E-038, E-090, E-130, E-155
Braunwald, Eugene, B-021, B-038, B-059, B-067, B-107, B-121; E-045, E-073, E-084, E-095, E-110, E-147; F-012, F-116, F-170; G-057, G-096
Bristow, Michael, A-001, A-064, A-112; E-019, E-041, E-042, E-053, E-060, E-077, E-081, E-084, E-102, E-108, E-111, E-119, E-147
Calkins, Hugh, B-080, B-101, B-152; E-080
Cannon, Christopher, B-038, B-102, B-144; F-018, F-019, F-025, F-078, F-099, F-125, F-130, F-167; H-021, H-038, H-047, H-067, H-075, H-102, H-107, H-144
Creager, Mark A., B-028, B-038, B-067, B-130, B-144, B-171; E-003, E-007, E-028, E-038, E-076, E-077, E-091, E-100, E-127, E-130, E-144, E-165; G-058; H-038, H-127, H-144
Dilsizian, Vasken, B-037, B-112, B-133; E-109; H-038, H-074
Douglas, Pamela S., E-012, E-014, E-102, E-119; F-012, F-014
Eagle, Kim A., C-021, C-034, C-130; E-012; F-114
Eisenhauer, Andrew C., B-84, B-101; E-101
Fleisher, Lee A., B-024; E-024
Gaziano, J. Michael, B-023, B-097, B-142, B-171; E-097; H-130
Genest, Jacques, E-019, E-103, E-130; H-019
Goldhaber, Sam, B-019, B-021; E-021, E-025, E-129, E-130, E-137
Gotto, Antonio M., E-019, E-025, E-038, E-102, E-119 E-130, E-139; F-069
Groh, William, B-067, B-084, B-101
Hayes, David, A-084, A-101; B-084, B-101, B-141; H-084, H-101, H-152
Hoffman, Gary, B-047; E-047; H-130, H-171
Isselbacher, Eric M., H-101, H-130
Kabbani, Samer, E-102, E-144; F-102, F-144
Kaplan, Norman, H-002, H-019, H-119, H-130, H-145, H-148
Karchmer, A. W., A-130; B-025, B-074, B-102, B-126, B-168; E-056, E-130, E-168
Klein, Irwin L., B-090, B-142; E-038
Konkle, Barbara A, B-006, B-025, B-046, B-120, B-122, B-171, B-172; E-025, E-078, E-082, E-120, E-171
Krauss, Ronald M., B-102, B-130; E-002, E-019, E-091, E-102, E-130; H-002, H-104
Libby, Peter, B-019, B-025, B-038, B-102, B-107, B-119, B-130, B-143, B-151; E-019, E-020, E-25, E-038, E-085, E-102, E-107, E-119, E-130, E-135, E-143, E-144, E-149, E-151; H-019, H-025, H-038, H-102, H-119, H-130
Linas, Stuart, E-019, E-062; E-102, E-130; H-019, H-102, H-130
Lipshultz, Steve, B-130, B-132, B-142; E-035
Lowes, Brian D, B-089; C-163; E-112; H-081, H-130
Mark, Daniel, B-008, B-101, B-130, B-137
McCullough, Peter A., E-002, E-015, E-033, E-119, E-124, E-147
McLaughlin, Vallerie, B-068, B-112, B-130; E-005, E-071, E-162; H-005, H-162
Miller, John, B-084, B-101; E-084, E-101
Morrow, David, B-021, B-026, B-061, B-107, B-142, B-154
Myerburg, Robert, E-137, E-144; H-028, H-084, H-137
Nabel, Elizabeth, E-036
Naka, Yoshifumi, E-157
Nesto, Richard W., H-081, H-102, H-130
Olgin, Jeffrey, A-101, A-102; E-036, E-101, E-171
Opie, Lionel, F-102
Pasternak, Richard C., E-019, E-038, E-088, E-091, E-102, E-130, E-144; H-038, H-091, H-102, H-104, H-130, H-144
Pennell, Dudley J., B-083, B-150, B-161; D-045; E-008, E-015, E-038, E-108; G-049
Popma, Jeffrey J., B-002, B-036, B-051, B-072, B-084, B-086, B-101, B-138; H-036, H-051, H-101, H-107, H-149
Port, J. David, A-001, A-112; F-013, F-128; G-112; H-019
Priori, Silvia, B-059, B-101, B-130
Pyeritz, Reed E., E-032, E-077, E-102, E-104; H-102, H-104
Rich, Stuart, A-162; C-162
Ridker, Paul M, B-019, B-038, B-119, B-131; E-002
Robertson, David, No information supplied.
Robertson, Rose Marie, No information supplied.
Roden, Dan, B-038; E-009, E-019, E-059, E-077, E-078, E-087; F-066
Rose, Eric, B-017, B-106, B-158
Rosenfield, Kenneth, A-123; B-002, B-036, B-051; E-002, E-036, E-051; H-067
Schwartz, Janice, A-136; E-054, E-140, E-160; G-096
Smallhorn, Jeffrey F., B-134
Sweitzer, Nancy K., B-147; H-078, H-147
Udelson, James E., B-038, B-090, B-127; E-038, E-076, E-090, E-109, E-127; H-038, H-081
Yancy, Clyde W. Jr., B-078, B-118, B-147; E-101; H-078, H-101, H-147
Zipes, Douglas P., A-043; B-101; D-105; E-004, E-040, E-043, E-059, E-077, E-079, E-093, E-101, E-156; F-012

INDEX

Note: Page numbers followed by f and t indicate figures and tables, respectively.